Oncology

Oncology

An Evidence-Based Approach

With 346 Figures in 501 Parts

Edited by

Alfred E. Chang, MD
Hugh Cabot Professor of Surgery; Chief, Division of Surgery Oncology; Department of Surgery, University of Michigan, Ann Arbor, Michigan

Patricia A. Ganz, MD
American Cancer Society Clinical Research Professor, Director, Division of Cancer Prevention and Control Research, Jonsson Comprehensive Cancer Center at UCLA, Professor, Schools of Public Health and Medicine, University of California, Los Angeles, Los Angeles, California

Daniel F. Hayes, MD
Clinical Director, Breast Oncology Program, University of Michigan Comprehensive Cancer Center, Ann Arbor, Michigan

Timothy J. Kinsella, MD
Vincent K. Smith Professor and Chairman, Department of Radiation Oncology, University Hospitals of Cleveland, Case Western Reserve University, Cleveland, Ohio

Harvey I. Pass, MD
Professor and Chief of Thoracic Surgery, Department of Cardiothoracic Surgery, Head, Thoracic Oncology, New York University School of Medicine and Comprehensive Cancer Center, New York, New York

Joan H. Schiller, MD
Melanie Heald Professor of Medical Oncology, Department of Medicine, University of Wisconsin Comprehensive Cancer Center, Madison, Wisconsin

Richard M. Stone, MD
Associate Professor, Department of Medicine, Harvard Medical School, Clinical Director, Adult Leukemia Program, Dana-Farber Cancer Institute, Boston, Massachusetts

Victor J. Strecher, PhD, MPH
Professor and Director, Health Media Research Laboratory, Department of Health Behavior and Health Education, University of Michigan School of Public Health, Associate Director, Cancer Prevention and Control, University of Michigan Comprehensive Cancer Center, Ann Arbor, Michigan

Foreword by Gabriel N. Hortobagyi, MD, FACP

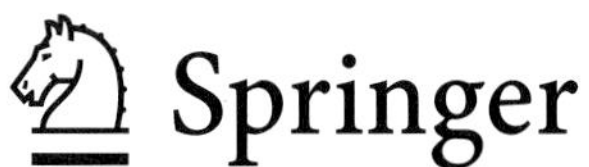
Springer

Alfred E. Chang, MD
Hugh Cabot Professor of Surgery
Chief, Division of Surgery Oncology
Department of Surgery
University of Michigan
Ann Arbor, MI, USA

Daniel F. Hayes, MD
Clinical Director, Breast Oncology Program
University of Michigan Comprehensive Cancer Center
Ann Arbor, MI, USA

Harvey I. Pass, MD
Professor and Chief of Thoracic Surgery
Department of Cardiothoracic Surgery
Head, Thoracic Oncology
New York University School of Medicine and Comprehensive Cancer Center
New York, NY, USA

Richard M. Stone, MD
Associate Professor, Department of Medicine
Harvard Medical School
Clinical Director, Adult Leukemia Program
Dana-Farber Cancer Institute
Boston, MA, USA

Patricia A. Ganz, MD
American Cancer Society Clinical Research Professor
Director, Division of Cancer Prevention and Control Research
Jonsson Comprehensive Cancer Center at UCLA
Professor, Schools of Public Health and Medicine
University of California, Los Angeles
Los Angeles, CA, USA

Timothy J. Kinsella, MD
Vincent K. Smith Professor and Chairman
Department of Radiation Oncology
University Hospitals of Cleveland
Case Western Reserve University
Cleveland, OH, USA

Joan H. Schiller, MD
Melanie Heald Professor of Medical Oncology
Department of Medicine
University of Wisconsin Comprehensive Cancer Center
Madison, WI, USA

Victor J. Strecher, PhD, MPH
Professor and Director, Health Media Research Laboratory
Department of Health Behavior and Health Education
University of Michigan School of Public Health
Associate Director, Cancer Prevention and Control
University of Michigan Comprehensive Cancer Center
Ann Arbor, MI, USA

Library of Congress Control Number: 2005926820

ISBN 10: 0-387-24291-0
ISBN 13: 978-0387-24291-0

Printed on acid-free paper.

Printed in the United States of America. (BS/MVY)

9 8 7 6 5 4 3 2 1

springeronline.com

I would like to dedicate this book to all of our cancer patients.
They are the ones who have taught us about living,
coping, and how to be better physicians.
AEC

Producing a new textbook is a little like designing
a clinical protocol by committee:
we had specific aims, with some proposed methods, and
we got a pretty good result. I appreciate the team work of my
co-editors, and especially the contributions of my colleagues
who helped to launch survivorship as a recognized
component of an oncology text.
PAG

To I. Craig Henderson, M.D., who first taught me the importance
of scientifically-based clinical evidence for decision-making, and
to my wife, Jane, who has provided so much so that I
can pursue my whim: academic medicine.
DFH

Dedicated to my wife Susan and children for their unending
support; also dedicated to my oncology mentors Sam Hellman,
George Canellos and Eli Glatstein.
TJK

To my family, Helen, Ally, and Eric, who always put up with my
tendency to get overextended, but always have time to make me
feel loved
HIP

To my parents, my husband George, and my children Quintin,
Craig, and Lindsey, all of whom have been incredibly supportive
over the years
JHS

To my wife Jane and my children Ben, Rebecca, Sarah, and Harry
RMS

For Jeri, Rachael, and Julia
VJS

Foreword

Compared to more traditional subspecialties, oncology is a young, vibrant, and progressive branch of medicine that has relatively few ties to a dogmatic past. Perhaps for this reason many innovations in oncology have occurred as a consequence of rapid cultural changes within the specialty, and continued change remains an accepted and integral part of our field. While most other practitioners of medicine learned a "standard of practice" and some dedicate their practice to clinical and/or basic research, research has been an integral and inseparable part of oncology since its inception. Consequently, virtually all oncologists consider clinical trials and experimental therapeutics as bread and butter and as necessary components of an ongoing progress. The broad acceptance of the necessity of prospective clinical trials and the continued testing of new drugs, strategies, and concepts highlights the need for differentiating hypothesis from fact, experience from experimental results, and opinion from fact. Such separation is the basis of evidence-based medicine, and oncology is one of the specialties with perhaps the richest tradition of practicing it. Considering that medicine has relied almost exclusively on clinical observation, anecdotal series, and uncontrolled personal experience for the past many centuries, such rapid adoption of evidence-based medicine is somewhat surprising and attests to the scientific orientation of our discipline.

For the past three decades several excellent textbooks on oncology were developed. The leading examples are multiauthored volumes that summarize the results of clinical trials placed in clinical context by experts on the field. These are encyclopedic textbooks in the best tradition of medicine, and several have progressed through multiple editions. In that context, what will the current textbook contribute to the field and how is it different from other volumes in the crowded field of oncology? Multiple answers to this question emerge from a careful review of this textbook. First, this book reflects a mature field of oncology; in addition to descriptions of natural history, clinical course, and the value of commonly used therapeutic strategies, much emphasis is placed on the cost, in terms of unwanted effects or toxicities associated with treatments. In addition to detailed presentations of acute side effects and their management, there is careful presentation of long-term effects, most of which are irreversible and some, potentially lethal. Only such careful assessment and tabulation of quantifiable therapeutic affects placed on the balance along with acute and long-term toxicities can provide a true picture of the therapeutic ratio of an intervention, which can then be translated in the context of each patient's clinical situation, risk of progression, recurrence, or death. Second, the book presents a systematic approach to issues of survivorship. Physicians with a major interest in survivorship describe some of these, while survivors themselves describe others, providing a poignant perspective not found in books entirely authored by medical specialists. This aspect is the logical consequence of the increasing integration of users in breast cancer research and allocation of resources. Patient perspectives have contributed in a major way to identification of research fund over the past decade, and their participation in the activities of multiple research groups have contributed to identification of important questions to be addressed and the prioritization of research activities in cancer centers, SPOREs, and other multi-investigator activities. Such contributions are irreplaceable and of great importance to reaching the ultimate goals of cancer research: improvements in quality and duration of life.

The third, and perhaps most important contribution of this volume, is the emphasis on determining the quality of evidence in the integration of research results into guidelines or recommendations for patient care or design of subsequent research. The first chapter is dedicated to the definitions of research quality, systematic approaches to quantify levels of evidence, and providing examples of such systematic approach to grading quality of cancer investigation. It is no accident that the editor in chief of the *Journal of the National Cancer Institute*, dedicated for many years to the assessment of the quality of research publications is the senior author of this chapter. In earlier decades, assessment of the quality of research was an intuitive process, and most seasoned oncologists based their enthusiasm for specific reports or research results on their subjective assessment of the research in question. Such subjective assessments were based, in part, on the name recognition of the reporting investigator(s), the reputation of the center or group behind the research, the sample size, and often the biases of those engaged in the assessment. The systematic approach to assigning specific levels of evidence to research reports goes a long way toward removing subjectivity from these assessments, focusing more on the methodology and the inherent strengths and weaknesses of any particular research approach than on the concordance of the results with preconceived biases or favored hypothesis. Identifying reports with the highest levels of evidence often clarifies seemingly confusing collections of data and often points out the glaring weaknesses or deficiencies of specific fields of interest. Sometimes it becomes apparent that despite decades of accepted treatment approaches, no evidence exists on which to base such approaches. It is apparent from such application of evidence-based scrutiny that modern medicine is still a hybrid filed, where evidence-based approaches coexist and often comingle with old observations, qualitative personal experiences, opinions, and anecdotes. It is amply clear that the generation of high-quality evidence requires time and resources, including the willing participation of users, in this case, research subjects and patients. It is also clear that in many situations, physicians will have to continue using clinical judgment, extrapolate from related evidence and utilize common sense in the day-to-day management of clinical problems, because only a relatively small proportion of oncological treatments have been subjected to strict, controlled, prospective clinical trials, and not every question will be the subject of high-quality clinical trials in the future. Limitations in time and resources and the ongoing supply of high-priority biological questions will always displace questions of lower priority.

Let us examine then other features of this remarkable book. The first few chapters review the basic approaches to treat cancer. Surgery, radiotherapy, and chemotherapy are carefully presented, with a clear description of mechanisms of action and in the context of modern biological understanding of the malignant process. The chapter about radiation therapy is an example of the enormous progress made in our understanding of this highly technological branch of cancer treatment and the major progress that has occurred in this specialty over the past few years. Targeted therapy is the latest addition to our armamentarium, but it is one of the most exciting aspects of systemic treatments because it is based on clear understanding of the molecular underpinnings of the biological advantage of certain malignant cells over their normal components, biological characteristics that drive the proliferation, invasion, metastasis, and survival of such cells. The recent success of specific forms of targeted therapies (imatinib, trastuzumab, bevacizumab, and the endocrine agents) emphasize the enormous potential of this approach in the development of more specific treatments with fewer expected consequences on nonmalignant tissue. This chapter also highlights the many challenges encountered in the development of targeted agents, such as the need to validate molecular targets, to demonstrate in vivo that the agent accomplishes its desired effect on the target and, in consequence, can be expected to produce a specific clinical effect. These challenges have proved to be major obstacles in the case of certain targets, yielding easily in the case of others.

Tumor markers are an inherently attractive concept. Would it not be desirable to have a marker of disease extent, activity or malignant potential that one can identify and quantify in a minimally invasive or noninvasive manner? Would it not be helpful to relay on such markers to determine the efficacy of therapy early in a therapeutic intervention? The author of Chapter 7 is a recognized expert in this field and has contributed to our conceptual systematization of the tumor marker field with the development of clear criteria for validating markers and guidelines for their utilization, as well as recommendations to avoid obvious pitfalls in this area.

Much of the high-level evidence we have today was derived from prospective clinical trials. The chapter describing these master tools is authored by enormously experienced clinical trials who have contributed both conceptually and practically to the definition, implementation and analysis of randomized clinical trials. This chapter provides an excellent roadmap for current and future investigators.

The ethics of human experimentation are a critical subject for all investigators and patients. Decades of controversy have refined our approach to randomized trials, no treatment or placebo controls, and defined optimal approaches for analysis and release of trial results. High-quality evidence can only be generated in the context of a highly ethical trial design. Screening and early diagnosis present particular challenges, largely because they relate to asymptomatic subjects, most of whom will not need nor benefit from these interventions. Therefore, these approaches benefit a few, while exposing many to potential risks. Trial design, ethics, and economics meet and often collide in this field.

As increasing emphasis has been placed on patient autonomy and as the population at large has gained increasing access to medical information, issues related to alternative and complementary therapies have also become prominent. This field includes IT, where assessment of levels of evidence can provide enormous benefits to our patients and also to healthcare providers, who often have only a passing knowledge of such popular, but often untested approaches, to the treatment of cancer or its symptoms. The lead author is clearly one of the most knowledgeable experts on this field and provides a broad overview of the issues.

Outstanding contributions cover the potential etiologies of cancer, as well as the basic biological principles of malignant transformation, invasion, and metastases. The role of the immune system is receiving increasing attention, as greater effort is being expended on the development of vaccines and other immunological approaches to cancer control.

One of the outstanding examples of the application of evidence-based medicine is Chapter 23. The authors describe the complexity of research that brings together epidemiology, basic sciences, and chemoprevention trials, in a field where isolated causes of cancer are seldom identified and where control of all variables is an unrealistic expectation. These issues are highlighted in examples of dietary intervention or the use of specific components of the human diet, such as vitamins, minerals, and other micronutrients.

The identification of genes involved in cancer predisposition has dramatically changed our approach to familial cancer syndromes. Our ability to precisely identify subjects at risk for certain malignant tumors has also placed in evidence complex social, psychological, financial, and ethical issues that need to be addressed with subjects potentially eligible for genetic screening or preventive interventions. Such advances have also uncovered potential leads for identifying other genes that influence the development of more common, apparently sporadic cancers in the population, and eventually point to future therapeutic strategies.

The chapters dedicated to specific malignant tumors bring together updated information about epidemiology, carcinogenesis, natural history, diagnostic procedures, and therapeutic interventions. The book highlights, in general, that optimal care requires close interdisciplinary collaboration, both in the diagnostic process and therapeutic strategies. There is much emphasis on the results of randomized trials, as the major theme of the book would indicate. It is painfully clear, however, that for common adult malignancies there is much evidence generated from prospective randomized trials that allows the development of evidence-based treatment guidelines; however, this is often not the case for less common tumors, especially those most resistant to systemic treatments. For these, treatment strategies are often based on observational or single-arm prospective trials. The recent identification of molecular targets for some of these tumors (renal cell or pancreatic cancers) has led to renewed interest and some notable successes in recent clinical trials.

Chapter 63 is an excellent example of how the editors envision the presentation of systematic knowledge about a specific disease condition. The authors synthesized an enormous body of information derived from clinical trials if patients with acute leukemia or myelodysplastic syndromes. The highest quality evidence, based on multiple phase III trials, is presented first, followed in descending order of quality by other types of evidence.

The stepwise development of therapeutic interventions, comparing the best "standard" to an investigational approach, is a logical candidate for evaluation in prospective randomized trials. Patient selection can be predetermined, and, in general, treatments can be compared on relatively homogeneous groups of patients. That is clearly not the case for complications of malignancy or treatment; such events occur at different times of the clinical course of the disease, and of course, patients cannot be selected a priori. Rather, the development of the complication selects the patients and treatments must be adjusted to the patients' circumstances.

For these reasons it is all the more satisfying to review Chapter 71 about acute CNS complications. Such complications are almost always dramatic and require prompt intervention. It is, therefore, all the more admirable to find level I evidence and Grade A recommendations for the management of an oncological emergency. The secondary message of these results is that appropriate controlled trials can be ethically developed in almost every circumstance in the oncological patient, and high level evidence can be generated for optimal management of subsequent patients.

Another excellent chapter, Chapter 76, summarizes current knowledge and therapeutic approaches to infectious complications of malignant disease and their treatments. While not presented with detailed assessment of levels of evidence, this chapter highlights current approaches to common and uncommon infections, the appropriate use of antibiotics and hematopoietic growth factors, and introduces methods to prevent or reduce the risk of infectious complications. It is gratifying how, from the number one cause of treatment-related mortality a few decades ago, infectious complications have become a much more manageable, and in fact, almost completely preventable complications of cancer treatment, especially in patients with solid tumors.

Chapter 83 focuses on a difficult field of research, the assessment, management, and prevention of nausea and emesis. While a common side effect of cancer treatment, especially chemotherapy and radiotherapy, nausea and emesis are difficult research subjects because of the major subjective component, interindividual variability, and the lack of external, validated, hard endpoints, short of counting the numbers of emetic episodes. Despite these obstacles, multiple prospective randomized have been conducted, comparing antiemetics with placebo or no treatment, or two antiemetics, or single antiemetics with combination therapy. The tables not only describe the results of such research, but list them in the order of higher to lower level of evidence. Such ranking facilitate the assessment of relative value of information derived from different clinical trials and also identifies opportunities to conduct additional research to clarify or complement existing evidence.

Other fields of research, especially those in the psychosocial and behavioral disciplines, have made less progress in the implementation of levels of evidence to research results. This observation is largely based on the predominantly "soft" endpoints utilized in many of these disciplines—endpoints that lend themselves less to easy quantification. As validated instruments are developed and employed in prospective research, this is also likely to change, and we can expect an increasing emphasis on evidence-based recommendations and guidelines in these fields too.

Much progress has been made since the War on Cancer was declared in 1971. Some of it was the result of the outstanding laboratory based research conducted with the support of the National Institutes of Health, National Cancer Institute, American Cancer Society, and multiple foundations, and resulted in marked improvement in our understanding of the basic biological underpinnings of malignant disease and the processes that give it its life-threatening characteristics. Some progress was derived from the technological progress in developing new diagnostic methods, refining our ability for early diagnosis, staging, and focusing of therapeutic interventions. Some progress was the result of successful drug development resulting in more effective therapeutic interventions that reduced markedly the probability of recurrence and mortality for patients diagnosed with several common human solid tumors and hematological malignancies. However, progress has been costly in financial terms, infrastructure building, and human resources. With more than 1800 new oncological drugs in the pipeline, and almost half of them at some stage of clinical development, resources are becoming even scarcer and more precious. It behooves us, as a community, to find or develop more effective and more cost-effective methods to assess the efficacy of drugs and procedures, to identify patients more and less likely to benefit from a specific intervention, and to minimize waste in the utilization of the multiple diagnostic and therapeutic approaches we have available to us today. Such urgent need for cost-effective approaches is even more dramatically highlighted by the plight of the majority of countries with limited resources around the globe. Squandering precious resources in poorly designed healthcare strategies limits access to life saving procedures. Our best hope is the increasingly stringent application of high-level evidence to decision making at the level of public health officials but also at the level of each individual physician. To enhance our probability of success, we need to speak in the language of evidence, think of levels of evidence in the design of research projects and clinical trials, and increasingly limit our recommendations to those interventions supported by the highest levels of evidence. Anything less will limit access to high-quality care and dilute our efforts to serve our patients. We hope that this textbook and subsequent editions of it will lead the way towards the implementation of evidence-based oncology and set the tone for future textbooks in other medical fields.

Gabriel N. Hortobagyi, MD, FACP
Professor and Chair
Department of Breast Medical Oncology
Director of the Multidisciplinary Breast Cancer Research Program
The University of Texas
M. D. Anderson Cancer Center

Preface

A new textbook in oncology?! What is different about this book compared to other established texts that have already been published? Why do we need a new book? For anyone in the market for a textbook, the main reason is to keep pace with the knowledge base that is growing ever so rapidly in oncology, a field that is evolving faster than all other medical fields. This book does not attempt to be an encyclopedic summary of that information. Rather, this textbook strives to organize that knowledge into a unified approach that categorizes and summarizes the evidence that is currently available. We realize that clinicians are too busy to keep up with the literature that is published in the many available journals. Therefore, a key feature of this book is the evidence-based tables that collate the best available evidence from the literature, enabling the reader to make decisions on the basis of data. We have chosen current experts to create evidence-based chapters on topics that span the field from basic and translational science to prevention to clinical practice, and ultimately to survivorship, totaling 113 chapters written by more than 250 contributors. The tone of this book is established in the first chapter, "Evidence-Based Approach to Oncology," which reviews the history of evidence-based medicine and describes the different levels of evidence. This book will be informative to residents, fellows, practicing clinicians, and allied health professionals.

This book has several unique features. Section One, "Principles of Oncology," contains several chapters that discuss areas that have only recently matured. The topics include the biologic principles of hematopoietic stem cell therapies; informatics infrastructure; economics of cancer care; and, patient decision making. The section on "Translational Basic Science," includes chapters that review the basic concepts of cancer biology; these are written from the perspective of clinical translational science and how it is relevant to the physician. The chapter entitled "Technologies in Molecular Biology: Diagnostic Applications" is both timely and concise, while exploring the application of genomics to daily clinical practice. In the section on "Cancer Prevention and Control," the chapter, "Behavioral Modification" is unique in the literature. Similarly, the section on "Cancer Imaging" has a chapter on the "Imaging of Gastrointestinal Stromal Tumor," which is not found in current oncology textbooks. The chapter on PET imaging investigates the promise of that modality. In the "Practice of Oncology" section, several chapters discuss the care of subpopulations of patients who pose different challenges to the clinician: immunosuppressed patients; elderly patients; patients with organ dysfunction; and pregnant women. Foremost, an entire section of 13 chapters is devoted to "Cancer Survivorship." These innovative chapters represent a broad and in-depth review of the long-term consequences of cancer treatment with respect to specific malignancies. A chapter on "Cancer Advocacy" from the perspectives of cancer survivors is in this section.

Most of the chapters fall into sections on Solid Tumors, Hematologic Malignancies, and the Practice of Oncology. These sections cover site-specific malignances, treatment toxicities, oncologic emergencies, and supportive care. They focus on the latest multimodality approach to the patient, with an emphasis on the best-available evidence from the literature. Where available, we have asked authors to include Level 1 clinical, treatment, and management data for each site-specific chapter. In those instances where Level 1 evidence may not be available, the best clinical practices based on published clinical experience are summarized. As opposed to review articles or standard textbook chapters, the evidence-based chapters presented in this book strive to present the reader with a thorough search of the evidence, judgment of the scientific quality of the evidence, and lastly a bias-free conclusion of the evidence.

This new book offers readers a user-friendly approach to the vast amount of information in the oncology literature. It is our intention that this book will become a useful tool for the improvement of readers' clinical practices. The Editorial Board would like to acknowledge the outstanding effort of the Springer staff for pulling this project together. In particular, we would like to thank Laura Gillan who initiated this book project, and Paula Callaghan who brought it to its completion.

Alfred E. Chang, MD
Patricia A. Ganz, MD
Daniel F. Hayes, MD
Timothy J. Kinsella, MD
Harvey I. Pass, MD
Joan H. Schiller, MD
Richard M. Stone, MD
Victor J. Strecher, PhD, MPH

Contents

Section Two Translational Basic Science

Section Three Cancer Prevention and Control

Section Four Cancer Imaging

Section Five Solid Tumors

Section Six Hematologic Malignancies

Section Seven Practice of Oncology

Section Eight Cancer Survivorship

Contributors

Alex A. Adjei, MD, PhD
Professor, Department of Oncology, Mayo Clinic Foundation, Rochester, MN, USA.

Manish Agrawal, MD
Staff Scientist, Department of Clinical Bioethics, Warren G. Magnuson Clinical Center and Medical Oncology Research Unit, National Cancer Institute, National Institutes of Health, Bethesda, MD, USA.

Daniel M. Albert, MD, MS
Chair Emeritus, F.A. David Professor, and Lorenz E. Zimmerman Professor, Department of Ophthalmology and Visual Sciences, University of Wisconsin-Madison, Madison, WI, USA.

Mark R. Albertini, MD
Associate Professor, Department of Medicine, University of Wisconsin-Madison; Chief of Oncology, William S. Middleton Memorial Veterans Hospital, Madison, WI, USA.

Steven Alberts, MD, MPH
Associate Professor, Department of Oncology, Mayo Clinic College of Medicine, Rochester, MN, USA.

Sarah W. Alexander, MD
Assistant Professor, Department of Pediatrics, Case Western University, Division of Pediatric Hematology and Oncology, Rainbow Babies and Children's Hospital, Cleveland, OH, USA.

Asim Amin, MD, PhD
Immunotherapy Co-Director, Blumenthol Cancer Center, Carolinas Medical Center, Charlotte, NC, USA.

Scott Antonia, MD, PhD
Medical Director, Cellular Therapies Core, Department of Interdisciplinary Oncology, H. Lee Moffitt Cancer Center & Research Institute, University of South Florida, Tampa, FL, USA.

Suzanne L. Aquino, MD
Assistant Professor, Department of Radiology, Harvard Medical School/Massachusetts General Hospital, Boston, MA, USA.

Meri Armour, RN, MSN
Senior Vice President, Ireland Cancer Center/University Hospitals of Cleveland, Cleveland, OH, USA.

David A. August, MD
Associate Professor, Department of Surgery; Chief, Division of Surgical Oncology, UMDNJ/Robert Wood Johnson Medical School and the Cancer Institute of New Jersey, New Brunswick, NJ, USA.

Noreen M. Aziz, MD, PhD, MPH
Senior Program Director, Office of Cancer Survivorship, Division of Cancer Control and Population Sciences, National Cancer Institute, Rockville, MD, USA.

Giuseppe Barbanti-Brodano, MD
Professor, Department of Experimental and Diagnostic Medicine, Section of Microbiology, University of Ferrara, Ferrara, Italy.

J. Carl Barrett, PhD
Director, Center for Cancer Research, National Cancer Institute, Bethesda, MD, USA.

Karen Basen-Engquist, PhD, MPH
Associate Professor, Department of Behavioral Science, The University of Texas at M. D. Anderson Cancer Center, Houston, TX, USA.

Wendie A. Berg, MD, PhD
Breast Imaging Consultant, Study Chair, American College of Radiology Imaging Network, Lutherville, MD, USA.

Smita Bhatia, MD, MPH
Director, Epidemiology and Outcomes Research, Department of Pediatric Oncology, City of Hope Cancer Center, Duarte, CA, USA.

Rina M. Bloch, MD
Assistant Professor, Department of Rehabilitation Medicine, Tufts-New England Medical Center, Boston, MA, USA.

David A. Bluemke, MD, PhD
Associate Professor, The Russell H. Morgan Department of Radiology and Radiological Science, The Johns Hopkins Hospital, Baltimore, MD, USA.

Diane C. Bodurka, MD
Associate Professor, Department of Gynecological Oncology, The University of Texas at M. D. Anderson Cancer Center, Houston, TX, USA.

Michael Boeckh, MD
Assistant Member, Program in Infectious Diseases, Fred Hutchinson Cancer Research Center; Assistant Professor of Medicine, University of Washington School of Medicine, Seattle, WA, USA.

Jeffrey P. Bond, PhD
Research Associate Professor, Department of Microbiology and Molecular Genetics, University of Vermont, Burlington, VT, USA.

Melissa L. Bondy, PhD
Professor, Department of Epidemiology, The University of Texas M. D. Anderson Cancer Center, Houston, TX, USA.

Louise J. Bordeleau, MD, FRCP(C), MSc
Attending, Department of Medical Oncology, Mount Sinai Hospital, Toronto, Ontario, Canada.

Kristin Bradley, MD
Assistant Professor of Human Oncology, University of Wisconsin, Madison, WI, USA.

Paul D. Brown, MD
Assistant Professor, Division of Radiation Oncology, Department of Oncology, Mayo Clinic College of Medicine, Rochester, MN, USA.

John Bryant, PhD
Professor, Associate Director, Departments of Biostatistics, National Surgical Adjuvant Breast and Bowel Project Biostatistical Center, Pittsburgh, PA, USA.

Julia W. Buchanan, BS
Associate in Research, Russell H. Morgan Department of Radiology and Radiological Science, Division of Nuclear Medicine, The Johns Hopkins University School of Medicine, Baltimore, MD, USA.

Jan C. Buckner, MD
Chair, Division of Medical Oncology, Professor of Oncology, Mayo Clinic College of Medicine, Rochester, MN, USA.

Susan V. Bukata, MD
Assistant Professor, Department of Orthopedics, University of Rochester Medical Center/Strong Memorial Hospital, Rochester, NY, USA.

Alan K. Burnett, MD, FRCPath, FRCP(Glasgow), FRCP(Edinburgh), FRCP(London), FMSci
Professor, Department of Haematology, University of Wales College of Medicine, Cardiff, Wales, UK.

John C. Byrd, MD
Associate Professor, Department of Internal Medicine, Division of Hematology and Oncology, The Ohio State University, The Arthur James Comprehensive Cancer Center, Columbus, OH, USA.

Michele Carbone, MD, PhD
Associate Professor, Department of Pathology, Cardinal Bernardin Cancer Center, Loyola University Chicago, Maywood, IL, USA.

Daniel B. Carr, MD, DABPM, FFPMANZCA(Hon)
Saltonstall Professor of Pain Research, Department of Anesthesia; Medical Director, Pain Management Program, Tufts-New England Medical Center, Boston, MA, USA.

Shamus R. Carr, MD
Surgical Resident, Department of Surgery, Thomas Jefferson University, Philadelphia, PA, USA.

Jacqueline Casillas, MD, MSHS
Assistant Professor, Department of Pediatrics, Division of Hematology/Oncology, David Geffen School of Medicine at UCLA, Los Angeles, CA, USA.

Barrie Cassileth, PhD
Chief, Integrative Medicine Service; Laurance S. Rockefeller Chair in Integrative Medicine, Department of Medicine, Memorial Sloan-Kettering Cancer Center, New York, NY, USA.

Mark S. Chambers, DMD
Associate Professor, Head & Neck Surgery; Deputy Chief, Section of Oncologic Dentistry and Prosthodontics, M. D. Anderson Cancer Center, Houston, TX, USA.

Alfred E. Chang, MD
Hugh Cabot Professor of Surgery; Chief, Division of Surgery Oncology; Department of Surgery, University of Michigan, Ann Arbor, MI, USA.

Shine Chang, PhD
Associate Director, Office of Preventive Oncology, National Cancer Institute, National Institutes of Health, Bethesda, MD, USA.

Daniel N. Chatzifotiadis, MD
Post Doctoral Research Fellow, Department of Radiology, Division of Nuclear Medicine, The Johns Hopkins Medical Institute, Baltimore, MD, USA.

Caroline Chiles, MD
Professor, Department of Radiology, Wake Forest University School of Medicine, Winston-Salem, NC, USA.

Hak Choy, MD
Nancy B. and Jake L. Hamon Distinguished Chair in Therapeutic Oncology Research, Professor and Chairman, Department of Radiation Oncology, Moncrief Radiation Oncology Center, University of Texas, Southwestern Medical Branch, Dallas, TX, USA.

Sue Chua, MBBS, FRACP
Senior Clinical Research Fellow, Breast Unit, Department of Medicine, Royal Marsden Hospital, Chelsea, London, UK.

Joseph I. Clark, MD
Associate Professor, Department of Medicine, Loyola University Chicago, Maywood, IL, USA.

Ezra E.W. Cohen, MD
Assistant Professor, Section of Hematology/Oncology, Department of Medicine, University of Chicago, Chicago, IL, USA.

Anne Coscarelli, PhD
Research Psychologist, Department of Public Health; Director, Ted Mann Family Resource Center, UCLA/David Geffen School of Medicine, Los Angeles, CA, USA.

Christopher J. Crnich, MD, MS
Research Fellow, Section of Infectious Diseases, Department of Medicine, University of Wisconsin, Madison, WI, USA.

Alvin A. Dahl, MD, PhD
Professor, Department of Clinical Cancer Research, National Hospital-Radium Hospital, Oslo, Norway.

Mary B. Daly, MD, PhD
Director, Cancer Prevention and Control Program, Department of Population Science, Fox Chase Cancer Center, Philadelphia, PA, USA.

Suzanne C. Danhauer, PhD
Assistant Professor and Associate Director, Psychosocial Oncology & Cancer Patient Support Programs, Department of Internal Medicine, Wake Forest University Baptist Medical Center, Winston-Salem, NC, USA.

Sarah Dash, MPH
Cancer Research Training Fellow, Applied Research Program, Division of Cancer Control and Population Sciences, National Cancer Institute, Bethesda, MD, USA.

Daniel J. De Angelo, MD, PhD
Assistant Professor, Department of Medicine, Harvard Medical School; Adult Leukemia Program, Dana-Farber Cancer Institute, Brigham and Women's Hospital, Boston, MA, USA.

James A. DeCaprio, MD
Associate Professor, Department of Medical Oncology, Dana-Farber Cancer Institute, Boston, MA, USA.

Joachim Deeg, MD
Member, Clinical Research Division, Fred Hutchinson Cancer Research Center; Professor of Medicine, University of Washington School of Medicine, Seattle, WA, USA.

George D. Demetri, MD
Clinical Director, Sarcoma Program, Dana-Farber Cancer Institute; Associate Professor, Department of Medicine, Harvard Medical School, Boston, MA, USA.

Sophie Dessureault, MD, PhD
Staff, Department of Interdisciplinary Oncology, H. Lee Moffitt Cancer Center & Research Institute, University of South Florida, Tampa, FL, USA.

Emily DeVoto, PhD, MSPH
Health Science Policy Analyst, Office of Medical Applications of Research, National Institutes of Health, Bethesda, MD, USA.

Kathleen M. Diehl, MD
Assistant Professor, Division of Surgical Oncology, Department of Surgery, University of Michigan, Ann Arbor, MI, USA.

James J. Dignam, PhD
Assistant Professor, Department of Health Studies, University of Chicago and University of Chicago Cancer Research Center, Chicago, IL, USA.

Gerard M. Doherty, MD
Norman W. Thompson Professor; Section Head, General Surgery; Chief, Division of Endocrine Surgery; Director, Department of Surgery, University of Michigan Health System, Ann Arbor, MI, USA.

Jessica S. Donington, MD
Assistant Professor, Department of Cardiothoracic Surgery, Stanford University School of Medicine, Stanford, CA, USA.

John H. Donohue, MD
Consultant in Surgery, Department of General Surgery, Mayo Clinic; Professor of Surgery, Mayo Graduate School of Medicine, Rochester, MN, USA.

Kristine A. Donovan, PhD, MBA
Assistant Professor, Department of Interdisciplinary Oncology, H. Lee Moffitt Cancer Center and Research Institute at the University of South Florida, Tampa, FL, USA.

Afshin Dowlati, MD
Assistant Professor, Department of Medicine, Case Western Reserve University, University Hospitals of Cleveland, Cleveland, OH, USA.

Faith M. Durden, MD
Assistant Professor, Department of Dermatology, Case Western Reserve University, University Hospitals of Cleveland, Cleveland, OH, USA.

Grace K. Dy, MD
Fellow, Department of Oncology, Mayo Clinic College of Medicine, Rochester, MN, USA.

Douglas B. Einstein, MD, PhD
Assistant Professor, Department of Radiation Oncology, Case Western Reserve University, Cleveland, OH, USA.

Ezekiel J. Emanuel, MD, PhD
Chair, Department of Clinical Bioethics, Warren G. Magnuson Clinical Center, National Institutes of Health, Bethesda, MD, USA.

Cathy Eng, MD
Assistant Professor, Department of Gastrointestinal Medical Oncology, The University of Texas M. D. Anderson Cancer Center, Houston, TX, USA.

Brad J. Erickson, MD
Associate Professor, Department of Radiology, Mayo Clinic Foundation, Rochester, MN, USA.

Scott E. Evans, MD
Instructor, Department of Pulmonary and Critical Care Medicine, Mayo Clinic College of Medicine, Mayo Clinic Foundation, Rochester, MN, USA.

Marni Feldmann, MD
Resident, Department of Ophthalmology and Visual Sciences, University of Wisconsin, Madison, WI, USA.

Elliot K. Fishman, MD
Professor, The Russell H. Morgan Department of Radiology and Radiological Science, The Johns Hopkins University School of Medicine, Baltimore, MD, USA.

Gini F. Fleming, MD
Associate Professor, Department of Medicine, University of Chicago, Chicago, IL, USA.

Michele R. Forman, PhD
Senior Investigator, Center for Cancer Research, National Cancer Institute, Bethesda, MD, USA

Sophie D. Fosså, PhD
Professor, Department of Long-term Studies, National Hospital-Radium Hospital, University of Oslo, Oslo, Norway.

Joseph S. Friedberg, MD
Chief, Division of Thoracic Surgery, Department of Surgery, Thomas Jefferson University, Philadelphia, PA, USA.

Shirish M. Gadgeel, MD
Assistant Professor, Department of Internal Medicine, Division of Hematology & Oncology, Karmanos Cancer Institute/Wayne State University, Detroit, MI, USA.

Evanthia Galanis, MD
Associate Professor, Division of Medical Oncology, Mayo Clinic College of Medicine, Rochester, MN, USA.

Patricia A. Ganz, MD
American Cancer Society Clinical Research Professor; Director, Division of Cancer Prevention and Control Research, Jonsson Comprehensive Cancer Center at UCLA, Professor, Schools of Public Health and Medicine, University of California, Los Angeles, Los Angeles, CA, USA.

Adam S. Garden, MD
Professor, Department of Radiation Oncology, The University of Texas M. D. Anderson Cancer Center, Houston, TX, USA.

Patrick J. Getty, MD
Assistant Professor, Department of Orthopaedic Surgery, Case Western Reserve University/University Hospitals of Cleveland, Cleveland, OH, USA.

Maged I. Gharib, MSc, MD, MRCP, MRCPath
Attending, Department of Haematology, Royal Manchester Children's Hospital, Manchester, UK.

Caterina Giannini, MD
Consultant, Department of Anatomic Pathology, Mayo Clinic Foundation, Rochester, MN, USA.

Paula Gill, MD
Fellow, Department of Oncology, Mayo Clinic Foundation, Rochester, MN, USA.

Montgomery Gillard, MD
Lecturer, Department of Dermatology, University of Michigan, Ann Arbor, MI, USA.

Timothy Gilligan, MD
Instructor in Medicine, Department of Medical Oncology, Harvard Medical School, Dana-Farber Cancer Institute, Boston, MA, USA.

Pamela J. Goodwin, MD, MSc, FBPC
Professor, Department of Medicine, University of Toronto; Senior Scientist, Samuel Lunenfeld Research Institute, Mount Sinai Hospital, Toronto, Ontario, Canada.

Gregory J. Gores, MD
Professor, Department of Medicine, Mayo Clinic College of Medicine, Rochester, MN, USA.

Leonidas C. Goudas, MD, PhD
Assistant Professor, Department of Anesthesiology, Tufts-New England Medical Center, Boston, MA, USA.

Annette Grambihler, MD
Staff, First Department of Internal Medicine, University of Mainz, Mainz, Germany.

Frederic W. Grannis, Jr., MD
Assistant Professor, Department of Thoracic Surgery, City of Hope National Medical Center, Duarte, CA, USA.

F. Anthony Greco, MD
Medical Director, Sarah Cannon Cancer Center, Nashville, TN, USA.

Axel Grothey, MD
Mayo Foundation Scholar, Division of Medical Oncology, Mayo Clinic Foundation, Rochester, MN, USA.

Steven Hahn, MD
Attending, Department of Surgery, Hospital of the University of Pennsylvania, Philadelphia, PA, USA.

John D. Hainsworth, MD
Director of Clinical Research, Sarah Cannon Cancer Center, Nashville, TN, USA.

Dima A. Hammoud, MD
Assistant Professor, Department of Diagnostic Radiology, Division of Neuroradiology, The Johns Hopkins University, Baltimore, MD, USA.

Lindsay A. Hampson, BS
Fellow, Department of Clinical Bioethics, Warren G. Magnuson Clinical Center, National Institutes of Health, Bethesda, MD, USA.

Paul M. Harari, MD
Associate Professor, Department of Human Oncology, University of Wisconsin Comprehensive Cancer Center, Madison, WI, USA.

Russell Harris, MD, MPH
Professor, Department of Medicine, University of North Carolina, Chapel Hill, NC, USA.

Lawrence E. Harrison, MD
Associate Professor, Chief, Division of Surgical Oncology, UMDNJ-New Jersey Medical School, Newark, NJ, USA.

Daniel F. Hayes, MD
Clinical Director, Breast Oncology Program, University of Michigan Comprehensive Cancer Center, Ann Arbor, MI, USA.

Craig Hofmeister, MD
Fellow, Division of Hematology-Oncology, Loyola University Chicago, Cardinal Bernadin Cancer Center, Maywood, IL, USA.

Brent Hollenbeck, MD
Lecturer, Department of Urology, University of Michigan, Ann Arbor, MI, USA.

Steven M. Horwitz, MD
Clinical Assistant Physician, Lymphoma Services, Department of Hematology, Department of Medicine, Memorial Sloan-Kettering Cancer Center, New York, NY, USA.

Thomas Huff, MD
Staff, Department of Orthopaedic Surgery, Case Western Reserve University, Cleveland, OH, USA.

Scott A. Hundahl, MD, FACS, FSSO, FAHNS
Professor, Department of Clinical Surgery, U.C. Davis; Chief of Surgery, VA Northern California Health Care System, Sacramento VA at Mather, Mather, CA, USA.

Stephen D. Hursting, PhD, MPH
Deputy Director, Office of Preventive Oncology, National Cancer Institute, Bethesda, MD, USA.

Jimmy Hwang, MD
Attending, Lombardi Comprehensive Cancer Center, Georgetown University Medical Center, Washington, DC, USA.

Paul B. Jacobsen, PhD
Professor and Program Leader, Health Outcomes and Behavioral Program, Department of Psychosocial and Palliative Care Program, H. Lee Moffitt Cancer Center and Research Institute, Tampa, FL, USA.

Timothy M. Johnson, MD
Professor, Departments of Dermatology, Otolaryngology, and Surgery, University of Michigan Medical School, University of Michigan, Ann Arbor, MI, USA.

Stephen R.D. Johnston, MA, PhD, FRCP
Consultant Medical Oncologist, Department of Medicine—Breast Unit, Royal Marsden Hospital, London, UK.

Stein Kaasa, MD, PhD
Professor, Department of Cancer Research and Molecular Medicine, Faculty of Medicine, The Norwegian University of Science and Technology and the Palliative Care Unit, St. Olavs Hospital, Trondheim, Norway.

Ihab R. Kamel, MD, PhD
Assistant Professor, The Russell H. Morgan Department of Radiology and Radiological Sciences, The Johns Hopkins Hospital, Baltimore, MD, USA.

Phillip W. Kantoff, MD, PhD
Professor, Department of Medicine; Chief, Division of Solid Tumor Oncology; Director, Lank Center for Genitourinary Oncology, Harvard Medical School, Dana-Farber Cancer Institute, Boston, MA, USA.

Theodore G. Karrison, PhD
Research Associate, Associate Professor, Department of Health Studies, University of Chicago and University of Chicago Cancer Research Center, Chicago, IL, USA.

Satomi Kawamoto, MD
Assistant Professor, The Russell H. Morgan Department of Radiology and Radiological Science, The Johns Hopkins Hospital, Baltimore, MD, USA.

Thomas Kearney, MD, FACS
Associate Professor, Department of Surgery, UMDNJ/Robert Wood Johnson Medical School; The Cancer Institute of New Jersey, New Brunswick, NJ, USA.

Vicki Keedy, MD
Fellow, Division of Hematology/Oncology, Vanderbilt University Medical Center, Nashville, TN, USA.

Michael L. Kendrick, MD
Assistant Professor, Department of Surgery, Mayo Clinic College of Medicine, Rochester, MN, USA.

Michael S. Kent, MD
Staff, Department of Cardiothoracic Surgery, Weill-Cornell Medical Center, New York, NY, USA.

James Khatcheressian, MD
Assistant Professor, Department of Internal Medicine, Division of Hematology/Oncology, Virginia Commonwealth University Health System, Richmond, VA, USA.

Timothy J. Kinsella, MD
Vincent K. Smith Professor and Chairman, Department of Radiation Oncology, University Hospitals of Cleveland, Case Western Reserve University, Cleveland, OH, USA.

Linda S. Kinsinger, MD, MPH
Assistant Director, VA National Center for Health Promotion and Disease Prevention, Durham, NC, USA.

Clifford Y. Ko, MD
Associate Professor, Department of Surgery, UCLA School of Medicine/West Los Angeles VA Medical Center, Los Angeles, CA, USA.

Jonathan E. Kolitz, MD
Director, Leukemia Service, Department of Medicine, North Shore University Hospital, New York University School of Medicine, Manhasset, NY, USA.

Barnett S. Kramer, MD, MPH
Associate Director for Disease Prevention, Office of Disease Prevention, National Institutes of Health, Bethesda, MD, USA.

Alexander S. Krupnick, MD
Fellow, Department of Surgery, Division of Cardiothoracic Surgery, Washington University, St Louis, MO, USA.

Tracey L. Krupski, MD
Resident, Department of Urology, David Geffen School of Medicine, University of California, Los Angeles, CA, USA.

Amit Kumar, MD
Resident, Department of Ophthalmology and Visual Sciences, University of Wisconsin, Madison, WI, USA.

Dan Laheru, MD
Assistant Professor, Department of Medical Oncology, The Sidney Kimmel Comprehensive Cancer Center at The Johns Hopkins, Baltimore, MD, USA.

Wendy Landier, RN, MSN, CPNP
Pediatric Nurse Practitioner, Division of Pediatrics, City of Hope Comprehensive Cancer Center, Duarte, CA, USA.

Joseph Lau, MD
Professor, Department of Medicine, Institute for Clinical Research and Health Policy Studies, Tufts-New England Medical Center, Boston, MA, USA.

Donald P. Lawrence, MD
Assistant Professor, Division of Hematology-Oncology, Tufts-New England Medical Center, Boston, MA, USA.

Cheryl T. Lee, MD
Assistant Professor, Department of Urology, The University of Michigan, Ann Arbor, MI, USA.

Julie Lemieux, MD
Attending, Department of Medicine, Mount Sinai Hospital, Toronto, Ontario, Canada.

Nathan Levitan, MD, MBA
Professor, Department of Medicine, Ireland Cancer Center/University Hospitals of Cleveland, Cleveland, OH, USA.

Andrew H. Limper, MD
Professor of Medicine, Biochemistry, and Molecular Biology, Department of Pulmonary & Critical Care Medicine, Mayo Clinic College of Medicine, Rochester, MN, USA.

Thomas S. Lin, MD, PhD
Assistant Professor, Department of Internal Medicine, Division of Hematology and Oncology, The Ohio State University, Columbus, OH, USA.

Andrew J. Lipman, MD
Clinical and Research Fellow, Division of Hematology-Oncology, Tufts-New England Medical Center, Boston, MA, USA.

Mark S. Litwin, MD, MPH
Professor, Department of Urology and Health Services, David Geffen School of Medicine, School of Public Health, Jonsson Comprehensive Cancer Center, University of California, Los Angeles, CA, USA.

Jon Håvard Loge, MD, PhD
Professor, Department of Behavioural Sciences in Medicine, University of Oslo and the Centre for Palliative Medicine, Ulleval University Hospital, Oslo, Norway.

B. Jack Longley, MD
Professor, Department of Dermatology, University of Wisconsin-Hospital and Clinics, Madison, WI, USA.

Charles Loprinzi MD
Professor, Division of Medical Oncology, Mayo Clinic Foundation, Rochester, MN, USA.

John R. Lurain, MD
John & Ruth Brewer Professor of Gynecology and Cancer Research, Department of Obstetrics and Gynecology; Director, John I. Brewer Trophoblastic Disease Center; Northwestern University Feinberg School of Medicine, Chicago, IL, USA.

Scott D. Luria, MD
Associate Professor, Department of Medicine, University of Vermont, Burlington, VT, USA.

John S. Macdonald, MD
Professor, Department of Medicine, New York Medical College; Medical Director, St. Vincent's Comprehensive Cancer Center, New York, NY, USA.

Cormac O. Maher, MD
Chief Resident Associate, Department of Neurosurgery, Mayo Clinic College of Medicine, Rochester, MN, USA.

Dennis G. Maki, MD
Chief, Section of Infectious Diseases, Department of Medicine, University of Wisconsin Medical School, Madison, WI, USA.

Karim S. Malek, MD
Assistant Professor, Department of Medicine, Section of Hematology and Oncology, Boston University School of Medicine, Boston, MA, USA.

Shakun Malik, MD
Chief, Center for Thoracic Medical Oncology, Director, Multidisciplinary Thoracic Oncology, Associate Professor, Division of Hematology/Oncology, Department of Medicine and Lombardi Cancer Center, Georgetown University Hospital, Washington, DC, USA.

Paul F. Mansfield, MD, FACS
Professor, Department of Surgical Oncology, The University of Texas M. D. Anderson Cancer Center, Houston, TX, USA.

John L. Marshall, MD
Associate Professor, Lombardi Cancer Center, Georgetown University, Washington, DC, USA.

Paul Martin, MD
Member, Clinical Research Division, Fred Hutchinson Cancer Research Center; Professor, Department of Medicine, University of Washington School of Medicine, Seattle, WA, USA.

Matthew J. Matasar, MD
Instructor, Department of Medicine, Columbia University Medical Center, New York, NY, USA.

Kevin McDonnell, MD, PhD
Fellow, Lombardi Cancer Center, Georgetown University, Washington, DC, USA.

Kevin P. McMullen, MD
Assistant Professor, Department of Radiation Oncology, Wake Forest University School of Medicine, Winston-Salem, NC, USA.

Richard P. McQuellon, PhD
Associate Professor and Director, Psychosocial Oncology & Cancer Patient Support Programs, Wake Forest University Health Sciences, Winston-Salem, NC, USA.

Fredric B. Meyer, MD
Professor, Department of Neurosurgery, Mayo Clinic College of Medicine, Rochester, MN, USA.

Laura C. Michaelis, MD
Fellow, Department of Medicine, Section of Hematology/Oncology, University of Chicago, Chicago, IL, USA.

Michael Milano, MD
Chief Resident, Department of Radiation and Cellular Oncology, University of Chicago, Chicago, IL, USA.

Paradi Mirmirani, MD
Assistant Professor, Department of Dermatology, Case Western Reserve University, University Hospitals of Cleveland, Cleveland, OH, USA.

Anthony C. Montag, MD
Associate Professor, Department of Pathology, University of Chicago Hospital, Chicago, IL, USA.

Craig H. Moskowitz, MD
Associate Professor, Department of Medicine, Lymphoma Service, Memorial Sloan-Kettering Cancer Center, New York, NY, USA.

Brooke T. Mossman
Professor, Department of Pathology, College of Medicine, University of Vermont, Burlington, VT, USA.

Kambiz Motamedi, MD
Assistant Professor, Department of Radiology, David Geffen School of Medicine at UCLA, Los Angeles, CA, USA.

Arno J. Mundt, MD
Associate Professor, Department of Radiation and Cellular Oncology, University of Chicago, Chicago, IL, USA.

David M. Nagorney, MD
Professor, Department of Surgery, Mayo Clinic College of Medicine, Rochester, MN, USA.

Alfred I. Neugut, MD, PhD
Professor, Department of Epidemiology, Mailman School of Public Health; Department of Medicine, Herbert Irving Comprehensive Cancer Center, College of Physicians and Surgeons, Columbia University Medical Center, New York, NY, USA.

Lisa A. Newman, MD, MPH
Associate Professor, Division of Surgical Oncology; Director, Breast Care Center, University of Michigan, Ann Arbor, MI, USA.

Jeffrey L. Nielsen, MD
Chief Resident, Department of Radiology, University Hospitals of Cleveland, Case Western Reserve University School of Medicine, Cleveland, OH, USA.

Jeffrey A. Norton, MD
Professor, Department of Surgery, Division of General Surgery, Stanford University Medical Center, Stanford, CA, USA.

Nomeli P. Nunez, PhD, MPH
Cancer Prevention Fellow, Center for Cancer Research, National Cancer Institute, Bethesda, MD, USA.

Olatoyosi M. Odenike, MD
Assistant Professor, Section of Hematology/Oncology, Department of Medicine, University of Chicago, Chicago, IL, USA.

Beth A. Overmoyer, MD, FACP
Assistant Professor, Department of Medicine, Case Western Reserve University, Cleveland, OH, USA.

Harpreet K. Pannu, MD
Consultant, The Russell H. Morgan Department of Radiology and Radiological Science, The Johns Hopkins Hospital, Baltimore, MD, USA.

Harvey I. Pass, MD
Professor and Chief of Thoracic Surgery, Department of Cardiothoracic Surgery; Head, Thoracic Oncology, New York University School of Medicine and Comprehensive Cancer Center, New York, NY, USA.

Martin G. Pomper, MD, PhD
Associate Professor, Department of Diagnostic Radiology, Division of Neuroradiology, The Johns Hopkins University, Baltimore, MD, USA.

Jeffrey L. Port, MD
Assistant Professor, Department of Cardiothoracic Surgery, Weill-Cornell Medical Center/New York Presbyterian Hospital, New York, NY, USA.

Heather Potter, MD
Resident, Department of Ophthalmology and Visual Sciences, University of Wisconsin, Madison, WI, USA.

Andrew Putnam, MD
Assistant Professor, Departments of Medicine and Oncology, Georgetown University, Washington, DC, USA.

M. Ramos-Nino, PhD
Research Assistant Professor, Department of Pathology, College of Medicine, University of Vermont, Burlington, VT, USA.

Ravi D. Rao, MBBS
Senior Associate Consultant, Division of Medical Oncology, Mayo Clinic College of Medicine, Rochester, MN, USA.

Douglas Reintgen, MD
Director, Department of Surgery, Lakeland Regional Cancer Center, Lakeland, FL, USA.

Mark R. Robbin, MD
Chief, Musculoskeletal and Emergency Radiology; Assistant Professor of Radiology, Department of Radiology, University Hospitals of Cleveland, Case Western Reserve University, Cleveland, OH, USA.

H. Ian Robins, MD, PhD
Professor, Department of Medicine, Human Oncology, and Neurology, University of Wisconsin, Madison, WI, USA.

Rafael Rosell, MD
Chief, Medical Oncology Service, Associate Professor, University of Barcelona; Scientific Director of Oncology Research, Catalan Institute of Oncology, Hospital Germans Trias i Pujol, Barcelona, Spain.

Randy N. Rosier, MD, PhD
Professor and Chairman, Department of Orthopaedics, The University of Rochester Medical Center/Strong Memorial Hospital, Rochester, NY, USA.

Julia H. Rowland, PhD
Director, Office of Cancer Survivorship, Division of Cancer Control and Population Sciences, National Cancer Institute, Bethesda, MD, USA.

Michael S. Sabel, MD
Assistant Professor, Division of Surgical Oncology, Department of Surgery, University of Michigan, Ann Arbor, MI, USA.

T. Sabo-Attwood, PhD
Fellow, Department of Pathology, College of Medicine, University of Vermont, Burlington, VT, USA.

Nasia Safdar, MD, MS
Clinical Instructor, Section of Infectious Diseases, Department of Medicine, University of Wisconsin Medical School, Madison, WI, USA.

Linda Sarna, RN, DNSc, FAAN
Professor, School of Nursing, University of California, Los Angeles, Los Angeles, CA, USA.

David T. Scadden, MD
Professor, Department of Medicine, Massachusetts General Hospital, Harvard Medical School, Boston, MA, USA.

Julian C. Schink, MD
Chief, Division of Gynecologic Oncology; Professor of Obstetrics and Gynecology, Northwestern University Medical School, Chicago, IL, USA.

Robert L. Schlossman
Dana-Farber Cancer Institute, Boston, MA, USA.

Leslie R. Schover, PhD
Professor, Department of Behavioral Science, University of Texas M. D. Anderson Cancer Center, Houston, TX, USA.

Roderich E. Schwarz, MD, PhD
Director, Pancreatic Cancer Program, Department of Surgery, UMDNJ-Robert Wood Johnson Medical School; The Cancer Institute of New Jersey, New Brunswick, NJ, USA.

Christopher N. Sciamanna, MD, MPH
Assistant Professor, Department of Community Health/Psychiatry, Brown University, Providence, RI, USA.

Leanne L. Seeger, MD, FACR
Professor and Chief, Musculoskeletal Imaging, Department of Radiology, David Geffen School of Medicine at UCLA, Los Angeles, CA, USA.

Edward G. Shaw, MD
Professor and Chair, Department of Radiation Oncology, Wake Forest University School of Medicine, Winston-Salem, NC, USA.

Joseph B. Shrager, MD
Associate Professor, Department of Surgery; Chief, Section of General Thoracic Surgery, Hospital of the University of Pennsylvania, Philadelphia, PA, USA.

Rebecca A. Silliman, MD, PhD
Professor, Department of Medicine and Public Health; Chief, Section of Geriatrics, Boston University School of Medicine, Boston Medical Center, Boston, MA, USA.

Paula Silverman, MD
Associate Professor, Clinical Program Director, Division of Hematology/Oncology, University Hospitals of Cleveland, Case Comprehensive Cancer Center, Case Western Reserve University, Cleveland, OH, USA.

Deepjot Singh, MD
Assistant Professor, Division of Hematology/Oncology, University Hospitals of Cleveland, Case Comprehensive Cancer Center, Case Western Reserve University, Cleveland, OH, USA.

Jeffrey R. Skaar
Graduate Student, Department of Medical Oncology, Harvard University, Dana-Farber Cancer Institute, Boston, MA, USA.

John M. Skibber, MD
Professor, Department of Surgical Oncology, The University of Texas M. D. Anderson Cancer Center, Houston, TX, USA.

Stephen R. Smalley, MD
Director, Department of Radiation Oncology, Olathe Medical Center, Olathe, KS, USA.

David L. Smith, MD
Chief, Department of Surgery, Wilford Hall Medical Center, Lackland AFB, TX, USA.

Thomas J. Smith, MD
Professor and Chairman, Department of Internal Medicine, Division of Hematology/Oncology, Virginia Commonwealth University Health System, Richmond, VA, USA.

Jason Sohn, PhD, DABR
Associate Professor, Associate Director of Medical Physics and Dosimetry, Department of Radiation Oncology, Division of Medical Physics and Dosimetry, University Hospitals of Cleveland, Case Western Reserve University, Cleveland, OH, USA.

Robert J. Soiffer, MD
Chief, Division of Hematologic Malignancies, Dana-Farber Cancer Institute, Associate Professor of Medicine, Harvard Medical School, Boston, MA, USA.

Vernon K. Sondak, MD
Professor, Department of Interdisciplinary Oncology, H. Lee Moffitt Cancer Center, Tampa, FL, USA.

Yukio Sonoda, MD
Assistant Attending Surgeon, Department of Surgery, Gynecology/Oncology, Memorial Sloan-Kettering Cancer Center, New York, NY, USA.

Jeffrey A. Sosman, MD
Professor, Division of Hematology/Oncology, Vanderbilt University Medical Center; Medical Director; Clinical Trials Office; Co-Leader, Signal Transduction and Cell Proliferation Program, Vanderbilt-Ingram Cancer Center, Nashville, TN, USA.

David Spriggs, MD
Head, Division of Solid Tumor Oncology, Winthrop Rockefeller Chair of Medical Oncology, Department of Medicine, Memorial Sloan-Kettering Cancer Center, New York, NY, USA.

Sandy Srinivas, MD
Assistant Professor, Department of Medicine, Stanford University, Palo-Alto, CA, USA.

Kerstin M. Stenson, MD, FACS
Associate Professor, Department of Surgery, Section of Otolaryngology-Head & Neck Surgery, Department of Surgery, University of Chicago, Chicago, IL, USA.

Volker W. Stieber, MD
Assistant Professor, Co-Director, Gamma Knife Unit, Department of Radiation Oncology, Comprehensive Cancer Center, Wake Forest University, Winston-Salem, NC, USA.

Wendy Stock, MD
Associate Professor, Department of Medicine, Section of Hematology/ Oncology; Director, Leukemia Program, University of Chicago, Chicago, IL, USA.

Ellen L. Stovall
President and CEO, National Coalition for Cancer Survivorship, Silver Spring, MD, USA.

Crawford J. Strunk, MD
Fellow, Department of Pediatric Hematology-Oncology, Case Western University, Division of Pediatric Hematology and Oncology, Rainbow Babies and Children's Hospital, Cleveland, OH, USA.

Zoë N. Swaine, Bsc (Hons)
Graduate Student, Department of Clinical and Health Psychology, University of Florida, College of Public Health and Health Professions, Gainesville, FL, USA.

Charles Swanton, MRCP, PhD
CR-UK Clinician Scientist, Department of Medicine, Royal Marsden Hospital, London, UK.

Karen L. Syrjala, PhD
Associate Member, Clinical Research Division, Fred Hutchinson Cancer Research Center, Associate Professor of Psychiatry and Behavioral Sciences, University of Washington School of Medicine, Seattle, WA, USA.

Kenneth K. Tanabe, MD
Associate Professor, Chief, Division of Surgical Oncology, Department of Surgery, Massachusetts General Hospital, Boston, MA, USA.

Stephen H. Taplin, MD, MPH
Senior Scientist, Applied Research Program, Division of Cancer Control and Population Sciences, National Cancer Institute, Rockville, MD, USA.

Marcie Tomblyn, MD
Assistant Professor, Department of Medicine/Hematology, Oncology, and Transplant, University of Minnesota, Minneapolis, MN, USA.

Lois B. Travis
Senior Investigator, National Institutes of Health, Department of Health and Human Services, Division of Cancer Epidemiology and Genetics, National Cancer Institute, Bethesda, MD, USA.

Anne Traynor, MD
Assistant Professor, Section of Medical Oncology, University of Wisconsin Comprehensive Cancer Center, University of Wisconsin Medical School, Madison, WI, USA.

Timothy J. Triche, MD, PhD
Professor, Department of Pathology & Pediatrics; Chair, Department of Pathology and Laboratory Medicine, Childrens' Hospital Los Angeles; Vice Chair, Pathology, Keck School of Medicine at USC, Los Angeles, CA, USA.

Peter A. Ubel, MD
Director, Program for Improving Health Care Decisions, Department of General Medicine, University of Michigan, Ann Arbor, MI, USA.

Asad Umar, DVM, PhD
Program Director, Gastrointestinal and Other Cancers Research Group, National Cancer Institute, Rockville, MD, USA.

John D. Urschel, MD, MA, FRCSC
Lecturer, Department of Surgery, McMaster University, Hamilton, Ontario, Canada.

David J. Vaughn, MD
Associate Professor, Department of Medicine, University of Pennsylvania, Philadelphia, PA, USA.

Andrew J. Vickers, PhD
Staff, Integrative Medicine Service, Memorial Sloan-Kettering Cancer Center, New York, NY, USA.

Nicholas Vogelzang, MD
Professor, Department of Medicine, University of Nevada School of Medicine; Director, Nevada Cancer Institute, Las Vegas, NV, USA.

Everett E. Vokes, MD
Director, Section of Hematology/Oncology, John E. Ultmann Professor of Medicine and Radiation and Cellular Oncology, University of Chicago, Chicago, IL, USA.

Richard L. Wahl, MD
Director, Nuclear Medicine/PET, Russell H. Morgan Department of Radiology and Radiological Sciences, The Johns Hopkins School of Medicine, Baltimore, MD, USA.

Timothy S. Wang, MD
Assistant Professor, Department of Dermatology, University of Michigan, Ann Arbor, MI, USA.

Iryna S. Watson, BA
Research Study Coordinator, Department of Psychosocial and Palliative Care, H. Lee Moffitt Research Center, Tampa, FL, USA.

Jeffrey Weber, MD, PhD
Chief, Division of Medical Oncology, Department of Medicine, USC/Norris Cancer Center, Los Angeles, CA, USA.

Daniel J. Weisdorf, MD
Professor, Director, Adult Blood and Marrow Transplant Program, Department of Medicine, University of Minnesota, Minneapolis, MN, USA.

Anton Wellstein, MD, PhD
Professor, Lombardi Cancer Center, Georgetown University, Washington, DC, USA.

Barry Wessels, PhD
Professor and Director, Department of Radiation Oncology, Division of Medical Physics and Dosimetry, University Hospitals of Cleveland, Case Western Reserve University, Cleveland, OH, USA.

Meir Wetzler, MD
Associate Professor, Department of Medicine, Leukemia Section, Roswell Park Cancer Institute, Buffalo, NY, USA.

Patrick Whelan, MD, PhD
Instructor in Pediatrics, Harvard Medical School, Boston, MA, USA.

Richard Whittington, MD
Professor, Department of Radiation Oncology, University of Pennsylvania, Philadelphia, PA, USA.

T. Christopher Windham, MD
Assistant Professor, Department of Interdisciplinary Oncology, H. Lee Moffitt Cancer Center and Research Institute, Tampa, FL, USA.

David P. Wood, Jr., MD
Professor and Chief of Urologic Oncology, Department of Urology, University of Michigan, Ann Arbor, MI, USA.

Antoinette J. Wozniak, MD
Professor, Department of Internal Medicine/Division of Hematology/Oncology, Karmanos Cancer Institute/Wayne State University, Detroit, MI, USA.

S.D. Yamada, MD
Assistant Professor, Department of Obstetrics and Gynecology, Section of Gynecologic Oncology, University of Chicago, Chicago, IL, USA.

Sam S. Yoon, MD
Assistant Professor, Division of Surgical Oncology, Department of Surgery, Massachusetts General Hospital, MA, USA.

Lydia B. Zablotska, MD, PhD
Assistant Professor, Department of Epidemiology, Mailman School of Public Health, Columbia University, New York, NY, USA.

Jane Zapka, ScD
Professor, Department of Biometry and Epidemiology, Medical University of South Carolina, Charleston, SC, USA.

Andrew D. Zelenetz, MD, PhD
Chief, Lymphoma Service, Memorial Sloan-Kettering Cancer Center, New York, NY, USA.

Paula Zeller, MA
Communications Consultant, Olney, MD, USA.

Lonnie Zeltzer, MD
Professor, Departments of Pediatrics, Anesthesiology, Psychiatry and Biobehavioral Sciences; Director, Pediatric Pain Program, David Geffen School of Medicine at UCLA; Associate Director, Patients and Survivors Program, Division of Cancer Prevention and Control Research; UCLA Jonsson Comprehensive Cancer Center, Los Angeles, CA, USA.

SECTION ONE

Principles of Oncology

1 Evidence-Based Approach to Oncology

Emily DeVoto and Barnett S. Kramer*

In the early years of the 21st century, clinicians and medical researchers often use the term *evidence-based medicine.* Cancer prevention, screening, diagnosis, and therapy, we hear, must be based on the best evidence to provide the best care. But is this approach new? And if it is, what have we been doing until now? In this chapter, we hope to provide perspectives on this question, by examining what evidence-based medicine (EBM)—oncology, in particular—is and is not, and by looking at the history of clinical inquiry, up to and including current research. We also hope to provide readers with a theoretical framework that will be useful in placing the results of new research into the context of existing knowledge, with the ultimate goal of improving clinical practice.

The principles of EBM were delineated by a working group in Canada (led by Gordon Guyatt of McMaster University) and published in JAMA in 1992.[1] According to Sackett and colleagues, some of the earliest promoters of the principles of the concept, EBM is "the integration of best research evidence with clinical expertise and patient values."[2] Thus, EBM is *not* cookbook practice performed by technicians without regard to experience, training, or independent clinical judgment. The practice of EBM has occurred with the recognition that up-to-date, scientifically valid medical information is needed on a regular basis; that traditional sources of information (such as textbooks, expert opinion, and the flood of new research) are either unreliable or overwhelming; and that patient and other demands limit clinicians' time available for keeping skills current and for identifying the most relevant information. In response, medicine has developed strategies and information systems for tracking down useful information quickly and mechanisms for stringent, systematic review and evaluation of clinical research.[2] The purpose of textbooks such as this, and other forums for EBM, is to empower practicing clinicians with the skills to evaluate the literature, to identify relevant clinical guidelines and recommendations, and to understand the study design factors that affect the quality of medical evidence, in support of sound clinical decision making.

Sackett and colleagues propose the following five steps for clinicians in making evidence-based decisions: "(1) Converting the need for information into an answerable question; (2) Tracking down the best evidence to answer the question; (3) Critically evaluating that evidence; (4) Integrating the critical evaluation with clinical expertise and knowledge of the patient; (5) Evaluating our effectiveness and efficiency in steps 1 to 4 and seeking ways to improve both for next time."[2]

Later in this chapter, we elaborate on these steps to provide a practical framework for clinical decision making. First, however, we attempt to place the development of the concept of medical evidence in a historical context, focusing on aspects of research that point to quality of evidence.

The History of *Evidence* in Medicine

Francois Joseph Victor Broussais (1772–1838) was a professor of General Pathology at Paris and one of the leading physicians in France. His central theoretical model of disease physiology was that vital processes depended on external stimuli, especially heat; these stimuli produced chemical changes, which modified normal tissue function. He conceived that if the stimuli are in balance, one is healthy, but if they are too weak or too strong, disease results. All disease is local, he held, but is transmitted to other organs by sympathy or via the gastrointestinal mucosa; he believed gastroenteritis was the basis of all pathology (Table 1.1).

P.C.A. Louis (1787–1872), a French contemporary of Broussais, agreed with Broussais that objective observation is central to medicine, but in their methods of observation and the conclusions they drew, their views diverged greatly, and this is why Louis has the more-lasting legacy in the annals of medicine. Louis devoted himself to the observation of inflammatory diseases such as typhoid fever and pneumonia. Until his time, bloodletting (using leeches) was the unchallenged treatment for inflammatory disease. Louis and a few contemporaries were the first to question explicitly whether full-force application of leeches was appropriate under all circumstances, and Louis was the first to test the hypothesis. To address this question, Louis examined the medical records of 79 pneumonia patients in his practice and analyzed their disease duration and mortality experience with respect to the time of their first bleeding relative to the course of the disease. He also took into account the number of bleedings and the subjects' ages. Of note, he started the investigation with a belief that bloodletting was effective. The finding of the study, that the beneficial effect of bloodletting was "much less than has been commonly believed," probably contributed to the demise of bloodletting as a widespread practice.[3]

*The opinions expressed in this manuscript are those of the authors and do not represent official opinions or positions of the National Institutes of Health, the Department of Health and Human Services, or the federal government.

TABLE 1.1. Historical landmarks in the development of evidence-based medicine.

1747	• First use of comparison groups in a clinical experiment	James Lind: experiments to treat scurvy in British sailors
1828	• First application of mathematical analysis to test a hypothesis • Introduction of concept of confounding (i.e., patients' response may vary for reasons other than treatment)	P.C.A. Louis: observations of the effect of timing of bloodletting on pneumonia outcomes
1853–1856	• First systematic use of statistics in medicine • Development of systematic data collection • Calculation of rates of morbidity and mortality, based on hospital intake and discharge data	Florence Nightingale presented data on mortality in field hospitals during Crimean War, leading to fundamental changes in patient hygiene
1920s–1930s	• Development of statistical methods: accounting for the role of chance in scientific studies • Development of experimental study design	Ronald Fisher, as described in his book *Design of Experiments* (1935)
1948	• First randomized clinical trial (RCT)	Sir Austin Bradford Hill assessed the use of streptomycin in treating tuberculosis
1970s	• U.S. 6th Circuit Court of Appeals grants RCTs status as a standard of evidence in the regulatory authority of the Food and Drug Administration	
1992	• Principles of evidence-based medicine delineated and published	Working group led by Gordon Guyatt, McMaster University

Louis was well ahead of his time in his use of standardized data collection and in his framing of research questions, but perhaps more importantly to the history of evidence-based medicine, Louis clearly recognized the limitations of his work. He wrote of the possibility that alternative, unmeasured factors (besides bloodletting) could explain his findings. He understood that his patients may have differed for reasons unrelated to treatment and that these differences might have had a more important influence on their outcomes than the treatment itself.[3] That is, Louis questioned the cause-and-effect relationship between bloodletting and increased survival, whether or not he articulated it as such.

The first historic example of the use of comparison control groups in clinical investigation comes from the well-known story of James Lind, an 18th-century British physician (1716–1794) who addressed the issue of scurvy in the British Navy. The value of fresh fruit in treating and preventing scurvy had been suggested by an earlier scholar, but Lind was the first to apply an experimental design to the investigation of this hypothesis. In 1747, he selected 12 patients/seamen on board a navy vessel, as he said, "as similar as I could have them," and then assigned 2 each to various treatments, one of which was to eat two oranges and one lemon per day (others were given cider or seawater). He found, of course, that the 2 who received the citrus fruits recovered the best, with those taking cider recovering next best. Although not a randomized design (he stated that "two of the worst" received the course of seawater), Lind at least attempted to start with a homogeneous group, reflecting his intent to reduce the effect of confounding. Although there was no formally declared untreated group, and each treatment group was quite small, the systematic, prospective construction of comparison groups was new to medical science.[4]

Florence Nightingale (1820–1910) collected data on the mortality experience of solders injured in the Crimean War (1853–1856). Her presentation of statistics on the vast improvement in patient outcomes following the introduction of hygienic practices into the field hospital led to widespread reforms in military medicine. Nightingale found, based on careful record keeping and comparisons to civilian populations, that infection among soldiers led to a doubling of expected mortality; this required development of new statistical methods. From this experience, Nightingale collaborated with other scientists to develop a systematic method for collecting data on disease and mortality in hospitals. The key data elements collected in this system were the counting of all patients entering and leaving the hospital, and the mean duration of stay, thus providing denominators for the reporting of true rates of morbidity and mortality.[5]

After scientists of the 19th century (such as Nightingale) developed their work in vital statistics, the growth of statistical theory, including ideas about randomization, flowered in the first half of the 20th century.[6] Ronald Fisher, an agricultural scientist, pioneered the theory and use of randomization in experiments. Fisher asserted that a "properly designed" experiment is one about which one can say that "Chance would so rarely cause such a large difference in outcome that I shall attribute the observed difference to the treatments," and that the only two possible explanations are chance and the treatments, that is, not bias or confounding. Another key feature of the randomized design is to vary the essential conditions only one at a time. In summary, the two main principles of the experimental method are numerical balance (equal numbers of subjects in the test and control group) and randomization of all the factors that are not being tested.[7]

In the area of observational medical science, or epidemiology, Austin Bradford-Hill developed a set of criteria to evaluate cause-and-effect relationships in disease. Around the same time, Bradford-Hill launched the first randomized clinical trial, investigating the efficacy of streptomycin in treating tuberculosis, which introduced the only clinical study design able to assess the question of cause and effect directly (more on this design follows). The introduction of the randomized trial to clinical cancer research followed a few years thereafter.

The design of clinical trials evolved in the 1950s and 1960s through the many trials that were initiated as a result of demand from the pharmaceutical industry, which wished to introduce to the market new drugs that met the standards of rigorous clinical testing. Despite struggles by research clinicians against rigorous randomized clinical trial designs (typically in the interest of providing all patients the opportunity of palliation or preventing disease progression), some important trials proceeded. In the 1970s, the U.S. 6th Circuit Court of Appeals granted randomized trials status as a standard of evidence toward the U.S. Food and Drug Administration's regulatory authority over the pharmaceutical industry.[8] Trials of chemotherapeutic agents and analgesics often gave disappointing results; however, a landmark randomized trial showing segmental mastectomy with axillary node dissection for breast cancer to be as effective as total mastectomy in demonstrating long-term survival was published by Bernard Fisher and colleagues in the National Surgical Adjuvant Breast and Bowel Program[9] and produced a demonstrable breakthrough in breast cancer care. At the same time, the results overturned centuries-old assumptions about the biology of breast cancer and how it spreads.

Evidence-Based Medicine as a Tool for Clinical Decision Making

Dr. A, a first-year oncology resident, sees patient X, a 47-year-old woman referred to the service with a 2-cm ductal carcinoma in situ found on a screening mammogram. How does Dr. A approach the management of patient X?

The classic approach Dr. A. might take is to consult someone who has treated similar patients before. She can also call on her knowledge from coursework. Finally, she can consult the literature, which might well be a daunting task in itself. The primary literature consists of scores of thousands of original research articles; the secondary literature consists of thousands of review articles.

Asking Answerable Clinical Questions

The first stage of evidence-based decision making is to look closely at the information available. When a clinical scenario is written down, the practitioner can scan it with regard to a set of central clinical issues to identify gaps in knowledge that need to be filled with additional clinical information, or by turning to the literature, or both. These issues are (1) clinical findings, (2) etiology, (3) clinical manifestations of disease, (4) differential diagnosis, (5) diagnostic tests, (6) prognosis, (7) therapy, (8) prevention, (9) patient experience and meaning, and (10) practitioner self-improvement.[2] Then, the questions can be formulated, and the questions should comprise four components: description of the patient or target disorder of interest, intervention, comparison intervention (relevant for therapy questions), and outcome.[10] Using the previous example, the clinician might ask, "For a 47-year-old woman with ductal carcinoma in situ, what is the likelihood that lumpectomy followed by radiation, compared to lumpectomy alone, will prevent recurrence?"

Research Design and Quality of Evidence

Central to the idea of evidence-based medicine is the idea that there is a hierarchy of quality of evidence that is related to the design and conduct of the study or studies from which it arose. It should be kept in mind as well that different study designs on the same topic often answer rather different questions from one another. The hierarchy of study designs is illustrated in the pyramid in Figure 1.1, which also reflects the relative numbers of studies in each category.

As described previously, P.C.A. Louis' writings were centuries ahead of his time in terms of suggesting the possibility of alternative explanations for his findings, or the concept of confounding, defined as a factor that tends to co-occur with the predictive (presumed causal) factor under study and that also tends to co-occur with the outcome. Louis, for example, found that bloodletting later in the disease process was associated with longer survival. To our knowledge, Louis did not make note of his patients' diet. It is possible that those who consumed more calories would have on the one hand received the bloodletting intervention later in their disease course, because they looked healthier to begin with, and on the other

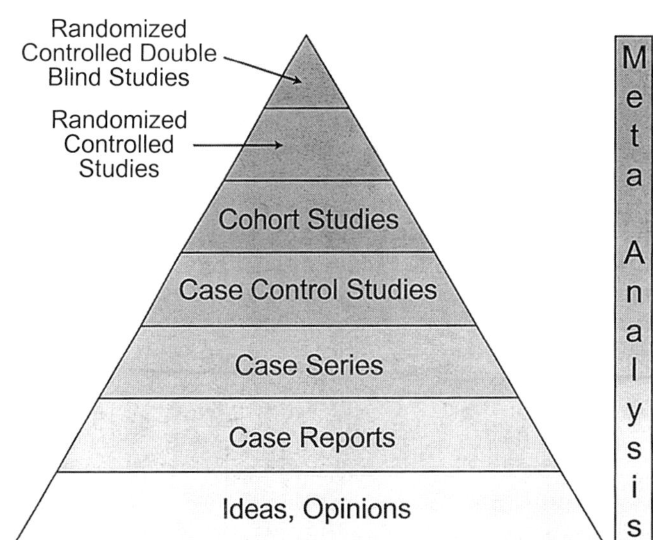

FIGURE 1.1. The pyramid of evidence represents levels of evidence as well as the relative numbers of studies at each level.

hand would have survived their disease better because in fact they *were* healthier. Diet would thus have been a *confounder* of the apparent association between timing of bloodletting and improved survival.

Unmeasured confounding is a central reason for distortion of study results, although it arises in different ways, which we discuss as they appear throughout this chapter. One of those is selection bias: in the case of Louis' work, patients may have been selected for late treatment as opposed to the early-treatment group for reasons other than random chance, thus leaving open the likelihood that factors (that is, the confounders) other than the treatment influenced the outcome.

Randomized Clinical Trials

Random allocation to a treatment or control group is the basis of all experimental design, and it is the only way to isolate the effect of a single factor under study on a given outcome and thus avoid the distorting effects of confounding. Even though potential confounding variables still exist among study subjects, randomization is designed to distribute them evenly between the test and control groups, thus removing their effects. The power of the randomized design is that it should provide equal balance not only of known confounding factors but also of unknown potential confounders. We discuss a few refinements to the randomized study design in the remainder of this chapter, but an entire chapter of this book is dedicated to randomized trials in cancer as well (see Chapter 8).

Another central (and related) tenet of scientific inquiry is the idea of a comparison or control group. In clinical research, in the absence of a control group similar in every way to the test group receiving an investigational intervention, it is impossible to discern how many subjects benefited from treatment as opposed to improving on their own.

An important factor to consider when evaluating oncology research, particularly studies of cancer therapy, is the choice of endpoints. Endpoints include health outcomes (total mortality, cause-specific mortality, quality of life) or indirect surrogates for any of these. Examples of surrogate endpoints are disease-free survival, progression-free survival, or tumor response rate. Studies of surrogate endpoints represent weaker, more indirect, evidence; however, a clinician may weigh studies differently depending on patient values.

The bulk of our understanding of risk factors and preventive factors for cancer comes from observational studies (that is, those described here). Recent research has moved toward testing hypotheses generated by observational studies in the context of clinical trials, sometimes with unexpected results, such as a study of prevention of cancer by beta-carotene in smokers that found that beta-carotene increased lung cancer incidence compared with placebo.[11] This finding stood in contrast to results from nonrandomized observational studies, which had suggested a benefit.

Cohort Studies in Oncology

A cohort study identifies a group of subjects on the basis of their naturally occurring exposure to an agent or agents of interest and follows them in time to observe their experience (incidence) of disease. Data can be collected from the present into the future (prospective cohort study) or use historic data, such as records of occupational exposure, to look from the present into the past (retrospective cohort study). For cancer, the cohort study design tends to be inefficient, because cancer is considered to be a relatively rarely occurring outcome requiring the following over time of rather large initial populations to observe statistically meaningful results. Most prospective cohorts that study cancer were constructed to study other diseases, such as heart disease (for example, the Framingham Heart Study), or a range of diseases (for example, the Nurses Health Study). The benefit of a prospective cohort design is that exposures are evaluated in individuals before their diagnosis of disease; thus, the disease cannot distort the measurement of exposure as in cross-sectional or retrospective study designs. Often cohort studies collect baseline exposure information in great detail that is highly useful (although imperfect) in controlling for confounding.

A drawback of prospective cohort studies is the attrition of participation over time, or *loss to follow-up*. Cohort studies often involve the repeated filling out of lengthy, detailed questionnaires on diet and other lifestyle factors, clinical examinations, and/or telephone interviews. Subjects remaining in such studies tend to be healthy relative to those who drop out, or the most motivated by health concerns, and may differ from those who drop out in other respects that are difficult to measure, which can result in confounding. Other reasons for attrition are illness, changing residence, and other changes in life circumstances that may be associated with unmeasured characteristics which differ between those who remain in a cohort study and those lost to follow-up and that are associated with disease risk. Such differences can distort the results or make study results less representative of the original target population.

In addition, cohort studies can be extremely expensive. Designing and implementing a cohort study that provides adequate richness of data and study outcomes and avoids issues of loss to follow-up is resource intensive, as are maintenance and analysis of the data, keeping track of the details of protocols, and many other administrative tasks.

Nested Case-Control Studies

A nested case-control study selects, from subjects in a cohort study, subjects who have the disease of interest (called *case subjects*) and a sample of subjects who are disease free at the time of sampling as controls. Similar to a conventional case-control study, this study design is efficient for studying rare diseases. It is a useful design if it is too expensive to measure a risk factor for every subject within a cohort study. It also shares with cohort studies the advantage of having subjects selected at baseline from the same population, so that case and control subjects chosen later are likely to be more comparable than those in a conventional case-control study.

It is possible, if the exposure of interest is not measured before subjects in the nested case-control study are selected, that such measurement will be essentially retrospective, for example, if a detailed dietary frequency questionnaire is administered, which results in the same limitations as a conventional case-control study. However, this design is useful for studying biologic markers of exposure that are measurable in blood or other tissue samples and that remain stable in storage, especially freezing. Often blood samples are taken from all subjects of a cohort at baseline and frozen for later analysis. As an example, the Kaiser Permanente Health Maintenance Organization collected and froze serum samples for all subjects on enrollment. Their record-keeping system provided longitudinal data on patients, including data on disease incidence. Researchers who wished to investigate the association between exposure to the pesticide DDT (dichlorodiphenyltrichloroethane) first selected, from the Kaiser cohort, breast cancer case subjects and a sample of control subjects who were disease free when the case was diagnosed. They then retrieved frozen serum samples that, for the case subjects, were taken at least several years before diagnosis with breast cancer, and measured the concentration of DDT in the samples to compare the concentrations in case and control subjects.[12]

Case-Control Studies

Many life-threatening diseases studied by epidemiologists are relatively rare. Consider, for example, the likelihood of being diagnosed with breast cancer in a given year, compared with that of coming down with a cold. If you only had the resources to study 500 women aged 50, with average risk factors, over a 5-year period, only 5 or 10 of them would be expected to be diagnosed with breast cancer during that time, whereas a large majority of them are likely to come down with a cold at least once in 5 years. The number of breast cancer cases is simply not adequate to allow valid comparisons among different hypothesized risk factors between women who are diagnosed with breast cancer and those who are not. On the other hand, if you set out to identify 250 women newly diagnosed with breast cancer (case subjects) in a given population, and simultaneously identified a suitable comparison group of 250 women (control subjects), you could substantially improve the statistical power (also called *efficiency*) of the study.

A study in which subjects are identified on the basis of their disease status has what is known as a *case-control* design. Once you identify the subjects, you can then interview them about hypothesized disease risk factors such as diet, pharmaceuticals, sun exposure, pregnancy history, and so on. This is the *bread-and-butter* design of the bulk of cancer epidemiology. However, it is particularly prone to sources of bias and confounding that randomized controlled trials and cohort studies are not.

The most important downside of case-control studies is potential bias from errors in recalling and reporting risk factors. For example, many people tend to underestimate or underreport their alcohol consumption. If people with and without a disease under study underestimate their consumption to a similar degree, then a true association between alcohol consumption and the disease would be more difficult to observe. In contrast, if someone diagnosed with a disease believes that his or her past alcohol consumption may have played a role in the disease, that consumption could either be further underreported or overreported relative to the true exposure. In any case, it is quite possible that the recall is different from that of someone without the disease. Just as it is difficult to predict which way someone is likely to misreport exposure, it is by extension difficult to predict the effect of such misreporting on estimates of disease association or risk.

Another drawback of case-control studies is the fact that exposures reported to occur at a given point in time might not represent the exposures that actually cause the disease. This consideration is important in diseases such as cancer that have a long latency period, that is, the time between a causal exposure and the diagnosis of disease. Conceivably, cancer itself could alter dietary or lifestyle patterns in the period before diagnosis, thus reversing the cause-and-effect sequence. In addition, if a marker of a hypothesized disease risk factor is measured in a body tissue, such as the concentration of a pesticide in blood, it is possible that the measurement could be affected by the disease, resulting in a spurious association or masking a true association.

Selection of an appropriate control group is particularly important, but also particularly difficult, for case-control studies. Bias, used here to mean systematic error in an estimate, can arise if case subjects and control subjects arise from populations with different underlying baseline characteristics. The more the case and control populations differ from one another, the more difficult it is to ensure that observed differences in risk factors are not due to extraneous, unmeasured factors, or *confounders*, that are associated with the factors under study and with the disease. For example, a study might find that people with lung cancer are more likely to drink alcohol than a group of control subjects similar in age. Rather than assuming that this finding indicates that alcohol is a risk factor for lung cancer, it is prudent to consider whether alcohol consumption is related to smoking, an established cause of lung cancer.

In summary, case-control studies are often more convenient to assemble than the preceding study designs when a rare disease or outcome is being studied, and they are less expensive than cohort (follow-up) or experimental studies. However, because exposure is assessed retrospectively, errors in recall are often a problem. In addition, it is sometimes difficult to generalize the results or to avoid bias from confounding because of the ways in which patient and control groups are selected. For these reasons, case-control studies tend to provide a lower level of evidence than cohort studies or experimental studies.

Cross-Sectional Studies

A cross-sectional study estimates the *prevalence* of disease (the number of cases of a disease) and possible disease risk factors in a given population at one point in time. Such studies are most usefully conducted by random sampling, which helps ensure that their results are representative of the larger population of interest. A special case of the cross-sectional design, which is, technically, a survey follow-up study because it is repeated on a regular basis, can be found in the Behavioral Risk Factor Surveillance System (http://www.cdc.gov/brfss/), an annual national survey that selects a representative sample of U.S. residents and interviews them about such behavioral factors as exercise, human immunodeficiency virus (HIV) awareness, drug use, and smoking. Statistics describing the prevalence of these factors can then be compared from year to year, and a new set of subjects is sampled each year.

Similar to cohort studies, subjects in cross-sectional studies are not selected for study on the basis of their disease status. Similar to case-control studies, however, measurement of risk factors is either nondirectional or retrospective, and the presence of risk factors cannot be shown to precede disease; that is, the temporality requirement for declaration of cause and effect is lost. Therefore, although cross-sectional studies are sometimes used to evaluate associations between risk factors and disease and to generate hypotheses, their ability to support evidence of causation is more limited than that of other observational studies.

Ecologic Studies

In studies of ecologic design, the number of people with an exposure is known, as is the number of people with a disease or outcome (mortality, for example), but the number of people with both the exposure and the disease is not known. In general, relevant information on individuals in the population is unknown. A study that is at least partly ecologic in design may be the only feasible option in the case of an environmental exposure experienced by an entire population. A well-known example of an ecologic study stemmed from the observation that the number of deaths in London increased sharply relative to average death rates during a period of particularly heavy smog and was closely proportional to the ambient temperature during that period.

Generally, however, the level of evidence provided by ecologic studies is considered quite weak, primarily because of the studies' inability to correct for other variables, that is, confounders, at the individual or aggregate level that could explain the observed associations. Indeed, such confounding remains a possibility in the London smog example, in which the agent that caused the excess deaths cannot be known with certainty. A commonly encountered example of ecologic data is the observation that rates of certain kinds of cancer, especially breast cancer, are high in countries with high consumption of dietary fat and that cancer rates are low in those countries reporting low dietary fat consumption. Such observations are useful in generating hypotheses for further study; however, as in the example of dietary fat and breast cancer, epidemiologic studies based on individual-level data with the ability to adjust for confounding factors often show little or no association between dietary fat and breast cancer.

Case Series and Case Reports

Reports of individual cases and case series represent the earliest known method of accumulating medical knowledge on most diseases. Although their importance is lower today given the availability of controlled studies, particularly clinical trials, they remain a popular mode of publication by clinicians of their investigations and observations. As evidence, however, case series and reports pose a number of problems and should be interpreted with substantial caution.

Many case series are collected retrospectively from medical records, and recording of information may be selective and subject to incompleteness or other forms of error compared to information collected according to a predefined plan. Selection bias can occur when the series is not representative of the general population, in particular when subjects with similar prognosis are selectively lost to follow-up. Case series based on medical records are also likely to lack adequate (if any) information on confounders. Finally, the decision as to which data to report may be selective, particularly if eligibility criteria are not established in advance. For example, striking results may lead to report of a case or a series of cases, distorting the sense of what would be expected in general. Unfortunately, for some exceedingly rare diseases, clinical knowledge rests on case series and case reports for lack of sufficient numbers to support more robust study designs (J. Lau, unpublished observation).

Preclinical Studies

Laboratory studies using immortalized cell lines, whole tumors, or some other system below the level of the organism are important in basic oncology, but their purpose is to isolate small subsets of the complex tumor biology machinery to elucidate mechanisms (Table 1.2). Rarely should they be taken in isolation as evidence for or against a given treatment strategy. They do represent a level of control that may never be attainable or ethical in whole humans; on the other hand, it is their very lack of organismal context that makes them unreliable to extrapolate to humans. Despite a tendency of some researchers and the media to tout breakthroughs in biomedical research on the basis of laboratory studies, they should be seen by practicing clinicians for their intent: mechanistic, preliminary, and hypothesis generating in relation to medical practice.

The toxic or beneficial effects of drugs, environmental agents, and foods are typically evaluated using laboratory rodents or other small mammals, according to stringent experimental and statistical analytic protocols. These protocols allow statistically efficient estimates of beneficial, safe, or toxic doses of chemicals in genetically homogeneous animals. Laboratory animals may also be used for mechanistic studies, for example, using gene *knockout* models. It is important to be able to test chemicals with uncertain safety on nonhumans. However, because mice and rats are not humans, assumptions must be made regarding the extrapolation of results to humans and again should not be used by the clinician in isolation for clinical decision making.

Expert Opinion

> Until modern times, 'facts' were deduced by arguments from premises approved by tradition and authority, without appeal to experimental validation. Even when observation ran counter to 'facts,' it was still believed that in some mysterious way authority must still be correct, particularly at a time in history when the fabric of society was such as to frown upon the challenge of authority. The modern therapeutic trial offers an alternative by relying upon impartial observance without regard for authoritarianism. Such an approach provides the foundation of scientific medicine."
>
> —Bernard Fisher[13]

In other words, the evidence of expert opinion is only as strong as the empiric evidence from which it is derived. As Albert Einstein pointed out: "Propositions arrived at purely by logical means are completely empty as regards reality. Because Galileo saw this, and particularly because he drummed it into the scientific world, he is the father of modern physics—indeed of modern science altogether." (From *Ideas and Opinions*, Modern Library, 1994)

The Role of Meta-Analyses and Literature Reviews

For many clinical questions, the practitioner will find that much of the work of reviewing and evaluating research has already been done, or at least addressed, and that summaries of literature exist. The end of this chapter offers a number of readily available sources of comprehensive literature reviews, along with other convenient sources of evidence-based medical knowledge. By way of definition, an overview or review of literature may be any type of summary, whereas the term *meta-analysis* describes a quantitative summary of results from different studies. Because a meta-analysis attempts to combine results from a number of studies into a summary statistic, it is important to be sure that the studies have a common outcome measure. Also, the underlying assumption is made that the studies are drawn from the same pool or universe of studies and can therefore be legitimately combined. Statistical tests for homogeneity are therefore often used to test this assumption. Also, the validity of a meta-analysis depends upon the assumption that there has not been substantial selective reporting of studies depending on their result (e.g., greater likelihood to report small positive studies than small negative studies). Funnel plots are used to assess this possibility graphically. In a funnel plot, the outcome variable for each study is graphed versus its variance.

Literature reviews may be systematic or rely on the recall of the author. In a systematic review, a complete computer search is made of the relevant literature using specific search terms and prospective rules for inclusion or exclusion of studies found in the systematic search.

To begin evaluating a review, the practitioner should ask two questions: does it ask a carefully focused clinical question, and is the method for including studies reasonable and appropriate? The latter question can be expanded as follows: are methodological standards articulated (for example, those laid out in this chapter), and do the studies chosen address the research question articulated by the reviewer? Stating inclusion criteria up front helps avoid any biases toward preconceived conclusions a reviewer might hold. Aspects of oncology studies to keep in mind when reviewing a review are outcomes (as described previously) and latency periods. Review writers should demonstrate that they exhaustively searched appropriate bibliographic databases (such as Medline), but also that they contacted experts in the area who might be aware not only of published studies not yet appearing in Medline, but of unpublished studies; this is important because studies with negative findings are less likely to reach publication.

Practitioners reading reviews should consider whether results of reasonably comparable studies are similar. Meta-analyses study formally and quantitatively whether results of similar studies differ more than would be expected by chance alone. If so, it is likely that study designs differ enough to account for observed differences in results.

A review should not simply compare the number of positive and negative studies of a given question to obtain an answer, as this fails to give different weight to large and small studies, large studies being more likely to show a positive result because of increased statistical power or efficiency. In addition, such a comparison ignores effects other than the primary outcome of interest, and says nothing about the magnitude of an effect, its clinical importance, or the relatively quality of individual studies.

Ranking the Evidence: The Role of Study Design and Study Quality

Looking at evidence in the field of oncology is similar to analogous processes in other fields of medicine. An example evidence rating system for research on cancer screening and prevention is used by the Physician's Data Query (PDQ) of the U.S. National Cancer Institute and can be found at http://cancer.gov. It rates evidence based on five domains of quality:

- Study design (evidence from the best studies available, ranked in descending order of strength)
- Internal validity ("quality" of execution within the study design)
- Consistency (coherence)/volume of the evidence
- Direction and magnitude of effects for health outcomes (both absolute and relative risks; as quantitative as possible; may vary for different populations)
- External validity/generalizability to other populations

When evaluating therapy studies, the strength of study endpoints (described under Randomized Clinical Trials) should be combined with the strength of the study design in ranking results (Table 1.3).

Illustration: Postmenopausal Hormone Therapy

Recently, the administration of hormones to postmenopausal women was brought into the spotlight. For decades, doctors had prescribed various combinations of estrogen and progesterone not only to relieve menopausal symptoms but also to reduce women's risk of osteoporosis, heart disease, and Alzheimer's disease. Consistent evidence for the beneficial effect of these hormones for prevention of several chronic diseases came from a large number of prospective cohort studies (as well as observational studies of other designs) comprising hundreds of thousands of women. In 2002, the practice of prescribing hormones returned abruptly to attention when results from the Women's Health Initiative, a large randomized controlled trial, showed that the drug PremPro (combined estrogen plus progestin) not only did not appear to protect women from heart disease and Alzheimer's disease but actually produced a modest increase in cardiovascular outcomes and cognitive disorders as well as breast cancer.[14] How is it possible that such a large, apparently authoritative body of evidence could give an answer at odds with that of a randomized trial, and the landscape of hormone therapy change so rapidly? In an observational cohort study, women are free to take postmenopausal hormones or not. Women who do choose hormone therapy tend to be more healthy and health conscious: they are more likely to see a physician on a regular basis, eat a healthful diet, and exercise. All these variables could affect the development and incidence of disease. Although an observational study can take such differences into account, there may remain other, unmeasured factors (confounding), or there may be systematic imprecision (bias) in the measurement of known factors, both of which

TABLE 1.2. Summary of study designs.

Study design	*Description*	+	–
Systematic reviews and meta-analyses	Summarize findings from a number of studies addressing a given clinical question; meta-analyses quantitatively estimate effects based on combining data from different studies.	Meta-analyses have greater statistical power than single studies to address questions. Convenient way to summarize findings from a range of studies.	Must meet assumption that studies can legitimately be combined (based on population, study design, etc.). Literature searches must be performed systematically and studies included without bias.
Randomized clinical trial	Subjects randomly assigned to an intervention or control group. Randomization ensures that the intervention is the only factor to vary between the comparison groups.	Represents true experiment. Randomization removes effects of confounding and bias. Considered gold standard among clinical studies. The most efficient method to test definitively for causal relationships between an intervention and health outcomes.	Expensive: requires extensive study infrastructure and training of staff. May be unethical or impracticable for some hypotheses.
Prospective cohort study (includes nested case-control study)	Exposures of subjects assessed at beginning of study; disease or other outcomes evaluated over time.	More efficient for common diseases. Allows assumption that exposure precedes disease. Allows consideration of a wide range of confounders.	Often expensive: requires large study infrastructure. Time consuming (subjects often followed for years). Subject to confounding (measured or unmeasured). Attrition of study population can affect generalizability.
Retrospective cohort study	Exposures of subjects assessed retrospectively, e.g., occupational exposures via historic job records.	Useful for assessing past exposures of large numbers of subjects over time.	Assumption that exposure precedes disease may be less strong than in prospective design. Confounders may have to be assessed at the present, and proxies for nonliving subjects may introduce bias.
Case-control study	Prior exposure and disease assessed at a point in time. Subjects selected on the basis of disease status (with or without); past exposures evaluated retrospectively.	More efficient for relatively rare diseases such as cancer. May allow consideration of a wide range of confounders.	Disease itself may affect evaluation of exposure (changes to biochemical measurement, selective recall). Subject to various types of error in evaluation of past exposure. Subject to confounding (measured or unmeasured). Exposure does not necessarily precede disease.

can distort estimates of risk and benefit. Such unmeasured confounding is believed to have resulted from the crucial bias (selection bias) that rather impressively provided such consistency of results among observational studies of combined hormone therapy. The Women's Health Initiative, in contrast, was able to eliminate whatever confounders were at play by virtue of its randomized placebo-controlled design.

Applying Research Evidence to the Individual

After identifying relevant studies, the clinician must think about their applicability to the individual patient, because even the best studies report estimates of effect in terms of an average. Study participants and real-world patients are likely to differ by degree, rather than grossly, in their response to treatment.[15] Individualizing treatment decisions involves estimation of the balance of risks and benefits, combined with a consideration of patient values. The number needed to treat (NNT) is the number of patients that need to be treated to prevent one additional adverse event, and it is the inverse of the absolute risk reduction, as described by McAlister et al.,[16] who provide a detailed guide to individualizing evidence from research. The number needed to harm (NNH), in contrast, is the number of patients treated who would be expected to experience one adverse event. NNT and NNH illustrate the balance between benefits and risks of a given intervention; in oncology, this is particularly relevant with regard to screening, which may result in harms from follow-up of false positives, and treatment, which often produces dose-dependent toxicity.

Clinicians should also consider the following levels of decision making when thinking about applying evidence to a particular patient, as conceptualized by Dr. Leon Gordis of Johns Hopkins University:

Level 1: "Would you have this done for yourself or for someone else in your immediate family?" Influenced by one's personal experience with the disease and capacity to deal with risk.

Level 2: "Would you make this recommendation for your own patients?" Also influenced by prior experience, but

TABLE 1.2. (continued)

Study design	*Description*	+	–
Nested case-control study	Analysis similar to case-control study, but subjects sampled from within cohort study.	For prospective studies, combines efficiency of case-control design with ability to demonstrate that exposure precedes disease.	See prospective cohort study.
Cross-sectional study (also called prevalence study)	Exposure and disease assessed at one point in time. May be repeated with different population samples at set time intervals (e.g., annual surveys).	Useful for measuring prevalence of an exposure or disease. Useful for generation of hypotheses and evaluating associations (as opposed to cause and effect). Repeated sampling design allows evaluation of population trends.	Exposure cannot be shown to precede disease. Inefficient for studying rare diseases.
Ecologic studies	Population-wide disease incidence or prevalence is compared with population-wide exposure estimates.	Useful for generating hypotheses. Useful for exposures that cannot be estimated on an individual level (e.g., ambient pollution).	Does not allow consideration of interindividual differences, which obscures confounding effects.
Case series or case reports	Descriptions of disease manifestations or therapy outcomes in single or multiple individual subjects, without controls; data often collected retrospectively.	May be the only feasible design for extremely rare diseases.	Lack control group. Subject to selection bias. Tend to lack information on confounders.
Preclinical studies: animal studies	Experimental design using animals, typically genetically homogeneous.	Large studies of animals (especially rodents) are useful for screening drugs and other chemicals for toxic or therapeutic effects.	May be inappropriate to extrapolate from rodent and other species to humans. Doses of chemicals used in toxicity studies may not be extrapolatable to doses likely to be experienced by humans.
Preclinical studies: laboratory studies below the whole-organism level	Experimental design utilizing controlled conditions, often involving effects of toxins or drugs on immortalized cancer cell lines or other cells.	Represent a level of control usually unattainable or unethical in humans. Generate hypotheses for human studies. Can elucidate biological mechanisms.	Lack organismal context, and therefore difficult to extrapolate to whole humans.

the strength of the scientific evidence may play a greater role.

Level 3: "Would you make an across-the-board recommendation for a population?" Must be based even more on rigorous assessment of the scientific evidence.

Level 1 is the level at which we all operate when we are making our own personal decisions regarding a procedure; it rests heavily on our own personal value systems and trade-offs. Nevertheless, it is important not to impose our own value systems on our patients. Level 2 is one in which clinicians engage in informed and shared decision making with patients. It is hoped that it involves reliance on strong evidence, although it is also heavily influenced by personal values of the patient if the decision is to be truly shared with the patient. Quick sound bites do not lend themselves to this format of informed decision making. By contrast, Level 3 involves an across-the-board recommendation for the entire population. Complexities are often sacrificed to strengthen the message. The messages are often sanitized of any mention of potential harms inherent in any test, procedure, or treatment. Here, therefore, recommendations should be based on particularly strong evidence.

TABLE 1.3. Levels of evidence.

I	Evidence obtained from at least one properly randomized controlled trial
II-1	Evidence obtained from well-designed controlled trials without randomization
II-2	Evidence obtained from well-designed cohort or case-control analytic studies, preferably from more than one center or research group
II-3	Evidence obtained from comparisons between times or places with or without the intervention; dramatic results in uncontrolled experiments (such as the results of treatment with penicillin in the 1940s) could also be included in this category
III	Opinions of respected authorities, based on clinical experience, descriptive studies, or reports of expert committees

From Canadian Task Force on the Periodic Health Examination. Can Med Assoc J 1979;121:1193–1254.

Are We Practicing Evidence-Based Medicine?

The goal of using evidence in medicine is to come closest to practice that represents best practice and to produce optimal health outcomes. Thus, it is desirable to evaluate the impact of medical knowledge on actual practice, in terms of both the practices themselves and, ultimately, their public health impact. On one level, the impact of evidence-based guidelines can be assessed by measuring practitioners' beliefs and knowledge over a time period relevant to the introduction of new knowledge by means of surveys. However, such surveys may not fully reflect actual practice and are an indirect surrogate for health outcomes.

The translation of knowledge into practice is often measured using administrative datasets such as Medicare claims data, which are assumed to reflect some robust proportion of procedures performed on enrollees, for example, screening mammography examinations. Such data are more objective than physician self-report, but may not capture all procedures of interest, as enrollees may undergo procedures outside the Medicare reimbursement system. For example, Medicare analyses are usually restricted to procedures in the age 65+ population for which the U.S. government is billed.

Looking at effects of guidelines on health outcomes (such as cancer incidence and mortality) is of great interest. However, these endpoints are often the most difficult to evaluate with confidence in terms of their link to new knowledge, because so many other factors are likely to influence rates of disease. For the United States, the most comprehensive data on disease incidence and mortality are compiled by the SEER program (Surveillance, Epidemiology, and End Results). SEER is a national dataset that is designed to reflect the total cancer experience of the U.S. population. Despite these caveats, occasionally a breakthrough in cancer medicine results in clearly measurable improvements in outcomes. Feuer et al.[17] reported on dramatic improvements in testicular cancer outcome statistics in SEER after the completion of a successful clinical trial of cisplatin, vinblastine, and bleomycin; improved survival rates then reached a plateau, apparently indicating the limits of diffusion of the results of the trial into medical practice.

Questions of impact of knowledge may be addressed by looking at rates of disease and mortality over a time frame relevant to the introduction of a given guideline, or to media coverage of, for example, a diagnosis of cancer in or a cancer screening or treatment procedure undergone by a celebrity. This approach is essentially an ecologic study design and is subject to the limitations described earlier. In one notable case, rates of breast-conserving surgery, which had been increasing (relative to mastectomies) in the 1980s, appeared to decline abruptly, albeit briefly, after widespread publicity about a mastectomy undergone by then First Lady Nancy Reagan. Nattinger et al.[18] carefully documented this change by analyzing news reports and the appropriate time period of subsequent SEER data.

Despite this evidence, other unmeasured factors affecting these rates are undoubtedly still at play, and outside of the context of a controlled trial it is extremely difficult to establish a causal effect that an intervening factor may have had on population mortality rates.

Progress in fighting cancer is often measured in terms of SEER-derived statistics; again, however, it is difficult to ascribe changes to a single factor. Recent reductions in deaths from breast cancer could be related to more widespread mammography screening, but improvements in breast cancer therapy are also likely to have an effect on mortality, and it is impossible to tease apart their effects on population-based mortality rates.

Another example of the use of national data to assess the impact of evidence-based medicine is that of colorectal cancer. The U.S. Preventive Services Task Force recommends screening for colorectal cancer by any of four methods; however, the reported prevalence of screening is below 50% in many states. As for the rates of disease, long-term declines in colorectal cancer incidence have slowed. Although screening is thought to play a role in reducing incidence and mortality, risk factors for colorectal cancer—physical inactivity and obesity—have increased in the population.[19] Although it is not possible to separate the effects of screening, improvements in therapy, and risk factors completely, they do act in different directions; the increase in physical obesity could conceivably explain the slowing of declines in incidence.

A common error in interpreting population cancer statistics is in the use of 5-year survival as a gauge of progress against a disease. Five-year survival is an appropriate outcome in a trial of a therapy, where all subjects in the numerator and denominator of the survival rate have the disease and a comparison is made between two groups randomly assigned to treatment after their diagnosis. In the general population, however, 5-year survival is much more likely to be a function of the date of diagnosis relative to the course of the disease. As a result, 5-year survival is unrelated to mortality and is ultimately a misleading statistic in this context.[20] For example, changes in screening patterns can advance the date of diagnosis without changing risk of death, thus artifactually lengthening survival time.

Other relevant outcomes beyond physician practice but shy of hard health outcomes include smoking rates, which are known to be closely related to rates of lung and oral cancer as well as a number of other health outcomes and total mortality. The Behavioral Risk Factor Surveillance Survey and National Household Survey on Drug Abuse measure the prevalence of smoking in the United States and can be used to estimate the impact of smoking-cessation programs and tobacco-related policies.

Evidence-Based Medicine and Societal Issues

Given finite resources, the medical system cannot provide every intervention no matter how small its potential benefit. From a societal perspective, it is therefore important for clinicians to judge interventions based on a balance between magnitude of benefit, quality of evidence, and resources. That is, one must keep in balance two questions: (1) Does it work? and (2) Should we do it? Otherwise, we could diminish the net health of the community by diverting resources from highly effective intervention to more marginally effective ones. The methods for such prioritization, however, are not yet well established. Cost-effectiveness analysis and cost-utility analysis are tools that can help, but many value judgments are necessary that go beyond quality of evidence. In the meantime, adhering to evidence-based principles of evaluating, for example, screening and diagnostic tools, may help eliminate ineffective redundancy and thus save costs while still achieving needed health outcomes.

Summary

This introduction has attempted to put evidence-based decision making in a useful, practical framework with special attention to issues relevant to the study and practice of oncology. We hope we have made it clear that evidence-based medicine is neither theoretical nihilism nor cookbook practice, in that it incorporates clinicians' knowledge and training with systematic methods for asking answerable questions, critically evaluating research, and taking into account patient values (thus marrying the tools of evidence-based medicine with the ethical concept of patient autonomy).

Resources

The landscape of medical research changes constantly, and thus the best resources for practitioners of evidence-based medicine are those that adapt databases, recommendations, and guidelines regularly to take into account new findings. Key online resources relevant to oncology are the Physicians' Data Query (PDQ) at http://cancer.gov, the public Website of the National Cancer Institute. The PDQ has several topical committees that meet regularly to develop and update Web-based resources and explicitly spell out their methodology for ranking evidence. The U.S. Agency for Healthcare Research and Quality (http://www.ahrq.gov) posts links to evidence-based guidelines, including their own U.S. Preventive Services Task Force, at the National Guidelines Clearinghouse (http://www.guideline.gov), and also offers access to comprehensive literature reviews on a wide variety of clinical questions. The Cochrane Library (http://www.cochrane.org) regularly updates its evidence-based databases on health care and publishes comprehensive literature reviews according to stringent rules of evidence.

Two journals relevant to general medicine and oncology exist to help summarize the vast sea of new research into a manageable format and according to an evidence-based approach: *ACP Journal Club* (published by the American College of Physicians) and *Cancer Treatment Reviews* (from Elsevier; this journal now incorporates the former *Evidence-Based Oncology*).

Further instruction in the general nuts and bolts of evidence-based medicine can be found in texts by the innovators of the field: David Sackett and colleagues *(Evidence-Based Medicine: How to Practice and Teach EBM*; Churchill Livingston, 2000) and the JAMA *Users' Guide to the Medical Literature: A Manual for Evidence-Based Clinical Practice.* The JAMA guides are a compilation of a previously published series of articles in JAMA and can also be accessed online by subscription.

References

1. Evidence-Based Medicine Working Group. Evidence-based medicine: a new approach to teaching the practice of medicine. JAMA 1992;268:2420–2425.
2. Sackett D, Straus SE, Richardson WS, et al. Evidence-Based Medicine: How to Practice and Teach Evidence-Based Medicine. Edinburgh: Churchill Livingston, 2000.
3. Morabia A. P.C.A. Louis and the birth of clinical epidemiology. J Clin Epidemiol 1996:49:1327–1333.
4. Dunn PM. James Lind (1716–94) of Edinburgh and the treatment of scurvy. Arch Dis Childhood 1997;76:F64–F65.
5. Keith JM. Florence Nightingale: statistician and consultant epidemiologist. Int Nurs Rev 1988;35:147–150.
6. Gehan E. The role of the biostatistician in cancer research. Biomed Pharmacother 2001;55:502–509.
7. Mainland D. The rise of experimental statistics and the problems of a medical statistician. Yale J Biol Med 1954;27:1–10.
8. Meldrum ML. A brief history of the randomized clinical trial: from oranges and lemons to the gold standard. In: Allegra CJ, Kramer BS (eds). Hematology/Oncology Clinics of North America: Understanding Clinical Trials. Philadelphia: Saunders, 2000.
9. Fisher B, Bauer M, Margolese R, et al. Five-year results of a randomized clinical trial comparing total mastectomy and segmental mastectomy with or without radiation in the treatment of breast cancer. N Engl J Med 1985;312:665–673.
10. Centre for Evidence-Based Medicine, http://www.cebm.utoronto.ca/practise/formulate/.
11. Albanes D, Heinonen OP, Taylor PR et al. α-Tocopherol and β-carotene supplements and lung cancer incidence in the Alpha-Tocopherol, Beta-Carotene Cancer Prevention Study: effects of base-line characteristics and study compliance. J Natl Cancer Inst 1996;88:1560–1570.
12. Krieger N, Wolff MS, Hiatt RA, et al. Breast cancer and serum organochlorines: a prospective study among white, black, and Asian women. J Natl Cancer Inst 1994;86(8):589–599.
13. Fisher B. Clinical trials for the evaluation of cancer therapy. Cancer (Phila) 1984;54:2609–2617.
14. Roussouw JE, Anderson GL, Prentice RL et al. Risks and benefits of estrogen plus progestin in healthy postmenopausal women: principal results from the Women's Health Initiative randomized clinical trial. JAMA 2002;288:321–333.
15. Dans AL, Dans LF, Guyatt GH, et al. Users' guides to the medical literature: XIV. How to decide on the applicability of clinical trial results to your patient. Evidence-Based Medicine Working Group. JAMA 1998;279:545–549.
16. McAlister FA, Straus SE, Guyatt GH et al. Users' guides to the medical literature. XX. Integrating research evidence with the care of the individual patient. JAMA 2000;283:2829–2836.
17. Feuer EJ, Frey CM, Brawley OW, et al. After a treatment breakthrough: a comparison of trial and population-based data for advanced testicular cancer. J Clin Oncol 1994;12:368–377.
18. Nattinger AB, Hoffmann RG, Howell-Pelz A, et al.. Effect of Nancy Reagan's mastectomy on choice of surgery for breast cancer by U.S. women. JAMA 1998;279:762–766.
19. Weir HK, Thun MJ, Hankey BF, et al. Annual report to the Nation on the status of cancer, 1975–2000, featuring the uses of surveillance data for cancer prevention and control. J Natl Cancer Inst 2003;95:1276–1299.
20. Welch HG, Schwartz SM, Woloshin S. Are increasing 5-year survival rates evidence of success against cancer? JAMA 2000; 283:2975–2978.

2

Principles of Chemotherapy

Grace K. Dy and Alex A. Adjei

During World War II, sailors who were accidentally exposed to nitrogen mustard following the explosion of a ship developed marrow and lymphoid hypoplasia.[1] This serendipitous discovery led to the first clinical trial conducted in 1942 using nitrogen mustard in patients with malignant lymphomas at Yale University.[2] This marked the beginning of a new era of research in the quest for effective and safe drugs used in cancer chemotherapy.

The term chemotherapy has been loosely applied to the myriad systemic therapeutic options in cancer treatment exclusive of irradiation and surgical approaches. In this chapter, we confine our discussion of chemotherapy to refer to the use of conventional cytotoxic agents. Use of targeted and biologic agents such as hormone or signal transduction manipulation and gene therapy is explored in other chapters.

Cancer Cell Population Kinetics

The discussion that follows briefly describes the various paradigms of tumor growth and response to cytotoxic agents to facilitate understanding of the rationale and basis for the approaches to cancer therapy with cytotoxic agents.

Skipper's Exponential Tumor Growth/Log-Kill Hypothesis

One of the pioneer investigations in tumor growth kinetics was made by Skipper and his colleagues,[3] who described the first model of tumor growth kinetics. Despite its flaws and oversimplified nature, the empiric observations derived from this model underlie many of the tenets in cancer chemotherapy. A conclusion derived from his L1210 mouse leukemia model was the exponential (logarithmic) growth of tumor cells. Doubling time of cancer cells was proposed to be constant, yielding a straight line on a semilog plot (Figure 2.1). Another conclusion generated from their experiments was the log-kill hypothesis, which proposes that anticancer drugs act with first-order kinetics, and hence, assuming homogeneous sensitivity to the drug, they will eliminate a constant proportion rather than a constant number of tumor cells regardless of the initial size of the tumor; that is, magnitude of tumor cell kill is a logarithmic function.[3] By this a posteriori reasoning, if sufficient drug is given, cure can be achieved when fewer than 1 tumor cell remains. Similarly, therapy against small-volume tumors or micrometastatic disease should be easily successful in effecting cures. However, clinical experience in adjuvant chemotherapy has not borne out this deductive assumption as successfully as hoped.

Gompertzian Model of Tumor Growth

With further studies, it became clear that Skipper's model was oversimplified and applied only to the proliferating segment within the tumor. Some early-stage malignancies, such as testicular germ cell tumor, may behave in such a way when they are composed of proliferating cells highly responsive to chemotherapeutic agents. However, most human solid tumors do not respond to chemotherapy, contrary to what would have been expected if tumor growth was exponential. Rather, the experimental data in human solid tumors support the Gompertzian kinetics of tumor growth, akin to the sigmoid curve seen in microbial kinetics under a controlled environment, where the initial growth phase is steep at smaller volumes, eventually plateauing and decreasing with time once a critical mass is reached[4] (Figure 2.2). As many anticancer agents are cell cycle specific and are usually most active against cells that are proliferating, a critical factor in drug responsiveness of tumors to cell-cycle-specific drugs depends on the particular phase the tumor is in its growth curve. This model also helps explain why, unless cure was effected, varying degrees of residual tumor volume result in similar relapse-free survival over time.

Norton–Simon Model

In Skipper's model, the exponential growth of tumors is presumed to be homogeneous. The Norton–Simon model takes into account the heterogeneity of a tumor cell population following the Gompertzian growth curve.[5,6] The log kill would be greater for very small cancers than for larger tumors. However, smaller cancers also regrow faster. The greater fractional kill, such as against micrometastases in the adjuvant setting, is offset by fractional repopulation of tumor cells at the same fast rate. Thus, tumors are difficult to eradicate under this model. As already stated, this model predicts the observation that adjuvant chemotherapy does not have much impact on overall survival, as opposed to the improvement in disease-free survival. Survival can thus be improved only when tumor cell populations are eradicated or rendered

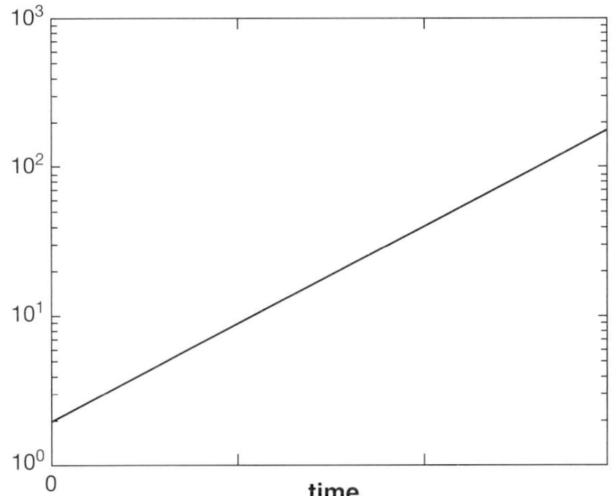

FIGURE 2.1. Skipper's model of tumor growth (*x*-axis, time for tumor growth; *y*-axis, tumor volume).

dormant during the early growth phase. Another implication is that effective therapy should be delivered at reduced intervals to maximize the chances of tumor eradication and to minimize tumor regrowth in between cycles of therapy.

Goldie and Coldman Hypothesis

An important corollary to tumor growth is the development of drug resistance resulting from spontaneous mutations that occur with cell proliferation, independent of the resistance inherent to the heterogeneity in cell kinetics described earlier. Goldie and Coldman had hypothesized that this occurs at a rate of 1 of 10^5 cells per gene.[7] If 1 g tumor, the minimum size for detection, contains 10^9 cells, then such a tumor might contain 10^4 clones resistant to any given drug. However, resistance to two drugs would be seen in fewer than 1 cell in a 10-g (10^{10} cells) tumor. This idea is consistent with the known observation that combination chemotherapy is more effective than single-agent regimens. Nevertheless, single agents have remained successful in the treatment of certain tumors, such as Burkitt's lymphoma at sizes greater than 1 g.[8] This hypothesis is one basis for the idea that chemotherapy should theoretically be started when tumor burden is smallest, to be effective; concomitant or alternating administration of noncross-resistant drugs is preferred to sequential chemotherapy. However, delaying therapy does not necessarily result in decreased responsiveness in many cases.[9,10] Similarly, administration of chemotherapy preoperatively, although it may be predicted to be more beneficial based on this model, does not confer any significant improvement in the clinical outcomes in resectable early-stage breast cancer. This model also assumes a stepwise development of resistance to individual agents and thus does not account for multidrug resistance patterns.

Tumor cell growth kinetics are complex and poorly understood. There are no available models that accurately describe all aspects of clinical behavior of solid tumors. The heterogeneous genetic abnormalities of different tumors underlie their behavior, making it impossible to make broad predictions.

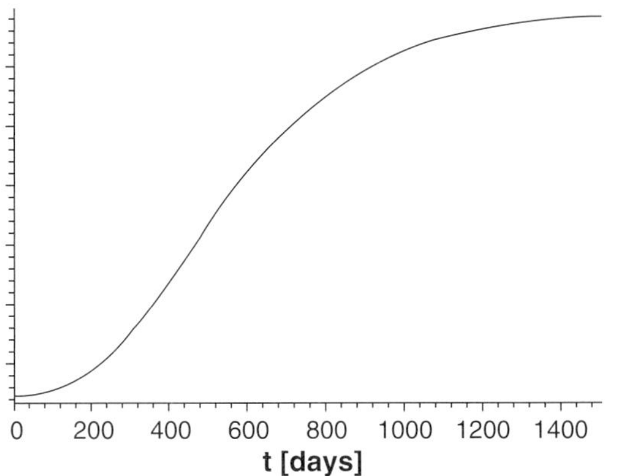

FIGURE 2.2. Gompertzian model of tumor growth (*x*-axis, time for tumor growth; *y*-axis, tumor volume).

Chemotherapy Approaches in the Management of Cancers

Cancer chemotherapy has principally been used in the management of advanced or metastatic disease, following failed local therapies, or in disease for which no alternative therapy is effective. Chemotherapy is curative for several advanced human cancers, such as gestational trophoblastic disease, certain hematologic malignancies, or germ cell testicular cancer. However, most common solid tumors are not curable with current chemotherapeutic regimens when metastatic (Table 2.1).

The roles of chemotherapy are manifold: *induction* chemotherapy denotes its use as primary therapy when there is no alternative treatment available or subsequently suitable even with tumor response, such as in hematologic malignancies, where disease is systemic. As an adjunct in *combined modality therapy*, chemotherapy is *adjuvant* when systemic treatment is applied after the tumor has been controlled by an alternative modality, such as surgery and/or radiotherapy, or *neoadjuvant* (*primary*) chemotherapy when localized cancer will otherwise not be optimally managed if systemic chemotherapy is not used before definitive local therapy.

Dose Intensity Versus Dose Density

Multiple laboratory experiments have established the proportionate dose–response curve, such that log kill is greater for the regimen with a higher dose intensity (i.e., by increasing the dose level delivered over a standard time interval). The slope of the curve is often steeper for tumors with a higher growth fraction. This observation underlies one of the principles in cancer chemotherapy—the administration of the highest possible dose of drugs in the shortest possible time intervals. The latter is typically limited by the recovery period of host organ function, such as the gastrointestinal tract and, in particular, the bone marrow, and thus explains the familiar 14- to 28-day intervals between cycles of therapy.

Progress in understanding of tumor growth kinetics has led to the emergence of new concepts in the schedules and

TABLE 2.1. Responses of tumors to chemotherapy.

Curable	*Prolonged survival*	*Palliative/minimal*
Hodgkin's lymphoma	Non-Hodgkin's lymphoma (e.g., follicular)	Multiple myeloma
Non-Hodgkin's lymphoma (e.g., Burkitt's, diffuse large cell)	Bladder cancer	Chronic leukemias
Acute leukemias	Breast cancer	Malignant melanoma
Testicular cancer	Lung cancer	Renal cell carcinoma
Ovarian cancer	Colorectal cancer	Glioblastoma multiforme
Choriocarcinoma	Oligodendrogliomas	Pancreatic carcinoma
Childhood cancers (e.g., rhabdomyosarcoma, Wilm's tumor, Ewing's sarcoma)		Hepatocellular carcinoma
		Head and neck cancers
		Esophageal carcinoma
		Gastric carcinoma
		Prostate carcinoma

dosing of cytotoxic agents. Dose intensity refers to the dose level or total amount of drug received over a fixed unit of time. It is a function of the magnitude of the dose level. Achieving a certain effective dose level is analogous to the concentration-dependent killing of some antibiotics, such as aminoglycosides, wherein increasing bactericidal activity is achieved with exposure to a higher dose until a threshold concentration of maximal efficacy is achieved. Dose intensity is an important concept derived from the well-observed steep dose–response effect of chemotherapy agents demonstrated in randomized trials such as in germ cell tumors.[11]

However, achieving a higher dose intensity by administration of higher dose levels of chemotherapy is hampered by concomitant increase in frequency and severity of toxicities. In addition, this concept may not be applicable in metastatic solid tumors, when tumor burden is largest. This restriction is illustrated by the negative results of myeloablative doses of chemotherapy compared to conventional chemotherapy in women with metastatic breast carcinoma.[12] Moreover, it has been observed in vitro that one of the important determinants of cytotoxicity is the duration of drug exposure beyond a threshold drug concentration. Indeed, there may be a readily tolerable minimal dose level for tumors, as implied in a recent trial by the Cancer and Leukemia Group B (CALGB) trial. In that study, there was no survival benefit to the administration of a more dose-intense regimen of 5-fluorouracil, adriamycin, and cyclophosphamide (FAC) in the adjuvant setting among women whose tumors did not express the HER/2 neu oncoprotein.[13]

In contrast, dose density refers to the total amount of drug received over a variable given period of time. To illustrate, giving 2x amount of drug in cycles of y days (A) is twice more dose intense than x drug in y days (B), whereas B is less dose dense than x drug given in y/2 days (C). C is as dose intense and dose dense as A. Simply, dose density is a function of frequency of dose administration within a treatment cycle. Dose density is analogous to the time-dependent killing activity of penicillins and cephalosporins wherein bactericidal activity is directly related to the time of exposure above the minimum inhibitory concentration (MIC), after which it becomes independent of drug concentration. A tumor thus relapses when subtotal eradication upon initial drug administration leads to tumor growth and development of drug resistance in between treatment cycles when the interval between therapy is prolonged. The dose-dense therapy may inhibit tumor regrowth between cycles and limit the emergence of malignant cell populations resistant to chemotherapy. Dose-dense strategy is the logical conclusion derived from the Norton–Simon model of tumor growth and drug response. Moreover, recent preclinical studies have shown that frequent administration in vivo of low doses of chemotherapeutic drugs, so-called "metronomic" dosing, may affect tumor endothelium and inhibit tumor angiogenesis, thus resulting in a better therapeutic index with reduced significant side effects (e.g., myelosuppression) involving other tissues. In solid tumors, this may be exemplified by the successful use of weekly paclitaxel in metastatic breast cancer.[14]

Chemotherapeutic Drugs

Anticancer drugs may be subdivided into two large groups based on the dependence of their mechanism of action on the cell cycle (Table 2.2). Cell-cycle-nonspecific drugs, which include alkylating agents and most antitumor antibiotics, kill tumor cells in both the resting and cycling phases. On the other hand, it was previously mentioned that cell-cycle-specific drugs are most effective when tumor cells are

TABLE 2.2. Drugs according to cell-cycle effects.

Cell cycle	*Agents*
Cell cycle nonspecific	Nitrogen mustards, aziridines, nitrosoureas, alkyl alkane sulfonates, nonclassic alkylating agents, anthracyclines, actinomycins, anthracenediones
Cell cycle specific	
S	Bleomycin, antimetabolites, camptothecins, epipodophyllotoxins
G_2	Bleomycin, epipodophyllotoxins
M	Vinca alkaloids, taxanes

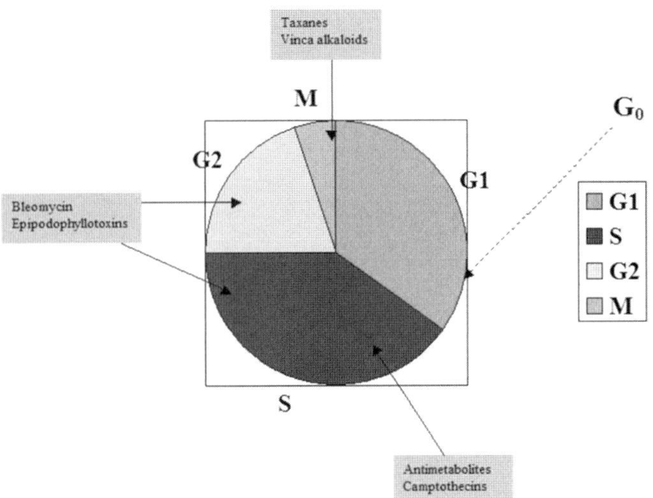

FIGURE 2.3. Cell-cycle-specific chemotherapeutic drugs and specific cell-cycle phase.

proliferating, that is, in cycles other than resting G0 phase (Figure 2.3). Moreover, these drugs are usually most active in a specific phase of the cell cycle. Cell-cycle-specific drugs include the antimetabolites, antitubulin agents, and drugs targeting topoisomerase. Tables 2.3 and 2.4 describe common toxicities for each drug that is discussed in more detail in the subsequent sections.

Classic Alkylating Agents

Alkylating agents were the first class of agents to be clinically tested for cancer therapeutics. The alkylating agents form covalent bonds with nucleophilic cellular molecules, such as oxygen-, nitrogen-, phosphorus-, or sulfur-containing sites, through their alkyl groups. As a class, alkylating agents lack tumor selectivity but are generally active at very low doses. The bifunctional alkylating agents (two alkylating groups) not only alkylate but also crosslink DNA, leading to DNA template damage, subsequent cessation of DNA synthesis, and initiation of apoptosis upon recognition by cell-cycle checkpoint proteins such as p53. Alkylating agents thus are cytotoxic, teratogenic, and carcinogenic. Most secondary malignancies resulting from their use are acute leukemias.

Dose-dependent myelosuppression is the usual toxicity common to alkylating agents. Dose-dependent nausea and vomiting are frequently encountered. Gonadal atrophy and alopecia are also common sequelae of alkylating agent treatment. Because of the steep dose–response curve, alkylating agents are standardly included in myeloablative high-dose chemotherapy regimens in various hematologic malignancies. In such cases, pulmonary toxicity, veno-occlusive disease of the liver (nitrosoureas, busulfan, thiotepa, cyclophosphamide, mitomycin C), and neurotoxicity (lipophilic agents such as ifosfamide, nitrosourea, thiotepa, busulfan, nitrosourea) may arise and are life threatening.

The classic alkylating agents typically contain a chloroethyl group. They are classified as nitrogen mustards, aziridines, nitrosoureas, and alkyl alkane sulfonates. Nonclassic monofunctional alkylating agents, on the other hand, feature a common N-methyl group, do not produce DNA crosslinks, and are essentially prodrugs requiring metabolic transformation into active intermediates. Included in this latter group are procarbazine, dacarbazine, hexamethylmelamine, and temozolomide.

Nitrogen Mustards

Mechlorethamine

Nitrogen mustards have been the most commonly used alkylating agents. The prototype is the vesicant mechlorethamine. It has an extremely short half-life of 15 to 20 minutes, as it undergoes rapid hydrolysis in the plasma to reactive metabolites. Its chief uses currently are in the treatment of lymphoma and mycosis fungoides (topical). Derivatives of mechlorethamine that have gained broader clinical use are the oxazaphosphorines cyclophosphamide and ifosfamide, chlorambucil, and melphalan.

Cyclophosphamide

Both cyclophosphamide and ifosfamide require metabolic transformation by the cytochrome P-450 mixed-function oxidases in hepatic microsomes into their reactive intermediates.[15] They are also capable of induction of the microsomal enzymes responsible for their metabolism. In the case of cyclophosphamide, the intermediates 4-hydroxycyclophosphamide and aldosphosphamide that escape oxidation by aldehyde dehydrogenase are converted by tumor cells into acrolein and phosphoramide mustard,[16] the active alkylating agent that is responsible for the biologic effects of cyclophosphamide; this reaction is similar for ifosfamide. Because these metabolites are renally cleared, accumulation of acrolein in urine is responsible for hemorrhagic cystitis unique to these two agents,[17] especially ifosfamide. Transitional cell carcinoma of the bladder developing as a late sequela has been described.[18] Bladder toxicity may be reduced by hydration, frequent bladder emptying, and the use of thiol-containing agents such as *N*-acetyl cysteine (NAC) and mercaptoethane sulfonate (MESNA). These protectants are rich in sulfhydryl groups that bind and inactivate the charged toxic metabolites.

Cyclophosphamide can be administered orally or intravenously. Nausea and vomiting are usually delayed, occurring hours after drug administration. Relative sparing of the platelet count at doses less than 30 mg/kg is very characteristic. Moreover, it exhibits a stem cell-sparing effect even at high doses, in contrast to busulfan and melphalan, because of the high levels of aldehyde dehydrogenase in the early bone marrow progenitor cells. Cyclophosphamide is the most immunosuppressive anticancer agent available. Cardiac toxicity is dose limiting in high-dose administration,[19] although no cumulative toxicity of low to moderate doses is evident. A toxic tubular effect has also been described wherein water retention, and an SIADH-like (syndrome of inappropriate antidiuretic hormone) picture can occur with the use of 50 mg/kg or higher doses.[20,21] Cyclophosphamide is used in various settings, such as in breast cancer, bone marrow transplant, and non-Hodgkin's lymphoma (NHL), to name a few.

Ifosfamide

Similar to cyclophosphamide, ifosfamide is well absorbed after oral administration. However, the oral metabolite chloracetaldehyde is highly neurotoxic and hence the oral form is not commercially available.[22,23] It has a lower affinity for its activating enzymes, and thus its transformation to alkylating

TABLE 2.3. Selected pharmacokinetic and toxicity features.

Chemotherapeutic agent		*Metabolism/ excretion*	*Toxicity*	*Administration*	*Dose reduction in renal or liver dysfunction*
Classic alkylating agents	Chlorambucil	Liver	Myelosuppression, hyperuricemia, mild N&V, pulmonary fibrosis, seizures, gonadal toxicity, secondary malignancies	Oral	
	Cyclophosphamide	Liver	Myelosuppression, hemorrhagic cystitis, N&V, alopecia, headache, nasal congestion with rapid infusion, SIADH, cardiomyopathy, immunosuppression, gonadal toxicity, pulmonary fibrosis (high-dose), secondary malignancy	Infusion or oral	Clcr < 10 mL/min: 25% reduction
	Ifosfamide	Liver	Myelosuppression, hemorrhagic cystitis, N&V, alopecia, metabolic acidosis, neurotoxicity (somnolence, hallucinations, ataxia, neuropathy), arrhythmias, CHF, SIADH, Fanconi syndrome, gonadal toxicity, azotemia, secondary malignancy	Infusion or slow IV push	Scr 2.1–3.0 mg/dL: 25% to 50% reduction
	Mechlorethamine	Plasma hydrolysis	Myelosuppression, severe N&V, dermatitis, thrombophlebitis, hyperuricemia, gonadal toxicity, secondary malignancy	Slow injection	
	Melphalan	Plasma hydrolysis, renal	Myelosuppression, mild N&V, vasculitis, mucositis, diarrhea, SIADH hypersensitivity reactions, gonadal toxicity, secondary malignancy	IV bolus, infusion or oral	Clcr 10–50 mL/min: 25% reduction Clcr < 10 mL/min: 50% reduction
	Mitomycin C	Liver	Myelosuppression, N&V, mucositis, HUS, DIC, microangiopathic hemolytic anemia, interstitial pneumonitis, thrombophlebitis, hepatic VOD, cardiomyopathy, bladder fibrosis (intravesical therapy)	Slow IV push or infusion, intravesical	Clcr < 10 mL/min: 25% reduction
	Thiotepa	Liver	Myelosuppression, mild N&V, hyperuricemia, dermatitis, secondary malignancy, hemorrhagic cystitis (intravesical therapy)	IV bolus or infusion, intrathecal, intravesical	
	Carmustine (BCNU)	Liver	Myelosuppression, severe N&V, thrombophlebitis, seizures (wafers), hepatotoxicity, nephrotoxicity, pulmonary fibrosis, infusion-related hypotension and arrhythmias at high doses, gonadal toxicity, secondary malignancy	IV infusion, wafer implant (glioblastoma)	
	Lomustine (CCNU)	Liver	Myelosuppression, severe N&V, gonadal toxicity, neurotoxicity (confusion, ataxia, dysarthria, lethargy), hepatotoxicity, nephrotoxicity, pulmonary fibrosis, secondary malignancy	Oral	Clcr 10–50 mL/min: 25% reduction Clcr < 10 mL/min: 50% reduction
	Streptozocin	Liver, renal	Nephrotoxicity, N&V, elevated transaminases and/or mild cholestasis, hypoglycemia, secondary malignancy	IV bolus or infusion	Clcr 10–50 mL/min: 25% reduction Clcr < 10 mL/min: 50% reduction
	Busulfan	Liver	Myelosuppression, gonadal toxicity, secondary malignancy, mild N&V, skin hyperpigmentation (oral), hyperuricemia, cholestasis, hepatic VOD, seizures, bronchopulmonary dysplasia with pulmonary fibrosis, adrenal insufficiency	Oral or IV infusion	
Nonclassic alkylating agents	Procarbazine	Liver	Myelosuppression; N&V, hemolysis (G6PD deficiency), MAOI crises, flu-like syndrome, disulfiram reactions with alcohol; neurotoxicity (paresthesias, neuropathies, ataxia, confusion, seizures), gonadal toxicity, secondary malignancy	Oral	Consider dose reduction if bilirubin >3 mg/dl
	Dacarbazine	Liver, renal	Myelosuppression, N&V, flu-like syndrome, photosensitivity	IV infusion	
	Altretamine	Liver, renal	N&V, myelosuppression, neurotoxicity (neuropathy, ataxia hallucinations), flu-like syndrome	Oral	
	Temozolomide	Plasma decomposition, renal	Myelosuppression, N&V, anorexia, headache, neurotoxicity (insomnia, somnolence, ataxia, hemiparesis, seizures), elevation of transaminases or cholestasis, peripheral edema	Oral	

Platinum compounds	Cisplatin	Renal	N&V, nephrotoxicity, electrolyte abnormalities, peripheral neuropathy, ototoxicity, myelosuppression, thromboembolic events, myocardial ischemia, ocular toxicity, thrombophlebitis, gonadal toxicity, mild elevation of transaminases or cholestasis, hypersensitivity reaction	IV infusion	Clcr 10–50 mL/min: 25% reduction Clcr < 10 mL/min: 50% reduction
	Carboplatin	Renal	Myelosuppression, N&V, nephrotoxicity, neuropathy, electrolyte abnormalities, mild elevation of transaminases or cholestasis, delayed hypersensitivity reaction	IV infusion	Calvert's formula
	Oxaliplatin	Renal	sensory > motor neuropathy, N&V, diarrhea, elevated liver transaminases, myelosuppression, nephrotoxicity, edema, hypersensitivity reaction	IV infusion	Consider in renal dysfunction
Antitumor antibiotics	Doxorubicin	Liver	Myelosuppression, mild N&V, mucositis, alopecia, cardiotoxicity, elevation of transaminases, radiation recall, hyperpigmentation, thrombophlebitis, urine discoloration	IV infusion, intraarterial, intravesical	Bilirubin 1.5–3 mg/dL: 50% reduction Bilirubin 3.1–5 mg/dL: 75% reduction
	Daunorubicin	Liver, renal	Myelosuppression, mild N&V, mucositis, alopecia, cardiotoxicity, elevation of transaminases, radiation recall, hyperpigmentation, urine discoloration	IV push or infusion	Bilirubin 2.1–3 mg/dL or AST 60–180 IU: 25% reduction Bilirubin 3.1–5 mg/dL or AST >180 IU: 50% reduction Bilirubin >5 mg/dL: omit use
	Idarubicin	Liver, renal	Myelosuppression, mild N&V, mucositis, alopecia, elevation of transaminases or cholestasis, GI hemorrhage, cardiotoxicity, radiation recall, hyperpigmentation, urine discoloration, thrombophlebitis	Oral, slow IV push or infusion	Serum creatinine ≥2 mg/dL: 25% reduction Bilirubin 1.5–5 mg/dL or AST 60–180 IU: reduce dose 50%. Bilirubin >5 mg/dL or AST >180 IU: do not administer
	Epirubicin	Liver, renal	Myelosuppression, mild N&V, mucositis, cardiotoxicity, radiation recall, alopecia, hyperpigmentation, urine discoloration, thrombophlebitis, gonadal toxicity	IV infusion	Serum creatinine >5 mg/dl: consider dose reduction Bilirubin 1.2–3 mg/dL or AST 2–4 times the upper limit of normal: 50% reduction Bilirubin >3 mg/dL or AST >4 times the upper limit of normal: 75% reduction
	Mitoxantrone	Liver	Myelosuppression, mucositis, N&V, arrhythmias, cardiotoxicity(cumulative doses >140–160 mg/m^2 cause CHF in ~10% of patients), elevated transaminases, urine discoloration, alopecia, secondary malignancy	IV infusion, intraperitoneal	Bilirubin 1.5–3 mg/dL: 50% reduction Bilirubin >3 mg/dl: 75% reduction
	Dactinomycin	Liver	Myelosuppression, severe N&V, mucositis, cardiotoxicity, radiation recall, fatigue, hyperpigmentation, elevated transaminases, thrombophlebitis, hypocalcemia, hepatic VOD	Slow IV push	
	Bleomycin	Kidney, renal	Skin reactions (erythema, peeling, etc.), pneumonitis, pulmonary fibrosis, anaphylactoid reactions, Raynaud's phenomenon, arterial thrombosis, myocardial ischemia	Slow IV bolus, IM, SC or intracavitary injection	Clcr 10–50 mL/min: 25% reduction Clcr <10 mL/min: 50% reduction
Antimetabolites	Methotrexate	Renal	Myelosuppression, mucositis, renal failure, uric acid nephropathy, elevation in transaminases or cholestasis, hepatic fibrosis, pneumonitis, serositis, neurotoxicity (high-dose or intrathecal), gonadal toxicity, vasculitis, thromboembolic disease	Oral, IV, IM, intrathecal	Clcr 61–80 mL/min: 25% reduction Clcr 51–60 mL/min: 30% reduction Clcr 10–50 mL/min: 50–70% reduction Clcr <10 mL/min: avoid use Bilirubin 3.1–5 mg/dL or AST >180 units: administer 75% of dose Bilirubin >5 mg/dL: do not use

(continued)

TABLE 2.3. Selected pharmacokinetic and toxicity features. (continued)

Chemotherapeutic agent	*Metabolism/ excretion*	*Toxicity*	*Administration*	*Dose reduction in renal or liver dysfunction*
Raltitrexed	Renal	Fatigue/asthenia, N&V, mucositis, severe diarrhea, myelosuppression, elevated liver transaminases or cholestasis, edema	IV infusion	Clcr 55–65 mL/min: 25% reduction Clcr 25–54 mL/min: 50–75% reduction Clcr <25 mL/min: do not administer
Pemetrexed	Renal	Myelosuppression, fatigue, mucositis, hand-foot syndrome, edema, elevated liver transaminases or cholestasis	IV infusion	Consider in renal dysfunction
5-Fluorouracil	Enzymatic catabolism	Myelosuppression, mucositis, hand-foot syndrome, acute coronary syndrome, GI ulcers, neurotoxicity, ocular symptoms	Slow IV bolus or infusion, topical, intraarterial	Bilirubin >5 mg/dL: omit use
5-FUDR	Enzymatic catabolism	Hepatotoxicity, hand-foot syndrome, myelosuppression, mucositis, neurotoxicity, edema, acute coronary syndrome, headache, ocular symptoms	IV, intra-arterial	
Capecitabine	Enzymatic catabolism	Diarrhea, hand-foot syndrome, myelosuppression, acute coronary syndrome, neurotoxicity, ocular symptoms; elevated transaminases or cholestasis	Oral	Clcr 30–50 mL/min: 25% reduction Clcr <30 mL/min: do not use
Cytarabine	Enzymatic deamination	Myelosuppression, N&V, GI ulcers, pancreatitis, cholestasis, hidradenitis, cerebellar dysfunction; with high-dose therapy: conjunctivitis, hand-foot syndrome, ARDS, elevated transaminases, hyperuricemia	IV infusion or bolus, IM, SC, intrathecal	Consider in hepatic dysfunction
Gemcitabine	Enzymatic deamination	Myelosuppression, N&V, flu-like symptoms, asthenia, fever, hemolytic-uremic syndrome, pneumonitis, elevated liver enzymes, somnolence, paresthesias	IV infusion	Consider in hepatic dysfunction
6-Mercaptopurine	Enzymatic; renal (with high-dose therapy)	Myelosuppression, mild N&V, mucositis, hepatotoxicity, crystalluria, hyperuricemia, pancreatitis	Oral	Consider in hepatic and renal dysfunction
6-thioguanine	Enzymatic; liver	Myelosuppression, N&V, mucositis, hepatotoxicity, hyperuricemia, crystalluria	Oral	Consider in hepatic and renal dysfunction
Fludarabine	Renal	Myelosuppression, autoimmune hemolytic anemia, edema, immunosuppression, fever, elevated liver enzymes, neurotoxicity (somnolence, neuropathy, confusion, cortical blindness, coma), tumor lysis syndrome	IV infusion	Clcr 30–70 mL/min: 20% reduction Clcr <30 mL/min: not recommended
Cladribine	Renal	Myelosuppression, immunosuppression, edema, fever, headache, dizziness, tumor lysis syndrome	IV infusion	
Pentostatin	Renal	Myelosuppression, immunosuppression, N&V, elevated liver enzymes, headache, lethargy, renal failure, acute pulmonary edema, ocular symptoms	IV infusion	Clcr <60 mL/min: administer 2 mg/m^2/dose

Antimicrotubule agents	Vincristine	Liver	Sensorimotor neurotoxicity, autonomic neuropathy(orthostatic hypotension/hypertension, ileus, constipation, bladder atony), seizures, alopecia, thrombophlebitis, hyperuricemia, SIADH, mild myelosuppression, ocular toxicity, ARDS	Bolus injection	Bilirubin 1.5–3.0 mg/dL or AST 60–180 units: 50% reduction. bilirubin 3.0–5.0 mg/dL: 75% reduction Serum bilirubin >5.0 mg/dL or AST >180 units: omit dose
	Vinblastine	Liver	Myelosuppression, mucositis, neurotoxicity, hypertension, myocardial ischemia(esp. in comb w/cisplatin bleomycin), Raynaud's phenomenon, hyperuricemia, thrombophlebitis, SIADH, neuropathy, ARDS	Slow IV push or infusion	bilirubin 1.5–3.0 mg/dL or AST 60–180 units: 50% reduction. bilirubin 3.0–5.0 mg/dL: 75% reduction Serum bilirubin >5.0 mg/dL or AST >180 units: omit dose
	Vinorelbine	Liver	Myelosuppression, N&V, mucositis, constipation/diarrhea, elevated liver enzymes, fatigue, mild neurotoxicity, thrombophlebitis, SIADH, rare hemorrhagic cystitis	IV push or short infusion	Serum bilirubin 2.1–3 mg/dL: 50% reduction Serum bilirubin >3 mg/dL: 75% reduction
	Paclitaxel	Liver	Myelosuppression, hypersensitivity, neuropathy, myalgias, alopecia, cardiac arrhythmias (most commonly bradyarrhythmias), myocardial ischemia, myocardial dysfunction (with trastuzumab), mild elevation in liver transaminases, mucositis and diarrhea	IV infusion	Liver
	Docetaxel	Liver	Myelosuppression, hypersensitivity, fluid retention, alopecia, skin rash, hand-foot syndrome, mucositis, diarrhea, fatigue, neuropathy, myalgia, arthralgias, mild elevation in liver transaminases, thrombophlebitis	IV infusion	Total bilirubin greater than or equal to the upper limit of normal (ULN), or AST (SGOT)/ALT (SGPT) >1.5 times the ULN concomitant with alkaline phosphatase >2.5 times the ULN: docetaxel should not be administered
Anti-topoisomerase agents	Topotecan	Renal	Myelosuppression, N&V, diarrhea, headache, fatigue, fever, alopecia, skin rash, hematuria, elevated liver enzymes	IV infusion	Clcr 20–39 mL/min: 50% reduction Clcr <20 mL/min: do not use
	Irinotecan	Liver	Myelosuppression, N&V, diarrhea, eosinophilia, elevated liver enzymes, fatigue, thrombophlebitis, cholinergic syndrome	IV infusion	
	Etoposide	Renal, liver	Myelosuppression, N&V, infusion-related hypotension, capillary leak syndrome, hypersensitivity, cerebral edema, elevation in liver transaminases, thrombophlebitis, secondary leukemias	IV bolus or infusion, oral	Clcr 10–50 mL/min: 25% reduction Clcr <10 mL/min: 50% reduction Bilirubin 1.5–3 mg/dL or AST 60–180 units: reduce dose by 50% Bilirubin >3 mg/dL or AST >180 units: reduce by 75%
	Teniposide	Liver	Myelosuppression, N&V, hypersensitivity, infusion-related hypotension, mild elevation in liver transaminases, secondary	IV infusion	

ARDS: acute respiratory distress syndrome
AST: aspartate transaminase
Clcr: creatinine clearance
DIC: disseminated intravascular coagulation
G6PD: glucose-6-phosphate dehydrogenase
HUS: hemolytic uremic syndrome
IM: intramuscular
IV: intravenous
MAOI: monoamine oxidase inhibitor
N&V: nausea and vomiting
SC: subcutaneous
SIADH: syndrome of inappropriate antidiuretic hormone secretion
VOD: veno-occlusive disease of the liver

TABLE 2.4. Frequency of adverse effects/toxicities.

Chemotherapeutic agent		*M*	*N&V*	*Mucositis*	*Constipation*	*Diarrhea*	*Liver*	*Pulm*	*Renal/ bladder*	*CVS*	*Neuro*	*Alopecia*	*Skin*	*Fever*	*Weakness /fatigue*	*HSR*
Classic alkylating agents	Chlorambucil	++++	+	+		±	±	±			±		+	±		±
	Cyclophosphamide	++++	++	+		+	±	±	+/+	+	+	+++	+			
	Ifosfamide	++++	+++		+	±	±	±	++/+++	+	+	++++	+			
	Mechlorethamine	++++	++++			+	±				+	+	+++	+		
	Melphalan	++++	+	++		±	+	+	±/+	+*		+	+			+
	Mitomycin C	++++	++	+			+§	+	+/±	+	+	+	+	+	+	
	Thiotepa	++++	+	±					+/+		+	+	+++	+	+	+
	Carmustine (BCNU)	++++	++++	+		+	++++‡	++§	+§/±	+§	+†	+	+			
	Lomustine (CCNU)	++++	++++	+		+	±	±	+		+	+	+			
	Streptozocin	+	++++			+	+		+++		±				±	
	Busulfan	++++	++++	+		+	+	+	/±	+	+	+	++		+	
Nonclassic alkylating agents	Procarbazine	++++	++++	+	+	+	+	±			++	+	+	+	++	
	Dacarbazine	++++	++++			±	±				+	+	+	+		
	Altretamine	+++	+++			+++	+		+		++	±	±			
	Temozolomide	++++	+++	+	++	+	++		/+		+++	+	+	+	++	
	cisplatin	++	++++				++		++	+	+++	+	±	±		+
	carboplatin	+++	+++		+	+	++		+		+	+	+			+
	oxaliplatin	+++	++++	+	++	++∞	+++	±	+	+	+++	±	+	++	+++	+
Antitumor antibiotics	Doxorubicin	++++	+++	++		+	+			+		++++	+			±
	Daunorubicin	++++	+++	+		+	±			+		++++	+			
	Idarubicin	++++	++++	+		++	++			+	+	++	+			
	Epirubicin	++++	++++	+++		++				+		++++	+		++	
	Mitoxantrone	++++	+++	++	+	++	++	±	+	+	+	++	+	+	++	±
	Dactinomycin	++++	+++	+		+	+	±				++	+	+	++	±
	Bleomycin	±	±	++				+		++		++	+++	++		+

Antimetabolites	Methotrexate	+++	+++	++		++	++	+	+	++	++	+	+			±
	Raltitrexed	+++	+++	++	+	++	++		+	+	+	+	++	++	+++	±
	Pemetrexed	+++	++	+	+	+	+++		++	++		±	+++		+++	
	5-Fluorouracil	++++	+	+++		++	±			+	+	+	++			
	5-FUDR	++	++	++		++	++++∫	±	+	±	+	+	+	+		±
	Capecitabine	++++	+++	++	+	+++	++			+	+	+	+++	+	++	
	Cytarabine	++++	++	+		+	+	±	±/±	+	+	+	+	+		
	Gemcitabine	++	+++	+	++	++	+++	±	++	+	+	+	++	++	++	+
	6-Mercaptopurine	+++	+	+		+	++	±	+			±	+	+		
	6-Thioguanine	+++	+	+		+	+				+		+			
	Fludarabine	+++	++	+		+	±	±	±	+	++	+	+		++	
	Cladribine	++	+		+	+			+	+	+	+	++	+++	+	
	Pentostatin	+++	+++	+		+	++		++	+	+	+	++	+	+	
Antimicrotubule agents	Vincristine	±	+	+	+	+	±		/+	+	+	+++	+		+	
	Vinblastine	++++	+	+	+	+	+		/+	+	+	++	+			
	Vinorelbine	++++	++	++	++	+	+		/±	±	++	++	+		++	±
	Paclitaxel	++++	+	+		+	+	±		++	+++	++++	+		+++	+
	Docetaxel	++++	+++	++		++	+	±		+++	++	++++	+++	++	+++	+
Antitopoisom-erase agents	Topotecan	++++	++++	+		++	+		+		+	++	++	++	+++	±
	Irinotecan	+++	++++		++	++++	++	±	±	+		+++		++	+++	
	Etoposide	++++	++	+		+	+	±		+	+	+++	+			+
	Teniposide	++++	++	+++		++	+			+		+	+			+

M, myelosuppression; N&V, nausea and vomiting; pulm, pneumonitis or pulmonary fibrosis; CVS, cardiovascular system; neuro, central and peripheral nervous system, HSR, serious hypersensitivity reactions.

*, Vasculitis.

§. High-dose or transplant setting.

†, Seizures occur in 54% of patients postoperatively after wafer implant.

‡, Elevated transaminases occur in 90% during the first week; hepatic veno-occlusive disease (VOD) of the liver occurs in up to 20% in transplant settings.

∞, Up to 80%–90% with 5-FU combination chemotherapy.

∫, With intraarterial therapy.

++++, 75%–100%.

+++, 40%–75%.

++, 15%–40%.

+, 1%–15%.

±, <1%.

metabolites proceeds more slowly than that of cyclophosphamide. Ifosfamide is more likely than cyclophosphamide to produce renal damage, and a Fanconi-like syndrome has been described after ifosfamide therapy. Central nervous system (CNS) toxicities of varying degrees such as hallucinations, cerebellar ataxias, weakness, aphasia, seizures, and coma are more likely to occur in patients with renal impairment or low serum albumin levels receiving high-dose chemotherapy.[25] It has greater activity against sarcomas and testicular cancer.

Aziridines

Thiotepa

Thiotepa is a representative agent of the class of analogues of the closed-ring intermediates of the nitrogen mustards called aziridines. Thiotepa inhibits not only DNA but RNA and protein synthesis as well. It is primarily administered intravenously because of variable oral absorption. Intrathecal treatment of meningeal carcinomatosis and intravesical instillation for superficial transitional cell carcinoma (TCC) of the bladder is also used. It is extensively metabolized by the mixed-function oxygenases of the cytochrome P-450 system in the liver into the active desulfurated metabolite triethylenephosphoramide (TEPA). Both thiotepa and TEPA have cytotoxic activity, although nadirs in leukocytes and platelets correlate best with the AUC (area under the drug concentration–time curve) of thiotepa. It is used in breast and ovarian cancer, as well as in the high-dose transplant settings for these two malignancies. Mucositis, skin changes (bronzing, rash, hyperpigmentation), and altered mental status may be seen at high doses.

Mitomycin C

Mitomycin C belongs to the family of related antibiotics from *Streptomyces caespitosus*,[26] and thus can also be classified under the antitumor antibiotic group. The mitomycins are the only known naturally occurring compounds containing an aziridine ring. Biochemical reduction of its quinone moiety transforms the drug into a highly reactive alkylator, thus the term bioreductive alkylation.[27] Both aerobic and anaerobic mechanisms of activation exist, each giving rise to different reactive species, although alkylation may be more likely to occur in a hypoxic environment.[28] Its role as a radiosensitizer arises from this cytotoxicity in hypoxic cells. Although it is not currently used in first-line therapy of any malignancy, it is used in combined modality treatment of squamous cell carcinoma of the anus and head and neck malignancies. It is also intravesically administered for superficial bladder cancer.

Nitrosoureas

Carmustine and Lomustine

Because of their lipophilicity and ability to cross the blood–brain barrier, chloroethylnitrosoureas such as carmustine (BCNU) and lomustine (CCNU) are used principally for the treatment of brain tumors. They may also be used in certain regimens for lymphomas. At physiologic pH, the chloroethyldiazonium hydroxide molecules and isocyanates that arise from the spontaneous decomposition of BCNU alkylate DNA, inhibit enzymes involved in DNA and RNA synthesis, respectively.[29–32] CCNU is relatively unionized at physiologic pH and is hepatically metabolized by the cytochrome P-450 system into active intermediates. In contrast to other agents, nitrosoureas exhibit a characteristic delayed myelosuppression.[33] Onset of leukocyte and platelet depression occurs 3 to 4 weeks after drug administration. Platelet counts may reach nadir before neutrophil counts. Nadir typically occurs at 4 to 6 weeks and may persist for an additional 1 to 3 weeks. Transient elevation of the serum transaminases develops in the majority of patients within 1 week of BCNU administration. Hepatic veno-occlusive disease may be observed in up to 20% of patients receiving high-dose BCNU therapy. Pulmonary fibrosis and renal toxicity may be evident when a cumulative dose of 1,000 to 1,400 mg/m^2 is exceeded for both nitrosoureas.

Streptozotocin

Unlike the other nitrosourea analogues, streptozotocin has no effect on RNA or protein synthesis. It does not form DNA crosslinks, although it can methylate DNA. This methylnitrosourea, isolated from *Streptomyces*, is remarkable for its lack of bone marrow toxicity.[34] When myelosuppression occurs, it is usually mild, with nadir occurring at 1 to 2 weeks. Nevertheless, when in combination with other cytotoxic agents, there is considerable synergism in regard to hematologic toxicity. Nausea and vomiting can be quite severe. Its diabetogenic effect in animals is correlated with its specific toxicity against pancreatic beta cells, hence its use in islet cell carcinoma of the pancreas. It has demonstrated clinically significant activity against islet cell carcinoma of the pancreas and carcinoid tumors.

Alkyl Alkane Sulfonates

Busulfan

Busulfan is the major representative of this class of agents. Its lipophilicity and low protein-binding affinity account for its penetration into the CNS.[35] It reacts more extensively with the thiol groups of amino acids and proteins than do the nitrogen mustards.[36] It is selectively more toxic against myeloid than lymphoid cells, in contrast to nitrogen mustards and nitrosoureas.[37] It is well absorbed orally and has a short duration of action because of extensive hepatic conjugation with glutathione. Consequently, acetaminophen may potentiate host toxicity when given 72 hours before busulfan due to interference with hepatic metabolism. Its metabolism exhibits circadian rhythmicity, especially in children.[38] Prolonged bone marrow aplasia may be seen after its administration, attributed to its cytotoxicity against hematopoietic stem cells. Hyperpigmentation of the skin, especially the palmar creases, is not uncommon. Seizures and hepatic veno-occlusive disease occur in a substantial proportion of patients with high-dose therapy in the transplant setting. Prophylactic anticonvulsant therapy is thus recommended with high-dose busulfan. It is used as a component of most regimens for chronic myelogenous leukemia, although it is no longer the frontline therapy.

Nonclassic Alkylating Agents

Procarbazine

Procarbazine (PCB) is widely distributed in most tissues, including the cerebrospinal fluid (CSF), with oral administration. It is a hydrazine analogue that inhibits DNA, RNA, and protein synthesis. An oral prodrug, its active end products and the mechanism of their cytotoxicity remain unclear, although the free radical species that arise from the decomposition of methyl- or benzylazoxy intermediates generated by the hepatic cytochrome P-450 system seem to be the most likely candidates. Current evidence favors its role as a methylating agent. The importance of first-pass hepatic metabolism is demonstrated by the neurotoxicity and lack of antitumor activity with intravenous administration.[39] In contrast, the most common dose-limiting toxicity of PCB given orally is myelosuppression. Nausea and vomiting often abate with continued administration. Because it inhibits monoamine oxidase (MAO) and is in turn extensively metabolized by the hepatic microsomes, the potential for drug and food interactions is increased. Gonadal toxicity resulting in azoospermia or ovarian failure is not uncommon. Its immunosuppressive property may contribute to increased risk of infections.[40] It is primarily used in the treatment of Hodgkin's disease (MOPP regimen) and brain tumors.

DACARBAZINE

Dacarbazine (DTIC) is a dimethyltriazene prodrug that is administered intravenously. It is hepatically demethylated by the cytochrome P-450 mixed-function oxidase to form 5-(3-methyltriazeno)imidazole-4-carboxamide (MTIC), which tautomerizes to the methyldiazonium ion species that acts as the active methylating agent. It was originally developed as a purine antimetabolite. However, it is not cell cycle specific. Evidence is also sufficient to suggest that its antitumor activity does not result from inhibition of purine synthesis. DTIC inhibits DNA, RNA, and protein synthesis in vitro.[41] Aside from its cytotoxicity, DTIC has antimetastatic properties in vivo, which may be related to its ability to enhance tumor immunogenicity.[42] Unlike procarbazine, it has poor CSF penetration. Myelosuppression is dose-limiting.[43] It is an active single agent used in the treatment of metastatic melanoma and Hodgkin's lymphoma.

TEMOZOLOMIDE

Temozolomide (TMZ) is an oral imidazotetrazinone whose ring structure spontaneously opens under physiologic conditions to generate the monomethyl triazine MTIC, the same methylating metabolite formed by metabolic dealkylation of DTIC.[44] The spontaneous conversion to MTIC, as opposed to the inefficient and variable demethylation of DTIC to MTIC in humans, accounts for its advantage over DTIC. This conversion is pH dependent, acidic conditions favoring the closed stable form of TMZ. In contrast, MTIC rapidly degrades to the methyldiazonium ion at pH less than 7.0.[45] TMZ's lipophilicity accounts for its CNS penetration. It is used in the treatment of metastatic melanoma, high-grade gliomas, and anaplastic astrocytoma. It is also being investigated for treatment of brain metastases from lung cancer and other tumors.

Platinum Compounds

Antitumor activity of platinum compounds was extrapolated and tested from the initial observations of Rosenberg and coworkers on the inhibition of *Escherichia coli* growth by a current delivered between platinum electrodes.[46] The core structure of the intravenously administered platinum analogues cisplatin, carboplatin, and oxaliplatin is based on the

Leaving group Carrier Ligand

cisplatin

carboplatin

oxaliplatin

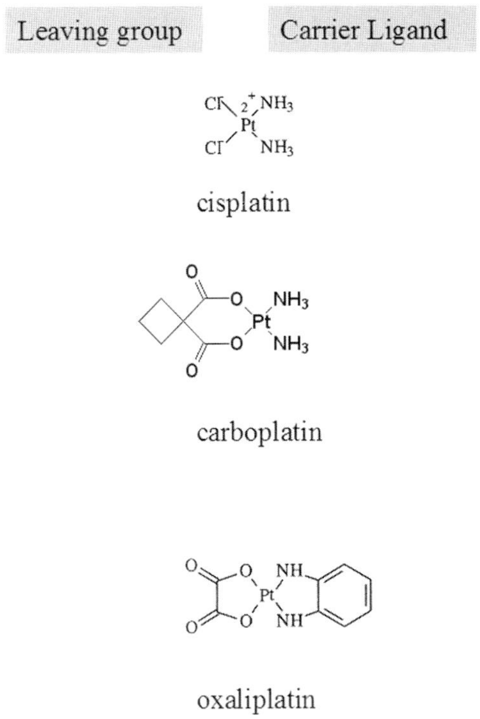

FIGURE 2.4. Structures of the platinum analogues.

cis configuration of platinum in its +2 oxidation state, designated as Pt(II). The cis isomers are cytotoxic whereas the trans isomers are much less potent. In addition to the oxidation state and isomeric configuration, clinical activity and toxicity of the platinum analogues seem to be related to the type of carrier ligand and leaving groups attached to the core *cis*-platinum structure. As shown in Figure 2.4, carboplatin differs from cisplatin by its cyclobutane dicarboxy leaving group, whereas oxaliplatin differs from carboplatin by its 1,2-diaminocyclohexane ring as its carrier ligand. Cisplatin undergoes an aquation reaction intracellularly wherein the chloride ions (the leaving groups) are displaced because of low intracellular chloride concentration. This reaction yields mono- and di-aquo platinum complexes that form strong covalent bonds with RNA as well as DNA and protein (in descending order of affinity), with intrastrand DNA crosslinks (also termed DNA adducts) being correlated with cytotoxicity and clinical outcomes.[47,48] In the case of cisplatin, detection of cisplatin-induced DNA adducts initiates a nucleotide excision DNA repair pathway (NER) as well as a signaling cascade that results in apoptosis mediated by the mismatch repair proteins (MMR). Consequently, increased NER or defective MMR protein is associated with resistance.

CISPLATIN

All three compounds are primarily cleared by the kidneys, although the extent of this clearance as well as their toxicity profiles differ. Platinum compounds, particularly cisplatin, appear to inhibit cytochrome P-450 activity, which may account for drug interactions in combination regimens with other chemotherapeutic agents. Cisplatin is generally administered with forced saline diuresis, as nephrotoxicity is dose limiting and cumulative. Its high emetogenic potential also warrants the maintenance of adequate fluid hydration.

Nephrotoxicity is manifested early as potassium and magnesium wasting, in addition to a reduction in glomerular filtration rate. The electrolyte derangements may be ascribed to inhibition of the Na^+/K^+ ATPase activity as well as the Ca^{2+} channel in renal tubular tissue.[49,50] Morphologic kidney damage is greatest in the renal tubules. Peripheral neuropathy, predominantly sensory, also commonly ensues after repeated administration and often may be irreversible. Approximately 85% of patients suffer this complication when cumulative dose exceeds $300\,mg/m^2$.[51] Cumulative and dose-dependent irreversible ototoxicity is not unusual. It is used as first-line agent in treating various malignancies, such as germ cell tumor, head and neck cancers, lung cancers, osteogenic sarcoma, genitourinary neoplasms, and upper gastrointestinal (GI) malignancies.[52]

Carboplatin

Carboplatin is 100 times less reactive than cisplatin in undergoing the intracellular aquation reaction. It requires 10-fold-higher drug concentrations and 7.5-fold-longer incubation time than cisplatin to induce the same degree of DNA damage. Unlike cisplatin, carboplatin is not significantly secreted by renal tubules. Its clearance is linearly related to the glomerular filtration rate (GFR). There is a good correlation between its AUC and dose-limiting thrombocytopenia. The AUC is the ratio of the amount of a drug that reaches the systemic circulation and the clearance of the drug. As carboplatin excretion has relatively simple pharmacokinetics, a formula relating the dose to AUC and renal function has been established. Calvert's formula [carboplatin dose (*mg*) = target AUC (*mg/mL* × *min*) × GFR (*mL/min*) + 25] uses the AUC and creatinine clearance to derive dose levels. Target AUC values of 5 and 7 mg/mL × minute are recommended for single-agent carboplatin in previously treated and untreated patients, respectively. The efficacy of carboplatin appears to be suboptimal at AUCs below 5 mg/mL × min and appears to plateau above an AUC of 7.5 mg/mL × minute. It is less emetogenic and neurotoxic than cisplatin, although more myelosuppressive.

As suggested previously, there is cross-reactivity between cisplatin and carboplatin and thus a similar reaction may be seen when one analogue is substituted for another. Carboplatin has confirmed activity for many of the diseases that are treated with cisplatin. It is of clinically equivalent efficacy as cisplatin in the treatment of non-small cell lung cancer (NSCLC), extensive-stage SCLC, and suboptimally debulked ovarian cancer. Cisplatin is clinically superior in treating germ cell, head and neck, and esophageal cancers.[52]

Oxaliplatin

Oxaliplatin is a third-generation platinum compound that undergoes spontaneous nonenzymatic conversion to its active metabolite. Oxaliplatin differs from both cisplatin and carboplatin by its unique carrier ligand, which is thought to cause reduced recognition and repair of oxaliplatin–DNA adducts.[53] It produces inter- and intrastrand DNA crosslinks more rapidly than cisplatin. It demonstrates both in vitro and in vivo activity against various tumor cell lines, even those resistant to cisplatin and carboplatin.[54] Although defects in certain MMR proteins, such as those seen in colorectal cancers, lead to cisplatin resistance, this is not the case with oxaliplatin, which remains effective. Oxaliplatin is synergistic with fluorouracil (5-FU)/leucovorin in vitro, and its activity in vivo is significantly enhanced by combination with 5-FU. It is not nephrotoxic and has minimal hematologic, auditory, or cardiac toxicity. Certain toxicities are unique to oxaliplatin. Neurotoxicity, chiefly sensory neuropathy, is exacerbated or triggered by exposure to cold. Although dose limiting, this effect is generally reversible on discontinuation of oxaliplatin. Acute dysesthesias in the upper extremities and laryngopharyngeal region with episodes of difficulty breathing or swallowing may be observed within hours or the first few days after therapy. Diarrhea is more marked with combination chemotherapy, usually given in the regimen with 5-FU and leucovorin in metastatic colon cancer.

Antitumor Antibiotics and Related Synethetic Compounds

Most of the antitumor antibiotics were initially isolated from various *Streptomyces* species. Central to their cytotoxic profile is the presence of numerous mechanisms by which each individual antibiotic interacts with DNA. The variety of chemical structures present in each compound participate in multiple mechanisms responsible for their activity against cells. The polycyclic chromophore structure intercalates with DNA and is also responsible for conferring the characteristic bright color of these drugs. Ring structures, such as the quinone group, not only interfere with electron transport, but also bind metal cations, intercalate into DNA and RNA, and generate reactive oxidant species, to name a few actions. DNA-modifying enzymes, such as topoisomerases and helicases, are common cellular enzymes targeted by these drugs.

Dose-limiting toxicities are related to myelosuppression and mucositis. Variable susceptibility to congestive cardiomyopathy is an associated complication from cumulative dose administration of anthracyclines. Emetogenic potential is considerable. Reversible alopecia is not unusual. They are also among the most potent vesicants available, and thus scrupulous attention should be given during the administration of these agents to prevent tissue extravasation. Photosensitivity, hyperpigmentation, and pigmentation of the nails and urine are common. Another interesting toxicity is the radiation recall phenomenon. As the term suggests, pain, erythema, and blistering or ulceration occur on previous radiation sites within 3 to 7 days of administration of the antitumor antibiotic. This phenomenon may be observed on any epithelial surface and may thus manifest as dermatitis, enteritis, pneumonitis, or stomatitis. The drugs most commonly implicated are the anthracyclines doxorubicin and daunorubicin, dactinomycin, and bleomycin.

Anthracyclines

The anthracyclines doxorubicin and daunorubicin are commonly incorporated into standard therapy regimens for multiple cancer types, given their broad antitumor activity over a wide range of doses and administration schedules as well as the lack of antagonistic interactions with other commonly used chemotherapy agents.

Anthracyclines exert pleiotropic mechanisms by which they effect cytotoxicity. Aside from DNA intercalation, anthracyclines inhibit DNA topoisomerase II, an enzyme that releases the torsional strain in DNA by actively inserting stable DNA strand breaks, facilitating the passage of one of the DNA strands through the other in the helix and then reannealing the strand break.[55] Anthracyclines form a ternary 'cleavable complex' with DNA topoisomerase II, which then 'traps' the DNA strand passage intermediates. This inhibition of topoisomerase II can be detected as protein-associated DNA single- and double-strand breaks linked to the enzyme. Another target is a group of nuclear enzymes, the helicases, that is critical in duplex DNA dissociation into single strands.[56] Their anthraquinone structure enables them to undergo one-electron reduction reactions catalyzed by flavin dehydrogenases or reductases. These reactions generate free radicals and other reactive oxidant species that damage intracellular macromolecules.[57] Moreover, certain signal transduction pathways, such as protein kinase C and the sphingomyelin pathway, can be modulated by anthracyclines, the end effects of which include apoptosis.[58,59]

Doxorubicin

Doxorubicin is primarily hepatically metabolized. The liposomal formulation has a small volume of distribution and hence is mainly confined to the intravascular compartment. It has a slower plasma clearance and prolonged terminal half-life compared to the regular formulation. Doxorubicin can induce histamine release, manifesting as facial flushing. Atrial and ventricular dysrhythmia may arise acutely with anthracycline administration, although these are usually not life threatening. Congestive cardiomyopathy is a late complication, occurring at less than 5% with cumulative dosage of greater than 400 mg/m^2 with intermittent schedules, 550 mg/m^2 with weekly, or up to 800 to 1,000 mg/m^2 with continuous infusion schedules. Risk factors that predispose to earlier development of congestive heart failure are old age; cardiovascular disorder associated with increased left ventricular outflow tract gradients, such as uncontrolled hypertension, aortic stenosis, or underlying cardiomyopathy; history of congestive heart disease; and mediastinal irradiation.

Epirubicin

Epirubicin is a derivative of doxorubicin. It is hepatically glucuronidated and its metabolites are excreted in bile. It was developed in efforts to reduce cardiotoxicity seen with doxorubicin. Epirubicin has a more favorable therapeutic index, with 30% less hematologic toxicity at equimolar doses. Risk of congestive heart failure, which may not differ from doxorubicin at equimyelosuppressive doses,[60] increases significantly with cumulative doses greater than 900 mg/m^2. Similar to doxorubicin, continuous infusion and weekly schedules are associated with decreased risk of cardiotoxicity. Epirubicin is used as a component of regimens used in adjuvant therapy in breast and gastric cancer.

Daunorubicin

Daunorubicin was the prototype anthracycline studied in the 1960s. It is more lipid soluble than doxorubicin, owing to the absence of one hydroxyl group. As compared to doxorubicin, there is a lower incidence of mucositis and colonic perforation. The renal clearance is approximately twice that for doxorubicin, thus making dose adjustments in patients with hepatic dysfunction unnecessary in many situations. Cardiac toxicity is likewise limiting. Its current use is mainly in the remission induction regimens for acute leukemias.

Idarubicin

Idarubicin is a 4-demethoxy derivative of daunorubicin that is orally bioavailable, has a longer half-life, and less potential for cardiotoxicity. Because of the alteration in its ring structure, it has a yellow color in aqueous solutions, as opposed to the characteristic red color of doxorubicin and daunorubicin. The primary metabolite of idarubicin, 13-idarubicinol, is cytotoxic and largely renally excreted. Although it has significant activity in the treatment of acute myelogenous leukemia (AML), it is less active against solid tumors.

Anthracenediones

Mitoxantrone

Mitoxantrone, a dark blue anthracenedione originally synthesized as a stable dye, intercalates nucleic acids and thus inhibits DNA and RNA synthesis. It also inhibits topoisomerase II by the formation of a cleavable complex, thus causing protein-associated single-strand DNA breaks.[61] In spite of its quinone structure, free radical production is limited, and in one model, mitoxantrone inhibited the rate of lipid peroxidation induced by doxorubicin.[62] This is clinically observed in the reduced severity of its cardiac effects in contrast to doxorubicin. It is used mainly in prostate and breast cancers, as well as leukemias and lymphomas.

Bleomycin

Bleomycin is a cell-cycle-specific polypeptide antibiotic that requires a metal ion cofactor for its activity, such as copper or iron, without which single- and double-strand breaks (approximately 10:1) in DNA cannot be produced.[63] Inhibition of cell growth occurs at the S phase, although it can also induce a G_2 arrest.[64] It is a mixture of multiple glycopeptides, the predominant active component of which is the A2 peptide, comprising 70% of the commercial preparation.

Bleomycin has a short half-life.[65] Renal excretion is the primary route of eliminating up to 70% of unchanged drug after a given dose. It is inactivated in the tissues by the enzyme bleomycin hydrolase, the concentrations of which are lowest in skin and lung,[66] thus explaining the clinical toxicities encountered. Fever within the first 12 hours of administration is almost universally observed. Hypotension is seen with rapid intravenous infusions of higher doses. Anaphylactoid reactions have been described, mostly in lymphoma patients receiving their first dose.[67] The most feared complication, however, is pulmonary interstitial fibrosis, which appears to be cumulatively dose dependent at 300 units total dose.[66] Pulmonary fibrosis appears earlier in those with impaired renal function. Exposure to high oxygen tensions even after prior therapy with bleomycin is associated with increased risk of developing this pulmonary toxicity. Onset is unpredictable, as it may occur during treatment or after cessation of therapy, and may progress even after discontinuation of the drug.[68] It is used in curative regimens for testicular cancer and Hodgkin's lymphoma.

Dactinomycin (Actinomycin D)

Actinomycin D has a tricyclic phenoxazone ring, which imparts its yellow color, attached to two symmetric cyclic polypeptides. It binds DNA, and also inhibits RNA and protein synthesis, by intercalating DNA through its chromophore structure between base pairs, whereas the peptide lactone rings lie in the minor groove of DNA.[69] Its rapid tissue uptake and long terminal half-life permit intermittent administration. The radiation recall phenomenon was first described in patients who received actinomycin, even years after irradiation. Toxicities are similar to the other antitumor antibiotics and seem to be of greater severity. It is used in curative regimens for several childhood tumors, refractory germ cell tumors.

Antimetabolites

Antimetabolites are structurally similar to natural compounds necessary for cell division. They act as competitive substrates for critical purine or pyrimidine nucleoside synthesis pathways. As expected from their mechanism of action through disruption of DNA synthesis, antimetabolites are most effective against tumors with a high growth fraction, and in particular during the S phase. In general, antimetabolites are not mutagenic, exhibit a plateau in cytotoxic effect, and require enzymatic conversion to an active form.

Folate Antagonists

Folates exist predominantly as polyglutamates within cells to facilitate intracellular retention in excess of the freely transportable monoglutamate form. They must first be reduced to tetrahydrofolate (FH_4) by the enzyme dihydrofolate reductase (DHFR) to become active coenzymes in one-carbon transfer reactions, among which are those required for the de novo purine synthesis mediated by glycineamide ribonucleotide formyltransferase (GARFT) and aminoimidazole carboxamide ribonucleotide transformylase (AICART), as well as the methylation of 2-deoxyuridylate for de novo synthesis of thymidylate through thymidylate synthetase (TS). Antifolates inhibit these reactions (Figure 2.5), which lead to formation of DNA strand breaks upon depletion of thymidylate and purine nucleotides, accumulation of deoxyuridine monophosphate (dUMP), and incorporation of deoxyuridine triphosphate (dUTP) into DNA. They are transported into the cell primarily via the reduced folate carrier (RFC) and to a smaller extent by the folate receptor protein (FRP). The primary toxicities seen with antifolates are myelosuppression and mucositis.

Methotrexate

Methotrexate (MTX) is the most commonly used antifolate agent in cancer chemotherapy. Cellular uptake of MTX is faster in rapidly dividing cells, with a concomitant decreased rate of efflux as opposed to slowly growing cells. It is then subsequently polyglutamated by the enzyme folylpolyglutamyl synthetase (FPGS), although less avidly and at slower rates compared to, in order of decreasing affinity, FH_2, FH_4, or

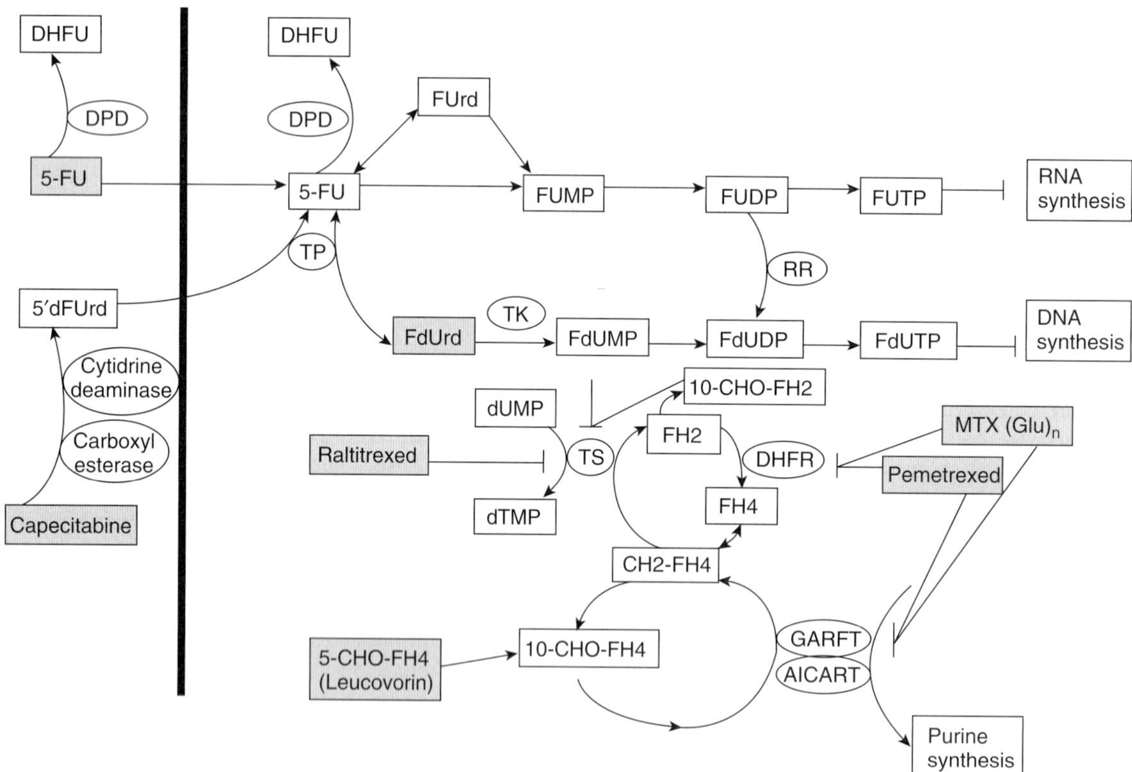

FIGURE 2.5. Mechanism of action of fluoropyrimidines and antifolates. AICART, aminoimidazole carboxamide ribonucleotide transformylase; dTMP, deoxythymidine monophosphate; dUMP, deoxyuridine monophosphate; DHFR, dihydrofolate reductase; DHFU, dihydrofluorouracil; CH_2-FH_4, 5,10-methylenetetrahydrofolate; 10-CHO-FH_2, 10-CHO-FH_4, 10-formyl-, -dihydro-, -tetrahydro-, -folate, respectively; DPD, dihydropyrimidine dehydrogenase; FH_2, FH_4, dihydro-, tetrahydro-, -folate, respectively; 5-FU, 5-fluorouracil; 5′-dFUrd, 5′-deoxy-5-fluorouridine; FUrd, 5-fluorouridine; FdUMP, FdUDP, FdUTP, fluorodeoxyuridine-, -mono-, -di-, -tri-, -phosphate, respectively; FUMP, FUDP, FUTP, fluorouridine-, -mono-, -di-, -tri-, -phosphate, respectively; GARFT, glycineamide ribonucleotide formyltransferase; MTX $(Glu)_n$, polyglutamated methotrexate; RR, ribonucleotide reductase; dTMP, deoxythymidine monophosphate; dUMP, deoxyuridine monophosphate; TK, thymidine kinase; TP, thymidine phosphorylase; TS, thymidylate synthase.

leucovorin. Polyglutamated MTX is a more potent and avid reversible inhibitor of DHFR than monoglutamated MTX. The ability to generate MTX polyglutamates seem to correlate with cytotoxicity in both murine and human tumor cells,[70,71] whereas increasing concentration of reduced folates can competitively reverse MTX toxicity.

MTX is rapidly absorbed orally, although incompletely at higher doses. It has a rather long terminal half-life, up to 27 hours.[72] CSF penetration at conventional doses is poor. It is thus administered intrathecally in prophylactic CNS therapy for ALL. MTX slowly penetrates third-space fluid collections such as pleural effusion and ascites. The half-life of MTX sequestered in these situations is further prolonged because of slow reentry into the bloodstream. Enhanced clinical toxicity may be observed if fluid collections are not drained before methotrexate therapy. MTX is primarily cleared by the kidneys within the first 12 hours after administration, mostly as unchanged drug. It should therefore be used cautiously in patients with renal insufficiency. In these circumstances, the enterohepatic circulation may assume a more important role in drug excretion,[73] and use of activated charcoal or cholestyramine may be tried to enhance plasma clearance through enhanced biliary excretion.[74,75] Carboxypeptidase G, an enzyme that removes the terminal glutamate residue from MTX, leads to MTX inactivation and is another effective alternative.

Standard Intravenous Administration

Major toxicities are myelosuppression and mucositis. Gastrointestinal epithelial cells are more sensitive to the effects of MTX, being inhibited at half the concentrations required to inhibit DNA synthesis in the bone marrow.[76] Mucositis typically appears 3 to 5 days after treatment and precedes the fall in leukocytes or platelets by several days. Unless drug clearance is severely impaired, such as in renal failure, myelosuppression and mucositis are usually reversed within 2 weeks.

High-Dose Therapy

High-dose MTX yields therapeutic concentrations in the CSF. Nephrotoxicity, manifested as oliguria and azotemia, is the major adverse effect of high-dose MTX therapy. Although MTX may be a direct tubular toxin per se, nephrotoxicity arising from high-dose therapy is mainly attributed to intratubular precipitation of MTX and its less-soluble metabolites, 7-OH MTX and 2,4-diamino-*N*-10-methyl pteroic acid (DAMPA), in acidic urine. Vigorous hydration and urine alkalinization can diminish such complication. Some myelosuppression and mucositis may occur. Leucovorin rescue (described next) reduces the likelihood of systemic toxicity. Acute transient transaminase elevations commonly occur after high-dose therapy, but late occurrence of liver failure or cirrhosis has not been reported. Repeated courses of high-dose MTX therapy can result in encephalopathy, dementia, paresis, and seizures.

Leucovorin Rescue

Methotrexate blood levels should be assayed every 24 hours with high-dose therapy in patients with impaired renal function as well as patients who have had excessive toxicity with prior MTX therapy. Leucovorin rescue is initiated at 12 to 24 hours after the start of high-dose drug infusion and should continue until MTX level is less than 50 nM/L. Leucovorin is typically administered as 10 mg/m^2 intravenously followed by oral doses given every 6 hours for 10 to 12 more doses. If MTX levels are above 500 nM/L, 1 μM/L, or 2 μM/L at 48 hours, a general guideline is that leucovorin should be administered at 15 mg/m^2, 100 mg/m^2, or 200 mg/m^2, respectively, every 6 hours over 48 more hours. Patients should be vigorously hydrated using bicarbonate-enriched fluids (2.5–3.5 L/m^2/day IV fluids + 45–50 mEq bicarbonate/L IV fluid) to maintain high urine output (more than 100 mL/h) and alkaline urine (above pH 7.0) for 12 hours before and 48 hours after high-dose therapy (more than 1 g/m^2) to avoid renal failure. MTX is used clinically in leukemia, lymphoma, breast cancer, head and neck cancer, osteogenic sarcoma, and choriocarcinoma.

Raltitrexed

Raltitrexed is a potent quinazoline analogue that selectively inhibits thymidylate synthase (TS). Similar to MTX, polyglutamation by folylpolyglutamyl synthetase (FPGS) is correlated with increasing cytotoxicity.[77] It is poorly absorbed orally. Its excretion, mostly as unchanged drug, is similarly correlated with creatinine clearance. Patients with insufficient folate intake may be at increased risk for clinical toxicity. Transient elevation of liver enzymes may be seen with its convenient IV dosing once every 3 weeks. It is an effective alternative to 5-FU-based therapy in patients with metastatic colorectal cancer. Another advantage over 5-FU is lesser frequency of mucositis. It also exhibits antitumor activity in non-small cell lung and breast cancers. It is approved in several countries in Europe, Canada, Asia, and Australia.

Pemetrexed

Pemetrexed is a pyrrolo-pyrimidine-based antifolate analogue whose main activity is inhibition of TS. It is transported into cells via the RFC, with transport kinetics similar to that of methotrexate. It binds to folate receptor-α with a very high affinity, similar to that of folic acid. Furthermore, cellular influx is also facilitated by the presence of high-affinity and highly specific transport systems for pemetrexed in malignant mesothelioma cell lines.[78] This transport system has a relatively low affinity for other inhibitors of DHFR or TS such as methotrexate and raltitrexed. Pemetrexed is likewise polyglutamated by FPGS to enhance intracellular concentration, and consequently, cytotoxicity. The polyglutamation reaction occurs 90- to 195-fold more efficiently with pemetrexed than methotrexate.[79] Polyglutamated pemetrexed is more than 60-fold more potent in its inhibition of TS than the monoglutamate. Its prolonged intracellular retention allows for bolus intermittent dosing schedules. At high concentrations, pemetrexed causes an S-phase block and apoptosis. Under the same conditions, it also exhibits multitarget inhibition of several crucial folate-requiring enzymes such as DHFR, GARFT, and, to a lesser extent, AICART and C1-FH_4 synthase.

Pemetrexed causes a rapid depletion of deoxythymidine-, deoxycytosine-, and deoxyguanosine triphosphates. Cells that rely on de novo purine synthesis and do not have purine salvage pathways are expected to be particularly sensitive to pemetrexed. It has been shown that pleural mesothelioma cells frequently (approximately 90%) exhibit codeletion of the gene coding for the enzyme methylthioadenosine phosphorylase (MTAP) with the CDKN2A gene.[80] Homozygous deletion of CDKN2A gene, which encodes for the cell-cycle regulatory proteins p16 and p14ARF, may be seen in 75% of pleural mesotheliomas.[80] As MTAP catalyzes an important purine salvage pathway, the frequency of its codeletion with CKDN2A, as well as the presence of highly specific transport systems for pemetrexed in malignant mesothelioma, may in part account for its efficacy in this tumor type.

Folic acid has been shown to be 100- to 1,000-fold less effective than leucovorin in protecting tumor cells against the cytotoxic effects of pemetrexed.[81] Nevertheless, folic acid reduces toxicity in mice while preserving the antitumor activity of pemetrexed. Myelosuppression and mucositis can be significantly ameliorated by folate and vitamin B_{12} supplementation without any demonstrable reduction in antitumor efficacy.

Pemetrexed has demonstrated broad antitumor activity in a wide variety of solid tumors, including mesothelioma, non-small cell lung, breast, cervical, colorectal, head and neck, and bladder cancers in a variety of Phase II trials. It exhibits synergistic antitumor activity with alkylating agents, irinotecan, and gemcitabine.[82] Promising activity has been demonstrated when pemetrexed is combined with cisplatin and gemcitabine.[82,83] A pivotal Phase III trial indicates the superiority of pemetrexed in combination with cisplatin versus cisplatin alone in malignant pleural mesothelioma.[84] Pemetrexed demonstrated equivalent efficacy to docetaxel, but with significantly less toxicity, in second-line NSCLC.[85]

Pyrimidine Antagonists

Pyrimidine antagonists comprise nucleic acid base analogues and their prodrugs as well as nucleoside analogues that generate substrates which ultimately become incorporated into the elongating DNA and RNA strand, thus inhibiting DNA, RNA, and ultimately protein, synthesis. All require intracellular anabolic conversion into active nucleotide substrates.

5-Fluorouracil

5-Fluorouracil (5-FU) is the simplest and most successful uracil derivative to date in clinical use. This fluoropyrimidine undergoes anabolic activation intracellularly into fluorodinated nucleosides and deoxynucleotides [fluorouridine monophosphate (FUMP); fluorouridine triphosphate, FUTP; fluorodeoxyuridine monophosphate, FdUMP; fluorodeoxyuridine triphosphate, FdUTP)] (see Figure 2.5). FdUMP inhibits TS and prevents formation of, and consequently depletes the available pool of, thymidylate necessary for generating dTTP; as a result, FdUTP and dUTP become the "preferred" substrates of reactions catalyzed by DNA polymerase, affecting DNA stability. Moreover, incorporation of FUTP in RNA interferes with proper RNA synthesis and function. 5-Flurodeoxyuridine (5-FUDR) or floxuridine is a fluoropyrimidine deoxynucleoside analogue that also undergoes similar metabolic conversion intracellularly to generate FUTP, FdUTP, and TS-inhibiting FdUMP. Genetic polymorphisms in TS may also affect treatment response. In vivo and in vitro studies have shown that lower TS activity is correlated with better antitumor response.

After intravenous administration, 5-FU readily penetrates the CSF and extracellular third-space fluid collections, such as ascites or pleural effusions. It has a short half-life (10–15 minutes). Both 5-FU and 5-FUDR are extensively catabolized (more than 85%). The initial rate-limiting step in degradation involves the enzyme dihydropyrimidine dehydrogenase (DPD), which is widely expressed in tissues including the liver, GI mucosa, leukocytes, and kidney. Thus, 5-FU is poorly absorbed orally. Because of its size, the liver has the highest total content of DPD and is a major site of 5-FU metabolism. DPD is subject to genetic polymorphisms, with 8- to 21-fold intersubject variability. Those with low DPD activity are susceptible to severe toxicity. Greater first-pass effect (more than 90%) through the liver results in lower systemic drug levels (and, consequently, fewer side effects) with FUDR, making it the preferred agent for hepatic arterial infusion (HAI). When administered with IV bolus schedules, FUDR is catabolized to the predominant 5-FU form.[86] Several important interactions between 5-FU and other agents have been described. Leucovorin expands the pool of reduced folates to enhance the inhibition of TS. Methotrexate pretreatment increases the formation of 5-FU nucleotides. 5-FU may interfere with the repair of platinum-associated DNA damage. Ionizing radiation augments DNA damage. All these agents demonstrate preclinical as well as Phase III trial evidence for improvement in clinical activity.

Meta-analysis of several randomized trials comparing various 5-FU schedules of administration has shown the superiority of continuous infusion of 5-FU over bolus administration when given as a single agent.[87] Moreover, bolus drug administration cannot achieve effective radiosensitization, as this requires constant drug exposure given the short half-life of 5-FU. Clinical toxicities also have some correlation with schedule of administration. Myelosuppression, especially leukopenia, is more pronounced with IV bolus schedules than with continuous infusion. Mucositis along the GI tract can be debilitating and dose limiting, especially with continuous infusion. Other GI symptoms, such as nausea, vomiting, and anorexia, can also be more severe with continuous infusion. With HAI regimens, systemic toxicities of 5-FU are dose limiting whereas hepatitis is usually mild. On the other hand, local-regional toxicities such as gastritis, gastric ulcers, enteritis, hepatitis, cholestasis, or cholecystitis predominate with HAI using 5-FUDR. 5-FU is currently used for GI malignancies and esophageal, head and neck, and breast cancers. 5-FUDR is principally used for HAI therapy of GI adenocarcinoma metastatic to the liver.

Capecitabine

Capecitabine is an oral fluropyrimidine carbamate precursor of 5-FU. It was developed to overcome the degradation of 5-FU in the GI tract when administered orally. With daily administration, it simulates continuous 5-FU IV infusion, without the inconvenience and morbidity associated with indwelling catheters. It is initially metabolized by hepatic carboxylesterase into 5′-deoxy-5-fluorocytidine, which in turn is converted to 5′-deoxy-5-fluorouridine (5′-dFUR) by the enzyme cytidine deaminase found in the liver as well as tumor tissues (Figure 2.6). The final step involves thymidine phosphorylase (TP), expressed at higher levels in tumor tissues than normal cells, which converts 5′-dFUR into 5′-FU. This preferential formation of 5-FU within tumor cells results in relatively low circulating plasma levels of 5-FU. Its current use is chiefly in the treatment of metastatic breast and colorectal cancer.

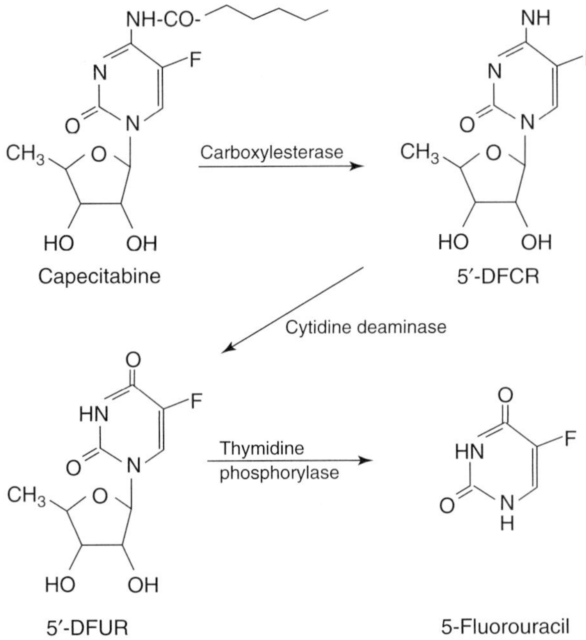

FIGURE 2.6. Metabolic activation of capecitabine (5′-DFCR, 5′-deoxy-5-fluorocytidine; 5′-DFUR, 5′-deoxy-5-fluorouridine).

Cytosine Arabinoside

Cytosine arabinoside (Ara-C) is one of the cornerstone agents in AML therapy. It was originally extracted from the sponge *Cryptothethya crypta*. This cytidine analogue differs from the native cytidine by the substitution of the sugar moiety arabinose for ribose. It is intracellularly activated after phosphorylation by different kinases into its triphosphate form (Ara-CTP) such as deoxycytidine kinase, deoxycytidine monophosphate kinase, and nucleoside dephosphate kinase. Deoxycytidine kinase activity is highest during the S phase of the cell cycle and is the rate-limiting step in the anabolic conversion of various other nucleoside analogues. Ara-CTP then competes with and depletes the dCTP pool and reversibly inhibits DNA polymerase. More importantly, the degree of incorporation of ara-CTP into DNA, leading to chain termination and inhibition of DNA synthesis, correlates with cytotoxicity.[76] It also inhibits ribonucleotide reductase, the enzyme that catalyzes the synthesis of other deoxynucleoside triphosphates. Likewise, ara-C inhibits the formation of CDP-choline integral to the synthesis of membrane glycoproteins and glycolipids. Balancing these are deaminating reactions, catalyzed by cytidine deaminase and dCMP deaminase, that degrade the active ara-C metabolites. Cytidine deaminase is widely distributed in normal cells, including the liver, GI mucosa, and mature granulocytes.

Ara-C enters cells by a saturable carrier-mediated transport system in common with physiologic nucleosides. It has been shown that the transport system is the rate-limiting factor in the formation ara-CTP.[88] At drug levels above 10 μmol/L, passive diffusion occurs and the ability to accumulate ara-CTP becomes saturated. Thus, high-dose regimens may overcome resistance in some cases associated with deficiencies in the transport system. In spite of its water solubility, ara-C penetrates the CNS quite effectively, 20% to 40% of plasma levels at steady state, to reach threshold cytotoxic levels for leukemia cells in the CSF at conventional doses. Because of the high concentrations of cytidine deaminase in the GI tract, oral administration yields significantly lower plasma levels, and therefore this route is precluded. Myelosuppression and GI toxicities are the major adverse effects of ara-C. Diarrhea and mucositis occur frequently. High-dose ara-C intensifies the severity of these toxicities. Moreover, certain syndromes unique to high-dose therapy are notable. Neurotoxicity in the form of cerebral-cerebellar dysfunction manifested as ataxia, dementia, slurred speech, and coma may lead to permanent disability in up to 40% of affected patients. An irreversible acute respiratory distress syndrome can occur in association with a high incidence of *Streptococcus viridans* pneumonia, especially in children. Steroid-responsive conjunctivitis is a frequent side effect. An unusual febrile state in conjunction with cutaneous eruption of plaques of nodules, termed neutrophilic eccrine hydradenitis, is also associated with high-dose therapy.

Gemcitabine

Gemcitabine (2,2-difluorodeoxycytidine, dFdC) is the most important cytidine analogue currently in use for solid tumors. Cellular influx also occurs via the nucleoside transport system. Intracellular activation by deoxycytidine kinase is the rate-limiting step necessary for antitumor activity. The diphosphate form (dFdCDP) inhibits ribonucleotide reductase more effectively than ara-C,[89] whereas the triphosphate dFdCTP not only inhibits DNA polymerase but also leads to DNA strand termination upon its incorporation into the elongating DNA strand. Similar to ara-C, cytidine deaminase catalyzes the major catabolic pathway in degrading gemcitabine to difluorodeoxyuridine (dFdU). Deamination requires activation by dCTP, whose level in turn is reduced upon inhibition of ribonucleotide reductase by dFdCDP. Moreover, dFdCTP directly inhibits cytidine deaminase. The preclinical finding that prolonged exposure to gemcitabine leads to dramatically greater antitumor effect is consistent with the concept of self-potentiation leading to prolonged intracellular concentrations of its primary cytotoxic metabolite, dFdCTP. Affinity of gemcitabine for deoxycytidine kinase and cytidine deaminase is much lower than deoxycytidine itself. Nevertheless, gemcitabine is a better substrate for the nucleoside transporter of tumor cells and has greater affinity for deoxycytidine kinase than ara-C. DFdCTP has a longer half-life than ara-CTP. Moreover, dFdCDP is a more potent inhibitor of ribonucleotide reductase than ara-CTP. Gemcitabine enhances the formation of DNA adducts, and thus cytotoxicity, by cisplatin. It also potently sensitizes cells to ionizing radiation. This radiosensitization is dose- and time-dependent and is maximal when radiation follows gemcitabine exposure. Because dFdCTP is present intracellularly for several days after drug administration, gemcitabine is able to radiosensitize cells for several days after bolus administration. However, this also underlies the unwanted side effect of increased treatment-related morbidity and, in some cases, mortality.[90] Gemcitabine is currently used in pancreatic and non-small cell lung cancers and is active in breast, bladder, and ovarian cancers, lymphomas, and head and neck cancers.

Purine Antagonists

These purine analogues, similar to their pyrimidine counterparts, require metabolic conversion before activation, which results in inhibition of de novo purine synthesis, and are consequently incorporated into DNA. Some also inhibit DNA polymerase and ribonucleotide reductase. These drugs enter cells via the nucleoside transport system. Myelosuppression is the major toxicity shared by all these agents.

6-Mercaptopurine and Thioguanine

6-Mercaptopurine (6-MP) and thioguanine (6-TG) are analogues of hypoxanthine and guanine, respectively, wherein there is a substitution of a sulfhydryl group for the endogenous 6-OH position. Both are intracellularly anabolized through the hypoxanthine-guanine phosphoribosyl transferase (HGPRT) pathway to form 6-thioinosine monophosphate (TIMP) and 6-thioguanylic acid (TGMP), respectively, which inhibit de novo purine synthesis mediated by 5-phosphoribosyl-1 pyrophosphate (PRPP) amidotransferase. Cytotoxicity arises from the incorporation of 6-thioguanosine triphosphate (6-TGTP) and the deoxytriphosphate form into DNA and RNA, which triggers the mismatch repair pathway leading into apoptosis. In spite of these similarities, cross-resistance between these two agents is not complete, as 6-TG remains active in HGPRT-deficient cells resistant to 6-MP.[91]

Both 6-MP and 6-TG are converted to inactive metabolites by the enzyme thiopurine methyltransferase (TPMT), with 6-TG being more extensively S-methylated than 6-MP. Genetic polymorphisms in the TPMT gene associated with reduced enzyme activity have been described. 6-TG is also inactivated upon deamination by the enzyme guanase. 6-MP, unlike 6-TG, is catabolized by xanthine oxidase, high concentrations of which can be found n the intestinal mucosa and liver. Both 6-MP and 6-TG have poor and variable oral bioavailability that is further reduced with food intake. In the case of 6-MP, this arises from the large first-pass effect as the drug is metabolized by xanthine oxidase. Allopurinol, a xanthine oxidase inhibitor, prevents catabolism of 6-MP. Moreover, concomitant allopurinol intake increases 6-MP bioavailability fivefold.[92] Dose reduction of 6-MP is thus warranted in patients taking allopurinol.

Anorexia, nausea, and vomiting may occur, especially among adults, more commonly with 6-MP than 6-TG. Hepatotoxicity, usually in the form of reversible cholestatic jaundice, has been reported for either drug. Acute hepatic necrosis may also ensue with high-dose 6-MP therapy, whereas fatal veno-occlusive disease has been reported with 6-TG. High-dose therapy with 6-MP or 6-TG can cause tubular precipitation and crystalluria. 6-MP is used in ALL whereas 6-TG is active in AML.

Fludarabine

Fludarabine is a 2-fluoromonophosphate derivative of adenosine arabinoside (ara-A) that is relatively water soluble and resistant to rapid deamination by adenosine deaminase (ADA). Upon dephosphorylation in plasma to 2-fluoro-ara-A, intracellular rephosphorylation by deoxycytidine kinase to its active form, 9-β-D-arabinofuranosyl-2-fluoroadenine triphosphate (F-ara-ATP), is necessary for cytotoxicity. F-ara-ATP inhibits several important enzymes in DNA replication, including DNA polymerase and ribonucleotide reductase. Its incorporation into DNA leads to DNA chain termination, primarily at the 3′-end, in contrast to ara-C, which is incorporated into 5′-termini. It demonstrates synergism with ara-C and cisplatin.[93,94]

Fludarabine is cleared primarily by the kidneys. Although it has good oral bioavailability, an oral formulation is not yet available for commercial use. Myelosuppression is dose related and may be cumulative. Development of autoimmune hemolytic anemia may occur most commonly during the first three cycles of treatment. Fever occurs in approximately 25% of patients, although about one-third of these patients have a serious documented infection. Increased risk for opportunistic infections is in consequence to significant and protracted reduction in CD4+ T cells; hence, prophylaxis against *Pneumocystis pneumonia* is required. Pulmonary toxicity, manifested as fever, cough, and interstitial pneumonitis, has also been associated with this drug. Fludarabine is active not only against actively dividing cells but also in malignancies with low growth fraction such as chronic lymphocytic leukemia (CLL) and low-grade lymphomas.

Cladribine

Cladribine (2-CdA) is a deoxyadenosine analogue with a chloride attached to the 2-position of the adenine ring that renders it resistant to breakdown by ADA. Intracellular phosphorylation by deoxycytidine kinase to the active 5′-triphosphate (2-CdATP) results in incorporation into DNA, leading to DNA chain termination and strand breaks; inhibition of DNA polymerases and ribonucleotide reductase ultimately results in inhibition of DNA synthesis. Cells with a high ratio of deoxycytidine kinase to deoxynucleotidase activity, such as lymphocytes, are particularly sensitive to the effects of cladribine. Similar to fludarabine, cladribine is cytotoxic to both actively dividing and nondividing cells. In resting cells, 2-CdATP seem to initiate the caspase cascade leading to apoptosis.[95]

Bioavailability of cladribine administered subcutaneously reaches nearly 100%. It can penetrate the blood–brain barrier, the CSF concentrations reaching about 25% of the plasma concentrations during continuous IV infusion. Cladribine is renally cleared and hence, should be used with caution in patients with renal insufficiency. Similar to fludarabine, it increases the intracellular concentrations of ara-CTP and probably other pyrimidine analogues as well. Immunosuppression results from prolonged suppression of CD4+ T lymphocytes; thus, opportunistic infections, in addition to myelosuppression, are the major adverse complications with this drug. Cladribine is highly active in the treatment of hairy cell leukemia, Waldenstrom's macroglobulinemia, indolent lymphomas, and leukemias. Its activity in fludarabine-resistant cases however, is much diminished.

Pentostatin

Pentostatin, or 2′-deoxycoformycin, is an adenosine analogue originally isolated from *Streptomyces antibioticus* but is now synthetically derived. It is a potent inhibitor of ADA, leading to high levels of deoxyadenosine and its triphosphate, which in turn inhibit ribonucleotide reductase in a negative feedback loop. Cells with high levels of deoxynucleoside kinase activity over 5-nucleotidase activity, such as lymphocytes, are most susceptible to the effects of ADA inhibition.[96] Postulated mechanisms of cytotoxicity are similar to the other adenosine analogues. In addition, it also prevents methylation reactions mediated by S-adenosylhomocyteine hydrolase.

Renal elimination accounts for most of the clearance of pentostatin (more than 90%). Pentostatin is per se a nephrotoxic agent, and renal failure is dose limiting. Opportunistic infections arising from immunosuppression may occur. Nausea and vomiting are the most common nonhematologic toxicities. It is highly active in hairy cell leukemia, Waldenstrom's macroglobulinemia, indolent lymphomas, and leukemias.

Microtubule-Targeting Drugs

Microtubules are integral components of the mitotic spindle apparatus during metaphase in dividing cells. They are also involved in many nonmitotic functions such as intracellular scaffolding, locomotion and chemotaxis, secretory processes, anchorage of subcellular organelles, and neurotransmission. They are composed of tubulin heterodimers that assemble into 13 protofilaments aligned side by side around a hollow central core. Posttranslation modification after tubulin polymerization accounts for the functional diversity of microtubules in various tissues.

There is a constant flux between the microtubule and the intracellular pool of tubulin. Each tubulin molecule is associated with two molecules of guanosine triphosphate (GTP). GTP is found only at the rapidly growing, or plus end, of the microtubule. Its hydrolysis after tubulin polymerization is not essential for microtubule growth at the plus end; however, hydrolysis of GTP does lower the concentration of the free tubulin subunit required for net polymerization at the plus end. The plus end switches spontaneously and rapidly between slow growth and rapidly shrinking states.[97] This "dynamic instability" occurs once the GTP "cap" is lost from the end of microtubule upon hydrolysis and depolymerization occurs. In contrast, the "minus end" is where net disassociation occurs because protofilaments align slowly at this end.

Vinca Alkaloids

Most antimicrotubules agents are alkaloids, structurally complex plant-derived organic bases. Vinca alkaloids are the first widely used class of antimicrotubule agents in cancer chemotherapy. They are cell-cycle-specific vesicants derived from the pink periwinkle plant, *Catharanthus roseus* (L.) G. Don. Vincristine and vinblastine are the two representative compounds. Vinorelbine is a vinblastine semisynthetic derivative with broad antitumor activity as a single agent that may not be completely cross-resistant with vincristine and vinblastine. Their antitumor and toxicity spectra vary significantly. This variability may arise from different tubulin isotypes, lipophilicity, or cellular retention.

Cytotoxicity of vinca alkaloids is principally related to the microtubular depolymerization by inhibiting microtubule assembly, resulting in metaphase arrest in G_2 and M cell-cycle phases in dividing cells. This explanation is oversimplified, as the lowest drug concentration that induces metaphase arrest and antiproliferative effects results in little or no disruption of the mitotic spindle apparatus or depolymerization. The vinca alkaloids have pleitropic biologic effects not necessarily related to their effects on microtubules, such as inhibiting purine, DNA, RNA, and protein synthesis. They are also potent inhibitors of angiogenesis. As microtubules function in cell processes other than mitosis, vinca alkaloids also affect cells in the nonmitotic phases of the cell cycle.

Thse vinca alkaloids are primarily eliminated by hepatic metabolism and biliary excretion. Hepatic metabolism is principally mediated by P-450 CYP3A. Agents that can increase toxicity include L-asparaginase and CYP3A inhibitors such as erythromycin. On the other hand, they can reduce the bioavailability of certain drugs such as digoxin and phenytoin. Vinca alkaloids are administered intravenously. Vinorelbine is orally bioavailable, although a commercial formulation is not yet available. Vincristine has the longest terminal half-life and the lowest clearance rate, whereas vinorelbine has the shortest half-life and the highest clearance rate. Vinca alkaloids should never be administered intrathecally, as the global dissolution of brain and spinal cord neurofilaments that ensues is fatal.

Vincristine

Vincristine has the greatest affinity for tubulin and has the highest degree of intracellular accumulation among the vinca alkaloids. These characteristics, together with its pharmacokinetic properties, are implicated in the associated neurotoxicity. Neurotoxicity is cumulative and the severity is related to total dose and duration of therapy. Motor dysfunction is usually irreversible. Autonomic neuropathy may be manifest as ileus, constipation, urinary retention, orthostatic hypotension, or hypertension. Central effects, such as seizure and blindness, have been reported. Aside from drug discontinuation or dose/schedule modification, approaches to prevent or reduce neuropathy include the use of folinic acid and glutamic acid. Severe myelosuppression is rare. In therapy, vincristine is unique in that a single maximum dose delivered is typically limited to 2 mg to prevent and/or delay the development of neurotoxicity. It is an integral component in chemotherapy regimens for lymphomas, Ewing's sarcoma, rhabdomyosarcoma, leukemias, and neuroblastoma.

Vinblastine and Vinorelbine

Neurologic effects are much less common and severe with vinblastine and least with vinorelbine. Myelosuppression, especially neutropenia, is the major dose-limiting toxicity of both vinblastine and vinorelbine. Mucositis and stomatitis happen more frequently with vinblastine than vincristine. Constipation, as with vincristine, occurs frequently. Vinblastine is an important component for regimens used in testicular carcinomas and lymphomas. Vinorelbine has demonstrated activity in advanced non-small cell lung cancer, breast cancer, and ovarian carcinomas as well as lymphomas.

Taxanes

Taxanes affect microtubules through a mechanism of action unique from the vinca alkaloids. Unlike the vinca alkaloids, which facilitate microtubule depolymerization, taxanes shift the dynamic equilibrium toward microtubule assembly, prevent depolymerization, and therefore suppress microtubular reorganization. The binding site for taxanes is different from that for vinca alkaloids, GTP, podophyllotoxins, and colchicine. Sustained mitotic arrest at the metaphase–anaphase boundary, apoptosis, and antiangiogenesis may be observed even at low concentrations where increase in microtubule bundling is not seen. Taxanes also exert inhibitory effects on nonmitotic cell-cycle phases, attesting to the myriad functions subserved by microtubules. They have also been shown to be effective radiosensitizers. This radiosensitizing effect is most likely related to their ability to cause cell-cycle arrest in the G_2 and M phases of the cell cycle, when tumor cells are highly susceptible to the effects of radiation. Taxanes are intravenously administered because of poor oral bioavailability, due in part to the constitutive overexpression of P-glycoprotein in enterocytes as well as the first-pass metabolism in the liver and/or intestines. They are widely distributed to almost all tissues and third-space fluid collections except the CNS. Plasma protein binding is high (more than 90%), and elimination half-lives are long. The principal route of metabolism is through the hepatic cytochrome P-450 system. Biliary excretion is the main route of elimination as renal clearance accounts for less than 10%. Dose reductions are therefore necessary in patients with hepatic dysfunction. Reversible and noncumulative neutropenia is the principal toxicity of the taxanes in clinical use.

Paclitaxel

The prototype taxane, paclitaxel, is a complex alkaloid ester initially isolated from the bark of the Pacific yew tree, *Taxus brevifolia*. It is currently a semisynthetic derivative from 10-deacetylbaccatin III and other precursors found in the needles of other more abundant *Taxus* species, such as the European yew, *Taxus baccata*. Paclitaxel binds to the N-terminal 31 amino acids of the β-tubulin subunit of the tubulin oligomers.[98] Aside from its effects on the microtubular system, in vitro experiments also showed inhibition of endothelial cell proliferation, motility, and invasiveness in a dose-dependent manner. Paclitaxel also inhibits the production of matrix metalloproteinases, which are enzymes that degrade matrix and thereby contribute to tumor invasiveness.

Clinical activity and toxicity of paclitaxel is highly dose- and schedule-dependent. Early clinical studies of paclitaxel were limited to 24-hour infusion schedules largely due to the severity of hypersensitivity reactions on shorter infusion schedules. However, the development of effective premedication regimens enabled reevaluation of shorter infusion schedules. The extensive distribution and high affinity of taxanes to peripheral tissue may explain the lack of significant differences in antitumor activity between the short and protracted infusion schedules. Patients treated with higher doses and/or shorter infusion schedules are more prone to neurotoxicity as compared to those treated with longer infusion. In contrast, both dose and duration of infusion are directly proportional to the degree of myelosuppression. Weekly treatment (80–100 mg/m^2/week), although more inconvenient than the conventional once every 3 weeks schedule (135 mg/m^2 over 24 hours or 175 mg/m^2 over 3 hours), has gained clinical acceptance. Weekly administration not only results in dose-dense therapy, it achieves a higher dose intensity, total cumulative dose over a 3-week period being higher than could be given in one dose. Weekly administration results in less myelosuppression and allows for better control of toxicities, as a dose may be omitted but treatment resumed the following week. This regimen results in sustained exposure of tumor cells to paclitaxel and simulates "metronomic" dosing as well that enhances its antiangiogenic activity.

The severity of myelosuppression seems to be related to prolonged infusions. Because of poor aqueous solubility, paclitaxel is formulated in polyoxyethylated castor oil (cremophor EL), which leaches the plasticizer out of polyvinylchloride containers and tubings. Cremophor, known to induce histamine release, is most likely responsible for the well-recognized hypersensitivity reactions seen with paclitaxel. Major anaphylactoid manifestations include bronchospasm, urticaria, and hypotension that usually occurs within 2 to 3 minutes after administration. The taxane structure itself may be contributory. Before the routine use of premedication with antihistamines and corticosteroids, severe acute hypersensitivity reactions occurred in 20% to 30% of patients treated with paclitaxel in early Phase I trials. With standard premedication, the incidence of major hypersensitivity reactions nowadays is low (less than 5%) and similar for the 3- or 24-hour infusion. Particularly pertinent to paclitaxel is its effect on atrioventricular conduction, as it causes bradyarrhythmias, which are mostly reversible and asymptomatic. A direct causal relationship observed between paclitaxel and ventricular and atrial tachycardias has yet to be proven. Combination of paclitaxel and doxorubicin results in a higher frequency of congestive heart failure than would have been expected from an equivalent cumulative dose of doxorubicin given alone.

Docetaxel

Docetaxel is a more water-soluble taxane semisynthetically derived from 10-deacetylbaccatin III, obtained from the needles of the European yew (*Taxus baccata*). It is more potent than paclitaxel and has nearly twofold-higher affinity for the β-tubulin subunit. In comparative studies, docetaxel has been found to be 1.3- to 12-fold more cytotoxic in vitro than paclitaxel. It has linear pharmacokinetics at clinically relevant doses, and its maximal activity can be achieved with fairly rapid infusion, in contrast to paclitaxel. Schedule-dependent activity thus seems not to be evident with docetaxel. It is highly protein bound, primarily to α-acid glycoprotein. CYP3A4 and CYP 3A5 constitute the major cytochrome P-450 isoforms responsible for the bulk of its metabolism.

Major anaphylactoid reactions induced by docetaxel are similar to those seen with paclitaxel although, unlike paclitaxel, docetaxel is suspended in a polysorbate 80 formulation. Whether the polysorbate or the taxane moiety itself or both are responsible for the hypersensitivity reactions is unclear. With corticosteroid and histamine antagonist premedication, incidence of major hypersensitivity reactions is reduced to 1% to 3%. Peripheral neuropathy is less common and less severe with docetaxel. Unlike paclitaxel, adverse cardiovascular events such as arrhythmias are rare with its use, and docetaxel can be combined with anthracyclines without excessive cardiac toxicity. On the other hand, fluid retention mimicking capillary leak syndrome characterized by edema, pleural effusions, ascites, or anasarca is noted with docetaxel, particularly at cumulative doses that exceed 400 mg/m². Docetaxel also causes an erythematous, pruritic maculopapular rash over the forearms and hands in up to 75% of patients. It is associated with palmar-plantar erythrodysesthesia that may respond to cooling or pyridoxine. Premedication with corticosteroids has been shown to reduce the incidence of dermatologic toxicities and fluid retention.

Drugs Targeting Topoisomerase

Unwinding of the DNA helix generates a torsional strain from supercoiling of the helix above and below the region of ongoing nucleic acid during DNA replication, transcription, or recombination. DNA topoisomerase I is a ubiquitous nuclear enzyme that relaxes this torsional strain by catalyzing a transient single-stranded nick in the DNA. This results in covalent linkage of the enzyme to the 3′-terminus of the cleaved DNA. It also reanneals the strand break after passage of the intact single strand through the gap in the cleaved DNA strand. Topoisomerase I is expressed in both mitotic and non-mitotic cells alike throughout the cell cycle, with higher levels of its mRNA and the topoisomerase protein found in malignant tumors than in their normal tissue counterparts.[99,100]

Topoisomerase II exists in two isoforms in mammalian cells. Although topoisomerase IIβ is expressed throughout the cell cycle, expression of topoisomerase IIα is cell cycle specific, highest during G_2–M phases of the cell cycle, and its concentrations are higher in rapidly proliferating cells. The α-isoenzyme is preferentially targeted by the topoisomerase II inhibitors at drug concentrations reached with standard doses. Unlike topoisomerase I, topoisomerase II is energy cofactor dependent, requiring ATP and magnesium for its catalytic activity. It becomes covalently attached to the 5′-terminus of the cleaved DNA. It then facilitates strand passage through another and thereafter religates the strand break. Furthermore, it can create double-stranded DNA gaps, orchestrate concerted strand passage, and can catalyze "unknotting" or decatenation of intertwined DNA, attesting to its role in mitosis.

Topoisomerase I-Targeting Agents

Camptothecin (CPT), a naturally occurring, relatively water-insoluble alkaloid extract from the bark and wood of the Chinese tree *Camptothecan acuminata*, is the prototype topoisomerase I-targeting agent. Its clinical development was halted early due to its toxicity and only upon the introduction of water-soluble forms was it reintroduced into clinical testing. The analogues have greater in vivo and in vitro activity and less severe and more predictable toxicity than camptothecin. All CPT analogues exhibit stereospecific-inhibition of topoisomerase I activity, with the naturally occurring S-isomer being up to 100 times more biologically active than the R-isomer. Nevertheless, they differ from classic enzyme inhibitors by not merely preventing the function of topoisomerase alone; CPTs trap the enzyme in a covalent complex bound to DNA, leading to persistence of single-strand breaks and accumulation of stabilized cleavable complexes, which by themselves are not lethal because the strand breaks are reversible upon drug removal. Active DNA synthesis is a crucial component to CPT-induced cytotoxicity,[101–103] making camptothecins relatively S-phase-specific agents, although non-S-phase-specific cytotoxicity has been described. According to the fork collision model,[102] lethal damage to DNA occurs once a DNA replication fork encounters a cleavable complex, resulting in a cytotoxic double-stranded break in DNA. CPTs thus are more aptly termed topoisomerase I-targeting agents.

All CPTs undergo a rapid, reversible, pH-dependent, nonenzymatic hydrolysis of the lactone ring to generate the less-active open-ring hydroxy carboxylate in aqueous solutions. The latter species predominate at physiologic or alkaline pH. This finding is clinically relevant because the low pH in the bladder favors the active closed lactone ring species that can cause severe hemorrhagic cystitis. Among the CPT analogues, irinotecan is structurally unique in that it lacks direct activity per se. It is a prodrug that must undergo cleavage of its bulky dipiperidino side chain by a carboxylesterase-converting enzyme to produce the metabolite SN-38 for biologic activity.

Topotecan

Topotecan was the first water-soluble CPT analogue approved for clinical use. It has a relatively higher CNS penetration than most other CPTs, due in part to its low plasma protein binding. Schedule-dependent synergism with radiation (concurrent, preradiation, or within 30 minutes after radiation) in vitro has been observed. Renal excretion is the main route of drug elimination. Dosage adjustments are recommended for patients with moderate renal impairment (20–39 mL/min). Hepatic metabolism by cytochrome P-450 enzymes is minimal. At the standard dose of 1.5 mg/m²/day for 5 consecutive days every 3 weeks, noncumulative and reversible neutropenia is the most common dose-limiting toxicity, with grade 4 neutropenia occurring in 81%, febrile neutropenia in 26%, grade 4 thrombocytopenia in 26%, and severe anemia (Hb less than 8 g/dL) in 40%. Topotecan is approved for use in cisplatin-refractory ovarian cancer, recurrent small cell lung cancer failing frontline chemotherapy, and leukemias.

Irinotecan

As mentioned earlier, irinotecan (CPT-11) has little inherent antitumor activity in vitro. Its water-insoluble deesterification metabolite SN-38 is 1,000-fold more potent than the parent compound. SN-38 has a longer half-life and high binding affinity to plasma proteins, especially albumin. In contrast with topotecan and other CPT analogues, the lactone form of SN-38 is preferentially stabilized by albumin, hence the equilibrium is shifted toward the formation of the lactone in physiologic conditions. Although SN-38 formation occurs in the plasma and intestinal mucosa, conversion of irinotecan to SN-38 predominates in the liver. Moreover, differential activity of carboxylesterase in malignant tissues may contribute to tumor sensitivity to this agent.[104] SN-38 undergoes glucuronidation in the liver mediated by UGT1A1 isoform of hepatic uridine diphosphate glucuronosyltransferase. UGT1A1 expression is highly variable, and its activity varies 17- to 52-fold among individuals. UGT1A1 activity is deficient in patients with Gilbert's syndrome, which can occur in up to 15% of the population. Biliary excretion of SN-

38 and irinotecan is the major route of elimination. Enterohepatic recirculation occurs as the glucuronidated SN-38 metabolite can be deconjugated by bacterial β-glucuronidases, thereby increasing exposure of the intestinal epithelium to SN-38. Ability to conjugate SN-38 and bilirubin, the endogenous substrate, is inversely related to myelosuppression, suggesting that agents that induce UGT activity, such as phenobarbital, may improve the therapeutic index of CPT-11. Certain polymorphisms of UGT1A1, such as in the promoter region with Gilbert's syndrome, have been correlated with decreased glucuronidating activity, resulting in increased risk for myelosuppression and diarrhea. Further elucidation of such polymorphisms and other pharmacogenetic variables will hopefully enable clinicians to better predict drug responses and toxicities. CPT-11 is approved for frontline therapy in metastatic colorectal carcinoma in combination with 5-FU and leucovorin.

DNA Topoisomerase II Inhibitors

The podophyllotoxins are extracts of the mayapple or mandrake plant, *Podophyllum peltatum*, long known in folk medicine. Two glycosidic derivates, etoposide (VP-16) and teniposide (VM-26), are currently in clinical use. The main mechanism of cytotoxicity was initially ascribed to tubulin-binding properties, at sites distinct from vinca alkaloids that result in inhibition of microtubule assembly and consequent S–G_2 phase block and cell death. However, new evidence demonstrates that the antimicrotubular effects occur only at concentrations severalfold higher that were not reached with clinically relevant doses. Moreover, the epipodophyllotoxins produce both single- and double-strand DNA breaks that were distinct from the cellular changes seen with antimicrotubule agents.[105] Epipodophyllotoxins, and anthracyclines as well, bind to topoisomerase II, stabilize the enzyme–DNA complex (termed cleavable or cleavage complex), and inhibit the reannealing of the cleaved DNA, thus resulting in both single- and double-stranded DNA strands. Similar to topoisomerase I inhibitors, replication fork collision with this cleavable complex increases the degree of lethal DNA fragmentation that ultimately leads to apoptosis.

Etoposide

VP-16 is available in both intravenous and oral formulations. Mean oral bioavailability is 50%, and nonlinear at doses beyond 200 to 250 mg/m^2. It exhibits high plasma protein binding such that patients with low serum albumin seem to be at risk for associated toxicities. It is eliminated by both renal and hepatic mechanisms. Up to 40% of unchanged drug is cleared through the kidneys. Dose reduction is recommended in patients with impaired creatinine clearance. Administration of cisplatin before VP-16 reduces VP-16 clearance, likely secondary to the effects on cytochrome P-450. Sequence-dependent synergism and reduced myelosuppression are also observed when paclitaxel administration precedes VP-16. VP-16 phosphate is a water-soluble prodrug that is completely and rapidly converted to VP-16. Its chief advantage lies in the reduced incidence of hypersensitivity reactions and better safety and tolerability profile. Pharmacokinetic, toxicity, and antitumor activity of VP-16 apply to VP-16 phosphate. Single-agent randomized studies demonstrate its marked schedule-dependent activity such that multiple daily divided-dose schedules result in higher rates of response and survival than continuous administration of the same total dose over 1 day. Antitumor activity seems to correlate with the duration of exposure above a threshold concentration; this is not seen in combination regimens.

Teniposide

VM-26 is more extensively metabolized by the liver, although its plasma clearance is slower than VP-16. It has an even higher degree of protein binding than VP-16 (99% versus 94%). Although CSF penetration is low, VM-26 is generally considered more clinically effective than VP-16 in the treatment of gliomas. Although it is only available for IV administration, this formulation may be administered orally, with a bioavailability of approximately 40%.

Noncumulative myelosuppression, chiefly neutropenia, is the principal dose-limiting toxicity of the epipodophyllotoxins. Nausea and vomiting are the main gastrointestinal toxicities, although usually mild to moderate in severity. Mucositis may be seen with high-dose VP-16 therapy. Other side effects seen with high-dose therapy are metabolic acidosis and reversible hepatotoxicity. Rapid infusion may result in transient hypotension. Hypersensitivity reactions, seen in less than 2% of patients receiving IV VM-26 and VP-16 but not oral VP-16, may result in part from the diluent used and occurs more frequently with rapid infusion. Incidence of secondary leukemias ranges from 0.37% to 4.7% and appears to be dose related. VP-16 is approved for use in small cell lung carcinoma and testicular carcinomas. VM-26 is used as part of the induction therapy of refractory childhood acute lymphoblastic leukemias.

Pharmacogenetics

One of the important factors affecting antitumor efficacy and clinical toxicity of cancer chemotherapeutic drugs and their complex interaction is an individual's genotype. It has been observed as early as the 1950s that responses to certain drugs may be heritable. The field of pharmacogenetics, which studies the genetic basis for interindividual variability in drug response, classically involved investigations on drug metabolism but currently also encompasses various pharmacokinetic and pharmacodynamic elements that participate in determining drug response. The ensuing discussion highlights selected pharmacogenetic variables well recognized in current clinical practice of cancer chemotherapy.

Thiopurine Methyltransferase

Thiopurine methyltransferase (TPMT) is a methylating enzyme whose gene is encoded on chromosome 6. It plays an important role in the catabolism of 6-MP and its prodrug azathioprine, thus preventing generation of thioguanine nucleotides. Early studies revealed that TPMT activity is inherited as an autosomal codominant trait.[106] About 1 in 300 individuals carry two mutant TPMT alleles, thus resulting in deficient activity. Approximately 10% of the population are heterozygotes with intermediate TPMT activity.[107] It has been shown that the various single-nucleotide polymorphisms do not result in altered levels of mRNA or TPMT protein. However, these mutations render the translated protein susceptible to degradation through the ubiquitin-proteasome system, decreasing the half-life to 30 minutes compared to 18 hours for the wild-type protein.[108] TPMT*3A, TPMT*3C, and TPMT*2 mutant alleles, which harbor point mutations resulting in amino acid substitutions, account for more than 95% of deficient TPMT activity among whites.

As there is no endogenous substrate for TPMT, individuals with defective enzyme activity are asymptomatic until exposure to thiopurine drugs results in severe myelosuppression that may be life threatening. On the other hand, individuals with high or high-normal TPMT are relatively resistant to the action of thiopurine drugs and thus may not achieve clinical remission if these drugs are used at standard dosages. An allele with increased TPMT activity has been described. TPMT activity can be influenced by various factors such as age and renal function. TPMT activity in red blood cells serves as a surrogate marker for TPMT activity in other tissues.

Dihydropyrimidine Dehydrogenase

Dihydropyrimidine dehydrogenase (DPD) catalyzes the initial rate-limiting step in the catabolism of endogenous pyrimidines and 5-FU. It is encoded on chromosome 1. DPD activity is inherited as an autosomal codominant trait. Approximately 0.1% of the population carry homozygous inactivating mutations whereas 3% are heterozygotes. DPD activity has a normal distribution in the population and there is manifold interindividual variability, although not obviously age- or gender-related. The most common mutant allele, DPYD*2A, results from a G to A transition that leads to deletion of exon 14 and thus ending with a truncated protein, which is subsequently degraded by the ubiquitin-proteasome system.

Individuals with deficient DPD activity experience profound systemic toxicity (myelosuppression, diarrhea, neurotoxicity) upon exposure to 5-FU, which may potentially result in fatalities. Assessment of DPD activity in human peripheral blood mononuclear cells correlates well with total body enzyme activity. On the other hand, high level of DPD mRNA expression in colorectal tumors confers resistance to 5-FU.[109]

Uridine Diphosphate Glucuronosyltransferase

Uridine diphosphate glucuronosyltransferase (UGT) is an enzyme that catalyzes the phase II catabolic reaction in which uridine diphosphate glucuronic acid is conjugated with drugs or poorly soluble endogenous substrates. There are two gene families (UGT1 and UGT2), each of which has various isoforms. The most important of these isoforms is UGT1A1, which is encoded on chromosome 2q37. Polymorphisms of the gene encoding UGT1A1 give rise to the hyperbilirubinemia phenotype of the rare Crigler–Najjar syndrome and the relatively common Gilbert syndrome.

UGT1A1 plays an important role in the metabolism of the active metabolite of irinotecan, SN38 by changing it into the more polar SN 38 glucuronide, which is mainly excreted in the bile. Reduced UGT1A1 expression, often associated with elevated levels of unconjugated bilirubin, is inherited in an autosomal-recessive pattern. Polymorphisms in the number of TA repeats in the promoter region, which is inversely related to UGT1A1 enzyme activity, constitute the most common abnormality. The wild-type promoter region has a $(TA)_6TAA$ sequence whereas the most common mutation results in an extra TA, thus the sequence becoming $(TA)_7TAA$ (UGT1A1*28). Patients with Gilbert syndrome are homozygous for this promoter variation, which leads to a 70% reduction in UGT1A1 expression. $(TA)_7TAA$ homozygosity occurs in about 0.5% to 23% in various populations. Other mutations in the promoter region of UGT1A1 gene alter transcription and have been associated with deficient or increased UGT1A1 activity.

Patients with the UGT1A1*28 allele are susceptible to severe, at times life-threatening, toxicities of irinotecan, mainly leukopenia and diarrhea.

References

1. Infield GB. Disaster at Bari. New York: Macmillan, 1971.
2. Gilman A, Philips FS. The biological actions and therapeutic applications of b-chloroethyl amines and sulfides. Science 1946; 103:409.
3. Skipper HE, Schabel FM, Wilcox WS. Experimental evaluation of potential anticancer agents. XIII: On the criteria and kinetics associated with curability of experimental leukemia. Cancer Chem Rep 1964;35:1–111.
4. Laird AK. Dynamics of growth in tumors and normal organisms. NCI Monogr 1969;30:15–28.
5. Norton L, Simor R. Growth curve of an experimental solid tumor following radiotherapy. J Natl Cancer Inst 1977;58:1735–1741.
6. Norton L, Simor R. Tumor size, sensitivity to therapy and the design of treatment schedules. Cancer Treat Rep 1977;61:1307–1317.
7. Goldie JH, Coldman AJ. A mathematic model for relating the drug sensitivity of tumors to their spontaneous mutation rate. Cancer Treat Rep 1979;63:1727–1733.
8. Iversen OH, Iversen U, Ziegler JL, Bluming AZ. Cell kinetics in Burkitt's lymphoma. Eur J Cancer 1974;10:144–163.
9. Frei E III, Freireich EJ, Gehan E, et al. Studies of sequential and combination antimetabolite therapy in acute leukemia: 6-mercaptopurine and methotrexate. Blood 1961;18:431–454.
10. Ludwig Breast Cancer Study Group. Combination adjuvant chemotherapy for node-positive breast cancer. Inadequacy of a single perioperative cycle. N Engl J Med 1988;319:677–683.
11. Samson MK, Rivlin SE, Jones SE, et al. Dose-response and dose-survival advantage for high- vs. low-dose cisplatin combined with vinblastine and bleomycin in disseminated testicular cancer. Cancer 1984;53:1029–1035.
12. Stadtmauer EA, O'Neill A, Goldstein LJ, et al., and the Philadelphia Bone Marrow Transplant Group. Conventional-dose chemotherapy compared with high-dose chemotherapy plus autologous hematopoietic stem-cell transplantation for metastatic breast cancer. N Engl J Med 2000;342(15):1069–1076.
13. Wood WC, Budman DR, Korzun AH, et al. Dose and dose intensity trial of adjuvant chemotherapy for stage II node-positive breast carcinoma. N Engl J Med 1994;330:1253–1259.
14. Seidman AD, Hudis CA, Albanel J, et al. Dose-dense therapy with weekly 1-hour paclitaxel infusions in the treatment of metastatic breast cancer. J Clin Oncol 1998;16:3353–3361.
15. Cohen JL, Jao JY. Enzymatic basis of cyclophosphamide activation by hepatic microsomes of the rat. J Pharmacol Exp Ther 1970;174:206.
16. Colvin M, Padgett CA, Fenselau C. A biologically active metabolite of cyclophosphamide. Cancer Res 1973;33(4):915–918.

17. Cox PJ. Cyclophosphamide cystitis: identification of acrolein as the causative agent. Biochem Pharmacol 1979;28(13):2045–2049.
18. Manoharan A. Carcinoma of the urinary bladder in patients receiving cyclophosphamide. Aust N Z J Med 1984;14(4):507.
19. Braverman AC, Antin JH, Plappert MT, et al. Cyclophosphamide cardiotoxicity in bone marrow transplantation: a prospective evaluation of new dosing regimens. J Clin Oncol 1991;9:1215–1223.
20. DeFronzo RA, Braine HG, Colvin M, et al. Water intoxication in man after cyclophosphamide therapy. Ann Intern Med 1973; 78:861–869.
21. Bressler RB, Huston DP. Water intoxication following moderate-dose intravenous cyclophosphamide. Arch Intern Med 1985; 145:548–549.
22. Klein HO, Wickramanayake PD, Coerper C, et al. High dose ifosfamide and mesna as continuous infusion over five days: a phase I/II trial. Cancer Treat Rev 1983;10(suppl A):167–173.
23. Goren MP, Wright RK, Pratt CB, Pell FE. Dechloroethylation of ifosfamide and neurotoxicity. Lancet 1986;2:1219–1220.
24. Moncrieff M, Foot A. Fanconi syndrome after ifosfamide. Cancer Chemother Pharmacol 1989;23(2):121–122.
25. Curtin JP, Koonings PP, Gutierrez M, et al. Ifosfamide-induced neurotoxicity. Gynecol Oncol 1991;42(3):193–196.
26. Wakaki S, Marumo H, Tomoka K. Isolation of new fractions of antitumor mitomycins. Antibiot Chemother 1958;8:228–240.
27. Lin AJ, Cosby LA, Shansky CW, et al. Potential bioreductive alkylating agents: 1. Benzoquinone derivatives. J Med Chem 1972;15:1247–1252.
28. Tomasz M, Chawla AK, Lipman R. Mechanism of monofunctional and bifunctional alkylation of DN by mitomycin C. Biochemistry 1988;27:3182–3187.
29. Colvin M, Bundrett RB, Cowens W, et al. A chemical basis for the antitumor activity of chloroethylnitrosorueas. Biochem Pharmacol 1976;25:695–699.
30. Baril BB, Baril EF, Lazlo J, et al. Inhibition of rat liver DNA polymerase by nitrosourea and isocyanates. Cancer Res 1975; 35(1):1–5.
31. Kann HE Jr, Kohn KW, Lyles JM. Inhibition of DNA repair by the 1,3-bis (2-choroethyl)-1-nitrosoureas breakdown product, 2-chloroethyl isocyanate. Cancer Res 1974;34(2):398–402.
32. Kann HE Jr, Kohn KW, Widerlite L, et al. Effects of 1,3-bis (2-chloroethyl)-1-nitrosourea and related compounds on nuclear RNA metabolism. Cancer Res 1974;34(8):1982–1988.
33. DeVita VT, Carbone PP, Owens AH, Jr, et al. Clinical trials with 1,3-bis (2-chloroethyl)-1-nitrosourea, NSC-409962. Cancer Res 1965;25:1876–1881.
34. Schein PS, O'Connell MJ, Blom J, et al. Clinical antitumor activity and toxicity of streptozotocin (NSC-85998). Cancer (Phila) 1974;34:993–1000.
35. Hassan M, Oberg G, Ehrsson H, et al. Pharmacokinetic and metabolic studies of high-dose busulphan in adults. Eur J Clin Pharmacol 1989;36:525–530.
36. Roberts JJ, Warwick GP. Mode of action of alkylating agents: formation of S-methylcysteine from ethyl methanesulphonate in vivo. Nature (Lond) 1957;179:1181.
37. Skinner WA, Gram HF, Greene MO, et al. Potential anticancer agents. XXXI. The relationship of chemical structure to antileukemic activity with analogues. J Med Pharmaceut Chem 1960;2:299.
38. Vassal G, Challine D, Koscielny S, et al. Chronopharmacology of high-dose busulfan in children. Cancer Res 1993;53:1534–1537.
39. Chabner BA, Sponzo R, Hubbard S, et al. High dose intermittent intravenous infusion of procarbazinde (NSC-77213). Cancer Chemother Rep 1973;57:361–363.
40. Liske R. A comparative study of cyclophosphamide and PCB on the antibody production in mice. Clin Exp Immunol 1973;15(2): 271–280.
41. Shirakawa S, Fre E III. Comparative effects of the antitumor agents 5-(dimethyltriazeno)imidazole-4-carboxamide and 1,3-bis (2-chloroethyl)-1-nitrosourea on cell cycle of L1210 leukemia cells in vivo. Cancer Res 1970;30:2173–2190.
42. Nicolin A, Bini A, Coronetti E, et al. Cellular immune responses to a drug treated L 51784 lymphoma subline. Nature (Lond) 1974;25(5476):654–655.
43. Buesa JM, Gracia M, Valle M, et al. Phase I trial of intermittent high-dose dacarbazine. Cancer Treat Rep 1984;68:499–504.
44. Tsang LL, Quarterman CP, Gescher A, Slack JA. Comparison of the cytotoxicity in vitro of temozolomide and dacarbazine, prodrugs of 3-methyl-(trizen-1-nyl) imidazole-4 carboxamide. Cancer Chemother Pharmacol 1991;27(5):342–346.
45. Denny BJ, Wheelhouse RT, Stevens MFG, et al. NMR and molecular modeling investigation of the mechanism of activation of the antitumor drug temozolomide and its interaction with DNA. Biochemistry 1994;33(31):9045–9051.
46. Rosenberg B, Van Camp L, Krigas T. Inhibition of cell division in *Escherichia coli* by electrolysis products from a platinum electrode. Nature (Lond) 1965;205:698.
47. Reed E, Ostchega Y, Steinberg S, et al. An evaluation of platinum-DNA adduct levels relative to known prognostic variables in a cohort of ovarian cancer patients. Cancer Res 1990;50: 2256–2260.
48. Buout JL, Mazard AM, Macquet JP. Kinetics of the reaction of cis-platinum compounds with DNA in vitro. Biochem Biophys Res Commun 1985;133:347–353.
49. Vassilev PM, Kanazirska MP, Charamella LJ, et al: Changes in calcium channel activity in membranes from cis-diamminedichloroplatinum(II)-resistant and -sensitive L1210 cells. Cancer Res 1987;47:519–522.
50. Uozumi J, Litterst CL. The effect of cisplatin on renal ATPase activity in vivo and in vitro. Cancer Chemother Pharmacol 1985;15:93–96.
51. Cersosimo RJ. Cisplatin neurotoxicity. Cancer Treat Rev 1989; 16:195–211.
52. Go RS, Adjei AA. Review of the comparative pharmacology and clinical activity of cisplatin and carboplatin. J Clin Oncol 1999; 17(1):409–422.
53. Scheeff ED, Briggs JM, Howell SB. Molecular modeling of the intrastrand guanin-guanine DNA adducts produced by cisplatin and oxaliplatin. Mol Pharmacol 1999;5:633–643.
54. Rixe O, Ortuzar W, Alvarez M, et al. Oxaliplatin, tetrapatin, cisplatin and carboplatin: spectrum of activity in drug-resistant cell lines and in the cell lines of the National Cancer Institute's Anticancer Drug Screen panel. Biochem Pharmacol 1996;52(12): 1855–1865.
55. Wang JC. Moving one DNA double helix through another by a type II DNA topoisomerase: the story of a simple molecular machine. Q Rev Biophys 1998;3:107–144.
56. Bachur NR, Yu F, Johnson R, et al. Helicase inhibition by anthracycline anticancer agents. Mol Pharmacol 1992;41(6):993–998.
57. Doroshow JH. Anthracycline antibiotic-stimulated superoxide, hydrogen peroxide and hydroxyl radical production by NADH dehydrogenase. Cancer Res 1983;43:4543–4551.
58. Donella-Deana A, Monti E, Pinna LA. Inhibition of tyrosine protein kinases by the antineoplastic agent adriamycin. Biochem Biophys Res Commun 1989;160(3):1309–1315.
59. Bose R, Verheij M, Haimovitz-Friedman A, et al. Ceramide synthase mediates daunorubicin-induced apoptosis: an alternative mechanism for generating death signals. Cell 1995;82(3):405–414.
60. Ryberg M, Nielsen D, Skovsgaard T, et al. Epirubicin cardiotoxicity: analysis of 469 patients with metastatic breast cancer. J Clin Oncol 1998;16:3502–3508.
61. Crespi MD, Ivanier SE, Genovese J, et al. Mitoxantrone affects topoisomerase activities in human breast cancer cells. Biochem Biophys Res Commun 1986;136(2):521–528.

62. Kharasch ED, Novak RF. Inhibition of adriamycin-stimulated microsomal lipid peroxidation by mitoxantrone and ametantrone. Biochem Biophys Res Commun 1982;108(3):1346–1352.
63. Lazo JS, Chabner BA. Bleomycin. In: Chabner BA, Longo DL (eds). Cancer Chemotherapy and Biotherapy: Principles and Practice. Philadelphia: Lippincott Williams & Wilkins, 2000:466–481.
64. Lazo JS, Sebti SM. Bleomycin. Cancer Chemother Biol Response Modif 94;15:44–50.
65. Dorr RT. Bleomycin pharmacology: mechanism of action and resistance and clinical pharmacokinetics. Semin Oncol 1992;19(2 suppl 5):3–8.
66. Umezawa H, Mada K, Takeuchi T, et al. New antibiotics, bleomycin A and B. J Antibiot 1966;19(5):200–209.
67. Chabner BA, Myers CE, Coleman CN, Johns DG. The clinical pharmacology of antineoplastic agents. N Engl J Med 1975;292:107–113, 1159–1168.
68. Ingrassia TS III, Rye JH, Trastek VG, Rosenow EC III. Oxygen-exacerbated bleomycin pulmonary toxicity. Mayo Clinic Proc 1991;66:173–178.
69. Muller W, Crothers D. Studies on the binding of actinomycin and related compounds to DNA. J Mol Biol 1968;35:251–290.
70. Samuels LL, Moccio DM, Sirotnak FM. Similar differential for total polyglutamylation and cytotoxicity among various folate analogues in human and murine tumor cells in vitro. Cancer Res 1985;45:1488–1495.
71. Matherly LH, Voss MK, Anderson LA, et al. Enhanced polyglutamylation of aminopterin relative to methotrexate in the Ehrlich ascites tumor cell in vitro. Cancer Res 1985;45:1073–1078.
72. Zaharko DS, Dedrick RL, Bischoff KB, et al. Methotrexate tissue distribution: prediction by a mathematical model. J Natl Cancer Inst 1971;46:775–784.
73. Steinberg SE, Campbell CL, Bleyer WA, et al. Enterohepatic circulation of methotrexate in rats in vivo. Cancer Res 1982;42:1279–1282.
74. Kepka L, De Lassence A, Ribrag V, et al. Successful rescue in a patient with high dose methotrexate-induced nephrotoxicity and acute renal failure. Leuk Lymph 1998;29(1–2):205–209.
75. Erttmann R, Landbeck G. Effect of oral cholestyramine on the elimination of high-dose methotrexate. J Cancer Res Clin Oncol 1985;110:48–50.
76. Chabner BA, Young RC. Threshold methotrexate concentration for in vivo inhibition of DNA synthesis in normal and tumorous target tissues. J Clin Invest 1973;52:1804–1811.
77. Cheradame S, Chazal M, Fischel JL, et al. Variable intrinsic sensitivity of human tumor cell lines to raltitrexed (Tomudex) and folylpolyglutamate synthetase activity. Anticancer Drugs 1999;10(5):505–510.
78. Wang Y, Zhao R, Chattopadhyay S, Goldman ID. A novel folate transport activity in human mesothelioma cell lines with high affinity and specificity for the new-generation antifolate, pemetrexed. Cancer Res 2002;62(22):6434–6437.
79. Shih C, Gosset L, Gates S, et al. LY231514 and its polyglutamates exhibit potent inhibition against both human dihydrofolate reductase (DHFR) and thymidylate synthase (TS): multiple folate enzyme inhibition. Ann Oncol 1996;7:85.
80. Illei PB, Rusch VW, Zakowski MF, Ladanyi M. Homozygous deletion of CDKN2A and codeletion of the methylthioadenosine phosphorylase gene in the majority of pleural mesotheliomas. Clin Cancer Res 2003;9:2108–2113.
81. Worzalla JF, Shih C, Schultz RM. Role of folic acid in modulating the toxicity and efficacy of the multitargeted antifolate, LY231514. Anticancer Res 1998;18(5A):3235–3239.
82. Teicher BA, Alvarez E, Liu P, et al. MTA (LY231514) in combination treatment regimens using human tumor xenografts and the EMT-6 murine mammary carcinoma. Semin Oncol 1999;26(2 suppl 6):55–62.
83. Tonkinson JL, Worzalla JF, Teng CH, et al. Cell cycle modulation by a multitargeted antifolate, LY231514, increases the cytotoxicity and antitumor activity of gemcitabine in HT29 colon carcinoma. Cancer Res 1999;59(15):3671–3676.
84. Vogelzang NJ, Rusthoven JJ, Symanowski J, et al. Phase III study of pemetrexed in combination with cisplatin versus cisplatin alone in patients with malignant pleural mesothelioma. J Clin Oncol 2003;21(14):2636–2644.
85. Hanna NH, Shepherd FA, Rosell R, et al. A phase III study of pemetrexed vs docetaxel in patients with recurrent c who were previously treated with chemotherapy. Proc Am Soc Clin Oncol 2003;22:622 (abstract 2503).
86. Ensminger WE, Rosowsky A, Raso V. A clinical-pharmacological evaluation of hepatic arterial infusions of 5-fluoro-2-deoxyuridine and 5-fluorouracil. Cancer Res 1978;38:3784–3792.
87. Efficacy of intravenous continuous infusion of fluorouracil compared with bolus administration in advanced colorectal cancer. Meta-analysis group in cancer. J Clin Oncol 1998;16:301–308.
88. Wiley JS, Jones SP, Sawyer WH, et al. Cytosine arabinoside influx and nucleoside transport sites in acute leukemia. J Clin Invest 1982;69(2):479–489.
89. Heinemann V, Hertel LW, Grindey GB, et al. Comparison of the cellular pharmacokinetics and toxicity of 2′2′-difluorodeoxycytidine and 1-beta-D-arabinofuranosylcytosine. Cancer Res 1988;48(14):4024–4031.
90. Scalliet P, Goor C, Galdermans D, et al. Gemzar (Gemcitabine) with thoracic radiotherapy: a phase II pilot study in chemonaive patients with advanced non-small cell lung cancer (NSCLC). Proc Am Soc Clin Oncol 1998;17:abstract 1923.
91. Morgan CJ, Chawdry RN, Smith AR. 6-Thioguanine-induced growth arrest in 6-mercapturine resistant human leukemia cells. Cancer Res 1994;4:5387–5393.
92. Zimm S, Collins JM, O'Neill D, et al. Chemotherapy: inhibition of first pass metabolism in cancer interaction of 6-mercaptopurine and allopurinol. Clin Pharmacol Ther 1983;34:810–817.
93. Li L, Keating MJ, Plunkett W, et al. Fludarabine mediated repair inhibition of cisplatin-induced DNA lesions in human chronic myelogenous leukemia-blast crisis K567 cells: induction of synergistic cytotoxicity independent of reversal of apoptosis. Mol Pharmacol 1997;52:798–806.
94. Gandhi V, Estey E, Du M, et al. Minimum dose of fludarabine for the maximal modulation of 1-beta-D-arabinofuranosylcytosine triphosphate in human leukemia blasts during therapy. Clin Cancer Res 1997;3:1539–1545.
95. Leoni LM, Chao Q, Cottam HB, et al. Induction of an apoptotic program in cell free extracts by 2-chloro-2′-deoxyadenosine 5′-triphosphate and cytochrome C. Proc Natl Acad Sci USA 1998;95:9567–9571.
96. Wortmann RL, Mitchell BS, Edwards NL. Biochemical basis for differential deoxyadenosine toxicity to T and B lymphoblasts: role for 5-nucleotides. Proc Natl Acad Sci USA 1979;76:2434–2437.
97. Mitchison T, Kirchner M. Dynamic instability of microtubule growth. Nature (Lond) 1984;312:237–242.
98. Rao S, Krauss NE, Heerding JM, et al. 3′-(*p*-Azidobenzamido) taxol photolabels the N-terminal 31 amino acids of β-tubulin. J Biol Chem 1994;269:3132–3134.
99. Van der Zee AG, Hollema H, de Jong S, et al. P-glycoprotein expression and DNA topoisomerase I and II activity in benign tumors of the ovary and in malignant tumors of the ovary, before and after platinum/cyclophosphamide chemotherapy. Cancer Res 1991;51:5915–5920.
100. Husain I, Mohler JL, Seigler HF, et al. Elevation of topoisomerase messenger RNA, protein and catalytic activity in human tumors: demonstration of tumor-type specificity and implications for cancer chemotherapy. Cancer Res 1994;54:539–546.
101. Holm C, Covey JM, Kerrigan D, et al. Differential requirement of DNA replication for the cytotoxicity of DNA topoisomerase

I and II inhibitors in Chinese hamster DC3F cells. Cancer Res 1989;49:6365–6368.

102. D'Arpa P, Beardmore C, Liu LF. Involvement of nucleic acid synthesis in cell killing mechanisms of topoisomerase poisons. Cancer (Phila) 1990;50:6919–6924.

103. Hsiang YH, Lihous MG, Liu LF. Arrest of replication forks by drug-stabilized topoisomerase I-DNA cleavable complexes as a mechanism of cell killing by camptothecin. Cancer Res 1989; 49:5077–5082.

104. Guichard S, Terret C, Hennebell I, et al. CPT-11 converting carboxylesterase and topoisomerase activities in tumor and normal colon and liver tissues. Br J Cancer 1999;80:364–370.

105. Wozniak AJ, Ross WE. DNA damage as a basis for 4′-demethylepipodophyllotoxin-9-(4,6-*O*-ethylidene-beta-D-glucopyranoside)(etoposide) cytotoxicity. Cancer Res 1983;43: 120–124.

106. Lilleyman JS, Lennard L. Mercaptopurine metabolism and risk of relapse in childhood lymphoblastic leukemia. Lancet 1994; 343:1188–1190.

107. Weinshilboum RM, Sladek SL. Mercaptopurine pharmacogenetics: monogenic inheritance of erythrocyte thiopurine methyltransferase activity. Am J Hum Genet 1980;32:651–662.

108. Tai HL, Krynetski EY, Schuetz EG, et al. Enhanced proteolysis of thiopurine S-methyltransferase (TPMT) encoded by mutant alleles in humans (TPMT*3A, TPMT*2): mechanisms for the genetic polymorphism of TPMT activity. Proc Natl Acad Sci USA 1997;94:6444–6449.

109. Salonga D, Danenberg KD, Johnson M, et al. Colorectal tumors responding to 5-fluorouracil have low gene expression levels of dihydropyrimidine dehydrogenase, thymidylate synthase and thymidine phosphorylase. Clin Cancer Res 2000;6(4):1322–1327.

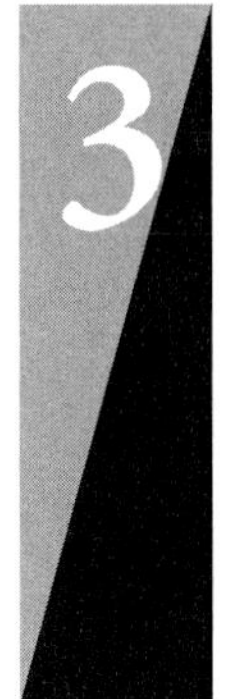

Principles of Radiation Oncology

Timothy J. Kinsella, Jason Sohn, and Barry Wessels

The medical specialty of radiation oncology has evolved significantly over the past 50 years, having begun as a subspecialty within diagnostic radiology in the 1930s and 1940s. Today, more than 50% of newly diagnosed cancer patients receive radiation therapy, typically as a part of curative combined modality treatment with surgery and/or chemotherapy. Additionally, a majority of patients who present with metastatic disease or who develop metastases following initial cancer treatment require palliative radiation therapy. As such, the radiation oncologist plays a major role in the management of most adult cancers and certain groups of pediatric and adolescent cancers. The intent of this chapter is to provide an overview of radiation biology, newer approaches to radiation treatment planning, the use of specialized applications of radiation therapy, and the mechanisms of drug–radiation interactions leading to radiosensitization, as well as the evolving area of *targeted* radiation therapy. It is hoped that this overview provides the necessary fundamental knowledge of radiation oncology for the reader (particularly nonradiation oncologists) to then better understand the rationale for the use of radiation therapy in specific cancers as detailed in other chapters throughout this textbook.

The Biologic Basis of Radiation Oncology

The Concept of Therapeutic Ratio

Shortly after the turn of the last century, radiation therapy began as a new modality for cancer treatment based on the discovery of X-rays by Roentgen and radium by the Curies. The pioneering use of X-rays and radium in the first two decades of the 20th century involved the use of large single doses of radiation therapy delivered in short treatment intervals, which, although resulting in a reduction of the tumor mass, was also associated with severe acute and late normal tissue toxicities. The concept of radiation dose fractionation (i.e., the use of smaller radiation doses given in multiple, typically daily, fractions) over several weeks evolved from an in vivo experiment in the 1920s using the testes of a rabbit as a model system for *tumor* proliferation.[1] These early French radiobiologists found that multiple radiation treatments compared to a large single dose of radiation resulted in sterility (the desired effect) without producing severe injury to the surrounding scrotum. The initial clinical use of radiation dose fractionation was then applied to patients with head and neck cancers as early as the 1930s, with improved tumor responses and reduced acute and late normal tissue toxicities.[2,3] Thus, the concept of a therapeutic ratio or index for radiation therapy was initially recognized more than 75 years ago.

The concept of the therapeutic ratio for radiation therapy, which compares the radiation dose–response curves for both tumor control rates and normal tissue(s) complication rates, is illustrated in three separate panels in Figure 3.1. The upper panel represents a theoretical optimal therapeutic ratio, where the tumor control curve lies always to the left of the normal tissue complication curve, whereas the middle panel shows an unacceptable therapeutic ratio in which the tumor control and normal tissue complication curves are reversed. Obviously, it would be easy to recommend the clinical use of radiation therapy for this idealized situation depicted in the upper panel. Conversely, in the middle panel, the radiation oncologist would need to carefully weight the type (acute, late) and grade (severity) of expected normal tissue(s) complications before recommending radiation therapy. Indeed, as illustrated in the section on radiation treatment planning (later in this chapter), the current use of three-dimensional conformal radiation treatment (3-D CRT), intensity-modulated radiation treatment (IMRT) planning, and image guided radiation therapy (IGRT) allows the radiation oncologist to quantitate the dose–volume histograms for each normal tissue included in the treatment volume so as to change an unacceptable therapeutic ratio (middle panel) to the bottom panel in Figure 3.1, which is the most realistic graph of tumor control and normal tissue injury as a function of radiation dose as found in many clinical settings. In actuality, for most common solid cancers the curves are not parallel, and the tumor control curve for most solid tumors is less steep than the normal tissue injury curves. Actual dose–response curves derived from in vivo experimental data or from clinical trials in humans are often more variable than the illustration in the bottom panel of Figure 3.1, particularly depending on the tumor type. Indeed, as is presented in other chapters on specific tumor types throughout this textbook, it is only by carefully designed and controlled clinical trials that the concept of a therapeutic ratio for radiation therapy can be quantitated for a specific tumor type.

Radiation Interactions with Biologic Materials

Ionizing radiation deposits energy as it trasverses various types of biologic materials or media (e.g., air, soft tissue, bone) within a human. The interaction of ionizing radiation with these biologics is a random process, with the frequency and density of energy deposition termed the linear energy transfer (LET). As human cells and tissues (as well as tumors) are principally considered to be dilute aqueous (water) solutions containing biomolecules, the localized but randomly distributed energy depositions from ionizing radiation can have either direct effects on important biomolecules such as DNA or indirect effects produced by intermediate radiation products resulting from interactions with water, which constitutes up to 90% of a cell or tissue as calculated on a weight basis. The most highly reactive species produced by the radiolysis of water is the hydroxyl radical (•OH), although there are many other types of free radicals produced by ionizing radiation, including DNA free radicals resulting from direct ionizations. These free radicals are generated within 10^{-2} to 10^{-12} seconds and subsequently cause chemical damage to DNA. It has been determined that ionizing radiation-induced cell killing in mammalian cells (including human tumor cells) results from a greater contribution (≅70%) of initial indirect ionizing effects on water than direct effects on essential biomolecules, principally DNA. These ionizing radiation-produced free radicals are highly reactive chemically within the cell and undergo a cascade of reactions to either acquire new electrons or to rid themselves of unpaired electrons, typically resulting in breakage of chemical bonds in DNA in very localized areas, called clusters, or multiply damaged sites. Because DNA is considered to be the most essential cellular biomolecule, the types of DNA damage caused by this sequence of initial energy deposition, production of free radicals and subsequent *clustered* breakage of chemical bonds can include DNA single-strand breaks (SSB), DNA double-strand breaks (DSB), DNA crosslinks, and DNA base damage. The creation of a DSB and, more specifically, an unrepaired DSB is considered the most cytotoxic DNA lesion resulting from ionizing radiation damage.[4,5] The molecular and biochemical processes involved in ionizing radiation damage and repair in human normal and malignant tissues are reviewed in the next section.

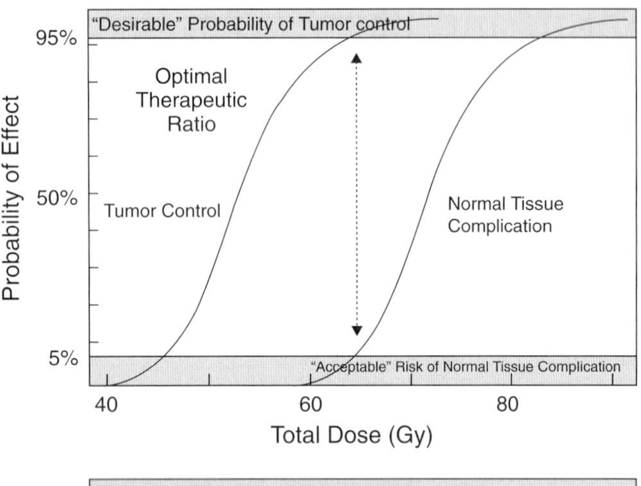

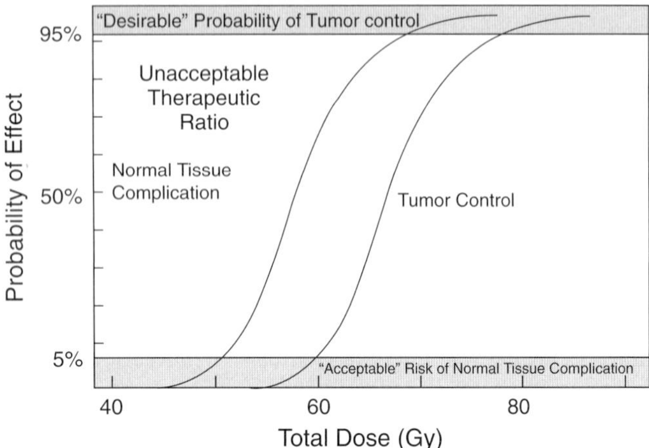

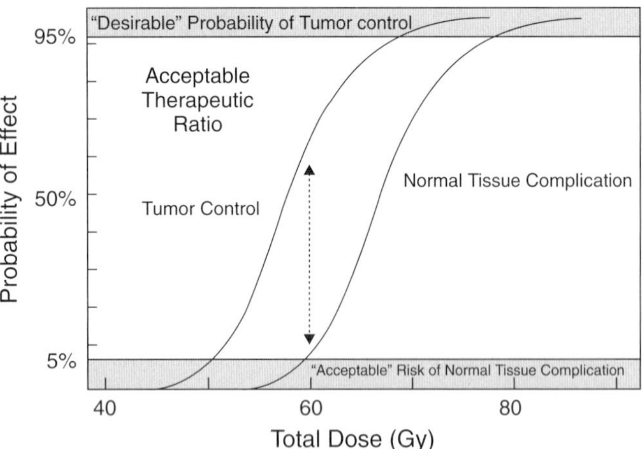

FIGURE 3.1. The concept of therapeutic ratio for radiation therapy under conditions in which the relationship between the normal tissue tolerance and tumor control dose–response curves is optimal (*upper panel*), unacceptable (*middle panel*), and acceptable (*lower panel*).

At the cellular level, the biologic effects of these initial physical interactions of ionizing radiation with biologic materials and the secondary chemical effects (i.e., DNA effects) can result in a cell's loss of reproductive capability. Functionally, the consequence of this reproductive loss can result in terminal differentiation, accelerated senescence, necrosis, or apoptosis.[6,7] A cell that has been lethally damaged by ionizing radiation may undergo a few cell divisions before death, and this lethally damaged cell's progeny are also destined to die. In the radiation biology laboratory, the radiation sensitivity of a cell (both normal and malignant) can be quantitated by analysis of cell survival curves. A radiation survival curve plots the fraction of cells surviving on a log scale against the radiation dose given (in cGy or Gy) on a linear scale (Figure 3.2). Survival is determined by the ability of a cell to form a macroscopic colony, usually defined as more than 50 cells (≅5–6 cell divisions). A typical radiation survival curve for a mammalian cell population has an initial "shoulder" in the low-dose region (up to 1–3 Gy), followed by a terminal exponential slope. The importance of this exponential relation is that, for a given radiation dose increment, a constant proportion (not a constant number) of cells are killed by ionizing radiation.[6,7] The *shoulder* region indicates a reduced efficiency of cell killing or, conversely, a higher efficiency of repair of sublethal or potentially lethal ionizing radiation damage. The resulting survival curve for mammalian cells based on a standard clonogenic survival assay is best described by a linear quadratic (LQ) model, according to the following formula:

$$S = e^{-(\alpha D + \beta D^2)}$$

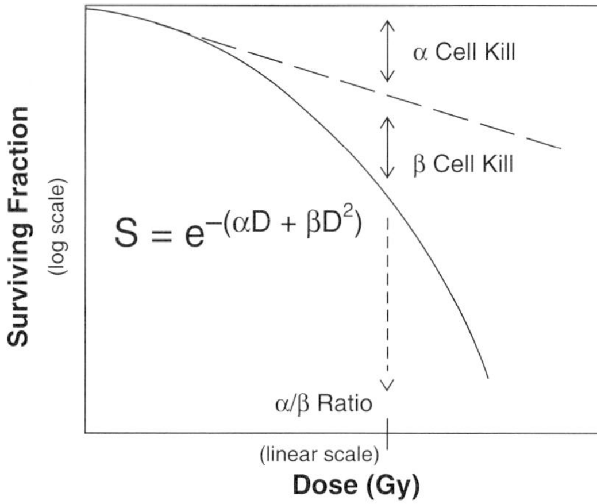

FIGURE 3.2. Log-linear illustration of in vitro radiation survival of a typical human cancer cell line showing an initial shoulder (a cell kill) at lower doses (usually 1–2 Gy) followed by a terminal slope (B-cell kill) at higher doses (≥3 Gy).

where S = surviving fraction, α = initial "repairable" radiation damage, β = irrepairable radiation damage, and D = ionizing radiation dose measured in grays (Gy).

Interestingly, this two-parameter (α, β) exponential model is reproduced when multiple fractions of ionizing radiation are given to either a normal or malignant cell population if the time interval between radiation doses (fractions) is sufficient to allow for initial radiation damage repair (usually 1–3 hours). However, the differential effects of ionizing radiation on cell kill in a malignant versus a normal cell population are not completely explained by this LQ model or any other mathematical model, as discussed later.

The discussion on radiation interactions at the cellular level so far has concerned sparsely ionizing radiation (low LET), such as produced by photons or high-energy electrons that are generated by linear accelerators used clinically for most cancers treated today. High linear energy transfer (high-LET) radiation can also be used clinically and involves the use of charged particles such as alpha particles and pi mesons. Additionally, intermediate-LET sources such as neutrons and protons are also used clinically, with a recent resurgence of interest in proton radiation therapy in the United States and Japan.[8,9] Because of these different LET radiation sources, the parameter of relative biologic effectiveness (RBE) is used in experimental radiation biology and clinical radiation therapy. The RBE is the dose ratio of different LET sources to produce the same biologic effect. Typically, with high- or intermediate-LET radiation, the radiation survival curve has a reduced or absent "shoulder" and a steeper exponential slope. The general explanation of the change in radiation survival (α, β parameters) with use of intermediate- to high- and intermediate-LET radiations compared to low-LET radiation is that the ionizing energy deposition is so dense with high- and intermediate-LET radiations that the DNA damage cannot be repaired as efficiently. There may also be less effect from the oxygenation state of a cell or tissue with high LET. However, as discussed later, the advantage of intermediate- and high-LET radiations in the radiation survival curve may not be easily translated to the clinic, as one must carefully weight the RBE of the tumor and the RBE of normal tissues. Thus, the therapeutic gain for a specific tumor and specific dose-limiting normal tissues may not be improved with high- or intermediate-LET radiation compared to low-LET radiation. Clinically, this is clearly the case for neutron beam irradiation, based on the past 20 years of human testing. As such, the recent renewed interest in proton beam irradiation should be tempered until prospective clinical data are available for specific patient groups in which proton beam treatments are compared to the standard of use of photons from conventional linear accelerators.[9]

Molecular and Cellular Radiation Biology

Repair of Ionizing Radiation Damage: Cellular and Molecular Mechanisms

As mentioned, ionizing radiation can cause a variety of lesions through direct interactions with DNA or, more commonly, through damage induced in adjacent water molecules within a cell or adjacent cells. These damages to DNA include damage to the deoxyribose backbone, base damage, single-strand breaks (SSBs), and double-strand breaks (DSBs).[4] Because exposure to ionizing radiation was inevitable during evolution, human cells have developed multiple repair pathways to handle the diverse types of DNA damage created by ionizing radiation.[5] Understanding these complex and sometimes redundant repair pathways in human cells has been a major focus in radiation biology during the past 10 to 15 years that will continue in the future.[10] These studies on radiation repair pathways also have many links to ionizing radiation effects on the cell cycle, which is discussed later in this chapter.

Repair of Base Damage and DNA Single-Strand Breaks

Repair of ionizing radiation-induced base damage involves a sequence of biochemical processes termed base excision repair (BER). DNA single-strand breaks (SSBs) are one of the most common lesions occurring in human cells, either spontaneously or as intermediates of enzymatic repair of base damage during BER. In BER, a single damaged base or locally multiply damaged bases are recognized and removed by specific glycosylases, resulting in apurinic or apyrimidinic (AP) sites that require cleavage by an AP endonuclease, followed by resynthesis using the complementary strand as a template, and finally by ligation of the repaired strand.[11,12] Ionizing radiation-induced DNA SSB repair is completed in steps similar to BER, in which a normal DNA strand serves as a template for repair. When DNA SSBs caused directly by ionizing radiation or arising as BER intermediates are not promptly and efficiently processed, the presence of clusters of damaged sites and of stalled replication forks can then result in DSBs.[4]

The availability of cellular models characterized by deficiencies in specific DNA repair proteins have proved to be good models to clarify the molecular mechanisms underlying BER and SSB repair.[10] For example, it has been shown that transfection of the human gene XRCC1 (X-ray repair cross-complementing gene 1) can correct mouse cells that have a deficiency in rejoining DNA SSB induced by ionizing radiation and alkylating agents. The XRCC1 protein acts as a scaffolding protein, which binds tightly to at least three other factors involved in BER and DNA SSB repair mechanisms including DNA ligase III, DNA polymerase β, and poly (ADP-ribose) polymerase (PARP).[12] The importance of XRCC1 in the response of a human cell population to DNA damage has been the subject recently of several studies evaluating whether polymorphism of the human XRCC1 gene contributes significantly to an increased cancer risk in selected populations.[12] Indeed, a genetic change in a single amino acid at codon 399 has been linked to an increased risk of several types of gastrointestinal cancers (gastric, pancreatic, colorectal) as well as breast cancer. Additionally, functional analysis of these polymorphisms suggest that these variants of XRCC1 may contribute to a hypersensitivity to ionizing radiation.[12]

Repair of DNA Double-Strand Breaks

It is well recognized that the most important lesion caused by ionizing radiation is a DSB.[4,5] Unrepaired or misrepaired DSBs can produce chromosomal deletions, translocations, and acentric/dicentric chromosomes, which result in cell lethality or genetic instability. Unlike repair of DNA SSB where the complementary normal DNA strand serves as a template, DSB repair is a more complicated process and can involve homologous recombination (HR) or nonhomologous end joining (NHEJ). Typically, ionizing radiation induces DNA DSBs where one or both DNA ends have a protruding DNA single-strand overhang. It is known from genetic and biochemical studies in radiosensitive yeast mutants that only one unrepaired (or misrepaired) DSB can result in cellular lethality.[5,10] The induction of DSBs by ionizing radiation shows a linear function with dose whereas the kinetics of unrepaired (unrejoined) DSBs has a linear quadratic (α, β) relationship with dose.[13] With low radiation doses, the quadratic component is insignificant. Thus, the survival curve for a DSB repair-proficient cell would have an initial "shoulder" (α component) at low radiation doses followed by a terminal exponential slope (β component), as previously illustrated in Figure 3.2. In contrast, the "shoulder" region is normally not observed in DSB repair-deficient cells, such as normal skin fibroblasts or normal lymphocytes from patients affected with the autosomal recessive disease ataxia telangiectasia (AT). DSB repair (including both HR and NHEJ) is presumably the fundamental process that mechanistically explains the previously described cellular responses to ionizing radiation damage termed sublethal damage repair (SLDR) and potentially lethal damage repair (PLDR).[4] However, in spite of numerous attempts to define DSB repair and survival following ionizing radiation in mathematical terms (such as the LQ model), other contributing factors such as cell-cycle checkpoints, hypoxia, genetic background diversity (polymorphism), induction of apoptosis, and bystander effects (e.g., autocrine or paracrine pathways) may significantly influence the survival response of a cell or tissue (including normal and malignant). These complex genetic and biochemical interactions are not easily simulated by mathematical modeling.

Homologous recombination (HR) is one of two major repair pathways in humans for repair of ionizing radiation-induced DSB. There are three general mechanisms for HR-mediated DSB repair.[5,14,15] Two of the HR mechanisms, termed gene conversion and break-induced homology, require homology with a separate DNA molecule (Figure 3.3). The other HR mechanism, single-strand annealing, requires only local homology on one end of the DSB (Figure 3.4). All three

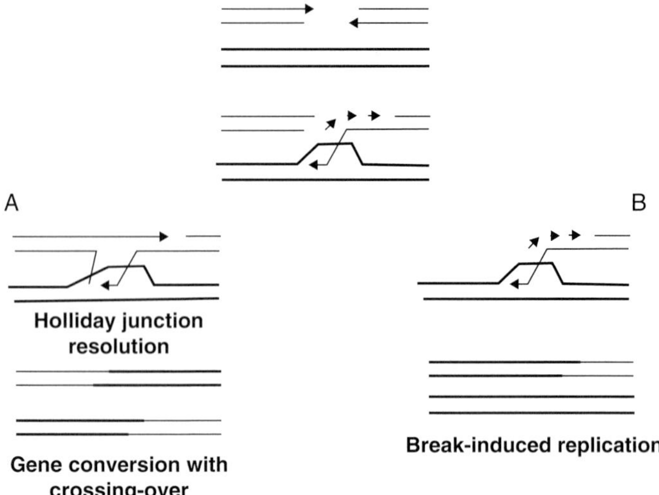

FIGURE 3.3. Various pathways of homologous recombination (HR). After 3′-Protruding DNA Single Strand (3′-PSS) are created (*arrowheads*), they invade a homologous region on another DNA molecule. Replication fork capture (A) results in the formation of a Holliday junction, with its subsequent resolution either with crossing-over (shown) or in the absence of cross-over events. When no replication fork capture occurs (B), the recombination follows the break-induced replication pathway.

HR mechanisms require a 3′-DNA single-strand overhang (3′-PSS). During gene conversion and break-induced replication, 3′-PSSs are created on both ends of a DSB. One then anneals to a homologous region on a sister chromatid, a homologous chromosome, or elsewhere to other chromosomes. New DNA synthesis is next initiated at the 3′-ends and proceeds to the 3′-PSS on the other end of the DSB. At this point, HR can proceed in two different directions, including (a) a Holliday junction (gene conversion), which results from the 3′-PSS annealing to the newly synthesized strand (Figure 3.3A), or (b) the replication fork proceeds until the end of the chromosome without encountering the other end of the DSB (break-induced replication; Figure 3.3B). The third HR mechanism, single-strand annealing, can be synthesis-dependent or

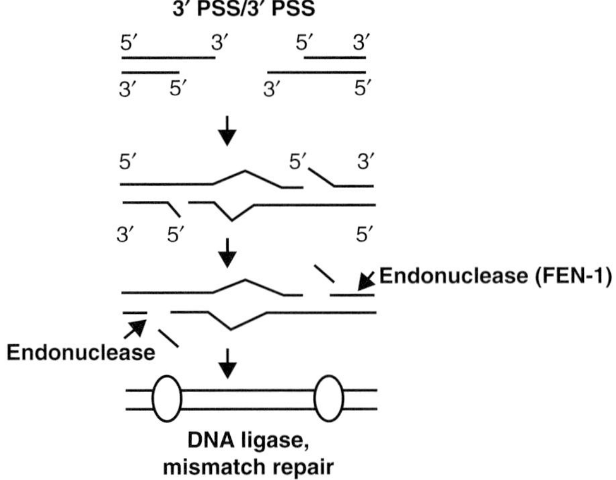

FIGURE 3.4. Single-strand annealing repairs double-strand breaks (DSBs) that contain both ends having 3′-PSS. Flap endonuclease (FEN-1) removes the misplaced DNA strand.

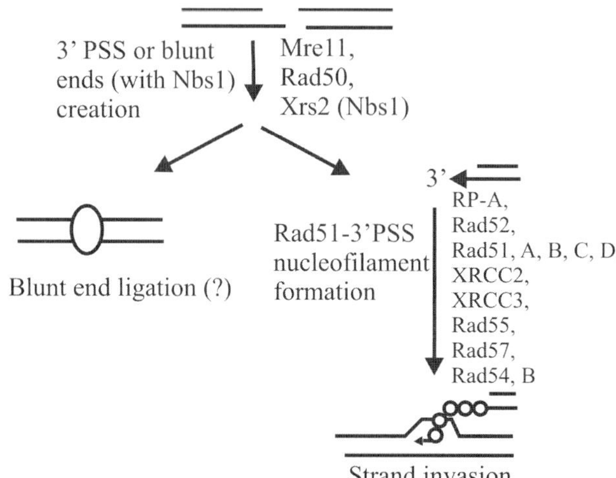

FIGURE 3.5. Proteins involved in the homologous recombination (HR) pathways of DSB repair: homology search and strand invasion. Taken from combined data obtained on yeast and vertebrate models.

-independent (Figure 3.4). Both types of single-strand annealing utilize local homology on the 3′-PSSs of both ends of the DSB. Annealing of the two 3′-PSSs results in a flap of one strand with synthesis-independent annealing or in a gap with synthesis-dependent annealing. The flap is subsequently removed by a 3′→5′ exonuclease or a flap endonuclease while a gap is filled by a DNA polymerase.

All three HR mechanisms require the gene products (proteins) of the RAD52 epistasis group (RAD50, 51, 52, 54, 57, 58, and 59) as well as participation of the gene products.[15] The Mre11 protein is thought to be a primary sensor of ionizing radiation induced DSB with subsequent recruitment of Rad50 and Xrs2 proteins in yeast and the Nijmegen breakage syndrome (Nbs1) protein in humans (Figure 3.5). The resulting complex of Mre11, Rad50, and Nbs1 is believed to generate 3′-PSS DNA lesions where several homologues of the yeast RAD51 gene (Figure 3.5) next interact with each other in a complex process to facilitate DNA strand migration, invasion, and finally repair.

In contrast, nonhomologous end joining (NHEJ) recombinational repair does not require extended homology between the ends of a DSB. DSB rejoining can proceed with a limited number of base pairings at the site of the break. In humans, the complex of repair proteins for NHEJ involves Ku70, Ku80, DNA-dependent protein kinase catalytic subunit (DNA PKcs), DNA ligase IV, and X-ray cross-complementation (XRCC) 4. According to a current model (Figure 3.6), the Ku70–Ku80 dimer initially binds to the ends of a DSB, and this dimer acts as a helicase to result in local unwinding at the DSB end.[15] DNA PKcs is then recruited near the sites of each end of the DSB followed by the XRCC4/DNA ligase IV complex to repair DSBs created by restriction enzymes. NHEJ can be divided into several pathways, depending on the type of DNA lesion detected. Rejoining of DNA DSB containing four base pair complementary ends created by restriction endonucleases is very efficient and precise. However, when the DSB ends are not complementary, repair is less efficient and may result in small insertions or deletions in the repair of noncomplementary (*difficult*) DSBs.

It is not clearly understood how human cells choose the pathway for DSB repair.[10] Two models have been proposed to explain how a cell might regulate whether HR or NHEJ pathways are used following ionizing radiation-induced DSBs. According to the first model, NHEJ is the major pathway active during the G_1 and early S phases of the cell cycle.[16] As sister chromatids occur during late S and G_2 phases, HR is the major DSB repair pathway at these cell-cycle phases.[5] The second model involves a direct competition for DNA DSB ends between the sensors of NHEJ and HR (see Figures 3.5, 3.6). Evidence for the first model is derived from murine *scid* cells, which lack NHEJ but can repair DSBs during the G_2 phase via HR pathways.[17] Evidence for the second model is found in human cells where the human Rad52 protein and the Ku70–Ku80 protein complex have been shown to compete to protect DNA DSB ends against exonuclease activity.[18] Additionally, the p53 tumor suppressor gene also appears to play a role in a human cell decision between NHEJ and HR following ionizing radiation damage.[10] It has been shown that human cells lacking functional p53 (either by null mutations or by mutant p53 expression) display up to 20-fold-higher rates of HR following ionizing radiation damage than cells expressing wild-type p53. Because p53 regulates the transcription and posttranslational activity of RAD51, it may be that the Rad51 protein plays a pivotal role in channeling DSB repair via the NHEJ pathway. Thus, these data suggest that the choice between NHEJ and HR is a function of cell-cycle phase, homologue availability, and the genetic background of a cell (e.g., p53 status).

The consequences of incomplete or faulty DNA repair of ionizing radiation damage may result in carcinogenesis in human normal cells or in the development of ionizing radiation resistance in human tumor cells. A number of genes whose products are involved in DSB repair have been found mutated in many different human cancers. For example, loss of heterozygosity (LOH) of RAD51, RAD52, and RAD54 have been found in human breast carcinomas. Additionally, nearly two-thirds of human pancreas cancers have overexpression of

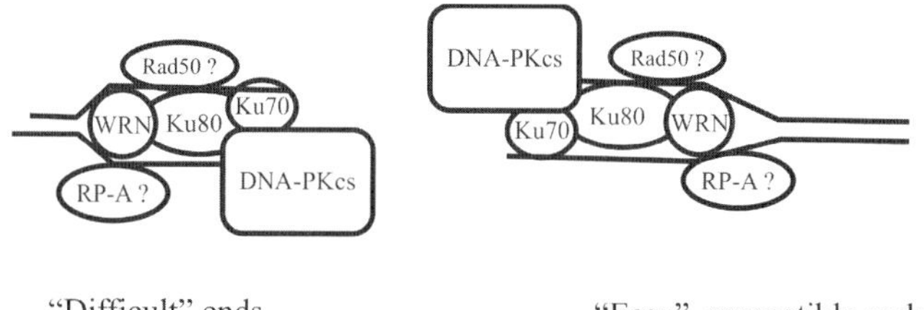

FIGURE 3.6. A model for nonhomologous end joining (NHEJ) involving DNA-PK. The Ku80/Ku70 complex senses and binds to DSB ends and recruits DNA-PKcs. Ku-associated helicase activity (WRN in the presence of RP-A?) is activated, and the Ku-complex migrates into the double helix with the Ku80 protein heading first in the 5′-direction of the broken end of DNA. It is speculated that, depending on the type of the DSB, either the XRCC4/DNA ligase IV complex or other proteins (i.e., nucleases and recombinases) are recruited to aid in the rejoining of the four broken ends of DNA.

the Rad51 protein, which could lead to cellular resistance to ionizing radiation damage and the development of tumor heterogeneity.

There is an ongoing search for new proteins responsible for ionizing radiation-induced DNA damage detection and repair.[10,15] During the past decade, several important DNA repair genes were discovered, mutations of which led to defects in DNA repair and extreme sensitivity to ionizing radiation. The X-ray cross-complementing (XRCC) genes were identified in humans and subsequently nine genetic complementation groups were recognized. As mentioned previously, the product of the XRCC1 gene was found to be important for DNA SSB repair. XRCC2 and XRCC3 gene products are part of the RAD51 family and are essential for the HR pathway in DNA DSB repair. XRCC4 to XRCC7 genes initially appeared to be involved in the NHEJ pathway for DNA DSB repair and were later sequenced to reveal that XRCC4 was DNA ligase IV, XRCC5 was Ku80, XRCC6 was Ku70, and XRCC7 was found to be DNA PKcs. Mutants within the XRCC8 complementation group show phenotypic similarities with ataxia telangiectasia (AT) and the Nijmegen breakage syndrome (NBS) with extreme sensitivity to ionizing radiation and to topoisomerase 1 inhibitors. Finally, the XRCC9 gene (also called Fanconi anemia G group) shows marked sensitivity to ionizing radiation and DNA crosslinking agents as well as spontaneous chromosome instability.

During the past few years, the RAD24 gene group members were identified to also include RAD9, RAD17, MEC3, and DDC1 genes. The products of this RAD24 epistaxis group appear to have regulatory roles that connect ionizing radiation-induced DNA repair and cell-cycle progression. It is also recognized that products of the tumor suppressor genes such as BRCA1, ATM, and p53 interact with RAD50 and RAD51 gene products to complete the complex process of DNA DSB damage recognition and repair.

Clearly, the field of DNA DSB repair is complex and is an area of intense research for the discipline of radiation oncology.[5,10,15] Although our knowledge of these complex interactions leading to DNA DSB repair is probably still quite rudimentary, translational radiation biologists/oncologists are beginning to explore how some of these genes or protein products might be therapeutic targets for modifying the ionizing radiation response in resistant human cancers. These translational approaches to novel "targeted" therapy in radiation oncology are discussed later in this chapter. The effects on ionizing radiation damage and repair on cell-cycle checkpoints are described in the next subsection.

Ionizing Radiation Effects on the Cell Cycle

It has been known for several decades that ionizing radiation leads to a prolongation of the cell cycle and can result in an arrest in the G_1, G_2, and S phases.[7,19,20] Because ionizing radiation causes a variety of DNA damage, it was initially inferred that these cell-cycle arrests (now called *checkpoints*) were essential for the repair of these different types of DNA damage. However, over the past 10 to 15 years, the biology of the cell cycle has become better understood as a complex but finely regulated process involving many factors, particularly the cyclins and cyclin-dependent kinases (CDKs).[19] Progression through the cell cycle is promoted by a number of CDKs that are complexed with specific regulatory proteins called cyclins, and these complexes drive the cell cycle. Additionally, there are a corresponding number of cell-cycle inhibitory proteins (CDKIs), which serve as negative regulators of the cell cycle. To date, at least nine structurally related CDKs have been identified along with more than 20 cyclins. The CDK–cyclin complexes themselves are activated by phosphorylation at specific sites, although not all these CDK–cyclin complexes have clearly defined cell-cycle regulatory roles. It is also now recognized that the G_0 phase is not a "quiescent" phase as initially termed. Indeed, cellular growth functions occur during G_0, and subsequent entry from G_0 into the cell cycle (G_1) is tightly regulated at the restriction point. This point is thought to divide the early and late G_1 phase of the cell cycle. A current model of the human cell cycle and the major cyclins, CDKs, and CDKIs is depicted in Figure 3.7.

The arrest of cells at the G_1 checkpoint following ionizing radiation damage is best understood at the present time. The retinoblastoma tumor suppressor gene product (Rb) governs the G_1–S phase transition.[21] In its active state, Rb is hypophosphorylated and forms an inhibitory complex with the E2F transcription factors. The activity of Rb is modulated by the sequential phosphorylation by CDK 4/6–cyclin D and CDK2–cyclin E. An ionizing radiation-induced G_1 arrest results from a specific CDKI, $p21^{waf1/cip1}$, which prevents key events such as the phosphorylation of RB and activation of E2F transcription factors. Importantly, $p21^{waf1}$ is induced at the transcriptional level by wild-type p53, which accumulates in irradiated cells and causes a cell-cycle arrest in both G_1 and G_2.[22,23] While the p53-mediated G_1 arrest is primarily due to the induction of p21, a p53-mediated G_2 arrest involves induction of both p21 and 14-3-3 σ, a protein that normally sequesters cyclin B–Cdc2 complexes in the nucleus.

Following recovery of a G_1 checkpoint, cyclin E binds to CDK2, and this active complex completely hyperphosphorylates Rb (pRb), which releases the E2F complex and fully activates the E2F transcription factors.[24] The irradiated cell then proceeds into S-phase transcription of a range of targets involved in chemotherapy-based radiosensitization. These drug–radiation targets include ribonucleotide reductase (RR), thymidylate synthase (TS), and thymidine kinase (TK). The interactions of radiosensitizing drugs such as RR inhibitors (gemcitabine, hydroxyurea) and TS inhibitors (fluoropyrimidines), as well as drugs activated by TK (fluoropyrimidines, halogenated pyrimidine analogues), are used clinically to enhance radiation cytotoxicity. These drug–radiation combinations are discussed later in this chapter (see following section on Mechanisms of Interaction with Conventional Chemotherapy).

Early in S phase, cyclins D and E are targeted by ubiquitination for proteasome degradation. The production of cyclin A and the subsequent complex of cyclin A–CDK2 enables S-phase progression, with the production of other enzymes and proteins involved in DNA synthesis, including histones and proliferating cell nuclear antigen (PCNA). Ionizing radiation can also induce an S-phase (or replication) checkpoint, which involves activation of ataxia telangiectasia mutated (ATM) and ATM and Rad-3 related (ATR) kinases with subsequent activation of Chk1 and Chk2.[25] The phosphorylation (activation) of Chk1 and Chk2 inhibits phorylation of Cdc2 and blocks progression into G_2 and entry into mitosis (M phase).

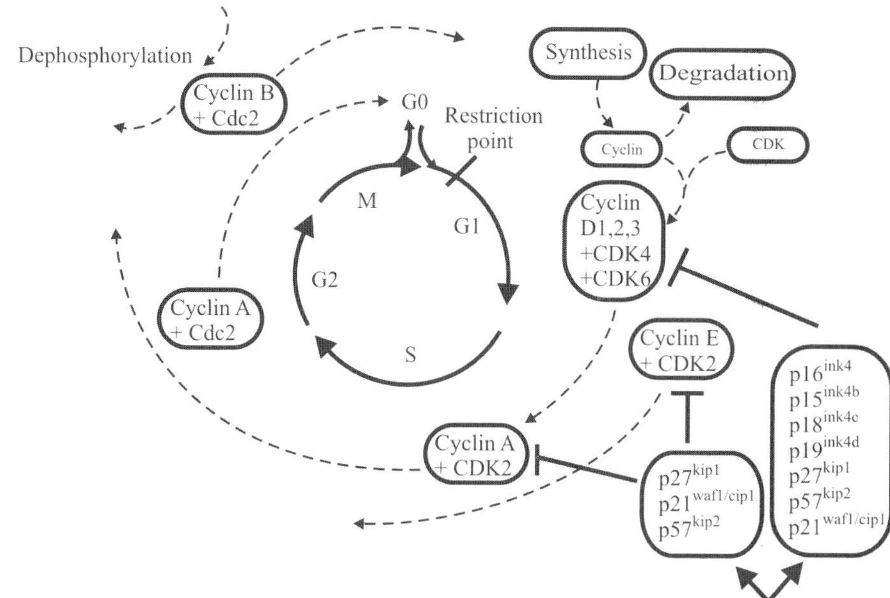

FIGURE 3.7. Current model of the cell cycle. The cell cycle is regulated by cyclins, cyclin-dependent kinases (CDKs), and cyclin-dependent kinase inhibitors (CDKIs). The cell cycle is divided into four distinct phases: G_1, S, G_2, and M. G_0 represents exit from the cell cycle in which the cell performs its routine functions, including the important function of cell growth. The progression of cell through the cell cycle is driven by CDKs, which are positively and negatively regulated by cyclins and CDKIs, respectively. The resection point governs the transition point beyond which a cell's progression through the cell cycle is independent of external stimuli.

A clear understanding of the role of the G_2 checkpoints to ionizing radiation damage and repair is lacking at the present time.[26] From genetic studies in yeast using *Saccharomyces cerevisiae*, the RAD9, RAD17, RAD24, and MEC3 genes are required for a G_2 arrest. In human cells, the DNA mismatch repair proteins MLH1 and MSH2 also appear to play a role in the G_2 arrest following ionizing radiation damage.[27] Based on the dramatic increase in our understanding of ionizing radiation effects on G_1 and S-phase checkpoints over the past few years, it is anticipated that the signaling pathways for recognition of ionizing radiation damage during G_2 and M will be better understood in the near future.[19]

Ionizing Radiation-Induced Apoptosis

It is well established that a principal mechanism of cell death following ionizing radiation damage involves necrosis.[6,7] More recently, radiation research has also focused on apoptosis as an alternative cell death mechanism following ionizing radiation.[6,7] Apoptosis is an active, energy-dependent process in which the cell participates in its own destruction (i.e., programmed cell death).[28] Apoptosis is characterized morphologically by cell shrinkage, cell membrane blebbing, chromatin condensation, and finally by fragmentation into apoptotic bodies. The molecular sequence or cascade of apoptosis involves the early release of cytochrome C from mitochondria, activation of an apoptotic protease-activating factor (Apaf-1), activation of caspase 9, and subsequent cleavage of downstream (effector) caspases in a self-amplifying cascade. The apoptotic cascade degrades several essential cellular proteins including β-actin, laminin, and polyadenosine 5′-diphosphate-ribosyl polymerase (PARP).[29] This cascade is regulated by members of the Bcl-2 family of proteins, which are either antiapoptotic (Bcl-2, Bcl-xL, Bcl-W) or proapoptotic (BAD, Bax, Bak).[28,29] Bcl-2 or Bcl-xL proteins bind and inhibit Apaf-1, which prevents the activation of caspases. However, in the presence of excess Bax, Bcl-2 may be displaced from Apaf-1, allowing caspase cleavage and activation.

The effects of ionizing radiation on apoptosis and cell-cycle arrests are interrelated, as evidenced by the central role of p53.[30] In addition to the effects of ionizing radiation-induced p53 protein expression on both the G_1 arrest and G_2 arrest as detailed in the prior section, p53 is also critical in the induction of apoptosis. For example, human tumor cells with certain mutations in the p53 gene are resistant to undergoing apoptosis following ionizing radiation. Another example of this interrelationship of cell-cycle arrest and apoptosis following ionizing radiation damage is demonstrated in isogenic human colon cancer cell lines that differ only in their p21 protein status. Wild-type p21 cells undergo a G_1 and G_2 cell-cycle arrest with enhanced clonogenic survival following ionizing radiation, whereas cells lacking the p21 protein do not undergo these cell-cycle arrests and proceed to apoptosis.

Ionizing Radiation Interaction with Oxygen

It has long been recognized that cellular and tissue oxygenation is a major determinant of radiosensitivity.[31,32] For several decades, oxygen was considered to be a radiation dose modifier as in vitro/in vivo radiobiology data suggested that the oxygen enhancement ratio (OER) is 2.5–3.0 for low-LET radiation (X-rays, photons) and 1.5–2.0 for intermediate-LET radiation (protons). More recently, experimental and limited clinical data suggest that the OER for both low- and intermediate-LET radiation are lower at lower doses typically used daily in treating human cancers. Although the underlying mechanism of the oxygen-modifying effect is not exactly known, the leading model suggests that cellular oxygen acts as a radiosensitizer by forming radicals such as peroxides in DNA, resulting in a fixation or persistence of ionizing radiation (IR) damage.

It is now known that two different forms of hypoxia exist in human cancers. Chronic hypoxia results from a tumor outgrowth of its blood supply, and variable levels or gradients of chronically low oxygen tension exist beyond the physiologic diffusion distance of oxygen through the interstitial (extravascular) tissue compartment.[33] It is hypothesized that these chronic hypoxic tumor areas (volumes) contain clonogenic and radioresistant hypoxic tumor cells. It is also recognized that reoxygenation of these chronically hypoxic tumor cells can occur, at least experimentally.[33,34] A second type of tumor hypoxia also exists and is termed acute or perfusion-limited hypoxia. Acute tumor hypoxia results from transient alterations in tumor vasculature.[34]

Over the past decade, several clinical studies have demonstrated that hypoxic tissue (defined as areas of oxygen tension less than 2.5 mmHg) exist in up to 50% to 60% of a wide range of locally advanced solid tumors including primary brain tumors, soft tissue sarcomas, and melanoma as well as carcinomas of the breast, head and neck, pancreas, and cervix.[35] Although trials of several hypoxic radiosensitizers have been negative, it is now realized that proper patient (tumor) selection was not performed in the design of these trials.[36] Current trials such as the accelerated radiotherapy, carbogen, and nicotinamide (ARCON) trials in Europe, particularly in head and neck cancer and bladder cancers, are selecting patients with biochemically confirmed hypoxic tumors for testing this approach.[37]

Hypoxia also causes altered gene expression in human tumors with associated changes in tumor microenvironment. The best characterized transcription factor is hypoxia-inducible factor 1 (HIF-1).[38] The changes in gene expression in hypoxic tumors are similar to changes in normal cells to adapt to a hypoxic stress such as trauma and subsequent wound healing. However, these hypoxia-regulated genes, when upregulated in human tumors, lead to resistance not only to radiation therapy but also to different types of chemotherapy.[39] The clinical targeting of HIF-1α to selectively kill or inhibit hypoxic tumor cells is now in early trials using drugs such as radamycin.[39] The advantage of targeting HIF-1 is the observed rapid response to changes in oxygenation, making it a good target for both acute and chronic hypoxic tumor cells. Such new targeted approaches in radiation oncology are discussed later in this chapter.

Radiation Treatment Planning

Three-Dimensional Conformal Radiation Therapy

Since computers were used for single plane treatment planning in the 1970s to 1980s, treatment planning systems have become further developed along with advances in computer hardware. These dramatic increases in computing power have allowed multiplane treatment planning to become practical. Once the planning systems became capable of handling large amounts of computed tomography (CT)-derived patient data, calculation algorithms were developed to account for the full scattering component of radiation transport in various human tissues.

The development of accurate three-dimensional dose calculations and 3-D rendering of patient anatomy provided the tool to sculpt a tumoricidal dose distribution conformed to a tumor (target) volume and to minimize dose to all other normal tissue (Figure 3.8). From these considerations, the term 3-D conformal radiation therapy (3-D CRT) gained rapid

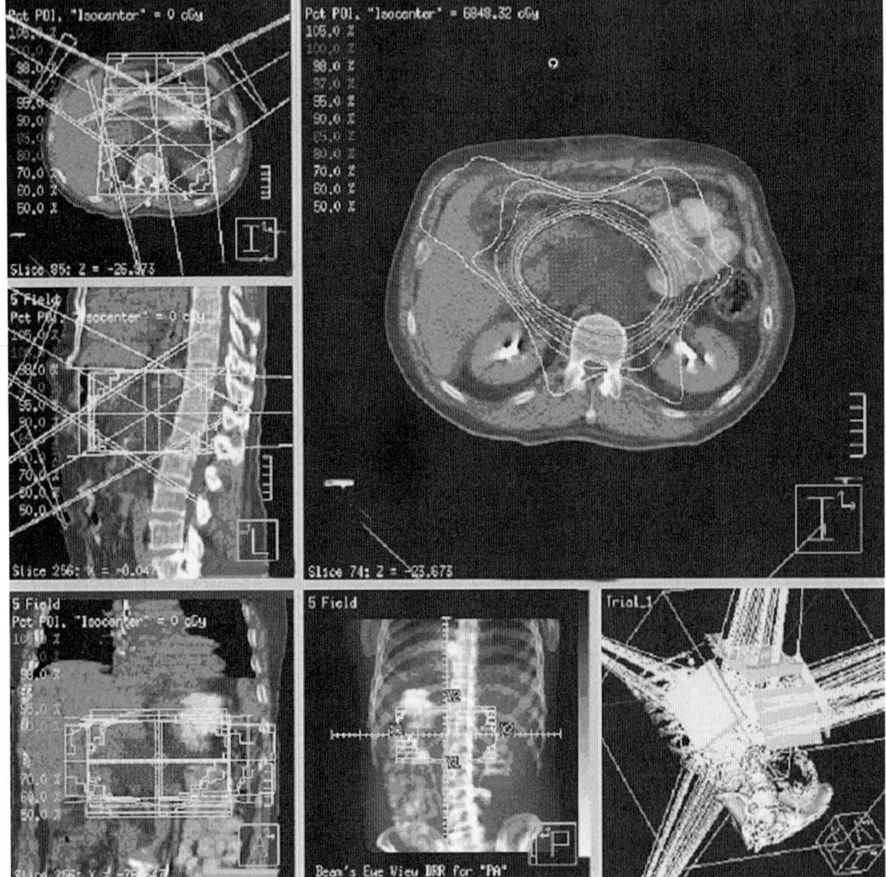

FIGURE 3.8. A tumor in the pancreas was treated with three-dimensional (3-D) conformal radiation therapy (CRT). Organs spared were kidneys, liver, spinal cord, and small bowel. Five noncoplanar beams were used for treatment. Each beam was conformed to the target volume with multileaf collimator as shown above to maximize the conformity. Three-dimensional rendering can assist the planner to optimize the beam angle.

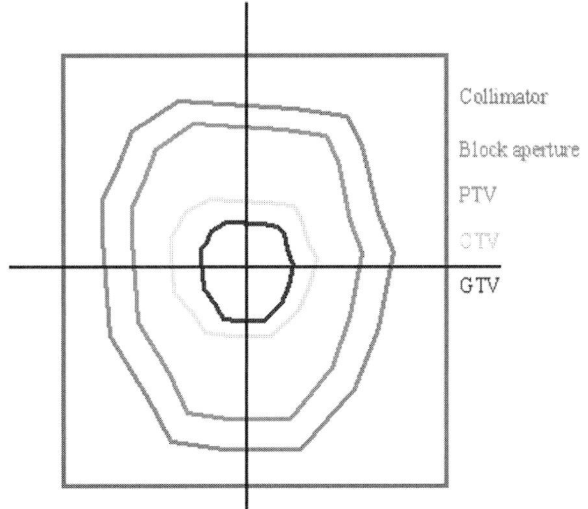

FIGURE 3.9. International Commission on Radiation Units and Measurements (ICRU) reports 50 and 62 introduced the volume definitions for radiation therapy treatment planning (see References 41, 42). Outer ring, block aperture; second from outer ring, planning target volume; third ring, clinical target volume; inside ring, gross target volume.

utility and acceptance.[40] Once dose could be highly conformed to the target volume, the margin of the target had to be more accurately determined; this has been accomplished by using multimodality imaging and carefully defining treatment and normal treatment volumes. The International Commission on Radiation Units and Measurements (ICRU) Reports 50 and 62 introduced the definition of volumes (Figure 3.9).[41,42] The gross target volume (GTV) is defined as the clinically palpable volume or, more typically, as visualized by imaging. It may consist of the primary tumor, metastatic lymphadenopathy, and local tumor extension. The clinical target volume (CTV) includes the tissue surrounding the GTV that might have microscopic malignant disease or "at-risk" regional lymph nodes. More than one CTV can be defined. The planning target volume (PTV) includes GTV and/or CTV plus a margin to account for variations in treatment delivery, including variations in treatment setup, patient motion during treatment, and organ motion. These ICRU reports also reviewed the definition of normal organs to be spared. Organs at risk (OAR) are defined as critical normal tissues, such as the spinal cord, whose radiation sensitivity may significantly influence treatment planning and/or the prescribed dose. After planning has been performed, a dose–volume histogram (DVH) can be generated from the plan (Figure 3.10). The DVH provides the information: dose versus volume of a specified organ. This information is very useful for radiobiologic studies. However, it does not provide spatial dose informa-

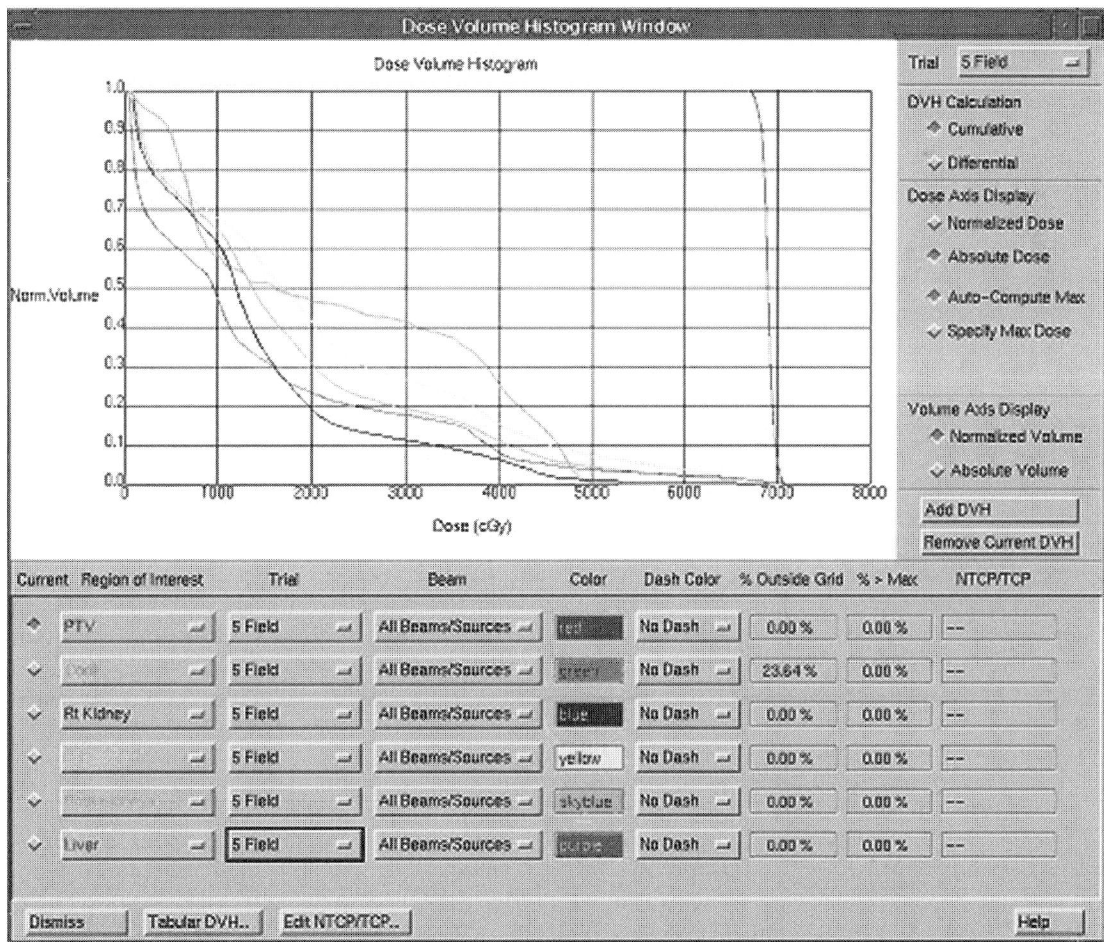

FIGURE 3.10. Three-dimensional treatment planning provided a tool for analyzing dose distribution in various organs interested. This tool is very useful in the analysis of the biologic consequences of the optimized irradiation.

tion. It can be used to complement the graphic isodose displays used in treatment planning by comparing the amount of dose given to specified organ volume. High dose conformity can enable the radiation oncologist to seek dose escalation to the target volume for possibly better radiobiologic advantages and an improved therapeutic gain, as previously described in Figure 3.1.

Intensity-Modulated Radiation Therapy

Three-dimensional CRT is used to optimize the radiation delivery to irregularly shaped volumes by manually setting individual beam angles. Intensity-modulated radiation therapy (IMRT) is a new approach to 3-D CRT. Clinical definition of complex treatment volumes often requires concave dose distributions. IMRT has been found to be most useful in this regard.[43] Radiation dose delivery to a target volume by IMRT is performed by the superposition of multiple "beamlets" from each treatment angle. Full dose uniformity is achieved by the summation of individual beams of small field size where the central axis is frequently blocked by complex multileaf collimator (MLC) patterns. The dose is figuratively painted in by discrete amounts wherever needed to maintain dose uniformity in a defined volume. Typically, in the optimization process using IMRT for radiation dose delivery, the relevant physical and geometric information of the irradiated object and radiation source serve as input data. Then, dose distribution may be calculated using the input data for volumes that have specific geometric characteristics. This dose calculation is known as a forward treatment planning process. However, an inverse treatment planning process is used to create IMRT plans. The inverse planning process essentially starts with a precise prescription of the goals of an ideal plan, and the planning system optimizes input data to meet these conditions. In addition to the availability of the physical parameters of the irradiated object (tumor volume), the relevant information about the capabilities and specifications of the available treatment machine may be inserted into the planning system. After the physician prescribes the desired doses to the different volumes including GTV, PTV, and adjacent dose-limiting normal tissues, the inverse planning system provides a delivery method to execute the prescription accurately with a specific treatment machine. The resultant computerized solutions appear as radiation intensities from the sources as a function of source location, which results in a dose function that is used in the delivery of targeted irradiation.

As shown in Figure 3.11, this head and neck treatment plan provides a sample of IMRT inverse planning process. This specific case shows a target volume for a patient with a base-of-tongue primary cancer where the GTV has been outlined and resulting in a corresponding PTV with expanded margins generated around it. The PTV has been prescribed to a uniform dose distribution of 7,200 cGy. Regional "at-risk" lymph nodes are also treated to the minimum dose of 5,400 cGy. Here, there are unique features of IMRT compared to the conventional radiation therapy, in that the IMRT can deliver different doses to multiple targets simultaneously. This method may eliminate the necessity of boost plans to deliver different doses to multiple targets. The fractional doses per day to physically defined target volumes can be made to vary. The daily doses should be selected carefully in view of the radiobiologic consideration. Most clinical experience is based on the same fractional doses, although total doses specific to multiple target sites and critical structures may be different.

Critical normal tissues such as the spinal cord and right parotid can be "spared" (see Figure 3.11) to doses of 4,300 and 2,200 cGy, which should result in no significant late toxicities. Once all objectives are determined, the inverse treatment planning system is able to optimize the dose distributions that satisfy the initial objectives. Most planning systems have used an intermediate step before giving a deliverable plan with a delivery machine. This intermediate step provides users with several options: which treatment delivery machine is being selected, how many intensity levels are to be used, and what is the basic prescription of multiple beam directions (gantry angles).

Current IMRT delivery methods have been implemented by MLCs installed on conventional linear accelerators, tomotherapy, and physical beam modulators.[44] Multileaf collimators include conventional MLCs that accompany the installation on most modern linear accelerators and specifically designed MLCs which have been attached to the gantry for IMRT use. There are two methods used for delivering modulated beams using MLCs: step-and-shoot and sliding window techniques.[44] The step-and-shoot method delivers dose to the target by a series of small beams. At each gantry angle, MLCs constantly form a series of segments to deliver a modulated beam. During the time of MLC movements between segments, the radiation beams are cycled to an off position automatically by the programmed accelerator software without further human interaction. However, the sliding window technique starts with all leaves closed from one side of a radiation field and opens the leaves in a dynamic pattern. The speed of each pair of leaves depends on the dose intensity desired. The radiation beams are continually on during the MLC movement.

Image-Guided Radiation Therapy

In the past, large target margins and treatment volume were used to accommodate the positioning error and organ motion associated with radiation therapy treatment. Because highly conformal radiation therapy can now be delivered, accurate target determinations (i.e., CTV, GTV, PTV) have become a very important issue. Various image modalities can now guide highly conformal therapy such as IMRT by locating the target before daily fractionated radiation therapy. Ultrasound imaging is often used for internal target positioning, mostly for localized prostate cancers.[45] However, because the ultrasound cannot penetrate air or bone, its use is limited to certain anatomic sites. Additionally, ultrasound, similar to CT, does not provide any functional information on tumor biology.

Traditionally, the determination of tumor volumes for radiation treatment planning, as well as determining responses following radiation therapy, has been limited to imaging techniques such as CT and magnetic resonance imaging (MRI) scanning. Based on these scanning techniques, we now can deliver higher radiation doses using 3-D CRT and IMRT techniques in certain situations such as localized prostate cancer[46] and head and neck cancers,[47] which translate into improved local tumor control and survival. With the

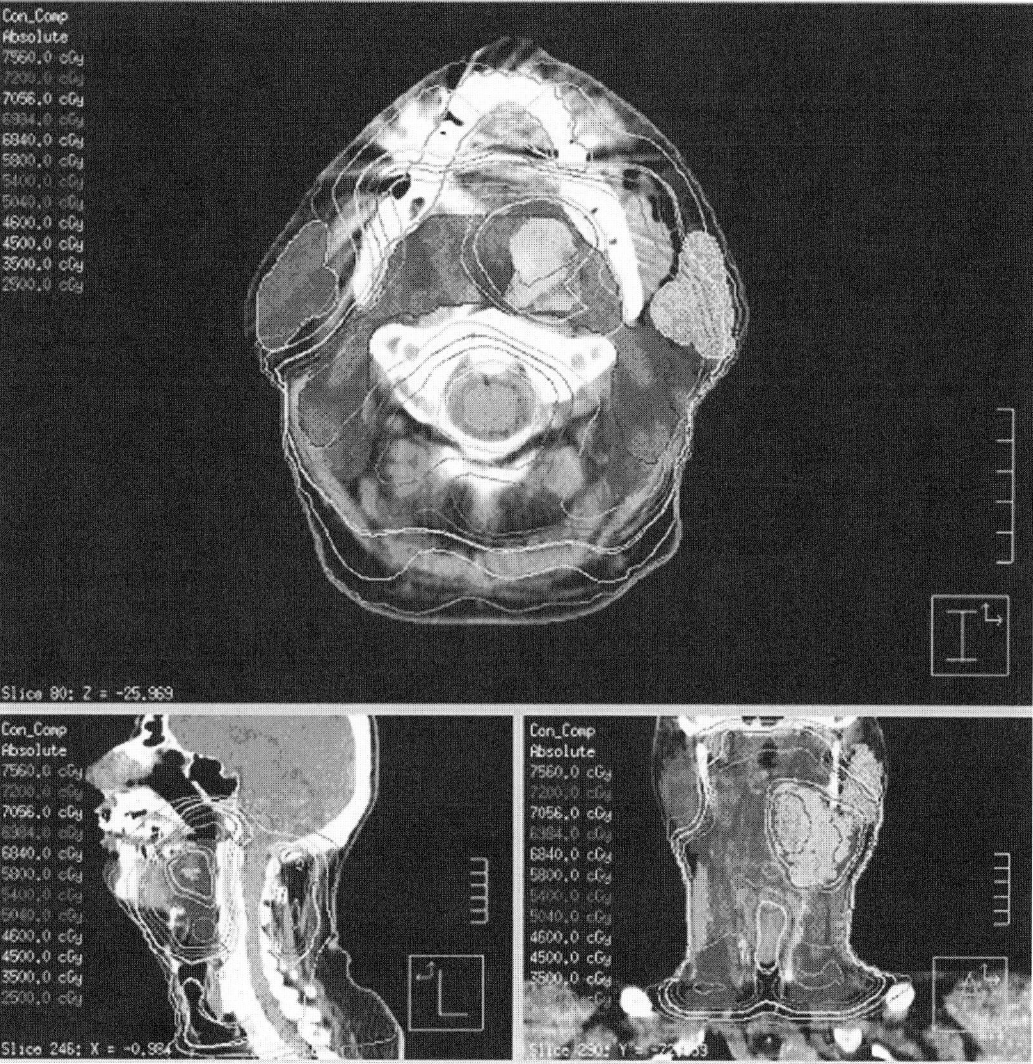

FIGURE 3.11. The orthogonal images for a head and neck cancer show the dose distribution from an intensity-modulated radiation treatment (IMRT) plan with nine beams at equally spaced gantry angles. Markedly reduced doses to the spinal cord (4,300 cGy) and the right parotid (2,200 cGy) are noted, while delivering 7,200 cGy to the primary tumor and 5,400 cGy to the at-risk lymph nodes.

clinical development of positron emission tomography (PET), single-photon emission computed tomography (SPECT), and magnetic resonance spectroscopy (MRS), radiation oncologists are attempting to integrate these function imaging techniques into radiation treatment planning. This evolving field of image-guided radiation therapy (IGRT) holds the potential to radically alter the way radiation therapy is used to treat cancer over the next decade. A comprehensive overview was recently published.[48]

Specialized Applications of Radiation Therapy

Systemic Radiation Therapy

Targeted radiation therapy combines principles of systemic and local therapy. Advantages of these approaches are to treat disease in multiple locations and to target microscopic subclinical disease. The rate of the uptake and retention of radioactivity to kill tumor cells relative to that of the normal tissues determines the efficiency of this treatment approach.

Systemic radiation therapy can be categorized into two forms: radioimmunotherapy and systemic unsealed radiation therapy.[49,50] Radioimmunotherapy uses antibodies, antibody fragments, or compounds as carriers to guide radiation to the target(s). The systemic unsealed radiation therapy can be administered by intravenous, oral, intratumoral, peritoneal, or intrathecal routes. These approaches are intended to concentrate the radioactivity into the target(s) and to deliver a therapeutic radiation dose. The applications of radioimmunotherapy are currently under way to treat lymphomas, leukemias, and some solid tumors with ^{131}I, ^{90}Y, ^{153}Lu, ^{186}Re, and several alpha-emitting radionuclides.[49] Other forms of systemic radiation therapy often use electron-emitting radioactive material. The most typical treatments using ^{131}I, ^{89}Sr, ^{32}P, and ^{153}Sm are for hyperthyroidism, differentiated thyroid cancer, painful skeletal metastases, polycythemia vera, malignant cysts, and neuroendocrine tumors.[50] These treatments are usually well tolerated without causing long-term effects, such as cancer or infertility. Several ongoing and new initiatives to explore the use of targeted therapy to be used as conditioning regimens for bone marrow transplant instead of nonspecific total-body irradiation show strong potential for reducing the side effects associated with the transplant process.[51]

Brachytherapy

Brachytherapy is the clinical procedure that inserts small encapsulated radioactive sources into the treatment (tumor) volume. Radioactive sources are continuously irradiating the treatment volume by an exponentially decaying dose rate. From each source, the therapeutic range is usually in the millimeter (mm) to centimeter (cm) range. Therefore, it provides a superior localization of dose to the tumor volume compared to the conventional external radiation therapy. There are two different methods in brachytherapy: an intracavitary approach where radioactive sources are implanted in body cavities in close proximity of the treatment volume, and an interstitial approach in which the sources are directly implanted in the treatment volume. Typically, the intracavitary implant is temporary. On the other hand, interstitial implant can be temporary or permanent. Most gynecologic tumors have been treated with brachytherapy using long-lived ^{137}Ce sources.[52] Recently, more brachytherapeutic applications to other anatomic sites have been introduced. These new applications include prostate seed implant for localized prostate cancers, intravascular irradiation to prevent coronary artery restenosis, and "mammo-site" breast irradiation as briefly discussed next.

Palladium-103 and ^{125}I seeds are used for the prostate seed implant procedure.[53,54] Accurate seed placement within the prostate, the most important task, is achieved by using transrectal ultrasonography, which provides accuracy and precision. The treatment procedure requires extensive treatment planning to localize each source and produce a combined plan for all sources. There are usually two steps to complete the treatment planning process for permanent seed implants: preplanning the target volume and intraoperative planning. Preplanning is performed with ultrasound images acquired before the surgery. Based on this plan, the strength of the seeds to be ordered, the number, and proposed seed placement may be preplanned. The premise of intraoperative planning is that preplanning is not necessary. All planning can be done in the operating room with real-time images. Advantages of the preplanning approach include: preevaluation of whether this treatment can be deliverable, more planning time to optimize the seed placement for ideal dose distribution, and minimization of ordering unnecessary seeds. The dosimetric goals of prostate cancer implant therapy are to deliver sufficient dose to the prostate and to spare the rectum, bladder, and other adjacent critical structures. These goals are achieved with optimizing the strength and the number of seeds.[54]

Intravascular brachytherapy has been introduced to treat coronary restenosis.[55,56] After a percutaneous coronary transluminal angioplasty (PCTA) is performed to reopen the blockage within the coronary artery, a radioactive source (^{192}Ir, ^{125}I, ^{90}Sr, or ^{32}P) may be positioned in the area of the restenosis. Depending on the selection of radioactive source, the treatment time varies from 3 to 25 minutes.[55] Due to the presence of the radiation-delivering catheter, minimizing the treatment time to restore maximum blood flow is a factor for consideration of source selection as well as other factors; other factors include the dose distribution in inhomogeneous tissue (calcified plaque versus normal tissue), and the artery diameter.[56]

Mammo-site brachytherapy is considered as an alternative to a standard 5-week external radiation therapy course for breast cancers.[57,58] This procedure shortens the treatment time to just 5 days. A specific device has been designed for this procedure, consisting of a hollow catheter to which an inflatable balloon is attached. It is temporarily implanted into the lumpectomy site. Beads of radioactive iridium are inserted into the catheter within the inflated balloon, which helps the catheter to be centered so that the dose can be uniformly delivered to the lumpectomy surface. The actual treatment takes typically two 15-minute sessions per day for 5 days. The catheter stays in place over the entire course of treatment. The preliminary clinical results with respect to local control and breast cosmesis are encouraging.[58]

Intraoperative Radiotherapy

Intraoperative radiation therapy (IORT) delivers a large single dose of 10 to 20 Gy to a tumor bed following surgical resection, during which the normal organs are physically moved out of the pathway of the radiation beam.[59] Intraoperative radiation therapy using X-ray beams was first described more than 80 years ago. However, refinements in techniques for IORT delivery and the generation of relevant large animal and human data on normal tissue tolerances to these large single doses of radiation therapy have ushered in a modern era for IORT.[60,61] It is now widely used for abdominal, pelvic, and retroperitoneal carcinomas and sarcomas as well as for some thoracic malignancies, extremity sarcomas, and head and neck cancers. The clinical experience to these tumor sites from large cancer centers throughout the world was recently summarized.[62] Linear accelerators designed for external radiation therapy have been adapted to deliver electron beams with IORT applicators, which collimate the electron beams according to the size and the slope of the treating area. Presently, dedicated mobile IORT machines are also used. These machines generate electron beams only. Therefore, shielding issues are minimal, and the machines are designed to be suitable for use in regular operating rooms.

Stereotactic Radiation Therapy

Stereotactic radiosurgery has been used worldwide as a primary or secondary procedure to treat both malignant and benign tumors. Typically, patients with brain metastases are treated following delivery of whole-brain irradiation.[63,64] The clinical results including appropriate patient selection are discussed in detail in the chapter on Brain Metastases. The target (tumor) volumes for this procedure are small, typically less than 30 cm^3 (less than 4 cm diameter). To achieve this goal, intracranial stereotactic positioning systems are designed to achieve accurate target localization and have also enabled effective nonsurgical treatment of arteriovenous malformations, acoustic neuromas, and primary brain tumors, in addition to brain metastases.

Stereotactic radiation therapy to well-defined intracranial lesions can be performed in single or multiple fractions. The type of tumor can determine the choice of fractionation.[63,64] Most centers perform radiosurgery on an outpatient basis. Treatment process starts with the fixation of a stereotactic frame on the patient's skull. Light sedation and local anesthetic applied before frame fixation are adequate for the patient's comfort throughout the treatment day. The patient with the frame goes through contrast-enhanced CT and/or MRI imaging with thin serial cuts (1–2 mm thick) taken in the region of the tumor. These scans are imported into a treatment planning software, where image segmentation is performed for volumetric evaluation and three-dimensional reconstruction.

There are two approaches for stereotactic radiosurgery: linear accelerator based and the gamma knife. With the first approach, tertiary micro-multileaf collimator and circular cones have been developed and adapted to a standard linear accelerator where 6 MV photons are typically used. The cone sizes for linear-based stereotactic radiosurgery range from 0.5 to 3.5 cm. The second technical approach to stereotactic radiosurgery uses the gamma knife (Elekta). This machine uses 201 cobalt sources (^{60}Co) and collimates the radiation beams using specially designed cranial helmets with 201 apertures and four different diameters (4, 8, 14, and 18 mm). The treatment is delivered with a combination of these helmets to conform the radiation distribution.

Whether a linear accelerator or a gamma knife is used, the radiation beams are arranged to intersect at a common point within the brain. The beam intersection volume is determined by the collimation system selected to encompass the target, and this produces a high-dose falloff just outside the intersection volume. Therefore, precise determination of the target volume is very important to deliver effective doses to the tumor(s). Noncoplanar arc beams are often used with linear accelerator-based stereotactic radiosurgery compared to stationary beams with the gamma knife.

Heavy Charged Particle Radiation Therapy

Heavy charged particles have two distinct characteristics compared to photons or electrons.[8] Dose distributions are highly localized, and the shallow depth sparing effect is significant due to the domination of the Bragg peak. This shallow depth sparing is much more significant than high-energy photons generated by linear accelerators. Additionally, the depth dose after the Bragg peak diminishes nearly to zero. As the Bragg peak depth depends on the incident energy, varying the energy of the primary beam can easily modulate the maximum dose depth. In addition to the advantage in depth dose distribution, the lateral dose gradient is significant at the beam edge.

As previously discussed, heavy charged particles also have a higher radiobiological effectiveness (RBE) and lower oxygen enhancement ratio (OER) because of higher linear energy transfer (LET). These factors may provide more radiobiologic advantages in addition to the physics described above. Recently, isocentrically mounted proton therapy machines are emerging as a competitive radiation therapy modality, as dose conformality has become more of a central issue.[8,9] It is possible that the new, clinically oriented proton therapy machines can deliver conformal radiation to the target that will be superior to the current IMRT methods using linear accelerators. However, carefully designed clinical trials are needed to evaluate these potential advantages to proton beam radiation therapy. For small targets, gamma knife irradiation with full frame immobilization represents the current "gold standard" by which other irradiation modalities are to be measured and compared.

Drug–Radiation Interactions and New Approaches to "Targeted" Radiation Therapy

Mechanisms of Interaction with Conventional Chemotherapy

The concomitant use of conventional chemotherapy agents such as the fluoropyrimidines and the platinum analogues during radiation therapy is the standard of care for neoadjuvant, postoperative adjuvant and definitive therapy in the treatment of locally advanced cancers of the head and neck, lung, and throughout the gastrointestinal tract, including esophageal, gastric, pancreas, rectal, and anal cancers. The results of various Phase 3 clinical trials of concomitant combined modality therapy using these drugs are reviewed throughout this textbook under the disease-specific sites. Indeed, the success of these concomitant combined modality treatments for the locally advanced cancers is probably the most significant advances in cancer therapy during the past 10 to 15 years.[65–67] Surprisingly, in spite of such success, the cellular and molecular mechanisms of interaction resulting in tumor radiosensitization remain poorly understood. Although an in-depth review of our current understanding of the greater than additive interactions of conventional chemotherapy drugs is beyond the scope of the chapter, the reader is referred to three recent reviews.[65–67] A brief overview of these drug–radiation interactions is summarized as follows.

5-Fluorouracil (5-FU) is clearly the most commonly used drug as a radiosensitizer, with the principal mechanism of sensitization related to inhibition of thymidylate synthase (TS) with subsequent progression through the G_1 checkpoint (restriction point) into S phase with altered (perturbed) triphosphate pools and reduced DNA repair.[68] As such, tumors with high levels (overexpression) of TS, which are known to be clinically resistant to 5-FU cytotoxicity, are probably also resistant to 5-FU-based radiosensitization. Two other enzymes involved in nucleoside metabolism including dihydropyrimidine dehydrogenase (DPD), a 5-FU catabolic enzyme, and thymidine phosphorylase (TP) may also be key regulators of fluoropyrimidine radiosensitization, including the use of oral prodrugs such as UFT and capecitabine.[66]

Chemotherapy drugs that target ribonucleotide reductase (RR), the rate-limiting enzyme in deoxynucleotide metabolism, can also result in clinical radiosensitization.[66,67] These drugs include hydroxyurea (HU) and gemcitabine (dFdCyd). It is known that ionizing radiation can cause a posttranscriptional overexpression of RR[69] and that the mechanism of radiosensitization appears to be progression into S phase under altered triphosphate pools (particularly dATP).[70]

The platinum analogues, including cisplatin, carboplatin, and oxaliplatin, are also commonly used as clinical radiosensitizers in head and neck cancers, non-small cell lung cancers, bladder cancers, and locally advanced cervical cancers. Several potential mechanisms of drug–radiation interactions with the platinum analogues have been proposed, including enhanced formation of toxic platinum–DNA adducts and crosslinks in the presence of IR free radicals; cell-cycle arrest at G_2/M with reduced DNA repair; and enhanced cellular platinum uptake by IR.[68]

Although the enhanced local control and improved survival rates have convinced the oncology community to consider these concomitant combined modality approaches as the current standard of care for many locally advanced solid tumors, there is also an enhancement in both acute (e.g., mucositis, myelosuppression) and late (e.g., esophageal, bowel strictures) normal tissue toxicities. Thus, more carefully designed clinical trials are still needed to measure the therapeutic gain and to test in patients the proposed mechanisms of these drug–radiation interactions leading to radiosensitization using noninvasive imaging techniques including PET and MR spectroscopy. Even in this era of molecularly targeted therapy, the oncology community should not overlook the success of these drug–radiation interactions and should continue to study the molecular targets of these leading to radiosensitization.

Mechanisms of Interaction with Bioreductive Drugs

As discussed earlier, hypoxic tumor cells exist in many common solid tumors and represent a therapeutically resistant tumor cell population that may limit the curability of these tumors to different chemotherapy drug classes as well as to radiation therapy. However, the presence of these hypoxic cell populations in tumors also represents an exploitable difference to enhance the therapeutic gain as normal tissues do not have such acute and/or chronically hypoxic cells. One approach to exploit hypoxia for a therapeutic gain is to use bioreductive drugs with radiation therapy to selectively kill the hypoxic cell population.

The development of bioreductive drugs has been an area of extensive preclinical research and clinical testing for more than 25 years, but even today there are no clinically proven bioreductive drugs approached in the United States for use with radiation therapy alone nor with chemoradiotherapy. Two recent review articles detailed the development and testing of these various nitroheterocyclic compounds.[71,72] At the present time, nimorazole is used in some European countries as a radiosensitizer in head and neck cancers based on a Phase III trial,[73] and tirapazamine is in Phase II and III testing combined with radiotherapy alone, cisplatin-based chemotherapy, and combined cisplatin/radiation therapy in the United States.[72]

Growth Factor Receptor Targeting for Radiosensitization

Over all the past several years, the potential therapeutic targeting of growth factor receptors on tumor cells is an area of active preclinical research and early clinical testing. Two key targets to enhance radiosensitization in human cancers are the epidermal growth factor (EGF) family and vascular endothelial growth factor (VEGF). For a comprehensive discussion of these approaches to radiosensitization, the reader is referred to two recent reviews.[74,75]

The epidermal growth factor receptor family has four transmembrane receptor tyrosine kinases, including HER2, HER3, HER4, and epidermal growth factor receptor (EGFR), which are involved in cell proliferation and survival responses, mediated through ligand binding. EGRF is known to be overexpressed in a majority of several tumors including non-small cell lung cancer, head and neck cancers, and glioblastoma multiforme. Clinical studies confirm that EGRF overexpression is associated with clinical radioresistance in these tumors. HER2 overexpression in breast cancer is also associated with clinical radioresistance. Thus, targeting the EGFR family clearly has the potential for radiosensitization. The preliminary results of a Phase III clinical trial comparing radiation therapy + the chimeric monoclonal antibody against EGRF (Cetuximab, Erbitux; ImClone Systems, New York, NY, and Bristol-Myers Squibb Company, Princeton, NJ, USA) were recently reported showing improved local control and survival at 2 and 3 years.[76] Although encouraging, several criticisms in trial design and the lower than expected local control and survival data in the radiation therapy alone, necessitate further clinical testing.

A second developmental area of tumor targeting involves targeting the tumor vasculature. It is recognized that tumor progression during radiation therapy is a major reason for radiation failures. The ability of a tumor to progress during radiation therapy is dependent on the continued formation of new tumor blood vessels. Consequently, by targeting tumor vasculature, one attempts to disrupt the proangiogenic balance between the tumor and its endothelial and vascular stromal cells.[75] Because VEGF is an important proangiogenic tumor growth factor, a considerable amount of emphasis has been placed on VEGF inhibition in preclinical testing with radiation therapy using protein- or receptor-targeted antibodies or using VEGF receptor signaling inhibitors including the cyclooxygenase 2 inhibitors.[77]

Two other approaches that attempt to target tumor growth and enhance tumor response to ionizing radiation involve targeting tumor oncogenes such as *Ras*[78] and the nuclear transcription factor NF-KB.[79] As no clinical data are available on these potential targeted therapies, the reader is referred to two recent reviews of the preclinical research and proposed clinical testing.[78,79]

Targeting DNA Repair for Tumor Radiosensitization

As reviewed previously in this chapter, recent advances in our understanding of DNA repair have shown genetic and epigenetic changes in several common human cancers, which result in alterations in IR damage recognition and damage repair processes. DNA mismatch repair (MMR) is a postreplicational process whose genes/proteins are not only capable of recognizing and processing single DNA base-pair mismatches and insertion-deletion loops during DNA replication, but also DNA adducts resulting from several types of chemotherapy drugs including the platinum analogues, alkylating/methylating drugs including procarbazine and temozolomide, and various nucleoside analogues including the fluoropyrimidines, gemcitabine, and the purine analogues, 6-thioguanine (6-TG) and 6-mercaptopurine (6-MP).[80] MMR is also involved in processing IR damage.[81] As such, MMR-deficient human tumors resulting from genetic defects [e.g., human nonpolyposis colorectal cancers (HNPCC)] or from epigenetic silencing (methylation) of hMLH1 and hMSH2 genes (e.g., found in 15%–30% of colon, gastric, endometrial, high-grade glioma, and ovarian and breast cancers) show clinical resistance to these chemotherapeutic agents as well as IR.[80–82] One approach to target these MMR-deficient human cancers for radiosensitization involves the use of the halogenated thymidine analogues such as iododeoxyuridine (IUdR), which are incorporated into DNA in place of thymidine and enhance DNA damage following IR exposure. MMR-deficient tumor cells fail to effectively remove IUdR DNA, unlike normal (MMR^+) cells, allowing for preferential tumor radiosensitization without enhancing normal tissue toxicity as recently shown in vivo.[83] A clinical trial of this approach using an oral prodrug of IUdR (IPdR) and radiation therapy in MMR-deficient ("resistant") human cancers is ongoing.

Another potential area for "targeted" radiosensitization involves the use of inhibitory drugs or proteins directed at double-strand break repair. As stated earlier, RAD51 is overexpressed in several clinically radioresistant tumors such as pancreas cancer. Additionally, ionizing radiation treatment can induce expression of RAD51 RNA and RAD51 protein-mediated homologous recombination of double-strand breaks in both normal and human tumor cells. At present, imatnib mesylate (Gleevac; Novartis) is a potential candidate for clinical testing of inhibiting RAD51 at its tyrosine 315 phosphorylating site.[84]

References

1. Regaud C. Sur Les Principles Radiophysiologiques De La Radiotherapie Des Cancers. Acta Radiol 1930;86:456–461.
2. Coutard H. Roentgen therapy of epitheliomas of the tonsillar region, hypopharynx and larynx from 1920 to 1926. Am J Roentgenol 1992;8:313–319.
3. Coutard H. Present conception of treatment of the larynx. Radiology 1940;34:136–145.
4. Ward JF. Mechanisms of DNA repair and their potential modification for radiotherapy. Int J Radiat Oncol Biol Phys 1986;12:1027–1032.
5. Haber JE. Partners and pathways repairing a double-strand break. Trends Genet 2000;16:259–264.
6. Cohen-Jonathan E, Bernhard E, McKenna GW. How does radiation kill? Curr Opin Chem Biol 1999;3:77–83.
7. Steel GG (ed). Clonogenic Cells and the Concept of Cell Survival in Basic Clinical Radiobiology. London: Arnold, 2002:52–54.
8. Cox JD. Proton beam radiation therapy in treatment of cancer. Clin Adv Hematol Oncol 2993;2:355–356.
9. Jagsi R, Delaney TF, Donelan K, Tarbell NJ. Real time rationing of scarce resources: the Northeast Proton Therapy Center experience. J Clin Oncol 2004;22:2246–2250.
10. Cline SD, Hanawalt PC. Who's on first in the cellular response to DNA damage? Nat Rev 2003;4:361–372.
11. Lindahl T, Wood RD. Quality control by DNA repair. Science 1000;286:1897–1905.
12. Caldecott KW. XRCC1 and DNA strand break repair. DNA Repair 2003;2:955–969.
13. Radivoyevitch T, Taverna P, Schupp JE, Kinsella TJ. The linear-quadratic log-survival radiation dose model: confidence ellipses, drug-drug interactions, and brachytherapeutic gains. Med Hypotheses Res 2004;1:23–28.
14. Valerie K, Povirk LF. Regulation and mechanisms of mammalian double-strand break repair. Oncogene 2003;22:5792–5812.
15. Leskov KS, Criswell T, Antonio S, Yang C-R, Kinsella TJ, Boothman DA. When x-ray inducible proteins meet DNA double strand break repair. Semin Radiat Oncol 2001;11:352–372.
16. Lee SE, Mitchell RA, Cheng A, et al. Evidence for DNA-PK-dependent and -independent DNA double-strand break repair pathways as a function of the cell cycle. Mol Cell Biol 1997;17:1425–1433.
17. Thompson LH. Evidence that mammalian cells possess homologous recombinational repair pathways. Mutat Res 1996;363:77–88.
18. Vandyck E, Stasiak AZ, Stasiak A, et al. Binding of double-strand breaks in DNA by human Rad 52 protein. Nature (Lond) 1999;398:728–731.
19. Pawlik TM, Keyomarsi K. Role of cell cycle in mediating sensitivity to radiotherapy. Int J Radiat Oncol Biol Phys 2004;59:928–942.
20. Sinclar W, Morton R. X-ray and ultraviolet sensitivity of synchronized Chinese hamster cells in culture. Nature (Lond) 1965;199:1158–1160.
21. Malumbres M, Baracid M. To cycle or not to cycle: a critical decision in cancer. Nat Rev Cancer 2001;1:222–231.
22. Nagasawa H, Li CY, Maki CG, et al. Relationship between radiation-induced G1 phase arrest and p53 function in human tumor cells. Cancer Res 1995;55:1842–1846.
23. Giaccia AJ, Kastan MB. The complexity of p53 modulation: emerging patterns from divergent signals. Genes Dev 1998;12:2973–2983.
24. Sherr CJ. The Pezcoller Lecture: Cancer cell cycles revisited. Cancer Res 2000;60:3689–3695.
25. Xu B, Kim SY, Lim DS, et al. Two molecularly distinct G(2)/M checkpoints are induced by ionizing radiation. Mol Cell Biol 2002;22:1049–1059.
26. Yamane K, Chen J, Kinsella TJ. Both DNA topoisomerase II-binding protein 1 and BRCA1 regulate the G2/M cell cycle checkpoint. Cancer Res 2003;63:3049–3053.
27. Yan T, Schupp JE, Hwang H-S, et al. Loss of DNA mismatch repair imparts defective cdc2 signaling and G2 arrest responses without altering survival after ionizing radiation. Cancer Res 2001;61:8290–8297.
28. Chao DT, Korsmeyer SJ. BCL-2 family: regulators of cell death. Annu Rev Immunol 1998;16:395–419.
29. Reed JC. Dysregulation of apoptosis in cancer. J Clin Oncol 1999;117:2941–2953.
30. Levin AJ. p53, the cellular gatekeeper for growth and division. Cell 1997;88:323–331.
31. Thomlinson R, Gray L. The histological structure of some human lung cancers and the possible implications for radiotherapy. Br J Cancer 1955;9:539–544.
32. Brown JM. Evidence for acutely hypoxic cells in mouse tumours and a possible mechanism for reoxygenation. Br J Radiol 1979;52:650–658.
33. Raleigh J, Dewhirst M, Thrall D. Measuring tumor hypoxia. Semin Radiat Oncol 1996;6:37–46.
34. Chaplin D, Olive P, Durand R. Intermittent blood flow in a murine tumor: radiobiological effects. Cancer Res 1987;47:597–604.
35. Vaupel P. Tumor microenvironmental physiology and its implications for radiation oncology. Semin Radiat Oncol 2004;14:198–206.
36. Kaanders J, Bussink J, van der Kogel AJ. Clinical studies of hypoxia modification in radiotherapy. Semin Radiat Oncol 2004;14:233–240.
37. Kaanders J, Wijffels KI, Marres , et al. Pomonidazole binding and tumor vascularity predict for treatment outcome in head and neck cancer. Cancer Res 2002;62:7066–7074.
38. Harris AL. Hypoxia—a key regulatory factor in tumour growth. Nat Rev Cancer 2002;2:38–47.

39. Semenza GL. Targeting HIF-1 for cancer therapy. Nat Rev Cancer 2003;3:721–732.
40. Purdy JA. Defining our goals: volume and dose specification for 3-D conformal radiation therapy. In: Meyer JL, Purdy JA (eds). Frontiers of Radiation Therapy and Oncology. 3-D Conformal Radiotherapy: A New Era in the Irradiation of Cancer. Basel: Karger, 1996:24–30.
41. Prescribing, Recording, and Reporting Photon Beam Therapy. International Commission on Radiation Units and Measurements (ICRU) Report 50, Bethesda, MD: ICRU Publications; 1993.
42. Prescribing, Recording, and Reporting Photon Beam Therapy. International Commission on Radiation Units and Measurements (ICRU) Report 62 (Supplement to ICRU Report 50), Bethesda, MD: ICRU Publications; 1999.
43. Purdy JA. Dose-volume specification: new challenges with intensity-modulated radiation therapy. Semin Radiat Oncol 2002;12:199–209.
44. Low DA. Quality assurance of intensity-modulated radiotherapy. Semin Radiat Oncol 2002;12:219–228.
45. Falco T, Shenouda G, Kaufman C, et al. Ultrasound imaging for external-beam prostate treatment setup and dosimetric verification. Med Dosim 2000;27:271–273.
46. Zelefsky MJ, Fuks Z, Leibel SA. Intensity-modulated radiation therapy for prostate cancer. Sem Radiat Oncol 2002;12:229–237.
47. Eisbruch A, Foote RL, O'Sullivan B, Beitler J, Vikram B. Intensity-modulated radiation therapy for head and neck cancer: emphasis on the selection and delineation of the targets. Semin Radiat Oncol 2002;12:238–249s.
48. Ling CC, Mitchell JB. Functional imaging and its application to radiation oncology. Semin Radiat Oncol 2001;11:1–92.
49. Knox SJ, Meredith RF. Clinical radioimmunotherapy. Semin Radiat Oncol 2000;10:73–93.
50. McDougall IR. Systemic radiation therapy with unsealed radionuclides. Semin Radiat Oncol 2000;10:94–102.
51. Houshmand P, Zlotnik A. Targetng tumor cells. Curr Opin Cell Biol 2003;15:640–644.
52. Hu KS, Enker WE, Harrison LB. High-dose rate intraoperative irradiation: current status and future directions. Semin Radiat Oncol 2002;12:62–80.
53. Blasko JC, Mate T, Sylvester JE, Grimm PD, Cavanaugh W. Brachytherapy for carcinoma of the prostate: techniques, patient selection and clinical outcomes. Semin Radiat Oncol 2002; 12:81–94.
54. Beaulieu L, Archambault L, Aubin S, et al. The robustness of dose distributions to displacement and migration of I-125 permanent seed implants over a wide range of seed number, activity, and designs. Int J Radiat Oncol Biol Phys 2004;58: 1298–1308.
55. Nguyen HP, Kaluza GL, Zymek PT, et al. Intracoronary brachytherapy. Catheter Cardiovasc Interv 2002;56:281–288.
56. Wang R, Li XA. Dosimetric comparison of two Sr-90/Y-90 sources for intravascular brachytherapy: an EGSnrc Monte Carlo calculation. Phys Med Biol 2002;47:4259–4269.
57. Streeter OE, Vicini FA, Keisch M, et al. MammoSite radiation therapy system. Breast 2003;12:491–496.
58. Keisch M, Vicini F, Kuske RR, et al. Initial clinical experience with the MammoSite breast brachytherapy applicator in women with early-stage breast cancer treated with breast-conserving therapy. Int J Radiat Oncol Biol Phys 2003;55:289–293.
59. Merrick HW, Dobelbower RR. Intraoperative radiation therapy in surgical oncology. Surg Oncol Clin N Am 2003;12:883–899.
60. Biggs PJ, Noyes RD, Willett CG. Clinical physics, applicator choice, technique, and equipment for electron intraoperative radiation therapy. Surg Oncol Clin N Am 2003;12:899–924.
61. Sindelar WF, Kinsella TJ. Normal tissue tolerance to intraoperative radiotherapy. Surg Oncol Clin N Am 2003;12:925–942.
62. Merrick HW, Thomas CR (eds). Intraoperative radiotherapy. Surg Oncol Clin N Am 2003;12:955–1078.
63. Sneed PK, Sun JN, Goetsch SJ, et al. A multi-institutional review of radiosurgery alone versus radiosurgery with whole brain radiotherapy as the initial management of brain metastases. Int J Radiat Oncol Biol Phys 2002;53:519–526.
64. Lorenzoni J, Deuriendt D, Massager N, et al. Radiosurgery for treatment of brain metastases: estimation of patient eligibility using three stratification systems. Int J Radiat Oncol Biol Phys 2004;60:218–224.
65. McGinn CJ, Lawrence TS. Recent advances in the use of radiosensitizing nucleosides. Semin Radiat Oncol 2001;11:270–280.
66. Lawrence TS, Blackstock G, McGinn CJ. The mechanisms of action of radiosensitization of conventional chemotherapeutic agents. Semin Radiat Oncol 2003;13:13–21.
67. Vallerga AK, Zarling D, Kinsella TJ. New radiosensitizing regimens, drugs, prodrugs and candidates: Capecitabine, Gemcitabine, Fludarabine, IPdR, Avastin, Veglin, Gleevac, Radvac, Erbitux or Iressa. Clin Adv Hematol Oncol 2004;2: 793–805.
68. Hwang H-S, Davis TW, Houghton JA, Kinsella TJ. Radiosensitivity of thymidylate synthase deficient human colon cancer cells is affected by progression through the G_1 restriction point into S-phase: implications for fluoropyrimidine radiosensitization. Cancer Res 2000;60:92–100.
69. Kuo M-L, Kinsella TJ. Expression of ribonucleotide reductase following ionizing radiation in human cervical carcinoma cells. Cancer Res 1998;58:2245–2252.
70. Kuo M-L, Hwang H-S, Sosnay PR, Kunugi KA, Kinsella TJ. Overexpression of the R_2 subunit of ribonucleotide reductase in human nasopharyngeal cancer cells reduces radiosensitivity. Cancer J (Boston) 2003;9:277–285.
71. Wouters BG, Weppler SA, Koritzinsky M, et al. Hypoxia as a target for combined modality treatments. Eur J Cancer 2002; 38:240–257.
72. Stratford IJ, Williams KJ, Cowen RL, Jaffar M. Combining bioreductive drugs and radiation for the treatment of solid tumors. Semin Radiat Oncol 2003;13:42–52.
73. Overgaard J, Hansen HS, Overgaard M, et al. A randomized double-blind phase III study of nimorazole as a hypoxic radiosensitized in supraglottic larynx and pharynx carcinoma. Results of the Danish Head and Neck Cancer Study Protocol 5-85. Radiother Oncol 1998;46:135–146.
74. Sartor CI. Epidermal growth factor family receptors and inhibitors: radiation response modulators. Semin Radiat Oncol 2003; 13:22–30.
75. Siemann DW, Shi W. Targeting the tumor blood vessel network to enhance the efficacy of radiation therapy. Semin Radiat Oncol 2003;13:53–61.
76. Bonner JA, Trigo J, Humblet Y, et al. Phase 3 trial of radiation therapy plus cetuximab versus radiation therapy alone in locally advanced squamous cell carcinomas of the head and neck. Proc ASCO 2004;23:487.
77. Milas L. Cyclooxygenase-2 (COX-2) enzyme inhibitors as potential enhancers of tumor radioresponse. Semin Radiat Oncol 2001;11:290–299.
78. McKenna WG, Muschell RJ, Gupta AK, Hahn SM, Bernhard EJ. Farinesyltransferase inhibitors as radiation sensitizers. Semin Radiat Oncol 2002;12(suppl 2):27–32.
79. Jung M, Dritschilp A. NF-kβ signaling pathway as a target for human tumor radiosensitization. Semin Radiat Oncol 2001; 11:346–351.
80. Karran P. Mechanisms of tolerance to DNA damaging therapeutic drugs. Carcinogenesis (Oxf) 2001;22:1921–1937.
81. Yan T, Schupp JE, Hwang H-S, et al. Loss of DNA mismatch repair imparts defective cdc2 signaling and G2 arrest responses

without altering survival after ionizing radiation. Cancer Res 2001;61:8290–8297.

82. Berry SE, Kinsella TJ. Targeting DNA mismatch repair for radiosensitization. Semin Radiat Oncol 2001;11:300–315.
83. Seo Y, Yan T, Schupp JE, Kinsella TJ. Differential radiosensitization in DNA mismatch repair proficient and deficient human colon cancer xenografts with 5-iodo-pyrimidinone-2′-deoxyribose. Clin Cancer Res 2004;10:7520–7528.
84. Russell JS, Brady K, Burgan WE, et al. Gleevac-mediated inhibition of RAD51 expression and enhancement of tumor cell radiosensitivity. Cancer Res 2003;63:7377–7383.

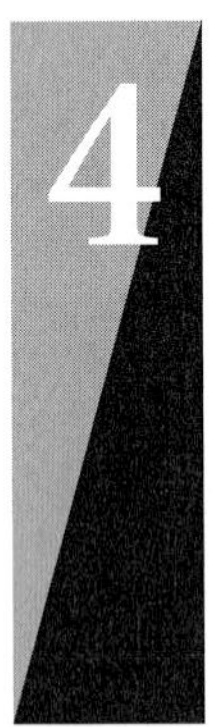

Principles of Surgical Therapy in Oncology

Michael S. Sabel, Kathleen M. Diehl, and Alfred E. Chang

History of Surgical Oncology

The role of surgery in the treatment of cancer has seen a dramatic change over the past century, from that of the only chance for cure to becoming one weapon in an armamentarium of oncologic therapies. As the role of surgery changes, so has the role of the surgeon, evolving from *cancer surgeon* to *surgical oncologist*. This role continues to evolve, as the management of cancer is altered by increased knowledge of genetics, molecular biology, and tumor immunology. Although surgery has historically been the first line of defense against a tumor, the escalating use of neoadjuvant therapies often shifts surgery to the second or third line. The role of surgery has expanded from that of purely therapeutic to include both palliation and prophylaxis. Inasmuch as surgeons are the ones with direct access to tumors, they have cemented their role as physician-scientists, investigating novel molecular and immunologic therapies. As new discoveries continue to transform our approach to cancer, the field of surgical oncology will continue to evolve (Table 4.1).

The surgical treatment of superficial cancers is clearly not a new concept. Some of the oldest medical records in existence, Egyptian papyri dating back to 1700 B.C., describe the cautery destruction of the breast.[1] Celsus and Galen, Roman physicians of the first and second centuries A.D., wrote about breast cancer operations, and the Greek physician Lenoidas described a mastectomy for breast cancer, including the use of cautery for hemostasis, in the 5th century A.D. Surgery was obviously limited to superficial tumors, and even that approach was halted throughout the dark ages of medicine. Ultimately the humoral theories of disease (blood, phlegm, white bile, and black bile) were replaced by scientific experimentation, and the principles of modern medicine began to take shape.

The principles of surgical oncology, along with several other fields, found their start with John Hunter (1728–1793), often referred to as the father of surgery. He first described many of the concepts of surgical oncology, including the idea that cancer could be a localized process that was potentially amenable to surgical cure. He stressed the need for total removal of the cancer along with the potential areas of lymphatic spread a century before Halsted's theory. These theories would not realize themselves, however, until the surgery itself became more feasible through a better understanding of anatomy and pathology through autopsies, the introduction of general anesthesia in 1842, and the principles of antisepsis, first described by Lister in 1867. This knowledge allowed surgical oncology to expand beyond superficial tumors, such as breast cancer, to the treatment of intraabdominal malignancies.

The next few decades would see the description of several major operations for cancer, including many by Theodore Billroth of Vienna, who could probably be considered the first surgical oncologist. He is most well known for the first successful partial gastrectomy for cancer (1881), but he also described the first total laryngectomy (1873), the first hemipelvectomy (1891), and the first suprapubic removal of a bladder tumor.[2] Other notable milestones include the resection of colon cancer (Weir, 1885),[3] the radical mastectomy (Halsted, 1891),[4] the radical hysterectomy for cancer (Kelly, 1895),[5] the first radical neck dissection (Crile, 1906),[6] and the first abdominoperineal resection for rectal cancer (Miles, 1908).[7]

Throughout the first half of the 20th century, surgery remained the mainstay of cancer treatment. Although these major operations were not without significant mortality and morbidity, the risks of surgery were still outweighed by the potential for cure or palliation of symptoms. It is during this time that the phrase *cancer surgeon* was popularized, as the only major advances in cancer care were surgical. Cancer surgeons were in abundance at the major medical centers and were the clinical leaders at the few dedicated cancer centers.

The mid-20th century saw advances in cancer therapies outside the realm of surgery. Roentgen's discovery of X-rays in 1896 ultimately led to radiation treatments for surface cancers such as those of the cervix, head and neck, or breast. Chemotherapy entered the scene with the discovery of the alkylating agent nitrogen mustard in WWII,[8] the folic acid antagonists reported by Farber in 1948,[9] and the concept of hormonal alteration proposed by Nobel laureate Charles Huggins in 1941.[10] It soon became apparent that cancer could be treated using more than one modality. It was at this time that the field of oncology began to mature, with clinical chemotherapists becoming known as oncologists. James Ewing, a pathologist who had experimented with immunotherapy, chemotherapy, and radium, established the multidisciplinary approach to the treatment of cancer with his book entitled *Neoplastic Diseases*.

In the mid-1960s, the term *surgical oncology* first arose; however, this phrase served to differentiate not between

TABLE 4.1. Important milestones in surgical oncology.

1600–1700 B.C.	Egyptians use cautery to destroy breast cancer.
400 B.C.	Hippocrates describes the clinical symptoms of cancer and coins the terms "carcinoma" and "sarcoma."
1st and 2nd century A.D.	Roman physicians use surgery to treat breast cancer.
5th century A.D.	The Greek physician Lenoidas first describes a mastectomy as a treatment of breast cancer.
1760s	John Hunter, the "Father of Scientific Surgery," describes principles of surgical oncology including cancer as local disease and lymphatic spread.
1775	Percival Pott describes scrotal cancer in chimney sweeps, first identifying a specific etiology of cancer.
1809	The first modern elective surgery for an abdominal cancer is performed: the removal of a 22-lb ovarian tumor by Ephraim MacDowell.
1829	Joseph Recamier first describes the principles of tumor metastasis.
1846	The first major cancer operation is performed under general anesthesia: the excision of the submaxillary gland and part of the tongue by John Collins Warren.
1867	Lister describes the principles of antisepsis and introduces carbolic acid, greatly reducing the morbidity of surgery.
1873	First total laryngectomy for laryngeal cancer by Theodore Billroth.
1881	First partial gastrectomy for cancer by Theodore Billroth.
1885	First colectomy for colon cancer by Robert Weir.
1887	New York Cancer Hospital becomes the first hospital in the United States specifically for cancer treatment.
1891	First hemipelvectomy by Theodore Billroth; first radical mastectomy for breast cancer by William Halsted.
1896	Roentgen discovers X-rays, ultimately leading to radiation oncology; G.T. Beason performs the first oophorectomy as hormonal treatment for breast cancer.
1906	First abdominoperineal resection for rectal cancer by W. Ernest Miles.
1909	Theodore Kocher first describes thyroid surgery.
1913	Both the American Association for the Advancement of Cancer (which would become the American Cancer Society) and the American College of Surgeons are established.
1919	James Ewing publishes *Neoplastic Diseases*, promoting the concept of the multidisciplinary treatment of cancer.
1927	First resection of pulmonary metastases by George Divis.
1935	First pancreaticoduodenectomy for pancreatic cancer by Allen O. Whipple.
1940	The James Ewing Society is established to "further our knowledge of cancer."
1940s	Chemotherapy begins with the discovery of nitrogen mustards and folic acid antagonists.
1957	The initiation of the National Surgical Adjuvant Breast Project (NSABP).
1960s	Dr. Walter Lawrence establishes a division of surgical oncology at the Medical College of Virginia.
1975	The Society of Surgical Oncology (SSO) is established.
1978	The term *surgical oncologist* is defined by the SSO and NCI, and the SSO formulates guidelines for postresidency surgical oncology training.
1998	The American Board of Surgery establishes the Advisory Council for Surgical Oncology. The American College of Surgeons Oncology Group (ACOSOG) is established.

cancer surgeons and general surgeons but rather between surgeons and oncologists. Although the fields of medical oncology and radiation oncology were quickly acknowledged as legitimate subspecialties, the field of surgical oncology had difficulty separating from general surgery. Most well-trained general surgeons felt capable of performing the majority of cancer operations, and so subspecialization was limited to university hospitals that allowed such a focus. In the mid-1960s, the Medical College of Virginia was the first university department of surgery to establish a formal division of surgical oncology under the auspices of Dr. Walter Lawrence. By 1986, 38% of university surgery departments had done the same.[11] Despite the territorial conflicts between general surgeons, whose workload continues to be devoted in large part to cancer, and the surgical oncologist, the field continued to emerge as a surgical subspecialty. In 1975, the Society of Surgical Oncology (SSO) was established from the James Ewing Society, a group of alumni who had trained at the Memorial Sloan-Kettering Cancer Center and gathered in New York for both scientific and social purposes. Although not a purely surgical society, it was dominated by surgeons and was established with the premise that its members would continue to be true to the inspiration of Dr. Ewing and his multidisciplinary approach to cancer. In conjunction with the National Cancer Institute (NCI), the SSO defined a surgical oncologist as an individual who is a fully qualified general surgeon who has had additional training and experience in all aspects of oncology, is capable of collaborating well with other oncology disciplines, has a full-time commitment to oncology, and serves the important role of leader of his fellow general surgeons in the care of the cancer patient.

Goals of Cancer Surgery

With the expansion of the multidisciplinary approach to cancer, the role of the surgeon has changed significantly. In addition to the well-established curative role, surgeons are often asked to obtain tissue for diagnosis and staging, debulk tumors as part of multimodality therapy, palliate incurable patients, or prevent cancer by the surgical removal of nonessential organs. As the management of cancer is altered by new discoveries in genetics, molecular biology, immunology, and improved therapeutics, so too will the functions of the surgical oncologist change. With our increased understanding of the genetic predisposition to cancer, the surgeon is increasingly being asked to remove healthy organs to prevent malignancy. However, as other effective methods of prevention are developed, such as chemoprevention or gene therapy, this role will certainly diminish. Improving imaging technologies may have diminished the need for surgical intervention for staging (such as in Hodgkin's lymphoma), but the expanded use of neoadjuvant therapies often requires interventions to accurately assess response to therapy. In addition, harvesting tumors may become increasingly important for molecular staging as well as identifying molecular targets for specific therapies. It is therefore imperative for surgical oncologists to remain up-to-date on the newest approaches to cancer therapy, both multidisciplinary and experimental, and be prepared to adapt to the changing requirements for surgery.

Curative Surgery

Surgery for Primary Cancers

The major objective for surgery of the primary cancer is to achieve optimal *local control* of the lesion. Local control is defined as the elimination of the neoplastic process and establishing a milieu in which local tumor recurrence is minimized. Historically, this was achieved with radical extirpative surgeries that shaped the surgical oncologists' major objective, namely, avoiding a local recurrence. Before William Halsted's description of the radical mastectomy, surgical treatment of breast cancer resulted in a dismal local control rate of less than 30%. The reason why Halsted's procedure was adopted as a standard approach was because he achieved greater than 90% local control, despite the fact that the overall survival of his patients was not improved.[4] The latter was due to the locally advanced stage of the patients who were treated in those days. This consideration ushered in the concept of en bloc removal of adjacent tissue when removing a primary cancer. Halsted's mastectomy involved the removal of adjacent skin (often necessitating a skin graft), underlying pectoral muscles, and axillary lymph nodes (Figure 4.1).

One of the major principles of surgical therapy of the primary tumor is to obtain adequate *negative margins* around the primary tumor, which could mean different operative approaches depending on the tumor type and its local involvement with adjacent structures. For example, the removal of a primary colon cancer that involves an adjacent loop of small bowel or bladder requires the en bloc resection of the primary tumor along with removal of the involved segment of small bowel and bladder wall. This approach avoids violation of the primary tumor margins that could lead to tumor spillage and possible implantation of malignant cells in the surrounding normal tissues. Aside from biopsies of the primary tumor, the lesion should not be entered during a definitive resection. In fact, any biopsy tract or incision that was performed before the tumor resection should be included in the procedure to reduce the risk of local recurrence (Figure 4.2).

The risk of local recurrence for all solid malignancies is clearly increased if negative margins are not achieved. The adequacy of the negative margin has been defined for most tumor types either from retrospective clinical experience or prospective clinical trials. For example, a 5-cm margin is an adequate bowel margin for primary colon cancers that has been established from clinical experience. Likewise, it is accepted that a 2-cm distal margin for rectal cancers results

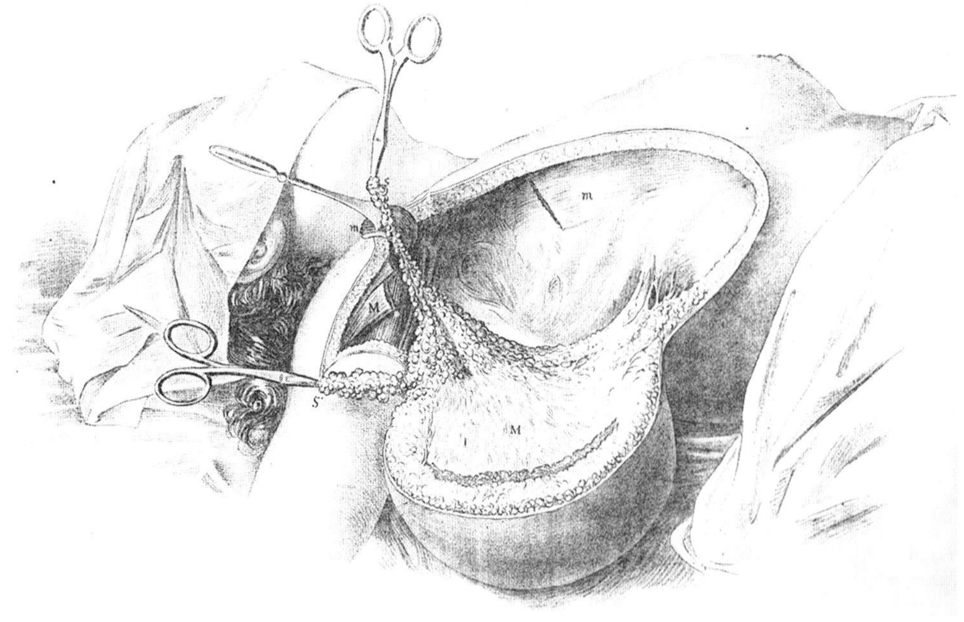

FIGURE 4.1. Original drawing of the radical mastectomy reported by William S. Halsted in 1894. Introduction of this operation led to improved local control in the treatment of breast cancer. (From Halsted,[4] by permission of *Annals of Surgery*.)

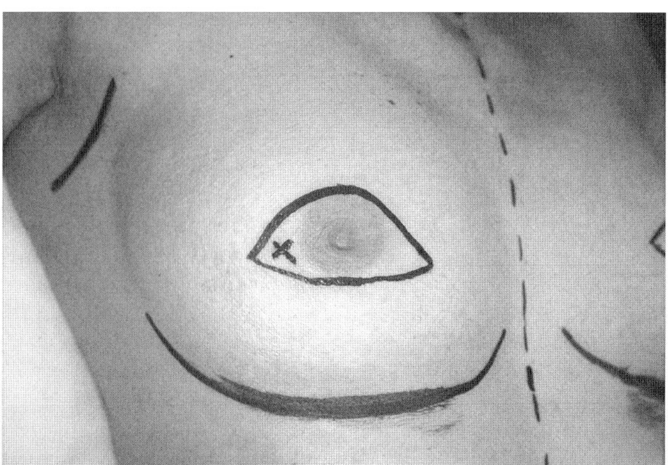

FIGURE 4.2. Location of core-needle biopsy site (*x*) in a patient undergoing a skin-sparing mastectomy for breast cancer. The biopsy site is incorporated in the elliptical skin incision to be removed en bloc with the specimen.

in adequate local control. Through several prospective, randomized clinical trials, the margins of excision for primary cutaneous melanomas differ according to the thickness of the primary (see Chapter 60). It was a commonly held notion that the development of a local recurrence would in itself result in metastatic disease with decreased overall survival. However, this has not been borne out in the context of prospective trials as described here.

The emergence of multimodal therapy has dramatically affected the surgical approach to many primary cancers, especially when surgical resection of the tumor is combined with radiotherapy. Local control is significantly improved after surgical resection of breast, rectal, sarcoma, head and neck, and pancreatic primary cancers. In fact, the addition of radiation therapy as an adjunctive therapy has allowed for less-radical procedures to be performed with an improvement in the quality of life of patients. A prime example of this is in breast cancer. Several clinical trials have demonstrated that the overall survival of patients with invasive breast cancer was comparable if treated by mastectomy versus lumpectomy plus adjuvant radiotherapy (see Chapter 55). This realization has resulted in better cosmesis and quality of life. In the National Surgical Adjuvant Breast and Bowel Project protocol, B-06, local recurrence in breast cancer patients did not affect overall survival.[12] In this seminal study, women with stage I or II breast cancer were randomized to total mastectomy with axillary node dissection, lumpectomy, and axillary node dissection followed by breast irradiation, or lumpectomy and axillary node dissection without irradiation. There was a significantly greater local relapse of tumor in women who underwent lumpectomy who did not receive breast irradiation versus those who received it (10% versus 39%, respectively, P less than 0.001). However, there was no difference in overall survival between any of the randomized groups. This study demonstrated the improved local control achieved with irradiation combined with lumpectomy.

Another example of how irradiation has altered surgical management of cancers is with extremity sarcomas. Before the 1970s, amputation was the standard surgical therapy of extremity soft tissue sarcomas because of the excessive local relapse rate with wide excisions. In a landmark trial conducted at the National Cancer Institute, subjects with high-grade soft tissue sarcomas were randomized to receive amputation versus limb-sparing surgery plus radiotherapy.[13] All subjects received postoperative chemotherapy. Despite a higher local recurrence rate in the limb salvage group, there were no significant differences in overall survival between the randomized groups. This study paved the way for offering limb salvage procedures for patients with soft tissue sarcomas.

As the field of multimodality therapy has developed, the role of surgery as primary therapy for certain solid malignancies has changed. The concept of neoadjuvant therapy where chemotherapy and/or radiation therapy is administered before surgical resection has become standard care for some tumors. A prime example of this is the treatment of anal squamous cell cancers. Before the 1970s, the primary therapy for this cancer was an abdominoperineal resection, which involves removal of the rectum and creation of a permanent colostomy. The discovery of effective chemoradiation therapy for this tumor has resulted in a high percentage of complete responses in many patients who then require having only excisional biopsies of residual scar.[14,15] This change has spared patients from having an abdominoperineal resection, which is now reserved for those who fail to completely respond to chemoradiation or who subsequently relapse. Another example is the treatment of childhood rhabdomyosarcomas. In breast cancer, the use of neoadjuvant chemotherapy has been able to render many more women to be candidates for breast-sparing surgery who may not have been initially because of large tumor size.[16,17] Postoperative adjuvant therapies involving chemotherapy and/or radiation therapy have also become standard approaches in many solid tumors, resulting in improved local control and overall survival.

Surgical Resection of Regional Lymph Nodes

The regional lymph nodes represent the most prevalent site of metastasis for solid tumors. Because of this, the involvement of the regional lymph nodes represents an important prognostic factor in the staging of the cancer patient. For this reason, the removal of the regional lymph nodes is often performed at the time of resection of the primary cancer. Besides staging information, a regional lymphadenectomy provides *regional control* of the cancer. Examples of this are patients with melanoma who have tumor metastatic to lymph nodes. It is well documented that the removal of these regional lymph nodes can result in long-term survival benefit in approximately 20% to 40% of individuals depending upon the extent of nodal involvement. Hence, the removal of regional lymph nodes can be therapeutic.

The controversies regarding regional lymphadenectomy for solid malignancies have related to the timing of the procedure as well as the extent of the procedure. For some visceral solid tumors such as gastric and pancreatic cancers, the extent of lymphadenectomy at the time of primary tumor resection has been hypothesized to be important in optimizing local and regional control and has an impact on improving overall survival. This concept has not been borne out in prospective randomized trials of gastric cancer in which the extent of lymphadenectomy has been examined (see Chapter

42). Based on these trials, the more-extended lymphadenectomy appears to result in more accurate staging of patients at a cost of increased morbidity. For nonvisceral solid tumors such as melanoma, breast cancers, and head and neck squamous cancers, the *elective* removal of regional lymph nodes at the time of primary tumor resection has been postulated to result in better survival outcomes compared to taking the wait-and-watch approach. The latter involves performing a lymphadenectomy only when the patient relapses in a nodal basin that would then necessitate a therapeutic lymph node dissection. In prospective randomized clinical studies evaluating elective versus therapeutic lymph node dissection in various tumor types, there was no survival advantage for performing elective lymph node dissections (Table 4.2).[18–25] It is apparent from these controversies that the initial removal of regional lymph nodes is most important for its staging impact, rather than its therapeutic effect. The introduction of *selective lymphadenectomy* based upon the concept of the *sentinel lymph node* has dramatically improved our ability to stage the regional lymph nodes of certain cancers. This is reviewed in more detail in the Diagnosis and Staging section of this chapter.

Surgical Resection of Metastatic Disease

The resection of *isolated* metastases in patients with solid malignancies should always be a consideration when technically feasible. The term *isolated* metastasis implies that there are no other sites of metastatic disease present as assessed by clinical and imaging modalities. Hence, the selection of candidate patients for surgical resection requires a thorough evaluation of the individual's disease status, preoperative medical status, and assessment of the feasibility of resecting the metastatic site with a negative margin. This process ends up identifying a small subset of patients who would be surgical candidates. Although there are no prospective randomized

TABLE 4.2. Randomized trials evaluating elective versus therapeutic lymphadenectomy (Level 1 evidence).

Author	*Reference*	*Cancer*	*Year*	*No. of patients*	*Randomized groups*	*F/U period*	*Results*
Fisher et al.	18, 19	Breast (clinical T1, T2, NO)	1977	1,079	Total mastectomy vs. total mastectomy and RT[a] vs. radical mastectomy	21 years	No significant differences between groups in overall or disease-free survival
Vandenbrouck et al.	20	Squamous cell cancer of oral cavity (clinical T1-3, NO)	1980	75	Elective neck dissection vs. therapeutic neck dissection	5 years	No significant differences between groups in overall or disease-free survival
Veronesi et al.	21, 22	Extremity melanoma (clinical NO)	1977	553	Elective lymphadenectomy vs. therapeutic lymphadenectomy	5 years	No significant differences between groups in overall or disease-free survival
Sim et al.	23	Melanoma (clinical NO)	1986	171	No lymphadenectomy vs. elective lymphadenectomy vs. delayed lymphadenectomy	4.5 years	No significant differences between groups in overall or disease-free survival
Balch et al.	24	Melanoma (intermediate thickness; clinical NO)	1996	740	Elective lymphadenectomy vs. therapeutic lymphadenectomy	7.4 years	No significant differences between groups in overall or disease-free survival
Cascinelli et al.	25	Truncal melanoma (>1.5 mm thickness; clinical NO)	1998	240	Elective lymphadenectomy vs. therapeutic lymphadenectomy	11 years	No significant differences between groups in overall or disease-free survival

F/U, follow-up.

[a]RT, radiation therapy to chest wall, internal mammary, axillary, and supraclavicular lymph nodes.

clinical studies documenting the survival benefit of surgical resection of isolated metastases, there is a significant body of retrospective evidence indicating that this approach can result in significant long-term benefit in patients with either lung or liver metastases. Aside from the regional lymph nodes, both lung and liver represent the next most common sites to which solid tumors metastasize.

The resection of metastases to the lung in patients with osteogenic or soft tissue sarcomas has been established from numerous retrospective reports. Both osteogenic and soft tissue sarcomas have a propensity to metastasize to the lung as the only site. Computed tomography studies of the lung are capable of identifying lesions that are a few millimeters in size. Multiple wedge excisions can be performed utilizing stapling devices without compromise of pulmonary function. Pulmonary metastasectomies for bone and soft tissue sarcoma can result in 5-year overall survival rates of approximately 35% if all disease is resected.[26,27] The resection of metastases for adenocarcinomas is not so well documented. Primary adenocarcinomas often metastasize to multiple sites and do not result in isolated lung metastases. When they are confined to the lung, the metastases are often too numerous to consider wedge resections. There are retrospective reports indicating that, in select patients with metastatic adenocarcinomas to the lung (i.e., colorectal primaries), resection can result in long-term survival benefit.[28,29]

A large body of retrospective evidence documents the benefit of resecting isolated liver metastases; this is especially the case for colorectal primary cancers. These cancers appear to have a pattern of spread that involves the liver as the initial site of metastasis. Resection of solitary or multiple colorectal liver metastases has resulted in a 25% to 40% overall 5-year survival rate, depending on the extent of liver involvement. Factors that have been associated with better survival are node-negative primary cancers, prolonged disease-free interval from time of primary resection to diagnosis of liver metastases, negative margins of hepatic resection, and fewer numbers of hepatic metastases (see Chapter 95). Current trials are under way to determine if adjuvant therapies given after hepatic metastasectomies further improve survival in this patient group. Besides colorectal liver metastases, the resection of noncolorectal liver metastases also can be therapeutic or palliative for selected individuals. For example, the resection of functional neuroendocrine metastases to the liver can result in palliation and prolonged survival of patients.[30] These tumors tend to be indolent in their growth rate; however, the symptoms associated with the metastatic lesion can often be detrimental to the quality of life of the patient. For other nonneuroendocrine, noncolorectal liver metastases, resection can result in survival benefit as well. Patients with isolated genitourinary or gynecologic primary malignancies with a prolonged disease-free interval have been reported to benefit from aggressive resection of hepatic metastases.[31]

Both liver and lung represent the majority of the evidence that resection of visceral metastases can result in long-term survival. These results have been observed usually in the absence of adjuvant systemic therapies. Our current concept that solid malignancies are systemic at their onset (i.e., breast cancer) would have us surmise that, with the presence of bulky visceral metastases, there must also be micrometastatic disease present at the time the bulky disease is resected. Nevertheless, approximately 20% to 25% of individuals remain disease free for many years. This finding begs the notion that perhaps an immune mechanism is involved in preventing disease relapse in a subset of these patients. Besides liver and lung sites, there are clearly anecdotes and published series indicating that the resection of isolated metastases to skin, bowel, adrenal glands, pancreas, and other sites can result in survival benefit. One of the roles of the surgical oncologist is to know when it is appropriate to offer surgical resection of metastatic disease as a palliative or therapeutic option.

Diagnosis and Staging

In addition to operating for curative purposes, the surgical oncologist will often operate for the purpose of obtaining tissue for diagnosis or staging or for monitoring response to therapy. Biopsies for diagnosis can be done with fine-needle aspiration, core-needle biopsy, or incisional or excisional biopsy.

Fine-Needle Aspiration

Fine-needle aspirations obtain cell suspensions suitable for cytology or flow cytometry. This technique can be helpful in aspirating a thyroid nodule, sometimes a breast lump, or a lymph node whenever lymphoma is not primary in the differential diagnosis. The advantages to fine-needle aspiration include the lack of a scar, lack of need for anesthetic, good patient tolerance of the procedure, and the relatively fast turnover of cytology in obtaining a diagnosis. Cell-surface receptors cannot be evaluated, and cytology cannot distinguish between invasive and noninvasive cancers. A fine-needle aspiration should be done only when the determination of atypical or malignant cells will help in diagnosis or treatment, such as proceeding with a thyroid lobectomy or documenting whether a lesion is recurrent cancer in a patient with a known history of the disease. Although a determination of cell abnormality and malignancy can be done, it is usually not sufficient for determining the definitive diagnosis of a primary neoplasm, with the possible exception of abnormal cytology on brushings from an endoscopic examination in a patient with a pancreatic head mass or bile duct stricture. Because of the possibility of false-positive results, cytology is not considered sufficient for proceeding with a major surgical resection such as a mastectomy. In such instances, a method of biopsy that yields definitive histology should be obtained.

Core-Needle Biopsy

Core-needle biopsies can be done percutaneously by palpating a mass or lymph node or by radiologic guidance. Core biopsy material yields tissue architecture, including the diagnosis of malignancy, the tissue of origin of the primary tumor, whether a tumor is noninvasive or invasive, and cell-surface receptors. Advantages include the ability to do the biopsy under local anesthesia, minimal scarring, and improved patient tolerance of the procedure. Care should be taken to keep the entry point for the needle in a location that can be incorporated in a definitive resection of the mass in the event the result shows a malignancy (Figure 4.2). A core-needle biopsy when diagnostic can allow planning for either neoadjuvant or adjuvant therapies or for surgical resection. For example, a core-needle biopsy of a large breast mass can allow neoadjuvant chemotherapy of a breast malignancy and possibly downstage the patient to being a breast conservation candidate, particularly when an excisional biopsy would be cosmetically unacceptable and obligate a mastectomy. Thus, it is usually the procedure of choice for making a pathologic diagnosis in many areas of oncology. For large soft tissue tumors or bone lesions, core biopsies should be the first method to consider to obtain a diagnosis.[32,33] However, core needle biopsies often do not yield sufficient tissue for making a diagnosis of primary lymphoma, which often requires incisional or excisional biopsies.

Incisional Biopsy

Incisional biopsies are usually done when a needle biopsy is nondiagnostic or technically not feasible. Common examples include a pancreatic mass in which attempts at obtaining cytology by endoscopic brushings or fine-needle aspiration via endoscopic ultrasound have been nondiagnostic, or for a retroperitoneal mass that is potentially a lymphoma. For these intraabdominal tumors, the minimally invasive laparoscopic approach offers advantages of obtaining adequate tissue material as well as staging information that might not be appreciated by imaging modalities. For tumors outside the abdomen, care should be taken in planning an incisional biopsy to keep the biopsy within the area of the definitive operation. Biopsies of the extremity should be done along the line of the long axis of the extremity (Figure 4.3). An improperly placed transverse incision on the extremity can lead to an unnecessarily morbid procedure because the definitive resection must achieve negative margins around the area of previous dissection (Figure 4.4). Impeccable hemostasis should be obtained during incisional biopsy procedures because the complication of a postoperative hematoma can lead to the dissemination of tumor cells into tissue planes well beyond the area that would be resected for definitive surgical therapy. For large cutaneous lesions, a *punch biopsy* represents a form of incisional biopsy that will sample all layers of the skin including the subcutaneous fat (Figure 4.5A). This procedure can be performed under local anesthesia in the outpatient setting using disposable punch biopsy tools (Figure 4.5B).

Excisional Biopsy

Smaller tumors are often more amenable to excisional biopsy. Excisional biopsy implies the removal of the entire skin lesion or lump. Small, particularly superficial, mobile tumors can be difficult to obtain with an adequate needle biopsy. Small masses or skin lesions on the extremity or trunk that are potentially malignant are often best approached with an excisional biopsy, as it allows definitive diagnosis without risking violation of tissue planes. Disadvantages include the resultant scar, the need for anesthetic, and the potential need for reexcision for margins. It is important to orientate excisional biopsy specimens in three dimensions for the pathologist to determine margins if surgical reexcision is needed. The precautions regarding orientation of incisions, not violating tissue planes, and hemostasis are the same as mentioned in the previous section on incisional biopsies.

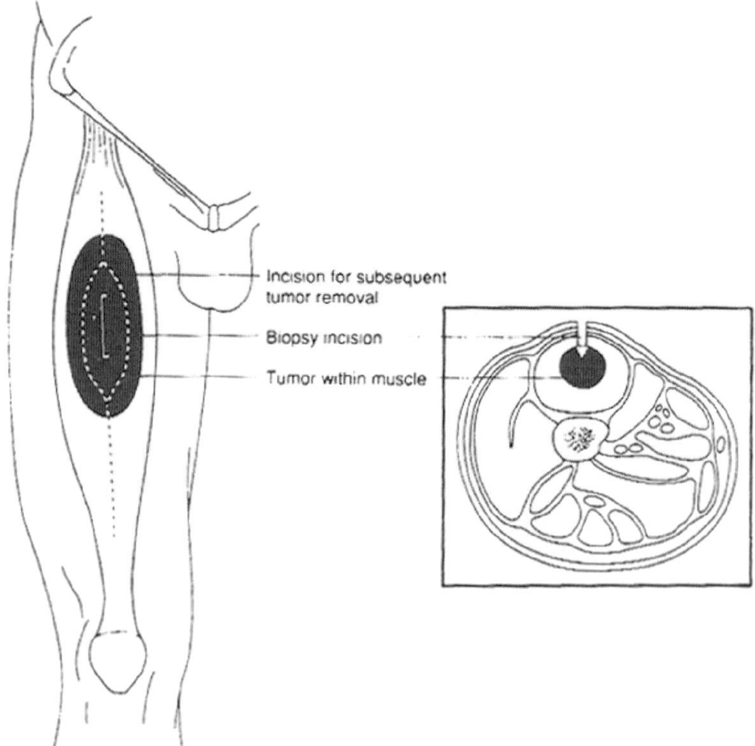

FIGURE 4.3. Placement of an incisional biopsy incision in a patient with an extremity soft tissue tumor. These incisions should be placed parallel to the long axis of the extremity. [By permission of Sondak VK. In: Greenfield LJ, et al. (eds). *Surgery Scientific Principles and Practice*. Philadelphia: Lippincott: Williams & Wilkins, 1993.]

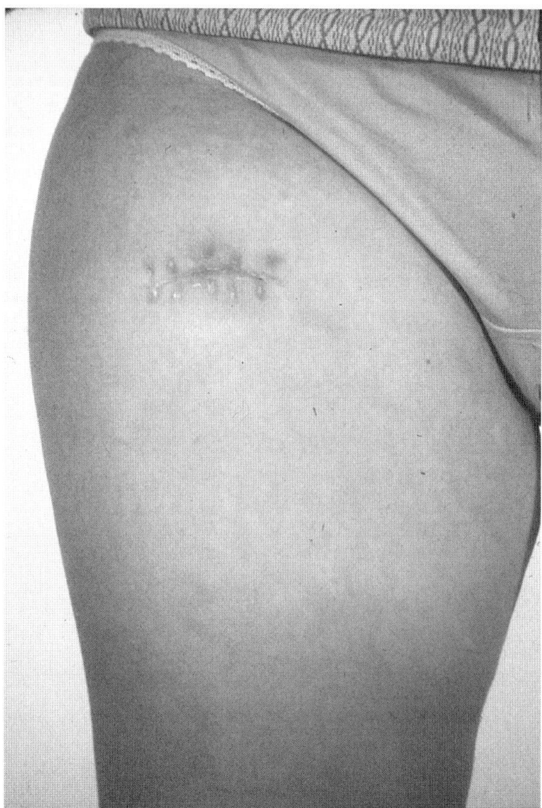

FIGURE 4.4. Improperly placed transverse incision of a large soft tissue tumor. The tumor proved to be a high-grade sarcoma, with the subsequent wide excision being compromised because of the initial procedure.

Care should be taken, when biopsying more then one lesion of the same patient, to use separate instrument setups between biopsies in the event that not all the lesions are malignant to avoid cross-contamination of malignant cells between surgical sites. In this setting, precise labeling of each biopsy specimen is needed in the event that only one of the biopsied lesions is malignant to correctly identify the area to be further treated. It is also important to ensure proper handling of specimens. For example, lymph node tissue obtained for the potential diagnosis of lymphoma should go to pathology fresh to procure part of the specimen for flow cytometry.

In addition to obtaining biopsies to make a diagnosis, the surgical oncologist is increasingly called on to do a biopsy to assess response to adjuvant therapy because routine imaging studies do not always reflect what is happening at the tissue level. For example, necrotic tumor may still show as a mass on CT or mammography. In some protocols, serial biopsies are obtained to access response to therapy; this is most often done as a core-needle biopsy.

Sentinel Lymph Node Biopsy

Increasingly, attempts at a more minimal approach to lymph node staging are being done with selective lymphadenectomy, also known as sentinel lymph node mapping or biopsy. The principle underlying this approach assumes that a cancer will metastasize to one or more *sentinel nodes* in the regional lymph node basin(s) as defined by the anatomic distribution of lymphatic vessels present within and adjacent to the tumor (Figure 4.6).[34] One can determine whether the lymph node basin is involved with tumor by removing the sentinel lymph nodes and performing careful histologic examination of the nodes. Negative sentinel nodes predict fairly accurately that the remaining nodes within that basin will also be uninvolved with tumor, thereby avoiding the need for a regional lymphadenectomy and its attendant complications. This method has become the standard of care for staging patients with invasive breast cancer or melanoma (greater than 1 mm thickness) and is increasingly being evaluated in other malignancies such as head and neck, lung, gynecologic (i.e., cervical cancer), and gastrointestinal malignancies (i.e., colorectal and gastric cancers). The sixth edition of the American Joint Commission on Cancer staging guidelines has been revised to reflect the identification of micrometastasis to lymph nodes in melanoma and breast cancer (see Chapters 55 and 60).

Complete lymph node dissections of the affected lymph node basin should be performed for positive sentinel lymph nodes. Continued questions remain regarding the incorporation of sentinel lymph node biopsy into melanoma treatment, including whether this method of staging and treating lymph node basins affects overall or disease-free survival (as is being evaluated in the Multicenter Selective Lymphadenectomy Trial), the natural history of microscopic sentinel node metastasis, and whether survival is affected by lymphadenectomy or treatments with interferon alpha-2b in these patients (as is being evaluated in the Sunbelt Melanoma Trial).[35] Sentinel lymph node biopsy has been accepted as accurately staging the clinically negative axilla in early-stage breast cancer patients with accuracy rates of 97% or greater. Currently, all patients with histologically proven metastasis to the sentinel node undergo completion axillary lymph node dissection.

Cancer Prevention

With the exponential increase in our understanding of inherited genetic mutations and the identification of patients who are predisposed to malignant transformation, surgical therapy has expanded beyond the therapy of established tumors and into the prevention of cancer. Prophylaxis is not a new concept in surgical oncology. Patients with chronic inflammatory diseases are known to be at high risk of subsequent malignant transformation. This realization typically prompts close surveillance and surgical resection at the first identification of premalignant changes. However, with the ability to perform genetic screening for relevant mutations, cancer prevention can be implemented before the onset of symptoms or histologic changes. With the decoding of the entire human genome, it is likely that more genes responsible for specific cancers will be identified, and the potential role for prevention will expand. Although many interventions may ultimately be nonsurgical (such as tamoxifen for the chemoprevention of breast cancer), the role of surgical therapy remains a primary option in the prevention of cancer. It is for this reason that all surgical oncologists must be aware of those high-risk situations that require surgery to prevent subsequent malignant disease (Table 4.3).

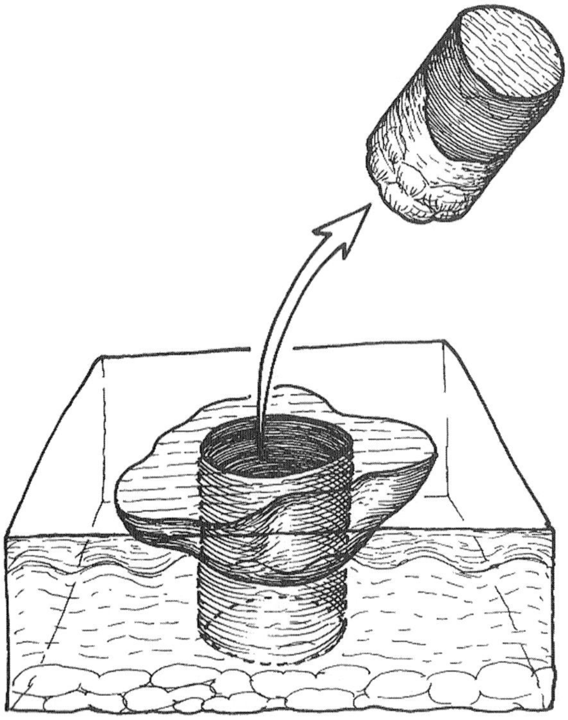

A

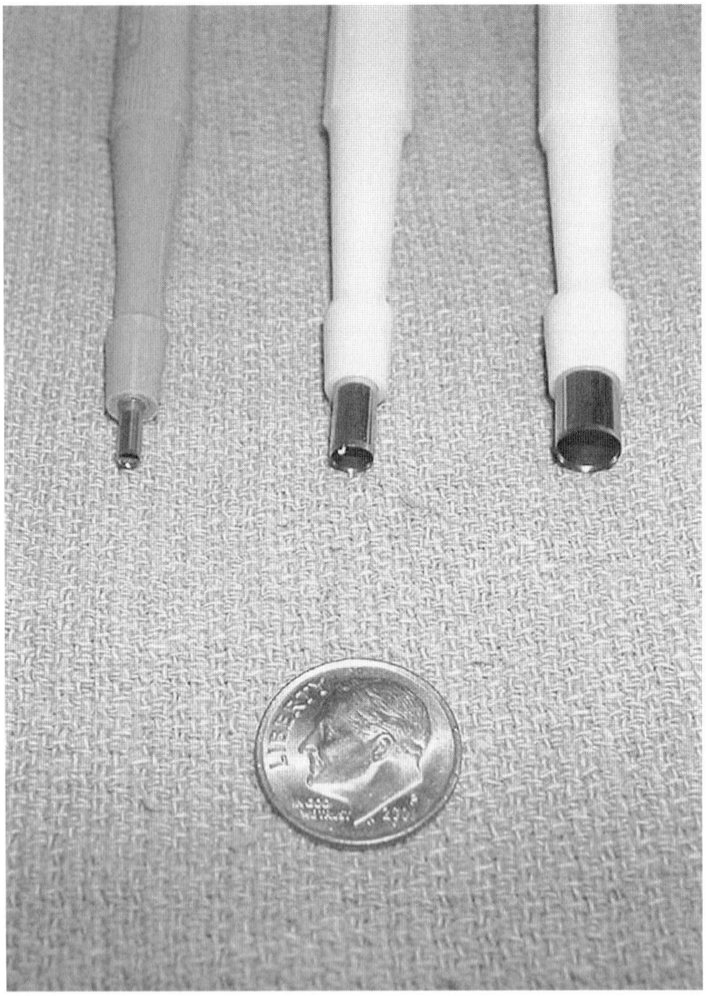

B

FIGURE 4.5. Punch biopsy of large cutaneous lesions. (A) Schematic view demonstrating that all layers of the skin can be sampled using this technique. (B) Different size punch biopsy tools that can be used. (A: From Arca MJ, Biermann JS, Johnson TM, et al.,[32] by permission of *Surgical Oncology Clinics of North America*.)

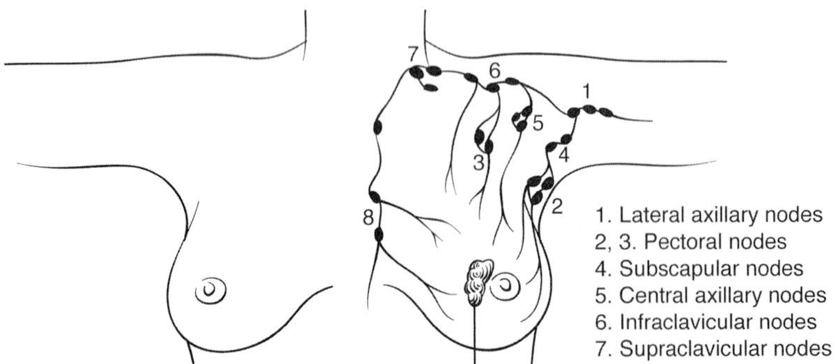

FIGURE 4.6. Schematic diagram illustrating the lymphatic drainage of the breast and sentinel lymph nodes.

TABLE 4.3. Potential indications for prophylactic organ removal.

Prophylactic surgery	*Potential indications*
Bilateral mastectomy (patients with no history of cancer)	BRCA1 or BRCA2 mutation Atypical hyperplasia or lobular carcinoma in situ (LCIS) Familial breast cancer
Bilateral mastectomy (patients with unilateral breast cancer)	BRCA1 or BRCA2 mutation Familial breast cancer or age of diagnosis less than 40 years History of atypical hyperplasia or LCIS followed by unilateral breast CA Difficult to evaluate contralateral breast
Bilateral oophorectomy in patients with no history of cancer	BRCA1 mutation Familial ovarian cancer Hereditary nonpolyposis colorectal cancer
Bilateral oophorectomy in addition to other abdominal cancer surgeries (postmenopausal women)	Hysterectomy for endometrial cancer Colon resection for colon cancer
Thyroidectomy	RET proto-oncogene mutation Multiple endocrine neoplasia type 2A (MEN 2A) Multiple endocrine neoplasia type 2B (MEN 2B) Familial non-MEN medullary thyroid carcinoma (FMTC)
Total proctocolectomy	Familial adenomatous polyposis (FAP) or APC mutation Ulcerative colitis Hereditary nonpolyposis colorectal carcinoma (HNPCC) germ-line mutation

Colorectal Cancer

One of the earliest examples of surgical prophylaxis is the recommendation for total proctocolectomy for subsets of patients with chronic ulcerative colitis. Patients with pancolitis, onset of disease at a young age, and a long duration of colitis are at high risk of developing colorectal cancer.[36] Other clinical diseases of the large intestine also illustrate the role of proctocolectomy in cancer prevention. Familial adenomatous polyposis coli (FAP) syndrome, defined by the diffuse involvement of the colon and rectum with adenomatous polyps often in the second or third decade of life, almost always predisposes to colorectal cancer if the large intestine is left in place. However, the role of screening and prophylactic proctocolectomy changed dramatically with the identification of the gene responsible for FAP, the adenomatous polyposis coli (APC) gene, located on the long arm of chromosome 5 (5q21).[37] Now, children of families in which an APC mutation has been identified can have genetic testing before polyps become evident. Carriers can have screening and surgical resection once polyps appear, usually in the late teens or early twenties. Although not ideal, the palatability of proctocolectomy in this population was furthered with the description of the total abdominal colectomy, mucosal proctectomy, and ileoanal pouch anastomosis.[38]

As we identify additional syndromes and genes that carry an increased risk of colorectal cancer, the potential role of screening and prophylactic surgery also expands. Hereditary nonpolyposis colorectal carcinoma (HNPCC), or Lynch syndrome, is an autosomal dominant disorder that is estimated to be responsible for 5% to 10% of all colorectal cancers. Although the carcinomas arise from benign adenomas, HNPCC is not characterized by a large number of polyps. Two Lynch syndromes have been described. Lynch syndrome I features an early age onset of cancer, often metachronous. Lynch syndrome II involves cancers not only of the small and large intestine but also endometrial, ovarian, renal, gastric, and hepatobiliary. Although the genes responsible for HNPCC have been identified, namely hMSH1, hMLH1, hPMS1, and hPMS2, these mutations do not have a 100% penetrance; thus, cancer will not develop in all carriers. Prophylactic surgery is recommended for some but not all carriers, but aggressive screening should be implemented and a subtotal colectomy should be performed if a cancer develops.[39,40]

Breast Cancer

Another example of prophylactic surgery is the bilateral mastectomy for women at high risk of developing breast cancer. Before the identification of the BRCA genes, prophylactic mastectomies were typically reserved as an option for women with lobular carcinoma in situ (LCIS). However, with the identification of BRCA1 and BRCA2, the role of prophylactic mastectomies has been greatly expanded. For women with BRCA1 or BRCA2 mutations, the lifetime probability of breast cancer is between 40% and 85%.[41–43] Because mastectomy cannot remove all breast tissue, women can expect a 90% to 94% risk reduction with prophylactic surgery.[44] Schrag et al. calculated the estimated gain in life expectancy after prophylactic surgery versus no operation in women with either a BRCA1 or BRCA2 mutation and found a 30-year-old woman would be expected to gain 2.9 to 5.3 years of life, depending on her family history.[45] However, potential benefits of prophylactic mastectomy must be weighed against quality of life issues and the morbidity of the surgery.[46] In addition, other methods for prophylaxis, such as tamoxifen chemoprevention or bilateral oophorectomy, must be considered. Along with the increased risk of breast cancer with BRCA1/2 mutations, the risk of ovarian cancer is also increased. Bilateral oophorectomy after childbearing is complete not only reduces the risk of ovarian cancer[47] but may also decrease the risk of breast cancer.[48] A detailed discussion must be held with each patient considering bilateral mastectomies regarding the risks and benefits, the knowns and unknowns. It is becoming increasingly important that today's surgical oncologist have a clear understanding of genetics and inherited risk.

Medullary Thyroid Cancer

Increased genetic knowledge has also changed our approach to thyroid cancer. Medullary thyroid cancer (MTC) is a well-established component of multiple endocrine neoplasia syndrome type 2a (MEN 2a) or type 2b (MEN 2b). Previously, family members at risk for MEN 2 underwent annual screening for elevated calcitonin levels; however, this only detected MTC after it developed. In 1993 it was identified that mutations in the RET proto-oncogene were present in almost all cases of MEN 2a and 2b. Now family members of MEN patients can be screened for the presence of a RET mutation. Those without the mutation need not undergo additional screening, whereas those with the mutation should undergo total thyroidectomy at a young age (6 years for MEN 2a, infancy for MEN 2b).[49]

Palliation

Surgical intervention is sometimes required in the patient with unresectable advanced cancer for palliative indications. The common indications for palliation in this setting are pain, bleeding, obstruction, malnutrition, or infection. The surgeon needs to consider several factors regarding each situation as to whether the surgical intervention will add significantly to the quality of life of the patient. These factors include the expected survival of the individual, the potential morbidity of the procedure, the likelihood that the procedure will palliate the patient, and whether there are alternative nonsurgical methods of palliation.

The acute onset of pain, bleeding, or obstruction represents a potential oncologic emergency. This topic is covered in more detail in Chapter 74 (Surgical Emergencies). Probably the most common oncologic emergency that the surgeon confronts is the obstruction of a hollow viscus, which can give rise to an acute abdomen, perforation of the viscus, and possibly bleeding. The hollow viscus could be the bowel, biliary tree, endobronchial tree, ureters, or bladder. There are surgical interventions that can be employed to address these problems, and in certain instances, nonsurgical approaches with stents that are effective.

Malnutrition is a common problem in the cancer patient, especially one with advanced, unresectable disease. Nutrition can be supplemented or replaced by intravenous hyperalimentation or enteral feedings via a gastrostomy or jejunostomy tube. Commonly, the surgeon is involved in placement of vascular access for hyperalimentation. If the gastrointestinal tract is functional, the surgeon may be called upon to place a feeding tube for enteral nutrition. The nutritional support of the cancer patient as well as aspects of vascular access are reviewed in more detail in Chapters 82 and 85.

Occasionally, the surgeon is involved in palliating pain caused by a metastatic lesion compressing an organ or adjacent nerves. Examples include cutaneous or subcutaneous melanoma metastases, a large ulcerating breast cancer, or a recurrent intraabdominal sarcoma mass. As indicated previously, the surgeon needs to assess the relative risk-to-benefit ratio in resecting a symptomatic mass, knowing that it will not affect the overall survival of the patient. If the quality of life of the individual can be improved at an acceptable operative risk, then the surgical intervention is warranted.

Surgical Considerations in the Cancer Patient

There are special considerations when planning operative procedures on cancer patients beyond the normal planning done for the same operation on a nononcologic patient (Table 4.4).

TABLE 4.4. Special considerations in the cancer patient.

Oncologic factors	*Potential associated problems*
Tumor-specific factors:	
Gastrointestinal	Obstruction and aspiration risk; gastrointestinal bleeding; bowel perforation
Head and neck/mediastinal	Reduced oral intake; superior vena cava obstruction; airway compromise; difficulty with ventilation or intubation
Cerebral tumors/brain metastasis	Decreased mental status; syndrome of inappropriate secretion of antidiuretic hormone; increased intracerebral pressures
Paraneoplastic syndromes	Syndrome of inappropriate secretion of antidiuretic hormone; hypercalcemia
Cancer factors:	
Cachexia/malnutrion	Increased infection; fluid and electrolyte management; wound healing
Hypercoagulability	Venous thrombosis; superior vena cava syndrome; pulmonary embolism
Bone metastasis	Hypercalcemia; increased fracture risk; potential for cord compression; potential for difficulty with intubation
Treatment-specific factors:	
Steroids	Gastritis and gastrointestinal bleeding; diabetes; adrenal insufficiency; difficulties with wound healing
Chemotherapy	Neutropenia and anemia; pulmonary fibrosis; cardiac dysfunction; stomatitis; alteration in mucosal integrity of the gastrointestinal tract; constipation; bowel perforation; nausea; vomiting; diarrhea; hypercoagulability
Radiation therapy	Pulmonary fibrosis; difficulty with wound healing
Tamoxifen	Hypercoagulability

These considerations include cancer syndromes affecting nutrition, debilitated performance status, hypercoagulability, paraneoplastic syndromes, tumor-specific effects, and effects of chemotherapy or radiation therapy.

Tumor-Specific Effects

Alteration of physiologic function or distortion of normal anatomy may occur due to specific tumor effects. For example, tumors of the mediastinum or neck may cause venous congestion, superior vena cava obstruction, airway compression, or tracheal deviation that may make establishment of an airway or ventilatory management difficult. Gastrointestinal tumors may cause obstruction, causing an aspiration risk. Cerebral tumors or brain metastases can cause changes in mental status, syndrome of inappropriate secretion of antidiuretic hormone making perioperative fluid management difficult, or may cause an increased intercerebral pressure that affects anesthesia management of the patient.

Paraneoplastic Syndromes

Paraneoplastic syndromes such as hyponatremia due to inappropriate secretion of antidiuretic hormone such as seen in small cell lung cancers, prostate, pancreas, and other cancers, or hypercalcemia such as seen in squamous cell carcinomas of the lung, breast, or kidney, will alter nutritional and fluid and electrolyte management. Although mild hyponatremia can be associated with mild symptoms such as nausea and headaches, severe, acute hyponatremia can lead to more severe symptoms, even seizures or coma. Hypercalcemia is most often associated with bone metastasis, but it may be related to a paraneoplastic syndrome and can lead to neuromuscular symptoms such as weakness and fatigue and gastrointestinal symptoms such as nausea, ileus, and abdominal pain. Severe hypercalcemia can disturb cardiac conductivity. Given the tendency to malnutrition and low serum albumin in cancer patients, serum calcium levels are often best determined by measuring ionized calcium.

Malnutrition

A hallmark warning sign of cancer is unexplained weight loss. Malnutrition has long been recognized in surgery as being related to an increased risk of infection, with difficulties in perioperative electrolyte and fluid management, and with difficulties in wound healing postoperatively. A large National Veterans Affairs Surgical Risk Study identified the preoperative serum albumin level as the single most important predictor of 30-day mortality.[50] Cancer cachexia is a syndrome of malnutrition with muscle wasting, protein malnutrition with myopathy, incomplete nutrient utilization, glucose intolerance, and anemia with decreased nutrient absorption. Its causes are multifactorial. Cancer, or its treatment, can cause alterations in taste, stomatitis, dysphagia, anorexia, nausea and vomiting, alterations in intestinal tract absorptive surface area, gastroparesis, constipation, pancreatic insufficiency, or pain, fatigue, and depression, which in turn can lead to impaired oral intake. Gastrointestinal tumor with associated obstruction or head and neck tumors can interfere with, or prohibit, oral intake. In addition, tumor- or treatment-associated diarrhea, fistulas, or nephrotic syndrome can lead to increased nutrient loss. An assessment of nutritional status can be done by assessing for a recent weight loss of 10% or more from prediagnosis weight, current caloric intake, or by measuring albumin, prealbumin serum transferrin, or cutaneous testing for anergy.

Hypercoagulability

Cancer is associated with hypercoagulability and an increased risk of venous thrombosis or pulmonary embolism. This susceptibility can be compounded by decreased mobility resulting from fatigue and diminished functional status, or by pain related to the operative procedure. Operations particularly of risk include operations of the abdomen, pelvis, hip, or leg. Surgery that is of long duration, which uses laparoscopy, or has a degree of postoperative immobilization adds additional risk. Cancer patients have twice the risk of postoperative venous thrombosis, and three times the risk of fatal pulmonary embolism, as noncancer patients undergoing the same procedure.[51] Patients at a higher risk are those with a history of previous myeloproliferative disorders such as polycythemia vera and primary thrombocytosis, or a history of obesity, varicose veins, cardiac dysfunction, indwelling central venous catheters, inflammatory bowel disease, nephrotic syndrome, pregnancy, or estrogen use, or treatment with tamoxifen or chemotherapy. Treatment with tamoxifen induces hypercoagulability with an associated two- to threefold greater risk of venous thrombosis. This risk is increased even more in women undergoing treatment with both chemotherapy and tamoxifen.[52,53] Chemotherapy has been shown to increase the risk of thromboembolism up to 7% in early-stage breast cancer patients.[52,54]

A history of hypercoagulable abnormalities should be ascertained, such as activated protein C resistance (factor V, Leiden); prothrombin variant 20210A; antiphospholipid antibodies (lupus anticoagulant and anticardiolipin antibody); deficiency or dysfunction of antithrombin, protein C, protein S, or heparin cofactor II; dysfibrinogenemia; decreased levels of plasminogen and plasminogen activators; heparin-induced thrombocytopenia; or hyperhomocystinemia.[55]

Cancer patients older than 40 years undergoing major surgery without prophylaxis have a risk of deep venous thrombosis of 10% to 20% and a risk of fatal pulmonary embolism of 0.2% to 5.0%.[10] Although most clinical trials show pneumatic compression devices to be similar in effectiveness to prophylactic doses of subcutaneous heparin, their effectiveness is directly dependent on compliance with their use, and most clinicians recognize that, in practice, pneumatic compression devices are only on the patient a portion of the time they are nonambulatory and therefore they are not as effective.[56] The sixth American College of Chest Physicians consensus conference in 2000 recommended the following: (1) oncology patients more than 40 years old undergoing major surgery, or nonmajor surgery in patients more than 60 years old, with no other risk factors, receive pneumatic compression devices or low molecular weight heparin; (2) oncology patients more than 40 years old undergoing major surgery and additional risk factors receive pneumatic compression devices and prophylactic low molecular weight heparin; and (3) low-dose coumadin for patients with central venous catheters. They did not recommend routine continuation of anticoagulation after discharge for surgical patients;

however, many clinical studies are under way regarding the efficacy of continued prolonged anticoagulation after discharge from a surgical procedure.

Chemotherapy Considerations

Agents such as adriamycin can affect cardiac function, and an assessment of functional status, a review of systems looking for decreased exercise tolerance, dyspnea, edema, orthopnea, etc., should be elicited. On physical examination, particular attention should be paid to signs of edema, tachycardia, or arrhythmias. At minimum, a 12-lead EKG should be done on any patient who has received adriamycin before undergoing a surgical procedure to look for conduction changes. An echocardiogram for an evaluation of function should be done for any symptomatic patients before any major surgical procedure in patients who have received an adriamycin-based chemotherapy. An evaluation of respiratory symptoms should be elicited in patients who have undergone radiation to the thorax or treatment with bleomycin-based chemotherapy to evaluate for pulmonary fibrosis. Treatment with corticosteroids can lead to diabetes or adrenal insufficiency requiring monitoring of glucose levels postoperatively and potential treatment with stress dose steroids and the implications for glucose control perioperatively. Treatment with steroids can also lead to gastritis and gastrointestinal bleeding or mask symptoms of peritonitis, making evaluation of abdominal pain difficult. Chemotherapy can also affect the gastrointestinal tract, with bowel perforation having been reported in patients undergoing treatment with cytosine arabinoside, taxol, and interleukin 2. In addition it should be remembered that oncology patients will still succumb to and need to be treated for the same illnesses as nononcologic patients such as cholecystitis and appendicitis; however, treatment with steroids, or immunosuppressive agents such as seen in patients after bone marrow transplantation, and the potential for neutropenic colitis in those undergoing chemotherapy can make evaluation of these more common diseases more difficult.[57]

Elderly Patient

In addition, the readers are reminded that older or elderly patients will increasingly make up the population of patients with cancer. Currently 60% of all malignancies, and 70% of all cancer deaths, occur in people over the age of 65.[58] In addition to the previously mentioned considerations, assessment of the older patient should include evaluation of activities of daily living, depression, cognitive function, current medications and potential medication interactions, and available social support.[59–62]

Clinical Trials: Role of the Surgical Oncologist

At the very heart of evidence-based medicine, and nowhere is this truer than in oncology, are clinical trials. Although the early trials initiated by the National Cancer Institute (NCI) in the mid-1970s primarily considered nonsurgical issues (leukemia, lymphoma, stage IV disease), surgeons quickly became involved in significant roles in clinical oncology trials, such as the National Surgical Adjuvant Breast Project (NSABP), which has answered, and continues to answer, many important questions regarding the optimal surgical and adjuvant therapy of breast and colon cancer. Today, most cooperative groups include surgery committees to address ongoing questions regarding the surgical management of a variety of malignancies. The prominent role of surgery in the design and implementation of clinical oncology trials is best exemplified by the establishment of the American College of Surgeons Oncology Group (ACOSOG) to evaluate the surgical management of patients with malignant solid tumors. Created in May 1998 under the leadership of Dr. Samuel Wells, the ACOSOG is 1 of 10 cooperative groups funded by the NCI to develop and coordinate multiinstitutional clinical trials.

As surgical oncologists, our obligation is not only to the patient who is sitting before us in the office, but to the progression of patients who will follow. The improved success and decreased morbidity of the treatments that we offer today are only possible because of the involvement of surgeons and their patients in clinical trials of the past. As the newest discoveries in all fields of oncology will have a direct impact on the surgical therapy, it is imperative that surgeons continue to play prominent roles as both leaders and participants in multidisciplinary cooperative group trials. All surgical oncologists should not only incorporate clinical trials into their practice but strongly encourage the participation of the general surgical community.

References

1. Lewison EF. Breast Cancer and Its Diagnosis and Treatment. Baltimore: Williams & Wilkins, 1955.
2. Rutledge RH. Theodore Billroth: a century later. Surgery (St. Louis) 1995;118:36–43.
3. Weir R. Resection of the large intestine for carcinoma. Ann Surg 1886;1886(3):469–489.
4. Halsted WS. The results of operations for the cure of cancer of the breast performed at the Johns Hopkins Hospital from June 1889 to January 1894. Ann Surg 1894;320(13):497–555.
5. Clark JG. A more radical method for performing hysterectomy for cancer of the cervix. Johns Hopkins Bull 1895;6:121.
6. Crile G. Excision of cancer of the head and neck. JAMA 1906; XLVII:1780.
7. Miles WE. A method for performing abdominoperineal excision for carcinoma of the rectum and terminal portion of the pelvic colon. Lancet 1908;2:1812–1813.
8. Krakoff IH. Progress and prospects in cancer treatment: the Karnofsky legacy. J Clin Oncol 1994;12:432–438.
9. Farber S, Diamond LK, Mercer RD, et al. Temporary regressions in acute leukemia in children produced by folic acid antagonist, aminopteroyl-glutamic acid. N Engl J Med 1948;238: 693.
10. Huggins CB, Hodges CV. Studies on prostatic cancer: the effect of castration, of estrogen and of androgen injection on serum phosphatases in metastatic carcinoma of the prostate. Cancer Res 1941;1:293–297.
11. Lawrence W Jr, Wilson RE, Shingleton WW, et al. Surgical oncology in university departments of surgery in the United States. Arch Surg 1986;121:1088–1093.
12. Fisher B, Remond C, Poisson R, et al. Eight-year results of a randomized clinical trial comparing total mastectomy and lumpectomy with or without irradiation in the treatment of breast cancer. N Engl J Med 1989;320:822–828.
13. Rosenberg SA, Tepper J, Glatstein E, et al. The treatment of soft-tissue sarcomas of the extremities: prospective randomized evaluations of (1) limb-sparing surgery plus radiation therapy

compared with amputation and (2) the role of adjuvant chemotherapy. Ann Surg 1982:196(3):305–315.
14. Nigro ND. Multidisciplinary management of cancer of the anus. World J Surg 1987;11(4):446–451.
15. Licitra L, Spinazze S, Doci R, Evans TR, Tanum G, Ducreux M. Cancer of the anal region. Crit Rev Oncol-Hematol 2002; 43(1):77–92.
16. Fisher B, Bryant J, Wolmark N, et al. Effect of preoperative chemotherapy on the outcome of women with operable breast cancer. J Clin Oncol 1998;16(8):2672–2685.
17. Bear HD, Anderson S, Brown A, et al. National Surgical Adjuvant Breast and Bowel Project Protocol B-27. The effect on tumor response of adding sequential preoperative docetaxel to preoperative doxorubicin and cyclophosphamide: preliminary results from National Surgical Adjuvant Breast and Bowel Project Protocol B-27. J Clin Oncol 2003;21(22):4165–4174.
18. Fisher B, Montague E, Redmond C, et al. (and other NSABP investigators). Comparison of radical mastectomy with alternative treatments for primary breast cancer: a first report of results from a prospective randomized clinical trial. Cancer (Phila) 1977; 39:2827–2839.
19. Fisher B, Jeong JH, Anderson S, Bryant J, Fisher ER, Wolmark N. Twenty-five-year follow-up of a randomized trial comparing radical mastectomy, total mastectomy, and total mastectomy followed by irradiation. N Engl J Med 2002:347(8):567–575.
20. Vandenbrouck C, Sancho-Garnier H, Chassagne D, Saravane D, Cachin Y, Micheau C. Elective versus therapeutic radical neck dissection in epidermoid carcinoma of the oral cavity: results of a randomized clinical trial. Cancer (Phila) 1980; 46:386–390.
21. Veronesi U, Adamus J, Bandiera DC, et al. Inefficacy of immediate node dissection in stage 1 melanoma of the limbs. N Engl J Med 1977;297(12):627–630.
22. Veronesi U, Adamus J, Bandiera DC, et al. Delayed regional lymph node dissection in stage I melanoma of the skin of the lower extremities. Cancer (Phila) 1982;49(11):2420–2430.
23. Sim F, Taylor WF, Pritchard DJ, Soule EH. Lymphadenectomy in the management of stage I malignant melanoma: a prospective randomized study. Mayo Clin Proc 1986;61:697–705.
24. Balch C, Soong SJ, Bartolucci AA, et al. Efficacy of an elective regional lymph node dissection of 1 to 4 mm thick melanomas for patients 60 years of age and younger. Ann Surg 1996; 224(3):255–266.
25. Cascinelli N, Morabito A, Santinami M, MacKie RM, Belli F. Immediate or delayed dissection of regional nodes in patients with melanoma of the trunk: a randomized trial. Lancet 1998; 351(9105):793–796.
26. van Geel AN, Pastorino U, Jauch KW, et al. Surgical treatment of lung metastases: the European Organization for Research and Treatment of Cancer – Soft Tissue and Bone Sarcoma Group study of 255 patients. Cancer (Phila) 1996;77:675–682.
27. Billingsley KG, Burt ME, Jara E, et al. Pulmonary metastases from soft tissue sarcoma: analysis of patterns of diseases and postmetastasis survival. Ann Surg 1999;229:602–612.
28. McAfee MK, Allen MS, Trastek VF, Ilstrup DM, Deschamps C, Pairolero PC. Colorectal lung metastases: results of surgical excision. Ann Thorac Surg 1992;53:780–786.
29. Ishikawa K, Hashiguchi Y, Mochizuki H, Ozeki Y, Ueno H. Extranodal cancer deposit at the primary tumor site and the number of pulmonary lesions are useful prognostic factors after surgery for colorectal lung metastases. Dis Colon Rectum 2003; 46:629–636.
30. Que FG, Nagorney DM, Batts KP, Linz LJ, Kvols LK. Hepatic resection for metastatic neuroendocrine carcinomas. Am J Surg 1995;169:36–43.
31. Harrison LE, Brennan MF, Newman E, et al. Hepatic resection for noncolorectal, nonneuroendocrine metastases: a fifteen-year experience with ninety-six patients. Surgery (St. Louis) 1997; 121:625–632.
32. Arca MJ, Biermann JS, Johnson TM, Chang AE. Biopsy techniques for skin, soft tissue, and bone neoplasms. Surg Oncol Clin N Am 1995;17:1–11.
33. Barth RJ Jr, Merino MJ, Solomon D, Yang JC, Baker AR. A prospective study of the value of core needle biopsy and fine needle aspiration in the diagnosis of soft tissue masses. Surgery (St. Louis) 1992;112:536–543.
34. Morton DL, Wen DR, Wong JH, et al. Technical details of intraoperative lymphatic mapping for early stage melanoma. Arch Surg 1992;127:392–399.
35. Reintgen D, Pendas S, Jakub J, et al. National trials involving lymphatic mapping for melanoma: the Multicenter Selective Lymphadenectomy Trial, the Sunbelt Melanoma Trial, and the Florida Melanoma Trial. Semin Oncol 2004;31:363–373.
36. Ekbom A, Helmick C, Zack M, et al. Ulcerative colitis and colorectal cancer: a population-based study. N Engl J Med 1990; 323:1228–1233.
37. Miyoshi Y, Nagase H, Ando H, et al. Somatic mutations of the APC gene in colorectal tumors: mutation cluster region in the APC gene. Hum Mol Genet 1992;1:229–233.
38. Ambroze W Jr, Dozois R, Pemberton J, et al. Familial adenomatous polyposis: results following ileal pouch-anal anastomosis and ileorectostomy. Dis Colon Rectum 1992;35:12–15.
39. Rodriguez-Bigas MA, Boland CR, Hamilton SR, et al. A National Cancer Institute workshop on Hereditary Nonpolyposis Colorectal Cancer Syndrome: meeting highlights and Bethesda guidelines. J Natl Cancer Inst 1997;89:1758–1762.
40. Lynch HT, Lynch J. Lynch syndrome: genetics, natural history, genetic counseling, and prevention. J Clin Oncol 2000;18(21a): 19s–31s.
41. Mann GB, Borgen PI. Breast cancer genes and the surgeon. J Surg Oncol 1998;67:267–274.
42. Eeles RA, Powles TJ. Chemoprevention options for BRCA1 and BRCA2 mutation carriers. J Clin Oncol 2000;18:93s–99s.
43. Anderson BO. Prophylactic surgery to reduce breast cancer risk: a brief literature review. Breast J 2001;7(5):321–330.
44. Hartmann LC, Schaid DJ, Woods JE, et al. Efficacy of bilateral prophylactic mastectomy in women with a family history of breast cancer. N Engl J Med 1999;340:77–84.
45. Schrag D, Kuntz KM, Garber JE, Weeks JC. Decision analysis: effects of prophylactic mastectomy and oophorectomy on life expectancy among women with BRCA1 or BRCA2 mutations. N Engl J Med 1997;336:1465–1471.
46. Newman LA, Keurer HM, Hunt KK, et al. Prophylactic mastectomy. J Am Cancer Soc 2000;191(3):322–330.
47. Rebbeck TR. Prophylactic oophorectomy in BRCA1 and BRCA2 mutation carriers. J Clin Oncol 2000;18(21s):100s–103s.
48. Rebbeck TR, Levin AM, Eisen A, et al. Breast cancer risk after bilateral prophylactic oophorectomy in BRCA1 mutation carriers. J Natl Cancer Inst 1999;91:1475–1479.
49. Phay JE, Moley JF, Lairmore TC. Multiple endocrine neoplasias. Semin Surg Oncol 2000;18:324–332.
50. Daley J, Khuri SF, Henderson W, et al. Risk adjustment of the postoperative morbidity rate for the comparative assessment of the quality of surgical care: results of the National Veterans Affairs Surgical Risk Study. J Am Coll Surg 1997;185:328–340.
51. Kakkar AK, Williamson RC. Prevention of venous thromboembolism in cancer patients. Semin Thromb Hemost 1999; 25:239–243.
52. Saphner T, Tormey DC, Gray R. Venous and arterial thrombosis in patients who received adjuvant therapy for breast cancer. J Clin Oncol 1991;9:286–294.
53. Deitcher SR, Gomes MP. The risk of venous thromboembolic disease associated with adjuvant hormone therapy for breast carcinoma: a systematic review. Cancer (Phila) 2004;101:439–449.

54. Levine MN, Gent M, Hirsh J, et al. The thrombogenic effect of anticancer drug therapy in women with stage II breast cancer. N Engl J Med 1988;318:404–407.
55. Geerts WH, Heit JA, Clagett GP, et al. Prevention of venous thromboembolism. Chest 2001;119:132S–175S.
56. Maxwell GL, Synan I, Dodge R, Carroll B, Clarke-Pearson DL. Pneumatic compression versus low molecular weight heparin in gynecologic oncology surgery: a randomized trial. Obstet Gynecol 2001;98:989–995.
57. Diehl KM, Chang AE. Acute abdomen, bowel obstruction, and fistula. In: Abeloff MD, Armitage JO, Niederhuber JE, Kastan MB, McKenna WG (eds). Clinical Oncology. Philadelphia: Elsevier Churchill Livingstone, 2004:1025–1045.
58. American Cancer Society: Cancer Facts and Figures 2003. Atlanta, GA: American Cancer Society, 2003.
59. Extermann M, Meyer J, McGinnis M, et al. A comprehensive geriatric intervention detects multiple problems in older breast cancer patients. Crit Rev Oncol Hematol 2004;49:69–75.
60. Chen CC, Kenefick AL, Tang ST, McCorkle R. Utilization of comprehensive geriatric assessment in cancer patients. Crit Rev Oncol Hematol 2004;49:53–67.
61. Extermann M. Studies of comprehensive geriatric assessment in patients with cancer. Cancer Control 2003;10:463–468.
62. Balducci L. Geriatric oncology. Crit Rev Oncol Hematol 2003; 46:211–220.

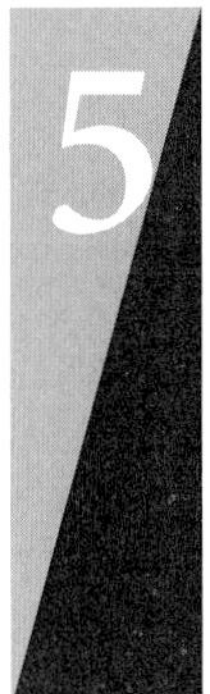

Principles of Targeted and Biological Therapies

Stephen R.D. Johnston, Sue Chua, and Charles Swanton

Development of Targeted Therapies

One of the characteristics of the malignant phenotype is the ability of cells to grow in an autonomous manner. Various components of the proliferative and/or survival signaling pathways can become constitutively activated or deregulated in human cancers.[1] Many studies have attempted to show that a given molecular change is the key event involved in the pathogenesis of a specific cancer. Such information may not only provide a better understanding of cancer but may allow a novel target to be identified for therapeutic intervention.

With our ever-increasing understanding of the pathogenesis of cancer, there are now a plethora of potential molecular targets in human cancer cells that are being utilized for the development of novel anticancer therapies (Table 5.1). Perhaps the oldest and most established targeted therapy is endocrine treatment for breast and prostate cancer, taking advantage of the estrogen receptor (ER) and androgen receptor (AR) that can readily be detected in many breast and prostate carcinomas, respectively. More recently, peptide growth factor receptors (EGFR and HER2) have become viable targets in human solid epithelial tumors such as lung, head and neck, breast, and colon cancer. The unraveling of the signal transduction cascade within cells has resulted in various small molecule signal transduction inhibitors (STIs) entering clinical development, whereas the complex protein interactions that regulate the cell cycle may allow various modulators to be developed to restore cell-cycle control in aberrantly behaving malignant cells. Likewise the ability to effectively trigger programmed cell death (apoptosis) in cancer cells adapted to prolonged survival is a promising new approach for the future. Finally, the capacity for malignant cells to acquire a blood supply is a key event in the growth of human tumors, and drugs are being developed that target either the endothelial cell or the vascular growth factor pathways. The principles and current status of targeted therapies in each of these six areas are reviewed in this chapter. However, a common theme to all these approaches is the need to confirm that a given molecular target is specifically involved in the pathogenesis of that cancer, to develop an assay to reliably detect the target in tumors, and to show that interrupting its function gives the desired anticancer effect.

Target Identification

Some of the problems of target identification in cancer are illustrated by considering kinases, regulatory enzymes that are integral to most signaling events inside cells. In cancer, these may be either pivotal or permissive for the pathogenesis of the malignant phenotype.[2] Pivotal kinases are often critical to tumor growth and maintenance and may be subject to activation by mutation, gene amplification, or translocation (i.e., p210BCR-ABL in chronic myeloid leukemia), whereas permissive kinases are not mutated or amplified but still may have a role in signal transduction pathways important in neoplastic growth. One of the challenges has been to identify pivotal kinases for anticancer drug development and to select patients with aberrations in these critical signaling pathways for inclusion in early clinical trials. To do this, robust biologic assays are required that will readily identify potential targets in cancer cells.

High-throughput screening using cDNA microarrays and techniques such as comparative genomic hybridization have been extensively employed to analyze gene expression in human tumors, thereby identifying novel targets for therapeutic drug development.[3] Target identification and validation have been supported by tissue microarray profiling that allows the analysis of DNA, RNA, or protein levels in thousands of tumor specimens at a time to identify the frequency of molecular alterations in a population of patients with a given cancer type. In future, complex proteomic techniques using mass spectrometry will allow the identification of potential protein drug targets that are differentially expressed between tumor and normal tissue. Preclinical studies are important to determine what a gene product–protein target does in the cell, and moreover what the consequences are of inhibiting its expression or function, respectively. The technique of synthetic short interfering RNAs (siRNA) that lead to the degradation of complementary mRNA, thereby silencing gene expression, is a helpful new tool in analyzing the functional significance of certain gene products. Similarly, high-throughput screens using siRNAs in mammalian cells are in progress to identify molecular regulators that are involved in the acquisition of the malignant phenotype and also in the development of drug resistance.

TABLE 5.1. Targets for the development of novel anticancer therapies.

Molecular target	*Anticancer therapeutic strategy*	*Tumor type and stage of clinical development*
Steroid hormone receptor		
ER	Antiestrogen (tamoxifen, fulvestrant),	Approved breast
AR	Aromatase inhibitor, LHRH agonist	Approved prostate
	Antiandrogen (flutamide), LHRH agonist	
Growth factor receptor		
EGFR	MoAb (cetuximab)	Approved colon; Phs III H&N, NSCLC.
	TKI (gefitinib, erlotinib)	Approved NSCLC; Phs III breast
	MoAb (trastuzumab)	Approved Breast
HER2	TKI (lapatinib, canertinib)	Phs III breast, renal
Oncogenic kinase		
BCR-ABL	TKI (imatinib)	Approved CML, GIST
Signal transduction pathway		
Ras	FTIs (tipifarnib, lonafarnib)	Phs III MDS, CML, breast, NSCLC
Raf	B-RAF Kinase Inhib (BAY43-9006)	Phs II Melanoma
MEK	MEK Kinase Inhib (PD0325901)	Phs I
m-TOR	mTOR Antag (temsirolimus, everolimus)	Phs III breast, renal
Cell cycle		
Cdk2	CDKI (flavopiridol, UCN-01, E7070)	Phs I
Proteosome	Proteosome Inhib (bortezomib)	Approved Myeloma
Histone deacetylase	HDACI (FR901228, MS-27-275)	Phs I
Apoptosis regulators		
TRAIL	MoAb	Phs I
Bcl-2	Antisense (G3139)	Phs II NHL
P53	P53 (ONXY-015, INGN201, Nutlin)	Phs II H&N, phs I
Caspase XIAP, FLIP	Sphingosine kinase (phenoxodiol)	Phs II breast, prostate
Angiogenesis		
Endothelial cell	Endo Inhib (thalidomide, TNP-740)	Phs II renal, H&N
VEGF	Endostatin, angiostatin Antisense	Phs I
	(angiozyme) MoAb (bevacizumab)	Phs I
VEGF-R	TKI (SU11248, PTK787) MoAb (2C7)	Approved Colon, phs
Integrins	Integrin Inhib (cilengitide) MMPI	II H&N
	(marimastat, BAY12-9566)	Phs I
		Phs I
		Phs I
		Phs III NSCLC, gastric

Approach to Targeting

Pharmacologic or biologic methods are usually employed in preclinical studies to establish the effect of altering the expression of the target gene or of interfering with the function of the target protein. Most approaches have utilized either small molecule inhibitors (often detected in screening assays) or monoclonal antibodies (MAbs) to interfere with the function of the target protein. In general, small molecule inhibitors have a short half-life and are orally delivered on a continuous long-term basis. However, side effects can be common and potentially troublesome, especially if there is a broader substrate for related cellular proteins/kinases. By contrast, MAbs have a longer half-life with a more acceptable toxicity profile, although they require regular intravenous administration. Monoclonal antibodies usually target surface receptors and may also lead to receptor downregulation, although there is the additional theoretical potential for direct tumor cell cytotoxicity via complement and antibody (antibody-mediated cellular cytotoxicity, ADCC). Side effects may relate to hypersensitivity reactions, with the potential also to develop human antimonoclonal antibodies (HAMAs) that may limit effectiveness. Other approaches to targeting include the use of antisense technology to inhibit target messenger RNA that is transcribed from a given gene, although a key limiting factor is appropriate delivery of nucleic acids to the tumor cell. The use of viral vectors in targeted therapy approaches to modify/replace or inhibit target genes has therefore attracted much attention, and this method has been used to replace or stabilize key tumor suppressor proteins that may regulate cell survival and apoptosis.

Targeted Therapies

Hormone Receptor-Targeted Therapies

Targeting hormonal growth pathways has been an effective strategy in the management of various tumors such as breast, prostate, and endometrial cancers. Early approaches were directed at surgical ablation of the glands supplying these hormonal stimuli (i.e., ovariectomy for breast cancer and orchiectomy for prostate cancer), but over the pst 30 years a large number of medical agents have become available based on an increasing understanding of molecular endocrinology.

Breast Cancer

Medical endocrine strategies in breast cancer are designed to counteract the proliferative effects of estrogen in ER-positive breast cancer, either with drugs that compete with estrogen for ER and block its effect (i.e., antiestrogens), or strategies that induce estrogen deprivation and remove the proliferative signal [i.e., oophorectomy or gonadotropin-releasing hormone (GnRH) agonists in premenopausal women, and aromatase inhibitors in postmenopausal women]. Tamoxifen is a nonsteroidal estrogen receptor (ER) antagonist that inhibits breast cancer growth by competitive antagonism of ER, although its actions are complex as a result of partial estrogenic agonist effects, which in some tissues (i.e., bone) can be beneficial but which in others may be harmful, increasing the risk of uterine cancer and thromboembolism. Oral aromatase inhibitors prevent conversion of adrenal androgens (androstenedione and testosterone) into estradiol (E_1) and estrone (E_2) by the cytochrome P-450 enzyme aromatase. Alternative endocrine approaches are also being developed, including steroidal antiestrogens that selectively downregulate expression of ER.[4]

Prostate Cancer

Normal prostate cells and tumor cells are sensitive to androgens, which are produced by two major sources: the testicles, which produce testosterone (95% of all androgens), and the adrenal glands, which produce dehydroandrosterone, dehydroandrosterone sulfate, and androstenedione. Both are under the influence of luteinizing hormone (LH), which in turn is controlled by GnRH produced by the hypothalamus. Testosterone levels have a negative feedback effect on GnRH release from the hypothalamus. Targeted endocrine medical treatment of prostate cancers aims to decrease the activity of androgens on the AR, either with antiandrogens (i.e., nonsteroidal agents such as flutamide, biclutamide) that competitively block dihydrotestosterone (DHT) binding to AR, and subsequent activation of AR-regulated genes, or by suppression of LH secretion (i.e., using specific LH agonists that ultimately inhibit LH secretion, thus reducing androgen production).

Growth Factor Receptor-Targeted Therapies

In human cancer cells, aberrant signaling through the epidermal growth factor receptor (EGFR) has been associated with neoplastic cell proliferation, resistance to apoptosis, migration and stromal invasion, and enhanced angiogenesis. The EGFR (or ErbB-1) is part of a subfamily of four closely related receptors that include HER-2/*neu* (ErbB-2), HER-3 (ErbB-3), and HER-4 (ErbB-4).[5] These receptors exist as inactive transmembrane monomers in cells, and dimerize after ligand activation either by homo- or heterodimerization between EGFR and another member of the ErbB receptor family. This dimerization results in activation of the intracellular tyrosine kinase domain through autophosphorylation, which in turn initiates a cascade of downstream signaling pathways that include Ras and mitogen-activated protein kinase (MAPK). In cancer cells, various mechanisms for activation of EGFR or related ErbB pathways include receptor overexpression (e.g., as a result of gene amplification in the case of HER-2), receptor mutation (e.g., truncated EGFR that lacks the extracellular domain but has a constitutively activated tyrosine kinase domain that functions independent of ligand), increased autocrine or paracrine expression of the various receptor ligands [e.g., transforming growth factor-alpha (TGF-α), amphiregulin, heparin-binding EGF], or decreased receptor turnover.

Studies have shown that EGFR or HER-2 overexpression in cancer is often associated with a poorer prognosis and resistance to conventional therapies including hormonal therapy, cytotoxic drugs, and radiotherapy.[6] Consequently, EGFR and related receptors represent an attractive target for the development of novel cancer therapeutics. The two most promising approaches have been MAbs against the extracellular ligand-binding domain of the receptor and small molecule inhibitors of the receptor intracellular tyrosine kinase enzymatic activity (TKIs).

Inhibition of Extracellular Domain Growth Factor Receptor: Monoclonal Antibodies

Cetuximab (C225 or Erbitux) is a chimeric antibody that binds to EGFR, inhibiting downstream signaling and promoting receptor internalization, and significant growth inhibition has been observed in a variety of human cancer xenograft models.[6] Additive effects were seen when cetuximab was combined with various cytotoxic agents and with ionizing radiation. The clinical development has focused on selecting patients with EGFR-overexpressing tumors, and Phase II/III trials have been conducted in head and neck cancer,[7] colorectal cancer,[8] and advanced non-small cell lung cancer[9] (Table 5.2). These latter studies have investigated whether addition of cetuximab can enhance the activity of conventional therapies for these tumor types. Recent data demonstrate that cetuximab, in addition to irinotecan in patients with irinotecan-refractory metastatic colorectal cancer, improves median survival and time to progression.[8]

HER2 gene amplification occurs in 25% to 30% of breast tumors and contributes to cell growth and malignant transformation, rendering tumors more resistant to both endocrine and conventional chemotherapies.[10] Trastuzumab (Herceptin) is a humanized MAb directed against HER2 and, when administered as a weekly intravenous infusion, gave clinical response rates of 35% as first-line therapy for patients with HER2+ve metastatic breast cancer.[11] One of the central principles is the appropriate selection of patients with HER2+ve tumors, and validated assays have been developed to identify either HER2 overexpression by immunohistochemistry or HER2 gene amplification by fluorescence in situ hybridization (FISH). The addition of trastuzumab to taxane- or anthracycline-based chemotherapy enhanced both objective response and time to disease progression, which in turn significantly improved overall survival in advanced breast cancer (median, 25 versus 20 months, $P < 0.046$).[12] As such, this represented one of the first examples of modern targeted therapies successfully modifying disease outcome.

TABLE 5.2. Clinical trials with monoclonal antibodies against epidermal growth factor receptor (EGFR).

Metastatic Colon Cancer Phase II Trial 329 EGFR-positive patients after irinotecan failure[9]	*Cetuximab alone*	*Irinotecan + Cetuximab*
Response rate	10.8%	22.9%
Median time to progression	1.5 months	4.1 months
Survival	6.9 months (NS)	8.6 months (NS)
Metastatic/Recurrent Head and Neck Cancer Phase III trial[8]	*Cisplatin*	*Cisplatin + Cetuximab*
Response rate	9.3%	22.6%
Progression-free survival	3.4 months	3.4 months
Advanced Non-Small Cell Lung Cancer EGFR positive 1st line[10]	*Vinorelbine + Cisplatin*	*Vinorelbine + Cisplatin + Cetuximab*
Response rate	32.2%	53.3%

Inhibition of Intracellular Signaling: Tyrosine Kinase Inhibitors

Imatinib Mesylate (STI-571 or Glivec)

When growth factor receptors are bound by their natural ligand, they undergo dimerization with subsequent activation of receptor tyrosine kinase activity, which in turn phosphorylates downstream signal transduction cascades. Small molecule tyrosine kinase inhibitors (TKIs) specifically target the receptor's internal tyrosine kinase domain. The first to prove effective in the clinic was imatinib mesylate (STI-571 or Gleevec), which targets a small family of tyrosine kinases including ABL, Kit, and platelet-derived growth factor receptor (PDGF), as well as certain oncogenic mutants of these proteins such as the *bcr-abl* oncogene found in chronic myeloid leukemia.[13] The success of this therapy relates to the dominant role that these pivotal kinases play in the pathogenesis of certain tumors; that is, 90% of gastrointestinal stromal tumors (GIST) exhibit aberrant signal transduction through KIT, primarily through activating point mutations in exon 11 that encodes the intracellular region of the protein, with evidence that KIT activation is an early tumorigenic event in most GIST tumors.[14] KIT mutations were a strong predictor of response to imatinib in early clinical trials and produced significantly prolonged survival.[15] The high level of efficacy appeared independent of tumor bulk and failure of prior chemotherapy, with objective responses in 54% of patients and stable disease in an additional 28% to 37%.[16,17] This molecularly targeted therapy has transformed the management of this previously intractable disease.

Gefitinib (Iressa)

Several small molecule inhibitors of EGFR tyrosine kinase are in development, including the synthetic anilinoquinazoline gefitinib (Iressa), which is an orally active, potent, and selective inhibitor of EGFR-TK. In experimental models gefitinib induced dose-dependent antiproliferative effects that delayed tumor growth.[18] The effects appeared mainly cytostatic, and additional studies suggested that, when given in combination with cytotoxic drugs, gefitinib could enhance their antitumor activity.[19] This interaction did not always appear to be dependent on overexpression of EGFR, and the mechanism for any enhanced cytotoxic effect remains unclear.

Evidence of efficacy in Phase II non-small cell lung cancer (NSCLC) studies led to the accelerated approval for gefitinib by the U.S. Food and Drug Administration (FDA) for the treatment of NSCLC in patients previously treated with chemotherapy[20,21] (Table 5.3). However, two Phase III randomized trials, INTACT-1 and INTACT-2 (Table 5.4), that compared platinum-based chemotherapy and gefitinib to chemotherapy alone in chemotherapy-naive NSCLC patients, failed to demonstrate a survival advantage for the addition of targeted therapy, despite the preclinical evidence for an additive benefit for gefitinib–chemotherapy combinations.[22] Several theories have been proposed to explain the failure of these trials, including the possibility that cytostatic effects of targeted therapy may abrogate the cytotoxic effects of cycle-dependent chemotherapy. Unlike the trastuzumab studies, where patients were selected based on HER2 status, there were insufficient data at the time to predict which biologic markers may correlate with response to gefitinib. This failing may have severely reduced the chance of success in the Phase III setting, which contained patients with a heterogeneous selection of tumor phenotypes.

Clinical trials have been undertaken with gefitinib in other tumor types, including breast cancer. There have been three Phase II monotherapy studies of gefitinib in patients with advanced breast cancer.[23–25] Overall, the data are relatively disappointing with low clinical response rates. The only trial to report a significant number of responses included patients with ER+ve tamoxifen-resistant breast cancer,[25] the setting in which preclinical models had shown evidence of

TABLE 5.3. Summary of Phase II studies in advanced platinum-refractory non-small cell lung cancer (NSCLC) with EGFR tyrosine kinase inhibitors (TKIs).

	IDEAL 1 Gefitinib 250/500 mg[25]	*IDEAL 2 Gefitinib 250/500 mg[24]*	*Erlotinib[36]*
Response rate	18/19%	12/9%	11%
1 year Survival	35/30%	29/24%	?
Median survival	7.6/8.1 months	6.1/6.0 months	?

TABLE 5.4. Phase III trials of gefitinib with chemotherapy as first-line treatment of NSCLC.

INTACT 1[26]	*Gem/Cis alone*	*Chemo + Gefitinib 250 mg*	*Chemo + Gefitinib 500 mg*
Response rate	44.8%	50.3%	49.7%
1-year survival	44%	41%	43%
Median survival	10.9 months	9.9 months	9.9 months
INTACT 2	*Carbo/Paclitaxel alone*	*Chemo + Gefitinib 250 mg*	*Chemo + Gefitinib 500 mg*
Response rate	28.7%	30.4%	30%
1-year survival	42%	41%	37%
Median survival	9.9 months	9.8 months	8.7 months

activity for gefitinib.[26] More research is required to establish tumor phenotypes in responding versus nonresponding patients.[27]

ERLOTINIB (TARCEVA)

Erlotinib is an ErbB1 TKI that binds reversibly to the adenosine triphosphate (ATP) hydrophobic pocket. Table 5.3 summarizes data from recent Phase II trials in advanced NSCLC with erlotinib. A Phase II study in 56 patients with EGFR-positive NSCLC refractory to platinum-based therapy gave a response rate of 11% for erlotinib 150 mg/day.[28] Results of Phase III combination studies of erlotinib with carboplatin and paclitaxel (TRIBUTE) or gemcitabine and cisplatin (TALENT) in NSCLC demonstrated no significant survival benefit or differences in time to progression.[29,30] However, the NCI Canadian BR21 placebo-controlled Phase III trial of erlotinib in NSCLC patients failing one or two prior chemotherapy regimens demonstrated prolonged survival in the erlotinib arm (6.7 versus 4.7 months).[31] Ongoing trials are investigating the activity for the combination of two targeted therapies in NSCLC, erlotinib and the VEGF antibody bevacizumab (avastin). Phase II data in other tumor types have revealed response rates in pretreated patients with ovary and head and neck tumors between 11% and 13%, although Phase II monotherapy trials in breast cancer have been relatively disappointing.[32] Important activity in previously treated glioblastoma multiforme was demonstrated in a Phase II study (with 8 of 49 patients achieving a partial response).

CANERTINIB DIHYDROCHLORIDE (CI-1033); LAPATINIB (GW 572016)

Canertinib dihydrochloride (CI-1033) is a selective and irreversible pan-erbB inhibitor. Activity has been demonstrated in Phase I studies with an acceptable side-effect profile, and Phase II studies are under way in breast and renal cancer.[33] Lapatinib (GW 572016) is a dual inhibitor of EGFR and HER2[34] that has shown responses in trastuzumab-resistant breast cancer patients.[35] Further studies of lapatinib in combination with either endocrine or cytotoxic therapy are ongoing in breast cancer.

Signal Transduction-Targeted Therapies

Elucidation of the signal transduction cascade downstream from growth factors and membrane receptor tyrosine kinases has revealed several key proteins involved in this malignant transformation, including the guanine nucleotide-binding proteins encoded by the *ras* proto-oncogene (Figure 5.1). Following posttranslational processing and addition of a hydrophobic 15-carbon farnesyl moiety, Ras is localized to the

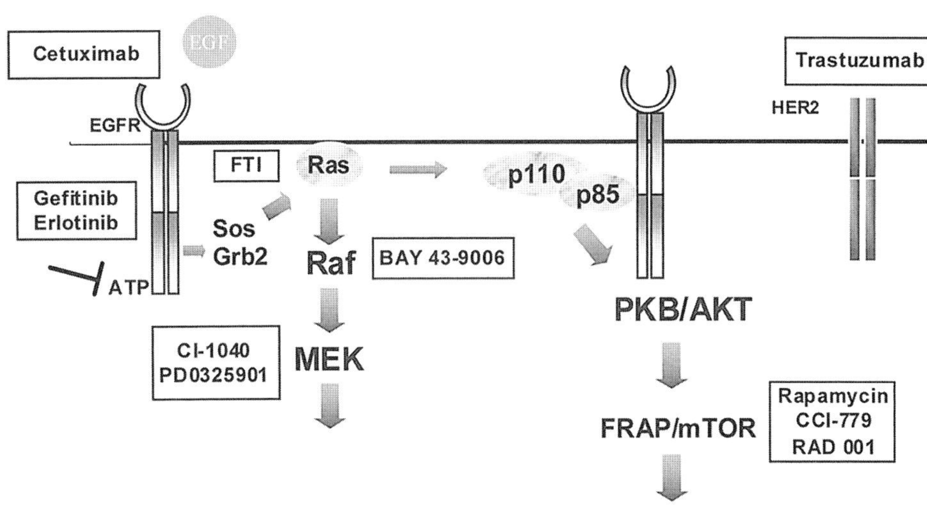

FIGURE 5.1. The signal transduction inhibitors.

inner plasma membrane and acts as a molecular switch that plays a crucial role in linking tyrosine kinase activation at the cell membrane to downstream cytoplasmic and nuclear targets, ultimately resulting in cell differentiation, proliferation, and survival.[36] Farnesylation has attracted attention because of its critical role for Ras signaling,[37] and farnsesyl transferase inhibitors (FTIs) were initially developed as a novel therapy to target aberrant Ras function in cancer.

Farnesyltransferase Inhibitors

As farnesyltransferase inhibitors (FTIs) have been developed and entered clinical trials, a fundamental research goal has been to understand their exact mechanism of action. Although FTIs clearly inhibit Ras farnesylation, it is unclear whether the antiproliferative effects of these compounds result exclusively from their effects on Ras alone. Other targets for FTIs include RhoB, a 21-kDa protein that regulates receptor trafficking and cell motility, and two centromere-associated proteins (CENP-E and CENP-F) that play a role in attaching centromeres to microtubules in early G_2 phase.[38]

The FTI lonafarnib (SCH66336 or sarasar) is a tricyclic compound that inhibits the growth of several tumor cell lines as well as K-*ras*-transformed xenografts in vivo.[39] In human xenograft studies a wide variety of tumors including colon, bladder, lung, prostate, and pancreas were growth inhibited in a dose-dependent manner, while prophylactic administration of SCH66336 delayed both tumor onset and growth.[40] In patients with solid tumors, efficacy has been reported in early Phase I clinical studies in a variety of tumor types including lung and head and neck cancer,[41] and confirmation of biologic efficacy has been demonstrated by inhibition of prenylation of prelamin A in buccal mucosa cells in treated patients[42] (Table 5.5). Based on promising preclinical evidence that lonafarnib may synergize with taxane-based chemotherapy,[43] randomized Phase II/III trials were initiated in NSCLC to investigate whether lonafarnib could further enhance the efficacy of standard taxane platinum-based chemotherapy. Tipifarnib (R115777 or zarnestra) is an imidazole-containing heterocyclic compound that is a potent and selective, orally active, nonpeptidomimetic inhibitor of the farnesyl protein transferase (FPTase) enzyme.[44] There is considerable evidence that tipifarnib may have promising activity in hematologic malignancies, in particular, newly diagnosed acute myelogenous leukemia (AML) and myelodysplasia (MDS)[45,46] (see Table 5.5).

In view of the higher incidence of Ras mutations in gastrointestinal malignancies, two randomized double-blind placebo-controlled Phase III trials of tipifarnib were conducted in colorectal and pancreatic cancer. There was no significant improvement in overall survival versus best supportive care for tipifarnib as monotherapy in advanced refractory colorectal cancer,[47] or for gemcitabine plus tipifarnib versus gemcitabine plus placebo in 688 patients with advanced pancreatic cancer.[48] Although several Phase I studies have assessed combinations of FTIs with various cytotoxic agents, it remains unclear whether they will significantly enhance the efficacy of standard cytotoxic regimens. Several issues have arisen, including competing toxicities (i.e., myelosuppression) and uncertainty on the optimal sequence/schedule for FTI–chemotherapy combinations. There may be more promise for combining FTIs with noncytotoxic therapies. In breast cancer, preclinical data have shown additive or synergistic interactions of FTIs with endocrine therapy,[49] and in view of this, randomized Phase II studies of both tipifarnib and lonafarnib with letrozole are in progress. Evidence has also emerged that FTIs may be radiosensitizers in selected cancer cell lines, and Phase I trials have investigated the feasibility of this combined modality in

TABLE 5.5. FTI Phase I/II clinical trials.

Drug	*Author*	*Dose range*	*Schedule*	*No. patients (pts)*	*Dose-limiting toxicities*	*Clinical/biological activity*
SCH 66336 Lonafarnib	Adjei et al.[51] Solid tumors	25–400 mg bid	7 days oral (q21)	20	Nausea, vomiting, diarrhea	Inhibition of prelamin A farnesylation in buccal mucosal cells; PR in 1 pt with non-small cell lung Ca; 8 pts stable for 5–10 cycles
	Eskens et al.[50] Head and neck cancer Lung cancer	25–300 mg bid	Continuous oral	24	Neutropenia, thrombocytopenia, vomiting, confusion	Stable disease lasting >9 months in 2 pts (thyroid Ca, pseudoyxoma peritonei)
R115777 Tipifarnib	Johnston et al.[56] Advanced breast cancer	Continuous dose (CD) of 300 or 400 mg bid $n = 41$) or intermittent dose (ID) of 300 mg bid for 21 days followed by 7 days rest ($n = 35$) 300 mg bid		76	Neutropenia, thrombocytopenia, neurotoxicity, and fatigue	CD: 4 partial responses (10%) lasting 4–12 months. 6 patients stable disease (15%) for at least 6 months ID: 5 partial responses (14%) and 3 patients with stable disease (9%)
	Kurzrock et al.[54] Myelodysplastic syndrome		21 days oral (q28)	21	Myelosuppression, fatigue and rash	1 complete remission 2 partial responses 3 pts with hematologic improvement
	Karp et al.[55] High-risk leukemias	100–1200 mg bid	21 days oral (q28)	34	Neurotoxicity	32% response rate in AML

both lung and head and neck cancer. The true role for FTIs in cancer therapy thus remains to be determined.

m-TOR Inhibitors: Targeting the PI3K/AKT Pathway

The mammalian target of rapamycin (mTOR) is a downstream effector of the phosphatidylinositol 3-kinase (PI3-K)/Akt (protein kinase B) signaling pathway that mediates cell survival, proliferation, and drug resistance (see Figure 5.1). The immunosuppressant rapamycin, together with the analogues CCI-779 (temsirolimus) and RAD-001 (everolimus), are specific inhibitors of mTOR that act by binding to the immunophilin FK506, thus blocking the action of p70S6 kinase and 4E-binding protein 1, which regulate transition through the G_1 phase of the cell cycle. In preclinical experiments, cell lines from breast, prostate, small cell lung cancer, melanoma, T-cell leukemia, and glioblastoma were especially sensitive to CCI-779.[50] In particular, breast cancer and prostate cell lines that had a constitutively activated PI3-K/Akt pathway due to either upstream HER2 overexpression, loss of the PTEN suppressor gene, or Akt overexpression were markedly more sensitive to CCI-779 than resistant lines that lacked these features.[51]

CCI-779 has an acceptable toxicity profile in Phase I studies with reports of neutropenia, rash, fever, hypertriglyceridemia, mucositis, and fatigue as the main toxicities, with clinical activity seen in patients with NSCLC, breast, and renal cell carcinoma.[52] Phase II studies in patients with advanced renal cell carcinoma demonstrated that CCI-779 was well tolerated with objective response rates of 7%, minor responses of 29%, and disease stabilized in 40% of patients.[53] This trial precipitated a randomized Phase III study comparing CCI-779 with interferon-alpha or the combination in poor prognosis renal cell carcinoma. Single-agent activity has also been documented in locally advanced or metastatic breast cancer in patients who have failed prior anthracyclines or taxanes.[54] Phase I studies of RAD-001 have demonstrated a similar toxicity profile to CCI-779.[55]

Raf Kinase Inhibitors: BAY 43-9006

RAF kinase is a critical signaling molecule downstream of RAS (see Figure 5.1). Activating mutations in BRAF (a RAF family member) occur in two-thirds of melanomas and at lower frequencies in other cancers.[56] Promising Phase I data with the orally active RAF kinase inhibitor BAY 43-9006 in combination with chemotherapy have been reported, with stable disease for at least 12 weeks in 38 of 115 (33%) patients. Toxicities included skin rash, hand-foot syndrome, diarrhea, and fatigue. Phase II trials are in progress in melanoma with continuous monotherapy dosing of 400 mg bid,[57] and in combination with carboplatin and paclitaxel.[58]

Intervention of the MAPK Pathway by Targeting MEK: CI-1040 and PD0325901

CI-1040 inhibits MEK allosterically at micromolar concentrations and is administered orally, thereby preventing activation of MAPK. The lack of sequence homology of the drug interaction site with other kinases increases the specificity of this small molecule inhibitor. CI-1040 is well tolerated in Phase I trials, with 98% of adverse events being only of grade 1 or 2 in severity (diarrhea, fatigue, rash, and vomiting).[59] Disappointing Phase II results were seen in patients with breast, lung, colon, and pancreatic carcinoma.[60] CI-1040 was limited by poor solubility, high metabolic clearance, and low bioavailability and was unable to consistently lead to more than 90% inhibition of the target in biopsied tumors. This result precipitated the development of PD0325901, a second-generation non-ATP-competitive allosteric MEK inhibitor. Preclinical studies have demonstrated promising activity with greater solubility, improved metabolic stability and bioavailability, and longer duration of MEK inhibition than its parent compound, and clinical trials are in progress.

Cell-Cycle-Targeted Therapies

The cell cycle is regulated by a number of key proteins that appear to be frequently inactivated or aberrantly expressed in human cancer. The cyclin D and E family of proteins, together with their cyclin-dependent kinase (cdk) partners (cdk4 and -6) phosphorylate the retinoblastoma (Rb) tumor suppressor protein, which regulates G_1/S transition and commitment to cell-cycle transition (Figure 5.2). Cyclin/cdk activity is restrained by cdk inhibitors (CKIs) of the $p16^{ink4a}$ and the $p21^{cip1}$ family of proteins. The appropriate interaction of the cyclin/cdk families and the CKIs regulate the cell-cycle checkpoints at the G_1/S and G_2/M transitions, ensuring faithful chromosome replication and separation to preserve genetic stability. Failure of these checkpoints to arrest cells in response to certain stimuli is characteristic of cancer cells and is due to the frequent genetic aberration in expression and function of cell-cycle regulatory proteins in transformed cells.

The greater understanding of the cell cycle has led to the development of a number of compounds that might restore the control of cell division in cancer cells. In particular, two strategies are now being explored in the clinic. First, compounds have been developed to mimic the action of CKIs by interfering with action of the cdk molecules.[61] Second, pharmacologic agents have been developed to target the proteosome or histone deacetylases, thereby interfering with the degradation and expression of key molecules that regulate the cell-cycle checkpoint.

Cdk Inhibitors

Flavopiridol

Flavopiridol targets the ATP-binding pocket of cdk2 and arrest cells at either the G_1/S or G_2/M checkpoints and may inhibit other cdks including cdk1, cdk7, and cdk9. The initial Phase I trial explored a 72-hour continuous infusion of flavopiridol, but dose-limiting toxicities included secretory diarrhea and symptomatic hypotension[62] (Table 5.6). In three separate phase II studies with this schedule, objective tumor responses were rare, although disease stabilization was seen in a number of patients.[63–65] Previous preclinical studies had shown synergy and induction of apoptosis when flavopiridol was combined with standard cytotoxic therapies,[66] and clinical activity using combination therapy has been seen in patients previously resistant to the given cytotoxic drug alone.[67,68] Preclinical evidence of synergism with paclitaxel therapy followed by flavopiridol in animal models further supported clinical studies of this combination,[69] and Phase I combination studies have demonstrated promising activity in lung, esophagus, and prostate cancer.[70] Thus, although cdk

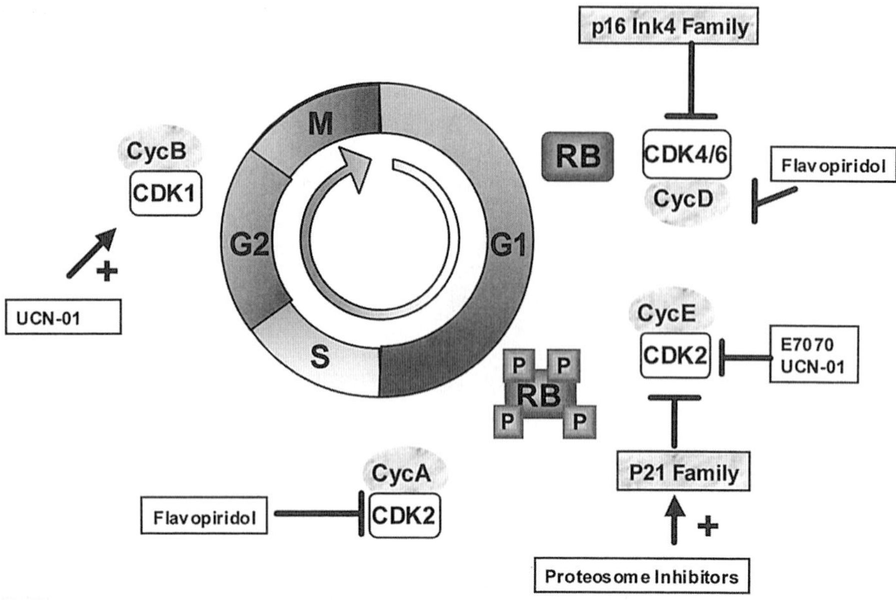

FIGURE 5.2. Cell-cycle-targeted therapies.

inhibitors alone may only have a cytostatic effect, combined therapy may prove more promising in enhancing their anticancer mode of action.

UCN-01

UCN-01 is a cell-cycle modulator with a number of complex effects resulting in both G_1/S arrest and aberrant entry into M phase. These cell-cycle kinetics are associated with an increased p27^{kip2}–cdk2 interaction, Rb hypophosphorylation, and cdk1 activation due to chk1 inhibition. Phase I trials examined a 72-hour continuous infusion schedule, with dose-limiting toxicities that included nausea, hypotension, hyperglycemia, and pulmonary toxicity, and evidence for activity was seen in two patients with melanoma and lymphoma.

E7070

E7070 is a novel sulphonamide compound that inhibits the activation of cyclin E–cdk2 complexes and in vitro has demonstrated activity against both colon and lung cancer xenografts. A number of Phase I studies have investigated different schedules. The main dose-limiting toxicity has been myelosuppression; alopecia, stomatitis, and diarrhea have also been reported.[71,72] Tumor stabilizations were seen in some of these studies, but documented tumor regressions

TABLE 5.6. Flavopiridol clinical trials.

Author	*Trial*	*Tumor type*	*Dose*	*Toxicity*	*Response*
Senderowicz[77]	Phase I *N* = 76	Refractory neoplasms	72h ivi q 2wk MTD 50–78 mg/m²/24h	Diarrhea (62.5 mg/m²/d × 3) ADP 98 mg/m²/d × 3 Hypotension Proinflammatory syndrome	1 partial response (PR) 3 minor responses
Schwartz[86]	Phase I Paclitaxel + FP	Advanced solid tumors	**P** Day 1 24h or 3h ivi **FP** Day 2 24h ivi	Neutropenia at P:FP doses of **P** 135 mg/m²/24h: **FP** 10 mg/m² & **P** 100 mg/m²/24h **FP** 20 mg/m²	Activity in lung, esophagus, prostate cancer
Bible[82]	Phase I 5-FU and LV *N* = 24	Advanced solid tumors	**FP** 40–100 mg/m²/24h Day 1 **5-FU** 350 mg/m²/day 1h ivi Days 2–5 **LV** 20 mg/m² Days 2–5	Diarrhea Headache Fatigue Hypotension Syncope Dehydration	1 PR (liver metastasis CRC) 13% SD
Stadler et al.[78]	Phase II *N* = 35	Advanced renal	50 mg/m²/d ivi over 72h q 2wk	Asthenia Diarrhea G3/420% Thrombosis (26%) (MI, PE, DVT, TIA)	Ineffective in metastatic renal cell carcinoma
Schwartz[80]	Phase II *N* = 16	Advanced gastric	50 mg/m²/d ivi over 72h q 2wk	Fatigue (93%) Diarrhea (73%) Venous thromboses (33%)	No major responses

FP, flavopiridol; P, paclitaxel; 5-FU, 5-fluorouracil; LV, leucovorin; *N*, number of patients; ADP, antidiarrhea prophylaxis.

were rare in phase II monotherapy trials conducted in non-small cell lung cancer[73] and in colorectal cancer[74] with E7070.

Proteosome Inhibitors

Protein concentrations within the cell may be altered by post-translational modification leading to polyubiquitination followed by proteasome-mediated degradation. Prevention of ubiquitination and proteasome-mediated degradation of cell-cycle proteins has been explored as a novel targeted anticancer therapy.[75] Bortezomib (PS-341 or velcade) is a potent and selective proteasome inhibitor that prevents the degradation of the CKIs p21 and p27. In addition, key apoptosis-related proteins are degraded by the proteasome such as IkappaB, an inhibitor of the transcription factor NFkappaB that regulates various apoptotic processes.

In 2003, the FDA approved the use of bortezomib in patients with multiple myeloma who have received two previous lines of treatment, partly due to the results of a large multicenter phase II trial in 202 patients with relapsed refractory multiple myeloma that demonstrated a 35% response rate with a median survival of 17.8 months.[76,77] A phase III trial comparing bortezomib with high-dose oral dexamethasone in relapsed or refractory multiple myeloma was terminated prematurely following the recommendation of an independent data monitoring committee to allow patients receiving high-dose dexamethasone to choose bortezomib therapy. Combination studies with cytotoxic agents are also under way, with promising activity already demonstrated.[77]

Histone Deacetylase (HDAC) Inhibitors

Inside the nucleus of cells, histone acetylation–deacetylation modifies the chromatin structure and association between DNA and nucleosomes, thus modulating access for nuclear transcription factors such as E_2F that are involved in initiating transcription of genes essential for S-phase entry. Inhibitors of histone deacetylase result in G_1 cell-cycle arrest and cell differentiation and appear to have anticancer effects including induction of apoptosis in transformed cells[79] and enhanced expression of the cdk inhibitor p21.[80] Two compounds have entered early clinical trials, depsipeptide (FR901228) and the synthetic benzamide derivative MS-27-275.

Apoptosis-Targeted Therapies

Apoptosis, or programmed cell death, in normal human tissues has an essential role in controlling overall cell number. In many human tumors apoptosis is impaired, contributing to cellular transformation. Triggering of apoptosis is determined by the ratio of pro- and antiapoptotic proteins, in particular, members of the Bcl2 family, the intracellular anti-apoptotic proteins (IAPs), tumor necrosis factor (TNF)-related apoptosis-inducing ligand (TRAIL), and the caspase family. Although cytotoxic chemotherapy drugs can induce apoptosis in malignant cells, resistance to chemotherapy may in some instances relate to alteration in the molecular pathways that regulate apoptosis.

There are two major apoptotic pathways that can be triggered in cells: the extrinsic death-receptor-induced extrinsic pathway, and the intrinsic mitochondrial apoptosome-mediated pathway (Figure 5.3). The extrinsic pathway is regulated by members of the TNF superfamily, FASL (FAS ligand), TNF, and TRAIL. These "death receptors" signal through the "death-inducing signaling complex" (DISC), leading to caspase activation and apoptosis. The intrinsic mitochondria apoptosome pathway is controlled by members of the Bcl2 family. The proapoptotic members of this family (e.g., BAX, BAK, BIM, and BID) precipitate the release of cytochrome *c* from mitochondria, which promotes the formation of the apoptosome (cytochrome *c*/APAF1/caspase 9) complex. Members of the Bcl2 family that inhibit the pathway include

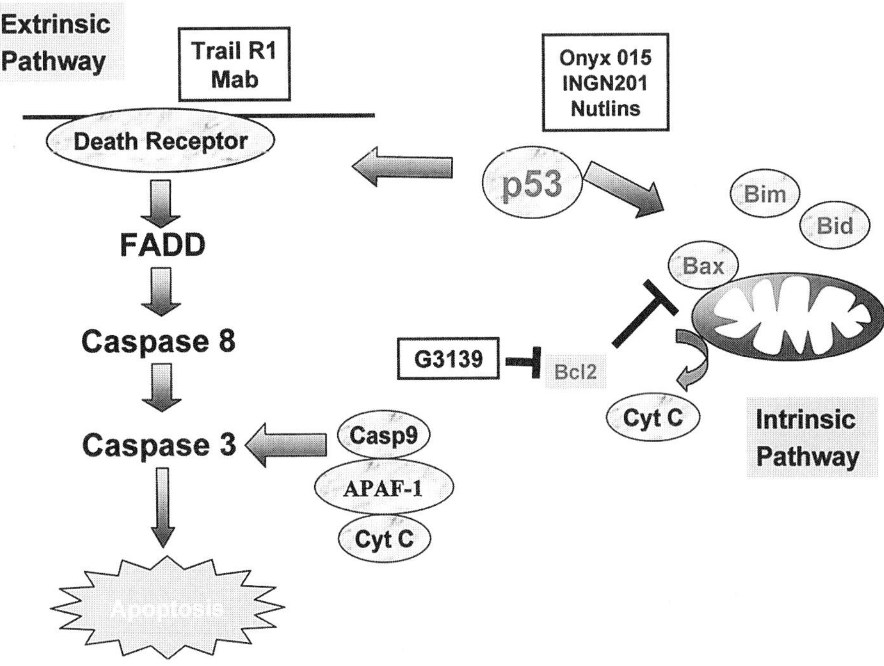

FIGURE 5.3. Apoptosis-targeted therapies.

Bcl2 itself, Bclxl, and Bclw. P53 can regulate both the intrinsic pathway by promoting the transcription of BAX and the extrinsic pathway through upregulation of the death receptor. Apoptosis is also suppressed by the IAPs (inhibitors of apoptosis). Members of this family include XIAP, IAP1, IAP2, and survivin. These proteins interact with and inhibit selected effector caspases. IAP suppressors have also been identified and include Smac/DIABLO and XAF1.

Many of the targeted therapies mentioned above act in part through the promotion of apoptosis; for example, the proteosome inhibitor bortezomib and the histone deacetylase inhibitor suberoylanilide hydroxamic acid (SAHA) precipitate apoptosis in tumor cells. Similarly, flavopiridol-mediated inhibition of the cell-cycle kinase, cdk1, enhances the cytotoxicity of doxorubicin in MCF7 human breast carcinoma xenografts through the suppression of survivin phosphorylation.[81] However, some of the more direct therapies targeting components of the apoptosis pathway are discussed next.

Strategies to Modulate Apoptosis

TRAILR1 Monoclonal Antibody

This MAb targets TRAILR1 expressed on human cancer cells and induces apoptosis in human tumor cell lines. Although initial studies suggested that TRAIL activation preferentially leads to apoptosis of tumor cells over normal cells, recent data suggest that human hepatocytes may also be sensitive to TRAIL activity.[82] Phase I studies are currently in progress.

Antisense Bcl2 Strategies: G3139

G3139 is an antisense phosphorothioate oligonucleotide that suppresses the expression of the antiapoptotic protein Bcl2. Results of a trial of 21 patients with non-Hodgkin's lymphoma treated with subcutaneous G3139 demonstrated a response rate of 14% with a further 43% exhibiting stable disease.[83] Phase III trials are in progress.

Strategies Targeting p53: ONYX-015, INGN 201, Nutlins

ONYX-015 is a mutant adenovirus with a loss-of-function mutation of the adenoviral E1B gene product. The wild-type viral gene product E1B inactivates p53. ONYX-015 selectively replicates in p53-deficient tumor cells leading to cytolysis. The virus is unable to replicate in cells with wild-type p53.[84] Promising results have been demonstrated in phase I and II trials, and also in combination with chemotherapy agents.[85] Regional delivery of ONYX-015 has been attempted in different tumor types. A Phase II trial of intratumoral ONYX-015 in combination with cisplatin and 5-fluorouracil in patients with recurrent head and neck cancer demonstrated objective tumor responses with an acceptable toxicity profile.[86] Furthermore, biopsies revealed selective adenoviral replication and necrosis within some tumor specimens. Intratumoral injection has also been attempted in patients with breast cancer chest wall recurrence. Hepatic artery infusion of ONYX-015 in a Phase I/II study of 35 patients with liver metastases secondary to colorectal carcinoma demonstrated antitumoral activity,[87] while a Phase I trial of intraperitoneal regional delivery of ONYX-015 was conducted in refractory ovarian cancer.[88]

INGN 201 is a replication incompetent adenovirus vector in which the E_1 region has been replaced by wild-type p53 gene under the control of a cytomegalovirus promoter. Preclinical studies demonstrated anticancer properties in head and neck tumor cell lines and xenografts. A Phase I trial of stereotactic intratumoral injection of INGN 201 into recurrent glioma demonstrated minimal toxicity and the transfer of p53 to astrocytic tumor cells that led to transcriptionally active p53, with upregulation of target genes such as $p21^{cip1}$ and apoptosis in subsets of cells. Phase II studies in patients with advanced recurrent squamous cell carcinoma of the head and neck treated with intralesional INGN 201 indicate that the virus is well tolerated.[89] Disease stabilized in 6 of 17 patients with nonresectable disease, and 2 of 17 patients exhibited partial responses. Paradoxically, efficacy appeared independent of p53 status.

Mdm2 inhibits p53 by promoting p53 nuclear export, impeding the interaction of transcription factors with the activation domain of p53 and triggering the degradation of p53 via the ubiquitin-proteosome pathway. Nutlins are a family of synthetic compounds that can successively displace Mdm2 from the N-terminus of p53, thereby promoting p53 activity.[90] This is an exciting technical development for the manipulation of protein–protein interactions by small molecules. Furthermore, it raises the possibility of activating p53 in tumors that retain normal p53, thereby promoting apoptotic pathways.

Targeting Sphingosine Kinase Activity: Phenoxodiol

Sphingosine kinase promotes the activity of the caspase inhibitory proteins XIAP and FLIP. The isoflavone phenoxodiol targets a regulator of sphingosine kinase thereby reducing XIAP and FLIP activity. Phase Ib/II data have recently been presented demonstrating promising activity of oral phenoxodiol in hormone refractory prostate cancer and late-stage ovarian cancer refractory to chemotherapy.[90,92]

Angiogenesis

Folkman first postulated that angiogenesis (the formation of new blood vessels from the preexisting vascular bed) is required for tumor progression.[93] Initially, malignant cells derive their nutrients from the normal host vessels by diffusion, but tumor growth is limited beyond 1 to 2 mm without new blood vessel growth.[94] Neovascularization is initiated by increased permeability of preexisting vessels in response to vascular endothelial growth factor (VEGF) produced by the tumor; this allows for the extravasation of plasma proteins that lay down the matrix upon which activated growth factor-secreting endothelial cells migrate. Proteolytic degradation of the extracellular matrix and basement membrane then enables endothelial cells to form new capillaries. Normally, perivascular cells are attracted and form basal lumina around the vessels, thus limiting endothelial cell proliferation and decreasing their dependence on VEGF-A. However, in tumors, pericytes have a decreased association with new blood vessels, which as a consequence are leaky due to an imbalance of appropriate proangiogenic and antiantigenic controls that control the so-called angiogenic switch. Hypoxia stimulates the tumor cells to generate proangiogenic factors, including vascular endothelial growth factor (VEGF), fibroblast growth factor (FGF), transforming growth factor-beta (TGF-β), and tumor necrosis factor-alpha (TNF-α). VEGF and FGF are considered the most important factors for tumor angiogenesis.

Tumor vascularization has been found to correlate with growth and metastatic potential in some tumor types, and microvessel density has been shown to be an adverse prognostic factor of distant disease and survival.[95] Consequently, antiangiogenesis has been a new strategy for the development of anticancer treatment. The characterization of natural inhibitors and promoters of angiogenesis has led to the development of novel compounds that potentially interfere with various steps required for angiogenesis (Table 5.6, Figure 5.4). In principle, these approaches involve either targeting the endothelial cell, targeting activators of angiogenesis, or targeting the extracellular matrix.

Targeting the Endothelial Cell (Thalidomide, TNP-740, Endostatin, Angiostatin)

Thalidomide has been found to have immunomodulating and antiangiogenic properties by impeding VEGF- and bFGF-dependent angiogenesis through inhibition of TNF, interleukin (IL)-12, and IL-6 and stimulation of IL-2, interferon, and CD8+ T cells. Clinical activity has been seen in refractory multiple myeloma, myelodysplasia, Kaposi's sarcoma, renal cell cancer, colorectal cancer, and recurrent glioblastomas. No benefit has been demonstrated in Phase III trials of metastatic breast and head and neck malignancies. The thalidomide analogue, CC-5013, has increased potency and efficacy with less sedation, constipation, and neuropathy and has demonstrated promising activity in Phase I trials of patients with advanced solid cancers.[96]

TNP-470 is a potent endothelial inhibitor in vitro, and animal models have demonstrated the broadest anticancer range of any known agent. In clinical trials, TNP-470 has shown evidence of antitumor effect both as monotherapy with responses observed in relapsed or refractory malignancies[97] and in combination with chemotherapy.[98]

The clinical observation that the removal of the primary tumor can lead to the rapid growth of previously dormant micrometastases led to the discovery of angiostatin and endostatin, two potent endogenous antiangiogenic agents. Endostatin is a 20-kDa C-terminal fragment of collagen XVIII found in vessel walls and basement membranes. Recombinant human endostatin inhibited endothelial cell proliferation and tumor growth in preclinical studies, and in a subsequent Phase II trial there were 23 patients with stable disease and 2 with minor responses of the 37 evaluable patients.[99] Angiostatin is a 38-kDa internal fragment of plasminogen, which has subsequently been shown to induce dormancy and regression of tumor models. Angiostatin binds to ATP synthase on the surface of human endothelial cells, induces apoptosis in endothelial cells and tumor cells, inhibits endothelial migration and tubule formation, and inhibits matrix-enhanced plasminogen activation. A Phase I trial in patients with advanced cancer demonstrated that it was well tolerated, with some patients (7 of 24) achieving long-term stable disease.[100]

Targeting Activators of Angiogenesis

Vascular endothelial growth factor (VEGF-A), a critical regulator of physiologic angiogenesis during embryogenesis and skeletal growth, is also important in the pathologic angiogenesis of tumor growth. VEGF-A is a multifunctional cytokine expressed by many tumor cells, promoting microvascular permeability, endothelial cell migration, division, and survival, and inhibiting apoptosis. Oxygen tension/hypoxia, growth factors, oncogenes, inflammatory cytokines, and various hormones regulate the level of VEGF-A. The effects of VEGF are mediated in part by two receptor tyrosine kinases (RTKs), VEGFR-1 (flt-1) and VEGFR-2 (flk-1), which are expressed on endothelial cells. The level of VEGF-A expression in cancer cells has been found to correlate with tumor size, metastasis, poor disease free-survival (DFS), and overall survival (OS).[101] Consequently, VEGF and its receptors

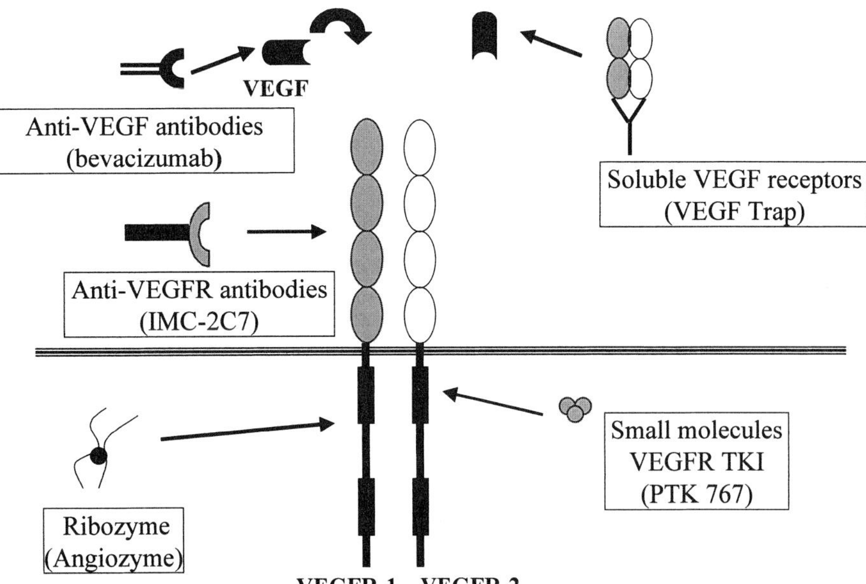

FIGURE 5.4. Inhibitors of angiogenesis.

have been investigated for antiangiogenesis therapies in various malignancies. Different strategies have been designed to inhibit VEGF function, including inhibition of endogenous tumor VEGF secretion (antisense), neutralizing VEGF in the microcirculation, or preventing VEGF binding to its receptor (antibodies), and targeting subsequent signal transduction by VEGF (small molecule receptor tyrosine kinase inhibitors) (see Figure 5.4).

Ribozymes are RNA molecules that can recognize RNA sequences and cleave specific sites on other RNA molecules. Angiozyme, a synthetic ribozyme that targets the VEGFR-1 mRNA, was well tolerated in a Phase I/II study of patients with refractory solid tumors,[102] and further trials are in progress. Bevacizumab (avastin) is a recombinant anti-VEGF humanized MAb,[103] which, in patients with untreated metastatic colorectal cancer given in combination with chemotherapy, showed a significant increase in response rate and time to progression compared with chemotherapy alone, with a 4.7-month prolongation of overall survival.[104] This result represents the first clinical validation for antiangiogenesis therapy as an effective cancer treatment, and recent similar studies in untreated advanced non-small cell lung cancer have demonstrated improved response rates and time to progression with the addition of bevacizumab.[105] Finally, several different small molecules targeting VEGF receptor tyrosine kinases have been developed, each with a different selectivity profile (Table 5.7); these include SU5416 (intravenously administered), SU6668, SU11248, and PTK 787.[106,107]

Targeting the Extracellular Matrix

The matrix metalloproteinases (MMPs) are a family of zinc-dependent endopeptidases that mediate degradation of extracellular matrix expressed by tumor cells or stroma.[108] They are synthesized as inactive zymogens (pro-MMP) and activated by proteinase cleavage. Their activity is regulated by endogenous inhibitors such as β2-macroglobulin, thrombospondin-2, tissue inhibitors of metalloproteinases (TIMPs), and small molecules with TIMP-like domains. MMPs can promote tumor progression by increasing cell growth, migration, invasion, metastasis, and angiogenesis. Several different approaches have been developed to inhibit the activity of MMPs, including antisense mRNA or ribozyme technology.[109] Integrins are a group of heterodimeric transmembrane receptors that mediate cell–cell and cell–ECM interactions. Vitaxin, a humanized derivative of a mouse LM609 MAb, was developed to inhibit the MMP-2 interaction with integrin $\alpha_v\beta_3$, although its instability precluded further development.[110] Cilengitide (EMD 121974) is a synthetic cyclic pentapeptide small molecule inhibitor of $\alpha_v\beta_3$ and $\alpha_v\beta_5$, which in a Phase I trial gave prolonged stable disease in 3 of 37 patients.[111] Finally, MMP enzymatic inhibitors (MMPI) have been developed. Marimastat was the first orally available MMPI and has been tested in several phase III trials in glioblastoma, breast, ovarian, and small and non-small cell lung cancers. These trials were discontinued because marimastat failed to demonstrate superiority over placebo or standard chemotherapy. However, in a Phase III placebo-controlled trial in patients with advanced gastric cancer, marimastat showed significant improvement in OS (2-year survival, 5% versus 18%) and PFS over placebo-treated patients. These benefits remained significant even after longer follow-up.[112] Other MMPIs in development are listed in Table 5.7.

Clinical Development of Targeted/Biologic Therapies

Clinical Trial Design

Clinical trials aim to identify effective drugs for further studies, while also allowing discontinuation of ineffective drugs in an ethical and efficient way. Traditional phase I/II/III clinical trials for cytotoxic agents assume that (1) the agent will reduce the size of the tumor in a dose-dependent manner; (2) the agent will have toxicities that are dose dependent; and (3) reduction in tumor size will lead to improved overall survival and/or improved quality of life. In contrast, newer targeted agents may not have an objective effect on tumor size other than tumor stabilization or metastasis prevention. There may not be a dose-dependent effect, and toxicities may only be modest.[113] Consequently, there are limitations in testing target-based agents with conventional trials designed for cytotoxic drugs, and alternative endpoints/trial designs are required.

Phase I: Biologic Endpoints and Surrogate Markers

Phase I trials are small studies aimed at finding the optimal dose of a drug using schedules determined from preclinical models. In conventional trials with cytotoxic agents, maximal tolerated dose (MTD) is often used to define the optimal dose rather than using the dose that has a quantifiable therapeutic effect. The dose of the agent is escalated in cohorts of three to six patients until there is unacceptable toxicity in two or more patients. The design of phase I trials is based on the assumption that the efficacy and toxicity of the drug increases as the dose increases and that the mechanism of toxicity and tumor effect are the same. Pharmacokinetic studies are included in Phase I trials but are not required to determine the optimal dose of a cytotoxic agent.

Due to their selective effect, targeted agents have the potential to achieve maximum biologic effect with minimal side effects. Therefore, the optimal dose in Phase I trials may need to be defined by a biologic endpoint rather than toxicity. Their wider therapeutic ratio may in some cases make it difficult to determine the MTD. Furthermore, the mechanisms of toxicity and biologic effect may differ, and therefore, MTD cannot be used to define the optimal dose. Conversely, others contend that unless the MTD and intratumoral pharmacodynamics of the novel agent are determined in Phase I and II clinical trials, Phase III trials run the risk of inadequate dosing and suboptimal target inhibition.[2]

Consequently, biologic endpoints in tumor and surrogate tissue rather than dose-limiting toxicity are often used to define the optimal dose of targeted agents for subsequent clinical trials. This characterization requires a biologic understanding of the target, a specific and reproducible assay for target inhibition, knowledge of the distribution of the target in the tissues of interest, accessibility of the appropriate tissue, and demonstration that the tissue is a valid surrogate for the tissue of interest. Phase I trials with targeted agents aim to define the dose or concentration of a drug that

TABLE 5.7. Antiangiogenesis therapies.

Agent	*Mechanism of action*	*Trial*	*Major toxicity*
TNP-740	Synthetic analogue of fumagillin; inhibition of Ets-1	Phase II advanced cancer, lymphomas and acute leukemia	Cerebellar dysfunction
Thalidomide	Unknown	Phase I malignant glioma & melanoma Phase II non-small cell lung cancer; phase II in CRC, lymphoma, MDS, liver, CLL, NSCLC Phase III prostate, myeloma, RCC	Fatigue, somnolence, myelosuppression, peripheral neuropathy, thromboembolism (in combination with chemotherapy)
Squalamine	Inhibition sodium-hydrogen exchanger, NHE3	Phase I solid tumors; phase II non-small cell lung cancer and solid tumors	
Combretastatin	Induction of apoptosis in proliferating endothelial cells	Phase I solid tumors; phase II to begin in mid-2000	
Endostatin		Phase I advanced neuroendocrine and melanoma	Rash
Angiostatin		Phase I advanced tumors	Erythema
Anti-VEGF antibody (bevacizumab)	Humanized mAb to VEGF	Phase II metastatic RCC, advanced prostate, NSCLC, colorectal and other solid tumours	Thrombosis, proteinuria, hypertension
Anti-VEGFR-2 (IMC-2C7)	Antibody to VEGFR-2	Preclinical	
Soluble VEGFR-1 (VEGF TRAP)	Inhibition of VEGF signaling by sequestration of VEGF and possibly formation of inactive heterodimers with cell-surface VEGF receptors	Phase I advanced tumors	Hypertension, fatigue, proteinuria
Ribozyme (angiozyme)	Cleavage of mRNA of VEGFR-1	Phase I/II refractory solid tumors	
SU11248	Small molecule inhibitor of VEGFR-2, PDGFR, KIT and FLT-3	Phase I advanced solid tumors	Asthenia, thrombocytopenia, neutropenia, skin discoloration, depigmentation
SU6668	Small molecule blocker of VEGF-receptor, FGF, and PDGF receptor signaling	Phase I in selected advanced tumors	Asthenia, thrombocytopenia, hypertension, diarrhea
PTK787/ZK22584	Inhibition of VEGFR-1,2,3 TKI	Phase I/ II with chemotherapy in CRC	Fatigue, neuropathy, diarrhea
Cilengitide (EMD121974)	Small molecule inhibitor of $\alpha_v\beta_3$ and $\alpha_v\beta_5$	Phase I advanced tumors	
Marimastat	Synthetic inhibitor that blocks TNF—a convertase; inhibitor of MMPs	Phase I pancreatic cancer; phase III NSCLC, small cell lung cancer and breast cancer; phase I GBM	Musculoskeletal pain and joint swelling
Prinomastat (AG-3340)	Synthetic MMP inhibitor	Phase III NSCLC, hormone refractory prostate, pancreatic, and small cell lung cancer	
Metastat (COL-3)	MMP inhibitor and tetracycline derivative	Phase I/II brain, Kaposi's sarcoma	Lupus, anemia
Neovastat (AE941)	Natural MMP inhibitor; derivative of shark cartilage	Phase II multiple myeloma, Phase III renal cell cancer, Phase III non-small cell lung cancer	
BMS-275291	Synthetic MMP inhibitor	Phase I	

provides maximal target inhibition.[114] Because determining target inhibition within the tumor is technically demanding, the sampling of normal or surrogate tissues has been an alternative approach. Examples of surrogate tissue use include the measurement of p70S6 kinase activity in peripheral blood mononuclear cells after treatment with an mTOR inhibitor, the assessment of EGFR and ERK/MEK phosphorylation status in skin biopsies after treatment with EGFR tyrosine kinase inhibitors, or assessment of prelamin A farnesylation in buccal mucosal cells following FTI treatment.[42] However, reliance on surrogate endpoints to determine the efficacy of these targeted therapies has attracted criticism because the pharmacodynamics within normal tissue may not reflect target inhibition within the tumor mass. For example, clinical trials investigating the activities of the EGFR inhibitors have failed to adequately assess the intratumoral pharmacodynamics before and after drug exposure.[2] Therefore, negative trial data may simply reflect inadequate drug dosage and tumor tissue concentrations of these agents rather than drug inactivity, which raises serious questions over the interpretation of negative clinical trial data unless proof of target inhibition is documented within tumor specimens rather than surrogate tissues.

Noninvasive functional imaging techniques that can quantify the level of target function in vivo are under investigation and include dynamic contrast-enhanced MRI (DCE MRI) for measuring tumor vascularization and vascular permeability with angiogenesis inhibitors and positron emission tomography (PET) to monitor metabolic changes in uptake of ^{18}F-fluoro-2-deoxy-D-glucose (^{18}FDG) within the tumor mass. Other functional modalities include doppler ultrasound and dynamic infrared imaging of vascular perfusion patterns.[115]

Phase II

The primary aim of a Phase II trial is to define the spectrum of antitumor activity for the new drug using the optimal dose and schedule determined from Phase I trials. With cytotoxic drugs, the traditional endpoint is response rate as measured by the percentage decrease in size of the tumor compared to the pretreatment size. However, objective response rate may not be an ideal endpoint for target-based agents because of their cytostatic properties. To overcome this difficulty, alternative endpoints have been used in Phase II clinical studies of targeted therapies. These include the following:

- Pharmacodynamic endpoints: for example, quantifying posttranslational changes in biological markers in either tumor or surrogate tissues
- Functional imaging studies to assess treatment response at the tumor site (FDG-PET or dynamic contrast-enhanced MRI)
- Assessment of time to disease progression and the proportion of patients with disease progression
- Quality of life (regarded as a secondary endpoint for cytotoxic agents)[113]

None of these endpoints has been well validated.[116,117] An alternative approach to clinical trials investigating the activity of targeted therapies is the use of the randomized discontinuation design. All patients are enrolled to receive the drug for an initial 2- to 4-month period. Patients with progressive disease, toxicity, or noncompliance during this period are removed from the study. The remaining patients are then randomized to continue the drug or a placebo. The endpoint is the percentage of patients that remain with stable disease in the randomized period. The advantages of this method are that it can overcome the slow accrual of trials that offer treatment or placebo upfront, eligibility criteria can be relatively broad, and enrichment of the randomized group may increase the efficiency of the trial.[118] Other Phase II trial designs include utilizing the patient as the internal control, whereby a single cohort of patients with progressive disease is treated with a cytostatic agent to determine whether the agent slows the rate of disease progression with reference to the pretreatment rate of progression. Similarly, neoadjuvant treatment can provide a valuable system with tumor sampling for molecular analysis that can be performed at progressive time points during treatment.

Phase III

The aim of Phase III trials is to determine efficacy or clinical benefit of a new regimen versus a standard therapy in a randomized study. Endpoints are usually progression-free survival or overall survival. With target-based agents, the traditional designs should remain relatively unchanged. It is important that the drug dose that optimally inhibits the target in question within patient tumor specimens be defined in advance of Phase III studies.

Patient Selection

The target should be critical to the biology of tumor [e.g., *bcr-abl* in chronic myeloid leukemia (CML)], and the targeted agent should be used in a biologically relevant population. Disease stage may also need to be considered in patient selection, as some agents may be less active in the advanced setting and more effective in patients with minimal disease. Many Phase III clinical trials conducted (with the exception of the trastuzumab and imatinib studies) have not selected patients based on target expression. It is noteworthy that had the Phase III study investigating the addition of trastuzumab to chemotherapy in patients with metastatic breast cancer not selected patients based on HER2 overexpression, the trial would have been negative.

At the same time, our understanding of the molecular profile in a tumor that may predict response to targeted therapies remains naive. Little is known about resistance to targeted therapies to guide appropriate strategies of combining different inhibitors together to inhibit redundant or parallel signaling pathways, thus maximizing clinical benefit. Future trials of targeted therapies must incorporate a prospective analysis of tumor tissue during treatment so that response can be correlated with the molecular phenotype (either through microarray or proteomic techniques), thus identifying predictive markers for future studies.

Conclusion: Challenges for the Future

Designing clinical trials to investigate the activity of these novel agents and optimize their use in a defined patient population are critical challenges to the success of targeted therapy. There remains much cause for optimism and enthusiasm, particularly following the notable successes in the past few years that have made it to the clinic, such as trastuzumab for breast cancer, bevacizumab for colorectal cancer, imatinib mesylate for CML and GIST, and gefitinib for lung cancer.

The field is moving fast, with an exploding knowledge base of molecular abnormalities in cancer and an increasing array of molecules that can target abnormal or overexpressed onco-proteins. As reviewed here, targeted therapies include a wide spectrum of approaches that are applicable to many different cancers, and the principles which govern their development are evolving as we learn how to utilize these novel agents. Within the next decade we should find out whether we make a paradigm shift in the treatment and prevention of cancer by translating scientific progress into clinical practice. Many truly believe that we will.

References

1. Hanahan D, Weinberg RA. The hallmarks of cancer. Cell 2000; 100(1):57–70.
2. Dancey J, Sausville EA. Issues and progress with protein kinase inhibitors for cancer treatment. Nat Rev Drug Discov 2003; 2(4):296–313.
3. Smith C. Drug target identification: a question of biology. Nature (Lond) 2004;428(6979):225–231.
4. Johnston SRD. Fulvestrant and the sequential endocrine cascade for advanced breast cancer. Br J Cancer 2004;90:15–18.
5. Hynes NE. ErbB2 activation and signal transduction in normal and malignant mammary cells. J Mammary Gland Biol Neoplasia 1996;1(2):199–206.
6. Ciardiello F, Tortora G. A novel approach in the treatment of cancer: targeting the epidermal growth factor receptor. Clin Cancer Res 2001;7(10):2958–2970.
7. Burtness BA, Li Y, Flood W, Mattar BI, Forastiere AA. Phase III trial comparing cisplatin (C) + placebo (P) to C + anti-epidermal growth factor antibody (EGF-R) C225 in patients (pts) with metastatic/recurrent head & neck cancer (HNC). Proc Am Soc Clin Oncol 2002;21:67 (abstract 901).
8. Cunningham D, Humblet Y, Siena S, et al. Cetuximab monotherapy and cetuximab plus irinotecan in irinotecan-refractory metastatic colorectal cancer. N Engl J Med 2004; 351(4):337–345.
9. Gatzemeier U, Rosell R, Ramlau R, et al. Cetuximab (C225) in combination with cisplatin/vinolrelbine vs. cisplatin/vinolrelbine alone in the first-line treatment of patients (pts) with epidermal growth factor receptor (EGFR) positive advanced non-small-cell lung cancer (NSCLC). Proc Am Soc Clin Oncol 2003;22 (abstract).
10. Slamon DJ, Clark GM, Wong SG, Levin WJ, Ullrich A, McGuire WL. Human breast cancer: correlation of relapse and survival with amplification of the HER-2/neu oncogene. Science 1987;235(4785):177–182.
11. Vogel CL, Cobleigh MA, Tripathy D, et al. First-line Herceptin monotherapy in metastatic breast cancer. Oncology 2001;61(suppl 2):37–42.
12. Slamon DJ, Leyland-Jones B, Shak S, et al. Use of chemotherapy plus a monoclonal antibody against HER2 for metastatic breast cancer that overexpresses HER2. N Engl J Med 2001; 344(11):783–792.
13. Druker BJ, Talpaz M, Resta DJ, et al. Efficacy and safety of a specific inhibitor of the BCR-ABL tyrosine kinase in chronic myeloid leukemia. N Engl J Med 2001;344(14):1031–1037.
14. Rubin BP, Singer S, Tsao C, et al. KIT activation is a ubiquitous feature of gastrointestinal stromal tumors. Cancer Res 2001; 61(22):8118–8121.
15. Heinrich MC, Corless CL, Demetri GD, et al. Kinase mutations and imatinib response in patients with metastatic gastrointestinal stromal tumor. J Clin Oncol 2003;21(23):4342–4349.
16. Demetri GD, von Mehren M, Blanke CD, et al. Efficacy and safety of imatinib mesylate in advanced gastrointestinal stromal tumors. N Engl J Med 2002;347(7):472–480.
17. Verweij J, van Oosterom A, Blay JY, et al. Imatinib mesylate (STI-571 Glivec, Gleevec) is an active agent for gastrointestinal stromal tumors, but does not yield responses in other soft-tissue sarcomas that are unselected for a molecular target. Results from an EORTC Soft Tissue and Bone Sarcoma Group phase II study. Eur J Cancer 2003;39(14):2006–2011.
18. Ciardiello F, Caputo R, Bianco R, et al. Antitumor effect and potentiation of cytotoxic drugs activity in human cancer cells by ZD-1839 (Iressa), an epidermal growth factor receptor-selective tyrosine kinase inhibitor. Clin Cancer Res 2000;6(5):2053–2063.
19. Sirotnak FM, Zakowski MF, Miller VA, Scher HI, Kris MG. Efficacy of cytotoxic agents against human tumor xenografts is markedly enhanced by coadministration of ZD1839 (Iressa), an inhibitor of EGFR tyrosine kinase. Clin Cancer Res 2000; 6(12):4885–4892.
20. Kris MG, Natale RB, Herbst RS, et al. A phase II trial of ZD 1839 (Iressa) in advanced non-small lung cancer patients who had failed platinum and docetaxel regimens (IDEAL 2). Proc Am Soc Clin Oncol 2002;21 (abstract).
21. Fukuoka M, Yano S, Giaccone G. Final results from a phase II trial of ZD1839 (Iressa) for patients with advanced non-small cell lung cancer (IDEAL 1). Proc Am Soc Clin Oncol 2002;21 (abstract).
22. Giaccone G, Herbst RS, Manegold C, et al. Gefitinib in combination with gemcitabine and cisplatin in advanced non-small-cell lung cancer: a phase III trial–INTACT 1. J Clin Oncol 2004;22(5):777–784.
23. Albain K, Elledge R, Gradishar WJ, et al. Open-label phase II multicentre trial of ZD1839(Iressa) in patients with advanced breast cancer. Breast Cancer Res Treat 2002;76.
24. Baselga J, Albanell J, Ruiz R, et al. Phase II and tumour pharmacodynamic study of gefitinib in patients with advanced breast cancer. Proc Am Soc Clin Oncol 2003;22 (abstract).
25. Robertson JFR, Gutteridge E, Cheung KL, et al. Gefitinib (ZD1839) is active in aquired tamoxifen-resistant oestrogen receptor positive and ER-negative breast cancer: results from a phase II study. Proc Am Soc Clin Oncol 2003:22 (abstract).
26. Knowlden JM, Hutcheson IR, Jones HE, et al. Elevated levels of epidermal growth factor receptor/c-erbB2 heterodimers mediate an autocrine growth regulatory pathway in tamoxifen-resistant MCF-7 cells. Endocrinology 2003;144(3):1032–1044.
27. Dancey JE, Freidlin B. Targeting epidermal growth factor receptor—are we missing the mark? Lancet 2003;362(9377):62–64.
28. Perez-Soler R, Chachoua A, Huberman M, et al. A phase II trial of the epidermal growth factor receptor (EGFR) tyrosine kinase inhibitor OSI-774, following platinum-based chemotherapy, in patients (pts) with advanced, EGFR-expressing, non-small cell lung cancer (NSCLC). Proc Am Soc Clin Oncol 2001:20.
29. Herbst RS, Prager D, Hermann R, et al. TRIBUTE— A phase III trial of erlotinib HCL (OSI-774) combined with carboplatin and paclitaxel chemotherapy in advanced non-small cell lung cancer. Proc Am Assoc Cancer Res 2004.
30. Gatzemeier U, Pluzanska A, Szczesna A, et al. Results of a phase III trial of erlotinib (OSI-774) combined with cisplatin and gemcitabine chemotherapy in advanced non-small cell lung cancer. Proc Am Assoc Cancer Res 2004.
31. Shepherd FA, Pereira J, Ciuleanu TE, et al. A randomised placebo controlled trial of erlotinib in patients with advanced non-small cell lung cancer (NSCLC) following failure of 1st line or 2nd line chemotherapy. Proc Am Assoc Cancer Res 2004.
32. Winer E, Cobleigh MA, Dickler M, et al. Phase II multicenter study to evaluate the efficacy and safety of Tarceva (erlotinib, OSI-774) in women with previously treated locally advanced or metastatic breast cancer. Breast Cancer Res Treat 2002;76.
33. Allen LF, Eiseman IA, Fry DW, Lenehan PF. CI-1033, an irreversible pan-erbB receptor inhibitor and its potential application for the treatment of breast cancer. Semin Oncol 2003;30(5 suppl 16):65–78.
34. Xia W, Mullin RJ, Keith BR, et al. Anti-tumor activity of GW572016: a dual tyrosine kinase inhibitor blocks EGF activation of EGFR/erbB2 and downstream Erb1/2 and AKT pathways. Oncogene 2002;21(41):6255–6263.
35. Spector NL, Raefsky E, Hurwitz H, et al. Safety, clinical efficacy, and biologic assessments from EGF10004: a randomized phase IB study of GW572016 for patients with metastatic carcinomas overexpressing EGFR or erbB2. Proc Am Soc Clin Oncol 2003: 22 (abstract).
36. Marshall CJ. Cell signalling. Raf gets it together. Nature (Lond) 1996;383(6596):127–128.

37. Kato K, Cox AD, Hisaka MM, et al. Isoprenoid addition to Ras protein is the critical modification for its membrane association and transforming activity. Proc Natl Acad Sci USA 1992;89(14):6403–6407.
38. Ashar HR, James L, Gray K, et al. Farnesyl transferase inhibitors block the farnesylation of CENP-E and CENP-F and alter the association of CENP-E with the microtubules. J Biol Chem 2000;275(39):30451–30457.
39. Bishop WR, Bond R, Petrin J, et al. Novel tricyclic inhibitors of farnesyl protein transferase. Biochemical characterization and inhibition of Ras modification in transfected Cos cells. J Biol Chem 1995;270(51):30611–30618.
40. Liu M, Bryant MS, Chen J, et al. Antitumor activity of SCH 66336, an orally bioavailable tricyclic inhibitor of farnesyl protein transferase, in human tumor xenograft models and wap-ras transgenic mice. Cancer Res 1998;58(21):4947–4956.
41. Eskens FA, Awada A, Cutler DL, et al. Phase I and pharmacokinetic study of the oral farnesyl transferase inhibitor SCH 66336 given twice daily to patients with advanced solid tumors. J Clin Oncol 2001;19(4):1167–1175.
42. Adjei AA, Erlichman C, Davis JN, et al. A Phase I trial of the farnesyl transferase inhibitor SCH66336: evidence for biological and clinical activity. Cancer Res 2000;60(7):1871–1877.
43. Shi B, Yaremko B, Hajian G, et al. The farnesyl protein transferase inhibitor SCH66336 synergises with taxanes in vitro and enhances their antitumor activity in vivo. Cancer Chemother Pharmacol 2000;46:387–393.
44. End DW, Smets G, Todd AV, et al. Characterization of the antitumor effects of the selective farnesyl protein transferase inhibitor R115777 in vivo and in vitro. Cancer Res 2001; 61(1):131–137.
45. Kurzrock R, Kantarjian HM, Cortes JE, et al. Farnesyltransferase inhibitor R115777 in myelodysplastic syndrome: clinical and biologic activities in the phase 1 setting. Blood 2003; 102(13):4527–4534.
46. Karp JE, Lancet JE, Kaufmann SH, et al. Clinical and biologic activity of the farnesyltransferase inhibitor R115777 in adults with refractory and relapsed acute leukemias: a phase 1 clinical-laboratory correlative trial. Blood 2001;97(11):3361–3369.
47. Cunningham D, De Gramont A, Scheithauer W, et al. Randomized double-blind placebo controlled trial of the farnesyltransferase inhibitor R-115777 (Zanestra) in advanced refractory colorectal cancer. Proc Am Soc Clin Oncol 2002;21.
48. Van Cutsem E, van de Velde H, Karasek P, A et al. Phase III trial of gemcitabine plus tipifarnib compared with gemcitabine plus placebo in advanced pancreatic cancer. J Clin Oncol 2004; 22(8):1430–1438.
49. Johnston SRD, Head J, Valenti M, Detre S, Dowsett M. Endocrine therapy combined with the farnesyltransferase inhibitor R115777 produces enhanced tumour growth inhibition in hormone-sensitive MCF-7 human breast cancer xenografts in vivo. Breast Cancer Res Treat 2002;76:A245.
50. Bjornsti MA, Houghton PJ. The tor pathway: a target for cancer therapy. Nat Rev Cancer 2004;4(5):335–348.
51. Yu K, Toral-Barza L, Discafani C, et al. mTOR, a novel target in breast cancer: the effect of CCI-779, an mTOR inhibitor, in preclinical models of breast cancer. Endocr Relat Cancer 2001; 8(3):249–258.
52. Raymond E, Alexandre J, Faivre S, et al. Safety and pharmacokinetics of escalated doses of weekly infusion of CCI-779, a novel mTOR inhibitor, in patients with cancer. J Clin Oncol 2004;22:2336–2347.
53. Atkins MB, Hidalgo M, Stadler WM, et al. Randomized phase II study of multiple dose levels of CCI-779, a novel mammalian target of rapamycin kinase inhibitor, in patients with advanced refractory renal cell carcinoma. J Clin Oncol 2004;22(5):909–918.
54. Chan S, Scheulen ME Johnston S, et al. Phase 2 study of two dose levels of CCI-779 in locally advanced or metastatic breast cancer (MBC) failing prior anthracycline and/or taxane regimens. Proc Am Soc Clin Oncol 2003.
55. O'Donnell A, Faivre S, Judson I, et al. A phase 1 study of the oral mTor inhibitor RAD001 as monotherapy to identify the optimal biological effective dose using toxicity, pharmacokinetic (PK) and pharmacodynamic (PD) endpoints in patients with solid tumours. Proc Am Soc Clin Oncol 2003 (abstract).
56. Davies H, Bignell GR, Cox C, et al. Mutations of the BRAF gene in human cancer. Nature (Lond) 2002;417(6892):949–954.
57. Strumberg D, Awada A, Piccart M, et al. Final report of the phase I clinical program of the novel raf kinase inhibitor BAY 43-9006 in patients with refractory solid tumors. Proc Am Soc Clin Oncol 2003;22.
58. Flaherty KT, Lee RJ, Humphries R, O'Dwyer PJ, Schiller JH. Phase I trial of BAY 43-9006 in combination with carboplatin (C) and paclitaxel (P). Proc Am Soc Clin Oncol 2003;22.
59. LoRusso PM, Adjei AA, Meyer MB, et al. A phase I clinical and pharmacokinetic evaluation of the oral MEK inhibitor, CI-1040, administered for 21 consecutive days, repeated every 4 weeks in patients with advanced cancer. Proc Am Soc Clin Oncol 2002;21.
60. Waterhouse DM, Rinehart J, Adjei AA, et al. A phase 2 study of an oral MEK inhibitor, CI-1040, in patients with advanced non-small-cell lung, breast, colon, or pancreatic cancer. Proc Am Soc Clin Oncol 2002;22.
61. Senderowicz AM, Sausville EA. Preclinical and clinical development of cyclin-dependent kinase modulators. J Natl Cancer Inst 2000;92(5):376–387.
62. Senderowicz AM, Headlee D, Stinson SF, et al. Phase I trial of continuous infusion flavopiridol, a novel cyclin-dependent kinase inhibitor, in patients with refractory neoplasms. J Clin Oncol 1998;16(9):2986–2999.
63. Stadler WM, Vogelzang NJ, Amato R, et al. Flavopiridol, a novel cyclin-dependent kinase inhibitor, in metastatic renal cancer: a University of Chicago Phase II Consortium study. J Clin Oncol 2000;18(2):371–375.
64. Shapiro GI, Supko JG, Patterson A, et al. A phase II trial of the cyclin-dependent kinase inhibitor flavopiridol in patients with previously untreated stage IV non-small cell lung cancer. Clin Cancer Res 2001;7(6):1590–1599.
65. Schwartz GK, Ilson D, Saltz L, et al. Phase II study of the cyclin-dependent kinase inhibitor flavopiridol administered to patients with advanced gastric carcinoma. J Clin Oncol 2001;19(7): 1985–1992.
66. Bible KC, Kaufmann SH. Cytotoxic synergy between flavopiridol (NSC 649890, L86–8275) and various antineoplastic agents: the importance of sequence of administration. Cancer Res 1997; 57(16):3375–3380.
67. Gries J-M, Kasimis B, Schwarzenberger P, et al. Phase I study of flavopiridol in non-small cell lung cancer patients after 24-hours IV administration combined with paclitaxel and carboplatin. Proc Am Soc Clin Oncol 2002;21 (abstract).
68. Shah MA, Kortmansky J, Gonen M. A phase I /pharmacological study of weekly sequential irinotecan and flavopiridol. Proc Am Soc Clin Oncol 2002 (abstract).
69. O'Connor DS, Wall NR, Porter AC, Altieri DC. A p34(cdc2) survival checkpoint in cancer. Cancer Cell 2002;2(1):43–54.
70. Schwartz GK, O'Reilly E, Ilson D, et al. Phase I study of the cyclin-dependent kinase inhibitor flavopiridol in combination with paclitaxel in patients with advanced solid tumors. J Clin Oncol 2002;20(8):2157–2170.
71. Punt CJ, Fumoleau P, van de Walle B, Faber MN, Ravic M, Campone M. Phase I and pharmacokinetic study of E7070, a novel sulfonamide, given at a daily times five schedule in patients with solid tumors. A study by the EORTC-early clinical studies group (ECSG). Ann Oncol 2001;12(9):1289–1293.
72. Raymond E, Bokkel Huinink WW, Taieb J, et al. Phase I and pharmacokinetic study of E7070, a novel chloroindolyl sulfonamide

cell-cycle inhibitor, administered as a one-hour infusion every three weeks in patients with advanced cancer. J Clin Oncol 2002;20(16):3508–3521.

73. Talbot D, Norbury C, Slade M, et al. A Phase II and pharmacodynamic study of E7070 in patients with non-small cell lung cancer (NSCLC) who have failed platinum-based chemotherapy. Proc Am Soc Clin Oncol 2002;21.
74. Mainwaring PN, Van Cutsem E, Van Laethem J-L, et al. A multicentre randomised phase II study of E7070 in patients with colorectal cancer who have failed 5-fluorouracil-based chemotherapy. Proc Am Soc Clin Oncol 2002;21 (abstract).
75. Adams J. The proteasome: a suitable antineoplastic target. Nat Rev Cancer 2004;4(5):349–360.
76. Richardson PG, Barlogie B, Berenson J, et al. A phase 2 study of bortezomib in relapsed, refractory myeloma. N Engl J Med 2003;348(26):2609–2617.
77. Berenson J, Jagannath S, Barlogie B, et al. Experience with long-term therapy using the proteosome inhibitor, bortezomib, in advanced multiple myelome (MM). Proc Am Soc Clin Oncol 2002;22 (abstract).
78. Orlowski RZ. Phase I study of the proteosome inhibitor bortezomib and pegylated doxorubicin in patients with refractory haematological malignanacies. Blood 2003;102 (abstract).
79. Marks PA, Richon VM, Rifkind RA. Histone deacetylase inhibitors: inducers of differentiation or apoptosis of transformed cells. J Natl Cancer Inst 2000;92(15):1210–1216.
80. Saito A, Yamashita T, Mariko Y, et al. A synthetic inhibitor of histone deacetylase, MS-27-275 with marked in vivo antitumour activity against human tumors. Proc Natl Acad Sci USA 1999; 96:4592–4597 (abstract).
81. Wall NR, O'Connor DS, Plescia J, Pommier Y, Altieri DC. Suppression of survivin phosphorylation on Thr34 by flavopiridol enhances tumor cell apoptosis. Cancer Res 2003;63(1):230–235.
82. Hu W, Kavanagh JJ. Anticancer therapy targeting the apoptotic pathway. Lancet Oncol 2003;4(12):721–729.
83. Waters JS, Webb A, Cunningham D, et al. Phase I clinical and pharmacokinetic study of bcl-2 antisense oligonucleotide therapy in patients with non-Hodgkin's lymphoma. J Clin Oncol 2000;18(9):1812–1823.
84. Bischoff JR, Kirn DH, Williams A, et al. An adenovirus mutant that replicates selectively in p53-deficient human tumor cells. Science 1996;274(5286):373–376.
85. Hall AR, Dix BR, O'Carroll SJ, Braithwaite AW. p53-dependent cell death/apoptosis is required for a productive adenovirus infection. Nat Med 1998;4(9):1068–1072.
86. Khuri FR, Nemunaitis J, Ganly I, et al. A controlled trial of intratumoral ONYX-015, a selectively-replicating adenovirus, in combination with cisplatin and 5-fluorouracil in patients with recurrent head and neck cancer. Nat Med 2000;6(8):879–885.
87. Reid TR, Sze D, Galanis E, Abbruzzese JL, Kirn DH, Freeman S. Intra-arterial administration of a replication-selective adenovirus ONYX-015 in patients with colorectal carcinoma metastatic to the liver: safety, feasibility and biological activity. Proc Am Soc Clin Oncol 2003 (abstract).
88. Vasey PA, Shulman LN, Campos S, et al. Phase I trial of intraperitoneal injection of the E1B-55-kd-gene-deleted adenovirus ONYX-015 (dl1520) given on days 1 through 5 every 3 weeks in patients with recurrent/refractory epithelial ovarian cancer. J Clin Oncol 2002;20(6):1562–1569.
89. Clayman GL, el Naggar AK, Lippman SM, et al. Adenovirus-mediated p53 gene transfer in patients with advanced recurrent head and neck squamous cell carcinoma. J Clin Oncol 1998; 16(6):2221–2232.
90. Vassilev LT, Vu BT, Graves B, et al. In vivo activation of the p53 pathway by small-molecule antagonists of MDM2. Science 2004;303(5659):844–848.
91. Davies R, Frydenberg M, Tulluch A, Kelly G. Interim results of a phase Ib/IIa study of a oral phenoxodiol in patients with late-stage, hormone-refractory prostate cancer. Proc Am Assoc Cancer Res 2004; LB-214 (abstract).
92. Rutherford T, O'Malley D, Makkenchery A, et al. Phenoxodiol phase Ib/II study in patients with recurrent ovarian cancer that are resistant to > *or* = second line chemotherapy. Proc Am Assoc Cancer Res 2004;4457 (abstract).
93. Folkman J. Tumor angiogenesis: therapeutic implications. N Engl J Med 1971;285(21):1182–1186.
94. Folkman J. Angiogenesis in cancer, vascular, rheumatoid and other disease. Nat Med 1995;1(1):27–31.
95. Weidner N. Angiogenesis in breast cancer. Cancer Treat Res 1996;83:265–301.
96. Sharma RA, Marriot JB, Clarke I, et al. Tolerability of the novel oral thalidomide analog CC-5013 demonstrating extensive immune activation and clinical response. Proc Am Soc Clin Oncol 2003 (abstract).
97. Bhargava P, Marshall JL, Rizvi N, et al. A Phase I and pharmacokinetic study of TNP-470 administered weekly to patients with advanced cancer. Clin Cancer Res 1999;5(8):1989–1995.
98. Herbst RS, Madden TL, Tran HT, et al. Safety and pharmacokinetic effects of TNP-470, an angiogenesis inhibitor, combined with paclitaxel in patients with solid tumors: evidence for activity in non-small-cell lung cancer. J Clin Oncol 2002; 20(22):4440–4447.
99. Kulke M, Bergsland E, Ryan DP, et al. A phase II, open-label, safety, pharmacokinetic, and efficacy study of recombinant endostatin in patients with advanced neuroendocrine tumours. Proc Am Soc Clin Oncol 2003 (abstract).
100. Voest EE, Beerepoot LV, Groenewegen G, et al. Phase I trial of recombinant human angiostatin by twice-daily subcutaneous injection in patients with advanced cancer. Proc Am Soc Clin Oncol 2002;21 (abstract).
101. Eppenberger U, Kueng W, Schlaeppi JM, et al. Markers of tumor angiogenesis and proteolysis independently define high- and low-risk subsets of node-negative breast cancer patients. J Clin Oncol 1998;16(9):3129–3136.
102. Weng DE, Weiss P, Kellackey C, et al. Angiozyme Pharmacokinetic and safety results: a phase I/II study in patients with refractory solid tumours. Proc Am Soc Clin Oncol 2001;20 (abstract).
103. Kim KJ, Li B, Houck K, Winer J, Ferrara N. The vascular endothelial growth factor proteins: identification of biologically relevant regions by neutralizing monoclonal antibodies. Growth Factors 1992;7(1):53–64.
104. Hurwitz H, Fehrenbacher L, Novotny W, et al. Bevacizumab plus irinotecan, fluorouracil, and leucovorin for metastatic colorectal cancer. N Engl J Med 2004;350(23):2335–2342.
105. Johnson DH, Fehrenbacher L, Novotny WF, et al. Randomized phase II trial comparing bevacizumab plus carboplatin and paclitaxel with carboplatin and paclitaxel alone in previously untreated locally advanced or metastatic non-small-cell lung cancer. J Clin Oncol 2004;22(11):2184–2191.
106. Raymond E, Faivre S, Vera C, et al. Final results of a phase I and pharmacokinetic study of SU11248, a novel multi-target tyrosine kinase, in patients with advanced cancers. Proc Am Soc Clin Oncol 2003;22 (abstract).
107. Steward WP, Thomas AL, Morgan B, et al. Extended phase I study of the oral vascular endothelial growth factor (VEGF) receptor inhibitor PTK787/ZK 222584 in combination with oxaliplatin/5-fluorouracil (5-FU)/leucovorin as first line treatment for metastatic colorectal cancer. Proc Am Soc Clin Oncol 2003;22 (abstract).
108. Stamenkovic I. Matrix metalloproteinases in tumor invasion and metastasis. Semin Cancer Biol 2000;10(6):415–433.
109. Yonemura Y, Endo Y, Fujita H, et al. Inhibition of peritoneal dissemination in human gastric cancer by MMP-7-specific antisense oligonucleotide. J Exp Clin Cancer Res 2001;20(2): 205–212.

110. Silletti S, Kessler T, Goldberg J, Boger DL, Cheresh DA. Disruption of matrix metalloproteinase 2 binding to integrin alpha v beta 3 by an organic molecule inhibits angiogenesis and tumor growth in vivo. Proc Natl Acad Sci USA 2001;98(1):119–124.
111. Eskens FA, Dumez H, Hoekstra R, et al. Phase I and pharmacokinetic study of continuous twice weekly intravenous administration of Cilengitide (EMD 121974), a novel inhibitor of the integrins alphavbeta3 and alphavbeta5 in patients with advanced solid tumours. Eur J Cancer 2003;39(7):917–926.
112. Bramhall SR, Hallissey MT, Whiting J, et al. Marimastat as maintenance therapy for patients with advanced gastric cancer: a randomised trial. Br J Cancer 2002;86(12):1864–1870.
113. Rowinsky EK. Challenges of developing therapeutics that target signal transduction in patients with gynecologic and other malignancies. J Clin Oncol 2003;21(suppl 10):175–186.
114. Gelmon KA, Eisenhauer EA, Harris AL, Ratain MJ, Workman P. Anticancer agents targeting signaling molecules and cancer cell environment: challenges for drug development? J Natl Cancer Inst 1999;91(15):1281–1287.
115. Janicek MJ, Janicek MR, Merriam P, et al. Imaging responses to Imatinib mesylate (Gleevec, STI571) in gastrointestinal stromal tumors (GIST): vascular perfusion patterns with Doppler ultrasound (DUS) and dynamic infrared imaging (DIRI). Proc Am Soc Clin Oncol 2002;21 (abstract).
116. Eisenhauer EA. Phase I and II trials of novel anti-cancer agents: endpoints, efficacy and existentialism. The Michel Clavel Lecture, held at the 10th NCI-EORTC Conference on New Drugs in Cancer Therapy, Amsterdam, 16–19 June 1998. Ann Oncol 1998;9(10):1047–1052.
117. Dent S, Zee B, Dancey J, Hanauske A, Wanders J, Eisenhauer E. Application of a new multinomial phase II stopping rule using response and early progression. J Clin Oncol 2001;19(3):785–791.
118. Kopec JA, Abrahamowicz M, Esdaile JM. Randomized discontinuation trials: utility and efficiency. J Clin Epidemiol 1993;46(9):959–971.

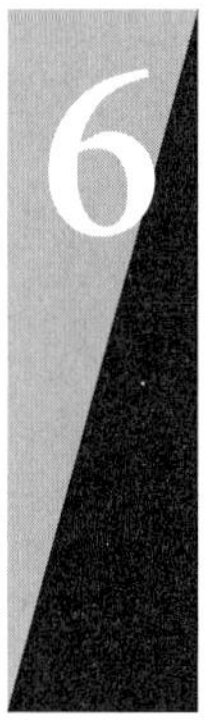

Biologic Principles of Hematopoietic Stem Cell Transplantation

Robert J. Soiffer

During the past 25 years, hematopoietic stem cell transplantation (HSCT) has become accepted as routine treatment for many patients with hematologic malignancies. Traditionally, the primary biologic objectives of HSCT for malignant disease and marrow disorders include the following:

- Delivery of chemotherapy/radiotherapy sufficient to destroy tumor cells
- Infusion of a source of hematopoietic stem cells to replace damaged lymphoid or myeloid progenitors
- Establishment of organ graft tolerance to prevent rejection of donor cells
- Induction of graft-versus-tumor (GVT) activity by allogeneic immune effector cells

Recent laboratory and clinical observations on the biology of transplantation have challenged many of the fundamental beliefs and practices established over the past quarter century. Insights into graft-versus-host disease (GVHD), graft-versus-leukemia (GVL) activity, stem cell engraftment, donor selection, minimal residual disease (MRD), infectious complications, and treatment-related organ dysfunction all have contributed to revisions and refinements in the current approach to potential transplant recipients.

Indications for Transplantation

For many diseases, the indications for transplantation were established in an era when standard treatment approaches had very little hope of producing cures or extended long-term survival. As both nontransplant therapeutic options and transplant-related methodologies have evolved, continued reassessment is needed to determine the place of transplantation in the design of treatment algorithms.

It is a common misconception that research in transplantation is bereft of comparative clinical trials. It is true that many reported Phase 2 trials are difficult to interpret in the absence of rigorously defined control groups. Single institution case-control studies are only of limited value. However, the establishment of well-organized data repositories such as the International Bone Marrow Transplant Registry (IBMTR) and the European Bone Marrow Transplant (EBMT) registry have led to large retrospective observational studies using standardized data collection tools across many centers. The reports emerging from these studies have proven useful in assessing the value of specific transplant strategies. However, these registry analyses do not take the place of rigorously conducted randomized trials. Indeed, there have been a number of randomized trials conducted in transplantation, although many have been underpowered to detect small, but significant, differences because of limited patient availability.

Transplant indications can be divided into three groups based on the objective evidence that supports its use. The first group includes those diseases for which results from prospective randomized trials are available to guide treatment decisions. The most definitive randomized study supporting transplantation was the PARMA trial, conducted in patients undergoing autologous HSCT for non-Hodgkin's lymphoma (Figure 6.1).[1] Patients with relapsed NHL were treated with two cycles of salvage chemotherapy upon study entry. Those patients exhibiting a response were randomized to receive either high-dose chemotherapy and autologous bone marrow transplantation or four more cycles of chemotherapy. With extended follow-up in each arm, both disease-free survival and overall survival were far superior for patients undergoing transplantation. In another randomized trial conducted in Europe at the same time, a survival advantage was demonstrated for patients with recurrent multiple myeloma randomized to autologous transplantation compared to conventional therapy. This finding was recently confirmed in another large randomized study.[2,3]

The importance of randomized trials is not limited to positive studies. The highly publicized randomized trials in breast cancer patients with metastatic disease or with more than 10 positive nodes failed to demonstrate any survival advantage for autologous transplantation.[4–6] Participation in these studies was critical in helping to determine that high-dose chemotherapy and autologous HSCT, which had become *standard* treatment for many patients with advanced disease, offered no clear-cut advantage to conventional therapy. Still, proponents of transplant point to the lower relapse rates in the transplant arm and argue that if toxicity could be eliminated, high-dose therapy might still offer advantages.

It is also important not to blindly extrapolate the results of positive studies to distinctly different clinical scenarios. For example, the encouraging results with autologous transplantation for intermediate-grade NHL in second remission prompted its use for patients thought to be at high risk for relapse in first remission. However, when a prospective randomized study was performed in these first remission patients, no clear benefit of transplantation could be demonstrated except perhaps in patients with very high international prognostic index (IPI) scores.[7–9]

There have also been circumstances in which different randomized studies have yielded conflicting results, as is most clearly the case for patients with acute myelogenous leukemia (AML) and acute lymphoblastic anemia (ALL) in first complete remission (CRI). Many of these trials were designed so that patients with HLA-identical donors were allocated (truly genetically selected) for allogeneic transplantation whereas those without donors were randomized to autologous transplantation or further chemotherapy. In some of these trials, allogeneic transplantation held a modest advantage when analyzed on an intention-to-treat basis. In other trials, no significant differences in disease-free survival (DFS) between the treatment arms could be found.[10–13] More recent data on the prognostic implications of certain chromosome abnormalities associated with AML and ALL have influenced thinking on who should undergo transplantation in first remission. General agreement exists that patients with adverse cytogenetics (such as monosomy 7 or multiple complex abnormalities in AML or the Philadelphia chromosome in ALL) should undergo HSCT in CRI. Patients with favorable cytogenetics [such as t(8;21) or inv16] are usually not offered transplantation in first remission. Transplant decisions for patients with intermediate-risk cytogenetics in AML and ALL are more difficult and require careful deliberation with the patient and his/her family.

The second group of transplant indications includes those diseases for which a cure rate has been established with HSCT that is superior to that obtained with conventional therapy but for which prospective randomized trials have not been conducted. This group includes patients with recurrent acute leukemia, recurrent Hodgkin's disease, low-grade lymphoma, chronic lymphocytic leukemia (CLL), aplastic anemia, and chronic myelogenous leukemia (CML).[14–24] CML deserves special consideration since the introduction of imatinib into practice in 2001.[25–27] In the pre-imatinib era, cure rates were less than 5% and median survival was 5 to 6 years with either hydroxyurea or interferon, the mainstays of therapy. In contrast, for patients under 50 years of age with an HLA-identical sibling donor, HSCT performed in the first year after diagnosis of stable-phase CML cures more than 70% of patients.[28,29] DFS for patients with unrelated donors appears to exceed 50% to 60% in identical circumstances.[16] For these younger patients with CML, it could be safely argued that HSCT offered the only hope for cure. However, this conclusion did not necessarily mean that HSCT was an obvious choice for all these patients, because there was a very real possibility that transplantation would dramatically shorten the lifespan of a subset of patients as a result of transplant-related complications. In the current imatinib era, the transplant decisions faced by physicians and patients cannot necessarily be based on a reproducible median survival of 5 to 6 years without HSCT. It is not known what the median survival will be for newly diagnosed patients treated with imatinib. Despite the early data that indicate imatinib is superior to interferon in inducing hematologic and cytogenetic remissions, the duration of these responses is not known.[30,31] Development of drug resistance has been identified in a number of patients.[32,33] At this point, it is too early to know how imatinib should change the approach to transplantation for CML.

The third group of transplant indications includes those diseases for which transplantation benefits some individuals but for which sufficient follow-up is not yet available in enough patients to determine the proper role of HSCT in disease management. Diseases that fall into this category include hemoglobinopathies, autoimmune disorders, and renal cell carcinoma.[34–36] Transplantation for these indications should be considered investigational.

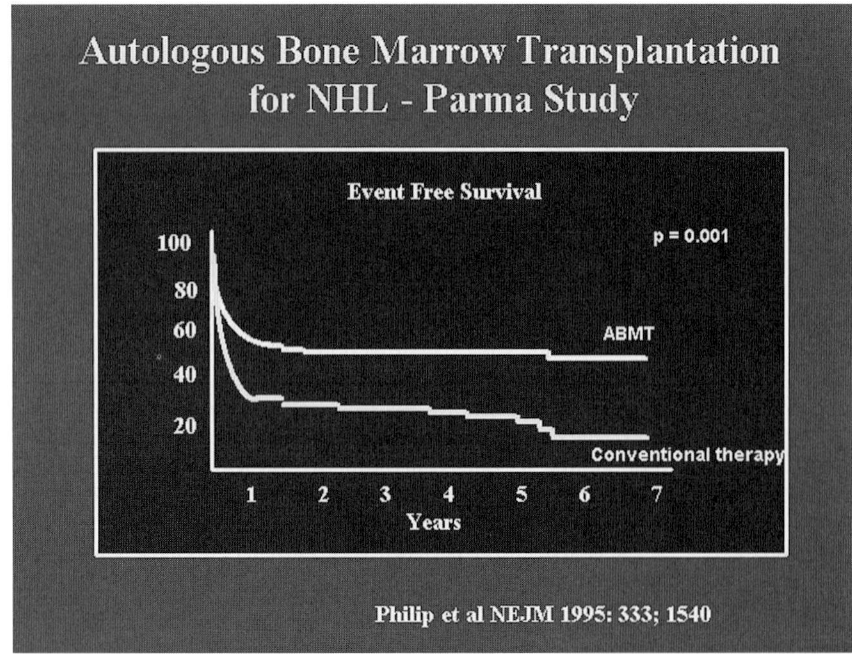

FIGURE 6.1. Randomized study of high-dose chemotherapy with autologous transplantation versus chemotherapy. Event-free survival in patients undergoing transplantation is superior to that in those receiving chemotherapy alone for recurrent chemotherapy-sensitive intermediate-grade non-Hodgkin's lymphoma. (Adapted from Philip et al.,[1] by permission of *New England Journal of Medicine*.)

Sources of Hematopoietic Stem Cells

Hematopoietic stem cells for transplantation can be obtained from bone marrow (BM) or peripheral blood (PB). Bone marrow was the traditional source for stem cells until the 1980s. At that time, antibodies were developed that could recognize CD34+ hematopoietic progenitors, and it was recognized that these CD34+ cells circulate in PB. Moreover, the number of these CD34+ cells in the periphery increased during recovery from myelosuppressive chemotherapy and after administration of growth factors, particularly granulocyte colony-stimulating growth factor (G-CSF).[37–39] Strategies to mobilize stem cells from the marrow out into PB with chemotherapy, growth factors, or a combination of the two were developed. Full lymphohematopoietic reconstitution was observed after ablation and infusion of these mobilized PB stem cells in the autologous transplant setting. Using mobilized PB containing a minimum of 2.0×10^6 CD34+ cells/kg, engraftment of both neutrophils and platelets is considerably more rapid than when BM is used.[40,41] For autologous transplantation, mobilized PB has replaced BM as the stem cell source in most centers. It is notable, however, that the use of peripheral blood stem cells (PBSCs) has not led to improved survival after autologous transplantation but has been associated with decreased duration of hospitalization.

Physicians were initially reluctant to use PB for allogeneic transplantation as it was feared that the increased number of T lymphocytes infused with PB would increase the incidence and severity of graft-versus-host-disease (GHVD). The first trials published in the 1990s demonstrated rapid engraftment without apparent increases in GVHD.[42,43] A number of randomized trials comparing allogeneic PBSC versus BM have been reported, as have a meta-analysis and registry data.[44–49] As in the autologous setting, neutrophil and platelet engraftment were more rapid with PBSCs. There have been conflicting reports on the risk of acute GVHD posed by PBSCs. In a randomized trial involving 350 patients, both acute GVHD (grade II–IV) and severe acute GVHD (grade III–IV) were significantly increased in the PBSCT group (52% versus 39%, $P = 0.014$ and 28% versus 16%, $P = 0.01$, respectively).[50] Other trials have found differences in acute GVHD that were not statistically significant. An IBMTR/EBMT retrospective review of 288 PBSC and 536 BM transplants revealed a borderline increase in grades II–IV acute GVHD [relative risk (RR), 1.19; 95% CI, 0.9–1.56].[51] A meta-analysis of 15 studies (9 cohorts, 5 randomized trials, and 1 database review) suggested that use of PBSCs did increase risk of acute GVHD (RR, 1.16; 95% CI, 1.04–1.28).[46]

A number of studies have suggested a higher incidence of chronic GVHD with PB.[44–46,51] An updated meta-analysis of the randomized trials demonstrated an overall relative risk of 1.57 (95% CI, 1.28–1.94) for chronic GVHD after PBSCT when compared with bone marrow transfer (BMT). The explanation for the increase in chronic GVHD may lie with the increase in the number of T cells infused, although there there may be an association between the development of chronic GVHD and the number of CD34 cells infused.[52,53]

It has been speculated that the larger number of T cells infused with mobilized peripheral blood might translate into improved immune reconstitution and a reduction in disease relapse posttransplant. In several studies, higher levels of B cells and T cells were noted after PBSCT compared to BMT,[54] with the increase in T-cell number associated with a lower incidence of confirmed infections (RR, 0.59; $P < 0.001$).[55] With regard to relapse, several randomized studies have demonstrated a decrease in the rate of relapse after PBSCT compared to BMT.[48,49] In the largest U.S. randomized trial, the hazard ratio for relapse was 0.49 (95% CI, 0.38–1.28) among patients transplanted with PBSCs.[44] Unfortunately, despite these effects on lymphoid recovery and disease relapse, most randomized studies have yet to demonstrate a convincing improvement in overall survival for PBSCs.

All the comparative studies of PBSCs and BM referenced previously have involved related donors. For unrelated donors, a single-arm cohort of PBSCT resulted in outcomes similar to that noted with BMT.[56] Comparative rates of engraftment, acute and chronic GVHD, and survival in the unrelated setting await completion of large multiinstitutional randomized studies now under way.

If there turns out to be no survival advantage to PBSCT compared with BMT in the allogeneic setting, policies regarding donor source may be determined by quality of life or economic issues. Donor preference for either PBSC or BM donation has been evaluated in one series of allogeneic donors with no differences in self-reported quality of life measures; however, patients randomized to donate autologous PBSC or BM have preferred PBSC collection.[57,58] Because of the reduction in hospital stay associated with PBSCT, costs have been lower in comparative analyses although these studies did not factor in the potentially added economic burden of a higher incidence of chronic GVHD.[59]

Conditioning Regimens

The conditioning regimen administered before stem cell infusion plays several potential roles in promoting the success of transplantation. Cytoreduction of the endogenous malignancy with high-dose chemo/radiotherapy has traditionally been central to transplantation and is the major mode by which autologous transplantation benefits patients. Typical conditioning regimens for autologous transplantation include cyclophosphamide/total-body irradiation (Cy/TBI), cyclophosphamide/busulfan (Bu/Cy), cyclophosphamide/BCNU/VP-16 (CBV), BCNU/etoposide, ara-C, melphalan (BEAM), VP-16/busulfan, and cyclophosphamide/thiotepa/carboplatin (CTCb). It is not clear if one particular regimen is superior in a particular clinical circumstance, although it is generally assumed that results with current standard regimens are reasonably equivalent.

For allogeneic transplantation, the conditioning regimen not only reduces the disease burden but also suppresses the host to facilitate donor engraftment. The most common ablative combinations have been cyclophosphamide/total-body irradiation or cyclosphosphamide/busulfan. Several randomized studies of Cy/TBI and Bu/Cy have been conducted in patients with AML and CML.[60–62] Socie et al. summarized the long-term results of four of these studies.[63] With more than 7 years of follow-up in each study, no differences in long-term outcome were noted for patients with CML. They noted a nonsignificant 10% improvement for AML patients receiving Cy/TBI compared to Bu/Cy. The development of intravenous busulfan and strict pharmacokinetic monitoring to target

TABLE 6.1. Comparison of autologous and allogeneic transplantation.

	Autologous	*Allogeneic*
Advantages	1. No HLA matching requirement 2. No graft-versus-host disease (GVHD) 3. No need for immunosuppression	1. Stem cells have not been exposed to chemotherapy 2. Stem cells free of tumor 3. Graft-versus-tumor activity
Disadvantages	1. ? Stem cell damage from prior therapy leading to delayed engraftment or myelodysplasia 2. ? Graft contamination with tumor 3. No graft-versus-tumor effect	1. Donor availability uncertain 2. GVHD 3. Infectious complications
	Lower risk of complications *Higher risk of relapse*	*Higher risk of complications* *Lower risk of relapse*

plasma levels of the drug has helped optimize efficacy and limit toxicity of the Bu/Cy regimen.[28,64]

Attempts to escalate doses of the conditioning have been disappointing. In several studies in which TBI dose intensity was increased to more than 1,500 cGy, modest decreases in relapse rates were offset by increases in regimen-related morbidity and mortality.[65–67] The introduction of monoclonal antibodies directed at marrow elements linked to radioisotopes in hopes of targeting only marrow and not vital organs may offer hope of providing truly selective myeloablation.[68]

The lack of benefit of conditioning regimen dose intensification and the recognition of the contribution of graft-versus-tumor activity to disease eradication prompted the development of low-dose, nonmyeloablative regimens. These regimens are designed not to have direct antitumor activity but rather to provide sufficient host suppression to permit engraftment of donor hematopoietic and lymphoid effector cells. Many regimens ranging from nearly myeloablative to minimally myelosuppressive have been piloted. Most regimens have combined a purine analogue, such as fludarabine, with an alkylating agent or low-dose TBI with or without anti-T-cell antibodies such as thymoglobulin or altemuzumab.[69–73] Studies indicate that these nonmyeloablative regimens can facilitate full donor engraftment with much decreased upfront toxicity, allowing transplantation to be performed in older patients or those with contraindications to high-dose therapy. Unfortunately, GVHD still is a problem. One-hundred-day transplant-related mortality is low in recipients of nonmyeloablative conditioning, but later morbidity and mortality, usually from GVHD, can be substantial.[74] Several retrospective comparative studies have suggested similar overall outcomes in recipients of myeloablative and nonmyeloablative transplants, but prospective randomized studies are needed to determine the impact of these less-intensive regimens on toxicity and disease control.

Potential Obstacles to Successful Transplantation

There are three major hurdles that must be overcome for HSCT to be successful: (1) identification of a suitable donor, (2) prevention and effective treatment of transplant-related complications, and (3) sustained eradication of underlying disease.

Identification of a Suitable Donor

Donor choice can have a profound influence on transplant outcome. Patients may receive either autologous or allogeneic stem cells. Pros and cons of each donor source are displayed in Table 6.1.

Autologous Transplantation

A major issue facing investigators surrounding autologous transplantation is the potential of tumor cell contamination. The aim of purging in autologous transplantation is to eliminate any contaminating malignant cells and leave intact the hematopoietic stem cells that are necessary for engraftment. Most clinical studies in lymphoma and myeloma have demonstrated that purging can deplete malignant cells in vitro without significantly impairing hematologic reconstitution,[75–77] but studies in AML using immunologic or chemical methods have been associated with delayed hematopoietic recovery (Figure 6.2).[78,79] The rationale for removing tumor cells from hematopoietic cells might therefore appear compelling, yet the issue of purging remains highly controversial. Both positive (CD34+ columns) and negative (exposure ex vivo to antibodies directed at tumor cells) selection techniques for tumor cell purging are available. However, purging has not as

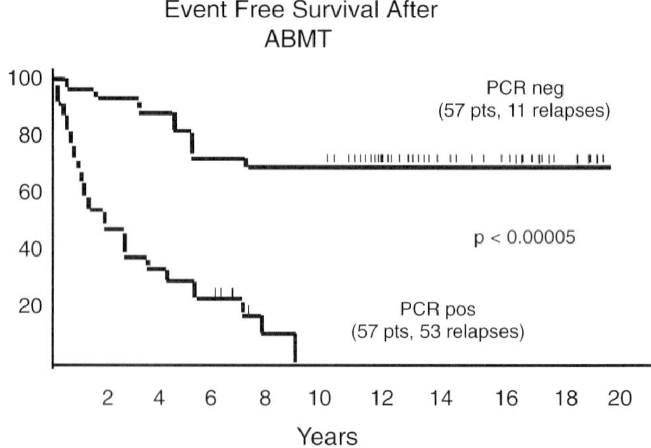

FIGURE 6.2. Successful purging of tumor cells from autologous marrow is associated with improved survival after transplantation. Patients whose marrows had no detectable lymphoma cells by polymerase chain reaction studies after immunologic purging had superior survival compared to patients with persistent evidence of disease. (Courtesy of J. Gribben.)

yet been universally adopted because there are no convincing data in Phase 2 trials that patients receiving purged marrow fare better than those receiving unpurged cells. A retrospective analysis of the European Blood and Marrow Transplant Lymphoma Registry compared the outcome of 270 patients whose BM had been purged and with the outcome of 270 case-matched control patients.[80] A variety of purging methodologies was used. Patients with low-grade lymphoma did not have a significantly improved progression-free survival if the BM was purged ($P = 0.18$), but they did have a significantly improved overall survival ($P = 0.0018$). In multiple myeloma, a Phase III randomized trial using purged versus unpurged autologous PBSC was performed using CD34 selection.[81] After CD34 selection, tumor burden was reduced by a median of 3.1 log, with 54% of CD34-selected products having no detectable tumor. There was no improvement in disease-free or overall survival.

Data indicate, however, that contamination of the stem cell inoculum with tumor cells contributes to posttransplant relapse. In studies at the Dana-Farber Cancer Institute, polymerase chain reaction (PCR) amplification of the t(14;18) was used to detect residual lymphoma cells in the BM before and after purging to assess whether efficient purging had any impact on disease-free survival.[82] In this study, patients with B-cell non-Hodgkin lymphoma and the bcl-2 translocation were studied. Residual lymphoma cells were detected in all patients in the harvested autologous BM. Following three cycles of immunologic purging using the anti-B-cell mAbs and complement-mediated lysis, PCR amplification detected residual lymphoma cells in 50% of patients. Patients who were infused with a source of hematopoietic cells that was free of detectable lymphoma cells had improved outcome compared to those who had residual detectable lymphoma (see Figure 6.2). This finding was independent of degree of BM infiltration at the time of BM harvest or remission status at the time of autologous BMT. Further evidence supporting the contribution of contaminating tumor cells to posttransplant relapse comes from gene marking studies in AML and neuroblastoma.[83–85]

Allogeneic Donors

When allogeneic transplantation is contemplated, an HLA-identical or closely matched donor must be found. The major HLA loci are located on chromosome 6 and are closely linked.[86] Because every individual inherits one chromosome 6 from their mother and one from their father, the chance of any one sibling being a match is one in four. A *complete* match between donor and recipient was considered identity of both alleles at HLA-A, HLA-B, and HLA-DR loci. Other major loci, such as HLA-C and HLA-DQ, can influence outcome and must be checked when performing a search for an unrelated donor. Indeed, HLA-C identity is now considered as important as a match at HLA-A, -B, and -DR.[87–90] Accurate HLA typing is essential. Serologic methods are no longer adequate. It is imperative that molecular techniques using site-specific oligonucleotide probes and direct sequencing be employed. The formation of the National Marrow Donor Registry (NMDR) has made possible thousands of unrelated transplants in the United States. More than 4 million people are registered as potential donors with the NMDP. The likelihood of finding an HLA-A, -B, and -DR match is 65% to 70%, although finding a donor is more difficult in minority populations. It can take weeks to many months between the time a search is initiated and a donor is identified, medically cleared, and ultimately donates.

Even when a "complete" match is found, complications such as GVHD can still be substantial. The reason for this is that minor HLA antigens, which can influence graft rejection or GVHD, cannot be easily typed.[91–93] Moreover, these minor antigens likely are not found on chromosome 6; therefore, a complete match of HLA major loci does not necessarily translate into a complete match of minor loci. Results of allogeneic transplantation using unrelated donors have been slightly worse than those of matched related transplants, but with improvements in typing, the gap has narrowed.[94]

Sometimes it is possible to identify more than one potential donor either within a family or through the NMDP. The most important characteristic in choosing a donor is HLA identity. The greater the HLA disparity, the greater the risk of GVHD, graft failure, and adverse outcome. Other factors that may increase GVHD include the use of female multiparous donors for male recipients (a minor HLA antigen located on the Y chromosome has recently been identified), older donor age, and prior cytomegalovirus (CMV) exposure.[95,96] ABO compatibility is desirable but is not a prerequisite for transplantation. ABO incompatibility may lead to hemolysis and delayed red cell engraftment.[97]

Transplantation of hematopoietic stem cells from haploidentical family members has been associated with increased risks of GVHD and graft failure.[98,99] Historically, outcome has been poor. Recent studies of infusion of large numbers of haploidentical peripheral blood stem cells exhaustively depleted of T cells through positive selection of CD34+ stem cells has been reported to result in high rates of engraftment and low rates of GVHD.[100] Despite T-cell depletion, relapse rates have been low, particularly in patients with AML. It now appears that mismatching of KIR receptor on donor NK cells and KIR ligand on recipient cells may actually promote cell-mediated destruction of AML cells and recipient antigen-presenting cells, leading to lower relapse rates without GVHD.[101,102]

Recent studies have demonstrated that umbilical cord blood (UCB) is very rich in stem cells but low in alloreactive T cells. As a consequence, it was hypothesized that these cells might support engraftment with less GVHD. A series of studies have confirmed that engraftment can be obtained with unrelated UCB with a reduced risk of GVHD, even when partially HLA-mismatched unrelated transplants donor cells used.[103–107] However, because the number of stem cells per kilogram recipient weight is relatively low in cord blood products, engraftment is slow. The number of cells available for transplantation from cord blood may make it difficult to utilize these products with large adult recipients. Strategies currently under investigation to address low cord blood cellularity include the use of multiple disparate products and expansion of stem cells ex vivo before infusion.[108] UCB transplantation should be considered for patients for whom traditional related or unrelated products are not available.

Transplant-Related Complications

When evaluating patients for potential complications of transplantation, it is critical to have a full understanding of the entire treatment course to assemble a reasonable differential diagnosis. Factors that must be taken into account include donor source (allogeneic or autologous), interval posttransplant (early versus late), type of GVHD prophylaxis, infectious prophylaxis, current use of immunosuppressive medications, ablative regimen, and duration of granulocytopenia. The three major categories of transplant-related toxicities are (1) treatment-related organ damage, (2) infectious complications, and (3) graft-versus-host disease.

Organ Damage

Damage can be manifested early or late after transplantation. Some of the more commonly recognized organ toxicities that are not clearly attributable to infection or GVHD are discussed next.

Idiopathic Pneumonia Syndrome (IPS)/Diffuse Alveolar Hemorrhage (DAH)/Engraftment Syndrome

These processes usually occur during the transplant hospitalization around the time of neutrophil recovery, more commonly after allogeneic HSCT.[109–111] These terms may represent slightly different manifestations of the same poorly understood entity. By definition, they have no clearly identified infectious etiology. Onset can be insidious, but decompensation can be sudden. Radiographic findings can be nonspecific. Mortality is extremely high in patients who require mechanical ventilation. Elevated circulating and bronchoalveolar lavage (BAL) levels of tumor necrosis factor (TNF) and other cytokines have been observed.[112,113] Early intervention with high-dose steroids (1 g IV solumedrol) even before diagnostic studies are performed may be lifesaving.[114] New agents, including TNF blockers such as etanercept (Enbrel), are being studied in clinical trials.[115]

Interstitial Pneumonitis (IP)

Interstitial pneumonitis (IP) often occurs 2 to 6 months after transplant. IP may present as a delayed inflammatory response to a conditioning agent, such as BCNU. In these circumstances, complete responses can be obtained with a steroid dose of 1 mg/kg. IP can be steadily progressive and fatal, particularly after allo-HSCT. IP must be distinguished from infectious pneumonitis.

Hepatic Veno-occlusive Disease (VOD)

VOD is a clinical syndrome characterized by painful hepatomegaly, jaundice, ascites, fluid retention, and weight gain.[116,117] The onset is usually before day + 35 after stem cell reinfusion, and other causes of these symptoms and signs are absent. VOD develops in 2% to 40% of patients after SCT and ranges in severity from mild, reversible disease to a severe syndrome associated with multiorgan failure and death, with established severe VOD shown to have a mortality rate approaching 100% by day + 100 post-SCT. VOD is believed to be caused by primary conditioning regimen-induced injury to sinusoidal endothelial cells and hepatocytes with subsequent damage to the central veins in zone 3 of the hepatic acinus.[118] Early changes include deposition of fibrinogen, factor VIII, and fibrin within venular walls and sinusoids. As the process of venular microthrombosis, fibrin deposition, ischemia, and fibrogenesis advances, widespread zonal disruption leads to portal hypertension, hepatorenal syndrome, multiorgan failure, and death. Despite therapeutic interventions, including the use of antithrombotic and thrombolytic agents such as prostaglandin E_1 and tissue-plasminogen activator (t-PA) with or without concurrent heparin, little success has been achieved in the treatment of severe VOD. Recently, the use of defibrotide (DF), a single-stranded polydeoxyribonucleotide that has specific aptameric-binding sites on vascular endothelium, has shown promise in the treatment of VOD.[119,120] DF upregulates the release of prostacyclin (PGI_2), prostaglandin E_2, thrombomodulin (TM), and t-PA both in vitro and in vivo. Moreover, it has been shown to decrease thrombin generation, tissue factor expression, plasminogen activator inhibitor (PAI)-1 release, and endothelin activity.

Hemolytic-uremic Syndrome (HUS)/ ThromboticThrombocytopenic Purpura (TTP)

Both HUS and, less commonly, TTP can occur after either allo- or autotransplant. HUS/TTP presents 2 to 12 months posttransplant. HUS is manifest by nonimmune-mediated hemolytic anemia characterized by schistocytes on smear, mild azotemia, and mild hypertension.[121,122] It is likely precipitated by endothelial damage caused by the ablative regimen or by medications such as cyclosporine, tacrolimus, or siroloimus. HUS is usually self-limited, and treatment is supportive. Plasmapheresis is generally not indicated but isolated reports have indicated some benefit.

Cardiomyopathy

Cardiac dysfunction can occasionally be observed after HSCT. It usually presents shortly after completion of conditioning and has been linked with cyclophosphamide.[123] It can present as myopericarditis. If patients can be managed through the acute episodes, there may not be permanent dysfunction. Long-term cardiac complications are uncommon and usually can be related to previous anthracycline exposure.

Neurologic Dysfunction

Neurologic dysfunction can be an unrecognized problem after HSCT. Potential issues include memory disturbance and learning disability secondary to irradiation, Guillain–Barre syndrome, limbic encephalitis, cyclosporine/tacrolimus-associated hypertensive encephalopathy and seizures, and peripheral neuropathies.[124]

Cataracts

Cataracts often develop in patients 1 to 5 years after transplant.[125] The incidence is increased in patients who received TBI and those on prolonged steroid therapy for GVHD.

Infection

Infection is a major cause of morbidity and mortality after transplantation. There are numerous predisposing factors that increase the risk of infection after HSCT, including the following:

- Prolonged granulocytopenia
- Disruption of mucosal barriers
- Extensive use of antibiotics
- Prolonged placement of indwelling venous access
- Delayed recovery of cellular immunity
- Impaired antibody production
- Use of immunosuppressive medications to treat or prevent GVHD

- Immune defects associated with underlying malignancy
- Suppression of immune responses by GVHD itself

It is important to have an understanding of the typical time course associated with risk of developing specific infections after HSCT.[126] It is critical to anticipate the development of infection, and considerable attention has been paid to prophylaxis and preemptive therapy. Examples are detailed here:

1. Bacterial: During the transplant hospitalization, gut decontamination with oral nonabsorbable antibiotics is often employed along with systemic agents such as a quinalone. If patients become febrile while neutropenic, typical broad-spectrum coverage is employed. For outpatients with chronic GVHD on steroids, oral antibiotics targeting encapsulated organisms are frequently prescribed on a chronic basis for suppression. Although routine immunoglobulin (IgG) administration is not recommended after transplant, it is recommended that patients whose IgG levels are consistently very low should receive replacement therapy.

2. Fungal: There are data indicating that prophylactic fluconazole can prevent *Candida* infections and may improve long-term survival after transplant.[127,128] Amphotericin B or a liposomal derivative has been routinely administered for fever and neutropenia unresponsive to antibacterial antibiotics. The newly available voriconazole may ultimately be substituted for amphotericin in this setting.[129,130] Moreover, its oral administration and activity against *Aspergillus* may lead to it being more widely adopted as fungal prophylaxis after discharge for patients on steroids for GVHD.

3. *Pneumocystis carinii*: *Pneumocystis carinii* pneumonia (PCP) can develop as early as 1 month after transplant. Prophylaxis should be instituted no later than 30 days post-HSCT and be continued for approximately a year or longer if the patient remains on steroids for GVHD. Trimethoprim-sulfamethoxazole is the most efficacious agent. For patients with allergies or cytopenias, atovoquone or other agents (dapsone, pentamidine) may be substituted, but coverage should never be omitted. Practitioners should be aware of development of PCP in the months after discontinuation of prophylaxis.

4. Viral: Herpesviruses (HSV, VZV, EBV, HHV-6, and, most importantly, CMV) present the largest viral problem after transplant. HSV-induced mucositis can be completely prevented with acyclovir administration during the transplant hospital stay. Many centers will continue acyclovir for 1 year to prevent varicella-zoster virus (VZV) infections, which occur in 30% to 40% of patients not receiving prophylaxis.[131] CMV usually occurs 2 to 6 months after transplant and is more common in allotransplant recipients. Patients at highest risk are those who are CMV seropositive and receive cells from a seronegative donor.[132] In this circumstance, no anti-CMV immunity is transferred. CMV-filtered, or better still, CMV-negative blood products are essential to prevent nosocomial transmission. Data exist that demonstrate that treatment of patients preemptively with gancyclovir when CMV reactivation can be detected in blood or BAL fluid (before actual development of invasive infection) will reduce the risk of subsequent CMV pneumonitis and improve survival.[133–136]

Vaccinations are routinely administered to patients 1 and 2 years after HSCT. Diptheria tetanus, inactivated polio, MMR (measles-mumps-rubella), hepatitis B, pneumococcal, and *Hemophilus influenzae* vaccine are often given.[137] The ability to make antibody is impaired post-HSCT and vaccinations are therefore usually delayed until the 1-year anniversary. Recent data suggest that vaccination of the donor before transplant may allow earlier transfer of immunity to the patient.[138]

Graft-Versus-Host Disease

GVHD causes complications after allogeneic HSCT as a direct result of organ damage and as a consequence of infectious complications prompted by GVHD therapy. GVHD can be classified as acute or chronic based on timing of onset and clinical features. Acute GVHD usually develops within the first 2 months of BMT and affects mainly the skin, gastrointestinal (GI) tract, and liver.[139] The current standard grading system for acute GVHD is based on the degree of involvement of these three organs (Table 6.2). When pharmacologic immunosup-

TABLE 6.2. Acute GVHD scoring.

Extent of organ involvement	*Skin*	*Liver*	*Gut*
Stage			
1	Rash on less than 25% of skin	Bilirubin 2–3 mg/dL	Diarrhea more than 500 mL/day or persistent nausea
2	Rash on 25%–50% of skin	Bilirubin 3–6 mg/dL	Diarrhea more than 1000 mL/day
3	Rash on more than 50% of skin	Bilirubin 6–15 mg/dL	Diarrhea more than 1500 mL/day
4	Generalized erythroderma with bullous formation	Bilirubin more than 15 mg/dL	Severe abdominal pain with or without ileus
Grade			
I	Stage 1–2	None	None
II	Stage 3 or 4	Stage 1 or 2	Stage 1
III	—	Stage 2–3 or	Stage 2–4
IV	Stage 4	Stage 4	—

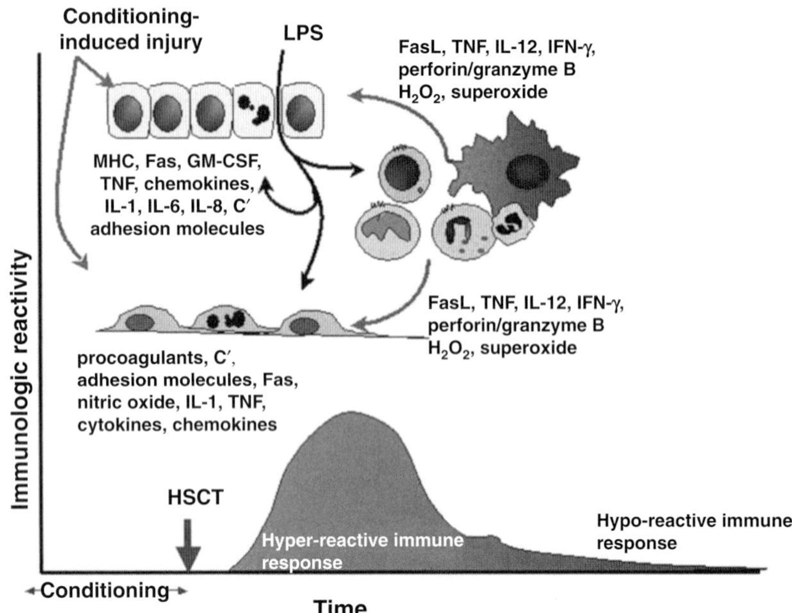

FIGURE 6.3. Pathophysiology of acute graft-versus-host disease (GVHD). The cytokine theory of acute GVHD pathogenesis involves release of proinflammatory cytokines after conditioning regimen-induced injury, which then leads to stimulation of alloreactive effector cells, which then leads to the further release of cytokines and tissue injury. (Courtesy of J. Antin.)

pression is used as GVHD prophylaxis after myeloablative transplant, moderate to severe acute GVHD (grades II–IV) occurs in 25% to 60% of matched related donor transplant recipients and up to 45% to 70% in unrelated donor recipients. Development of grade II–IV acute GVHD is associated with decreased survival in patients after allogeneic BMT.[140–143]

Chronic GVHD has a later onset than acute GVHD and is often clinically distinct.[144] Chronic GVHD may resemble an autoimmune collagen vascular disease. Patients can manifest sclerodermatous skin changes, keratoconjunctivitis, sicca syndrome, lichenoid oral mucosal lesions, esophageal and vaginal strictures, liver disease, and pulmonary insufficiency. Despite immunosuppresive agents, approximately 30% to 50% of patients develop chronic GVHD after conventional myeloablative HLA-identical sibling BMT. The incidence of chronic GVHD may be even higher after allogeneic transplantation using unmanipulated peripheral blood stem cells.[45,46,51,52] Chronic GVHD may be classified as subclinical or clinical, limited or extensive. Although subclinical or clinically limited chronic GVHD often resolves spontaneously with minimal intervention, extensive chronic GVHD requires prolonged immunosuppressive treatment and is associated with significant morbidity and mortality. More than 50% of patients with extensive chronic GVHD will die, mostly secondary to infections resulting from severe immune dysfunction.

Large single-institution and registry series have identified factors that place patients at higher risk for the development of GVHD. For acute GVHD, these include HLA incompatibility, use of an unrelated donor, prior donor allosensitization through pregnancy or blood transfusion, older patient or donor age, recipient CMV seropositivity, and increased intensity of the ablative regimen. For chronic GVHD, prior acute GVHD is the major risk factor, but also important are use of peripheral blood stem cells, histoincompatibility, and the prior use of corticosteroids.[95,145–147]

GVHD Pathophysiology

The pathophysiology of GVHD has received extensive attention. It is recognized that donor T cells are critical mediators in the graft-versus-host reaction. However, recent animal research suggests that the pathophysiology of acute GVHD is far more complex and that it involves intricate interactions between cellular and cytokine components of the immune system (Figure 6.3).[148,149] Acute GVHD is now believed to occur in three phases: (1) tissue damage from conditioning regimen, (2) donor T-cell activation phase, and (3) inflammatory effector phase. In the earliest phase of GVHD, inflammatory cytokines are released from host tissue in response to damage by the pretransplant conditioning regimen. These cytokines, including interleukin 1 (IL-1) and tumor necrosis factor-alpha, upregulate the expression of adhesion molecules and host major histocompatibility complex (MHC) antigens and enhance recognition of the host tissue by mature donor T lymphocytes. During the second phase, donor T cells of the T-helper 1 (Th1) subset are activated upon recognition of alloantigens and secrete cytokines such as interleukin 2 and interferon-alpha. IL-2 plays a central role in the recruitment of other T cells, cytotoxic T lymphocytes (CTLs), natural killer (NK) cells, monocytes, and macrophages.

GVHD Prophylaxis

T cells remain the prime target for most current therapeutic strategies in GVHD prophylaxis in humans. Effective approaches for the prevention and treatment of GVHD involve direct blockade of T-cell function. These methods have included the downregulation of T lymphocytes by inhibiting cellular proliferation (methotrexate), inhibition of de novo purine synthesis (mycophenolate mofetil), suppression of IL-2 secretion by blocking calcineurin activity (cyclosporine, tacrolimus), interfering with downstream growth signaling pathways (rapamycin), reduction of T-cell responsiveness by blocking the IL-2 receptor (dacluzimab), and generation of immunosuppressive cytokines (extracorporeal photopheresis).[150–156] Combination therapy with methotrexate and a calcineurin inhibitor, albeit flawed, remains the gold standard for GVHD prophylaxis.[157–160] The recent combination of tacrolimus and sirilimus (rapamycin) has shown significant promise in recipients of HLA-matched unrelated and related transplants.[161]

The most effective means for GVHD prophylaxis has been ex vivo depletion of T cells from the donor inoculum.[162] Donor T-cell depletion (TCD), when it was first introduced in the early 1980s, offered the potential for prevention of GVHD without the morbidity associated with immunosuppressive drugs such as methotrexate and cyclosporine. Numerous TCD methods have been utilized over the past two decades; these have included negative selection techniques using monoclonal antibody(ies) plus complement, immunotoxins, counterflow centrifugal elutriation, soybean lectin agglutination, and, more recently, positive selection through CD34+ columns.[163–166] Most early trials documented that TCD could substantially limit acute and chronic GVHD. However, this reduction in GVHD did not translate into improved overall survival because of unexpected high rates of graft failure, Epstein–Barr virus (EBV)-associated lymphoproliferative disorders (EBV-LPD), and disease recurrence following TCD-BMT (Table 6.3).[167–170] It is believed that certain sets of donor cells removed in the purging process are also important for graft maintenance, viral surveillance, and elimination of residual leukemia cells that have survived the high-dose ablative conditioning regimen. Despite the problems associated with T-cell depletion, there remains great interest in developing and improving this technology, particularly for recipients of mismatched or unrelated grafts. Reasonable applications for TCD may include those patients at high risk for GVHD (unrelated or mismatched grafts) or patients with comorbid medical conditions who might have a high risk of complications after conventional BMT. TCD may be ideal for patients with diseases where GVL activity is less critical, such as first remission acute leukemia. In the future, studies need to assess the potential role of T-cell depletion when mobilized PBSCs are used for allogeneic transplantation, particularly with respect to its effect on chronic GVHD. It would be ideal to be able to manipulate different lymphoid subgroups responsible for GVHD and GVL, but whether these processes can be effectively separated at a clinical level remains unknown.

GVHD Treatment

Once established, administration of corticosteroids is the most effective approach to the treatment of both acute and chronic GVHD. Complete responses occur in 25% to 40% of patients. Addition of other agents to corticosteroids or increasing the steroid dose has not improved response rates or outcomes.[171,172] A comparative trial of 2 and 10 mg/kg/day of methylprednisolone demonstrated no advantage of the higher dose in terms of response or survival.[173] For acute GVHD, calcineurin inhibitors such as cyclosporine and tacrolimus are useful in patients who did not receive these agents initially as prophylaxis.[174] Serotherapy with antithymocyte globulin (ATG) can produce responses, although subsequent infection rates are high and survival does not appear to be improved. Other anti-T-cell antibodies with distinct specficities have been studied. Responses have been reported, but these antibodies have not proven superior to steroids alone. Medications aimed at blocking T-cell proliferation (mycophenxlate mofetil) or activation (rapamycin) appear to induce responses in single-arm trials, but these agents have not yet been studied fully in randomized trials. Targeting cytokine receptors such as IL-2 (dacluzimab, denileukin difitox), IL-1 (IL-1RA), and tumor necrosis factor-alpha (TNF-α) (infliximab) have yielded promising results in small uncontrolled trials but have not proven to add benefit in randomized trials.[150–156,175,176]

Treatment of extensive chronic GVHD with immunosuppressive therapy has been even less rewarding than that of acute GVHD. Although the combination of cyclosporine and prednisone is the treatment of choice in many centers, a recent randomized trial failed to show any survival advantage.[177] Encouraging uncontrolled trials with thalidomide have been reported, but subsequent randomized studies did not demonstrate significant benefit.[178,179] Both psoralen plus ultraviolet A (PUVA) therapy and extracorporeal photopheresis (ECP) have been reported to be effective in acute and particularly chronic GVHD.[180,181] Randomized studies are currently under way to evaluate the value of ECP. The overall disappointing results of immunosuppressive therapy for chronic GVHD make other efforts, such as prevention of infection and physical therapy, even more critical to maintenance of patient well-being.

Sustained Eradication of Disease

The goal of HSCT for malignant disease or marrow disorders is sustained eradication of disease. This result can be obtained in certain circumstances with high-dose chemotherapy. However, it is clear from preclinical models and clinical studies that immune-mediated allogeneic effects, termed graft-versus-tumor (GVT) or graft-versus-leukemia (GVL) effects, are central to the therapeutic effect of allogeneic

TABLE 6.3. Pros and cons of T-cell depletion.

Advantages	*Disadvantages*
Decreased incidence of acute and chronic GVHD	Higher incidence of graft failure
Reduced or no requirement for posttransplant immunosuppression as GVHD prophylaxis	Loss of GVL activity (higher incidence of disease relapse, especially with CML)
Decreased organ toxicity	Delayed immune reconstitution
Lower early transplant-related mortality	Increased risk for posttransplant EBV-associated lymphoproliferative disorder

HSCT.[182] Evidence to support the existence of GVL activity has come from several sources. First, a higher relapse rate has been noted in recipients of syngeneic transplants compared with allogeneic transplants from sibling donors, suggesting that the genetic/immunologic discrepancy between donor and host plays a role in disease control.[140,183] Second, a reduced risk of relapse is observed in patients who develop GVHD after HSCT.[184] Third, relapse rates are higher in recipients of T-cell-depleted grafts where alloreactive T cells are removed.[167] Fourth, withdrawal of immunosuppression in some patients who have relapsed after transplant can induce a remission.[185] All these lines of evidence still only provided indirect evidence of the existence of GVL activity. Direct evidence was finally obtained when donor lymphocyte infusions (DLI) were successfully used to treat patients with CML who had relapsed after BMT.

Many reports confirmed the efficacy of DLI in inducing remissions in patients who have relapsed after transplant, particularly in patients with CML.[186–188] DLI induces complete cytogenetic remissions in more than 70% in patients with CML when treated in either cytogenetic or hematologic relapse. Responses are noted in other diseases, including multiple myeloma, MDS, CLL, and low-grade lymphoma. Acute leukemia and advanced CML may be less sensitive to DLI. DLI can cause GVHD. However, it is exciting to note that DLI can induce remissions in the absence of GVHD, demonstrating that GVL and GVHD can be separable.[189] The dramatic activity of DLI is what has led to the exploration of nonmyeloablative conditioning regimens in clinical situations that rely predominantly on GVL activity for therapeutic benefit. It is hoped that current efforts to identify targets of DLI will lead to generation of vaccines that can be tested in clinical trials.[190,191]

References

1. Philip T, Guglielmi C, Hagenbeek A, et al. Autologous bone marrow transplantation as compared with salvage chemotherapy in relapses of chemotherapy-sensitive non-Hodgkin's lymphoma [see comments]. N Engl J Med 1995;333:1540–1545.
2. Attal M, Harousseau JL, Stoppa AM, et al. A prospective, randomized trial of autologous bone marrow transplantation and chemotherapy in multiple myeloma. Intergroupe Francais du Myelome [see comments]. N Engl J Med 1996;335:91–97.
3. Child JA, Morgan GJ, Davies FE, et al. High-dose chemotherapy with hematopoietic stem-cell rescue for multiple myeloma. N Engl J Med 2003;348:1875–1883.
4. Stadtmauer EA, O'Neill A, Goldstein LJ, et al. Conventional-dose chemotherapy compared with high-dose chemotherapy plus autologous hematopoietic stem-cell transplantation for metastatic breast cancer. Philadelphia Bone Marrow Transplant Group. N Engl J Med 2000;342:1069–1076.
5. Rodenhuis S, Bontenbal M, Beex LV, et al. High-dose chemotherapy with hematopoietic stem-cell rescue for high-risk breast cancer. N Engl J Med 2003;349:7–16.
6. Tallman MS, Gray R, Robert NJ, et al. Conventional adjuvant chemotherapy with or without high-dose chemotherapy and autologous stem-cell transplantation in high-risk breast cancer. N Engl J Med 2003;349:17–26.
7. Haioun C, Lepage E, Gisselbrecht C, et al. Survival benefit of high-dose therapy in poor-risk aggressive non-Hodgkin's lymphoma: final analysis of the prospective LNH87-2 protocol—a groupe d'Etude des lymphomes de l'Adulte study. J Clin Oncol 2000;18:3025–3030.
8. Santini G, Salvagno L, Leoni P, et al. VACOP-B versus VACOP-B plus autologous bone marrow transplantation for advanced diffuse non-Hodgkin's lymphoma: results of a prospective randomized trial by the non-Hodgkin's Lymphoma Cooperative Study Group. J Clin Oncol 1998;16:2796–2802.
9. Kluin-Nelemans HC, Zagonel V, Anastasopoulou A, et al. Standard chemotherapy with or without high-dose chemotherapy for aggressive non-Hodgkin's lymphoma: randomized phase III EORTC study. J Natl Cancer Inst 2001;93:22–30.
10. Zittoun RA, Mandelli F, Willemze R, et al. Autologous or allogeneic bone marrow transplantation compared with intensive chemotherapy in acute myelogenous leukemia. European Organization for Research and Treatment of Cancer (EORTC) and the Gruppo Italiano Malattie Ematologiche Maligne dell'Adulto (GIMEMA) Leukemia Cooperative Groups. N Engl J Med 1995;332:217–223.
11. Cassileth PA, Harrington DP, Appelbaum FR, et al. Chemotherapy compared with autologous or allogeneic bone marrow transplantation in the management of acute myeloid leukemia in first remission. N Engl J Med 1998;339:1649–1656.
12. Burnett AK. Transplantation in first remission of acute myeloid leukemia. N Engl J Med 1998;339:1698–1700.
13. Thiebaut A, Vernant JP, Degos L, et al. Adult acute lymphocytic leukemia study testing chemotherapy and autologous and allogeneic transplantation. A follow-up report of the French protocol LALA 87. Hematol Oncol Clin N Am 2000;14:1353–1366.
14. Clift RA, Buckner CD, Appelbaum FR, et al. Long-term follow-up of a randomized trial of two irradiation regimens for patients receiving allogeneic marrow transplants during first remission of acute myeloid leukemia [letter]. Blood 1998;92:1455–1456.
15. Szydlo R, Goldman JM, Klein JP, et al. Results of allogeneic bone marrow transplants for leukemia using donors other than HLA-identical siblings. J Clin Oncol 1997;15:1767–1777.
16. Hansen JA, Gooley TA, Martin PJ, et al. Bone marrow transplants from unrelated donors for patients with chronic myeloid leukemia. N Engl J Med 1998;338:962–968.
17. Horning SJ. High-dose therapy and transplantation for low-grade lymphoma. Hematol Oncol Clin N Am 1997;11:919–935.
18. Yuen AR, Rosenberg SA, Hoppe RT, Halpern JD, Horning SJ. Comparison between conventional salvage therapy and high-dose therapy with autografting for recurrent or refractory Hodgkin's disease. Blood 1997;89:814–822.
19. Horning SJ, Chao NJ, Negrin RS, et al. High-dose therapy and autologous hematopoietic progenitor cell transplantation for recurrent or refractory Hodgkin's disease: analysis of the Stanford University results and prognostic indices. Blood 1997;89:801–813.
20. Freedman AS, Neuberg D, Mauch P, et al. Long-term follow-up of autologous bone marrow transplantation in patients with relapsed follicular lymphoma. Blood 1999;94:3325–3333.
21. Georges GE, Storb R. Stem cell transplantation for aplastic anemia. Int J Hematol 2002;75:141–146.
22. Rabinowe SN, Soiffer RJ, Gribben JG, et al. Autologous and allogeneic bone marrow transplantation for poor prognosis patients with B-cell chronic lymphocytic leukemia. Blood 1993:1366–1376.
23. Michallet M, Archimbaud E, Bandini G, et al. HLA-identical sibling bone marrow transplantation in younger patients with chronic lymphocytic leukemia. Ann Intern Med 1996;124:311–315.
24. Deeg HJ, Amylon ID, Harris RE, et al. Marrow transplants from unrelated donors for patients with aplastic anemia: minimum effective dose of total body irradiation. Biol Blood Marrow Transplant 2001;7:208–215.
25. Druker BJ. Chronic myeloid leukemia in the imatinib era. Semin Hematol 2003;40:1–3.

26. Kantarjian H, Sawyers C, Hochhaus A, et al. Hematologic and cytogenetic responses to imatinib mesylate in chronic myelogenous leukemia. N Engl J Med 2002;346:645–652.
27. Sawyers CL, Hochhaus A, Feldman E, et al. Imatinib induces hematologic and cytogenetic responses in patients with chronic myelogenous leukemia in myeloid blast crisis: results of a phase II study. Blood 2002;99:3530–3539.
28. Radich JP, Gooley T, Bensinger W, et al. HLA-matched related hematopoietic cell transplantation for chronic-phase CML using a targeted busulfan and cyclophosphamide preparative regimen. Blood 2003;102:31–35.
29. Sehn LH, Alyea EP, Weller E, et al. Comparative outcomes of T-cell-depleted and non-T-cell-depleted allogeneic bone marrow transplantation for chronic myelogenous leukemia: impact of donor lymphocyte infusion. J Clin Oncol 1999;17:561–568.
30. O'Brien SG, Guilhot F, Larson RA, et al. Imatinib compared with interferon and low-dose cytarabine for newly diagnosed chronic-phase chronic myeloid leukemia. N Engl J Med 2003; 348:994–1004.
31. O'Dwyer ME, Mauro MJ, Blasdel C, et al. Clonal evolution and lack of cytogenetic response are adverse prognostic factors for hematologic relapse of chronic phase CML patients treated with imatinib mesylate. Blood 2004;103:451–455.
32. Heinrich MC, Corless CL, Demetri GD, et al. Kinase mutations and imatinib response in patients with metastatic gastrointestinal stromal tumor. J Clin Oncol 2003;21:4342–4349.
33. Druker BJ. Overcoming resistance to imatinib by combining targeted agents. Mol Cancer Ther 2003;2:225–226.
34. Gaziev J, Lucarelli G. Stem cell transplantation for hemoglobinopathies. Curr Opin Pediatr 2003;15:24–31.
35. Childs R, Drachenberg D. Allogeneic stem cell transplantation for renal cell carcinoma. Curr Opin Urol 2001;11:495–502.
36. Burt RK, Traynor AE, Craig R, Marmont AM. The promise of hematopoietic stem cell transplantation for autoimmune diseases. Bone Marrow Transplant 2003;31:521–524.
37. Bensinger WI, Price TH, Dale DC, et al. The effects of daily recombinant human granulocyte colony-stimulating factor administration on normal granulocyte donors undergoing leukapheresis. Blood 1993;81:1883–1888.
38. Demirer T, Ayli M, Ozcan M, et al. Mobilization of peripheral blood stem cells with chemotherapy and recombinant human granulocyte colony-stimulating factor (rhG-CSF): a randomized evaluation of different doses of rhG-CSF. Br J Haematol 2002; 116:468–474.
39. Gazitt Y. Comparison between granulocyte colony-stimulating factor and granulocyte-macrophage colony-stimulating factor in the mobilization of peripheral blood stem cells. Curr Opin Hematol 2002;9:190–198.
40. Siena S, Schiavo R, Pedrazzoli P, Carlo-Stella C. Therapeutic relevance of CD34 cell dose in blood cell transplantation for cancer therapy. J Clin Oncol 2000;18:1360–1377.
41. Hartmann O, Le Corroller AG, Blaise D, et al. Peripheral blood stem cell and bone marrow transplantation for solid tumors and lymphomas: hematologic recovery and costs. A randomized, controlled trial. Ann Intern Med 1997;126:600–607.
42. Schmitz N, Dreger P, Suttorp M, Rohwedder EB, Haferlach T, Loffler H, Hunter A, Russell NH. Primary transplantation of allogeneic peripheral blood progenitor cells mobilized by filgrastim (granulocyte colony-stimulating factor). Blood 1995; 85:1666–1672.
43. Bensinger WI, Weaver CH, Appelbaum FR, et al. Transplantation of allogeneic peripheral blood stem cells mobilized by recombinant granulocyte colony-stimulating factor. Blood 1995;85:1655–1658.
44. Bensinger WI, Martin PJ, Storer B, et al. Transplantation of bone marrow as compared with peripheral-blood cells from HLA-identical relatives in patients with hematologic cancers. N Engl J Med 2001;344:175–181.
45. Couban S, Simpson DR, Barnett MJ, et al. A randomized multicenter comparison of bone marrow and peripheral blood in recipients of matched sibling allogeneic transplants for myeloid malignancies. Blood 2002;100:1525–1531.
46. Cutler C, Giri S, Jeyapalan S, Paniagua D, Viswanathan A, Antin JH. Acute and chronic graft-versus-host disease after allogeneic peripheral-blood stem-cell and bone marrow transplantation: a meta-analysis. J Clin Oncol 2001;19:3685–3691.
47. Schmitz N, Bacigalupo A, Hasenclever D, et al. Allogeneic bone marrow transplantation vs filgrastim-mobilised peripheral blood progenitor cell transplantation in patients with early leukaemia: first results of a randomised multicentre trial of the European Group for Blood and Marrow Transplantation. Bone Marrow Transplant 1998;21:995–1003.
48. Powles R, Mehta J, Kulkarni S, et al. Allogeneic blood and bone-marrow stem-cell transplantation in haematological malignant diseases: a randomised trial. Lancet 2000;355:1231–1237.
49. Blaise D, Kuentz M, Fortanier C, et al. Randomized trial of bone marrow versus lenograstim-primed blood cell allogeneic transplantation in patients with early-stage leukemia: a report from the Societe Francaise de Greffe de Moelle. J Clin Oncol 2000;18:537–546.
50. Schmitz N, Beksac M, Hasenclever D, et al. Transplantation of mobilized peripheral blood cells to HLA-identical siblings with standard-risk leukemia. Blood 2002;100:761–767.
51. Champlin RE, Schmitz N, Horowitz MM, et al. Blood stem cells compared with bone marrow as a source of hematopoietic cells for allogeneic transplantation. IBMTR Histocompatibility and Stem Cell Sources Working Committee and the European Group for Blood and Marrow Transplantation (EBMT). Blood 2000;95:3702–3709.
52. Przepiorka D, Anderlini P, Saliba R, et al. Chronic graft-versus-host disease after allogeneic blood stem cell transplantation. Blood 2001;98:1695–1700.
53. Zaucha JM, Gooley T, Bensinger WI, et al. CD34 cell dose in granulocyte colony-stimulating factor-mobilized peripheral blood mononuclear cell grafts affects engraftment kinetics and development of extensive chronic graft-versus-host disease after human leukocyte antigen-identical sibling transplantation. Blood 2001;98:3221–3227.
54. Tayebi H, Tiberghien P, Ferrand C, et al. Allogeneic peripheral blood stem cell transplantation results in less alteration of early T cell compartment homeostasis than bone marrow transplantation. Bone Marrow Transplant 2001;27:167–175.
55. Storek J, Dawson MA, Storer B, et al. Immune reconstitution after allogeneic marrow transplantation compared with blood stem cell transplantation. Blood 2001;97:3380–3389.
56. Remberger M, Ringden O, Blau IW, et al. No difference in graft-versus-host disease, relapse, and survival comparing peripheral stem cells to bone marrow using unrelated donors. Blood 2001; 98:1739–1745.
57. Rowley SD, Donaldson G, Lilleby K, Bensinger WI, Appelbaum FR. Experiences of donors enrolled in a randomized study of allogeneic bone marrow or peripheral blood stem cell transplantation. Blood 2001;97:2541–2548.
58. Nishimori M, Yamada Y, Hoshi K, et al. Health-related quality of life of unrelated bone marrow donors in Japan. Blood 2002; 99:1995–2001.
59. Bennett C, Waters T, Stinson T, et al. Valuing clinical strategies early in development: a cost analysis of allogeneic peripheral blood stem cell transplantation. Bone Marrow Transplant 1999; 24:555–560.
60. Devergie A, Apperley JF, Labopin M, et al. European results of matched unrelated donor bone marrow transplantation for chronic myeloid leukemia. Impact of HLA class II matching. Chronic Leukemia Working Party of the European Group for Blood and Marrow Transplantation. Bone Marrow Transplant 1997;20:11–19.

61. Clift RA, Buckner CD, Thomas ED, et al. Marrow transplantation for chronic myeloid leukemia: a randomized study comparing cyclophosphamide and total body irradiation with busulfan and cyclophosphamide. Blood 1994;84:2036–2943.
62. Blaise D, Maraninchi D, Archimbaud E, et al. Allogeneic bone marrow transplantation for acute myeloid leukemia in first remission: a randomized trial of a busulfan-Cytoxan versus Cytoxan-total body irradiation as preparative regimen: a report from the Group d'Etudes de la Greffe de Moelle Osseuse. Blood 1992;79:2578–2582.
63. Socie G, Clift RA, Blaise D, et al. Busulfan plus cyclophosphamide compared with total-body irradiation plus cyclophosphamide before marrow transplantation for myeloid leukemia: long-term follow-up of 4 randomized studies. Blood 2001; 98:3569–3574.
64. Andersson BS, Thall PF, Madden T, et al. Busulfan systemic exposure relative to regimen-related toxicity and acute graft-versus-host disease: defining a therapeutic window for i.v. BuCy2 in chronic myelogenous leukemia. Biol Blood Marrow Transplant 2002;8:477–485.
65. Clift RA, Buckner CD, Appelbaum FR, et al. Allogeneic marrow transplantation in patients with acute myeloid leukemia in first remission: a randomized trial of two irradiation regimens. Blood 1990;76:1867–1871.
66. Clift RA, Buckner CD, Appelbaum FR, et al. Allogeneic marrow transplantation in patients with chronic myeloid leukemia in the chronic phase: a randomized trial of two irradiation regimens. Blood 1991;77:1660–1665.
67. Alyea E, Neuberg D, Mauch P, et al. Effect of total body irradiation dose escalation on outcome following T-cell-depleted allogeneic bone marrow transplantation. Biol Blood Marrow Transplant 2002;8:139–144.
68. Matthews DC, Appelbaum FR, Eary JF, et al. Development of a marrow transplant regimen for acute leukemia using targeted hematopoietic irradiation delivered by 131I-labelled anti-CD45 antibody, combined with cyclophosphamide and total body irradiation. Blood 1995;85:1122–1131.
69. Giralt S, Khouri I, Champlin R. Nonmyeloablative "mini transplants." Cancer Treat Res 1999;101:97–108.
70. Slavin S, Nagler A, Naparstek E, et al. Nonmyeloablative stem cell transplantation and cell therapy as an alternative to conventional bone marrow transplantation with lethal cytoreduction for the treatment of malignant and nonmalignant hematologic diseases. Blood 1998;91:756–763.
71. Feinstein LC, Sandmaier BM, Hegenbart U, et al. Non-myeloablative allografting from human leucocyte antigen-identical sibling donors for treatment of acute myeloid leukaemia in first complete remission. Br J Haematol 2003;120: 281–288.
72. Feinstein LC, Sandmaier BM, Maloney DG, et al. Allografting after nonmyeloablative conditioning as a treatment after a failed conventional hematopoietic cell transplant. Biol Blood Marrow Transplant 2003;9:266–272.
73. Perez-Simon JA, Kottaridis PD, Martino R, et al. Nonmyeloablative transplantation with or without alemtuzumab: comparison between 2 prospective studies in patients with lymphoproliferative disorders. Blood 2002;100:3121–3127.
74. Mielcarek M, Martin PJ, Leisenring W, et al. Graft-versus-host disease after nonmyeloablative versus conventional hematopoietic stem cell transplantation. Blood 2003;102:756–762.
75. Freedman AS, Gribben JG, Neuberg D, et al. High-dose therapy and autologous bone marrow transplantation in patients with follicular lymphoma during first remission. Blood 1996;88: 2780–2786.
76. Freedman A, Gribben J, Kuhlman C, et al. Effective purging of autologous hematopoietic stem cell (HSC) transplants for non-Hodgkin's lymphoma (NHL) using high density microparticles coated with anti-CD19 and anti-CD20 monoclonal antibodies: elimination of B cells, high CD34+ cell yield and rapid engraftment. Blood 1999;94(suppl 1):638a.
77. Vescio R, Schiller G, Stewart AK, et al. Multicenter phase III trial to evaluate CD34(+) selected versus unselected autologous peripheral blood progenitor cell transplantation in multiple myeloma. Blood 1999;93:1858–1868.
78. Miller CB, Rowlings PA, Zhang MJ, et al. The effect of graft purging with 4-hydroperoxycyclophosphamide in autologous bone marrow transplantation for acute myelogenous leukemia. Exp Hematol 2001;29:1336–1346.
79. Robertson MJ, Soiffer RJ, Freedman AS, et al. Human bone marrow depleted of CD33-positive cells mediates delayed but durable reconstitution of hematopoiesis: clinical trial of MY9 monoclonal antibody-purged autografts for the treatment of acute myeloid leukemia. Blood 1992;79:2229–2236.
80. Williams CD, Goldstone AH, Pearce RM, Pet al. Purging of bone marrow in autologous bone marrow transplantation for non-Hodgkin's lymphoma: a case-matched comparison with unpurged cases by the European Blood and Marrow Transplant Lymphoma Registry. J Clin Oncol 1996;14:2454–2464.
81. Stewart AK, Vescio R, Schiller G, et al. Purging of autologous peripheral-blood stem cells using CD34 selection does not improve overall or progression-free survival after high-dose chemotherapy for multiple myeloma: results of a multicenter randomized controlled trial. J Clin Oncol 2001;19:3771–3779.
82. Gribben JG, Freedman AS, Neuberg D, et al. Immunologic purging of marrow assessed by PCR before autologous bone marrow transplantation for B-cell lymphoma. N Engl J Med 1991;325:1525–1533.
83. Brenner MK, Rill DR, Moen RC, et al. Gene-marking to trace origin of relapse after autologous bone-marrow transplantation. Lancet 1993;341:85–86.
84. Rill DR, Buschle M, Foreman NK, et al. Retrovirus-mediated gene transfer as an approach to analyze neuroblastoma relapse after autologous bone marrow transplantation. Hum Gene Ther 1992;3:129–136.
85. Rill DR, Moen RC, Buschle M, et al. An approach for the analysis of relapse and marrow reconstitution after autologous marrow transplantation using retrovirus-mediated gene transfer. Blood 1992;79:2694–2700.
86. Rhodes DA, Trowsdale J. Genetics and molecular genetics of the MHC. Rev Immunogenet 1999;1:21–31.
87. Petersdorf EW, Longton GM, Anasetti C, et al. Association of HLA-C disparity with graft failure after marrow transplantation from unrelated donors. Blood 1997;89:1818–1823.
88. Petersdorf EW, Gooley TA, Anasetti C, et al. Optimizing outcome after unrelated marrow transplantation by comprehensive matching of HLA class I and II alleles in the donor and recipient. Blood 1998;92:3515–3520.
89. Petersdorf EW, Hansen JA, Martin PJ, et al. Major-histocompatibility-complex class I alleles and antigens in hematopoietic-cell transplantation. N Engl J Med 2001;345:1794–1800.
90. Sasazuki T, Juji T, Morishima Y, et al. Effect of matching of class I HLA alleles on clinical outcome after transplantation of hematopoietic stem cells from an unrelated donor. Japan Marrow Donor Program. N Engl J Med 1998;339:1177–1185.
91. Goulmy E, Schipper R, Pool J, et al. Mismatches of minor histocompatibility antigens between HLA-identical donors and recipients and the development of graft-versus-host disease after bone marrow transplantation. N Engl J Med 1996;334:281–285.
92. Miklos DB, Kim HT, Zorn E, et al. Antibody response to DBY minor histocompatibility antigen is induced after allogeneic stem cell transplantation and in healthy female donors. Blood 2004;103:353–359.

93. Behar E, Chao NJ, Hiraki DD, et al. Polymorphism of adhesion molecule CD31 and its role in acute graft-versus-host disease. N Engl J Med 1996;334:286–291.
94. Petersdorf E, Anasetti C, Servida P, Martin P, Hansen J. Effect of HLA matching on outcome of related and unrelated donor transplantation therapy for chronic myelogenous leukemia. Hematol Oncol Clin N Am 1998;12:107–121.
95. Gale RP, Bortin MM, Van Bekkum DW, et al. Risk factors for acute graft-versus-host disease. Br J Haematol 1987;67:396–406.
96. Kollman C, Howe CW, Anasetti C, et al. Donor characteristics as risk factors in recipients after transplantation of bone marrow from unrelated donors: the effect of donor age. Blood 2001; 98:2043–2051.
97. Klumpp TR, Fairclough D, Ritz J, Soiffer R. The effect of minor ABO mismatches on the incidence of graft-versus-host disease after allogeneic bone marrow transplantation. Transplantation 1994;57:780.
98. Henslee-Downey PJ, Gluckman E. Allogeneic transplantation from donors other than HLA-identical siblings. Hematol Oncol Clin N Am 1999;13:1017–1039.
99. Beatty PG, Clift RA, Mickelson EM, et al. Marrow transplantation for related donors other than HLA-identical siblings. N Engl J Med 1985;313:765–771.
100. Aversa F, Tabilio A, Velardi A, et al. Treatment of high-risk acute leukemia with T-cell-depleted stem cells from related donors with one fully mismatched HLA haplotype. N Engl J Med 1998;339:1186–1193.
101. Ruggeri L, Capanni M, Casucci M, et al. Role of natural killer cell alloreactivity in HLA-mismatched hematopoietic stem cell transplantation. Blood 1999;94:333–339.
102. Ruggeri L, Capanni M, Urbani E, et al. Effectiveness of donor natural killer cell alloreactivity in mismatched hematopoietic transplants. Science 2002;295:2097–2100.
103. Wagner JE, Kernan NA, Steinbuch M, Broxmeyer HE, Gluckman E. Allogeneic sibling umbilical-cord-blood transplantation in children with malignant and non-malignant disease. Lancet 1995;346:214–219.
104. Wagner JE, Rosenthal J, Sweetman R, et al. Successful transplantation of HLA-matched and HLA-mismatched umbilical cord blood from unrelated donors: analysis of engraftment and acute graft-versus-host disease. Blood 1996;88:795–802.
105. Kurtzberg J, Laughlin M, Graham ML, et al. Placental blood as a source of hematopoietic stem cells for transplantation into unrelated recipients. N Engl J Med 1996;335:157–166.
106. Laughlin MJ, Barker J, Bambach B, et al. Hematopoietic engraftment and survival in adult recipients of umbilical-cord blood from unrelated donors. N Engl J Med 2001;344:1815–1822.
107. Wagner JE, Barker JN, DeFor TE, et al. Transplantation of unrelated donor umbilical cord blood in 102 patients with malignant and nonmalignant diseases: influence of CD34 cell dose and HLA disparity on treatment-related mortality and survival. Blood 2002;100:1611–1618.
108. Shpall EJ, Quinones R, Giller R, et al. Transplantation of ex vivo expanded cord blood. Biol Blood Marrow Transplant 2002; 8:368–376.
109. Kantrow SP, Hackman RC, Boeckh M, Myerson D, Crawford SW. Idiopathic pneumonia syndrome: changing spectrum of lung injury after marrow transplantation. Transplantation 1997; 63:1079–1086.
110. Ho VT, Weller E, Lee SJ, Alyea EP, Antin JH, Soiffer RJ. Prognostic factors for early severe pulmonary complications after hematopoietic stem cell transplantation. Biol Blood Marrow Transplant 2001;7:223–229.
111. Lewis ID, DeFor T, Weisdorf DJ. Increasing incidence of diffuse alveolar hemorrhage following allogeneic bone marrow transplantation: cryptic etiology and uncertain therapy. Bone Marrow Transplant 2000;26:539–543.
112. Cooke KR, Hill GR, Gerbitz A, et al. Tumor necrosis factor-alpha neutralization reduces lung injury after experimental allogeneic bone marrow transplantation. Transplantation 2000; 70:272–279.
113. Clark JG, Mandac JB, Dixon AE, Martin PJ, Hackman RC, Madtes DK. Neutralization of tumor necrosis factor-alpha action delays but does not prevent lung injury induced by alloreactive T helper 1 cells. Transplantation 2000;70:39–43.
114. Metcalf JP, Rennard SI, Reed EC, et al. Corticosteroids as adjunctive therapy for diffuse alveolar hemorrhage associated with bone marrow transplantation. University of Nebraska Medical Center Bone Marrow Transplant Group. Am J Med 1994;96:327–334.
115. Yanik G, Hellerstedt B, Custer J, et al. Etanercept (Enbrel) administration for idiopathic pneumonia syndrome after allogeneic hematopoietic stem cell transplantation. Biol Blood Marrow Transplant 2002;8:395–400.
116. Bearman SI. The syndrome of hepatic veno-occlusive disease after marrow transplantation. Blood 1995;85:3005–3020.
117. McDonald GB, Sharma P, Matthews DE, Shulman HM, Thomas ED. Venocclusive disease of the liver after bone marrow transplantation: diagnosis, incidence, and predisposing factors. Hepatology 1984;4:116–122.
118. Richardson P, Guinan E. The pathology, diagnosis, and treatment of hepatic veno-occlusive disease: current status and novel approaches. Br J Haematol 1999;107:485–493.
119. Richardson PG, Murakami C, Jin Z, et al. Multi-institutional use of defibrotide in 88 patients after stem cell transplantation with severe veno-occlusive disease and multisystem organ failure: response without significant toxicity in a high-risk population and factors predictive of outcome. Blood 2002;100:4337–4343.
120. Richardson PG, Elias AD, Krishnan A, et al. Treatment of severe veno-occlusive disease with defibrotide: compassionate use results in response without significant toxicity in a high-risk population. Blood 1998;92:737–744.
121. Rabinowe SN, Soiffer RJ, Tarbell NJ, et al. Hemolytic-uremic syndrome following bone marrow transplantation in adults for hematologic malignancies. Blood 1991;77:1837–1844.
122. Ruutu T, Hermans J, Niederwieser D, et al. Thrombotic thrombocytopenic purpura after allogeneic stem cell transplantation: a survey of the European Group for Blood and Marrow Transplantation (EBMT). Br J Haematol 2002;118:1112–1119.
123. Murdych T, Weisdorf DJ. Serious cardiac complications during bone marrow transplantation at the University of Minnesota, 1977–1997. Bone Marrow Transplant 2001;28:283–287.
124. Graus F, Saiz A, Sierra J, et al. Neurologic complications of autologous and allogeneic bone marrow transplantation in patients with leukemia: a comparative study. Neurology 1996; 46:1004–1009.
125. Deeg HJ, Flournoy N, Sullivan KM, et al. Cataracts after total body irradiation and marrow transplantation: a sparing effect of dose fractionation. Int J Radiat Oncol Biol Phys 1984;10:957.
126. Leather HL, Wingard JR. Infections following hematopoietic stem cell transplantation. Infect Dis Clin N Am 2001;15:483–520.
127. Marr KA, Seidel K, Slavin MA, et al. Prolonged fluconazole prophylaxis is associated with persistent protection against candidiasis-related death in allogeneic marrow transplant recipients: long-term follow-up of a randomized, placebo-controlled trial. Blood 2000;96:2055–2061.
128. Marr KA, Seidel K, White TC, Bowden RA. Candidemia in allogeneic blood and marrow transplant recipients: evolution of risk factors after the adoption of prophylactic fluconazole. J Infect Dis 2000;181:309–316.
129. Herbrecht R, Denning DW, Patterson TF, et al. Voriconazole versus amphotericin B for primary therapy of invasive aspergillosis. N Engl J Med 2002;347:408–415.

130. Walsh TJ, Pappas P, Winston DJ, et al. Voriconazole compared with liposomal amphotericin B for empirical antifungal therapy in patients with neutropenia and persistent fever. N Engl J Med 2002;346:225–234.
131. Koc Y, Miller KB, Schenkein DP, et al. Varicella zoster virus infections following allogeneic bone marrow transplantation: frequency, risk factors, and clinical outcome. Biol Blood Marrow Transplant 2000;6:44–49.
132. Ljungman P, Brand R, Einsele H, Frassoni F, Niederwieser D, Cordonnier C. Donor CMV serologic status and outcome of CMV-seropositive recipients after unrelated donor stem cell transplantation: an EBMT megafile analysis. Blood 2003;102: 4255–4260.
133. Einsele H, Ehninger G, Hebart H, et al. Polymerase chain reaction monitoring reduces the incidence of cytomegalovirus disease and the duration and side effects of antiviral therapy after bone marrow transplantation. Blood 1995;86:2815–2820.
134. Zaia JA, Schmidt GM, Chao NJ, et al. Preemptive ganciclovir administration based solely on asymptomatic pulmonary cytomegalovirus infection in allogeneic bone marrow transplant recipients: long-term follow-up. Biol Blood Marrow Transplant 1995;1:88–93.
135. Reusser P, Einsele H, Lee J, et al. Randomized multicenter trial of foscarnet versus ganciclovir for preemptive therapy of cytomegalovirus infection after allogeneic stem cell transplantation. Blood 2002;99:1159–1164.
136. Hebart H, Muller C, Loffler J, Jahn G, Einsele H. Monitoring of CMV infection: a comparison of PCR from whole blood, plasma-PCR, pp65-antigenemia and virus culture in patients after bone marrow transplantation. Bone Marrow Transplant 1996;17: 861–868.
137. Guidelines for preventing opportunistic infections among hematopoietic stem cell transplant recipients. Biol Blood Marrow Transplant 2000;6:659–713; 715; 717–627; quiz 729–633.
138. Molrine DC, Antin JH, Guinan EC, et al. Donor immunization with pneumococcal conjugate vaccine and early protective antibody responses following allogeneic hematopoietic cell transplantation. Blood 2003;101:831–836.
139. Ringden ODH. Clinical spectrum of graft-versus-host disease. In: Ferrara JLM DH, Burakoff S (eds) Graft-vs-Host Disease, 2nd ed. New York: Dekker, 1997:525–559.
140. Horowitz MM, Gale RP, Sondel PM, et al. Graft-versus-leukemia reactions after bone marrow transplantation. Blood 1990; 75:555–562.
141. Nash RA, Pepe MS, Storb R, et al. Acute graft-versus-host disease: analysis of risk factors after allogeneic marrow transplantation and prophylaxis with cyclosporine and methotrexate. Blood 1992;80:1838–1845.
142. Sullivan K. Graft-versus-host disease. In: Thomas E, Blume K, Forman S (eds) Hematopoietic Cell Transplantation, 2nd ed. Malden: Blackwell, 1999:515–536.
143. Sullivan KM, Weiden PL, Storb R, et al. Influence of acute and chronic graft-versus-host disease on relapse and survival after bone marrow transplantation from HLA-identical siblings as treatment of acute and chronic leukemia. Blood 1989;73: 1720–1728.
144. Sullivan KM, Shulman HM, Storb R, et al. Chronic graft versus host disease in 52 patients: adverse natural course and successful treatment with combination immunosuppression. Blood 1981;57:267.
145. Weisdorf DJ, Haake R, Blazar B, et al. Risk factors for acute graft-versus-host disease in histocompatible donor bone marrow transplantation. Transplantation 1991;51:1197–1203.
146. Clark JG, Schwartz DA, Flournoy N, et al. Risk factors for airflow obstruction in recipients of bone marrow transplants. Ann Intern Med 1987;107:648.
147. Atkinson K, Horowitz MM, Gale RP, et al. Risk factors for chronic graft-versus-host disease after HLA-identical bone marrow transplantation. Blood 1990;75:2459–2464.
148. Ferrera JLM, Antin JH. Pathophysiology of graft-versus-host disease. In: Thomas ED, Blume KG, Forman SJ (eds). Hematopoietic Stem Cell Transplantation. Boston: Blackwell, 1999: 305–315.
149. Ferrara JL. Pathogenesis of acute graft-versus-host disease: cytokines and cellular effectors. J Hematother Stem Cell Res 2000;9:299–306.
150. Anasetti C, Hansen JA, Waldmann TA, et al. Treatment of acute graft-versus-host disease with humanized anti-Tac: an antibody that binds to the interleukin-2 receptor. Blood 1994;84:1320–1327.
151. Przepiorka D, Kernan NA, Ippoliti C, et al. Daclizumab, a humanized anti-interleukin-2 receptor alpha chain antibody, for treatment of acute graft-versus-host disease. Blood 2000; 95:83–89.
152. Castagna L. Mycophenolate mofetil (MMF) for refractory chronic graft versus host disease (cGvHD). Haematologica 2003;88:ELT28; author reply ELT29.
153. Apisarnthanarax N, Donato M, Korbling M, et al. Extracorporeal photopheresis therapy in the management of steroid-refractory or steroid-dependent cutaneous chronic graft-versus-host disease after allogeneic stem cell transplantation: feasibility and results. Bone Marrow Transplant 2003;31: 459–465.
154. Bisaccia E, Palangio M, Gonzalez J, Adler KR, Rowley SD, Goldberg SL. Treating refractory chronic graft-versus-host disease with extracorporeal photochemotherapy. Bone Marrow Transplant 2003;31:291–294.
155. Kiehl MG, Schafer-Eckart K, et al. Mycophenolate mofetil for the prophylaxis of acute graft-versus-host disease in stem cell transplant recipients. Transplant Proc 2002;34:2922–2924.
156. Benito AI, Furlong T, Martin PJ, et al. Sirolimus (rapamycin) for the treatment of steroid-refractory acute graft-versus-host disease. Transplantation 2001;72:1924–1929.
157. Ruutu T, Volin L, Parkkali T, Juvonen E, Elonen E. Cyclosporine, methotrexate, and methylprednisolone compared with cyclosporine and methotrexate for the prevention of graft-versus-host disease in bone marrow transplantation from HLA-identical sibling donor: a prospective randomized study. Blood 2000;96:2391–2398.
158. Chao NJ, Schmidt GM, Niland JC, et al. Cyclosporine, methotrexate, and prednisone compared with cyclosporine and prednisone for prophylaxis of acute graft-versus-host disease. N Engl J Med 1993;329:1225–1230.
159. Deeg HJ, Lin D, Leisenring W, et al. Cyclosporine or cyclosporine plus methylprednisolone for prophylaxis of graft-versus-host disease: a prospective, randomized trial. Blood 1997;89:3880–3887.
160. Nash RA, Antin JH, Karanes C, et al. Phase 3 study comparing methotrexate and tacrolimus with methotrexate and cyclosporine for prophylaxis of acute graft-versus-host disease after marrow transplantation from unrelated donors. Blood 2000; 96:2062–2068.
161. Antin JH, Kim HT, Cutler C, et al. Sirolimus, tacrolimus, and low-dose methotrexate for graft-versus-host disease prophylaxis in mismatched related donor or unrelated donor transplantation. Blood 2003;102:1601–1605.
162. Ho VT, Soiffer RJ. The history and future of T-cell depletion as graft-versus-host disease prophylaxis for allogeneic hematopoietic stem cell transplantation. Blood 2001;98:3192–3204.
163. Waldmann HG, Hale G, Cividalli G, et al. Elimination of graft-versus-host disease by in vitro depletion of alloreactive lymphocytes with a monoclonal rat anti-human lymphocyte antibody (Campath-1). Lancet 1984;2:483–486.

164. Filipovich AH, Vallera D, McGlave P, et al. T cell depletion with anti-CD5 immunotoxin in histocompatible bone marrow transplantation. Transplantation 1990;50:410–415.
165. Soiffer RJ, Murray C, Mauch P, et al. Prevention of graft-versus-host disease by selective depletion of CD6-positive T lymphocytes from donor bone marrow. J Clin Oncol 1992;10: 1191–1200.
166. Reisner Y, Kapoor N, Kirkpatrick D, et al. Transplantation for acute leukemia with HLA-A and B nonidentical parental marrow cells fractionated with soybean agglutinin and sheep red blood cells. Lancet 1981;2:327.
167. Marmont A, Horowitz MM, Gale RP, et al. T-cell depletion of HLA-identical transplants in leukemia. Blood 1991;78: 2120–2130.
168. Kernan NA, Bordignon C, Heller G, et al. Graft failure after T-cell-depleted leukocyte antigen identical marrow transplants for leukemia: I. analysis of risk factors and results of secondary transplants. Blood 1989;74:2227–2236.
169. Goldman JM, Gale RP, Horowitz MM, et al. Bone marrow transplantation for chronic myelogenous leukemia in chronic phase. Increased risk for relapse associated with T-cell depletion. Ann Intern Med 1988;108:806–814.
170. Zutter MM, Martin PJ, Sale GE, et al. Epstein-Barr virus lymphoproliferation after bone marrow transplantation. Blood 1988;72:520.
171. Martin PJ, Schoch G, Fisher L, et al. A retrospective analysis of therapy for acute graft-versus-host disease: initial treatment. Blood 1990;76:1464–1472.
172. Martin PJ, Schoch G, Fisher L, et al. A retrospective analysis of therapy for acute graft-versus-host disease: secondary treatment. Blood 1991;77:1821–1828.
173. Van Lint MT, Uderzo C, Locasciulli A, et al. Early treatment of acute graft-versus-host disease with high- or low-dose 6-methylprednisolone: a multicenter randomized trial from the Italian Group for Bone Marrow Transplantation. Blood 1998;92: 2288–2293.
174. Ohashi Y, Minegishi M, Fujie H, Tsuchiya S, Konno T. Successful treatment of steroid-resistant severe acute GVHD with 24-h continuous infusion of FK506. Bone Marrow Transplant 1997; 19:625–627.
175. Antin JH, Weinstein HJ, Guinan EC, et al. Recombinant human interleukin-1 receptor antagonist in the treatment of steroid-resistant graft-versus-host disease. Blood 1994;84:1342–1348.
176. Antin JH, Weisdorf D, Neuberg D, et al. Interleukin-1 blockade does not prevent acute graft-versus-host disease: results of a randomized, double-blind, placebo-controlled trial of interleukin-1 receptor antagonist in allogeneic bone marrow transplantation. Blood 2002;100:3479–3482.
177. Koc S, Leisenring W, Flowers ME, et al. Therapy for chronic graft-versus-host disease: a randomized trial comparing cyclosporine plus prednisone versus prednisone alone. Blood 2002;100:48–51.
178. Koc S, Leisenring W, Flowers ME, et al. Thalidomide for treatment of patients with chronic graft-versus-host disease. Blood 2000;96:3995–3996.
179. Arora M, Wagner JE, Davies SM, et al. Randomized clinical trial of thalidomide, cyclosporine, and prednisone versus cyclosporine and prednisone as initial therapy for chronic graft-versus-host disease. Biol Blood Marrow Transplant 2001;7: 265–273.
180. Dall'Amico R, Rossetti F, Zulian F, et al. Photopheresis in paediatric patients with drug-resistant chronic graft-versus-host disease. Br J Haematol 1997;97:848–854.
181. Besnier DP, Chabannes D, Mussini JM, Dupas B, Esnault VL. Extracorporeal photochemotherapy for secondary chronic progressive multiple sclerosis: a pilot study. Photodermatol Photoimmunol Photomed 2002;18:36–41.
182. Truitt RL, Johnson BD. Principles of graft-vs.-leukemia reactivity. Biol Blood Marrow Transplant 1995;1:61–68.
183. Gale RP, Horowitz MM, Ash RC, et al. Identical-twin bone marrow transplants for leukemia. Ann Intern Med 1994;120: 646–652.
184. Weiden PL, Flournoy N, Sanders JE, et al. Anti-leukemic effect of graft-versus-host disease contributes to improved survival after allogeneic marrow transplantation. Transplant Proc 1981; 13:248–251.
185. Collins RH, Rogers ZR, Bennett M, Kumar V, Nikein A, Fay JW. Hematologic relapse of chronic myelogenous leukemia following allogeneic bone marrow transplantation. Apparent graft-versus-leukemia effect following abrupt discontinuation of immunosuppression. Bone Marrow Transplant 1992;10:391–395.
186. Collins RH Jr, Shpilberg O, Drobyski WR, et al. Donor leukocyte infusions in 140 patients with relapsed malignancy after allogeneic bone marrow transplantation [see comments]. J Clin Oncol 1997;15:433–444.
187. Kolb HJ, Schattenberg A, Goldman JM, et al., the European Group for Blood and Marrow Transplantation Working Party Chronic Leukemia. Graft-versus-leukemia effect of donor lymphocyte transfusions in marrow grafted patients. Blood 1995;86:2041–2050.
188. Porter DL, Antin JH. Adoptive immunotherapy for relapsed leukemia following allogeneic bone marrow transplantation. Leuk Lymphoma 1995;17:191–197.
189. Alyea EP, Soiffer RJ, Canning C, et al. Toxicity and efficacy of defined doses of CD4(+) donor lymphocytes for treatment of relapse after allogeneic bone marrow transplant. Blood 1998; 91:3671–3680.
190. Yang XF, Wu CJ, Chen L, et al. CML28 is a broadly immunogenic antigen, which is overexpressed in tumor cells. Cancer Res 2002;62:5517–5522.
191. Yang XF, Wu CJ, McLaughlin S, et al. CML66, a broadly immunogenic tumor antigen, elicits a humoral immune response associated with remission of chronic myelogenous leukemia. Proc Natl Acad Sci USA 2001;98:7492–7497.

Evaluation of Tumor Markers: An Evidence-Based Guide for Determination of Clinical Utility

Daniel F. Hayes

A tumor marker is clinically useful if its results serve to separate a large heterogeneous population into smaller populations with more precisely predictable outcomes. In theory, if this separation is both reliable and disparate, one can apply therapy more efficiently to the population by exposing those most likely to need and benefit from the therapy while ensuring that the other group avoids needless toxicities. In essence, the term *tumor marker* has come to describe a variety of molecules or processes that differ from the norm in either malignant cells, tissues, or fluids in patients with malignancies. Assessing these alterations from normal can be used to place patients into categories that are distinguished by different outcomes, either in the absence of specific therapy or after various treatments are applied.

Tumor markers can include changes at the genetic level (for example, mutations, deletions, or amplifications), at the transcriptional level (for example, over- or underexpression), at the translational or posttranslational level (for example, increased or decreased quantities of protein, or abnormal glycosylation of proteins), and/or at the functional level (for example, histologic description of cellular grade or presence of neovascularization). Each of these can be assessed by one or more assays, which can be performed using one or more methods with differing reagents. This enormous heterogeneity of approaches is the root of considerable confusion regarding the true value, in clinical terms, of a given tumor marker.

The *molecular revolution* is now well into its fourth decade. Yet, in spite of impressive advances in our understanding of the biology of human malignancy and in the technology of investigating molecular processes, the number of clinically useful products from these advances is disappointing. For example, in 1995, the American Society of Clinical Oncology (ASCO) convened a panel of experts to establish guidelines for the use of tumor markers in colon and breast carcinoma. Although the Expert Panel reviewed many putative markers (including both tissue-based and circulating markers), their ultimate recommendations were surprisingly sparse (Table 7.1).[1–3]

Why are the ASCO guidelines so conservative? In reviewing the available literature, the Panel recognized that the science of clinical tumor marker investigation has been haphazard and relatively chaotic. Too often, studies of tumor markers are more inclined to be "fishing expeditions" with the hope that something interesting will be detected with statistical significance, rather than being prospective, hypothesis-driven investigations. In light of this confusion, several authors of the Guidelines separately developed a proposal for a framework in which previously published tumor marker studies might be critically evaluated in an evidence-based manner.[4] The rest of this chapter reviews the generic concepts and policies related to tumor marker evaluation. Specific marker evaluation for a given disease are reviewed in the relevant chapter pertaining to that malignancy.

Critical Elements of a Clinically Useful Tumor Marker

The first and most obvious element of evaluating a tumor marker is to determine its stated use. Tumor markers can be valuable for risk assessment, screening, diagnosis, prognosis, prediction of benefit from therapy, and monitoring disease course (Table 7.2). The most commonly accepted uses are for prognosis and prediction, as well as monitoring. The first two of these require more detailed understanding.

What Is the Question: Prognosis Versus Prediction?

Estimating a patient's prognosis requires a complicated set of evaluations, which includes the propensity of a malignancy to expand in volume (proliferative capacity), its ability to escape its natural site of origin and establish growth in a foreign tissue (metastatic potential), and its relative sensitiv-

TABLE 7.1. American Society of Clinical Oncology clinical practice guidelines for use of tumor markers in breast and colon cancer (tissue factors only).

Disease	*Factor*	*Use*	*Guideline*
Breast cancer	Estrogen and progesterone receptors	Predictive factors for endocrine therapy	Measure on every primary breast cancer and on metastatic lesions if results influence treatment planning
	DNA flow cytometrically derived parameters	Prognosis or prediction	Data are insufficient to recommend obtaining results
	c-erbB-2 (HER-2/neu)	Prognosis	Data are insufficient to recommend obtaining results for this use
		Prediction for: trastuzumab CMF-like regimens doxorubicin taxanes endocrine Rx	c-erbB-2 should be evaluated on every primary breast cancer at time of diagnosis or at time of recurrence for use as predictive factor for trastuzumab; Committee could not make definitive recommendations regarding CMF-like regimens; c-erbB-2 may identify patients who particularly benefit from anthracyline-based therapy but should not be used to exclude anthracycline; treatment c-erbB-2 should not be used to prescribe taxane-based therapy or endocrine therapy
	P53	Prognosis or prediction	Data are insufficient to recommend use of p53
	Cathepsin-D	Prognosis	Data are insufficient to recommend use of cathepsin-D
Colorectal cancer	Circulating carcinoembryonic antigen	Screening	Not recommended
		Preoperative	Recommended to guide surgical planning
		Postoperative	Recommended to monitor for early, asymptomatic, and resectable metastases
		Metastatic setting	Recommended to monitor benefit from therapy
	Lipid-associated sialic acid	Monitoring	Not recommended for screening, diagnosis, staging, or monitoring
	CA19-9	Monitoring	Not recommended for screening, diagnosis, staging, or monitoring
	DNA ploidy and flow cytometry	Prognosis	Data are insufficient to recommend use of DNA ploidy or flow cytometry
	P53	Prognosis	Data are insufficient to recommend use of p53
	Ras	Prognosis	Data are insufficient to recommend use of ras

Source: Adapted from Bast RC Jr, Ravdin P, Hayes DF, et al.,[3] by permission of *J of Clinical Oncology*.

ity or resistance to therapy. Therapies for most solid tumors include surgery, radiation, and systemic therapies such as hormone therapies or chemotherapies. In this regard, the terms "prognostic" and "predictive" have taken on separate meanings.[5,6] The prognostic factor designation is usually reserved for those markers that specifically provide an estimate of the odds of the recurrence of a given cancer after local therapy only. It is usually a measure of both proliferation and metastatic potential, and it usually implies the odds of systemic recurrence and/or death in a patient who does not receive systemic therapy. If the factor is associated with a poor prognosis, patients who are "positive" for the prognostic factor have a worse outcome than those who are "negative" in the absence of systemic therapy. Therapy may be effective, but it is equally so (in relative terms) for both factor-positive and factor-negative patients. The best examples of prognostic factors for most solid tumors are the TNM staging systems.

A predictive factor helps select therapies most likely to work against that patient's tumor. A predictive factor may be the precise target of the therapy, an associated molecule or pathway that modifies the effectiveness of the therapy, or simply an alteration that is an epiphenomenon linked to the target or pathway of the therapy (such as coamplification of a neighboring gene). If the factor is a pure predictive factor, prognosis in the absence of therapy is the same for factor-negative and -positive patients (it has no prognostic effects). However, assuming it predicts *for* benefit from therapy, factor-positive patients have a much better prognosis than factor-negative patients in the presence of the therapy for which the factor is predictive. For example, it is now clearly established that the level of estrogen receptor (ER) content in breast cancer tissue is positively related to the odds of response and benefit from antiestrogen hormonal therapy, such as ovarian ablation, tamoxifen, or aromatase inhibitors, because the ER plays a fundamental role in estrogen-dependent tumor growth and biology.[7] In contrast, *p*-glycoprotein content is a negative predictive factor for resistance to certain drugs, because this protein modulates multidrug resistance by increasing efflux of the antineoplastic agent from the cancer cell.[8]

TABLE 7.2. Potential uses of tumor markers.

Determination of risk
Screening
Differential diagnosis
Benign vs. malignant
Known malignant: tissue of origin
Prognosis
Prediction
Monitoring disease course
Detect recurrence in patient free of obvious disease
Patient with established recurrence

Many, in fact most, factors may be both prognostic and predictive. For example, in addition to serving as a predictive factor, ER is also a favorable prognostic factor. Breast cancers with high ER content have generally slower growth potentials, and patients with ER-"positive" tumors have a better prognosis, even if they receive no treatment.[9,10]

To further complicate this discussion, some markers may be associated with a *poor* prognosis independent of therapy, but they may predict for an *improved* outcome related to specific treatment modalities. For example, in breast cancer, amplification and/or overexpression of HER-2 is a marker of poor prognosis in the absence of any systemic therapy.[11–14] However, HER-2 serves as the target for a humanized monoclonal antibody, trastuzumab (herceptin), and response and benefit from trastuzumab are tightly linked to HER-2 amplification and/or overexpression.[15,16] Thus, untreated HER-2-positive patients have a worse prognosis than HER-2-negative patients if they do not receive trastuzumab, but they may actually have a more favorable prognosis if they do.

These considerations are often ignored in many "prognostic factor" studies. Often, a population of patients is studied with a new, putative prognostic factor simply because the samples to be assayed happen to be available and the outcome for the patients is known. Indeed, a prognostic factor can only be evaluated in the absence of systemic therapy, or at least in the absence of any therapy with which it interacts. A predictive factor can only be evaluated in the context of an untreated control group, preferably one that is prospectively identified and followed, as in prospective randomized trials. It is not surprising that studies of a marker that might have both prognostic and predictive capabilities, especially if these effects are in opposition (as may be the case with HER-2), will provide relatively random and conflicting results if not carefully planned with appropriate consideration of treatment effects control groups and satisfactory control groups.

What Is the Strength of the Marker?

A marker is only helpful if it separates an entire population into two different groups whose outcome is likely to be so different that one group might be treated differently from another. Again using breast cancer as an example, both ER and HER2 are good examples of strong predictive markers that are clinically useful. Patients with ER-negative tumors appear very unlikely to benefit from hormone therapy,[17] and, likewise, it appears that patients with HER2-low or -negative cancers are very unlikely to benefit from trastuzumab.[4,18] It is important to recognize that clinical utility of a marker is not justified simply because a tumor marker may separate two populations of patients whose outcomes differ with statistical significance. A P value less than 0.05 simply implies it is likely that those two populations are different (see following). Rather, for a marker to be clinically useful, it must not only separate the two populations with reliability, the separation must be of sufficient magnitude that one would treat the two groups differently.

How large this magnitude needs to be for a tumor marker to be acceptable for clinical use is an arbitrary decision, and it depends on the perspectives of the patient, the caregiver, and the societal elements that pay for the care. Several studies have been performed in which patients are queried regarding how much benefit they would require to accept a given level of toxicity.[19–21] Not surprisingly, results from these studies are heterogeneous, although in general a decreasing proportion of patients is willing to accept therapy as the absolute odds of benefit decrease. However, for a few patients, any benefit is worth the risk of toxicities, and for a few others therapy is never acceptable, even if the odds of benefit are enormous. Sophisticated tools are now available on paper and on the Internet to help patients understand and quantify the relative odds of benefit and toxicities of certain therapies in selected situations, such as for adjuvant therapy of primary breast cancer.[22–24] These tools are based on clinical and pathologic prognostic and predictive factors, such as the T, N, and M status, and a few classic markers, such as ER. However, these tools are potentially flexible enough to be modified to permit incorporation of new prognostic factors if the estimate of magnitude between positive and negative subgroups is sufficiently reliable.

Is the Magnitude of Difference Between the Two Groups Reliable?

The hallmark of any scientific observation is, of course, reproducibility. With few exceptions, tumor markers seem to pass through a "life cycle" in which the original report is extraordinarily positive with great acclaim, but subsequent studies fail to live up to the promise. There are several elements regarding both technical variability of the assay and clinical trial design that account for this phenomenon, and these may hinder acceptance of the assay for routine clinical use. There are fundamentally three reasons for this conundrum: (1) technical variability of the assay; (2) variations in the manner in which different assays for the same marker are performed; and (3) inadequate and variable study designs.

The assay must be technically reliable and reproducible. Assay reproducibility is critical for any clinical test. Reproducibility hinges on several factors, all of which must be standardized and validated. Too often, an assay is developed in an individual investigator's laboratory based on personal preferences and subjective techniques that are not easily transported to other investigators and laboratories. For an assay to be useful clinically, it must be shown to be accurate throughout a broad dynamic range of values and reproducible at each of these levels as well. Concern must be taken regarding fixatives and other processing of samples, because these can have an enormous impact on the results of an assay from one laboratory to the next, resulting in false positives or negatives.

Analysis and Quantitation of Results

How the assay is "scored" or "read" is also critical for reproducibility. For example, when immunohistochemistry is performed, does the reader report the results as percent cells that stained, the intensity of staining, or a combination of both? Are the results reported as such, or in an index, such as 0–3+? Furthermore, selection of the cutoff that distinguishes positive from negative populations can give incredibly different results for the same assay. Several means of establishing a cutoff are employed, and there is no consensus regarding the optimal method.[25] One method is to arbitrarily select a cutoff, based on some preconceived reason, such as the mean level of the assay in an affected population or the mean plus two standard deviations (2 SD) of the level in an unaffected population. A second method is to test several potential cutoffs in one population, selecting the one that appears most robust relative to separation of the outcomes of the two groups or to apparent statistical significance. Regardless of the method used, it is essential to validate the results in a separate group of patients.[26] Thus, even if the same assay using the same reagents is applied in two different studies, use of different cutoffs will substantially affect the results.

Do Two Studies Use the Same Assay?

Because of competition among scientists and commercial interests, different assays are often developed to evaluate the same marker. Thus, when reading what appears to be a confirmatory study of a given marker, one must be certain that the same assay was used in both studies. For example, HER2 status can be determined by examination of cancer tissue amplification of the erbB2 gene using a variety of techniques including Southern blotting, slot-blot quantification, or fluorescence in situ hybridization, and by evaluation of the protein using Western blotting, immunohistochemistry, immunofluorescence, or enzyme-linked immunosorbent assays (ELISA). Moreover, the circulating extracellular domain of HER2 can be quantified in human serum using ELISA.[27] Although they are all correlated, each of these assays, which in one way or another provides an indication of overproduction of HER2, appears to differ from the other and to provide different results in regard to prediction of outcome. Furthermore, even if the assay format is the same, use of different reagents or conditions may affect results. For example, it has been clearly shown that different antibodies against HER-2 can provide very different results in immunohistochemical (IHC) assays.[28] Thus, it is not surprising that results from study to study are not validated, if the assays that are being compared are not identical.

Was the Study Design Appropriate to Address the Hypothesis?

The results of a tumor marker are most likely to be valid if they are studied in the context of a plausible hypothesis that is prospectively addressed; for example, a study of prognosis in the absence of the therapy being considered or prediction that the specific therapy will be beneficial. Many published studies report results related to hypotheses that are retrospectively derived from the observed data. Although such studies are valuable to generate hypotheses, these observations must be prospectively validated in subsequent, well-designed studies.[4,25] Unfortunately, most tumor marker studies are performed using archived specimens collected for reasons unrelated to the study under question. Therefore, it is difficult to validate exciting but preliminary observations, which requires time-consuming prospective studies. Nonetheless, failure to do so often leaves the reader unable to draw definitive conclusions and, in the long run, delays acceptance of the marker for clinical use.

How Should Tumor Markers Be Selected for Clinical Use?

To summarize the preceding paragraphs, a good tumor marker study should provide accurate estimate of the magnitude of difference in outcomes between subgroups of patients who are positive or negative for the marker, using a reliable, accurate, and reproducible assay. Do prognostic and predictive factors exist that permit such elegant selection of patients for treatment? Sadly, in most solid tumors, the answer is no. For patients with newly diagnosed solid malignancies, there is no example of a prognostic factor that predicts subsequent recurrence and death with absolute certainty. Therefore, when these markers are applied in the clinic, both physician and patient must accept some margin of error. These decisions involve both the tumor marker results, as already discussed, and also a careful assessment of the magnitude of effectiveness of therapy for the patient's condition (proportional reduction in risk of events), the degree of toxicity of that therapy, and the patient's willingness (as well as the caregiver's and society's) to either forgo potential benefit to avoid toxicity or to accept toxicity and cost to gain benefit.

Therefore, part of the art, and science, of medicine is to determine which markers are most reliable in separating groups of patients into those that will do well from those that will not, and into those that will benefit from therapy from those that will not. If performed appropriately, tumor marker analysis should permit delivery of therapy as efficiently as possible, providing benefit to the greatest number of patients while avoiding exposure to toxicities as much as possible.

Levels of Evidence (LOE) to evaluate tumor markers have been proposed, again by the American Society of Clinical Oncology Expert Panel on Tumor Markers (Table 7.3).[4] LOE I data are generated from either a prospective, highly powered study that specifically addresses the issue of tumor marker utility or from an overview or meta-analysis of studies, each of which provides lower levels of evidence. LOE II data are derived from companion studies in which specimens are collected prospectively as part of a therapeutic clinical trial, with preestablished endpoints and statistical evaluation for the marker as well as for the therapeutic intervention.

Ideally, the estimate of the relative strength of a marker for clinical utilities should be determined within the context of LOE I (or at worse II) studies. In these studies, the marker is the primary objective of a well-designed, highly powered, hypothesis-driven prospective clinical trial, or it is the objective of a statistically rigorous overview of LOE II and/or III studies. Furthermore, the strength of new prognostic or predictive factors can only be estimated by multivariate analytical methods, including preexisting accepted factors such as TNM staging and histopathology. It is possible that a marker may be quite prognostic or predictive when considered in a univariate fashion but that it is, in fact, only reflecting information already achieved through other, established methods. In this case, acceptance of the new marker would only occur if it can be performed more easily or reliably or less expensively.

TABLE 7.3. Levels of evidence for grading clinical utility of tumor markers.

Level	Type of Evidence
I	Evidence from a single high-powered prospective study that is specifically designed to test marker or evidence from meta-analysis and/or overview of Level II or III studies. In the former case, the study must be designed so that therapy and follow-up are dictated by protocol. Ideally, the study is a prospective randomized trial in which diagnostic and/or therapeutic clinical decisions in one arm are determined based at least in part on marker results, and diagnostic and/or therapeutic clinical decisions in control arm are made independently of marker results. However, may also include prospective but not randomized trials with marker data and clinical outcome as primary objective.
II	Evidence from study in which marker data are determined in relationship to prospective therapeutic trial that is performed to test therapeutic hypothesis but not specifically designed to test marker utility (i.e., marker study is secondary objective of protocol). However, specimen collection for marker study and statistical analysis are prospectively determined in protocol as secondary objectives.
III	Evidence from large but retrospective studies from which variable numbers of samples are available or selected. Therapeutic aspects and follow-up of patient population may or may not have been prospectively dictated. Statistical analysis for tumor marker was not dictated prospectively at time of therapeutic trial design.
IV	Evidence from small retrospective studies which do not have prospectively dictated therapy, follow-up, specimen selection, or statistical analysis. May be matched case controls, etc.
V	Evidence from small pilot studies designed to determine or estimate distribution of marker levels in sample population. May include "correlation" with other known or investigational markers of outcome, but not designed to determine clinical utility.

Source: From Hayes et al.,[4] by permission of *Journal of the National Cancer Institute.*

Summary

In summary, the field of tumor marker generation is evolving rapidly, with a convergence of molecular biology and technology and understanding of clinical trial design and analysis. Several of the large cooperative trialists' groups have now established separate correlative/biologic committees that are charged with designing hypothesis-driven LOE I and II studies, based on results from pilot studies. The emergence of erbB-2 in breast cancer as a predictive factor, in a manner similar to ER, may serve as a model of directed studies that lead to determination of the relative strength of the marker and determination of whether it should be used clinically. One hopes that careful and thoughtful consideration of study design will considerably shorten the life cycle required to being a tumor marker from the laboratory to the clinic.

Acknowledgment. Supported in part by NIH grant CA64057 and by the Fashion Footwear Association of New York (FFANY)/QVC Presents/Shoes on Sale.

References

1. ASCO Expert Panel. Clinical Practice Guidelines for the Use of Tumor Markers in Breast and Colorectal Cancer: Report of the American Society of Clinical Oncology Expert Panel. J Clin Oncol 1996;14:2843–2877.
2. ASCO Expert Panel. 1997 update of recommendations for the use of tumor markers in breast and colorectal cancer. J Clin Oncol 1998;16:793–795.
3. Bast RC Jr, Ravdin P, Hayes DF, et al. 2000 Update of recommendations for the use of tumor markers in breast and colorectal cancer: clinical practice guidelines of the American Society of Clinical Oncology. J Clin Oncol 2001;19(6):1865–1878.
4. Hayes DF, Bast R, Desch CE, et al. A tumor marker utility grading system (TMUGS): a framework to evaluate clinical utility of tumor markers. J Natl Cancer Inst 1996;88:1456–1466.
5. McGuire WL, Clark GM. Prognostic factors and treatment decisions in axillary-node-negative breast cancer. N Engl J Med 1992;326(26):1756–1761.
6. Gasparini G, Pozza F, Harris AL. Evaluating the potential usefulness of new prognostic and predictive indicators in node-negative breast cancer patients. J Natl Cancer Inst 1993; 85(15):1206–1219.
7. Osborne CK. Receptors. In: Harris J, Hellman S, Henderson I, Kinne D (eds). Breast Diseases, 2nd ed. Philadelphia: Lippincott; 1991:301–325.
8. Trock B, Leonessa F, Clarke R. Multidrug resistance in breast cancer: a meta-analysis of MDR1/gp170 expression and its possible functional significance. J Natl Cancer Inst 1997;89: 917–931.
9. Fisher B, Costantino J, Redmond C, et al. A randomized clinical trial evaluating tamoxifen in the treatment of patients with node-negative breast cancer who have estrogen-receptor-positive tumors. N Engl J Med 1989;320:479–484.
10. Fisher B, Redmond C, Dimitrov N, et al. A randomized clinical trial evaluating sequential methotrexate and fluorouracil in the treatment of patients with node-negative breast cancer who have estrogen-receptor-negative tumors. N Engl J Med 1989;320: 473–478.
11. Ravdin PM. Should HER2 status be routinely measured for all breast cancer patients? Semin Oncol 1999;26(4 suppl 12): 117–123.
12. Press MF, Bernstein L, Thomas PA, et al. HER-2/neu gene amplification characterized by fluorescence in situ hybridization: poor prognosis in node-negative breast carcinomas. J Clin Oncol 1997; 15(8):2894–2904.
13. Hayes DF. Tumor markers for breast cancer. Ann Oncol 1993; 4:807–819.
14. Trock BJ, Yamauchi H, Brotzman M, Stearns V, Hayes DF. c-erbB-2 as a prognostic factor in breast cancer: a meta-analysis. Proc Am Soc Clin Oncol 2000;2000:97a.
15. Slamon DJ, Leyland-Jones B, Shak S, et al. Use of chemotherapy plus a monoclonal antibody against HER2 for metastatic breast cancer that overexpresses HER2. N Engl J Med 2001; 344(11):783–792.
16. Mass R. The role of HER-2 expression in predicting response to therapy in breast cancer. Semin Oncol 2000;27(6 suppl 11):46–52; discussion 92–100.
17. Early Breast Cancer Trialist's Collaborative Group. Tamoxifen for early breast cancer: an overview of the randomised trials. Lancet 1998;351:1451–1467.
18. Vogel CL, Cobleigh MA, Tripathy D, et al. Efficacy and safety of trastuzumab as a single agent in first-line treatment of HER2-

overexpressing metastatic breast cancer. J Clin Oncol 2002; 20(3):719–726.
19. Coates AS, Simes RJ. Patient assessment of adjuvant treatment in operable breast cancer. New York: Wiley, 1992.
20. Lindley C, Vasa S, Sawyer T, Winer E. Quality of life and preferences for treatment following systemic adjuvant therapy for early stage breast cancer. J Clin Oncol 1998;16:1380–1387.
21. Siminoff LA, Ravdin P, Colabianchi N, Sturm CM. Doctor-patient communication patterns in breast cancer adjuvant therapy discussions. Health Expect 2000;3(1):26–36.
22. Ravdin PM, Siminoff LA, Davis GJ, et al. Computer program to assist in making decisions about adjuvant therapy for women with early breast cancer. J Clin Oncol 2001;19(4):980–991.
23. Loprinzi CL, Thome SD. Understanding the utility of adjuvant systemic therapy for primary breast cancer. J Clin Oncol 2001; 19(4):972–979.
24. Whelan T, Levine M, Willan A, et al. Effect of a decision aid on knowledge and treatment decision making for breast cancer surgery: a randomized trial. JAMA 2004;292(4):435–441.
25. Simon R, Altman DG. Statistical aspects of prognostic factor studies in oncology. Br J Cancer 1994;69:979–985.
26. Clark GM. Prognostic and predictive factors. In: Harris J, Lippman M, Morrow M, Osborne CK (eds). Diseases of the Breast, 2nd ed. Philadelphia: Lippincott Williams & Wilkins, 2000:489–515.
27. Yamauchi H, Stearns V, Hayes DF. When is a tumor marker ready for prime time? A case study of c-erbB-2 as a predictive factor in breast cancer. J Clin Oncol 2001;19(9):2334–2356.
28. Press M. Sensitivity of HER-2/neu antibodies in archival tissue samples: potential source of error in immunohistochemical studies of oncogene expression. Cancer Res 1994;54(10): 2771–2777.

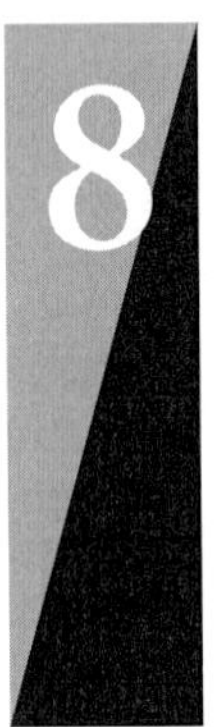

Design and Analysis of Oncology Clinical Trials

James J. Dignam, Theodore G. Karrison, and John Bryant

In this chapter, we discuss the design and analysis of oncology clinical trials. Because analysis follows naturally from design and is specified a priori in any well-planned trial, it is appropriate to discuss these topics together. We review clinical trial designs and associated analytical methods used in the different phases of therapy development. Along the way we identify areas in which the methodology is adapting to new approaches to therapeutic intervention. This chapter provides only a brief sketch of the main concepts and current research areas, and we refer the reader to primary sources and comprehensive texts on clinical trials in oncology for further details. Two excellent recent texts in particular, the *Handbook of Statistics in Clinical Oncology*[1] and *Clinical Trials in Oncology*,[2] provide the fundamentals of trial design, conduct, and analysis, as well as up-to-date discussion of new challenges and active research in statistical methods for oncology clinical trials.

Some General Statistical Concepts

Although we assume some familiarity with basic statistical concepts and space does not permit a detailed account, we review here some concepts vital to the design and analysis of clinical trials and associated studies. In the classical (e.g., frequentist) statistical hypothesis testing paradigm, a quantity referred to as *type II* or *β error* equals the probability that a statistical test fails to produce a decision in favor of a treatment effect when in fact the effect is manifest in the population. The complement of this probability $(1 - \beta)$ is referred to as *statistical power*, and equals the probability of correctly detecting a treatment effect. Statistical power depends on the other principal parameters in hypothesis testing, specifically, the probability of incorrectly finding in favor of an effect when none exists (discussed in a following section), the sample size, and the size of the treatment effect. It is imperative that clinical trials be designed with adequate statistical power, typically 0.80 or greater for anticipated treatment effects that are both realistic and clinically material, so as not to obtain equivocal findings concerning the potential worth of a new treatment under consideration. Studies with low statistical power can cause delay in development or even abandonment of promising treatments and waste valuable resources, not least of which is the participation and goodwill of patients.[3] In contrast, an adequately powered trial that does not find a new treatment to be superior *is* informative, and resources can then appropriately be directed into other more promising alternatives.

In statistical hypothesis testing, *type I* or *α error* refers to the probability of incorrectly deciding in favor of a treatment difference when in fact none exists. Typically, the α probability is fixed at some small value, such as 0.05 or 0.01. When hypothesis tests are repeated, the probability increases that at least one test result will be erroneous. A particular complication arising in clinical trials is the need to periodically evaluate the primary hypothesis as information accumulates. These *interim analyses* are conducted to ensure that if definitive evidence of benefit or harm emerges before the anticipated end of the trial, then actions can be taken for the protection and benefit of trial participants. Appropriate statistical methodology to accommodate multiple serial analyses is discussed later.

Types of Trials and the Evolution of Treatment

In this section we review design, conduct, and analysis of the three phases of therapy development. We also follow one clinical trial statistician's recommendation that more descriptive names be used that reflect the goals of each study phase.[4]

Phase I or Dose Evaluation Trials

Objectives

The primary objective of a Phase I oncology trial is to determine the maximum tolerated dose (MTD) of a new experimental regimen. The general assumption is that as dose is increased, greater efficacy will be achieved; hence, the search for the highest dose level compatible with an acceptable toxicity profile. This assumption is certainly reasonable, particularly for cytotoxic drugs, although it need not always be the case. For example, the maximum beneficial effect of immunomodulating agents may occur at intermediate dosages, or the degree of efficacy may plateau so that little is gained by increasing the dose beyond a certain level. These situations create further design and analytical challenges that are probably best addressed in a randomized comparative setting. For the remainder of this section, we assume that the primary aim of a Phase I trial is to determine the MTD, under the assumption that the highest dose will produce the greatest beneficial effects. Secondary objectives may be to conduct pharmacokinetic studies in individual patients or detect evidence of antitumor activity. More recently, a better knowledge of drug metabolic pathways and pharmacogenomics is beginning to be incorporated into some trial designs, with the goal being to evaluate the relationship between toxicity and genotype.[5]

Clinical Issues

Key clinical issues to be addressed when designing a Phase I trial include patient selection, the starting and subsequent dose levels to be evaluated, and the specification of dose-limiting toxicities. The obvious ethical requirement when selecting patients for a Phase I trial is that no other effective treatment is available, although for a given patient there may be more than one experimental trial for which he/she is eligible. Most Phase I studies are conducted in adults with solid tumors; patients with leukemia and children are usually excluded or studied separately.[6,7] Because assessment of activity is not the main objective of the trial, patients need not have measurable disease and multiple tumor types may be included. Life expectancy should be at least 3 months, the interval from any prior treatment should be sufficient to ensure that toxicities occurring over the course of the trial are due to the new agent and not prior therapy, and patients should generally have normal organ function and biochemical profiles.

The manner in which a starting dose and subsequent dose levels are chosen, and the historical development behind the various recommendations for doing so, have been described.[1–8] We simply note here that the starting dose is generally chosen to be low enough that there is a very small likelihood of severe toxicity. With regard to dose escalation, the increments are typically rapid initially, followed by smaller increases as one presumably approaches the toxic range. For example, the highly cited *modified Fibonacci* scheme begins by doubling the first dose, then increasing by factors of 1.67, 1.5, 1.4, and 1.33.

The determination of the MTD is based on the toxicities (adverse events) observed in individual patients and is greatly facilitated by the U.S. National Cancer Institute's Common Toxicity Criteria (CTC) system. In the CTC, adverse events (AEs) are grouped into various organ/symptom categories, with each AE graded as 0 (none), 1 (mild), 2 (moderate), 3 (serious/severe), 4 (life threatening), or 5 (fatal). Typically, any grade 3 or higher AE is deemed a "dose-limiting toxicity" (DLT) (although certain grade 3 AEs may be excluded). A second grading scale may be used to indicate whether, in the physician's judgment, the AE is likely to have been related to the investigational treatment, and only those AEs scored to be at least "possibly" related to the agent are regarded as DLTs. Note that while common toxicities can be detected in Phase I trials, the sample sizes are far too small to detect less-frequent adverse events.

The criteria for a DLT should be clearly specified in the protocol, along with the time interval over which each patient will be observed for the occurrence of a DLT (typically one therapy cycle). With appropriately defined criteria, each patient's outcome can be regarded as a binary random variable Y taking the value 0 if the patient did not have a DLT and 1 if the patient had a DLT within the specified time frame.

Trial Design Types

The first issue to clarify is what, specifically, is meant by the MTD, for as Storer[9] points out, "a strict quantitative definition of the MTD is rarely acknowledged in clinical protocols." As discussed previously, a dose given to an individual patient is deemed "tolerable" in that patient if he/she does not experience a DLT, but in statistical terms the MTD must be defined with reference to the patient population. By virtue of the traditional and still frequently used "3 + 3" design, described below, the MTD is usually defined as the highest dose level for which the incidence of DLT is less than 33%. Thus, when employing this design, we are saying that we want to determine the dose that will be tolerable in at least 2/3 of the patients, and therefore are accepting that serious toxicity will be produced in up to 1/3 of the patients. Given that most cancers carry an appreciable risk of mortality, this seems an appropriate percentile to target, but it should not be used unthinkingly. There may be some patient populations, for example, in whom a lower percentile would be more appropriate; conversely, patients at a *very* high risk of mortality or morbidity may be willing to accept a greater chance of serious side effects for potential therapeutic benefits.

"3 + 3"

In the traditional "3 + 3" design[11] (Table 8.1), groups of three patients are treated. If none experiences a DLT, the dose is escalated, whereas if two or more experience a DLT, dose escalation is terminated and the previous dose level is provisionally defined as the MTD. If one of three has a DLT, three more patients are added at the same dose level, and if none of these has dose-limiting toxicity, dose escalation continues; otherwise, the previous dose level is considered the MTD. Once a presumed MTD is reached, however, if only three patients have been studied at that dose, three more are added and if two or more of these patients experience a DLT (yielding greater than one of six), further dose reduction occurs. Thus, it is intuitive that this design is targeting a dose that is close to but less than the 33rd percentile. Simulations conducted by Storer[9] and others indicate that it is nearer to the 25th percentile.

Accelerated Titration

One criticism of the traditional design, particularly when accompanied by a conservative starting dose, is that too many patients are treated at subtherapeutic levels. Simon et al.[12] have therefore proposed a variant of the "3 + 3" algorithm, known as the *accelerated titration design*, to overcome this problem. Essentially, only one patient is treated at each dose level, and the dose is doubled for each subsequent patient until either a DLT is observed or two patients experience grade 2 or higher toxicity. At this point the design reverts to the traditional "3 + 3" with subsequent dose increments of 40%. *Intrapatient* dose escalation is also permitted if the patient had no worse than grade 1 toxicity at the previous

TABLE 8.1. Design features for three "classic" statistical designs for Phase I trials.

Design	*Description*	*Pros*	*Cons*
"3 + 3"	1) Begin at lowest dose, treating 3 patients. If DLT rate is —0/3, escalate (to next pre-specified dose level) —1/3, add 3 more: then if 1/6, escalate ≥2/6, go to step 2) —≥2/3, go to step 2) 2) If 6 patients studied at the previous dose level (1/6 AEs), declare —that dose to be the MTD; otherwise, add 3 more: Then if —<1/6, declare MTD —≥2/6, decrease dose and continue	Easy to implement Conservative dose levels	Many patients may be treated at subtherapeutic Targeted percentile not explicit
Accelerated titration	1) Begin at lowest dose. Treat one patient at a time and double 2) the dose until DLT observed or two patients have experienced 3) grade 2 or higher AE; then go to step 2) 4) Revert to "3 + 3" design with dose increments of 40% (intrapatient) 5) Dose escalation permitted in if no worse than grade 1 AE)	Easy to implement Moves quickly to therapeutic dose levels	More high-grade toxicities will occur Targeted percentile not explicit
Storer's BD design (up and down)	1) (Stage B) Begin at lowest dose. Treat one patient at a time and 2) escalate until DLT, then deescalate until first nontoxic response; 3) go to step 2 4) (Stage D). If DLT rate is —0/3, escalate (to next prespecified dose level) —1/3, add 3 more at same dose —≥2/3, deescalate Sampling continues until fixed number, n_D, patients treated at stage D	Easy to implement Moves quickly to therapeutic dose levels Targeted percentile is explicit (33rd percentile)	More high-grade toxicities will occur

treatment course. As would be expected, this design reduces the number of patients in the trial who are undertreated, at the expense of a slightly higher percentage experiencing grade 3 or higher toxicity. The authors also describe a statistical model for estimating the MTD that takes into account not just whether or not a patient has experienced a DLT but the full range of toxicity data from all treatment courses. Legedza and Ibrahim describe a related longitudinal model that incorporates the effects of current dose, cumulative dose, and clearance rate on cumulative toxicity.[13] In this design, dose administration within a patient is tailored over successive treatment courses in an attempt to treat all patients at more-efficacious dose levels.

Up and Down

To provide a more solid inferential basis for estimating the MTD, Storer[9,14] proposed and evaluated the properties of a number of "up-and-down" designs, including two-stage versions to allow more rapid dose escalation, as in the accelerated titration design. His BD design, for example, explicitly targets the 33rd percentile of the tolerance distribution. Initially (stage B), a single patient is treated at each dose level, escalating sequentially from the starting dose until a DLT is observed. Deescalation then occurs until the first nontoxic response, at which point the second stage (stage D) begins and cohorts of three patients are enrolled. Then, if none of the three has a DLT, the dose is escalated; if two or more have a DLT, the dose is deescalated; and if one of three has a DLT, the next cohort is treated at the same dose level. Sampling continues in this manner until a fixed number of second stage patients (for example, $n_D = 24$) are treated. The total number of patients, $n = n_B + n_D$, is therefore variable, depending upon when the second stage is reached. After the trial is completed, a logistic regression model

$$p(x) = \Pr(Y = 1|x) = \frac{\exp(\alpha + \beta x)}{1 + \exp(\alpha + \beta x)} \qquad (1)$$

is fit to the n pairs of points $(x_1, y_1), (x_2, y_2), \ldots (x_n, y_n)$ where x_i is the dose and y_i the response (0 or 1) of the ith patient. The method provides not only a point estimate of the MTD, but a means to derive confidence intervals as well. However, for the small sample sizes typically used in Phase I trials, computationally demanding "exact" methods may be required to obtain these confidence intervals. The method is easily modified to estimate other percentiles of the tolerance distribution (i.e., the 25th percentile). Korn et al.[15] found stage B too aggressive and recommended treating two patients at a time, increasing dose levels until the first DLT is observed. Other useful variations of up-and-down designs are discussed by Ivanova et al.[16]

Continual Reassessment Method (CRM)

An alternative to the classic designs is the Bayesian approach developed by O'Quigley et al.,[17] who called it the "continual reassessment method" or CRM (Table 8.2). This method is based on a one-parameter model for the dose—toxicity curve, for example, the logistic model (Eq. 1) with the α parameter fixed at a suitably chosen constant a_0. Within the Bayesian framework, a *prior* probability distribution is assigned to the parameter β, data are collected, and knowledge about this parameter is updated by constructing the *posterior* probability distribution for β. Thus, in the CRM, a prior distribution for β is specified and the first patient is assigned to the dose level whose probability of toxicity as given by Eq. 1 is closest to the 33rd (or other desired) percentile. After observing the outcome in this patient, the posterior distribution for β is formed, toxicity probabilities updated, and the next patient assigned the dose closest to the desired percentile. This process is repeated until a fixed number of patients have been studied. The method tends to converge to the correct target level, even if the original model is incorrectly specified.[18]

Modified CRM

Although it is clearly an attractive approach, some problems with the CRM were immediately recognized. First, there was discomfort about starting the first patient at too high a dose. Second, escalating more than one dose level at a time was thought to be too risky. Finally, there were concerns that trial durations would be extended unduly because of the need to await the outcome in each individual patient before enrolling the next patient. This concern led to the so-called modified CRM[10,19] whereby the trial starts at the lowest dose level, the dose is increased no more than one level at a time, and the cohort size is increased to three patients. Results of a simulation study comparing the modified CRM to the original CRM and the traditional "3 + 3" design showed that the "3 + 3" design generally placed more patients at dose levels below the MTD; consequently, the CRM designs were more likely to assign patients to therapeutic dose levels and to arrive at the correct estimate of the MTD, although there were exceptions.[10]

A method that maintains the simplicity of the classic design, but, as in the CRM, makes better use of the cumulative data, has recently been proposed.[20] The method capitalizes on the assumption that toxicity is nondecreasing with dose, using a technique known as isotonic regression to estimate the dose–toxicity curve at each step, essentially pooling and averaging outcomes from adjacent dose levels to maintain a nondecreasing curve. For example, if the current data were 1 toxicity in 6 patients treated at dose level x_1, 1 in 6 at dose level x_2, and 0 of 3 at dose level x_3 ($x_1 < x_2 < x_3$), the algorithm would first pool the data at x_2 and x_3 to maintain monotonicity, replacing each estimate with $1/9 = (1 + 0)/(6 + 3)$. As 1/9 also is less than 1/6 from the first dose, the data would be pooled again, and all three estimates would be changed to $2/15 = (1 + 1)/(6 + 9)$. Additional patients are added at the current, higher, or lower dose level depending on the current DLT rate in relation to a specified target. The trial is terminated when the same dose level is indicated in three consecutive cohorts, or when some prespecified number of patients have been evaluated. A simulation study comparing the method with the traditional "3 + 3," modified CRM, and up-and-down designs found similar performance to the modified CRM and fewer patients underdosed compared to the "3 + 3" design, but on average more patients were required and were treated above the true MTD.[20]

TABLE 8.2. Design features for three Bayesian statistical designs for Phase I trials.

Design	*Description*	*Pros*	*Cons*
Continual reassessment method (CRM)	1) Choose prior distribution for β parameter of logistic family 2) Assign first patient to dose level for which prior probability of DLT is closest to the desired percentile 3) Observe outcome and update posterior distribution Assign next patient to dose level with probability of DLT closest to desired percentile; go to step 3) Sampling continues until fixed number *N* patients are treated	More patients treated at therapeutic dose levels Utilizes all information available to choose next dose level Targeted percentile is explicit	Requires software to implement First patient could be assigned any dose and dose escalation can jump more than one level leading to higher observed toxicity rates
Modified CRM	1) Choose prior distribution for β parameter of logistic family 2) Begin at lowest dose. Enroll 3 patients, observe outcomes and update posterior distribution 3) Determine dose level with probability of DLT closest to desired percentile, but *escalate no more than one level*; go to step 3) Sampling continues until fixed number *N* patients are treated	Less aggressive escalation than CRM Utilizes all available information to choose next dose level Targeted percentile is explicit	Requires software to implement
TITE-CRM	1) Choose prior distribution for β parameter of logistic family 2) Choose T, duration of time over which toxicity will be monitored for each patient and t_{int}, interval between dose cohorts (e.g., half-*month*) 3) Begin at lowest dose. Enroll 3 patients, follow for t_{int} and observe outcomes 4) For *all* patients enrolled thus far, calculate $g(x, u)$ (see text); then update posterior distribution Determine dose level with probability of DLT closest to desired percentile, but *escalate no more than one level*; go to step 4) Sampling continues until fixed number *N* of patients are treated	Incorporates late toxicities Reduces trial duration Utilizes all information available to choose next dose level Targeted percentile is explicit	Requires software to implement More toxicities will be observed, particularly if they occur toward end of monitoring period T

TITE-CRM

All the previously mentioned designs require that the toxicity outcome in each patient, or cohort of patients, be observed before more patients are entered. However, in certain situations such as radiotherapy or chemoprevention studies, interest may focus on late-onset toxicities as well as short-term effects, and the current designs would require an inordinate period of time to complete the study. Cheung and Chappell[21] have therefore proposed an extension of the CRM that incorporates the time to toxicity in each patient, which they termed TITE-CRM. The main idea is as follows. Suppose toxic events occurring anywhere up to T time units from administration of therapy are of interest. Rather than waiting for each cohort of patients to be followed for this length of time ($T = 6$ months in their example), one could enter new patients at, say, half-month intervals. As in the CRM, the first patient is assigned to a dose level based on prior information or, as in the modified CRM, to the lowest candidate dose. The single-parameter logistic model or other suitable dose–response model is assumed, with $p(x)$ corresponding to the probability that an individual receiving dose x will experience a DLT by time T. Then, if an individual has been followed for u less than T time units, the probability of a toxic event is simply taken to be $g(x, u) = u/T \cdot p(x)$ At the time the next patient(s) is (are) to be enrolled, the observed toxicities and follow-up times of patients already entered are used to form the posterior estimate of β, and the dose level for the next patient(s) is selected according to the usual CRM or modified CRM criteria. Simulation studies showed that TITE-CRM produced results comparable to its CRM counterpart, while significantly reducing the average trial duration.[21] The only downside was that TITE-CRM tended to generate slightly more AEs. As might be expected, differences were greatest for situations in which AEs tend to occur near the end of the observation period, because escalation may occur before any such events are observed.

Phase II or Pilot Efficacy and Safety Evaluation Trials

Objectives and Clinical Issues

Phase II clinical trials are conducted to determine whether a new agent or regimen has sufficient antitumor activity, usually measured in terms of reduction in tumor size, to warrant further study. Secondary objectives are to collect additional safety and toxicity data, and correlative studies to evaluate the effects of treatment on specific biomarkers or other intermediate endpoints may be included. It is assumed that the drug dose and administration schedule will have been determined from prior Phase I trials.

Unlike Phase I studies, Phase II trials should be performed in a single, well-defined tumor type and patient population. The extent of disease, patient performance status, and the amount of prior therapy are usually highly prognostic, and therefore, it is important to weigh the eligibility criteria carefully, as these parameters will define the population for which findings may pertain. This is particularly important, as in most phase II trials the observed level of activity will be compared not to a concurrent control group, but rather to a historical probability of response to standard treatment for patients presumed to be comparable in terms of stage of disease, performance status, and other characteristics.

Trial Design

Endpoints

For most Phase II trials, drug activity is defined in terms of reduction in tumor burden. The most recent criteria for measuring activity, known as the Response Evaluation Criteria in Solid Tumors or RECIST,[22] are based on unidimensional measurements. The criteria require the identification of target lesions and nontarget lesions at baseline. A complete response (CR) is the disappearance of all target and nontarget lesions, provided no new lesions have developed. A partial response (PR) is a 30% or greater decrease in the sum of the longest diameter (LD) of all target lesions, provided no nontarget lesions have progressed and no new lesions have developed. Progressive disease (PD) is defined as a 20% or greater increase in the sum of the LD of target lesions, progression of nontarget lesions, or the occurrence of new lesions. If there has been neither sufficient shrinkage to qualify for PR nor sufficient increase to qualify for PD, the patient is classified as having stable disease (SD). A patient who achieves either a CR or PR is defined as an objective responder, and the proportion of patients responding, that is, the *response rate*, has become the primary endpoint of interest in the design and analysis of phase II cancer clinical trials. While it is conceptually straightforward and can be assessed within a shorter time frame, there has been concern that the response rate is an inadequate substitute for more clinically relevant endpoints such as extension of survival. Some studies have shown that less than 25% of agents that show positive tumor response are eventually found to extend survival in comparative trials,[23] whereas other studies suggest that tumor response is a reasonable surrogate for survival extension.[24] Moertel[25] and others have raised additional problems with the use of response rates in Phase II trials, such as subjectivity and lack of reproducibility in assessment. Other possible choices for endpoints are discussed later in this section.

Sample Size

In a typical Phase II study, the objective is to compare the observed response rate for the new agent to some level, p_0 which is usually set equal to or slightly below the response rate achievable with standard therapy in the target patient population. The value for p_0 must be chosen carefully, using information from previously reported trials and investigator knowledge, because the main objective will be to determine whether there is sufficient evidence to conclude that the response rate for the new regimen is greater than p_0. In formal terms, if we let p denote the probability of response, the problem can be formulated as a test of the null hypothesis $H_0 : p = p_0$, against the alternative hypothesis $H_A : p = p_A$ where p_A is a response rate that, if true, would be clinically material. The value of p_A, along with the sample size, will determine the power of the study and therefore, two points should be noted. First, to detect a small improvement (say, 10% or less) requires a large sample size. For example, to detect an improvement from 20% to 30% with 85% power, more than

100 subjects are required, which may be undesirable for a Phase II trial, where there are limited efficacy data thus far. Second, the value for p_A must be realistic; it is of little value to design and carry out a study to detect an effect size $p_A - p_0$ that is unlikely to be realized, simply because it is compatible with the number of patients that can be recruited in a reasonable time period. Most Phase II clinical trials aim for a response rate improvement of 15% to 20%.

For a specified significance level and power, it is straightforward to determine the number of patients needed for the trial (see Fleming,[26] for example) and to test H_0. It should be noted that, in the context of Phase II trials, hypothesis tests are *one-sided* in the sense that we are only interested if the new treatment improves the response rate and not in establishing whether it could be worse. Statistical power should be high (85% or 90%), because if the drug is rejected as inactive it may never undergo further study. It is not uncommon to relax the α level from the usual 5% to 10%, because if the drug is falsely declared active, its lack of efficacy would likely be uncovered in subsequent trials.

Trial Design Types

Multistage Designs

Because it is ethically undesirable to expose patients unnecessarily to an ineffective agent, Phase II studies are usually designed to allow early stopping in the event that the drug appears inactive. This idea goes back to Gehan,[27] and one of the most popular designs incorporating early stopping is Simon's optimal two-stage design.[28] For a specified p_0, p_A, α, and β, this design calls for enrollment of n_1 patients in the first stage. If r_1 or fewer responses are observed, the trial is terminated due to lack of activity. Otherwise, an additional n_2 patients are entered for a total $n = n_1 + n_2$. Then, if r or fewer total responders among the n patients are observed, the regimen is rejected, whereas if more than r responses are observed, the regimen is declared sufficiently active to warrant further study. The optimal design is the one that minimizes the expected sample size under the null hypothesis. For example, if $p_0 = 0.10$, $p_A = 0.25$ and $\alpha = \beta = 0.10$ (90% power), then 21 patients would be enrolled in the first stage and if 2 or fewer responses were observed, the trial would be terminated. Otherwise, an additional 29 patients would be accrued for a total of 50, and if 7 or fewer responses were observed, the drug would be rejected, whereas 8 or more responses (an observed response rate of 16% or more) would be sufficient to deem it worthy of further investigation. The probability of stopping at the first stage if, in fact, the true response rate is only 10%, is fairly high, 0.65; hence, the attraction of the two-stage design.

Simon also provides tables for a *minimax* design, which is that having the smallest total sample size that satisfies the design constraints, although it often requires a relatively large sample size in the first stage. Jung et al.[29] note that there are typically many designs that satisfy the design constraints, and present graphical software that allows one to easily search for a trial design that is a good compromise between different options. Green et al.,[2] on the other hand, prefer a more flexible two-stage approach in which an approximately equal number of patients are recruited in each stage and the power is set to 90%. In a typical example, if, after the first stage the *alternative hypothesis* (e.g., that a response of some specified size exists) is rejected at significance level $\alpha = 0.02$, the trial is discontinued for lack of activity. Otherwise, the study proceeds through the second stage where the null hypothesis is tested at $\alpha = 0.055$. Roughly, this design will stop early if the observed response rate after the first stage is less than p_0 and will declare the agent sufficiently active to warrant further study if, after the second stage, the observed response rate exceeds $(p_0 + p_A)/2$. Three-stage designs have also been proposed.[30,31] The logistic difficulties of suspending recruitment between stages, as well as the increase in study duration that this entails, lead most investigators to opt for two-stage designs. However, in situations in which it is highly desirable to minimize the number of patients exposed to an inactive therapy, a three-stage design may be attractive. Some have argued that complete and partial responses should not necessarily be combined, because complete responses are far rarer and are much more likely to confer a survival advantage.[32,33] They propose two-stage designs that distinguish complete from partial responses, giving more weight to the former.

As mentioned previously, a secondary objective of Phase II trials is the collection and reporting of toxicity data. Usually, toxicity analyses are carried out separately from the analysis of response rates, but designs have been proposed that incorporate toxicity and response simultaneously. Conaway and Petroni[34] and Bryant and Day,[35] for example, consider trials to establish whether a new drug is "sufficiently promising" in the sense that it has both a response rate that is greater *and* a toxicity rate that is no worse than standard treatment. If we let p_R denote the true response rate of the new treatment and p_T the true rate of DLT, the null and alternative hypotheses can be written:

$$H_0: p_R \le p_{R_0} \quad \text{or} \quad p_T > p_{T_0}$$
$$H_A: p_R > p_{R_0} \quad \text{and} \quad p_T \le p_{T_0}$$

where p_{R_0} and p_{T_0} are the response and toxicity rates associated with standard therapy. Thus, the null hypothesis is rejected only if the response rate is sufficiently high and the toxicity rate is not unacceptably high. One must model the association between response and toxicity by introducing another parameter, θ, corresponding to the odds ratio for toxicity among responders relative to nonresponders. Fortunately, however, the design characteristics are fairly insensitive to the assumed value for θ. Finally, as one might be willing to accept greater toxicity with higher response rates and vice versa, Conaway and Petroni[36] propose a related design that incorporates such trade-offs.

Bayesian Trial Designs

The previously mentioned designs are frequentist in nature, in that power and significance probabilities refer to the probability of events under given hypotheses about the parameters of interest. A Bayesian approach offers an alternative inferential framework, for which proponents argue is particularly suited to situations involving accumulating data.[37] For example, Thall and Simon[38] present a Bayesian design for Phase II trials in which a "moderately informative" prior distribution is assigned to p_S, the response rate associated with standard therapy. A flat or "weakly informative" prior is assigned to p_E, the response rate for the experimental treatment, to reflect the limited knowledge available for p_E before the study is begun. A maximum sample size for the trial, n_{max}, is specified, patients are enrolled, and the trial is continued until the new drug is shown with high posterior probability to be either promising or not promising or until n_{max} is reached, in which case the study is deemed inconclusive. Thus, if X_n denotes the number of responders observed among the first n patients enrolled, $n = 1,2, \ldots n_{max}$, the posterior probability that p_E exceeds p_S by some minimally interesting amount, δ, is computed. If this probability is very high (say, greater than 0.95) or very low (say, less than 0.05), the trial is terminated and the drug is declared promising or not promising, respectively. Otherwise, the study is continued provided n_{max} has not been reached.

Thall and Simon[38] evaluate the frequentist operating characteristics of this design under continuous monitoring and a maximum sample size of $n_{max} = 65$. They also suggest setting a minimum sample size, n_{min}, of 10 patients so that, in effect, monitoring does not begin until the 10th patient is enrolled. Results show, for example, that under a fairly informative prior for p_S centered, say, at 0.20, a weak prior for p_E, and a minimally interesting difference of $_\delta = 0.15$, that if $p_E = p_S$ there is a 7.1% chance that the outcome would erroneously lead to a conclusion that the experimental drug is promising, an 83.5% chance that it will correctly be declared nonpromising, and a 9.4% chance that the results will be inclusive. If the true effect is positive ($p_E = 0.40$), there is an 87.5% chance that the drug will be declared promising, a 7.7% chance that it will be declared nonpromising, and a 4.8% chance that the trial would be inconclusive. Subsequent work describes a Bayesian sequential design for more complicated situations involving multiple outcomes, such as response and toxicity.[39]

Another proponent of the Bayesian approach is Heitjan,[40] who points out that in multistage, frequentist designs, the evidence required for terminating the trial is not the same at all analysis times, and that a drug can be rejected as inactive even though there is no strong evidence that the response rate is any less than that of the standard. He describes a Bayesian approach designed either to convince a *skeptic* that the drug is beneficial or to convince an *enthusiast* that it is not. This is accomplished by using different prior probabilities corresponding to these two states of belief and, after outcomes have been observed, calculating the posterior probability that (a) the new drug is better than the standard given the skeptic's prior (the "persuade-the-pessimist probability") and (b) the standard is better than the new drug given the enthusiast's prior (the "persuade-the-optimist probability"). Thus, this method requires that the evidence be sufficient "to choose between hypotheses [favorable or unfavorable] to the satisfaction of all interested parties" and, if not, the results are regarded as inconclusive.[40]

Randomized Phase II Trial

When there are multiple candidate agents to consider advancing to further development, randomized Phase II trials, sometimes called selection designs, provide a means to select agents for further study.[41–43] These trials, which allocate patients to different treatments under consideration by random assignment and compare outcomes between groups, have several advantages with respect to patient selection and other biases present in studies without parallel comparison groups (discussed in detail in the next section). However, as a means to determine efficacy in any absolute sense, these trials lack statistical power and α error control at the sample sizes typically envisaged for Phase II trials. Nonetheless, the initial intended use of randomized Phase II trials as "selection designs" has been broadened to encompass small-scale randomized trials with a standard therapy comparison group. Although this approach has some advantages, positive results emerging from these trials cannot be deemed sufficiently conclusive as to preclude Phase III investigation (see Liu in Reference 1 for discussion). Table 8.3 illustrates advantages and disadvantages of one-arm and randomized comparative Phase II trials.

Recent Design Concepts

For cytostatic agents, where frank tumor shrinkage is not anticipated, there may be a need for alternative Phase II designs based on endpoints other than response rates. For trials enrolling patients who have failed prior therapy, Mick et al.[44] propose a method that uses each patient as his/her own control, comparing the time to progression under the new agent with the time to progression under prior therapy. Rosner et al.[45] propose a *randomized discontinuation* design, in which all patients are initially treated with the experimental agent. After a specified interval, responders remain on

TABLE 8.3. Advantages and disadvantages of single-arm versus randomized Phase II trials.

	Single-arm trial	*Pilot randomized trial*
Advantages	• Maximum adverse event information for new agent • Can offer new agent to all participants • Simple endpoint that is rapidly ascertained	• Concurrent control group • Randomization provides for rigorous ancillary studies of tumor response markers • Can use time to event endpoints more readily in this comparative setting
Disadvantages	• Historical control group response rate must be used • Tumor response endpoint may be poor surrogate for survival extension • Time to event endpoints may be difficult to define and do not fit into multistage framework	• Low power, high α for feasible sample sizes • Necessity to randomize patients in terminal disease situation • Quantity of adverse event information for experimental agent is reduced • Positive findings may interfere with conduct of appropriately powered Phase III trial

Here, we are considering a randomized phase II trial as a relatively small (100 patients or fewer) study intended to serve as a pilot trial for potential efficacy. Note that the original proposal for use of randomized phase II trials was for selection of potentially superior candidates from among multiple new agents (see Simon et al.[41] and Liu et al.[42]), and *not* to compare new therapies to existing standards. More recently, Bayesian designs for phase II randomized selection design trials have been proposed (see Esty and Thall[43]).

treatment and those who progress discontinue, while those patients with stable disease are randomized to either continued treatment with the drug or placebo. The idea behind this design is that the randomized comparison allows one to assess whether the drug is truly slowing the rate of growth of the tumor, as opposed to having simply selected patients for study with slow-growing tumors. Because the patients with stable disease form a more homogeneous subgroup, this design also generally requires a smaller sample size than would a trial that randomized all patients at entry. It is important to bear in mind—and the authors also emphasize this point—that the purpose of this design is mainly to determine whether the drug is active in an explanatory sense. Obviously, it matters a great deal whether the initial percentage of patients exhibiting stable disease is high or low, as in the latter case the total sample size required may be quite large and a demonstration of activity in the randomized component would mean only that there is benefit in a small subset of the population. Korn et al.[46] point out other caveats with this design. For example, patients may find it unattractive to potentially discontinue a treatment that appears to be working. They describe a number of other approaches, including single-arm trials with time to progression as an endpoint and trials with appropriately validated biologic response markers as surrogates for tumor response.

Phase III or Comparative Efficacy Trials

General Description and Objectives

The term *Phase III trial* is synonymous with a prospective comparison under randomized treatment assignment [alternately called a randomized controlled trial or randomized clinical trial (RCT)] of two or more treatment regimens, conducted for the purpose of establishing which is *superior* or, in some cases, to establish *equivalence* (in the sense that any difference in outcome is smaller than that considered clinically material) between different treatment regimens. Thus, two key features that distinguish RCTs are the inclusion of a concurrent control group and the use of randomization to assign treatment. The main purpose of concurrently evaluating individuals receiving the standard and test treatment(s) is to eliminate temporal trends in diagnosis, characterization of the disease, and ancillary care that would likely be present in any comparison with a historical control group. Concurrent evaluation also provides implicit control over the commonly seen phenomenon of research participation itself having a positive effect on outcomes, regardless of the type of intervention. Randomization, which disassociates treatment assignment from any and all extraneous factors on the part of the patient or the physician, is the fundamental means by which bias is removed from measures of treatment effect.

The obvious alternative to randomization is a nonrandomized comparative trial, but this design is generally insufficient for definitive evaluation of treatments for the purpose of choosing one over another. While differences in characteristics between treatment groups can be addressed to various degrees in other ways, typically by comparing "like with like" through matching, stratification into homogeneous groups, or statistical modeling or adjustment, only randomization will reliably eliminate bias in treatment comparisons. Furthermore, it is often not the *known* potential confounding factors that we must concern ourselves with, but rather *unknown* or uncollected factors, where these methods are not relevant. Nonetheless, primarily due to ethical concerns, some advocate relying on observational studies with reference to historical experience, coupled with the use of statistical methods to account for potential confounding of treatment effects and other factors, to evaluate new treatments.[47,48] Numerous problems with the validity of historically controlled comparative studies have been demonstrated specifically in cancer research, including temporal changes in disease definition,[49,50] data quality issues,[51] diagnostic bias in assessing treatment response,[25] and out-of-date historical control comparisons that tend to inflate effects for new therapies.[23] The RCT in and of itself represents a significant medical research advance, and, as the recognized gold standard evaluative tool in therapy development, is integral to the evidence-based medicine paradigm.

Trial Design Issues

Endpoints and Sample Size

Phase III trial design begins with specification of a primary endpoint, which is typically a simple binary event such as survived/died or recurred/remained recurrence free, but usually with one important difference relative to Phase II trials; for each patient the time from randomization until occurrence of this event will be recorded, rather than the event status at some fixed time landmark. These time-to-event endpoints are particularly suited for adjuvant therapy trials, where because the number of patients participating is appreciably larger than in Phase II trials, recruitment takes place over a lengthy interval and each patient will have a different follow-up duration at any given time from trial initiation. Use of follow-up time per patient is more efficient than waiting until all patients have reached some fixed time. The treatment effect measure is usually specified in terms of *hazards*, which can be thought of as failure probabilities or failure rates per unit of time, between two treatment groups. Hypotheses are thus usually formulated in terms of the hazard ratio (HR) as $H_0: \lambda_A/\lambda_B = HR = 1.0$ where λ_A and λ_B are the hazards for treatments A and B, versus alternative $H_A: HR < 1.0$, for some value of the HR that represents a clinically material difference in outcomes. In the case of an equivalence trial, one might test a null hypothesis that the HR does not differ from 1.0 by more than some specified amount such that the two treatments would be considered equivalent (hence, this difference must be small) versus the alternative that a greater difference exists (see References 1, 2 for more on equivalence trials). Under the assumption that this ratio is relatively constant over time, a given HR can be converted to an absolute difference between groups in proportions remaining event free at a given follow-up time. For example, a new/standard HR equal to 0.75, or a 25% reduction in failure rate in the new relative to the standard group, may translate into an absolute difference in the proportion of patients remaining free of the event between groups of 4.6% at 5 years, given that the standard group 5-year survival percentage is 80% (Table 8.4).

TABLE 8.4. Absolute difference in 5-year survival and number of events required for a two-arm Phase III trial.

Reduction in hazard of failure for new treatment	*Standard group proportion event free at 5 years* .50	.60	.70	.80	.90	.95	*No. of events required*
20%	.074	.065	.052	.037	.019	.010	630
25%	.095	.082	.065	.046	.024	.012	379
33%	.130	.111	.088	.062	.032	.016	191
40%	.160	.136	.107	.075	.039	.020	128
50%	.207	.175	.137	.094	.049	.025	65

Table entries show the absolute difference (new – standard) in 5-year survival for the hazard reduction due to the new treatment on the left-hand column and the 5-year survival in the standard treatment group (middle columns, top), assuming exponential survival patterns. The right-most column shows the number of events required (Eq. 2) for 80% power at a two-sided $\alpha = 0.05$. The number of *patients* required for the trial to obtain results in some specified time period will depend on the standard group failure rate and the rate at which patients can be accrued.

From the specification of difference of interest or effect size, the sample size in terms of number of *events* required to detect this difference with desired statistical power and significance level can be determined. Depending on the anticipated accrual rate and the prognosis (e.g., rapidity of failure events) in the control treatment group, the number of *patients* required can then be approximated. Typically, the required number of events is based on the normal theory approximation of the natural logarithm of the hazard ratio. For a two-arm trial, the total number of events is

$$D = \frac{(Z_{1-\beta} + Z_{\alpha/2})^2}{[\log_e(HR)]^2 \, p_A \cdot p_B} \qquad (2)$$

where $Z_{1-\beta}$ and $Z_{\alpha/2}$ are the values from the standard normal distribution associated with the power and significance level desired, and p_A and p_B are the proportions of total patients to be allocated to the two arms, respectively (e.g., 0.5 for equal allocation). One can see from this equation that the number of events required depends strongly on the HR, becoming dramatically larger as the HR approaches 1.0 (see Table 8.4). The number of patients required and total duration of the trial depend on the rate of patient accrual and the failure rate in the control group, both of which contribute to the determination of how rapidly the requisite events will be observed. The accrual rate is typically estimated from previous experience and may also involve querying potential investigators to project the accrual rate per unit of time. Similarly, the failure rate for patients under standard therapy is derived from past observations and available literature estimates. The computations are straightforward but generally require computer programs (see Shuster in Reference 1, or commercial programs) or under certain assumptions, tabled values.[52] Sample size methods have been extended to take into account other factors that will influence power, such as patients withdrawing from the study while it is ongoing (dropout), switching from the assigned treatment to the other group (cross-over), or deviating from protocol treatment (noncompliance).[53–56]

Another important design aspect concerns the desire to ensure that factors associated with outcomes, called prognostic factors, are balanced between treatment arms. Although random allocation to treatments naturally provides equal distribution of characteristics, using key prognostic variables as *stratification* factors, and incorporating these into the randomization process (by randomizing within strata or other means discussed in the next section), imbalances that can arise by chance can essentially be prevented. The number of stratification factors needs to be limited to a few key factors, because the strata increase multiplicatively with the number of factors and factor levels. For example, the use of four factors [say, age groups (less than 50 years, 50–64 years, 65 years or older), lymph node status (positive, negative), performance status (0–1, more than 1), and surgical procedure (procedure A or B)] produces $3 \times 2 \times 2 \times 2 = 24$ strata in which to balance treatment assignments. As the number of strata becomes large relative to the number of patients to be entered, the efficiency of stratification as a means to balance treatment arms diminishes.[57]

Trial Conduct

Randomization

Because randomization is the signifying characteristic of Phase III trials, correct implementation and maintenance of this feature is vital. In the simplest case, a series of treatment assignments are generated from a random mechanism such as a random number table or computer program. Sequential assignments should only be revealed one at a time (to avoid compromising the randomness with respect to the next assignment), and thus it is preferable to have a secure centralized randomization procedure, via telephone or computer contact. To balance the number of patients in each arm, *block randomization*, in which an equal number of assignments on each treatment arm of the trial occurs after each block of patients is enrolled, can be used (for example, assigning ABABBA, AABABB, etc., for randomly ordered strings of assignments brings the number on each arm into balance after each set of six patients; note that the size of the block is not revealed and can also be varied to make the process unpredictable). To incorporate stratification factors to be balanced between treatment arms, blocked randomization can be used within each stratum. When the number of strata is large, and in particular in multicenter trials, this type of assignment scheme can become unwieldy and cannot necessarily assure balance. In this case, some type of *dynamic allocation* scheme can be used whereby the current assignment is generated based on previous assignments. This type of randomization must be centralized, as stratification factor data for all previously enrolled patients must be available when randomizing the current patient. Rather than deterministic assignments to balance the arms, often "biased-coin" randomization is used, in which the assignment probability is weighted toward the arm for which assignments are needed to achieve balance. The minimization algorithm is frequently used for dynamic balancing taking stratification factors into account.[58] This allocation scheme balances treatment arms for each stratification factor singly, but not necessarily for every combination of factors, as in fully stratified randomization. However, it is much easier to manage over multicenter studies and performs well for multiple stratification factors.[57]

There are several ways in which the benefits of randomization can be eroded or nullified. Of course, any breach of the random assignment process has an irreparable effect on the validity of the trial. Second, a large number (or differential number per arm) of patients "canceled" or withdrawn from the trial calls into question the validity of the comparison for the remaining participants. Differential follow-up and ascertainment of status per arm can have a similar effect. Third, bias in assessment of outcomes can have a major impact on the estimated treatment effect, and thus, objective outcome measures and blinding of treatment assignment come into play. Treatment assignment blinding is not feasible for many oncology trials (e.g., radiotherapy and most chemotherapy regimens), but has been used with great success in others (e.g., tamoxifen). In either case, and in particular for studies that cannot be blinded (among patients or caregivers), unambiguous, objectively defined endpoints are essential. In cases where determination of the endpoint involves possible observer subjectivity, such as when reading a diagnostic scan to determine disease progression, keeping assessors unaware of treatment assignment may be necessary.

TRIAL MONITORING

As in earlier trials, Phase III trials include provisions for formal oversight of risks and benefits to ensure patient welfare and use resources efficiently. Interim monitoring consists of both continuous oversight of adverse events and periodic interim tests (a predetermined number) of primary study hypotheses. With respect to these interim tests, a large body of statistical developments has addressed how to conduct tests to determine if an early determination of treatment superiority is warranted while at the same time controlling for inflation of α error (e.g., false-positive findings) resulting from repeatedly performing statistical hypothesis tests. Caution is also warranted because early results from time-to-event data tend to be unstable and change as more information accumulates. In essence, these problems are addressed by simply requiring a stricter criterion than the typical P less than 0.05 "significance" for interim analyses, and early approaches to this problem used either a smaller constant significance criterion throughout interim and definitive analyses, chosen such that the significance level for the entire set of sequential tests does not exceed α, or a constant but much more stringent criterion early in interim analyses and a more conventional significance level after the trial has accumulated the requisite information for definitive analysis. Figure 8.1 shows these and some other examples of early stopping boundaries, which when exceeded at any of the interim analyses shown on the x-axis would prompt consideration of early stopping. These boundaries are symmetric with respect to superiority for either the new or standard treatment group, reflecting the fact that two-sided hypothesis tests remain the convention. In reality, it is unlikely that a trial tending toward a significant difference in favor of the standard treatment would be continued until such a result was realized. Thus, an additional rule that allows for stopping early for "futility" with respect to the new treatment is usually also specified. Alternatively, asymmetric boundaries that more easily allow stopping early for evidence that the new treatment may actually be inferior to the standard (evidence de facto that the new treatment will not ultimately prevail) can be used. More comprehensive treatment of this topic can be found in clinical trials texts[1,2] or books on group sequential monitoring.[59] Regardless of the specific approach adopted, an interim analysis plan should be devised during trial design and adhered to throughout trial conduct because failure to account for multiplicity of analyses can result in spurious *positive* findings. Also, a specified plan may help to avoid diminished influence of a trial even when results are decidedly positive, which can occur if there is a perception by others that the trial had been terminated prematurely due to favorable results at a particular analysis time.[60]

The decision to discontinue the trial (accrual and/or treatment, depending on its current state) and release findings is typically vested in an independent Data and Safety Monitoring Committee (DSMC). However, in addition to evaluating according to the monitoring rule, the DSMC considers a broader body of information regarding the trial as well as external information that bears on treatment for the disease under study. Table 8.5 outlines the membership, aspects of trial conduct over which the DSMC has oversight, and recommendations that might arise from trial review and DSMC

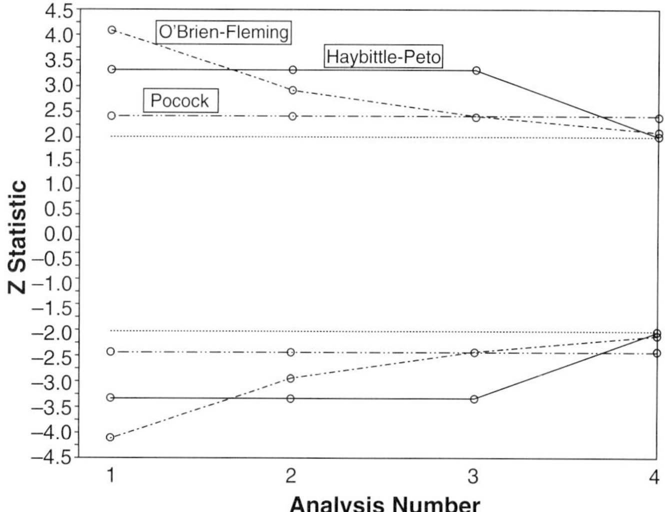

FIGURE 8.1. Different types of stopping boundaries for monitoring a Phase III trial. The upper and lower boundaries represent statistical test values on the vertical axis (on a standard normal scale), which, if exceeded at a given analysis indicated on the horizontal axis, would prompt stopping of the trial (the fourth analysis is the definitive analysis at the predetermined requisite number of events). The horizontal lines at ±1.96 represent the standard P greater than 0.05 boundary. Note that the Pocock boundary uses a fixed, modestly more extreme value, but the final test result must then also be more extreme than the conventional 0.05 test to be considered significant. The Haybittle–Peto method uses a conventional final test value but is very conservative through the penultimate hypothesis test. The O'Brien–Fleming boundaries begin very conservatively, but change as more information accrues, and also allow that the final test be performed using the conventional significance level.

TABLE 8.5. Prototypical Phase III trial data and safety monitoring committee.

Membership (voting members, external to trial)	*Additional attendees*
Physicians	Trial statistician
Statisticians	Trial coordinator
Patient advocate	Trial chair[a]
Medical ethicist	Sponsor representatives[a]

Review Scope:

— Patient accrual, reporting delinquency and patient withdrawals, treatment compliance, data quality
— Adverse events
— Treatment efficacy endpoints
— Other relevant materials, including confidential reports provided by other investigators

Decision to stop/alter trial conduct and/or release findings may be based on:

— Evidence of benefit or harm according to monitoring guidelines or adverse events (expected or otherwise) observed in the trial
— Evidence of little likelihood that treatment difference will be realized
— External information that raises concerns regarding the scientific, clinical, or ethical assumptions on which the current trial was based
— Poor likelihood of trial yielding meaningful findings due to problems with accrual, compliance, or patient retention

[a]Note that these individuals are typically excluded from discussions of interim efficacy data, although there is currently some debate regarding this issue.

deliberations. The policies and procedures for U.S. National Cancer Institute-sponsored Cooperative Group trials provide a good overview of DSMC structure and function for Phase III trials.[61]

Analysis

Definitive analysis commences when either the requisite number of events indicated in the trial design has been observed, or the DSMC has deemed that the trial results should be disclosed due to early stopping conditions being met.

An important aspect of Phase III trial analysis is the definition of the analysis cohort. The concept of analysis by *intention-to-treat* is often discussed, but the definition of this term can sometimes be unclear, so it is best to explicitly describe which patients are included.[62] In the strictest sense, the intention-to-treat cohort includes all patients randomized, irrespective of eligibility, acceptance of and adherence to assigned treatment, and any and all other postrandomization deviations from protocol. However, it is often the case that patients found ineligible for the trial after randomization due to having been incorrectly staged or for other reasons are excluded from the primary analysis, and this practice (used with caution) is sometimes advocated, as it allows for evaluation of the therapy in the population for which it was intended.[2] A more controversial and rarely acceptable form of patient exclusion involves removal of patients who did not or could not comply with assigned therapy regimens or received nonprotocol therapy. Such exclusions can easily lead to biased comparisons, and in general, any post hoc analysis of treatment benefit in relation to dose received is fraught with interpretational difficulties and should be avoided in primary analysis.[63]

For time-to-event data, the principal summaries are the survival distribution (or survival curve) and the estimated hazard ratio. The survival curve $S(t)$ represents the probability of remaining event free until at least time t, or $S(t) = \Pr(T > t)$. This function is plotted from randomization (e.g., at $t = 0$, $S(t) = 1.0$) to some follow-up time that a remaining fraction of patients has reached. This points to an important feature of time-to-event data, that is, *censoring*, where it is known that a patient is event free as of some follow-up time, but the (potential) failure time is not yet observed. Censoring is a natural consequence of staggered enrollment into the trial, so that at any given time, some patients have less follow-up than others (administrative censoring), but also may occur because patients may withdraw from or be lost to follow-up before experiencing the event of interest. Administrative censoring can be reasonably assumed to be independent of failure risk except in cases where characteristics of participants enrolled changes over time (which is why well-defined entry criteria are necessary). Any censoring associated with propensity for failure (e.g., sicker patients more often withdrawing) that results in different rates of loss per treatment arm can bias treatment comparisons.

In the case in which censoring is assumed independent of probability of failure, then estimating $S(t)$ using available information per patient, including follow-up to censoring, is straightforward. For a set of ordered observed times where one or more patients had an event $t_1 < t_2 < t_3 < \ldots < t_J$, define d_j as the number of events at time t_j and Y_j as the number of patients available to possibly fail (all those who have not yet failed and were not censored before t_j; by convention, those censored exactly at t_j are considered at risk to fail). The Kaplan–Meier (KM) estimator[64] is the product of the quantities $(1 - d_j/Y_j)$ over the J failure times

$$S(t) = \prod_{j=1}^{J}\left(1 - \frac{d_j}{Y_j}\right) \tag{3}$$

Although the KM curve is the typical graphical summary, the relative hazard of failure between groups is the principal measure of efficacy. The HR (and associated statistical tests) pertains to the entire span of follow-up, as opposed to a test of difference in the survival curves at a specific time point, in which case the result would depend on which time was chosen. The *log-rank test*, which frequently accompanies the KM curve, in fact compares underlying failure probabilities between groups over the J failure times.[65] Issues related to this and other tests for comparing survival time distributions are discussed here.

The HR can be estimated by computing the incidence density or *average failure rate* in each treatment group. For two treatment arms with n_A and n_B patients, respectively, the average failure rate for treatment arm A is $I_A = D_A/\bar{T}_A$, where $\bar{T}_A = \Sigma_{i=1}^{n_A} T_i$, the sum of times to event or censoring for each patient, and D_A is the total number of events in arm A. For I_B similarly computed, $HR = I_A/I_B$. More commonly, the HR is estimated via the Cox proportional hazards model,[66] which relates the hazard of failure to covariates through the equation

$$\lambda(t, x) = \lambda_0(t) \cdot \exp(\beta_1 \cdot x_1 + \beta_2 \cdot x_2 + \ldots \beta_p \cdot x_p) \tag{4}$$

where $\lambda_0(t)$ is an unspecified "baseline hazard" and the x's represent covariates, which may include indicators for treatment group and other factors. For example, for a single covariate, x_1, representing treatment group with $x_1 = 0$ for the standard treatment and $x_1 = 1$ for the new treatment, $\lambda_0(t)\exp(\beta_1)/\lambda_0(t) = \exp(\beta_1)$ equals the HR. From this model, a significance test for HR = 1.0 and confidence interval for the HR are obtained. With additional prognostic factors included in the model, $\exp(\beta_1)$ gives the HR *adjusted* or *controlling* for these factors. Prognostic factor analysis using this model or other techniques often follows primary analysis of Phase III trials. The modeling process, which entails deciding which factors to include, determining the correct way to represent a given factor (i.e., in categories, on a continuous scale, and so forth), consideration of interrelationships (e.g., interactions) among factors, and many other issues, can be complex, as can using model results for prediction of individual patient outcomes or classification into prognostic risk classes. A comprehensive review of current modeling methods applied to oncology data is provided by Schumacher et al. in Reference 1.

One important issue concerning the HR and tests used to compare hazards pertains to how failure events occur over time in the groups being compared. The *proportional hazards* condition, whereby the HR is constant over time, is implicit in the previously described model (hence the name). Under this condition, the quantity $\log_e(S^A(t))/\log_e(S^B(t))$, where S^A and S^B are the KM estimates at time t in the two treatment groups, will be approximately the same at different time points on the survival curves. Note, however, that under this condition the absolute difference in proportions event free from the KM curve will not be constant, but in fact the curves will diverge over time. The log-rank test[65] gives equal weight to failure events across the time span and is the optimal test under proportional hazards. For failure patterns that deviate from proportional hazards, there are a number of alternatives to the log-rank test that are more sensitive to differences between survival curves. The Wilcoxon[67] test places more weight on failures occurring early, and so is more sensitive to the case where survival curves separate early but may later converge. Other tests also tend to weight earlier failures,[68,69] and a generalized class of tests exists that encompass the standard log-rank and Wilcoxon test as well as tests with other weighting schemes.[70] Choice of test should be determined by whether there is specific interest in or expectation that differences will emerge under some pattern other than proportional hazards. In any case, when different tests differ, it is usually the case that the treatment effect is changing over time and thus a single HR may be an inadequate summary, and separate HR estimates for specific time intervals may be more appropriate. One of several formal tests for proportionality can be used when there is empirical evidence of nonproportionality from the KM curve plot. Heuristically, a single HR under strongly nonproportional hazards is akin to the mean of a highly skewed distribution, in that it may be computed but does not serve as a readily interpretable summary of the data. Figure 8.2 illustrates how statistical tests may differ under some different patterns of failure among survival cures being compared.

Another issue with KM survival curve displays relates to the follow-up period shown. Often the curves are plotted until a time point for which very few patients are under observation. This practice can create the misleading illusion of a large expanse between the curves, when in fact variability on the estimated proportion event free when few patients remain is very large, and if a few patients or even one patient were to fail, the estimate would change substantially. It is more

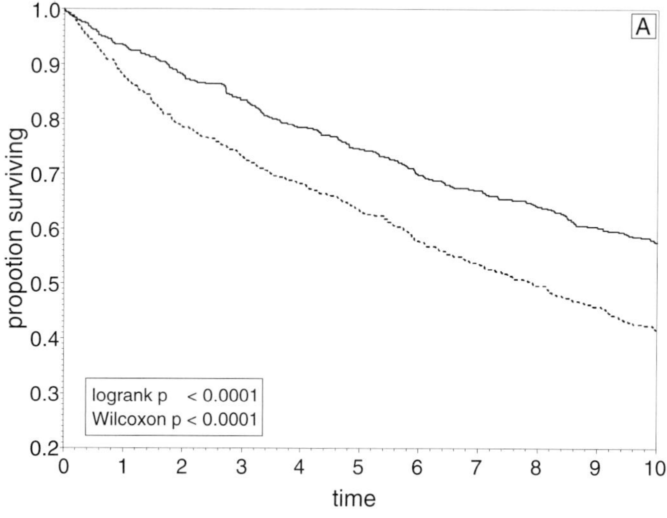

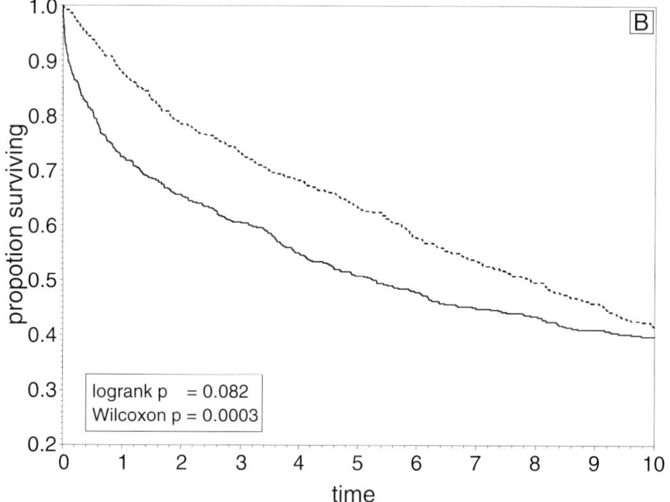

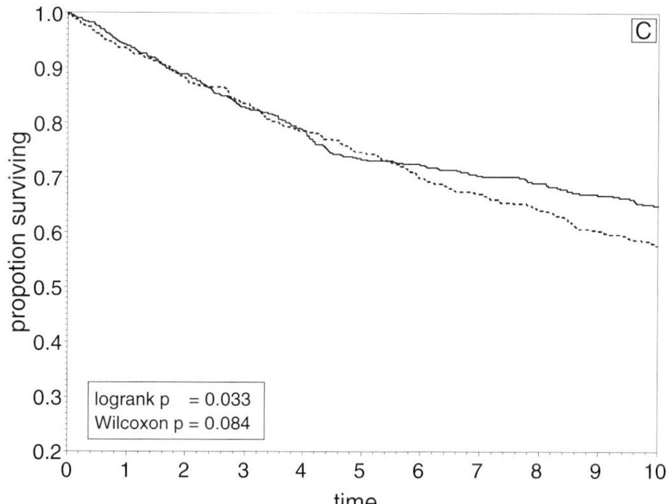

FIGURE 8.2. Examples of survival curves exhibiting different failure patterns. Data are generated from hypothetical data with 500 subjects per group. In comparing curves, the Wilcoxon test gives greater weight to earlier failures, whereas the log-rank test weights failures equally throughout follow-up. (A) Curves follow the proportional hazards pattern. The hazard ratio is constant (HR = 2.0). (B) Curves show a violation of proportional hazards, converging over time as the hazard ratio becomes smaller. (C) These curves also are nonproportional, separating later in follow-up.

appropriate to plot the curves and cite proportions event free only at time landmarks that most of the patients who remain event free have reached.

Some Additional Topics

Confirmatory Trials and Meta-Analyses

Because of the planning, infrastructure, cost, and time required, Phase III trials are carefully designed to avoid equivocal findings, and thus provide definitive evidence for or against changes in therapy standards. Nonetheless, questions regarding the treatments under evaluation will invariably remain unanswered, and thus there is an important role for replicated (referred to as confirmatory) trials and the synthesis of similar trials into a coherent body of evidence. This is particularly important for clinical decision making, where evidence from trials must be weighed in relation to an individual patient's utility for various treatment options. For the small to moderate benefits seen for most cancer treatment advances, these confirmatory trials may in fact be necessary to effect change.[71,72] Although costly to obtain, such corroborating evidence can contribute greatly to practice changes, as the qualitative value of multiple trials with similar findings cannot be understated. It is also not uncommon that replicated trials fail to obtain similar results, providing an opportunity for closer scrutiny of differences between trials and their potential breadth of applicability.

A more formal quantitative means of combining evidence from trials is by meta-analysis, a widely used analytic tool in many areas of social and medical science. Meta-analysis refers to a process whereby data from independent studies are combined to form a quantitative summary estimate of a given effect. Randomized trials are in fact more suited to meta-analysis than nearly all other research designs, as there is likely to be considerable similarity in disease definitions, study design features, classes of therapeutic agents or procedures, and endpoints, and this information is increasingly well documented in trial reports.[73] Meta-analyses were initially carried out by extracting effect estimates from published literature and combining these into a single estimate using statistical techniques, but in medical meta-analysis studies, it is usually considered necessary to obtain patient-level data from each trial, a laborious process that necessarily includes seeking data from unpublished trials to avoid the "publication bias" toward positive findings. Once these data are acquired and standardized for a common endpoint, the individual trial effect measures (i.e., hazard ratios) may be combined using an appropriate statistical model into a summary effect estimate. Results of each trial are also presented, as well as tests for evidence of significant heterogeneity among trials, in which case a single summary measure may be inappropriate and thus omitted. Often, a quality weight measure based on design features is assigned to each trial, providing a natural opportunity to evaluate trial quality.

A principal advantage of meta-analyses is the ability to evaluate consistency among trial findings and possibly uncover small but clinically meaningful treatment effects that were not statistically significant in any one trial (although the meta-analysis is generally not considered the equivalent of an adequately powered RCT). One disadvantage is that combined trial estimates based on heterogeneous treatment regimens may be able to illustrate only a proof of principle (for example, "multidrug chemotherapy is effective"), which may be of limited use for specific clinical questions, such as which regimen to use. Furthermore, comparisons of different regimens from data aggregated across trials are subject to all attendant limitations and biases of observational studies. Despite these and other limitations and pitfalls,[74,75] meta-analyses are a valuable complementary research strategy that has been influential in cancer treatment. An excellent example of the methods and data summaries used in meta-analysis in oncology can be found in the reports of the Early Breast Cancer Trialists' Collaborative Group.[76]

Bayesian Approach

As in the case of Phase I and II trials, Bayesian statistical methodology is increasingly being applied to various aspects of Phase III trials. In study design, a Bayesian approach to formulating the sample size in terms of the questions (1) "what treatment effect might realistically be realized with a new regimen?" and (2) "what magnitude of effect would prompt the current standard to be supplanted?" provides a useful framework that more closely resembles clinical practice.[77,78] In trial monitoring, the use of "skeptical" and "optimistic" prior distributions introduced earlier, considered in conjunction with accumulating trial results, provides a rational means to determine whether current results are sufficiently convincing to justify early stopping.[79]

References

1. Crowley J (ed). Handbook of Statistics in Clinical Oncology. New York: Dekker, 2001.
2. Green S, Benedetti J, Crowley JJ. Clinical Trials in Oncology, 2nd ed. Boca Raton: Chapman & Hall/CRC, 2003.
3. Halpern SD, Karlawish JHT, Berlin JA. The continuing unethical conduct of underpowered clinical trials. JAMA 2002;288:358–362.
4. Piantadosi S. Clinical Trials: A Methodologic Perspective. New York: Wiley, 1997.
5. Iyer L, Das S, Janisch L, et al. UGT1A1*28 polymorphism as a determinant of irinotecan disposition and toxicity. Pharmacogenomics J 2002;2:43–47.
6. Leventhal BG, Wittes RE. Phase I trials. In: Leventhal BG, Wittes RE (eds). Research Methods in Clinical Oncology. New York: Raven Press, 1988:41–59.
7. Von Hoff DD, Rozencweig M, Muggia FM. Variation in toxicities of anticancer drugs in children and adults. Clin Pharmacol Ther 1977;21:121.
8. Von Hoff DD, Kuhn J, Clark GM. Design and conduct of phase I trials. In: Buyse ME, Staquet MJ, Sylvester RJ (eds). Cancer Clinical Trials, Methods and Practice. Oxford: Oxford University Press, 1984:210–220.
9. Storer B. Design and analysis of phase I clinical trials. Biometrics 1989;45:925–937.
10. Goodman SN, Zahurak ML, Piantadosi S. Some practical improvements in the continual reassessment method for phase I studies. Stat Med 1995;14:1149–1161.
11. Carter SK. Study design principles for the clinical evaluation of new drugs as developed by the chemotherapy programme of the National Cancer Institute. In: Staquet MJ (ed). The Design of Clinical Trials in Cancer Therapy. Brussels: Editions Scientique Europe, 1973:242–389.

12. Simon R, Freidlin B, Rubinstein I, et al. Accelerated titration designs for phase I clinical trials in oncology. J Natl Cancer Inst 1997;89:1138–1147.
13. Legedza AT, Ibrahim J. Longitudinal design for phase I clinical trials using the continual reassessment method. Control Clin Trials 2000;21:574–588.
14. Storer B. Small-sample confidence sets for the MTD in a phase I clinical trial. Biometrics 1993;49:1117–1125.
15. Korn EL, Midthune D, Chen TT, et al. A comparison of two phase I trial designs. Stat Med 1994;13:1799–1806.
16. Ivanova A, Montazer-Haghighi A, Mohanty SG, Durham SD. Improved up-and-down designs for phase I trials. Stat Med 2003; 22:69–82.
17. O'Quigley J, Pepe M, Fisher L. Continual reassessment method: a practical design for phase I clinical trials in cancer. Biometrics 1990;48:853–862.
18. Shen LZ, O'Quigley. Consistency of continual reassessment method in dose finding studies. Biometrika 1996;83:395–406.
19. Faries D. Practical modifications of the continual reassessment method for phase I cancer clinical trials. J Biopharm Stat 1994;4: 147–164.
20. Leung DH, Wang Y. Isotonic designs for phase I trials. Control Clin Trials 2001;22:126–138.
21. Cheung YK, Chappell R. Sequential designs for phase I clinical trials with late-onset toxicities. Biometrics 2000;56:1177–1182.
22. Therasse P, Arbuck SG, Eisenhauer EA, et al. New guidelines to evaluate the response to treatment in solid tumors. J Natl Cancer Inst 2000;92:205–216.
23. Chen TT, Chute JP, Feigal E, et al. A model to select chemotherapy regimens for phase III trials for extensive-stage small-cell lung cancer. J Natl Cancer Inst 2000;92:1601–1607.
24. Buyse M, Thirion P, Carlson RW, et al. Relation between tumour response to first-line chemotherapy and survival in advanced colorectal cancer: a meta-analysis. Meta-Analysis Group in Cancer. Lancet 2000;356:373–378.
25. Moertel CG. Improving the efficiency of clinical trials: a medical perspective. Stat Med 1984;3:455–465.
26. Fleming TR. One sample multiple testing procedures for phase II clinical trials. Biometrics 1982;38:143–151.
27. Gehan E. The determination of the number of patients required in a follow-up trial of a new chemotherapeutic agent. J Chron Dis 1961;13:346–353.
28. Simon R. Optimal two-stage designs for phase II clinical trials. Control Clin Trials 1989;10:1–10.
29. Jung S-H, Carey M, Kim K. Graphical search for two-stage designs for phase II clinical trials. Control Clin Trials 2001;22: 367–372.
30. Ensign LG, Gehan E, Kamen DS, et al. An optimal three-stage design for phase II clinical trials. Stat Med 1994;13:1727–1736.
31. Chen TT. Optimal three-stage designs for phase II cancer clinical trials. Stat Med 1997;16:2701–2711.
32. Panageas KS, Smith A, Gonen M, et al. An optimal two-stage phase II design utilizing complete and partial response information separately. Control Clin Trials 2002;23:367–379.
33. Lin SP, Chen T. Optimal two-stage designs for phase II clinical trials with differentiation of complete and partial responses. Comm Stat A-Theory Methods 2000;29:923–940.
34. Conaway MR, Petroni GR. Bivariate sequential designs for phase II trials. Biometrics 1995;51:656–664.
35. Bryant J, Day R. Incorporating toxicity considerations into the design of two-stage phase II clinical trials. Biometrics 1995;51: 1372–1383.
36. Conaway MR, Petroni GR. Designs for phase II trials allowing for trade-off between response and toxicity. Biometrics 1996;52: 1375–1386.
37. Berry DA. Decision analysis and Bayesian methods in clinical trials. In: Thall PF (ed). Recent Advances in Clinical Trial Design and Analysis. Boston: Kluwer, 1995:125–154.
38. Thall PF, Simon R. Practical Bayesian guidelines for phase IIB clinical trials. Biometrics 1994;50:337–349.
39. Thall PF, Simon R, Estey EH. Bayesian sequential monitoring designs for single-arm clinical trials with multiple outcomes. Stat Med 1995;14:357–379.
40. Heitjan DF. Bayesian interim analysis of phase II cancer clinical trials. Stat Med 1997;16:1791–1802.
41. Simon R, Wittes RE, Ellenberg SS. Randomized phase II clinical trials. Cancer Treat Rep 1985;69:1375–1381.
42. Liu PY, Dahlberg S, Crowley J. Selection designs for pilot studies based on survival. Biometrics 1993;49:391–398.
43. Estey EH, Thall PF. New designs for phase 2 clinical trials. Blood 2003;102:442–448.
44. Mick R, Crowley JJ, Carroll RJ. Phase II clinical trial design for noncytotoxic anticancer agents for which time to disease progression is the primary endpoint. Control Clin Trials 2000;21: 343–359.
45. Rosner GL, Stadler W, Ratain MJ. Randomized discontinuation design: application to cytostatic antineoplastic agents. J Clin Oncol 2002;20:4478–4484.
46. Korn EL, Arbuck SG, Pluda JM, et al. Clinical trial designs for cytostatic agents: are new approaches needed? J Clin Oncol 2001; 19:265–272.
47. Gehan E. The evaluation of therapies: historical control studies. Stat Med 1984;3:315–324.
48. Hellman S, Hellman DS. Of mice but not men. Problems of the randomized clinical trial. N Engl J Med 1991;324:1585–1589.
49. Dupont WD. Randomized vs. historical clinical trials: Are the benefits worth the costs? Am J Epidemiol 1985;122:940–947.
50. Micciolo R, Valagussa P, Marubini E. The use of historical controls in breast cancer. An assessment in three consecutive trials. Control Clin Trials 1985;6:259–270.
51. Byar DP. Why databases should not replace randomized clinical trials. Biometrics 1980;36:337–342.
52. Freedman LS. Tables of the number of patients required in clinical trials using the log-rank test. Stat Med 1982;1:121–129.
53. Lachin JM, Foulkes MA. Evaluation of sample size and power for analysis of survival with allowance for nonuniform patient entry, losses to follow-up, noncompliance, and stratification. Biometrics 1986;42:507–519.
54. Lagakos E. Sample size based on the log-rank statistic in complex clinical trials. Biometrics 1988;44:229–241.
55. Shih JH. Sample size calculation for complex clinical trials with survival endpoints. Control Clin Trials 1995;16:395–407.
56. Ahnn S, Anderson SJ. Sample size determination in complex clinical trials comparing more than two groups for survival endpoints. Stat Med 1998;17:2525–2534.
57. Therneau TM. How many stratification factors are "too many" to use in a randomization plan? Control Clin Trials 1993;14:98–108.
58. Pocock SJ, Simon R. Sequential treatment assignment with balancing for prognostic factors in the controlled clinical trial. Biometrics 1975;31:103–115.
59. Jennison C, Turnbull J. Group Sequential Methods with Applications to Clinical Trials. London: Chapman & Hall/CRC, 2000.
60. George SL, Li C, Berry D, et al. Stopping a clinical trial early: frequentist and Bayesian approaches applied to a CALGB trial in non-small-cell lung cancer. Stat Med 1996;13:1313–1327.
61. Smith MA, Ungerleider RS, Korn EL, et al. Role of independent data-monitoring committees in randomized clinical trials sponsored by the National Cancer Institute. J Clin Oncol 1997;15: 2736–2743.
62. Gail MH. Eligibility exclusions, losses to follow-up, removal of randomized patients, and uncounted events in cancer clinical trials. Cancer Treat Rep 1985;69:1107–1113.
63. Redmond C, Fisher B, Wieand HS. The methodologic dilemma in retrospectively correlating the amount of chemotherapy received in adjuvant therapy protocols with disease-free survival. Cancer Treat Rep 1983;67:519–526.

64. Kaplan EL, Meier P. Nonparametric estimation from incomplete observations. J Am Stat Assoc 1958;53:457–481.
65. Mantel N. Evaluation of survival data and two rank order statistics in its consideration. Cancer Chemother Rep 1966;50: 163–170.
66. Cox DR. Regression models and life tables (with discussion). J R Stat Soc Ser B 1972;34:187–220.
67. Gehan EA. A generalized Wilcoxon test for comparing arbitrarily single-censored samples. Biometrika 1965;52:203–223.
68. Peto R, Peto J. Asymptotically efficient rank invariant test procedures. J R Stat Soc A 1972;135:189–198.
69. Prentice RL. Linear rank tests with right censored data. Biometrika 1978;65:167–179.
70. Harrington DP, Fleming TR. A class of rank test procedures for censored survival data. Biometrika 1982;69:553–566.
71. Parmar MK, Ungerleider RS, Simon R. Assessing whether to perform a confirmatory randomized clinical trial. J Natl Cancer Inst 1996;88:1645–1651.
72. Berry DA. When is a confirmatory randomized clinical trial needed? (editorial) J Natl Cancer Inst 1996;88:1606–1607.
73. Moher D, Schulz KF, Altman D; CONSORT Group (Consolidated Standards of Reporting Trials). The CONSORT statement: revised recommendations for improving the quality of reports of parallel-group randomized trials. JAMA 2001;285:1987–1991.
74. Rockette HE, Redmond CK. Limitations and advantages of meta-analysis in clinical trials. Recent Results Cancer Res 1988; 111:99–104.
75. Pignon JP, Hill C. Meta-analyses of randomized clinical trials in oncology. Lancet Oncol 2001;2:475–482.
76. Early Breast Cancer Trialists' Collaborative Group. Tamoxifen for early breast cancer: an overview of the randomised trials. Lancet 1998;351:1451–1467.
77. Parmar MKB, Spiegelhalter DJ, Freedman LS, et al. The CHART trials: Bayesian design and monitoring in practice. Stat Med 1994;13:1297–1312.
78. Stenning SP, Parmar MKB. Designing randomized trials: both large and small trials are needed. Ann Oncol 2002;13:131–138.
79. Parmar MKB, Griffiths GO, Spiegelhalter DJ, et al. Monitoring of large randomized clinical trials: a new approach with Bayesian methods. Lancet 2001;358:375–381.

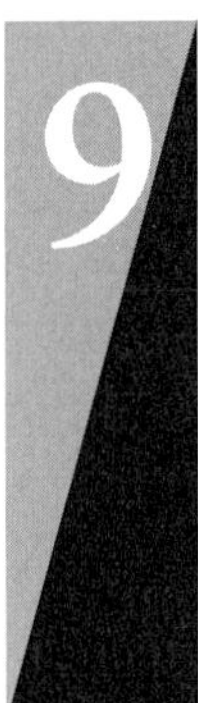

Ethics of Clinical Oncology Research

Manish Agrawal, Lindsay A. Hampson, and Ezekiel J. Emanuel

Ever since the earliest days of cancer research, ethical issues have been integral. In 1891, a French physician, Victor Cornil, reported that to determine whether cancer was contagious, a small section of breast tumor removed from the breast of one woman was implanted in her contralateral noncancerous breast. The surgical resection and implant were conducted when the patient was anesthetized and without the patient's consent. When this research study was initially reported it was condemned "as criminal."[1] In 1892, another cancer surgeon, William Coley, was conducting studies to determine whether "artificial erysipelas" (induced inflammation) would have antineoplastic effects. In describing one patient with a sarcoma, he noted that initially the patient was most reluctant to undergo the treatment. But "after some deliberation he consented, and on the 21st of April 1892 I began inoculations." Since that time, there has been substantial thought about the ethical issues involved in clinical oncology research, producing both more systematic analyses and important empirical data relevant to these issues. We delineate a general framework for analyzing the ethics of clinical research studies and then examine ethical issues involved in individual topics: (1) randomization and clinical equipoise; (2) informed consent; (3) Phase I oncology research; (4) stored biologic samples; (5) genetic testing; and (6) conflict of interest.

General Framework

Clinical oncology research must fulfill eight ethical requirements (Table 9.1).[2,3] First, research must reflect a collaborative partnership between researchers and the community from which participants are drawn.[4] Typically, a collaborative partnership is manifest in support from patient advocacy groups and the public for research funding, as well as inclusion of lay or patient representatives in research advisory and oversight boards such as institutional review boards (IRBs). Second, the research must be socially valuable, addressing meaningful gaps in therapy or scientific understanding.[5] "Me-too" studies confirming well-known findings are unethical. Third, the study must be conducted to generate reliable and valid data so that there is a reasonable chance the data will be able to advance therapy or contribute knowledge. Trivial questions, invalid or biased methods, and poor statistical techniques are unethical because worthless science cannot justify any risk or inconvenience to research participants. Consequently, there is no conflict between science and ethics. For research to be ethical, it must be good science.

Fourth, subject selection must be fair.[6,7] The eligibility requirements and recruitment strategies must be defined by the scientific objectives of the research study, not by social vulnerability or status. After scientific objectives, individuals likely to experience lower risks and greater benefits should be considered for recruitment and enrollment. It is not permissible to enroll privileged individuals preferentially in studies that are perceived to be especially promising. It is unreasonable to recruit individuals of a certain group into a study for convenience alone, when the conduct or results of that study would not benefit that group. Fortunately, unfair subject selection is rarely a problem in cancer research, where recruitment is necessarily tied to the disease under study. Fifth, the research must have a favorable risk-to-benefit ratio. Although risks can rarely be eliminated, they should be minimized. Similarly, the potential benefits to the participants and to future patients should be enhanced. When the benefits to individual participants are minimal, the risks are justified by the benefits of advancing knowledge for society. Sixth, research must also undergo independent review by a committee of peers and laypersons, such as an institutional review board (IRB). Such review is intended to provide unbiased evaluation of the scientific and ethical aspects of research as well as institutional and public accountability for that research.

Seventh, subjects must offer their informed consent to participate in research.[8,9] Informed consent has four requirements: (1) competence of the research participant to make decisions; (2) disclosure of relevant information by the researcher; (3) understanding of the information by the participant; and (4) voluntary consent by the participant to enroll. When participants lack competence, such as in pediatric research, permission from a surrogate is generally required. Finally, respect for persons does not end with informed consent. Researchers must respect the participants' rights to privacy and to relevant new findings and recognize the continued voluntary nature of participation in the study. Most importantly, researchers must monitor the health and well-being of research participants and intervene when it is threatened.

Each of these eight requirements must be satisfied; that is, all are necessary, although in particular circumstances,

TABLE 9.1. What makes oncology research ethical?

Requirement	*Underlying ethical values*	*Explanation*	*Benchmarks for fulfillment*
Collaborative partnership	Nonexploitation and respect for community's self-determination	Inclusion of the patients, representatives of advocacy groups, and other community members in determining research funding, research priorities, ethical oversight, and strategies for studies.	1) Ensure appropriate representation of researchers, health policymakers, and the community. 2) Involve researchers, health policymakers, and the community to share responsibilities for determining the importance of health problem, assessing the value of the research, planning, conducting, and overseeing the research, and integrating the research into the healthcare system. 3) Respect the community's values, culture, traditions, and social practices. 4) Contribute to developing the capacity for researchers, health policymakers, and the community to become full and equal partners in the research enterprise. 5) Ensure recruited participants and communities receive benefits from the conduct and results of research. 6) Share fairly the financial and other rewards of the research.
Social or scientific value	Scarce resources and nonexploitation	Evaluation of a treatment, intervention, or hypothesis with the aim of improving health and well-being or increasing knowledge.	1) Specify the beneficiaries of the research. 2) Assess the importance of the health problems being investigated and the prospect of value of the research for each of the beneficiaries. 3) Enhance the value of the research for each of the beneficiaries through dissemination of knowledge, product development, long-term research collaboration, and/or health system improvements. 4) Prevent supplanting the extant health system infrastructure and services.
Scientific validity	Scarce resources and nonexploitation	Use of accepted scientific principles and methods, including statistical techniques, to produce reliable and valid data.	1) Ensure the scientific design of the research realizes social value for the primary beneficiaries of the research. 2) Ensure the scientific design realizes the scientific objectives while guaranteeing research participants the healthcare interventions they are entitled to. 3) Ensure the research study is feasible given the social, political, and cultural environment and with sustainable improvements in the local healthcare and physical infrastructure.

Fair subject selection	Distributive justice	Selection of research participants so that stigmatized and vulnerable individuals are not targeted for risky research and favored or privileged individuals not preferentially enrolled in potentially beneficial research.	1) Select the study population to ensure scientific validity of the research. 2) Select the study population to minimize the risks of the research and enhance other principles, especially collaborative partnership and social value. 3) Identify and protect vulnerable populations.
Favorable risk–benefit ratio	Nonmaleficence, beneficence, and nonexploitation	Minimization of risks; enhancement of potential benefits. Risks to the individual participants are proportionate to the benefits to the individual participants and to society.	1) Assess the potential risks and benefits of the research to the study population in the context of its health risks. 2) Assess the risk–benefit ratio by comparing the net risks of the research project with the potential benefits derived from collaborative partnership, social value, and respect for study populations.
Independent review	Public accountability, minimizing influence of potential conflicts of interest	Review of the design of the research trial, its proposed subject population, and risk-to-benefit ratio by individuals unaffiliated with the research.	1) Ensure public accountability through reviews mandated by laws and regulations. 2) Ensure public accountability through transparency and reviews by other international and nongovernmental bodies. 3) Ensure independence and competence of the reviews.
Informed consent	Respect for persons, autonomy	Provision of information to participants about purpose of the research, its procedures, potential risks, benefits, and alternatives so that the individual understands this information and can make a voluntary decision whether to enroll and continue to participate.	1) Involve the community in establishing recruitment procedures and incentives. 2) Disclose information in culturally and linguistically appropriate formats. 3) Implement supplementary community and familial consent procedures where culturally appropriate. 4) Obtain consent in culturally and linguistically appropriate formats. 5) Prevent penalization for withdrawal from the research.
Respect for potential and enrolled subjects	Respect for persons, autonomy, and welfare	1. Permitting withdrawal from the research 2. Protecting privacy through confidentiality 3. Informing of newly discovered risks or benefits 4. Informing about results of clinical research 5. Monitoring of the health and well-being of participants and providing treatments for adverse reactions from the research.	1) Develop and implement procedures to protect the confidentiality of recruited and enrolled participants. 2) Ensure participants know they can withdraw without penalty. 3) Provide enrolled participants with information that arises in the course of the research study 4) Monitor and develop interventions for medical conditions, including research related injuries, of enrolled participants that are at least as good as existing local norms. 5) Inform participants and the study community of the results of the research.

such as mental incompetence or emergency research, the consent of the individual research participant can be waived. Furthermore, these principles are universal; they apply to research in all countries, although precisely how they are fulfilled may vary depending on the particular economic, social, and cultural circumstances. For instance, in cultures in which signatures are not the common form of consenting, other mechanisms may be used.[10] Finally, in designing any particular research study, tensions between the principles may arise. Different principles may have to be balanced against other principles; for some studies, lowering risk may have to be balanced against scientific validity or social value. Such balancing is inevitable. It means that there can be several different ethically acceptable ways to conduct a research study.

Randomization and Clinical Equipoise

Randomized controlled trials (RCTs) permit the comparison of standard care with one or more new interventions. RCTs are the gold standard of clinical research. Controls and some form of randomization have been used for about 100 years,[11] although the first modern randomized, placebo-controlled trial was conducted only in 1948 to evaluate streptomycin for pulmonary tuberculosis.[12] There are many concerns about the ethics of randomization, including the need for researchers to suspend their suspicions about what treatment is superior and to follow a protocol rather than provide individualized care.[13] In addition, randomization is probably the aspect of informed consent most commonly misunderstood by research participants.

Controlling for factors that are unknown but might influence outcomes is the scientific justification for randomization. Clinical equipoise is the dominant ethical justification for randomization.[14–16] Originally, the concept of *theoretical equipoise* was articulated as a justification for RCTs.[17] Theoretical equipoise held that it was ethical to conduct a randomized research study when there was exactly balanced evidence for the various interventions being tested. Theoretical equipoise has many problems. Rarely is the evidence exactly balanced. It is "overwhelmingly fragile . . . balanced on a knife's edge [because] it is disturbed by a slight accretion of evidence" for one intervention or the other.[14] Furthermore, it relies on the personal views of individual physicians; it requires each physician who enrolls a patient to be in a state of uncertainty about which intervention is better—a situation that rarely occurs.

In 1987, as an alternative, Freedman proposed *clinical equipoise*.[14] It is based on the recognition that the purpose of a clinical trail is *social*, to change standards of medical practice within the community. Consequently, clinical equipoise exists when there is uncertainty or disagreement among *the expert medical community* about which intervention is better. An RCT is conducted to resolve this uncertainty within the medical community. Clinical equipoise is the ethical manifestation of the statistical dictum that an RCT must begin with an honest null hypothesis.[14] More importantly, "clinical equipoise is consistent with a decided treatment preference on the part of the investigators. [Physicians] must simply recognize that their less-favored treatment is preferred by colleagues whom they consider to be responsible and competent."[14] Thus, it is the absence of consensus among the medical experts about the best intervention that ethically justifies the research study.

One virtue of clinical equipoise is that it rejects special ethical significance for any individual physician's hunch or intuitions about what is best. It relies on data, not on emotions. This approach can help convince patients that a trial is just as good an option as any alternative. Indeed, when there is clinical equipoise, then, at the start of the trial, whatever arm the patient is randomized to, should be as good as any other arm; all arms could be said to be in the patients' best interest. The recent experience with the trial of bone marrow transplantation for breast cancer should emphasize to the oncology community the dangers—ethical, scientific, as well as for individual patients—of relying on feelings rather than data from RCTs to choose what treatment to receive.

One important empirical question is whether clinical research does adhere to clinical equipoise. If it did, we should find that in many trials there is no difference between the new intervention and standard care, and that the numbers of trials demonstrating that the intervention arm is superior to standard care should be comparable with the number of trials demonstrating the superiority of standard care. The few meta-analyses that exist suggest that intervention arms are shown to be superior more frequently than standard care arms (Table 9.2).[18,19] Indeed, at least some data suggest that there is an equal balance between studies that show superiority of the intervention arm and those showing superiority of standard therapy when research is sponsored by government agencies. However, when sponsored by commercial organizations, the innovative interventions were significantly more likely to be proven superior. These data suggest that at least when commercially sponsored, there may be too high a threshold for testing a new intervention in an RCT; that is, researchers initiate a new RCT when there is more than sufficient evidence favoring the new intervention's effectiveness. This choice may be explained by the fact that launching an RCT is costly both in terms of effort and resources. Because of the costs, the research community may hesitate to initiate RCTs except when there is substantial evidence supporting the new intervention.[20]

Although clinical equipoise seems to solve many ethical problems with randomized control trials, some residual problems remain. For instance, why is a P value of 0.05 the level at which the community of medical experts is convinced that one intervention is better than another? Similarly, when the trial is nearing full accrual, clinical equipoise may not hold as data may suggest one arm is better than another. In such circumstances, there may be questions about the ethics of enrolling additional participants, even if the P value is not 0.05.

Informed Consent

Informed consent is an important element of ethical clinical research and is the most extensively empirically studied aspect of research ethics.[21–27] As noted earlier, to have valid informed consent requires fulfilling four elements: (1) competence, (2) disclosure, (3) understanding, and (4) voluntari-

TABLE 9.2. Data on adherence to clinical equipoise in randomized controlled trials.

Author	*Year published*	*Disease(s)*	*Studies*	*% favoring innovative therapy*	*% showing equality between innovation and standard therapy*	*% favoring standard therapy*	*Comments*
Djulbegovic et al.[18]	2000	Multiple Myeloma	136 reported between 1996 and 1998	29%	59%	12%	Commercially sponsored trials were significantly more likely to favor new innovative therapy arms (74% vs. 26%; $P = 0.004$). Studies funded by nonprofit organizations showed no difference (53% vs. 47%; $P = 0.61$)
Joffe et al.[19]	2004	Adult cancers	103 from two U.S. cooperative cancer groups between 1981 and 1995	29%	68%	3%	Mean effect size = 1.19 (95% CI, 1.12–1.27), favoring innovative therapy arm.

ness.[2] The published studies have predominantly focused on understanding, by evaluating what research participants understand and what are their motivations (Table 9.3).[26,28] Disclosure of information and voluntariness are less well studied.[27,29–31]

Limitations of the Empirical Data on Informed Consent

Despite the emphasis placed on informed consent and the numerous empirical studies, the reliability of conclusions is limited by five serious methodologic problems. First, there are no standard instruments to measure the domains of informed consent. Thus, there are varying and inconsistent methods and outcome measures, and the questions asked vary considerably from study to study. Although there are some proposed measures, none are widely accepted, such as the SF-36 for measuring quality of life.[32,33] This limits the comparability and generalizability of the available data. Second, there is confusion as to what should be measured. Studies claiming to assess understanding are often measuring motivations, recall, or voluntariness, none of which are understanding. For example, questions asking about the purpose of a study do not distinguish between the investigator's purpose for conducting the study from the purpose a particular individual may have for participating in the study. Third, the studies tend to be small; they usually involve fewer than 100 participants and are from single institutions.

Fourth, there is important variability in the timing of the assessment of understanding. Measuring understanding on the day a research participant decides to enroll in a study assesses understanding at the ethically key moment of decision making. Conversely, measurements made a week or more after signing consent assesses memory or recall rather than understanding. Such assessments may result in differences that could be completely due to the delay in assessment and have nothing to do with the quality of the informed consent process. Finally, insufficient attention has been given to the diversity of study contexts. Issues pertinent for informed consent in a randomized control trial for cancer differ from than those for a Phase I cancer trial, or an epidemiologic study, yet these differences are rarely addressed.[28] For example, asking a person their understanding of the chances they might benefit by enrolling in a randomized control trial of adjuvant therapy for breast cancer is not comparable to asking a person enrolling in a Phase II study of a single agent for metastatic breast cancer. In the adjuvant situation, the goal is cure, whereas in the metastatic setting the goal is palliation. Thus, a single study attempting to evaluate understanding in patients in these different research contexts is difficult to interpret.

Data on Informed Consent

Despite these limitations, three consistent results emerge from the published studies on informed consent. First, some problems exist with the informed consent process as it is currently practiced.[23,34] In some cases, disclosure seems to be inadequate. Several studies have suggested that although regulations are being followed, informed consent documents have become increasingly unreadable, lengthy, and uninformative.[22,35,36] These studies have found the forms written at the level of scientific journals rather than at an acceptable 8th-grade reading level.[35,36] Another study evaluating disclosure by asking European investigators their practice of obtaining consent found that 12% failed to inform their patients about the trial before randomization, 38% reported not always telling patients that they had been assigned their treatment randomly, and 5% never sought consent.[37] However, in the Phase I setting the available data suggest disclosure may be better. The only study evaluating the substantive content of Phase I oncology consent forms found that 99% of 272 forms explicitly stated the study was research and that in 86% this statement was prominent.[38] Furthermore, 92% indicated safety testing was the research goal. Overall, the mean length of the risks section was 35 lines in contrast with 4 lines as the average length of the benefit section; and 67% of the forms mentioned death as a potential consequence of participation in the study, whereas only 5% mentioned cure as a possible benefit. Only 1 consent form indicated that any benefits were expected. In a different study, evaluating disclosure during the physician-patient discussion in the Phase I setting, Tomamichel et al. reported that the lack of known treatments and the investigational nature of the Phase I

TABLE 9.3. Studies evaluating the quality of informed consent in Phase I oncology trials.

Author	Year	Sample size	Methods of evaluation	Reasons for participating	Awareness of study purpose and design	Confidence in benefit from enrolling in study	Satisfied with informed consent process	Would participate again
Rodenhuis et al.[40]	1984	10	Interview 1 week after treatment begun	50% hope for improvement of their diseases; 30% pressure of family	60%–80% recalled, "experimental," "so far only animal studies," "effect uncertain"	—	—	—
Itoh et al.[41,65]	1996	32	Questionnaire after enrollment but before drug administration	19% treatment benefit; 63% no benefit but participate anyway	43% knew goal is to determine recommended dose	63% did not expect to benefit	81% said understood almost all information given to them	—
Yoder et al.[44]	1997	37	Quantitative and qualitative interviews at entry and exit of study	70% to get best medical care; 85% decreased tumor size	—	—	—	100%
Hutchison et al.[45]	1998	28	Interviews 2–4 weeks after consenting to participate	Majority hope for benefit	—	"Most important reason . . . was hope it might help them"	89%	—
Daugherty et al.[9]	2000	144[a]	Interviews within 1 week of receiving drug	73% seeking anticancer response	31% knew purpose	73% thought there may be psychologic benefit	96%	
Tomamichel et al.[39]	1995	31	Quantitative and qualitative analysis of taped interviews	59% possibility of medical benefit	—	—	96%	—
Moore et al.[75]	2001	15	Pre- and posttreatment questionnaire and structured interviews	Three themes: 1) need to try everything 2) maintaining hope 3) help others	—	Described "living with the reality of incurable disease whilst still hoping for a miracle cure"	—	—
Schutta et al.[75a]	2000	8	Quantitative and qualitative analysis of taped focus group	Hope for therapeutic benefit	—	—	—	—
Joffe et al.[28]	2001	50[b]	Mail survey 1–2 weeks after consent		75% knew trials done to improve treatment of future patients; 71% knew may be no medical benefit to themselves	71% knew may not be direct medical benefit to them from participating	90%	77%
Meropol et al.[48]	2003	328[c]	Questionnaire after enrollment	60% expect to benefit	—	64% "unsure" or "maybe"	—	—

[a]The initial publication by Daugherty et al.[19] of 27 patients is included in the 144 patients.

[b]Survey of patients participating in phase I, II, and III studies. Total number of patients was 207 of which 50 were enrolled in phase I studies. Unfortunately, the analysis of the responses failed to stratify according to phase.

[c]The initial publication by Cheng et al. of 30 patients, included in the 328 patients.

oncology study were verbally stated by physicians to cancer patients in more than 90% of consultations and the lack of sufficient knowledge of toxicity of the drug in more than 80%.[39] Two other studies report similar findings.[40,41]

Several studies have focused on evaluating understanding by the research participant and found that the participants did not understand various aspects of the study.[28,42] For example, a study by Penman et al. of 144 cancer patients participating in trials at academic cancer centers found that participants did not fully understand toxicity;[42] participants recalled an average of 3 risks when the consent forms mentioned an average of 11 risks. More importantly, participants tended to recall the minor toxicities, such as hair loss, rather than major potential toxicities.

Studies evaluating understanding have consistently found that participants most frequently fail to understand details of research design. In a study of 299 Finnish patients with breast cancer enrolled in a randomized control trial of hormonal treatment, 51% thought the doctor had chosen the therapy.[43] More recently, Joffe et al. reported on 207 patients enrolled in Phase I, II, and III oncology studies surveyed 3 to 14 days after consent.[19] Overall, 75% of participants knew that the main reason cancer trials are done is to improve the treatment of future cancer patients, while 71% reported that they may not experience direct medical benefit from participating in the clinical trial, yet 48% thought the treatments and procedures were standard for their type of cancer. The understanding aspect of informed consent in Phase I oncology trials has been the most extensively studied area of Phase I ethics research. Most participants in Phase I oncology studies are motivated to participate by hopes for stabilization, improvement, or even cure of their cancer (see Table 9.3).[44–48] This observation has been widely interpreted to suggest patients have deficient understanding of the objectives, benefits, and risks of Phase I research. However, the data also show that patient decisions to participate may reflect a motivation to maintain hope in a difficult situation rather than misunderstanding of the information.[44] For example, although Daugherty et al. found that 85% of patients were motivated to participate for possible therapeutic benefit, 78% were either unwilling or unable to state whether they believed they personally would receive benefit from participating in a Phase I trial.[49] Similarly, Itoh et al. found 63% of the participants did not expect any benefit but wished to participate anyway.[41] The largest study evaluating understanding by Meropol et al., which asked Phase I participants how confident they were being among those who would benefit, found only 27% thought they would definitely benefit from participating in research.[48]

Second, several intervention studies have been conducted in an attempt to improve the informed consent process. Three broad types of interventions have been tried: (1) modifying the consent form, (2) augmenting the discussion between research participants and investigators, and (3) using a multimedia or computer-based intervention.[22,50] Regardless of the approach, the majority of the studies have not shown meaningful improvements in the understanding of research participants. The major exception is by Aaronson et al., finding that using a telephone-based nursing intervention could improve participants' understanding.[50] About 15% to 20% of participants in the intervention group showed improvements in the level of their understanding of side effects, trial objectives, and randomization. It should be noted that although studies using consent forms have failed to show a consistent and substantial improvement in understanding, they may still be important to research participants. Joffe et al. found that 84% read the consent carefully and 86% found it easy to understand.[28]

Finally, despite deficiencies, virtually all the studies report that research participants are generally satisfied with the informed consent process.[23,42,51–53] Hietanen et al. reported that of 299 breast cancer patients, 68% thought they had enough time for decision making and 87% were happy with their decision to participate.[43] Similarly, Verheggen et al. evaluated 198 research participants in 26 clinical trials, finding that the majority of participants were "quite satisfied with the oral and written information disclosure."[51] Daugherty et al., Tomamichel et al., and others report more than 95% satisfaction in the informed consent process by research participants of Phase I oncology trials.[28,39,49]

Future Directions in Research on Informed Consent

That a discrepancy seems to exist between what patients understand and their satisfaction with the informed consent process poses several research issues. First, what individuals should understand when they decide to participate in research needs to be clearly delineated and justified. As there is not agreement of what constitutes good informed consent, it is difficult to judge the current informed consent process. Some argue understanding of purpose, methods, risks, benefits, and alternatives to the research are essential components of valid informed consent. Others lessen the importance of understanding and argue good faith effort at disclosure in nontechnical language is all that is required for valid informed consent even if patients ultimately do not fully understand. Furthermore, the standards of valid informed consent need to be defined in different research contexts, because what is required for patients to understand may be different depending on the context of the particular study. For example, in a natural history trial studying factors leading to health disparities, good disclosure may be all that is required. Conversely, in a study involving bone marrow transplant with high-dose chemotherapy, total-body irradiation, and a high chance for peritransplant mortality with a potential for prolonged and numerous hospital admissions, a more complete understanding may be more important. Second, what information matters to individuals when making decisions about participating in research needs to be further studied. One reason research participants may not understand certain aspects covered in informed consent is that the details are not that important to or salient for them. If research design is unimportant to research participants' decision making, then it may be difficult, and even unnecessary, to improve their understanding of it.

Besides those discussed previously, in the Phase I context, two issues are particularly important for further research. Studies that delineate between issues of understanding and those of motivation are needed. More importantly, research that evaluates the role hope plays in patients' decisions to participate and whether this hope should be fostered or damped is needed.

Phase I Oncology Studies

Phase I oncology studies are critical to the development of drugs that fight cancer because they are the primary process by which basic research is translated into clinical applications that could potentially lead to larger clinical trials and effective cancer therapies. There are two fundamental ethical concerns about Phase I cancer research: the risk–benefit ratio and quality of informed consent.[30,31,42,54–56] Data regarding the risk–benefit ratio are reviewed here, whereas the data on informed consent in Phase I studies were discussed earlier under the section on informed consent.

Risks and Benefits of Phase I Oncology Studies

The risks and benefits of Phase I oncology studies have been primarily derived from meta-analyses looking at response rates and mortality.[57,58] The two largest published meta-analyses of Phase I studies report on trials conducted between 1970 and 1987; they reveal response rates of approximately 5% and mortality of 0.5% (Table 9.4).[57,58] Although there have been a few other meta-analyses, they are limited by including only single-institution studies, evaluating only a few trials, and not evaluating trials published in the past decade (Table 9.4).[59–63] Consequently, neither the newer compounds currently being evaluated, such as antibodies, vaccines, immunotoxins, and antiangiogenesis factors, nor improved supportive care measures are reflected in the commonly cited response rate of 5%. More recent data suggest that the response rates may be higher. A recent meta-analysis of 477 Phase I studies sponsored by the Cancer Therapy Evaluation Program (CTEP) at the National Cancer Institute between 1991 and 2002, including 10,867 participants, reported a response rate of 4% for trials with one investigational agent but an overall response rate of 12.2% for all types of Phase I trials, including those escalating doses of proven therapies.[64] In addition, another meta-analysis looking at all studies published in 2002, reports an overall response rate of 18%.[65] With the exception of a few agents such as cis-platinum for testicular cancer and imatinib mesylate for chronic myeloid leukemia, which produced a complete hematologic response rate of 98%, of which 96% lasted beyond 1 year, there are few data on the impact of Phase I oncology studies on other clinical parameters of benefit such as overall survival or symptom control.[66–68]

In regard to risks, the published meta-analyses report a mortality of 0.5% and the more recent meta-analyses report a slightly higher mortality of 0.7% to 1.3%.[57,58,64,65] Besides traditional risks such as mortality, toxicity, and survival, non-medical risks are raised as risks that should be factored in the risk–benefit ratio; these include frequent blood draws, radiologic evaluations, physician visits, and biopsies, all of which require a substantial commitment of time and resources from the patients and their families. However, it is unknown whether such factors adversely affect outcomes and quality of life of Phase I research participants. Similarly, there is a concern that nausea, vomiting, and other debilitating side effects are common; however, their overall frequency, severity, and impact on quality of life have been poorly documented. The few data that do exist on the quality of life effect suggest that despite the time commitment and side effects, participating in Phase I oncology studies may actually improve patients' quality of life compared with the alternative of receiving supportive care.[69–74]

This result seems paradoxical. The improvement in quality of life of cancer patients in Phase I trials may be due to receiving psychologic benefit from participating in Phase I studies.[49] For some participants, the routine and regular physician contacts reduce psychologic distress during a time of great uncertainty. For others, it may allow them to exercise their willpower in a situation they did not choose.[45,75] In addition, some also receive comfort from knowing they are helping future patients with cancer.[28,75,76] More clinical data besides response rates and mortality are needed to fully characterize the risks and benefits of participating in Phase I oncology studies.

Besides obtaining a more complete picture of the risk–benefit ratio of Phase I oncology trials, there are several other research challenges. What criteria should we use to define a favorable risk–benefit ratio for Phase I oncology

TABLE 9.4. Response rates and death rates of Phase I oncology trials.

Author	Trial years	Total no. of research agents evaluated	Total no. of trials evaluated	No. of patients evaluated	Total response rate	Toxic death rate	Other
Decoster et al.[57]	1972–1987	87	211	6,639	4.5%	0.5%	No
Estey et al.[58]	1974–1982	54	187	6,447	4.2%		No
Smith et al.[58a]	1984–1992	NR	23	610	3%	1%	Single institution
Von Hoff et al.[59]	1970–1983	113	228	7,960	6.3%	NR	No
Itoh et al.[60]	1981–1991	38	56	2,200	4%	NR	Japanese studies only
Sekine et al.[63]	1976–1993		399	12,076	4.1%		Single-agent studies only
Bachelot et al.[62]	1986–1993		9	154	6%	0.6%	
Han et al.[61]	1991–2000	16	16	420	15%		UK studies only
Horstman et al.[64]	1991–2002		477	10,687	12.2%	0.68%	
Agrawal et al.[56]	2002		125	2,830	18%	1.3%	

studies? Who should decide what criteria to use to define a favorable risk–benefit ratio?

To determine when a risk–benefit ratio is favorable or unfavorable requires a standard of evaluation, and one appropriate for patients with advanced cancer whose health will most likely deteriorate and who will die, yet no standard has been explicitly articulated. Indeed, determining risk–benefit ratios is one of the most important, but least developed, areas of determining the ethics of research trials.[2,77–79] One approach could be to elucidate a standard based on socially accepted determinations of risk–benefit ratios already used for cancer treatments, such as in FDA approval of cancer agents. For example, high-dose interleukin 2 (IL-2) is the only FDA-approved treatment for metastatic renal cell carcinoma. This IL-2 regimen has a response rate of 14% (5% complete responses, 9% partial responses), with a median response duration of 20 months.[80] The possible toxicities of IL-2 are substantial, including a sepsis-like syndrome, requiring judicious use of fluids and vasopressor support to maintain blood pressure while avoiding pulmonary edema from capillary leak. Other chemotherapy treatments, such as gemcitabine, are the FDA-approved treatment of choice for metastatic pancreatic cancer, despite a 5.4% response rate, because of demonstrated quality of life benefits.[81] Thus, an explicit standard, or at least a reasonable approach by which to judge a risk–benefit ratio of Phase I studies, is needed to meaningfully discuss whether a particular risk–benefit ratio is favorable or unfavorable.

Research with Stored Biologic Samples

As information about activation of genes and expression of proteins in cancer tissues becomes more central to oncology, use of stored biologic samples has become an ever more important aspect of clinical oncology research. Over the past decade or so there has been great controversy about when and under what conditions it is ethical to conduct research with stored biologic samples. In 1995, the ELSI-DOE Working Group suggested that all research with stored biologic samples be reviewed by an IRB and that, to show respect for persons, consent should be obtained to use the sample even if not strictly required by the federal research regulations.[82] Subsequently, other groups have advanced other positions. The American Society of Human Genetics argues recontact for consent is unnecessary for research using previously stored samples, provided the risks are minimal.[83]

In addition to the disagreements about whether consent should be obtained at all, there are disagreements about what individuals should have to consent to. The National Action Plan on Breast Cancer recommends asking individuals to consent to future research on the disease being studied and separately to consent to research on other diseases.[84] The National Bioethics Advisory Commission (NBAC) argues that individuals should be offered six choices, including allowing individuals to authorize future research on the same disease, but requiring recontact for consent for research on other diseases.[85]

This disagreement has produced uncertainty about what the ethical requirements are and worries that research is being stymied. Regarding samples to be prospectively collected, the ethical principle of respect for persons suggests that consent should be obtained. However, there is a further question of what the person should consent to. Respect for persons alone does not determine *how many* or *which* choices individuals should be asked to consent to. For these issues, we need empirical data revealing which choices individuals find as expressions of respect. Similarly, for previously collected samples that lack consent, the question is, what procedures demonstrate respect for persons. Given these questions, empirical research is essential to determining when and how to obtain consent for research with stored samples.

Although the available data are limited, they indicate that research participants are willing to have their biologic samples used for all kinds of research (Table 9.5).[86–89] Indeed, these data suggest multiple questions on the consent form are unnecessary. Based on these data, it has been suggested that it is sufficient to prospectively ask research subjects to consent to any type of research with their stored biologic sample.[86] It has also been suggested that previously collected clinical samples can be used in research when anonymized, based on presumed consent with an opt-out when feasible.

Genetic Testing

Rapid advances in molecular biology resulting from new analytical techniques combined with detailed knowledge of the human genome, offer the opportunity of discovering the genetic basis of many cancers.[90] As basic research into the genetic basis of cancer progresses, the clinical testing of cancer genes is becoming more common.[91] Two ethical issues with genetics testing research are particularly relevant: confidentiality and informed consent.

A fundamental aspect of respect for human persons is protecting confidentiality. The available research suggests that maintaining confidentiality is a real concern of potential research participants. For example, in a study in which Hadley et al. offered genetic testing to 111 eligible first-degree relatives of patients with hereditary nonpolyposis colon cancer (HNPCC), 51% chose to participate.[92] Fears of discrimination and concerns about psychologic issues were major barriers to testing. A study by Armstrong et al. of BRCA1/2 testing found similar concerns about job and insurance discrimination.[93] Worries about job and insurance discrimination are concerns for family members, and safeguards should be in place to protect confidentiality. Research on how valid these concerns are and how frequent breaches of confidentiality involving genetic tests in research occur would be helpful. If they are uncommon, dissemination of such information might increase enrollment into genetic testing research studies, and if they are common, it would help develop safeguards to protect confidentiality.

A second important issue surrounds informed consent and genetics testing. In the context of genetics testing research, it is particularly important for research participants to understand the implications about genetic testing because of its potential psychologic impact on individuals.[94] Indeed, the data suggest individuals with depressive symptoms are less likely to participate in genetic testing. A study by Lerman et al. of 208 members of four extended (HNPCC) families reported that those with symptoms of depression were four

TABLE 9.5. Data on attitudes toward conducting research with stored biologic samples.

Author	*Year*	*Population*	*Data source*	*Percent permitting research with their research-derived stored biologic samples*	*Comment*
Wendler and Emanuel[86]	2002	504 Americans; 246 enrolled in Alzheimer's research and 258 Medicare beneficiaries	Survey of attitudes	87.9% (for anonymized samples collected as part of research) anonymized	27.3% would require consent for research on clinically derived samples that are
Stegmayr and Asplund[87]	2002	1,311 people 11 years after blood sample collection in the MONICA project	Permission for genetic research	93.0%	22.3% wanted information about each use of their sample
Malone et al.[88]	2002	5,411 individuals in ECOG cancer studies	Permission as part of informed consent	89.4%	
		2,154 individuals in ECOG cancer studies	Permission as part of informed consent; more detailed form based on National Action Plan for Breast Cancer model requiring three questions	93.7% (cancer) 86.9% (other, noncancer kinds of research)	
Chen et al.[89]	2004	1,060 individuals enrolled in NIH studies	Permission as part of informed consent	87.1%	6.7% refused future research with stored samples

times less likely to obtain testing.[95] Biesecker et al. reported similar findings in a study of psychosocial factors effecting genetics testing decisions among BRCA1/BRCA2 families.[94] Furthermore, informed consent is also exceptionally important in genetics testing research because there is no real option of *going back* once the results of the test are known. Thus, individuals who do not really understand the potential impact of knowing they are carriers of a gene that predisposes them to cancer could potentially suffer long-term consequences. However, with the current emphasis on genetic counseling and the importance placed on it, valid informed consent may already be in place.

Data on risks and benefits of genetic testing would be helpful in genetics testing research. For example, there is a perception of a potential tremendous psychologic burden from knowing the results of genetic tests, but there are few long-term data on how such knowledge affects quality of life, the impact of increased interaction with physicians, and potentially more testing and follow-up. Data on the effects on other family members and family dynamics would also be helpful.

Conflict of Interest

After the Gelsinger case at the University of Pennsylvania and multiple cases at Fred Hutchinson Cancer Center, much attention has been focused on the financial conflicts of interest of clinical researchers in general and of oncology researchers in particular.[96,97] This controversy raises five fundamental questions: What is a conflict of interest? How frequently do researchers have a financial interest in their own clinical research? Do financial interests distort the design, conduct, or dissemination of research data or compromise patient safety and well-being? How should they be regulated? How well do the safeguards work?

What is a conflict of interest? All professionals have primary interests that define and orient their professional activities. Teachers' primary interest is to educate their students. Judges' primary interest is to ensure justice is served for plaintiffs and defendants. Physicians' primary interests are to promote patient well-being and to teach medical students. The primary interests of clinical researchers are to produce and disseminate generalizable knowledge that will improve health care for future patients and to ensure the health and well-being of their research participants. In addition to these primary interests, professionals also have secondary interests. For a researcher, these could include publishing, gaining recognition and fame, spending time with his or her family, and obtaining a good income. These secondary interests are not in themselves illegitimate or nefarious; in fact, secondary interests can often be praiseworthy. What makes them problematic is their ability to unduly influence decisions about an individual's primary interest.[98]

A conflict of interest occurs when a secondary interest distorts or appears to distort a judgment related to a primary interest. In other words, a conflict of interest occurs when a reasonable person could "believe that professional judgment has been improperly influenced, whether or not it has."[98] Mere suspicion by a reasonable person that a professional judgment is biased or unduly influenced is sufficient reason for a conflict of interest to exist, regardless of whether an undue influence has actually occurred. Conflict of interest rules are meant both to ensure objectivity in professional judgments by minimizing the likelihood such judgments will be compromised and to minimize any harms that might result from the bias if it does exist. Thus, the aim of conflict of interest regulations is not to prevent secondary interests altogether, but to prevent the secondary interest from influencing or appearing to influence judgments concerning the primary interest.[98]

How frequently do researchers have financial interest in their own clinical research? With the passage of the Bayh–Dole Act in 1980, which granted universities and medical schools the exclusive licensing rights to intellectual property developed through federally funded research conducted at their institutions, industry support of research grew significantly.[99] In 1986, 46% of all biotechnology firms supported research at universities; by 1996, the proportion had doubled to 92%. As a result, universities' share of new gene patents increased from 53% to 73% between 1990 and 1999, and at least 2,900 companies have been formed around an innovation licensed from researchers at an academic institution since 1980.[100,101] Consequently, from 1991 to 2000, the income to universities from licensing grew from $121 million to $997 million per year.[99] Similarly, the fraction of clinical research supported by industry grew from 32% in 1980 to approximately 62% in 2000 while the federal government's share fell.[102] This expansion by industry has many positive effects for research and researchers, including providing access to industrial facilities and databases, increased financial support for research, and use of industrial expertise.[103] However, this increase in industry support and involvement in research has also resulted in further opportunities for financial conflicts of interest in clinical research.

Financial relationships between industry and researchers are common; studies suggest that between 23% and 28% of academic investigators in biomedical research receive funding from industry.[104,105] Probably the most well documented rates of researcher-industry relations are those of the UCSF faculty, which consists of 900 PIs (principal investigators) in an institution with $374 million in National Institutes of Health (NIH) grants, placing it in the top five institutions receiving NIH funding.[106] In 1999, 7.6% of the faculty reported having personal financial ties to their research sponsors.[106] Of these, 34% had occasional speaking engagements, 33% had paid consultancy arrangements, 32% served on boards of directors or scientific advisory boards, and 14% had equity in a company, with the mean value of the equity being $100,000. Thus, although the prevalence of faculty with financial ties to industry was relatively low, those with financial interests often had multiple ties, some of which involved substantial sums.

Do financial interests distort the design, conduct, or dissemination of research data or compromise patient safety and well-being? In one bone marrow protocol at the Fred Hutchinson Cancer Center, 80 of 82 enrolled research subjects died and the study investigators had $294 million of holdings in a drug company sponsoring part of the research.[97] Importantly, this does not prove that the patients' well-being was compromised by the potential conflict of interest, but it does raise questions. In fact, the researchers were cleared of conflict of interest allegations in a lawsuit that was brought against them and Fred Hutchinson Cancer Research Center by the patient's families.[107,108] Unfortunately, there are no data substantiating whether the financial interests of investigators compromise the safety of research subjects. This conjecture is difficult to establish, especially as there are no data on the overall safety of clinical research.

Regarding the link between financial interests and research design, the data indicate that industry-sponsored research is certainly no worse methodologically than clinical research sponsored by nonprofit organizations, such as the NIH.[109–112] Indeed, the data indicate that industry-sponsored research studies may well be more methodologically rigorous.[18,113] In one study, industry-sponsored trials were more likely to be double blind than trials with other sources of funding.[114] In another study that used a 100-point scale to evaluate five criteria for methodological rigor—randomization, outcome, inclusion/exclusion criteria, statistical analysis, and report of the interventions—industry-sponsored trials scored 73.1 while nonindustry-sponsored studies averaged 53.4 ($P < 0.0001$).[115] Recently, Lexchin et al. comprehensively reviewed studies that assessed sponsorship, design, and conduct of research.[116] They found that "none of the 13 [assessments in the literatures] reported that industry funded studies had poorer methodological quality . . . Of nine [out of 13 assessments] that provided statistical analyses, four found that drug company sponsored research had better quality scores." Thus, it appears that financial interests do not compromise research design.

Financial interests may, however, adversely affect data collection and interpretation. Many studies have reported that research funded by industry is more likely to be favorable to the industry's experimental interventions than if the research was funded by a nonindustry source. Of 11 meta-analyses, 9 reported that industry-sponsored trials were significantly more likely to give pro-industry results.[102] Indeed, when all studies were aggregated, having industry sponsorship was associated with an odds ratio of 3.60 (95% CI, 2.63–4.91) for having a pro-industry conclusion. For instance, Als-Nielsen et al. reported that among studies funded by for-profit entities, 51% reported results favorable to industry, whereas only 16% of studies funded by nonprofits generated results favorable to industry.[117] Furthermore, one report summarizing a number of randomized studies conducted in multiple myeloma, found that 74% of industry-sponsored trials produced results favorable to the industry's new treatment, whereas only 53% of trials funded by nonprofit entities generated results favorable to the experimental treatments.[18] Specifically regarding oncology studies, Friedberg et al. reported that drug company-sponsored studies were much less likely to report unfavorable qualitative outcomes than studies funded by nonprofit sources (5% versus 38%).[118]

Importantly, such data do not necessarily demonstrate bias or compromised studies. The fact that industry-sponsored studies generate pro-industry results may reflect a "pipeline" issue; that is, because conducting large research trials is very expensive, industry tends to only undertake drug trial studies when it is reasonably sure the results will be positive. Experimental interventions that are more uncertain or may not generate huge profits may be terminated before large randomized studies because of industry's caution about expending resources. This decision may ultimately deprive society of important new interventions, but it does not constitute a financial conflict of interest that might compromise the integrity of the research design or the data collection and interpretation. However, none of the reported studies links industry funding to biased scientific judgments, which, in turn, produce too many study outcomes favorable to the funding industry. Just showing that industry-sponsored studies generate pro-industry conclusions is insufficient to demonstrate that financial conflicts of interest actually bias the conduct of studies.

Nevertheless, there are data suggesting that industry financial support does distort the judgment of researchers. Stelfox and colleagues analyzed all published studies in 1995–1996 regarding the safety of calcium channel blockers

TABLE 9.6. Support of calcium channel antagonists and financial interest.[119]

	Support Ca blockers	*Neutral*	*Critical of Ca blockers*	*P value*
No. of respondents	24 (69%)	15 (83%)	30 (91%)	0.02
Financial interest in Ca blocker manufacturer	23 (96%)	9 (60%)	11 (37%)	<0.001
Financial interest in any manufacturer	24 (100%)	10 (67%)	13 (43%)	<0.001
Honorarium from any pharmaceutical manufacturer	75%	40%	17%	<0.001
Research funding from any pharmaceutical manufacturer	87%	40%	20%	<0.001
Employment or consultation for any pharmaceutical manufacturer	25%	33%	17%	0.45

in postmyocardial infarction patients.[119] They found 70 publications: 5 original research papers, 32 reviews, and 33 letters to the editor. As Table 9.6 shows, researchers with a financial interest in a manufacturer of calcium channel antagonist, or even those with a financial interest in *any* manufacturer, were significantly more likely to support the safety of calcium channel blockers than researchers without a financial interest. Indeed, this trend held true for researchers with any type of financial interest in any pharmaceutical manufacturer, including receiving honoraria and research funding. The only time there was no association between having a financial interest in any pharmaceutical manufacturer and supporting the safety of calcium channel blockers, was when the researchers' financial interest was to have been employed by or served as a consultant to manufacturers.

Finally, there are data showing that financial interests do alter dissemination of research results. A study of 42 placebo-controlled trials of selective serotonin reuptake inhibitors (SSRI) submitted to Swedish regulators found that, of the 21 studies showing positive effects of the drug over placebo, 19 were published, with the results frequently appearing in more than 1 article. Conversely, of the 21 studies that showed no difference between the experimental SSRI drug and placebo, only 6 were published.[120] Whether this is a result of the publication bias against negative studies at major journals or the result of industry withholding negative data was not determined. However, a 1993 survey of 2,167 life science faculty from the 50 universities receiving the most NIH funding found that one-fifth of the faculty had delayed publication for more than 6 months during the past 3 years to allow for patent application or negotiation, to resolve intellectual property rights disputes, to protect their scientific lead over competitors, or to slow the distribution of undesired results. Delays in publication were associated with participation in a research relationship with industry [odds ratio (OR) = 1.34] and with commercialization of one's own research results (OR = 3.15).[104,121] More importantly, there have been a number of high-profile cases in which industry has actively and explicitly tried to prevent the dissemination of negative findings about drugs. In the Olivieri case in Toronto, Apotex, the company that funded Dr. Olivieri's research on their drug, tried to prevent her from publishing findings suggesting that the drug was not only *not beneficial* for patients with iron overload, but may actually be *harmful* to them.[122] Similarly, the manufacturers of Synthroid brand thyroid replacement, Boots Co., funded a study to compare Synthroid with generic thyroid replacement drugs.[123] The results showed no difference in patient outcomes. Boots then tried to prevent the UCSF researchers who conducted the study from publishing the data.

These data suggest that financial interests probably do not have an adverse effect on the *conduct* of clinical research and may actually be beneficial in terms of study design. Conversely, in terms of data interpretation and dissemination, the data suggest that "money does talk."

How can we protect against this distorting influence of conflicts of interest? In general, there are three types of safeguards for conflicts of interest. First, and most commonly, is for researchers to disclose their financial interest. In addition, the financial interest is managed by instituting data safety and monitoring boards (DSMBs) or independent consent monitors. Finally, when financial interests are too extensive, prohibitions can be implemented.

Disclosure of researchers' financial interests in journal articles is becoming routine and more comprehensive. However, the data about intrainstitutional disclosure and the communication of the disclosed information to the various research oversight groups and committees indicates a flawed system. A recent General Accounting Office (GAO) study of five major research institutions found that the rules regarding disclosure and prohibitions of financial interests varied widely.[124] Furthermore, the disclosed information was not well recorded by the institutions and was not readily available to the institutions' IRBs when they considered protocols. Of the 111 cases in which researchers had substantial financial interests, the GAO found that in only 3 did the researchers divest and in no cases were they told to do so by their universities.

There are other data indicating that disclosure may not be an adequate safeguard even if institutions do have conflict of interest (COI) disclosure policies in place, researchers frequently lack knowledge about such policies. For instance, at UCSF and Stanford, 58% of researchers surveyed could not accurately describe the COI policy of their institution.[125] In addition, COI policies lack specificity and there are inconsistent standards for disclosure across institutions.[126–128]

Importantly, while there have been vociferous calls for disclosure of financial interests to research subjects, there have been almost no data on whether patients can understand these data and how they might react.[129] Indeed, some highly regarded commentators have worried that disclosure to patients would only reveal the problem without providing them any mechanism to address it, thereby increasing anxiety but not solving the underlying conflict of interest.[130]

To address problems about conflict of interest, the Board of Directors of American Society of Clinical Oncology (ASCO) voted to revise its conflict of interest policy in 2002.

The new policy requires disclosure of all financial payments or interests from entities "having an investment, licensing, or other commercial interest in the subject matter under consideration," including (1) executive or leadership positions, (2) ownership of stock or equity in companies, (3) consultancy or service on an advisory board, (4) honoraria for speeches, (5) royalty payments on a patent, (6) nonresearch-related travel or gifts, and (7) expert testimony.[131] The policy does not view research-related funding, funding to attend investigators' meetings, or funding as part of a grant to present research results at a widely attended open meeting (such as the ASCO annual meeting) as a conflict of interest; therefore, ASCO does not require disclosure of this type of information.

In addition to disclosure, ASCO has also implemented restrictions on researchers' "finder's fees," payments for recruiting goals or recruiting speed, and payments for certain data results. Similarly, ASCO believes that because principal investigators or individuals on the executive committees of large multicenter studies as well as those on data safety and monitoring boards have such extensive decision-making authority over the conduct, analysis, and dissemination of study results, these individuals should have none of the listed financial interests in a commercial sponsor.

There are two important exceptions to these restrictions. Because of the extensive oversight provided through study sections, DSMBs, and other independent review mechanisms, these restrictions do not apply to NIH-supported research studies that might "involve products of specific commercial interests." Furthermore, recognizing the importance of translational research and the reality that the developer of a new technology is probably the best person to conduct the initial research studies, the ASCO policy recognizes that when there is limited worldwide expertise and when "an inventor of a unique technology or treatment being evaluated in a trial," these restrictions might be relaxed. In these cases, there must be a data safety and monitoring board in place to ensure the safety of the research participants.

Ethics is a key area of oncology research, and current ongoing empirical research on many ethical issues—such as how to improve informed consent, the role hope plays in patients' decisions to participate in Phase I studies, and patients perceptions of COI—may well change the answers to these ethical questions.

References

1. Lederer SE. Subjected to science: human experimentation in America before the Second World War. Baltimore: Johns Hopkins University Press, 1995.
2. Emanuel EJ, Wendler D, Grady C. What makes clinical research ethical? JAMA 2000;283(20):2701–2711.
3. Emanuel EJ, Wendler D, Killen J, Grady C. What makes clinical research in developing countries ethical? The benchmarks of ethical research. J Infect Dis 2004;189(5):930–937.
4. International ethical guidelines for biomedical research involving human subjects. In: Council for International Organizations of Medical Sciences (CIOMS). Geneva: CIOMS, 1993.
5. Freedman B. Scientific value and validity as ethical requirements for research: a proposed explication. IRB 1987;9(6):7–10.
6. The Belmont Report. In: The National Commission for the Protection of Human Subjects of Biomedical and Behavioral Research; 1979. Washington, DC: U.S. Government Printing Office, 1979.
7. World Medical Association, Declaration of Helsinki: Ethical Principles for Medical Research Involving Human Subjects (Tokyo 2004). http://www.wma.net/e/policy/b3.htm. Accessed 2005.
8. The Nuremberg Code. JAMA 1996;276(20):1691.
9. Berg JW, Appelbaum PS, Lidz CW, Parker LS. Informed consent: legal theory and clinical practice. New York: Oxford University Press, 2001.
10. Wendler D, Rackoff JE. Informed consent and respecting autonomy: what's a signature got to do with it? IRB 2001;23(3):1–4.
11. Lilienfeld AM. The Fielding H. Garrison Lecture: Ceteris paribus: the evolution of the clinical trial. Bull Hist Med 1982; 56(1):1–18.
12. Medical Research Council: Streptomycin treatment of pulmonary tuberculosis. Br Med J 1948;2:769–782.
13. Hellman S, Hellman DS. Of mice but not men. Problems of the randomized clinical trial. N Engl J Med 1991;324(22):1585–1589.
14. Freedman B. Equipoise and the ethics of clinical research. N Engl J Med 1987;317(3):141–145.
15. Bracken MB. Clinical trials and the acceptance of uncertainty. Br Med J (Clin Res Ed) 1987;294(6580):1111–1112.
16. Lilford RJ, Jackson J. Equipoise and the ethics of randomization. J R Soc Med 1995;88(10):552–559.
17. Fried C. Medical Experimentation: Personal Integrity and Social Policy. New York: American Elsevier, 1974.
18. Djulbegovic B, Lacevic M, Cantor A, et al. The uncertainty principle and industry-sponsored research. Lancet 2000;356(9230): 635–638.
19. Joffe S, Harrington DP, George SL, Emanuel EJ, Budzinski LA, Weeks JC. Satisfaction of the uncertainty principle in cancer clinical trials: retrospective cohort analysis. BMJ 2004; 328(7454):1463.
20. Roberts TG Jr, Lynch TJ Jr, Chabner BA. The phase III trial in the era of targeted therapy: unraveling the "go or no go" decision. J Clin Oncol 2003;21(19):3683–3695.
21. Verheggen FW, van Wijmen FC. Informed consent in clinical trials. Health Policy 1996;36(2):131–153.
22. Daugherty CK. Impact of therapeutic research on informed consent and the ethics of clinical trials: a medical oncology perspective. J Clin Oncol 1999;17(5):1601–1617.
23. Subject Interview Study. In: Advisory Committee on Human Radiation Experiments Final Report. New York: Oxford University Press, 1996.
24. Albrecht TL, Blanchard C, Ruckdeschel JC, Coovert M, Strongbow R. Strategic physician communication and oncology clinical trials. J Clin Oncol 1999;17(10):3324–3332.
25. Taylor KM, Feldstein ML, Skeel RT, Pandya KJ, Ng P, Carbone PP. Fundamental dilemmas of the randomized clinical trial process: results of a survey of the 1,737 Eastern Cooperative Oncology Group investigators. J Clin Oncol 1994;12(9):1796–1805.
26. Simes RJ, Tattersall MH, Coates AS, Raghavan D, Solomon HJ, Smartt H. Randomised comparison of procedures for obtaining informed consent in clinical trials of treatment for cancer. Br Med J (Clin Res Ed) 1986;293(6554):1065–1068.
27. Sugarman J, McCrory DC, Powell D, et al. Empirical research on informed consent. An annotated bibliography. Hastings Cent Rep 1999;29(1):S1–S42.
28. Joffe S, Cook EF, Cleary PD, Clark JW, Weeks JC. Quality of informed consent in cancer clinical trials: a cross-sectional survey. Lancet 2001;358(9295):1772–1777.
29. Annas GJ. The changing landscape of human experimentation: Nuremberg, Helsinki, and beyond. Health Matrix Clevel 1992; 2(2):119–140.
30. Lipsett MB. On the nature and ethics of phase I clinical trials of cancer chemotherapies. JAMA 1982;248(8):941–942.

31. Kodish E, Stocking C, Ratain MJ, Kohrman A, Siegler M. Ethical issues in phase I oncology research: a comparison of investigators and institutional review board chairpersons. J Clin Oncol 1992;10(11):1810–1816.
32. Joffe S, Cook EF, Cleary PD, Clark JW, Weeks JC. Quality of informed consent: a new measure of understanding among research subjects. J Natl Cancer Inst 2001;93(2):139–147.
33. Miller CK, O'Donnell DC, Searight HR, Barbarash RA. The Deaconess Informed Consent Comprehension Test: an assessment tool for clinical research subjects. Pharmacotherapy 1996;16(5): 872–878.
34. Riecken HW, Ravich R. Informed consent to biomedical research in Veterans Administration Hospitals. JAMA 1982;248(3):344–348.
35. Morrow GR. How readable are subject consent forms? JAMA 1980;244(1):56–58.
36. Grossman SA, Piantadosi S, Covahey C. Are informed consent forms that describe clinical oncology research protocols readable by most patients and their families? J Clin Oncol 1994; 12(10):2211–2215.
37. Williams CJ, Zwitter M. Informed consent in European multicentre randomised clinical trials—are patients really informed? Eur J Cancer 1994;30A(7):907–910.
38. Horng S, Emanuel EJ, Wilfond B, Rackoff J, Martz K, Grady C. Descriptions of benefits and risks in consent forms for phase I oncology trials. N Engl J Med 2002;347(26):2134–2140.
39. Tomamichel M, Sessa C, Herzig S, et al. Informed consent for phase I studies: evaluation of quantity and quality of information provided to patients. Ann Oncol 1995;6(4):363–369.
40. Rodenhuis S, van den Heuvel WJ, Annyas AA, Koops HS, Sleijfer DT, Mulder NH. Patient motivation and informed consent in a phase I study of an anticancer agent. Eur J Cancer Clin Oncol 1984;20(4):457–462.
41. Itoh K, Sasaki Y, Fujii H, et al. Patients in phase I trials of anticancer agents in Japan: motivation, comprehension and expectations. Br J Cancer 1997;76(1):107–113.
42. Penman DT, Holland JC, Bahna GF, et al. Informed consent for investigational chemotherapy: patients' and physicians' perceptions. J Clin Oncol 1984;2(7):849–855.
43. Hietanen P, Aro AR, Holli K, Absetz P. Information and communication in the context of a clinical trial. Eur J Cancer 2000; 36(16):2096–2104.
44. Yoder LH, O'Rourke TJ, Etnyre A, Spears DT, Brown TD. Expectations and experiences of patients with cancer participating in phase I clinical trials. Oncol Nurs Forum 1997;24(5):891–896.
45. Hutchison C. Phase I trials in cancer patients: participants' perceptions. Eur J Cancer Care (Engl) 1998;7(1):15–22.
46. Cheng JD, Hitt J, Koczwara B, et al. Impact of quality of life on patient expectations regarding phase I clinical trials. J Clin Oncol 2000;18(2):421–428.
47. Meropol NJ, Schulman KA, Weinfurt K, et al. Discordant perceptions of patients and their physicians regarding phase I trials. ASCO Annual Meeting, 2002.
48. Meropol NJ, Weinfurt KP, Burnett CB, et al. Perceptions of patients and physicians regarding phase I cancer clinical trials: implications for physician–patient communication. J Clin Oncol 2003;21(13):2589–2596.
49. Daugherty C, Ratain MJ, Grochowski E, et al. Perceptions of cancer patients and their physicians involved in phase I trials. J Clin Oncol 1995;13(5):1062–1072.
50. Aaronson NK, Visser-Pol E, Leenhouts GH, et al. Telephone-based nursing intervention improves the effectiveness of the informed consent process in cancer clinical trials. J Clin Oncol 1996;14(3):984–996.
51. Verheggen FW, Jonkers R, Kok G. Patients' perceptions on informed consent and the quality of information disclosure in clinical trials. Patient Educ Couns 1996;29(2):137–153.
52. Verheggen FW, Nieman FH, Reerink E, Kok GJ. Patient satisfaction with clinical trial participation. Int J Qual Health Care 1998;10(4):319–330.
53. Ferguson PR. Patients' perceptions of information provided in clinical trials. J Med Ethics 2002;28(1):45–48.
54. Emanuel EJ. A phase I trial on the ethics of phase I trials. J Clin Oncol 1995;13(5):1049–1051.
55. Miller M. Phase I cancer trials. A collusion of misunderstanding. Hastings Cent Rep 2000;30(4):34–43.
56. Agrawal M, Emanuel EJ. Ethics of phase 1 oncology studies: reexamining the arguments and data. JAMA 2003;290(8):1075–1082.
57. Decoster G, Stein G, Holdener EE. Responses and toxic deaths in phase I clinical trials. Ann Oncol 1990;1(3):175–181.
58. Estey E, Hoth D, Simon R, Marsoni S, Leyland-Jones B, Wittes R. Therapeutic response in phase I trials of antineoplastic agents. Cancer Treat Rep 1986;70(9):1105–1115.
58a. Smith TL, Lee JJ, Kantariian HM, et al. Design and result of phase I cancer clinical trials: three-year experience at MD Anderson Cancer Center. J Clin Oncol 1996;14(1):287–295.
59. Von Hoff DD, Turner J. Response rates, duration of response, and dose response effects in phase I studies of antineoplastics. Invest New Drugs 1991;9(1):115–122.
60. Itoh K, Sasaki Y, Miyata Y, et al. Therapeutic response and potential pitfalls in phase I clinical trials of anticancer agents conducted in Japan. Cancer Chemother Pharmacol 1994;34(6): 451–454.
61. Han C, Braybrooke JP, Deplanque G, et al. Comparison of prognostic factors in patients in phase I trials of cytotoxic drugs vs new noncytotoxic agents. Br J Cancer 2003;89(7):1166–1171.
62. Bachelot T, Ray-Coquard I, Catimel G, et al. Multivariable analysis of prognostic factors for toxicity and survival for patients enrolled in phase I clinical trials. Ann Oncol 2000; 11(2):151–156.
63. Sekine I, Yamamoto N, Kunitoh H, et al. Relationship between objective responses in phase I trials and potential efficacy of non-specific cytotoxic investigational new drugs. Ann Oncol 2002;13(8):1300–1306.
64. Horstmann E, McCabe MS, Grochow L, et al. Risks and benefits of phase 1 oncology trials, 1991 through 2002. N Engl J Med 2005;352(9):895–904.
65. Agrawal M, Grady C, Fairclough D, Emanauel E. Patients? Decision-making process of participating in phase I oncology studies. ASCO Annual Meeting, 2005.
66. Higby DJ, Wallace HJ Jr, Albert DJ, Holland JF. Diaminodichloroplatinum: a phase I study showing responses in testicular and other tumors. Cancer (Phila) 1974;33(5):1219–1215.
67. Druker BJ, Talpaz M, Resta DJ, et al. Efficacy and safety of a specific inhibitor of the BCR-ABL tyrosine kinase in chronic myeloid leukemia. N Engl J Med 2001;344(14):1031–1037.
68. Druker BJ. Inhibition of the Bcr-Abl tyrosine kinase as a therapeutic strategy for CML. Oncogene 2002;21(56):8541–8546.
69. Berdel WE, Knopf H, Fromm M, et al. Influence of phase I early clinical trials on the quality of life of cancer patients. A pilot study. Anticancer Res 1988;8(3):313–321.
70. Melink TJ, Clark GM, Von Hoff DD. The impact of phase I clinical trials on the quality of life of patients with cancer. Anticancer Drugs 1992;3(6):571–576.
71. Cohen L, de Moor C, Parker PA, Amato RJ. Quality of life in patients with metastatic renal cell carcinoma participating in a phase I trial of an autologous tumor-derived vaccine. Urol Oncol 2002;7(3):119–124.
72. Cox K. Enhancing cancer clinical trial management: recommendations from a qualitative study of trial participants' experiences. Psychooncology 2000;9(4):314–322.
73. Campbell S, Whyte F. The quality of life of cancer patients participating in phase I clinical trials using SEIQoL-DW. J Adv Nurs 1999;30(2):335–343.

74. Hope-Stone LD, Napier MP, Begent RH, Cushen N, O'Malley D. The importance of measuring quality of life in phase I/II trials of cancer therapy: the effects of antibody targeted therapy: Part I. Eur J Cancer Care (Engl) 1997;6(4):267–272.
75. Moore S. A need to try everything: patient participation in phase I trials. J Adv Nurs 2001;33(6):738–747.
75a. Schutta KM, Burnett CB. Factors that influence a patient's decision to participate in a phase I cancer clinical trial. Oncol Nurs Forum 2000;27(9):1435–1438.
76. Daugherty CK, Siegler M, Ratain MJ, Zimmer G. Learning from our patients: one participant's impact on clinical trial research and informed consent. Ann Intern Med 1997;126(11):892–897.
77. Weijer C. The ethical analysis of risk. J Law Med Ethics 2000; 28(4):344–361.
78. King NM. Defining and describing benefit appropriately in clinical trials. J Law Med Ethics 2000;28(4):332–343.
79. Meslin EM. Protecting human subjects from harm through improved risk judgments. IRB 1990;12(1):7–10.
80. Fyfe G, Fisher RI, Rosenberg SA, Sznol M, Parkinson DR, Louie AC. Results of treatment of 255 patients with metastatic renal cell carcinoma who received high-dose recombinant interleukin-2 therapy. J Clin Oncol 1995;13(3):688–696.
81. Burris HA III, Moore MJ, Andersen J, et al. Improvements in survival and clinical benefit with gemcitabine as first-line therapy for patients with advanced pancreas cancer: a randomized trial. J Clin Oncol 1997;15(6):2403–2413.
82. Clayton EW, Steinberg KK, Khoury MJ, et al. Informed consent for genetic research on stored tissue samples. JAMA 1995; 274(22):1786–1792.
83. ASHG report. Statement on informed consent for genetic research. The American Society of Human Genetics. Am J Hum Genet 1996;59(2):471–474.
84. National Action Plan on Breast Cancer. Executive summary: model consent form for biological tissue banking: focus group report. Available at: http://www.4woman.gov/napbc/catalog.wci/napbc/model_consent.htm.
85. Research involving human biological materials: ethical issues and policy guidance. In: National Bioethics Advisory Commission, 1999. Rockville, MD: U.S. Government Printing Office, 1999.
86. Wendler D, Emanuel E. The debate over research on stored biological samples: what do sources think? Arch Intern Med 2002;162(13):1457–1462.
87. Stegmayr B, Asplund K. Informed consent for genetic research on blood stored for more than a decade: a population based study. BMJ 2002;325(7365):634–635.
88. Malone T, Catalano PJ, O'Dwyer PJ, Giantonio B. High rate of consent to bank biologic samples for future research: the Eastern Cooperative Oncology Group experience. J Natl Cancer Inst 2002;94(10):769–771.
89. Chen DT, Rosenstein DL, Muthappan PG, et al. Research with stored biological samples: what do research participants want? Arch Intern Med 2005;165(6):652–655.
90. Kataki A, Konstadoulakis MM. Reflections of the European Conference "Molecular Screening of Individuals at High Risk for Developing Cancer: Medical, Ethical, Legal, and Social Issues." Genet Test 2000;4(1):79–84.
91. Calzone KA, Biesecker BB. Genetic testing for cancer predisposition. Cancer Nurs 2002;25(1):15–25; quiz 6–7.
92. Hadley DW, Jenkins J, Dimond E, et al. Genetic counseling and testing in families with hereditary nonpolyposis colorectal cancer. Arch Intern Med 2003;163(5):573–582.
93. Armstrong K, Calzone K, Stopfer J, Fitzgerald G, Coyne J, Weber B. Factors associated with decisions about clinical BRCA1/2 testing. Cancer Epidemiol Biomarkers Prev 2000;9(11):1251–1254.
94. Biesecker BB, Ishibe N, Hadley DW, et al. Psychosocial factors predicting BRCA1/BRCA2 testing decisions in members of hereditary breast and ovarian cancer families. Am J Med Genet 2000;93(4):257–263.
95. Lerman C, Hughes C, Trock BJ, et al. Genetic testing in families with hereditary nonpolyposis colon cancer. JAMA 1999; 281(17):1618–1622.
96. Nelson D, Weiss R. Penn researchers sued in gene therapy death: teen's parents also name ethicist as defendant. Washington Post 2000;A3.
97. Wilson DHD. Uninformed consent. The Seattle Times 2001; March 11–15:Sect. 1–14.
98. Thompson DF. Understanding financial conflicts of interest. N Engl J Med 1993;329(8):573–576.
99. Blumenthal D. Academic-industrial relationships in the life sciences. N Engl J Med 2003;349(25):2452–2459.
100. Kelch RP. Maintaining the public trust in clinical research. N Engl J Med 2002;346(4):285–287.
101. Moses H III, Martin JB. Academic relationships with industry: a new model for biomedical research. JAMA 2001;285(7):933–935.
102. Bekelman JE, Li Y, Gross CP. Scope and impact of financial conflicts of interest in biomedical research: a systematic review. JAMA 2003;289(4):454–465.
103. Is the university-industrial complex out of control? Nature (Lond) 2001;409(6817):119.
104. Blumenthal D, Campbell EG, Causino N, Louis KS. Participation of life-science faculty in research relationships with industry. N Engl J Med 1996;335(23):1734–1739.
105. Blumenthal D, Gluck M, Louis KS, Stoto MA, Wise D. University-industry research relationships in biotechnology: implications for the university. Science 1986;232(4756):1361–1366.
106. Boyd EA, Bero LA. Assessing faculty financial relationships with industry: a case study. JAMA 2000;284(17):2209–2214.
107. Marshall E. Hutchinson's mixed win. Science 2004;304:371.
108. Stromberg I. Clinical trials beat the rap. Wall Street Journal 2004:A18.
109. Kjaergard LL, Nikolova D, Gluud C. Randomized clinical trials in hepatology: predictors of quality. Hepatology 1999;30(5): 1134–1138.
110. Cho MK, Bero LA. The quality of drug studies published in symposium proceedings. Ann Intern Med 1996;124(5):485–489.
111. Anderson JJ, Felson DT, Meenan RF. Secular changes in published clinical trials of second-line agents in rheumatoid arthritis. Arthritis Rheum 1991;34(10):1304–1309.
112. Rochon PA, Gurwitz JH, Cheung CM, Hayes JA, Chalmers TC. Evaluating the quality of articles published in journal supplements compared with the quality of those published in the parent journal. JAMA 1994;272(2):108–113.
113. Massie BM, Rothenberg D. Publication of sponsored symposiums in medical journals. N Engl J Med 1993;328(16):1196–1197; author reply 7–8.
114. Davidson RA. Source of funding and outcome of clinical trials. J Gen Intern Med 1986;1(3):155–158.
115. Liebeskind DS, Kidwell CS, Saver JL. Empiric evidence of publication bias affecting acute stroke clinical trials. Stroke 1999;30(1):268.
116. Lexchin J, Bero LA, Djulbegovic B, Clark O. Pharmaceutical industry sponsorship and research outcome and quality: systematic review. BMJ 2003;326(7400):1167–1170.
117. Als-Nielsen B, Chen W, Gluud C, Kjaergard LL. Association of funding and conclusions in randomized drug trials: a reflection of treatment effect or adverse events? JAMA 2003;290(7): 921–928.
118. Friedberg M, Saffran B, Stinson TJ, Nelson W, Bennett CL. Evaluation of conflict of interest in economic analyses of new drugs used in oncology. JAMA 1999;282(15):1453–1457.
119. Stelfox HT, Chua G, O'Rourke K, Detsky AS. Conflict of interest in the debate over calcium-channel antagonists. N Engl J Med 1998;338(2):101–106.

120. Melander H, Ahlqvist-Rastad J, Meijer G, Beermann B. Evidence b(i)ased medicine: selective reporting from studies sponsored by pharmaceutical industry: review of studies in new drug applications. BMJ 2003;326(7400):1171–1173.
121. Blumenthal D, Campbell EG, Anderson MS, Causino N, Louis KS. Withholding research results in academic life science. Evidence from a national survey of faculty. JAMA 1997;277(15): 1224–1228.
122. Bonetta L. Inquiry into clinical trial scandal at Canadian research hospital. Nat Med 1998;4(10):1095.
123. A duty to publish. Nat Med 1998;4(10):1089.
124. General Accounting Office. Biomedical Research: HHS Direction Needed to Address Financial Conflicts of Interest. Report No. GAO-02-89. Washington, DC: United States General Accounting Office, 2001.
125. Boyd EA, Cho MK, Bero LA. Financial conflict-of-interest policies in clinical research: issues for clinical investigators. Acad Med 2003;78(8):769–774.
126. Bero LA. Disclosure policies for gifts from industry to academic faculty. JAMA 1998;279(13):1031–1032.
127. Lo B, Wolf LE, Berkeley A. Conflict-of-interest policies for investigators in clinical trials. N Engl J Med 2000;343(22):1616–1620.
128. McCrary SV, Anderson CB, Jakovljevic J, et al. A national survey of policies on disclosure of conflicts of interest in biomedical research. N Engl J Med 2000;343(22):1621–1626.
129. Kim SY, Millard RW, Nisbet P, et al. Potential research participants views regarding researcher and institutional financial conflicts of interest. J Med Ethics 2004;30(1):73–79.
130. Foster RS. Conflicts of interest: recognition, disclosure, and management. J Am Coll Surg 2003;196(4):505–517.
131. American Society of Clinical Oncology: revised conflict of interest policy. J Clin Oncol 2003;21(12):2394–2396.

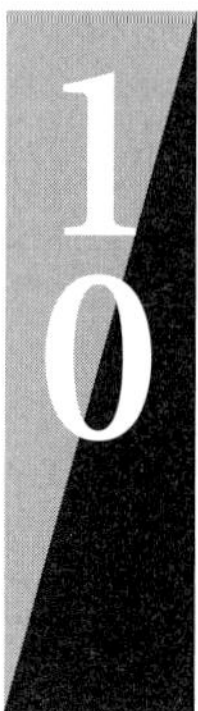

Informatics Infrastructure for Evidence-Based Cancer Medicine

Jeffrey P. Bond and Scott D. Luria

An old man, and pale: anemia. Also thin: first thought, cancer. Second thought, tuberculosis, alcoholism, some other chronic process . . . the computer provided him with a differential, complete with probabilities of diagnosis. From *The Andromeda Strain* (1969),[1] by Michael Crichton

How is cancer information exchanged among laypersons, clinical professionals, and medical researchers? High hopes for the role of computers in medical information exchange have been reflected in science fiction for decades. After at least two information technology paradigm shifts (personal computers and the Internet) and countless successful implementations of, for example, shared electronic records, knowledge bases, decision support systems, speech-to-text tools, natural language processing tools, or remote monitoring devices in a variety of medical and nonmedical settings, we are in the process of realizing these high hopes. An important component of cancer information exchange infrastructure is support for the *use of knowledge derived from medical research in combination with patient data to guide cancer-related decisions, that is, support for evidence-based cancer medicine*, the central focus of this chapter.

We focus on three classes of scenarios that require informatics support: a healthcare professional making a cancer-related decision about a patient, someone (referred to here as a layperson) making a cancer-related decision without medical training and without consulting a healthcare professional, and a researcher making a decision regarding a cancer-related experiment. Each such decision involves a collection of potential actions, information that describes the context of the action, and knowledge derived from scientific experiments that constitutes evidence bearing the merit of the potential actions given the context (Figure 10.1).

The purpose of this chapter is to describe how clinicians, patients, and researchers can find information related to cancer prevention, diagnosis, treatment, and research on the World Wide Web. (Although WWW resources will not necessarily behave as they did at the time this chapter was written, we think it is important to include numerous specific examples.) Here *infrastructure*, then, refers to standards, software, and digital information rather than hardware. We emphasize digital media but do not intend to imply that other media (such as printed textbooks, classroom lectures, handwritten notes, pamphlets, posters in subways, radio/television spots, or phone support lines) cannot be preferable to computer-related infrastructure for accomplishing particular goals. Currently the support for integration of knowledge bases and context data available to most clinicians is poor; in nearly all examples below, this integration is manual.

We do not attempt comprehensive coverage of medical informatics (for example, electronic medical records,[2] HIPAA,[3] or telemedicine,[4]), which includes cancer informatics. Readers interested in resources describing broader aspects of bioinformatics or medical informatics might consult one of the more comprehensive resources listed in Table 10.1. Readers interested in a variety of online bioinformatics databases and software might consider one of the URLs given in Table 10.2.

We focus on two structures that facilitate information exchange: indexes and graphs, analogous to the index and table of contents of a book or the index accessed using a search box and the directory of a Web resource. Given a set of objects, *indexes* associate words or phrases with subsets, which can be combined using set algebra. For example, one can search for clinical trials at http://clinicaltrials.gov with a query such as disease="breast cancer", experimental treatment="surgery", and state="Vermont." *Graphs* consist of *nodes* and relationships between nodes. In the cases described here, the nodes are Web pages and the relationships are represented by links or buttons. An example of such a graph is a collection of Web pages including directory pages that support browsing. Graphs need not be hierarchical like a physical filing system because there may be multiple paths between Web pages.

One of the primary difficulties in developing informatics support for cancer-related decisions results from the level of detail we expect. Informatics support for book purchases necessarily includes rudimentary support for cancer informatics in that it serves to identify books on cancer. Searches based on author, title, or keywords from a simple vocabulary (for

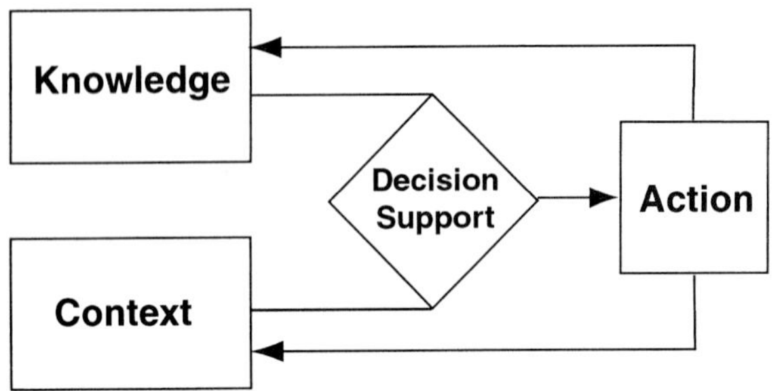

FIGURE 10.1. Schematic describing how potential actions are based on and inform knowledge derived from scientific experiments and the information that describes the context of the action.

example, *breast cancer*) often serve to identify sets of book records that can either be browsed manually or productively ranked (for example, the number of times a book has been purchased is evidence related to the quality of the book). We expect cancer informatics support to do better than simply finding books that will answer questions, we expect to identity chapters or paragraphs that answer our questions. Ideally, informatics resources should answer questions directly.

Such fine granularity requires, relative to the task of simply identifying of books on cancer, a complex vocabulary and a query syntax that supports context data. In this chapter, we focus on four components of such a solution: vocabulary resources that support intelligent indexing, manually created graphs for browsing, manual indexing of documents based on their generalilty and usefulness, and integration of the search with patient data.

Laypersons' Decisions

A variety of cancer information portals and sources of information exist on the World Wide Web for laypersons (Table 10.3). We focus on two comprehensive resources: Cancer.gov, which is maintained by the U.S. National Cancer Institute (NCI), and Cancer.org, which is maintained by the American Cancer Society (ACS).

Cancer.gov Features

Cancer.gov is a source of general cancer information as well as information on NCI research programs, NCI research funding, cancer statistics, and clinical trials. The cancer information section, http://cancer.gov/cancerinfo, includes a variety of information that is intended for laypersons seeking information about cancer etiology, diagnosis, and treatment. Below we highlight certain features of Cancer.gov.

"What You Need to Know About Cancer" (WYNTK) documents. http://cancer.gov/cancerinfo/wyntk provides a starting point for obtaining information about cancer in general and more than 20 specific cancers. Each such document includes information about symptoms, diagnosis, and treatment. An overview document provides a general and readable introduction to cancer with pointers to other NCI resources.

Dictionary. http://cancer.gov/dictionary/ provides *non-technical* definitions of cancer-related terms. There are currently more than 4,000 terms, with approximatly 40 terms added each month. For example:

metastasis (meh-TAS-ta-sis) The spread of cancer from one part of the body to another. A tumor formed by cells that have spread is called a *metastatic tumor* or a *metastasis*. The metastatic tumor contains cells that are like those in the original (primary) tumor. The plural form of metastasis is metastases (meh-TAS-ta-seez).

Physician Data Query (PDQ). http://cancer.gov/cancerinfo/pdq is "NCI's comprehensive cancer database, containing peer-reviewed summaries on cancer treatment, screening, prevention, genetics, and supportive care" and also provides information on clinical trials and directories. Although most of this information is directed at healthcare professionals, many of the topics have links to pages written specifically for patients and linked to dictionary entries. Compared to the WYNTK documents, "PDQ patient" documents are more specific; for example, there is a single WYNTK document on

TABLE 10.1. General biomedical informatics resources.

Resource	*Scope*
Bioinformatics: A Practical Guide to the Analysis of Genes and Proteins[53]	Sequences, structures, genomes, alignments, phylogenetic trees
Bioinformatics Sequence and Genome Analysis[54]	Sequences, structures, genomes, alignments, phylogenetic trees
NCBI Handbook[23]	NCBI databases (sequence, structure, journal publication, gene expression, textbook, and taxonomy databases) as well as BLAST and genome browsing tools
Nucleic Acids Research Database Issues[55]	Peer-reviewed set of articles about biological databases
Nucleic Acids Research Software Issue[56]	Peer-reviewed set of articles about computational biology software
Cancer Informatics[57]	Cancer informatics
Medical Informatics[6]	Medical informatics
Public Health Informatics and Information Systems[58]	Public Health Informatics
Informatics in Primary Care[59]	Includes chapters on electronic medical, records, clinical decision support, and knowledge bases

TABLE 10.2. General WWW resources for biomedical informatics.

Name or supporting organization	*URL*	*Scope*
Nucleic Acids Research Database Issue	nar.oupjournals.org	Comprehensive database of biological databases
Nucleic Acids Research Software Issue	nar.oupjournals.org	Comprehensive database of computational biology software
EBI	ebi.ac.uk	Bioinformatics
NCBI	ncbi.nlm.nih.gov	Bioinformatics
SEER	seer.cancer.gov	Cancer Statistics
NCI	cancer.gov	Cancer Information
ACS	cancer.org	Cancer Information
SDSC Biology Workbench	workbench.sdsc.edu	Bioinformatics
Cancer Biomedical Informatics Grid	cabig.nci.nih.gov	Cancer informatics

leukemia while there are seven PDQ documents for patients on leukemia, each focused on a different leukemia.

Search box. A search box allows users to identify pages relevant to a set of keywords. The search may return both "Best Bets," NCI pages that Cancer.gov staff have judged most likely to provide the desired information based on the query, as well as a list of pages matching the set of keywords. An advanced search page allows users to restrict the scope of the search based on NCI organization (e.g., to the Division of Cancer Control and Population Sciences), to a database of clinical trials, to subsets of the PubMed publication database, to specific cancer topics (for example, tobacco), or to a database of genetics services.

Browsing support. A directory allows the same documents to be browsed from different points of view, for example, by type of cancer, by treatment, or by etiology.

Examples. Certainly laypersons are encouraged to consult health professionals on cancer-related questions, but laypersons should have many more questions than their physicians have time to answer. We describe how to obtain information related to typical questions by browsing or using the search box.

Example 1. Should I limit use of my cell phone to reduce my risk of cancer?

By browsing:
- Go to http://cancer.gov/cancerinfo
- Follow the link to "Prevention, Genetics, Causes"
- Follow the link to "Cancer Causes and Risk Factors"
- Follow the link to "Cellular Telephone Use and Cancer"

By searching:
- Enter "cell phone" in the search box.
- Follow the link to, for example, "Cellular Telephone Use and Cancer"

Example 2. One of my moles looks a little different than it did 5 years ago. Should I make an appointment to see my doctor?
- Enter "mole" in the search box
- Follow the link to "What You Need To Know About Moles and Dysplastic Nevi"
- Follow the link to "Pictures of Melanoma"

Cancer.org Features

Cancer.org is a source of general cancer information for a variety of interest groups: patients, families or friends of patients, survivors, health care information seekers, healthcare professionals, and supporters. Below we highlight certain features of Cancer.org.

Context data and private data management. Users can create accounts and set preferences that include interest groups, type of cancer, location, and language. Users can also manage a "Planner," which includes a calendar, to-do list, e-mail groups, and bookmarks.

Cancer-related information based on context data. The cancer.org home page points to directories for each of the interest groups listed above. For example, the "health information seeker" category points to information about risk, prevention, detection, myths, and statistics. The "patients, family, and friends" directory points to treatment decision support as well as information useful in preparation for or during treatment. The "survivor" directory includes information about healthy lifestyles as well as tapping into the cancer survivor community. If a user selects an interest group, then by default they are directed to the appropriate directory.

"In My Community" boxes present regional information based on the specified zip code. "Getting Specific" boxes

TABLE 10.3. WWW Cancer information resources for laypersons.

Source	*URL*
Open Directory Project	dmoz.org/Health/Conditions_and_Diseases/Cancer
Yahoo	dir.yahoo.com/Health/Diseases_and_Conditions/Cancers
Association of Cancer Online Resources	**www.acor.org**
National Cancer Institute	www.cancer.gov
American Cancer Society	***www.cancer.org***
American Society of Clinical Oncology	www.plwc.org
University of Pennsylvania	www.oncolink.upenn.edu

present information specific to the specified type of cancer. For example, if a user specifies "health information seeker" as their interest group and "colon and rectal cancer" as the type of cancer of interest, selecting the "Who is at Risk?" link will return a page with general information about cancer risk (for example, "Tobacco and Cancer") as well as a box that includes information on risk factors for colon and rectal cancer.

Interactive decision support tools. Cancer.org links to NexCura decision support tools, which are designed to be used by laypersons to help them work more effectively with clinicians to make better decisions, and to National Comprehensive Cancer Network[5] treatment guidelines.

News. An "ACS News Center" box on the home page provides indexed news updates and inspirational stories.

Example. My father had cancer in his sixties and I am 35. What family history information should I collect before an appointment with my doctor?

- Go to cancer.org
- Follow the link to "Cancer Information Seekers"
- Follow the link to "Who is at Risk?"
- If "colon and rectal cancer has been specified in the users preferences, then a link to "What are the Risk Factors for Colon and Rectal Cancer?" will appear. Otherwise, the user can manually choose this type of cancer.

Locating Support Resources, Clinical Trials, or Oncologists

After diagnosis, most cancer patients require more emotional support than a doctor can realistically provide. Although most such emotional support is beyond the capabilities of computer infrastructure, digital infrastructure can help patients find and communicate with other cancer patients. At the NCI site, http://cancer.gov/cancerinfo/support/ points to information about support, support organizations, finding an oncologist, finances, insurance, and hospice care. For example, the "Taking Time" document includes "Cancer will change your life," "Your feelings: learning you have cancer," and "Living each day" sections.

At the ACS site, the "survivors" interest group also includes a variety of support resources for survivors and patients. ClinicalTrials.gov provides a database of federally and privately supported clinical research as well as background information. The American Society of Clinical Oncology Web resources include "People Living With Cancer," http://www.peoplelivingwithcancer.org," which has resources for finding clinical trials and oncologists.

Clinician Decisions

The importance of evidence-based decision support at the point of service is firmly established,[6] and many commercial medical informatics support products are available (Table 10.4). Many of these currently offer free limited term trials and support handheld devices. Below we describe some of the information resources that are components of a typical clinical knowledge base.

Technical summaries. In addition to summary text, technical summaries include links to other knowledge resources (including other technical summaries, guidelines, primary literature, and drug information). Such summaries may include information about authors, document status, and the last modification date. Free technical summaries can be found in the PDQ section of Cancer.gov (http://cancer.gov/pdq). Technical summaries related to cancer genetics can be found in the Online Mendelian Inheritance in Man (http://www.ncbi.nlm.nih.gov/OMIM). Appending "AND review[Publication Type]" to a PubMed query restricts the search to review articles.

TABLE 10.4. Commercial clinical information products.

Product	*URL*
UpToDate	uptodate.com
First Consult	firstconsult.com
MD Consult	mdconsult.com
InfoPOEMs	infopoems.com
WebMD	webmd.com

Guidelines. Computer interpretable guidelines[7–11] can provide formal and compact support for evidence-based decision making. Freely available cancer diagnosis and treatment guidelines are available at NGC[12] and NCCN.[5]

Directory. Users unfamiliar with the model of data in a clinical knowledge base benefit from manually curated sets of links to information resources. For example, the Physician Data Query (PDQ)[13,14] home page points to cancer information summary classes (adult treatment, pediatric treatment, supportive care, prevention, genetics, etc.) and clinical trials resources (search page, user's guide, or support for clinical trials submission) as well as help documentation that includes an annotated directory (which has extensive text along with headings).

Index. Most cancer information knowledge bases include a search box. After users enter a text string in a search box, a formal query is constructed, the formal query is compared against the documents in the database, and the matches are ordered. Formal queries may be constructed by interpreting "and" or "or" as Boolean operators rather than keywords, by default addition of Boolean operators, by stemming[15] words (so that, for example, "neoplasms" will match "neoplasm"), identifying approximate matches that catch spelling errors (for example, "endometril cancer" will match "endometrial cancer"), considering the semantic role of the words (for example, interpreting "Li" as an author name or as an element), expanding queries based on synonyms (so that, for example, "tumor" will match "neoplasm"), or expanding queries based on generalization/specialization relationships among vocabulary words (so that, for example, "surgery" in a query will match "mastectomy" in a document). Some resources allow subsequent queries to be applied only to the current results.

Drug information. Knowledge bases should include information on dosage, drug-drug interactions, and side effects. The U.S. Food and Drug Administration maintains a database of approved cancer drugs[16] that includes generic drug name, trade name, sponsor, pointers to sudy details, and dosage. Some PDQ entries are indexed by drugs; for example, entering "tamoxifen" in the search box returns a variety of relevant documents.

Clinical trials. It is important to access clinical trials databases to identify trials for which a patient is eligible and evidence bearing on treatment (evidence that may be preliminary from an ongoing study or final). http://clinicaltrials.gov supports identification of ongoing clinical trials based on facility, location, disease, and age group. Appending "AND clinical trials[Publication Type]" to a PubMed query restricts the scope of the search to reports on clinical trials.

Documents for laypersons. Although several knowledge bases for laypersons are described previously, a clinician's knowledge base should provide direct links from pages aimed at specialists to documents directed at laypersons.

Researchers' Decisions

Cancer researchers may act based on a collection of information that includes, for example, clinical trials, population data, scientific publications, nucleic acid or protein sequences, genes, genomes, human genetic variation, protein structures, protein domains, gene expression data, or taxonomy. Cancer information also includes relationships between these objects. For example, a gene may be related to a DNA sequence, a protein sequence, a somatic mutation database, publications describing the gene, and summary information about cancers related to genetic variation. Supporting navigation of such a heterogeneous colletion of objects based on relationships between them is a difficult problem.

NCBI

The U.S. National Center for Biotechnology Information,[17] or NCBI, was created by the U.S. Congress in 1988 as a division of the National Library of Medicine of the National Institutes of Health. The prescience of the architects of the NCBI and its resources is illustrated by the fact that NCBI resources, including GenBank,[18] PubMed,[19] and BLAST,[18,20–22] are perhaps the most widely known informatics tools for biologists and are used effectively by a wide variety of scientists and educators. Information relating the biologic objects listed above can be accessed through an intuitive search engine, Entrez, that allows users to identify subsets of entries matching search criteria. NCBI developed a programmer's toolkit and tools for remote data access before the emergence of the World Wide Web. NCBI declared its data model and described data using a formal exchange syntax (ASN.1) before the development of XML.

We do not have the space to cover NCBI tools comprehensively, so instead focus on a few key tools and an example that integrates use of several tools. Comprehensive and regularly updated documentation about NCBI resources is available online in the NCBI Handbook.[23]

Keyword-based searches. Entrez provides a consistent interface for querying a wide variety of NCBI databases, including publications, sequences, structures, genomes, genes, inherited disorders, and protein domains. The search box supports an unusually intelligent parser based on a controlled vocabulary (Medical Subject Heading, or MeSH[24]). For example, a naive query string such as "gene expression tumor treatment fibroblast 2004" is interpreted as ((((("gene expression"[MeSH Terms] OR gene expression[Text Word]) AND ((tumor[Text Word] OR tumour[Text Word]) OR "neoplasms"[MeSH Terms])) AND (("therapy"[MeSH Subheading] OR "therapeutics"[MeSH Terms]) OR treatment[Text Word])) AND ("fibroblasts"[MeSH Terms] OR fibroblast[Text Word])) AND 2004.[25]). The resulting query is sufficiently precise to retrieve a small number of publications, including, for example, a paper[26] on the use of microarrays for predicting the clinical course of several common carcinomas. Selecting the "Details" button shows explicitly how the query is interpreted. A "Preview/Index" button provides support for construction of precise Boolean queries based on the NCBI data model and controlled vocabularies. Additional "Links" provide additional features, including the addition of hypertext links from words or phrases in PubMed abstracts to related textbook entries.

Sequence-based searches. The BLAST family of tools[20–22,27] allows certain types of objects, nucleotide sequences (including genomes), protein sequences, and position-specific models of protein or protein domains, to be searched based on sequence features in addition to annotation. The BLAST tools have proven useful because of their ease of use, speed, and reliable statistics. These tools return not only matches to the query, but expectation values that provide an estimate of the number of matches of similar or greater similarity that would have been obtained under a null hypothesis (no related sequences are in the database). Thus, users need not rely on expert knowledge to judge the relevance of a match and can rely on common knowledge from probability and statistics.

Example. What is Li Fraumeni syndrome?

- Select the **OMIM** link from the menu bar http://www.ncbi.nlm.nih.gov. OMIM refers to the Online Mendelian Inheritance in Man,[28] a manually curated catalog of genes and genetic disorders. Enter "Li Fraumeni in the search box and execute the search.
- Follow the link to "Li Fraumeni syndrome LFS". This page includes a wide variety of text description of Li Fraumeni sydrome; for example, it indicates that LFS is a familial cancer syndrome of diverse tumors caused by certain mutations in the TP53 gene.
- Follow the link to the "TP53 gene," which indicates, among other useful information, that the p53 protein binds to and activates the expression of genes that inhibit growth or invasion.
- Following the "Allelic variants" link indicates that an Arg 248 to Trp mutation causes Li Fraumeni syndrome.
- Follow the link to "Cho et al"[29] to find an abstract of the paper describing the solution of the p53 structure. Selecting "Links/Books" adds hyperlinks from terms in the abstract to textbook entries describing the linked terms.
- Select "Links/Structure" and follow the link to 1TSR. If you have a structure viewer installed then selecting "View 3D structure" allows you to see that interactions of Arg 248 with the DNA binding site would be disrupted by an Arg248 to Trp mutation.

In this example, NCBI resources took us from the name of a syndrome to an atomic level hypothesis about the cause of the syndrome with a very small number of operations. The infrastructure developed by NCBI provides outstanding capacity for browsing sets of publications, sequences, structures, genes, and syndromes by traversing relationsihps between them.

European Bioinformatics Institute

Similar to the NCBI, the European Bioinformatics Institute,[30,31] part of the European Molecular Biology Laboratory, provides support for a wide variety of databases that include sequence, structure, protein family, mutations, and literature databases. Notable features include a uniform interface to germline and somatic locus-specific mutation databases, including APC, CDKN2a, RB1, and TP53 database, suppport for private management of queries and results, and the Universal Protein Knowledge Base.[15,32,33]

caBIG

The National Cancer Institute of the U.S. National Institutes of Health has undertaken construction of comprehensive cancer informatics infrastructure, the cancer Biomedical Informatics Grid (caBIG). caBIG includes data, vocabulary, standards, software infrastructure, and applications. Although the intial focus of this effort is on cancer, much of the infrastructure is generally useful in the biomedical sciences.

caBIG data currently include the Gene Expression Data Portal (GEDP[34]), Cancer Gene Anatomy Project (CGAP[35–38]), the Cancer Molecular Anatomy Project (CMAP[39]), and the cancer Model Organisms Databases (caMOD[40]). These resources integrate data describing the molecular anatomic changes that accompany tranformation of a cell from normal to cancerous. Users can approach these data from the perspective of microarray experiments, genes, tissues, pathways, chromosomes, cancer targets, targeted agents, trials, or cancer models.

The NCI Enterprise Vocabulary Service (EVS[41]) provides cancer-specific vocabulary in the context of mature vocabulary resources such as National Library of Medicine's Unified Medical Language System (UMLS[42–46]). EVS includes the NCI Thesaurus[47] and the NCI Metathesaurus.[48] The NCI Thesaurus provides a graph that can be browsed to find NCI Thesaurus concepts. Concept pages contain technical definitions, synonyms, more general concepts that include the current concept, and relationships to other concepts. For example, browsing from the top level to "Gene," to "DNA Repair Gene," and finally to "OGG1" yields the OGG1 concept entry. Browsing the entry reveals that OGG1 is a gene that encodes a protein that incises DNA at 8-oxoguanine residues, that it is also known as "8-Oxoguanine DNA Glycosylase," that it is included within the concept "DNA Repair Gene," and that it exhibits the "Gene_Found_In_Organism" relationship with the concept "Human." The power of such a vocabulary is not in such manual browsing, however, but in computer inference. A cancer researcher might be interested in finding human genes involved in DNA repair. The NCI Thesaurus would allow a computer to infer, for example, that something pertaining to OGG1, such as a gene expression level, also pertains to "DNA Repair Enzymes," or to include "OGG1" in a response to the question "Which DNA repair genes are found in humans?"

SEER-Medicare

Presumably standards for sharing electronic medical records will eventually allow virtual clinical trials, for example, researchers will identify patients satisifying specified characteristics based on shared medical records and compare the outcomes by treatment regimen. The Surveillance, Epidemiology and End Results (SEER) program of the NCI collects and distributes cancer incidence and survival data from cancer registries (representing about 14% of the U.S. population at the time of writing). Medicare records provide information about treatment claims for health care services. By linking these two datasets into the SEER-Medicare Linked Database,[49,50] investigators can evaluate diagnosis and treatment methods without having to recruit patients. More than 100 publications have made use of the SEER-Medicare database. For example, Potosky et al.[51] used the SEER-Medicare-linked database to assess reasons for a dramatic rise in prostate cancer incidence.

Summary

There is currently a wide variety of detailed cancer information available on the World Wide Web. We look forward to the integration of these resources into point-of-service support that integrates with patient data and will further reduce cancer-related pain and suffering (see Figure 10.1).

Acts are chosen based on data describing the context of the decision and evidence/knowledge bearing on the relative merit of acts based on the given context. Figure 10.1 is very general in that many acts that are not cancer related are based on evidence and context data (it is similar to a model of an agent,[52] a basic entity in the study of artificial intelligence). For example, e-business transactions include product information, evidence about purchasing patterns, context data that include a consumer's transaction history as well as highly sensitive (e.g., credit card) information, alerts, and sophisticated decision support tools that suggest transactions. Below, we provide examples of three classes of decisions that require informatics support: clinicians' decisions, laypersons' decisions, and researchers' decisions.

Clinicians' Decisions. Clinicians act based on patient information and medical knowledge. Rectangles in Box 1 represent classes of information, not individual information sources. For example, "Context Data" for a clinician decision include patient medical information in electronic medical records, handwritten notes, a patient's observations communicated verbally to the clinician, and unrecorded observations based on a physical exam. Scientific evidence comes from training, experience and medical literature. "Scientific evidence" is used here to include a broad range of evidence-based information that includes, for example, the seven warning signs of cancer and DNA mutation databases.

- How will estrogen therapy affect a particular patient's cancer risk?
- Does a patient's family history of cancer warrant genetic testing?
- A patient being seen for an aneuryism is otherwise healthy but a has spot on a chest X-ray. Should I refer for a biopsy, refer to take out a lobe of the lung, or follow noninvasively?

Laypersons' Decisions. Like clinicians, laypersons act based on their medical history and medical knowledge, but in practice these decisions are very different. Clinicians' and laypersons' acts may be of different types; for example, a clinician's act may be an order for a laboratory test, an act that is unavailable to laypersons. In practice, important acts of laypersons include finding an oncologist, finding a clinical trial, making an appointment with a clinician, identifying a question or observation to present to a clinician, gathering information before a visit to a clinician, a change in lifestyle, and worrying.

Even when clincians and laypersons are evaluating the same actions, however, clinicans' and laypersons' decisions are, in practice, made with very different informatics support. Clinicians make decisions based on formal medical records, years of professional training and experience, and peer-reviewed medical literature. Laypersons make decisions without such detailed and reliable support, because they may act based on an incomplete understanding of their medical history, limited medical knowledge, hearsay, and information they find on the World Wide Web that is not peer reviewed.

- Should I reduce my cell phone use to reduce my cancer risk?
- I have an unusual mole; do I have skin cancer?
- I have been diagnosed with cancer. How do I find an oncologist, clinical trial, or support group?

Researchers' Decisions. Researchers' acts include the design of experiments, including identification of hypotheses, and inference based on experimental results. For researchers the context data include their experimental data. Scientific evidence includes primary databases (for example, DNA sequence and clinical trials databases), primary literature, and technical synopses.

- Why did prostate cancer incidence increase dramatically in the late 1980s?
- What is the molecular cause of Li Fraumeni syndrome?
- Given gene expression data from a tumor, what is the course of a particular carcinoma?

References

1. Crichton M. The Andromeda Strain, 1st ed. New York: Knopf, 1969.
2. American College of Physicians–American Society of Internal Medicine. Carter JH (ed). Electronic Medical Records: A Guide for Physicians and Administrators, 1st ed. Philadelphia: American College of Physicians–American Society of Internal Medicine, 2001.
3. Health Insurance Portability and Accountability Act (HIPAA), http://www.hhs.gov/ocr/hipaa/
4. London JW, Morton DE, Marinnucco D, et al. The implementation of telemedicine within a community cancer network. J Am Med Inform Assoc 1997;4(1):18–24.
5. National Comprehensive Cancer Network, http://www.nccn.org/
6. Shortliffe EH. Medical Informatics: Computer Applications in Health Care and Biomedicine, 2nd ed. New York: Springer, 2001.
7. Tu SW, Campbell J, Musen MA. The structure of guideline recommendations: a synthesis. Proc AMIA Symp 2003;679–683.
8. Peleg M, Boxwala AA, Ogunyemi O, et al. GLIF3: the evolution of a guideline representation format. Proc AMIA Symp 2000; 645–649.
9. Ohno-Machado L, Gennari JH, Murphy SN, et al. The guideline interchange format: a model for representing guidelines. J Am Med Inform Assoc 1998;5(4):357–372.
10. Peleg M, Boxwala AA, Tu S, et al. The InterMed approach to sharable computer-interpretable guidelines: a review. J Am Med Inform Assoc 2004;11(1):1–10.
11. Peleg, M, Tu S, Bury J, et al. Comparing computer-interpretable guideline models: a case-study approach. J Am Med Inform Assoc 2003;10(1):52–68.
12. National Guideline Clearinghouse, http://www.guideline.gov/
13. Hubbard SM, et al. The Physician Data Query (PDQ) cancer information system. J Cancer Educ 1986;1(2):79–87.
14. Physician Data Query, http://www.cancer.gov/cancer_information/pdq/
15. Leinonen R, Diez FG, Binns D, et al. UniProt Archive. Bioinformatics 2004.
16. U.S. Food and Drug Administration: Oncology Tools.0
17. National Center for Biotechnology Information, http://www.ncbi.nlm.nih.gov/
18. Wheeler DL, Church DM, Edgar R, et al. Database resources of the National Center for Biotechnology Information: update. Nucleic Acids Res 2004;32(database issue):D35–D40.
19. NCBI PubMed, http://www.ncbi.nlm.nih.gov/PubMed
20. NCBI BLAST family of tools, http://www.ncbi.nlm.nih.gov/blast/
21. Altschul SF, Gish W, Miller W, et al. Basic local alignment search tool. J Mol Biol 1990;215(3):403–410.
22. Altschul SF, Madden TL, Schaffer AA, et al. Gapped BLAST and PSI-BLAST: a new generation of protein database search programs. Nucleic Acids Res 1997;25(17):3389–3402.
23. The NCBI Handbook, http://www.ncbi.nlm.nih.gov/books/bv.fcgi?call=bv.View..ShowSection&rid=handbook
24. Medical Subject Headings, http://www.nlm.nih.gov/mesh/meshhome.html
25. Herwig S, Strauss M. The retinoblastoma protein: a master regulator of cell cycle, differentiation and apoptosis. Eur J Biochem 1997;246(3):581–601.
26. Chang HY, Sneedon JB, Alizadeh AA, et al. Gene expression signature of fibroblast serum response predicts human cancer progression: similarities between tumors and wounds. PLoS Biol 2004;2(2):E7.
27. Wheeler DL, Church DM, Edgar R, et al. Database resources of the National Center for Biotechnology Information: 2002 update. Nucleic Acids Res 2002;30(1):13–16.
28. Hamosh A, Scott AF, Amberger J, et al. Online Mendelian Inheritance in Man (OMIM), a knowledgebase of human genes and genetic disorders. Nucleic Acids Res 2002;30(1): 52–55.
29. Cho Y, Sharma V, Sacchettini JC, et al. Crystal structure of a p53 tumor suppressor-DNA complex: understanding tumorigenic mutations. Science 1994;265(5170):346–355.
30. European Bioinformatics Institute.
31. Brooksbank C, Camon E, Harris MA, et al. The European Bioinformatics Institute's data resources. Nucleic Acids Res 2003;31(1):43–50.
32. Camon E, Barrell D, Lee V, et al. The Gene Ontology Annotation (GOA) Database: sharing knowledge in Uniprot with Gene Ontology. Nucleic Acids Res 2004;32(database issue):D262–D266.
33. Apweiler R, Bairoch A, Wu CH, et al. UniProt: the Universal Protein knowledgebase. Nucleic Acids Res, 2004;32(database issue):D115–D119.
34. Gene Expression Data Portal, http://gedp.nci.nih.gov/
35. Cancer Gene Anatomy Project, http://cgap.nci.nih.gov/
36. Strausberg RL, Ruetow KH, Greenhut SF, et al. The cancer genome anatomy project: building an annotated gene index. Trends Genet 2000;16(3):103–106.
37. Strausberg RL, Beutow KH, Greenhut SF, et al. The cancer genome anatomy project: online resources to reveal the molecular signatures of cancer. Cancer Invest 2002;20(7–8):1038–10-50.

38. Strausberg RL. The Cancer Genome Anatomy Project: new resources for reading the molecular signatures of cancer. J Pathol 2001;195(1):31–40.
39. Cancer Molecular Anatomy Project, http://cmap.nci.nih.gov/
40. Cancer Model Organisms Database, http://cancermodels.nci.nih.gov
41. NCI Enterprise Vocabulary Service, http://ncicb.nci.nih.gov/core/EVS
42. Unified Medical Language System, http://www.nlm.nih.gov/research/umls/
43. Browne AC, Divita G, Aronson AR, et al. UMLS Language and Vocabulary Tools. Proc AMIA Symp 2003;798.
44. Kashyap V. The UMLS Semantic Network and the Semantic Web. Proc AMIA Symp 2003;351–355.
45. Bangalore A, Thorn KE, Tilley C, et al. The UMLS Knowledge Source Server: an object model for delivering UMLS data. Proc AMIA Symp 2003;51–55.
46. Bodenreider O. The Unified Medical Language System (UMLS): integrating biomedical terminology. Nucleic Acids Res 2004; 32(database issue):D267–D270.
47. NCI Thesaurus, http://nciterms.nci.nih.gov/
48. NCI Metathesaurus.
49. SEER-Medicare Linked Database, http://healthservices.cancer.gov/seermedicare/
50. Warren JL, Klabunde CN, Schrag D, et al. Overview of the SEER-Medicare data: content, research applications, and generalizability to the United States elderly population. Med Care 2002; 40(suppl 8):IV-3–IV-18.
51. Potosky AL, Miller BA, Albertsen PC, et al. The role of increasing detection in the rising incidence of prostate cancer. JAMA 1995;273(7):548–552.
52. Russell SJ, Norvig P. Artificial Intelligence: A Modern Approach, 2nd ed. Upper Saddle River, NJ: Prentice Hall, 2003.
53. Baxevanis AD, Ouellette BFF. Bioinformatics: A Practical Guide to the Analysis of Genes and Proteins, 2nd ed. Methods of Biochemical Analysis, vol 43. New York: Wiley, 2001.
54. Mount DW. Bioinformatics : Sequence and Genome Analysis. Cold Spring Harbor, NY: Cold Spring Harbor Laboratory Press, 2001.
55. Nucleic Acids Research Database Issue, http://www3.oup.co.uk/nar/database/c/
56. Nucleic Acids Research Web Server Issue, http://nar.oupjournals.org/cgi/content/full/31/13/3289
57. Silva JS. Cancer Informatics: Essential Technologies for Clinical Trials. Health informatics. New York: Springer, 2000.
58. O'Carroll PW. Public Health Informatics and Information Systems. New York: Springer, 2003.
59. Norris TE. Informatics in Primary Care: Strategies in Information Management for the Healthcare Provider. New York: Springer, 2002.

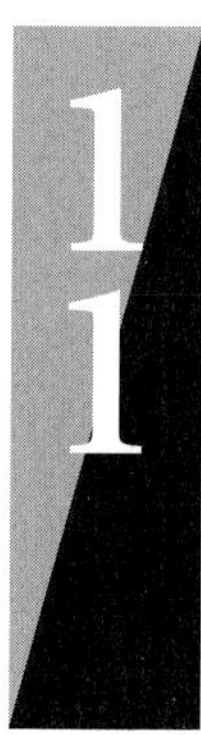

Economics of Cancer Care

James Khatcheressian and Thomas J. Smith

The Standard Principles of Economics and Oncology

Several major issues emerge when combining the "dismal science" of economics[1] with the science of oncology. With rising healthcare costs yet limited resources, it becomes important to know how to factor economic considerations into the medical decision-making process. This task is made more difficult by the paucity of comparative studies of costs and outcomes (under the general term of cost-effectiveness) and quality of life; as a result, clinicians are left on their own to decide "who does what to whom, at what cost, and with whose money."

The Cost of Care Is Increasing Rapidly at an Unsustainable Rate

Cancer care is second only to cardiovascular disease in terms of yearly cost to the healthcare system; expenditures for diagnosis, supportive care, and treatment are rising and pose an increasingly severe economic burden on society. Estimates from 2001 reveal that the United States spends $56 billion yearly on cancer treatment; additionally, $16 billion yearly is attributed to indirect morbidity costs and $85 billion for indirect mortality costs. To put this into perspective, medical care costs now are 15% and education now less than 5% of U.S. Gross National Product (GNP) (*New York Times*, January 9, 2004), whereas 30 years ago both medical care and education had 6% of the GNP[2]; additionally, these costs have risen over the past several years at an annual rate of 10% or higher. Medicare cancer drug costs *tripled* from $1.2 billion in 1998 to $3.8 billion in 2002 (Association of Community Cancer Centers Website, accessed August 20, 2003). Precise figures for private insurance, Medicaid, and direct patient costs are not available, but practice patterns are similar. Furthermore, as the baby boomer generation begins to reach retirement age, a time when they are most likely to develop cancer, the economic burden of cancer care and treatment will continue to rise.

How to Factor Economics into Medical Decision Making

With the increasing demand for expanded services, new technologies, and a growing elderly population, conflicts must arise between payers, clinicians, and patients regarding what services to provide, to whom, and on what basis. Our health economist colleague, Dr. Bruce Hillner, calls this the "What to do to whom, with whose money, at what cost?" question. There are several ways to factor economic costs and treatment effectiveness into decision making. The most informative types of analyses are cost-minimization, cost-effectiveness, and cost-utility; the methods are listed in Table 11.1. We briefly discuss each with regard to its advantages, liabilities, and possible application to clinical practice.

A significant problem is the reluctance of some clinicians and patients to accept limitation of resources or rationing by cost-effectiveness or any other method.[3] Although a full discussion of the thorny ethical, legal, and economic issues is beyond the scope of this chapter, some overriding factors based on our experience are listed in Table 11.2. Ethicists,[4,5] and now clinicians,[6] have argued that the least ethical way to allocate resources is to continue in the usual unexamined mode and that ignoring the economic issues is not morally defensible. Until there is general consensus in society on "what to do to whom, with whose money, at what cost," these issues will continue under debate. Concurrently, all payers have limited budgets, so they are doing some form of implicit or explicit rationing now.

Cost or Effectiveness Alone

Clinical Outcomes Alone

This type of study is concerned solely with clinical efficacy such as improved response rates, survival, and symptom management; it ignores treatment costs entirely. This is the easiest method by which to make decisions for treatments that are clearly superior to any others available. A good example of a medication that fits into this category is imatinab mesylate (gleevec) in the treatment of chronic myelogenous leukemia (CML). It clearly has better response rates, time to disease progression, and toxicity profile than the traditional treatment of interferon and cytarabine and has become the standard of care as first-line treatment for CML.[7] The decision to use imatinib mesylate is quite easy for physicians given the lack of any other similarly effective agents. But at $24,000/year (www.drugstore.com), an obvious economic consequence of this method is that some patients will not be able obtain a medication due to prohibitive costs, for instance, a 20% co-payment or lack of insurance.

TABLE 11.1. **Types of studies and application to oncology.**

Type of study	*Advantages and disadvantages*	*Application to oncology*
Clinical outcomes alone	Easy to perform. Ignores costs.	Traditional way to make decisions, e.g., imitinab mesylate (gleevec) works for chronic myelogenous leukemia (CML). Use it. Pay what the manufacturer demands.
Cost only	Ignores clinical outcomes.	Often used by insurers as first reaction to "sticker shock" of new drugs, e.g., zevalin at \$22,000–\$28,000/dose.
Costs and clinical outcomes together Cost minimization: assumes two strategies are equal; lowest cost strategy is preferred.	Easy to do if there are direct comparisons.	For instance, if darbopoietin is equivalent to epoietin for chemotherapy-associated anemia, choose the least expensive drug.
Cost-effectiveness: Compares two strategies; assigns \$ per additional year of life (LY) saved by strategy.	Requires a trial that directly compares strategies, and economic analysis alongside that trial. "Only accept treatments that gain a year of life for under \$100,000/life year."	There are very few direct comparisons of drugs and strategies. The trials typically must be large to detect small differences, are unexciting compared to new drug trials, and have no willing sponsor.
Cost-utility: assigns \$ per additional year of life (LY) saved by strategy, then estimates the quality of that benefit in \$/quality adjusted (QALY).	Compares two strategies, with their quality of life comparisons converted to utility, or the value placed on time in a health state, e.g., time spent on chemo = 0.7 compared to a healthy individual whose utility = 1.0.	There are few interventions that make a large difference in utility. Also, there is rarely one simple yardstick of utility that covers all health states.
Cost-benefit: Compares two strategies but converts the clinical benefits to money, e.g., a year of life is worth \$100,000.	Possible but rarely done due to difficulty in assigning \$ value to human life.	Would almost certainly be unfavorable to most palliative interventions, as patients rarely work or generate income.

The standard cost-effectiveness equation is $\Delta C/\Delta E = (C_2 - C_1)/(E_2 - E_1)$ where C = costs and E = effectiveness of treatment measured in time. For intervention 2, as its cost decreases or effectiveness improves, its CE ratio improves, i.e., decreased cost per year of life gained. When utility, or (life year gained) × (utility factor), is calculated, the equation becomes $\Delta C/\Delta U$ where $\Delta U = U_2 - U_1$. For example, a therapy that does not improve survival but decreases utility factor to 10% will decrease U by (1 year) × (0.10) = 0.1 year. If this treatment costs an additional \$10,000/year, then the cost-utility ratio is $\Delta C = C_2 - C_1$ = \$10,000 = \$100,000/QALY (the intervention is "less effective" because it adversely affects morbidity).

TABLE 11.2. **Difficulties in application of cost-effectiveness analysis or rationing by any method.**

Factor	*Pros, cons, and comment*
We should not ration health care at all.	Avoids the issues—for those able to afford unlimited care. Unsustainable, and not morally defensible in the current high-cost environment.[6] Rationing goes on all the time now, based on ability to pay.
There are no accepted guidelines to use.	This is one of the most daunting tasks: to have a uniform standard. For many years, an unwritten rule has been that technologies that cost \$50,000/LY or less were acceptable, based on the incremental cost of dialysis vs. no dialysis.[3] The great majority of published studies referenced that standard.[45] Laupacis and colleagues in Canada proposed that therapies under \$20,000/LY (\$ Canadian, 1992) be automatically accepted, that therapies \$20,000–\$100,000 be considered, and that therapies over \$100,000 be rejected.[46]
The cost-effectiveness ratio of \$50,000/LY is too low.	Recently, Ubel and colleagues have proposed that one of the main reasons cost-effectiveness is not more widely used is that \$50,000 is too low, and that with inflation and the affluence of the United States, a benchmark of \$100,000–\$200,000 is more appropriate.[45]
There are no unbiased studies.	Initial evidence was that industry-sponsored studies were more likely to be published if positive for their product[47] and that industry sponsored more cost-minimization studies, to show that their product was as cost-effective as the competition, but not to address the issue of whether the therapy was a good buy for society.[48] A comprehensive review suggests that quality control in most studies was low regardless of funding source and that industry-sponsored trials have improved.[49]
Clinicians should not ration at the bedside.	Clinicians have no training in this aspect of care, no framework for decisions, and were not able to adequately judge the appropriateness of their patient for care versus others.[50] Others argue that the healthcare budget should not be balanced by denying services to vulnerable groups such as the elderly.[51,52] Although clinicians may elect to not do these tasks, a more reasonable view is that clinicians should at least be involved, because someone must do it, and the decisions should be best informed.[5]
The individual always comes first.	Hadorn gave the name "the rule of rescue" to the compelling need of one visible patient (in this case, a 7-year-old with relapsed acute leukemia who might have a small chance of cure with a matched unrelated stem cell transplant) to the less-visible needs of many others who might also need those same healthcare dollars.[53] This rule nearly collapsed the Oregon expansion of Medicaid services to the uninsured; a mechanism for appeals of individual decisions is always necessary, but some services cannot be provided.

Cost Only

This type of study ignores clinical outcomes and relies exclusively upon the expense of a treatment or strategy. Many newer and more expensive agents improve quality and quantity of life (cetuximab, bevicizimab, irinotecan, or oxaliplatin in metastatic colon cancer; all at $2,000–$4,000 per treatment).[6] This type of method is often used by insurers as a rationale to not cover particular medications that may be efficacious but do not have enough supporting data to become a requisite standard of care. Ibritumomab tiuxetan (zevalin), an yttrium-90 antibody to CD20, is an active agent against non-Hodgkins lymphoma (NHL), but may register acute "sticker-shock" effect with many payers at $22,000–$28,000 per dose. And although it appears to have definite activity in NHL, it has not yet evolved into a definitive treatment choice in the algorithm of salvage therapy, at least in part because payers may not reimburse for its use. Unfortunately, cost alone does not help clinicians choose among a variety of therapeutic strategies, unless out-of-pocket expenses for patients make treatment unattainable.

Combining Cost and Effectiveness

Cost Minimization

Simply put, with cost minimization two equally effective strategies are compared in terms of cost, and the less-expensive strategy is chosen. Oftentimes, an assumption of equivalent efficacy of the two interventions must be made based on indirect evidence, that is, drug A and B are shown to have similar response rates, but in separate Phase II trials rather than head-to-head studies. Manufacturers are reluctant to design direct comparative studies for fear of losing market share should their product appear inferior.[8] For example, darbepoietin and erythropoietin have not been directly compared in a large randomized trial until now, but available data indicate they are likely equivalent in the treatment of anemia; therefore, by the cost-minimization method, the less-expensive drug is preferable. This method is most useful when trying to choose between drugs in the same class, such as the hematopoietic growth factors just mentioned. However, assuming equivalent efficacy of drugs from different classes based on noncomparative studies would be fraught with bias.

Cost-Effectiveness

This method compares two known but not equally efficacious strategies and assigns a cost per additional year of life (LY) saved by the best ("dominant") strategy. Treatment A, which gains 1 month of survival at a cost of $2,000, has a cost-effectiveness ratio of $24,000/LY. This cost per unit of effectiveness fosters a reasonable basis of comparison and can be put into a "League Table" (like team standings) so that decision makers can compare alternative uses of the same money. The gold standard way to get this information is to append a concurrent economic analysis to the trial, but such trials can also be done retrospectively after the trial has closed, so long as the assumptions and conclusions are justifiable ("robust").

For this type of study to be clinically applicable, a limit must be set on the cost that society will pay for the additional year of life saved; otherwise, there is no reason to do the study or impetus for making the strategy more efficient. For example, a typical limit often used is in the range of $50,000 to $100,000 per additional year of life saved. By setting this limit, one can then reanalyze the intervention to determine how to improve the cost-effectiveness ratio. There are only two ways to improve the ratio: increase effectiveness or lower costs. Most studies use only the published cost of a drug or intervention. Health economists would argue that the cost of an intervention, including drug price, hospital cost, and physician fees, should always be on the bargaining table. A therapy that costs $4,000 to save a month of life looks a lot more attractive to payers if the drug cost is reduced to $1,000 to save that same month! Clinicians should note that the current gold standard for studies is that 1 month of added survival for 12 people is as important as 12 months for 1 person or a chance at cure for a small percentage of people.

Cost Utility

Cost-effectiveness looks only at survival: quantity rather than quality of life gained. Morbidity associated with diagnosis, treatment, or complications is not factored into the calculation for effectiveness. In cost utility, the quality of life in a given state of disease or treatment is converted to a utility ratio where 1.0 equals perfect health and 0 equals death. For example, a patient without evidence of disease after breast-conserving surgery may have a utility range of 0.90 to 1.00, whereas a patient with progressive metastatic breast cancer may have a utility range of 0.40 to 0.60. The utility ratio converts "cost-effectiveness" into cost per quality-adjusted life-year (QALY). For example, an intervention that costs $10,000 per year of life gained would be converted to $20,000 per QALY if the treatment's toxicity lowered the patient's utility from 1.0 to 0.5 so that only half of a quality-adjusted year was gained. Because utility can be assigned to any disease state, it can be used to compare different strategies across a variety of clinical conditions; survival and quality of life (which may be affected by the treatment, disease state, or both) are combined to arrive at a more realistic cost per year of life gained or, more specifically, cost per QALY.

One difficulty with this method is assigning proper utility ratios. Quality of life assessments are, by nature, subjective and lack a single, standard reference as a guide. Attributes tested usually include, but are not limited to, variables such as emotion, mobility, cognition, and pain. Controversy exists as to the most appropriate source for such testing, whether patients, healthcare workers, or the general population (society) due to differences in perspective. Patients and clinicians view the medical process differently and consequently place greater emphasis on the issues (such as life, morbidity, expense) that matter most to them. For example, patients are more likely than clinicians expect, to accept toxic treatments in exchange for minor clinical benefits,[9–15] although there is variability,[16] whereas a clinician may place more emphasis on functional status than a patient would. The most objective source and that least prone to personal bias is probably lay people (jurors) as recommended by national consensus panels.[17] The difficulty in this lies in properly educating the jurors in all aspects of a patient's experience: emotional

TABLE 11.3. **Examples of utility ranges.**

Disease state	*Utility range: 0 = dead 1 = perfect health*
Last month of life with acute leukemia	0.00
Metastatic breast cancer, last month of life	0.16–0.54
Extensive small cell lung cancer (SCLC), progressive disease	0.31
Metastatic prostate, depending on symptoms	0.42–0.58
Advanced ovarian cancer, responding to chemotherapy	0.71
Anxiety/discomfort from thoracoscopy	0.88
Induction interferon for stage II/III melanoma	0.94
Extensive SCLC, complete remission	0.99
Hydroxyurea for CML	1.00

turmoil, treatment toxicity, inconvenience, and other physical and psychosocial stressors. Quality of life scores can also be converted to utility values[18] using validated methods, but oftentimes quality of life scores are so high that there is little discrimination between treatments. We have listed some representative utility values for time spent in various cancer states in Table 11.3.

Cost Benefit

This method compares two interventions but assigns the clinical benefit a monetary value; for example, a year of life is worth $100,000. The figure is usually based on factors related to the overall economic productivity of an individual. Therefore, a treatment that costs $10,000 to prolong life 1 year might be valued if the person generates $100,000/year of value to society but not valued if the person is not productive. This kind of analysis, although common in the areas of business, insurance adjustment, and economics, is rarely used in clinical studies because of the difficulties in assigning a monetary value to a human life, especially if that value is tied into an individual's socioeconomic status. Additionally, this method would almost certainly have a negative impact on most palliative care interventions because these patients rarely generate income.

We have listed a summary of cost-utility studies in Table 11.4 for comparison. Although many of these studies were performed over a number of years with disparate means of analysis and ranges of utility values factored into their equation, they are more likely to be accurate than no data at all and can form the basis of discussion.

How to Apply Cost-Effectiveness Data

The question of how to apply cost and effectiveness data to clinical practice is difficult to answer, as there is no one standard that is universally accepted. A Canadian schema has been widely accepted as one reasonable approach, but it is not used in the United States.[19] Some benchmarks, and representative cost-effectiveness analyses, are listed in Table 11.5. The difficulty in developing a single accepted standard of what is explicit "healthcare rationing" lies in the varied and conflicting motives, points of view, and concerns of the three P's of the healthcare system: patients, physicians, and payers. The perspectives of each are listed in Table 11.6.

The perspective of cancer *patients* is different from that of well people; they are more willing to accept toxic treatments, for perceived minor benefits, than most would imagine. Generally, from studies available, these patients are willing to undergo toxic chemotherapy for a less than 10% chance of cure, 3 months of life prolongation, or greater than 10% chance of symptom relief,[9–12] although there is variation among patients.[16] Furthermore, there is no reason for a patient to be concerned with treatment costs until their out-of-pockets expenses become prohibitive; until they reach this limiting threshold, they may feel entitled to treatment regardless of the cost.

Physicians may find themselves trapped in the uncomfortable middle ground between their patients' desire for all possible treatment alternatives and societal, or payer, demand to limit treatment costs. For most physicians there is no

TABLE 11.4. **Cost-effectiveness of representative cancer treatments.**

Intervention	*Cost/year of life added*
Immunoglobulin for chronic lymphocytic leukemia	$7,900,000
Autologous bone marrow transplant (ABMT) for all relapsed Hodgkins disease	$421,000
Antiemesis with ondansetron vs. metoclopramide in cisplatin regimens	$190,000–$460,000
IDDS vs. CMM, "as randomized"	$239,000–$297,000
First-line fluorouracil (5-FU)-based chemotherapy vs. best supportive care, pancreas/biliary cancer	$120,000
Pamidronate to reduce skeletal complications in breast cancer	$119,000
Breast cancer screening, elderly	$70,000–$140,000
Adjuvant CMF, 75-year-old woman	$58,000
5-FU-based treatment for GI cancers	$31,000
Adjuvant tamoxifen + CMF, ER + women	$14,000–$33,000
Breast conservation vs. mastectomy	$21,000
Biopsy versus no biopsy for 50-year-old man with elevated prostate-specific antigen (PSA) levels	Less than $0

TABLE 11.5. **Barriers to use of cost and cost-effectiveness data.**

Group	*Barrier*
Patients	—Patients are more willing to receive toxic treatments for small benefits than well people —Patients may feel entitled to treatment regardless of cost —Cost may not become an issue for patients until out-of-pocket expenses are prohibitive —Strict effectiveness data may not reflect improved quality of life seen with palliative treatments
Physicians	—Physicians may be trapped between patient demands for all possible treatment and societal demand to limit care —For most physicians, there are no rewards to limiting care —For many oncologists, the supportive care drugs with high incremental cost-effectiveness ratios may be the most lucrative to the practice
Payers/government	—Payers may not want to antagonize their secondary constituents, consumers, by not covering some desired services based on cost-effectiveness data —The lawsuits about high-dose chemotherapy with stem cell transplant for metastatic breast cancer make some payers leery of confrontation

incentive to limit a patient's access to care; in fact, for many oncologists the supportive care drugs such as erythropoietin, filgrastim, and bisphosphonates help support their practice. Physicians may also be hesitant to set limits on cancer care of their own accord outside of widely accepted professional standards; this is both uncomfortable for the physician and probably inappropriate bedside medical rationing that may not be based on sound evidence. For example, a physician may decide that palliative radiation therapy for painful bone metastases should be replaced by opioid medication alone because costs of radiotherapy are assumed to be very high. In fact, studies tell us that radiotherapy in such settings is indeed cost-effective and falls well within accepted ratio standards.[20] In the interest of balancing the appropriate delivery of care with responsible financial prudence, clinical guidelines addressing these issues should continue to be examined by appropriate consensus groups.[21]

Payers often need to balance their need to cut costs by limiting coverage for certain diagnostic or therapeutic interventions with the image they must present to the public, their secondary constituents, and consumers: that of an organization that is primarily concerned with the medical well-being of their clients, rather than their own fiscal health. The federal government, in the form of Medicare and Medicaid, shares the same concerns of private payers.[19]

TABLE 11.6. **A framework on how to apply cost-effectiveness data.**

Category	*Consideration*	*Comment*
Treatment A is more effective and saves money compared with treatment B	Use treatment A	Hypofractionated (single-dose) radiation for bone metastases vs. multiple dose schemes[32] PET scans before thoracotomy prevent 21% of futile thoracotomies[26]
Incremental cost-effectiveness of treatment A $0–$50,000	Use treatment A, as likely appropriate use of societal resources	Several widely used interventions fall here: —Guideline-based pain management vs. oncology-based care[55] —Adjuvant therapy for breast cancer —Adjuvant therapy for colon cancer —Stem cell transplantation vs. melphalan and prednisone for myeloma patients under 65[56]
Incremental cost-effectiveness of treatment A $50,000–$100,000	Consider treatment A	Routine preoperative head CT (vs. none) for resectable lung cancer with no evidence of CNS disease[57] Breast cancer screening (vs. none) in women older than 75[58]
Incremental cost-effectiveness of treatment A more than $100,000	Do not use treatment A	Several widely used interventions fall here: —Bisphosphonates for breast and myeloma cancer[59] —Selective 5-HT3 antagonists for antiemesis (reviewed by Earle et al.[54]) —Radiotherapy boost to whole breast radiation as part of primary therapy[60] —Trastuzamab for metastatic breast cancer[61]

The Lack of Studies

There are a small number of recent studies looking at the issue of cost-effectiveness and cost utility. Barriers to performing such studies include, but are not limited to (1) lack of sponsorship; (2) cooperative group efforts to accrue large enough sample sizes to detect the small differences seen; and (3) the lack of glamour associated with studies that seek to limit resource utilization and possibly come to uncomfortable conclusions regarding how to ration health care.

These studies generate little enthusiasm as they require large patient populations to detect relatively small differences in cost-effectiveness, and there are rarely additional funds to support them. Cooperative groups are more interested in spending money on trials of new therapies than showing cost-effectiveness (partly because there is no ready market for the results), and sponsors are not willing to spend money that puts their product at risk. Several pharmacoeconomic trials that made perfect sense to perform in the cooperative group setting, based on preliminary data, generated no support. The first suggested trial tested 2 μg/kg filgrastim instead of 5 μg/kg filgrastim for prevention of neutropenia, based on a small randomized trial that showed equivalence.[22,23] The second trial would have used bisphosphonates to prevent skeletal complications from metastatic breast cancer every 3 months rather than monthly, as monthly pamidronate had a cost-effectiveness ratio outside the usually accepted bounds.[24] Both trials were turned down by the cooperative group for similar reasons: the job of the cooperative group is to cure cancer, not to save money; someone else should concentrate on saving money; and there are more important questions to answer from the same budget. Drug or device companies may not have much reason to do this, either: the only aspect of a large randomized clinical trial in cancer pain management[24] that was not funded by the company was the cost-effective analysis.

Comfort levels of this type of healthcare rationing may also depend on where a clinician practices. In general, Americans spend more on heroic end-of-life intervention than their European counterparts, who are more likely to divert healthcare dollars into preventive strategies. In the United States, more than 20% of all medical expenditures are spent on the last year of a patient's life.[25]

Studies That Have Changed—or Could Change—Practice

There are a number of studies that would seem appropriate for economic evaluation because of high costs, small benefit, large societal impact, or some combination of these (Table 11.7). Cost or cost-minimization analysis showed that positron emission tomography (PET) scans prevented 21% of futile thoracotomies for resectable small cell lung cancer[26]; one could argue that PET scans would be used anyway, but they appear to lower costs overall by preventing more expensive surgery. The nonplatinum combination of gemcitabine-paclitaxel was no better or less toxic than other regimens in a large randomized trial and cost 25% more.[27] Our own analysis of inpatient palliative care units showed a 60% cost savings in a matched case-control set and prospective clinical-financial analysis.[28] Many other studies were done, but in general, they would not be expected to have either a clinical or economic impact, so are not included.

Cost-effectiveness studies showed that some commonly used treatments were within the range of accepted cost-effectiveness ratios but some were not. Postmastectomy radiation in premenopausal women improved survival at a cost of $24,900/LY. Capecitabine/docetaxel in metastatic breast cancer, compared to docetaxel alone, improved survival by 3 months[29] at a cost-effectiveness ratio[30] of approximately $3,700/LY (Canadian), well within accepted standards of treatment. In this study, utility was not included but the magnitude of survival benefit would likely offset the negative effects of toxicity associated with capecitabine. Of note, the alternative strategies of sequential therapies were not tested, so no conclusion can be drawn. A more expensive initial strategy, autologous stem cell transplant for myeloma instead of melphalan and prednisone, had longer survival that offset the cost, so the incremental cost-effectiveness was acceptable. One recent study[31] looked at cost-effectiveness through a spreadsheet-based model comparing three strategies for treating pain caused by cancer: guideline-based care, oncology-based care, and usual care. Treatment strategies included medications and procedure-based interventions. The effectiveness unit used was "additional patient relieved of cancer pain," rather than the typical additional year of life gained. Guideline-based care (GBC) was more effective at relieving cancer pain compared to oncology-based care (OBC) or usual care (UC): 80% versus 55% and 30%, respectively. The incremental cost-effectiveness for GBC compared to OBC was $452 per additional patient relieved of cancer pain, whereas the cost-effectiveness of OBC compared to UC was $601 per additional patient relieved of cancer pain.

Several cost-utility studies produced noteworthy results. Single fraction radiation for painful bone metastases instead of the usual six treatments was as effective and cost substantially less.[32] Gordois and colleagues analyzed the impact of imatinib mesylate (gleevec) in the treatment of accelerated-phase CML and blast crisis CML compared to conventional chemotherapy and palliative care in hospital or at home.[33] Imitinab mesylate improved QALYs in accelerated-phase CML of 2.09 years at $45,000/QALY and in blast crisis CML of approximately 0.58 months at $63,000/QALY. An analysis of imitinab mesylate in chronic-phase CML, a much more common and costly treatment, compared with interferon and cytarabine, or bone marrow transplantation, has not yet been published in the English literature. Testing for HER-2 positivity by various methods, and treatment with trastuzamab if HER-2 positive, gave better survival by a few months; however, the cost was always over $100,000/LY.[34] The more common and economically important question, at what cost does trastuzamab gain a year of life, especially in second- or third-line treatment, was not addressed.

Many important advances of the past years have not been studied, including the cost-effectiveness of adjuvant therapy for non-small cell lung cancer, dose-dense therapy of breast cancer, and the effectiveness and cost-effectiveness of most palliative chemotherapy regimens.

TABLE 11.7. Evidence-based new data.

Trial	*Reference*	*Year*	*No. of patients*	*Randomized*	*Stage*	*Intervention*	*Median follow-up*	*Outcome of interest*	*Conclusion*
Cost or cost minimization									
PET scan in resectable NSCLC	Verboun[26]	2002	188	Y	I-IV	Conventional workup vs. PET scan preop	1 year after surgery	21% of futile thoracotomies vs. 41% with CWU; avoided 1 in 5; cost saving	PET scan improves preop screening, lowers costs
Cisplatin-paclitaxel, P-gemcitabine, vs. PG	Smit[27]	2003	480	Y	IIIB-IV	C + P vs. C + G vs. P + G	1 year	OS similar; no differences except P + G, cost 25% more	No advantage, higher cost for nonplatinum combinations
Palliative care inpatient units	Smith[28]	2003	180	N	End of life	High-volume expert providers, standardized care, algorithms	NA	60% reduction in cost of care compared to usual care, health outcomes similar	Inpatient palliative care units may improve care at less cost
Cost-effectiveness									
Post-mastectomy radiation therapy in premenopausal women	Lee[61]	2002	DA	Y	I-III	Postmastectomy radiation therapy in premenopausal women vs. none	15 years	Relative risk of death reduced to 0.69; adds 0.29 LY at $24,900/LY	Cost-effectiveness ratio acceptable
Capecitabine + docetaxol vs. docetaxol alone	Verma[29,30]	2003		Y	IV	Capecitabine + docetaxol vs. docetaxol alone	NS	Combination gives additional 3 months at cost of $3,700/LY (Canadian)	Cost-effectiveness ratio acceptable; with improved survival, utility not likely to be important; trial did not have Capecitabine-alone arm for comparison, or test sequential therapy
Autologous stem cell transplant vs. chemotherapy in myeloma	Kouraoukis[56]	2003	36 ASCT, 16 M & P	N	Advanced	ASCT vs. M & P patients < 65, single center		Increased OS by 19.3 months, cost-effectiveness $13,000–$64,000/LY (Can)	Cost-effectiveness acceptable under best and worst case scenarios
Pain control	Abernathy[31]	2003	DA using published data	Some		Pain control with guidelines (G), oncology (O), usual care (U)		Pain control achieved at 1 month in 80%, 55%, and 30%, respectively ICE for guideline-based care $452/patient.	Acceptable cost per outcome using guidelines to improve pain control
Cost-utility									
Single vs. 6 fractions radiation for painful bone metastases	Van den Hout[32]	2003	Y						
Testing for HER-2 positivity		2004	DA using published data			Testing strategies of immunotesting first, with FISH after, or FISH		All dominant strategies over $100,000/LY	Authors suggest if society willing to pay for trastuzamab, should be willing to pay for optimal testing; avoids question of whether trastuzamab cost-effectiveness is acceptable

CWU, conventional workup; NSCLC, non small cell lung cancer; P, paclitaxel; G. gemcitabine; NA, not available; NS, not stated; DA, decision analysis; FISH, fluorescence in situ hybridization; ICE, ifosfamide (Ifex®), carboplatin (Paraplatin®), and etoposide (VP-16, VePesid®).

The 2004 Clinical and Research Challenges in Economics and How the Principles and Practice of Oncology May Be Changing

Continued increases in patient demands coupled with escalating costs, without subsequent raises in insurance premiums, will ensure some means of rationing in the future. Cost and effectiveness analyses offer some way to set a level playing field for old and new technologies and competing interests.

Cost-effectiveness analyses can be done successfully either alongside a clinical trial, when economic interests are especially prominent,[35] or retrospectively, after a therapy is shown to be effective, but the cost is high. Cooperative groups, industry groups, or individual researchers can do such trials. There is always a potential for publication bias, or industry supporting only those trials that are likely to show their product is within the fundable range of cost-effectiveness ratios, as with clinical trials. Funding for these trials will remain problematic as long as these trials are competing for the same funds as regular clinical or quality of life trials.

The impact of cost-effectiveness studies has been hard to gauge. Reflecting over the past years, we can think of only several examples of the importance of cost-effectiveness studies. When adjuvant chemotherapy for women with node-negative breast cancer was first endorsed, a major objection was the cost, estimated at $300 million or more yearly in the United States.[36] Subsequent studies showed that adjuvant treatments had similar cost-effectiveness ratios to the treatment of hypertension, and were clearly acceptable.[37,38] Similar objections were raised to the use of chemotherapy for advanced non-small cell lung cancer, with only a few months of time gained compared to best supportive care, but subsequent analyses showed that chemotherapy could actually be cost saving[39] or have very acceptable cost-effectiveness ratios.[40] Chemotherapy with mitoxantrone in advanced prostate cancer showed no survival benefit[41] but actual cost savings due to avoided radiation and hospitalizations.[42] Royle and Waugh showed that a relatively simple strategy of searching Medline and similar databases is sufficient for finding cost-effectiveness studies,[43] so the process of updates should not be difficult. It is important to factor in the cost of the intervention, if a change in prescribing practices is sought, as some interventions may cost more than the cost savings generated, especially with low-cost drugs; this is not likely to be the case in cancer treatment.[44]

Summary

In the United States, the cost of health care is now equal to 15% of the Gross National Product, the highest ever, and is growing at more than 10% annually. Costs rise in response to increased demand for new therapeutic and diagnostic technologies, and as the population ages. Given the limited resources of payers, an evidence-based and practical method is needed to mesh our desire for expanded treatment choices with the reality of limited healthcare dollars. Cost-effectiveness, defined as the amount of money spent to gain an additional year of life (LY) by treatment A compared to treatment B, is one accepted method of analysis and allocation of resources. Cost-utility assessments, which generate quality-adjusted life-years (QALY), adjust cost-effectiveness to account for the morbidity associated with treatment and illness. We review recent data supporting evidence-based decision making, some high-profile studies that have changed clinical practice, and the economic implication of such changes.

Few studies have integrated cost-effectiveness into their design for a variety of economic and logistic reasons, but such studies are needed if we are to make treatment decisions that are both clinically sound and economically prudent. Once the data are published, clinicians need commonly agreed-upon standards to make treatment decisions that account for cost and effectiveness, such as "Use therapies that cost $100,000/LY or less and do not use therapies that cost $200,000/LY and more." If the cost-effectiveness ratio is too high, then the cost of the therapy could be lowered, such as by convincing pharmaceutical manufacturers to lower the cost of a drug.

There are examples of cost-minimization and cost-effectiveness analysis helping in the decision to allocate resources. Hospital-based palliative care consultation teams and inpatient units provide equal or better care and can save as much as 60% per day compared to standard hospital care, and such programs are growing rapidly. PET scanning, although very expensive, reduces futile thoracotomies of potentially resectable non-small cell lung cancer for one of five patients and can be cost saving; however, it would still be used even if it cost additional money. Chemotherapy for metastatic prostate cancer improves symptoms but has limited impact on survival; surprisingly, to many, the cost of chemotherapy is more than offset by avoided complications, such that the cost-effectiveness is acceptable. Imitinab mesylate for CML, bisphosphonates used to prevent skeletal complication in breast cancer and multiple myeloma, trastuzamab for breast cancer, and expensive antiemetics, such as serotonin antagonists, have a cost-effectiveness ratio of more than $100,000/LY, well outside the $50,000/LY parameters normally accepted as appropriate for cost-effectiveness. However, the treatments are widely used and accepted as the standard of care. Other effective strategies that use costly interventions such as dose-dense chemotherapy in the adjuvant setting for breast cancer, supported by filgrastim at $1,000 to $2,000/cycle, clearly have benefit but have not even been studied.

Cost-effectiveness studies offer an objective method by which to base resource allocation decisions, rather than solely relying on the response rate or survival benefit of a particular strategy. Few new cost-effectiveness or cost-utility studies have changed practice, and many expensive accepted strategies have been adopted without any consideration of cost. The rapid growth of new and expensive strategies with rapid cost escalation increases the need for unbiased cost-effectiveness studies and generally accepted guidelines with which to apply the results.

References

1. Smith A. An inquiry into the nature and causes of the wealth of nations. In: Cannan E (ed). London: Methuen, 1904:1723–1790.
2. Lamm RD. The ghost of health care future. Inquiry 1994;31:365–367.

3. Smith TJ, Hillner BE, Desch CE. Efficacy and cost-effectiveness of cancer treatment: rational allocation of resources based on decision analysis. JNCI 1993;85:1460–1474.
4. Bochner F, Martin ED, Burgess ND, Somogyi AA, Misan GM: How can hospitals ration drugs? Drug rationing in a teaching hospital: a method to assign priorities. Drug Committee of the Royal Adelaide Hospital. BMJ 1994;308:901–905.
5. Smith TJ, Bodurtha JN. Ethical considerations in oncology: balancing the interests of patients, oncologists, and society. J Clin Oncol 1995;13(9):2464–2470.
6. Schrag D. The price tag on progress: chemotherapy for colorectal cancer. N Engl J Med 2004;351(4):317–319.
7. Druker BJ. Imatinib alone and in combination for chronic myeloid leukemia. Semin Hematol 2003;40(1):50–58.
8. Bennett CL, Smith TJ, George SL, Hillner BE, Fleishman S, Niell HB. Free-riding and the prisoner's dilemma: problems in funding economic analyses of phase III cancer clinical trials. J Clin Oncol 1995;13:2457–2463.
9. Tamburini M, Buccheri G, Brunelli C, Ferrigno D. The difficult choice of chemotherapy in patients with unresectable non-small cell lung cancer. Support Care Cancer 2000;8(3):223–228.
10. Slevin ML, Stubbs L, Plant HJ, et al. Attitudes to chemotherapy: comparing views of patients with cancer with those of doctors, nurses, and general public. BMJ 1990;300:1458–1460.
11. Balmer CE, Thomas P, Osborne RJ. Who wants second-line, palliative chemotherapy? Psycho-Oncology 2001;10:410–418.
12. Bremnes RM, Andersen K, Wist EA. Cancer patients, doctors and nurses vary in their willingness to undertake cancer chemotherapy. Eur J Cancer 1995;31A(12):1917–1918.
13. Davies E, Clarke C, Hopkins A. Malignant cerebral glioma. I: Survival, disability, and morbidity after radiotherapy. BMJ 1996;313:1507–1512.
14. Davies E, Clarke C, Hopkins A. Malignant cerebral glioma. II: Perspectives of patients and relatives on the value of radiotherapy. BMJ 1996;313:1512–1516.
15. Meystre CJN, Burley NMJ, Ahmedzai S. What investigations and procedures do patients in hospices want? Interview based survey of patients and their nurses. BMJ 1997;315:1202–1203.
16. Silvestri G, Pritchard R, Welch HG. Preferences for chemotherapy in patients with advanced non-small cell lung cancer: descriptive study based on scripted interviews. BMJ 1998; 317(7161):771–775.
17. Siegel JE, Weinstein MC, Russell LB, Gold MR. Recommendations for reporting cost-effectiveness analyses. JAMA 1996; 276(16):1339–1341.
18. O'Leary JF, Fairclough DL, Jankowski MK, Weeks JC. Comparison of time-trade-off utilities and rating scale values of cancer patients and their relatives: evidence for a possible plateau relationship. Med Decis Making 1995;15:132–137.
19. Tunis SR. Why Medicare has not established criteria for coverage decisions. N Engl J Med 2004;350:2196–2198.
20. Barton MB, Jacob SA, Gebsky V. Utility-adjusted analysis of the cost of palliative radiotherapy for bone metastases. Australas Radiol 2003;47:274–278.
21. Russell LB, Gold MR, Siegel JE, Daniels N, Weinstein MC. The role of cost-effectiveness analysis in health and medicine. JAMA 1996;276(14):1172–1177.
22. Toner GC, Shapiro JD, Laidlaw CR, et al. Low-dose versus standard-dose lenograstim prophylaxis after chemotherapy: a randomized, crossover comparison. J Clin Oncol 1998;16:3874–3879.
23. Juan O, Campos JM, Caranana V, Sanchez JJ, Casan R, Alberola V. A randomized, crossover comparison of standard-dose versus low-dose lenograstim in the prophylaxis of post-chemotherapy neutropenia. Support Care Cancer 2001;9(4):241–246.
24. Smith TJ, Staats PS, Deer T, et al. Randomized clinical trial of an implantable drug delivery system compared with comprehensive medical management for refractory cancer pain: impact on pain, drug-related toxicity, and survival. J Clin Oncol 2002; 20:4040–4049.
25. Hoover DR, Crystal S, Kumar R, Sambamoorthi U, Cantor JC. Medical expenditures during the last year of life: findings from the 1992–1996 Medicare Current Beneficiary Survey. Health Serv Res 2002;37(6):1625–1642.
26. Verboom P, van Tinteren H, Hoekstra OS, et al. PLUS study group. Cost-effectiveness of FDG-PET in staging non-small cell lung cancer: the PLUS study. Eur J Nucl Med Mol Imaging 2003;30(11):1444–1449.
27. van Smit EF, Meerbeeck JP, Lianes P, et al. Three-arm randomized study of two cisplatin-based regimen and paclitaxel plus gemcitabine in advanced non-small-cell lung cancer: a phase III trial of the European Organization for Research and Treatment of Cancer Lung Cancer Group–EORTC 08975. J Clin Oncol 2003;21(21):3909–3917.
28. Smith TJ, Cassel JB, Coyne PJ, Hager MA. Quality of care and cost savings associated with an inpatient high volume, standardized-care palliative care unit. J Palliat Med 2003; (in press).
29. O'Shaughnessy J, Miles D, Vukelja S, et al. Superior survival with capecitabine plus docetaxel combination therapy in anthracycline-pretreated patients with advanced breast cancer: Phase III trial results. J Clin Oncol 2002;20:2812–2823.
30. Verma S, Ilersich AL. Population-based pharmacoeconomic model for adopting capecitabine/docetaxel combination treatment for anthracycline-pretreated metastatic breast cancer. Oncologist 2003;8:232–240.
31. Abernethy AP, Samsa GP, Matchar DB. A clinical decision and economic analysis model of cancer pain management. Am J Manag Care 2003;9(10):651–664.
32. Van den Hout W, van der Linden YM, Steenland E, et al. Single versus multiple-fraction radiotherapy in patients with painful bone metastases: cost-utility analysis based on a randomized trial. JNCI 2003;95:222–229.
33. Gordois A, Schuffham P, Warren E, Ward S: Cost-utility analysis of imatinib mesilate for the treatment of advanced stage chronic myeloid leukaemia. Br J Cancer 2003;89:634–640.
34. Elkin EB, Weinstein MC, Winer EP, Kuntz KM, Schnitt SJ, Weeks JC. HER-2 testing and trastuzumab therapy for metastatic breast cancer: a cost-effectiveness analysis. J Clin Oncol 2004;22(5):854–863.
35. Hillner BE, Smith TJ. Does a clinical trial warrant an economic analysis? JNCI 1998;90(10):724–725.
36. McGuire WL, Abeloff MD, Fisher B, Glick JH, Henderson IC, Osborne CK. Adjuvant therapy in node-negative breast cancer. A panel discussion. Breast Cancer Res Treat 1989;13:97–115.
37. Hillner BE, Smith TJ. Efficacy and cost-effectiveness of adjuvant chemotherapy in women with node-negative breast cancer. A decision analysis model. N Engl J Med 1991;324:160–168.
38. Smith TJ, Hillner BE. The efficacy and cost-effectiveness of adjuvant therapy of early breast cancer in premenopausal women. J Clin Oncol 1993;11:771–776.
39. Jaakimainen L, Goodwin PJ, Pater J, Warde P, Murray N, Rapp E. Counting the costs of chemotherapy in a National Cancer Institute of Canada randomized trial in non-small cell lung cancer. J Clin Oncol 1990;8:1301–1309.
40. Smith TJ, Hillner BE, Neighbors DM, McSorley PA, Le Chevalier T. An economic evaluation of a randomized clinical trial comparing vinorelbine, vinorelbine plus cisplatin and vindesine plus cisplatin for non-small cell lung cancer. J Clin Oncol 1995;13:2166–2173.
41. Tannock IF, Osoba D, Stockler MR, et al. Chemotherapy with mitoxantrone plus prednisone or prednisone alone for symptomatic hormone-resistant prostate cancer: a Canadian randomized trial with palliative end points. J Clin Oncol 1996;14(6): 1756–1764.
42. Bloomfield DJ, Krahn MD, Neogi T et al. Economic evaluation of chemotherapy with mitoxantrone plus prednisone for symp-

tomatic hormone resistant prostate cancer, based on a Canadian randomized trial with palliative endpoints. J Clin Oncol 1997; 16:2272–2279.
43. Royle P, Waugh N. Literature searching for clinical and cost-effectiveness studies used in health technology assessment reports carried out for the National Institute for Clinical Excellence appraisal system. Health Technol Assess 2003;7(34):1–51.
44. Mason J, Drummond M, Torrance G. Some guidelines on the use of cost-effectiveness league tables. BMJ 1993;306:570–572.
45. Ubel PA, Hirth RA, Chernew ME, et al. What is the price of life and why doesn't it increase at the rate of inflation? Arch Intern Med 2003;163:1637–1641.
46. Laupacis A, Feeny D, Detsky AS, Tugwell PX. How attractive does a new technology have to be to warrant adoption and utilization? Tentative guidelines for using clinical and economic evaluation. Can Med Assoc J 1992;146:473–481.
47. Friedman E. Capitation, integration, and managed care. Lessons from early experiments. JAMA 1996;275:957–962.
48. Hartman M, Knoth H, Schulz D, Knoth S. Industry-sponsored economic studies in oncology versus studies sponsored by non-profit organizations. Br J Cancer 2003;89(8):1405–1408.
49. Knox KS, Adams JR, Djulbegovic B, Stinson TJ, Tomor C, Bennett CL. Reporting and dissemination of industry versus non-profit sponsored economic analyses of six novel drugs used in oncology. Ann Oncol 2000;11:1591–1595.
50. Sulmasy DP. Physicians, cost control, and ethics. Ann Intern Med 1992;116:920–926.
51. Callahan D. Controlling the costs of health care for the elderly—fair means and foul. N Engl J Med 1996;335:744–746.
52. Levinsky NG. The purpose of advance medical planning—autonomy for patients or limitation of care? N Engl J Med 1996;335:741–743.
53. Hadorn DC. The Oregon priority-setting exercise: quality of life and public policy. Hastings Cent Rep 1991;21(suppl):11–16.
54. Earle CC, Chapman R, Baker C, et al. Systematic overview of cost-utility assessments in oncology. J Clin Oncol 2000;18:3302–3317.
55. Drummond M, Stoddart G, Labelle R, Cushman R. Health economics: an introduction for clinicians. Ann Intern Med 1987;107:88–92.
56. Kouroukis CT, O'Brien BJ, Benger A, et al. Cost-effectiveness of a transplantation strategy compared to melphalan and prednisone in younger patients with multiple myeloma. Leuk Lymphoma 2003;44(1):29–37.
57. Fuchs VR, Garber AM. The new technology assessment. N Engl J Med 1990;323:673–677.
58. Evans RW. Cost-effectiveness analysis of transplantation. Surg Clin N Am 1986;66:603–616.
59. Hillner BE, Weeks JC, Desch CE, Smith TJ. Pamidronate in prevention of bone complications in metastatic breast cancer: a cost-effectiveness analysis. J Clin Oncol 2000;18:72–79.
60. Hayman JA, Hillner BE, Harris JR. Cost-effectiveness of routine radiation therapy following conservative surgery for early-stage breast cancer. J Clin Oncol 1998;16:1022–1029.
61. Lee JH, Glick HA, Hayman JA, et al. Decision-analytic model and cost-effectiveness evaluation of postmastectomy radiation therapy in high-risk premenopausal breast cancer patients. J Clin Oncol 2002;20:2713–2725.

12 Principles of Screening for Cancer

Russell Harris and Linda S. Kinsinger

Screening is defined as testing for a condition when the person has no recognized signs or symptoms of that condition. The purpose of screening is not to merely detect a condition, but rather to help people live better or longer. This is an important distinction: the detection of earlier disease by itself is insufficient to justify a screening program. The program must additionally demonstrate that people live longer or better because of the earlier detection.

A positive screening test result does not indicate that a person has the condition, but rather that he or she has a higher probability of having the condition. People with positive screening tests usually undergo diagnostic testing to determine whether the condition is present. For example, a woman with a positive mammogram result does not necessarily have breast cancer, but she may undergo a needle localization biopsy to determine whether she has breast cancer.

Screening is not a single test, but rather a cascade of events that can lead to either benefits or harms (see The Cascade of Screening, later in this chapter). Potential benefits include living better or living longer and are usually experienced some years after screening. Potential harms include the effects of false-positive or false-negative screening tests and problems that result from overdiagnosis and overtreatment. Harms are usually suffered soon after screening.

Because screening programs may lead to either net benefit or net harm, decision makers must carefully evaluate proposed programs. Eight criteria distinguish effective programs:

1. Disease: The disease should cause a sufficient burden of suffering to warrant attention and should have a detectable preclinical phase of sufficient length to allow early detection (see The Critical Point in Cancer Treatment, later in this chapter).
2. Test: The screening test should be sufficiently sensitive to detect those cancers that could benefit from earlier treatment. Note that the test does not need to be maximally sensitive but rather "sensitive enough" to detect those cancers that it is important to detect. Cancers that are important to detect are those which are treatable when detected by screening but not when detected clinically.
3. Test: There are usually many more false-positive test results than true-positive results. The screening test should be specific enough to minimize the number of false-positive test results so as to minimize their negative consequences.
4. Availability and acceptability: The screening test, workup, and resultant treatment should be available to all and acceptable both to clinicians and to the people being screened.
5. Treatment: There must be a treatment for the disease that is more effective when applied to screening-detected cancers than clinically detected cancers. By "more effective," we mean that people will live longer or better as a result of this earlier treatment.
6. Harms of overtreatment: Often earlier detection includes detection of people with intermediate lesions that would never progress to invasive cancer. Screening may lead many people with these lesions to be subjected to treatment that they do not need and which causes harm. To minimize harms, people with lesions that will not progress to clinically important disease should rarely be subjected to potentially harmful and unnecessary treatment.
7. Benefits and harms: Overall benefits (in terms of people living longer or better) must outweigh overall harms (including harms from the screening test, harms from the workup, the adverse effects of earlier treatment and overtreatment, the psychologic effects of labeling, and the downstream effects of surveillance).
8. Costs: The net health benefits must come at a reasonable cost.

Screening for cancer is a popular idea, but this popularity may be based more on intuition than on understanding. Studies show that the great majority of Americans are convinced that being screened is part of being a responsible citizen.[1] What is less certain is how well the public comprehends the magnitude of the potential benefits of cancer screening; even less certain is whether the public appreciates the magnitude of the potential harms. Further, one could wonder whether the public has a reasonable grasp of the gaps in our knowledge of the effects of screening.

One might argue that whether the public understands these issues is irrelevant. The fact is that the public has decided that cancer screening is a good that it desires. We suggest that there are several important reasons for the public to better understand screening. The first is that screening consumes resources, such as money and the time of medical personnel. In a system strapped for resources to appropriately care for all our people, expending resources on services that offer little benefit and risk greater harm reduces the contribution medical care can make to the health of the public. The second reason is that if widespread screening fails to reduce the rate at which people die of cancer, ultimately the public will ask why it does not. If the medical care system has not informed the public of the limitations of cancer screening as a strategy to reduce cancer mortality, its credibility will be damaged. Finally, if the public pins all its hopes for cancer control on screening, this attitude may inhibit creative new ideas and research that could develop alternative strategies for cancer control.

The public needs to have a clear idea of both sides of the cancer screening coin: benefits and harms. Clinicians must play a large role in this educational effort. This chapter attempts to help clinicians better understand these issues so that they can appropriately advise the public.

The Idea of Cancer and the Idea of Screening

The public's understanding of how cancer works is central to its understanding of how screening works and thus to its strong interest in screening. Especially relevant is the public's perception of the development and progression of cancer and of the degree of homogeneity of cancers with the same name (e.g., breast cancer) in their malignant potential.

Although the process of cancer development is not completely understood, it is clear that a normal cell does not become cancer suddenly, all at once. Rather, cells undergo a number of assaults over time, with various results.[2] Some of these assaulted cells develop various abnormal forms, or "intermediate lesions," such as cervical intraepithelial neoplasia (CIN), colonic polyps, or ductal carcinoma in situ of the breast (DCIS). Although not cancer themselves, these intermediate lesions do at times develop into cancer.

As screening frequently detects intermediate lesions, their natural history is important. If nearly all intermediate lesions progress to malignant cancer, then early detection and treatment would appear to be an effective strategy for cancer control. The detection of intermediate lesions would be a triumph. By interdicting the developing cancer at this early point (i.e., even before it can be called a *cancer*), treatment could eradicate a lesion that would have caused major health problems in the years to come.

With many intermediate lesions, however, the majority (most often, the great majority) never progress to invasive cancer. Thus, screening often results in detecting and treating intermediate lesions that do not need to be detected or treated. If there are any harms to this early detection and treatment, the magnitude of these harms must be counted against the magnitude of the benefit. It is doubtful if many people understand this result of screening, or at least the frequency with which it occurs.

After cancer develops, a critical issue is the extent to which it uniformly progresses in a linear and inevitable manner to cause symptoms and death. If cancer is always an inexorably progressive condition, it is intuitively appealing to think that early detection is an effective strategy for cancer control. The experiences of people who have cancer with the same name (e.g., breast cancer) would vary little; all would be destined for a difficult death because the cancer had progressed too far for effective treatment. Again, the facts are otherwise.

Cancers, even cancers with the same name (e.g., breast cancer), vary widely in their growth rate and malignant potential. Studies have found that cancers that vary with respect to certain cell markers have different prognoses.[3] Gene expression profiling using DNA microarrays[4,5] has shown the genetic heterogeneity of individual breast cancers. There is not one type of breast (or colorectal or prostate) cancer, but a number of types, each with a different natural history. Together with the probable but largely unknown ways in which individual susceptibility varies, these cancer types produce great variation in the ways a particular cancer is expressed. Some cancers in certain individuals grow rapidly and are lethal within a short time, regardless of our best treatments. Screening is unlikely to make a difference for people with such cancers, which may metastasize from the first cell.

Other cancers with the same name grow more slowly, or not at all. People with some of these latter cancers may be greatly helped by early detection and treatment; others have cancers that do not need to be detected and treated at all. In some cases, lesions that clearly meet histologic criteria for cancer do not cause important clinical problems. Experts have termed this last group *pseudodisease*, lesions that appear to be cancer but do not progress to clinically important disease. It is the existence of this type of cancer, less malignant and less requiring of treatment, that gives pause to the push for screening. Here are cancers that do not need to be found early; some of them do not need to be found at all.

Much of the public has another conception of how cancer works. The word *cancer* usually means a condition that universally and inevitably progresses, a condition that is potentially fatal in every case. The fact that some people have long-term survival after cancer diagnosis is attributed to some exceptional characteristic of the individual or to effective treatment. Intermediate lesions are called *premalignant*; the popular conception is that they too inexorably progress to cause major clinical problems. This incorrect view of the nature of cancer is an important underlying reason for the popularity of cancer screening. As people have commented to the authors, cancer screening "simply makes sense." Given this view of cancer, one can understand their thinking.

The Critical Importance of Treatment Effectiveness in Determining the Benefits of Screening

The purpose of screening is not simply to detect disease earlier, but rather to help people live better or longer (i.e., improve health outcomes) because of early detection. Thus, the question we need to ask ourselves in considering a screening situation is not how many early cancers we find but how many people avoid poor health outcomes.

Although many people and their clinicians view the potential benefits of screening as primarily a function of the accuracy (especially the sensitivity) of a screening test, in fact, the factor that most commonly limits the benefit from screening is the treatment. For a screening program to improve health outcomes, it must include a treatment that is not only effective but which is more effective if applied earlier than if applied later. That is, the critical issue with screening is the *timing* of treatment. If the treatment is not effective at any time, obviously screening is not useful. If treatment is excellent and just as effective for clinically detected cancer as screening-detected cancer, then again early detection by screening is not helpful. Screening is only useful in improving health outcomes when the treatment is effective for screening-detected cancer but not clinically detected cancer.

This treatment criterion for a screening program is often misunderstood. The important question is this: where in the natural history of this cancer is the critical point (see following discussion) at which a particular treatment becomes ineffective? Theoretically, at least, many treatments may be effective when a potentially fatal cancer is only a few cells in size. As this cancer grows, however, there comes a point at which treatment is no longer effective in altering its natural history and helping the person to live better or longer. It is the location of this *critical point*, and especially its relationship with the point of detection by the screening test, that determines the effectiveness of the screening-and-early-treatment program. If the critical point is earlier than the point at which the cancer can be detected by screening, then screening cannot be helpful. If the critical point is during the "lead time" produced by the screening test, then screening will be helpful. If the treatment is very effective and the critical point is after the point at which regular, competent medical care would detect the cancer, then screening is not useful because treatment after usual clinical detection is as effective as treatment after screening detection.

When treatment is particularly effective, the critical point for some potentially fatal cancers may be at a far-advanced stage. Even very effective treatments may become ineffective for far-advanced stage cancers. Far advanced stage cancers at diagnosis may occur in several situations: in people who neglect their health; in people without access to regular, competent medical care; or in people without understanding that early signs or symptoms should be evaluated. In the past, for example, some women presented with breast tumors that were the size of a lemon or even an orange. It would be difficult to deny that many such cancers could have been treated more successfully had they been evaluated at an earlier stage. Few women present with such advanced tumors now, at least partly, because most women in this country recognize that breast lumps of any size should be examined by a physician.

The treatment requirement for a screening program is that the treatment must be more effective after detection by screening than after usual clinical detection. It does not require that the treatment be effective for far-advanced stage cancers. One does not need to implement a screening program to prevent the development of far-advanced cancers by helping people understand that new symptoms and signs should be reported to one's physician. This educational effort is different from screening.

The issue of the effectiveness of treatment at different points in the natural history of cancer is made more complex by the marked variation in cancers and individuals, as just discussed. It is not surprising, for example, that early detection and treatment rarely reduce mortality by 100%. For example, in the overviews of the randomized controlled trials of breast cancer screening, mortality is reduced by less than 20%.[6] This finding would imply that about 20% of women destined to die of breast cancer have a type of cancer that is better treated earlier than later. The other 80% of women destined to die of breast cancer have a type of cancer for which earlier treatment is not useful. These women may have a particularly malignant form of cancer in which metastasis occurs at an early stage, too early to be detected by screening.

Many other women are detected by breast cancer screening, of course, but these may be women not destined to die of breast cancer. They may have either a less-malignant form of the disease for which later treatment is as effective as earlier treatment or a benign form of cancer that would never have caused major adverse health outcomes even without treatment.

The Critical Point in Cancer Treatment

As shown in Figure 12.1, cancer begins as a small number of cells. If it were possible to detect every cancer at this point, and accurately distinguish the potentially fatal ones from the nonfatal, then our treatments would have a high rate of success. As the cancer grows, however (moving to the right in the figure), the potentially fatal cancers reach a point at which they are less effectively treated. This critical point varies between cancers and within cancers with the same name. It also varies between treatments. An important advance in treatment may mean that cancers can be effectively treated at a later stage in their development (i.e., farther toward the right of the figure).

The relationship of the critical point to the point at which a screening test can detect a cancer helps determine the potential benefits of screening. If the critical point is between points A and B in the figure (i.e., before the screening test can detect the cancer), then screening with the present test will not reduce the burden of suffering of the cancer. If the critical point is between points B and C (i.e., within the detectable preclinical phase of the cancer), then screening may well be helpful in reducing mortality and/or morbidity. If the critical point is to the right of point C in the figure, then the treatment is effective for even advanced cancers, and earlier detection is not needed.

Sensitivity of the Screening Test: A Less Important Criterion

In contrast to effective treatment, the sensitivity of the screening test, that is, its ability to detect early cancer, may or may not be an important factor in determining the benefit from a screening program. If a screening test is made more sensitive (for example, by reducing the cut-point for defining "abnormal"), it is likely that the test will detect more cancers. However, if these additional cancers are either more

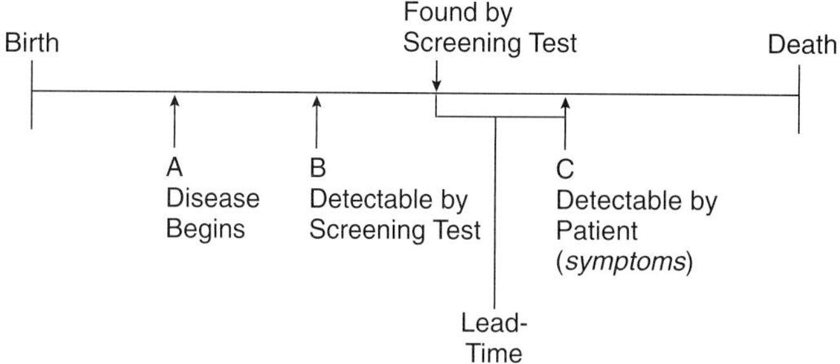

FIGURE 12.1. Natural history of cancer. *Critical Point*, point at which treatment becomes less effective; could be between *A* and *B*, between *B* and *C*, or after *C*.

benign (and would never cause problems) or more malignant (and thus have already metastasized), then the extra sensitivity would not have made a contribution to improving health outcomes. The operative question is not how many more cancers are found by a more sensitive test but rather whether screening has moved detection for at least some potentially fatal cancers back to a more treatable stage. If this has not occurred, then the more sensitive test has not been a useful addition to the screening program. This rationale includes such strategies as screening more frequently (i.e., reducing the screening interval), which may increase sensitivity but may or may not improve health outcomes.

For this reason, the sensitivity of a screening test may not be related to its ability to improve health outcomes. For example, screening for cervical cancer with the Pap smear probably has a fairly low sensitivity,[7,8] yet screening every 3 years apparently reduces cervical cancer mortality by more than 80%.[9] Developments in the technology of screening tests that seek to improve screening programs by increasing the sensitivity of the screening test may increase sensitivity without improving health outcomes. Such approaches may increase the cost of screening without providing additional health benefit.

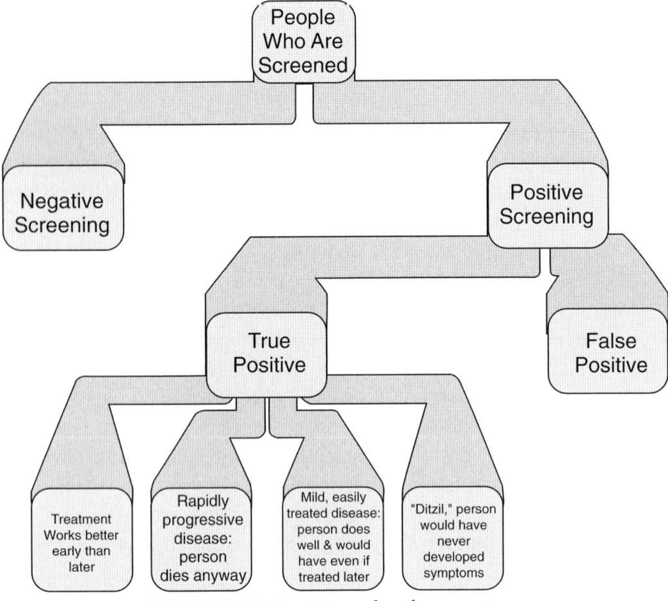

FIGURE 12.2. Cascade of screening.

Potential Harms of Screening: False-Positive Results and Overtreatment

It is difficult to understand how finding cancer earlier could cause harm. In the popular paradigm of cancer being an inexorably progressive disease, the idea of harms from screening makes little sense. It is not difficult to understand why people report having little concern about being harmed by a screening test. But in a real world in which not every cancer is an enemy, most of the intermediate lesions never progress to invasive cancer, workups and diagnostic tests have side effects, and cancer treatments can cause suffering of their own, the possibility of doing harm with screening is easier to understand.

The Cascade of Screening

Screening is not a single test, but rather a cascade of events that can result in either benefit or harm (Figure 12.2). The first step is the screening test itself. Although some diagnostic tests can have useful intermediate results, with a screening test the result is either positive or negative. If a recommendation for anything other than continued routine screening comes from the screening test, it is a positive test. The patient is notified that all is not well and that further evaluation of some kind is needed.

Typically, with cancer screening, many more people have a negative screening test than a positive. After a positive test, further workup is required to determine whether the screening test is a true positive or a false positive. The workup may vary depending on the degree of positivity of the screening test or other circumstances. Some people with false-positive tests have ongoing anxiety related to the experience of screening whereas others do not.

People with a true-positive test do not all benefit from earlier detection of their cancer. These people fall into four categories. Category 1 includes people with fast-growing, malignant disease for which treatment is ineffective. These people do not benefit from earlier detection. Category 2 includes people whose cancer is easily treated regardless of when it is detected. These people also do not benefit from earlier detection. Category 3 includes people whose cancer would never have caused important clinical problems and does not need to be treated. These people have "pseudodisease" and do not benefit from earlier detection. Category 4 includes people whose cancer is more effectively treated earlier, after screening detection, than later, after clinical detection. These are the people who benefit from earlier detection. Treatment of people from category 3 is overtreatment; any adverse effects from treatment of this group must be counted as among the harms of screening. This situation happens frequently because category 3 cancers cannot always be accurately distinguished from other categories.

We next consider two categories of potential harms from screening: false-positive screening tests and overtreatment. Although false-negative tests could also theoretically cause harm by false reassurance, we know of little evidence to substantiate this potential harm.

False-Positive Test Results

False-positive screening test results can cause harm both psychologically and by adverse effects from unnecessary workups. Although a positive screening test does not mean that one has the disease in question, it does mean a person has been placed into a higher risk group than previously. That is, the risk of having breast cancer is higher among women with a positive mammogram than among women who have not yet had a mammogram. The individual may experience the uncertainty of not knowing whether she has breast cancer. This occurrence usually causes stress to the individual involved; any delay in the diagnostic workup adds to the person's concern.

The psychologic trauma from a false-positive screening test can be increased by incomplete resolution of the situation. For example, women with an abnormal mammogram are sometimes asked to return for follow-up mammograms every 6 months (rather than annually). Similarly, some men with a high prostate-specific antigen (PSA) value and a negative prostate biopsy are asked to return in 3 to 6 months for a second set of biopsies because the cancer may have been missed in the first set. People who have had benign colonic polyps removed are sometimes asked to have repeat colonoscopy at more frequent intervals. Some of these people may suffer psychologic stress as a result of prolonging the experience of uncertainty.

Some people who have had seemingly complete resolution of the false-positive screening test (e.g., a woman with an abnormal mammogram who had a negative biopsy and was told she does not have cancer) still have lasting concerns. A study of women after having a false-positive mammogram found that many still had lingering doubts that interfered with sleep or function 6 months after a negative biopsy.[10] A recent study found a similar result among men with a high PSA screening test and a negative biopsy for prostate cancer.[11]

Because false-positive tests lead to workups without clinical benefit, any complication from the workup of a false-positive screening test (e.g., colonic perforation from a false-positive fecal occult blood test) is also a harm from screening. Most workups for positive screening tests will be negative.

Although these psychologic effects and complications from workups may seem of little consequence when compared with the potential for extending life by screening, the weighing of these effects on a population level must take into account that the actual number of false-positive screening tests is far larger than the number of true-positive tests, and larger still then the number of true-positive tests that lead to extended life.

The rate at which a screening test yields false positives is determined by its specificity. Many screening tests have specificities above 90%. Although this sounds very high, specificity in the 90% range guarantees a large number of false-positive tests. This is because specificity is the percentage of all people without the cancer who are classified correctly as having a negative test; 1-specificity is the percentage of people without disease who are incorrectly classified as having cancer (i.e., false positive). In a screening program, however, the number of people without cancer is very large; thus, even 10% (or even 5%) of a large number is still a large number.

In most cases, the number of false-positive screening tests outnumbers true-positive tests by a factor of from 4:1 (e.g., prostate cancer) to 10:1 (e.g., breast cancer) or higher. If we consider the proportion of people who have at least one false-positive screening test over a period of years of repeated screening, the ratio of false-positive to true-positive tests is even larger. In one study, nearly 50% of women had at least one abnormal mammogram over 10 years of annual screening.[12]

Because the prevalence of cancer in a screening population is low, the number of true-positive tests is usually low. If, as noted previously (see Figure 12.2), only a fraction of the true-positive tests lead to extended life, then the number of people who could, over a period of years, potentially suffer the harms of a false positive screening test so far outnumbers the people who may reap the benefits that weighing benefit and harm overall is not straightforward.

As noted previously, improving the sensitivity of a screening test may or may not lead to increased benefits from screening. However, improving the specificity of a screening test often leads to less harm because there are fewer false-positive tests. A smaller number of false-positive tests gives less opportunity for adverse psychologic effects of screening and for adverse effects of negative workups. Thus, improving the specificity of screening tests should often be a priority.

For most tests, whether screening or diagnostic, sensitivity and specificity are inversely related. Thus, increasing the specificity of a screening test may well reduce the sensitivity. The optimal screening test, then, may be neither the most sensitive nor the most specific test, but rather the test (or test cut-point) that gives the optimal trade-off between benefits and harms.

Overdiagnosis and Overtreatment

In addition to false-positive tests, harms may also follow from true-positive tests. Not all people with true-positive screening tests benefit from the earlier detection of cancer. One can think of people with true-positive tests as having cancers in one of four categories.

Category 1: People with an aggressive, malignant cancer may not benefit from screening because the cancer has already metastasized before it can be detected. We are learning, in fact, that some cancers may metastasize within the first few cell divisions, too early to be the target of screening.

Category 2: Other people with slower-growing cancers may be highly treatable even after clinical detection. Testicular cancer may be such a tumor; our treatments are highly effective without the need of early detection. People with such cancers do not benefit from screening.

Category 3: Some people may have pseudodisease, cancers that do not need treatment at all. These people either have intermediate lesions that would not progress but are still considered positive tests (e.g., small colonic adenomas) or have cancer that would not cause clinically important problems for the person in his/her lifetime. These are lesions that appear to be cancer but do not act as we think cancer usually acts. These people cannot benefit from early detection of their "cancer."

Category 4: These are people who can benefit from earlier detection. These people have cancers that are potentially lethal but which can be treated more effectively because they were found earlier. In this case, the criterion is met that the treatment must be more effective if applied after screening detection than later, after clinical detection. Usually, this group of true-positive cancers is a minority of all true positives. The randomized controlled trials of breast cancer screening, for example, tell us that less than 20% of potentially lethal breast cancers (categories 1 and 4) belong to group 4.

A problem with this formulation, however, is that many cancers can only be placed in their proper category retrospectively. That is, the people in category 3, who do not need to be detected or treated, are often initially difficult to distinguish from the other groups. Thus, people in this category are still treated. An example is men with prostate cancer detected by screening. The majority of men with screening-detected prostate cancer have tumors that are moderately differentiated. Some cancers of this type are potentially lethal whereas others will never cause clinical problems. Because it is impossible to distinguish these cancers with high confidence at the time of diagnosis, virtually all men with this type of cancer are treated. This constitutes overdiagnosis, as we are diagnosing some men with cancer who do not need to be diagnosed, and overtreatment, as we are treating some men who do not need treatment.

The fact of overtreatment is undeniable and likely occurs with many cancers. The most important question is how often it occurs. Determining the number of people in category 3 (the primary group that is affected by overtreatment), however, is not simple. One can consider the issue in either of two ways: pathologically or epidemiologically. These different approaches explain much of the debate about the frequency of "clinically important" prostate cancers.

The pathologic approach to determining the frequency of cancers that do not need treatment uses grade and other cellular prognostic characteristics to determine prognosis at the time of diagnosis. People who are at risk of overtreatment have cancers with more benign characteristics. The problem with this approach is that none of the known prognostic characteristics is able to separate benign from malignant cancers with a high degree of accuracy. For example, one population-based study found that from 40% to 70% of men (depending upon age) with localized Gleason score 7 prostate cancer died of prostate cancer within 15 years of diagnosis.[13] This finding also means that 30% to 60% of men with this type of cancer did not die of prostate cancer in that time. As these men were diagnosed before widespread PSA screening, it is likely that these survival figures would be higher today, independent of any changes in the effectiveness of treatment. Thus, the Gleason score and extent of tumor only give partial information about prognosis, and we are uncertain about whether an individual man will die of prostate cancer.

Another approach is based on the epidemiology of the cancer. This approach examines such issues as the difference between incidence and mortality; trends over time; changes in the effectiveness of treatment; and the lead time produced by the screening test. Using these assumptions with statistical modeling, investigators can calculate an approximation of the proportion of cancers that would not have caused problems during the person's lifetime. The problem with this approach is that it is based on a number of assumptions, at least some of which may be incorrect.

The best way to calculate the percentage of cancers that would never become clinically apparent is an analysis of results from a randomized controlled trial (RCT) of screening, comparing invited and control groups. If the trial screens people in the invited group for several years and then stops screening, the initial increase in incidence usually seen in the invited group compared with the control group should gradually decrease after the end of screening, as the cancers in the control group are detected at a later time. If the cumulative incidence of cancer in the control group never catches up with the invited group, this is evidence of detection by screening (in the invited group) of cancers that would never become clinically apparent. This approach may theoretically underestimate the true frequency of overdiagnosis, however, as it does not count cancers that produce only minimal symptoms (but symptoms sufficient to be diagnosed) in the overdiagnosis category. Although such cancers do cause some symptoms, they may grow so slowly that they would never progress to important clinical problems within the lifetime of the individual. The extent to which such cancers exist is unknown, but they do not need to be diagnosed early.

Overtreatment causes harm in a number of ways. First, the individual has been labeled as a "cancer patient," with likely important consequences for the person's life. Second, most cancer treatments have some side effects, some of which may be long lasting. Thus, in attempting to gain additional life in the future, people must undergo immediate harm from treatment. Finally, the large number of people being treated leads to an exaggerated view by professionals and the public of the true frequency of the cancer and the effectiveness of treatment.[14] Further, *5-year survival* statistics, which improve as more benign cancers are detected and treated, provide an erroneous overestimate of the efficacy of treatment (15) (see following discussion), and many "cancer survivors" are actually people who had either benign-type cancers (category 2) or pseudodisease (category 3) (see Cancer Survivors, later in this chapter).

The Fallacy of 5-Year Survival in Indicating the Effectiveness of a Screening Program

The 5-year survival rate is frequently cited as evidence for the effectiveness of screening in reducing cancer mortality. Nearly every cancer has a longer 5-year survival for early-stage disease than late-stage disease. It should then follow that finding the cancer at an earlier stage leads to improved outcomes and lower mortality.

Factors other than the effectiveness of screening, however, are important determinants of the 5-year survival rate.[15] As survival is defined as the time from diagnosis to death, it is heavily influenced by early detection, even if death is not postponed. Thus, improved 5-year survival for early-stage cancers could simply reflect the stage at which the cancer is found, with no effect of screening on the natural history of the cancer.

A second problem with the 5-year survival rate as a measure of the effectiveness of screening is related to the heterogeneity of cancers with the same name. Cancers diagnosed at an early stage may be pathologically different from cancers diagnosed at a later stage. Screening may have little to do with the higher 5-year survival rate for early-stage cancers: they would have lower malignant potential regardless of how (or when) they were detected.

Biases in Cancer Screening

Several biases may lead one to believe that screening is effective even in situations where it is not. The first of these is "lead time bias" (Figure 12.3). As shown in the figure, lead time is the time by which earlier detection advances diagnosis. If treatment is ineffective, however ("situation 2" in Figure 12.3), then the patient will die at the same time he/she would have without earlier detection ("situation 1"). The patient's "survival," measured from diagnosis, has been prolonged but the patient has not benefited. Thus, studies that compare survival between people whose cancers were

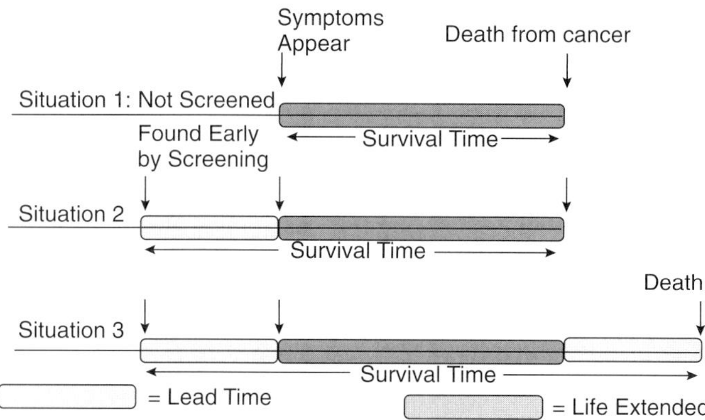

FIGURE 12.3. Lead time bias.

detected by screening with those whose cancer was detected clinically are flawed. The important issue with screening is whether there is a "situation 3," in which people's lives have actually been extended. The best study design to avoid this bias is the randomized controlled trial.

A second bias also may cause people to conclude that screening is useful when it is not. This bias, termed "length-biased sampling" (or "length-time bias"), is associated with the heterogeneity of cancer growth rates and malignant potential (Figure 12.4). Patients 1 and 4 in the figure have rapidly progressive tumors that spend relatively little time in the "detectable preclinical phase" area. As a result, these cancers are often missed by screening tests. Patients 2 and 3, however, have slower-growing, less-malignant cancers that are less likely to be fatal. These cancers spend a longer time in the detectable preclinical phase area and thus are more likely to be detected by screening. Thus, length-biased sampling makes us believe that screening is effective because people with screening-detected cancers do better than people with clinically detected cancers. Slower-growing and less-malignant cancers are preferentially detected by screening programs.

Interestingly, patient 4, whose cancer was detected at a later age, does not die of his or her cancer, even though the cancer is faster growing and malignant, because of competing risks: he or she is more likely to die of another cause at this older age. Patient 4 is not helped by screening.

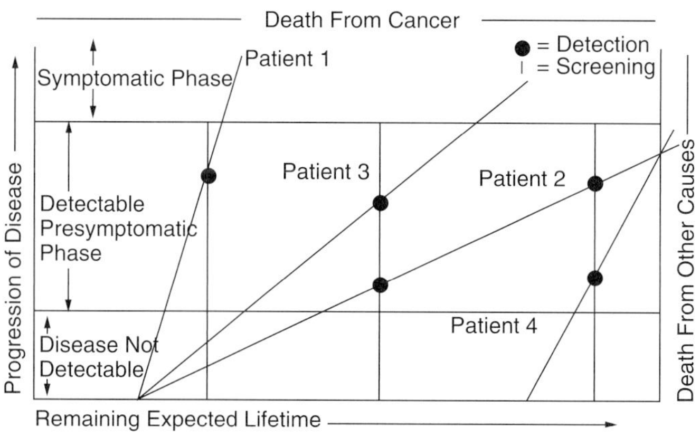

FIGURE 12.4. Length-biased sampling.

Cancer Survivors

The prominence of cancer survivors is a factor in the public's strong interest in cancer screening. A number of people who appear to have been cured of cancer attribute their well-being to detection of their cancer by screening and resultant early treatment. Their testimony to the power of screening contributes to the public's perception that cancer screening is a responsibility. However, at least some of these people likely had either an easily treated benign-type cancer (category 2) or pseudodisease (category 3). Neither of these cancers requires earlier detection. Easily treated cancers are slower growing and can be treated as well after clinical detection as after screening detection. Pseudodisease cancers would never have caused important problems and thus do not need treatment at all. Because it is often difficult to distinguish these cancers at diagnosis from more malignant forms, people who do well after treatment tend to attribute their well-being to screening and early detection. Because many of these people choose to have high public visibility, this creates a bias in favor of the public's view that screening is highly effective in reducing mortality from cancer.

Weighing Benefits and Harms: Decision Making About Screening

Weighing the benefits and harms of screening programs is difficult. First, one must determine the presence and magnitude of the benefits and harms. Benefits seem intuitive, but closer inspection shows that they are easy to overestimate. Evidence about the accuracy or yield of screening tests by itself is inadequate, as is evidence about the effectiveness of treatment in people detected clinically. Etiologic data about trends in mortality over time are open to multiple interpretations. To avoid the strong biases involved, the ideal study design is a randomized controlled trial (RCT) of screening. Even this design, however, is open to criticism, as has been shown by the controversy over the breast cancer screening trials.[16,17] In the end, the determination of the benefits of screening depends on examining evidence from many sources with different designs, and then considering the relevance of the studies to the community setting.[18] One should consider not only whether there are benefits, but how many people benefit and by how much. Judgment is involved in this complex process.

The same process is involved in determining the harms of screening. This part of the equation is often forgotten: a screening program is justified if, and only if, the benefits outweigh the harms of the program. Even RCTs of screening often do not report on the adverse effects caused by screening.

After determining the magnitude of benefits and harms, decision makers need to consider whether one outweighs the other. A problem is that the benefits and harms are usually in different metrics. Benefits should be stated in terms of the estimated number of lives extended in 1,000 people screened over a given time period. Some have claimed reassurance from negative screening tests as a benefit, but careful examination shows that such reassurance is based on questionable assumptions. The actual reduction in the probability of cancer after a negative cancer screening test is very small. Harms should include the number of people in 1,000 screened with false-positive tests, people who are referred for workups and may suffer psychologic distress. Ideally, one should also estimate the number of people who were overtreated and the consequences of overtreatment.

Weighing the (usually) small number of lives extended against the larger number of people with various types of harms requires a value judgment. What value is placed on the experience of the people suffering harms and what value is placed on the people whose lives are extended? Currently, our culture seems to have decided that even a small number of lives extended by cancer screening outweighs a larger number of people having problems with false positives and overtreatment. It is not clear whether this concept will change as the public becomes more aware of the magnitude of the benefits and harms from cancer screening.

For many cancer screening decisions, some have suggested that the people undergoing the screening should be informed of the potential harms as well as the potential benefits and should be involved in the decision.[19] This approach is called shared decision making (SDM). Research is currently exploring ways of making SDM more feasible and effective in the clinical setting, using decision aids and other decision support resources.

The benefits and harms of cancer screening usually vary by age. The incidence and mortality of most cancers usually associated with screening increase with age. If screening leads to a constant relative reduction in mortality risk, then the absolute reduction in risk (i.e., mortality benefit) increases with age. Thus, younger people with a low probability of having cancer may receive few benefits and expose themselves to important harms by having screening. For example, women in their forties probably receive some benefit from mammography screening for breast cancer, but the magnitude of benefit is small. These women do, however, have a higher probability of having a false-positive mammogram. Given this information, some women will choose to have mammography in their forties and some will not. The age at which the benefits of screening overcome the harms depends on personal values. In general, however, screening is not offered to people at a younger age who have a very low probability of having cancer.

In considering an upper age limit for screening, it is important to remember that any life extension from screening does not occur immediately after screening but rather some years in the future. Thus, to realize the benefit from screening one must live a certain period into the future. As people age, however, the risk of dying of a cause other than cancer increases. Some older people, then, do not live long enough to benefit from screening. Clearly, people with a limited life expectancy have little to gain from screening.

The harms of screening may or may not vary by age. In some cases (e.g., mammography), the screening test may yield fewer false positives in older people, thus decreasing the harms of this finding. In other cases (e.g., PSA for prostate cancer), the screening test may yield more false positives and thus potentially increase the probability of harms. Harms should be carefully considered in every screening decision; the weight they are given by the patient may vary by age. Interventions to reduce psychologic harms by educating people about false positives before screening may be useful but need more research.

An important decision for people who have decided to be screened is the frequency of repeat screening. It is unusual to have RCT evidence about the relative benefits and harms of various screening intervals. More commonly, we reason about this issue with indirect evidence, including our understanding of the natural history of the cancer and measurements of cancer incidence in people who have waited different times to be rescreened.

In general, cancer detection is greatest with the first screening round, the so-called prevalence screen, because there are more asymptomatic cancers to be detected initially than on later screening rounds. Cancers detected in a previous round of screening have been removed from the pool of remaining asymptomatic cancers. Thus, a short screening interval will likely find fewer cancers than a longer interval. The longer the interval, the closer cancer detection will revert to the initial round.

The balance of benefits and harms from various screening intervals is more complex. A shorter screening interval usually means increased sensitivity, but specificity may be reduced. In deciding the most appropriate screening interval, one must consider the trade-offs between finding all appropriate cancers (i.e., increased sensitivity) and increasing the rate of harms related to false positives.

The value of cancer screening after previously negative screening tests is uncertain and needs further study. It is possible that various results from previous screening tests (e.g., men with very low PSA values or women with benign types of parenchymal findings on a mammogram) may be markers of people at decreased risk of developing cancer. These markers may help us define a group of people who do not need further screening, thus allowing us to target screening to people who have the greatest possibility of benefit. If by defining a low-risk population (rather than a high-risk population) we could reduce the number of people requiring screening (thus reducing costs and potential false positives and overtreatment), the balance between the benefits and harms of screening could be improved.

The Costs and Cost-Effectiveness of Screening

Even after gathering the evidence about the benefits and harms of screening, policy makers must still ask the question of whether the net benefits are worth the costs and resource utilization. It may be, for example, that annual abdominal computed tomography (CT) scans detect unsuspected cancers of several types and even sometimes extend a life. But the costs of such a strategy (leaving aside the likely harms for the large number of false positives) may be prohibitive. In other words, the benefits may not be worth the cost.

Opportunity costs are also important. That is, if clinicians spend large amounts of time discussing cancer screening that has little probability of benefit, this may take away from time that could be used, for example, to counsel people about stopping tobacco use, or spending more time on SDM for potentially beneficial cancer screening.

Cancer Screening Examples

To illustrate these principles, we have included examples of screening from four different cancers (cervical, prostate, breast, and colorectal) among those most commonly considered for screening. In each case, there is the clear potential for benefits and harms. In each case, the benefits are not large in an absolute sense, whereas the harms are not inconsequential. Rational people may decide to have or not to have screening for these cancers based on the same understanding of the evidence. It is important for the public to come to a better understanding of the potential benefits and harms of cancer screening.

Example of Cervical Cancer Screening

Incidence and Mortality

In 2004, an estimated 10,520 new cases of and 3,900 deaths from invasive cervical cancer were expected.[20] In 2000, the age-adjusted incidence rate in nine Surveillance, Epidemiology, and End Results Program (SEER) registries was 8 per 100,000 women; the age-adjusted mortality rate was 3 per 100,000.[21] From 1950 to 1970, the incidence and mortality rates of invasive cervical cancer fell impressively by more than 70%. From 1970 to 2000, the rates continued to decrease by more than 40%.[22] This trend has been attributed largely to screening with the Papanicolaou (Pap) test.

Screening Tests

The Pap test, the standard screening test for cervical cancer, has never been studied in an RCT. A large body of consistent observational data, however, supports its effectiveness in reducing mortality from cervical cancer. Both incidence and mortality from cervical cancer have sharply decreased in a number of large populations following the introduction of well-run screening programs.[23–26] Reductions in cervical cancer incidence and mortality were proportional to the intensity of screening.[22,27]

Case-control studies have found that the risk of developing invasive cervical cancer is 3 to 10 times greater in women who have not been screened.[28–32] Risk also increases with longer duration following the last normal Pap test, or similarly, with decreasing frequency of screening.[33,34] Screening every 2 to 3 years, however, has not been found to increase significantly the risk of finding invasive cervical cancer above the risk expected with annual screening.[34,35]

The precise sensitivity and specificity of Pap tests has been difficult to determine because of the methodological limitations of studies.[36] Studies that compare the Pap test with repeat Pap testing have found that the sensitivity of any abnormality on a single test for detecting high-grade lesions is 55% to 80%.[7,8] Because of the usual slow-growing nature of cervical cancer, the sensitivity of a program of regular Pap testing is likely higher.

Specificity of the Pap test is probably above 90%; it seldom categorizes a woman without any degree of cervical intraepithelial neoplasia (CIN) as having anything more than a mild cytologic abnormality. Specificity is lower, however, for women with mild, clinically unimportant degrees of dysplasia, who are often categorized as having cytologic abnormalities that require further testing and even treatment. Women with such cytologic findings as atypical squamous cells of undetermined significance (ASCUS) are often shown on further evaluation to have neither severe dysplasia nor invasive cancer. If these women are counted as false positives, then specificity will be calculated as lower.[7]

Newer techniques that employ liquid-based cytology (e.g., ThinPrep) have been developed to improve the sensitivity of screening. As with the Pap test, the optimal studies to determine the sensitivity and specificity of these technologies have not been done. Some less than optimal studies show that sensitivity is modestly higher for detecting any degree of CIN, with modestly lower specificity.[37,38] One careful study, however, showed that conventional Pap testing was slightly more sensitive and specific than liquid-based cytology.[39]

The evidence is also mixed about whether liquid-based techniques improve rates of test adequacy.[37,38] One advantage of liquid-based cytology is that human papillomavirus (HPV) testing can be done on the same preparation; one disadvantage is that liquid-based approaches are more expensive than conventional Pap testing. No study has examined whether liquid-based cytology actually reduces the number of women dying of cervical cancer compared with conventional Pap testing.

Rationale for Screening

Invasive squamous carcinoma of the cervix results from the progression of preinvasive precursor lesions called cervical intraepithelial neoplasia (CIN), or dysplasia. Not all these lesions progress to invasive cancer; many mild and moderate lesions regress. The rate at which invasive cancer develops from CIN is usually slow, measured in years and perhaps decades.[40] This long natural history provides the opportunity for screening to effectively detect this process during the preinvasive phase, thus allowing early treatment and cure. Because many of these preinvasive lesions (especially low-grade lesions) would have never progressed to invasive cancer,[41–43] screening also runs the risk of leading to treatment of women who do not need to be treated. This approach leads to harms of screening by overtreatment.

The leading etiologic factor in the development of preinvasive and invasive cervical cancer is infection with specific types of HPV transmitted by sexual contact. Thus, women who are not sexually active rarely develop cervical cancer, whereas sexual activity at an early age with multiple sexual partners is a strong risk factor. About 95% of women with invasive cervical cancer have evidence of HPV infection.[44–47] Many women with HPV infection, however, never develop cervical cancer; thus, this infection is necessary but not sufficient for the development of cancer.[48]

Harms of Screening

The major potential harm of screening for cervical cancer lies in the detection of many lesions [such as most cases of low-grade squamous intraepithelial lesions (LSIL)] that would never progress to cervical cancer. Women with abnormal LSIL or high-grade squamous intraepithelial lesions (HSIL) on Pap testing are usually referred for colposcopy and treated with cryotherapy or loop electrosurgical excision procedure (LEEP), which permanently alters the cervix and has unknown fertility and pregnancy consequences. As younger women have the highest incidence of acquisition of HPV and LSIL, they are disproportionately at risk of receiving intervention for a condition that often spontaneously resolves.

The cost of newer screening methods is also problematic. A cost-effectiveness analysis found little effect on life expectancy with the new technologies when used for annual screening.[49] They may be more cost-effective when used on a less frequent (e.g., every 3 years) basis.

Balance of Benefits and Harms

Based on an analysis of screening records from nearly 350,000 women in Bristol, England, investigators projected that 1,000 women would need to be screened for cervical cancer for 35 years to prevent 1 death from the disease.[50] For each death prevented, the authors estimated that more than 150 women have an abnormal result, more than 80 are referred for investigation, and more than 50 receive treatment.

Annually in the United States, 50 million women undergo screening; about 3.5 million (7%) will be referred for further evaluation. Of these, more than 2 million will be referred for further evaluation of atypical squamous cells of undetermined significance (ASCUS).[51] Fewer than 11,000 cases of invasive cervical cancer were expected in 2004. Thus, Pap test screening results in a large number of colposcopies for benign conditions. Strategies to improve the specificity of the cervical cytopathology test are being evaluated by the ASCUS/LSIL Triage Study (ALTS).[52] Improved specificity, even at the cost of sensitivity, will likely improve the balance between benefits and harms, given the large burden of false positives, abnormalities that do not represent risk for invasive cancer or death.

Improved cervical cancer screening practices may also favor a more positive benefit-to-harm balance. Such practices include not screening women who have had hysterectomies (with removal of the cervix) for benign disease. More than one-third of U.S. women have had hysterectomies by age 65, more than 90% of which are done for noncancer indications.[53] These women rarely have important abnormalities on Pap testing.[54,55] In addition, continued Pap test screening for women over age 65 who previously have had regular cervical cancer screening with normal test results provides little benefit. The risk of cervical cancer and yield of screening decline steadily through middle age.[56] The majority of older women who are found to have invasive cervical cancer have not been screened recently, if at all.[53] Thus, the focus of cervical cancer screening practices should be on finding and screening women at increased risk because of inadequate past screening rather than continuing to screen women at low risk.

Example of Prostate Cancer Screening

Incidence and Mortality

The American Cancer Society estimated that, in 2004, 230,110 men would be diagnosed with prostate cancer; 29,900 men would die of this disease.[20] The age-adjusted prostate cancer incidence in nine Surveillance, Epidemiology, and End Results (SEER) registries between 1996 and 2000 was about 173 per 100,000 men.[21] The mortality during that period was about 33 per 100,000 men. The probability at birth of being diagnosed with prostate cancer by age 80 is about 14%; the probability at birth of dying of this disease by age 80 is about 1.26%.[22] The difference between prostate cancer incidence and mortality is one of largest for any cancer; this difference increased greatly after PSA screening became widespread. This is a strong indication that at least some prostate cancers now detected by screening would never become clinically important.

The incidence of prostate cancer increased dramatically after the beginning of PSA screening in the late 1980s and then stabilized in the later 1990s. Mortality from prostate cancer decreased after about 1992, a total reduction of about 20% by 2000. Screening is one of several possible interpretations of this reduction in mortality.[57]

Screening Tests

The two most common screening tests for prostate cancer are prostate-specific antigen (PSA) and digital rectal exam (DRE). No well-conducted RCT of prostate cancer screening has been completed; two large studies are under way.

Because of the uncertainty about which prostate cancers are clinically important, the sensitivity and specificity of screening is difficult to determine. DRE detects fewer cancers than PSA. Various approaches have been suggested for increasing the sensitivity and specificity of screening, but whether these approaches improve detection of clinically important cancers and reduce detection of unimportant cancers is unknown.[58]

Rationale for Screening

Because of the absence of clear evidence that screening reduces mortality from prostate cancer, the rationale for screening is not established. However, many men are still being screened.[59] Many believe that the ecologic evidence (showing a reduction in mortality after the start of PSA screening) justifies screening; others find that screening has a strong intuitive appeal.

A single well-conducted RCT compared radical prostatectomy and watchful waiting in men with clinically detected prostate cancer.[60] After 8 years, fewer men in the prostatectomy group had died of prostate cancer [13.6% versus 7.1%; absolute difference, 6.6% (2.1%–11.1%)]. The groups did not differ in all-cause mortality. As the cancers in this study were more advanced than those usually detected by screening PSA, this study does not provide adequate evidence about the effectiveness of screening.

Harms of Screening

Two major sources of the harms of prostate cancer screening are false positives and overdiagnosis and overtreatment. False-positive tests are common. On the initial screening round, from 5% to 27% of men (depending on age) have a PSA greater than 4.0 (the traditional cut-point); about 30% of these men will have prostate cancer diagnosed by biopsy.[57] A problem for men with a negative biopsy is that biopsies often miss some prostate cancers; thus, even a negative biopsy does not assure a man that he does not have cancer,[61] and this uncertainty could increase anxiety.

The frequency of overdiagnosis and overtreatment of prostate cancer caused by screening is uncertain. Surveillance data show a large increase in the number of new cases of prostate cancer, with only a small absolute reduction in mortality, after the introduction of PSA screening in the late 1980s.

If, as seems likely, most of the new cases detected would never have been fatal, then more than half of screening-detected prostate cancers do not require major treatment.

Although a small percentage of prostate cancers have histologic characteristics that reliably predict either a very small or a very large malignant potential, most prostate cancers have intermediate histology, leaving us uncertain about the likely prognosis. Because of the inability to determine prognosis from clinical and histologic data, most men under age 70 years receive aggressive treatment: either radical prostatectomy or radiation therapy. These treatments have important adverse effects, including impotence and incontinence, for some 50% of men being treated.[57] Thus, if there are a substantial number of men who do not need treatment but receive it, many of them will be harmed unnecessarily. The exact magnitude of this problem is uncertain, but it may be quite large.

Balance of Benefits and Harms

For screening for prostate cancer, the benefits are not clear whereas the harms are very clear. Thus, the net balance between the two is currently impossible to determine. Given this information, some men will choose to have screening while others will choose not to be screened. Several professional associations and expert groups recommend shared decision making (SDM), informing men of the pros and cons of screening and encouraging them to participate in the decision about whether to be screened.[62–67]

Example of Breast Cancer Screening

Incidence and Mortality

The American Cancer Society estimated that, in 2004, 215,990 women would be newly diagnosed with breast cancer; 40,110 would die of this disease.[20] About 59,390 women will be diagnosed with carcinoma in situ of the breast, primarily by mammography.[20] From 1996 to 2000, the age-adjusted incidence in nine Surveillance, Epidemiology, and End Results (SEER) registries was about 137 per 100,000 women; the age-adjusted mortality during this period was about 28 per 100,000.[21] The probability at birth of being diagnosed with breast cancer in 80 years of life is about 11%; the probability at birth of dying of breast cancer by age 80 is about 2%.[21] Breast cancer incidence for all women increased from 1980 to 2000, although the increase slowed considerably in the late 1990s. Between 1990 and 2000, breast cancer mortality for all women decreased by about 2.3% per year.[22,68] The reasons for this decrease are not clear and may be due to a combination of screening and improved treatment.[69]

Screening Tests

Three primary tests are currently in use for breast cancer screening. Although still controversial, the overall evidence shows that mammography results in a reduction in breast cancer mortality by less than 20%.[6] Indirect evidence suggests that clinical breast examination (CBE), when well conducted, may also lead to a small reduction in mortality, but uncertainty about this remains.[70,71] Breast self-examination (BSE) has been shown in a large RCT to be ineffective in reducing mortality.[72]

The accuracy of mammography depends on a number of factors. One large prospective cohort study of 329,495 women of ages 40 to 89 years from seven population-based mammography registries found sensitivity ranged from 62.9% in women with dense breasts to 87% in women with fatty breasts. Specificity ranged from 89.1% in women with dense breasts to 96.9% in women with fatty breasts.[73]

The accuracy of mammography varies among radiologists and among countries.[74–78] In general, North American radiologists tend to interpret a higher percentage of mammograms as positive than radiologists in other countries, without evident additional benefit. In one study of community radiologists in New England, false-positive rates ranged from 2.6% to 15.9%.[76] The accuracy of CBE also varies widely among clinicians.[79]

Newer approaches to breast cancer screening are being studied, targeted especially to increasing sensitivity.[80] Interestingly, although earlier mammography from the 1970s and 1980s was certainly less sensitive than present-day mammography, the Health Insurance Project (HIP) study from this era found a similar reduction in breast cancer mortality as more recent studies.[81,82] Thus, it is not clear whether increasing sensitivity will provide additional reduction in breast cancer mortality.

Rationale for Screening

The primary rationale for screening comes from the RCTs of screening that have been conducted over the past 30 years.[17,83] Although the overall evidence suggests that breast cancer mortality is reduced by mammographic screening, the reduction is less than 20%[6]; this means that 80% of the women who have potentially fatal cancers are not helped by screening and earlier treatment. Clearly, some breast cancers are aggressive and metastasize before they can be detected by mammography. Some, however, respond better to earlier treatment than to later, thus reducing mortality.

Given the relatively low reduction in mortality from breast cancer from screening, the absolute number of women whose lives would be extended is small. From one to two women in their forties and from two to six women in their fifties and sixties would have their lives extended by screening annually for 10 years.[84]

Harms of Screening

The two major potential harms of screening for breast cancer are false-positive tests and overtreatment of ductal carcinoma in situ (DCIS). One study estimated that 49% of women would have at least one false-positive mammogram after 10 rounds of screening; almost 19% would undergo a biopsy as a result of the false positive.[12] False-positive mammograms sometimes lead to a recommendation of a short-interval follow-up (e.g., 6 months rather than a year), despite the evidence that such a policy rarely leads to increased cancer detection.[85] False-positive mammograms do lead to increased anxiety, both in the short run and after 6 to 12 months, for some women.[10,86]

Ductal carcinoma in situ (DCIS) is a heterogeneous intermediate lesion with an uncertain prognosis. This lesion was rare before screening mammography but has increased dramatically as the number of women undergoing mammograms has increased. About 1 in 1300 mammograms detects DCIS;

from 16% to 28% of all breast "cancers" are DCIS.[87] Probably less than 50% of untreated women with DCIS ever develop invasive breast cancer.[88–90] Treatment is often surgical; some women have mastectomy whereas others have breast conservation surgery. Few women treated for DCIS eventually die of breast cancer.[91]

Because DCIS is so common (an estimated 59,000 cases in 2004)[1] and because its prognosis is so uncertain, many women undergo unnecessary surgery because of its diagnosis. This is an important area of overtreatment. One modeling study found that detection of DCIS plays a minor role in the reduction in breast cancer mortality from screening.[92]

Balance of Benefits and Harms

Screening for breast cancer is an important example of the trade-offs involved in the decision to be screened. On the one hand, screening likely does extend some women's lives. On the other hand, screening also leads to many women having workups for false-positive screening tests, and other women having treatment for DCIS, a lesion that would never develop into invasive breast cancer for many women. It is important for women to understand these trade-offs; women should be offered the opportunity to participate in the decision about screening.

Improving screening programs should seek not only to improve sensitivity. Improved sensitivity may or may not further reduce mortality. Improved specificity should also be a priority. If the number of women with false-positive tests can be reduced, potential harms could be decreased, thus improving the balance between benefits and harms.

Another way of improving breast cancer screening programs would involve finding ways of determining which women with DCIS are truly at risk of invasive cancer, allowing some women to avoid unnecessary surgery.

Example of Colorectal Cancer Screening

Incidence and Mortality

In 2004, an estimated 146,940 new cases of and 56,730 deaths from colon and rectal cancers were expected.[20] Colorectal cancer (CRC) is the third leading cause of new cancer cases (11% of all new cases) and cancer deaths (10% of all cancer deaths) in both men and women.[20] In 2000, the age-adjusted incidence rate in nine Surveillance, Epidemiology, and End Results Program (SEER) registries was 55 per 100,000; the age-adjusted mortality rate was 21 per 100,000.[21] The lifetime risk from birth of being diagnosed with CRC is about 6%; the lifetime risk of dying from CRC is about 2%. Thus, about 1 in 3 people who develop CRC die of this disease. Between 1992 and 2001, mortality from CRC declined by 1.8% per year[93] and incidence declined by 0.8% annually in the United States.[94] The early detection and removal of precancerous colorectal polyps may have contributed to the decline in CRC incidence and mortality.[95]

Screening Tests

The major screening tests currently available for CRC screening are the fecal occult blood test, sigmoidoscopy, colonoscopy, and double-contrast barium enema. These tests are used to identify precancerous or cancerous lesions in the colon and rectum. No one screening strategy has been shown to be superior to the others, although they differ in regard to accuracy, effectiveness, and potential harms.

Fecal occult blood testing (FOBT) has been examined in three RCTs involving more than 250,000 people followed for up to 18 years.[96,97] All three trials found a reduction in CRC mortality from 15% to 33%, with an absolute risk reduction for CRC deaths ranging from 0.8 per 1000 with biennial screening in the United Kingdom over 8 years of follow-up[98] to 4.6 per 1000 with annual screening in Minnesota during 18 years of follow-up.[99] The Minnesota study also noted a 17% to 20% decrease in incidence of CRC.[99] The sensitivity of a single test is approximately 30% to 50%, with a specificity of 90% to 98%, depending on how the test is done. Fecal occult blood tests find about 25% to 50% of patients with colorectal cancer, but only 2% of patients with a positive test had cancer in the Minnesota trial.

The effectiveness of sigmoidoscopy to reduce CRC deaths has been examined in three well-designed case-control studies.[100–102] These studies showed a mortality reduction of 60% to 80%.[97] In a small, randomized trial of sigmoidoscopy, in which persons with polyps were followed up with colonoscopy, the incidence of colorectal cancer was decreased by 80% but no decrease in mortality was found.[103] Using full examination of the colon as the "gold standard," sigmoidoscopy has been found to identify 70% to 80% of patients with advanced adenomas or cancer.[104,105] The sensitivity and specificity of sigmoidoscopy are difficult to determine, because all visible polyps are typically removed, many of which may have little to no malignant potential.

The ability of screening colonoscopy to reduce colorectal cancer morbidity or mortality has not been directly studied to date. Data from studies of other modalities have been extrapolated to support the effectiveness of colonoscopy. Because it is often used as the gold standard, determining its sensitivity and specificity has been difficult. A recent study by Pickhardt et al., comparing optical colonoscopy with CT virtual colonoscopy,[106] in which 1,233 patients underwent both procedures, found the sensitivity of optical colonoscopy for adenomatous polyps to be 88% to 92%, depending on the size of the polyps. As with sigmoidoscopy, the natural history of many polyps found on colonoscopic examination is not known; thus, the potential for identifying false positives must be considered.

No screening studies of double-contrast barium enema with a mortality outcome have been published; thus, the accuracy and effectiveness of this procedure are unknown.[96] Its sensitivity is likely lower than that of endoscopic procedures, but if it misses primarily polyps that are small and not likely to progress to invasive cancer, its effectiveness for screening may be adequate.

Rationale for Screening

A variety of different types of polyps occur in the colon and rectum. Hyperplastic polyps are the most common of those that have little potential for becoming malignant. They cannot be distinguished visually from adenomatous polyps, so biopsy is required for diagnosis. Whether the presence of distal hyperplastic polyps increases the risk of proximal neoplastic polyps is uncertain.[107] A systematic review of 18 studies[108] estimated a 21% to 25% risk for any proximal neoplasia in patients with a distal hyperplastic polyp, including a 4% to 5% risk of an advanced neoplasm (cancer or polyp with severe dysplasia or villous histology). In 4 of the studies in which colonoscopy was performed regardless of distal findings, however, the relative risk of finding any proximal neoplasia was 1.3 (95% confidence interval, 0.9–1.8).

Two-thirds of all colonic polyps are adenomatous, which are defined as dysplastic and thus have malignant potential. Most colorectal cancers arise from adenomatous polyps. Some proportion of these grow from small (less than 5 mm) to large (greater than 1.0 cm) to cancer, generally over a period of 10 years or longer. The proportion that makes this transition is thought to be small; adenomatous polyps occur in 30% to 40% of adults over the age of 50, but the risk of developing colorectal cancer is only about 6%.[107] However, removal of adenomatous polyps is associated with a reduced risk of colorectal cancer incidence and mortality.

Harms of Screening

The harms of screening for colorectal cancer include the risk of the screening tests themselves, the risks of the subsequent workup from positive screening tests, the potential for false-negative screening results, and the potential for overdiagnosis and treatment of lesions that would not have become malignant over the person's lifetime. No direct adverse effects of FOBT exist (other than the inconvenience and some patients' distaste for performing the test). Both sigmoidoscopy and colonoscopy are associated with low risks for major complications, including bleeding and perforation of the colon during the examination. A large population-based study of Medicare beneficiaries aged 65 and older found perforation rates of nearly 1 per 1,000 for sigmoidoscopy and 2 per 1,000 for colonoscopy.[109] The risk of death following colonic perforation was 52 to 65 per 1,000 perforations.

Fecal occult blood tests may miss small adenomas, as these lesions frequently do not bleed. Whether that represents a true negative or a false negative is uncertain, as these small adenomas may not be likely to develop into neoplastic lesions. Even though some consider colonoscopy to be the optimal examination of the colon and rectum for detection of precancerous and cancerous lesions, studies have shown that significant lesions (i.e., those larger than 1 cm) may be missed. The Pickhardt study comparing virtual with optical colonoscopy found that virtual colonoscopy missed 5 of 59 advanced neoplasms (defined as adenomatous polyps 10 mm or more in diameter or demonstrating high-grade dysplasia, villous changes, or cancer) and optical colonoscopy missed 7 of the 59 lesions.[106]

The risk of overdiagnosis and treatment of lesions that do not have long-term malignant potential (false-positive lesions) is more difficult to quantify. Most adenomas (60%–75%) are smaller than 1 cm on endoscopic examination.[107] The risk for high-grade dysplasia increases from 1% in small adenomas (less than 5 mm) to 6% for medium-sized adenomas (5–10 mm) to 21% for large adenomas (greater than 1 cm).[107]

Balance of Benefits and Harms

In a recent study of a screening colonoscopy program at a work site,[110] the authors created a clinical index to stratify risk for advanced proximal neoplasia (defined as an adenoma 1 cm or larger or one with villous histology, severe dysplasia, or cancer) and to identify a subgroup at low risk for whom screening sigmoidoscopy alone might be sufficient. Scores were based on age, sex, and distal findings. In the validation arm of the study, the 47% of the cohort determined to be in the low-risk subgroup had a risk for advanced proximal neoplasia of 0.4%. Use of the index in this population identified 92% of persons with advanced proximal neoplasia. The number needed to screen (NNS) to detect advanced proximal neoplasia among patients with any distal polyp was 16 and, among everyone, the NNS was 36. The NNS to extend one life from colorectal cancer mortality was not calculated and would be higher.

Colorectal cancer screening reduces death from colorectal cancer and decreases the incidence of invasive cancer by finding and removing adenomatous polyps. These benefits of screening, however, are tempered somewhat by the effort involved, the harms of the screening procedures themselves, and the possibility of overdiagnosis and overtreatment of small lesions with low malignant potential. As tests with greater sensitivity are developed, the risk of overdiagnosis increases.

References

1. Schwartz LA, Woloshin S, Fowler FJ, Welch HG. Enthusiasm for cancer screening in the United States. JAMA 2004;291: 71–78.
2. Hahn WC, Weinberg RA. Rules for making human tumor cells. N Engl J Med 2002;347:1593–1603.
3. Keyomarsi K, Tucker SL, Buchholz TA, et al. Cyclin E and survival in patients with breast cancer. N Engl J Med 2002; 347:1566–1575.
4. van de Vijver MJ, He YD, van't Veer LJ, et al. A gene-expression signature as a predictor of survival in breast cancer. N Engl J Med 2002;347(25):1999–2009.
5. Ramaswamy S, Perou CM. DNA microarrays in breast cancer: the promise of personalised medicine. Lancet 2003;361:1576–1577.
6. Nystrom L, Andersson I, Bjurstam N, et al. Long-term effects of mammography screening: updated overview of the Swedish randomized trials. Lancet 2002;359:909–919.
7. Soost HJ, Lange HJ, Lehmacher W, et al. The validation of cervical cytology. Sensitivity, specificity, and predictive values. Acta Cytol 1991;35:8–14.
8. Benoit AG, Krepart GV, Lotocki RJ. Results of prior cytologic screening in patients with a diagnosis of Stage I carcinoma of the cervix. Am J Obstet Gynecol 1984;148:690–694.
9. Peto J, Gilham C, Fletcher O, Matthews FE. The cervical cancer epidemic that screening has prevented in the UK. Lancet 2004; 364:249–356.
10. Lerman C, Trock B, Rimer B, et al. Psychological and behavioral implications of abnormal mammograms. Ann Intern Med 1991; 114:657–661.
11. McNaughton-Collins M, Fowler FJ, Caubert J-F, et al. Psychological effects of a suspicious prostate cancer screening test followed by a benign biopsy result. Am J Med 2004;117:719–725.
12. Elmore J, Barton M, Moceri V, et al. Ten-year risk of false positive screening mammograms and clinical breast examinations. N Engl J Med 1998;338:1089–1096.
13. Albertsen PC, Hanley JA, Gleason DF, Barry MJ. Competing risk analysis of men aged 55 to 74 years at diagnosis managed conservatively for clinically localized prostate cancer. JAMA 1998;280:975–980.
14. Black WC, Welch HG. Advances in diagnostic imaging and overestimations of disease prevalence and the benefits of therapy. N Engl J Med 1993;328:1237–1243.

15. Welch HG, Schwartz LM, Woloshin S. Are increasing 5-year survival rates evidence of success against cancer? JAMA 2000; 283:2975–2978.
16. Olsen O, Gotzsche PC. Cochrane review on screening for breast cancer with mammography. Lancet 2001;358:1340–1342.
17. Fletcher SW, Elmore JG. Mammographic screening for breast cancer. N Engl J Med 2003;348:1672–1680.
18. Harris RP, Helfand M, Woolf SH, et al. Current methods of the U.S. Preventive Services Task Force: a review of the process. Am J Prev Med 2001;20(3S):21–35.
19. Sheridan SL, Harris RP, Woolf SH, et al. Shared decision making about screening and chemoprevention. Am J Prev Med 2004;26: 56–66.
20. Jemal A, Tiwani RC, Murray T, et al. Cancer statistics, 2004. CA Cancer J Clin 2004;54:8–29.
21. Surveillance, Epidemiology, and End Results (SEER) Program (www.seer.cancer.gov) SEER* Stat Database: Incidence: SEER 9 Regs Public-Use, Nov 2002 Sub (1973–2000). National Cancer Institute, DCCPS, Surveillance Research Program, Cancer Statistics Branch, released April 2003, based on the November 2002 submission.
22. Ries LAG, Eisner MP, Kosary CL, et al. (eds). SEER Cancer Statistics Review, 1975–2000. National Cancer Institute. Bethesda, MD, http://seer.cancer.gov/csr/1975_2000, 2003.
23. Laara E, Day NE, Hakama M. Trends in mortality from cervical cancer in the Nordic countries: association with organised screening programmes. Lancet 1987;1(8544):1247–1249.
24. Christopherson WM, Lundin FE Jr, Mendez WM, et al. Cervical cancer control: a study of morbidity and mortality trends over a twenty-one-year period. Cancer 1976;38:1357–1366.
25. Miller AB, Lindsay J, Hill GB. Mortality from cancer of the uterus in Canada and its relationship to screening for cancer of the cervix. Int J Cancer 1976;17:602–612.
26. Johannesson G, Geirsson G, Day N. The effect of mass screening in Iceland, 1965–1974, on the incidence and mortality of cervical carcinoma. Int J Cancer 1978;21:418–425.
27. Sigurdsson K. Effect of organized screening on the risk of cervical cancer. Evaluation of screening activity in Iceland, 1964–1991. Int J Cancer 1993;54:563–570.
28. Benedet JL, Anderson GH, Matisic JP. A comprehensive program for cervical cancer detection and management. Am J Obstet Gynecol 1992;166:1254–1259.
29. Aristizabal N, Cuello C, Correa P, et al. The impact of vaginal cytology on cervical cancer risks in Cali, Colombia. Int J Cancer 1984;34:5–9.
30. Clarke EA, Anderson TW. Does screening by "Pap" smears help prevent cervical cancer? A case-control study. Lancet 1979; 2(8132):1–4.
31. La Vecchia C, Franceschi S, Decarli A, et al. "Pap" smear and the risk of cervical neoplasia: quantitative estimates from a case-control study. Lancet 1984;2(8406):779–782.
32. Herrero R, Brinton LA, Reeves WC, et al. Screening for cervical cancer in Latin America: a case-control study. Int J Epidemiol 1992;21:1050–1056.
33. Celentano DD, Klassen AC, Weisman CS, et al. Duration of relative protection of screening for cervical cancer. Prev Med 1989;18:411–422.
34. Screening for squamous cervical cancer: duration of low risk after negative results of cervical cytology and its implication for screening policies. IARC Working Group on evaluation of cervical cancer screening programmes. Br Med J (Clin Res Ed) 1986;293(6548):659–664.
35. Kleinman JC, Kopstein A. Who is being screened for cervical cancer? Am J Public Health 1981;71:73–76.
36. Nanda K, McCrory DC, Myers ER, et al. Accuracy of the Papanicolaou test in screening for and follow-up of cervical cytologic abnormalities: a systemic review. Ann Intern Med 2000;132: 810–819.
37. Hartmann KE, Hall SA, Nanda K, et al. Screening for Cervical Cancer. Rockville, MD: Agency for Health Research and Quality, 2002.
38. McCrory DC, Matchar DB, Bastian L, et al. Evaluation of Cervical Cytology. Evidence Report/Technology Assessment No. 5. AHCPR Publication No. 99-E010. Rockville, MD: Agency for Health Research and Quality, 1999.
39. Coste J, Cochand-Priollet B, de Cremoux P, et al. Cross sectional study of conventional cervical smear, monolayer cytology, and human papillomavirus DNA testing for cervical cancer screening. BMJ 2003;326(7392):733.
40. Holowaty P, Miller AB, Rohan T, et al. Natural history of dysplasia of the uterine cervix. J Natl Cancer Inst 1999;91:252–258.
41. Nasiell K, Roger V, Nasiell M. Behavior of mild cervical dysplasia during long-term follow-up. Obstet Gynecol 1986;69: 665–669.
42. Nash JD, Burke TW, Hoskins WJ. Biologic course of cervical human papillomavirus infection. Obstet Gynecol 1987;69:160–162.
43. Melnikow J, Nuovo J, Willan AR, et al. Natural history of cervical squamous intraepithelial lesions: a meta-analysis. Obstet Gynecol 1998;92(4 pt 2):727–735.
44. Bosch FX, Manos, MM, Muñoz N, et al. Prevalence of human papillomavirus in cervical cancer: a worldwide perspective. International biological study on cervical cancer (IBSCC) Study Group. J Natl Cancer Inst 1995;87:796–802.
45. Wallin KL, Wiklund F, Angström T, et al. Type-specific persistence of human papillomavirus DNA before the development of invasive cervical cancer. N Engl J Med 1999;341:1633 1638.
46. Alani RM, Münger K. Human papillomaviruses and associated malignancies. J Clin Oncol 1998;16:330–337.
47. Walboomers JM, Jacobs MV, Manos MM, et al. Human papillomavirus is a necessary cause of invasive cervical cancer worldwide. J Pathol 1999;189:12–19.
48. Ho GY, Bierman R, Beardsley L, et al. Natural history of cervicovaginal papillomavirus infection in young women. N Engl J Med 1998;338:423–428.
49. Fox J, Remington P, Layde P, Klein F. The effect of hysterectomy on the risk of an abnormal screening Papanicolaou test result. Am J Obstet Gynecol 1999;180:1104–1109.
50. Raffle AE, Alden B, Quinn M, et al. Outcomes of screening to prevent cancer: analysis of cumulative incidence of cervical abnormality and modeling of cases and deaths prevented. BMJ 2003;326:901–905.
51. Solomon D, Schiffman M, Tarone R, et al. Comparison of three management strategies for patients with atypical squamous cells of undetermined significance: baseline results from a randomized trial. J Natl Cancer Inst 2001;93:293–299.
52. Schiffman M, Adrianza MF. ASCUC-LSIL Triage Study. Design, methods, and characteristics of trial participants. Acta Cytol 2000;44:726–742.
53. Sawaya GF. Should routine screening Papanicolaou smears be done for women older than 65 years? Arch Intern Med 2004; 164:243–245.
54. Fox J, Remington P, Layde P, et al. The effect of hysterectomy on the risk of an abnormal screening Papanicolaou test result. Am J Obstet Gynecol 1999;180:1104–1109.
55. Pearce KF, Haefner HK, Sarwar SF, et al. Cytopathological findings on vaginal Papanicolaou smears after hysterectomy for benign gynecologic disease. N Engl J Med 1996;335:1559–1562.
56. US Preventive Services Task Force. Screening for Cervical Cancer: Recommendations and Rationale. Accessed at http://www.ahrq.gov/clinic/uspstf/uspscerv.htm on Feb. 29, 2004.
57. Harris R, Lohr KN. Screening for prostate cancer: an update of the evidence for the US Preventive Services Task Force. Ann Intern Med 2002;137:917–929.

58. Barry MJ. Prostate-specific-antigen testing for early diagnosis of prostate cancer. N Engl J Med 2001;344:1373–1377.
59. Sirovich BE, Schwartz LM, Woloshin S. Screening men for prostate and colorectal cancer in the United States. JAMA 2003;289:1414–1420.
60. Holmberg L, Bill-Axelson A, Helgesen F, et al. A randomized trial comparing radical prostatectomy with watchful waiting in early prostate cancer. N Engl J Med 2002;347:781–789.
61. Djavan B, Ravery V, Zlotta A, et al. Prospective evaluation of prostate cancer detected on biopsies 1, 2, 3 and 4: when should we stop? J Urol 2001;166:1679–1683.
62. Prostate-specific antigen (PSA) best practice policy. American Urological Association (AUA). Oncology 2002;14:267–272.
63. American Cancer Society. ACS Cancer Detection Guidelines: Cancer-Related Checkup. Accessed at www.cancer.org on November 23, 2004.
64. American Medical Association. Policy H-425.980 Screening and Early Detection of Prostate Cancer. Accessed at www.ama-assn.org on November 23, 2004.
65. US Preventive Services Task Force. Screening for prostate cancer: recommendations and rationale. Ann Intern Med 2002;137:915–916.
66. Periodic Health Examinations. Revision 5.6, August 2004. American Academy of Family Physicians. Accessed at www.aafp.org on November 23, 2004.
67. American College of Physicians. Screening for prostate cancer. Ann Intern Med 1997;126:480–484.
68. Ghafoor A, Jemal A, Ward E, Cokkinides V, Smith R, Thun M. Trends in breast cancer by race and ethnicity. CA Cancer J Clin 2003;53:342–355.
69. Jatoi I, Miller AB. Why is breast cancer mortality declining? Lancet Oncol 2003;4:251–254.
70. Barton MB, Harris R, Fletcher SW. Does this patient have breast cancer? JAMA 1999;282:1270–1280.
71. Harris R, Kinsinger LS. Routinely teaching breast self-examination is dead. What does this mean? J Natl Cancer Inst 2002;94:1420–1421.
72. Thomas DB, Gao DL, Ray RM, et al. Randomized trial of breast self-examination in Shanghai: final results. J Natl Cancer Inst 2002;94:1445–1457.
73. Carney PA, Miglioretti DL, Yankaskas BC, et al. Individual and combined effects of age, breast density, and hormone replacement therapy use on the accuracy of screening mammography. Ann Intern Med 2003;138:168–175.
74. Smith-Bindman R, Chu PW, Miglioretti DL, et al. Comparison of screening mammography in the United States and the United Kingdom. JAMA 2003;290:2129–2137.
75. Elmore JG, Nakano CY, Koepsell TD, Desnick LM, D'Orsi CJ, Ransohoff DF. International variation in screening mammography interpretations in community-based programs. J Natl Cancer Inst 2003;95:1384–3193.
76. Elmore JG, Miglioretti DL, Reisch LM, et al. Screening mammograms by community radiologists: variability in false-positive rates. J Natl Cancer Inst 2002;94:1373–1380.
77. Beam CA, Conant EF, Sickles EA. Association of volume and volume-independent factors with accuracy in screening mammogram interpretation. J Natl Cancer Inst 2003;95:282–290.
78. Esserman L, Cowley H, Eberle C, et al. Improving the accuracy of mammography: volume and outcome relationships. J Natl Cancer Inst 2002;94:369–375.
79. Fletcher SW, O'Malley MS, Bunce LA. Physicians' abilities to detect lumps in silicone breast models. JAMA 1985;253:2224–2228.
80. Liberman L. Breast cancer screening with MRI: what are the data for patients at high risk? N Engl J Med 2004;351:497–500.
81. Shapiro S, Venet W, Strax P, Venet L. Periodic Screening for Breast Cancer: The Health Insurance Plan Project and Its Sequelae, 1963–1986. Baltimore: Johns Hopkins University Press, 1988.
82. Fletcher SW, Black W, Harris R, Rimer BK, Shapiro S. Report of the International Workshop on Screening for Breast Cancer. J Natl Cancer Inst 1993;85:1644–1656.
83. Humphrey LL, Helfand M, Chan BK, Woolf SH. Breast cancer screening: a summary of the evidence for the U.S. Preventive Services Task Force. Ann Intern Med 2002;137:347–360.
84. Harris R, Leininger L. Clinical strategies for breast cancer screening: weighing and using the evidence. Ann Intern Med 1995;122:539–547.
85. Yasmeen S, Romano PS, Pettinger M, et al. Frequency and predictive value of a mammographic recommendation for short-interval follow-up. J Natl Cancer Inst 2003;95:429–436.
86. Yasmeen S, Romano PS, Pettinger M, et al. Re: Short-interval follow-up mammography: are we doing the right thing? J Natl Cancer Inst 2003;95:1175–1176.
87. Barton MB, Moore S, Polk S, Shtatland E, Elmore JG, Fletcher SW. Increased patient concern after false-positive mammograms: clinician documentation and subsequent ambulatory visits. J Gen Intern Med 2001;16:150–156.
88. Ernster VL, Ballard-Barbash R, Barlow WE, et al. Detection of ductal carcinoma in situ in women undergoing screening mammography. J Natl Cancer Inst 2002;94:1546–1554.
89. Page DL, Dupont WD, Rogers LW, Landenberger M. Intraductal carcinoma of the breast: follow-up after biopsy only. Cancer (Phila) 1982;49:751–758.
90. Page DL, Jensen RA. Ductal carcinoma in situ of the breast: understanding the misunderstood stepchild. JAMA 1996;275:948–949.
91. Welch HG, Black WC. Using autopsy series to estimate the disease "reservoir" for ductal carcinoma in situ of the breast: how much more breast cancer can we find? Ann Intern Med 1997;127:1023–1028.
92. Ernster VL, Barclay J, Kerlikowske K, Wilkie H, Ballard-Barbash R. Mortality among women with ductal carcinoma in situ of the breast in the population-based surveillance, epidemiology and end results program. Arch Intern Med 2000;160:953–958.
93. Surveillance, Epidemiology, and End Results (SEER) Program (www.seer.cancer.gov) SEER* Stat Database: Mortality: All COD, Public-Use With State, Total U.S. (1969–2001). National Cancer Institute, DCCPS, Surveillance Research Program, Cancer Statistics Branch, released April 2004. Underlying mortality data provided by NCHS (www.cdc.gov/nchs).
94. Surveillance, Epidemiology, and End Results (SEER) Program (www.seer.cancer.gov) SEER* Stat Database: Incidence: SEER 9 Regs Public-Use, Nov 2003 Sub (1973–2001). National Cancer Institute, DCCPS, Surveillance Research Program, Cancer Statistics Branch, released April 2004, based on the November 2003 submission.
95. Weir HK, Thun MJ, Hankey BF, et al. Annual report to the nation on the status of cancer, 1975–2000, featuring the uses of surveillance data for cancer prevention and control. J Natl Cancer Inst 2003;95:1276–1299.
96. Pignone M, Rich M, Teustch SM, Berg AO, Lohr KN. Screening for colorectal cancer in adults at average risk: a summary of the evidence for the U.S. Preventive Services Task Force. Ann Intern Med 2002;137:132–141.
97. Walsh JME, Terdiman JP. Colorectal cancer screening. Scientific review. JAMA 2003;289:1288–1296.
98. Hardcastle JD, Chamberlain JO, Robinson MH, et al. Randomized controlled trial of faecal-occult-blood screening for colorectal cancer. Lancet 1996;348:1472–1477.
99. Mandel JS, Bond JH, Church TR, et al. Reducing the mortality from colorectal cancer by screening for fecal occult blood. Minnesota Colon Cancer Screening Study. N Engl J Med 1993;328:1365–1371.
100. Selby JV, Friedman GD, Quesenberry CP Jr, Weiss NS. A case-control study of screening sigmoidoscopy and mortality from colorectal cancer. N Engl J Med 1992;326:653–657.

101. Newcomb PA, Norfleet RG, Storer BE, Surawicz TS, Marcus PM. Screening sigmoidoscopy and colorectal cancer mortality. J Natl Cancer Inst 1992;84:1572–1575.
102. Muller AD, Sonnerberg A. Prevention of colorectal cancer by flexible endoscopy and polypectomy: a case-control study among veterans. Arch Intern Med 1995;123:904–910.
103. Thiis-Everson E, Hoff GS, Sauar J, Langmark F, Majak BM, Vatn MH. Population-based surveillance by colonoscopy: effect on the incidence of colorectal cancer. Telemark Polyp Study I. Scand J Gastroenterol 1999;34:414–420.
104. Lieberman DA, Weiss DG, Bond JH, Ahnen DJ, Garewal H, Chejfec G. Use of colonoscopy to screen asymptomatic adults for colorectal cancer. Veterans Affairs Cooperative Study Group 380. N Engl J Med 2000;343:162–168.
105. Imperiale TF, Wagner DR, Lin CY, Larkin GN, Rogge JD, Ransohoff DF. Risk of advanced proximal neoplasms in asymptomatic adults according to the distal colorectal findings. N Engl J Med 2000;343:169–174.
106. Pickhardt PJ, Choi JR, Hwang I, et al. Computed tomographic virtual colonoscopy to screen for colorectal neoplasia in asymptomatic adults. N Engl J Med 2003;349:2191–2200.
107. Lawrence SP, Ahnen DJ. Approach to the patient with colonic polyps. In: Rose BD (ed) UpToDate. Wellesley: UpToDate, 2004.
108. Dave S, Hui S, Kroenke K, Imperiale TF. Is the distal hyperplastic polyp a marker for proximal neoplasia? A systematic review. J Gen Intern Med 2003;18:128–137.
109. Gatto NM, Frucht H, Sundararajan V, Jacobson JS, Grann VR, Neugut AI. Risk of perforation after colonoscopy and sigmoidoscopy: a population-based study. J Natl Cancer Inst 2003; 95:230–236.
110. Imperiale TF, Wagner DR, Lin CY, Larkin GN, Rogge JD, Ransohoff DF. Using risk for advanced proximal colonic neoplasia to tailor endoscopic screening for colorectal cancer. Ann Intern Med 2003;139:959–965.

13 Patient Decision Making

Peter A. Ubel

- A 73-year-old man requests a prostate-specific antigen (PSA) test from his primary care physician, but the physician does not believe the test is in the patient's best interest.
- A woman with metastatic colon cancer has continued to progress on standard therapy. She asks her oncologist whether she should enter a Phase I trial or, instead, enter a hospice program.
- A woman with a strong family history of breast cancer, and a BRCA-1 mutation, asks her genetic counselor to explain the pros and cons of a prophylactic mastectomy.
- A 55-year-old man with myelodysplasia comes to a cancer referral center to see whether they think a bone marrow transplant is feasible in someone his age.

Patients interact with a wide range of clinicians, seeking help in deciding how to prevent, detect, or treat cancer. Many of these decisions are difficult—sometimes because there is not great evidence about the risks and benefits of specific healthcare interventions, such as the role of PSA testing in preventing mortality and morbidity from prostate cancer; sometimes because the evidence, although solid, is so complex that it is difficult for patients to process the information in the time they have to make a decision; and oftentimes, because the decisions involve difficult value judgments, in which there is no right or wrong decision for all patients, because the best choice varies depending on patient preferences.

How should clinicians handle these difficult situations? When should they make clinical recommendations and when should they let patients decide what is best? How can they explain uncertainty to patients in ways that they can understand? Or should they even bother to do so?

A Paradigm Shift: Involving Patients in Healthcare Decisions

A generation ago, clinicians did not struggle with these questions, because patients played a limited role in their healthcare decisions. For example, a 1961 survey revealed that the majority of patients undergoing cancer treatments did not know that they had cancer; their oncologists withheld such information because of fear that patients could not emotionally handle it.[1] Many physicians did not discuss treatment alternatives with patients, because they, the physicians, would be making the decisions. For example, it was not uncommon for a woman to wake up from a breast biopsy procedure to learn not only that she had breast cancer but that the surgeon had gone ahead and performed a mastectomy.[2]

A paradigm shift has occurred over the past several decades. Most physicians now recognize that patients deserve information about their health, and few think it is appropriate to withhold cancer diagnosis from patients, except in the most extreme circumstances.[1] This shift was spurred on in part by the legal community, who encouraged patients to sue physicians for not informing them about their treatment alternatives; by the growth of the bioethics movement and its emphasis on patient autonomy; and by larger societal changes, with consumer groups and community organizations becoming more involved in decision making that was previously left to experts.

Accompanying this shift has been a change in clinicians' attitudes. Many clinicians now recognize that healthcare decisions often involve trade-offs that require value judgments. For example, oncology trials used to measure survival rates while paying little attention to quality of life issues. As the science of quality of life measurement matured, however, such measures have been incorporated into the vast majority of trials, thereby providing important information to guide oncologic decision making. But at the same time, quality of life information has made these decisions more complex. In the past, a study might simply have shown that the median survival for chemotherapy A was 3 months greater than chemotherapy B, making the decision about which chemotherapy to choose relatively straightforward. Now, however, a trial might show that chemotherapy A, although leading to longer survival, also leads to a lower quality of life. Now, the *best* choice depends on patients' preferences for longevity versus quality of life.[3]

Many clinical decisions are not purely scientific matters, but also involve value judgments that vary from person to person. For example, the right choice, for a patient choosing between surgical and radiation treatment of his prostate cancer, depends on how much he thinks he would be bothered by surgical complications such as impotence or incontinence and on how important he feels it is to have the cancer physically removed from his body. Similarly, whether a woman should begin receiving annual mammography at age 40 or 50 depends on how she feels about the inconvenience and discomfort of mammography, the financial costs of screening, the consequences of false-positive testing, and the benefits of receiving more aggressive screening.

Patients deserve a role in medical decisions, not only because those decisions often hinge on patients' values but also because higher levels of patient involvement in healthcare decision making leads to better health outcomes. Patients who are more involved in decisions about their care are more likely to adhere to their treatment regimens, to report higher levels of satisfaction with medical care, and to have better functional and clinical outcomes.[4–7] For example, a randomized trial demonstrated that a brief intervention to increase patient involvement in medical decision making among diabetic patients significantly lowered their HgbA1C levels.[8]

Clinicians used to leave patients in the dark about their healthcare decisions. Those days are long gone. Part of the art of medicine now includes knowing how and when to involve patients in healthcare decisions.

How to Involve Patients in Healthcare Decisions

It is one thing to recognize that choices between healthcare interventions often hinge on patients' values and quite another to find a practical and useful way to involve patients in their healthcare decisions. So how can physicians go about doing this?

Clinicians could simply play the role of information providers, giving patients all the information (ideally in a comprehensible manner) that patients need to make their decisions. Genetic counselors often take this approach, seeing their role as educators but not advisors. They help patients understand information, but believe it is beyond their purview to make clinical recommendations. The decision, they believe, is up to the patient. Alternatively, clinicians could give patients information in conjunction with a clinical recommendation, involving patients in decisions by giving them the final say, but guiding them with their recommendations.

More often, physicians reside somewhere between those extremes. Across physicians, then, there is a continuum of decision-making styles, with some physicians leaving decisions completely up to patients, with others sharing decision-making authority with patients, and with yet others taking the decision-making role on themselves by making strong clinical recommendations to their patients. Although the use of some level of participatory decision making has been correlated with higher levels of patient satisfaction and better clinical outcomes, there is little empirical evidence about differences in outcomes across the continuum of participatory decision making.[9] Many physicians benefit from tailoring their decision-making style to the individual patient and the specific clinical context.

As do physicians, patients vary in their decision-making styles. Some patients prefer to completely defer decisions to their physician. Others see themselves as the primary decision maker and do not want physicians to give them a recommendation. Many patients want to share decision-making roles with their clinicians.[10–13]

Moreover, a given patient's decision-making style varies depending on the clinical situation. When situations are more complex and alternatives do not create value-laden trade-offs, patients often want physicians to play a more significant role in making decisions.[14,15] For example, oncology patients being evaluated for possible pulmonary embolisms would rarely feel any need to discuss the relative merits of Doppler testing versus *d*-dimer testing.[16] These kinds of decisions are seen as medical decisions that require a clinician's training to make and which do not lead to the kinds of trade-offs that require patients to be heavily involved in the decision. Other decisions are less clinically complex and involve important trade-offs, such as those described previously between quality of life and quantity of life. In these cases, more patients express an interest in being involved in the decision. For similar reasons, patients express more interest in being involved in decisions for nonacute conditions than emergent ones.

Clinicians should not be expected to know how likely the average patient would be to desire a specific decision-making role in every clinical context they encounter. There would be little reason, in other words, for clinicians to remember that 13% of patients want a physician's recommendation in one specific clinical context whereas 53% want one in another context. As interesting as these statistics are, they are not relevant to the one-on-one decisions that clinicians and patients make. Rather than familiarize themselves with these statistics, clinicians should find out whether *this* patient wants to be involved in *this* decision. And that is best handled by talking with the patient. Such conversations are crucial, because clinicians typically underestimate how involved cancer patients want to be in their decisions.[17,18]

Although there is significant variance, across patients and across situations, in how involved patients want to be in their healthcare decisions, one desire is almost universal: patients want to be thoroughly informed about their treatment alternatives, even when they want their clinicians to decided what alternative they should take.[10,19,20] This situation, then, creates another challenge for clinicians, that is, providing their patients with comprehensible information about their healthcare alternatives to help them make good decisions.

Challenges to Helping Patients Make Good Decisions

Emotion

Many physicians fear that patients are so overwhelmed by the emotional content of their situations that they are unable to truly comprehend their medical alternatives. For example, patients often experience strong emotions when they receive cancer diagnoses. Extreme emotions can interfere with good decision making. Patients with terminal metastatic cancers may be so afraid of dying that they grasp at nonexistent straws. Elderly patients with localized prostate cancer may be so distressed at the thought of cancer cells residing in their bodies that they will not even consider watchful waiting.

Clinicians should recognize, however, that emotions are not necessarily antithetical to optimal decision making. For example, neurologists have determined that many patients with frontal lobe injuries have completely intact reasoning abilities; they can process information about risks and benefits normally but make bad decisions about their lives. They make bad decisions because they lack emotional feedback to guide their decisions.[21] In some contexts, in fact, intuitive *gut* decision making leads to better outcomes than highly reasoned decision making.[22,23]

Moreover, even when emotions interfere with optimal decision making, the emotions may still deserve a role in decision making. For example, imagine a patient who is prey to what decision scientists call an *omission bias*; he would rather accept a 10% chance of some terrible outcome from natural causes than a 5% chance of the same outcome resulting as a complication of treatment because he believes he will blame himself for making a choice that leads to a treatment complication.[24] Rationally speaking, a 5% chance of something bad happening is better than a 10% chance of the same thing happening. But if this person would truly torture himself if he experienced the complication following treatment, and would not do so if he experienced the outcome naturally, then he should probably not receive treatment.

Similarly, the need to maintain hope and provide accurate information is a central challenge to physician–patient communication in oncology.[25,26] On one hand, patients report a strong desire to have physicians encourage hope and optimism about their cancer, often in settings where there is little chance of long-term survival.[27] On the other hand, overly optimistic communication can lead to a misplaced focus on aggressive treatment and is often regretted by patients when they reach later stages of their illness.[28] Furthermore, providing patients with accurate information about a prognosis with and without treatment is necessary for their participation in medical decision making. Concern about how best to balance accuracy and hope can lead many clinicians to avoid participatory decision making.[29]

Numeracy and Literacy

Patients can also struggle with decisions because they have difficulty processing numerical information. Many people have a difficult time understanding concepts such as percentages or frequencies.[30,31] They do not know how to interpret imprecise medical information ("the test indicates you have somewhere between a 60% and 80% chance of . . ."). They also have difficulty with medical lingo; even seemingly simple words such as *recurrence* confuse many patients.[32,33] To make matters worse, physicians are frequently unaware that patients do not understand the information the physicians have communicated to them.[34,35]

Folklore and Prior Beliefs

Patients' decisions are often guided by folklore and prior beliefs. A patient who believes that cancer can spread through the air may be reluctant to have a surgical resection of his cancer for fear that the surgery will spread the cancer.[36] Culturally based models of disease and illness can clash with biomedical models, hindering participatory decision making.[37] These clashes are often evident in patient skepticism about the efficacy of certain biomedical treatments and interest in alternative and complementary approaches.[38,39] In addition, patients often have false beliefs about their risks of specific cancers. For example, the average woman's lifetime risk of breast cancer is about 13% and yet the average woman thinks her risk is closer to 40%.[40] Physicians need to negotiate a common understanding among these divergent beliefs, bringing together respect for the individual cultural background of a patient with the need to help patients understand their true clinical situations.

Distrust

Distrust of the medical profession and other components of the healthcare system may interfere with a patient's ability to make a good decision. Distrust arises when physicians are no longer seen as committed to acting in their patients' best interest.[41] This situation may occur when patients are concerned about physician motives, for example, cost-containment, or have had prior experiences of failed expectations.[42] Largely anecdotal evidence suggests that distrust is most prevalent among minority groups in the United States, in part because of both historical and current examples of racism within the medical system.[43] Although some level of skepticism may encourage patients to become involved in their medical decisions, high levels of distrust of the healthcare system may lead patients to discount the potential benefits of medical treatment and avoid medical care. Low levels of trust may also interfere with effective physician–patient relationships, making it more difficult and less rewarding for physicians to devote time and energy to effective participatory decision making.

Desire to Avoid Difficult Decisions

Even in dispassionate moments, people can make irrational decisions—decisions that conflict with their own preferences. For example, imagine the following admittedly hypothetical situation: you were recently diagnosed with colon cancer, and there are two surgical treatments available. Surgery 1 cures 80% of patients without complications, but the remaining 20% die of colon cancer. Surgery 2 also cures patients without complications 80% of the time, but only 16% die of colon cancer. The remaining 4% are cured of their colon cancer, but experience one of four surgical complications: a permanent colostomy, chronic diarrhea, intermittent abdominal pain, or a wound infection that takes 1 year to heal. More than 90% of people say that the four side effects of surgery 2 are preferable to dying of colon cancer. And yet, 50% of people still choose surgery 1 over surgery 2.[44] It appears that people are so overwhelmed by the sheer number and graphicness of the four complications of surgery 2 that they choose surgery 1. People minimize the survival difference between these two treatments ("the difference is only 4%") while fixating on the different rate of complications. This seemingly irrational choice does not go away when people are shown, in writing, the inconsistency of their views. Avoiding such decisions probably requires face-to-face conversations.

People do not need to be scared by graphic side effects to shy away from what seem like superior alternatives. For example, in one study, when physicians were presented with a hypothetical patient with severe osteoarthritis, many said they would prescribe a new nonsteroidal antiinflammatory drug (NSAID) for the patient if it were available at the same time that they referred the patient to an orthopedic specialist. But when physicians were told that two new NSAIDs were available, many decided not to prescribe *either* NSAID and simply referred the patient to a specialist without any new medication. Addition of the second NSAID put physicians in a position where they had to make a slightly more difficult choice, and many physicians acted as if they were unwilling to make that choice.[45] A similar phenomenon likely explains why people are more likely to purchase jams from a grocery store displaying 6 of the jams than one displaying 24; when there is too much to think about, people are averse to making tough choices.[46]

Anecdotal Reasoning

Perhaps one of the most powerful influences on patients' decisions is their anecdotal experiences. It might be hard to interest a patient in chemotherapy whose aunt had a bad experience with chemotherapy. Anecdotal information is very powerful and can draw people's attention away from much more representative evidence. For example, even when informed of the success rates of treatment alternatives, people's choices can be influenced by uninformative anecdotes. A treatment alternative that is described as curing an illness 75% of the time is looked on less favorably if people are exposed to hypothetical anecdotes of patients who did not improve with treatment.[47]

Emotional Mispredictions

Good decisions rely on good predictions. When choosing what television show to watch, what flavor of yogurt to eat, or what house to buy, people try to think about which alternative will best help them reach their goal of being happy or healthy or safe or whatever. And yet, people frequently mispredict how alternatives will make them feel. They spend piles of money on a big new house, expecting it to make them happy, and find out that they miss their cozy, old neighborhood.[48]

Such mispredictions are common in health settings.[49] For example, patients with inflammatory bowel disease expect that having a colostomy would make them miserable, and yet patients emotionally adapt to colostomies relatively quickly.[50] People predict that they would be miserable if they had kidney failure, and yet most dialysis patients are happy.[51] Such mispredictions could influence patients' healthcare decisions. If a prostate cancer patient overestimates how much he will be bothered by impotence or incontinence, he may forgo potentially beneficially treatments.

Clinician Resources and Training

Despite the multiple patient factors that hinder effective decision making, clinicians may still be the greatest obstacle to involving patients in their healthcare decisions. Although clinicians rarely withhold cancer diagnoses from patients anymore, they still often fail to give patients enough information to be fully involved in their healthcare decisions. Analyzing audiotapes of visits between clinicians and patients, researchers have found that physicians rarely give patients thorough and comprehensible information about their treatment alternatives.[52] In addition, clinicians often do a poor job of giving patients an opportunity to express their concerns, interrupting them frequently throughout the visits, and not giving them a chance to ask questions.

Physicians' poor communication results partly from remnants of paternalism. Many physicians still believe that healthcare decisions are primarily theirs to make. Nevertheless, even those physicians who reject this view often have difficulty communicating to patients. Most physicians do not receive extensive training on how to communicate effectively with patients.[53] Medical school curricula are still dominated by the basic sciences. Also, clinical teaching, although emphasizing the importance of conducting thorough histories and physical examinations, rarely uses the latest advances in the communication sciences. This is unfortunate, because communication skills can be taught, and medical schools that have integrated communication skills into their curricula have found that their medical students are better communicators.[54]

In addition, clinicians face time pressures and fiscal constraints that reduce their incentive to discuss issues at length with their patients. Perhaps more importantly, clinicians recognize that patients are not always emotionally or intellectually prepared to absorb a great deal of information about their healthcare alternatives. Consequently, clinicians may feel that it is a waste of time and money to embark on lengthy discussions of treatment alternatives with their patients.

Helping Patients to Make Better Decisions

It would be easy for clinicians to conclude that, if patients are going to make bad decisions because of emotions, mispredictions, or an inability to make difficult choices, then they should give up on involving patients in their healthcare decisions. But this would be a mistake. It would violate legal and ethical norms, it would reduce patient satisfaction and treatment adherence, and it would leave patients vulnerable to physicians' own biases. Physicians make many of the same mistakes patients make, for example, avoiding difficult decisions and mispredicting the emotional consequences of health problems. In addition, physicians are prone to specialty biases; urologists, for example, have very different attitudes toward radical prostectectomy from radiation oncologists[55] and different attitudes toward PSA testing from primary care physicians.[56]

For these reasons, we think clinicians should not abandon the idea of involving patients in their healthcare decisions. Instead, we recommend the use of several strategies to facilitate this task.

Being Selective

Patients do not need to be involved in every healthcare decision. When decisions are low stake, and do not involve trade-offs (where patient preferences are important in deciding what is best), clinicians do not need to involve patients in the decisions. For example, patients suffering from chemotherapy-related nausea probably do not want a lengthy discussion of the merits of one class of medication versus another. Instead, they want relief from their nausea.

When deciding how much to involve patients in a decision, clinicians should think about whether reasonable clinicians could disagree about the course of action, not just clinicians from one's own specialty but also those from other specialties. The greater the medical consensus, the less need to talk at great length to patients about inferior alternatives.[16]

Clinicians should think about how quickly a decision needs to be made. In emergency situations, it is often difficult to involve patients in treatment decisions. Furthermore, if emotions are running high, patients are often most likely to rely on clinicians for advice. Patients still need and deserve information about their treatment alternatives, but when patients are too emotional to make decisions, they will often be happy to receive recommendations from their physician. When decisions are not so urgent, however, there is more opportunity to involve patients. Decisions in oncology span the spectrum from the emergent to the elective and clinicians should tailor their decision-making style to this spectrum.

Taking Advantage of Time

Clinicians should remind themselves that strong emotions often dissipate over time. Furthermore, the ability to retain and process information about a cancer diagnosis increases over time. When possible, clinicians should rely on time as a useful clinical intervention. For example, men with new diagnoses of localized prostate cancer often find out about their diagnosis at the same clinic visit that they decide how to treat the cancer. It is doubtful that these patients have had time to absorb all the information in one sitting, especially given their likely shock at receiving a cancer diagnosis. Perhaps a better goal at such a visit is to communicate their diagnosis and prognosis to patients, and let them know that good treatment options are available, which they can decide about over the next few weeks. When delivering bad news to patients, clinicians should expect that many patients will not be able to process much clinical information during the initial visit, and will usually be more capable on subsequent visits of doing so, when the shock has subsided.

Time may also provide an important context for balancing the need for hope and the need for accurate information. The object of a patient's hope should vary as his or her disease progresses. Initially, most patients focus on long-term survival, whereas later patients may be encouraged to move to short-term goals, and finally many terminal patients will shift to hoping for a *good* or peaceful death.[57,58] Clinicians should understand where a patient is in this timeline and help the patient to reframe his or her object of hope to match their clinical circumstance.[59] Realistic information can be focused on what is needed to negotiate the decisions at each step.

Using Tools for Providing Information

In helping patients make good decisions, clinicians should give patients written information to help them comprehend their clinical alternatives, when possible, or refer them to appropriate Websites. Providing audiotapes of visits where important decisions are discussed may increase patient satisfaction and retention of information and is nearly universally preferred by patients.[60–62] Clinicians should encourage patients to review all materials with loved ones, and arrange for an opportunity to answer any questions that arise. Use of these tools may provide additional benefits by facilitating caregiver support during the decision process.[63]

Risk communication is an important component of providing information to patients about their medical decisions. Thus, the use of specific strategies for improving risk communication may have substantial benefits for involving patients in their decisions. Presentation of frequencies with specific reference groups (25 of 1,000 people who undergo chemotherapy will die of the treatment) instead of percentages (0.25%) may reduce confusion and facilitate understanding of small risks.[64] Furthermore, the use of the same denominator (i.e., 1,000 people) for different risks (e.g., risk of dying of chemotherapy and risk of cancer recurrence) simplifies the comparison of these risks.[64] Presentation of both negative (25 of 1,000 people who undergo chemotherapy will die of the treatment) and positive framing (975 of 1,000 people who undergo chemotherapy will not die of the treatment) can reduce biases in decision making.[65,66] Furthermore, when possible, the use of visual aids, such as bar graphs or pie charts, can increase the comprehension and saliency of risk information[28] and can even reduce the influence of anecdotal information.[67]

Building Trust

Trust is a critical component of the physician–patient relationship and necessary for patients to participate effectively in their medical decisions. Open communication is one of the key factors that establishes and reinforces trust.[68] Thus, even relatively basic steps toward participatory decision making, such as providing adequate information to patients and listening to their opinions and concerns, may serve to increase trust in the relationship and further improve decision outcomes. Trust is greatest in relationships where the patient believes that physician values are compatible with their own.[69] Such perceptions of value congruence are determined in part by the physician's behavior, practice circumstances, and payment structure, but may also be fostered by the physician demonstrating interest in and respect for the patient's life outside of their cancer diagnosis.[6,70] Trust erodes when physicians fail to meet patients' expectations for communication and competency.[71] Developing systems to minimize errors in either the process or outcomes of care helps to ensure that patients' expectations are met, thereby also increasing trust and facilitating participatory decision making.

Tailoring the Approach to the Individual Patient

Clinicians should remember that one size does not fit all. Some patients depend on your clinical recommendations while others will only want you to lay out their clinical alternatives. Giving recommendations is part of being a good doctor. Recommendations may seem odd in some contexts; if a patient is choosing, for example, between two treatments that yield identical survival rates but different complications, it would seem that the choice entirely depends on the patient's views of the various complications. And yet, may patients expect their doctors to tell them what to do and will be anxious if too much of the decision is laid at their feet.[72] In such cases, physicians might do best to talk to patients about their various complications, to find out how patients feel about the complications, and then to make recommendations that seem to fit best with patients' values.

Conclusion

Under pressure to see more patients in less time, it is difficult for busy clinicians to always find enough time to involve patients in their healthcare decisions. Fortunately, with the growth of the Internet, with the increasing use of group visits, and with the expanding use of healthcare teams to take care of oncology patients, there are lots of creative ways clinicians can help patients understand their medical choices. And given the high stakes of so many oncologic decisions, involving patients in their healthcare decisions can be one of the most rewarding aspects of practicing the art of medicine.

References

1. Novack DH, Plumer R, Smith RL, Ochitill H, Morrow GR, Bennett JM. Changes in physicians' attitudes toward telling the cancer patient. JAMA 1979;241(9):897–900.
2. Lerner BH. The Breast Cancer Wars. New York: Oxford, 2001.
3. Singer PA, Tasch ES, Stocking C, Rubin S, Siegler M, Weichselbaum R. Sex or survival: trade-offs between quality and quantity of life. J Clin Oncol 1991;9(2):328–334.
4. Hall JA, Roter DL, Katz NR. Meta-analysis of correlates of provider behavior in medical encounters. Med Care 1988;26(7): 657–675.
5. Robbins JA, Bertakis KD, Helms LJ, Azari R, Callahan EJ, Creten DA. The influence of physician practice behaviors on patient satisfaction. Fam Med 1993;25(1):17–20.
6. Bertakis KD, Roter D, Putnam SM. The relationship of physician medical interview style to patient satisfaction. J Fam Pract 1991;32(2):175–181.
7. Greenfield S, Kaplan S, Ware JE Jr. Expanding patient involvement in care. Effects on patient outcomes. Ann Intern Med 1985;102(4):520–528.
8. Greenfield S, Kaplan SH, Ware JE Jr, Yano EM, Frank HJ. Patients' participation in medical care: effects on blood sugar control and quality of life in diabetes. J Gen Intern Med 1988; 3(5):448–457.
9. Kaplan SH, Greenfield S, Gandek B, Rogers WH, Ware JE Jr. Characteristics of physicians with participatory decision-making styles. Ann Intern Med 1996;124(5):497–504.
10. Blanchard CG, Labrecque MS, Ruckdeschel JC, Blanchard EB. Information and decision-making preferences of hospitalized adult cancer patients. Soc Sci Med 1988;27(11):1139–1145.
11. Degner LF, Sloan JA. Decision making during serious illness: what role do patients really want to play? J Clin Epidemiol 1992;45(9):941–950.
12. Sutherland HJ, Llewellyn-Thomas HA, Lockwood GA, Tritchler DL, Till JE. Cancer patients: their desire for information and participation in treatment decisions. J R Soc Med 1989;82(5): 260–263.
13. Gattellari M, Butow PN, Tattersall M. Sharing decisions in cancer care. Soc Sci Med 2001;52:1865–1878.
14. Deber RB, Kraetschmer N, Irvine J. What role do patients wish to play in treatment decision making? Arch Intern Med 1996; 156(13):1414–1420.
15. Nease RF Jr, Brooks WB. Patient desire for information and decision making in health care decisions: the Autonomy Preference Index and the Health Opinion Survey. J Gen Intern Med 1995; 10(11):593–600.
16. Whitney SN. A new model of medical decisions: exploring the limits of shared decision making. Med Decis Making 2003; 23:275–280.
17. Bruera E, Sweeney C, Calder K, Palmer L, Benisch-Tolley S. Patient preferences versus physician perceptions of treatment decisions in cancer care. J Clin Oncol 2001;19:2883–2885.
18. Bruera E, Willey JS, Palmer JL, Rosales M. Treatment decisions for breast carcinoma: patient preferences and physician perceptions. Cancer (Phila) 2002;94:2076–2080.
19. Cassileth BR, Zupkis RV, Sutton-Smith K, March V. Information and participation preferences among cancer patients. Ann Intern Med 1980;92(6):832–836.
20. Jenkins V, Fallowfield L, Saul J. Information needs of patients with cancer: results from a large study in UK cancer centers. Br J Cancer 2001;84:48–51.
21. Damasio AR. Descartes' Error: Emotion, Reason, and the Human Brain. New York: Putnam's, 1994.
22. Wilson TD, Schooler JW. Thinking too much: introspection can reduce the quality of preferences and decisions. J Personality Soc Psychol 1991;60(2):181–192.
23. Ubel PA, Loewenstein G. The role of decision analysis in informed consent: choosing between intuition and systematicity. Soc Sci Med 1997;44(5):647–656.
24. Spranca M, Minsk E, Baron J. Omission and commission in judgement and choice. J Exp Soc Psychol 1991;27(1):76–105.
25. Kodish E, Post SG. Oncology and hope. J Clin Oncol 1995;13(7): 1817.
26. Ubel PA. Truth in the most optimistic way. Ann Intern Med 2001;134(12):1142–1143.
27. Butow PN, Dowsett S, Hagerty R, Tattersall MH. Communicating prognosis to patients with metastatic disease: what do they really want to know? Support Care Cancer 2002;10(2):161–168.
28. Edwards A, Elwyn G, Mulley A. Explaining risks: turning numerical data into meaningful pictures. Br Med J 2002;324:827–830.
29. Baile WF, Lenzi R, Parker PA, Buckman R, Cohen L. Oncologists' attitudes toward and practices in giving bad news: an exploratory study. J Clin Oncol 2002;20(8):2189–2196.
30. Schwartz LM, Woloshin S, Black WC, Welch HG. The role of numeracy in understanding the benefit of screening mammography. Ann Intern Med 1997;127(11):966–972.
31. Lipkus IM, Samsa G, Rimer BK. General performance on a numeracy scale among highly educated samples. Med Decis Making 2001;21(1):37–44.
32. Lerman C, Daly M, Walsh WP, et al. Communication between patients with breast cancer and health care providers: determinants and implications. Cancer (Phila) 1993;72:2612–2620.
33. Lobb EA, Butow PN, Kenny DT, Tattersall MH. Communicating prognosis in early breast cancer: do women understand the language used? Med J Aust 1999;171:290–294.
34. Chaitchik S, Kreitler S, Shaked S, Schwartz I, Rosin R. Doctor–patient communication in a cancer ward. J Cancer Educ 1992; 7(1):41–54.
35. Gattellari M, Butow PN, Tattersall MHN, Dunn SM, Macleod CA. Misunderstanding in cancer patients: why shoot the messenger. Ann Oncol 1999;10:39–46.
36. Margolis ML, Christie JD, Silvestri GA, Kaiser L, Santiago S, Hansen-Flaschen J. Racial differences pertaining to a belief about lung cancer surgery: results of a multicenter survey. Ann Intern Med 2003;139(7):558–563.
37. Kleinman A, Eisenberg L, Good B. Culture, illness, and care: clinical lessons from anthropologic and cross-cultural research. Ann Intern Med 1978;88(2):251–258.
38. Paltiel O, Avitzour M, Peretz T, et al. Determinants of the use of complementary therapies by patients with cancer. J Clin Oncol 2001;19(9):2439–2448.
39. Iwu MM, Gbodossou E. The role of traditional medicine. Lancet 2000;356(suppl):s3.
40. Fagerlin A, Zikmund-Fisher BJ, Ubel PA. Communicating the list time risk of prostate cancer to patients: does this information create undue anxiety or unjustifiable optimism? In submission 2003.
41. Hall MA, Dugan E, Zheng B, Mishra AK. Trust in physicians and medical institutions: What is it, can it be measured, and does it matter? Milbank Q 2001;79(4):613–639.
42. Kao AC, Green DC, Zaslavsky AM, Koplan JP, Cleary PD. The relationship between method of physician payment and patient trust. JAMA 1998;280(19):1708–1714.
43. Gamble VN. Under the shadow of Tuskegee: African Americans and health care (public health then and now). Am J Public Health 1997;87(11):1773–1778.

44. Ubel PA. Is information always a good thing? Helping patients make "good" decisions. Med Care 2002;40(suppl 9):V39–V44.
45. Redelmeier DA, Shafir E. Medical decision making in situations that offer multiple alternatives. JAMA 1995;273(4):302–305.
46. Iyengar SS, Lepper MR. When choice is demotivating: can one desire too much of a good thing? J Personality Soc Psychol 2000; 79(6):995–1006.
47. Ubel PA, Jepson C, Baron J. The inclusion of patient testimonials in decision aids: effects on treatment choices. Med Decis Making 2001;21(1):60–68.
48. Gilbert DT, Wilson TD. Miswanting: some problems in the forecasting of future affective states. In: Forgas JP (ed). Feeling and Thinking: The Role of Affect in Social Cognition. New York: Cambridge University Press, 2000:178–197.
49. Ubel PA, Loewenstein G, Jepson C. Whose quality of life? a commentary exploring discrepancies between health state evaluations of patients and the general public. Qual Life Res 2003; 12(6):599–607.
50. Boyd NF, Sutherland HJ, Heasman KZ, Tritchler DL, Cummings BJ. Whose utilities for decision analysis? Med Decis Making 1990;10(1):58–67.
51. Riis J, Loewenstein G, Baron J, Jepson C, Fagerlin A, Ubel PA. Ignorance of hedonic adaptation to hemodialysis: a study using ecological momentary assessment. J Exp Psychol Gen 2005; 134(1):3–9.
52. Braddock CH III, Edwards KA, Hasenberg NM, Laidley TL, Levinson W. Informed decision making in outpatient practice: time to get back to basics. JAMA 1999;282(24):2313–2320.
53. Lurie SJ. Raising the passing grade for studies of medical education. JAMA 2003;290(9):1210–1212.
54. Yedidia MJ, Gillespie CG, Kachur E, et al. Effect of communications training on medical student performance. JAMA 2003; 290(9):1157–1165.
55. Fowler FJ Jr, McNaughton Collins M, Albertsen PC, Zietman A, Elliott DB, Barry MJ. Comparison of recommendations by urologists and radiation oncologists for treatment of clinically localized prostate cancer. JAMA 2000;283(24):3217–3222.
56. Chan ECY, Vernon SW, Haynes MC, O'Donnell FT, Ahn C. Physician perspectives on the importance of facts men ought to know about prostate-specific antigen testing. J Gen Intern Med 2003;18:350–356.
57. Benzein E, Norberg A, Saveman BI. The meaning of the lived experience of hope in patients with cancer in palliative home care. Palliat Med 2001;15(2):117–126.
58. Hegarty M. The dynamic of hope: hoping in the face of death. Prog Palliat Care 2001;9:42–46.
59. Abrahm JL. Update in palliative medicine and end-of-life care. Annu Rev Med 2003;54:53–72.
60. Ong LM, Visser MR, Lammes FB, van Der Velden J, Kuenen BC, de Haes JC. Effect of providing cancer patients with the audiotaped initial consultation on satisfaction, recall, and quality of life: a randomized, double-blind study. J Clin Oncol 2000;18(16): 3052–3060.
61. Bruera E, Pituskin E, Calder K, Neumann CM, Hanson J. The addition of an audiocassette recording of a consultation to written recommendations for patients with advanced cancer: a randomized, controlled trial. Cancer (Phila) 1999;86(11):2420–2425.
62. Scott JT, Entwistle VA, Sowden AJ, Watt I. Giving tape recordings or written summaries of consultations to people with cancer: a systematic review. Health Expect 2001;4(3): 162–169.
63. Speice J, Harkness J, Laneri H, et al. Involving family members in cancer care: focus group considerations of patients and oncological providers. Psycho-Oncology 2000;9(2):101–112.
64. Paling J. Strategies to help patients understand risks. Br Med Bull 2003;327(7417):745–748.
65. McNeil BJ, Pauker SG, Sox HC Jr, Tversky A. On the elicitation of preferences for alternative therapies. N Engl J Med 1982; 306(21):1259–1262.
66. Malenka DJ, Baron JA, Johansen S, Wahrenberger JW, Ross JM. The framing effect of relative and absolute risk. J Gen Intern Med 1993;8(10):543–548.
67. Fagerlin A, Wang C, Ubel PA. Reducing the influence of anecdotal reasoning on people's health care decisions: is a picture worth a thousand statistics? In submission 2003.
68. Thom DH. Physician behaviors that predict patient trust. J Fam Pract 2001;50(4):323–328.
69. Sitkin SB, Roth NL. Explaining the limited effectiveness of legalistic remedies for trust/distrust. Organiz Sci 1993;4:367–392.
70. Alaszewski A, Horlick-Jones T. How can doctors communicate information about risk more effectively? Br Med J 2003;327: 728–731.
71. Keating NL, Green DC, Kao AC, Gazmararian JA, Wu VY, Cleary PD. How are patients' specific ambulatory care experiences related to trust, satisfaction, and considering changing physicians? J Gen Intern Med 2002;17(1):29–39.
72. Ubel PA. "What should I do, doc?" Some psychologic benefits of physician recommendations. Arch Intern Med 2002;162(9): 977–980.

14

Establishing an Interdisciplinary Oncology Team

Nathan Levitan, Meri Armour, and Afshin Dowlati

In recent decades, cancer treatment has evolved from a purely surgical approach to the complex coordination of sophisticated surgery, radiotherapy, and chemotherapy. The technology associated with pain and nutrition management has improved,[1–3] and the importance of psychosocial factors in the treatment of cancer patients has been recognized.[4] The knowledge base pertaining to cancer treatment has become so vast that many physicians have developed subspecialty expertise in a focused aspect of cancer care. Quality of care analyses have indicated that the improved outcomes of certain cancer treatments occur when they are provided at high-volume facilities.[5]

One response to the challenges inherent in the provision of state-of-the-art cancer care has been the formal coordination of multiple disciplines in the planning and implementation of a treatment program. The American College of Surgeons, which certifies hospital-based cancer programs, requires the interaction of medical oncologists, radiation oncologists, and surgeons at prospective treatment planning conferences.[6] Patient advocacy organizations such as the R.A. Bloch Cancer Foundation strongly advocate this approach to care as well.[7]

The interaction of multiple disciplines in cancer care has variably been referred to as *multidisciplinary* or *interdisciplinary*. In *The Helper's Journal*, Larson draws a distinction between these two terms. He defines *multidisciplinary care* as that which involves clinicians with multiple different areas of expertise, although not necessarily in a coordinated fashion. In contrast, he defines *interdisciplinary care* as the formal collaboration of these clinicians in each patient's treatment planning, "where the interaction of the team is necessary to produce the final product."[8] Henceforth, we use the term interdisciplinary with the aforementioned intended meaning.

The purpose of this chapter is to review the scientific basis for and the logistic challenges involved in the delivery of interdisciplinary cancer care. Noting at the outset that currently there is a paucity of data in the medical literature pertaining to the impact of this type of care in comparison to conventional treatment, we explore closely related issues. The following questions are addressed: (1) How has cancer care evolved in recent years, and why is there a need for a coordinated approach to care? (2) Can cancer care be standardized on the basis of clinical trials outcomes, or must all treatment decisions be individualized? (3) How much variability exists in the delivery of cancer care, and when does this represent a lapse in quality? (4) How can physician behavior be modified to provide patients with the best care? (5) How does the establishment of an interdisciplinary treatment team increase the likelihood that uniform, high-quality, state-of-the-art cancer care will be delivered?

The Historical Evolution of Individual Cancer Treatment Modalities

Surgery

The earliest attempts at surgical treatment for cancer occurred in London in the early 1800s and were described by John Abernethy.[9] Limited by pain and infection, the outcomes of these operative procedures were poor. With the availability of general anesthesia and antiseptics in the mid-1800s,[10,11] early procedures for the surgical treatment of breast cancer were developed.[12] In the late 1800s, William Halsted developed an aggressive surgical approach to breast cancer treatment.[13] The "radical mastectomy" resulted in a fourfold increase in the cure rate for breast cancer.[13,14] Subsequent advances in opioid pain management and blood banking permitted even more extensive surgical procedures in the 1950s.[15,16] Breast-sparing surgery became widespread by the 1980s, and axillary sentinel node sampling was developed in the 1990s.[17,18] By the end of the 20th century, liver transplantation became feasible for selected cases of hepatocellular carcinoma. Additional examples of state-of-the-art cancer surgery include complex reconstruction for hand and neck cancers, bone grafting for resection of pediatric osteosarcomas, nerve-sparing retroperitoneal surgery for prostate and testicular cancer, resection of isolated pulmonary,[19] hepatic,[20] or intracranial metastases, minimally invasive abdominal surgery, and video-assisted thoracoscopy.[21]

Radiation Therapy

The origins of radiation therapy for cancer date back to the discovery of the X-ray by Roentgen in 1895.[22] The properties of radium were reported by the Curies in 1898.[23] The effectiveness of therapeutic radiation was established in the 1920s,[24,25] and radiation therapy for cancer treatment became established as a medical specialty within the American Board of Radiology in 1934. Between the 1930s and the 1950s, radiation therapy became a well-established treatment for cancer of the head and neck.[26–28] By 1950, radiation therapy had also become the treatment of choice for patients with Hodgkin's disease.[29,30] Brachytherapy became widely used in the 1980s.[31] By the late 1990s, progress in computer technology facilitated the wide availability of computed tomography (CT) scan-guided computerized treatment planning,[32] as well as conformal and intensity-modulated radiation therapy.[33]

Chemotherapy

The birth of cancer chemotherapy occurred in the early 1940s, when nitrogen mustard was shown to be effective in the treatment of patients with lymphoid malignancies.[34] In 1949, methotrexate was used as curative therapy for patients with metastatic choriocarcinoma.[35] Combination chemotherapy became well established in the 1970s, when the effectiveness of the MOPP (nitrogen mustard, oncovin, procarbazine, prednisone) regimen was shown for patients with Hodgkin's disease.[36] Widespread use of newer cytotoxic chemotherapeutic agents including anthracyclines, vinca alkaloids, and platinum compounds occurred in the 1980s. The taxanes and the camptothecins were shown to be effective either alone and in combination with other drugs during the 1990s.[37–40] Effective new antinausea drugs as well as biologic agents for the treatment of neutropenia and anemia have reduced the toxicity associated with cytotoxic chemotherapy and have facilitated the development of high-dose chemotherapy strategies.[41–45] The newest developments in chemotherapy include monoclonal antibodies directed against lymphoid cell-surface antigens,[46] drugs that act at the signal transduction pathway to impair cell proliferation,[47–49] and antiangiogenesis agents.[50,51]

Combined Modality Therapy

As surgery, radiotherapy, and chemotherapy treatments for cancer have become individually more sophisticated over time, strategies for combining these modalities have evolved as well. In 1977, the National Surgical Adjuvant Breast and Bowel Protocol Group (NSABP) demonstrated that women who underwent breast-conserving surgery (lumpectomy) followed by radiation achieved rates of long-term survival equivalent to those who underwent mastectomy. Subsequent trials by this and other cooperative groups have proven, in Phase III trials, that postoperative adjuvant chemotherapy can improve long-term survival rates in breast cancer by approximately one-third.[52,53] Chemotherapy, radiotherapy, and surgery have all been applied in the treatment of locally advanced breast cancer.[54]

Adjuvant therapy for colon cancer patients with nodal involvement can improve 5-year survival rates by approximately 30%.[55] Patients with rectal cancer or gastric cancer benefit from postoperative concurrent chemoradiotherapy.[56] Carefully selected patients with non-Hodgkin's lymphoma or Hodgkin's disease are treated with chemotherapy followed by radiotherapy.[57] The use of concurrent chemoradiotherapy without surgery for patients with limited-stage small cell lung cancer has been associated with previously unattainable cure rates of more than 20%.[58] Patients with stage III superior sulcus non-small cell lung cancers benefit from concurrent chemoradiotherapy followed by surgery.[59]

Organ preservation can be achieved with concurrent chemoradiotherapy for patients with cancers of the larynx, hypopharynx, and nasopharynx.[60,61] Nigro demonstrated that patients with anal cancer can achieve improved cure rates (75% versus 30%) and also avoid surgical resection of the anus when they are treated with this bimodality approach.[62] In treating pediatric patients with osteosarcoma, the use of initial chemotherapy and radiation followed by limb-sparing surgery for those who respond to induction therapy can reduce the incidence of amputation to 17%.[63,64]

Controversies in Multimodality Treatment

Phase III clinical trials have demonstrated the superiority of combined modality treatment over surgery, chemotherapy, or radiotherapy alone for several types and stages of cancer. However, the emergence of new data with potential relevance to treatment decisions is a dynamic process. Just as one issue is addressed by clinical research, the next question is asked by investigators involved in the design of future trials. In addition, clinical trials may produce confusing or contradictory data. Accordingly, if one attempts to define "state-of-the-art" multimodality cancer therapy, there may be disagreement among treating physicians in many clinical situations. Several examples are presented next.

Lung cancer is the most common cause of cancer deaths among men and women in the United States. Patients with this disease are common in the practices of medical and radiation oncologists as well as thoracic surgeons. The importance of surgical resection in the treatment of stage I and II non-small cell lung cancer is well established, as is the role of chemotherapy for patients with symptomatic metastatic disease. The efficacy of postoperative adjuvant chemotherapy following lung cancer resection has recently been demonstrated.[65,66] However, it is unclear which chemotherapy regimen is optimal, and whether patients should be treated if they have a small stage IA cancer, if more than 6 weeks have elapsed since surgery, or if patients are advanced in age. Postoperative radiotherapy has been shown to reduce local recurrence without a clear prolongation of survival for patients with stage II and III disease. The decision to use this treatment in the immediate postoperative period versus at the time of tumor recurrence must be individualized.

There are strong data to indicate that patients with clinical stage III lung cancer should undergo careful mediastinal staging before surgery. If multistation nodal involvement is evident, based on radiographic procedures or surgical nodal evaluation, tumor resection should not be carried out. This practice is not followed by many physicians across the United States. The role of preoperative chemotherapy for patients with clearly resectable stage IIIA lung cancer is not well defined, nor is the optimal combination of chemotherapy, radiotherapy, and surgery for patients with advanced IIIA disease.

Breast cancer is the second most common cause of cancer death among women in the United States. The efficacy of hormonal and radiation therapy following resection of in situ cancer has been established, although the use of one or both modalities must be considered for each patient.[67] Adjuvant chemotherapy following resection of node-positive disease for pre- and postmenopausal women is well established, although the optimal combination of chemotherapy drugs and the role of consolidation therapy are unclear.[68] Radiotherapy to the chest wall following resection of breast cancer with multiple positive nodes can prolong survival. However, the utilization of this treatment is highly variable.[69]

Patients with locally advanced breast cancer are generally treated with induction chemotherapy. The optimal role and sequence of radiation and surgical resection are not clear.[70,71] Finally, although a multitude of chemotherapy drugs have been shown to be effective in the treatment of metastatic breast cancer, there is disagreement concerning the use of sequential single agents versus combination chemotherapy.[72]

Esophageal cancer that invades at least into the muscularis propria is often treated with concurrent chemoradiotherapy followed by surgery. If one examines the results of Phase III clinical trials, the efficacy of this combined modality therapy is questionable.[73,74] In the management of *rectal cancer*, the use of a mesorectal excision has been shown to be superior to conventional resection.[75] It is not clear how to determine which surgeons are properly trained to perform this procedure.[76] Induction chemoradiotherapy is used in selected patients in an effort to minimize the extent of resection and, in some cases, to permit a sphincter-sparing approach.

For patients with muscle-invasive *bladder cancer*, chemoradiotherapy can be used selectively to achieve bladder preservation.[77] However, the application of limited surgery, chemoradiotherapy, and radical cystectomy remains highly variable.[78] The management of *prostate cancer* is complex, as options often include observation, hormonal therapy, surgery, or radiation (external beam or brachytherapy).[79] Clinically node-negative nonseminomatous *testicular cancer* can be managed with initial chemotherapy or with observation; treatment varies with the preference of the treating physician and the details of the patient's disease.[80]

Variability in Clinical Practice

The preceding examples highlight the complexity of cancer care, the absence of a single correct approach to the management of many patients, and the need to individualize treatment decisions. However, one could also ask to what extent variability in cancer care is the result of justifiable differences in the interpretation of clinical trials outcomes versus a lack of familiarity on the part of physicians with state-of-the-art medical information. Several investigators have attempted to address this question, largely in reference to nonmalignant conditions.

Ellerbeck demonstrated wide variation in the use of aspirin and beta blockers following myocardial infarction during 1992–1993 in several states in the United States.[81] This study was conducted at a time when the benefit of these medications was widely recognized. Patients for whom there existed a possible contraindication to these medications were excluded from the study. At the time of hospital discharge, 77% of patients received aspirin and 45% of patients received beta blockers.[82] Schein showed that the selection of the type of procedure utilized by ophthalmologists for cataract excision varied with their surgical volume and with the number of years in practice.[83] Carey studied the use of radiographs in the evaluation of patients with low back pain. He found that chiropractors and orthopedic surgeons in private practice were more likely than those employed by a large institution to order radiographs.[84] Wennberg reported marked differences in the use of coronary angiography and revascularization in different regions of New England. He demonstrated that the number of stress tests performed in a region correlated with the number of invasive procedures that were subsequently performed.[85]

Guadagnoli showed that Medicare beneficiaries with a strong medical indication for coronary angiography following myocardial infarction were more likely to be referred by their physicians for this procedure if they were enrolled in a fee-for-service rather than a managed care insurance plan (46% versus 37%).[86] Hemingway showed that among 908 patients in London with a strong medical indication for coronary angioplasty, 34% were not referred for this procedure; and among 908 patients with a strong medical indication for coronary artery bypass graft, 26% were treated medically.[87] These studies suggest that, although some examples of variability in treatment recommendations reflect the need to individualize patient management, others indicate a lapse in the quality of care.

Variability in Cancer Care

If one attempts to assess the variability of cancer care across the United States, or the extent to which physicians adhere to established standards of cancer care, there are few data available.[88] Perez developed a questionnaire containing five different lung cancer case scenarios.[89] Primary care physicians, pulmonologists, medical oncologists, radiation oncologists, and thoracic surgeons were asked to complete the survey. Questions pertained to prognosis, recommended treatment, and the expected impact of treatment on outcome. For all stages of lung cancer, the recommended treatments varied greatly among the different specialists. Differences of opinion pertained not only to complex and controversial treatment decisions, but also to issues for which a clear standard of care had been established.

Emanuel and colleagues[90] used data from the Centers for Medicare and Medicaid Services to retrospectively study the use of chemotherapy in the final months of life for patients over the age of 65 (Figure 14.1). They found that, in the state of Massachusetts, 33%, 23%, and 9% of patients received chemotherapy in the last 6 months, 3 months, and 1 month of life, respectively. These data are among the first large-scale outcomes analyses of the practice of chemotherapy administration in the Unites States.

An initiative is currently under way to retrospectively analyze the use of adjuvant chemotherapy for patients with

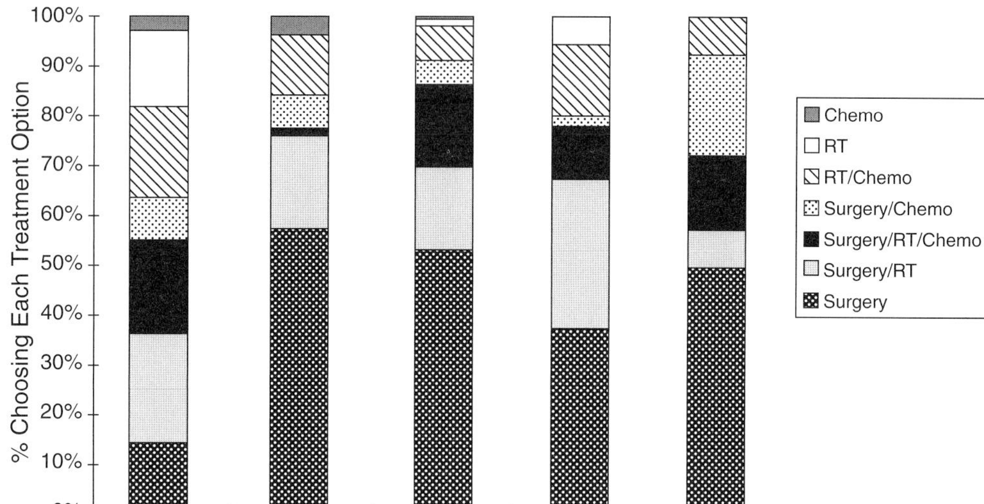

FIGURE 14.1. Percentage of physicians (by specialty) choosing each treatment option for the treatment of stage II non-small cell lung cancer. Specialty by column, from *left*: primary care physicians (PCPs), pulmonary physicians, oncologists, radiation oncologists, and thoracic surgeons. (From Emanuel et al.,[91] by permission of *Annals of Internal Medicine*.)

colon and lung cancer.[91] This study, jointly sponsored by the Rand Corporation and the American Society of Clinical Oncology, will document the compliance of medical oncologists in the United States with two practice recommendations that are well supported in the medical literature and are considered standard care.

Alteration of Physician Practice Patterns

Thus far, we have described the complexity of many cancer treatment decisions. We have reviewed some of the data pertaining to variability in treatment patterns for multiple medical conditions, including cancer. We have shown that in some situations this variability reflects the absence of a single correct evidence-based approach, whereas in other situations the deviation from an established standard practice constitutes a lapse in quality of care.

In an effort to encourage uniformity of care when a *best practice* does exist, several strategies have been employed. These include the following:[92]

Didactic continuing medical education presentations
Distribution of consensus conference recommendations
Individualized physician education (academic detailing)
Active participation in guideline development
Physician feedback specific to his/her prior treatment decisions
Reminders encountered by physicians in the course of active patient care

Several studies have shown that neither traditional didactic continuing education programs nor the dissemination of patient care guidelines is effective in altering physician behavior.[93–97] Following the national distribution in Canada of a consensus statement pertaining to the use of cesarean section, physician acceptance was measured.[98] Surveys demonstrated that only 67% of targeted physicians were aware of the recommendations, and rates of cesarean section declined only slightly. Following the dissemination of the Joint National Committee VI Hypertension Treatment Guidelines in the state of New York, physician compliance was found to be approximately 52%.[99] The distribution of guidelines for the management of community-acquired pneumonia to physicians at the Massachusetts General Hospital resulted in a 56% rate of compliance.[100] Poor adherence of surgeons to guidelines concerning breast cancer management has been demonstrated.

Several other interventions have been shown to be more effective. When physicians are used individually to educate colleagues, some change in behavior has been observed.[101–103] Reminders in the chart specific to individual patients have been shown to be more effective than general reminders or lectures.[104–106] Recruitment of local physician opinion leaders to advocate a particular change and/or provision of specific feedback concerning their compliance with guidelines can also alter behavior.[107–111] Involvement of physicians in the process of local guideline development can be effective as well.[112]

Several authors have attempted to explain the difficulties that are encountered in attempting to change physician practice.[113] Smith suggests that the many years of formal education and postgraduate training to which physicians are exposed, as well as their own practice experience, result in the establishment of somewhat rigid practice patterns that are difficult to alter.[114] He notes that the multitude of printed materials to which physicians are exposed may actually desensitize them to new educational content.

Grol proposes that the most effective strategy for altering physician practice patterns should include the integration of several techniques (Table 14.1).[115] These methods include (a) provision of scientific evidence in the development of guidelines, (b) interactive rather than "top down" physician education, (c) ongoing monitoring of clinical performance and provision of feedback to physicians, and (d) patient empowerment. Greco adds that physician opinion leaders, financial incentives, financial penalties, and administrative rules are influential as well.[116]

TABLE 14.1. Effects of different strategies to improve patient care.

Strategy	*No. of reviews*	*No. of studies*	*Conclusions*
Educational materials, mailed information	9	3–37	Limited effects
Continuing medical education	4	3–17	Limited effects
Interactive educational meetings	4	2–6	Few studies, mostly effective
Educational outreach visits	8	2–8	Particularly affects prescribing and prevention
Use of opinion leaders	3	3–6	Mixed effects
Feedback on performance	7	16–37	Mixed effects, effect on test ordering
Reminders	5	5–68	Mostly effective
Substitution or delegation of tasks	7	2–14	Pharmacist, effect on prescribing; nurse, no effect
Use of computer (systems)	4	7–21	Computerized decision support, mostly effective
Total quality management and continuous quality improvement	1	55	Limited effects, weak study designs
Patient-oriented interventions	7	2–34	Mixed effects, reminding patients mostly effective in prevention
Combined and multifaceted interventions	16	2–39	Mostly very effective

Source: From Grol R.[115] Improving the quality of medical care: building bridges among professional pride, payer profit, and patient satisfaction. JAMA 2001;286:2578–2585.

The Case for Interdisciplinary Treatment Teams in Cancer Treatment Planning

Information presented heretofore in this chapter can be summarized as follows:

The knowledge base necessary to provide state-of-the-art cancer care is extensive.

The cancer treatment literature resides in journals specific to several different medical specialties, and no single physician is likely to be familiar with all aspects of this scientific evidence.

A familiarity with active clinical trials and emerging scientific data for each type of cancer is needed.

Physicians from different cancer-related specialties often have divergent opinions concerning cancer treatment and prognosis.

For most major types of malignancy, some treatment recommendations are established as standard care whereas many others remain controversial.

Although data are not available to quantify the extent to which physicians involved in cancer care adhere to standard treatment recommendations, studies pertaining to several other fields of medicine suggest that compliance may be suboptimal.

When emerging medical knowledge is presented to physicians in a didactic fashion, they are slow to integrate such information into their patterns of practice.

The mere dissemination of treatment guidelines to physicians does not alter their treatment decisions.

To alter physician practice patterns, necessary steps include interactive learning, engagement of physicians in the process of guideline development, involvement of "thought leaders," and provision of ongoing outcomes data.

If one accepts these conclusions, then the need for a collaborative approach to cancer care is clear. When physicians from multiple cancer-related specialties meet to discuss new cancer patients and to prospectively plan the optimal treatment plan, several important events occur.

1. Specialty-specific knowledge is shared among participating physicians.
2. New information from the medical literature possessed by any member of the group is shared and likely integrated into the treatment planning process.
3. Disagreements among specialists are discussed until a unified opinion is formulated, thus providing the patient with clear and consistent information.
4. Locally applicable treatment guidelines are developed by participating physicians. The fact of their involvement in the process increases the likelihood of adherence.
5. The interdisciplinary team is an ideal forum for the identification of key outcome measures. These same physicians can review the data and modify the process of treatment as needed; this constitutes a *total quality management* cycle.[117]
6. Medical institutions involved in clinical research can utilize these meetings to determine patient eligibility for clinical trials and to inform the treating physicians accordingly.

Models for the Delivery of Interdisciplinary Care

As noted previously, there is broad support on the part of both medical professional organizations and patient advocacy groups for an interdisciplinary approach to cancer care. It is generally accepted that care labeled as such is characterized by the participation of multiple specialists in the formulation of an individualized treatment plan for each patient. However, beyond this definition, the optimal structure for such a process has not been clearly defined.

Three models for the provision of interdisciplinary gastrointestinal cancer care have been described in a 2002 monograph prepared by The Advisory Board Company.[118] The simplest model consists of a prospective treatment planning conference. Next, in order of increasing complexity, is the *virtual clinic*, in which a coordinator facilitates movement of the patient through his/her multiple physician visits and testing procedures. The highest level of integration is achieved by the establishment of a "comprehensive clinic," in which all physicians involved in the care of the patient practice in a single location (Table 14.2). There are no available data to indicate either the number of institutions that are providing interdisciplinary cancer care or the specific model(s) in use at these intuitions.

Beyond Surgery, Radiation Therapy, and Chemotherapy

Thus far, our discussion of integrated care has focused on the coordination of physicians from multiple cancer-related specialties. One can broaden the definition of interdisciplinary treatment to include several other components of care. Ko reviewed the records of 301 cancer patients and 6,745 controls and found that oncology patients frequently had coexistent pulmonary and cardiac conditions, thus requiring the participation of primary care physicians, cardiologists, and pulmonologists in the process of treatment planning and delivery.[119] A model of interdisciplinary care for hepatocellular carcinoma published by Van Cleave and colleagues includes (in addition to physicians) nurses, social workers, pharmacists, and a chaplain.[120]

To what extent do psychosocial and/or nutritional services alter outcomes in cancer care? Several clinical trials have tested the hypothesis that psychologic treatment can prolong survival in cancer patients.[121–123] The results of these studies are contradictory, and no firm conclusions can be drawn. More uniform data suggest that this type of intervention can favorably affect quality of life.[122,124–126] Arguably, relief of distress and enhancement of quality of life may be more appropriate metrics with which to evaluate the efficacy of psychosocial services for cancer patients than prolongation of survival.

Potential nutritional interventions range from oral to parenteral and from cancer prevention to the support of patients with metastatic disease.[126–128] Some investigators have found that oral intake of fish oil can reverse cancer anorexia and weight loss while others have observed no benefit.[129,130] Although the use of parenteral nutrition for patients with end-stage cancer can prolong survival, the associated cost and adverse effect on quality of life add complexity to the decision to undertake this therapy.[131]

A detailed review of the data pertaining to psychologic and nutritional intervention in cancer care is beyond the scope of this manuscript (see Chapter 85). However, there exists a broad body of literature pertaining to these treatments with which physician members of the interdisciplinary team are unlikely to be familiar. Mental health professionals and nutritionists can bring this expertise to the interdisciplinary team.

A demonstration project entitled Safe Conduct has been implemented as a component of care for patients with advanced lung cancer at the Ireland Cancer Center at University Hospitals of Cleveland. For participating patients, in addition to physician services from several cancer-related specialties, the interdisciplinary team includes a spiritual counselor, a social worker, and a nurse practitioner. In addition to careful attention to pain and symptom control, this team addresses the spiritual, emotional, and logistic needs of participating patients throughout the continuum of care.

Project Safe Conduct's positive impact on patients and caregivers emerges in several areas, based on preliminary data comparing these patients to lung cancer patients receiving care at ICC 1 year before the introduction of the Safe Conduct Team (SCT) (Figure 14.2):

The number of hospice referrals increased from 13% to 80%.
The hospice length of stay increased from an average of 10 days to 43 days.
The hospital admission rate (number of hospitalizations per patient per year) was 3.20 before Project Safe Conduct and dropped to 1.05 for SCT patients.
Unplanned hospitalizations and emergency room visits dropped from 6.3 per patient to 3.1.

TABLE 14.2. Models of interdisciplinary care.

Model	*Interdisciplinary clinic setup*	*Collaborative treatment planning*
Prospective treatment planning conference	Clinic visits not formally coordinated	Interdisciplinary treatment planning conference
Virtual gastrointestinal (GI) clinic	Patients see multiple specialists during separate but coordinated visits	Interdisciplinary treatment planning conference on separate day
Comprehensive GI clinic	Patients meet with multiple specialists during a single clinic visit	GI specialists confer on treatment planning during clinic visit

Source: Courtesy of the Advisory Board Company.

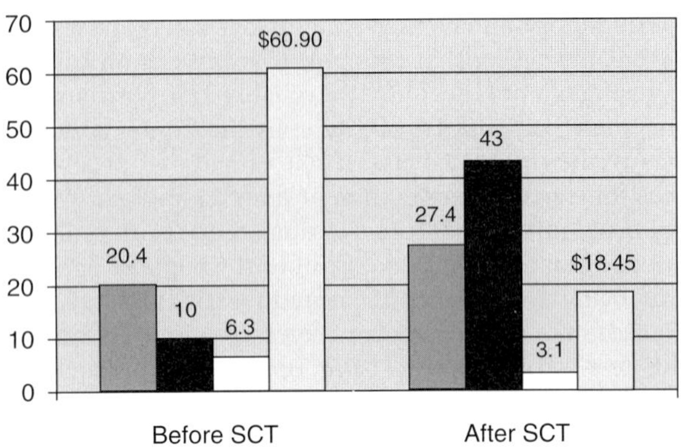

FIGURE 14.2. The positive impact on patients and caregivers of Project Safe Conduct emerges in several areas, based on preliminary data comparing these patients with lung cancer patients receiving care at Ireland Cancer Center (ICC) 1 year before the introduction of the Safe Conduct Team (SCT).

Seventy-five percent of SCT patients died at home, where most patients prefer to be at the end of life.

Average per-day pharmaceutical costs dropped from $60.90 per patient to $18.45.

Caregivers of SCT patients reported reduced burdens in interviews conducted after the death of their loved one.

Economic Implications

Quality of care considerations aside, the existing fee-for-service model of medical care in the United States (including the traditional Medicare plan) does not provide a strong economic incentive for the provision of interdisciplinary cancer care. Administrative costs associated with the establishment and support of these teams cannot be passed on to insurers. Although Medicare has developed a modifier that provides reimbursement if a patient is seen by several physicians in the same clinic in 1 day, physicians cannot bill for time spent at treatment planning conferences.

Theoretically, there are economic advantages that could result from an interdisciplinary approach to cancer treatment. In *Market Driven Health Care*, Dr. Regina Helzlinger predicts that consumers are increasingly demanding integrated disease-focused care.[132] If so, then institutions providing such services may have an advantage in the medical marketplace regardless of the reimbursement model.[133] In addition, the interdisciplinary team may contribute to optimal resource utilization and efficient work flow. Data do not exist to facilitate a more rigorous return-on-investment analysis pertaining to interdisciplinary cancer care.

Future Directions

In this chapter, we have shown that there exists in the medical literature strong justification for the establishment of interdisciplinary teams for cancer treatment. Several potential models with differing levels of complexity have been described, although the optimal structure for the delivery of such care has not been defined. The incremental cost involved in establishing these teams, as well as the impact on reimbursement, resource utilization, clinical trials participation, and patient satisfaction, remain unclear. Most important, the effects of interdisciplinary care on disease-free survival, overall survival, and quality of life have not been measured. Carefully designed outcomes studies are needed to address these issues.

References

1. Evans WK, Nixon DW, Daly JM, et al. A randomized study of oral nutritional support versus ad lib nutritional intake during chemotherapy for advanced colorectal and non-small cell lung cancer. J Clin Oncol 1987;5:113–124.
2. Tandon S, Gupta S, Sinha S. Nutritional support as an adjunct therapy of advanced cancer patients. Indian J Med Res 1984; 80:180–188.
3. Foley K. Advances in cancer pain. Arch Neurol 1999;56:413–417.
4. Spiegel D. Effects of psychotherapy on cancer survival. Nat Rev Cancer 2002;2:383–389.
5. Adams D, Johansen K, Brand R, Rennie D, Milstein A. Selective referral to high-volume hospitals: estimating potentially avoidable deaths. JAMA 2000;283:1159–1166.
6. Standards of the Commission on Cancer. Volume I: Cancer Program Standards. Chicago, IL: American College of Surgeons, 1996.
7. Bloch R. Cancer . . . there's hope. R.A. Bloch Cancer Foundation, 1982:9–106.
8. Larson D. The Helper's Journal. Champaign, IL: Research Press, 1993:200–202.
9. Abernethy J. Surgical Observations on the Constitutional Origin and Treatment of Local Diseases. London: Longman, Hurst, Rees, Orm, and Brown, 1814:180–200.
10. Moore C. On the influence of inadequate operations on the theory of cancer. Med Chir Trans 1867;50:245–280.
11. Lister J. On the antiseptic principles in the practice of surgery. Lancet 1867;2:353–356.
12. Moore C. On the influence of inadequate operations on the theory of cancer. Med Chir Trans 1867;50:245–280.
13. Halsted W. The results of operations for the cure of cancer of the breast performed at Johns Hopkins Hospital from June 1, 1889 to January 1894. Ann Surg 1894;20:497–555.
14. Halsted W. The results of radical operation for the cure of carcinoma of the breast. Ann Surg 1907;46:1–19.
15. Martin H. Radical surgery in the cancer of the head and neck. Surg Clin N Am 1958;33:329–350.
16. Kruskall M. Autologous blood transfusion. In: Hoffman R, Banz E, Shattil S (eds) Hematology: Basic Principles and Practice. New York: Churchill Livingstone, 1995:2063–2067.
17. Fisher B, Montague E, Redmond C. Comparison of radical mastectomy with alternative treatments for primary breast cancer. Cancer (Phila) 1977;29:2827–2838.
18. Noguchi M. Is it necessary to perform prospective randomized studies before sentinel node biopsy can replace routine axillary dissection? Breast Cancer 2003;10:179–187.
19. McCormack P. Surgical resection of pulmonary metastasis. Semin Surg Oncol 1990;6(5):297–302.
20. Wanebo H, Chu Q, Vezerdis M, Soderberg C. Patient selection for hepatic resection of colorectal metastasis. Arch Surg 1996; 131:322–329.
21. Cox C, Pendas S, Cox J. Guidelines for lymphatic mapping of patients with breast cancer. Ann Surg 1998;227:645–651.

22. Roentgen W. On a new kind of rays (preliminary communication). [Translation of a paper read before the Physikalische-medicinischen Gesellschaft of Wurzburg on December 28, 1895.] Br J Radiol 1931;4:32.
23. Curie P, Curie M, Bemont G. Sur une nouvelle substance fortement radioactive continue dans la pechblende (note presented by M. Becquerel). C R Acad Sci (Paris) 1898;127:1215–1217.
24. Janeway H. Radium Therapy in Cancer at the Memorial Hospital, NY. New York: Hoeber, 1917.
25. Ewing J. Early experiences in radiation therapy. Janeway Memorial Lecture, 1933. Am J Roentgenol Radium Ther 1934; 31:153–183.
26. Martin H. Radical surgery in the cancer of the head and neck. Surg Clin N Am 1958;33:329–3350.
27. Coutard H. Roentgen therapy of epitheliomas of the tonsillar regional hypopharynx and larynx from 1920 to 1926. Am J Roentgenol 1932;28:313–331.
28. Coutard H. Principles of x-ray therapy of malignant diseases. Lancet 1934;2:1–8.
29. Easson E, Russell M. The cure of Hodgkin's disease. Br Med J 1963;1:1704–1707.
30. Peters M, Middlemiss K. A study of Hodgkin's disease treated by irradiation. Am J Roentgenol 1958;79:114–121.
31. Downs T, Sadetsky N, Pasta D, et al. Health related quality of life patterns in patients treated with interstitial prostate brachytherapy for localized prostate cancer—data from CaPSURE. J Urol 2003;170:1822–1827.
32. Mackie T. Radiation therapy treatment optimization. Semin Radiat Oncol 1999;9:1–3.
33. Grills I, Yan D, Martinez A, Vicini F, Wong J, Kestin L. Potential for reduced toxicity and dose escalation in the treatment of inoperable non-small-cell lung cancer: a comparison of intensity-modulated radiation therapy (IMRT), 3D conformal radiation, and elective nodal irradiation. Int J Radiat Oncol Biol Phys 2003;57:875–890.
34. Gilman A, Philips F. The biological actions and therapeutic applications of the B-chloroethyl amines and sulfides. Science 1946;103:409–436.
35. Hertz R, Lewis J, Lipsett M. Five years' experience with the chemotherapy of metastatic choriocarcinoma in acute leukemia in children produced by folic acid antagonist, 4-aminopteroylglutamic acid (Aminopterin). N Engl J Med 1948;238:787–793.
36. DeVita V, Serpick A. Combination chemotherapy in the treatment of Hodgkin's disease. Ann Intern Med 1970;73:881–895.
37. Weiss R, Sarosy G, Clagett-Carr K, Russo M, Leyland-Jones B. Anthracycline analogs: the past, present, and future. Cancer Chemother Pharmacol 1986;18:185–197.
38. Rosenberg B. Fundamental studies with cisplatin. Cancer (Phila) 1985;55:2303–2316
39. Rowinsky E, Donehower R. Drug therapy: paclitaxel (Taxol). N Engl J Med 1995;332:1004–1014.
40. Wall M, Wani M, Cook C. Plant antitumor agents. I. The isolation and structure of camptothecin, a novel alkaloidal leukemia and tumor inhibitor from *Camptotheca accuminata*. J Am Chem Soc 1966;88:3888.
41. Kovac A. Benefits and risks of newer treatments for chemotherapy-induced and postoperative nausea and vomiting. Drug Saf 2003;26(4):227–259.
42. Vansteenkiste J, Rossi G, Foote M. Darbepoetin alfa: a new approach to the treatment of chemotherapy-induced anaemia. Expert Opin Biol Ther 2003;3:501–508.
43. Bedell C. Pegfilgrastim for chemotherapy-induced neutropenia. Clin J Oncol Nurs 2003;7:55–56, 63–64.
44. Stockerl-Goldstein A, Blume K, Allogeneic hematopoietic cell transplantation for adult patients with acute myeloid leukemia. In: Thomas E, Blume K, Forman S (eds) Hematopoietic Cell Transplantation. Malden, MA: Blackwell, 1999: 823.
45. McSweeney P, Storb R. Bone marrow transplantation for malignant disease. In: Rick R, Fleisher T, Schwartz B (eds) Clinical Immunology: Principles and Practice. St. Louis: Mosby-Year Book, 1995:1831–1851.
46. Kaminski M, Zasady K, Francis I. Radioimmunotherapy of B-cell lymphoma with ^{131}I-anti-B$_1$ (anti-CD20) antibody. N Engl J Med 1993;329:459–465.
47. Sepp-Lorenzino L, Ma Z, Rands E. A peptidomimetic inhibitor of farnesyl protein transferase blocks the anchorage-dependent and -independent growth of human tumor cell lines. Cancer Res 1995;55:5302–5309.
48. Drucker B, Talpaz M, Resta D. Clinical efficacy of an abl specific tyrosine kinase inhibitor as targeted therapy for chronic myelogenous leukemia. Blood 1999;94(suppl 10, pt 1) (abstract 1639).
49. Cobleigh M, Voel D, Tripathy N. Efficacy and safety of Herceptin (humanized anti-HER2 antibody) as a single agent in 222 women with HER2 overexpression who relapsed following chemotherapy for metastatic breast cancer. Proc Am Soc Clin Oncol 1998;17:97a (abstract 376).
50. Bower M, Howard M, Gracie F. A phase II study of thalidomide for Kaposi's sarcomas: activity and correlation with KSVH DNA load. J AIDS Hum Retrovirol 1995;14:A35 (abstract 76).
51. Politi P, Reboredo M, Losso C. Phase I trial of thalidomide in AIDS-related Kaposi sarcoma. Proc Am Soc Clin Oncol 1998;17:161 (abstract).
52. Fisher B, Redmond C, Legault-Poisson S. Postoperative chemotherapy and tamoxifen compared with tamoxifen alone in the treatment of positive-node breast cancer patients aged 50 years and older with tumors responsive to tamoxifen: results from the National Surgical Adjuvant Breast and Bowel Project B-16. J Clin Oncol 1990;8:1005–1018.
53. Early Breast Cancer Trialists' Collaborative Group. Systemic treatment of early breast cancer by hormonal, cytotoxic, or immune therapy: 133 randomized trials involving 31,000 recurrences and 24,000 deaths among 75,000 women. Lancet 1992;339:1–15, 71–85.
54. Zambetti M, Oriana S, Quattrone P. Combined sequential approach in locally advanced breast cancer. Ann Oncol 1999; 10:305–310.
55. Moertel C, Fleming T, Macdonald J. Levamisole and fluorouracil for adjuvant therapy of resected colon cancer. N Engl J Med 1990;322:352–358.
56. Wolmark N, Wieand H, Hyams D, et al. Randomized trial of postoperative adjuvant chemotherapy with or without radiotherapy for carcinoma of the rectum: National Surgical Adjuvant Breast and Bowel Project Protocol R-02. J Natl Cancer Inst 2000;92:388–396.
57. HD and NHL xrt with chemo seq.
58. Johnson D. Evolution of cisplatin-based chemotherapy in non-small cell lung cancer: a historical perspective and the Eastern Cooperative Oncology Group experience. Chest 2000;117: 133S–137S.
59. Rusch V, Giroux D, Kraut M, et al. Induction chemoradiation and surgical resection for non-small cell lung carcinomas of the superior sulcus: initial results of Southwest Oncology Group Trial 9416 (Intergroup Trial 0160). J Thorac Cardiovasc Surg 2001;121:472–483.
60. Forastiere A. Larynx preservation trials: a critical appraisal. Semin Radiat Oncol 1998:8:254–261.
61. Dimery I, Peters L, Goepfert H. Effectiveness of combined induction chemotherapy and radiotherapy in advanced nasopharyngeal carcinoma. J Clin Oncol 1993;11:1919–1928.
62. Nigro N. An evaluation of combined therapy for squamous cell cancer of the anal canal. Dis Colon Rectum 1984;27:763–781.

63. Brennan M, Casper E, Harrison L. Soft tissue sarcoma. In: DeVita V, Hellman S, Rosenberg S (eds) Cancer: Principles and Practice of Oncology, 5th ed. Philadelphia: Lippincott, 1996: 1738.
64. Winkler K, Beron G, Delling G, et al. Neoadjuvant chemotherapy of osteosarcoma: results of randomized cooperative trial (COSS-82) with salvage chemotherapy based on histological tumor response. J Clin Oncol 1988;6:329–637.
65. Scagliotti G, Fossati R, Torri V, et al. Adjuvant Lung Project Italy/European Organisation for Research Treatment of Cancer-Lung Cancer Cooperative Group Investigators. Randomized study of adjuvant chemotherapy for completely resected stage I, II, or IIIA non-small-cell lung cancer. J Natl Cancer Inst 2003; 95:1453–1461.
66. Johnson B. Adjuvant chemotherapy for non-small-cell lung cancer: the end of the beginning. J Natl Cancer Inst 2003;95:1422–1424.
67. Nakhlis F, Morrow M. Ductal carcinoma in situ. Surg Clin N Am 2003;83:821–839.
68. Nabholtz J, Vannetzel J, Llory J, Bouffette P. Advances in the use of taxanes in the adjuvant therapy of breast cancer. Clin Breast Cancer 2003;4:187–192.
69. Price F, Mendenhall N, Benda R, Morris C. Postmastectomy radiotherapy: patterns of recurrence and long-term disease control using electrons. Int J Radiat Oncol Biol Phys 2003; 56:716–725.
70. Anderson WF, Chu CC, Chang S. Inflammatory breast carcinoma and noninflammatory locally advanced breast carcinoma: distinct clinicopathologic entities? J Clin Oncol 2003; 21:2254–2259.
71. Therasse P, Mauriac L, Welnicka-Jaskiewicz M, et al. Final results of a randomized Phase III trial comparing cyclophosphamide, epirubicin, and fluorouracil with a dose-intensified epirubicin and cyclophosphamide + filgrastim as neoadjuvant treatment in locally advanced breast cancer: an EORTC-NCIC-SAKK Multicenter Study. J Clin Oncol 2003;21:843–850.
72. Seidman A. Sequential single-agent chemotherapy for metastatic breast cancer: therapeutic nihilism or realism? J Clin Oncol 2003;21:577–579.
73. Leonard G, McCaffrey J, Maher M. Optimal therapy for esophageal cancer. Cancer Treat Rev 2003;29:275–282.
74. Makary M, Kiernan P, Sheridan M, et al. Multimodality treatment for esophageal cancer: the role of surgery and neoadjuvant therapy. Am Surg 2003;69:693–700.
75. Kapiteijn E, van de Velde C. The role of total mesorectal excision in the management of rectal cancer. Surg Clin N Am 2002;82:995–1007.
76. Kapiteijn E, Putter H, van de Velde C. Impact of the introduction and training of total mesorectal excision on recurrence and survival in rectal cancer in The Netherlands. Br J Surg 2002; 89:1142–1149.
77. Kim H, Steinberg G. The current status of bladder preservation in the treatment of muscle invasive bladder cancer. J Urol 2000; 164:627–632.
78. Rödel C, Grabenbauer G, Kühn R, et al. Combined-modality treatment and selective organ preservation in invasive bladder cancer: long-term results. J Clin Oncol 2002;20:3061–3071.
79. Clark J, Inui T, Silliman R, et al. Patients' perceptions of quality of life after treatment for early prostate cancer. J Clin Oncol 2003;21:3777–3784.
80. Oliver RT. Emerging controversies in the management of stage 1 germ cell cancers. BJU Int 2003;92(1):1–2.
81. Ellerbeck E, Jencks S, Radford M, Kresowik T, Craig A, Gold J. Quality of care for Medicare patients with acute myocardial infarction. A four-state pilot study from the Cooperative Cardiovascular Project. JAMA 1995;273:1509–1514.
82. Wennberg D. Variation in the delivery of health care: the stakes are high. Ann Intern Med 1998;128:866–868.
83. Schein O, Steinberg E, Javitt J, Cassard S, Tielsch J, Steinwachs D. Variation in cataract surgery practice and clinical outcomes. Ophthalmology 1994;101:1142–1152.
84. Carey T, Garrett J. Patterns of ordering diagnostic tests for patients with acute low back pain. The North Carolina Back Pain Project. Ann Intern Med 1996;125:807–814.
85. Wennberg D, Kellett M, Dickens J, Malenka D, Keilson L, Keller R. The association between local diagnostic testing intensity and invasive cardiac procedures. JAMA 1996;275: 1161–1164.
86. Guadagnoli E, Landrum M, Peterson E, Gahart M, Ryan T, McNeil B. Appropriateness of coronary angiography after myocardial infarction among Medicare beneficiaries: managed care versus fee for service. N Engl J Med 2000;343: 1460–1406.
87. Hemingway H, Crook A, Feder G, et al. Underuse of coronary revascularization procedures in patients considered appropriate candidates for revascularization. N Engl J Med 2001;344: 645–654.
88. Hewitt H, Simone J (eds) Ensuring Quality Cancer Care. National Cancer Policy Board, Institute of Medicine and Commission of Life Sciences, National Research Council. Washington, DC: National Academy Press, 1999:26–27, 1–17.
89. Perez E. Perceptions of prognosis, treatment, and treatment impact on prognosis in non-small cell lung cancer. Chest 1998; 114:593–604.
90. Emanuel E, Young-Xu Y, Levinsky N, Gazelle G, Saynina O, Ash A. Chemotherapy use among Medicare beneficiaries at the end of life. Ann Intern Med 2003;138:639–643.
91. Epstein A, Schneider E, Kahn K, Malin J. National Initiative on Cancer Care Quality (NICCQ): project protocol and human subject protection guidelines. 2001;3.
92. Use of treatment guidelines surges as urge to manage care increases. J Natl Cancer Inst 1995;87:1044–1047.
93. Davis D, Thomson M, Oxman A, Haynes R. Evidence for the effectiveness of CME: a review of 50 randomized controlled trials. JAMA 1992;268:1111–1117.
94. White C, Albanese M, Brown D, Caplan R. The effectiveness of continuing medical education in changing the behavior of physicians caring for patients with acute myocardial infarction: a controlled randomized trial. Ann Intern Med 1985;102: 686–692.
95. Kosecoff J, Kanouse D, Rogers W, McCloskey L, Winslow C, Brook R. Effects of the National Institutes of Health Consensus Development Program on physician practice. JAMA 1987; 258:2708–2713.
96. Lomas J. Words without action? The production, dissemination, and impact of consensus recommendations. Annu Rev Public Health 1991;12:41–65.
97. Mor V, Laliberte L, Petrisek A, et al. Impact of breast cancer treatment guidelines on surgeon practice patterns: results of a hospital-based intervention. Surgery (St. Louis) 2000;128: 847–861.
98. Lomas J, Anderson G, Domnick-Pierre K, Vayda E, Enkin M, Hannah W. Do practice guidelines guide practice? The effect of a consensus statement on the practice of physicians. N Engl J Med 1989;321:1306–1311.
99. Clause S, Hamilton R. Medicaid prescriber compliance with Joint National Committee VI Hypertension Treatment Guidelines. Ann Pharmacother 2002;36:1505–1511.
100. Halm E, Atlas S, Borowsky L, et al. Understanding physician adherence with a pneumonia practice guideline: effects of patient, system, and physician factors. Arch Intern Med 2000; 160:98–104.
101. Schaffner W, Ray W, Federspiel C, Miller W. Improving antibiotic prescribing in office practice: a controlled trial of three educational methods. JAMA 1983;250:1728–1732.

102. Ray W, Blazer D, Schaffner W, Federspiel C, Fink R. Reducing long-term diazepam prescribing in office practice: a controlled trial of educational visits. JAMA 1986;256:2536–2539.
103. Ray W, Schaffner W, Federspiel C. Persistence of improvement in antibiotic prescribing in office practice. JAMA 1985;253: 1774–1776.
104. Headrick L, Speroff T, Pelecanos H, Cebul R. Efforts to improve compliance with the National Cholesterol Education Program guidelines: results of a randomized controlled trial. Arch Intern Med 1992;152:2490–2496.
105. McPhee S, Bird J, Jenkins C, Fordham D. Promoting cancer screening: a randomized, controlled trial of three interventions. Arch Intern Med 1989;149:1866–1872.
106. Tierney W, Hui S, McDonald C. Delayed feedback of physician performance versus immediate reminders to perform preventive care: effects on physician compliance. Med Care 1986;24: 659–666.
107. Lomas J, Enkin M, Anderson G, Hannah W, Vayda E, Singer J. Opinion leaders vs. audit and feedback to implement practice guidelines: delivery after previous cesarean section. JAMA 1991; 265:2202–2207.
108. Everitt D, Soumerai S, Avorn J, Klapholz H, Wessels M. Changing surgical antimicrobial prophylaxis practices through education targeted at senior department leaders. Infect Control Hosp Epidemiol 1990;11:578–583.
109. Spiegel J, Shapiro M, Berman B, Greenfield S. Changing physician test ordering in a university hospital: an intervention of physician participation, explicit criteria, and feedback. Arch Intern Med 1989;149:549–553.
110. Mertens W, Higby D, Brown D, et al. Improving the care of patients with regard to chemotherapy-induced nausea and emesis: the effect of feedback to clinicians on adherence to antiemetic prescribing guidelines. J Clin Oncol 2003;21: 1373–1378.
111. Berwick D, Coltin K. Feedback reduces test use in a health maintenance organization. JAMA 1986;255:1450–1454.
112. Wachtel T, O'Sullivan P. Practice guidelines to reduce testing in the hospital. J Gen Intern Med 1990;5:335–341.
113. Cabana M, Rand C, Powe N, et al. Why don't physicians follow clinical practice guidelines? A framework for improvement. JAMA 1999;282:1458–1465.
114. Smith W. Evidence for the effectiveness of techniques to change physician behavior. Chest 2000;118:8S–17S.
115. Grol R. Improving the quality of medical care: building bridges among professional pride, payer profit, and patient satisfaction. JAMA 2001;286:2578–2585.
116. Greco P, Eisenberg J. Changing physicians' practices. N Engl J Med 1993;329:1271–1273.
117. Berwick D, Blanton G, Roessner J. Curing Health Care. San Francisco: Wiley, 1990:31.
118. The Advisory Board Company. Interdisciplinary Gastrointestinal Cancer Programs. Practice Brief #30, February 11, 2002.
119. Ko C, Chaudhry S. The need for a multidisciplinary approach to cancer care. J Surg Res 2002;105:53–57.
120. Van Cleave J, Devine P, Odom-Ball P. Multidisciplinary care of hepatocellular carcinoma. Cancer Pract 1999;7:302–308.
121. Fawzy F, Canada A, Fawzy N. Malignant melanoma: effects of a brief, structured psychiatric intervention on survival and recurrence at 10-year follow-up. Arch Gen Psychiatry 2003;60: 100–103.
122. Goodwin P, Leszcz M, Ennis M, et al. The effect of group psychosocial support on survival in metastatic breast cancer. N Engl J Med 2001;345:1719–1726.
123. Ross L, Boesen E, Dalton S, Johansen C. Mind and cancer: does psychosocial intervention improve survival and psychological well-being? Eur J Cancer 2002;38:1447–1457.
124. Greer S. Psychological intervention. The gap between research and practice. Acta Oncol 2002;41:238–243.
125. Butler L, Koopman C, Cordova M, Garlan R, DiMiceli S, Spiegel D. Psychological distress and pain significantly increase before death in metastatic breast cancer patients. Psychosom Med 2003;65:416–426.
126. Talamini R, Franceschi S, La Vecchia C, Serraino D, Barra S, Negri E. Diet and prostatic cancer: a case-control study in northern Italy. Nutr Cancer 1992;18:277–286.
127. Persson C, Johansson B, Sjoden P, Glimelius B. A randomized study of nutritional support in patients with colorectal and gastric cancer. Nutr Cancer 2002;42:48–58.
128. Cohen L, Rose D, Wynder E. A rationale for dietary intervention in postmenopausal breast cancer patients: an update. Nutr Cancer 1993;19:1–10.
129. Barber M, Ross J, Voss A, Tisdale M, Fearon K. The effect of an oral nutritional supplement enriched with fish oil on weight-loss in patients with pancreatic cancer. Br J Cancer 1999;81: 80–86.
130. Bruera E, Strasser F, Palmer J, et al. Effect of fish oil on appetite and other symptoms in patients with advanced cancer and anorexia/cachexia: a double-blind, placebo-controlled study. J Clin Oncol 2003;21:129–134.
131. Okusaka T, Okada S, Ishii H, Ikeda M, Kosakamoto H, Yoshimori M. Prognosis of advanced pancreatic cancer patients with reference to calorie intake. Nutr Cancer 1998;32:55–58.
132. Herzlinger R. Market driven health care. Cambridge: Perseus, 1997:8–96.
133. The Advisory Board Company. The Oncology Watch, October 3, 2003, p 3.

15

Principles of Complementary and Alternative Medicine for Cancer

Andrew J. Vickers and Barrie Cassileth

Complementary and alternative medicine (CAM) is a general term used to describe techniques as diverse as chiropractic and yoga, iridology and meditation, colonic irrigation and spiritual healing. As such, it resists simple definition. Most published definitions describe CAM simply as practices outside of mainstream care.[1] A more fundamental issue concerns the difference between *complementary* and *alternative* approaches. Alternative therapies are used in place of mainstream care. Conversely, complementary therapies are used as adjuncts to mainstream care for symptom management and to enhance quality of life. This distinction is especially important in oncology, where treatment choices can be literally a matter of life and death.

CAM is widely used by the general public in the United States[2,3] and in other industrialized countries.[4–7] CAM use is markedly prevalent among cancer patients: a systematic review located 26 surveys of cancer patients from 13 countries, including 5 from the United States. The average prevalence across all studies was 31%, with prevalence rates as high as 64% in published reports.[8] Research published subsequent to the systematic review showed similar or slightly increased rates of CAM use.[9–15] Particularly popular today among cancer patients is the use of herbs, vitamins, and other dietary supplements. For example, more than one in four prostate cancer patients at a Canadian cancer clinic[16] and at a veterans' affairs medical center[17] used supplements or herbal treatments. A review of several studies reporting CAM product use in breast cancer patients found rates as high as 50% for herbs and 60% for other supplements.[18]

Given such widespread use, the first principle of CAM for cancer is that health professionals should ask patients about their use of CAM. This information helps to complete the clinical picture and to alert clinicians to potentially harmful interactions with conventional therapy. Keeping an open dialogue with patients is also likely to reduce the risk that they abandon conventional care to pursue unproven alternative cures.

In this chapter, we review data on alternative cancer treatments, botanical (herbal) anticancer agents, and interactions between CAM therapies and conventional oncologic care. We then review the evidence supporting the use of complementary therapies for symptom control.

Alternative Cancer Therapies

This section reviews *alternative therapies*, anticancer therapies offered outside of mainstream cancer treatment programs. Most of these methods are based on unfounded theories and involve considerable travel or expense; many are also known to incur significant risks of adverse events. It is common for advocates of alternative therapies to promote their treatment instead of conventional care. For example, Nicholas Gonzalez, a private physician in New York who treats cancer with a regimen that involves diet, vitamins, enzymes, and enemas, has stated that "You don't do chemotherapy and [my regimen]. You do one or the other."[19] This feeling raises the possibility that patients may be harmed by postponing care of proven benefit, an especially important consideration given that alternative cancer therapies are shown to be ineffective when subjected to clinical trial.

The related principle is the importance of trying to dissuade patients from using unproven cancer therapies. These therapies are typified by one or more of the following characteristics:

1. Promoted as effective against a wide range of ailments
2. The government or medical profession is said to conspire to suppress the therapy
3. Use of testimonials instead of facts and figures
4. Product is available from only one source
5. Credibility based on having been available for years and on anecdotal reports
6. New laws of nature are used to explain how it works
7. Promoted as "less toxic" than mainstream cancer treatment
8. Recommended for use instead of mainstream cancer treatments

Burzynski and Antineoplastons

An alternative cancer therapy popular for over a decade is that of Stanislaw Burzynski, who treats cancer with what he terms "antineoplastons." These are mixtures of peptides, amino acids, and other simple organic substances that he claims promote the body's natural defenses against cancer. Although he has published several studies of his own, these are of a rather unclear design.[20] A Phase II trial in glioma conducted under the auspices of the National Cancer Institute (NCI) was halted due to poor accrual and a failure of Burzynski to agree with the investigators on possible expansion of the eligibility criteria. Nine patients were accrued, six of whom were evaluable for response. There were no objective responses, and all six patients showed evidence of tumor progression after treatment durations between 16 and 66 days. The mean time to treatment failure (progression or discontinuation due to toxicity) was 29 days. All nine patients died before the study closed, all but one death resulting from tumor progression.[21] Despite the absence of data in support of Burzynski's regimen, it remains heavily promoted, especially as a treatment for pediatric brain tumors.

High-Dose Vitamin C

High-dose vitamin C was originally popularized as a cancer therapy by Linus Pauling. His claim that vitamin C potentiated the body's ability to fight off cancer garnered intense public interest and prompted two randomized trials in the late 1970s and early 1980s. Both trials found no difference between vitamin C and placebo, with short survival times regardless of allocation.[22,23] Interest in vitamin C as a cancer therapy recurred as researchers argued that early investigations were based on incomplete understanding of the vitamin C mode of action and that the oral doses used were inadequate.[24] Intravenous vitamin C with arsenic is currently under investigation as a treatment for myeloma at Sylvester Cancer Center.[25]

Laetrile

Laetrile is a substance derived from the pits of apricots and other fruits. It was a popular alternative cancer cure throughout the 1970s until research documented its lack of benefit[26] and its sale was banned in the United States. Following a two-decade hiatus, promotional activity resumed. Often termed "vitamin B_{17}" or sold as amygdalin, laetrile currently is available via the Internet and in Tijuana, Mexico.

Metabolic Therapies: Gerson and Gonzalez

Metabolic therapies are based on the belief that cancer is a symptom of the accumulation of toxins. The aim of treatment is therefore "detoxification" using coffee enemas or high colonics, special diets, raw juices, enzymes, and supplements. A retrospective study of melanoma patients treated by Gerson therapy, conducted by physicians working at the clinic where study patients were treated, concluded that 5-year survival of patients receiving Gerson therapy was higher than reported in large cohort studies.[27] This analysis was flawed by the use of unadjusted comparisons to nonrandomized controls and the exclusion of 40% of the Gerson therapy patients from analysis. In response to detailed criticisms, the authors accepted that a nonrandomized study such as the one published did not provide strong evidence of a treatment effect.[28] A more promising result has been reported from a cohort study of 11 pancreatic cancer patients treated by Nicholas Gonzalez using a metabolic regimen. Gonzalez reported 81% survival at 1 year and 45% survival at 2 years and claimed such results were far superior to national averages.[29] The study was small and obviously prone to several biases: not only is the comparison to national average unadjusted for confounders, but the principal results are based on patient selection; 12 patients who did not comply with treatment were excluded from analysis. Nonetheless, the generally positive results reported by Gonzalez were sufficient to prompt an NIH-funded Phase III trial, which remains under way.

Psychotherapy as a Cancer Cure

The theory that changing mental state can affect the course of cancer has been popularized by authors such as Bernie Siegel and Deepak Chopra. A support group program called Exceptional Cancer Patients (ECaP), developed by Dr. Bernie Siegel, was evaluated in a matched cohort study. Thirty-four women with breast cancer attending the ECaP program were matched 1:3 with comparable patients identified from tumor registries. At 10 years of follow-up, there were no differences in survival between the two groups, with approximately 40% of patients in both groups alive at the end of the study.[30]

Several other studies, however, appear to show survival advantages in cancer patients receiving psychologic treatment. In the late 1970s, David Spiegel conducted a randomized trial that aimed to examine the effects of a psychosocial support group on quality of life and symptoms in women with metastatic breast cancer. As a post hoc analysis, the investigators looked at survival differences and reported a statistically significant prolongation of survival in the group receiving psychosocial support.[31] This trial has been extremely widely publicized and extensively cited, despite an unplanned survival analysis and subsequent randomized replications that failed to support Spiegel's results.[32,33]

Electromagnetic Therapies

Some practitioners claim that cancer and other diseases are caused by disruptions of the body's electromagnetic fields. They believe that disease can be treated using pulsed, high-frequency electromagnetic waves. "BioResonance Therapy" is a relatively new version of the many alternative "energy therapies" that predominated in the 1930s. For example, Royal R. Rife developed an energy machine to destroy the microbes that he believed were the cause of cancer. Electromagnetic therapies today are costly treatments, offered mainly in Tijuana, Mexico, and in some European countries, despite their lack of value.

Oxygen and Ozone Therapies

Oxygen therapy refers to treatments based on the idea that cancer and other disease cannot survive in an oxygen-rich environment. Such therapies purport to kill cancer cells by delivering high levels of oxygen to tissues. Methods include intravenous infusion, ingestion, colonic administration, or dermal application of hydrogen; "ozone autohemotherapy," in which blood is bubbled with ozone and reinjected; and "oxygenated" water, pills, and solutions. Oxygen therapies are popular today despite the absence of supportive data and reports of serious side effects, including death.[34–36]

Botanical (Herbal) Medicines Used Against Cancer

Medicines derived from whole plant extracts, and which therefore contain many different types of molecules, are generally described as herbal medicines. The term botanical is used here to reflect that such agents are obtained from a wide variety of natural products, not just from herbs. Medicinal botanicals are minimally toxic, particularly when compared with plant-derived chemotherapeutic agents, and they are readily available without prescription. Described next are some botanicals commonly used by cancer patients. No botanical product has been proven effective against cancer, despite Internet claims of herbal remedy cures.

A principle of CAM for cancer is therefore that patients should not be advised to pursue anticancer therapy with botanicals.

Essiac. Essiac was popularized by a nurse, Rene Caisse, who claims to have derived the formula from a traditional native healer. This product consists of four herbs: burdock root, Turkey rhubarb, sorrel, and slippery elm. A review in the *Canadian Medical Association Journal* reported no published research on Essiac.[37]

Mistletoe. Mistletoe extracts, which are more widely known by the trade names Iscador, Helixor, and Eurixor, are popular cancer treatments in Europe and are available in some mainstream European cancer clinics. Unlike many botanical treatments, mistletoe extracts have been subjected to randomized trials in cancer patients. A systematic review of early trials revealed small sample sizes and serious methodologic shortcomings in most studies.[38] In subsequent larger studies, no survival benefit was found in patients with malignant melanoma[39] or head and neck cancer.[40] A small trial in glioma reported possible benefit in a subgroup, but there were no overall differences between groups.[41]

Noni. This popular botanical product is typical of many unproven therapies: it is a natural product used for "thousands of years" by "traditional Polynesian healers." The discovery of its use against cancer is colorful, involving the miraculous cure of a pet dog. Claims made for noni are ambiguous and implausible, as it is promoted as a "blood purifier" to "cleanse the body of harmful bacteria." Its value for cancer is based on a mouse study[42] that used a polysaccharide fraction of the fruit. There are no published human studies of noni.

Pau d'arco tea. Pau d'arco tea is said to be an old Incan remedy for many illnesses, including cancer. Made from the bark of an indigenous South American evergreen tree, its putative active ingredient, lapachol, has been isolated. In a Phase I trial, the blood levels of lapachol that were achieved without toxicity were far below those predicted to be effective on the basis of cell culture studies.[43]

PC-SPES. PC-SPES (PC for prostate cancer; spes is Latin for hope), a botanical treatment for prostate cancer, consists of eight herbs, all but two from Traditional Chinese Medicine. Laboratory research supports the activity of PC-SPES against prostate cancer, and antiproliferate and proapoptotic effects on tumor lines in vitro[44] have been demonstrated.[45,46] In rat models, PC-SPES decreased the incidence of spontaneous tumors and reduced tumor weight of implanted tumors.[47] PC-SPES also demonstrated estrogenic activity in a yeast assay and in mice.[44]

Phase II studies with PC-SPES show prostate-specific antigen (PSA) declines and improvements in pain and quality of life.[48–50] In a single-arm study of PC-SPES involving 70 patients with prostate cancer, no patient progressed objectively or in terms of PSA at median 64-week follow-up. PC-SPES was associated with a number of endocrine side effects[51] and with increased risk of thromboembolic events.[52–54] A randomized trial comparing PC-SPES to DES in 90 patients with androgen-independent prostate cancer found that 17 of 38 PC-SPES patients, versus 8 of 39 DES patients, achieved a PSA response ($P = 0.023$).[55]

Despite these encouraging results, a survival advantage for PC-SPES has yet to be demonstrated. More importantly, the product is no longer available for clinical use: PC-SPES was found to contain warfarin (and SPES, a more generic version for all cancers, to contain alprazolam) and was withdrawn by the manufacturer in February 2002.

β-Glucans. Many mushrooms used in Oriental botanical medicine contain β-glucans, a class of polysaccharide molecule. These agents have been widely studied for their anticancer effects. Most human Phase III trials of mushroom-derived β-glucans have used the polysaccharide Kureha (PSK), an extract of *Coriolus versicolor*, or an extract from the culture medium of *Schizophyllum commune* Fries known as SPG. Trials typically compared chemotherapy or radiotherapy plus β-glucan versus conventional treatment alone, finding superior survival for PSK compared to controls following colectomy,[56,57] gastrectomy,[58,59] and esophagectomy.[60] In a typical trial, 120 patients with Dukes' C colorectal cancer undergoing curative resection were randomized to PSK or placebo and followed for up to 10 years. Significant differences between groups for both disease-free and overall survival emerged, with median survival in the PSK group approximately 5 years compared to just over 4 years in controls.[56] SPG was slightly but not significantly superior to control for gastrectomy, although improved survival was seen in patients with curative resection in a subgroup analysis.[61,62] Results have been less encouraging in breast cancer[63,64] and leukemia.[65] The most promising results for SPG are seen in cervical cancer, with trials demonstrating improvements in survival[66] and increased rates of tumor response.[67]

In Phase II trials, an extract of Shiitake mushroom given to 61 patients with prostate cancer found that no patient experienced PSA decline, 4 showed some evidence of disease stabilization, and 23 patients progressed.[68] In a "preference" study, 269 consecutive patients undergoing liver resection for hepatocellular carcinoma were offered active hexose correlated compound (AHCC), an extract of several different fungi. Overall survival in the 113 patients who selected AHCC was superior to that of nonusers (hazard ratio, 0.64; $P < 0.001$).

Green tea. Interest in green tea as an anticancer botanical stemmed originally from epidemiologic research that demonstrated lower rates of various cancers, particularly colorectal cancer, in Chinese and Japanese green tea drinkers.[69] Typically, tea consumption was compared in cancer patients and matched local controls. Odds ratios for colon and rectal cancer among the highest consumers were 0.6 to 0.8 compared to those who did not consume tea regularly.[70] Green tea prevents induced colorectal tumors in animal models[71,72] and appears to have moderate inhibitory effects on cell growth.[73,74] Although green tea is under study as a possible chemopreventive agent,[75] its viability as a cancer treatment has yet to be documented.

Interactions Between CAM and Conventional Oncologic Therapy

Concurrent use of botanicals with conventional treatments raises the risk of interactions,[76] including herb–drug interactions that reduce the effectiveness of chemotherapy.

The relevant principle of CAM for cancer is that patients should avoid botanical products and other dietary supplements during and for a 2-week washout period before chemotherapy, radiotherapy, or surgery. Botanicals with hormonal effects should not be used concurrently with hormonal therapy.

Metabolic interactions: Many botanicals are known to modify the activity of cytochrome CYP450 3A4, affecting the blood levels of drugs metabolized on this pathway.[77] St. John's wort, for example, induces CYP450 3A4 in vitro,[77] and in a randomized cross-over study, the plasma concentration of SN-38, irinotecan's active metabolite, was dramatically reduced when patients concurrently used St. John's wort.[78] Several other popular botanicals, such as *Echinacea* and goldenseal, also were shown to modify CYP450 3A4 activity by an in vitro screen.[77]

Antioxidants: Many cytotoxic therapies, notably radiotherapy, depend on producing oxidative damage within the cancer cell. The activity of radiotherapy depends at least in part on the production of free radicals. Many botanicals, such as grape seed extract and ginseng, contain antioxidant constituents. Patients may unwittingly exacerbate the problem by taking additional antioxidants in the form of other dietary supplements. It is widely thought that concurrent administration of antioxidant supplements may, at least in theory, compromise the effectiveness of radiation therapy and some chemotherapeutic agents.[79] Although some researchers believe that concurrent use of antioxidants and cytotoxic therapy[80] can produce benefits, suppression of chemotherapy-induced apoptosis by antioxidants has been demonstrated in vitro.[81] Moreover, a nonrandomized comparative study recently found poorer survival in patients taking high doses of vitamins, including antioxidants, concurrent with systemic therapy.[82] At the very least, caution is advised.

Hormonal interactions: Many botanicals, including soy, chasteberry, dong quai, ginseng, and red clover, contain phytoestrogens, or plant-based estrogen-like substances. These compounds may interfere with antiestrogen therapies such as tamoxifen or raloxifene, or promote the growth of estrogen-sensitive tumors.[83,84] Indeed, genistein, the predominant isoflavone in soy products, reduced the inhibitory effect of tamoxifen in a mouse model of breast cancer.[85] Similarly, black cohosh increased the proliferation of MCF-7 breast cancer cells in vitro.[86,87] Although some authors claim the opposite effect, that is, that botanicals containing phytoestrogens can inhibit breast tumor cell growth or potentiate antiestrogen therapy,[88] the possibility of harmful interactions will remain a concern until studies are conducted.

Other chemotherapy interactions: CAM products may interact with chemotherapeutic agents through a number of other mechanisms. In vitro study has shown that berberine, a component of a number of herbs, upregulates the expression of pgp-170, a multidrug-resistant transporter protein, in a number of cancer cell lines, resulting in decreased paclitaxel cytotoxicity.[89] Botanicals can also interfere with the conversion of chemotherapy prodrugs to the active form[90] or with apoptotic pathways.[81]

Surgical interactions: Over-the-counter remedies interfere with blood coagulation, posing a risk of bleeding complications in the perioperative period.[91] Garlic and vitamin E are common examples. Psychoactive herbs, such as valerian or kava kava, are reported to potentiate the sedative effects of anesthetics.[91]

Complementary Therapies for Symptom Control

Therapies such as acupuncture, massage, relaxation therapy, and hypnosis are widely used for symptom control by the general public. Acupuncture, for example, is widely used in the United States to treat conditions such as back pain, and massage therapy is sought to help treat for anxiety disorders. Similarly, complementary therapies are increasingly used to treat symptoms of cancer or its treatment. A description of the most important complementary therapies is given below, followed by a review of the evidence for their effects against cancer-related symptoms. On the basis of this evidence, the following principles apply to the use of complementary modalities for cancer symptoms:

- Hypnosis or relaxation therapy should be considered for acute or chronic cancer pain, particularly when pain is poorly controlled with medication or when medication causes unacceptable adverse effects.
- Acupuncture is indicated to help control chronic cancer pain that remains severe despite medication or when medication causes unacceptable adverse effects.
- Mild or moderate mood disorders can be alleviated with therapies such as relaxation, imagery, meditation, and massage. Music therapy is available for inpatients at some cancer centers and appears effective for mood disorder in this population.
- Hypnosis or acupuncture is often effective for poorly controlled acute or subacute nausea in cancer patients.
- Botanicals do not relieve hot flashes.

Types of Complementary Therapies

Mind–body medicine. A wide variety of complementary therapies are used to relieve stress and enhance quality of life by producing relaxation. Hypnosis is the induction of a deeply relaxed state during which the therapist works to increase suggestibility and to help patients suspend critical faculties. Once in this state, sometimes called a hypnotic trance, patients are given therapeutic suggestions to encourage changes in behavior or symptom relief. Visualization and imagery techniques involve the induction of a relaxed state followed by use of a visual image, such as a pastoral scene, that enhances the sense of relaxation. Progressive relaxation involves sequential tensing and relaxing of muscles.

Acupuncture. Acupuncture is the insertion of very fine needles at special points on the body. Although details of practice may differ between individual schools, all traditional Chinese medical theory is based in the Taoist concept of *yin* and *yang* and the flow of *Qi* (energy) along hypothesized channels in the body. Stimulating acupuncture points situated on these channels provides one way of altering the flow of energy. Modern scientific understanding views acupuncture points as corresponding to physiologic and anatomic features such as peripheral nerve junctions.

Massage. Therapeutic massage involves manipulation of the soft tissue of whole or partial body areas to induce general improvements in health, such as relaxation or improved sleep, or specific physical benefits, such as relief of muscular aches and pains.

Music therapy. Music therapy is the controlled use of music to effect clinical change. Music therapists select and play live music according to patient mood and preference. They may involve patients in music making by having them develop lyrics, sing, or play a drum.

Pain

The most commonly used complementary therapies for pain include mind–body techniques, acupuncture, and massage. Both a systematic review[92] and a National Institutes of Health (NIH) technology assessment panel[93] have supported the use of hypnosis for cancer-related pain. There is also randomized trial evidence that relaxation and imagery reduce pain in cancer patients.[94] There is good evidence that acupuncture is effective for both chronic and acute nonmalignant pain.[95] Support for its use in oncology comes from a recent randomized trial involving 90 patients with refractory neuropathic cancer pain: pain scores at 60 days fell by more than a third in the acupuncture group compared to little change in patients receiving placebo ($P < 0.001$ for the difference between groups).[96] Several small randomized trials indicate that massage can reduce pain in cancer patients at varying stages of disease.[97,98] In the largest study to date, 87 hospitalized cancer patients were randomized to massage or to control on a crossover basis. Pain and anxiety scores fell by approximately 40% during massage compared with little or no change during control sessions.[99] National Comprehensive Cancer Network (NCCN) guidelines currently recommend consideration of massage and acupuncture for refractory cancer pain.[100]

Anxiety and Depression

Many complementary therapies modulate levels of arousal. The most obvious examples are hypnosis and relaxation therapies. A systematic review included 15 randomized trials that assessed the effects of relaxation therapies on acute, treatment-related anxiety and depression in cancer patients. Scores of patients receiving relaxation therapy were approximately half a standard deviation better than controls, with differences between groups being statistically significant.[101] Several randomized trials have explored the effects of relaxation treatments on anxiety and depression in out-patients. In a typical study, 109 cancer patients with varying diagnoses and different stages of disease were randomized to receive seven weekly 90-minute meditation classes and were encouraged to practice meditation at home. Anxiety and depression scores fell by nearly 50% in the meditation group with little change in controls ($P < 0.01$ for difference between groups on reanalysis).[102]

The broad perception that massage is relaxing has now been documented in randomized trials.[103–106] Several studies examined the effects of massage on psychologic endpoints in cancer patients. In a high-quality trial, 35 patients undergoing autologous bone marrow transplant were randomized to receive up to nine 20-minute massages during inpatient stay or to standard care control. Massage was superior to control for anxiety, fatigue, and general well-being, although differences for depression did not reach statistical significance.[107] A randomized cross-over study of 87 hospitalized cancer patients found that foot massage reduced anxiety scores substantially whereas the control procedure produced little change.[99]

Music therapy has been shown to reduce mood disturbance in patients undergoing autologous bone marrow transplant: 69 patients were randomized either to receive a course of treatments from music therapists during their inpatient stay or to standard care alone. Total mood disturbance scores fell by approximately two-thirds immediately following music therapy compared to only about 15% in controls ($P = 0.0003$ for the difference between groups). When measured over the course of the inpatient stay, anxiety scores were approximately 33% lower in the music therapy group ($P = 0.014$).[108]

Nausea and Vomiting

A variety of cognitive behavioral techniques address chemotherapy-related nausea and vomiting; many include hypnosis and relaxation techniques.[109] Most randomized trials show clinically and statistically significant improvements in nausea and vomiting in patients assigned to relaxation or hypnosis compared to controls (Table 15.1).

There is solid evidence that acupuncture reduces postoperative nausea and vomiting. A meta-analysis of 19 studies involving 1,679 patients showed that acupuncture reduced both nausea (relative risk compared to placebo control, 0.4; 95% CI, 0.2–0.7; 5 trials) and vomiting (relative risk compared to placebo control, 0.5; 95% CI, 0.35–0.65; 8 trials) in the immediate postoperative period. These findings were robust to sensitivity analyses of study size and quality.[110]

The results for chemotherapy-associated nausea are less clear. In one study, women undergoing myeloablative chemotherapy were randomized to acupuncture, placebo acupuncture, or antiemetic medication. The mean number of vomiting episodes in the three groups was 6.3, 10.7, and 13.4, respectively, with highly significant differences between acupuncture and placebo.[111] The effects of acupuncture on nausea and vomiting, however, do not appear to persist. One estimate is that the effects of treatment do not last more than approximately 8 hours.[112] Wristbands that provide continuous electrical or pressure stimulation to an acupuncture point on

TABLE 15.1. Randomized controlled trials (RCTs) of hypnosis or relaxation versus control.

Author	*Year*	*Patients*	*Intervention*	*Result*
Jacknow[123]	1994	20 children with chemotherapy nausea/vomiting	Hypnosis versus standard care control	No difference in nausea/vomiting but fewer antiemetics in hypnosis group; less anticipatory nausea in hypnosis group at follow-up
Zeltzer[124]	1991	54 children starting chemotherapy	Hypnosis versus relaxation versus standard care control	Hypnosis superior to nonhypnotic relaxation for control of both anticipatory and posttreatment nausea; both treatments superior to control
Vasterling[125]	1993	60 adults starting chemotherapy	Relaxation versus distraction versus standard care control	Relaxation and distraction equally effective and superior to control for anticipatory nausea
Morrow[126]	1982	60 patients experiencing anticipatory nausea	Systematic desensitization (including relaxation) versus standard care control	Decreased anticipatory nausea in the treatment group compared to control
Troesch[127]	1993	28 newly diagnosed patients about to start chemotherapy	Guided imagery and relaxation versus standard care control	Less nausea and vomiting in the treatment group but no statistically significant differences from controls
Cotanch[128]	1987	60 patients receiving in-patient chemotherapy	Relaxation versus music tapes versus standard care control	Decreased vomiting in relaxation group compared to controls; trend toward decreased nausea
Holli[129]	1993	67 patients receiving chemotherapy	Relaxation therapy versus standard care control	No differences in vomiting between groups
Syrjala[130]	1992	45 patients undergoing bone marrow transplant	Hypnosis versus cognitive behavioral training versus "therapist contact" control versus standard care control	Nausea and vomiting did not differ between groups
Syrjala[94]	1995	94 patients undergoing bone marrow transplant	Hypnosis versus cognitive behavioral training versus "therapist contact" control versus standard care control	Nausea did not differ between groups
Burish[131]	1981	16 patients undergoing chemotherapy	Hypnosis and relaxation training versus standard care control	Lower nausea scores in treated patients; very low levels of vomiting in both groups
Lyles[132]	1982	50 patients undergoing chemotherapy	Relaxation therapy and hypnosis versus standard care control	Lower nausea in group receiving relaxation therapy and hypnosis
Zeltzer[133]	1984	19 children with chemotherapy nausea/vomiting	Hypnosis versus supportive counseling	Large reductions in symptoms in both groups; no difference between groups
Burish[134]	1987	24 patients undergoing chemotherapy	Relaxation therapy versus standard care control	Less nausea and vomiting in relaxation therapy group
Lerman[135]	1990	48 patients undergoing chemotherapy	Relaxation therapy versus standard care control	Relaxation therapy reduced postchemotherapy nausea; effects on anticipatory nausea depended on patient's predominant coping style
Feldman[136]	1990	60 patients undergoing chemotherapy	Hypnosis versus standard care control	No difference between groups

the wrist are promoted for purported antiemetic effects, but studies do not support their value.[113–116] Wristbands may not provide adequately strong stimulation to the acupuncture point.[117]

Hot Flashes

Botanicals such as soy and black cohosh are promoted to reduce treatment-related hot flashes in cancer patients. However, evidence suggests that they are not effective. Randomized, placebo-controlled trials show no benefit for black cohosh[118] or soy[119,120] in reducing the frequency of hot flashes in breast cancer patients. Vitamin E decreases hot flashes only minimally,[121] but its low cost and lack of toxicity have led at least some authorities to recommend its use.[122]

Complementary and Alternative Medicine for Cancer: Summary

Current data suggest that many patients use CAM therapies. The use of complementary therapies for symptom control can be encouraged. These therapies are noninvasive, pleasant, and effective. Randomized trials support their value. Conversely, alternative methods, promoted for use instead of conventional oncologic therapy, should be discouraged. These methods are not effective. Moreover, they are invasive, typically biologically active, expensive, and potentially harmful, as patients may delay timely receipt of beneficial care while trying a nonviable "alternative."

The provision of evidence-based complementary therapies along with mainstream cancer treatment is a relatively recent development. Termed "integrative oncology" to emphasize the integration of complementary and mainstream care, this synthesis seeks to provide optimal overall management of cancer patients. High-quality research, an integral aspect of integrative oncology, is enabled when the expertise available in cancer programs is applied to the study of complementary therapies. Because research supports the value of complementary modalities in the control of symptoms associated with cancer and its treatment, these modalities should increasingly become part of oncologic care.

References

1. Zollman C, Vickers A. ABC of complementary medicine. What is complementary medicine? BMJ 1999;319(7211):693–696.
2. Eisenberg DM, Davis RB, Ettner SL, et al. Trends in alternative medicine use in the United States, 1990–1997: results of a follow-up national survey. JAMA 1998;280:1569–1575.
3. Druss BG, Rosenheck RA. Association between use of unconventional therapies and conventional medical services. JAMA 1999;282:651–656.
4. Thomas KJ, Nicholl JP, Coleman P. Use and expenditure on complementary medicine in England: a population based survey. Complementary Ther Med 2001;9:2–11.
5. Fisher P, Ward A. Complementary medicine in Europe. BMJ 1994;309:107–111.
6. MacLennan AH, Wilson DH, Taylor AW. The escalating cost and prevalence of alternative medicine. Prev Med 2002; 35(2):166–173.
7. Millar WJ. Use of alternative health care practitioners by Canadians. Can J Public Health 1997;88:154–158.
8. Ernst E, Cassileth BR. The prevalence of complementary/alternative medicine in cancer: a systematic review. Cancer (Phila) 1998;83(4):777–782.
9. Rees RW, Feigel I, Vickers A, et al. Prevalence of complementary therapy use by women with breast cancer. a population-based survey. Eur J Cancer 2000;36(11):1359–1364.
10. Crocetti E, Crotti N, Feltrin A, et al. The use of complementary therapies by breast cancer patients attending conventional treatment. Eur J Cancer 1998;34(3):324–328.
11. Miller M, Boyer MJ, Butow PN, et al. The use of unproven methods of treatment by cancer patients. Frequency, expectations and cost. Support Care Cancer 1998;6(4):337–347.
12. Gray RE, Fitch M, Goel V, et al. Utilization of complementary/alternative services by women with breast cancer. J Health Soc Policy 2003;16(4):75–84.
13. Chrystal K, Allan S, Forgeson G, et al. The use of complementary/alternative medicine by cancer patients in a New Zealand regional cancer treatment centre. N Z Med J 2003; 16(1168):U296.
14. Diefenbach MA, Hamrick N, Uzzo R, et al. Clinical, demographic and psychosocial correlates of complementary and alternative medicine use by men diagnosed with localized prostate cancer. J Urol 2003;170(1):166–169.
15. Yoshimura K, Ichioka K, Terada N, et al. Use of complementary and alternative medicine by patients with localized prostate carcinoma: study at a single institution in Japan. Int J Clin Oncol 2003;8(1):26–30.
16. Jewett MA, Fleshner N, Klotz LH, et al. Radical prostatectomy as treatment for prostate cancer [comment]. CMAJ Can Med Assoc J 2003;168(1):44–45.
17. Kao GD, Devine P. Use of complementary health practices by prostate carcinoma patients undergoing radiation therapy. Cancer (Phila) 2000;88(3):615–619.
18. Richardson MA. Biopharmacologic and herbal therapies for cancer: research update from NCCAM. J Nutr 2001; 131(11):3037S.
19. Specter M. The outlaw doctor. New Yorker 2001;48.
20. Burzynski SR, Kubove E, Burzynski B. Phase I clinical studies of antineoplaston A5 injections. Drugs Exp Clin Res 1987;13(suppl 1):37–43.
21. Buckner JC, Malkin MG, Reed E, et al. Phase II study of antineoplastons A10 (NSC 648539) and AS2-1 (NSC 620261) in patients with recurrent glioma. Mayo Clin Proc 1999; 74(2):137–145.
22. Creagan ET, Moertel CG, O'Fallon JR, et al. Failure of high-dose vitamin C (ascorbic acid) therapy to benefit patients with advanced cancer. A controlled trial. N Engl J Med 1979; 301(13):687–690.
23. Moertel CG, Fleming TR, Creagan ET, et al. High-dose vitamin C versus placebo in the treatment of patients with advanced cancer who have had no prior chemotherapy. A randomized double-blind comparison. N Engl J Med 1985;312(3):137–141.
24. Drisko JA, Chapman J, Hunter VJ. The use of antioxidant therapies during chemotherapy. Gynecol Oncol 2003;88(3):434–439.
25. Bahlis NJ, McCafferty-Grad J, Jordan-McMurry I, et al. Feasibility and correlates of arsenic trioxide combined with ascorbic acid-mediated depletion of intracellular glutathione for the treatment of relapsed/refractory multiple myeloma. Clin Cancer Res 2002;8(12):3658–3668.
26. Moertel CG, Fleming TR, Rubin J, et al. A clinical trial of amygdalin (Laetrile) in the treatment of human cancer. N Engl J Med 1982;306(4):201–206.
27. Hildenbrand GL, Hildenbrand LC, Bradford K, et al. Five-year survival rates of melanoma patients treated by diet therapy after the manner of Gerson: a retrospective review. Altern Ther Health Med 1995;1(4):29–37.
28. Zollman C, Rees R. Disputes conclusions in Hildenbrand study. Altern Ther Health Med 1997;2(4):14–15.
29. Gonzalez NJ, Isaacs LL. Evaluation of pancreatic proteolytic enzyme treatment of adenocarcinoma of the pancreas, with nutrition and detoxification support. Nutr Cancer 1999; 33(2):117–124.
30. Gellert GA, Maxwell RM, Siegel BS. Survival of breast cancer patients receiving adjunctive psychosocial support therapy: a 10-year follow-up study. J Clin Oncol 1993;11(1):66–69.
31. Spiegel D, Bloom JR, Kraemer HC, et al. Effect of psychosocial treatment on survival of patients with metastatic breast cancer. Lancet 1989;2(8668):888–891.
32. Cunningham AJ, Edmonds CV, Jenkins GP, et al. A randomized controlled trial of the effects of group psychological therapy on survival in women with metastatic breast cancer. Psycho-Oncology 1998;7(34):508–517.
33. Goodwin PJ, Leszcz M, Ennis M, et al. The effect of group psychosocial support on survival in metastatic breast cancer. N Engl J Med 2001;345(24):1719–1726.
34. Sherman SJ, Boyer LV, Sibley WA. Cerebral infarction immediately after ingestion of hydrogen peroxide solution. Stroke 1994; 25(5):1065–1067.
35. Meyer CT, Brand M, DeLuca VA, et al. Hydrogen peroxide colitis: a report of three patients. J Clin Gastroenterol 1981; 3(1):31–35.
36. Hirschtick RE, Dyrda SE, Peterson LC. Death from an unconventional therapy for AIDS. Ann Intern Med 1994;120(8):694.
37. Kaegi E. Unconventional therapies for cancer: 1. Essiac. The Task Force on Alternative Therapies of the Canadian Breast Cancer Research Initiative. Can Med Assoc J 1998;158(7): 897–902.
38. Kleijnen J, Knipschild P. Mistletoe treatment for cancer. Review of controlled trials in humans. Phytomedicine 1994;1:255–260.
39. McNamee D. Mistletoe extract ineffective in melanoma. Lancet 1999;354:1101.
40. Steuer-Vogt MK, Bonkowsky V, Ambrosch P, et al. The effect of an adjuvant mistletoe treatment programme in resected head

and neck cancer patients: a randomised controlled clinical trial. Eur J Cancer 2001;37(1):23–31.
41. Lenartz D, Dott U, Menzel J, et al. Survival of glioma patients after complementary treatment with galactoside-specific lectin from mistletoe. Anticancer Res 2000;20(3B):2073–2076.
42. Hirazumi A, Furusawa E, Chou SC, et al. Anticancer activity of *Morinda citrifolia* (noni) on intraperitoneally implanted Lewis lung carcinoma in syngeneic mice. Proc West Pharmacol Soc 1994;37:145–146.
43. Block JB, Serpick AA, Miller W, et al. Early clinical studies with lapachol (NSC-11905). Cancer Chemother Rep [2] 1974; 4(4):27–28.
44. DiPaola RS, Zhang H, Lambert GH, et al. Clinical and biologic activity of an estrogenic herbal combination (PC-SPES) in prostate cancer. N Engl J Med 1998;339(12):785–791.
45. Hsieh T, Chen SS, Wang X, et al. Regulation of androgen receptor (AR) and prostate specific antigen (PSA) expression in the androgen-responsive human prostate LNCaP cells by ethanolic extracts of the Chinese herbal preparation, PC-SPES. Biochem Mol Biol Int 1997;42(3):535–544.
46. de la Taille A, Hayek OR, Buttyan R, et al. Effects of a phytotherapeutic agent, PC-SPES, on prostate cancer: a preliminary investigation on human cell lines and patients. BJU Int 1999; 84(7):845–850.
47. Tiwari RK, Geliebter J, Garikapaty VP, et al. Anti-tumor effects of PC-SPES, an herbal formulation in prostate cancer. Int J Oncol 1999;14(4):713–719.
48. de la Taille A, Buttyan R, Hayek O, et al. Herbal therapy PC-SPES: in vitro effects and evaluation of its efficacy in 69 patients with prostate cancer. J Urol 2000;164(4):1229–1234.
49. Oh WK, George DJ, Hackmann K, et al. Activity of the herbal combination, PC-SPES, in the treatment of patients with androgen-independent prostate cancer. Urology 2001;57(1):122–126.
50. Pfeifer BL, Pirani JF, Hamann SR, et al. PC-SPES, a dietary supplement for the treatment of hormone-refractory prostate cancer. BJU Int 2000;85(4):481–485.
51. Small EJ, Frohlich MW, Bok R, et al. Prospective trial of the herbal supplement PC-SPES in patients with progressive prostate cancer. J Clin Oncol 2000;18(21):3595–3603.
52. Schiff JD, Ziecheck WS, Choi B. Pulmonary embolus related to PC-SPES use in a patient with PSA recurrence after radical prostatectomy. Urology 2002;59(3):444.
53. Weinrobe MC, Montgomery B. Acquired bleeding diathesis in a patient taking PC-SPES. N Engl J Med 2001;345(16):1213–1214.
54. Lock M, Loblaw DA, Choo R, et al. Disseminated intravascular coagulation and PC-SPES: a case report and literature review. Can J Urol 2001;8(4):1326–1329.
55. Small EJ, Kantoff PW, Weinberg S, et al. A prospective multicenter randomized trial of the herbal supplement, PC-SPES vs diethylstilbestrol (DES) in patients with advanced, androgen independent prostate cancer (AiPCa.). Proc Am Soc Clin Oncol 2002;21:178a.
56. Torisu M, Hayashi Y, Ishimitsu T, et al. Significant prolongation of disease-free period gained by oral polysaccharide K (PSK) administration after curative surgical operation of colorectal cancer. Cancer Immunol Immunother 1990;31(5):261–268.
57. Mitomi T, Tsuchiya S, Iijima N, et al. Randomized controlled study on adjuvant immunochemotherapy with PSK in curatively resected colorectal cancer. The Cooperative Study Group of Surgical Adjuvant Immunochemotherapy for Cancer of Colon and Rectum. Gan To Kagaku Ryoho 1989;16(6):2241–2249.
58. Niimoto M, Hattori T, Tamada R, et al. Postoperative adjuvant immunochemotherapy with mitomycin C, futraful and PSK for gastric cancer. An analysis of data on 579 patients followed for five years. Jpn J Surg 1988;18(6):681–686.
59. Nakazato H, Koike A, Saji S, et al. Efficacy of immunochemotherapy as adjuvant treatment after curative resection of gastric cancer. Study Group of Immunochemotherapy with PSK for Gastric Cancer. Lancet 1994;343(8906): 1122–1126.
60. Ogoshi K, Satou H, Isono K, et al. Immunotherapy for esophageal cancer. A randomized trial in combination with radiotherapy and radiochemotherapy. Cooperative Study Group for Esophageal Cancer in Japan. Am J Clin Oncol 1995; 18(3):216–222.
61. Fujimoto S, Furue H, Kimura T, et al. Clinical evaluation of schizophyllan adjuvant immunochemotherapy for patients with resectable gastric cancer—a randomized controlled trial. Jpn J Surg 1984;14(4):286–292.
62. Fujimoto S, Furue H, Kimura T, et al. Clinical outcome of postoperative adjuvant immunochemotherapy with sizofiran for patients with resectable gastric cancer: a randomised controlled study. Eur J Cancer 1991;27(9):1114–1118.
63. Toi M, Hattori T, Akagi M, et al. Randomized adjuvant trial to evaluate the addition of tamoxifen and PSK to chemotherapy in patients with primary breast cancer. 5-Year results from the Nishi-Nippon Group of the Adjuvant Chemoendocrine Therapy for Breast Cancer Organization. Cancer (Phila) 1992;70(10): 2475–2483.
64. Iino Y, Yokoe T, Maemura M, et al. Immunochemotherapies versus chemotherapy as adjuvant treatment after curative resection of operable breast cancer. Anticancer Res 1995;15(6B): 2907–2911.
65. Ohno R, Yamada K, Masaoka T, et al. A randomized trial of chemoimmunotherapy of acute nonlymphocytic leukemia in adults using a protein-bound polysaccharide preparation. Cancer Immunol Immunother 1984;18(3):149–154.
66. Okamura K, Suzuki M, Chihara T, et al. Clinical evaluation of sizofiran combined with irradiation in patients with cervical cancer. A randomized controlled study; a five-year survival rate. Biotherapy 1989;1(2):103–107.
67. Noda K, Takeuchi S, Yajima A, et al. Clinical effect of sizofiran combined with irradiation in cervical cancer patients: a randomized controlled study. Cooperative Study Group on SPG for Gynecological Cancer. Jpn J Clin Oncol 1992;22(1):17–25.
68. deVere White RW, Hackman RM, Soares SE, et al. Effects of a mushroom mycelium extract on the treatment of prostate cancer. Urology 2002;60(4):640–644.
69. Kohlmeier L, Weterings KG, Steck S, et al. Tea and cancer prevention: an evaluation of the epidemiologic literature. Nutr Cancer 1997;27(1):1–13.
70. Ji BT, Chow WH, Hsing AW, et al. Green tea consumption and the risk of pancreatic and colorectal cancers. Int J Cancer 1997;70(3):255–258.
71. Hirose M, Hoshiya T, Akagi K, et al. Effects of green tea catechins in a rat multi-organ carcinogenesis model. Carcinogenesis (Oxf) 1993;14(8):1549–1553.
72. Hirose M, Takahashi S, Ogawa K, et al. Chemoprevention of heterocyclic amine-induced carcinogenesis by phenolic compounds in rats. Cancer Lett 1999;143(2):173–178.
73. Yang GY, Liao J, Kim K, et al. Inhibition of growth and induction of apoptosis in human cancer cell lines by tea polyphenols. Carcinogenesis (Oxf) 1998;19(4):611–616.
74. Chen ZP, Schell JB, Ho CT, et al. Green tea epigallocatechin gallate shows a pronounced growth inhibitory effect on cancerous cells but not on their normal counterparts. Cancer Lett 1998;129(2):173–179.
75. Kelloff GJ, Crowell JA, Steele VE, et al. Progress in cancer chemoprevention: development of diet-derived chemopreventive agents. J Nutr 2000;130(suppl 2S):467S–471S.
76. Cassileth BR, Lucarelli C. Herb Drug Interactions in Oncology. Hamilton, Ontario: Decker, 2003.
77. Budzinski JW, Foster BC, Vandenhoek S, et al. An in vitro evaluation of human cytochrome P450 3A4 inhibition by selected commercial herbal extracts and tinctures. Phytomedicine 2000; 7(4):273–282.

78. Mathijssen RH, Verweij J, de Bruijn P, et al. Effects of St. John's wort on irinotecan metabolism. J Natl Cancer Inst 2002; 94(16):1247–1249.
79. Labriola D, Livingston R. Possible interactions between dietary antioxidants and chemotherapy. Oncology (Huntingt) 1011; 13(7):1003–1008.
80. Prasad KN, Kumar B, Yan XD, et al. Alpha-tocopheryl duccinate, the most effective form of vitamin E for adjuvant cancer treatment: a review. J Am Coll Nutr 2003;22(2):108–117.
81. Somasundaram S, Edmund NA, Moore DT, et al. Dietary curcumin inhibits chemotherapy-induced apoptosis in models of human breast cancer. Cancer Res 2002;62(13):3868.
82. Lesperance ML, Olivotto IA, Forde N, et al. Mega-dose vitamins and minerals in the treatment of non-metastatic breast cancer: an historical cohort study. Breast Cancer Res Treat 2002; 76(2):137–143.
83. Smolinske SC. Dietary supplement-drug interactions. J Am Med Womens Assoc 1999;54(4):191–192, 195.
84. Boyle FM. Adverse interaction of herbal medicine with breast cancer treatment. Med J Aust 1997;167(5):286.
85. Ju YH, Doerge DR, Allred KF, et al. Dietary genistein negates the inhibitory effect of tamoxifen on growth of estrogen-dependent human breast cancer (MCF-7) cells implanted in athymic mice. Cancer Res 2002;62(9):2474–2477.
86. Liu ZP, Yu B, Huo JS, et al. Estrogenic effects of *Cimicifuga racemosa* (black cohosh) in mice and on estrogen receptors in MCF-7 cells. J Med Food 2001;4(3):171–178.
87. Hsieh CY, Santell RC, Haslam SZ, et al. Estrogenic effects of genistein on the growth of estrogen receptor-positive human breast cancer (MCF-7) cells in vitro and in vivo. Cancer Res 1998;58(17):3833–3838.
88. Bodinet C, Freudenstein J. Influence of *Cimicifuga racemosa* on the proliferation of estrogen receptor-positive human breast cancer cells. Breast Cancer Res Treat 2002;76(1):1–10.
89. Lin HL, Liu TY, Wu CW, et al. Berberine modulates expression of mdr1 gene product and the responses of digestive track cancer cells to paclitaxel. Br J Cancer 1999;81(3):416–422.
90. Yokoi T, Narita M, Nagai E, et al. Inhibition of UDP-glucuronosyltransferase by aglycons of natural glucuronides in kampo medicines using SN-38 as a substrate. Jpn J Cancer Res 1995;86(10):985–989.
91. Ang-Lee MK, Moss J, Yuan CS. Herbal medicines and perioperative care. JAMA 2001;286(2):208–216.
92. Sellick SM, Zaza C. Critical review of 5 nonpharmacologic strategies for managing cancer pain. Cancer Prev Control 1998; 2(1):7–14.
93. NIH Technology Assessment Panel on Integration of Behavioral and Relaxation Approaches into the Treatment of Chronic Pain and Insomnia. Integration of behavioral and relaxation approaches into the treatment of chronic pain and insomnia. NIH Technology Assessment Panel on Integration of Behavioral and Relaxation Approaches into the Treatment of Chronic Pain and Insomnia. JAMA 1996;276(4):313–318.
94. Syrjala KL, Donaldson GW, Davis MW, et al. Relaxation and imagery and cognitive-behavioral training reduce pain during cancer treatment: a controlled clinical trial. Pain 1995;63(2): 189–198.
95. Linde K, Vickers A, Hondras M, et al. Systematic reviews of complementary therapies: an annotated bibliography. Part 1: Acupuncture. BMC Complement Altern Med 2001;1(1):3.
96. Alimi D, Rubino C, Pichard-Leandri E, et al. Analgesic effect of auricular acupuncture for cancer pain: a randomized, blinded, controlled trial. J Clin Oncol 2003;21(22):4120–4126.
97. Weinrich SP, Weinrich MC. The effect of massage on pain in cancer patients. Appl Nurs Res 1990;3(4):140–145.
98. Ferrell-Torry AT, Glick OJ. The use of therapeutic massage as a nursing intervention to modify anxiety and the perception of cancer pain. Cancer Nurs 1993;16(2):93–101.
99. Grealish L, Lomasney A, Whiteman B. Foot massage. A nursing intervention to modify the distressing symptoms of pain and nausea in patients hospitalized with cancer. Cancer Nurs 2000; 23(3):237–243.
100. Mock V, Atkinson A, Barsevick A, et al. NCCN Practice Guidelines for Cancer-Related Fatigue. Oncology (Huntingt) 2000;14(11A):151–161.
101. Luebbert K, Dahme B, Hasenbring M. The effectiveness of relaxation training in reducing treatment-related symptoms and improving emotional adjustment in acute non-surgical cancer treatment: a meta-analytical review. Psycho-Oncology 2001; 10(6):490–502.
102. Speca M, Carlson LE, Goodey E, et al. A randomized, wait-list controlled clinical trial: the effect of a mindfulness meditation-based stress reduction program on mood and symptoms of stress in cancer outpatients. Psychosom Med 2000;62(5):613–622.
103. Field T, Morrow C, Valdeon C, et al. Massage reduces anxiety in child and adolescent psychiatric patients. J Am Acad Child Adolesc Psychiatry 1992;31(1):125–131.
104. Stevensen C. The psychophysiological effects of aromatherapy massage following cardiac surgery. Complement Ther Med 1994;2(1):27–35.
105. Fraser J, Kerr JR. Psychophysiological effects of back massage on elderly institutionalized patients. J Adv Nurs 1993; 18(2):238–245.
106. Field T, Seligman S, Scafidi F, et al. Alleviating posttraumatic stress in children following Hurricane Andrew. J Appl Dev Psychol 1996;17(1):37–50.
107. Ahles TA, Tope DM, Pinkson B, et al. Massage therapy for patients undergoing autologous bone marrow transplantation. J Pain Symptom Manag 1999;18(3):157–163.
108. Cassileth BR, Vickers AJ, Magill LA. Music therapy for mood disturbance during hospitalization for autologous stem cell transplantation: a randomized controlled trial. Cancer (Phila) 2003;98(12):2723–2729.
109. Redd WH, Montgomery GH, DuHamel KN. Behavioral intervention for cancer treatment side effects. JNCI Cancer Spectrum 2001;93(11):810.
110. Lee A, Done ML. The use of nonpharmacologic techniques to prevent postoperative nausea and vomiting: a meta-analysis. Anesth Analg 1999;88(6):1362–1369.
111. Shen J, Wenger N, Glaspy J, et al. Electroacupuncture for control of myeloablative chemotherapy-induced emesis: a randomized controlled trial. JAMA 2000;284(21):2755–2761.
112. Dundee J. Acupuncture/acupressure as an antiemetic: studies of its use in postoperative vomiting, cancer chemotherapy and sickness of early pregnancy. Complement Med Res 1988; 3(1):2–14.
113. Roscoe JA, Morrow GR, Bushunow P, et al. Acustimulation wristbands for the relief of chemotherapy-induced nausea. Altern Ther Health Med 2002;8(4):56–63.
114. Roscoe JA, Morrow GR, Hickok JT, et al. The efficacy of acupressure and acustimulation wrist bands for the relief of chemotherapy-induced nausea and vomiting. A University of Rochester Cancer Center Community Clinical Oncology Program multicenter study. J Pain Symptom Manag 2003; 26(2):731–742.
115. Pearl ML, Fischer M, McCauley DL, et al. Transcutaneous electrical nerve stimulation as an adjunct for controlling chemotherapy-induced nausea and vomiting in gynecologic oncology patients. Cancer Nurs 1999;22(4):307–311.
116. Treish I, Shord S, Valgus J, et al. Randomized double-blind study of the Reliefband as an adjunct to standard antiemetics in patients receiving moderately-high to highly emetogenic chemotherapy. Support Care Cancer 2003;11(8):516–521.
117. Dundee JW, Ghaly RG, Bill KM, et al. Effect of stimulation of the P6 antiemetic point on postoperative nausea and vomiting. Br J Anaesth 1989;63(5):612–618.

118. Jacobson JS, Troxel AB, Evans J, et al. Randomized trial of black cohosh for the treatment of hot flashes among women with a history of breast cancer. J Clin Oncol 2001;19(10):2739–2745.
119. Quella SK, Loprinzi CL, Barton DL, et al. Evaluation of soy phytoestrogens for the treatment of hot flashes in breast cancer survivors: a North Central Cancer Treatment Group Trial. J Clin Oncol 2000;18(5):1068–1074.
120. Van Patten CL, Olivotto IA, Chambers GK, et al. Effect of soy phytoestrogens on hot flashes in postmenopausal women with breast cancer: a randomized, controlled clinical trial. J Clin Oncol 2002;20(6):1449–1455.
121. Barton DL, Loprinzi CL, Quella SK, et al. Prospective evaluation of vitamin E for hot flashes in breast cancer survivors. J Clin Oncol 1998;16(2):495–500.
122. Loprinzi CL, Barton DL, Rhodes D. Management of hot flashes in breast-cancer survivors. Lancet Oncol 2002;2:199–204.
123. Jacknow DS, Tschann JM, Link MP, et al. Hypnosis in the prevention of chemotherapy-related nausea and vomiting in children: a prospective study. J Dev Behav Pediatr 1994;15(4):258–264.
124. Zeltzer LK, Dolgin MJ, LeBaron S, et al. A randomized, controlled study of behavioral intervention for chemotherapy distress in children with cancer. Pediatrics 1991;88(1):34–42.
125. Vasterling J, Jenkins RA, Tope DM, et al. Cognitive distraction and relaxation training for the control of side effects due to cancer chemotherapy. J Behav Med 1993;16(1):65–80.
126. Morrow GR, Morrell C. Behavioral treatment for the anticipatory nausea and vomiting induced by cancer chemotherapy. N Engl J Med 1982;307(24):1476–1480.
127. Troesch LM, Rodehaver CB, Delaney EA, et al. The influence of guided imagery on chemotherapy-related nausea and vomiting. Oncol Nurs Forum 1993;20(8):1179–1185.
128, Cotanch PH, Strom S. Progressive muscle relaxation as antiemetic therapy for cancer patients. Oncol Nurs Forum 1987;14(1):33–37.
129. Holli K. Ineffectiveness of relaxation on vomiting induced by cancer chemotherapy. Eur J Cancer 1993;29(13):1915–1916.
130. Syrjala KL, Cummings C, Donaldson GW. Hypnosis or cognitive behavioral training for the reduction of pain and nausea during cancer treatment: a controlled clinical trial. Pain 1992;48(2):137–146.
131. Burish TG, Lyles JN. Effectiveness of relaxation training in reducing adverse reactions to cancer chemotherapy. J Behav Med 1981;4(1):65–78.
132. Lyles JN, Burish TG, Krozely MG, et al. Efficacy of relaxation training and guided imagery in reducing the aversiveness of cancer chemotherapy. J Consult Clin Psychol 1982;50(4):509–524.
133. Zeltzer L, LeBaron S, Zeltzer PM. The effectiveness of behavioral intervention for reduction of nausea and vomiting in children and adolescents receiving chemotherapy. J Clin Oncol 1984;2(6):683–690.
134. Burish TG, Carey MP, Krozely MG, et al. Conditioned side effects induced by cancer chemotherapy: prevention through behavioral treatment. J Consult Clin Psychol 1987;55(1):42–48.
135. Lerman C, Rimer B, Blumberg B, et al. Effects of coping style and relaxation on cancer chemotherapy side effects and emotional responses. Cancer Nurs 1990;13(5):308–315.
136. Feldman CS, Salzberg HC. The role of imagery in the hypnotic treatment of adverse reactions to cancer therapy. J S C Med Assoc 1990;86(5):303–306.

SECTION TWO

Translational Basic Science

16 Fundamental Aspects of the Cell Cycle and Signal Transduction

Jeffrey R. Skaar and James A. DeCaprio

During normal cycles of cell growth and division, cells are exquisitely sensitive to their environment, responding to many stimuli ranging from nutrient availability, growth factors, and cell density with either increased proliferation or growth arrest. The cell's ability to sense and respond to these environmental cues is lost on the progression of cells to a malignant state, rendering cancer cells resistant to growth inhibition by growth factor withdrawal, contact inhibition, or irradiation. These cancerous cells acquire many genetic and epigenetic mutations that can constitutively activate signaling pathways to mimic growth factor signaling, block growth inhibitory signals, and fundamentally alter core components of the cell-cycle machinery, removing key inhibitors or increasing amounts and activity of key activators. Although the genetic alterations of many upstream genes of diverse function have been shown to lead to malignancy, in the end these upstream factors feed into a core network that governs cell-cycle progression.

The Cell Cycle

The cell cycle can be divided into four phases: G_1, S, G_2, and M. G_1 refers to the gap between the mitosis (M) of the previous cell division and the DNA synthesis (S) stage of the upcoming cell, and G_2 refers to the gap between DNA synthesis and mitosis. Additionally, quiescent cells, which are nondividing but metabolically active and terminally differentiated, such as muscle cells or neurons, are considered to be in G_0 phase.

The control of cell-cycle progression from G_1 to S to G_2 to M is tightly controlled by the activities of a small number of heterodimeric kinase complexes (Figure 16.1). The regulatory subunit of each dimer is required for kinase function, and the levels of these regulatory proteins oscillate throughout the cell cycle in response to upregulation by transcription factors and downregulation by the ubiquitin proteosome system. Because of the cyclic behavior of these regulatory subunits, they are called cyclins, and the kinases they regulate are called cyclin-dependent kinases (cdks).

In general, expression of G_1 cyclins activates the G_1-specific cyclin–cdk complex, allowing transcription of genes required for entry into S phase, including the DNA synthesis machinery; S-phase-specific cyclins; and proteins that remove inhibitors of S-phase cyclin/cdk activity. The increase in S-phase cyclin expression and function causes activation of the DNA synthesis machinery as well as the transcription of genes required for M phase, including cyclins and the mitosis machinery. Finally, M-phase cyclin–cdk complexes activate the mitotic machinery to break down the nuclear envelope, assemble the mitotic spindle to align the chromosomes during metaphase, and divide the cell during anaphase.

Because the cyclins in each phase of the cell cycle are degraded by the ubiquitin proteosome system on phase progression, once a cell enters the cell cycle, it is obligated to attempt complete cell division. Therefore, the primary control of cell-cycle entry occurs in G_0 cells, when cyclins are not expressed. Exposure of G_0 cells to mitogens induces the expression of cyclins and other proteins required for the cell cycle. After a certain period of exposure to mitogens, the cell reaches the restriction point, and it is irrevocably committed to entering the cell cycle. If mitogens are removed before the restriction point, the cell will exit the cell cycle and reenter G_0.

When G_0 mammalian cells are stimulated with mitogens, receptor tyrosine kinases transduce signals to activate immediate early transcription factors such as c-Fos and c-Jun, causing expression of the D-type cyclins, the E_2F family of transcription factors, and other early genes required for progression through G_1.[1–3] The activities of these early gene products ultimately control the passage of the cell through the restriction point and into the cell cycle. During G_1, E_2F family transcription factors are bound by the retinoblastoma protein, pRb, which converts E_2F from a transcriptional activator to a transcriptional repressor via its association with histone deacetylase complexes. As cyclin D levels rise through G_1 in response to mitogenic stimuli, the cyclin forms an active cyclin–cdk complex with either of the two related D-type cyclin cdks, Cdk4 or Cdk6; these active kinase complexes drive the cell through the restriction point by phosphorylating pRb, allowing E_2F to activate transcription of cyclin E (Figure 16.2). As the amount of cyclin D–Cdk complex increases, it acts as a sink for the Cip/Kip family of cdk inhibitors.[4]

The Cip/Kip inhibitors, including p21, p27, and p57, act as potent inhibitors of cyclin E/Cdk2 activity. Cyclin D–Cdk complexes contribute to increasing cyclin E/Cdk2 activity through E_2F-mediated transcription as well as the sequestra-

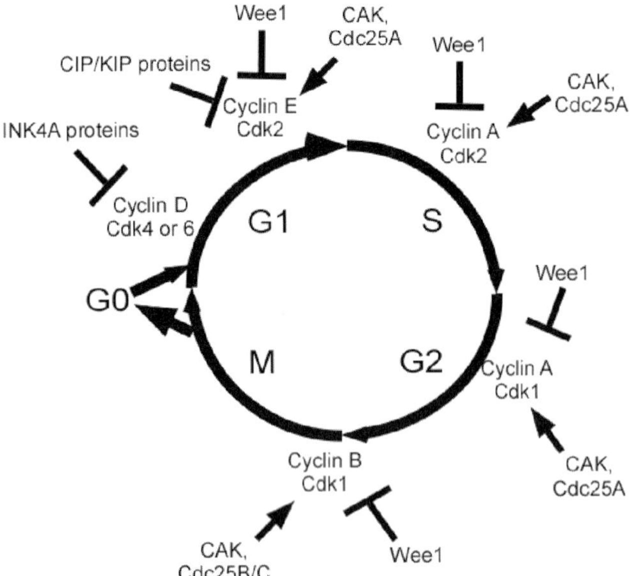

Figure 16.1. The human cell cycle. The cell cycle is divided into four phases: G_1, S, G_2, and M. Cyclin D–Cdk4/6 controls early G_1, cyclin E–Cdk2 controls late G_1, cyclin A–Cdk2/1 controls S and G_2, and cyclin B–cdk1 controls G_2 and entry into M phase. Activators and inhibitors of these cyclin–cdk complexes are shown. G_0 is a state defined by quiescent, nondividing cells that have exited the cell cycle.

tion of the Cip/Kip inhibitors. The production of robust cyclin E/Cdk2 activity supplants cyclin D/Cdk4/6 activity as the driving force of progression from G_1 phase to S phase.[4] At this point, the cell has passed the restriction point, as cyclin D/Cdk4/6 activity is no longer required. Cyclin E/Cdk2 serves to hyperphosphorylate pRb, completely removing its inhibition of E_2F, allowing transcription of genes required for S phase, including cyclin A, the S-phase cyclin.

Cyclin A, similar to the D-type cyclins, can bind two distinct cdks, Cdk2 and Cdk1. Currently, any differences in the function between the two cyclin A–Cdk complexes are unknown. The active cyclin A–Cdk2/1 complex has a nuclear localization and is thought to control DNA replication, controlling initiation and restricting replication to once per cell cycle, by phosphorylation of substrates. RPA, Mcm4, and the DNA polymerase α-primase are known cyclin A substrates that are involved in DNA replication.[5] In addition to a role in regulating DNA replication, cyclin A plays a key role in allowing cell-cycle progression through G_2 phase into M.

During S phase, cyclin B levels begin to increase, and by G_2 phase, two cdk complexes, cyclin A–Cdk1 and cyclin B–Cdk1, are active. The accumulation of active cyclin B/Cdk1 is strictly dependent on cyclin A/Cdk1 activity. During the S and G_2 phases, cyclin A/Cdk1 phosphorylates Cdh1, preventing it from targeting cyclin B to the anaphase-promoting complex (APC) for ubiquitination and degradation.[5] Active cyclin B/Cdk1 first accumulates in the cytoplasm, where it is thought to prepare structural components of the cell for the upcoming cell division. Cyclin B/cdk1 activity reorganizes the cell's microtubules and microfilaments, and phosphorylates proteins in the nuclear lamina, resulting in this structure's breakdown.[6] Just before the breakdown of the nuclear membrane, cyclin B/Cdk1 translocates to the nucleus to target further substrates, including those that control the shutdown of RNA polymerase III-mediated transcription.[6] Finally, cyclin B and cyclin A are rapidly degraded by the APC before the end of mitosis. The APC also mediates the transition from metaphase to anaphase by degrading securin, the inhibitor of separase. Separase then proceeds to cleave Scc1, a protein found in the cohesin complex of proteins that holds the newly replicated chromosomes together, allowing anaphase to ensue.

In addition to being regulated by their cyclin partners, mammalian cdks are subject to regulation by a number of different inhibitors throughout the cell cycle. These inhibitors can arrest or slow the cell cycle in response to many signals including nutrient depletion, failures in DNA replication, and DNA damage. During the G_1 to S transition, two distinct inhibitor classes function to inhibit Cdk4/6 and Cdk2 activity. The INK4 family of proteins (p16INK4A, p15INK4B, p18INK4C, and p19INK4D) are noncompetitive inhibitors of Cdk4 and Cdk6, binding to these kinases and causing allosteric changes that weaken binding to both cyclin D and adenosine triphosphate (ATP).[4] With the exception of p19INK4D, the expression of the INK4 family does not appear to be cell-cycle dependent, and p16INK4A, which appears to be the most important of the INK4 proteins, has been shown to increase with age and population doubling. However, the exact mechanism of regulation of this family of proteins remains under investigation.

The Cip/Kip family of cdk inhibitors, which includes p21, p27, and p57, also function at the G_1 to S transition. Cip/Kip inhibitors can inhibit multiple cyclin–cdk complexes with varying efficiencies, but, important for the G_1 to S transition, as already mentioned, they inhibit cyclin E/Cdk2 strongly while inhibiting cyclin D/Cdk4/6 poorly.[4] When bound to the cyclin E–Cdk2 complex, the Cip/Kip proteins bind the catalytic site of the cdk, blocking ATP from binding. In addition to being inactivated by titration away from cyclin E–Cdk2 complexes by cyclin D/Cdk4/6, p27 is subject to ubiquitin-mediated degradation during S phase. Although the regulation of all the Cip/Kip proteins is not completely understood, the gene for p21, *CDKN1A*, in particular, is subject to upregulation by the p53 tumor suppressor (see following) in response to DNA damage, allowing p53 to block cell-cycle progression.[3,7–9] p21 is a particularly potent protein for inducing cell-cycle arrests, as it can also inhibit cyclin A/Cdk2 and, indirectly, cyclin A/cyclin B/Cdk1.[6]

During the S, G_2, and M phases of the cell cycle, cyclin–cdk complexes containing Cdk2 and Cdk1 are also regulated by activating and inhibiting phosphorylations. All the cdks require an activating phosphorylation provided by a Cdk-activating kinase (CAK) composed of cyclin H, Cdk7,

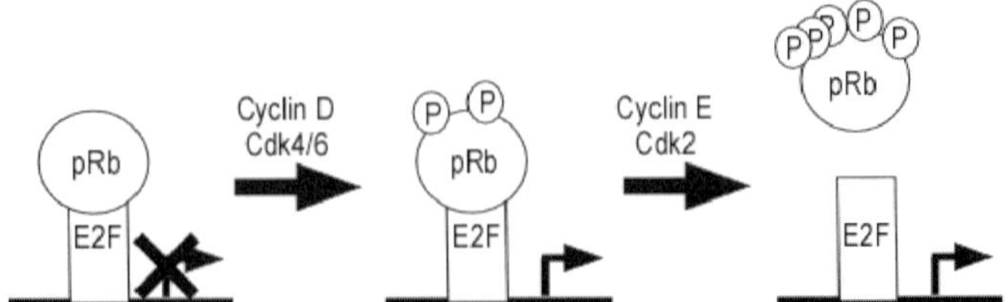

Figure 16.2. Inactivation of pRb by cyclin–Cdk complexes in G_1. Phosphorylation of pRb by cyclin D/Cdk4/6 in early G_1 partially inactivates pRb, allowing some E_2F-mediated transcription. Hyperphosphorylation of pRb by cyclin E–sCdk2 in late G_1 phase completely inactivates pRb, allowing uninhibited E_2F-mediated transcription.

and MAT1.[5,6] Because the cyclin H–Cdk7 complex can be inhibited by the Cip/Kip inhibitor p21, p21 upregulation by DNA damage can induce a G_1 arrest by direct inhibition of cyclin E/Cdk2 and a G_2–M arrest by indirect inhibition of cyclin B/A/Cdk1 via cyclin H/Cdk7 inactivation. However, the most potent control over Cdk2 and Cdk1 activity comes from the inhibitory phosphorylation of two amino-terminal tyrosine residues by the Wee1 kinase.[6] Phosphorylation of these residues blocks not only the ability of the kinase to transfer phosphate but also the ability to bind ATP. Removal of these inhibitory phosphorylations is accomplished by the actions of a Cdc25 phosphatase member. Cdc25A specifically dephosphorylates Cdk2 and Cdc25B and Cdc25C specifically dephosphorylates Cdk1.[6,10] The effects of Cdc25B and Cdc25C on Cdk1 are additive, and after activation by Cdc25B, cyclin B/Cdk1 activates Cdc25C by phosphorylation in a positive feedback loop. By regulating the levels and activities of Wee1 kinase activity and Cdc25 phosphatase activity, the cell can stop or promote cell-cycle progression as required. For example, the detection of DNA damage during S phase results in the rapid degradation of Cdc25A and increased expression of Wee1, causing a cell-cycle arrest.[10]

Finally, cell-cycle progression can be blocked by other pathways not directly involving cdks and cdk inhibitors. The mitotic spindle checkpoint monitors the proper attachment of chromosomes to the mitotic spindle and the proper alignment of these chromosomes along the metaphase plate. Failures in the mitotic spindle activate a mitotic checkpoint complex (MCC) that includes Mad2, BubR1, and Bub3. Mad2 and BubR1 both can bind and inhibit Cdc20, the subunit of the APC that targets securin, as well as cyclin B, for degradation.[11] Inhibition of APC-mediated degradation of securin prevents cleavage of the cohesin complex holding replicated sister chromosomes together, preventing mitosis.

The Cell Cycle and Cancer

With all the growth-promoting and -inhibiting signals that are integrated into the core cell-cycle controllers, it is surprising that the majority of cancers, although arising from mutations in many different genes, result from the improper activation or inactivation of relatively few pathways. Recent research in cell culture systems coupled with genetic analysis has shown that human cells acquire changes to as few as five distinct pathways, mainly controlling protein phosphatase 2A (PP2A) function, telomere maintenance, RAS activation, the pRb pathway, and the p53 pathway.[1] Currently the contribution of PP2A inactivation to cancer is unknown, although it has been suggested that only the inactivation of a particular subtype of PP2A complexes is required for transformation of human cells. However, significantly more is known about telomere maintenance, RAS activation, the pRb pathway, and p53 pathway in human cancer.

Telomerase

Telomeres, the repetitive, structured regions of DNA at the end of chromosomes, are required elements for chromosome integrity. These regions are not synthesized by the normal replicative DNA polymerases, but they are instead added to the end of chromosomal DNA by the telomerase ribonuclear protein, composed of an RNA template and the telomerase reverse transcriptase (TERT) protein.[1] The telomeres form a unique structure that allows for linear DNA chromosomes to persist without the activation of DNA damage pathways. After expression of telomerase ceases during the differentiation of a cell, subsequent DNA replications cause a progressive shortening of telomeric regions of DNA as a result of the inability of normal replicative DNA polymerases to completely copy the end of chromosomes. Over time, the loss of telomeric DNA to the "end replication problem" results in the activation of a checkpoint similar to DNA damage responses.[1,12] In normal cells, this telomeric checkpoint activation results in senescence, but mutations in the pRb pathway and the p53 pathway can allow these cells to continue to cycle.[1,12] Although these cells can escape senescence, the shortening of telomeres continues with each replication, reducing overall telomere length to a critical level. At this crisis point, telomeres fail to protect chromosome ends, activating DNA damage responses that result in chromosome fusion, leading to breakage, genomic instability, and massive amounts of cell death.[12] Rare escape mutants of crisis either reactivate telomerase to maintain telomere length or acquire mutations that activate the alternative lengthening of telomeres (ALT) pathway. For cancer cells to gain infinite replicative capacity, they must maintain telomere length via one of these two methods, most commonly reactivation of telomerase expression.

The pRb Pathway

The ability of a cancerous cell to break through senescence is governed by mutations affecting the pRb pathway, the p53 pathway, and the activation of Ras. As already discussed, pRb acts as the ultimate inhibitor of the G_1 to S transition by binding and converting the E_2F transcription factor into a repressor. Hyperphosphorylation of pRb, initially by cyclin D/Cdk4/6 and then cyclin E/Cdk2, dissociates pRb from E_2F, allowing E_2F-mediated transcription to occur. The importance of pRb in cancer is documented in hereditary retinoblastoma, which originally defined pRb as a tumor suppressor protein. In hereditary retinoblastoma, patients inherit one wild type and one mutant allele of *RB1*. The normal allele of *RB1* is lost in a somatic cell, leading to the development of an *RB1*–/– tumor. This loss of heterozygosity (LOH) defines the classic tumor suppressors.[3] Although mutation of *RB1* itself leads mainly to retinoblastoma and some osteosarcomas, the importance of the pRb pathway to all cancers has been confirmed by mutation of pRb or pRb pathway modifiers in other tumors. Nearly all known tumors contain a mutation that activates Cdk4, amplifies cyclin D, or eliminates the Cdk4/6 inhibitor p16INK4A. In particular, a high percentage of breast cancers exhibit overexpression of cyclin D1, whereas p16INK4A is often inactivated in melanomas and pancreatic cancer.[4] Even more strikingly, known human tumor viruses, such as human papilloma virus, the causative agent of most cervical cancers, and Kaposi's sarcoma-associated herpesvirus, the causative agent of Kaposi's sarcoma, target the pRb pathway specifically through direct pRb inactivation or by expression of a constitutively active D-type viral cyclin, respectively. Finally, mutations in the pRb pathway appear to be mutually exclusive, with tumors containing mutations in only one gene in the pathway. Of special note, mutations within p16INK4A are especially potent because it shares its second exon, read in a different frame, with the p14ARF (alternate reading frame) tumor suppressor, which functions in the regulation of p53.[2,13] The two proteins are both considered products of one gene, *CDKN2A*.

The p53 Pathway

Mutations in the p53 pathway allow cancerous cells to avoid senescence by preventing cell-cycle arrest at the G_1 to S and G_2 to M transitions. *TP53* is a canonical tumor suppressor gene and is subject to LOH in tumors. Germ-line mutation of p53 causes Li Fraumeni syndrome, an early-onset cancer syndrome, resulting in a broad spectrum of tumors, including cancers of the brain, breast, and blood.[14] Additionally, Wilm's tumors often have germ-line mutations in *TP53*. Mutations in *TP53* are found in more than 50% of all sporadic tumors, and, in some capacity, p53 appears to be dysregulated in every cancer. p53 functions as a tetrameric transcription factor, promoting the expression of cell-cycle arrest genes and proapoptotic genes in response to signals of DNA damage, aberrant growth signaling, heat shock, and other cellular stresses.[7] Tumors commonly contain point mutants in the p53 DNA-binding domain, and mutations often result in the abnormal stabilization of p53. Additionally, heterozygous mutations of *TP53* can function as dominant negatives for p53 function because of the tetramerization functions of p53.[3,9] Finally, p53 is also a target for inactivation by human papilloma virus in cervical cancer, affirming its importance in the development of cancer.

Functional inactivation of p53 is advantageous for tumor formation because it affects two cell-cycle transition points as well as apoptotic pathways. The dual function of p53 allows the cell to stop cycling to attempt to repair damage and to undergo apoptosis if the damage is irreparable. When induced by cellular stress, p53 activates transcription of the gene for the Cip/Kip inhibitor p21 to induce both a G_1 and G_2–M arrest.[7,9] Additional products of p53 target genes, including GADD45 and 14–3-3σ, also aid in arresting the cell cycle.[9] Proapoptotic p53 target genes include the genes for PUMA, Apaf-1, and Bax, a critical inhibitor of the antiapoptotic protein Bcl-2.[9,15] A negative feedback loop is also initiated by p53-mediated transcription, increasing levels of the p53 ubiquitin ligase Hdm2, potentially allowing resumption of the cell cycle following repair of damage.

Under normal conditions, p53 is extremely unstable, but upon exposure to genotoxic stress, it is stabilized by phosphorylation of serine residue 15 (Figure 16.3). Depending on the genotoxic stress, the kinase responsible for this phosphorylation is either the ataxia telangiectasia-mutated (ATM) kinase or the ataxia telangiectasia and Rad3-related (ATR) kinase.[3,9] Notably, inherited mutations in *ATM* result in cancer, although not all the ATM cancer-relevant functions involve p53. Phosphorylation of serine 15 interferes with p53 binding to the ubiquitin ligase Hdm2, blocking ubiquitination of p53 and resulting in stabilization of p53. As noted earlier, stabilized p53 induces the expression of genes involved in arresting the cell cycle to allow for DNA repair but also induces proapoptotic genes if the cell cannot repair the damage. Transcriptional activation by p53 is dependent on binding to the transcriptional coactivators p300/CBP that activate p53 by acetylation of C-terminal lysines and func-

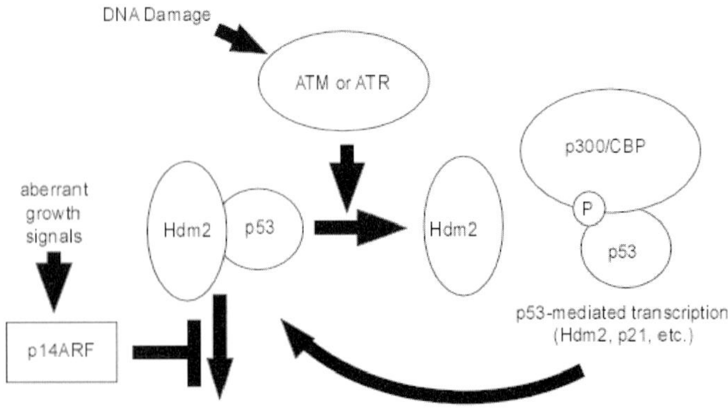

Figure 16.3. Regulation of p53 activity. Phosphorylation of p53 by ataxia telangiectasia-mutated (ATM) or ataxia telangiectasia and Rad3-related (ATR) in response to DNA damage leads to the dissociation of the p53–Hdm2 complex, resulting in p53 stabilization. p14ARF inhibits the ubiquitin ligase activity of Hdm2 toward p53, resulting in p53 stabilization.

tion as a histone acetyltransferase for transcription. p53 can also be activated in response to aberrant growth signals, such as inappropriate inactivation of pRb, through a distinct pathway involving p14ARF.[13] p14ARF binds to Hdm2 and prevents the polyubiquitination of p53 independent of p53 phosphorylation.[2] Activation or overexpression of E_2F or c-Myc induces apoptosis through p14ARF-mediated stabilization of p53, creating a link between the pRb and p53 pathways.

Because of their functional significance to the p53 pathway, Hdm2 and p14ARF are often dysregulated in human cancer, and it is thought that the majority of tumors with wild-type p53 overexpress *HDM2* or inactivate *CDKN2A*, the gene encoding p14ARF. In particular, p14ARF mutations are common in melanoma. Although it is not strictly required to inactivate both p53 and pRb through the same mutation event, both Hdm2 and p14ARF can become dysregulated by mechanisms that also inactivate the pRb pathway. Hdm2 is often amplified in human cancers as part of an amplicon with Cdk4, and p14ARF is often lost by deletions that affect p16INK4.[2,4] The role of other proteins intimately associated with p53 in human cancer, such as p300/CBP, is less clear, although they remain a target of investigation.

Signal Transduction

The mitogenic signals that a cell receives are transmitted through receptor-associated tyrosine kinases (RTKs) to RAS, which in turn activates a multitude of cellular pathways leading to cell growth and proliferation. Therefore, a broad class of oncogenic mutations that occur in signal transduction pathways can generally be considered RAS pathway activators. Oncogenic mutations in the RAS pathway can occur upstream of RAS, downstream of RAS, or in RAS itself. Activated mutants of all three RAS proteins can promote oncogenesis, and, although their functions are not entirely overlapping, a generic RAS signaling pathway is described next (Figure 16.4).[16]

The RAS proteins are small, farnesylated GTPases. Farnesylation, the attachment of a 15-carbon lipophilic chain, is required for proper localization of RAS to the cell membrane in close proximity to RTKs.[16,17] When mitogens bind to an

RTK, the receptor dimerizes and becomes autophosphorylated, allowing the SH_2 domain of an adapter protein known as growth factor receptor-bound protein 2 (GRB2) to bind, which in turn recruits the son of sevenless (SOS) protein to the cell membrane, where RAS is anchored.[17] SOS functions as a guanine nucleotide exchange factor (GEF), facilitating the ability of inactive RAS to become active RAS by exchanging bound guanosine diphosphate (GDP) for guanosine triphosphate (GTP). RAS in the GTP bound state remains active until a GTPase-activating protein (GAP) allows the hydrolysis of GTP to GDP.[17]

GTP-bound RAS can activate a multitude of pathways, but two are particularly relevant to our understanding of cancer. First, RAS activates the serine/threonine kinase RAF, which subsequently activates the mitogen-activated protein kinase (MAPK) pathway.[17] The end effect of the activation of this pathway is the activation of c-Fos and c-Jun by phosphorylation, resulting in the upregulation of gene expression required for the G_1 phase of the cell cycle, including the D-type cyclins. A second pathway activated by RAS is the phosphatidylinositol 3-kinase (PI-3) pathway.[17] Activated PI-3 kinase phosphorylates phosphatidylinositol 4,5-bisphosphate to produce the second messenger phosphatidylinositol 3,4,5-triphosphate. This second messenger lipid can activate numerous other proteins including the kinase Akt. Phosphorylation by Akt promotes growth by inactivating many proapoptotic proteins such as Bad and the forkhead family of transcription factors. The PI-3 kinase pathway also affects levels of the Cip/Kip protein p27, most likely through upregulation of the proteins required for p27 degradation. Finally, the functions of the PI-3 kinase pathway are antagonized by the phosphatase and tensin homologue (PTEN) protein that removes a phosphorylation from the PI-3 kinase-generated secondary messengers.

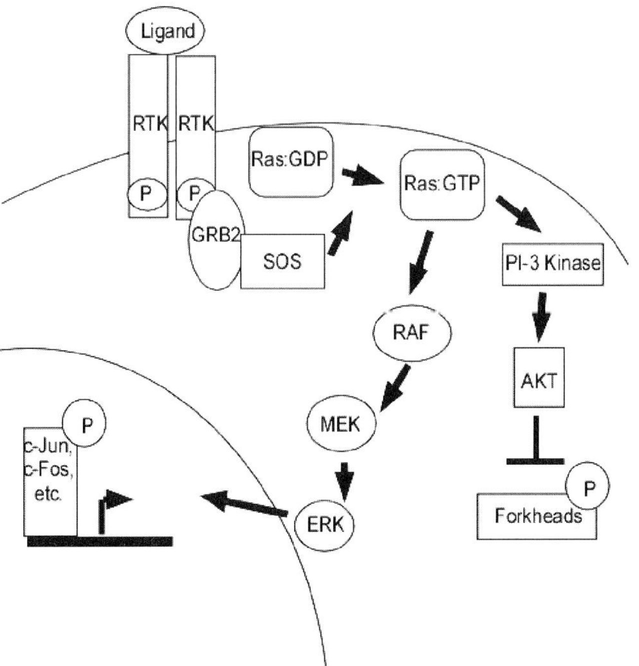

Figure 16.4. The RAS pathway. Mitogenic stimuli from growth factors are transmitted through receptor tyrosine kinases (RTKs) to RAS, which becomes active by exchanging guanosine diphosphate (GDP) for guanosine triphosphate (GTP). GTP-bound RAS can activate many pathways, including the RAF and phosphatidylinositol 3-kinase (PI-3) kinase pathways.

The RAS pathway and various subpathways are subject to activation at many points in cancer. Activating mutations in the epidermal growth factor receptor (EGFR), platelet-derived growth factor receptor (PDGFR), c-Kit, and FMS-like tyrosine kinase 3 (FLT3). RTKs are common in cancer, as well as simple overexpression of normal proteins.[18–21] Mutations in RAS that maintain the GTP-bound state are also found in tumors, and the inactivation of RAS GAPs, such as the NF1 tumor suppressor, can lead to RAS activation through decreased rates of hydrolysis of GTP.[16] Additionally, several downstream RAS effectors have links to cancer. BRAF activations have been observed in many patients, and the PTEN tumor suppressor is also subject to inactivation in multiple cancers. Finally, RTKs are not the only RAS activators. Other tyrosine kinases such as the translocation product BCR-Abl can bind GRB2 and activate RAS. *BCR-Abl* is the oncogene found on the Philadelphia chromosome, and activation of RAS by BCR-Abl is required for its oncogenic function.[22]

Targeted Therapy

Historically, cancers have been treated with nonspecific genotoxic agents and antimitotic drugs such as cisplatin and taxol. Such chemotherapeutic agents are successful in killing cancerous cells; however, their lack of specificity can result in increased toxicity for normal cells as well. Knowing the pathways required for the transformation of human cells allows not only the rational design of drugs against specific pathways in cancer, but also the correct application of treatment based on the mutations present in individual tumors. In particular, the pRb pathway and Ras pathway have been examined for potential small molecule drugs that are effective and easily delivered. Both these pathways contain enzymes that catalyze posttranslation modifications required for functional activity, and these enzymes are particularly important for small molecule inhibitor approaches.

CDK Inhibition

Although designing drugs for restoring pRb binding to, and repression of, E_2F would be extremely difficult, the G_1 cyclin–cdk complexes appear to be good candidates for rational drug design. Preventing hyperphosphorylation of pRb should block the cell from breaching the restriction point, preventing cell-cycle progression. The inhibition of the G_1 cyclin–cdk complexes can be targeted in two distinct ways. The most obvious method of inhibition is the direct inhibition of the desired cyclin–cdk complex, but a second method of cyclin/cdk inhibition, analogous to the effect of the Cip/Kip p21 on cyclin B/Cdk1, seeks to inhibit the cyclin/cdk activation by CAK or prevent inhibition by Wee1.[23] Many cdk inhibitors have been developed, with varying degrees of specificity for individual cdks. In general, these inhibitors tend to inhibit other cellular kinases as well as cdks, and the design of absolutely specific cdk inhibitors is not imperative, providing that nonspecific inhibitors are effective treatments. Currently the most promising cdk inhibitors in clinical trials are flavopiridol and UCN-01, both of which are nonspecific cdk inhibitiors.

Flavopiridol inhibits a broad spectrum of cdks by acting as a competitive inhibitor of ATP for the binding pocket of cdks.[23] Although the inhibitory effect of flavopiridol on most cdks can be competed away by the addition of excess ATP, the inhibitory effect of flavopiridol on cyclin T/Cdk9 cannot be competed away by the addition of excess ATP, making the exact mechanism of inhibition of cyclin T/Cdk9 unclear. Additionally, flavopiridol appears to be more specific for a subset of cdks because it is less potent in its inhibition of cdk7 (CAK). Cell-cycle arrests from flavopiridol can result at either the G_1–S transition or the G_2–M transition. As expected, the G_1–S transition results in part from the direct inactivation of Cdk4/6/2, but flavopiridol also reduces *CYCLIN D1* expression and inhibits activation of G1 cdks by CAK.[23] The inhibition of CAK can also result in the G_2–M arrest.

UCN-01 causes cell-cycle arrest in a different manner from flavopiridol, regulating the activity of cdks indirectly at low concentrations.[23] Created by rational design from staurosporine, a nonspecific kinase inhibitor, UCN-01 affects several kinase targets, including PKC, cdks, Wee1, and PDK1.[23] Although UCN-01 only directly inhibits cdks at high concentrations, it has an antiproliferative effect that functions in part through its inhibition of Wee1. Blocking Wee1 activity leads to increased activation of Cdk1, causing premature entry into mitosis and apoptosis. Recent research also indicates that UCN-01 can inhibit PDK1, which may contribute to the antiproliferative effects. PDK1 activates Akt by phosphorylation, so inhibition of PDK1 would prevent Akt from inactivating the forkhead family of transcription factors. Although UCN-01 affects cdk regulation through Wee1, the drug clearly has off targets, such as PDK1, which may contribute to its success or failure as a chemotherapeutic agent.

Ras Inhibition

The RAS pathway offers many possibilities for the small molecule approach, including the targeting of RAS itself, modifiers of RAS activity, upstream activators, or downstream effectors. Of these approaches to inhibition of RAS activity, targeting of RAS itself has been the least successful. The development of drugs that block GTP binding and do not result in the activation of RAS has been difficult. Because of the high concentrations of GTP in a cell, it is likely that such a drug would have to be used at very high concentrations.[24] Instead, most attempts to target RAS pathways have focused on RAS modifiers, downstream effectors, and upstream activators.

The modification of RAS by farnesyltransferase is essential for the proper membrane localization and activation of RAS. Farnesyltransferase adds a 15-carbon chain to a cysteine near the C-terminus of RAS, which is then cleaved by an endopeptidase before the new C-terminus is methylated by a methyltransferase.[17] After these reactions, RAS localizes to the plasma membrane, where K-RAS and N-RAS, but not H-RAS, undergo an additional palmitoylation. Soon after the discovery of this pathway, inhibitors of the farnesyltransferase were developed. These inhibitors are quite successful in inhibiting farnesyltransferase activity in vitro and in vivo, but they have been ineffective in inhibiting RAS in patients because of the alternative pathways for targeting K-RAS and N-RAS to the membrane.[24,25] In the presence of farnesyltransferase inhibitor, K-RAS and N-RAS become substrates for geranylgeranylation, the addition of a 20-carbon group that substitutes for farnesylation. Inhibitors of this process were also generated, but the combination of farnesylation and geranylgeranylation inhibitors results in high levels of cytotoxicity, most likely because of other targets of farnesylation and geranylgeranylation.[25] Despite the lack of success of farnesyltransferase inhibitors, the endopeptidase and methyltransferase involved in RAS localization remain possible targets for this approach.

The inhibition of downstream RAS pathways has also been an area of active research for chemotherapeutic agents. The signal transduction machinery of the BRAF and PI-3 kinase pathways appears suitable for the development of small molecule inhibitions. In fact, inhibitors of the BRAF and MEF kinases have been developed and used in clinical trials, and although the compounds are successful in inhibiting their kinases, they generate only partial responses.[24] More recent attempts to target downstream pathways are focusing on the PI-3 kinase pathway, but these attempts remain in their infancy.

Receptor Tyrosine Kinase Inhibition

By far the most successful approach to targeting the RAS pathway in cancer has been to develop inhibitors of upstream activators of RAS. The development of inhibitors for specific RTKs limits the utility of these drugs to cancers where that particular RTK is overactive, but given these constraints, this class of drugs seems highly effective. RTKs play prominent roles in many cancers, ranging from non-small cell lung cancer to breast cancer to gastrointestinal stromal tumors, which often feature activation/overexpression of EGFR, ErbB2/HER-2, and c-Kit, respectively.[22,26] Additionally, the Bcr-Abl oncoprotein, which causes chronic myelogenous leukemia, can mimic RTK signaling. The fusion of Bcr to c-Abl redistributes the normally nuclear c-Abl activity to the cytoplasm, where it can activate RAS.

Drugs using two different mechanisms of action have been used successfully against the upstream activators. First, herceptin, a humanized antibody against the extracellular domain of Erb2, has been used in treating Erb2/HER2/Neu-positive breast cancers. Erb2 is the most highly active EGFR family member, and although there is no known ligand for Erb2, activation of other EGFR family receptors by ligand binding results in their heterodimerization with Erb2 and increased signaling potential.[21,26] The antibody stops the transmission of signals to RAS before they start by binding Erb2, blocking dimerization and activation, and stimulating internalization and degradation of the receptor.[26] Herceptin may also contribute to immune responses against tumors, as demonstrated by the increased effectiveness of herceptin with a complete Fc region of the antibody. Several other humanized antibodies have been approved for use in targeting RTKs; erbitux targets EGFR, whereas avastin targets vascular endothelial growth factor receptor (VEGFR).

The second class of drugs is small molecule inhibitors of the tyrosine kinase activity of receptors such as PDGFR and EGFR, which have been targeted for inhibition successfully with gleevec and iressa.[26] Gleevec is the final product of a screen that began looking at modified ATP competitive inhibitors of PKC-α for the inhibition of PDGFR, which is activated in many tumors. Although it was designed as an inhibitor or PDGFR, it functions against RTKs related to PDGFR, such as c-Kit. Surprisingly, it also was found to be effective against the Bcr-Abl fusion protein. When used in the treatment of cancers resulting specifically from activations of c-Kit and Bcr-Abl, such as gastrointestinal stromal tumors and chronic myelogenous leukemia, respectively, gleevec has been wildly successful.[26] Iressa, a small molecule inhibitor of EGFR, has also been a successful treatment in non-small cell lung cancer, and inhibitors of several other RTKs involved in cancer, such as FLT3, are under development.[20]

Although antibodies and small molecules targeting RTKs are effective, they have limited utility for the treatment of multiple cancers, as the targeted RTK must be activated in a tumor for the drugs to have an effect. For instance, herceptin is only beneficial in breast cancers expressing Erb2, which encompass only 30% of all breast cancers.[26] Even further specificity has recently been shown with non-small cell lung cancers and iressa. The target of iressa, EGFR, is expressed in the tumors of multiple patients, but the best response is seen only in a subset of patients who have somatic mutations in the kinase domains of EGFR.[18,19] This exquisite sensitivity has also been reported for gleevec treatment of tumors containing c-Kit mutations. Taken together, the examples of herceptin, iressa, and gleevec, show that inhibition of RTKs is extremely effective only when the expression pattern and mutations of the receptors in any given tumor are known.

Although much is known about the core cell-cycle machinery and the alterations of the machinery in cancer, many modifiers of these proteins, either upstream or downstream, and their connection to the core cell-cycle machinery remain a mystery. Further research into these areas will present new targets for the rational design of drugs to combat cancer. The continued development of effective cancer treatments is dependent upon a further understanding of the pathways that lead to cancer, the development of drugs that inhibit these pathways, and the ability to determine which drugs to use against specific cancers or even the tumors of specific patients.

References

1. Hahn WC, Weinberg RA. Modelling the molecular circuitry of cancer. Nat Rev Cancer 2002;2:331–341.
2. Sherr CJ, McCormick F. The RB and p53 pathways in cancer. Cancer Cell 2002;2:103–112.
3. Vogelstein B, Kinzler KW. Cancer genes and the pathways they control. Nat Med 2004;10:789–799.
4. Ortega S, Malumbres M, Barbacid M. Cyclin D-dependent kinases, INK4 inhibitors and cancer. Biochim Biophys Acta 2002;1602:73–87.
5. Yam CH, Fung TK, Poon RY. Cyclin A in cell cycle control and cancer. Cell Mol Life Sci 2002;59:1317–1326.
6. Smits VA, Medema RH. Checking out the G(2)/M transition. Biochim Biophys Acta 2001;1519:1–12.
7. Prives C, Hall PA. The p53 pathway. J Pathol 1999;187:112–126.
8. Taylor WR, Stark GR. Regulation of the G_2/M transition by p53. Oncogene 2001;20:1803–1815.
9. Vogelstein B, Lane D, Levine AJ. Surfing the p53 network. Nature (Lond) 2000;408:307–310.
10. Bartek J, Lukas C, Lukas J. Checking on DNA damage in S phase. Nat Rev Mol Cell Biol 2004;5:792–804.
11. Bharadwaj R, Yu H. The spindle checkpoint, aneuploidy, and cancer. Oncogene 2004;23:2016–2027.
12. Maser RS, DePinho RA. Connecting chromosomes, crisis, and cancer. Science 2002;297:565–569.
13. Sherr CJ. Tumor surveillance via the ARF-p53 pathway. Genes Dev 1998;12:2984–2991.
14. Chompret A. The Li-Fraumeni syndrome. Biochimie (Paris) 2002;84:75–82.
15. Fridman JS, Lowe SW. Control of apoptosis by p53. Oncogene 2003;22:9030–9040.
16. Malumbres M, Barbacid M. RAS oncogenes: the first 30 years. Nat Rev Cancer 2003;3:459–465.
17. Coleman ML, Marshall CJ, Olson MF. RAS and RHO GTPases in G_1-phase cell-cycle regulation. Nat Rev Mol Cell Biol 2004;5:355–366.
18. Lynch TJ, Bell DW, Sordella R, et al. Activating mutations in the epidermal growth factor receptor underlying responsiveness of non-small-cell lung cancer to gefitinib. N Engl J Med 2004;350:2129–2139.
19. Paez JG, Janne PA, Lee JC, et al. EGFR mutations in lung cancer: correlation with clinical response to gefitinib therapy. Science 2004; 304:1497–1500.
20. Stirewalt DL, Radich JP. The role of FLT3 in haematopoietic malignancies. Nat Rev Cancer 2003;3:650–665.
21. Vlahovic G, Crawford J. Activation of tyrosine kinases in cancer. Oncologist 2003;8:531–538.
22. Wong S, Witte ON. The BCR-ABL story: bench to bedside and back. Annu Rev Immunol 2004;22:247–306.
23. Senderowicz AM. Small-molecule cyclin-dependent kinase modulators. Oncogene 2003;22:6609–6620.
24. Downward J. Targeting RAS signalling pathways in cancer therapy. Nat Rev Cancer 2003;3:11–22.
25. Sebti SM. Blocked pathways: FTIs shut down oncogene signals. Oncologist 2003;3(suppl 8):30–38.
26. Madhusudan S, Ganesan TS. Tyrosine kinase inhibitors in cancer therapy. Clin Biochem 2004;37:618–635.

17

Viral Carcinogenesis

Michele Carbone and
Giuseppe Barbanti-Brodano

Important causes of human tumors are biologic and environmental agents, mostly of a chemical and physical nature, that act by genotoxic mechanisms which induce alterations in the cell genome such as chromosomal deletions, rearrangements, and mutations. In the complex multifactorial pathogenesis of cancer, viruses often participate as biologic cofactors that cooperate with chemical and physical agents in both the initiation and progression of tumors. Thus, the detection of a tumor virus in a given tumor does not establish causation. Moreover, the genetic background of an individual and his/her immune status at the time of infection or during viral latency may influence susceptibility to various carcinogens, especially viral carcinogens. Often, it appears that oncogenic viruses act at the beginning of tumor development, inducing in the host cell a number of genetic alterations and immortalizations that can lead to tumor growth. Viruses at other times can be oncogenic only upon infection of cells that already contain genetic alterations. For example, BKV can transform human mesothelial cells that overexpress Notch-1 and which express telomerase activity, whereas in the absence of these alterations, mesothelial cells were not transformed. Oncogenic viruses may act directly, as the combined effects of viral sequences or gene products within the target cell lead to transformation. In other circumstances, the role of viruses may be more subtle, that is, predominantly indirect. Examples of this condition are liver cancer, arising during hepatocyte regeneration that follows hepatitis B and C virus infection, and acquired immunodeficiency syndrome (AIDS)-associated neoplasms, favored by loss of antitumor immune surveillance as a result of human immunodeficiency virus (HIV) infection of the immune system and consequent immunosuppression. HIV-induced immunosuppression allows the emergence of oncogenic viruses such as Epstein–Barr virus (EBV), which causes B-cell lymphomas in AIDS patients. Thus, in AIDS, two viruses cooperate independently to cause human cancer. It is also argued that the regenerative process associated with liver cirrhosis, which is caused by hepatitis B virus (HBV) and hepatitis C virus (HCV) infection, and the release of cytokines by the inflammatory infiltrate in the regenerating liver favor tumor development. In this latter scenario, the role of HBV and HCV in causing hepatocellular carcinoma would be indirect yet critical.

Viruses are important causes of cancer in several animal species, and they are increasingly implicated in human neoplasia. Because oncogenic viruses are generally involved in the initial phases of tumor development, control of viral infection should prevent or reduce the incidence of those tumors linked to viral infection. Cancer-associated viruses belong to several families of deoxyriboviruses and riboviruses (Table 17.1). The International Agency for Research on Cancer (IARC) so far has identified six viruses—human papillomavirus (types 16 and 18), Epstein–Barr virus, hepatitis B virus, hepatitis C virus, human T-cell lymphotropic virus type I, and human immunodeficiency virus type 1 (also, KSHV is a likely candidate)—as group 1 carcinogens, that is, agents that have been shown to be carcinogenic in humans. Together, these viruses may cause or contribute to about 15% of human malignancies.[1] However, if other viruses for which the evidence is suggestive but not definitive, and the group 2 carcinogens are included, this value would almost double.[1] Ment in SV-40 as an emerging carcinogenic agent.

The classic Koch's postulates, formulated to demonstrate the etiologic role of microorganisms in infectious diseases, cannot be applied directly to prove the viral etiology of human tumors for various reasons: (1) several tumor-associated viruses are ubiquitous in humans, and (2) they produce a persistent or latent infection in many human tissues, making epidemiologic studies difficult. Viruses are seldom complete carcinogens, and their carcinogenic potential becomes apparent only when studied together with those carcinogens associated with a specific tumor type. For example, skin carcinomas in patients infected with cutaneous human papillomavirus (HPV) develop in sun-exposed areas because of the cocarcinogenicity of UV light; SV-40 infection may carry a higher risk of mesothelioma development in individuals exposed to asbestos, etc. Furthermore, cooperation among different viruses may be required for cocarcinogenesis, such as HIV-1 and EBV in lymphomas that develop in AIDS patients. In this case, HIV causes immunosuppression that facilitates EBV lymphomagenesis. Thus, because Koch's postulates do not address these issues, new rules should be considered to establish the oncogenic role of viruses in humans.[2-4] To address this problem, the National Cancer Institute (NCI) organized (December 11–12, 2003), an international workshop with some of the leading experts in various disciplines. The recommendations of this workshop concerning the identification of human cocarcinogens appeared in an issue of *Seminars in Cancer Biology* in 2004, edited by M. Carbone and M. Wong.

TABLE 17.1. Human tumor viruses.

Virus family	*Virus*	*Genome type*	*Associated tumors*
Herpesviridae	Epstein–Barr virus	DNA	Burkitt's lymphoma B-cell and T-cell lymphomas Nasopharyngeal carcinoma Gastric cancer Leiomyomas and leiomyosarcomas Breast cancer (?)
	Human herpesvirus 8	DNA	Kaposi's sarcoma Primary effusion lymphoma Castleman's disease Multiple myeloma (?)
Papovaviridae	BK virus	DNA	Brain, bone, pancreatic, and urinary tract tumors
	JC virus	DNA	Brain tumors, mainly medulloblastoma, colorectal tumors
	Simian virus 40	DNA	Mesothelioma, brain and bone tumors, lymphomas
	Human papillomavirus	DNA	Skin, anogenital, oral, and laryngeal papillomas and carcinomas
Hepadnaviridae	Hepatitis B virus	DNA	Hepatocellular carcinoma
Flaviviridae	Hepatitis C virus	RNA	Hepatocellular carcinoma Lymphoproliferative diseases (?)
Retroviridae	Human T-cell lymphotropic virus I	RNA	Adult T-cell leukemia and lymphoma
	Human T-cell lymphotropic virus II	RNA	Hairy cell leukemia
	Human immunodeficiency virus 1	RNA	Kaposi's sarcoma B-cell lymphoma Anogenital carcinoma (?) Hepatocellular carcinoma (?)

Oncogenic Deoxyriboviruses

Herpesviruses

Epstein–Barr Virus

Epstein–Barr virus (EBV) is a member of the human herpesvirus subfamily Gammaherpesviridae. EBV is an enveloped virus with a double-stranded DNA genome of 172 kilobases (kb) containing more than 100 genes. EBV is a ubiquitons virus that infects and persists in about 90% of the world's human population. EBV selectively infects mature B lymphocytes, the only cells bearing the CD21 receptor for virus attachment, recognized by the viral envelope glycoprotein gp350.[5] However, natural killer (NK) cells can also be infected with EBV and are associated with unusual malignancies of these cell types. Primary infection with EBV usually occurs in childhood. In most cases, the clinical course is unapparent. In a subset of infected individuals, primary EBV infection can result in infectious mononucleosis, a self-limited lymphoproliferative disease. The syndrome of mononucleosis is more frequent when primary infection is delayed into adolescence. Once infected, individuals become lifelong virus carriers and, when the virus has gained access to the B-cell compartment, it is disseminated to many organs including liver, Bm, and central nervous system (CNS). B cells are eliminated by specific cytotoxic T cells, and T-cell immunosuppression can lead to the development of EBV-associated malignant lymphomas. However, EBV is also associated with the development of lymphoid and epithelial malignancies in apparently immunocompetent hosts.[6]

After infection, EBV enters a latent state, with or without a minimal production of viral progeny. During latency the viral genome remains in an episomal state, sometimes with rare viral DNA molecules integrated into the cell genome.[5] Latent infection by EBV causes the immortalization of B lymphocytes, which lose the ability to achieve terminal differentiation. EBV-infected B lymphocytes produce antibodies but never reach the stage of plasma cells.[5] During latency, EBV expresses only some of its genes: six proteins localized in the nucleus and called Epstein–Barr nuclear antigens (EBNA) 1, -2, -3A, -3B, -3C, and leader protein (LP); three proteins localized in the cytoplasmic membrane, called latent membrane proteins (LMPs) 1, -2A, -2B; two small noncoding RNAs (EBER-1 and EBER-2); and the *BARF1* gene, located in the *Bam*HI-A region of the viral genome.[5] Several of these genes are expressed in EBV-immortalized lymphoblastoid cell lines and in EBV-associated malignancies.[5,6] These genes have activities that may contribute to the deregulation of normal cell growth and to oncogenesis. EBNA-1 is a DNA-binding protein that is postulated to act as a transcriptional activator of the cellular recombinase-activating genes RAG-1 and RAG-2,[7] which in turn lead to chromosomal translocations within the host cell. The main function of EBNA-1 is maintenance of the EBV episome during cell division. EBNA-2 (in concert with EBNA-LP) also functions as a transcriptional activator that induces the expression of *CD21*, which encodes the cellular EBV receptor, and *CD23*, the tyrosine kinase c-*fgr*, *cyclin D2*, and all the other latent EBV genes, including the LMP-1, LMP-2A, and LMP-2B.[5,6,8] LMP-4 by itself cannot transform human cells. LMP-1 transforms rodent cells and is necessary for transformation of human cells; it has multiple effects, including increased expression of cellular adhesion molecules, upregulation of lymphocyte activation antigens, and stimulation of the transcription factors, such as AP1 and NF-kB.[5,6]

The human lymphoid malignancies associated with EBV infection are Burkitt's lymphoma, B-cell lymphomas in immunocompromised individuals, T-cell lymphomas, the X-linked lymphoproliferative disease, and Hodgkin's disease.[9–15] Lymphocyte immortalization induced by EBV and the acquisition of an indefinite life span may increase the probability of accumulating genetic alterations that can lead to malignancy. In fact, EBV-positive lymphomas typically develop specific chromosomal translocations involving the regulatory sequences of the immunoglobulin genes on chromosome 14q32 (76% of cases), 22q11 (16% of cases), or 2p11 (8% of cases), which are joined to the c-*myc* proto-oncogene on chromosome 8q24.[16] These translocations cause the deregulated activation of c-*myc* expression and are the basis for oncogenicity in BL. c-*myc* activation renders the proliferation of EBV-immortalized cells independent of *LMP1* and *EBNA2* expression.[17] EBV infection may favor, but is not a necessary prerequisite, for the rearrangement of c-*myc* and for lymphoma development, because rare cases of endemic Burkitt's lymphoma (BL) in equatorial Africa are EBV negative.[18,19] Moreover, only 15% to 20% sporadic BL in the Western world are EBV positive whereas all BL contain the typical c-*myc* translocations.[20] EBV-associated B-cell lymphomas occur with notable frequency in patients with acquired immunodeficiency syndrome (AIDS), and 65% to 100% of AIDS lymphomas, especially brain lymphomas, contain EBV DNA. These tumors, in addition to c-*myc* translocations, often contain c-*ras* mutations, p53 inactivation by deletion or point mutation, and *bcl-6* rearrangements.[21,22] A similar set of molecular alterations was described in EBV-positive lymphoproliferative disorders and lymphomas arising in immunosuppressed transplant patients.[23] I think EBV by itself is able to drive these proliferative conditions. They are initially polyclonal, and through selection become monoclonal and autonomous, that is, no longer responsive to reduction of immunosuppressive drugs. These findings support the notion that multiple genetic alterations are required for the development of the transformed phenotype. EBV, by contributing to some of these genetic changes, increases the risk of these tumors in infected individuals.

The X-linked lymphoproliferative disease (XLP) or Duncan's disease is a hereditary syndrome caused by the alteration of a gene located at chromosome region Xq25.[24,25] The XLP gene, called SH2D1A, was recently cloned,[25] and its product regulates the interaction between B and T lymphocytes. Mutations in the SH2D1A gene, detected in XLP patients, generate a state of immune dysfunction that induces an altered response to viral infections, especially to EBV. XLP patients, when infected with EBV, develop in approximately 65% of cases a severe form of infectious mononucleosis that is fatal in 70% of children less than 10 years of age.[25] Most surviving patients develop a lymphoproliferative disorder or a lymphoma, and a few develop aplastic anemia or vasculitis.[25] The pathogenesis of the disease is related to an enhanced response to EBV infection.[25] Following infection with EBV, normal individuals develop a T-cell response to EBV-infected B cells with elevated serum levels of TH-1 cytokines, such as interferon-γ and IL-2. This response is greatly increased in XLP patients,[26] and the dysregulated TH-1 response is considered the most important pathogenetic event that causes fulminant infectious mononucleosis. The malignant lymphomas arising in XLP patients are non-Hodgkin's B-cell lymphomas of the Burkitt's type and diffuse large cell lymphomas.[24] The expression of EBV genes has not been studied in detail in XLP lymphomas, and the pathogenic role of EBV in these tumors is under investigation.

In Hodgkin's disease (HD), EBV involvement is supported by the presence of EBV DNA in 26% to 67% of sporadic cases and in 100% of HD arising in AIDS patients.[13,27] Episomal EBV DNA is detected in the multinucleated Reed–Sternberg cells, the malignant neoplastic giant cells of HD that are required for the histopathologic diagnosis of the disease. The EBV genome is detected also in Hodgkin cells, the mononuclear giant cells that are considered the precursors of Reed–Sternberg cells. In HD, Reed–Sternberg and Hodgkin cells represent clonal expansions of EBV-infected cells. The oncogene EBV LMP-1 is expressed within Reed–Sternberg cells and their precursors, whereas EBNA-2 is not expressed.[13,27] The function of EBNA-1 is to maintain the EBV episome, from which the various EBV onco-proteins are expressed. LMP-1, the most potent EBV oncogene, seems to play an important role in the pathogenesis of HD.[13] In addition to the EBV-infected Hodgkin and Reed–Sternberg cells, the pathologic tissue contains macrophages, B and T-lymphocytes that outnumber the malignant cells. In this context, the EBV antigens expressed in HD neoplastic cells may stimulate the reactive cellular component of the disease to secrete cytokines and other biologic mediators that could favor the growth and the expansion of tumor cells.[13]

EBV can also infect nonlymphoid cells, such as epithelial and, in children with AIDS, muscle cells, which are devoid of the CD21 receptor. EBV probably infects these cells by fusion or cell-to-cell contact with EBV-infected lymphocytes.[5,28] Thus, EBV can contribute to the development of some types of epithelial cancers, such as nasopharyngeal carcinoma (NPC).[9,14,15] Undifferentiated NPC accounts for up to 80% of all NPC and occurs with high prevalence in certain regions of East Asia, such as Southern China. Clustering of this tumor in these specific geographic areas is probably a result of a combination of genetic predisposition and lifestyle factors.[14,15] Detection of IgA antibodies against the EBV viral capsid antigen, a rare finding in the normal population, has been successfully employed as a marker of increased tumor risk in screening programs in high-incidence areas.[14,15] Multiple copies of monoclonal EBV episomes are present in every cell of NPCs,[14,15] whereas integrated EBV DNA has been detected only in a fraction of NPC.[28,29] Immunoblotting demonstrates LMP-1 protein in 65% or more NPC, and LMP-1 transcripts are detectable in virtually all cases by polymerase chain reaction (PCR) analysis.[14,15,30] EBNA-1 is expressed in essentially all NPC cells. Other nonlymphoid malignancies possibly associated with EBV are gastric carcinoma, leiomyoma, and leiomyosarcoma. In gastric carcinoma, the viral DNA is found in approximately 90% of the rare gastric lymphoepithelioma-like carcinomas and in about 10% of the common gastric ade-

TABLE 17.2. Mechanisms of transformation by Epstein–Barr virus.

First phase	*Second phase*	*Third phase*
Expression of viral antigens	Transactivation and expression of cellular and viral genes	Chromosome translocations
EBNA1, EBNA2	*RAG1, RAG2, CD21, CD23, c-fgr, cyclin D2, LMP1, LMP2A, LMP2B*	t(8;14), t(2;8), t(8;22)
LMP1	*LFA1, LFA3, HLAII, ICAM1, blc-2, vimentin*	Increased expression of the oncogene c-*myc*, directed by the promoter-enhancer of the immunoglobulin genes

nocarcinomas.[28,31,32] EBV is present in clonal, episomal form in the malignant epithelial cells that express *EBNA1* but not other *EBNA* genes or *LMP1*.[28,30–32] Recently, it was shown that the EBV *BARF1* gene, which acts as an oncogene,[33] is expressed in EBV-positive gastric adenocarcinomas,[32,34] suggesting that *BARF1* contributes to gastric cancer. Leiomyomas and leiomyosarcomas are rare smooth muscle cell tumors whose frequency is increased in immunocompromised patients, especially in HIV-positive patients and in organ transplant recipients.[35,36] Leiomyomas and leiomyosarcomas developing in immunocompromised patients, but not in immunocompetent individuals, are associated with EBV, and the tumor cells harbor episomal monoclonal EBV genomes.[35] EBV is the likely cause of oral hairy leukoplakia,[28] an EBV cytolytic lesion not known, and is associated with undifferentiated parotid carcinoma.[37] The possible association of EBV with some aggressive forms of breast cancer has been suggested by some investigators,[38] but presently the weight of evidence does not support a pathogenic role of EBV in breast cancer. The mechanisms of cellular transformation by EBV are reported in Table 17.2. LMP-1 also induces a variety of invasiveness, metastasis, and angiogenic factors including matrix metalloproteinase (MMP)-9, cyclooxygenase (COX)-2, vascular endothelial growth factor (VEGF), fibroblast growth factor (FGF)-2, and HIFIX.

Human Herpesvirus 8

Human herpesvirus 8 (HHV-8) is a herpesvirus recently isolated from Kaposi's sarcoma (KS) tissue[39] using the technique of representational difference analysis.[40] HHV-8 is a gammaherpesvirus, showing sequence homology to EBV and to herpesvirus saimiri, a squirrel monkey virus that induces lymphoproliferative disorders in monkeys and transforms human T cells.[41] HHV-8 is associated with KS, primary effusion lymphoma (PEL), and Castleman's disease. PELs are AIDS-associated lymphomas characterized by malignant lymphocyte effusions in the pleural, pericardial, and peritoneal cavities, usually without significant tumor masses or lymphadenopathy. All PELs contain HHV-8 DNA and most, but not all, are coinfected by EBV,[42–44] suggesting that the two viruses may cooperate in neoplastic transformation. Multicentric Castleman's disease (MCD) is a rare polyclonal lymphoproliferative disorder[45] appearing in both immunocompromised and immunocompetent individuals. HHV-8 is present in nearly 100% of HIV-1-positive patients with MCD. Among MCD immunocompetent patients, HHV-8 is detected in about 40% of cases.[44]

KS occurs in four epidemiologic forms[46]: (1) classic KS, a rare tumor of elderly men, usually of Mediterranean origin, with a mild clinical course; (2) endemic KS, developing in HIV-1-negative individuals in equatorial Africa; (3) iatrogenic KS, occurring in immunosuppressed transplant recipients; and (4) epidemic KS, presently the most common form of KS, developing in patients with AIDS. KS lesions exhibit a complex morphology and contain a variety of cell types, including malignant spindle cells, probably of endothelial origin.[47–49] KS cells release various lymphokines, including IL-6 genome, interferon-γ (IFN-γ), basic fibroblast growth factor (bFGF), tumor necrosis factor-γ (TNF-γ), and VEGF. KS growth is enhanced by inflammatory cytokines of the Th1 type and by the HIV-1 Tat protein.[47] These observations suggest that the local dysregulation of cytokines plays an important role in the development of KS lesions. HHV-8 DNA was detected in 89% to 100% of KS biopsies and in only 2% of non-KS biopsies, except for blood (8%–25%), from the same individual,[43,44] indicating that the viral load is highest in KS lesions. Seroepidemiology demonstrates that HHV-8 antibody prevalence is low (2%–3%) in the United States and in England, and that it is greater and increases steadily with age in Mediterranean Europe and in Africa. HHV-8 seroprevalence reaches 85% in KS patients and 35% in homosexual men. Moreover, in this latter category the prevalence of HHV-8 antibodies rises with the increasing number of homosexual partners in the previous 2 years,[44] suggesting that HHV-8 could be the sexually transmitted agent previously suggested to be associated with KS.[48,49] HHV-8 is not present in other vascular tumors, including angiomas, hemangiomas, and angiosarcomas, and is only rarely detected in other forms of skin tumors, such as squamous cell carcinomas and melanomas.[44] The presence of HHV-8 DNA in peripheral blood cells of HIV-1-positive individuals and HHV-8 reactivation from a latency stage correlates with a greater risk of developing KS.[44,50,51] PCR in situ hybridization, RNA in situ hybridization, and immunohistochemistry showed HHV-8 in nearly all spindle cells of KS lesions.[44,51,52]

The oncogenic mechanisms of HHV-8 are not fully understood. Sequence analysis of the viral genome[53] yielded clues to the transforming activity of HHV-8.[44,52,50] Several HHV-8 genes have significant sequence homology to human genes,[44,50,52,54] suggesting that the virus has captured cellular genes during evolution. The viral homologues are similar to cellular genes involved in apoptosis, growth control, cell-cycle regulation, and chemokine and cytokine signaling. HHV-8 contains a gene homologous to *bcl-2* that inhibits apoptosis.[55] The viral antiapoptotic activity is supported by two other cellular homologues: FLIP, which interferes with apoptosis signaled through the FLICE death; and LANA, which binds p53, inhibiting p53-mediated apoptosis.[44,50,52] HHV-8 also codes for a *cyclin D*-like gene whose protein product participates in pRb phosphorylation.[56,57] Another HHV-8 protein that is involved in cell proliferation is the G protein-coupled receptor (GPCR), which is constitutively active for downstream signaling in the absence of the chemokine ligands.[58] GPCR shows a high sequence homology to the cellular IL-8 receptor, transforms NIH3T3 mouse fibroblasts in vitro, and induces VEGF expression.[59] Transgenic mice expressing HHV-8 GPCR in hematopoietic cells develop angioproliferative KS-like lesions in multiple organs.[60] The viral MIP-I, MIP-II, and MIP-III proteins exhibit homology to the cellular chemokine MIP-1-α. MIP-I and MIP-II possess strong angiogenic potential and may therefore contribute to the marked vascularization characteristic of KS.[61] The K1 protein of KSHV, the homologue of EBV LMP-1, also induces MMP-9 and VEGF expression (John Pagano, personal communication). Furthermore, the virus encodes a homologue of cellular IL-6, a possible growth factor for KS cells, and up to four proteins related to cellular interferon-regulatory factors (IRF)[52,54,62] that may confer resistance to the antiproliferative effects of IFN-α. Because KS growth appears to be supported by a variety of cytokines,[47] it is interesting that HHV-8 codes for homologues of cellular cytokines and cytokine receptors that may function as growth factors for the proliferation of KS cells. HHV-8 has also been linked to the development of multiple myeloma,[63] but this association is not established.

Papovaviruses

BK Virus, JC Virus, and Simian Virus 40

BK virus (BKV), JC virus (JCV), and simian virus 40 (SV-40) belong to the family of Papovaviridae. The three viruses are similar in structural and functional properties.[64,65] Nucleotide sequence homology of the three viruses is 68% to 72%, and protein sequence homology is 76% to 90% in different regions of the viral genomes.[64] Primary infection by BKV and JCV occurs in childhood and is usually unapparent. During primary infection, the virus spreads by viremia to several organs and establishes a latent infection in the kidneys. Reactivation from latency can be induced by immunologic impairment. BKV and JCV are ubiquitous in the human population worldwide, and seroprevalence in adults is 80% to 100%. Both viruses are probably transmitted by the respiratory and the orofecal route.[4,66,67] BKV and JCV cause posttransplantation interstitial nephritis in renal transplant recipients and BKV causes hemorrhagic cystitis in bone marrow transplant patients.[4,64–66] JCV is the etiologic agent of progressive multifocal leukoencephalopathy, a severe degenerative neurologic disease affecting immunosuppressed individuals.[64,65] SV-40, which is a monkey virus, was introduced only recently into the human population when polio vaccines, produced in SV-40-contaminated monkey kidney cell cultures, were massively administered to millions of individuals between 1955 and 1963.[68] Soon it was shown that people vaccinated with SV-40-contaminated polio vaccines shed infectious SV-40 in stools for at least 5 weeks after vaccination.[69] This observation suggested that SV-40 could be transmitted from recipients of contaminated polio vaccines to contacts by the orofecal route and could spread in humans by horizontal infection. This hypothesis is supported by some experimental results. First, SV-40 DNA sequences have been detected in normal and neoplastic tissues of persons too young (1 to 30 years) to have been vaccinated with SV-40-contaminated polio vaccines.[3,70–74] Second, SV-40 sequences have been found in blood specimens of neoplastic and healthy individuals[72,74,75–79] and SV-40 virions were detected in urine and sewage samples,[68,80] suggesting that the hematalogic and orofecal routes of transmission might be responsible for SV-40 horizontal infection in humans. An alternative or additional hypothesis is that some polio vaccines continued to be contaminated by SV-40 after 1963.[81] Third, infectious SV-40 was rescued by transfection of monkey cells with the DNA of an SV-40-positive human choroid plexus carcinoma in an individual too young to have received a contaminated vaccine.[82] Finally, antibodies to SV-40 capsid antigens were found in sera of children and of both normal and HIV-1-infected adults.[83–86]

The early region of the BKV, JCV, and SV-40 genomes, which is expressed in the initial phase of the replicative cycle, encodes the two viral oncoproteins: the large T antigen (Tag) and the small t antigen (tag). The Tag displays multiple functions that alter the normal physiologic metabolism of cells, ultimately leading to immortalization and neoplastic transformation.[64,65,87–89] An important property of Tag in relation to transformation and oncogenicity is its ability to bind and block the functions of the tumor suppressors p53 and the pRb family proteins (p105 Rb1, p107, and p130 Rb2).[88–91] Polyomavirus Tag induces chromosomal damage in human cells characterized by numerical and structural chromosomal aberrations such as DNA gaps, breaks, dicentric and ring chromosomes, deletions, duplications, and translocations.[92–95] The molecular mechanism of the clastogenic effect of Tag may reside in its ability to bind topoisomerase I[96] and in its helicase activity,[97] which could induce chromosome damage when Tag promotes the unwinding of the two strands of cellular DNA. Moreover, Tag inhibition of p53-induced apoptosis allows DNA-damaged cells to survive, increasing their probability of becoming transformed and acquiring immortality.[89] Small tag[98] cooperates with large Tag in transformation by reducing serum dependence of transformed cells and binds protein phosphatase 2A (PP-2A).[99] PP-2A is a serine/threonine phosphatase that regulates the phosphorylation signaling activated by protein kinases,[100] and it has recently been shown to function as a tumor suppressor gene involved in some lung, colon, and breast carcinomas and melanoma.[101,102] In addition, SV-40 small tag is able to enhance transcription of E_2F-activated early growth response genes.[103]

BKV, JCV, and SV-40 transform to neoplastic phenotypes and are highly oncogenic in rodent and human cells.[3] The spectrum of experimentally induced tumors is similar but distinct for each of the three viruses.[3] BKV, JCV, and SV-40 DNA were detected in human tumors by PCR, and occasionally by Southern hybridization of the whole cell genome, indicating the presence of relatively low amounts of viral sequences. Expression of virus-specific RNA and Tag was often observed in virus-positive tumors. The histotype of the human tumors positive for viral sequences corresponds to that of the tumors induced by the three viruses in experimental animals. BKV has been associated to human brain tumors, tumors of pancreatic islets, osteosarcomas, and tumors of the urinary tract.[3,4,64–66,104] BKV DNA sequences were also detected in primary KS and in KS cell lines.[105] JCV has been associated with human brain tumors, especially astrocytoma and medulloblastoma,[64,65,106–109] and possibly with colorectal carcinoma.[109–112] In colorectal cancers, negative for mutations in the APC gene, JCV Tag activates the Wnt pathway, with consequent constitutive expression of β-catenin,[113] which leads to continuous cell proliferation. SV-40 is associated with human mesothelioma, with brain tumors, and possibly with osteosarcoma and non-Hodgkin's B-cell lymphoma.[114–117] Human brain tumors can be coinfected by SV-40 and BKV or by SV-40 and JCV,[107] suggesting a possible interaction between polyomaviruses in oncogenesis. In three human brain tumors, one of the authors (G.B.B.) detected the simultaneous presence of the DNA sequences of BKV, JCV, and SV-40.[4,66] It remains to be demonstrated whether in these tumors the viruses coexist in the same cells. Some studies, however, did not detect SV-40 in human tumors.[118] Three independent panels have reviewed the association of SV-40 with human tumors: one organized by the National Cancer Institute,[28] one by the Institute of Medicine,[119] and one at an international SV-40 mesothelioma consensus conference held at the University of Chicago.[120] All three panels concluded that there is compelling evidence that SV-40 is present in some human tumors, especially mesothelioma and brain tumors, and that SV-40 is a potent cocarcinogen.

Because BKV and JCV are ubiquitous in humans,[3] their DNA sequences are often detected not only in tumors but also in normal tissues.[72,74] The viral load in BKV-, JCV-, and SV-40-positive human tumors is usually low (10^{-2} to 10^{-4} genome equivalents per cell), and Tag is expressed only in a fraction of tumor cells.[3,75] This is a general characteristic of polyomavirus-induced tumors: for example, only a fraction of tumor cells in SV-40 transgenic tumors is Tag positive. However, BKV, JCV, and SV40 induce chromosome aberrations[92,95] that can affect the functions of genes important in tumorigenesis.[121] Once the genetic damage has been triggered in tumors and chromosomal alterations have reached a threshold, genomic instability ensues[122,123] as a result of the functional alteration of DNA repair genes, especially in the presence of Tag-mediated inactivation of cellular p53, which prevents DNA repair or apoptosis of damaged cells. These events lead to accumulation of genetic lesions and to tumor progression.[122,123] A similar course of events may occur in some polyomavirus-positive human tumors, where the clastogenic activity of Tag, similarly to a chemical or physical carcinogen, initiates the tumorigenic process by causing DNA damage, and then becomes dispensable; it may be lost during tumor progression when the accumulation of genetic alterations renders the presence of viral transforming genes unnecessary. Immunoselection may select against persistently polyomavirus-infected cells, whereas genetically mutated cells that have lost the viral genome may have a proliferative advantage and become the prevalent population in the tumor. This "hit-and-run" mechanism has been demonstrated in SV-40-mediated transformation of some rodent cells.[124,125] In human mesothelial cells, SV-40 Tag activates an autocrine-paracrine loop involving the hepatocyte growth factor (HGF) and its cellular receptor, the oncogene c-*met*,[126] as well as VEGF and its cellular receptor.[127,128] It has been suggested that HGF and VEGF, released from SV-40-positive cells, bind their receptors in neighboring SV-40-negative cells, driving them into proliferation and tumorigenesis.[126–129]

There is strong evidence in support of a causative association between SV40 and mesothelioma, including (1) the ability of SV-40 Tag to bind and inactivate p53 and Rb family proteins in primary human mesotheliomas[130,131]; (2) the induction of growth arrest and apoptosis in mesothelioma cell lines transfected with antisense DNA to the SV-40 early region gene[132]; (3) the presence of SV40 in malignant mesothelioma cells and not in nearby stromal cells microdissected from the same slide[133]; and (4) the activation, in primary human mesothelial cells, of *Notch-1*, a gene promoting cell-cycle progression and cell proliferation,[134] considered a general requirement for the maintenance of the neoplastic phenotype in human cells.[135] Also, (5) human mesothelial cells are resistant to SV-40-induced cell lysis and are particularly susceptible to SV-40-mediated transformation[126,136] because human mesothelial cells limit SV-40 replication thanks to the endogenous high levels of wild-type p53.[136,137] Therefore, SV-40 DNA remains episomal, the viral oncogenes are expressed, cell lysis is limited, and the frequency of transformation is high ($1–5 \times 10^{-3}$ transformed foci in human mesothelial cells compared to $1 \times 10^{-7}–1 \times 10^{-8}$ transformed foci in human fibroblasts).[136,137] (6) Human mesothelial cells are specifically susceptible to SV-40 infection compared to the human polyomavirus JCV, which does not infect mesothelial cells, and BKV, which causes mesothelial cell lysis.[138] (7) Asbestos, which is the main cause of human mesothelioma, cooperates with SV-40 in transformation of human mesothelial cells,[136] suggesting that asbestos and SV-40 are cocarcinogens in the pathogenesis of mesothelioma. (8) SV-40 tumor antigens induce telomerase activity in human mesothelial cells,[138] a requirement for cellular immortalization and tumor growth. (9) SV-40 induces promoter methylation and inactivation of the RASSF1A tumor suppressor gene in both SV-40-positive mesothelioma and in SV-40-transformed human mesothelial cells.[137] Most of the conflicting arguments concerning the role of SV-40 in human tumors have been extensively discussed in a recent critical review[139] that points out the unique features of SV-40 infection in humans and emphasizes the limitations of the conventional studies of descriptive epidemiology which cannot reliably distinguish among infected and noninfected cohorts.[119,139]

Human Papillomaviruses

Papillomaviruses belong to the family Papovaviridae and are small (55 nm), nonenveloped viruses with a double-stranded circular DNA genome of about 8 kb. Papillomaviruses infect several animal species and are highly species specific and epitheliotropic. The human papillomavirus (HPV) species comprises more than 140 different types, but only a few types are prevalent in human neoplasia.[140,141] HPV is associated with both benign and malignant proliferative epithelial lesions affecting the genital organs and skin.[142] The mucosal HPV types infect the anogenital tract. Low-risk HPVs, with HPV-6 and HPV-11 as classic representatives, induce benign proliferations such as condylomata acuminata and papillomas that often regress and only rarely progress to malignancy. High-risk HPVs are associated to cervical cancer and other anogenital malignancies, such as vulva, vagina, penis, and anal cancer. Six HPV types, HPV-16, -18, -31, -33, -35, and

-39, are associated with more than 90% of cervical carcinomas.[140,141] The cutaneous HPV types are involved in skin warts and in epidermodysplasia verruciformis (EV), a hereditary autosomal recessive disease associated with a state of immunodeficiency and characterized by a great number of skin warts, often disseminated and confluent. In up to half of the affected patients, the warts of EV progress to skin carcinomas,[140–143] usually in sun-exposed sites because of the effect of UV irradiation, a clear example of cooperation in human carcinogenesis between a physical agent and viral infection and genetic predisposition. The HPV types most commonly involved in skin warts and EV lesions are HPV-5, -8, -9, -12, -14, -20, -23, -38, -49, and -75, but the squamous cell carcinomas arising from EV lesions contain mostly HPV-5, -8, -20, -23, and -38.[140–143]

The role of HPV in human neoplasia involves complex mechanisms.[140–144] Of great importance in the pathogenesis of both genital and cutaneous HPV-associated tumors is host immunosuppression, especially loss of cell-mediated immunity. Skin warts and cutaneous squamous cell carcinomas are common in immunosuppressed transplant recipients, and the frequency of condylomata acuminata and cervical cancer is enhanced in HIV-1-infected patients.[140,141] Most of the information about the role of HPV in anogenital tumorigenesis has been obtained from studies of cervical cancer.[144] While the genome of the low-risk HPV-6 and HPV-11 remains episomal in benign genital papillomas, the DNA of high-risk HPV-16, -18, -31, and -33 becomes integrated into the DNA of the tumor cells in cervical cancer.[144,145] Despite frequent loss of much of the viral genome in cervical cancer cells, the regions encoding the early viral proteins E6 and E7 are always maintained and expressed in HPV-positive cervical cancers.[140–145] Analysis of the high-risk HPV genomes in a variety of in vitro systems and in primary tumors indicated that the *E6* and *E7* genes are the primary oncogenes of HPV. HPV cannot be grown in vitro, possibly because virus maturation specifically requires differentiated epidermal cells. However, in vitro studies using retrovirus-mediated gene transfer and other transfection techniques demonstrated that HPV-16 or HPV-18 *E6* and *E7* genes in combination were able to efficiently immortalize and transform primary human foreskin keratinocytes (which resemble the normal in vivo target cells of HPV), whereas *E7* alone immortalized genital keratinocytes at a reduced efficiency and *E6* alone was ineffective.[146–148] HPV-16- and HPV-18-transformed keratinocytes showed aberrant differentiation patterns that made them almost indistinguishable from cells of low-grade cervical intraepithelial neoplasia, a precursor of cervical cancer.[146–148] Retrovirus constructs encoding low-risk HPV-6 E7 alone or both HPV-6 E6 and E7 failed to immortalize genital keratinocytes.[148]

Subsequent molecular analysis of the transforming activities of E6 and E7 oncoproteins has elucidated their role in the pathogenesis of genital cancer. The E6 protein of high-risk HPV types binds the p53 tumor suppressor protein with high affinity and mediates its degradation via the ubiquitin pathway.[149,150] The E6 protein also activates telomerase[151] and binds E6BP or ERC55, a calcium-binding protein[152,153] that may influence keratinocyte differentiation. Moreover, E6 binds paxillin,[154] which mediates a variety of signals from the cytoplasmic membrane to focal adhesion molecules and the actin cytoskeleton and binds, and possibly inactivates the hDLG protein,[155,156] the human homologue of the *Drosophila* large tumor suppressor protein. E6 transactivates TATA containing heterologous promoters through a mechanism unrelated to p53 binding.[157] The observation that although the E6 proteins encoded by several other papillomaviruses, such as bovine papillomavirus, HPV-1, and HPV-8, do not interact with p53 yet show strong transforming activity,[158] emphasizes the biologic relevance of these additional E6 activities.

The E7 oncoprotein binds p105Rb. The affinity of high-risk E7 proteins for pRb is severalfold higher than that of low-risk E7 proteins.[145,159] pRb plays an important role in cell-cycle control by coordinating entry of cells from G_1 into S phase.[89,160] Unphosphorylated pRb binds members of the E_2F family of transcription factors[89,145,161] in early G_1. E_2F proteins transcriptionally activate c-*myb*, c-*myc*, c-*fos*, c-*jun*, *cyclin A*, and *cyclin E* genes and other genes involved in DNA replication and stimulation of cell proliferation.[89,145] By binding to E_2F, pRb inhibits E_2F-mediated transcriptional activation and thus blocks cell-cycle progression from G_1 to S. In normal cells this block is relieved by phosphorylation of pRb through the action of the cyclin-dependent kinases (CDKs), resulting in the dissociation of the E_2F–pRb complex. Free E_2F is then able to transactivate its cell-cycle-promoting target genes, triggering progression into S phase.[89,145,160,161] The E7 oncoprotein can disrupt the pRb-mediated control of the cell cycle through at least three different mechanisms, leading to release of E_2F and to unregulated activation of E_2F target genes: (1) the direct binding of E7 to pRb results in a competitive interference with pRb–E_2F complex formation,[89,145,162] (2) E7-induced degradation of pRb,[145,163] and (3) E7-mediated interference with regulatory pathways upstream of pRb, such as blocking the activity of the $p21^{WAF1}$ CDK inhibitor.[164,165] The interaction with pRb is not the only activity through which E7 can contribute to cell transformation, as the transformation potential of mutant E7 proteins does not necessarily correlate with their ability to bind pRb.[166–168] E7 also interacts with the pRb-related proteins p107 and p130,[89,145] and it has been found in complexes with the cell-cycle regulatory proteins cyclin A, cyclin E, $p21^{WAF1}$, and $p27^{KIP1}$.[30] E7-induced alterations of the molecular pathways controlled by these cell-cycle regulatory proteins further contribute to the dysregulation of cell growth. E7 interferes with $p21^{WAF1}$-mediated regulation of DNA methylation[30] and with the $p21^{WAF1}$-induced DNA replication arrest in cells with DNA damage,[30] thus favoring the accumulation of DNA damage.[169] E7 has transcriptional modulatory activities and can influence transcription of cellular genes in an E_2F-independent fashion by interacting with proteins of the AP1 family of transcription factors[170] or with general transcription factors, such as the TATA box binding protein (TBP).[171]

The functional inactivation of the p53 and pRb family gene products by the oncoproteins of high-risk HPV types substitutes for mutations in these tumor suppressor genes. Indeed, it was shown that primary genital tumors and tumor cell lines infected with HPV do not carry mutations in *p53* and *Rb* genes,[172,173] although mutations may subsequently occur during tumor progression toward an invasive and metastatic phenotype. Conversely, p53 mutations are detected only in the rare HPV-negative cervical cancers.[174] In contrast to high-risk anogenital HPV infections, cutaneous HPV infections may contribute indirectly and in a less complex way to skin squamous cell carcinoma: the presence of HPV may simply protect cells from apoptosis after genetic damage induced by solar exposure, thus resulting in increased survival of the genetically altered cells.[141] Besides their involvement in genital and cutaneous carcinogenesis, HPVs are also linked to head and neck cancers and to esophageal carcinoma.[141,143,175] Although the transforming functions of HPV E6 and E7 proteins are important pathogenetic factors in human tumorigenesis, they are probably not sufficient to induce malignancy. In animals, human papillomavirus often cooperates with other carcinogens to cause cancer.[144] An outstanding example of the synergism between papillomaviruses and environmental factors is bovine papillomavirus, which induces papillomas and carcinomas of the alimentary tract in cattle in cooperation with dietary carcinogens.[176] Some metabolites of the vaginal microbial flora, alcohol, and smoke are considered relevant risk factors for the development of cervical, oropharyngeal, and laryngeal cancers.[141,143,175] Sexual hormones may enhance the oncogenic effect of HPV on genital tissues, because the promoter of high-risk HPV types harbors consensus sequences responding to transcriptional activation by estrogens and progesterone.[30] Herpes simplex virus infection may cooperate with HPV by promoting DNA mutations in genital tissues.[177] Physical carcinogens also have a cooperative role, as shown by transition to malignancy of the EV lesions exposed to UV light[140–143] and by the frequent conversion of laryngeal papillomas to carcinomas following X-ray treatment.[141]

Hepadnaviruses

Hepatitis B Virus

Hepatitis B virus (HBV) is the prototype of a new family of closely related DNA viruses, the Hepadnaviruses. This family comprises the woodchuck hepatitis virus (WHV), the ground squirrel hepatitis virus, and the duck hepatitis B virus as well as several other avian and mammalian strains. As in humans infected with HBV, chronic hepatitis and hepatocellular carcinoma (HCC) are commonly observed in persistently infected woodchucks and less frequently in infected ground squirrels and ducks.[178] All the hepadnaviruses show hepatotropism and similar life cycles in their hosts. They all start the replication cycle by reverse transcription of viral RNA to form DNA within core particles of the virus. The partially double-stranded circular DNA encodes four overlapping open reading frames[179]: *S* for the surface or envelope gene, *C* for the core gene, *P* for the polymerase gene, and *X* for the *X* gene. The *S* and *C* genes have upstream regions designated pre-*S* and pre-*C*. The whole virion, or Dane particle, is a 42-nm spherical body that contains the nucleocapsid. The viral envelope, coded by the *S* gene, contains three distinct components (large, middle, and small proteins) that are synthesized by beginning transcription within the pre-*S* or *S* gene, respectively. HBV can produce a large excess of the envelope surface antigen (HBsAg), consisting of both rods and small spheres with an average diameter of 22 nm, that can be found in patients' blood. The hepatitis B core antigen (HBcAg) is the nucleocapsid that encloses the viral DNA. When HbcAg-derived peptides are processed and expressed on the surface of hepatocytes, a T-cell-mediated immune response is induced to kill infected cells and eliminate the virus. The hepatitis B antigen (HbeAg) is a circulating peptide derived from the core gene and secreted by liver cells. Its presence in serum is a marker of active viral replication. The *X* gene encodes two proteins that have transactivating activity on the HBV enhancer to support viral replication. The X proteins can also transactivate cellular genes that may play a role in hepatocellular carcinoma.

Chronic HBV infection and cirrhosis are conditions leading to the development of HCC.[180–183] This concept emerged from evidence that (1) the greatest incidence of HCC is detected in areas of the world (tropical and equatorial regions) where HBV infection is widespread and (2) most patients affected by HCC bear markers of a long-lasting HBV infection. Based on prospective epidemiologic studies, it is estimated that chronic HBV carriers exhibit a 100-fold-increased risk for HCC development.[184] In sub-Saharan Africa with a high incidence of HCC, endemic infection by HBV cooperates in HCC together with exposure to aflatoxins derived from fungi of the *Aspergillus* genus, which grow on improperly stored foods.[181,185] The mechanisms of hepatocarcinogenesis by HBV are both direct and indirect. The direct mechanisms are related to integration of the HBV genome into cellular DNA and to potential oncogenic functions expressed by some viral genes (Figure 17.1). The role of HBV integration is most clearly observed in animal models. In more than 50% of HCCs arising in woodchucks, the WHV sequences specifically integrate 5′ or 3′ to the proto-oncogenes c-*myc* or n-*myc*, inducing a steady-state level overexpression of their mRNA, due to near insertion of the WHV enhancers.[180] In human HCC, the HBV DNA integrates randomly in the cellular genome, and direct effects of insertional mutagenesis on oncogene activation were observed. In one such rare case, HBV DNA was integrated within an exon of the gene of the retinoic acid receptor β,[180,186] disrupting the gene sequence. Because retinoic acid is important in inducing terminal cell differentiation, the inappropriate expression of one of its receptors may disturb the normal control of cell growth. In a second HCC, HBV DNA integration occurred in an intron of the *cyclin A* gene,[180,185,187] leading to its truncation and to the production of a *cyclin A*/HBV fusion gene. The N-terminus of the cyclin A protein, containing the signal for protein degradation, was deleted and replaced by HBV pre-S sequences (including the strong pre-S2/S promoter). The resulting fusion protein was expressed in a high amount, and it was resistant to degradation.[180,185,187] Constitutive expression of this chimeric form of cyclin A may lead to cell-cycle deregulation, uncontrolled DNA synthesis, and cell proliferation. In human HCC, deletions, rearrangements, and mutations at several chromosomal loci are frequently observed,[180,185] inducing overexpression of c-*myc* and c-*fos* oncogenes and reduced expression of the most common tumor suppressor genes, such as p53, pRb, and p16^{INK4}.[185] None of these chromosomal alterations, however, seems to be a direct consequence of HBV DNA integration.

A more relevant direct viral mechanism of human hepatocyte transformation is related to the expression of the HBV *X* gene.[183] Its products, the X protein, transform NIH3T3 and other immortalized mouse cells to the neoplastic phenotype,[188,189] and transgenic mice expressing the HBV *X* gene from the HBV promoter develop HCC.[190] HBV X can transcriptionally activate a broad array of cellular genes, including epidermal growth factor and cellular proto-oncogenes, such as c-*myc*, c-*fos*, and c-*jun*. Because HBV X does not bind to DNA, HBV X-mediated transcriptional alterations may

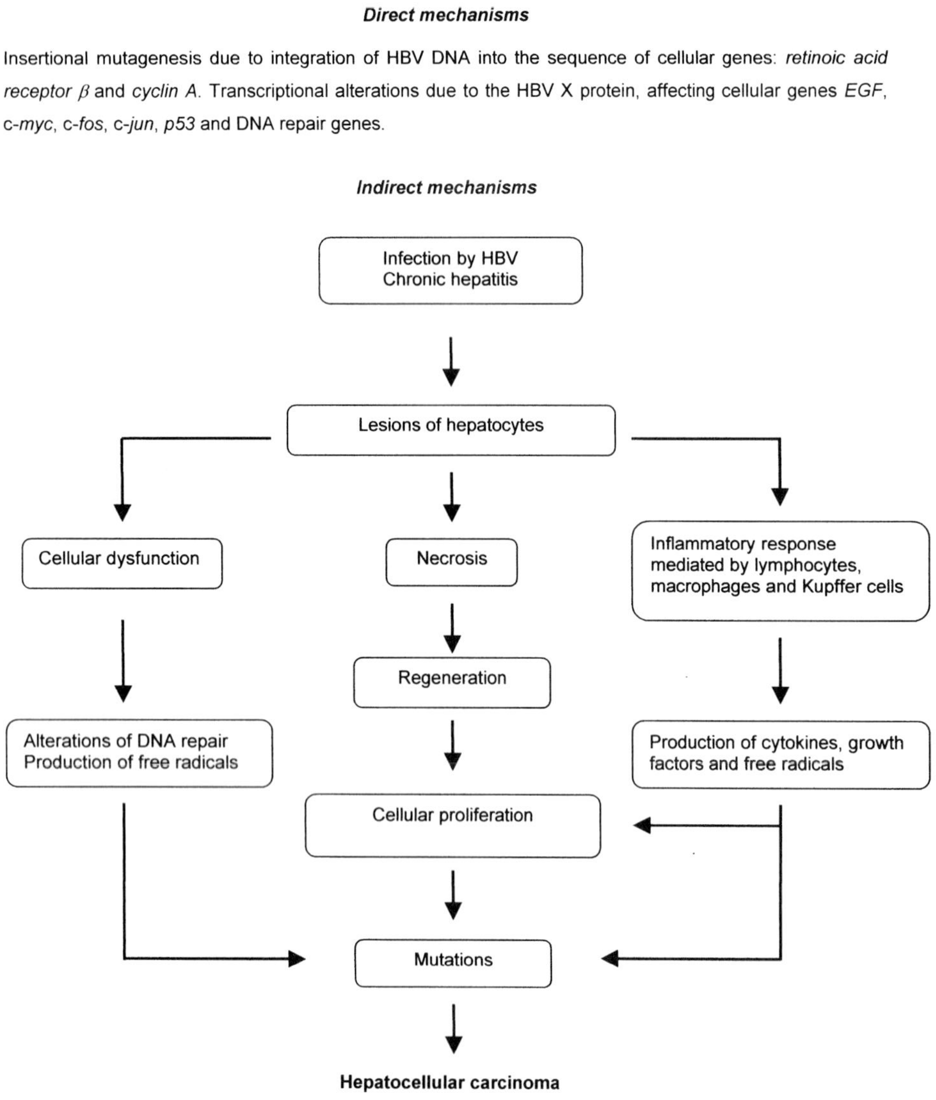

Direct mechanisms

Insertional mutagenesis due to integration of HBV DNA into the sequence of cellular genes: *retinoic acid receptor β* and *cyclin A*. Transcriptional alterations due to the HBV X protein, affecting cellular genes *EGF*, c-*myc*, c-*fos*, c-*jun*, *p53* and DNA repair genes.

Indirect mechanisms

Infection by HBV
Chronic hepatitis
↓
Lesions of hepatocytes
→ Cellular dysfunction → Alterations of DNA repair / Production of free radicals → Mutations
→ Necrosis → Regeneration → Cellular proliferation → Mutations
→ Inflammatory response mediated by lymphocytes, macrophages and Kupffer cells → Production of cytokines, growth factors and free radicals → Cellular proliferation; Mutations
Mutations
↓
Hepatocellular carcinoma

FIGURE 17.1. Indirect and direct mechanisms and the integration of the HBV genome into cellular DNA.

occur through the interaction with cellular transcription factors in the nucleus, through posttranscriptional modulation of their activities or through affecting signal transduction cascades in the cytoplasm.[26] HBV X binds p53,[191] inhibiting p53-mediated transcriptional transactivation[192] and apoptosis.[193] A close correlation has been observed between the HBV X–p53 interaction and the development of HCC in a transgenic mouse model.[194] The mechanism of p53 inhibition by HBV X is unique, because p53 is sequestered by HBV X in the cytoplasm of hepatocytes,[195] thereby blocking entry of p53 into the nuclear compartment. A further mechanism by which the HBV X protein could influence HCC development is through binding to components of DNA repair complexes. For example, the X protein binds to a human homologue of a UV light-damaged DNA-binding protein in monkeys.[196] The X protein also blocks binding of p53 to a transcription factor, ERCC3, involved in DNA repair.[192] The disruption of the fidelity of DNA repair, mediated by the X protein, may contribute to the genetic alterations observed in infected hepatocytes. HBV DNA integration in some HCCs can result in the deletion of the 3′-end of the HBV *X* and pre-*S/S* genes. This deletion leads to the synthesis of truncated pre-S/S proteins, which exhibit transactivation potential for a wide range of cellular genes involved in cell proliferation such as PKC, c-*raf*, AP-1, and NF-kB.[197]

HBV may also elicit an indirect promoting effect in liver cancer. This effect is related to the immunopathogenesis of chronic HBV infection. The T-cell-mediated immune response to HBV antigens, mostly derived from HBcAg epitopes located on the surface of hepatocytes, normally kills infected cells in the liver and clears the organ from HBV infection. When this cellular immune response is ineffective, the HBV infection progresses from acute to chronic hepatitis and, in some patients, to liver cirrhosis. During this process, the coexistent inflammation and hepatocyte regeneration increase the risk of HCC development. Liver cell proliferation in the presence of inflammation and of inflammatory mediators favors accumulation of genomic alterations, which can lead to hepatocyte transformation. During the inflammatory response, lymphocytes and macrophages produce cytokines and growth factor that stimulate hepatocyte proliferation. The phagocytic cells release products of the oxidative metabolism such as H_2O_2 and hydroxyl radicals.[180,183] Oxygen free radicals, produced by activated Kupffer cells, lead to the formation of

8-hydroxyguanosine adducts, which are promutagenic DNA lesions inducing G to T transversion.[180,183] The role of hepatocyte necrosis and regeneration in hepatocarcinogenesis is best illustrated by Chisari's model of *HbsAg* transgenic mice.[198,199] These mice overproduce the HBV large envelope polypeptide, accumulate toxic quantities of HBsAg within the hepatocytes, and develop a severe, prolonged hepatocellular injury. This lesion triggers inflammation, regenerative hyperplasia, transcriptional deregulation, and aneuploidy, finally progressing to neoplasia. These results are supported by the evidence that mice transgenic for the *TGF-α* gene, showing continuous mitogenic stimulation of hepatocytes, develop liver cancer.[200] In human chronic hepatitis, liver injury may be due to either the immune response during HBV infection or the toxic effects of alcohol.[30,181,201] In summary, severe prolonged cellular injury and persistent growth stimulation induce a proliferative response, which leads to genetic damage that can lead to tumor development. It should be noted that HBV also replicates in extrahepatic sites, such as bone marrow, lymphoid cells, pancreas, and kidneys.[202,203] Therefore, clearance of the virus from hepatocytes may not cure the disease, and HBV moving from these extrahepatic locations may reinfect the liver after transplant.[202]

Oncogenic Riboviruses

Flaviviruses

Hepatitis C Virus

The hepatitis C virus (HCV) belongs to a genus of the family Flaviviridae. The virion is spherical and enveloped. The genome is a single-stranded linear RNA molecule of about 9.5 kb encoding a single large polyprotein precursor of about 3,000 amino acids from which three structural and seven nonstructural proteins are generated by specific cleavage. The capsid protein or core protein is located at the amino-terminus of the polyprotein precursor. Similarly to HIV-1, HCV shows a great genomic variability, thus representing a quasi-species, that is, a population of closely related, yet heterogeneous, viral genomes.[204–206] Nevertheless, HCV can be subdivided into six major genotypes. HCV genetic heterogeneity may have important implications because it could influence the immunologic and therapeutic responses as well as represent a major obstacle in the preparation of an effective anti-HCV vaccine.[30,204–207] Epidemiologic studies have shown that HCC is associated with HCV infection, but the proportion of cases related to HCV varies considerably.[208] In countries of southern Europe such as Italy, Spain, and Portugal, as well as in Japan, HCV infection appears to be the most frequent underlying cause of HCC, because from 50% to 70% of patients with HCC show anti-HCV antibodies. In the United States, the proportion of patients with HCC who are seropositive for anti-HCV antibodies is much lower, about 30%,[208,209] but still very significant.

The process of hepatocarcinogenesis caused by HCV results mainly from indirect mechanisms.[183] Similar to HBV infection, when the cell-mediated immune response fails to eradicate HCV infection, the acute hepatitis may evolve toward chronic persistent hepatitis, cirrhosis, and HCC. As for HBV infection, the host immune response plays the major role in causing the hepatocellular damage.[182,205,206,208,210] During the evolution from acute infection to chronic hepatitis and cirrhosis, the repeated bouts of inflammation, necrosis, and hepatocyte regeneration favor the emergence of a neoplastic liver cell population. Cirrhosis is found in about 90% of HCC patients with HCV markers,[182,205] although there are patients with HCV-related HCC without liver cirrhosis.[211] This observation suggests a possible direct role of HCV in hepatocarcinogenesis. Various mechanisms appear possible. The HCV nonstructural protein NS3 transforms to the neoplastic phenotype in the NIH3T3 mouse fibroblasts.[212] Moreover, the HCV core protein suppresses apoptosis[183,213] and, in cooperation with the human activated c-H-*ras* oncogene, causes malignant transformation of primary rat embryo fibroblasts.[214] Finally, HCV core gene transgenic mice develop HCC.[215] The HCV genotype 1b has been associated with more severe and rapidly progressive liver disease and a higher risk of HCC.[182,208]

HCV infects other tissues besides the liver, and it is associated with several diseases,[216,217] such as sialadenitis, membranoproliferative glomerulonephritis, and mixed cryoglobulinemia, a disorder characterized by the presence in the serum of a mixture of polyclonal immunoglobulins of various isotypes that reversibly precipitate at temperatures below 37°C. Most of these immunoglobulins are complexes of polyclonal IgG and polyclonal rheumatoid factor that are mainly IgM.[216,217] Because mixed cryoglobulinemia is considered the expression of a low-grade malignant lymphoproliferative disease, an association was postulated between HCV and lymphoproliferative disorders. Epidemiologic studies showed a significant association between HCV infection and B-cell non-Hodgkin's lymphoma (NHL).[217] HCV-related markers (HCV RNA and anti-HCV antibodies) were detected in 34% of B-cell NHL, compared to 3% Hodgkin's lymphomas and 1.5% healthy controls.[217] Comparable values of association between B-cell NHL and HCV infection were confirmed in subsequent studies,[217,218] although HCV markers were not detected in NHL cells in HCV-infected patients.[216,219,220] A case-control study demonstrated that HCV infection increases by 50-fold the risk of B-cell NHL involving the liver and the major salivary glands (the most common sites of HCV infection) and by four fold the risk of lymphomas at other sites.[221] Although HCV has been widely detected in peripheral blood mononuclear cells of patients with mixed cryoglobulinemia and B-cell NHL with HCV infection, the virus replicates poorly in lymphoid cells.[216,219] Therefore, the postulated oncogenic role of HCV in lymphoproliferative disorders is presently unclear. According to other models of B-cell lymphomagenesis,[13] HCV may act as an exogenous prolonged antigenic stimulus inducing a mitogenic effect and proliferation of B lymphocytes in HCV-infected patients.[219] Treatment with IFN of HCV infection in patients with splenic lymphomas led to strikingly complete responses of the lymphomas, but not in noninfected patients.

Retroviruses

Human T-Cell Leukemia Virus Types I and II

Human T-cell leukemia viruses type I (HTLV-I) and type II (HTLV-II) belong to the subfamily Oncovirinae of the family Retroviridae. HTLV-I infection is endemic in Japan, other regions of Asia such as the Philippines, the Caribbean region, central Africa, and some areas of Australia and New Guinea. In these areas of the world, the seroprevalence rate of antibodies to HTLV-I is 5% to 33% in the normal human population.[207] HTLV-I is associated with adult T-cell leukemia and lymphoma (ATL),[222,223] as well as with its cutaneous variants, mycosis fungoides and Sézary's syndrome. HTLV-I is also the etiologic agent of HTLV-I-associated myelopathy or tropical spastic paraparesis. HTLV-II is associated with an atypical form of hairy cell leukemia.[30,222,224] Monoclonal integration of HTLV-I proviral DNA was demonstrated in ATL neoplastic cells, and all individuals with ATL have antibodies to HTLV-I.[225,226] HTLV-I, at variance from the avian and rodent retroviruses, immortalizes T lymphocytes much like the oncogenic deoxyriboviruses, that is, through the product of a viral oncogene, the *tax* gene. The Tax protein has pleiotropic effects because it is able to activate or repress the expression of a wide array of cellular genes.[227] Tax does not bind directly to DNA, but it interacts with cellular transcription factors or modulators of cellular functions. Binding of Tax to NF-KB results in transcriptional activation of *IL-2α* and *IL-2α* receptor genes, leading to autocrine stimulation of T-cell proliferation.[228,229] Interaction of Tax with serum responsive factor (SRF) activates the expression of c-*fos* and of the early growth response genes *egr*-1 and *egr*-2.[230] Other cellular genes activated by Tax include the *GM-CSF, IL-1, IL-3, IL-6, PDGF, TGF-β1, TNF-β*, and *NGF*.[231] Conversely, Tax represses transcription of the *DNA polymerase β* gene[232] encoding a cellular enzyme involved in host cell DNA repair. This finding suggests a possible correlation between HTLV-I infection and host cell chromosomal damage, which is often observed in ATL. Tax inhibits the expression of the *lck* gene,[233] encoding a tyrosine kinase of the *src* family, which plays a major role in the regulation of T-cell activation.[233] Tax also dysregulates the cell cycle by binding and inactivating $p16^{INK4}$, a key inhibitor of CDK4 and CDK6.[234] In HTLV-I-infected cells, Tax is responsible for the stabilization and inactivation of p53 protein by phosphorylation at Ser15, which blocks p53 interaction with transcription factors.[227,235] Tax also targets the mitotic checkpoint protein MAD-1, an important control protein for the formation of the mitotic spindle.[227,236] The block of p53 and MAD-1 functions may be responsible for the genetic instability, aneuploidy, and chromosomal rearrangements that have been reported in ATL cells,[226,227] and may affect oncogenes, tumor suppressor and DNA repair genes. Also, Tax expression enhances the mutation frequency in chromosomal DNA after transfection of the *tax* gene into the rat fibroblastic cell line Rat 2.[237] These diverse effects of Tax suggest a scenario where ATL cells are initially dependent on Tax expression for proliferation. After the appearance of chromosomal aberrations and mutations involving genes crucial in oncogenesis, the neoplastic cells grow independently from Tax and ATL progresses toward a more malignant phenotype.

Human Immunodeficiency Virus Type 1

Human immunodeficiency virus type 1 (HIV-1) belongs to the subfamily Lentivirinae of the family Retroviridae. In the course of HIV-1 infection, an opportunistic neoplastic pathology develops that is mainly due to immunosuppression, leading to decrease of the immune surveillance against tumors and latent viruses. Indeed, most cancers arising during AIDS are associated with oncogenic viruses (Table 17.3), because HIV-1 infection provides the immunologic background on which other viruses can escape immune control and induce tumors.[238] However, a large body of evidence indicates that HIV-1 itself may be oncogenic through the expression of the Tat protein, the product of the early HIV-1 *tat* gene.[239,240] The Tat protein of HIV-1 is a small polypeptide of 14 to 15 kDa containing 86 to 102 amino acids, depending on the viral strains. Tat is a potent transactivator of the HIV-1 LTR and is also able to activate the expression of many cellular genes, thereby affecting cellular functions and inducing angiogenesis, cell proliferation, inhibition of apoptosis, and oncogenesis.[239,240] A remarkable property of Tat protein is that it is released from HIV-1-infected cells, circulates in the bloodstream and in extracellular fluids, and is taken up by uninfected cells where it exerts its biologic effects.[241–243] Tat induces neoangiogenesis in vivo[240,244] and has a synergic effect with bFGF on the induction of KS-like lesions in nude mice.[245] During neoangiogenesis and cell growth, Tat activates the expression of cytokines, chemokines, and growth factors (IL-1α, IL-1β, IL-2, IL-6, IL-8, IFN-γ, TNF-α, TNF-β, MCP-1, bFGF, VEGF, GM-CSF, PDGF, SF/HGF, and TGF-β) by KS cells and induces the activity of urokinase and collagenase IV, which allow endothelial cells to invade underlying tissues.[239] The multiple angiogenic and growth-stimulating effects of Tat, together with the profound immunodeficiency associated with AIDS, may be responsible for the more aggressive and invasive behavior of AIDS-KS compared to the other forms of this tumor.[46,49] When Tat is transfected under the control of the HIV-1 long terminal repeat, it efficiently transforms immortalized keratinocytes to a neoplastic phenotype.[246] Moreover, Tat inhibits expression of the manganese-dependent superoxide dismutase (*Mn-SOD*) gene by direct interaction with *Mn-SOD* transcripts,[247] thereby contributing to the establishment and maintenance

TABLE 17.3. Tumors with increased incidence in acquired immunodeficiency syndrome (AIDS).

Tumor	*Associated virus*
Kaposi's sarcoma[a]	Human herpesvirus 8 and HIV-1 Tat
Primary effusion lymphoma	Human herpesvirus 8
Multiple myeloma	Human herpesvirus 8 (?)
B-cell non-Hodgkin's lymphoma[a] (mostly systemic and brain lymphomas)	Epstein–Barr virus
Hodgkin's disease	Epstein–Barr virus
Leiomyoma and leiomyosarcoma (in children)	Epstein–Barr virus
Cervical carcinoma and squamous cell neoplasia of oropharynx and anus	Human papillomavirus

[a]Tumors whose frequency is significantly increased in AIDS patients.

of oxidative stress. *Mn-SOD* has been shown to control cell proliferation by regulation of the oxidative metabolism[248] and is a candidate tumor suppressor gene involved in the pathogenesis of melanoma and other human tumors.[249] The oncogenic activity of Tat may be related also to its ability to downregulate p53 expression[250,251] as well as to upregulate *IL-2*, *bcl*-2, and *IL-6* gene transcription.[252–255] The angiogenic and tumorigenic effects of Tat are confirmed and recapitulated in *tat*-transgenic mice.[256,257] These animals develop angiogenic proliferation in the derma, resembling the early phases of KS. In addition, they develop skin papillomas and carcinomas, adenocarcinomas of subcutaneous glands, lymphoid hyperplasia and lymphomas, liver dysplasia and hepatocarcinomas, polyps of the rectum, and squamous cell hyperplasia of the anal orifice and adjacent perianal skin. Liver dysplasia affects about 40% of *tat*-transgenic mice[256,257] and represents a preneoplastic state, predisposing to liver tumorigenesis induced by chemical carcinogens.[258,259] In conclusion, the HIV-1 Tat protein is oncogenic and may be a cofactor in AIDS-related malignancies, especially in KS and PELs where Tat may cooperate with HHV-8 in the angiogenic and oncogenic effects.[46–49,239]

Conclusions and Perspectives

There has been notable progress in recent years in identifying the causative roles of viruses in human tumors and elucidating the molecular mechanisms of virus-induced cellular transformation. Because of the multifactorial and multistep nature of human carcinogenesis, infection with a tumor virus is usually not sufficient for malignant transformation and tumor growth. Human tumor viruses must therefore be studied in the context of the cofactors that cause a specific tumor type susceptibility. Exposure to exogenous and endogenous carcinogens, genetic alterations of the host cells, and the patient's immunologic status determine, among infected individuals, those who will develop a malignancy. Great efforts are under way to set up effective therapeutic and prophylactic interventions against tumor viruses.[30] Vaccines against tumor viruses have both prophylactic and therapeutic applications and may protect from viral infection or may control tumor growth by eliciting a cell-mediated immune response against infected tumor cells. Excellent results have been obtained with an anti-HBV prophylactic vaccine, prepared with HBsAg expressed in yeasts. The report of a national HBV vaccination program in children of Taiwan indicates that the incidence of HCC is declining,[182,260] and a similar trend is observed in other areas of the world with endemic HBV infection, where the anti-HBV vaccine has been administered on a mass scale. This is the first example of prevention of a human cancer by vaccination. Recently, the introduction of a new oral HBV recombinant vaccine constituted by HBsAg produced in transgenic potatoes and production of HbsAg in transgenic tomatoes and bananas is under way.[261] Oral immunization, because of its simplicity of use, ease of administration, and increased compliance, represents the ideal mode of delivery for implementation of large-scale vaccination programs in poor areas of the world where HBV infection is endemic and the incidence of HCC is high.

Vaccination against HCV faces more difficult problems because of the genetic heterogeneity virus and its great antigenic variability. Therefore, an HCV vaccine is not yet available. Vaccines against HPV have been prepared by using the nonstructural proteins E6 and E7 as well as virus-like particles made of the structural proteins L1 and L2 from HPV-16 and HPV-18. Rodents immunized with these proteins become resistant to papillomavirus tumorigenesis.[30,262,263] These HPV vaccines are currently being tested in clinical trials. A vaccine against EBV was prepared with the major envelope glycoprotein gp350, the main component of the EBV envelope antigen, which functions as a viral receptor for virus attachment to susceptible cells. This vaccine protected cottontop tamarin monkeys from B-cell lymphomas induced by EBV,[264,265] but it has not been adopted for use. A recombinant vaccinia vector containing a safety-modified SV-40 Tag sequence was constructed.[266] Such modified Tag excludes the p53 and Rb protein binding sites as well as the amino-terminal oncogenic CRI and J domains,[267] but preserves the immunogenic regions. Tumorigenesis studies carried out in mice indicated that this vector can efficiently prime the immune response to provide effective, antigen-specific prophylactic and therapeutic protection against SV-40 Tag-expressing lethal tumors.[266] This vaccine is currently being produced for testing in clinical trials and would be used, as a prophylactic measure, in individuals exposed to asbestos, at risk for mesothelioma. Although truncation of Tag at the carboxyl terminus, where the p53 binding sites are located, produces unstable products,[267] such types of vaccines may represent in the future a useful immunoprophylactic and immunotherapeutic intervention against human tumors associated with SV40.[268]

A vaccine against HIV-1 has long been sought. Several vaccine preparations, based on the two envelope glycoproteins gp120 and gp160 as well as on the core capsid antigen, have been tested, but the results were generally disappointing.[239] The evidence that both the intracellular and the extracellular Tat protein is crucial for HIV-1 replication[239,240] prompted the preparation of anti-Tat vaccines. These vaccines protected monkeys from a letal challenge with the SHIV virus,[269,270] a recombinant virus containing the HIV-1 *tat* gene within the simian immunodeficiency virus (SIV) genome. It seems reasonable, therefore, to include the Tat protein within the polyvalent vaccine that will be used in the future to prevent and cure the HIV-1 infection. As a result of the oncogenic properties of Tat, anti-Tat immunization may also reduce the incidence of Tat-related tumors arising in the course of AIDS.

References

1. zur Hausen H. Viral oncogenesis. In: Parsonnet J (ed). Microbes and Mal. New York: Oxford Press, 1999:107–130.
2. zur Hausen H. Viruses in human cancers. Science 1991; 254:1167–1173.
3. Barbanti-Brodano G, Martini F, De Mattei M, et al. BK and JC human polyomaviruses and simian virus 40: natural history of infection in humans, experimental oncogenicity, and association with human tumors. Adv Virus Res 1998;50:69–99.
4. Tognon M, Corallini A, Martini F, et al. Oncogenic transformation by BK virus and association with human tumors. Oncogene 2003;22:5192–5200.
5. Rickinson AB, Kieff E. Epstein–Barr virus. In: Knipe DM, Howley PM (eds). Fields Virology. Philadelphia: Lippincott Williams & Wilkins, 2001:2575–2627.

6. Knecht H, Berger C, al-Homsi AS, et al. Epstein-Barr virus oncogenesis. Crit Rev Oncol Hematol 1997;26:117–135.
7. Srinivas SK, Sixbey JW. Epstein-Barr virus induction of recombinase-activating genes RAG1 and RAG2. J Virol 1995;69: 8155–8158.
8. Wilson JB, Levine AJ. The oncogenic potential of Epstein-Barr virus nuclear antigen 1 in transgenic mice. Curr Top Microbiol Immunol 1992;182:375–384.
9. zur Hausen H, Schulte-Holthausen H, Klein G, et al. EBV DNA in biopsies of Burkitt tumours and anaplastic carcinomas of the nasopharynx. Nature (Lond) 1970;228:1056–1058.
10. Pallesen G, Hamilton-Dutoit SJ, Zhou X. The association of Epstein-Barr virus (EBV) with T cell lymphoproliferations and Hodgkin's disease: two new developments in the EBV field. Adv Cancer Res 1993;62:179–239.
11. Meijer CJ, Jiwa NM, Dukers DF, et al. Epstein-Barr virus and human T-cell lymphomas. Semin Cancer Biol 1996;7:191–196.
12. Herbst H. Epstein-Barr virus in Hodgkin's disease. Semin Cancer Biol 1996;7:183–189.
13. Boiocchi M, Dolcetti R, DeRe V, et al. Association of Epstein-Barr virus with Hodgkin's disease. In: Barbanti-Brodano G, Bendinelli M, Friedman H (eds). DNA Tumor Viruses: Oncogenic Mechanisms. New York: Plenum Press, 1995:375–393.
14. Niedobitek G, Agathanggelou A, Nicholls JM. Epstein-Barr virus infection and the pathogenesis of nasopharyngeal carcinoma: viral gene expression, tumour cell phenotype, and the role of the lymphoid stroma. Semin Cancer Biol 1996;7:165–174.
15. Young LS, Murray PG. Epstein-Barr virus and oncogenesis: from latent genes to tumours. Oncogene 2003;22:5108–5121.
16. Croce CM. Chromosome translocations and human cancer. Cancer Res 1986;46:6019–6023.
17. Polack A, Hortnagel K, Pajic A, et al. c-myc activation renders proliferation of Epstein-Barr virus (EBV)-transformed cells independent of EBV nuclear antigen 2 and latent membrane protein 1. Proc Natl Acad Sci USA 1996;93:10411–10416.
18. Klein G, Klein E. Evolution of tumours and the impact of molecular oncology. Nature (Lond) 1985;315:190–195.
19. Lenoir G, Bornkamm GW. Burkitt's lymphoma: a human cancer model for the study of the multistep development of cancer: proposal for a new scenario. In: Klein E (ed). Advances in Viral Oncology, vol 7. New York: Raven Press, 1986:173–206.
20. Razzouk BI, Srinivas S, Sample CE, et al. Epstein-Barr virus DNA recombination and loss in sporadic Burkitt's lymphoma. J Infect Dis 1996;173:529–535.
21. Brooks L, Crook T, Crawford D. Epstein-Barr virus and lymphomas. In: Newton R, Beral V, Weiss I (eds). Infections and Human Cancer. Cold Spring Harbor, NY: Cold Spring Harbor Laboratory Press, 1999:99–123.
22. Gaidano G, Pastore C, Gloghini A, et al. AIDS-related non-Hodgkin's lymphomas: molecular genetics, viral infection and cytokine deregulation. Acta Haematol 1996;95:193–198.
23. Swinnen L. Posttransplant lymphoproliferative disorder. In: Goedert J (ed). Infectious Causes of Cancer. Totowa, NJ: Humana Press, 2000:63–76.
24. Purtilo DT, Cassel CK, Yang JP, et al. X-linked recessive progressive combined variable immunodeficiency (Duncan's disease). Lancet 1975;1:935–940.
25. Seemayer T, Greiner T, Gross T, et al. X-linked lymphoproliferative disease. In: Goedert J (ed). Infectious Causes of Cancer. Totowa, NJ: Humana Press, 2000:51–61.
26. Gross TG, Davis JR, Baker KS, et al. Exaggerated IL-2 response to Epstein-Barr virus (EBV) in X-linked lymphoproliferative disease (XLP). Clin Immunol Immunopathol 1995;75:280–281.
27. O'Connor P, Scadden D. Hodgkin's disease. In: Goedert J (ed). Infectious Causes of Cancer. Totowa, NJ: Humana Press, 2000: 113–127.
28. Wong M, Pagano JS, Schiller JT, et al. New associations of human papillomavirus, simian virus 40, and Epstein-Barr virus with human cancer. J Natl Cancer Inst 2002;94:1832–1836.
29. Kripalani-Joshi S, Law HY. Identification of integrated Epstein-Barr virus in nasopharyngeal carcinoma using pulse field gel electrophoresis. Int J Cancer 1994;56:187–192.
30. Hoppe-Seyler F, Butz K. Viral mechanisms of human carcinogenesis. In: Coleman W, Tsongalis G (eds). The Molecular Basis of Human Cancer. Totowa, NJ: Humana Press, 2002:233–247.
31. Osato T, Imai S. Epstein-Barr virus and gastric carcinoma. Semin Cancer Biol 1996;7:175–182.
32. Takada K. Epstein-Barr virus and gastric carcinoma. J Clin Pathol Mol Pathol 2000;53:255–261.
33. Wei MX, Ooka T. A transforming function of the BARF1 gene encoded by Epstein-Barr virus. EMBO J 1989;8:2897–2903.
34. zur Hausen A, Brink AA, Craanen ME, et al. Unique transcription pattern of Epstein-Barr virus (EBV) in EBV-carrying gastric adenocarcinomas: expression of the transforming BARF1 gene. Cancer Res 2000;60:2745–2748.
35. Jenson H. Leiomyoma and leiomyosarcoma. In: Goedert J (ed). Infectious Causes of Cancer. Totowa, NJ: Humana Press, 2000: 145–159.
36. Granovsky MO, Mueller BU, Nicholson HS, et al. Cancer in human immunodeficiency virus-infected children: a case series from the Children's Cancer Group and the National Cancer Institute. J Clin Oncol 1998;16:1729–1735.
37. Raab-Traub N, Rajadurai P, Flynn K, et al. Epstein-Barr virus infection in carcinoma of the salivary gland. J Virol 1991;65: 7032–7036.
38. Bonnet M, Guinebretiere JM, Kremmer E, et al. Detection of Epstein-Barr virus in invasive breast cancers. J Natl Cancer Inst 1999;91:1376–1381.
39. Chang Y, Cesarman E, Pessin MS, et al. Identification of herpesvirus-like DNA sequences in AIDS-associated Kaposi's sarcoma. Science 1994;266:1865–1879.
40. Lisitsyn N, Wigler M. Cloning the differences between two complex genomes. Science 1993;259:946–951.
41. Biesinger B, Muller-Fleckenstein I, Simmer B, et al. Stable growth transformation of human T lymphocytes by herpesvirus saimiri. Proc Natl Acad Sci USA 1992;89:3116–3119.
42. Cesarman E, Chang Y, Moore PS, et al. Kaposi's sarcoma-associated herpesvirus-like DNA sequences in AIDS-related body-cavity-based lymphomas. N Engl J Med 1995;332:1186–1191.
43. Sarid R, Olsen SJ, Moore PS. Kaposi's sarcoma-associated herpesvirus: epidemiology, virology, and molecular biology. Adv Virus Res 1999;52:139–232.
44. Boshoff C. Kaposi's sarcoma associated herpesvirus. In: Newton R, Beral V, Weiss RA (eds). Infections and Human Cancer. Cancer Surveys, vol 33. Cold Spring Harbor, NY: Cold Spring Harbor Laboratory Press, 1999:157–190.
45. Castleman B, Iverson L, Menendez VP. Localized mediastinal lymph-node hyperplasia resembling thymoma. Cancer (Phila) 1956;9:822–830.
46. Ensoli B, Sgadari C, Barillari G, et al. Biology of Kaposi's sarcoma. Eur J Cancer 2001;37:1251–1269.
47. Ensoli B, Sturzl M, Monini P. Cytokine-mediated growth promotion of Kaposi's sarcoma and primary effusion lymphoma. Semin Cancer Biol 2000;10:367–381.
48. Monini P, de Lellis L, Fabris M, et al. Kaposi's sarcoma-associated herpesvirus DNA sequences in prostate tissue and human semen. N Engl J Med 1996;334:1168–1172.
49. Ganem D. KSHV and Kaposi's sarcoma: the end of the beginning? Cell 1997;91:157–160.
50. Ensoli B, Sturzl M, Monini P. Reactivation and role of HHV-8 in Kaposi's sarcoma initiation. Adv Cancer Res 2001;81:161–200.
51. Russo JJ, Bohenzky RA, Chien MC, et al. Nucleotide sequence of the Kaposi sarcoma-associated herpesvirus (HHV8). Proc Natl Acad Sci USA 1996;93:14862–14867.

52. Sturzl M, Zietz C, Monini P, et al. Human herpesvirus-8 and Kaposi's sarcoma: relationship with the multistep concept of tumorigenesis. Adv Cancer Res 2001;81:125–159.
53. Neipel F, Albrecht JC, Fleckenstein B. Cell-homologous genes in the Kaposi's sarcoma-associated rhadinovirus human herpesvirus 8: determinants of its pathogenicity? J Virol 1997;71: 4187–4192.
54. Cheng EH, Nicholas J, Bellows DS, et al. A Bcl-2 homolog encoded by Kaposi sarcoma-associated virus, human herpesvirus 8, inhibits apoptosis but does not heterodimerize with Bax or Bak. Proc Natl Acad Sci USA 1997;94:690–694.
55. Chang Y, Moore PS, Talbot SJ, et al. Cyclin encoded by KS herpesvirus. Nature (Lond) 1996;382:410.
56. Swanton C, Mann DJ, Fleckenstein B, et al. Herpes viral cyclin/Cdk6 complexes evade inhibition by CDK inhibitor proteins. Nature (Lond) 1997;390:184–187.
57. Arvanitakis L, Geras-Raaka E, Varma A, et al. Human herpesvirus KSHV encodes a constitutively active G-protein-coupled receptor linked to cell proliferation. Nature (Lond) 1997;385:347–350.
58. Bais C, Santomasso B, Coso O, et al. G-protein-coupled receptor of Kaposi's sarcoma-associated herpesvirus is a viral oncogene and angiogenesis activator. Nature (Lond) 1998;391:86–89.
59. Yang TY, Chen SC, Leach MW, et al. Transgenic expression of the chemokine receptor encoded by human herpesvirus 8 induces an angioproliferative disease resembling Kaposi's sarcoma. J Exp Med 2000;191:445–454.
60. Boshoff C, Endo Y, Collins PD, et al. Angiogenic and HIV-inhibitory functions of KSHV-encoded chemokines. Science 1997;278:290–294.
61. Moore PS, Boshoff C, Weiss RA, et al. Molecular mimicry of human cytokine and cytokine response pathway genes by KSHV. Science 1996;274:1739–1744.
62. Rettig MB, Ma HJ, Vescio RA, et al. Kaposi's sarcoma-associated herpesvirus infection of bone marrow dendritic cells from multiple myeloma patients. Science 1997;276:1851–1854.
63. Imperiale MJ. The human polyomaviruses: an overview. In: Khalili K, Stoner G (eds). Human Polyomaviruses. New York: Wiley-Liss, 2001:53–71.
64. Imperiale MJ. Oncogenic transformation by the human polyomaviruses. Oncogene 2001;20:7917–7923.
65. Corallini A, Tognon M, Negrini M, et al. Evidence for BK virus as a human tumor virus. In: Khalili K, Stoner G (eds). Human Polyomaviruses. New York: Wiley-Liss, 2001:431–460.
66. Bofill-Mas S, Formiga-Cruz M, Clemente-Casares P, et al. Potential transmission of human polyomaviruses through the gastrointestinal tract after exposure to virions or viral DNA. J Virol 2001;75:10290–10299.
67. Carbone M, Rizzo P, Pass HI. Simian virus 40, poliovaccines and human tumors: a review of recent developments. Oncogene 1997;15:1877–1888.
68. Melnick JL, Stinebaugh S. Excretion of vacuolating SV-40 virus (papova virus group) after ingestion as a contaminant of oral poliovaccine. Proc Soc Exp Biol Med 1962;109:965–968.
69. Bergsagel DJ, Finegold MJ, Butel JS, et al. DNA sequences similar to those of simian virus 40 in ependymomas and choroid plexus tumors of childhood. N Engl J Med 1992;326:988–993.
70. Carbone M, Rizzo P, Procopio A, et al. SV40-like sequences in human bone tumors. Oncogene 1996;13:527–535.
71. Martini F, Iaccheri L, Lazzarin L, et al. SV40 early region and large T antigen in human brain tumors, peripheral blood cells, and sperm fluids from healthy individuals. Cancer Res 1996; 56:4820–4825.
72. Lednicky JA, Stewart AR, Jenkins JJ III, et al. SV40 DNA in human osteosarcomas shows sequence variation among T-antigen genes. Int J Cancer 1997;72:791–800.
73. Martini F, Lazzarin L, Iaccheri L, et al. Different simian virus 40 genomic regions and sequences homologous with SV40 large T antigen in DNA of human brain and bone tumors and of leukocytes from blood donors. Cancer (Phila) 2002;94:1037–1048.
74. Martini F, Dolcetti R, Gloghini A, et al. Simian-virus-40 footprints in human lymphoproliferative disorders of HIV– and HIV+ patients. Int J Cancer 1998;78:669–674.
75. Yamamoto H, Nakayama T, Murakami H, et al. High incidence of SV40-like sequences detection in tumour and peripheral blood cells of Japanese osteosarcoma patients. Br J Cancer 2000;82: 1677–1681.
76. David H, Mendoza S, Konishi T, et al. Simian virus 40 is present in human lymphomas and normal blood. Cancer Lett 2001; 162:57–64.
77. Li RM, Branton MH, Tanawattanacharoen S, et al. Molecular identification of SV40 infection in human subjects and possible association with kidney disease. J Am Soc Nephrol 2002; 13:2320–2330.
78. Li RM, Mannon RB, Kleiner D, et al. BK virus and SV40 co-infection in polyomavirus nephropathy. Transplantation 2002; 74:1497–1504.
79. Vastag B. Sewage yields clues to SV40 transmission. JAMA 2002;288:1337–1338.
80. Kops SP. Oral polio vaccine and human cancer: a reassessment of SV40 as a contaminant based upon legal documents. Anticancer Res 2000;20:4745–4749.
81. Lednicky JA, Garcea RL, Bergsagel DJ, et al. Natural simian virus 40 strains are present in human choroid plexus and ependymoma tumors. Virology 1995;212:710–717.
82. Shah KV. Neutralizing antibodies to simian virus 40 (SV40) in human sera from India. Proc Soc Exp Biol Med 1966;121: 303–307.
83. Jafar S, Rodriguez-Barradas M, Graham DY, et al. Serological evidence of SV40 infections in HIV-infected and HIV-negative adults. J Med Virol 1998;54:276–284.
84. Butel JS, Jafar S, Wong C, et al. Evidence of SV40 infections in hospitalized children. Hum Pathol 1999;30:1496–1502.
85. Rollison DE, Helzlsouer KJ, Alberg AJ, et al. Serum antibodies to JC virus, BK virus, simian virus 40, and the risk of incident adult astrocytic brain tumors. Cancer Epidemiol Biomarkers Prev 2003;12:460–463.
86. Simmons DT. SV40 large T antigen functions in DNA replication and transformation. Adv Virus Res 2000;55:75–134.
87. Ali SH, DeCaprio JA. Cellular transformation by SV40 large T antigen: interaction with host proteins. Semin Cancer Biol 2001; 11:15–23.
88. Testa JR, Giordano A. SV40 and cell cycle perturbations in malignant mesothelioma. Semin Cancer Biol 2001;11:31–38.
89. Dyson N, Buchkovich K, Whyte P, et al. The cellular 107K protein that binds to adenovirus E1A also associates with the large T antigens of SV40 and JC virus. Cell 1989;58:249–255.
90. Dyson N, Bernards R, Friend SH, et al. Large T antigens of many polyomaviruses are able to form complexes with the retinoblastoma protein. J Virol 1990;64:1353–1356.
91. Ray FA, Peabody DS, Cooper JL, et al. SV40 T antigen alone drives karyotype instability that precedes neoplastic transformation of human diploid fibroblasts. J Cell Biochem 1990; 42:13–31.
92. Stewart N, Bacchetti S. Expression of SV40 large T antigen, but not small t antigen, is required for the induction of chromosomal aberrations in transformed human cells. Virology 1991; 180:49–57.
93. Neel JV, Major EO, Awa AA, et al. Hypothesis: "Rogue cell"-type chromosomal damage in lymphocytes is associated with infection with the JC human polyoma virus and has implications for oncogenesis. Proc Natl Acad Sci USA 1996;93: 2690–2695.
94. Trabanelli C, Corallini A, Gruppioni R, et al. Chromosomal aberrations induced by BK virus T antigen in human fibroblasts. Virology 1998;243:492–496.

95. Simmons DT, Melendy T, Usher D, et al. Simian virus 40 large T antigen binds to topoisomerase I. Virology 1996;222:365–374.
96. Dean FB, Bullock P, Murakami Y, et al. Simian virus 40 (SV40) DNA replication: SV40 large T antigen unwinds DNA containing the SV40 origin of replication. Proc Natl Acad Sci USA 1987;84:16–20.
97. Rundell K, Parakati R. The role of the SV40 small t antigen in cell growth promotion and transformation. Semin Cancer Biol 2001;11:5–13.
98. Pallas DC, Shahrik LK, Martin BL, et al. Polyoma small and middle T antigens and SV40 small t antigen form stable complexes with protein phosphatase 2A. Cell 1990;60:167–176.
99. Baysal BE, Farr JE, Goss JR, et al. Genomic organization and precise physical location of protein phosphatase 2A regulatory subunit A beta isoform gene on chromosome band 11q23. Gene Amst 1998;217:107–116.
100. Wang SS, Esplin ED, Li JL, et al. Alterations of the PPP2R1B gene in human lung and colon cancer. Science 1998;282: 284–287.
101. Calin GA, di Iasio MG, Caprini E, et al. Low frequency of alterations of the alpha (PPP2R1A) and beta (PPP2R1B) isoforms of the subunit A of the serine-threonine phosphatase 2A in human neoplasms. Oncogene 2000;19:1191–1195.
102. Beck GRJ, Zerler BR, Moran E. Introduction to DNA tumor viruses: adenovirus, simian virus 40, and polyomavirus. In: McCance DJ (ed). Human Tumor Viruses. Washington, DC: Ameican Society for Microbiology (ASM) Press, 1998:51–86.
103. Flaegstad T, Andresen PA, Johnsen JI, et al. A possible contributory role of BK virus infection in neuroblastoma development. Cancer Res 1999;59:1160–1163.
104. Monini P, Rotola A, de Lellis L, et al. Latent BK virus infection and Kaposi's sarcoma pathogenesis. Int J Cancer 1996;66: 717–722.
105. Rencic A, Gordon J, Otte J, et al. Detection of JC virus DNA sequence and expression of the viral oncoprotein, tumor antigen, in brain of immunocompetent patient with oligoastrocytoma. Proc Natl Acad Sci USA 1996;93:7352–7357.
106. Krynska B, Del Valle L, Croul S, et al. Detection of human neurotropic JC virus DNA sequence and expression of the viral oncogenic protein in pediatric medulloblastomas. Proc Natl Acad Sci USA 1999;96:11519–11524.
107. Del Valle L, Gordon J, Ferrante P, et al. Jc virus in experimental and clinical brain tumorigenesis. In: Khalili K, Stoner G (eds). Human Polyomaviruses. New York: Wiley-Liss, 2001:409–430.
108. Khalili K, Del Valle L, Otte J, et al. Human neurotropic polyomavirus, JCV, and its role in carcinogenesis. Oncogene 2003; 22:5181–5191.
109. Laghi L, Randolph AE, Chauhan DP, et al. JC virus DNA is present in the mucosa of the human colon and in colorectal cancers. Proc Natl Acad Sci USA 1999;96:7484–7489.
110. Ricciardiello L, Chang DK, Laghi L, et al. Mad-1 is the exclusive JC virus strain present in the human colon, and its transcriptional control region has a deleted 98-base-pair sequence in colon cancer tissues. J Virol 2001;75:1996–2001.
111. Ricciardiello L, Baglioni M, Giovannini C, et al. Induction of chromosomal instability in colonic cells by the human polyomavirus JC through a hit and run mechanism. Cancer Res 2003;63(21):7256–7262.
112. Enam S, Del Valle L, Lara C, et al. Association of human polyomavirus JCV with colon cancer: evidence for interaction of viral T-antigen and beta-catenin. Cancer Res 2002;62: 7093–7101.
113. Jasani B, Cristaudo A, Emri SA, et al. Association of SV40 with human tumours. Semin Cancer Biol 2001;11:49–61.
114. Garcea RL, Imperiale MJ. Simian virus 40 infection of humans. J Virol 2003;77:5039–5045.
115. Vilchez RA, Butel JS. SV40 in human brain cancers and non-Hodgkin's lymphoma. Oncogene 2003;22:5164–5172.
116. Barbanti-Brodano G, Sabbioni S, Martini F, et al. Simian virus 40 infection in humans and association with human diseases: results and hypotheses.Virology, 2004;318(1):1–9.
117. Shah KV. Does SV40 infection contribute to the development of human cancers? Rev Med Virol 2000;10:31–43.
118. Stratton K, Almario DA, McCormick MC, eds. Immunization safety review: SV40 contamination of polio vaccine and cancer. Institute of Medicine of the National Academies. Washington, DC: National Academic Press, 2002.
119. Klein G, Powers A, Croce C. Association of SV40 with human tumors. Oncogene 2002;21:1141–1149.
120. Reinartz JJ. Cancer genes. In: Coleman W, Tsongalis GJ (eds). The Molecular Basis of Human Cancer. Totowa, NJ: Humana Press, 2002:45–64.
121. Lengauer C, Kinzler KW, Vogelstein B. Genetic instabilities in human cancers. Nature (Lond) 1998;396:643–649.
122. Coleman W, Tsongalis GJ. The role of genomic instability in the development of human cancer. In: Coleman W, Tonsgalis GJ (eds). The Molecular Basis of Human Cancer. Totowa, NJ: Humana Press, 2002:115–142.
123. Tzeng YJ, Zimmermann C, Guhl E, et al. SV40 T/t-antigen induces premature mammary gland involution by apoptosis and selects for p53 missense mutation in mammary tumors. Oncogene 1998;16:2103–2114.
124. Salewski H, Bayer TA, Eidhoff U, et al. Increased oncogenicity of subclones of SV40 large T-induced neuroectodermal tumor cell lines after loss of large T expression and concomitant mutation in p53. Cancer Res 1999;59:1980–1986.
125. Cacciotti P, Libener R, Betta P, et al. SV40 replication in human mesothelial cells induces HGF/Met receptor activation: a model for viral-related carcinogenesis of human malignant mesothelioma. Proc Natl Acad Sci USA 2001;98:12032–12037.
126. Cacciotti P, Strizzi L, Vianale G, et al. The presence of simian-virus 40 sequences in mesothelioma and mesothelial cells is associated with high levels of vascular endothelial growth factor. Am J Respir Cell Mol Biol 2002;26:189–193.
127. Catalano A, Romano M, Martinotti S, et al. Enhanced expression of vascular endothelial growth factor (VEGF) plays a critical role in the tumor progression potential induced by simian virus 40 large T antigen. Oncogene 2002;21:2896–2900.
128. Carbone M, Pass HI, Miele L, et al. New developments about the association of SV40 with human mesothelioma. Oncogene 2003;22:5173–5180.
129. Carbone M, Rizzo P, Grimley PM, et al. Simian virus-40 large-T antigen binds p53 in human mesotheliomas. Nat Med 1997; 3:908–912.
130. De Luca A, Baldi A, Esposito V, et al. The retinoblastoma gene family pRb/p105, p107, pRb2/p130 and simian virus-40 large T-antigen in human mesotheliomas. Nat Med 1997;3:913–916.
131. Waheed I, Guo ZS, Chen GA, et al. Antisense to SV40 early gene region induces growth arrest and apoptosis in T-antigen-positive human pleural mesothelioma cells. Cancer Res 1999;59: 6068–6073.
132. Shivapurkar N, Wiethege T, Wistuba II, et al. Presence of simian virus 40 sequences in malignant mesotheliomas and mesothelial cell proliferations. J Cell Biochem 1999;76:181–188.
133. Bocchetta M, Miele L, Pass HI, et al. Notch-1 induction, a novel activity of SV40 required for growth of SV40-transformed human mesothelial cells. Oncogene 2003;22:81–89.
134. Weijzen S, Rizzo P, Braid M, et al. Activation of Notch-1 signaling maintains the neoplastic phenotype in human Ras-transformed cells. Nat Med 2002;8:979–986.
135. Bocchetta M, Di Resta I, Powers A, et al. Human mesothelial cells are unusually susceptible to simian virus 40-mediated transformation and asbestos cocarcinogenicity. Proc Natl Acad Sci USA 2000;97:10214–10219.
136. Gazdar AF, Butel JS, Carbone M. SV40 and human tumours: myth, association or causality? Nat Rev Cancer 2002;2:957–964.

137. Foddis R, De Rienzo A, Broccoli D, et al. SV40 infection induces telomerase activity in human mesothelial cells. Oncogene 2002;21:1434–1442.
138. Vilchez RA, Kozinetz CA, Butel JS. Conventional epidemiology and the link between SV40 and human cancers. Lancet Oncol 2003;4:188–191.
139. Cerni C, Seelos C. Papillomaviruses as promoting agents in human epithelial tumors. In: Barbanti-Brodano G, Bendinelli M, Friedman H (eds). DNA Tumor Viruses: Oncogenic Mechanisms. New York: Plenum Press, 1995:123–155.
140. zur Hausen H. Papillomaviruses in human cancers. In: Goedert J (ed). Infectious Causes of Cancer. Totowa, NJ: Humana Press, 2000:245–261.
141. Bosch FX, Lorincz A, Munoz N, et al. The causal relation between human papillomavirus and cervical cancer. J Clin Pathol 2002;55:244–265.
142. Leigh IM, Brener JA, Buchanan JAG. Human papilloma viruses and cancers of the skin and oral mucosa. In: Goedert J (ed). Infectious Causes of Cancer. Totowa, NJ: Humana Press, 2000: 289–309.
143. zur Hausen H. Papillomaviruses and cancer: from basic studies to clinical application. Nat Rev Cancer 2002;2:342–350.
144. Phillips AC, Vousden KH. Human papillomavirus and cancer: the viral transforming genes. In: Newton R, Beral V, Weiss RA (eds). Infections and Human Cancer. Cold Spring Harbor, NY: Cold Spring Harbor Laboratory Press, 1999:55–74.
145. Munger K, Phelps WC, Bubb V, et al. The E6 and E7 genes of the human papillomavirus type 16 together are necessary and sufficient for transformation of primary human keratinocytes. J Virol 1989;63:4417–4421.
146. Hawley-Nelson P, Vousden KH, Hubbert NL, et al. HPV16 E6 and E7 proteins cooperate to immortalize human foreskin keratinocytes. EMBO J 1989;8:3905–3910.
147. Woodworth CD, DiPaolo JA. Immortalization of keratinocytes by human papillomaviruses. In: Barbanti-Brodano G, Bendinelli M, Friedman H (eds). DNA Tumor Viruses: Oncogenic Mechanisms. New York: Plenum Press, 1995:91–109.
148. Scheffner M, Werness BA, Huibregtse JM, et al. The E6 oncoprotein encoded by human papillomavirus types 16 and 18 promotes the degradation of p53. Cell 1990;63:1129–1136.
149. Scheffner M, Huibregtse JM, Vierstra RD, et al. The HPV-16 E6 and E6-AP complex functions as a ubiquitin-protein ligase in the ubiquitination of p53. Cell 1993;75:495–505.
150. Klingelhutz AJ, Foster SA, McDougall JK. Telomerase activation by the E6 gene product of human papillomavirus type 16. Nature (Lond) 1996;380:79–82.
151. Keen N, Elston R, Crawford L. Interaction of the E6 protein of human papillomavirus with cellular proteins. Oncogene 1994;9: 1493–1499.
152. Chen JJ, Reid CE, Band V, et al. Interaction of papillomavirus E6 oncoproteins with a putative calcium-binding protein. Science 1995;269:529–531.
153. Tong X, Howley PM. The bovine papillomavirus E6 oncoprotein interacts with paxillin and disrupts the actin cytoskeleton. Proc Natl Acad Sci USA 1997;94:4412–4417.
154. Kiyono T, Hiraiwa A, Fujita M, et al. Binding of high-risk human papillomavirus E6 oncoproteins to the human homologue of the Drosophila discs large tumor suppressor protein. Proc Natl Acad Sci USA 1997;94:11612–11616.
155. Lee SS, Weiss RS, Javier RT. Binding of human virus oncoproteins to hDlg/SAP97, a mammalian homolog of the Drosophila discs large tumor suppressor protein. Proc Natl Acad Sci USA 1997;94:6670–6675.
156. Desaintes C, Hallez S, Van Alphen P, et al. Transcriptional activation of several heterologous promoters by the E6 protein of human papillomavirus type 16. J Virol 1992;66:325–333.
157. Elbel M, Carl S, Spaderna S, et al. A comparative analysis of the interactions of the E6 proteins from cutaneous and genital papillomaviruses with p53 and E6AP in correlation to their transforming potential. Virology 1997;239:132–149.
158. Munger K, Phelps WC. The human papillomavirus E7 protein as a transforming and transactivating factor. Biochim Biophys Acta 1993;1155:111–123.
159. Weinberg RA. The retinoblastoma protein and cell cycle control. Cell 1995;81:323–330.
160. La Thangue NB. DRTF1/E2F: an expanding family of heterodimeric transcription factors implicated in cell-cycle control. Trends Biochem Sci 1994;19:108–114.
161. Huang PS, Patrick DR, Edwards G, et al. Protein domains governing interactions between E2F, the retinoblastoma gene product, and human papillomavirus type 16 E7 protein. Mol Cell Biol 1993;13:953–960.
162. Boyer SN, Wazer DE, Band V. E7 protein of human papilloma virus-16 induces degradation of retinoblastoma protein through the ubiquitin-proteasome pathway. Cancer Res 1996;56:4620–4624.
163. Funk JO, Waga S, Harry JB, et al. Inhibition of CDK activity and PCNA-dependent DNA replication by p21 is blocked by interaction with the HPV-16 E7 oncoprotein. Genes Dev 1997;11: 2090–2100.
164. Jones DL, Alani RM, Munger K. The human papillomavirus E7 oncoprotein can uncouple cellular differentiation and proliferation in human keratinocytes by abrogating p21Cip1-mediated inhibition of cdk2. Genes Dev 1997;11:2101–2111.
165. Edmonds C, Vousden KH. A point mutational analysis of human papillomavirus type 16 E7 protein. J Virol 1989;63:2650–2656.
166. Banks L, Edmonds C, Vousden KH. Ability of the HPV16 E7 protein to bind RB and induce DNA synthesis is not sufficient for efficient transforming activity in NIH3T3 cells. Oncogene 1990;5:1383–1389.
167. Phelps WC, Munger K, Yee CL, et al. Structure-function analysis of the human papillomavirus type 16 E7 oncoprotein. J Virol 1992;66:2418–2427.
168. White AE, Livanos EM, Tlsty TD. Differential disruption of genomic integrity and cell cycle regulation in normal human fibroblasts by the HPV oncoproteins. Genes Dev 1994;8: 666–677.
169. Antinore MJ, Birrer MJ, Patel D, et al. The human papillomavirus type 16 E7 gene product interacts with and transactivates the AP1 family of transcription factors. EMBO J 1996; 15:1950–1960.
170. Massimi P, Pim D, Storey A, et al. HPV-16 E7 and adenovirus E1a complex formation with TATA box binding protein is enhanced by casein kinase II phosphorylation. Oncogene 1996; 12:2325–2330.
171. Choo KB, Chong KY. Absence of mutation in the p53 and the retinoblastoma susceptibility genes in primary cervical carcinomas. Virology 1993;193:1042–1046.
172. Lee YY, Wilczynski SP, Chumakov A, et al. Carcinoma of the vulva: HPV and p53 mutations. Oncogene 1994;9:1655–1659.
173. Crook T, Wrede D, Tidy JA, et al. Clonal p53 mutation in primary cervical cancer: association with human-papillomavirus-negative tumours. Lancet 1992;339:1070–1073.
174. Herrero R, Munoz N. Human papillomavirus and cancer. In: Newton R, Beral V, Weiss RA (eds). Infections and Human Cancer. Cancer Surveys, vol 33. Cold Spring Harbor, NY: Cold Spring Harbor Laboratory Press, 1999:75–98.
175. Jackson ME, Campo MS. Cooperation between bovine papillomaviruses and dietary carcinogens in cancers of cattle. In: Barbanti-Brodano G, Bendinelli M, Friedman H (eds). DNA Tumor Viruses: Oncogenic Mechanisms. New York: Plenum Press, 1995:111–122.
176. Di Luca D, Caselli E, Cassai E. Herpes simplex virus as a cooperating agent in human genital carcinogenesis. In: Barbanti-Brodano G, Bendinelli M, Friedman H (eds). DNA Tumor

Viruses: Oncogenic Mechanisms. New York: Plenum Press, 1995:281–293.
177. Lee WM. Hepatitis B virus infection. N Engl J Med 1997;337: 1733–1745.
178. Lau JY, Wright TL. Molecular virology and pathogenesis of hepatitis B. Lancet 1993;342:1335–1340.
179. Buendia MA, Pineau P. The complex role of hepatitis B virus in human hepatocarcinogenesis. In: Barbanti-Brodano G, Bendinelli M, Friedmam H (eds). DNA Tumor viruses: oncogenic Mechanisms. New York: Plenum Press, 1995:171–193.
180. Wild CP, Hall AJ. Hepatitis B virus and liver cancer: unanswered questions. In: Newton R, Beral V, Weiss RA (eds). Infections and Human Cancer. Cold Spring Harbor, NY: Cold Spring Harbor Laboratory Press, 1999:35–54.
181. Kao JH, Chen DS. Overview of hepatitis B and C viruses. In: Goedert JJ (ed). Infectious Causes of Cancer. Totowa, NJ: Humana Press, 2000:313–330.
182. Block TM, Mehta AS, Fimmel CJ, et al. Molecular viral oncology of hepatocellular carcinoma. Oncogene 2003;22:5093–5107.
183. Beasley RP. Hepatitis B virus. The major etiology of hepatocellular carcinoma. Cancer (Phila) 1988;61:1942–1956.
184. Grisham JW. Molecular genetic alterations in primary hepatocellular neoplasms. In: Coleman W, Tsongalis GJ (eds). The Molecular Basis of Human Cancer. Totowa, NJ: Humana Press, 2002:269–346.
185. Dejean A, Bougueleret L, Grzeschik KH, et al. Hepatitis B virus DNA integration in a sequence homologous to v-erb-A and steroid receptor genes in a hepatocellular carcinoma. Nature (Lond) 1986;322:70–72.
186. Wang J, Zindy F, Chenivesse X, et al. Modification of cyclin A expression by hepatitis B virus DNA integration in a hepatocellular carcinoma. Oncogene 1992;7:1653–1656.
187. Shirakata Y, Kawada M, Fujiki Y, et al. The X gene of hepatitis B virus induced growth stimulation and tumorigenic transformation of mouse NIH3T3 cells. Jpn J Cancer Res 1989;80: 617–621.
188. Hohne M, Schaefer S, Seifer M, et al. Malignant transformation of immortalized transgenic hepatocytes after transfection with hepatitis B virus DNA. EMBO J 1990;9:1137–1145.
189. Kim CM, Koike K, Saito I, et al. HBX gene of hepatitis B virus induces liver cancer in transgenic mice. Nature (Lond) 1991;351:317–320.
190. Feitelson MA, Zhu M, Duan LX, et al. Hepatitis B X antigen and p53 are associated in vitro and in liver tissues from patients with primary hepatocellular carcinoma. Oncogene 1993;8:1109–1117.
191. Wang XW, Forrester K, Yeh H, et al. Hepatitis B virus X protein inhibits p53 sequence-specific DNA binding, transcriptional activity, and association with transcription factor ERCC3. Proc Natl Acad Sci USA 1994;91:2230–2234.
192. Wang XW, Gibson MK, Vermeulen W, et al. Abrogation of p53-induced apoptosis by the hepatitis B virus X gene. Cancer Res 1995;55:6012–6016.
193. Ueda H, Ullrich SJ, Gangemi JD, et al. Functional inactivation but not structural mutation of p53 causes liver cancer. Nat Genet 1995;9:41–47.
194. Takada S, Kaneniwa N, Tsuchida N, et al. Cytoplasmic retention of the p53 tumor suppressor gene product is observed in the hepatitis B virus X gene-transfected cells. Oncogene 1997;15: 1895–1901.
195. Lee TH, Elledge SJ, Butel JS. Hepatitis B virus X protein interacts with a probable cellular DNA repair protein. J Virol 1995; 69:1107–1114.
196. Hildt E, Hofschneider PH, Urban S. The role of hepatitis B virus (HBV) in the development of hepatocellular carcinoma. Semin Virol 1996;7:333–347.
197. Chisari FV, Klopchin K, Moriyama T, et al. Molecular pathogenesis of hepatocellular carcinoma in hepatitis B virus transgenic mice. Cell 1989;59:1145–1156.
198. Chisari FV, Ferrari C. Hepatitis B virus immunopathogenesis. Annu Rev Immunol 1995;13:29–60.
199. Jhappan C, Stahle C, Harkins RN, et al. TGF alpha overexpression in transgenic mice induces liver neoplasia and abnormal development of the mammary gland and pancreas. Cell 1990; 61:1137–1146.
200. Lieber CS, Garro A, Leo MA, et al. Alcohol and cancer. Hepatology 1986;6:1005–1019.
201. Luscombe CA, Locarnini SA. The mechanism of action of antiviral agents in chronic hepatitis B. Virol Hepatol Rev 1996;2:1–35.
202. Fiume L, Di Stefano G, Busi C, et al. Liver targeting of antiviral nucleoside analogues through the asialoglycoprotein receptor. J Viral Hepatol 1997;4:363–370.
203. Hayashi J, Kishihara Y, Yamaji K, et al. Hepatitis C viral quasispecies and liver damage in patients with chronic hepatitis C virus infection. Hepatology 1997;25:697–701.
204. Purcell R. The hepatitis C virus: overview. Hepatology 1997; 26:11S–14S.
205. Bendinelli M, Vatteroni ML, Maggi F, et al. Hepatitis C virus. In: Specter S (ed). Viral Hepatitis: Diagnosis, Therapy, and Prevention. Totowa, NJ: Humana Press, 1999:65–127.
206. Farci P, Alter HJ, Govindarajan S, et al. Lack of protective immunity against reinfection with hepatitis C virus. Science 1992; 258:135–140.
207. Di Bisceglie AM. Hepatitis C and hepatocellular carcinoma. In: Hoofnagle JH (ed). Hepatitis C. New York: Academic Press, 2000:265–275.
208. Di Bisceglie AM, Order SE, Klein JL, et al. The role of chronic viral hepatitis in hepatocellular carcinoma in the United States. Am J Gastroenterol 1991;86:335–338.
209. Nelson DR, Lau JYN. Pathogenesis of hepatocellular damage in chronic hepatitis C virus infection. Clin Liver Dis 1997;1: 515–527.
210. De Mitri MS, Poussin K, Baccarini P, et al. HCV-associated liver cancer without cirrhosis. Lancet 1995;345:413–415.
211. Sakamuro D, Furukawa T, Takegami T. Hepatitis C virus nonstructural protein NS3 transforms NIH 3T3 cells. J Virol 1995; 69:3893–3896.
212. Ray RB, Meyer K, Ray R. Suppression of apoptotic cell death by hepatitis C virus core protein. Virology 1996;226:176–182.
213. Ray RB, Lagging LM, Meyer K, et al. Hepatitis C virus core protein cooperates with ras and transforms primary rat embryo fibroblasts to tumorigenic phenotype. J Virol 1996;70: 4438–4443.
214. Moriya K, Fujie H, Shintani Y, et al. The core protein of hepatitis C virus induces hepatocellular carcinoma in transgenic mice. Nat Med 1998;4:1065–1067.
215. Agnello V. Mixed cryoglobulinemia and other extrahepatic manifestations of hepatitis C virus infection. In: Hoofnagle JH (ed). Hepatitis C. New York: Academic Press, 2000:295–313.
216. Ferri C, Pileri S, Zignego AL. Hepatitis C virus, B-cell disorders and non-Hodgkin's lymphoma. In: Goedert J (ed). Infectious Causes of Cancer. Totowa, NJ: Humana Press, 2000:349–368.
217. De Vita S, Sacco C, Sansonno D, et al. Characterization of overt B-cell lymphomas in patients with hepatitis C virus infection. Blood 1997;90:776–782.
218. De Vita S, Sansonno D, Dolcetti R, et al. Hepatitis C virus within a malignant lymphoma lesion in the course of type II mixed cryoglobulinemia. Blood 1995;86:1887–1892.
219. Ascoli V, Lo Coco F, Artini M, et al. Extranodal lymphomas associated with hepatitis C virus infection. Am J Clin Pathol 1998; 109:600–609.
220. De Vita S, Zagonel V, Russo A, et al. Hepatitis C virus, non-Hodgkin's lymphomas and hepatocellular carcinoma. Br J Cancer 1998;77:2032–2035.
221. Tajima K, Takezaki T. Human T cell leukemia virus type I. In: Newton R, Beral V, Weiss RA (eds). Infections and Human

Cancer. Cancer Surveys, vol 33. Cold Spring Harbor, NY: Cold Spring Harbor Laboratory Press, 1999:191–211.

222. Matsuoka M. Human T-cell leukemia virus type I and adult T-cell leukemia. Oncogene 2003;22:5131–5140.
223. Rosenblatt JD, Golde DW, Wachsman W, et al. A second isolate of HTLV-II associated with atypical hairy-cell leukemia. N Engl J Med 1986;315:372–377.
224. Yoshida M, Miyoshi I, Hinuma Y. Isolation and characterization of retrovirus from cell lines of human adult T-cell leukemia and its implication in the disease. Proc Natl Acad Sci USA 1982;79:2031–2035.
225. Matsuoka M. Adult T-cell leukemia/lymphoma. In: Goedert J (ed). Infectious Causes of Cancer. Totowa, NJ: Humana Press, 2000:211–229.
226. Gatza ML, Watt JC, Marriott SJ. Cellular transformation by the HTLV-I Tax protein, a jack-of-all-trades. Oncogene 2003;22:5141–5149.
227. Greene WC, Leonard WJ, Wano Y, et al. Trans-activator gene of HTLV-II induces IL-2 receptor and IL-2 cellular gene expression. Science 1986;232:877–880.
228. Maruyama M, Shibuya H, Harada H, et al. Evidence for aberrant activation of the interleukin-2 autocrine loop by HTLV-1-encoded p40x and T3/Ti complex triggering. Cell 1987;48:343–350.
229. Fujii M, Tsuchiya H, Chuhjo T, et al. Interaction of HTLV-1 Tax1 with p67SRF causes the aberrant induction of cellular immediate early genes through CArG boxes. Genes Dev 1992;6:2066–2076.
230. Franchini G. Molecular mechanisms of human T-cell leukemia/lymphotropic virus type I infection. Blood 1995;86:3619–3639.
231. Jeang KT, Widen SG, Semmes OJ 4th, et al. HTLV-I trans-activator protein, tax, is a trans-repressor of the human beta-polymerase gene. Science 1990;247:1082–1084.
232. Lemasson I, Robert-Hebmann V, Hamaia S, et al. Transrepression of lck gene expression by human T-cell leukemia virus type 1-encoded p40tax. J Virol 1997;71:1975–1983.
233. Suzuki T, Kitano S, Matsushime H, et al. HTLV-I Tax protein interacts with cyclin-dependent kinase inhibitor p16 INK4A and counteracts its inhibitory activity towards CDK4. EMBO J 1995;7:1607–1614.
234. Pise-Masison CA, Choi KS, Radonovich M, et al. Inhibition of p53 transactivation function by the human T-cell lymphotropic virus type 1 Tax protein. J Virol 1998;72:1165–1170.
235. Jin DY, Spencer F, Jeang KT. Human T cell leukemia virus type 1 oncoprotein Tax targets the human mitotic checkpoint protein MAD1. Cell 1998;93:81–91.
236. Miyake H, Suzuki T, Hirai H, et al. Trans-activator Tax of human T-cell leukemia virus type 1 enhances mutation frequency of the cellular genome. Virology 1999;253:155–161.
237. Scadden DT. AIDS-related malignancies. Annu Rev Med 2003;54:285–303.
238. Caputo A, Betti M, Boarini C, et al. Mutiple functions of human immunodeficiency virus type 1 Tat protein in the pathogenesis of AIDS. Recent Res Dev Virol 1999;1:753–771.
239. Barillari G, Ensoli B. Angiogenic effects of extracellular human immunodeficiency virus type 1 Tat protein and its role in the pathogenesis of AIDS-associated Kaposi's sarcoma. Clin Microbiol Rev 2002;15:310–326.
240. Helland DE, Welles JL, Caputo A, et al. Transcellular transactivation by the human immunodeficiency virus type 1 tat protein. J Virol 1991;65:4547–4549.
241. Ensoli B, Buonaguro L, Barillari G, et al. Release, uptake, and effects of extracellular human immunodeficiency virus type 1 Tat protein on cell growth and viral transactivation. J Virol 1993;67:277–287.
242. Chang HC, Samaniego F, Nair BC, et al. HIV-1 Tat protein exits from cells via a leaderless secretory pathway and binds to extracellular matrix-associated heparan sulfate proteoglycans through its basic region. AIDS 1997;11:1421–1431.
243. Corallini A, Campioni D, Rossi C, et al. Promotion of tumour metastases and induction of angiogenesis by native HIV-1 Tat protein from BK virus/tat transgenic mice. AIDS 1996;10:701–710.
244. Ensoli B, Gendelman R, Markham P, et al. Synergy between basic fibroblast growth factor and HIV-1 Tat protein in induction of Kaposi's sarcoma. Nature (Lond) 1994;371:674–680.
245. Kim CM, Vogel J, Jay G, et al. The HIV tat gene transforms human keratinocytes. Oncogene 1992;7:1525–1529.
246. Flores SC, Marecki JC, Harper KP, et al. Tat protein of human immunodeficiency virus type 1 represses expression of manganese superoxide dismutase in HeLa cells. Proc Natl Acad Sci USA 1993;90:7632–7636.
247. Church SL, Grant JW, Meese EU, et al. Sublocalization of the gene encoding manganese superoxide dismutase (MnSOD/SOD2) to 6q25 by fluorescence in situ hybridization and somatic cell hybrid mapping. Genomics 1992;14:823–825.
248. Church SL, Grant JW, Ridnour LA, et al. Increased manganese superoxide dismutase expression suppresses the malignant phenotype of human melanoma cells. Proc Natl Acad Sci USA 1993;90:3113–3117.
249. Li CJ, Wang C, Friedman DJ, et al. Reciprocal modulations between p53 and Tat of human immunodeficiency virus type 1. Proc Natl Acad Sci USA 1995;92:5461–5464.
250. Longo F, Marchetti MA, Castagnoli L, et al. A novel approach to protein–protein interaction: complex formation between the p53 tumor suppressor and the HIV Tat proteins. Biochem Biophys Res Commun 1995;206:326–334.
251. Westendorp MO, Li-Weber M, Frank RW, et al. Human immunodeficiency virus type 1 Tat upregulates interleukin-2 secretion in activated T cells. J Virol 1994;68:4177–4185.
252. Zauli G, Gibellini D. The human immunodeficiency virus type-1 (HIV-1) Tat protein and Bcl-2 gene expression. Leuk Lymphoma 1996;23:551–560.
253. Scala G, Ruocco MR, Ambrosino C, et al. The expression of the interleukin 6 gene is induced by the human immunodeficiency virus 1 TAT protein. J Exp Med 1994;179:961–971.
254. Ambrosino C, Ruocco MR, Chen X, et al. HIV-1 Tat induces the expression of the interleukin-6 (IL6) gene by binding to the IL6 leader RNA and by interacting with CAAT enhancer-binding protein beta (NF-IL6) transcription factors. J Biol Chem 1997;272:14883–14892.
255. Corallini A, Altavilla G, Pozzi L, et al. Systemic expression of HIV-1 tat gene in transgenic mice induces endothelial proliferation and tumors of different histotypes. Cancer Res 1993;53:5569–5575.
256. Altavilla G, Trabanelli C, Merlin M, et al. Morphological, histochemical, immunohistochemical, and ultrastructural characterization of tumors and dysplastic and non-neoplastic lesions arising in BK virus/tat transgenic mice. Am J Pathol 1999;154:1231–1244.
257. Altavilla G, Caputo A, Lanfredi M, et al. Enhancement of chemical hepatocarcinogenesis by the HIV-1 tat gene. Am J Pathol 2000;157:1081–1089.
258. Altavilla G, Caputo A, Trabanelli C, et al. Prevalence of liver tumours in HIV-1 tat-transgenic mice treated with urethane. Eur J Cancer 2004;40(2):275–283.
259. Chang MH, Chen CJ, Lai MS, et al. Universal hepatitis B vaccination in Taiwan and the incidence of hepatocellular carcinoma in children. Taiwan Childhood Hepatoma Study Group. N Engl J Med 1997;336:1855–1859.
260. Kong Q, Richter L, Yang YF, et al. Oral immunization with hepatitis B surface antigen expressed in transgenic plants. Proc Natl Acad Sci USA 2001;98:11539–11544.
261. Schiller JT, Lowy DR. Papillomavirus-like particles and HPV vaccine development. Semin Cancer Biol 1996;7:373–382.

262. Tindle RW. Human papillomavirus vaccines for cervical cancer. Curr Opin Immunol 1996;8:643–650.
263. Epstein MA, Morgan AJ, Finerty S, et al. Protection of cotton-top tamarins against Epstein-Barr virus-induced malignant lymphoma by a prototype subunit vaccine. Nature (Lond) 1985;318:287–289.
264. Morgan AJ. The development of Epstein-Barr virus vaccines. In: Barbanti-Brodano G, Bendinelli M, Friedmam H (eds). DNA Tumor Viruses: Oncogenic Mechanisms. New York: Plenum Press, 1995:395–419.
265. Xie YC, Hwang C, Overwijk W, et al. Induction of tumor antigen-specific immunity in vivo by a novel vaccinia vector encoding safety-modified simian virus 40 T antigen. J Natl Cancer Inst 1999;91:169–175.
266. Saenz-Robles MT, Sullivan CS, Pipas JM. Transforming functions of simian virus 40. Oncogene 2001;20:7899–7907.
267. Imperiale MJ, Pass HI, Sanda MG. Prospects for an SV40 vaccine. Semin Cancer Biol 2001;11:81–85.
268. Cafaro A, Caputo A, Fracasso C, et al. Control of SHIV-89.6P-infection of cynomolgus monkeys by HIV-1 Tat protein vaccine. Nat Med 1999;5:643–650.
269. Pauza CD, Trivedi P, Wallace M, et al. Vaccination with tat toxoid attenuates disease in simian/HIV-challenged macaques. Proc Natl Acad Sci USA 2000;97:3515–3519.

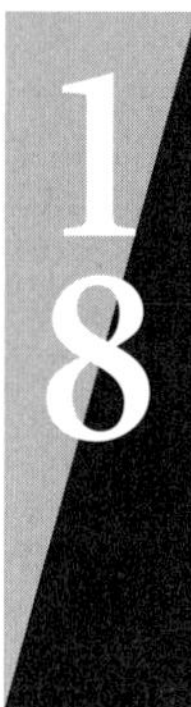

Environmental Carcinogenesis

T. Sabo-Attwood, M. Ramos-Nino, and Brooke T. Mossman

Environmental carcinogens are broadly defined as compounds that humans are exposed to through diet, lifestyle, infectious agents, and occupation.[1] They are considered as nongenetic factors that contribute to cancer risk. A subset of *known* and *reasonably anticipated* human carcinogens can be classified as environmental carcinogens and include such compounds as dioxins, metals, components of pesticides, the polyaromatic hydrocarbon (PAH) benzo(*a*)pyrene (BaP), and mineral fibers such as erionite and asbestos[2] (Table 18.1). These contaminants are major constituents of indoor and outdoor air pollution, water, soil, and food products.

Criteria for deciding whether a substance is a carcinogen are constantly being modified as technology and our understanding of carcinogenesis evolve. Definitively linking exposure to environmental contaminants and cancer is difficult because parameters such as dose, duration, composition, and routes of exposure are indeterminate. Currently, the U.S. Environmental Protection Agency (EPA) relies on data from human epidemiologic, animal, and mechanistic studies to classify compounds as carcinogens. Individually, these approaches have limitations, and therefore, these assays should complement each other in defining which compounds have the ability to cause cancer in humans.

One of the major hurdles in assessing the ability of environmental contaminants to cause disease is defining the dose of exposure. Contact with suspected compounds is commonly at low levels over long periods of time. In many cases, the latency period can last decades, masking our ability to realize the cancerous potential of compounds until many people are already sick; this is the case for asbestos-related diseases that have latency periods of greater than 20 to 40 years.[3] Thus, a causal link between exposure to asbestos and malignancies was not realized until long after thousands of people were exposed.

Another difficulty in assessing the exposure dose of compounds found in the environment is their ability to bioaccumulate in both environmental media and human tissues. Many potential carcinogens have lipophilic properties whereby smaller doses accumulate in human tissues over time.[4] Biomagnification through the food chain is also another way small doses of chemicals are amplified. For example, there is increasing concern regarding compounds termed hormonally active agents (HAA) that have the ability to act as natural hormones such as estrogen, androgens, and thyroidal proteins. Although much controversy exists regarding the carcinogenic potential of HAAs, they have been implicated in a variety of reproductive diseases including breast and prostate cancers.[5,6] Enough scientific data have convinced the EPA to mandate the testing of all active ingredients of pesticides for endocrine disrupting effects through the Food Quality Protection Act (P.L. 104–170, 1996).

It is also difficult to causally link carcinogenesis to a single compound because environmental contaminants are frequently present as complex mixtures. Interactions of a single compound with other chemicals and elements may greatly increase or decrease the carcinogenic potential to human populations.

As exposure to target compounds can vary greatly among individuals, much of the information available today regarding human cancer risk stems from occupational and accidental exposures. In these situations, information regarding the dose, composition, and duration of the exposure is readily available. A classic example is the industrial accident in Seveso, Italy, where in 1976 an explosion at an industrial plant released large quantities of 2,3,7,8-tetrachlorodibenzo-*p*-dioxin (TCDD) into the air.[7] Populations residing in the vicinity of the plant have been studied to try and elucidate the direct effect of TCDD exposure on human health, specifically the development of cancers. Although controversial, evidence from epidemiologic, animal, and mechanistic studies support the National Toxicology Program (NTP) classification of TCDD as a known human carcinogen.[8]

Mechanisms of Action of Environmental Carcinogens

Cancer is a multistage process that involves tumor initiation, promotion, and progression. Environmental carcinogens can initiate and/or advance this process by altering the expression and activity of genes crucial to biologic processes that maintain cell growth, differentiation, DNA repair, cell-cycle control, and apoptosis, among others.

In many cases, these compounds act through genetic mechanisms, interacting directly with DNA. Some are metabolically activated to reactive molecules that form covalent adducts with DNA, causing mutations in genes important to processes such as cell-cycle regulation and DNA repair.[9] Polyaromatic hydrocarbons were the first compounds shown

TABLE 18.1. **A partial list of *known* and *reasonably anticipated* human carcinogens.**

Aflatoxins
Arsenic compounds, inorganic
Asbestos
Benzene
Benzo(*a*)pyrene[a]
Cadmium and cadmium compounds
Chromium hexavalent compounds
Coal tars and coal tar pitches
Coke oven emissions
Diethylstilbestrol
Environmental tobacco smoke
Erionite
Ethylene oxide
Nickel compounds
Pesticide components: dichlorodiphenyltrichloroethane (DDT)[a]
Radon
Silica, crystalline (respirable size)
Solar radiation
Soots
2,3,7,8-Tetrachlorodibenzo-*p*-dioxin (TCDD); dioxin
Thiotepa
Wood dust

[a]All compounds that are "reasonably anticipated" human carcinogens. Compounds focused on in this chapter are denoted in boldface type.

Source: Data from the National Institute for Environmental Health Sciences NTP. Tenth Report on Carcinogens, 2002.[2]

to cause cancer (at least in part) by forming covalent adducts with DNA. The most notorious PAH historically is BaP, a compound that was isolated from coal tar in 1930 and shown to induce tumors in rodent models. It was later discovered that a reactive metabolite of BaP could form covalent adducts with DNA, resulting in altered cell growth and repair.[10]

Compounds may also act through epigenetic mechanisms whereby they do not directly alter the genome, but cause mitogenic expansion of initiated cells by modifying the expression of genes that control cell proliferation and death.[11] Changes in DNA methylation, growth factor signaling pathways, oxidative stress, and cellular communication are thought to contribute to carcinogenesis.[12,13]

Certain genes are thought to be major targets of chemical carcinogens. These genes, termed *proto-oncogenes* and *tumor repressor genes*, when mutated, allow cells to grow uncontrollably. Alterations in these types of genes have been discovered in many different types of cancers including breast, colon, and lung cancer.[9,14]

The proto-oncogenes that have been identified so far, such as *ras* and *myc*, have many different cellular functions including regulation of the cell cycle and apoptosis.[15] Mutations in these genes contribute to dysregulated cell division. The mutant proteins retain their normal functions but are no longer sensitive to the controls that regulate these processes. *ras* gene products are involved in kinase signaling pathways that regulate cell growth and differentiation. Mutations in *ras* have been implicated in organochlorine pesticide and polychlorinated biphenyl (PCB)-induced human cancers[16] and in Syrian hamster embryo cells (SHE) exposed to arsenic.[17]

One of the most well recognized tumor suppressors is *p53*. In general, tumor suppressors produce products that inhibit cell division under suboptimal conditions for growth such as DNA damage and loss of growth factors. This gene is found to be defective in about half of all tumors, regardless of their type or origin.[18,19] The mutations that inactivate *p53* may be inherited or acquired sporadically during an individual's life span.[20]

Mutations in *p53* have been observed in various cell lines exposed to environmental contaminants. For example, an increase in *p53* mutations was discovered in human breast epithelial cells (MCF) exposed to organophosphorous pesticides,[21] and in human bronchial epithelial cells by PAHs.[14] Whether environmental compounds contribute to the development of these types of cancers in humans by directly mutating *p53* or similar types of genes remains to be elucidated.

The propensity to develop cancer following environmental exposure to compounds can be increased by genetic factors. Gene polymorphisms can render individuals more susceptible to developing cancer in comparison to the average population.[22] Many of these mutations arise in metabolizing enzymes that can increase the formation of reactive compounds in the body. One of the best studied populations is cigarette smokers. Mutations in cytochrome P-450 enzymes increase the formation of reactive metabolites of BaP, a major component in cigarettes. Additionally, phase II enzymes that are required for elimination of reactive compounds have also been shown to contain mutations; this leads to DNA damage that contributes to the development of lung cancer.[23] Therefore, individuals with these mutations are at greater risk to develop cancer from cigarette smoke. Studying populations with specific polymorphisms gives us important information regarding the mechanism of action of environmental carcinogens.

Occupational Carcinogens

Occupational carcinogens, a subset of environmental carcinogens that are generally encountered at higher doses due to workplace use, are more easily detected, and exposures can be regulated. As illustrated previously, a person's risk of developing cancer is influenced by a combination of factors including genetics, the presence of certain medical conditions, diet, and personal habits (cigarette smoking and alcohol consumption). Occupational hazards, particularly coal tar fumes, asbestos, and aromatic amines, have been linked historically to cancer development.[22] According to the National Institute for Occupational Safety and Health, an estimated 20,000 cancer deaths and 40,000 new cases of cancer each year in the United States are attributable to occupation (less than 8% of all cancers). Many U.S workers are exposed to substances that have tested as carcinogens in animal studies, but less than 2% of chemicals (of a total of approximately 80,000 chemicals) in commerce have been tested for carcinogenicity.[24] When new chemicals are introduced into the U.S. market, the Toxic Substances Control Act (TSCA) requires a manufacturer or distributor to submit a premanufacture notice to the EPA 90 days before marketing. The EPA may order additional testing, including cancer bioassays. In general, chemicals are selected for testing when there is a significant human exposure or evidence suggesting potential carcinogenicity.

Identification of occupational cancers often depends on the observation of a cluster of cases. Following these initial observations, it is necessary to establish a link between the agent and the development of cancers. This phase normally is followed by a cohort study, which compares the incidence of cancers in people exposed to the suspected agent with an unexposed population or a case-controlled epidemiologic study. In the case-control study, populations with cancer are compared to those without it to determine if exposure to the suspect carcinogen occurs more frequently among people with cancers. The strengths and limitations of occupational cancer epidemiology are highlighted by Ward et al.[25] As of 1999, the International Agency for Research on Cancer (IARC) classified 38 chemicals with industrial uses as Group 1 (known human carcinogens). In addition, many other industrial chemicals are in IARC Groups 2A and 2B, indicating "probably" or "possibly" carcinogenic to humans. These classifications indicate that there is sufficient evidence for carcinogenicity in animals but less than sufficient evidence from epidemiologic studies. Most insufficient evidence is the result of appropriate cohorts for accurate epidemiologic studies.[25]

More than 3 million U.S. workers are estimated to have potential occupational exposure to agents classified by IARC as Group 1 or Group 2A or 2B.[8] Doll and Peto estimated that occupational exposures accounted for 4% of human cancers, and the majority of these cases involved lung cancers and mesotheliomas caused by asbestos exposure.[26] Other estimates range as high as 10%.[27,28] The contribution of occupational carcinogens to human cancers is exceeded only by cigarette smoking and diet.[25]

In light of the multiplicity of compounds considered environmental or occupational carcinogens, we have chosen to review a few select compounds and information on their carcinogenic potential. Initially, we discuss contaminants to which the general population is exposed in food products, water, and air pollution; these include PAHs, dioxins, pesticides, and arsenic. We then concentrate on naturally occurring durable fibers to which humans are primarily exposed in environmental and occupational settings, namely asbestos.

Polyaromatic Hydrocarbons

Polyaromatic hydrocarbons are a group of more than 100 ubiquitous environmental contaminants that occur naturally in coal, crude oil, and gasoline and are produced mainly from incomplete combustion of fossil fuels. PAHs are found in tobacco smoke, smoke from wood-burning stoves and fireplaces, and motor vehicle exhaust.[2] Additionally, smoking or charbroiling meat can increase the formation of PAHs.[29] Aside from occupational exposure, humans can potentially come into contact with PAHs through contaminated air, food, and water sources.[2]

One of the major routes of exposure to PAHs is via air pollution. It has been estimated that the daily intake for the general population of total PAHs inhaled is $207\,ng/m^3$.[30] PAHs are believed to be present in urban air absorbed to respiratory particles.[23] Once inhaled, these compounds can form covalent adducts with DNA, or are metabolized to quinones by CYP450 enzymes, namely CYP1A1, that initiates the formation of reactive oxygen species (ROS). The formation of ROS can also be stimulated by particle-induced inflammation.[31] The consequence of these actions is thought to contribute to carcinogenesis via damage to DNA, initiation of cell proliferation, or alterations in cell-cycle control.

The carcinogenic potential of PAHs has been well established for decades, and evidence to date has resulted in many of these compounds being labeled as reasonably carcinogenic.[2] The most striking data come from animal and in vitro studies of BaP, as well as occupationally exposed populations and cigarette smokers. Epidemiologic data supporting the development of cancer in the general (nonsmoking) population by inhaling these compounds is not as robust, but recent studies in conjunction with previous occupational exposure data suggest that exposure to PAHs in ambient air is a current concern. Presently, increases in markers of genotoxicity such as PAH–DNA adducts, PAH–protein adducts, cytogenetic damage, and urinary metabolites[30] have been detected in several populations exposed to air pollution containing PAHs as a major contaminant in comparison to control regions.[31] Lung tumors have also been detected in animals exposed to PAH-containing diesel exhaust.[32] Data from in vitro studies show that *c-myc* expression, adduct formation, and cell-cycle progression are altered in lung epithelial cells exposed to PAHs[33] and particulate matter containing PAH compounds.[34] Li et al.[35] showed a positive correlation between PAH content of particulate matter and the generation of ROS in rodent macrophages, whereas arsenic caused oxidative stress-induced apoptosis in rat lung epithelial cells.[36]

PAHs are also found in groundwater, usually as a result of industrial runoff into raw water supplies, and in leachates from coal tar and asphalt linings in water storage tanks and distribution lines. Overall, the levels of PAHs in drinking water supplies have been relatively low and, in general, are more abundant in food than water. A study by Kazerouni et al.[29] showed the presence of PAHs in charbroiled meats and vegetables. They suggest that PAHs in plants are directly acquired from contaminated soil and air. Although animals that ingest PAHs in their diet get stomach cancers, future studies are required to determine if human populations are at increased risk for PAH-induced cancer through dietary exposures.[2]

The genotoxic mechanisms by which PAHs initiate cancer have been extensively explored since the discovery years ago that reactive metabolites of BaP could form DNA adducts. Based on this information, current biomarkers of PAH exposure have been limited to the detection of PAH metabolites and PAH–DNA adducts in blood, urine, and various tissues.[37,38] Epigenetic mechanisms are not as well defined; however, recent studies indicate PAHs can alter cell signaling cascades that control cell communication, growth, and immune functions, which may lead to additional targets that would be useful as biomarkers of exposure. The expression of key signaling pathways including mitogen-activated protein kinase (MAPK), activator protein 1 (AP-1), nuclear factor kappa beta (NFκβ), and protein kinase C (PKC) have all been shown to be affected by PAHs. More specifically, PAH-induced activation of MAPK, which resulted in altered cellular communication via gap junctions,[39] suppressed various PKC isoforms,[40] suppressed humoral and cell-mediated immunity,[41] and induced AP-1 and NFκβ, which may be involved in tumor-promoting effects.[35] Additionally, PAHs have been shown to act through nuclear receptors, including estrogen receptors and the aryl hydrocarbon (Ah) receptor.[42,43] Deciphering which signaling pathways are involved in PAH-induced carcinogenesis is a complex task that is a current focus of researchers in the field.

Pesticides

Pesticides are a group of both natural and synthetic compounds that are used to control unwanted insects, plants, fungi, and rodents. All pesticides contain biologically active compounds that are purposely designed to interfere with normal biologic processes in target organisms. The activity of these compounds may target specific plants or animals, or they may be toxic to a wide range of species. Therefore, humans exposed to certain pesticides may be at risk to the toxic effects of these compounds, including the development of certain cancers.

Aside from individuals who come into contact with pesticides through occupational exposures, the general population is exposed to pesticides through the ingestion of food and water, by absorption through the skin, or by inhalation during application. Assessing exposure through these routes is extremely difficult because many of these factors rely on lifestyle and vary tremendously on an individual basis.

The EPA's pesticide program and other national and international bodies have classified approximately 165 pesticide chemicals as known, probable, or possible human carcinogens. Currently, there is a lack of human data to support most pesticides as being definitively carcinogenic to humans (except arsenic and ethylene oxide). However, data from animal and in vitro mechanistic studies suggest many of the main components of pesticides have the potential to cause cancer in humans and are therefore classified as probable carcinogens.[2]

Many pesticides may cause tumors by disrupting cell proliferation, apoptosis, and cell communication and inducing oxidative stress through nongenotoxic mechanisms.[12] For example, glycophosphate-based pesticides alter cell-cycle parameters in human lymphocytes.[44] In another study, different chemical classes of pesticides were shown to alter cellular proliferation by activation of erbB-2/MAPK signaling pathways.[45]

1,1,1-Trichloro-2,2-bis(*p*-chlorophenyl)-ethane (DDT) is one of the most well-studied organochlorine pesticides reasonably anticipated to be a human carcinogen.[2] Despite the banning of DDT in the United State in the early 1970s because of its adverse effects on wildlife, it is still produced in other countries.[46] DDT is an environmentally persistent compound that has been detected at high levels in air, water, soil, plants, animals, and human tissues. A great deal of controversy surrounds the carcinogenic potential of DDT. There is an abundance of in vitro data to suggest DDT is carcinogenic; however, data from human and animal studies have been inconsistent.

DDT can interfere with normal endocrine pathways and so it is suspected to contribute to the increasing incidence of breast and prostate cancers. There is also evidence of DDT-induced tissue damage through oxidative mechanisms.[47] More recently, DDT has also been shown to alter cell signaling pathways (MAPK) that regulate growth through the AP-1 transcription factor.[48] DDT also activated the oncogene *erb-B2* and MAPK phosphorylation in human prostate[45] and breast epithelial cells,[49] which correlated with cell proliferation. These results provide evidence of signaling pathways whereby environmental chemicals may alter tumorigenesis.

Arsenic

Inorganic arsenic has been known as a human carcinogen for decades. The first evidence suggesting arsenic could cause cancer occurred in 1977.[50] During this time, arsenic was being applied directly to the skin as a treatment for psoriasis, which resulted in the development of skin cancers.[51] Arsenic is released into the atmosphere from both natural and anthropogenic sources, the latter being responsible for the majority of emissions released.[51] The production of arsenic in the Unites States has been banned since 1985; however, it is still imported for use. The current concern lies in being exposed to arsenic through food and drinking water. Additionally, individuals may be exposed to arsenic compounds through air emissions from industrial facilities that manufacture pesticides, glass, and cigarette tobacco, smelting operations, and the burning of fossil fuels.[2]

Studies from around the world have linked exposure to arsenic with the formation of skin, lung, and bladder cancers. There is also increasing evidence that arsenic increases the risk of developing cancers of the kidney, liver, and colon. The majority of epidemiologic studies have focused on populations with contaminated groundwater/drinking water. Many of these populations have higher incidences of lung cancers in comparison to control populations.[52,53] More recently, there is concern that ingestion of arsenic through contaminated food sources and ambient air pollution may be additional routes of exposure.

The means by which arsenic causes cancer is not well understood. Multiple mechanisms have been proposed and include both genotoxic and nongenotoxic modes of action.[51] Arsenic does not interact with DNA, but indirectly causes chromosome aberrations, genomic instability, and aberrant DNA methylation in promoter regions of genes. In animal studies, arsenic induces the formation of ROS, which may alter regulation of DNA repair and cell-cycle progression.[54,55] The generation of ROS by arsenic can have a profound effect on signal transduction pathways. Growth factor receptors [epidermal growth factor receptor (EGFR), platelet-derived growth factor (PDGF), vascular endothelial growth factor (VEGF)], G proteins (Ras, C-src), kinases [extracellular regulated kinase (ERK), c-Jun NH_2-terminal kinase (JNK), p38], and nuclear transcription factors [NFκβ, AP-1, hypoxia-inducible factor 1 (HIF-1)] have all been suggested as targets of arsenic-induced oxidative damage through mechanisms that are still poorly understood.[56] Arsenic can also affect these pathways independent of free radical generation by direct interaction with these proteins. Alterations in these signaling pathways can have profound effects on cell proliferation, apoptosis, differentiation, and transformation.[57]

Dioxins

Dioxins are a collective group of structurally related compounds that are by-products of industrial and combustion activities such as smelting, bleaching of paper and pulp, the manufacture of some pesticides, waste incineration, and burning fuels such as wood, coal, or oil. They are also released from natural processes such as volcanic eruptions and forest fires.[2] Dioxins are found throughout the world in air, soil, water, and food sources. These compounds break down very slowly and therefore tend to bioaccumulate in the environment. Dioxins also tend to accumulate in the tissues of both mammalian and aquatic species. The major route of exposure is now thought to be via food sources.[2]

Environmental exposure to dioxins has been a concern for decades. Two of the best publicized accounts of dioxin exposure include the industrial accident in Seveso, Italy, in 1976[7] and the use of Agent Orange during the Vietnam War in the 1960s and 1970s.[58] Epidemiologic data from these incidents imply that there is sufficient evidence of an association between dioxins and various cancers including soft tissue sarcomas, lymphomas, leukemias, and Hodgkin disease.

TCDD is the most well-studied dioxin. TCDD is regarded by the NTP as a known human carcinogen (Ninth Report on Carcinogens, 2001) based on sufficient evidence from human epidemiologic and mechanistic studies. Experimental animal studies also support TCDD as a carcinogen because it produces tumors in multiple species including mice, rats, and hamsters. Mutations in the proto-oncogene *H-ras* have also been observed in TCDD-exposed animals.[59] Despite the decision of the National Institute of Environmental Health Sciences (NIEHS) to add TCDD to the list of known carcinogens, scientists argue that current scientific data suggesting the carcinogenic potential of TCDD in humans are weak and inconsistent.[60]

The best-studied mode of action of TCDD-induced carcinogenesis is via the aryl hydrocarbon (Ah) receptor. The Ah receptor controls the expression of genes containing a xenobiotic response element (XRE) in their promoters. Studies have shown activation of the Ah receptor by TCDD produces a wide spectrum of biologic responses, including altered metabolism, growth, differentiation,[61] stress, DNA repair, and motility,[62] that may contribute to carcinogenesis.

The effect of TCDD on specific signaling pathways has recently been studied. For example, the MAPK-ERK pathway has been implicated in TCDD-induced carcinogenesis through activation of tumor necrosis factor-alpha (TNF-α) and epidermal growth factor (EGF).[62] Whether activation of this pathway by dioxins is independent of the Ah receptor remains to be elucidated. New scientific approaches including gene arrays are currently being employed to gain a better understanding of the mechanisms responsible for dioxin-mediated carcinogenesis. Recently, Martinez et al.[63] showed that TCDD alters multiple integrated cell signaling pathways associated with lung cancer in human airway epithelial cells using a gene array approach.

Asbestos: General Aspects of Exposure

Asbestos, a group of naturally occurring, fibrous silicate minerals, include the serpentine mineral, chrysotile, and five amphibole minerals (actinolite, amosite, anthophyllite, crocidolite, and tremolite)[64] (Table 18.2). Chrysotile, anthophyllite, amosite, and crocidolite are the only forms that have been used commercially.[65] However, tremolite can be a contaminant in chrysotile and talc deposits, and actinolite is a common contaminant in amosite deposits.[2] Occupational exposure to chrysotile, amosite, anthophyllite, and mixtures containing crocidolite has resulted in lung carcinomas, and mesothelioma has been observed after occupational exposure to crocidolite, amosite, and, to a lesser extent, chrysotile asbestos.[66–68] Due to asbestos-related cancers in occupational settings, consumption of asbestos in the United States has been declining since 1973.[2]

Asbestos is released into the environment from natural and man-made sources and has been detected in indoor and outdoor air, soil, drinking water, food, and medicines. Significant exposure to any type of asbestos increases the risk of lung cancer, mesothelioma, and nonmalignant lung and pleural disorders, including asbestosis, pleural plaques, pleural thickening, and pleural effusions. This conclusion is based on observations of these diseases in workers with cumulative exposures ranging from about 5 to 1,200 fibers-year/mL, which results from 40 years of occupational exposure to air concentrations of 0.125 to 30 fibers/mL. These conclusions are supported by results from animal and mechanistic studies.[69]

Evidence for asbestos carcinogenicity in humans comes from epidemiologic studies as well as from numerous clinical reports on workers exposed to asbestos in a variety of occupational settings.[68,70] Most recently, tremolite asbestos exposure has been associated with an increased incidence of disease in vermiculite miners and millers from Libby, Montana. Vermiculite is a clay mineral used in concrete aggregate, fertilizer carriers, insulation, potting soil, and soil conditioners. The Libby mine opened in 1921 and at one point accounted for 80% of the world's vermiculite production. The Libby vermiculite deposit is unique in the sense that it contains an average amphibole asbestos content of 4% to 6%,[71] including tremolite and actinolite.[69] Miners, millers, and some residents of Libby were exposed to high levels of asbestos-containing dust and developed nonmalignant respi-

TABLE 18.2. Types and physicochemical properties of asbestos fibers (defined as having at least a 3:1 length-to-diameter ratio).

Type	*Composition*	*Morphology*	*Sources*
Chrysotile	$(Mg)_6(OH)_8Si_4O_{10}$ (±Fe)	Curly	95% of asbestos usage historically
Crocidolite	$Na_2(Fe^{3+})_2(Fe^{2+})_3(OH)_2Si_8O_{22}$ (±Mg)	Straight/rodlike	Mined in Australia and South Africa
Amosite	$Fe_7(OH)_2Si_8O_{22}$ (± Mg, Mn)	Straight/rodlike	Mined in Australia and South Africa
Tremolite	$Ca_2Mg_5(OH)_2Si_8O_{22}$ (± Fe)	Straight/rodlike	Contaminant of certain chrysotile deposits
Anthophyllite	$(Mg, Fe)_7(OH)_2Si_8O_{22}$	Straight/rodlike	Mined in northern Europe
Actinolite	$Ca_2Fe_5(OH)_2Si_8O_{22}$ (± Mg)	Straight/rodlike	Contaminant of certain chrysotile deposits

Source: Data from Guthrie,[64] by permission of BookCrafters, Inc.; 1993.

ratory diseases, lung cancer, and mesothelioma.[69] A mortality review that compared asbestos-related deaths in Libby versus Montana versus the United States found that, for the 20-year period examined (1979–1998), mortality from asbestosis was approximately 40 times higher than the rest of Montana and 60 times higher than the rest of the U.S. population. Lung cancer mortality was 1.2 to 1.3 times higher than expected compared to Montana and the United States, and the mesothelioma mortality was also elevated.[72] The Libby vermiculite mine closed in 1990, but its products are still on the market.[71] In a recent medical testing program to identify and quantify asbestos-related radiographic abnormalities among persons exposed to vermiculite in Libby, cross-sectional interview and medical testing was conducted in 7,307 persons who have lived, worked, or played in Libby for at least 6 months before December 31, 1990. Of these, 6,668 participants received chest radiographs to assess the prevalence of pleural and interstitial abnormalities. The study showed 17.8% of pleural abnormalities and less than 1% interstitial abnormalities.

Tremolite asbestos, a hydrated calcium magnesium silicate [$Ca_2Mg_5Si_8O_{22}(OH)_2$], is also a known contaminant of chrysotile and fibrous talc.[73–75] The differences in cancer potential between chrysotile asbestos, a serpentine mineral, and amphibole asbestos have been debated extensively. Many studies show that chrysotile is cleared from the lungs more rapidly than amphiboles.[76] Due to the clearance and dissolution of chrysotile, it has been suspected that contaminating tremolite might be responsible for mesotheliomas occurring in chrysotile miners and millers.[75] It also has been suggested that processed chrysotile contains little or no tremolite.[77] Amosite asbestos was the most common fiber type found in the lungs of asbestos-exposed mesothelioma patients.[78] In a more recent study by Roggli et al.,[75] 312 cases of mesothelioma were analyzed for fiber types in lung parenchyma by scanning electron microscopy. Tremolite was identified in 53% of the cases and was increased in 26% of the cases. Fibrous talc was identified in 62% and correlated strongly with the tremolite content ($P = 0.0001$). Chrysotile was only identified in 10% of the cases, and amounts correlated with the proportion of tremolite. In 4.5% of the cases, noncommercial amphibole fibers (tremolite, actinolite, and/or anthophyllite) were the only fiber types found existing above background (control individual) levels. They concluded that tremolite in lung tissue samples from mesothelioma victims were derived from contamination of talc and chrysotile, and that tremolite accounted for a considerable fraction of the excess fiber burden in end-users of asbestos products.

Asbestos-Induced Malignant Disease

Bronchogenic Carcinoma/Lung Cancers

Heavy occupational exposure to asbestos has been associated with developing lung cancer, and a dose–response relationship between asbestos exposure and cancer incidence has been well documented.[79,80]

Cigarette smoking and asbestos exposure have additive or synergistic interactions in inducing cancer of the lung.[68,81] Compared to cigarette smokers with no asbestos exposure, there is a substantial increase in mortality rate in cigarette-smoking asbestos workers.[81,82]

Mesothelioma

Malignant mesothelioma is a rare tumor that is derived from mesothelial cells of the serosal surface of a body cavity. The most important causal factor for the development of human mesothelioma is exposure to asbestos, primarily to amphibole asbestos. After Wagner et al.[83] reported 33 cases of pleural mesothelioma in a crocidolite-mining area in South Africa, increasing attention has been given to this disease. Although mesothelioma is a rare disease with an annual incidence in the United States of 2,000 to 3,000 cases, a steady rise in cases has been reported.[84,85] In Europe, the incidence of malignant pleural mesothelioma has risen for decades and is expected to peak between the years 2010 and 2020.[86] In a recent study on 1,445 cases of mesothelioma in the United States, it was determined that commercial amphiboles were responsible for most of the mesothelioma cases observed.[75] Chrysotile asbestos may produce mesothelioma in man, but the number of cases is small, and the required exposures are large.[87] A recent report suggests that heavy exposures to chrysotile asbestos alone or with negligible amphibole contamination can cause malignant mesothelioma and other lung cancers in man.[88] However, studies evaluating worker populations that are transient and may be exposed to different types of fibers over a lifetime are difficult to interpret.

Mechanisms of Action of Asbestos Fibers

The potential of asbestos fibers to cause cancer has been linked to their geometry, size, and chemical composition. Long (more than $5\,\mu m$), thin (diameter less than $3\,\mu m$) fibers are a health concern[89] and have been found to cause mesothelioma and fibrosis after intrapleural or intraperitoneal administration to rodents.[90] In addition to size, the chemical composition of fibers plays an important role in determining the durability, biopersistence, and biodegradability of asbestos types. The greater durability of amphiboles compared to chrysotile appears to be one of the principal reasons for their greater carcinogenic potential. Amphibole fibers persist at sites of tumor development and may serve as stimuli for neoplastic growth of cells.[91,92] The persistence of the amphibole fibers at the site of tumor formation is important to both tumor induction and promotion because the mean latency period between initial exposure to asbestos and the development of mesothelioma is around 30 to 40 years.[67,93]

An important unresolved issue is whether asbestos fiber carcinogenicity is through direct effects of asbestos on mesothelial cells or through indirect mechanisms involving oxidative stress.[94,95] A ramification of interaction of long (more than $5\,\mu m$) fibers with cells is frustrated phagocytosis and a prolonged oxidative burst.[96] The increased durability and high iron content of the amphiboles, crocidolite, and amosite also may contribute to their higher carcinogenic potential through oxidants catalyzed by iron and/or surface reactions occurring on the fiber. The cytotoxicity of crocidolite fibers in human lung carcinoma cells is directly linked to iron mobilization and is followed by increased ferritin synthesis, a perpetual feedback system for uptake of iron by cells.[97,98] Studies on animal models and cell cultures have confirmed that asbestos fibers generate ROS and reactive nitrogen species (RNS).[67,95,99] These effects may be potentiated by the inflammation associated with fiber exposures.[100]

A complex profile of somatic genetic changes has been revealed in human malignant mesotheliomas. These changes implicate a multistep process of tumorigenesis. The occurrence of multiple, recurrent cytogenetic deletions suggests that loss and/or inactivation of tumor suppressor genes are critical to the development and progression of mesothelioma. Deletions of specific regions in the short (p) arms of chromosomes 1, 3, and 9 and long (q) arms of 6, 13, 15, and 22 are repeatedly observed, and loss of a copy of chromosome 22 is the single most consistent numerical change.[101]

Asbestos fibers in vitro cause the production of DNA damage either via production of ROS or by direct damage to chromosomes after phagocytosis of fibers.[90,102] The consequences of such DNA damage could be the loss of tumor suppressor genes, activation of proto-oncogenes, or unregulated generation of growth factors through paracrine/autocrine mechanisms.[103] Asbestos also causes alterations in cell signaling pathways linked to abnormal growth control in pulmonary epithelial cells, mesothelial cells, endothelial cells, and fibroblasts.[3,104] Asbestos also activates redox-sensitive transcription factors such as NF-κβ[105] and AP-1,[106] which leads to increased cell survival, inflammation, and, paradoxically, the upregulation of antioxidant enzymes such as manganese superoxide dismutase.[100] This enzyme is also overexpressed in asbestos-related mesotheliomas,[107,108] rendering them highly resistant to oxidative stress in comparison to normal mesothelial cells.

Carcinogenesis was classically thought to be a proliferation-driven process. However, it is now recognized that neoplastic growth is an imbalance between apoptosis and proliferation. In support of this concept, a dynamic balance between apoptosis and cell proliferation is observed in mesothelial cells exposed to crocidolite asbestos.[109] Studies in vitro indicate that asbestos can induce apoptosis in mesothelial cells through formation of ROS[110,111] and by mitochondrial pathways.[94,112]

Studies in our group have found that the EGFR is an important initial target of asbestos fibers at the cell membrane (Figure 18.1). This growth factor is required for proliferation of human mesothelial cells[113] and is produced in an autocrine fashion in mesotheliomas.[114] Autophosphorylation of the EGFR occurs in mesothelial cells after in vitro exposures to asbestos. Moreover, aggregation and phosphorylation of the EGFR by long fibers initiates cell signaling cascades linked to asbestos-induced injury and mitogenesis.[115,116] Increased expression of EGFR in rat pleural mesothelial cells correlates with the carcinogenicity of mineral fibers.[117]

We have also shown that the EGFR is causally linked to activation of the MAPK cascade and increased expression of the proto-oncogenes c-*fos* and c-*jun* (see Figure 18.1).[116,118] Expression of both *fos* and *jun* family members (components of the transcription factor AP-1 complex) is required for transition through the G_1 phase and entry into the S phase of the cell cycle.[119] Most recently, ERK 1/2-induced activation by asbestos has been linked to the induction of *fra-1*, an important component of the AP-1 complex that is causally related to anchorage-independent growth in mesothelioma.[107] Microarray analyses have shown increased expression of *fra-1* in rat and human mesotheliomas.[120] Other growth factors and their receptors also are important in malignant mesothelioma including transforming growth factor-alpha (TGF-α), which binds to the EGFR,[121] insulin growth factor II,[122] and PDGF.[123] Increased levels of hepatocyte growth factor (HGF)

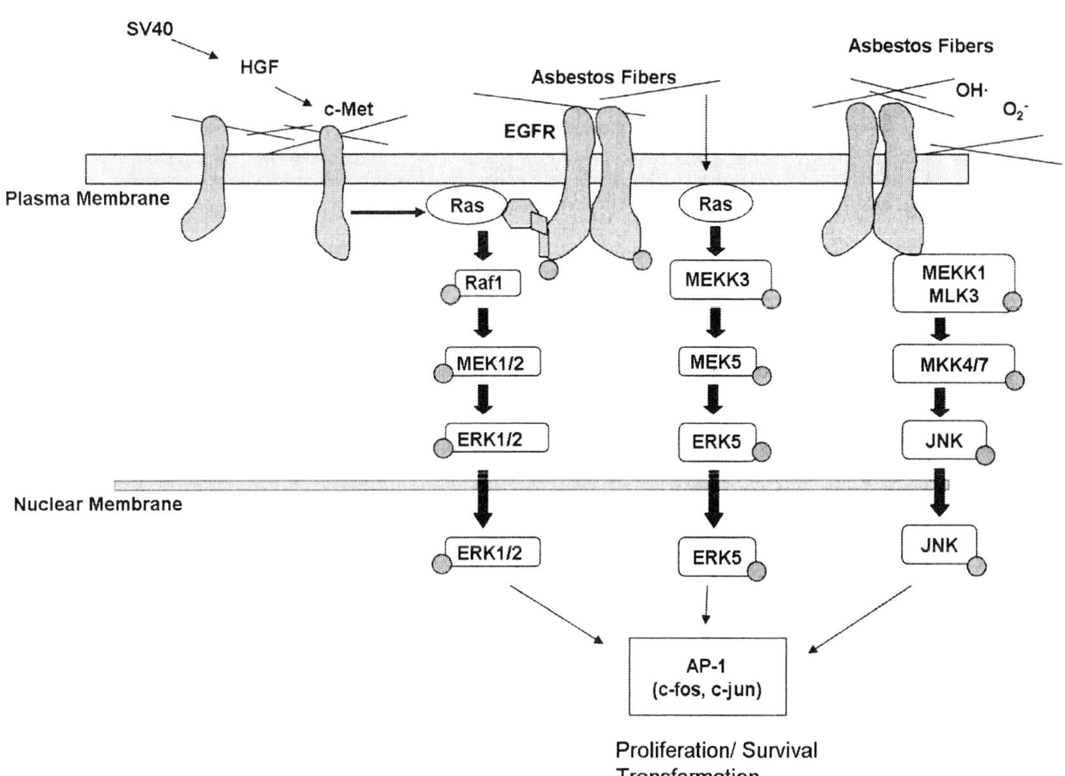

Figure 18.1. Schematic showing some of the major cell signaling events thought to be involved in asbestos-induced carcinogenesis.

TABLE 18.3. Summary of important environmental/occupational carcinogens and their modes of action

	DNA adducts	*Elaboration of ROS*	*Cell-cycle progression*	*Cell signaling/altered transcription factors*	*Mutations in proto-oncogenes/ tumor suppressors*
PAHs (BaP)	X[33]	X[31]	X[33]	X[39]	X[14]
DDT		X[47]	X[49]	X[48]	X[45]
Arsenic		X[55]	X[55]	X[56]	
TCDD			X[62]	X[61]	X[59]
Asbestos		X[95]	X[119]	X[106]	

Superscript numbers are references to support these mechanisms.

and keratinocyte growth factor (KGF), known growth factors for mesothelial cells, have been detected in pleural lavage fluids in rodents exposed to asbestos.[124] The HGF receptor, c-Met, a proto-oncogene product whose activation leads to cell growth and altered morphogenesis, is activated in SV-40-positive human mesothelioma cells.[125] High expression levels of *c-met* have been detected in rat mesothelioma cells and are *fra-1* dependent.[126]

Conclusions

Identification and understanding the mechanisms of cancer induction and/or development induced by environmental carcinogens are critical for both cancer prevention and therapeutic approaches. As emphasized at a recent workshop,[127] removal or reduction of carcinogens in the environment is the most effective way to reduce future cancer risks. In this regard, clinicians and basic scientists should be advocates in the public health arena.

This chapter illustrates the complexities of action of diverse groups of environmental/occupational carcinogens, but also indicates common modes of action that might be modeled in bioassays using human cells to predict carcinogenicity (Table 18.3); these include assays for DNA damage or repair and carcinogenic adduct formation and assays for activation of key proto-oncogenes or inhibition of tumor suppressor genes. It is important to realize that agents in combination, for example, asbestos and cigarette smoke, may be more carcinogenic than individual agents; thus, modeling and revealing additive or multiplicative risks from mixtures of carcinogens are critical future tasks. Defining gene–environment interactions will also be important in defining genetic predisposition to suspect agents.

A recent volume[128] presents the challenges of diagnosis and treatment of occupational cancers to the physician, which include the necessity for thorough patient questionnaires emphasizing smoking habits and working histories. The identity of prototypic cancers, such as mesothelioma, may pinpoint asbestos exposures, but these tumors are difficult to diagnose. A multidisciplinary clinical team is advocated to address genetic factors, diagnosis of tumors, treatment options, and follow-up of patients.

References

1. Boffetta P, Nyberg F. Contribution of environmental factors to cancer risk. Br Med Bull 2003;68:71–94.
2. National Institute for Environmental Health Sciences (NTP). Tenth Report on Carcinogens. Washington, DC: NTP, 2002.
3. Mossman BT, Churg A. Mechanisms in the pathogenesis of asbestosis and silicosis. Am J Respir Crit Care Med 1998;157 (5 pt 1):1666–1680.
4. Bounias M. Etiological factors and mechanism involved in relationships between pesticide exposure and cancer. J Environ Biol 2003;24(1):1–8.
5. Alavanja MC, Samanic C, Dosemeci M, et al. Use of agricultural pesticides and prostate cancer risk in the Agricultural Health Study cohort. Am J Epidemiol 2003;157(9):800–814.
6. Duell EJ, Millikan RC, Savitz DA, et al. A population-based case-control study of farming and breast cancer in North Carolina. Epidemiology 2000;11(5):523–531.
7. Bertazzi PA, Zocchetti C, Guercilena S, et al. Dioxin exposure and cancer risk: a 15-year mortality study after the "Seveso accident." Epidemiology 1997;8(6):646–652.
8. National Institute for Environmental Health Sciences (NTP). Ninth Report on Carcinogens. Washington, DC: NTP, 2001.
9. Sarasin A. An overview of the mechanisms of mutagenesis and carcinogenesis. Mutat Res 2003;544(2–3):99–106.
10. Rubin H. Synergistic mechanisms in carcinogenesis by polycyclic aromatic hydrocarbons and by tobacco smoke: a bio-historical perspective with updates. Carcinogenesis (Oxf) 2001; 22(12):1903–1930.
11. Barrett JC, Shelby MD. Mechanisms of human carcinogens. Prog Clin Biol Res 1992;374:415–434.
12. Rakitsky VN, Koblyakov VA, Turusov VS. Nongenotoxic (epigenetic) carcinogens: pesticides as an example. A critical review. Teratog Carcinog Mutagen 2000;20(4):229–240.
13. Sutherland JE, Costa M. Epigenetics and the environment. Ann NY Acad Sci 2003;983:151–160.
14. Smith LE, Denissenko MF, Bennett WP, et al. Targeting of lung cancer mutational hotspots by polycyclic aromatic hydrocarbons. J Natl Cancer Inst 2000;92(10):803–811.
15. Vermeulen K, Berneman ZN, Van Bockstaele DR. Cell cycle and apoptosis. Cell Prolif 2003;36(3):165–175.
16. Porta M, Malats N, Jariod M, et al. Serum concentrations of organochlorine compounds and K-ras mutations in exocrine pancreatic cancer. PANKRAS II Study Group. Lancet 1999; 354(9196):2125–2129.
17. Takahashi M, Barrett JC, Tsutsui T. Transformation by inorganic arsenic compounds of normal Syrian hamster embryo cells into a neoplastic state in which they become anchorage-independent and cause tumors in newborn hamsters. Int J Cancer 2002;99(5):629–634.
18. Cooper K. p53 mutations in human papillomavirus-associated oesophageal squamous cell carcinoma. Br J Cancer 1995; 72(5):1337.
19. Lane DP, Lain S. Therapeutic exploitation of the p53 pathway. Trends Mol Med 2002;8(suppl 4):S38–S42.
20. Hung J, Anderson R. p53: functions, mutations and sarcomas. Acta Orthop Scand Suppl 1997;273:68–73.

21. Cabello G, Juarranz A, Botella LM, Calaf GM. Organophosphorous pesticides in breast cancer progression. J Submicrosc Cytol Pathol 2003;35(1):1–9.
22. Doll R. Nature and nurture: possibilities for cancer control. Carcinogenesis (Oxf) 1996;17(2):177–184.
23. Sorensen M, Autrup H, Moller P, et al. Linking exposure to environmental pollutants with biological effects. Mutat Res 2003;544(2–3):255–271.
24. NIOSH safety and health topic: occupational cancer, CDC, 2004. (Accessed June 2004 at http://www.cdc.gov/niosh/topics/cancer/).
25. Ward EM, Schulte PA, Bayard S, et al. Priorities for development of research methods in occupational cancer. Environ Health Perspect 2003;111(1):1–12.
26. Doll R, Peto R. The causes of cancer: quantitative estimates of avoidable risks of cancer in the United States today. J Natl Cancer Inst 1981;66(6):1191–1308.
27. Landrigan PJ, Markowitz S. Current magnitude of occupational disease in the United States. Estimates from New York State. Ann NY Acad Sci 1989;572:27–45; discussion 55–60.
28. Leigh JP, Markowitz SB, Fahs M, Shin C, Landrigan PJ. Occupational injury and illness in the United States. Estimates of costs, morbidity, and mortality. Arch Intern Med 1997;157(14): 1557–1568.
29. Kazerouni N, Sinha R, Hsu CH, Greenberg A, Rothman N. Analysis of 200 food items for benzo[a]pyrene and estimation of its intake in an epidemiologic study. Food Chem Toxicol 2001;39(5):423–436.
30. Georgiadis P, Kyrtopoulos SA. Molecular epidemiological approaches to the study of the genotoxic effects of urban air pollution. Mutat Res 1999;428(1–2):91–98.
31. Farmer PB, Singh R, Kaur B, et al. Molecular epidemiology studies of carcinogenic environmental pollutants. Effects of polycyclic aromatic hydrocarbons (PAHs) in environmental pollution on exogenous and oxidative DNA damage. Mutat Res 2003;544(2–3):397–402.
32. McClellan RO. Health effects of exposure to diesel exhaust particles. Annu Rev Pharmacol Toxicol 1987;27:279–300.
33. Fields WR, Desiderio JG, Leonard RM, Burger EE, Brown BG, Doolittle DJ. Differential c-myc expression profiles in normal human bronchial epithelial cells following treatment with benzo[a]pyrene, benzo[a]pyrene-4,5 epoxide, and benzo[a]pyrene-7,8–9,10 diol epoxide. Mol Carcinog 2004;40(2):79–89.
34. Pohjola SK, Lappi M, Honkanen M, Rantanen L, Savela K. DNA binding of polycyclic aromatic hydrocarbons in a human bronchial epithelial cell line treated with diesel and gasoline particulate extracts and benzo[a]pyrene. Mutagenesis 2003;18(5): 429–438.
35. Li J, Chen H, Ke Q, et al. Differential effects of polycyclic aromatic hydrocarbons on transactivation of AP-1 and NF-kappaB in mouse epidermal cl41 cells. Mol Carcinog 2004;40(2): 104–115.
36. Lau AT, He QY, Chiu JF. A proteome analysis of the arsenite response in cultured lung cells: evidence for in vitro oxidative stress-induced apoptosis. Biochem J 2004;382:641–650.
37. Castano-Vinyals G, D'Errico A, Malats N, Kogevinas M. Biomarkers of exposure to polycyclic aromatic hydrocarbons from environmental air pollution. Occup Environ Med 2004; 61(4):e12.
38. Rappaport SM, Waidyanatha S, Serdar B. Naphthalene and its biomarkers as measures of occupational exposure to polycyclic aromatic hydrocarbons. J Environ Monit 2004;6(5):413–416.
39. Rummel AM, Trosko JE, Wilson MR, Upham BL. Polycyclic aromatic hydrocarbons with bay-like regions inhibited gap junctional intercellular communication and stimulated MAPK activity. Toxicol Sci 1999;49(2):232–240.
40. Yu D, Kazanietz MG, Harvey RG, Penning TM. Polycyclic aromatic hydrocarbon o-quinones inhibit the activity of the catalytic fragment of protein kinase C. Biochemistry 2002; 41(39):11888–11894.
41. Burchiel SW, Luster MI. Signaling by environmental polycyclic aromatic hydrocarbons in human lymphocytes. Clin Immunol 2001;98(1):2–10.
42. Saeki K, Matsuda T, Kato TA, et al. Activation of the human Ah receptor by aza-polycyclic aromatic hydrocarbons and their halogenated derivatives. Biol Pharm Bull 2003;26(4):448–452.
43. Vondracek J, Kozubik A, Machala M. Modulation of estrogen receptor-dependent reporter construct activation and G0/G1-S-phase transition by polycyclic aromatic hydrocarbons in human breast carcinoma MCF-7 cells. Toxicol Sci 2002;70(2):193–201.
44. Marc J, Mulner-Lorillon O, Belle R. Glycophosphate-based pesticides affect cell cycle regulation. Biol Cell 2004;96(3):245–249.
45. Tessier DM, Matsumura F. Increased ErbB-2 tyrosine kinase activity, MAPK phosphorylation, and cell proliferation in the prostate cancer cell line LNCaP following treatment by select pesticides. Toxicol Sci 2001;60(1):38–43.
46. Colborn T, Dumanoski D, Myers J. Our Stolen Future. New York: Penguin, 1997.
47. Hassoun E, Bagchi M, Bagchi D, Stohs SJ. Comparative studies on lipid peroxidation and DNA-single strand breaks induced by lindane, DDT, chlordane and endrin in rats. Comp Biochem Physiol C 1993;104(3):427–431.
48. Frigo DE, Tang Y, Beckman BS, et al. Mechanism of AP-1-mediated gene expression by select organochlorines through the p38 MAPK pathway. Carcinogenesis (Oxf) 2004;25(2):249–261.
49. Shen K, Novak RF. DDT stimulates c-erbB2, c-met, and STATS tyrosine phosphorylation, Grb2-Sos association, MAPK phosphorylation, and proliferation of human breast epithelial cells. Biochem Biophys Res Commun 1997;231(1):17–21.
50. Tseng WP. Effects and dose–response relationships of skin cancer and blackfoot disease with arsenic. Environ Health Perspect 1977;19:109–119.
51. Rossman TG. Mechanism of arsenic carcinogenesis: an integrated approach. Mutat Res 2003;533(1–2):37–65.
52. Guo HR, Wang NS, Hu H, Monson RR. Cell type specificity of lung cancer associated with arsenic ingestion. Cancer Epidemiol Biomarkers Prev 2004;13(4):638–643.
53. Nakadaira H, Endoh K, Katagiri M, Yamamoto M. Elevated mortality from lung cancer associated with arsenic exposure for a limited duration. J Occup Environ Med 2002;44(3):291–299.
54. Shukla A, Gulumian M, Hei TK, Kamp D, Rahman Q, Mossman BT. Multiple roles of oxidants in the pathogenesis of asbestos-induced diseases. Free Radic Biol Med 2003;34(9):1117–1129.
55. Shi H, Shi X, Liu KJ. Oxidative mechanism of arsenic toxicity and carcinogenesis. Mol Cell Biochem 2004;255(1–2):67–78.
56. Harris GK, Shi X. Signaling by carcinogenic metals and metal-induced reactive oxygen species. Mutat Res 2003;533(1–2):183–200.
57. Barchowsky A, O'Hara KA. Metal-induced cell signaling and gene activation in lung diseases. Free Radic Biol Med 2003; 34(9):1130–1135.
58. Frumkin H. Agent Orange and cancer: an overview for clinicians. CA Cancer J Clin 2003;53(4):245–255.
59. Watson MA, Devereux TR, Malarkey DE, Anderson MW, Maronpot RR. H-ras oncogene mutation spectra in B6C3F1 and C57BL/6 mouse liver tumors provide evidence for TCDD promotion of spontaneous and vinyl carbamate-initiated liver cells. Carcinogenesis (Oxf) 1995;16(8):1705–1710.
60. Cole P, Trichopoulos D, Pastides H, Starr T, Mandel JS. Dioxin and cancer: a critical review. Regul Toxicol Pharmacol 2003; 38(3):378–388.
61. Mimura J, Fujii-Kuriyama Y. Functional role of AhR in the expression of toxic effects by TCDD. Biochim Biophys Acta 2003;1619(3):263–268.

62. Matsumura F. On the significance of the role of cellular stress response reactions in the toxic actions of dioxin. Biochem Pharmacol 2003;66(4):527–540.
63. Martinez JM, Afshari CA, Bushel PR, Masuda A, Takahashi T, Walker NJ. Differential toxicogenomic responses to 2,3,7,8-tetrachlorodibenzo-p-dioxin in malignant and nonmalignant human airway epithelial cells. Toxicol Sci 2002;69(2):409–423.
64. Guthrie GDJ, Mossman BT. Health effects of mineral dusts. In: Ribbe PH (ed). Mineralogical Society of America. Washington, DC: BookCrafters, 1993.
65. Hazardous Substance Data Bank: Asbestos. National Library of Medicine, NIEHS, 2000. (Accessed June 2004 at http://www.nlm.nih.gov/pubs/factsheets/hsdbfs.html).
66. MacDonald L. The health hazards of asbestos removal. JAMA 1992;267(1):52–53.
67. Mossman BT, Bignon J, Corn M, Seaton A, Gee JB. Asbestos: scientific developments and implications for public policy. Science 1990;247(4940):294–301.
68. Mossman BT, Gee JB. Asbestos-related diseases. N Engl J Med 1989;320(26):1721–1730.
69. Asbestos: Health effects of exposure to asbestos. ATSDR, 2003. (Accessed June 2004 at http://www.atsdr.cdc.gov/asbestos/asbestos_effects.html).
70. Craighead JE, Mossman BT. The pathogenesis of asbestos-associated diseases. N Engl J Med 1982;306(24):1446–1455.
71. Fact Sheet FS-012–01, USGS, March 2001. (Accessed June 2003 at http://pubs.usgs.gov/fs/fs012–01/).
72. Asbestos: Asbestos exposure in Libby, Montana. ASTDR, 2003. (Accessed June 2004 at http://www.atsdr.cdc.gov/asbestos/asbestos_study.html).
73. McDonald JC, Armstrong B, Case B, et al. Mesothelioma and asbestos fiber type. Evidence from lung tissue analyses. Cancer (Phila) 1989;63(8):1544–1547.
74. Langer AM, Nolan RP, Addison J. On talc, tremolite, and tergiversation. Br J Ind Med 1991;48(5):359–360.
75. Roggli VL, Vollmer RT, Butnor KJ, Sporn TA. Tremolite and mesothelioma. Ann Occup Hyg 2002;46(5):447–453.
76. Bernstein DM, Chevalier J, Smith P. Comparison of Calidria chrysotile asbestos to pure tremolite: inhalation biopersistence and histopathology following short-term exposure. Inhal Toxicol 2003;15(14):1387–1419.
77. Craighead J. Airways and lung. In: Pathology of Environmental and Occupational Disease. St. Louis: Mosby, 1995.
78. Roggli VL, Pratt PC, Brody AR. Asbestos fiber type in malignant mesothelioma: an analytical scanning electron microscopic study of 94 cases. Am J Ind Med 1993;23(4):605–614.
79. McDonald JC. Cancer risks due to asbestos and man-made fibres. Recent Results Cancer Res 1990;120:122–131.
80. McDonald JC, McDonald AD, Armstrong B, Sebastien P. Cohort study of mortality of vermiculite miners exposed to tremolite. Br J Ind Med 1986;43(7):436–444.
81. Hammond EC, Selikoff IJ, Seidman H. Asbestos exposure, cigarette smoking and death rates. Ann NY Acad Sci 1979;330:473–490.
82. Saracci R. The interactions of tobacco smoking and other agents in cancer etiology. Epidemiol Rev 1987;9:175–193.
83. Wagner JC, Sleggs CA, Marchand P. Diffuse pleural mesothelioma and asbestos exposure in the North Western Cape Province. Br J Ind Med 1960;17:260–271.
84. Grondin SC, Sugarbaker DJ. Malignant mesothelioma of the pleural space. Oncology (Huntingt) 1999;13(7):919–926; discussion 26, 31–32.
85. Grondin S, Sugarbaker D. Malignant mesothelioma of the pleural space. Oncology 1999;13(7):919–926.
86. Boutin C, Schlesser M, Frenay C, Astoul P. Malignant pleural mesothelioma. Eur Respir J 1998;12(4):972–981.
87. Churg A. Chrysotile, tremolite, and malignant mesothelioma in man. Chest 1988;93(3):621–628.
88. Yano E, Wang ZM, Wang XR, Wang MZ, Lan YJ. Cancer mortality among workers exposed to amphibole-free chrysotile asbestos. Am J Epidemiol 2001;154(6):538–543.
89. Vu VT, Lai DY. Approaches to characterizing human health risks of exposure to fibers. Environ Health Perspect 1997; 105S(suppl 5):1329–1336.
90. Asbestos in public and commercial buildings: a literature reviewed synthesis of current knowledge. Cambridge, MA: Health Effects Institute-Asbestos Research, 1991. (Accessed June 2003 at http://www.asbestos-institute.ca/reviews/hei-ar/hei-ar.html).
91. Jaurand MC, Gaudichet A, Halpern S, Bignon J. In vitro biodegradation of chrysotile fibres by alveolar macrophages and mesothelial cells in culture: comparison with a pH effect. Br J Ind Med 1984;41(3):389–395.
92. Woodworth CD, Mossman BT, Craighead JE. Induction of squamous metaplasia in organ cultures of hamster trachea by naturally occurring and synthetic fibers. Cancer Res 1983;43(10):4906–4912.
93. Mossman BT, Kamp DW, Weitzman SA. Mechanisms of carcinogenesis and clinical features of asbestos-associated cancers. Cancer Invest 1996;14(5):466–480.
94. Shukla A, Jung M, Stern M, et al. Asbestos induces mitochondrial DNA damage and dysfunction linked to the development of apoptosis. Am J Physiol Lung Cell Mol Physiol 2003;285(5):L1018–L1025.
95. Kamp DW, Graceffa P, Pryor WA, Weitzman SA. The role of free radicals in asbestos-induced diseases. Free Radic Biol Med 1992;12(4):293–315.
96. Hansen K, Mossman BT. Generation of superoxide (O_2^-.) from alveolar macrophages exposed to asbestiform and nonfibrous particles. Cancer Res 1987;47(6):1681–1686.
97. Fang R, Aust AE. Induction of ferritin synthesis in human lung epithelial cells treated with crocidolite asbestos. Arch Biochem Biophys 1997;340(2):369–375.
98. Chao CC, Lund LG, Zinn KR, Aust AE. Iron mobilization from crocidolite asbestos by human lung carcinoma cells. Arch Biochem Biophys 1994;314(2):384–391.
99. Janssen YM, Van Houten B, Borm PJ, Mossman BT. Cell and tissue responses to oxidative damage. Lab Invest 1993;69(3):261–274.
100. Kinnula VL. Oxidant and antioxidant mechanisms of lung disease caused by asbestos fibres. Eur Respir J 1999;14(3):706–716.
101. Murthy SS, Testa JR. Asbestos, chromosomal deletions, and tumor suppressor gene alterations in human malignant mesothelioma. J Cell Physiol 1999;180(2):150–157.
102. Fung H, Kow YW, Van Houten B, Mossman BT. Patterns of 8-hydroxydeoxyguanosine formation in DNA and indications of oxidative stress in rat and human pleural mesothelial cells after exposure to crocidolite asbestos. Carcinogenesis (Oxf) 1997; 18(4):825–832.
103. Pass HI, Mew DJ. In vitro and in vivo studies of mesothelioma. J Cell Biochem Suppl 1996;24:142–151.
104. Churg A. The uptake of mineral particles by pulmonary epithelial cells. Am J Respir Crit Care Med 1996;154(4 pt 1):1124–1140.
105. Janssen YM, Barchowsky A, Treadwell M, Driscoll KE, Mossman BT. Asbestos induces nuclear factor kappa B (NF-kappa B) DNA-binding activity and NF-kappa B-dependent gene expression in tracheal epithelial cells. Proc Natl Acad Sci USA 1995;92(18):8458–8462.
106. Ramos-Nino ME, Haegens A, Shukla A, Mossman BT. Role of mitogen-activated protein kinases (MAPK) in cell injury and proliferation by environmental particulates. Mol Cell Biochem 2002;234–235(1–2):111–118.

107. Ramos-Nino ME, Timblin CR, Mossman BT. Mesothelial cell transformation requires increased AP-1 binding activity and ERK-dependent Fra-1 expression. Cancer Res 2002;62(21): 6065–6069.
108. Kahlos K, Pitkanen S, Hassinen I, Linnainmaa K, Kinnula VL. Generation of reactive oxygen species by human mesothelioma cells. Br J Cancer 1999;80(1–2):25–31.
109. Goldberg JL, Zanella CL, Janssen YM, et al. Novel cell imaging techniques show induction of apoptosis and proliferation in mesothelial cells by asbestos. Am J Respir Cell Mol Biol 1997; 17(3):265–271.
110. Broaddus VC, Yang L, Scavo LM, Ernst JD, Boylan AM. Asbestos induces apoptosis of human and rabbit pleural mesothelial cells via reactive oxygen species. J Clin Invest 1996;98(9):2050–2059.
111. BeruBe KA, Quinlan TR, Fung H, et al. Apoptosis is observed in mesothelial cells after exposure to crocidolite asbestos. Am J Respir Cell Mol Biol 1996;15(1):141–147.
112. Kamp DW, Panduri V, Weitzman SA, Chandel N. Asbestos-induced alveolar epithelial cell apoptosis: role of mitochondrial dysfunction caused by iron-derived free radicals. Mol Cell Biochem 2002;234–235(1–2):153–160.
113. Laveck MA, Somers AN, Moore LL, Gerwin BI, Lechner JF. Dissimilar peptide growth factors can induce normal human mesothelial cell multiplication. In Vitro Cell Dev Biol 1988; 24(11):1077–1084.
114. Mossman BT, Gruenert DC. SV40, growth factors, and mesothelioma: another piece of the puzzle. Am J Respir Cell Mol Biol 2002;26(2):167–170.
115. Pache JC, Janssen YM, Walsh ES, et al. Increased epidermal growth factor-receptor protein in a human mesothelial cell line in response to long asbestos fibers. Am J Pathol 1998;152(2): 333–340.
116. Zanella CL, Posada J, Tritton TR, Mossman BT. Asbestos causes stimulation of the extracellular signal-regulated kinase 1 mitogen-activated protein kinase cascade after phosphorylation of the epidermal growth factor receptor. Cancer Res 1996;56(23): 5334–5338.
117. Faux SP, Houghton CE, Hubbard A, Patrick G. Increased expression of epidermal growth factor receptor in rat pleural mesothelial cells correlates with carcinogenicity of mineral fibres. Carcinogenesis (Oxf) 2000;21(12):2275–2280.
118. Heintz NH, Janssen YM, Mossman BT. Persistent induction of c-fos and c-jun expression by asbestos. Proc Natl Acad Sci USA 1993;90(8):3299–3303.
119. Reddy SP, Mossman BT. Role and regulation of activator protein-1 in toxicant-induced responses of the lung. Am J Physiol Lung Cell Mol Physiol 2002;283(6):L1161–L1178.
120. Sandhu H, Dehnen W, Roller M, Abel J, Unfried K. mRNA expression patterns in different stages of asbestos-induced carcinogenesis in rats. Carcinogenesis (Oxf) 2000;21(5):1023–1029.
121. Walker C, Everitt J, Ferriola PC, Stewart W, Mangum J, Bermudez E. Autocrine growth stimulation by transforming growth factor alpha in asbestos-transformed rat mesothelial cells. Cancer Res 1995;55(3):530–536.
122. Rutten AA, Bermudez E, Stewart W, Everitt JI, Walker CL. Expression of insulin-like growth factor II in spontaneously immortalized rat mesothelial and spontaneous mesothelioma cells: a potential autocrine role of insulin-like growth factor II. Cancer Res 1995;55(16):3634–3639.
123. Metheny-Barlow LJ, Flynn B, van Gijssel HE, Marrogi A, Gerwin BI. Paradoxical effects of platelet-derived growth factor-A overexpression in malignant mesothelioma. Antiproliferative effects in vitro and tumorigenic stimulation in vivo. Am J Respir Cell Mol Biol 2001;24(6):694–702.
124. Adamson IY, Bakowska J. KGF and HGF are growth factors for mesothelial cells in pleural lavage fluid after intratracheal asbestos. Exp Lung Res 2001;27(7):605–616.
125. Cacciotti P, Libener R, Betta P, et al. SV40 replication in human mesothelial cells induces HGF/Met receptor activation: a model for viral-related carcinogenesis of human malignant mesothelioma. Proc Natl Acad Sci USA 2001;98(21):12032–12037.
126. Ramos-Nino ME, Scapoli L, Martinelli M, Land S, Mossman BT. Microarray analysis and RNA silencing link fra-1 to cd44 and c-met expression in mesothelioma. Cancer Res 2003;63(13): 3539–3545.
127. Mossman B, Klein G, zur Hausen H. Modern criteria to determine the etiology of human carcinogens. Semin Cancer Biol (in press).
128. Chase K, Whysner J, Shields P. Clinics in Occupational and Environmental Medicine. Carcinogens in the Workplace. Philadelphia: Saunders, 2003.

Cancer Metastasis

Kevin McDonnell and Anton Wellstein

Cancer metastasis, the spread of cancer from its primary location to secondary sites, heralds the progression to a fundamentally distinct oncologic disease. Metastatic infiltration often disrupts the integrity and physiologic functioning of the target organ, giving rise to the pain, morbidity, and mortality that make metastatic disease such a devastating illness.[1–11]

Molecular Origins of the Metastatic Phenotype

The biologic process by which a primary tumor escapes the vicinity of its original environment and colonizes remote destinations is complex, involving a cascade of pathophysiologic events. Such events, it has been suggested, occur through a sequence of stochastic genetic alterations[12] fostered by an inherent genetic instability.[13–15] These mutations are perpetuated by a mechanism of evolutionary selection, which confers a survival advantage on the metastasizing cell.[16–18] In contrast to the idea of random molecular occurrences spawning the metastatic phenotype, some investigators have proposed that metastasis derives from activation of preexisting genetic scripts, for example, RAS- and/or MYC-mediated mechanisms,[19,20] that promote metastasis. Alternately, cells may acquire the ability to metastasize via the silencing of metastatic suppressor genes.[21,22] The first metastatic suppressor was identified as the "non-metastatic clone 23" (NM23) gene,[23] whose suppressive effects are believed to be mediated via influences upon ERK-MAPK signaling.[24] Subsequently, additional metastatic suppressor genes have been characterized, including, among others, KAI-1,[25] KISS-1,[26] tissue inhibitors of metalloproteinases (TIMPs),[27] MKK4,[28,29] BRMS1,[30] SSeCKs,[31] RhoGD12,[32] and Drg-1.[33] This collection of metastasis suppressor genes are unified mechanistically insofar as they inhibit the spread of primary tumors via modulation of cellular growth and adhesion properties and cytoskeletal architecture.[29] Whether the metastatic phenotype ultimately develops from a series of random mutations, activation of preprogrammed genetic scripts, or inhibition of suppressive mechanisms, further investigations of the molecular origins of this phenotype may yield important insights into the specific targeting and/or control of cancer metastases.

The Tumor Microenvironment

The metastasizing cancer cell is endowed with a constellation of properties that permits it to successfully translocate to secondary tumor sites. Among these properties is the ability to sustain uncontrolled primary growth.[12] Such primary growth takes place by virtue of the cell's own genetic programming, but it also may be abetted by a permissive microenvironment.[34–38] Microenvironmental biologic status may have a dramatic effect on the capability of the tumor to expand and ultimately metastasize. For example, the microenvironment provides a rich source of tumor growth stimulatory molecules. Microenvironmental expression of these factors permits primary tumor expansion and induces tumor metastasis.[39–42] Other microenvironmental influences are important with regard to tumor growth and metastasis as well. For example, the immunologic status of the microenvironment mirrors the immunologic integrity of the organism as a whole, and this integrity exerts a dramatic influence on tumor growth.[43] Immunodeficient states are associated with increases in the incidence of cancer,[44,45] and ultraviolet irradiation-induced compromise of immune function results in increased malignant growth.[46–49] Conversely, there has been demonstrated an inverse relationship between the occurrence of cancer and metastasis and activation of microenvironmental immunity.[50–53]

The Tumor Microenvironment: Blood Vessel Formation

Microenvironmental vascular status also exerts a profound impact on the ability of the primary tumor to grow and metastasize. Expression of blood vessel growth-promoting molecules is generally a poor prognostic factor associated with cancer[54,55] and specifically with breast cancer,[56–58] cancer of the central nervous system,[59–61] gynecologic cancers,[62–64] gastrointestinal cancer,[65–67] and prostate cancer.[68,69] Proclivity for metastasis correlates with the degree of tumor-associated blood vessel formation.[70–78] Such tumor-associated blood vessel formation promotes metastasis in two ways: blood vessels function to transport growth-stimulating nutrients to the burgeoning primary tumor and as a conduit by which metastasizing cells travel toward their secondary tumor destinations.

The formation of blood vessels is regulated by the cumulative effects of a variety of molecules; the roles of these molecules typically are defined during the period of embryonic blood vessel formation and later reprised in the context of pathologic tumor-associated vessel genesis. During embryonic development, blood vessels arise via a number of distinct mechanisms including vasculogenesis, angiogenesis, and vessel intussusception.

Vasculogenesis is the de novo construction of the vasculature. During this process, embryonal mesoderm is stimulated to differentiate into precursor hemangioblasts and then endothelial cells. Fibroblast growth factors (FGFs)[79] and vascular endothelial growth factor (VEGF)[80] provide key differentiation signals initiating the mesodermal to endothelial transition. VEGF, together with other molecular factors, cue endothelial cells to proliferate further and assemble into linear aggregates that subsequently reorganize to form a tubular vascular reticulum.[81–83] Additional molecules play more specialized roles; for example, the integrins induce lumen formation,[84] and angiopoietin 1 acts to promote the entrenchment and stabilization of the nascent vasculature by modulating endothelial cell adherence to nearby tissue and extracellular components.[85–87]

Following incipient vasculogenic establishment of the original blood vessel system, the vasculature may continue to expand via ancillary mechanisms including angiogenesis or vessel intussusception. Angiogenesis entails proliferation of the previously established endothelial cell population, permitting collateral expansion from the nascent vascular reticulum. VEGF is a primary molecular promoter of angiogenesis. However, for efficient collateral expansion to occur, angiopoietin 1-mediated fortification of the vasculature must be abrogated. Such reversal is mediated through the antagonistic actions of angiopoietin 2, which inhibits the actions of angiopoietin 1 at the Tie 2 receptor, permitting the disruption of endothelial cell–extracellular matrix stabilizing interactions.[88] An additional mechanism that may allow expansion of the extant blood vessel system is the process of intussusception in which blood vessels are split by VEGF-stimulated growth and interposition of an endothelial tissue barrier across the lumen of the vessel.[89–92]

The pathologic formation of blood vessels during tumor growth and metastasis reactivates many of the mechanisms operating during embryonic blood vessel formation. Reminiscent of embryonic vasculogenesis, endothelial precursor hemangioblastic cells are activated from the bone marrow. These cells incorporate into the newly forming tumor vasculature,[93–96] frequently comprising more than one-third of the blood vessels.[97] Both FGF and VEGF have been demonstrated to function as molecular mediators of tumor-associated vasculogenesis.[98–102] Angiogenic sprouting, as well, contributes to pathologic blood vessel formation, and this mechanism is also modulated by FGFs and VEGF[103] in addition to angiopoietin 2.[104]

Tumors may also achieve vascularization via specialized mechanisms. Tumors may "co-opt" existing blood vessels by associating with previously established vasculature and, in so doing, satisfying their own metabolic needs by allowing themselves access to the nutrients and oxygen transported through these vessels. Intriguingly, in a mechanism referred to as "vascular mimicry," tumor cells may functionally imitate the endothelial cell itself by forming tumor cell-lined channels that accommodate blood flow.[90,91,105]

The Angiogenic Switch

Generally, blood vessel formation takes place when the stimulatory effects of proangiogenic molecules surpass the inhibitory effects of antiangiogenic molecules. More specifically, the magnitude and actual pattern of the blood vessel formation depends upon the precise timing, distribution, and absolute and relative expression levels of these angiogenic factors. In turn, expression of these factors is initiated by various genetically programmed triggers that have been designated "angiogenic switches."[106,107] Within the pathophysiologic context of tumor-associated blood vessel formation, these switches are clinically and phenotypically important insofar as their activation is one hallmark of an aggressive, metastatic phenotype.

Within the tumor microenvironment, an angiogenic switch may be activated in response to an altered physiologic milieu. For example, when a burgeoning tumor outgrows its blood supply and creates a circumstance of tissue hypoxia, there occurs a reactive increased expression of multiple genes including, among others, hypoxia-inducible factor 1 (HIF-1).[108,109] HIF-1, in turn, modulates an angiogenic cascade involving expression of a multitude of proangiogenic factors including VEGF[110–112] and FGF.[113] Other physiologic perturbations such as hypoglycemia[114] and ischemia[115] may also lead to activation of an angiogenic switch.

The angiogenic switch, in addition to the increased levels of VEGF and FGF, may also comprise increased expression of proangiogenic matrix metalloproteinases,[116,117] the downregulation of antiangiogenic factors,[118] activation of oncogenes, or inactivation of tumor suppressor genes.[114,115,119,120] Activation of angiogenesis may also derive from the cumulative acquisition of proangiogenic genetic elements over time, for example, through the horizontal transfer of DNA among neighboring tumor cells.[121] Ultimately, elucidation of the molecular basis of the angiogenesis activation will yield additional insight into mechanisms of tumor progression and allow for effective targeting of tumor metastasis.[122]

The Importance and Role of the Lymphatic System During Metastasis

The lymphatic system functions as a key microenvironmental adjunct to the vascular system for the spread of metastasizing cells to their secondary sites.[123,124] The importance of the lymphatic system as an avenue of metastatic dispersion is underscored by the prognostic value associated with the spread of cancers to regional lymph nodes[125,126] and the impact of the removal of such lymph nodes on the prevention of metastasis and overall survival.[127,128]

That peritumoral lymphatics play an integral role in metastatic spread is established[129,130]; what is more controversial is the role that intratumoral lymphatics play.[131–134] This controversy has been fueled by the recent discovery of lymphatic-specific molecules such as VEGF C,[135–137] VEGF D,[138,139] and VEGFR-3.[140,141] An association between tumor expression of these lymphatic-specific factors and metastasis has been established, suggesting that tumor lymphangiogenesis is an important prognostic indicator in the same fashion as is tumor angiogenesis.[142,143] It is anticipated that the metastatic significance of intratumoral lymphatics and lymphangiogenesis will be more firmly defined as additional lymphatic-specific molecules are identified and the mechanism of tumor-associated lymphangiogenesis is further examined.

Intravasation

Following proliferation, metastasizing cells exit from the primary tumor site into the bloodstream or the lymphatic circulation via the process of intravasation.[8] Woodhouse et al. observed that intravasating cells recapitulate the peripatetic cell phenotype characterizing embryonal physiologic processes that are dependent upon migrating, invading cells such as the primordial establishment of the original vascular and nervous systems.[144,145]

The migratory aspects of intravasation entail specific cellular capabilities. The cell must exhibit the mechanical ability for translocation; the development and advancement of pseudopodia permit such locomotion.[146] A variety of motility factors promote pseudopodia-mediated translocation; these include autocrine molecules, for example, insulin-like growth factor II[147] and autotaxin,[148] paracrine molecules such as insulin-like growth factor I,[149] and the extracellular matrix molecules laminin, fibronectin,[150] and collagen.[151]

For the metastatic cell to transit successfully beyond its microenvironment, it must traverse the extracellular matrix. Abetting this penetration, metalloproteinases degrade the extracellular matrix,[152,153] with expression levels of metalloproteinase expression correlating with the proclivity of cells to metastasize.[154,155]

Tumor-associated blood vessel formation furthers the intravasation process. Extracellular matrix degradation takes place via the degradative effects of endothelial cell-released collagenases and urokinases.[156] As well, VEGF expression accompanies the expansion of the tumor vascular network. VEGF, which is also known as vascular permeability factor,[157] causes the formation of leaky permeable vessels. Such leakiness, important for the expansion of the tumor vasculature,[158] also contributes to the successful intravasation of metastasizing tumor cells.

End-Organ Arrest: Organ-Directed Metastasis

Postintravasation, tumor cells migrate to the sites of metastasis. Clinical and experimental observations suggest that metastatic destinations are selective for specific tissues[159]; for example, among others, breast and prostate cancers preferentially metastasize to bone,[160] colorectal cancer to the liver,[161] and skin cancer to the lung.[162]

Mechanisms proposed to account for directed metastasis are controversial. The British surgeon Stephen Paget retrospectively investigated the metastatic destinations of a variety of cancers by examining autopsy records and documented organ-specific metastasis patterns.[163] He attributed this proclivity for organ-specific metastasis to a salutary interaction between the metastasizing cell and the end organ. He likened the metastasizing cell to a seed that thrives in the growth-promoting "soil" of the target organ.

An alternative mechanism explaining directed metastasis was proposed in the early 20th century by another surgeon, James Ewing. Ewing also documented a nonrandom pattern of metastatic cancer spread; in contrast to Paget, however, Ewing suggested that metastatic patterns could be attributed to an anatomic, circulatory bias[164]; that is, metastasizing cells tend to lodge and secondarily proliferate at the first vascular bed distal from the primary tumor site.

Analyses of patterns of metastatic spread provide support for Ewing's hypothesis. Weiss et al., in extensive studies of colon cancer metastasis, observed generalized proximal organ metastasis correlating with the magnitude of target organ flow.[165] Weiss' analyses, however, do not wholly vitiate the "seed and soil" hypothesis of Paget. To the contrary, in these same studies, Weiss observes that patterns of secondary metastasis do not perfectly correlate with the magnitude of blood flow. In some organs, the tendency for metastasis is greater than or less than what would be predicted solely on the basis of the magnitude of blood flow. These findings suggest that some specific interaction between the circulating metastatic cell and the target organ influences the likelihood of that cell metastasizing to that organ. Additional observations corroborate this notion; patients with ovarian cancer frequently develop malignant abdominal ascites, necessitating placement of peritoneovenous shunts. In these circumstances, malignant cells are drained from the abdomen back into the circulation via the jugular vein whence they pass through the capillary bed of the lungs. Ewing would predict that these patients would develop pulmonary metastases, and yet autopsy results reveal an overwhelming absence of such growths.[166,167]

Hart and Fidler examined the organ biases of B16 melanoma metastases. In the whole animal, B16 cells spontaneously form metastases within the lung and ovaries. The investigators intravenously injected B16 cells into mice bearing syngeneic pulmonary, ovarian, and renal subcutaneous implants.[168] Hart and Fidler found that B16 tumors do not develop randomly; rather, they formed selectively within the implanted lung and ovarian tissue, and not within the kidney tissue. Thus, it would seem that some special interaction between circulating B16 cells and the pulmonary and ovarian tissue dictates the metastatic bias.

A number of recent investigators, including Binacone et al., have sought to elucidate the mechanistic basis of organ-selective metastasis.[169] E-selectins are adhesion molecules expressed on the surface of endothelial cells. Binacone demonstrated that the destination of metastasizing B16 cells could be efficiently directed by controlling cell-surface expression of E-selectin. This demonstration suggested that organ-directed metastasis may be defined, in part, by an interaction between proteins expressed on the surface of the target organ endothelium and those expressed on the surface of metastasizing cells. In support of this hypothesis, the metastatic destination of Chinese hamster ovary cells can be altered by transfecting these cells to express $\alpha_4\beta_1$ integrin on their surface.[170]

In agreement with the idea of metastasizing cell–organ endothelium interactions providing a basis for organ-selective metastasis, a number of different lines of evidence have suggested the uniqueness of organ endothelia.[171–173] Ruoslahti and his coworkers have suggested that the uniqueness of the organ endothelia derives from signature endothelial cell-surface proteins that comprise an *address system* and ensure delivery of the metastasizing cell to a designated target tissue.[174–176] For example, specific proteins have been identified that mediate the binding of metastatic breast and prostate cancer cells to lung tissue[177–179] and colon cancer cells to the liver.[180]

Taken as a whole, the evidence supports both a circulatory, anatomic bias, as proposed by Ewing, and unique end-organ properties, as theorized by Paget, underlying the ultimate site of metastasis. Recent investigative initiatives have sought to further define the molecular basis and relative contributions of the circulatory, anatomic, and "seed and soil" mechanisms toward organ-directed metastasis.

Extravasation

Having arrested at their target organ, metastasizing cells must extravasate from the circulation by traversing the endothelium and underlying basement membrane to achieve successful secondary metastatic growth. This success derives to a significant degree from the same locomotive and tissue penetrative capacities that were required to complete intravasation.

Novel insights into the molecular and mechanical aspects of extravasation have been garnered by the development and implementation of innovative experimental and investigative techniques such as in vivo video microscopy[181–183] and laser scanning confocal microscopy.[184] The ability of metastasizing cells to translocate beyond the endothelium significantly relies upon the inherent locomotive potential of the metastasizing cell and has been correlated with the expression of, among other molecules, transforming growth factor-beta[185] and activation of promotogenic pathways involving, for example, protein kinase 2/p38[186] and c-erbB-2.[187] To complete its transendothelial migration, the extravasating cell may also require a permeable endothelial cell layer[188,189] as well as activation of transendothelial migratory mechanisms.[190–192]

Beyond the endothelial layer, the metastasizing cell must penetrate the underlying basement membrane. Mechanistically, this process has been compared with the process of inflammation-associated leukocyte infiltration[193–198] requiring, reminiscent of intravasation, metalloproteinase expression to degrade the basement membrane.[199–201] Once the extravasation process is complete, the metastasizing cell faces its final obstacle of secondary proliferation at the metastatic site.

Growth and Expansion of the Tumor at the Secondary Site

Expansion of the tumor at its secondary site represents perhaps the most clinically significant of the metastatic steps, for it is this growth and colonization at the target organ that causes the physical disruption and physiologic derangement of that organ, ultimately giving rise to the morbidity and mortality characterizing metastatic disease.

Factors influencing expansion of the metastatic mass are similar to those modulating growth at the primary tumor site. These factors include properties inherent to the metastatic cell itself such as accelerated and uninhibited growth, as well as the ability to co-opt the resources of the secondary target site for the cell's own metabolic requirements.

In addition to its inherent characteristics, the metastasizing cell also relies on a receptive microenvironmental *soil* to achieve optimal growth at the secondary site. As the site of the primary tumor location, the immunologic, angiogenesis-promoting and growth-stimulatory milieu of the secondary site modulates the extent of metastatic tumor expansion.[202–206] Further understanding of those variables that promote successful completion of this last metastatic step may afford new insights into strategies directed at preventing and vanquishing metastatic disease.

Discovery of Tumor Metastasis-Related Genes

Ultimately, conquering metastatic disease will likely derive from a more thorough characterization of the genes expressed during each step of metastasis. Transcriptional and functional analysis of metastatic gene products may provide new insights into the molecular mechanisms underlying the process of metastasis and identify potential targets for therapeutic intervention.

Molecular technologic advances have made it possible to discover genes that are differentially expressed between normal physiologic and aberrant pathologic states. Two of the more versatile techniques that permit identification of variably expressed genes are differential display and microarray analysis.[207] Differential display employs reverse transcription and the polymerase chain reaction using mRNA derived from different cellular states, allowing, for example, the identification of genes that are expressed during the process of metastasis and not expressed during nonpathologic states. Another technique used to examine differential gene expression, microarray analysis, characterizes gene expression based on the relative hybridization of reversed transcribed gene products to a prefabricated, nucleic acid-containing matrix. Demonstrating their power and utility, these techniques have been used to discover metastasis suppressor genes[208] and metastatic molecular signatures.[209–211]

The endeavor to discover metastasis-related genes has inspired innovative investigative approaches including the use of phage display technology. Ngaiza and colleagues[212] employed this technique to identify colon cancer genes mediating metastasis to the liver. The gene products from a highly metastatic colon cancer cell line were expressed on the surface of the phage. Genes involved directly in the process of liver metastasis were identified by in vivo biopanning, that is, by injecting the phage into the circulation and selecting those phages that specifically bound to the liver. One theoretical advantage of this technique is that it identifies genes whose expression is not merely correlated with the process of metastasis but rather those whose function is directly integral to the mechanism itself.

As more novel and precise methods for metastasis gene discovery are developed and consequently, more specific metastatic gene products are identified, so also, ideally, will the therapeutic targeting of the metastatic process become more focused and efficacious.

Antimetastasis-Directed Therapies

Investigations of metastatic genes and the mechanisms driven by these genes have afforded new therapeutic modalities for the treatment of cancer. Novel therapies have been directed against specific molecules implicated in the metastatic process, for example, erb-B2,[213,214] the epidermal growth factor receptor,[215] and caveolin 1.[216] New treatments have sought to modulate the expression of classes of metastatic-related molecules such as the metalloproteinases[217,218] and metalloproteinase inhibitors.[219] To reduce metastatic tumor growth, innovative approaches such as activating the transcription of metastasis suppressor genes[220] and deactivating putative metastatic switches, for example, hypoxia-inducible factor,[221] have also been employed. Therapies have also been directed against specific steps of the metastatic cascade. One primary target has been angiogenesis,[222] with focused approaches aimed at neutralizing the effects of proangiogenic molecules such as VEGF[223–225] to curtail tumor growth and metastasis and increase patient survival. Phage display technologies have made possible the identification of tumor vascular homing peptides, and these peptides have been employed to exploit tumor-associated angiogenesis and to selectively deliver anticancer agents to tumor sites.[226,227] Accompanying the further clarification of the molecular biology of the metastatic process is the development of potentially more effective and potent antimetastatic clinical interventions.

Summary and Conclusions

The ravaging sequelae of metastatic disease underscore the eminent need for effective therapies. The metastatic process comprises an intricate sequence of complex events. Current research initiatives aimed at defining the molecular basis of these events are providing new insights into the targeting and prevention of cancer metastasis. Future research efforts, it is anticipated, will contribute to the optimization of current and introduction of innovative antimetastasis therapeutic modalities.

References

1. Chang HM. Cancer pain management. Med Clin N Am 1999; 83:711–736.
2. Cleeland CS, et al. Pain and its treatment in outpatients with metastatic cancer. N Engl J Med 1994;330:592–596.
3. Perron V, Schonwetter RS. Assessment and management of pain in palliative care patients. Cancer Control 2001:8:15–24.
4. El Kamar FG, Grossbard ML, Kozuch PS. Metastatic pancreatic cancer: emerging strategies in chemotherapy and palliative care. Oncologist 2003;8:18–34.
5. Brescia FJ, Portenoy RK, Ryan M, Krasnoff L, Gray G. Pain, opiod use, and survival in hospitalized patients with advanced cancer. J Clin Oncol 1992;10:149–155.
6. Sporin MB. The war on cancer. Lancet 1996;347:1377–1381.
7. Woodhouse EC, Chuaqui RF, Liotta LA. General mechanisms of metastasis. Cancer (Phila) 1997;80:1529–1537.
8. Fidler IJ. Critical determinants of metastasis. Cancer Biol 2002; 12:89–96.
9. Weir HK, et al. Annual report to the nation on the status of cancer, 1975–2000, featuring the uses of surveillance data for cancer prevention and control. JNCI 2003;95:1276–1299.
10. Glare P, et al. A systemic review of physician's survival predictions in terminally ill cancer patients. BMJ 2003;327:1–6.
11. Chambers AF, Groom AC, MacDonald IC. Dissemination and growth of cancer cells in metastatic sites. Nat Rev Cancer 2002; 2:563–572.
12. Hanahan D, Weinberg A. The hallmarks of cancer. Cell 2000; 100:57–70.
13. Hahn WC, Weinberg RA. Rules for making human tumor cells. N Engl J Med 2002;347:1593–1603.
14. Lengauer C, Kinzler KW, Vogelstein B. Genetic instabilities in human cancers. Nature (Lond) 1998;396:643–649.
15. Papadopoulos S, et al. Assessment of genomic instability in breast cancer and uveal melanoma by random amplified polymorphic DNA analysis. Int J Cancer 2002;99:193—200.
16. Vineis P, Matullo G, Manuguerra M. An evolutionary paradigm for carcinogenesis. J Epidemiol Community Health 2003; 57:89–95.
17. Gatenby RA, Vicent TL. An evolutionary model of carcinogenesis. Cancer Res 2003;63:6212–6220.
18. Vineis P. Cancer as an evolutionary process at the cell level: an epidemiological perspective. Carcinogenesis (Oxf) 2003;24:1–6.
19. Pozzatti R, et al. Primary rat embryo cells transformed by one or two oncogenes show different metastatic potentials. Science 1986;232:223–227.
20. Wyllie A, et al. Rodent fibroblast tumors expressing human *myc* and *ras* genes: growth, metastasis and endogenous oncogene expression. Br J Cancer 1987;56:251–259.
21. Steeg PS. Metastatic suppressors alter the signal transduction of cancer cells. Nat Rev Cancer 2002;3:55–63.
22. Shevde LA, Welch DR. Metastasis suppressor pathways—an evolving paradigm. Cancer Lett 2003;198:1–20.
23. Steeg PS, et al. Evidence for a novel gene associated with low tumor metastatic potential. J Natl Cancer Inst 1988;80:200–204.
24. Steeg PS, Palmieri T, Ouatas M, Salerno M. Histidine kinases and histidine phosphorylated proteins in mammalian cell biology, signal transduction and cancer. Cancer Lett 2003;190: 1–12.
25. Chikawa T, et al. Localization of metastasis suppressor gene(s) for prostatic cancer to the short arm of human chromosone 11. Cancer Res 1992;52:3486–3490.
26. Lee JH, et al. KiSS-1, a novel human malignant melanoma metastasis-suppressor gene. J Natl Cancer Inst 1996;88: 1731–1737.
27. Egeblad M, Werb Z. New functions for the matrix metalloproteinases in cancer progression. Nat Rev Cancer 2002;2:161–174.
28. Yamada SD, et al. Mitogen-activated protein kinase kinase 4 (MKK4) acts as a metastasis suppressor gene in human ovarian carcinoma. Cancer Res 2002;62:6717–6723.
29. Kauffman EC, Robinson VL, Stadler WM, Sokoloff MH, Rinker-Schaeffer CW. Metastasis suppression: the evolving role of metastasis suppressor genes for regulating cancer cell growth at the secondary site. J Urol 2003;169:1122–1133.
30. Seraj MJ, Samant RS, Verderame MF, Welch DR. Functional evidence for a novel human breast carcinoma metastasis suppressor, BRMS1, encoded at chromosome 11q13. Cancer Res 2000;60:2764–2769.
31. Xia W, Unger P, Miller L, Nelson J, Gelman IH. The Src-suppressed C kinase substrate, SSeCKS, is a potential metastasis inhibitor in prostate cancer. Cancer Res 2001;61:5644–5651.
32. Gildea JJ, et al. RhoGD12 is an invasion and metastasis supressor gene in human cancer. Cancer Res 2002;62:6418–6423.
33. Bandyopadhyay S, et al. The Drg-1 gene suppresses tumor metastasis in prostate cancer. Cancer Res 2003;63:1731–1736.
34. Fidler IJ. The organ microenvironment and cancer metastasis. Differentiation (Camb) 2002;70:498–505.
35. Park CC, Bissell MJ, Baecellos-Hoff MH. The influence of the microenvironment on the malignant phenotype. Mol Med Today 2000;6:324–329.
36. Roskelley CD, Bissell MJ. The dominance of the microenvironment in breast and ovarian cancer. Cancer Biol 2002;12:97–104.

37. Kinzler KW, Vogelstein B. Landscaping the cancer terrain. Science 1998;280:1036–1037.
38. Wang F, et al. Phenotypic reversion or death of cancer cells by altering signaling pathways in three dimensional contexts. JNCI 2002;94:1494–1503.
39. Bissell MJ, Radisky D. Putting tumors in context. Nat Rev Cancer 2001;1:46–54.
40. Tisty TD, Hein PW. Know thy neighbor: stromal cells can contribute oncogenic signals. Curr Opin Genet Dev 2001;11: 54–59.
41. Skobe M, Fusenig NE. Tumorigenic conversion of immortal human keratinocytes through stromal cell activation. Proc Natl Acad Sci USA 1998;95:1050–1055.
42. Olumi AF, et al. Carcinoma-associated fibroblasts direct tumor progression of initiated human prostatic epithelium. Cancer Res 1999;59:5002–5011.
43. Pardoll DM. Does the immune system see tumors as foreign or self? Annu Rev Immunol 2003;21:807–839.
44. Hadden JW. Immunodeficiency and cancer: prospects for correlation. Int Immunopharmacol 2003;3:1061–1071.
45. Mbulaiteye SM, Biggar RJ, Goedert JJ, Engels EA. Immune deficiency and risk for malignancy among persons with AIDS. J AIDS 2003;32:527–533.
46. Gruijl FR. Ultraviolet radiation and tumor immunity. Methods 2002;28:122–129.
47. Mudgil AD, et al. Ultraviolet B irradiation induces expansion of intraepithelial tumor cells in a tissue model of early cancer progression. J Invest Dermatol 2003;121:191–197.
48. Fisher MS, Kripke ML. Systemic alteration induced in mice by ultraviolet light irradiation and its relationship to ultraviolet carcinogenesis. Proc Natl Acad Sci USA 1977;74:1688–1692.
49. Jiang W, et al. UV irradiation augments lymphoid malignancies in mice with one functional copy of wild-type p53. Proc Natl Acad Sci USA 2001;98:9790–9795.
50. Schwartzbaum J, et al. Cohort studies of association between self-reported allergic conditions, immune-related diagnoses and glioma and meningioma risk. Int J Cancer 2003;106:423–428.
51. Holly EA, Eberle CA, Bracci PM. Prior history of allergies and pancreatic cancer in the San Francisco Bay Area. Am J Epidemiol 2003;158:432–441.
52. Maria DA, et al. Resistance to melanoma metastases in mice selected for high acute inflammatory response. Carcinogenesis (Oxf) 2001;22:337–342.
53. Cui Z, et al. Spontaneous regression of advanced cancer: identification of a unique genetically determined, age-dependent trait in mice. Proc Natl Acad Sci USA 2003;100:6682–6687.
54. Weidner N. Angiogenesis as a predictor of clinical outcome in cancer patients. Hum Pathol 2000;31:403–405.
55. Thompson WD. Tumour versus patient: vascular and tumour survival versus prognosis. J Pathol 2001;193:425–426.
56. Weidner N, Folkman J, Pozza F. Tumor angiogenesis: a new significant and independent prognostic indicator in early-stage breast carcinoma. J Natl Cancer Inst 1992;84:1875–1887.
57. Toi M, Inada K, Suzuki H. Tumor angiogenesis in breast cancer: its importance as a prognostic indicator and association with vascular endothelial growth factor suppression. Breast Cancer Res Treat 1995;36:193–204.
58. Eppenberger U, Kueng W, Schlaeppi JM. Markers of tumor angiogenesis and proteolysis independently define high- and low-risk subsets of node-negative breast cancer patients. J Clin Oncol 1998:16:3129–3136.
59. Bian XW, Du LL, Shi JQ. Correlation of bFGF, FGF-1 and VEGF expression with vascularity and malignancy of human astrocytomas. Anal Quant Cytol Histol 2000;22:267–274.
60. Eggert A, Ikegaki N, Kwiatkowski J. High-level expression of angiogenic factors is associated with advanced tumor stage in human neuroblastomas. Clin Cancer Res 1999;6:1900–1908.
61. Stockhammer G, Obwegeser A, Kostron H. Vascular endothelial growth factor (VEGF) is elevated in brain tumor cysts and correlates with tumor progression. Acta Neuropathol (Berl) 2000;100:101–105.
62. Loncaster JA, Cooper RA, Logue JP. Vascular endothelial growth factor (VEGF) expression is a prognostic factor for radiotherapy outcome in advanced carcinoma of the cervix. Br J Cancer 2000; 83:775–781.
63. Hollingsworth HC, Kohn EC, Steinberg SM, Rothenberg ML, Meriono MJ. Tumor angiogenesis in advanced stage ovarian carcinoma. Am J Pathol 1995;147:33.
64. Sivridis E, Giatromanolaki A, Gatter KC, Harris AL, Koukourakis MI. Association of hypoxia inducible factor 1-alpha and 2-alpha with activated angiogenic pathways and prognosis in patients with endometrial carcinomas. Cancer (Phila) 2002;95: 1055–1063.
65. Yoshikawa T, Tsuburaya A, Kobayashi O. Plasma concentrations of VEGF and bFGF in patients with gastric carcinoma. Cancer Lett 2000;153:7–12.
66. Cascinu S, Staccioli MP, Gasparini G. Expression of vascular endothelial growth factor can predict event-free survival in stage II colon cancer. Clin Cancer Res 2000:2803–2807.
67. Maeda K, Chung Y, Takatsuka S. Tumour angiogenesis and tumour cell proliferation as prognostic indicators in gastric carcinoma. Br J Cancer 1995;72:319.
68. Weidner N, Carroll PR, Flax J. Tumor angiogenesis correlates with metastasis in invasive prostate carcinoma. Am J Pathol 1993;143:401–409.
69. Fregene TA, Khanuja PS, Noto AC. Tumor-associated angiogenesis in prostate cancer. Anticancer Res 1993;13:2377.
70. Liotta LA, Kleinerman J, Saidel G. Quantitative relationships of intravascular tumor cells, tumor vessels and pulmonary metastases following tumor implantation. Cancer Res 1974;34: 997–1004.
71. Folkman J. Role of angiogenesis in tumor growth and metastasis. Semin Oncol 2002;29:15–18.
72. Carmeliet P. Angiogenesis in cancer and other diseases. Nature (Lond) 2000;407:249–257.
73. Detmar M, Velasco P, Richard L. Expression of vascular endothelial growth factor induces an invasive phenotype in human squamous cell carcinomas. Am J Pathol 2000;156:159–167.
74. Ribatti D, Vacca A, Dammacco F. The role of vascular phase in solid tumor growth: a historical review. Neoplasia 1999;1: 293–302.
75. Folkman J. Angiogenesis and apoptosis. Semin Cancer Biol 2003; 13:159–167.
76. Zetter BR. Angiogenesis and tumor metastasis. Annu Rev Med 1998;49:407–424.
77. Fidler IJ, Ellis LM. The implications of angiogenesis for the biology and therapy of cancer metastasis. Cell 1994;79:185–188.
78. Folkman J. Tumor angiogenesis: therapeutic implications. N Engl J Med 1971;285:1–7.
79. Krah K, Mironov V, Risau W, Flamme I. Induction of vasculogenesis in quail blastodisc-derived embryoid bodies. Dev Biol 1994;164:123–132.
80. Shalaby F, et al. Failure of blood-island formation and vasculogenesis in Flk-1-deficient mice. Nature (Lond) 1995; 6535(376):62–66.
81. Ferrara N. Vascular endothelial growth factor and the regulation of angiogenesis. Recent Prog Horm Res 2000;55:15–35.
82. Veikkola T, Karkkainen MJ, Claesson-Welsh L, Alitalo K. Regulation of angiogenesis via vascular endothelial growth factor receptors. Cancer Res 2000;60:203–212.
83. Ferrara N, Davis-Smyth T. The biology of vascular endothelial growth factor. Endocr Rev 1997;18:4–25.
84. Bayless KJ, Salazar R, Davis GE. RGD-dependent vacuolation and lumen formation observed during endothelial cell morphogenesis in three-dimensional fibrin matrices involves the

alpha(v)beta(3) and alpha(5)beta(1) integrins. Am J Pathol 2000; 156:1673–1683.
85. Thurston G, Rudge JS, Ioffe E. Angiopoietin-1 protects the adult vasculature against plasma leakage. Nat Med 2000;6:1–4.
86. Thurston G, et al. Leakage-resistant blood vessels in mice transgenically overexpressing angiopoietin-1. Science 1999;286:2511–2514.
87. Suri C, Jones PF, Patan S. Requisite role of angiopoietin-1, a ligand for the TIE2 receptor, during embryonic angiogenesis. Cell 1996;87:1171–1180.
88. Maisonpierre PC, Suri C, Jones PF, et al. Angiopoietin-2, natural antagonist for Tie2 that disrupts in vivo angiogenesis. Science 1997;277:55–60.
89. Patan S, Munn LL, Jain RK. Intussusceptive microvascular growth in a human colon adenocarcinoma xenograft: a novel mechanism of tumor angiogenesis. Microvasc Res 1996;51: 260–272.
90. Maniotis AJ, et al. Vascular channel formation by human melanoma cells in vivo and in vitro: vasculogenic mimicry. Am J Pathol 1999;155:739–752.
91. Folberg R, Hendrix MJ, Maniotis AJ. Vasculogenic mimicry and tumor angiogenesis. Am J Pathol 2000;156:361–381.
92. Djonov V, Schmid M, Tschanz SA, Burri PH. Intussusceptive angiogenesis: its role in embryonic vascular network formation. Circ Res 2000;86:286–292.
93. Rafii M. Circulating endothelial precursors: mystery, reality and promise. J Clin Invest 2000;105:17–19.
94. Asahara T, Kalka C, Isner JM. Stem cell therapy and gene transfer for regeneration. Gene Ther 2000;7:451–457.
95. Takahashi T, Kalka C, Masuda H. Ischemia- and cytokine-induced mobilization of bone marrow-derived endothelial progenitor cells for neovascularization. Nat Med 1999;5:434–438.
96. Rafii S. Efficient mobilization and recruitment of marrow-derived endothelial and hematopoietic cells by adenoviral vectors expressing factors. Gene Ther 2002;9:631–641.
97. Lyden D, et al. Impaired recruitment of bone marrow-derived endothelial cells blocks tumour angiogenesis and growth. Nat Med 2001;7:1194–1201.
98. Asahara T, Takahashi T, Masuda H. VEGF contributes to postnatal neovascularization by mobilizing bone marrow-derived endothelial progenitor cell precursors. EMBO J 1999;18: 3964–3972.
99. Kalka C, Masuda H, Takahashi T. Vascular endothelial growth factor (165) gene transfer augments circulating endothelial progenitor cells in human subjects. Circ Res 2000;86:1198–1202.
100. Hattori K. Vascular endothelial growth factor and angiopoietin-1 stimulate postnatal hematopoiesis by recruitment of vasculogenic and hematopoietic stem cells. J Exp Med 2001;193: 1005–1014.
101. Reyes M, et al. Origin of endothelial progenitors in human postnatal bone marrow. J Clin Invest 2002;109:337–346.
102. Hattori K. Placental growth factor reconstitutes hematopoiesis by recruiting VEGFR1(+) stem cells from bone-marrow microenvironment. Nat Med 2002;8:841–849.
103. Mandriota SJ, Pepper MS. Vascular endothelial growth factor-induced in vitro angiogenesis and plasminogen activator expression are dependent on endogenous basic fibroblast growth factor. J Cell Sci 1997;110:2293–2302.
104. Lobov IB, Brooks PC, Lang RA. Angiopoietin-2 displays VEGF-dependent modulation of capillary structure and endothelial cell survival in vivo. Proc Natl Acad Sci USA 2002;99:11205–11210.
105. McDonald DM, Munn LL, Jain RK. Vasculogenic mimicry: how convincing, how novel, and how significant. Am J Pathol 2000; 156:383–388.
106. Liotta LA, Steeg PS, Stetler-Stevenson WG. Cancer metastasis and angiogenesis: an imbalance of positive and negative regulation. Cell 1991;64:327–336.
107. Hanahan D, Folkman J. Patterns and emerging mechanisms of the angiogenic switch during tumorigenesis. Cell 1996;86: 353–364.
108. Maxwell PH, Dachs GU, Gleadle JM. Hypoxia-inducible factor-1 modulates gene expression in solid tumors and influences both angiogenesis and tumor growth. Proc Natl Acad Sci USA 1997; 94:8104–8109.
109. Shweiki D, Itin A, Soffer D, Keshet E. Vascular endothelial growth factor induced by hypoxia may mediate hypoxia-initiated angiogenesis. Nature (Lond) 1992;359:843–845.
110. Semenza GL. Surviving ischemia: adaptive responses mediated by hypoxia-inducible factor 1. J Clin Invest 2000;106:809–812.
111. Semanza GL. Regulation of hypoxia-induced angiogenesis: a chaperone escorts VEGF to the dance. J Clin Invest 2001;108: 39–40.
112. Dvorak HF. Vascular permeability factor/vascular endothelial growth factor: a critical cytokine in tumor angiogenesis and a potential target for diagnosis and therapy. J Clin Oncol 2002;20: 4368–4380.
113. Pugh CW, Ratcliffe PJ. Regulation of angiogenesis by hypoxia: role of the HIF system. Nat Med 2003;9:677–684.
114. Shweiki D, Neeman M, Itin A. Induction of vascular endothelial growth factor expression by hypoxia and by glucose deficiency in multicell spheroids: implications for tumor angiogenesis. Proc Natl Acad Sci USA 1995;92:768–772.
115. Banai S, et al. Upregulation of vascular endothelial growth factor expression induced by myocardial ischaemia: implications for coronary angiogenesis. Cardiovasc Res 1994;28:1176–1179.
116. Bergers G, Brekken R, McMahon G. Matrix metalloproteinase-9 triggers the angiogenic switch during carcinogenesis. Nat Cell Biol 2000;2:737–744.
117. Wang H, Keiser JA. Vascular endothelial growth factor upregulates the expression of matrix metalloproteinases in vascular smooth muscle cells: role of flt-1. Circ Res 1998;83:832–840.
118. Arbiser JL, Moses MA, Fernandez CA. Oncogenic H-ras stimulates tumor angiogenesis by two distinct pathways. Proc Natl Acad Sci USA 1997;94: 861–866.
119. Laughner E, Taghavi P, Chiles K. HER2 (neu) signaling increases the rate of hypoxia-inducible factor 1 alpha (HIF-1alpha) synthesis: novel mechanism for HIF-1-mediated vascular endothelial growth factor expression. Mol Cell Biol 2001;21:3995–4004.
120. Ravi R, Mookerjee B, Bhujwalla ZW. Regulation of tumor angiogenesis by p53-induced degradation of hypoxia-inducible factor 1alpha. Genes Dev 2000;14:34–44.
121. Bergsmedh A, et al. Horizontal transfer of oncogenes by uptake of apoptotic bodies. Proc Natl Acad Sci USA 2001;98:6407–6411.
122. Rosen L. Antiangiogenic strategies and agents in clinical trials. Oncologist 2000;5:20–27.
123. Stacker SA, Achen MG, Jussila L, Baldwin ME, Alitalo K. Lymphangiogenesis and cancer metastasis. Nat Rev Cancer 2002;2:573–583.
124. Jussila L, Alitalo K. Vascular growth factors and lymphangiogenesis. Physiol Rev 2002;82:673–700.
125. Karkkainen MJ, Makinen T, Alitalo K. Lymphatic endothelium: a new frontier of metastasis research. Nat Cell Biol 2002; 4:E2–E5.
126. Fisher B, et al. relation of number of positive axillary nodes to the prognosis of patients with primary breast cancer. An NSABP update. Cancer (Phila) 1983;52:1551–1557.
127. Hein DW, Moy RL. Elective lymph node dissection in stage I malignant melanomas: a meta-analysis. Melanoma Res 1992; 2:273.
128. Enker E, Laffer UT, Block GE. Enhanced survival of patients with colon and rectal cancer is based upon wide anatomic resection. Ann Surg 1979;190:350.
129. Beasley NJ, et al. Intratumoral lymphangiogenesis and lymph node metastasis in head and neck cancer. Cancer Res 2002; 62:1315–1320.

130. Pepper MS. Lymphangiogenesis and tumor metastasis: myth or reality. Clin Cancer Res 2001;7:462–468.
131. Leu AJ, Berk DA, Lymboussaki A, Alitalo K, Jain RK. Absence of functional lymphatics within a murine sarcoma: a molecular and functional evaluation. Cancer Res 2000;60:4324–4327.
132. Stacker SA, Baldwin ME, Achen MG. The role of tumor lymphangiogenesis in metastatic spread. FASEB J 2002;16:922–934.
133. Padera TP, et al. Lymphatic metastasis in the absence of functional intratumor lymphatics. Science 2002;296:1883–1886.
134. Jain RK, Fenton BT. Intratumoral lymphatic vessels: a case of mistaken identity or malfunction? J Natl Cancer Inst 2002;94: 417–421.
135. Oh S, et al. VEGF and VEGF-C specific induction of angiogenesis and lymphangiogenesis in the differentiated avian chorioallantoic membrane. Dev Biol 1997;188:96–109.
136. Jeltsch M, et al. Hyperplasia of lymphatic vessels in VEGF-C transgenic mice. Science 1997;276:1423–1425.
137. Skobe M, et al. Induction of tumor lymphangiogenesis by VEGF-C promotes breast cancer metastasis. Nat Med 2001;7:192–198.
138. Achen MG, et al. Vascular endothelial growth factor D (Vegf-D) is a ligand for the tyrosine kinases VEGF receptor 2 (Flk-1) and VEGF receptor 3 (Flt-4). Proc Natl Acad Sci USA 1998;95: 548–553.
139. Stacker SA, et al. VEGF-D promotes the metastatic spread of tumor cells via the lymphatics. Nat Med 2001;7:186–191.
140. Veikkola T, et al. Signalling via vascular endothelial growth factor receptor-3 is sufficient for lymphangiogenesis in transgenic mice. EMBO J 2001;20:1223–1231.
141. Kukk E, et al. VEGF-C receptor binding and pattern of expression with VEGFR-3 receptor binding suggests role in lymphatic vascular development. Development (Camb) 1996;122:3829–3837.
142. Cassella M, Skobe M. Lymphatic vessel activation in cancer. Ann NY Acad Sci 2002;979:120–130.
143. Mandriota SJ, et al. Vascular endothelial growth factor-C-mediated lymphangiogenesis promotes tumour metastasis. EMBO J 2001;20:672–682.
144. Woodhouse EC, Chuaqui RF, Liotta LA. General mechanisms of metastasis. Cancer (Phila) 1997;80:1529–1537.
145. Comoglio PM, Trusolino L. Invasive growth: from development to metastasis. J Clin Invest 2992;109:857–862.
146. Stossel TP. On the crawling of animal cells. Science 1993;260: 1086–1094.
147. El-Badry OM, et al. Insulin-like growth factor II acts as an autocrine growth and motility factor in human rhabdomyosarcoma tumors. Cell Growth Differ 1990;1325–351.
148. Stracke ML, et al. Identification, purification and partial sequence analysis of autoaxin, a novel motility-stimulating protein. J Biol Chem 1992;267:2524–2529.
149. Stracke ML, et al. Insulin-like growth factors stimulate chemotaxis in human melanoma cells. Biochem Biophys Res Commun 1988;153:1076–1083.
150. McCarthy JB, Furcht LT. Laminin and fibronectin promote the haptotoactic migration of B16 mouse melanoma cells in vitro. J Cell Biol 1984;98:1474–1480.
151. Tchao R. Novel forms of epithelial cell motility on collagen and on glass surfaces. Cell Motil 1982;2:333–341.
152. Ray JM, Stetler-Stevenson WG. The role of matrix metalloproteases and their inhibitors in tumor invasion, metastasis, and angiogenesis. Eur Respir J 1994;7:2062–2072.
153. Sledge GW Jr, Miller KD. Exploiting the hallmarks of cancer: the future conquest of breast cancer. Eur J Cancer 2003;39: 1668–1675.
154. Morikawa K, et al. Influence of organ microenvironment on extracellular matrix degradative activity and metastasis of human colon carcinoma cells. Cancer Res 1988;48:6863–6871.
155. Stetler-Stevenson M. Type IV collagenase in tumor invasion and metastases. Cancer Metastasis Rev 1990;9:289–303.
156. Weidner N. New paradigm for vessel intravasation by tumor cells. Am J Pathol 2002;160:1937–1939.
157. Dvorak HF, et al. Vascular permeability factor/vascular endothelial growth factor: an important mediator of angiogenesis in malignancy and inflammation. Int Arch Allergy Immunol 1955; 107:233–235.
158. Dvorak HF, et al. Distribution of vascular permeability factor (vascular endothelial growth factor) in tumors: concentration in tumor blood vessels. J Exp Med 1991;174:1275–1278.
159. Poste G, Fidler IJ. The pathogenesis of cancer metastasis. Nature (Lond) 1980;283:139–146.
160. Lee Y. Breast carcinoma: pattern of metastasis at autopsy. J Surg Oncol 1983;23:175–180.
161. Welch JP, Donaldson GA. The clinical correlation of an autopsy study of recurrent colorectal cancer. Ann Surg 1979;189:496–502.
162. Lee Y. Malignant melanoma: patterns of metastasis. CA Cancer J Clin 1980;30:137.
163. Paget S. The distribution of secondary growths in cancer of the breast. Cancer Metastasis Rev 1989;8:98–101.
164. Ewing J. Neoplastic Diseases. Philadelphia: Saunders, 1928: 77–89.
165. Weiss L, et al. Haematogenous metastatic patterns in colonic carcinoma: an analysis of 1541 necropsies. J Pathol 1986;150: 195–203.
166. Tarin D, et al. Mechanism of human tumor metastasis studied in patients with peritoneovenous shunts. Cancer Res 1984; 44:3584–3592.
167. Tarin D, Vass ACR, Kettlewell MGW, Price JE. Absence of metastatic sequelae during long-term treatment of malignant ascites by perito-venous shunting. Invasion Metastasis 1984;4: 1–12.
168. Hart IR, Fidler IJ. Role of organ selectivity in the determination of metastatic patterns of B16 melanoma. Cancer Res 190; 40:2281–2287.
169. Biancone L, Araki M, Araki K, Vassalli P, Stamenkovic I. Redirection of tumor metastasis by expression of E-selectin in vivo. J Exp Med 1996;183:581–587.
170. Matsura N, et al. Induction of experimental bone metastasis in mice by transfection of integrin alpha 4 beta 1 into tumor cells. Am J Pathol 1996;148:55–61.
171. Auerbach R, Alby L, Morrissey LW, Tu M, Joseph J. Expression of organospecific antigens on capillary endothelial cells. Microvasc Res 1985;29:401–411.
172. Rajotte D, et al. Molecular heterogeneity of the vascular endothelium revealed by in vivo phage display. J Clin Invest 1998;102:430–437.
173. Auerbach R, et al. Specificity of adhesion between murine tumor cells and capillary endothelium: an in vitro correlate of preferential metastasis in vivo. Cancer Res 1987;47:1492–1496.
174. Ruoslahti E, Rajotte D. An address system in the vasculature of normal tissues and tumors. Annu Rev Immunol 2000;18:813–827.
175. Pasqualini R, Ruoslahti E. Organ targeting in vivo using phage display peptide libraries. Nature (Lond) 1996;380:364–366.
176. Arap W, et al. Steps towards mapping the human vasculature by phage display. Nat Med 2002;8:121–127.
177. Johnson RC, Zhu DX, Augustin-Voss HG, Pauli BU. Lung endothelial dipeptidyl peptidase IV is an adhesion molecule for lung-metastatic rat breast and prostate carcinoma cells. J Cell Biol 1993;121:1423–1432.
178. Rajotte D, Ruoslahti E. Membrane dipeptidase is the receptor for a lung-targeting peptide indentified by in vivo phage display. J Biol Chem 1999;274(17):11593–11598.
179. Essler M, Ruoslahti E. Molecular specialization of breast vasculature: a breast-homing phage-displayed peptide binds to

aminopeptidase P in breast vasculature. Proc Natl Acad Sci USA 2002;99:2252–2257.
180. Ngaiza JR, Walter S, Barghava P, Malerczyk C, Wellstein A. Pa28alpha: a liver homing protein identified from a colon cancer cell line by in vivo phage display. In: AACR Meeting, New Orleans, 2001;42:261 (abstract).
181. Koop S, et al. Independence of metastatic ability and extravasation: metastatic ras-transformed and control fibroblasts extravasate equally well. Proc Natl Acad Sci USA 1996;93: 11080–11084.
182. Morris VL, Schmidt EE, MacDonald IC, Groom AC, Chambers AF. Sequential steps in hematogenous metastasis of cancer cells studied by in vivo videomicroscopy. Invasion Metastasis 1997; 17:281–296.
183. Groom AC, MacDonald IC, Schmidt EE, Morris VL, Chambers AF. Tumor metastasis to the liver, the roles of proteinases and adhesion molecules: new concepts from in vivo videomicroscopy. Can J Gastroenterol 1999;13:733–743.
184. Heyder C, et al. Real time visualization of tumor cell/endothelial cell interactions during transmigration across the endothelial barrier. J Cancer Res Clin Oncol 2002;128:533–538.
185. Siegel PM, Shu W, Cardiff RD, Muller WJ, Massague J. Transforming growth factor beta signaling impairs neu-induced mammary tumorigenesis while promoting pulmonary metastasis. Proc Natl Acad Sci USA 2003;100:8430–8435.
186. Laferriere J, Houle F, Huot J. Regulation of the metastatic process by E-selectin and stress-activated protein kinase-2/p38. Ann NY Acad Sci 2002;973:562–572.
187. Roetger A, et al. Selection of potentially metastatic subpopulations expressing c-erbB-2 from breast cancer tissue by use of an extravasation model. Am J Pathol 1998;153:1797–1806.
188. Satoh H, et al. Localization of 7H6 tight junction-associated antigen along the cell border of vascular endothelial cells correlates with paracellular barrier function against ions, large molecules and cancer cells. Exp Cell Res 1996;222:269–274.
189. Tobioka H, Sawada N, Zhong Y, Mori M. Enhanced paracellular barrier function of rat mesothelial cells partially protects against cancer cell penetration. Br J Cancer 1996;74:439–445.
190. Osani M, et al. Hepatocyte nuclear factor (HNF)-4alpha induces expression of endothelial fas ligand (fasl) to prevent cancer cell migration: a novel defense mechanism of endothelium against cancer metastasis. Jpn J Cancer Res 2002;93:532–541.
191. Lewalle JM, Cataldo D, Bajou K, Lambert CA, Foidart JM. Endothelial cell intracellular Ca2+ concentration is increased upon breast tumor cell contact and mediates tumor cell transendothelial migration. Clin Exp Metastasis 1998;16:21–29.
192. Voura EB, Sandig M, Kalnins VI, Siu C. Cell shape changes and cytoskeletal reorganization during transendothelial migration of human melanoma cells. Cell Tissue Res 1998;293:375–387.
193. Madri JA, Graesser D. Cell migration in the immune system: the evolving inter-related roles of adhesion molecules and proteinases. Dev Immunol 2000;7:103–116.
194. Faveeuw C, Preece G, Ager A. Transendothelial migration of lymphocytes across high endothelial venules into lymph nodes is affected by metalloproteinases. Immunobiology 2001;98: 688–695.
195. Leppert D, et al. Stimulation of matrix metalloproteinase-dependent migration of T cells by eicosanoids. FASEB J 1995;9: 1473–1481.
196. Leppert D, Waunbant E, Galardy R, Bunnett N, Hauser SL. T-cell gelatinases mediate basement membrane transmigration in vitro. J Immunol 1995;154:4379–4389.
197. Madri JA, Graesser D, Haas T. The roles of adhesion molecules and proteinases in lymphocyte transendothelial migration. Biochem Cell Biol 1996;74:749–757.
198. Klier CM, Nelson PJ. Chemokine-induced extravasation of MonoMac 6 cells: chemotaxis and MMP activity. Ann NY Acad Sci 1999;878:575–577.
199. Robinson SC, Scott KA, Balkwill FR. Chemokine stimulation of monocyte matrix metalloproteinase-9 requires endogenous TNF-alpha. Eur J Immunol 2002;32:404–412.
200. Yoon SO, Park SJ, Yun CH, Chung AS. Roles of matrix metalloproteinases in tumor metastasis and angiogenesis. J Biochem Mol Biol 2003;36:128–137.
201. Kuittinen O, Savolainen E, Koisten P, Mottonen M, Turpeenniemi-Hujanen T. MMP-2 and MMP-9 expression in adult and childhood acute lymphatic leukemia (ALL). Leukemia Res 2001;25:125–132.
202. Roberts AB, Wakefield LM. The two faces of transforming growth factor beta in carcinogenesis. Proc Natl Acad Sci USA 2003;15:8621–8623.
203. Stamenkovic I. Matrix metalloproteinases in tumor invasion and metastasis. Cancer Biol 2000;10:415–433.
204. Cairns RA, Khokha R, Hill RP. Molecular mechanisms of tumor invasion and metastasis: an integrated view. Curr Mol Med 2003;3:659–671.
205. Fidler IJ. Seed and soil revisited: contribution of the organ microenvironment to cancer metastasis. Surg Oncol Clin N Am 2001;10:257–269.
206. Berman RS, Portera CA, Ellis LM. Biology of liver metastases. Cancer Treat Res 2001;209:183–206.
207. Bashyam MD. Understanding cancer metastasis. Cancer (Phila) 2002;94:1821–1829.
208. Duncan LM, Deeds J, Hunter J. Down-regulation of the novel gene melastatin correlates with potential for melanoma metastasis. Cancer Res 1998;58:1515–1520.
209. Ince TA, Weinberg RA. Functional genomics and the breast cancer problem. Cancer Cell 2002;1:15–17.
210. van't Veer LJ, et al. Gene expression profiling predicts clinical outcome of breast cancer. Nature (Lond) 2002;415:530–536.
211. Ramaswamy S, Ross KN, Lander ES, Golub TR. A molecular signature of metastasis in primary solid tumors. Nat Genet 2003;33:49–54.
212. Ngaiza JR, Walter S, Barghava P, Malerczyk C, Wellstein A. Pa28alpha: a liver homing protein identified from a colon cancer cell line by in vivo phage display. In: AACR Meeting, New Orleans, 2001;42:261 (abstract 1411).
213. Yu D, Hung M. Overexpression of ErbB2 in cancer and ErbB2-targeting strategies. Oncogene 2000;19:6115–6121.
214. Rowinsky EK. Signal events: cell signal transduction and its inhibition in cancer. Oncologist 2003;8:5–17.
215. Ciardielli F, Tortora G. A novel approach in the treatment of cancer: targeting the epidermal growth factor receptor. Clin Cancer Res 2001;7:2958–2970.
216. Thompson TC, Timme TL, Goltsov A. Caveolin-1, a metastasis-related gene that promotes cell survival in prostate cancer. Apoptosis 1999;4:233–237.
217. Kraiem Z, Korem S. Matrix metalloproteinases and the thyroid. Thyroid 2000;10:1061–1069.
218. Elkin M, et al. Inhibition of matrix metalloproteinase-2 expression and bladder carcinoma metastasis by halofuginone. Clin Cancer Res 1999;5:1982–1988.
219. Tremont-Lukats IW, Gilbert MR. Advances in molecular therapies in patients with brain tumors. Cancer Control 2003;10:125–137.
220. Ouatas M, Salerno M, Palmieri T, Steeg PS. Basic and translational advances in cancer metastasis: Nm23. J Bioenerg Biomembr 2003;35:73–79.
221. Welsh SJ, Powis G. Hypoxia inducible factor as a cancer drug target. Curr Cancer Drug Targets 2003;3:391–405.
222. Chambers AF, MacDonald IC, Schmidt EE, Morris VL, Groom AC. Clinical targets for anti-metastasis therapy. Adv Cancer Res 2000;79:91–121.
223. Kim JA. Targeted therapies for the treatment of cancer. Am J Surg 2003;186:264–268.

224. Niethammer AG, et al. A DNA vaccine against VEGF receptor 2 prevents effective angiogenesis and inhibits tumor growth. Nat Med 2002;8:1369–1375.
225. Willett CG, et al. Direct evidence that the VEGF-specific antibody bevacizumab has antivascular effects in human rectal cancer. Nat Med 2003;10:145–147.
226. Arap W, et al. Targeting the prostate for destruction through a vascular address. Proc Natl Acad Sci USA 2002;99:1527–1531.
227. Ruoslahti E. Targeting tumor vasculature with homing peptides from phage display. Cancer Biol 2000;10:435–442.

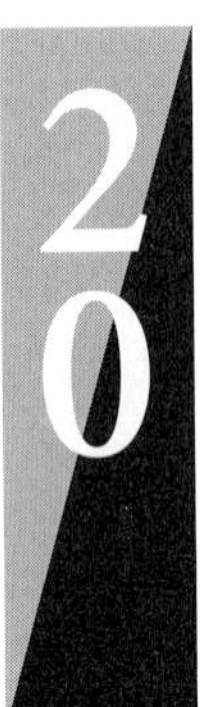

Tumor Immunology and Immunotherapy

Jeffrey Weber, Sophie Dessureault, and Scott Antonia

The principles of basic cellular immunology as elucidated during the past decade include a much greater understanding of the way cytolytic T cells and helper T cells are generated in the host, how immune tolerance mechanisms lead to the deletion of reactive T cells centrally within the thymus or peripherally within the tissues, and the molecular mechanisms by which T cells recognize cognate antigen and transduce signals to become activated effector cells. A significant level of attention has been paid in recent years to how those principles of basic immunology may be applied to the generation of immunotherapy strategies for cancer. In this chapter, we review recent data on the existence of tumor-specific and tumor-associated antigens that might be recognized by immune effector cells; discuss the development of immune molecules and cytokines that might be effective in mediating tumor regression by an immunologic mechanism; mention new developments on mechanisms of immunosuppression in cancer patients; and review the most recent data on the use of nonspecific and antigen-specific immunotherapies that have promise in the treatment of human malignancy.

Tumor Antigens Recognized by Immune Cells

Melanoma Tumor Antigens

Tumor-reactive lymphocytes derived from patient peripheral blood or found to infiltrate metastatic melanoma lesions have been grown in vitro,[1] permitting the cloning of melanoma antigens recognized by T cells[2,3] (Table 20.1, Figure 20.1). The antigen called MAGE (melanoma antigen E) defined a family of antigens not previously identified. MAGE-1 and members of its multigene family were present on melanomas and other tumors as well as testis and placenta but no other normal tissue.[4]

A second group of antigens is the melanosome-related differentiation proteins. MART-1/Melan A was defined via recognition by cytotoxic T lymphocyte (CTL) clones from melanoma patient peripheral blood and by tumor-infiltrating lymphocytes (TIL).[5] MART-1 is expressed by virtually all metastatic melanoma lesions, and also by melanocytes, but not normal tissue. The nonamer sequence AAGIGILTV and decamer EAAGIGILTV, representing amino acid residues 27–35 and 26–35 of MART-1, respectively, bound most strongly to human leukocyte antigen (HLA)-A2.[6] These peptides stimulated the growth of specific CTL from peripheral blood mononuclear cells (PBMC) of HLA-A2-positive melanoma patients and normals.[7] In a clinical study of patients with melanoma who had resected lymph nodal disease, class I peptide tetramers were employed to detect MART-1 and tyrosinase-specific CTL in tumor-infiltrating lymph nodal tissue. From 0.1% to 3% of CD8+ lymphocytes infiltrating tumor-involved lymph nodes were MART-1 specific. In contrast, the proportion of MART-1-specific cells in nontumor-containing lymph nodes was not different from background.[8,9]

Antigen pMel17/gp100 was defined via recognition by CTL clones from melanoma patient peripheral blood and by TIL. This 100-kilodalton (100-kDa) transmembrane glycoprotein is recognized by the HMB-45 and NKI-beteb monoclonal antibodies on melanocytes and melanoma cells.[10,11] CTL clones derived from melanoma patients, and TIL grown from a melanoma patient, recognized melanoma cells that expressed gp100 in association with HLA-A2.1.[12] Multiple peptides derived from gp100 that fit the consensus motif for binding to HLA-A2 were recognized by TIL from melanoma patients, including gp100 209–217 (ILDQVPSFV) and gp100 154–162 (TKTWGQYWQV), as well as gp100 457–466 (LLDGTAATLRL).[13,14] TIL specific for gp100 have been reported to induce regression of metastatic melanoma in patients also receiving interleukin (IL)-2) therapy.[14] These data suggest that gp100 may be a relevant tumor regression antigen.

Tyrosinase is a membrane-bound protein involved in melanin synthesis[15] that is expressed by virtually all primary cutaneous melanomas and by up to 90% of metastatic lesions. It encodes several epitope peptides that are presented by HLA-A2 to CTL reactive with human melanomas.[16] A peptide derived from tyrosinase, amino acids 368–376, YMNGTMSQV, was shown to be posttranslationally modified by deamidation of asparagine to aspartic acid, resulting in a sequence recognized by human CTL, YMDGTMSQV, known as tyrosinase 368–376 (370D).[17] The tyrosinase 368–376 (370D) peptide encodes a biologically important epitope and can induce CTL in vitro and in vivo[18] (also Weber et al., unpublished data).

Recently, "cancer-testis" antigens distinct from the MAGE family, called NY-ESO-1 and SSX-2, were discovered that both elicit a strong humoral response yet encode epitope peptides recognized by CTL clones, TIL, and T helper cells

TABLE 20.1. Tumor antigens.

Tumor antigen	*Specificity*	*Immunogenicity*	*Reference*
Melanoma antigen E (MAGE)	Melanoma; other tumors; testis; placenta	MAGE-specific T cells derived from peripheral blood mononuclear cells (PBMC) of melanoma patients and from melanoma tumor specimens	1–4
MART-1/Melan A	Melanoma; melanocytes	MART-1/Melan A-specific cytotoxic T lymphocytes (CTLs) derived from PBMC and tumor-infiltrating lymphocytes (TILs) of melanoma patients	5–9
pMel17/gp100	Melanoma; melanocytes (recognized by the HMB-45 antibody)	CTL clones generated from PBMC and TIL of melanoma patients; TILs specific for gp100 induce regression of metastatic melanoma in patients also receiving interleukin (IL)-2 therapy	10–14
Tyrosinase	Melanoma	Tyrosinase 370D can induce CTL activity in vitro and in vivo	15–18
"Cancer testis antigen" (NY-ESO-1 and SSX-2)	Melanoma; a number of adenocarcinomas (breast, prostate, lung, esophagus); testis; placenta	Elicits a strong humoral response; recognized by CTL clones, TIL, and T helper cells from patients with melanoma and breast cancer	19–23
Carcinoembryonic antigen (CEA) differentiation antigen	Gastric, pancreatic, colorectal, breast, and non-small cell lung cancers; epithelial surface of the colon and some fetal tissue	CEA-specific CTL responses can be detected after immunization, but they are difficult to generate	31–33
HER-2/neu	Breast cancer; normal breast epithelial cells	CTL responses detected by ELISPOT after immunization	34–39
Alpha fetoprotein (AFP)	Hepatocellular carcinoma	Peptides defined from AFP glycoprotein have been pulsed onto dendritic cells and shown to be immunogenic in patients who are HLA A*0201 positive	40
MUC-1	Normal epithelial cells in the gut, pancreas, gallbladder, and mammary tissue	Both major histocompatibility complex (MHC) restricted and unrestricted effector cells have been shown to recognize the MUC-1 repeat backbone	41

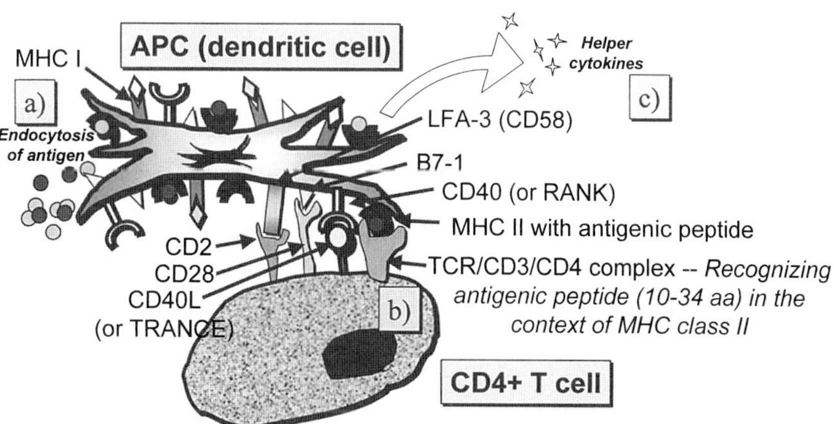

FIGURE 20.1. Schematic indicating the cellular events involved with processing and presenting antigens to T cells. (a) Specificity: Antigen uptake and presentation by antigen-presenting cells (APC) with peptide in the groove of a major histocompatibility complex (MHC) class II molecule (e.g., DR, DP, or DQ) to a naïve CD4+ T cell. (b) Activation: APC–T cell interaction: cross-talk and mutual activation. In addition to TCR ligation with antigenic peptide in the context of MHC (signal 1), costimulatory molecules such as B7 (signal 2) on the APC must interact with CD28 to achieve full T-cell activation. CTLA-4 (not shown) competitively binds B7 and results in downregulation of the T-cell response. Interaction of adhesion molecules such as LFA-3 and CD2 assists during MHC–TCR ligation. Interaction of activating signals to the APC such as CD40–CD40L interaction results in activation of the APC. (c) Differentiation: T-cell activation by an activated APC. Interleukins (IL-12, IFN-gamma, IL-2, TNF-alpha versus IL-4, IL-5, IL-10, TNF-gamma) are produced and help determine T-cell differentiation. Expression of APC surface molecules is increased. In the absence of signals 1 and 2 (antigenic peptide and costimulatory molecule), T-cell antigen receptor (TCR) ligation results in anergy rather than activation.

from patients with melanoma and breast cancer.[19,20] These antigens were expressed by a variety of adenocarcinomas (breast, prostate, and lung), as well as esophageal cancers and melanomas, suggesting wide potential utility. NY-ESO-1 is immunogenic, inducing spontaneous serologic and T-cell responses in 50% of patients whose tumors express it.[21–23] NY-ESO-1 is expressed only by tumors and tissues lacking class I major histocompatibility complex (MHC) (testis, placenta), suggesting that it may not induce tolerance. CD4 T-cell responses have been seen to bind NY-ESO-1, as well as other melanoma differentiation antigens.[24–30]

Although many tumor antigens have been defined in patients with melanoma, a number of self-"differentiation" antigens from epithelial cancers have been shown to be immunogenic. Carcinoembryonic antigen (CEA) is a glycoprotein normally expressed in low levels on the epithelial surface of the colon and in some fetal tissue that functions as an intercellular adhesion molecule.[31,32] Increased expression of CEA on tumor cells mediates attachment of tumor cells to normal cells and promotes metastasis.[31,32] It is expressed in a majority of gastric and pancreatic carcinomas and colorectal, breast, and non-small cell lung cancers.[31] Early clinical studies of peptide-based vaccination with CEA antigen involved the use of autologous dendritic cell (DC) to deliver the CEA-derived peptides.[33] The results of these studies indicate that peptide-specific CTL responses against the CEA peptides were difficult to generate. Heteroclitic peptides that contain a substitution of one or more amino acids in the site of T-cell receptor contact may cause enhanced proliferation and cytotoxic activity directed toward cells bearing the native antigen. A known and commonly targeted CTL epitope of CEA has been designated as CAP1, and studies have shown that the peptide CAP1-6D, which has asparagine substituted for aspartic acid at position 6, greatly enhances CEA-specific CTL activity compared to the CAP1 epitope.[31] A trial using this epitope pulsed onto DC is described next.

HER-2/neu is a transmembrane protein that is expressed on most breast epithelial cells and tumor cells and overexpressed on 20% to 30% of invasive breast cancers. HER-2/neu functions as an epidermal growth factor receptor consisting of an extracellular domain (ECD) and an intracellular cytoplasmic domain (ICD).[34] HER-2 is weakly expressed on the epithelial surfaces of normal tissues in adulthood but highly overexpressed on the surface of tumor cells in many cancers.[34,35] The HER-2/neu p369–377 moiety is an immunodominant, HLA class I-binding peptide that is part of the ECD of the HER-2/neu protein.[35] After immunization, CTL responses detected by ELISPOT assay were apparent in some patients, but the responses were undetectable after 5 months. Combined with a previous study, the results indicate that CD4+ T-cell help is required for lasting immunity to the p369–377 epitope.[36]

A HER-2/neu ECD vaccine containing subdominant peptides p42–56, p98–114, and p328–345, and ICD peptides p776–790, p927–941, and 1166–1180, was administered intradermally monthly for 6 months with granulocyte macrophage-colony-stimulating factor (GM-CSF) adjuvant and shown to be immunogenic in 94% of patients.[37,38] A recent Phase I/II clinical study examined the efficacy of peptide-pulsed DC vaccinations in 10 patients suffering from metastatic breast or ovarian cancer utilizing HER-2/neu and Muc-1 peptides.[39] They identified and used two HLA-A2 restricted HER-2/neu peptides designated as E75 and GP2[38,39] and two novel Muc1 peptides, M1.1 and M1.2.[39] After vaccinations, the major CTL response in vivo was induced with the immunodominant E75 and M1.2 peptides.

The alpha fetoprotein is elevated in patients with hepatocellular carcinoma, and peptides defined from that glycoprotein have been pulsed onto dendritic cells in vitro and in vivo and shown to be immunogenic in patients who are HLA A*0201 positive.[40] A unique antigen found on many different tumors of epithelial origin is MUC-1,[41] which is a polypeptide repeat core peptide derived from a transmembrane glycoprotein from which many branched sugars are bound on normal epithelial cells in the gut, pancreas, gallbladder, and mammary tissue. The sugar side chains are truncated in many tumors, exposing the core polypeptide for recognition by T cells. Both MHC-restricted and -unrestricted effector cells have been shown to recognize the MUC-1 repeat backbone, suggesting that it might serve as a tumor-specific target.

Cytokines and Activation Molecules as Cancer Therapy

Interferon-Alpha: A Cytokine That Is an Effective Adjuvant Treatment for Melanoma

Interferon-alpha, a biologic compound that has both antiproliferative and immune modulatory activity in vitro and in vivo, has been tested in a number of Phase II studies in metastatic melanoma, yielding response rates of 10% to 25% with a small proportion of complete responses (CRs) and median survival of 6 to 9 months.[42,43] Response rates appeared to be dose related. These modest results, however, have led to a number of trials of high-, moderate-, and low-dose interferon as adjuvant treatment in patients with resected intermediate (stage IIB and IIC) and high-risk (stage III lymph nodal) melanoma. In Europe, low-dose extended-duration regimens have been tested with fixed doses of 3 million units/m^2 for up to 3 years. A total of seven well-conceived randomized trials have compared low-dose interferon to a control arm, usually observation (Table 20.2). For patients with high-risk disease, no differences in overall and relapse-free survival were observed in those six European and one American studies.[44–48] For those with intermediate-risk disease, there is no clear survival benefit, but with brief follow-up, several studies have shown a relapse-free survival advantage to the low-dose interferon arm. However, in the most recently published and largest trial to date, the "AIM-HIGH" trial in the UK, which compared low-dose interferon for 3 years with observation, did not show any difference in either overall survival or time to relapse.[49,50] In that study, 674 patients with stage IIB or III disease received either interferon at a dose of 3 million units subcutaneously three times a week for 2 years or observation. There was no difference in overall survival (odds ratio, 0.94; $P = 0.6$) or in relapse-free survival (odds ratio, 0.91; $P = 0.3$). The overall survival at 5 years was 44%, interestingly, considerably better than the 37% figure for the interferon arm of the EST 1684 trial that resulted in U.S. Food and Drug Administration (FDA) approval for high-dose interferon.[51] In an editorial that accompanied the recent publication of the results of the AIM-HIGH trial, it was concluded that except for the nearly mature EORTC 18952

TABLE 20.2. Low-dose interferon-alpha trials for adjuvant therapy of melanoma.

Reference	*Cooperative group (PI)*	*N*	*Eligibility*	*Study summary: dosage, schedule, duration*	*Outcome DFS*	*OS*
44	Austrian (Pehamberger et al.)	311	T3–4, N0	Interferon (IFN)-2a 3 MU/d SC × 3 weeks then TIW × 11 months	+	–
45	French (Grob et al.)	499	T3, N0	IFN-2a 3 MU SC TIW × 18 months	+	–
46	WHO-16 (Cascinelli et al.)	444	N1–2	IFN-2a 3 MU SC TIW × 3 years	–	–
47	Scottish (Cameron et al.)	95	T3–4, N1	IFN-2a 3 MU SC BIW × 6 months	–	–
48	EORTC 18871 (Kleeberg et al.)	830	T3–4, N1	IFN-2a 1 MU/d SC × 1 year versus IFN-0.2 mg/day SC × 1 year	–	–
49	UK "AIM-HIGH" (Hancock et al.)	674	Stage IIB–III	FN-2a 3 MU SC TIW × 2 years	–	–
56	EORTC 18952 (Eggermont)	1418	T4, N1	Intermediate-dose IFN: IFN-2b 10 MU/d SC × 1 month; then TIW × 11 months or 5 MU SC TIW × 23 months	–	–

intermediate-dose interferon trial, the end had been reached for low-dose interferon in Europe. In the United States, low-dose interferon has never been routinely employed for melanoma. It is noteworthy that low-dose interferon has been licensed in the European Community for intermediate-risk primary melanoma, based on early data suggesting a relapse-free survival advantage for that regimen.

In the United States, a number of large cooperative group studies have compared a regimen of intravenous high-dose induction therapy followed by maintenance high-dose interferon with observation or vaccine therapy for high-risk disease (Table 20.3). The only equivalent trial in Europe is the EORTC 18952 trial, which we discuss later. Three well-powered trials have tested high-dose interferon as adjuvant therapy for resected high-risk melanoma, although the best quality data suggesting an advantage in relapse-free and overall survival are derived from the smallest and oldest trial, the EST 1684 trial of 280 patients.[51] In that trial, patients were randomized to either observation or the by now standard high-dose regimen of 20 million units/m^2 intravenously daily times five for 4 weeks in the induction phase. The maintenance phase ensued in which interferon was administered at a dose of 10 million units/m^2 subcutaneously three times a week for 11 months. In that trial, one-third of the patients either discontinued the regimen or required a dose modification because of toxicity. The differences in relapse-free and overall survival significantly favored the interferon arm, with 5-year survival of 37%, median survival of 2.78 years, and $P = 0.04$. Interestingly, over time the advantage for overall survival has diminished with $P = 0.09$ at 12 years follow-up, although other causes of death in that aging cohort may obscure the results. Following the EST 1684 study, the U.S. Intergroup performed two subsequent trials of high-dose interferon. In the EST 1690 trial, 683 patients were randomly allocated to receive either observation, high-dose interferon, or the European regimen of a fixed low interferon dose of 3 million units three times a week for 2 years.[52] No differences in overall or even relapse-free survival were seen in that larger trial. As accrual to that trial ended, a follow-up trial comparing high-dose interferon with a ganglioside vaccine for 2 years in high-risk patients was initiated. In that EST 1694 trial, 780 patients were accrued, and the study was stopped prematurely, because there was a significant difference in relapse-free survival favoring the interferon arm with a very low P value of 0.01 that met the monitoring committee requirement for early closure.[53] A statistically significant difference in overall survival was also observed in that trial, with a relatively brief period of follow-up. A fourth smaller trial of high-dose interferon, interferon with ganglioside, and ganglioside alone was conducted, with relapse-free survival data similar to the 1694 trial, albeit with small numbers and brief follow-up.[54] The conclusion from an analy-

TABLE 20.3. High-dose interferon-alpha trials for adjuvant therapy of melanoma.

Reference	*Cooperative group (PI)*	*N*	*Eligibility*	*Study summary: dosage, schedule, duration*	*Outcome DFS*	*OS*
51	ECOG EST 1684 (Kirkwood et al.)	287	T4, N1	IFN-2b 20 MU/m^2/day IV × 1 month (induction phase) then 10 MU/m^2 SC TIW × 11 months (maintenance phase)	+	+
52	ECOG 1690 (Kirkwood et al.)	683	T4, N1	IFN-2b 20 MU/m^2/day IV × 1 month (induction phase) then 10 MU/m^2 SC TIW × 11 months (maintenance phase) versus 3 MU/day SC TIW × 2 years	–	–
53	ECOG EST 1694 / SWOG 9512 (Kirkwood et al.)	780	T4, N1	IFN-2b 20 MU/m^2/day IV × 1 month (induction phase) then 10 MU/m^2 SC TIW × 11 months (maintenance phase) versus GM2-KLH/QS-21 vaccine	+	+

TIW, three times per week; BIW, twice a week.

sis of these four trials was that all four demonstrated a relapse-free survival benefit for high-dose interferon, but any overall survival benefit was unclear and could only unequivocally be claimed for the trial with the most premature follow-up.

A meta-analysis of the randomized high-dose interferon trials has been conducted to increase the number of patients accrued and the statistical power to perceive small differences in survival.[55] The results of that meta-analysis indicate that the relapse-free survival advantage of high-dose interferon is significant and reproducible but that the data suggesting a survival advantage are much weaker. This brings us to the EORTC 18902 trial, in which patients with high-risk disease were randomly assigned to receive an intermediate-dose induction regimen of interferon. The induction consisted of 10 million units/m^2 of interferon administered subcutaneously every day for 4 weeks, followed by 1 year of 10 million units/m^2 three times a week, compared with 5 million units/m^2 three times a week for 2 years. The results of that study have been presented publicly, first at ASCO in 2001, with the final summary presented in 2003.[56] The data do not suggest that there is any difference in overall survival between the groups, although a modest difference in relapse-free survival was observed. If the high-dose regimen of EST 1684 truly resulted in a significant overall survival difference, why would that difference not be seen with a similarly dose intense, although subcutaneous regimen, in the EORTC 18902 trial? The answer is likely that there is no reproducible, significant, and biologically important overall survival difference for high-risk melanoma patients who receive the high-dose interferon regimen. Significant differences in relapse-free survival were observed in all four trials and were maintained in the meta-analysis after adjustment for prognostic variables, suggesting that the difference is genuine.

What conclusions can be drawn about recommending high-dose interferon to patients with resected high-risk melanoma? One is that it is likely to confer a moderate benefit in relapse-free survival, postponing the time to disease recurrence but not changing overall survival significantly. Is the acknowledged toxicity and cost of the year-long regimen justified by the relapse-free survival benefit? Admittedly, the Q-TWIST quality of life analysis, which assumed the level of survival benefit found in the EST 1684 trial, indicated that in spite of the side effects the use of high-dose interferon was justified.[57] However, the relapse-free survival advantage without the likelihood of ever observing a clear overall survival benefit renders interferon an acceptable but hardly desirable option. It should be offered to patients with resected high-risk melanoma but should not be a clearly superior option to a well-designed randomized Phase III or even a Phase II study. Given the difficulty and lack of acceptance of a randomized trial in high-risk melanoma that includes an observation arm, high-dose interferon is a reasonable and proper control arm against which new therapies in development may be measured.

Activity of Recombinant Interleukin 2 (IL-2) for Metastatic Melanoma

Given at high doses as a single agent, IL-2 produces significant clinical responses in some cancers, and it is now being tested in combination with tumor vaccines.[58–60] IL-2 was shown to mediate regression of melanoma and renal cell cancer and has activity in patients with non-Hodgkin's lymphoma. It was approved by the FDA for metastatic melanoma due to a multicenter Phase II experience of 270 patients with a 16% response rate and a median survival of 12.2 months.[61,62] Survival of metastatic melanoma after treatment with high-dose IL-2 is associated with development of autoimmune thyroiditis and vitiligo, as well as the height of the lymphocyte rebound that occurs after cessation of treatment with IL-2 (Table 20.4). When given at the FDA-approved dosage and schedule of 600,000 international units/kg every 8 hours as an intravenous bolus, IL-2 was quite toxic, and it is not recommended for use in an inpatient hospital setting unless given by medical and nursing personnel experienced in its use. IL-2 could be beneficial in a variety of different ways. It could drive the expansion of tumor-specific T cells that are activated by the vaccine. It may also be beneficial during the effector phase of an antitumor T-cell response. For example, it has recently been shown that B7-H1, a member of the B7 family of costimulatory molecules, can be expressed by carcinomas and result in the induction of apoptosis of activated T cells.[63] This B7-H1-mediated negative effect on T cells is prevented in the presence of exogenous IL-2.[64] A very low dose IL-2 regimen has been shown to result in the prolonged persistence of transferred T cells in melanoma patients.[65] This dose of IL-2 is sufficient to saturate IL-2 receptors in vivo. Therefore, the vaccine augmentation effect can potentially be achieved with minimal toxicity.

TABLE 20.4. Known toxicities of interleukin 2 (IL-2).

Common toxicities (occur in 30% or more of patients)	• Low platelet levels; increases risk of bleeding • Low blood pressure • Flushing or rash of the face and body • Chills • Nausea and vomiting • Diarrhea • Tachycardia • Fluid retention • Changes in liver function tests • Arthralgias and myalgias • Reduced volumes of urine • Weight gain • Breathing problems • Fever • Dry skin
Less common toxicities (occur in 10% to 29% of patients)	• Weakness • Low levels of white blood cells; increases risk of infection • Low levels of red blood cells; increases risk of anemia • Mental changes, such as confusion or memory loss • Congestion • Itching • Loss of appetite • Dizziness • Mouth sores • Fatigue or weakness • Enlargement of the abdomen • Changes in electrolyte levels • Cardiac arrhythmias

Recombinant Interleukin 12 (IL-12)

Secreted by activated dendritic cells, IL-12 produces several effects that could enhance an antitumor T-cell response, including the induction of a T helper cell type 1 (Th1) response and the production of γ-interferon.[66] Recombinant IL-12 protein given to cancer patients at the maximum tolerated dose (MTD) in a Phase II trial produced unacceptable toxicity.[67] However, based on animal models, the administration of doses well below the MTD should be sufficient for use of this agent as a tumor vaccine augmentation strategy.[68,69] Gajewski and colleagues conducted Phase I[69] and Phase II clinical trials[70] in melanoma patients combining subcutaneously injected IL-12 with a peptide-pulsed PBMC-based tumor vaccine. The IL-12 was given at a dose well below the MTD three times every other day after each vaccine. Toxicity was acceptable, and two patients (10%) had CRs. In other trials reported by Cebon et al.,[71] melanoma patients were treated with IL-12 in combination with a tumor vaccine (Melan-A peptide vaccine). Cohorts of patients were treated with escalating doses of IL-12 given subcutaneously or intravenously on the day the first vaccine was given and once again 3 weeks later, with five vaccines given over an 8-week period. Toxicity was acceptable, and 1 of 21 patients had a partial response (PR). Before significant efficacy can be realized with this approach, considerable work needs to be done to determine the optimal dose and schedule of IL-12 administration as well as the optimal vaccine with which to combine it.

Recombinant Flt3 Ligand

Flt3 ligand stimulates progenitor cells in the bone marrow, resulting in an increase in DC in the peripheral blood when administered to normal subjects and to patients with metastatic cancer.[72–74] This property of Flt3 ligand makes it a candidate for use as a vaccine augmentation strategy, making available an increased number of DC that could possibly respond and contribute to a tumor vaccine in vivo. Disis et al. recently reported the results of a clinical trial involving 10 patients with HER-2/neu-overexpressing breast or ovarian cancer.[75] Patients were given Flt3 ligand subcutaneously daily for 14 days of 28-day cycles and received a HER-2/neu peptide-based vaccine on day 7 of each cycle. Patients were treated for up to 6 cycles. Clinical responses were not assessable, as 9 of the 10 patients had no evidence of disease. However anti-HER-2/neu T-cell responses were induced in most of the patients. The clinical effectiveness of this approach needs to be tested.

Recombinant CD40 Ligand

Signaling through CD40 on dendritic cells is a potent activation stimulus.[76] Also, Mellman's group recently showed that CD40 ligation results in the activation of cross-presentation of exogenous antigens taken up by DCs on MHC class I molecules.[77] There is evidence to suggest that one target of the immunosuppressive mechanisms of tumor cells is CD40-expressing antigen-presenting cells (APC). Sotomayor et al. have reported, using a murine model, that the in vivo delivery of an activating anti-CD40 antibody prevented tumor cell-induced T-cell unresponsiveness.[78] In addition, others have previously reported that CD40 ligand can prevent inhibition of DC function mediated by IL-10 (which is produced by some tumors)[79] and DC apoptosis that can be induced by tumors.[80,81] Finally, Dotti et al. have shown that the bystander production of CD40 ligand at a tumor vaccine site improved the efficacy of the vaccine.[82] These observations all support the use of CD40-activation strategies to enhance the development of antitumor T-cell responses in cancer patients.

A clinical trial has been reported using recombinant human CD40 ligand protein systemically in cancer patients[83]; this was a Phase I, single-agent trial. Cohorts of patients with refractory cancer were treated with escalating doses of the CD40 ligand protein injected subcutaneously each day for 5 consecutive days. Patients without significant toxicity and no evidence of progression received additional courses at 4-week intervals. Thirty-two patients were treated, with the dose-limiting toxicity found to be liver transaminase elevation. This toxicity was transient in all but 2 patients, and no deaths attributed to this toxicity were reported. Interestingly, 2 patients had significant tumor regressions, with 1 patient developing a sustained CR.

Activating DCs in the setting of tumor vaccination by signaling through CD40 remains an attractive strategy that needs to be developed, with attempts to reduce the incidence of hepatic toxicity and to combine this approach with the use of tumor vaccines to improve therapeutic efficacy.

CpG Oligonucleotides

Signaling through toll-like receptors (TLR) can produce effects in DC that are similar to CD40 ligation.[84] Several TLR exist; however, TLR-9 may be one of the more important TLR involved in the induction of a relevant antitumor T-cell response.[85] The ligands for TLR-9 are immunostimulatory DNA sequences that contain unmethylated CpG sequences.[86] Among other actions, CpG oligonucleotide binding to TLR-9 increases DC surface expression of T-cell costimulatory molecules and secretion of TH1-promoting cytokines including IL-12.[87–89] These compounds are quite effective in augmenting T-cell-mediated tumor rejection in a variety of murine models.[90–95] When administered to humans, they have been found to be safe,[94] and there are indications that they can enhance the effectiveness of vaccines for certain infectious diseases.[96] Clinical trials involving cancer patients are ongoing. To date, only one trial has been briefly reported.[97] Patients with metastatic melanoma were immunized with a MAGE-3 protein-based vaccine, using a CpG compound as an adjuvant. One PR was reported in this Phase I trial. Considerable work remains to be done to determine if CpG oligonucleotides will augment the effectiveness of tumor vaccines, but the approach is promising.

Blocking Anti-CTLA.4 Antibody

CTLA.4 binding to its ligand, CD28, delivers an inhibitory signal to T cells.[98,99] Removal of this potential inhibition is the rationale for administering a blocking anti-CTLA.4 monoclonal antibody in combination with tumor vaccines. Phan et al. conducted a clinical trial involving patients with metastatic melanoma.[100] Patients were treated systemically with an anti-CTLA.4 antibody just before receiving a gp100 peptide-based vaccine every 3 weeks. Individual patients were treated with one to six cycles. Two of the 14 patients had CRs and 1 had a PR. Six of the patients developed significant autoimmune toxicities, all of which resolved spontaneously or with steroid treatment.

Hodi et al. also tested the anti-CTLA.4 antibody in melanoma and ovarian cancer patients, observing no objective tumor regressions.[101] However, this was a single-dose trial and was not combined with a tumor vaccine. Tumor biopsies from three of the patients obtained after antibody administration revealed extensive tumor necrosis, providing compelling evidence that the antibody has the potential to produce a clinical effect. Interestingly, the tumor necrosis was only observed in patients who had previously been immunized with a GM-CSF-modified vaccine.

Antigen-Specific and Nonspecific Therapies

Evidence That Cell Vaccines Might Be Beneficial in Melanoma

Cell-based vaccines for melanoma have been evaluated in trials since the 1970s (Table 20.5). Melacine, consisting of two lyophilized melanoma cell line lysates administered with the Ribi adjuvant, and Canvaxin, consisting of three irradiated and frozen intact cell lines administered with bacille Calmette–Guérin (BCG), have been shown to mediate regression in a small proportion of patients with stage IV disease, in the range of 5% to 10%.[102–105] Melacine was shown to have a 7% response rate in a small Phase II randomized trial with a survival no different from multiagent chemotherapy[102] and has been tested in a large randomized Phase III trial as adjuvant therapy for patients with resected stage II melanoma compared with an observation arm.[104,105] For all patients as randomized, there was no difference in overall and disease-free survival, but for patients who were HLA-A2 positive, a relapse-free survival advantage was seen, indicating that the HLA-A2 population might be appropriate for further testing of that cell vaccine.

More current developments in this field include the use of cytokine gene-transduced tumor cells as vaccines. Dranoff and colleagues have pioneered the use of autologous GM-CSF gene-engineered tumor cell vaccines for cancer, a treatment strongly supported by preclinical murine experiments.[106] In a recent published trial in patients with stage IV melanoma treated with adenovirally transduced GM-CSF-secreting tumor cells, most subcutaneous lesions exhibited significant necrosis, and tumor regression [1 CR, 1 PR, and 1 mixed response (MR)] was seen in 3 of 26 evaluable patients.[107] Thirty-five patients were selected for the trial; 34 had sufficient tumor cells to generate vaccine, but 8 progressed and could not receive vaccine. A similar strategy in non-small cell lung cancer yielded 5 patients with stable disease and 1 mixed response of 25 evaluable patients.[108] As in the melanoma trial, 8 patients progressed before receiving vaccine, indicating that patients selected for this promising therapy must be carefully selected, limiting its applicability. Fourteen patients with pancreatic cancer who had a curative resection and were free of disease received an allogeneic GM-CSF-transduced cell vaccine as well as chemoradiotherapy.[109] Their 1- and 3-year survival was surprisingly favorable, with 3 patients alive 25 months after diagnosis, suggesting that the vaccine regimen, albeit in a heterogeneous group of patients, might have potential as adjuvant treatment.

Heat Shock Proteins

Several clinical trials have tested the notion that heat shock proteins (Hsp), which have been shown to bind tumor antigen peptides, can be extracted from fresh tumor and used to vaccinate patients. Parmiani described a trial of 42 patients treated with four weekly injections of tumor cell-derived Hsp gp96 in which 28 patients were assessable for response.[110] There were 2 CRs as well as 3 patients with prolonged stable disease. All five had evidence of an immune response to autol-

TABLE 20.5. Types of vaccines.

Type of vaccine	*Advantages*	*Disadvantages*	*Examples*
Whole tumor cell-based vaccines	Diverse Ags without knowing the exact Ag(s) that may be responsible for tumor rejection	Limited immunogenicity	Melacine; CancerVax
Cytokine gene-transduced tumor cell-based vaccines	Same as for whole tumor cell vaccines, but more immunogenic	Cell culture and individualized gene transfer is expensive, labor intensive, and limited by variable levels of gene expression	GM-CSF; IL-2
Peptide-based vaccines	No need for patient-derived tissue; can monitor immune response	Limited number of Ags; patient selection based on HLA type; posttranslational modification; MHC class I versus class II	MAGE; MART; gp100; tyrosinase; gp75
Antigen-pulsed or gene-modified dendritic cell-based vaccines	Efficient and safe method of inducing antitumor immune response	Expensive, labor intensive	Tyrosinase-pulsed DCs; gp100-pulsed DCs
DNA and RNA-based vaccines	Genetic material delivered without the difficulties associated with the development of immune reactivity against viral vectors	Variable gene transfer efficiencies	B7-1; melanoma-associated antigens

AG, antigen; DC, dendritic cell; GM-CSF, granulocyte macrophage colony-stimulating factor.

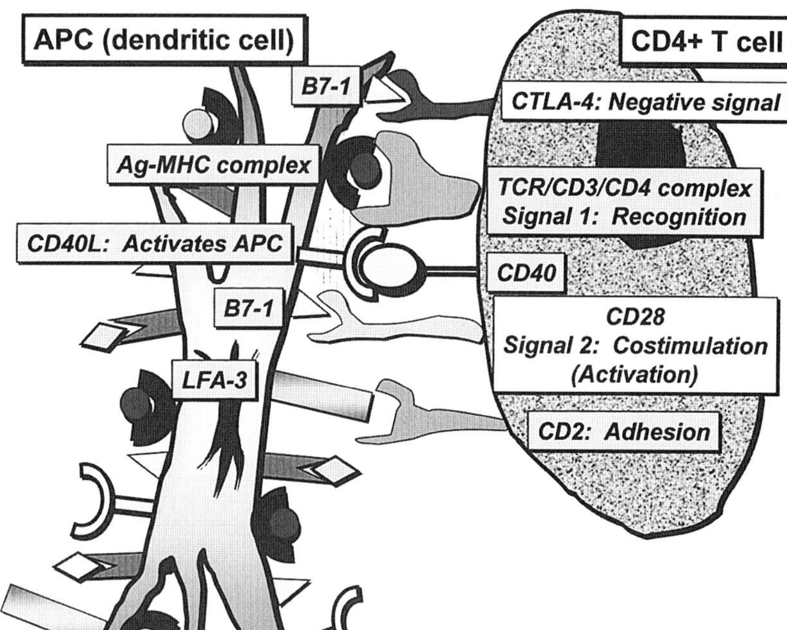

FIGURE 20.2. CTLA-4 binding leads to immunosuppression. T cells require two signals for activation. Signal 1 is the recognition of antigenic peptide in the context of MHC molecules; signal 2 can be provided by cell-surface molecules CD80 or CD86 (B7-1 and B7-2, respectively). CTLA-4 competitively binds B7 molecules and results in a damping of the T-cell response.

ogous tumor cells, and toxicity was minimal. The same group published a trial of autologous Hsp 96 therapy after resection of liver metastases from stage IV colorectal cancer patients.[111] There was a correlation between immune response to autologous tumor cells and overall as well as relapse-free survival, which was quite favorable compared to historical controls.

Development of Peptide Vaccines for Melanoma

Peptides of 8 to 10 amino acids are derived by intracellular cleavage of a variety of proteins, and are selectively conducted by the TAP transporter mechanism to the endoplasmic reticulum where they bind nascent class I molecules and are presented on the surface of the cell in association with class I molecules for interrogation by T cells. Because peptides are the smallest unit recognized by T cells, they might be useful as vaccine immunogens in the proper MHC class I context for recognition by T cells. A MAGE-3 HLA-A1-restricted peptide in aqueous solution was used to treat 39 patients with metastatic melanoma, of whom 26 finished four treatments every 4 weeks.[112] Four PR as well as 3 CR were seen, often with a prolonged time to attain response; 2 complete responders had a duration beyond 2 years. The full-length MAGE-3 gene encoding the same peptide was chimerically linked to an H. Flu protein as adjuvant and used to vaccinate 35 patients in a Phase I trial with adjuvant AS-02B.[113] Two objective responses were observed in that trial, one in a patient with bladder cancer and one with melanoma. In both trials, no immune responses to the MAGE-3 peptide were observed. Jager and colleagues showed that 6 of 26 patients treated with MAGE-1, MAGE-3, MART-1/Melan A, and tyrosinase peptides exhibited tumor regression.[114] Disease was stabilized in 22 of 26 evaluable patients with metastatic melanoma. A correlation was seen between strong MHC class I staining and response; there was also a correlation between the presence of skin/subcutaneous disease, low tumor burden, immune response, and clinical response.

Rosenberg's group has tested a gp100 peptide incorporating a single amino acid change to increase class I binding with IFA to which intravenous IL-2 was added, in patients with stage IV melanoma. A 41% response rate was observed, which was much higher than prior trials with the gp100 vaccine or with high-dose IL-2 alone. However, this result has not been confirmed in a subsequent multicenter study. The same substituted gp100 peptide vaccine was combined with an antibody that abrogated CTLA-4 signaling to augment T-cell reactivity (Figure 20.2). In that trial there were 3 responses (2 CR, 1 PR) in 14 patients with stage IV melanoma that were maintained beyond 12 months, with regression of a brain metastasis. Significant levels of reversible autoimmune side effects were observed that correlated with response. Slingluff and colleagues immunized 26 patients with stage IV melanoma who received multiple peptides including adjuvant and GM-CSF or with dendritic cells pulsed with the same peptides.[115] Two PRs and 2 patients with stable disease (SD) were observed in the peptide/GM-CSF group, compared with 1 PR and 1 SD in the DC group. Immunity to the peptides was correlated with clinical response. The HLA-Cw*0702 restricted MAGE-A12:170–178 peptide emulsified in IFA was given to 9 patients with metastatic melanoma.[116] One of 9 patients demonstrated a PR, but no systemic immune responses to the MAGE-A12 peptide by tetramer or gamma interferon polymerase chain reaction (PCR) assay were seen. A MART-1/Melan-A peptide without adjuvant but with IL-12 was administered intradermally to 28 patients with stage IV melanoma. Of 24 evaluable patients, there was 1 CR, 1 PR, and 2 patients with SD. Many of the aforementioned peptides have been tested as adjuvant treatment for their ability to promote a T-cell response in patients with resected high- or intermediate-risk melanoma and thereby prevent or prolong time to relapse. Interleukin-12 and GM-CSF are effective vaccine adjuvants in mice and have been tested for their ability to augment immunity in resected melanoma patients. Both cytokines were shown to increase immunity to a multipeptide vaccine with toil-based adjuvant Montanide ISA 51, with favorable median survival in high-risk disease of greater than 48 months, similar to the latest trials including high-dose interferon. Multipeptide vaccines for melanoma are currently being tested in larger Phase II trials and represent the next logical experimental arm of a randomized clinical trial for high-risk melanoma.

Dendritic Cell-Based Vaccines

Dendritic cells (DC) are the most potent cells known in humans that prime and stimulate T-cell responses, and they are highly specialized cells which process and present antigens to immune cells. DCs have been grown from a variety of precursors, including peripheral blood monocytes, as well as selected CD34+ progenitors, and a number of cytokines and maturing stimuli have been used to generate human DC ex vivo for clinical trials of adoptive transfer after pulsing with antigen. Nestle and colleagues intravenously administered mature monocyte-derived DC cultured in vitro with IL-4 and GM-CSF and pulsed with tumor antigen peptides and/or tumor lysate to patients with stage IV melanoma.[117] Five CR or PR were observed in 16 patients,[118] and the trial has been extended to a larger multicenter Phase II trial.

Seven patients with metastatic melanoma received gp100 and MART-1 peptide-pulsed monocyte-derived DC.[119] DC were administered intravenously four times at 3-week intervals in escalating doses. Only one of seven patients evaluated demonstrated an objective PR. Enhancement of CTL reactivity was seen in one of five patients who completed all four vaccines.

Eleven stage IV melanoma patients received mature monocyte-derived DC loaded with a MAGE-3A1 peptide.[120] The patients received five vaccinations at 2-week intervals. The first three vaccinations were administered subcutaneously and the last two were administered intradermally. Six of 11 patients had regression of their disease. ELISPOT assays indicated that peptide-specific CTL precursors were expanded in 8 of 11 patients. Intriguingly, immune responses declined after the regimen of injections.

Fourteen patients with malignant melanoma were given four intravenous injections of DC derived from CD34+ stem cells and matured with tumor necrosis factor (TNF)-α then pulsed with HLA-A1+ MAGE-1 and MAGE-3 peptides or with HLA-A2+ Melan-A, gp100, and tyrosinase peptides.[121] Antitumor responses were observed in 2 patients and peptide-specific DTH reactions were found in 4.

Banchereau et al. immunized 11 patients with CD34+ progenitor-derived mature DC and achieved 3 CR. They showed that clinical response correlated with immune responses detected in the peripheral blood,[122] and they have continued to treat patients with mature CD34-derived DC with excellent clinical results.

The CEA CAP1-6D-substituted peptide was pulsed onto DC in the presence of Flt3 ligand, a DC growth factor, in 12 patients with lung or colorectal cancer who were HLA A*0201+. Patients received subcutaneous cytokine for 10 days before immunization with escalating doses of intravenous peptide-pulsed DC. Lytic activity against target cells bearing CAP1-6D, as well as native CEA peptide, was observed in 7 of 12 patients. Five patients showed evidence of tumor regression, with 1 CR, 1 PR, 1 MR, and 2 with SD. Evidence of clinical response correlated with the expansion of antigen-specific CTL by tetramer analysis. Dendritic cells that have been pulsed with autologous tumor lysates have been shown to mediate regression of pediatric tumors, including neuroblastoma and Ewing's sarcoma.[123,124]

Adoptive Transfer of CTL

CD8+ T-cell clones specific for MART1MelanA or gp100 were administered to 10 stage IV melanoma patients by Yee and colleagues.[125] Adoptively transferred T-cell clones persisted in vivo in response to low-dose IL-2 treatment, trafficked to tumor sites, and eliminated antigen-positive tumor cells. Mixed response or stable disease was observed in 8 of 10 patients for up to 21 months.

Selected peptide-specific, tumor-reactive CD8+ T-cell clones derived from tumor-infiltrating lymphocytes were administered intravenously to 12 patients with stage IV melanoma after a nonmyeloablative conditioning regimen, followed by differing doses of IL-2.[126] Although no objective responses were seen, the same authors then administered oligoclonal populations of mixed CD4 and CD8 T cells to 13 patients after treatment with the same nonmyeloablative chemotherapy regimen.[127] Persistence of the transferred T cells for up to 7 months occurred and was associated with their proliferation in vivo and trafficking to tumor sites. Seven PR or CR were observed, with 3 patients having SD. Autoimmune vitiligo was associated with response. Ten HLA-A2+ patients with tyrosinase-positive melanomas received intravenous infusions of tyrosinase 369 < n.377 peptide-primed CTL on day 1 and 5 days later for four cycles.[128] Two patients experienced disease regression, but CTL were undetectable in the circulation within 5 minutes after injection. The T cells concentrated in the liver and the spleen but did not especially target tumor tissues.

Mechanisms of Immunosuppression in Cancer Patients

Cancers have multiple mechanisms that prevent the activation of, and evade, the immune response, as described next (Table 20.6). It is likely that a therapeutic vaccine may not be an adequate immunotherapy without the means to overcome immunosuppression. With adequate knowledge of how tumors evade T-cell-mediated rejection, strategies are being developed that should improve the efficacy of cancer immunotherapy.

TABLE 20.6. Mechanisms of immunosuppression in cancer patients.

- Downmodulation of MHC
- Tumor-derived immune inhibition (e.g., transforming growth factor (TGF)-beta, IL-10)
- Th2 dominant T-cell response
- APC dysfunction [e.g., as a result of tumor-derived vascular endothelial growth factor (VEGF)]
- Treg cells (including CD25+ CD4+ and CD25-CD4+ cells), both via direct contact and via secreted factors (such as IL-10 and TGF-beta)

Downmodulation of MHC

A number of small-scale assessments of MHC class I expression and its loss by metastatic melanomas have been conducted using IHC staining, indicating that loss of class I expression confers a worse prognosis.[129–134] The majority of melanomas show normal staining for the nonpolymorphous class I A, B, C determinants, without evidence for allele-specific deletion or downregulation. Less than 10% of tumors show deletion of the beta-2 microglobulin gene, resulting in complete loss of class I expression. Approximately 10% to 40% of tumors demonstrate a decrease in class I staining or with antibody MA 2.1 recognizing class I allele A2 due to downregulation of mRNA expression or gene deletion causing absent expression of that allele. Fourteen primary melanomas were examined in one study, with MHC allele loss seen by IHC in 20%.[131] In a study of 48 metastatic lesions from 39 patients, loss of HLA class I expression of more than 50% was seen and was associated with a poorer clinical outcome.[132] Loss of HLA class I diminished immune recognition by melanoma-specific T cells in vitro,[134] although the effects on immune response to a vaccine are unclear.

The Tumor Microenvironment Is Toxic to T Cells

Tumors are known to express "tumor-rejection" antigens, and T cells specific for these tumor antigens are present either in the circulation or within tumors. If circulating T cells become activated and extravasate into the tumor parenchyma, they often encounter immunosuppressive molecules either secreted by or expressed on the surface of the tumor cells. For example, B7-H1, a member of the B7 family of costimulatory molecules, can be expressed by carcinomas and result in the induction of apoptosis of activated T cells.[135] Also, many tumors are known to secrete transforming growth factor (TGF)-β, or IL-10,[136] two cytokines known to downmodulate T-cell function. Regulatory T cells that function to suppress Th1 immune responses normally secrete both these cytokines.[137,138] Ectopic secretion of those cytokines by tumor cells can suppress Th1 cell-mediated rejection of tumors.

Blocking tumor-specific B7-H1 molecules from binding to their ligands on activated T cells improved the efficacy of antitumor T cells in preclinical models,[139,140] suggesting a therapeutic approach. IL-2 at high doses produces significant clinical responses in some cancers and is being tested in combination with tumor vaccines.[59,60] The B7-H1-mediated negative effect on T-cell function is overcome in the presence of exogenous IL-2.[64] A very low dose IL-2 regimen has been shown to result in the prolonged persistence of transferred T cells in melanoma patients.[65] This dose of IL-2 is sufficient to saturate IL-2 receptors in vivo.[141] Therefore an "immune augmenting" effect of IL-2 can potentially be achieved with minimal toxicity.

Th2 Skewing of the T-Cell Repertoire

The T helper cell subset that mediates tumor cell rejection are Th1 cells. A skewing of the tumor cell-specific Th population to Th2, which mediates antibody responses, would be expected to limit T-cell-mediated rejection of tumors. Tumor antigen-specific Th2 cells predominate in cancer patients[142] and can be found in the tumor parenchyma; this may be caused by the presence of plasmacytoid DC (DC2) recruited into tumors,[143] which favor a Th2 response.

IL-12 secreted by activated dendritic cells produces several effects that could enhance an antitumor T-cell response, including the support of a Th1 response; this suggests a possible approach to preventing the Th2 switch induced by tumors. Recombinant IL-12 protein given to cancer patients at the maximum tolerated dose (MTD) in a Phase II trial produced unacceptable toxicity.[66] However, based on animal models, the administration of doses well below the MTD should be sufficient for use of this agent as a tumor vaccine augmentation strategy, as previously suggested.[67,68] Gajewski et al. conducted phase I[69] and Phase II clinical trials[144] in melanoma patients combining subcutaneously injected IL-12 with a peptide-pulsed PBMC-based tumor vaccine. The IL-12 was given at a dose well below the MTD, every other day after each vaccine for three injections. Toxicity was acceptable, and 2 patients (10%) had complete responses. In other trials reported by Cebon et al.,[71] melanoma patients were treated with IL-12 in combination with a tumor vaccine (Melan-A peptide vaccine). Toxicity was acceptable, and 1 of 21 patients had a partial response. The optimal dose and schedule of IL-12 as well as the optimal vaccine to choose have yet to be defined, but well-tolerated doses of subcutaneous IL-12 has a clear immune-potentiating effect with peptide vaccines (Weber et al., unpublished data).

Antigen-Presenting Cell Dysfunction

Antigen-presenting cells in cancer patients are dysfunctional. Tumor-derived vascular endothelial growth factor (VEGF) can interfere with the differentiation of DCs,[145] as can IL-6 and MCS-F.[146] Also, IL-10 has been shown to interfere with dendritic cell function.[147–149] Tumor cells are also capable of inducing DCs to undergo apoptosis.[150,151] There is evidence that this tumor-induced APC dysfunction can be rescued by signaling through CD40. Signaling through CD40 on dendritic cells is a potent activation stimulus.[78,152] The in vivo delivery of an activating anti-CD40 antibody prevented tumor cell-induced T-cell unresponsiveness.[79] In addition, CD40 ligand can prevent the inhibition of DC function mediated by IL-10[153] and tumor-induced DC apoptosis.[81] Finally, the bystander production of CD40 ligand at a tumor vaccine site improved the efficacy of that vaccine in an animal model.[82] These observations all support the use of CD40-activation strategies to circumvent tumor-induced DC dysfunction and augment antitumor T-cell responses in cancer patients.

A Phase I clinical trial has been reported using recombinant human CD40 ligand protein systemically in cancer patients. Cohorts of patients with refractory cancer were treated with escalating doses of the CD40 ligand protein injected subcutaneously each day for 5 consecutive days. Patients without significant toxicity and no evidence of progression received additional courses at 4-week intervals. Thirty-two patients were treated with the dose-limiting toxicity, which was found to be liver transaminase elevation. This toxicity was transient in all but 2 patients, and no deaths attributed to this toxicity were reported. Interestingly, 2 patients had significant tumor regressions, with 1 patient developing a sustained complete response. Activating DCs in the setting of tumor vaccination by signaling through CD40 remains an attractive strategy that needs to be developed, with attempts to reduce the incidence of hepatic toxicity, and to combine this approach with the use of tumor vaccines to improve efficacy.

References

1. Topalian SL, Solomon D, Rosenberg SA. Tumor specific cytolysis by lymphocytes infiltrating human tumors. J Immunol 1989;142:3714–3725.
2. Van Der Bruggen P, Traversari C, Chomez P, et al. A gene encoding an antigen recognized by cytolytic T lymphocytes on a human melanoma. Science 1991;254:1643–1647.
3. Traversari C, van der Bruggen P, Luescher I, et al. A nonpeptide encoded by human gene MAGE-1 is recognized on HLA-A1 by cytolytic T lymphocytes directed against tumor antigen MZ2-E. J Exp Med 1992;176:1453–1457.
4. Gauler B, van den Eynde B, van der Bruggen P, et al. Human gene MAGE-3 codes for an antigen recognized on melanoma cells by autologous lymphocytes. J Exp Med 1994;179:921–929.
5. Kawakami Y, Eliyahu S, Delgado C, et al. Cloning of the gene coding for a shared melanoma antigen recognized by autologous T cells infiltrating into tumor. Proc Natl Acad Sci USA 1994; 96:3515–3519.
6. Coulie PG, Brichard V, Van Pel A, et al. A new gene coding for a differentiation antigen recognized by autologous cytolytic T lymphocytes on HLA-A2 melanomas. J Exp Med 1994; 180:35–42.
7. Kawakami Y, Eliyahu S, Sakaguchi K, et al. Identification of the immunodominant peptides of the MART-1 human melanoma antigen recognized by the majority of HLA-A2-restricted tumor-infiltrating lymphocytes. J Exp Med 1994;180:347–352.
8. Romero P, Gervois N, Schneider J, et al. Cytolytic T lymphocyte recognition of the immunodominant HLA-A*0201-restricted Melan-A/MART-1 antigenic peptide in melanoma. J Immunol 1997;159:2366–2374.
9. Romero P, Dunbar PR, Valmori D, et al. Ex vivo staining of metastatic lymph nodes by class I major histocompatibility complex tetramers reveals high numbers of antigen-experienced tumor specific cytolytic T lymphocytes. J Exp Med 1998; 188:1641–1650.
10. Jimenez M, Maloy WL, Hearing VJ. Specific identification of an authentic clone for mammalian tyrosinase. J Biol Chem 1989;264:3397–3403.
11. Adema GJ, DeBoer AJ, Vogel AM, et al. Molecular characterization of the melanocyte lineage specific antigen gp100. J Biol Chem 1994;269:20126–20133.
12. Bakker ABH, Schreurs WJ, de Boer AJ, et al. Melanocyte lineage specific antigen gp100 is recognized by melanoma-derived tumor-infiltrating lymphocytes. J Exp Med 1994;179:1005–1011.
13. Bakker ABH, Schreurs MWJ, Tafazzul G, et al. Identification of a novel peptide derived from the melanocyte specific gp100 antigen as the dominant epitope recognized by an HLA-A2.1 restricted anti-melanoma CTL line. Int J Cancer 1995;62:97–102.
14. Kawakami Y, Eliyahu S, Delgado C, et al. Identification of a human melanoma antigen recognized by tumor-infiltrating lymphocytes associated with in vivo tumor rejection. Proc Natl Acad Sci USA 1994;91:6458–6462.
15. Brichard V, Van Pel A, Wolfel T, et al. The tyrosinase gene encodes for an antigen recognized by autologous cytolytic T lymphocytes on HLA-A2 melanomas. J Exp Med 1993;178: 489–495.
16. Wolfel T, Van Pel A, Brichard V, et al. Two tyrosinase nonpeptides recognized on HLA-A2 melanomas by autologous cytolytic T lymphocytes. Eur J Immunol 1994;24:759–764.
17. Skipper JCA, Hendrickson RC, Gulden PH, et al. An HLA-A2 restricted tyrosinase antigen on melanoma cells results from post-translational modification and suggests a novel processing pathway for membrane proteins. J Exp Med 1996;183:527–534.
18. Weber J, Sondak VK, Scotland R, et al. Granulocyte-macrophage-colony-stimulating factor added to a multipeptide vaccine for resected Stage II melanoma. Cancer (Phila) 2003;97(1):186–2003.
19. Wang R-F, Parkhurst MR, Kawakami Y, et al. Utilization of an alternative open reading frame of a normal gene in generating a human cancer antigen. J Exp Med 1996;183:1131–1138.
20. Lang KS, Caroli CC, Muhm A, et al. HLA-A2 restricted melanocyte specific CD8(+) T lymphocytes detected in vitiligo patients are related to disease activity and are predominantly directed against MART-1. J Invest Dermatol 2001;116:891–897.
21. Jaeger E, Chen Y-T, Drijfhout JW, et al. Simultaneous humoral and cellular immune response against cancer testis antigen NY-ESO-1: definition of human histocompatibility leucocyte antigen (HLA)-A2 binding peptide epitopes. J Exp Med 1998; 187:265–274.
22. Wang R-F, Johnston SL, Zeng G, et al. A breast and melanoma-shared tumor antigen: T cell responses to antigenic peptides translated from different open reading frames. J Immunol 1998; 161:3596–3606.
23. Jager E, Chen YT, Drijfhout JW, et al. Simultaneous humoral and cellular immune response against cancer-testis antigen NY-ESO-1: definition of human histocompatibility leukocyte antigen (HLA)-A2-binding peptide epitopes. J Exp Med 1998;187(2): 265–270.
24. Manici S, Sturniolo T, Imro MA, et al. Melanoma cells present a MAGE-3 epitope to CD4+ cytotoxic T cells in association with histocompatibility leukocyte antigen DR11. J Exp Med 1999;189:871.
25. Chaux P, Vantomme V, Stroobant V, et al. Identification of MAGE-3 epitopes presented by HLA-DR molecules to CD4(+) T lymphocytes. J Exp Med 1999;189(5):767–778.
26. Schultz ES, Lethe B, Cambiaso CL, et al. A MAGE-A3 peptide presented by HLA-DP4 is recognized on tumor cells by CD4+ cytolytic T lymphocytes. Cancer Res 2000;60(22):6272–6275.
27. Toulokian CE, Leitner WW, Topalian SL, et al. Identification of a MHC class II restricted human gp100 epitope using DR4-IE transgenic mice. J Immunol 2000;164:3535–3542.
28. Zeng G, Touloukian CE, Wang X, et al. Identification of CD4+ T cell epitopes from NY-ESO-1 presented by HLA-DR molecules. J Immunol 2000;165(2):1153–1159.
29. Kobayashi H, Lu J, Celis E. Identification of helper T-cell epitopes that encompass or lie proximal to cytotoxic T-cell epitopes in the gp100 melanoma tumor antigen. Cancer Res 2001; 61(20):7577–7584.
30. Zeng G, Wang X, Robbins PF, et al. CD4(+) T cell recognition of MHC class II-restricted epitopes from NY-ESO-1 presented by a prevalent HLA DP4 allele: association with NY-ESO-1 antibody production. Proc Natl Acad Sci USA 2001;98(7):3964–3969.
31. Schlom J. Carcinoembryonic antigen (CEA) peptides and vaccines for carcinoma. In: Kast M (ed). Peptide-Based Cancer Vaccines. Georgetown: Landes Bioscience, 2000:90–105.
32. Marshall J. Carcinoembryonic antigen-based vaccines. Semin Oncol 2003;30:30–36.
33. Morse MA, Deng Y, Coleman D, et al. A Phase I study of active immunotherapy with carcinoembryonic antigen peptide (CAP-1)-pulsed, autologous human cultured dendritic cells in patients with metastatic malignancies expressing carcinoembryonic antigen. Clin Cancer Res 1999;5:1331–1338.
34. Peoples GE, Goedegebuure PS, Smith R, et al. Breast and ovarian cancer-specific cytotoxic T lymphocytes recognize the same HER2/neu-derived peptide. Proc Natl Acad Sci USA 1995;92: 432–436.
35. Fisk B, Blevins TL, Wharton JT, et al. Identification of an immunodominant peptide of HER-2/neu protooncogene recognized by ovarian tumor-specific cytotoxic T lymphocyte lines. J Exp Med 1995;181:2109–2117.

36. Knutson KL, Schiffman K, Disis ML. Immunization with a HER-2/neu helper peptide vaccine generates HER-2/neu CD8 T-cell immunity in cancer patients. J Clin Invest 2001;107:477–484.
37. Disis ML, Grabstein KH, Sleath PR, et al. Generation of immunity to the HER-2/neu oncogenic protein in patients with breast and ovarian cancer using a peptide-based vaccine. Clin Cancer Res 1999;5:1289–1297.
38. Knutson KL, Schiffman K, Cheever MA, et al. Immunization of cancer patients with a HER-2/neu, HLA-A2 peptide, p369–377, results in short-lived peptide-specific immunity. Clin Cancer Res 2002;8:1014–1018.
39. Disis ML, Gooley TA, Rinn K, et al. Generation of T-cell immunity to the HER-2/neu protein after active immunization with HER-2/neu peptide-based vaccines. J Clin Oncol 2002;20:2624–2632.
40. Butterfield L, Meng W, Koh A, et al. T cell responses to HLA-A0201 restricted peptides derived from human alpha fetoprotein. J Immunol 2001;166:5300–5308.
41. Brossart P, Heinrichs KS, Stuhler G, et al. Identification of HLA-A2-restricted T-cell epitopes derived from the MUC1 tumor antigen for broadly applicable vaccine therapies. Blood 1999;93:4309–4317.
42. Legha SS, Papadopoulos NE, Plager C, et al. Clinical evaluation of recombinant interferon alfa-2a (Roferon-A) in metastatic melanoma using two different schedules. J Clin Oncol 1987;5:1240–1246.
43. Kirkwood JM, Ibrahim JG, Sondak VK, et al. Interferon alfa-2a for melanoma metastases. Lancet 2002;359:978–979.
44. Pehamberger H, Soyer HP, Steiner A, et al. Adjuvant interferon alfa-2a treatment in resected primary stage II cutaneous melanoma. J Clin Oncol 1998;16:1425–1429.
45. Grob JJ, Dreno B, Salmoniere P, et al. Randomised trial of interferon α-2a as adjuvant therapy in resected primary melanoma thicker than 1.5 mm without clinically detectable node metastases. Lancet 1998;351:1905–1910.
46. Cascinelli N, Belli F, Mackie RM, et al. Effect of long-term adjuvant therapy with interferon alpha-2a in patients with regional node metastases from cutaneous melanoma: a randomised trial. Lancet 2001;358:866–869.
47. Cameron DA, Cornbleet MC, Mackie RM, et al. Adjuvant interferon alpha 2b in high risk melanoma: the Scottish study. Br J Cancer 2001;84:1146–1149.
48. Kleeberg UR, Bröcker EB, Lejeune F, et al. Adjuvant trial in melanoma patients comparing rIFNα to IFNγ to Iscador to a control group after curative resection of high risk primary (>3 mm) or regional lymph node metastasis (EORTC 18871). Eur J Cancer 1999;35:582 (abstract 24).
49. Hancock BW, Wheatley K, Harriss S, et al. Adjuvant interferon in high-risk melanoma: the AIM HIGH Study—United Kingdom Coordinating Committee on Cancer Research Randomized Study of Adjuvant Low-Dose Extended-Duration Interferon Alfa-2a in High-Risk Resected Malignant Melanoma. J Clin Oncol 2004;22(1):53–61.
50. Creagan ET, Dalton RJ, Ahmann DL, et al. Randomized, surgical adjuvant clinical trial of recombinant interferon alfa-2a in selected patients with malignant melanoma. J Clin Oncol 1995;13:2776–2783.
51. Kirkwood JM, Strawderman MH, Ernstoff MS, et al. Interferon alfa-2b adjuvant therapy of high-risk resected cutaneous melanoma: the Eastern Co-operative Oncology Group trial EST1684. J Clin Oncol 1996;14:7–17.
52. Kirkwood JM, Ibrahim JG, Sondak VK, et al. High and low-dose interferon alpha-2b in high risk melanoma: first analysis of Intergroup trial E1690/S9111/C9190. J Clin Oncol 2000;18:2444–2458.
53. Kirkwood JM, Ibrahim JG, Sosman JA, et al. High-dose interferon alfa-2b significantly prolongs relapse-free and overall survival compared with the GM2-KLH/QS-21 vaccine in patients with resected stage IIB-III melanoma: results of Intergroup Trial E1694/S9512/C509801. J Clin Oncol 2001;19:2370–2380.
54. Kirkwood JM, Manola J, Ibrahim J, et al. A pooled analysis of Eastern Cooperative Oncology Group and intergroup trials of adjuvant high-dose interferon for melanoma. Clin Cancer Res 2004;10(5):1670–1677.
55. Wheatley K, Ives N, Hancock BW, et al. Does adjuvant interferon α for high risk melanoma provide a worthwhile benefit? A meta-analysis of the randomised trials. Cancer Treat Rev 2003;29:241–252.
56. Eggermont AM, Punt CJ. Does adjuvant systemic therapy with interferon-alpha for stage II-III melanoma prolong survival? Am J Clin Dermatol 2003;4(8):531–536.
57. Cole BF, Gelber RD, Kirkwood JM, et al. Quality-of-life adjusted survival analysis of interferon alfa-2b adjuvant treatment of high-risk resected cutaneous melanoma: an Eastern Co-operative Oncology Group study. J Clin Oncol 1996;14:2666–2673.
58. Overwijk WW, Theoret MR, Restifo NP. The future of interleukin-2: enhancing therapeutic anticancer vaccines. Cancer J Sci Am 2000;6(suppl 1):S76–S80.
59. Shimizu K, Fields RC, Giedlin M, et al. Systemic administration of interleukin 2 enhances the therapeutic efficacy of dendritic cell-based tumor vaccines. Proc Natl Acad Sci USA 1999;96:2268–2273.
60. Rosenberg SA, Yang JC, Schwartzentruber DJ, et al. Immunologic and therapeutic evaluation of a synthetic peptide vaccine for the treatment of patients with metastatic melanoma. Nat Med 1998;4:321–327.
61. Atkins MB, Lotze MT, Dutcher JP, et al. High-dose recombinant interleukin 2 therapy for patients with metastatic melanoma: analysis of 270 patients treated between 1985 and 1993. J Clin Oncol 1999;17(7):2105–2116.
62. Atkins MB, Kunkel L, Sznol M, et al. High-dose recombinant interleukin-2 therapy in patients with metastatic melanoma: long-term survival update. Cancer J Sci Am 2000;6(suppl 1):S11–S14.
63. Dong H, Strome SE, Salomao DR, et al. Tumor-associated B7-H1 promotes T-cell apoptosis: a potential mechanism of immune evasion. Nat Med 2002;8:793–800.
64. Carter L, Fouser LA, Jussif J, et al. PD-1:PD-L inhibitory pathway affects both CD4(+) and CD8(+) T cells and is overcome by IL-2. Eur J Immunol 2002;32:634–643.
65. Yee C, Thompson JA, Byrd D, et al. Adoptive T cell therapy using antigen-specific CD8+ T cell clones for the treatment of patients with metastatic melanoma: in vivo persistence, migration, and antitumor effect of transferred T cells. Proc Natl Acad Sci USA 2002;99:16168–16173.
66. Trinchieri G. Interleukin-12 and the regulation of innate resistance and adaptive immunity. Nat Rev Immunol 2003;3:133–146.
67. Leonard JP, Sherman ML, Fisher GL, et al. Effects of single-dose interleukin-12 exposure on interleukin-12-associated toxicity and interferon-gamma production. Blood 1997;90:2541–2548.
68. Noguchi Y, Richards EC, Chen YT, et al. Influence of interleukin 12 on p53 peptide vaccination against established Meth A sarcoma. Proc Natl Acad Sci USA 1995;92:2219–2223.
69. Fallarino F, Uyttenhove C, Boon T, et al. Improved efficacy of dendritic cell vaccines and successful immunization with tumor antigen peptide-pulsed peripheral blood mononuclear cells by coadministration of recombinant murine interleukin-12. Int J Cancer 1999;80:324–333.
70. Peterson AC, Harlin H, Gajewski TF. Immunization with Melan-A peptide-pulsed peripheral blood mononuclear cells plus recombinant human interleukin-12 induces clinical activity and T-cell responses in advanced melanoma. J Clin Oncol 2003;21:2342–2348.

71. Cebon J, Jager E, Shackleton MJ, et al. Two phase I studies of low dose recombinant human IL-12 with Melan-A and influenza peptides in subjects with advanced malignant melanoma. Cancer Immunol 2003;3:7–17.
72. Morse MA, Nair S, Fernandez-Casal M, et al. Preoperative mobilization of circulating dendritic cells by Flt3 ligand administration to patients with metastatic colon cancer. J Clin Oncol 2000;18:3883–3893.
73. Rini BI, Paintal A, Vogelzang NJ, et al. Flt-3 ligand and sequential FL/interleukin-2 in patients with metastatic renal carcinoma: clinical and biologic activity. J Immunother 2002; 25:269–277.
74. Fong L, Hou Y, Rivas A, et al. Altered peptide ligand vaccination with Flt3 ligand expanded dendritic cells for tumor immunotherapy. Proc Natl Acad Sci USA 2001;98:8809–8814.
75. Disis ML, Rinn K, Knutson KL, et al. Flt3 ligand as a vaccine adjuvant in association with HER-2/neu peptide-based vaccines in patients with HER-2/neu-overexpressing cancers. Blood 2002; 99:2845–2850.
76. Grewal IS, Flavell RA. CD40 and CD154 in cell-mediated immunity. Annu Rev Immunol 1998;16:111–135.
77. Delamarre L, Holcombe H, Mellman I. Presentation of exogenous antigens on major histocompatibility complex (MHC) class I and MHC class II molecules is differentially regulated during dendritic cell maturation. J Exp Med 2003;198:111–122.
78. Sotomayor EM, Borrello I, Tubb E, et al. Conversion of tumor-specific CD4+ T-cell tolerance to T-cell priming through in vivo ligation of CD40. Nat Med 1999;5:780–787.
79. Brossart P, Zobywalski A, Grunebach F, et al. Tumor necrosis factor alpha and CD40 ligand antagonize the inhibitory effects of interleukin 10 on T-cell stimulatory capacity of dendritic cells. Cancer Res 2000;60:4485–4492.
80. Pirtskhalaishvili G, Shurin GV, Esche C, et al. Cytokine-mediated protection of human dendritic cells from prostate cancer-induced apoptosis is regulated by the Bcl-2 family of proteins. Br J Cancer 2000;83:506–513.
81. Esche C, Gambotto A, Satoh Y, et al. CD154 inhibits tumor-induced apoptosis in dendritic cells and tumor growth. Eur J Immunol 1999;29:2148–2155.
82. Dotti G, Savoldo B, Yotnda P, et al. Transgenic expression of CD40 ligand produces an in vivo antitumor immune response against both CD40(+) and CD40(−) plasmacytoma cells. Blood 2002;100:200–207.
83. Vonderheide RH, Dutcher JP, et al. Phase I study of recombinant human CD40 ligand in cancer patients. J Clin Oncol 2001; 19:3280–3287.
84. Krieg AM. CpG motifs in bacterial DNA and their immune effects. Annu Rev Immunol 2002;20:709–760.
85. Krieg AM. CpG motifs: the active ingredient in bacterial extracts? Nat Med 2003;9:831–835.
86. Hemmi H, Takeuchi O, Kawai T, et al. A Toll-like receptor recognizes bacterial DNA. Nature (Lond) 2000;408:740–745.
87. Jakob T, Walker PS, Krieg AM, et al. Activation of cutaneous dendritic cells by CpG-containing oligodeoxynucleotides: a role for dendritic cells in the augmentation of Th1 responses by immunostimulatory DNA. J Immunol 1998;161:3042–3049.
88. Sparwasser T, Koch ES, Vabulas RM, et al. Bacterial DNA and immunostimulatory CpG oligonucleotides trigger maturation and activation of murine dendritic cells. Eur J Immunol 1998; 28:2045–2054.
89. Hartmann G, Weiner GJ, Krieg AM. CpG DNA: a potent signal for growth, activation, and maturation of human dendritic cells. Proc Natl Acad Sci USA 1999;96:9305–9310.
90. Brunner C, Seiderer J, Schlamp A, et al. Enhanced dendritic cell maturation by TNF-alpha or cytidine-phosphate-guanosine DNA drives T cell activation in vitro and therapeutic anti-tumor immune responses in vivo. J Immunol 2000;165:6278–6286.
91. Sandler AD, Chihara H, Kobayashi G, et al. CpG oligonucleotides enhance the tumor antigen-specific immune response of a granulocyte macrophage colony-stimulating factor-based vaccine strategy in neuroblastoma. Cancer Res 2003;63: 394–399.
92. Rieger R, Kipps TJ. CpG oligodeoxynucleotides enhance the capacity of adenovirus-mediated CD154 gene transfer to generate effective B-cell lymphoma vaccines. Cancer Res 2003; 63:4128–4135.
93. Davila E, Kennedy R, Celis E. Generation of antitumor immunity by cytotoxic T lymphocyte epitope peptide vaccination, CpG-oligodeoxynucleotide adjuvant, and CTLA-4 blockade. Cancer Res 2003;63:3281–3288.
94. Stern BV, Boehm BO, Tary-Lehmann M. Vaccination with tumor peptide in CpG adjuvant protects via IFN-gamma-dependent CD4 cell immunity. J Immunol 2002;168:6099–6105.
95. Merad M, Sugie T, Engleman EG, et al. In vivo manipulation of dendritic cells to induce therapeutic immunity. Blood 2002;99:1676–1682.
96. Halperin SA, Van Nest G, Smith B, et al. A phase I study of the safety and immunogenicity of recombinant hepatitis B surface antigen co-administered with an immunostimulatory phosphorothioate oligonucleotide adjuvant. Vaccine 2003;21:2461–2467.
97. Van Ojik H, Bevaart L, Dahle CE, et al. Phase I/II study with CpG 7909 as adjuvant to vaccination with MAGE-3 protein in patients with MAGE-3 positive tumors. Ann Oncol 2003;13:157.
98. Walunas TL, Lenschow DJ, Bakker CY, et al. CTLA-4 can function as a negative regulator of T cell activation. Immunity 1994; 1:405–413.
99. Chambers CA, Krummel MF, Boitel B, et al. The role of CTLA-4 in the regulation and initiation of T-cell responses. Immunol Rev 1996;153:27–46.
100. Phan GQ, Yang JC, Sherry RM, et al. Cancer regression and autoimmunity induced by cytotoxic T lymphocyte-associated antigen 4 blockade in patients with metastatic melanoma. Proc Natl Acad Sci USA 2003;100:8372–8377.
101. Hodi FS, Mihm MC, Soiffer RJ, et al. Biologic activity of cytotoxic T lymphocyte-associated antigen 4 antibody blockade in previously vaccinated metastatic melanoma and ovarian carcinoma patients. Proc Natl Acad Sci USA 2003;100:4712–4717.
102. Hsueh EC, Gupta RK, Qi K. Correlation of specific immune responses with survival in melanoma patients with distant metastases receiving polyvalent melanoma cell vaccine. J Clin Oncol 1998;16:2913–2920.
103. Mitchell MS. Cancer vaccines, a critical review: part I. Curr Opin Invest Drugs 2002;3:140–149.
104. Sosman JA, Unger JM, Liu PY, et al. Southwest Oncology Group. Adjuvant immunotherapy of resected, intermediate-thickness, node-negative melanoma with an allogeneic tumor vaccine: impact of HLA class I antigen expression on outcome. J Clin Oncol 2002;20:2067–2075.
105. Sondak VK, Liu PY, Tuthill RJ, et al. Adjuvant immunotherapy of resected, intermediate-thickness, node-negative melanoma with an allogeneic tumor vaccine: overall results of a randomized trial of the Southwest Oncology Group. J Clin Oncol 2002; 20:2058–2066.
106. Dranoff G, Jaffee E, Lazenby A, et al. Vaccination with irradiated tumor cells engineered to secrete GM-CSF stimulates potent, specific, and long lasting anti-tumor immunity. Proc Natl Acad Sci USA 1993;90:3539–3543.
107. Soiffer R, Hodi FS, Haluska F, et al. Vaccination with irradiated, autologous melanoma cells engineered to secrete granulocyte-macrophage colony-stimulating factor by adenoviral-mediated gene transfer augments antitumor immunity in patients with metastatic melanoma. J Clin Oncol 2003;21:3343–3350.
108. Salgia R, Lynch T, Skarin A, et al. Vaccination with irradiated autologous tumor cells engineered to secrete granulocyte-macrophage colony-stimulating factor augments antitumor

immunity in some patients with metastatic non-small-cell lung carcinoma. J Clin Oncol 2003;21:624–630.
109. Jaffee EM, Hruban RH, Biedrzycki B, et al. Novel allogeneic granulocyte-macrophage colony-stimulating factor-secreting tumor vaccine for pancreatic cancer: a phase I trial of safety and immune activation. J Clin Oncol 2001;19:145–156.
110. Belli F, Testori A, Rivoltini L, et al. Vaccination of metastatic melanoma patients with autologous tumor-derived heat shock protein gp96-peptide complexes: clinical and immunologic findings. J Clin Oncol 2002;20:4169–4180.
111. Mazzaferro V, Coppa J, Carrabba MG, et al. Vaccination with autologous tumor-derived heat-shock protein gp96 after liver resection for metastatic colorectal cancer. Clin Cancer Res 2003;9:3235–3245.
112. Marchand M, van Baren N, Weynants P, et al. Tumor regressions observed in patients with metastatic melanoma treated with an antigenic peptide encoded by gene MAGE-3 and presented by HLA-A1. Int J Cancer 1999;80:219–230.
113. Marchand M, Punt CJ, Aamdal S, et al. Immunisation of metastatic cancer patients with MAGE-3 protein combined with adjuvant SBAS-2: a clinical report. Eur J Cancer 2003;39:70–77.
114. Jager E, Ringhoffer M, Karbach J, et al. Inverse relationship of melanocyte differentiation antigen expression in melanoma tissues and CD8+ cytotoxic-T-cell responses: evidence for immunoselection of antigen-loss variants in vivo. Int J Cancer 1996;66:470–476.
115. Slingluff CL Jr, Petroni GR, Yamshchikov GV, et al. Clinical and immunologic results of a randomized phase II trial of vaccination using four melanoma peptides either administered in granulocyte-macrophage colony-stimulating factor in adjuvant or pulsed on dendritic cells. J Clin Oncol 2003;21:4016–4026.
116. Bettinnotti MP, Panelli MC, Ruppe E, et al. Clinical and immunological evaluation of patients with metastatic melanoma undergoing immunization with the HLA-Cw*0702-associated epitope MAGE-A12:170–178. Int J Cancer 2003;105:210–216.
117. Nestle FO, Alijagic S, Gilliet M, et al. Vaccination of melanoma patients with peptide- or tumor-lysate pulsed dendritic cells. Nat Med 1998;4:328–332.
118. Panelli MC, Wunderlish J, Jeffries J, et al. Phase 1 study in patients with metastatic melanoma of immunization with dendritic cells presenting epitopes derived from the melanoma-associated antigens MART-1 and gp100. J Immunother 2000;23:487–498.
119. Sadanaga N, Nagashima H, Mashino K, et al. Dendritic cell vaccination with MAGE peptide is a novel therapeutic approach for gastrointestinal carcinomas. Clin Cancer Res 2001;7:2277–2284.
120. Thurner B, Haendle I, Roder C, et al. Vaccination with Mage-3A1 peptide-pulsed mature monocyte-derived dendritic cells expands specific cytotoxic T-cells and induces regression of some metastases in advanced stage IV melanoma. J Exp Med 1999;190:1669–1678.
121. Mackensen A, Herbst B, Chen JL, et al. Phase I study in melanoma patients of a vaccine with peptide-pulsed dendritic cells generated in vitro from CD34(+) hematopoietic progenitor cells. Int J Cancer 2000;86:385–392.
122. Banchereau J, Palucka AK, Dhodapkar M, et al. Immune and clinical responses in patients with metastatic melanoma to CD34(+) progenitor-derived dendritic cell vaccine. Cancer Res 2001;61:6451–6458.
123. Geiger J, Hutchinson R, Hohenkirk L, et al. Treatment of solid tumors in children with tumour-lysate-pulsed dendritic cells. Lancet 2000;356:1163–1164.
124. Chang AE, Redman BG, Whitfield JR, et al. A phase I trial of tumor lysate-pulsed dendritic cells in the treatment of advanced cancer. Clin Cancer Res 2002;8:1021–1032.
125. Yee C, Thompson JA, Byrd D, et al. Adoptive T cell therapy using antigen-specific CD8+ T cell clones for the treatment of patients with metastatic melanoma: in vivo persistence, migration, and antitumor effect of transferred T cells. Proc Natl Acad Sci USA 2002;99(25):16168–16173.
126. Dudley ME, Wunderlich JR, Yang JC, et al. A phase I study of nonmyeloablative chemotherapy and adoptive transfer of autologous tumor antigen-specific T lymphocytes in patients with metastatic melanoma. J Immunother 2002;25:243–251.
127. Dudley ME, Wunderlich JR, Robbins PF, et al. Cancer regression and autoimmunity in patients after clonal repopulation with antitumor lymphocytes. Science 2002;298:850–854.
128. Mitchell MS, Darrah D, Yeung D, et al. Phase I trial of adoptive immunotherapy with cytolytic T lymphocytes immunized against a tyrosinase epitope. J Clin Oncol 2002;20:1075–1086.
129. Kageshita T, Wang Z, Calorini L, et al. Selective loss of human leukocyte class I allospecificities and staining of melanoma cells by monoclonal antibodies recognizing monomorphic determinants of class I human leukocyte antigens. Cancer Res 1993;53:3349–3354.
130. van Duinen SG, Ruiter DJ, Broecker EB, et al. Level of HLA antigens in locoregional metastases and clinical course of the disease in patients with melanoma. Cancer Res 1988;48(4):1019–1025.
131. Natali PG, Nicotra MR, Bilgotti A, et al. Selective changes in expression of HLA class I polymorphic determinants in human solid tumors. Proc Natl Acad Sci USA 1989;6:6719–6723.
132. Marincola FM, Shamamian P, Alexander RB, et al. Loss of HLA haplotype and B locus down-regulation in melanoma cell lines. J Immunol 1994;153:1225–1237.
133. Kageshita T, Hirai S, Ono T, et al. Down-regulation of HLA class I antigen-processing molecules in malignant melanoma: association with disease progression. Am J Pathol 1999;154(3):745–754.
134. Geertsen R, Boni R, Blasczyk R, et al. Loss of single HLA class I allospecificities in melanoma cells due to selective genomic abbreviations. Int J Cancer 2002;99(1):82–87.
135. Dong H, Strome SE, Salomao DR, et al. Tumor-associated B7-H1 promotes T-cell apoptosis: a potential mechanism of immune evasion. Nat Med 2002;8(8):793–800.
136. Sato T, McCue P, Masuoka K, et al. Interleukin 10 production by human melanoma. Clin Cancer Res 1996;2(8):1383–1390.
137. Zuany-Amorim C, Sawicka E, Manlius C, et al. Suppression of airway eosinophilia by killed *Mycobacterium vaccae*-induced allergen-specific regulatory T-cells. Nat Med 2002;8(6):625–629.
138. Kitani A, Fuss I, Nakamura K, et al. Transforming growth factor (TGF)-beta 1-producing regulatory T cells induce Smad-mediated interleukin 10 secretion that facilitates coordinated immunoregulatory activity and amelioration of TGF-beta1-mediated fibrosis. J Exp Med 2003;198(8):1179–1188.
139. Curiel TJ, Wei S, Dong H, et al. Blockade of B7-H1 improves myeloid dendritic cell-mediated antitumor immunity. Nat Med 2003;9(5):562–567.
140. Strome SE, Dong H, Tamura H, et al. B7-H1 blockade augments adoptive T-cell immunotherapy for squamous cell carcinoma. Cancer Res 2003;63(19):6501–6505.
141. Overwijk WW, Theoret MR, Restifo NP. The future of interleukin-2: enhancing therapeutic anticancer vaccines. Cancer J Sci Am 2000;6(suppl 1):S76–S80.
142. Tatsumi T, Kierstead LS, Ranieri E, et al. Disease-associated bias in T helper type 1 (Th1)/Th2 CD4(+) T cell responses against MAGE-6 in HLA-DRB10401(+) patients with renal cell carcinoma or melanoma. J Exp Med 2002;196(5):619–628.
143. Zou W, Machelon V, Coulomb-L'Hermin A, et al. Stromal-derived factor-1 in human tumors recruits and alters the function of plasmacytoid precursor dendritic cells. Nat Med 2001;7(12):1339–1346.
144. Peterson AC, Harlin H, Gajewski TF. Immunization with Melan-A peptide-pulsed peripheral blood mononuclear cells plus

recombinant human interleukin-12 induces clinical activity and T-cell responses in advanced melanoma. J Clin Oncol 2003; 21(12):2342–2348.

145. Gabrilovich DI, Chen HL, Girgis KR, et al. Production of vascular endothelial growth factor by human tumors inhibits the functional maturation of dendritic cells. Nat Med 1996;2(10): 1096–1103.

146. Menetrier-Caux C, Montmain G, Dieu MC, et al. Inhibition of the differentiation of dendritic cells from CD34(+) progenitors by tumor cells: role of interleukin-6 and macrophage colony-stimulating factor. Blood 1998;92(12):4778–4791.

147. Steinbrink K, Wolfl M, Jonuleit H, et al. Induction of tolerance by IL-10-treated dendritic cells. J Immunol 1997;159(10): 4772–4780.

148. Koch F, Stanzl U, Jennewein P, et al. High level IL-12 production by murine dendritic cells: upregulation via MHC class II and CD40 molecules and downregulation by IL-4 and IL-10. J Exp Med 1996;184(2):741–746.

149. Steinbrink K, Jonuleit H, Muller G, et al. Interleukin-10-treated human dendritic cells induce a melanoma-antigen-specific anergy in CD8(+) T cells resulting in a failure to lyse tumor cells. Blood 1999;93(5):1634–1642.

150. Esche C, Shurin GV, Kirkwood JM, et al. Tumor necrosis factor-alpha-promoted expression of Bcl-2 and inhibition of mitochondrial cytochrome c release mediate resistance of mature dendritic cells to melanoma-induced apoptosis. Clin Cancer Res 2001;7(suppl 3):974s–979s.

151. Kiertscher SM, Luo J, Dubinett SM, et al. Tumors promote altered maturation and early apoptosis of monocyte-derived dendritic cells. J Immunol 2000;164(3):1269–1276.

152. Grewal IS, Flavell RA. CD40 and CD154 in cell-mediated immunity. Annu Rev Immunol 1998;16:111–135.

153. Delamarre L, Holcombe H, Mellman I. Presentation of exogenous antigens on major histocompatibility complex (MHC) class I and MHC class II molecules is differentially regulated during dendritic cell maturation. J Exp Med 2003;198(1): 111–122.

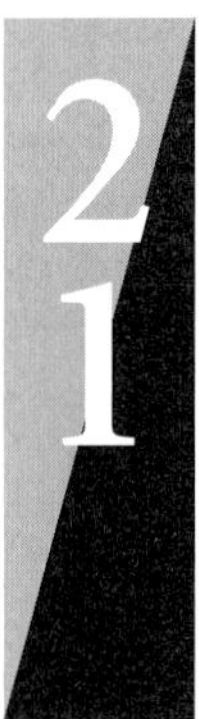

Technologies in Molecular Biology: Diagnostic Applications

Timothy J. Triche

For more than 100 years, cancer has been diagnosed by empirical, largely subjective means, not unlike clinical medicine itself. A consequence of this is that universal acceptance of a diagnosis, particularly any beyond benign versus malignant, has been an elusive goal. In one published study of rhabdomyosarcoma diagnosis involving more than 800 blinded cases and more than a dozen pathologists working in teams of two at eight institutions, with a 20% resampling, concordance between groups for subclassification (with clinical and therapeutic consequences) was no better than 60%. (The figure for individual reproducibility was marginally better, of the order of 70%.)[1] It should be noted that these pathologists were acknowledged to be the world's experts in the diagnosis of this disease at the time. Thus, it is reasonable to conclude that cancer diagnosis is less than a perfectly objective science.

On the other hand, it is also important to note that there is no better alternative, at least until recently. This situation is changing rapidly, as new, relatively objective, and certainly dichotomous or quantitative methods are introduced into practice as diagnostic tools in cancer. This in turn is progressively rendering the diagnosis of cancer more precise, reproducible, and yes, objective. To be clear, *the initial diagnosis of cancer of any type remains a histologic diagnosis.* That said, all further refinement (and even as a factor in the initial decision of benign versus malignant) increasingly relies on an ever-enlarging panoply of diagnostic tools, most rooted in biotechnology and disparate medical fields such as immunology, biochemistry, molecular genetics, and bioinformatics. This chapter describes these methods and illustrates how they augment and clarify the diagnosis of cancer. Of note is the further benefit of these methods: they frequently also provide information about prognosis and potential therapy, as is shown.

Cancer Diagnosis

"Subjective" Versus "Objective" Cancer Diagnosis

The towering achievements in histologic diagnosis of cancer, as evidenced by treatises such as *Ackerman's Surgical Pathology*, are testimony to the remarkable ability of the human mind for pattern recognition. The issue is not knowledge or insight, but consistency and reproducibility, as noted previously. Further, it is self-evident that no form of morphologic diagnosis, nor its practitioners, can hope to identify genomic alterations that bear directly on diagnosis, prognosis, and potential therapy by histologic examination. The consequences of genomic alterations may in some way be evident, but that is not direct or objective evidence. For example, anaplasia is often considered a marker of higher-grade malignancy in cancer diagnosis and has been linked to mutations in p53, the most commonly mutated gene in human cancer.[2–5] However, the correlation between anaplasia and p53 mutations detected by DNA sequencing or similar methods is poor[4]; rather, multiple genes may contribute to the phenotype.[6] Thus, morphology is not a surrogate of genomic analysis. The goal, then, of the diagnostic technologies discussed here is to provide objective evidence of class, character, genotype, phenotype, prognosis, and potential therapy, but *not* a diagnosis of cancer per se. That remains the domain of morphologic diagnosis. Nonetheless, the certainty of such diagnoses, and especially their value to the practice of oncology, can be markedly enhanced by these methods.

Diagnosis Versus Prognosis and Therapy

As intimated previously, the real value of sophisticated molecular technologies is their potential impact on precise, objective, unambiguous cancer diagnosis. To place this in context, however, it is important to remember that the only reason to establish a diagnosis of cancer in the first place is to determine prognosis and therefore therapy. In the first instance, a diagnosis of any form of cancer (specifically, solid tumors) implies that the tumor must be completely removed and potentially treated systemically with chemotherapy and/or radiotherapy. If benign, or a pseudoneoplastic condition (fibromatosis, for example), these issues do not apply. Function, cosmetic effect, interference with normal bodily function, and similar concerns dominate such diagnoses; life-threatening consequences are rarely part of the dialogue. Thus, the first and paramount issue in cancer diagnosis, whether a tissue is or is not cancerous, relates directly to therapy. However, as cancer therapy has become progressively more sophisticated and multimodal, a simple diagnosis of "cancer" is obviously inadequate. Furthermore, a diagnosis of "high grade" or "grade III" is fraught with some degree of uncertainty. One need only consider the conflicting grading of brain tumors espoused by WHO versus other authors (notably, the existence of three versus four grades of astrocytic brain tumors) to appreciate the conundrum. Clearly, a glioblastoma multiforme is a deadly tumor. But what of a grade II astrocytoma, and in which diagnostic scheme? This, then, is the sole purpose of diagnosis, and of the methods described herein: to establish the best possible course of action based on the best available diagnostic and prognostic information. The purpose of the diagnostic technologies discussed here is therefore to *augment* the precision and utility of a cancer diagnosis and its direct relevance to treatment.

Integration of Diagnostic Information with Therapy

As appealing as extensive data on a given tumor may be, the ultimate test of the relevance of such data is whether these can be integrated into patient management. It is of no value to determine that a given tumor has a p53 mutation, for example, unless there is a body of literature that suggests that such mutations are associated with more aggressive clinical behavior.[2] Fortunately, for many tumors, this is the case,[5] and p53 mutational analysis is now a commercially available test, offered by Roche Diagnostics. However, for most genes, there is little or no such compelling information, and mutational analysis of, for example, RB, MDM2, E2, or any other cell-cycle control gene, while of research interest, is at present of little or no clinical value.[7]

Despite the need to distinguish between clinical research and practice, there are a number of assays that are, or are becoming, the standard of care. Some examples include HER2/neu in breast cancer, p53 analysis in many forms of cancer, gene translocation analyses in leukemia, MYCN amplification in childhood neuroblastoma, and c-KIT and platelet-derived growth factor receptor (PDGFR) mutational analysis in gastrointestinal stromal tumor (GIST). The latter is of particular interest because it is primarily of importance as a predictor of response to targeted therapy with gleevec (imatinib), a kinase inhibitor that inhibits not only its original target, the cytosolic kinase ABL, in chronic myelogenous leukemia (CML), but also c-KIT and PDGFR, both receptor tyrosine kinases often mutated and constitutionally activated in GIST. This is an important paradigm shift as well: here, for the first time, a diagnostic assay is performed specifically to determine eligibility for therapy, or at least to predict the likelihood of response to, a targeted cancer therapeutic agent of a new type, a kinase inhibitor. This pairing of agent with target, and its mutational status, is rapidly emerging as a major change in approach to cancer chemotherapy: response to targeted agents is predicated on the presence in the tumor of a suitable target, in this case, a mutated phosphokinase. This specificity also explains the narrow therapeutic response window (e.g., mutated versus wild type) for agents such as iressa (gefitinib). This kinase inhibitor is specific for epidermal growth factor receptor (EGFR), another RTK that is commonly actively overexpressed or overactive in a wide variety of cancers. However, enthusiasm for iressa has been tempered by the reality that only about 10% of patients with lung cancer, for example, respond to therapy. Recently, it was shown that this is precisely the group with mutations in their EGFR RTK; those with wild-type EGFR fail to respond and do not benefit from therapy with iressa.[8] Interestingly, it appears that this is true of other types of lung cancer (e.g., nonsmokers) and other kinase inhibitors.[9] It will be interesting to see if this becomes a standard of care, whereby eligibility for treatment with a selective agent such as iressa or gleevec will require diagnostic assay for a specific mutation in the tyrosine kinase domain of the receptor or cytosolic kinase.[10]

Therapeutic Targets

The examples cited previously of directed therapies specific for a particular protein or a mutation therein are likely to grow rapidly in number as new agents and new targets are identified. One consequence of the widespread use of molecular biologic methods in the analysis of cancer tissue is the increasing awareness of recurring patterns of genes or proteins preferentially expressed by certain types or classes of tumors. Examples are illustrated in more detail later in the discussion of technologies used to identify these genes, but here we focus instead on the consequence of their identification.

Although identification of mutated kinases has captured the imagination of oncologists and cancer biologists, the reality is that mutations are commonplace in cancer, and the consequences of these mutations are widespread in all forms of cancer. As a general rule, proliferation in cancer cells is increased for lack of cell-cycle control, and apoptosis is inhibited for lack of a viable apoptotic pathway in many cancer cells. The causes of this are too numerous (and often unknown) to document in detail here. Rather, it is fair to state that no one defect explains enhanced cell proliferation and diminished apoptosis in cancer. Thus, a comprehensive analysis of contributing genes to both processes, both promoting and suppressing, can identify potential therapeutic targets, if the gene or its protein product is a *druggable target*. Receptor tyrosine kinases are obvious examples, based on prior comments, and so are cell-cycle regulatory genes such as MDM2 and P53, as well as a huge number of other genes involved in one or another aspect of these two basic defects in cancer cell control. Thus, adenoviral-mediated p53 replacement therapy has been explored in lung and head and neck cancer for many years,[11,12] and recently Roche has developed an MDM2 inhibitor for those tumors with unopposed MDM2 activity.[13] In a broader sense, gene targets identified by a variety of biologic and genomic studies have also promoted development of agents that selectively inhibit tumor characteristics, such as their ability to promote angiogenesis to develop a vascular supply necessary for growth beyond microscopic tumorlets. In this case, at least five compounds that target the vascular endothelial growth factor, VEGF, or its receptor, FLT1, have been developed to specifically inhibit angiogenesis in cancer.[14,15] Early clinical results are promising but it is too early to draw conclusions.

In general, it should be apparent that the more one knows about a given cancer, the more precisely it can be targeted with therapeutics intended to exploit features unique to that tumor. In the future, the list of candidate targets is likely to expand far beyond the current short list of kinase inhibitors, monoclonal antibodies against receptor tyrosine kinases (e.g., Herceptin for HER/neu amplified breast cancer), and angiogenesis inhibitors. Proteasome inhibitors are currently being evaluated, for example,[16,17] while many other candidate targets remain to be exploited, individually (integrins such as the vitronectin receptor, alpha V beta 3, for example)[18] or as a class (of which there are many).[19]

In view of these concerns, it is reasonable to examine the contributions of molecular technologies to the characterization of cancer, and ultimately the choice of therapy, based on knowledge of candidate targets amenable to targeted therapies such as these.

Diagnostic Technologies

In general, all the methods to be described here can be characterized as analytic tools for the characterization of DNA, RNA, or protein, paralleling the sequence of genomic function, from archival information in DNA, its encoding in mRNA, and its translation into a functional molecule, protein (Figure 21.1). However, this simple schema, although largely correct, overlooks great complexity in the structure, organization, function, and modification of genetic information. To note only a few examples, only about 3% of the genome is associated with genes; the function of the rest is largely unknown, although there is clear evidence that this is not just "junk" DNA, as has been supposed.[20] Similarly, although only 40,000 genes, more or less, are known, thousands more noncoding RNA transcripts have been detected in expressed RNA pools in cells.[21] Thus, genetic and epigenetic controls over DNA replication, RNA expression, and even nuclear chromatin structure are also relevant to cancer origins, grade, and outcome, but are not explored here. Instead, we examine the proven and widely used methods for analysis of the functional genome, starting with proteins, known in aggregate as the proteome.

Protein Based

Immunohistochemistry

By far the most established method of detecting protein in cancer cells is immunohistochemistry (IHC) (Figure 21.2). This technique is widely employed in routine cancer diagnosis in surgical pathology, but it is also used for a number of assays to determine eligibility for directed therapy, or at least to assess the likelihood of efficacy for such therapies. A typical example of this is HER2/neu. Even though HER2

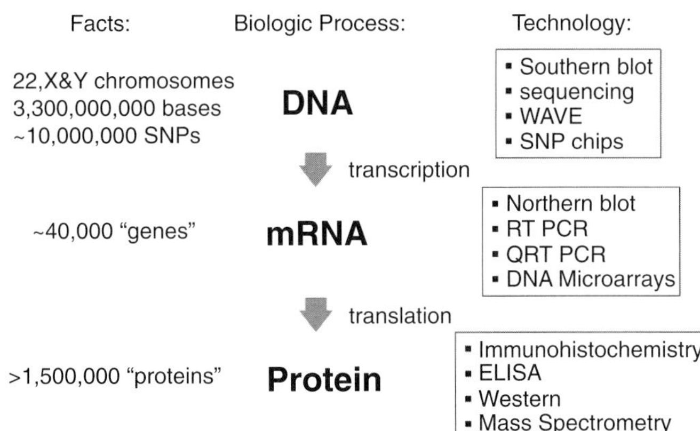

FIGURE 21.1. Diagram: DNA to RNA to protein.

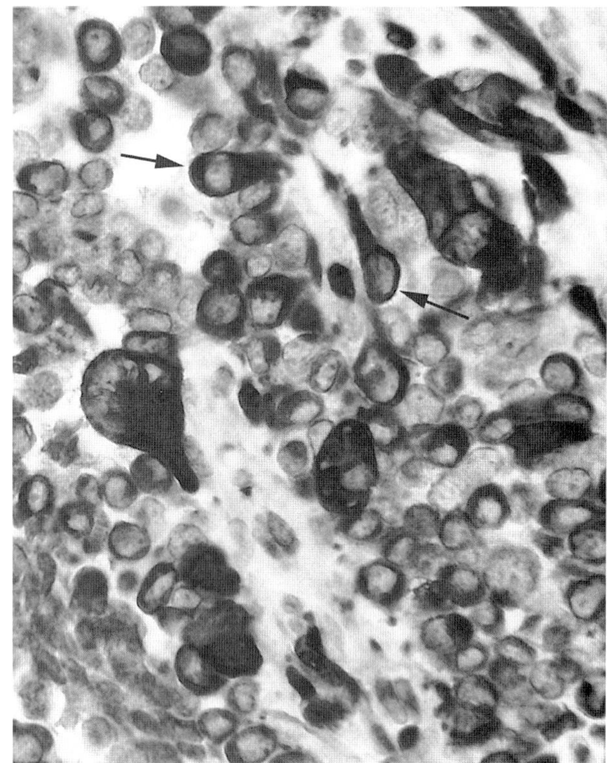

FIGURE 21.2. Immunohistochemistry (IHC) photomicrograph.

amplification is most significantly associated with prognosis in breast cancer, because there is a close association between amplification and elevated protein expression, it is generally sufficient to simply detect the protein by IHC. However, there is significant disagreement as to the superiority of IHC (e.g., protein detection) as opposed to FISH (fluorescent in situ hybridization to detect DNA copy number), and whether DNA amplification is more important than protein expression. A similar controversy surrounds childhood neuroblastoma, where MYCN amplification detected by FISH is the standard diagnostic procedure for MYCN determination; polymerase chain reaction (PCR) for elevated MYCN expression levels is occasionally misleading and not a reliable marker for genomic amplification. Similarly, detection of MYCN protein by IHC is not a reliable surrogate either.

Despite these potential limitations, IHC is far and away the most common technique employed to augment morphologic diagnosis. It is enjoying something of a resurgence, as genes detected by other methods (as described next) need to be validated at the protein level. To serve this burgeoning need, innumerable biotechnology companies producing vast numbers of antibodies specific for a given gene product have arisen and increasingly supply the specific antibody paired with the gene of interest. Two benefits accrue: protein staining is considered the diagnostic gold standard (as not all expressed genes necessarily result in expressed protein), and the technology is simple, cheap, reproducible (with some caveats), and technically straightforward.

Western Blots and Immunoprecipitation

Historical problems with nonspecificity of antibody staining on tissue sections, coupled with a relative lack of quantitation, led to the development of a method to detect protein and confirm identity based on objective criteria such as molecular mass and reactivity with an allegedly specific antibody. In this method, the crude protein extract is incubated with an antibody and the antigen–antibody complex is precipitated from solution, then separated into antigen and antibody by gel electrophoresis. Conversely, the mixture can be electrophoresed and separated by molecular mass, then transferred to a filter membrane (the "Western" blot, as opposed to a DNA Southern blot or RNA Northern blot) and incubated with the antibody. Either way, the protein can be identified by its reactivity with antibody and its relative mass, or molecular weight. An example of a comparative Western analysis of the same protein from a series of Ewing's tumors is illustrated in Figure 21.3. It is immediately apparent that the relative amount of the protein in erstwhile identical tumors is in reality markedly different, thereby documenting a quantitative difference in protein content that would be difficult to assess by IHC, for example, where only degrees of antibody staining can be assessed, generally nonquantitatively.

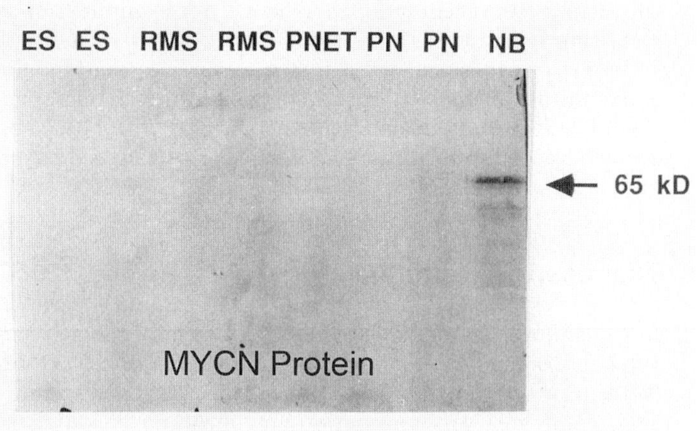

FIGURE 21.4. Enzyme-linked immunosorbent assay (ELISA).

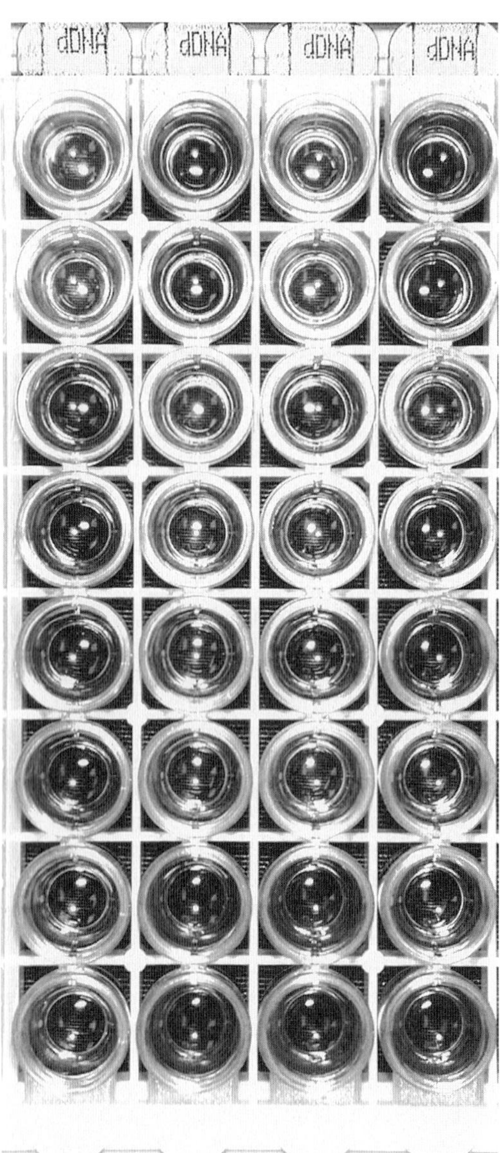

FIGURE 21.3. Western blot, same protein.

ELISA

Enzyme-linked immunosorbent assay, or ELISA, is a widely used laboratory procedure for identifying proteins or other antigens present at concentrations as low as one part in a billion within complex mixtures such as serum and urine. As such, the assay has been employed to detect viral antigens, tumor antigens, and many other protein moieties for years. Two basic methods are commonly used: (1) the specimen containing the suspected target antigen is coated on the substrate, then detected by enzyme-linked specific antibody, or (2), in the sandwich ELISA assay, the plate is coated with specific antibody and washed, the serum, urine, or similar complex protein mixture is added then eluted, and finally an enzyme-linked version of the same antibody is added and subsequently detected by chromogenic or fluorescent methods. The latter method presumes the existence of more than one epitope on the antigen; otherwise, the second antibody will not bind and no antigen is detected. Thus, either multiples of the same epitope must be present on the antigen, or two different antibodies directed against two epitopes must be used in the assay. Quantitation is readily performed when dilutions of the target mixture are performed and assayed, as the optical density of the mixture following enzymatic chromogen generation (as with horseradish peroxidase, a commonly used enzyme) increases linearly with increasing concentration of the target antigen. When suitable positive controls are performed in parallel, the concentration of the antigen in the serum or urine can be readily calculated from a simple $y = mx + b$ graph of optical density (OD) versus dilution. A typical result performed in a 96-well format is illustrated in Figure 21.4.

ELISA assays are probably the most common laboratory procedure performed for immunodetection of protein antigens. However, the confluence of several factors has lent a new life to this venerable assay: as genomic methods increasingly identify gene targets, their protein end product can be predicted with accuracy and a suitable ELISA assay established. This method is of particular value in serum-based diagnostics, where the presence of enormous concentrations of albumin and immunoglobulins vastly overshadows the relatively rare tumor cell products. However, by virtue of the remarkable ability of solid-phase immunoabsorption to retain even rare proteins on an immobilized immunoglobulin-coated solid substrate, it is possible to both detect and quantitate such proteins. The presence in serum and urine of many tumor-associated proteins or peptides makes detection and quantitation of these antigens by ELISA an attractive means of early detection and monitoring of tumor persistence or recurrence. The marked sensitivity of the assay, coupled with its low cost, proven sensitivity and specificity, and amenability to rigorous laboratory quality control procedures, has made it the method of choice for such assays. However, successful use presumes both knowledge of the antigen, as well as the availability of a suitably specific antibody. Initially, these requirements are rarely satisfied, and tumor antigens must be identified by other methods. This process has been markedly enhanced in the past decade by rapid progress in mass spectrometry and related methods, well suited to detection, characterization, and even quantitation of unknown proteins and peptides.

Proteomics and Mass Spectrometry

Although antibody-based protein detection methods are preferred when the antigen is known and a suitable antibody to detect it is available, such methods are of no value with unknown antigens, which is the more common situation when searching for novel tumor antigens. Although a high index of suspicion may derive from preliminary gene expression analyses on expressed mRNA, the ultimate identification requires detection and at least partial sequence identification. By far the most common method of doing so currently is mass spectrometry. However, mass spectrometry is not a single method; rather, there are many variations, too many to discuss here. Suffice it to say that increasingly, sample preparation methods that mimic ELISA or affinity capture methods are coming to dominate clinical proteomics, while rather more demanding, tedious, expensive, but ultimately unequivocal methods, such as tandem mass spectrometry are finding wide acceptance as research tools. Here, we focus on mass spectrometry with suitable interface for specimen complexity reduction coupled with high throughput.

Clinical proteomics, as opposed to research proteomics, necessitates high throughput, reproducibility, and reasonable cost. Most research methods that utilize preparative columns for sample cleanup before mass spectrometry are not suitable for clinical use. The columns are expensive and must be replaced frequently. However, raw serum or urine cannot be successfully analyzed by mass spectrometry because of the vast difference in concentration between target protein or peptide compared to contaminating proteins such as albumin. However, depletion methods that selectively remove albumin and serum globulins may have an untoward effect: a very high percentage of serum proteins, likely including tumor antigens, are in fact bound to albumin. Removal of albumin may thus remove a large amount of the target antigen. Thus, methods which selectively immobilize target proteins or peptides from complex mixtures are to be preferred, not unlike the solid-phase adsorption of ELISA assays discussed previously.

SELDI TOF is a currently popular method of preisolating a vast variety of proteins or peptides before mass spectrometry. This method relies on the selective elution with laser desorption and ionization of proteins, followed by time of flight mass spectrometry. Marketed by Ciphergen, this technology has been used for the majority of clinical proteomics publications to date.[22–32] In essence, this method utilizes a specimen target immobilization using a "protein chip," the characteristics of which vary widely, from strong anion or cation exchangers to immobilized antibody bases. Each spot is repeated several times in a row, and the adsorbed target is selectively eluted under varying elution conditions, from weak to strong. Each step is ionized and separated on the basis of the mass to charge (m/z) ratio. The resultant peaks are recorded and conditions optimized to identify the peak or peaks of interest. A typical example is illustrated in Figure 21.5. For identification, the same protein chip can be incubated with one or more proteases, such as trypsin and the resultant peptides spectrographed. The peptide pattern is highly reproducible and by definition identifies partial sequences within the intact protein. When compared to the vast online libraries of peptide fragments that result from any protein treated with any common protease, it is possible to make an identification from peptide mapping more than 90% of the time. If any doubt remains, the same specimen can be subjected to tandem mass spectrometry with quadrapole-based, collision-induced dissociation of individual amino acids, which can then be readily identified and the amino acid sequence deduced. This finding is then easily compared to genomic or protein library data for a positive identification, regardless of whether prior knowledge exists.

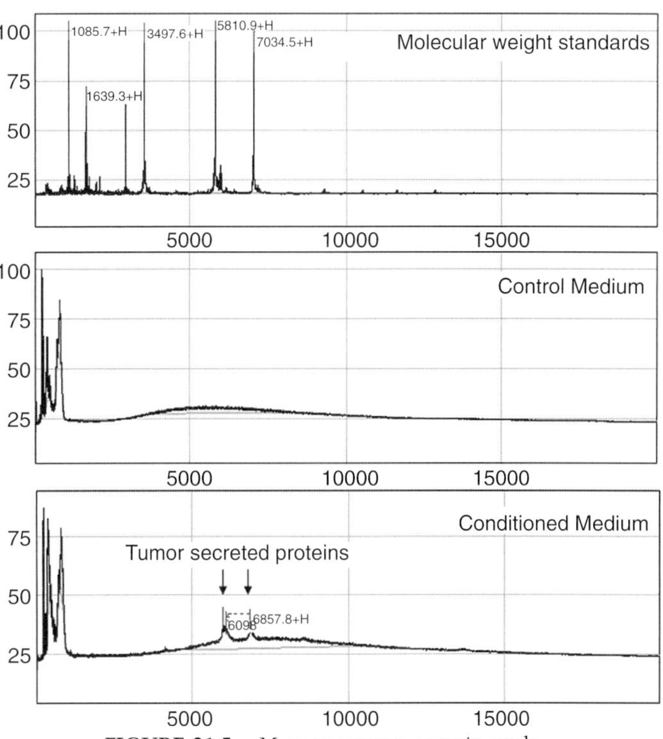

FIGURE 21.5. Mass spectrum, protein peak.

RNA Based

All protein is ultimately the product of mRNA coding information translated into amino acid sequences that constitute proteins, which then undergo a vast number of posttranslational modifications, resulting in more than a million identifiable proteins from fewer than 50,000 genes. In part, it is the potential to reduce this posttranslational complexity to manageable levels, as well as the precision and unambiguous result of RNA assays as compared to protein assays, which has driven the rapid development of RNA-based assays of interest to both biomedical research and clinical medicine. Nucleic acids are intrinsically more manageable; there are no issues with antibody specificity or ambiguous peaks on mass spectrometry. Even a single base is readily detected. Thus, many of the current methods for characterizing tumor or tissue gene expression use mRNA assays as surrogates for predicted protein gene product. Although it is true that mRNA assays fail to reflect the vast number of protein moieties that exist within a cell, many derived from the same gene, it is also true that all these proteins ultimately track back to mRNA message: if there is no message, there is no protein. The converse, of course, is not always correct: message may not result in protein, or the levels of protein may not parallel message levels, as a result of truncated or prolonged protein half-life, or even a failure of reliable translation without immediate proteasomal degradation, as occurs, for example, with mutated genes producing codon changes that result in premature stop codons and truncated protein. These are usually rapidly degraded, and in this case, abundant mRNA is not reflected in abundant detectable protein, which is rapidly degraded to undetectable peptides and amino acids. Despite these caveats, RNA assays are perhaps the most widely used assay for gene expression in cancer today. It is therefore useful to review the various methods used to identify and quantify mRNA expression.

RNA Blots (Northern Blot)

The oldest method to identify and roughly quantitate RNA is the Northern blot, named for its similarity to the DNA blot described by E.M. Southern.[33] Many variations have subsequently been described, including simple transfer without electrophoretic separation of RNA samples to nitrocellulose or nylon filters followed by detection with a suitably specific radioactive or fluorescently labeled probe. A virtue of this method is its ability to both determine relative molecular mass and quantify the amount of mRNA present in the sample, based on density (or fluorescence) measurements of the hybridized, labeled probe. However, a major shortcoming is the large amount of RNA required, the need for extensive laboratory handling (purification, electrophoresis, etc.), and the time required for a result. Most human tissues, and especially tumor biopsies, rarely provide sufficient material for Northern blots. Consequently, alternative methods of RNA detection and quantitation have been developed.

RNA Amplification: Polymerase Chain Reaction

a. Basic PCR: Polymerase chain reaction, or PCR, has become the method of choice for detecting even minute amounts of RNA or DNA, even in contaminated, impure, degraded, or otherwise unsatisfactory specimens. It is thus ideally suited to the small biopsies, cytology specimens, body fluids, or even laser-captured cells that are commonly used for nucleic acid assays. With suitable amplification (e.g., numbers of cycles), it is possible to detect the RNA from even single cells. A typical result for PCR amplification of MYCN in neuroblastoma after varying numbers of rounds of amplification is illustrated in Figure 21.6. Note that in this example, the MYCN-amplified and overexpressing specimen (from a needle biopsy) shows detectable product long before the single-copy control, indicating high-level expression. Despite the difference, this method is generally not used for absolute quantitation. Instead, quantitative real-time PCR has become the method of choice.

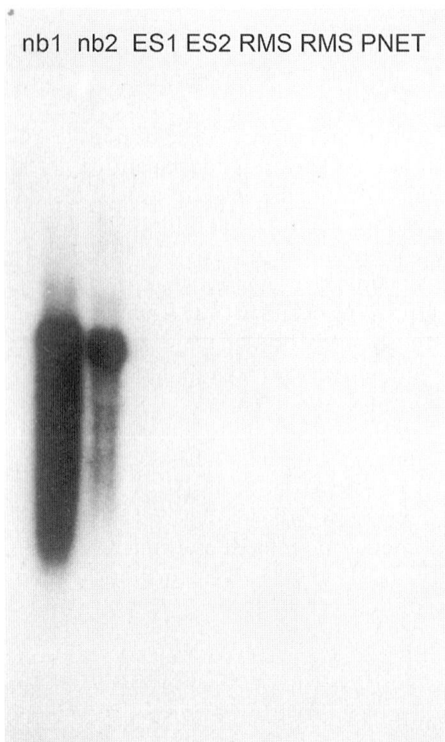

FIGURE 21.6. Polymerase chain reaction (PCR).

b. Quantitative PCR: Quantitative real-time PCR has become a standard laboratory diagnostic technology by virtue of its extraordinary sensitivity, amenability to quality control and reproducibility, speed, and cost. Although the product amplified is DNA, this is generally a cDNA produced by reverse transcriptase of mRNA. At least three manufacturers (e.g., Roche, ABI, and Cepheid) make devices and numerous reagent suppliers make various chemistries for DNA detection, including TaqMan (Roche, Basel, Switzerland) and Molecular Beacons probes, Amplifluor (Chemicon, Temecula, CA) and Scorpion primers (DxS, Ltd., Manchester, UK), and intercalating dyes such as SYBR Green (Finnzymes, Espoo, Finland). All have been used successfully. Regardless of the chemistry, in each case the point at which there is a detectable change in fluorescence intensity during the course of multiple cycles of DNA amplification is noted and termed the cycle threshold, Ct, the point termed the log-linear phase

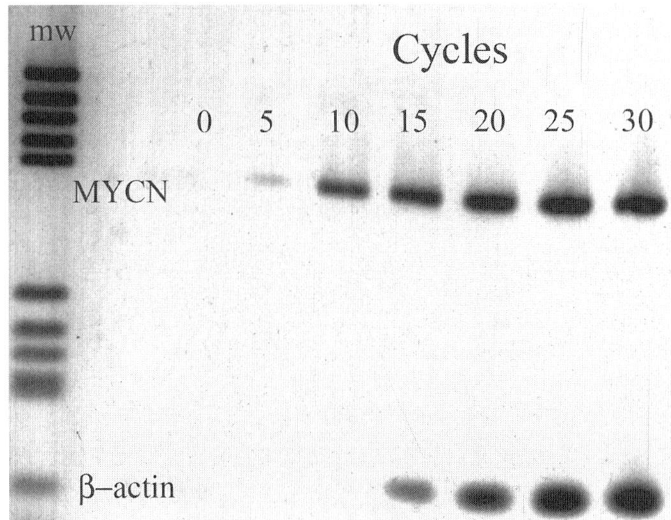

FIGURE 21.7. Quantitative real-time (QRT) PCR.

of amplification. This is a sensitive index of how much target is present in the sample, and is thus a highly reproducible measurement of the amount of RNA (or DNA) present in a sample. A typical result for detection of a chimeric oncogene in a Ewing's sarcoma (e.g., EWS-FLI1) is illustrated in Figure 21.7, where it is clear that the unknown sample shows a cycle threshold and subsequent amplification virtually indistinguishable from the positive control and quite distinct from the negative control.

Microarrays

By far the most dramatic advance in the detection of mRNA has been the development of microarray technology during the past decade. These arrays, whether constructed of cDNA, oligomeric DNA, or in situ synthesized 25-mer oligomeric DNA, share the ability to detect thousands of RNA transcripts simultaneously. From a few hundred "spots" a decade ago, the current generation of arrays routinely assays all known, and many unknown, genes from the entire transcriptome. For example, the current generation of Affymetrix (Santa Clara, CA) GeneChips, the U133 plus 2, assesses the expression of 47,000 unique RNA transcripts, a number considerably larger than the estimated number of genes in the human genome. The identity of more than half is unknown. The major impact of these arrays has been their ability to simultaneously measure the gene expression activity of any and all genes, and deliver a quantitative value, resulting in a vast number of gene by gene measurements. These gene expression profiles are markedly different for different tissues and tumors and have been shown to provide powerful diagnostic information that in many cases is superior to any antecedent diagnostic technology, on a par with an expert pathologist, and far more reproducible.

a. cDNA: The first-generation microarrays were created by spotting cDNAs of specific sequence, complementary to known genes, usually by fine-tipped metal probes held in physical arrays. The arrays were then "stamped" with the same cDNA in the same position, one after another. The resultant arrays are then incubated with a dual sample: a mixture of control and tumor, for example, in balanced proportion, each with a different color fluor (typically Cy3 and Cy5). The result is either red, green, yellow, or black, or variations thereon. A typical result is illustrated in Figure 21.8a. Red or green denotes 100% hybridization by only one of the RNA moieties in the mix (e.g., control or tumor, for example); yellow indicates balanced competitive hybridization of both in about equal proportion; and black indicates no hybridization by either. By calculating the ratios of red to green, the "fold change," or multiples of greater or lesser expression of sample versus control, can be calculated.

Although this method is still in use, it has become considerably less popular with recognition that cDNA clones are prone to cross-hybridization, are often not monoclonal, and may in fact be mislabeled. This intrinsic lack of control over the actual sequence present on the array has prompted the search for more precise nucleotide probes for arrays.

b. Spotted oligomeric DNA: In an effort to improve the reproducibility of spotted arrays, most laboratories are increasingly using defined oligomers (usually 50-mers or 60-mers) of known sequence. Advantages of this approach include the ability to precisely replicate arrays from newly synthesized oligomers and achieve the same results, the

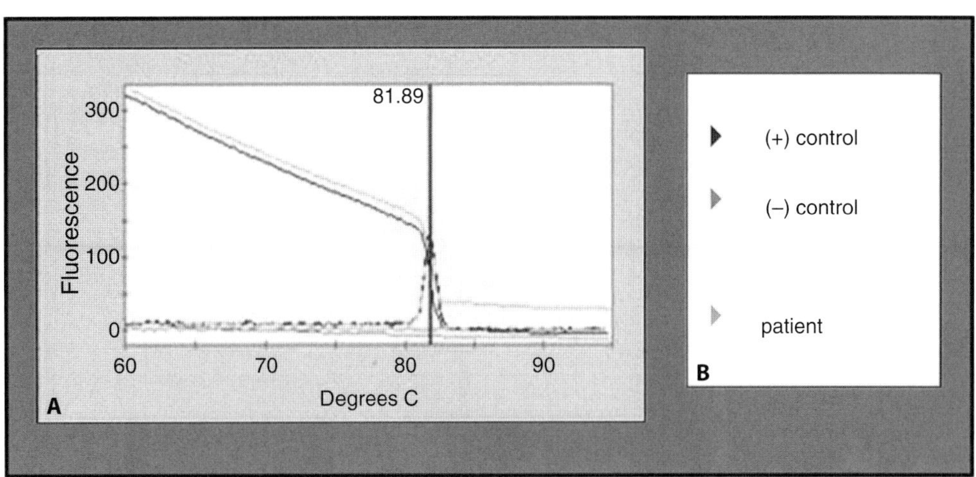

FIGURE 21.8. Microarrays: (a) spotted; (b) GeneChip.

ability to compare data from one lab to another, and the absence of cross-hybridization caused by mixed clones or conserved sequences within large cDNAs that result in non-specific cross-hybridization. In addition, variations in expressed gene sequence due to alternative exon usage, truncated message, and even mutations can be readily detected with custom arrays that are otherwise difficult to create from standard UNIGEN database information. Thus, the user is free to generate highly specific custom arrays to interrogate expressed in detail. Several commercial vendors, such as Agilent, have entered the field, which will result in standardization of arrays and results that would otherwise be difficult to achieve in "home brew" microarray facilities. This in turn will enhance their utility for clinical use, where reproducibility and reliability are of paramount importance.

c. Synthesized oligomeric DNA: Figure 21.8b illustrates the physical appearance of a typical commercial oligonucleotide array (Affymetrix GeneChip), where 25-mer segments of a gene are arrayed from 6′ to 3′ in "tiles," or areas containing that probe. Typically, 11 to 16 such 25-mers are generated across the coding sequence of the gene, paired with a one-nucleotide mismatch (below) (e.g., PM versus MM, or perfect match versus mismatch). The PM minus MM signal intensity for each pair is calculated, and the mean value for all tiles within a gene is calculated and reported as an expression value. A variety of correction algorithms are then applied to calculate a normalized value for each of the genes on the array, using values from internal standards on the array. In a typical analysis, the values for each gene in each sample are compared one to another in high-dimensional space, and the nearest neighbors, based on any of a number of criteria, are calculated and the patient samples "clustered" to identify those most similar to one another. When done well, very obvious clusters of "like" and "unlike" are readily appreciated, thereby establishing classes of tumor (Figure 21.9). Surprisingly, these clusters typically match known tumor groupings closely. Cases that do not frequently have subsequently been shown to be misdiagnosed. In other cases, the method identifies previously unrecognized subsets within tumor groups, many of which may have important clinical or therapeutic features of value for patient management in the future. In general, whole-transcriptome expression profiling has had an enormous impact on biomedical research and is poised to enter the clinical practice of medicine, particularly in oncology, where gene dysregulation is a regular feature of most cancers. Finding which genes has been the challenge. Microarray technology appears to accomplish that, rapidly and facilely, to great effect.

DNA Based

Analysis of DNA takes many forms. Methods to do so span virtually the entire history of molecular biology, more so than RNA or protein (at least as defined by modern sequencing and characterization methods). Progress in DNA analysis has been remarkable: from crude biochemical methods to coarse RFLP (restriction fragment polymorphism analysis) to modern methods that embody rapid sequence determination and identification of DNA from virtually any source, the ability to obtain precise, voluminous DNA sequence information is now virtually unlimited. The achievements of the human genome sequencing project seem to pale in the face of potential individual whole-genome sequencing within days at minimal cost: all 3.3. billion bases, times two (sense and antisense), times two (both haplotypes). In this context, it also worth mentioning that about one-third of the DNA extracted from a cell is mitochondrial in origin, and mitochondria undergo mutational damage over time, with resultant disease onset as well. Analysis of this DNA, too, will be of importance. It is likely that as highly automated, inexpensive methods of doing so become commonplace, broad DNA sequencing will likely become central to analysis of genetic anomalies in cancer and other diseases. At present, however, assays of more limited scope are the norm, as is illustrated here.

Southern Blot

The first widely used method for DNA identification without resort to laborious manual DNA sequencing methods was developed by E.M. Southern in 1975.[33] This method is based

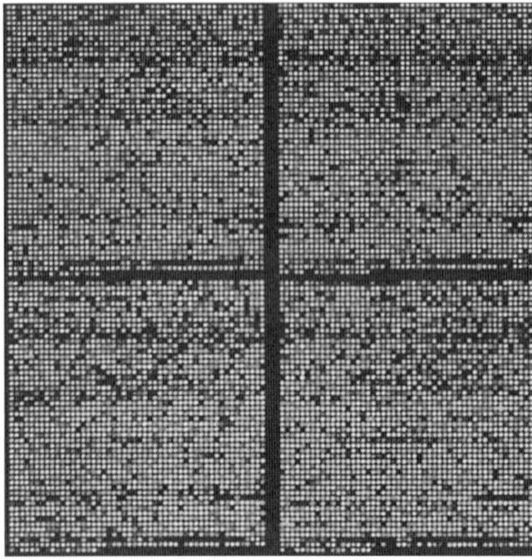

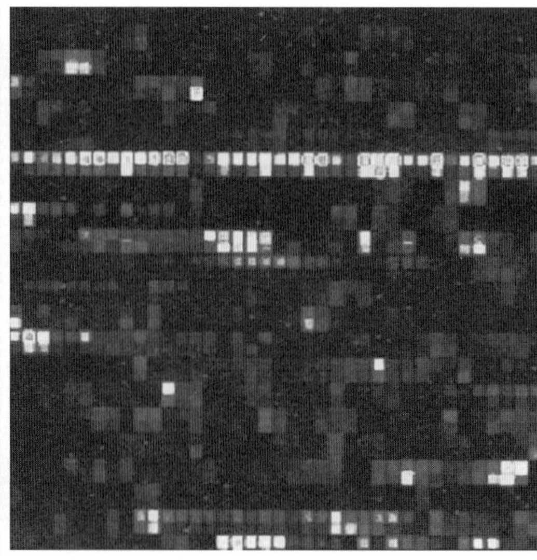

FIGURE 21.9. GEP clustering.

on the remarkable specificity of binding between nucleotides in the DNA helix. If the double helix is denatured ("melted"), the single-stranded DNA is then readily annealed with complementary DNA sequences. By denaturing DNA, electrophoresing it to separate different fragments by molecular weight, transferring the gel to a solid substrate such as nylon or nitrocellulose membranes, and incubating these filters with radioactive or fluorescently labeled complementary DNA probes (e.g., short sequences sufficient to establish absolute identity), it is possible to identify any sequence from the mix of genomic DNA. A side benefit is that loss or gain of chromosomal DNA can also be ascertained; comparison of a single-copy DNA probe with an amplified gene, for example, allows ready determination of copy number. An example from an MYCN-amplified childhood neuroblastoma is illustrated in Figure 21.10. Here, a variety of tumors with a single copy of the gene show comparably dense bands at the appropriate molecular weight. In contrast, the amplified tumor shows a marked increase in signal strength. Scintigraphy of radioactive DNA probes, fluorography of fluorescently labeled DNA, or densitometry of chromogen-labeled DNA allows precise quantitation of the signal, and therefore a ratio that defines copy number.

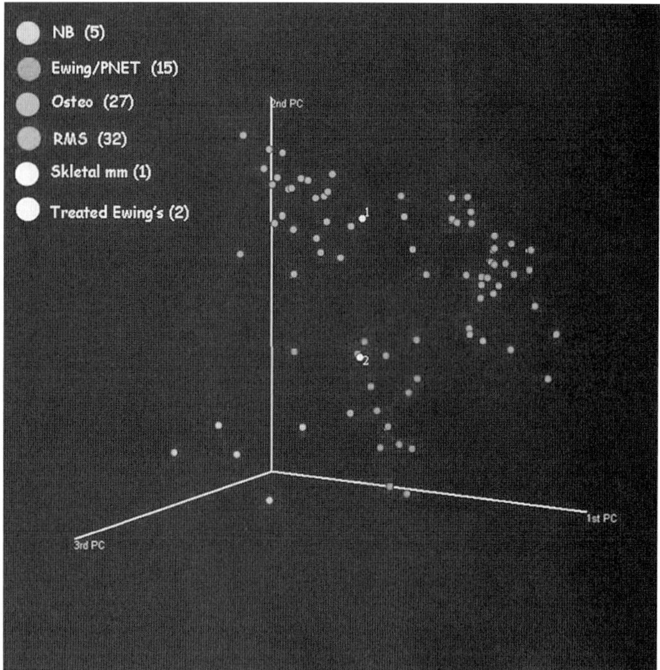

FIGURE 21.10. Southern blot.

Fluorescent In Situ Hybridization (FISH)

The remarkable specificity of DNA hybridization has given rise to many variations on DNA assays. One particularly useful method for clinical purposes is fluorescent in situ hybridization (FISH). In this method, fluorescently or affinity-tagged DNA probes some hundreds to several thousand bases in size are applied to tumor sections, cytospins, or imprints, for example, and hybridized under denaturing then reannealing conditions, conditions similar to those developed for Southern blots. The labeled DNA is now bound to target DNA and readily detected. This method can be used for a variety of purposes, such as detecting amplified genes, as in MYCN amplification in neuroblastoma (Figure 21.11) or, more commonly, to detect HER2/neu amplification in breast

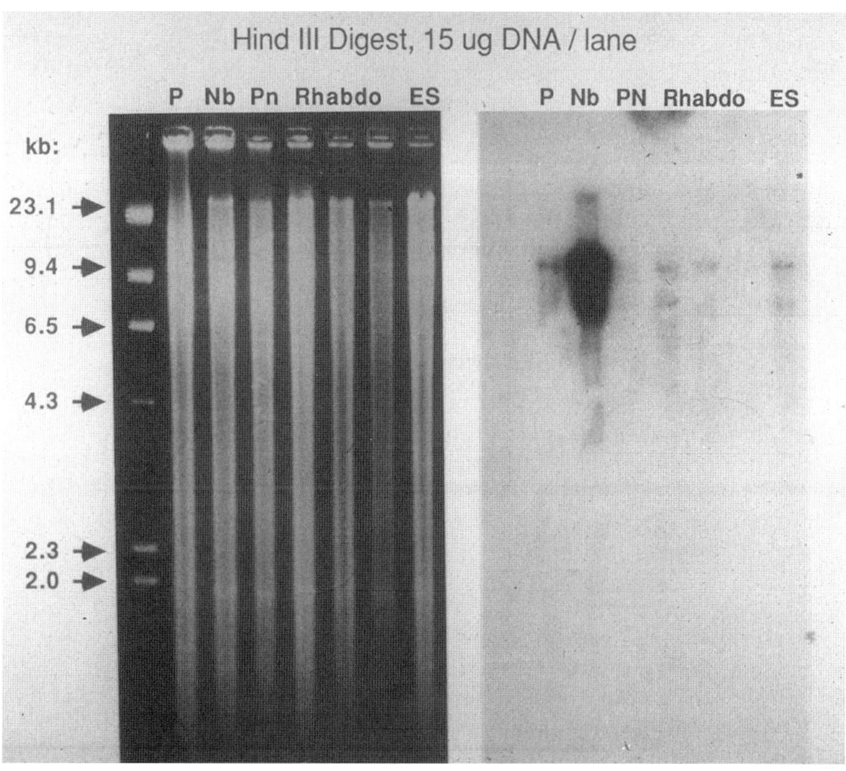

FIGURE 21.11. Fluorescent in situ hybridization (FISH); MYCN; tissue section.

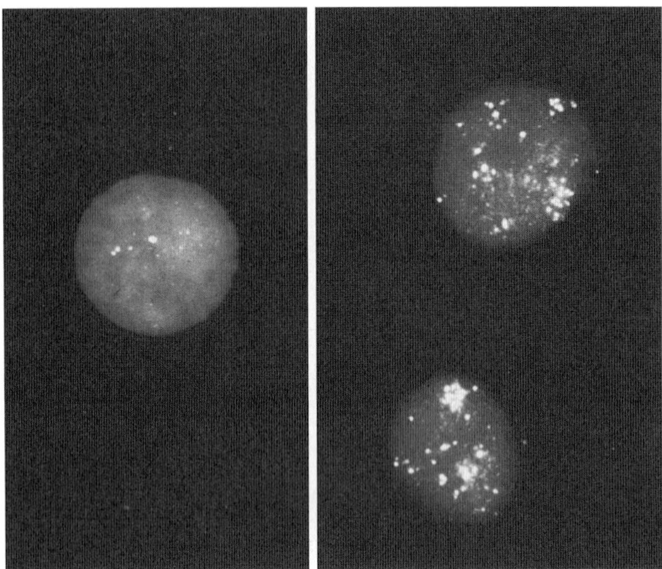

FIGURE 21.12. DNA sequence.

cancer. Both are of great prognostic importance, imparting a graver prognosis than would otherwise be the case, and establishing the basis for more-aggressive therapy. FISH, then, is a valuable diagnostic and prognostic tool that begets more aggressive therapy when an amplified gene is detected.

DNA Sequencing

Direct detection of sequence variation in DNA has been greatly facilitated by the advent of high-throughput, automated, multichannel DNA sequencers. These machines were in fact responsible for the rapid progress made in the human genome sequencing project. The technology is now routinely used in research and diagnostic laboratories to determine the identity of, for example, PCR-amplified DNA, and to detect mutations or polymorphisms in genomic DNA. An example of heterozygous mutation of a gene is illustrated in Figure 21.12, where both G and C peaks are identified at the same location, indicating that there is a mutation in one allele of the gene, whereas the other allele remains wild type. Most often in cancer cells the wild-type allele is subsequently lost, resulting in unopposed function of the mutant and total loss of wild-type functionality, common in oncogenes such as p53.

Mutation Detection (WAVE, and Similar Methods)

Indirect means of DNA sequence detection have proliferated, especially before the availability of cheap, fast DNA sequencing. Several of the methods are based on aberrant migration in a gel due to conformational changes in the DNA double helix that results from base mismatches. They retain their importance as screening methods in particular, due to their low cost, high sensitivity, and high throughput, superior even to DNA sequencing. Their value stems from the fact that most mutation or polymorphisms screening assays presume a low incidence of positives. Rather than laboriously sequencing all samples, a prescreen that detects the rare anomalous case is used. When an anomaly is detected, it is simple to confirm the anomaly by direct DNA sequencing of the anomalous case. This is the principle behind SSCP (single-strand conformation polymorphism) and its many derivatives such as dHPLC (denaturing high performance liquid chromatography).[34] A particularly useful method has been commercialized by Transgenomics, the so-called WAVE technology. In this method, homo- and hetero-DNA dimers are formed after denaturing and renaturing conditions and immobilization on a hydrophobic column matrix. Increasing concentrations of acetonitrile selectively elute triethylaminoethyl (TEAA)-bound DNA duplexes; heteroduplexes elute first, followed by homoduplexes. Mismatched dimers elute aberrantly, reflected in peak height and shape. Samples that show such anomalies are then subjected to confirmatory DNA sequencing, as described earlier. In this way, a large number of clinical samples can be screened, and only those showing anomalous elution patterns need be confirmed by DNA sequencing. A typical example of mutation detection by WAVE dHPLC is illustrated in Figure 21.13.

Polymorphisms

An interesting aspect of genomic DNA organization is the presence throughout the genome of millions of single-base variations between individuals, called SNPs, for single-nucleotide polymorphisms. The HapMap project (http://www.hapmap.org/index.html.en) estimates there are 10 million such variants that occur with sufficient frequency as to warrant designation as polymorphisms. An example is illustrated in Figure 21.14, from the HapMap home page. These SNPs are not mutations; mutations occur rarely and are usually either inherited in the germ line from one parent

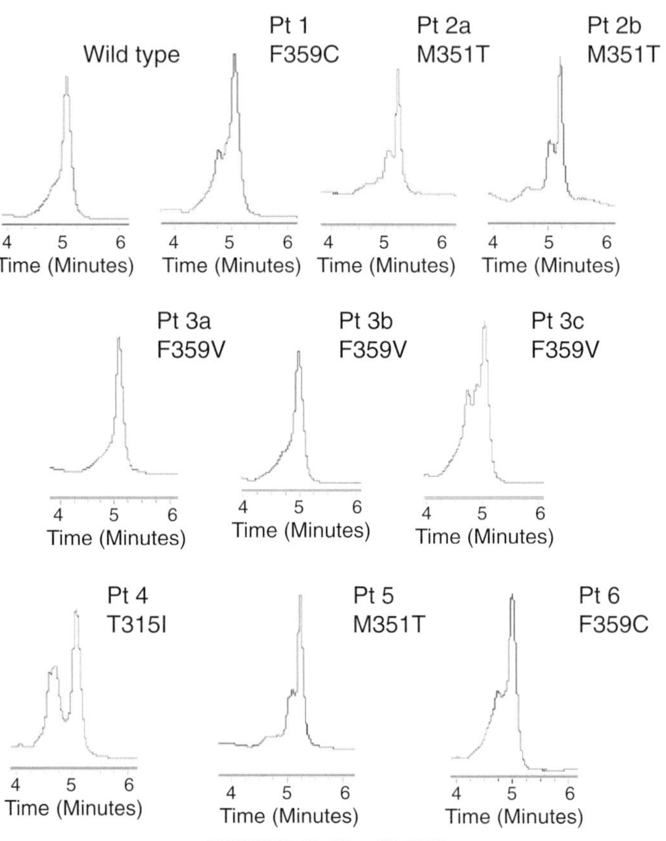

FIGURE 21.13. WAVE?

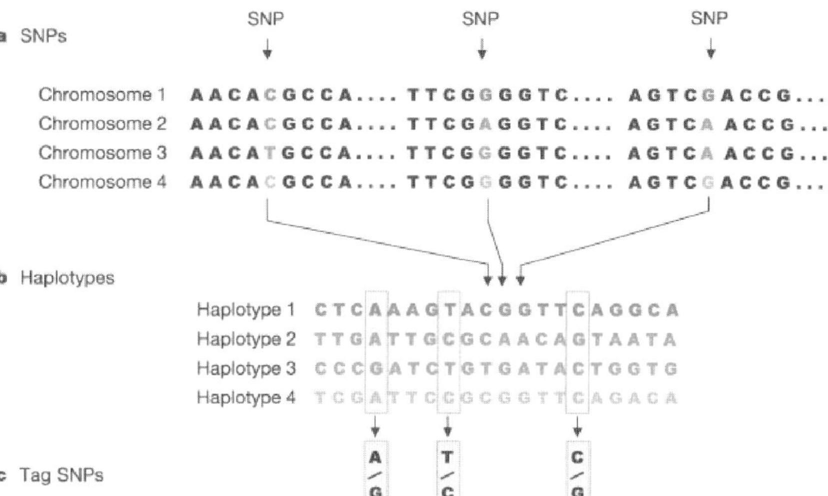

FIGURE 21.14. Single nucleotide polymorphisms (SNPs): illustration from HapMap.

or arise de novo as a somatic mutation. In contrast, polymorphisms reflect human genetic variation between individuals. During sexual reproduction, chromosomal cross-over events result in the creation of mosaics of large blocks of DNA ("haplotype blocks") inherited from one or the other parent (Figure 21.15, also from the HapMap home page). This overall pattern is called a haplotype. Because these blocks of DNA are inherited as blocks, each individual inherits two haplotypes, one from each parent. These haplotypes have generally arisen as much as 150,000 years ago in the human germ line in Africa and have undergone further diversification with the spread of humanity over the globe. They show marked ethnic variation, resulting from expansion of isolated groups of humans, and variable age, due to additional polymorphisms that arose subsequent to dispersion of ethnic populations. The aggregate effect is a *fingerprint* of genetic diversity that can be used to identify the genetic background of any individual and, further, to associate that genetic makeup with disease propensity, severity, response to drugs, and many other parameters. Polymorphic variants of CYP450, for example, are powerful tools to predict drug metabolism in individuals, potentially guiding dosage for the individual as opposed to the "average." In oncology, idiosyncratic responses to drugs such as cyclophosphamide are linked to specific polymorphic variants of CYP450.[35,36] This burgeoning field, termed "pharmacogenetics," is likely to increasingly dictate individualized therapy based on haplotype variants of critical genes such as CYP450 and many others that in aggregate dictate an individual's disease susceptibility and likely response to therapy.[37–42]

Whole-Genome Assays for SNPs

Given the apparent importance of polymorphic variation among individuals to important clinical issues such as disease susceptibility and response to therapy and prognosis, a practical method for genotyping individuals is needed for clinical use. The HapMap project referenced earlier is providing the data, including tag SNPs that will enable identification of haplotype blocks and therefore the individual's haplotype; only about 500,000 of these are needed to predict an individual's genotype, as opposed to direct detection of all 10 million SNPs, or any large fraction thereof. A variety of methods for large-scale detection of SNPs are being developed. At present, two approaches merit discussion, as both are used for whole-genome SNP analysis.

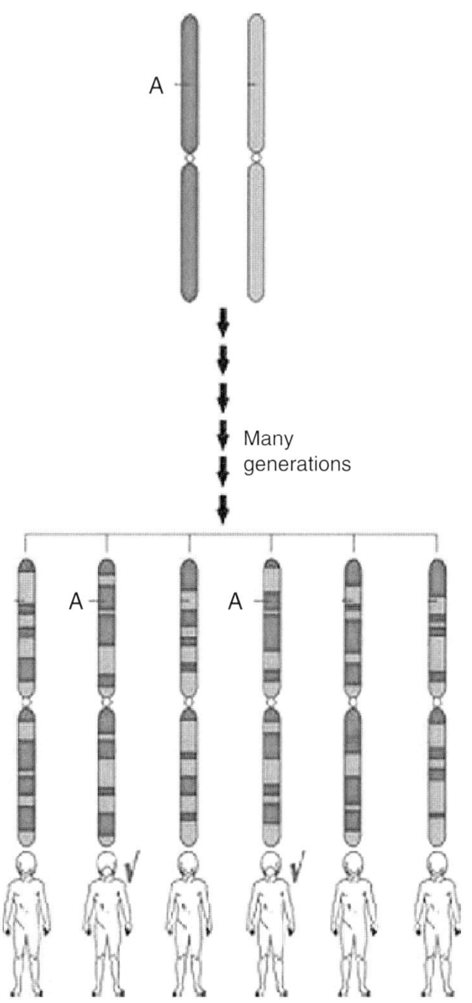

FIGURE 21.15. Genomic mosaicism.

a. Bead Arrays: The first, a multiplex bead assay developed by Michael et al.[43] and commercialized by Illumina, Inc. (San Diego, CA), termed Beadarray, is capable of identifying up to approximately 1,500 SNPs per assay, by adsorbing a random bead mixture (~1,000 to ~1,500 types, specific for one SNP) onto the etched ends of approximately 50,000 optical fiber complexes. Each fiber binds a bead; with 1,500 bead types, each is represented with about 30-fold redundancy. A unique decoding scheme, based on unique "address" sequences incorporated into PCR-amplified genomic DNA sequences, is then used to identify each bead and assign a call value for each SNP.[44,45] The result is about a 90+% successful call for SNPs from dbSNP. High-quality, validated SNPs results in more than 95% calls. SNPs can be drawn from the entire genome, or regionally at high density. This flexibility lends itself to disease association studies, where a locus is first identified, then probed in detail with regional SNP beads. However, there is a significant design and validation component for each SNP, and the cost per SNP is higher than SNP arrays (see following). Nonetheless, this technology has been widely used by the HapMap project, with great success.

b. SNP photolithography arrays: The second high-throughput method, available commercially from Affymetrix, is based on the same technology employed for the GeneChips discussed earlier. For SNP detection, the region of interest for a specific allele, termed "A" (e.g., the SNP and 14 surrounding nucleotides, designated −7 through +7) is represented by 25-mer oligonucleotide sequences, with the specific nucleotide of interest represented in position 13. Target sequences bind most stably to such sequences and yield the brightest signal. The brightest signal should thus occur for the 25-mer representing the SNP at position 0. To further control for nonspecific hybridization, a one-base mismatch sequence is tiled on the array immediately below the perfect match, yielding a 2 × 7 matrix of 14 tiles. This is then doubled, to include the same setup for the alternate allele ("B"), yielding a 4 × 7 matrix. Finally, this is replicated in the antisense direction, for a grand total of 56 tiles. To detect the target DNA on these probes, genomic DNA is fragmented by one or more restriction endonucleases, PCR primer adapters ligated to the ends, and preferentially PCR amplified by fragment size (e.g., 400–800 bp). These PCR products are then fragmented, denatured, end labeled, and hybridized to the SNP arrays, resulting in the hybridization pattern illustrated in Figure 21.16. With suitable software, the genotype for any given SNP can be called with greater than 95% confidence.[46,47] At present, arrays capable of interrogating up to 126,000 SNPs are available, and the number is expected to rise to 500,000 and more in the near future. With reasonable selection of SNPs, this density will allow haplotyping with unprecedented precision and sensitivity across the entire genome. The disadvantage is that, unlike the bead array system already described, the user cannot specify specific SNPs for analysis.

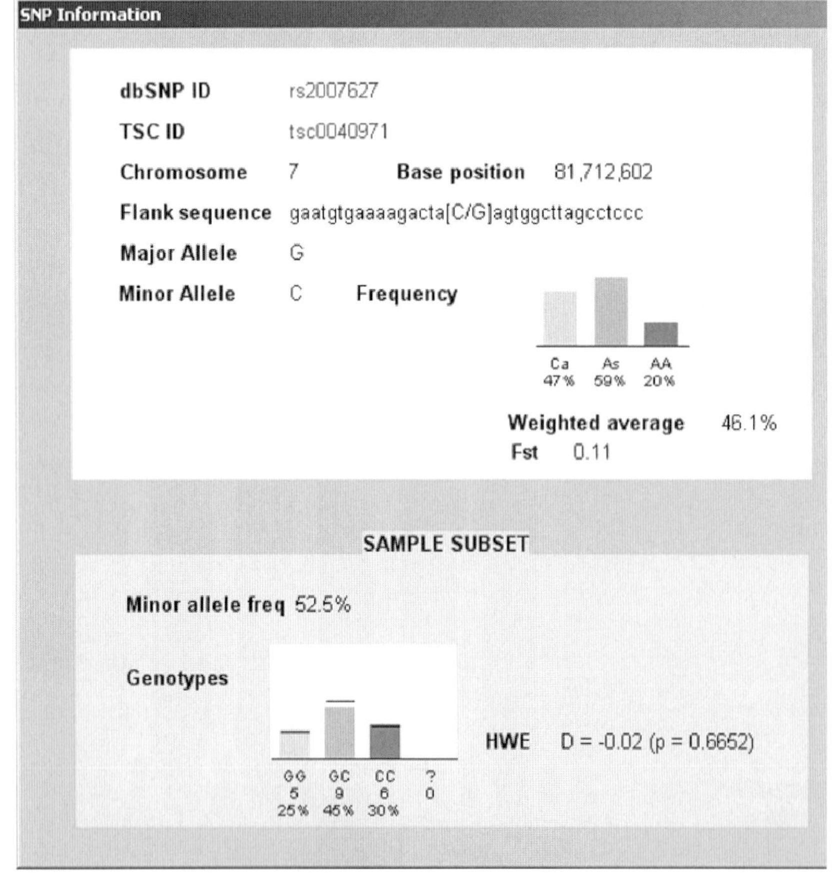

FIGURE 21.16. SNP: chip.

These methods may thus be complementary technologies for very high density SNP haplotyping.

Although high-density SNP haplotyping will ultimately be of value in oncology as a means to identify patient subpopulations with greater or lesser tolerance for certain cytotoxic drugs and perhaps even disease susceptibility, the immediate value of SNPs, particularly as high-density microarrays, is their phenomenal ability to detect DNA copy loss and gain, and to map these genomic alterations to very precisely defined regions of chromosomes.[48–50] In one respect, this can be considered a logical extension of cytogenetic analysis, SKY, CGH, and even array CGH, none of which approach the power of this technology to detect DNA loss and gain by as few as 1,000 bases within specific regions of the genome. This approach is of enormous potential value for identifying recurring genomic abnormalities in cancer that is currently beyond the limits of detection by current technology. Wider use of this technology for this purpose is inevitable. Initial publications, including use of laser-captured and amplified DNA, have already appeared.[49] Many more are expected.

Bioinformatics in Medicine

An inevitable consequence of the use of large-scale genomic technologies in biology and medicine is the accumulation of vast amounts of data that must be reduced to useful knowledge. Each of the newer technologies discussed (e.g., mass spectrometry-based proteomics, microarray-based gene expression analysis, and SNP-based genotyping) of necessity create this challenge. This in turn has spawned an urgent need for those skilled in both biology and quantitative analyses. Unfortunately, the methods required for data management go far beyond data archiving and statistical analysis. Bioinformatics is the broadly defined discipline that has resulted from this need. Many different tools have and continue to be developed to meet this need. National Institutes of Health (NIH) sponsors NCBI, the National Center for Biotechnology Information, which both hosts genomic data and provides suitable browser and analytic tools. The HapMap project noted earlier offers similar tools for inspection and analysis of SNP data. Numerous commercial sources of software for analysis of gene expression data and linkage analysis are also available. The full scale of the endeavor is far beyond the scope of this chapter. It is fair to say, however, that as the technology advances rapidly, so does the need for analytical methods, but also the need for tools to integrate these data sets with one another and with other types of data that bear on the problem, such as clinical, biologic, and other molecular data. As a general comment, the steady intrusion of genomic methods on the practice of medicine, and especially in cancer, the most common genetic disease of all, will inevitably require different training for its practitioners in the future. At a minimum, the future oncologist, and allied disciplines, will likely need to concurrently deal with clinical, biologic, laboratory, genomic, and statistical data in the evaluation of a patient. Whether responsible for the primary analysis, or accepting or rejecting the result, this future oncologist will need to be conversant with at least a basic understanding of the quantitative analytical methods used for genomic studies.

Clinical Impact

Evidence of Efficacy

Whenever a new procedure or technology is introduced into medicine, there is inevitably a rush of enthusiasm, usually followed by unwarranted skepticism, in response to the inevitable failures that accompany any new method. The difference with genomic technologies is already apparent, however: although sequencing the human genome may have had little or no direct impact on the practice of medicine, the derivative information and technology are responsible, to a greater or lesser degree, for nearly all the technologies discussed in this chapter. The characteristic of all these newer methods is that all have resulted in publications that document their actual or potential efficacy in patient management, most notably in oncology. This, then, is the real value of these technologies: they enhance our ability to both understand and treat cancer, in ways unheard of a short time ago. The impact going forward can hardly be less.

Integration with Morphologic Diagnosis

As powerful and promising as genomic technology is for the field of oncology, it is also important to place this enthusiasm in context. Osler allegedly admonished his students to be neither the first to adopt new medications nor the last to abandon them. A similar comment can be made with reference to diagnostics and technology: new and unproven technologies are no substitute for older methods with proven efficacy. Even new technologies that offer more precise diagnoses or better indications for therapy may not be warranted when viewed in context with cost-versus-benefit considerations. Is a $3,000 genetic test that indicates you have a 60% lifetime risk to develop cancer of value, when 33% of the population will develop cancer in their lifetime? In a similar vein, is a diagnostic genetic test with 90% reliability that costs $1,000 preferable to a pathologic review of a glass slide for a total of $150? Further, what genetic test determines whether the submitted specimen is in fact cancer?

The real value of genetic tests is the enormous contribution they can make to refined, objective, reproducible diagnoses. Most of the methods discussed here are in actual use, some as clinical research tools, other as ancillary diagnostics, to be considered in aggregate with other methods, starting with routine histologic examination. When the innate precision and scope of genomic testing is paired with basic pathologic evaluation for the presence of cancer, diagnoses result that are far more likely to be replicated and to direct optimal therapy. Thus, in actual practice, morphologic and genetic methods are overwhelmingly synergistic, and should be employed whenever possible, when there is clinical need and the result will likely aid therapy.

Implications for Directed Therapy

The most direct impact of precise diagnostic methods is, of course, to tailor therapy for patients most likely to benefit, the "Holy Grail" of "personalized medicine."[40,42,51] As laudable as these goals may be, the reality is that to date very few examples of this exist. Herceptin for HER2/neu amplified

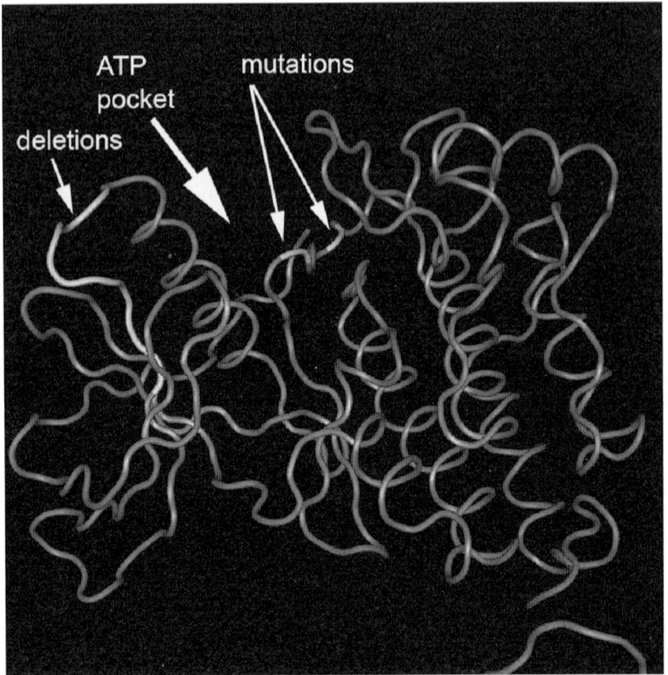

FIGURE 21.17. Three-dimensional (3-D) structure of TK domain of epidermal growth factor receptor (EGFR).

breast cancer, gleevec for GIST, and ATRA for APL are clear exceptions, but broad-based "personalized medicine" remains an unattained goal. This reality may change rapidly, however, as suitable genomic profiling methods become readily available at reasonable cost. A striking example of this is the recent recognition that iressa (gefitinib), which has only a 10% response rate in most solid tumors, is in fact 100% effective in inducing a dramatic reduction in tumor size in non-small cell lung cancer patients.[8] The fact that response is directly linked to mutations in the ATP-binding pocket of the tyrosine kinase domain of the EGFR (Figure 21.17), and that these mutations can be detected by any of a number of methods, will almost certainly revolutionize the selective use of iressa for this tumor.[10,52] In fact, pairing of a routine diagnostic test with therapy has already been proposed by the authors of this landmark study, and several national commercial labs are apparently in negotiations with that group to license the intellectual property and offer widespread testing. It is likely this paradigm will be repeated many times as many new selective agents (kinase inhibitors, growth factor receptor blockers, proteasomal inhibitors, angiostatins, etc.) go into clinical trials. It is worth remembering in this regard that iressa might not have been FDA approved if the response rate had been any lower. One wonders how many drugs that showed little efficacy in an unselected population are in fact highly efficacious in selected patient populations. Diagnostic testing using the methods described herein will likely answer that question, at least in some cases.

Integration Within Evidence-Based Medicine

To put the preceding information within the broad context of evidence-based oncology, it is useful to observe that, although Osler observed that medicine was an art based on science, it is increasingly driven by that science, which inexorably seeks to mechanistically define human disease. As the basic biology of cancer is increasingly understood, the opportunity to employ that knowledge to diagnostic and therapeutic advantage will increase in direct proportion. Given the rapid increase in our knowledge of the functions of the human genome in health and disease, it is incumbent on the practitioner to incorporate this knowledge into the daily practice of oncology. This is no small task; the rate of accumulation of new and relevant knowledge of cancer mechanisms, diagnostic tests, and potential new therapies is set to increase exponentially, as the true value of research on the human genome is realized. Ideally, as in the iressa and lung cancer example noted previously, this new knowledge should be applied as soon as practical. In reality, the need for convincing evidence will limit the rate at which this knowledge and its associated therapies become standard of care. In between is a vast landscape of clinical research that will be required to provide this evidence. The need for targeted translational and clinical research to move discovery from the basic science laboratory to the patient has never been more acute, a point recognized and well articulated by the current director of the NIH.[53]

Concluding Remarks

The preceding discussion attempts to place the many useful technologies derived from molecular biology within a clinical context. While the technology is powerful, it is no substitute for clinical acumen and experience. One need only consider the results of the most cutting edge technology applied to cancer diagnosis and therapy, when the starting material is breast adipose tissue instead of tumor, to appreciate that it is the basic oversights that most commonly result in equivocal or flatly erroneous information. Thus, technology is no substitute for common sense and clinical judgment.

The reverse is also true: untoward affection for historical norms has no place in the future of medicine. Evidence-based medicine demands objective evidence of diagnoses and information used for clinical management. The obvious consequence of this is a need for integration of new technologies within diagnostic evaluations of cancer. However, too often proponents of one or another technology overlook the valid and potentially more efficacious and cost-effective contributions of established or alternative technologies to clinical diagnosis. As a general rule, any diagnostic technology that cannot be delivered for less than a few hundred dollars will not be accepted as a routine diagnostic modality. Consequently, many if not most of the technologies discussed in this chapter are not yet ready for "prime time" within the context of clinical medicine, as opposed to clinical research. Despite this caveat, there is no question that with increasing appreciation of the power of these technologies, coupled with relentless reductions in cost, genomic methods in general will progressively augment the diagnostic armamentarium of clinical oncology.

References

1. Asmar L, et al. Agreement among and within groups of pathologists in the classification of rhabdomyosarcoma and related childhood sarcomas. Report of an international study of four

pathology classifications. Cancer (Phila) 1994;74(9):2579–2588.
2. Overgaard J, et al. TP53 mutation is an independent prognostic marker for poor outcome in both node-negative and node-positive breast cancer. Acta Oncol 2000;39(3):327–333.
3. La Perle KM, Jhiang SM, Capen CC. Loss of p53 promotes anaplasia and local invasion in ret/PTC1-induced thyroid carcinomas. Am J Pathol 2000;157(2):671–677.
4. Malkin D, et al. Mutations of the p53 tumor suppressor gene occur infrequently in Wilms' tumor. Cancer Res 1994;54(8):2077–2079.
5. Soussi T, Beroud C. Assessing TP53 status in human tumours to evaluate clinical outcome. Nat Rev Cancer 2001;1(3):233–240.
6. Frank AJ, et al. The TP53-ARF tumor suppressor pathway is frequently disrupted in large/cell anaplastic medulloblastoma. Brain Res Mol Brain Res 2004;121(1–2):137–140.
7. Nishimura Y, et al. Cyclin D1 expression in endometrioid-type endometrial adenocarcinoma is correlated with histological grade and proliferative activity, but not with prognosis. Anticancer Res 2004;24(4):2185–2191.
8. Lynch TJ, et al. Activating mutations in the epidermal growth factor receptor underlying responsiveness of non-small-cell lung cancer to gefitinib. N Engl J Med 2004;350(21):2129–2139.
9. Pao W, et al. EGF receptor gene mutations are common in lung cancers from "never smokers" and are associated with sensitivity of tumors to gefitinib and erlotinib. Proc Natl Acad Sci USA 2004;101(36):13306–13311.
10. Stratton MR, Futreal PA. Cancer: understanding the target. Nature (Lond) 2004;430(6995):30.
11. McCormick F. Cancer therapy based on p53. Cancer J Sci Am 1999;5(3):139–144.
12. McCormick F. Cancer-specific viruses and the development of ONYX-015. Cancer Biol Ther 2003;2(4 suppl 1):S157–S160.
13. Vassilev LT, et al. In vivo activation of the p53 pathway by small-molecule antagonists of MDM2. Science 2004;303(5659):844–848.
14. Verheul HM, Pinedo HM. Vascular endothelial growth factor and its inhibitors. Drugs Today (Barc) 2003;39(suppl C):81–93.
15. Davidoff AM, Kandel JJ. Antiangiogenic therapy for the treatment of pediatric solid malignancies. Semin Pediatr Surg 2004;13(1):53–60.
16. Adams J. The development of proteasome inhibitors as anticancer drugs. Cancer Cell 2004;5(5):417–421.
17. Ravi R, Bedi A. NF-kappaB in cancer—a friend turned foe. Drug Resist Update 2004;7(1):53–67.
18. Hoekstra WJ, Poulter BL. Combinatorial chemistry techniques applied to nonpeptide integrin antagonists. Curr Med Chem 1998;5(3):195–204.
19. Owa T, et al. Cell cycle regulation in the G_1 phase: a promising target for the development of new chemotherapeutic anticancer agents. Curr Med Chem 2001;8(12):1487–1503.
20. Gaffney DJ, Keightley PD. Unexpected conserved non-coding DNA blocks in mammals. Trends Genet 2004;20(8):332–337.
21. Morey C, Avner P. Employment opportunities for non-coding RNAs. FEBS Lett, 2004;567(1):27–34.
22. Sellers TA, Yates JR. Review of proteomics with applications to genetic epidemiology. Genet Epidemiol 2003;24(2):83–98.
23. Kozak KR, et al. Identification of biomarkers for ovarian cancer using strong anion-exchange ProteinChips: potential use in diagnosis and prognosis. Proc Natl Acad Sci USA 2003;100(21):12343–12348.
24. Yip TT, Lomas L. SELDI ProteinChip array in oncoproteomic research. Technol Cancer Res Treat 2002;1(4):273–280.
25. Merchant M, Weinberger SR. Recent advancements in surface-enhanced laser desorption/ionization-time of flight-mass spectrometry. Electrophoresis 2000;21(6):1164–1177.
26. Petricoin EF, et al. Use of proteomic patterns in serum to identify ovarian cancer. Lancet 2002;359(9306):572–577.
27. Yanagida M, et al. Matrix assisted laser desorption/ionization-time of flight-mass spectrometry analysis of proteins detected by anti-phosphotyrosine antibody on two-dimensional-gels of fibroblast cell lysates after tumor necrosis factor-alpha stimulation. Electrophoresis 2000;21(9):1890–1898.
28. Nelson RW, Nedelkov D, Tubbs KA. Biosensor chip mass spectrometry: a chip-based proteomics approach. Electrophoresis 2000;21(6):1155–1163.
29. Berndt P, Hobohm U, Langen H. Reliable automatic protein identification from matrix-assisted laser desorption/ionization mass spectrometric peptide fingerprints. Electrophoresis 1999;20(18):3521–3526.
30. Conrads TP, et al. Cancer diagnosis using proteomic patterns. Expert Rev Mol Diagn 2003;3(4):411–420.
31. Wulfkuhle JD, et al. Proteomic approaches to the diagnosis, treatment, and monitoring of cancer. Adv Exp Med Biol 2003;532:59–68.
32. Rosenblatt KP, et al. Serum proteomics in cancer diagnosis and management. Annu Rev Med 2004;55:97–112.
33. Southern EM. Detection of specific sequences among DNA fragments separated by gel electrophoresis. J Mol Biol 1975;98(3):503–517.
34. Frueh FW, Noyer-Weidner M. The use of denaturing high-performance liquid chromatography (DHPLC) for the analysis of genetic variations: impact for diagnostics and pharmacogenetics. Clin Chem Lab Med 2003;41(4):452–461.
35. Yule SM, et al. Cyclophosphamide pharmacokinetics in children. Br J Clin Pharmacol 1996;41(1):13–19.
36. Jain KK. Applications of biochips: from diagnostics to personalized medicine. Curr Opin Drug Discov Dev 2004;7(3):285–289.
37. Cardon LR, Abecasis GR. Using haplotype blocks to map human complex trait loci. Trends Genet 2003;19(3):135–140.
38. Loktionov A. Common gene polymorphisms, cancer progression and prognosis. Cancer Lett 2004;208(1):1–33.
39. Kohn EC, et al. Molecular therapeutics: promise and challenges. Semin Oncol 2004;31(1 suppl 3):39–53.
40. Ulrich CM, Robien K, McLeod HL. Cancer pharmacogenetics: polymorphisms, pathways and beyond. Nat Rev Cancer 2003;3(12):912–920.
41. Oscarson M. Pharmacogenetics of drug metabolising enzymes: importance for personalised medicine. Clin Chem Lab Med 2003;41(4):573–580.
42. Onyango P. Genomics and cancer. Curr Opin Oncol 2002;14(1):79–85.
43. Michael KL, et al. Randomly ordered addressable high-density optical sensor arrays. Anal Chem 1998;70(7):1242–1248.
44. Fan JB, et al. Highly parallel SNP genotyping. Cold Spring Harb Symp Quant Biol 2003;68:69–78.
45. Gunderson KL, et al. Decoding randomly ordered DNA arrays. Genome Res 2004;14(5):870–877.
46. Kennedy GC, et al. Large-scale genotyping of complex DNA. Nat Biotechnol 2003;21(10):1233–1237.
47. Matsuzaki H, et al. Parallel genotyping of over 10,000 SNPs using a one-primer assay on a high-density oligonucleotide array. Genome Res 2004;14(3):414–425.
48. Wong KK, et al. Allelic imbalance analysis by high-density single-nucleotide polymorphic allele (SNP) array with whole genome amplified DNA. Nucleic Acids Res 2004;32(9):e69.
49. Lieberfarb ME, et al. Genome-wide loss of heterozygosity analysis from laser capture microdissected prostate cancer using single nucleotide polymorphic allele (SNP) arrays and a novel bioinformatics platform dChipSNP. Cancer Res 2003;63(16):4781–4785.

50. Bignell GR, et al. High-resolution analysis of DNA copy number using oligonucleotide microarrays. Genome Res 2004;14(2): 287–295.
51. McLeod HL, Yu J. Cancer pharmacogenomics: SNPs, chips, and the individual patient. Cancer Invest 2003;21(4):630–640.
52. Minna JD, et al. Cancer. A bull's eye for targeted lung cancer therapy. Science 2004;304(5676):1458–1461.
53. Zerhouni E. Medicine. The NIH roadmap. Science 2003; 302(5642):63–72.

SECTION THREE

Cancer Prevention and Control

22

Cancer Epidemiology

Melissa L. Bondy and
Shine Chang

With examples from the literature, this chapter clarifies aspects of epidemiology, including study designs and prevention or correction of potential biases. This chapter provides insight to clinicians and other health professionals on cancer epidemiology and helps them communicate and interpret research findings to patients. In addition, the chapter reviews the epidemiologic literature, discussing examples and the magnitude of cancer-related risk factors.

Central Concepts of Cancer Epidemiology

Cancer epidemiology is the comparative study of the *distribution* and *determinants* of health-related conditions, especially disease, within defined human populations. *Distribution* of disease means identification, description, and interpretation of patterns of cancer occurrence; determinants are causative or contributing factors to that occurrence, or to the prevention, control, and outcome of cancer.[1,2] Historically, epidemiology strove to identify and control sources of infectious diseases, but now, especially in industrialized countries, it focuses on chronic diseases such as cancer. Its studies of smoking and lung cancer in the 1950s developed strategies and statistical methods of current cancer research. More recently, the Human Genome Project included studies classified as "molecular epidemiology" that make use of molecular genetic markers, now of interest in cancer and other epidemiologic studies.

Although research capabilities grow and change, cancer epidemiology relies on the historical principles of the general discipline. Epidemiology incorporates research from biologic, clinical, social, and statistical sciences to explore the patterns and causes of disease within a defined population to show influences from patterned, and measurable (i.e., nonrandom), factors. Many (not single) endogenous and exogenous factors cause disease. Analytical epidemiology concentrates on identifying and measuring the relative contribution and interaction of these factors.

Surveillance and Descriptive Studies in Cancer Epidemiology

Public health surveillance, a major aspect of epidemiology, requires systematic gathering and analysis of data related to health outcomes. This gathering and analysis, crucial to public health efforts, is enabled by surveillance systems such as the Surveillance, Epidemiology, and End Results (SEER) Program established by the National Cancer Institute in 1973. The SEER program includes 14 population-based cancer registries invaluable to epidemiologists (http://www-seer.ims.nci.nih.gov).[3]

SEER collects cancer information on about 26% of the U.S. population and, offering more data than other surveillance projects, now serves as the primary source of insight into U.S. cancer incidence and trends. SEER verifies and describes virtually every new case of cancer in its reporting area, and thus its population-based data span the disease spectrum and are more representative of cancer trends in the United States than reports from individual hospitals. These reports are limited by referral patterns, specialized patient populations, and small case sizes and do not permit accurate analysis of trends and incidence patterns. For epidemiologists, SEER, and SEER-type registries, indispensably delineate case-originating populations for calculating reliable incidence rates.[4]

Public health and epidemiologic research also gain from the efforts of other agencies. Annually, the American Cancer Society publishes *Cancer Statistics*, available on its Website (http://www.cancer.org/). It estimates the U.S. rates of cancer occurrence, the numbers of deaths, newly diagnosed cases, and survival rates, and describes behaviors affecting risk of cancer and use of screening tests. A resource available for international cancer incidence, prevalence, mortality, and survival data is the International Agency for Research on Cancer (IARC) at http://www-dep.iarc.fr/.[5] Several IARC-designed software packages permit online calculation of cancer trends by geographic location, age, and gender. IARC also has on its Website the Automated Childhood Cancer Information Systems, a database of childhood cancer in Europe.

Analytical Study Designs

Some epidemiologic studies, such as randomized intervention trials and randomized controlled clinical trials, follow the principles of scientific experimentation in which a treatment or intervention of interest and the control condition are randomly assigned.[2] Although such studies attempt to minimize systematic or methodological errors through randomization, other well-designed and well-conducted nonexperimental (observational) studies also can provide accurate estimates of treatment effects.[5–8]

Nonexperimental analytical studies assess the causal influence of potential risk factors, which, because of ethical or practical issues, cannot be evaluated experimentally. Observation of *naturally* occurring exposures identifies risk factors and their weight in disease incidence. A subtle point is that such exposures must show a difference between healthy and diseased participant groups of such quantity to make comparison possible and useful. Exploring them, epidemiologists often employ cohort and case-control studies.

Cohort studies: Cohort studies evaluate participants initially free of a specific disease of interest whose exposure status can be quantified. Subjects are followed for a defined time period to ascertain endpoints, such as new events in, or death from, disease. The disease rate in the exposed group is then compared statistically to the rate in an unexposed group to generate a relative rate ratio or relative risk that indicates the increase or reduction in risk associated with the exposure of interest. A prospective cohort study resembles a clinical trial in which subjects are not randomly allocated to an exposure arm. Rather, as already mentioned, exposure (or lack of exposure) occurs "naturally" and the investigator uses variations in the levels of exposure to evaluate differences in the risk of disease during some follow-up period.

An example of a notable cohort, the Nurses' Health Study, began in 1976 to track 120,000 U.S. registered nurses. The initial goal of the cohort was to evaluate the effect of oral contraceptives and risk of breast cancer,[9] but data from the Nurses' Health Study have also provided insights into health outcomes such as heart disease and other types of cancer and important clues about estrogens and the etiology of breast cancer. Because they trace subjects over time, cohorts permit efficient study of relatively common diseases with a reasonably long latency period from exposure to disease onset. They may be impractical for the study of rare cancers because, in studies of rare cancers, statistically meaningful results can be achieved only by assembling and long-term following of higher than average risk individuals, whereas cohorts used in studies include people of average risk and experience. Cohort studies may be forward looking or *prospective*, as in clinical trials following up subjects in real time, or historical or *retrospective*, using records to identify the study population and then reconstructing their exposure and subsequent disease experience.

Case-control studies: To evaluate potential causal associations of rare cancers, *case-control studies* are more efficient than cohort studies. They identify and recruit individuals diagnosed with cancer from a defined population, location, and time period. These subjects are compared to a group with identical characteristics as the case but without the disease. The investigators employ comprehensive and carefully analyzed self-reports, health records, and biologic specimens to reconstruct the cases' prediagnosis exposure experience. They assign a "reference" date substituting for a diagnosis date to each control, whose exposure experience before that date is reconstructed. The exposure frequency of the case group is then compared statistically to the exposure frequency among the control group. The resultant statistic, known as an odds ratio (OR), is analogous to a relative risk and serves as a measure of the strength of the association between the exposure and the disease.[10]

Cluster investigations: Clinicians often encounter concern in their communities about multiple cancer occurrences (i.e., a cancer cluster) that are feared to have resulted from a shared environmental exposure. Cluster investigations use standard epidemiologic study designs, primarily case-control studies, to ascertain the existence of area-specific excess of cancer cases (i.e., spatial cluster) or in a limited time period (i.e., temporal cluster) or both (space-time cluster).[11–13] Public health agencies must investigate cancer clusters and communicate findings to the public,[10] and in the United States, clinicians should refer cluster inquiries to local health departments or the U.S. Centers for Disease Control and Prevention (http://www.cdc.gov or http://www.atsdr.cdc.gov). Such investigations, however, seldom verify cancer clusters.[10]

Statistical Measures in Epidemiology

Epidemiologic analyses generally focus on the strength or magnitude of an exposure–disease association, rather than on statistical hypothesis testing using a *P* value.[2] *P* values provide a measure of probability for observing the study results, or results more extreme than those observed, if indeed no true association exists. *P* values provide limited information on the strength, direction, or precision of an effect measure or on the extent to which confounding or other bias explains an association (or lack of an association) between exposure and disease.

One of several measures of *relative risk* is often used to estimate either/or, or dichotomous, outcomes, such as disease occurrence versus no disease.[2] In a cohort study, where disease rates can be calculated directly, the ratio of incidence of those exposed to an agent can be compared with the rate of those unexposed. If the rates are the same in the two groups, the ratio is 1:1, or the relative risk is 1.0, indicating no association between exposure and disease. A ratio larger than 1, for example, 2:1, shows the exposed group has a higher rate of disease than the unexposed group. If the rate is lower in the exposed than the unexposed group, the ratio will be less than 1, suggesting exposure provides protection.

The further the effect measure is away from the "null" value of 1.0 in either direction, the stronger the association. Notice that a relative risk of 2.0 (2-fold-increased risk compared with the reference group) is equivalent in strength to a relative risk of 0.5 (half the risk of the reference group). In case-control studies, in which rates of disease are not calculated directly, the *odds ratio* used is an effect measure on a ratio scale and, as mentioned previously, is functionally equivalent to a relative risk. Other types of ratio-based relative risks are rate ratios, hazard ratios, standardized mortality ratios (SMR), standardized incidence ratios (SIR), and proportional mortality ratios.

Confidence intervals measure the precision of an effect measure, such as relative risk and odds ratios. As with *P* values, confidence intervals are functions of the variability of the data and the sample size. For example, a confidence interval provides a likely range in which the true effect measure lies within some level of confidence, often calculated as 95% confidence intervals.

Relative risks are important to help judge whether an association is causal and to estimate the degree that exposures increase or decrease risk. Relative risks, however, are comparative measures, not "absolute" measures of risk from exposure.

Attributable risk measures (expressed as a number or percentage) provide estimates of the actual rate of cases "due to" exposure, assuming there is a causal relationship.[10] Attributable risks indicate the proportion of the disease possibly preventable if an exposure were removed from a specified population at risk. Estimating attributable risk for specific exposures helps understand the importance of some exposure in a larger public health context.

Bias and Its Control in Epidemiologic Studies

To varying degrees, all human studies are susceptible to bias, that is, inaccurate measures of the effect of a treatment or exposure on disease. An important goal of any study is to make every effort feasible to minimize the effect of bias.

Three general types of bias can occur: (1) *confounding bias*, when an extraneous factor distorts (increases or decreases) the true magnitude of the exposure–disease association; (2) *information (misclassification) bias*, when information collected on exposure, treatment, disease, or other study factors is inaccurate or incomplete; (3) *selection bias*, when subjects who are sampled, recruited, enrolled, and complete the study are unrepresentative of the population at risk, and inaccurately reflect the exposure–disease relationship in the target population or population at risk.

Confounding: In clinical trials, investigators use randomization to reduce the probability that an extraneous factor will cause bias in the results because "nuisance" factors should be randomly and evenly distributed among treatment groups. In the absence of randomization, however, confounding particularly threatens the validity of results derived from observational studies. For a factor to exert a confounding influence requires that factor to be associated with, or a marker for, the disease of interest and for it to occur at a differing frequency between the exposure (or treatment) groups. When these two conditions hold, the extraneous factor (i.e., the confounder) may bias the exposure–disease association.

Statistical methods to correct (i.e., control or adjust for) confounding, such as pooled stratified analysis or multivariate regression analysis, are available but are effective only if data on the potentially confounding variables are collected and accurate. Thus, observational studies often collect data on many factors for statistical analysis that are not directly related to the cause–effect relationship being investigated. Design strategies can also minimize or eliminate confounding. For example, a study of asbestos exposure and lung cancer could avoid confounding from smoking status by recruiting only nonsmokers. In many instances, confounders are adjusted to correct for residual error based on reports from other investigations that have demonstrated notable associations between the confounder and the outcome. Such an approach may guard against potential error from that confounder but, in cases of limited sample size, overadjusting, or adjusting for too many confounders, can also introduce error as well. In such circumstances, a more conservative approach to the statistical analysis of data may be preferred.

Information bias: The major concern for the validity of epidemiologic research of cancer is inaccurate or incomplete information on study participants' exposure relevant to etiology. It is usually impossible, especially in retrospective studies, to measure exposure dose and duration during a time thought to be biologically relevant to cancer initiation. In lieu of direct measures, indirect or surrogate measures of exposure are used. For instance, a proxy for blood levels of cotinine, a biomarker of tobacco use, could be self-reported recall of smoking behavior. Such proxy measures may be useful to approximate real exposure, but they provide only imprecise information on dose, duration, and exposure time. When exposure measures are equally inaccurate between study groups (i.e., nondifferential error), the cause–effect relationship may be attenuated or completely obscured. Nondifferential misclassification of exposure has no doubt been one reason why few environmental agents have been firmly established as known risk factors for cancer.

Differential information bias occurs when comparison groups show differences in the accuracy and completeness of exposure information. Recall bias in case-control studies, for example, can occur when cases are more likely to remember exposures differently from controls. Cases may be more likely to remember relatives having a disease of interest compared with controls, leading to a biased estimate of the effect of the family history. However, some investigators suggest that recall bias may be more theoretical than factual.[2]

Selection bias: Because human studies include investigation of samples of people from larger populations of interest (i.e., target populations), they potentially include sample selection bias. This problem occurs when exposure or disease frequency in the sample, the study participants, is unrepresentative of that experienced by the target population. Case-control studies are vulnerable to this bias because it is difficult to identify and recruit healthy controls who accurately reflect the baseline exposure in the population that gave rise to the cases. Cohort studies and randomized trials, on the other hand, are susceptible to selection bias from attrition. If participants who are lost during the follow-up period have a different outcome experience from those who remain in the study, final results may also be biased. For this reason, great effort must be expended in prospective studies to ensure the most complete follow-up possible of study participants.

Determining Causality

Epidemiologic studies strive to provide accurate and precise risk estimates of an exposure–disease association. Widely applied concepts originally derived from two papers by Sir Austin Bradford Hill, describing the philosophy and epidemiologic reasoning in causal inference,[2] include the following criteria to evaluate study results and guide judgments on the likelihood that an association is indeed causal and not merely a random or chance finding.

1. *Strength of the exposure–disease association.* Although their existence does not preclude other sources of error, large relative risks are less likely than small relative risks to result from chance or uncontrolled confounding.
2. *Temporal relationship between exposure and disease onset.* Studies gain strength if they can establish that an exposure preceded onset of disease.
3. *Biologic coherence.* When a plausible biologic mechanism and/or when experimental evidence from animal studies supports the hypothesized relation, more confidence may be placed in the observed relationship.
4. *Dose–response gradient.* If exposure intensity or duration is associated with increased disease frequency, the results appear coherent and believable.
5. *Consistency of results within and across studies.* If multiple reports evaluating the same type of exposure show

similar effects, and/or if multiple studies using different target populations and study designs report consistent results, there is greater evidence to favor a true relationship.

Molecular Epidemiology

Classic or traditional epidemiology, as discussed previously, permits epidemiologists to evaluate risks and environmental causality in cancer. Molecular epidemiology, a hybrid of epidemiology and molecular genetics, enables researchers to assess biologic characteristics influencing cancer susceptibility. The combination of epidemiologic approaches and bench science has effectively "broken open the black box of epidemiology," a discipline historically left to speculate as to the biologic mechanisms underlying its detected exposure–disease associations.[14,15] The concept that risk of cancer from a given exposure differs between subgroups of a population is an example of what is known in the epidemiologic vernacular as *effect modification*. Biostatisticians often refer to this heterogeneity of effect as *interaction*. With the advent of polymerase chain reactions and other advanced laboratory methods, epidemiologists incorporating molecular markers into their studies can begin to identify specific suspect endogenous or exogenous host factors at the biochemical or molecular level that put individuals at considerably higher (or lower) cancer risk.[16]

Molecular epidemiologic studies aim to determine the roles, including interactions, of environmental and genetic factors in the initiation and progression of cancer. Incorporating genetic markers in epidemiologic studies of cancer etiology shows promise for revealing details of carcinogenic pathways that can provide strategies for prevention and, ultimately, reduce cancer risk. Although the promise for critical advances in understanding cancer is great, molecular epidemiology faces important challenges, such as ensuring the appropriate interpretation of molecular testing and resolving associated ethical, legal, and social concerns.

The use of molecular epidemiology to identify biomarkers also may provide useful information on the extent of exposure to carcinogens and cancer risk. Perera and Weinstein[15] delineated four characteristics important for biomarkers to predict risk: internal dose, biologically effective dose, response, and susceptibility. Describing and determining the occurrence of such suitably selected biomarkers has already advanced research on the mechanisms of cancer initiation and promotion and enabled improved assessment of the cancer risk of healthy individuals. Moreover, the knowledge that gene mutations and changes in their expression underlie carcinogenesis has spurred the hunt for aberrant genes and their associated proteins.

Molecular parameters added to population-based studies should help to identify genes, proteins, and pathways involved in cancer development caused by environmental exposures and susceptible or resistant subpopulations. The exponential growth of scientific technology and information promises rapid expansion of knowledge about the identity of potentially mutant genes and cancer pathways.

As a hypothetical framework for dissecting the development of cancer in individuals, current studies of molecular epidemiology consider both the complex, multistage process of carcinogenesis and heterogeneous responses to carcinogenic exposures. Improving continuously, measurements of human exposure to carcinogens have been successfully applied in a number of molecular epidemiologic studies. Inherited and acquired genetic predispositions to cancer have been, and continue to be, identified. Correlating inherited genetic polymorphisms with other cancer risk factors shows considerable promise that molecular epidemiologists will gain in their ability to assess multiple biomarkers and to predict an individual's risk for specific diseases. The field has the near-term potential to impact regulatory quantitative risk assessments, useful in the determination of allowable exposures, and molecular epidemiologic data may also help identify individuals most apt to benefit from cancer prevention strategies.

Molecular epidemiology investigators employ traditional epidemiologic study designs, including case-control and cohort studies that focus on one or more biologic markers that may show an association between exposure and disease outcome. Molecular studies often raise the "nature versus nurture" question, with evidence supporting consensus that gene–environment interplay explains many chronic diseases, including cancer: "Genetics is the loaded gun, and the environment pulls the trigger." Among studies supporting such a statement is a recent large, although statistically limited, study of twins concluding that environment plays a substantial role but requires genetic potential in causing sporadic cancers.[16]

Molecular epidemiology studies also face the methodological challenges to traditional epidemiologic studies, such as precise measurement of exposure and effects, appropriate selection of study samples, and reduction of the influence of confounders and potential competing risk factors. One important issue is assuring an adequate sample size for study because the prevalence of a specific genetic polymorphism or other biomarker under investigation is often either very rare or quite high, either of which situations require a large number of cases to detect an association.[17] One approach to this problem is to combine data from several studies, particularly of rare cancers, to obtain adequate statistical power for meaningful conclusions. When sample sizes are modest, especially, caution in interpretation of data or linking findings with further implications is in order.

The Global Cancer Burden

Estimates of the global cancer burden have been made for 1975, 1980, 1985, and 2000.[18] These estimates include all forms of cancer except nonmelanoma skin cancer, poorly registered on incidence statistics and infrequently fatal. In 2000, cancer deaths among men totaled 4.7 million, and an estimated 5.3 million new cases were diagnosed, an increase of 1.5 million from 1985, lung cancer being the most common form of cancer in men, with an estimated 902,000 new cases in 2000. The estimated number of lung cancer cases has increased by 35% over the 5-year period covered by these estimates. Other cancers showing notable increases are colorectal, prostate, bladder, melanoma, and lymphoma, particularly non-Hodgkin's lymphoma. Some increases may be due to better surveillance or impaired precision in the estimation of rates but likely have a real etiologic component.

In 2000, it was estimated that 4.7 million new cases of cancer occurred in women, an increase of almost 1 million new cases over the previous 5 years. Breast cancer, the most common form of female cancer, has shown an increase of 94% in the past 25 years, nearly doubling, with an estimated 1 million new cases in 2000. A similar increase has taken place in oral cavity and colorectal cancers and in lymphoma. The largest relative increase of cancer in women has been in lung cancer, up from 126,700 new cases in 1975 to 337,000 in 2000, an increase of 26%, almost entirely explainable by women's increase in smoking.[19]

The number of new cases of cancer worldwide apparently doubled between 1970 and 2000 and should show even further rates of increase. The estimated number of new cases of cancer was 5.9 million in 1975, 6.4 million in 1980, and 7.6 million in 1985. If age-specific rates remain constant at the 1985 levels, 8.4 million new cases would occur in 1990 and 10.3 million new cases in the year 2000. Beyond 2000, the absolute number of cancer cases should continue to rise as the post-World War II generation crosses the age–risk threshold. In many countries, this generation is the first whose numbers were not reduced by a great war and the first to have benefited from the advances in medical care and treatment witnessed in the second half of this century. In contrast to earlier populations, most members of this generation are still alive at ages where cancer risk rises.

Geographic and Temporal Variation in Cancer Risk

The notable international variation of cancer rates and types has led to the growing interest in geographic pathology or cancer mapping as a tool in cancer epidemiology. These descriptive studies offering data on disease in varied groups in multiple locations are important for generating hypotheses in epidemiology, as in-migrant or ecologic studies evaluate exposure and disease on a population rather than individual level. For example, one can look at general exposures, such as smoking, sunlight, or dietary fat intake, and plot them against the incidence of the disease. If one plots dietary fat consumption by country with the incidence of breast cancer, for example, one finds greater rates of breast cancer in countries with high dietary fat intake. Because the dietary intake for a country reflects intake of its people en masse and is not directly measured and linked to each individual cancer patient's intake, this association might be false. However, such associations can help investigators identify new avenues for further investigations.

Cancer mapping produces other data useful for hypothesis-generating studies. Geographic variation can be seen from cancer mortality or incidence maps using computer-generated mapping programs for areas as small as a county and used to uncover spatial clusters or geographic variation of common tumor types. The National Cancer Institute (NCI) has published an atlas of cancer mortality maps at the county and state level, available for viewing on the NCI Website (http://www-seer.ims.nci.nih.gov). These maps revealed high rates of oral cancer among rural Southern women and prompted investigators to conduct case-control studies into a long-standing practice of snuff dipping among the cases, leading to implementation of smokeless tobacco prevention programs.

Cancer Risk Factors

Epidemiology shows that, because different world populations show different types of levels of disease, much human cancer may be avoidable. For example, immigrants take on the cancer pattern of their new home, as immigrants to Australia have within decades, or Japanese immigrants experience higher breast cancer rates after a few decades in the United States than in comparative populations in Japan. Further, groups with unique and differentiating cultural or lifestyle characteristics such as Seventh Day Adventists, Mormons, or African-Americans in parts of the United States have cancer patterns distinct from those of the general community. Comparisons support the generally agreed-upon estimate that upward of 80% to 90% of cancer may be attributable to environmental factors such as dietary, social, and cultural practices.[19]

However, such factors have not been clearly delineated, nor has it been made clear how individuals are affected by combination or accretion of factors. Cancer prevention efforts have focused on efforts to reduce exposures or behaviors suspect in incidence, such as smoking, and to promote those with protective effects, such as physical exercise, and, as well, to reduce concerns over exposures or acts that may have trivial or no impact on cancer, such as cell phone use. Cancer control studies thus embrace a variety of elements and approaches and aim to reduce the incidence of cancer, and failing which, to reduce mortality, either by finding disease at an early and curable stage or by improving survival rates stage-for-stage by therapeutic improvements. Cancer prevention, control, and education programs bring epidemiologists into contact and cooperation with several other disciplines including clinical science, behavioral science, and health education and communication.

Tobacco

Tobacco smoking, the single most lethal human carcinogen, remains the largest single avoidable cause of premature death worldwide.[20] Estimates connect at least 16% of all cancers in developed countries to tobacco use, with a higher proportion of tobacco-related cancers among men (25%) than women (4%). Tobacco-related cancers include those of the oral cavity, pharynx, larynx, lung, bladder, pancreas, kidney, renal pelvis, and endometrium. However, in the last case, reduced rather than increased risk is thought to result from antiestrogenic effects of tobacco use rather than exposure to the more than 55 carcinogenic compounds identified by the International Agency for Research on Cancer.[21] For more than 40 years, it has been clear that prevention of smoking would lead to substantial reductions in death associated with lung and other cancers and heart disease, bronchitis, emphysema, and other conditions. Nonetheless, tobacco-related disease has increased in many parts of the world, especially in developing countries where tobacco use has started within the past 30 years and involves 80% of the world's daily smokers, now estimated at 1.1 billion.

Tobacco addiction mechanisms are complex. As suggested by reports of associations between smoking quit-rates and specific polymorphisms in the dopamine receptor gene (DRD2),[22] a key receptor in the mesolimbic dopaminergic reward system, the genetic susceptibility of individuals to tobacco addiction varies considerably. Just as multiple factors affect behavior, multiple factors likely influence susceptibility to tobacco-related cancers, which helps explain why not all tobacco users get cancer.

Important smoking outcomes appear to be related to gender, ethnicity, and life experiences. Women, relative to men, and African-Americans, compared to white Americans, appear to have higher risk of bladder cancer associated with tobacco use. Age is also an important factor because smokers usually begin during their teens or early adult years. Early-start smokers persist and smoke higher amounts than late starters, increasing their risks over time. Synergistic effects with tobacco use have been observed with asbestos and crystalline silica in occupational settings, and with alcohol acting as a solvent, probably facilitating absorption of smoking by-products, whereas a diet high in intake of fruits and vegetables may impede the formation of smoking-related DNA adducts, reduce the DNA damage from tobacco carcinogens, and promote other mechanisms that prevent cellular damage and reduce risk.

Recent tobacco research includes the evaluation of exposure to environmental tobacco smoke and outcomes of exposure-related adverse health events, including lung cancer. Based on 30 epidemiologic studies, the United States Environmental Protection Agency (EPA) concluded that environmental tobacco smoke was a human lung carcinogen and that nonsmokers who are exposed to environmental tobacco smoke faced increased risk of lung cancer.[23] Although diluted with ambient air, environmental tobacco smoke tends to have more carcinogens than smoke inhaled through filters. However, the current emphasis of research and health policy in Western countries on passive smoke inhalation should not divert attention from the major public health issue of active cigarette smoking: smokers are at much higher risk of cancer than others involuntarily inhaling cigarette smoke. Therefore, any program of cancer control should put control of smoking first; such control is likely to have greater impact on reducing cancer incidence and cancer mortality than any other current strategy.

Viruses and Infection

The contribution of viruses to the public health burden of cancer incidence is greatest in young to middle-aged individuals, the age–incidence curve peaking before middle age.[24] The estimated attributable risk associated with viruses and cancer is about 15% worldwide.[25] However, to date, only five viruses have been firmly established associated with increased cancer risk: human papilloma virus (HPV), with an increased risk of cervix cancer in women; Epstein–Barr virus (EBV) with an increased risk of nasopharyngeal cancer and Burkitt's and Hodgkin's lymphoma; human T-lymphotropic virus type 1 (HTLV-1), with adult T-cell leukemia and some types of non-Hodgkin's lymphoma; hepatitis B and C with an increased risk of primary liver cancer; and human herpesvirus 8 (HHV-8) infection with Kaposi's sarcoma and some forms of non-Hodgkin's lymphoma (Table 22.1).[24] Advances in technology and laboratory techniques, such as polymerase chain reaction (PCR) have facilitated research, but because the mechanisms by which viruses cause cancer may leave little evidence of infection and because some viruses can remain latent for many years, definitive implication of specific viruses in carcinogenesis has been difficult.

Long latency periods between infection and cancer diagnosis, and the fact that only a portion of people who are infected develop cancer, suggest that although viral agents may increase the risk of individuals for developing cancer they are not the sole determinant for developing the disease.

TABLE 22.1. Known viral risk factors for selected human cancers.

Viral risk factor	*Cancer type*	*Other factors that influence risk*
Epstein–Barr virus (EBV)	Burkitt's lymphoma Nasopharyngeal carcinoma B-cell lymphoma Hodgkin's disease Breast cancer[a]	Malaria Nitrosamines Immunodeficiency, human immunodeficiency virus (HIV)-1
Hepatitis B virus (HBV)	Liver cancer	Aflatoxin, alcohol
Hepatitis C virus (HCV)	Liver cancer Splenic lymphoma	Aflatoxin, alcohol
Human herpesvirus-8 (HHV-8)	Kaposi's sarcoma Primary effusion lymphoma Multicentric Castleman disease	HIV-1 EBV, HIV-1 HIV-1
Human papillomavirus (HPV)	Cancer of the cervix, vulva, vagina, penis, anus, skin, and oropharyngeal region	Smoking, oral contraceptive use, multiparity, other sexually transmitted diseases
Human T-cell lymphotrophic virus type 1 (HTLV-1)	Adult T-cell leukemia/lymphoma (ATL)	
Simian virus 40 (SV40)	Mesothelioma Non-Hodgkin's lymphoma, brain and bone tumors, B-cell lymphomas[a]	Asbestos
Helicobactor pylori[b]	Gastric cancer	Smoking, chronic inflammation, poor diet

[a] Unconfirmed, but suspected.

[b] Bacterial risk factor.

However, great geographic variation in rates of infection and virally related cancer worldwide suggests that much infection-related cancer could be prevented by control of viral infection. This is no trivial matter, because viral infection rates are high in many parts of the world and the types of cancers associated with them often have poor prognoses and few successful treatment options. Obviously, effective vaccination programs against these viral infections would considerably reduce the burden of these forms of cancer and the global problem.

Bacterial infection has also been linked to cancer risk in the example of *Helicobacter pylori (H. pylori)* infection and increased risk of gastric cancer, the second leading cause of cancer mortality in the world.[24,25] Incidence rates of gastric cancer vary geographically, particularly for the intestinal type, which is typically accompanied by chronic atrophic gastritis and intestinal metaplasia. Both chronic atrophic gastritis and intestinal metaplasia, possible precursors to gastric cancer, are thought to result from *H. pylori* infection, suggesting an important role for *H. pylori* infection in gastric carcinogenesis.[26] Other evidence comes from epidemiologic investigations linking areas with high rates of *H. pylori* infection to regions with high rates of gastric cancer, although the consistency of such findings is hampered by multiple bacterial strains that vary in virulence and promotion of conditions that enhance carcinogenesis, such as chronic inflammation and decreased stomach acid secretion.[27–29] Risk factors for *H. pylori* infection are associated more with socioeconomic factors, such as overcrowding, family size, and bed-sharing rather than lifestyle behaviors, such as tobacco use, or diet. Despite the apparent complexity of the relationship between *H. pylori* infection and gastric cancer, increasing evidence supports efforts to control and reduce *H. pylori* infection as a means to reduce cancer risk, particularly among children, for whom infection rates are high and reach nearly 100% by adulthood in areas of high infection rates.

Sunlight Exposure

Exposure to sunlight has been well established as the major agent in the development of skin cancer, particularly solar ultraviolet (UV) A and B wavelengths. Exposure to UVA can result in DNA base damage, strand breaks, and DNA–protein cross-links, whereas exposure of DNA to UVB mainly results in dimerizations between adjacent pyrimidines, which may predispose for *p53* mutation hotspots.[30] Knowledge of the underlying molecular mechanisms for sunlight's role in skin carcinogenesis contributes to efforts in prevention and control in human populations, but for successful public health interventions, other information is necessary.

The rapid rise in the worldwide incidence of skin cancer in the past decade is hypothesized to result in part from the migration of Caucasian populations to areas for which their skin is not well adapted. This hypothesis is supported by reports linking skin cancer incidence with solar radiation at different geographic latitudes.[31] Locales with greater annual sun exposure tend to have higher incidence of skin cancer, but many other factors also contribute to skin cancer risk, such as age at exposure, ethnicity, skin color, lifestyle, occupation, and individual genetic susceptibility.

Important differences between the subtypes of skin cancer suggest differences in carcinogenic pathways. Squamous cell cancer (SCC) develops from stem cells in the follicular and interfollicular region of the dermis; basal cell carcinoma (BCC) arises from basal cells in the skin and follicular infundibulum; and melanoma develops mainly from melanocytic nevi. Most lesions develop on the face in BCC, the most common form of human skin cancer worldwide, but nearly a third of BCC lesions occur on skin typically protected from the sun. It rarely appears on sun-exposed sites such as the forearms and the backs of hands, as SCC does. Some research suggests childhood or adolescent exposure during childhood and adolescence, both intermittent sun exposure and severe sunburns, predisposes for adult BCC and melanoma and associates adult sunlight exposure with SCC risk.[32]

During the past 30 years melanoma incidence, particularly for lesions appearing on women's legs and men's torsos, where sunlight exposure tends to be intermittent, has increased worldwide. Melanoma is the rarest type of skin cancer, but its mortality rates can be high without early detection and treatment. Such efforts can be directed toward groups at high risk, such as those with pale skin, or red or blond hair, who freckle easily, particularly those with higher numbers of nevi from sun exposure during childhood.

Two major hypotheses have emerged to explain variation in skin cancer incidence related to sun exposure: first, that the pattern of exposure (i.e., intermittent or steady) and total accumulated exposure contribute to risk independently; and second, that exposure before age 10 strongly determines lifetime risk, although sun exposure in adulthood may influence the manifestation of outright cancer. Major support for the importance of childhood sun exposure comes from Australian studies, where early age at immigration predicts increased risk of skin cancer.[33] Intermittent sun exposure with sunburn in childhood has been associated with later increased BCC risk, and other research suggests that adult exposures may promote skin carcinogenesis through response to short-term exposure to sunlight.

The main factor responsible for the dramatic increases in skin cancer rates is generally held to be the increased levels of recreational sun exposure (as during sunbathing sessions or outdoor recreational activities), a result of the economic improvement of many white communities. Since 1980, the sun tanning fashion has fostered marketing of sunbeds and their use,[32] as in Sweden where nearly half of women 15 to 35 years old reported regular sunbed exposure.[34] This habit is suspected to increase the risk of skin cancers, but further studies are needed to correctly assess the magnitude of risk associated with the so-called "UVA sun tanning."[34] The important message is to avoid overexposure to sunlight and, in particular, to avoid sunburns at all times and to be particularly careful to protect children.[35] Australia and New Zealand, where sun exposure can be intense and of high annual duration, have effectively mounted solar protection campaigns that suggest the possibility of achieving population-wide success in skin cancer prevention and control.

Diet

Diet and nutritional factors became the focus of serious attention in the etiology of cancer after the 1940s.[36] Initially dealing with the effect of feeding specific diets to animals receiving chemical carcinogens, research turned to the potential of associations with human cancer risk. Estimated national per capita food intake data and cancer mortality rates were compared, and data established risk with diet, particularly associating higher dietary fat intake and increased rates of breast cancer. Improved dietary assessment methods and the identification and correction of certain methodological difficulties gave rise to the science of nutritional epidemiology.[37]

As the complexity of the association with cancer for fats and fatty acids has unfolded, research interest has broadened to include other foods and food compounds. In general, high consumption of fruits and vegetables is associated with a reduced risk of a number of forms of cancer including lung, oral, pancreatic, laryngeal, esophageal, bladder, and gastric cancer, with three major exceptions being the lack of strong association with hormonally related cancers, such as those of the prostate, breast, ovary, and endometrium.[38]

Investigation into reduced risk associated with consumption of dark green, leafy vegetables and red and yellow fruits and vegetables with high levels of micronutrients thought to have antioxidant and other anticarcinogenic properties, have identified components of interest. Compounds, such as phytoestrogens in soybean products and lycopene and other carotenoids in high concentrations in tomatoes and other fruits and vegetables, have been the subject of recent studies developing interest in testing these food compounds as chemopreventive agents in prevention trials.[38] Investigators are showing interest not only in the micronutrient compounds but also in how foods may be metabolized (e.g., glycemic index) and prepared (e.g., grilled meats have become suspect). Interest in the potential for diet and nutrition to help determine cancer risk is flourishing.

Alcohol Consumption

The strongest evidence of a causal role for alcohol consumption in carcinogenesis comes from investigations of cancers of the oral cavity, pharynx, larynx, and esophagus.[39] To assess alcohol's effect independently from the strong confounding effect of tobacco use, another important risk factor for these cancers, studies have evaluated risk associated with alcohol consumption among groups of nonsmokers, although carefully conducted studies among smokers suggest a synergistic effect for alcohol consumption linked to tobacco use.[40] Another confounding factor associated with alcohol consumption is poor diet, particularly low fruit and vegetable consumption. Modification of alcohol's effect on cancer risk suggests the importance of antioxidant or other anticancer components of fruits and vegetables, such as vitamin A, depleted from liver stores by alcohol.

For risk of liver cancer, evidence suggests a modest effect of alcohol, but risk appears to be synergistically enhanced by viral hepatitis infection. The literature is unclear about whether alcohol-induced liver cirrhosis increases risk of liver cancer because not all alcoholics with liver cancer have cirrhosis. Epidemiologic studies that rely on self-reports may include underreporting of intake by alcoholics and neglect physiologic differences between alcoholics and others consuming alcohol, but it is plausible that heavy, but not moderate, drinkers may consume quantities of alcohol necessary to demonstrate an association with liver cancer.

A number of investigations suggest a role for alcohol in the development of pancreatic and colon cancers, as well as hormonally responsive cancers of the breast and prostate for which the mechanistic pathways may differ from those of cancers of the oral cavity, pharynx, larynx, and esophagus.[41–43] Both acute and chronic intake have been shown to increase circulating estrogens and to decrease circulating androgens in both men and women, consistent with the increased breast cancer risk observed for higher consumption of alcohol.[43] However, only heavy alcohol intake, not moderate consumption, has been associated with increased prostate cancer risk, suggesting an alternative pathway rather than the putative increased androgen exposure mechanism.

The influence of the type of alcohol and its metabolites remains of interest but unclear. Mouthwash with more than 25% alcohol has been associated with higher risk of mouth cancer, and studies for some cancers suggest that distilled liquors have more potent effects than other types of alcohol. Other studies suggest some compounds in alcoholic beverages heighten or lessen carcinogenic effects. Ethyl carbamate and acetaldehyde, by-products of alcohol metabolism, are both animal carcinogens; conversely, resveratrol, a compound in wines, beer, and grape skins, has received much recent attention for several of its anticarcinogenic properties.[43] Although high consumption of alcohol is clearly not recommended in regard to cancer risk, it remains unresolved whether consumption that is more moderate increases risk sufficiently to cause concern.

Obesity

Large-scale prospective studies assessing the long-term effects of obesity have shown that obesity increases cancer risk. The American Cancer Society Study described the pattern of mortality related to relative body size for 900,000 subjects followed for 16 years.[44] Obese women had an increased risk of cancer of the endometrium, cervix, ovary, and breast; obese men had an increased risk of stomach and prostate cancer; and both obese women and men had increased risk of esophageal, colorectal, liver, gallbladder, pancreatic, and kidney cancer, as well as non-Hodgkin's lymphoma and multiple myeloma. The Danish Record-linkage Study comparison of a cohort of nearly 44,000 obese persons with the whole Danish population found the obese had an increased incidence of cancers of the esophagus, liver, pancreas, colon, prostate, and kidney.[45] More recent studies indicate in women a clear relationship between obesity and increased risk of endometrium, renal cell, gallbladder, and colorectal cancer, and among men, greater risk of colon cancer, renal cell cancer, gallbladder cancer, and esophageal and gastric cardia adenocarcinoma. Lung cancer is the one neoplasm that the obese may be less prone to develop than leaner individuals, possibly because of smoking-related effects on resting energy expenditure, although some have argued that residual confounding by smoking or weight loss due to presymptomatic disease may bias findings.

The relationship between breast cancer and obesity is less clear. Among postmenopausal women, the obese have a greater risk of breast cancer than their leaner counterparts, whereas among premenopausal women, the obese appear to experience modest protection from breast cancer compared to leaner women.[46] For postmenopausal women, the effect of obesity and breast cancer risk appears to be greater in those who have never used hormone replacement therapy, supporting the hypothesis that in the absence of ovarian sources of estrogens, increased risk is derived from excess estrogen converted from adrenal hormones in the fat tissue of heavier women.

For prostate cancer, no strong relationship for either risk or mortality has been consistently demonstrated with adult obesity, usually measured as body mass index (BMI) equal to or greater than 30 kg/m^2. BMI, the most widely used measure of body composition in epidemiologic studies, serves as the basis for the NHLBI/NIH and WHO clinical definitions for underweight, normal, overweight, and obesity.[47,48] The components of BMI, height and weight, are easy to recall accurately, easy and inexpensive to measure, and generally recorded in a variety of documents, all considerations for conducting research in large populations. However, using BMI to quantify obesity and body composition has drawbacks because the same BMI result will be found in people with vastly different height and weight, BMI is correlated with both lean mass and fat mass, and it provides no information about the ratio of lean to fat mass or about body fat distribution, which has metabolic implications for steroid hormone balance. Characterizing body composition using only BMI thus may mask associations between carcinogenesis and specific components of obesity.

Other measures of body composition, particularly the ratio of waist and hip circumferences and skin-fold thickness, have also been used in epidemiologic research. Ratio measures must be interpreted carefully within the context of underlying body size distributions of the study sample, whereas assessing body composition using skin-fold thicknesses requires special training for accurate measurement. Recent work identifying hormones, growth factors, and cytokines that are associated with specific components of body composition present new opportunities for better mechanistic investigations. Overall, although the mechanisms underlying the obesity–carcinogenesis relationship are not fully understood, they are likely to be complex, because both obesity and cancer are multifactorial diseases involving many genetic pathways.

Physical Activity

The most consistent evidence supporting a role for physical activity in the prevention of cancer comes from studies of colon cancer. As reviewed by Colditz et al., nine of nine case-control studies and six of seven cohort studies across different populations consistently reported significantly reduced risk of colon cancer as a result of physical activity independent of BMI effects.[49] In general, a dose–response pattern exists for levels of physical activity and colon cancer; increases in intensity, frequency, or duration show an inverse relationship to risk. Hypothesized mechanisms include reduced exposure time in those whose physical activity increases gut motility and reduces the bowel transit time of potential carcinogens. For breast cancer, a protective effect of physical activity in premenopausal and postmenopausal women measured at different intensities and times is indicated by a growing number of studies in the United States and abroad, as reviewed by McTiernan et al.[50] Likewise, but in far fewer studies than for colon or breast cancer, is emerging a pattern of reduced risk of pre- and postmenopausal endometrial cancer associated with physical activity. Other investigations report protective effects associated with physical activity for prostate and testicular cancer, albeit less consistently so than for colon and breast cancer.

The beneficial impact of physical activity on cancer risk may result from its direct influence on biochemical factors important in the carcinogenic pathway, such as growth factors, hormones, and immune function. Physical activity lowers levels of insulin, glucose, and triglycerides, and raises HDL cholesterol, which may protect against proliferation of colon and breast cancer lesions. Exercise appears to increase the number and/or the activity of macrophages, natural killer cells, and their regulating cytokines, although epidemiologic data on immune function are limited. Physical activity may also prevent cancer indirectly by prevention and control of obesity and producing physiologic changes in hormone profiles suspect in tumorigenesis. High levels of exercise delay menarche and reduce the number of ovulatory cycles, thereby reducing lifetime exposure to endogenous estrogen and the risk for estrogen-dependent cancers.[51] Exercise may also reduce the risk of hormone-dependent cancers by increasing the production of sex hormone-binding globulin (SHBG) in men and women, lowering levels of circulating bioavailable testosterone and estradiol.

Epidemiologic research on physical activity has been limited in the past by poor quantification. Recent studies have improved efforts to capture, at a minimum, the intensity level, frequency, and duration of physical activities and to factor in nonrecreational or formal exercise. Increasing data have permitted derivation of standardized expenditure values that may serve as a basis for calculating metabolic—and health—values of specific activities. Other approaches include direct measurement devices or even biologic markers, such as doubly labeled water, to quantify physical activity. Ultimately, because it is a modifiable lifestyle factor, physical activity holds great promise for a large positive impact on public health, in addition to reducing cancer incidence.

Occupational Exposures

Occupational exposures have been estimated to account for approximately 4% of all cancers.[52] Many occupational risk factors for cancer have been identified through epidemiologic research, particularly carcinogenic chemicals commonly used in industry. The International Agency for Research on Cancer furnishes a comprehensive source of occupational exposures associated with cancer in its series of monographs, and the U.S. National Toxicology Program's annual report on carcinogens offers another useful resource. These reports reflect a considerable body of work conducted by scientific researchers in many disciplines including toxicology, carcinogenesis, and epidemiology.

Epidemiologic studies, including retrospective cohort and nested case-control studies, identify increased cancer risk associated with single occupational exposures, particularly when the exposure–disease relationships are clear,[53] as for benzene exposure in rubber hydrochloride workers. Studies of rare histopathologic types of cancer in occupational settings have also revealed occupational carcinogens, as, for example, studies relating exposure to vinyl chloride to angiosarcoma of the liver,[54] a rare (less than 1% of all hepatic cancers) subtype of hepatic cancers. The impact of mixtures suspected to be occupational carcinogens is harder to characterize because their precise makeup may resist description or be unknown and may vary between exposures. Exposure duration may be short and/or transient.[55] These issues impede research on the relationships between cutting and lubricating oils and bladder cancer and between diesel exhaust and lung cancer, the first and second most common occupation-related cancers, respectively. Useful research has resulted from the evaluation of large occupational cohorts, such as farmers, laundry and dry-cleaning workers, and painters. However, cohort studies require long follow-up for development of disease and sufficiently large numbers so that enough numbers of cancers of the same organs can be analyzed.[52,56] Moreover, results from cohort studies may be influenced by secular trends during follow-up, and workers with the same job titles may experience different levels of exposure.

Today, with an improved safety profile in the workforce apparent in many industrialized countries, it is important to ensure that exposure to known carcinogenic hazards in the workplace is not transferred to the preindustrialized countries, whose workers deserve at least the standards of protection achieved in industrialized countries. Specifically, for identified carcinogens, enforced legislation that clearly defined exposure restrictions and dose limits could reduce occupational cancers.

Radiation

Ionizing radiation can damage DNA directly or indirectly by causing the formation of highly reactive free radicals that can damage DNA or induce chromosomal instability in nearby cells not directly damaged by radiation (i.e., the "bystander" effect). Unlike other types of exposures, radiation exposure tends to induce DNA strand breaks that then lead to chromosomal rearrangements, such as translocations, inversions, additions, and deletions. Exposure to ionizing radiation in humans has been consistently associated with leukemia and cancers of the breast, thyroid, and lung.[57] Evidence comes from studies of radiotherapy-treated patients, residents exposed to environmental radon, workers with occupational exposure to radiation, and, for the largest part, survivors of the Japanese atomic bomb (UNSCEAR) and the nuclear accident at Chernobyl in 1986.[58]

Some studies have focused on children, as excess risk of cancer appears inversely related to age at exposure. From long-term studies of the Japanese atomic bomb survivors, a linear dose–response pattern has emerged for exposure to ionizing radiation and risk of solid cancers, and a linear quadratic dose–response relationship has appeared for leukemia except for the highest levels of exposure.[59] However, findings from the atomic bomb survivors are based on a single, acute radiation exposure unreflective of the low-level, chronic, or fractionated exposures occurring more commonly in contemporary occupational and environmental settings, for which epidemiologic data often lack good dosimetry information, or show inadequate ascertainment of cancer outcomes, possible screening biases, short length of follow-up for cancer development, and small sample sizes.[59]

With increasing numbers of cancer patients experiencing longer survival, interest has grown in the possible long-term effects and interplay between radiotherapy and chemotherapy drugs and the effect of radiation exposure in patients with altered immune function. Elevated risk of cancers, such as Hodgkin's lymphoma, leukemia, and cancers of the skin and lung, has been associated in some studies with previous radiotherapy and chemotherapy treatment for cancer. In such reports, the strength of association has been modified by other risk factors, including smoking and Epstein–Barr virus infection.

Hormones

Initially, evidence from many studies seemed to support an increased risk of breast cancer in young women (less than 35 or perhaps less than 45 years of age) associated with current prolonged use (more than 5 years) of oral contraceptives. However, a recent study by Marchbanks et al.[60] of findings of the Women's Contraceptive and Reproductive Experiences (Women's CARE) study found no association between past or present use of oral contraceptives and breast cancer. The findings of this well-conducted, population-based study of 4,575 women with breast cancer and 4,682 controls has enormous importance because more than 75% of the women in the study had used oral contraceptives. Thus, even a small risk associated with such a common exposure could account for a substantial number of new breast cancer cases. The study also reported no difference by dose of estrogen (low or high).

A 1996 meta-analysis of 54 epidemiologic studies of oral contraceptives and risk of breast cancer showed a slightly increased risk of breast cancer to those who took oral contraceptives, compared to nonusers [relative risk (RR), 1.24; 95% confidence interval (CI), 1.15–1.33].[61] The risk diminished steadily after cessation of use, with no excess after 10 years. This meta-analysis had the virtues of large size and inclusion of data from published and unpublished studies conducted around the world, and its finding strongly supports two main conclusions. First, breast cancers diagnosed in women who had used combined oral contraceptives were clinically less advanced than those diagnosed in women who had never used these contraceptives: long-term users, compared to women who never used contraceptives, had lower relative risk for tumors that had spread beyond the breast compared to localized tumors (RR, 0.88; 95% CI, 0.81–0.95). No obvious association appeared in the results for recency of use by women with different background risks of breast cancer, from different countries and ethnic groups, with different reproductive histories, and those with or without a family history of breast cancer.

Other features of hormonal contraceptive use, such as duration of use, age at first use, and the dose and type of the hormone within the contraceptives, had little additional effect on breast cancer risk once recency of use had been taken into account. Further reassuring news is that the relative risks are small and the period at risk appears confined to times of life when the incidence of breast cancer, although not negligible, has not reached the highest levels attained in the latter part of the sixth and seventh decades of life.

In 1995, approximately 38% of postmenopausal women in the United States were using hormone replacement therapy (HRT) consisting of either estrogen or estrogen and progesterone. Although data from both case-control and cohort studies suggested that HRT may increase the risk of breast cancer, similar studies suggested that HRT decreased the risk of cardiac disease among postmenopausal women. The results from these observational studies led to randomized controlled clinical trials evaluating the safety and efficacy of HRT for primary or secondary prevention of cardiac disease, which, so far, it has not been shown to be.

The Women's Health Initiative (WHI) study, a primary prevention trial, has focused on strategies for preventing cardiac disease, breast and colorectal cancer, and osteoporosis in postmenopausal women.[62] The 15-year study had several research arms, including an intervention arm of combined HRT with estrogen and progesterone that found combined HRT increased risk of breast cancer and cardiovascular disease. For other medical problems, such as menopausal symptoms or osteoporosis, it was recommended that its use be minimized and that physicians counsel their patients about the potential benefits and risks of combined HRT. The estrogen-only arm of the WHI study ended, so it is more difficult to make recommendations for these women, but women should be aware that the results from the observational studies have consistently suggested that estrogen alone may also be a risk factor for breast cancer, especially after use for more than 5 years.

Other important recent studies have shown support for the association of breast cancer risk and HRT use. The Nurses' Health Study follow-up was extended to 1992, recording 1,935 cases of invasive breast cancer in the 725,550 woman-years of postmenopausal women tracked.[63] The risk of breast cancer was significantly increased among women using estrogen alone (RR, 1.32; 95% CI, 1.14–1.54), compared to postmenopausal women who had never used hormones. The risk of breast cancer was also significantly increased among women using estrogen plus progestin (RR, 1.41; 95% CI, 1.15–1.74). Among current HRT users, such therapy for 5 to 9 years was associated with higher risk (RR, 1.46; 95% CI, 1.22–1.74), with a similar risk for 10 years of use. This effect of duration of use for 5 or more years was greater among older women (RR for women aged 60 to 64, 1.71; 95% CI, 1.34–2.18). The relative risk of death from breast cancer was also increased among women who had taken estrogen for 5 or more years (RR, 1.45; 95% CI, 1.01–2.09).

Previous studies of postmenopausal ovarian cancer risk disagree, with some reporting increased risk with estrogen use and others finding either a protective or null effect. Most of these studies were relatively small and limited by incomplete information about ovarian cancer risk factors, but two recent large studies linked hormone use and ovarian cancer. A large prospective study[63] associated postmenopausal estrogen use for 10 or more years with increased risk of ovarian cancer mortality, and a recent Swedish study[64] reported that estrogen use alone and estrogen-progestin used sequentially (progestin used on the average of 10 days/month) may add to risk for ovarian cancer. In contrast, estrogen-progestin used continuously (progestin used on average 28 days/month) seemed to confer no increased ovarian cancer risk.

A study of ovarian cancer risk of women in the Breast Cancer Detection and Demonstration Project, who used estrogen-only replacement therapy, particularly for 10 or more years, found them at significantly increased risk of ovarian cancer.[65] Women using short-term estrogen-progestin-only replacement therapy were not at increased risk, but risk associated with short-term and longer-term estrogen-progestin replacement therapy warrants further investigation.

Risk Factors for Childhood Cancer Occurrence

Environmental risk factors for adult cancer generally involve long latency periods from exposure start to clinical onset of disease. Cigarette smoking illustrates this point; smoking usually begins during adolescence, but associated malignancies become apparent only after many decades. However, the genetic processes that go awry and lead to childhood cancer are likely different from that of adult malignancies, as suggested by a shorter time for the carcinogenic process to occur in children. Infancy, when embryonal neoplasms such as neuroblastoma predominate, is when childhood cancer incidence rates are highest.[66] One may reasonably surmise, therefore, that many childhood cancers result from aberrations in early developmental processes.

To our dismay, from a prevention standpoint, little current evidence supports a major etiologic role for environmental or other exogenous factors in childhood cancer. A comprehensive review of epidemiologic studies of childhood cancer is available elsewhere.[66] The major types of childhood cancer and risk factors that are reasonably well documented are shown in Table 22.2. Many other factors, suspected to raise or lower increase or decrease risk, are not well established, and even the known risk factors shown in the table explain only a small proportion of childhood cancer cases.

Concluding Remarks

Cancer is, and will be for the immediate future, a major public health problem; but several already-identified causes suggest many human cancers may be avoidable. Cancer rates would be lowered dramatically by reduction of tobacco smoking and factors influencing breast cancer. Although tobacco control could be achieved by government and societal actions, prospects for the prevention of breast cancer are more remote. In this regard, ongoing intervention trials of selective estrogen receptor modulators (SERMs), such as tamoxifen and raloxifene, in healthy women have a unique role in being the only available intervention with a reasonable probability of prevention. Other important reductions could be brought about by vaccination against hepatitis B and human papilloma virus and control of *H. pylori*. A growing concern, not just for cancer but for other chronic diseases, such as diabetes and heart disease, is the impact of epidemic rates of overweight and obesity. As evidence accumulates for a role of excess weight and lack of physical activity in both the etiology of and survival from cancer, strategies to prevent and effectively treat obesity and to promote increased physical activity and other healthy lifestyle behaviors are likely to be critical for improving public health. However, greater efforts in behavioral research and development of successful interventions are integral to such an effort. Failing primary prevention, screening for cancers of the breast, cervix, and colon could reduce mortality

TABLE 22.2. Known risk factors for selected childhood cancers.

Cancer type	*Risk factor*	*Comments*
Acute lymphoid leukemia	Ionizing radiation	Although primarily of historical significance, prenatal diagnostic X-ray exposure increases risk. Therapeutic irradiation for cancer treatment also increases risk.
	Race	White children have a 2-fold higher rate than black children in the U.S.
	Genetic conditions	Down syndrome is associated with an estimated 20-fold increased risk. Neurofibromatosis type 1, Bloom syndrome, ataxia telangiectasia, and Langerhans cell histiocytosis, among others, are associated with an elevated risk.
Acute myeloid leukemias	Chemotherapeutic agents	Alkylating agents and epipodophyllotoxins increase risk.
	Genetic conditions	Down syndrome and neurofibromatosis 1 are strongly associated. Familial monosomy 7 and several other genetic syndromes are also associated with increased risk.
Brain cancers	Therapeutic ionizing radiation to the head	With the exception of cancer radiotherapy, higher risk from radiation treatment is essentially of historical importance.
	Genetic conditions	Neurofibromatosis 1 is strongly associated with optic gliomas, and, to a lesser extent, associated with other CNS tumors. Tuberous sclerosis and several other genetic syndromes are associated with increased risk.
Hodgkin's disease	Family history	Monozygotic twins and siblings of cases are at increased risk.
	Infections	Epstein–Barr virus is associated with increased risk.
Non-Hodgkin's lymphoma	Immunodeficiency	Acquired and congenital immunodeficiency disorders, and immunosuppressive therapy, increase risk.
	Infections	Epstein–Barr virus is associated with Burkitt's lymphoma in African countries.
Osteosarcoma	Ionizing radiation	Cancer radiotherapy and high radium exposure increase risk.
	Chemotherapy	Alkylating agents increase risk.
	Genetic conditions	Increased risk is apparent with Li–Fraumeni syndrome and hereditary retinoblastoma.
Ewing's sarcoma	Race	White children have about a 9-fold higher incidence rate than black children in the U.S.
Neuroblastoma		No known risk factors.
Retinoblastoma		No known nonhereditary risk factors.
Wilms' tumor	Congenital anomalies	Aniridia and Beckwith–Wiedemann syndrome, as well as other congenital and genetic conditions, increase risk.
	Race	Asian children reportedly have about half the rates of white and black children.
Rhabdomyosarcoma	Congenital anomalies and genetic conditions	Li–Fraumeni syndrome and neurofibromatosis 1 are believed to be associated with increased risk. There is some concordance with major birth defects.

from these common diseases, and screening for other forms of cancer will emerge as public health strategies are given proper evaluation. Cancer cases are expected to rise in the new millennium, so cancer control strategies will increase in importance. Implementing current knowledge could prevent thousands, if not millions, of premature deaths.

References

1. Szklo M, Nieto FJ. Epidemiology: Beyond the Basics. Gaithersburg, MD: Aspen, 2000.
2. Rothman KJ, Greenland S. Modern Epidemiology, 2nd ed. Philadelphia: Lippincott-Raven, 1998.
3. http://www.cdc.gov or http://www.atsdr.cdc.gov.
4. Ries LAG, Kosary CL, Hankey BF, Miller BA, Harras A, Edwards BK (eds). SEER Cancer Statistics Review, 1973–1994. NIH Publication 97-2789. Bethesda, MD: National Cancer Institute, 1997.
5. http://www-dep.iarc.fr/.
6. Weiss NS. Clinical Epidemiology: The Study of the Outcome of Illness, 2nd ed. New York: Oxford University Press, 1996.
7. Benson K, Hartz AJ. A comparison of observational studies and randomized, controlled trials. N Engl J Med 2000;342:1878–1886.
8. Concato J, Shah N, Horwitz RI. Randomized, controlled trials, observational studies, and the hierarchy of research designs. N Engl J Med 2000;342:1887–1892.
9. Colditz GA, Stampfer MJ, Willett WC, et al. Type of postmenopausal hormone use and risk of breast cancer: 12-year follow-up from the Nurses' Health Study. Cancer Causes Control 1992;5:433–439.
10. Adami HO, Hunter D, Trichopoulos D. Textbook of Cancer Epidemiology. New York: Oxford University Press, 2002.
11. Brownson RC. Outbreak and cluster investigations In: Brownson RC, Petitti DB (eds). Applied Epidemiology. New York: Oxford University Press, 1998:71–104.
12. Rothman KJ. A sobering start for the cluster busters' conference. Am J Epidemiol 1990;132(suppl 1):S6–S13.
13. Alexander FE. Clusters and clustering of childhood cancer: a review. Eur J Epidemiol 1999;15:847–852.
14. Perera FP. Molecular epidemiology: on the path to prevention? J Natl Cancer Inst 2000;92:602–612.
15. Perera FP, Weinstein IB. Molecular epidemiology and carcinogen-DNA adduct detection: new approaches to studies of human cancer causation. J Chronic Dis 1982;35:581–600.
16. Lichtenstein P, Holm NV, Verkasalo PK, et al. Environmental and heritable factors in the causation of cancer: analyses of cohorts of twins from Sweden, Denmark, and Finland. N Engl J Med 2000;343:78–85.
17. Vineis P, Malats N, Lang M, et al (eds). Metabolic Polymorphisms and Susceptibility to Cancer. Lyon: IARC, 1999.
18. Parkin DM. Global cancer statistics in the year 2000. Lancet Oncol 2001;9:533–543.

19. Doll R, Peto R. The causes of cancer: quantitative estimates of avoidable risks of cancer in the United States today. J Natl Cancer Inst 1991;66:1191–1308.
20. Kuper H, Adami HO, Boffetta P. Tobacco use, cancer causation and public health impact. J Intern Med 2002;251:455–466.
21. International Agency for Research on Cancer. Tobacco: A Major International Health Hazard. Lyon: IARC, 1986.
22. Wu X, Hudmon KS, Detry MA, Chamberlain RM, Spitz MR. D2 dopamine receptor gene polymorphisms among African-Americans and Mexican-Americans: a lung cancer case-control study. Cancer Epidemiol Biomarkers Prev 2000;9:1021–1026.
23. USDHHS (United States Department of Health and Human Services). Reducing the health consequences of smoking: 25 years of progress. A report of the Surgeon General. Washington, DC: U.S. Government Printing Office, 1989.
24. Lancaster WD, Piccardo JC. Viral agents. In: Bertino JR (ed). Encyclopedia of Cancer, 2nd ed. San Diego: Academic Press, 2002.
25. Doll R. Prevention: some future perspectives. Prev Med 1978; 7:486–497.
26. Yamaguchi N, Kakizoe T. Synergistic interaction between *Helicobacter pylori* gastritis and diet in gastric cancer. Lancet Oncol 2001;2:84–94.
27. Kelley JR, Duggan JM. Gastric cancer epidemiology and risk factors. J Clin Epidemiol 2003;56(1):1–9.
28. National Cancer Institute. Prevention of Gastric Cancer, Health Professional Version. 2003. Retrieved on April 22, 2004, http://www.nci.nih.gov/cancerinfo/pdq/prevention/gastric/healthprofessional/#Section_21.
29. Correa P. *Helicobacter pylori* and gastric carcinogenesis. Am J Surg Pathol 1995;19(suppl 1):S37–S43.
30. Tommasi S, Denissenko MF, Pfeifer GP. Sunlight induces pyrimidine dimers preferentially at 5-methylcytosine bases. Cancer Res 1997;57:4727–4730.
31. Giles GG, Marks R, Foley P. The incidence of nonmelanomic skin cancer in Australia. Br Med J 1988;296:13–17.
32. Rosso S, Zanetti R, Martinez C, et al. The multicentre south European study 'Helios' II: Different sun exposure patterns in the aetiology of basal cell and squamous cell carcinomas of the skin. Br J Cancer 1996;73:1447–1454.
33. Elwood M, Jopson J. Melanoma and sun exposure: an overview of published studies. Int J Cancer 1997;73:198–203.
34. Autier P, Dore JF, Lejeune F, et al. Cutaneous malignant melanoma and exposure to sunlamps or sunbeds: an EORTC multicenter case-control study in Belgium, France and Germany. Int J Cancer 1994;58:809–813.
35. Autier P, Dore JF, Lejeune D, et al. Recreational exposure to sunlight and lack of information as risk factors for cutaneous malignant melanoma. Results of a European Organisation for Research and Treatment of Cancer (EORTC) case-control study in Belgium, France and Germany. Melanoma Res 1994;4:79–85.
36. Armstrong B, Doll R. Environmental factors and cancer incidence and mortality in different countries, with special reference to dietary practices. Int J Cancer 1975;15:617–631.
37. Willett WC. Nutritional Epidemiology. Oxford: Oxford University Press, 1990.
38. Steinmetz KA, Potter JD. Vegetable, fruit, and cancer I. Epidemiology. Cancer Causes Control 1991;2:325–358.
39. International Agency for Research on Cancer. Monographs on the Evaluation of Carcinogenic Risk of Chemicals to Humans, vol 44. Alcohol Drinking. Lyon: IARC, 1988.
40. Longnecker MP. Alcohol consumption and risk of cancer in humans: an overview. Alcohol 1995;12:87–96.
41. Dennis LK, Hayes RB. Alcohol and prostate cancer. Epidemiol Rev 2001;23:110–114.
42. Sarkar DK, Liehr JG, Singletary KW. Role of estrogen in alcohol promotion of breast cancer and prolactinomas. Alcoholism Clin Exp Res 1995;25:230S–236S.
43. Bhat KP, Pezzuto JM. Cancer chemopreventive activity of resveratrol. Ann NY Acad Sci 2002;957:210–229.
44. Calle EE, Rodriquez C, Walker-Thurmond K, Thun MJ. Overweight, obesity, and mortality from cancer in a prospectively studied cohort of U.S. adults. N Engl J Med 2003;348:1625–1638.
45. Moller H, Mellemgaard A, Lindvig K, Olsen J. Obesity and Cancer Risk: A Danish record-linkage study. Eur J Cancer 1994; 30:344–350.
46. Ballard-Barbash R. Anthropometry and breast cancer: body size—a moving target. Cancer (Phila) 1994;74:1090–1100.
47. NCI/NHLBI Obesity Education Initiative Task Force Members. Clinical Guidelines on the Identification, Evaluation, and Treatment of Overweight and Obesity in Adults. Washington, DC: NHLBI, 1998:1–137.
48. WHO Consultation on Obesity. Global Prevalence and Secular Trends in Obesity. Obesity. Preventing and Managing the Global Epidemic. Geneva: WHO, 1998:17n>40.
49. Colditz GA, Cannuscio CC, Frazier AL. Physical activity and reduced risk of colon cancer: implications for prevention. Cancer Causes Control 1997;8:649–667.
50. McTiernan A, Ulrich C, Slate S, Potter J. Physical activity and cancer etiology: associations and mechanisms. Cancer Causes Control 1998;9:487–509.
51. Bernstein L, Ross RK, Lobo RA, Hanisch R, Krailo MD, Henderson BE. The effects of moderate physical activity on menstrual cycle patterns in adolescence: implications for breast cancer prevention. Br J Cancer 1987;55:681–685.
52. Doll R, Peto R. The Causes of Cancer. Oxford: Oxford University Press, 1981.
53. Ward E. Overview of preventable industrial causes of occupational cancer. Environ Health Perspect 1995;103(suppl 8):197–203.
54. Doll R. Effects of exposure to vinyl chloride. An assessment of the evidence. Scand J Work Environ Health 1988;14:61–78.
55. Zaebst D, Clapp D, Blade LM, et al. Quantitative determination of trucking industry workers' exposures to diesel exhaust particles. Am Indust Hyg Assoc J 1991;52:529–541.
56. Carpenter L, Roman E. Cancer and occupation in women: identifying associations using routinely collected national data. Environ Health Perspect 1999;107(suppl 2):299–303.
57. Boice JD Jr, Land CE, Preston DL. Ionizing radiation. In: Schottenfeld D, Fraumeni JF (eds). Cancer Epidemiology and Prevention, 2nd ed. New York: Oxford University Press, 1996:319–354.
58. Moysich KB, Menezes RJ, Michalek AM. Chernobyl-related ionizing radiation exposure and cancer risk: an epidemiologic review. Lancet Oncol 2002;3:269–279.
59. United Nations Scientific Committee on the Effects of Atomic Radiation (UNSCEAR). Report to the General Assembly. Sources and Effects of Ionizing Radiation, vol 1, Sources; vol 2, Effects. Washington, DC: United Nations, 2002.
60. Marchbanks PA, McDonald JA, Wilson HG, et al. Oral contraceptives and the risk of breast cancer. N Engl J Med 2002; 346:2025–2032.
61. Collaborative Group on Hormonal Factors in Breast Cancer. Breast cancer and hormonal contraceptives: collaborative reanalysis of individual data on 53,297 women with breast cancer and 100,239 women without breast cancer from 54 epidemiological studies. Lancet 1996;347:1713–1727.
62. Writing Group for the Women's Health Initiative Investigators. Risks and benefits of estrogen plus progestin in healthy postmenopausal women: principal results from the Women's Health Initiative randomized controlled trial. JAMA 2002:288:321–333.
63. Rodriguez C, Patel AV, Calle EE, Jacob EJ, Thun MJ. Estrogen replacement therapy and ovarian cancer mortality in a large prospective study of US women. JAMA 2001;285(11):1460–1465.

64. Riman T, Dickman PW, Nilsson S, et al. Hormone replacement therapy and the risk of invasive epithelial ovarian cancer in Swedish women. J Natl Cancer Inst 2002;94:497–504.
65. Lacey JV Jr, Mink PJ, Lubin JH, et al. Menopausal hormone replacement therapy and risk of ovarian cancer. JAMA 2002; 288:334–341.
66. Ries LAG, Smith MA, Gurney JG, et al (eds). Cancer Incidence and Survival Among Children and Adolescents: United States SEER program 1975–1995. NIH 99-4649. Bethesda, MD: National Cancer Institute, SEER Program, 1999. The publication and additional data available on the SEER Website: http://www-seer.ims.nci.nih.gov/publications.

23

Evidence-Based Cancer Prevention Research: A Multidisciplinary Perspective on Cancer Prevention Trials

Stephen D. Hursting, Michele R. Forman, Asad Umar, Nomeli P. Nunez, and J. Carl Barrett

More than 1 million Americans were expected to be diagnosed with cancer in 2004. This fact is especially tragic given that many cancers are preventable. The ongoing challenge to the medical, scientific, and public health communities is to formulate evidence-based decisions and implement effective and safe interventions for cancer prevention.

Randomized controlled clinical trials remain the gold standard to test cause and effect in human research and inform evidence-based medical decisions. The era of cancer prevention trials began with the seminal paper by Peto in 1981,[1,2] who examined the role of β-carotene and vitamin A in cancer prevention. Since 1981, there have been numerous cancer prevention trials of nutritional interventions and pharmacologic agents. Some of these prevention trials reported clearly positive results while other trials reveal mixed results, null findings, and even unsuspected adverse effects.

A comprehensive review of all cancer prevention trials is beyond the scope of this chapter. We present here a brief review of multistage carcinogenesis and possible molecular targets for cancer prevention. We then discuss examples of randomized, controlled clinical trials that examine the effects of five different cancer prevention modalities. These *case studies* of human trials in cancer prevention were selected to explore the reasons why several trials did not achieve the expected cancer preventive outcomes, whereas others reached their goals. We describe the state of the art before each series of trials followed by the design, some background on the preventive agent or dietary intervention used, primary endpoints, results, and future directions. Reflections on the results are threaded with investigations of the complexities inherent to prevention trials and mechanisms underlying the adverse or null endpoints. Finally, we explore the lessons learned from the trials to identify achievable goals and the underpinnings to, and the relevant criteria for, future human research in the prevention of cancer.

Multistage Carcinogenesis Process and Targets for Prevention

Humans are exposed to a wide variety of endogenous and exogenous carcinogenic insults, including chemicals, radiation, physical agents, bacteria, and viruses. Recent progress in the study of the multistep process of carcinogenesis, particularly on the mechanisms of chemically and virally induced cancer, has revealed several points along the carcinogenesis pathway that may be amenable to cancer prevention strategies. The classic view of experimental carcinogenesis, in which tumor initiation is followed by tumor promotion and progression in a sequential fashion, has undergone significant revision as our understanding of cancer-related genes and the biosystem has evolved. However, the concepts and underlying processes of initiation, promotion, and progression remain theoretically important. Tumor initiation begins in cells with DNA alterations resulting from inherent genetic mutations or, more commonly, from spontaneous or carcinogen-induced genetic or epigenetic changes. Alterations in specific genes modify the responsiveness of the initiated cell to its microenvironment, eventually providing a growth advantage relative to normal cells. The tumor promotion stage is characterized by clonal expansion of initiated cells caused by alterations in the expression of genes whose products are associated with hyperproliferation, apoptosis, tissue remodeling, and inflammation.[3] During the tumor progression stage, preneoplastic cells develop into invasive tumors through further clonal expansion, usually associated with alterations in gene expression

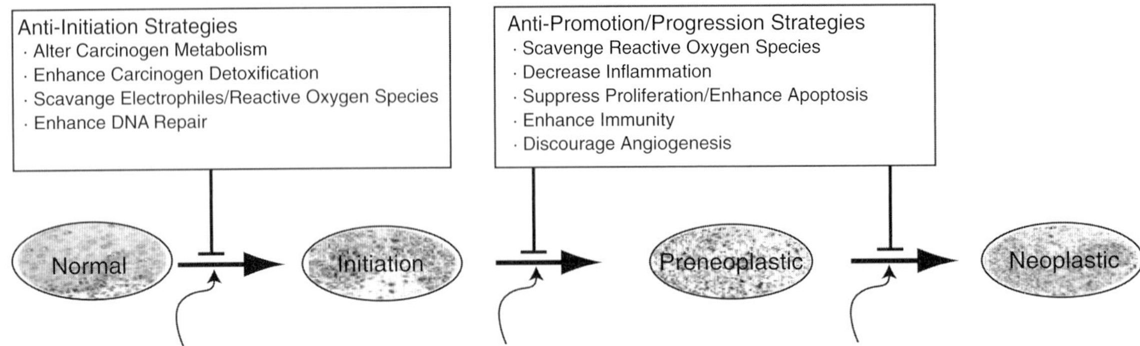

FIGURE 23.1. Multistage carcinogenesis model: a schematic presentation of stage-specific prevention strategies. The initiation stage is characterized by the conversion of a normal cell to an initiated cell in response to genetic or epigenetic changes in the cell's DNA. The conversion of an initiated cell to a preneoplastic population of cells and ultimately to a tumor is determined by additional genetic/epigenetic changes that affect the balance between growth and death in these cells. Strategies to intervene in these processes to decrease rates of mutation epigenetic change and maintain the growth–death balance in cancer cells are listed in the boxes.

and additional genetic damage due to progressive genomic instability.[3]

As depicted in Figure 23.1, possible ways of interfering with tumor initiation events include (i) modifying carcinogen activation by inhibiting the enzymes responsible for that activation or by directly scavenging DNA-reactive electrophiles and free radicals; (ii) enhancing carcinogen detoxification by altering the activity of detoxifying enzymes; and (iii) modulating certain DNA repair processes. Possible ways of blocking the processes involved in the promotion and progression stages of carcinogenesis include (i) scavenging reactive oxygen species; (ii) altering the expression of genes involved in cell signaling, particularly those regulating cell proliferation, apoptosis, and differentiation; (iii) decreasing inflammation; (iv) enhancing immune function; or (v) suppressing angiogenesis.

We now appreciate that the nature of initiation, promotion, and progression events is complex. For instance, we know from the work of Fearon and Vogelstein and others that multiple mutational and epigenetic events are involved in the formation of cancers.[4] Furthermore, humans are generally exposed to mixtures of agents that can simultaneously act at different stages of the carcinogenesis process. Thus, rather than three discrete stages occurring in a predictable order, human carcinogenesis is best characterized as an accumulation of alterations in genes regulating cellular growth, death, and malignant properties. These alterations occur through a series of clonal selections influenced by endogenous and exogenous factors. Epigenetic changes often develop in a cancer or the microenvironment and may also drive this multistep process.[5] Nonetheless, the processes involved in cancer initiation, promotion, and progression already described remain important and relevant targets for cancer prevention. Interventions that increase or decrease rates of mutation, rates of epigenetic change, or the balance between growth and death in cancer cells can significantly influence the ultimate development of cancer. One of the most important questions in contemporary cancer research is this: What safe and effective interventions should be recommended to prevent cancer?

Case Study I: Trials of β-Carotene Supplementation and Lung Cancer Chemoprevention

In 1976, Sporn defined the term chemoprevention as the use of natural or synthetic agents to reverse or suppress multistage carcinogenesis.[6,7] There are numerous examples in the literature demonstrating that bioactive food components or chemopreventive agents can influence one or more of these targets and interfere with the carcinogenesis process.[3] In the oft-cited paper entitled "Can dietary β-carotene materially reduce human cancer rates?," Peto described the role of retinol and the retinoids in later-stage carcinogenesis and recommended β-carotene, rather than vitamin A, chemoprevention trials in the general population aged 50 years or older, because high doses of β-carotene for treatment of erythropoietic protoporphyia were not associated with toxicity as was the case for vitamin A.[1,8]

Following Peto's paper, four large-scale randomized placebo-controlled clinical trials of β-carotene (summarized in Table 23.1) revealed no protection but rather adverse effects or no difference in rates of lung cancer among participants in the β-carotene arm compared to the placebo arm. Two trials enrolled high-risk individuals while the other two enrolled apparently healthy individuals. The Alpha-Tocopherol β-Carotene Trial (ATBC) in Finland included male smokers at high risk of lung cancer (mean, 36 years of smoking) who were administered β-carotene, α-tocopherol, both, or a placebo for 6 years on average. The β-Carotene Retinol Efficacy Trial (CARET) in the United States enrolled men and women who were either smokers (mean, 49 years) or asbestos-exposed workers, and administered β-carotene, retinyl palmitate, both, or a placebo for 4 years on average. In these two trials, the β-carotene-supplemented group experienced an increased risk of lung cancer (by 18% in ATBC and 36% in CARET) compared to the placebo group, and the effect appeared stronger in participants who drank greater than average amounts of alcohol daily (i.e., a 35% versus 3% increase in lung cancer risk, respectively, in ATBC).[9–11] Also, more of a systemic effect appeared in subsequent analysis, as illustrated by a 23% and 25% increase in prostate and in stomach cancers, respectively, in the supplemented (versus placebo) group in ATBC, and an 18% and 26% increase in total mortality and in cardiovascular deaths among the β-carotene group in CARET.

In contrast, participants in the Physicians Health Trial and the Women's Health Study were apparently healthy, had a low rate of smokers, and were administered an alternate-day schedule of β-carotene for 12 and 2 years of follow-up, respectively. Compared with the placebo group, β-carotene supplementation in these participants was not associated with an increased risk of lung cancer; rates of lung cancer did not differ by treatment arm. In all four trials, participants in the β-carotene-supplemented arm compared to the placebo arm had significantly higher concentrations of β-carotene in blood, indicating uptake of the supplement but not necessarily efficacy. The search for reasons why β-carotene supplementation was associated with adverse effects occurred in several areas of study, including a reevaluation of the epidemiologic results, animal experiments, and clinical nutrition research.

Evidence from Observational Epidemiology

A review of epidemiologic studies covering the period before, during, and soon after the four trials revealed more significant inverse associations between serum concentrations of and dietary intake of β-carotene and lung cancer in case-control than cohort studies.[12] Methodological differences in estimation of intake and blood values may have complicated comparisons and contributed to the inconsistent results.

Evidence from Animal Research

A few experimental studies had been conducted examining the effect of β-carotene on skin cancer before the randomized clinical trials in humans. Two research groups subsequently addressed major questions arising from the trials. The USDA-Tufts group focused on research to explain the "apparent exacerbation of lung carcinogenesis by β-carotene supplementation in smokers."[13] In a study of ferrets with and without exposure to cigarette smoke and with and without β-carotene supplementation for 6 months, a strong proliferative response in lung tissue and squamous metaplasia was observed in the β-carotene-supplemented animals without smoke exposure and was especially enhanced in the smoking +β-carotene group. In vitro incubation of lung tissue from smoke-exposed ferrets with all-*trans*-β-carotene revealed that the β-carotene molecule is unstable. It forms oxidative byproducts that induce cytochrome P-450 enzymes, interfere with retinoic acid metabolism, and downregulate retinoic acid receptor (RAR)-β.[13] Indeed, the downregulation of RAR-β expression observed in the lungs of ferrets who were receiving both β-carotene supplementation and smoke exposure suggests this modulation of RAR-β may play a role in the enhancement of lung tumorigenesis in response to β-carotene.

In contrast, a recent follow-up study showed that lycopene, a carotenoid found chiefly in tomato products, has protective activity in the same ferret model. Ferrets were either exposed to a smoking chamber at levels of cigarette smoke comparable to one to two packs/day, or not exposed to smoke, and administered supplements of lycopene at either 15 or 60 mg/day for 9 weeks.[14] Both low- and high-dose lycopene supplementation inhibited lung squamous metaplasia in this model. Compared with ferrets exposed to smoke alone, ferrets supplemented with lycopene and exposed to smoke had significantly higher plasma insulin-like growth factor-binding protein 3 (IGFBP-3) and lower insulin-like growth factor 1 (IGF-1)/IGFBP-3 ratio, thereby reducing serum levels of bioavailable IGF-1. In addition, cigarette smoke exposure increased phosphorylation of the apoptosis protein BAD and significantly decreased cleaved caspase 3 (an apoptosis-related

TABLE 23.1. Beta carotene supplementation trials of lung cancer.

Trial	*Agent(s)*	*Population*	*N*	*Follow-up*	*Risk effect*
ATBC	β-Carotene (20 mg/day)	Male smokers	29,133	5–8 years	876 cases
(Finland)	Vitamin E (50 mg/day) (2 × 2 design)	50–69 years (μ = 57 years) 36 years of smoking		μ = 6 years	RR = 1.18 (1.03, 1.36)*
CARET	β-Carotene (30 mg/day)	Men and women	18,314	4–7 years	286 cases
(U.S.)	Retinyl palmitate (25,000 IU) (2 × 2 design)	Smokers (μ = 58 years) 49 years of smoking	14,254	μ = 4 years	RR = 1.36 (1.07 – 1.73) β-carotene supplement RR = 1.28 (1.04, 1.57)* β-carotene + retinyl palmitate
		Asbestos (μ = 57 years) 43 years of smoking	4,060		RR = 1.40 (0.95 – 2.07) asbestos exposed RR = 1.23 (0.96 – 1.56) heavy smokers
PHS I	β-Carotene (50 mg/ alternate/day)	Male MDs	22,071	12 years	82 cases in β-carotene
(U.S.)		40–84 years 11% smokers			88 cases in placebo RR = 0.98 (0.91, 1.06)*
WHS	β-Carotene (50 mg/ alternate/day) of 8 groups	Women	39,876	2.1 years	30 cases in β-carotene
(U.S.)		45 years + 13% smokers			21 in placebo*

protease) in the lungs of ferrets; however, lycopene supplementation reversed the smoke-induced suppression of apoptosis and prevented the smoke-induced elevation of BAD phosphorylation.[14] These findings, along with other recent studies,[15] begin to elucidate the potential chemopreventive capacity and limitations of carotenoids, as well as the mechanisms underlying the effects of β-carotene on lung cancer observed in human trials.

Evidence from Pharmacokinetic and Pharmacodynamic Research

Limited pharmacokinetic research was conducted before the trials, and determinations of an optimal dose and the duration of supplementation were not established. Single-dose studies of β-carotene that demonstrated peak plasma response within 24 to 48 hours were conducted in healthy young men before the trials.[16] Chronic-dose studies, ranging from 15 to 180 mg/day β-carotene, were conducted in healthy participants at the same time as the trials.[17–19] The chronic-dose studies began to reveal large interindividual variation in response to the varying dosages. Along with limited information on the bioavailability of β-carotene was the issue of identifying responders from nonresponders, a phenomenon later reported in trial participants.[20] Human nutrition research was not conducted to test the effects of β-carotene supplementation in high-risk groups such as smokers and drinkers of alcohol in the ATBC and CARET. The publication of adverse effects in human trials led to animal research as the only ethical approach to examine the interaction of multiple risk behaviors and a pharmaceutical dose supplementation as well as the complex molecular pathways leading to lung carcinogenesis.

Case Study II: High-Fiber, Fruit, and Vegetable Interventions and Colon Polyp Recurrence

During the 1980s, three lines of evidence suggested that certain aspects of lifestyle, especially dietary factors, were associated with colon carcinogenesis. First, mortality rates for colorectal cancer (CRC) varied across regions of the world. The variation in worldwide rates of CRC was a recognized "ecologic" association. The second line of evidence appeared in the rapid changes in CRC incidence within a country. During a 40-year period in Japan, for example, CRC incidence rose at a dramatic rate, in men more than women. The third line of evidence came from migration studies demonstrating that risk of CRC changed with adoption of a new diet. For example, the CRC incidence rate for American-born Japanese approached or was higher than the rate in Japan.[21] Indeed, in most cases, migrants adopted the CRC rates of their new country within a generation. Moreover, animal evidence overwhelmingly revealed a protective effect of fiber on colon carcinogenesis.[22–24] Thus, by 1988, the *Surgeon General's Report on Nutrition: Diet and Colorectal Cancer (CRC) Risk* and the 1989 *National Academy of Sciences Diet and Health Report* summarized the field by concluding there was sufficient evidence that a high-fat diet increased risk and a high-fiber, high-fruit-and-vegetable diet decreased CRC risk.

During this era, the progression of colorectal carcinogenesis was depicted as a series of sequential steps from normal epithelium to development of aberrant crypts, followed by early adenomatous polyps, the formation of advanced adenomas, and finally cancer.[4] Population-based incidence rates of adenomatous polyps were not available, and identification of a high-risk group other than those with familial adenomatous polyposis syndrome (FAP) was difficult. Therefore, investigators in cancer prevention focused on trials of dietary interventions to reduce recurrence of adenomatous polyps in individuals with prior adenomatous polyps.

High-Fiber, Fruit, and Vegetable Trials of Polyp Recurrence

In the early 1990s, several cancer prevention trials tested the effect of a low-fat and high-fiber intervention on adenomatous polyp recurrence.[25–30] In each trial, summarized in Table 23.2, individuals had a complete colonoscopy and removal of at least one adenomatous polyp. Eligibility criteria differed by trial according to polyp size, number, and time interval from polypectomy to enrollment. The intervention plan varied as well from a wheat bran or fiber supplement, to combinations of low-fat diet plus wheat bran supplements, to an overall dietary plan of a high-fiber, high-fruit-and-vegetable, low-fat regimen. Actual percent of calories from fat on the intervention ranged from 20% to 25%, compared to the usual dietary regimen of 33% to 37% of calories from fat. The approach to fat reduction ranged from removal of butter and/or visible fat from meat to use of low-fat dairy products through to major changes in categories of food intake. In addition, several trials included a supplement of 20 mg/day β-carotene or a placebo.[27] Given the randomization schema, as many as eight distinct combinations (including the placebo + usual diet group) of the trial might be tested in a factorial design.

The length of the trials ranged from 1 to 4 years, with assessment of polyp recurrence by colonoscopists who were blinded to the patient's group status. The randomized trial design was followed according to strict guidelines established at the beginning of the studies, including random assessment of dietary compliance by dietitians,[27] annual completion of (previously validated) dietary food frequency questionnaires, and multiple-day food records in randomly selected subcohorts of the Polyp Prevention Trial (PPT) participants.[30] In addition, blood specimens were collected in the fasting state to measure micronutrient levels as biomarkers of dietary change.[27] Rates of recurrence in the intervention and control/usual dietary regimen groups did not differ at the end of each trial, thereby revealing no significant prevention of adenomatous polyp recurrence by dietary intervention.

In an effort to explain why recurrence was not prevented or lowered in those randomized to an intervention scheme compared to those on the placebo/usual diet, several possibilities were presented, including (1) the wrong endpoint; (2) inadequate trial length for the study population; and (3) wrong intervention.

The Wrong Endpoint

By the time the trials were completed, it was recognized that less than 10% of adenomas developed into CRC and not all CRC developed through the adenoma pathway. In several trials, secondary outcomes such as the rates of large adeno-

TABLE 23.2. Colorectal neoplasia prevention trials evaluating dietary fat and fiber.

Reference	*Sample size*[a]	*Design/cohort*[b]	*Intervention*	*Primary results*
DeCosse[108]	58	DBRCT in familial adenomatous polyposis (FAP) patients	Wheat bran fiber (2.2 g/day) + placebo vs. wheat bran fiber (2.2 g/day) + vitamin C (4 g/day) + vitamin E (400 mg/day) vs. wheat bran fiber (22.5 g/day) + vitamins C + E × 48 months	Rectal adenoma number: nonsignificant reduction with high-dose fiber + vitamins
McKeown-Eyssen[29]	201	Partially blinded RCT in patients with prior adenoma	Low fat (50 g/day or 20% of total calories) + fiber (≥50 g/day) vs. customary diet × 24 months (average)	Adenoma incidence/recurrence: no effect
MacLennan[27]	424	Factorial, partially DBRCT in patients with prior adenoma	Low fat intake (<25% of total calories) vs. wheat bran (25 g/day) vs. beta-carotene (20 mg/day): 7-arm factorial trial × 24–48 months	Adenoma incidence/recurrence: no overall effect; reduction in large (≤1 cm) adenomas with combination of wheat bran + low-fat diet*
Alberts[26,109,110]	1,429	DBRCT in patients 40–80 years old with prior adenoma (≥3 mm)	Wheat bran fiber 2 g/day vs. 13.5 g/day × 36 months	Adenoma number: 1% reduction (NS); persons with adenomas: 12% reduction (NS)
Schatzkin[25]	2,079	Partially blinded RCT in patients 35 years or older with prior adenoma	Low fat (≤20% of total calories), fiber (18 g/1,000 kcal), fruits and vegetables (5–8 servings/day) vs. typical U.S. diet × 48 months	Adenoma incidence/recurrence: no effect (RR =1.00)
Faivre[28,111]	655	DBRCT in patients 35–75 years old with prior adenoma	Fiber 3.8 g/day (ispaghula husk) vs. calcium 2 g/day vs. placebo	Adenoma incidence/recurrence: 34% reduction with calcium (NS); 67% increase* with fiber
Women's Health Initiative[92]	45,000–48,000	Complex factorial, 3 × 2 × 2 factorial DBRCT in postmenopausal women 50–79 years old	Low-fat diet vs. calcium + vitamin D vs. hormone replacement therapy × 9 years	Colorectal cancer incidence: ongoing

NS, nonsignificant.
[a] Number randomized.
[b] Trial designs: RCT, randomized, controlled trial; SBRCT, single-blind, randomized controlled trial; DBRCT, double-blind, randomized, controlled trial.
*Statistically significant result ($P < 0.05$).

mas (10 mm or larger), which have a greater malignant potential than small adenomas, were reduced by an intervention such as low-fat diet plus wheat bran supplement[27] and the overall dietary intervention (high-fiber, high-fruit-and-vegetable, low-fat) in the study.[25] However, the numbers of participants were too small to indicate whether the observed effects on this secondary endpoint were significant.

Inadequate Trial Length

Trial participants were adults with a history of at least one polyp before enrollment and therefore already at risk of another polyp. While they were at high risk of a recurrence, their mean age was typically in the sixties, and their colonic mucosa might be less amenable to (molecular, cellular, or tissue) modulations from diet than a younger, healthier group. The duration of the intervention(s) was not tested before the trials to define the time interval for optimal effect. Therefore, questions arose regarding the adequacy of the trial length, with passive follow-up of trial participants frequently occurring postintervention.[25,26] Dietary instruments to assess intake have limitations, including measurement error contributed by degree of completion based on instrument length and the number of days reporting, as well as the respondent's accuracy in estimation of portion size and frequency, which varied by the participant's education and age.[31] In the trials providing high-fiber supplements, adverse side effects were rarely mentioned, but attrition due to the inability to continue on the high-fiber regimen is a potential factor. Across trials, some patients refused to have the follow-up colonoscopy, thereby leading to selective subcohorts with endpoint ascertainment.[29]

Wrong Intervention

Dietary change from a high-fat, low-fiber diet to a low-fat, high-fiber and/or -fruit-and-vegetable plan offers choice of food substitutes and therefore more opportunity for long-term compliance. The downside of this broad application of dietary change is the difficulty in identifying which phytochemicals were eaten; their frequency and amount of intake; and whether food preparation and processing enhances or reduces absorption. For example, the length of time cooking dark green leafy vegetables modifies folate concentrations and the amount of insoluble fiber, whereas reducing water content from tomatoes increases lycopene concentrations from raw tomato to sauce to paste.

Fruit and vegetables contain more than 25,000 recognized phytochemicals. The search for the protective constituents in plants involves identifying the major sources of variation. For example, seasonality and soil content can alter the concentration of plant phytochemicals, and inter- and intraindividual variability in intake of phytochemicals modifies concentrations in human sera. Phytochemical databases to estimate intakes are limited to a few components such as carotenoids.[32] Thus, the effects of food constituents on cancer endpoints are difficult to determine.

Prior Evidence

Reviews of earlier research revealed a fairly consistent inverse association between fiber intake and CRC in case-control studies, whereas large population-based, prospective cohort studies such as the Nurses' Health and Health Professional Studies[33,34] did not demonstrate an association. Questions arose whether biases inherent to the case-control design led to spurious associations. For example, dietary reporting by patients *after* colon cancer diagnosis and telescoping of exposure assessment might bias the estimate of the effect of dietary fiber intake on cancer risk. Specifically, patients report dietary intake during the period of appearance of symptoms and illness rather than before this period, which could lead to an effect when indeed it did not exist.

An Update

Two articles in *The Lancet* in 2003 presented data from observational, prospective research suggesting a significant inverse association between dietary fiber intake and risk of polyps[35] or CRC.[36] Both studies had a larger and more varied range in dietary fiber intake (i.e., from 12 to 36 g/day) than in earlier cohort studies of more homogeneous populations.[33,34] The major protective dietary source was fiber from grains, cereals, and fruit,[35] and no food source of fiber was significantly more protective than another in the European Prospective Investigation into Cancer and Nutrition (EPIC) study.[36] Interestingly, use of fiber supplements was not associated with reduced risk. The adenomatous polyp study was based on sigmoidoscopy rather than colonoscopy for detection of polyps, reducing the area of the colon that was screened and therefore the potential to identify all polyps. A major strength of both studies was that participants were reporting intake potentially reflective of chronic, long-term habits. Identifying the duration and phases of the life cycle during which the intake occurred would be a major contribution to elucidate the timing of mechanisms of action in polyps and CRC. Thus, the dietary intervention trials had not determined the optimal range in intake for reduction in polyp recurrence, as evidenced by the breadth of dietary exposures in the two recent observational studies. Further analysis of the trials to explore the subset of individuals who met or went beyond the dietary goals of the trials might elucidate whether the duration of the trial was adequate to confer reduction in risk of polyp recurrence.

Case Study III: Chemoprevention Studies of Retinoids and Second Primary Cancers of the Upper Aerodigestive Tract

One of the first definitive proofs of principle for chemoprevention came from the translational studies of Kim and Hong and colleagues, who have studied retinoids and other chemopreventive agents in upper aerodigestive tract cancers since the early 1980s. Clinical, epidemiologic, and animal studies in the 1970s and 1980s had suggested that vitamin A could positively influence epithelial cell differentiation and thus, retinoids may be effective agents for preventing epithelial cancers in the upper aerodigestive tract.[37]

Chemoprevention Trials of Upper Aerodigestive Tract Cancers by Retinoids

As summarized in Table 23.3, Hong et al. established that high-dose 13-*cis* retinoic acid (13-CRA) is more effective than placebo in reversing oral premalignant lesions (OPLs)[38] and later showed that low-dose 13-CRA is more effective than β-carotene and less toxic than high-dose 13-CRA.[39,40] These studies demonstrate that retinoids can indeed be used to reverse OPLs, as suggested by several reports in animal models.[41–43] Further explorations of less toxic and more effective agents and regimens were accomplished by incorporating multidisciplinary studies of biomarkers into their trials and the development of statistical methodologies for analyzing multiple biomarkers for the prediction of cancer development in patients with OPLs,[44] Studies by Hong and colleagues demonstrate the importance of conducting parallel basic and translational studies. They observed that the synthetic retinoid fenretinide induces apoptosis through retinoic acid receptor-independent mechanisms and induces cell death in cell lines resistant to all-*trans* retinoic acid, 13-CRA, 9-CRA, and other nuclear receptor-dependent retinoids.[45] These findings have led to an ongoing trial of fenretinide in patients with retinoid-resistant OPLs and to the characterization of several novel retinoids with even more potent apoptosis-inducing effects than fenretinide.[46] Further studies are needed to determine whether these agents reduce mortality after treatment is completed.

The Hong group, along with many groups studying chemoprevention of OPLs, are currently moving away from retinoids toward less toxic agents, including bioactive food components, such as vitamin E and green tea polyphenols, or pharmacologic agents that target specific pathways, such as inhibitors of farnesyl transferase, cyclooxygenase 2, or the epidermal growth factor receptor. However, these initial studies of retinoids were critical to establish the feasibility of developing a translational chemoprevention strategy.

These translational research findings also led to new combination approaches to preventing OPLs. Retinoid resistance was shown to be associated with higher levels of genetic instability and mutant p53 expression.[47] Combination regimens of 13-CRA, α-tocopherol, and interferon-γ have been very effective in reversing laryngeal premalignant lesions but not OPLs,[48] probably because some, but not all, of the p53-mutated OPL clones can be eliminated, suggesting that some genotypically altered clones can regrow and manifest as phenotypic lesions after treatment is discontinued.[49,50]

TABLE 23.3. Prevention trials evaluating chemoprevention of upper aerodigestive tract cancers by retinoids.

Reference	*Sample Size*	*Design*	*Intervention*	*Primary results*
Papadimitrakopoulou[48]	36	Prospective nonrandomized trial	Oral isotretinoin (100 mg/m^2 per day), oral alpha-tocopherol (1,200 IU/day), and subcutaneous interferon-α (3 megaunits/m^2 twice weekly) for 12 months	A striking difference in response was observed in favor of laryngeal lesions 9/19 [47%] complete response rate at 6 months and 7/14 [50%] at 12 months vs. 1/11 [9%] and 0/7 [0%], respectively, for oral lesions)
Papadimitrakopoulou[40]	59	RCT	30 mg/day beta-carotene, or 0.5 mg/kg/day isotretinoin for 12 months	Isotretinoin 8% reduction Beta-carotene 55% reduction in oral premalignant lesions (OPL)
Lippman[47]	40	RCT	1.5 mg/kg/day isotretinoin for 3 months	Inverse relation of levels of p53 protein and response to isotretinoin in OPL
Lippman[39]	70	Phase I, RCT in Phase II	1.5 mg/kg/day isotretinoin for 3 months: patients with stable lesions given 1.5 mg/kg/day isotretinoin (n = 26) or 30 mg/day beta-carotene (n = 33) for 9 months	55% response in Phase I of 59 in the RCT, 92% vs. 45% response in isotretinoin vs. β-carotene arms
Hong[51]	103	RCT	Oral isotretinoin (100 mg/m^2/day) or placebo for 12 months	No significant difference between groups in the number of local, regional, or distance recurrences of the primary cancers, but second primary tumors were 4% for isotretinoin vs. 24% for the placebo
Hong[38]	44	RCT	13-*cis*-Retinoic acid (n = 24) or placebo (n = 20), 1–2 mg/kg/day for 3 months, and followed them for 6 months	Decrease in lesion size in 67% of those given the drug and in 10% of those given placebo (P = 0.0002); dysplasia reversed in 54% (13 patients) of the drug group vs. 10% (2 patients) of the placebo group (P = 0.01)

RCT, randomized controlled clinical trial.

The Hong group also established that second primary tumors (SPTs), the leading cause of cancer-related death among individuals cured of an initial primary head and neck tumor, can be prevented by retinoid treatment. Patients definitively treated for an initial head and neck cancer showed a marked decrease in SPTs in response to a high-dose 13-CRA regimen for 1 year.[51] However, significant side effects were associated with the high-dose 13-CRA treatment. Also, the effectiveness of the retinoid treatment diminished over time; in fact, the SPT rate by 3 years after cessation of 13-CRA treatment was the same as the placebo group.[52] A follow-up study of the effect of low-dose 13-CRA for 3 years for preventing SPTs is nearing completion.[53] Again, linking laboratory studies with these clinical trials has proven beneficial. For example, Hong, in collaboration with Margaret Spitz and colleagues, showed that susceptibility of peripheral blood lymphocytes to chromosomal breaks induced by the mutagens bleomycin or benzo[*a*]pyrene diol epoxide is an independent risk factor for head and neck cancer.[54,55] The mutagen-sensitive phenotype has also been shown to be a significant predictor of SPT risk.[56] Thus, the Hong group illustrates the model of the multidisciplinary approach to cancer prevention that takes advantage of conducting basic research on biomarkers and clinical research on pharmacokinetics of the agent in the prevention of OPL and SPT. This model is elaborated in Figure 23.2.

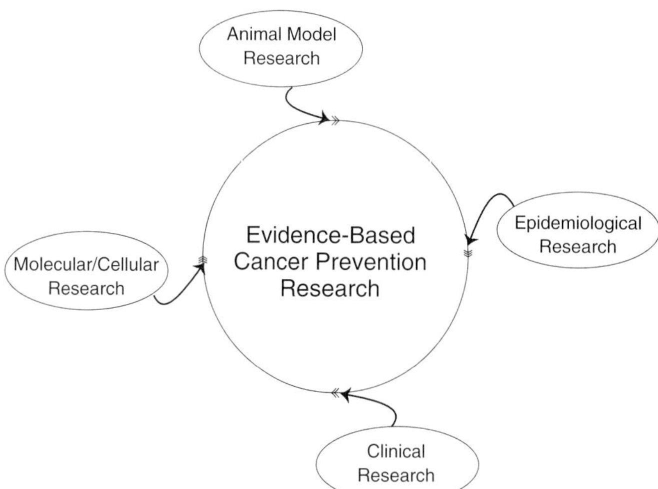

FIGURE 23.2. The transdisciplinary nature of evidence-based cancer prevention research. Research progress in the principles and practice of cancer prevention will increasingly require the integration of observational epidemiologic and clinical findings, the development and use of relevant animal models, the characterization of basic mechanisms at the molecular and cellular level, and the ultimate test of an hypothesis in clinical research.

Case Study IV: Tamoxifen and Breast Cancer

Breast cancer is the most common noncutaneous cancer among women in the United States.[57] Although breast cancer mortality has declined in the United States over the past decade, it remains the second leading cause of cancer-related deaths in women, after lung cancer.[58] Approximately 211,300 women in the United States were diagnosed with invasive breast cancer in 2004, and about 39,800 women will have died of the disease.[57]

Hormonal therapy has an important place in the treatment and prevention of breast cancer. Because the antiestrogen drug tamoxifen decreased contralateral breast cancer incidence, in 1992, the National Surgical Adjuvant Breast Cancer and Bowel Project (NSABP) started the Breast Cancer Prevention Trial (NSABP P-1) to test the hypothesis that tamoxifen could be used for the prevention of breast cancer in a group of healthy women at high risk for the disease.[59–63] Before the Breast Cancer Prevention Trial, anecdotal evidence suggested that primary breast cancer could be prevented by tamoxifen chemotherapy; however, there was no evidence from a randomized clinical trial to support this notion.[59–63] In the NSABP P-1 trial, women considered at high risk for breast cancer were (1) more than 60 years of age; or (2) aged 35 to 59 years with a 5-year predicted risk for breast cancer of 1.66% or more based on the Gail model risk for breast cancer (this risk is equivalent to that of a 60-year old woman[64]); or (3) having a history of lobular carcinoma in situ. In this trial, 13,388 women were randomized to receive tamoxifen 20mg/day (n = 6,681) or placebo for 5 years (n = 6,707). The main objective of the trial was to determine whether tamoxifen prevented invasive breast cancers; secondary aims were to determine whether tamoxifen would lower the incidence of fatal and nonfatal myocardial infarctions and the incidence of bone fractures. Results from this trial, summarized in Table 23.4, showed that tamoxifen reduced the risk of invasive breast cancer by 49% and the risk of noninvasive breast cancers by 50%. These effects were observed in estrogen receptor positive (ER+), not estrogen receptor negative (ER–), breast cancers. Women on the tamoxifen arm had 19% fewer bone fractures, but this reduction was not statistically different from the placebo group. With respect to vascular events and endometrial cancer, tamoxifen increased the risk of endometrial cancer (risk ratio = 2.93; 95% CI = 1.35–4.97) and increased the rates of stroke, pulmonary embolism, and deep-vein thrombosis.

Overall, this trial showed that tamoxifen use was associated with fewer ER+ breast cancers in pre- and post-menopausal women with a high-risk profile.[61] However, there is a cautionary note for sexually active premenopausal women taking tamoxifen, because tamoxifen was initially developed as a fertility drug.[65] Also, results from the Breast Cancer Prevention Trial showed that tamoxifen does not increase the risk of other cancers (besides endometrial), but may increase the risk of cataracts. Similar findings to the Breast Cancer Prevention Trial have appeared in other trials (Table 23.4), such as the Italian Randomized Trial of Tamoxifen and The International Breast Cancer Intervention Study 1.[66,67] Preliminary analysis of the Italian study revealed no difference between the tamoxifen and placebo groups[68]; however, by the end of the trial, women in the tamoxifen arm did have a lower risk of breast cancer.[66] On the other hand, the Royal Marsden Hospital Tamoxifen Chemoprevention trial reported no differences in the tamoxifen and placebo groups.[69] Women recruited for the latter trial had a strong family history of breast cancer; because of this, it is likely that carriers of familial breast cancer genes have an intrinsically different response to estrogen antagonism. For example, a subsequent study in the same population by the NSABP group found that tamoxifen reduced breast cancer incidence by 62% in BRCA2, not BRCA1, carriers.[70] The reason why tamoxifen did not decrease breast cancer incidence among women with BRCA1 mutations may be that *BRCA1* tumors are frequently ER negative.[71] As the Royal Marsden Hospital Tamoxifen Chemoprevention Trial included women with a strong family history of breast cancer, it is possible that many of them could have been ER negative.

Because tamoxifen increases the incidence of stroke and endometrial cancers, and long-term tamoxifen treatment may eventually lead to tamoxifen-resistant breast cancers, a search for alternative agents for breast cancer prevention and therapy, such as aromatase inhibitors, is under way. Aro-

TABLE 23.4. Breast cancer prevention trials with tamoxifen and raloxifene.

Reference	*Trial*	*Sample size*	*Design*	*Intervention*	*Primary results*
Fisher[61]	Breast Cancer Prevention Trial	13,388	Randomized Trial	Tamoxifen (20mg) for 5 years	Tamoxifen reduced the risk of invasive breast cancer by 49% and the risk of noninvasive breast cancers by 50%; these effects were observed in estrogen receptor positive (ER+), not estrogen receptor negative (ER–)
Cuzick[67]	International Breast Cancer Intervention Study	7,152	Randomized Trial	Tamoxifen (20mg) for 5 years	Tamoxifen reduces the risk of breast cancer by about a third
Veronesi[68]	Italian Randomized Trial of Tamoxifen	5,408	Randomized Trial	Tamoxifen (20mg) for 5 years	Tamoxifen reduces the risk of breast cancer
Powles[69]	Royal Marsden Hospital Tamoxifen Chemoprevention Trial	2,494	Randomized Trial	Tamoxifen (20mg) up to 8 years	No differences in the tamoxifen and placebo groups
Dickler[78]	Multiple Outcomes of Raloxifene Evaluation (MORE) Trial	7,705	Randomized Trial	Raloxifene (60mg) for 4 years	65% reduction in risk of both in situ and invasive breast cancer

matase is a cytochrome P-450 enzyme that catalyzes the rate-limiting step in the synthesis of estradiol from androgens.[72] The aromatase inhibitors represent a new class of agents in the treatment and prevention of breast cancer. Recent evidence suggests that aromatase inhibitors have several advantages over tamoxifen for the prevention and treatment of breast cancer.[73–75] For example, aromatase inhibitors are effective in treating tamoxifen-resistant cancers as second-line agents, and they do not increase the risk of endometrial cancers.[76] It is likely that the aromatase inhibitors may replace tamoxifen in the management of metastatic breast cancer.[77] However, there is concern that these estrogen-lowering drugs may promote osteoporosis or decrease bone density and, in turn, increase the risk of bone fractures. Because aromatase inhibitors cannot prevent the production of estrogen by the ovaries, the use of aromatase inhibitors may be limited to postmenopausal women.

Another potential alternative to tamoxifen that prevents bone loss and does not appear to increase the risk of endometrial cancer is raloxifene.[78] Results from the Multiple Outcomes of Raloxifene Evaluation Trial showed that raloxifene has positive estrogenic effects on bone and lipid metabolism and antiestrogenic effects on breast tissue.[78] Even though this trial was designed to assess raloxifene's effect on bone density, results showed a 65% reduction in risk of both in situ and invasive breast cancer in women taking raloxifene[78]; moreover, raloxifene did not appear to increase risk of endometrial cancer. These results have led to further evaluation of raloxifene as a possible alternative to tamoxifen. Currently, raloxifene is being evaluated in the Study of Tamoxifen and Raloxifene (STAR) trial.[65]

Case Study V: Finasteride and Prostate Cancer

The Prostate Cancer Prevention Trial (PCPT) is a double-blind chemoprevention trial of prostate cancer in 18,882 nonsymptomatic, healthy men who were randomized to 5 mg/day of finasteride or placebo for 7 years.[79] Finasteride is an inhibitor of (~90% of) 5-α-reductase, an enzyme involved in hormone metabolism of testosterone to dihydrotestosterone (DHT), the most active androgen in the prostate. Intraprostatic DHT is thought to be a major stimulus for prostate cancer cell growth, as evidenced by in vitro and in vivo studies.[80,81] Thus, reducing DHT by inhibiting 5-α-reductase activity is a plausible strategy for preventing prostate cancer development.

There was significant preclinical and clinical experience with finasteride before the initiation of the PCPT. Numerous animal model studies suggested finasteride had prostate cancer preventive activity in several rats,[82] and finasteride had been approved and was in wide clinical use as treatment for benign prostatic hyperplasia.[83] The toxicity profile for finasteride was well characterized as being low and well tolerated by healthy subjects.

At the end of the 7-year trial, an endpoint biopsy was performed in all men, demonstrating a 24.8% lower cumulative incidence of prostate cancer in the finasteride compared to the placebo group.[79] However, the finasteride group also had a higher rate of high-grade cancers (higher Gleason scores) than the placebo group. In addition, men in the finasteride group reported more problems with sexual function but fewer urinary problems than men in the placebo group. Thus, this prevention trial identified multiple issues, including (1) a significantly higher detection rate in both arms of the study compared to earlier studies[84] and (2) a 27% increase in high-grade Gleason scores in the treatment arm based on central review by pathologists blinded to treatment assignment, whereas the proportion in the placebo group was similar to other series.[85] Fortunately, this was a well-designed trial with well-planned tissue collection and storage, so despite the mixed results the trial will certainly yield tremendous information about prostate carcinogenesis. Another large trial (8,000 men) using the 5-α-reductase inhibitor dutasteride for a 4-year intervention is also currently under way.[86]

Case Study VI: Calcium Supplementation and Colon Polyp Recurrence

The epidemiologic data on colon cancer incidence rates around the world, as well as the increase in rates among recent Japanese migrants to Hawaii, provide supporting evidence to the trials of high-fiber and fruit and vegetable as well as calcium supplementation and adenomatous polyp recurrence.[87] In addition, separate epidemiologic observations consistently demonstrate an inverse relation between dietary intake of calcium and incidence of colon cancer, as summarized by Sorenson et al.[88] Animal experimental research led by M. Lipkin and colleagues was the forerunner to the approach of identifying colon cell proliferation kinetics in mouse models and human subjects.[89] This team moved back and forth between the two biosystems to develop the first multistage model of colonic tumor development in 1974. Lipkin and Newmark have also demonstrated that calcium supplementation reduced cell proliferation in the mouse and in human subjects at high risk of colon cancer.[89]

Calcium Supplementation Reduces Polyp Recurrence

As summarized in Table 23.5, three trials of calcium supplementation alone (or with other micronutrients) were reported in the 1990s with the endpoint of polyp recurrence.[28,90,91] Calcium carbonate was the form of supplement administered in doses ranging from 1.6 to 3 g/day, with participants having a follow-up colonoscopy at 1 and 3 years on trial, similar to the design of the fiber, fruit, and vegetable trials. Participants in two of the three trials experienced a reduction in recurrence of 15% to 34%,[28,91] but no significant difference was found in the third trial.[90] Secondary data analysis of the third trial revealed a reduction in recurrence in patients aged less than 65 years and in those with one adenoma at baseline. There are other ongoing trials with calcium supplementation arms such as the Women's Health Initiative.[92]

Lipkin and colleagues recently completed a series of animal model experiments demonstrating the carcinogenic role of diet alone in de novo development of colon tumors, using rodents unexposed to a carcinogen but administered a "Western-style diet" of high fat, low fiber, and low calcium and other micronutrients associated with cancer prevention. This same team reported the protective effects of dietary calcium add-back to the Western-style diet to reduce risk of colon tumors in mice relative to rodents who remained on

TABLE 23.5. Colorectal neoplasia prevention trials evaluating calcium.

Reference	*Sample size*[a]	*Design/cohort*[b]	*Intervention*[c]	*Primary results*[d]
Hofstad[90]	116	DBRCT in patients with current adenomas (those <1 cm were retained)	1.6 g/day + beta-carotene 15 mg + vitamin C 150 mg + vitamin E 75 mg + selenium 101 µg/day × 36 months	Growth of small adenomas: no effect, Adenoma incidence/recurrence: increased* Fecal bile acids: no effect
Baron[91]	930	DBRCT in patients with prior adenoma	3.0 g/day × 48 months	Patients with adenoma recurrence, 19% reduction*; adenoma number, 24% reduction*
Faivre[28,111]	655	RDBCT in patients with prior adenoma; 35–75 years old	2.0 g/day (vs. 3.8 g/day ispaghula husk) vs. placebo × 36 months	Adenoma incidence/recurrence, 34% reduction (NS)
Women's Health Initiative[92]	45,000–48,000	Complex factorial, DBRCT in postmenopausal women 50–79 years old	Calcium + vitamin D; hormone replacement therapy; low-fat diet × approximately 9 years	Colorectal cancer incidence (among many others): ongoing

[a] Number randomized.

[b] Trial designs: SBRCT, single-blind, randomized, controlled trial; DBRCT, double-blind, randomized, controlled trial; DBRCXT, double-blind, randomized, controlled cross-over trial; RCXT, unblinded, randomized, controlled cross-over trial.

[c] Calcium carbonate unless noted otherwise.

[d] Proliferation assessed via random biopsies of normal appearing mucosa. NS, nonsignificant.

*Statistically significant result ($P < 0.05$).

the Western diet alone.[89] The challenges rest in how well the Western-style rodent diet is mirrored in the complex arrays of current Western-style human diets and the identification of the windows of human development that are sensitive to their reported dietary modulations.

Case Study VII: Nonsteroidal Antiinflammatory Drugs, Selective Cyclooxygenase 2 Inhibitors, and Cancer Prevention

As a class, nonsteroidal antiinflammatory drugs (NSAIDs) are structurally diverse, yet seem to share several common activities that might be relevant to the prevention of cancer. Antineoplastic effects may include modulation of cell cycle, apoptosis, proliferation, and invasion. Although many of these effects are linked to cyclooxygenase (COX) inhibitory activity, a number of COX-independent effects are well established. COX inhibition by NSAIDs is exerted on at least two distinct isoforms: COX-1 and COX-2. COX-1 is constitutively expressed in most tissues, whereas COX-2 is found generally at low levels of expression unless induced by inflammatory factors, growth factors, or tumor promoters. Most NSAIDs, including aspirin or sulindac, suppress the activities of both isozymes. This indiscriminate inhibition causes anticancer effects as well as collateral damage, including gastric ulceration and renal toxicity. COX-2-selective inhibitors (COXIBs), including celecoxib (Celebrex) and rofecoxib (Vioxx), burst on the scene in 1999 with the potential to revolutionize the relief of inflammation and pain arthritis, without the collateral side effects of aspirin and the other nonselective NSAIDs. It was soon discovered that these agents also had tremendous potential as safe and effective chemopreventive agents for some cancers. However, Vioxx was withdrawn from the market on September 30, 2004, because of concern that it increases the risk of heart attacks and strokes in patients taking it longer than 18 months.[93] Although recent findings suggest a higher risk of admission for congestive heart failure in users of rofecoxib but not celecoxib, relative to non-NSAID controls,[94] further studies and analyses are imperative to determine if the increased cardiovascular risks are limited to Vioxx or are characteristic of the entire class of COXIBs.

Evidence from Animal Studies

COX-2 is commonly overexpressed in many cancers, including many stages of colorectal carcinogenesis; some studies report overexpression in more than 50% of adenomas and more than 80% of adenocarcinomas, but it is rarely expressed in normal colorectal epithelium. The role of NSAIDs in cancer prevention was first investigated in rodent models in the early 1980s.[95] NSAIDs, such as aspirin, indomethacin, piroxicam, and sulindac, exhibited inhibitory effects on tumors of the colon; however, tumor growth often resumed when NSAIDs were discontinued. Overwhelming preclinical data suggest that COX-2 is functionally important for neoplastic progression, as evidenced by the regression of intestinal polyps in rodent models of colorectal cancer prevention as well as in COX-2-deficient mice. As recently reviewed,[96] almost 400 reports in PubMed are published on rodent models of both genetic and carcinogen-induced carcinogenesis that used NSAIDs or their derivatives. The majority of these studies demonstrate NSAIDs are relatively effective against most stages of colon cancer, including aberrant crypt foci; adenoma and adenocarcinoma multiplicity, incidence, and size; metastasis; and survival.

Nine studies of COXIBs—two with NS-398, one with MF tricyclic, two with nimesulide, one with rofecoxib, and three with celecoxib—have proved this class of chemopreventive agents is promising in reducing aberrant crypts and colorectal tumors in carcinogen-induced and genetically driven rodent models of intestinal neoplasia.[96] COX-2 is overexpressed at very early stages of colorectal carcinogenesis in animals, as reported by Oshima et al.[97] This study also showed that the COX-2-selective agent MF tricyclic was as effective as the nonselective COX inhibitor sulindac. This study further provided direct evidence of the mechanistic importance and significance of COX-2 inhibition, as COX-2 knockout (+/–, and –/–) mice had a reduction in adenomas in a dose-dependent (COX-2 gene) manner.[98]

Evidence from Epidemiologic Studies and Randomized Clinical Trials

Among 21 retrospective and 9 prospective observational studies, all but 2 reported statistically significant inverse associations between use of NSAIDs or COXIBs and colorectal neoplasia risk.[96] Reductions in neoplastic lesions by NSAIDs use ranged from 16% to 92% with an average reduction in adenomas of about 40% to 50%. In contrast, a prospective study of 12,180 individuals for 8.5 years reported an association between daily aspirin use and increased CRC risk for men (RR = 1.38) and women (RR = 1.10).[98] A major difference in this from other observational studies is that the median age of participants was 73 years. In a report from the Physicians' Health Trial and Follow-Up Study (n = 22,071 healthy men aged 40–84 years in 1982), aspirin was not associated with risk of colorectal cancer in those randomized to 325 mg every other day for the first 6 years [RR = 1.03 (95% CI = 0.83–1.28)] nor associated with risk in the postrandomization interval in men who used aspirin frequently [RR = 1.07 (95% CI = 0.75–1.53)].[99] A much larger number of studies show a positive cancer preventive effect of NSAIDs and COXIBs. In nested case-control analysis of a population-based cohort study of 940,000 individuals in the UK, a significant 40% reduction in colorectal cancer risk was reported in long-term aspirin users of 300 mg daily, but no significant benefit appeared in users of 75 or 150 mg daily.[100]

Numerous clinical trials showing protective effects of NSAIDs against colon polyp formation or colon cancer are summarized in Table 23.6. In 2003, three studies reported dramatic findings that reveal aspirin as a major player in the defense against cancer. Two randomized controlled studies considered patients at risk of colorectal cancer. Both studies found a clear reduction in polyp recurrence from aspirin use. In one study, 1,084 patients with a history of polyps were followed with a colonoscopy 3 years after their entry into the study.[101] The greatest benefit was observed in the low-dose (81 mg daily) group, who experienced an unadjusted risk ratio of 0.81 (95% CI = 0.69–0.96) whereas those in the high-dose (325 mg daily) group experienced a RR of 0.96 (95% CI = 0.81–1.13). When large or malignant polyps were considered separately, the benefits were clearer; risk ratios of 0.59 (95% CI = 0.38–0.92) in the low-dose group, and to some extent in the high-dose group (RR = 0.83; 95% CI = 0.55–1.23). The second study followed 517 patients with previous malignant CRC for a year and reported the RR for new polyps of 0.65 (95% CI = 0.46–0.91) in the 325 mg daily aspirin treatment group.[102] Meanwhile, a third study, which combined three earlier case-control studies into a cancer patient base of 965 and 1,779 controls,[103] showed a dramatic reduction in the incidence of tumors of the mouth, throat, and esophagus with long-term use of aspirin. After controlling for factors, such as smoking and diet, the incidence of the three types of cancer in people who had taken aspirin regularly for at least 5 years was a third that in nonusers [OR = 0.33 (95% CI = 0.13–0.82)]. Similarly, more than 15 case series and reports have described the benefits of NSAIDs for prevention of prevalent adenomas in persons with familial adenomatous polyposis (FAP).

Selective COX-2 inhibitors (COXIBs) recently approved for treatment and management of pain and arthritis provide a unique opportunity in terms of sparing COX-1 beneficial functions while inhibiting COX-2 in the process. On the basis of preclinical and observational studies just described, COXIBs have now advanced to human clinical trials in cancer prevention. A recent randomized, placebo-controlled trial of celecoxib administered over 6 months to 77 individuals with FAP showed significant regression and reduction in colorectal adenoma number and size. As an added benefit, celecoxib treatment also decreased duodenal polyps, suggesting a dual-organ benefit in this cohort. The importance of this study is underscored by FDA's approval of celecoxib to complement the endoscopic surveillance and prophylactic surgery in FAP individuals. Furthermore, based on these preliminary but landmark results, celecoxib is now under study in several clinical trials involving persons at elevated risk for CRC because of either a genetic predisposition or a history of prior sporadic neoplasia.

Summary and Lessons Learned

Randomized clinical trials remain the most robust test of an intervention, and a review of cancer prevention trials provides valuable lessons. In this chapter, we discussed examples of trials that highlight the effects of several prevention modalities on different stages of cancer, from late-stage intermediate endpoints (such as colon polyps) through second primary cancers (such as head and neck tumors). Of the five modalities discussed (diet, pharmacologic agents, selective hormone therapies/modulators, nonsteroidal antiinflammatory drugs, and vitamin and mineral supplements), two of the modalities, notably the NSAIDs and calcium supplements, were true successes without significant side effects. Both these interventions were effective at reducing risk of colonic malignancies, perhaps because the colon is an organ with higher cellular turnover in the adult years than other targeted organ sites.[104] The other case studies provided examples of either null results, mixed results (i.e., some preventive activity accompanied by significant adverse effects), or, in the case of the β-carotene-lung cancer trials, a small but significant cancer-enhancing effect that could only have been detected by conducting a clinical trial.

What have we learned from the failures and successes in the prevention trials? In the lung cancer prevention trials, we learned that β-carotene supplementation was the wrong intervention for individuals at high risk for lung cancer. Nonhuman primates administered β-carotene supplements had squamous metaplasia of the lungs that was markedly enhanced in the smoke exposed. In vitro work revealed that β-carotene molecules increased radical oxygen intermediates and reduced apoptosis, thereby defying the oft-cited role of β-carotene as an antioxidant and increasing its provitamin A capacity for cellular proliferation. In contrast, administration of another carotenoid, lycopene, in several doses inhibited

TABLE 23.6. Nonsteroidal antiinflammatory drugs (NSAIDs) in the prevention/treatment of sporadic colorectal adenomas or colorectal cancer prevention.

Reference	*Sample size*	*Design*	*NSAID*	*Dose and duration (months)*	*Primary result(s)*
Matsuhashi, 1997[112]	15	CS	Sulindac	300 mg po qd × 4	13 of 20 polyps in 15 patients shrank or disappeared*
Ladenheim, 1995[113]	44	DBRCT	Sulindac	150 mg po bid vs. placebo × 4	8% probability of >50% sporadic adenoma regression
Hixson, 1993[114]	9	CS	Sulindac or piroxicam	200 mg po bid (sulindac) or 20 mg po qd (piroxicam) × 6	Discontinued due to toxicity in 2; piroxicam more toxic than sulindac; no dramatic adenoma regression
Carbone, 1998[115]	Step 1 = 12 Step 2 = 31	Steps 1 & 2: CS	Piroxicam	Step 1: 10 mg po qd or qod Step 2: 10 mg po qod + DFMO 0.5 gm/m² × 6	Step 1: 10 mg qod tolerable; no changes in ODC or urinary polyamine concentrations Step 2: combination is tolerable; possible synergistic effects
Calaluce, 2000[116]	96	DBRCT	Piroxicam	7.5 mg po qd vs. placebo × 24	Reduced mucosal prostanoid concentrations*; significant GI side effects*
Chow, 2000[117]	27	DBRCT	Ibuprofen	300 or 600 mg po qd vs. placebo × 1	Reduced mucosal prostanoid concentrations*; 300 mg po qd recommended for future studies
Barnes, 1999[118]	10	DBRCXT	Aspirin	81 mg po qd vs. placebo × 3	Reduced mucosal prostanoid concentrations*; reduced TGF-α staining*; both effects returned to baseline levels following 3 months off aspirin
Ruffin, 1997[119]	65	DBRCT	Aspirin	40.5, 81, 162, 324, or 648 mg po qd vs. placebo × 2 weeks	Reduced mucosal PGE_2* with 81 mg po qd; reduced mucosal PGF_2-alpha with 40.5 mg po qd
Gann, 1994[120]	22,071	DBRCT	Aspirin	325 mg po qod vs. placebo ×60	CRC RR = 1.15 (95% CI = 0.80–1.65); In situ cancer or adenoma RR = 0.86 (95% CI = 0.68–1.10)
Baron, 2002[121]	1,121	DBRCT	Aspirin	80 mg po QD vs. 325 mg po QD vs. placebo × 48	Adenoma recurrence: all and advanced 80 mg: RR (all) = 0.81* (0.68–0.96); RR (advanced) = 0.60 (0.35–1.03) 325 mg: RR (all) = 0.96 (0.82–1.13); RR (advanced) = 0.81 (0.49–1.32)
Benamouzig, 2002[122]	291	DBRCT	Aspirin	160–300 mg po QD vs. placebo × 48	Interim adenoma recurrence at 1 year (preliminary result): OR = 0.56* (95% CI = 0.31–1.01)

Sample size is the number of subjects evaluated at study completion. Intervention is the duration of agent administration until described effect.

po, administered by mouth; qd, once per day; qod, every other day; bid, twice per day; CR, case report; CS, case series; DBRCT, double-blind, randomized, controlled trial; DBRCXT, double-blind, randomized, controlled, cross-over trial; CCTRL, case-control.

*Statistically significant result ($P < 0.05$).

bioavailable IGF-1 and reduced risk of lung cancer.[14] Baboons administered β-carotene supplements and given alcohol suffered from hepatotoxicity. Therefore, β-carotene supplementation in the presence of carcinogens—smoking and alcohol intake—increased risk, whereas lycopene reduced risk.

The finasteride and tamoxifen trials illustrate the risks and benefits of long-term pharmacologic manipulations of the sex hormones. Finasteride reduced the incidence of low- and intermediate-grade prostate cancer but increased the incidence of high-grade prostate cancer, possibly by enhancing clonal expansion of prostate cancer cells in an androgen-deficient environment. Tamoxifen reduced risk for ER+ breast cancers, but had no effect on ER– breast cancers and increased endometrial cancer risk. Side effects from an intervention may limit acceptance, as illustrated by problems in sexual function reported in the finasteride group and hot flashes in women on tamoxifen.

The timing of the intervention is an important factor, especially for the prevention of early or intermediate steps in the carcinogenesis process. From our trial examples, lung epithelium with 20–30 person-years of cigarette smoke exposure (as was the case in the β-carotene trials) might be too far along the carcinogenesis process to expect a relatively brief period of β-carotene supplementation, or other interventions that target early or intermediate cancer processes, to prevent cancer. Similarly, in the Polyp Prevention Trial, the effects of relatively brief period of dietary change late in life on polyp recurrence may have also been a case of too little too late.[27]

What have we learned from the successes? The successful trials have demonstrated proof of principle that nutritional interventions or chemopreventive agents can reduce the risk of carcinogenesis across the entire cancer spectrum, from precursor lesions to second primary tumors. The successful trials were able to avoid the pitfalls discussed above and use what turned out to be the right intervention, the right at-risk population, and the right dose and timing to hit an appropriate target for cancer prevention. Another key lesson learned from these trials is the utility of combinations of drug regimens to reduce toxicity, for example, the addition of α-tocopherol to 13-*cis* retinoic acid in the upper aerodigestive tract cancer prevention trials.

As mentioned previously, an important predictor of a successful prevention trial was the identification of the right intervention for the appropriate high-risk group or tumor type. An illustrative example is the inhibition of COX-2 activity by NSAIDs or COXIBS; these agents appear to hold great promise for the prevention of colon cancer and possibly many other cancers. It is important to note, however, that the *right* intervention does not have to be a pharmacologic agent developed to hit a specific molecular target. The example from the trials of calcium supplements to reduce polyp recurrence reminds us that a safe, inexpensive lifestyle intervention could have a large-scale public health impact. Several lifestyle interventions, including physical activity, prudent dietary change in total calories or reduction in fat intake, and increased fruit and vegetable intake, may significantly reduce the risk of many cancers.

Opportunities for tool refinement arise from the conduct of these trials. For example, dietary change from a high-fat, low-fiber to a low-fat, high-fiber, fruit and vegetable plan offered individual choice of food substitutes. However, food composition databases were not available to examine which bioactive food components reduced polyp recurrence. One of the challenges for breast cancer prevention is that 30% to 40% of breast cancer cases can be attributed to a major risk factor(s) (e.g., early age at menarche, family history), but the remainder of breast cancer patients will not be identified in the high-risk groups.[105] Risk assessment tools are important since they are used to counsel women about their disease management and to identify individuals at high risk who may be eligible for chemoprevention therapies. Risk assessment models such as the Gail model, which uses known risk factors to estimate breast cancer risk in women, may not be suitable for specific ethnic groups, such as African-Americans.[103] Indeed, few African-American women participated in the Breast Cancer Detection and Demonstration Project (BCDDP), which was the data source for the Gail model.[106] No such tools exist to assess breast cancer risk in Hispanic-white women nor are there algorithms to identify the at-risk for prostate cancer.

Concomitant with increasing longevity, a plethora of comorbidities appear in the aging population. Prescriptives, such as statins, are now being advocated for use in all Type 2 diabetics by the American College of Physicians, while over-the-counter medications, such as NSAIDs, are frequently taken in these same individuals for arthritis and other pain relief. However, the effective dose of each agent may be dependent on the disease and vary by age, gender, and the presence of other drugs. Simultaneous use of multiple therapies creates the challenge to identify appropriate dosages in combination for efficacy. An understanding of their beneficial or adverse effects in early or late stage chronic disease is essential.

A final lesson learned from the successful trials is the importance of integrating animal and human research into translational science. This approach involves linking clinical, behavioral, epidemiologic, animal, and molecular studies for a tremendously powerful approach to cancer prevention.[107] Three aspects of this integrated approach include (1) testing the efficacy and safety of the particular agent and identifying potential targets for other agents or combinations of agents; (2) having the tools available to test the efficacy of an agent at the same time as examining whether the agent confers protection from cancer and/or also increases risk of another disease; and (3) having the ability to accelerate the pace at which interventions are moved from the bench to bedside. Through the interface of animal and human explorations, calcium supplementation arose as a successful intervention for polyp recurrence and colon neoplasia with benefits for the overall biosystem. Similarly, an interdisciplinary approach led to the approval of the COX-2 inhibitor celecoxib for the prevention of familial adenomatous polyposis. Thus, perhaps the clearest lesson from this brief review of several cancer prevention trials is that future progress in cancer prevention will depend on the confluence of energies and expertise from a multidisciplinary team, as illustrated in Figure 23.2.

References

1. Peto R, Doll R, Buckley JD, Sporn MB. Can dietary beta-carotene materially reduce human cancer rates? Nature (Lond) 1981; 290(5803):201–208.
2. Peto R. Cancer, cholesterol, carotene, and tocopherol. Lancet 1981;2(8237):97–98.
3. Hursting SD, Slaga TJ, Fischer SM, DiGiovanni J, Phang JM. Mechanism-based cancer prevention approaches: targets, examples, and the use of transgenic mice. J Natl Cancer Inst 1999; 91(3):215–225.
4. Fearon ER, Vogelstein B. A genetic model for colorectal tumorigenesis. Cell 1990;61(5):759–767.
5. Stanley LA. Molecular aspects of chemical carcinogenesis: the roles of oncogenes and tumour suppressor genes. Toxicology 1995;96(3):173–194.
6. Sporn MB. Approaches to prevention of epithelial cancer during the preneoplastic period. Cancer Res 1976;36(7 pt 2):2699–2702.
7. Sporn MB, Dunlop NM, Newton DL, Smith JM. Prevention of chemical carcinogenesis by vitamin A and its synthetic analogs (retinoids). Fed Proc 1976;35(6):1332–1338.
8. Mathews-Roth MM. Beta-carotene therapy for erythropoietic protoporphyria and other photosensitivity diseases. Biochimie (Paris) 1986;68(6):875–884.
9. The effect of vitamin E and beta carotene on the incidence of lung cancer and other cancers in male smokers. The Alpha-Tocopherol, Beta Carotene Cancer Prevention Study Group. N Engl J Med 1994;330(15):1029–1035.
10. Albanes D, Heinonen OP, Taylor PR, et al. Alpha-tocopherol and beta-carotene supplements and lung cancer incidence in the alpha-tocopherol, beta-carotene cancer prevention study: effects of base-line characteristics and study compliance. J Natl Cancer Inst 1996;88(21):1560–1570.
11. Omenn GS, Goodman GE, Thornquist MD, et al. Effects of a combination of beta carotene and vitamin A on lung cancer and cardiovascular disease. N Engl J Med 1996;334(18):1150–1155.
12. Koo LC. Diet and lung cancer 20+ years later: more questions than answers? Int J Cancer 1997;10(suppl):22–29.
13. Wang XD, Liu C, Bronson RT, et al. Retinoid signaling and activator protein-1 expression in ferrets given beta-carotene supplements and exposed to tobacco smoke. J Natl Cancer Inst 1999; 91(1):60–66.
14. Liu C, Lian F, Smith DE, et al. Lycopene supplementation inhibits lung squamous metaplasia and induces apoptosis via up-

regulating insulin-like growth factor-binding protein 3 in cigarette smoke-exposed ferrets. Cancer Res 2003;63(12):3138–3144.
15. Martin KR, Saulnier MJ, Kari FW, et al. Timing of supplementation with the antioxidant *N*-acetyl-L-cysteine reduces tumor multiplicity in novel, cancer-prone p53 haploinsufficient Tg.AC (v-Ha-ras) transgenic mice but has no impact on malignant progression. Nutr Cancer 2002;43(1):59–66.
16. Brown ED, Micozzi MS, Craft NE, et al. Plasma carotenoids in normal men after a single ingestion of vegetables or purified beta-carotene. Am J Clin Nutr 1989;49(6):1258–1265.
17. Dimitrov NV, Meyer C, Ullrey DE, et al. Bioavailability of beta-carotene in humans. Am J Clin Nutr 1988;48(2):298–304.
18. Micozzi MS, Brown ED, Taylor PR, Wolfe E. Carotenodermia in men with elevated carotenoid intake from foods and beta-carotene supplements. Am J Clin Nutr 1988;48(4):1061–1064.
19. Mathews-Roth MM. Plasma concentrations of carotenoids after large doses of beta-carotene. Am J Clin Nutr 1990;52(3):500–501.
20. Albanes D, Virtamo J, Taylor PR, et al. Effects of supplemental beta-carotene, cigarette smoking, and alcohol consumption on serum carotenoids in the Alpha-Tocopherol, Beta-Carotene Cancer Prevention Study. Am J Clin Nutr 1997;66(2):366–372.
21. Locke FB, King H. Cancer mortality risk among Japanese in the United States. J Natl Cancer Inst 1980;65(5):1149–1156.
22. Reddy BS. Dietary fat and cancer: specific action or caloric effect. J Nutr 1986;116(6):1132–1135.
23. Reddy BS. Dietary fiber and colon cancer: animal model studies. Prev Med 1987;16(4):559–565.
24. Reddy BS. Prevention of colon carcinogenesis by components of dietary fiber. Anticancer Res 1999;19(5A):3681–3683.
25. Schatzkin A, Lanza E, Corle D, et al. Lack of effect of a low-fat, high-fiber diet on the recurrence of colorectal adenomas. Polyp Prevention Trial Study Group. N Engl J Med 2000;342(16):1149–1155.
26. Alberts DS, Martinez ME, Roe DJ, et al. Lack of effect of a high-fiber cereal supplement on the recurrence of colorectal adenomas. Phoenix Colon Cancer Prevention Physicians' Network. N Engl J Med 2000;342(16):1156–1162.
27. MacLennan R, Macrae F, Bain C, et al. Randomized trial of intake of fat, fiber, and beta carotene to prevent colorectal adenomas. The Australian Polyp Prevention Project. J Natl Cancer Inst 1995;87(23):1760–1766.
28. Bonithon-Kopp C, Kronborg O, et al. Calcium and fibre supplementation in prevention of colorectal adenoma recurrence: a randomised intervention trial. European Cancer Prevention Organisation Study Group. Lancet 2000;356(9238):1300–1306.
29. McKeown-Eyssen GE, Bright-See E, Bruce WR, et al. A randomized trial of a low fat high fibre diet in the recurrence of colorectal polyps. Toronto Polyp Prevention Group. J Clin Epidemiol 1994;47(5):525–536.
30. Lanza E, Schatzkin A, Daston C, et al. Implementation of a 4-y, high-fiber, high-fruit-and-vegetable, low-fat dietary intervention: results of dietary changes in the Polyp Prevention Trial. Am J Clin Nutr 2001;74(3):387–401.
31. Willett WC. Nutritional Epidemiology. New York: Oxford University Press, 1999.
32. Mangels AR, Holden JM, Beecher GR, et al. Carotenoid content of fruits and vegetables: an evaluation of analytic data. J Am Diet Assoc 1993;93(3):284–296.
33. Michels KB, Edward G, Joshipura KJ, et al. Prospective study of fruit and vegetable consumption and incidence of colon and rectal cancers. J Natl Cancer Inst 2000;92(21):1740–1752.
34. Fuchs CS, Giovannucci EL, Colditz GA, et al. Dietary fiber and the risk of colorectal cancer and adenoma in women. N Engl J Med 1999;340(3):169–176.
35. Peters U, Sinha R, Chatterjee N, et al. Dietary fibre and colorectal adenoma in a colorectal cancer early detection programme. Lancet 2003;361(9368):1491–1495.
36. Bingham SA, Day NE, Luben R, et al. Dietary fibre in food and protection against colorectal cancer in the European Prospective Investigation into Cancer and Nutrition (EPIC): an observational study. Lancet 2003;361(9368):1496–1501.
37. Kim ES, Hong WK, Khuri FR. Chemoprevention of aerodigestive tract cancers. Annu Rev Med 2002;53:223–243.
38. Hong WK, Endicott J, Itri LM, et al. 13-cis-Retinoic acid in the treatment of oral leukoplakia. N Engl J Med 1986;315(24):1501–1505.
39. Lippman SM, Batsakis JG, Toth BB, et al. Comparison of low-dose isotretinoin with beta carotene to prevent oral carcinogenesis. N Engl J Med 1993;328(1):15–20.
40. Papadimitrakopoulou VA, Hong WK, Lee JS, et al. Low-dose isotretinoin versus beta-carotene to prevent oral carcinogenesis: long-term follow-up. J Natl Cancer Inst 1997;89(3):257–258.
41. Tsiklakis K, Papadakou A, Angelopoulos AP. The therapeutic effect of an aromatic retinoid (RO-109359) on hamster buccal pouch carcinomas. Oral Surg Oral Med Oral Pathol 1987;64(3):327–332.
42. Alam BS, Alam SQ. The effect of different levels of dietary beta-carotene on DMBA-induced salivary gland tumors. Nutr Cancer 1987;9(2–3):93–101.
43. Stich HF, Tsang SS. Promoting activity of betel quid ingredients and their inhibition by retinol. Cancer Lett 1989;45(1):71–77.
44. Lee JJ, Hong WK, Hittelman WN, et al. Predicting cancer development in oral leukoplakia: ten years of translational research. Clin Cancer Res 2000;6(5):1702–1710.
45. Sun SY, Yue P, Wu GS, et al. Implication of p53 in growth arrest and apoptosis induced by the synthetic retinoid CD437 in human lung cancer cells. Cancer Res 1999;59(12):2829–2833.
46. Sun SY, Yue P, Kelloff GJ, et al. Identification of retinamides that are more potent than N-(4-hydroxyphenyl)retinamide in inhibiting growth and inducing apoptosis of human head and neck and lung cancer cells. Cancer Epidemiol Biomarkers Prev 2001;10(6):595–601.
47. Lippman SM, Shin DM, Lee JJ, et al. p53 and retinoid chemoprevention of oral carcinogenesis. Cancer Res 1995;55(1):16–9.
48. Papadimitrakopoulou VA, Clayman GL, Shin DM, et al. Biochemoprevention for dysplastic lesions of the upper aerodigestive tract. Arch Otolaryngol Head Neck Surg 1999;125(10):1083–1089.
49. Mao L, El-Naggar AK, Papadimitrakopoulou V, et al. Phenotype and genotype of advanced premalignant head and neck lesions after chemopreventive therapy. J Natl Cancer Inst 1998;90(20):1545–1551.
50. Shin DM, Mao L, Papadimitrakopoulou VM, et al. Biochemopreventive therapy for patients with premalignant lesions of the head and neck and p53 gene expression. J Natl Cancer Inst 2000;92(1):69–73.
51. Hong WK, Lippman SM, Itri LM, et al. Prevention of second primary tumors with isotretinoin in squamous-cell carcinoma of the head and neck. N Engl J Med 1990;323(12):795–801.
52. Benner SE, Pajak TF, Lippman SM, et al. Prevention of second primary tumors with isotretinoin in patients with squamous cell carcinoma of the head and neck: long-term follow-up. J Natl Cancer Inst 1994;86(2):140–141.
53. Khuri FR, Kim ES, Lee JJ, et al. The impact of smoking status, disease stage, and index tumor site on second primary tumor incidence and tumor recurrence in the head and neck retinoid chemoprevention trial. Cancer Epidemiol Biomarkers Prev 2001;10(8):823–829.
54. Spitz MR, Fueger JJ, Beddingfield NA, et al. Chromosome sensitivity to bleomycin-induced mutagenesis, an independent risk factor for upper aerodigestive tract cancers. Cancer Res 1989;49(16):4626–4628.
55. Wu X, Gu J, Hong WK, et al. Benzo[*a*]pyrene diol epoxide and bleomycin sensitivity and susceptibility to cancer of upper aerodigestive tract. J Natl Cancer Inst 1998;90(18):1393–1399.

56. Spitz MR, Hoque A, Trizna Z, et al. Mutagen sensitivity as a risk factor for second malignant tumors following malignancies of the upper aerodigestive tract. J Natl Cancer Inst 1994;86(22): 1681–1684.
57. Jemal A, Murray T, Samuels A, et al. Cancer statistics, 2003. CA Cancer J Clin 2003;53(1):5–26.
58. Weir HK, Thun MJ, Hankey BF, et al. Annual report to the nation on the status of cancer, 1975–2000, featuring the uses of surveillance data for cancer prevention and control. J Natl Cancer Inst 2003;95(17):1276–1299.
59. Tamoxifen for early breast cancer: an overview of the randomised trials. Early Breast Cancer Trialists' Collaborative Group. Lancet 1998;351(9114):1451–1467.
60. Cuzick J, Baum M. Tamoxifen and contralateral breast cancer. Lancet 1985;2(8449):282.
61. Fisher B, Jeong JH, Dignam J, et al. Findings from recent National Surgical Adjuvant Breast and Bowel Project adjuvant studies in stage I breast cancer. J Natl Cancer Inst Monogr 2001(30):62–66.
62. Effects of adjuvant tamoxifen and of cytotoxic therapy on mortality in early breast cancer. An overview of 61 randomized trials among 28,896 women. Early Breast Cancer Trialists' Collaborative Group. N Engl J Med 1988;319(26):1681–1692.
63. Controlled trial of tamoxifen as adjuvant agent in management of early breast cancer. Interim analysis at four years by Nolvadex Adjuvant Trial Organisation. Lancet 1983;1(8319):257–261.
64. Dunn BK, Ford LG. From adjuvant therapy to breast cancer prevention: BCPT and STAR. Breast J 2001;7(3):144–157.
65. Jordan VC, Fritz NF, Langan-Fahey S, et al. Alteration of endocrine parameters in premenopausal women with breast cancer during long-term adjuvant therapy with tamoxifen as the single agent. J Natl Cancer Inst 1991;83(20):1488–1491.
66. Veronesi U, Maisonneuve P, Rotmensz N, et al. Italian randomized trial among women with hysterectomy: tamoxifen and hormone-dependent breast cancer in high-risk women. J Natl Cancer Inst 2003;95(2):160–165.
67. Cuzick J, Forbes J, Edwards R, et al. First results from the International Breast Cancer Intervention Study (IBIS-I): a randomised prevention trial. Lancet 2002;360(9336):817–824.
68. Veronesi U, Maisonneuve P, Costa A, et al. Prevention of breast cancer with tamoxifen: preliminary findings from the Italian randomised trial among hysterectomised women. Italian Tamoxifen Prevention Study. Lancet 1998;352(9122): 93–97.
69. Powles T, Eeles R, Ashley S, et al. Interim analysis of the incidence of breast cancer in the Royal Marsden Hospital tamoxifen randomised chemoprevention trial. Lancet 1998;352(9122): 98–101.
70. King MC, Wieand S, Hale K, et al. Tamoxifen and breast cancer incidence among women with inherited mutations in BRCA1 and BRCA2: National Surgical Adjuvant Breast and Bowel Project (NSABP-P1) Breast Cancer Prevention Trial. JAMA 2001; 286(18):2251–2256.
71. Couzin J. Choices—and uncertainties—for women with BRCA mutations. Science 2003;302(5645):592.
72. Coombes RC, Hall E, Gibson LJ, et al. A randomized trial of exemestane after two to three years of tamoxifen therapy in postmenopausal women with primary breast cancer. N Engl J Med 2004;350(11):1081–1092.
73. Mouridsen H, Gershanovich M, Sun Y, et al. Superior efficacy of letrozole versus tamoxifen as first-line therapy for postmenopausal women with advanced breast cancer: results of a phase III study of the International Letrozole Breast Cancer Group. J Clin Oncol 2001;19(10):2596–2606.
74. Goss PE, Ingle JN, Martino S, et al. A randomized trial of letrozole in postmenopausal women after five years of tamoxifen therapy for early-stage breast cancer. N Engl J Med 2003;349(19): 1793–1802.
75. Long BJ, Jelovac D, Handratta V, et al. Therapeutic strategies using the aromatase inhibitor letrozole and tamoxifen in a breast cancer model. J Natl Cancer Inst 2004;96(6):456–465.
76. Brodie A. Aromatase inhibitors and the application to the treatment of breast cancer. In: Pasqualini J (ed). Breast Cancer: Prognosis, Treatment and Prevention. New York: Dekker, 2002: 251–270.
77. Mouridsen H, Gershanovich M. The role of aromatase inhibitors in the treatment of metastatic breast cancer. Semin Oncol 2003; 30(4 suppl 14):33–45.
78. Dickler MN, Norton L. The MORE trial: multiple outcomes for raloxifene evaluation—breast cancer as a secondary end point: implications for prevention. Ann NY Acad Sci 2001;949:134–142.
79. Thompson IM, Goodman PJ, Tangen CM, et al. The influence of finasteride on the development of prostate cancer. N Engl J Med 2003;349(3):215–224.
80. Kadohama N, Karr JP, Murphy GP, Sandberg AA. Selective inhibition of prostatic tumor 5 alpha-reductase by a 4-methyl-4-azasteroid. Cancer Res 1984;44(11):4947–4954.
81. Petrow V, Padilla GM, Mukherji S, Marts SA. Endocrine dependence of prostatic cancer upon dihydrotestosterone and not upon testosterone. J Pharm Pharmacol 1984;36(5):352–353.
82. Huynh H. Induction of apoptosis in rat ventral prostate by finasteride is associated with alteration in MAP kinase pathways and Bcl-2 related family of proteins. Int J Oncol 2002;20(6): 1297–1303.
83. Doggrell SA. Combination of finasteride and doxazosin for the treatment of benign prostatic hyperplasia. Expert Opin Pharmacother 2004;5(5):1209–1211.
84. Punglia RS, D'Amico AV, Catalona WJ, et al. Effect of verification bias on screening for prostate cancer by measurement of prostate-specific antigen. N Engl J Med 2003;349(4):335–342.
85. Scardino PT. The prevention of prostate cancer—the dilemma continues. N Engl J Med 2003;349(3):297–299.
86. Barqawi A, Thompson IM, Crawford ED. Prostate cancer chemoprevention: an overview of United States trials. J Urol 2004; 171(2 pt 2):S5–S8; discussion S9.
87. Holt PR. Dairy foods and prevention of colon cancer: human studies. J Am Coll Nutr 1999;18(5 suppl):379S–391S.
88. Sorenson AW, Slattery ML, Ford MH. Calcium and colon cancer: a review. Nutr Cancer 1988;11(3):135–145.
89. Lipkin M. Early development of cancer chemoprevention clinical trials: studies of dietary calcium as a chemopreventive agent for human subjects. Eur J Cancer Prev 2002;11(suppl 2): S65–S670.
90. Hofstad B, Almendingen K, Vatn M, et al. Growth and recurrence of colorectal polyps: a double-blind 3-year intervention with calcium and antioxidants. Digestion 1998;59(2):148–156.
91. Baron JA, Beach M, Mandel JS, et al. Calcium supplements for the prevention of colorectal adenomas. Calcium Polyp Prevention Study Group. N Engl J Med 1999;340(2):101–107.
92. Design of the Women's Health Initiative clinical trial and observational study. The Women's Health Initiative Study Group. Control Clin Trials 1998;19(1):61–109.
93. FitzGerald GA. Coxibs and cardiovascular disease. N Engl J Med 351:1709–1711.
94. Mamdani M, Juurlink DN, Lee DS, et al. Cyclo-oxygenase-2 inhibitors versus non-selective non-steroidal anti-inflammatory drugs and congestive heart failure outcomes in elderly patients: a population-based cohort study. Lancet 2004;363(9423):1751–1756.
95. Pollard M, Luckert PH. Indomethacin treatment of rats with dimethylhydrazine-induced intestinal tumors. Cancer Treat Rep 1980;64(12):1323–1327.
96. Hawk ET, Viner JL, Umar A, et al. Cancer and the cyclooxygenase enzyme: implications for the treatment and prevention. Am J Cancer 2003;2(1):27–55.

97. Oshima M, Dinchuk JE, Kargman SL, et al. Suppression of intestinal polyposis in Apc delta716 knockout mice by inhibition of cyclooxygenase 2 (COX-2). Cell 1996;87(5):803–809.
98. Paganini-Hill A, Hsu G, Ross RK, Henderson BE. Aspirin use and incidence of large-bowel cancer in a California retirement community. J Natl Cancer Inst 1991;83(16):1182–1183.
99. Sturmer T, Glynn RJ, Lee IM, et al. Aspirin use and colorectal cancer: post-trial follow-up data from the Physicians' Health Study. Ann Intern Med 1998;128(9):713–720.
100. Garcia Rodriguez LA, Huerta-Alvarez C. Reduced incidence of colorectal adenoma among long-term users of nonsteroidal antiinflammatory drugs: a pooled analysis of published studies and a new population-based study. Epidemiology 2000;11(4):376–381.
101. Baron JA, Cole BF, Sandler RS, et al. A randomized trial of aspirin to prevent colorectal adenomas. N Engl J Med 2003;348(10): 891–899.
102. Sandler RS, Halabi S, Baron JA, et al. A randomized trial of aspirin to prevent colorectal adenomas in patients with previous colorectal cancer. N Engl J Med 2003;348(10):883–890.
103. Bosetti C, Talamini R, Franceschi S, et al. Aspirin use and cancers of the upper aerodigestive tract. Br J Cancer 2003;88(5): 672–674.
104. Iyngkaran N, Yadav M, Boey CG, Lam KL. Severity and extent of upper small bowel mucosal damage in cow's milk proteinsensitive enteropathy. J Pediatr Gastroenterol Nutr 1988;7(5): 667–674.
105. Helzlsouer KJ. Early detection and prevention of breast cancer. In: Greenwald P, Kramer BS, Weed DL (eds). Cancer Prevention and Control. New York: Dekker, 1995:509–535.
106. Bondy ML, Newman LA. Breast cancer risk assessment models: applicability to African-American women. Cancer (Phila) 2003; 97(suppl 1):230–235.
107. Tsao AS, Kim ES, Hong WK. Chemoprevention of cancer. CA Cancer J Clin 2004;54(3):150–180.
108. DeCosse JJ, Miller HH, Lesser ML. Effect of wheat fiber and vitamins C and E on rectal polyps in patients with familial adenomatous polyposis. J Natl Cancer Inst 1989;81(17):1290–1297.
109. Martinez ME, Reid ME, Guillen-Rodriguez J, et al. Design and baseline characteristics of study participants in the Wheat Bran Fiber trial. Cancer Epidemiol Biomarkers Prev 1998;7(9):813–816.
110. Earnest DL, Sampliner RE, Roe DJ, et al. Progress report: the Arizona phase III study of the effect of wheat bran fiber on recurrence of adenomatous colon polyps. Am J Med 1999;106(1A): 43S–45S.
111. Faivre J, Couillault C, Kronborg O, et al. Chemoprevention of metachronous adenomas of the large bowel: design and interim results of a randomized trial of calcium and fibre. ECP Colon Group. Eur J Cancer Prev 1997;6(2):132–138.
112. Matsuhashi N, Nakajima A, Fukushima Y, et al. Effects of sulindac on sporadic colorectal adenomatous polyps. Gut 1997;40(3): 344–349.
113. Ladenheim J, Garcia G, Titzer D, et al. Effect of sulindac on sporadic colonic polyps. Gastroenterology 1995;108(4):1083–1087.
114. Hixson LJ, Earnest DL, Fennerty MB, Sampliner RE. NSAID effect on sporadic colon polyps. Am J Gastroenterol 1993;88(10): 1652–1656.
115. Carbone PP, Douglas JA, Larson PO, et al. Phase I chemoprevention study of piroxicam and alpha-difluoromethylornithine. Cancer Epidemiol Biomarkers Prev 1998;7(10):907–912.
116. Calaluce R, Earnest DL, Heddens D, et al. Effects of piroxicam on prostaglandin E2 levels in rectal mucosa of adenomatous polyp patients: a randomized phase IIb trial. Cancer Epidemiol Biomarkers Prev 2000;9(12):1287–1292.
117. Chow HH, Earnest DL, Clark D, et al. Effect of subacute ibuprofen dosing on rectal mucosal prostaglandin E2 levels in healthy subjects with a history of resected polyps. Cancer Epidemiol Biomarkers Prev 2000;9(4):351–356.
118. Barnes CJ, Hamby-Mason RL, Hardman WE, et al. Effect of aspirin on prostaglandin E2 formation and transforming growth factor alpha expression in human rectal mucosa from individuals with a history of adenomatous polyps of the colon. Cancer Epidemiol Biomarkers Prev 1999;8(4 pt 1):311–315.
119. Ruffin MT, Krishnan K, Rock CL, et al. Suppression of human colorectal mucosal prostaglandins: determining the lowest effective aspirin dose. J Natl Cancer Inst 1997;89(15):1152–1160.
120. Gann PH, Manson JE, Glynn RJ, Buring JE, Hennekens CH. Lowdose aspirin and incidence of colorectal tumors in a randomized trial. J Natl Cancer Inst 1993;85(15):1220–1224.
121. Baron JA, Cole BF, Mott LA, et al. Aspirin chemoprevention of colorectal adenomas. Proc AACR 2002;43:669.
122. Benamouzig R, Deyra J, Martin A, et al. Efficacy of lysin acetylsalicylate to prevent colorectal adenomas: one year results of the APACC Randomized Trial. Gastroenterology 2002;122:A70 (abstract).

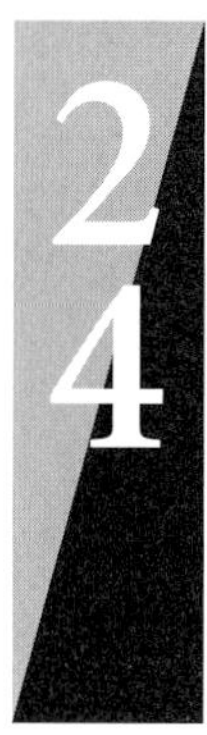

Screening

Stephen H. Taplin, Sarah Dash, Paula Zeller, and Jane Zapka

Proving the Efficacy of Screening Tests Is Only the Beginning

Primary care providers, including physicians, nurse practitioners, physician assistants, and the people who work with them, operate at the interface of the medical and lay communities. It is frequently stated that one in eight women gets breast cancer sometime in her lifetime. Oncologists consider the care of that one woman and others like her, whereas primary care physicians work with all eight, seven of whom will not get cancer. Oncologists deal directly with the consequences of delayed diagnoses and the morbidity of late-stage diagnoses while primary care physicians see the effects of false-positive tests. The difference in populations affects how each healthcare provider judges the evidence regarding cancer screening and may tip decisions in different directions in the face of ambiguity. However, ultimately the decision to encourage screening does depend on evidence. This chapter is about the evidence-based daily practice of screening in the primary care setting, where providers discuss screening, cancer, and the consequences of each.

Screening looks for cancers or precancerous lesions before the disease has had a chance to appear symptomatically. Some call this *early detection*. Because the idea that early detection saves lives has become so intuitively appealing, cancer screening captures the imagination and emotions of individuals, their families, and their physicians.[1] The appeal is so high that 87% of U.S. adults surveyed in 2002 believed that routine screening is almost always good, and 74% believe that finding cancer early saves lives most or all of the time.[1]

The medical community operates from a different paradigm and does not have such faith in screening.[1,2] Clinicians must "first, do no harm" and are compelled to identify an overall benefit before offering a test. Much of the controversy regarding screening is about whether it offers a net benefit—and by that we mean whether it reduces mortality. To reduce mortality, screening must meet at least two conditions: (1) that the test can find a cancer or precursor to cancer before it becomes symptomatic; and (2) that treating an early lesion changes the natural history of the disease and gains additional life for the patient. For example, at the center of the debate about prostate cancer screening is the fact that many men die of other causes even when prostate cancer is present, so it is not clear that all prostate cancer treatment contributes to additional life.

Even if it can be shown that cancer screening saves lives, there are serious concerns about its potentially negative impact on people who will never get the disease. Unnecessary biopsies, additional tests, and the treatment of conditions that do not represent disease are common concerns. These concerns have generated major debates and a careful approach by the medical community to deciding whether and how often to recommend cancer screening[3–5] (see Chapter 12). The medical community's approach to screening recommendations includes identifying that the cancer has a substantial impact on society, there is a presymptomatic stage, the cancer can be found by screening during this stage, finding the cancer early leads to additional life compared with waiting for symptomatic detection, and the benefit of screening is worth the risk.[6] Using such an approach, the U.S. Preventive Services Task Force (USPSTF) sorted through the evidence and reached the conclusion that screening for cervical, colon, and breast cancers is beneficial.[7–9] The American Cancer Society agrees.[10] Prostate cancer is more controversial.[11] This chapter summarizes the evidence regarding the benefit of currently available screening tests for breast, cervical, colon, and prostate cancers among average-risk individuals. Genetic screening (which is covered in Chapter 26) is not discussed here because it is not recommended for average-risk people. Similarly, screening for new cancers or recurrence after a cancer diagnosis is a special case that is not considered here; however, it is covered in Chapter 102.

Screening Is a Process

Understanding the literature on the benefit of screening in average-risk populations is a necessary step toward evidence-based practice, but it is only the beginning. Although there is a great deal of discussion about the various screening tests, it is really the entire screening process that matters. The test is only one part of a screening process that begins with the recruitment of eligible people and continues by conducting the screening test, evaluating those with positive results, and treating those with disease (Figure 24.1).[12] A successful screening process means mortality is reduced because those steps and transitions occur. For example, the proportion of people who make the transition from a positive test to evaluation and treatment varies between 27% and 93%, depending upon the screening test, the person's insurance status, patient and provider factors, and the organization of the healthcare setting in which the test is administered.[13] Making sure that transition occurs is the final subject of this chapter, and it is clear that without it screening cannot have an impact on mortality.

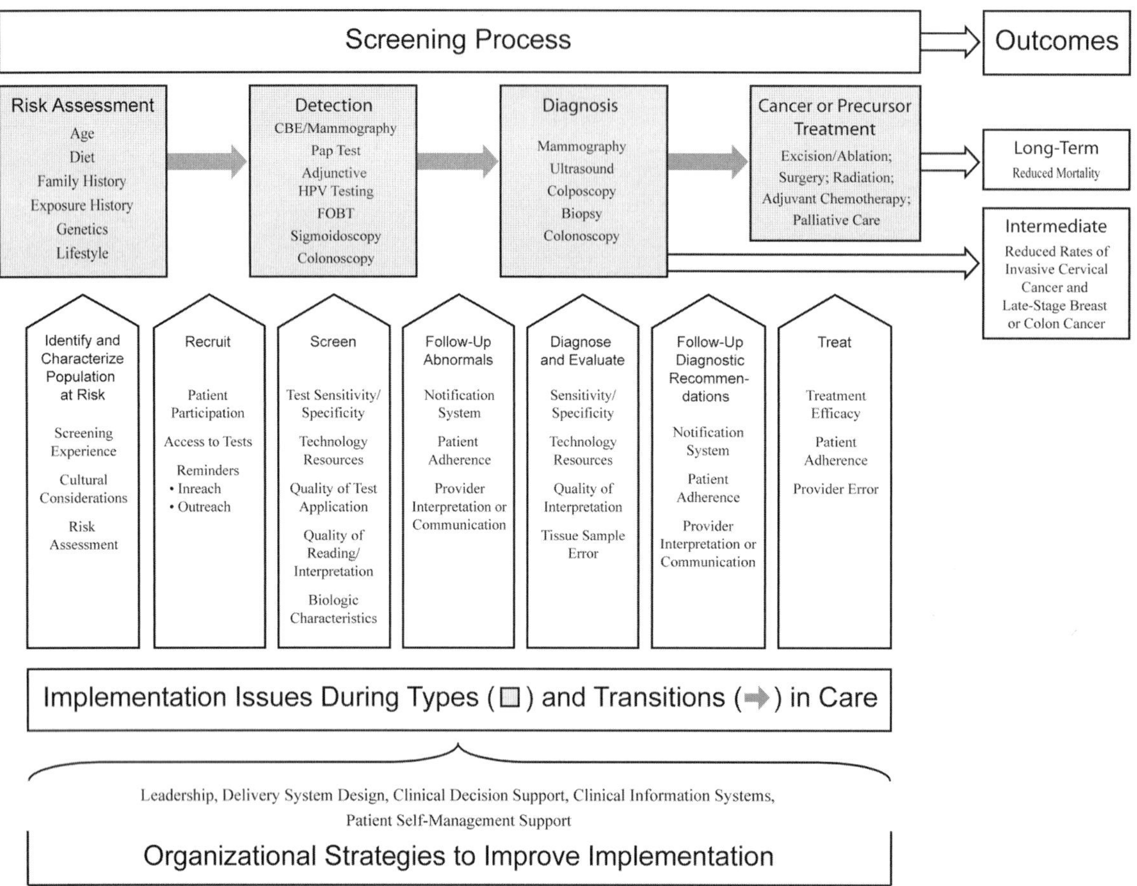

FIGURE 24.1. The screening process involves types of care and the transitions between them. (Adapted from Zapka et al.,[12] by permission of *Cancer Epidemiology Biomarkers & Prevention*.)

The Evidence for Screening

Clinicians and scientists have difficulty proving the intuitive notion that early detection results in longer life, because the observation of selected cases is deceiving and ascertainment of all relevant data for an entire population is difficult. Collections of cancer cases from a practice or screening center do not represent the full spectrum of the disease, so conclusions are not valid for the condition as a whole. Furthermore, watching cases from the day of diagnosis forward almost always makes survival look better for those at early cancer stages because there is more observation time, not necessarily because the process adds years to patients' lives.

People evaluating screening tests hope to minimize bias by designing and conducting studies carefully. Randomized trials reduce concerns about the inference drawn because it is more likely that the intervention and control populations are comparable, but how the study is implemented also influences its quality. Randomization, cause-of-death assessment, selection bias, and population characteristics all can affect inferences drawn from a study, and these factors can also affect whether the conclusions apply to the general population. The risk of these biases differs with study designs and has led the medical community to rank the design types based on the ability to draw valid conclusions. The highest quality results are likely to come from well-conducted randomized trials because they create similar groups and allow the assignment of an intervention to one of the groups so that selection bias is avoided.[14] One persistent concern, however, is that people willing to be in a randomized trial differ from people in the general population. Data from case-control studies are rated below randomized trials but allow for assessment of factors associated with rare conditions. The limitation of this design is that conclusions are affected by how well the cases and controls reflect similar populations and whether all potential confounders and effect modifiers have been identified.[15] Despite being considered of lower quality, observational studies can provide powerful insights when conducted where comprehensive data are collected for entire populations.[16–19] Such studies are especially important for evaluating whether the impact of screening in practice is consistent with expectations from randomized trials. In fact, some recent analyses show that well-designed and carefully conducted observational studies of interventions may obtain results that are indistinguishable from randomized trials.[19,20] Given the rapid progression of technology, observational studies are a necessary part of evaluating new technologies that may be implemented in practice before randomized trials can be conducted.

The following section summarizes the evidence on screening for breast, cervical, colon, and prostate cancers, covering the following topics: (1) epidemiology and natural history; (2) screening test characteristics; (3) review of the literature on benefit; and (4) summary recommendations from the American Cancer Society (ACS) and the U.S. Preventive Services Task Force (USPSTF), the organizations to which U.S. primary care practitioners look most often for recommendations.[6,10] Specialty societies such as the American Academy of Family Physicians, American Academy of Obstetrics and Gynecology, American Academy of Physicians, and American College of Gastroenterology have also reviewed the evidence. We have included the recommendations that most strongly influence primary care, recognizing that providers are also strongly influenced by their patients and colleagues.[21]

The test characteristics discussed in this chapter include sensitivity, specificity, and positive predictive value. "Sensitivity" is the ability of a test to find the screened-for condition when it is present. "Specificity" is the ability of the test to determine that the screened-for condition is absent when the screened person is disease free. The "positive predictive value" (PPV) of a test is the proportion of positive tests due to the condition of interest.

Breast Cancer Screening

Epidemiology and Natural History

New invasive breast cancer was expected to affect 215,990 U.S. women in 2004; an additional 59,390 will have had in situ disease.[22,23] One in 8.3 women will have breast cancer sometime in her lifetime, assuming she lives to age 85.[24] The incidence of invasive breast cancer rises from about 43.5 in 100,000 among women aged under 40 to more than 468 in 100,000 among women aged over 75 years.[25] Breast cancer incidence is lower among African-Americans than Caucasian-Americans (121.7 versus 140.8 in 100,000), but higher than in Asian-Americans (121.7 versus 97.2 in 100,000).[26] An estimated 40,580 women in the United States will have died of breast cancer in 2004. Although the risk of death due to breast cancer for all races has decreased since the 1970s, African-Americans are more likely to die of breast cancer today than in 1969.[26]

An important factor in screening is the *sojourn time*, defined as the length of time from when a cancer can be found in humans by a particular technology to when it has grown enough to cause symptoms.[27]By contrast, *lead time* is the length of time between when a cancer is actually found by a screening test and when it would become symptomatic. Screening must occur at intervals that are the same or shorter than the sojourn time.

The heterogeneity of breast cancer biology poses challenges for screening. Although the estimated sojourn time for a breast cancer is about 2 years among women ages 40 to 49, it may be as long as 4 years among women ages 60 to 69.[28,29] Although some ductal carcinoma in situ (DCIS) progresses to invasive disease, some does not,[30] and much invasive cancer arises in the ducts and lobules of the breast without an in situ component being apparent.[27] Investigators are evaluating whether biologic markers such as high- and low-grade nuclear changes, rather than morphology, would clarify whether some of what we call DCIS is actually a benign condition that does not need treatment.[27] This important issue is at the heart of some people's concern about screening, because fully 16% of cancers found at screening in the United States are DCIS.[31]

Screening Tests

There are four tests commonly discussed for breast cancer screening: clinical breast examination, breast self-examination, film-screen mammography, and digital mammography. Table 24.1 summarizes the characteristics of these tests. Breast self-examination has been encouraged for years and consists of women systematically searching their own breasts in both supine and upright positions. Clinical breast examination is a similar systematic search by the healthcare provider.[32]

TABLE 24.1. Summary of screening test characteristics: breast cancer.

Test	*Sensitivity*	*Specificity*	*Who administers*	*% Positive in practice*	*Recommended follow-up*	*Comment*
Film-screen mammography[7,43]	77%–96%	94%–97%	Radiologists	10%–12%	Additional mammography Ultrasound Clinical evaluation Biopsy	By definition, only cancers that are referred for biopsy will be identified and make up the denominator for these estimates. This verification bias results in an overestimate of the sensitivity.
Digital mammography[43]	64%	86%	Radiologists	12%	Additional mammography Ultrasound Clinical evaluation Biopsy	A randomized trial of digital mammography compared with film-screen mammography began in 2001.
Clinical breast examination[32,194,195]	17%–58%	94%	Clinicians	7%	Mammography Surgical evaluation	Testing sensitivity of clinical breast examination (CBE) is often done against mammography so the distribution of cancer sizes includes very small tumors.
Breast self-examination[53]	42%–72%	N/A	Women	N/A	Clinical evaluation	These estimates are based on testing women on silicone models.

Film-screen mammography uses low-dose radiation, radiographic film, and equipment dedicated to breast imaging. Two plates on the machine compress the breast so that the radiation dosage is minimized. The process is highly regulated by the Mammography Quality Standards Act (MQSA), which specifies parameters for technical (radiation exposure, development, etc.) and clinical (positioning, contrast, etc.) image quality. Since the passage of the Act in 1992, technical image quality in the United States has improved,[33] but there are persistent concerns about the quality of the clinical image and reader's interpretations.[34–36]

The American College of Radiology has created guidelines for the terminology used to describe and summarize findings on film-screen mammography.[37] These guidelines encourage consistent assessments and explain how to measure interpretive performance using the following terminology: 0, need additional imaging and/or prior mammogram for comparison; 1, normal; 2, benign finding; 3, probably benign finding—initial short-interval follow-up suggested; 4, suspicious abnormality—biopsy should be considered; and 5, highly suggestive of malignancy—appropriate action should be taken.[38] The American College of Radiology updated their assessment categories in 2003 and added a sixth category for images done after a breast cancer has been identified by biopsy.

Film-screen mammography sensitivity varies between 77% and 96%, although most healthcare providers expect a sensitivity of approximately 80% in clinical practice.[39,40] Many factors influence the sensitivity of film-screen mammography, including younger age of patients, dense breast parenchyma, and having been screened within 1 or 2 years of the current mammogram.[7,40,41] Specificity varies between 94% and 97% and is also influenced by these factors. For film-screen mammography, PPV is between 2% and 12% when a positive test is defined as one that leads to any additional evaluation with more mammograms, ultrasound, or visits to a clinician. The proportion of women found to have cancer among those referred to biopsy is higher (20% to 75%) because those women frequently have already been evaluated by ultrasound or additional mammographic imaging.[7]

Digital mammography uses equipment dedicated to breast imaging similar to film-screen mammography, but with a different receptor that creates the potential for a dynamic image.[42] Photons that pass through the breast are collected by the receptor and counted. The information is digitized to allow display as a function of the photon count associated with a square micrometer of breast tissue. Unlike film-screen mammograms, which are preserved as fixed images similar to photographs, digital mammography stores data that can be manipulated by the radiologist.

The challenge in digital mammography is how to record and display the wealth of data that can be collected. For example, one receptor in digital mammography can detect and record up to 246 shades of gray. Designers make trade-offs between information devoted to recording this contrast and information needed to establish spatial relationships.[42] The radiologist can print a hard-copy image or review the image on a cathode-ray tube display (soft copy).

Digital mammography is not widely used because its advantages over film-screen techniques have not been proven.[43] Recent work from a randomized trial suggests that digital and film-screen mammography have comparable accuracy, but the number of women recalled for additional imaging is lower with digital mammography.[4] A randomized trial comparing digital mammography with film-screen mammography began in 2001.[44]

Computer-assisted reading uses software to analyze the output of digital mammography or the digitized image from equipment that scans a film-screen mammogram. The computer analysis identifies and marks areas of concern and displays them on an image shown on a cathode-ray tube adjacent to the view box where the original image is reviewed. Some, but not all, evaluations have shown that its use increases detection,[45,46] and it has been approved by the U.S. Food and Drug Administration (FDA) for the second reading of films.[45]

Other technologies, such as ultrasound, are used for breast imaging but are not approved for screening use by the FDA. Ultrasound's application involves scanning the breast with a hand-held transducer that projects sound waves and captures them bouncing off the tissue. This information is processed to provide two-dimensional images that can be recorded on film and displayed on a lighted box as with any radiologic image.[47] Ultrasound is time intensive and subject to some subjectivity because the operator must decide which images to record and how carefully to scan the breast, limiting this technology's effectiveness for screening. On the other hand, it is used effectively for the diagnostic workup of palpable lesions or abnormalities found via mammography.[48]

Although it is possible to identify individuals at high risk for breast cancer due to genetic defects, this is not recommended for the general population.[49,50] As noted in Chapter 19, the search for genetic defects usually begins with the affected individual and then proceeds to the family if a defect is found. Currently, less than 10% of breast cancers are estimated to be associated with a genetic defect.[50]

Summary of the Evidence for the Benefit of Breast Cancer Screening Tests

Among the three screening tests commonly considered for breast cancer, only one has been shown to be efficacious: film-screen mammography. Clinical breast examination has never been studied as the sole intervention in a randomized trial.[32] One randomized trial of film-screen mammography compared its benefit to regular screening with clinical breast examination and found no advantage for film-screen mammography.[51] Some argue that the lack of film-screen mammography benefit in this trial supports the belief that clinical breast examination is effective. At present, however, no evidence-based guideline recommends clinical breast examination as the sole screening approach, even in countries with low resources.[52] The systematic teaching of breast self-examination was examined in a large study conducted among women working in China. Groups of factory workers were trained in breast self-examination and brought back regularly for retraining. Despite demonstrating that women receiving the intervention had a higher sensitivity for finding lumps in silicone models, cumulative breast cancer mortality after 10 years was no different between the intervention and control populations.[53]

The evidence for the benefit of film-screen mammography, which has been collected in randomized clinical trials since the 1960s, is summarized in Table 24.2. The American Cancer Society and the USPSTF both recommend screening beginning at age 40 based on evidence for a 16% reduction in

TABLE 24.2. Evidence for the efficacy of film-screen mammography.

Study name	*Years of intervention*	*Longest follow-up*	*Site of study*	*Age group (years)*	*Study design*	*Exposure (intervention vs. control)*	*Screening rounds*	*Screening interval (months)*	*Views*	*% Exposed to intervention (round)*	*Contamination*	*Relative risk (*odds ratio) of breast cancer mortality*	*Comment*
HIP[196]	1963–1966	18	Staff-model managed care plan	40–64	Randomized controlled trial (RCT)	Mammography + CBE vs. usual care	4	12	2	67% (1); 54% (2); 50% (3); 46% (4)	Unknown	0.83 (0.7–1.0)	The first study to test mammography and have surgeons operate based on nonpalpable lesions.
CNBSS-1[197]	1980–1985	11–16	National healthcare system	40–49	RCT	Mammography + CBE vs. usual care [all women prescreened and instructed in breast self-examination (BSE)]	4–5	12	2	100% (1); 85%-89% (2–4)	25%	0.98 (0.73–1.31)	Used community radiologists; all women screened by CBE at baseline.
CNBSS-2[51]	1980–1985	13	National healthcare system	50–59	RCT	Mammography + CBE vs. usual care (all women prescreened and instructed in BSE)	4–5	12	2	100 (1); 90.4% (2); 86.5% (5)	16%	1.14 (0.83–1.56)	Used community radiologists; all women screened by CBE at baseline.
Edinburgh[198]	1978–1985	14	Primary care practices in Scotland	45–64	RCT	Mammography + CBE vs. usual care	4	24	1–2	66% (1); 44% (7)	Not reported	0.71 (0.53–0.95)	Randomization by physician practice resulted in population differences. Recent meta-analyses exclude this study.
Gothenburg[17,199]	1983–1984	12	Clinics in county health system	39–59	RCT	Mammography vs. usual care; controls offered screening after year 5, completed screening at approx. year 7	5	18	1–2	85% (1); 75%–78% (2–5)	20%	0.86 (0.54–1.37)	
Stockholm[200]	1981	11	Clinics in county health system	40–64	RCT	Mammography vs. usual care; controls offered screening after year 5	2	24–28	1	81% (1); 81% (2)	Not reported	0.71 (0.4–1.2)	
Malmo[201]	1976–1994	11–13	Screening clinic outside main hospital	45–70	RCT	Mammography vs. usual care; controls offered screening after year 14	9	18–24	1–2	74% (1); 70% (2–5)	25%	0.81 (0.62–1.07)	
Swedish 2-County Trial[202]	1977	20	Mobile vans managed by county health system	40–74	RCT	Mammography vs. usual care; controls offered screening after year 7	3	24–33	1	89% (1); 83% (2); 84% (3)	13%	0.68 (0.5–0.93)	Most commonly cited study. Used 2-year interval for women 40–49 and 3-year interval for women 50–74.

breast cancer mortality over 14 years of follow-up among women aged 40 to 49 years and 22% breast cancer mortality reduction over 14 years among women ages 50 to 74.[7] Although the difference in cumulative mortality appears to increase with follow-up among intervention women ages 40 to 49 compared with controls, the benefit decreases with time among women ages 50 to 74.[7] Some have suggested that screening may actually result in higher breast cancer mortality based on the cumulative mortality for the first 3 to 4 years among intervention women compared with control women.[4] Whether that difference is real or not, it disappears with time. Because film-screen mammography technology has improved since the randomized trials began, some groups believe that the benefit is greater for those seeking screening today.[54]

Despite the consensus in the United States to begin screening at age 40, there is some controversy about the findings on which this recommendation is based.[4,5,55,56] In all randomized trials, the number of cancers found within a particular age group is relatively small, so there are advantages to combining results from several trials. However, each trial has unique characteristics and was implemented by different teams. Most of the controversy has to do with the internal validity of the trials and whether their results can be combined to provide an overall estimate of film-screen mammography's impact[7,27]

Two investigators, Olsen and Gotzsche, reviewed eight trials and raised questions about randomization, comparability of the cases and controls, assessment of cause of death, and exclusions after randomization.[55] These investigators concluded that only two trials met standards of research quality that justify inclusion in meta-analysis; neither trial showed a benefit. The USPSTF reviewed the same list of trials and kept all but one in its analysis.[7] A separate meta-analysis by an international group produced the same conclusion as the USPSTF regarding which trials to exclude from meta-analyses, and estimated a 19% mortality reduction at 14 years among women ages 40 to 49 and a 25% mortality reduction among women ages 50 to 69, but only the latter was statistically significant.[27]

Because of the controversies surrounding mammography, there is widespread agreement that the determination of whether to screen should be based on an informed decision that acknowledges that any benefit among populations of younger women is evident only after many years and that the overall benefit for all women is modest.[4,5] Part of the informed decision-making process should include the information that one reason for the modest benefit is that many women diagnosed with breast cancer do well when detected in the course of usual care.[57] To show a benefit, screening must perform better than usual care. Furthermore, because the effect on mortality is moderate, a high quality of screening implementation is important to reproduce the impact demonstrated in the trials.

There are persistent questions regarding the optimal frequency with which to screen, and there is no randomized trial comparing 1- versus 2-year screening intervals. There has been a trial to compare film-screen mammography intervals every 1 versus 3 years among women aged 50 to 62 years.[58] In this trial, the investigators estimated expected deaths based on the observed stage differences between two screening groups and concluded there was no advantage to annual film-screen mammography compared to triennial screening.[58] However, because the sojourn time for young women is close to 2 years, some argue that the screening interval for this age group should be 1 year.[28,59]

Recommendations

The ACS recommends annual film-screen mammography and clinical breast examination beginning at age 40.[59] They recommend individualizing decisions about when to stop screening.

The USPSTF recommends screening film-screen mammography, with or without clinical breast examination, every 1 to 2 years for women aged 40 and older and also recognizes the need to individualize when to stop screening.[7]

Cervical Cancer Screening

Epidemiology and Natural History

Cervical cancer was the most common cause of cancer death among women during the early part of the 19th century. It is now uncommon in the United States, but it is second after lung cancer as the cause of cancer death for women worldwide.[60] In 2004, an estimated 10,520 cases were expected to be diagnosed in the United States.[22,25] Incidence and death rates differ by race: incidence is higher among African-Americans (13.6 in 100,000)[25] than among Caucasian-Americans (8.1 in 100,000; ACS). In 2004, an estimated 3,900 cervical cancer deaths were expected (2.7 in 100,000), and there is concern that mortality will be highest among recent immigrants to the United States, among whom screening rates are lowest.[23,25,61]

Cervical cancer is directly related to the presence of an infectious disease. Some 93% to 100% of cervical squamous cell carcinomas contain DNA from human papillomavirus (HPV). Thirteen types of HPV (16, 18, 31, 33, 35, 39, 45, 41, 52, 56, 58, 59, and 68) are associated with increased risk for cervical cancer and are transmitted during sexual intercourse.[62] The transformation of cervical cells from atypical squamous cells of unknown significance (ASCUS) through low-grade squamous intraepithelial (LSIL) to high-grade intraepithelial lesions (HSIL), cervical intraepithelial neoplasia (CIN), and invasive cancer takes 10 or more years. The terminology for these changes is described next. The transformation process may be reversible in the early stages.[63] Ninety percent of LSILs in adolescents and 50% to 80% of LSILs in adults regress to normal tissue. However, some lesions progress to CIN and invasive cancer.[63] Once a cervical intraepithelial grade 2 (CIN2) lesion exists, it progresses to cervical cancer over a period of about 41 months.[9]

Several factors increase women's risk of cervical cancer, including sexual intercourse, smoking, a history of multiple sexual partners, immunosuppression, and in utero exposure to diethylstilbestrol (DES).[64] Based on a representative sample of U.S. women in the mid-1990s, 23% reported having unprotected intercourse in the previous 3 months, including 25% of unmarried women ages 15 to 18.[65] Smoking is associated with the secretion of nicotine and cotinine in cervical mucus, but the mechanism through which this facilitates cancer development in the presence of HPV is not clear.[66] Women with high-grade squamous intraepithelial lesions are more likely to be current smokers who are HPV positive compared with women with LSIL (OR 3.0; 95% CI, 1.2, 7.7)[67] Women with multiple sexual partners in their lifetime may have as high as a threefold increased risk for cervical cancer, which is likely due to acquisition of HPV.[64,68] Finally, immunosuppressed women are at increased risk of developing CIN.[69]

As we acquire more information about genetics, we gain insights into why not all women who harbor high-risk HPV types develop invasive cancer. There are specific DNA mutations associated with increased risk, but the mechanism is not yet clear. For example, one study found two mutations associated with a three- to fourfold increase in risk of invasive cervical disease. The author of that study suggested that the mutations affected how cigarette smoke was metabolized into compounds that facilitated cell transformation in the presence of HPV.[70]

Screening Tests

Cervical cancer screening has been available for many years. This section reviews the Papanicolaou (Pap) test, first used in the 1940s, and other tests used for cervical cancer screening. The purpose of these tests is to identify precursor lesions that can be treated to prevent the subsequent development of invasive cervical cancer. Two tests, the Pap smear and liquid-based cytology, sample cells shed from the cervix. The other tests look directly at the cervix to evaluate abnormalities.

For the Pap test, a clinician takes a sample of endocervical cells by scraping a flat spatula around the surface of the cervix and sampling within the cervical entrance using a swab or brush. The endocervical brush is now suggested as an alternative to the cotton swab, although there has been some evidence that it does not improve sensitivity over the standard technique.[9,71] The cell sample is spread on a glass slide and fixed with a preservative so that a cytopathology technician and/or pathologist can review it for abnormalities. Detection errors occur when cells from the transformation zone between the endo- and ectocervix are not captured, the cells dry on the slide before they are preserved, or abnormal cells are not recognized at the time of the cytology review. Liquid-based cytology (LBC) uses the same collection technique as a conventional Pap smear, but the cells are immediately placed in a receptacle with fixative solution rather than spread on a glass slide. The solution is filtered, and the collected cells are then spread on a slide for review.

Ratings of cervical cell abnormalities evolved to the current Bethesda System through a consensus process and review of the literature between 1988 and 2001.[72] This system rates specimen adequacy (satisfactory or unsatisfactory) and then provides three summary categories: negative for intraepithelial lesion or malignancy, epithelial cell abnormality (see interpretation), and other (see interpretation). The interpretation of epithelial lesions falls into four major categories (one with subcategories): (1) atypical squamous cells, with the subcategories "of undetermined significance" (ASCUS) and "cannot exclude HSIL" (ASCH); (2) LSILs, encompassing mild dysplasia and low-grade CIN1; (3) HSILs, which include moderate and severe dysplasia, carcinoma in situ, CIN2, and CIN3; and (4) squamous cell carcinoma. The source of the specimen (i.e., LBC or conventional Pap) is also reported, because LBC specimens may be used for subsequent HPV testing as indicated.[72] If glandular cells are present, they also are described.

Although the purpose of cervical cancer screening seems clear, the many precursor lesions and neoplasias that may occur influence the evaluation and comparison of screening tests. Screening test sensitivity and specificity will vary depending upon what condition investigators choose to identify. For example, HPV testing may have high sensitivity for the high-risk HPV virus (types 16 and 18), but there may not be any squamous cell change of the cervix, which is the primary concern. For squamous cell changes, HPV screening specificity is low because many women harbor the virus for prolonged periods before any cellular changes are visible. In a meta-analysis by Nanda and colleagues, the standard was to use an interpretation of LSIL or worse as the definition of a positive test and presence of CIN2 or CIN3 as histologic confirmation of disease.[71] As shown in Table 24.3, Pap sensitivity is 30% to 87% (mean, 47%) and specificity is 46% to 100% (mean, 95%) in low-prevalence populations.[71,73]

TABLE 24.3. Summary of screening test characteristics: cervical cancer.

Test	*Sensitivity*	*Specificity*	*Who administers*	*% Positive in practice*	*Recommended follow-up*	*Comment*
Papanicolaou screen[73,76,203,204]	30%–87% (mean 47%)	86%–100% (mean 95%)	Clinician	8%–13%	Repeat testing of ASCUS, HPV testing of ASCUS in which HSIL cannot be excluded, and colposcopy of anyone with LSIL or higher lesions	Follow-up is based on consensus guidelines.[205]
Thin-Prep[76]	80%*	98%	Clinician	NA	Same as above	*Based on abnormalities of LSIL or greater.
HPV DNA testing[73,206,207]	83%–100%	46%–89%	Clinician	5%–40% depending upon age	Pap smear and/or colposcopy and biopsy as indicated by either	Sensitivity based on ≥LSIL. Specificity based on <LSIL. Risk of positive HPV is higher in younger women.
Acetic acid and direct visualization[77]	80%£	81%	Clinician	NA	Biopsy of abnormalities at the time they are identified	£Based on abnormalities of HSIL or greater.

Follow-up is based on consensus guidelines.[205]

Specificity based on <LSIL. Risk of positive HPV is higher in younger women.

*Based on abnormalities of LSIL or greater. Sensitivity based on ≥LSIL.

£Based on abnormalities of HSIL or greater.

The true-positive rate was reported by some investigators as 13% higher for LBC compared with conventional Pap, but the false-positive rate was also increased by 12%. These findings suggest that LBC has a higher sensitivity and lower specificity than the conventional Pap smear.[71,74]

Because detection errors limit the efficacy of Pap and LBC techniques, there has been an effort to automate the interpretive process and improve detection.[74] Studies are under way to use computer software to analyze images of LBC preparations, but these systems are not yet in widespread use.[74–76]

Although cytology remains the accepted screening method in the United States, other methods exist, including direct visualization of the cervix and analysis of intrinsic or reflected light emission from the cervix. Direct visual inspection (DVI) is a technique first used in the 1930s and then abandoned with the introduction of the Pap smear. However, DVI is reappearing in the developing world because it has the advantage that when an abnormality is identified, it can be dealt with during the same visit.[77] Sensitivity for CIN appears comparable between DVI and Pap smear, but specificity is lower with DVI. An alternative to DVI is to use a photograph that can be analyzed by a physician (cryptography). However, this technique appears to have lower sensitivity than either Pap or DVI and is, therefore, not recommended. Finally, new technologies are being developed that involve the spectroscopic evaluation of light reflected from the cervix. Although this technology is in its infancy, it holds promise for the detection of CIN2 and CIN3 because the early neoplastic cells present with these conditions reflect light differently from normal tissue.[77]

HPV testing may someday be an alternative to cytologic screening for cervical cancer, but current knowledge is inadequate to adopt it as the primary screening tool.[64] HPV testing involves identifying and typing HPV in cervical mucus. It appears most useful in managing women with ASCUS as only those with HPV may need monitoring.[78]

Summary of the Evidence for the Benefit of Cervical Screening Tests

Evidence for the benefit of cervical cancer screening comes from cohort studies conducted in countries with active screening programs. This evidence is summarized in Table 24.4; it shows a 24% to 70% reduction in invasive cervical cancer incidence and a 22% reduction in mortality with the implementation of screening programs. The evidence is so convincing across published studies that virtually no one advocates for randomized trials or questions the impact of cervical cancer screening by cytology.

One area of controversy, however, is the frequency with which cervical cancer screening should occur. As our understanding of the slow progression of this disease has grown, screening intervals recommended by U.S. organizations have widened. As noted above, even change from HSIL to invasive cancer takes an estimated mean of 41 months, so most now believe that screening may occur successfully at intervals as infrequent as every 3 years with a low risk of invasive cancer development.[9] One group of investigators estimates that after three negative Pap smears, the risk associated with screening every 3 years, compared with annually, is as low as 3 in 100,000.[79] Others suggest that setting a fixed screening rate for all women does not make sense. Because the risk varies with age and sexual history, they recommend varying the frequency from 1 to 5 years depending upon risk.[80]

Recommendations

The ACS recently reviewed the new data on cervical cancer and updated its recommendations. ACS now recommends that screening begin 3 years after onset of sexual activity or by age 21 and may stop at age 70 if the low-risk status of the woman is established (i.e., three or more negative screens within 10 years and no high-risk conditions such as HIV, in utero DES exposure, immunocompromise by organ transplantation, chemotherapy, or chronic corticosteroid treatment). The ACS recommends an annual Pap up to age 30, and then every 2 to 3 years after three successive adequate negative Pap smears. Because of the greater sensitivity of LBC, the Society recommends screening every 2 years to age 30 if LBC is used, then every 2 to 3 years if it has been established by history and Pap results that the woman is at low risk.

Based on indirect evidence, the USPSTF recommends that screening begin within 3 years of onset of sexual activity or by age 21 and that it end at age 65 if women have had negative Pap smears and are otherwise at low risk. They recommend screening at least every 3 years.[81,82]

Colorectal Cancer Screening

Epidemiology and Natural History

In 2004, an estimated 146,940 people in the United States were expected to be diagnosed with colorectal cancer (CRC), and an estimated 56,730 were expected to die of the disease.[22] African-Americans are more likely to be diagnosed with and die of CRC than Caucasian-Americans (62 in 100,000 versus 55 in 100,000 and 29 in 100,000 versus 21 in 100,000, respectively).[25] Data on other groups, such as American Indian/Alaska Natives, Asian/Pacific Islanders, and Hispanics, are limited, but individuals in these populations are less likely to die of CRC than Caucasian-Americans (14.8 in 100,000, 13.1 in 100,000, and 14.2 in 100,000, respectively).[25]

As with other cancers, the estimated length of time for the development of CRC from normal tissue has implications for screening. Unlike other cancers, the sequence of mutations occurring with CRC is well described and provides a model for cancer progression, from abnormal cell through polyp to invasive cancer. This knowledge of CRC mutations holds promise for diagnosing and determining prognosis in screening and treatment programs.[83–89] The time it takes for CRC to develop varies from as little as 2 years for individuals with the hereditary nonpolyposis colorectal cancer (HNPCC) gene to 10 or more years for individuals at average risk for CRC.[85,90] Recommended screening intervals are, therefore, shorter for people at higher CRC risk.[10]

Most CRC arises from adenomatous polyps (adenomas). The potential of adenomas to progress to CRC varies; in general, larger polyps have a higher potential for malignancy. The goal of CRC screening is to detect adenomas that are likely to become CRC. A minority of cancers may not progress through the adenoma-to-carcinoma sequence; in these cases, existing screening tests are relied upon to detect early-stage cancers rather than adenomas.[8,91]

TABLE 24.4. Evidence for the efficacy of cervical cancer screening.

Study name	*Years of intervention*	*Longest follow-up (years)*	*Site of study*	*Age group (years)*	*Study design and screening comparison*	*Exposure (intervention)*	*Screening rounds*	*Screening interval (months)*	*% Exposed to intervention (round)*	*Measure of effect*	*Comment*
Finland[16]	1960–1987	27	Entire country	30–55 (60)	Obs	Pap smear	Up to 5 screens	60	80%	60%–70% reduction in incidence	Women ages >60 added in 1987. An evaluation of outcomes in the population as a whole without individual-level data.
Norway 1[208]	1959	20	Ostfold county	25–29	Obs	Pap smear	4	24	80% (1) 66% (4th)	38% reduction in incidence	Screening through primary care began in early 1960s.
Norway 2[204]	1995–2000	5	Entire country	25–69 w/o screens in 3 years	Obs	Pap smear	2	36	8% more than without exception system	24% decreased incidence 1999–2000	The most recent study showed an additional reduction in incidence with outreach reminders added to the program. Total population screening went from 65.2% to 70.7%.
Denmark[209,210]	1967–1982	8	Entire country	30–54 vs. >54	Obs	Pap smear	0–13	24	88%	22% lower mortality	Implemented screening in the 1960s by counties. Full implementation of organized program with mailed reminders in the late 1980s. National recommendation is screen every 3 years.
Sweden[208]	1967	5	Entire country	30–49	Obs	Pap smear	NA	48		72% reduction in incidence (30–54 years)	Population-based analysis without individual-level data.

Screening Tests

Available screening tests for CRC are fecal occult blood testing (FOBT), sigmoidoscopy, and colonoscopy.[92] Barium enema also remains an option for CRC screening and is discussed briefly. Digital rectal examination (DRE) has been used but is not effective and is not recommended as a CRC screening tool.[10,93]

Fecal occult blood testing requires that a person collect three stool samples and place them on a special card that is mailed or taken to the laboratory for processing to identify whether the sample contains blood. A reagent placed on the card identifies hemoglobin in the stool through two main mechanisms: guaiac-based tests that detect blood through the pseudoperoxidase activity of heme (FOBT; not specific for human blood) and immunochemical techniques (IFOBT; immunochemical FOBT) that use antibody reactions to identify human hemoglobin.[89,90,94–96] Guaiac-based tests generally require the patient to eliminate nonsteroidal antiinflammatory medications, red meat, and certain vitamins for 3 to 5 days before testing.[89,96–98]

The disadvantages of FOBT are its low sensitivity for CRC (approximately 25% to 50% for Dukes stage A or B) and the precursors to CRC (10% to 20% for most polyps 1.0cm or larger), and its low specificity (approximately 88% to 98% for single use).[88,99,100] Rehydration of test slides may increase sensitivity by 2% to 4%, but it also substantially increases the false-positive rate from 8% to 16%.[100–103] Median completion and return rates of FOBT (when individuals are given the test to take home) vary between 40% and 50%.[104] Adherence depends upon the population studied, the test type, and the level of dietary restriction required.[88,90,97–99,105–107] One recent randomized trial demonstrated a 40% completion rate when a two-sample brush approach was used in people without dietary restriction compared to 23% and 30% for two three-sample techniques among people on peroxidase-restricted diets before testing.[97] The distinct advantage of FOBT, however, is that the test is inexpensive and it is the one technique demonstrated to reduce mortality in randomized trials.[8,96]

IFOBT may improve on the sensitivity and specificity of guaiac-based tests and does not require dietary restrictions.[108,109,110] However, the cost of IFOBT is two to five times higher than that of FOBT, and at least one study comparing IFOBT and FOBT showed no improvement in the rate of completion of tests.[59,89,94,96,108,110] At present, evidence suggests that sensitivity of IFOBT is 66% to 69% and specificity is 95% to 97%.[94,95]

Sigmoidoscopy is the direct visual examination of the rectum and lower colon using a flexible lighted tube (sigmoidoscope). It requires 1% to 2% saline enemas for preparation and takes about 10 minutes to perform.[111] Administration of the test requires special training, but it is routinely performed by primary care physicians, physician assistants, and nurses, as well as by specialists such as gastroenterologists.[111] Sigmoidoscopy is estimated to detect 68% to 78% of advanced neoplasia in the distal colon.[8] However, its effectiveness is reduced compared to colonoscopy because it cannot reach the proximal part of the colon and, therefore, misses 40% to 50% of advanced neoplasms.[18,112] In addition, its sensitivity may be reduced in women because they are more likely than men to have a shorter, more limited examination.[113]

Colonoscopy uses a flexible scope to visualize the entire colon. Preparation for colonoscopy is more extensive than for sigmoidoscopy, typically involving 1 day of clear liquids and laxative preparation.[111] The test itself requires sedation, skilled support personnel, and a trained endoscopist. It takes about 30 minutes to perform colonoscopy and 2 to 3 hours of patient recovery time.[111] It is the most accurate test currently available for detecting CRC or adenomas, with sensitivity of a single test ranging from 75% to 92%, depending on the size of the lesion detected and training of the operator.[114,115] However, colonoscopy is not a perfect test, missing on average 13% to 27% of adenomas less than 1 centimeter in diameter.[116]

The disadvantages of both endoscopic procedures are that they carry a risk of perforation (1.96 per 1,000 colonoscopies, 0.88 per 1,000 sigmoidoscopies) or bleeding and require that the bowel be completely cleared.[117] Patients may also experience pain or discomfort during the procedure, particularly with sigmoidoscopy, which is not performed under sedation.[111,113,118] In general, rates of endoscopic evaluation after a positive FOBT are suboptimal. In a study of 24,246 Medicare beneficiaries who underwent FOBT, only 34% of those with positive results underwent a complete colonic evaluation consisting of either colonoscopy or flexible sigmoidoscopy with air-contrast barium enema; an additional 34% underwent either flexible sigmoidoscopy or a barium enema.[119] Rates of recommended follow-up testing (colonoscopy or flexible sigmoidoscopy with air-contrast barium enema) in other studies have ranged from 21% to 90%, with the highest rates of follow-up achieved in randomized trials.[119] Low follow-up rates may be due to a lack of follow-through on the part of physicians—in one study, primary care physicians ordered a complete diagnostic evaluation of the colon for only 70% of patients with positive FOBT[120]—and of patients, who need to schedule the colonoscopy upon physician recommendation.

Double-contrast barium enema (DCBE) provides a radiographic image of the entire colon and rectum. It does not require sedation, although it does require full colon cleansing and has occasionally been associated with anaphylactic reactions to the latex bulb used to administer the contrast agent.[121–123] Table 24.5 contains sensitivity and specificity estimates for DCBE.

Emerging screening methods: Screening methods currently in development include virtual colonoscopy [also known as spiral computed tomography (CT) or CT colonography] and tests for altered DNA in the stool.[88,89,114,124,125] A new technology called capsule video endoscopy, approved in 2001 by the FDA for diagnosing small-intestine disorders, may prove useful for CRC screening in the future.[89] Cost-effectiveness, system capacity, and other issues relating to these technologies are also important and remain to be demonstrated.[114,126,127]

Summary of the Evidence for the Benefit of CRC Screening Tests

Table 24.5 summarizes the test characteristics of the technologies used for CRC screening.[8,10,90,92,128,129] As noted in Table 24.5, FOBT is the only CRC screening method that has been evaluated in randomized clinical trials. These trials have demonstrated that annual FOBT reduces CRC mortality by 15% to 33%.[102,106,130] Biennial (every 2 years) FOBT screening

TABLE 24.5. **Summary of screening test characteristics: colorectal cancer.**

Test	Sensitivity (%) CRC**	Sensitivity (%) Large adenoma	Specificity (%) CRC	Specificity (%) Large adenoma	Who administers	% Positive in practice	Recommended follow-up for positive test	Proportion of positives evaluated In practice*	Comment
Fecal occult blood test (FOBT): unrehydrated[90,96,110,119,211,212]	11–86	21–30	91–99	91–92	Patient (at home)	2.4%–9%	Colonoscopy or DCBE with flexible sigmoidoscopy	34%–50%	Annual repetition of FOBT yields higher sensitivity than single FOBT. Screening FOBT in physician's office is not recommended.
FOBT: rehydrated[96,102,110,119,212]	50–92	22–53	94	94	Patient (at home)	8%-10%	Colonoscopy or DCBE with flexible sigmoidoscopy	34%–50%	In RCT by Mandel et al., rehydration increased positive test from 2.4% to 9.8%.
Immunochemical fecal occult blood test (IFOBT)[95,110,211,213]	69–100	25–79	86	86–95	Patient (at home)	9%	Colonoscopy or DCBE with flexible sigmoidoscopy	50%	Combination FOBT/IFOBT tests may have higher sensitivity than either type of test alone.
Double Contrast Barium Enema (DCBE)[115,214]	65–85	48	Not reported	85	Radiologist	N/A	Colonoscopy	N/A	Sensitivity of barium enema has been shown to vary by hospital & practitioner.[115]
Sigmoidoscopy[111,116,136,137,215,216]	50–70 for advanced neoplasms	75% for polyps <1 cm	Not reported	Not reported	Primary care physician, physician's assistant, nurse, gastroenterologist	17%	Colonoscopy	74%-85%	Positive rate includes all adenomas.
Sigmoidoscopy + FOBT[134,137,212]	76 for advanced neoplasias**	Not reported	Not reported	Not reported	Primary care physician, physician's assistant, nurse, gastroenterologist (patient for FOBT)	10%–17%	Colonoscopy + or DCBE	77%	The addition of FOBT increased the sensitivity by 0.05% in the one study with a direct of Sig vs. Sig plus FOBT.[137]
Colonoscopy[114–116]	95	88–94	Not reported	Not reported	Gastroenterologist	>5%	Endoscopic or surgical resection	Not reported	Sensitivity of colonoscopy has been shown to vary by hospital and practitioner.[115] Sensitivity for high-risk lesions and cancer.
Virtual colonoscopy[114]	100% (2 of 2) malignant polyps were detected	94	Not reported	96	Radiologist/CT technician	7%–8%	Optical colonoscopy	Not on market	
Stool-based DNA testing (Multi-Target Assay Panel)[127,217,218]	44–91	48–86	Not reported	93–96	Not on market	Not available	Not on market	Not on market	

*This represents the proportion of positives followed up with the recommended procedure (e.g., colonoscopy). In the Lurie study, close to 100% of Medicare recipients with a positive FOBT were followed up, but only 34% had either colonoscopy or FS with barium enema, which were considered the recommended procedures for follow-up.

**Advanced neoplasias defined as cancer or high-risk adenomas ≥1 cm or with villous/dysplastic features.

reduces mortality by 15% to 21%.[102,106,130,131] Although research has suggested that CRC screening by IFOBT would also reduce mortality from CRC,[132] more needs to be done to evaluate its cost, accuracy, and adherence to its use by people to whom it is recommended.[94,132]

Evidence for the benefit of sigmoidoscopy has been demonstrated in two case-control studies showing that people who died of CRC were 59% to 79% less likely than controls to have been screened even once by sigmoidoscopy.[18,133] Research also suggests that using FOBT in conjunction with sigmoidoscopy could confer additional benefit compared with sigmoidoscopy alone because it may detect cancers in the proximal sigmoid colon that are missed by sigmoidoscopy.[134] Two ongoing randomized clinical trials (RCTs) to evaluate flexible sigmoidoscopy will report their initial results within the next several years,[135,136] and an ongoing trial in Norway is evaluating the benefit of flexible sigmoidoscopy and flexible sigmoidoscopy combined with FOBT.[137] Consistent with the reduction in mortality conferred by screening endoscopy, several studies have shown reductions of 42% to 76% in CRC incidence among those offered endoscopy compared with those who were not offered the test.[133,138,139]

There is little direct evidence of the efficacy of colonoscopy in reducing CRC incidence and mortality, although there is indirect evidence of its benefit from studies of other CRC screening methods (Table 24.6).[90,112,140] The direct evidence to date consists of a case-control study of U.S. veterans that found that people who died of colon cancer were less likely than controls to have had colonoscopy (OR, 0.43; 95% CI, 0.30–0.63).[138] In this study, people with either colon or rectal cancer were also less likely to have had colonoscopy (OR, 0.47; 95% CI, 0.37–0.58; OR, 0.61; 95% CI, 0.48–0.77).[138] Colonoscopic polypectomy has been found to reduce the incidence of CRC, suggesting that the removal of polyps is the proximal reason for screening-based reductions in CRC incidence and mortality.[140,141]

Emerging technologies such as virtual colonoscopy or stool DNA screening have not been demonstrated to reduce CRC incidence or mortality. Studies suggest that these methods hold promise for the future, and ongoing research is comparing emerging to current screening methods.

Recommendations

The ACS, USPSTF, U.S. Multisociety Task Force on Colorectal Cancer, and American College of Gastroenterology (ACG) agree that CRC screening is effective in reducing CRC incidence and mortality, and each has developed recommendations.[8,10,112] The USPSTF strongly recommends screening for men and women 50 years of age and older but has concluded that there are insufficient data to determine which strategy is best in terms of the balance between benefits and potential harms.[8,112]

Similar to the USPSTF, the ACS[10] and U.S. Multisociety Task Force on Colorectal Cancer[90] recommend a range of options for screening average-risk individuals beginning at age 50. Both recommend annual FOBT, flexible sigmoidoscopy every 5 years, annual FOBT plus flexible sigmoidoscopy every 5 years, DCBE every 5 years, or colonoscopy every 10 years.

Despite strong expert consensus on the benefits of screening for colorectal cancer, actual screening rates in the population remain low for all available CRC screening tests. In general, individuals at higher risk, such as those with familial adenomatous polyposis (FAP) or HNPCC, should be screened more aggressively than those at average risk.[8,10,90,112] Genetic tests exist for individuals suspected to have a hereditary syndrome such as HNPCC or FAP. Chapter 26 covers genetic screening and counseling for high-risk populations.

Prostate Cancer Screening

Prostate cancer is a challenge in clinical care because 1 in every 6 men will be diagnosed with it in his lifetime but only 1 in 29 will die of it.[11] Therefore, prostate cancer will not affect the life expectancy of many men diagnosed with the disease, even if they were never screened. Because it is impossible for an individual to know the effect of the diagnosis on his life expectancy, many men diagnosed with prostate cancer overestimate the benefit they gain from screening.[1,142] A smaller proportion (48%) of men who went untreated for prostate cancer were satisfied with their therapy compared with men treated with androgen (63%), radiation (70%), or radical prostatectomy (59%).[143] Although individuals may be satisfied with therapy, its effect has implications for morbidity and quality of life for those who are told they have the disease.[1,144]

Epidemiology and Natural History

In 2004, an estimated 230,110 new cases of prostate cancer were diagnosed in the United States and 29,900 men will have died of the disease.[22,25] The overall incidence peaked in 1992 at about 230 in 100,000 men, but the rate has dropped since that time to the current rate of about 173 in 100,000.[25] The incidence in Caucasian-Americans is lower (168 in 100,000) than it is among African-Americans (277 in 100,000), as is the mortality (30 in 100,000 versus 73 in 100,000). Overall, prostate cancer mortality has been falling since 1991, but the reason is not clear. Some have attributed the reduction to increased screening[145] but others conclude that cannot be the explanation because the decline is disproportionate to the change in incidence and too early in relation to increased use of prostate screening tests.[146,147] Prostate cancer is a slow-growing tumor, with a lead time ranging from 5 to 11 years depending upon what test and criteria are used to determine a positive screen.[148] Mortality differences would therefore not be expected to closely follow increases in screening.

Screening Tests

Prostate-specific antigen (PSA) is an organ-specific protein secreted by the luminal epithelial cells of the prostatic ducts, acini, and periurethral glands. It may be found floating free or bound to a complex of proteins.[149] Levels of PSA are measured in blood and are elevated by benign prostatic hypertrophy, inflammation, and the presence of neoplastic prostatic tissue (Table 24.7). Recent work suggests that measuring PSA bound in a protein matrix (cPSA) may be more specific than measuring serum totals.[149] In practice, digital rectal examination (DRE) and transrectal ultrasound are often conducted before to PSA testing, but this does not cause increased serum PSA levels.[150] A positive test for prostate cancer is generally

TABLE 24.6. Evidence for the efficacy of colorectal cancer screening.

Study	Years of intervention	Longest follow-up	Site of study	Age group	Study design	Exposure or intervention and screening rounds	Screening interval (months)	% Exposed to intervention	Contamination	Relative risk (RR) or odds ratio (OR) of colon cancer mortality	Comment
Mandel[102]	1975–1992	13 years	Minnesota	50–80	RCT	FOBT annually or biennially (two intervention groups)	12 or 24	90% completed at least one screening. 46% of annual FOBT group completed all tests. 60% of biennial group completed all tests.	1.8% of colorectal cancer in controls had cancer detected by FOBT.	33% (annual); RR = 0.67 (95% CI, 0.50–0.87) 21% (biennial); RR = 0.94 (95% CI, 0.68–1.31)	The cumulative incidence of colorectal cancer was nearly identical in both intervention and control groups, suggesting all cancers were found in each; 28%–38% of 1- and 2-year group, respectively, had colonoscopy.
Hardcastle[130]	1981–1995	Median 7.8 years, but varied by time of enrollment. All follow-up stopped June 1995.	UK	45–74	RCT	FOBT without rehydration (3–6 rounds)	24	60% completed at least one screening.	Not reported.	15	4% of intervention group had colonoscopy.
Kronborg[106]	1985–1995	10 years	Funen, Denmark	45–75	RCT	FOBT without rehydration (5 rounds)	24	67% for round 1; more than 90% for repeat screenings.	Controls continued to seek usual care.	RR = 0.82 (95% CI, 0.68–0.99)	Predictive value of positive FOBT: 17% in first round tp, 9% in final round; PPV for large adenomas was 32% at first round, 21% at final round.

(*continued*)

TABLE 24.6. Evidence for the efficacy of colorectal cancer screening. (*continued*)

Study	*Years of intervention*	*Longest follow-up*	*Site of study*	*Age group*	*Study design*	*Exposure or intervention and screening rounds*	*Screening interval (months)*	*% Exposed to intervention*	*Contamination*	*Relative risk (RR) or odds ratio (OR) of colon cancer mortality*	*Comment*
Selby[18]	n/a	n/a	Kaiser Permanente Medical Care Program, Oakland, CA	45 or older	Case-control	Rigid sigmoidoscopy (single exposure)	n/a	8.8% of cases; 24.2% of controls.	n/a	For cancer of rectum and distal colon: adjusted OR = 0.41 (95% CI, 0.25–0.69) For cancer of rest of colon (out of reach of sigmoidoscope): adjusted OR = 0.96 (95% CI, 0.61–1.50)	Landmark case-control study that raised possibility of mortality reduction through use of sigmoidoscopy.
Newcomb[133]	n/a	n/a	Greater Marshfield Community Health Plan members (Wisconsin)	20–75	Case-control	Sigmoidoscopy (single exposure)	n/a	10% among cases; 30% among controls.	n/a	OR = 0.21 (95% CI, 0.08–0.52)	Reduction in risk appeared to be limited to rectum and distal colon.
Winawer[134]	1975–1979	9 years	Recipients of self-paid comprehensive medical examinations, Strang Clinic	40 and older	Prospective cohort	FOBT + rigid sigmoidoscopy compared with rigid sigmoidoscopy alone	12 months	80% for round 1; 20% for round 2; 16% for round 3; 28% for round 6.	?	50% reduction in mortality with FOBT + sigmoidoscopy compared with sigmoidoscopy alone	
Muller[138]	n/a	n/a	US military veterans	Mean age 57	Case-control	Endoscopy (sigmoidoscopy, colonoscopy) and/or tissue removal (at least one exposure)	n/a	2.7% among cases; 10.1% among deceased controls.	n/a	OR = 0.44 (95% CI, 0.36–0.53) (for any colorectal procedure)	

TABLE 24.7. Summary of screening test characteristics: prostate cancer.

Test	*Sensitivity*	*Specificity*	*Who administers*	*% Positive in practice*	*Recommended follow-up*	*Comment*
Prostate-specific antigen (PSA)[219]	63%–83%	81%-98% depending upon age	Laboratory test ordered by clinician	4%–27% depending upon age	Urology evaluation and consideration of 6-quadrant biopsy	Using PSA level >4ng/mL as positive and "clinically significant disease" as outcome of detection.
Digital rectal examination (DRE)[219]	59%–64%	NA	Clinician	NA	PSA, consideration of urology evaluation	Specificity figures are ambiguous because biopsy of any prostate in men >50 years may find cancer, but not necessarily disease.

defined as 4 nanograms per milliliter (ng/L). Using that definition, sensitivity of the PSA test for cancer occurring within 2 years is about 73%.[11] Between 4% of men in their fifties and 27% of men in their seventies will test positive based on this definition.[11] DRE finds localized cancer only 50% to 60% of the time.[11] Although investigators are looking for proteins that may provide more sensitive and specific prostate cancer screening tests, none have been found and reported to date.

Summary of the Evidence for the Benefit of Prostate Screening Tests

According to the USPSTF, the evidence that prostate cancer screening with either DRE or PSA testing is beneficial for reducing prostate cancer mortality is not convincing.[11,150] The only published study of PSA designed as a randomized trial reported a screening benefit but did not maintain the randomized groups (screen, control) in their analysis (Table 24.8).[151] When other authors reanalyze the data maintaining the original randomized groups intended for screening and control populations, the benefit is not apparent.[11] In observational studies, several factors make it difficult to determine whether finding prostate cancer early truly increases the length of life for men who are diagnosed: (1) the long lead time for prostate cancer, (2) the significant proportion of men who will develop some form of the disease, and (3) biases inherent in following cancer cases.

Demonstrating a benefit for prostate cancer screening is important because serious consequences are associated with overtreatment. Radical prostatectomy has a significant morbidity, including total incontinence (10%), partial incontinence (14%), requiring pads to stay dry (28%), diarrhea (21%), erection insufficient for intercourse (80%), and being bothered by sexual dysfunction (53% to 59%, depending upon age).[144] Radiation therapy also has a substantial morbidity that includes total incontinence (3%), partial incontinence (2%), requiring pads to stay dry (3%), diarrhea (37%), erection insufficient for intercourse (62%), and being bothered by sexual dysfunction (40% to 47%, depending upon age).[152] Large randomized trials are currently under way in the United States, Austria, and Canada to evaluate the benefits of screening with PSA.[153]

Recommendations

The USPSTF report concludes that there is insufficient evidence to recommend either for or against screening with PSA. The ACS recommends offering PSA and DRE annually beginning at age 50 among men who have a life expectancy of at least 10 additional years, but only after appropriate discussion of risks and benefits.[10]

Screening for Other Cancers

The USPSTF recommends against routine screening for bladder, thyroid, ovarian, and pancreatic cancers in the general population, even for individuals at higher risk for ovarian and thyroid cancers, because the available tests are either inadequate or have not been proven beneficial.

For testicular, skin, and oral cancers, the USPSTF has determined that there is insufficient evidence to recommend for or against screening in the primary care setting, although discussions of screening options with selected patients at high risk for testicular cancer may be appropriate.[14]

Screening Is a Process

While screening trials fund teams of specially trained individuals to ensure that recruitment, screening, and follow-up occur, these resources do not exist in daily clinical practice.[12] In primary care practice, a number of organizations, institutions, and individuals must share responsibility for making sure that the entire screening process occurs. The number and complexity of steps in the screening process may lead to confusion or breakdowns in communication.[12] These breakdowns may result in failure to follow up on a positive test or to treat diagnosed cancer.[13,154,155] Factors outside the doctor–patient relationship, such as healthcare insurance and the clinical setting itself, influence individual propensity to seek screening and the likelihood that the screening process will be complete.[12] This section summarizes some of what has been learned about the five major phases of the screening process: (1) identifying and understanding the population at risk; (2) identifying the method of recruitment; (3) clarifying the screening approach; (4) developing the follow-up approach; and (5) referring patients for treatment.

Identifying and Understanding the Population at Risk

The populations that should be screened for specific cancers are now easily identifiable from a strictly demographic

TABLE 24.8. Evidence for the efficacy of prostate cancer screening.

Study name	Years of intervention	Longest follow-up (years)	Site of study	Age group	Study design and screening comparison	Exposure (intervention)	Screening rounds	Screening interval (months)	% Exposed to intervention (round)	Measure of effect	Comment
Labrie[151]	1988–1996	8	Quebec City	45–80 years	RCT	31,300 intervention (PSA & DRE), 15,432 control	Up to 7	Annual	23.00%	"Intention to treat" 4.6 vs. 4.8 deaths/1,000	Control group had 6.5% screened. Reported benefit was not based on intention to treat.
Friedman[220]	10 years before diagnosis in 1979–1985	NA	HMO	Mean age 69.5 years	Case-control; cases were men with metastatic (stage D) prostate cancer dx	DRE in 10 years prior	N/A	N/A	2.45 exams among cases, 2.52 exams among controls	OR of DRE in cases vs. controls, 0.9 (95% CI 0.5–1.7)	
Jacobsen[221]	10 years before diagnosis in 1976–1991	NA	Olmstead County, Minnesota	Mean age at death 79 years	Case-control; cases were men with prostate cancer listed on death certificate; age-matched controls	DRE in 10 years prior	N/A	N/A	84% controls, 75% cases any DRE	OR of DRE in cases vs. controls, 0.51 (95% CI, 0.31–0.84)	No difference in timing of DRE exposure.
Richert-Boe[222]	2–10 years before death in 1981–1990	NA	HMO	Mean age at death 70.3 years	Case-control: cases were men who died of prostate cancer	DRE in 10 years prior	N/A	N/A	Screen DRE; 77% cases, 80% controls	OR of DRE in cases vs. controls, 0.84 (95% CI, 0.4–1.46)	Results unchanged when looked at exposure within 5 years.
Lu-Yao[223]	1987–1990	11 years	Two separate geographic areas: Seattle-Puget Sound and Connecticut	65–80	Ecologic study: cohort comparison	Relative PSA rate, prostate Bx rate, radical prostatectomy rate, mortality rate	N/A		Seattle to Connecticut: relative PSA 5.4 (95% CI, 4.76–6.1), Bx 2.2 (95% CI, 1.8–2.7)	Mortality 1.03 (0.95–1.1)	Radical prostatectomy was more common in Seattle: 2.7% vs. 0.5% of population.
Bartsch[224]	1993 onward		One state in Austria compared with surrounding states	45–75	Ecologic study: cohort comparison	PSA screening			32%	Test of trend in deaths due to prostate cancer: 0.011e per year decrease in Tyrol compared with 0.0057 decrease in rest of Austria	

standpoint. For women, screening begins 3 years after onset of sexual activity or by age 21 to look for precursors to cervical cancer, by age 40 for breast cancer, and by age 50 for colorectal cancer. Screening for men begins at age 50 for colon cancer; a discussion of prostate cancer should also occur at that time so that men understand the strengths and weaknesses of current knowledge.[10]

However, identifying the population at risk involves more than specifying gender or age range. It is also important to understand the cultural characteristics of populations, their interest in screening, and their understanding of screening tests so that those at risk understand the recommendations and seek the appropriate tests.[104,156,157] Those at highest risk of late-stage cancers after screening are those who have not been screened before.[155]

Figure 24.2 shows that screening rates in the United States vary from as low as 10% of women having had a recent endoscopic evaluation of colorectal cancer to as high as 81% having had a recent Pap smear.[158] The figure shows that, as of the year 2000, less than 30% of men or women had undergone FOBT within the previous 2 years, and fewer had undergone endoscopy. Men are more likely to report having had a PSA test than either FOBT or endoscopic screening.[159] Because the potential mortality reduction among individuals screened for colon cancer is promising, encouraging CRC screening is becoming a high priority.[10,160]

Although Figure 24.2 demonstrates rising rates of mammographic screening and sustained cervical cancer screening, women with lower incomes are less likely to have access to care and are less likely to be screened for these two cancers, even though programs are in place to reach low-income women in all 50 states.[161,162] Across the United States, an estimated 15% of individuals are without insurance coverage at any given time, and a much higher percentage is without coverage some time during the year.[163] Lack of insurance and lack of a regular source of health care are highly correlated with lack of screening.[158,164,165] For example, African-Americans are less likely to have health insurance than Caucasians and are therefore less likely to undergo screening tests for CRC.[162,166] It is estimated that cancer mortality is 19% higher in the lowest socioeconomic groups than in the highest.[167] Recently, levels of cancer screening among racial minorities have improved to the point that they approach the levels of screening among Caucasians; people without health insurance or a regular source of health care continue to be underscreened.[168] As a nation, we cannot achieve the maximum mortality reduction afforded by cancer screening if some populations go unscreened or untreated.

Identifying the Method of Recruitment

Reaching individuals, however, is not only a function of income and access. Even when they have access to care, not all people seek recommended screening.[155,169,170] Providers may work with their teams, practices, health plans, third-party payers, and community to develop recruitment methods for screening. There is evidence that changes in practice that affect multiple levels of health care, including reimbursement, records systems, and tailoring of recruitment messages, have the strongest impact.[171,172]

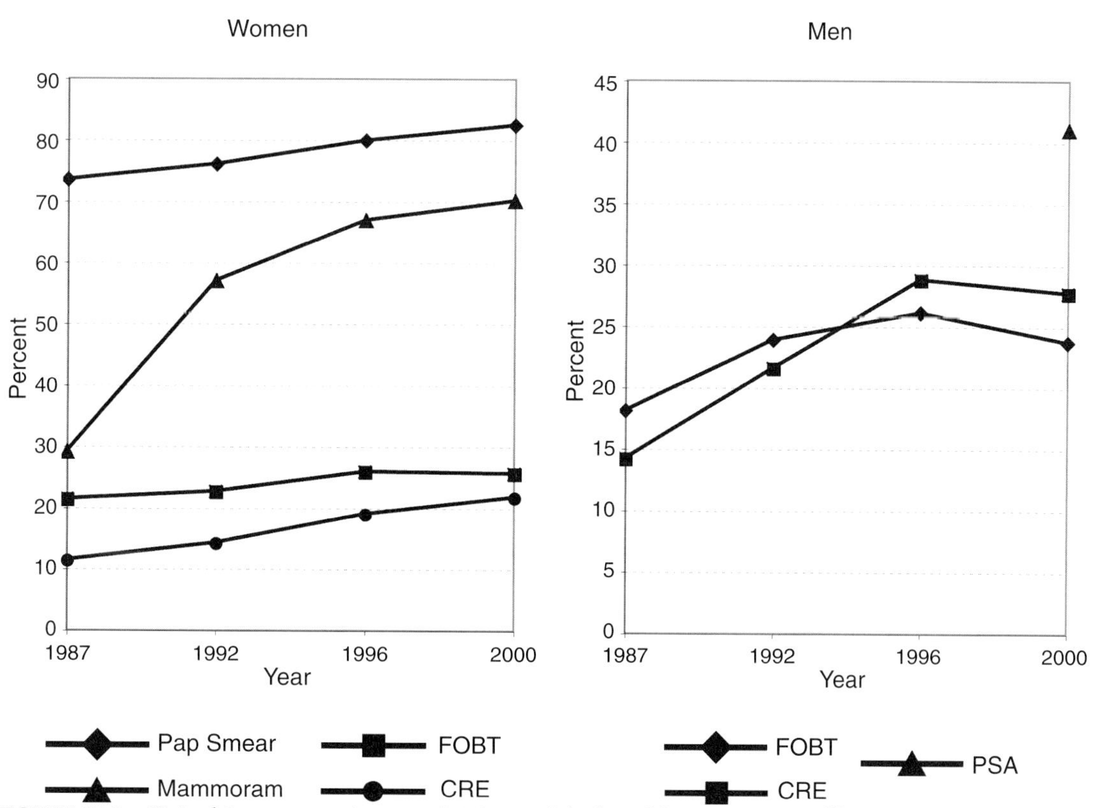

FIGURE 24.2. United States screening rates (1987–2000). (Adapted from Swan et al.,[158] by permission of *Cancer*.)

Ultimately, practitioners must make choices about how to reach individuals with appropriate recommendations and encourage them to consider screening. This is a crucial step in the screening process; for example, a recommendation from a primary care physician is a primary predictor of whether women seek colorectal cancer screening.[173] However, physicians' recommendations are not always consistent with screening guidelines; for example, a nationwide survey of primary care physicians suggested the presence of knowledge gaps and suboptimal screening delivery for CRC screening.[160] Primary care physicians also face substantial time limitations with regard to making all necessary and appropriate screening recommendations in light of their other prevention and treatment obligations[174]; therefore, systematic changes may have the largest impact on making the screening recommendation.[172]

One key systematic change is the implementation of clinical reminder systems, as there is strong evidence that issuing reminders leads to increased screening rates for film-screen mammography and cervical cancer.[172,175–178] The two major types of reminders are inreach and outreach. Inreach reminders involve notifying a provider that a patient is due for a screening test while he or she is in the office. Systems to provide inreach reminders may be as simple as a chart review and paper alert or as sophisticated as an electronic note on an automated medical record. Overall, inreach reminders and physician feedback have been shown to result in the mammography screening of an additional 5% to 20% of the study population compared with "usual care" controls.[179] Outreach reminders consist of contacting individuals outside of an office visit. Studies involving telephone calls from a cancer registry, mailed recommendations, and motivational telephone calls addressing specific barriers to screening have shown that such reminders result in the Pap and mammography screening of an additional 15% to 31% of the study population compared with usual care.[175,177]

Even after recommendations are made, ensuring that individuals seek screening may require adopting and adapting new strategies to encourage women to follow through on the recommendation. For example, McPhee and colleagues have shown that having female lay leaders discuss screening at gatherings in women's homes promotes the use of film-screen mammography among Cambodians.[180] Understanding factors that affect use of screening tests will help providers work with members of their organizations and communities to plan effective education and recruitment strategies for the populations they serve. The process of understanding and enabling individuals to manage their care has been called "self-management support" by some, and it may be critical to successful screening implementation.[181]

Clarifying the Screening Approach

In addition to ordering the screening test, the primary care provider may be responsible for conduct the screening. Organizing the care within a practice is therefore critical to getting screening accomplished. How that screening occurs, however, differs by the organizational setting of healthcare delivery, the cancer site, the set of screening tests recommended, and which test or set of tests the patient prefers. For example, screening mammography and colonoscopy depend upon referrals whereas cervical cancer screening, FOBT, and sigmoidoscopy can be conducted by the primary care team. To incorporate cancer screening into a busy practice, primary care providers need to organize their approach and clarify who is talking with the patient, what is being said, and how tests are ordered. This is all part of organizing the approach to screening, and it has been shown to increase screening rates when implemented systematically in practice using the entire healthcare team.[172,182–184]

Developing the Follow-Up Approach

When testing requires a referral, a tracking system to document the patient's progress through the care continuum can be helpful. The proportion of positive screening tests varies with the type of test but, in general, is about 10% (see Tables 24.1, 24.3, 24.5, 24.7). Follow-up for these individuals is not automatic, and failure to ensure successful follow-up compromises the mortality reduction achievable.[178] For example, follow-up for positive FOBT has been estimated to range between 49% and 79%,[185] and follow-up after a mammogram was as low as 35% women in one HMO even though access to care was assured.[186] In a review of published evaluations of follow-up after positive screening tests, Yabroff and colleagues found that two-thirds of reported studies had follow-up rates below 75%.[13] Among the 45 observational studies in her review, only 1 showed follow-up greater than 90%.[13] Factors that improved follow-up of abnormal tests included addressing the lack of health insurance for a patient, using peer counselors, making system-wide changes in a health plan or clinic, and more actively encouraging patients to manage their care.[13,172]

Because of apparent problems with follow-up of abnormal tests, a framework has been outlined for thinking through the issues and developing methods to ensure follow-up of positive tests.[13] Healthcare team members can use the work of Yabroff and others to guide their design of a system to ensure follow-up. Studies indicate that several elements are necessary for a successful follow-up system. First, a mechanism to ensure communication between the person performing the screening and the providers responsible for follow-up is necessary. Even if the provider conducts the test, as is usually the case with cervical cancer screening, clinicians need some method of ensuring that they receive the test results. Second, the provider team needs to have a plan for dealing with a positive result once it is received, because not all positive results need to be acted upon and the primary care provider is not always the responsible party. For example, radiology facilities are obligated by the MQSA to report mammography results to all women screened. Yet even in this case, a woman notified by the radiologist may not respond.

Communication with the patient about the follow-up plan is the next critical step in the implementation process. Such communication should clarify which tests are needed and what those tests involve for the patient. Research shows that communication from the provider to the patient about the importance of follow-up and the details about further workup will influence whether follow-up occurs.[13,187] Women with fears of painful procedures or fatalistic views regarding cancer diagnosis are less likely to comply with follow-up recommendations.[13] As shown in Tables 24.1, 24.3, 24.5, and

24.7, evaluations needed after a positive test vary from repeating the test or ordering additional mammograms or colonoscopy to surgical consultation. Incorporating the patient into the care plan has become an important part of follow-up care and may increase adherence to the plan.[13] For example, telephone contact addressing women's perceptions of the cervical cancer screening test and educating them before or after the Pap test through interactive discussion improved follow-up by 24% to 26%.[178] Ultimately, improving follow-up requires the coordinated effort of providers, staff working with them, and patients.

Referring for Treatment

After developing the follow-up approach, the next critical step is ensuring that patients are referred to and receive appropriate specialty care. Referral to oncology specialists by primary care providers (PCPs) depends on some degree of coordinated care. Developing this coordination was highlighted in the National Cancer Policy Board's 1999 analysis as a key step toward improving the quality of America's health care. They concluded that optimal cancer care delivery should ensure, among other things, a "mechanism to coordinate services."[188] Also, a committee of the Institute of Medicine selected care coordination as one of 20 "priority areas" requiring concerted effort if the nation's healthcare system is to be transformed.[188]

Literature is sparse regarding referral barriers relevant to screened cancers, but access and reimbursement for the uninsured are a clear challenge.[162] However, difficulties are not confined to those traditionally considered underserved by the healthcare system. Access to quality cancer treatment in general is subject to numerous barriers, including patient characteristics such as old age, low SES,[162] minority race or ethnicity,[189] and lack of health insurance. Researchers studying older cancer patients concluded that patient preference is a "major determinant in the referral decisions of primary care providers." Another potential issue is that PCPs might be unaware of cancer treatment options available to seniors.[190] Recent work raises questions regarding referral patterns and points out that the majority of patients are not seen by an oncologist who might help them with decisions.[191]

Although treatment options and systems are not a focus of this chapter, clinicians need to be mindful of the institutional and insurance barriers that may limit access. Successful referrals in any cancer patient depend on factors such as physician characteristics (e.g., specialty, training, experience, age), quality of patient–provider communication, and complexity and constraints of the current healthcare environment.[188]

Steps are being taken to improve the coordination of cancer treatment after a positive screening. A pilot project that tested the effects of patient navigators ("proactive patient advocates") on removing barriers to diagnosis and state-of-the-art treatment found the concept promising.[192] At the public policy level, Congress passed legislation in 2000 to fill the "treatment gap" in the National Breast and Cervical Cancer Early Detection Program by giving states the option to extend Medicaid benefits to uninsured women diagnosed through the program.[193] To date, the U.S. Department of Health and Human Services has approved proposals from 48 states and the District of Columbia to implement the act (CDC).

Summary and Conclusion

This chapter has reviewed the evidence related to the epidemiology, natural history, and screening of four common cancers (breast, cervical, colorectal, and prostate). It presents this evidence within the context of the challenges of primary care practice and emphasizes the need to view cancer screening as a process of care. Ensuring access to screening and treatment for all is necessary to achieve the potential for mortality reduction afforded by current screening technologies. Regardless of healthcare coverage, organized systems are needed to ensure progress throughout the continuum of care. Implementation of the numerous steps and transitions in this continuum requires the interest, commitment, and collaborative action of patients, primary care providers, specialty care providers, administrators, and public health officials. Only through this collaboration can mortality reduction be maximized.[171]

References

1. Schwartz LM, Woloshin S, Fowler FJ Jr, Welch HG. Enthusiasm for cancer screening in the United States. JAMA 2004;291:71–78.
2. Prorok PC. Evaluation of screening programs for the early detection of cancer. In: Cornell RG (ed). Statistical Methods for Cancer Studies. New York: Dekker, 1984:267–328.
3. Ernster VL. Mammography screening for women aged 40 through 49: a guidelines saga and a clarion call for informed decision making. Am J Public Health 1997;87:1103–1106.
4. Baines CJ. Mammography screening: are women really giving informed consent? J Natl Cancer Inst 2003;95:1508–1511.
5. Berg AO. Mammography screening: are women really giving informed consent? (Counterpoint). J Natl Cancer Inst 2003;95:1511–1512.
6. U.S. Preventive Services Task Force. Guide to Clinical Preventive Services, 2nd ed. Report of the U.S. Preventive Services Task Force. Baltimore: U.S. Preventive Services Task Force, 1996.
7. Humphrey LL, Helfand M, Chan BKS, Woolf SH. Breast cancer screening: a summary of the evidence for the U.S. Preventive Services Task Force. Ann Intern Med 2002;137:347–360.
8. Pignone M, Rich M, Teutsch SM, Berg AO, Lohr KN. Screening for colorectal cancer in adults at average risk: a summary of the evidence for the U.S. Preventive Services Task Force. Ann Intern Med 2002;137:132–141.
9. Saslow D, Runowicz CD, Solomon D, et al. American Cancer Society guideline for the early detection of cervical neoplasia and cancer. CA Cancer J Clin 2002;52:342–362.
10. Smith RA, Cokkinides V, Eyre HJ. American Cancer Society guidelines for the early detection of cancer, 2003. CA Cancer J Clin 2003;53:27–43.
11. Harris R, Lohr KN. Screening for prostate cancer: an update of the evidence for the U.S. Preventive Services Task Force. Ann Intern Med 2002;137:917–929.
12. Zapka JG, Taplin SH, Solberg LI, Manos MM. A framework for improving the quality of cancer care: the case of breast and cervical cancer screening. Cancer Epidemiol Biomarkers Prev 2003;12:4–13.
13. Yabroff KR, Washington KS, Leader A, Neilson E, Mandelblatt J. Is the promise of cancer-screening programs being compromised? Quality of follow-up care after abnormal screening results. Med Care Res Rev 2003;60:294–331.
14. U.S. Preventive Services Task Force (ed) Guide to Clinical Preventive Services. Baltimore: Williams & Wilkins, 1996:xxvi.

15. Weiss NS. Control definition in case-control studies of the efficacy of screening and diagnostic testing. Am J Epidemiol 1983;118:457–460.
16. Hakama M, Louhivuori K. A screening programme for cervical cancer that worked. Cancer Surv 1988;7:403–416.
17. Nystrom L, Andersson I, Bjurstam N, et al. Long-term effects of mammography screening: updated overview of the Swedish randomised trials. Lancet 2002;359:909–919.
18. Selby JV, Friedman GD, Quesenberry CP, Weiss NS. A case-control study of screening sigmoidoscopy and mortality from colorectal cancer. N Engl J Med 1992;326:653–657.
19. Concato J, Shah N, Horwitz RI. Randomized, controlled trials, observational studies, and the hierarchy of research designs. N Engl J Med 2000;342:1887–1892.
20. Benson K, Hartz AJ. A comparison of observational studies and randomized controlled trials. N Engl J Med 2004;342:1878–1885.
21. Tudiver F, Guibert R, Haggerty J, et al. What influences family physicians' cancer screening decisions when practice guidelines are unclear or conflicting? J Fam Pract 2002;51:760.
22. Cancer facts and figures 2004. Atlanta, GA: American Cancer Society, 2004. (Accessed February 2, 2004, at http://www.cancer.org/downloads/STT/CAFF2004PWSecured.pdf.)
23. Breast cancer facts & figures 2003–2004. Atlanta, GA: American Cancer Society, 2004. (Accessed January 21, 2004, at http://www.cancer.org/docroot/STT/content/STT_1x_Breast_Cancer_Facts__Figures_2003–2004.asp.)
24. Probability of developing or dying of cancer: breast cancer (DEVCAN). Bethesda, MD: National Cancer Institute, SEER, 2003. (Accessed January 21, 2004, at http://seer.cancer.gov/faststats/html/dev_breast.html.)
25. SEER 12 Registries Incidence and Mortality (2002 submission). Bethesda, MD: National Cancer Institute, SEER, 2002. (Accessed January 21, 2004, at http://seer.cancer.gov/faststats/html/dev_breast.html.)
26. Cancer facts and figures 2003. Atlanta, GA: American Cancer Society, 2003. (Accessed December 30, 2003, at http://www.cancer.org/downloads/STT/CAFF2003PWSecured.pdf.)
27. International Agency for Research on Cancer. Breast Cancer Screening, vol 7. Lyon, France: IARC Press, 2002.
28. Duffy SW, Day NE, Tabar L, Chen HH, Smith TC. Markov models of breast tumor progression: some age-specific results. J Natl Cancer Inst Monogr 1997;22:93–97.
29. Shen Y, Zelen M. Screening sensitivity and sojourn time from breast cancer early detection clinical trials: mammograms and physical examinations. J Clin Oncol 2001;19:3490–3499.
30. Kerlikowske K, Molinaro A, Cha I, et al. Characteristics associated with recurrence among women with ductal carcinoma *in situ* treated by lumpectomy. J Natl Cancer Inst 2003; 95:1692–1702.
31. Ernster VL, Ballard-Barbash R, Barlow WE, et al. Detection of ductal carcinoma in situ in women undergoing screening mammography. J Natl Cancer Inst 2002;94:1546–1554.
32. Barton MB, Harris RH, Feltcher SW. Does this patient have breast cancer? The screening clinical breast examination: should it be done? How. JAMA 1999;282:1270–1280.
33. Hendrick RE, Chrvala CA, Plott CM, et al. Improvement in mammography quality control: 1987–1995. Radiology 1998;207: 663–668.
34. Beam CA, Layde PM, Sullivan DC. Variability in the interpretation of screening mammograms by US radiologists. Arch Intern Med 1996;156:209–213.
35. Elmore JG, Wells CK, Lee CH, Howard DH, Feinstein AR. Variability in radiologists' interpretations of mammograms. N Engl J Med 1994;331:1493–1499.
36. Taplin SH, Rutter CM, Finder C, et al. Screening mammography: clinical image quality and the risk of interval breast cancer. AJR 2002;178:797–803.
37. American College of Radiology (ACR). Breast Imaging Reporting and Data System (BI-RADS™), 3rd ed. Reston, VA: American College of Radiology, 1998.
38. Bi-Rads®-Mammography: Assessment Categories. Reston, VA: American College of Radiology, 2003. (Accessed February 2, 2004, at http://www.acr.org/departments/stand_accred/birads/mammo_assess.pdf.)
39. Kerlikowske K, Grady D, Barclay J, Sickles EA, Ernster V. Effect of age, breast density, and family history on the sensitivity of first screening mammography. JAMA 1996;276:33–38.
40. Yankaskas BC, Taplin SH, Ichikawa L, et al. Association between mammography timing and measures of screening performance in the U.S. Radiology (in press).
41. Carney PA, Miglioretti DL, Yankaskas BC, et al. Individual and combined effects of age, breast density, and hormone replacement therapy use on the accuracy of screening mammography. Ann Intern Med 2003;138:168–175.
42. Pisano ED, Kuzmiak C, Koomen M, Cance W. What every surgical oncologist should know about digital mammography. Semin Surg Oncol 2001;20:181–186.
43. Lewin JM, D'Orsi CJ, Hendrick RE, et al. Clinical comparison of full-field digital mammography and film-screen mammography for detection of breast cancer. AJR Am J Roentgenol 2002; 179:671–677.
44. James JJ. The current status of digital mammography. Clin Radiol 2004;59:1–10.
45. Roque AC, Andre TC. Mammography and computerized decision systems: a review. Ann N Y Acad Sci 2002;980:83–94.
46. Gur D, Sumkin JH, Rockette HE, et al. Changes in breast cancer detection and mammography recall rates after the introduction of a computer-aided detection system. J Natl Cancer Inst 2004; 96:185–190.
47. Teaching Atlas of Breast Ultrasound, 2nd ed. New York: Thieme, 1996.
48. Kerlikowske K, Smith-Bindman R, Ljung BM, Grady D. Evaluation of abnormal mammography results and palpable breast abnormalities. Ann Intern Med 2003;139:274–284.
49. Sevilla C, Moatti JP, Julian-Reynier C, et al. Testing for BRCA1 mutations: a cost-effectiveness analysis. Eur J Hum Genet 2002; 10:599–606.
50. Burke W, Daly M, Garber J, et al. Recommendations for follow-up care of individuals with an inherited predisposition to cancer. II. BRACA1 and BRCA2. JAMA 1997;27:997–1003.
51. Miller AB, To T, Baines CJ, Wall C. Canadian National Breast Screening Study 2: 13-year results of a randomized trial in women aged 50–59 years. J Natl Cancer Inst 2000;92:1490–1499.
52. Anderson BO, Braun S, Lim S, et al. Early detection of breast cancer in countries with limited resources. Breast J 2003; 9:S51–S59.
53. Thomas DB, Gao DL, Ray RM, et al. Randomized trial of breast self-examination in Shanghai: final results. J Natl Cancer Inst 2002;94:1445–1457.
54. Duffy SW, Tabar L, Chen HH, et al. The impact of organized mammography service screening on breast carcinoma mortality in seven Swedish counties. Cancer (Phila) 2002;95:458–469.
55. Olsen O, Gotzsche PC. Systematic review of screening for breast cancer with mammography. Lancet 2001;358:9290.
56. Green BB, Taplin SH. Breast cancer screening controversies. J Am Board Fam Pract 2003;16:233–241.
57. Breast Cancer Screening Among Women in Their Forties: An Overview of the Issues. Bethesda MD: National Institutes of Health, 1997.
58. Breast Screening Frequency Trial Group. The frequency of breast cancer screening: results from the UKCCCR Randomised Trial. Eur J Cancer 2002;38:1458–1464.
59. Smith RA, Saslow D, Sawyer KA, et al. American Cancer Society guidelines for breast cancer screening: update 2003. CA Cancer J Clin 2003;53:141–169.

60. World Health Organization and International Agency for Research on Cancer. World Cancer Report. Lyon, France: International Agency for Research on Cancer, 2003.
61. Taylor VM, Jackson JC, Schwartz SM, Tu SP, Thompson B. Cervical cancer among Asian American women: a neglected public health problem? Asian Am Pac Isl J Health 1996;4:327–342.
62. Franco EL. Primary screening of cervical cancer with human papillomavirus tests. J Natl Cancer Inst Monogr 2003;31:89–96.
63. IARC Working Group on Evaluation of Cervical Cancer Screening Programmes. Screening for squamous cervical cancer: duration of low risk after negative results of cervical cytology and its implication for screening policies. Br Med J 1986;293:659–664.
64. Franco EL, Duarte-Franco E, Ferenczy A. Cervical cancer: epidemiology, prevention and the role of human papillomavirus infection. Can Med Assoc J 2001;164:1017–1025.
65. Levine PB. Parental involvement laws and fertility behavior. J Health Econ 2003;22:861–878.
66. McCann MF, Irwin DE, Walton LA, et al. Nicotine and cotinine in the cervical mucus of smokers, passive smokers, and nonsmokers. Cancer Epidemiol Biomarkers Prev 1992;1:125–129.
67. Coker AL, Bond SM, Williams A, Gerasimova T, Pirisi L. Active and passive smoking, high-risk human papillomaviruses and cervical neoplasia. Cancer Detect Prev 2002;26:121–128.
68. Brinton LA, Hamman RF, Huggins GR, et al. Sexual and reproductive risk factors for invasive squamous cell cervical cancer. J Natl Cancer Inst 1987;79:23–30.
69. Ferenczy A, Coutlee F, Franco E, Hankins C. Human papillomavirus and HIV coinfection and the risk of neoplasias of the lower genital tract: a review of recent developments. Can Med Assoc J 2003;169:431–424.
70. Sierra-Torres CH, Au WW, Arrastia CD, et al. Polymorphisms for chemical metabolizing genes and risk for cervical neoplasia. Environ Mol Mutagen 2003;41:69–76.
71. Nanda K, McCrory DC, Myers ER, et al. Accuracy of the Papanicolaou test in screening for and follow-up of cervical cytologic abnormalities: a systematic review. Ann Intern Med 2000; 132:810–819.
72. Davey DD. Cervical cytology classification and the Bethesda System. Cancer J 2003;9:327–334.
73. Sasieni P, Cuzick J. Could HPV testing become the sole primary cervical screening test? J Med Screen 2002;9:49–51.
74. Sherman ME. Future directions in cervical pathology. J Natl Cancer Inst Monogr 2003;31:72–79.
75. Ronco G, Vineis C, Montanari G, et al. Impact of the AutoPap (currently Focalpoint) primary screening system location guide use on interpretation time and diagnosis. Cancer (Phila) 2003; 99:83–88.
76. Hartmann KE, Nanda K, Hall S, Myers E. Technologic advances for evaluation of cervical cytology: is newer better? Obstet Gynecol Surv 2001;56:765–774.
77. Wright TC Jr. Cervical cancer screening using visualization techniques. J Natl Cancer Inst Monogr 2003;31:66–71.
78. Sherman ME, Lorincz AT, Scott DR, et al. Baseline cytology, human papillomavirus testing, and risk for cervical neoplasia: a 10-year cohort analysis. J Natl Cancer Inst 2003;95:46–52.
79. Sawaya GF, McConnell KJ, Kulasingam SL, et al. Risk of cervical cancer associated with extending the interval between cervical-cancer screenings. N Engl J Med 2003;349:1501–1509.
80. Sasieni P, Adams J, Cuzick J. Benefit of cervical screening at different ages: evidence from the UK audit of screening histories. Br J Cancer 2003;89:88–93.
81. Cervical cancer—screening. Rockville, MD: U.S. Preventive Services Task Force, 2003. (Accessed January 14, 2004, at http://www.ahrq.gov/clinic/uspstf/uspscerv.htm.)
82. U.S. Preventive Services Task Force. Screening for cervical cancer. In: DiGuiseppi C, Atkins D, Woolf S (eds). Guide to Clinical Preventive Services: Report of the US Preventive Services Task Force. Baltimore: Williams & Wilkins, 1996:105–117.
83. Pasche B, Mulcahy M, Benson AB III. Molecular markers in prognosis of colorectal cancer and prediction of response to treatment. Best Pract Res Clin Gastroenterol 2002;16:331–345.
84. Kinzler KW, Vogelstein B. Lessons from hereditary colorectal cancer. Cell 1996;87:159–170.
85. Chung DC, Rustgi AK. The hereditary nonpolyposis colorectal cancer syndrome: genetics and clinical implications. Ann Intern Med 2003;138:560–570.
86. Hofstad B, Vatn M. Growth rate of colon polyps and cancer. Gastrointest Endosc Clin N Am 1997;7:345–363.
87. Vogelstein B, Fearon ER, Hamilton SR, et al. Genetic alterations during colorectal-tumor development. N Engl J Med 1988; 319:525–532.
88. Ahlquist DA, Shuber AP. Stool screening for colorectal cancer: evolution from occult blood to molecular markers. Clin Chim Acta 2002;315:157–168.
89. Levin B, Brooks D, Smith RA, Stone A. Emerging technologies in screening for colorectal cancer: CT colonography, immunochemical fecal occult blood tests, and stool screening using molecular markers. CA Cancer J Clin 2003;53:44–55.
90. Winawer S, Fletcher R, Rex D, et al. Colorectal cancer screening and surveillance: clinical guidelines and rationale—update based on new evidence. Gastroenterology 2003;124: 544–560.
91. Chen CD, Yen MF, Wang WM, Wong JM, Chen TH. A case-cohort study for the disease natural history of adenoma-carcinoma and de novo carcinoma and surveillance of colon and rectum after polypectomy: implication for efficacy of colonoscopy. Br J Cancer 2003;88:1866–1873.
92. Anderson WF, Guyton KZ, Hiatt RA, et al. Colorectal cancer screening for persons at average risk. J Natl Cancer Inst 2002; 94:1126–1133.
93. Herrinton LJ, Selby JV, Friedman GD, Quesenberry CP, Weiss NS. Case-control study of digital-rectal screening in relation to mortality from cancer of the distal rectum. Am J Epidemiol 1995;142:961–964.
94. Young GP, St John DJ, Winawer SJ, Rozen P. Choice of fecal occult blood tests for colorectal cancer screening: recommendations based on performance characteristics in population studies: a WHO (World Health Organization) and OMED (World Organization for Digestive Endoscopy) report. Am J Gastroenterol 2002;97:2499–2507.
95. Allison JE, Tekawa IS, Ransom LJ, Adrian AL. A comparison of fecal occult-blood tests for colorectal-cancer screening. N Engl J Med 1996;334:155–159.
96. van Ballegooijen M, Habbema JDF, Boer R, Zauber AG, Brown ML. Report to the Agency for Healthcare Research and Quality. A comparison of the cost-effectiveness of fecal occult blood tests with different test characteristics in the context of annual screening in the Medicare population. Baltimore, MD: Centers for Medicare and Medicaid Services, 2003.
97. Cole SR, Young GP, Esterman A, Cadd B, Morcom J. A randomised trial of the impact of new faecal haemoglobin test technologies on population participation in screening for colorectal cancer. J Med Screen 2003;10:117–122.
98. Pignone M, Campbell MK, Carr C, Phillips C. Meta-analysis of dietary restriction during fecal occult blood testing. Eff Clin Pract 2001;4:150–156.
99. Ahlquist DA, Wieand HS, Moertel CG, et al. Accuracy of fecal occult blood screening for colorectal neoplasia. A prospective study using Hemoccult and HemoQuant tests. JAMA 1993; 269:1262–1267.
100. Ransohoff DF, Lang CA. Improving the fecal occult-blood test. N Engl J Med 1996;334:189–190.
101. Levin B, Hess K, Johnson C. Screening for colorectal cancer. A comparison of 3 fecal occult blood tests. Arch Intern Med 1997;157:970–976.

102. Mandel JS, Bond JH, Church TR, et al. Reducing mortality from colorectal cancer by screening for fecal occult blood. N Engl J Med 1993;328:1365–1371.
103. Ransohoff DF, Lang CA. Part I: Suggested technique for fecal occult blood testing and interpretation in colorectal cancer screening. Ann Intern Med 1997;126:808–810.
104. Vernon S. Adherence to colorectal cancer screening. Ann NY Acad Sci 1995;768:292–295.
105. Hardcastle JD, Chamberlain JO, Robinson MH, et al. Randomised controlled trial of faecal-occult-blood screening for colorectal cancer. Lancet 1996;348:1472–1477.
106. Kronborg O, Fenger C, Olsen J, Jorgensen OD, Sondergaard O. Randomised study of screening for colorectal cancer with faecal-occult-blood test. Lancet 1996;348:1467–1471.
107. Mandel JS, Church TR, Bond JH, et al. The effect of fecal occult-blood screening on the incidence of colorectal cancer. N Engl J Med 2000;343:1603–1607.
108. Robinson MH, Pye G, Thomas WM, Hardcastle JD, Mangham CM. Haemoccult screening for colorectal cancer: the effect of dietary restriction on compliance. Eur J Surg Oncol 1994;20:545–548.
109. Cole SR, Young GP. Effect of dietary restriction on participation in faecal occult blood test screening for colorectal cancer. Med J Aust 2001;175:195–198.
110. Ko CW, Dominitz JA, Nguyen TD. Fecal occult blood testing in a general medical clinic: comparison between guaiac-based and immunochemical-based tests. Am J Med 2003;115:111–114.
111. Walsh JM, Terdiman JP. Colorectal cancer screening: scientific review. JAMA 2003;289:1288–1296.
112. Rex DK, Johnson DA, Lieberman DA, Burt RW, Sonnenberg A. Colorectal cancer prevention 2000: screening recommendations of the American College of Gastroenterology. Am J Gastroenterol 2000;95:868–877.
113. Eloubeidi MA, Wallace MB, Desmond R, Farraye FA. Female gender and other factors predictive of a limited screening flexible sigmoidoscopy examination for colorectal cancer. Am J Gastroenterol 2003;98:1634–1639.
114. Pickhardt PJ, Choi JR, Hwang I, et al. Computed tomographic virtual colonoscopy to screen for colorectal neoplasia in asymptomatic adults. N Engl J Med 2003;349:2191–2200.
115. Rex DK, Rahmani EY, Haseman JH, et al. Relative sensitivity of colonoscopy and barium enema for detection of colorectal cancer in clinical practice. Gastroenterology 1997;112:17–23.
116. Rex DK, Cutler CS, Lemmel GT, et al. Colonoscopic miss rates of adenomas determined by back-to-back colonoscopies. Gastroenterology 1997;112:24–28.
117. Gatto NM, Frucht H, Sundararajan V, et al. Risk of perforation after colonoscopy and sigmoidoscopy: a population-based study. J Natl Cancer Inst 2003;95:230–236.
118. Schoen RE, Weissfeld JL, Bowen NJ, Switzer G, Baum A. Patient satisfaction with screening flexible sigmoidoscopy. Arch Intern Med 2000;160:1790–1796.
119. Lurie JD, Welch HG. Diagnostic testing following fecal occult blood screening in the elderly. J Natl Cancer Inst 1999;91:1641–1646.
120. Turner B, Myers ME, Hyslop T, et al. Physician and patient factors associated with ordering a colon evaluation after a positive fecal occult blood test. J Gen Intern Med 2003;18:357–363.
121. Sussman GL, Beezhold DH. Latex allergy—a clinical perspective. J Long Term Eff Med Implants 1994;4:95–101.
122. Misselbeck WJ, Gray KR, Uphold RE. Latex induced anaphylaxis: a case report. Am J Emerg Med 1994;12:445–447.
123. Ownby DR, Tomlanovich M, Sammons N, McCullough J. Anaphylaxis associated with latex allergy during barium enema examinations. AJR Am J Roentgenol 1991;156:903–908.
124. Johnson CD, Ahlquist DA. Computed tomography colonography (virtual colonoscopy): a new method for colorectal screening. Gut 1999;44:301–305.
125. Dong SM, Traverso G, Johnson C, et al. Detecting colorectal cancer in stool with the use of multiple genetic targets. J Natl Cancer Inst 2001;93:858–865.
126. Traverso G, Shuber A, Olsson L, et al. Detection of proximal colorectal cancers through analysis of faecal DNA. Lancet 2002;359:403–404.
127. Ahlquist DA, Skoletsky JE, Boynton KA, et al. Colorectal cancer screening by detection of altered human DNA in stool: feasibility of a multitarget assay panel. Gastroenterology 2000;119:1219–1227.
128. Walsh JM, Terdiman JP. Colorectal cancer screening: clinical applications. JAMA 2003;289:1297–1302.
129. Helm J, Choi J, Sutphen R, et al. Current and evolving strategies for colorectal cancer screening. Cancer Control 2003;10:193–204.
130. Hardcastle JD, Armitage NC, Chamberlain J, et al. Fecal occult blood screening for colorectal cancer in the general population. Cancer (Phila) 1986;58:397–403.
131. Mandel JS, Church TR, Ederer F, Bond JH. Colorectal cancer mortality: effectiveness of biennial screening for fecal occult blood. J Natl Cancer Inst 1999;91:434–437.
132. Saito H, Soma Y, Koeda J, et al. Reduction in risk of mortality from colorectal cancer by fecal occult blood screening with immunochemical hemagglutination test. A case-control study. Int J Cancer 1995;61:465–469.
133. Newcomb PA, Storer BE, Morimoto LM, Templeton A, Potter JD. Long-term efficacy of sigmoidoscopy in the reduction of colorectal cancer incidence. J Natl Cancer Inst 2003;95:622–625.
134. Winawer SJ, Flehinger BJ, Schottenfeld D, Miller DG. Screening for colorectal cancer with fecal occult blood testing and sigmoidoscopy. J Natl Cancer Inst 1993;85:1311–1318.
135. Prorok PC, Andriole GL, Bresalier RS, et al. Design of the prostate, lung, colorectal and ovarian (PLCO) cancer screening trial. Controlled Clin Trials 2000;21:273S–309S.
136. Atkin WS, Hart A, Edwards R, et al. Uptake, yield of neoplasia, and adverse effects of flexible sigmoidoscopy screening. Gut 1998;42:560–565.
137. Gondal G, Grotmol T, Hofstad B, et al. The Norwegian Colorectal Cancer Prevention (NORCCAP) screening study: baseline findings and implementations for clinical work-up in age groups 50–64 years. Scand J Gastroenterol 2003;38:635–642.
138. Muller AD, Sonnenberg A. Prevention of colorectal cancer by flexible endoscopy and polypectomy. A case-control study of 32,702 veterans. Ann Intern Med 1995;123:904–910.
139. Kavanagh AM, Giovannucci EL, Fuchs CS, Colditz GA. Screening endoscopy and risk of colorectal cancer in United States men. Cancer Causes Control 1998;9:455–462.
140. Winawer SJ, Zauber AG, Ho MN, et al. Prevention of colorectal cancer by colonoscopic polypectomy. N Engl J Med 1993;329:1977–1981.
141. Muller AD, Sonnenberg A. Protection by endoscopy against death from colorectal cancer. A case-control study among veterans. Arch Intern Med 1995;155:1741–1748.
142. Ransohoff DF, McNaughton CM, Fowler FJ. Why is prostate cancer screening so common when the evidence is so uncertain? A system without negative feedback. Am J Med 2002;113:663–667.
143. Hoffman RM, Hunt WC, Gilliland FD, Stephenson RA, Potosky AL. Patient satisfaction with treatment decisions for clinically localized prostate carcinoma. Results from the Prostate Cancer Outcomes Study. Cancer (Phila) 2003;97:1653–1662.
144. Potosky AL, Reeve BB, Clegg LX, et al. Quality of life following localized prostate cancer treated initially with androgen deprivation therapy or no therapy. J Natl Cancer Inst 2002;94:430–437.
145. Cookson MS. Prostate cancer: screening and early detection. Cancer Control 2004;8:133–140.

146. Potosky AL, Feuer EJ, Levin DL. Impact of screening on incidence and mortality of prostate cancer in the United States. Epidemiol Rev 2001;23:181–186.
147. Perron L, Moore L, Bairati I, Bernard PM, Meyer F. PSA screening and prostate cancer mortality. C Med Assoc J 2002; 166:586–591.
148. Tornblom M, Eriksson H, Franzen S, et al. Lead time associated with screening for prostate cancer. Int J Cancer 2004;108: 122–129.
149. Partin AW, Brawer MK, Bartsch G, et al. Complexed prostate specific antigen improves specificity for prostate cancer detection: results of a prospective multicenter clinical trial. J Urol 2003; 170:1787–1791.
150. Caplan A, Kratz A. Prostate-specific antigen and the early diagnosis of prostate cancer. Am J Clin Pathol 2002;117:S104–S108.
151. Labrie F, Candas B, Dupont A, et al. Screening decreases prostate cancer death: first analysis of the 1988 Quebec prospective randomized controlled trial. Prostate 1999;38:83–91.
152. Potosky AL, Legler J, Albertsen PC, et al. Health outcomes after prostatectomy or radiotherapy for prostate cancer: results from the Prostate Cancer Outcomes Study. J Natl Cancer Inst 2000;92:1582–1592.
153. Schmid HP, Prikler L, Semjonow A. Problems with prostate-specific antigen screening: a critical review. Recent Results Cancer Res 2003;163:226–231.
154. McCarthy BD, Ulcickas-Yood M, Boohaker EA, et al. Inadequate follow-up of abnormal mammograms. Am J Prev Med 1996; 12:282–288.
155. Sung HY, Kearney KA, Miller M, et al. Papanicolaou smear history and diagnosis of invasive cervical carcinoma among members of a large prepaid health plan. Cancer (Phila) 2000;88:2283–2289.
156. Hiatt RA, Pasick RJ, Stewart S, et al. Community-based cancer screening for underserved women: design and baseline findings from the Breast and Cervical Cancer Intervention Study. Prev Med 2001;33:190–203.
157. Hiatt RA, Klabunde C, Breen N, Swan J, Ballard-Barbash R. Cancer screening practices from National Health Interview Surveys: past, present, and future. J Natl Cancer Inst 2002;94: 1837–1846.
158. Swan J, Breen N, Coates RJ, Rimer BK, Lee NC. Progress in cancer screening practices in the United States: results from the 2000 National Health Interview Survey. Cancer (Phila) 2003;97:1528–1540.
159. Sirovich BE, Schwartz LM, Woloshin S. Screening men for prostate and colorectal cancer in the United States: does practice reflect the evidence? JAMA 2003;289:1414–1420.
160. Klabunde CN, Frame PS, Meadow A, et al. A national survey of primary care physicians' colorectal cancer screening recommendations and practices. Prev Med 2003;36:352–362.
161. Lawson HW, Henson R, Bobo JK, Kaeser MK. Implementing recommendations for the early detection of breast and cervical cancer among low-income women. MMWR Morbid Mortal Wkly Rep 2000;49(RR02):35–55.
162. Mandelblatt JS, Yabroff KR, Kerner JF. Equitable access to cancer services: a review of barriers to quality care. Cancer (Phila) 1999; 86:2378–2390.
163. Hidden costs, value lost: uninsurance in America. Washington, DC: Institute of Medicine, 2003. (Accessed February 2, 2004, at http://www.nap.edu/openbook/030908931X/html/2.html.)
164. Breen N, Wagener DK, Brown ML, Davis WW, Ballard-Barbash R. Progress in cancer screening over a decade: results of cancer screening from the 1987, 1991, and 1998 National Health Interview Surveys. J Natl Cancer Inst 2001;93:1704–1713.
165. Cokkinides V, Chao A, Smith RA, Vernon SW, Thun MJ. Correlates of underutilization of colorectal cancer screening among U.S. adults, age 50 years and older. Prev Med 2003;36: 85–91.
166. Cooper GS, Koroukian SM. Racial disparities in the use of and indications for colorectal procedures in Medicare beneficiaries. Cancer (Phila) 2004;100:418–424.
167. Singh GK, Miller BA, Hankey BF, Feuer EJ, Pickle LW. Changing area socioeconomic patterns in U.S. cancer mortality, 1950–1998: Part I. All cancers among men. J Natl Cancer Inst 2002;94:904–915.
168. Sambamoorthi U, McAlpine DD. Racial, ethnic, socioeconomic, and access disparities in the use of preventive services among women. Prev Med 2003;37:475–484.
169. Jackson JC, Taylor VM, Chitnarong K, et al. Development of a cervical cancer control intervention program for Cambodian American women. J Community Health 2000;25:359–375.
170. Tu SP, Taplin SH, Barlow WE, Boyko EJ. Breast cancer screening by Asian-American women in a managed care environment. Am J Prev Med 1999;17:55–61.
171. Zapka JG. Interventions for patients, providers, and health care organizations. Cancer 2004;101(suppl 5):1165–1187.
172. Stone EG, Morton SC, Hulscher ME, et al. Interventions that increase use of adult immunization and cancer screening services: a meta-analysis. Ann Intern Med 2002;136:641–651.
173. Stockwell DH, Woo P, Jacobson BC, et al. Determinants of colorectal cancer screening in women undergoing mammography. Am J Gastroenterol 2003;98:1875–1880.
174. Yarnall KS, Pollak KI, Ostbye T, Krause KM, Michener JL. Primary care: is there enough time for prevention? Am J Public Health 2003;93:635–641.
175. Yabroff KR, Mandelblatt JS. Interventions targeted toward patients to increase mammography use. Cancer Epidemiol Biomarkers Prev 1999;8:749–757.
176. Mandelblatt JS, Yabroff KR. Effectiveness of interventions designed to increase mammography use: a meta-analysis of provider-targeted strategies. Cancer Epidemiol Biomarkers Prev 1999;8:759–767.
177. Wagner TH. The effectiveness of mailed patient reminders on mammography screening: a meta-analysis. Am J Prev Med 1998; 14:64–70.
178. Yabroff KR, Kerner JF, Mandelblatt JS. Effectiveness of interventions to improve follow-up after abnormal cervical cancer screening. Prev Med 2000;31:429–439.
179. Mandelblatt J, Kanetsky PA. Effectiveness of interventions to enhance physician screening for breast cancer. J Fam Pract 1995; 40:162–171.
180. Lam TK, McPhee SJ, Mock J, et al. Encouraging Vietnamese-American women to obtain Pap tests through lay health worker outreach and media education. J Gen Intern Med 2003; 18:516–524.
181. Glasgow RE, Orleans CT, Wagner EH. Does the chronic care model serve also as a template for improving prevention? Milbank Q 2001;79:579–612.
182. Dietrich AJ, Carney PA, Winchell CW, Sox CH, Reed SC. An office systems approach to cancer prevention in primary care. Cancer Pract 1997;5:375–381.
183. Carney-Gersten P, Keller A, Landgraf J, Dietrich AJ. Tools, teamwork, and tenacity: an office system for cancer prevention. J Fam Pract 1992;35:388–394.
184. Taplin SH, Galvin MS, Payne T, Coole D, Wagner E. Putting population-based care into practice: real option or rhetoric? J Am Board Fam Pract 1998;11:116–126.
185. Myers RE, Turner B, Weinberg D, et al. Complete diagnostic evaluation in colorectal cancer screening: research design and baseline findings. Prev Med 2001;33:249–260.
186. Burack RC, Simon MS, Stano M, George J, Coombs J. Follow-up among women with an abnormal mammogram in an HMO: is it complete, timely, and efficient? Am J Manag Care 2000; 6:1102–1113.
187. Paskett E, Rimer B. Psychosocial effects of abnormal pap tests and mammograms: a review. J Womens Health 1995;4:73–82.

188. Institute of Medicine, Commission on Life Sciences National Research Council. Ensuring Quality Cancer Care. Washington, DC: National Academy Press, 1999.
189. Institute of Medicine. Unequal Treatment: Confronting Racial and Ethnic Disparities in Healthcare. Washington, DC: National Academies Press, 2003.
190. Townsley CA, Naidoo K, Pond GR, et al. Are older cancer patients being referred to oncologists? A mail questionnaire of Ontario primary care practitioners to evaluate their referral patterns. J Clin Oncol 2003;21:4627–4635.
191. Earle CC, Neumann PJ, Gelber RD, Weinstein MC, Weeks JC. Impact of referral patterns on the use of chemotherapy for lung cancer. J Clin Oncol 2002;20:1786–1792.
192. Freeman HP, Muth BJ, Kerner JF. Expanding access to cancer screening and clinical follow-up among the medically underserved. Cancer Pract 1995;3:19–30.
193. Lantz PM, Weisman CS, Itani Z. A disease-specific Medicaid expansion for women. The Breast and Cervical Cancer Prevention and Treatment Act of 2000. Womens Health Issues 2003; 13:79–92.
194. Bobo J, Lee N. Factors associated with accurate cancer detection during a clinical breast examination. Ann Epidemiol 2000; 10:463.
195. Oestreicher N, White E, Lehman CD, et al. Predictors of sensitivity of clinical breast examination (CBE). Breast Cancer Res Treat 2002;76:73–81.
196. Shapiro S, Benet W, Strax P, Venet L. Periodic Screening for Breast Cancer: The Health Insurance Plan Project and Its Sequelae, 1963–1986. Baltimore: Johns Hopkins University Press, 1988:55.
197. Miller AB, To T, Baines CJ, Wall C. The Canadian National Breast Screening Study. 1: Breast cancer mortality after 11 to 16 years of follow-up. Ann Intern Med 2002;137:E305–E315.
198. Alexander FE, Anderson TJ, Brown HK, et al. 14 years of follow-up from the Edinburgh randomised trial of breast-cancer screening. Lancet 1999;353:1903–1908.
199. Bjurstam N, Bjorneld L, Duffy SW, et al. The Gothenburg breast screening trial: first results on mortality, incidence, and mode of detection for women ages 39–49 years at randomization. Cancer (Phila) 1997;80:2091–2099.
200. Frisell J, Lidbrink E, Hellstrom L, Rutqvist LE. Follow-up after 11 years: update of mortality results in the Stockholm mammographic screening trial. Breast Cancer Res Treat 1997; 45:263–270.
201. Andersson I, Aspegren K, Janzon L, et al. Mammographic screening and mortality from breast cancer: the Malmo mammographic screening trial. Br Med J 1988;297:943–948.
202. Tabar L, Vitak B, Chen HH, et al. The Swedish Two-County Trial twenty years later. Updated mortality results and new insights from long-term follow-up. Radiol Clin N Am 2000;38:625–651.
203. Wright TC Jr, Cox JT, Massd LS, Twiggs LB, Wilkinson EJ. 2001 Consensus guidelines for the management of women with cervical cytological abnormalities. JAMA 2002;278:2120–2129.
204. Nygard JF, Skare GB, Thoresen SO. The cervical cancer screening programme in Norway, 1992–2000: changes in Pap smear coverage and incidence of cervical cancer. J Med Screen 2002; 9:86–91.
205. Wright TC, Cox JT, Massad LS, et al. 2001 consensus guidelines for the management of women with cervical intraepithelial neoplasia. J Lower Genital Tract Dis 2003;7:154–167.
206. Manos M, Kinney WK, Hurley LB, et al. Identifying women with cervical neoplasia: using human papillomavirus DNA testing for equivocal Papanicolaou results. JAMA 1999;281:1605–1610.
207. Wright JC, Weinstein MC. Gains in life expectancy from medical interventions: standardizing data on outcomes [see comments]. N Engl J Med 1998;339:380–386.
208. Day NE. Effect of cervical cancer screening in Scandinavia. Obstet Gynecol 1984;63:714–718.
209. Lynge E. Effect of organized screening on incidence and mortality of cervical cancer in Denmark. Cancer Res 1989;49: 2157–2160.
210. Bigaard J. Cervical cancer screening in Denmark. Eur J Cancer 2000;36:2198–2204.
211. Greenberg PD, Bertario L, Gnauck R, et al. A prospective multicenter evaluation of new fecal occult blood tests in patients undergoing colonoscopy. Am J Gastroenterol 2000;95: 1331–1338.
212. Lieberman DA, Weiss DG. One-time screening for colorectal cancer with combined fecal occult-blood testing and examination of the distal colon. N Engl J Med 2001;345:555–560.
213. van den Akker-van Marle ME, van Ballegooijen M, van Oortmarssen GJ, Boer R, Habbema JD. Cost-effectiveness of cervical cancer screening: comparison of screening policies. J Natl Cancer Inst 2002;94:193–204.
214. Winawer SJ, Fletcher RH, Miller L, et al. Colorectal cancer screening: clinical guidelines and rationale. Gastroenterology 1997;112:594–642.
215. Wherry DC, Thomas WM. The yield of flexible fiberoptic sigmoidoscopy in the detection of asymptomatic colorectal neoplasia. Surg Endosc 1994;8:393–395.
216. Rex DK. Current colorectal cancer screening strategies: overview and obstacles to implementation. Rev Gastroenterol Disord 2002;2:S2–S11.
217. Tagore KS, Lawson MJ, Yucaitis JA. Sensitivity and specificity of a stool DNA multitarget assay panel for the detection of advanced colorectal neoplasia. Clin Colorectal Cancer 2004; 3:47–53.
218. Mulhall BP. Recent findings on test performance. Washington, DC: Walter Reed Army Medical Center, 2003 (unpublished work).
219. U.S. Preventive Services Task Force. Screening for prostate cancer: recommendations and rationale. Am Fam Physician 2003;67:787–792.
220. Friedman GD, Hiatt RA, Quesenberry CP Jr, Selby JV. Case-control study of screening for prostatic cancer by digital rectal examinations. Lancet 1991;337:1526–1529.
221. Jacobsen SJ, Bergstralh EJ, Katusic SK, et al. Screening digital rectal examination and prostate cancer mortality: a population-based case-control study. Urology 1998;52:173–179.
222. Richert-Boe KE, Humphrey LL, Glass AG, Weiss NS. Screening digital rectal examination and prostate cancer mortality: a case-control study. J Med Screen 1998;5:99–103.
223. Lu-Yao G, Albertsen PC, Stanford JL, et al. Natural experiment examining impact of aggressive screening and treatment on prostate cancer mortality in two fixed cohorts from Seattle area and Connecticut. BMJ 2002;325:740.
224. Bartsch G, Horninger W, Klocker H, et al. Prostate cancer mortality after introduction of prostate-specific antigen mass screening in the Federal State of Tyrol, Austria. Urology 2001;58:417–424.

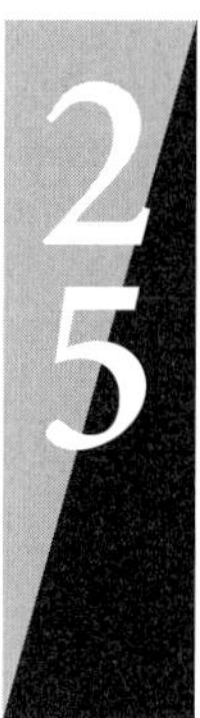

Genetic Screening and Counseling for High-Risk Populations

Mary B. Daly

As we enter the 21st century, we are witnessing a historic transition in science that will reveal the genetic basis of common medical conditions and have an enormous impact on biology, medicine, health care, and society. The role of genetics in understanding and treating cancer has traditionally been limited to the observation of cytogenetic abnormalities in certain tumor types. With the recent stimulus of the Human Genome Project, new opportunities to define all cancer in genetic terms are emerging. Efforts to characterize the several classes of genes involved in the transformation and growth of cancer cells have not only advanced knowledge of the genetic basis of cancer but also stimulated the development of sophisticated high throughput technologies that open a new generation of opportunities for the next decade of clinical research and application. Molecular genetic analysis will permit the identification of cancer susceptibility patterns decades before the onset of symptoms or the appearance of disease. The impact of this genetic revolution will shape the practice of medicine, and in particular, the practice of oncology, in many ways. The growing appreciation of the molecular basis of carcinogenesis will have clinical applications in understanding cancer etiology and assigning more precise estimates of risk; in tailoring screening and prevention approaches to populations at defined levels of risk; in improving accuracy of diagnosis and prognosis based on molecular profiles; and in the rational design of therapeutic modalities based on molecular targets.

Although the grouping of site-specific cancer clusters in some families has been recognized for decades, it was not until the past few decades, with the identification of genes such as *BRCA1* and *BRCA2*, that hereditary patterns of cancer could be definitively linked to discrete germ-line mutations. Although hereditary cancers account for only 10% of all cancers, the identification of these genes and the attention devoted to these discoveries have heightened awareness of the genetic contribution to cancer in general among both the medical profession and the lay community and have provided a means to begin to recognize individuals and families with an increased genetic risk of cancer.

Because deleterious mutations in genes associated with hereditary cancer syndromes diagnose a *risk* for cancer, not the disease itself, knowledge of germ-line cancer susceptibility genes has stimulated intense interest in preventive strategies that may be employed to alter an individual's risk and that of his or her family members. Studies are under way to understand the functions of cancer susceptibility genes and how their alteration contributes to carcinogenesis. Gene–gene and gene–environment interactions are being explored to understand the significant variation in penetrance of these genes. This work is likely to elucidate the causal mechanisms of the traditional epidemiologic factors associated with cancer that will have implications for the more common sporadic forms.

This chapter explores the application of the rapidly expanding field of genetics to genetic screening and counseling for hereditary cancer syndromes in the clinical setting.

Kinds of Assays

One component of the success of the Human Genome Project, in concert with the realization that all diseases have a genetic basis, is the advent of rapid and relatively inexpensive molecular genetic technologies that can be run at high throughput. There are different technologies for different types of mutations, and most are limited to specialized genetic laboratories or cancer research settings. The technologies for detecting mutations in the major cancer susceptibility genes are constantly evolving but can basically be divided into tests of gene function, such as protein truncation tests, gel shift assays, enzymatic mutations screens, and methods to directly sequence the genes.

Because many of the genetic mutations associated with cancer syndromes result in premature truncation of the protein product, protein truncation tests have been widely used. This approach uses in vitro transcription and translation to produce a radiolabeled protein. Truncated forms can be detected when electrophoresed against normal controls on an agarose gel.[1] Protein truncation tests are misleading when the gene length is normal, but its function is altered, or when the protein products produced by the mutated gene are too small for detection by this method.[2]

Gel shift assays compare the mobility through a gel matrix of a test DNA sample to that of a control sample. The motility of DNA in a gel matrix is determined by its length, base composition, single- and double-strand characteristics, and double-strand mobility in the presence of mismatched controls. Examples of gel shift assays are single-strand conformation polymorphism (SSCP) analysis, denaturing gradient gel electrophoresis (DGGE), heteroduplex analysis (HA), and conformation-sensitive gel electrophoresis (CSGE). Although gel shift assays are relatively easy to perform and inexpensive, their sensitivity is lower than other types of assays, making them less appropriate for clinical genetic testing.

Based on the principle that heteroduplexes form between wild-type and mutant genetic sequences, enzymatic mutation detection (EMD) methods use enzymes with high specificity for insertions, deletions, and base–substitution mismatches. Normal and mutant alleles of the target gene are amplified and labeled with fluorescent dyes. The enzyme scans the double-stranded DNA until it detects a structural distortion, where it cleaves the genetic material, forming two shorter, radiolabeled fragments. These products are analyzed on an automated DNA sequencer for relative mobility. EMD is easy to use and highly specific for all types of alterations and has the advantage of detecting multiple sequence variants in the same polymerase chain reaction (PCR) product.[2]

Direct sequencing of the gene is the gold standard for mutation scanning. All the coding regions, as well as the intron–exon boundaries of a gene, are amplified by PCR and sequenced, either manually or by automated techniques, in 250 to 400 base pairs. This approach is costly and labor intensive. Direct sequencing can miss certain types of mutations or large deletions or can detect mutations of unknown clinical significance. Many of these technical limitations will most likely be eliminated as the technology is improved and as clinical correlations are established for each mutation.

Clinicians considering using a genetic testing facility for clinical purposes should consider the quality control circumstances of the testing facility being considered. All laboratories doing clinical genetic testing should be certified by the Clinical Laboratory Improvement Act (CLIA) and the College of American Pathology (CAP). Access to a medical geneticist is helpful to assist in test interpretation for difficult cases.

Hallmarks of Hereditary Cancers

A list of known inherited cancer syndromes and their associated genes is shown in Table 25.1.[3] This chapter discusses in more detail the hereditary patterns of breast/ovarian cancer, colorectal cancer, and multiple endocrine neoplasias, syndromes for which there are clinically available tests and which comprise a large portion of all hereditary cancer syndromes.

The features of a pedigree that characterize hereditary patterns of cancer include early age of onset, high penetrance, bilaterality in paired organs, vertical transmission through either parent, and an association with other cancers.[4] The actual prevalence of mutations leading to hereditary cancers varies considerably in the population and is sometimes related to ethnic ancestry. It is known that certain mutations, the "founder mutations," are more common in families who are all traced to a certain ancestor believed to be the founder of the original mutation. In these cases, knowing the ethnicity of an individual may guide which mutations to explore.

Penetrance refers to the proportion of individuals carrying the mutation who actually develop the associated disease(s). The observation that there are mutation carriers who never develop disease suggests that there are genetic, metabolic, and/or environmental events that can modify the effect of a mutation. A better understanding of these modifiers is likely to provide opportunities for prevention of the involved disease. There are also emerging data to suggest that the location of the mutation within the gene may influence the type and severity of the disease that is manifest.

Rationale for Genetic Screening

Screening for cancer susceptibility genes has the potential to reduce the burden of cancer by providing opportunities for tailored early detection or primary prevention interventions to at-risk individuals. It can also spare those who receive true-negative results the burden of unnecessary screening and prevention procedures. The success of this approach is dependent upon the availability of surveillance measures and preventive strategies with documented efficacy and limited risk. The widespread clinical application of genetic testing, however, also poses specific challenges, including the implications for other family members who may not be involved or interested in the receipt of genetic risk information, the consequences of labeling healthy individuals with a disease predisposition, and the profound social and cultural significance awarded to genetic traits. Our understanding of the genetic basis of disease, and the rapid evolution in the science of human genetics, is moving at such a pace as to challenge the ability of both families and medical professionals to process and communicate the information becoming available.

Several advisory bodies have issued guidelines for the application of genetic testing for cancer susceptibility to the clinical setting. In a statement adopted on March 1, 2003, the American Society of Clinical Oncology (ASCO) reaffirmed its commitment to the integration of cancer risk assessment and management into the practice of oncology. In this update of earlier guidelines, the society set forth a set of *indications* for clinical genetic testing, recommendations for counseling to accompany genetic testing, and a commitment to maintaining confidentiality of genetic information. At the same time, ASCO underscored the responsibility of the patient to communicate genetic test results to other family members. The ASCO statement supports the establishment of federal legislation to prevent discrimination on the basis of genetic status and urged public and private health insurance providers to cover genetic testing and counseling services. ASCO maintains its commitment to providing educational opportunities in genetics for healthcare providers.[5]

The American Society of Human Genetics (ASHG) also stated the importance of public and professional education to develop a responsible approach to genetic testing and supported the need for further research to determine optimal preventive strategies for individuals with a genetic predisposition to cancer.[6] A position paper from the National Society of Genetic Counselors (NSGC) spells out in detail the components of the genetic testing process and stresses the need for a multidisciplinary approach, including genetic counselors, physicians, nurses, social workers, and behavioral scientists.[7] As this field is moving so quickly, these recommendations continue to evolve, but constant is the need to protect the health and well-being of genetically susceptible individuals.

TABLE 25.1. Inherited cancer syndromes for which clinical testing is available.

Syndrome	*Involved gene(s)*	*Associated cancers*
Beckwith–Wiedemann syndrome	*BWS* critical region 11p15 Genes involved: *KCNQ1OT1* *IGF2* *H19* *CDKN2C*	Embryonal tumors, Wilms' tumor, adrenocortical carcinoma, hepatoblastoma, rhabdomyosarcoma, neuroblastoma, gastric teratoma
Bloom syndrome	*BLM (RECQL3)* at 15q26.1	Leukemia, lymphoma, aerodigestive tract, skin, breast, cervix
Breast ovarian cancer (BOC) syndrome	*BRCA1* at 17q21, *BRCA2* at 13q12	Breast, ovary, prostate, pancreas
Cowden syndrome	*PTEN* at 10q23	Breast, uterus, thyroid, kidney, melanoma, glioblastoma
Familial adenomatous polyposis (FAP)	*APC* at 5q21	Colorectal, upper digestive tract, thyroid, hepatoblastoma
Fanconi anemia	*FANCA* at 16q24.3 *FANCC* at 9q22.3 *FANCD2* at 3p25.3 *FANCF* at 11p15 *FANCG* at 9p13 *FANCE* at 6p22 *BRCA2* at 13q12.3	Leukemia, squamous cell cancers, hepatocellular, brain tumors
Hereditary nonpolyposis colon cancer	*MSH2* at 2p22, *MLH1* at 3p21, *PMS1* at 2q31, *PMS2* at 7p22, *MSH6* at 2p16	Colorectal cancer, endometrial, ovarian, gastric, small intestine, ureter and kidney cancers
Li–Fraumeni syndrome	*TP53* at 17p13.1	Sarcoma, breast cancer, leukemia, adrenocortical cancer, brain tumor
Familial melanoma	*CMM1* at 1p36, *TP16* at 9p21, *CDK4* at 12q14	Multiple melanomas
Multiple colorectal adenomas	*MYH*, 1p34	Multiple colorectal adenomas (15–100), autosomal recessive
Multiple endocrine neoplasia type 1 (MEN-1)	*MEN1* at 11q13	Parathyroid, pancreatic islet, and pituitary cancers
Multiple endocrine neoplasia type 2 (MEN-2)	*RET* at 10q11.2	Medullary thyroid cancer, pheochromocytoma, benign parathyroid tumors
Neurofibromatosis type 1	*NF1* at 17q11.2	Optic glioma, neurofibrosarcoma
Neurofibromatosis type 2	*NF2* at 22q12	Meningioma, astrocytoma, acoustic neuroma, spinal schwannoma, ependymoma, neurofibroma
Nevoid basal cell syndrome (Gorlin syndrome)	*PTC* at 9q22.3	Basal cell cancer, ovarian fibroma, medulloblastoma
Peutz–Jeghers syndrome	*STK11* at 19p13.3	Colon, breast, pancreas, uterus, lung, testis, and ovarian cancer
Retinoblastoma syndrome	*RB1* at 13q14.1	Retinoblastoma, osteosarcoma, Ewing sarcoma, leukemia, lymphoma, melanoma, lung and bladder cancer
Tuberous sclerosis	*TSC1* at 9q34, *TSC2* at 16p13.3	Childhood brain tumors, Wilms' tumor, renal cell cancer
Von Hippel–Lindau syndrome	*VHL* at 3p25	Renal cell cancer, pheochromocytoma, hemangiomas
Down's syndrome	Trisomy 21	Leukemia
Klinefelter syndrome	47XXY	Male germ cell and breast cancer
Turner syndrome	45X	Wilms' tumor, neurogenic tumors, uterine tumor, leukemia, and gonadal tumors

Source: Data from Schneider.[3]

Ethical, Legal, and Social Issues

The exciting potential of the work emanating from the Human Genome Project has led to unbounded enthusiasm about our ability to affect the health of the population through population screening for genetic cancer predisposition, through a more sophisticated understanding of the molecular profile of the cancer phenotype, and through new gene-targeted drug development. However, the recent expansion of technology into the field of medical genetics has outstripped our ability to conceptualize the ethical and moral dimensions of the application of molecular genetics to the clinical setting of oncology. There are outstanding ethical issues that concern patients and their families, the healthcare profession, and society at large.

Most of the ethical debate for the public has centered on the ability to genetically characterize individuals for inherited cancer susceptibility syndromes. Limitations of test accuracy and the relative uncertainties about effective preventive strategies for those who test positive have led many to advise caution about the widespread adoption of genetic testing in the clinical setting. In fact, concern about the potential adverse consequences of genetic testing for cancer susceptibility has led to the view that genetic information is *qualitatively* different from other medical information because of its potential to be used in a discriminatory manner and its unique implications for family members. The public has expressed concern that the explosion of genetic information may result in an environment in which people will be labeled and disadvantaged in the workplace and in their ability to obtain insurance based on genetic information. In fact, the most common reason cited for not considering genetic testing for mutations in the *BRCA1/2* genes is fear of insurance discrimination.[8] Legislation for protection against discrimination based on genetic test results is incomplete and has not been thoroughly challenged in the court system. Responsibility to other family members is another concern voiced by individuals who undergo genetic testing. Privacy and confidentiality issues place the burden of communicating genetic test results with the proband, who may not have a sophisticated medical background and who may face difficult family dynamics in the communication process. The application of the new genetics to the diagnosis, characterization, and treatment of cancer has not generated as much concern and attention among cancer patients, who are often overwhelmed by their situation and the details of the treatments proposed to them. A good example of this is the increasing use of microsatellite instability (MSI) testing of colon tumors in the clinical setting without full disclosure to the patient that the testing may uncover a hereditary cancer syndrome in their family.

The promise of the new genetic technologies is emerging at a time when healthcare resources are shrinking and when access to care is not shared by all members of society. Although advances in technology will most likely lead to more cost-effective assays, the costs will still put a significant strain on the healthcare budget. Disparities in cancer care will grow as more advanced technologies are introduced into the treatment setting. The role of insurance companies in providing coverage for these new costs is unclear. The magnitude of insurance and/or employment risks from discrimination on the basis of genetic risk information is also a major concern for state and federal government agencies and the insurance industry.

There has been considerable debate about the issue of "genetic exceptionalism," that is, whether genetic testing is sufficiently different from other types of medical tests to warrant special considerations. Because of some of the unique aspects of genetic information, the standard of care has evolved to obtain formal informed consent for the conduct of a specific genetic test, even when done strictly for clinical management and not in the context of research. Unique components of the consent process are the acknowledgment of potential social and family implications of the test results, including the potential for discrimination based on genetic risk status, the symbolic meaning of heritage in our culture, the probabilistic nature of the test results, and the potential for lifetime classification of an individual as "at risk."[9,10] Suggested components of the informed consent process are shown in Table 25.2. This process should take into account the participant's prior experiences, beliefs, attitudes, concerns, expectations, and motivations concerning genetic risk and should be handled with attention to confidentiality and the needs of other family members.

One special circumstance is the issue of genetic testing of children and adolescents. The ASHG and the American College of Medical Genetics, as well as ASCO, have suggested a series of points to consider in confronting this situation. The primary indication for genetic testing of a minor should be the provision of timely medical benefit. If the cancer occurs predominantly in childhood and risk reduction strategies and therapies are available, such as medullary thyroid cancer, there is justification for testing. Psychosocial benefits to competent adolescents, including reduction of uncertainty and anxiety, and contribution to life decisions may also be an indication. For those diseases, such as adult-onset cancers for which the medical and/or psychosocial benefits will not occur until adulthood, genetic testing should generally be deferred. The involvement and preparation of the family should be an integral part of this process. It is the responsibility of the provider to weigh the interests of the children and their families in their delivery of responsible genetic services.[5,11]

The ability to characterize individuals genetically facilitates the application of this technology on a global scale and, in addition to creating typologies of cancer susceptibility in the population, will permit the molecular definition of ancestry, ethnicity, intelligence, and other human features with the potential for misuse. All these issues call for public education about the issues the genetic revolution is raising and a general discourse on the use of genetics in the oncology setting.

TABLE 25.2. Components of informed consent for genetic testing.

Purpose of the test	The purpose of the genetic test must be clearly described.
Practical aspects of the test	Amount of blood to be drawn, length of time to receive results, other information to be collected, cost of testing, and a contact person should be included.
Interpretation of results	The potential types of test results should be clarified, including true-positive, true-negative, indeterminant, and inconclusive results.
Potential risks	Risks to be described are psychosocial, threats to family dynamics and health, and insurance discrimination.
Potential benefits	The use of genetic test information may provide both psychologic benefit as well as guidance in medical management interventions.
Privacy and confidentiality	Measures used to assure privacy and confidentiality of the test results should be described.
Alternatives	A description of alternatives to genetic testing, including risk assessment based on clinical history, should be provided.

Education of the Healthcare Providers

As the genetic contribution to cancer continues to evolve, primary care providers will assume a more pivotal role in the provision of clinical genetic services, including providing education to patients and their families about genetic information in general, genetic testing in particular, and the use of genetic technologies in cancer risk reduction surveillance, diagnosis, and treatment. The involvement of the entire healthcare team will be critical to assess the outcomes of family decisions regarding genetic information and to guide individuals and their families through the complex world of cancer genetics. There are data to suggest, however, that among members of the healthcare profession, knowledge regarding the criteria for hereditary cancer syndromes, the indications for associated genetic testing, and the role that molecular genetics plays in the prevention, diagnosis, and treatment of cancer is limited. A nationally representative random sample of physicians in primary and tertiary care specialties found that fewer than one-third of physicians had recommended cancer genetic testing to a patient. Barriers to the use of genetic tests in their patient populations included lack of confidence in their ability to recommend testing and lack of access to counseling and testing services.[12] Healthcare providers are often at a loss about how to understand and communicate genetic test results to individuals, about what is their responsibility to inform other at-risk relatives of their potential genetic risk, and about how to assure confidentiality and privacy of genetic information in the medical record system. Limited physician knowledge of genetics may pose a barrier to the referral of appropriate candidates for genetic testing and the standard utilization of genetic predictive testing in clinical practice for increased cancer surveillance, screening, and prevention. Based on the potential for identification, classification, prevention, and treatment for a wide variety of cancer types, physicians and other healthcare providers and their patients would greatly benefit from training in interpretation and use of genetic predisposition testing as part of their clinical practice.

Genetic Counseling

The development of technology to locate and isolate cancer susceptibility genes has brought together the fields of oncology, cancer control, genetics, and genetic counseling to create a new specialty of cancer risk counseling whose goal is to communicate more accurate information about personal cancer risk profiles based on personal and family histories.[13] The field of genetic counseling has evolved and plays a growing role in the evaluation and risk estimation of families with known or suspected genetic conditions. The traditional elements of genetic counseling have included (1) an accurate diagnosis of the genetic condition or predisposition; (2) an estimate of the probable cause of the disorder; (3) an estimation of risk of future occurrences of the condition within the family based on the pattern of inheritance of the disease; (4) communication of an understanding of the genetic and medical facts of the disorder; (5) an exploration of appropriate courses of action to manage the genetic risk and to alter the risk of occurrence; and (6) ways of coping with the disorder or risk of the disorder.[14,15] Building on this tradition, *cancer risk* counseling is an interactive education and communication process whose purpose is to evaluate an individual's potential risk of developing specific forms of cancer based on inherited susceptibilities, physiologic modulators, and lifestyle and environmental factors that contribute to cancer risk and to communicate this information in a comprehensible and sensitive way (Table 25.3). Familial cancer risk counseling uses a broad approach to place genetic risk in the context of other related risk factors, thereby customizing it to the experiences of the individual. In addition to addressing genetic risk and the clinical management of that risk, cancer risk counseling also considers the psychosocial needs of the individual and the family. Typically, the process involves the collection of pertinent medical, familial, and lifestyle information, the documentation of cancer diagnoses, the delivery of background information about cancer risks and cancer genetics, the identification of specific hereditary cancer syndromes, and the transmission of personalized risk estimates.[16] The ultimate goal of the education and communication process is to help the individual and other family members make informed and appropriate decisions about genetic testing options and strategies for cancer prevention and/or early detection.

TABLE 25.3. Basic elements of cancer genetic counseling.

- Documentation of extended family medical history
- Development of a family pedigree
- Collection of medical records from proband and appropriate family members
- Collection of information about other risk factors (biologic, environmental, lifestyle)
- Careful assessment of risk
- Education about cancer, genetics, and preventive options
- Communication of risk estimate in clear and simple language
- Development of individualized prevention and surveillance strategy
- Attention to emotional and social needs and concerns of proband and family
- Long-term follow-up and support

Genetic counseling for genetic cancer risk represents a new direction in genetics and has raised some particularly interesting and difficult issues. Risk estimates for cancer may be either empirical or based on actual gene identification but are typically complex and sophisticated, challenging the communication skills of the counseling team. The nature of the counseling situation often requires the involvement of other family members to supply missing information or even for genetic screening, a situation that may compromise privacy and confidentiality within the family. The options offered by the counseling team, including genetic testing, may involve emotional and ethical dilemmas for which there are no clear answers. Despite these problematic issues, cancer risk counseling is a growing field that has tremendous potential to assist families in understanding their risk for cancer and in making informed choices for prevention.

Components of a Counseling Program

Target Population

Individuals who seek cancer risk counseling are often highly motivated by a personal experience with cancer in their family and by concern for the risks faced by themselves and their offspring. Participants in cancer risk counseling are often self-referred, but as physicians become more aware of the importance of family history in determining an individual's risk for cancer, they are increasingly referring their patients for genetic evaluation. Although the general indication for participation in a cancer risk counseling program is a perception of increased risk for cancer based on family history and/or other recognized risk exposures, individual participants come to the process with a wide variety of experiences, health beliefs, expectations, and needs. An assessment of individual differences that can influence comprehension and compliance with appropriate health recommendations, therefore, is one of the primary goals of the counseling team.

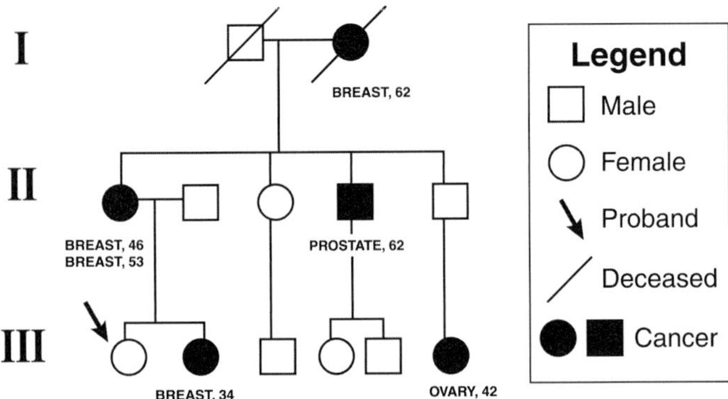

FIGURE 25.1. Sample pedigree with standard nomenclature to illustrate family relationships and disease information.

The Counseling Team

Traditionally, the medical genetics counseling team has included a medical geneticist, a genetic counselor, and often the referring primary care physician, usually an obstetrician or pediatrician. Genetic counselors typically earn a Master of Science degree at an accredited institution and are certified by the American Board of Genetic Counselors. Dedicated training in the field of cancer genetics has recently been added to the curricula of genetic counseling education programs. There is also a growing interest in genetics on the part of nurses, many of whom are beginning to seek specialized training in the field. As the field of genetic counseling has expanded to include adult diseases such as cancer, other disciplines, including oncology, molecular genetics, social work, and psychology have joined the team to provide the multidisciplinary approach needed. Originally, cancer risk counseling programs were mainly situated in cancer centers and academic institutions, but increasingly these services are expanding to community hospitals, worksites, and health centers where they are often one component of a more broadly based health promotion program.

Information Collection

The very first step in evaluating an individual's risk for cancer is to assess the individual's concerns and reasons for seeking counseling to guarantee that personal needs and priorities will be met in the counseling process. The next step is to collect the pertinent medical, family, and personal information to assemble a risk profile and begin to explore options for dealing with the risk. A detailed family history is the cornerstone of effective genetic counseling. The counselor begins with the health of the proband and proceeds outward to include first-, second-, and third-degree relatives on both the maternal and paternal side. In addition to cancer diagnoses by primary site, age at onset, bilaterality when appropriate, and current age or age at death are recorded. Cancer diagnoses are validated by obtaining medical records, pathology reports, or death certificates when possible. Other medical and genetic conditions that may predispose individuals to cancer risk (e.g., Crohn's disease and colon cancer, atypical ductal hyperplasia, and breast cancer) should also be noted. It is important to include information about family members unaffected with cancer to appreciate the penetrance of the disease and overall patterns of inheritance. Information about possible consanguinity is also valuable, particularly in the consideration of recessive disorders. Ancestry and ethnicity should be recorded, as some inherited conditions are more common in certain ethnic groups (founder effects).

Family history data are graphically represented on a pedigree, which follows standard nomenclature to illustrate family relationships and disease information[17] (Figure 25.1). Factors that limit the informativeness of the pedigree are small family size, early deaths in family members precluding the possibility of developing adult diseases, prophylactic surgeries that remove an organ from subsequent risk of cancer (e.g., total hysterectomy for uterine fibroids where the ovaries are also removed), and incomplete information about the health of family members. The degree of accuracy of reporting cancer diagnoses in relatives varies by how close the relatives are to the proband, with lack of information about specific cancer diagnoses in older second and/or third generations being a particularly common problem encountered in pedigree generation.

The collection of a targeted medical history of the proband serves two purposes: (1) the identification of premalignant conditions associated with subsequent cancer progression and (2) the estimation of other risk factors that may interact with or modify familial cancer risk. A careful reproductive history is pertinent to a number of common cancers in women. Exogenous hormone use and other medication history is also of value. The knowledge of other medical conditions may affect the management recommendations for reducing cancer risk. Caution about the use of exogenous estrogens in women with a familial predisposition of breast cancer, for example, may be tempered by a strong personal or family history of osteoporosis.

Environmental exposures and lifestyle factors, such as smoking, diet and alcohol use, and type of occupation may contribute to the overall estimation of risk, and their identification may offer opportunities for lifestyle changes to alter risk. Although occupational exposures to carcinogens such as benzene or asbestos account for a relatively small proportion of cancer, their recognition is very important in elucidating patterns of cancer and in eliminating other causes among exposed individuals. Environmental exposures and lifestyles are often shared by family members and must be recognized when assessing hereditary patterns of cancer. Finally, a record of past cancer screening practices establishes a history of health promotion behavior and will help guide the counselor in making reasonable and appropriate health recommendations.

The Education Component

Genetic risk information cannot be effectively communicated in the absence of general information about cancer risk, cancer genetics, and risk estimation. Individuals faced with a familial risk of cancer must assimilate complex and often highly technical information to make informed decisions about genetic testing, cancer screening, and preventive actions for themselves and to communicate that information to other family members. An integral part of the genetic counseling process is an educational preparation, provided either in a group or individual setting, to help the proband develop the understanding necessary to make informed decisions about his or her cancer risk. The basic educational components of cancer risk information include the following.

The Concepts of Cancer and Cancer Risk Factors

The multifactorial nature of cancer is explored with an emphasis on the pathways of cancer formation and expression. Persons seeking counseling who are affected with cancer may be particularly interested in information about the presentation, diagnosis, and treatment of cancer. The basics of cancer epidemiology can be presented, and examples, such as the importance of hormonal regulation in breast cancer and the importance of diet in colon cancer, can be used to illustrate the role of both external factors and internal metabolism in changing normal cells to premalignant and malignant tissue.

The Role of Family History in Cancer Risk Assessment

The interaction of shared environmental and genetic backgrounds among family members in determining risk is explored. Sample pedigrees can be used to illustrate the types of family cancer patterns (Table 25.4), and to demonstrate the concepts of vertical transmission through maternal or paternal lines, the significance of age at onset, and bilaterality of disease and penetrance issues. With this background, the counselor can then review the proband's own pedigree for the patterns expressed and for the identification of pertinent risk factors.

TABLE 25.4. Family cancer patterns.

Sporadic: A single occurrence of a cancer occurring on one side of the family.

Familial: A pattern of cancers on one side of the family, seen in one or more generations, that does not fit an autosomal dominant pattern of inheritance of cancer. The cancers on that side of the family do not fit a known cancer family syndrome. The pattern seen may represent a clustering of incidental cancers or may be the result of shared environmental or lifestyle factors.

Hereditary: A pattern of cancers on one side of the family, seen in two or more generations, in several members of the family, that fits an autosomal dominant pattern of cancers. The cancers on that side of the family may fit a known cancer family syndrome:
OR
Genetic testing performed on the proband or the proband's family member has detected a mutation in a cancer predisposition gene (e.g., *BRCA1*) and inheritance of this mutation has been established.

The Role of Genes in Cancer Development

The counselor introduces the concepts and language of chromosomes, genes, DNA, and how genetic alterations can lead to cancer. It is particularly important for the proband to understand the difference between the acquisition of genetic alterations during his/her lifetime that may affect his/her risk for cancer, and the inheritance of cancer-related genetic alterations from a parent, which can also be passed on to his/her offspring. Within this context, the counselor can introduce information about the recently identified cancer susceptibility genes, such as *BRCA1*, *BRCA2*, *APC*, the hereditary nonpolyposis colorectal cancer (HNPCC) genes, etc., and the cancer syndromes associated with each, with an emphasis on those syndromes that appear to be most consistent with the proband's family history. The educational component of cancer risk counseling is meant to be interactive with ample opportunity for the proband to ask questions and to tailor the information to the needs of the individual.

The Assignment of Risk

Cancer risk assessment is an attempt to quantify the probability of an individual's risk for a particular cancer using empirical models that account for a variety of personal, familial, and environmental risk factors. It is a complex process, both because it is based on imperfect and often conflicting data and because it involves probabilistic statements about the *chance* of an event occurring, concepts that are difficult to convey and to understand. The concept of risk can be presented in a variety of ways, each of which has a different interpretation. *Absolute risk* refers to the rate of cancer occurrence in the population and often serves as the background risk to which individuals compare themselves. *Relative risk* is the comparison of risk in an individual with a particular set of risk factors at a particular point in time to that of an individual without those risk factors, thus implying some magnitude of vulnerability.[18] *Cumulative risk* is the risk over a defined time period calculated by accumulating relative risks over time.

Cancer risk counselors attempt to place the proband's risk of cancer within the context of population risk, both in quantitative and qualitative terms, to provide a rationale for recommended health behaviors. The majority of families do not exhibit the features of hereditary cancer syndromes but rather represent the effect of a combination of multiple genetic and environmental factors that interact to increase cancer risk to a moderate degree. For these families, counselors often use empirical approaches based on epidemiologic data that provide age-specific risks of cancer in tabular formats which can incorporate several pertinent risk factors. For some cancers, these empirical data have actually been integrated into mathematical models that can predict cumulative risk estimates of developing a cancer over a defined time period in an individual's lifetime. The Gail model, for example, predicts breast cancer risk from age 20 to 80 years, using a model that includes current age, age at menarche, age at first live birth, number of first-degree relatives with breast cancer, and number of breast biopsies.[19] It has recently been validated by the Breast Cancer Prevention Trial[20] and is most accurate in predicting breast cancer among women who are being screened with regular mammograms.[21] This model is now available from the National Cancer Institute on a floppy disk, the "Risk Disc," that can easily be used in the clinical setting.

For families in whom a hereditary pattern of cancer is suspected, the recent cloning of rare but highly penetrant cancer susceptibility genes, such as *BRCA1* and *BRCA2*, has made available the direct assessment of mutation status, thus obviating the need for empirical risk models. Other parameters, such as the Amsterdam Criteria and the Bethesda Guidelines for HNPCC,[22,23] have been established to identify families who are candidates for genetic testing. In addition to these sets of criteria, mathematical models are appearing that, based on features of the family history, predict the likelihood of being a mutation carrier and help the counselor and clinician further refine genetic testing decisions.[24,25] BRCAPRO is a statistical model based on published estimates of penetrance that uses information on personal and familial cancer status to calculate an individual's probability of carrying a deleterious mutation on *BRCA1* or *BRCA* and is used in the clinical setting to guide decisions about whether to undergo genetic testing.[26]

Genetic Testing: Interpretation of Test Results

Genetic testing for cancer and its role, benefits, and limitations are discussed in the counseling session both in terms of the scientific merits of understanding the genetic basis of cancer and, when appropriate, as it may apply to further characterizing the cancer risk within the proband's family. When possible, it is best to first consider testing an affected family member who meets the criteria for a hereditary cancer, as that individual is the one most likely to test positive. When a mutation is found, additional family members can be tested with an assay that specifically tests for that particular mutation.

There are four possible interpretations of a genetic test result (Table 25.5). If a known risk-associated mutation is found within a family, those family members who test positive for the mutation are considered "true positives." They are counseled that they are at increased risk for a spectrum of cancers, and options for risk management are discussed (see following). It must be emphasized that a positive mutation result is not a positive cancer test but rather a susceptibility estimate. A positive test result does, however, confirm a 50% chance of passing on the mutation to each biologic child of the carrier. A second outcome of a positive test result is the discovery of a variant of the gene of *unknown clinical significance*. These genes are truly altered but have not yet been clearly linked to disease risk and may represent neutral alterations in the gene structure that do not compromise its function. Over time, as more families are studied, most of these variants most likely can be separated into disease-related changes and benign changes, known as polymorphisms. Until then, families found to carry one of these variants must be counseled about the uncertain meaning of the result, and recommendations will be based on their family and personal history of disease. When a disease-related mutation has been identified in a family, subsequent family members who test negative for that mutation are thought to be "true negatives" whose risks for the relevant cancers are *not* increased over those of the general population. These family members may be spared the increased surveillance and/or consideration of prophylactic surgery offered to carriers. They can also be reassured that they will not pass on the deleterious mutation to their offspring. Finally, when no mutation is found in any family member (which is the most common situation), the meaning of a negative test result is ambiguous. It may mean that there truly is no mutation in the family and that the family history represents a clustering of sporadic cancers, it may mean a known disease-related mutation does exist in the family but no informative family members were available for testing, or it may mean that a mutation exists but cannot be detected by current technology. Again, counseling must emphasize the ambiguous nature of the test results. These families may still face a significantly increased risk of cancer and management should be based on other factors. A clear distinction is made between the probability of being a mutation carrier and the probability of developing cancer. Estimates of penetrance of the gene, that is, the chance that a mutation will actually result in cancer in a person, are also typically derived from small studies among narrowly defined families and are difficult to apply to any particular individual unless he or she matches the characteristics of the families studied. Information on other factors that may modify gene expression is rudimentary at this point for most of the genes identified.

TABLE 25.5. Genetic test results.

True positive	The person is a carrier of an alteration in a known cancer-predisposing gene.
True negative	A person is not a carrier of a known cancer-predisposing gene that has been positively identified in another family member.
Indeterminant	A person is not a carrier of a known cancer-predisposing gene and the carrier status of other family members is either also negative or is unknown.
Inconclusive	A person is a carrier of an alteration in a gene that currently has no known significance.

Psychosocial Support

Just as important as a careful risk factor analysis and interpretation of risk to family members is attention to the psychosocial issues raised by the enhanced risk and the emotional needs of those involved.[27] This consideration is especially critical in the setting of counseling for cancer risk, which deals with the complexity of probabilities, which involves the entire family, and which may provide risk information that can become a source of discrimination. Cancer is one of the most feared diseases of modern times. Cultural beliefs about cancer, painful memories of relatives' experiences with cancer, high levels of mental stress associated with cancer-related anxiety, unresolved grief, feelings of denial, guilt, and other family dynamics can all interfere with the receipt and understanding of risk information and with the formulation of strategies for risk reduction and can have a negative impact on quality of life. Both the information received during the process of genetic counseling and the information-seeking coping style of the individual may elicit further emotional reactions, especially if the counseling involves the receipt of genetic test results. The counselor takes an active role in helping the counselee identify his/her risk status, confront fears and anxieties about the meaning of that risk, develop coping strategies to deal with both the emotional and medical components of his/her unique situation and coping style, and facilitate decision making. The counselor can also assist the counselee in communicating cancer risk information to other family members, in dealing with their potential reactions, and in enrolling them in a counseling program. Follow-up genetic counseling sessions have been found to reinforce the information communicated in the original sessions, to solidify decisions made, to assess adjustment to risk status, and to make referrals for specialty consultations if needed.[28]

General Management Strategies

One of the primary motivations for seeking cancer risk counseling is to identify ways to reduce or delay the risk of developing cancer or to enhance the possibility of detecting cancer at an early, curable stage. Individuals who seek these services clearly want recommendations for the medical management of their risk from their providers. By achieving a reliable estimate of cancer risk, either by considering personal and family history or by performing genetic testing, the cancer risk counselor, working with the medical team, can help to tailor primary and secondary prevention strategies to the individual. Although there are presently limited data on the long-term efficacy of prevention strategies directed at individuals with a familial or hereditary risk, clinical management decisions are being made based on the best available evidence. Recommendations fall into four general categories: increased screening, pharmacologic interventions (chemoprevention), surgical prophylaxis, and lifestyle changes. Screening recommendations are problematic for cancers, such as ovarian and pancreatic cancer, for which no early detection method has been found to be sufficiently sensitive and specific, and for situations such as the Li–Fraumeni syndrome, in which individuals are at risk for a wide spectrum of cancers during their lifetime. On the other hand, members of high-risk families are ideal candidates to participate in trials of newer imaging technologies and intermediate biomarkers to improve the early detection of cancer in younger individuals.

There is intense interest on the part of high-risk individuals to learn about opportunities to reduce their cancer risk by changes in diet, exercise, or other lifestyle modifications that may minimize their exposure to carcinogens. Preliminary data suggest, for instance, that the use of exogenous estrogens, including oral contraceptives and estrogen replacement, may confer an increased risk for breast cancer among women with a hereditary predisposition[29] and that limiting exposure to these agents may be beneficial. The exact role of diet and exercise remains elusive for most cancers, although recommendations can be made on the basis of general health and ideal weight maintenance. Dietary supplementation with micronutrients and other natural products to reduce cancer risk is so far unsupported by scientific data. Long-term studies are needed to assess the role of any of these strategies in the setting of familial risk for cancer. (See following for specific management options.) It is important that clinicians play an active role, in partnership with the genetic counselors, in the counseling of individuals predisposed to familial cancers to review current medical management strategies and to tailor recommendations to the unique needs of each individual.

Effectiveness of Cancer Risk Counseling

Several studies have attempted to assess the effectiveness and efficacy of genetic counseling and have identified a number of common predictors of response. Utilization of genetic counseling services is associated with higher socioeconomic status and educational level and, in the setting of prenatal genetic conditions, with intention to have children.[30] Understanding and retention of the information received have been found to be higher among individuals who are self-referred, those with higher educational levels, and among those families at the higher risk levels. Multiple counseling sessions have been shown to boost understanding and information retention.[31] Another consistent observation has been that, although it is important, the information obtained at a genetic counseling session is not the only factor contributing to risk-related decisions. Rather, perception of risk is a concept formed over a person's lifetime and is a result of internalizing personal experiences and beliefs. Decisions made in the genetic counseling setting, therefore, reflect a complicated interplay of expectations, emotions, and value judgments. As a result, the genetic counselor is likely to be most successful when the information shared during genetic counseling is provided in the context of the counselee's personal orientation and belief system.

Risk Management for Hereditary Cancer Syndromes

Hereditary Breast/Ovarian Cancer

Approximately 5% to 10% of all breast cancer demonstrates an autosomal dominant pattern of inheritance. Hereditary breast cancer is characterized by early age at onset (5 to 15 years earlier than sporadic cases), bilaterality, vertical transmission through both maternal and paternal lines, and association with tumors of other organs, particularly the ovary and prostate gland.[4,32,33] Syndromes most often associated with hereditary breast cancer are the hereditary breast ovarian cancer (HBOC) syndrome associated with mutations in the *BRCA1* and *BRCA2* genes, the Li–Fraumeni syndrome associated with p53 mutations, and Cowden's syndrome associated with mutations in PTEN. The clinical evidence of an autosomal dominant inherited predisposition to breast cancer was originally supported by segregation analysis, a quantitative method to determine if a particular trait is distributed in the population in a Mendelian manner of inheritance. Applied to the CASH data set, segregation analysis and goodness-of-fit tests of genetic models provided evidence for the existence of a rare autosomal dominant allele associated with increased susceptibility to breast cancer.[34]

In 1990, a susceptibility gene for breast cancer was mapped by genetic linkage to the long arm of chromosome 17, in the interval 17q12–21.[35] The linkage between breast cancer and genetic markers on chromosome 17q was soon confirmed by others, and evidence for the coincident transmission of both breast and ovarian cancer susceptibility in linked families was observed.[4] The *BRCA1* gene was subsequently identified by positional cloning methods and has been found to encode a protein of 1,863 amino acids. This susceptibility gene appears to be responsible for disease in 45%

of families with multiple cases of breast cancer only and up to 90% of families with both breast and ovarian cancer.[36] A second breast cancer susceptibility gene, *BRCA2*, was localized through linkage studies of 15 families with multiple cases of breast cancer to the long arm of chromosome 13. Germ-line mutations in *BRCA2* are thought to account for approximately 35% of multiple case breast cancer families and are also associated with male breast cancer, ovarian cancer, prostate cancer, and pancreatic cancer.[37,38] The risk for breast cancer in female *BRCA2* mutation carriers appears similar to that for *BRCA1* carriers, but the age of onset is shifted to an older age distribution.[39]

Of the several hundred mutations described in these genes, most lead to a frame shift resulting in missing or nonfunctional proteins.[40] In addition, tumors from individuals with *BRCA1/2* mutations show deletion of the wild-type allele, supporting speculation that these genes play a role in tumor suppression. Both *BRCA1* and *BRCA2* also are involved in the control of meiotic and mitotic recombination and in the maintenance of genomic stability, suggesting an additional role in the DNA repair process.[41–43] The growing body of data elucidating the functions of these genes suggests a gatekeeper role, characterized by interactions with other genes in the regulation of the cell cycle and DNA repair, which may provide novel opportunities to develop genotype-based therapeutic approaches to treatment and prevention. Although sporadic mutations of *BRCA1/2* are rarely described, inactivation or decreased expression of these genes by epigenetic phenomena, such as hypermethylation, may account for some cases of breast and ovarian cancer in the population.[44]

The frequency of mutations in *BRCA1* in the general population has been estimated to be 0.0006, which corresponds to a carrier frequency of 1 in 800. Carrier rates are not distributed evenly, however, and tend to concentrate in families with multiple cases of breast and/or breast/ovarian cancer. *BRCA1* and *BRCA2* also demonstrate differential prevalence rates in certain ethnic groups. Most notably, in the United States, three specific founder mutations, the 185delAG mutation and the 5382insC mutation on *BRCA1* and the 6174delT mutation on *BRCA2*, have been found to be common in Ashkenazi Jews. The frequency of these three mutations approximates 1 in 40 in this population and accounts for up to 25% of early-onset breast cancer and up to 90% of families with both breast and ovarian cancer.[45] Additional founder effects have been described in the Netherlands (*BRCA1* 2804 delAA and several large deletion mutations), in Iceland (*BRCA2* 995 del5), and Sweden (*BRCA1* 3171 ins5).[46–49]

The actual expression of disease in gene mutation carriers is estimated to range from 36% to 85% for breast cancer and from 16% to 60% for ovarian cancer. Male carriers of *BRCA* mutations are also at increased risk for breast cancer, with lifetime estimates of approximately 6%.[50,51] Among female *BRCA1* carriers who have already developed a primary breast cancer, estimates for a second contralateral breast cancer are as high as 64% by age 70 and for ovarian cancer as high as 44% by age 70.[52] It is not generally known whether the specific location of mutations confer differential rates of penetrance, or what other genetic and/or environmental or lifestyle factors may interact with the presence of a mutation to determine expressivity. One region of *BRCA2*, however, the "ovarian cancer cluster region" in exon 11, appears to be associated with an increased risk of ovarian cancer and decreased risk of breast cancer.[53] Ongoing studies are addressing the role of reproductive factors, endogenous and exogenous hormone exposure, diet, and lifestyle factors in the modulation of risk among carriers.

The clinical presentation of *BRCA1/2*-associated breast cancer indicates distinctive pathologic features. Historically, medullary, tubular, and lobular histologic findings and improved survival have been associated with familial breast cancer.[54] The Breast Cancer Linkage Consortium examined histopathologic features of breast cancer in women with *BRCA1/2* mutations and, when compared to controls, they showed an excess of high-grade tumors in *BRCA1* carriers and a relative lack of in situ component adjacent to invasive lesions.[55] High mitotic and total grade, as well as higher rates of aneuploidy, estrogen receptor (ER) negativity, and high proliferative fractions were also reported for *BRCA1* carriers in kindreds followed by Henry Lynch, who also noted higher rates of medullary histology.[56] The phenotype for *BRCA2*-related tumors appears to be more heterogeneous and may include an excess of lobular histology.[57] Recently, differential gene expression profiles have been described for *BRCA1*, *BRCA2*, and sporadic breast cancers, suggesting functional differences in tumors depending on their genetic characterization.[58] In accordance with the poor prognostic features noted histologically for *BRCA1*-related breast cancer, two European studies recently reported survival rates that were similar to or worse than sporadic cases, with a significantly increased risk of contralateral breast cancer.[59,60]

Breast cancer is also a component of the rare Li–Fraumeni syndrome in which germ-line mutations of the p53 gene on chromosome 17p have been documented.[61] First reported by Bottomley et al.,[62] this syndrome is characterized by premenopausal breast cancer in combination with childhood sarcoma, brain tumors, leukemia and lymphoma, and adrenocortical carcinoma. A germ-line mutation in the p53 gene has been identified in more than 50% of families exhibiting this syndrome, and inheritance is autosomal dominant with a penetrance of at least 50% by age 50. Although highly penetrant, the Li–Fraumeni gene is thought to account for less than 1% of breast cancer cases.[63]

One of the more than 50 cancer-related genodermatoses, Cowden's syndrome is characterized by an excess of breast cancer, gastrointestinal and gynecologic malignancies, and thyroid disease, both benign and malignant.[64] Skin manifestations include multiple trichilemmomas, oral fibromas and papillomas, and acral, palmar, and plantar keratoses. Germ-line mutations in PTEN, a protein tyrosine phosphatase with homology to tensin, located on chromosome 10q23, are responsible for this syndrome. Loss of heterozygosity observed in a high proportion of related cancers suggests that PTEN functions as a tumor suppressor gene. Its defined enzymatic function indicates a role in maintenance of the control of cell proliferation.[65] Disruption of PTEN appears to occur late in tumorigenesis and may act as a regulatory molecule of cytoskeletal function. Although it accounts for a small fraction of hereditary breast cancer, the characterization of PTEN function will provide valuable insights into signal pathways and the maintenance of normal cell physiology.[66]

Ataxia telangiectasia (AT) is an autosomal recessive disorder characterized by neurologic deterioration, telangiectasias, immunodeficiency states, and hypersensitivity to ionizing radiation. It is estimated that approximately 1% of the general population may be heterozygous carriers of the mutated gene, ataxia telangiectasia-mutated (ATM), which has been localized to chromosome 11q22–23.[67] The ATM gene encodes for a member of the phosphatidylinositol-3-kinase-like enzymes that are involved in cell-cycle control, meiotic recombination, telomere length monitoring, and DNA damage response pathways. AT cells are sensitive to ionizing radiation and radiomimetic drugs and lack cell-cycle regulatory properties after exposure to radiation.[68] In vitro studies of AT carrier-derived lymphoblastoid cell lines have demonstrated defective control of apoptosis and mitotic spindle checkpoint control.[69] Several epidemiologic studies have suggested a statistically increased risk of breast cancer among female heterozygote carriers, with estimated relative risks ranging from 3.9 to 5.1.[70,71] ATM gene mutations associated with cancer in heterozygote carriers tend to be dominant negative missense mutations.[72] Breast cancer among AT heterozygotes is characterized by early age at onset, bilateral disease, and prolonged survival.[73] A comparative analysis of ATM transcripts in invasive breast cancers, benign lesions, and normal breast tissue found decreased expression of the ATM gene in the invasive tumors compared to the other tissues, suggesting a dominant negative effect of the mutation on breast carcinogenesis.[74] Recently, two recurrent ATM mutations, T7271G and IVS10→G, were associated with an increased risk of breast cancer in multicase families in a population-based case-control study.[75] Given the high heterozygote carrier rate in the population, this association could account for a significant proportion of hereditary breast cancer and poses a potential risk related to diagnostic radiation exposure in these individuals.

Breast and/or ovarian cancer may also be a feature of Peutz–Jeghers syndrome, basal cell nevus (Gorlin) syndrome, multiple endocrine neoplasia type 1 (MEN1), and HNPCC. The identification and location of these and other breast/ovarian cancer genes will permit further investigation of the precise role they play in cancer progression and allow us to determine the percentage of total breast cancer caused by the inheritance of mutant genes. This development, in turn, will ultimately enrich our understanding of all breast and ovarian cancer, sporadic as well as hereditary, and will facilitate the identification of high-risk individuals.

Tailored management strategies for hereditary breast ovarian cancer (HBOC) are beginning to emerge. Individuals who appear to meet criteria for one of the BOC syndromes should be offered the opportunity to participate in clinical genetic counseling delivered by a team of trained healthcare professionals. Women who have tested positive for a *BRCA1* or *BRCA2* mutation are advised to start annual mammography between the ages of 25 and 35 years and to have clinical breast exams every 6 to 12 months.[76] Because of the very early onset of breast cancer in women with germ-line p53 mutations, routine screening is recommended starting at age 20 to 25 for this group.[77] There are preliminary data that magnetic resonance imaging (MRI) of the breast may be more sensitive in detecting early lesions in young women with dense breast tissue, although specificity is generally lower,[78] and several trials are under way to determine the role of this imaging modality, especially in the setting of familial risk. Men testing positive for a *BRCA1/2* mutation should also consider annual screening with mammography and clinical breast exam as well as annual prostate cancer screening with digital rectal exam and prostate-specific antigen (PSA) testing.[76]

Screening recommendations are problematic for ovarian cancer, for which no test or series of tests have been found to be sufficiently sensitive and specific. Despite the limitations, however, many practitioners have begun screening with the combination of pelvic exam, transvaginal ultrasound, and CA-125 in women with a family history of ovarian cancer. Although it is an important component of complete gynecologic care, the pelvic exam alone is clearly insufficient to detect most limited, early-stage epithelial ovarian tumors. Tumor markers, such as CA-125, lack the sensitivity and specificity to serve as the sole form of screening. Transvaginal ultrasound is currently being studied in a large screening trial nationwide and may prove to offer the best alternative to detect early-stage ovarian cancers. A recent report of the use of proteomics to identify early-stage ovarian cancer may represent a breakthrough for ovarian cancer screening. Proteomics is a new and emerging technology that can identify low molecular weight molecules in a high-throughput, nonbiased discovery approach using patient serum, plasma, urine, or tissue specimens. Petricoin et al.[79] identified a small set of key protein values from patient serum that discriminated ovarian cancer cases from unaffected controls with a sensitivity of 100% and a specificity of 95%. Ultimately, a complementary series of markers may be combined for use in conjunction with ultrasonography to improve the predictive value of the screening process.

Outcome data from chemoprevention trials are just beginning to emerge. The recently completed Breast Cancer Prevention Trial, which randomized more than 13,000 high-risk women to the antiestrogen tamoxifen or placebo found a 49% reduction in the incidence of breast cancer among women in the tamoxifen arm.[80] The reduction in risk was limited to estrogen receptor-positive tumors. A very limited subset analysis of these data indicated that women with *BRCA1* mutations (who are more likely to develop hormone receptor-negative breast tumors) did not benefit from tamoxifen whereas those with *BRCA2* mutations did.[81] A second large trial comparing tamoxifen to the selective estrogen receptor modulator raloxifene is under way.

To date, there have been no Phase III randomized chemoprevention trials for ovarian cancer. However, because of the strong epidemiologic association between oral contraceptive (OC) use and a reduction in ovarian cancer rates,[82] many gynecologists are recommending their use in women with an increased risk from either family history or nulliparity. Preliminary data from studies of women with *BRCA1/2* mutations suggest that they enjoy the same degree of protection (approximately 40% reduction) from OCs as do women in the general population. Small pilot studies are now under way to determine the chemopreventive role of other agents, including members of the retinoid family as well as progestational agents.

Prophylactic oophorectomy is being considered by women with a family history of ovarian cancer, particularly those who are *BRCA1/2* mutation carriers, because of the uncertain nature of screening and the high case-fatality rate of advanced-stage cancer. Two large recent studies demonstrated an 85% to 96% reduction in ovarian cancer and a 50% reduction in breast cancer among women undergoing oophorectomy for prophylaxis.[83,84] Prophylactic surgery does not, however, eliminate the risk for primary peritoneal cancer, which is estimated to range from 1.9% to 10.7%.[85] Furthermore, premenopausal women choosing this option must consider the long-term consequences of surgically induced menopause. Similarly, prophylactic mastectomy does not completely eliminate the risk of subsequent breast cancer, although a recent retrospective review of 2,029 women who had elected the procedure for a variety of reasons estimates a greater than 90% reduction in risk.[86] This finding was supported by a prospective study of *BRCA1/2* carriers in which no breast cancers were observed in the 76 women who underwent prophylactic mastectomy.[87] This consideration occurs most commonly among women from high-risk families or those with known *BRCA1/2* mutations who are making treatment choices for their first primary breast cancer, given the increased rate of second cancers in the same breast as well as the contralateral breast in that setting. Another indication for the procedure among high-risk women is extremely dense breast tissue, which renders both clinical breast examination and standard mammography less reliable. Studies are now under way to prospectively follow women who elect prophylactic oophorectomy or mastectomy to monitor long-term disease reduction as well as to document the variables influencing the decision to pursue prophylactic surgery and the medical and psychologic consequences of the surgery.

Hereditary Colorectal Cancer Syndromes (FAP, HNPCC)

The adenomatous polyposis coli (*APC*) gene on chromosome 5q21 encodes a protein that is important in cell adhesion, signal transduction, and transcriptional activation. Germ-line mutations in *APC* are associated with familial adenomatous polyposis (FAP), a syndrome whose clinical phenotype includes hundreds to thousands of adenomatous polyps in the colon and rectum developing after the first decade of life and a 90% risk of developing colorectal cancer by the fourth decade of life.[88] Additional features include extracolonic tumors including thyroid, periampullary, pancreatic, and gastric, hepatoblastoma in children, and congenital hypertrophy of retinal pigment epithelium (CHRPE). In some variants of FAP, the disease presentation may include fewer polyps and later onset of disease. One variant, called Gardner's syndrome, includes osteomas, epidermoid cysts, fibromas, odontomas, and desmoid cysts.[89] These attenuated forms of FAP are often associated with distinct locations of the mutation on the gene, supporting a genotype–phenotype correlation in this syndrome. For example, a FAP mutation at I1307K, prevalent in 6% of people of Ashkenazi Jewish descent, appears to effect a modest (twofold) increase in colon cancer in that population.[90] Although highly penetrant, FAP accounts for less than 1% of all colon cancer. Genetic tests for FAP include protein truncation tests and full gene sequencing. The most common use of genetic testing for FAP is to determine if an unaffected relative of a patient with clinical manifestations of FAP has inherited the genetic mutation. Genetic testing is recommended at ages 10 to 12 years. Alternatively, at-risk individuals can pursue endoscopic screening for the phenotypic features of the syndrome. Annual endoscopic screening usually begins at puberty, with decreasing frequency with increasing decades of life. Some recommend screening for hepatoblastoma with alpha fetoprotein levels in children starting at age 5 years. For primary prevention of FAP, the recommended strategy is colectomy, usually in the second decade of life. Subtotal colectomy with ileorectal anastomosis, total protocolectomy with Brooke ileostomy, or protcolectomy and ileoanal pull-through are acceptable surgical options. Those who choose subtotal colectomy require frequent endoscopic evaluation of the rectum because of the persistent risk of rectal adenomas and carcinomas. The use of specific or nonspecific cyclooxygenase (COX)-2 inhibitors, such as celecoxib, has been recommended as an adjunct to endoscopic surveillance following subtotal colectomy.[91] Upper endoscopic surveillance, as well as thyroid examination, are also recommended by some.

HNPCC is an autosomal dominant condition caused by the germ-line mutation of one of several DNA mismatch repair genes, *hMSH2* on chromosome 2p16, *hMLH1* on chromosome 3p21, *hPMS1* and *hPMS2* on chromosomes 2q31 and 7q11, respectively, *hMSH6* on chromosome 2p16, and *hMSH3* on chromosome 5q11.2–q13.2.[92] The function of these genes is to maintain the fidelity of DNA during replication. When mismatch repair is faulty, somatic mutations occur throughout the genome that can ultimately trigger the carcinogenic pathway.[89] It is estimated that germ-line mutations in the HNPCC account for 3% to 5% of all colorectal cancers.[93]

Individuals with HNPCC have a lifetime risk of developing colorectal cancer of 70%, with a mean age at diagnosis of 44 years. Both synchronous and metachronous tumors are common, and both tumors and polyps are often right sided. Extracolonic cancers, including endometrial, ovarian, gastric, urinary tract, kidney, biliary tract, central nervous system, and small bowel, are also increased.[89] Criteria for HNPCC, the Amsterdam criteria, were developed by the International Collaborative Group in 1990 and subsequently revised to include other HNPCC-associated cancers, such as endometrial cancer, small bowel cancers, and ureteral or renal pelvis cancers, whose relative risk ranges from 3 to 25 times that of the general population (Table 25.6).[22,94]

Because tumor DNA from individuals with HNPCC often have a distinct phenotype with changes in the length of nucleotide repeat sequences, termed MSI, the analysis of MSI in the tumor specimens is often recommended as the first step of evaluation before proceeding to full genetic sequencing for *MLH1* or *MSH2*. Clinical indications for testing a

TABLE 25.6. The Amsterdam criteria for hereditary nonpolyposis colorectal cancer (HNPCC).

The Amsterdam Criteria I:
Histologically confirmed colorectal cancer in at least three relatives, one of whom is a first-degree relative of the other two.
Occurrence of disease in at least two successive generations.
Age at diagnosis below 50 years in at least one individual.
Exclusion of familial adenomatous polyposis.
Amsterdam Criteria II:
Histologically confirmed HNPCC-related cancers (colorectal cancer, or cancer of the endometrium, small bowel, ureter, or renal pelvis) in at least three relatives, one of whom is a first-degree relative of the other two.
Occurrence of disease in at least two successive generations.
Age at diagnosis below 50 years in at least one individual.
Exclusion of familial adenomatous polyposis.

Source: From Vasen et al.,[94] by permission of *Gastroenterology*.

TABLE 25.7. The revised Bethesda guidelines.

Tumors from individuals should be tested for MSI in the following situations:
Colorectal cancer diagnosed in a patient who is less than 50 years of age.
Presence of synchronous, metachronous colorectal, or other HNPCC-associated tumors, regardless of age.
Colorectal cancer with the MSI-H histology diagnosed in a patient who is less than 60 years of age.
Colorectal cancer diagnosed in one or more first-degree relatives with an HNPCC-related tumor, with one of the cancers being diagnosed under age 50 years.
Colorectal cancer diagnosed in two or more first- or second-degree relatives with HNPCC-related tumors, regardless of age.

Source: By permission of A Umar, C Boland, J Terdiman, et al., *Journal of the National Cancer Institute* 96:261, 2004.

colonic tumor for MSI are outlined in the Bethesda criteria (Table 25.7) and include early age at onset (less than 50 years), an individual with multiple primary cancers, and a family history of colorectal and/or endometrial cancer.[23,89] Of note, tumors that are positive for MSI (MSI high) are characterized by a better clinical outcome compared to tumors with low or no expression of MSI.[95] Newer assays include immunohistochemistry staining of tumors using antibodies to the *MLH1* and *MSH2* protein products. Histopathologic features of HNPCC-related colorectal cancer include mucinous or signet-ring types, poor cellular differentiation, and peritumoral lymphocytic infiltration.[96] The polyps that precede cancer are more often villous with areas of high-grade dysplasia than sporadic polyps.[93] Other rare genetic syndromes associated with an increased risk for colon polyps and cancers are Turcot syndrome, Peutz–Jeghers sysndrome, and juvenile polyposis.

Management strategies for HNPCC are based on the observed natural history of the diseases included in the syndrome. Because of the early age of onset of colorectal cancers, it is recommended that annual screening colonoscopy be initiated by age 25, or 5 years younger than the youngest affected individual in the family, and continued at frequent intervals for known mutation carriers. Those relatives who have a 50% chance of being a mutation carrier, but have not undergone genetic testing, are recommended to begin colonoscopy every 1 to 2 years, starting between 20 and 30 years, and annually after age 40. Because of the predominance of right-sided tumors in HNPCC, flexible sigmoidoscopy is not a sufficient screening tool. Because of the significantly increased risk for endometrial cancer in women with an HNPCC mutation, some form of screening of the uterus is recommended starting at age 25, although the optimal screening tool is not clear.[93] Current options include annual transvaginal ultrasound or endometrial aspirates.[97] Because of the high rate of metachronous tumors seen with HNPCC mutations (25%–40%), subtotal colectomy with ileorectal anastomosis rather than standard colectomy is recommended for individuals at the time of diagnosis of colon cancer.[93] As in the case of *BRCA1/2*, oophorectomy (with hysterectomy) may be presented as an option for women with HNPCC.

Multiple Endocrine Neoplasias (MEN) Types 1 and 2

The familial MEN syndromes are characterized by clustering of benign and malignant endocrine tumors and other systemic manifestations. MEN type 1 includes combinations of more than 20 different types of tumors, but the most characteristic are tumors of the parathyroid, pituitary, and pancreatic glands. The term multiple refers both to the occurrence of multiple tumors in the same gland and to multiple different kinds of tumors in the same individual and/or family. MEN1 is inherited as an autosomal dominant disease with variable penetrance and a prevalence of 1 in 30,000 to 1 in 50,000.[98] The MEN1 gene has been localized to chromosome 11q13 and encodes a protein called menin. Menin is thought to interact with one or more transcription factors in the nucleus, and loss of its function is thought to be the mechanism of tumor formation in the syndrome.[99] Much of the morbidity associated with this syndrome is attributable to the excess production of hormones. Hyperparathyroidism from parathyroid tumors is the most common (more than 90%) and earliest manifestation of the syndrome, occurring in the third decade of life and involving three or all four parathyroid glands. Enteropancreatic islet cell tumors occur in 30% to 75% of MEN1-affected individuals and usually present with symptoms of hormone excess after age 40 years. Tumors occur both in the pancreas and in the duodenum and are commonly multicentric. Hormones secreted by pancreatic islet cell tumors can include chromogranin A and B, pancreatic polypeptide, glucagons, insulin, proinsulin, somatostatin, gastrin vasoactive intestinal polypeptide (VIP), serotonin, calcitonin, growth hormone (GH)-releasing factor, and neurotensin.[99] The prevalence of pituitary adenomas in MEN1 ranges from 10% to 60%, and most are less than 1 cm in diameter. Other rare manifestations of MEN1 include carcinoid tumors, adrenal cortical hyperplasias, lipomas, and angiofibromas.

MEN1 germ-line mutation testing is recommended for index cases with clinical MEN1 manifestations and their at-risk relatives. Periodic biochemical testing for hormone excess is a less efficient alternative. Management of MEN1 tumors includes surgery as well as medical management of hormone-secreting tumors. The treatment of choice for primary hyperparathyroidism is total parathyroidectomy, with immediate autotransplantation of parathyroid tissue to an accessible site, usually the forearm.[100] Subtotal parathyroidectomy is associated with a high rate of subsequent recurrence. Insulinomas are often treated with surgical resection because of the difficulty in achieving medical management. Surgery for other islet cell tumors is controversial, as most are multicentric and can often be managed medically. Treatment of pituitary tumors depends on the type of adenoma but does not differ from that for sporadic pituitary tumors. Regular screening for hormone excess in known or suspected mutation carriers is controversial. If elected, annual biochemical screening should begin in early childhood and continue for life. Tumor imaging [e.g., magnetic resonance imaging (MRI) of the pancreas and pituitary] are recommended every 3 to 5 years.[99]

As in MEN1, the MEN2 syndromes represent several variants of benign and malignant tumors, all of which, however, show a high penetrance for medullary thyroid cancer (MTC), a rare calcitonin-producing tumor of the parafollicular cells of the thyroid gland.[99] All MEN2 syndromes are caused by germ-line mutations that activate the *RET* proto-oncogene, located on chromosome 10q11.2, which encodes the RET (rearranged during transfection) protein, a tyrosine kinase receptor expressed in tumors of neural crest origin.[101] RET activates several downstream pathways involved in cell growth, survival, and differentiation.[102] MEN2A, which accounts for 90% of all MEN2 cases, is characterized by MTC in 90% of mutation carriers, unilateral or bilateral pheochromocytomas, tumors of the adrenal chromaffin cells, in 50% of carriers, and multicentric parathyroid tumors in 20% to 30%. MEN2B accounts for 5% of MEN2 cases and is characterized by MTC, pheochromocytoma, and developmental abnormalities including mucosal and intestinal ganglioneuromatosis, marfanoid habitus, neurofibromas, and medullated corneal nerve fibers. MTC in MEN2b occurs at an earlier age and is thought to have a more aggressive course. MTC in multiple family members (four cases or more) is the only manifestation of familial MTC (FMTC) and is thought to have a more benign course. Other rare variants include MEN2A with cutaneous lichen amyloidosis and MEN2A or FMTC with Hirschsprung's disease.

DNA sequencing for *RET* mutations is clinically available and is indicated for all index cases and their at-risk relatives. Approximately 2.5% to 7% of mutations in RET are spontaneous new mutations, and therefore, genetic screening is recommended for all individuals with MTC, regardless of family history. *RET* mutations exhibit a characteristic genotype–phenotype correlation, with specific mutations associated with each variant of the syndrome. Because C cell hyperplasia is a precursor lesion to MTC, serum calcitonin levels provide an excellent tumor marker, particularly to monitor the tumor status of those diagnosed with MTC. Primary prevention is recommended in mutation carriers, however, with total thyroidectomy in childhood (before age 5 years in MEN2a and before 1 year in MEN2B). Pheochromocytomas usually present at a later age than MTC (between 30 and 40 years) with intractable hypertension and/or hypertensive crisis. Screening for pheochromocytoma is done by measurement of plasma metanephrines or 24-hour urinary catecholamines or metanephrines.[99] Abdominal MRI is performed to confirm the diagnosis in suspected cases. Prophylactic adrenalectomy is not recommended because of the dangers of adrenal insufficiency. Hyperparathyroidism may present with hypercalciuria or renal calculi but is often asymptomatic. MEN2-associated hyperparathyroidism is managed in a manner similar to sporadic forms.

There are several other rare genetic syndromes associated with cancer susceptibility, including basal cell nevus syndrome, von Hippel–Lindau syndrome, retinoblastoma, and neurofibromatosis (see Table 25.1), which are described in depth by Offit.[1]

Future Directions

The rapidly evolving insights into the molecular genetic pathways of carcinogenesis will have broad application to the future of clinical oncology. The availability of predictive genetic testing to extend beyond the small number of highly penetrant genes will depend on the identification of an increased number of low penetrant genes that alter susceptibility to cancer in all individuals. Although the genes involved in complex carcinogenic pathways are likely to have a small individual effect on risk, their attributable risk can be high because they affect a large segment of the population.

The relatively new field of molecular epidemiology is capitalizing on the existence of genetic polymorphisms to identify genetic clues of exposure to carcinogens or particular vulnerabilities to carcinogens. Genetic variation in the metabolism of carcinogens can alter response to environmental carcinogens by changing the rate of metabolism of procarcinogens or the catabolism of carcinogens. Genetic polymorphisms can also result in DNA damage or alterations in signal transduction pathways and represent an important component to cancer susceptibility.[103] In addition to their role in carcinogenesis, genetic polymorphisms may also contribute to treatment toxicities and are likely to explain why some patients suffer severe adverse reactions to chemotherapy and/or radiation therapy. Furthermore, drug-metabolizing enzymes may also determine patterns of response in individual patients. A better understanding of the role of these polymorphisms and their complex interactions will ultimately permit individualized estimates of risk and lead to targeted prevention as well as therapeutic strategies.

The application of a genetic approach to cancer diagnosis not only will lead to a better understanding of the pathophysiology of cancer, it will also provide tools for more accurate diagnosis and prognosis that will translate into more appropriate and targeted therapeutic approaches. Microarray technology is beginning to emerge as a powerful tool that allows both qualitative and quantitative screening for sequence variations in genomic DNA for thousands of genes in a biologic sample. Current tools for diagnosing cancer rely heavily on the histopathologic appearance of a tissue specimen, resulting in a limited classification scheme with inherent tumor heterogeneity. Microarray technology has the potential to create a taxonomy of tumors that will reflect their molecular diversity.

Microarray technology is being applied in the area of cancer prognosis to better classify tumors and to predict outcome.[104] The ability to create a genetic taxonomy for each cancer will greatly enhance our ability to match patients to appropriate treatment regimens.[105] In breast cancer, for example, both the overexpression of HER2/neu and abnormal p53 expression are associated with decreased survival. In colon cancer, the presence of high-frequency microsatellite instability in the tumor is associated with early age of onset, a predominance of tumors in the proximal colon, increased sensitivity to chemotherapy, and improved survival.

In addition to cancer prevention and early detection, genetic status will provide clinicians with the possibility of suitable, novel therapeutic options. Historically, cytotoxic therapies have been designed to capitalize on the increased cell proliferation rates generally manifested by cancer cells, a feature also shared by many benign cells, thus resulting in significant, dose-limiting toxicities. To improve the current state of cancer treatment, therapies specifically designed to reverse the specific genetic defect(s) expressed by a tumor are needed. The relatively new field of pharmacogenomics applies genome-based technologies to identify genetically determined targets for new drug development and to tailor drug regimens and schedules to individual genetic profiles.[106]

Cancer treatment resistance, a major barrier to effective therapy, is still poorly understood but is acknowledged to be largely attributable to gene expression variability. This is another area where microarray technology will be applied to stimulate progress in understanding cellular and subcellular resistance mechanisms. These and other targeted therapeutic advances likely represent the tip of the iceberg for rational drug design and will be followed by gene-based strategies using ribozymes, other growth factor receptor antibodies, immunotoxins, signal transduction inhibitors, and antiangiogenic molecules, to name a few.

Finally, as we move from the setting of single gene identification, the possibility of whole-genome screening looms large on the horizon. The possibility of complete genomic sequencing as a routine clinical test on every individual to be used for predictive and preventive medicine will become feasible as the work of the Human Genome Project proceeds. However, its adoption as a part of routine medical practice must consider the criteria for the adoption of population screening on a public health basis. Widespread genetic screening for a disease should be restricted to those diseases that are relatively common and serious, for which the natural history is defined and consistent, and for which effective primary and/or secondary prevention interventions exist. The associated gene(s) must be well characterized and accurately identified through existing detection methods. Genetic testing must be relatively inexpensive, acceptable to the population, and associated with pre- and posttest counseling. Genetic screening for diseases that selectively affect a segment of the population should be targeted specifically to that group and not offered to the population as a whole. As we move into an era characterized by genetic identity, ethical and social concerns must be carefully considered.[107]

Conclusions

As the importance of cancer prevention and control grows in recognition, cancer risk counseling services are becoming a standard component of primary health care. Individuals are becoming increasingly aware of the role of their family history in their own personal cancer risk. The growing sophistication in the process of risk identification, including the use of genetic tests for cancer susceptibility genes, is stimulating research to develop risk modification and cancer prevention strategies. Several registries of high-risk families are being assembled to provide prospective data on the epidemiology and natural history of familial cancers and the effectiveness of a variety of cancer control interventions. Optimal screening protocols for members of high-risk families are being developed and evaluated. Long-term follow-up of mutation carriers will help to define the spectrum of cancer risk, the clinical course of hereditary cancer, and response to treatment. Central to these research efforts are ongoing studies of the short- and long-term effects of cancer risk counseling on health behaviors and quality of life. Coincidental with this are the many new educational initiatives to prepare healthcare professionals to become part of the cancer risk counseling team.

References

1. Offit K. Clinical Cancer Genetics: Risk Counseling and Management, 1st ed. New York: Wiley-Liss, 1998.
2. Andrulis IL, Anton-Culver H, Beck J, et al. Comparison of DNA- and RNA-based methods for detection of truncating *BRCA1* mutations. Hum Mutat 2002;20:65–73.
3. Schneider K. Counseling About Cancer. Strategies for Genetic Counseling, 2nd ed. New York: Wiley-Liss, 2002.
4. Narod S, Feunteun J, Lynch H, et al. Familial breast-ovarian locus on chromosome 17q12–23. Lancet 1991;338:82.
5. American Society of Clinical Oncology. American Society of Clinical Oncology policy statement update: genetic testing for cancer susceptibility. J Clin Oncol 2003;21(12):2397–2406.
6. American Society of Human Genetics. Statement of the American Society of Human Genetics on genetic testing for breast and ovarian cancer predisposition. Am J Hum Genet 1994;55:i–iv.
7. National Society of Genetic Counselors. Predisposition genetic testing for late-onset disorders in adults: a position paper of the National Society of Genetic Counselors. JAMA 1997;278(15): 1217–1220.
8. Armstrong K, Calzone K, Stopfer J, et al. Factors associated with decisions about clinical *BRCA1/2* testing. Cancer Epidemiol Biomarkers Prev 2000;9:1251–1254.
9. Burke W. Genetic testing. N Engl J Med 2002;347(23):1867–1875.
10. Geller G, Botkin JR, Green MJ, et al. Genetic testing for susceptibility to adult-onset cancer: the process and content of informed consent. JAMA 1997;277:1467–1474.
11. American Society of Human Genetics, American College of Medical Genetics. ASHG/ACMG report. Points to consider: ethical, legal, and psychosocial implications of genetic testing in children and adolescents. Am J Hum Genet 1995;57:1233–1241.
12. Wideroff L, Freedman AN, Olson L, et al. Physician use of genetic testing for cancer susceptibility: results of a national survey. Cancer Epidemiol Biomarkers Prev 2003;12:295–303.
13. Baty B, Venne V, McDonald J, et al. BRCA1 testing: genetic counseling protocol development and counseling issues. J Genet Counsel 1997;6(2):223–244.
14. Peters J. Familial cancer risk. Part I: Impact on today's oncology practice. J Oncol Manage 1994;3:18–30.
15. Muller H. Genetic counseling and cancer. In: Weber W, Laffer U, Durig M (eds). Hereditary Cancer and Preventive Surgery. Basel: Karger, 1990:12–18.
16. Peters J. Familial cancer risk. Part II: Breast cancer risk counseling and genetic susceptibility testing. J Oncol Manag 1994; 3:14–22.
17. Bennett R, Steinhaus K, Uhrich S, et al. Recommendations for standardized human pedigree nomenclature. Am J Human Genet 1995;56:745–752.
18. Mahon S, Casperson D. Hereditary cancer syndrome: part 1. Clinical and educational issues. Oncol Nurs Forum 1995; 22(5):763–771.
19. Gail MH, Brinton LA, Byar DP, et al. Projecting individual probabilities of developing breast cancer for white females who are being examined annually. J Natl Cancer Inst 1989;81(24):1879–1886.
20. Costantino JP, Gail MH, Pee D, et al. Validation studies for models projecting the risk of invasive and total breast cancer incidence. J Natl Cancer Inst 1999;91:1541–1548.
21. Hoskins KF, Stopfer JE, Calzone KA, et al. Assessment and counseling for women with a family history of breast cancer. A guide for clinicians. JAMA 1995;273(7):577–585.
22. Vasen H, Mecklin J, Khan P, et al. The international collaborative group on hereditary non-polyposis colorectal cancer (ICG-HNPCC). Dis Colon Rectum 1991;34:424–425.
23. Rodriguez-Bigas M, Boland C, et al. A National Cancer Institute workshop on hereditary nonpolyposis colorectal cancer syndrome: meeting highlights and Bethesda guidelines. JNCI 1997; 89(23):1758–1762.
24. Shattuck-Eidens D, Oliphant A, McClure M, et al. BRCA1 sequence analysis in women at high risk for susceptibility muta-

tions, risk factor analysis and implications for genetic testing. JAMA 1997;278(15):1242–1250.
25. Berry D, Parmigiani G, Sanchez J, et al. Probability of carrying a mutation of breast-ovarian cancer gene BRCA1 based on family history. JNCI 1997;89(3):227–238.
26. Berry DA, Iversen ES, Gudbjartsson DF, et al. BRCAPRO validation, sensitivity of genetic testing of *BRCA1/BRCA2*, and prevalence of other breast cancer susceptibility genes. J Clin Oncol 2002;20:2701–2712.
27. Lynch H, Harris R, Organ C, et al. Management of familial breast cancer. Arch Surg 1978;113:1061–1067.
28. Kessler S. The process of communication, decision making and coping in genetic counseling. In: Kessler S (ed). Genetic Counseling, Psychological Dimensions. New York: Academic Press, 1979.
29. Ursin G, Henderson B, Halle R, et al. Does oral contraceptive use increase the risk of breast cancer in women with *BRCA1/BRCA2* mutations more than in other women? Cancer Res 1997;57(17):3678–3681.
30. Tambor E, Bernhardt B, Chase G, et al. Offering cystic fibrosis carrier screening to an HMO population: factors associated with utilization. Am J Hum Genet 1997;55:626–637.
31. Evers-Kiebooms G, van den Berghe H. Impact of genetic counseling: a review of published follow-up studies. Clin Genet 1979;15:465–474.
32. Phipps RF, Perry PM: Familial breast cancer. Postgrad Med J 1988;64:847–849.
33. Sellers TA, Potter JD, Rich SS, et al. Familial clustering of breast and prostate cancers and risk of postmenopausal breast cancer. J Natl Cancer Inst 1994;86:1860–1865.
34. Claus EB, Risch N, Thompson WD. Genetic analysis of breast cancer in the cancer and steroid hormone study. Am J Hum Genet 1991;48:232–242.
35. Hall J, Lee M, Newman B, et al. Linkage of early onset familial breast cancer to chromosome 17q21. Science 1990;250:1684–1689.
36. Easton DF, Bishop DT, Ford D, et al. Genetic linkage analysis in familial breast and ovarian cancer: results from 214 families. Am J Hum Genet 1993;52:678–701.
37. Wooster R, Neuhausen SL, Mangion J, et al. Localization of a breast cancer susceptibility gene, BRCA2, to chromosome 13q12-13. Science 1994;265:2088–2090.
38. Gayther SA, Mangion J, Russell P, et al. Variation of risks of breast and ovarian cancer associated with different germline mutations of the BRCA2 gene. Nat Genet 1997;15:103–105.
39. Schubert EL, Lee MK, Mefford HC, et al. BRCA2 in American families with four or more cases of breast or ovarian cancer: recurrent and novel mutations, variable expression, penetrance, and the possibility of families whose cancer is not attributable to BRCA1 or BRCA2. Am J Hum Genet 1997;60:1031–1040.
40. Miki Y, Swensen J, Shattuck-Eidens D, et al. A strong candidate for the breast and ovarian cancer susceptibility gene BRCA1. Science 1994;266:66–71.
41. Scully R, Chen J, Plug A. Association of *BRCA1* with Rad51 in mitotic and meiotic cells. Cell 1997;88(2):265–275.
42. Sharan SK, Morimatsu M, Albrecht U, et al. Embryonic lethality and radiation hypersensitivity mediated by Rad51 in mice lacking BRCA2. Nature (Lond) 1997;386:804–810.
43. Blackwood A, Weber B. *BRCA1* and *BRCA2*: from molecular genetics to clinical medicine. J Clin Oncol 1998;16(5):1969–1977.
44. Fraser JA, Reeves JR, Stanton PD, et al. A role for BRCA1 in sporadic breast cancer. Br J Cancer 2003;88:1263–1270.
45. Neuhausen S, Gilewski T, Norton L, et al. Recurrent *BRCA2* 6174delT mutations in Ashkenazi Jewish women affected by breast cancer. Nat Genet 1998;13(1):126–128.
46. Peelen T, van Vliet M, Petrij-Bosch A, et al. A high proportion of novel mutations in *BRCA1* with strong founder effects among Dutch and Belgian hereditary breast and ovarian cancer families. Am J Hum Genet 1997;60(5):1041–1049.
47. Thorlacius S, Olafsdottir G, Kryggvadottir L, et al. A single BRCA2 mutation in male and female breast cancer families from Iceland with varied cancer phenotypes. Nat Genet 1996;13:117–119.
48. Arason A, Jonasdottir A, Barkardottir RB, et al. A population study of mutations and LOH at breast cancer gene loci in tumours from sister pairs: two recurrent mutations seem to account for all BRCA1/BTCA2 linked breast cancer in Iceland. J Med Genet 1998;35(6):446–449.
49. Einbeigi Z, Bergman A, Kindblom LG, et al. A founder mutation of the BRCA1 gene in Western Sweden associated with a high incidence of breast and ovarian cancer. Eur J Cancer 2001;37(15):1904–1909.
50. Brose MS, Rebbeck TR, Calzone KA, et al. Cancer risk estimates for BRCA1 mutation carriers identified in a risk evaluation program. J Natl Cancer Inst 2002;94:1365–1372.
51. Easton DF, Steele L, Fields P, et al. Cancer risks in two large breast cancer families linked to BRCA2 on chromosome 13q12-13. Am J Hum Genet 1997;61:120–128.
52. Greene MH. Genetics of breast cancer. Mayo Clin Proc 1997;72:54–65.
53. Ford D, Easton DF, Stratton M, et al. Genetic heterogeneity and penetrance analysis of the BRCA1 and BRCA2 genes in breast cancer families. Am J Hum Genet 1998;62:676–689.
54. Malone KE, Daling JR, Weiss NS, et al. Family history and survival of young women with invasive breast carcinoma. Cancer (Phila) 1996;78:1417–1425.
55. Breast Cancer Linkage Consortium. Pathology of familial breast cancer: differences between breast cancers in carriers of BRCA1 and BRCA2 mutations and sporadic cases. Lancet 1997;349:1505–1510.
56. Marcus JN, Page DL, Watson P, et al. BRCA1 and BRCA2 hereditary breast carcinoma phenotypes. Cancer (Phila) 1997;80:543–556.
57. Marcus JN, Watson P, Page DL, et al. Hereditary breast cancer: pathobiology, prognosis, and BRCA1 and BRCA2 gene linkage. Cancer (Phila) 1996;77:697–709.
58. Hedenfalk I, Duggan D, Chen Y, et al. Gene-expression profiles in hereditary breast cancer. N Engl J Med 2001;344:539–548.
59. Verhoog LC, Brekelmans CTM, Seynaeve C, et al. Survival and tumour characteristics of breast-cancer patients with germline mutations of BRCA1. Lancet 1998;351:316–321.
60. Johannsson OT, Ranstam J, Borg A, et al. Survival of BRCA1 breast and ovarian cancer patients: a population-based study from southern Sweden. J Clin Oncol 1998;16:397–404.
61. Garber JE, Goldstein AM, Kantor AF, et al. Follow-up study of twenty-four families with Li-Fraumeni syndrome. Cancer Res 1991;51(22):6094–6097.
62. Bottomley R, Condit P. Cancer families. Cancer Bull 1968;20:22.
63. Ford D, Easton DF. The genetics of breast and ovarian cancer. Br J Cancer 1995;72:805–812.
64. Tsou HC, Teng DHF, Ping XL, et al. The role of MMAC1 mutations in early-onset breast cancer: causative in association with Cowden syndrome and excluded in BRCA1-negative cases. Am J Hum Genet 1997;61:1036–1043.
65. Lynch ED, Ostermeyer EA, Lee MK, et al. Inherited mutations in PTEN that are associated with breast cancer, Cowden disease, and juvenile polyposis. Am J Hum Genet 1997;61:1254–1260.
66. Myers MP, Tonks NK: Invited editorial: PTEN: sometimes taking it off can be better than putting it on. Am J Hum Genet 1997;61:1234–1238.
67. Savitsky K, Bar-Shira A, Gilad S, et al. A single ataxia telangiectasia gene with a product similar to PI-3 kinase. Science 1995;268:1749–1753.

68. Gilad S, Chessa L, Khosravi R, et al. Genotype–phenotype relationships in ataxia-telangiectasia and variants. Am J Hum Genet 1998;62:551–561.
69. Shigeta T, Takagi M, Delia D, et al. Defective control of apoptosis and mitotic spindle checkpoint in heterozygous carriers of *ATM* mutations. Cancer Res 1999;59:2602–2607.
70. Swift M, Morrell D, Massey RB, et al. Incidence of cancer in 161 families affected by ataxia-telangiectasia. N Engl J Med 1991;325:1831–1836.
71. Easton DF. Cancer risks in A-T heterozygotes. Int J Radiat Biol 1994;66(suppl 6):S177–S182.
72. Khanna KK. Cancer risk and the ATM gene: a continuing debate. J Natl Cancer Inst 2000;92:795–802.
73. Broeks A, Urbanus JH, Floore AN, et al. ATM-heterozygote germline mutations contribute to breast cancer susceptibility. Am J Hum Genet 2000;66:494–500.
74. Waha A, Sturne C, Kessler A, et al. Expression of the *ATM* gene is significantly reduced in sporadic breast carcinomas. Int J Cancer 1998;78:306–309.
75. Chenevix-Trench G, Spurdle AB, Gatei M, et al. Dominant negative ATM mutations in breast cancer families. J Natl Cancer Inst 2002;94:205–215.
76. Burke W, Daly M, Garber J, et al. Recommendations for follow-up care of individuals with an inherited predisposition to cancer II. *BRCA1* and *BRCA2*. JAMA 1997;277(12):997–1003.
77. Daly M. NCCN practice guidelines: genetics/familial high-risk cancer screening. Oncology 1999;13(11A):161–183.
78. Warner E, Plewes DB, Shumak RS, et al. Comparison of breast magnetic resonance imaging, mammography, and ultrasound for surveillance of women at high risk for hereditary breast cancer. J Clin Oncol 2001;19(15):3524–3531.
79. Petricoin EF, Ardekani AM, Hitt, BA, et al. Use of proteomic patterns in serum to identify ovarian cancer. Lancet 2002;359: 572–577.
80. Fisher B, Costantino J, Wickerham L, et al. Tamoxifen for prevention of breast cancer: report of the national surgical adjuvant breast and bowel project P-1 study. J Natl Cancer Inst 1998; 90(18):1371–1388.
81. King MC, Wieand S, Hale K, et al. Tamoxifen and breast cancer incidence among women with inherited mutations in BRCA1 and BRCA2: National Surgical Adjuvant Breast and Bowel Project (NSABP-P1) Breast Cancer Prevention Trial. JAMA 2001;286(18):2251–2256.
82. Ness RB, Grisso JA, Klapper J, et al. Risk of ovarian cancer in relation to estrogen and progestin dose and use characteristics of oral contraceptives. Am J Epidemiol 2000;152:233–241.
83. Rebbeck TR, Lynch HT, Neuhausen SL, et al. Prophylactic oophorectomy in carriers of BRCA1 or BRCA2 mutations. N Engl J Med 2002;346(21):1616–1622.
84. Kauf ND, Satagopan JM, Robson ME, et al. Risk-reducing salpingooophorectomy in women with a BRCA1 or BRCA2 mutation. N Engl J Med 2002;346(21):1609–1615.
85. Eisen A, Weber B. Primary peritoneal carcinoma can have multifocal origins: implications for prophylactic oophorectomy. J Natl Cancer Inst 1998;90(11):797–799.
86. Hartmann L, Jenkins R, Schaid D, et al. Prophylactic mastectomy: preliminary retrospective cohort analysis. Proc Am Assoc Cancer Res 1997;38:1123.
87. Meijers-Heijboer H, van Geel B, van Putten WL, et al. Breast cancer after prophylactic bilateral mastectomy in women with a BRCA1 or BRCA2 mutation. N Engl J Med 2001;345(3):159–164.
88. Herrera L. Familial Adenomatous Polyposis. New York: Liss, 1990.
89. Solomon CH, Pho LN, Burt RW. Current status of genetic testing for colorectal cancer susceptibility. Oncology 2002;16(2): 161–171.
90. Laken SJ, Petersen GM, Gruber SB, et al. Familial colorectal cancer in Ashkenazim due to a hypermutable tract in APC. Nat Genet 1997;17:70–83.
91. Higuchi T, Iwama T, Yoshinaga K, et al. A randomized, double-blind, placebo-controlled trial of the effects of Rofecoxib, a selective cyclooxygenase-2 inhibitor, on rectal polyps in familial adenomatous polyposis patients. Clin Cancer Res 2003;9: 4756–4760.
92. Marra G, Boland CR. Hereditary nonpolyposis colorectal cancer: the syndrome, the genes, and historical perspectives. J Natl Cancer Inst 1995;87:1114–1125.
93. AGA technical review on hereditary colorectal cancer and genetic testing. Gastroenterology 2001;121:198–213.
94. Vasen HF, Watson P, Mecklin JP, et al. New criteria for hereditary non-polyposis colorectal cancer (HNPCC, Lynch syndrome) proposed by the International Collaborative Group on HNPCC (ICG HNPCC). Gastroenterology 1999;116:1453–1456.
95. Gafà R, Maestri I, Matteuzzi M, et al. Sporadic colorectal adenocarcinomas with high-frequency microsatellite instability. Cancer (Phila) 2000;89:2025–2037.
96. Messerini L, Mori S, Zampi G. Pathologic features of hereditary non-polyposis colorectal cancer. Tumori 1996;82:114–116.
97. Burke W, Petersen G, Lynch P, et al. Recommendations for follow-up care of individuals with an inherited predisposition to cancer I. Hereditary nonpolyposis colon cancer. JAMA 1997; 277(11):915–919.
98. Giruad S, Zhang CX, Serova-Sinilnikove O, et al. Germ-line mutation analysis in patients with multiple endocrine neoplasia type 1 and related disorders. Am J Hum Genet 1998; 63:455–467.
99. Brandi ML, Gagel RF, Angeli A, et al. Guidelines for diagnosis and therapy of MEN type 1 and type 2. J Clin Endocrinol Metab 2001;86(12):5658–5671.
100. Marx S, Spiegel AM, Skarulis MC, et al. Mulitple endocrine neoplasia type 1: clinical and genetic topics. Ann Intern Med 1998;129:484–494.
101. Eng C. *RET* proto-oncogene in the development of human cancer. J Clin Oncol 1999;17:380–393.
102. Bryant J, Farmer F, Kessler LJ, et al. Pheochromocytoma: the expanding genetic differential diagnosis. JNCI 2003;95:1196–1204.
103. Nebert DW. Polymorphisms in drug-metabolizing enzymes: what is their clinical relevance and why do they exist? Am J Hum Genet 1997;60:265–271.
104. Ahr A, Holtrich U, Solbach C, et al. Molecular classification of breast cancer patients by gene expression profiling. J Pathol 2001;195:312–320.
105. Rosell R, Monzo M, O'Brate A, et al. Translational oncogenomics: toward rational therapeutic decision-making. Curr Opin Oncol 2002;14:171–179.
106. Herrmann J, Rastelli L, Burgess C, et al. Implications of oncogenomics for cancer research and clinical oncology. Cancer J 2001; 7:40–51.
107. Grody WW. Molecular genetic risk screening. Annu Rev Med 2001;54:473–490.

26

Behavior Modification

Christopher N. Sciamanna

There is no question at this point in our medical knowledge that health behaviors play a prominent role in morbidity and mortality from cancer and other diseases. The seminal paper by McGinnis and Foege "Actual causes of death in the United States" in 1993 did a great deal to put health behaviors on the map as significant public health problems. In their analysis, the authors concluded that approximately half of all deaths are due to health behaviors. The three most prominent behaviors in their analysis, tobacco (19%), diet and physical activity patterns (14%), and alcohol (5%), could be linked to more than one-third of all deaths in 1990.[1] A reanalysis of the same question reached basically the same conclusions using data from the year 2000.[2] This chapter takes a similar examination of the available evidence for the most common health behaviors that are implicated as contributing to cancer. We focus the analysis on tobacco use, diet, physical activity, being overweight, and sun exposure, as each is quite common and has been the subject of significant study. For each behavior, this chapter discusses one or more cancers with which the behavior is purported to be associated, yet the discussion focuses on behaviors, rather than cancers. For each behavior, this chapter examines (1) the evidence linking changes in the health behaviors to reducing cancer morbidity and mortality, (2) the effectiveness of physician counseling as a commonly used method of behavior modification, (3) the recommendations of professional groups regarding what individuals can do to improve these health behaviors, and (4) methods for improving the quality of physician counseling for behavior modification.

Efficacy of Risk Reduction

The contributions of adverse health behaviors to cancer morbidity and mortality are substantial and well documented. A World Cancer Research Fund panel estimated that 30% to 40% of all cancers are attributable to inappropriate diet, physical activity, and high body weight.[3] In this section, we review the evidence linking changes in several established cancer risk behaviors to changes in cancer morbidity and mortality. This review is not meant to be exhaustive, but intends to review the most common cancers, primarily those for which the most data exist.

Efficacy of Risk Reduction: Tobacco Use

There is a large body of evidence from prospective cohort and case-control studies showing that many of the health risks of tobacco use can be reduced by smoking cessation. As compared with smokers, the excess risk of lung cancer decreases sharply in ex-smokers after approximately 5 years since quitting. Although an excess risk from smoking most likely persists through life, the excess risk approaches that of a never smoker after 15 to 20 years since quitting.[4] After quitting, the risk of oral, pharyngeal, and laryngeal cancers decreases, approaching that of a never smoker in approximately 15 years.[5,6] Also, within 2 years of quitting, the risk of pancreatic cancer decreases by approximately 50%.[7–9]

Efficacy of Risk Reduction: Diet

Differences in dietary intake are thought to account for approximately 30% of cancers in Western countries, although less in developing countries.[10] Although many studies have examined the association of different dietary components on cancer risk, very few have examined the likely effect of changing the diet on subsequent risk or survival from cancer.

Early data showed that an increase in the polyunsaturated fatty acid concentration in membranes stimulated the oxidation of precarcinogens to reactive intermediates.[11] The largest study to date, however, a pooled analysis on roughly 350,000 women, found no association between replacing monounsaturated, polyunsaturated fats with carbohydrates on the incidence of breast cancer.[12] In this same study, a weak positive association was identified between replacing saturated fats with carbohydrates on breast cancer incidence. There is little evidence linking dietary fat to the incidence of colorectal cancer. A single large randomized trial, however, showed no effect of a diet low in fat and high in fiber, fruit, and vegetables on the recurrence of colorectal adenomas.[13]

Fruit and vegetable intake is negatively associated with incidence of many cancers, including those of the oral cavity, esophagus, pharynx,[14] stomach,[15] colorectal region,[16–18] lung,[19] cervix,[14] and kidney.[14] Intervention trials, however, in which fiber and fruit and vegetable intake have been augmented, have failed to slow the recurrence of colorectal adenomas.[13,20,21] Similarly, a study of beta-carotene supplementation failed to decrease the incidence of lung cancer.[22] Similar to other food groups, very little evidence exists to understand the effect of changes of fruit and vegetable intake on cancer incidence. The three studies that have examined increases in fruit and vegetable intake, including the Polyp Prevention Trial as mentioned previously, have not found decrease in the recurrence of colorectal adenomas.[13,20,21] An ongoing randomized trial, the Women's Healthy Eating and Living Study, will add to our understanding of the effect of a diet high in vegetables, fruits, and fiber and low in fat on breast cancer survival.[23]

Efficacy of Risk Reduction: Physical Inactivity

In the United States, fewer than half of adults attain recommended levels of physical activity.[24] There is conflicting evidence supporting a link between physical inactivity and cancers of the prostate, endometrium, and lung,[25] and there have been no intervention trials showing a decrease in the incidence or recurrence of any cancer. Furthermore, little evidence exists examining the effect of changes in physical activity level on risk of cancer.

Efficacy of Risk Reduction: Alcohol Abuse

Nearly one-third of U.S. adults drink an excessive amount of alcohol.[26] Excessive alcohol use appears to be associated with cancers of the breast, oropharynx, pharynx, esophagus, and liver.[27–31] Little evidence exists examining the effect on changes in alcohol consumption on the risk of breast or other cancers. Two studies from Italy observed that, although stopping smoking decreased the risk of laryngeal cancer within only a few years, stopping drinking led to a much smaller decline in laryngeal and esophageal cancer risk after more than a decade.[32,33]

Efficacy of Risk Reduction: Overweight and Obesity

There is no end in sight for the epidemic of overweight and obesity in the United States. In 2001, a national survey observed more than 67% of adult men and 50% of adult women to be overweight [body mass index (BMI) greater than 25], and of those an equal number of men and women (21%) were classified as obese (BMI greater than 30).[34] Although overweight and obesity are associated with breast cancer incidence, few studies have examined the effect of weight loss on the incidence of cancer, which precludes any firm conclusions.[35,36] Although firm conclusions are not possible, some evidence can be found in the Nurses' Health Study, in which women who gained more than 20 pounds from age 18 to midlife doubled their risk for breast cancer, compared to women who maintained a stable weight.[37]

Efficacy of Risk Reduction: Sun Exposure

Exposure to the sunlight has been implicated in the high incidence of skin cancers, which most commonly include cutaneous melanoma, basal cell carcinoma, and squamous cell carcinoma.[38–40] There is no direct evidence, however, that personal sun protection behaviors can reduce the incidence of melanoma, and evidence that sun protection behaviors modify the incidence of other skin cancers is mixed.[41,42] For example, a randomized controlled trial of daily sunscreen use in a general population in Australia showed no effect on risk of basal cell carcinoma over 5 years of intervention and follow-up.[43] Another randomized controlled trial, however, of sunscreen applied daily to the head, neck, hands, and arms reduced the number of new squamous cell carcinomas over a 5-year period.[44] A third randomized trial observed that sunscreen use decreased the incidence of, and increased the regression rate of, solar keratoses.[45,46]

Effectiveness of Physician Counseling

This section highlights the evidence, and the strength of that evidence, regarding the efficacy of physicians in bringing about changes in health behaviors (intermediate outcomes) and in changing cancer incidence or survival (distal outcomes).

Effectiveness of Physician Counseling: Tobacco Use

Of all the health behaviors, the most agreement exists regarding the efficacy of physician counseling. Several well-designed randomized controlled trials have established that physician counseling helps smokers quit.[47] Providing self-help brochures without clinical advice has limited efficacy, but physician advice alone can increase quit rates by as much as 10%.[48,49] Cummings and colleagues observed that training internists for 3 hours and providing self-help books to smokers increased smoking cessation rates by approximately 2%.[48] The 1996 and 2000 Clinical Practice Guidelines contain a summary of this evidence.[47,50] The guidelines emphasized the role of (1) identification of smokers in practice, such as using smoking as a "vital sign,"[51] (2) physician advice to quit, and (3) the use of medications to assist smokers in their quitting attempts. Several studies have also shown that feedback about smoking-specific risk factors such as pulmonary function and carbon monoxide testing by physicians can double smoking cessation rates.[52–54]

Effectiveness of Physician Counseling: Poor Diet

There is inconclusive evidence that physician counseling can lead to dietary changes.[55–59] In one such study, physicians gave patients a self-help booklet and a brief motivational message, which led to significant changes in the intake of fat and fiber, compared with a usual care comparison group.[56] Most studies, however, have included several hours of physician education and training on diet counseling, as other studies have shown that physicians receive little training on diet and may often not be aware of the effect of dietary modifications.[60–63] Similar studies have observed that brief training of physicians can lead to changes in blood cholesterol,[64] saturated fat intake,[65] and fruit and vegetable intake.[55] Some studies, however, have found no effect of physician counseling, and many primary care-based studies have also employed office systems, computer-tailored print messages, and counseling by nutritionists and nurses, which make it difficult to understand the independent effects of physician counseling.[55,57,65–67]

Effectiveness of Physician Counseling: Physical Inactivity

There is inconclusive evidence that physician intervention counseling can also lead to changes in physical activity, as studies have shown the effects to be mixed.[57,68–72] A 2002 review by the United States Preventive Services Task Force identified only eight studies on which to base their conclusion.[73] Most studies have tested low-intensity interventions such as 3 to 5 minutes of counseling in a routine outpatient visit and included several hours to several days of provider training. In some of the studies, the patients completed a self-report tool on physical activity levels or answered questions from a validated survey in the office waiting room or at home. In many of the studies, a research assistant or nurse conducted a baseline assessment and placed it in the chart for the physician to use during the clinical encounter. As such, it is difficult from many of the studies to understand the independent effects of physician counseling. In the six studies that compared an intervention condition, including physician counseling to a usual care control group, the effects on physical activity were mixed. Only one of the studies met all the methodological criteria for a quality rating of "good."[73] The U.S. Preventive Services Task Force (USPSTF) study found the available evidence to be inconclusive.[73]

Effectiveness of Physician Counseling: Alcohol Abuse

There is a reasonable amount of evidence that physician counseling can decrease drinking in patients who abuse alcohol. At least three randomized trials have been conducted, all showing that counseling led to a decreased amount of drinking.[74–76] In one such study, providers were trained to provide a brief (5 to 10 minutes) counseling intervention, and an office support system was used that screened patients and cued providers to intervene, in addition to making patient education materials available.[76] The intervention led to a decrease of 5.8 drinks per week compared with a usual care condition.[76,77] Two other large studies showed decreases in the range of 10 drinks per week in the intervention condition, compared to the control condition.[74,75] Although not all studies have shown positive effects,[78] two meta-analyses have shown that brief interventions, typically conducted by physicians, are effective at decreasing alcohol intake among heavy drinkers in outpatient settings.[79,80]

Effectiveness of Physician Counseling: Overweight and Obesity

There is inconclusive evidence about the effects of physician counseling to help patients lose weight.[65,81–85] In one such study, physicians counseled patients and incorporated meal replacements and nurse visits, which led to losses of approximately 4% of body weight, equal to the effects of two nutritionist-led intervention conditions.[81] There have been few studies, however, and many studies that showed an effect on weight loss were actually designed to improve dietary patterns, such as decreasing saturated fat intake.[64,65,86] A significant barrier to physician counseling for overweight and obesity is the apparent complexity of counting calories, which is the basis of all weight loss recommendations.[87] Training programs have been developed and user-friendly reminder cards have been developed, but many barriers remain and conclusions based on the available evidence are difficult to make.[87,88]

Effectiveness of Physician Counseling: Sun Exposure

Very little evidence exists to understand the effects of physician counseling on sun protection behaviors. At least one intervention has been shown to increase healthcare provider counseling, but the effects of physician counseling on patient's use of sun protection behaviors or on subsequent development of skin cancer is not yet known.[89] A randomized trial of a community-based, multiintervention program, including office-based counseling by physicians, showed that the intervention increased sun protection behaviors in the intervention towns.[90] More parents recalled receiving advice to use sun protection behaviors in the intervention towns, giving some indirect evidence that the increased use of sun protection behaviors was due to more physician counseling. The United States Preventive Services Task Force concluded, in October 2003, that there was insufficient evidence to recommend for or against routine counseling by primary care clinicians to prevent skin cancer.[91]

Recommendations of Professional Groups

This section attempts to summarize the recommendations, including the similarities and differences, of recommendations from guidelines published by professional groups, such as the USPSTF, American Lung, American Heart, and health insurance companies, regarding the expected standards of care and reimbursement for behavioral counseling.

Recommendations of Professional Groups: Tobacco Use

Professional groups are in broad agreement that tobacco use in any form and in any amount is not safe and should be discontinued. No safe level of smoking has ever been identified.[10] Groups agree that tobacco use in the form of cigarette smoking, cigar smoking, snuff, and chewing are all carcinogenic and should be discontinued.[47,50,92,93] Professional groups agree that physicians should advise their patients to discontinue tobacco use and to use pharmacotherapy as appropriate.[47,50,92,93]

Recommendations of Professional Groups: Poor Diet

Professional groups differ on some of the specifics of diet, but generally recommend that patients limit the intake of high-fat (especially saturated and trans-unsaturated fat) and high-sugar foods and eat a sufficient amount of fruits and vegetables (e.g., five or more servings) and whole grains. There are differences, however, in the specifics. For example, the United States Department of Agriculture's 2000 "Dietary Guidelines for Americans" suggests eating no more than 30% of calories from fat, while the American Heart Association suggests eating between 25% and 35% of calories from fat.[94,95] The American Cancer Society guidelines, released in 2002, are less specific but generally recommend the same above changes as other groups.[96]

Recommendations of Professional Groups: Physical Inactivity

Professional groups generally agree that physical activity is an important part of staying healthy. The American College of Sports Medicine and the Centers for Disease Control released joint recommendations in 1995, suggesting that most Americans could benefit from regular physical activity, defined as at least 30 minutes of moderate or vigorous activity on most, or at least 5, days of the week.[97] These recommendations have not changed in any significant manner since 1995. The 2002 American Cancer Society Guidelines are consistent with these recommendations.[96] The USPSTF also recommends that lower amounts of vigorous activity, 20 minutes for 3 days each week, are acceptable levels of activity.[73,98]

Recommendations of Professional Groups: Alcohol Abuse

Recommendations for alcohol use differ in several ways between organizations, mainly based on the group toward which the recommendations are targeted. No safe level of alcohol intake has been identified, as the epidemiologic studies typically compared high versus low intake, rather than examining a possible threshold effect.[27] Given the data supporting the cardiac benefits of moderate alcohol and the effects of alcohol on blood pressure, the American Heart Association recommends a limit of one drink per day for women and a limit of two drinks per day for men.[99] The American Cancer Society is less specific, noting only "if you drink alcoholic beverages, limit consumption."[96]

Recommendations of Professional Groups: Overweight and Obesity

In the year 2000, the National Heart, Lung and Blood Institute, in partnership with the North American Association for the Study of Obesity, released "The Practical Guide: Identification, Evaluation and Treatment of Overweight and Obesity in Adults."[100] These guidelines defined a healthy body weight, based on the body mass index (BMI) [weight in kilograms/(height in meters)^2] between 18.5 and 25.0.[100] According to these guidelines, individuals are considered to be overweight if the BMI is between 25 and 30 and obese if the BMI is greater than 30.[100] The guidelines contain specific recommendations, including thresholds for considering various weight loss methods, such as caloric restriction, physical activity, medications, and surgery. These BMI recommendations are consistent with those of the American Heart Association,[101] which also recommend that children and adolescents maintain a BMI less than the 85th percentile, according to age-appropriate growth charts. The American Cancer Society guidelines are less specific, suggesting to "maintain a healthful weight throughout life," "balance caloric intake with physical activity," and "lose weight if currently overweight or obese."[96]

Recommendations of Professional Groups: Sun Exposure

The American Cancer Society,[102] the American Academy of Dermatology,[103] the American Academy of Pediatrics,[104] and the American College of Obstetricians and Gynecologists[105] all recommend patient education about sun protection behaviors (SPBs), such as sun avoidance, clothing, hats, and sunscreens. The American Academy of Family Physicians recommends sun protection for all with increased sun exposure.[106] The American College of Preventive Medicine (ACPM) concluded that sun-protective behaviors are probably effective in reducing skin cancer but that the evidence does not support physician counseling about SPBs with every patient.[107] ACPM concluded that evidence does not support advising patients to use chemical sunscreens and that their use may actually increase the risk of malignant melanoma.[108]

Improving the Quality of Physician Counseling for Behavior Modification

Although little direct evidence exists from randomized trials to inform us of the best ways to counsel patients to modify health behaviors, much can still be learned and applied from the available evidence. The way that a doctor communicates with a patient has a strong influence on patient satisfaction and patient adherence. There are several communication patterns in particular that appear to lead to positive outcomes. First, patients whose physicians encourage them to participate actively in their medical treatment decisions have improved health outcomes.[109–112] Second, building rapport, through a discussion of psychosocial issues that help the physician understand the "whole person," is associated with improved patient satisfaction and adherence to physicians' recommendations.[113,114] Third, providers who support motivations that are initiated by patients, also known as being "patient centered," have patients who are more satisfied with their care and who take a more active role in their care and have better outcomes.[110,114,115] Regardless of the interaction, these communication patterns are best to employ whenever possible. This is particularly true of health behavior counseling, which can be stressful for both the doctor and the patient, given patient resistance to change and the overall low likelihood of success of behavior change.

A commonly used framework for organizing brief behavior counseling is the "5 A's"[116,117]: "Address the Agenda," "Assess," "Advise," "Assist," and "Arrange."[47] We try to highlight these five activities and the previously mentioned communication patterns in a case study, adapted and reprinted with permission.[63] This case study is related to diet, but the process (the 5 A's) are the same for changing any health behavior.[47,117–119]

Case

Mrs. R is a 55-year-old woman whom you have seen in your practice for the past 3 years. She has a history of previous cholecystectomy, and had a stage 2 infiltrating ductal carcinoma of the breast treated 2 years ago. She also has high blood cholesterol with the following profile 1 month ago: total cholesterol = 255, LDL = 176, HDL = 48, triglycerides = 155. She has no hypertension, no diabetes, no family history of myocardial infarction, and a BMI of 29. She is returning today to discuss the results of her lipid profile.

1. Address the Agenda:
   Express the desire to talk about the patient's eating habits. For example, "I'd like to talk with you about how you are eating, because it can affect your blood cholesterol, your weight, and may affect the chance that your breast cancer returns." Sometimes, behavior modification discussions can seem as if they come out of nowhere—this helps to get it on the table in a friendly way that makes no assumptions as to the quality of their diet.

2. Assess:
   a. Behavior level

   Before giving nutrition advice, you need to know the patient's current eating pattern. Just because someone has high blood cholesterol or is overweight does not necessarily mean that they eat the wrong foods. It is difficult to accurately assess someone's diet with a question or set of questions. One approach is to ask patients to describe their dietary pattern with a question such as "What do you eat in a typical day?" However, there are several formal written self-assessments that patients can complete in the waiting room that provide more detailed information to help you understand what changes, if any, are needed.[88,120–124] One specific example is "Rate Your Plate," developed by researchers at the Center for Primary Care and Prevention (CPCP) at Memorial Hospital of Rhode Island. This instrument assesses eating patterns by asking about 21 food habits (e.g., intake of meat, milk, sweets, etc.).[88,124] This tool can be used for counseling and goal setting as well as assessment and has accompanying patient education materials.

   Based on your diet assessment, you learn that Mrs. R. eats a diet high in saturated fat (e.g., fatty cuts of red meat several times a week, cheese daily, high-fat snacks and desserts daily), and eats fewer than two servings of vegetables and fewer than two servings of fruits each day. Given the possible link between dietary fat and breast cancer, it seems prudent to counsel Mrs. R about decreasing her dietary fat to lower her risk of breast cancer recurrence. In addition, her cholesterol is high, so there may be more than one behavioral target for dietary counseling. It is important to discuss the results of the diet assessment with her as it will form the basis of much of the behavioral counseling to follow.

   b. Readiness to change
      - "Have you thought about changing your diet at all?"
      - "How much do you want to change your diet right now, on a scale of 1 to 10?"

   An open-ended question such as the first will often lead to an eye-opening discussion about the patient's attitudes toward behavior change, their experience with past behavior change, and their plans for future behavior change. A closed-ended question such as the second can also be useful and can be later followed up by asking "What would make you more ready to change your diet right now?"

   c. History of change efforts
      - "Have you ever tried to cut down on the amount of fat you eat?"
      - "What was that like?"

   Behavior change is a process where repeated trial and error provides the learning necessary to change for good. If you find that, for example, the patient ate lower-fat snacks and desserts for 6 months, you should congratulate them (build their confidence), and ask how they did it and what led to them to change back to higher-fat choices. If, for example, the patient went back to eating more fatty snacks and sweets after the holiday season of eating out at parties and restaurants, this is a great chance to do problem solving and help them overcome a barrier that could impede their progress toward a healthy eating pattern.

   d. Knowledge of risks
      - "What do you know about the link between what you eat and breast cancer?"
      - "I see that your cholesterol is high. What do you know about how your eating habits can affect your cholesterol?"

   Nutrition knowledge varies widely. Data from 1994 showed that 60% of people knew about the dietary fat–heart disease link, although less than 10% knew about the saturated fat–heart disease link.[125] The recent emphasis on dietary fat restriction has covered up the important differences between types of fat, and this is a chance to make those clear. In counseling, every opportunity to personalize the message to the patient should be taken, so including a discussion about cholesterol and weight, two issues specific to Mrs. R, is very useful.

   e. Reasons for changing or maintaining behavior.
      - "What are the positive (negative) things about the way you eat now?"
      - "What are the positive (negative) things about making a change in your eating habits?"

   Understanding the patient's attitudes and motivations are important. Mrs. R may have had a brother who had been diagnosed with heart disease or another incentive for changing her diet that you could not have imagined but is critical to her. Many people are aware that they have unhealthy eating habits but are ambivalent about it. Allowing them to discuss both sides of the issue can help them to convince themselves to change, but it can also uncover barriers to changing (e.g., someone who eats many meals away from home) or opportunities to changing (e.g., has trouble affording cholesterol medications) that may not have been revealed otherwise. Letting the patient discover these issues is much more powerful than preaching them yourself.

3. Advise:
   - "As your doctor, I need you to know that reducing the fat, saturated fat, and calories you eat is important for your health because it will help you decrease your cholesterol, maintain a healthy weight, and may decrease the chance that your breast cancer returns."

   Strong, clear, and personalized advice is best.[47] Personalizing the message plays to the strengths of the clinician who knows the patient and his or her medical history well. Given the frequency of diseases related to diet, most patients in adult practice will have a specific reason for changing their diet.

4. Assist:
   a. Offer to correct misunderstandings and provide new information.
      - "Would you like to talk about food choices that would be better for your health?"

   The above quote may seem too passive for many physicians, but it helps to keep the focus of the counseling on the patient instead of on the physician. Although the word *physician* means teacher, you must first know whether you have a willing pupil in front of you. If the answer is "yes," you may use it as a chance to explain the differences between saturated and unsaturated fats and how replacing high-fat snacks and sweets with lower-fat substitutes or using vegetable oils such as canola or olive oil, or liquid or tub margarine, would be better choices than butter or stick margarine. If they say "no," then this may not be the right time for a detailed discussion. Keeping the door open for future discussions then becomes the goal.

b. Express empathy
   - "It's understandable that you might not want to take steps to change right now."
   - "Changing your diet can be very difficult."

Empathy is one of the most critical skills toward building a strong doctor–patient relationship.[110,114] Some people believe that empathy may give the patient an "easy way out"; that is, if you prepare them for the possibility of failure, they will fail. If Mrs. R tries to change her eating habits, and fails, she may feel uncomfortable the next time she comes to see you or might cancel her appointment altogether. This discomfort is a barrier to the therapeutic doctor–patient relationship. Empathy for the human condition and the difficulty of behavior change is a part of successful behavior counseling.

c. Address barriers to change.
   - "What might make it difficult for you to eat less fat?"
   - "Can you think of ways to overcome your craving for sweets, or choose sweets that may be lower in fat?"

Problem solving is a critical part of behavior change, either done at home or with the doctor in the office. Two important skills in problem solving are to identify two types of barriers to making the change: (1) attitudes that maintain the problem behavior (e.g., "I don't like vegetables") and (2) triggers, that is, situations or feelings that lead to the problem behavior (e.g., "When I go out to dinner, I always eat too much."). After helping to identify the problems, discuss ways that the patient may overcome the barrier. It is not critical that you have all the answers: remember that the patient has many of them. In this capacity, the physician may serve as a "facilitator" rather than a "lecturer." People who have more positive attitudes about dietary change or who feel more confident about dealing with their triggers are more likely to go on to change their behavior and, ultimately, to succeed in making behavior changes.

d. Consider smaller steps toward the ultimate goal
   - "It is difficult to make big changes in how you eat all at once. Can you think of any small changes you can make now?"

This is especially true for people who are not ready to change. For them, simply thinking about the reasons they have for changing would qualify as a step forward, as they are most likely still defending their habits. For someone like Mrs. R, with five separate behaviors to consider for diet counseling alone (meat, cheese, sweets, fruit and vegetable intake, and calorie intake), focusing on more than one behavior may be counterproductive. Encouraging more fruits and vegetables is often a good first step, as this is a positive change rather than a sacrifice. Increases in fruits and vegetables can lead to decreases in other higher-fat foods such as sweets and meats. Be as specific as possible: "How do you think you could eat more fruits and vegetables?" For example, eating a larger portion of vegetables at dinner, adding a fruit at breakfast and for a snack, etc.

e. Make goal(s) clear
   - "Now I'd like us to set a goal for what you will do before you see me again. From what you have told me, you are going to add fruit to your breakfast, eat fruit for a snack, and eat a larger portion of vegetables at dinner. Does that sound like a reasonable goal?" Again, be as specific as possible, so the next time you see the patient, you'll know exactly where to start and won't have to go through a lengthy assessment a second time. You'll be able to say: "When I last saw you, you agreed to work on adding a serving of fruit to your breakfast, eat fruit for a snack, and eat a larger portion of vegetables at dinner. How did that go?" In addition, when the goal is clear, you can give targeted patient information, instead of a generic guide to healthy eating. The patient will be more likely to listen, believing that it is more specific to their situation.

f. Refer interested patients
   - "It seems that you're eating too much saturated fat, which may be the reason why your cholesterol is high. First, I would like to help you try to improve your eating habits, before I consider giving you medications. Medications may have side effects and you may have to take them for the rest of your life. A nutritionist can really help you make changes in your eating habits. Do you think you would be interested in seeing a nutritionist?" For patients who have health problems that can be improved via a dietary change, strong consideration should be given to referral to a qualified dietitian. Given the fact that many patients will not follow through with referrals, asking about their interest in a nonjudgmental way allows you to save time and keep the patient feeling involved in the decision process.

5. Arrange follow-up:

a. Keep the door open for further dialogue.
   - "Is this something you are willing to talk about again at your next visit?" Setting the stage for future discussions is critical to maintaining a therapeutic doctor–patient relationship. Repeated "doses" of behavioral counseling are often necessary over months or years and on a variety of topics aside from nutrition. Thus, neither the patient nor physician should view the counseling session as particularly stressful. This approach also reminds patients that they are an active member of their care team, thereby encouraging autonomy.[115]

b. Schedule follow-up appointment or phone call to further discussion.
   - "Would you be willing to schedule another appointment to talk about how your dietary changes are going and recheck your cholesterol?" Scheduling a return visit will help the patient to understand the importance of making dietary changes and, like a student held accountable for homework, will encourage the patient to follow through on the goals set above.

Providing counseling or advice to your patients takes time, but it is worth the effort in helping your patient to achieve better health as well as improving the doctor–patient relationship. Even if you cannot do everything this chapter suggests, physician advice alone has been shown to be more effective that no intervention at all,[47] and these strategies are likely to improve patient adherence and satisfaction.

References

1. McGinnis JM, Foege WH. Actual causes of death in the United States [see comments]. JAMA 1993;270(18):2207–2212.
2. Mokdad AH, Marks JS, Stroup DF, et al. Actual causes of death in the United States, 2000. JAMA 2004;291(10):1238–1245.
3. Adami HO, Day NE, Trichopoulos P, et al. Primary and secondary prevention in the reduction of cancer morbidity and mortality. Eur J Cancer 2001;37(suppl 8):S118–S127.
4. Tobacco: A Major International Health Hazard. Lyon: International Agency for Research on Cancer, 1986.
5. Ahrens W, Jockel KH, Patzak W, et al. Alcohol, smoking, and occupational factors in cancer of the larynx: a case-control study. Am J Indust Med 1991;20(4):477–493.
6. De Stefani E, Boffetta P, Oreggia F, et al. Smoking patterns and cancer of the oral cavity and pharynx: a case-control study in Uruguay. Oral Oncol 1998;34(5):340–346.
7. Fuchs CS, Colditz GA, Stampfer MJ, et al. A prospective study of cigarette smoking and the risk of pancreatic cancer. Arch Intern Med 1996;156(19):2255–2260.
8. Boyle P, Maisonneuve P, Bueno de Mesquita B, et al. Cigarette smoking and pancreas cancer: a case control study of the search programme of the IARC. Int J Cancer 1996;67(1):63–71.
9. Chiu BC, Lynch CF, Cerhan JR, et al. Cigarette smoking and risk of bladder, pancreas, kidney, and colorectal cancers in Iowa. Ann Epidemiol 2001;11(1):28–37.
10. Doll R, Peto R. The causes of cancer: quantitative estimates of avoidable risks of cancer in the United States today. J Natl Cancer Inst 1981;66(6):1191–1308.
11. Gower JD. A role for dietary lipids and antioxidants in the activation of carcinogens. Free Radic Biol Med 1988;5(2):95–111.
12. Missmer SA, Smith-Warner SA, Spiegelman D, et al. Meat and dairy food consumption and breast cancer: a pooled analysis of cohort studies. Int J Epidemiol 2002;31(1):78–85.
13. Schatzkin A, Lanza E, Corle D, et al. Lack of effect of a low-fat, high-fiber diet on the recurrence of colorectal adenomas. Polyp Prevention Trial Study Group. N Engl J Med 2000;342(16): 1149–1155.
14. Food, Nutrition, and the Prevention of Cancer: A Global Perspective. Washington, DC: American Institute for Cancer Research, 1997.
15. Palli D. Epidemiology of gastric cancer: an evaluation of available evidence. J Gastroenterology 2000;35(suppl 12):84–89.
16. Investigators E. Fruit and vegetables and colorectal cancer. In: Proceedings of the European Conference in Nutrition and Cancer. Lyons: IARC, 2003.
17. Fuchs CS, Giovannucci EL, Colditz GA, et al. Dietary fiber and the risk of colorectal cancer and adenoma in women. N Engl J Med 1999;340(3):169–176.
18. Michels KB, Giovannucci E, Joshipura KJ, et al. Prospective study of fruit and vegetable consumption and incidence of colon and rectal cancers. J Natl Cancer Inst 2000;92(21):1740–1752.
19. Ruano-Ravina A, Figueiras A, Barros-Dios JM. Diet and lung cancer: a new approach. Eur J Cancer Prev 2000;9(6):395–400.
20. Alberts DS, Martinez ME, Roe DJ, et al. Lack of effect of a high-fiber cereal supplement on the recurrence of colorectal adenomas. Phoenix Colon Cancer Prevention Physicians' Network. N Engl J Med 2000;342(16):1156–1162.
21. Bonithon-Kopp C, Kronborg O, Giacosa A, et al. Calcium and fibre supplementation in prevention of colorectal adenoma recurrence: a randomised intervention trial. European Cancer Prevention Organisation Study Group. Lancet 2000;356(9238): 1300–1306.
22. Omenn GS, Goodman GE, Thornquist MD, et al. Effects of a combination of beta carotene and vitamin A on lung cancer and cardiovascular disease. N Engl J Med 1996;334(18):1150–1155.
23. Pierce JP, Faerber S, Wright FA, et al. A randomized trial of the effect of a plant-based dietary pattern on additional breast cancer events and survival: the Women's Healthy Eating and Living (WHEL) Study. Control Clin Trials 2002;23(6):728–756.
24. Brown DW, Brown DR, Heath GW, et al. Associations between recommended levels of physical activity and health-related quality of life. Findings from the 2001 Behavioral Risk Factor Surveillance System (BRFSS) survey. Prev Med 2003;37(5): 520–528.
25. Friedenreich CM, Courneya KS, Bryant HE. Influence of physical activity in different age and life periods on the risk of breast cancer. Epidemiology 2001;12(6):604–612.
26. Foster SE, Vaughn RD, Foster WH, et al. Alcohol consumption and expenditures for underage drinking and adult excessive drinking. JAMA 2003;289(8):989–995.
27. Singletary KW, Gapstur SM. Alcohol and breast cancer: review of epidemiologic and experimental evidence and potential mechanisms. JAMA 2001;286(17):2143–2151.
28. Chhabra SK, Souliotis VL, Kyrtopoulos SA, et al. Nitrosamines, alcohol, and gastrointestinal tract cancer: recent epidemiology and experimentation. In Vivo 1996;10(3):265–284.
29. Longnecker MP, Paganini-Hill A, Ross RK. Lifetime alcohol consumption and breast cancer risk among postmenopausal women in Los Angeles. Cancer Epidemiol Biomarkers Prev 1995;4(7):721–725.
30. Harnack LJ, Anderson KE, Zheng W, et al. Smoking, alcohol, coffee, and tea intake and incidence of cancer of the exocrine pancreas: the Iowa Women's Health Study. Cancer Epidemiol Biomarkers Prev 1997;6(12):1081–1086.
31. Makimoto K, Higuchi S. Alcohol consumption as a major risk factor for the rise in liver cancer mortality rates in Japanese men. Int J Epidemiol 1999;28(1):30–34.
32. Altieri A, Bosetti C, Talamini R, et al. Cessation of smoking and drinking and the risk of laryngeal cancer. Br J Cancer 2002; 87(11):1227–1229.
33. Bosetti C, et al. Smoking and drinking cessation and the risk of oesophageal cancer. Br J Cancer 2000;83(5):689–691.
34. Ahluwalia IB, et al. State-specific prevalence of selected chronic disease-related characteristics: Behavioral Risk Factor Surveillance System, 2001. MMWR Surveill Summ 2003;52(8):1–80.
35. Ballard-Barbash R, Swanson CA. Body weight: estimation of risk for breast and endometrial cancers. Am J Clin Nutr 1996; 63(suppl 3):437S–441S.
36. Vainio H, Kaaks R, Bianchini F. Weight control and physical activity in cancer prevention: international evaluation of the evidence. Eur J Cancer Prev 2002;11(suppl 2):S94–S100.
37. Huang Z, et al. Dual effects of weight and weight gain on breast cancer risk. JAMA 1997;278(17):1407–1411.
38. Harmful effects of ultraviolet radiation. Council on Scientific Affairs. JAMA 1989;262(3):380–384.
39. Koh HK. Cutaneous melanoma [see comments]. N Engl J Med 1991;325(3):171–182.
40. Preston DS, Stern RS. Nonmelanoma cancers of the skin [see comments]. N Engl J Med 1992;327(23):1649–1662.
41. Rigel DS. The effect of sunscreen on melanoma risk. Dermatol Clin 2002;20(4):601–606.
42. Bastuji-Garin S, Diepgen TL. Cutaneous malignant melanoma, sun exposure, and sunscreen use: epidemiological evidence. Br J Dermatol 2002;146(suppl 61):24–30.
43. Green A, et al. Daily sunscreen application and beta carotene supplementation in prevention of basal-cell and squamous-cell carcinomas of the skin: a randomised controlled trial. Lancet 1999;354(9180):723–729.

44. Staples M, Marks R, Giles G. Trends in the incidence of non-melanocytic skin cancer (NMSC) treated in Australia 1985–1995: are primary prevention programs starting to have an effect? Int J Cancer 1998;78(2):144–148.
45. Thompson SC, Jolley D, Marks R. Reduction of solar keratoses by regular sunscreen use. N Engl J Med 1993;329(16):1147–1151.
46. Naylor MF, et al. High sun protection factor sunscreens in the suppression of actinic neoplasia. Arch Dermatol 1995;131(2): 170–175.
47. Fiore M, et al. Treating Tobacco Use and Dependence. Clinical Practice Guideline. Washington, DC: Public Health Service, U.S. Department of Health and Human Services, 2000.
48. Cummings SR, et al. Training physicians in counseling about smoking cessation. A randomized trial of the "Quit for Life" program. Ann Intern Med 1989;110(8):640–647.
49. Strecher VJ, et al. Can residents be trained to counsel patients about quitting smoking? Results from a randomized trial [see comments]. J Gen Intern Med 1991;6(1):9–17.
50. Fiore MC, Bailey WC, Cohen SJ. Smoking Cessation. Clinical Practice Guideline No. 18. AHCPR Publication No. 96-0692. Washington, DC: U.S. Department of Health and Human Services, Public Health Service, Agency for Health Care Policy and Research, 1996.
51. Ahluwalia JS, et al. Smoking status as a vital sign. J Gen Intern Med 1999;14(7):402–408.
52. Jamrozik K, et al. Controlled trial of three different antismoking interventions in general practice. Br Med J Clin Res Ed 1984; 288(6429):1499–1503.
53. Richmond RL, Webster IW. A smoking cessation programme for use in general practice. Med J Aust 1985;142(3):190–194.
54. Risser NL, Belcher DW. Adding spirometry, carbon monoxide, and pulmonary symptom results to smoking cessation counseling: a randomized trial. J Gen Intern Med 1990;5(1):16–22.
55. Delichatsios HK, et al. EatSmart: efficacy of a multifaceted preventive nutrition intervention in clinical practice. Prev Med 2001;33(2 pt 1):91–98.
56. Beresford SA, et al. A dietary intervention in primary care practice: the Eating Patterns Study [see comments]. Am J Public Health 1997;87(4):610–616.
57. Calfas KJ, et al. Preliminary evaluation of a multicomponent program for nutrition and physical activity change in primary care: PACE+ for adults. Prev Med 2002;34(2):153–161.
58. Ockene IS, et al. Effect of training and a structured office practice on physician-delivered nutrition counseling: the Worcester-Area Trial for Counseling in Hyperlipidemia (WATCH). Am J Prev Med 1996;12(4):252–258.
59. Caggiula AW, et al. Cholesterol-lowering intervention program. Effect of the step I diet in community office practices. Arch Intern Med 1996;156(11):1205–1213.
60. Flynn MM, Sciamanna CN, Vigilante KC. Inadequate physician knowledge of the effects of diet on blood lipids and lipoproteins. Nutr J 2003;2(1):19.
61. National Nutrition Monitoring and Related Research Act of 1990, Public Law 101-445. 1990. Washington, DC: U.S. Congress.
62. Position of the American Dietetic Association: nutrition—an essential of medical education. J Am Diet Assoc 1994;94(5): 555–557.
63. Sciamanna C, Gans K, Goldstein M. Physician-delivered nutrition counseling: why and how? Med Health Rhode Island 2000; 83(11):351–355.
64. Reid R, et al. Dietary counselling for dyslipidemia in primary care: results of a randomized trial. Can J Diet Pract Res 2002; 63(4):169–175.
65. Ockene IS, et al. Effect of physician-delivered nutrition counseling training and an office-support program on saturated fat intake, weight, and serum lipid measurements in a hyperlipidemic population: Worcester Area Trial for Counseling in Hyperlipidemia (WATCH). Arch Intern Med 1999;159(7): 725–731.
66. Steptoe A, et al. The impact of behavioral counseling on stage of change in fat intake, physical activity, and cigarette smoking in adults at increased risk of coronary heart disease. Am J Public Health 2001;91(2):265–269.
67. Evans AT, et al. Teaching dietary counseling skills to residents: patient and physician outcomes. The CADRE Study Group. Am J Prev Med 1996;12(4):259–265.
68. Petrella RJ, Lattanzio CN. Does counseling help patients get active? Systematic review of the literature. Can Fam Physician 2002;48:72–80.
69. Bull FC, Jamrozik K. Advice on exercise from a family physician can help sedentary patients to become active. Am J Prev Med 1998;15(2):85–94.
70. Calfas KJ, et al. A controlled trial of physician counseling to promote the adoption of physical activity. Prev Med 1996; 25(3):225–233.
71. Norris SL, et al. Effectiveness of physician-based assessment and counseling for exercise in a staff model HMO. Prev Med 2000;30(6):513–523.
72. Goldstein MG, et al. Physician-based physical activity counseling for middle-aged and older adults: a randomized trial. Ann Behav Med 1999;21(1):40–47.
73. Berg AO. U.S. Preventive Services Task Force. Behavioral counseling in primary care to promote physical activity: recommendation and rationale. Am J Nurs 2003;103(4):101–107; discussion 109.
74. Wallace P, Cutler S, Haines A. Randomised controlled trial of general practitioner intervention in patients with excessive alcohol consumption. Br Med J 1988;297(6649): 663–668.
75. Fleming MF, et al. Brief physician advice for problem alcohol drinkers. A randomized controlled trial in community-based primary care practices. JAMA 1997;277(13):1039–1045.
76. Adams A, et al. Alcohol counseling: physicians will do it. J Gen Intern Med 1998;13(10):692–698.
77. Ockene JK, et al. Provider training for patient-centered alcohol counseling in a primary care setting. Arch Intern Med 1997; 157(20):2334–2341.
78. Fiellin DA, Reid MC, O'Connor PG. New therapies for alcohol problems: application to primary care. Am J Med 2000;108(3): 227–237.
79. Bien TH, Miller WR, Tonigan JS. Brief interventions for alcohol problems: a review. Addiction 1993;88(3):315–335.
80. Wilk AI, Jensen NM, Havighurst TC. Meta-analysis of randomized control trials addressing brief interventions in heavy alcohol drinkers. J Gen Intern Med 1997;12(5):274–283.
81. Ashley JM, et al. Weight control in the physician's office. Arch Intern Med 2001;161(13):1599–1604.
82. Bowerman S, et al. Implementation of a primary care physician network obesity management program. Obes Res 2001;9(suppl 4):321S–325S.
83. Stamps PL, Catino DC, Feola AC. Treatment of obesity in three rural primary care practices. J Fam Pract 1983;17(4): 629–634.
84. Molokhia M. Obesity wars: a pilot study of very low calorie diets in obese patients in general practice. Br J Gen Pract 1998; 48(430):1251–1252.
85. Lanza E, et al. Implementation of a 4-y, high-fiber, high-fruit-and-vegetable, low-fat dietary intervention: results of dietary changes in the Polyp Prevention Trial. Am J Clin Nutr 2001; 74(3):387–401.
86. Olivarius NF, et al. Randomised controlled trial of structured personal care of type 2 diabetes mellitus. Br Med J 2001; 323(7319):970–975.
87. Simkin-Silverman LR, Wing RR. Management of obesity in primary care. Obesity Res 1997;5(6):603–612.

88. Gans KM, et al. REAP and WAVE: new tools to rapidly assess/discuss nutrition with patients. J Nutr 2003;133(2): 556S–562S.
89. Dietrich AJ, et al. Sun protection counseling for children: primary care practice patterns and effect of an intervention on clinicians. Arch Fam Med 2000;9(2):155–159.
90. Dietrich AJ, et al. Persistent increase in children's sun protection in a randomized controlled community trial. Prev Med 2000;31(5):569–574.
91. Counseling to prevent skin cancer: recommendations and rationale of the U.S. Preventive Services Task Force. MMWR Recomm Rep 2003;52(RR-15):13–17.
92. The State of Health Care Quality 2003: Industry Trends and Analysis. Washington, DC: National Committee for Quality Assurance, 2003:1–61.
93. U.S. Preventive Services Task Force. Guide to Clinical Preventive Services, 2nd ed. Alexandria, VA: International Medical, 1996.
94. Pearson TA, et al. AHA Guidelines for Primary Prevention of Cardiovascular Disease and Stroke: 2002 Update: Consensus Panel Guide to Comprehensive Risk Reduction for Adult Patients Without Coronary or Other Atherosclerotic Vascular Diseases. American Heart Association Science Advisory and Coordinating Committee. Circulation 2002;106(3):388–391.
95. Dietary Guidelines for Americans, 2000. Washington, DC: United States Department of Agriculture, 2000:1–44.
96. Byers T, et al. American Cancer Society guidelines on nutrition and physical activity for cancer prevention: reducing the risk of cancer with healthy food choices and physical activity. CA Cancer J Clin 2002;52(2):92–119.
97. Pate RR, et al. Physical activity and public health. A recommendation from the Centers for Disease Control and Prevention and the American College of Sports Medicine [see comments]. JAMA 1995;273(5):402–407.
98. Increasing physical activity. A report on recommendations of the Task Force on Community Preventive Services. MMWR Recomm Rep 2001;50(RR-18):1–14.
99. Goldberg IJ, et al. AHA Science Advisory: Wine and your heart: a science advisory for healthcare professionals from the Nutrition Committee, Council on Epidemiology and Prevention, and Council on Cardiovascular Nursing of the American Heart Association. Circulation 2001;103(3):472–475.
100. Clinical Guidelines on the Identification, Evaluation and Treatment of Overweight and Obesity in Adults. Bethesda, MD: National Heart, Lung, and Blood Institute, 2000.
101. Kavey RE, et al. American Heart Association guidelines for primary prevention of atherosclerotic cardiovascular disease beginning in childhood. J Pediatr 2003;142(4):368–372.
102. Cancer Prevention & Early Detection: Facts & Figures 2003. Washington, DC: American Cancer Society, 2003.
103. Lim HW, Cooper K. The health impact of solar radiation and prevention strategies: report of the Environment Council, American Academy of Dermatology. J Am Acad Dermatol 1999;41(1):81–99.
104. Ultraviolet light: a hazard to children. American Academy of Pediatrics. Committee on Environmental Health. Pediatrics 1999;104(2 pt 1):328–333.
105. Primary and preventive care: periodic assessments. ACOG Committee on Primary Care. Int J Gynaecol Obstet 2000;70(3): 393–399.
106. "Safe-Sun" Guidelines. Washington, DC: American Academy of Family Physicians, 2000.
107. Ferrini RL, Perlman M, Hill L. American College of Preventive Medicine practice policy statement: skin protection from ultraviolet light exposure. The American College of Preventive Medicine. Am J Prev Med 1998;14(1):83–86.
108. Ferrini RL, Perlman M, Hill L. Skin protection from ultraviolet light exposure: American College of Preventive Medicine Practice Policy Statement. Am J Prev Med 1998;14(1):83–86.
109. Greenfield S, Kaplan S, Ware JE Jr. Expanding patient involvement in care. Effects on patient outcomes. Ann Intern Med 1985;102(4):520–528.
110. Kaplan SH, Greenfield S, Ware JE Jr. Assessing the effects of physician-patient interactions on the outcomes of chronic disease. Med Care 1989;27(suppl 3):S110–S127.
111. Rost K, Flavin M, Cole K. Change in metabolic control and functional status after hospitalization: impact of patient activation intervention in diabetic patients. Diabetes Care 1991;14: 881.
112. Bertakis KD, et al. Physician practice styles and patient outcomes: differences between family practice and general internal medicine. Med Care 1998;36(6):879–891.
113. Safran DG, et al. Linking primary care performance to outcomes of care. J Fam Pract 1998;47(3):213–220.
114. Paasche-Orlow M, Roter D. The communication patterns of internal medicine and family practice physicians. J Am Board Fam Pract 2003;16(6):485–493.
115. Williams GC, Freedman ZR, Deci EL. Supporting autonomy to motivate patients with diabetes for glucose control. Diabetes Care 1998;21(10):1644–1651.
116. Glynn TJ, Manley MW. How to Help Your Patients Stop Smoking. Bethesda, MD: National Institutes of Health, National Cancer Institute, 1997.
117. Goldstein MG, et al. Models for provider-patient interaction: applications to health behavior change. In: Shumaker SA, et al (eds). The Handbook of Health Behavior Change. New York: Springer, 1998:85–113.
118. Pinto BM, Goldstein MG. Physician-delivered physical activity counseling. Med Health Rhode Island 1997;80(9): 303–304.
119. Sciamanna CN, et al. Nutrition counseling in the promoting cancer prevention in primary care study. Prev Med 2002; 35(5):437–446.
120. Retzlaff BM, et al. The Northwest Lipid Research Clinic Fat Intake Scale: validation and utility [see comments]. Am J Public Health 1997;87(2):181–185.
121. Kris-Etherton P, et al. Validation for MEDFICTS, a dietary assessment instrument for evaluating adherence to total and saturated fat recommendations of the National Cholesterol Education Program Step 1 and Step 2 diets. J Am Diet Assoc 2001;101(1):81–86.
122. Subar AF, et al. Fruit and vegetable intake in the United States: the baseline survey of the Five A Day for Better Health Program. Am J Health Promot 1995;9(5):352–360.
123. Thompson FE, et al. Evaluation of 2 brief instruments and a food-frequency questionnaire to estimate daily number of servings of fruit and vegetables. Am J Clin Nutr 2000;71(6): 1503–1510.
124. Gans KM, et al. Rate Your Plate: An eating pattern assessment and educational tool used at cholesterol screening and education programs. J Nutr Educ 1993;25:29–36.
125. Fogel RW. Continuing Survey of Food Intakes: Diet and Knowledge Health Survey Questionnaire. Rockville, MD: United States Department of Agriculture, 1996.

SECTION FOUR

Cancer Imaging

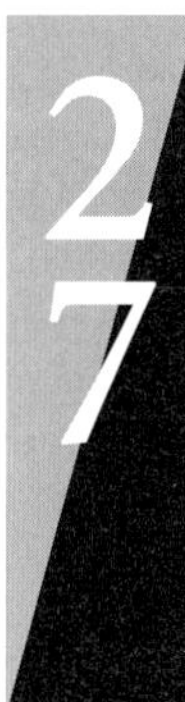

Central Nervous System Imaging

Dima A. Hammoud and Martin G. Pomper

Brain tumor imaging has four main goals, namely, evaluating lesion extent, estimating tumor grade, identifying associated complications, and defining a comprehensive differential diagnosis. It assesses the relationship of the lesion to various brain structures and identifies associated findings, such as increased intracranial pressure, impending herniation, hydrocephalus, hemorrhagic transformation, and mass effect. A comprehensive differential diagnosis is usually established based on the patient's age, tumor location, and specific imaging findings.

Cross-sectional imaging with computed tomography (CT) or magnetic resonance imaging (MRI) is necessary for accurate brain tumor characterization. Plain film imaging has virtually no role. Before the advent of CT scan and MRI, imaging techniques, such as pneumoencephalography and plain film X-rays of the skull, were the only options for neurosurgeons in the preoperative evaluation of brain tumors. Cross-sectional imaging has significantly facilitated the task of preoperative evaluation and planning of brain tumor surgery.

Computed Tomography

Since its introduction in the 1970s, CT has enjoyed wide application within all the radiologic subspecialties. In fact, CT has effectively replaced conventional tomography and many other radiologic procedures (e.g., lymphangiography and pneumoencephalography). CT has undergone major changes in the past few years, with incremental improvements in hardware and software technologies, including refinement of spiral CT systems, overcoming limitations. In a typical modern spiral or "helical" CT scan, instead of obtaining data using sequential single exposures by moving the gantry, the patient is moved through a rotating, continuous fan-beam exposure, and a block of data in the form of a corkscrew or helix is obtained.[1] Improvements, such as the introduction of higher heat capacity X-ray tubes, subsecond X-ray tube rotation times, detector technologies, and real-time image reconstruction computer hardware and software, transformed CT scan into a very fast, large-volume, multi-beam acquisition technology.

CT, however, currently plays a limited role in brain tumor imaging. Its availability in the emergency department makes it the first-line technique for evaluating patients presenting with signs and symptoms of increased intracranial pressure, seizures, and other neurologic symptoms that could be caused intracranial neoplasms. Inevitably, if a tumor is discovered on CT, the patient will need further imaging, usually with contrast-enhanced MRI for adequate evaluation. Patients with contraindications to MRI, such as severe claustrophobia, a pacemaker, or severe obesity may have to undergo a contrast-enhanced CT scan instead of MRI.

One of the advantages of CT is its ability to depict hemorrhagic and calcific findings, which could narrow the differential diagnosis of a detected lesion in certain cases (Figure 27.1). It also provides information about bony lesions, such as metastatic disease to the skull and hyperostotic changes associated with meningiomas. Detailed anatomy of the base of the skull, provided by CT imaging, can provide precious information in specific cases, such as intracranial extension of nasopharyngeal tumors and metastatic disease. Currently, CT is not routinely used in the evaluation of patients with brain tumors either pre- or postoperatively, with few exceptions.

Magnetic Resonance Imaging

Magnetic resonance imaging has become the mainstay of diagnosis in the evaluation of primary and metastatic brain tumors. Unfortunately, MRI is very sensitive but not very specific. Although it provides excellent anatomic detail, MRI remains incapable of accurately grading tumors. Extension of T_2 signal abnormalities, involvement of the corpus callosum, enhancement pattern, cortical involvement, intra- versus extraaxial localization, mass effect, and the age of the patient are some of the factors that allow the radiologist to narrow the differential diagnosis of a brain lesion.

New techniques are constantly being developed to increase the specificity of MRI. Among the most promising of those new techniques are fast fluid-attenuated inversion recovery (FLAIR) imaging, diffusion-weighted imaging (DWI), perfusion imaging, and magnetic resonance spectroscopy (MRS). Functional MRI (fMRI), diffusion tensor imaging, magnetization transfer (MT) imaging, and perfusion imaging with arterial spin labeling are applied clinically only infrequently.

Fast Fluid-Attenuated Inversion Recovery (FLAIR) Imaging

FLAIR is an MRI sequence that produces heavily T_2-weighted images with cerebrospinal fluid (CSF) signal suppression by employing a specific inversion pulse placed at the CSF null point.[2] Suppression of the CSF signal leads to better lesion-to-CSF contrast, allowing better delineation of masses adja-

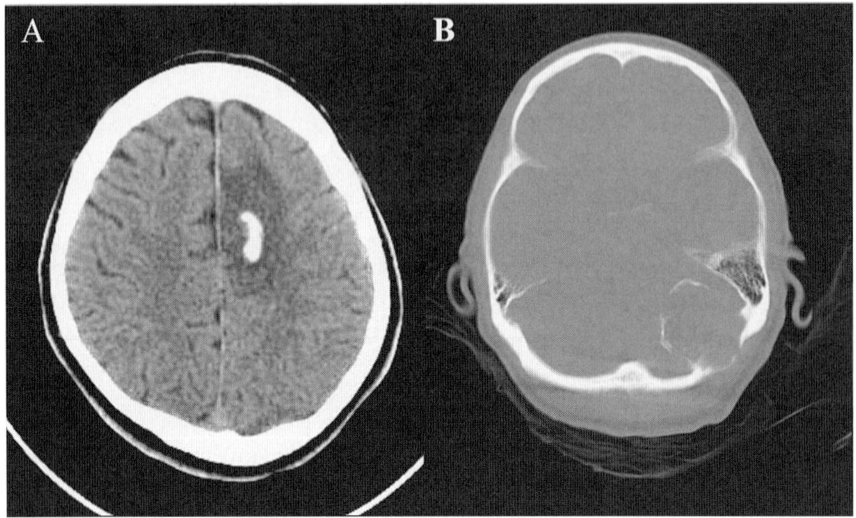

FIGURE 27.1. (A) Oligodendroglioma: nonenhanced computed tomography (CT) scan showing left frontal hypodense mass with calcifications. (B) Intradiploic epidermoid cyst: nonenhanced CT scan showing bony erosion and expansion.

cent to ventricles and sulci (Figure 27.2); however, that is true only for relatively large lesions, as small tumors may be lost among the periventricular gliosis that appears bright on FLAIR.[3] Based on multiple studies, FLAIR was found to be superior to both proton density (PD)- and T_2-weighted images in delineating intraparenchymal lesions. In a large prospective, blinded analysis, Maubon et al. evaluated 102 patients with a multitude of neurologic presentations, including brain tumors, using turbo spin echo (TSE), turbo FLAIR, and gradient and SE (GRASE) images. They found that FLAIR was significantly superior to both GRASE and turbo SE for white matter disease (P less than 0.05), superior only to TSE (P less than 0.05) for vascular disease, but not superior to either gradient SE or TSE for tumors.[4] Multiple descriptive studies with smaller numbers of patients showed more encouraging results: increased sensitivity of detection and better conspicuity of lesions using FLAIR sequences compared to T_2-weighted images,[5] better appreciation of peritumoral edema, and better definition between edema and tumor than T_2-weighted and proton density-weighted images.[6] In a retrospective analysis including only 18 patients, Bynevelt et al. found FLAIR to be superior for appreciation of the lesion (91% of studies) and for demonstration of its margin (92%) and suggested that FLAIR can replace PD- and T_2-weighted spin-echo imaging in radiologic follow-up of low-grade glioma.[7] All three studies, however, relied on the subjective evaluation of the quality of images by different readers.

FLAIR imaging has also been used in the differentiation of intracranial epidermoid from other pathologies, related mostly to the incomplete signal suppression due to the presence of keratin and cholesterol crystals in epidermoids (Figure 27.3B). In a series of eight patients with a surgically confirmed diagnosis of epidermoid, Chen et al. compared conventional MR sequences with fast fluid-attenuated inversion recovery (fast-FLAIR) and echo-planar diffusion-weighted (DW) MR imaging. On fast-FLAIR imaging, the mean signal intensity of epidermoid tumors was significantly higher than that of CSF but significantly lower than that of the brain. The authors concluded that fast-FLAIR imaging is superior to conventional MR imaging in depicting intracranial epidermoid

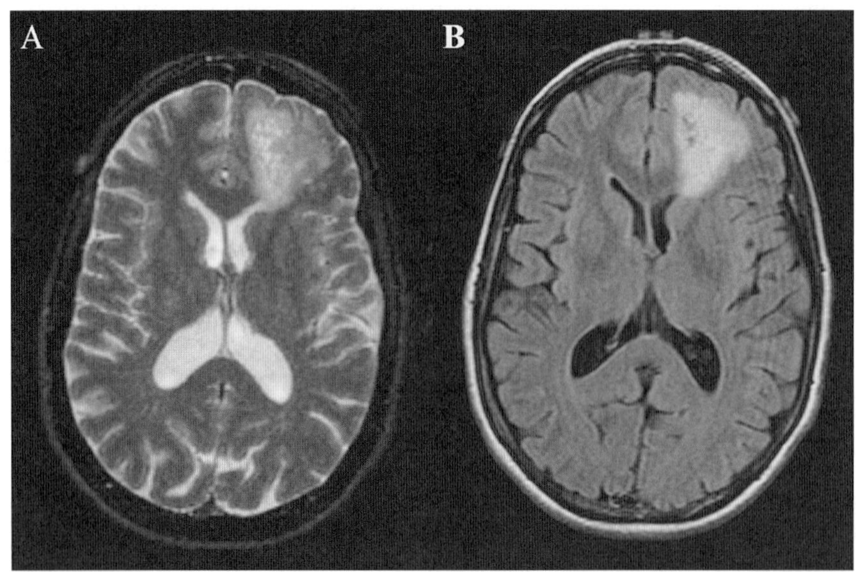

FIGURE 27.2. (A) T_2-weighted and (B) fast fluid-attenuated inversion recovery (FLAIR) image of left frontal lobe anaplastic astrocytoma. FLAIR delineates the tumor border more clearly as a result of inherent cerebrospinal fluid (CSF) signal suppression.

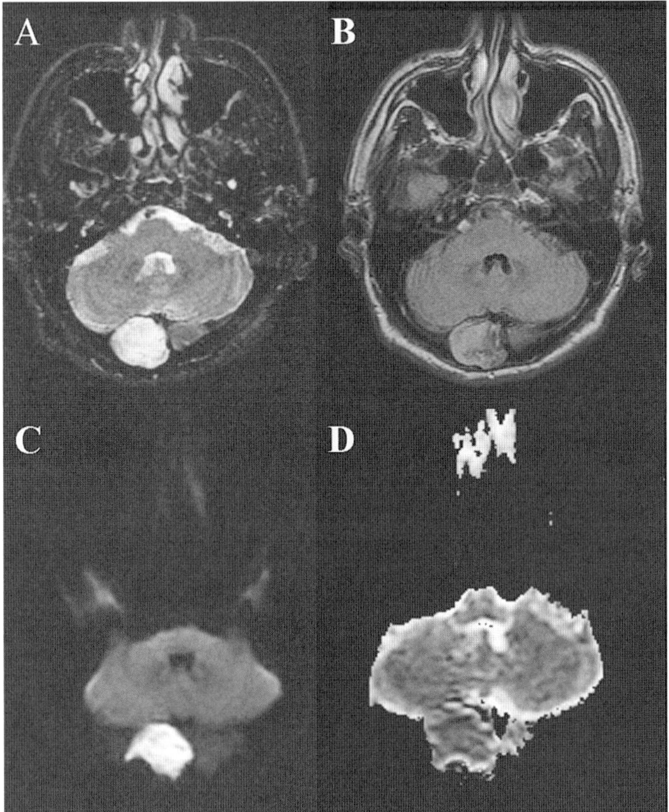

FIGURE 27.3. (A) T_2-weighted images, (B) FLAIR images, (C) diffusion-weighted image (DWI), and (D) apparent diffusion coefficient (ADC) maps of posterior fossa epidermoid cyst eroding the bone. Note incomplete suppression of signal on FLAIR images and restricted diffusion on DWI and corresponding ADC maps.

cysts.[8] Similar results confirming the superiority of FLAIR to other sequences in the evaluation of epidermoid cysts were reached by Ikushima et al.[9]

A recent application of FLAIR imaging is the evaluation of leptomeningeal spread of tumors, whether primary or metastatic. High signal intensity in the sulci and fissures is suggestive of tumor involvement (Figure 27.4A). In one study evaluating 70 patients with cytologically proven leptomeningeal metastases, FLAIR imaging was found to have a sensitivity of only 34% for disease detection, compared to 66% for gadolinium-enhanced MR[10] (Figure 27.4B). So, although FLAIR can help support the diagnosis, it alone cannot be used for the exclusion of leptomeningeal metastases, and contrast-enhanced T_1-weighted imaging remains essential for that diagnosis. Contrast-enhanced FLAIR imaging, on the other hand, can improve detection of leptomeningeal disease in pediatric patients when compared to routine contrast-enhanced T_1-weighted imaging, partly because of suppression of signal intensity from normal vascular structures on the surface of the brain, allowing easier visualization of abnormal leptomeninges.[11] That study, however, was limited by the small number of patients with a history of medulloblastoma ($n = 6$).

The lack of definite proof of the usefulness of enhanced FLAIR images has hampered the routine implementation of this sequence in the clinical evaluation of brain tumor patients.

Diffusion-Weighted Imaging

Diffusion-weighted imaging (DWI) relies on the detection of the Brownian motion of water molecules between the intracellular and extracellular spaces in the brain. Such motion through tissue is a random event, the speed and direction of which is dictated by the presence of barriers such as macromolecules, cell membranes, and cellular organelles. Contrast is generated on DWI through background suppression and changes in signal intensity between images obtained at different gradient strengths (b values) that are sensitive to diffusion. Apparent diffusion coefficient (ADC) maps are then generated as the slopes of the lines derived from plotting the natural log of the signal intensity (SI) versus gradient strength. These apparent diffusion coefficient maps are essential for the visual evaluation of diffusion because the signal intensity (SI) of DWI is prone to T_2 shine-through effects from heavy T_2 weighting. ADC maps are independent of T_1 and T_2 effects, with decreased ADC values indicative of decreased diffusion.[3]

DWI has been evaluated for its potential in the differentiation of necrotic brain tumors from abscesses, of infiltrat-

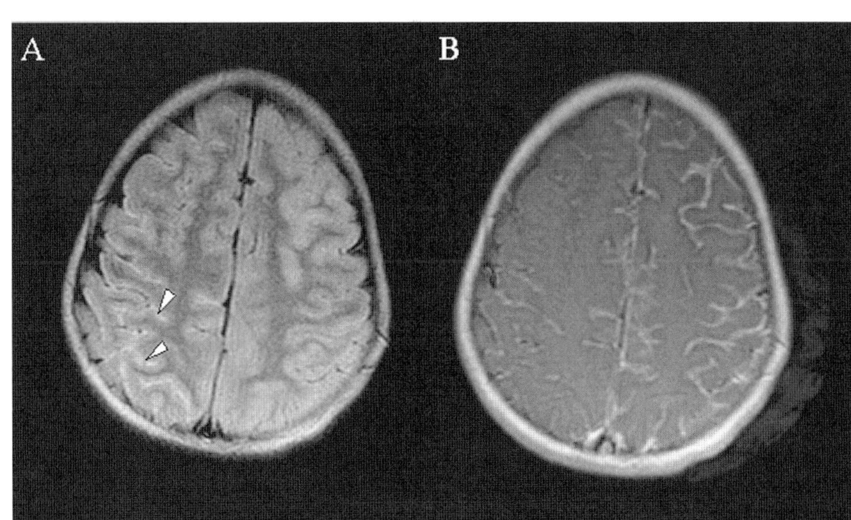

FIGURE 27.4. 10 year-old patient with leukemic meningeal infiltration. (A) FLAIR shows increased signal in the sulci at the brain convexity, more on the right side (*arrowheads*). (B) Corresponding enhanced T_1-weighted images show marked meningeal enhancement compatible with the diagnosis of diffuse leukemic involvement.

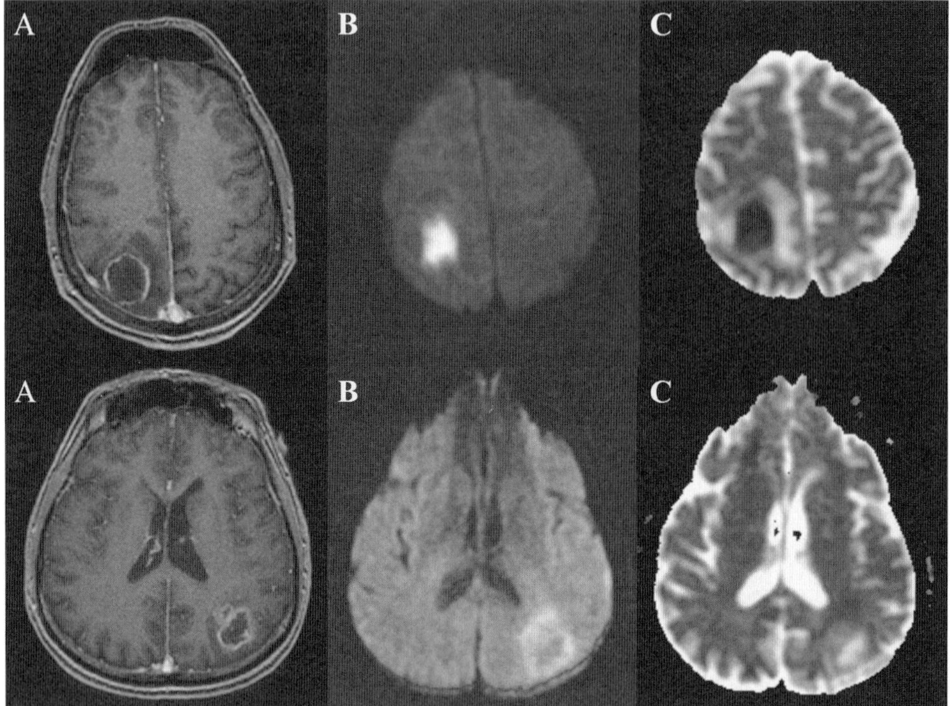

FIGURE 27.5. Enhanced T_1-weighted images, DWI images, and ADC maps of (A) right parietal abscess and (B) left parietoocipital glioblastoma multiforme (GBM). Note restricted diffusion in the abscess cavity (increased signal on DWI and decreased signal on ADC maps) in A compared to nonrestricted diffusion of the necrotic tumor (decreased signal on DWI and increased signal on ADC maps) in B.

ing tumor from vasogenic edema, and in tumor grading. Resembling free water, necrotic or cystic portions of tumors display high ADCs whereas abscess cavities, consisting of necrotic debris, neutrophils, and bacteria, which impede free water diffusion, tend to have low ADCs[12] (Figure 27.5). However, although Dorenbeck et al. found overlapping ADC values between tumors and abscesses,[13] multiple other studies demonstrated the opposite. In a case-control designed study, Guzman et al. found that the ADC values in patients with brain abscesses were significantly lower than those in patients with neoplastic lesions (P less than 0.05).[14] Similar confirmatory results were reached by other investigators.[15–17]

Besides the differences seen within the cystic/necrotic portions, Chan et al. found that the tumor wall of cystic or necrotic brain tumors had significantly lower ADCs relative to those of the abscess wall (P less than 0.005).[18]

In a more quantitative study in which the authors calculated ADC values based on eight gradient (b) values, the specificity of DWI in differentiating tumor from abscess was 100% using a threshold ADC value of $1.10 \times 10^{-3}\,mm^2/s$. Unfortunately, those results cannot currently be applied clinically because most available commercial systems calculate ADC based on two b values only.[19]

Another application of DWI is the differentiation of epidermoid tumors from arachnoid cysts, a classic diagnostic problem on conventional MRI sequences. Because cysts contain more free water than solid masses, they tend to have more restricted diffusion and higher ADC values (see Figure 27.3C,D), which proved to be the case for arachnoid cyst versus epidermoid, as proven in two preliminary studies.[20,21] DWI was found to provide the best lesion conspicuity of epidermoid in comparison to FLAIR and conventional sequences.[8] By implementing both FLAIR (see foregoing) and DWI, epidermoid and arachnoid cysts can be fairly easily differentiated without cisternography, the previous clinical standard, in the majority of cases.[3]

The ability of DWI to differentiate between high- and low-grade tumors has been evaluated by several groups. Sugahara et al. found that the cellularity of a variety of histologically verified gliomas correlated well with the minimum calculated ADC value of these tumors ($P = 0.007$) but not with the signal intensity on T_2-weighted images.[22] They hypothesized that the highly cellular (higher-grade) gliomas would have smaller intercellular space than tumors of lower cellularity and consequently would display lower ADCs; this is similar to the case for lymphoma and medulloblastoma, both being highly cellular CNS tumors and known to display low ADC values.[23] Further support for the utility of DWI in tumor grading comes from the work of Bulakbasi et al., who evaluated 49 patients with malignant tumors. They found that ADCs were effective for grading malignant tumors (P less than 0.001) but not for distinguishing different tumor types with the same grade. In this study, high-grade malignant tumors had significantly lower ADC values than did low-grade malignant and benign tumors.[24] Two more studies further supported the previous results, showing that ADC values are significantly higher in low-grade than in high-grade tumors.[25,26] As far as tumor extension is concerned, however, DWI provided no clear advantage over the conventional methods. ADC values could not separate high-grade gliomas from surrounding edema.[25,27,28]

Perfusion Imaging

The most common MR perfusion imaging techniques exploit the spin dephasing ($T_2{}^*$) effect from the passage of contrast through the parenchymal capillary bed. The SI loss engendered by the passage of gadolinium-based contrast enables calculation of contrast concentration within each pixel over time, which in turn provides relative measurements of regional cerebral blood volume (rCBV). Rapid imaging is necessary to gather as much data as possible from the entire brain during the first-pass of a bolus injection of gadolinium.[3]

Perfusion imaging likely reflects tumor angiogenesis, a strong indicator of tumor grade. Studies employing perfusion techniques with histologic correlation agree that high rCBVs mean higher tumor grade (Figure 27.6). Specifically, rCBV correlated with areas highest in mitotic activity and vascularity but not with areas of cellular atypia or high cellularity.[29] Sugahara et al. found a significant correlation between rCBV ratios of gliomas and vascularity of the tumors determined both by angiography and histology (*P* less than 0.001).[30] In a series of 160 patients, Law et al. demonstrated increased sensitivity of detection of high-grade gliomas with rCBV values when compared to conventional imaging only. They also demonstrated a significant difference in the values of rCBV between high-grade and low-grade gliomas (*P* less than 0.0001).[31] Similar results were reached in three other studies.[32–34]

Perfusion imaging has proved helpful in the preoperative diagnosis of and differentiation between different brain lesions. Recently, Hartmann et al. found significantly lower rCBVs in primary CNS lymphoma (PCNSL) compared to glioblastoma multiforme (GBM) (*P* less than 0.0001).[35] Similarly, low rCBV measurements were found in 17 patients with gliomatosis cerebri, which is in concordance with the lack of vascular hyperplasia found at histopathologic examination in those tumors. The authors concluded that perfusion MR imaging provides useful adjunctive information to conventional MR imaging techniques in the evaluation of this relatively rare but important entity.[32] In the classic problem of differentiating toxoplasmosis from lymphoma in patients with acquired immunodeficiency syndrome (AIDS), rCBV was decreased throughout the toxoplasmosis lesions whereas all active lymphomas displayed areas of increased rCBV. The difference in rCBV between those two entities was significant (*P* less than 0.005). Reduced rCBV in toxoplasmosis lesions is probably due to a lack of vasculature within the abscess compared to the hypervascularity of lymphomas, especially within foci of active tumor growth.[36]

Finally, in a series of 51 patients, Law et al. found that peritumoral rCBV values in high-grade gliomas were significantly higher than in metastases (*P* less than 0.001). Mean maximum rCBV in high-grade gliomas was also significantly higher than in low-grade gliomas in a study by Yang et al.[32] Whether perfusion imaging can be used to define tumor borders remains an attractive concept to be investigated.

Magnetic Resonance Spectroscopy

Chemists have relied on nuclear magnetic resonance (NMR) spectroscopy for 50 years for molecular structure elucidation; magnetic resonance spectroscopy (MRS) is an in vivo extension of NMR. More than for structure determination, however, MRS is applied in medicine to determine the concentrations of a relatively few metabolites that are altered in disease. In MRS, the high-resolution morphologic imaging capabilities of MR are sacrificed to provide metabolic data that, in many cases, precede structural abnormality.[3]

Proton MRS is the most commonly applied technique for brain tumors because of the high natural abundance of protons in tissue. For brain tumor proton spectroscopy, the metabolites of interest include *N*-acetylaspartate (NAA), choline (Cho), creatine (Cr), lactate, lipids, and certain amino acids, such as alanine and succinate.[37] MRS imaging (MRSI) and chemical shift imaging (CSI) provide phase encoding of spatial information and generate metabolite maps. Multislice MRSI competes with single-voxel MRS, in which a small portion of the lesion is interrogated rather than the whole tumor volume, which is more easily implemented, with brief imaging times (less than 10 min/volume element, or voxel) and commercially available software. Nevertheless MRSI, with its smaller voxel size (less than 1 cm^3) and superior brain coverage, is necessary for complete characterization of heterogeneous brain tumors.

The key metabolite in brain tumor MRSI is choline (Cho), the underlying causes for the alteration of which remain controversial. The majority of choline in the brain is, in normal

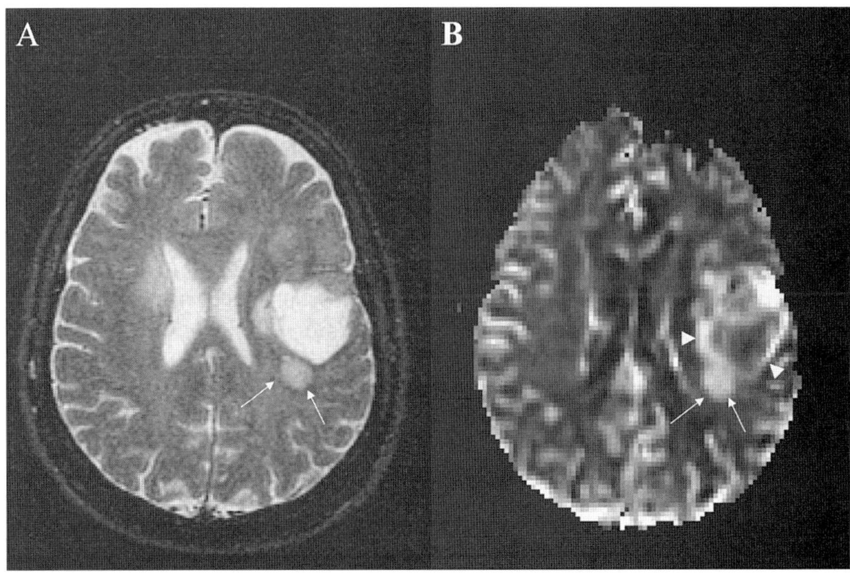

FIGURE 27.6. (A) T_2-weighted image of glioblastoma multiforme showing necrotic changes with well-defined areas of abnormal signal intensity, compatible with tumor, anterior, medial and posterior to the cystic component as well as in the right centrum semiovale. (B) Corresponding regional cerebral blood volume (rCBV) maps show marked increased values in the posterior component (*arrows*) and in the wall of the necrotic tumor (*small arrowheads*), suggestive of a higher-grade component of the tumor.

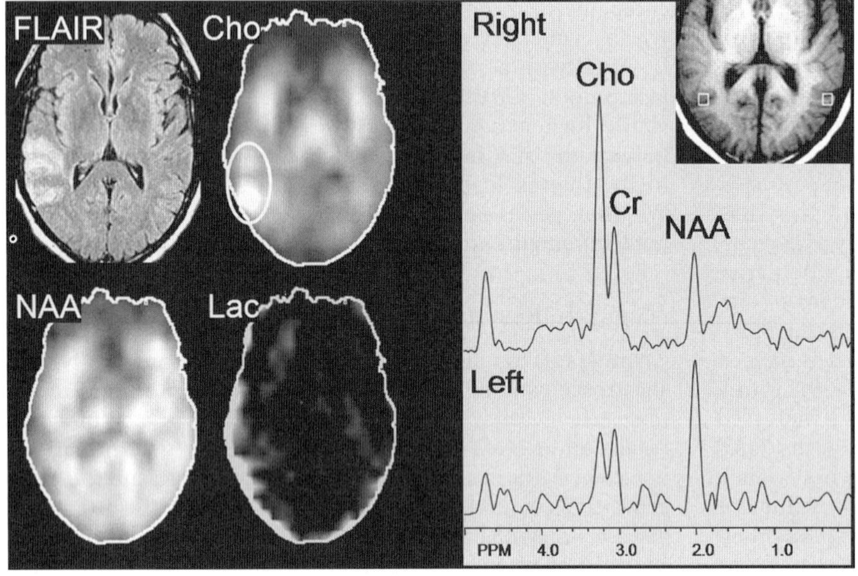

FIGURE 27.7. Patient with right temporal lobe glioblastoma multiforme. Metabolite maps on the right side are notable for increased choline (Cho) in the lesion (*circle*). Note decreased *N*-acetylaspartate (NAA) peak and marked increased Cho peak in the right temporal lobe (*upper spectrum*) when compared to the normal contralateral temporal lobe (*lower spectrum*).

conditions, bound to cell membranes, myelin, and complex brain lipids. In pathologic conditions, Cho is thought to reflect cell membrane, myelin, and lipid turnover, leading to release of MRS-visible Cho.[38] Cho is present primarily within glia.[39] Because malignant brain tumors are glial neoplasms, it seems reasonable that Cho would be elevated within them, as is usually reported (Figure 27.7). In fact, in one study by Gupta et al., a statistically significant linear correlation between tumor to contralateral normalized Cho signal ratio (nCho) and cell density was found, although nCho did not significantly correlate with proliferative index.[40]

Low NAA levels in brain tumors are believed to be the result of the lack of neurons in what are essentially glial neoplasms (Figure 27.7). Increased lactate and lipids are found in brain tumors, the former believed to be associated with high tumor glycolytic rates and the latter caused by cellular breakdown and necrosis.[3]

Originally, MRSI was evaluated in the differentiation of normal from neoplastic tissue and its impact on decision making and surgical planning. Rand et al. found that the prospective accuracy of MRSI in the nonblinded and retrospective accuracy in the blinded discrimination of neoplastic from nonneoplastic disease were 0.96 and 0.83, respectively.[41]

However, preoperative diagnosis and grading remain the goals of brain tumor MRSI. Despite the stunning results obtained in one study in which Preul et al. accurately graded 90 of 91 brain tumors,[42] most studies report such overlap as to make spectroscopy of marginal utility for tumor grading. In a study by Bulakbasi et al., MR spectroscopy could differentiate benign from malignant tumors but was not useful in grading malignant tumors. However, in the same study, ADC values were effective for grading malignant tumors (P less than 0.001) but not for distinguishing different tumor types with the same grade, as previously mentioned. The authors concluded that the two modalities can have a complementary effect in the differentiation and grading of brain tumors.[24]

Law et al. proved that the combination of rCBV, Cho/Cr, and Cho/NAA resulted in increased specificity for the detection of high-grade gliomas from 57.5% with rCBV alone to 60.0% with both modalities. No increased sensitivity, positive predictive value (PPV), or negative predictive value (NPV) was achieved, however, when the MRS findings were combined with perfusion.[31] In a series of 176 patients, however, Moller-Hartmann et al. were able to establish that the additive information of proton MRSI led to a 15.4% higher number of correct diagnoses, 6.2% fewer incorrect, and 16% fewer equivocal diagnoses than with structural MRI data alone, in a multitude of pathologies, including brain tumors.[43]

Perhaps more clinically useful than tumor grading is the role of MRS in the planning of guided biopsies. In 29 patients in whom the preoperative metabolite levels were correlated with the histologic findings, it was found that with abnormally increased Cho and decreased NAA, biopsy invariably was positive for tumor.[44] Similar results were reached by Martin et al.[45]

In the evaluation of tumor borders in 31 patients with diffusely infiltrating gliomas, Croteau et al. tried to determine a correlation between different proton MRS/I metabolic ratios and the degree of tumor infiltration. They correlated the metabolite ratios with the histopathologic analyses of biopsies obtained at the same location and found that the Cho to normal contralateral Cr and Cho to normal contralateral Cho ratios (Cho/nCr and Cho/nCho) were positively correlated with the degree of tumor infiltration, whereas the NAA to normal contralateral Cr ratio (NAA/nCr) was negatively correlated, for all tumor grades combined.[46] The strength of this study resides in the coregistration of the biopsy sites with the metabolite values obtained from the same voxels. The potential of MRSI in the accurate delineation of tumor borders requires further investigation.

Another use for MRSI is in the differentiation of primary from metastatic brain tumors. In a recent study, a significant increase in Cho concentration was found in both the peritumoral and tumoral regions of malignant gliomas, compared with metastases. Similarly, a prominent difference in the Cho/Cr ratio between gliomas and metastases (P less than 0.05) and elevated myo-inositol levels (MI/Cr) within the enhancing foci of gliomas but not in the metastases were also found (P less than 0.05). That study, however, was limited by the small number of patients (22).[47]

Functional Magnetic Resonance Imaging

The main use for functional magnetic resonance imaging (fMRI) in neuroimaging has been for the noninvasive study of brain activation. The most common fMRI method detects signals based on the blood oxygen level dependence (BOLD) effect. During brain activation, there is increased blood flow to the area of activation, which appears to be a direct consequence of neurotransmitter activity. Blood flow increases over a wider volume and to a greater extent than is necessary simply to provide oxygen and glucose for increased metabolism, so oxygen extraction decreases with greater neuronal activity. Consequently, the ratio of oxygenated (diamagnetic oxyhemoglobin) to deoxygenated (paramagnetic deoxyhemoglobin) blood near the corresponding areas of neuronal activation will increase, resulting in lower T_2^* (dephasing) effect and increased signal.[48] Statistical techniques are employed or baseline images are subtracted from images obtained during activation to generate activation maps that are superimposed on MR images.

In brain tumor imaging, fMRI is generally used for the preoperative localization of sensorimotor cortex, hemispheric language dominance, and other eloquent (essential) regions, locations that can be perturbed in the presence of a tumor. Cerebral reorganization (plasticity) is defined as the capacity of ipsilateral and contralateral brain regions to assume functions that are normally assumed by the damaged brain. That reorganization puts critical motor regions at risk if the standard anatomic techniques are used to locate motor cortex preoperatively. Functional MRI can preemptively locate that reorganized cortex (Figure 27.8).

Neurosurgeons routinely perform cortical mapping intraoperatively. Cortical mapping is just that; that is, it determines function only in the cortex, which is a peripheral brain structure. Functional MRI can evaluate subcortical structures in areas far removed from the limited amount of cortex that is exposed and therefore available for intraoperative mapping.[3]

Functional MRI, however, is incompletely validated. Good, but not perfect, correlation between fMRI and cortical electrical stimulation has been demonstrated in several studies.[49,50] Studies comparing PET and fMRI have shown much lower degrees of correlation, usually around 50%, with some patients showing no correlation of activation between the two techniques.[51,52] Additionally, it remains unclear whether nonactivated brain regions may be safely resected, in part because of that spatial and temporal dispersion of blood oxygen level changes. Schreiber et al. found that the BOLD contrast can be reduced in the proximity of gliomas, but not affected by nonglial space-occupying lesions, such as vascular malformations, leading to overinterpretation of the interhemispheric reorganization in gliomas.[53] Similar results were reached by Holodny et al., who suggested that this could result from loss of autoregulation in the tumor vasculature of glioblastomas and venous compression.[54]

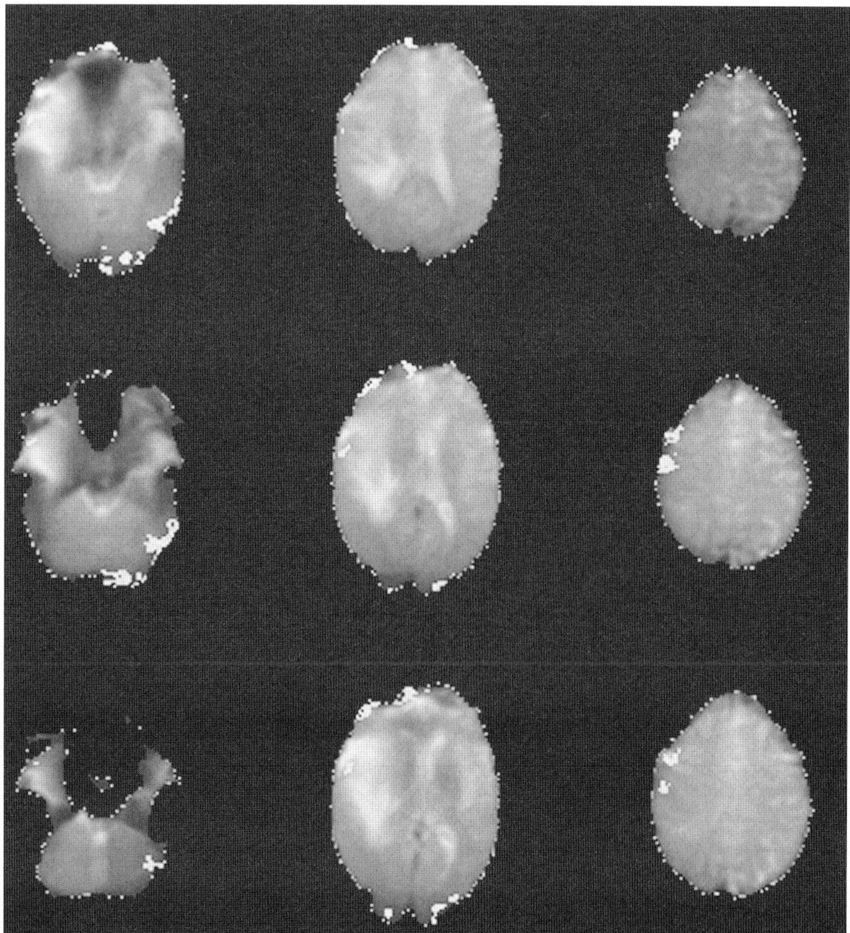

FIGURE 27.8. Cerebral reorganization in right-handed patient with right paracavernous meningioma. Functional magnetic resonance imaging (MRI) demonstrates that the task of reading words activates superiorly displaced speech areas in the right hemisphere. The patient was informed of the risk of losing speech postoperatively.

Although fMRI is a noninvasive technique with high spatial and temporal resolution, short examination time, and wide availability, it will likely not replace intraoperative cortical mapping.

Diffusion Tensor Imaging

Diffusion tensor imaging (DTI) is a magnetic resonance technique that is sensitive to the diffusion of water in brain tissue, thus revealing the anisotropy and orientation of white matter tracts in the brain. Myelin or protein fibers likely account for diffusion anisotropy. Measurement of ADCs along six independent axes of the tensor provides the shape of the diffusion ellipsoid, that is, fully characterizes diffusion in three dimensions. Mean diffusivity (MD) and fractional anisotropy (FA) can be calculated for each pixel, representing the magnitude and directionality of water diffusion within that pixel. Once fiber direction is known in each pixel, a three-dimensional (3-D) map can be generated that depicts patterns of connectivity throughout the brain. Display of the effects of mass lesions on large nerve fiber tracts by DTI can be used for preoperative planning. Specifically, fiber mapping enables visualization of subcortical fiber tracts that are important in motor function.

Although many studies have demonstrated the usefulness of diffusion tensor imaging in the delineation of tumor infiltration, vascularity, and cellularity[55–57] (Figure 27.9), in the differentiation between peritumoral edema and tumor infiltration,[58] and in the differentiation between metastasis and primary brain tumors,[59] more studies and well-organized clinical trials need to be performed before fiber tracking can be integrated into a neurosurgical planning system. Newer techniques decreasing the time of acquisition and minimizing image distortion are being investigated[60] and could help in making diffusion tensor imaging applicable for routine clinical practice.

Positron Emission Tomography and Single-Photon Emission Tomography

Positron emission tomography (PET) exploits the annihilation of positrons and electrons into photons to achieve the nuclear imaging analog of X-ray computed tomography (CT). In the decay of a positron-emitting radionuclide, the positron interacts with an electron, yielding two photons that travel in (nearly) opposite directions. By detecting those photons in coincidence, the projection data required for tomographic reconstruction are obtained. ^{18}F-Fluorodeoxyglucose (FDG) is the most commonly used tracer in the clinic. Similar to glucose, FDG is transported into cells by a glucose transporter, but remains trapped within the cell, thus reflecting the energy metabolism within tissues. Highly malignant brain tumors usually show increased FDG uptake in comparison to the surrounding brain parenchyma (Figure 27.10). However, because of inherent limitations, such as low resolution and high background glucose metabolism of normal gray matter structures, ^{18}F-fluorodeoxyglucose positron emission tomography (FDG-PET) use is not a part of the routine diagnostic evaluation of brain tumor patients. Other potential uses for PET in brain tumor evaluation include grading, localization for biopsy, differentiating radiation necrosis from tumor

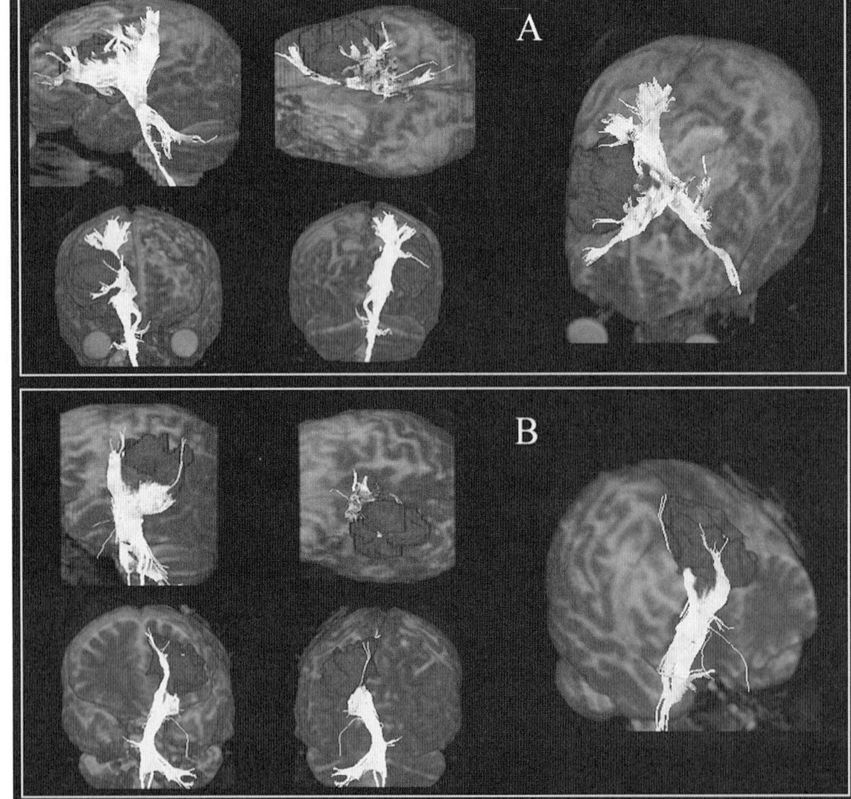

FIGURE 27.9. Fiber tracking in brain tumors with diffusion tensor imaging (DTI). The three-dimensional (3-D) relationship of the corona radiata with the tumor can be clearly appreciated. The corona radiata of the first patient (A) surrounds the surface of the tumor because of mechanical compression rather than infiltration. In the second patient's case (B), the trajectory of the corona radiata was not changed. Instead, it projected into the core of the infiltrative tumor. (From Mori et al.,[57] by permission of *Annals of Neurology*.)

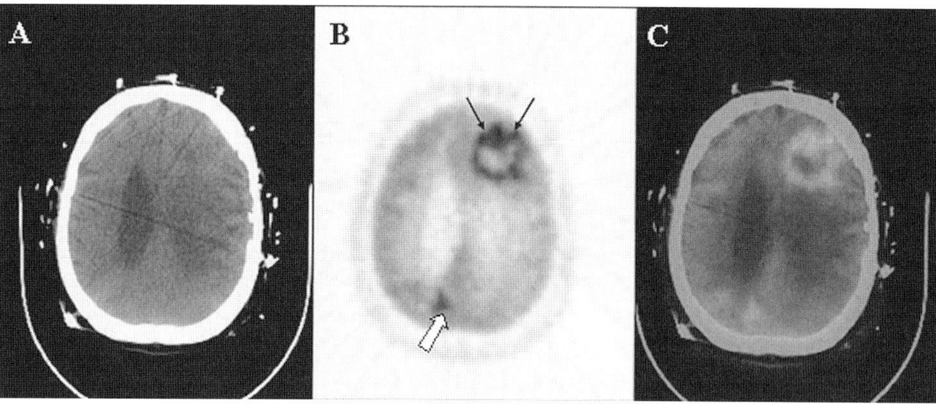

FIGURE 27.10. (A) CT scan, (B) ^{18}F-fluorodeoxyglucose positron emission tomography (FDG-PET) scan, and (C) fused CT and PET scan images of left frontal lobe recurrent GBM. Note increased FDG uptake in the periphery of the necrotic mass (*black arrows*), compatible with tumor recurrence rather than radiation necrosis. Note the presence of another focus of increased uptake (*white arrow*) in the right parietal region consistent with the diagnosis of multifocal GBM.

necrosis, assessing response to therapy, predicting survival, and assessing malignant transformation of low-grade gliomas. In 47 patients with different brain tumors, the sensitivity of FDG-PET for differentiating tumor from radiation necrosis was 75% and the specificity was 81%.[61] In another study yielding even lower sensitivity and specificity values, the authors concluded that the ability of ^{18}F-fluorodeoxyglucose positron emission tomography (FDG-PET) to differentiate recurrent tumor from radiation necrosis is limited.[62] FDG-PET was found to be of prognostic importance in multiple studies.[63,64] However, in the assessment of response to chemotherapy or radiotherapy, the role of FDG-PET remains of limited clinical utility.[65]

Newer tracers such as methyl-[^{11}C]-L-methionine (MET) for measurement of amino acid transport and incorporation and ^{18}F-3-deoxy-3-fluorothymidine (FLT) for evaluation of DNA synthesis, among others, seem to be promising in further characterization of brain tumors; however, they remain of limited clinical use currently.

The use of single-photon emission tomography (SPECT) in brain tumors is limited. Thallium (Tl) is the most studied radiotracer with the longest track record. Some studies have shown a relationship between ^{201}Tl uptake and tumor grade.[66] Due to the overlap between tumor uptake and histologic grades, ^{201}Tl cannot be used as the sole noninvasive diagnostic or prognostic tool in brain tumor patients.[67,66] However, it may help in differentiating a high-grade tumor recurrence from radiation necrosis. ^{99m}Tc-Sestamibi is theoretically a better imaging agent than ^{201}Tl, but it has not convincingly been shown to differentiate tumors according to grade.[68]

Intraoperative Imaging and Navigation

Stereotactic Navigation

Rapid 3-D MR techniques that provide thin sections (1.5 mm) can be merged with a frameless stereotactic system to improve the safety and accuracy of neurosurgical procedures. Using this technique, the surgeon's "view" is expanded to include structures deep to the region that he or she is resecting in real time. Accurate delineation of the boundaries of the lesion is the goal with this technique, as the completeness of resection is highly correlated with survival for both low- and high-grade tumors. The usefulness and reliability of the method was immediately recognized and allowed its widespread use. In a large series of 325 cases, the use of the frameless stereotactic viewing system was associated with minimal additional effort or time spent in setting up the procedure. The system was found to be reliable, achieving a useful registration in 95.4% of cases.[69] In another case-control study, the impact of neuronavigation on glioblastoma surgery regarding time consumption, extent of tumor removal, and survival was evaluated, with and without the use of neuronavigation, in 52 cases and in 52 corresponding controls. Radical tumor resection based on radiologic evaluation was achieved in 31% of navigation cases versus 19% in conventional operations. The absolute and relative residual tumor volumes were significantly lower with neuronavigation. Radical tumor resection was associated with a highly significant prolongation in survival (P less than 0.0001). Survival was longer in patients who underwent surgery using neuronavigation (median, 13.4 versus 11.1 months).[70]

Similarly, stereotactic techniques have improved the efficiency of postoperative radiation of brain tumors. In stereotactic conformal radiotherapy, a computer-generated plan guides the use of a variable collimator to distribute the radiation field in such a way that the tumor may receive a very large dose, a surrounding area a moderate dose, and radiosensitive structures a minimal dose of radiation.[71]

Problems arise with techniques that use preoperative image coregistration, however, because the brain tends to move during the procedure due to swelling or to the introduction of air. Intraoperative acquisition of data sets eliminates the problem of brain shift in conventional navigational systems.

Intraoperative MRI Techniques

Intraoperative MR devices, either with an upright double doughnut configuration or that require the patient to be moved to a magnet adjacent to the operating suite, have been developed to avoid potential image misregistration. Intraoperative MR techniques enable continual, near real-time visual feedback during the procedure.[3] In one study evaluating 38 patients with high-grade gliomas, intraoperative MR imaging significantly increased the rate of complete tumor removal.[72] Other uses for intraoperative MR, besides guidance to the site of an abnormality, include minimization of the size of the craniotomy, identification of adjacent structures, thus maximizing preservation of normal tissue, determination of the completeness of tumor resection, and surveillance for intraoperative complications.[73,74–76]

Postoperative Evaluation

The differentiation of tumor recurrence from radiation necrosis in patients with malignant gliomas who have been treated previously remains a challenge. Multiple imaging modalities were evaluated to address the problem, including FDG-PET, MRS, and perfusion imaging, in view of the limitations of conventional MRI in these cases. FDG-PET has been traditionally used in the differentiation of recurrence from radionecrosis. Sensitivities for detection of recurrent tumor ranged from as low as 43% to as high as 86%.[61,62,77,78] Lower specificity values, however, were found, and most investigators considered the modality insufficient for the evaluation of tumor recurrence.[62,77]

MRS/I is finding a niche in therapeutic monitoring and has recently been applied with success to the classic problem of differentiating recurrent tumor from radiation injury. In one study ($n = 56$), a significant difference in metabolite ratios (Cho/Cr and Cho/NAA) emerged between neoplastic and nonneoplastic lesions after stereotactic radiotherapy.[79] In another prospective study involving 27 patients, MRSI spectral patterns allowed reliable differential diagnostic statements to be made when the tissues are composed of either pure tumor or pure necrosis; however, these were less definitive in tissues composed of varying degrees of mixed tumor and necrosis.[80] Perfusion imaging is also helpful in the prognostic evaluation and postoperative follow-up of patients with brain tumors. Although tumors that recur after radiation therapy tend toward lower rCBV values than native lesions, earlier diagnosis of recurrent tumor has been suggested using perfusion imaging than with serial MR imaging or with nuclear imaging techniques. In a series of 59 patients, perfusion imaging (rCBV maps) was found to predict tumor progression earlier than MR imaging in 32%, earlier than ^{201}Tl-SPECT in 63%, and earlier than clinical assessment in 55% of the studies.[81] Sugahara et al. evaluated 20 patients with the diagnosis of recurrent tumor versus radionecrosis by a combination of perfusion imaging and thallium single-photon emission tomography (^{201}Tl-SPECT). The rCBV values overlapped between neoplastic and nonneoplastic lesions, and the authors suggested that ^{201}Tl-SPECT may be useful in making the differentiation.[82] In view of an improved spatial resolution in comparison to SPECT and PET,[83] perfusion MRI is a promising technique that needs to be evaluated further in clinical studies.

Conclusion

Clinical neuroimaging is undergoing a transformation from the purely anatomic techniques of CT and MRI to those that are functional, such as perfusion imaging and BOLD fMRI, as well as to molecular imaging techniques including MRSI and PET. Complementing the already widely available MR-based methods, the advent of PET-CT and the likely emergence of PET-MR suggest a prominent role for PET in functional brain imaging in the near future. The ultimate goal of this work is to combine multimodality and multiparametric imaging to gain the most relevant physiologic information for diagnosis, prognosis, and therapeutic monitoring of patients with CNS-related cancer. An early goal is to define the true extent of tumor infiltration within the brain, that is, that which extends beyond that seen on conventional contrast-enhanced MR images. The rational combination of the parameters discussed here will likely enable that definition in the short term, with the potential to affect positively the way brain tumors are currently treated, and ultimately survival, from this now uniformly devastating disease.

References

1. Padhani AR, Dixon AK. Whole body computed tomography: recent developments. In: Grainger RG, Allison D (eds). Grainger & Allison's Diagnostic Radiology: A Textbook of Medical Imaging, vol 1. New York: Churchill Livingstone, 2001:81–82.
2. Okuda T, Korogi Y, Shigematsu Y, et al. Brain lesions: when should fluid-attenuated inversion-recovery sequences be used in MR evaluation? Radiology 1999;212(3):793–798.
3. Pomper MG, Port JD. New techniques in MR imaging of brain tumors. Magn Reson Imaging Clin N Am 2000;8(4):691–713.
4. Maubon AJ, Pothin A, Ferru JM, Berger VM, Daures JP, Rouanet JP. Unselected brain 0.5-T MR imaging: comparison of lesion detection and characterization with three T_2-weighted sequences. Radiology 1998;208(3):671–678.
5. De Coene B, Hajnal JV, Gatehouse P, et al. MR of the brain using fluid-attenuated inversion recovery (FLAIR) pulse sequences. AJNR Am J Neuroradiol 1992;13(6):1555–1564.
6. Tsuchiya K, Mizutani Y, Hachiya J. Preliminary evaluation of fluid-attenuated inversion-recovery MR in the diagnosis of intracranial tumors. AJNR Am J Neuroradiol 1996;17(6):1081–1086.
7. Bynevelt M, Britton J, Seymour H, MacSweeney E, Thomas N, Sandhu K. FLAIR imaging in the follow-up of low-grade gliomas: time to dispense with the dual-echo? Neuroradiology 2001; 43(2):129–133.
8. Chen S, Ikawa F, Kurisu K, Arita K, Takaba J, Kanou Y. Quantitative MR evaluation of intracranial epidermoid tumors by fast fluid-attenuated inversion recovery imaging and echo-planar diffusion-weighted imaging. AJNR Am J Neuroradiol 2001;22(6): 1089–1096.
9. Ikushima I, Korogi Y, Hirai T, et al. MR of epidermoids with a variety of pulse sequences. AJNR Am J Neuroradiol 1997;18(7): 1359–1363.
10. Singh SK, Agris JM, Leeds NE, Ginsberg LE. Intracranial leptomeningeal metastases: comparison of depiction at FLAIR and contrast-enhanced MR imaging. Radiology 2000;217(1):50–53.
11. Griffiths PD, Coley SC, Romanowski CA, Hodgson T, Wilkinson ID. Contrast-enhanced fluid-attenuated inversion recovery imaging for leptomeningeal disease in children. AJNR Am J Neuroradiol 2003;24(4):719–723.
12. Ebisu T, Tanaka C, Umeda M, et al. Discrimination of brain abscess from necrotic or cystic tumors by diffusion-weighted echo planar imaging. Magn Reson Imaging. 1996;14(9):1113–1116.
13. Dorenbeck U, Butz B, Schlaier J, Bretschneider T, Schuierer G, Feuerbach S. Diffusion-weighted echo-planar MRI of the brain with calculated ADCs: a useful tool in the differential diagnosis of tumor necrosis from abscess? J Neuroimaging 2003;13(4): 330–338.
14. Guzman R, Barth A, Lovblad KO, et al. Use of diffusion-weighted magnetic resonance imaging in differentiating purulent brain processes from cystic brain tumors. J Neurosurg 2002; 97(5):1101–1107.
15. Chang SC, Lai PH, Chen WL, et al. Diffusion-weighted MRI features of brain abscess and cystic or necrotic brain tumors: com-

parison with conventional MRI. Clin Imaging 2002;26(4):227–236.
16. Lai PH, Ho JT, Chen WL, et al. Brain abscess and necrotic brain tumor: discrimination with proton MR spectroscopy and diffusion-weighted imaging. AJNR Am J Neuroradiol 2002;23(8):1369–1377.
17. Kim YJ, Chang KH, Song IC, et al. Brain abscess and necrotic or cystic brain tumor: discrimination with signal intensity on diffusion-weighted MR imaging. AJR Am J Roentgenol 1998;171(6):1487–1490.
18. Chan JH, Tsui EY, Chau LF, et al. Discrimination of an infected brain tumor from a cerebral abscess by combined MR perfusion and diffusion imaging. Comput Med Imaging Graph 2002;26(1):19–23.
19. Nadal Desbarats L, Herlidou S, de Marco G, et al. Differential MRI diagnosis between brain abscesses and necrotic or cystic brain tumors using the apparent diffusion coefficient and normalized diffusion-weighted images. Magn Reson Imaging 2003;21(6):645–650.
20. Tsuruda JS, Chew WM, Moseley ME, Norman D. Diffusion-weighted MR imaging of the brain: value of differentiating between extraaxial cysts and epidermoid tumors. AJNR Am J Neuroradiol 1990;11(5):925–931; discussion 932–924.
21. Tsuruda JS, Chew WM, Moseley ME, Norman D. Diffusion-weighted MR imaging of extraaxial tumors. Magn Reson Med 1991;19(2):316–320.
22. Sugahara T, Korogi Y, Kochi M, et al. Usefulness of diffusion-weighted MRI with echo-planar technique in the evaluation of cellularity in gliomas. J Magn Reson Imaging 1999;9(1):53–60.
23. Kotsenas AL, Roth TC, Manness WK, Faerber EN. Abnormal diffusion-weighted MRI in medulloblastoma: does it reflect small cell histology? Pediatr Radiol 1999;29(7):524–526.
24. Bulakbasi N, Kocaoglu M, Ors F, Tayfun C, Ucoz T. Combination of single-voxel proton MR spectroscopy and apparent diffusion coefficient calculation in the evaluation of common brain tumors. AJNR Am J Neuroradiol 2003;24(2):225–233.
25. Kono K, Inoue Y, Nakayama K, et al. The role of diffusion-weighted imaging in patients with brain tumors. AJNR Am J Neuroradiol 2001;22(6):1081–1088.
26. Yang D, Korogi Y, Sugahara T, et al. Cerebral gliomas: prospective comparison of multivoxel 2D chemical-shift imaging proton MR spectroscopy, echoplanar perfusion and diffusion-weighted MRI. Neuroradiology 2002;44(8):656–666.
27. Castillo M, Smith JK, Kwock L, Wilber K. Apparent diffusion coefficients in the evaluation of high-grade cerebral gliomas. AJNR Am J Neuroradiol 2001;22(1):60–64.
28. Stadnik TW, Chaskis C, Michotte A, et al. Diffusion-weighted MR imaging of intracerebral masses: comparison with conventional MR imaging and histologic findings. AJNR Am J Neuroradiol 2001;22(5):969–976.
29. Aronen HJ, Gazit IE, Louis DN, et al. Cerebral blood volume maps of gliomas: comparison with tumor grade and histologic findings. Radiology 1994;191(1):41–51.
30. Sugahara T, Korogi Y, Kochi M, et al. Correlation of MR imaging-determined cerebral blood volume maps with histologic and angiographic determination of vascularity of gliomas. AJR Am J Roentgenol 1998;171(6):1479–1486.
31. Law M, Yang S, Wang H, et al. Glioma grading: sensitivity, specificity, and predictive values of perfusion MR imaging and proton MR spectroscopic imaging compared with conventional MR imaging. AJNR Am J Neuroradiol 2003;24(10):1989–1998.
32. Yang S, Wetzel S, Law M, Zagzag D, Cha S. Dynamic contrast-enhanced T_2*-weighted MR imaging of gliomatosis cerebri. AJNR Am J Neuroradiol 2002;23(3):350–355.
33. Shin JH, Lee HK, Kwun BD, et al. Using relative cerebral blood flow and volume to evaluate the histopathologic grade of cerebral gliomas: preliminary results. AJR Am J Roentgenol 2002;179(3):783–789.
34. Lam WW, Chan KW, Wong WL, Poon WS, Metreweli C. Preoperative grading of intracranial glioma. Acta Radiol 2001;42(6):548–554.
35. Hartmann M, Heiland S, Harting I, et al. Distinguishing of primary cerebral lymphoma from high-grade glioma with perfusion-weighted magnetic resonance imaging. Neurosci Lett 2003;338(2):119–122.
36. Ernst TM, Chang L, Witt MD, et al. Cerebral toxoplasmosis and lymphoma in AIDS: perfusion MR imaging experience in 13 patients. Radiology 1998;208(3):663–669.
37. Grand S, Passaro G, Ziegler A, et al. Necrotic tumor versus brain abscess: importance of amino acids detected at ^{1}H MR spectroscopy: initial results. Radiology 1999;213(3):785–793.
38. Burtscher IM, Holtas S. Proton magnetic resonance spectroscopy in brain tumours: clinical applications. Neuroradiology 2001;43(5):345–352.
39. Fulham MJ, Bizzi A, Dietz MJ, et al. Mapping of brain tumor metabolites with proton MR spectroscopic imaging: clinical relevance. Radiology 1992;185(3):675–686.
40. Gupta RK, Cloughesy TF, Sinha U, et al. Relationships between choline magnetic resonance spectroscopy, apparent diffusion coefficient and quantitative histopathology in human glioma. J Neurooncol 2000;50(3):215–226.
41. Rand SD, Prost R, Haughton V, et al. Accuracy of single-voxel proton MR spectroscopy in distinguishing neoplastic from nonneoplastic brain lesions. AJNR Am J Neuroradiol 1997;18(9):1695–1704.
42. Preul MC, Caramanos Z, Collins DL, et al. Accurate, noninvasive diagnosis of human brain tumors by using proton magnetic resonance spectroscopy. Nat Med 1996;2(3):323–325.
43. Moller-Hartmann W, Herminghaus S, Krings T, et al. Clinical application of proton magnetic resonance spectroscopy in the diagnosis of intracranial mass lesions. Neuroradiology 2002;44(5):371–381.
44. Dowling C, Bollen AW, Noworolski SM, et al. Preoperative proton MR spectroscopic imaging of brain tumors: correlation with histopathologic analysis of resection specimens. AJNR Am J Neuroradiol 2001;22(4):604–612.
45. Martin AJ, Liu H, Hall WA, Truwit CL. Preliminary assessment of turbo spectroscopic imaging for targeting in brain biopsy. AJNR Am J Neuroradiol 2001;22(5):959–968.
46. Croteau D, Scarpace L, Hearshen D, et al. Correlation between magnetic resonance spectroscopy imaging and image-guided biopsies: semiquantitative and qualitative histopathological analyses of patients with untreated glioma. Neurosurgery 2001;49(4):823–829.
47. Fan G, Sun B, Wu Z, Guo Q, Guo Y. In vivo single-voxel proton MR spectroscopy in the differentiation of high-grade gliomas and solitary metastases. Clin Radiol 2004;59(1):77–85.
48. Matthews PM, Jezzard P. Functional magnetic resonance imaging. J Neurol Neurosurg Psychiatry 2004;75(1):6–12.
49. Fandino J, Kollias SS, Wieser HG, Valavanis A, Yonekawa Y. Intraoperative validation of functional magnetic resonance imaging and cortical reorganization patterns in patients with brain tumors involving the primary motor cortex. J Neurosurg 1999;91(2):238–250.
50. Lurito JT, Lowe MJ, Sartorius C, Mathews VP. Comparison of fMRI and intraoperative direct cortical stimulation in localization of receptive language areas. J Comput Assist Tomogr 2000;24(1):99–105.
51. Paulesu E, Connelly A, Frith CD, et al. Functional MR imaging correlations with positron emission tomography. Initial experience using a cognitive activation paradigm on verbal working memory. Neuroimaging Clin N Am 1995;5(2):207–225.
52. Krings T, Schreckenberger M, Rohde V, et al. Functional MRI and ^{18}F FDG-positron emission tomography for presurgical planning: comparison with electrical cortical stimulation. Acta Neurochir (Wien) 2002;144(9):889–899; discussion 899.

53. Schreiber A, Hubbe U, Ziyeh S, Hennig J. The influence of gliomas and nonglial space-occupying lesions on blood-oxygen-level-dependent contrast enhancement. AJNR Am J Neuroradiol 2000;21(6):1055–1063.
54. Holodny AI, Schulder M, Liu WC, Wolko J, Maldjian JA, Kalnin AJ. The effect of brain tumors on BOLD functional MR imaging activation in the adjacent motor cortex: implications for image-guided neurosurgery. AJNR Am J Neuroradiol 2000;21(8):1415–1422.
55. Gauvain KM, McKinstry RC, Mukherjee P, et al. Evaluating pediatric brain tumor cellularity with diffusion-tensor imaging. AJR Am J Roentgenol 2001;177(2):449–454.
56. Beppu T, Inoue T, Shibata Y, et al. Measurement of fractional anisotropy using diffusion tensor MRI in supratentorial astrocytic tumors. J Neurooncol 2003;63(2):109–116.
57. Mori S, Frederiksen K, van Zijl PC, et al. Brain white matter anatomy of tumor patients evaluated with diffusion tensor imaging. Ann Neurol 2002;51(3):377–380.
58. Sinha S, Bastin ME, Whittle IR, Wardlaw JM. Diffusion tensor MR imaging of high-grade cerebral gliomas. AJNR Am J Neuroradiol 2002;23(4):520–527.
59. Lu S, Ahn D, Johnson G, Cha S. Peritumoral diffusion tensor imaging of high-grade gliomas and metastatic brain tumors. AJNR Am J Neuroradiol 2003;24(5):937–941.
60. Yamada K, Kizu O, Mori S, et al. Brain fiber tracking with clinically feasible diffusion-tensor MR imaging: initial experience. Radiology 2003;227(1):295–301.
61. Chao ST, Suh JH, Raja S, Lee SY, Barnett G. The sensitivity and specificity of FDG PET in distinguishing recurrent brain tumor from radionecrosis in patients treated with stereotactic radiosurgery. Int J Cancer 2001;96(3):191–197.
62. Ricci PE, Karis JP, Heiserman JE, Fram EK, Bice AN, Drayer BP. Differentiating recurrent tumor from radiation necrosis: time for re-evaluation of positron emission tomography? AJNR Am J Neuroradiol 1998;19(3):407–413.
63. De Witte O, Levivier M, Violon P, et al. Prognostic value positron emission tomography with [^{18}F]fluoro-2-deoxy-D-glucose in the low-grade glioma. Neurosurgery 1996;39(3):470–476; discussion 476–477.
64. Barker FG JR, Chang SM, Valk PE, Pounds TR, Prados MD. 18-Fluorodeoxyglucose uptake and survival of patients with suspected recurrent malignant glioma. Cancer (Phila)1997;79(1):115–126.
65. Spence AM, Mankoff DA, Muzi M. Positron emission tomography imaging of brain tumors. Neuroimaging Clin N Am 2003;13(4):717–739.
66. Sun D, Liu Q, Liu W, Hu W. Clinical application of ^{201}Tl SPECT imaging of brain tumors. J Nucl Med 2000;41(1):5–10.
67. Oriuchi N, Tamura M, Shibazaki T, et al. Clinical evaluation of thallium-201 SPECT in supratentorial gliomas: relationship to histologic grade, prognosis and proliferative activities. J Nucl Med 1993;34(12):2085–2089.
68. Benard F, Romsa J, Hustinx R. Imaging gliomas with positron emission tomography and single-photon emission computed tomography. Semin Nucl Med 2003;33(2):148–162.
69. Golfinos JG, Fitzpatrick BC, Smith LR, Spetzler RF. Clinical use of a frameless stereotactic arm: results of 325 cases. J Neurosurg 1995;83(2):197–205.
70. Wirtz CR, Albert FK, Schwaderer M, et al. The benefit of neuronavigation for neurosurgery analyzed by its impact on glioblastoma surgery. Neurol Res 2000;22(4):354–360.
71. Gildenberg PL, Woo SY. Multimodality program involving stereotactic surgery in brain tumor management. Stereotact Funct Neurosurg 2000;75(2–3):147–152.
72. Knauth M, Wirtz CR, Tronnier VM, Aras N, Kunze S, Sartor K. Intraoperative MR imaging increases the extent of tumor resection in patients with high-grade gliomas. AJNR Am J Neuroradiol 1999;20(9):1642–1646.
73. Tuominen J, Yrjana SK, Katisko JP, Heikkila J, Koivukangas J. Intraoperative imaging in a comprehensive neuronavigation environment for minimally invasive brain tumour surgery. Acta Neurochir Suppl 2003;85:115–120.
74. Kanner AA, Vogelbaum MA, Mayberg MR, Weisenberger JP, Barnett GH. Intracranial navigation by using low-field intraoperative magnetic resonance imaging: preliminary experience. J Neurosurg 2002;97(5):1115–1124.
75. Wirtz CR, Knauth M, Staubert A, et al. Clinical evaluation and follow-up results for intraoperative magnetic resonance imaging in neurosurgery. Neurosurgery 2000;46(5):1112–1120; discussion 1120–1121.
76. Lewin JS, Metzger A, Selman WR. Intraoperative magnetic resonance image guidance in neurosurgery. J Magn Reson Imaging 2000;12(4):512–524.
77. Thompson TP, Lunsford LD, Kondziolka D. Distinguishing recurrent tumor and radiation necrosis with positron emission tomography versus stereotactic biopsy. Stereotact Funct Neurosurg 1999;73(1–4):9–14.
78. Kahn D, Follett KA, Bushnell DL, et al. Diagnosis of recurrent brain tumor: value of ^{201}Tl SPECT vs. ^{18}F-fluorodeoxyglucose PET. AJR Am J Roentgenol 1994;163(6):1459–1465.
79. Schlemmer HP, Bachert P, Herfarth KK, Zuna I, Debus J, van Kaick G. Proton MR spectroscopic evaluation of suspicious brain lesions after stereotactic radiotherapy. AJNR Am J Neuroradiol 2001;22(7):1316–1324.
80. Rock JP, Hearshen D, Scarpace L, et al. Correlations between magnetic resonance spectroscopy and image-guided histopathology, with special attention to radiation necrosis. Neurosurgery 2002;51(4):912–919; discussion 919–920.
81. Siegal T, Rubinstein R, Tzuk-Shina T, Gomori JM. Utility of relative cerebral blood volume mapping derived from perfusion magnetic resonance imaging in the routine follow-up of brain tumors. J Neurosurg 1997;86(1):22–27.
82. Sugahara T, Korogi Y, Tomiguchi S, et al. Posttherapeutic intraaxial brain tumor: the value of perfusion-sensitive contrast-enhanced MR imaging for differentiating tumor recurrence from nonneoplastic contrast-enhancing tissue. AJNR Am J Neuroradiol 2000;21(5):901–909.
83. Bitzer M, Klose U, Nagele T, et al. Echo planar perfusion imaging with high spatial and temporal resolution: methodology and clinical aspects. Eur Radiol 1999;9(2):221–229.

28

Breast Imaging

Wendie A. Berg

In this chapter, the current status of breast imaging for both screening and diagnosis is reviewed. Mammography remains the standard for screening; however, moderate evidence supports the use of ultrasound (US) or magnetic resonance imaging (MRI) for supplemental screening of certain subgroups of women. Evaluation of a lump is highly accurate when both mammography and US are used. For the patient with nipple discharge, US appears to be an acceptable, noninvasive alternative to ductography.

MRI and US also play a role in evaluating disease extent in both ipsilateral and contralateral breasts. No imaging test is sufficiently accurate compared to sentinel lymphadenectomy to preoperatively identify metastatic nodes, although US-guided fine-needle aspiration can confirm metastatic adenopathy. Positron emission tomography plays a role in restaging recurrent breast cancer.

Screening

The goal of screening is early detection that will alter the natural history of the disease without harming healthy individuals. Such an intervention should also be cost-effective and practical to implement. Tabar et al.[1] retrospectively examined the prognosis of breast cancers by histologic type, grade, size, and node status in the Swedish Two-County trial. Cancers were divided into those with good, intermediate, and poor prognosis. Those with good prognosis showed 20-year survival of 91%, compared to 72% for those of intermediate prognosis and 40% for those with poor prognosis. "Good" prognosis cancers had more than 90% 20-year survival and included all ductal carcinoma in situ (DCIS) as well as node-negative invasive cancers of small size: less than 20mm if grade I invasive ductal, less than 15mm if grade II, less than 10mm if grade III, and less than 10mm invasive lobular.[1] All tubular cancers had good or intermediate prognosis.[1] "Poor" prognosis cancers were larger in size and node positive but fundamentally of the same histology as those of good prognosis. Mammographic screening shifts the distribution of cancers toward those with better prognosis. In the Swedish Two-County trial,[1] 50% of mammographic screen-detected cancers had good prognosis and 18% had poor prognosis, whereas 19% of clinically detected cancers had good prognosis and 47% poor prognosis.

A report commissioned by the United States Preventive Services Task Force[2] reviewed eight randomized, controlled trials of mammography and two of breast self-examination (BSE). The Edinburgh trial was excluded for reasons of lower socioeconomic status and higher all-cause mortality in the control group and the lack of masking when evaluating cause of death. Across the seven remaining trials, in women 50 years or older, a 22% reduction in breast cancer mortality was found among women screened [95% confidence interval (CI), 13%–30%] at 14 years of observation.[2] In women 40 to 49 years of age, the summary risk reduction was 15% (95% CI, 1%–27%) at 14 years of observation.[2]

Cancer is detected in 5 to 7 of every 1,000 women on the initial mammogram and in 2 to 3 per 1,000 on each incidence (annual) screen,[3–5] with the incidence increasing with advancing age.[4] In one practice, cancer detection rates on screening mammography were 6 per 1,000 when breast imaging specialists performed the interpretation and only 3.4 per 1,000 when interpreted by generalists.[6]

Some of the reduction in breast cancer mortality after the introduction of mammographic screening is attributable to improved treatments. In an analysis of population-based service screening in Sweden, Tabar et al.[7] reported a 16% reduction in breast cancer mortality in the period 1978–1997 compared to the period 1958–1977 among women not screened, by 44% in all women 40 to 69 years of age who were screened with mammography, and by 48% in women 40 to 49 years of age who were not screened.

Randomized controlled trials have not demonstrated a mortality reduction from breast self-examination (BSE). The Shanghai trial of 133,000 Chinese women randomized to receive instruction in BSE or not, found no difference in mortality; indeed, women in the BSE group were 84% more likely to undergo an unnecessary benign breast biopsy.[8] Importantly, the combination of clinical breast examination (CBE, by the woman's care provider) and mammography is more effective in lowering breast cancer mortality than mammography alone.[9]

Despite its effectiveness in reducing mortality from breast cancer, mammography is less sensitive when the breast tissue is dense. Breast density is classified into four categories[10]: fatty (less than 25% dense); minimal scattered fibroglandular density (25%–49% dense); heterogeneously dense (50%–74% dense); and extremely dense (75% or more dense). Dense tissue is especially common in younger women. Stomper et al.[11] reviewed mammograms from 1,353 women and reported that approximately 62% of women in their thirties, 56% of women in their forties, 37% of women in their fifties, and 27% of women in their sixties had at least 50% parenchymal density on mammography. Kerlikowske et al.[12] reported results on 27,281 screening mammograms and found the sensitivity to cancer was 98.4% in women 50 years of age or older with fatty breasts and 83.7% in dense breasts ($P = 0.01$). In women under 50, the sensitivity was 81.8% in fatty breasts and 85.4% in dense breasts (NS), although the numbers of cancers were small.[12] In women under 50 with a family history of breast cancer, sensitivity decreased to 68.8%.[12] Mandelson et al.[13] reported sensitivity as low as 30% among women with extremely dense breasts in a Seattle screening mammography program. Among women with mutations in BRCA-1 or -2, mammography depicts fewer than half of cancers.[14–17] Thus, in women with dense breasts, and particularly those at increased risk because of a family or personal history of breast cancer or atypia, methods to supplement mammography are sought.

Screening does not assure a benefit to all women.[18] The most aggressive cancers are often not detectable at screening but have metastasized by the time they are clinically detected. Detecting breast cancer when it is small and node negative does not assure improved survival; some of these cancers will still metastasize. Tabar[1] noted that cancers manifested as branching, casting calcifications were often lethal even when less than 15 mm in size at detection. Women treated for breast cancer may still die of other causes; treatment can be unnecessary, particularly in older women as competing risks of death increase. Such "overtreatment" may even increase all-cause mortality.[19,20] Without treatment, the majority of DCIS will progress to invasive carcinoma, but this may occur over a period of 20 years or more.[21,22] Yen et al.[23] analyzed the results of the Swedish Two-County trial and estimate that at the first (prevalent) baseline screen, 37% of DCIS is nonprogressive, but at subsequent (incidence) screens, only 4% of new DCIS would not progress. This finding suggests that "overtreatment" may occur at the first (prevalent) screen with any given screening test but would be uncommon if the test were performed annually. In other words, cancers that are new on subsequent (incidence) screens are almost always biologically relevant. Randomized controlled trials with death as the endpoint are considered the gold standard for assessing the impact of any screening modality on survival.[24] Mammography is the only screening test to date that has been shown to reduce deaths due to breast cancer.

Supplemental screening with ultrasound (US) and magnetic resonance imaging (MRI), in addition to mammography, are being considered, particularly in women with heterogeneously dense or extremely dense (hereafter referred to as dense) breast tissue who are at high risk. Indeed, dense breast tissue itself is an indicator of elevated risk of 1.8- to 6-fold, averaging 4-fold across multiple series.[25] As recently reviewed,[26] in single-center studies of screening US totaling 42,838 examinations in average-risk women,[27–32] 150 cancers had been identified (3.5 per 1,000 exams) only sonographically in 126 women (Table 28.1). Of 126 women with sonographically depicted cancers, 114 (90.5%) had dense or heterogeneously dense parenchyma. Of the 150 cancers, 141 (94%) were invasive, and 99 (70%) were 1 cm or smaller in size. More than 90% were node negative. Although these results are encouraging, these studies were not blinded to results of mammography, and variable equipment, performance, and interpretive criteria were used. Publication of minimum equipment standards for breast US,[33] as well as a standardized lexicon for description of lesions and reporting

TABLE 28.1. Summary of studies of screening breast ultrasound, biopsies prompted by US, positive predictive value of biopsy, and prevalence of cancers seen only sonographically.

Investigator	*N*	*No. of biopsies*[a] *(%)*	*No. malignant (%)*[b]	*Prevalence (%)*
Gordon 1995[27]	12,706	279 (2.2)[c]	44/279 (16)	44/12,706 (0.35)[c]
Buchberger[28d]	8,103	362 (4.5)	32/362 (8.8)	32/8,103 (0.39)[e]
	867[d]	43	8/43 (19)	8/867 (0.9)[e]
Kaplan 2001[29]	1,862	102 (5.5)	6/91 (6.6)	6/1,862 (0.3)
Kolb 2002[30]	13,547[g]	358 (2.6)	37/358 (10)	37/13,547 (0.27)[g]
Crystal 2003[32]	1,517	38 (2.5)[h]	7/38 (18)	7/1,517 (0.46)[h]
Leconte 2003[31]	4,236[i]	NS[f]	16/NS	16/4,236 (0.38)
Overall	42,838	1,182/38,602 (3.1)	134/1,171 (11.4)	150/42,838 (0.35)

[a] Biopsies or aspirations prompted by screening sonography.

[b] Refers to cancers seen only on breast sonography, expressed as percent of biopsies (PPV).

[c] All women had clinical or mammographic abnormalities. Diagnosis was by fine-needle aspiration biopsy. Numbers refer to solid masses. Sixteen cancers were found in 15 women with ipsilateral cancer.

[d] In this series, 867 women were evaluated because of palpable or mammographic abnormalities; 5 cancers seen only on sonography were in patients with another mammographically or clinically evident cancer.

[e] Cancer was found only on sonography in 0.54% of women with a personal history of cancer compared to 0.26% of women with no personal history of cancer.

[f] NS, not stated.

[g] Includes patients described in 1998 series.[9] Number of studies, not women, as some women had more than one study. Cancer was found only on sonography in 0.48% of high-risk women compared to 0.16% of normal risk women.

[h] Cancer was found only on sonography in 4/318 (1.3%) women with first-degree family history or personal history of breast cancer and 3/1,199 (0.25%) women of average risk; biopsies includes 17 aspirations of which 13 yielded clear fluid.

[i] 1,016 had a personal history of breast cancer and 136 a palpable lesion (with the palpable lesions themselves excluded), although the number of cancers seen in women at high risk was not specified. Sixteen cancers were identified, but the number of biopsies induced by sonography was not specified: results of this study were not included in calculating the biopsy rate or the malignancy rate of biopsies.

Source: Adapted from Reference 26, with permission.

TABLE 28.2. Rates of detection of cancer by magnetic resonance imaging (MRI) only in women at high risk of breast cancer.

Investigator	*Mean age (years)*	*N (patients)*	*Bx*[a] *(%)*	*PPV*[b] *(%)*	*Cancers on MRI only (% of patients)*	*No. of DCIS only on MRI*[c] *(%)*	*MRI sensitivity*[d]	*MRI + mammography sensitivity*[d]	*Mammography sensitivity*[d]
Kuhl[39]*	39	192	14/293 (5)	9/14 (64)	6 (3)	1 (17)	9/9 (100)	9/9 (100)	3/9 (33)
Tilanus-Linthorst[140]	43	109	9 (8)	3/9 (33)	3 (3)	0 (0)	NA[e]	NA	NA
Stoutjesdijk[50]*	NS	179	30/258 (17)	13/30 (43)	6 (3)	2 (25)	13/13 (100)	13/13 (100)	6/13 (46)
Podo[41]	46	105	9 (9)	8/9 (89)	7 (7)	3 (43)	8/8 (100)	8/8 (100)	1/8 (13)
Leach[141]	<50	1,236	NS[e]	NS	15 (1)	NS	NS	NS	NS
Morris[142]	50	367	64/367 (17)	14/59 (24)	14 (4)	8 (57)	NA	NA	NA
Kriege[38]*	40	1,909[f]	56/4,169 (1.7)	32/56 (57)	20 (1)	1 (5)[d]	29/45 (64)[g]	41/45 (91)[g]	15/45 (33)[g]
Warner[143]*	47	236	37/457 (8.1)	17/37 (46)	7 (3)	2 (29)	17/22 (77)	19/22 (86)	8/22 (36)
Total	—	4,333	219/5,758 (3.8)	96/214 (45)	78 (1.8)	17/63 (27)	76/97 (78)	90/97 (93)	33/97 (34)

Numbers in parentheses represent percentages.

*Results of MRI and mammography were blinded to each other. Not stated in Leach et al.[141]

[a] Biopsies prompted by MRI per number of screenings.

[b] PPV, positive predictive value; number of malignancies of total number of biopsies.

[c] Of cancers seen only on MRI, number (%) that were ductal carcinoma in situ (DCIS).

[d] MRI and mammographic sensitivity reported only when results of MRI and other imaging modalities and clinical follow-up are described.

[e] NA, not applicable; all participants had negative mammography and clinical breast examination; NS, not stated.

[f] A total of 4,169 rounds of screening were performed. Of 6 DCIS lesions in this patient population, 5 were seen on mammography and only 1 on MRI.

[g] 41 cancers were classified as BI-RADS category 3 or higher on either mammography or MRI, with 3 cancers classified as BI-RADS 3 on each, but overlap not specified. Sensitivity numbers for each of MRI and mammography do not include category 3 lesions.

criteria,[34] will help decrease variability in this technique, although there remains a shortage of highly qualified radiologists and technologists. To better assess the generalizability of breast US, a 3-year multicenter trial of screening sonography in high-risk women, blinded to the results of mammography, opened in April 2004, funded by the Avon Foundation and National Cancer Institute through the American College of Radiology Imaging Network (ACRIN Protocol 6666; www.acrin.org).[35] The ACRIN protocol provides training materials for investigators, and standardizes equipment and interpretive criteria, to better assess generalizability of screening US. Sonography is widely available and inexpensive, and it is easy to accurately biopsy lesions seen only on sonography with core biopsy technique.[36]

Importantly, DCIS is not well seen on US: it should be seen as complementary to mammography. When results of mammography were also reported,[28,30,31] across 26,753 examinations another 56 cancers were seen only mammographically, of which 42 (75%) were DCIS and 14 (25%) were invasive.

Across eight published series (Table 28.2), 4,293 very high risk women have been screened with MRI, with 77 (1.8%) of women having cancer depicted only on MRI. The median size of cancers was 7 to 20 mm, and in all but one series, more than 80% of MRI-only depicted cancers had negative nodes.[37] Where detailed, 15 of 62 (24%) of the cancers seen only on MRI were DCIS (see Table 28.2). In the largest single series of MRI screening to date,[38] mammographic and MRI interpretations were blinded to each other, and 51 cancers were detected in 1,909 women. Sensitivity to invasive cancer was 33% for mammography and 80% for MRI, with specificities of 95% and 90%, respectively; sensitivity to DCIS was 83% for mammography and 17% for MRI.[38]

When both US and MRI have been performed in the same high-risk patients, MRI has shown superior sensitivity.[39–41] Liberman[42] summarized results across these series, which found 7 of 24 (29%) of cancers on mammography, 7 of 23 (30%) on US, and 23 of 24 (91%) on MRI. MRI is limited, however, by high cost, relative lack of availability, variable patient tolerance, the requirement for contrast injection, and relative lack of availability and expertise to biopsy lesions found only on MRI.

False Positives

False positives are a risk of any screening test. For mammography, Elmore et al.[43] estimated that after 10 annual screening mammograms, nearly 24% of women had had a false-positive result at least once, with a cumulative risk of a false-positive mammogram of 49.1%. Of women who did not have breast cancer, 18.6% underwent biopsy after 10 mammograms.[43] Short-interval follow-up of specific lesions, such as nonpalpable circumscribed masses and focal asymmetries has been validated,[44–46] with risk of malignancy less than 2% among appropriately classified lesions. Importantly, the prognosis is not adversely affected by short-interval follow-up in this setting.

Biopsy of benign lesions seen only sonographically, and induced short-interval follow-up, are risks of screening ultrasound. Across the five series where specifics are detailed,[27–30,32] after 38,602 screening sonograms, 1,137 (2.9%) resulted in biopsy and 134 (11.8%) biopsies showed malignancy. In the four series with details,[27,29,30,32] short-interval follow-up was recommended in another 6.6% of women. Criteria for classifying a lesion seen only sonographically as probably benign have been proposed[47,48] but require broader validation. Follow-up is generally performed only for nonpalpable lesions, although one recent study suggests the combination of benign-appearing features on both mammography and sonography may allow follow-up of even palpable lesions[49]; further validation of such an approach is required. It should be noted that in all but one series[30] only a single prevalence screen was performed: these rates of false positives are likely higher than would be seen on annual incidence screens.

With MRI, from 2% to 17% of women screened were recommended for biopsy based on MRI, and 24% to 89% of MRI-prompted biopsies proved malignant (see Table 28.2). Short-interval follow-up was recommended in 5% to 24% of women on the first screening round where specified[38,39,50–52] and decreased to 3% to 7% when results of subsequent screening rounds were detailed.[39,52] With MRI, the criteria for follow-up and risk of malignancy in lesions followed have not been widely studied. Liberman et al.[51] report 7% of lesions seen only on MRI that were followed proved malignant, and another 3% of patients developed cancer elsewhere in their breasts during short-interval follow-up. It is encouraging that, in the series of Kriege et al.,[38] 275 of 4,169 (6.6%) of examinations were recommended for short-interval follow-up, with only 3 of 275 (1.1%) of those proving malignant. MRI-guided core and vacuum-assisted biopsy are becoming more widely available[53,54] but require availability of scanner time and personnel. A facility that offers breast MRI should observe standardized technique and interpretive criteria[55] and offer MRI-guided biopsy.

Screening Guidelines

There is persuasive evidence that greater reductions in mortality result from annual screening compared with screening every 2 years, particularly in younger women.[2,56,57] Modeling data also suggest that shorter screening intervals are associated with fewer cases diagnosed with distant metastases[58] and smaller tumor size at detection. Further, smaller tumor size is highly correlated with survival time, independent of method of detection.[59] Annual mammography is therefore recommended for women beginning at age 40.[60,61] Screening should be continued as long as a woman is in good health, with at least 5-year life expectancy,[62] and as long as she would be a candidate for treatment.[60,61,63–65] If there is a first-degree relative with premenopausal breast cancer, annual screening should begin 10 years before the age of diagnosis of the relative.[66] Any woman with a personal history of cancer, atypia, or lobular carcinoma in situ should begin annual screening. Women who have had mantle irradiation to the chest, as for Hodgkin's disease, are at increased risk of breast cancer if the radiation was received before age 31, with increased rates of breast cancer beginning 8 years after the radiation treatment[67–69]: annual screening should begin 8 years after treatment if the radiation was before age 31.

As already discussed, there is moderate supporting evidence for supplemental screening with US or MRI in certain situations, although further study is warranted. Using MRI to screen women at high genetic risk of breast cancer is approved by the Blue Cross-Blue Shield Technology Evaluation Center (www.bluecares.com/tec/vol18/18_15.html). No data support the use of MRI to screen women at normal risk. US is more widely available and less expensive and has been shown to increase detection of cancers in women of average risk with dense breast tissue in single-center studies. Insurance does not generally cover screening US, and not all centers have the appropriate equipment or personnel to offer this service. A woman needs to understand the risk of false positives with any screening test. The detection of early breast cancer is critical in reducing mortality due to breast cancer, and both US and MRI depict early invasive breast cancers. Some DCIS is depicted on US and more on MRI, but mammography remains the standard for detection of DCIS. While the natural history of breast cancer should be independent of the method of detection, a survival benefit has not been proven for any screening test other than mammography.

Lump

Ultrasound is the initial test of choice in evaluating a lump in a young woman (under 30 years old).[70] The most common cause of a palpable mass in a woman under age 30 is a fibroadenoma.[71] A palpable, circumscribed, oval mass with no posterior features or minimal posterior enhancement is most likely a fibroadenoma. If such a mass, in a woman under 30 years of age, has clinically been known to the patient and stable for a period of at least 6 to 12 months, then follow-up is a reasonable alternative to biopsy. Because 15% of fibroadenomas are multiple, bilateral whole breast ultrasound is reasonable in initial imaging evaluation. Many women prefer excision of a palpable lump, and direct excision of a probable fibroadenoma is reasonable in a young woman. The finding of a sonographically suspicious mass should prompt bilateral mammographic evaluation to better define the extent of presumed malignancy. A clinically suspicious mass without a sonographic correlate merits further evaluation with mammography.

At age 30 and over, breast cancer is increasingly common, and mammography is the initial test of choice for symptomatic women. When a lump appears highly suggestive of malignancy on mammography, US is useful in guiding biopsy, with 95% sensitivity on initial core biopsy and no delayed false negatives.[36,72,73] A spot compression tangential mammographic view over a palpable mass can improve visibility of the mass and demonstrate overlying skin thickening or retraction.[74] Moderate evidence supports the use of US in addition to mammography in the evaluation of women with palpable masses or thickening (Table 28.3). In the multiinstitutional study of Georgian-Smith et al.,[75] 616 palpable lesions were evaluated sonographically and all 293 palpable cancers were depicted sonographically. Across several series (see Table 28.3), of 545 cancers in women with symptoms, 529 (97.1%) were depicted with the combination of mammography and US. A negative result after both mammographic and sonographic evaluation of a palpable abnormality is highly predictive of benign outcome, with 98.6% negative predictive value across these series.[75–79] Nevertheless, final management of a clinically suspicious mass must be based on clinical grounds.

TABLE 28.3. Sensitivity and negative predictive value (NPV) of combined mammography and US in symptomatic women.

	N (cancers)	Sensitivity	NPV	Purpose of study/patient population	Detection of misses	Cancers missed
Georgian-Smith et al. 2000[75]	293	293 (100)	Na	Palpable, sensitivity of US to cancers	Biopsy	None
Dennis et al. 2001[76]	0	Na	600/600 (100%)	Palpable, biopsy avoidance	Biopsy or 2-year follow-up	None
Moy et al. 2002[77]	6	0	227/233 (97.4)	Palpable	Tumor registry, 2-year follow-up	2 DCIS, 1 ILC, 3 IDC[a]
Kaiser et al. 2002[78]	6	6 (100)	117/117 (100%)	Thickening	Biopsy or 14-month follow-up	na
Houssami et al. 2003[79]	240	230 (95.8)[b]	174/184 (94.6)	Symptoms[b]	Tumor registry, 2-year follow-up	na
Overall	545	529 (97.1)	1,118/1,134 (98.6)			

[a] DCIS, ductal carcinoma in situ; ILC, invasive lobular carcinoma; IDC, invasive ductal carcinoma.

[b] In the series of Houssami et al.,[79] 157 women with cancer had a lump and 114 without cancer had a lump.

Nipple Discharge

Bloody nipple discharge and spontaneous unilateral clear nipple discharge merit imaging and clinical evaluation, with malignancy found in 13% of patients on average (range, 1% to 23%) across multiple series.[80] Papilloma is the most common cause of nipple discharge, found in 44% to 45% of patients,[80,81] with fibrocystic changes accounting for the rest. Milky discharge is almost always physiologic or due to hyperprolactinemia[80] and does not warrant imaging workup. Injection of contrast into the discharging duct, followed by magnification craniocaudal and true lateral mammographic views (galactography), has been the standard for imaging evaluation of nipple discharge.[82] US is an alternative method for evaluating nipple discharge and has the advantage of being noninvasive. A few studies have compared US and galactography (Table 28.4), with promising but limited evidence for the utility of US in this setting. The visualization of intraductal masses on US is facilitated by distension of the duct. Whether the full extent of multiple intraductal lesions is well depicted on US has not been systematically studied. MRI has also been used to evaluate nipple discharge with some success,[83] and further study is warranted.

Extent of Disease

From 73% to 98% of DCIS evident mammographically is manifest as microcalcifications.[84–86] The extent of calcifications on mammography can underestimate the area involved by DCIS, although Holland and Hendriks[87] showed this discrepancy was less than 2cm in 80% to 85% of cases. When the original tumor is manifest as calcifications mammographically, a postlumpectomy mammogram is advocated before radiation therapy, even when clear margins have been achieved.[88] Residual calcifications on postoperative mammograms do predict residual tumor, with 10 (71%) of 14 patients having residual DCIS in the series of Gluck et al.[89]

Several series have demonstrated a detection benefit of sonography after mammography and clinical examination in evaluating the preoperative extent of breast cancer (Table 28.5), particularly in dense breasts.[90] On average, 48% of breasts with cancer will have additional tumor foci not depicted on mammography or clinical examination.[91] If US is being used to guide biopsy, there is an advantage to at least scanning the quadrant containing the cancer, because 93% of additional tumor foci are within the same quadrant as the index lesion,[92] and more than 90% of malignant foci will be detected by combined mammography and US in this setting. When considering extent of disease, imaging of the contralateral breast should always be performed; 4% to 6% of patients are found to have unsuspected contralateral cancer on supplemental US or MRI.[90,93–95]

As with screening, MRI depicts additional tumor foci not seen on US, mammography, or clinical breast examination. Fischer et al.[93] reported results in a series of 463 patients, including 405 cancers, where preoperative mammography, clinical breast examination, sonography, and MR imaging had been performed: multifocality in 30 of 42 patients, multicentricity in 24 of 50 patients, and additional contralateral carcinomas in 15 of 19 patients were depicted with MR imaging alone. As a result of the MR imaging findings, therapy was

TABLE 28.4. Results of evaluation of nipple discharge with galactography and ultrasound (US).

	N	Detection of lesion at galactography (%)	Detection of lesion at US (%)	Detection by combined galactography and US (%)
Hild et al. 1998[144]	28 ducts with d/c with pathologic findings	19 (68)	26 (93)	28 (100)
Yang and Tse 2004[145]	12 DCIS	8/12 (75) successful, all positive	11 (92)	12 (100)
Overall	40	27/36 (75) where able to be performed	37 (93)	40 (100)

TABLE 28.5. Use of combined mammography and ultrasound (US) and magnetic resonance imaging (MRI) in evaluating local extent of breast cancer.

	N (cancers or breasts)	*Sensitivity mammography + US (%)*	*Detection of misses*	*Cancers missed on mammography + US*	*Sensitivity MRI alone (%)*
Fischer et al. 1999[93]	405 cancers	366[a] (90.4)	MRI	4 DCIS, 3 ILC, 32 IDC[a]	377 (93)
Berg et al. 2000[146]	64 cancers	62 (97)	Some surgery, details not specified	2 ILC	Not performed
Hlawatsch et al. 2002[96]	105 breasts with cancer	95 (90) accurate extent[b]	MRI	7 invasive NOS, 1 DCIS	97 (92)
Moon et al. 2002[147]	289 cancers	276 (95.5)[c]	Some surgery, details not specified	5 IDC, 1 ILC, 7 DCIS	Not performed
Berg et al. 2004[90]	96 breasts with cancer	81 (84)[c]	MRI, 2-year follow-up	7 DCIS, 6 IDC, 2 ILC	91 (95)
Berg et al. 2004[90]	177 cancers	162 (91.5)	MRI, 2-year follow-up	8 DCIS, 4 ILC, 3 IDC	167 (94)

[a] DCIS, ductal carcinoma in situ; ILC, invasive lobular carcinoma; IDC, invasive ductal carcinoma; NOS, not otherwise specified.

[b] Of 105 index lesions, 96 were identified on mammography and 9 only on US. Of 27 breasts with multifocal or multicentric tumor, 48% were identified on mammography, 63% with combined mammography + ultrasound (US), and 81% via magnetic resonance imaging (MRI).

[c] Includes clinical breast examination.

changed in 66 of 463 (14%) of patients.[93] In the series of Berg et al.,[90] of 96 breasts anticipating conservation after mammography and CBE, 30 (31%) were found to have additional tumor: 17 (57%) of those with greater extent were identified by supplemental US and 29 (97%) by MRI; however, disease was then overestimated by at least 2 cm or additional foci in 12 of 96 (13%) of breasts by US and 20 of 96 (21%) of breasts by MRI. After combined mammography, CBE, and US, MRI depicted additional tumor in another 12 of 96 (13%) of breasts and overestimated extent in another 6 (6%); US showed no detection benefit after MRI.[90] The impact of supplemental US or MRI in evaluating disease extent increases with increasing breast density.[90] In a study of 104 patients with cancer by Hlawatsch et al.,[96] US depicted additional tumor in 13 and produced 2 false positives; MRI depicted additional tumor in another 7 and produced 8 false positives.

In particular, an extensive intraductal component (EIC) is often underestimated without MRI.[90] The presence of an EIC correlates with increased risk of positive margins[97] and increased risk of recurrence.[98] Importantly, if clear margins are achieved, even when an EIC is present, Hurd et al.[99] failed to show an adverse effect on disease-free or overall survival or local control.

Initial detection and extent of invasive lobular carcinoma are also especially problematic on mammography as the single file cells typically infiltrate without associated calcifications or discrete mass. In the series of Butler et al.,[100] 81 of 208 (39%) of invasive lobular carcinomas were mammographically subtle or occult and 71 of 81 (88%) were well depicted sonographically. In several series,[91,101–103] MRI has been shown to be significantly more accurate than mammography, CBE, or US in determining the extent of invasive lobular carcinoma.

Although the frequency of residual tumor at pathology averages 48%,[91] the risk of recurrence after lumpectomy and radiation is generally 1% to 2% per year for the first 5 years, averaging 5% to 13% at 5 years.[104–106] Approximately half of this discrepancy may be attributed to cases that would have positive margins if lumpectomy were based on mammography and CBE[90]: supplemental imaging with MRI or US will decrease the need for reexcision. Of the other half with residual tumor, representing 20% to 25% of patients, roughly half of the residual tumor will be successfully treated with radiation and/or chemotherapy.[107] Distinction of those who will benefit from preoperative additional imaging with US or MRI from those who will undergo unnecessary additional surgery and even mastectomy for tumor that would have resolved in conventional treatment, is not clear at this time, although those with invasive lobular cancer, an EIC, and/or dense breasts appear to be more likely to benefit.

US is insensitive to DCIS, as described, as DCIS is often manifest as microcalcifications. US is not particularly sensitive to lesions manifest solely as calcifications due to their small size and similarity to speckle artifact present in tissue. Nevertheless, US can help identify the invasive component of malignant calcifications. Soo et al.[108] evaluated 111 cases of suspicious calcifications and only 26 (23%) could be seen sonographically. Of those seen on US, 69% were malignant compared to only 21% of those not seen on US.[108] Those cancers seen on US were more likely invasive (72% versus 28%), and underestimation of disease was less common when biopsies were performed with US guidance than stereotactic guidance. Similarly, Moon et al.[109] showed 45 of 100 (45%) of suspicious microcalcifications were sonographically visible, including 31 of 38 (82%) of malignant calcifications and 14 of 62 (23%) of benign calcifications.

MRI is particularly indicated in cases of breast cancer presenting as an axillary metastasis.[110,111] Identification of the primary usually allows breast conservation. In patients with positive margins at initial excision, MRI is also appropriate to assess for residual tumor.[112,113] There is no need to delay imaging in this setting, as was suggested by Frei et al.,[114] as excision of the area immediately around the lumpectomy site will be performed in any event and false positives due to granulation tissue at the lumpectomy site are not of particular clinical import. The purpose of MRI in the setting of positive margins is to evaluate the rest of the breast(s) and determine the possible need for mastectomy versus wider excision.

In patients with locally advanced breast cancer, in whom neoadjuvant chemotherapy is planned, strong evidence supports the use of MRI in accurately sizing and evaluating the extent of tumor before and after treatment to assess response and plan appropriate surgery.[115–117] A multicenter trial is currently under way to further evaluate the use of MRI in this setting (ACRIN Protocol 6652, www.acrin.org). Chest wall invasion can accurately be determined by MRI.[118]

Positron emission tomography (PET) using ^{18}F-deoxyglucose (FDG) can predict response to treatment within as little as 8 days.[119] After a single course of treatment, Schelling et al.[120] correctly identified all responders by a decrease in the standardized uptake value to below 55% of baseline. At that threshold, histopathologic response was predicted with an accuracy of 88% after the first course of treatment and 91% after the second course. It has been suggested, therefore, that ineffective chemotherapy as determined by PET might be discontinued and new treatments instituted.[120] Further study of PET in this context is warranted.

Axillary Node Status

Unfortunately, no reliable noninvasive imaging method has been developed that accurately predicts axillary or internal mammary nodal status. Most lymph nodes are not included on mammographic imaging. In the setting of a known breast cancer, loss of the fatty hilum or indistinct borders to a node seen mammographically can suggest metastatic nodal involvement.[121] Mammographically spiculated borders of axillary nodes in the patient with breast cancer predict extranodal extension and poor prognosis.[122] Isolated nodal enlargement without a known cancer is usually due to benign, reactive conditions.[121] When a metastatic node is identified and the primary cannot be found clinically or mammographically, MR imaging has been shown to be highly efficacious, depicting the occult primary in 70% to 75% of patients[110,123,124] and thereby facilitating breast conservation.[125]

On sonography, loss of the fatty hilum, an irregularly thickened cortex, indistinct margins, and a long-to-short-axis ratio less than 1.5 suggest metastatic involvement,[126] although the accuracy of this approach is not well established.

Enhancement of lymph nodes in the axilla and internal mammary chains is frequently seen on MR imaging. Using a threshold of greater than 100% increase in signal intensity on the first postcontrast series, Kvistad et al.[127] showed a sensitivity of 83% to axillary metastases, specificity of 90%, and accuracy of 88%. Similar results were found by Yoshimura et al.[128]: using morphologic parameters of long-axis dimension greater than 1 cm and long-to-short-axis ratio less than 1.6, they found a sensitivity of 79%, specificity of 93%, and accuracy of 88% in identifying metastatic axillary nodes on MR imaging. When a suspicious node is identified on MRI or US, fine-needle aspiration can confirm the presence of metastatic adenopathy preoperatively, allowing full axillary dissection at the time of treatment surgery.[129]

Current staging of breast cancer includes identification of the presence of micrometastases (less than 2 mm) in the sentinel node (first draining lymph node). As such, the challenge of imaging is to equal that level of sensitivity and to detect foci of metastatic disease ranging from 2 mm down to even a few cells. This is below the threshold of morphologic imaging. Uptake of FDG in axillary lymph nodes can be used to identify metastatic disease. When the status of the axilla as a whole is considered, across seven single-center studies,[130] whole-body PET with FDG successfully predicted the status in 113 of 132 (86%) of axillae with metastatic disease by hematoxylin and eosin (H&E) staining. Another 143 of 174 (82%) of negative axillae were correctly predicted.

Results from a prospective multicenter study were recently published[131] evaluating PET in axillary nodal staging in 308 assessable axillae, 109 (35%) of which had tumor involvement. The mean sensitivity was 61% (range, 54% to 67%), positive predictive value (PPV) 62% (range, 60% to 64%), and negative predictive value (NPV) 79% (range, 76% to 81%).[131] The average sensitivity was lower when there was only one tumor-involved node in the axilla (46%) than when more than one node was involved (64%, $P = 0.005$).[131] Lower sensitivity was seen for metastases from invasive lobular carcinoma (25%) than from invasive ductal carcinoma (64%, P less than 0.005).[131] At this time, PET does not appear to be sufficiently accurate to triage patients to full axillary dissection versus sentinel lymph node biopsy.[132,133]

Metastatic Disease and Recurrence

The differentiation of scar from recurrent tumor can be problematic on mammography and US. MRI may be helpful in this setting, although further study is warranted. Heywang-Kobrunner et al.[134] found that in 30 of 32 (94%) cases postsurgical scar did not enhance beyond 18 months after surgery, although delayed development of enhancement in fat necrosis can occur.[135]

PET is approved for restaging breast cancer and evaluating for recurrence. Bender et al.[136] found all 16 local recurrences and 28 axillary nodal recurrences in their series using FDG-PET. Further study of this issue is needed. Moon et al.[137] assessed the accuracy of whole-body PET for detection of recurrent or metastatic breast cancer in 57 patients. Sensitivity for individual lesions was 85% and specificity was 79%.[137] Muscle uptake and inflammation were sources of false positives. Bone metastases are a common source of false negatives.[137] Indeed, FDG-PET and bone scintigraphy have been shown to be complementary in the detection of bone metastases, with lytic metastases well depicted by PET and blastic metastases by bone scintigraphy.[138] FDG-PET has no role in detection of brain metastases because of the high normal uptake of FDG in the brain.

Summary

Screening mammography remains the standard. In high-risk women, supplemental screening with MRI is being considered, and further study is warranted. In women of average risk with dense breast tissue, single-center studies support elective supplemental screening with ultrasound, and further study is both needed and ongoing.

At this time, indications for ultrasound include the following:

Initial evaluation of a breast lump in a woman less than 30 years of age. (Note: Mammography should also be performed if the sonogram is suspicious or if there is strong clinical suspicion and the sonogram is negative.)

Evaluation and biopsy guidance of a clinically suspicious lump in a woman of any age.
Evaluation and biopsy guidance of lesions manifest as highly suspicious microcalcifications over a large (greater than 2 cm) area, to identify any associated mass that may represent an invasive component.
Evaluation of bloody or spontaneous clear nipple discharge.
Evaluation of both breasts in women with newly diagnosed breast cancer and dense breast tissue.

Indications for contrast-enhanced breast MRI include the following:

Metastatic axillary node with unknown primary.
Evaluation of the local extent of breast cancer bilaterally, particularly if the breasts are dense, tumor is invasive lobular, or there is suspicion for extensive intraductal component.
Positive margins after lumpectomy.
Initial sizing and assessment of response to neoadjuvant chemotherapy
Suspicious abnormality on mammography, one view only, not able to be localized for biopsy after full workup with additional views and ultrasound.[139]

References

1. Tabar L, Vitak B, Chen HH, et al. The Swedish Two-County Trial twenty years later. Updated mortality results and new insights from long-term follow-up. Radiol Clin N Am 2000;38(4):625–651.
2. Humphrey LL, Helfand M, Chan BK, Woolf SH. Breast cancer screening: a summary of the evidence for the U.S. Preventive Services Task Force. Ann Intern Med 2002;137(5 part 1):347–360.
3. Thurfjell EL, Lindgren JA. Population-based mammography screening in Swedish clinical practice: prevalence and incidence screening in Uppsala County. Radiology 1994;193(2):351–357.
4. Kan L, Olivotto IA, Warren Burhenne LJ, Sickles EA, Coldman AJ. Standardized abnormal interpretation and cancer detection ratios to assess reading volume and reader performance in a breast screening program. Radiology 2000;215(2):563–567.
5. Sohlich RE, Sickles EA, Burnside ES, Dee KE. Interpreting data from audits when screening and diagnostic mammography outcomes are combined. AJR Am J Roentgenol 2002;178(3):681–686.
6. Sickles EA, Wolverton DE, Dee KE. Performance parameters for screening and diagnostic mammography: specialist and general radiologists. Radiology 2002;224(3):861–869.
7. Tabar L, Yen MF, Vitak B, Chen HH, Smith RA, Duffy SW. Mammography service screening and mortality in breast cancer patients: 20-year follow-up before and after introduction of screening. Lancet 2003;361(9367):1405–1410.
8. Thomas DB, Gao DL, Ray RM, et al. Randomized trial of breast self-examination in Shanghai: final results. J Natl Cancer Inst 2002;94(19):1445–1457.
9. Alexander FE, Anderson TJ, Brown HK, et al. 14 years of follow-up from the Edinburgh randomised trial of breast-cancer screening. Lancet 1999;353(9168):1903–1908.
10. American College of Radiology. Illustrated Breast Imaging Reporting and Data System (BI-RADS): Mammography, 4th ed. Reston, VA: American College of Radiology, 2003.
11. Stomper PC, D'Souza DJ, DiNitto PA, Arredondo MA. Analysis of parenchymal density on mammograms in 1353 women 25–79 years old. AJR Am J Roentgenol 1996;167(5):1261–1265.
12. Kerlikowske K, Grady D, Barclay J, Sickles EA, Ernster V. Effect of age, breast density, and family history on the sensitivity of first screening mammography [see comments]. JAMA 1996; 276(1):33–38
13. Mandelson MT, Oestreicher N, Porter PL, et al. Breast density as a predictor of mammographic detection: comparison of interval- and screen-detected cancers. J Natl Cancer Inst 2000;92(13): 1081–1087.
14. Meijers-Heijboer H, van Geel B, van Putten WL, et al. Breast cancer after prophylactic bilateral mastectomy in women with a BRCA1 or BRCA2 mutation. N Engl J Med 2001;345(3):159–164.
15. Brekelmans CT, Seynaeve C, Bartels CC, et al. Effectiveness of breast cancer surveillance in BRCA1/2 gene mutation carriers and women with high familial risk. J Clin Oncol 2001;19(4):924–930
16. Scheuer L, Kauff N, Robson M, et al. Outcome of preventive surgery and screening for breast and ovarian cancer in BRCA mutation carriers. J Clin Oncol 2002;20(5):1260–1268.
17. Komenaka IK, Ditkoff BA, Joseph KA, et al. The development of interval breast malignancies in patients with BRCA mutations. Cancer (Phila) 2004;100(10):2079–2083.
18. Welch HG. Informed choice in cancer screening. JAMA 2001; 285(21):2776–2778.
19. Gotzsche PC, Olsen O. Is screening for breast cancer with mammography justifiable? Lancet 2000;355(9198):129–134.
20. Olsen O, Gotzsche PC. Cochrane review on screening for breast cancer with mammography. Lancet 2001;358(9290):1340–1342.
21. Page DL, Lagios MD. Pathology and clinical evolution of ductal carcinoma in situ (DCIS) of the breast. Cancer Lett 1994;86(1):1–4.
22. Feig SA. Ductal carcinoma in situ. Implications for screening mammography. Radiol Clin N Am 2000;38(4):653–668, vii.
23. Yen MF, Tabar L, Vitak B, Smith RA, Chen HH, Duffy SW. Quantifying the potential problem of overdiagnosis of ductal carcinoma in situ in breast cancer screening. Eur J Cancer 2003; 39(12):1746–1754.
24. Kopans DB, Monsees B, Feig SA. Screening for cancer: when is it valid? Lessons from the mammography experience. Radiology 2003;229(2):319–327.
25. Harvey JA, Bovbjerg VE. Quantitative assessment of mammographic breast density: relationship with breast cancer risk. Radiology 2004;230(1):29–41.
26. Berg WA. Supplemental screening sonography in dense breasts. Radiol Clin N Am 2004;42(5):845–851.
27. Gordon PB, Goldenberg S. Malignant breast masses detected only by ultrasound. A retrospective review [see comments]. Cancer (Phila) 1995;76(4):626–630.
28. Buchberger W, Niehoff A, Obrist P, DeKoekkoek-Doll P, Dunser M. Clinically and mammographically occult breast lesions: detection and classification with high-resolution sonography. Semin Ultrasound CT MR 2000;21(4):325–336.
29. Kaplan SS. Clinical utility of bilateral whole-breast US in the evaluation of women with dense breast tissue. Radiology 2001; 221(3):641–649.
30. Kolb TM, Lichy J, Newhouse JH. Comparison of the performance of screening mammography, physical examination, and breast US and evaluation of factors that influence them: an analysis of 27,825 patient evaluations. Radiology 2002;225(1):165–175.
31. Leconte I, Feger C, Galant C, et al. Mammography and subsequent whole-breast sonography of nonpalpable breast cancers: the importance of radiologic breast density. AJR Am J Roentgenol 2003;180(6):1675–1679.
32. Crystal P, Strano SD, Shcharynski S, Koretz MJ. Using sonography to screen women with mammographically dense breasts. AJR Am J Roentgenol 2003;181(1):177–182.
33. American College of Radiology. ACR Standards 2000–2001. Reston, VA: American College of Radiology, 2000.
34. American College of Radiology. Illustrated Breast Imaging Reporting and Data System (BI-RADS): Ultrasound, 4th ed. Reston, VA: American College of Radiology, 2003.

35. Berg WA. Rationale for a trial of screening breast ultrasound: American College of Radiology Imaging Network (ACRIN) 6666. AJR Am J Roentgenol 2003;180:1225–1228.
36. Berg WA. Image-guided breast biopsy and management of high-risk lesions. Radiol Clin N Am 2004;42(5):935–946, vii.
37. Morris EA. Screening breast MRI in high-risk women. In: Berg WAJ (ed). Women's Imaging: Strategies for Clinical Practice: Categorical Course Syllabus. Leesburg, VA: American Roentgen Ray Society, 2004:139–144.
38. Kriege M, Brekelmans CT, Boetes C, et al. Efficacy of MRI and mammography for breast-cancer screening in women with a familial or genetic predisposition. N Engl J Med 2004;351(5):427–437.
39. Kuhl CK, Schmutzler RK, Leutner CC, et al. Breast MR imaging screening in 192 women proved or suspected to be carriers of a breast cancer susceptibility gene: preliminary results. Radiology 2000;215(1):267–279.
40. Warner E, Plewes DB, Shumak RS, et al. Comparison of breast magnetic resonance imaging, mammography, and ultrasound for surveillance of women at high risk for hereditary breast cancer. J Clin Oncol 2001;19(15):3524–3531.
41. Podo F, Sardanelli F, Canese R, et al. The Italian multi-centre project on evaluation of MRI and other imaging modalities in early detection of breast cancer in subjects at high genetic risk. J Exp Clin Cancer Res 2002;21(suppl 3):115–124.
42. Liberman L. Breast cancer screening with MRI: what are the data for patients at high risk? N Engl J Med 2004;351(5):497–500.
43. Elmore JG, Barton MB, Moceri VM, Polk S, Arena PJ, Fletcher SW. Ten-year risk of false positive screening mammograms and clinical breast examinations. N Engl J Med 1998;338(16):1089–1096.
44. Sickles EA. Nonpalpable, circumscribed, noncalcified solid breast masses: likelihood of malignancy based on lesion size and age of patient. Radiology 1994;192:439–442.
45. Vizcaino I, Gadea L, Andreo L, et al. Short-term follow-up results in 795 nonpalpable probably benign lesions detected at screening mammography. Radiology 2001;219(2):475–483.
46. Varas X, Leborgne JH, Leborgne F, Mezzera J, Jaumandreu S. Revisiting the mammographic follow-up of BI-RADS category 3 lesions. AJR Am J Roentgenol 2002;179(3):691–695.
47. Stavros AT, Thickman D, Rapp CL, Dennis MA, Parker SH, Sisney GA. Solid breast nodules: use of sonography to distinguish between benign and malignant lesions. Radiology 1995;196:123–134.
48. Berg WA. Breast ultrasonography: cystic lesions and probably benign findings. In: Berg WA (ed). Women's Imaging: Strategies for Clinical Practice. Categorical Course Syllabus. Leesburg, VA: American Roentgen Ray Society, 2004:95–102.
49. Graf O, Helbich TH, Fuchsjaeger MH, et al. Follow-up of palpable, circumscribed, non-calcified solid breast masses with mammography and ultrasound: can biopsy be averted? Radiology 2004;233:850–856.
50. Stoutjesdijk MJ, Boetes C, Jager GJ, et al. Magnetic resonance imaging and mammography in women with a hereditary risk of breast cancer. J Natl Cancer Inst 2001;93(14):1095–1102.
51. Liberman L, Morris EA, Benton CL, Abramson AF, Dershaw DD. Probably benign lesions at breast magnetic resonance imaging: preliminary experience in high-risk women. Cancer (Phila) 2003;98(2):377–388.
52. Warner E, Plewes DB, Hill KA, et al. Surveillance of BRCA1 and BRCA2 mutation carriers with magnetic resonance imaging, ultrasound, mammography, and clinical breast examination. JAMA 2004;292(11):1317–1325.
53. Perlet C, Schneider P, Amaya B, et al. MR-Guided vacuum biopsy of 206 contrast-enhancing breast lesions. Rofo Fortschr Geb Rontgenstr Neuen Bildgeb Verfahr 2002;174(1):88–95.
54. Liberman L, Morris EA, Dershaw DD, Thornton CM, Van Zee KJ, Tan LK. Fast MRI-guided vacuum-assisted breast biopsy: initial experience. AJR Am J Roentgenol 2003;181(5):1283–1293.
55. American College of Radiology. Illustrated Breast Imaging Reporting and Data System (BI-RADS): Magnetic Resonance Imaging. Reston, VA: American College of Radiology, 2003.
56. Andersson I, Janzon L. Reduced breast cancer mortality in women under age 50: updated results from the Malmo Mammographic Screening Program. J Natl Cancer Inst Monogr 1997;22:63–67.
57. Bjurstam N, Bjorneld L, Duffy SW, et al. The Gothenburg breast screening trial: first results on mortality, incidence, and mode of detection for women ages 39–49 years at randomization. Cancer (Phila) 1997;80(11):2091–2099.
58. Michaelson JS, Halpern E, Kopans DB. Breast cancer: computer simulation method for estimating optimal intervals for screening. Radiology 1999;212(2):551–560.
59. Michaelson JS, Silverstein M, Wyatt J, et al. Predicting the survival of patients with breast carcinoma using tumor size. Cancer (Phila) 2002;95(4):713–723.
60. Smith RA, Saslow D, Sawyer KA, et al. American Cancer Society guidelines for breast cancer screening: update 2003. CA Cancer J Clin 2003;53(3):141–169.
61. Smith RA, Cokkinides V, Eyre HJ. American Cancer Society guidelines for the early detection of cancer, 2004. CA Cancer J Clin 2004;54(1):41–52.
62. Walter LC, Covinsky KE. Cancer screening in elderly patients: a framework for individualized decision making. JAMA 2001;285(21):2750–2756.
63. Yancik R, Wesley MN, Ries LA, Havlik RJ, Edwards BK, Yates JW. Effect of age and comorbidity in postmenopausal breast cancer patients aged 55 years and older. JAMA 2001;285(7):885–892.
64. McPherson CP, Swenson KK, Lee MW. The effects of mammographic detection and comorbidity on the survival of older women with breast cancer. J Am Geriatr Soc 2002;50(6):1061–1068.
65. Mandelblatt J, Saha S, Teutsch S, et al. The cost-effectiveness of screening mammography beyond age 65 years: a systematic review for the U.S. Preventive Services Task Force. Ann Intern Med 2003;139(10):835–842.
66. Dershaw DD. Mammographic screening of the high-risk woman. Am J Surg 2000;180(4):288–289.
67. Hancock SL, Tucker MA, Hoppe RT. Breast cancer after treatment of Hodgkin's disease. J Natl Cancer Inst 1993;85(1):25–31.
68. Aisenberg AC, Finkelstein DM, Doppke KP, Koerner FC, Boivin JF, Willett CG. High risk of breast carcinoma after irradiation of young women with Hodgkin's disease. Cancer (Phila) 1997;79(6):1203–1210.
69. Clemons M, Loijens L, Goss P. Breast cancer risk following irradiation for Hodgkin's disease. Cancer Treat Rev 2000;26(4):291–302.
70. Bassett LW. Imaging of breast masses. Radiol Clin N Am 2000;38(4):669–691.
71. Bartow SA, Pathak DR, Black WC, Key CR, Teaf SR. Prevalence of benign, atypical, and malignant breast lesions in populations at different risk for breast cancer. A forensic autopsy study. Cancer (Phila) 1987;60(11):2751–2760.
72. Parker SH, Jobe WE, Dennis MA, et al. US-guided automated large-core breast biopsy. Radiology 1993;187(2):507–511.
73. Liberman L, Feng TL, Dershaw DD, Morris EA, Abramson AF. US-guided core breast biopsy: use and cost-effectiveness. Radiology 1998;208(3):717–723.
74. Sickles EA. Practical solutions to common mammographic problems: tailoring the examination. AJR Am J Roentgenol 1988;151(1):31–39.
75. Georgian-Smith D, Taylor KJ, Madjar H, et al. Sonography of palpable breast cancer. J Clin Ultrasound 2000;28(5):211–216.

76. Dennis MA, Parker SH, Klaus AJ, Stavros AT, Kaske TI, Clark SB. Breast biopsy avoidance: the value of normal mammograms and normal sonograms in the setting of a palpable lump. Radiology 2001;219(1):186–191.
77. Moy L, Slanetz PJ, Moore R, et al. Specificity of mammography and US in the evaluation of a palpable abnormality: retrospective review. Radiology 2002;225(1):176–181.
78. Kaiser JS, Helvie MA, Blacklaw RL, Roubidoux MA. Palpable breast thickening: role of mammography and US in cancer detection. Radiology 2002;223(3):839–844.
79. Houssami N, Irwig L, Simpson JM, McKessar M, Blome S, Noakes J. Sydney Breast Imaging Accuracy Study: comparative sensitivity and specificity of mammography and sonography in young women with symptoms. AJR Am J Roentgenol 2003; 180(4):935–940.
80. Paterok EM, Rosenthal H, Sabel M. Nipple discharge and abnormal galactogram. Results of a long-term study (1964–1990). Eur J Obstet Gynecol Reprod Biol 1993;50(3):227–234.
81. Leis HP Jr, Greene FL, Cammarata A, Hilfer SE. Nipple discharge: surgical significance. South Med J 1988;81(1):20–26.
82. Cardenosa G, Doudna C, Eklund GW. Ductography of the breast: technique and findings. AJR Am J Roentgenol 1994;162(5):1081–1087.
83. Orel SG, Dougherty CS, Reynolds C, Czerniecki BJ, Siegelman ES, Schnall MD. MR imaging in patients with nipple discharge: initial experience. Radiology 2000;216(1):248–254.
84. Ikeda DM, Andersson I. Ductal carcinoma in situ: atypical mammographic appearances. Radiology 1989;172(3):661–666.
85. Stomper PC, Margolin FR. Ductal carcinoma in situ: the mammographer's perspective. AJR Am J Roentgenol 1994;162(3):585–591.
86. Dershaw DD, Abramson A, Kinne DW. Ductal carcinoma in situ: mammographic findings and clinical implications. Radiology 1989;170(2):411–415.
87. Holland R, Hendriks JH. Microcalcifications associated with ductal carcinoma in situ: mammographic-pathologic correlation. Semin Diagn Pathol 1994;11(3):181–192.
88. Aref A, Youssef E, Washington T, et al. The value of postlumpectomy mammogram in the management of breast cancer patients presenting with suspiciouis microcalcifications. Cancer J Sci Am 2000;6(1):25–27.
89. Gluck BS, Dershaw DD, Liberman L, Deutch BM. Microcalcifications on postoperative mammograms as an indicator of adequacy of tumor excision. Radiology 1993;188(2):469–472.
90. Berg WA, Gutierrez L, NessAiver M, et al. Diagnostic accuracy of mammography, clinical breast examination, ultrasound, and magnetic resonance imaging in preoperative assessment of the local extent of breast cancer. Radiology 2004;233(3):830–849.
91. Liberman L, Morris EA, Dershaw DD, Abramson AF, Tan LK. MR imaging of the ipsilateral breast in women with percutaneously proven breast cancer. AJR Am J Roentgenol 2003; 180(4):901–910.
92. Holland R, Veling SH, Mravunac M, Hendriks JH. Histologic multifocality of Tis, T1–2 breast carcinomas. Implications for clinical trials of breast-conserving surgery. Cancer (Phila) 1985; 56(5):979–990.
93. Fischer U, Kopka L, Grabbe E. Breast carcinoma: effect of preoperative contrast-enhanced MR imaging on the therapeutic approach. Radiology 1999;213(3):881–888.
94. Lee SG, Orel SG, Woo IJ, et al. MR imaging screening of the contralateral breast in patients with newly diagnosed breast cancer: preliminary results. Radiology 2003;226(3):773–778.
95. Liberman L, Morris EA, Kim CM, et al. MR imaging findings in the contralateral breast of women with recently diagnosed breast cancer. AJR Am J Roentgenol 2003;180(2):333–341.
96. Hlawatsch A, Teifke A, Schmidt M, Thelen M. Preoperative assessment of breast cancer: sonography versus MR imaging. AJR Am J Roentgenol 2002;179(6):1493–1501.
97. Wazer DE, Schmidt-Ullrich RK, Schmid CH, et al. The value of breast lumpectomy margin assessment as a predictor of residual tumor burden. Int J Radiat Oncol Biol Phys 1997;38(2):291–299.
98. Fourquet A, Campana F, Zafrani B, et al. Prognostic factors of breast recurrence in the conservative management of early breast cancer: a 25-year follow-up. Int J Radiat Oncol Biol Phys 1989;17(4):719–725.
99. Hurd TC, Sneige N, Allen PK, et al. Impact of extensive intraductal component on recurrence and survival in patients with stage I or II breast cancer treated with breast conservation therapy. Ann Surg Oncol 1997;4(2):119–124.
100. Butler RS, Venta LA, Wiley EL, Ellis RL, Dempsey PJ, Rubin E. Sonographic evaluation of infiltrating lobular carcinoma. AJR Am J Roentgenol 1999;172(2):325–330.
101. Rodenko GN, Harms SE, Pruneda JM, et al. MR imaging in the management before surgery of lobular carcinoma of the breast: correlation with pathology. AJR Am J Roentgenol 1996;167(6): 1415–1419.
102. Weinstein SP, Orel SG, Heller R, et al. MR imaging of the breast in patients with invasive lobular carcinoma. AJR Am J Roentgenol 2001;176(2):399–406.
103. Bedrosian I, Mick R, Orel SG, et al. Changes in the surgical management of patients with breast carcinoma based on preoperative magnetic resonance imaging. Cancer (Phila) 2003; 98(3):468–473.
104. Fisher ER, Anderson S, Tan-Chiu E, Fisher B, Eaton L, Wolmark N. Fifteen-year prognostic discriminants for invasive breast carcinoma. Cancer (Phila) 2001;91(S8):1679–1687.
105. Fisher B, Dignam J, Wolmark N, et al. Lumpectomy and radiation therapy for the treatment of intraductal breast cancer: findings from National Surgical Adjuvant Breast and Bowel Project B-17. J Clin Oncol 1998;16(2):441–452.
106. Bartelink H, Horiot J-C, Poortmans P. Recurrence rates after treatment of breast cancer with standard radiotherapy with or without additional radiation. N Engl J Med 2001;345:1378–1387.
107. Broet P, de la Rochefordiere A, Scholl SM, et al. Contralateral breast cancer: annual incidence and risk parameters. J Clin Oncol 1995;13(7):1578–1583.
108. Soo MS, Baker JA, Rosen EL. Sonographic detection and sonographically guided biopsy of breast microcalcifications. AJR Am J Roentgenol 2003;180(4):941–948.
109. Moon WK, Myung JS, Lee YJ, Park IA, Noh DY, Im JG. US of ductal carcinoma in situ. Radiographics 2002;22(2):269–280; discussion 280–281.
110. Orel SG, Weinstein SP, Schnall MD, et al. Breast MR imaging in patients with axillary node metastases and unknown primary malignancy. Radiology 1999;212(2):543–549.
111. Chen C, Orel SG, Harris E, Schnall MD, Czerniecki BJ, Solin LJ. Outcome after treatment of patients with mammographically occult, magnetic resonance imaging-detected breast cancer presenting with axillary lymphadenopathy. Clin Breast Cancer 2004;5(1):72–77.
112. Soderstrom CE, Harms SE, Farrell RS Jr, Pruneda JM, Flamig DP. Detection with MR imaging of residual tumor in the breast soon after surgery [see comments]. AJR Am J Roentgenol 1997;168(2): 485–488.
113. Lee JM, Orel SG, Czerniecki BJ, Solin LJ, Schnall MD. MRI before reexcision surgery in patients with breast cancer. AJR Am J Roentgenol 2004;182(2):473–480.
114. Frei KA, Kinkel K, Bonel HM, Lu Y, Esserman LJ, Hylton NM. MR imaging of the breast in patients with positive margins after lumpectomy: influence of the time interval between lumpectomy and MR imaging. AJR Am J Roentgenol 2000;175(6):1577–1584.
115. Abraham DC, Jones RC, Jones SE, et al. Evaluation of neoadjuvant chemotherapeutic response of locally advanced breast cancer by magnetic resonance imaging. Cancer (Phila) 1996; 78(1):91–100.

116. Rieber A, Brambs HJ, Gabelmann A, Heilmann V, Kreienberg R, Kuhn T. Breast MRI for monitoring response of primary breast cancer to neo-adjuvant chemotherapy. Eur Radiol 2002;12(7):1711–1719.

117. Partridge SC, Gibbs JE, Lu Y, Esserman LJ, Sudilovsky D, Hylton NM. Accuracy of MR imaging for revealing residual breast cancer in patients who have undergone neoadjuvant chemotherapy. AJR Am J Roentgenol 2002;179(5):1193–1199.

118. Morris EA, Schwartz LH, Drotman MB, et al. Evaluation of pectoralis major muscle in patients with posterior breast tumors on breast MR images: early experience. Radiology 2000;214(1):67–72.

119. Wahl RL, Zasadny K, Helvie M, Hutchins GD, Weber B, Cody R. Metabolic monitoring of breast cancer chemohormonotherapy using positron emission tomography: initial evaluation. J Clin Oncol 1993;11(11):2101–2111.

120. Schelling M, Avril N, Nahrig J, et al. Positron emission tomography using [^{18}F]fluorodeoxyglucose for monitoring primary chemotherapy in breast cancer. J Clin Oncol 2000;18(8):1689–1695.

121. Dershaw DD. Isolated enlargement of intramammary lymph nodes. AJR Am J Roentgenol 1996;166(6):1491.

122. Dershaw DD, Selland DG, Tan LK, Morris EA, Abramson AF, Liberman L. Spiculated axillary adenopathy. Radiology 1996;201(2):439–442.

123. Mahfouz AE, Sherif H, Saad A, et al. Gadolinium-enhanced MR angiography of the breast: is breast cancer associated with ipsilateral higher vascularity? Eur Radiol 2001;11(6):965–969.

124. Morris EA, Schwartz LH, Dershaw DD, van Zee KJ, Abramson AF, Liberman L. MR imaging of the breast in patients with occult primary breast carcinoma. Radiology 1997;205(2):437–440.

125. Olson JA Jr, Morris EA, Van Zee KJ, Linehan DC, Borgen PI. Magnetic resonance imaging facilitates breast conservation for occult breast cancer. Ann Surg Oncol 2000;7(6):411–415.

126. Feu J, Tresserra F, Fabregas R, et al. Metastatic breast carcinoma in axillary lymph nodes: in vitro US detection. Radiology 1997;205(3):831–835.

127. Kvistad KA, Rydland J, Smethurst HB, Lundgren S, Fjosne HE, Haraldseth O. Axillary lymph node metastases in breast cancer: preoperative detection with dynamic contrast-enhanced MRI. Eur Radiol 2000;10(9):1464–1471.

128. Yoshimura G, Sakurai T, Oura S, et al. Evaluation of axillary lymph node status in breast cancer with MRI. Breast Cancer 1999;6(3):249–258.

129. Krishnamurthy S, Sneige N, Bedi DG, et al. Role of ultrasound-guided fine-needle aspiration of indeterminate and suspicious axillary lymph nodes in the initial staging of breast carcinoma. Cancer (Phila) 2002;95(5):982–988.

130. Wahl RL. Current status of PET in breast cancer imaging, staging, and therapy. Semin Roentgenol 2001;36(3):250–260.

131. Wahl RL, Siegel BA, Coleman RE, Gatsonis CG. Prospective multicenter study of axillary nodal staging by positron emission tomography in breast cancer: a report of the Staging Breast Cancer with PET Study Group. J Clin Oncol 2004;22(2):277–285.

132. Guller U, Nitzsche EU, Schirp U, et al. Selective axillary surgery in breast cancer patients based on positron emission tomography with ^{18}F-fluoro-2-deoxy-D-glucose: not yet! Breast Cancer Res Treat 2002;71(2):171–173.

133. Guller U, Nitzsche E, Moch H, Zuber M. Is positron emission tomography an accurate non-invasive alternative to sentinel lymph node biopsy in breast cancer patients? J Natl Cancer Inst 2003;95(14):1040–1043.

134. Heywang-Kobrunner SH, Schlegel A, Beck R, et al. Contrast-enhanced MRI of the breast after limited surgery and radiation therapy. J Comput Assist Tomogr 1993;17(6):891–900.

135. Solomon B, Orel S, Reynolds C, Schnall M. Delayed development of enhancement in fat necrosis after breast conservation therapy: a potential pitfall of MR imaging of the breast. AJR Am J Roentgenol 1998;170(4):966–968.

136. Bender H, Kirst J, Palmedo H, et al. Value of 18-fluoro-deoxyglucose positron emission tomography in the staging of recurrent breast carcinoma. Anticancer Res 1997;17(3B):1687–1692.

137. Moon DH, Maddahi J, Silverman DH, Glaspy JA, Phelps ME, Hoh CK. Accuracy of whole-body fluorine-18-FDG PET for the detection of recurrent or metastatic breast carcinoma. J Nucl Med 1998;39(3):431–435.

138. Cook GJ, Houston S, Rubens R, Maisey MN, Fogelman I. Detection of bone metastases in breast cancer by 18-FDG PET: differing metabolic activity in osteoblastic and osteolytic lesions. J Clin Oncol 1998;16(10):3375–3379.

139. Lee CH, Smith RC, Levine JA, Troiano RN, Tocino I. Clinical usefulness of MR imaging of the breast in the evaluation of the problematic mammogram. AJR Am J Roentgenol 1999;173(5):1323–1329.

140. Tilanus-Linthorst MM, Obdeijn IM, Bartels KC, de Koning HJ, Oudkerk M. First experiences in screening women at high risk for breast cancer with MR imaging. Breast Cancer Res Treat 2000;63(1):53–60.

141. Leach MO, Eeles RA, Turnbull LW, et al. The UK national study of magnetic resonance imaging as a method of screening for breast cancer (MARIBS). J Exp Clin Cancer Res 2002;21(suppl 3):107–114.

142. Morris EA, Liberman L, Ballon DJ, et al. MRI of occult breast carcinoma in a high-risk population. AJR Am J Roentgenol 2003;181(3):619–626.

143. Warner E. Intensive radiologic surveillance: a focus on the psychological issues. Ann Oncol 2004;15(suppl 1):I43–I47.

144. Hild F, Duda VF, Albert U, Schulz KD. Ductal orientated sonography improves the diagnosis of pathological nipple discharge of the female breast compared with galactography. Eur J Cancer Prev 1998;7(suppl 1):S57–S62.

145. Yang WT, Tse GM. Sonographic, mammographic, and histopathologic correlation of symptomatic ductal carcinoma in situ. AJR Am J Roentgenol 2004;182(1):101–110.

146. Berg WA, Gilbreath PL. Multicentric and multifocal cancer: whole-breast US in preoperative evaluation. Radiology 2000;214(1):59–66.

147. Moon WK, Noh DY, Im JG. Multifocal, multicentric, and contralateral breast cancers: bilateral whole-breast US in the preoperative evaluation of patients. Radiology 2002;224(2):569–576.

29

Imaging of Thoracic Malignancies

Caroline Chiles and Suzanne L. Aquino

Radiologic imaging of malignancy has evolved over the past 20 years. It not only provides better detection with superior anatomic resolution through computed tomography (CT) and magnetic resonance (MR) imaging, but it also provides physiologic information through positron emission tomography (PET). Today's technology incorporates the use of image modality fusion for even better disease localization and characterization. By fusing data from PET and CT studies, radiologic imaging brings together the superior resolution of CT with the low resolution of PET, thereby providing important information on tumor metabolism and replication. Tumor imaging is at the forefront of this technology explosion and is the focus of most cutting-edge research, as well as clinical applications. This chapter reviews current imaging of primary and metastatic malignancies of the thorax.

Tumors of the Bronchus

Bronchogenic Carcinoma

Non-Small Cell Lung Cancer

Detection

A patient with bronchogenic carcinoma may report symptoms including cough, sputum production, or hemoptysis at first presentation for evaluation by a physician. Other patients have advanced disease and nonspecific systemic symptoms, including weight loss and weakness, at initial examination. Chest radiographs may show findings that suggest lung cancer. Still other patients report no symptoms related to lung cancer, and abnormal results on chest radiographs prompt further workup. In almost 40% of patients with lung cancer, the disease has spread outside the thorax.[1]

Whether earlier detection of lung cancer improves outcomes remains controversial. Randomized, controlled lung cancer screening studies performed in the 1970s did not show a reduction in the number of deaths from lung cancer in patients screened with chest radiography and sputum cytology when compared with controls who received either less-frequent chest radiography or advice that chest radiography and sputum cytology be performed once a year.[2–4] This failure to demonstrate a reduction in lung cancer mortality occurred despite an increase in the detection of early-stage, resectable lung cancers and improved lung cancer survival in the experimental group screened every 4 months. Criticisms of these studies included insufficient statistical power, contamination of the control group, and a 25% noncompliance rate among the screened group.[5] In the Mayo Lung Project and the Czechoslovak screening studies, the incidence of lung cancer in the experimental groups was significantly higher than in the control population, suggesting that the two groups were not balanced with regard to important variables that affect lung cancer risk.[6] This discrepancy in incidence adversely affected calculated lung cancer mortality. The failure of screening chest radiography to improve the outcome in lung cancer occurred in multiple studies. A meta-analysis of screening studies enrolling a total of 245,610 subjects showed an 11% higher mortality from lung cancer when compared with less-frequent radiographic screening.[7]

A newer approach to lung cancer screening is low-dose helical CT, rather than conventional chest radiography. The Early Lung Cancer Action Project (ELCAP) recruited 1,000 high-risk individuals for baseline and annual repeat screening with low-dose helical CT.[8,9] In 1999, Henschke et al. reported the results of 1,000 baseline screening CT examinations.[8] Bronchogenic carcinoma was diagnosed in 27 individuals. Twenty-three of these patients had stage I disease; only 1 patient had unresectable disease. In 1,184 annual repeat screening examinations, malignancy was diagnosed in 7 individuals: 5 stage IA, 1 stage IIIA, and 1 small cell carcinoma.[9]

The conflicting analyses of earlier lung cancer screening trials and the advent of new technology capable of detecting early-stage lung cancer prompted the National Cancer Institute to fund a large-scale randomized, controlled lung cancer screening trial, the National Lung Screening Trial (NLST). In this trial, low-dose helical CT was compared with chest radiography in 50,000 participants at increased risk for lung cancer. Inclusion criteria required that participants be 55 to 74 years old and have at least a 30-pack/year cigarette-smoking history. Enrollment and incidence screening occurred between 2002 and 2004. Participants were randomized to either CT (experimental arm) or chest radiography (control arm) and received screening examinations once a year for 3 years. Follow-up will continue through 2009. In a subset of 10,000 participants, samples of blood, urine, and sputum were collected and archived to be available for further study using biomarkers for early detection of lung cancer.

Imaging Appearance

Bronchogenic carcinomas have a variety of appearances on imaging studies, ranging from a solitary pulmonary nodule to lobar consolidation. Some of these appearances strongly suggest specific cell types, despite considerable overlap.

Solitary Pulmonary Nodule

A solitary pulmonary nodule is defined radiographically as an opacity measuring less than 3 cm in diameter and surrounded by air-containing lung. Opacities that are larger than 3 cm in diameter are considered masses. The solitary pulmonary nodule presents a diagnostic challenge. Although most such nodules are benign, each must be further evaluated as a possible neoplasm. The interface between malignant nodules and the surrounding lung may appear smooth, lobulated, irregular, or spiculated. The margins of the solitary pulmonary nodule have been correlated with the incidence of malignancy.[10] A nodule with spiculated margins has a higher likelihood of malignancy than does the smoothly marginated nodule. A peripheral solitary pulmonary nodule is a common presentation for adenocarcinoma of the lung. The nodule may be round or oval, with smooth, lobulated, or irregular margins (Figure 29.1). The nodule may cause distortion of the surrounding pulmonary architecture and retraction of the overlying pleura. The concept of *scar carcinoma* suggests that some lung cancers, particularly adenocarcinomas, may arise in preexisting lung scars. Fibrosis observed microscopically, however, may represent a desmoplastic reaction of the host tissue to the neoplasm.

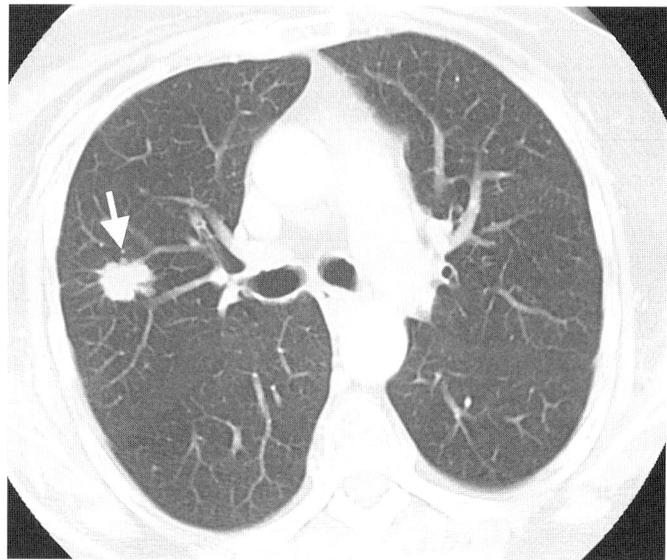

FIGURE 29.1. Axial computed tomography (CT) image (lung window setting) in a 69-year-old woman shows a spiculated, solid attenuation nodule (*arrow*) in the right upper lobe, typical for non-small cell bronchogenic carcinoma.

CT screening for lung cancer has helped to clarify the early appearances and growth rates of malignant primary tumors in the lung.[11] Nodules seen on high-resolution CT (HRCT), with 1.0- to 1.25-mm slice thicknesses, can be categorized on the basis of their CT attenuation as ground-glass opacity, mixed ground-glass and solid attenuation, and solid (Figure 29.2).[12,13] Volume-doubling rates have been calculated as fastest for solid nodules at 149 days, intermediate for mixed ground-glass/solid nodules at 457 days, and prolonged for ground-glass opacities at 813 days.[11]

Henschke et al. report a higher malignancy rate in nodules of mixed or ground-glass attenuation than in solid nodules found with screening CT.[14] Ground-glass attenuation correlates with bronchioloalveolar cell carcinoma histology and with a more favorable prognosis.[15] For this reason, some authorities recommend limited (wedge) resection for nodules of ground-glass attenuation and lobectomy for solid nodules.[16]

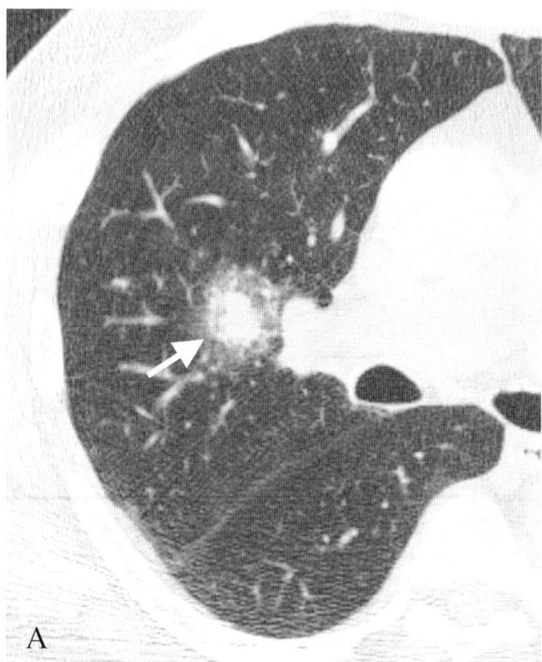

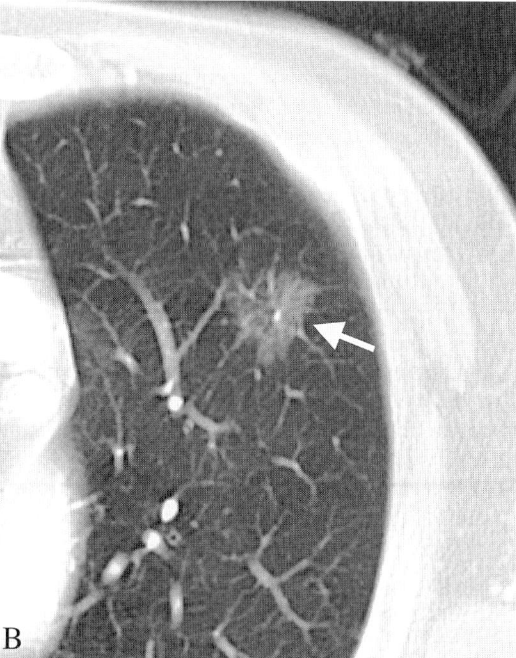

FIGURE 29.2. Axial CT images (lung window settings) show solitary pulmonary nodules in two different patients. (A) The solitary pulmonary nodule (*arrow*) in the right upper lobe demonstrates a mixed ground-glass and solid attenuation. (B) The solitary pulmonary nodule (*arrow*) in the left upper lobe of a different patient shows a ground-glass attenuation nodule. The ground-glass attenuation is suggestive of a bronchioloalveolar cell histology.

Atelectasis and Postobstructive Pneumonitis

Atelectasis results from endobronchial obstruction or extrinsic compression of a bronchus. Atelectasis is a common presenting appearance of squamous cell carcinoma.[17] Two-thirds of squamous cell carcinomas arise within main, lobar, or segmental bronchi.[18] Although the atelectasis is most often segmental, it may be lobar or may involve the entire lung.[17] The chest radiograph may demonstrate secondary signs of volume loss, with shift of the mediastinum to the involved side and elevation of the diaphragm. The central mass is often obscured by the collapsed lung.

When the upper lobe is collapsed, the trachea is deviated to the affected side, and the ipsilateral hilum is retracted superiorly. In atelectasis of the right upper lobe resulting from bronchogenic carcinoma, the minor fissure is classically distorted into a reverse S, the "S" sign of Golden.[19] The lateral aspect of the minor fissure migrates cephalad, whereas the medial aspect of the fissure is tethered beneath the central neoplasm.

In some patients, the obstructed lobe is filled with inflammatory debris, and the classic signs of volume loss are not present. In these patients, the opacified lobe represents postobstructive pneumonitis, in which air bronchograms are typically absent. This radiographic finding can help to differentiate postobstructive pneumonitis from infectious pneumonia.[17] All cases of pneumonia occurring in adults should be followed radiographically to confirm resolution after antibiotic therapy and to exclude the presence of an underlying endobronchial lesion. Although squamous cell carcinoma is the neoplasm typically associated with lobar atelectasis, adenocarcinoma may also arise centrally. Enlarged hilar or mediastinal lymph nodes from any of the bronchogenic carcinomas, including both small cell and non-small cell, can extrinsically compress the bronchi and produce obstructive pneumonitis and atelectasis.

Airspace Opacification

The radiographic appearance of airspace opacification, mimicking pneumonia, can be caused by bronchioloalveolar cell carcinoma (BAC), a subtype of adenocarcinoma. BAC may be either focal (nodular) or diffuse disease. The diffuse form includes lobar or segmental consolidation, as well as multiple poorly defined pulmonary nodules. The pneumonic appearance of BAC is unique to this neoplasm. A diagnosis of BAC should be considered when a peripheral pneumonia seen on chest radiographs fails to clear after antibiotic therapy.

The consolidative form of BAC is seen on CT images as peripheral, segmental, or lobar airspace opacification with air bronchograms (Figure 29.3). The CT angiogram sign was first described with BAC and was initially thought to be useful in the distinction of BAC from pneumonia.[20] The CT angiogram sign describes the CT appearance of enhancing pulmonary vessels within an area of homogeneously hypoattenuating pulmonary consolidation. Subsequent reports determined that the CT angiogram sign occurred in postobstructive pneumonitis and pneumonia as well and therefore, was not a useful discriminator for the consolidative form of BAC.[21,22] Aquino et al. and Jung et al. determined several CT features that were significant in the differentiation of pneumonic-type BAC from pneumonia.[23,24] Features that suggest BAC include peripheral distribution, coexisting nodules, elongation and narrowing of the bronchi, widening of the bronchial angle, and bulging of the interlobar fissure.

Pancoast Tumor

Pancoast tumors make up less than 5% of all lung cancers. Their radiographic appearance and clinical presentation are unique. The tumor arises in the lung apex and typically involves, through direct extension, the parietal pleura and chest wall.[25] The clinical syndrome described by Pancoast results from invasion of the tumor into the lower trunks of the brachial plexus and sympathetic chain. Patients experience shoulder pain, which may radiate down the arm, with eventual numbness and weakness in the C8 and T1 distribution, and atrophy of the muscles of the hand. Horner syndrome occurs in 20% of patients with Pancoast tumors and is caused by invasion of the paravertebral sympathetic chain by the tumor.[25] The tumor may also invade the vertebral body and ribs.

A Pancoast tumor is suggested radiographically by a thickening of the pleura of at least 5 mm at the lung apex or by asymmetry of the apical caps of more than 5 mm.[26,27] The tumor is sometimes detected when the lung apex is seen on images of the shoulder or cervical spine obtained to investigate a complaint of shoulder pain. Although Pancoast tumors can be visualized on axial CT images, MR imaging is the preferred modality.[28,29] The coronal and sagittal planes of MR provide more accurate information for determining the extent of tumor invasion into the chest wall, including involvement of the brachial plexus, vertebral body, and neural foramen (Figure 29.4). MR angiography is complementary to MR imaging and can demonstrate displacement and encasement of the subclavian and brachiocephalic artery and vein.[30]

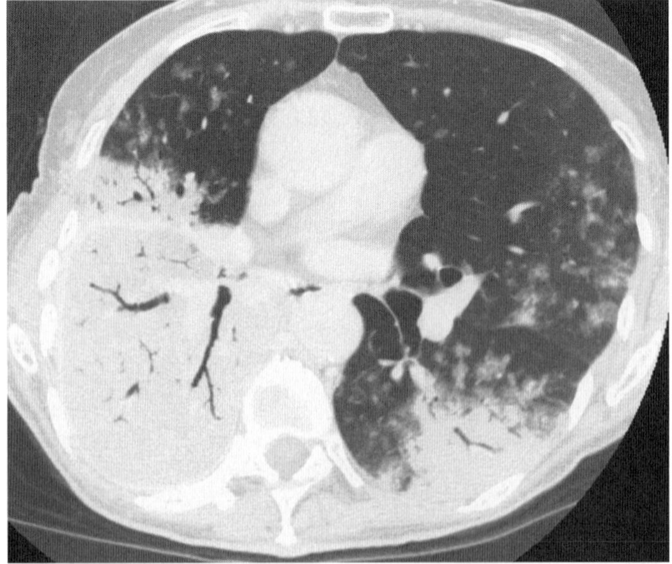

FIGURE 29.3. Axial CT (lung window settings) in a 63-year-old woman with the consolidative form of bronchioloalveolar cell carcinoma shows consolidation of the right lower lobe. The air bronchograms in the right lower lobe appear stretched. Focal areas of consolidation and ground-glass attenuation are also present in the right middle lobe, lingula, and left lower lobe.

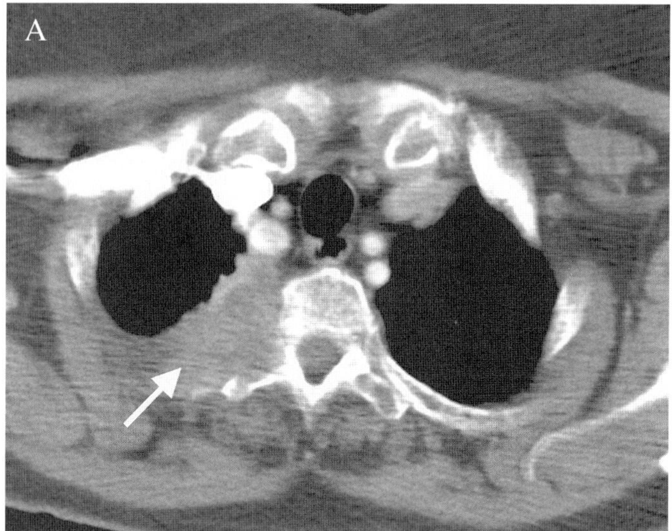

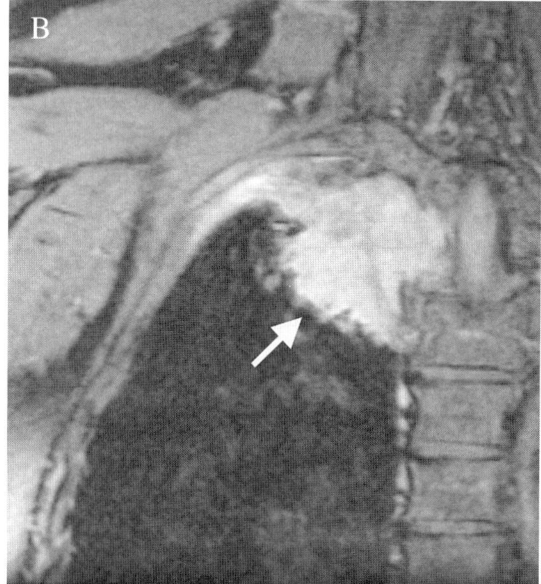

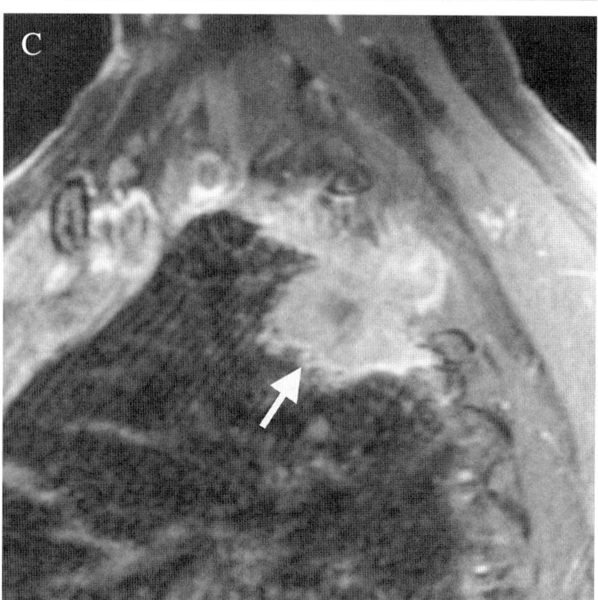

FIGURE 29.4. An 82-year-old woman with a Pancoast tumor. (A) Axial CT (soft tissue windows) shows a mass (*arrow*) at the right lung apex, consistent with a Pancoast tumor. Coronal (B) and sagittal (C) magnetic resonance (MR) images more clearly identify the invasion of the chest wall and the vertebral body by the tumor (*arrow*).

Staging

Imaging Modalities

Chest radiography remains the most frequently ordered radiographic examination. Its relatively low cost and widespread availability make it a very useful tool in the detection and diagnosis of thoracic disease. A chest radiograph with abnormal findings suggesting bronchogenic carcinoma typically prompts CT examination of the chest. The anatomic detail visible on CT images makes CT the examination of choice in such situations, as well as for patients with strong clinical evidence of thoracic disease despite normal chest radiographic results. CT is also useful to guide percutaneous transthoracic needle aspiration of thoracic masses. Although lacking the spatial resolution of CT, MR imaging allows imaging in coronal and sagittal planes and therefore is especially useful in the evaluation of patients with suspected invasion of the chest wall or diaphragm. In addition, MR imaging can be helpful in evaluating mediastinal invasion and vascular involvement by tumor.

Positron emission tomography (PET) with fluorodeoxyglucose (FDG) uses the higher glucose consumption of hypermetabolic tumors to assist in differentiating between benign and malignant lesions and to determine the extent of disease. Because it relies on increased metabolism, FDG-PET imaging has improved the radiologic staging of lung cancer.[31] Some of the limitations of PET, including spatial resolution and visual correlation with CT anatomy, are addressed in the newer dual PET/CT scanners. The addition of fusion imaging shows even better sensitivity and specificity for the detection of lymph node metastases and recurrent tumor.[32,33]

Primary Tumor (T)

The high spatial resolution of CT makes it an excellent modality for assessing the size and extent of the primary

TABLE 29.1. TNM definitions.

T = primary tumor	
T1	Tumor less than or equal to 3 cm in greatest diameter, surrounded by lung or visceral pleura without bronchoscopic evidence of invasion more proximal than the lobar bronchus
T2	Tumor with any of the following: greatest diameter more than 3 cm; involvement of main bronchus, at least 2 cm distal to the carina; invasion of visceral pleura; atelectasis or obstructive pneumonitis extending to the hilum but without involvement of entire lung
T3	Tumor of any size that directly invades any of the following: chest wall (includes superior sulcus tumors), diaphragm, mediastinal pleura, parietal pericardium; Tumor in the main bronchus less than 2 cm distal to the carina but without involvement of the carina; Tumor with associated atelectasis or obstructive pneumonitis of the entire lung
T4	Tumor of any size that invades any of the following: mediastinum, heart, great vessels, trachea, esophagus, vertebral body, or carina; Tumor with a malignant pleural or pericardial effusion; Tumor with satellite tumor nodules in the ipsilateral primary-tumor lobe of the lung
N = regional lymph nodes	
N0	No regional lymph node metastasis
N1	Metastasis to ipsilateral peribronchial and/or hilar lymph nodes
N2	Metastasis to ipsilateral mediastinal and/or subcarinal lymph nodes
N3	Metastasis to contralateral mediastinal or hilar lymph nodes; metastasis to ipsilateral or contralateral scalene or supraclavicular lymph nodes
M = distant metastasis	
M0	No distant metastasis
M1	Distant metastasis present

Source: Adapted from Mountain,[40] by permission of *Chest*.

tumor (T). The diameter of the tumor determines its categorization as T1 and T2 (Tables 29.1, 29.2). Nodules 3 cm or smaller in greatest dimension are classified as T1 tumors. Masses larger than 3 cm are considered T2 tumors. A lesion that measures 3 cm or smaller and involves a bronchus is classified as T1 if it does not extend more centrally than the lobar bronchus. T2 tumors can involve a main bronchus but must be at least 2 cm distal to the carina. The 2-cm distance allows a surgeon to clamp the bronchus at the time of lobectomy. A T1 tumor must be surrounded by lung or visceral pleura without invasion of the visceral pleura; a T2 tumor may invade the visceral pleura. Involvement of the visceral pleura is a difficult determination with any imaging modality, as the visceral and parietal pleurae are not readily distinguishable in the absence of pleural effusion or pneumothorax. Visceral pleural invasion is associated with a higher frequency of mediastinal nodal involvement and a poorer prognosis.[34,35] T2 tumors may also be characterized by lobar collapse or postobstructive pneumonitis extending to the hilum. T3 tumors are those that invade, by direct extension, the chest wall, diaphragm, mediastinal pleura, or pericardium. Endobronchial tumors within 2 cm of the carina, but without involvement of the carina, are also classified as T3 tumors. Invasion of the chest wall can be evaluated with CT or MR imaging, although the patient's description of chest wall pain may be just as accurate as an indicator of chest wall invasion.[36,37] CT criteria for chest wall invasion include rib destruction, contact of 5 cm or more with the chest wall, obtuse (greater than 90°) angle of the mass with the chest wall, increase in attenuation of the subpleural fat plane, and visualization of tumor in the intercostal space or deeper chest wall tissue.[36,38–41] When chest wall invasion is suggested on CT images, thin-section CT or MR imaging may be helpful. Uhrmeister et al. acquired 1-mm collimation CT images to evaluate 39 patients who had tumor contact with the chest wall and who underwent surgical exploration. Soft tissue invasion and abnormalities in the fat plane were more accurately identified on 1-mm CT images reconstructed by means of a standard soft tissue algorithm than with 10-mm collimation.[42]

TABLE 29.2. International system for staging lung cancer.

Stage	*TNM subset*
IA	T1 N0 M0
IB	T2 N0 M0
IIA	T1 N1 M0
IIB	T2 N1 M0 T3 N0 M0
IIIA	T3 N1 M0 T1–3 N2 M0
IIIB	T4 N0–2 M0 T1–4 N3 M0
IV	Any T any N M1

Source: Adapted from Mountain,[40] by permission of *Chest*.

On MR images, the most accurate indicator of parietal pleura invasion is signal intensity within the parietal pleura that is identical to that of tumor on T_1-weighted images.[37] This sign was present in 17 of 20 patients with chest wall invasion, with no false-positive errors, for an overall accuracy of 91%. In this series, Padovani et al. found that T_2-weighted images and gadolinium-enhanced T_1-weighted images provided no additional information.[37] Shiotani et al. recommended breathing dynamic echoplanar MR imaging of the thorax to look for movement of the tumor against the pleura or fixation of the tumor to the chest wall.[43] Sakai et al. pointed out, however, that benign pleural adhesions cannot be distinguished from chest wall invasion on MR images.[44]

T4 tumors are the most extensive, invading the mediastinum, heart, great vessels, trachea, esophagus, vertebral body, or carina. The presence of a malignant pleural effusion indicates a T4 tumor. Satellite tumor nodules within the same lobe as the primary lesion are also categorized as T4

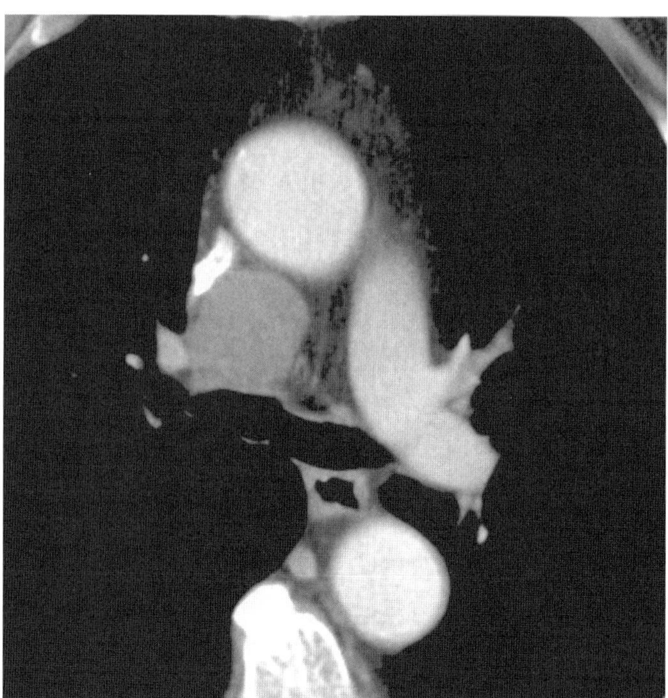

FIGURE 29.5. Axial CT (soft tissue window). A right lower paratracheal node is greater than 1.0 cm in short axis, meeting the CT criterion for abnormality.

disease. Surgical treatment is not appropriate for T4 tumors, which are considered stage IIIB or stage IV disease, depending on the presence or absence of distant metastases.

Nodal Involvement (N)

The most widely used CT criterion for the evaluation of hilar and mediastinal lymph nodes is the short-axis diameter. Lymph nodes larger than 1 cm in the short axis on axial CT images are considered abnormal; lymph nodes with diameters up to and including 1 cm are considered normal (Figure 29.5). Because normal-sized lymph nodes can harbor microscopic metastases, CT results can be falsely negative. Conversely, lymph nodes that are enlarged because of inflammatory disease can lead to a false-positive interpretation. In 2003, Toloza et al. published a meta-analysis of 20 studies comparing CT with mediastinoscopy in the staging of lung cancer. The data pooled from a total of 3,438 patients suggest that CT for staging mediastinal disease has a sensitivity of 57%, specificity of 82%, positive predictive value of 56%, and negative predictive value of 83%.[45] These investigators concluded that, despite a decade of advances in CT technology, the accuracy of CT scanning for staging mediastinal disease was not significantly better than results reported in a meta-analysis by Dales et al. in 1990.[45,46] These limitations notwithstanding, CT remains valuable in that it can guide the selection of nodes for mediastinoscopy or transbronchial needle aspiration.

In 2003, Gould et al. published a meta-analysis of 39 studies that were reported between 1994 and 2003, evaluating FDG-PET for mediastinal lymph node staging in patients with known or suspected non-small cell lung cancer. They determined that PET with 18-FDG was more accurate than CT for mediastinal staging.[47] The median sensitivity and specificity of CT for identifying mediastinal nodal (N2 and N3) disease were 61% and 79%, respectively, whereas median sensitivity and specificity were 85% and 90%, respectively, for PET. When CT showed enlarged lymph nodes, PET was more likely to yield both true positives and false positives. False-positive PET interpretations most commonly occur when acute inflammation is present within lymph nodes, particularly in patients with sarcoidosis, silicosis, and tuberculosis.[48–50] False-positive PET results can also occur when there is direct extension of the primary tumor into the mediastinum, as nodal glucose uptake contiguous with the primary lesion may not be distinguishable from direct tumor extension into the node.[51] False-negative interpretations of PET scans can occur as a result of misalignment of the PET findings to the American Thoracic Society (ATS) nodal map, so that FDG uptake is not localized correctly.[49,52] Other false negatives with PET scan interpretation are due to small malignant lymph nodes that are below the spatial resolution limits of the scanner or enlarged lymph nodes with subtotal tumor replacement.[49,51] Cerfolio et al. reported that false-negative FDG-PET results were most common in evaluating the subcarinal (ATS station 7) and aortopulmonary window (ATS stations 5 and 6) nodal stations.[53]

Positive findings on PET studies should be confirmed by biopsy. Some authors believe that negative findings on PET studies should be considered in light of the patient's pretest probability of mediastinal metastasis and whether enlarged mediastinal nodes are demonstrated by CT.[47] Graeter et al. reported a negative predictive value of 98.4% in their series and suggested that the negative predictive value of PET is sufficient to omit mediastinoscopy.[48] The American Society of Clinical Oncology (ASCO) recommends biopsy of lymph nodes that are either greater than 1.0 cm in short axis on CT or positive on PET scanning (Figure 29.6). Their 2003 recom-

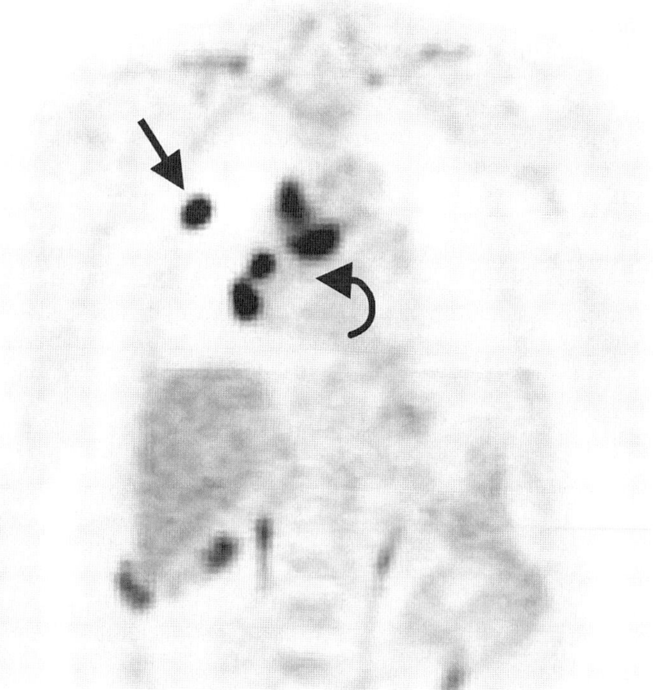

FIGURE 29.6. A 60-year-old man with non-small cell lung cancer. Coronal reconstruction of a positron emission tomography (PET) scan shows increased uptake within the primary tumor (*arrow*) as well as ipsilateral hilar and mediastinal lymph nodes (*curved arrow*).

mendations are that a lymph node that is enlarged on CT should still undergo biopsy even if the FDG-PET scan is negative.[54]

Staging is also more accurate with PET than with CT for predicting the likelihood of long-term survival.[55,56] Dunagan et al. suggested that staging with PET may prove especially worthwhile in patients with comorbid illnesses or poor functional status, in whom the risk from invasive diagnostic procedures or surgery is accelerated.[55]

Some of the errors encountered in visual correlation of PET and CT images can be altered with coregistration of CT and PET data sets.[32,57,58] A dual PET/CT scanner allows precise coregistration of the functional images of PET with the anatomic images of CT.[59] Antoch et al. reported a slight, but not statistically significant, improvement in the assessment of lymph node involvement with dual PET/CT when compared with PET.[60] The positive and negative predictive values were 89% and 94%, respectively, for dual PET/CT, 80% and 94% for PET, and 50% and 77% for CT. Lardinois et al. found that nodal staging with integrated PET/CT was significantly more accurate than with PET alone. Integrated CT-PET provided additional information in 20 (41%) of 49 patients with non-small cell bronchogenic carcinoma beyond that provided by conventional visual correlation of PET and CT.[32]

Small Cell Lung Cancer

Because of its rapid growth and early metastatic spread, small cell lung carcinoma is considered separately from non-small cell carcinoma. One in seven patients with lung cancer has small cell lung cancer. In 2000, the age-adjusted incidence of small cell lung cancer in the United States was 8.6 cases per 100,000 population, whereas the incidence of non-small cell lung cancer was 53.8 cases per 100,000.[61] The typical radiographic appearance of small cell lung cancer is that of a hilar or perihilar mass, which may represent a combination of the primary tumor and lymphadenopathy, and bulky mediastinal lymphadenopathy. Tracheobronchial and vascular compression are often present. Bronchial compression is frequently associated with obstructive atelectasis, which is demonstrated radiographically in 22% of patients.[62] Although chest radiography and CT suggest complete compression of the bronchus, bronchoscopy usually demonstrates a detectable lumen.[62] Small cell lung cancer is the most common primary tumor to cause superior vena cava syndrome, which results from mass effect on the superior vena cava, brachiocephalic veins, or both. The enlarged lymph nodes may also compress the pulmonary artery, producing oligemia in the involved lung.

The Veterans Administration Lung Cancer Study Group recommended a two-stage system for lung cancer: limited stage, which includes tumor that is confined to the thorax and can be encompassed in a tolerable radiation field, and extensive stage, which extends beyond those confines. A majority of patients (65% to 90%) have extensive-stage disease at presentation. Use of the TNM system has been recommended for those few patients with small cell lung cancer that is potentially surgically resectable. The clinical staging of small cell lung cancer focuses on the most common sites of metastatic disease: the liver, adrenal glands, retroperitoneal lymph nodes, brain, skeleton, and bone marrow. Staging with MR imaging or CT of the brain and abdomen, radionuclide bone scan, and bone marrow aspiration is routine, as patients may have distant metastases without clinical signs or symptoms. PET scanning may prove to be a worthwhile replacement for this combination of studies. FDG-PET imaging was compared with the sum of other staging procedures in 30 patients with histologically proven small cell lung cancer.[63] FDG-PET and the conventional staging system showed identical results in 23 of 36 examinations. Discordant results were observed in the examinations of 5 patients, but the overall staging of limited versus extensive disease was not affected. A retrospective analysis of PET in 46 patients with both treated and untreated small cell lung cancer demonstrated that PET had prognostic value.[64] Overall survival rates were significantly lower in patients with positive PET results than in those with negative PET results. Survival also showed a significant negative correlation with the maximum standardized uptake value (SUV).

Small cell lung cancer is somewhat unusual in its rapid response to therapy. Within 1 month of initiation of therapy, follow-up chest radiographs show a decrease in mediastinal and hilar lymphadenopathy and often return to their normal baseline appearance. In patients with obstructive atelectasis at presentation, partial or complete reexpansion of the lung is evident radiographically in 85% of patients within 1 month of initiation of therapy.[62] Contrast enhancement of the mediastinal lymph nodes on CT images has been suggested as predictive of response to chemotherapy. Enhancement of the nodes by 30 Hounsfield units (HU) or more predicted a reduction of at least 80% in tumor volume.[65] PET may also provide prognostic information in follow-up of treated patients with small cell lung cancer.[64] Routine radiographic follow-up is not currently recommended, however, to detect recurrence in these patients. Recurrences are signaled by clinical histories in 71% of patients and by chest radiographs in only 12%.[66]

Carcinoid

Bronchial carcinoid is a neuroendocrine neoplasm with behavior that can vary from that of a low-grade typical carcinoid to a more aggressive atypical carcinoid. Pulmonary carcinoid tumors account for 1% to 2% of all lung neoplasms. The patient with carcinoid tumor is usually symptomatic, typically in the fifth decade of life, and likely to describe symptoms related to bronchial obstruction such as cough, hemoptysis, dyspnea, or recurrent pneumonia.[67,68] Chest radiographs may show signs related to the bronchial obstruction, including lobar atelectasis, or postobstructive pneumonitis.[69,70] Bronchial obstruction may also produce hypoxic vasoconstriction of the affected lung, resulting in a hyperlucent, oligemic appearance.[69] A hilar or perihilar mass may also be visible radiographically. With CT, the tumor can be localized within a lobar, segmental, or large subsegmental bronchus. Volume loss of the lobe or lung segment is characterized by displacement of fissures and crowding of the bronchi and pulmonary vessels. In many patients, postobstructive pneumonitis predominates, with consolidation of the lung and little evidence of volume loss. The presence of air-trapping can facilitate recognition of an endobronchial lesion. Air-trapping is usually visible on inspiratory images but is more marked on images obtained in expiration. Mucoid impaction may also be seen distal to the endobronchial obstruction, signaled by the gloved-finger appearance of mucus-filled bronchi. On noncontrast-enhanced CT images, calcification may be seen within the carcinoid tumor. CT

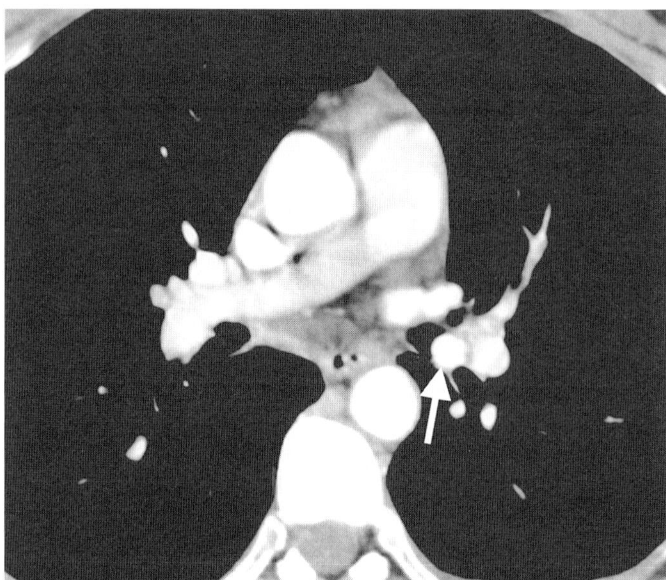

FIGURE 29.7. A 44-year-old woman with atypical chest pain and cough. Axial chest CT (soft tissue window) shows an intensely enhancing nodule in the left lower lobe bronchus (*arrow*) that proved to be typical carcinoid at resection.

demonstrates calcification in 43% of central carcinoids but in only 10% of peripheral carcinoids.[71,72] Because of their vascular nature, carcinoid tumors often enhance intensely after the intravenous administration of contrast material. The enhancement can be so intense that the tumor is mistaken for a vascular abnormality, such as a pulmonary varix or an arteriovenous malformation (Figure 29.7).[73]

One third of patients with carcinoid tumors are asymptomatic, and a solitary peripheral pulmonary nodule or mass is discovered incidentally on a chest radiograph. These patients are typically a decade older than symptomatic patients with a central carcinoid tumor. Peripheral carcinoids are usually round or ovoid, with smooth, lobulated margins. The size of these tumors ranges from 1 to 10 cm.[74] Peripheral carcinoids are occasionally multiple; a larger tumor may be accompanied by one or more tumorlets. The peripheral carcinoid is likely to be found in the right upper lobe, right middle lobe, or lingula. On CT images, the peripheral carcinoid is of homogeneous attenuation. On MR images, bronchial carcinoids have high signal intensity on T_2-weighted images and short-inversion-time inversion recovery images.[75]

Erasmus et al. reported PET imaging of seven carcinoid tumors, including three central endobronchial lesions, three peripheral pulmonary nodules (1.5–3.0 cm), and one 10-cm lung mass.[76] The endobronchial lesions had SUV measurements of 1.6 to 2.3 and were indistinguishable from mediastinal activity. SUVs were 2.2 to 2.4 in the peripheral nodules and 6.6 in the large lung mass. Currently, PET imaging is not useful in distinguishing carcinoid tumors from benign nodules.

Although the histologic distinction between typical and atypical carcinoid is important for therapeutic decisions and prognosis, no radiographic features distinguish the two.[77] Both typical and atypical carcinoid tumors can metastasize to regional lymph nodes or to distant sites, including liver, bone, and skin. Hilar and mediastinal lymph node enlargement can be readily identified with CT. CT is also superior to imaging with radiolabeled somatostatin analogues (^{123}I-Tyr-3-octreotide) in the detection of metastases from carcinoid tumors.[78]

Tumors of the Pleura

Malignant Mesothelioma

According to Kawahima and Libshitz, who evaluated the CT scans of 50 patients with malignant pleural mesothelioma (MPM), the most common finding on CT is pleural thickening (92%), followed by tumor involvement of the interlobar fissures (86%) and pleural fluid (74%) (Figure 29.8).[79] Similar findings were reported by Metintas et al., who found a rind-

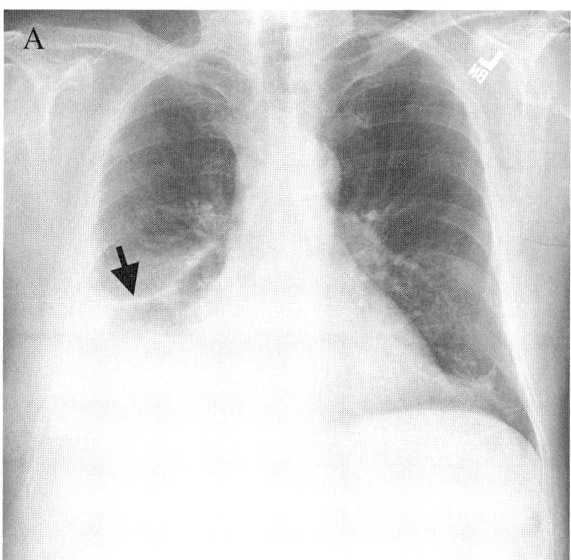

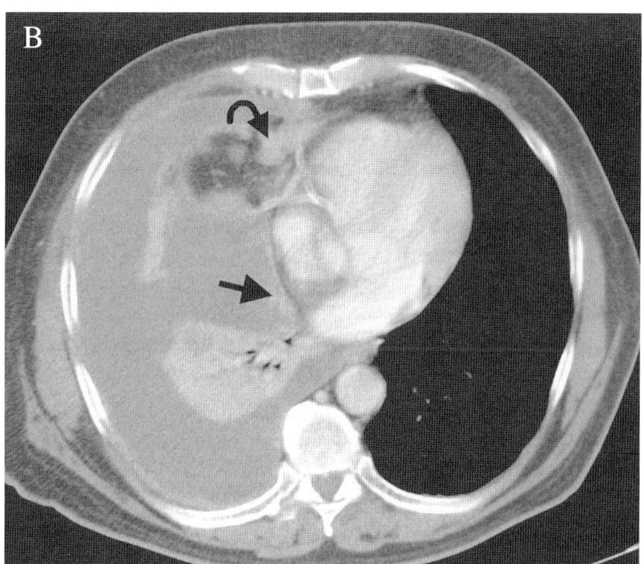

FIGURE 29.8. A 70-year-old man with malignant mesothelioma. (A) Initial chest radiograph shows an asymmetric right pleural effusion that extends into the minor fissure (*arrow*). (B) CT scan shows irregular thickening and enhancement of the parietal pleura (*arrow*), including the mediastinal pleura. The lymph nodes in the paradiaphragmatic fat are enlarged (*curved arrow*).

like extension tumor on the pleura in 70% of the 99 patients they imaged with MPM.[80] Other findings suggesting MPM were multiple nodules encasing the lung, pleural thickening with an irregular pleuropulmonary margin, and pleural thickening with superimposed separate nodules. However, these findings were also seen with metastatic pleural disease, which was frequently indistinguishable. Rindlike thickening and thickness greater than 1 cm strongly suggested MPM, but other sources for pleural malignancy should be considered.

Knuuttila et al. reported that MR imaging was superior to CT in evaluating MPM. They found that MR imaging improved the detection of tumor involvement in the interlobar fissures, diaphragm, peritoneum, and bony structures (Figure 29.9). The two modalities were equal, however, in detecting invasion of the chest wall, mediastinum, and adjacent lung.[81] In a separate report, Knuutila et al. found that contrast-enhanced T_1 fat-suppression was the most useful sequence for displaying invasion of adjacent anatomic structures, including the diaphragm, lung, mediastinum, pericardium, chest wall, and skeleton by mesothelioma, as well as pleural metastases.[82]

Heelan et al. also found MR imaging superior to CT in displaying tumor involvement in the diaphragm and chest wall (as extension through endothoracic fascia or solitary

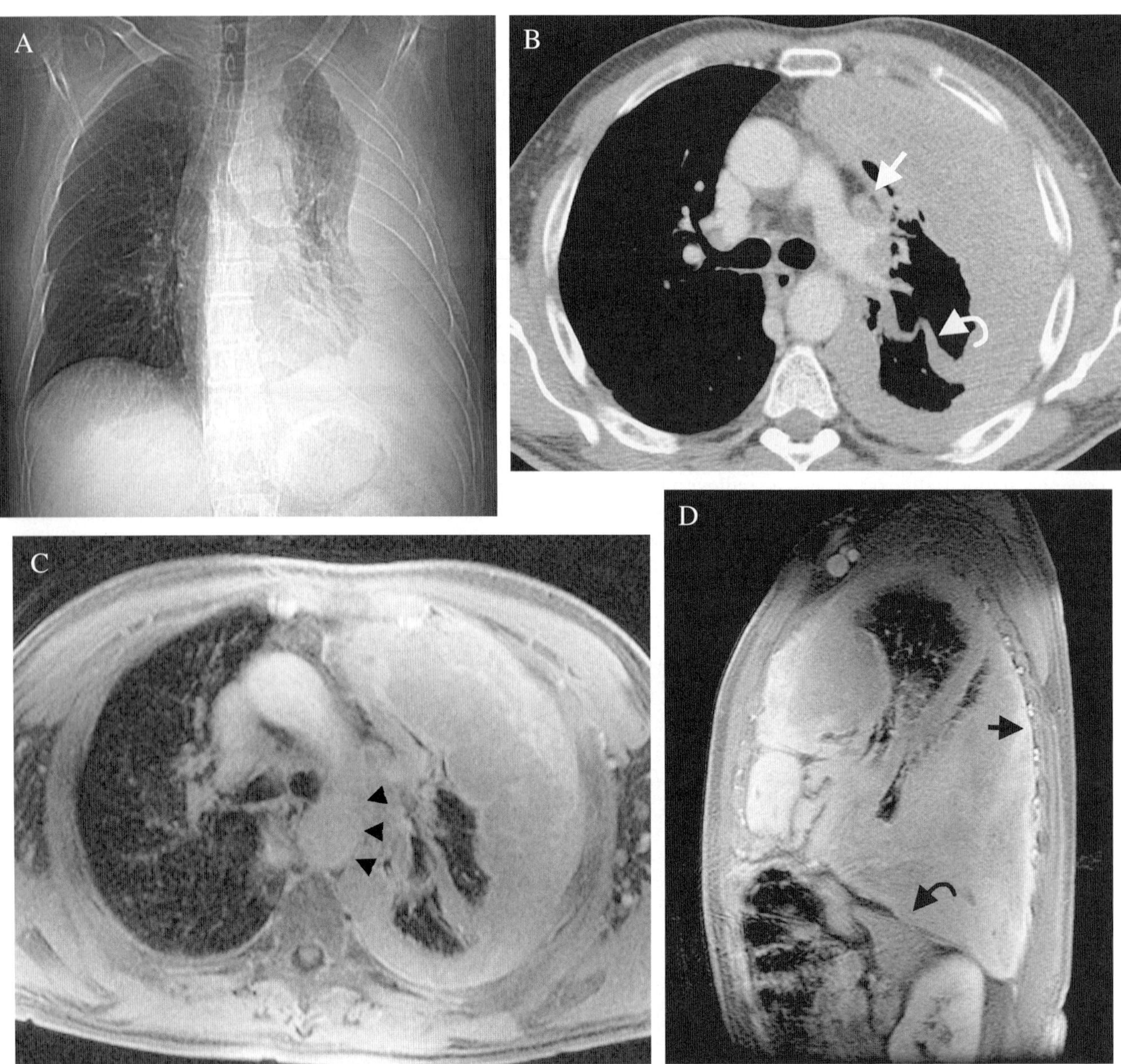

FIGURE 29.9. A 52-year-old man with malignant mesothelioma. (A) Chest radiograph shows loculated pleural effusion in left pleural space with compression of the left lung medially. (B) CT scan of the thorax with intravenous contrast shows large soft tissue mass in the pleural space that involves the pleura along the mediastinum (*arrow*) and fissure (*curved arrow*). (C) T_1-weighted MR image with fat saturation following gadolinium administration shows no evidence for chest wall invasion, although mediastinal fat planes are obliterated (*arrowheads*). (D) Sagittal image of same sequence shows diffuse pleural tumor that involves the pleura (*arrow*). The mass displaces the diaphragm inferiorly without invasion (*curved arrow*).

chest wall foci).[83] The difference between CT and MR imaging in detecting visceral pleural tumor, invasion of lung, and mediastinal and pericardial involvement was not statistically significant. Therefore, CT is recommended as the standard diagnostic choice and MR imaging as an additional study in patients for whom diaphragmatic and chest wall invasion is highly probable.

As with most malignant diseases in the thorax, FDG-PET has shown improved sensitivity in detecting MPM; however, limitations arise with the false detection of tumor in patients with benign inflammatory pleural disease and infection.[84,85] Sensitivity in the detection of tumor as areas of increased uptake in pleural thickening and nodules identified on CT ranges from 91% to 100%. Although PET is sensitive in detecting tumor, Flores et al. found PET limited in specific tumor and local nodal staging; sensitivities were 19% and 11%, respectively.[86] However, they concluded, as did Gerbaudo et al., that FDG-PET is very helpful in detecting distant metastases in supraclavicular lymph nodes and abdomen that were not identified with CT.[85,86]

Metastatic Disease to the Thorax

Pulmonary Metastases

Radiologic applications for imaging of metastases are useful in initial staging as well as assessment of a patient's response to neoadjuvant therapy for restaging before planned definitive surgical treatment and follow-up imaging for tumor recurrence. CT has evolved as the routine choice in staging, restaging, and detection of recurrence. Its superior anatomic resolution, combined with widespread availability and applications, contributes to its popularity. CT is superior to chest radiography for the detection of pulmonary metastases, although with limitations. Because of its excellent spatial resolution, CT demonstrates small lesions that mimic metastatic foci but are frequently benign. Limitations come into play especially in the initial diagnosis of patients with extrathoracic malignancies and no prior radiographic studies to document preexisting parenchymal disease.[87] For instance, although Chalmers and Best found pulmonary nodules on CT in 20% of patients with extrathoracic malignancies and normal chest radiographs, 80% of these nodules were benign.[88] Similar results were found by Kronawitter et al., who found, in routine preoperative workup for liver metastatectomy in patients with colon cancer, that the majority of nodules seen on chest CT images were benign.[89] Only 5% of patients had true metastases. Povoski et al. reported that CT demonstrated pulmonary metastases in 4 of 100 patients with colon cancer whose results on chest radiographs before hepatectomy were normal.[90] Picci et al. reported that, in 51 children with osteosarcoma, CT was sensitive but not specific in detecting pulmonary metastases.[91] They found, however, that the likelihood of metastases increased with the number of nodules detected. Four of 13 patients with a single nodule had a true metastasis. All patients with more than seven nodules had metastases.

Other reports have demonstrated that the stage of an extrathoracic malignancy should be considered when determining whether CT should be included in the workup.[92–94] Lim and Carter found that the detection of metastases from renal cell carcinoma with CT was low, especially with small primary tumors.[93] With increasing tumor stage or with the demonstration of a nodule on a radiograph, however, they found CT more useful in detecting pulmonary metastases. Similarly, Heaston et al. reported that CT improved the detection of metastases in patients with locally advanced melanoma, as well as helping to identify extrapulmonary metastases.[95] Reiner et al. found that routine chest CT was essential in the management of newly diagnosed squamous cell carcinoma of the head and neck.[96] In 66 of 189 patients, CT demonstrated significant abnormalities, whereas only 23% were detected on chest radiographs. Thirty-six patients had 41 tumors, of which 13 were additional primaries and 28 were metastases. Conventional radiographs showed only 12 (29%) of these tumors. Reiner and colleagues therefore recommended routine thoracic CT before treatment for this patient population, which has a significant cigarette-smoking history and risk for bronchogenic carcinoma.

In the follow-up management of patients who have been treated for cancer and who undergo surveillance for recurrence, CT is very useful for detecting new pulmonary metastases.[89] Follow-up CT imaging to detect early metastases can improve survival rates for patients with certain malignancies, such as sarcomas and colon cancer.[91,97,98]

Most pulmonary metastases reach the lungs through the pulmonary arterial system.[99–101] The most common manifestation of pulmonary metastases is multiple nodules.[99,100,102,103] Association of a nodule with a pulmonary vessel, the "mass-vessel sign" on high-resolution CT (HRCT), has been correlated with a hematogeneous origin.[101] Although pulmonary metastases are generally multiple, a few tumors can manifest with a single pulmonary metastasis.[95,104] Metastatic nodules can range from miliary to several centimeters in size. Miliary nodules are more likely to occur in association with tumors, such as thyroid carcinoma, renal cell carcinoma, and melanoma.[105,106] Their distribution with respect to the interstitial compartments is typically random.[107,108] Larger nodules are more likely to be seen with sarcomas and tumors from the colon and kidney. Metastases can be characterized not only by size but also by density and composition. For instance, metastases may have a solid, ground-glass, or mixed solid and ground-glass appearance. Others can calcify or cavitate.

Ground-glass nodules or nodules with surrounding ground-glass opacities are consistent with either hemorrhage or airspace disease into the adjacent lung (Figure 29.10). Metastatic nodules with surrounding hemorrhage have been described with choriocarcinoma, melanoma, renal cell carcinoma, angiosarcoma, and Kaposi's sarcoma.[109–111] Bronchioloalveolar cell carcinoma nodules may have a ground-glass appearance or may have a surrounding ground-glass pattern.[112] This pattern has been attributed to lining of adjacent airspaces by tumor through a lepidic growth pattern or to filling of airspaces with mucinous material.[113] Nonmalignant processes with similar patterns may mimic metastases and should be included in the differential diagnosis. Infections, such as viral pneumonias, tuberculosis, fungal infections including invasive aspergillosis, arteriovenous malformations, and Wegener granulomatosis with local hemorrhage, can be very similar in appearance.[109,112]

The diagnosis of calcified metastases is straightforward when new nodules develop in a patient with osteosarcoma (Figure 29.11) or chondrosarcoma. However, in the absence of

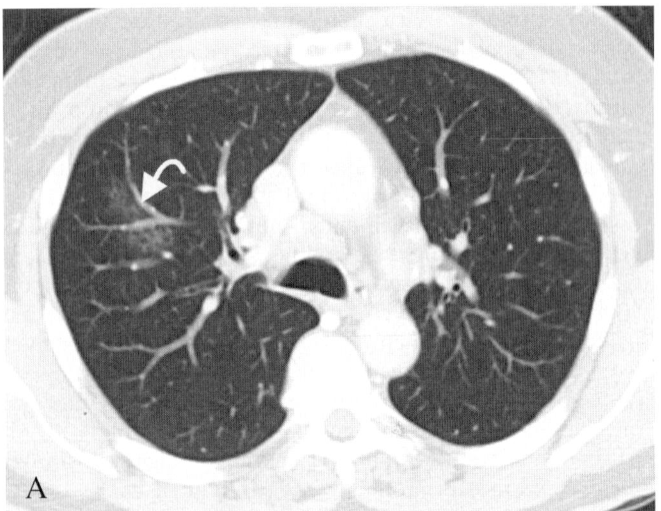

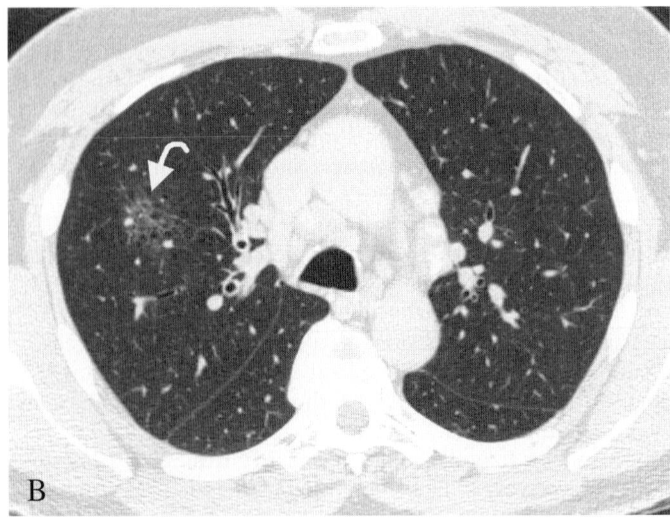

FIGURE 29.10. A 72-year-old man with history of metastatic melanoma involving the lungs. (A) CT scan image in lung windows at 5-mm slice thickness shows one of multiple ground-glass foci in the lungs (*curved arrow*). (B) High-resolution image at 1.25-mm slice thickness better displays the ground-glass (*curved arrow*) and associated thickened interlobular septa.

prior radiographs to show that a nodule is new, other considerations should include granuloma, amyloid, or hamartoma. Metastatic mucinous adenocarcinoma originating from the pancreas, small bowel, or ovary; thyroid carcinoma; and on rare occasions soft tissue sarcomas and choriocarcinoma may also contain calcifications.[114–119]

Multiple cavitary metastases are more likely to result from squamous cell carcinoma but may also be seen with transitional cell carcinoma, adenocarcinoma, sarcoma, and lymphoma.[120–125] Cavitation of metastases may be seen before therapy but may also reflect response after chemotherapy (Figure 29.12).[122,126] The initial finding of multiple cavitary nodules does not necessarily suggest tumor.[127–129] Inflammatory disease, such as Wegener granulomatosis, rheumatoid arthritis, eosinophilic granulomatosis, and amyloid, may be characterized by numerous cavitary nodules. Pulmonary infections, such as fungal infection, mycobacterial disease, septic emboli, and tracheobronchial papillomatosis, should also be considered.

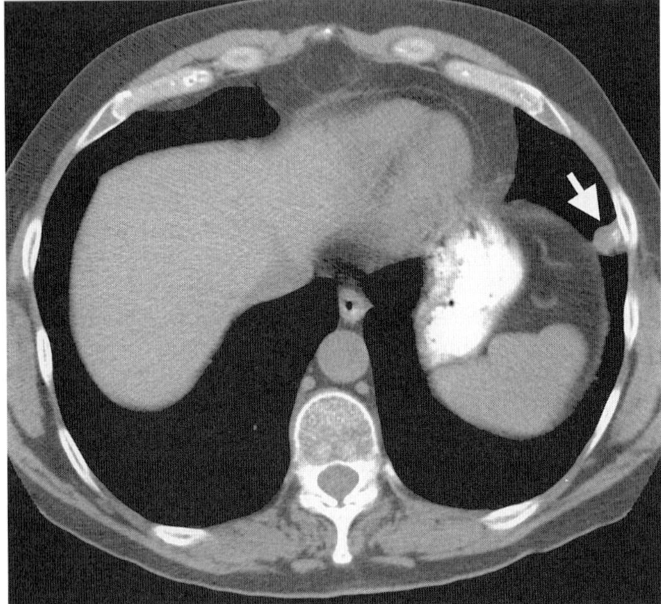

FIGURE 29.11. A 19-year-old man with history of osteosarcoma of the femur. CT scan of the thorax in soft tissue windows shows a pulmonary nodule (*arrow*) with central calcification that was a metastasis on resection.

Tumor emboli are the result of hematogenous metastases that occlude and enlarge within the pulmonary arteries. On CT images they appear as branching lobulated enlargement of the small- to medium-sized vessels (Figure 29.13).[130] This unusual pattern of metastasis is seen with tumors that spread hematogeneously, such as sarcoma, renal cell carcinoma, hepatoma, and melanoma. Distal infarction may result, with distal ground-glass pattern or consolidation.[130,131] Microscopic emboli, which may manifest as idiopathic cor pulmonale, are rare complications associated with tumors from the breast, liver, and gastrointestinal tract. Frequently, the lungs are clear on chest radiographs and CT images.[108] On rare occasions, CT may show evidence of interstitial disease consistent with associated lymphangitic involvement.[132] Angiography results may be normal or may show delayed vessel filling.[133] Ventilation-perfusion scanning may demonstrate multiple subsegmental perfusion defects.[133,134]

Endobronchial Metastases

Endobronchial obstruction of an airway by metastasis is rare; the reported incidence is 2%.[135] The most common tumor to metastasize to the airways is renal cell carcinoma.[125,136,137] Other tumors that spread to the airways include melanoma, lymphoma, and tumors of the breast, larynx, thyroid, and colon.[125,135–138] Patients with tumor involving the airways frequently have metastases to other areas of the thorax, including the lymph nodes and pulmonary parenchyma.[136] The proximal airways, rather than the small airways, are generally involved. Complete occlusion results in mucous filling of the distal occluded airways. On CT images, these occluded airways appear as arborizing opaque structures that are separate from the vasculature. Called the *finger-in-glove sign* on

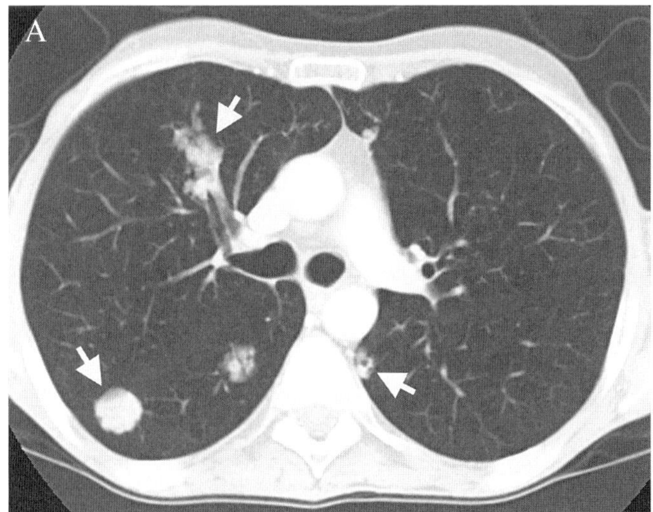

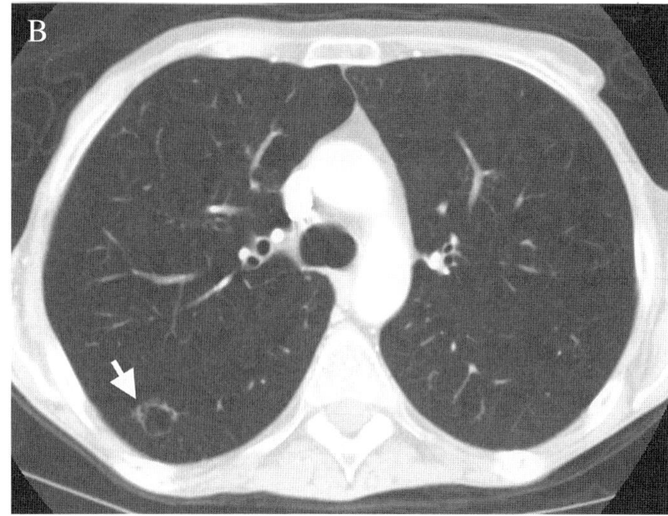

FIGURE 29.12. A 55-year-old man with pharyngeal carcinoma of the lungs. (A) CT scan in lung windows demonstrates multiple pulmonary metastases (*arrows*). (B) Following chemotherapy, CT scan shows interval decrease in size of the nodules with cavitation (*arrow*).

chest radiographs, the branching plugged airways resemble white-gloved fingers. If airway plugging extends into the subpleural distribution, a tree-in-bud pattern can be seen.

Lymphangitic Carcinomatosis

Lymphangitic tumor involvement of the lungs predominantly affects the pulmonary lymphatics and the investing perilymphatic connective tissue. The patterns most frequently described on HRCT are thickened interlobular septae and bronchovascular interstitium, reticular lines, and polygonal structures.[139,140] Thickened interstitial compartments can be smooth or nodular.[140,141] A smooth pattern may be the result of direct tumor infiltration in the interstitium and lymphatics or of interstitial edema from a more proximal tumor of the lymphatics (i.e., with hilar or mediastinal lymphadenopathy).[142,143] Nodular lymphangitic disease is more indicative of direct tumor deposition in the interstitium (Figure 29.14). Malignancies commonly associated with a lymphangitic carcinomatosis pattern in the lungs include adenocarcinoma from lung, breast, and gastrointestinal tract, melanoma, lymphoma, and leukemia.[108,142–145] Disease may initially reach the lungs by either embolic spread or direct extension from hilar lymphatic disease.[132,146] On chest radiographs the pattern frequently resembles edema, with thickening of the perihilar bronchovasculature and subpleural Kerley B lines (see Figure 29.14). Frequently, however, the distribution is asymmetric and therefore suggestive of neoplasm. Alternatively, if a patient appears febrile, a lobar or segmental pattern may mimic pneumonia.

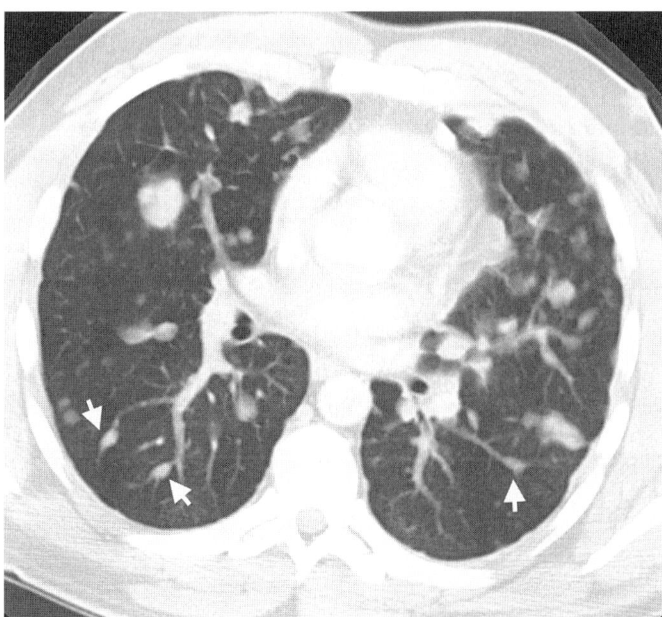

FIGURE 29.13. A 24-year-old man with metastatic soft tissue sarcoma, axial chest CT (lung windows). Some of the nodules appear as focal symmetric enlargement of the small pulmonary arteries (*arrows*) consistent with tumor emboli.

CT and HRCT are more sensitive and specific in identifying lymphangitic involvement. However, Hirakata et al. showed that detection of pulmonary involvement with HRCT is limited in comparison to that of histopathology.[108] Interstitial involvement can extend from the perihilar axial interstitium to the subpleural interlobular septa and also may involve the subpleural interstitium leading to thickened fissures.[143,147] Johkoh et al. correlated HRCT findings to those of histopathology and found that the distribution in most patients with lymphangitic carcinomatosis was in the perihilar axial interstitium.[147] Other interstitial diseases may resemble lymphangitic carcinomatosis, including sarcoidosis and lymphoma. The distribution of disease and pattern of associated nodules may help to distinguish between disorders. Honda et al. found that lymphangitic carcinomatosis tended to involve the subpleural interstitial spaces, whereas sarcoidosis tended to be more symmetric and to occur in the upper lungs.[148]

Metastases of Mixed Parenchymal Patterns

Lymphoma involvement of the lungs may be mixed, manifesting as a combination of consolidative, nodular, or interstitial involvement (Figure 29.15).[144] The latter form

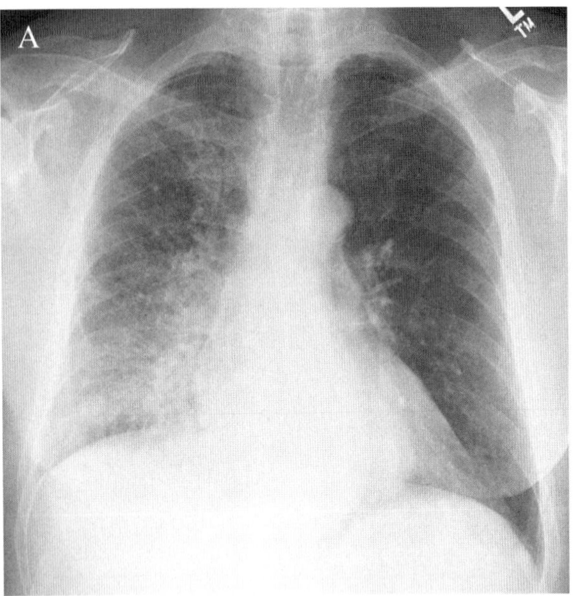

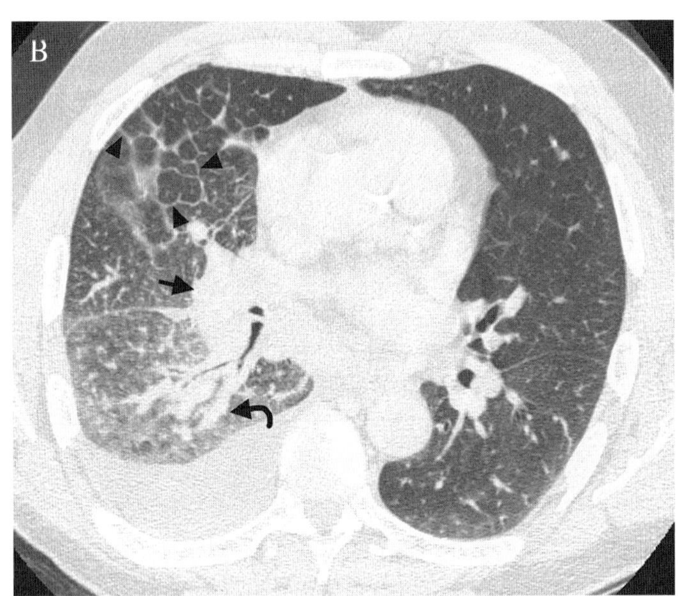

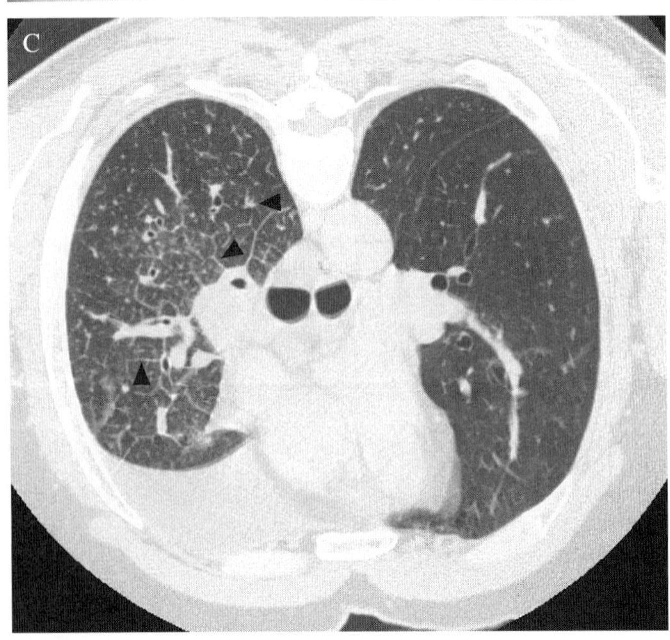

FIGURE 29.14. A 68-year-old woman who presented with weight loss and a dry cough. (A) Chest radiograph shows asymmetric opacities in the right lung and hilum. The right hilum is enlarged, and there are diffuse reticular opacities. (B) CT scan of the thorax at 2.5-mm slice thickness in lung windows shows enlargement of the right hilum (*arrow*), thickening of the bronchovasculature (*curved arrow*), and diffuse thickened interlobular septa (*arrowheads*). There is also a dependent right pleural effusion. (C) Prone images at 1.25-mm slice thickness better display the thickened interlobular septa (*arrowheads*). The pleural effusion is free flowing and collects in the dependent anterior pleural space.

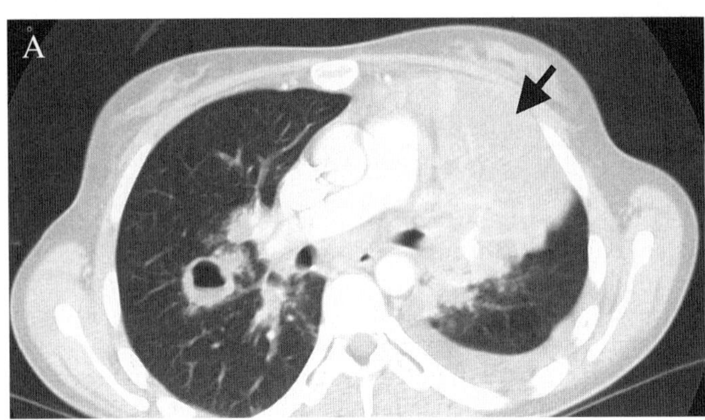

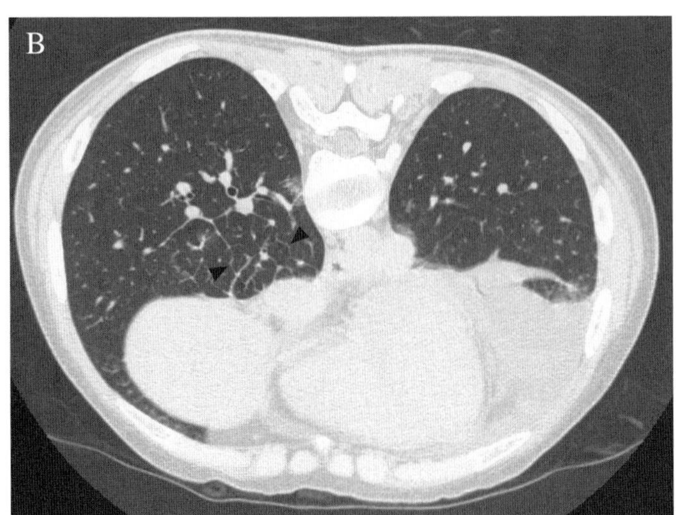

FIGURE 29.15. A 19-year-old woman with recurrent Hodgkin's lymphoma in the thorax. (A) CT scan in lung windows demonstrated a consolidative mass (*large arrow*) in the left upper lobe and left pleural effusion. In the right thorax, there is perihilar lymphadenopathy (*curved arrow*) and cavitary nodules (*arrow*). (B) High-resolution CT, 1.25-mm slice thickness, prone images show thickened interlobular septa (*arrowheads*) consistent with lymphangitic spread.

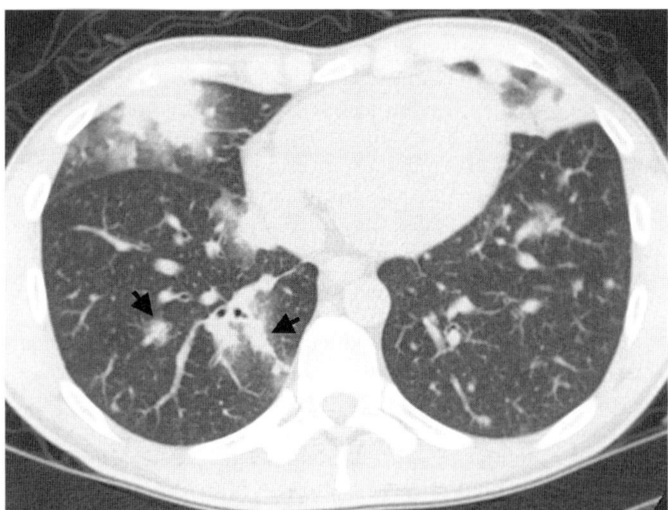

FIGURE 29.16. A 36-year-old man with Kaposi's sarcoma of the lungs. CT scan in lung windows shows multiple airspace nodules and masses with surrounding ground-glass appearance. The nodules in the right lower lobe are distributed along the bronchovasculature (*arrows*).

commonly is seen as an extension of tumor along the axial bronchovascular interstitium from hilar lymphatic disease or from an adjacent pulmonary mass. An air bronchogram is commonly seen in consolidative and nodular forms. Nodules also may cavitate. The presence of lymphadenopathy may help in the differential diagnosis, especially in patients with Hodgkin disease. However, lymphadenopathy is not necessarily present in involvement of the lungs by primary non-Hodgkin lymphoma.[144,149]

The consolidative form of adenocarcinoma and its subtype, bronchoalveolar cell carcinoma, are often initially misdiagnosed as lobar pneumonia. Presenting symptoms include fever, cough, and systemic symptoms consistent with infection that may accompany tumor.[23] Coexisting pulmonary findings, such as associated subcentimeter nodules (possibly with a ground-glass appearance, and cavitary) or scattered areas of ground-glass pattern should signal possible malignancy. On rare occasions, cystlike changes in the consolidation may develop.[150] These changes may be mistaken for bronchiectasis or cavitation from necrosis. A ground-glass appearance with septal thickening mimicking a crazy-paving pattern is unusual for metastatic adenocarcinoma but is well described.[23,151]

Involvement of the lungs by Kaposi's sarcoma commonly includes mediastinal and hilar lymphadenopathy. Tumor tends to extend along the bronchovasculature into the parenchyma (Figure 29.16). Multiple flame-shaped lesions or nodules with poorly defined borders or ground-glass pattern develop in the same distribution and commonly contain an air bronchogram.[109,152] Other manifestations, however, include a single pulmonary nodule, pleural effusion, or tracheal and bronchial lesions.[152]

FDG-PET Detection of Pulmonary Metastases

The detection of thoracic metastases from all tumor sources with FDG-PET has not been completely evaluated in the current literature. However, available results show that PET can be useful in the detection of thoracic metastases for melanoma and tumors of the colon and breast. The major weakness of PET imaging is the nodule size threshold for detection. Limitations exist with metastases smaller than 1 cm. Therefore, PET imaging should be accompanied by an imaging modality with excellent anatomic resolution, such as CT.

Lymph Node Metastases in the Thorax

The detection of unsuspected distant lymph node disease has a significant impact on tumor staging and patient prognosis. On chest radiographs, multiple pulmonary nodules are the most common manifestation of intrathoracic metastases; lymph node disease is second.[124,153–155] Tumors that most frequently have metastases identifiable on chest radiographs include renal and other genitourinary tumors, melanoma, breast tumors, and head and neck tumors (Figure 29.17). Distribution of lymphadenopathy most commonly identified on radiographs is in the mediastinal, especially the right paratracheal, region.[153]

Numerous studies of lung cancer imaging have demonstrated that CT is superior to chest radiography in detecting lymph node metastases. Williams et al.[156] demonstrated that CT is superior to chest radiography in the detection of metastatic testicular seminoma. With chest radiography, metastases were found in 25 of 200 patients. These results included mediastinal lymph nodes in 17 patients, pulmonary metastases in 7, pleural effusions in 5, and pleural masses in 2. With CT, however, metastases were found in 30 patients, including 21 with mediastinal nodes, 12 with lung metastases, 6 with pleural effusions, and 2 with pleural masses. CT showed disease in 5 patients whose chest radiography results were normal and revealed additional metastases in 4 patients with abnormal findings on chest radiographs.

The characterization of lymph node disease by means of CT is limited by the size threshold for detecting abnormal nodes. Lymph nodes are generally interpreted as abnormal if their short-axis diameter exceeds 1 cm. For this reason, lymph node enlargement due to inflammatory or infectious disease

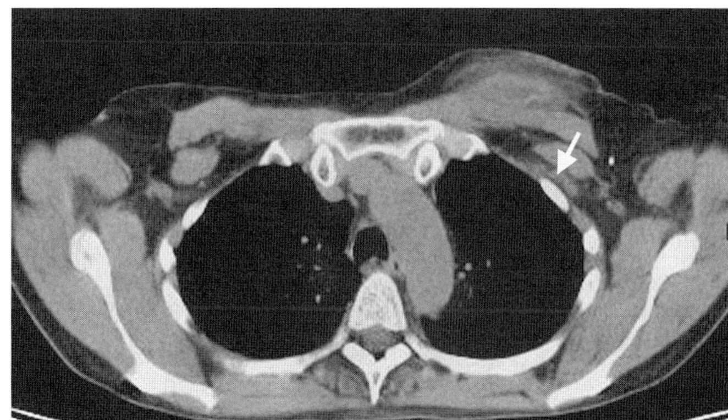

FIGURE 29.17. A 52-year-old man with esophageal carcinoma. Dual fluorodeoxyglucose-positron emission tomography (FDG-PET)/CT scan of the thorax shows increased uptake in paraesophageal lymph node (*white arrow*). Subcarinal lymph node (*black arrow*) of the same caliber shows no evidence of FDG uptake, suggesting the absence of metastases.

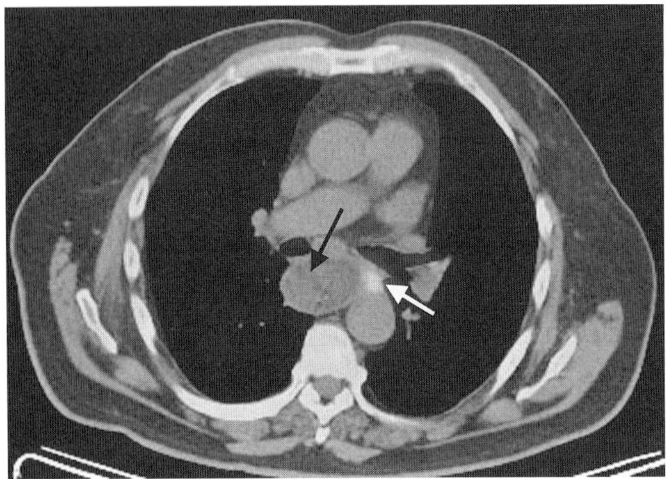

FIGURE 29.18. A 56-year-old woman with previous left mastectomy for breast cancer. Dual FDG-PET/CT scan images show increased uptake of FDG in small subpectoral lymph nodes (*arrow*), indicating metastatic nodal disease. These lymph nodes are normal in size by CT criteria.

is frequently misinterpreted as neoplastic. Early metastases to small nodes are often overlooked. FDG-PET improves specificity by better identifying lymph node disease on the basis of tumor glycolysis rather than visual size criteria (Figure 29.18). Eubank et al. found PET more accurate than CT (88% and 73%, respectively) for detecting metastatic breast cancer to the mediastinum and internal mammary lymph nodes.[32] Other studies have demonstrated the usefulness of PET in detecting metastases from the abdomen and lung.[157] However, PET also has limitations with regard to lymph node size. The size threshold for tumor detection in metastatic foci is limited with PET because of camera resolution constraints. Lymph nodes with metastases that measure 5 mm or less can be missed.[32] For instance, although FDG-PET is useful for detecting distant metastases in patients with breast cancer, it should not be the study of choice for axillary lymph node staging. Numerous studies have shown the sensitivity of PET for the detection of sentinel node disease to be as low as 20%.[158,159]

Pleural Metastatic Disease

In adult patients, 22% of newly diagnosed pleural effusions identified on chest radiographs are caused by malignancy.[160] The likelihood that a newly diagnosed unilateral pleural effusion is malignant increases with a patient's age and the size of the effusion.[160,161] Even the presence of bilateral pleural effusions should warrant further evaluation, especially if the patient's heart is of normal size. According to Blackman et al., 50% of patients with such findings have a malignancy.[162] Metastatic adenocarcinoma is responsible for 80% of malignant pleural effusions; however, in 7% to 10%, the primary site remains unknown.[163–165] Overall, bronchogenic cancer accounts for 36% to 43% of malignant pleural effusions, followed by breast cancer at 9% to 25% and lymphoma at 7% to 10%.[164,165]

The upright chest radiograph is of limited value in detecting small volumes of fluid in the pleural space. According to Blackmore et al., the smallest amount of fluid detected is 50 mL when a meniscus sign at the costophrenic angle is identified on a lateral chest film.[166] The approximate volume of fluid identified on a posteroranterior radiograph is 200 mL when a meniscus sign is present. At a volume of 500 mL, fluid typically obscures the diaphragm. Lateral decubitus films can reveal as little as 5 mL fluid; however, this technique can be limited by soft tissues, bedding, and clothing that may overlie the dependent thorax.[167]

As determined with chest radiographs, the incidence of pleural effusion in patients with primary Hodgkin disease is 7% to 13%.[168–170] It is approximately 10% in patients with primary non-Hodgkin lymphoma.[169,171] With the use of cross-sectional imaging modalities, such as CT, the sensitivity for detecting additional metastases in the thorax increases. Filly et al. reported that 80% of patients with primary Hodgkin disease and pleural effusion had lymphadenopathy that was demonstrated on chest radiographs.[169] However, Castellino et al. reported a higher incidence (100%) on the basis of CT results.[170]

Ultrasonography is sensitive in the detection and quantification of pleural effusions.[172,173] Yang et al. found ultrasound useful in characterizing the nature of pleural effusions.[174] Transudates were usually anechoic. Although exudative effusions could also appear anechoic, fluid that was complex, homogenously echogenic, or that contained complex septations was specific for an exudate. Associated findings, including a thickened pleura or underlying pulmonary lesions, also indicated an exudate. Only the presence of pleural nodules was useful in detecting malignancy in the pleural space (Figure 29.19). Similar results were reported by Gorg et al., who also reported that only the presence of pleural masses was specific for malignancy.[175] According to Bradley et al., imaging of the pleura with ultrasonography was useful in evaluating malignant effusions to distinguish benign from

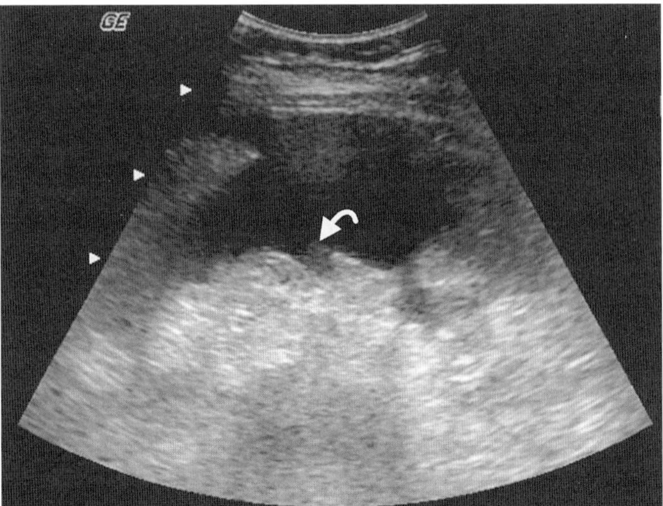

FIGURE 29.19. A 55-year-old man with metastatic adenocarcinoma and a pleural effusion. Ultrasound image shows lobulated soft tissue tumor (*curved arrow*) in the pleural space consistent with malignancy.

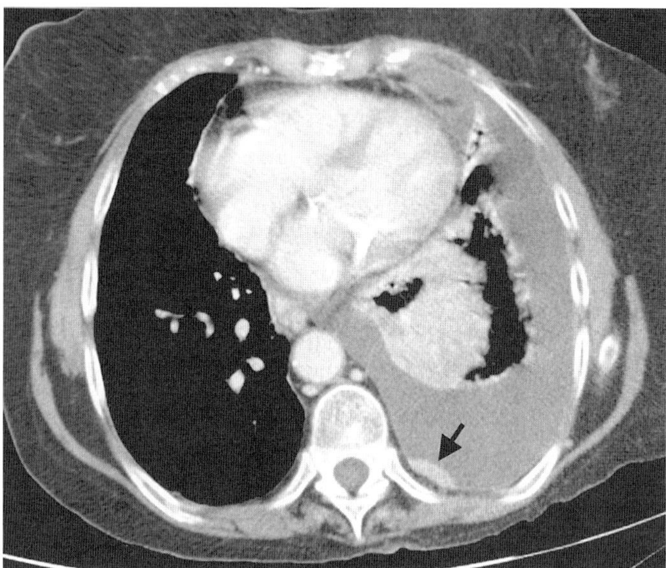

FIGURE 29.20. A 75-year-old woman with lung cancer. CT scan of the thorax (soft tissue windows) demonstrates an enhancing pleural nodule (*arrow*) consistent with tumor deposit.

malignant pleural masses and to provide real-time guidance for needle placement during percutaneous biopsy.[176] Vascular abnormalities and other benign masses were readily identified as anechoic and pulsatile. Malignant tumors showed varied echogenicity indicating soft tissue, interruption of the pleural line (90%), and decreased motion with respiration.

Although the spatial resolution of CT is excellent, small tumor deposits on the pleura can be missed.[177] According to Akaogi et al., small nodules in the interlobar fissures in a patient with lung cancer without an effusion may be the only indication of pleural involvement.[178] Malignant effusions frequently do not demonstrate any pleural changes on contrast-enhanced CT studies. Approximately 50% of malignant effusions resemble simple transudative effusions without pleural changes.[177,179] Therefore, the absence of associated pleural thickening or nodularity does not preclude a malignant effusion. Several studies have evaluated the use of CT in establishing criteria for detecting malignant pleural disease.[177,179–182] Arenas-Jimenez et al. found that pleural nodules and nodular pleural thickening were the most sensitive and specific findings for malignant pleural effusion (Figure 29.20).[177] The finding of mediastinal and circumferential pleural thickening was also more frequent in malignant disease but could be seen with an empyema. Associated findings such as a pulmonary mass or nodules, enlarged mediastinal lymph nodes, a chest wall mass, or liver nodules helped to confirm radiologic evidence. In patients with lymphoma, ancillary findings of extrapleural tumor or enlarged lymph nodes in the extrapleural space demonstrated with CT may also help to explain the source of pleural disease. Aquino et al. found that 41% of patients with lymphoma and pleural effusion had abnormal pleural or extrapleural disease or both. Ninety-five percent of patients with extrapleural tumors had adjacent paraspinal and posterior mediastinal lymph node disease.[183]

MR imaging is useful in the detection of pleural malignancy; however, because of the duration of scan time, limitations in whole-body imaging due to the need for varying sequences for specific organs, limited fields of view, and high costs, this modality is the second choice, after CT. Falaschi et al. found that MR imaging was equal to CT in the detection of morphologic changes suggesting malignant pleural disease.[184] They also found that MR imaging provided additional information as a result of changes in signal intensity with malignancy. In six patients, CT results were equivocal, whereas benign disease was distinguishable from malignant disease on the basis of MR imaging information. The most useful findings on MR images were high signal intensity on proton-density-weighted and T_2-weighted studies and the use of lesion-to-muscle ratio in each sequence. Similar results were found by Hierholzer et al.[185] Both CT and MR imaging were sensitive (93% and 96%, respectively) in detecting morphologic changes of malignant pleural disease (i.e., mediastinal pleural thickening, nodularity, irregular pleural contour, and infiltration of the chest wall or diaphragm). MR images displayed increased signal indicating malignancy in T_2-weighted and contrast-enhanced T_1-weighted series, with sensitivities of 91% and 93%, respectively. No significant features were found on noncontrast-enhanced T_1-weighted images.

As a general imaging tool for routine pretreatment evaluation of thoracic malignancy, CT is more practical and cost-effective. However MR imaging is more sensitive in detecting tumor involvement of the chest wall and diaphragm. As mentioned earlier in the chapter, MR imaging is superior to CT in the assessment of chest wall and mediastinal involvement by superior sulcus tumors. Carlsen et al. also found MR imaging useful in the pretreatment assessment of patients with mediastinal lymphoma and suspected involvement of the chest wall and pleura.[186] MR imaging detected chest wall or pleural malignancy or both in 22 of 57 patients; by comparison, with CT, disease was detected in only 2 patients.

FDG-PET is more sensitive than CT for the detection of malignant pleural disease. Bury et al. described an increase in FDG uptake in the pleura in all 16 patients with malignant pleural disease in their study group.[187] As in most FDG-PET studies, infection could mimic malignancy. In the study by Bury and colleagues, two patients with pleural empyema also showed abnormal uptake, which mimicked tumor. Gupta et al. reported a sensitivity and specificity of 88.8% and 94.1%, respectively, for FDG-PET in correctly distinguishing benign from malignant pleural disease in patients with lung cancer.[188] Extra care should be taken when interpreting any FDG-PET image of a patient with malignant pleural disease who was previously treated by means of talc pleurodesis. Talc, which causes a chronic granulomatous response in the pleural space, appears intensely hot on FDG-PET images and mimics tumor.[189] Careful correlation of PET findings with those of CT is necessary to distinguish abnormal foci of increased attenuation on PET from true neoplasm (Figure 29.21). This abnormal uptake will not resolve over time; therefore, areas of new increased FDG uptake suggest recurrent disease.

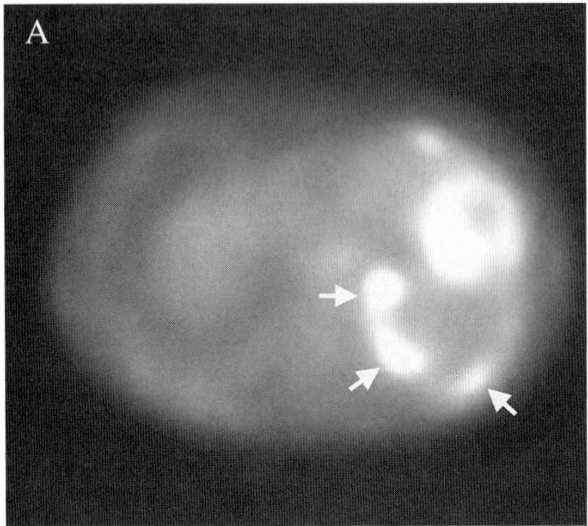

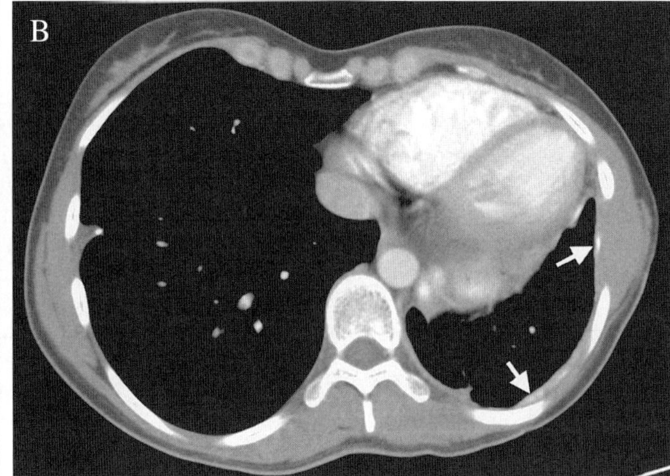

FIGURE 29.21. A 26-year-old woman with previous history of talc pleurodesis for malignant pleural effusion. (A) FDG-PET scan shows areas of increased uptake in the pleural space (*arrows*). (B) Correlative CT scan (soft tissue windows) shows increased attenuation (*arrows*) in the pleural space consistent with talc deposits. The patient had no clinical evidence for recurrence, and her PET and CT scans were stable over 3 years.

References

1. Fry WA, Menck HR, Winchester DP. The National Cancer Data Base report on lung cancer. Cancer (Phila) 1996;77:1947–1955.
2. Berlin NI, Buncher CR, Fontana RS, et al. The National Cancer Institute Cooperative Early Lung Cancer Detection Program. Am Rev Respir Dis 1984;130:545–549.
3. Frost JK, Ball WC Jr, Levin ML, et al. Early lung cancer detection: results of the initial (prevalence) radiologic and cytologic screening in The Johns Hopkins study. Am Rev Respir Dis 1984; 130:549–554.
4. Melamed MR, Flehinger BJ, Zaman MB, et al. Screening for early lung cancer: results of the initial (prevalence) radiologic and cytologic screening in the Memorial Sloan-Kettering study. Chest 1984;86:44–53.
5. Fontana RS, Sanderson DR, Woolner LB, et al. Screening for lung cancer. A critique of the Mayo lung project. Cancer (Phila) 1991; 67:1155–1164.
6. Strauss GM, Gleason RE, Sugarbaker DJ. Screening for lung cancer re-examined. A reinterpretation of the Mayo lung project randomized trial on lung cancer screening. Chest 1993;103:337S–341S.
7. Manser RL, Irving LB, Byrnes G, et al. Screening for lung cancer: a systematic review and meta-analysis of controlled trials. Thorax 2003;58:784–789.
8. Henschke CI, McCauley DI, Yankelevitz DF, et al. Early lung cancer action project: overall design and findings from baseline screening. Lancet 1999;354:99–105.
9. Henschke CI, Maidich DP, Yankelevitz DF, et al. Early lung cancer action project: initial findings on repeat screenings. Cancer (Phila) 2001;92:153–159.
10. Siegelman SS, Khouri NF, Leo FP, et al. Solitary pulmonary nodules: CT assessment. Radiology 1986;160:307–312.
11. Hasegawa M, Sone S, Takashima S, et al. Growth rate of small lung cancers detected on mass CT screening. Br J Radiol 2000; 73:1252–1259.
12. Mirtcheva RM, Vazquez M, Yankelevitz DF, et al. Bronchioloalveolar carcinoma and adenocarcinoma with bronchioloalveolar features presenting as ground-glass opacities on CT. J Clin Imaging 2002;26:95–100.
13. Gaeta M, Caruso R, Barone M, et al. Ground-glass attenuation in nodular bronchioloalveolar carcinoma: CT patterns and prognostic value. J Comput Assist Tomogr 1998;22:215–219.
14. Henschke CI, Yankelevitz DF, Mirtcheva R, et al. CT screening for lung cancer: frequency and significance of part-solid and nonsolid nodules. AJR Am J Roentgenol 2002;178:1053–1057.
15. Kim EA, Johkoh T, Lee KS, et al. Quantification of ground-glass opacity on high-resolution CT of small peripheral adenocarcinoma of the lung: pathologic and prognostic implications. AJR Am J Roentgenol 2001;177:1417–1422.
16. Asamura H, Suzuki K, Watanabe S, et al. A clinicopathological study of resected subcentimeter lung cancers: a favorable prognosis for ground glass opacity lesions. Ann Thorac Surg 2003; 76:1016–1022.
17. Sider L. Radiographic manifestations of primary bronchogenic carcinoma. Radiol Clin N Am 1990;28:583–597.
18. Rosado de Christenson ML, Templeton PA, Moran CA. Bronchogenic carcinoma: radiologic-pathologic correlation. RadioGraphics 1994;14:429–446.
19. Golden R. The effect of bronchostenosis upon the roentgen-ray shadows in carcinoma of the bronchus. Am J Roentgenol 1925; 13:21–30.
20. Im JG, Hann MC, Yu EJ, et al. Lobar bronchioloalveolar carcinoma: "angiogram sign" on CT scans. Radiology 1990;176:749–753.
21. Shah RM, Friedman AC. CT angiogram sign: incidence and significance in lobar consolidations evaluated by contrast-enhanced CT. AJR Am J Roentgenol 1998;170:719–721.
22. Murayama S, Onitsuka H, Murakami J, et al. "CT angiogram sign" in obstructive pneumonitis and pneumonia. J Comput Assist Tomogr 1993;17:609–612.
23. Aquino SL, Chiles C, Halford P. Distinction of consolidative bronchioloalveolar carcinoma from pneumonia: do CT criteria work? AJR Am J Roentgenol 1998;171:359–363.
24. Jung JI, Kim H, Park SH, et al. CT differentiation of pneumonic-type bronchioloalveolar cell carcinoma and infectious pneumonia. Br J Radiol 2001;74:490–494.
25. Johnson DE, Goldberg M. Management of carcinoma of the superior pulmonary sulcus. Oncology 1997;11:781–765; discussion 785–786.
26. O'Connell RS, McLoud TC, Wilkins EW. Superior sulcus tumor: radiographic diagnosis and workup. AJR Am J Roentgenol 1983; 140:25–30.
27. Renner RR, Pernice NJ. The apical cap. Semin Roentgenol 1977; 12:299–302.

28. Takasugi JE, Rapoport S, Shaw C. Superior sulcus tumors: the role of imaging. J Thorac Imaging 1989;4:41–48.
29. Heelan RT, Demas BE, Caravelli JF, et al. Superior sulcus tumors: CT and MR imaging. Radiology 1989;170:637–641.
30. Laissy JP, Soyer P, Sekkal SR, et al. Assessment of vascular involvement with magnetic resonance angiography (MRA) in Pancoast syndrome. Magn Reson Imaging 1995;13:523–530.
31. Pieterman RM, van Putten JWG, Meuzelaar JJ, et al. Preoperative staging of non-small-cell lung cancer with positron-emission tomography. N Engl J Med 2000;343:254–261.
32. Lardinois D, Weder W, Hany TF, et al. Staging of non-small cell lung cancer with integrated positron-emission tomography and computed tomography. N Engl J Med 2003;348:2500–2507.
33. Aquino SL, Asmuth JC, Moore RH, et al. Improved image interpretation with registered thoracic CT and positron emission tomography data sets. AJR Am J Roentgenol 2002;178:939–944.
34. Kang JH, Kim KD, Chung KY. Prognostic value of visceral pleura invasion in non-small cell lung cancer. Eur J Cardiothorac Surg 2003;23:865–869.
35. Manac'h D, Riquet M, Medioni J, et al. Visceral pleura invasion by non-small cell lung cancer: an underrated bad prognostic factor. Ann Thorac Surg 2001;71:1088–1093.
36. Glazer HS, Duncan-Meyer J, Aronberg DJ, et al. Pleural and chest wall invasion in bronchogenic carcinoma: CT evaluation. Radiology 1985;157:191–194.
37. Padovani B, Mouroux J, Seksik L, et al. Chest wall invasion by bronchogenic carcinoma: evaluation with MR imaging. Radiology 1993;187:33–38.
38. Ratto GB, Piacenza G, Frola C, et al. Chest wall involvement by lung cancer: computed tomographic detection and results of operation. Ann Thorac Surg 1991;51:182–188.
39. Pennes DR, Glazer GM, Wimbish KJ, et al. Chest wall invasion by lung cancer: limitations of CT evaluation. AJR Am J Roentgenol 1985;144:507–511.
40. Pearlberg JL, Sandler MA, Beute GH, et al. Limitations of CT in evaluation of neoplasms involving chest wall. J Comput Assist Tomogr 1987;11:290–293.
41. Scott IR, Müller NL, Miller RR, et al. Resectable Stage III lung cancer: CT, surgical, and pathologic correlation. Radiology 1988;166(1 pt 1):75–79.
42. Uhrmeister P, Allmann KH, Wertzel H, et al. Chest wall infiltration by lung cancer: value of thin-sectional CT with different reconstruction algorithms. Eur Radiol 1999;9:1304–1309.
43. Shiotani S, Sugimura K, Sugihara M, et al. Diagnosis of chest wall invasion by lung cancer: useful criteria for exclusion of the possibility of chest wall invasion with MR imaging. Radiat Med 2000;18:283–290.
44. Sakai S, Murayama S, Murakami J, et al. Bronchogenic carcinoma invasion of the chest wall: evaluation with dynamic cine MRI during breathing. J Comput Assist Tomogr 1997;21:595–600.
45. Toloza EM, Harpole L, McCrory DC. Noninvasive staging of non-small cell lung cancer. Chest 2003;123(suppl 1):137S–146S.
46. Dales RE, Stark RM, Raman S. Computed tomography to stage lung cancer. Approaching a controversy using meta-analysis. Am Rev Respir Dis 1990;141:1096–1101.
47. Gould MK, Kuschner WG, Rydzak CE, et al. Test performance of positron emission tomography and computed tomography for mediastinal staging in patients with non-small-cell lung cancer. Ann Intern Med 2003;139:879–892.
48. Graeter TP, Hellwig D, Hoffmann K, et al. Mediastinal lymph node staging in suspected lung cancer: comparison of positron emission tomography with F-18-fluorodeoxyglucose and mediastinoscopy. Ann Thorac Surg 2003;75:231–236.
49. Vansteenkiste JF, Stroobants SG, DeLeyn De Leyn PR, et al. Lymph node staging in non-small-cell lung cancer with FDG-PET scan: a prospective study on 690 lymph node stations from 68 patients. J Clin Oncol 1998;16:2142–2149.
50. Albes JM, Lietzenmayer R, Schott U, et al. Improvement of non-small-cell lung cancer staging by means of positron emission tomography. Thorac Cardiovasc Surg 1999;47:42–47.
51. Berlangieri SU, Scott AM, Knight SR, et al. F-18 fluorodeoxyglucose positron emission tomography in the non-invasive staging of non-small cell lung cancer. Eur J Cardiothorac Surg 1999;16(suppl 1):S25–S30.
52. Chin R Jr, Ward R, Keyes JW, et al. Mediastinal staging of non-small-cell lung cancer with positron emission tomography. Am J Respir Crit Care Med 1995;152:2090–2096.
53. Cerfolio RJ, Ojha B, Bryant AS, et al. The role of FDG-PET scan in staging patients with nonsmall cell carcinoma. Ann Thorac Surg 2003;76:861–866.
54. Pfister DG, Johnson DH, Azzoli CG, et al. American Society of Clinical Oncology treatment of unresectable non-small-cell lung cancer guideline: update 2003. J Clin Oncol 2004;22:330–353.
55. Dunagan DP, Chin R Jr, McCain TW, et al. Staging by positron emission tomography predicts survival in patients with non-small cell lung cancer. Chest 2001;119:333–339.
56. Hicks RJ, Kalff V, MacManus MP, et al. 18F-FDG PET provides high-impact and powerful prognostic stratification in staging newly diagnosed non-small cell lung cancer. J Nucl Med 2001;42:1596–1604.
57. Vansteenkiste JF, Stroobants SG, Dupont RJPJ, et al. FDG-PET scan in potentially operable non-small cell lung cancer: do anatometabolic PET–CT fusion images improve the localization of regional lymph node metastases? The Leuven Lung Cancer Group. Eur J Nucl Med 1998;25:1495–1501.
58. Magnani P, Carretta A, Rizzo G, et al. FDG/PET and spiral CT image fusion for mediastinal lymph node assessment on non-small cell lung cancer patients. J Cardiovasc Surg 1999;40:741–748.
59. Beyer T, Townsend DW, Brun T, et al. A combined PET/CT scanner for clinical oncology. Results of the initial screen (prevalence). Early lung cancer detection: introduction. J Nucl Med 2000;41:1369–1379.
60. Antoch G, Stattaus J, Nemat AT, et al. Non-small cell lung cancer: dual-modality PET/CT in preoperative staging. Radiology 2003;229:526–533.
61. Ries LAG, Eisner MP, Kosary CL, et al. (eds). SEER Cancer Statistics Review, 1975–2000. Bethesda, MD: National Cancer Institute. http://seer.cancer.gov/csr/1975_2000, 2003.
62. Vaaler AK, Forrester JM, Lesar M, et al. Obstructive atelectasis in patients with small cell lung cancer. Incidence and response to treatment. Chest 1997;111:115–120.
63. Schumacher T, Brink I, Mix M, et al. FDG-PET imaging for the staging and follow-up of small cell lung cancer. Eur J Nucl Med 2001;28:483–488.
64. Pandit N, Gonen M, Krug L, et al. Prognostic value of [^{18}F] FDG-PET imaging in small cell lung cancer. Eur J Nucl Med 2003;30:78–84.
65. Choi JB, Park CK, Park DW, et al. Does contrast enhancement on CT suggest tumor response for chemotherapy in small cell carcinoma of the lung. J Comput Assist Tomogr 2002;26:797–800.
66. Perez EA, Loprinzi CL, Sloan JA, et al. Utility of screening procedures for detecting recurrence of disease after complete response in patients with small cell lung carcinoma. Cancer (Phila) 1997;80:676–680.
67. Rea F, Binda R, Spreafico G, et al. Bronchial carcinoids: a review of 60 patients. Ann Thorac Surg 1989;47:412–414.
68. Harpole DH Jr, Feldman JM, Buchanan S, et al. Bronchial carcinoid tumors: a retrospective analysis of 126 patients. Ann Thorac Surg 1992;54:50–54; discussion 54–55.
69. Jeung MY, Gasser B, Gangi A, et al. Bronchial carcinoid tumors of the thorax: spectrum of radiologic findings. RadioGraphics 2002;22:351–365.

70. Forster BB, Muller NL, Miller RR, et al. Neuroendocrine carcinomas of the lung: clinical, radiologic, and pathologic correlation. Radiology 1989;170:441–445.
71. Magid D, Siegelman SS, Eggleston JC, et al. Pulmonary carcinoid tumors: CT assessment. J Comput Assist Tomogr 1989;13:244–247.
72. Zwiebel BR, Austin JH, Brimes MM. Bronchial carcinoid tumors: assessment with CT of location and intratumoral calcification in 31 patients. Radiology 1991;179:483–486.
73. Aronchick JM, Wexler JA, Christen B, et al. Computed tomography of bronchial carcinoid. J Comput Assist Tomogr 1986;10:71–74.
74. Choplin RH, Kawamoto EH, Dyer RB, et al. Atypical carcinoid of the lung: radiographic features. AJR Am J Roentgenol 1986;146:665–668.
75. Douek PC, Simoni L, Revel D, et al. Diagnosis of bronchial carcinoid tumor by ultrafast contrast-enhanced MR imaging. AJR Am J Roentgenol 1994;163:563–564.
76. Erasmus, JJ, McAdams HP, Patz EF Jr, et al. Evaluation of primary pulmonary carcinoid tumors using FDG PET. AJR Am J Roentgenol 1998;170:1369–1373.
77. Gould PM, Bonner JA, Sawyer TE, et al. Bronchial carcinoid tumors: importance of prognostic factors that influence patterns of recurrence and overall survival. Radiology 1998;208:181–185.
78. King CM, Reznek RH, Bomanji J, et al. Imaging neuroendocrine tumours with radiolabelled somatostatin analogues and x-ray computed tomography: a comparative study. Clin Radiol 1993;48:386–391.
79. Kawashima A, Libshitz HI. Malignant pleural mesothelioma: CT manifestations in 50 cases. AJR Am J Roentgenol 1990;155:965–969.
80. Metintas M, Ucgun I, Elbek O, et al. Computed tomography features in malignant pleural mesothelioma and other commonly seen pleural diseases. Eur J Radiol 2002;41:1–9.
81. Knuuttila A, Halme M, Kivisaari L, et al. The clinical importance of magnetic resonance imaging versus computed tomography in malignant pleural mesothelioma. Lung Cancer 1998;22:215–225.
82. Knuuttila A, Kivisaari L, Kivisaari A, et al. Evaluation of pleural disease using MR and CT. With special reference to malignant pleural mesothelioma. Acta Radiol 2001;42:502–507.
83. Heelan RT, Rusch VW, Begg CB, et al. Staging of malignant pleural mesothelioma: comparison of CT and MR imaging. AJR Am J Roentgenol 1999;172:1039–1047.
84. Benard F, Sterman D, Smith R, et al. Metabolic imaging of malignant pleural mesothelioma with fluorodeoxyglucose positron emission tomography. Chest 1998;114:713–722.
85. Gerbaudo VH, Sugarbaker DJ, Britz-Cunningham S, et al. Assessment of malignant pleural mesothelioma with 18F-FDG dual-head gamma-camera coincidence imaging: comparison with histopathology. J Nucl Med 2002;43:1144–1149.
86. Flores RA, Akhurst TB, Gonen MC, et al. Positron emission tomography defines metastatic disease but not locoregional disease in patients with malignant pleural mesothelioma. J Thorac Cardiovasc Surg 2003;126:11–16.
87. Kim YH, Lee KS, Primack SL, et al. Small pulmonary nodules on CT accompanying surgically resectable lung cancer: likelihood of malignancy. J Thorac Imaging 2002;17:40–46.
88. Chalmers N, Best JJ. The significance of pulmonary nodules detected by CT but not by chest radiography in tumour staging. Clin Radiol 1991;44:410–412.
89. Kronawitter U, Kemeny NE, Heelan R, et al. Evaluation of chest computed tomography in the staging of patients with potentially resectable liver metastases from colorectal carcinoma. Cancer (Phila) 1999;86:229–235.
90. Povoski SP, Fong Y, Sgouros SC, et al. Role of chest CT in patients with negative chest x-rays referred for hepatic colorectal metastases. Ann Surg Oncol 1998;5:9–15.
91. Picci P, Vanel D, Briccoli A, et al. Computed tomography of pulmonary metastases from osteosarcoma: the less poor technique. A study of 51 patients with histological correlation. Ann Oncol 2001;12:1601–1604.
92. Fernandez EB, Colon E, McLeod DG, et al. Efficacy of radiographic chest imaging in patients with testicular cancer. Urology 1994;44:243–248; discussion 248–249.
93. Lim DJ, Carter MF. Computerized tomography in the preoperative staging for pulmonary metastases in patients with renal cell carcinoma. J Urol 1993;150:1112–1114.
94. Warner G, Cox G. Evaluation of chest radiography versus chest computed tomography in screening for pulmonary malignancy in advanced head and neck cancer. J Otolaryngol 2003;32:107–109.
95. Heaston DK, Putman CE, Rodan BA, et al. Solitary pulmonary metastases in high-risk melanoma patients: a prospective comparison of conventional and computed tomography. AJR Am J Roentgenol 1983;141:169–174.
96. Reiner B, Siegel E, Sawyer R, et al. The impact of routine CT of the chest on the diagnosis and management of newly diagnosed squamous cell carcinoma of the head and neck. AJR Am J Roentgenol 1997;169:667–671.
97. Yamada H, Katoh H, Kondo S, et al. Surgical treatment of pulmonary recurrence after hepatectomy for colorectal liver metastases. Hepatogastroenterology 2002;49:976–979.
98. Koong HN, Pastorino U, Ginsberg RJ. Is there a role for pneumonectomy in pulmonary metastases? Ann Thorac Surg 1999;68:2039–2043.
99. Al-Mehdi AB, Tozawa K, Fisher AB, et al. Intravascular origin of metastasis from the proliferation of endothelium-attached tumor cells: a new model for metastasis. Nat Med 2000;6:100–102.
100. Wong CW, Song C, Grimes MM, et al. Intravascular location of breast cancer cells after spontaneous metastasis to the lung. Am J Pathol 2002;161:749–753.
101. Milne EN, Zerhouni EA. Blood supply of pulmonary metastases. J Thorac Imaging 1987;2:15–23.
102. Stackpole CW. Intrapulmonary spread of established B16 melanoma lung metastases and lung colonies. Invasion Metastasis 1990;10:267–280.
103. Alterman AL, Fornabaio DM, Stackpole CW. Metastatic dissemination of B16 melanoma: pattern and sequence of metastasis. J Natl Cancer Inst 1985;75:691–702.
104. Cahan WG, Shah JP, Castro EB. Benign solitary lung lesions in patients with cancer. Ann Surg 1978;187:241–244.
105. Schlumberger M, Arcangioli O, Piekarski JD, et al. Detection and treatment of lung metastases of differentiated thyroid carcinoma in patients with normal chest X-rays. J Nucl Med 1988;29:1790–1794.
106. Piekarski JD, Schlumberger M, Leclere J, et al. Chest computed tomography (CT) in patients with micronodular lung metastases of differentiated thyroid carcinoma. Int J Radiat Oncol Biol Phys 1985;11:1023–1027.
107. Lee K, Kim T, Han J, et al. Diffuse micronodular lung disease: HRCT and pathologic findings. J Comput Assist Tomogr 1999;23:99–106.
108. Hirakata K, Nakata H, Haratake J. Appearance of pulmonary metastases on high-resolution CT scans: comparison with histopathologic findings from autopsy specimens. AJR Am J Roentgenol 1993;161:37–43.
109. Primack SL, Hartman TE, Lee KS, et al. Pulmonary nodules and the CT halo sign. Radiology 1994;190:513–515.
110. Patel A, Ryu J. Angiosarcoma in the lung. Chest 1993;103:1531–1535.
111. Benditt JO, Farber HW, Wright J, et al. Pulmonary hemorrhage with diffuse alveolar infiltrates in men with high-volume choriocarcinoma. Ann Intern Med 1988;109:674–675.
112. Gaeta M, Blandino A, Scribano E, et al. Computed tomography halo sign in pulmonary nodules: frequency and diagnostic value. J Thorac Imaging 1999;14:109–113.

113. Sidhu GS, Wieczorek R, Cassai ND, et al. The concept of bronchioloalveolar cell adenocarcinoma: redefinition, a critique of the 1999 WHO classification, and an ultrastructural analysis of 155 cases. Int J Surg Pathol 2003;11:89–99.
114. de Santos LA, Lindell MM Jr, Goldman AM, et al. Calcification within metastatic pulmonary nodules from synovial sarcoma. Orthopedics 1978;1:141–144.
115. Cockshott WP, Hendrickse JP. Pulmonary calcification at the site of trophoblastic metastases. Br J Radiol 1969;42:17–20.
116. Hall FM, Frank HA, Cohen RB, et al. Ossified pulmonary metastases from giant cell tumor of bone. AJR Am J Roentgenol 1976; 127:1046–1047.
117. Jimenez JM, Casey SO, Citron M, et al. Calcified pulmonary metastases from medullary carcinoma of the thyroid. Comput Med Imaging Graph 1995;19:325–328.
118. Franchi M, La Fianza A, Babilonti L, et al. Serous carcinoma of the ovary: value of computed tomography in detection of calcified pleural and pulmonary metastatic implants. Gynecol Oncol 1990;39:85–88.
119. Rosenfield AT, Sanders RC, Custer LE. Widespread calcified metastases from adenocarcinoma of the jejunum. Am J Dig Dis 1975;20:990–993.
120. Chaudhuri MR. Cavitary pulmonary metastases. Thorax 1970; 25:375–381.
121. Dodd GD, Boyle JJ. Excavating pulmonary metastases. Am J Roentgenol Radium Ther Nucl Med 1961;85:277–293.
122. Thalinger AR, Rosenthal SN, Borg S, et al. Cavitation of pulmonary metastases as a response to chemotherapy. Cancer (Phila) 1980;46:1329–1332.
123. Rovirosa A, Salud A, Felip E, et al. Cavitary pulmonary metastases in transitional cell carcinoma of the urinary bladder. Urol Int 1992;48:102–104.
124. Shin MS, Shingleton HM, Partridge EE, et al. Squamous cell carcinoma of the uterine cervix. Patterns of thoracic metastases. Invest Radiol 1995;30:724–729.
125. Alexander PW, Sanders C, Nath H. Cavitary pulmonary metastases in transitional cell carcinoma of urinary bladder. AJR Am J Roentgenol 1990;154:493–494.
126. Charig MJ, Williams MP. Pulmonary lacunae: sequelae of metastases following chemotherapy. Clin Radiol 1990;42:93–96.
127. Lee KS, Kim TS, Fujimoto K, et al. Thoracic manifestation of Wegener's granulomatosis: CT findings in 30 patients. Eur Radiol 2003;13:43–51.
128. Ohdama S, Akagawa S, Matsubara O, Yoshizawa Y. Primary diffuse alveolar septal amyloidosis with multiple cysts and calcification. Eur Respir J 1996;9:1569–1571.
129. Essadki O, Chartrand-Lefebvre C, Finet JF, Grenier P. Cystic pulmonary metastasis simulating a diagnosis of histiocytosis X. J Radiol 1998;79:886–888.
130. Shepard J, Moore E, Templeton P, et al. Pulmonary intravascular tumor emboli: dilated and beaded peripheral pulmonary arteries at CT. Radiology 1993;187:797–801.
131. Kang C, Choi J, Kim H, et al. Lung metastases manifesting as pulmonary infarction by mucin and tumor embolization: radiographic, high-resolution CT, and pathologic findings. J Comput Assist Tomogr 1999;23:644–646.
132. Odeh M, Oliven A, Misselevitch I, et al. Acute cor pulmonale due to tumor cell microemboli. Respiration 1997;64:384–387.
133. Chan CK, Hutcheon MA, Hyland RH, et al. Pulmonary tumor embolism: a critical review of clinical, imaging, and hemodynamic features. J Thorac Imaging 1987;2:4–14.
134. Schriner RW, Ryu JH, Edwards WD. Microscopic pulmonary tumor embolism causing subacute cor pulmonale: a difficult antemortem diagnosis. Mayo Clin Proc 1991;66:143–148.
135. Braman SS, Whitcomb ME. Endobronchial metastasis. Arch Intern Med 1975;135:543–547.
136. Litle VR, Christie NA, Fernando HC, et al. Photodynamic therapy for endobronchial metastases from nonbronchogenic primaries. Ann Thorac Surg 2003;76:370–375.
137. Baumgartner WA, Mark JB. Metastatic malignancies from distant sites to the tracheobronchial tree. J Thorac Cardiovasc Surg 1980;79:499–503.
138. Mason AC, White CS. CT appearance of endobronchial non-Hodgkin lymphoma. J Comput Assist Tomogr 1994;18:559–561.
139. Zerhouni EA, Naidich DP, Stitik FP, et al. Computed tomography of the pulmonary parenchyma. Part 2: Interstitial disease. J Thorac Imaging 1985;1:54–64.
140. Ren H, Hruban RH, Kuhlman JE, et al. Computed tomography of inflation-fixed lungs: the beaded septum sign of pulmonary metastases. J Comput Assist Tomogr 1989;13:411–416.
141. Ikezoe J, Godwin JD, Hunt KJ, et al. Pulmonary lymphangitic carcinomatosis: chronicity of radiographic findings in long-term survivors. AJR Am J Roentgenol 1995;165:49–52.
142. Munk PL, Muller NL, Miller RR, Ostrow DN. Pulmonary lymphangitic carcinomatosis: CT and pathologic findings. Radiology 1988;166:705–709.
143. Stein MG, Mayo J, Muller N, Aberle DR, Webb WR, Gamsu G. Pulmonary lymphangitic spread of carcinoma: appearance on CT scans. Radiology 1987;162:371–375.
144. Berkman N, Breuer R, Kramer M, Polliack A. Pulmonary involvement in lymphoma. Leuk Lymphoma 1996;20:229–237.
145. Tanaka N, Matsumoto T, Miura G, et al. CT findings of leukemic pulmonary infiltration with pathologic correlation. Eur Radiol 2002;12:166–174.
146. Heyneman LE, Johkoh T, Ward S, et al. Pulmonary leukemic infiltrates: high-resolution CT findings in 10 patients. AJR Am J Roentgenol 2000;174:517–521.
147. Johkoh T, Ikezoe J, Tomiyama N, et al. CT findings in lymphangitic carcinomatosis of the lung: correlation with histologic findings and pulmonary function tests. AJR Am J Roentgenol 1992;158:1217–1222.
148. Honda O, Johkoh T, Ichikado K, et al. Comparison of high resolution CT findings of sarcoidosis, lymphoma, and lymphangitic carcinoma: is there any difference of involved interstitium? J Comput Assist Tomogr 1999;23:374–379.
149. Lewis E, Caskey C, Fishman E. Lymphoma of the lung: CT findings in 31 patients. AJR Am J Roentgenol 1991;156:711–714.
150. Strollo DC, Rosado-de-Christenson ML, Franks TJ. Reclassification of cystic bronchioloalveolar carcinomas to adenocarcinomas based on the revised World Health Organization Classification of Lung and Pleural Tumours. J Thorac Imaging 2003;18:59–66.
151. Akira M, Atagi S, Kawahara M, et al. High-resolution CT findings of diffuse bronchioloalveolar carcinoma in 38 patients. AJR Am J Roentgenol 1999;173:1623–1629.
152. Wolff SD, Kuhlman JE, Fishman EK. Thoracic Kaposi sarcoma in AIDS: CT findings. J Comput Assist Tomogr 1993;17:60–62.
153. McLoud TC, Kalisher L, Stark P, et al. Intrathoracic lymph node metastases from extrathoracic neoplasms. AJR Am J Roentgenol 1978;131:403–407.
154. Chen JT, Dahmash NS, Ravin CE, et al. Metastatic melanoma in the thorax: report of 130 patients. AJR Am J Roentgenol 1981; 137:293–298.
155. Kutty K, Varkey B. Incidence and distribution of intrathoracic metastases from renal cell carcinoma. Arch Intern Med 1984; 144:273–276.
156. Williams MP, Husband JE, Heron CW. Intrathoracic manifestations of metastatic testicular seminoma: a comparison of chest radiographic and CT findings. AJR Am J Roentgenol 1987;149: 473–475.
157. Schirrmeister H, Kuhn T, Guhlmann A, et al. Fluorine-18 2-deoxy-2-fluoro-D-glucose PET in the preoperative staging of breast cancer: comparison with the standard staging procedures. Eur J Nucl Med 2001;28:351–358.

158. Barranger E, Grahek D, Antoine M, et al. Evaluation of fluorodeoxyglucose positron emission tomography in the detection of axillary lymph node metastases in patients with early-stage breast cancer. Ann Surg Oncol 2003;10:622–627.
159. van der Hoeven JJ, Hoekstra OS, Comans EF, et al. Determinants of diagnostic performance of [F-18]fluorodeoxyglucose positron emission tomography for axillary staging in breast cancer. Ann Surg 2002;236:619–624.
160. Marel M, Zrustova M, Stasny B, et al. The incidence of pleural effusion in a well-defined region. Epidemiologic study in central Bohemia. Chest 1993;104:1486–1489.
161. Salyer WR, Eggleston JC, Erozan YS. Efficacy of pleural needle biopsy and pleural fluid cytopathology in the diagnosis of malignant neoplasm involving the pleura. Chest 1975;67:536–539.
162. Blackman NS, Rabin CB. Bilateral pleural effusion; its significance in association with a heart of normal size. J Mt Sinai Hosp NY 1957;24:45–53.
163. Monte SA, Ehya H, Lang WR. Positive effusion cytology as the initial presentation of malignancy. Acta Cytol 1987;31:448–452.
164. Sahn SA. Malignant pleural effusions. Clin Chest Med 1985; 6:113–125.
165. O'Donovan PB, Eng P. Pleural changes in malignant pleural effusions: appearance on computed tomography. Cleve Clin J Med 1994;61:127–131; quiz 162.
166. Blackmore CC, Black WC, Dallas RV, et al. Pleural fluid volume estimation: a chest radiograph prediction rule. Acad Radiol 1996; 3:103–109.
167. Moskowitz H, Platt RT, Schachar R, et al. Roentgen visualization of minute pleural effusion. An experimental study to determine the minimum amount of pleural fluid visible on a radiograph. Radiology 1973;109:33–35.
168. Castellino RA, Filly R, Blank N. Routine full-lung tomography in the initial staging and treatment planning of patients with Hodgkin's disease and non-Hodgkin's lymphoma. Cancer (Phila) 1976;38:1130–1136.
169. Filly R, Bland N, Castellino RA. Radiographic distribution of intrathoracic disease in previously untreated patients with Hodgkin's disease and non-Hodgkin's lymphoma. Radiology 1976;120:277–281.
170. Castellino RA. Diagnostic imaging evaluation of Hodgkin's disease and non-Hodgkin's lymphoma. Cancer (Phila) 1991;67: 1177–1180.
171. Das DK, Gupta SK, Ayyagari S, Bambery PK, Datta BN, Datta U. Pleural effusions in non-Hodgkin's lymphoma. A cytomorphologic, cytochemical and immunologic study. Acta Cytol 1987; 31:119–124.
172. Kocijancic I, Vidmar K, Ivanovi-Herceg Z. Chest sonography versus lateral decubitus radiography in the diagnosis of small pleural effusions. J Clin Ultrasound 2003;31:69–74.
173. Eibenberger KL, Dock WI, Ammann ME, et al. Quantification of pleural effusions: sonography versus radiography. Radiology 1994;191:681–684.
174. Yang PC, Luh KT, Chang DB, Wu HD, Yu CJ, Kuo SH. Value of sonography in determining the nature of pleural effusion: analysis of 320 cases. AJR Am J Roentgenol 1992;159:29–33.
175. Gorg C, Restrepo I, Schwerk WB. Sonography of malignant pleural effusion. Eur Radiol 1997;7:1195–1198.
176. Bradley MJ, Metreweli C. Ultrasound in the diagnosis of the juxta-pleural lesion. Br J Radiol 1991;64:330–333.
177. Arenas-Jimenez J, Alonso-Charterina S, Sanchez-Paya J, et al. Evaluation of CT findings for diagnosis of pleural effusions. Eur Radiol 2000;10:681–690.
178. Akaogi E, Mitsui K, Onizuka M, et al. Pleural dissemination in non-small cell lung cancer: results of radiological evaluation and surgical treatment. J Surg Oncol 1994;57:33–39.
179. Aquino SL, Webb WR, Gushiken BJ. Pleural exudates and transudates: diagnosis with contrast-enhanced CT. Radiology 1994; 192:803–808.
180. Leung AN, Muller NL, Miller RR. CT in differential diagnosis of diffuse pleural disease. AJR Am J Roentgenol 1990;154:487–492.
181. Mori K, Hirose T, Machida S, et al. Helical computed tomography diagnosis of pleural dissemination in lung cancer: comparison of thick-section and thin-section helical computed tomography. J Thorac Imaging 1998;13:211–218.
182. Traill ZC, Davies RJ, Gleeson FV. Thoracic computed tomography in patients with suspected malignant pleural effusions. Clin Radiol 2001;56:193–196.
183. Aquino SL, Chen MY, Kuo WT, Chiles C. The CT appearance of pleural and extrapleural disease in lymphoma. Clin Radiol 1999;54:647–650.
184. Falaschi F, Battolla L, Mascalchi M, et al. Usefulness of MR signal intensity in distinguishing benign from malignant pleural disease. AJR Am J Roentgenol 1996;166:963–968.
185. Hierholzer J, Luo L, Bittner RC, et al. MRI and CT in the differential diagnosis of pleural disease. Chest 2000;118:604–609.
186. Carlsen SE, Bergin CJ, Hoppe RT. MR imaging to detect chest wall and pleural involvement in patients with lymphoma: effect on radiation therapy planning. AJR Am J Roentgenol 1993;160: 1191–1195.
187. Bury T, Paulus P, Dowlati A, et al. Evaluation of pleural diseases with FDG-PET imaging: preliminary report. Thorax 1997;52: 187–189.
188. Gupta NC, Rogers JS, Graeber GM, et al. Clinical role of F-18 fluorodeoxyglucose positron emission tomography imaging in patients with lung cancer and suspected malignant pleural effusion. Chest 2002;122:1918–1924.
189. Kwek B, Aquino SL, Fischman AJ. Fluorodeoxyglucose positron emission tomography and CT after talc pleurodesis. Chest 2004; 125:2356–2360.

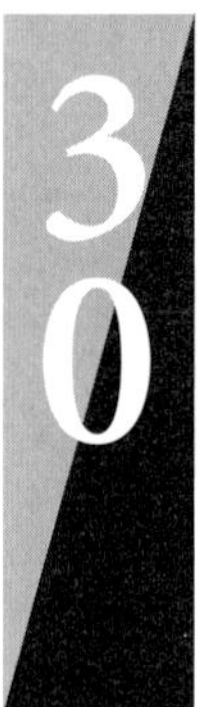

Imaging of Gastrointestinal Stromal Tumor

Ihab R. Kamel and Elliot K. Fishman

Gastrointestinal stromal tumor (GIST) is a rare stromal neoplasm that accounts for 5% of all soft tissue sarcomas.[1] It is the most common mesenchymal neoplasm of the gastrointestinal tract.[2,3] Before the advent of immunohistologic methods, most spindle cell sarcomas of the gastrointestinal tract were considered to be leiomyomas or leiomyosarcomas, with occasional examples of neurogenic tumors. GIST defines a distinct group of gastrointestinal tumors that originate from the intestinal cells of Cajal. These cells act as regulators of bowel peristalsis and therefore are also called *pacemaker cells*.[4–6] Cajal cells normally express cKIT (CD 117), which is a tyrosine kinase growth factor receptor. This cKIT immunoreactivity is the best defining feature of GISTs, distinguishing them from true smooth muscle tumors (i.e., leiomyomas and leiomyosarcomas) and tumors arising from neural crest derivatives (i.e., schwannomas and neurofibromas)[6,7]; this is considered the most specific criterion for the diagnosis of GIST. In addition, targeting the cKIT receptor with a cKIT tyrosine kinase inhibitor [STI-571, imatinib (gleevec); Novartis, Basel, Switzerland] has been successfully utilized in treating patients with GIST.[8,9]

General Features

GISTs may occur anywhere throughout the gastrointestinal tract, from the esophagus to the anus. They may also occur in the mesentery, omentum, and retroperitoneum. The estimated prevalence of GISTs is 10 to 20 cases per million population.[10] Up to 70% of GISTs arise in the stomach and approximately 20% to 30% arise from the small bowel. Incidence in the esophagus, colon, and rectum is rare.[11,12] In the esophagus, leiomyomas are more common than GIST, accounting for approximately 75% of mesenchymal tumors.[13] However, in the stomach, small bowel, colon, and anorectum, GISTs account for almost all mesenchymal tumors because other tumors, such as leiomyoma and leiomyosarcoma in these sites are rare.[10,14,15] Most GISTs exhibit an exophytic growth pattern, growing along the bowel wall. For small lesions, the overlying mucosa is typically intact, but mucosal ulceration may occur in large and aggressive tumors. Surrounding organ invasion may occur in approximately one-third of cases.[16] Metastatic disease is common and was reported in nearly 50% of patients in one study.[1] The liver is the most common site of metastases (65%), followed by the peritoneum (21%). Metastases to the lymph nodes, lungs, and bones are considered rare. Most patients eventually develop recurrence after complete surgical resection. The liver and peritoneum are the two most common sites for recurrence.[17]

Most GISTs are sporadic, and the majority of cases present with a solitary lesion. However, patients with type I neurofibromatosis have an increased prevalence of GIST. Typically, these patients are children or young adults with multiple small intestinal GISTs.[18,19] Gastric GISTs may rarely occur in association with pulmonary chondromata and extraadrenal paraganglioma in Carney's syndrome,[20,21] which has a predilection for young women.

Clinical Presentation

At presentation, most patients are in their fifth and sixth decade of life, and GISTs are rarely seen in patients younger than 40 years of age.[11] No gender predilection has been established,[22,23] although some data showed male predominance.[1,24] There is no association between race, ethnicity, occupation, or geographic location.[25]

The clinical manifestation of GIST is widely variable, depending on tumor location and size. The most frequent location for GIST is in the stomach (70%), followed by the small bowel (20% to 30%).[10] Tumor size is extremely variable, ranging from small lesions to large masses. Small tumors are usually asymptomatic and are diagnosed incidentally during imaging, endoscopy, or surgery. GISTs may remain clinically silent because of their submucosal origin and tendency to grow exophytically. Symptomatic GISTs are usually large and may present with gastrointestinal bleeding from mucosal ulceration.[26] Patients may present with hematemesis, melena, or symptoms and signs of anemia resulting from occult bleeding.[27] Other symptoms include abdominal fullness and pain. A palpable mass may also be present. The submucosal location of the tumor may cause obstruction or perforation, especially those arising form the esophagus or small intestine. Tumors in the esophagus may present with dysphagia, and those arising in the duodenum may compress the adjacent pancreatic head, resulting in fever and jaundice. Rectal GISTs may present with symptoms of mass effect such as frequency, hesitancy, or poor urinary stream due to invasion of the urinary bladder.[26]

Pathologic, Histologic, and Immunohistochemical Features

GISTs usually involve the outer muscular layer and therefore, are predominantly exophytic. They usually project into the abdominal cavity. Mucosal ulceration may be seen in up to 50% of cases.[28] Tumor size ranges from several millimeters to larger than 30 cm. Typically, tumors are well circumscribed but lack a true capsule. They may result in significant mass effect on surrounding organs. Cut sections are pink, tan, or gray with focal areas of hemorrhage, cystic degeneration, and necrosis, especially if large. Extensive hemorrhage and necrosis may result in cavity formation, which may communicate with the gastrointestinal lumen.

GISTs usually present with moderate to high cellularity, and tumor cells vary from spindle (70% to 80%) to epithelioid (20% to 30%).[16,27] Spindle cell GISTs exhibit spindle cells that have elongated nuclei with tapered, blunt, or rounded ends and eosinophilic or basophilic cytoplasm. Epithelioid GISTs are composed of round or polygonal cells with central or slightly eccentric nuclei; they may show mitosis, but typically, they have a more benign clinical course than spindle cell GISTs. Histologically, GISTs with spindle-shaped cells may simulate smooth muscle tumors or nerve sheath tumors. They may also have prominent vascularity, hemorrhage, extensive hyalinization, or myxoid degeneration.

The biologic behavior of GISTs ranges between benign and malignant, and the differentiation is based on size, location, cellularity, and the degree of mitotic activity. Generally, malignant GISTs are large and more cellular than benign GISTs. However, the critical size is not agreed upon. Tumor behavior varies significantly by location, and the cutoff tumor size also varies by location. GISTs arising from the stomach are more likely to be benign than malignant.[10] Gastric GISTs that are smaller than 5 cm in maximum diameter, with five or fewer mitoses per 50 consecutive high-power fields, have a low risk for metastasis, and are considered benign. Gastric GISTs that are larger than 10 cm and with more than five mitoses per 50 high-power fields are considered malignant. Tumors that fall between these two categories have indeterminate malignant potential. Tumors with high mitotic activity (more than 50 mitoses per 50 high-power fields) are considered aggressive with high-grade malignant potential.[29] GISTs that arise from the small intestine tend to be more aggressive than those arising from the stomach. Most esophageal, colonic, and anorectal GISTs are malignant. Because benign-appearing GISTs may recur or metastasize, it has been recently suggested to classify GISTs into very low, low-, intermediate-, and high-risk categories rather than as benign or malignant.[30] Careful clinical and imaging follow-up is therefore advised for all patients.[30,31]

The diagnosis of GIST requires confirmation with immunostaining for CD 117, which is expressed by all GIST, both spindle and epithelioid type,[6] regardless of their anatomic site or clinical behavior. The presence and expression of CD 117 is also found in the interstitial cells of Cajal, which are the pacemaker cells of the gastrointestinal tract. This association suggests that these cells are the common origin of GISTs.[4] The expression of CD 117 is the most specific marker for GIST.[30] However, it is not pathognomonic, as other malignant neoplasms, including malignant melanoma, seminoma, sarcoma, and some leukemias, may also express CD 117.[6] Fortunately, the distinction between GISTs and other tumors that express CD 117 can be made histologically. Approximately 70% to 80% of GISTs also express CD34, which is a hemopoietic progenitor cell antigen. GIST may also express smooth muscle antigen in approximately one-third of cases, but it is rarely reactive to desmin, present in true smooth muscle tumors, and S-100 immunostaining, present in schwannoma.

Computed Tomography Protocol and Image Processing Technique

Many cross-sectional imaging modalities are available for the evaluation of patients with GISTs, including ultrasound, computed tomography (CT), magnetic resonance imaging (MRI), and positron emission tomography (PET). CT is the mainstay of abdominal imaging. It is widely available and highly accurate, particularly in assessing liver metastases.[32,33] If properly performed, CT will adequately address most clinical concerns in patients with GISTs. CT features provide information that may help in differentiating GISTs from lymphoma and epithelial gastrointestinal tumors. With the introduction of new targeted medical therapy for GISTs, CT is increasingly utilized to assess tumor response and to evaluate for disease recurrence. In addition, CT is currently the first imaging modality requested in patients with suspected bowel obstruction, which is reported in up to 30% of GISTs.[34–36] Occasionally a small bowel neoplasm may be detected in these cases. CT may also be utilized to guide tissue biopsy.

The recent introduction of multidetector row CT, combined with multiplanar reconstructions and high-fidelity volume rendering, can provide comprehensive evaluation of the abdomen, particularly the vascular anatomy[37–39]; this is particularly useful in determining the origin of large exophytic GISTs, which may be difficult to determine in an axial plane. Multiplanar volume rendering and maximum intensity projection techniques are also used to accurately delineate small mucosal lesions, to better characterize the morphology of the lesion, and to detect hepatic and peritoneal metastases.

Although CT may detect an incidental GIST, patients are more commonly referred for accurate tumor localization, characterization, staging, and surveillance for metastases or recurrence after surgery. For routine scanning of the abdomen and pelvis, a detector configuration of 4×2.5 mm, table speed of 15 mm, and pitch of 6 : 1 allow for adequate coverage in a single breath-hold of 20–25 seconds. Image reconstruction of 5 mm, with optional 2.5-mm overlap, can be performed in such cases. Newer 16-slice multidetector CT scanners allow the use of 1.5-mm detectors with 2-mm-thick slices at 1-mm intervals. Contrast enhancement is typically achieved using 120 mL (2 mL/kg) nonionic contrast media injected intravenously, with a power injector, at a rate of 3 ml/s. Depending on the clinical indication, arterial and/or portal venous imaging is performed using a 25-second and 60- to 65-second scan delay, respectively. In patients undergoing dual-phase CT of the liver, in addition to CT of the chest, abdomen, and pelvis, arterial-phase images of the liver should be obtained in the first breath-hold at 25 seconds, followed by scans through the chest, abdomen, and pelvis in the second breath-hold at 65 seconds. For the evaluation of the abdominal vascular anatomy before possible resection, a detector configuration of 16 × 0.75-mm collimation and 0.5-mm intervals will result in superior three-dimensional image reconstruction and volume rendering techniques.

Positive oral contrast is not administered when imaging GIST because it may degrade image reconstruction and obscure small mucosal lesions. Positive oral contrast agents may also mix unevenly with gastric and intestinal fluid, resulting in pseudotumor.[40,41] When imaging the stomach and small bowel, 750 mL water is recommended as a negative contrast agent, given to the patient approximately 15 minutes before imaging. Patients also receive an additional 250 mL immediately before the study to ensure adequate distention of the stomach. Water is well tolerated and results in good gastric and proximal small bowel distension as well as excellent visualization of the enhancing gastric wall.[42] One disadvantage of using water as oral contrast is the suboptimal distension of the distal small bowel. Some authors have advocated using positive contrast initially, followed by water to allow adequate distension of the stomach and small bowel.[43] Alternatively, oral metoclopramide can be administered to improve ileal distension and reduce bowel peristalsis.[44] GISTs that are detected incidentally may be seen on a routine CT scan of the abdomen, which is usually performed with high-density oral contrast.

At our institution, CT scanning is performed using a multislice variable detector array (Sensation 16; Siemens Medical Solutions, Malvern, PA). Multidetector row CT images are acquired as a volume data set during a single breath-hold. All CT imaging data, in the original resolution of 512 × 512, are sent from the scanner to a freestanding workstation for postprocessing (Leonardo with In Space software; Siemens). Volume rendering allows the best approach to visualize the stomach and small bowel compared to other rendering algorithms.[42,45] Volume rendering utilizes all the attenuation information in any given slab of tissue, and real-time adjustments can be performed to accentuate the stomach and small bowel. Histograms of the relative density values are manipulated through trapezoid control of variables, such as width, level, opacity, and brightness. This function assigns opacity and color to each voxel and can be instantaneously adjusted to alter the final display. It is often helpful to start with two-dimensional multiplanar reconstructions and then proceed to the three-dimensional volume rendering. Initial two-dimensional multiplanar reconstructions allow for quick assessment of the abdomen in the axial, coronal, and sagittal planes. The main advantage of three-dimensional volume rendering is the enhanced depth perception, which improves visualization of a complex mass or tortuous vessels. Interactive application of different orientations and cut planes enhance the visualization of the bowel and the display of tumor in any plane that is necessary for the surgeon or referring physician.

General CT Features

General features of GISTs depend on the organ of origin and tumor size. Most tumors arise from the muscularis propria of the stomach or small intestine, and the submucosal origin of these tumors explains their typical CT features. They commonly manifest as a dominant exophytic mass. Less common CT findings include dominant intramural and intraluminal masses. Small tumors are typically homogeneous, well defined, and sharply marginated. Contrast enhancement is usually moderate. Large tumors tend to have central necrosis and mucosal ulceration. Enhancement of large tumors is typically heterogeneous, although this feature cannot reliably predict tumor behavior or malignant potential.[27] Peripheral contrast enhancement indicates viable tumor, whereas central areas of low attenuation may appear due to hemorrhage, necrosis, or cystic degeneration. Cavitary lesions may develop, which often communicate with the bowel lumen. They may contain air, air–fluid level, or food residue. Calcification is unusual and may be mottled or extensive. Ascites has rarely been reported in patients with GISTs, suggesting that these tumors do not incite local inflammatory reaction. Vessels are often stretched over large tumors, but vascular encasement of the mesenteric and retroperitoneal vessels is rare.[24]

Regardless of the site of GIST, differentiation of benign tumors from their malignant counterparts is difficult on CT. Distinguishing between low-grade and high-grade malignant GISTs by CT has been recently reported.[46] CT features favoring a diagnosis of high-grade GIST and, associated with poor survival, included large tumor size (larger than 11.1 cm), irregular surface, unclear boundary, mesenteric or bowel wall invasion, heterogeneous enhancement, distant metastases, and peritoneal dissemination.

CT is the most common technique in evaluating hepatic metastases.[32,33] These are typically hypodense on unenhanced CT, with occasional hyperdensities resulting from hemorrhage or proteinaceous material. Contrast-enhanced CT metastases are heterogeneous in enhancement, likely because of cystic degeneration. Following treatment with imatinib, metastases to the liver commonly become hypodense, appearing cystlike with a well-defined margin.[47,48] Decrease in attenuation of the treated lesions may be due to myxomatous change resulting in small pyknotic nuclei in an eosinophilic myxoid background.[49]

Stomach

Most GISTs arise from the stomach, accounting for 2% to 3% of all gastric tumors. According to a recently published study, 28 of 64 GISTs (44%) were located in the stomach.[27] At CT, most tumors are large with an exogastric extension into the gastrohepatic ligament, gastrosplenic ligament, or the lesser sac.[27] Most tumors have rim enhancement, with central areas of low attenuation due to hemorrhage, necrosis, or cystic degeneration (Figures 30.1–30.3). These findings have no correlation with malignant potential. Large tumors may also cavitate, and the cavities may communicate with the gastric lumen and become filled with food residue, fluid, or air–fluid

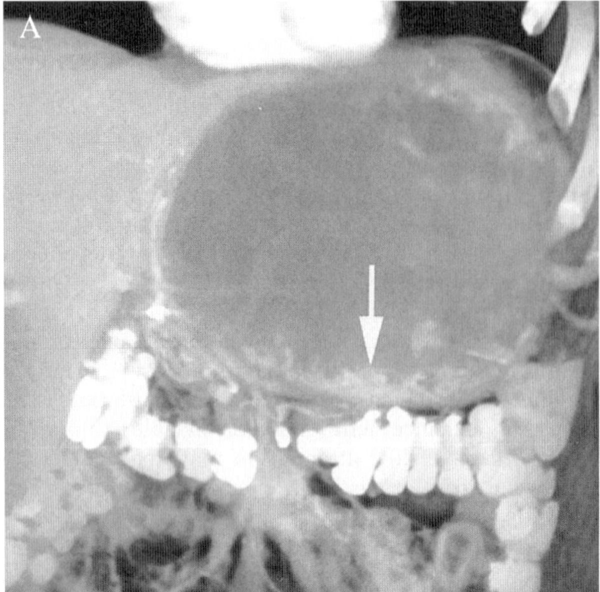

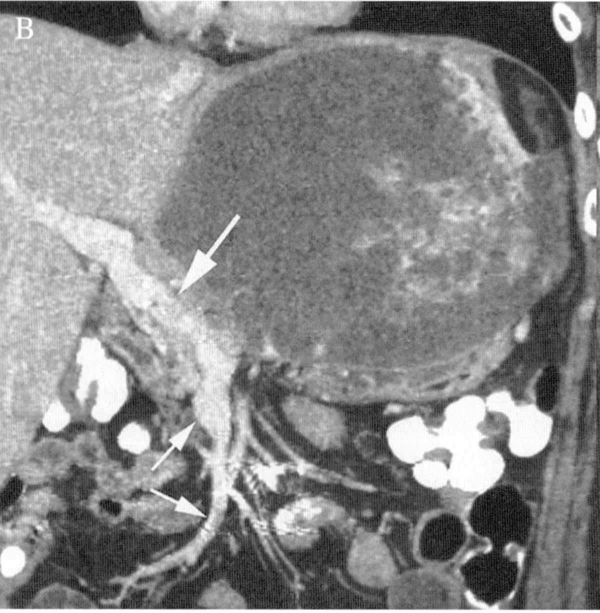

FIGURE 30.1. Large gastric gastrointestinal stromal tumor (GIST) in a 45-year-old man with history of abdominal pain and weight loss. (A) Coronal volume-rendered image through the upper abdomen reveals a large heterogeneous cystic and/or necrotic mass in the left upper quadrant that is inseparable from the stomach. Notice peripheral solid component with heterogeneous enhancement (*arrow*). The mass abuts the liver without evidence of invasion. Oral contrast is seen in the large bowel from a prior computed tomography (CT) scan. (B) Coronal reconstruction reveals patency of portal vein (*arrow*) and superior mesenteric vein (*small arrows*). These findings are important for surgical planning.

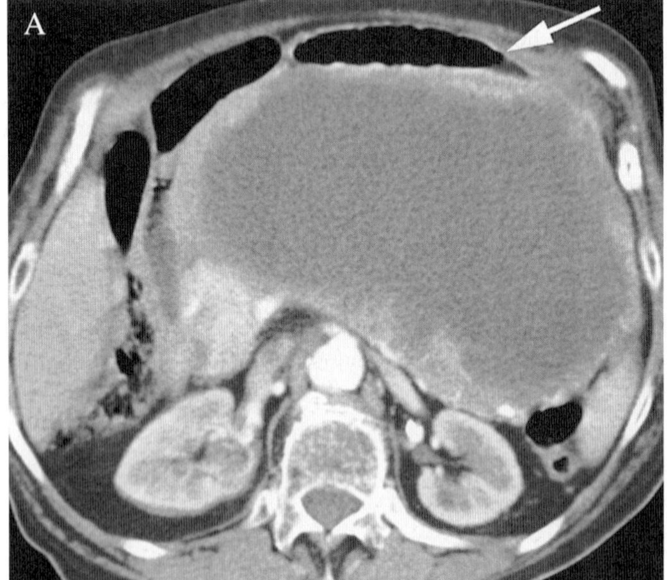

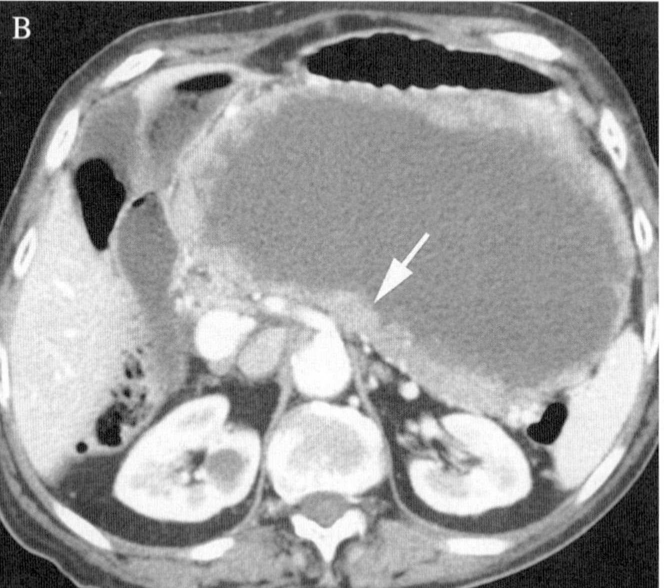

FIGURE 30.2. Gastric GIST in a 92-year-old woman with early satiety, abdominal pain, and anemia. (A) Axial CT of the abdomen in the arterial phase reveals a large cystic/necrotic mass in the left upper quadrant, extending into the gastrosplenic ligament. The mass appears to arise from the posterior aspect of the stomach, which is displaced anteriorly (*arrow*). (B) Axial CT at the same level as (A) in the portal venous phase shows irregular enhancing peripheral solid components (*arrow*) and central necrosis. (C) Coronal volume-rendered image demonstrates the craniocaudal extension of the mass to the pelvis. (D) Sagittal reconstruction better reveals the extraluminal nature of the mass. The mass is related to the posterior aspect of the stomach (*arrow*), which contains an air–fluid level.

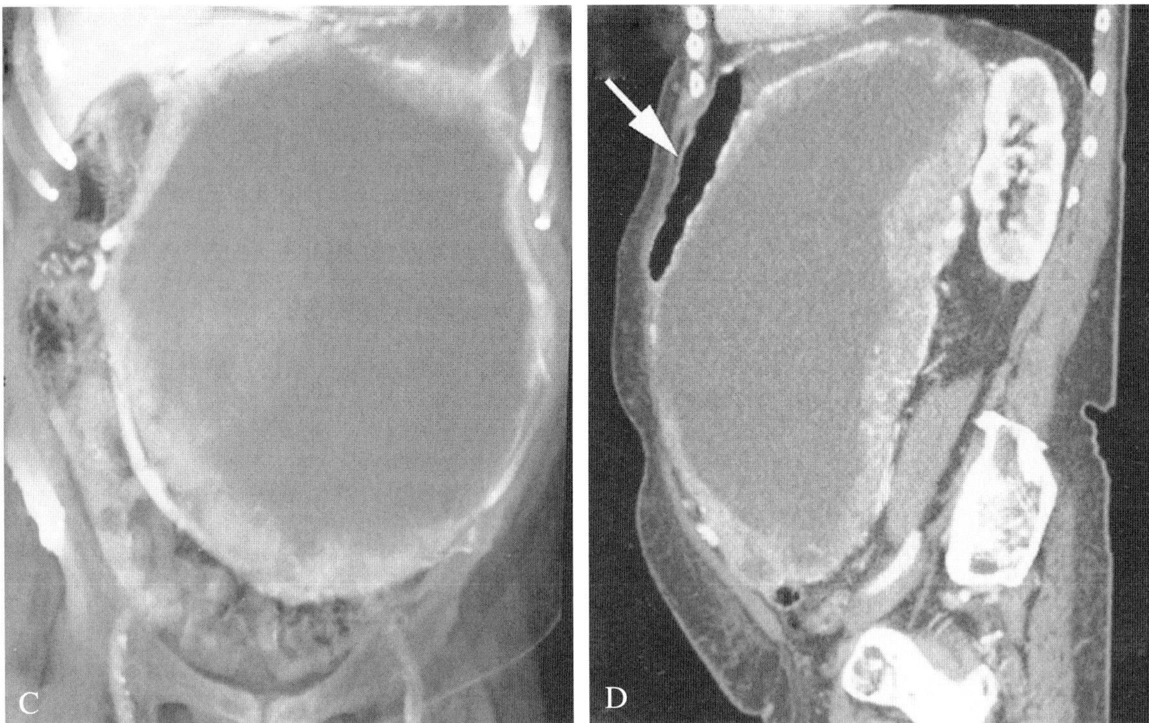

FIGURE 30.2. (continued)

level (Figure 30.4). Homogeneous enhancement of the tumor is uncommon, accounting for 8% of cases according to one study.[27] Calcifications are unusual and were reported in 3% of cases. Multidetector row CT with volume rendering allows for accurate delineation of the tumor outline and subtle gastric wall thickening at the site of tumor attachment to the gastric wall. These features help in determining the organ of origin in large tumors and their relationship to surrounding organs. CT may also demonstrate extragastric extension into the gastrohepatic ligament, gastrosplenic ligament, and lesser sac. It can demonstrate invasion of surrounding organs, ascites, or peritoneal carcinomatosis. Liver metastases may also be detected; these are usually hypovascular and best seen in the portal venous phase. Metastatic lymph node involvement is not observed in patients with GIST.

The differential diagnosis for gastric GISTs includes other mesenchymal neoplasms that arise in the gastric wall, including leiomyomas (Figure 30.5), leiomyosarcomas, schwanno-

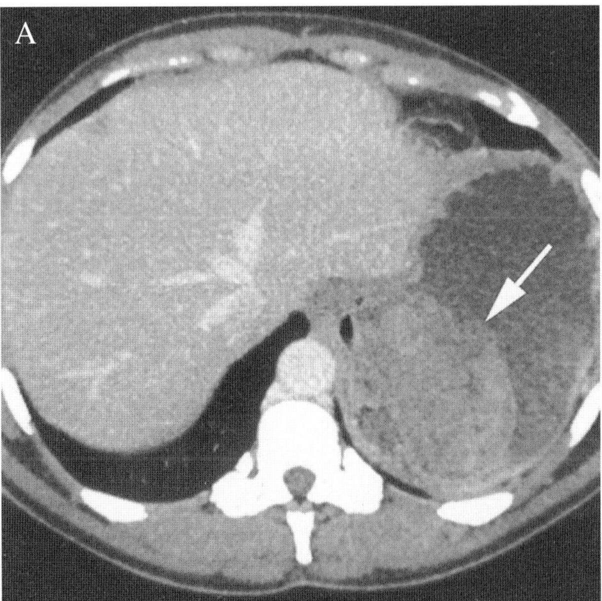

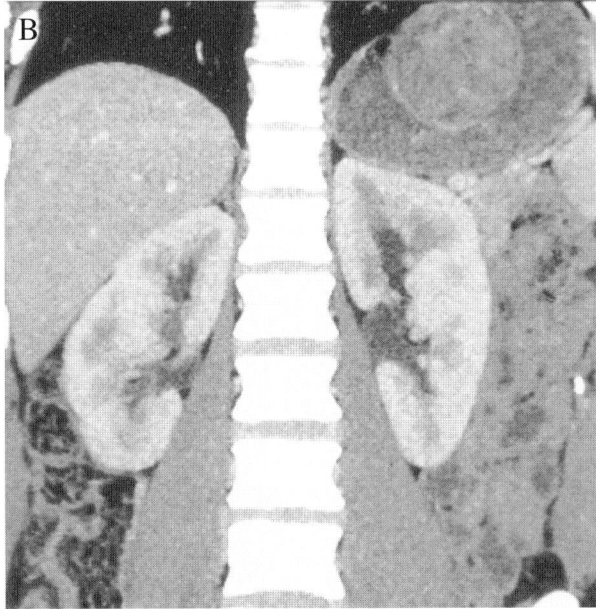

FIGURE 30.3. Gastric GIST in a 48-year-old woman presenting with upper gastrointestinal bleeding. (A) Axial CT of the abdomen reveals a large mass (*arrow*) in the fundus of the stomach. The mass is entirely projecting into the gastric lumen, with no exophytic components. This finding is somewhat atypical because most GISTs have an exophytic component. (B) Coronal reconstruction confirms the intraluminal nature of the mass. No extragastric extension was seen.

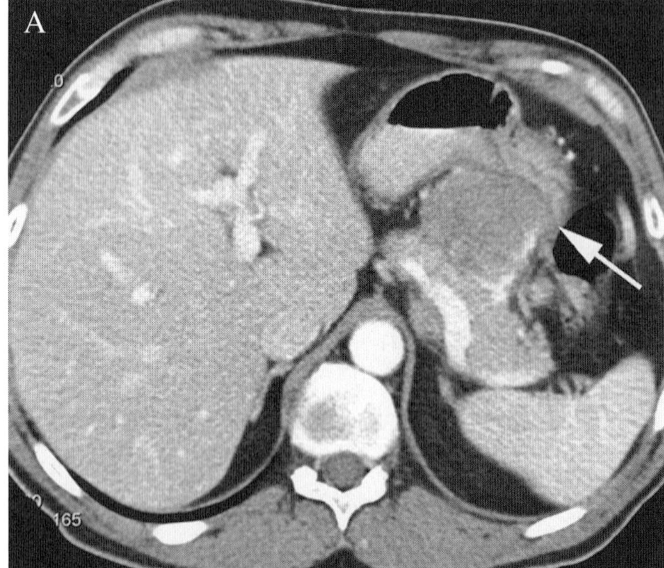

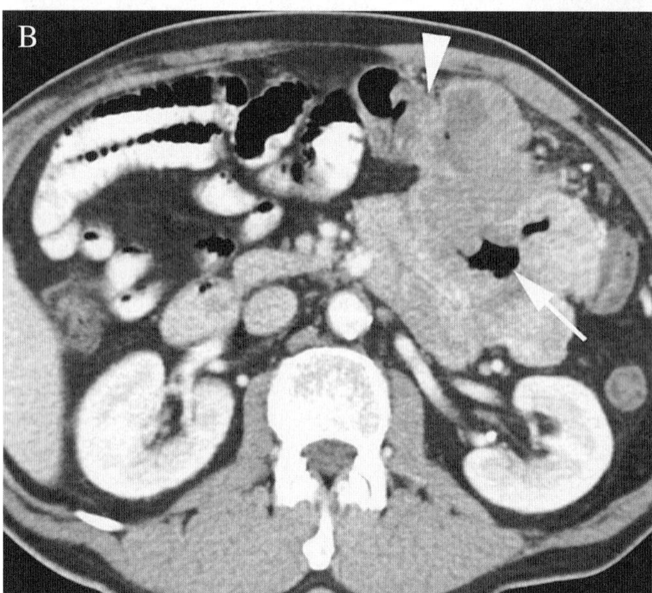

FIGURE 30.4. Malignant gastric GIST in a 49-year-old man. (A) Axial CT of the abdomen with oral and intravenous contrast reveals an exophytic mass arising from the posterior aspect of the stomach (*arrow*) and extending along the gastrosplenic ligament. Note marked thickening of the gastric mucosal folds posteriorly. (B) Axial CT of the abdomen at a level lower than (A) reveals extensive central necrosis and a cavity (*arrow*) that is air filled. The mass invades the wall of the transverse colon (*arrowhead*).

mas, and neurofibromas. The imaging features of these tumors may be similar to GISTs. Gastric adenocarcinoma and lymphoma may also have a radiologic appearance similar to GISTs. However, they rarely demonstrate large exophytic growth, and when advanced are commonly associated with bulky adenopathy, a feature that is not seen in malignant GISTs.

Small Intestine

GIST may occur anywhere throughout the small intestine, and these patients usually present with signs and symptoms of bowel obstruction. At CT, GISTs may appear as an intramural polyp or intraluminal mass. Tumor margins are typically well defined, unless they have mucosal ulcerations. Tumors may also cavitate and form fistulous communication with surrounding bowel loops. Similar to gastric GISTs, tumors typically enhance with central areas of low attenuation due to hemorrhage, necrosis, or cyst formation (Figure 30.6). Homogeneous pattern of enhancement is less common. Tumors may encase or invade surrounding small bowel, colon, urinary bladder, or ureter. Patients may also present

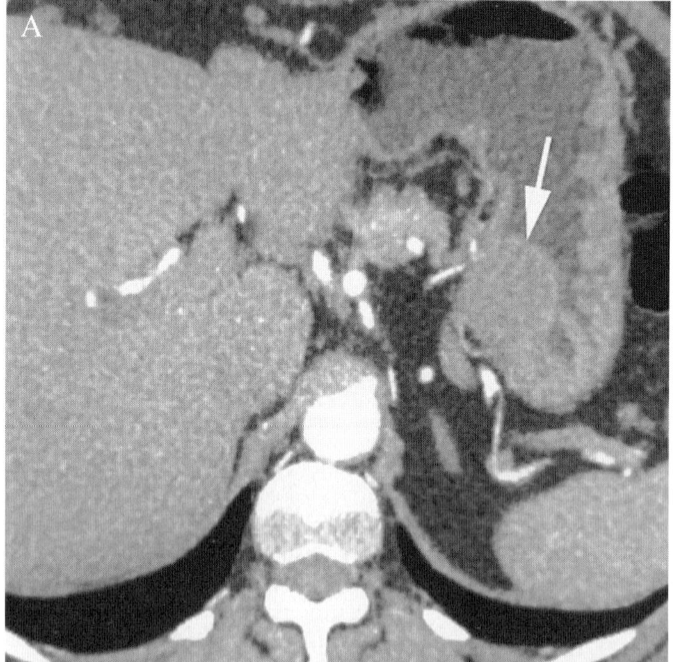

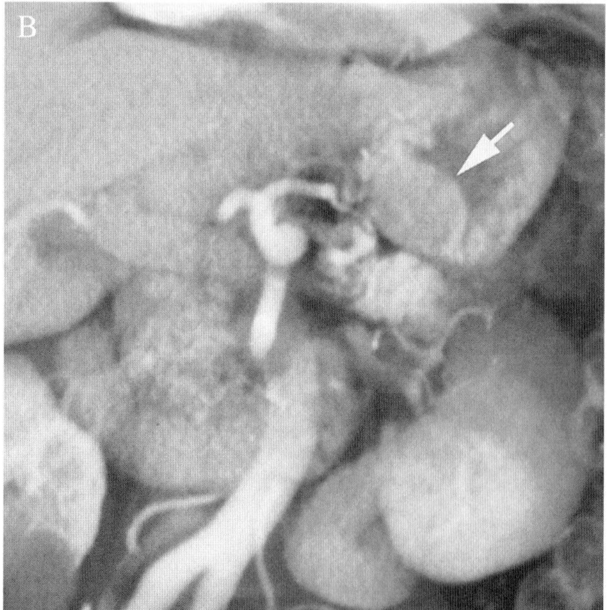

FIGURE 30.5. Incidental submucosal gastric leiomyoma simulating GIST in a 56-year-old man. (A) Axial contrast-enhanced CT of the abdomen reveals a small submucosal soft tissue mass in the fundus of the stomach (*arrow*). The homogeneous enhancement and lack of exophytic component favor the diagnosis of leiomyoma over GIST. (B) Coronal volume-rendered image better demonstrates the smooth contour of the lesion (*arrow*) and the intact overlying mucosa.

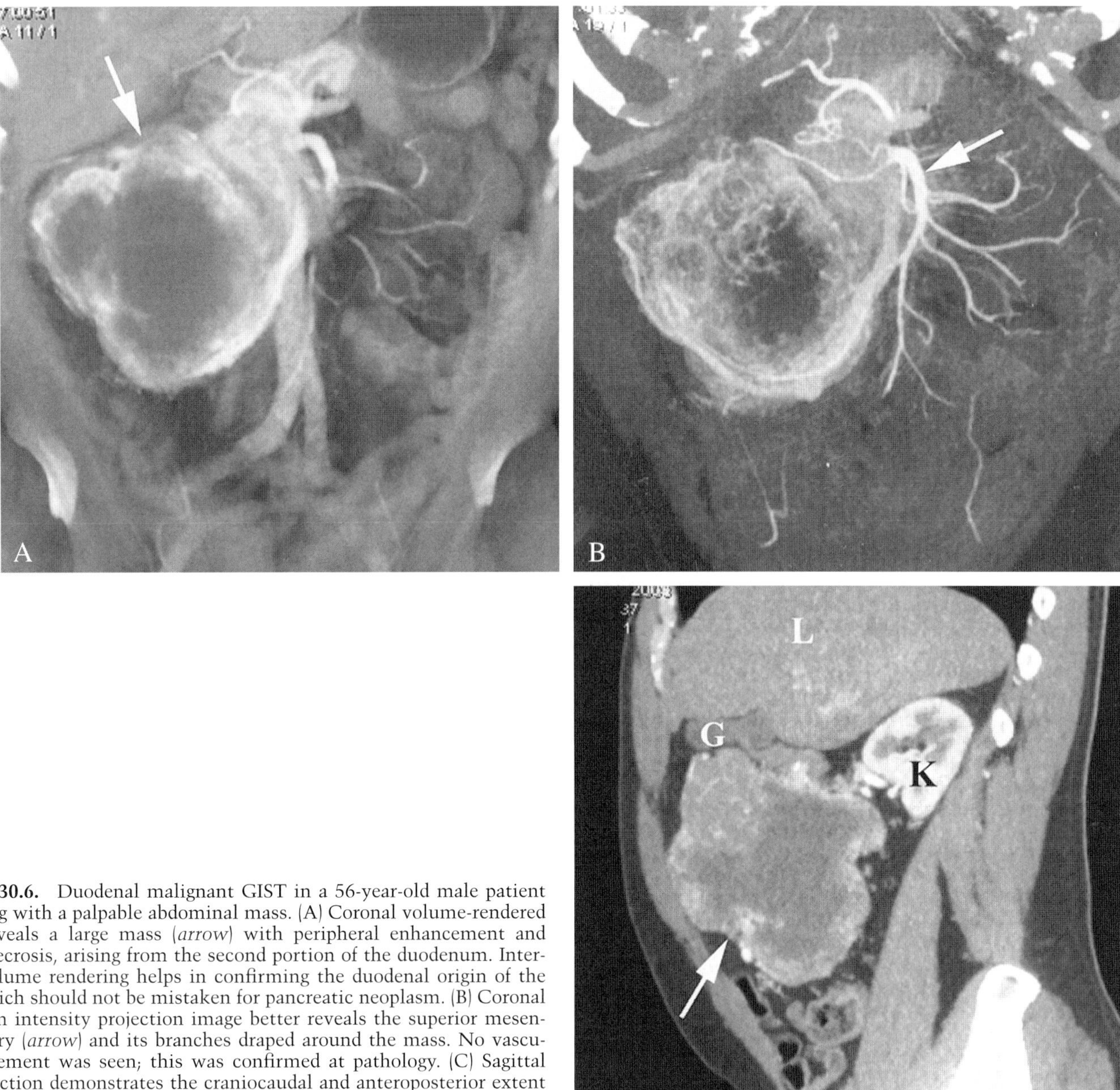

FIGURE 30.6. Duodenal malignant GIST in a 56-year-old male patient presenting with a palpable abdominal mass. (A) Coronal volume-rendered image reveals a large mass (*arrow*) with peripheral enhancement and central necrosis, arising from the second portion of the duodenum. Interactive volume rendering helps in confirming the duodenal origin of the mass, which should not be mistaken for pancreatic neoplasm. (B) Coronal maximum intensity projection image better reveals the superior mesenteric artery (*arrow*) and its branches draped around the mass. No vascular encasement was seen; this was confirmed at pathology. (C) Sagittal reconstruction demonstrates the craniocaudal and anteroposterior extent of the mass (*arrow*) and the relation to the surrounding organs, including the liver (*L*), gallbladder (*G*), and right kidney (*K*). These findings are important for surgical planning.

with metastases to the liver, peritoneum, or omentum. Ascites may occur but is uncommon. Patients with neurofibromatosis (type I) may have multiple small intestinal GISTs[18,19] (Figure 30.7).

Differential diagnosis for small intestinal GISTs includes adenocarcinoma, which is the most common primary malignancy of the proximal small bowel. However, adenocarcinoma typically manifests as an annular lesion in the proximal small bowel, which is not a feature of GISTs. Lymphoma may be indistinguishable from GISTs, especially when it produces large masses that may cavitate, ulcerate, and extend into the mesentery. However, the presence of lymphadenopathy favors the diagnosis of lymphoma. Tumors of the duodenum and proximal small bowel may cause a significant mass effect on the pancreas or simulate a pancreatic primary[50,51] (Figure 30.8). Judicious application of image postprocessing may help in avoiding this pitfall.

Anorectum

Anorectal GISTs account for 9% of 64 GISTs, according to a recently published series.[27] Unlike GISTs in other locations, a male predominance has been reported.[14,52] Clinical presentation includes rectal pain, bleeding, and rectal mass. Anorectal GISTs present as eccentric mural masses that invade the rectal wall. The most common finding at CT is a focal well-circumscribed mural mass, which expands the rectal wall and

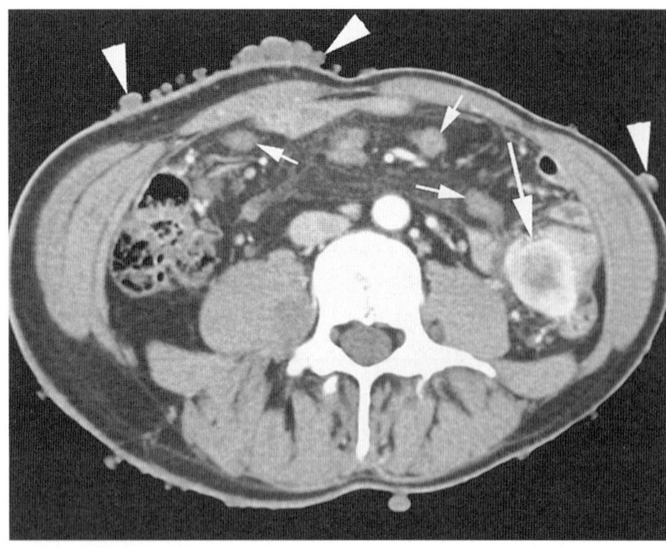

FIGURE 30.7. Multiple GISTs in a 42-year-old man with history of neurofibromatosis (type I) and lower gastrointestinal bleeding. Axial CT of the lower abdomen in the arterial phase reveals multiple pedunculated skin lesions (*arrowhead*) and within the abdomen (*small arrows*) compatible with neurofibromas. In addition, there is an enhancing soft tissue mass in the distal jejunum (*arrow*), which was proven to be a GIST at small bowel resection.

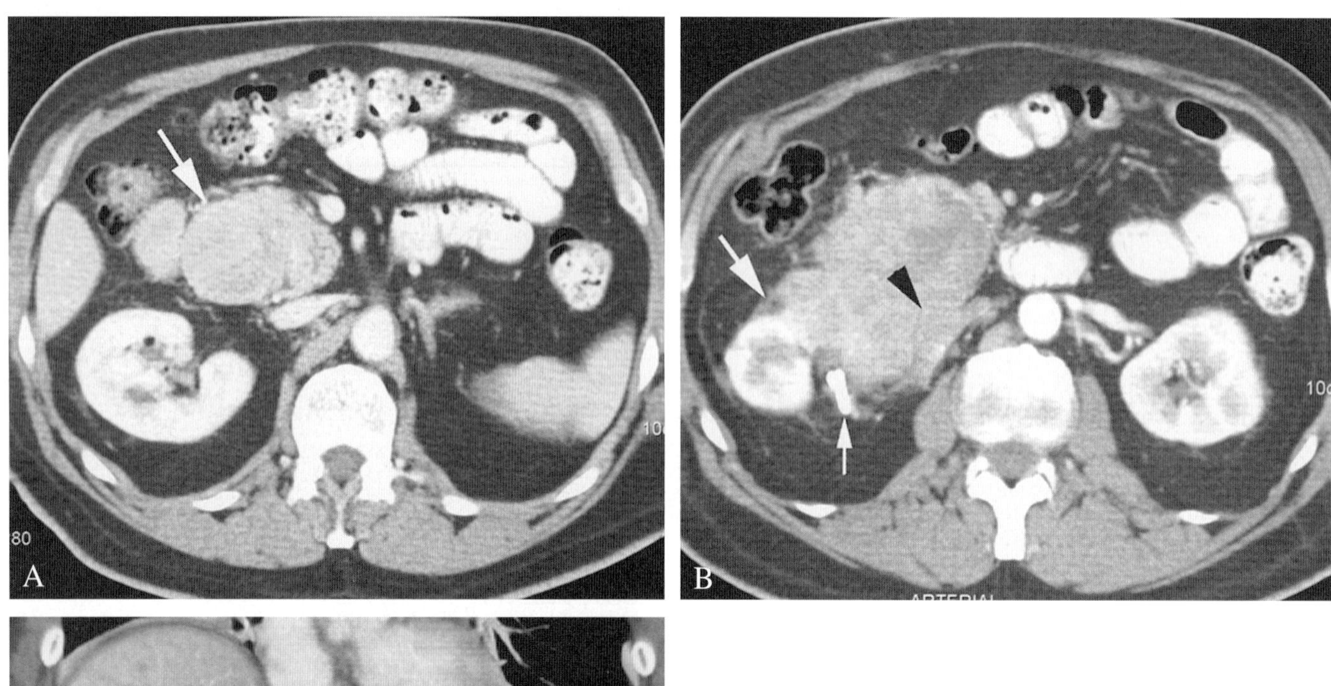

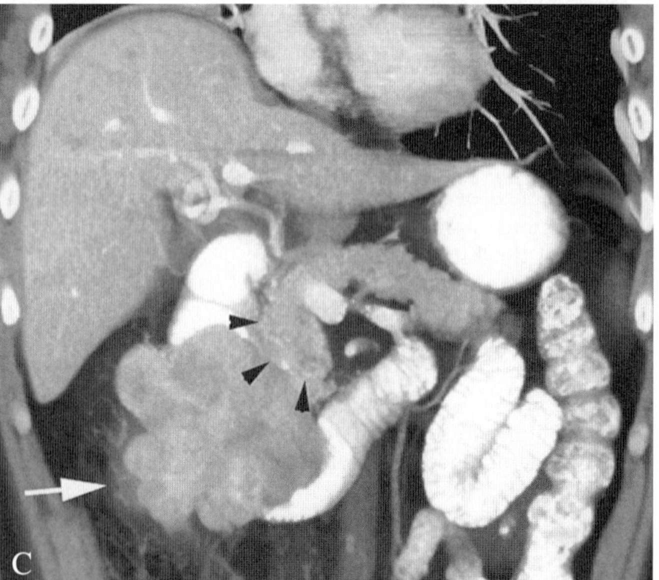

FIGURE 30.8. Poorly differentiated high-grade duodenal sarcoma in a 61-year-old man. (A) Axial CT of the abdomen with oral and intravenous contrast reveals a soft tissue mass in the region of the pancreatic head (*arrow*), involving the descending portion of the duodenum. This mass could be mistaken for pancreatic neoplasm. (B) Axial CT of the abdomen at a level lower than (A) shows invasion of the right renal hilum (*arrow*) and the inferior vena cava (*arrowhead*). A ureteric stent is seen in place (*small arrow*). (C) Coronal volume-rendered image shows the epicenter of the lobulated mass along the descending portion of the duodenal mass, with surrounding mesenteric fat stranding (*arrow*) indicating peritumoral spread of disease. The pancreas is well visualized (*arrowheads*) and is normal.

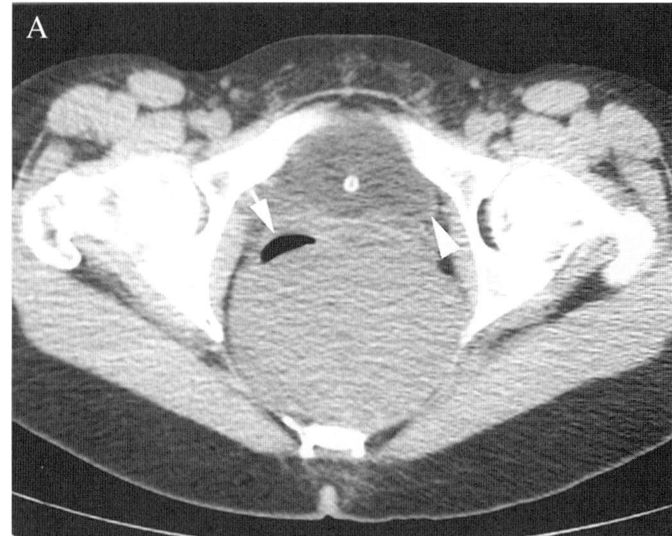

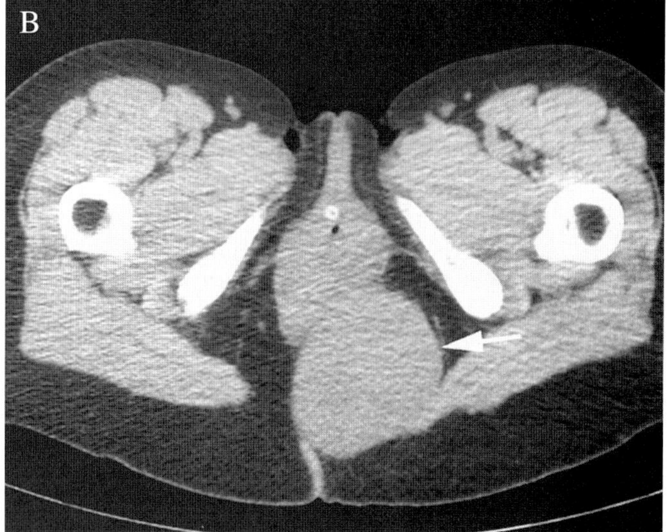

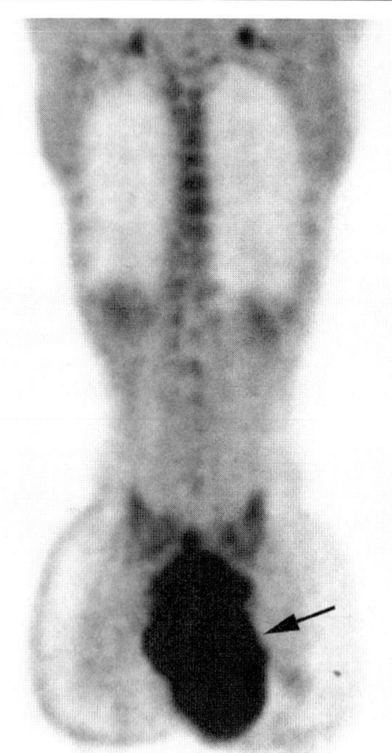

FIGURE 30.9. Malignant GIST in a 40-year-old woman presenting with rectal mass. (A) Axial noncontrast CT of the pelvis performed as part of positron emission tomography (PET)/CT reveals a large pelvic soft tissue mass displacing the air-filled rectum (*arrow*) and urinary bladder (*arrowhead*) anteriorly. (B) Axial noncontrast CT at a level lower than (A) reveals extension of the mass into the left ischiorectal fossa (*arrow*). (C) Coronal whole-body PET image reveals intense fluorodeoxyglucose (FDG) uptake indicating increased metabolic activity of the tumor (*arrow*), which is common in patients with untreated GISTs.

may ulcerate (Figure 30.9). The mass may extend into the ischiorectal fossa and may invade surrounding pelvic organs, including the vagina, prostate, or urinary bladder. These findings may result in difficulty identifying the organ of origin on cross-sectional imaging. Similar to GISTs in other locations of the gastrointestinal tract, enhancement is heterogeneous with areas of low attenuation from hemorrhage or necrosis. Calcification and adenopathy are rare. GISTs in the anorectal region show malignant behavior even when small (less than 2 cm in maximum dimension) and have no more than five mitoses per 50 high-power fields. These tumors are also associated with significant mortality rates.[53]

Rectal adenocarcinoma, anal squamous cell carcinoma, leiomyoma, leiomyosarcoma, lymphoma, and malignant melanoma may have a CT appearance similar to anorectal GIST and are in the differential diagnosis. Leiomyosarcoma may have a dominant polypoid mass while adenocarcinoma may have an irregular margin, soft tissue invasion into ischiorectal fossa, and perirectal adenopathy.[14] Primary anorectal lymphoma may be seen in patients with acquired immunodeficiency syndrome and may be associated with mucosal ulceration or perianal fistula. Other features that may be seen in primary anorectal lymphoma, include tumor heterogeneity, concentric wall thickening, intraluminal polypoid masses, and thickening of adjacent levator ani muscle.[27]

Colon

Primary colonic GISTs are much less common than gastric, small bowel, and anorectal GISTs. These transmural tumors may involve the intraluminal and extraserosal surfaces of the colon.[15] They are smooth or multinodular in contour with areas of low attenuation due to hemorrhage, necrosis, or cystic degeneration. Circumferential involvement of the colon with aneurysmal dilatation of the involved segment of the colon has been described.[15]

At CT, small lesions are confined to the wall of the colon and appear as mural or submucosal masses, which may ulcerate. Differential diagnosis includes adenocarcinoma, lymphoma, leiomyosarcoma, and metastatic melanoma. Tumors arising adjacent to the colon, such as retroperitoneal sarcomas, may involve the colon and may be mistaken for GISTs.

Esophagus

The most common neoplasm of the esophagus is leiomyoma, accounting for 75% of tumors. They occur in a younger population (median age, 35 years) compared to GISTs, which are relatively uncommon in the esophagus and occur in older patients (median age, 63 years).[15] Esophageal GISTs are most commonly located in the distal third of the esophagus and may extend into the stomach. These lesions may be homogeneous or heterogeneous with central areas of low attenuation due to hemorrhage, necrosis, or cystic degeneration. Most esophageal GISTs are benign, unlike the trend seen elsewhere in the gastrointestinal tract where most GISTs are malignant.

The differential diagnosis of esophageal GISTs include leiomyoma, duplication cysts, lipoma, neurofibroma, schwannoma, and hemangioma. GISTs may also simulate other lesions that have a polypoid appearance such as papilloma, adenoma, fibrovascular polyp, and inflammatory polyp. Large GISTs may invade the mediastinum, simulating advanced carcinoma, lymphoma, leiomyosarcoma, and malignant melanoma.

Omentum and Mesentery

Primary GISTs rarely may arise from the omentum or mesentery[54]; these are usually large multilobulated masses with areas of low attenuation due to hemorrhage, necrosis, or cystic degeneration. Trace amount of free fluid in the abdomen may be present.[55] CT findings of GISTs arising in these locations are not characteristic, and they are indistinguishable from other sarcomas including liposarcoma, fibrosarcoma, leiomyosarcoma, inflammatory pseudopolyp, and mesenteric fibromatosis. Therefore, presumptive diagnosis before biopsy or surgery may be difficult.

GISTs from the gastrointestinal tract may metastasize to the omentum and mesentery, resulting in multiple peritoneal masses (Figure 30.10). Patients may also develop peritonitis secondary to tumor rupture. In these cases, the differential diagnosis includes peritoneal carcinomatosis and lymphoma.

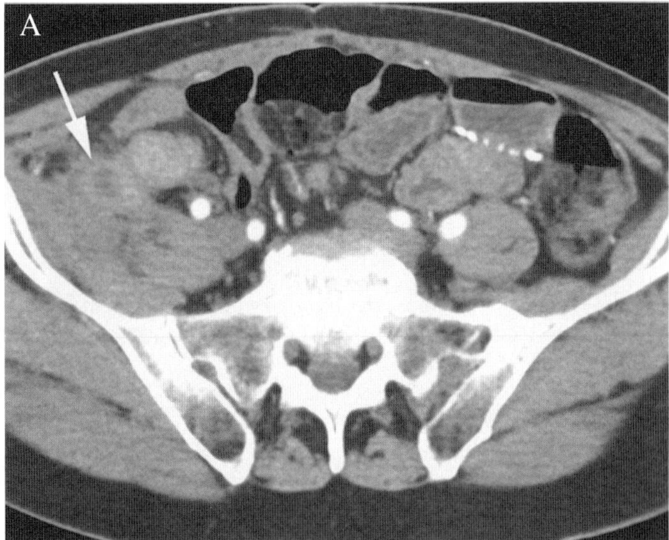

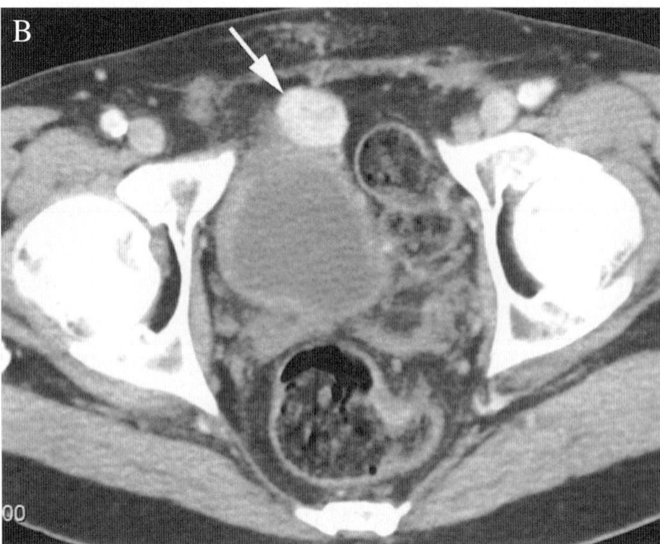

FIGURE 30.10. Tumor recurrence in a 75-year-old man 14 months after resection of malignant mesenteric GIST. (A) Axial CT of the pelvis reveals a rim-enhancing soft tissue mass along the right iliopsoas muscle (*arrow*) suspicious for tumor recurrence. Surgical sutures from prior bowel resection are identified in the left lower quadrant. (B) Axial CT of the pelvis at a level more inferior than (A) reveals a hypervascular mass (*arrow*) anterior to the urinary bladder compatible with tumor recurrence.

Treatment and Prognosis

Surgical resection of the primary disease followed by observation is the conventional treatment for patients with GISTs and offers the best cure rate.[48,56] For resectable GISTs, preoperative histologic confirmation is usually not necessary as these tumors may bleed, rupture, or disseminate as a result of biopsy.[17] For the same reasons, the tumor should be removed en bloc during surgery.[57] A safety margin of normal surrounding soft tissue or bowel should be included if possible to reduce the risk of recurrence.[48,58] Because lymph node metastases are rare, extensive lymphadenectomy is not routinely performed.

Because of the unpredictable behavior of GIST, follow-up by imaging is performed to assess for disease recurrence, even though there is no proof that early detection of recurrent GIST results in survival benefit.[31] Disease recurrence has been reported in up to 80% of cases despite complete resection with pathologically proven negative margins.[57] Although most recurrences occur within 2 years, tumors with low mitotic index may take more than 10 years to metastasize.[35] Recurrence is commonly local and peritoneal, often associated with liver metastases (Figure 30.11). Lymph node involvement is unusual. Most metastatic GISTs are confined to the abdomen, unlike other soft tissue sarcomas, which metastasize to the lungs.[59]

Patients with recurrence have a poor prognosis.[30] Arterial embolization, surgery, and irradiation have been ineffective in treating patients with metastases and recurrent disease. Until recently, drug therapy for patients with GISTs has also been ineffective. However, a promising new drug, STI 571 (imatinib mesylate, gleevec) has been recently introduced. This new drug inhibits tyrosine kinase and was first reported in a case of recurrent metastatic GIST that failed extensive surgery and chemotherapy.[56] The authors reported favorable response to therapy after 1 month of treatment, using MRI and PET. The safety and effectiveness of this new therapy were subsequently demonstrated in patients with advanced unresectable or metastatic disease.[60,61] Current studies demonstrate up to 69% of patients showing favorable response to therapy.[61] However, it is still unclear how long the response to therapy will last and whether maintenance therapy is required.

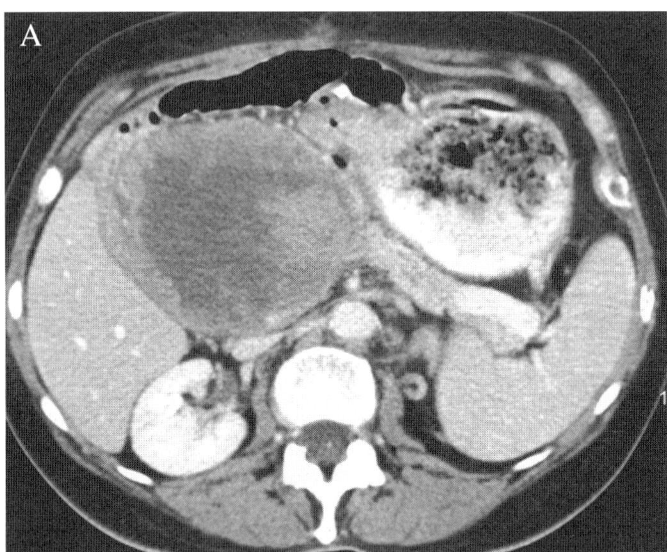

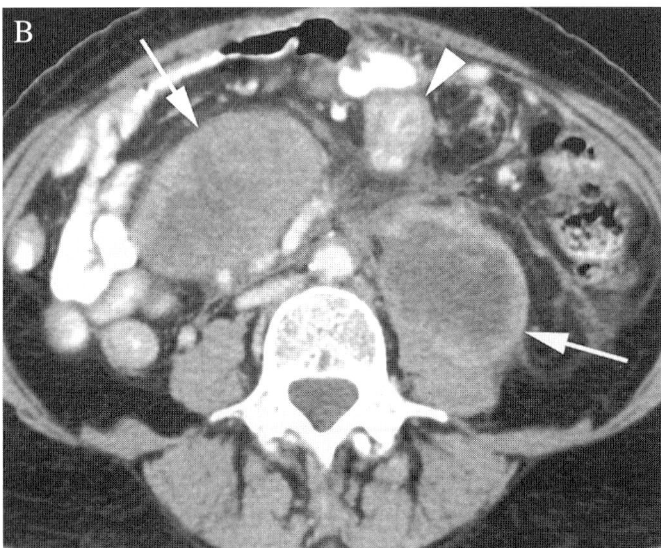

FIGURE 30.11. Recurrent malignant GIST of the small bowel in a 62-year-old woman. (A) Axial CT of the upper abdomen in the portal venous phase reveals a large partially necrotic liver mass, with peripheral enhancement and central low attenuation. (B) Axial CT at a level lower than (A) reveals additional enhancing paraaortic (*arrows*) and mesenteric root (*arrowhead*) masses, with central necrosis. These findings are consistent with peritoneal recurrence.

References

1. DeMatteo RP, Lewis JJ, Leung D, Mudan SS, Woodruff JM, Brennan MF. Two hundred gastrointestinal stromal tumors: recurrence patterns and prognostic factors for survival. Ann Surg 2000;231:51–58.
2. Stelow EB, Stanley MW, Mallery S, Lai R, Linzie BM, Bardales RH. Endoscopic ultrasound-guided fine-needle aspiration findings of gastrointestinal leiomyomas and gastrointestinal stromal tumors. Am J Clin Pathol 2003;119:703–708.
3. Miettinen M, Sobin LH, Sarlomo-Rikala M. Immunohistochemical spectrum of GISTs at different sites and their differential diagnosis with a reference to CD117 (KIT). Mod Pathol 2000;13:1134–1142.
4. Kindblom LG, Remotti HE, Aldenborg F, Meis-Kindblom JM. Gastrointestinal pacemaker cell tumor (GIPACT): gastrointestinal stromal tumors show phenotypic characteristics of the interstitial cells of Cajal. Am J Pathol 1998;152:1259–1269.
5. Sircar K, Hewlett BR, Huizinga JD, Chorneyko K, Berezin I, Riddell RH. Interstitial cells of Cajal as precursors of gastrointestinal stromal tumors. Am J Surg Pathol 1999;23:377–389.
6. Sarlomo-Rikala M, Kovatich AJ, Barusevicius A, Miettinen M. CD117: a sensitive marker for gastrointestinal stromal tumors that is more specific than CD34. Mod Pathol 1998;11:728–734.
7. Miettinen M, Virolainen M, Maarit Sarlomo R. Gastrointestinal stromal tumors—value of CD34 antigen in their identification and separation from true leiomyomas and schwannomas. Am J Surg Pathol 1995;19:207–216.
8. Bauer S, Corless CL, Heinrich MC, et al. Response to imatinib mesylate of a gastrointestinal stromal tumor with very low expression of KIT. Cancer Chemother Pharmacol 2003;51:261–265.
9. Dagher R, Cohen M, Williams G, et al. Approval summary: imatinib mesylate in the treatment of metastatic and/or unresectable malignant gastrointestinal stromal tumors. Clin Cancer Res 2002;8:3034–3038.
10. Miettinen M, Lasota J. Gastrointestinal stromal tumors: definition, clinical, histological, immunohistochemical, and molecular genetic features and differential diagnosis. Virchows Arch 2001;438:1–12.
11. Miettinen M, Sarlomo-Rikala M, Lasota J. Gastrointestinal stromal tumors: recent advances in understanding of their biology. Hum Pathol 1999;30:1213–1220.
12. Greenson JK. Gastrointestinal stromal tumors and other mesenchymal lesions of the gut. Mod Pathol 2003;16:366–375.
13. Miettinen M, Sarlomo-Rikala M, Sobin LH, Lasota J. Esophageal stromal tumors: a clinicopathologic, immunohistochemical, and molecular genetic study of 17 cases and comparison with esophageal leiomyomas and leiomyosarcomas. Am J Surg Pathol 2000;24:211–222.
14. Miettinen M, Furlong M, Sarlomo-Rikala M, Burke A, Sobin LH, Lasota J. Gastrointestinal stromal tumors, intramural leiomyomas, and leiomyosarcomas in the rectum and anus: a clinicopathologic, immunohistochemical, and molecular genetic study of 144 cases. Am J Surg Pathol 2001;25:1121–1133.
15. Miettinen M, Sarlomo-Rikala M, Sobin LH, Lasota J. Gastrointestinal stromal tumors and leiomyosarcomas in the colon: a clinicopathologic, immunohistochemical, and molecular genetic study of 44 cases. Am J Surg Pathol 2000;24:1339–1352.
16. Logrono R, Jones DV, Faruqi S, Bhutani MS. Recent advances in cell biology, diagnosis, and therapy of gastrointestinal stromal tumor (GIST). Cancer Biol Ther 2004;3:251–258.
17. DeMatteo RP. The GIST of targeted cancer therapy: a tumor (gastrointestinal stromal tumor), a mutated gene (c-kit), and a molecular inhibitor (STI571). Ann Surg Oncol 2002;9:831–839.
18. Fuller CE, Williams GT. Gastrointestinal manifestations of type 1 neurofibromatosis (von Recklinghausen's disease). Histopathology (Oxf) 1991;19:1–11.
19. Boldorini R, Tosoni A, Leutner M, et al. Multiple small intestinal stromal tumours in a patient with previously unrecognised

neurofibromatosis type 1: immunohistochemical and ultrastructural evaluation. Pathology 2001;33:390–395.
20. Carney JA. The triad of gastric epithelioid leiomyosarcoma, pulmonary chondroma, and functioning extra-adrenal paraganglioma: a five-year review. Medicine (Baltim) 1983;62:159–169.
21. Carney JA. Gastric stromal sarcoma, pulmonary chondroma, and extra-adrenal paraganglioma (Carney Triad): natural history, adrenocortical component, and possible familial occurrence. Mayo Clin Proc 1999;74:543–552.
22. Ueyama T, Guo KJ, Hashimoto H, Daimaru Y, Enjoji M. A clinicopathologic and immunohistochemical study of gastrointestinal stromal tumors. Cancer (Phila) 1992;69:947–955.
23. Crosby JA, Catton CN, Davis A, et al. Malignant gastrointestinal stromal tumors of the small intestine: a review of 50 cases from a prospective database. Ann Surg Oncol 2001;8:50–59.
24. Burkill GJ, Badran M, Al-Muderis O, et al. Malignant gastrointestinal stromal tumor: distribution, imaging features, and pattern of metastatic spread. Radiology 2003;226:527–532.
25. Licht JD, Weissmann LB, Antman K. Gastrointestinal sarcomas. Semin Oncol 1988;15:181–188.
26. Lau S, Tam KF, Kam CK, et al. Imaging of gastrointestinal stromal tumour (GIST). Clin Radiol 2004;59:487–498.
27. Levy AD, Remotti HE, Thompson WM, Sobin LH, Miettinen M. Gastrointestinal stromal tumors: radiologic features with pathologic correlation. Radiographics 2003;23:283–304, 456; quiz 532.
28. Suster S. Gastrointestinal stromal tumors. Semin Diagn Pathol 1996;13:297–313.
29. Franquemont DW. Differentiation and risk assessment of gastrointestinal stromal tumors. Am J Clin Pathol 1995;103:41–47.
30. Fletcher CD, Berman JJ, Corless C, et al. Diagnosis of gastrointestinal stromal tumors: a consensus approach. Hum Pathol 2002;33:459–465.
31. Dematteo RP, Maki RG, Antonescu C, Brennan MF. Targeted molecular therapy for cancer: the application of STI571 to gastrointestinal stromal tumor. Curr Probl Surg 2003;40:144–193.
32. Kamel IR, Fishman EK. Recent advances in CT imaging of liver metastases. Cancer J 2004;10:104–120.
33. Kamel IR, Choti MA, Horton KM, et al. Surgically staged focal liver lesions: accuracy and reproducibility of dual-phase helical CT for detection and characterization. Radiology 2003;227:752–757.
34. Ludwig DJ, Traverso LW. Gut stromal tumors and their clinical behavior. Am J Surg 1997;173:390–394.
35. Pidhorecky I, Cheney RT, Kraybill WG, Gibbs JF. Gastrointestinal stromal tumors: current diagnosis, biologic behavior, and management. Ann Surg Oncol 2000;7:705–712.
36. McGrath PC, Neifeld JP, Lawrence W Jr, Kay S, Horsley JS III, Parker GA. Gastrointestinal sarcomas. Analysis of prognostic factors. Ann Surg 1987;206:706–710.
37. Kamel IR, Lawler LP, Corl FM, Fishman EK. Patterns of collateral pathways in extrahepatic portal hypertension as demonstrated by multidetector row computed tomography and advanced image processing. J Comput Assist Tomogr 2004;28:469–477.
38. Johnson PT, Heath DG, Hofmann LV, Horton KM, Fishman EK. Multidetector-row computed tomography with three-dimensional volume rendering of pancreatic cancer: a complete preoperative staging tool using computed tomography angiography and volume-rendered cholangiopancreatography. J Comput Assist Tomogr 2003;27:347–353.
39. Nino-Murcia M, Tamm EP, Charnsangavej C, Jeffrey RB Jr. Multidetector-row helical CT and advanced postprocessing techniques for the evaluation of pancreatic neoplasms. Abdom Imaging 2003;28:366–377.
40. Springer P, Dessl A, Giacomuzzi SM, et al. Virtual computed tomography gastroscopy: a new technique. Endoscopy 1997;29:632–634.
41. Raptopoulos V, Davis MA, Davidoff A, et al. Fat-density oral contrast agent for abdominal CT. Radiology 1987;164:653–656.
42. Horton KM, Fishman EK. Current role of CT in imaging of the stomach. Radiographics 2003;23:75–87.
43. Matsuoka Y, Masumoto T, Koga H, et al. Positive and negative oral contrast agents for combined abdominal and pelvic helical CT: first iodinated agent and second water. Radiat Med 2000;18:213–216.
44. Thoeni RF, Filson RG. Abdominal and pelvic CT: use of oral metoclopramide to enhance bowel opacification. Radiology 1988;169:391–393.
45. Horton KM, Fishman EK. Multidetector-row computed tomography and 3-dimensional computed tomography imaging of small bowel neoplasms: current concept in diagnosis. J Comput Assist Tomogr 2004;28:106–116.
46. Tateishi U, Hasegawa T, Satake M, Moriyama N. Gastrointestinal stromal tumor. Correlation of computed tomography findings with tumor grade and mortality. J Comput Assist Tomogr 2003;27:792–798.
47. Chen MY, Bechtold RE, Savage PD. Cystic changes in hepatic metastases from gastrointestinal stromal tumors (GISTs) treated with Gleevec (imatinib mesylate). AJR Am J Roentgenol 2002;179:1059–1062.
48. Joensuu H, Fletcher C, Dimitrijevic S, Silberman S, Roberts P, Demetri G. Management of malignant gastrointestinal stromal tumours. Lancet Oncol 2002;3:655–664.
49. Berman J, O'Leary TJ. Gastrointestinal stromal tumor workshop. Hum Pathol 2001;32:578–582.
50. Pope TL Jr, Buschi AJ, Brenbridge AN. Leiomyosarcoma of the duodenum simulating pancreatic carcinoma: case report. Va Med 1982;109:398–400.
51. Lawler LP, Horton KM, Fishman EK. Peripancreatic masses that simulate pancreatic disease: spectrum of disease and role of CT. Radiographics 2003;23:1117–1131.
52. Tworek JA, Goldblum JR, Weiss SW, Greenson JK, Appelman HD. Stromal tumors of the anorectum: a clinicopathologic study of 22 cases. Am J Surg Pathol 1999;23:946–954.
53. Miettinen M, El-Rifai W, L HLS, Lasota J. Evaluation of malignancy and prognosis of gastrointestinal stromal tumors: a review. Hum Pathol 2002;33:478–483.
54. Miettinen M, Monihan JM, Sarlomo-Rikala M, et al. Gastrointestinal stromal tumors/smooth muscle tumors (GISTs) primary in the omentum and mesentery: clinicopathologic and immunohistochemical study of 26 cases. Am J Surg Pathol 1999;23:1109–1118.
55. Zighelboim I, Henao G, Kunda A, Gutierrez C, Edwards C. Gastrointestinal stromal tumor presenting as a pelvic mass. Gynecol Oncol 2003;91:630–635.
56. Joensuu H, Roberts PJ, Sarlomo-Rikala M, et al. Effect of the tyrosine kinase inhibitor STI571 in a patient with a metastatic gastrointestinal stromal tumor. N Engl J Med 2001;344:1052–1056.
57. Ng EH, Pollock RE, Munsell MF, Atkinson EN, Romsdahl MM. Prognostic factors influencing survival in gastrointestinal leiomyosarcomas. Implications for surgical management and staging. Ann Surg 1992;215:68–77.
58. Lehnert T. Gastrointestinal sarcoma (GIST): a review of surgical management. Ann Chir Gynaecol 1998;87:297–305.
59. Mudan SS, Conlon KC, Woodruff JM, Lewis JJ, Brennan MF. Salvage surgery for patients with recurrent gastrointestinal sarcoma: prognostic factors to guide patient selection. Cancer (Phila) 2000;88:66–74.
60. Demetri GD, von Mehren M, Blanke CD, et al. Efficacy and safety of imatinib mesylate in advanced gastrointestinal stromal tumors. N Engl J Med 2002;347:472–480.
61. van Oosterom AT, Judson I, Verweij J, et al. Safety and efficacy of imatinib (STI571) in metastatic gastrointestinal stromal tumours: a phase I study. Lancet 2001;358:1421–1423.

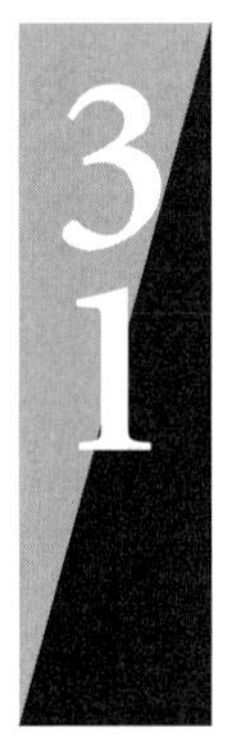

Genitourinary Imaging

Satomi Kawamoto, Harpreet K. Pannu, David A. Bluemke, and Elliot K. Fishman

Kidney

Renal Cell Carcinoma

With the increased availability of abdominal ultrasound, computed tomography (CT), and magnetic resonance imaging (MRI), many renal cell carcinomas are now incidentally discovered, which has resulted in detection of such tumors at an early stage in asymptomatic patients.

CT is currently the method of choice for evaluation of suspected renal masses and for preoperative staging of renal cell carcinoma (Figure 31.1).[1–3] The advent of spiral CT has had a significant impact on evaluation of renal masses. With the use of spiral CT, the sensitivity of CT in detecting renal cell carcinoma approaches 100% and specificity is 88% to 95%,[4,5] or evaluation of known or suspected renal masses, both pre- and postcontrast images with intravenous contrast medium, should be obtained because small renal cell carcinomas are difficult to diagnose without intravenous contrast and diagnosis of masses requires assessment of enhancement.[1,6] Spiral CT allows a high-quality scan dedicated to the kidneys during various phases of contrast enhancement after a rapid bolus of intravenous contrast material.[4,7,8] In addition, reformatted and three-dimensional images created from volumetric data sets obtained by spiral CT, particularly with recently introduced multidetector CT, can help assessment of the tumor extent and accurate staging (Figure 31.2).[9] For detection of renal masses, nephrographic phase images obtained with scan delay, at least 90 seconds after the start of intravenous contrast medium injection, are important because of a higher sensitivity than corticomedullary phase images to detect renal masses.[6–8,10]

MRI can also be used as an alternative imaging modality to CT for patients allergic to iodine or patients with an inconclusive CT study.[11] Gadolinium (Gd)-containing contrast material has been shown to be remarkably safe and is well tolerated in patients with a history of iodinated contrast allergy. Recent studies showed MRI is considered equivalent to CT in accuracy for the detection and characterization of renal masses.[12–14] A high-quality MR examination can be performed with torso phased-array coils and a variety of breath-hold sequences. Imaging protocols generally include T_1-weighted images obtained with spin-echo and/or breath-hold spoiled gradient echo images and T_2-weighted images obtained with fat-suppressed fast spin-echo images or breath-hold half Fourier single-shot fast spin-echo images. Gadolinium-containing intravenous contrast material is necessary to detect and characterize small lesions (Figure 31.3).[15,16] An advantage of MRI gadolinium contrast (as opposed to CT contrast) is lack of nephrotoxicity.

Staging of the tumor by radiologic examination is relevant because prognosis and surgical planning largely depends on preoperative imaging delineation of disease extent. Reported accuracy of CT and MRI for staging of renal cell carcinoma is similar, ranging from 67% to 95% for CT and from 67% to 96% for MRI.[9,11–13] It may be difficult to distinguish stage I (confined within the renal capsule) from stage II (extending into the perinephric fat) disease. Thickening of the renal fascia and dilated tortuous vessels in the perinephric space are not reliable signs of tumor extension into the perinephric fat and may be caused by edema, inflammation, or engorgement of vessels due to increased blood flow through a vascular tumor. Perinephric fat stranding has been detected in up to 50% of stage I tumors on CT (see Figure 31.1). The presence of an enhancing nodule of 1 cm or greater in the perinephric space has been reported to be highly specific (98%) but only 46% sensitive on CT. MRI has been reported to be slightly more accurate compared to CT to predict invasion of perirenal fat.[11,12]

Tumor thrombus within the renal vein, inferior vena cava (IVC), or right atrium can be directly visualized by CT or MRI. Using spiral CT and electron beam CT, sensitivity and specificity of tumor thrombus in the renal vein were 85% and 98%.[17] In a recent study using multidetector CT with dedicated protocol and thin collimation, 100% accuracy of tumor thrombus in the renal vein and IVC has been reported.[9] MRI and MR angiography also achieved high sensitivity of 89% to 100%, with specificity of 96% to 100%, in assessment of tumor thrombus in the renal vein and IVC.[16,18,19] A recent study showed tumor invasion of the IVC wall was imaged by MRI with three-dimensional (3-D) gadolinium-enhanced MR angiography and venography with sensitivity and specificity of 100% and 89%, respectively.[20]

Distinction between metastatic and hyperplastic lymph nodes is limited for both CT and MRI because size remains the only criterion for diagnosis of lymph node metastasis. Studer et al. reported that CT is sensitive for the detection of enlarged lymph nodes in patients with renal cell carcinoma (95%), but more than 50% of enlarged nodes were caused by benign inflammatory changes, probably the result of tumoral necrosis or venous thrombosis.[21] They also reported that when using a size criteria of 1 cm or greater for regional lymph node metastasis there is a 4% false-negative rate for lymph node staging.[21]

A variety of complex or complicated cystic masses occur in the kidney. Bosniak has described a classification system

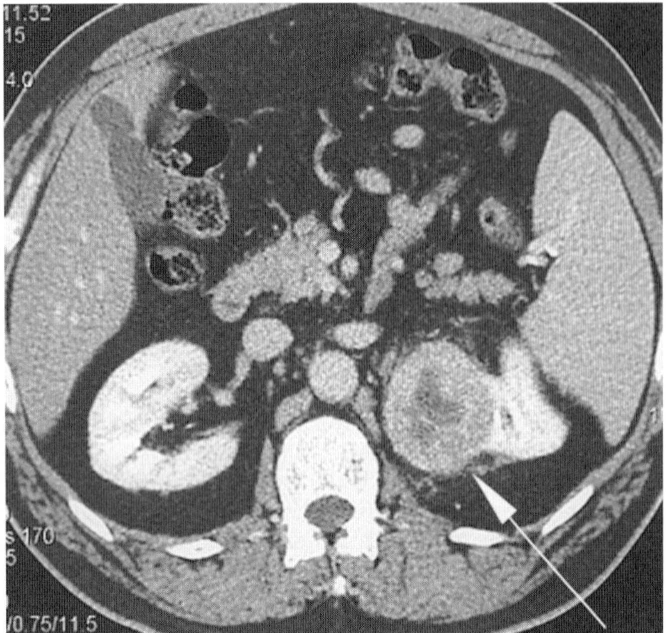

FIGURE 31.1. Renal cell carcinoma. Contrast-enhanced computed tomography (CT) scan shows heterogeneous mass in the left kidney (*arrow*). There is stranding around the mass, which is caused by peritumoral inflammation found by pathologic specimen. There was no capsular invasion. The pathologic stage was T2 Nx Mx.

in which CT features are used to classify cystic masses into four types to determine the likelihood of malignancy and aid in the management of complicated cystic lesions.[22] CT and MRI with intravenous contrast material are equivalent for distinguishing cysts from neoplasms.[1] Image subtraction is commonly used for MRI and aids in complex cases. Images without gadolinium are subtracted from those obtained after gadolinium contrast agent. Complex cystic lesions that may otherwise appear to enhance are subtracted from the resulting image. The method is particularly important for patients with polycystic kidneys.

With increased detection of renal tumors at an earlier stage, more limited or less invasive surgical procedures, such as nephron-sparing and laparoscopic surgery, have evolved as effective alternatives to radical nephrectomy.[23] Nephron-sparing surgery is increasing in frequency because excellent preliminary results have been reported with small, low-stage renal cell carcinoma. More recently, less invasive nephron-sparing procedures have been applied to the treatment of renal cell carcinoma including laparoscopic surgery, radiofrequency ablation, and cryoablation. CT and MRI can play an important role to assess the precise location of the tumor in relation to the major vessels and the renal collecting system and to determine whether nephron-sparing surgery can be performed (see Figure 31.2).[24–27]

Other solid renal masses include oncocytoma, lymphoma, angiomyolipoma, pseudotumor, and metastatic tumor to the kidney (Figure 31.4). Oncocytoma requires surgical resection because it is not radiographically distinguished from renal cell carcinoma, but other tumors are generally not treated by surgery. Percutaneous renal biopsy may be useful in several clinical situations: (a) lesions that do not have the typical radiologic features of renal cell carcinoma, (b) lesions that are unresectable, (c) lesions that are of uncertain histology, (d) possibly metastatic lesions, (e) lesions for which lymphoma is a diagnostic consideration, and (f) lesions for which treatment may be altered by histologic diagnosis.[28] In these populations, the accuracy of biopsy of 87% to 89% without significant complications has been reported.[28,29]

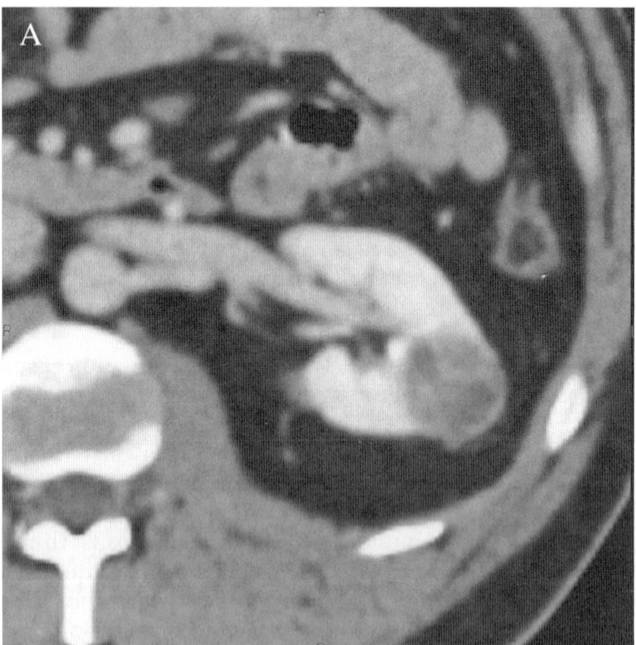

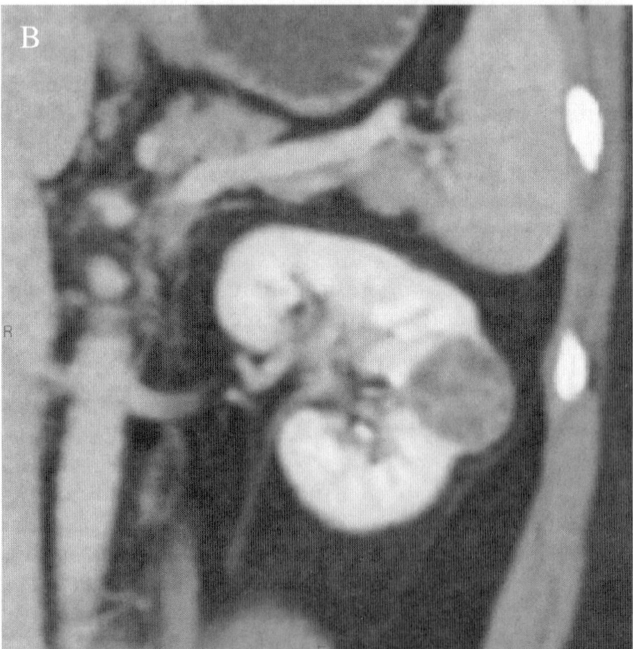

FIGURE 31.2. Renal cell carcinoma. (A) Contrast-enhanced CT scan obtained during nephrographic phase shows a 3-cm mass in the left kidney. (B) Coronal reformatted CT image shows the mass is located in the periphery and is partially exophytic. There is no evidence of vascular or collecting system involvement. The patient underwent nephron-sparing nephrectomy. The pathologic stage was T1 Nx Mx.

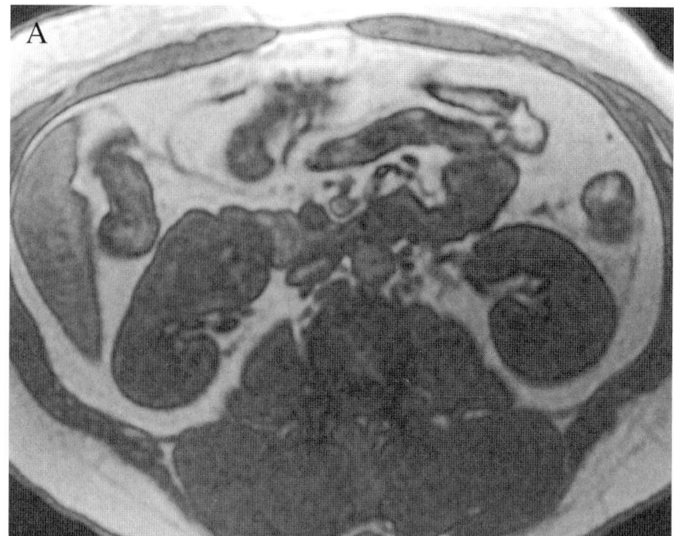

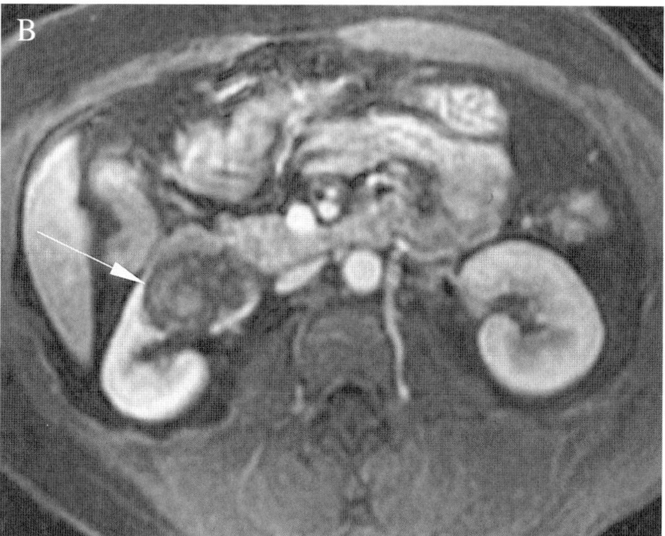

FIGURE 31.3. Renal cell carcinoma. (A) Axial T_1-weighted image shows right renal mass isointense to the kidney, which is difficult to appreciate without contrast enhancement. (B) Postcontrast T_1-weighted image with fat suppression shows the minimal enhancement of the mass, which is much less than the adjacent renal cortex. The mass abuts the pancreatic head (*arrow*). The patient underwent right nephrectomy. Pathologically, it was papillary renal cell carcinoma with the pathologic stage of T1 Nx Mx.

Urothelial Carcinoma

Collecting System and Ureter

Transitional cell carcinoma (TCC) of the renal pelvis accounts for approximately 7% of primary malignancies of the kidney. TCC is often multifocal. Two percent to 4% of patients with TCC of the bladder develop upper urinary tract tumors, and metachronous upper tract tumors develop in 19% of upper tract TCC. Urography, sonography, or retrograde pyelography is often the initial study for suspected upper tract urothelial tumors.[1] The most sensitive imaging modality for detecting and delineating tumors in the upper urinary tract is retrograde pyelography,[30] with sensitivity of 72% and specificity of 85%.[31]

Transitional carcinoma of the upper urinary tract may be seen on CT as an intraluminal soft tissue mass (Figure 31.5), diffuse or eccentric thickening or irregularity of the wall, or with obstruction of the collecting system proximal to a soft tissue mass.[32,33] On noncontrast CT, it is seen as soft tissue density of 10 to 40 Hounsfield units (HU), and there is minimal increase in density after intravenous contrast medium administration.[1] With multidetector CT, a ureteral mass as small as 5 mm can be detected. It may displace and compress the renal sinus fat or infiltrate the renal parenchyma (Figure 31.6).[32,33] A focal obstructive nephrogram may be seen with a delayed and late persistent dense nephro-

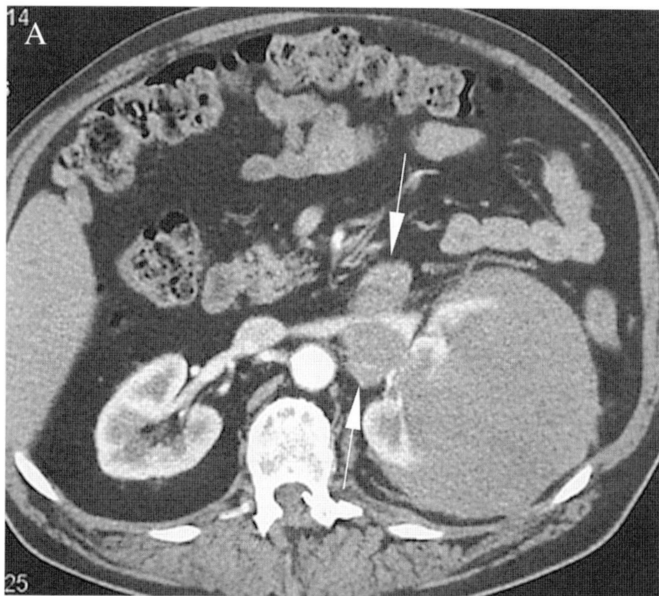

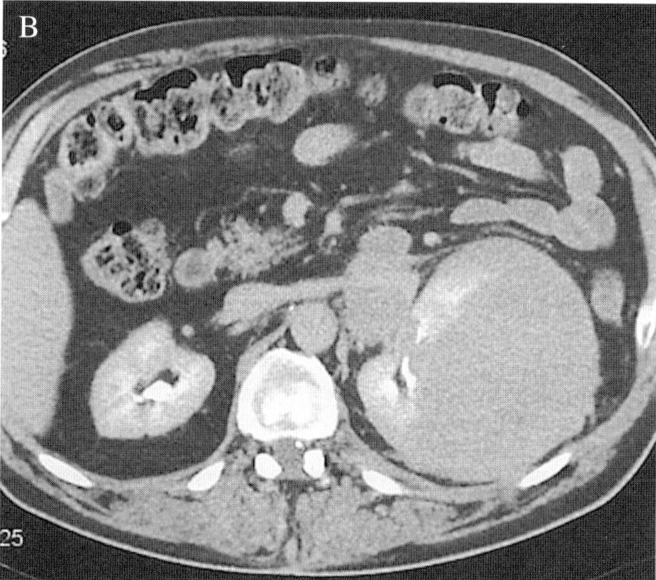

FIGURE 31.4. Malignant lymphoma of the kidney. (A) Contrast-enhanced CT obtained during corticomedullary phase shows large soft tissue mass involving the left kidney. Lymphadenopathy is also seen along the left renal vein (*arrow*). (B) Contrast-enhanced CT obtained during excretory phase shows minimal, homogeneous contrast enhancement of the mass. The patient underwent ultrasound-guided percutaneous biopsy, which revealed malignant lymphoma.

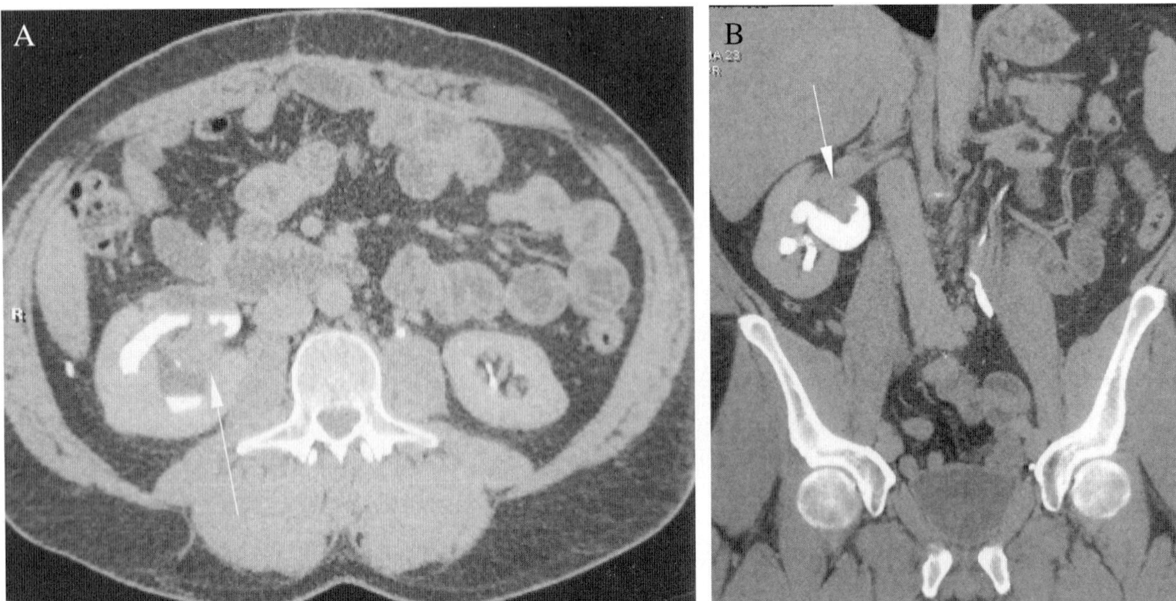

FIGURE 31.5. Transitional cell carcinoma of the right renal pelvis. (A) Contrast-enhanced CT scan obtained during excretory phase. There is a soft tissue mass within the right renal pelvis. Right hydronephrosis is caused by the accessory right renal artery crossing the ureterovesical junction seen on arterial phase images (not shown). (B) Coronal reformatted CT image obtained during excretory phase. Soft tissue mass causes filling defect within the dilated right renal pelvis. The patient underwent laparoscopic nephrectomy. Pathologically, it was superficially invasive low-grade transitional cell carcinoma, and the pathologic stage was T1 Nx Mx.

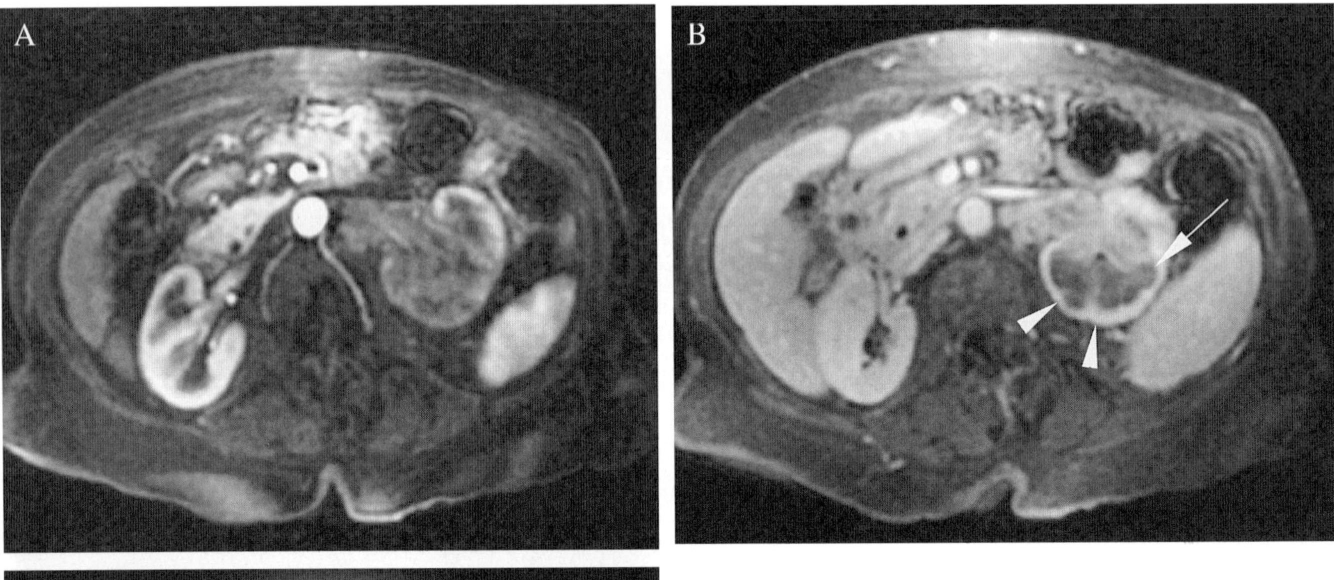

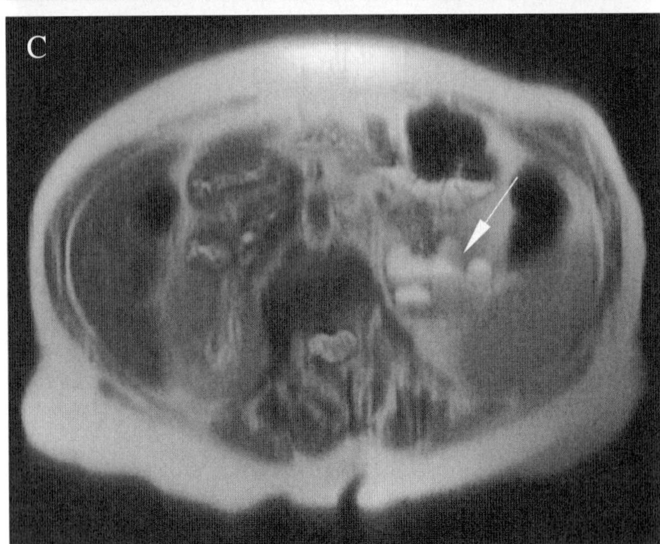

FIGURE 31.6. Transitional cell carcinoma of the left renal pelvis. (A) Axial T_1-weighted gradient echo image with fat suppression obtained at early phase after gadolinium contrast agent injection shows poorly defined mass in the left renal hilum infiltrating the renal parenchyma. (B) Axial T_1-weighted gradient echo image with fat suppression obtained at nephrographic phase shows focal dilatation of the collecting system (*large arrow*) with delayed cortical nephrogram (*small arrows*) in the posterior aspect of the left kidney. (C) Axial T_2-weighted breath-hold half Fourier single-shot fast spin-echo image shows the mass in the left renal hilum infiltrating the renal parenchyma. There is focal dilatation of the left collecting system (*arrow*). Pathologically, it was infiltrating high-grade transitional cell carcinoma involving the renal pelvis. There was extensive infiltration into the peripelvic fat and invasion of renal parenchyma. Metastatic carcinoma was present in the lymph nodes. The pathological stage was pT4 N2 Mx.

gram.[34] CT can differentiate tumor from other causes of filling defects such as stone or blood clot by measurements of density.[35]

Although CT is the most accurate imaging procedure available for staging of urothelial tumors,[1] it is generally agreed that CT cannot distinguish Ta to T2 lesions (Ta, limited to mucosa; T1, tumor involves the submucosa; T2, muscle invasive tumor).[36] Overstaging localized disease as T3 (deep invasion into the renal parenchyma or peripelvic soft tissue) is common, particularly when hydronephrosis is present. However, to detect invasion beyond the pelvic wall or metastatic disease, conventional CT has 85% accuracy,[37] and CT plays an important role in defining adjacent organ invasion.[38] In the detection of lymph node involvement, CT has specificity of 94% to 100% but variable sensitivity of 47% to 88%.[38–40] With use of spiral CT, improved T staging is expected due to better resolution, but no publications are available to date.

MRI is not commonly used for diagnosis and staging of the upper tract TCC. However, MRI is useful for patients who cannot tolerate iodinated contrast material (see Figure 31.6).[33] In a study of MRI with nine patients with upper urinary tract transitional cell carcinoma, including gadolinium-enhanced sequences, MRI achieved accuracy of 89% for staging.[41] There was understaging of direct tumor invasion into the renal parenchyma in one case.[41]

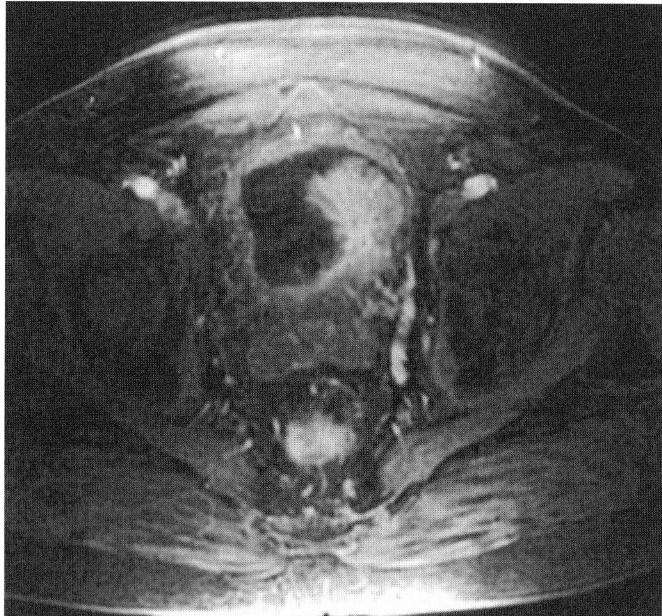

FIGURE 31.7. Bladder cancer. Axial T_1-weighted magnetic resonance (MR) image with fat suppression obtained after gadolinium contrast agent injection shows a large papillary mass arising from the left posterior wall projecting into the bladder lumen. There is contrast enhancement in the central portion of the tumor.

Bladder Carcinoma

Cystoscopy is the primary diagnostic procedure for diagnosis and follow-up of bladder carcinomas and is very sensitive in detecting small bladder neoplasms. The stage of tumor at diagnosis determines management and is an important prognostic factor. Clinical staging by cystoscopy, biopsy, and bimanual examination under anesthesia is accurate for superficial tumors (T1 and lower), but a significant error has been shown in staging muscle-invasive tumors (T2a and higher).[42,43]

CT and MRI are performed for tumor staging once the diagnosis of bladder carcinoma has been established. Bladder tumors are seen as focal or diffuse wall thickening, or a sessile or pedunculated soft tissue mass protruding into the bladder lumen on CT and MR imaging (Figures 31.7, 31.8). Transitional cell carcinoma of the bladder enhances immediately and intensely after bolus injection of iodinated contrast material compared to uninvolved bladder wall on CT or MRI (Figures 31.7, 31.8). In some instances, MRI can differentiate superficial (T2a) and deep muscle invasion (T2b). MRI also allows detection of extravesical spread more readily than with other imaging modalities because of its superior soft tissue differentiation and multiplanar imaging capability. On MRI, transitional cell carcinoma tends to have an intermediate signal intensity, greater than normal muscle on T_2-weighted images, and is significantly more intense than muscle on gadolinium-enhanced T_1-weighted images. If the inner aspect of the low-intensity bladder wall is irregular, superficial muscle invasion is suspected. If the low-intensity bladder line is disrupted, deep muscle invasion is diagnosed.[44–47] Reported overall accuracy of MR imaging in staging of bladder cancer ranges from 73% to 96%, which is 10% to 33% higher than that obtained with CT.[47] With the use of gadolinium-containing contrast material, improved detection of small tumors and an increase in accuracy of local staging were reported.[46] Therefore, MRI is the staging modality of choice for invasive tumors. The use of phased-array external surface coils or endorectal surface coils allows higher signal-to-noise ratio and higher spatial resolution images of the bladder, and these are successfully applied to the imaging of bladder cancer.[48]

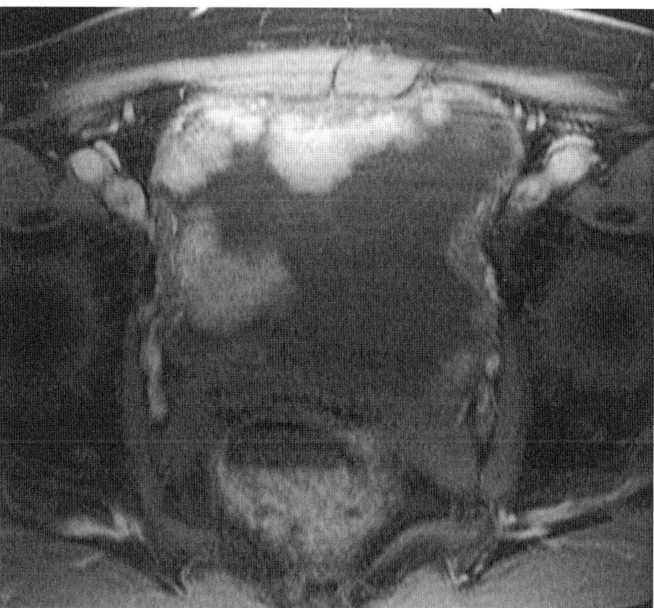

FIGURE 31.8. Bladder cancer. Axial T_1-weighted MR image with fat suppression obtained after gadolinium contrast agent injection shows multifocal masses arising from the anterior and right lateral wall of the bladder projecting into the bladder lumen.

Patients with bladder cancer and lymph node metastases have a worse prognosis than those without metastatic nodes. Reported accuracy of CT and MRI in detecting lymph node metastasis is similar, ranging from 70% to 98%.[49] Three-dimensional magnetization prepared rapid acquisition gradient echo (MP-RAGE) images have improved the detection of suspicious lymph nodes.[50,51] Lymphotrophic contrast agents, such as ultrasmall superparamagnetic iron oxide (USPIO) may improve distinguishing between benign and malignant lymph nodes.[52]

Inflammation of the bladder wall after radiotherapy or other causes may be indistinguishable from neoplastic infiltration as both may enhance substantially. A study showed that early-phase dynamic gadolinium-enhanced imaging improved distinction of tumor and postbiopsy changes of the bladder wall because bladder cancer enhanced earlier (6.5 seconds) than postbiopsy inflammation and granulation tissue (13.6 seconds) after gadolinium contrast administration.[53]

Virtual cystoscopy created with CT or MR data has recently been used to detect bladder cancer. Recent studies of virtual cystoscopy created with CT data showed a sensitivity of 89% to 100% compared with fiberoptic cystoscopy.[54–56] Most tumors not detected by virtual cystoscopy were reported to be less than 1 cm.

Adrenal Gland

Adrenal Adenoma and Differentiation from Other Adrenal Masses

Incidental discovery of adrenal masses is a common clinical problem as a result of the widespread use of imaging procedures, occurring in up to 5% of patients who have undergone abdominal CT.[57] Most adrenal masses are benign nonhyperfunctioning adenomas even in patients with a known extra-adrenal malignancy (Figure 31.9).[57] Primary adrenal carcinoma is rare, with a reported incidence of 2 cases per million (Figure 31.10). Differentiation of benign and malignant adrenal masses is critical to determine appropriate treatment. With advances in CT and MR imaging with dedicated imaging protocols, characterization of these adrenal masses has greatly increased in accuracy.

CT is generally considered the modality of choice for initial characterization of the adrenal mass. A noncontrast scan should be first performed, and a contrast-enhanced CT scan may be necessary if the noncontrast scan is not conclusive.[58] MRI is reserved for cases that have indeterminate findings on CT.[58,59]

Generally, larger adrenal lesions have a greater likelihood of being malignant (see Figure 31.10). In 39 patients with extraadrenal malignancy, 87% of lesions smaller than 3 cm were benign and 95% of lesions greater than 3 cm were malignant.[60] In another study, among 45 adrenal masses greater than 5 cm found by imaging studies, 33% were malignant.[61] Because of significant overlap of benign and malignant lesions based on size criteria alone, most authorities recommend that masses greater than 4 or 5 cm should be biopsied or surgically excised. Increase in size of the lesion during follow-up can be helpful in predicting malignancy. Adenomas tend to have smooth margins and a homogeneous density, whereas metastases can be heterogeneous and have an irregular shape. However, these are not specific signs of malignancy.[58]

The presence and amount of lipid in many adrenal adenomas accounts for their low attenuation on unenhanced CT scans and their loss in relative signal intensity on chemical shift MR images (see Figure 31.9). There is an inverse linear relationship between the percentage of lipid-rich cortical cells

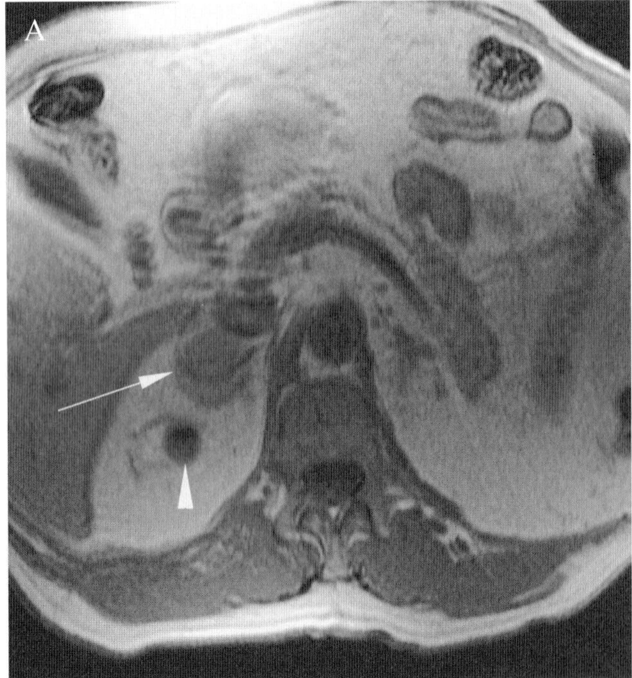

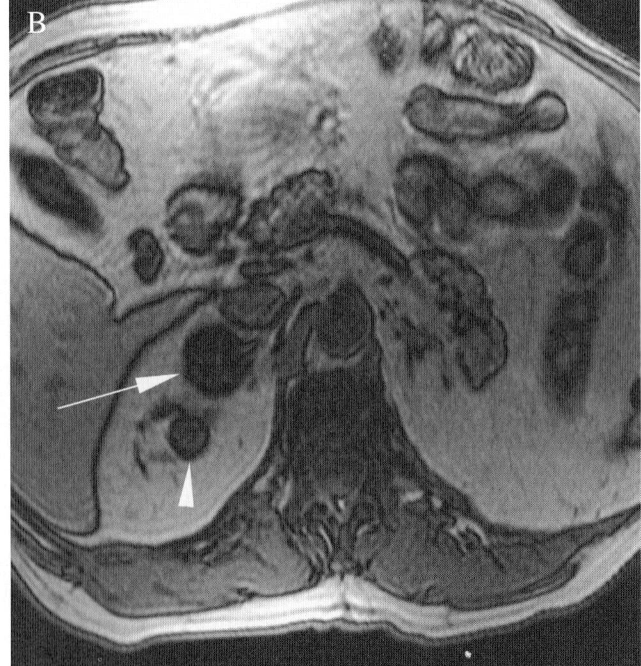

FIGURE 31.9. Adrenal adenoma. (A) Axial T_1-weighted in-phase MR image shows right adrenal mass (*large arrow*). There is a small cyst in the upper pole of the right kidney (*small arrow*). (B) Axial T_1-weighted out-of phase image shows significant signal dropoff in the lesion (*large arrow*), which is diagnostic of an adenoma.

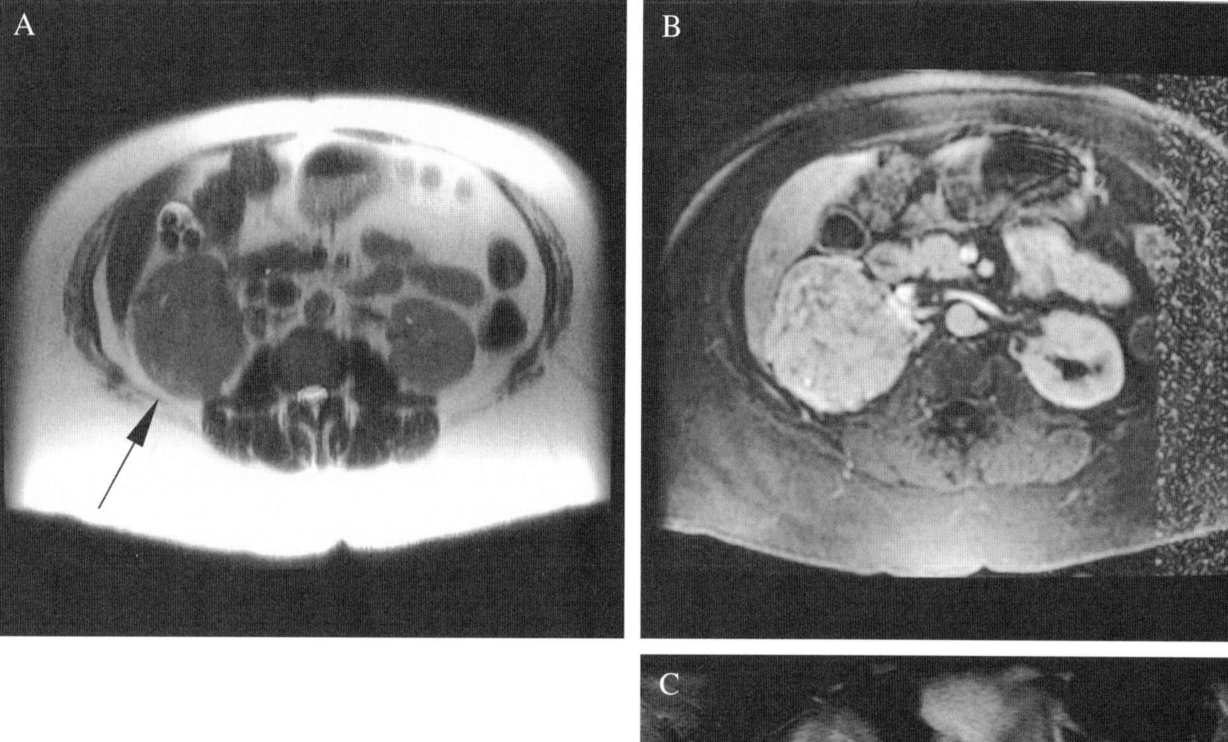

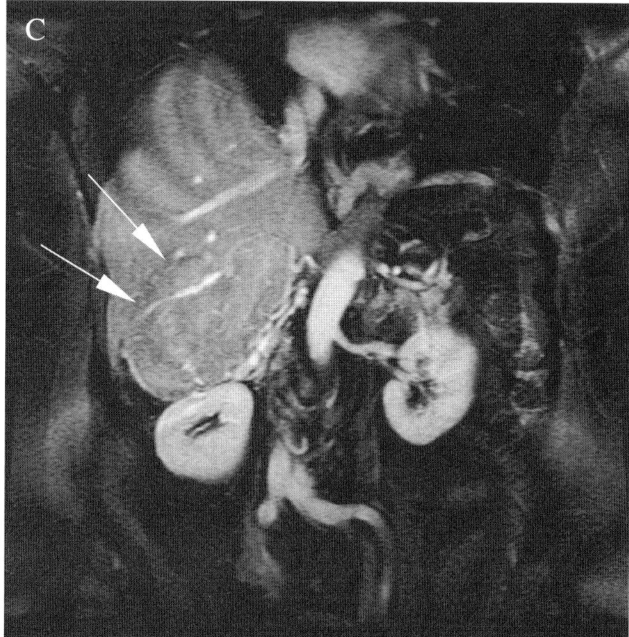

FIGURE 31.10. Adrenal carcinoma. (A) Axial T_2-weighted breath-hold half Fourier single-shot fast spin-echo image shows 8-cm mass in the right adrenal gland (*large arrow*). There are gallstones (*small arrows*). (B) Axial T_1-weighted gradient echo image with fat suppression obtained after gadolinium intravenous contrast material shows enhancement of the adrenal mass. (C) Coronal T_1-weighted gradient echo image with fat suppression obtained after gadolinium intravenous contrast agent injection shows the mass clearly above the right kidney (*arrow*), displacing the right kidney medially and laterally.

in adrenal adenomas and the unenhanced CT attenuation number and a similar inverse linear relationship to the relative change in MR signal intensity on chemical shift images. Metastases, on the other hand, have little intracytoplasmic fat and therefore do not have low attenuation at nonenhanced CT.[58] Similarly, metastases do not lose signal on chemical shift MR images.

Studies have been performed to determine an adequate threshold to differentiate benign versus malignant adrenal masses on nonenhanced CT. Boland et al. performed a meta-analysis of 10 studies to determine an optimal density threshold to differentiate benign from malignant lesions, and reported that using 10 HU as a threshold, noncontrast CT has 71% sensitivity and 98% specificity for characterizing adrenal masses.[62]

If the adrenal mass is more than 10 HU at noncontrast CT, CT with intravenous contrast material should be performed to evaluate enhancement washout characteristics. Adenomas lose enhancement more rapidly than nonadenomas, and delayed CT attenuation value was used to differentiate adenomas from nonadenomas. Using an attenuation measurement of less than 30 to 40 HU at 10 to 30 minutes after contrast injection, the adrenal mass is almost always an adenoma.[63] A relative percentage enhancement washout of greater than 50% calculated by (1 − delayed enhanced HU value/initial enhanced HU value) × 100 has a sensitivity of 98% and specificity of 100% for benign disease.[64] Other investigators used percentage enhancement washout calculated by (initial enhanced HU value − delayed enhanced HU value)/(initial enhanced HU value − unenhanced HU value) with a threshold of 60% at 50 to 80 seconds after administration of contrast material for the initial scan and 15 minutes for the delayed scan, and achieved 86% to 98% sensitivity and 92% to 96% specificity.[65,66]

When CT with intravenous contrast is equivocal, chemical shift MR imaging should be performed as chemical shift MR imaging is the most sensitive technique for differentiating adenomas from metastases of the adrenal gland.[58] With the chemical shift MR technique, the sensitivity and specificity for differentiating adenomas from metastasis ranges from 81% to 100% and 94% to 100%, respectively.[67–70] Reported cases of nonadenomas that met these CT or MRI criteria for adenoma, included pheochrcomocytoma,[71] metastasis from renal cell carcinoma, and adrenocortical carcinoma.[66,72]

Pheochromocytoma

Pheochromocytoma is usually benign, but approximately 10% of these lesions are malignant. CT is the study of choice to confirm the diagnosis when a pheochromocytoma is suspected on clinical and laboratory grounds.[58] On CT, pheochromocytoma appears as a well-defined mass with marked enhancement after intravenous contrast administration. MR findings may enable characterization of pheochromocytoma because the signal intensity of these tumors may be very high on T_2-weighted images, probably caused by cystic components. However, there is considerable overlap between the MR appearance of pheochromocytoma and other adrenal lesions. The sensitivity and specificity of MR imaging for diagnosing pheochromocytoma were 64.7% and 88.0%, respectively.[73]

Adrenal Biopsy

Adrenal biopsy is required when imaging studies cannot accurately characterize an adrenal mass. Harisinghani et al. analyzed 225 oncologic patients who had undergone CT-guided biopsies of an adrenal mass that were indeterminate at CT or MRI and reported that a negative or benign pathology can be regarded as a true-negative evaluation with no necessity to repeat the biopsy.[59]

Prostate Cancer

Accurate staging of prostate cancer is essential for the prognosis and treatment planning. In particular, it is crucial to determine the local extent of prostate cancer (extracapsular extension and seminal vesicle infiltration) and the presence of metastatic disease (lymphatic or hematogenous), because radical prostatectomy is the preferred method of treatment for patients with disease confined to the capsule. Patients with disease outside the prostate are generally not surgical candidates and may be offered an alternative therapy. Clinical staging based on digital rectal examination, transrectal ultrasound, Gleason score, sextant biopsy, and prostate-specific antigen (PSA) has limited accuracy and may underestimate the extent of disease. Previous studies indicated that digital rectal examination underestimates the local extent of cancer in 40% to 60% of the cases.[74] The purpose of preoperative imaging evaluation is to increase the accuracy of the assigned clinical stage.[49]

The current major clinical role of MRI is to detect disease outside the capsule, including extracapsular extension, seminal vesicle infiltration, nodal metastasis, and bone marrow metastasis once cancer has been diagnosed (Figure 31.11).[74] Detection of such extracapsular disease eliminates unnecessary surgical procedures.[49,74] A decision analysis model suggested that preoperative MRI was cost-effective for men with moderate or high probability of extracapsular disease.[75]

On T_2-weighted images, prostate cancer is typically seen as an area of decreased signal intensity within the normally high-signal-intensity peripheral zone. The presence of decreased T_2 signal intensity in the peripheral zone is of limited sensitivity as some tumors are isointense and of limited specificity because other causes, such as hemorrhage, prostatitis, scarring, radiotherapy, cryosurgery, and hormonal therapy can cause low T_2 signal intensity. Overall, the sensitivity of MRI for detecting prostate cancer is approximately 60%.[76] A more-recent study indicated that in patients with an elevated PSA and negative transurethral sonography-guided quadrant or sextant biopsy results, MRI had a sensitivity of 83% and a positive predictive value of 50% for detection of prostate cancer.[76] Extracapsular tumor extension is seen as asymmetry or invasion of the neurovascular bundle, obliteration of the rectoprostatic angle, and bulging of the prostate capsule, which may be irregular with a square or rectangular edge or, less commonly, a smooth curvilinear bulge. Accuracy of staging extracapsular extension with MRI ranges

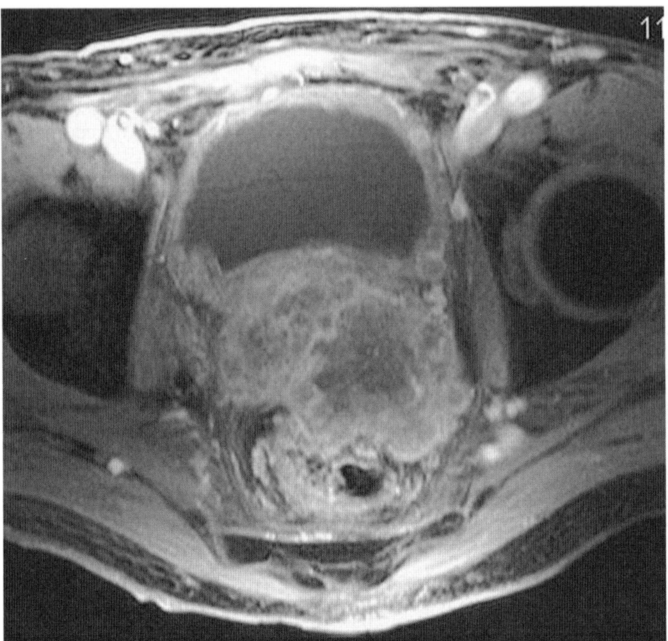

FIGURE 31.11. Prostate cancer. Axial T_1-weighted gradient echo image with fat suppression obtained after gadolinium contrast agent injection. There is a large heterogeneously enhancing mass involving the prostate gland, with involvement of the bladder wall and rectal wall. Pathologically, it was poorly differentiated carcinoma with small cell neuroendocrine features.

from 51% to 92%. It remains impossible to detect microscopic extracapsular extension.[74] Seminal vesicle invasion is seen as enlargement of one seminal vesicle with abnormal asymmetric low signal intensity within the lumen on T_2-weighted images, although low signal intensity of the seminal vesicles can be caused by other reasons including hemorrhage, radiation, hormonal therapy, and amyloid deposits.[49] The accuracy of detection of seminal vesicle invasion with endorectal coil ranges between 54% and 96%.[77–80] A meta-analysis suggested that turbo spin echo, endorectal coil, and multiple imaging planes improve staging performance by MRI.[81]

By combining diagnostic variables (age, PSA level, and Gleason tumor grade) with MRI findings, the accuracy of staging can be increased.[82] It has been shown that the addition of MRI improves the prediction of seminal vesicle invasion and extracapsular extension in patients with intermediate risk, as indicated by PSA levels of 10 to 20 ng/mL and Gleason scores of 5 to 7.[83]

CT is not recommended for local staging because of its inability to differentiate among normal, hyperplastic, and cancerous glands.[49] Sensitivity in detection of extracapsular extension of prostate carcinoma is low, especially in early clinical stages. However, it provides useful information for clinically suspected advanced disease with apparent extracapsular extension and extrapelvic involvement.[49] Guidelines for the use of CT in patients with PSA greater than 20 ng/mL have been reported and are in clinical use.[84]

CT and MRI are useful to detect nodal metastasis in a select group of patients with high risk for nodal metastasis, predicted by digital rectal examination, serum PSA, and biopsy Gleason score.[74] A study showed that identification of enlarged lymph nodes with subsequent biopsy using CT guidance was shown to identify lymph nodes metastases and thus prevent unnecessary surgery in more than 10% of patients.[85] In this study, nodes 6 mm or greater in cross-sectional diameter were considered pathologic and were biopsied. CT-guided aspiration biopsy improved the specificity and accuracy of CT in diagnosing lymph node metastases from 96.7% and 93.7% to 100% and 96.5%, respectively. The overall accuracy of CT in detecting pelvic lymph node metastases from prostate cancer is in the range of 67% to 93%.[49] MRI with a three-dimensional technique has revealed an accuracy of 90% in the detection of nodal metastasis in bladder and prostate cancer.[51] Use of ultrasmall superparamagnetic iron oxide particles (USPIO) was investigated to detect clinically occult lymph node metastases in prostate cancer and significantly improved the detection of small and otherwise undetectable lymph node metastasis compared to conventional MRI. It increased sensitivity and specificity of nodal metastasis from 35.4% and 90.4% to 90.5% and 97.8%, respectively.[86]

MR spectroscopic imaging (^{1}H-MRSI) is a method that demonstrates normal and altered tissue metabolism. It has been shown that prostate cancer is characterized at MRSI by increased choline and/or decreased levels of citrate.[87] The addition of MRSI to MRI has been shown to increase staging accuracy[88] and have potential for more accurate tumor localization.[89] MRSI, interventional MRI-guided biopsy, and therapy are currently under investigation[90,91] and not considered to be routine.

Uterus

Cervical Cancer

Cervical carcinoma is staged according to the International Federation of Gynecology and Obstetrics (FIGO) staging system. Accurate staging of cervical cancer is crucial in determining the mode of treatment. Routine clinical staging incorporates gynecologic pelvic examination under anesthesia, chest X-ray, lesion biopsies, cystoscopy, and, if indicated, renal sonography for detection of hydronephrosis.[92] In most centers, stage IB (confined to the cervix) and stage IIA (extends beyond the cervix but within upper two-thirds of the cervix, no parametrial invasion) disease are treated with hysterectomy with pelvic lymph node dissection. Radiation therapy is the treatment of choice with parametrial involvement (stage IIB or higher).[49] However, clinical staging was shown to be inaccurate, and discrepancy between clinical staging and surgical staging, ranging from 34% to 39%, has been reported.[92]

MRI is the modality of choice to image cervical masses that are greater than 1.5 cm or presumed to extend beyond the cervix.[93] On MRI, cervical carcinoma most often appears as an intermediate signal or high-signal-intensity mass distorting or disrupting the normal cervical zonal anatomy of the cervix (Figure 31.12). The size of the tumor measured by MRI correlates well with surgical measurement of the tumor size. When the hypointense ring of the cervical stroma is preserved on MRI, parametrial extension can be virtually excluded.[93] Parametrial extension is suggested when there is full-thickness invasion of the cervical stroma associated with irregularity or asymmetry of the lateral cervical margin, parametrial mass, or stranding within the parametrial fat (Figure 31.12). However, when full-thickness stromal invasion occurs, microscopic parametrial extension may be present despite a smooth lateral cervical margin and the absence of abnormality in the parametrial fat.

Boss et al. performed meta-analysis of 12 studies published between 1986 and 1995 describing the staging accuracy of MRI in cervical carcinoma.[92] The mean percentage of overall staging accuracy of MRI without use of contrast agents was 79% (range, 47%–90%), in comparison with the accuracy of the clinical examination of 72% (range, 55%–85%) and that of CT of 62% (range, 32%–80%). The mean percentage of accuracy in detecting parametrial invasion with MRI was 88%, with clinical examination 86%, and with CT 72%. Some studies indicated higher staging accuracy of gadolinium-enhanced T_1-weighted[94] or dynamic enhancement studies.[95–97] Another meta-analysis study including 57 articles from 1985 to 2002 showed higher sensitivity and specificity in evaluating bladder invasion by MRI (75% and 91%) compared to CT (64% and 73%), but the specificity of rectal invasion was comparable between MRI and CT.[98]

CT has been used to assess patients with tumors of advanced cervical cancer and evaluating patients for recurrence.[49] The use of CT in early disease has been limited due to prior reports of low sensitivity and specificity for local invasion.[99] However, major advances in CT technology during the past few years may broaden the use of CT.[99] Accuracy of

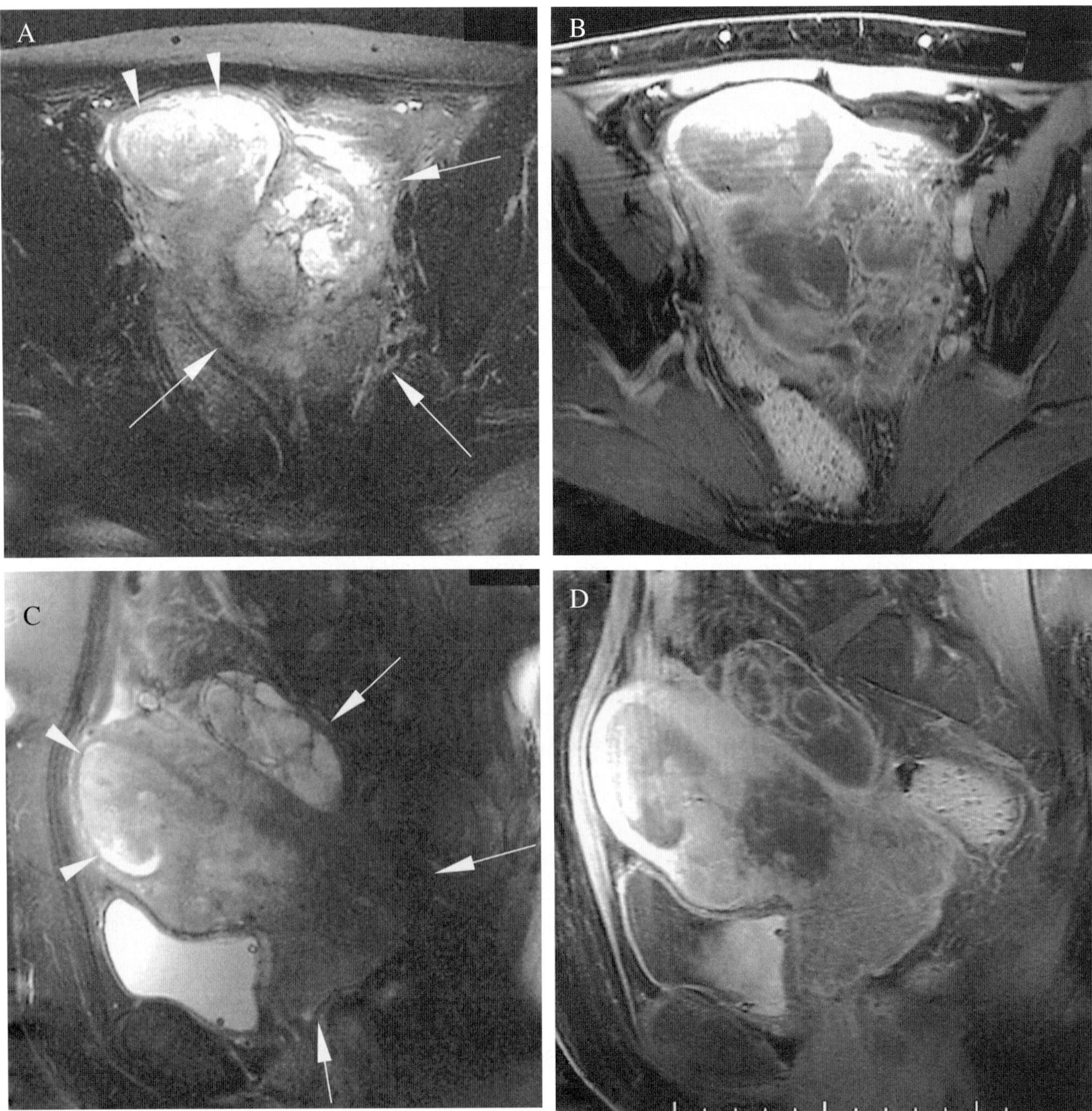

FIGURE 31.12. Cervical cancer. (A) Axial T_2-weighted image with fat suppression shows a large mass obliterating the entire cervix, extending anteriorly into the myometrium and the left pelvic side wall (*large arrow*). The mass obstructs the endometrial canal, which is dilated and filled with secretion and debris (*small arrows*). (B) Axial T_1-weighted gradient echo image with fat suppression obtained after gadolinium contrast agent injection. There is heterogeneous contrast enhancement of the mass. The central area is not enhanced, representing necrosis. (C) Sagittal T_2-weighted image with fat suppression shows large mass arising from the cervix, extending superiorly into the myometrium (*large arrow*). The mass obstructs the endometrial canal, which is dilated and filled with secretion and debris (*small arrows*). (D) Sagittal T_1-weighted gradient echo image with fat suppression obtained after gadolinium contrast agent injection. There is heterogeneous contrast enhancement of the mass with areas of necrosis. The International Federation of Gynecology and Obstetrics (FIGO) staging was IIIB.

CT staging is greater with advanced disease and is reported as 92% for stage IIIB to IVB cervical cancers.[100]

The presence of pelvic lymph node metastases is not part of the FIGO staging criteria; however, it is the most important prognostic factor and findings may be crucial for treatment planning.[92] Yang et al. reported that central necrosis of pelvic lymph nodes had a positive predictive value of 100% in the diagnosis of metastastic adenopathy in patients with cervical cancer.[101] They reported that spiral CT and MRI are roughly equivalent with accuracy in detecting metastatic pelvic lymph nodes, with accuracy rate of spiral CT and MRI being 89.5% and 85.5%, respectively, when a node of greater than 10 mm in maximal axial diameter or a node with central necrosis was defined as a metastasic node.[101] Meta-analysis studies also showed similar performance in the detection of lymph node metastasis from cervical cancer,[102] with mean accuracy of detection of lymph node metastasis being 86% with nonenhanced MRI and 81% with CT.[92]

Local recurrence of cervical cancer occurs centrally in the pelvis or at the side wall. CT is an effective diagnostic tool for detection of recurrent cervical cancer, but it may be difficult to differentiate recurrence from postoperative and postirradiation fibrosis.[103] Gadolinium-enhanced MRI is useful to detect recurrent tumor, which shows increased signal intensity on T_1-weighted images, whereas radiation fibrosis remains low in signal intensity if imaged more than 12 months after radiation therapy.[103] Dynamic contrast-enhanced MRI has been reported to be more accurate in depicting postoperative recurrent tumor compared to pre- and postcontrast T_1-weighted images and T_2-weighted images.[104]

Endometrial Cancer

Endometrial carcinoma is staged according to the FIGO staging system. The prognosis is related to the histologic tumor grade, depth of myometrial invasion, stage of the tumor, and presence of lymph node metastasis. Metastasis to the paraaortic and paracaval lymph nodes may occur without involvement of pelvic lymph nodes if the tumor spreads along the lymphatics accompanying the ovarian vessels. The probability of extrauterine disease and risk of nodal involvement is related primarily to tumor grade and depth of myometrial invasion.

Endometrial carcinoma often presents with vaginal bleeding in postmenopausal women and is usually diagnosed by a combination of ultrasound and endometrial biopsy, which provides the tumor grade and histologic type. Most women with endometrial carcinoma do not require imaging studies[93] as surgical staging with the FIGO staging system is performed. However, knowledge of the extent of endometrial cancer spread before undertaking surgery can be of value because myometrial invasion of more than 50% may require more extensive surgery, including pelvic and paraaortic lymphadenectomy.[105] MRI is recommended when locally advanced disease is expected based on physical examination findings and in patients with a difficult physical examination because of obesity or prior radiation or surgery.[106] Hardesty et al. performed a cost analysis study and reported that staging with MRI has similar cost and accuracy compared to the current method of staging with intraoperative gross dissection of the uterus and that MRI decreases the number of unnecessary lymph node dissections.[107]

Kinkel et al. performed a meta-analysis in the preoperative assessment of myometrial invasion and demonstrated that contrast-enhanced MRI of the pelvis performed significantly better than ultrasound, CT, and noncontrast MRI.[108] Because MRI can more clearly demonstrate the primary neoplasm and more accurately determine the depth of myometrial invasion than CT, MRI is often used as the imaging procedure of choice in the preoperative evaluation of patients with high-grade endometrial carcinoma,[49] although advanced extrauterine disease may be assessed with either MRI or contrast-enhanced CT scan.[93]

Noninvasive endometrial carcinoma may be identified within the uterine cavity on T_2-weighted MR images and is seen as a signal intensity mass intermediate between that of normal endometrium and that of myometrium.[49] In some cases, the endometrial stripe may appear homogeneously widened. Preservation of the low-signal-intensity junctional zone usually implies the absence of myometrial invasion, with negative predictive value close to 100%. When myometrial invasion occurs, the interruption of the low-signal-intensity junctional zone on T_2-weighted images[109] or the interruption of the subendometrial enhancing line on early dynamic T_1-weighted images[110] is seen. The depth of myometrial invasion can also be assessed to differentiate stage IB and IC disease. The accuracy of MRI in differentiating noninvasive carcinoma (stage 1A) from invasive carcinoma has been reported to range from 74% to 85%, and in distinguishing deep invasion (stage 1C) from superficial disease (stage 1A and 1B) accuracy ranges from 75% to 95%. Dynamic contrast-enhanced MRI improved the accuracy of assessing myometrial invasion from about 83% to 91%.[108] When patients have thinning of the myometrium due to distension of the endometrial cavity,[111] when the junctional zone is not entirely visualized, or when the zonal anatomy is distorted by uterine abnormalities, such as leiomyoma or adenomyosis, MRI is less accurate for assessing myometrial invasion.[49] For patients with a thickened or indistinct junctional zone from adenomyosis or other reasons, dynamic contrast-enhanced MRI improves the accuracy of staging.[112,113]

Ovarian Cancer

Because of paucity of symptoms in early stages, approximately 60% to 75% of patients with ovarian cancer present with advanced disease.[93,114] Ovarian cancer is staged surgically according to the FIGO staging system. The FIGO system reflects the three primary mechanisms of disease spreads of ovarian cancer, including local, peritoneal, and lymphatic.

In most centers, endovaginal ultrasound is the primary imaging modality used for screening for ovarian cancer and evaluation of an adnexal mass. Because most patients with ovarian cancer present with adnexal or pelvic masses and the majority of adnexal and pelvic masses are benign, differentiation between benign and malignant ovarian tumor is clinically important.

In patients with ovarian cancer, imaging can be used to determine the extent of primary disease before surgical staging and debulking. Imaging is also used to assess for recurrence, especially in symptomatic patients. The primary disease can be staged with CT or MRI, which are equivalent for detecting peritoneal metastases.[115–118] In a study of 118 women with pelvic malignancies, the sensitivity for peritoneal disease was 92% for CT and 95% for MRI.[118]

The major role of MRI in evaluation of adnexal masses includes determining if a mass is truly ovarian in origin, to accurately diagnose certain benign lesions, such as dermoid cyst and endometrial cyst, and to more precisely define the internal architecture of ovarian masses. MRI is reported to be a cost-effective next step when the results of the ultrasound are indeterminate.[114]

On MRI, the presence of solid components or nodules in a cystic tumor, necrosis in a solid tumor, thick, irregular walls or septations, larger lesion size, enhancement of internal structure as well as presence of ascites, peritoneal disease, or adenopathy increase the possibility of malignancy.[119] The

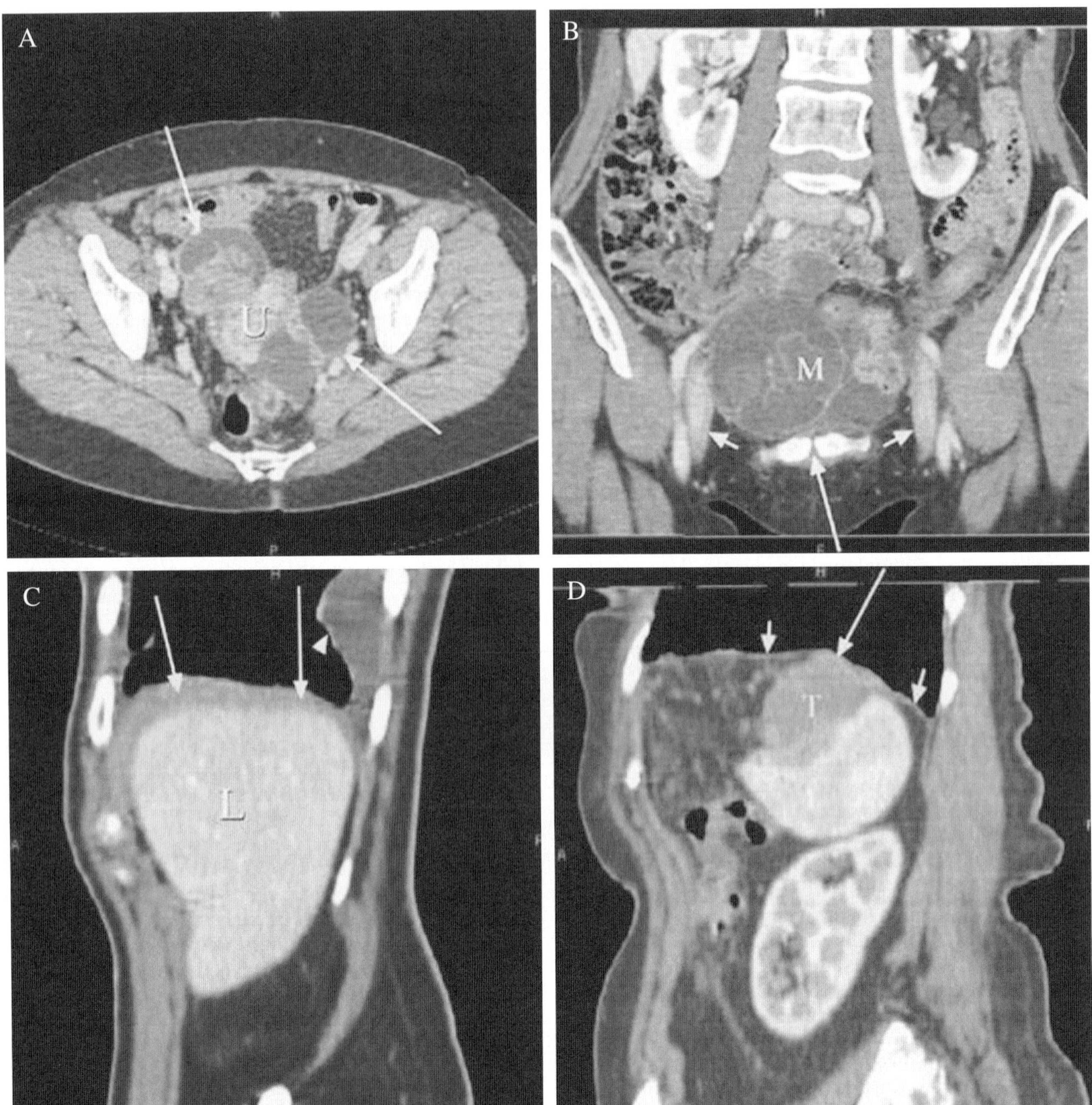

FIGURE 31.13. Ovarian cancer. (A) Axial CT of the pelvis obtained after intravenous contrast material injection shows mixed cystic and solid masses in the bilateral adnexae. *U*, uterus. (B) Coronal reformatted image obtained after intravenous contrast material injection shows cystic ovarian masses abutting the bilateral external iliac veins (*short arrows*). *Large arrow* indicates the pubic symphysis. (C) Sagittal reformatted image of the right upper abdomen obtained after intravenous contrast material injection shows thickening of the right hemidiaphragm by tumor deposits along the liver surface (*large arrows*). *Arrowhead* indicates a right pleural effusion. (D) Sagittal reformatted image of the left upper abdomen obtained after intravenous contrast material injection shows tumor (*T*) invading the superior portion of the spleen. *Short arrows* indicate left hemidiaphragm. (From Pannu et al.,[124] by permission of *RadioGraphics*.)

accuracy of MRI for the diagnosis of malignancy has been reported to range from 83% to 86% without contrast enhancement and from 78% to 95% with contrast enhancement.

CT is usually performed as it is a rapid test and readily available. The peritoneum, retroperitoneum, and viscera are assessed for metastases. Evaluation includes sites that are difficult to evaluate at surgery, such as the diaphragm, splenic hilum, stomach, lesser sac, liver, mesenteric root, and suprarenal paraaortic nodes (Figure 31.13).[120,121] Optimal debulking of disease at sites, such as the bowel mesentery and porta hepatis may also be difficult. With a successful debulking procedure, residual tumor implants are subcentimeter in size. Preoperative localization of the sites of peritoneal metastases and retroperitoneal adenopathy aids in surgical planning. Preoperative imaging also helps identify patients who may benefit from neoadjuvant chemotherapy to reduce disease volume before surgical debulking. CT and clinical parameters have been used to develop scoring systems to predict the success of surgery.[116,120,122]

A study performed in the late 1990s on 64 patients presenting with ovarian cancer found that the overall sensitivity of single-detector CT for detecting peritoneal metastases was 85% to 93% and the sensitivity for subcentimeter lesions was 25% to 50%.[123] There have been significant improvements in CT technology in the past few years with newer multidetector row scanners replacing older single-detector scanners and increasing number of detector rows. These changes allow thin slices of large volumes of anatomy to be obtained in a few seconds. Thin slices optimize visualization of subcentimeter structures and can be used to generate images in multiple planes to evaluate structures, such as the diaphragm and pelvis (see Figure 31.13).[124,125]

Patients who are suspected to have recurrent disease based on symptoms or biochemical markers can be imaged with CT, MRI, or PET. Detection of lesions on all modalities is dependent on size. For CT, detection is greater for implants greater than 5 to 10mm than for smaller lesions.[123,126] Sensitivity of single-detector CT is more than 50% for detecting implants at most sites, except the small bowel and mesentery, where lesions can be difficult to appreciate because of partial volume averaging.[116] Implants are easier to visualize when surrounded by ascites. The sensitivity of multidetector row CT for detecting tumor recurrence is not established. The sensitivity of MRI was 91% for detecting recurrence in 64 women with ovarian cancer.[127] Implants less than 2cm were present in false-negative cases. Peritoneal, mesenteric, and bowel metastases can be effectively detected with MRI.[128]

Although CT and MRI are usually performed to evaluate patients for recurrence, small implants can be difficult to detect on visceral surfaces by anatomic imaging. The lesions may not be appreciated because of lack of significant contrast difference between tumor and normal viscera. An advantage of functional imaging with PET is that lesions are conspicuous as there is increased uptake in tumor and minimal background activity. The sensitivity of PET for recurrent tumor is higher in patients with suspected relapse compared with those without clinical disease.[129] Sensitivities ranging from 80% to 100% have been reported in four series with a total of 113 patients.[129–132] However, similar to CT and MRI, lesion detection is dependent on size and is less likely for lesions less than 1 to 2cm in size than for larger masses.[129,130,133,134] Omental carcinomatosis with subcentimeter lesions may not show sufficient uptake to be detected on PET although it is evident on CT.[134] In 22 patients with primarily subcentimeter lesions, including microscopic disease, the sensitivity of PET for detecting tumor recurrence was 10%.[135] In a study of 31 patients with a mean lesion size of 1.1cm, the patient-based sensitivity of PET for disease recurrence was 81% and lesion-based sensitivity was 45%.[134] The specificity of PET for recurrent ovarian cancer ranges from 42% to 100%.[129–132,134,135] Three studies that compared PET findings with surgery found specificities of 93%, 42%, and 50%, respectively.[130,134,135] High specificities of 83% and 100% were reported in two studies comparing PET with surgical or clinical follow-up.[129,131] Increased uptake can be seen in postsurgical inflammation and in normal bowel and urinary tract.

However, PET may play a role in assessing patients when CT and MRI are negative and tumor markers are rising.[131,136–138] It has been suggested as a complementary test to anatomic imaging.[131,134,138,139] Sensitivity is improved when both CT and PET are performed.[140] There is also improved correlation with surgical findings if the findings on CT and PET are combined.[141] Detection of omental implants and malignant retroperitoneal nodes is improved. PET/CT scanners may play a more significant role in the future in evaluating patients with ovarian cancer. CT images as well as PET images are generated and fused for localization of abnormal activity on PET and characterization of malignant potential in masses seen on CT.[142,143] However, as currently performed, the CT obtained as part of a PET/CT study is technically limited as the tube current is lower and images are noisier, there is respiratory motion artifact, there is artifact from the patient's arms, and bowel or intravenous contrast are typically not given.

In summary, CT or MRI can be used to detect extraovarian spread of primary tumor and recurrent disease. CT is usually performed due to ease of study and ready availability. Lesion conspicuity is high on PET, and it has been suggested as a complementary test to anatomic imaging for detecting tumor spread. The new fused PET/CT scanners combine the benefits of functional and anatomic imaging and have the potential to more accurately determine disease extent. Subcentimeter lesions are difficult to detect by all imaging modalities.

References

1. Kenny PJMB. The kidney. In: Lee JKT, Stanley RJ, Heiken JP (eds). Computed Body Tomography with MRI Correlation. Philadelphia: Lippincott-Raven, 1998:1087–1170.
2. Silverman SG, Lee BY, Seltzer SE, Bloom DA, Corless CL, Adams DF. Small (≤3cm) renal masses: correlation of spiral CT features and pathologic findings. AJR Am J Roentgenol 1994;163: 597–605.
3. Zagoria RJ, Wolfman NT, Karstaedt N, Hinn GC, Dyer RB, Chen YM. CT features of renal cell carcinoma with emphasis on relation to tumor size. Invest Radiol 1990;25:261–266.
4. Kopka L, Fischer U, Zoeller G, Schmidt C, Ringert RH, Grabbe E. Dual-phase helical CT of the kidney: value of the corticomedullary and nephrographic phase for evaluation of renal lesions and preoperative staging of renal cell carcinoma. AJR Am J Roentgenol 1997;169:1573–1578.
5. Garant M, Bonaldi VM, Taourel P, Pinsky MF, Bret PM. Enhancement patterns of renal masses during multiphase helical CT acquisitions. Abdom Imaging 1998;23:31–36.
6. Birnbaum BA, Jacobs JE, Ramchandani P. Multiphasic renal CT: comparison of renal mass enhancement during the corticomedullary and nephrographic phases. Radiology 1996;200: 753–758.
7. Cohan RH, Sherman LS, Korobkin M, Bass JC, Francis IR. Renal masses: assessment of corticomedullary-phase and nephrographic-phase CT scans. Radiology 1995;196:445–451.
8. Szolar DH, Kammerhuber F, Altziebler S, et al. Multiphasic helical CT of the kidney: increased conspicuity for detection and characterization of small (<3-cm) renal masses. Radiology 1997; 202:211–217.
9. Catalano C, Fraioli F, Laghi A, et al. High-resolution multidetector CT in the preoperative evaluation of patients with renal cell carcinoma. AJR Am J Roentgenol 2003;180:1271–1277.
10. Zeman RK, Zeiberg A, Hayes WS, Silverman PM, Cooper C, Garra BS. Helical CT of renal masses: the value of delayed scans. AJR Am J Roentgenol 1996;167:771–776.

11. Fein AB, Lee JK, Balfe DM, et al. Diagnosis and staging of renal cell carcinoma: a comparison of MR imaging and CT. AJR Am J Roentgenol 1987;148:749–753.
12. Walter C, Kruessell M, Gindele A, Brochhagen HG, Gossmann A, Landwehr P. Imaging of renal lesions: evaluation of fast MRI and helical CT. Br J Radiol 2003;76:696–703.
13. Ergen FB, Hussain HK, Caoili EM, et al. MRI for preoperative staging of renal cell carcinoma using the 1997 TNM classification: comparison with surgical and pathologic staging. AJR Am J Roentgenol 2004;182:217–225.
14. Kreft BP, Muller-Miny H, Sommer T, et al. Diagnostic value of MR imaging in comparison to CT in the detection and differential diagnosis of renal masses: ROC analysis. Eur Radiol 1997; 7:542–547.
15. Semelka RC, Hricak H, Stevens SK, Finegold R, Tomei E, Carroll PR. Combined gadolinium-enhanced and fat-saturation MR imaging of renal masses. Radiology 1991;178:803–809.
16. Narumi Y, Hricak H, Presti JC Jr, et al. MR imaging evaluation of renal cell carcinoma. Abdom Imaging 1997;22:216–225.
17. Welch TJ, LeRoy AJ. Helical and electron beam CT scanning in the evaluation of renal vein involvement in patients with renal cell carcinoma. J Comput Assist Tomogr 1997;21:467–471.
18. Choyke PL, Walther MM, Wagner JR, Rayford W, Lyne JC, Linehan WM. Renal cancer: preoperative evaluation with dual-phase three-dimensional MR angiography. Radiology 1997;205: 767–771.
19. Laissy JP, Menegazzo D, Debray MP, et al. Renal carcinoma: diagnosis of venous invasion with Gd-enhanced MR venography. Eur Radiol 2000;10:1138–1143.
20. Aslam Sohaib SA, Teh J, Nargund VH, Lumley JS, Hendry WF, Reznek RH. Assessment of tumor invasion of the vena caval wall in renal cell carcinoma cases by magnetic resonance imaging. J Urol 2002;167:1271–1275.
21. Studer UE, Scherz S, Scheidegger J, et al. Enlargement of regional lymph nodes in renal cell carcinoma is often not due to metastases. J Urol 1990;144:243–245.
22. Bosniak MA. The current radiological approach to renal cysts. Radiology 1986;158:1–10.
23. Russo P. Renal cell carcinoma: presentation, staging, and surgical treatment. Semin Oncol 2000;27:160–176.
24. Smith PA, Marshall FF, Urban BA, Heath DG, Fishman EK. Three-dimensional CT stereoscopic visualization of renal masses: impact on diagnosis and patient treatment. AJR Am J Roentgenol 1997;169:1331–1334.
25. Urban BA, Fishman EK. Helical CT with multiplanar display: role in evaluation and clarification of complex renal pathology. J Comput Assist Tomogr 1998;22:548–554.
26. Coll DM, Herts BR, Davros WJ, Uzzo RG, Novick AC. Preoperative use of 3D volume rendering to demonstrate renal tumors and renal anatomy. Radiographics 2000;20:431–438.
27. Wunderlich H, Reichelt O, Schubert R, Zermann DH, Schubert J. Preoperative simulation of partial nephrectomy with three-dimensional computed tomography. BJU Int 2000;86:777–781.
28. Lechevallier E, Andre M, Barriol D, et al. Fine-needle percutaneous biopsy of renal masses with helical CT guidance. Radiology 2000;216:506–510.
29. Niceforo J, Coughlin BF. Diagnosis of renal cell carcinoma: value of fine-needle aspiration cytology in patients with metastases or contraindications to nephrectomy. AJR Am J Roentgenol 1993; 161:1303–1305.
30. Torres GMRP. Kidney. In: Stark DDBW (ed). Magnetic Resonance Imaging. St. Louis: Mosby, 1999:517–528.
31. Chen GL, El-Gabry EA, Bagley DH. Surveillance of upper urinary tract transitional cell carcinoma: the role of ureteroscopy, retrograde pyelography, cytology and urinalysis. J Urol 2000;164:1901–1904.
32. Gatewood OM, Goldman SM, Marshall FF, Siegelman SS. Computerized tomography in the diagnosis of transitional cell carcinoma of the kidney. J Urol 1982;127:876–887.
33. Wong-You-Cheong JJ, Wagner BJ, Davis CJ Jr. Transitional cell carcinoma of the urinary tract: radiologic-pathologic correlation. Radiographics 1998;18:123–142; quiz 148.
34. Breatnach ES, Stanley RJ, Lloyd K. Focal obstructive nephrogram: an unusual CT appearance of a transitional cell carcinoma. J Comput Assist Tomogr 1984;8:1019–1022.
35. Pollack HM, Arger PH, Banner MP, Mulhern CB Jr, Coleman BG. Computed tomography of renal pelvic filling defects. Radiology 1981;138:645–651.
36. McCoy JG, Honda H, Reznicek M, Williams RD. Computerized tomography for detection and staging of localized and pathologically defined upper tract urothelial tumors. J Urol 1991;146: 1500–1503.
37. Nyman U, Oldbring J, Aspelin P. CT of carcinoma of the renal pelvis. Acta Radiol 1992;33:31–38.
38. Planz B, George R, Adam G, Jakse G, Planz K. Computed tomography for detection and staging of transitional cell carcinoma of the upper urinary tract. Eur Urol 1995;27:146–150.
39. Bretheau D, Lechevallier E, Uzan E, Rampal M, Coulange C. Value of radiologic examinations in the diagnosis and staging of upper urinary tract tumors. Prog Urol 1994;4:966–973.
40. Millan-Rodriguez F, Palou J, de la Torre-Holguera P, Vayreda-Martija JM, Villavicencio-Mavrich H, Vicente-Rodriguez J. Conventional CT signs in staging transitional cell tumors of the upper urinary tract. Eur Urol 1999;35:318–322.
41. Weeks SM, Brown ED, Brown JJ, Adamis MK, Eisenberg LB, Semelka RC. Transitional cell carcinoma of the upper urinary tract: staging by MRI. Abdom Imaging 1995;20:365–367.
42. Robinson P, Collins CD, Ryder WD, et al. Relationship of MRI and clinical staging to outcome in invasive bladder cancer treated by radiotherapy. Clin Radiol 2000;55:301–306.
43. Levy DA, Grossman HB. Staging and prognosis of T3b bladder cancer. Semin Urol Oncol 1996;14:56–61.
44. Kim B, Semelka RC, Ascher SM, Chalpin DB, Carroll PR, Hricak H. Bladder tumor staging: comparison of contrast-enhanced CT, T_1- and T_2-weighted MR imaging, dynamic gadolinium-enhanced imaging, and late gadolinium-enhanced imaging. Radiology 1994;193:239–245.
45. Rholl KS, Lee JK, Heiken JP, Ling D, Glazer HS. Primary bladder carcinoma: evaluation with MR imaging. Radiology 1987;163: 117–121.
46. Tanimoto A, Yuasa Y, Imai Y, et al. Bladder tumor staging: comparison of conventional and gadolinium-enhanced dynamic MR imaging and CT. Radiology 1992;185:741–747.
47. Barentsz JO, Jager GJ, Witjes JA, Ruijs JH. Primary staging of urinary bladder carcinoma: the role of MRI and a comparison with CT. Eur Radiol 1996;6:129–133.
48. Hayashi N, Tochigi H, Shiraishi T, Takeda K, Kawamura J. A new staging criterion for bladder carcinoma using gadolinium-enhanced magnetic resonance imaging with an endorectal surface coil: a comparison with ultrasonography. BJU Int 2000; 85:32–36.
49. Lee JKT WA, Semelka RC. Pelvis. In: Lee JKTSS, Stanley RJ, Heiken JP (eds). Computed Body Tomography with MRI Correlation. Philadelphia: Lippincott-Raven, 1998:1209–1274.
50. Barentsz JO, Jager G, Mugler JP III, et al. Staging urinary bladder cancer: value of T_1-weighted three-dimensional magnetization prepared-rapid gradient-echo and two-dimensional spin-echo sequences. AJR Am J Roentgenol 1995;164:109–115.
51. Jager GJ, Barentsz JO, Oosterhof GO, Witjes JA, Ruijs SJ. Pelvic adenopathy in prostatic and urinary bladder carcinoma: MR imaging with a three-dimensional T_1-weighted magnetization-prepared-rapid gradient-echo sequence. AJR Am J Roentgenol 1996;167:1503–1507.

52. Bellin MF, Roy C, Kinkel K, et al. Lymph node metastases: safety and effectiveness of MR imaging with ultrasmall superparamagnetic iron oxide particles: initial clinical experience. Radiology 1998;207:799–808.
53. Barentsz JO, Jager GJ, van Vierzen PB, et al. Staging urinary bladder cancer after transurethral biopsy: value of fast dynamic contrast-enhanced MR imaging. Radiology 1996;201:185–193.
54. Bernhardt TM, Schmidl H, Philipp C, Allhoff EP, Rapp-Bernhardt U. Diagnostic potential of virtual cystoscopy of the bladder: MRI vs. CT. Preliminary report. Eur Radiol 2003;13: 305–312.
55. Song JH, Francis IR, Platt JF, et al. Bladder tumor detection at virtual cystoscopy. Radiology 2001;218:95–100.
56. Kim JK, Ahn JH, Park T, Ahn HJ, Kim CS, Cho KS. Virtual cystoscopy of the contrast material-filled bladder in patients with gross hematuria. AJR Am J Roentgenol 2002;179:763–768.
57. Korobkin M, Francis IR, Kloos RT, Dunnick NR. The incidental adrenal mass. Radiol Clin N Am 1996;34:1037–1054.
58. Mayo-Smith WW, Boland GW, Noto RB, Lee MJ. State-of-the-art adrenal imaging. Radiographics 2001;21:995–1012.
59. Harisinghani MG, Maher MM, Hahn PF, et al. Predictive value of benign percutaneous adrenal biopsies in oncology patients. Clin Radiol 2002;57:898–901.
60. Candel AG, Gattuso P, Reyes CV, Prinz RA, Castelli MJ. Fine-needle aspiration biopsy of adrenal masses in patients with extraadrenal malignancy. Surgery (St. Louis) 1993;114:1132–1136; discussion 1136–1137.
61. Khafagi FA, Gross MD, Shapiro B, Glazer GM, Francis I, Thompson NW. Clinical significance of the large adrenal mass. Br J Surg 1991;78:828–833.
62. Boland GW, Lee MJ, Gazelle GS, Halpern EF, McNicholas MM, Mueller PR. Characterization of adrenal masses using unenhanced CT: an analysis of the CT literature. AJR Am J Roentgenol 1998;171:201–204.
63. Dunnick NR, Korobkin M. Imaging of adrenal incidentalomas: current status. AJR Am J Roentgenol 2002;179:559–568.
64. Pena CS, Boland GW, Hahn PF, Lee MJ, Mueller PR. Characterization of indeterminate (lipid-poor) adrenal masses: use of washout characteristics at contrast-enhanced CT. Radiology 2000;217:798–802.
65. Korobkin M, Brodeur FJ, Francis IR, Quint LE, Dunnick NR, Londy F. CT time-attenuation washout curves of adrenal adenomas and nonadenomas. AJR Am J Roentgenol 1998;170:747–752.
66. Caoili EM, Korobkin M, Francis IR, et al. Adrenal masses: characterization with combined unenhanced and delayed enhanced CT. Radiology 2002;222:629–633.
67. Mayo-Smith WW, Lee MJ, McNicholas MM, Hahn PF, Boland GW, Saini S. Characterization of adrenal masses (<5 cm) by use of chemical shift MR imaging: observer performance versus quantitative measures. AJR Am J Roentgenol 1995;165:91–95.
68. Bilbey JH, McLoughlin RF, Kurkjian PS, et al. MR imaging of adrenal masses: value of chemical-shift imaging for distinguishing adenomas from other tumors. AJR Am J Roentgenol 1995; 164:637–642.
69. Tsushima Y, Ishizaka H, Matsumoto M. Adrenal masses: differentiation with chemical shift, fast low-angle shot MR imaging. Radiology 1993;186:705–709.
70. Heinz-Peer G, Honigschnabl S, Schneider B, Niederle B, Kaserer K, Lechner G. Characterization of adrenal masses using MR imaging with histopathologic correlation. AJR Am J Roentgenol 1999;173:15–22.
71. Blake MA, Krishnamoorthy SK, Boland GW, et al. Low-density pheochromocytoma on CT: a mimicker of adrenal adenoma. AJR Am J Roentgenol 2003;181:1663–1668.
72. Yamada T, Saito H, Moriya T, et al. Adrenal carcinoma with a signal loss on chemical shift magnetic resonance imaging. J Comput Assist Tomogr 2003;27:606–608.
73. Varghese JC, Hahn PF, Papanicolaou N, Mayo-Smith WW, Gaa JA, Lee MJ. MR differentiation of phaeochromocytoma from other adrenal lesions based on qualitative analysis of T_2 relaxation times. Clin Radiol 1997;52:603–606.
74. Barentsz JO, Engelbrecht MR, Witjes JA, de la Rosette JJ, van der Graaf M. MR imaging of the male pelvis. Eur Radiol 1999;9: 1722–1736.
75. Jager GJ, Severens JL, Thornbury JR, de La Rosette JJ, Ruijs SH, Barentsz JO. Prostate cancer staging: should MR imaging be used? A decision analytic approach. Radiology 2000;215:445–451.
76. Ellis JH, Tempany C, Sarin MS, Gatsonis C, Rifkin MD, McNeil BJ. MR imaging and sonography of early prostatic cancer: pathologic and imaging features that influence identification and diagnosis. AJR Am J Roentgenol 1994;162:865–872.
77. Rorvik J, Halvorsen OJ, Albrektsen G, Ersland L, Daehlin L, Haukaas S. MRI with an endorectal coil for staging of clinically localised prostate cancer prior to radical prostatectomy. Eur Radiol 1999;9:29–34.
78. Hricak H, White S, Vigneron D, et al. Carcinoma of the prostate gland: MR imaging with pelvic phased-array coils versus integrated endorectal-pelvic phased-array coils. Radiology 1994;193: 703–709.
79. Bartolozzi C, Menchi I, Lencioni R, et al. Local staging of prostate carcinoma with endorectal coil MRI: correlation with whole-mount radical prostatectomy specimens. Eur Radiol 1996; 6:339–345.
80. Chelsky MJ, Schnall MD, Seidmon EJ, Pollack HM. Use of endorectal surface coil magnetic resonance imaging for local staging of prostate cancer. J Urol 1993;150:391–395.
81. Engelbrecht MR, Jager GJ, Laheij RJ, Verbeek AL, van Lier HJ, Barentsz JO. Local staging of prostate cancer using magnetic resonance imaging: a meta-analysis. Eur Radiol 2002;12:2294–2302.
82. Getty DJ, Seltzer SE, Tempany CM, Pickett RM, Swets JA, McNeil BJ. Prostate cancer: relative effects of demographic, clinical, histologic, and MR imaging variables on the accuracy of staging. Radiology 1997;204:471–479.
83. D'Amico AV, Whittington R, Schnall M, et al. The impact of the inclusion of endorectal coil magnetic resonance imaging in a multivariate analysis to predict clinically unsuspected extraprostatic cancer. Cancer (Phila) 1995;75:2368–2372.
84. Huncharek M, Muscat J. Serum prostate-specific antigen as a predictor of staging abdominal/pelvic computed tomography in newly diagnosed prostate cancer. Abdom Imaging 1996;21:364–367.
85. Oyen RH, Van Poppel HP, Ameye FE, Van de Voorde WA, Baert AL, Baert LV. Lymph node staging of localized prostatic carcinoma with CT and CT-guided fine-needle aspiration biopsy: prospective study of 285 patients. Radiology 1994;190:315–322.
86. Harisinghani MG, Barentsz J, Hahn PF, et al. Noninvasive detection of clinically occult lymph-node metastases in prostate cancer. N Engl J Med 2003;348:2491–2499.
87. Kurhanewicz J, Vigneron DB, Hricak H, Narayan P, Carroll P, Nelson SJ. Three-dimensional ^{1}H-MR spectroscopic imaging of the in situ human prostate with high (0.24–0.7 cm^3) spatial resolution. Radiology 1996;198:795–805.
88. Yu KK, Scheidler J, Hricak H, et al. Prostate cancer: prediction of extracapsular extension with endorectal MR imaging and three-dimensional proton MR spectroscopic imaging. Radiology 1999;213:481–488.
89. Scheidler J, Hricak H, Vigneron DB, et al. Prostate cancer: localization with three-dimensional proton MR spectroscopic imaging: clinicopathologic study. Radiology 1999;213:473–480.
90. Hata N, Jinzaki M, Kacher D, et al. MR imaging-guided prostate biopsy with surgical navigation software: device validation and feasibility. Radiology 2001;220:263–268.
91. Kooy HM, Cormack RA, Mathiowitz G, Tempany C, D'Amico AV. A software system for interventional magnetic resonance

image-guided prostate brachytherapy. Comput Aided Surg 2000;5:401–413.
92. Boss EA, Barentsz JO, Massuger LF, Boonstra H. The role of MR imaging in invasive cervical carcinoma. Eur Radiol 2000;10:256–270.
93. Fielding JR. MR imaging of the female pelvis. Radiol Clin N Am 2003;41:179–192.
94. Hricak H, Hamm B, Semelka RC, et al. Carcinoma of the uterus: use of gadopentetate dimeglumine in MR imaging. Radiology 1991;181:95–106.
95. Hawighorst H, Knapstein PG, Weikel W, et al. Cervical carcinoma: comparison of standard and pharmacokinetic MR imaging. Radiology 1996;201:531–539.
96. Abe Y, Yamashita Y, Namimoto T, et al. Carcinoma of the uterine cervix. High-resolution turbo spin-echo MR imaging with contrast-enhanced dynamic scanning and T_2-weighting. Acta Radiol 1998;39:322–326.
97. Van Vierzen PB, Massuger LF, Ruys SH, Barentsz JO. Fast dynamic contrast enhanced MR imaging of cervical carcinoma. Clin Radiol 1998;53:183–192.
98. Bipat S, Glas AS, van der Velden J, Zwinderman AH, Bossuyt PM, Stoker J. Computed tomography and magnetic resonance imaging in staging of uterine cervical carcinoma: a systematic review. Gynecol Oncol 2003;91:59–66.
99. Pannu HK, Fishman EK. Evaluation of cervical cancer by computed tomography: current status. Cancer (Phila) 2003;98:2039–2043.
100. Walsh JW, Goplerud DR. Prospective comparison between clinical and CT staging in primary cervical carcinoma. AJR Am J Roentgenol 1981;137:997–1003.
101. Yang WT, Lam WW, Yu MY, Cheung TH, Metreweli C. Comparison of dynamic helical CT and dynamic MR imaging in the evaluation of pelvic lymph nodes in cervical carcinoma. AJR Am J Roentgenol 2000;175:759–766.
102. Scheidler J, Hricak H, Yu KK, Subak L, Segal MR. Radiological evaluation of lymph node metastases in patients with cervical cancer. A meta-analysis. JAMA 1997;278:1096–1101.
103. Jeong YY, Kang HK, Chung TW, Seo JJ, Park JG. Uterine cervical carcinoma after therapy: CT and MR imaging findings. Radio Graphics 2003;23:969–981; discussion 981.
104. Yamashita Y, Harada M, Torashima M, et al. Dynamic MR imaging of recurrent postoperative cervical cancer. J Magn Reson Imaging 1996;6:167–171.
105. Frei KA, Kinkel K. Staging endometrial cancer: role of magnetic resonance imaging. J Magn Reson Imaging 2001;13:850–855.
106. Hricak H, Rubinstein LV, Gherman GM, Karstaedt N. MR imaging evaluation of endometrial carcinoma: results of an NCI cooperative study. Radiology 1991;179:829–832.
107. Hardesty LA, Sumkin JH, Nath ME, et al. Use of preoperative MR imaging in the management of endometrial carcinoma: cost analysis. Radiology 2000;215:45–49.
108. Kinkel K, Kaji Y, Yu KK, et al. Radiologic staging in patients with endometrial cancer: a meta-analysis. Radiology 1999;212:711–718.
109. Hricak H, Stern JL, Fisher MR, Shapeero LG, Winkler ML, Lacey CG. Endometrial carcinoma staging by MR imaging. Radiology 1987;162:297–305.
110. Seki H, Kimura M, Sakai K. Myometrial invasion of endometrial carcinoma: assessment with dynamic MR and contrast-enhanced T1-weighted images. Clin Radiol 1997;52:18–23.
111. Lien HH, Blomlie V, Trope C, Kaern J, Abeler VM. Cancer of the endometrium: value of MR imaging in determining depth of invasion into the myometrium. AJR Am J Roentgenol 1991;157:1221–1223.
112. Tanaka YO, Nishida M, Tsunoda H, Ichikawa Y, Saida Y, Itai Y. A thickened or indistinct junctional zone on T_2-weighted MR images in patients with endometrial carcinoma: pathologic consideration based on microcirculation. Eur Radiol 2003;13:2038–2045.
113. Utsunomiya D, Notsute S, Hayashida Y, et al. Endometrial carcinoma in adenomyosis: assessment of myometrial invasion on T_2-weighted spin-echo and gadolinium-enhanced T_1-weighted images. AJR Am J Roentgenol 2004;182:399–404.
114. Togashi K. Ovarian cancer: the clinical role of US, CT, and MRI. Eur Radiol 2003;13(suppl 4):L87–L104.
115. Prayer L, Kainz C, Kramer J, et al. CT and MR accuracy in the detection of tumor recurrence in patients treated for ovarian cancer. J Comput Assist Tomogr 1993;17:626–632.
116. Forstner R, Hricak H, Occhipinti KA, Powell CB, Frankel SD, Stern JL. Ovarian cancer: staging with CT and MR imaging. Radiology 1995;197:619–626.
117. Kurtz AB, Tsimikas JV, Tempany CM, et al. Diagnosis and staging of ovarian cancer: comparative values of Doppler and conventional US, CT, and MR imaging correlated with surgery and histopathologic analysis. Report of the Radiology Diagnostic Oncology Group. Radiology 1999;212:19–27.
118. Tempany CM, Zou KH, Silverman SG, Brown DL, Kurtz AB, McNeil BJ. Staging of advanced ovarian cancer: comparison of imaging modalities. Report from the Radiological Diagnostic Oncology Group. Radiology 2000;215:761–767.
119. Sohaib SA, Sahdev A, Van Trappen P, Jacobs IJ, Reznek RH. Characterization of adnexal mass lesions on MR imaging. AJR Am J Roentgenol 2003;180:1297–1304.
120. Bristow RE, Duska LR, Lambrou NC, et al. A model for predicting surgical outcome in patients with advanced ovarian carcinoma using computed tomography. Cancer (Phila) 2000;89:1532–1540.
121. Forstner R, Chen M, Hricak H. Imaging of ovarian cancer. J Magn Reson Imaging 1995;5:606–613.
122. Meyer JI, Kennedy AW, Friedman R, Ayoub A, Zepp RC. Ovarian carcinoma: value of CT in predicting success of debulking surgery. AJR Am J Roentgenol 1995;165:875–878.
123. Coakley FV, Choi PH, Gougoutas CA, et al. Peritoneal metastases: detection with spiral CT in patients with ovarian cancer. Radiology 2002;223:495–499.
124. Pannu HK, Bristow RE, Montz FJ, Fishman EK. Multidetector CT of peritoneal carcinomatosis from ovarian cancer. Radio Graphics 2003;23:687–701.
125. Pannu HK, Horton KM, Fishman EK. Thin section dual-phase multidetector-row computed tomography detection of peritoneal metastases in gynecologic cancers. J Comput Assist Tomogr 2003;27:333–340.
126. Buy JN, Moss AA, Ghossain MA, et al. Peritoneal implants from ovarian tumors: CT findings. Radiology 1988;169:691–694.
127. Low RN, Saleh F, Song SY, et al. Treated ovarian cancer: comparison of MR imaging with serum CA-125 level and physical examination: a longitudinal study. Radiology 1999;211:519–528.
128. Low RN, Semelka RC, Worawattanakul S, Alzate GD, Sigeti JS. Extrahepatic abdominal imaging in patients with malignancy: comparison of MR imaging and helical CT, with subsequent surgical correlation. Radiology 1999;210:625–632.
129. Zimny M, Siggelkow W, Schroder W, et al. 2-[Fluorine-18]-fluoro-2-deoxy-D-glucose positron emission tomography in the diagnosis of recurrent ovarian cancer. Gynecol Oncol 2001;83:310–315.
130. Kubik-Huch RA, Dorffler W, von Schulthess GK, et al. Value of (18F)-FDG positron emission tomography, computed tomography, and magnetic resonance imaging in diagnosing primary and recurrent ovarian carcinoma. Eur Radiol 2000;10:761–767.
131. Torizuka T, Nobezawa S, Kanno T, et al. Ovarian cancer recurrence: role of whole-body positron emission tomography using 2-[fluorine-18]-fluoro-2-deoxy-D-glucose. Eur J Nucl Med Mol Imaging 2002;29:797–803.
132. Yen RF, Sun SS, Shen YY, Changlai SP, Kao A. Whole body positron emission tomography with ^{18}F-fluoro-2-deoxyglucose

for the detection of recurrent ovarian cancer. Anticancer Res 2001;21:3691–3694.

133. Karlan BY, Hawkins R, Hoh C, et al. Whole-body positron emission tomography with 2-[18F]-fluoro-2-deoxy-D-glucose can detect recurrent ovarian carcinoma. Gynecol Oncol 1993;51: 175–181.
134. Cho SM, Ha HK, Byun JY, Lee JM, Kim CJ, Nam-Koong SE. Usefulness of FDG PET for assessment of early recurrent epithelial ovarian cancer. AJR Am J Roentgenol 2002;179:391–395.
135. Rose PG, Faulhaber P, Miraldi F, Abdul-Karim FW. Positive emission tomography for evaluating a complete clinical response in patients with ovarian or peritoneal carcinoma: correlation with second-look laparotomy. Gynecol Oncol 2001;82:17–21.
136. Bristow RE, Simpkins F, Pannu HK, Fishman EK, Montz FJ. Positron emission tomography for detecting clinically occult surgically resectable metastatic ovarian cancer. Gynecol Oncol 2002;85:196–200.
137. Bristow RE, del Carmen MG, Pannu HK, et al. Clinically occult recurrent ovarian cancer: patient selection for secondary cytoreductive surgery using combined PET/CT. Gynecol Oncol 2003; 90:519–528.
138. Nakamoto Y, Saga T, Ishimori T, et al. Clinical value of positron emission tomography with FDG for recurrent ovarian cancer. AJR Am J Roentgenol 2001;176:1449–1454.
139. Woodward PJ, Hosseinzadeh K, Saenger JS. From the archives of the AFIP: radiologic staging of ovarian carcinoma with pathologic correlation. Radiographics 2004;24:225–246.
140. Turlakow A, Yeung HW, Salmon AS, Macapinlac HA, Larson SM. Peritoneal carcinomatosis: role of 18F-FDG PET. J Nucl Med 2003;44:1407–1412.
141. Yoshida Y, Kurokawa T, Kawahara K, et al. Incremental benefits of FDG positron emission tomography over CT alone for the preoperative staging of ovarian cancer. AJR Am J Roentgenol 2004;182:227–233.
142. Pannu HK, Bristow RE, Cohade C, Fishman EK, Wahl RL. PET-CT in recurrent ovarian cancer: initial observations. Radio Graphics 2004;24:209–223.
143. Makhija S, Howden N, Edwards R, Kelley J, Townsend DW, Meltzer CC. Positron emission tomography/computed tomography imaging for the detection of recurrent ovarian and fallopian tube carcinoma: a retrospective review. Gynecol Oncol 2002;85:53–58.

32 Musculoskeletal Imaging

Leanne L. Seeger and Kambiz Motamedi

Musculoskeletal tumors often present an imaging dilemma to the clinician. This dilemma occurs not only because primary musculoskeletal malignancies are less common than tumors of other organ systems, such as lung or gastrointestinal, but also because of the vast array of possible pathologies reflecting the many different types of mesenchymal tissue. This chapter concentrates on imaging neoplasia of the extremities (see Chapter 58 for Soft Tissue Sarcoma).

It should be kept in mind that distinguishing between benign neoplasia and low-grade malignancy can be challenging, even for the pathologist[1]; this is especially true for tumors composed of cartilage (enchondroma or osteochondroma versus chondrosarcoma)[2,3] and fat (lipoma versus liposarcoma).[4] The key to the diagnosis and treatment of musculoskeletal neoplasia is best accomplished by a team approach, with close interaction between the oncologist, oncologic surgeon, radiologist, and pathologist.[5–7]

Tissue Type

Musculoskeletal tumors may originate from any mesenchymal tissue, including bone (osteoid), cartilage (chondroid), fat (lipoid), connective tissue (fibrous), or vessels (endothelium). The primary cell of origin for some musculoskeletal tumors is unknown; for example, the spectrum of Ewing sarcoma–primitive neuroectodermal tumor (PNET).[8]

Quite often, in cases of benign or low-grade malignant tumors where the principal architectural structure of the underlying cell type is preserved, the tumor origin can be determined with imaging because of the distinct imaging properties of each cell type. In contrast, for the moderate- and higher-grade malignancies, the imaging appearance is generally nonspecific because of alteration of the cells of origin. Plain films show only a mass or a destructive lesion of bone, computed tomography (CT) shows a density similar to muscle, and magnetic resonance imaging (MRI) shows a low to intermediate signal on T_1-weighted images and a high signal on T_2 images.[9]

Tumors that make an osteoid (e.g., osteosarcoma) or chondroid matrix (e.g., chondrosarcoma) are usually mineralized on plain film, and the calcification will almost always show on CT. Osteoid mineralization is amorphous and cloudlike, whereas chondroid mineralization is usually punctate, often in small circles and arcs (Figures 32.1, 32.2).

Osteoid

Calcified lesions can be recognized as such by the high density seen on plain film and CT. On MRI, calcification will be low signal on both T_1- and T_2-weighted images.[10,11] Ossification, on the other hand, will show a peripheral rim of low signal similar to cortex, representing the calcified surface, and an internal signal characteristic of fat, similar to marrow.[12,13]

Chondroid

Cartilage lesions are usually lobulated in appearance, with typical chondroid mineralization. As a result of the high inherent water content of hyaline cartilage, the density on CT is greater than that of fat but less than that of muscle. On MRI, cartilage will show low signal on T_1 images and very high signal with T_2 imaging.[3,14] Chondrosarcomas are often secondary tumors, arising from an underlying benign lesion, such as enchondroma or osteochondroma.[15,16] Tissue sampling with percutaneous biopsy can be misleading as only a portion of the tumor may contain malignant cells. Thus, imaging plays an important role in evaluating for more aggressive behavior of the lesion, such as cortical thinning (endosteal scalloping), cortical destruction, and a soft tissue mass.[17] The biopsy should then be directed toward these areas. If doubt exists, the entire lesion must be removed.[18]

Fat

Low-grade lesions composed of fat will appear as a lucent mass on plain film and show a density equal to subcutaneous fat on CT. The MR appearance will also follow that of subcutaneous fat, appearing high signal (white) on conventional T_1 spin-echo images and low signal (black) with fat suppression.[19]

If a soft tissue mass contains both areas of fat and areas that are clearly different by either MR or CT, this is usually a liposarcoma.[20] The regions that appear to be muscle on CT or show high signal on T_2 MRI images, should be targeted for biopsy as these are more likely to contain cells of a higher malignant grade. Lipomatous lesions may sometimes display areas of chunky ossification, indicating a nonaggressive behavior.[21]

Fibrous

Fibrous tumors have a density similar to muscle on plain film and CT. With MRI, low-grade fibrous lesions are

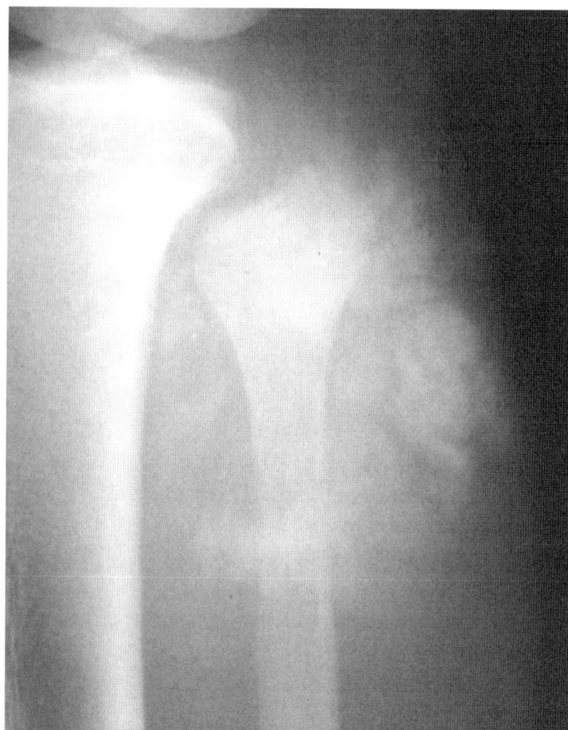

FIGURE 32.1. Osteoid matrix in an osteosarcoma of the proximal fibula. The mineralization is amorphous and cloudlike.

characteristically low signal on both T_1- and T_2-weighted images.[22] In addition to low-grade fibrous lesions, low T_1 and T_2 signal can also be seen with osteoid and hemosiderin. An osteoid-forming lesion can be excluded by plain film evaluation.

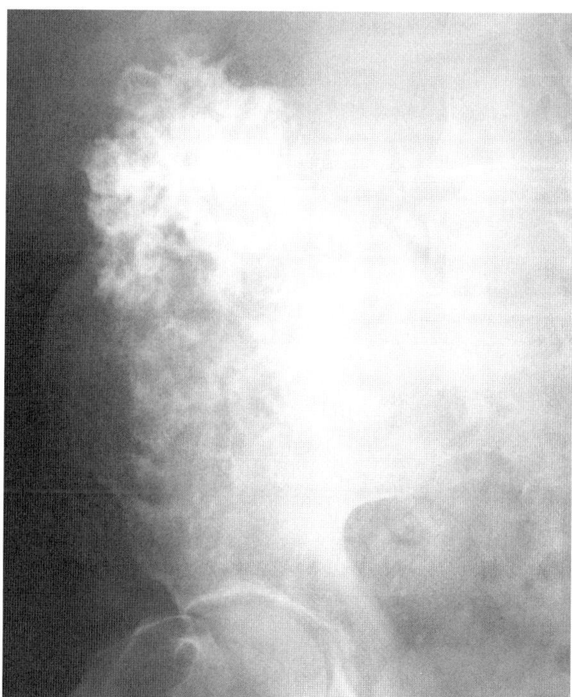

FIGURE 32.2. Chondroid matrix in a chondrosarcoma. The mineralization is punctate and forms circles and arcs.

Vascular

Benign vascular lesions of soft tissue may display phleboliths on plain film or CT (Figure 32.3). With MRI, the vessels can be recognized as serpentine tubular structures that may show signal voids from flowing blood. The mass usually contains fat interspersed between the vessels, another finding suggestive of a low-grade vascular lesion.[10]

Although hemangiomas of the skull and vertebra have a classic imaging appearance,[23] vascular tumors of bone in the extremities have no typical appearance, and even benign

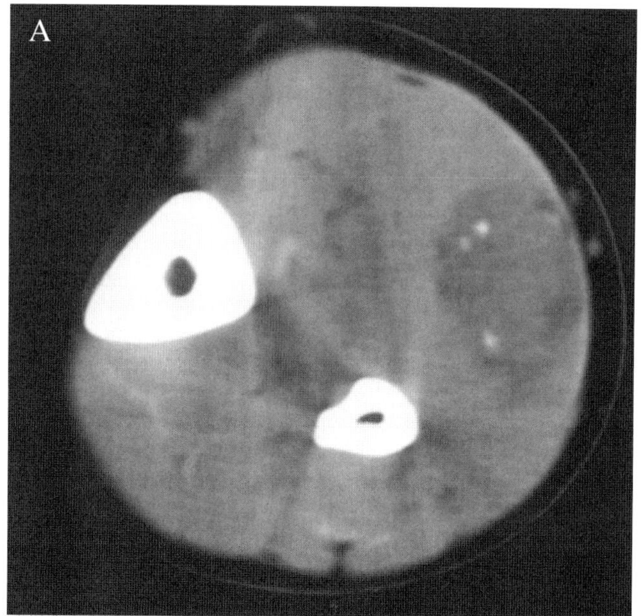

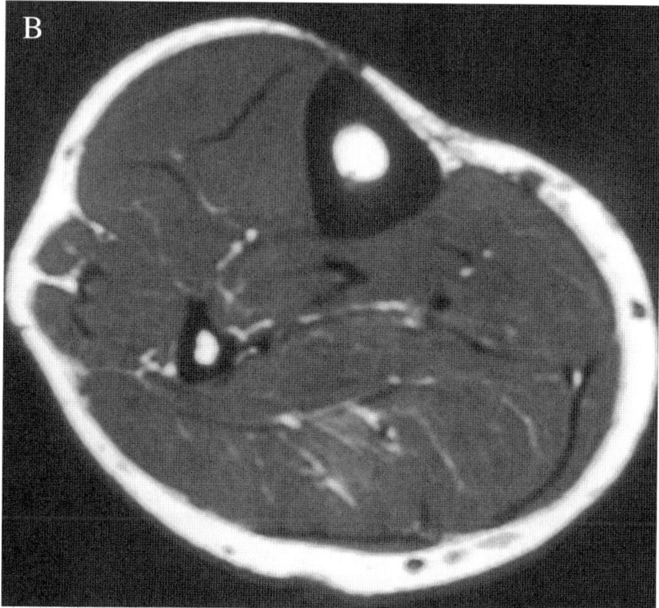

FIGURE 32.3. Soft tissue hemangioma of the calf. (A) Computed tomography (CT) image shows a mass that is lower density than muscle, suggesting the presence of fat. The punctate densities represent phleboliths, a classic finding with benign hemangiomas. (B) T_1-weighted magnetic resonance (MR) scan shows signal intensity equal to subcutaneous fat around and within the mass. Note that the phleboliths are not evident on MR.

hemangioma can look extremely aggressive. Angiosarcomas appear similar to sarcomas of other tissue types, but may be multifocal and cross joints, a behavior unusual for other sarcomas. It is therefore important to image the entire extremity when dealing with this tumor.[24]

Tumor Location

As indicated, certain bone tumors have a typical appearance with imaging, especially if low grade. Certain tumors also have predilection for specific bones and a specific location along a bone (epiphysis, metaphysis, diaphysis) (Figure 32.4). Most of these are benign.

In the realm of malignancy, the round cell tumors stand out in that they have both favorite locations and a typical appearance[25,26]; this includes both primary lymphoma of bone and Ewing sarcoma–PNET. These tumors are characteristically found along the shaft (diaphysis) of long bones, or on flat bones including the ilium, scapular body, and ribs. Their appearance is that of a lesion that permeates the cortex circumferentially in a manner similar to a sieve rather than causing focal cortical destruction. These tumors are almost uniformly associated with a large soft tissue mass, another feature not typically seen with other malignant bone tumors.

Imaging Modalities

Many imaging techniques are now at the disposal of the oncologist, not only for diagnosing musculoskeletal tumors but also for evaluating the response to radiation or chemotherapy and for posttreatment follow-up. The choice of modality will reflect the cell of origin for the diagnosis and the type of treatment undertaken for long-term surveillance.

Plain Radiography

Whether a bone or soft tissue neoplasia is the concern, the initial evaluation of a mass should be performed with plain radiography.[27] For bone lesions, plain films will show the aggressiveness of the tumor, and these remain the most specific modality for developing a differential diagnosis. For soft tissue masses, plain films can narrow the differential diagnoses by displaying or excluding the presence of mineralization in or around the lesion and detect changes in adjacent bone.[28]

When evaluating plain films, it is important to search for periosteal new bone and, if present, characterize it (Figure 32.5). This feature, which is often overlooked, can be extremely helpful in determining the behavior of a lesion. Periosteal new bone that is unilaminar or multilaminar but uninterrupted, is associated with benign processes, including low-grade neoplasia, trauma, or indolent infection. Periosteal new bone that is interrupted signifies an aggressive process, which may be either neoplastic or inflammatory.

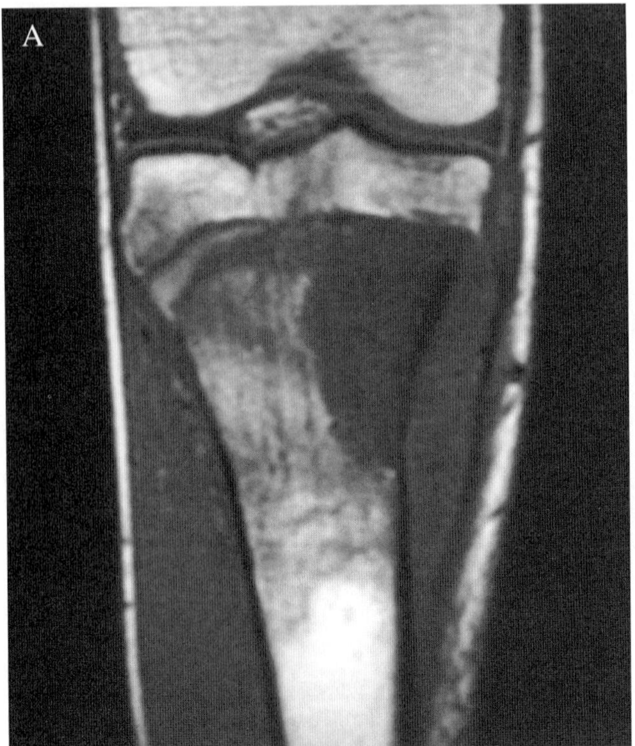

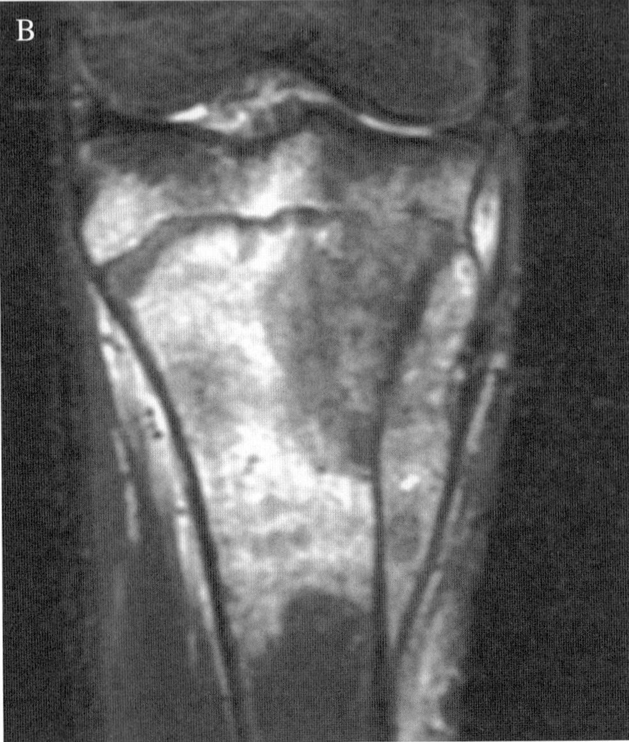

FIGURE 32.4. Edema around a proximal tibia osteosarcoma. (A) The tumor is confined to the focal low signal area in the medial metaphysis. The heterogeneous marrow signal lateral and distal to the tumor represents edema. (B) With inversion recovery imaging (similar to fat-suppressed T_2), edema in the surrounding marrow becomes high signal; this could be mistaken for tumor, significantly overestimating the size of the lesion. Note that the soft tissue mass extends further distal than the marrow involvement; this is important to recognize for surgical planning.

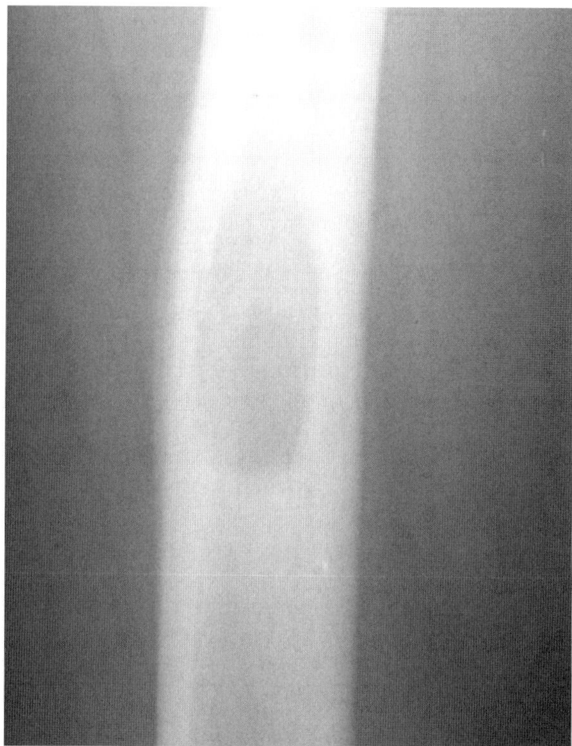

FIGURE 32.5. Benign periosteal new bone overlying a hemangioma of the femoral shaft. It is delicate and bilaminar, but continuous. Periosteal new bone associated with a more aggressive process would be interrupted.

Computed Tomography

Following plain films, CT is indicated for imaging primary tumors of bone and soft tissue lesions that are mineralized. For bone lesions, CT is superior to MRI in characterizing changes, including subtle areas of cortical thinning or destruction, and in providing information that may assist in planning an approach for biopsy.[29,30] CT easily displays the relationship of soft tissue masses to neurovascular structures and joints, assisting in determining the choice of surgical procedure (resection versus amputation) and the surgical approach.

CT is excellent for showing architectural detail in small bones, including ribs. An area where CT remains underutilized is in evaluation of bone scan abnormalities in cases where plain films fail to demonstrate the pathology; this is especially true for focal tracer uptake in ribs in the patient with a known primary malignancy. Thin-section scans targeted to the area of concern can almost always differentiate between a traumatic etiology (often forgotten by the patient) and metastatic disease.

CT guidance is commonly used for percutaneous biopsy.[31] With skin markers over the area of concern, the exact area of interest can be accurately localized with respect to depth and proximity to vital structures. This method is especially useful for core biopsies where precise needle localization might be essential.[32]

One argument for using MRI rather than CT has been the multiplanar imaging capability of MR imaging, allowing scan acquisition in the sagittal, coronal, or oblique plane. This situation is no longer the case. The advent and popularity of multidetector row CT has placed this technique again in the forefront of diagnostic imaging.[33] Especially for bone tumors, rapid acquisition of slices at submillimeter increments and the ability to reformat in any plane displays anatomy and pathology to an advantage never before possible with CT.[34,35]

Magnetic Resonance Imaging

Not uncommonly, when a person complains of a new mass or bone pain, an MRI is the first study ordered. Although this is frequently diagnostic for traumatic lesions, the appearance of malignancy with MRI is generally nonspecific.[36] Plain films are far superior for characterizing bone lesions. MRI may overestimate the extent of a lesion if it is fractured and will almost uniformly overlook foci of mineralization. The role of MRI is thus primarily one of staging rather than diagnosis.[29,37,38]

Although the radiology literature initially advocated the use of intravenous gadolinium for imaging musculoskeletal tumors, subsequent work has shown that the contrast agent generally adds nothing to the diagnosis or local staging of musculoskeletal neoplasia. Attempts within the past decade to add specificity to MRI with use of dynamic contrast imaging have been popular overseas but have not added diagnostic information at a clinically significant level.[39] The advantage of contrast enhancement, as originated in imaging of the central nervous system, reflects the destruction of the blood–brain barrier by a pathologic process. There is no corollary for such a barrier in the musculoskeletal system. Contrast enhancement thus reflects local vascularity and the size of the extracellular fluid compartment. As these features significantly overlap for benign and malignant processes, the technique adds nothing to tumor conspicuity, diagnosis, or staging.[40]

Technetium 99m medronate (^{99m}Tc-MDP) remains the mainstay for detection of bone metastatic disease. This may, however, not remain the case. Research using total-body MRI has suggested that this modality may not only be more sensitive than bone scintigraphy but also allows simultaneous imaging of solid organs, including the brain and liver.[41] One caveat is that evaluation of ribs with MRI is limited because of both the small size of the bone and respiratory motion. Another possible problem with whole-body MRI is the common detection of incidental lesions in both bone and soft tissues throughout the body. Studies with whole-body CT screening have shown that significant financial resources go into workup of these findings, often with invasive procedures, for confirmation of a benign diagnosis.

There is a recent trend for utilizing molecular imaging in conjunction with cross-sectional imaging, specifically MRI. Recent published research appears very promising, likely opening new chapters specifically in musculoskeletal tumor imaging.[42,43]

Radionuclide Imaging

Aside from its role in routine screening and detection of metastatic disease, the ^{99m}Tc-MDP bone scan can serve other purposes.[44,45] Not uncommonly, metastatic disease may present as a solitary symptomatic lesion in an area that is not readily amenable to biopsy for technical reasons.[46] In this instance, a bone scan may show that the process is actually multifocal and plain film correlation might display another focus that is more readily approachable. Radionuclide bone scans are also useful for evaluation of primary bone lesions that might be multifocal, such as brown tumors from hyperparathyroidism.[47] Bone lesions are often incidentally discovered on imaging studies obtained for unrelated reasons. In cases where the diagnosis is in question, a radionuclide scan will show the activity of the lesion. If tracer uptake is normal, the lesion can generally be disregarded. If the area is either photopenic or shows increased activity, further workup is warranted.

Thallium (^{201}Tl chloride) single photon emission computed tomography (SPECT) scanning has been used for determining a tumor's response to therapy as well as searching for metastatic disease.[48] The concept is quite attractive, because CT and MRI show only morphology, not tumor metabolism. Unfortunately, thallium uptake is nonspecific, with activity seen not only in malignancy but also in benign neoplasia and traumatic and inflammatory disorders. Its use has thus declined, being replaced by positron emission tomography (PET).[49]

Positron Emission Tomography

PET imaging is addressed in depth in Chapter 33. Suffice to say here that trials are now under way to define the exact role of PET in diagnosis and screening for a variety of tumors, including various types of sarcoma.[50] Although relatively recent, the advent of PET/CT has had a great impact on musculoskeletal oncology, as foci of abnormal activity can be precisely localized on the CT image and evaluated for their significance.[51]

Ultrasound

Ultrasound plays little role in the routine diagnosis, staging, and follow-up of sarcomas. Although it can be used for image guidance for biopsy,[52] this is usually more easily accomplished with CT. Ultrasound may be useful for detecting suspected tumor recurrence in the patient with implanted hardware, where artifact precludes other means of cross-sectional imaging.[53,54]

Occasionally ultrasound may be used for the diagnosis of vascular lesions by using color Doppler imaging mode.[55] In addition, ultrasound is helpful in differentiating fluid collections from solid masses.

Which Modality to Use When

Primary musculoskeletal malignancies are often treated initially with chemotherapy and/or radiation therapy, followed by surgical resection. Surgical choices include en bloc resection, resection and reconstruction (endoprosthesis, allograft, arthroplasty or arthrodesis), and amputation. The surgical procedure is determined by the histologic type of tumor, its location, and the extent of local involvement.

Preoperative Local Staging

Evaluation of bone tumors should begin with plain films.[56] If the tumor needs to be further characterized for either diagnosis or biopsy, CT is usually the modality of choice. If there is a possibility of multifocality in bone, a radionuclide bone scan is in order.[48] Although marrow involvement can be easily seen with CT, many surgeons prefer MRI to assess the length of marrow disease to determine the level of resection.

Bone tumors should be evaluated for location, length of intramedullary involvement, areas of cortical destruction, and any soft tissue mass. For both bone and soft tissue tumors, the relationship or involvement of major neurovascular structures or joints should be determined.

If endoprosthetic or allograft reconstruction is under consideration, measurements need to be made from the end of the tumor to the proximal and distal joints[57]; this is important not only for determining the level of osteotomy but also for sizing the prosthesis or allograft. This step is most easily accomplished with MRI, where a longitudinal T_1 scan can be acquired that includes both the proximal and distal joint. Accurate measurements may then be made at the console or on a workstation.

For soft tissue neoplasia, either CT or MRI may be used for local staging. Both accurately show the relationship of the mass to neurovascular structures and may be used to determine compartmentalization of the tumor.

Posttreatment Evaluation

Following chemotherapy and/or radiotherapy, one indicator of tumor response is obviously a reduction in size of the mass. This evaluation may be done with equal accuracy with either CT or MRI, where cross-sectional measurements are easily achieved.[58]

Long-Term Surveillance

The modality for long-term monitoring will depend on the type of treatment undertaken. If a patient has undergone en bloc resection or amputation, cross-sectional imaging with CT or MRI may be used for follow-up.[59] In certain cases of postsurgical treatment, intravenous contrast may be useful to differentiate between a residual or recurrent mass and a fluid collection, such as a seroma.[40] If an endoprosthesis, arthroplasty, or allograft has been placed, artifact from the metal components will render both these modalities basically useless. Plain films are useful to evaluate for mechanical complications but are of limited use for local recurrence unless mineralization is present. If a mass is highly suspected and hardware is present, imaging with ultrasound or PET may be useful. If ultrasound is used and a mass lesion is seen, it could be biopsied under ultrasound guidance at the time of the scan.

When follow-up studies are requested, it is important for the individual responsible for image interpretation to have access to prior examinations, both preoperative and especially, postoperative. Small foci of residual or recurrent disease may be easily overlooked without the advantage of direct comparison for subtle architectural changes.

Conclusion

Imaging plays a crucial role in musculoskeletal oncology. In cooperation with the functions of the other members of the team, it provides for detection and characterization of the tumor. It is capable of producing a useful list of differential diagnoses for initial workup and approach. It directs the biopsy toward the areas of interest within a lesion. It further assists in staging the disease, planning the therapy and follow-up.

The imaging of musculoskeletal sarcomas of the extremities should commence with plain radiography to evaluate for matrix mineralization and bone erosion/destruction. The next step should include a CT scan (for bone lesions) or MRI to further characterize the imaging characteristics. CT is commonly used for image-guided biopsy. Either CT or MRI may be used for staging of the tumor. The radionuclide bone scan and PET are used as an adjunct to detect polyostotic lesions. Ultrasound plays a limited role, usually for cases with hardware where other modalities are of limited value, and in guidance for biopsies. Both MRI and CT are frequently used for posttherapy follow-up if hardware is not present.

References

1. Murphey MD, Kransdorf MJ, Smith SE. Imaging of soft tissue neoplasms in the adult: malignant tumors. Semin Musculoskeletal Radiol 1999;3(1):39–58.
2. Kocher MS, Jupiter JB. Enchondroma versus chondrosarcoma of the phalanx. Orthopedics 2000;23(5):493–494.
3. Murphey MD, Flemming DJ, Boyea SR, Bojescul JA, Sweet DE, Temple HT. Enchondroma versus chondrosarcoma in the appendicular skeleton: differentiating features. RadioGraphics 1998; 18(5):1244–1245.
4. Gaskin CM, Helms CA. Lipomas, lipoma variants, and well-differentiated liposarcomas (atypical lipomas): results of MRI evaluations of 126 consecutive fatty masses. Am J Roentgenol 2004;182(3):733–739.
5. Frassica FJ, Khanna JA, McCarthy EF. The role of MR imaging in soft tissue evaluation: perspective of the orthopedic oncologist and musculoskeletal pathologist. Magn Reson Imaging Clin N Am 2000;8(4):915–927.
6. Lee SH, Kim DJ, Oh JH, et al. Validation of a functional evaluation system in patients with musculoskeletal tumors. Clin Orthop 2003;1(411):271–226.
7. Kawai S. An interdisciplinary and comprehensive approach for treatment of musculoskeletal tumors in the bone and joint decade. J Orthop Sci 2002;7(3):285–286.
8. Kransdorf MJ, Smith SE. Lesions of unknown histogenesis: Langerhans cell histiocytosis and Ewing sarcoma. Semin Musculoskeletal Radiol 2000;4(1):113–125.
9. Siegel MJ. Magnetic resonance imaging of musculoskeletal soft tissue tumors. Radiol Clin N Am 2001;39(4):701–720.
10. Nagira K, Yamamoto T, Marui T, Akisue T, Yoshiya S, Kurosaka M. Ossified intramuscular hemangioma: multimodality imaging findings. Clin Imaging 2001;25(5):368–372.
11. Mulligan SA, Schwartz ML, Broussard MF, Andrews JR. Heterotopic calcification and tears of the ulnar collateral ligament: radiographic and MR imaging findings. Am J Roentgenol 2000; 175(4):1099–1102.
12. Ledermann HP, Schweitzer ME, Morrison WB. Pelvic heterotopic ossifications: MR imaging characteristics. Radiology 2002; 222(1):189–195.
13. De Smet AA, Norris MA, Fisher DR. Magnetic resonance imaging of myositis ossificans: analysis of seven cases. Skeletal Radiol 1992;21(8):503–507.
14. De Beuckeleer LH, De Schepper AM, Ramon F. Magnetic resonance imaging of cartilaginous tumors: is it useful or necessary? Skeletal Radiol 1996;25(2):137–141.
15. Ahmed AR, Tan TS, Unni KK, Collins MS, Wenger DE, Sim FH. Secondary chondrosarcoma in osteochondroma: report of 107 patients. Clin Orthop 2003;1(411):193–206.
16. Marco RA, Gitelis S, Brebach GT, et al. Cartilage tumors: evaluation and treatment. J Am Acad Orthop Surg 2000;8(5):292–304.
17. Murphey MD, Walker EA, Wilson AJ, Kransdorf MJ, Temple HT, Gannon FH. From the Archives of the AFIP: imaging of primary chondrosarcoma: radiologic-pathologic correlation. RadioGraphics 2003;23(5):1245–1278.
18. Yao L, Nelson SD, Seeger LL, et al. Primary musculoskeletal neoplasms: effectiveness of core-needle biopsy. Radiology 1999; 212(3):682–686.
19. Bancroft LW, Kransdorf MJ, Peterson JJ, Sundaram M, Murphey MD, O'Connor MI. Imaging characteristics of spindle cell lipoma. Am J Roentgenol 2003;181(5):1251–1254.
20. Kooby DA, Antonescu CR, Brennan MF, Singer S. Atypical lipomatous tumor/well-differentiated liposarcoma of the extremity and trunk wall: importance of histological subtype with treatment recommendations. Ann Surg Oncol 2004;11(1):78–84.
21. Kransdorf MJ, Bancroft LW, Peterson JJ, Murphey MD, Foster WC, Temple HT. Imaging fatty tumors: distinction of lipoma and well-differentiated liposarcoma. Radiology 2002;224(1):99–104.
22. Smith SE, Kransdorf MJ. Primary musculoskeletal tumors of fibrous origin. Semin Musculoskelet Radiol 2000;4(1):73–88.
23. Amaral L, Chiuriu M, Almeida JR, Ferreira NF, Mendonca R, Lima SS. MR imaging for evaluation of lesions of the cranial vault: a pictorial essay. Arq Neuropsiquiatr 2003;61(3A):521–532.
24. Choi JJ, Murphey MD. Angiomatous skeletal lesions. Semin Musculoskelet Radiol 2000;4(1):103–112.
25. Ghanem I, Tolo VT, D'Ambra P. Malogalowkin MH. Langerhans cell histiocytosis of bone in children and adolescents. J Pediatr Orthop 2003;23(1):124–130.
26. Porn U, Howman-Giles R, Onikul E, Uren R. Langerhans cell histiocytosis of the lumbar spine. Clin Nucl Med 2003;28(1): 52–53.
27. Priolo F, Cerase A. The current role of radiography in the assessment of skeletal tumors and tumor-like lesions. Eur J Radiol 1998;27(suppl 1):S77–S85.
28. Davies AM, Wellings RM. Imaging of bone tumors. Curr Opin Radiol 1992;4(6):32–38.
29. Woertler K. Benign bone tumors and tumor-like lesions: value of cross-sectional imaging. Eur Radiol 2003;13(8):1820–1835.
30. Robbin RM, Murphey MD. Benign chondroid neoplasms of bone. Semin Musculoskeletal Radiol 2000;4(1):45–58.
31. Bickels J, Jelinek JS, Shmookler BM, et al. Biopsy of musculoskeletal tumors. Current concepts. Clin Orthop 1999;1(368): 212–219.
32. Anderson MW, Temple HT, Dussault RG, et al. Compartmental anatomy: relevance of staging and biopsy of musculoskeletal tumors. Am J Roentgenol 1999;173(6):1663–1671.
33. Rydberg J, Buckwalter KA, Caldemeyer KS et al. Multi-section CT: scanning techniques and clinical applications. RadioGraphics 2000;20(6):1787–1806.
34. Buckwalter KA, Rydberg J, Kopecky KK, Crow K, Yang EL. Musculoskeletal imaging with multi-slice CT. Am J Roentgenol 2001;176(4):979–986.
35. Kopecky KK, Buckwalter KA, Sokiranski R. Multi-slice CT spirals past single-slice CT in diagnostic efficacy. Diagn Imaging 1999;21(4):36–42.
36. Azouz EM. Magnetic resonance imaging of benign bone lesions: cysts and tumors. Top Magn Reson Imaging 2002;13(4):219–229.
37. Ma LD. Magnetic resonance imaging of musculoskeletal tumors: skeletal and soft tissue masses. Curr Probl Diagn Radiol 1999;28(2):29–62.
38. Temple HT, Bashore CJ. Staging of bone neoplasms: an orthopedic oncologist's perspective. Semin Musculoskeletal Radiol 2000;4(1):17–23.
39. Geirnaerdt MJ, Bloem JL, van der Woude HJ, Taminiau AH, Nooy MA, Hogendoorn PC. Chondroblastic osteosarcoma: characterization by gadolinium-enhanced MR imaging correlated with histopathology. Skeletal Radiol 1998;27(3):145–153.

40. van der Woude HJ, Bloem JL, Verstraete KL, Taminiau AH, Nooy MA, Hogendoorn PC. Osteosarcoma and Ewing's sarcoma after neoadjuvant chemotherapy: value of dynamic MR imaging in detecting viable tumor before surgery. Am J Roentgenol 1995; 165(3):593–598.
41. Iizuka-Mikami M, Nagai K, Yoshida K, et al. Detection of bone marrow and extramedullary involvement in patients with non-Hodgkin's lymphoma by whole-body MRI: comparison with bone and ^{67}Ga scintigraphies. Eur Radiol 2004;14:1074–1081.
42. Graadt van Roggen JF, Bovee JV, van der Woude HJ, et al. An update of diagnostic strategies using molecular genetic and magnetic resonance imaging techniques for musculoskeletal tumors. Curr Opin Rheumatol 2000;12(1):77–83.
43. Uchida A, Seto M, Hashimoto N, et al. Molecular diagnosis and gene therapy in musculoskeletal tumors. J Orthop Sci 2000; 5(4):418–423.
44. Pneumaticos SG, Chatziioannou SN, Moore WH, et al. The role of radionuclides in primary musculoskeletal tumors beyond the 'bone scan'. Crit Rev Oncol Hematol 2001;37(3):217–226.
45. Yahara J, Noguchi M, Noda S. Quantitative evaluation of bone metastases in patients with advanced prostate cancer during systemic treatment. BJU Int 2003;92(4):379–384.
46. Othman S, El-Desouki M. Bone scan appearance in aggressive osteogenic sarcoma with pleural, lung, bone and soft-tissue metastases. Clin Nucl Med 2003;28(11):926.
47. Solav S. Bone scintiscanning in osteolytic lesions. Clin Nucl Med 2004;29(1):12–20.
48. Abdel-Dayem HM. The role of nuclear medicine in primary bone and soft tissue tumors. Semin Nucl Med 1997;27(4):355–363.
49. Aoki J, Endo K, Watanabe H, et al. FDG-PET for evaluating musculoskeletal tumors: a review. J Orthop Sci 2003;8(3):435–441.
50. Ioannidis JP, Lau J. ^{18}F-FDG PET for the diagnosis and grading of soft-tissue sarcoma: a meta-analysis. J Nucl Med 2003;44(5): 717–724.
51. Peterson JJ, Kransdorf MJ, O'Connor MI. Diagnosis of occult bone metastases: positron emission tomography. Clin Orthop 2003;1(415S):S120–S128.
52. Torriani M, Etchebehere M, Amstalden E. Sonography-guided core needle biopsy of bone and soft tissue tumors. J Ultrasound Med 2002;21(3):275–281.
53. Jacobson JA, Lax MJ. Musculoskeletal sonography of the postoperative orthopedic patient. Semin Musculoskeletal Radiol 2002; 6(1):67–77.
54. Khuu H, Moore D, Young S, et al. Examination of tumor and tumor-like conditions of bone. Ann Diagn Pathol 1999;3(6):364–369.
55. Bodner G, Schocke MF, Rachbauer F, et al. Differentiation of malignant and benign musculoskeletal tumors: combined color and power Doppler US and spectral wave analysis. Radiology 2002;223(2):410–416.
56. Taljanovic MS, Hunter TB, Fitzpatrick KA, et al. Musculoskeletal magnetic resonance imaging: importance of radiography. Skeletal Radiol 2003;32(7):403–411.
57. Massengill AD, Seeger LL, Eckardt JJ. The role of plain radiography, computed tomography, and magnetic resonance imaging in sarcoma evaluation. Hematol Oncol Clin N Am 1995;9(3): 571–604.
58. van de Woude HJ, Bloem JL, Hogendoorn PC. Preoperative evaluation and monitoring chemotherapy in patients with high-grade osteogenic and Ewing's sarcoma: a review of current imaging modalities. Skeletal Radiol 1998;27(2):57–71.
59. Panicek DM, Schwartz LH. MR imaging after surgery for musculoskeletal neoplasm. Semin Musculoskeletal Radiol 2002;6(1): 57–66.

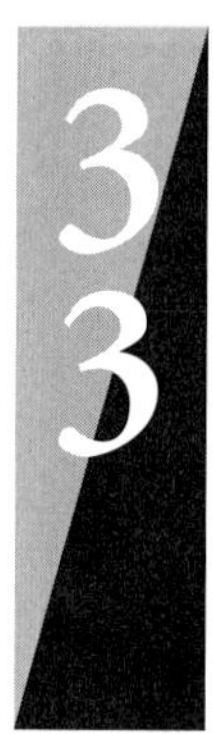

Positron Emission Tomography and Cancer

Daniel N. Chatzifotiadis, Julia W. Buchanan, and Richard L. Wahl

Positron emission tomography, PET, is a potent imaging tool in the management of a diverse array of cancers. This chapter briefly discusses the rationale for PET imaging and describes how it differs from more typical anatomic imaging, reviews the principles of metabolic targeting with the radiolabeled glucose analogue ^{18}F-fluoro-2-deoxy-D-glucose (FDG), and then describes the clinical results of PET imaging in several types of common cancers. Although there are detailed descriptions of tumor imaging with other modalities in several areas of this textbook, the discussion here focuses on the role of PET.

PET imaging was originally introduced as a functional tool for quantitatively imaging metabolic activity in the brain. PET is a nuclear medicine technique in which positron-emitting radiopharmaceuticals with short half-lives are injected intravenously into patients and then imaged with a PET scanner. The readers are referred to a textbook that describes in detail the chemistry and physics of positron emission tomographic imaging.[1] It should be noted that the most commonly used positron emitter is ^{18}F-fluoride, which is cyclotron produced and has a 109-minute half-life. This radioisotope is most commonly used in clinical PET imaging as ^{18}F-fluoro-2-deoxy-D-glucose (FDG), which traces the early steps of glucose metabolism.

Cancers typically have accelerated glucose metabolism, and FDG traces the initial accumulation of the radiotracer into the cancer via membrane transport, and also its initial phosphorylation by hexokinase to FDG-6-phosphate. This latter substance is polar and typically retained in most cancers.

Glucose utilization is accelerated in most cancers, but some cancers do not have high glucose uptake; these include many prostate cancers, renal cancers (primary), hepatomas and mucinous tumors, and some low-grade lymphomas. Some cancers, such as some brain tumors, that have high glucose uptake may also be difficult to image because the background FDG uptake is high in normal brain. This condition makes defining brain tumors more problematic as the target/background uptake ratios are often lower than elsewhere in the body where there is less normal FDG uptake.

Normal tissues using glucose include the brain, heart, kidneys, testes, exercising skeletal muscle, and the kidneys. FDG is excreted unchanged via the kidneys, which can make detection of lesions in the renal area problematic as well as in the bladder region. PET is a "molecular imaging" tool and, in contrast to single photon emission computed tomography (SPECT) imaging, is capable of providing quantitative data based on the amount of radioactivity in a tissue in the human body noninvasively. It is highly accurate in such quantitation and is able to detect lesions smaller than 1 cm in size. However, PET is not a microscope tool and can often fail to detect lesions in the subcentimeter range. With current available equipment, PET typically loses considerable sensitivity for lesions in the 5-mm range and smaller, but lesion detectability is dependent on many factors, most importantly, the absolute uptake of radiotracer into the lesion as well as the lesion/background ratio. The higher the lesion uptake and the lower the background, the better the chance of lesion detection.

In general, lesions smaller than 5 mm are not detected well with PET in its current form. As a functional imaging tool, PET quantifies the tracer uptake well and displays it in an anatomically correct manner. Unfortunately, if the lesion/background ratio is high, the PET scan can show a "hot spot" but only provide general information as to the precise lesion location. Thus, there has been a great deal of interest in using PET to provide fused images with anatomy, so-called anatometabolic images, which combine form and function into a single image. This merge can be done with software fusion methods, fusing PET and CT or PET and magnetic resonance imaging (MRI) images, but the most common approach is to use dedicated PET/CT scanning devices, which are both PET and CT scanners in a single device.

PET/CT imaging is quickly replacing PET imaging alone as the preferred tool for PET imaging in cancer. This approach was developed by Townsend and colleagues and has been rapidly disseminated throughout the world, with PET/CT scanners representing nearly the entire marketplace for PET imaging equipment at this time. Such devices acquire a CT scan and then a PET scan as part of the same imaging procedure. Because the scanners are linked together, they generate PET, CT, and then PET/CT fused image data. This approach is the new standard for PET imaging of cancer, is the routine procedure for clinical PET at the authors' institution, and is quickly replacing PET alone as an imaging tool. Of interest is that PET alone is a superb imaging tool in many cancers, and PET/CT, while often better and more easily interpreted, is not necessarily dramatically more accurate than PET in all cancers. Nonetheless, PET/CT quite consistently has fewer equivocal diagnoses, fewer equivocal lesion localizations, and greater accuracy than PET. However, much of the evidence for PET is based on the PET literature and is not yet based on PET/CT data. Although only PET/CT images are shown in this chapter, PET imaging represents the foundation for most of the conclusions presented. The use of PET, which has clear advantages over CT or MRI as a functional imaging tool, remains a very valid technique for tumor imaging in clinical practice.

The use of PET has expanded widely in the United States and the world since the approval by the Center for Medicare Services for reimbursement of PET imaging in several common situations. Broadly, Medicare will reimburse for tumor diagnosis, staging, and restaging at present, with more limited reimbursement for PET assessments of early responses to treatment. However, these rules have been in rapid evolution. Currently, the most common uses for PET imaging in our center are for tumor staging, assessment of treatment response, and restaging for recurrence after treatment or with rising serum markers.

The use of PET in several disease types is discussed in detail in the following sections, covering several major types of cancer.

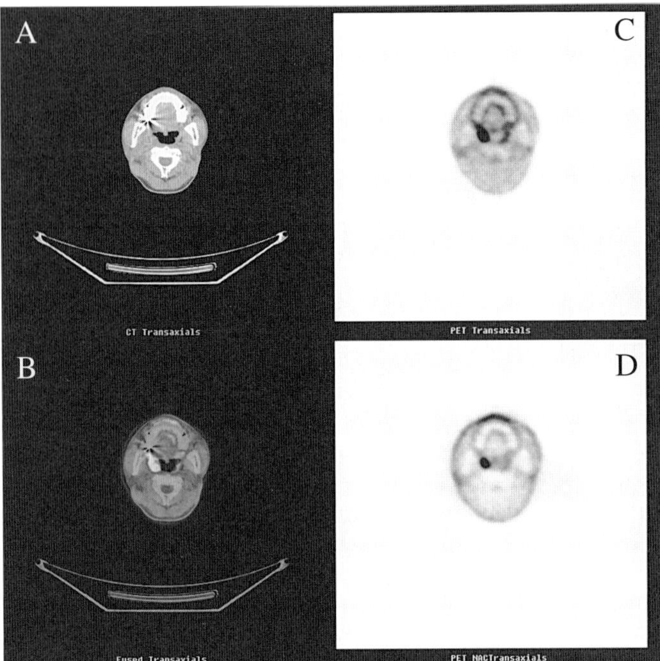

FIGURE 33.1. A transverse ^{18}F-fluoro-2-deoxy-D-glucose (FDG)-positron emission tomography (PET) scan in a middle-aged patient who had a history of an enlarged right neck lymph node at level 7 that had been excused and demonstrated squamous cell carcinoma. PET/computed tomography (CT) images were obtained with FDG to determine if there was evidence of a primary squamous cell carcinoma. Transverse PET images (with (C) and without (D) attenuation correction) and CT (A), and fused PET/CT (B) images, are displayed. Focal increased FDG is seen in the right palatine tonsil region; this is greater than the normal FDG uptake expected in the lymphocyte-rich tonsils. Biopsy of the right tonsil demonstrated a primary squamous cell carcinoma. PET has been reported to detect between 15% and 35% of unknown primary squamous cell carcinomas in the head and neck.

Head and Neck Cancer

FDG-PET, is considered to be a useful technique in the evaluation of primary head and neck small cell carcinoma (HNSCC). The imaging technique can be performed either 50 minutes after the injection of FDG injection or up to 90 minutes after, because of the continuing improved target-to-background ratios. Normal variants of uptake in adenoidal, palatine, and lingual tonsils, in laryngeal and neck musculature (scalene, vocalis, cricoarytenoid), or in glands (salivary and parotids) need to be kept in mind.

Staging of the primary tumor was tried by some investigators,[2] but CT and physical examination remain the mainstay in tumor staging. FDG-PET has a role in only 5% of patients, but it can identify the unknown primary in about 20% to 50% of these cases.[3–6]

Routine panendoscopy can identify the small lesions that may not be seen by PET;[7] however, FDG-PET seems to predict tumor curability with radiotherapy.[8]

Adams et al.[9] reported that FDG-PET has a sensitivity of 90% and a specificity of 94%, which are better than MRI (80% and 79%, respectively) and CT (82% and 85%, respectively).

Kau et al.[10] studied 70 patients suspicious for lymph node metastases and found that the sensitivity and specificity of FDG-PET for detecting lymph nodes were 87% and 94%, respectively, compared with those of CT (65% and 47%) and MRI (88% and 41%) (Figure 33.1).

Several studies have compared the sensitivity and the specificity of all imaging modalities (FDG-PET and conventional imaging).[11–14] False-negative PET studies are found because of small tumor burden in nodes, cystic degenerations of metastatic nodes that are only surrounded by a small rim of viable tumor, low tracer uptake in a metastatic node, imaging artifacts, and proximity to the primary tumor. Additionally, in distant metastases or in synchronous second primary tumors, which are present in 8% of the cases,[15] the rate of PET detection is very high[16] (Table 33.1).

FDG-PET in Evaluation of Recurrent Head and Neck Cancer

Most recurrences occur in the first 24 months after therapy for HNSCC. Distant recurrences are more common in patients with locally recurrent disease than distant metastases at initial staging, with the lungs the most common site of distant recurrence.[17]

Early detection of recurrent head and neck cancer has a crucial role in predicting the clinical outcome, because patients with early-stage HNSCC who undergo salvage surgery have a 70% 2-year relapse-free survival (RFS), whereas those with recurrent advanced-stage disease undergoing salvage surgery have a 22% 2-year RFS.[18]

FDG-PET is more sensitive, specific, and accurate in the detection of local recurrent head and neck cancer[19–21] and in the detection of recurrent HNSCC, regardless of the primary treatment modality (surgery versus radiation therapy)[21–25] than CT or MRI (Table 33.2).

The negative predictive value of FDG-PET is very high, but the positive predictive value is somewhat lower for local recurrence in the region of the primary tumor because of false-positive findings (i.e., laryngeal muscle uptake, adipose tissue uptake, or radioactive saliva in the floor of the mouth, throat, or vallecula).

TABLE 33.1. Studies comparing CT, MRI, US, and PET for nodal staging in head and neck cancer.

Author	Year	No. of patients	CT/MRI/US	Sens	Spec	PET Sens	Spec
Hannah et al.[12]	2002	40	CT	81	81	82	94
Di Martino et al.[13]	2000	50	CT	84	96	84	90
			US	88	88		
Stokkel et al.[16]	1999	54	CT	84	96	84	90
			US	84	88		
Stuckensen et al.[14]	2000	106	CT	66	74	70	82
			MRI	64	69		
			US	84	68		
Kau et al.[10]	1999	70	CT	65	47	87	94
			MRI	88	41		

CT, computed tomography; MRI, magnetic resonance imaging; US, ultrasonography; PET, positron emission tomography; Sens, sensitivity; Spec, specificity.

A positive PET scan requires a biopsy, and if this is not positive, a repeat biopsy or close clinical follow-up may be required 2 to 3 months later. Standard uptake value (SUV) measurements have a wide overlap between disease recurrence versus nontumor-related FDG accumulation (SUV range, 2.1–36.9 versus 1.5–9.3, respectively).

Role of FDG-PET in Monitoring Therapy

Brun et al.,[26] in a study of 47 patients, with two-thirds of these in stage IV disease, showed that the pretreatment SUV was lower in patients with a complete response (8.0 versus 12.0), the 5-year overall survival (OS) was 72% in those who had low FDG activity after 1 to 3 weeks of treatment, and the 5-year OS was only 35% in those who had high FDG uptake in the same period.

Kitagawa et al.[27] studied 15 patients who were treated with neoadjuvant chemotherapy and showed that lesions with a pretreatment SUV greater than 7 had residual viable tumor in 3 of 8 cases, whereas all lesions with SUV less than 7 were treated successfully. All 7 tumors with posttreatment SUV less than 4 did not show residual disease and 3 of the 7 tumors with posttreatment SUV greater than 4 did. The same group calculated the sensitivity, specificity, and accuracy of PET-FDG, MRI, and CT in primary lesions and in neck metastases, finding FDG-PET to be more specific (89%) compared with MRI (41%) and CT (59%) in primary lesions but not in nodal metastases (74% versus 85% and 76%, respectively).[28]

Goerres et al.[29] evaluated the detection of residual disease in 26 patients with stage III–IV HNSCC, and PET was performed 6 weeks after the end of combined chemotherapy and radiation therapy. The sensitivity, specificity, and accuracy were 91%, 93%, and 92%, respectively. They also showed that the PET study at 6 weeks often revealed a second primary tumor or a distant metastasis that had not been detected at the time of initial staging.

Kubota et al.[30] also concluded that the high negative predictive value of FDG-PET (91%) may be used to prevent additional invasive procedures for the detection of recurrent head and neck cancers after combined radiochemotherapy in most clinical settings.

Radiation Therapy Alone

Greven et al.[31] demonstrated, in a study of 45 patients who had FDG-PET before and at 1, 4, 12, and 24 months after high-dose radiation therapy, that imaging at 4 months was more reliable than at 1 month. It seems that an interval of 6 to 8 weeks after radiation treatment is most appropriate, but it must be kept in mind that FDG uptake can be significantly high in regions of radiation therapy up to 12 to 16 months after treatment.[32]

Other PET Tracers

Radiolabeled amino acids, ^{11}C-methionine, radiolabeled tyrosine, ^{11}C-choline, ^{18}F-thymidine, ^{64}Cu-ATSM [copper (II)-dia-cetyl-bis (*N*-4-methylthiosemicarbazone)], ^{18}F-fluoromisonidazole, and ^{18}F-2-nitroimidazole (EF5), have been studied as potential imaging agents for head and neck tumors.[33–40] Several of these show promise and may be introduced into clinical practice in the future.

Thyroid

Since the early 1950s, the whole-body scan (WBS) using a tracer dose of iodine-131 (^{131}I) has been widely used for detection of metastases of differentiated thyroid cancer (DTC). Some studies have investigated the role of FDG-PET in thyroid nodules, based on the hypothesis that malignant lesions would be more FDG avid[41,42] than the benign ones.

TABLE 33.2. Imaging of recurrent head and neck cancer.

Author	Year	No. of patients	CT/MRI Sens	Spec	Acc	PET Sens	Spec	Acc	Remarks
Li et al.[22]	2001	43	53	79	66	91	86	88	
Terhaard et al.[23]	2001	75				92	63		
Lowe et al.[24]	2000	44	38	85		100	93		$P < 0.002$
Kunkel et al.[25]	2003	97				83	81		For all findings
						87	67		Local metastases
						87	99		Nodal >>
						71	93		Distant >>

This is clearly not true, as shown by Kresnik et al.,[43] who demonstrated that many malignant nodules were not FDG avid, most likely because they were well differentiated. Additionally, other studies have shown that multimodular goiter[44,45] or thyroiditis,[46,47] predominantly lymphocytic, may have increased FDG uptake.

In patients who underwent FDG-PET for some other reason, Kang et al.[48] reported that thyroid incidentallomas were found in 2.2%, and among these, 27% proved to be cancer. In a larger group of patients (4,525) Cohen et al.[49] reported that incidentallomas were found in 2.3% and 47% were thyroid cancers.

FDG-PET in Evaluation of Differentiated Thyroid Cancer

In a large multicenter study of unselected thyroid cancer patients ($n = 222$), Grunwald et al.[50] found that the sensitivity of FDG-PET for localizing metastatic disease in patients with DTC was 75% and that it was 85% for the group with a negative WBS ($n = 166$).

Feine et al.[51] noticed that there were tumors that accumulated only FDG, others only ^{131}I, and some both FDG and iodine. He named this alternating pattern of either ^{131}I or FDG uptake in thyroid cancer metastases as the "flip-flop" phenomenon. Thus, some thyroid tumors without functional differentiation for iodine (^{123}I or ^{131}I) uptake showed high glucose metabolism, and many differentiated papillary and follicular thyroid cancers did not have increased FDG uptake.

Wang et al.[52] reported that progressive dedifferentiation of thyroid cancer cells results in a loss of their ability to concentrate iodine, which results in a negative WBS in 20% of originally differentiated thyroid cancers. Thyroid cancer cells that lose their ability to concentrate radioactive iodine may exhibit increased metabolic activity, which results in enhanced glucose uptake. Many studies showed that FDG-PET is more sensitive than WBS in high-grade tumors, whereas an iodine scan is more commonly positive in low-grade carcinomas.[53–55] Expression of the GLUT-1 transporter on the cell membrane is closely related to the grade of malignancy in thyroid neoplasms, with anaplastic tumors and widely invasive follicular or metastatic tumors showing a high-level of GLUT-I glucose transporter expression.[56]

Some studies have reported that increased TSH levels stimulate FDG uptake by thyroid cancer cells.[57,58] A case report by Sisson demonstrated increased FDG uptake in a thyroid cancer metastasis imaged both before and then after withdrawal from thyroid hormone therapy. Helal et al.[59] studied 37 patients with DTC who had undergone resection and ablation with radioactive iodine. He found a sensitivity of 76% in these patients and concluded that FDG-PET should be a first-line investigation in patients with elevated thyroglobulin and a negative WBS (Figure 33.2).

Schluter et al.[60] studied 64 patients with thyroid cancer with either elevated serum thyroglobulin or clinical suspicion of metastases and negative WBS and reported that the positive predictive value (PPV) was 83% whereas the negative predictive value (NPV) was 25%. The true positive FDG-PET findings were correlated positively with increasing thyroglobulin levels. The FDG-PET was true positive in 11%, 50%, and 93% of patients with thyroglobulin levels less than 10, 10 to 20, and more than 100 ng/dL, respectively. This finding suggests that the mass of thyroid cancer tissue is related to detectability, which is not surprising.

The use of recombinant human thyrotropin (rhTSH) has recently been proposed to increase the sensitivity of FDG-PET in the diagnosis of recurrent and metastatic cancer versus the unstimulated setting. Moog et al.[61] compared imaging findings in 10 patients who were either under TSH suppression and were hyperthyroid, or were hypothyroid with stimulated TSH. Increases of 63% in the tumor-to-background ratios were observed in the latter case. Petrich et al.[62] reported that in 30 patients they found more suspicious lesions for cancer in more patients when they received rhTSH. These observations were also supported by an in vitro culture experiment.[63]

Wang et al.[64] evaluated 125 patients with a mean of 41 months of follow-up who had a negative WBS, a positive FDG-PET study, and elevated thyroglobulin. They concluded that the single strongest predictor of survival was the volume of FDG-avid disease. Detection of tumor with FDG-PET is a volume-dependent phenomenon.

In another study, the same authors[65] evaluated the ability of an ablation dose of ^{131}I to destroy FDG-avid metastatic lesions in patients with thyroid cancer who had FDG-PET scans pre- and post-^{131}I treatment. The authors found that the total volume of FDG-avid metastases rose from a mean of 159 mL to 235 mL after ^{131}I ablation therapy and the post-^{131}I thyroglobulin level rose 132% above the value at baseline. In patients with a negative FDG-PET scan, the serum thyroglobulin levels decreased to 38% of baseline after ^{131}I

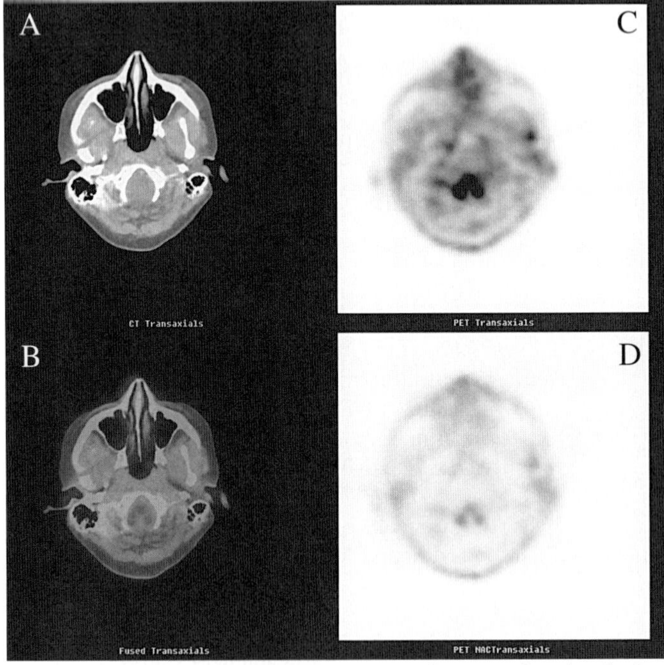

FIGURE 33.2. Transverse FDG-PET scan of a young female who had a history of follicular thyroid carcinoma with lymph node and capsular involvement 3 years before this scan. She had developed an elevated serum thyroglobulin level, and her iodine scan was negative. This PET scan was performed to look for a recurrent noniodine-avid tumor. This scan was performed without recombinant thyroid-stimulation hormone (rhTSH) stimulation and demonstrates increased radiotracer uptake in the left neck in level 2 lymph nodes, which were subsequently proven to be metastatic thyroid cancer (A) CT scan. (B) Fused PET/CT image. (C) Attenuation corrected PET image. (D) Nonattenuation corrected PET image.

TABLE 33.3. Studies comparing PET findings in different types of thyroid cancer.

Author	*Year*	*Type of thyroid cancer*	*Sens*	*Spec*	*Acc*	*PPV*	*NPV*	*Remarks*
Plotkin et al.[67]	2002	Hürthle	92	80	89	92	80	
Lowe et al.[66]	2003	Hürthle	92					
Diehl et al.[69]	2001	Medullary	78	79				
Schluter et al.[60]	2001	Papillary/follicular or mixed				83	25	↑ Tg level ^{131}I WBS(−)

Acc, accuracy; PPV, positive predictive value; NPV, negative predictive value; WBS, whole-body scan.

therapy. High-dose ^{131}I therapy does not appear to have a tremendously beneficial effect on the viability of metastatic FDG-avid lesions. Nonresectable regional disease can be treated with external-beam irradiation or, if limited, with surgery, while widespread disease may be amenable to experimental chemotherapy.

Hürthle Cell Carcinoma

Hürthle cell cancer is a histologic subtype of DTC that is clinically more aggressive and has little or no iodine uptake. In a study of 12 patients Lowe et al.[66] described a sensitivity of 92% for FDG-PET. Plotkin et al.[67] reported a sensitivity of 92%, a specificity of 80%, a PPV of 92%, a NPV of 80%, and an accuracy of 89% (Table 33.3).

Medullary Thyroid Cancer

Medullary thyroid cancer (MTC) is a rare calcitonin-secreting tumor originating from the parafollicular C cells. At the time of initial diagnosis, most of the patients with this malignancy are noted to have lymph node metastases. The primary treatment modality is surgical resection of all malignant lesions. Brandt-Mainz et al.[68] studied 20 patients and found the overall sensitivity to be 76%. In another study, Diehl et al.[69] demonstrated, in 55 cases, that FDG-PET had a sensitivity of 78% and a specificity of 79%, in comparison with ^{131}In-pentetreotide, 25% and 92%, with dimercaptosuccinic acid (DMSA), 33% and 78%, with ^{99m}Tc-MIBI (hexakis-2-methoxy-2-isobutyl isonitrile), 25% and 100%, with CT, 50% and 20%, and with MRI, 82% and 67%. A reasonable imaging approach in the staging and follow-up of MTC would be a combination of FDG-PET and MRI.

Novel, more-specific PET tracers, such as ^{18}F-dihydroxyphenylalanine and 6-^{18}F-DOPAv (dopamine), have been proposed by Hoegerle et al.[70] and Courgiotis et al.,[71] respectively, with promising results, especially in lymph node staging. Nonetheless, FDG-PET has assumed an increasingly important role in the management of thyroid cancer. The ability of this method to detect many non-iodine-avid tumor foci is of considerable practical utility and is changing the practice of thyroidology. Our own experience suggests that, in patients with thyroid cancer with possible recurrence of non-iodine-avid disease, FDG-PET/CT (ideally under TSH stimulation) is an excellent method to precisely locate recurrent tumors and to direct the surgeon to their precise location if surgical intervention is being considered.

Esophagus

Esophageal cancer is relatively infrequent, with 14,000 new cases reported in the United States in 2003. The 5-year survival rate is not more than 14%.[72] The incidence of the disease is much higher in Asia and Northern France and in some regions of the world where esophageal cancer is endemic.

FDG-PET in Staging Esophageal Carcinoma

The accuracy of endoscopic ultrasonography (EUS) is lower for evaluation of T1 and T2 tumor than for T3 and T4, and the CT scan is inaccurate for identifying nonbulky lymphadenopathy. Neither EUS nor CT is able to distinguish tumor from inflammation. The introduction of FDG-PET has greatly improved the staging of esophageal carcinoma. Squamous cell and adenocarcinomas of the esophagus are both generally characterized by high FDG uptake.[73,74] FDG uptake in esophageal cancer is greater than that in the normal uninflamed esophagus, and the primary tumor can be distinguished easily from background activity in most cases.[75]

FDG-PET false-positive results in the esophagus and nearby tissues can be caused by inflammation (reflux esophagitis), radiation-induced esophagitis, benign tumors, skeletal and adipose tissue uptake, and heterogeneous uptake in the primary, simulating periesophageal nodal metastases.

FDG-PET false-negative results are the result of small tumor volume, well-differentiated tumor, and close proximity to the primary tumor. Histologic confirmation of PET findings is necessary before a patient is denied potentially curative surgery. PET is very useful in identifying a site suitable for biopsy.

FDG-PET has been shown to detect primary esophageal cancer with a higher sensitivity than that of CT (95% to 100% versus 81% to 92%).[73,76–78] Himeno et al.[79] reported that FDG-PET has a sensitivity of 100% for the detection of primary tumors extending to the submucosa (TIb) or deeper, but cannot detect lesions confined to the mucosa (Tis or T1a). Kato et al.[80] described that there is a significant relationship between FDG uptake and the depth of tumor invasion; this is most likely a relationship between tumor volume and invasion (Figure 33.3).

Although PET detects most primary esophageal cancers, it is not as sensitive for nodal metastases. Yoon et al.[81] evaluated 82 patients with squamous cell carcinoma and 677 lesions and found the sensitivity for PET was 30% and that for CT was 11%. This result shows the extent of the problem of nodal staging with both methods. Although PET was more sensitive than CT, both techniques failed to detect small nodal metastases that are often under 1 cm in size. There is considerable variability in the literature concerning nodal staging in esophageal cancer.

The 5-year survival without lymph node involvement is 42% to 72% versus only 10% to 12%[82] for patients with disease that has spread to the lymph nodes. Metastatic lymph node size was the strongest independent predictor of survival among several prognostic factors, such as primary tumor size, histopathologic type, number of metastatic lymph nodes.[83]

The combined accuracy of EUS and CT (70% to 90%) in the detection of mediastinal nodal metastases was reported to be greater than that of each modality alone,[84] but limitations remained because of inability to detect tumor involvement in normal-sized lymph nodes and to differentiate metastatic from inflammatory disease.

Kim et al.[74] compared FDG-PET with CT and histopathologic results from esophagectomy and extensive lymph node dissection. The sensitivity, specificity, and accuracy for FDG-PET to detect metastatic lymph nodes were 52%, 94%, and 84%, respectively, and those for CT were 15%, 97%, and 77%, respectively. That study showed that FDG-PET had greater sensitivity and accuracy than CT, with equal specificity in nodal staging.

Flamen et al.[73] compared FDG-PET (attenuation corrected with spiral CT) and EUS in 74 patients with potentially resectable esophageal cancer and showed that EUS was more sensitive (81% versus 33%) but less specific (67% versus 89%) than PET for detection of regional nodal metastases. Combined EUS and CT were more sensitive (62% versus 33%) and less specific (67% versus 89%) in the same setting. The findings from PET resulted in upstaging in 15% of patients and in downstaging in 7% of patients. PET is a better method for detection of distant metastatic disease than any other method available, but it is not as robust for locoregional disease. PET is routinely recommended before surgery for esophageal carcinoma.

A curative surgical approach is not appropriate in patients with metastases to distant foci. Distant metastatic disease most commonly occurs in distant lymph nodes, liver, and lung. FDG-PET is superior to CT and MRI for detection of distant metastatic disease.[73,74,85–89] FDG-PET uncovered 3% to 37% of findings that were unsuspected. Kinkel et al.[87] reported that at the specificity level of 85% the mean sensitivities of FDG-PET, ultrasound, CT, and MRI were 90%, 55%, 63%, and 76%, respectively.

Flamen et al.[73] demonstrated that the accuracy of FDG-PET in 74 patients with stage IV disease was 82%, whereas it was only 64% for a combination of CT and EUS (*P* less than 0.01). The sensitivity and specificity were 74% and 90% for FDG-PET, 41% and 83% for CT, and 42% and 94% for EUS.

Luketich et al.[88] found, in 35 patients with potentially resectable esophageal cancer, that distant metastatic disease was identified by PET in 20% with an accuracy of 91%. The same group[89] found that the sensitivity and specificity of FDG-PET for detection of distant disease were 69% and 93% for FDG-PET and 46% and 74% for CT.

PET prevents ineffective radical therapies by detection of occult stage IV disease and identification of the local or distant metastases that are most accessible to confirmation by directed tissue sampling using minimally invasive procedures. Wallace et al.[90] found that the combination of PET and EUS with fine-needle aspiration biopsy is the most effective strategy for staging.

Table 33.4 summarizes the results of studies evaluating the sensitivity, specificity, and accuracy of CT, EUS, and FDG-PET for detecting local tumor extension (T and N stages) and systemic disease (M).[73,74,81,89,91–93]

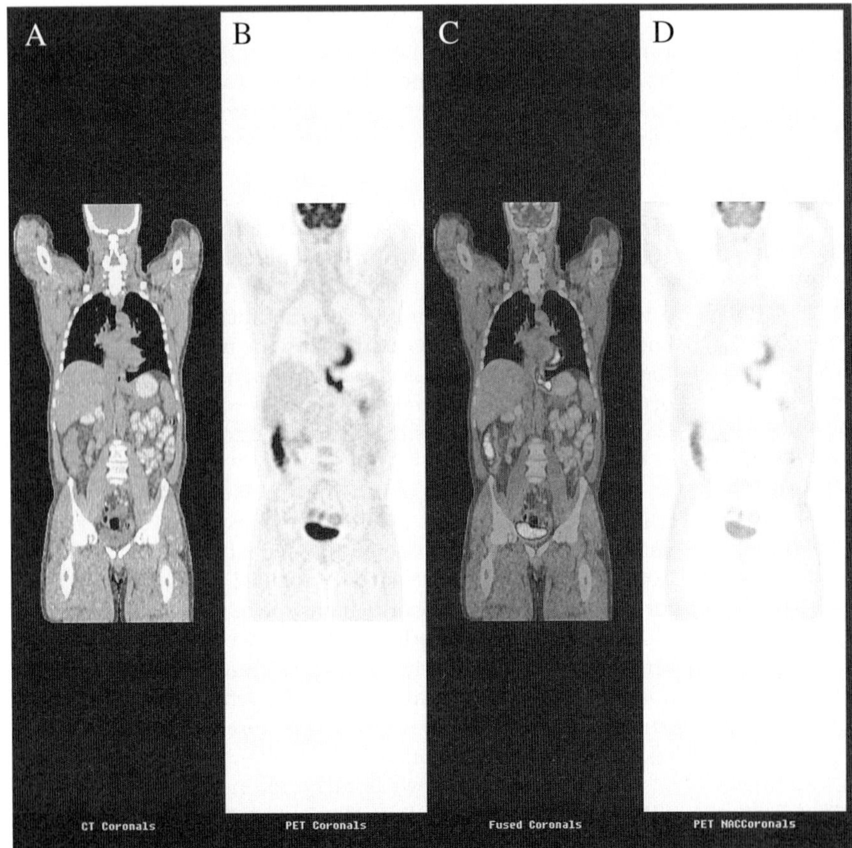

FIGURE 33.3. Coronal PET/CT images obtained from a middle-aged male with a history of gastroesophageal reflux and biopsy-proven esophageal carcinoma. These images show intense tracer uptake in the primary lesion located at the gastroesophageal junction and extending downward into the stomach. No metastatic disease is identified. (A) CT scan. (B) Fused PET/CT image. (C) Attenuation corrected PET image. (D) Nonattenuation corrected PET image.

TABLE 33.4. Comparison of various modalities (CT/EUS with PET) for initial staging of esophageal cancer.

		Sens			*Spec*			*Acc*			
Author	*Year*	*EUS*	*CT*	*PET*	*EUS*	*CT*	*PET*	*EUS*	*CT*	*PET*	*Remarks*
Wren et al.[91] T/N	2002	90 (T) 75 (N)	50 (T) 73 (N)					85 (T) 75 (N)			
Hustinx et al.[92] (M)	2000		46 (M)	69 (M) (NAC)		74 (M)	93 (M) (NAC)				
Flamen et al.[73] (N) Reanalysis	2000	81 (RN)	62 (+ EUS)	33 (RN)	67	67 (+ EUS)	89				
Kim et al.[74] (surgical extent L/N dissection)	2001		15	52		97	94		77	84	
Wu et al.[93] (N)	2003	68	77		75	79					$P < 0.01$
Yoon et al.[81] (N)	2003		11	30		95	82				$P < 0.01$
Luketich et al.[89] (M)	1999		46	69		74	93				$P < 0.01$
Flamen et al.[105] (M)	2000	42	41	74	94	83	90		64 (CT + EUS)	82	22% change of stage
Reanalysis by Lerut[84]	2000		46 (+ EUS)	77		69 (+ EUS)	90				

EUS, endoscopic ultrasound; T, evaluation of T-stage; NAC, nonattenuation corrected images; N, evaluation of lymph nodes; SCT, spiral computed CT; M, distant metastases; RN, regional lymph nodes.

Luketich et al.[89] also demonstrated the 30-month survival rate was 60% in patients with localized disease on PET, as compared with 20% in patients with PET evidence of distant disease. The same numbers for CT, 52% and 38%, respectively, were not significantly different.

Assessment of Response to Treatment

Complete macroscopic and microscopic resection of the primary tumor is a strong independent prognostic factor. Patients with locally advanced disease (T3–T4) after complete resection have a 20% to 31% chance of 5-year survival, whereas there is essentially no chance of a 5-year survival in those with an incomplete resection.[82]

Randomized trials compared patients who received preoperative chemotherapy or chemoradiotherapy followed by surgery with patients who received surgical treatment alone. The results were conflicting,[94] and this was attributed to the fact that the response to chemoradiotherapy was probably not uniform. Nonresponders had a poor prognosis, not only because of their disease but also because of therapy-induced side effects and the delay in surgical treatment. Anatomic imaging modalities cannot differentiate viable tumor from posttherapeutic effects in many instances. The accuracy of EUS for determination of tumor stage after therapy is less than 50%.[95,96]

Several studies demonstrated the usefulness of FDG-PET to predict response either shortly after initiation of therapy or after its completion. Weber et al.[97] studied 40 patients with locally advanced adenocarcinomas of the gastroesophageal junction. PET imaging was performed before preoperative chemotherapy and on day 14 of the first chemotherapy cycle. Changes in tumor FDG uptake at these early time points were correlated with the clinical and histopathologic response after 3 months of chemotherapy. In clinical responders, defined as a decrease of tumor length and wall thickness by more than 50%, FDG uptake at day 14 had decreased by 54% ± 17%, compared with nonresponders, at 15% ± 21%.

Using a threshold of a 35% decrease in the SUV from the baseline metabolic activity, FDG uptake predicted subsequent clinical response with a sensitivity and specificity of 93% and 95%, respectively. Sensitivity and specificity for predicting histopathologic response were 89% and 75%, respectively. The 2-year survival rate of "PET responders" was 49% whereas it was only 9% for "PET nonresponders."

The same authors studied[98] 27 patients with locally advanced squamous cell carcinomas of the esophagus before neoadjuvant chemoradiotherapy and 3 to 4 weeks after completion of therapy. Therapy-induced reduction of tumor FDG uptake was significantly higher for histopathologic responders (72% ± 11%) than for nonresponders (42% ± 22%). Using a threshold of a 51% decrease in the SUV from the baseline metabolic activity for prediction of a response to therapy resulted in a sensitivity of 100% and a specificity of 52%. Brucher et al.[99] and Flamen et al.[100] showed similar results, with the latter using only visual analysis (sensitivity, 71% and specificity, 81%).

Downey et al.[101] studied 24 patients with esophageal cancer who received induction therapy before esophagectomy. The 2-year disease-free survival (DFS) was greater when the tumor showed more than a 60% decrease in FDG uptake. Arslan et al.[102] failed to distinguish residual tumor from postchemoradiation esophagitis using SUV measurements in 24 patients 4 weeks after treatment completion. PET appears to have a greater role in assessing early response than it does in assessing residual tumor (Table 33.5).

Detection of Recurrent Disease

Recurrence is common despite a presumed cure after resection because of micrometastatic disease at distant sites, which can then proliferate. Fukunaga et al.[103] first reported the increased FDG uptake in patients with recurrence. Yeung et al.[104] and Flamen et al.[105] studied recurrent disease. The latter study showed that FDG-PET was comparable to or somewhat inferior to conventional imaging. The sensitivity, specificity, and accuracy for FDG-PET were 100%, 57%, and 74%, respectively, and 100%, 93%, and 96% for conventional imaging. In the detection of regional or distant recurrence, the sensitivity, specificity, and accuracy were 94%, 82%, and

TABLE 33.5. PET in the evaluation of response to therapy for esophageal cancer.

Author	*Year*	*No. of patients*	*Sens*	*Spec*	*PPV*	*NPV*	*DFS (2 years)*	*Remarks*
Brucher et al.[99]	2001	27	100	55	72	100		52% ↓ SUV 3 weeks ($P < 0.0001$)
Weber et al.[98]	2004	27	100	52				51% ↓ SUV 3–4 weeks after therapy
Flammen et al.[100]	2002	36	71	81				Visual 3–4 weeks
Weber et al.[97]	2001	40	93	95				35% ↓ SUV
Downey et al.[101]	2003	24					67%	SUV ↓ 60% (OS same)

SUV, standard uptake value; DFS, disease-free survival; OS, overall survival;

87% for FDG-PET and 81%, 82%, and 81%, respectively, for conventional imaging. In practice PET has been useful for detecting recurrent disease and is complementary to CT.

In summary, PET with FDG is a useful diagnostic tool for esophageal carcinoma. It is generally used at initial diagnosis to perform whole-body staging and to determine the baseline metabolic rate of the tumors. It then can be used to follow the response to locoregional or systemic therapies. Large declines in FDG uptake after therapy are associated with a better response than a modest decline in tracer uptake. PET cannot detect microscopic disease or even disease under a few millimeters in size with current technology. This is a continuing limitation as is the uptake of FDG into inflammatory cells after treatment. Nonetheless, FDG-PET is established as an important tool at several points in the management of patients with esophageal carcinoma. PET/CT is the preferred embodiment of this application at present, but literature to strongly support the superiority of PET/CT over PET is limited at this time.

Lung

Non-small cell lung cancer (NSCLC) is the leading cause of cancer death in men and women in the United States. It has surpassed breast cancer as the number one cancer killer of women. When it is diagnosed early, the prognosis is relatively good, with greater than a 60% 5-year survival for stage I disease compared to only 14% for all patients.[106] The primary treatment of lung cancer is surgery (if it is indicated), but once nodal or distant metastases have developed, the correct type of therapy is adjuvant chemotherapy or radiation therapy. Correct staging is the mainstay of appropriate clinical management.

FDG-PET is a valuable noninvasive imaging test for detecting malignancy in solitary pulmonary nodules (SPNs), for staging or restaging NSCLC, for monitoring therapy, and for detecting residual or recurrent disease, and, finally, it provides prognostic information that is independent of lesion size, clinical stage, and cell type. It contributes to better informed medical decision making and more cost-effective medical care.

Diagnosis of NSCLC and Evaluation of Pulmonary Nodules

In the United States, approximately 150,000 indeterminate pulmonary nodules are discovered each year and between 30% and 50% of these are malignant.[107,108] The incidence of cancer is not low enough to ignore it, nor is it high enough to decide to resect all nodules.

Chest radiography and CT scan can establish the benign nature of a lesion. Certain patterns of calcification (likelihood ratio, 0.07) or the presence of fat within the nodule or a low growth rate over 2 years (likelihood ratio, 0.01) are diagnostic of a benign etiology.[109] CT provides some assessment of the likelihood of malignancy based on morphology and the presence of secondary findings, such as hilar or mediastinal adenopathy, but the vast majority of SPNs are indeterminate by radiographic or CT criteria.[110]

Biopsy by CT-guided transthoracic needle aspiration and bronchoscopy are helpful when positive, but because of sampling error, a benign result cannot exclude tumor. On the other hand, more invasive procedures, such as thoracoscopic or surgical biopsy, are associated with increased cost and morbidity.[111] FDG-PET and contrast-enhanced dynamic CT (dCT) are accurate, noninvasive methods for diagnosing lung cancer.

Lowe et al.[112] showed that FDG-PET has an overall sensitivity of 92% and a specificity of 90% in a study of 89 patients with nodules between 0.7 and 4.0 cm in diameter using a SUV cutoff of 2.5 or greater. Another criterion is if nodules are hyperintense compared to the mediastinum. With application of these two criteria, FDG-PET is approximately 96% sensitive and 80% specific for malignancy.

False-positive results may be caused by the increased glycolytic activity within activated macrophages. Active granulomatous diseases can be FDG avid, such as tuberculosis,[113] sarcoidosis,[114] aspergillosis,[115] histoplasmosis,[116] or lipoid pneumonia and talc granulomata after pleurodesis,[117] and pneumonitis and necrosis after high-dose radiation therapy.[118] False-negative results can occur in some low-grade tumors, including bronchoalveolar carcinoma[119] and bronchial carcinoid.[120] Lesions that are near the limiting spatial resolution of the PET scanner (about 6 mm on newer systems) may be falsely negative because of the effect of the volume averaging (partial volume effect).

In a meta-analysis of 40 studies of 1,474 focal pulmonary lesions, Gould et al.[121] reported a sensitivity of FDG-PET of 92% (95% confidence interval, range 89%–93%). They noted that in practice the sensitivity of 97% and a specificity of 78% decrease false-negative results. A nodule less than 1 cm should be considered worrisome for malignancy if any FDG accumulation is seen.

Dynamic CT uses intravenous iodinated contrast material to measure nodule perfusion, and this information provides an estimate of the likelihood of malignancy. A pre-

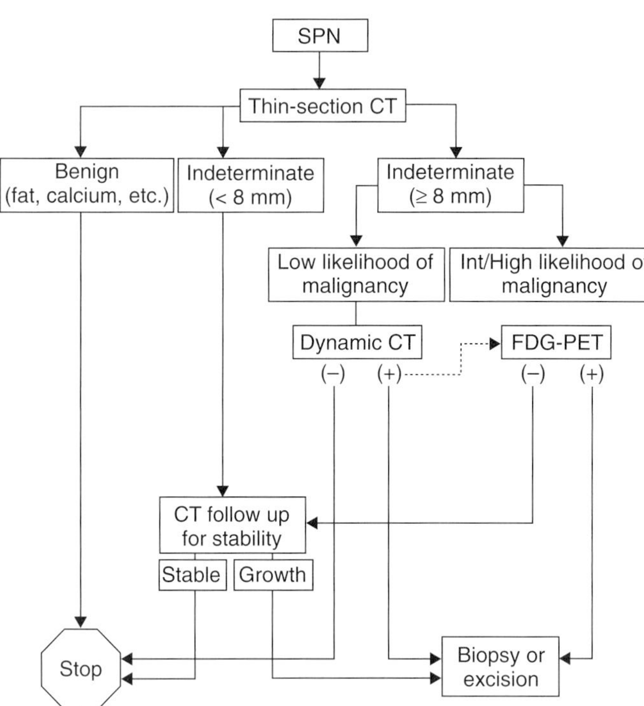

FIGURE 33.4. Diagnostic algorithm for lung nodules.

contrast density measurement in Hounsfield units (HU) is obtained after a bolus injection of contrast material, and density measurements are performed at 1, 2, 3, and 4 min. Enhancing nodules are presumed to be malignant and nonenhancing nodules are presumed to be benign. Using a threshold of 15 HU, this technique has a sensitivity of 98%, a specificity of 58%, an accuracy of 77%, and a very high negative predictive value (Swensen et al.[122]).

Nathan et al.,[123] in a recent study of 36 patients, evaluated pulmonary nodules larger than 8 mm with both FDG-PET and dCT. The overall sensitivity and specificity for FDG-PET were 95% and 80%, respectively (using the criteria referred to above), and for dCT (with a cutoff of 15 HU) were 100% and 27%, respectively.

Rohren et al.[124] suggested a diagnostic algorithm as is shown in Figure 33.4. A negative dCT scan can confidently exclude malignancy, but after a positive dCT the patients should be followed with an FDG-PET study, because one-half of them can be shown to be truly negative with PET imaging. All this staging information can be used to plan subsequent diagnostic strategies (percutaneous needle biopsy or mediastinoscopy) and to guide appropriate therapy.

One in 10 to 1 in 20 pulmonary nodules that are negative by FDG-PET imaging may, in fact, be malignant. One approach is to follow patients with a negative PET scan with serial CT examinations. A negative PET scan excludes high-grade lung carcinoma, so the risk of following patients over 1 to 2 years for nodule growth is low. Most of them are T1N0M0 at the time of surgery.[125]

Zhuang et al.[126] and Matthies et al.[127] proposed dual-time PET imaging and thought this was suitable for nodules near the level of the cutoff value of 2.5 for SUV.

Relative FDG uptake in malignant nodules tends to increase between the scans, whereas the relative FDG uptake in benign nodules tends to remain stable or decrease slightly. Using a threshold of a 10% increase in SUV between 1 and 3 hours led to an increase in sensitivity for FDG-PET from 80% to 100%. The specificity, however, declined from 94% to 89% (Table 33.6). Demura et al.[128] reported the significance of dual time point PET imaging in the staging of disease of the mediastinum.

Staging NSCLC

The most standardized staging system is the TNM system. T denotes features of the primary mass, including size, location, and invasion, N denotes regional lymph node status, and M the presence or absence of metastatic disease.[124]

Because most patients have had a diagnostic CT before referral for FDG-PET, the PET scan is used mainly for assigning T stage (1) for the evaluation of the likelihood of malignancy in additional pulmonary nodules and to direct a confirmatory biopsy to them and (2) for the identification of malignant pleural effusions, which may be reactive or malignant, as CT cannot distinguish them.

In a study of 100 patients with newly diagnosed bronchogenic carcinoma, Marom et al.[129] compared staging with FDG-PET to staging obtained with a chest CT scan, a bone scan, and contrasted brain CT or MRI. For overall staging FDG-PET had an accuracy of 83%, whereas with conventional imaging it was 65% (*P* less than 0.005) (Table 33.7).

For mediastinal lymph nodes, PET had an accuracy of 85% and for conventional imaging it was 58%. The important point here was that 9% of PET-positive studies were CT negative and 10% of PET-negative studies were CT false positive. In N3 stage disease, the sensitivity and specificity of PET were 92% and 93%, respectively, and for CT they were 25% and 98% (*P* less than 0.005). In M stage, the PET scan

TABLE 33.6. Representative literature of FDG-PET findings in initial diagnosis of non-small cell lung cancer (NSCLC).

Author	Year	No. of patients	PET criteria (SUV or visual)	Sens		Spec		Acc	
				PET	CT	PET	CT	PET	CT
Swensen et al.[122] (Dynamic CT/threshold 15 HU)	2000	356			38		58		77
Nathan et al.[123]	2003	36	SUV > 2.5 + visual	95	100	80	27		
Matthies et al.[127] (dual time point PET)	2002	36	↑SUV (10%)	100		89			
Gould et al.[121] (meta-analysis)	2001	1474 lesions		97		78			

HU, Hounsfield units; FDG, ^{18}F-fluoro-2-deoxy-D-glucose.

Dual time point PET 1 and 3 hours after injection of FDG-PET.

TABLE 33.7. Studies comparing PET/CI/bone scan in staging of non-small cell lung cancer (NSCLC).

Author	Year	No. of patients	Modality (PET/CI bone scan)	Sens			Spec			Acc			PPV			NPV			Remarks
				PET	CI	BS	PET	CI	BS	PET	CI	BS	PET	CI	BS	PET	CI	BS	
Marom et al.[129]	1999	100	PET/CI							83	65								Overall ($P < 0.001$)
			PET/CI							85	58								Mediastinal ($P < 0.001$)
			PET/CI	92	25		93	98											N3 stage ($P < 0.001$)
			PET/CI							91	80								M stage
			PET/BS	92		50	99		92				92		50	99		92	Osseous metastases
Dwamena et al.[131] (meta-analysis)	1999	514	PET/CI	79	60		91	77		92	75								
Bury et al.[136] (recurrent or residual)	1999	126	PET/CI	100	72		92	95		96	84		92	93		100	79		

BS, bone scan; CI, conventional imaging.

was 91% accurate and conventional imaging was 80%. FDG PET also was superior to bone scintigraphy for evaluating osseous metastases from lung cancer: sensitivity, specificity, PPV, and NPV for FDG-PET were 92%, 99%, 92%, and 99%, respectively, and for bone scintigraphy these were 50%, 92%, 50%, and 92%.

Erasmus et al.[130] showed that FDG-PET was very sensitive and specific for evaluating adrenal metastases.

Metastatic disease to regional lymph nodes is categorized by location in relationship to the tumor. For N0 disease, the 5-year survival is 60%, for N2 it is 20%, and for N3 it is very poor.[106]

The "gold standard" method for mediastinal lymph node staging is supposed to be mediastinoscopy. The overall sensitivity of the "gold standard" is approximately 90%, and it has the disadvantage of sampling errors and the technical difficulty of obtaining overall coverage with a single entry port (i.e., inaccessibility in the aortopulmonary window lymph nodes).[124]

On the other hand, CT uses size criteria to assess nodal metastases (1 cm in the short axis dimension). The limitation of this approach is that enlarged nodes may reflect inflammatory changes rather than metastatic involvement and small nodes may contain tumor deposits. Dwamena et al.,[131] in a meta-analysis of 514 patients, reported that the sensitivity, specificity, and accuracy of FDG-PET were 79%, 91%, and 92%, respectively, and those of CT were 60%, 77%, and 75%. The average sensitivity of PET for nodal disease from a variety of studies[132–135] was 88% as compared with 63% for CT, and the average specificity was 91% for PET and 76% for CT.

The most common sites of metastases from lung carcinoma include lung (additional pulmonary lobes or to the contralateral lung), brain, adrenals, bone, and, less commonly, in liver and soft tissue.

Monitoring Therapy and Detection of Residual or Recurrent Disease

FDG-PET provides metabolic rather than anatomic information and allows functional assessment of lung tumors during or shortly after therapy. Patients with a complete resolution of FDG uptake in their tumor following therapy have been shown to have a good prognosis, as compared to those who have residual FDG uptake in their tumors. After treatment it is not necessary to find visible alterations in gross anatomic structure, but some posttreatment effects do occur. Tissue necrosis and concomitant macrophage-mediated inflammation after radiotherapy usually lead to the delay of a follow-up PET scan for 3 to 6 months. Radiographic findings usually peak within 6 to 12 weeks following completion of therapy and resolve by 6 months. The typical appearance on PET is diffuse low-grade or intermediate-grade FDG activity confined to a geographic field corresponding to the radiation port.

Bury et al.,[136] in a study of 126 patients with stage I to IIIB NSCLC treated with radiation therapy, showed that in detection of residual or recurrent disease FDG-PET had a sensitivity, specificity, accuracy, PPV, and NPV of 100%, 92%, 96%, 92%, and 100%, respectively, and the values for CT were 72%, 95%, 84%, 93%, and 79%. Because of its high sensitivity and negative predictive value, the investigators concluded that FDG-PET was a useful adjunct to CT in monitoring the effects of radiation therapy.

Prognostic Information and Future Trends in PET Imaging

FDG-PET is used in determining planning target volumes (PTV), target coverage, and critical organ dose for radiotherapy. In one study, inclusion of a PET scan resulted in a change in PTV in approximately 30% of the patients[137] because of more accurate delineation of metabolically active tumor. In another study, PTV was changed in all patients after inclusion of a PET scan in the preprocedure evaluation.[138] It has been shown that FDG uptake in NSCLC correlates with the grade of the primary tumor, but it is an independent risk factor.[139]

Ahuja et al.[140] showed that FDG-PET provides prognostic information that is entirely independent of a tumor's size and clinical stage at the time of diagnosis. When the SUV in the primary tumor was less than 10, the median patient survival was 24.6 months. If it was greater than 10, survivals fell to 11.4 months. If the SUV was greater than 10 and the primary lesion was larger than 3 cm, survival was only 5.7 months. Dhital et al.[141] reported that the 1-year survival of patients with tumor SUV_{max} less than 10 was 75% and with SUV_{max} greater than 20 it was only 17%.

Radiolabeled thymidine, a marker of DNA synthesis, choline agents (for the evaluation of membrane synthesis and turnover), and radiolabeled amino acids (for the evaluation of protein catabolism), are many of the agents that are under investigation for potential utility in patients with NSCLC.[142,143]

Breast

Breast cancer is the most common malignancy in women in the United States and is the second leading cause of cancer death in women. It represents 31% of all cancers in women. It is estimated that nearly 190,000 new cases appear every year and that 40,000 women die of breast cancer yearly.[144,145] Brown et al.[146] described the marked overexpression of the GLUT-1 glucose transporter in human breast cancer and the correlation between tumor FDG uptake and the number of viable tumor cells. Biochemical imaging using PET offers significant advantages and provides unique information about the physiologic processes associated with cancer.

Early studies[147–149] in patients with locally advanced breast cancer (LABC) or metastatic disease reported that FDG-PET detected the majority of the lesions, but the selection bias of patients with advanced disease did not allow determination of the specificity. Several subsequent clinical studies have shown that FDG-PET has a sensitivity ranging from 63% to 93% and specificity ranging from 73% to 94%[150–154] (Table 33.8).

Adler et al.[155] reported a sensitivity of 96% in 27 primary lesions. Using a standard uptake value (SUV) threshold of 2 to 2.5, they were able to differentiate malignant from benign lesions with approximately 90% accuracy. Dehdashti et al.[156] found a sensitivity of 88% and specificity of 100% using a SUV of 2.0 as the cutoff number to discriminate malignancy. In a recent meta-analysis[154] of the PET literature, data from 606 patients indicated that FDG-PET had a sensitivity of 88% [95% confidence interval (CI), 83%–92%] and a specificity of 79% (95% CI, 71%–85%) (Figure 33.5).

FDG-PET has limitations in detecting (1) tumors smaller than 1 cm), (2) more well-differentiated histologic subtypes of tumors (tubular carcinoma and in situ carcinoma), and (3) lobular carcinomas.

Avril et al.[150] demonstrated that the sensitivity for detecting tumors larger than 1 cm using sensitive imaging reading criteria (definite and probable FDG uptake) was 57%, compared with 91% (with conventional image reading) for tumors larger than 1 cm. The sensitivity for detecting carcinoma in situ was even lower at 25%, and there was a significantly higher false-negative rate with infiltrating lobular carcinoma (65%) than with infiltrating ductal carcinoma (24%). In the same study, they showed that the overall sensitivity of FDG-PET for detecting breast cancer was improved by using a more sensitive threshold for image interpretation compared to a conventional threshold (80% versus 64%), although the overall specificity was significantly poorer (75% versus 94%). They also reported a sensitivity of 50% for the identification of multifocal or multicentric breast cancer. Although breast conservation therapy has become standard for treating early breast cancer, it cannot be applied in these subsets of patients because up to 41% of breast cancers are multifocal or multicentric.[157]

Schirrmeister et al.[151] demonstrated that PET was twofold more sensitive (63%) than combined mammography and ultrasound (32%) to detect multifocal lesions. The specificity was not different between these approaches.

The disadvantages of FDG-PET, such as high expense, modest whole-body radiation exposure, and a low accuracy in general screening, have prompted the development of high-resolution PET scanners dedicated to breast imaging with the capability of coregistering PET and mammographic images.[158–160] The spatial resolution of these scanners is 2.8 mm full width at half maximum, about half that of current whole-body PET instruments, and they can utilize a lower dose of radiotracer and decreased acquisition time.

The level of FDG uptake in an untreated breast cancer has prognostic information that may help to (1) stratify patients according to risk for recurrence or treatment failure and (2) target the aggressiveness of therapy for an individual patient to the aggressiveness of her tumor.

FDG uptake has a strong correlation with the histologic type (higher in ductal versus lobular),[161–163] tumor histologic grade,[161,164,165] indices of proliferation (higher uptake with higher levels of proliferation),[162,163] microscopic tumor growth

TABLE 33.8. FDG-PET results in initial diagnosis of breast cancer.

			Sensitivity		*Specificity*	
Author	*Year*	*No. of patients*	*PET*	*CT/MRI*	*PET*	*CT/MRI*
Avril et al.[150]	2000	22 (<1 cm) 170 (>1 cm) 12 (in situ)	57% (SIR) 91% (SIR) 25% (SIR)		90	
Schirrmeister et al.[151]	2001	117	93		75	
Walter et al.[152]	2003	40	63	89	91	74
Heinisch et al.[153]	2003	36	76	95	73	73
Samson et al.[154]	2001	606	88		79	
Meta-analysis (size, 2–4 cm diameter)	(1993–2000)		(95% CI: 83%–92%)		(95% CI: 71%–85%)	
Avril et al.[150]	2000	144 (all sizes)	64 (CIR) 80 (SIR)		94 (CIR) 75 (SIR)	

SIR, sensitive image reading; CIR, conventional image reading.

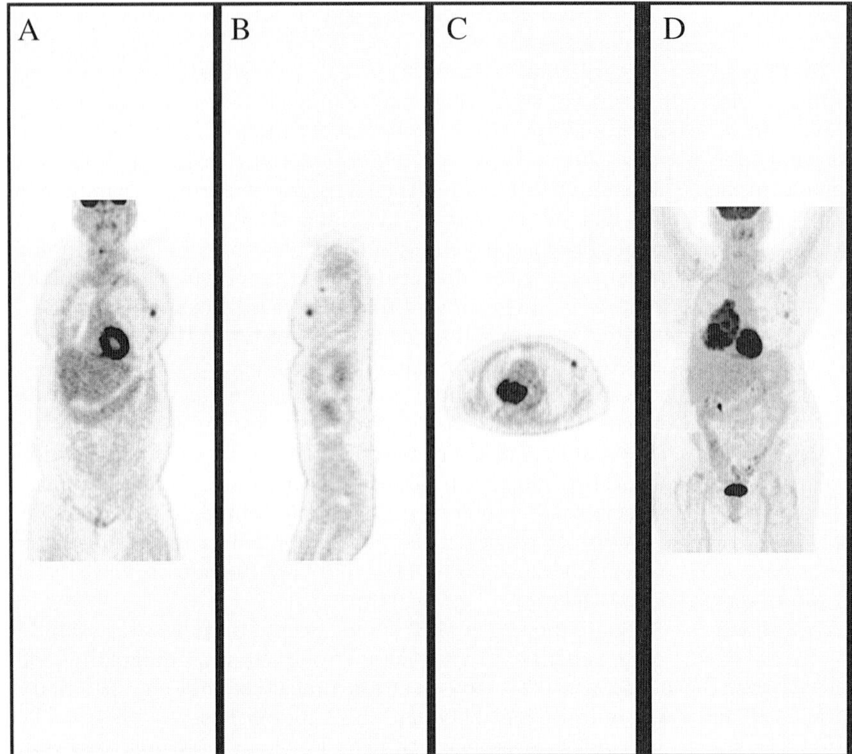

FIGURE 33.5. Transverse (C), coronal (A), sagittal (B), and maximum image projection (MIP) (D) (projection) PET images that demonstrate intense uptake of FDG in primary lung cancer (small cell). A previously unsuspected primary breast carcinoma is seen in the left breast.

pattern[162] (nodular versus diffuse), and S phase.[164,165] A weaker correlation with FDG has been reported for microvessel density, a surrogate of angiogenesis,[166,167] and tumor cell density.[162,167]

No correlation was found between FDG uptake and tumor size,[162,163,168] axillary node status,[161,162,163] steroid receptor status,[162,163,168,169] the presence of inflammatory cells,[162] percentage of necrotic, fibrotic, and cystic components,[162] or the thymidine labeling index (LI).[168]

Oshida et al.[166] and Mankoff et al.[171] found that FDG uptake in the primary tumor is predictive of response to treatment and patient outcome, even when they are treated with a variety of different protocols.

Eubank et al.[170] assumed that FDG uptake may be a marker of tumor cell resistance to apoptosis, and this was supported by other studies.[172,173] Intermediates in the glucolytic pathway are key factors in initiating apoptosis, and alterations in these pathways limit apoptosis. Overexpression of some genes is associated with high glucolytic rates and resistance to apoptosis. An example is the P13K/Akt pathway.

Lymph Node Staging

The single most important prognostic factor in early stage breast cancer is the status of the axillary lymph nodes. The 10-year survival rate of patients with histologically negative axillary nodes (65% to 80%) is significantly higher than that of those with involvement of one to three nodes (38% to 63%) or more than three axillary nodes (13% to 27%).[174] The extent of axillary disease influences the choice of the therapeutic regimen for individual patients. Many studies using FDG-PET for axillary staging showed a sensitivity of 40% to 94% and a specificity of 80% to 100%.[154,175–180]

Because neither physical examination nor conventional imaging can detect axillary nodal metastases, lymph node dissection (either conventional or limited with the use of sentinel node localization) is routinely performed to assess axillary nodal status in all patients with invasive cancers of 20mm or less (80% or more of these patients have negative axillary lymph nodes). The risk of axillary nodal metastases is reported to be less than 5% in patients with tubular carcinoma less than 1cm in diameter, grade I tumors less than 5mm in diameter, or tumors with a single focus of microinvasion.

With the introduction of step sectioning and immunohistochemical staining, micrometastases can be detected in up to 45% of cases.[181] Microscopic nodal involvement may be important for prognosis and treatment planning, and FDG-PET will miss this.[182]

Avril et al.[180] found that the sensitivity of FDG-PET for detecting axillary disease in patients with T1 tumors (33%) was significantly less than for patients with tumors larger than 2cm (94%). The specificity (100%) was the same for both subgroups. It has also been shown that the number of nodes involved with tumor at dissection influenced the sensitivity of PET (Table 33.9).

In preclinical studies of several types of tumors, including rat mammary tumors, Wahl et al.[183] showed that FDG uptake in lymph nodes involved by metastatic tumor is greater than FDG uptake in normal lymph nodes. In a recent multicenter study involving 308 axilla sites, the same investigators reported a moderate accuracy of FDG-PET and a

TABLE 33.9. FDG-PET results for detection of axillary lymph node metastases.

Study	*Year*	*No. of patients*	*Sens*	*Spec*
Wahl et al.[175]	2004	308	61	80
Kumar et al.[176]	2004	49	40	100
Zornoza et al.[177]	2004	100	84	98
Greco et al.[178]	2001	167	94 [68/72]	86 [82/95]
Schrirrmeister et al.[179]	2001	113	79 [27/34]	92 [73/79]
Avril et al.[180]	1996 all sizes	51	79 [19/24]	96 [26/27]
Stage T1		18	33 [2/6]	100 [12/12]
Stage >T1		23	94 [17/18]	100 [5/5]

Numbers in brackets are patient numbers used to derive sensitivity and specificity values.

mean sensitivity and specificity of 61% and 80%, respectively, when at least one focus of abnormal axillary uptake was detected.[185]

A recent meta-analysis found that FDG-PET has a higher sensitivity for predicting lymph node metastases in the axilla of patients with palpable axillary nodes, 90%, than for those having nonpalpable nodes, 69%, but lower specificity, 88% versus 94%.[154] Greco et al.[178] showed that in primary breast cancers, the detection rate for axillary nodal disease by FDG-PET depended on the size of the primary lesion, with an overall sensitivity and specificity of 94% and 86%, respectively.

Sentinel lymph node mapping is now a validated, minimally invasive technique that includes histologic analysis of the primary draining nodes in the axilla identified at surgery after perilesional injection of ^{99m}Tc-sulfur colloid and/or blue dye.[186]

FDG-PET has been reported to have a sensitivity in the range of 20% to 50%[185–187] in patients with pathologic results from sentinel lymph node (SLN) biopsy. In more advanced disease, however, especially with palpable axillary nodes, a large volume of disease ("packed" SLN) may not be visualized at mapping because lymph flow is diverted around it, and this may potentially result in a false-negative examination.[188]

Lymphatic spread of tumor to the internal mammary (IM) nodes occurs in up to 25% of patients at the time of initial diagnosis and more commonly in recurrence.[189] IM nodes are not as accessible as axillary nodes, and radiotherapy and lymphadenectomy did not seem to improve patient survival.[157] For these reasons, they are not sampled, although the presence of IM-FDG uptake predicts treatment failure.

Detection of Distant Metastatic Disease and Recurrence

The most common sites of locoregional recurrence among patients following mastectomy, axillary node dissection, and radiation therapy are the chest wall and supraclavicular nodes.[190] FDG-PET is a sensitive method for detecting metastases in the brachial plexus in patients with breast cancer.[191,192] Eubank et al.,[193] in a study of 73 patients with recurrent or metastatic breast cancer, demonstrated that FDG uptake in mediastinal or IM nodes was two times more prevalent than suspiciously enlarged nodes by CT. The sensitivity of FDG-PET was 85%, much higher than CT (50%), with nearly the same specificity (90% for PET and 83% for CT). Of these, 30% of patients suspected of having only locoregional recurrence by conventional imaging and clinical examination had mediastinal or IM-FDG uptake. Moon et al.[194] reported an overall lesion-by-lesion sensitivity of 85% for FDG-PET and a specificity of 79%.

Gallowitsch et al.[195] reported sensitivity, specificity, PPV, NPV, and accuracy of 97%, 82%, 87%, 96%, and 90%, respectively, for FDG-PET, compared with 84%, 60%, 73%, 75%, and 74%, respectively, for CT. Lonneux et al.,[196] in a study of 39 patients (asymptomatic) with a rise in tumor makers, showed that FDG-PET detected recurrences with 94% sensitivity, whereas conventional imaging had a sensitivity of 18%. Kamel et al.,[197] in a study of 60 similar patients, found an overall sensitivity, specificity, and accuracy of 89%, 84%, and 87%, respectively, for locoregional recurrence and found it more sensitive than the serum tumor marker CA15-3 (Table 33.10). Inoue et al.[198] demonstrated that the patients

TABLE 33.10. FDG-PET results for detection of recurrent/distant metastases.

			Sens		*Spec*		*Acc*		*PPV*		*NPV*	
Study	*Year*	*No. of patients*	*PET*	*CT/MRI*	*PET*	*CT/MRI*	*PET*	*CT/MRI*	*PET*	*CT/MRI*	*PET*	*CT/MRI*
Moon et al.[194]	1998	57	85	—	79	—	—	—	82	—	92	—
Eubank et al.[193]	2001	73	85	50	90	83	88	73				
Gallowitch et al.[195]	2003	62	97	84	82	60	90	74	87	73	96	75
Lonneux et al.[196] (clinical suspected recurrence)	2000	39	94	18	50							
Kamel et al.[197]	2003	60	89		84		87					

with a higher SUV had a significantly poorer prognosis than those patients with lower values.

The skeleton is the most common site of distant metastases in breast cancer. Bone scintigraphy is considered the most sensitive method for detecting and determining the extent of skeletal metastases. However, purely lytic lesions or metastases confined to the marrow cavity may be difficult to detect on a bone scan, due to the lack of a sufficient osteoblastic response.[199] Cook et al.[200] reported that the level of FDG uptake in lytic lesions was significantly greater compared with osteoblastic lesions and that the prognosis of patients with predominantly lytic disease was significantly worse.

Osseous metastases are a frequent finding in breast cancer; approximately 70% of patients with advanced disease have an osseous metastasis, which is a major contributor to morbidity and treatment cost.[201] The median survival for these patients is 24 months and the 5-year survival is 20%. Breast cancer causes osteolytic more often than osteoblastic metastatic lesions, although osteoblastic changes often develop after treatment.

The reported higher sensitivity of FDG-PET for detection of osteolytic lesions likely reflects the ability of FDG-PET to detect metastatic deposits in the bone marrow before the development of a significant reactive bone formation that is necessary for detection by bone scintigraphy. FDG-PET detection of osseous metastatic disease appears to be unrelated to reactive bone formation, but rather is related to detection of the metabolic activity of the tumor cells.

^{18}F-Fluoride PET may provide improved detection of bone metastases in breast cancer, and in other tumors, because its concentration is approximately twofold greater than that of ^{99m}Tc-methylene disphosphonate (^{99m}Tc-MDP) and its clearance is faster, resulting in a higher bone to background ratio. Schirrmeister et al.[202] compared a whole-body ^{18}F-PET scan with a whole body ^{99m}Tc-MDP scan and demonstrated that the former detected more lesions in more patients than the conventional bone scan. Finally, it was found that FDG-PET changed the clinical stage in 36% of patients with breast cancer and the management in 58%.[203]

Monitoring Treatment Response

Neoadjuvant chemotherapy (NACT) is the standard therapy for patients with locally advanced breast cancer (LABC). NACT is associated with a good response rate in more than 70% of the patients, including a complete pathologic remission in about 10% to 15%.[204] It has been used to improve primary tumor resectability (including the use of breast-conserving surgery) and to assess chemosensitivity to selected chemotherapeutic agents. It can also be used as an alternative therapy for patients who are unresectable or chemoresistant.

Conventional imaging methods are limited in assessing response to therapy, and often a delay of several weeks after completion of therapy is required before the effectiveness of the treatment can be assessed. Wahl et al.[205] reported that metabolic changes could be detected as early as 8 days post-treatment in responders. Persistent FDG uptake is seen in nonresponding patients.

Schelling et al.[206] and Smith et al.[207] were able to separate responders from nonresponders with sensitivities of 90% and 100% and specificities of 74% and 85% after the first course of chemotherapy. Their results were similar although they used a different SUV cutoff.

In assessing the response to chemotherapy, Vranjesevic et al.[208] noted, in a study of 61 patients using FDG-PET and conventional imaging (CT/MRI/US), that the former was more accurate (90% versus 75%).

Other biologic and physiologic tumor properties may be responsible for clinical prognosis. For example, imaging with ^{15}O-water can estimate regional blood flow within a tumor. Low perfusion may be responsible for a poor response to intravenous chemotherapy.[209] Mankoff et al.[210] showed that blood flow declined an average of 32% in responders and increased an average of 48% in nonresponders. The posttherapy blood flow measurement was the only statistically significant variable associated with improved disease-free survival. Using PET in this way may help to identify the physiologic manifestations of drug resistance.

Patients with breast cancer undergoing chemotherapy often receive the hematopoietic cytokines, granulocyte colony-stimulating factor (G-CSF) or granulocyte macrophage colony-stimulating factor (GM-CSF). The use of these agents results in an increase in bone marrow uptake of FDG, which may be misinterpreted as diffuse bone marrow involvement by breast cancer. The higher bone marrow background activity after cytokine therapy may make it more difficult to detect osseous metastases.

Sugawara et al.[211] studied the effects of G-CSF and GM-CSF on the biodistribution of FDG in rats and found that SUV_{lean} (SUV corrected for lean body mass) of the bone marrow was greater during G-CSF treatment than the baseline level. Markedly increased FDG uptake is also often seen in the spleen because of extramedullary hematopoiesis in the spleen.[211,212]

Smith et al.[213] and Gennari et al.[214] showed by quantitative methods that a significant reduction in axillary nodal FDG uptake after neoadjuvant chemotherapy could predict a complete microscopic pathologic response, and that may be an even more important marker for prognosis because nodal disease is thought to reflect the presence of occult disseminated disease.

Stafford et al.[215] evaluated the response of skeletal metastases to therapy using serial FDG-PET and found a strong correlation between the quantitative change in FDG SUV and the overall clinical assessment of response, assessed with physical examination, conventional imaging, and change in tumor markers.

Mortimer et al.[216] reported a series of 40 patients who underwent FDG-PET for the evaluation of response to tamoxifen 7 to 10 days after institution of therapy. FDG uptake predicted a subsequent response to therapy consistent with a "metabolic flare."

Other PET Tracers

Energy metabolism is associated not only with tumor growth, but also with a variety of other biologic processes, such as inflammation or tissue repair. Other PET tracers have been used for staging and guiding treatment by identifying therapeutic targets, by identifying factors associated with resistance to therapy, and by making early assessments of therapeutic response.

Decreased tumor proliferation is an early event in response to successful treatment.[217] Thymidine is incorporated into

DNA but not RNA, so its uptake and retention in the tumor serves as a specific marker of cell growth. Shields et al.[218] showed that ^{11}C-thymidine could be used in assessing early response to treatment. The ^{18}F analogue of thymidine (FLT) has been used because its longer half-life is an advantage.[219–221] FLT has been used to measure the response to treatment in several different tumor types, including breast cancer.

Tumor hypoxia has been established as a resistance factor for radiotherapy, and evolving evidence indicates that it promotes tumor aggressiveness and resistance to a variety of systemic treatment modalities.[222,223] Hypoxia could not be reliably predicted by FDG uptake,[224] although it contributes to increased rates of glycolysis, as was shown by Clavo et al.[225] The most widely used PET agent for imaging hypoxia is ^{18}F-fluoromisonidazole.[226] PET imaging of hypoxia holds great promise for identifying the subset of breast cancers with significant hypoxia, where alternative therapeutic strategies that can overcome the resistance associated with hypoxia will likely be needed.

The majority of breast cancers express estrogen receptors (ER) and progesterone receptors (PR), and their expression is an indicator of prognosis and predicts the likelihood of responding to antiestrogen therapy.[227] Most breast cancers are hormone sensitive, requiring estrogen for proliferation. Currently, tumor ERs and PRs are evaluated by in vitro assays, but these assays provide limited information about the functional status of the receptors and the likely responsiveness of the tumor to hormone therapy. Only 55% to 60% of patients with ER(+) disease actually respond to hormonal therapy [versus fewer than 10% of patients with ER(−) disease].[228,229] Furthermore, ER expression can be heterogeneous in large or metastatic breast cancers, and biopsy can be misleading as a result of sampling error.

The most extensively studied compound is 16α-^{18}F-fluoro-17β-estradiol (FES), which showed an excellent correlation between tumor FES uptake measured on PET images and the ER concentration of the tumor determined by conventional quantitative ligand binding assays[230] or by immunohistochemistry,[231] either in the primary tumor or in metastatic lesions. FES-PET has been shown to be highly sensitive (93%) for detection of ER(+) metastatic foci[232] at an acceptable radiation dose to the patient.[233] Mankoff et al.[234] showed heterogeneous FES uptake within the same tumor and between metastatic lesions, both qualitatively and quantitatively, which can help in establishing prognosis and in guiding treatment selection.

In patients with known metastatic breast cancer, FES uptake decreased after the initial therapeutic dose of tamoxifen, and this is presumably related to the nonavailability of ERs to interact with FES because the receptors were occupied by tamoxifen and its bioactive metabolites. This finding shows that the tumor uptake of FES appears to be a receptor-mediated process.

Dehdashti et al.[235] found no significant relationship between FDG uptake and either ER status or FES uptake. FES-PET and in vitro ER assays agreed in 88% of patients. Mortimer et al.[236] reported that patients with FES(+) disease had longer survival than those with FES(−) tumors. When there is a high degree of ER blockade in the primary tumor (about 50% decrease in SUV from baseline), a good response to therapy is predicted.[237]

Within 7 to 10 days after the initiation of hormonal treatment, a small number of patients (5% to 20%) experience a phenomenon known as the hormonal flare reaction, with pain in osseous metastatic lesions, pain and erythema in soft tissue lesions, hypocalcemia, and apparent disease progression on bone scintigraphy.[237]

The percent change in FDG uptake and the baseline FES uptake were the best predictors of response to therapy. The PPV for response to tamoxifen with a metabolic flare (an increase in tumor FDG uptake of 10% or more as the cutoff criterion) was 91% and the NPV was 94%. The PPV and NPV for the baseline FES uptake (with a cutoff SUV of 2.0) were 79% and 88%, respectively.[237]

The flare reaction is a strong predictor of response because nearly 80% of the patients who develop this reaction respond to hormonal therapy.[238] Hormonal flare is presumed to represent an initial agonist effect of the drug on the tumor before its antagonist effects supervene.[239]

PET can be used to guide therapy by showing characteristics of the tumor at the biochemical level before therapy or early during therapy.

Gastric Cancer

Gastric cancer is the second most common cause of cancer death in the world, with an overall 5-year survival rate less than 25%.[240] The leading cause for the development of gastric cancer is repeated infection with *Helicobacter pylori*.

There two different types: the intestinal type, which predominantly involves the distal stomach (most common in Asia), and the diffuse or signet-ring type, which mainly involves the proximal stomach (most common in Western countries).

Tumors consisting of signet-ring cells or with large amounts of mucin are frequently false negative by FDG-PET, probably because of a lower expression of glucose transporters in these types of tumors and a lower tumor cell density.[241,242] Even large tumors with a diameter of several centimeters can be falsely negative on FDG-PET if the tumor cells demonstrate low metabolic activity.[243]

Yeung et al.[244] studied 23 patients with gastric cancer and found that FDG-PET had a sensitivity of 93% for detection of gastric cancer, a specificity of 100% for detection of local recurrence, but low sensitivity (22%) and high specificity (97%) for detection of metastatic disease in intraabdominal lymph mode stations.

Stahl et al.[241] reported higher detection rates in the intestinal type (83%) compared with the nonintestinal type (41%). The SUV was greater in the intestinal type (6.7 ± 3.4) than in the nonintestinal type (4.8 ± 2.8). Nonmucinous tumors had higher SUVs (7.2 ± 3.2) than the mucinous ones (3.9 ± 2.1), and the same was true for grade 2 tumors, which had higher FDG uptake than the grade 3 tumors.

Mochiki et al.[245] described the existence of a relationship between the intensity of FDG uptake and survival, which did not agree with the results of Stahl and coworkers.[241] Yoshioka et al.[246] demonstrated the usefulness of FDG-PET in detecting metastatic disease in the liver, lungs, and lymph nodes, but it was not useful for detection of osseous metastases and peritoneal or pleural carcinomatosis. De Potter et al.[243] reported in a study of 33 patients that the sensitivity, speci-

TABLE 33.11. Representative literature of PET findings in the initial diagnosis, recurrence, and response to therapy for gastric cancer.

Author	*Year*	*No. of patients*	*Sens*	*Spec*	*PPV*	*NPV*	*SR (2-year)*	*Remarks*
Yeung et al.[244]	1999	23	22	97				Abdominal lymph node detection
Stahl et al.[241]	2003	40	83 41	(intestinal type) (nonintestinal type)				$P < 0.01$
De Potter et al.[243] (recurrence)	2002	33	70	69	78	60		
Ott et al.[247] (prediction of response)	2003	35	77	86			90	SUV ↓ 35% (cutoff)

SR, survival rate.

ficity, PPV, and NPV of FDG-PET were 70%, 69%, 78%, and 60%, respectively, in the detection of recurrent disease.

Ott et al.[247] have used a 35% decrease from the baseline metabolic activity on day 14 of preoperative chemotherapy to predict tumor response in patients with gastric cancer (Table 33.11). The sensitivity and specificity of FDG-PET for prediction of histopathologic response were 77% and 86%, respectively, and the 2-year overall survival of "responders" compared with that of "nonresponders" was 90% and 25%, respectively.

Colorectal Carcinoma

Colorectal cancer is the third most common cause of cancer in men and women, and it affects 5% of the population in the United States and other Western countries. Approximately 106,000 new cases of colon cancer, 40,570 new cases of rectal cancer, and 57,000 deaths (10% of all cancer deaths) were expected to occur in 2004 in the United States.[248] Most patients (70%) diagnosed with colorectal cancer undergo surgery with curative intent, and the overall survival of 5 years is less than 60%.

The recurrence rate is close to 40% within the 5 years following surgery, with up to 80% of the recurrence appearing in the first 2 years. The most common sites of recurrence are in the liver (20%), in the original local site (12.5%), and in the lungs (8%). Only 20% of patients are amenable to a second surgery with curative intent, and long-term survival is expected in only 30% of these.[249,250]

The diagnosis of colorectal carcinoma is based on colonoscopy and biopsy. Most follow-up strategies include carcinoembryonic antigen (CEA) testing and liver imaging. The use of frequent colonoscopy is still being investigated.

FDG-PET in the Diagnosis and Initial Staging of Colorectal Carcinoma

FDG-PET can usually differentiate benign from malignant lesions (hepatic and pulmonary lesions, indeterminate lymph nodes) and can play an important role in the evaluation of patients with rising tumor markers in the absence of a known source of disease. When these lesions (or metastases) are found with FDG-PET, they may lead to a cancellation of surgery in these patients.

Abdel-Nabi et al.[251] and Kantorova et al.[252] demonstrated that FDG-PET had a high sensitivity for detection of distant metastases, particularly in the liver, but neither FDG-PET nor CT was sensitive enough to reliably detect local lymph node involvement. FDG-PET was, however, superior to CT for detecting hepatic metastases, with a sensitivity and specificity of 88% and 100%, respectively, compared with 38% and 97% for CT.[251]

Mukai et al.[253] reported that FDG-PET changed the treatment modality in 8% of patients and the extent of surgery in 13%. In a study of 110 patients, Yasuda et al.[254] showed that precancerous adenomatous polyps could be detected with a sensitivity of 24% for lesions from 5 to 30 mm in size and of 90% for lesions greater than 13 mm.

Although there are false-positive findings such as abscesses, fistulas, diverticulitis, and adenomas, the identification of focal uptake should not be ignored. However, the impact on patient management is not high because most patients will undergo surgery anyway, and staging is usually performed with preoperative liver ultrasound and during surgery. PET results may have a role in changing the type of surgery (curative versus palliative or concomitant liver metastases resection).

FDG-PET in the Diagnosis and Staging of Recurrent Colorectal Cancer

Early detection of recurrent disease is of primary importance because it may lead to a cure in up to 25% of patients. Surgical or medical treatment with the intent to improve survival and the quality of life should be guided by the accurate staging of disease. The size and number of hepatic metastases and the presence of extrahepatic disease affect the prognosis. The prognosis is poor if extrahepatic metastases are present, and this is believed to be a contraindication to hepatic resection.[255]

Iterative measurement of CEA is a useful, albeit imperfect, method to monitor the detection of recurrence, with a sensitivity of 59% and specificity of 84%.[256] Barium studies have been reported to be only 49% sensitive, 85% specific, and 80% accurate for overall recurrence.[257] A strategy in which increased CEA levels trigger the ordering of a PET study is limited by the diagnostic performance of CEA itself, which is far from optimal.

CT has an accuracy of 25% to 73% for localizing recurrence, but it fails to demonstrate hepatic metastases in up to 7% of patients and underestimates the number of lobes involved in up to 33% of patients. Metastases to the peritoneum, mesentery, and lymph nodes are commonly missed on CT, as well as the differentiation of postsurgical changes from local tumor recurrence.[258,259] CT portography (superior mesenteric arterial portography) is more sensitive (80% to 90%) than CT (70% to 80%) for detection of hepatic metastases, but there are many false-positive findings, which lower the positive predictive value.[260,261] There are also limitations in accurate operative staging because of adhesions or the site of the surgical incision (transverse upper abdominal for liver resection). Shiepers et al.[262] studied 76 patients and found that the accuracy of FDG-PET and CT were 95% and 65%, respectively, for differentiation of scar from local recurrence.

Huebner et al.,[263] in a meta-analysis review of 11 articles, reported that the sensitivity and specificity for detecting recurrent colorectal cancer with FDG-PET were 97% and 76%, respectively, and for liver and local pelvic recurrences FDG-PET had specificities of 99% and 98%. Whiteford et al.[264] demonstrated that the sensitivity of FDG-PET imaging for detection of mucinous adenocarcinoma was significantly lower than for nonmucinous adenocarcinoma, 58% and 92%, respectively, mainly because of the relative hypocellularity of these tumors.[265]

The high diagnostic accuracy of FDG-PET for detecting liver metastases was confirmed by Kinkel et al.,[266] who compared noninvasive imaging modalities (US, CT, MRI, and FDG-PET) for the detection of hepatic metastases from colorectal, gastric, and esophageal cancers. They found that FDG-PET had the highest sensitivity (90%), compared with 76% for MRI, 72% for CT, and 55% for US. Delbeke et al.[267] reported that FDG-PET had a higher accuracy (92%) than CT (78%) and CT portography (80%) for detection of hepatic metastases. Although the sensitivity of FDG-PET (91%) was lower than that of CT portography (97%), the specificity was much higher, particularly at postsurgical sites.

Ogunbiyi et al.[268] compared the sensitivity of FDG-PET and CT in local recurrence (91% versus 52%) and in hepatic lesions (95% versus 74%). Rydzewski et al.[269] found that the PPV of FDG-PET for characterizing liver lesions was similar to that of intraoperative ultrasonography (US) (93% and 89%, respectively) and superior to CT and MRI imaging (Table 33.12).

A major advantage of FDG-PET is its ability to detect extrahepatic disease not discovered by the other modalities. Valk et al.[270] compared the sensitivity of FDG-PET and CT for specific anatomic locations and found that FDG-PET was more sensitive than CT in all locations except the lung, where the two modalities were equivalent. The largest difference between PET and CT was found in the abdomen, pelvis, and retroperitoneum, where more than one-third of PET positive lesions were negative by CT. PET was also more specific than CT at all sites except the retroperitoneum.

Delbeke et al.[267] concluded that, outside of the liver, FDG-PET was especially helpful in detecting nodal involvement, differentiating local recurrence from postsurgical changes, evaluating the malignancy of indeterminate pulmonary nodules, and detecting distant metastases in the chest, abdomen, or pelvis.

Gambhir et al.,[271] in a review of 2,244 patient studies, reported that the sensitivity and specificity for FDG-PET were 94% and 87%, respectively, compared with 79% and 73% for CT. Flanagan et al.[272] reported the use of FDG-PET in 22 patients with unexplained elevation of CEA serum levels after resection of colorectal carcinoma with no abnormal findings on conventional workup, including CT. The sensitivity of FDG-PET in these patients was 100%, the specificity 71%, and the PPV 89%. Valk et al.[270] reported a sensitivity of 93% and a specificity of 92% in a similar group of 18 patients.

Flamen et al.[273] used FDG-PET to study 50 patients with elevated CEA and negative ($n = 31$) or equivocal ($n = 19$) findings on conventional imaging and found a sensitivity of 79% for the patients and 75% for the lesions. Cohade et al.,[274] in a study of 45 patients, showed that PET/CT integrated imaging reduced the frequency of equivocal and probable lesion characterization by 50% compared with PET alone. This hybrid modality increased the number of definite locations by 25% and increased the overall correct staging from 78% to 89%.

Impact of FDG-PET on Patient Management

FDG-PET imaging allows the detection of unsuspected metastases in 13% to 36% of patients and has a clinical impact in 14% to 65%.[267,268,270,272,273,275–279]

In the study by Delbeke et al.,[267] PET altered surgical management in 28% of the patients, in one-third by initiating surgery and in two-thirds by avoiding surgery.

Meta et al.[280] analyzed the answers to questionnaires that were sent to 60 referring physicians and concluded that PET had an impact on the clinical management in 65% of their patients (80% upstaged and 20% downstaged). In a study of 51 patients Ruers et al.[281] found that clinical management decisions based on conventional diagnostic methods were changed in 20% of patients based on the findings of FDG-PET imaging, especially by detecting unsuspected extrahepatic disease.

Strasberg et al.[282] demonstrated a higher long-term overall survival (OS) at 3 years (70%) and higher disease-free rates in patients selected for curative resection who had a PET study than those who did not have PET included in their workup (30% to 64%).

Current PET/CT fusion images can further affect clinical management[283–287] by guiding therapy toward a less invasive and more efficient surgical procedure or by guiding a biopsy to an FDG-avid region of the tumor. Additionally, it can provide better maps than CT alone to modulate the field and dose of radiation therapy.

Monitoring Therapy

The ability of PET to differentiate scar tissue from recurrent tumor in the pelvis was recognized very early.[288,289] Increased FDG uptake can be present immediately after radiation because of inflammatory changes, and this is not always associated with residual tumor. Moore et al.[290] found a sensitivity of 84% and specificity of 88% for the detection of local pelvic recurrence 6 months after external-beam radiation therapy for rectal cancer. In contrast, Schiepers et al.[291] concluded that there was no correlation between FDG uptake and cell kinetics in patients with primary rectal cancer treated by irradiation. Guillem et al.[292] demonstrated in a study of 15 patients treated with combined chemoradiation that FDG-PET added useful information. In a study of 25 patients with rectal cancer, Calvo et al.[293] described SUVs that were significantly decreased after treatment, but no correlation was found between postradiation metabolic activity and the 3-year survival rate.

Hepatic metastases can be treated with either systemic chemotherapy or regional therapy to the liver. A variety of

TABLE 33.12. FDG-PET results in detection and staging recurrent colorectal carcinoma.

			Sens			Spec			Acc			PPV			
Author	*Year*	*No. of patients*	*PET*	*CT*	*Others*	*PET*	*CT*	*Others*	*PET*	*CT*	*Others*	*PET*	*CT*	*Others*	*Remarks*
Moertel et al.[256]	1993	417			59 (CEA)			34 (CEA)							
Whiteford et al.[264]	2000	109													
Mucinous			58												
Nonmucinous			92												$P < 0.005$
Ogunbiyi et al.[268]	1997	58													For detection of hepatic metastases CEA↑/CI(−)
Local recurrence			91	52		100	80								
Hepatic			95	74		100	85		92	78	80 (CT portography)				
Delbeke et al.[267]	1997	52	91		97 (CT portography)										
Valk et al.[270]	1999	18	93			92									
Heubner et al.[263] (meta-analysis)	2000	577	97			76									
Gambhir et al.[271] (review)	2001	2244	94	79		87	73								
Rydzewski et al.[269]	2002	47										93	78	89 (intra-operative US)	
Kinkel et al.[266] (hepatic metastasis)	2002	54	90	72	76 (MRI) 55 (US)										Specificity >85% Colorectal, gastric, and esophageal cancers

CI, conventional imaging.

regional therapies exist, including chemotherapy administered through the hepatic artery using infusion pumps, selective chemoembolization, radiofrequency ablation, cryoablation, alcohol ablation, and radiolabeled ^{90}Y-microspheres.

Findlay et al.[294] showed that, in patients with hepatic metastases, responders can be discriminated from nonresponders after 4 to 5 weeks of chemotherapy with fluorouracil by measuring FDG uptake before and during therapy. Some results reported by Vitola et al.,[295] Torizuka et al.,[296] and Langenhoff et al.,[297] showed that 3 weeks after radiofrequency ablation and cryoablation, 51 of the 56 metastatic sites became FDG negative and there was no recurrence during 16 months follow-up.

Wong et al.[298] compared FDG-PET imaging, CT, MRI, and serum levels of CEA to monitor the therapeutic response of hepatic metastases to ^{90}Y-glass microspheres. They found that FDG uptake correlated best with the changes in serum levels of CEA.

New PET Tracers for Clinical Use

^{18}F-Fluoride has a mechanism of uptake similar to that for other bone imaging radiopharmaceuticals, but because of the better spatial resolution and routine acquisition of tomographic images, ^{18}F-fluoride PET imaging offers potential advantages over conventional bone scintigraphy for detecting metastases. Schirrmeister et al.[299] demonstrated that twice as many benign and malignant lesions were detected with ^{18}F-fluoride PET compared to planar scintigraphy.

Higashi et al.[300] demonstrated that the in vitro uptake of ^{11}C-thymidine or ^{18}F-fluorothymidine correlates with the tumor proliferation rate and that these radiopharmaceuticals are assessing the rate of DNA synthesis. Dittman et al.[301] compared FDG with FLT uptake and showed that FLT-PET accurately visualized thoracic tumors and cerebral metastases, but that high physiologic uptake in the liver and bone marrow prevents detection of metastases in these locations.

Summary

FDG-PET is indicated as the initial test for diagnosis and staging of recurrence, for preoperative staging (N and M) of known recurrence, for the differentiation of benign from malignant lesions (indeterminate lymph nodes, hepatic and pulmonary lesions), for the differentiation of posttreatment changes from recurrent tumor, for the evaluation of patients with rising tumor markers in the absence of a known source, for a subgroup of patients at high risk (elevated CEA levels), for patients with a normal CT in whom surgery could be avoided if FDG-PET shows metastases, and for screening for recurrence in patients at high risk. It also affects the clinical management by guiding further procedures (biopsy, surgery, and radiation therapy) and excluding the need for additional procedures.

Lymphoma

Lymphoma is a general term that refers to a group of malignancies originating in the lymphoid tissue, including Hodgkin's disease (HD) and non-Hodgkin's lymphoma (NHL).[302] The first evaluations of PET for staging in large cohorts of patients with lymphoma were performed by Moog et al.[303,304] (mixed populations with HD and NHL). For nodal staging, Moog et al.[303] evaluated 60 patients with CT and PET and verified discordant results by biopsy whenever possible. A total of 160 nodal regions were positive by both modalities, and 25 were positive by PET alone. Nine of these were verified histologically, and PET was true positive in 7 cases and false positive in 2 cases. Six regions were positive by CT only, and in the 3 in which verification was obtained, the CT result was false positive. There was a change in management in 10% to 15% of the patients.

For extranodal staging, Moog et al.[304] also evaluated 81 patients. Forty-two disease sites were detected by both modalities, and PET detected an additional 24 sites, of which 15 were verified pathologically, including 9 sites in bone marrow, 3 in the spleen, and 2 elsewhere, and in 14 sites PET was true positive. Six of 7 lesions detected only by CT were verified, and 5 of these were false positive.

FDG-PET was found to be of value in the diagnosis of HD and aggressive NHL.[305,306] It is generally accepted that FDG-PET may have a role in diagnosis and staging of low-grade follicular NHL. For other subtypes of low-grade lymphoma (small cell lymphocytic and probably mantle cell lymphoma), it seems that FDG-PET has no value for staging and follow-up.[305,307] Similar discouraging results have been demonstrated in a small group of patients with follicular lymphoma of the duodenum.[308] In contrast, marginal zone B-cell lymphoma, an entity that was initially considered to originate from mucosa-associated lymphoid tissue (MALT) lymphoma, but in recent reports is classified as a distinctive histologic type, was shown to take up FDG only in the involved lymph nodes.

From the studies of Moog et al.[309] and Carr et al.,[310] it appears that both PET and iliac crest biopsy should be performed to stage the bone marrow. It is probable that some patients with diffuse involvement have homogeneous uptake on PET, whereas some patients with focal involvement are missed by random biopsy. FDG-PET can be useful in guiding the biopsy to a site of active disease.

An additional study evaluated FDG-PET as a predictor of prognosis. Aggressive and treatment resistant tumors showed a trend toward higher uptake of FDG, with an inverse relationship between the survival rate of patients and the degree of FDG uptake.[311]

The complementary role of FDG-PET to conventional staging of 45 patients with newly diagnosed HD and NHL was investigated by Delbeke et al.[312] In addition to the positive impact of PET, these authors report that false-negative FDG imaging understaged 3 patients (7%), including 2 patients with low-grade NHL and 1 with HD. They concluded that FDG-PET is an efficient method for staging of lymphoma but should be used in conjunction with conventional staging as a complementary modality.

Recently, Hong et al.[313] evaluated the clinical value of FDG-PET for the staging of malignant lymphoma. The sensitivities and specificities for detection of nodal involvement for PET, CT, and ^{67}Ga scanning were determined to be 93.3%, 98.9%, and 25.8%, and 100%, 99.1%, and 99.8%, respectively. In detecting extranodal lymphoma, the sensitivities and specificities of the PET, CT and ^{67}Ga scanning were 87.5%, 87.5%, and 37.5%, and 100%, 100%, and 100%, respectively. Sasaki et al.[314] showed a specificity of 99% for

TABLE 33.13. Representative recent literature of PET findings in lymphoma.

Author	*Year*	*No. of patients*	*No lesions*	*Sens*			*Spec*		
				PET	*CT*	^{67}*Ga*	*PET*	*CT*	^{67}*Ga*
Hong et al.[313]	2003	30	—	93	98	26	100	99	100
Nodal evaluation				88	88	38	100	100	100
Extranodal evaluation									
Sasaki et al.[314]	2002	46	152	92	65		99	99	
Wirth et al.[319]	2002	50	117	82	68	69	—	—	
Stumpe et al.[315]	1998	50		86	81		96	41	
HD									
NHL				89	86		100	67	
Shen et al.[318]	2002	25	111	96		72			
Rini et al.[320] (HD + splenic involvement)	2003	32		92		50	100		95

HD, Hodgkin's disease; NHL, non-Hodgkin's lymphoma.

both CT and PET, whereas the sensitivity of CT was 65% and that of PET was 92%. An older study including 50 patients compared FDG-PET for staging of HD and NHL to CT.[315] The sensitivity and specificity of PET were 86% and 96% for HD and 89% and 100% for NHL. The sensitivity and specificity of CT were 81% and 41% for HD and 86% and 67% for NHL.

In comparison to ^{67}Ga, PET showed better performance than ^{67}Ga, as was reported by Paul et al.[316] (the first report on FDG uptake in five patients with lymphomas) and Okada et al.[317] Of course, their mechanism of uptake by malignant tissue is based on different principles. FDG, as mentioned before, is incorporated into malignant cells with a high glucolytic metabolism due to intracellular trapping of FDG phosphate. ^{67}Ga is taken up by malignant cells, lymphoma in particular, probably based on an intracellular transferrin-related transport mechanism. Inside the cells, the tracer is incorporated in lysosome-like granules and shows a slower clearance from malignant as compared with normal tissues.

A study comparing PET and ^{67}Ga evaluated 111 sites of disease in 25 patients with different types of lymphoma at diagnosis and relapse.[318] The sensitivity of PET was 96% versus 72% for ^{67}Ga. The false-negative ^{67}Ga studies were attributed to poor detection of low-grade NHL, bone and bone marrow involvement, and lesions smaller than 12 mm in diameter.

The differences in the performance rate of PET, ^{67}Ga, and CT for staging of HD and NHL were evaluated in 50 patients.[319] On a site-based analysis, PET showed superior values, 82%, as compared with both ^{67}Ga, 69%, and CT, 68%.

Diagnosis of splenic involvement is difficult using nuclear medicine techniques, because both ^{67}Ga and FDG are physiologically taken up in variable amounts by the normal spleen. Lymphomatous splenic involvement is, as a rule, diffuse, thus increasing the diagnostic challenge. The sensitivity, specificity, and accuracy of PET were 92%, 100%, and 97%, respectively, as compared with 50%, 95%, and 78% for ^{67}Ga[320] (Table 33.13).

Buckmann et al.[321] found that PET is 10% to 20% more accurate than CT in detecting and staging of malignant lymphoma. They also reported that PET is better than CT in detecting bone marrow involvement and is useful as a guide for bone marrow biopsy.

A change in staging is more likely to result in a change in treatment strategy for lymphoma subtypes in which treatment is given with a curative intent. For example, upstaging from an early (stage I–II) to an advanced stage (III–IV) in HD or large cell lymphoma will probably result in the selection of a longer course of chemotherapy as the exclusive treatment, as opposed to a shorter course of chemotherapy followed by radiation therapy (Figure 33.6).

A similar upstaging in patients with follicular lymphoma will also influence treatment and follow-up of the disease. Schoder et al.[322] demonstrated that PET findings led to a change in the clinical stage in 44% of 46 patients: in patients with NHL and HD, 21% were upstaged and 23% were downstaged. In a recent prospective study of 88 patients with HD, Naumann et al.[323] demonstrated a change in staging in 18 patients (20%).

FDG-PET appears to be a noninvasive, efficient, and cost-effective whole body imaging modality with a high sensitivity, specificity, and accuracy for staging patients with most histologic types of HD and NHL (Figure 33.7). It is generally

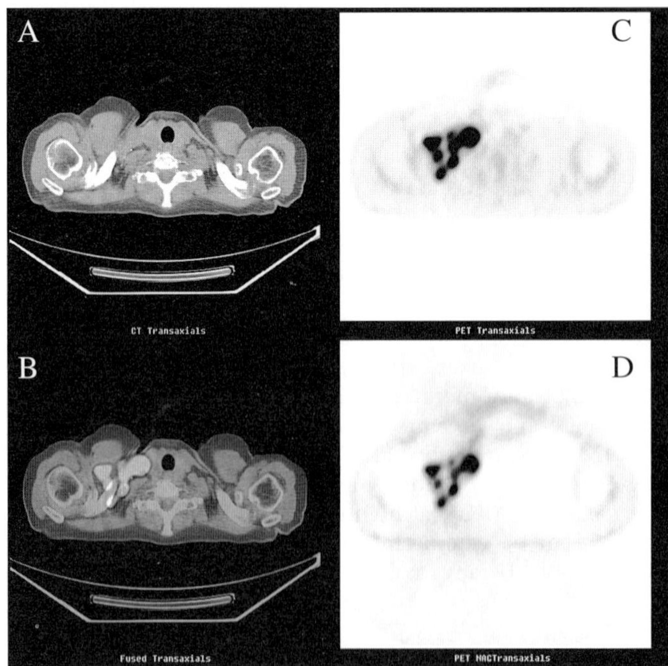

FIGURE 33.6. Transaxial PET/CT images obtained with FDG in a patient in the mid-twenties with a new diagnosis of Hodgkin's lymphoma. Intense focal tracer uptake is seen in multiple lymph nodes in the right neck and axillary region. (A) CT scan. (B) Fused PET/CT image. (C) Attenuation corrected PET image. (D) Nonattenuation corrected PET image.

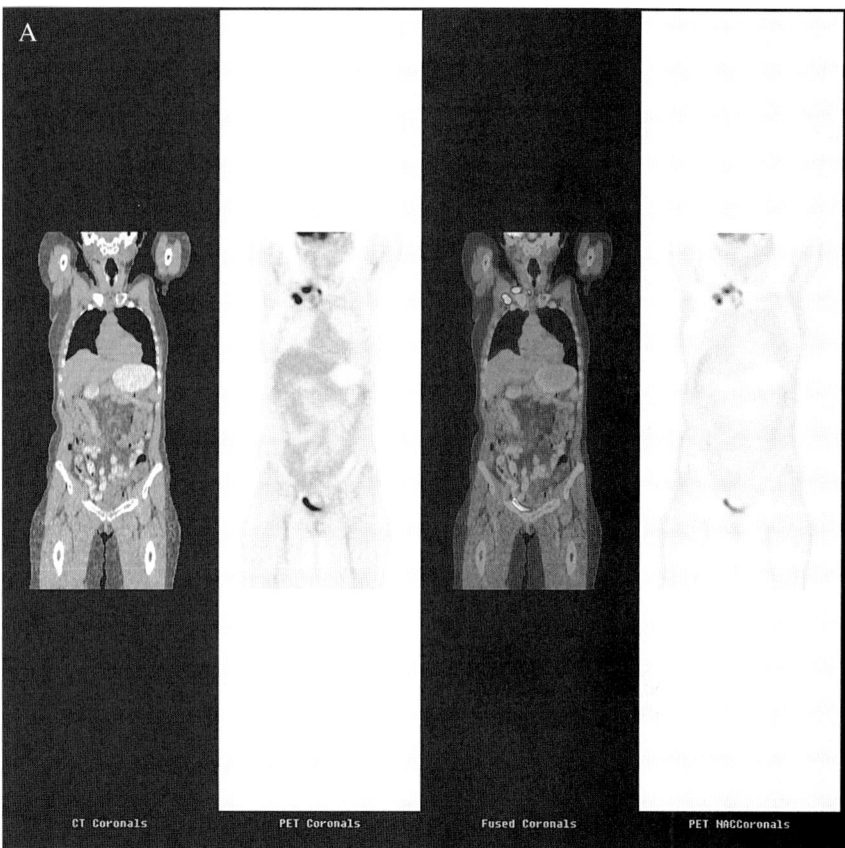

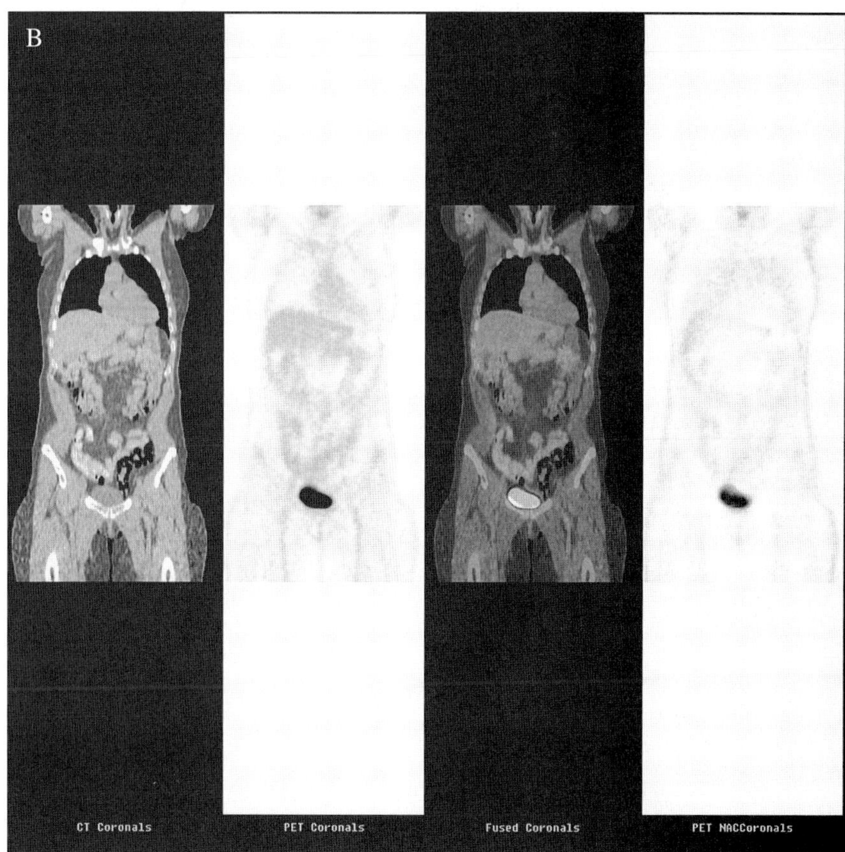

FIGURE 33.7. (A) Coronal PET/CT images of a 60+-year-old woman with recurrent follicular non-Hodgkin's lymphoma. Intense focal uptake is noted in the right supraclavicular area that is attributed to recurrent disease. (B) Coronal PET/CT images of the patient noted in (A) at 12 weeks after radioimmunotherapy with Bexxar (^{131}I-tositumomab and unlabeled tositumomab therapy). The dramatic decrease in FDG uptake in the right supraclavicular area indicates an excellent response to therapy.

TABLE 33.14. Representative literature of PET in monitoring response to treatment of lymphoma.

Authors	*Year*	*No. of patients*	*Type of disease*	*PPV (%)*	*NPV (%)*	*DFS*		*OS*	
						(−) PET	*(+) PET*	*(−) PET*	*(+) PET*
FDG evaluation after first-line treatment:									
Kostakoglu et al.[331]	2002	30	NHL + HD	83	65	65	17	—	—
Spaepen et al.[336]	2003	93	NHL	100	83	85	4	—	—
Weihrauch et al.[329]	2001	28	HD	60	100	95	40	—	—
Spaepen et al.[343]	2003	60	HD	—	—	91	4	—	—
FDG evaluation during treatment:									
Torizuka et al.[337]	2004	20 (1–2 cycles)	NHL + HD	63	100	24–34 mo	8–16 mo		
Zijlstra et al.[335]	2003		NHL			64	25		
Spaepen et al.[336]	2003	26 (2nd cycle) 70 (3–4 cycles)	NHL	—	—	92	10	100	60
FDG evaluation before stem cell transplantation:									
Spaepen et al.[343]	2003	60	NHL + HD	—	—	96	23	100	55
Filmont et al.[342]	2003	43	NHL + HD	92%	88%	—	—	—	—
Schot et al.[341]	2003	46	NHL + HD			62	32	— —	—

Cycles, cycles of chemotherapy.
Mo = months.

accepted today that FDG-PET is a clinically valuable tool that should be added to conventional staging modalities.[329,330]

FDG-PET for Predicting Treatment Response

Evaluation of PET for assessment of treatment response has been studied more extensively in HD and NHL than in any other tumor. Differentiation of viable tumor from fibrosis in a residual posttreatment mass is a common problem in lymphoma that is seen in more than 85% of patients with HD and approximately 40% of the patients with NHL.

Initial studies have assessed response to treatment in heterogeneous populations including both HD and NHL patients. Cremerius et al.[324] reported better specificity and positive predictive value (PPV) for FDG-PET (92% and 94%, respectively) as compared with that of CT (17% and 60%) in 27 patients.

Zinzani et al.[325] studied 44 patients with HD or aggressive NHL who had residual abdominal disease and showed that the 2-year progression-free survival (PFS) rate was 95% for the PET-negative group and 0% for the PET-positive group.

A PPV of 100% for PET, as compared with 42% for CT, was found in 54 patients with HD and aggressive NHL assessed after therapy by Jerusalem et al.[326] The negative predictive values (NPV) of PET (83%) and CT (87%) were not significantly different. Recurrence was noticed in the same study, with both positive PET and CT in 26% of patients and with negative PET and positive CT in only 10%. The PFS (2-year) rate with negative PET and negative CT was 87%, with positive CT and negative PET only 60%, and finally, with positive PET regardless of the CT, 0%.

Mikhaeel et al.[327] also found in 45 patients with aggressive NHL that the relapse rate was 17% for PET-negative patients and 100% for PET-positive patients compared with 25% for CT-negative patients and 41% for CT-positive patients. The progression-free survival (PFS) for 1 year was 83% for PET-positive and 0% for PET-negative patients.

Spaepen et al.[328] evaluated 93 patients with NHL and reported that all patients who had persistent FDG uptake relapsed, with a 2-year PFS rate of 85% of patients with negative PET findings. The 2-year PFS rate was 4% in patients with positive PET findings. Weihrauch et al.[329] studied the predictive value of PET in 28 patients with HD who had residual masses after treatment. The 1-year PFS was 95% for the PET-negative group as compared with 40% for the positive group. Spaepen et al.[330] evaluated 60 patients with HD with or without masses at the end of first-line treatment; the 2-year disease free survival (DFS) rate was 4% for the PET-positive group and 85% for the PET-negative group.

Kostakoglu et al.[331] compared FDG-PET after the first cycle of chemotherapy and after completion of chemotherapy. PET had greater sensitivity and PPV for predicting relapse after the first cycle. PET after the first cycle had a lower false-negative rate (13%) than the posttherapy PET (35%), possibly reflecting the presence of a small but still detectable tumor load of resistant cells early, but not late, in the therapy course (Table 33.14).

In general, in NHL and high-grade HD, a positive PET at the end of first-line therapy is highly suggestive of disease and requires intensive confirmatory investigation. A negative PET does not exclude the presence of minimal residual disease or future relapse and requires close follow-up. However, in early HD, a negative PET can be used to define complete response (CR) with favorable prognosis, even in the presence of residual masses on CT (see Figure 33.7A,B). A positive PET, especially if located in a site different from the residual mass, should be assessed with caution, and benign or inflammatory etiologies should also be considered in the differential diagnosis of persistent disease.[330]

Evaluation During Treatment

Many studies have been conducted to evaluate the extent and time course of changes in FDG metabolism in response to chemotherapy. The rapidity of response during treatment appears to be an accurate predictor of overall response, with early tumor regression indicating higher cure rates.[332] Accurate early assessment of response allows for timely institution of aggressive second-line protocols. If resistant tumor burden is identified, additional treatment-related toxicity might be prevented.

Romer et al.[333] found that a single PET study performed after two cycles of chemotherapy was predictive of long-term prognosis. Mikhaeel et al.[334] reported the results of 23 patients with NHL who had FDG-PET after two to four cycles of chemotherapy. No relapse was seen in patients with minimal or no FDG uptake, whereas 88% of patients who had persistent FDG uptake relapsed. The same group also found that in 23 patients with HD during treatment, the relapse rate was 100% in the PET-positive group and 8% in the PET-negative group.

Zijlstra et al.[335] studied the prognostic value of FDG-PET in 26 patients with aggressive NHL after two cycles of chemotherapy. At a median follow-up of 16 months, the PFS rate was 64% in patients who had negative FDG-PET findings and was 25% in patients who had positive FDG-PET findings. Spaepen et al.[336] evaluated 70 patients with aggressive NHL and found that visual interpretation of FDG-PET, performed after three to four cycles of first-line chemotherapy, predicted PFS and OS independently from and better than the international prognostic index.

Torizuka et al.[337] reported that FDG-PET may be predictive of clinical outcome and could differentiate short-term responders from nonresponders in a group of 17 patients, most of them with advanced-stage lymphoma.

Prognostic value of FDG-PET Before Stem Cell Transplantation

High-dose chemotherapy (HDT) with autologous stem cell transplantation (ASCT) has been shown to improve survival in patients with relapsed aggressive NHL or HD.[338] A number of studies indicate that FDG-PET performed during or after salvage chemotherapy has a high predictive value for relapse after HDT/ASCT.[339,340] Schot et al.[341] evaluated 46 patients with recurrent or persistent NHL/HD lymphoma after HDT/ASCT. The PFS for 2 years was 62% for PET-negative studies versus 32% for PET-positive patients.

Filmont et al.[342] showed that PPV (92%) and NPV (88%) in 43 patients with NHL/HD were very similar if the PET study was obtained 2 to 5 weeks after initiation of salvage chemotherapy, before ASCT, or within a median interval of 2.4 months. Spaepen et al.[343] assessed the prognostic value of FDG-PET after salvage chemotherapy before HDT/ASCT in 60 patients with NHL and HD. The 2-year PFS and OS rates for patients with negative FDG-PET scans were 96% and 100%, respectively, as compared with 23% and 55% for those with positive FDG-PET results.

FDG-PET for the Detection of Recurrence

Although early diagnosis of relapse will lead to early administration of salvage therapy, the crucial question is whether a lesion is metabolically active, because two-thirds of patients with HD present with fibrotic or recurrent mass lesions, and 20% of these relapse.[344] Fifty percent of patients with high-grade NHL present with a mass lesion and only 25% of them relapse.[344] ^{67}Ga will not accurately indicate whether a tumor is metabolically active, and it has limitations in detection of intraabdominal and low-grade lymphoma.[345]

False-positive PET studies may be the result of FDG uptake in a hyperplastic thymus, in the gastrointestinal tract, or in an inflamed lung lesion.[346] False-negative results may also arise from the absence of an FDG-avid lesion within small tumor lesions, possibly because of low glucose metabolism after therapy or acquisition problems, such as spatial resolution and partial volume effect.

The value of the sensitivity and specificity of FDG-PET and CT to predict the relapse of malignant lymphoma were described in several studies.[347,348] Jerusalem et al.[349] evaluated the recurrence rate in 45 NHL/HD patients with residual tumor masses and positive FDG-PET results, and it was only 26% in patients with residual tumors and negative FDG-PET results. The 1-year PFS and OS rates were 86% and 92%, respectively, for the PET-negative group, and only 0% and 55%, respectively, for the PET-positive group.

Guay et al.[350] compared the diagnostic accuracy of FDG-PET and CT in detecting residual disease or relapse during the posttherapy period in 48 patients with HD. The sensitivity, specificity, PPV, and NPV of FDG-PET for predicting relapse were 79%, 97%, 92%, and 92%, respectively. The accuracy of FDG-PET was 92%, higher than the accuracy of CT (56%). Freudenberg et al.[351] described the advantages of PET/CT fusion imaging in 27 patients with lymphoma and evaluated the clinical significance of combined PET/CT and compared the staging results of PET/CT with those of FDG-PET and CT alone (Table 33.15).

Summary

FDG-PET provides an excellent tool in the initial staging of lymphomas, in restaging lymphoma after initial treatment, in predicting response during and at the end of therapy, and during follow-up for diagnosis of recurrence.

A pretreatment FDG-PET study is essential for accurate assessment of residual masses and early monitoring of response to the treatment. A baseline PET will help detect

TABLE 33.15. Recent literature of PET findings in recurrence of lymphoma.

			Sens		*Spec*		*PPV*		*NPV*		*ACC*	
Authors	*Year*	*No. of patients*	*PET*	*CT*	*PET*	*CT*	*PET*	*CT*	*PET*	*CT*	*PET*	*CT*
Freudenberg et al.[351]	2004	27	86	78	100	54	100	65	87	70	93	67
Guay et al.[350]	2003	48	79	—	97	—	92	—	92	—	92	56
Filmont et al.[342]	2003	78	87	94	80	56	95	72	83	67	90	71

relapse or residual disease, because relapse occurs most often in the region of previous disease.[352]

Melanoma

Cutaneous melanoma is the seventh most common newly diagnosed cancer in the United States: 55,100 new cases were diagnosed in 2004 and 7,910 patients will have died of systemic disease.[353] Wahl et al.[354] and Kern et al.[355] demonstrated that radiolabeled glucose analogues were preferentially taken up in murine melanomas and human melanoma xenografts, establishing the rationale for the potential use of FDG in patients with melanoma.

There is no defined role for PET in the initial diagnosis of melanoma, as has been shown by Wagner et al.,[356] because the inherent spatial resolution of PET reduces the sensitivity for detection of lesions less than 80 mm² and it is unlikely that this technique (as currently performed) will ever be effective in the initial diagnosis of small, surgically curable melanoma in situ.

Initial Staging of Clinically Localized Disease

In intermediate- and high-risk lesions greater than 1 mm in thickness, assessment of the SLN draining the tumor site is very important. Rinne et al.[357] studied 52 patients with primary melanoma greater than 1.5 mm in depth who had no evidence of local or distant metastases; they found that the accuracy of PET for identification of regional or distant metastases was 95% per lesion and 94% per patient and that for CT was 68% per lesion and 77% per patient.

Macfarlane et al.[358] found that PET accurately predicted regional nodal status in 88% of 23 patients with primary melanoma more than 1.5 mm thick. Wagner et al.[359] performed a large prospective trial containing 70 patients with primary thick melanoma (more than 1.0 mm) and 4 patients with recurrent melanoma in or adjacent to the surgical scar who underwent PET and SLN biopsy. They demonstrated a sensitivity of 11% to 17% (depending on reading threshold) and a specificity of 94% to 100%. This is one of the first articles to suggest that PET is not sensitive for staging regional nodes in patients with newly diagnosed thick melanomas.

Acland et al.[360] found that FDG-PET failed to identify all 14 positive SLNs found in 50 patients who underwent sentinel node biopsy for primary melanomas more than 1 mm in thickness. Fink et al.[361] found, in 48 patients with stage I or II disease, that FDG-PET identified only one metastatic node, and they concluded that this result was likely "due to the small size of the metastatic deposits in the sentinel node."

There is now strong evidence that FDG-PET is not useful in the initial staging of primary melanoma when there is no clinical evidence of local or distant metastatic spread. This finding is attributed to the small size of most nodal metastases and the low prevalence of nodal disease in patients with primary melanoma.

Local Recurrence and Satellite or In-Transit Metastases

There are no studies that specifically examine the efficacy of FDG-PET in the evaluation of patients with locally recurrent primary melanoma tumors, and there are only two studies that evaluated satellite and in-transit metastases. Acland et al.[362] studied 9 patients with satellite metastases adjacent to the primary tumor excision site and found a sensitivity of 93% and a specificity of 50% for the ability of FDG-PET to detect locoregional metastatic disease. Stas et al.[363] described a change in clinical management in patients with varying types of recurrent melanoma with adjacent metastases or distant in-transit lesions. These findings suggest a possible role for PET in this population, but very small tumor volume of disease will not be detected.

The sensitivity of FDG-PET may be low in patients with small metastases in adjacent lymph nodes,[379,380] but patients with suspected regional metastases based on physical examination or other imaging modalities may have greater detectability with PET. The majority of patients (80% or greater) with clinically localized tumors never develop distant disease. Blessing et al.[364] found a sensitivity of 74% and a specificity of 93% for the evaluation of 20 clinically suspicious lymph node basins imaged with FDG-PET.

Crippa et al.,[365] in a study of 38 patients, found the accuracy of FDG PET to be 91% for clinically or radiographically enlarged lymph nodes. Sensitivity dropped off rapidly for lymph nodes less than 5 mm, but was 100% and 83% for nodes that were greater than or equal to 10 mm and 6 to 10 mm, respectively.

Tyler et al.[366] attempted to show the utility of FDG-PET in a study of 95 patients with clinically evident stage III lymph node and/or in-transit melanoma. The sensitivity was 87%, the PPV (with the integration of pertinent clinical information) was 91%, the specificity was 44% (although few prophylactic lymph node dissections were performed), and the findings led to a change in clinical management in 15% of the patients. These findings argue that FDG-PET has a useful role in the patient with suspected regional lymph node metastases (Table 33.16).

In the case of confirmed lymph node metastases beyond the SLN, the value of FDG-PET is to localize occult distant metastases that might be amenable to surgical resection or to exclude metastatic disease in patients with equivocal findings on conventional anatomic images. Wagner et al.[367] and Acland et al.[362] showed that in this group of patients it was unknown distant disease that may have altered patient management.

Identification of Distant Metastases

FDG-PET can be used in patients with recently diagnosed melanoma and those who have clinical, laboratory, or radiologic evidence of distant metastases, in patients with previously resected melanoma with findings suspicious for recurrent disease in the form of distant metastases, and, finally, in patients with previously treated distant metastases requiring restaging to plan future surgical or medical management.

Gritters et al.[368] studied 12 patients with various stages of melanoma (thick primaries, palpable lymph nodes, or presumed metastases on CT), and they found intraabdominal visceral and lymph node metastases that were not seen on CT. Steinert et al.[369] found a 92% sensitivity for FDG-PET in 33 patients with known metastatic melanoma or high-risk primaries (greater than 1.5 mm).

TABLE 33.16. Representative literature of FDG-PET findings in melanoma.

Author	Year	No. of patients	Sensitivity			Specificity			Accuracy		Remarks
			PET	CI	SNB	PET	CI	SNB	PET	CI	
Wagner et al.[359]	1999	70	11–17	95		94–100		100			Stage I–II
Crippa et al.[365]	2000	38	100 (10 mm diameter) 83 (6–10 mm diameter) 23 (<5 mm diameter)						91		Regional lymph metastasis
Wagner et al.[356]	2001	45	90 (>5.3 mm diameter) 14 (<5.3 mm diameter.)								Stage I–II
Eigtved et al.[371]	2000	38	97	62		56	22				Generally
Swetter et al.[372]	2002	104	84	58		97	70				Distant (all foci)
Hafner et al.[377]	2004	100	8			100					Regional lymph nodes
Havengna et al.[378]	2003	53	15			88					Regional lymph nodes
Rinne et al.[370]	1998	48	92	58		95	45		92	56	Distant (all foci)
Tyler et al.[366]	2000	95	87			41					PPV: 90% Stage III

SNB, sentinel node biopsy.

Rinne et al.[370] examined 48 patients with clinical or CT findings suggesting local or distant metastatic disease, and FDG-PET was found to be 92% sensitive, 95% specific, and 93% accurate, compared with 58%, 45%, and 56% for sensitivity, specificity, and accuracy, respectively, for CT.

Eigtved et al.[371] confirmed the superiority of FDG-PET in a study of 38 patients with either local recurrence, in-transit recurrence, regional lymph node metastases, or distant metastases, with sensitivity and specificity of 97% and 56%, respectively, compared with 62% and 22% for conventional imaging.

It is obvious now that PET is indeed superior for localization of distant metastases outside of the lungs and brain, independent of the particular stage of the high-risk patient. Swetter et al.,[372] in a study of 104 patients, reported a sensitivity and specificity for PET of 84% and 97% and for CT of 58% and 70%, respectively, for the detection of metastatic disease.

Gulec et al.[373] studied 49 patients and found that FDG-PET identified more metastatic sites in 55% of the patients and changed the management in 49% of them. Dietlein et al.[374] and Krug et al.[375] reported that FDG-PET was inferior in the detection of pulmonary and liver metastases, but these studies suffered from various methodologic weaknesses. Distant metastases can be identified by FDG-PET either in patients with locoregional disease or in patients with known distant lesions, and these findings can change their clinical management.

Response to Therapy

The usefulness of FDG-PET in evaluating response to therapy was shown by Mercier et al.,[376] who studied three patients who underwent a FDG-PET scan before and 1 month after treatment (isolated limb perfusion therapy with melphalan) and found a reduction in the number of lesions and diffuse radiotracer uptake, most likely because of posttreatment inflammation.

^{11}C-Methionine,[379] ^{125}I-alpha-methyl-tyrosine (AMT), ^{18}F-DOPA,[380] ^{18}F-FLT,[381] ^{11}C-*N*-methylspiperone,[382] and radiolabeled alpha-melanocyte-stimulating hormone[383] are some of the new promising radiopharamaceuticals in the field of melanoma.

In conclusion, FDG-PET is the modality of choice for evaluating patients who fit in one of these four categories:

1. Individuals at high risk for distant metastases based on the extent of locoregional disease
2. Patients with findings that are suspicious for distant metastases
3. Individuals with known distant tumor deposits who still stand to benefit from customized therapies if new lesions are discovered or treated lesions regress
4. Patients at high risk for systemic relapse who are considering aggressive medical therapy

References

1. Wahl RL, Buchanan JW (eds). In: Principles and Practice of Positron Emission Tomography. Philadelphia: Lippincott Williams & Wilkins, 2002.
2. Laubenbacher C, Saumweber D, Wagner MC, et al. Comparison of fluorine-18-fluorodeoxyglucose PET, MRI and laryngoscopy for staging head and neck squamous cell carcinomas. J Nucl Med 2995;36:1747–1757.
3. Wong WL, Chevretton EB, McGurk M, et al. A prospective study of PET-FDG imaging for the assessment of head and neck squamous cell carcinoma. Clin Otolaryngol Appl Sci 1997;22:209–214.
4. Braams JW, Pruim J, Kole AC, et al. Detection of unknown primary head and neck tumors by positron emission tomography. Int J Oral Maxillofac Surg 1997;26:112–115.
5. Safa AA, Tran LM, Rege S, et al. The role of positron emission tomography in occult primary head and neck cancers. Cancer J Sci Am 1999;5:214–218.
6. Jungehulsing M, Scheidhauer K, Damm M, et al. 2 [F]-Fluoro-2-deoxy-D-glucose positron emission tomography is a sensitive tool for the detection of occult primary cancer (carcinoma of

unknown primary syndrome) with head and neck lymph node manifestation. Otolaryngol Head Neck Surg 2000;123:294–301.
7. Greven KM, Keyes JJ, Williams DR, et al. Occult primary tumors of the head and neck: lack of benefit from positron emission tomography imaging with 2-[F-18]fluoro-2-deoxy-D-glucose. Cancer (Phila) 1999;86:114–118.
8. Rege S, Safa AA, Chaiken L, et al. Positron emission tomography: an independent indicator of radiocurability in head and neck carcinomas. Am J Clin Oncol 2000;23:164–169.
9. Adams S, Baum RP, Stuckensen T, Bitter K, Hor G. Prospective comparison of F-18-FDG-PET with conventional imaging modalities (CT, MRI, US) in lymph node staging of head and neck cancer. Eur J Nucl Med 1998;25:1255–1260.
10. Kau RJ, Alexiou C, Laubenbacher C, Werner M, Schwaiger M, Arnold W. Lymph node detection of head and neck squamous cell carcinomas by positron emission tomography with fluorodeoxyglucose F-18 in a routine clinical setting. Arch Otolaryngol Head Neck Surg 1999;125:1322–1328.
11. Stokkel MP, ten Broek FW, Hordjk GJ, et al. Preoperative evaluation of patients with primary head and neck cancer using dual-head 18-fluorodeoxyglucose positron emission tomography. Ann Surg 2000;231:229–234.
12. Hannah A, Scott AM, Tochon-Danguy H, et al. Evaluation of ^{18}F-fluorodeoxyglucose position emission tomography and computed tomography with histopathologic correlation in the initial staging of head and neck cancer. Ann Surg 2002;236:208–217.
13. Di Martino E, Nowak B, Hassan HA, et al. Diagnosis and staging of head and neck cancer: a comparison of modern imaging modalities (positron emission tomography, computed tomography, color-coded duplex sonography) with penendoscopic and histopathologic findings. Arch Otolaryngol Head Neck Surg 2000;126:1457–1461.
14. Stuckensen T, Kovacs AF, Adams S, et al. Staging of the neck in patients with oral cavity squamous cell carcinomas: a prospective comparison of PET, ultrasound, CT and MRI. J Craniomaxillofac Surg 2000;28:319–324.
15. Schwartz LH, Ozsahin M, Zhang GN, et al. Synchronous and metachronous head and neck carcinomas. Cancer (Phila) 1994;74:1933–1938.
16. Stokkel MP, Moons KG, ten Broek FW, et al. ^{18}F-Fluorodeoxyglucose dual-head positron emission tomography as a procedure for detecting simultaneous primary tumors in cases of head and neck cancer. Cancer (Phila) 1999;86:2370–2377.
17. Lowe VJ, Stack BC Jr. Esophageal cancer and head and neck cancer. Semin Roentgenol 2002;37(2):140–150.
18. Goodwin WJ Jr. Salvage surgery for patients with recurrent squamous cell carcinoma of the upper aerodigestive tract: when do the ends justify the means? Laryngoscope 2000;110:1–18.
19. Goerres GW, Schmid DT, Bandhauer F, et al. Positron emission tomography in the early follow-up of advanced head and neck cancer. Arch Otolaryngol Head Neck Surg 2004;130:105–109.
20. Wax MK, Myers LL, Gona JM, Husain SS, Nabi HA. The role of positron emission tomography in the evaluation of the N-positive neck. Otolaryngol Head Neck Surg 2003;129:163–167.
21. Lapela M, Eigtved A, Jyrkkio S, et al. Experience in qualitative and quantitative FDG-PET in follow-up of patients with suspected recurrence from head and neck cancer. Eur J Cancer 2000;36:858–867.
22. Li P, Zhuang H, Mozley PD, et al. Evaluation of recurrent squamous cell carcinoma of the head and neck with FDG positron emission tomography. Clin Nucl Med 2001;26:131–135.
23. Terhaard CH, Bongers V, van Rijk PP, et al. F-18-fluorodeoxy-glucose positron-emission tomography scanning in detection of local recurrence after radiotherapy for laryngeal/pharyngeal cancer. Head Neck 2001;23:933–941.
24. Lowe VJ, Boyd JH, Dunphy FR, et al. Surveillance for recurrent head and neck cancer using positron emission tomography. J Clin Oncol 2000;18:651–658.
25. Kunkel M, Forster GJ, Reichert TE, et al. Detection of recurrent oral squamous cell carcinoma by [^{18}F]-2-fluorodeoxyglucose-positron emission tomography. Implications for prognosis and patient management radiation treatment planning with an integrated positron emission and computer tomography (PET/CT): a feasibility study. Cancer (Phila) 2003;98:2257–2265.
26. Brun E, Kjellen E, Tennval J, et al. FDG-PET studies during treatment: prediction of therapy outcome in head and neck squamous cell carcinoma. Head Neck 2002;24:127–135.
27. Kitagawa Y, Sadato N, Azuma H, et al. FDG-PET to evaluate combined intra-arterial chemotherapy and radiotherapy of head and neck neoplasms. J Nucl Med 1999;40:1132–1137.
28. Kitagawa Y, Nishizawa S, Sano K, et al. Prospective comparison of F-18-FDG-PET with conventional imaging modalities (MRI, CT, and Ga-67 scintigraphy) in assessment of combined intra-arterial chemotherapy and radiotherapy for head and neck carcinoma. J Nucl Med 2003;44:198–206.
29. Goerres GW, Schmid DT, Bandhauer F, et al. Positron emission tomography in the early follow-up of advanced head and neck cancer. Arch Otolaryngol Head Neck Surg 2004;130:105–109; discussion 120–121.
30. Kubota K, Yokoyama J, Yamaguchi K, et al. FDG-PET delayed imaging for the detection of head and neck cancer recurrence after radio-chemotherapy: comparison with MRI/CT. Eur J Nucl Med Mol Imaging 2004;31:590–595.
31. Greven KM, Williams DW III, McGuirt WF Sr, et al. Serial positron emission tomography scans following radiation therapy of patients with head and neck cancer. Head Neck 2001;23: 942–946.
32. Lowe VJ, Heber ME, Anscher MS, et al. Chest wall FDG accumulation in serial FDG-PET images in patients being treated for bronchogenic carcinoma with radiation. Clin Positron Imaging 1998;1:185–191.
33. Leskinen-Kallio S, Nagren K, Lehikoinen P, Ruotsalainen U, Teras M, Joensuu H. Carbon-11-methionine and PET is an effective method to image head and neck cancer. J Nucl Med 1992; 33:691–695.
34. Braams JW, Pruim J, Nikkels PGJ, Roodenburg JLN, Vaalburg W, Vermey A. Nodal spread of squamous cell carcinoma of the oral cavity detected with PET-tyrosine, MRI and CT. J Nucl Med 1996;37:897–901.
35. Nonomiya H, Oriuchi N, Kahn N, et al. Diagnosis of tumor in the nasal cavity and paranasal sinuses with [11]choline PET; comparative study with 2-F-18 fluoro-2-deoxy-D-glycose (FDG) PET. Ann Nucl Med 2004;18:29–34.
36. Cobben DCP, van der Laan B, Maas B, et al. F-18-FLT PET for visualization of laryngeal cancer: comparison with F-18-FDG-PET. J Nucl Med 2004;45:226–231.
37. Lewis JS, Herrero P, Sharp TL, et al. Delineation of hypoxia in canine myocardium using PET and copper (II)-diacetyl-bis(*N*(4)-methylthiosemicarbazone). J Nucl Med 2002;43:1557–1569.
38. Maurer RI, Blower PJ, Dilworth JR, Reynolds CA, Zheng Y, Mullen GE. Studies on the mechanism of hypoxic selectivity in copper bis (thiosemicarbazone) radiopharmaceuticals. J Med Chem 2002;45:1420–1431.
39. Nunn A, Linder K, Strauss HW. Nitroimidazoles and imaging hypoxia. Eur J Nucl Med 1995;22:265–280.
40. Piert M, Machulla HJ, Becker G, Aldinger P, Winter E, Bares R. Dependency of the [F-18]fluoromisonidazole uptake on oxygen delivery and tissue oxygenation in the porcine liver. Nucl Med Biol 2000;27:693–700.
41. Adler LP, Bloom AD. Positron emission tomography of thyroid masses. Thyroid 1993;3:195–200.
42. Bloom AD, Adler LP, Shuck JM. Determination of malignancy of thyroid nodules with positron emission tomography. Surgery (St. Louis) 1993;114:728–734.
43. Kresnik E, Gallowitsch HJ, Mikosch P, et al. Fluorine-18-fluorodeoxyglycose positron emission tomography in the preop-

erative assessment of thyroid nodules in an endemic goiter area. Surgery (St. Louis) 2003;133:294–299.
44. Borner AR, Voth E, Wienhard K, Wagner R, Schicha H. F-18-FDG-PET in autonomous goiter. Nuklear-medizin 1999;38:1–6.
45. Gianoukakis AG, Karam M, Cheema A, Cooper JA. Autonomous thyroid nodules visualized by positron emission tomography with F-18-fluorodeoxyglucose: a case report and review of the literature. Thyroid 2003;13:395–399.
46. Yasuda S, Shohtsu A, Ide M, Takagi S, Suzuki Y, Tajima T. Diffuse F-18 FDG uptake in chronic thyroiditis. Clin Nucl Med 1997;22:341.
47. Schmid DT, Kneifel S, Stoeckli SJ, Padberg BC, Merrill G, Goerres GS. Increased 18F-FDG uptake mimicking thyroid cancer in a patient with Hashimoto's thyroiditis. Eur Radiol 2003;13:2119–2121.
48. Kang KW, Kim SK, Kang HS, et al. Prevalence and risk of cancer of focal thyroid incidentaloma identified by F-18-fluorodeoxyglucose positron emission tomography for metastasis evaluation and cancer screening in healthy subjects. J Clin Endocrinol Metab 2003;88:4100–4104.
49. Cohen MS, Arslan N, Dehdashti F, et al. Risk of malignancy in thyroid incidentalomas identified by fluorodeoxyglucose-positron emission tomography. Surgery (St. Louis) 2001;130: 941–946.
50. Grunwald F, Kalicke T, Feine U, et al. Fluorine-18-fluorodeoxyglucose positron emission tomography in thyroid cancer: results of a multicentre study. Eur J Nucl Med 1999;26:1547–1552.
51. Feine U, Lietzenmayer R, Hanke JP, Held J, Whorle H, Muller-Schauenburg W. Fluorine-18-FDG and iodine-131-iodide uptake in thyroid cancer. J Nucl Med 1996;37:1468–1472.
52. Wang WP, Macapinlac H, Larson SM, et al. F-18–2-fluoro-2-deoxy-D-glucose positron emission tomography localizes residual thyroid cancer in patients with negative diagnostic I-131 whole body scans and elevated serum thyroglobulin levels. J Clin Endocrinol Metab 1999;84:2291–2302.
53. Altenvoerde G, Lerch H, Kuwert T, Matheja P, Schafers M, Schober O. Positron emission tomography with F-18-deoxyglucose in patients with differentiated thyroid carcinoma, elevated thyroglobulin levels, and negative iodine scans. Langenbecks Arch Surg 1998;383:160–163.
54. Grunwald F, Menzel C, Bender H, et al. Comparison of 18FDG-PET with 131 iodine and 99mTc-sestamibi scintigraphy in differentiated thyroid cancer. Thyroid 1997;7:327–335.
55. Maxon HR. Detection of residual and recurrent thyroid cancer by radionuclide imaging. Thyroid 1999;9:443–446.
56. Schonberger J, Ruschoff J, Grimm D, et al. Glucose transporter I gene expression is related to thyroid neoplasms with an unfavorable prognosis: an immunohistochemical study. Thyroid 2002;12:747–754.
57. Chin BB, Patel P, Cohade C, Ewertz M, Wahl R, Ladenson P. Recombinant human thyrotropin stimulation of fluoro-D-glucose positron emission tomography uptake in well-differentiated thyroid carcinoma. J Clin Endocrinol Metab 2004;89:91–95.
58. Moog F, Linke R, Manthey N, et al. Influence of thyroid-stimulating hormone levels on uptake of FDG in recurrent and metastatic differentiated thyroid carcinoma. J Nucl Med 2000;41:1989–1995.
59. Helal BO, Merlet P, Toubert ME, et al. Clinical impact of (18)F-FDG-PET in thyroid carcinoma patients with elevated thyroglobulin levels and negative (131) I scanning results after therapy. J Nucl Med 2001;42:1464–1469.
60. Schluter B, Bohuslavizki KH, Beyer W, et al. Impact of FDG-PET on patients with differentiated thyroid cancer who present with elevated thyroglobulin and negative 131 I scan. J Nucl Med 2001;42:71–76.
61. Moog F, Linke R, Manthey N, et al. Influence of thyroid-stimulating hormone levels on uptake of FDG in recurrent and metastatic differentiated thyroid carcinoma. J Nucl Med 2000;41:1989–1995.
62. Petrich T, Borner AR, Otto D, et al. Influence of rhTSH on [(18)F]fluorodeoxyglucose uptake by differentiated thyroid carcinoma. Eur J Nucl Med Mol Imaging 2002;29:641–647.
63. Deichen JT, Schmidt C, Prante O, Maschauer S, Papadopoulos T, Kuwert T. Influence of TSH on uptake of F-18 fluorodeoxyglucose in human thyroid cells in vitro. Eur J Nucl Med Mol Imaging 2004;31:507–512.
64. Wang WP, Larson SM, Fazzari M, et al. Prognostic value of [F-18] fluorodeoxyglucose positron emission tomographic scanning in patients with thyroid cancer. J Clin Endocrinol Metab 2000;85:1107–1113.
65. Wang WP, Larson SM, Tuttle RM, et al. Resistance of F-18-fluorodeoxyglucose-avid metastatic thyroid cancer lesions to treatment with high-dose radioactive iodine. Thyroid 2001; 11:1169–1175.
66. Lowe VJ, Mullan BP, Hay ID, Mclver B, Kasperbauer JL. F-18-FDG-PET of patients with Hurthle cell carcinoma. J Nucl Med 2003;44:1402–1406.
67. Plotkin M, Hautzel H, Krause BJ, et al. Implication of 2-(18)fluoro-2-deoxyglucose positron emission tomography in the follow-up of Hurthle cell thyroid cancer. Thyroid 2002; 12:155–161.
68. Brandt-Mainz K, Muller SP, Gorges R, Saller B, Bocksch A. The value of fluorine-18 fluorodeoxy-glucose PET in patients with medullary thyroid cancer. Eur J Nucl Med 2000;27:490–496.
69. Diehl M, Risse JH, Brandt-Mainz K, et al. Fluorine-18 fluorodeoxyglucose positron emission tomography in medullary thyroid cancer. Results of a multicentre study. Eur J Nucl Med 2001;28:1671–1676.
70. Hoegerle S, Altehoefer C, Ghanem N, Brink I, Moser E, Nitzsche E. F-18-DOPA positron emission tomography for tumour detection in patients with medullary thyroid carcinoma and elevated calcitonin levels. Eur J Nucl Med 2001;28:64–71.
71. Courgiotis L, Sarlis NJ, Reynolds JC, et al. Localization of medullary thyroid carcinoma metastasis in a multiple endocrine neoplasia type 2A patient by 6-[^{18}F]-fluorodopamine positron emission tomography. J Clin Endocrinol Metab 2003;88: 637–641.
72. Enzinger PC, Mayer RJ. Esophageal cancer. N Engl J Med 2003;349:2241–2252.
73. Flamen P, Lerut A, Van Cutsem E, et al. Utility of positron emission tomography for the staging of patients with potentially operable esophageal carcinoma. J Clin Oncol 2000;18:3202–3210.
74. Kim K, Park SJ, Kim BT, et al. Evaluation of lymph node metastases in squamous cell carcinoma of the esophagus with positron emission tomography. Ann Thorac Surg 2001;71:290–294.
75. Fukunaga T, Okazumi S, Koide Y, et al. Evaluation of esophageal cancers using fluorine-18-fluorodeoxyglucose PET. J Nucl Med 1998;39:102–107.
76. Flanagan FL, Dehdashti F, Siegel BA, et al. Staging of esophageal cancer with FDG-PET. AJR 1997;168:417–424.
77. Mc Ateer D, Wallis F, Couper G, et al. Evaluation of ^{18}F-FDG positron emission tomography in gastric and esophageal carcinoma. Br J Radiol 1999;72:525–529.
78. Yeung HWD, Macapinlac HA, Mazumdar M, et al. FDG-PET in esophageal cancer: incremental value over computed tomography. Clin Positron Imaging 1999;5:255–260.
79. Himeno S, Yasuda S, Shimada H, et al. Evaluation of esophageal cancer by positron emission tomography. Jpn J Clin Oncol 2002;32:340–346.
80. Kato H, Kuwano H, Nakijima M, Miyareki T. Comparison between positron emission tomography in the use of the assessment of esophageal carcinoma. Cancer 2002;94(4):921–928.

81. Yoon YC, Lee KS, Shim YM, Kim BT, Kim K, Kim TS. Metastasis to regional lymph nodes in patients with esophageal squamous cell carcinoma: CT versus FDG PET for presurgical detection prospective study. Radiology 2003;227:764–770.
82. Lerut T, Coosemans W, Decker G, et al. Cancer of the esophagus and gastro-esophageal junction: potentially curative therapies. Surg Oncol 2001;10:113–122.
83. Dehdashti F, Siegel BA. Neoplasms of the esophagus and stomach. Semin Nuclear Med 2004;34(3):198–208.
84. Lerut T, Flamen P, Ectors N, et al. Histopathologic validation of lymph node staging with FDG-PET scan in cancer of esophagus and gastroesophageal junction: a prospective study based on primary surgery with extensive lymphadenectomy. Ann Surg 2000;232:743–752.
85. Giovagnoni A, Valeri G, Ferrara C. MRI of esophageal cancer. Abdom Imaging 2002;27:361–366.
86. Motohara T, Semelka RC. MRI in staging of gastric cancer. Abdom Imaging 2002;27:376–383.
87. Kinkel K, Lu Y, Both M, et al. Detection of hepatic metastases from cancers of the gastrointestinal tract by using noninvasive imaging methods (US, CT, MR imaging, PET): a meta-analysis. Radiology 2002;224:748–756.
88. Luketich JD, Schauer P, Meltzer CC, et al. The role of positron emission tomography in staging esophageal cancer. Am Thorac Surg 1997;64:765–769.
89. Luketich JD, Friedman DM, Weigel TL, et al. Evaluation of distant metastases in esophageal cancer: 100 consecutive positron emission tomography scans. Ann Thorac Surg 1999;68: 1133–1137.
90. Wallace MB, Nietert RJ, Earle C, et al. An analysis of multiple staging management strategies for carcinoma of the esophagus: computed tomography, endoscopic ultrasound, positron emission tomography, and thoracoscopy/laparoscopy. Ann Thorac Surg 2002;74:1026–1032.
91. Wren SM, Stijns P, Srinivas S. Positron emission tomography in the initial staging of esophageal cancer. Arch Surg 2002;137: 1001–1006.
92. Hustinx R, Dolin RJ, Benard F, et al. Impact of attenuation correction on the accuracy of FDG-PET in patients with abdominal tumors: a free-response ROC analysis. Eur J Nucl Med 2000;27:1365–1371.
93. Wu LF, Wang BZ, Feng JL, et al. Preoperative TN staging of esophageal cancer: comparison of miniprobe ultrasonography, spiral CT and MRI. World J Gastroenterol 2003;9:219–224.
94. MRC, Oesophageal Cancer Working Group. Surgical resection with or without preoperative chemotherapy in oesophageal cancer: a randomized controlled trial. Lancet 2002;359:1727–1733.
95. Beseth BD, Bedford R, Isacoff WH, et al. Endoscopic ultrasound does not accurately assess pathologic stage of esophageal cancer after neoadjuvant chemoradiotherapy. Am Surg 2000;66: 827–831.
96. Laterza E, de Manzoni G, Guglielmi A, et al. Endoscopic ultrasonography in the staging of esophageal carcinoma after preoperative radiotherapy and chemotherapy. Ann Thorac Surg 1999;67:1466–1469.
97. Weber WA, Ott K, Becker K, et al. Prediction of response to preoperative chemotherapy in adenocarcinomas of esophagogastric junction by metabolic imaging. J Clin Oncol 2001;19:3058–3065.
98. Weber WA, Ott K. Imaging of esophageal and gastric cancer. Semin Oncol 2004;31(4):530–541.
99. Brucher BL, Weber W, Bauer M, et al. Neoadjuvant therapy of esophageal squamous cell carcinoma: response evaluation by positron emission tomography. Ann Surg 2001;233:300–309.
100. Flamen P, Van Cutsem E, Lerut A, et al. Positron emission tomography for assessment of the response to induction chemotherapy in locally advanced esophageal cancer. Ann Oncol 2002;13:361–368.
101. Downey RJ, Akhurst T, Ilson D, et al. Whole body [18]FDG-PET and the response of esophageal cancer to induction therapy: results of a prospective trial. J Clin Oncol 2003;21:428–432.
102. Arslan N, Miller TR, Dehdashti F, Battafarano RJ, Siegel BA. Evaluation of response to neoadjuvant therapy by quantitative 2-deoxy-2-[^{18}F] fluoro-D-glucose with positron emission tomography in patients with esophageal cancer. Mol Imaging Biol 2002;4:301–310.
103. Fukunaga T, Enomoto K, Okazumi S, et al. Analysis of glucose metabolism in patients with esophageal cancer by PET: estimation of hexokinase activity in the tumor and usefulness for clinical assessment using FDG. Nippon Geka Gakka Zasshi 1994;95:317–325.
104. Yeung HW, Macapinlac HA, Mazumdar M, Bains M, Finn RD, Larson SM. FDG-PET in esophageal cancer, incremental value over computed tomography. Clin Positron Imaging 1999;2: 255–260.
105. Flamen P, Lerut A, Van Cutsem E, et al. The utility of positron emission tomography for the diagnosis and staging of recurrent esophageal cancer. J Thorac Cardiovasc Surg 2000;120: 1085–1092.
106. Boring CC, Squires TS, Tong T. Cancer statistics, 1992. CA Cancer J Clin 1992;42(1):19–38.
107. Stoller JK, Ahmad M, Rice W. Solitary pulmonary module. Cleve Clin J Med 1988;55(I):68–74.
108. Dewan NA, Gupta NC, Redepenning LS, et al. Diagnostic efficacy of PET-FDG imaging in solitary pulmonary modules. Potential role in evaluation and management. Chest 1993; 104(4):997–1002.
109. Erasmus JJ, Connolly JE, McAdams HP, et al. Solitary pulmonary nodules: Part I. Morphologic evaluation for differentiation of benign and malignant lesion. Radiographics 2000;20:43–58.
110. Gurney JW, Lyddon DM, McKay JA. Determining the likelihood of malignancy in solitary pulmonary nodules with Bayesian analysis. Part II. Application. Radiology 1993;186(2):415–422.
111. Winning AJ, Mclvor J, Seed WA, et al. Interpretation of negative results in fine needle aspiration of discrete pulmonary lesions. Thorax 1986;41(11):875–879.
112. Lowe VJ, Duhaylongsod FD, Patz EF, et al. Pulmonary abnormalities and PET data analysis: a retrospective study. Radiology 1997;202(2):435–439.
113. Goo JM, Im JG, Do KH, et al. Pulmonary tuberculoma evaluated by means of FDG PET: findings in 10 cases. Radiology 2000;216:117–121.
114. Lewis PJ, Salama A. Uptake of fluorine-18-fluorodeoxyglucose in sarcoidosis. J Nucl Med 1994;35:1647–1649.
115. Wilkinson MD, Fulham MJ, Mc Caughan BC, et al. Invasite aspergillosis mimicking stage IIIA non-small-cell lung cancer on FDG positron emission tomography. Clin Nucl Med 2003;28: 234–235.
116. Croft DR, Trapp J, Kernstine K, et al. FDG-PET imaging and the diagnosis of non-small cell lung cancer in a region of high hitoplasmosis prevalence. Lung Cancer 2002;36:297–301.
117. Bender H, Palmedo H, Biersack HJ, et al. Atlas of Clinical PET in Oncology: PET Versus CT and MRI. Berlin: Springer, 2000.
118. Frank A, Lefkowitz D, Jaeger J, et al. Decision logic for retreatment of asymptomatic lung cancer recurrence based on positron emission tomography findings. Int J Radiat Oncol Biol Phys 1995;32(5):1495–1512.
119. Yap CS, Schiepers C, Fishbein MC, et al. FDG-PET imaging in lung cancer: how sensitive is it for bronchoalveolar carcinoma? Eur J Nucl Med Mol Imaging 2002;29:1166–1173.
120. Erasmus JJ, McAdams HP, Patz EF Jr, et al. Evaluation of primary pulmonary carcinoid tumors using FDG PET. AJR Am J Roentgenol 1998;170:1369–1373.
121. Gould MK, Maclean CC, Kuschner WG, et al. Accuracy of positron emission tomography for diagnosis of pulmonary modules and mass lesions. JAMA 2001;285(7):914–924.

122. Swensen SJ, Viggiano RW, Midthun DE, et al. Lung nodule enhancement at CT: multicenter study. Radiology 2000;214: 73–80.
123. Nathan MA, Mullan BP, Hartman TE. Characterization of the solitary pulmonary module ^{18}F-FDG PET versus nodule enhancement CT. Eur J Nucl Med 2003;30(suppl 2):S151.
124. Rohren EM, Lowe VJ. Update in PET imaging of non-small cell lung cancer. Semin Nucl Med 2004;34(2):134–153.
125. Marom EM, Sarvis S, Herndon JE, et al. T1 lung cancers: sensitivity of diagnosis with fluorodeoxyglucose PET. Radiology 2002;223:453–459.
126. Zhuang H, Pourdehnad M, Lambright ES, et al. Dual time point ^{18}F-FDG PET imaging for differentiating malignant from inflammatory processes. J Nucl Med 2001;42:1412–1417.
127. Matthies A, Hickeson M, Cuchiara A, et al. Dual time point ^{18}F-FDG PET for the evaluation of pulmonary nodules. J Nucl Med 2002;43:871–875.
128. Demura Y, Tsuchida T, Ishizaki T, et al. ^{18}F-FDG accumulation with PET for differentiation between benign and malignant lesions in the thorax. J Nucl Med 2003;44:540–548.
129. Marom EM, McAdams HP, Erasmus JJ, et al. Staging non-small cell lung cancer with whole-body PET. Radiology 1999;212(3): 803–809.
130. Erasmus JJ, Patz EF, McAdams HP, et al. Evaluation of adrenal masses in patients with bronchogenic carcinoma using ^{18}F-fluorodeoxyglucose positron emission tomography. AJR Am J Roentgenol 1997;168(5):1357–1360.
131. Dwamena BA, Seema SS, Angobaldo JO, et al. Metastases from non-small cell lung cancer: mediastinal staging in the 1990s. Meta-analytic comparison of PET and CT. Radiology 1999; 213(2):530–536.
132. Wahl RL, Quint LE, Greenough RL, et al. Staging of mediastinal non-small cell lung cancer with FDG PET, CT, and fusion images: preliminary prospective evaluation. Radiology 1994; 191:371–377.
133. Steinert HC, Hauser M, Allemann F, et al. Non-small cell lung cancer: nodal staging with FDG PET versus CT with correlative lymph node mapping and sampling. Radiology 197;202:441–446.
134. Vansteenkiste JF, Mortelmans LA. FDG-PET in the locoregional lymph node staging of non-small cell lung cancer. A comprehensive review of the Leuven lung cancer group experience. Clin Positron Imaging 1999;2:223–231.
135. Pieterman RM, van Putten JW, Meuzelaar JJ, et al. Preoperative staging of non-small-cell lung cancer with positron-emission tomography. N Engl J Med 2000;343:254–261.
136. Bury T, Corhay JL, Duysinx B, et al. Value of FDG-PET in detecting residual or recurrent non-small cell lung cancer. Eur Respir J 1999;14(6):1376–1380.
137. Mah K, Cladwell CB, Ung YC, et al. The impact of ([18])F-FDG-PET on target and critical organs in CT-based treatment planning of patients with poorly defined non-small-cell lung carcinoma: a prospective study. Int J Radiat Oncol Biol Phys 2002;52:339–350.
138. Erdi YE, Rosenzweig K, Erdi AK, et al. Radiotherapy treatment planning for patients with non-small cell lung cancer using positron emission tomography (PET). Radiother Oncol 2002;62: 51–60.
139. Jeong HJ, Min JJ, Park JM, et al. Determination of the prognostic value of (^{18}F)fluorodeoxyglucose uptake by using positron emission tomography in patients with non-small cell lung cancer. Nucl Med Commun 2002;23:865–870.
140. Ahuja V, Coleman RE, Herndon J, et al. The prognostic significance of fluorodeoxyglucose positron emission tomography imaging for patients with nonsmall cell lung carcinoma. Cancer (Phila) 1998;83:918–924.
141. Dhital K, Saunders CA, Seed PT, et al. [^{18}F]Fluorodeoxyglucose positron emission tomography and its prognostic value in lung cancer. Eur J Cardiothorac Surg 2000;18:425–428.
142. Yasukawa T, Yoshikawa K, Aoyagi H, et al. Usefulness of PET with ^{11}C-methionine for the detection of hilar and mediastinal lymph node metastasis in lung cancer. J Nucl Med 2000;41: 283–290.
143. Hustinx R, Lemaire C, Jerusalem G, et al. Whole-body tumor imaging using PET and 2–[18]F-fluoro-L-tyrosine: preliminary evaluation and comparison with ^{18}F-FDG. J Nucl Med 2003;44:533–539.
144. Greenlee RT, Murray T, Hill-Harmon MB, et al. Cancer statistics 2001. CA Cancer J Clin 2001;51:15–35.
145. Wingo PA, Cardinez CJ, Landis SH, et al. Long-term trends in cancer mortality in the United States, 1930–1998. Cancer (Phila) 2003;97(suppl 12):3133–3175.
146. Brown RS, Wahl RL. Overexpression of Glut-1-glucose transporter in human breast cancer: an immunohistochemical study. Cancer (Phila) 1993;72:2979–2985.
147. Minn H, Soini I. [^{18}F]Fluorodeoxyglucose scintigraphy in diagnosis and follow-up of treatment in advanced breast cancer. Eur J Nucl Med 1989;15(2):61–66.
148. Wahl RL, Cody RL, Hutchins GD, Mudgett EE. Primary and metastatic breast carcinoma: initial clinical evaluation with PET with the radiolabeled glucose analogue 2-[F-18]-fluoro-2-deoxy-D-glucose. Radiology 1991;179(3):765–770.
149. Kuota K, Matsuzawa T, Amemiya A, et al. Imaging of breast cancer with [^{18}F] fluorodeoxyglucose and positron emission tomography. J Comput Assist Tomogr 1989;13(6):1097–1098.
150. Avril N, Rose CA, Schelling M, et al. Breast imaging with positron emission tomography and [fluorine-18]-fluorodeoxyglucose: use and limitations. J Clin Oncol 2000;18:3495–3502.
151. Schirrmeister H, Kuhn T, Guhlmann A, et al. Fluorine-18-2-deoxy-2-fluoro-D-glucose PET in the preoperative staging of breast cancer: comparison with the standard staging procedures. Eur J Nucl Med 2001;28(3):351–358.
152. Walter C, Scheidhauer K, Scharl A, et al. Clinical and diagnostic value of preoperative MR mammography and FDG-PET in suspicious breast lesions. Eur Radiol 2003;13(7):1651–1656.
153. Heinisch M, Gallowitsch HJ, Mikosch P, et al. Comparison of FDG-PET and dynamic contrast-enhanced MRI in the evaluation of suggestive breast lesions. Breast 2003;121(1):17–22.
154. Samson D, Flamm CR, Aronson N. FDG positron emission tomography for evaluation of breast cancer. Washington, DC: Blue Shield and Blue Cross Association, 2001:1–93.
155. Adler LP, Crowe JP, al-Kaisi NK, Sunshine JL. Evaluation of breast masses and axillary lymph nodes with [F-18] 2-deoxy-2-fluoro-D-glucose PET. Radiology 1993;187(3):743–750.
156. Dehdashti F, Mortimer JE, Siegel BA, et al. Positron tomographic assessment of estrogen receptors in breast cancer: comparison with FDG-PET and in vitro receptor assays. J Nucl Med 1995;36(10):1766–1774.
157. Morrow M, Harris JR. Local management of invasive breast cancer. In: Harris JR, Lippman ME, Morrow M, Osborne CK (eds). Diseases of the Breast, 2nd ed. Philadelphia: Lippincott Williams & Wilkins, 2000:515–560.
158. Weinberg I, Majewski S, Weisenberger A, et al. Preliminary results for positron emission mammography: real-time functional breast imaging in a conventional mammography gantry. Eur J Nucl Med 1996;23:804–806.
159. Murthy K, Aznar M, Thompson CJ, et al. Results of preliminary clinical trials of the positron emission mammography system PEM-I: a dedicated breast imaging system producing glucose metabolic images using FDG. J Nucl Med 2000;41:1851–1858.
160. Murthy K, Aznar M, Bergman AM, et al. Positron emission mammographic instrument: initial results. Radiology 2000; 215:280–285.
161. Crippa F, Seregni E, Agresti R, et al. Association between [^{18}F]-fluorodeoxyglucose uptake and postoperative histopathology, hormone receptor status, thymidine labeling index and p53 in

primary breast cancera preliminary observation. Eur J Nucl Med 1998;25:1429–1434.
162. Avril N, Menzel M, Dose J, et al. Glucose metabolism of breast cancer assessed by ^{18}F-FDG-PET: histologic and immunohistochemical tissue analysis. J Nucl Med 2001;42:9–16.
163. Buck A, Schirrmeister H, Kuhn T, et al. FDG uptake in breast cancer: correlation with biological and clinical prognostic parameters. Eur J Nucl Med Mol Imaging 2002;29:1317–1323.
164. Adler LP, Crowe JP, Al-Kaisi NK, et al. Evaluation of breast masses and axillary lymph nodes with [F-18] 2-deoxy-2-fluoro-D-glucose PET. Radiology 1993;187:743–750.
165. Crowe JP Jr, Adler LP, Shenk RR, et al. Positron emission tomography and breast masses: comparison with clinical, mammographic, and pathological findings. Ann Surg Oncol 1994;1:132–140.
166. Oshida M, Uno K, Suzuki M, et al. Predicting the prognoses of breast carcinoma patients with positron emission tomography using 2-deoxy-2-[^{18}F] fluoro-D-glucose. Cancer (Phila) 1998;82:2227–2234.
167. Bos R, van Der Hoeven JJ, van Der Wall E, et al. Biologic correlates of [^{18}F]-fluorodeoxyglucose uptake in human breast cancer measured by positron emission tomography. J Clin Oncol 2002;20:379–387.
168. Crippa F, Agresti R, Seregni E, et al. Prospective evaluation of [fluorine-18]-FDG-PET in presurgical staging of the axilla in breast cancer. J Nucl Med 1998;39:4–8.
169. Dehdashti F, Mortimer JE, Siegel BA, et al. Positron tomographic assessment of estrogen receptors in breast cancer: Comparison with FDG-PET and *in vitro* receptor assays. J Nucl Med 1995;36:1766–1774.
170. Eubank WB, Mankoff DA. Current and future uses of positron emission tomography in breast cancer imaging. Semin Nucl Med 2004;34(3):224–240.
171. Mankoff DA, Dunnwald LK, Gralow JR, et al. Blood flow and metabolism in locally advanced breast cancer (LABC): relationship to response to therapy. J Nucl Med 2002;43:500–509.
172. Gottleib E, Heiden MV, Thompson CB. Bcl-x_l prevents the initial disease to mitochondrial membrane potential and subsequent reactive oxygen species production during tumor necrosis factor alpha-induced apoptosis. Mol Cell Biol 2000;20:5680–5689.
173. West KA, Castillo SS, Dennis PA. Activation of the P13K/Akt pathway and chemotherapeutic resistance. Drug Resist Update 2002;6:234–248.
174. Hellman S, Harris JR. Natural history of breast cancer. In: Harris JR, Lippman ME, Marrow M, Osborne CK (eds). Diseases of the Breast, 2nd ed. Philadelphia: Lippincott Williams & Wilkins, 2000:407–423.
175. Wahl RL, Siegel BA, Coleman RE, Gatsonis CG. Prospective multicenter study of axillary nodal staging by positron emission tomography in breast cancer: a report of the staging breast cancer with PET Study Group. J Clin Oncol 2004;22(2):277–285.
176. Kumar R, Potenta S, Loving VA, et al. FDG-PET positive lymph modes are highly predictive of metastasis in breast cancer. J Nucl Med 2004;45(suppl):154 (abstract).
177. Zornoza G, Garcia-Velloso MJ, Sola J, Regueira FM, Pina L, Beorlegui C. ^{18}F-FDG PET complemented with sentinel lymph node biopsy in the detection of axillary involvement in breast cancer. Eur J Surg Oncol 2004;30(1):15–19.
178. Greco M, Crippa F, Agresti R, et al. Axillary lymph node staging in breast cancer by 2-fluoro-2-deoxy-D-glucose-positron emission tomography: clinical evaluation and alternative management. J Natl Cancer Inst 2001;93(8):630–635.
179. Schirrmeister H, Kuhn T, Guhlmann A, et al. Fluorine-18-2-deoxy-2-fluoro-D-glucose PET in the preoperative staging of breast cancer: comparison with the standard staging procedures. Eur J Nucl Med 2001;28(3):351–358.
180. Avril N, Dose J, Janicke F, et al. Assessment of axillary lymph node involvement in breast cancer patients with positron emission tomography using radiolabeled 2(fluorine-18)-fluoro-2-deoxy-D-glucose. J Natl Cancer Inst 1996;88(17):1204–1209.
181. Freneaux P, Nos C, Vincent-Salomon A, et al. Histological detection of minimal metastatic involvement in axillary sentinel nodes: a rational basis for a sensitive methodology usable in daily practice. Mod Pathol 2002;15(6):641–646.
182. Yeatman TJ, Cox CE. The significance of breast cancer lymph node micrometastases. Surg Oncol Clin N Am 1999;8:481–496.
183. Wahl Rl, Kaminski MS, Either SP, et al. The potential of 2-deoxy-2-fluoro-D-glucose (FDG) for detection of tumor involvement in lymph nodes. J Nucl Med 1990;31:1831–1835.
184. Albertini JJ, Lyman GH, Cox C, et al. Lymphatic mapping and sentinel node biopsy in the patient with breast cancer. JAMA 1996;276:1818–1822.
185. Barranger E, Grahek D, Antoine M, et al. Evaluation of fluorodeoxyglucose positron emission tomography in the detection of axillary lymph node metastases in patients with early stage breast cancer. Ann Surg Oncol 2003;10:622–627.
186. Guller U, Nitzsche EU, Schirp U, et al. Selective axillary surgery in breast cancer patients based on positron emission tomography with ^{18}F-fluoro-2-deoxy-D-glucose: not yet! Breast Cancer Res Treat 2002;71:171–173.
187. Kelemen PR, Lowe V, Phillips N. Positron emission tomography and sentinel lymph node dissection in breast cancer. Clin Breast Cancer 2002;3:73–77.
188. Wagner JD, Schauwecker D, Davidson D, et al. Prospective study of fluorodeoxyglucose: positron emission tomography imaging of lymph node basins in melanoma patients undergoing sentinel node biopsy. J Clin Oncol 1999;17:1508–1515.
189. Cody HS III, Urban JA. Internal mammary node status: a major prognosticator in axillary node-negative breast cancer. Ann Surg Oncol 1995;2:32–37.
190. Katz A, Strom EA, Buchholz TA, et al. Locoregional recurrence patterns after mastectomy and doxorubicin-based chemotherapy: Implications for postoperative irradiation. J Clin Oncol 2000;18:2817–2827.
191. Hathaway PB, Mankoff DA, Maravilla KR, et al. Value of combined FDG PET and MR imaging in the evaluation of suspected recurrent local-regional breast cancer: preliminary experience. Radiology 1999;210(3):807–814.
192. Ahmad A, Barrington S, Maisey M, Rubens RD. Use of positron emission tomography in evaluation of brachial plexopathy in breast cancer patients. Br J Cancer 1999;79(3–4):478–482.
193. Eubank WB, Mankoff DA, Takasugi J, et al. [18]Fluorodeoxyglucose positron emission tomography to detect mediastinal or internal mammary metastases in breast cancer. J Clin Oncol 2001;19:3516–3523.
194. Moon DH, Maddahi J, Silverman DH, Glaspy JA, Phelps ME, Hoh CK. Accuracy of whole-body fluorine-18-FDG PET for the detection of recurrent or metastatic breast carcinoma. J Nucl Med 1998;39(3):431–435.
195. Gallowitsch HJ, Kresnik E, Gasser J, et al. F-18 fluorodeoxyglucose positron emission tomography in the diagnosis of tumor recurrence and metastases in the follow-up of patients with breast carcinoma: a comparison to conventional imaging. Invest Radiol 2003;38(5):250–256.
196. Lonneux M, Borbath I, Berliere M, et al. The place of whole-body PET FDG for the diagnosis of distant recurrence of breast cancer. Clin Positron Imaging 2000;3:45–49.
197. Kamel EM, Wyss MT, Fehr MK, von Schulthess GK, Goerres GW. [^{18}F]-Fluorodeoxyglucose positron emission tomography in patients with suspected recurrence of breast cancer. J Cancer Res Clin Oncol 2003;129(3):147–153.
198. Inoue T, Yutani K, Taguchi T, Tamaki Y, Shiba E, Noguchi S. Preoperative evaluation of prognosis in breast cancer patients by

[18F]2-deoxy-2-fluoro-D-glucose-positron emission tomography. J Cancer Res Clin Oncol 2004;130(5):273–278.
199. Nielsen OS, Munro AJ, Tannock IF. Bone metastases: pathophysiology and management policy. J Clin Oncol 1991;9:509–524.
200. Cook GJ, Houston S, Rubens R, et al. Detection of bone metastases in breast cancer by 18FDG-PET: differing metabolic activity in osteoblastic and osteolytic lesions. J Clin Oncol 1998;16:3375–3379.
201. Mundy GR, Guise TA, Yoneda T. Biology of bone metastases. In: Harris JR, Lippman ME, Marrow M, Osborne CK (eds). Diseases of the Breast, 2nd ed. Philadelphia: Lippincott Williams & Wilkins, 2000:911–920.
202. Schirrmeister H, Guhlmann A, Kotzerke J, et al. Early detection and accurate description of extent of metastatic bone disease in breast cancer with fluoride ion and positron emission tomography. J Clin Oncol 1999;17:2381–2389.
203. Yap CS, Seltzer MA, Schieppers C, et al. Impact of whole body of FDG-PET on the staging and managing patients with breast cancer: the referring physicians perspective. J Nucl Med 2001;42:1334–1337.
204. Eubank WB, Mankoff DA, Takasugi J, et al. 18-Fluorodeoxyglucose positron emission tomography to detect mediastinal or internal mammary metastases in breast cancer. J Clin Oncol 2001;19(15):3516–3523.
205. Wahl RL, Zasadny K, Helvie MA, et al. Metabolic monitoring of breast cancer chemohormonotherapy using positron emission tomography: initial evaluation. J Clin Oncol 1993;11:2101–2111.
206. Schelling M, Avril N, Nahrig J, et al. Positron emission tomography using [18F] fluorodeoxyglucose for monitoring primary chemotherapy in breast cancer. J Clin Oncol 2000;18(8):1689–1695.
207. Smith IC, Welch AE, Hutcheon AW, et al. Positron emission tomography using [18F]-fluorodeoxy-D-glucose to predict the pathologic response of breast cancer to primary chemotherapy. J Clin Oncol 2000;18(8):1676–1688.
208. Vranjesevic D, Filmont JE, Meta J, et al. Whole-body (18)F-FDG PET and conventional imaging for predicting outcome in previously treated breast cancer patients. J Nucl Med 2002;43(3):325–329.
209. Jain RK. Haemodynamic and transport barriers to the treatment of solid tumors. Int J Radiat Biol 1991;60:85–100.
210. Mankoff DA, Dunnwald LK, Gralow JR, et al. Changes in blood flow and metabolism in locally advanced breast cancer treated with neoadjuvant chemotherapy. J Nucl Med 2003;44:1806–1814.
211. Sugawara Y, Fisher SJ, Zasadny KR, et al. Preclinical and clinical studies of bone marrow uptake of fluorine-18-fluorodeoxyglucose with or without granulocyte colony-stimulating factor during chemotherapy. J Clin Oncol 1998;16:173–180.
212. Abdel-Dayem HM, Rosen G. El-Zeftawy H, et al. Fluorine-18 fluorodeoxyglucose splenic uptake from extramedullary hematopoiesis after granulocyte colony-stimulating factor stimulation. Clin Nucl Med 1999;24:319–22.
213. Smith IC, Welch AE, Hutcheon AW, et al. Positron emission tomography using [18F]-fluorodeoxy-D-glucose to predict the pathologic response of breast cancer to primary chemotherapy. J Clin Oncol 2000;18:1676–1688.
214. Gennari A, Donati S, Salvadori B, et al. Role of 2-[18F]-fluorodeoxyglucose (FDG) positron emission tomography (PET) in the early assessment of response to chemotherapy in metastatic breast cancer patients. Clin Breast Cancer 2000;1:156–161.
215. Stafford SE, Gralow JR, Schubert EK, et al. Use of serial FDG-PET to measure the response of bone-dominant breast cancer to therapy. Acad Radiol 2001;9:913–921.
216. Mortimer JE, Dehdashti F, Siegel BA, et al. Metabolic flare: indicator of hormone responsiveness in advanced breast cancer. J Clin Oncol 2001;19:2797–2803.
217. Tannock IF. Cell proliferation. In: Tannock IF, Hill RP (eds). The Basic Science of Oncology. New York: McGraw-Hill, 1992.
218. Shields AF, Mankoff DA, Link JM, et al. [Carbon-11]-thymidine and FDG to measure therapy response. J Nucl Med 1998;39:1757–1762.
219. Shields AJ, Grierson J, Dohmen BM, et al. Imaging proliferation in vivo with [F-18]FLT and positron emission tomography. Nat Med 1998;4:1334–1336.
220. Grierson JR, Shields AF. Radiosynthesis of 3′-deoxy-3′-[18F]fluorothymidine[18F]FLT for imaging of cellular proliferation in vivo. Nucl Med Biol 2000;27:143–156.
221. Vesselle H, Grierson J, Muzi M, et al. In vivo validation of 3′-deoxy-3′-[18F]fluorothymidine[18F]FLT) as a proliferation imaging tracer in humans: correlation of [18F]FLT uptake by positron emission tomography with Ki-67 immunohistochemistry and flow cytometry in human lung tumors. Clin Cancer Res 2002;8:3315–3323.
222. Sutherland RM. Tumor hypoxia and gene expression- implications for malignant progression and therapy. Acta Oncol 1998;37:567–574.
223. Teicher BA. Hypoxia and drug resistance. Cancer Metastasis Rev 1994;13:139–168.
224. Rajendran JG, Mankoff DA, O'Sullivan F, et al. Hypoxia and glucose metabolism in malignant tumors: evaluation by FMISO and FDG-PET imaging. Clin Cancer Res 2004;10:2245–2252.
225. Clavo AC, Wahl RL. Effects of hypoxia on the uptake of tritiated thymidine, L-leucine, L-methionine and FDG in cultured cancer cells. J Nucl Med 1996;37:502–506.
226. Rajendran JG, Krohn KA. Imaging tumor hypoxia. In: Bailey DL, Townsend DW, Valk PE, Maisey MN (eds). Positron Emission Tomography: Principles and Practice. London: Springer Verlag, 2002:689–696.
227. Sledge GJ, McGuire W. Steroid hormone receptors in human breast cancer. Adv Cancer Res 1983;38:61–75.
228. Elledge RM, Fuqua SAW. Estrogen and progesterone. In: Harris JR, Lippman ME, Marrow M, Osborne CK (eds). Diseases of the Breast, 2nd ed. Philadelphia: Lippincott Williams & Wilkins, 2000:471–488.
229. Ravdin PM, Green S, Dorr TM, et al. Prognostic significance of progesterone receptor levels in estrogen receptor-positive patients with metastatic breast cancer treated with tamoxifen: results of a prospective Southwest Oncology Group study. J Clin Oncol 1992;10:1284–1291.
230. Mintum MA, Welch MJ, Siegel BA, et al. Breast cancer: PET imaging of estrogen receptors. Radiology 1988;169:45–48.
231. Mankoff DA, Peterson LM, Petra PH, et al. Factors affecting the level and heterogeneity of uptake of [18F]fluoroestradiol (FES) in patients with estrogen receptor positive (ER+) breast cancer. J Nucl Med 2002;43:287P (abstract).
232. McGuire AH, Dehdashti F, Siegel BA, et al. Positron tomographic assessment of 16alpha-[F-18]-fluoro-17beta-estradiol uptake in metastatic breast carcinoma. J Nucl Med 1991;32:1526–1531.
233. Mankoff DA, Peterson LM, Tewson TJ, et al. [18F]-Fluoroestradiol radiation dosimetry in human PET studies. J Nucl Med 2001;42:679–684.
234. Mankoff DA, Peterson LM, Tewson TJ, et al. Noninvasive PET imaging of ER expression in breast cancer: sex steroid binding protein (SBP or SHBG) interaction and ER expression heterogenicity. Proc AACR 2001;42:6 (abstract).
235. Dehdashti F, Morimer JE, Siegel BA, et al. Positron tomographic assessment of estrogen receptors in breast cancer. Comparison with FDG-PET and in vitro receptor assays. J Nucl Med 1995;36:1766–1774.
236. Mortimer JE, Dehdashti F, Sieger BA, et al. Clinical correlation of FDG-PET imaging with estrogen receptor and response to systemic therapy. Clin Cancer Res 1996;2:933–939.

237. Mortimer JE, Dehdashti F, Siegel BA, et al. Metabolic flare: indicator of hormone responsiveness in advanced breast cancer. J Clin Oncol 2001;19:2797–2803.
238. Vogel C, Schoenfelder J, Shemano I, et al. Worsening bone scan in the evaluation of antitumor response during hormonal therapy of breast cancer. J Clin Oncol 1995;13:1123–1128.
239. Legha S. Tamoxifen in the treatment of breast cancer. Ann Intern Med 1988;109:219–228.
240. Chan AO, Wong BC, Lam SK. Gastric cancer: past, present and future. Can J Gastroenterol 2001;15:469–474.
241. Stahl A, Ott K, Weber WA, et al. FDG PET imaging of locally advanced gastric carcinomas: correlation with endoscopic and histopathological findings. Eur J Nucl Med Mol Imaging 2003;30:288–295.
242. Kawamura T, Kusakabe T, Sugino T, et al. Expression of glucose transporter-1 in human gastric carcinoma: association with tumor aggressiveness, metastases and patient survival. Cancer 2001;92:634–641.
243. De Potter T, Flamen P, Van Cutsem E, et al. Whole-body PET with FDG for the diagnosis of recurrent gastric cancer. Eur J Nucl Med Mol Imaging 2002;29:525–529.
244. Yeung HWD, Macapinlac HA, Karpeh M, et al. Accuracy of FDG-PET in gastric cancer: preliminary experience. Clin Positron Imaging 1999;4:213–221.
245. Mochiki E, Kuwano H, Katoh H, Asao T, Oriuchi N, Endo K. Evaluation of ^{18}F-2-deoxy-2-fluoro-D-glucose positron emission tomography for gastric cancer. World J Surg 2004;28:247–253.
246. Yoshioka T, Yamaguchi K, Kubota K, et al. Evaluation of ^{18}F-FDG PET in patients with advanced, metastatic, or recurrent gastric cancer. J Nucl Med 2003;44:690–699.
247. Ott K, Fink U, Becker K, et al. Prediction of response to preoperative chemotherapy in gastric carcinoma by metabolic imaging: results of a prospective trial. J Clin Oncol 2003;21:4604–4610.
248. Jemal A, Tiwari RC, Murray T, et al. Cancer statistics, 2004. CA Cancer J Clin 2004;54:8–29.
249. Kievit J. Follow-up of patients with colorectal cancer: numbers needed to test and treat. Eur J Cancer 2002;38:986–999.
250. Longo WE, Johnson FE. The preoperative assessment and postoperative surveillance of patients with colon and rectal cancer. Surg Clin N Am 2002;82:1091–1108.
251. Abdel-Nabi H, Doerr RJ, Lamonica DM, et al. Staging of primary colorectal carcinomas with fluorine-18 fluoro-deoxyglucose whole-body PET: correlation with histopathologic and CT findings. Radiology 1998;206:755–760.
252. Kantorova I, Lipska L, Belohlavek O, Visokai V, Trubac M, Schneiderova M. Routine (18)F-FDG PET preoperative staging of colorectal cancer: comparison with conventional staging and its impact on treatment decision making. J Nucl Med 2003;44:1784–1788.
253. Mukai M, Sadahiro S, Yasuda S, et al. Preoperative evaluation by whole-body ^{18}F-fluorodeoxyglucose positron emission tomography in patients with primary colorectal cancer. Oncol Rep 2000;7:85–87.
254. Yasuda S, Fujii H, Nakahara T, et al. 18F-FDG PET detection of colonic adenomas. J Nucl Med 2001;42:989–992.
255. Hughes KS, Simon R, Songhorabodi S, et al. Resection of liver for colorectal carcinoma metastases: a multi-institutional study of indications for resection. Surgery (St. Louis) 1988;103:278–288.
256. Moertel CG, Fleming TR, McDonald JS, et al. An evaluation of the carcinoembryonic antigen (CEA) test for monitoring patients with resected colon cancer. JAMA 1993;270:943–947.
257. Chen YM, Ott DJ, Wolfman NT, et al. Recurrent colorectal carcinoma: evaluation with barium enema examination and CT. Radiology 1987;163:307–310.
258. Charnsangavej C, Whitley NO. Metastases to the pancreas and peripancreatic lymph nodes from carcinoma of the right colon: CT findings in 12 patients. AJR 1993;160:49–52.
259. McDaniel KP, Charnsangavej C, Dubrow R, et al. Pathways of nodal metastases in carcinoma of the cecum, ascending colon and transverse colon: CT demonstration. AJR 1993;161:61–64.
260. Small WC, Mehard WB, Langmo LS, et al. Preoperative determination of the resectability of hepatic tumors: efficacy of CT during arterial portography. AJR 1993;161:319–322.
261. Petrson MS, Baron RL, Dodd GD III, et al. Hepatic parenchymal perfusion detected with CTPA: imaging–pathologic correlation. Radiology 1992;183:149–155.
262. Schiepers C, Penninckx F, De Vadder N, et al. Contribution of PET in the diagnosis of recurrent colorectal cancer: comparison with conventional imaging. Eur J Surg Oncol 1995;21:517–522.
263. Huebner RH, Park KC, Shepherd JE, et al. A meta-analysis of the literature for whole-body FDG PET detection of recurrent colorectal cancer. J Nucl Med 2000;41:1177–1189.
264. Whiteford MH, Whiteford HM, Yee LF, et al. Usefulness of FDG-PET scan in the assessment of suspected metastatic or recurrent adenocarcinoma of the colon and rectum. Dis Colon Rectum 2000;43:759–767; discussion 767–770.
265. Berger KL, Nicholson SA, Dehdashti F, et al. FDG PET evaluation of mucinous neoplasms: correlation of FDG uptake with histopathologic features. Am J Roentgenol 2000;174:1005–1008.
266. Kinkel K, Lu Y, Both M, et al. Detection of hepatic metastases from cancers of the gastrointestinal tract by using noninvasive imaging methods (US, CT, MR imaging, PET): a meta-analysis. Radiology 2002;224:748–756.
267. Delbeke D, Vitola J, Sandler MP, et al. Staging recurrent metastatic colorectal carcinoma with PET. J Nucl Med 1997;38:1196–1201.
268. Ogunbiyi OA, Flanagan FL, Dehdashti F, et al. Detection of recurrent and metastatic colorectal cancer: comparison of positron emission tomography and computed tomography. Ann Surg Oncol 1997;4:613–620.
269. Rydzewski B, Dehdashti F, Gordon BA, Teefey SA, Strasberg SM, Siegel BA. Usefulness of intraoperative sonography for revealing hepatic metastases from colorectal cancer in patients selected for surgery after undergoing FDG PET. AJR Am J Roentgenol 2002;178:353–358.
270. Valk PE, Abella-Columna E, Haseman MK, et al. Whole-body PET imaging with F-18-fluorodeoxyglucose in management of recurrent colorectal cancer. Arch Surg 1999;134:503–511.
271. Gambhir SS, Czernin J, Schimmer J, et al. A tabulated review of the literature. J Nucl Med 2001;42(suppl):9S–12S.
272. Flanagan FL, Dehdashti F, Ogunbiyi OA, et al. Utility of FDG PET for investigating unexplained plasma CEA elevation in patients with colorectal cancer. Ann Surg 1998;227:319–323.
273. Flamen P, Hoekstra OS, Homans F, et al. Unexplained rising carcinoembryonic antigen (CEA) in the postoperative surveillance of colorectal cancer: the utility of positron emission tomography (PET). Eur J Cancer 2001;37:862–869.
274. Cohade C, Osman M, Leal J, et al. Direct comparison of FDG PET and PET-CT imaging in colorectal carcinoma. J Nucl Med 2003;44:1797–1803.
275. Strasberg SM, Dehdashti F, Siegel BA, et al. Survival of patients evaluated by FDG PET before hepatic resection for metastatic colorectal carcinoma: a prospective database study. Ann Surg 2001;33:320–321.
276. Ruers TJ, Langenhoff BS, Neeleman N, et al. Value of positron emission tomography with [F-18] fluorodeoxyglucose in patients with colorectal liver metastases: a prospective study. J Clin Oncol 2002;20:388–395.
277. Imdahl A, Reinhardt MJ, Nitzsche EU, et al. Impact of ^{18}F-FDG-positron emission tomography for decision making in colorectal cancer recurrences. Arch Surg 2000;385:129–134.
278. Staib L, Schirrmeister H, Reske SN, et al. Is (18)F-fluorodeoxyglucose positron emission tomography in recurrent

colorectal cancer a contribution to surgical decision making? Am J Surg 2000;180:1–5.
279. Kalff VV, Hicks R, Ware R. F-18 FDG PET for suspected or confirmed recurrence of colon cancer. A prospective study of impact and outcome. Clin Positron Imaging 2000;3:183.
280. Meta J, Seltzer M, Schiepers C, et al. Impact of ^{18}F-FDG PET on managing patients with colorectal cancer: the referring physicians perspective. J Nucl Med 2001;42:586–590.
281. Ruers TJ, Langenhoff BS, Neeleman N, et al. Value of positron emission tomography with [F-18] fluorodeoxyglucose in patients with colorectal liver metastases: a prospective study. J Clin Oncol 2002;20:388–395.
282. Strasberg SM, Dehdashti F, Siegel BA, et al. Survival of patients evaluated by FDG PET before hepatic resection for metastatic colorectal carcinoma: a prospective database study. Ann Surg 2001;33:320–321.
283. Delbeke D, Martin WH, Patton JA, et al. Value of iterative reconstruction, attenuation correction, and image fusion in the interpretation of FDG PET images with an integrated dual-head coincidence camera and x-ray-based attenuation maps. Radiology 2001;218:163–171.
284. Martinelli M, Townsend D, Meltzer C, et al. Survey of results of whole body imaging using the PET/CT at the University of Pittsburgh Medical Center PET facility. Clin Positron Imaging 2000;3:161.
285. Yeung HW, Schoder H, Larson SM. Utility of PET/CT for assessing equivocal PET lesions in oncology: initial experience. J Nucl Med 2002;43:32P.
286. Bar-Shalom R, Yefremov N, Guralnik L, et al. Clinical performance of PET/CT in the evaluation of cancer: additional value for diagnostic imaging and patient management. J Nucl Med 2003;44:1200–1209.
287. Roman CD, Delbeke D. Incremental diagnostic value of fusion imaging with integrated PET–CT in oncology compared to PET alone. RSNA Scientific Program 2003:487.
288. Beets G, Penninckx F, Schiepers C, et al. Clinical value of whole-body positron emission tomography with [^{18}F] fluorodeoxyglucose in recurrent colorectal cancer. Br J Surg 1994;81:1666–1670.
289. Strauss LG, Clorius JH, Schlag P, et al. Recurrence of colorectal tumors: PET evaluation. Radiology 1989;170:329–332.
290. Moore HG, Akhurst T, Larson SM, et al. A case controlled study of 18-fluorodeoxyglucose positron emission tomography in the detection of pelvic recurrence in previously irradiated rectal cancer patients. J Am Coll Surg 2003;197:22–28.
291. Schiepers C, Haustermans K, Geboes K, Filez L, Bormans G, Penninckx F. The effect of preoperative radiation therapy on glucose utilization and cell kinetics in patients with primary rectal carcinoma. Cancer (Phila) 1999;85:803–811.
292. Guillem JG, Puig-La Calle J Jr, Akhurst T, et al. Prospective assessment of primary rectal cancer response to preoperative radiation and chemotherapy using 18-fluorodeoxyglucose positron emission tomography. Dis Colon Rectum 2000;43:18–24.
293. Calvo FA, Domper M, Matute R, et al. ^{18}F-FDG positron emission tomography staging and restaging in rectal cancer treated with preoperative chemoradiation. Int J Radiat Oncol Biol Phys 2004;58:528–535.
294. Findlay M, Young H, Cunningham D, et al. Noninvasive monitoring of tumor metabolism using fluorodeoxyglucose and positron emission tomography in colorectal cancer liver metastases: correlation with tumor response to fluorouracil. J Clin Oncol 1996;14:700–708.
295. Vitola JV, Delbeke D, Meranze SG, et al. Positron emission tomography with F-18-fluorodeoxyglucose to evaluate the results of hepatic chemoembolization. Cancer (Phila) 1996;78: 2216–2222.
296. Torizuka T, Tamaki N, Inokuma T, et al. Value of fluorine-18-FDG PET to monitor hepatocellular carcinoma after interventional therapy. J Nucl Med 1994;35(12):1965–1969.
297. Langenhoff BS, Oyen WJ, Jager GJ, et al. Efficacy of fluorine-18-deoxyglucose positron emission tomography in detecting tumor recurrence after local ablative therapy for liver metastases: a prospective study. J Clin Oncol 2002;20:4453–4458.
298. Wong CY, Salem R, Raman S, et al. Evaluating ^{90}Y-glass microsphere treatment response of unresectable liver metastases by FDG-PET: a comparison with CT and MRI. Eur J Nucl Med Mol Imaging 2002;29:815–820.
299. Schirrmeister H, Gulhman A, Elsner K, et al. Sensitivity in detecting osseous lesions depends on anatomic location: planar scintigraphy versus ^{18}F PET. J Nucl Med 1999;40:1623–1629.
300. Higashi K, Clavo AC, Wahl RL. In vitro assessment of 2-fluoro-2-deoxy-D-glucose, L-methionine, and thymidine as agents to monitor early response of a human adenocarcinoma cell line to radiotherapy. J Nucl Med 1993;34:773–780.
301. Dittman H, Dohman BM, Paulsen F, et al. [^{18}F] FLT PET for diagnosis and staging of thoracic tumors. Eur J Nucl Med Mol Imaging 2003;30:1407–1412.
302. Boring C, Squires T, Tong T, et al. Cancer statistics. CA Cancer J Clin 1994;44:7–26.
303. Moog F, Bangerter M, Diederichs CG, et al. Lymphoma role of whole-body 2-deoxy-2-[F-18] fluoro-D-glucose (FDG) PET in nodal staging. Radiology 1997;203:795–800.
304. Moog F, Bangerter M, Diederichs CG, et al. Extranodal malignant lymphoma: detection with FDG PET versus CT. Radiology 1998;206:475–481.
305. Jerusalem GH, Beguin YP. Positron emission tomography in non-Hodgkin's lymphoma (NHL): relationship between tracer uptake and pathological findings, including preliminary experience in the staging of low-grade NHL. Clin Lymphoma 2002; 3:56–61.
306. Friedberg JW, Chengazi V. PET scans in the staging of lymphoma: current status. Oncologist 2003;8:438–447.
307. Hoffmann M, Kletter K, Diemling M, et al. Positron emission tomography with fluorine-18-2-fluoro-2-deoxy-D-glucose (F18-FDG) does not visualize extranodal B-cell lymphoma of the mucosa-associated lymphoid tissue (MALT)-type. Ann Oncol 1999;10:1185–1189.
308. Hoffmann M, Chott A, Puspok A, et al. ^{18}F-Fluorodeoxyglucose positron emission tomography (^{18}F-FDG-PET) does not visualize follicular lymphoma of the duodenum. Ann Hematol 2004;83:276–281.
309. Moog F, Bangerter M, Kotzerke J, et al. ^{18}F-Fluorodeoxy-glucose positron emission tomography as a new approach to detect lymphomatous bone marrow. J Clin Oncol 1998;16:603–609.
310. Carr R, Barrington SF, Madan B, et al. Detection of lymphoma in bone marrow by whole-body positron emission tomography. Blood 1998;91:3340–3346.
311. Okada J, Oonish H, Yoshikawa K, et al. FDG-PET for predicting the prognosis of malignant lymphoma. Ann Nucl Med 1994;8: 187–191.
312. Delbeke D, Martin WH, Morgan DS, et al. 2-Deoxy-2-[F-18] fluoro-D-glucose imaging with positron emission tomography for initial staging of Hodgkin's disease and lymphoma. Mol Imaging Biol 2002;4:104–114.
313. Hong SP, Hahn JS, Lee JD, Bae SW, Youn MJ. ^{18}F-Fluorodeoxyglucose-positron emission tomography in the staging of malignant lymphoma compared with CT and ^{67}Ga scan. Yonsei Med J 2003;44(5):779–786.
314. Sasaki M, Kuwabara Y, Koga H, et al. Clinical impact of whole body FDG-PET on staging and therapeutic decision making for malignant lymphoma. Ann Nucl Med 2002;16(5): 337–345.
315. Stumpe KDM, Urbinelli M, Steinert HC, et al. Whole-body positron emission tomography using fluorodeoxyglucose for staging of lymphoma: effectiveness and comparison with computed tomography. Eur J Nucl Med 1998;25:721–729.

316. Paul R. Comparison of fluorine-18-2-fluorodeoxyglucose and gallium-67 citrate imaging for detection of lymphoma. J Nucl Med 1987;28:288–292.
317. Okada J, Yoshikawa K, Imazeki K, et al. The use of FDG-PET in the detection and management of malignant lymphoma. Correlation of uptake with prognosis. J Nucl Med 1991;32:686–691.
318. Shen YY, Kao A, Yen RF. Comparison of ^{18}F-fluoro-2-deoxyglucose positron emission tomography and gallium-67 citrate scintigraphy for detecting malignant lymphoma. Oncol Rep 2002;9:321–325.
319. Wirth A, Seymour JF, Hicks RJ, et al. Fluorine-18 fluorodeoxyglucose positron emission tomography, gallium-67 scintigraphy and conventional staging for Hodgkin's disease and non-Hodgkin's lymphoma. Am J Med 2002;112:262–268.
320. Rini JN, Manalili EY, Hoffman MA, et al. F-18 FDG versus Ga-67 for detecting splenic involvement in Hodgkin's disease. Clin Nucl Med 2002;27:572–527.
321. Buckmann I, Reinhardt M, Elsner K, et al. 2-(Fluorine-18) fluoro-2-deoxy-D-glucose positron emission tomography in the detection and staging of malignant lymphoma. A bicenter trial. Cancer (Phila) 2001;91(5):889–899.
322. Schoder H, Meta J, Yap C, et al. Effect of whole-body (18)F-FDG-PET imaging on clinical staging and management of patients with malignant lymphoma. J Nucl Med 2001;42(8):1139–1143.
323. Naumann R, Beuthien-Baumann B, Reiss A, et al. Substantial impact of FDG-PET imaging on the therapy decision in patients with early-stage Hodgkin's lymphoma. Br J Cancer 2004; 90(3):620–625.
324. Cremerius U, Fabry U, Neuerburg J, et al. Positron emission tomography with ^{18}F-FDG to detect residual disease after therapy for malignant lymphoma. Nucl Med Commun 1998; 19:1055–1063.
325. Zinzani PL, Magagnoli M, Chierichetti F, et al. The role of positron emission tomography (PET) in the management of lymphoma patients. Ann Oncol 1999;10:1181–1184.
326. Jerusalem G, Beguin Y, Fassotte MF, et al. Whole-body positron emission tomography using ^{18}F-fluorodeoxyglucose for post-treatment evaluation in Hodgkin's disease and non-Hodgkin's lymphoma has higher diagnostic and prognostic value than classical computed tomography scan imaging. Blood 1999;94: 429–433.
327. Mikhaeel NG, Timothy AR, Odoherty MJ, Hain S, Maisey MN. 18-FDG-PET as a prognostic indicator in the treatment of aggressive non-Hodgkin's lymphoma, comparison with CT. Leuk Lymphoma 2000;39:543–553.
328. Spaepen K, Stroobants S, Dupont P, et al. Prognostic value of positron emission tomography (PET) with fluorine-18 fluorodeoxy-glucose [18F]FDG after first-line chemotherapy in non-Hodgkin's lymphoma: is (18F) FDG-PET a valid alternative to conventional diagnostic methods? J Clin Oncol 2001;19(2): 414–419.
329. Weihrauch MR, Re D, Scheidhauer K, et al. Thoracic positron emission tomography using ^{18}F-fluorodeoxyglucose for the evaluation of residual mediastinal Hodgkin disease. Blood 2001;98(10):2930–2934.
330. Spaepen K, Stroobants D, Dupont P, et al. Can positron emission tomography using ^{18}F-fluorodeoxyglucose (18)F-FDG PET) after first line treatment distinguish Hodgkin's disease patients who need additional therapy from others where additional therapy would mean avoidable toxicity? Br J Haematol 2001;115(2):272–278.
331. Kostakoglu L, Coleman M, Leonard JP, Kuji I, Zoe H, Goldsmith SJ. PET predicts prognosis after 1 cycle of chemotherapy in aggressive lymphoma and Hodgkin's disease. J Nucl Med 2002;43(8):1018–1027.
332. Armitage JO, Wisenburger DD, Hutchins M, et al. Chemotherapy for diffuse large cell hymphoma: rapidly responding patients have more durable remissions. J Clin Oncol 1986;4:160–164.
333. Romer W, Schwaiger M. Positron emission tomography in diagnosis and therapy monitoring of patients with lymphoma. Clin Positron Imaging 1998;1:101–110.
334. Mikhaeel NG, Timothy AR, Odoherty MJ, Hain S, Maisey MN. 18-FDG-PET as a prognostic indicator in the treatment of aggressive non-Hodgkin's lymphoma: comparison with CT. Leuk Lymphoma 2000;39:543–553.
335. Zijlstra JM, Hoekstra OS, Raijmakers PG, et al. ^{18}FDG positron emission tomography versus ^{67}Ga scintigraphy as prognosis test during chemotherapy for non-Hodgkin's lymphoma. Br J Haematol 2003;123(3):454–462.
336. Spaepen K, Stroobants S, Dupont P, et al. Early restaging positron emission tomography with (18)-F-fluorodeoxyglucose predicts outcome in patients with aggressive non-Hodgkin's lymphoma. Ann Oncol 2003;13:1356–1363.
337. Torizuka T, Nakamura F, Kanno T, et al. Early therapy monitoring with FDG-PET in aggressive non-Hodgkin's lymphoma and Hodgkin's lymphoma. Eur J Nucl Med Mol Imaging 2004; 31(1):22–28.
338. Carr R, Barrington SF, Madan B, et al. Detection of lymphoma in bone marrow by whole-body positron emission tomography. Blood 1998;91(9):3340–3346.
339. Becherer A, Mitterbauer M, Jaeger U, et al. Positron emission tomography with [^{18}F]2-fluoro-D-2-deoxyglucose (FDG-PET) predicts relapse of malignant lymphoma after high-dose therapy with stem cell transplantation. Leukemia 2002;16(2): 260–267.
340. Cremerius U, Fabry U, Wildberger JE, et al. Pre-transplant positron emission tomography (PET) using fluorine-18-fluorodeoxyglucose (FDG) predicts outcome in patients treated with high-dose chemotherapy and autologous stem cell transplantation for non-Hodgkin's lymphoma. Bone Marrow Transplant 2002;30(2):103–111.
341. Schot B, van Imhoff G, Pruim J, Sluiter W, Vaalburg W, Vellenga E. Predictive value of early ^{18}F-fluorodeoxyglucose positron emission tomography in chemosensitive relapsed lymphoma. Br J Haematol 2003;123(2):282–287.
342. Filmont JE, Czermin J, Yap C, Silverman DH, Quon A, Phelps ME, et al. Value of F 18-fluorodeoxyglucose positron emission tomography for predicting the clinical outcome of patients with aggressive lymphoma prior to and after autologous stem-cell transplantation. Chest 2003;124(2):608–613.
343. Spaepen K, Stroobants S, Dupont P, Vandenberghe P, Maertens J, Bormans G, et al. Prognostic value of pretransplantation positron emission tomography using fluorine 18-fluorodeoxyglucose in patients with aggressive lymphoma treated with high-dose chemotherapy and stem cell transplantation. Blood 2003;102(1):53–59.
344. Hoskin P. FDG-PET in management of lymphoma: a clinical perspective. Eur J Nucl Med 2002;29(4):449–451.
345. Front D, Bar-Shalom R, Mor M, Haim N, Epelbaum R, Frenkel A, et al. Aggressive non-Hodgkin lymphoma: early prediction of outcome with 67Ga scintigraphy. Radiology 2000;214:253–257.
346. Jerusalem G, Beguin Y, Fassotte MF, et al. Early detection of relapse by whole-body positron emission tomography in the follow-up of patients with Hodgkin's disease. Ann Oncol 2003;14:123–130.
347. Bangerter M, Moog F, Griesshammer M, et al. Role of whole body FDG-PET imaging in predicting relapse of malignant lymphoma in patients with residual masses after treatment. Radiography 1999;5:155–163.
348. Cremerius U, Fabry U, Kroll U, Zimny M, Neuerburg J, Osieka R, et al. Clinical value of FDG-PET for therapy monitoring of malignant lymphoma: results of a retrospective study in 72 patients. Nuklearmedizin 1999;38(1):24–30.
349. Jerusalem G, Beguin Y, Fassotte MF, Najjar F, Paulus P, Rigo P, et al. Whole body emission tomography using F-18-fluorodeoxyglucose for post treatment evaluation in Hodgkin's

disease and non-Hodgkin's lymphoma has a higher diagnostic and prognostic value than classical computed tomography scan imaging. Blood 1999;94(2):429–433.
350. Guay C, Lepine M, Verreault J, Benard F. Prognostic value of PET using 18F-FDG in Hodgkin's disease for posttreatment evaluation. J Nucl Med 2003;44(8):1225–1231.
351. Freudenberg LS, Antoch G, Schutt P, Beyer T, Jentzen W, Muller SP, et al. FDG-PET/CT in restaging patients with lymphoma. Eur J Nucl Med Mol Imag 2004:31(3):325–329.
352. Ora Israel, Zohar Keidar, and Rachel Bar-Shalom: Seminars in Nuclear Medicine, Vol XXXIV, No 3 (July), 2004:166–179.
353. Cancer Facts & Figures 2004, in American Cancer Society, Survellance Research, Atlanta, GA: American Cancer Society, 2004.
354. Wahl RL, Hutchins GD, Buchsbaum DJ, et al. 18F-2-deoxy-2-fluoro-D-glucose uptake into human tumor xenografts. Feasibility studies for cancer imaging with positron emission tomography. Cancer 1991;67:1544–1550.
355. Kern KA. [14C] deoxyglucose uptake and imaging in malignant melanoma. J Surg Res 1991;50:643–647.
356. Wagner JD, Schauwecker DS, Davidson D, et al. FDG-PET sensitivity for melanoma lymph node metastases is dependent on tumor volume. J Surg Oncol 2001;77:237–242.
357. Rinne D, Baum RP, Hor G, et al. Primary staging and follow-up of high risk melanoma patients with whole-body 18F-fluorodeoxyglucose positron emission tomography: results of a prospective study of 100 patients. Cancer 1998;82:1664–1671.
358. Macfarlane DJ, Sondak V, Johnson T, et al. Prospective evaluation of 2-[18F]-2-deoxy-D-glucose positron emission tomography in staging of regional lymph nodes in patients with cutaneous malignant melanoma. J Clin Oncol 1998;16:1770–1776.
359. Wagner JD, Schauwecker D, Davidson D, et al. Prospective study of fluorodeoxyglucose-positron emission tomography imaging of lymph node basins in melanoma patients undergoing sentinel nodebiopsy. J Clin Oncol 1999;17:1508–1515.
360. Acland KM, Healy C, Calonje E, et al. Comparison of positron emission tomography scanning and sentinel node biopsy in the detection of micrometastases of primary cutaneous malignant melanoma. J Clin Oncol 2001;19:2674–2678.
361. Fink AM, Holle-Robatsch S, Herzog N, et al. Positron emission tomography is not useful in detecting metastasis in the sentinel lymph node in patients with primary malignant melanoma stage I and II. Melanoma Res 2004;14:141–145.
362. Acland KM, O'Doherty MJ, Russel-Jones R. The value of positron emission tomography scanning in the detection of subclinical metastatic melanoma. J Am Acad Dermatol 2000;42:606–611.
363. Stas M, Stroobants S, Dupont P, et al. 18-FDG PET scan in the staging of recurrent melanoma: additional value and therapeutic impact. Melanoma Res 2002;12:479–490.
364. Blessing C, Feine U, Geiger L, et al. Positron emission tomography and ultrasonography: a comparative retrospective study assessing the diagnostic validity in lymph node metastases of malignant melanoma. Arch Dermatol 195;131:1394–1398.
365. Crippa F, Leutner M, Belli F, et al. Which kinds of lymph node metastases can FDG PET detect? A clinical study in melanoma. J Nucl Med 2000;41:1491–1494.
366. Tyler DS, Onaitis M, Kherani A, et al. Positron emission tomography scanning in malignant melanoma. Cancer (Phila) 2000;89:1019–1025.
367. Wagner JD, Schauwecker D, Hutchins G, et al. Initial assessment of positron emission tomography for detection of nonpalpable regional lymphatic metastases in melanoma. J Surg Oncol 1997;64:181–189.
368. Gritters LS, Francis IR, Zasadny KR, et al. Initial assessment of positron emission tomography using 2-fluorine-18-fluoro-2-deoxy-D-glucose in the imaging of malignant melanoma. J Nucl Med 1993;34:1420–1427.
369. Steinert HC, Huch Boni RA, Buck A, et al. Malignant melanoma: staging with whole-body positron emission tomography and 2-[F-18]-fluoro-2-deoxy-D-glucose. Radiology 1995;195:705–709.
370. Rinne D, Baum RP, Hor G, et al. Primary staging and follow-up of high risk melanoma patients with whole-body ^{18}F-fluorodeoxyglucose positron emission tomography: results of a prospective study of 100 patients. Cancer (Phila) 1998; 82:1664–1671.
371. Eigtved A, Andersson AP, Dahlstrom K, et al. Use of fluorine-18-fluorodeoxyglucose positron emission tomography in the detection of silent metastases from malignant melanoma. Eur J Nucl Med 2000;27:70–75.
372. Swetter SM, Carroll LA, Johnson DL, et al. Positron emission tomography is superior to computed tomography for metastatic detection in melanoma patients. Ann Surg Oncol 2002;9: 646–653.
373. Gulec SA, Faries MB, Lee CC, et al. The role of fluorine-18 deoxyglucose positron emission tomography in the management of patients with metastatic melanoma: impact on surgical decision making. Clin Nucl Med 2003;28:961–965.
374. Dietlein M, Krug B, Groth W, et al. Positron emission tomography using ^{18}F-fluorodeoxyglucose in advanced stages of malignant melanoma: a comparison of ultrasonographic and radiological methods of diagnosis. Nucl Med Commun 1999;20:255–261.
375. Krug B, Dietlein M, Groth W, et al. Fluoro-18-fluorodeoxyglucose positron emission tomography (FDG-PET) in malignant melanoma: diagnostic comparison with conventional imaging methods. Acta Radiol 2000;41:446–452.
376. Mercier GA, Alavi A, Fraker DL. FDG positron emission tomography in isolated limb perfusion therapy in patients with locally advanced melanoma: preliminary results. Clin Nucl Med 2001;26:832–836.
377. Hafner J, Schmid MH, Kempf W, et al. Baseline staging in cutaneous malignant melanoma. Br J Dermatol 2004;150:677–686.
378. Havenga K, Cobben DC, Oyen WJ, et al. Fluorodeoxyglucose — positron emission tomography and sentinel lymph node biopsy in staging primary cutaneous melanoma. Eur J Surg Oncol 2003;29:662–664.
379. Lindholm P, Leskinen S, Nagren K, et al. Carbon-11-methionine PET imaging of malignant melanoma. J Nucl Med 1995;36: 1806–1810.
380. Mishima Y, Imahori Y, Honda C, et al. In vivo diagnosis of human malignant melanoma with positron emission tomography using specific melanoma-seeking ^{18}F-DOPA analogue. J Neurooncol 1997;33:163–169.
381. Gobben DC, Jager PL, Elsinga PH, et al. 3′-^{18}F-fluoro-3′-deoxy-L-thymidine: a new tracer for staging metastatic melanoma? J Nucl Med 2003;44:1927–1932.
382. Sadzot B, Sheldon J, Flesher J, et al. Tracers for imaging melanin with positron emission tomography. Synapse 1999;31:5–12.
383. Froidevaux S, Calame-Christe M, Schuhmacher J, et al. A gallium-labeled DOTA-alpha-melanocyte-stimulating hormone analog for PET imaging of melanoma metastases. J Nucl Med 2004;45:116–123.

SECTION FIVE

Solid Tumors

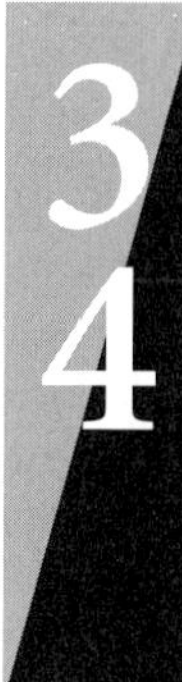

Central Nervous System Tumors

Ravi D. Rao, Paul D. Brown, Caterina Giannini, Cormac O. Maher, Fredric B. Meyer, Evanthia Galanis, Brad J. Erickson, and Jan C. Buckner

The term *primary central nervous system tumors* refers to a heterogeneous group of tumors characterized by their location in the central nervous system (CNS). These tumors exhibit a wide range of clinical behavior from extremely lethal (e.g., glioblastoma) to potentially curable (e.g., germ cell tumors and medulloblastomas). The occurrence of these tumors has devastating effects on patients, and their management can be major challenge to physicians. By virtue of their location, brain tumors cause a disproportionate amount of disability and pose a threat to a patient's sense of self that is unparalleled by any other disease. The currently available therapies for most primary CNS tumors have limited activity with significant toxicity. Survivors of these tumors often have significant residual neurologic and cognitive deficits that limit their functioning for the rest of their lives.

Epidemiology

The incidence of primary CNS tumors is between 4 and 5 cases per 100,000 per year. They represent about 2% of all cancers, but account for a disproportionate amount of morbidity and mortality. They may occur in any age group from infancy to old age, with a slight male preponderance. Half of all CNS tumors are diffuse gliomas. CNS tumors are the third leading cause of cancer-related death in adolescents and adults between the ages of 15 and 34 years. The peak age of incidence is between 60 and 80 years. The incidence appears to be increasing among the elderly,[1] although this finding may be the result of increased availability of better imaging technology.

Etiology of Primary Central Nervous System Tumors

Most malignant CNS tumors arise as a consequence of acquired somatic mutations in genes that are responsible for control of cell growth and proliferation. Genetic predisposition to these tumors appears relatively uncommon. Gliomas are more common in patients with type 1 neurofibromatosis, Turcot's syndrome, and Li–Fraumeni syndrome.

Although the etiology of most primary CNS tumors is unknown, a few environmental factors have been identified as being important in causation, such as ionizing radiation and human immunodeficiency virus (HIV) infection. Currently, the role of several other putative environmental links (e.g., artificial sweeteners and cell phones) in the causation of gliomas remains speculative.

Pathology of Primary Central Nervous System Tumors

The spectrum of primary CNS tumors includes a wide variety of neoplasms and includes tumors of primary neuroectodermal derivation and those derived from the supportive elements and brain coverings. Classic histopathologic techniques during the past century have resulted in the accumulation of a large amount of information regarding morphologic characteristics and patterns of growth of a variety of tumors, which have resulted in the present approach to CNS tumor classification and grading. During the past 15 years, advances in molecular genetics have led to the delineation of some of the molecular mechanisms underlying tumorigenesis and tumor progression. Although histopathologic diagnosis is (and will most likely remain for a long time) the gold standard in the approach to classification and grading of a large variety of CNS tumors, molecular genetics data are now being added as complementary data to tumor diagnosis.

Prognostic Factors and Markers

It has been long recognized that several patient-related factors (age, performance status, disease-related symptoms, and mental status), tumor variables (histologic tumor type and grade, contrast enhancement, size, location, and biologic markers of proliferation rate, apoptosis, and genetic abnormalities), and treatment variables (extent of surgical resection, radiation dose, and chemotherapy) influence outcomes.

Age has been most consistently shown to influence the survival in multiple studies. Another important factor appears to be the performance score (PS). In multiple clinical trial settings, a favorable PS has been shown to positively influence outcomes. In addition, normal versus abnormal mental status has been shown to be a significant prognostic. In nearly all models tested, baseline Mini-Mental Status Exam (MMSE) score correlated more strongly with both time to progression and survival than did the performance status, suggesting that mental status may be a more important determinant of clinical outcome than physical functioning in patients with high-grade glioma. Some symptoms, specifically seizures that have occurred for longer than 6 months, are associated with a favorable survival prognosis.[2,3] Abnormalities in the epidermal growth factor receptor (EGFR), p53, and phosphatase and tensin analogue (PTEN, a tumor suppressor gene) have been long recognized as having a pathogenetic role in astrocytoma. The prognostic value of these markers is a subject of much ongoing research. In one study, EGFR amplification was found to be associated with a good prognosis in one subset of patients [those over age 60 with glioblastoma multiforme (GBM)]. Several of these markers are closely linked to several other clinical covariables, making analyses of benefits of individual effects difficult. Multiple reports have attested to the association between 1p and 19q deletions in oligodendrogliomas and responsiveness to chemotherapy and a better outcome. Analyses of these mutations are now being used to guide therapy.[4,5] Evaluation of the relative expression levels of DNA and RNA of several tumor suppressor genes and oncogenes (by techniques such as gene expression analysis and comparative genomic hybridization) has identified the existence of subgroups of tumors with distinct clinical behaviors.[6,7] Differences in patterns of gene expression can be found to occur between gliomas of different grades, as well as in other tumor types. More interestingly, these analyses can identify subtypes among tumors within a single diagnostic category that have different outcomes. Research is currently under way to develop prognostic models and markers that may be clinically useful.

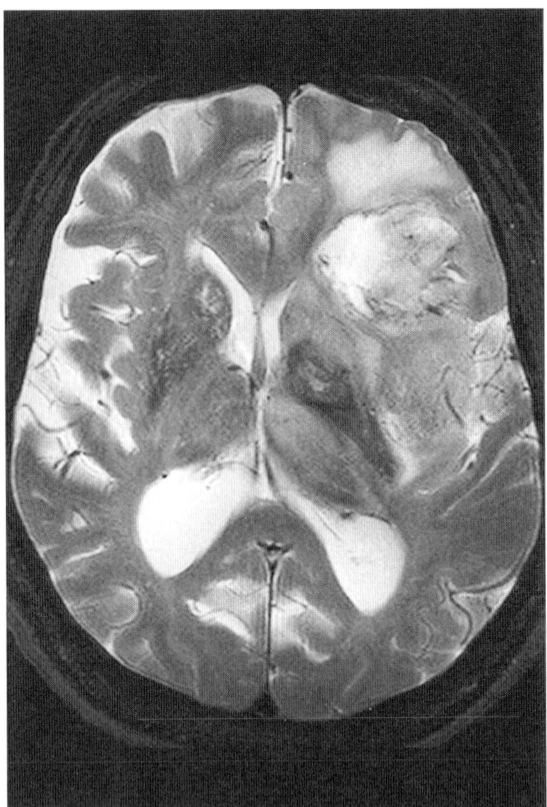

FIGURE 34.1. Head magnetic resonance imaging (MRI) demonstrates a grade 3 astrocytoma as it appears on T2-weighted images. Note the presence of a mass effect and edema in the frontal lobe.

Clinical Presentation of Central Nervous System Tumors

Patients with primary CNS tumors can present with a variety of neurologic symptoms and signs. The clinical symptomatology is variable and depends on a number of patient- and tumor-related factors, such as age, histology, location, rate of growth, and presence of cerebral edema (Figure 34.1). The spectrum of symptoms seen at presentation has changed considerably over the past few decades as advanced imaging techniques have become increasingly available.

The symptoms caused by CNS tumors are typically progressive, with evolution of newer symptoms over time. Headaches are the most common symptom of primary brain tumors in general and have been noted to occur in half of patients at presentation.[8] Over the course of their illness, a majority of patients have headaches. The features of a headache thought to be "classic" for brain tumors (i.e., association with nausea and vomiting and being worse in the morning) occur only in one-fifth of patients.[8] Most commonly, headaches have features associated with tension, migraine, or sinus headaches. Primary brain tumors are the most feared diagnosis in someone with a new seizure. The incidence of seizures as a presenting feature appears to depend upon the rate of growth of the tumor and the location. Mental status alterations ranging from subtle to severe deficits in cognition, personality, and perception commonly occur in patients with brain tumors. These symptoms may be present at diagnosis in 15% to 20% of patients. Patients may present with several focal neurologic signs such as cranial nerve deficits, hormonal deficiencies, visual field deficits, papilledema, weakness, aphasia, and alterations in sensation.

Therapy of these symptoms in patients with CNS tumors presents a challenge. Anticonvulsants can be used to treat those patients who develop seizures. There is no proven benefit to using prophylactic anticonvulsant medications in patients who have not yet had a seizure.[9] Cerebral edema occurs commonly and is treated with steroids. Increases in intracranial pressure (ICP) necessitate additional measures such as fluid restriction, use of osmotic agents and diuretics, hyperventilation, elevation of the head of the bed, and placement of ventriculoperitoneal shunts.

Imaging in CNS Tumors

Patients suspected of having CNS tumors based on symptoms need imaging studies performed for diagnostic reasons. Over the past few decades, major advances in diagnostic imaging technology have taken place. More importantly, this technology has become widely available. These imaging studies provide digital cross-sectional images of the brain and surrounding structures based on differences in physical properties between various structures. There are many similarities in the appearance of brain tumors (primary or secondary) on computed tomography (CT) and magnetic resonance imaging (MRI), but there are some unique features that can allow a specific tumor type to be suggested as the likely candidate.

Computerized Tomography

On nonenhanced CT, tumors may have intensity similar to or slightly lower than brain tissue. Some tumors (e.g., metastases and high-grade gliomas) may have gross hemorrhage, recognized as amorphous moderately hyperdense areas typically within tumors. The presence of a fluid–fluid level in a mass may be useful in differentiating benign hemorrhages from malignant. Calcification occurs in some tumors, and the pattern can be of diagnostic importance.

Magnetic Resonance Imaging

MRI has been a substantial advance over CT for intracranial tumors. MRI provides direct multiplanar acquisitions, which can be useful for differentiating some intra- and extraaxial masses. However, the biggest advantage is the many different tissue properties that MRI can identify. Early "sequences" (images are created by broadcasting sequences of radiofrequency pulses into the patients, and then "listening" to how the hydrogen protons of the patient react) could show the T_1 and T_2 relaxation properties (so-called T_1- and T_2-weighted images) and proton density. MRI imaging studies based on the flow of blood have also been developed. More recently, techniques for looking at non-water chemicals of the brain (spectroscopy), the diffusion of water (diffusion-weighted imaging, DWI), and perfusion imaging, as well as the ability to suppress the signal from specific classes of protons (e.g., fat suppression, magnetization transfer suppression, and bulk water suppression, known as fluid-attenuated inversion recovery or FLAIR) have been developed.

Contrast Enhancement

Both CT and MRI have intravenous agents that can demonstrate blood–brain barrier (BBB) breakdown, which is referred to as enhancement. Higher-grade tumors enhance whereas most lower-grade tumors do not. However, there are many notable exceptions to this generalization, including meningiomas, most metastases, and some low-grade gliomas such as pilocytic astrocytomas and gangliogliomas (GG). Generally, MRI has more sensitivity to contrast enhancement. When CT was the primary evaluation tool, so-called double-dose delayed scanning was performed to improve the detection of enhancement. Although sensitivity with MRI is usually adequate, the use of three times the standard dose ("triple dose") has been shown to demonstrate enhancement when the standard dose does not.

T_1-Weighted Imaging

T_1-weighted images are bright in areas where the protons quickly realign with the main magnetic field after being "perturbed" by the radiofreqency (RF) pulses. Protons found in lipids have this property and are bright, whereas bulk water (similar to cerebrospinal fluid, CSF) does not and is dark. Gadolinium has paramagnetic properties and causes change in the property of water protons, making them realign faster and thus become bright. Hemorrhage, calcium, and protein breakdown products can have a variable appearance.

T_2/Proton Density/Fluid-Attenuated Inversion Recovery

T_2, proton density (PD), and FLAIR images have a similar appearance, except for the appearance of bulk water. Bulk water (e.g., CSF) is bright on T_2, similar to white matter on PD, and dark on FLAIR. Abnormal tissue (tumor, edema, gliosis, and necrosis) is bright on all three sequences whereas normal brain is intermediate, with gray matter being brighter than white matter. Because tumor and edema are bright on these images, this presents a problem when trying to precisely demarcate tumor boundary.

Perfusion-Weighted Imaging

Perfusion-weighted imaging (PWI) uses the effect of flow on MRI signal to measure perfusion of tissue. The most common clinical tool for this uses a bolus injection of gadolinium, which produces a reduction in signal on T_2-weighted images. Integrating the signal reduction over the course of the bolus produces an image that is proportional to the cerebral blood volume. Areas of treatment-related necrosis tend to have low blood volume; this may be helpful in differentiating recurrent tumor from necrosis.[10]

Magnetic Resonance Spectroscopy

Magnetic resonance spectroscopy (MRS) measures the concentration of chemicals other than water. Because water is about 10,000 times more concentrated than these chemicals, it requires long acquisition time and/or low resolution to obtain reasonable spectra. The most prevalent form of MRS is to select a single sample of tissue that typically measures about $2\,cm^3$. The chemicals of greatest interest for brain tumors are choline, *N*-acetylaspartate (NAA), creatine, and lactate. Creatine is not a metabolite specific for brain tumors, but tends to be fairly constant in concentration in the brain, and because the other chemicals are typically not measured as absolute concentrations, they are expressed as ratios of the creatine concentration. NAA is a chemical that is quite specific for axons and is highest in areas of healthy brain. Any process that replaces or destroys axons reduces NAA levels. Choline is a marker of cell membranes. It is increased in areas of high membrane activity (such as tumors) and decreased in areas of necrosis or atrophy.[11,12] Lactate is a marker of anaerobic metabolism; as such, it is not detectable in normal brain (Figure 34.2). It is often elevated in tumors, particularly the higher-grade tumors, and in necrotic tissue.

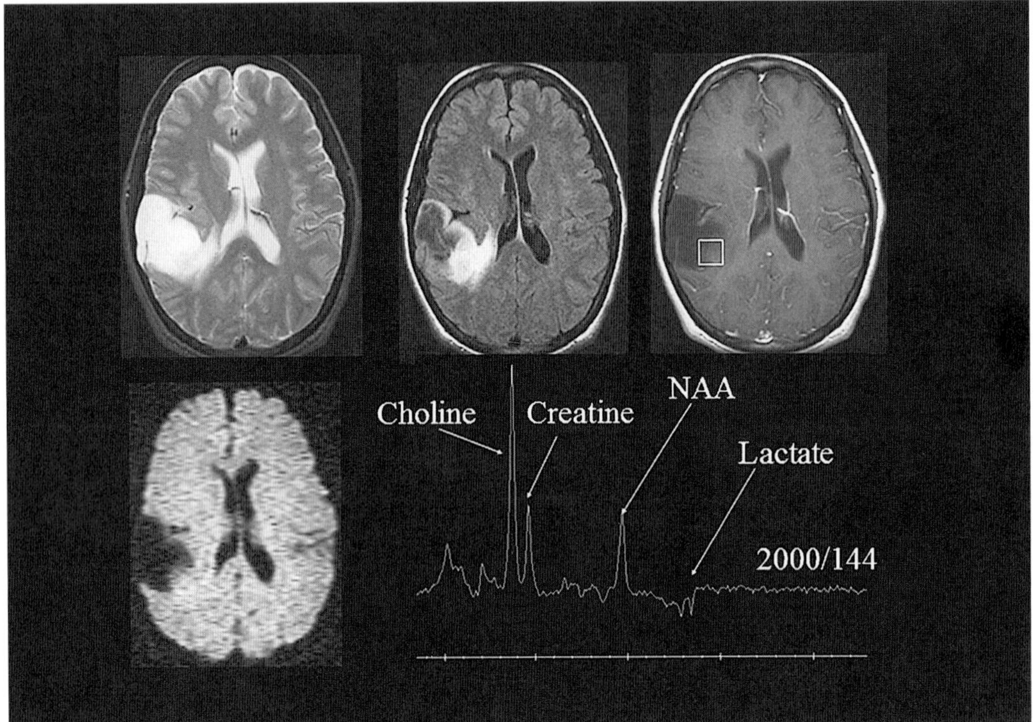

FIGURE 34.2. T2 and post-gadolinium (Gd) images in a patient with a grade 2 astrocytoma. The spectrum shown is obtained from the region shown on the post-gadolinium image. This particular spectrum was obtained with an echo time of 144 milliseconds (ms), which inverts the lactate peak, allowing one to be certain that lactate is present and is not hidden by other chemical species.

Special Considerations in Management of CNS Tumors

Thromboembolism

Patients with primary CNS tumors (especially gliomas) have an increased incidence of thromboembolic phenomena. Several hypotheses have been proposed to explain this predisposition, including elevated prothrombotic clotting factor levels, presence of a consumptive coagulopathy, and venous stasis due to paresis of extremities. The incidence of thrombotic phenomenon in patients undergoing therapy for high-grade gliomas is 20% to 30%.[13] Risk factors for development of thrombotic events include increased age, previous history of thromboembolism, higher-grade tumors, hemiparesis, use of chemotherapy, prolonged neurosurgery, and AB blood group.[14] The recommended therapy for diagnosed venous thromboembolic in these patients is similar to that in other situations.

Cognitive Deficiencies in Patients Treated for CNS Tumors

The deleterious effect of radiotherapy (RT) on the long-term cognitive performance of patients with CNS tumors is a major concern. As more effective treatments for intracranial lesions have become available and long-term survival has increased in some diseases, attention has been placed on identifying and quantifying the adverse effects of RT on cognition and neuropsychiatric functioning. Studies of neurocognitive function in patients treated for various intracranial tumors are confounded by differences in distribution of factors such as age at therapy, surgery, chemotherapy, tumor characteristics, tumor progression, concurrent medical illnesses, neurologic comorbidity, insensitivity of tools used (e.g., MMSE) and medications. In several disease states, the risks of neurocognitive deficits caused by therapy are quite small and are greatly overshadowed by deficits caused by the tumor itself. There appears a clear relationship between age at therapy, dose of radiation, and the extent of the deficiency.[15] The effect of radiation is of greatest concern in young patients (e.g., medulloblastomas)[16,17] and in diseases in which therapy leads to long disease-free survival. These patients are in their most productive years, and cognitive deficits that occur have a larger impact on their capacity to function socially and to be gainfully employed. Several pharmacologic strategies are currently being studied to minimize neurocognitive dysfunction associated with therapy in patients with CNS tumors.[18–22]

Retrospective studies of patients treated for low-grade glioma (LGG) with whole-brain radiotherapy (WBRT) have detected an increased incidence of neurocognitive difficulties when compared to controls (e.g., those treated with surgery or focal RT).[23] Patients treated with higher doses of WBRT have greater deficits than those receiving lower doses.[24] Patients with high-grade glioma (HGG) have also been found to have cognitive impairments after completion of therapy in retrospective studies.[25] However, in this particular group of patients, the dominant cause of neurocognitive deficits appears to be largely the effect of the tumor, and not that of therapy.[26,27] Long-term neurotoxicity remains a major problem in patients treated for primary CNS lymphoma (PCNSL), especially in those older than 60 years.

Diffuse Gliomas

Gliomas include a variety of neuroectodermal tumors that show morphologic and immunohistochemical evidence of their glial lineage, primarily glial fibrillary acidic protein (GFAP) positivity. These tumors include astrocytomas, oligodendrogliomas, ependymomas, and tumors with mixed differ-

TABLE 34.1. World Health Organization (WHO) classification and grading of diffuse gliomas.

Tumor type	*WHO grade*
Infiltrating astrocytomas:	
Astrocytoma	II
Protoplasmic	
Fibrillary	
Gemistocytic	
Anaplastic astrocytoma (AA)	III
Glioblastoma multiforme (GBM)	IV
Giant cell astrocytoma	
Gliosarcoma	
Oligodendrogliomas:	
Oligodendroglioma	II
Anaplastic oligodendroglioma	III
Mixed oligoastrocytomas:	
Oligoastrocytoma	II
Anaplastic oligoastrocytoma	III

Pilocytic astrocytoma, pleomorphic xanthoastrocytoma, subependymal giant cell astrocytoma, and the rare desmoplastic infantile astrocytoma represent distinct clinicopathologic entities, distinct from diffuse astrocytomas and characterized by a relatively circumscribed pattern of growth and a favorable prognosis.

entiation, generally oligoastrocytomas (Table 34.1). A fundamental distinction among different glial tumors is based on their pattern of growth; they can be circumscribed and relatively demarcated from surrounding parenchyma, or diffuse and widely infiltrative of brain parenchyma. Ependymomas represent the best example among gliomas of tumors with a solid, noninfiltrative growth pattern. Infiltration is virtually absent in intracranial ependymomas. Diffuse gliomas include diffuse astrocytomas, oligodendrogliomas, and mixed oligoastrocytomas. These tumors are characterized by their marked tendency to grow through preexisting gray and white matter, resulting in the formation of distinctive "secondary structures." These structures include perivascular aggregation, when neoplastic cells cluster around preexisting small vessels; perineuronal satellitosis, in which neoplastic cells grow into cortex surrounding the cell body of cortical neurons; and subpial aggregation, with neoplastic cells clustering in the molecular layer just below the pia. Common to diffuse gliomas is also the tendency to progress into higher grades of malignancy over time. These tumors are classified and graded in the most recent World Health Organization (WHO) classification as grade II to IV. Fundamental in distinguishing grade of malignancy of diffuse gliomas are histologic features such as presence of mitotic activity, endothelial vascular changes (endothelial proliferation), and necrosis with or without presence of pseudopalisading (Figure 34.3). These same morphologic features may be of no importance in different tumor types such as pilocytic astrocytoma, hence the absolute necessity of identifying tumor type *before* grading them.

High-Grade Diffuse Gliomas

High-grade diffuse glioma refers to a group of diffusely infiltrative tumors that are characterized by a somewhat variable but relatively poor prognosis; these include grade 3 and 4 astrocytomas [anaplastic astrocytoma (AA) and GBM],

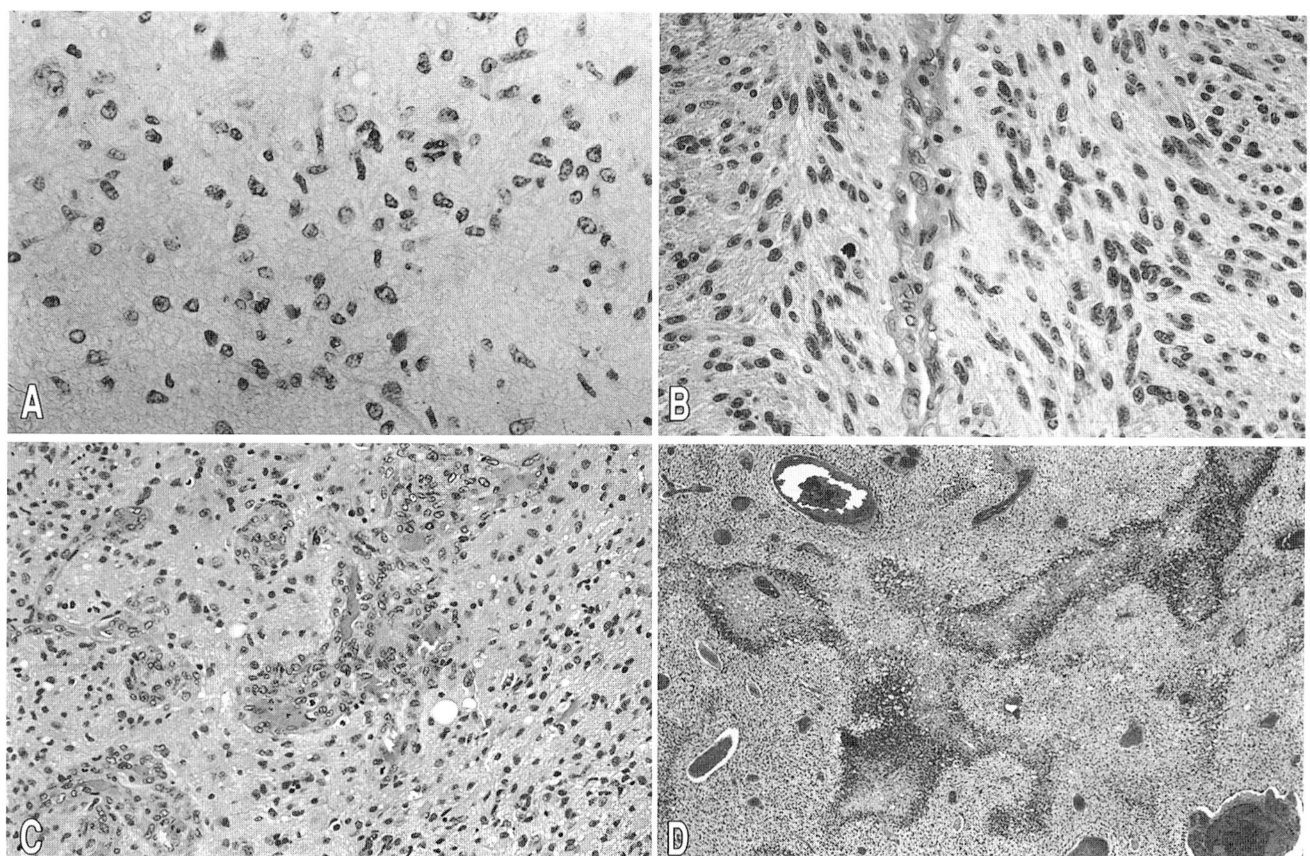

FIGURE 34.3. Morphologic features used in the diagnosis and grading of diffuse/infiltrating astrocytomas include atypia (A), mitotic activity (B), endothelial proliferation (C), and necrosis (D). Necrosis may be serpiginous and occur in association with pseudopalisading of neoplastic cells (as shown in this picture), or it may involve large areas of tumor.

anaplastic oligodendroglioma, and anaplastic oligoastrocytoma mixed tumors. Because of the infiltrative nature of these tumors, surgical resection alone is insufficient to cure patients. These tumors are resistant to radiation and chemotherapy, and long-term survival is rare. Outcomes are poor, with median survivals of 1 to 2 years.

Surgery

Surgical resection of hemispheric gliomas is indicated when it may be performed without significant morbidity, when it will improve preoperative symptoms such as increased intracranial pressure and seizures, and when it might improve the long-term prognosis. The relative indications for resection of gliomas therefore vary according to tumor location, preoperative symptoms, and the specific histologic diagnosis. The role of surgical resection in improving prognosis is controversial.[28]

Radiation

The role of RT in the treatment of newly diagnosed high-grade gliomas was firmly established by two prospective randomized trials conducted in the 1960s and 1970s. Brain Tumor Study Group (BTSG) 69–01 randomized high-grade glioma patients in the postoperative setting to supportive care or RT (60 Gy WBRT).[29] Median survival was 14 weeks in the supportive care group and significantly improved to 35 weeks in the RT group. The significant survival benefit of postoperative RT has been confirmed in other studies and in a number of meta-analyses.[30] Unfortunately for the majority of high-grade glioma patients, the benefit from RT is only temporary, with eventual tumor recurrence, progression, and ultimately death. Therefore, a number of studies have prospectively tested multiple RT parameters (e.g., treatment volume, total dose, dose fractionation, dose escalation, special radiation procedures) to further improve the therapeutic ratio for these patients. Presently, complex radiation treatment plans (e.g., three-dimensional conformal RT) deliver high doses of radiation to the tumor volume with margin (e.g., 2-cm margins) while significantly sparing surrounding normal structures from these high doses of radiation. This approach is supported by studies demonstrating that focal RT was not inferior to WBRT.[31,32] This paradigm shift in treatment volumes has occurred in an effort to reduce acute and late toxicity and the recognition that the vast majority of tumor progressions recur locally. Other strategies that have been investigated include dose escalation, various fractionation schedules, and brachytherapy (Table 34.2). Various modifications that have been studied include hyperfractionation (delivery of multiple smaller-sized fractions at shorter intervals), accelerated fractionation (decreases the overall treatment time), brachytherapy, radiosurgery, and particle. Each of these strategies has some theoretical advantage beyond conventional radiation. Unfortunately, none of these techniques has resulted in an improvement in the therapeutic ratio compared to standard conventional focal RT. Elderly patients, especially those with a poor PS, constitute a subset that may derive benefit even with a shortened RT course, an important consideration for patients with a short survival. A number of prospective trials have shown equivalent results for elderly patients with shortened course of RT (e.g., 30 Gy in 10 fractions) compared to a more protracted course of RT (e.g., 60 Gy in 30 fractions).[33,34]

In summary, postoperative RT to 55–60 Gy in 1.8- to 2-Gy fractions results in a significant survival benefit, albeit temporarily, and is the standard of care. To date, radiation dose escalation has not shown to result in improved outcomes despite extensive study.

Chemotherapy

Chemotherapy has a limited role in the therapy of high-grade astrocytomas. One of the earliest trials to test the role of chemotherapy was a BTSG phase III four-arm randomized trial comparing best supportive care, BCNU (carmustine) alone, RT alone, and a combination of BCNU and RT. The median survival of the patients in the groups was as follows:

TABLE 34.2. A selected review of randomized radiotherapy (RT) studies in newly diagnosed high-grade gliomas.

Study and reference	*Therapies tested*	*RT dose (Gy/fr)*	*Chemotherapy*	*Median survival (weeks)*
Hyperfractionation Scott (RTOG 9006)[145]	EBRT Hyperfxn	60/30 72/60	BCNU BCNU	48.5 (GBM) 44.2 (GBM) $P = 0.44$
Accelerated RT Prados[146]	EBRT Accelerated RT	59.4/33 70.4/44 (1.6 Gy BID)	±DFMO ±DFMO	42 41 $P = 0.75$
Brachytherapy Laperriere[147]	EBRT ^{125}I + EBRT	50/25 60 Gy + 50/25	CCNU at discretion of oncologists	57.2 59.8 $P = 0.49$
Selker[148]	EBRT ^{125}I + EBRT	60.2/35 60 Gy + 60.2	BCNU BCNU	58.8 68.1 $P = 0.10$
Radiosurgery Souhami (RTOG 93–05)[149]	EBRT EBRT + SRS	60/30 60/30 + 15–24	BCNU BCNU	60.6 58.9 $P = 0.53$
Particle therapy Griffin (RTOG)[150]	EBRT EBRT + Neut.	65/33 50 + 15	None None	37.0 42.1 NS

RT, radiotherapy; RTOG, Radiation Therapy Oncology Group; GBM, glioblastoma multiforme; Hyperfxn, hyperfractionation; EBRT, conventional external-beam radiotherapy; DFMO, difluromethylornithine; BTCG, Brain Tumor Cooperative Group; SRS, stereotactic radiosurgery; Neut, Neutrons; NS, not statistically significant.

TABLE 34.3. Important randomized clinical trials testing adjuvant chemotherapy in high-grade gliomas.

Study	*Concept/therapy tested*	*Conclusions*
BTSG trial 6901[151]	Compared best supportive care; BCNU alone; BCNU + RT and RT alone	All treatment groups had longer survival than the best supportive care group
BTSG trial 7201[29]	Compared MeCCNU alone; radiotherapy; BCNU + RT and MeCCNU + RT	MeCCNU-alone arm did the worst; RT is an essential component of therapy
BTCG trial 7501[152]	Compared combination of RT (60Gy) with one of four therapies: BCNU; high-dose steroids; procarbazine; or BCNU + high-dose steroids	High-dose steroids-only group had the worst outcome; no advantage to adding steroids to BCNU
BTCG trial 7702[153]	Compared RT + BCNU; RT + streptozocin; hyperfractionated RT (twice daily) + BCNU; RT + misonidazole (radiation sensitizer) + BCNU	Outcomes similar in all arms; no advantage to using streptozocin, misonidazole, or hyperfractionation
BTCG trial 8001[31]	Compared use of BCNU alone with combinations of BCNU + procarbazine; BCNU + hydroxyurea; BCNU + procarbazine + epipodophyllotoxin	Combination chemotherapy did not improve survival
BTCG trial 8301[123]	Compared IA to IV BCNU, in a four-arm trial that also tested benefit of adding 5-FU to regimens; all patients received RT	IA BCNU worsened survival in those with AA and was more toxic; 5-FU did not impact on outcomes
RTOG/ECOG trial 7401[154]	Compared 60Gy RT alone; 60Gy RT followed by a 10-Gy boost; 60-Gy RT + BCNU and RT + methyl-CCNU + DTIC	No advantage to using multiagent therapy or RT boost
CNS Cancer Consortium[155]	Comparing BCNU with alternative chemotherapy agent diaziquone (AZQ); all patients received RT	No difference between the two arms
NCCTG[156]	Compared BCNU with an alternative nitrosourea PCNU; all received RT	PCNU more toxic and did not improve outcomes
ECOG/SWOG[157]	Pre-RT chemotherapy with three cycles of BCNU and cisplatin compared with RT + concurrent BCNU; GBM patients only	Pre-RT chemotherapy was significantly more toxic and did not improve outcomes

BCNU, carmustine; RT, radiation therapy; MeCCNU, semustine; IA, intraarterial; IV, intravenous; Gy, gray; 5-FU, 5-fluorouracil; PCNU, 1-(2-chloroethyl)-3-(2,6-dioxo-3-piperidyl-1-nitrosourea; GBM, glioblastoma multiforme; DTIC, dacarbazine; BTSG, Brain Tumor Study Group; BTCG, Brain Tumor Cooperative Group; RTOG, Radiation Therapy Oncology Group; ECOG, Eastern Cooperative Oncology Group; NCCTG, North Central Cancer Treatment Group; SWOG, South West Oncology Group.

best supportive care, 14 weeks; BCNU alone, 19 weeks; RT alone, 36 weeks; and combined therapy arm, 35 weeks. Although survival distribution curves were identical for the first 12 months from initiation of treatment, there was a higher survival rate at 18 months among the patients receiving the combination therapy, with 10% still alive at that time, as compared to only 4% of patients in the radiation-alone group.[29] Several other studies have been conducted to address the role of chemotherapy in high-grade gliomas, with most having failed to demonstrate an advantage of adding chemotherapy to radiation in the adjuvant setting (Table 34.3). To address this issue further, two meta-analyses have been performed. Fine et al. evaluated 16 randomized trials of patients with high-grade astrocytomas. The estimated increase in survival for patients treated with combination radiation and chemotherapy was 10.1% at 1 year and 8.6% at 2 years.[35] In another meta-analysis, the use of chemotherapy (all received a nitrosourea compound, alone or in combination) was associated with a 15% relative decrease in the risk of death; this translated into an absolute increase in 1-year survival of 6%.[36] The median survival was prolonged by 2 months with chemotherapy. One potential explanation for the negative results in several of the clinical trials may be that they were not adequately powered to detect the benefit of chemotherapy. More recently, Stupp et al. reported results of a randomized phase III trial of radiation alone (standard therapy arm) compared with the combination of temozolomide ($75\,mg/m^2$/day for 42 days) and concomitant radiation followed by six additional cycles of temozolomide (150–$200\,mg/m^2$/day × 5 days every 28 days). Temozolomide therapy resulted in an increase in the median survival by 3 months (from 12 to 15 months); the 2-year survival was 26% in the study arm, which was statistically superior to 8% in the control arm. Therapy with concomitant temozolomide and radiation appears to be well tolerated in this setting.[37] Consequently, it is appropriate to use either temozolomide or BCNU in addition to RT for patients with glioblastoma multiforme.

Several investigators have evaluated the potential benefits of using combinations of drugs over single-agent chemotherapy (usually BCNU). However, based on the data available currently, the benefit of using any combination regimen over single-agent therapy is questionable at this time.

Currently available data suggest that, similar to their low-grade counterparts, high-grade oligodendrogliomas (both pure and mixed) are relatively chemotherapy sensitive when compared to pure astrocytomas. The use of combination therapy with PCV (a combination of procarbazine (PCBZ), lomustine (CCNU) and vincristine) or single agent TMZ appears to lead to responses in large proportions of patients with progressive high-grade oligodendroglial tumors, though in some of the studies, confirmatory biopsies were not obtained at time of progression.[4,38,39] Until recently, there has been a paucity of randomized trial data on which to base decisions. In June 2004, the first report of R9402 was released. Patients with anaplastic oligodendroglioma or oligoastrocytoma were randomized to immediate radiation therapy, or four cycles of PCV, followed by radiation. Although there was no difference in overall survival in the two groups, disease-free survival was prolonged in the group receiving chemotherapy. Regardless of treatment, patients with chromosome 1p and/or 19q deletion had longer survival. These preliminary data suggest that adjuvant PCV may be appropriate for patients with anaplastic oligodendroglial-containing tumors.[40]

Therapy for recurrent gliomas remains a challenge in spite of much research evaluating different agents, combinations, and strategies (including high-dose chemotherapy with stem cell rescue). Response rates are generally low (10% to 30%) and time to progression is short, varying from a few to several months.[41,42] Given the minimal efficacy of standard treatments, investigational therapies are appropriate as initial treatment for these patients.

Chemotherapy Implants

An approach that has been tested in HGG with some evidence of benefit is the use of biodegradable BCNU-impregnated wafers (Gliadel). These wafers are composed of a complex of BCNU and a polymer. After implantation into a tumor cavity at the time of surgical resection, the complex degrades over a period of a few weeks, delivering high local concentrations of BCNU. Data from trials in both newly diagnosed and recurrent GBM patients demonstrated a small but significant benefit in both these groups.[43,44]

Low-Grade Diffuse Glioma

Low-grade glioma (LGG) is a term applied to members of a group of tumors that have a more indolent clinical course than high-grade astrocytomas (Figure 34.4). The term LGG encompasses a number of disease entities that are predominantly characterized by their clinical behavior: slow growth and tendency for local recurrences. Patients with diffuse infiltrative LGGs have a median survival of around 5 to 10 years, depending upon histology.[45] These tumors occur in young adults (twenties and thirties) and typically present with seizures.[46] Favorable prognostic features include oligodendroglial histology, younger age at diagnosis, tumor size less than 5 cm, and, possibly, greater extent of tumor resection. Late recurrences are relatively common, and patients should be followed lifelong for recurrences. When these tumors do recur, they may recur either as low-grade or as higher-grade tumors. Management of these patients includes symptomatic therapy of symptoms (e.g., seizures). Therapy of the tumors includes a combination of surgery and radiation. Most of the data on which to base treatment decisions in LGGs are derived from retrospective studies; very few prospective randomized trials have been performed in patients with this disease.

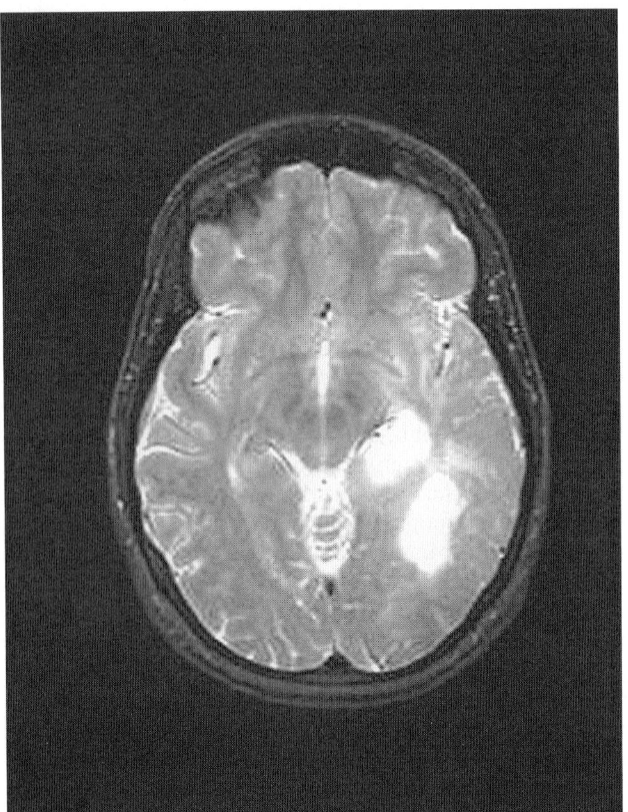

FIGURE 34.4. Brain MRI of patient with a low-grade oligoastrocytoma in the left temporoparietal region demonstrates area of enhanced T2 signal. This tumor had decreased T1 intensity and did not enhance with Gd contrast (not shown). This 31-year-old patient had stable disease for 2 years before requiring therapy for her tumor.

Symptom Control

Deferring therapy until there an unequivocal need for antitumor therapy appears to be a reasonable option in LGGs. Retrospective[47,48] data suggest that patients who have radiologically suspected LGGs and are observed have outcomes similar to those who underwent immediate therapy. This strategy, which has the advantage of avoiding therapy-related toxicity, has been supported by the results of a recent randomized prospective study.[49]

Surgery

Most patients with low-grade gliomas require at least a diagnostic brain biopsy. In some cases, more-extensive resections may be indicated. The surgical decision is guided by the location of the tumor, age and the functional status of the patient. Gliomas that extensively involve eloquent cortex or deep tracts or nuclei are usually not candidates for a large resection. Specialized surgical techniques with functional imaging and awake resections may allow for a greater amount of tumor resection. The therapeutic benefit of more-aggressive resection remains controversial.

Radiation Therapy

A prospective randomized trial has shown RT at diagnosis delays tumor recurrence in comparison to delayed radiation at the time of tumor progression.[49] However, in the absence of data demonstrating a survival benefit to this approach, it is acceptable to defer irradiation until there is evidence of symptomatic tumor growth. The rationale for delaying radiation is to reduce the risk of radiation-induced neurocognitive deficits. Two prospective randomized trials between intermediate- and high-dose RT have failed to demonstrate a benefit for the higher dose[49,50] (Table 34.4). Typically, at the present time, doses between 45 and 54 Gy delivered in 180- to 200-Gy fractions are considered acceptable.

Chemotherapy

The role of chemotherapy in the therapy of the majority of adult LGG remains under investigation. Interpretation of data

TABLE 34.4. Randomized radiotherapy trials for newly diagnosed low-grade gliomas.

Study	*No. enrolled*	*Therapy*	*Five-year PFS (%)*	*Five-year OS (%)*
Karim[49]	290	54 Gy	44	63
		Observation	37	66
			$P = 0.02$	NS
Karim[50]	343	45 Gy	47	58
		59.4 Gy	50	59
			NS	NS
Shaw[158]	203	50.4 Gy	55	72
		64.8 Gy	52	64
			NS	NS

PFS, progression-free survival; OS, overall survival; NS, not significant.

from retrospective studies on the use of chemotherapy is confounded somewhat by the fact that some of the series describe the use of chemotherapy at the time of recurrence and others at initial treatment. There are two situations in which chemotherapy has a role in the therapy of LGG: children and patients with oligodendroglial components.

Chemotherapy has a definite role in the therapy of children with LGG. A study testing a combination of carboplatin and vincristine in children with unresectable low-grade gliomas demonstrated prolonged periods of progression-free survival (68% at 3 years). The benefit was far greater in those younger than 5 years when compared to older patients.[51] Similar encouraging results were seen in a study using single-agent carboplatin in children with optic pathway tumors.[52] Other studies have confirmed the observation about chemotherapy responsiveness in children with LGG to some agents.[53–55] Areas of ongoing investigation in children include benefits of multidrug therapy (as compared to single-agent therapy) and the role of adjuvant chemotherapy.

Oligodendroglial tumors are chemotherapy sensitive. Because high-grade oligodendroglial tumors were shown to respond to PCV,[4,41] several investigators have evaluated the role of this regimen in LGG with oligodendroglial elements. The data from these reports are difficult to interpret, as the patient population tested is heterogeneous. A Phase II trial that evaluated this combination postoperatively (and before RT) found that a substantial minority of patients (up to half) attains objective responses with this regimen.[56] Other investigations into PCV use in oligodendroglial tumors have confirmed that there is a definite substantial objective response rate (~60%), with a median duration of response of approximately 1 to 1.5 years.[57,58] However, PCV has a high rate of hematologic toxicity, which limits its use. More recent investigations have demonstrated that temozolomide (TMZ) may be an active agent in this disease as well.[59] A recent European Phase II trial demonstrated a 52% response rate with a median duration of response of 13 months.[38] Oligodendroglial tumors that progress after initial therapy with radiation or PCV seem to maintain responsiveness to other chemotherapeutic agents (e.g., TMZ).[60] The implications of a response to either of these regimens on overall neurologic status, long-term disease-free survival, or overall survival remain to be evaluated. Another area of interest in oligodendroglial tumors is the correlation between responses and genetic markers (1p and 19q deletions), which may allow for better patient selection.[56] Other approaches under investigation are the use of chemotherapy before radiation (in an effort to delay the use of radiation), based on data that suggest that this may be a viable strategy.[61] The role of adjuvant chemotherapy for these patients is also under investigation. A Phase III trial of radiation alone compared with radiation followed by procarbazine, CCNU, and vincristine (PCV) has completed accrual (RTOG-9802), and outcome results are pending.

At present, the role of chemotherapy in the primary therapy of adult low-grade gliomas remains to be defined. There has been only one randomized study to evaluate the benefit of adding chemotherapy (CCNU) to RT (55 Gy) in the adjuvant setting; this study failed to show any improvements in the CCNU arm.[62] A more-recent Phase II trial testing the use of TMZ in patients with progressive LGG demonstrated response rates of 73% in patients with astrocytomas, with most of these responses lasting more than a year.[59] Phase III trials to test the utility of TMZ are planned and will help clarify the role of this agent in LGGs.

Circumscribed Astrocytomas

Pilocytic Astrocytoma

Pilocytic astrocytome (PA) is a distinct clinical entity that occurs generally in children and young adults, hence the old name of *juvenile pilocytic astrocytoma*. It represents the most common childhood glioma, with the cerebellar location being the most frequent. These tumors have a distinct radiologic appearance; they are well circumscribed, are frequently cystic, and enhance significantly with contrast administration (Figure 34.5). Histologically, PA is frequently a biphasic tumor with densely fibrillated areas rich in Rosenthal fibers and loosely arranged, often microcystic areas in which eosinophilic granular bodies can be found. Cellular pleomorphism and hyperchromasia can be marked. Therapy is mainly surgical, with excellent outcomes with a gross total resection (GTR).[63]

Pleomorphic Xanthoastrocytoma

Pleomorphic xanthoastrocytoma (PXA) is a rare tumor representing less than 1% of all astrocytic tumors. Its most frequent location is the temporal lobe, where it occurs frequently as a cystic lesion with a mural nodule, superficially located and involving the leptomeninges. PXA is typically a tumor of children and young adults, who typically present with seizures. PXA frequently demonstrates immunohistochemical expression of neuronal markers; however, it is fundamentally a glial astrocytic tumor.[64] Morphologically, PXA is characterized by marked cellular pleomorphism with frequent presence of giant cells. Xanthic changes with cell vacuolation are frequent, but not invariable, as the name would appear to suggest. This tumor has a relatively favorable prognosis when compared to diffuse astrocytomas. Ability to achieve a GTR is the stronger predictor of disease-free and overall survival. Increased mitotic activity and presence of necrosis have been associated with frequency of recurrence and survival. In a small proportion of patients, PXAs progress to higher-grade tumors.[64] Factors that underlie such a transformation are unknown.

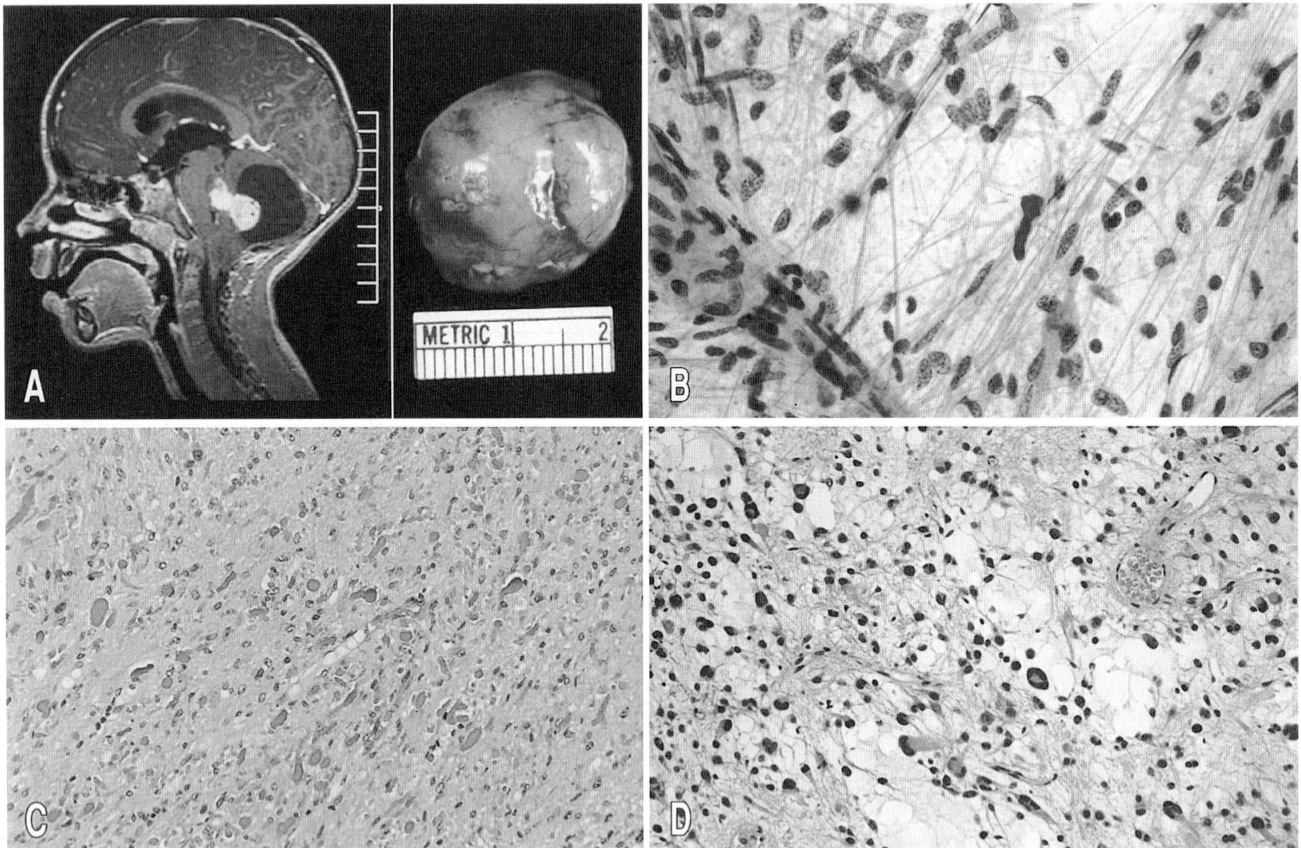

FIGURE 34.5. Typical example of pilocytic astrocytoma. The tumors typically occur in young adults. The most typical location is in the cerebellum, frequently in the midline. Pilocytic astrocytomas may often have a cystic component as demonstrated on the MRI (A). A strongly enhancing mural nodule is characteristic, which grossly appears as a well-demarcated, glistening hypervascular nodule. Morphologically, the tumor is characteristically biphasic, with densely fibrillated areas rich in Rosenthal fibers (C) and loosely arranged microcystic areas with eosinophilic granular bodies (D). Characteristic long bipolar cells and Rosenthal fibers can often be recognized on smear preparations (B).

Meningioma

Meningiomas are tumors of the meninges that are believed to arise from the arachnoidal cap cells. According to the most recent WHO classification (2000), meningiomas are classified in three grades: grade I (classic), grade II (atypical), and grade III (anaplastic or malignant). Grade I meningiomas include a variety of characteristic histomorphologic patterns, but none of these has prognostic significance. Classic meningiomas, following GTR, have a very low frequency of recurrence. Grade II meningiomas (including two morphologic variants, clear cell and chordoid meningioma) are associated with a more-aggressive biologic behavior. Atypical meningiomas, despite GTR, tend to recur at increased frequency, up to 50% to 60% at 5 years. Atypical tumors are defined by the presence of an increased mitotic index (more than 4 mitoses/mm^2) and/or at least three among the following criteria: presence of macronucleoli, pattern-less growth, small cell appearance, and necrosis. Grade III meningiomas are tumors with a very high mitotic index (more than 20 mitoses/10 high-power field, HPF) and/or have a frankly malignant appearance resembling carcinoma, melanoma, or sarcoma. Independent of their morphologic appearance, meningiomas may show invasion of the underlying brain parenchyma.

Although most (90%) meningiomas are slow-growing low-grade tumors, even low-grade tumors can be "biologically malignant" if their location makes treatment impossible. In most cases, the diagnosis can be made using imaging studies such as CT and MRI (Figure 34.6). Most patients are completely asymptomatic and are diagnosed incidentally at autopsy. Asymptomatic meningiomas that are discovered incidentally can be observed,[65,66] as the majority of them do not require therapy. Patients treated with GTR have longer disease-free survival.[67] Features that have been found to be associated with postoperative recurrences are: incomplete resections, age less than 40 years, male sex, and presence of anaplastic features. Several retrospective reviews have shown that external-beam and stereotactic radiation can reduce and delay recurrences in those with residual disease.[68–70] Cytotoxic chemotherapy and biologic agents (e.g., hydroxyurea, interferon, and antiprogestational agents) have not been shown to have any benefit.

Craniopharyngiomas

Craniopharyngiomas are midline tumors that typically arise in the sellar or suprasellar region from residual nests of epithelial cells from Rathke's pouch. They occur most commonly in infants and children. They account for 5% to 10% of all pediatric primary intracranial malignancies and are the third most common intracranial tumors in children.

The symptoms and signs caused by craniopharyngiomas can be explained by the displacement of surrounding struc-

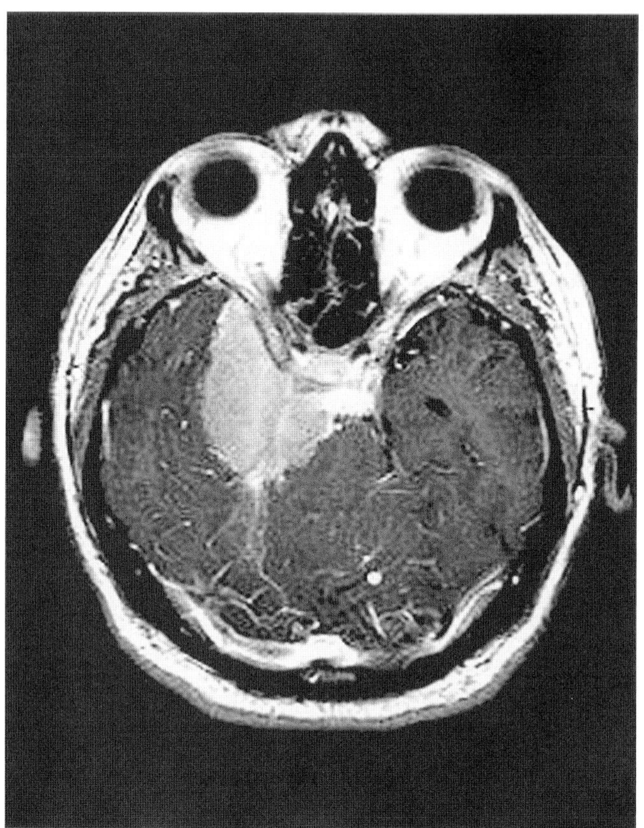

FIGURE 34.6. Post-Gd enhancing images from a head MRI study of a patient with a skull base meningioma. This homogeneously enhancing mass involved the right cavernous sinus, right suprasellar cistern, medial aspect of the right middle cranial fossa, right prepontine cistern, right petrous ridge, and right tentorium. Therapy was necessitated by neurologic dysfunction caused by tumor-associated cerebral edema.

tures, primarily the pituitary gland and optic chiasm. In a majority of cases the diagnosis can be made by radiologic studies, such as, CT or MR scanning. The present of a calcified, cystic, suprasellar mass is diagnostic of craniopharyngioma (Figure 34.7). Poor prognostic factors include severe hydrocephalus, intraoperative adverse events, mucoid epithelial type,[71] and young age (less than 5 years).

The optimal goal of treatment is to achieve a total resection,[72] as recurrences are uncommon after complete resections. No adjuvant therapy is required if a complete resection is achieved.[73,74] However if a complete resection is not technically feasible, or significant morbidity (e.g., visual loss) is expected with an aggressive resection, a more-limited debulking followed by RT is the preferred approach. Patients treated with postoperative RT after subtotal resections have local control rates comparable, or superior, to those achieved by GTR. Other supplemental and sometimes alternative treatment modalities are intracavitary irradiation (with ^{32}P), stereotactic radiosurgery, and intracystic chemotherapy (bleomycin).

Ependymoma

Ependymomas are uncommon intracranial tumors that arise from ependymal cells which line the ventricles in the brain and spinal cord. They occur primarily in children, with most patients being less than 5 years of age at diagnosis. The symptoms at diagnosis correlate with the location of the tumor. As these tumors involve the central canal, and interrupt the normal flow of CSF, patients present with signs of raised ICP.[75] Surgical removal is the preferred initial treatment of choice for posterior fossa ependymomas in children. The extent of resection is a significant factor in prognosis; in several studies the presence of residual tumor was the most important factor that predicts for relapse.[76,77] Although debulking may extend symptom-free survival, it is clear that only a GTR confers any chance for a cure.[76,78] Therefore, aggressive surgical strategies are often justified for patients with this diagnosis. Factors that prevent the GTR of an ependymoma are adherence to the floor of the fourth ventricle, extension out of the foramina of Luschka, or invasion of the surrounding brain.[79–81] Some subsets of patients may do well without any additional therapy following surgery.[82,83] On the other hand, radiation (greater than 50 Gy) is indicated for the therapy of patients with residual disease and for those with posterior fossa tumors. Routine prophylactic radiation to the entire craniospinal axis is not recommended, as this strategy does not improve outcomes[84,85] and is toxic.

Chemotherapy agents such as carboplatin, vincristine, and ifosfamide appear to have some activity in children with ependymoma. A Pediatric Oncology Group (POG) trial in patients younger than 3 years demonstrated that prolonged chemotherapy (up to, but not beyond, 1 year) with delayed radiation was a viable option.

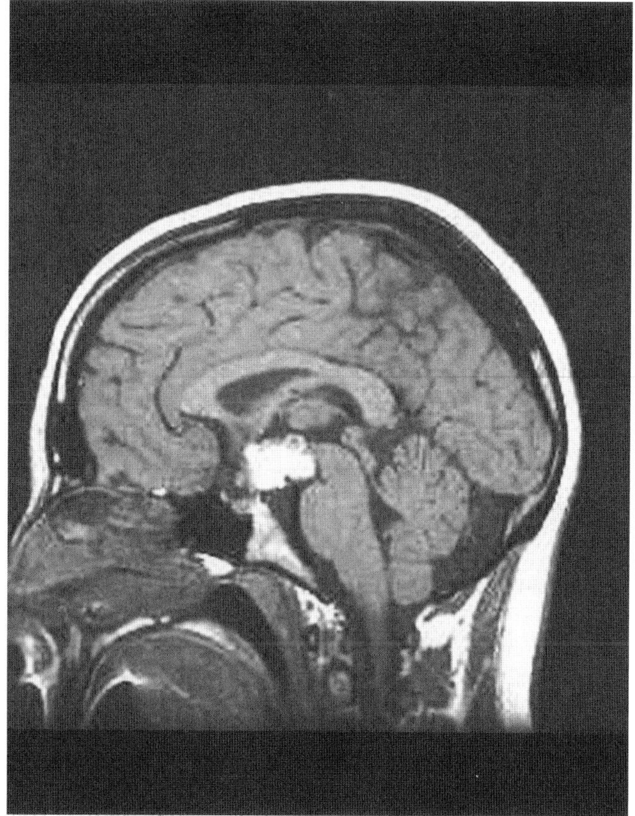

FIGURE 34.7. MRI of head and sella demonstrating a craniopharyngioma. The image demonstrates a large multilobulated mass in the suprasellar cistern. This 21-year-old patient had stable disease for many years before requiring surgery.

Primary Central Nervous System Germ Cell Tumors

Primary intracranial germ cell tumors (GCTs) occur in the brain, in the absence of any disease outside the CNS. These tumors occur predominantly in late childhood, with two-thirds occurring in the second decade of life, with a slight male predominance.

Histologically, GCTs are analogous to their extra-CNS counterparts.[86] Histology is the primary determinant of outcome, with patients with pure germinomas having higher rates of cure (5-year survival greater than 90%), whereas those with nongerminomatous components do much worse.[82,86–88] These tumors occur predominantly in the midline, with the most favored location being the pineal gland (Figure 34.8). The symptoms depend upon location, with the most common presenting features being nausea, vomiting, pituitary hormonal deficiencies, hydrocephalus, and visual disturbances. Tumor markers [beta-human chorionic gonadotropin (beta-HCG), alpha fetoprotein (AFP), or lactic dehydrogenase (LDH)] can be elevated in the CSF and sometimes in the serum as well.[89] The presence of elevated tumor markers is sufficient to make the diagnosis in the presence of an appropriate radiologic image. Cytologic evaluation of the CSF for malignant cells is an essential part of the initial diagnostic workup.

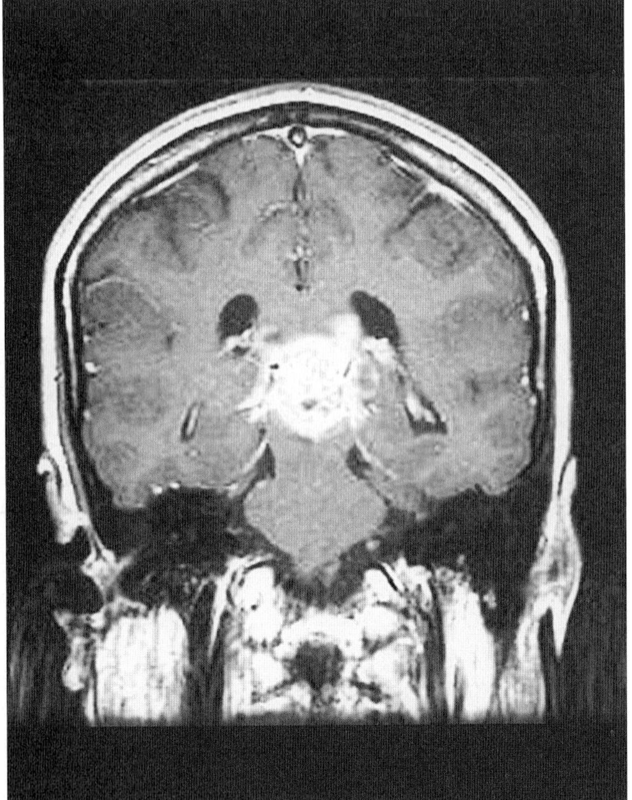

FIGURE 34.8. Brain MRI study demonstrating a sellar tumor. This 19-year-man presented with hormonal imbalances and was found to have a germinoma on biopsy. MRI spine (not shown) demonstrated multiple meningeal metastases. He was cured with multimodality therapy.

The marked efficacy of RT and chemotherapy (with active agents such as cisplatin, etoposide, bleomycin, and ifosfamide) has led to the development of multimodality therapy for these patients. Patients with negative serum and CSF markers require an open exploration of the mass. If the intraoperative biopsy is consistent with the diagnosis of germinoma, it is not necessary or indicated to remove the tumor. Patients with germinoma achieve excellent results achieved with RT alone, which can achieve high cure rates (greater than 90%). Because of concerns about long-term toxicity of RT, attempts are under way to reduce the toxicity by reducing the radiation dose and fields[88,90–92] and by using neoadjuvant chemotherapy followed by lower radiation doses.[93] Patients with evidence of disseminated germinoma are treated with craniospinal radiation. The standard approach in nongerminomas that cannot be completely resected is to administer chemotherapy and to perform a "second-look" surgery for persistent masses. Residual masses may consist of benign elements (e.g., mature teratoma) that have not responded to therapy. Trials using chemotherapy as the sole adjuvant therapy in GCTs have demonstrated impressive (greater than 75%) response rates to chemotherapy. However, because most of these patients relapse, this approach is clearly inadequate.

Medulloblastoma

Medulloblastoma is the most common among the embryonal tumors (a group that includes supratentorial PNET, ependymoblastoma, and medulloepithelioma). They account for 20% to 25% of all childhood tumors. The peak incidence is between 5 and 9 years, with a second peak in the late teens. This tumor is rare beyond 40 years of age. Medulloblastomas occur predominantly in the midline (cerebellar vermis).[94] Under the WHO classification, medulloblastomas are listed as grade IV tumors. Histologically a classic variant of medulloblastoma is described; in addition, there are other well-defined morphologic variants that have prognostic significance, including desmoplastic medulloblastoma, medulloblastoma with extensive nodularity, and large cell medulloblastoma.

Patients with medulloblastomas typically present because of symptoms and signs of raised intracranial pressure. Imaging studies demonstrate midline tumors in the cerebellum that are typically contrast enhancing. The enhancement can often be heterogeneous, with cysts, hemorrhage, or necrosis (Figure 34.9).[95] Appropriate staging at diagnosis includes imaging of the entire neuraxis and CSF sampling. The best identified prognostic features have been taken into account in the Chang staging system.[96] Outcomes of patients with medulloblastomas have improved dramatically in the past few decades.

An attempt at surgical removal of a medulloblastoma is almost always indicated as the initial therapy; the extent of surgical resection has prognostic significance.[97–101] Medulloblastoma is a radioresponsive disease with a propensity for dissemination throughout the CSF. Hence, craniospinal axis radiation is a requirement for all patients. Attempts at developing regimes that exclude radiation have been unsuccessful, with the majority of patients failing in the CNS.[102,103] Craniospinal radiation remains one of the most technically complex treatments in radiation oncology in spite of improved technology. Using reduced radiation doses in conjunction with chemotherapy appears to be a more-promising strategy.[104] The results of these studies are of great importance for the pediatric population, yet they have little bearing on the treatment of adults with medulloblastoma because the concerns for late toxicity are not as great. Therefore, even with the addition of chemotherapy to the treatment regimen of adults with medulloblastoma, the craniospinal dose is not typically lowered.

Prospective randomized trials in children have demonstrated that delaying RT (until after chemotherapy) is detrimental.[105,106] Because the majority of failures occur locally after chemotherapy and craniospinal radiation followed by posterior fossa boost, there is growing interest in boosting only the tumor bed and not the entire posterior fossa.[107]

Medulloblastomas are chemotherapy-sensitive tumors, with the most active regimens containing CCNU (lomustine), vincristine, cyclophosphamide, etoposide, and cisplatin. Subsequent studies revealed that although adjuvant chemotherapy (with CCNU and vincristine) did not benefit patients with medulloblastomas as a group, patients with high-risk features (i.e., young age, presence of residual disease, brainstem involvement, and T3–T4 disease) had a survival advantage.[99,108] As noted previously, the use of chemotherapy may allow for reductions to be made in the dose of RT.[104] One recently reported randomized trial testing chemotherapy in the adjuvant setting found a benefit in event-free survival even in average-risk patients; at the same time, overall survival was not any different between the groups.[109] The use of preradiation chemotherapy has some theoretical advantages and led to a high proportion of responses. However, as noted earlier, this strategy leads to delays in institution of RT, which can be detrimental.[106] One other indication to use chemotherapy may be in the setting of an autologous stem cell transplant and as a strategy to avoid radiation in some young children, with some success.[110–112]

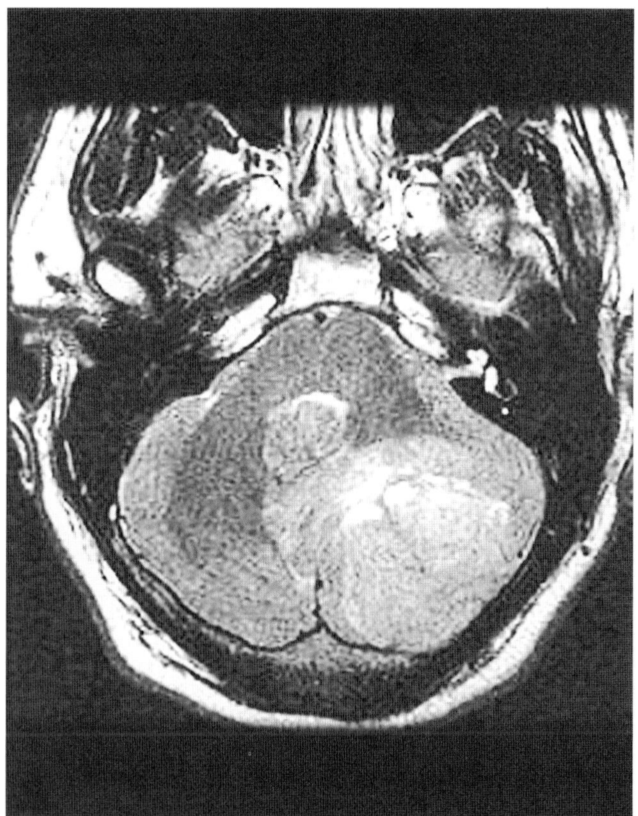

FIGURE 34.9. MRI of head of a patient with cerebellar medulloblastoma demonstrates a large mass lesion with indistinct borders. This lesion had a low T1 signal and a high T2 signal with hazy Gd enhancement. Note areas of necrosis, hemorrhage, and effacement of the fourth ventricle. At the time of this study, the patient had cerebellar tonsillar herniation. This patient was successfully treated with multimodality therapy.

Outcomes are very poor for patients with recurrent medulloblastoma, with very few long-term survivors. High-dose chemotherapy with stem cell rescue (i.e., autologous stem cell transplant) is currently under investigation for therapy of relapsed disease.[113]

Primary Central Nervous System Lymphoma

Primary CNS lymphoma (PCNSL) is a relatively rare disorder whose incidence has been increasing. Most patients are between 40 and 70 years, with the median age at diagnosis being 60 years. These tumors remain localized to the CNS and only rarely metastasize to the outside. Epstein–Barr virus (EBV) is associated with PCNSL, especially in immunosuppressed patients The increased incidence during the past few decades seems to be independent of HIV disease.[114]

PCNSL can present in almost any location in the CNS, including the meninges, vitreous, and the spinal cord. These tumors appear as hyperintense lesions on T_2-weighted MRI images that enhance with contrast (Figure 34.10). Edema is usually minimal, and hemorrhage, necrosis, calcification, and cysts are unusual. Resolution with the use of steroids suggests (but does not confirm) the diagnosis of PCNSL. A biopsy is required to confirm the diagnosis and to differentiate PCNSL from metastatic lesions and rule out other etiologies (e.g., infections in HIV-infected patients).

Untreated patients with PCNSL have a median survival of 1.5 months. Therapy with steroids and radiation improves the quality of life and prolongs survival of these patients. The response rate to radiation therapy alone is greater than 90%.[115] However, prognosis is extremely poor, with 1-, 2-, and 5-year survival rates being 48%, 28%, and less than 5%, respectively. Almost all patients have relapses and eventually die of the disease. The use of combination chemotherapy regimens leads to high response rates, with small improvements in survival. However, the benefits seemed to be limited to those younger than 60 years. In older patients, the toxicity is significant, with a very high risk of dementia (greater than 80%).[116,117] Currently the most effective regimens are those that incorporate high-dose systemic methotrexate (MTX) as initial therapy.[118] Response rates noted have ranged from 80% to 90%,[119,120] the median survival of patients has been between 32 and 54 months, and the 5-year survival has been in the range of 30% to 40%.[121,122] Radiation may be used as salvage therapy in those with relapses.

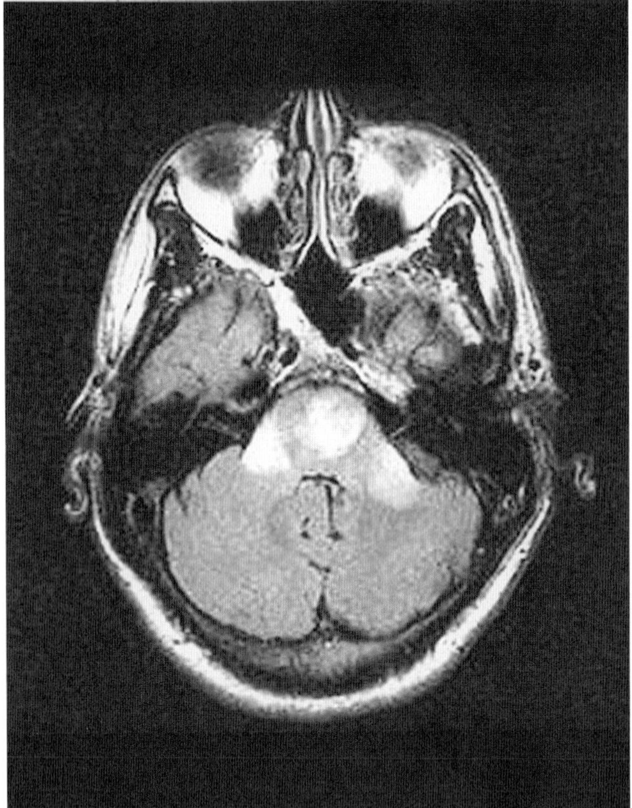

FIGURE 34.10. Fluid-attenuated inversion-recovery (FLAIR) image from a head MRI image of a patient with primary central nervous system (CNS) lymphoma. Note areas of hyperintense signal in the pons, adjacent to the cerebellum. This patient responded to initial therapy (with high-dose methotrexate) and recurred, but was successfully salvaged by therapy with high-dose therapy and autologous stem cell rescue. He subsequently relapsed in the vitreous humor bilaterally.

Novel Therapeutic Approaches

To improve outcomes in patients with high-grade astrocytomas, various novel therapies and drug delivery methods for conventional therapies have been employed. Some of these are discussed here.

Intraarterial Chemotherapy

The use of intraarterial (IA) chemotherapy (into the carotid artery) was first investigated in the 1980s and found to be feasible, albeit with a certain degree of neurotoxicity (ocular pain, visual impairment, and leukoencephalopathy). A Phase III randomized trial in patients with high-grade gliomas comparing intraarterial and intravenous BCNU[123] demonstrated significant toxicity (ipsilateral visual loss in 15%) and *decreased* survival in the patients with AA. A similar high rate of toxicity was seen with the use of IA cisplatin.[124–126] This approach to therapy of CNS tumors using currently available chemotherapeutic agents is not justified in view of the excessive neurotoxicity noted in these studies.

Blood–Brain Barrier Disruption

The value of blood–brain disruption (BBB) disruption by osmotic agents (e.g., mannitol) with chemotherapy to increase drug delivery to gliomas remains under investigation. In one such study, patients with GBM were treated with IA mannitol and combination chemotherapy (a regimen of MTX, cyclophosphamide, and PCBZ). Significant neurotoxicity was noted, with 3 (of 38) patients experiencing strokelike events during therapy,[127] although survival seemed to be better than historic controls.

Studies using positron emission tomography (PET) scanning have demonstrated that although IA administration of mannitol can increase the permeability of the BBB in the tumor, the increase is even greater (and lasts longer than) in the normal brain.[128] Thus, although BBB disruption can enhance drug delivery to the tumor, this is accompanied by an even greater increase in the drug delivered into the normal brain. These factors may explain the high rate of toxic events. Based on the toxicity data, and the lack of confirmatory clinical evidence that BBB modification in conjunction with chemotherapy improves the outcome of patients with glioma, this approach should be considered investigational at this time.

Immune Therapies for CNS Tumors

The role of immunologic therapies in CNS tumors is currently experimental. It is now recognized that GBMs are immunogenic and have several tumor-specific antigens [such as interleukin 13 receptor-α-2 chain, PHD finger protein 3, and glioma-expressed antigen 2 (GLEA2)], which can be exploited for therapeutic purposes. Several immune-based therapies are currently being investigated, including tumor vaccines, conjugated antibody therapies, adoptive immunotherapy, and intracavitary cytokine plus antigen therapy.

Ongoing areas of research include attempts at identifying tumor-specific antigens, mechanisms of immune tolerance, and appropriate methods to deliver immune effector cells or antibodies to the tumor. A few early clinical trials have been reported and have demonstrated the feasibility and safety of these approaches.[129–134]

Convection-Enhanced Delivery of Agents to Brain Tumors

Convection-enhanced delivery (CED) is a method of delivering therapeutic agents to the tumor cavity directly using implantable catheters. Catheters are left in the tumor cavity at the time of surgery, and therapeutic agents are perfused into the tumor cavity through the catheter under pressure using pumps. This technique has the advantage of completely bypassing the BBB, achieving high volumes of distribution, and achieving local concentrations of the agent that would be impossible to achieve by any other method of delivery. Various kinds of therapeutic agents are currently being tested for their safety and utility when administered in this manner; these include traditional chemotherapeutic agents, antibodies, fusion products of toxins with antibodies, viral vectors carrying genes, and labeled cytokines.[135]

Gene Therapy

Gliomas are ideal targets for gene transfer approaches because of their limited ability to metastasize and have been among the earliest tumor types to be included in clinical gene transfer trials. The gene most extensively used in gene therapy of gliomas is the herpes simplex virus thymidine kinase (HSV-tk), a gene that does not normally exist in mammalian cells. Transferring HSV-tk gene into tumor cells renders them able to phosphorylate ganciclovir into an active form that is lethal to tumor cells. Several retroviral and adenoviral vectors have been studied as vehicles for transferring the HSV-tk gene in gliomas.[136,137] A multicenter Phase III trial testing the delivery of this gene, in conjunction with RT, did not demonstrate any survival advantage to this therapy over RT alone.[138] A different gene transfer approach under investigation consists of tumor suppressor gene (p53) reconstitution. Early clinical studies of Adp53 a non-replicating adenoviral vector encoding the p53 gene administration in patients with recurrent glioma have been conducted and have demonstrated excellent tolerance.[139] Major limitations to the further development of this strategy include lack of adequate dissemination of the virus, low expression of viral receptors on tumor cells, lack of animal models that adequately replicate the behavior of human tumors, and inability to adequately monitor the effects of therapy.[140]

Signal Transduction Inhibitors

During the past few years, research into the biology of CNS tumors has led the identification of several aberrant signaling pathways that appear to be important in the causation of, and in the maintenance of, the malignant phenotype. Several new agents have been developed designed to target key members of these pathways. Examples of agents that may potentially be used in CNS tumor (mainly glioma) patients are EGFR inhibitors such as ZD1839 (gefitinib, Iressa), OSI-774 (erlotinib, Tarceva), CI-1033 and EKB-569, mTOR inhibitors (such as rapamycin, RAD-001, and CCI-779), and inhibitors of platelet-derived growth factor (PDGF) such as imatinib mesylate (STI-571, Gleevec). Recent released results of clinical trials using CCI-779,[141] OSI-774,[142,143] and imatinib[144] have demonstrated a small but definite degree of anticancer activity in high-grade gliomas. Ongoing trials with these agents will demonstrate if these signal transduction inhibitors have enough activity to make an impact on the overall outcome of these patients. However, based on currently available data, it appears unlikely that signal transduction inhibitors would have enough anticancer activity on their own to impact the natural history of these tumors. Combinations of these agents with other therapies (such as cytotoxic agents or radiation) need to be investigated.

References

1. Greig NH, Ries LG, Yancik R, Rapoport SI. Increasing annual incidence of primary malignant brain tumors in the elderly. J Natl Cancer Inst 1990;82(20):1621–1624.
2. Curran WJ Jr. Recursive partitioning analysis of prognostic factors in three Radiation Therapy Oncology Group malignant glioma trials. J Natl Cancer Inst 1993;85:704–710.
3. Shaw EG, Seiferheld W, Scott C, et al. Reexamining the Radiation Therapy Oncology Group (RTOG) Recursive Partitioning Analysis (RPA) for Glioblastoma Multiforme (GBM) patients. Proceedings, Annual ASTRO Meeting. Int J Radiat Oncol Biol Phys 2003;57(2):S135–S136.
4. Cairncross G, Macdonald D, Ludwin S, et al. Chemotherapy for anaplastic oligodendroglioma. National Cancer Institute of Canada Clinical Trials Group. J Clin Oncol 1994;12(10):2013–2021.
5. Ino Y, Betensky RA, Zlatescu MC, et al. Molecular subtypes of anaplastic oligodendroglioma: implications for patient management at diagnosis. Clin Cancer Res 2001;7(4):839–845.
6. Fuller GN, Hess KR, Rhee CH, et al. Molecular classification of human diffuse gliomas by multidimensional scaling analysis of gene expression profiles parallels morphology-based classification, correlates with survival, and reveals clinically-relevant novel glioma subsets. Brain Pathol 2002;12(1):108–116.
7. Pomeroy SL, Tamayo P, Gaasenbeek M, et al. Prediction of central nervous system embryonal tumour outcome based on gene expression. Nature (Lond) 2002;415(6870):436–442.
8. Forsyth PA, Posner JB. Headaches in patients with brain tumors: a study of 111 patients. Neurology 1993;43(9):1678–1683.
9. Glantz MJ, Cole BF, Forsyth PA, et al. Practice parameter: anticonvulsant prophylaxis in patients with newly diagnosed brain tumors. Report of the Quality Standards Subcommittee of the American Academy of Neurology. Neurology 2000;54(10):1886–1893.
10. Sugahara T, Korogi Y, Tomiguchi S, et al. Posttherapeutic intraaxial brain tumor: the value of perfusion-sensitive contrast-enhanced MR imaging for differentiating tumor recurrence from nonneoplastic contrast-enhancing tissue. AJNR Am J Neuroradiol 2000;21(5):901–909.
11. Speck O, Thiel T, Hennig J. Grading and therapy monitoring of astrocytomas with ^{1}H-spectroscopy: preliminary study. Anticancer Res 1996;16(3B):1581–1585.
12. Gupta R, Sinha U, Cloughesy T, Alger J. Inverse correlation between choline magnetic resonance spectroscopy signal intensity and the apparent diffusion coefficient in human glioma. Magn Reson Med 1999;41(1):2–7.
13. Quevedo JF, Buckner JC, Schmidt JL, Dinapoli RP, O'Fallon JR. Thromboembolism in patients with high-grade glioma. Mayo Clin Proc 1994;69(4):329–332.
14. Streiff MB, Weir EG, Kickler TS, Htut M, Grossman SA. ABO blood group is a risk factor for venous thromboembolism in patients with malignant gliomas. Proc Am Soc Clin Oncol 2003;22:113.
15. Silber JH, Radcliffe J, Peckham V, et al. Whole-brain irradiation and decline in intelligence: the influence of dose and age on IQ score. J Clin Oncol 1992;10(9):1390–1396.
16. Chin HW, Maruyama Y. Age at treatment and long-term performance results in medulloblastoma. Cancer (Phila) 1984;53(9):1952–1958.
17. Silverman CL, Palkes H, Talent B, Kovnar E, Clouse JW, Thomas PR. Late effects of radiotherapy on patients with cerebellar medulloblastoma. Cancer (Phila) 1984;54(5):825–829.
18. Catania MA, Marciano MC, Parisi A, et al. Erythropoietin prevents cognition impairment induced by transient brain ischemia in gerbils. Eur J Pharmacol 2002;437(3):147–150.
19. Fike JR, Gobbel GT, Marton LJ, Seilhan TM. Radiation brain injury is reduced by the polyamine inhibitor alpha-difluoromethylornithine. Radiat Res 1994;138(1):99–106.
20. Kondziolka D, Mori Y, Martinez AJ, McLaughlin MR, Flickinger JC, Lunsford LD. Beneficial effects of the radioprotectant 21-aminosteroid U-74389G in a radiosurgery rat malignant glioma model. Int J Radiat Oncol Biol Phys 1999;44(1):179–184.
21. Weitzner MA, Meyers CA, Valentine AD. Methylphenidate in the treatment of neurobehavioral slowing associated with cancer and cancer treatment. J Neuropsychiatry Clin Neurosci 1995;7(3):347–350.
22. Plafki C, Carl UM, Glag M, Hartmann KA. The treatment of late radiation effects with hyperbaric oxygenation (HBO). Strahlenther Onkol 1998;174(suppl 3):66–68.
23. Surma-aho O, Niemela M, Vilkki J, et al. Adverse long-term effects of brain radiotherapy in adult low-grade glioma patients. Neurology 2001;56(10):1285–1290.

24. Kiebert GM, Curran D, Aaronson NK, et al. Quality of life after radiation therapy of cerebral low-grade gliomas of the adult: results of a randomised phase III trial on dose response (EORTC trial 22844). EORTC Radiotherapy Co-operative Group. Eur J Cancer 1998;34(12):1902–1909.
25. Hochberg FH, Slotnick B. Neuropsychologic impairment in astrocytoma survivors. Neurology 1980;30(2):172–177.
26. Torres IJ, Mundt AJ, Sweeney PJ, et al. A longitudinal neuropsychological study of partial brain radiation in adults with brain tumors. Neurology 2003;60(7):1113–1118.
27. Taylor BV, Buckner JC, Cascino TL, et al. Effects of radiation and chemotherapy on cognitive function in patients with high-grade glioma. J Clin Oncol 1998;16(6):2195–2201.
28. Laws ER, Parney IF, Huang W, et al. Survival following surgery and prognostic factors for recently diagnosed malignant glioma: data from the Glioma Outcomes Project. J Neurosurg 2003;99(3):467–473.
29. Walker MD, Green SB, Byar DP, et al. Randomized comparisons of radiotherapy and nitrosoureas for the treatment of malignant glioma after surgery. N Engl J Med 1980;303(23):1323–1329.
30. Laperriere N, Zuraw L, Cairncross G. The Cancer Care Ontario Practice Guidelines Initiative Neuro-Oncology Disease Site G. Radiotherapy for newly diagnosed malignant glioma in adults: a systematic review. Radiother Oncol 2002;64(3):259–273.
31. Shapiro WR, Green SB, Burger PC, et al. Randomized trial of three chemotherapy regimens and two radiotherapy regimens in postoperative treatment of malignant glioma. Brain Tumor Cooperative Group Trial 8001. J Neurosurg 1989;71(1):1–9.
32. Kita M, Okawa T, Tanaka M, Ikeda M. Radiotherapy of malignant glioma: prospective randomized clinical study of whole brain vs local irradiation. Gan No Rinsho (Japanese Journal of Cancer Clinics) 1989;35(11):1289–1294.
33. Bauman GS, Gaspar LE, Fisher BJ, Halperin EC, Macdonald DR, Cairncross JG. A prospective study of short-course radiotherapy in poor prognosis glioblastoma multiforme. Int J Radiat Oncol Biol Phys 1994;29(4):835–839.
34. Hoegler DB, Davey P. A prospective study of short course radiotherapy in elderly patients with malignant glioma. J Neuro-Oncol 1997;33(3):201–204.
35. Fine HA, Dear KB, Loeffler JS, Black PM, Canellos GP. Meta-analysis of radiation therapy with and without adjuvant chemotherapy for malignant gliomas in adults. Cancer (Phila) 1993;71(8):2585–2597.
36. Stewart LA. Chemotherapy in adult high-grade glioma: a systematic review and meta-analysis of individual patient data from 12 randomised trials. Lancet 2002;359(9311):1011–1018.
37. Stupp R, Mason WP, Van Den Bent MJ, et al. Concomitant and adjuvant temozolomide (TMZ) and radiotherapy (RT) for newly diagnosed glioblastoma multiforme (GBM). Conclusive results of a randomized phase III trial by the EORTC Brain & RT groups and NCIC Clinical Trials Group. Proc Am Soc Clin Oncol 2004;23:1 (abstract 2).
38. van den Bent MJ, Taphoorn MJ, Brandes AA, et al. Phase II study of first-line chemotherapy with temozolomide in recurrent oligodendroglial tumors: the European Organization for Research and Treatment of Cancer Brain Tumor Group Study 26971. J Clin Oncol 2003;21(13):2525–2528.
39. Chinot OL, Honore S, Dufour H, et al. Safety and efficacy of temozolomide in patients with recurrent anaplastic oligodendrogliomas after standard radiotherapy and chemotherapy. J Clin Oncol 2001;19(9):2449–2455.
40. Cairncross G, Seiferhel WS, E., Jenkins R, et al. An intergroup randomized controlled clinical trial (RCT) of chemotherapy plus radiation (RT) versus RT alone for pure and mixed anaplastic oligodendrogliomas: initial report of RTOG 94-02. Proc Am Soc Clin Oncol 2004;23:107 (abstract 1500).
41. Buckner JC, Brown LD, Kugler JW, et al. Phase II evaluation of recombinant interferon alpha and BCNU in recurrent glioma. J Neurosurg 1995;82(3):430–435.
42. Yung WK, Prados MD, Yaya-Tur R, et al. Multicenter phase II trial of temozolomide in patients with anaplastic astrocytoma or anaplastic oligoastrocytoma at first relapse. Temodal Brain Tumor Group. J Clin Oncol 1999;17(9):2762–2771.
43. Brem H, Piantadosi S, Burger PC, et al. Placebo-controlled trial of safety and efficacy of intraoperative controlled delivery by biodegradable polymers of chemotherapy for recurrent gliomas. The Polymer-brain Tumor Treatment Group. Lancet 1995;345(8956):1008–1012.
44. Westphal M, Hilt DC, Bortey E, et al. A phase 3 trial of local chemotherapy with biodegradable carmustine (BCNU) wafers (Gliadel wafers) in patients with primary malignant glioma. Neuro-Oncology 2003;5(2):79–88.
45. Shaw EG, Daumas-Duport C, Scheithauer BW, et al. Radiation therapy in the management of low-grade supratentorial astrocytomas. J Neurosurg 1989;70(6):853–861.
46. Lote K, Stenwig AE, Skullerud K, Hirschberg H. Prevalence and prognostic significance of epilepsy in patients with gliomas. Eur J Cancer 1998;34(1):98–102.
47. Recht LD, Lew R, Smith TW. Suspected low-grade glioma: is deferring treatment safe? Ann Neurol 1992;31(4):431–436.
48. Olson JD, Riedel E, DeAngelis LM. Long-term outcome of low-grade oligodendroglioma and mixed glioma. Neurology 2000;54(7):1442–1448.
49. Karim AB, Afra D, Cornu P, et al. Randomized trial on the efficacy of radiotherapy for cerebral low-grade glioma in the adult: European Organization for Research and Treatment of Cancer Study 22845 with the Medical Research Council study BRO4: an interim analysis. Int J Radiat Oncol Biol Phys 2002;52(2):316–324.
50. Karim AB, Maat B, Hatlevoll R, et al. A randomized trial on dose-response in radiation therapy of low-grade cerebral glioma: European Organization for Research and Treatment of Cancer (EORTC) Study 22844. Int J Radiat Oncol Biol Phys 1996;36(3):549–556.
51. Packer RJ, Ater J, Allen J, et al. Carboplatin and vincristine chemotherapy for children with newly diagnosed progressive low-grade gliomas. J Neurosurg 1997;86(5):747–754.
52. Mahoney DH Jr, Cohen ME, Friedman HS, et al. Carboplatin is effective therapy for young children with progressive optic pathway tumors: a Pediatric Oncology Group phase II study. Neuro-Oncology 2000;2(4):213–220.
53. Massimino M, Spreafico F, Cefalo G, et al. High response rate to cisplatin/etoposide regimen in childhood low-grade glioma. J Clin Oncol 2002;20(20):4209–4216.
54. Packer RJ, Lange B, Ater J, et al. Carboplatin and vincristine for recurrent and newly diagnosed low-grade gliomas of childhood. J Clin Oncol 1993;11(5):850–856.
55. Castello MA, Schiavetti A, Varrasso G, Clerico A, Cappelli C. Chemotherapy in low-grade astrocytoma management. Childs Nerv Syst 1998;14(1-2):6–9.
56. Buckner JC, Gesme D Jr, O'Fallon JR, et al. Phase II trial of procarbazine, lomustine, and vincristine as initial therapy for patients with low-grade oligodendroglioma or oligoastrocytoma: efficacy and associations with chromosomal abnormalities. J Clin Oncol 2003;21(2):251–255.
57. Soffietti R, Ruda R, Bradac GB, Schiffer D. PCV chemotherapy for recurrent oligodendrogliomas and oligoastrocytomas. Neurosurgery 1998;43(5):1066–1073.
58. van den Bent MJ. New perspectives for the diagnosis and treatment of oligodendroglioma. Expert Rev Anticancer Ther 2001;1(3):348–356.
59. Quinn JA, Reardon DA, Friedman AH, et al. Phase II trial of temozolomide in patients with progressive low-grade glioma. J Clin Oncol 2003;21(4):646–651.

60. van den Bent MJ, Chinot O, Boogerd W, et al. Second-line chemotherapy with temozolomide in recurrent oligodendroglioma after PCV (procarbazine, lomustine and vincristine) chemotherapy: EORTC Brain Tumor Group phase II study 26972. Ann Oncol 2003;14(4):599–602.
61. Streffer J, Schabet M, Bamberg M, et al. A role for preirradiation PCV chemotherapy for oligodendroglial brain tumors. J Neurol 2000;247(4):297–302.
62. Eyre HJ, Crowley JJ, Townsend JJ, et al. A randomized trial of radiotherapy versus radiotherapy plus CCNU for incompletely resected low-grade gliomas: a Southwest Oncology Group study. J Neurosurg 1993;78(6):909–914.
63. Burkhard C, Di Patre PL, Schuler D, et al. A population-based study of the incidence and survival rates in patients with pilocytic astrocytoma. J Neurosurg 2003;98(6):1170–1174.
64. Giannini C, Scheithauer BW, Lopes MB, Hirose T, Kros JM, VandenBerg SR. Immunophenotype of pleomorphic xanthoastrocytoma. Am J Surg Pathol 2002;26(4):479–485.
65. Olivero WC, Lister JR, Elwood PW. The natural history and growth rate of asymptomatic meningiomas: a review of 60 patients. J Neurosurg 1995;83(2):222–224.
66. Go RS, Taylor BV, Kimmel DW. The natural history of asymptomatic meningiomas in Olmsted County, Minnesota. Neurology 1998;51(6):1718–1720.
67. Stafford SL, Perry A, Suman VJ, et al. Primarily resected meningiomas: outcome and prognostic factors in 581 Mayo Clinic patients, 1978 through 1988. Mayo Clinic Proc 1998;73(10):936–942.
68. Barbaro NM, Gutin PH, Wilson CB, Sheline GE, Boldrey EB, Wara WM. Radiation therapy in the treatment of partially resected meningiomas. Neurosurgery 1987;20(4):525–528.
69. Taylor BW Jr, Marcus RB Jr, Friedman WA, Ballinger WE Jr, Million RR. The meningioma controversy: postoperative radiation therapy. Int J Radiat Oncol Biol Phys 1988;15(2):299–304.
70. Hakim R, Alexander E III, Loeffler JS, et al. Results of linear accelerator-based radiosurgery for intracranial meningiomas. Neurosurgery 1998;42(3):446–453; discussion 53–54.
71. Petito CK, DeGirolami U, Earle KM. Craniopharyngiomas: a clinical and pathological review. Cancer (Phila) 1976;37(4): 1944–1952.
72. Fahlbusch R, Honegger J, Paulus W, Huk W, Buchfelder M. Surgical treatment of craniopharyngiomas: experience with 168 patients. J Neurosurg 1999;90(2):237–250.
73. Kalapurakal JA, Goldman S, Hsieh YC, Tomita T, Marymont MH. Clinical outcome in children with craniopharyngioma treated with primary surgery and radiotherapy deferred until relapse. Med Pediatr Oncol 2003;40(4):214–218.
74. Merchant TE, Kiehna EN, Sanford RA, et al. Craniopharyngioma: the St. Jude Children's Research Hospital experience 1984–2001. Int J Radiat Oncol Biol Phys 2002;53(3):533–542.
75. Prayson RA. Clinicopathologic study of 61 patients with ependymoma including MIB-1 immunohistochemistry. Ann Diagn Pathol 1999;3(1):11–18.
76. Healey EA, Barnes PD, Kupsky WJ, et al. The prognostic significance of postoperative residual tumor in ependymoma. Neurosurgery 1991;28(5):666–671; discussion 71–72.
77. Robertson PL, Zeltzer PM, Boyett JM, et al. Survival and prognostic factors following radiation therapy and chemotherapy for ependymomas in children: a report of the Children's Cancer Group. J Neurosurg 1998;88(4):695–703.
78. Evans AE, Anderson JR, Lefkowitz-Boudreaux IB, Finlay JL. Adjuvant chemotherapy of childhood posterior fossa ependymoma: cranio-spinal irradiation with or without adjuvant CCNU, vincristine, and prednisone: a Childrens Cancer Group study. Med Pediatr Oncol 1996;27(1):8–14.
79. Lyons MK, Kelly PJ. Posterior fossa ependymomas: report of 30 cases and review of the literature. Neurosurgery 1991;28(5): 659–664; discussion 64–65.
80. van Veelen-Vincent ML, Pierre-Kahn A, Kalifa C, et al. Ependymoma in childhood: prognostic factors, extent of surgery, and adjuvant therapy. J Neurosurg 2002;97(4):827–835.
81. Ikezaki K, Matsushima T, Inoue T, Yokoyama N, Kaneko Y, Fukui M. Correlation of microanatomical localization with postoperative survival in posterior fossa ependymomas. Neurosurgery 1993;32(1):38–44.
82. Salazar OM. A better understanding of CNS seeding and a brighter outlook for postoperatively irradiated patients with ependymomas. Int J Radiat Oncol Biol Phys 1983;9(8):1231–1234.
83. Goldwein JW, Leahy JM, Packer RJ, et al. Intracranial ependymomas in children. Int J Radiat Oncol Biol Phys 1990; 19(6):1497–1502.
84. Kovalic JJ, Flaris N, Grigsby PW, Pirkowski M, Simpson JR, Roth KA. Intracranial ependymoma long term outcome, patterns of failure. J Neuro-Oncol 1993;15(2):125–131.
85. Rousseau P, Habrand JL, Sarrazin D, et al. Treatment of intracranial ependymomas of children: review of a 15-year experience. Int J Radiat Oncol Biol Phys 1994;28(2):381–386.
86. Matsutani M, Sano K, Takakura K, et al. Primary intracranial germ cell tumors: a clinical analysis of 153 histologically verified cases. J Neurosurg 1997;86(3):446–455.
87. Schild SE, Haddock MG, Scheithauer BW, et al. Nongerminomatous germ cell tumors of the brain. Int J Radiat Oncol Biol Phys 1996;36(3):557–563.
88. Shirato H, Nishio M, Sawamura Y, et al. Analysis of long-term treatment of intracranial germinoma. Int J Radiat Oncol Biol Phys 1997;37(3):511–515.
89. Allen JC, Nisselbaum J, Epstein F, Rosen G, Schwartz MK. Alpha fetoprotein and human chorionic gonadotropin determination in cerebrospinal fluid. An aid to the diagnosis and management of intracranial germ-cell tumors. J Neurosurg 1979;51(3):368–374.
90. Allen JC, DaRosso RC, Donahue B, Nirenberg A. A phase II trial of preirradiation carboplatin in newly diagnosed germinoma of the central nervous system. Cancer (Phila) 1994;74(3):940–944.
91. Calaminus G, Bamberg M, Baranzelli MC, et al. Intracranial germ cell tumors: a comprehensive update of the European data. Neuropediatrics 1994;25(1):26–32.
92. Matsutani M, Sano K, Takakura K, Fujimaki T, Nakamura O. Combined treatment with chemotherapy and radiation therapy for intracranial germ cell tumors. Childs Nerv Syst 1998;14 (1-2):59–62.
93. Buckner JC, Peethambaram PP, Smithson WA, et al. Phase II trial of primary chemotherapy followed by reduced-dose radiation for CNS germ cell tumors. J Clin Oncol 1999;17(3):933–940.
94. Tamayo P, Gaasenbeek M, Sturla LM, et al. Medulloblastoma: clinical presentation and management. Experience at the Hospital for Sick Children, Toronto, 1950–1980. J Neurosurg 1983; 58(4):543–552.
95. Bourgouin PM, Tampieri D, Grahovac SZ, Leger C, Del Carpio R, Melancon D. CT and MR imaging findings in adults with cerebellar medulloblastoma: comparison with findings in children. AJR Am J Roentgenol 1992;159(3):609–612.
96. Harisiadis L, Chang CH. Medulloblastoma in children: a correlation between staging and results of treatment. Int J Radiat Oncol Biol Phys 1977;2(9-10):833–841.
97. del Charco JO, Bolek TW, McCollough WM, et al. Medulloblastoma: time-dose relationship based on a 30-year review. Int J Radiat Oncol Biol Phys 1998;42(1):147–154.
98. Raimondi AJ, Tomita T. Medulloblastoma in childhood. Acta Neurochir 1979;50(1-2):127–138.
99. Evans AE, Jenkin RD, Sposto R, et al. The treatment of medulloblastoma. Results of a prospective randomized trial of radiation therapy with and without CCNU, vincristine, and prednisone. J Neurosurg 1990;72(4):572–582.
100. Jenkin D, Goddard K, Armstrong D, et al. Posterior fossa medulloblastoma in childhood: treatment results and a proposal for a

new staging system. Int J Radiat Oncol Biol Phys 1990;19(2): 265–274.

101. Cervoni L, Cantore G. Medulloblastoma in pediatric age: a single-institution review of prognostic factors. Childs Nerv Syst 1995;11(2):80–84; discussion 5.
102. Bouffet E, Bernard JL, Frappaz D, et al. M4 protocol for cerebellar medulloblastoma: supratentorial radiotherapy may not be avoided. Int J Radiat Oncol Biol Phys 1992;24(1):79–85.
103. Thomas PR, Deutsch M, Kepner JL, et al. Low-stage medulloblastoma: final analysis of trial comparing standard-dose with reduced-dose neuraxis irradiation. J Clin Oncol 2000;18(16): 3004–3011.
104. Packer RJ, Goldwein J, Nicholson HS, et al. Treatment of children with medulloblastomas with reduced-dose craniospinal radiation therapy and adjuvant chemotherapy: a Children's Cancer Group Study. J Clin Oncol 1999;17(7):2127–2136.
105. Zeltzer PM, Boyett JM, Finlay JL, et al. Metastasis stage, adjuvant treatment, and residual tumor are prognostic factors for medulloblastoma in children: conclusions from the Children's Cancer Group 921 randomized phase III study. J Clin Oncol 1999;17(3):832–845.
106. Kortmann RD, Kuhl J, Timmermann B, et al. Postoperative neoadjuvant chemotherapy before radiotherapy as compared to immediate radiotherapy followed by maintenance chemotherapy in the treatment of medulloblastoma in childhood: results of the German prospective randomized trial HIT '91. Int J Radiat Oncol Biol Phys 2000;46(2):269–279.
107. Carrie C, Muracciole X, Gomez F, et al. Conformal radiotherapy, reduced boost volume, hyperfractionated radiotherapy and online quality control in standard risk medulloblastoma without chemotherapy, results of the French M-SFOP 98 protocol. Int J Radiat Oncol Biol Phys 2003;57(suppl 2):S195.
108. Tait DM, Thornton-Jones H, Bloom HJ, Lemerle J, Morris-Jones P. Adjuvant chemotherapy for medulloblastoma: the first multicentre control trial of the International Society of Paediatric Oncology (SIOP I). Eur J Cancer 1990;26(4):464–469.
109. Taylor RE, Bailey CC, Robinson K, et al. Results of a randomized study of preradiation chemotherapy versus radiotherapy alone for nonmetastatic medulloblastoma: The International Society of Paediatric Oncology/United Kingdom Children's Cancer Study Group PNET-3 Study. J Clin Oncol 2003; 21(8):1581–1591.
110. Mason WP, Grovas A, Halpern S, et al. Intensive chemotherapy and bone marrow rescue for young children with newly diagnosed malignant brain tumors. J Clin Oncol 1998;16(1):210–221.
111. Bailey CC, Gnekow A, Wellek S, et al. Prospective randomised trial of chemotherapy given before radiotherapy in childhood medulloblastoma. International Society of Paediatric Oncology (SIOP) and the (German) Society of Paediatric Oncology (GPO): SIOP II. Medical & Pediatric Oncology 1995;25(3):166–178.
112. Hartsell WF, Gajjar A, Heideman RL, et al. Patterns of failure in children with medulloblastoma: effects of preirradiation chemotherapy. Int J Radiat Oncol Biol Phys 1997;39(1): 15–24.
113. Graham ML, Herndon JE II, Casey JR, et al. High-dose chemotherapy with autologous stem-cell rescue in patients with recurrent and high-risk pediatric brain tumors. J Clin Oncol 1997;15(5):1814–1823.
114. Olson JE, Janney CA, Rao RD, et al. The continuing increase in the incidence of primary central nervous system non-Hodgkin lymphoma: a surveillance, epidemiology, and end results analysis. Cancer (Phila) 2002;95(7):1504–1510.
115. Nelson DF, Martz KL, Bonner H, et al. Non-Hodgkin's lymphoma of the brain: can high dose, large volume radiation therapy improve survival? Report on a prospective trial by the Radiation Therapy Oncology Group (RTOG): RTOG 8315. Int J Radiat Oncol Biol Phys 1992;23(1):9–17.
116. Abrey LE, DeAngelis LM, Yahalom J. Long-term survival in primary CNS lymphoma. J Clin Oncol 1998;16(3):859–863.
117. Bessell EM, Graus F, Punt JA, et al. Primary non-Hodgkin's lymphoma of the CNS treated with BVAM or CHOD/BVAM chemotherapy before radiotherapy. J Clin Oncol 1996;14(3): 945–954.
118. DeAngelis LM. Primary CNS lymphoma: treatment with combined chemotherapy and radiotherapy. J Neuro-Oncol 1999; 43(3):249–257.
119. Schlegel U, Pels H, Glasmacher A, et al. Combined systemic and intraventricular chemotherapy in primary CNS lymphoma: a pilot study. J Neurol Neurosurg Psychiatry 2001;71(1):118–122.
120. Freilich RJ, Delattre JY, Monjour A, DeAngelis LM. Chemotherapy without radiation therapy as initial treatment for primary CNS lymphoma in older patients. Neurology 1996;46(2):435–439.
121. Maher EA, Fine HA. Primary CNS lymphoma. Semin Oncol 1999;26(3):346–356.
122. Ferreri AJ, Reni M, Villa E. Therapeutic management of primary central nervous system lymphoma: lessons from prospective trials. Ann Oncol 2000;11(8):927–937.
123. Shapiro WR, Green SB, Burger PC, et al. A randomized comparison of intra-arterial versus intravenous BCNU, with or without intravenous 5-fluorouracil, for newly diagnosed patients with malignant glioma. J Neurosurg 1992;76(5):772–781.
124. Newton HB, Page MA, Junck L, Greenberg HS. Intra-arterial cisplatin for the treatment of malignant gliomas. J Neuro-Oncol 1989;7(1):39–45.
125. Mortimer JE, Crowley J, Eyre H, Weiden P, Eltringham J, Stuckey WJ. A phase II randomized study comparing sequential and combined intraarterial cisplatin and radiation therapy in primary brain tumors. A Southwest Oncology Group study. Cancer (Phila) 1992;69(5):1220–1223.
126. Hiesiger EM, Green SB, Shapiro WR, et al. Results of a randomized trial comparing intra-arterial cisplatin and intravenous PCNU for the treatment of primary brain tumors in adults: Brain Tumor Cooperative Group trial 8420A. J Neuro-Oncol 1995; 25(2):143–154.
127. Neuwelt EA, Howieson J, Frenkel EP, et al. Therapeutic efficacy of multiagent chemotherapy with drug delivery enhancement by blood-brain barrier modification in glioblastoma. Neurosurgery 1986;19(4):573–582.
128. Zunkeler B, Carson RE, Olson J, et al. Quantification and pharmacokinetics of blood-brain barrier disruption in humans. J Neurosurg 1996;85(6):1056–1065.
129. Schneider T, Gerhards R, Kirches E, Firsching R. Preliminary results of active specific immunization with modified tumor cell vaccine in glioblastoma multiforme. J Neuro-Oncol 2001;53(1): 39–46.
130. Cokgor I, Akabani G, Kuan CT, et al. Phase I trial results of iodine-131-labeled antitenascin monoclonal antibody 81C6 treatment of patients with newly diagnosed malignant gliomas. J Clin Oncol 2000;18(22):3862–3872.
131. Reardon DA, Akabani G, Coleman RE, et al. Phase II trial of murine ^{131}I-labeled antitenascin monoclonal antibody 81C6 administered into surgically created resection cavities of patients with newly diagnosed malignant gliomas. J Clin Oncol 2002;20(5):1389–1397.
132. Kikuchi T, Akasaki Y, Irie M, Homma S, Abe T, Ohno T. Results of a phase I clinical trial of vaccination of glioma patients with fusions of dendritic and glioma cells. Cancer Immunol Immunother 2001;50(7):337–344.
133. Yu JS, Wheeler CJ, Zeltzer PM, et al. Vaccination of malignant glioma patients with peptide-pulsed dendritic cells elicits systemic cytotoxicity and intracranial T-cell infiltration. Cancer Res 2001;61(3):842–847.
134. Becker R, Eichler MK, Jennemann R, Bertalanffy H. Phase I clinical trial on adjuvant active immunotherapy of human gliomas with GD2-conjugate. Br J Neurosurg 2002;16(3):269–275.

135. Dunn IF, Black PM. The neurosurgeon as local oncologist: cellular and molecular neurosurgery in malignant glioma therapy. Neurosurgery 2003;52(6):1411–1422; discussion 22–24.
136. Prados MD, McDermott M, Chang SM, et al. Treatment of progressive or recurrent glioblastoma multiforme in adults with herpes simplex virus thymidine kinase gene vector-producer cells followed by intravenous ganciclovir administration: a phase I/II multi-institutional trial. J Neuro-Oncol 2003;65(3): 269–278.
137. Sandmair AM, Loimas S, Puranen P, et al. Thymidine kinase gene therapy for human malignant glioma, using replication-deficient retroviruses or adenoviruses. Hum Gene Ther 2000; 11(16):2197–2205.
138. Rainov NG. A phase III clinical evaluation of herpes simplex virus type 1 thymidine kinase and ganciclovir gene therapy as an adjuvant to surgical resection and radiation in adults with previously untreated glioblastoma multiforme. Hum Gene Ther 2000;11(17):2389–2401.
139. Lang FF, Bruner JM, Fuller GN, et al. Phase I trial of adenovirus-mediated p53 gene therapy for recurrent glioma: biological and clinical results. J Clin Oncol 2003;21(13):2508–2518.
140. Miller CR, Buchsbaum DJ, Reynolds PN, et al. Differential susceptibility of primary and established human glioma cells to adenovirus infection: targeting via the epidermal growth factor receptor achieves fiber receptor-independent gene transfer. Cancer Res 1998;58(24):5738–5748.
141. Galanis E, Buckner J, Maurer M, et al. NCCTG Phase II trial of CCI-779 in recurrent glioblastoma multiforme (GBM). Proc Am Soc Clin Oncol 2004;23:107.
142. Raizer JJ, Abrey LE, Wen P, et al. A phase II trial of elotinib (OSI-774) in patients with recurrent malignant gliomas not on EIAEDs. Proc Am Soc Clin Oncol 2004;23:107 (abstract 1502).
143. Prados M, Chang S, Burton E, et al. Phase I study of OSI-774 alone or with temozolomide in patients with malignant glioma. Proc Am Soc Clin Oncol 2003;22(2003):99 (abstract 394).
144. Raymond E, Brandes A, Van Oosterom A, et al. Multicentre Phase II study of imatinib mesylate in patients with recurrent glioblastoma: an EORTC NDDG/BTG intergroup Study. Proc Am Soc Clin Oncol 2004;23:107 (abstract 1505).
145. Scott C, Curran WJ, Yung WK, et al. Long term results of RTOG 9006: a randomized trial of hyperfractionated radiotherapy (RT) to 72.0 Gy and carmustine vs. standard RT and carmustine for malignant glioma patients with emphasis on anaplastic astrocytoma (AA) patients. Proc Am Soc Clin Oncol 1998;17:401 (abstract 1546).
146. Prados MD, Wara WM, Sneed PK, et al. Phase III trial of accelerated hyperfractionation with or without difluromethylornithine (DFMO) versus standard fractionated radiotherapy with or without DFMO for newly diagnosed patients with glioblastoma multiforme. Int J Radiat Oncol Biol Phys 2001;49(1):71–77.
147. Laperriere NJ, Leung PM, McKenzie S, et al. Randomized study of brachytherapy in the initial management of patients with malignant astrocytoma. Int J Radiat Oncol Biol Phys 1998; 41(5):1005–1011.
148. Selker RG, Shapiro WR, Burger P, et al. The Brain Tumor Cooperative Group NIH Trial 87-01: a randomized comparison of surgery, external radiotherapy, and carmustine versus surgery, interstitial radiotherapy boost, external radiation therapy, and carmustine. Neurosurgery 2002;51(2):343–355; discussion 55–57.
149. Souhami L, Scott C, Brachman D, et al. Randomized prospective comparison of stereotactic radiosurgery (SRS) followed by conventional radiotherapy (RT) with BCNU to RT with BCNU alone for selected patients with supratentorial glioblastoma multiforme (GBM): report of RTOG 93-05 protocol. Int J Radiat Oncol Biol Phys 2002;54(2S):94–95 (abstract 158).
150. Griffin TW, Davis R, Laramore G, et al. Fast neutron radiation therapy for glioblastoma multiforme. Results of an RTOG study. Am J Clin Oncol 1983;6(6):661–667.
151. Walker MD, Alexander E Jr, Hunt WE, et al. Evaluation of BCNU and/or radiotherapy in the treatment of anaplastic gliomas. A cooperative clinical trial. J Neurosurg 1978;49(3):333–343.
152. Green SB, Byar DP, Walker MD, et al. Comparisons of carmustine, procarbazine, and high-dose methylprednisolone as additions to surgery and radiotherapy for the treatment of malignant glioma. Cancer Treat Rep 1983;67(2):121–132.
153. Deutsch M, Green SB, Strike TA, et al. Results of a randomized trial comparing BCNU plus radiotherapy, streptozotocin plus radiotherapy, BCNU plus hyperfractionated radiotherapy, and BCNU following misonidazole plus radiotherapy in the postoperative treatment of malignant glioma. Int J Radiat Oncol Biol Phys 1989;16(6):1389–1396.
154. Chang CH, Horton J, Schoenfeld D, et al. Comparison of postoperative radiotherapy and combined postoperative radiotherapy and chemotherapy in the multidisciplinary management of malignant gliomas. A joint Radiation Therapy Oncology Group and Eastern Cooperative Oncology Group study. Cancer (Phila) 1983;52(6):997–1007.
155. Schold SC Jr, Herndon JE, Burger PC, et al. Randomized comparison of diaziquone and carmustine in the treatment of adults with anaplastic glioma. J Clin Oncol 1993;11(1):77–83.
156. Dinapoli RP, Brown LD, Arusell RM, et al. Phase III comparative evaluation of PCNU and carmustine combined with radiation therapy for high-grade glioma. J Clin Oncol 1993;11(7): 1316–1321.
157. Grossman SA, O'Neill A, Grunnet M, et al. Phase III study comparing three cycles of infusional carmustine and cisplatin followed by radiation therapy with radiation therapy and concurrent carmustine in patients with newly diagnosed supratentorial glioblastoma multiforme: Eastern Cooperative Oncology Group Trial 2394. J Clin Oncol 2003;21(8):1485–1491.
158. Shaw E, Arusell R, Scheithauer B, et al. Prospective randomized trial of low- versus high-dose radiation therapy in adults with supratentorial low-grade glioma: initial report of a North Central Cancer Treatment Group/Radiation Therapy Oncology Group/Eastern Cooperative Oncology Group study. J Clin Oncol 2002; 20(9):2267–2276.

35

Eye, Orbit, and Adnexal Structures

Daniel M. Albert, Marni Feldmann, Heather Potter, and Amit Kumar

Primary Ocular Tumors: Melanoma

Two distinct populations of pigmented cells can be found in the eye. The pigmented epithelial cells of the iris, ciliary body, and retina are derived from the neural tube. These cells undergo reactive hyperplasia in response to a variety of stimuli, but they only rarely undergo malignant transformation. The other population consists of the stromal melanocytes, which can be found in the skin, conjunctiva, and uveal tract. These are neural crest in origin and do not undergo reactive hyperplasia, but they are the source of the most common primary intraocular tumor: uveal melanoma. The uveal melanocytes are considered the counterpart of dermal melanocytes, the source of cutaneous melanoma. (Dermal melanoma is discussed elsewhere in this text. This chapter focuses on eye-related melanomas.)

Difference From Skin Melanoma

Melanoma of the eye differs from melanoma of the skin in several respects. (1) It is much less common, occurring with an incidence that is approximately one-eighth that of skin melanoma.[1] (2) As a result of the ocular anatomy, the clinical appearance of uveal melanoma is different from that of skin melanoma. (3) The genetics, histology, and growth pattern of the two tumors are different as well.

Uveal melanoma is the most common primary intraocular malignancy in Caucasians, accounting for nearly 70% of all primary intraocular tumors.[2] Melanomas may occur in the conjunctiva as well, but these make up only 2% of ocular melanomas.

The uvea is defined as the vascular layer of the globe and includes the iris, ciliary body, and choroid. The uveal melanocytes are distributed within the stroma of this layer. Pigmented tumors of the iris are usually slow growing and metastasize infrequently. Melanomas of the ciliary and choroid are more common, more aggressive, and of greater concern to the clinician.

Much of the information in this chapter is derived from the recent Collaborative Ocular Melanoma Study (COMS) sponsored by the National Eye Institute and National Cancer Institute. This investigation was a very large study involving approximately 9,000 patients with choroidal melanomas.[3] In addition to gaining insight into the natural history and identifying prognostic factors, the COMS evaluated treatment modalities, its primary focus.

Epidemiology

The Third National Cancer Survey found that melanoma accounted for 70%, or most, of all primary ocular malignancies, followed by the childhood tumor retinoblastoma.[2] The incidence of ocular melanoma has been reported to be between 5 and 7.3 cases per 1,000,000 persons.[2,4–7] In several of these studies, the precise site of origin was not identified; however, melanoma arising from the posterior uveal tract accounted for the majority.

The incidence of ocular melanoma increases with age and peaks in the seventh decade; however, the median age at diagnosis is 56 years.[1,4] Melanoma, in rare instances, does occur in young persons. In an analysis of the cases seen at the Armed Forces Institute of Pathology and Wills Eye Hospital, between 1.08% and 1.59% of uveal melanoma cases were in patients younger than 20 years old.[1]

There appears to be no gender predilection;[8] however, there is a large discrepancy among races. In the 3,586 patients encountered at Wills Eye Hospital, only 0.39% were African-American.[1] In addition, among Caucasians, uveal melanoma is more prevalent in lightly pigmented individuals with lightly pigmented irides.[9] Other populations in which there is a greater prevalence include patients with dysplastic nevus syndrome, melanosis oculi, and oculodermal melanocytosis.[10–12]

Presenting Symptoms

Many uveal melanomas are asymptomatic and are found on screening examinations, but some patients present with decreased vision, positive visual phenomena such as flashing lights, or a red eye with prominent sentinel vessels. Occasionally melanoma presents as a mass visible on the sclera or in the pupil (Figure 35.1). The latter is much more likely if the tumor is located anteriorly or reaches a large size. The mechanisms producing decreased visual acuity or a visual field defect include localized lens cataract or subluxation from an anterior ciliary body tumor. Choroidal tumors produce retinal detachment, bleeding into the vitreous, and

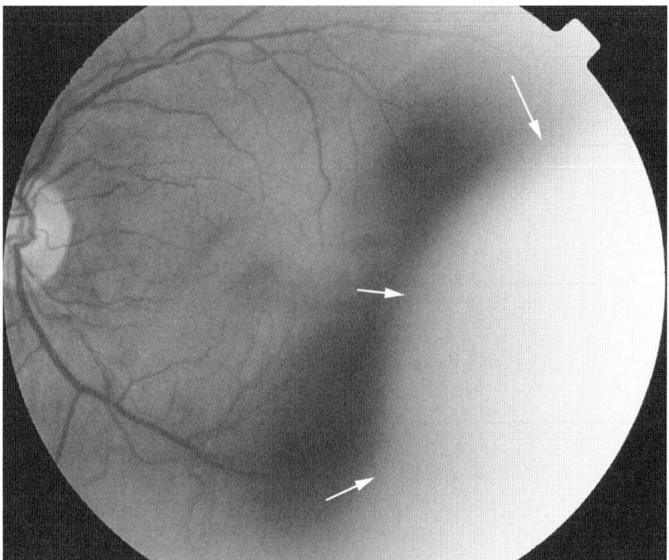

FIGURE 35.1. Choroidal mass representing choroidal melanoma as seen on indirect ophthalmoscopy. Edge is marked with *arrows*.

direct obscuration due to the mass (Figure 35.2). Large tumors can also present with glaucoma caused by anatomic crowding of the anterior chamber angle or neovascularization secondary to ischemia or inflammation induced by the tumor. There may or may not be associated pain.

Etiology

The genetic basis for uveal melanoma is unknown. The etiology of melanoma, however, involves both genetic predisposition (described previously) and predisposing environmental stimuli. Cigarette smoking[13] and ultraviolet radiation (UV)[14] appear to increase the risk.

Pathology

From the pathologic characteristics of melanoma, including location, structure, size, and cellular phenotype, much can be inferred about the prognosis in each case.

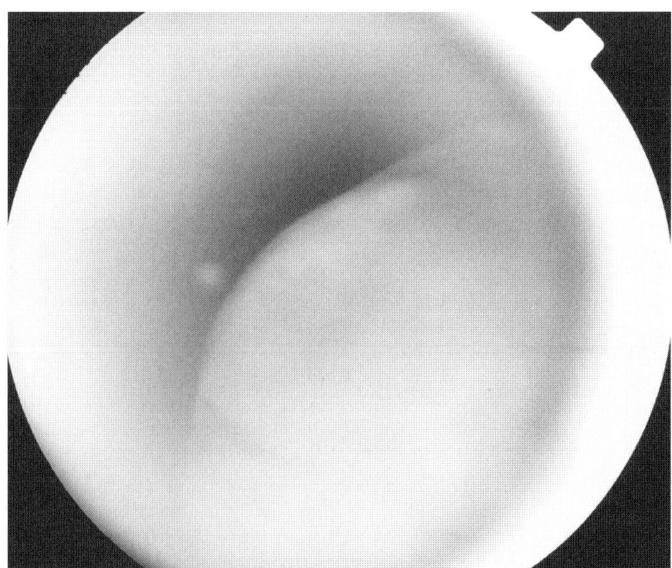

FIGURE 35.2. Higher-magnification view of choroidal melanoma.

Metastasis

About 2.5% of patients with choroidal and ciliary body melanomas have metastases at the time of diagnosis.[15] Obviously, if a secondary tumor is found at a distant location, the patient will have a greatly worsened prognosis. Metastases result from hematogenous dissemination, and the liver is the most frequent site of spread. In the large choroidal melanomas study, the COMS data showed that in tumor-related death, liver metastases were extremely common (93%); these were followed in frequency by lung metastases (24%) and bone metastases (16%).[16]

Extrascleral Extension

Extension of the tumor through the outer layer of the eye is termed extrascleral extension (Figure 35.3). Large extrascleral extensions (greater than 4 mm) drastically worsen the prognosis.[3] The overall incidence is 13% in patients with uveal melanoma.[17] It is generally detected anteriorly at the limbus or posteriorly adjacent to or within the optic nerve. The tumor spreads typically along the vortex veins and ciliary vessels or nerves, and extensions occur more frequently in larger tumors.[17] The COMS showed that 55.7% of enucleated eyes had scleral invasion on histologic examination and 8.2% had extrascleral extension.[18]

Location

The location of the tumor within the globe is an important factor with regard to time of diagnosis. Ciliary body tumors are often obscured from direct visualization by the irides and often are not detected until they are quite large. Ciliary body melanomas occasionally grow in a ringlike fashion to encompass the entire 360° of the ciliary body, making tumor resection impossible. For posterior choroidal tumors, those adjacent to the optic nerve have a worse prognosis, and there is a suspicion that proximity to the foveal avascular zone also worsens prognosis.[3]

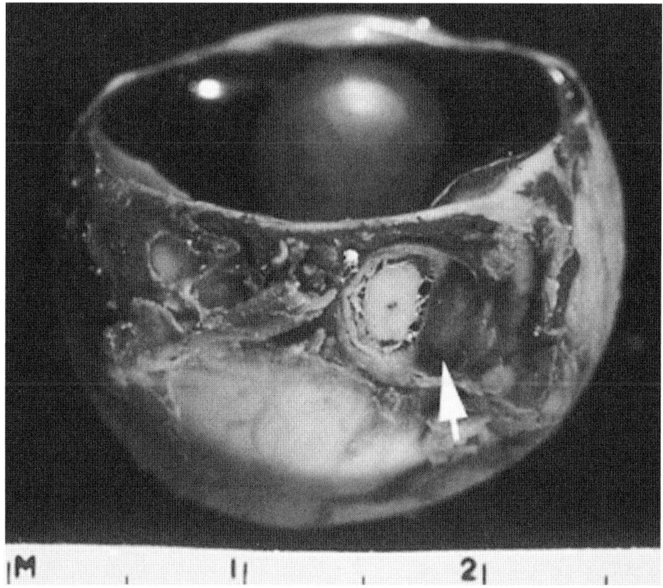

FIGURE 35.3. Extrascleral extension of choroidal melanoma evident as pigmented mass (*arrow*) adjacent to the optic nerve.

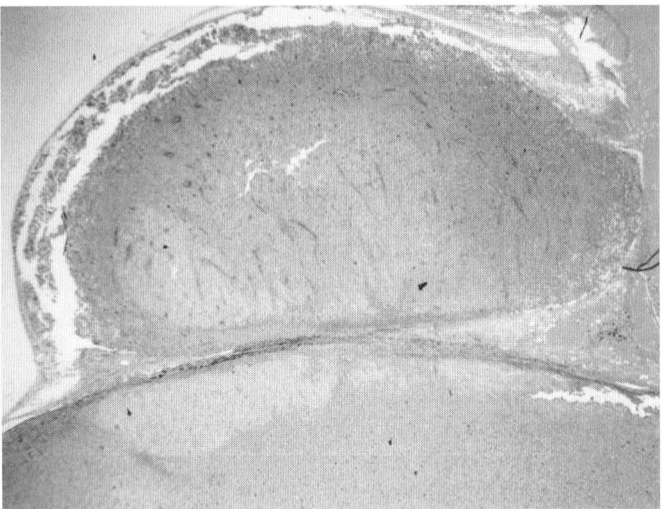

FIGURE 35.4. Dilated blood vessels seen in a choroidal melanoma internal to Bruch's membrane, secondary to the bottleneck effect of Bruch's membrane. 4×.

Intraocular Involvement

Evidence of intraocular spread also worsens the prognosis. Small melanomas generally begin as discoid lesions and grow thicker to assume an almond-like shape while progressively displacing Bruch's membrane and the retina inward. When Bruch's membrane is disrupted, the tumor begins to grow in the subretinal space and assumes more of a mushroom configuration. The portion of the tumor internal to Bruch's membrane can be seen to have dilated blood vessels as it is squeezed by the collar of Bruch's membrane, limiting outflow (Figure 35.4). Some tumors extend through the retina and seed the vitreous. Conversely, other tumors do not follow this pattern of forming a bulky, clinically obvious mass, but rather spread within the plane of the uvea diffusely, thickening this coat and making detection more difficult.

Tumor Size

Size of tumor as it affects prognosis has been studied extensively; tumor size served as the basis for the classification of patients in the COMS. The dimensions of these categories, along with the 5-year melanoma-associated mortality rate, are given in Table 35.1.

TABLE 35.1. Classification of tumor size according to boundary lines.

Type	*Apical height*	*Basal diameter*	*Five-year mortality*
Small	1–3 mm	More than 5 mm	1%
Medium	3.1–8 mm	Less than 16 mm	10%
Large	More than 8 mm	More than 16 mm	30%–35%

Data from Collaborative Ocular Melanoma Study Group. Mortality in patients with small choroidal melanoma. COMS report no 4. Arch Ophthalmol 1997;115:886–893; The Collaborative Ocular Melanoma Study Group. The Collaborative Ocular Melanoma Study (COMS) randomized trial of iodine-125 brachytherapy for choroidal melanoma. III: Initial mortality findings. COMS report no. 18. Arch Ophthalmol 2001;119:969–982; Collaborative Ocular Melanoma Study Group. The Collaborative Ocular Melanomoa Study (COMS) randomized trial of pre-enucleation radiation of large choroidal melanoma. II: Initial mortality findings. COMS report no. 10. Am J Opthalmol 1998;125:779–796.

Tumor Cell Type

In 1931, Callender recognized certain distinguishing cellular characteristics of melanomas and found that they correlated with prognosis after enucleation. These characteristics were subsequently modified slightly by the Armed Forces Institute of Pathology (AFIP), but they are still routinely evaluated and are described in Table 35.2.

Tumors were characterized as spindle cell (A, B, or a combination); mixed (when less than one-half of the tumor is composed of epithelioid cells); or epithelioid (when greater than one-half of the tumor is composed of these cells). Spindle cell tumors carry the best prognosis and epithelioid the worst. Large tumors and more anterior tumors tend to be of the epithelioid type more commonly than do smaller tumors.

Other Classification Methods

Folberg and coworkers have extensively studied the vascular pattern in melanoma. They hypothesized that the blood vessels within the melanoma may be tumor derived. They demonstrated that certain vascular patterns have a strong correlation with the presence of metastatic disease.[18,19] Sorenson et al. and Gamel et al. attempted to objectify the histopathologic nuclear characteristics by basing a measurement on the 10 largest nucleoli identified in the tumor.[20,21] This, in conjunction with largest tumor diameter, is among the best objective cytologic measures of a tumor's malignant poten-

TABLE 35.2. Armed Forces Institute of Pathology (AFIP) modification of the Callender classification.

Cell type	*Size/shape*	*Cytoplasm*	*Nucleus*	*Nucleolus*	*Other*
Spindle A	Elongated and small with indistinct cell membrane	Sparse	Elongated, but plumper than nevus cells, fine chromatin pattern, ± line in chromatin	Not present or indistinct	Cohesive, mitoses rare
Spindle B	Plumper spindle with indistinct cell membrane	Relatively sparse	Larger and plumper than spindle A, more coarse and clumped chromatin	Sharper definition, small, round, deeply stained, eccentric	Less cohesive, ± fascicular arrangement, occasional mitosis
Epithelioid	Larger, polygonal, pleomorphic, distinct cell border	Abundant, eosinophilic	Largest, round, ± multiple, pleomorphic, chromatin margination	Largest, multiple, eosinophilic, central, distinct	Loss of cohesiveness, more mitoses

Source: Collaborative Ocular Melanoma Study Group,[29] by permission of *American Journal of Ophthalmology*.

tial.[21] Marcus et al. counted nucleolar organizing regions and achieved similar results.[22] According to Whelchel et al., the presence of tumor-infiltrating lymphocytes is associated with death from metastasis.[23] On the molecular level, researchers have shown that metastases are more likely to occur from growing tumors,[24,25] so cell-cycle studies are being performed[26] and markers of cell division are being tested. DNA ploidy analysis is another important way to gather information relevant to prognosis.[26–28]

Diagnosis and Workup

Differential Diagnosis

Misdiagnoses of melanoma are uncommon in recent years and are generally less than 2% at most clinical centers in the United States. The diagnostic accuracy of the COMS study was 99.7%.[29] Nevertheless, the differential diagnosis of uveal neoplasms must be considered when evaluating a patient with suspected melanoma.

The differential diagnosis includes retinal detachment, choroidal detachment, metastatic tumor to the choroid, exudative age-related macular degeneration, ectopic disciform degeneration, localized choroidal hemangioma, large choroidal nevus, and congenital hypertrophy of the retinal pigment epithelium (CHRPE). The principal distinguishing features of melanoma are described next.

Clinical Evaluation and Imaging

More than 90% of the time melanoma can be diagnosed by clinical evaluation and imaging. Indirect ophthalmoscopy is the most important and widely used diagnostic technique, allowing a wide field of view and good stereopsis. Oftentimes, skilled observers can make accurate estimates of the tumor size and height by visualization; however, the most reliable measurements are obtained by ultrasound imaging. Examination of the uninvolved eye may reveal lesions there as well. Such findings make the likelihood of a primary choroidal melanoma less likely.

A transilluminatron can be a useful adjunct to indirect ophthalmoscopy. Solid lesions such as melanoma and organized hemorrhage do not transilluminate light, whereas lesions associated with relatively clear fluid such as retinal detachment and choroidal effusion do.

Lenses with mirrors, or goniolenses, are particularly helpful in determining the anterior borders of tumors in the posterior choroid and in visualizing the far periphery of the retina, the ciliary body, and the anterior chamber angle. Melanoma appears on ophthalmoscopy or gonioscopy most often as a fairly well circumscribed, brownish-gray, elevated subretinal mass. It is important to remember, however, that approximately 25% of melanomas are relatively amelanotic. Oftentimes there is associated pathology of the overlying retina, such as a detachment or a retinopathy producing orange lipofuscin exudates.

Choroidal nevi, in contrast to most melanomas, are flat, being rarely greater than 3mm in height and infrequently greater than 10mm in basal diameter. The overlying subretinal fluid, orange pigment, and clinical symptoms associated with melanomas are not normally present with nevi. Metastases to the choroid differ from melanomas in that there are often multiple foci metastases and they tend to be flat with indistinct margins. CHRPE is generally not difficult to distinguish from melanoma because it is flat and darker black in color. The borders of CHRPE are distinct, and nonpigmented spots or lacunae are often seen centrally. Advanced age-related macular degeneration (ARMD) can produce lesions with characteristics similar to melanoma. These lesions tend to be symmetric and occur in the known setting of ARMD. Also, there is a much greater tendency to have associated subretinal hemorrhage with ARMD.

Ultrasound Imaging

Different types of tissue have characteristic reflectivities on ultrasound. The A mode is used to distinguish melanoma from other tumors that can be very similar in ophthalmoscope appearance, such as choroidal hemangioma. The A mode can also be used to measure tumor height. The B mode generates an image of the globe and is therefore helpful in measuring the greatest basal diameter as well as tumor height (Figure 35.5). It can also be used to look for an underlying tumor in the setting of a retinal detachment or cloudy media. Finally, B mode ultrasonography is used to look for evidence of extrascleral extension.

Fluorescein Angiography

Fundus fluorescein angiography has limited usefulness in the diagnosis of uveal melanomas because there is no diagnostic staining pattern for these tumors. Typically there is mottled hyperfluorescence with "hot spots" and a double circulation. A clinical situation in which angiography may be helpful is when attempting to differentiate a choroidal melanoma, which will show mottled fluorescence with late staining, from exudative ARMD with hemorrhage, which would block fluorescence.

Photography

Serial clinical photographs are a standard method for following the growth of a melanoma and are useful for distinguishing it from other suspicious lesions. The photographs allow for observation of the lesion over time and for documenting growth. Fundus photography is also useful for monitoring the tumor during and after therapeutic intervention.

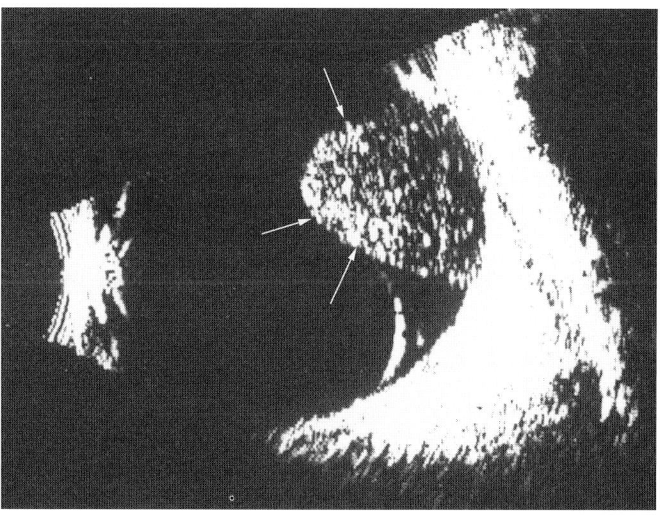

FIGURE 35.5. B-scan ultrasound of a choroidal melanoma (*arrows*).

Chest Radiography/Computed Tomography (CT)/Magnetic Resonance Imaging (MRI)

These modalities are used to rule out potential primary tumors such as carcinomas of the lung and breast if a secondary eye metastasis is a concern. Imaging studies, particularly of the liver, help to determine whether distant metastases are present in a patient with known uveal melanoma. When there is clinical suspicion of extrascleral extension, MRI imaging of the orbits may also be of benefit; this is particularly true as current imaging sequences allow a detailed view of anatomy.

Blood Testing

Liver enzymes are monitored to help detect hepatic metastases. Immunologic testing is not yet reliable. Folberg showed that 78% of patients with melanoma tested positive for tumor-associated antibodies (TAA), but 24% of controls tested positive as well.

Treatment and Prognosis

The management of uveal melanoma has long been the subject of considerable controversy, and enucleation of any tumor was the accepted therapy in all cases for many years. This choice was the result of two factors: (1) the data regarding the natural history of these tumors were (and remain) limited; and (2) there was a lack of an organized, reliable clinical trial. The aforementioned COMS trial is the largest of its type and has set the treatment standards of today.

There are certain variables a clinician must consider before generating a treatment protocol: these are (1) size, location, and extent of tumor; (2) visual status of the affected and fellow eye; and (3) age and general health of the patient. The ultimate goal should be to destroy or inactivate the neoplasm, to maintain useful vision in the involved eye, to employ a treatment with as few side effects as possible, and, most importantly, to provide the patient with the best prognosis and quality of life. The different modalities are discussed in the following section with the general indications for each.

Observation

Serial observation is acceptable if the tumor is small and dormant, if the patient is seriously ill or elderly, or if the tumor is in the patient's only useful eye and is growing slowly. Appropriate observations consist of ophthalmoscopic examination with ultrasound measurements with or without photographic documentation every 3 months.

The COMS study found growth in 21% of small tumors at 3 years and 31% at 5 years. Because of the positive correlation between tumor size and occurrence of metastases, the risk factors for growth were identified by several different researchers, and these were formalized into an algorithm by Shields and colleagues. The five risk factors predictive of growth are tumors with thicknesses greater than 2 mm, posterior tumor margin touching the optic disc, visual symptoms, orange pigment, and subretinal fluid. Shields and colleagues, in the same paper, suggest "timely treatment" of some small melanomas that show substantial risk of growth.[30]

Photocoagulation

Photocoagulation has been employed in the treatment of small melanomas. Its effectiveness has been debated. It uses laser energy to destroy the lesion. The criteria for selecting patients with melanoma for photocoagulation were suggested by Meyer-Schwickerath and Vogel[31,32] and were adapted by Shields:[33]

1. The diagnosis of melanoma and evidence of growth should be documented thoroughly.
2. The tumor should not be greater than 5 diopters in elevation and 6 disc diameters in greatest diameter.
3. It must be possible to completely surround the tumor without damage to the fovea or optic disc.
4. There must be sufficient mydriasis and clear ocular media for the procedure.
5. The tumor surface should not have large retinal vessels.

In a 54-patient series by Vogel at 20 years, 63% of patients treated with photocoagulation were alive, although not all these patients were considered cured by photocoagulation.[32,33]

Transpupillary thermotherapy (TTT) is a related technique and consists of delivering heat to the tumor via infrared light; this is intended to induce necrosis of the tumor tissues. Shields et al. had a 14-month follow-up of 100 patients, and in 94% there was local tumor control. There was, however, worsening of visual acuity in 42%.[34] A longer follow-up is necessary to properly assess this modality.

Episcleral Radioactive Plaque

This highly specialized multidisciplinary approach is much more widely available than charged-particle therapy (discussed later). Based on preoperative tumor measurements, tumor shape, and tumor location, a concave plaque housing several small radioactive beads is fashioned to fit over the tumor while avoiding treatment of uninvolved areas. Although iodine-125 is the most commonly used isotope, ruthenium-106 is used frequently in Europe, and other isotopes such as palladium-103 are being tried.[35,36]

Under general or retrobulbar anesthesia, this plaque is sutured onto the sclera overlying the tumor. The tumor location and plaque placement are confirmed by transillumination, ophthalmoscopic observation, and intraoperative ultrasonography. This plaque remains in place 2 to 5 days and is then removed.

The COMS study specifically evaluated iodine-125 plaque therapy versus enucleation for 1,317 medium-sized melanomas. The outcome was no difference between the two modalities in survival at 5 and 12 years.[37] Of the patients who received plaque therapy, 50% lost substantial vision in 3 years.

Charged-Particle Beam Therapy

Cyclotrons and synchrotrons produce hydrogen or helium ion beams that have been successfully used to treat ocular melanomas. Only a handful of centers have these capabilities, and this is a comparatively costly form of treatment.[38] Wilson and Hungerford found no better local tumor control with proton beam as compared to iodine-125 brachytherapy. Tumor recurrences at 5 years were 5% and 4%, respectively.[39] In addition, although the procedure involves sophisticated planning techniques and precise tumor mapping, damage to the adjacent retina and optic nerve are still problematic. Finger et al. reported that 32% of patients maintained visual acuity better than 20/100.[36]

Enucleation

Enucleation or resection of the globe and proximal optic nerve continues to be recommended in selected cases. Current indications include large ciliary body or choroidal melanomas, melanoma associated with significant visual loss or secondary glaucoma, and any melanoma invading the optic nerve.[40]

In the COMS medium-size tumor trial,[37] patients with medium-size tumors were given the option of enucleation. It was found in 1,317 patients randomized to enucleation or iodine-125 brachytherapy that neither mortality rates at 12 years nor quality of life differed between the two groups.[41,42]

For the 1,003 large-melanoma patients enrolled in the COMS, there was another query, whether preenucleation radiation of 2,000 cGy was associated with a more favorable outcome. It was determined that such treatment neither favorably nor unfavorably influenced outcomes in terms of 5-year survival or local orbital complications. Thus, enucleation should not normally be preceded by radiation.[43,44]

Local Surgical Excision

Sclerouvectomy, developed by Peyman et al.,[45] is a surgical excision of the melanoma in which the tumor is approached from the scleral surface. Normally this surgery follows multiple sessions of photocoagulation therapy. This treatment has limited usefulness due to the concern of incomplete resection. Damato and Foulds[46] found that residual tumor was seen in a significant number of cases. This rate appears to be reduced by the use of adjunctive brachytherapy.

Still in an experimental stage is a procedure called transvitreal endoresection. In this technique, the tumor is approached from the retina. Obviously, this technique carries risk of tumor dissemination and incomplete resection.[3]

Primary Ocular Tumors: Retinoblastoma

Epidemiology

Retinoblastoma is the most common primary malignant intraocular tumor of infancy and early childhood. It is the third most common intraocular malignancy, second to choroidal melanoma and metastases. Retinoblastoma has an incidence of from 1 in 14,000 to 1 in 20,000 live births, therefore affecting approximately 350 children each year in the United States. It is responsible for approximately 1% of all cancer deaths under the age of 15.[47,48] Its distribution is worldwide; however, there is a higher incidence in Haiti, Jamaica, Nigeria, South Africa, Africa, Asia, and parts of Latin America.[49] There is no gender predilection. Retinoblastoma is one of the most common congenital tumors, and approximately 90% present before age 3. Retinoblastoma affects each eye equally. Sixty percent to 70% of cases are unilateral, with mean age at diagnosis being 24 months. Thirty percent to 40% are bilateral, with mean age at diagnosis of 14 months. For small tumors, there are some potentially vision-sparing treatments, including radiation therapy, photocoagulation, and cryotherapy. With larger tumors, treatment includes chemoreduction and/or enucleation. It was formerly considered fatal when it spread beyond the eye and optic nerve. However, with recent advances in combined chemotherapy, there are reports of cure even with distant spread.[50]

Presenting Symptoms

Presenting signs include leukocoria (56.2%); strabismus (23.6%); poor vision (7.7%); and family history of retinoblastoma (6.8%). Leukocoria has been found to correlate to advanced disease, and strabismus is associated with macular disease[51] (Figure 35.6). Less frequently, children may have a wide variety of presentations: pain, hypopyon, hyphema, heterochromia, spontaneous globe perforation, proptosis, cataract, glaucoma, nystagmus, tearing, or anisocoria.

Basic Science: Genetics

Retinoblastoma arises from defects in the retinoblastoma gene at the Rb 1 locus located at the q14 band of chromosome 13.[52] The gene is large, containing 180 kb DNA. The initial mutation of the gene inactivates one copy of the gene. This initial mutation can be of any size, even as small as a point mutation. It should be noted that all retinoblastoma tumors have other mutational events, and additional unknown stochastic events may be required for full malignant transformation. Both hereditary and sporadic forms of retinoblastoma arise as a consequence of mutations in both alleles at the Rb1 locus. In other words, to give rise to retinoblastoma, a second mutation is required in the second, homologous copy of the Rb gene so that no functional gene product is produced.[53,54] The loss of the second copy of the gene is always somatic. There is a high rate of spontaneous mutation at this locus, and 94% of all cases are considered sporadic. Only 6% have a positive family history, but 30% to 40% of cases are hereditary. The differences between hereditary and nonhereditary retinoblastoma are of great importance for prognosis and genetic counseling for family members because there is an increased risk of second malignancies with the hereditary form.

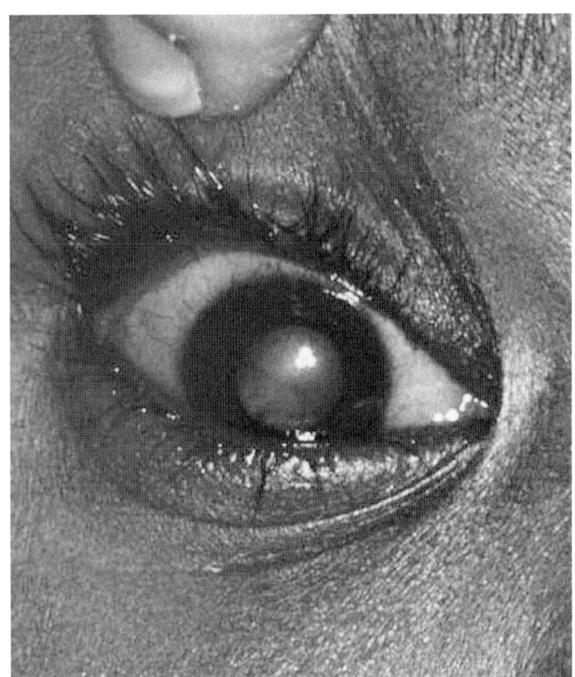

FIGURE 35.6. Leukocoria in the right eye of patient with retinoblastoma.

If the initial mutation occurs in a germ-line cell, the patient has *hereditary retinoblastoma.* Each tumor arises from a distinct retinal cell that independently loses the second copy of the retinoblastoma gene through a deletion or mutation. In this instance, the mutation is transmitted as a dominant trait with virtually complete penetrance; carriers are at high risk (greater than 90%) of developing retinoblastoma in childhood and other primary cancers such as osteosarcoma later in life.[55,56] The cumulative risk of developing a second primary malignancy is 1% per year; this risk is increased in patients treated with radiation.[55] In addition, other family members may be at high risk. Forty percent of retinoblastoma cases are hereditary; the majority of patients with hereditary retinoblastoma have bilateral disease.[56] Almost every case with multifocal disease is hereditary, and approximately 10% to 20% of unilateral cases are hereditary. Most patients have a new germ-line mutation and therefore have no previous family history of retinoblastoma. These patients may also have multifocal, unilateral, or unifocal retinoblastoma associated with additional independently arising tumors, *trilateral retinoblastoma,* in the central nervous system (pineal gland or in the supersellar/parasellar region). There are still a small number of carriers that remain unaffected. Carriers may be unaffected for a variety of reasons, including incomplete penetrance, balanced carriers, and 13q14 trisomics.

If the mutation occurs in a somatic cell, the patient has *nonhereditary retinoblastoma,* and relatives are not at an increased risk for developing retinoblastoma. Sixty percent of retinoblastoma cases are nonhereditary. Almost all cases of nonhereditary retinoblastoma have a single primary tumor in only one eye. These patients are not at increased risk of developing other cancers later in life.

Pathology

Location and Growth Pattern

The origin of retinoblastoma has been widely debated. The most widely accepted view is that retinoblastoma arises from a multipotential precursor cell that may develop into nearly any type of inner or outer retinal cell.[47] As a result, there is heterogeneity of the histopathologic, ultrastructural, and immunohistochemical features.

Spread of the tumor into the vitreous (vitreous "seeds") can give rise to viable tumor implants throughout the eye. Tumor cells may disseminate through the choroidal vasculature, spread extraocularly through the substance of the optic nerve, and grow into the orbit in advanced cases. The tumor may also extend into the subarachnoid space and gain access to the cerebrospinal fluid. Following overt extraocular extension, there are frequently palpable preauricular and cervical lymph nodes. In advanced cases, there may be distant metastatic spread to the central nervous system, skull and distal bones, and lymph nodes.[48]

There are two main patterns of growth of retinoblastoma tumors: endophytic and exophytic. Endophytic retinoblastomas tend to originate on the inner surface of the retina (and accordingly can be viewed directly with ophthalmoscopy) and grow toward the vitreous (Figure 35.7). Exophytic retinoblastomas originate from the outer retinal surface and grow toward the choroid, producing elevation of the retina and possibly retinal detachment (Figure 35.8). Most commonly, the two types of growth patterns coexist in the same eye. Characteristically, retinoblastoma outgrows its blood supply, leading to ischemic coagulative necrosis and marked apoptosis.

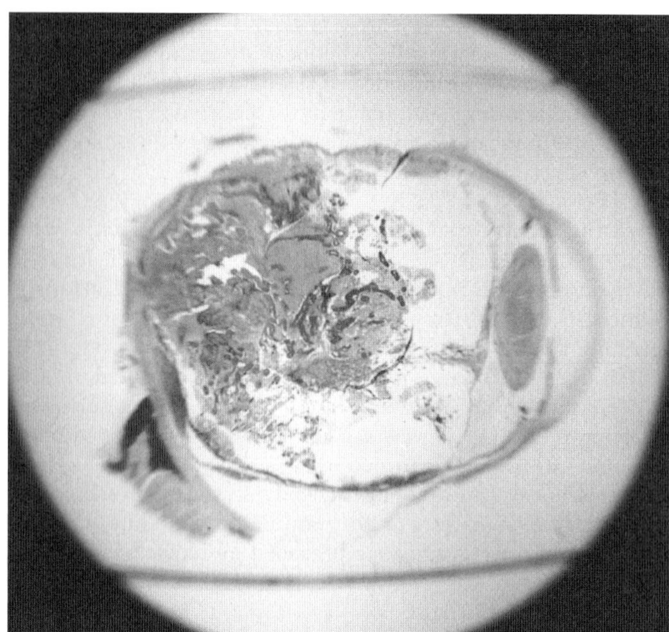

FIGURE 35.7. Endophytic retinoblastoma replacing retina with invasion of vitreous. 1×.

Histologic Features

Retinoblastomas are typically nodular masses with frequent satellite seedings. On macroscopic view, smaller tumors appear as translucent, gray to white intraretinal tumors that are fed and drained by dilated tortuous retinal vessels. More-advanced tumors appear chalky white and can fill a large portion of the eye (Figure 35.9). On light microscopic examination, there may be areas of undifferentiated tumor together with tumor containing differentiated structures. Undifferentiated areas are composed of cells resembling embryonic retinoblasts, small round cells with large hyperchromatic

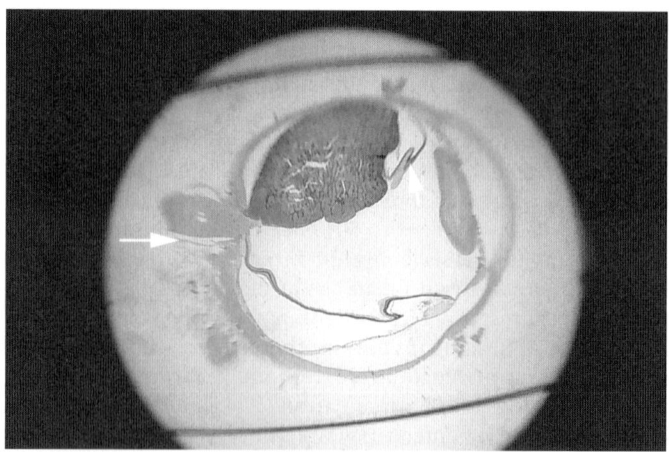

FIGURE 35.8. Exophytic retinoblastoma limited to the subretinal space. Retina marked with *arrow.* 1×.

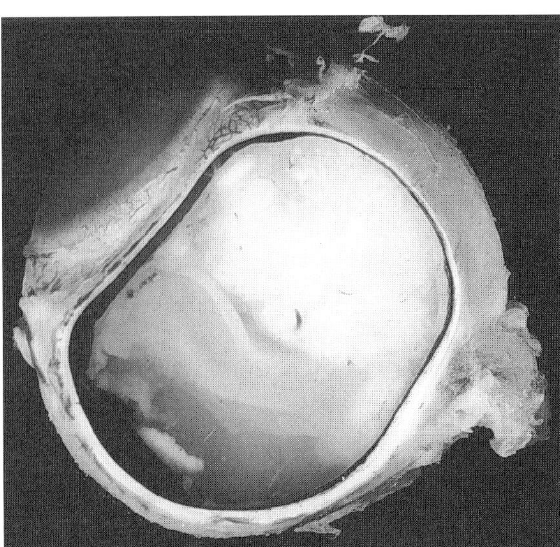

FIGURE 35.9. Retinoblastoma filling almost the entire vitreous cavity. Extensive calcification contributes to the chalky-white appearance.

nuclei and scant cytoplasm. Differentiated structures include Flexner–Wintersteiner rosettes, Homer–Wright rosettes, and fleurettes (Figure 35.10).

Flexner–Wintersteiner rosettes are the most common distinguishing feature and are specific for retinoblastoma. They consist of clusters of cuboidal or short columnar cells with peripherally displaced nuclei surrounding a central lumen. The lumen has a limiting membrane, resembling the external limiting membrane of the retina, through which photoreceptor-like elements protrude; some photoreceptor elements taper into fine filaments.

Less common are Homer–Wright rosettes, which have radially arranged cells around the central tangle of fibrils. These are also seen in neuroblastoma and medulloblastoma. The fleurette is present in a small percentage of tumors. It represents the tumor cells' attempt at photoreceptor differentiation.

Regression

Retinoblastoma is unusual in that it may undergo spontaneous necrosis or regression; this has been estimated to occur in about 1 of 100 tumors. The mechanism is unknown. Eyes with tumors that undergo spontaneous necrosis may develop phthisis marked by calcification and severe inflammation. Histologically, the eyes are filled with islands of calcified cells embedded in a mass of fibroconnective tissue. There also may be proliferation of retinal pigment epithelium.

Staging and Prognostic Indicators

The Reese–Ellsworth classification system[47] (Table 35.3) is the most frequently employed method of staging retinoblastoma. It classifies the tumors into five groups based on tumor size and location and predicts the likelihood of local tumor control and preservation of vision. In general, group I is considered very favorable whereas group V is considered very unfavorable. There are new international classification criteria for intraocular retinoblastoma (Table 35.4).

The more numerous and highly differentiated the rosettes, the better the prognosis. Smaller tumors have a better prognosis, and they are more likely to have a greater concentration of well-formed rosettes than are larger, more-advanced tumors. Larger tumors, especially those with extraocular extension, tend to have smaller, less-differentiated rosettes. The most important prognostic indicator is optic nerve invasion.[47,49]

Relation to Retinocytoma

Retinocytoma, also called retinoma, is clinically indistinguishable from retinoblastoma; however, retinoblastoma is histologically malignant whereas retinocytoma is histologically benign. Retinoblastoma cells are histologically different from retinocytoma cells. They are larger, with scanty cytoplasm and more hyperchromatic nuclei with frequent mitotic figures and necrosis with calcification. Retinocytoma cells, in contrast, are smaller, with abundant cytoplasm and intercellular matrix and more evenly displaced nuclear chromatin with no evidence of mitotic figures, and although there may be some calcification, there is no necrosis in retinoma. Retinocytomas have numerous fleurettes admixed with individual cells that demonstrate varying degrees of photoreceptor differentiation. Histologically, the fleurette is composed

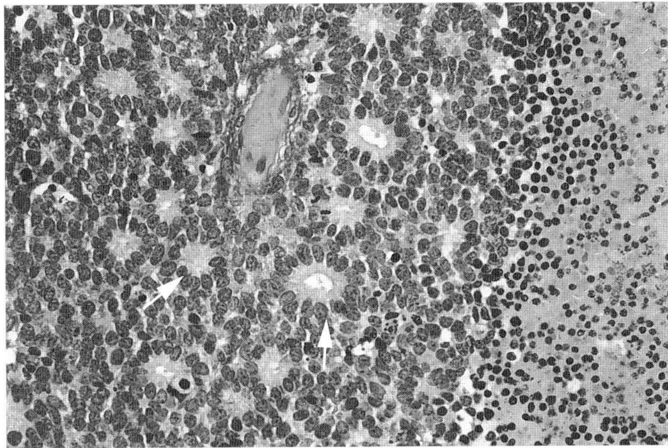

FIGURE 35.10. Retinoblastoma histology with Flexner–Winterstein rosettes (*arrows*). 20×.

TABLE 35.3. The Reese–Ellsworth system of predicting success by external-beam radiation therapy.

Group	*Criteria*
I	a. Solitary tumor less than 4 dd, at or behind the equator b. Multiple tumors, none larger than 4 dd, all at or behind equator
II	a. Solitary tumor 4–10 dd, at or behind the equator b. Multiple tumors, 4–10 dd, at or behind the equator
III	a. Any lesion anterior to the equator b. Solitary tumor larger than 10 dd, at or behind the equator
IV	a. Multiple tumors, some larger than 10 dd b. Any lesion extending anterior to the ora serrata
V	a. Massive tumors involving more than half the retina b. Vitreous seeding

dd, disc diameter (1 dd ≅ 1.5 mm).

Source: Sahel,[47] by permission of W.B. Saunders.

TABLE 35.4. International classification of intraocular retinoblastoma.

Group	Criteria
A	Small intraretinal tumors away from foveola and disc • All tumors are 3 mm or smaller in greatest dimension, confined to the retina • All tumors are located farther than 3 mm from the foveola and 1.5 mm from the optic disc
B	All remaining discrete tumors confined to the retina • All tumors confined to the retina not in group A • Tumor-associated subretinal fluid less than 3 mm from the tumor with no subretinal seeding
C	Discrete local disease with minimal subretinal or vitreous seeding • Tumor(s) are discrete • Subretinal fluid, present or past, without seeding, involving up to one-fourth of retina • Local subretinal seeding, less than 3 mm (2 dd) from the tumor • Local fine vitreous seeding close to discrete tumor
D	Diffuse disease with significant vitreous or subretinal seeding • Tumor(s) may be massive or diffuse. • Subretinal fluid, present or past, without seeding, involving up to total retinal detachment • Diffuse subretinal seeding; may include subretinal plaques or tumor nodules • Diffuse or massive vitreous disease may include "greasy" seeds or avascular tumor masses
E	Presence of any one or more of these poor prognosis features • Tumor touching the lens • Neovascular glaucoma • Tumor anterior to anterior vitreous face involving ciliary body or anterior segment • Diffuse, infiltrating retinoblastoma • Opaque media from hemorrhage • Tumor necrosis with aseptic orbital cellulitis • Phthisis bulbi

Source: http://eyecancer.com/Organizations/RBinternational.html, by permission.

of cells with prominent eosinophilic cellular processes that are filled with mitochondria.

Clinical characteristics of retinocytomas include a functional eye with clear media and no evidence of retinal detachment. There is proliferation and migration of retinal pigment epithelial cells. Retinocytomas have a cottage-cheese appearance: opaque with white calcified flecks. They are also comparatively small, homogeneous, translucent, gray, slightly elevated placoid masses that have functional retinal blood vessels looping into the mass. Although histologically benign, retinocytomas can be locally invasive. Typically, retinocytomas are found admixed with retinoblastomas, although there may be cases of pure retinocytoma. In contrast to retinoblastomas, retinocytomas are radioresistant.

Diagnostic Workup

The differential diagnosis of retinoblastoma is essentially the differential diagnosis of leukocoria and includes persistent hyperplastic primary vitreous, cataract, retinopathy or prematurity, toxocariasis, colobomas of choroid and disc, uveitis, Coats' disease, vitreous hemorrhage, retinal dysplasia, retinal detachment, Norrie's disease, and other tumors.[59]

A patient who has any of the aforementioned presenting signs needs prompt workup for possible retinoblastoma. It is extremely important for any child with strabismus to have a dilated fundoscopic examination. It is important to get a careful family history, specifically asking about family history of retinoblastoma, eye tumors, childhood cancer, or history of enucleations. Further workup entails documenting the existence of retinoblastoma and determining if there is any evidence of metastasis. A complete eye examination, including dilated fundus examination bilaterally, is performed. Frequently an examination under anesthesia needs to be performed if the child is over 2 months of age. Fundus photographs and detailed retinal drawings should be made to help follow the effects of treatment. Ultrasonography may help distinguish retinoblastomas from other noncancerous tumors.[58,59] Orbital CT and ultrasound may reveal characteristic calcific densities within the tumor (Figure 35.11).

Several methods are employed to determine if metastases are present. Computed tomography (CT) and magnetic resonance imaging (MRI) are used to evaluate orbital and central nervous systems (CNS) anatomy for extraocular disease. Head CT may reveal an early pinealoblastoma,[60] and this may help to provide more treatment options. CT generally does not reveal optic nerve spread because this is usually infiltrative and does not enlarge the nerve. Consultation with a pediatric

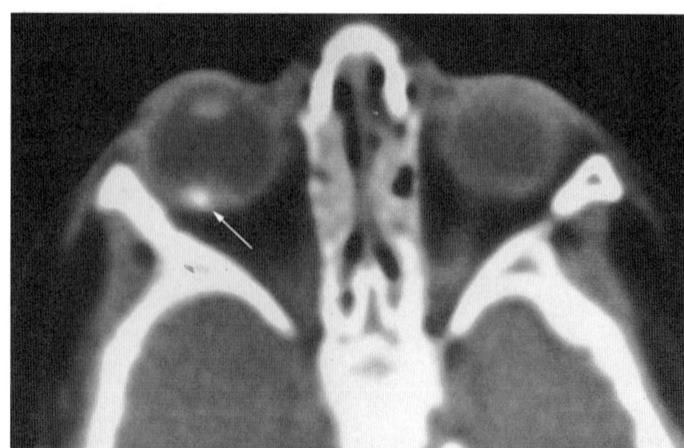

FIGURE 35.11. Calcification in retinoblastoma (*arrow*) seen on computerized tomography scan.

oncologist affords bone marrow aspiration and biopsy along with lumbar puncture for the evaluation of tumor cells. With smaller tumors, the need for the routine use of these methods has been questioned.[61] Bone marrow biopsy and lumbar puncture are often reserved for patients with neurologic abnormalities or evidence of extraocular extension. Given the possible hereditary component, parents and siblings should obtain DNA analysis to assist in genetic counseling. It is recommended that children at risk for familial hereditary retinoblastoma be screened until age 4 years to detect early disease.[62]

Therapy, Prognosis, and Complications

The goal of treatment is complete control of the tumor while preserving useful vision. Although enucleation was at one time extensively employed, recent advances in other treatment options yielding globe salvage rates of 66% to 78% have been reported.[63–65] Currently, the mainstays of treatment are enucleation, laser therapy, cryogenics, radiation therapy, and chemotherapy. The visual prognosis is excellent in most cases. A study by Abramson and associates in children with bilateral retinoblastoma revealed visual acuity of 20/20 to 20/40 in 58%, visual acuity of 20/50 to 20/400 in 31%, and visual acuity worse than 20/400 in only 9%.[66] Five-year survival is greater than 90% after successful treatment of ocular disease when there is no evidence of metastasis.[67] If there is metastatic disease, the prognosis is quite poor.[68]

Enucleation

Enucleation is the treatment of choice only when the eye cannot be salvaged by other means of treatment. It is considered appropriate in eyes with large tumors (involving more than 50% of the globe); where there is no expectation for useful vision; and where long-standing retinal detachment, neovascular glaucoma, pars plana tumor seeding, anterior chamber or choroidal involvement, and optic nerve or orbital tumor extension exist.[69,70] Care must be taken during the procedure to avoid penetrating the globe and to resect the greatest amount of optic nerve possible (usually more than 10mm).

Chemoreduction with Local Tumor Ablation

Local/systemic chemotherapy is used to reduce tumor volume to allow for more focused (and less-damaging) consolidative ablative therapies such as laser, cryotherapy, or radiotherapy in an effort to avoid enucleation and external-beam radiation therapy (EBRT). The appropriate regimen is debated; however, the current standard includes carboplatin, either etopside or teniposide, and vincristine with or without cyclosporine. Chemoreduction has improved the ocular salvage rate. At 5-year follow-up, the globe salvage rate is 85% for Reese–Ellsworth groups I through IV and 47% for group V.[71] More recent studies prove chemoreduction to be successful in treatment and avoidance of enucleation or EBRT without significant systemic toxicity in Reese–Ellsworth eye groups I, II, and III.[72] More-effective methods of treatment are required for groups IV and V. Chemotherapy produces a mean decrease in tumor base by 35% and a nearly 50% decrease in thickness.[73] Although chemotherapy is effective at reducing tumor volume, it is not curative. Focal therapy is necessary for complete eradication.[70] It is extremely important to note that all these chemicals are mutagenic and may contribute to the development of second tumors in patients with hereditary retinoblastoma.

Laser Photocoagulative Ablation

Laser therapy is used for small, posteriorly located tumors that are less than 4.5mm in basal diameter and less than 2.5mm in thickness. The current method employs direct confluent treatment with argon or xenon lasers over the entire tumor to coagulate the entire blood supply. There is a 70% tumor control rate and a 30% recurrence rate.[69] Complications include retinal vascular occlusions, retinal traction, retinal hole formation, and preretinal fibrosis.

Cryotherapy

Similar to laser therapy, cryotherapy is used to treat small tumors that are less than 3.5mm in basal diameter and less than 2.0mm in thickness.[69] It uses a triple freeze-thaw technique under direct visualization. Most commonly, it is administered before chemotherapy to enhance the likelihood of cure. This procedure may be associated with rhegmatogenous retinal detachment.[70]

Thermotherapy and Chemothermotherapy

The use of heat alone for treatment of retinoblastoma is controversial. Heat has been found to have a synergistic effect with chemotherapy and radiation therapy.[69] It is useful for tumors in the posterior pole, within 6mm of the fovea or optic disc, that are 6mm or less in basal diameter and 3mm or less in thickness.[69] Complete tumor regression is found in 86%; predictors of local tumor recurrence were male sex and previous use of chemoreduction (and therefore larger tumor).[74] Complications include focal iris atrophy, peripheral focal lens opacity, retinal traction, retinal vascular occlusion, and transient localized serous retinal detachment.[74]

Brachytherapy (Plaque Radiotherapy)

Brachytherapy is typically used for small-to-medium-sized tumors (less than 16mm basal diameter and less than 8mm in thickness) and also as a salvage therapy when the other globe-conserving strategies have failed. The use of intraoperative ultrasound can enhance local tumor control. Brachytherapy involves the placement of a radioactive implant over the base of the tumor to irradiate transclerally. The average length of treatment is 2 to 4 days. Overall, there is approximately 90% tumor control.[75] Given that the plaque therapy limits the radiation dose to periocular structures, the incidence of secondary radiation-induced malignancies may be lower than with EBRT. However, there is a higher incidence of radiation optic neuropathy and retinopathy. Visual outcome varies with tumor size and location, but it is considered good in 62% (visual acuity of 20/20 to 20/30 in more than half of the cases).[76]

External-Beam Radiation Therapy

Retinoblastoma tumors are responsive to radiation. The current standard of treatment for groups I, II, and III is chemotherapy plus local therapy as described previously. Groups IV and V require EBRT or enucleation. Current techniques involve megavoltage radiation treatments, often lens sparing, with 4,000 to 4,500cGy over 4 to 6 weeks. The ocular salvage rate depends on the stage of the disease. The

Reese–Ellsworth criteria are employed to help determine the success of therapy based on the stage of the tumor (see Table 35.3). Group I has a very favorable prognosis of eye preservation when treated with external beam radiation, whereas group V has a very unfavorable prognosis. Nearly all children in groups I through IV will be cured of retinoblastoma using this technique; in group V, the cure rate is 85% to 90%.[77] Recurrence continues to be problematic; retinoblastoma typically recurs within the first 1 to 2 years after treatment. The potential side effects of radiation that limit its use are increased risk of secondary or independent primary malignancies in a population with germ-line alterations of a tumor suppressor gene in addition to radiation-induced cataracts, optic neuropathy, and vasculopathy or hypoplasia of bone and soft tissues. Overall, 58% of patients with hereditary disease receiving EBRT developed second malignancies compared to only 27% in the group not treated with radiation.[55] There is controversy over the role of prophylactic radiation in children with heritable retinoblastoma.[69]

Chemotherapy

The role of systemic chemotherapy as monotherapy is controversial. Although systemic chemotherapy has not been successful in treating intraocular retinoblastoma, there has been some success in treating metastatic disease.[78–80] Systemic chemotherapy may be considered when there is metastatic disease or extension into the optic nerve, choroid, or orbit. Concern exists over the leukemogenic and mutagenic effects of chemotherapy.

Metastatic Tumors of the Eye

Metastatic cancers of the eye and adnexa are now being recognized with much greater frequency as a result of earlier detection of malignancies and increasing patient survival. In fact, metastatic tumors are the most common malignancies to involve the eye and orbit.[81–84]

It is therefore imperative that oncologists keep this diagnosis in mind when considering eye symptoms that may be experienced by their patients. Metastatic hematopoietic tumors that also commonly affect the eye are discussed in a subsequent chapter.

Epidemiology

In patients with known malignancy, 4.7% to 12% have been shown at autopsy to have involvement of the eye or orbit.[83,85] Shields et al., in a study of 520 eyes, found that there is a gender difference in the incidence of ocular metastases. Women are affected two times as often as men.[86] After the identification of a metastatic tumor in the uvea or orbit, the prognosis for survival is uniformly bad, and few patients survive more than 1 year.[81]

Location

The most frequent site of metastases in the eye, orbit, and adnexa is the uveal tract, specifically the choroid, with the orbit being the second most frequent site. In children this is reversed, with the orbit the most common site. Freedman and Folk[87] reviewed 112 patients presenting with ocular and orbital metastases who were evaluated clinically with modern methods and found that 56 had choroidal involvement, 49 had orbital involvement, and 5 had involvement of both sites. The remaining 2 patients had lesions involving the optic nerve and retina.

Tumor Type

In a large study performed by the Shields and their associates, the site or origin of globe metastases was evaluated. Breast (47%) and lung (21%) represented more than two-thirds of the primary tumor sites. There was a gender difference in tumor type. The three most common primary tumors in women were breast (68%), lung (12%), and gastrointestinal tract (2%). In men, 40% of primary sites were lung, followed by (and to a much lesser extent) gastrointestinal tract and kidney. In breast carcinoma metastases to the eye, 90% of the patients had a known history of breast cancer.[86] The figure was less than this for lung and renal tumors.

Presenting Symptoms

Choroidal Metastasis

According to Stephens and Shields, choroidal metastases most often present with blurry vision (80%); pain (14%); photopsias or flashes of light (13%); red eye (6%); floaters (6%); and visual field defects (3%).[84] Most often the tumors are flat, creamy, yellow choroidal lesions with overlying retinal pigment epithelial changes, specifically with breast metastases having a peau d'orange pattern of pigmentary changes.[86,88,89] Oftentimes a small lesion can be associated with a relatively large serous retinal detachment. Multiple foci in one eye occur in approximately 20% of patients, and 20% to 40% of cases are bilateral.[90] Metastatic carcinomas grow rapidly and spread quickly. Often tumors develop in the second eye within 1 month after the diagnosis of a clinically unilateral tumor.[91]

Orbital Metastasis

Orbital metastases may present with unilateral or bilateral symptoms of pain, periocular redness, double vision, or eyelid malposition. In addition, the patient or the patient's family might note a progressive bulging or sinking in of the eye. Examination of patients with orbital metastases may reveal periorbital inflammation, restricted extraocular movements, ptosis, lid retraction, exophthalmos, or enophthalmos.

Diagnosis and Workup

Workup of patients with suspected ocular or orbital metastases includes a detailed clinical history, review of systems, and physical examination. In addition, to further support the diagnosis of ocular metastases, fluoroscein angiography can be employed. The typical staining pattern for choroidal metastases includes early hypofluorescence, followed by mottled fluorescence with pinpoint foci, and increasing hyperfluorescence late in the study.[88] Other useful imaging methods are ultrasonography (A scan and B scan) and MRI to look for transscleral extension or optic nerve involvement. Transocular fine-needle aspiration and wedge biopsy may be performed when noninvasive methods have failed to establish the diagnosis.

In a patient with suspected orbital metastasis, imaging studies and history alone can sometimes establish the diagnosis. For example, it may be unnecessary to perform a biopsy in a patient with known metastatic breast cancer who develops enophthalmos and has findings consistent with metastatic orbital carcinoma on MRI. In many situations, however, an orbitotomy with biopsy may be necessary to determine the site of the primary or determine the presence or absence of receptor sites or other features pertinent to decisions regarding therapy.

Pathology

The pathologic descriptions of primary tumors are provided elsewhere in this text. In general, metastatic lesions usually appear more anaplastic than the primary tumor. Oftentimes the tumor is so anaplastic that special immunohistochemical staining and/or electron microscopy is required to reach a diagnosis when the primary is undetected.

Treatment

A multidisciplinary team approach is required in the treatment of metastases to the eye. The ophthalmologist or oculoplastic surgeon is involved in identifying the tumor by examination or biopsy, defining the extent of the tumor, and monitoring its activity. In addition, the ophthalmologist can monitor changes in visual acuity, visual field, or orbital symptoms. Observation is acceptable for small, peripheral ocular lesions or lesions in terminally ill patients.[88] External-beam radiation is the most common method of treating uveal and orbital metastases.[92,93] Many times this is combined with systemic chemotherapy, although both can be used alone as well. Other modes of treatment for choroidal metastases are brachytherapy, laser photocoagulation, local excision, and enucleation.

Visual acuity may remain quite good. Even in cases of vision loss, most patients show complete (26% to 50%) or partial (33% to 67%) return of their visual signs and symptoms.[94] Unfortunately, the prognosis for survival is very poor. The mean survival period is approximately 8 months.[84,87,90–92] This period is increasing for breast cancer and now is reported to be 31 months.[90]

The Phakomatoses

The term *phakomatosis* was originally described by Brouwer in 1917 and van der Hoeve in 1923 to classify hereditary diseases with tumorous growths arising in disparate organ systems, some of which have the potential for malignant transformation. The tumorous growths are classified as *hamartomas*, an abnormal proliferation of tissue normally present in the involved site, and *choristomas*, an abnormal proliferation of tissue not normally present at the involved site. The original three disorders characterized as phakomatoses include von Recklinghausen's neurofibromatosis; tuberous sclerosis (Bourneville's syndrome); and von Hippel–Lindau disease (cerebellar-retinal angiomatosis). All the original phakomatoses are inherited in an autosomal dominant fashion and have been linked to mutations in recessive tumor suppressor genes. Brouwer and Van der Hoeve added a fourth disorder, Sturge–Weber syndrome, to the phakomatoses in 1937. Sturge–Weber syndrome, unlike the primary phakomatoses, has no established pattern of inheritance and can occur sporadically. There are several other disorders that have occasionally been included in the classification of phakomatoses: Wyburn–Mason syndrome; ataxia telangiectasia (Louis–Bar syndrome); linear nevus sebaceous syndrome; Klippel–Trenaunay–Weber syndrome; and encephalooculoangiomatosis.[95]

Neurofibromatosis 1

Neurofibromatosis type 1 (NF-1), also known as von Recklinghausen disease or peripheral neurofibromatosis, is an inherited disorder of the neuroectoderm resulting in hamartomas of the skin, eyes, central nervous system, and viscera. These hamartomas increase in both size and number throughout life. Inheritance is autosomal dominant, with nearly 100% penetrance, with highly variable expressivity even among affected siblings.[96,97] NF-1 occurs in approximately 1 in 3,000 to 5,000 of the population with no predilection for race or sex. The NF-1 gene has been mapped to the long arm of chromosome 17 (17q11.2).[98] The gene is large (more than 300 kilobases, kb) and therefore has a high rate of mutation, approximately 1 in 10,000 live births.[96,97] Approximately 30% to 50% of cases arise from new mutations, typically paternal in origin.[99]

The diagnosis of NF-1 is made when two or more of the following seven criteria established by the NIH are met:[100]

1. Six or more café-au-lait spots greater than 5 mm in diameter in prepubescents or greater than 15 mm in diameter in postpubescents
2. Two or more neurofibromas of any type or one plexiform neurofibroma
3. Freckling of axillary, inguinal, or other intertriginous areas
4. Optic nerve glioma
5. Two or more Lisch nodules of the iris
6. A distinctive osseous lesion, such as sphenoid bone dysplasia or thinning of the long-bone cortex, with or without pseudarthrosis
7. A first-degree relative with NF-1 according to the preceding criteria

There are many abnormalities associated with NF-1: café-au-lait spots; axillary/inguinal freckling; pigmented iris nodules (Lisch nodules) (Figure 35.12); fibroma molluscum (nodular cutaneous/subcutaneous neurofibromas); plexiform neurofibromas of eyelid and orbit resulting in a characteristic S-shaped lid fissure; retinal and optic nerve gliomas; congenital glaucoma; and dysplasia of orbital bones resulting in pulsating exophthalmos. Mild mental retardation is present in approximately 45%.[101] Café-au-lait spots, axillary freckling, and Lisch nodules are all melanocytic in origin, whereas neurofibromas are derived from Schwann cells.[97] There are also many hamartomas present in the central and peripheral nervous system and the gastrointestinal (GI) tract.[101] It is important to note that malignant transformation is possible. There is a 3% to 15% lifetime risk of malignancy; these are most commonly neurofibrosarcoma and optic nerve gliomas.[102,103]

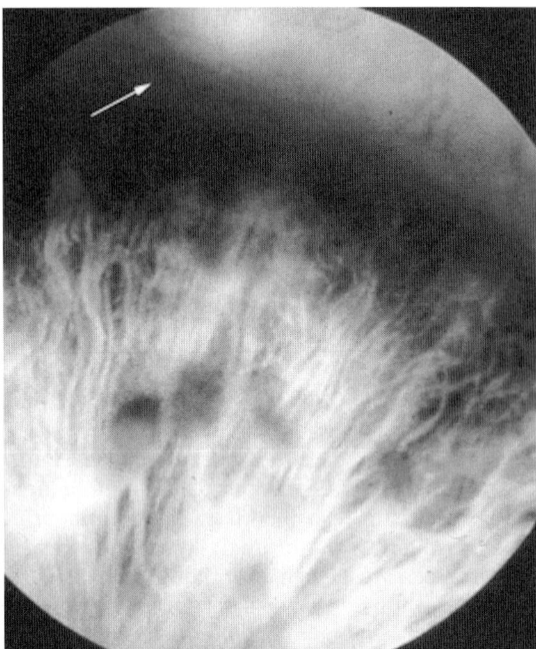

FIGURE 35.12. Lisch nodules on iris of patient with neurofibromotosis type 1. Limbus indicated by the *arrow*.

The most common presenting sign is the café-au-lait spot, a flat, hyperpigmented macule, which is present in 94% to 100% of affected adults.[104] Typically, a few lesions are present at birth, and they increase in size and number during the first decade of life. Histologically, there is hyperpigmentation of the basal cell layer secondary to a nonspecific increase in the number of dopa-positive melanocytes.[105,106] On electron microscopy, giant pigment granules in the melanocytes known as macromelanosomes are found; this finding, however, is not specific for NF-1.[107] Axillary/intertriginous freckling is frequently seen and is relatively unique to NF-1. Although freckling is common in the general population, in contrast to NF-1, it does not occur in areas of skin apposition. The freckles seen in NF-1 generally appear in late childhood and are approximately 1 to 3 mm in diameter. The freckles are histologically similar to café-au-lait spots. Neither freckles nor café-au-lait spots have malignant potential.[105] Neurofibromas, in contrast, do have malignant potential.

There are three types of neurofibromas in NF-1: dermal neurofibromas (fibroma molluscum); nodular neurofibromas; and plexiform neurofibromas. Dermal neurofibromas can be widely distributed throughout the body and appear as pedunculated pigmented nodules. Histologically, they are composed of enlarged cutaneous nerves surrounded by a proliferation of Schwann cells and connective tissue[101] (Figure 35.13). Appearing in late childhood and increasing in number throughout adulthood, they are present in nearly all patients with NF-1 and can cause severe disfigurement.[97] Nodular neurofibromas are similar to dermal neurofibromas, but they are only present in approximately 5% of patients with NF-1 and can occur in patients without the disease. They are firmer lesions with better defined margins located along deeper peripheral nerves. Plexiform neurofibromas occur in approximately 10% of patients and are pathognomonic for NF-1. They are extensive subcutaneous swellings of prominently enlarged nerves in deeper nerve trunks. Plexiform neurofibromas are diffuse masses with indistinct borders that have extensive interdigitations and occasionally feel like a "bag of worms." They are associated with surrounding hyperpigmentation and hypertrophy of underlying soft tissues and bone, leading to regional gigantism.[97] Gross pathology reveals a myxoid gelatinous appearance. Histologically, there is a thickened perineural sheath surrounding each enlarged nerve. Plexiform neurofibromas are often present at birth. They may develop in infancy or early childhood and may enlarge significantly over time, causing severe disfigurement. The upper eyelid exhibits a characteristic S shape when affected by a plexiform neurofibroma, and 25% of eyelid plexiform neurofibromas extend to involve the orbit.[97] When there is a neurofibroma of the upper lid in association with ipsilateral hemifacial hypertrophy, there may also be obstruction of the channels for aqueous outflow; approximately 50% of patients with plexiform neurofibromas develop glaucoma in the ipsilateral eye.[97,101,108] Other mechanisms of congenital glaucoma in patients with neurofibromatosis include infiltration of the angle by a neurofibroma; closure of the angle secondary to neurofibromas thickening the ciliary body and choroid; and secondary fibrovascularization and synechial closure of the angle.[108] Nodular and plexiform neurofibromas in 1% to 4% of patients may undergo malignant degeneration with development of a neurofibrosarcoma.[109] This transformation is frequently accompanied by rapid tumor growth and pain.[103]

Optic nerve gliomas are low-grade pilocytic astrocytomas typically presenting in the first decade of life. They occur in approximately 15% of NF-1 patients but are only symptomatic in 1% to 5%.[97,110] Although usually considered to be benign tumors, optic nerve gliomas can behave as low-grade malignancies (Figure 35.14). If the glioma involves the optic chiasm, mortality is at least 50%. On CT or MRI imaging,

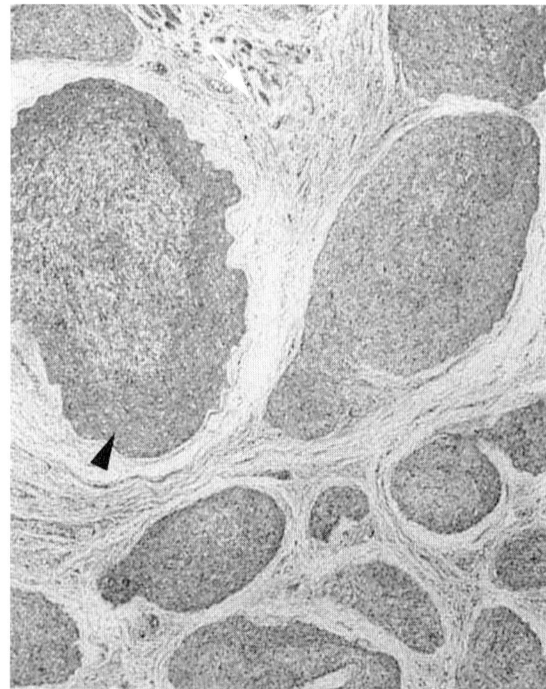

FIGURE 35.13. Enlarged cutaneous nerves (*arrowhead*) in a fibrous matrix (*arrow*) of a neurofibroma. 20×.

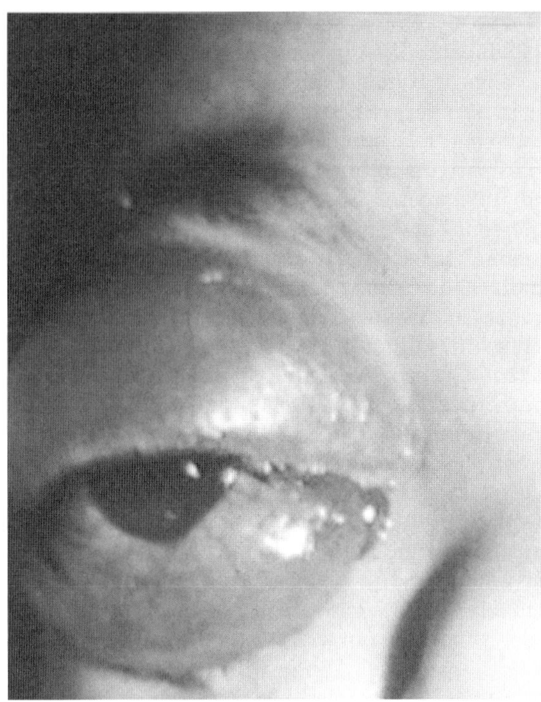

FIGURE 35.14. Proptosis and conjunctival chemosis secondary to optic nerve glioma.

optic nerve gliomas appear as cylindrical or fusiform enlargements of the optic nerve[97] (Figure 35.15). In general, because the great majority of optic nerve gliomas are self-limited with slow growth, the recommendation is for observation. If there is evidence of rapid progression, various treatment methods may be used, including surgical excision, radiotherapy, or chemotherapy.

Lisch nodules are the most common ocular finding (see Figure 35.12). Rarely present earlier than the age of 3 years, Lisch nodules occur in nearly 100% of affected adults. The number of nodules per iris increases with age.[96] The presence of Lisch nodules in a patient with café-au-lait spots confirms the presence of NF-1. Lisch nodules are melanocytic hamartomas of the iris pigment epithelium presenting as sharply demarcated, elevated, dome-shaped lesions with a gelatinous appearance.[97] They typically arise from the anterior border of the iris and protrude into the anterior chamber, but they may also be located deep in the stroma.[101] Histologically, they consist of uniform, spindle-shaped melanin-containing cells within the anterior layers of iris stroma and are similar to iris nevi.[97,111]

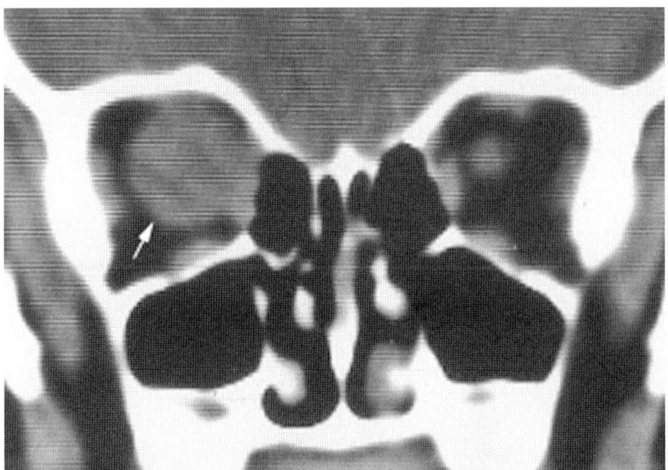

FIGURE 35.15. Computerized tomography scan of optic nerve glioma (*arrow*) in patient in Figure 35.14.

Choroidal lesions are present in 30% to 50% of adults.[112,113] These are flat, hyperpigmented, avascular proliferations with indistinct borders and are located in the posterior pole.[97] There may be single or multiple lesions. Histologically, these are composed of melanocytic and neuronal elements. A characteristic finding is layers of proliferated Schwann cell processes arranged in contact with axons (the ovoid body).[114,115] The various ocular lesions of NF-1 typically do not produce symptoms or affect vision.

Less-common manifestations of NF-1 include enlarged corneal nerves (6%–22%);[112,113] seizure disorder (3%–13%);[97,116] scoliosis (10%); pseudoarthroses; and mild intellectual impairment. Of great concern is the association of NF-1 with certain malignant tumors: neurofibrosarcoma, optic pathway gliomas, Wilms' tumor, rhabdomyosarcoma, pheochromocytoma (5%),[101] astrocytomas, and several types of leukemia.[97] There is also an association with juvenile xanthogranuloma and capillary hemangiomas. Patients with NF-1 have been stated to have an increased risk of uveal melanoma.[117]

Treatment of lid and orbital neurofibromas is surgical excision because the tumors are radioresistant. Surgical treatment improves cosmesis, but the lesions tend to recur.[89] Life expectancy is substantially reduced in patients with NF-1 secondary to systemic hypertension, expansive growth of intracranial neoplasms and associated cancers, sarcomas, leukemias, and lymphomas.[111]

Neurofibromatosis 2

Neurofibromatosis type 2 (NF-2), or central neurofibromatosis, is an inherited disorder clinically distinct from NF-1, characterized by bilateral schwannomas of the eighth cranial nerve (frequently termed acoustic neuromas). The mode of inheritance is autosomal dominant with high penetrance, although it can occur sporadically.[101,118] NF-2 is much less common than NF-1, occurring in approximately 1 in 50,000 live births.[119] The gene has been mapped to an area near the center of the long arm of chromosome 22 and encodes for a cytoskeletal protein and a tumor suppressor gene.[120] Patients with NF-2 typically present in their teens to early adulthood with decreased hearing or tinnitus secondary to acoustic neuromas.

The characteristic acoustic neuromas become symptomatic with tinnitus, hearing loss, and balance problems around the second or third decade of life. There is a high rate of CNS spinal cord gliomas (67.4%); meningiomas (49.2%); and neurofibromas of the vestibular (98.4%) or optic nerve roots (4.8%).[118] The gliomas are typically low-grade astrocytomas with little malignant potential, but they can result in disabling pain and neurologic deficits. The relentless progression of these gliomas can lead to loss of vision, paresis, and even death secondary to brainstem compression.[119] Presenile cataracts are present in 67% to 85%; the majority are posterior subcapsular cataracts or cortical cataracts occurring before age 30.[118,121] Other findings in NF-2 are optic nerve meningioma (4.8%);[118,119] epiretinal membranes;[122] and retinal hamartomas (9%–21%)[118] in the form of combined hamartomas of retinal pigment epithelium and retina[123] or bilateral retinal hamartomas.[124]

Treatment options for vestibular schwannomas include surgical excision (total or subtotal), irradiation, and observation. Surgical excision is the preferred treatment, but it may be associated with perioperative complications, including loss of hearing in the operated ear, air embolism, intracranial hemorrhage, and stroke. Radiotherapy is reserved for patients unable or unwilling to undergo surgical excision.[125] As with NF-1, patients with NF-2 also have substantially reduced life expectancy secondary to growth of the CNS neoplasms.[111]

Tuberous Sclerosis

Tuberous sclerosis (TS) is also an autosomal dominant disorder. It has been mapped to chromosome 9q34 and 16p13.3. Inheritance is autosomal dominant, with high penetrance but variable expressivity. However, at least two-thirds of cases occur as a result of new mutations.[126] Prevalence estimates range from 1 in 6,000 to 1 in 100,000. There is no racial or sex predilection. TS is characterized by benign tumor growth in multiple organ systems, specifically skin, brain, eye, heart, and kidney.

Gomez established criteria for the diagnosis of TS in 1979. This scheme included primary and secondary criteria. Diagnosis was made on the presence of one primary criterion or two secondary criteria. The primary criteria included facial angiofibromas, ungual fibromas, cortical "tubers," subependymal hamartomas, and multiple retinal hamartomas. The secondary criteria included infantile spasms, hypopigmented macules, shagreen patches, single retinal hamartoma, bilateral renal angiomyolipomas or cysts, cardiac rhabdomyoma, or a first-degree relative with a primary diagnosis of TS.[127] The criteria for diagnosis of TS were updated in 1998. Currently, diagnosis of TS requires the presence of two major criteria or one major criterion along with two minor criteria. The major diagnostic criteria for TS include facial angiofibroma, nontraumatic ungual fibromas, three or more hypomelanotic macules, shagreen patch, multiple retinal nodular hamartomas, cortical tubers, subependymal nodules, cardiac rhabdomyoma, lymphangiomyomatosis, and renal angiomyolipomas. Minor criteria include multiple dental pits, hamartomatous rectal polyps, bone cysts, cerebral white matter radial migration lines, gingival fibromas, nonrenal hamartomas, retinal achromic patch, "confetti" skin lesions, and multiple renal cysts.[128,129] The classic triad of TS (the *Vogt triad*) consists of epilepsy, mental retardation, and adenoma sebaceum (angiofibromas of the face). However, the Vogt triad is only present in about 30% of cases.[130]

The most common neurologic symptom of TS is seizures, which are present in approximately 85% of patients. The seizures of patients with TS are usually infantile spasms or partial seizures with rapid secondary generalization. Mental retardation and autism are also common, affecting 50% to 60% of TS patients. Seizures and mental retardation are associated with benign periventricular brain tumors, astrocytic hamartomas, and "tuber"-like areas of sclerosis in the brain.[128]

Adenoma sebaceum is one of the hallmarks of TS. Present in approximately 50% to 80% of cases, this is a reddish-brown papular rash on the malar region of the face and on the chin.[127,128] Frequently mistaken for acne, these lesions are actually angiofibromas that first appear in childhood and increase in number with age.[131] The earliest skin finding is an "ash leaf" spot, a hypopigmented macule present in at least 90% of TS patients at birth or in early infancy.[127] This lesion is sharply demarcated in the shape of an ash leaf. Histologically, the spots have normal numbers of melanosomes, but they are smaller with decreased melanin. UV light may help to visualize the spots in lightly pigmented individuals. Another classic lesion is a shagreen patch, or collagenoma. Shagreen patches occur in about 20% to 35% of cases.[127] They are thickened, yellowish plaques of skin that typically appear in the lumbosacral area. Less common are café-au-lait spots, nevi, and fibromas.

Retinal phakomas are present in 50% of cases.[132] These lesions are bilateral in 30% to 50%. Arising from the innermost layer of the retina, they are composed of nerve fibers and undifferentiated cells that appear glial in origin and are frequently referred to as astrocytic hamartomas. Phakomas rarely affect vision significantly. There are three distinct forms of retinal phakomas. One type occurs in young children and is translucent, gray-white in color, with a flat, smooth surface with indistinct margins in the nerve fiber layer. It is not calcified. The more common retinal hamartoma is calcified, giving the lesion a yellow-white, glistening appearance (Figure 35.16). The lesion is elevated, with sharply demarcated borders and an irregular surface, giving rise to the classic *mulberry* appearance. This type of lesion is occasionally referred to as giant drusen because it is located on or near the optic disc. A third type is intermediate between the first two, with a plaque-like appearance. Histologically, the retinal phakomas consist of elongated, fibrous astrocytes with small oval nuclei and long processes forming a meshwork and containing relatively large blood vessels.[95] The giant drusen may

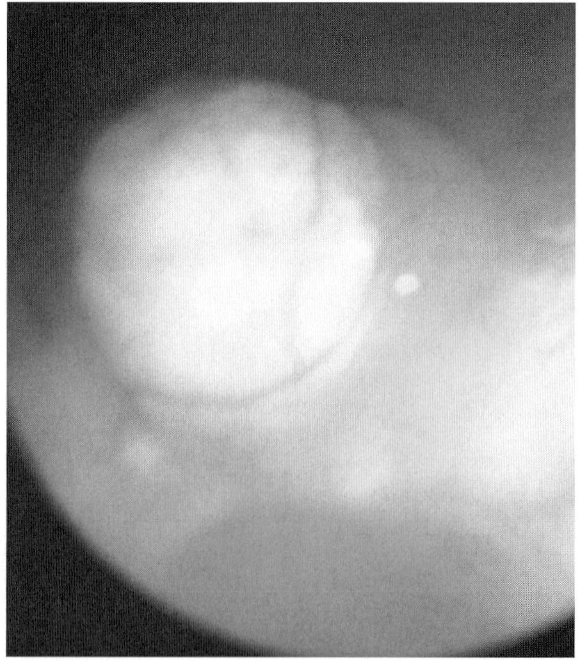

FIGURE 35.16. Retinal hamartoma as seen on indirect ophthalmoscopy.

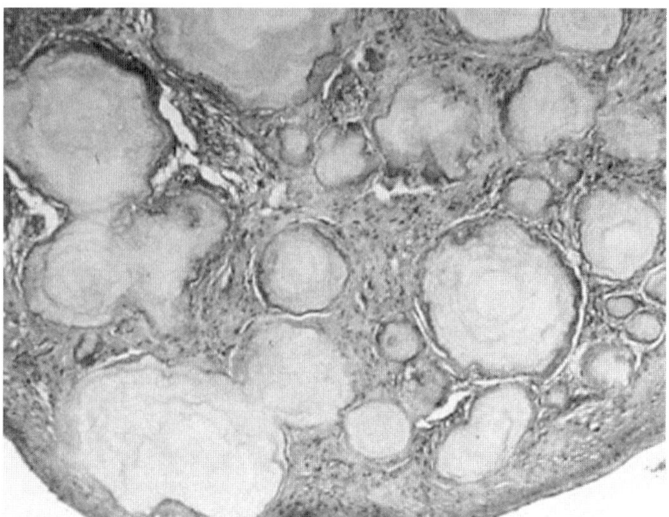

FIGURE 35.17. Giant drusen adjacent to optic nerve seen in retinal phakomas. 20×.

contain hyaline and calcium deposits (Figure 35.17). The retinal phakomatoses can be confused with retinoblastoma or a retinal detachment.

Currently, treatment is merely symptomatic. Patients undergo periodic physical examinations along with imaging modalities to identify potentially treatable conditions such as cardiac rhabdomyosarcomas, enlarging astrocytomas, or renal tumors. Life expectancy is substantially reduced in patients with TS, most commonly secondary to renal failure or problems from enlarging CNS tumors such as obstructive hydrocephalus.[111] Approximately 2% of patients with TS develop renal cell carcinoma.[109] Less-common causes of mortality include cardiac conduction defects, heart failure from cardiac rhabdomyoma, or pulmonary insufficiency from lymphangioleiomyomatosis of the lung.[111]

von Hippel–Lindau Disease

von Hippel–Lindau (VHL) disease, also known as retinal angiomatosis, is an autosomal dominant disorder with irregular penetrance caused by germ-line mutations in the von Hippel–Lindau tumor suppressor gene, located on chromosome 3p25; 20% to 25% are familial cases. Incidence is approximately 1 in 36,000. There is no sex or racial predilection.[111] VHL disease is associated with multiple benign and malignant tumors of many organ systems: the central nervous system, eyes, kidneys (renal cell carcinoma), pancreas, liver, epididymis, and adrenal glands (pheochromocytoma). The origin of the lesions is primarily from the mesoderm, unlike TS and NF, which arise from the ectoderm.

The diagnosis of VHL was originally made only in individuals with both retinal and cerebellar hemangioblastomas, or with either entity alone if the patient had a positive family history. Melmon and Rosen expanded the diagnostic criteria in 1964 to include patients with any single manifestation of the syndrome complex, provided that a CNS hemangioblastoma had been proved in the family.[133]

VHL is characterized by hemangioblastomas of the central nervous system, cerebellum, and retina. Hemangioblastomas are tumors composed of capillaries and lipidized stromal cells. The most common abnormality is the Lindau tumor, a cerebellar hemangioblastoma. It is present in approximately 60% of cases; the majority are cystic, and 20% are solid.[134] Patients typically develop symptoms, typically headache or signs of cerebellar dysfunction, in their mid-thirties. The tumors are typically located in the lateral and posterior cerebellum and are clearly demarcated from surrounding normal tissue, making complete surgical removal possible. Twenty-five percent of patients develop renal cell carcinoma, and 75% of cases are bilateral: 5% by age 30, and more than 40% by age 60.[134–136] The diagnosis of renal cell carcinoma associated with VHL occurs in the fifth decade of life, earlier than the sporadic form, which is diagnosed typically in the sixth decade of life. Three percent to 10% of patients develop pheochromocytomas, which are often bilateral. However, it appears pheochromocytomas are present only within certain families because these cases are typically clustered within few family groups. On electron microscopy, pheochromocytomas have predominantly norepinephrine granules with characteristic eccentrically located electron-dense cores. This histology differs from pheochromocytomas present in patients with multiple endocrine neoplasia 2 (MEN-2) syndrome, which have both epinephrine and norepinephrine secretory granules.[137] There are many other visceral disease manifestations: renal cysts or adenomas, pancreatic cysts, epididymal adenomas or cysts, hepatic cysts, or cystic lesions of the lung, adrenals, bone, omentum, and mesocolon.[134,138] Unlike the other phakomatoses, VHL rarely has cutaneous manifestations, although café-au-lait spots, melanocytic nevi, and port-wine stains (nevus flammeus) can occur.

Ocular involvement occurs in nearly all cases of VHL. Ocular lesions are typically among the first VHL lesions to be diagnosed, occurring about 10 years before the cerebellar disease. Fifty percent to 60% develop retinal capillary hemangiomas.[133] These retinal angiomas are typically located in the peripheral fundus; they may be present at birth but are often not detected until the second or third decade of life. Thirty percent of cases have multiple tumors in one eye and 50% have lesions bilaterally.[139] Initially, the retinal lesions are focal collections of capillaries that appear clinically as small, reddish nodules that are flat or slightly elevated and associated with normal-sized vessels. They enlarge to form mature pink globular masses that are each characteristically supplied by a single, markedly dilated and tortuous artery and a similar-appearing venule running between the lesion and the optic disc. Histologically, retinal angiomas consist of relatively well-formed, thin-walled capillaries forming an anastomosing pattern that are separated by large nodules of plump vacuolated cells which contain birefringent material.[101] Although these capillaries histologically appear well formed, they are leaky and lead to lipid accumulation in the subretinal space and retinal detachments. As a result, vision may be lost, and there may be secondary degenerative changes, including glaucoma or cataracts.

Early diagnosis and treatment are crucial for the preservation of vision, although there have been occasional reports of spontaneous regression of tumors that were left untreated. The typical course of untreated tumors is continued exudation beneath the retina, which leads to extensive retinal detachment along with neovascularization of the retina and iris, peripheral anterior synechiae, intractable secondary glaucoma, and phthisis.[101]

Treatment includes surrounding the angiomas with photocoagulation or cryotherapy.[101] It is extremely important to examine all family members. The median age of death is 45 to 50 years of age secondary to associated renal and intracranial tumors.[140]

Sturge–Weber Syndrome

Sturge–Weber syndrome (SWS), also known as encephalofacial or encephalotrigeminal angiomatosis, involves lesions of the eye, skin, and brain that are always present at birth.[111] Unlike the primary phakomatoses, SWS occurs sporadically. How often the entire triad of symptoms involving the skin, brain, and eye occurs in more than one family member is still unknown.[101] SWS is apparently not familial and does not follow a clear pattern of genetic inheritance. In the few familial clusters described, patients do not have clear-cut autosomal inheritance as is seen in NF, TS, and VHL. The lesions of SWS result from an abnormality of the primordial vascular system during early embryogenesis, likely at 4 to 8 weeks, involving the development of the cephalic neuroectoderm, a neural crest derivative.[141] The prevalence is unknown, and there is no racial or sex predilection.

The diagnosis of SWS established by Reese involves at least two of the following: facial hemangioma (port-wine stain) with ipsilateral intracranial hemangioma, ipsilateral choroidal hemangioma, or congenital glaucoma. The ipsilateral leptomeningeal vascular malformations result in multiple abnormalities: cerebral calcification, seizures, hemianopia, hemiparesis, or mental retardation.[142]

The port-wine stain of SWS can be very disfiguring. It is well demarcated and consists of an abnormally large number of dilated, well-formed capillaries in the dermis. The lesion is deep purple in color and partially blanches with pressure. It typically follows the distribution of the first and second divisions of the trigeminal nerve and is located in the forehead and upper eyelid; it may also involve the lower eyelid and maxillary/mandibular regions[143] (Figure 35.18). If the lesion does not extend to the supraorbital portion of the face, there is no associated epilepsy or intracranial calcification.[115] There may be hypertrophy of the underlying soft tissues and bone along with thickening of the affected skin. Histologically, the dermal angioma is composed of a flat to moderately thick zone of dilated, telangiectatic, cutaneous capillaries lined by a single layer of endothelial cells.[143]

Leptomeningeal hemangiomas occur ipsilateral to the facial angiomas in the parieto-occipital region. They consist of a cluster of small, uniform-caliber venules. There is progressive calcification of cerebral blood vessels and cortical gyri. The characteristic calcium deposits in the brain parenchyma form after birth and are evident by skull radiographs at age 1, and also by CT scan, by the "railroad-track sign," a curvilinear, double-contoured density that parallels cerebral convolutions that are most prominent in the occipital and temporal lobes. Mental retardation occurs in 50% of SWS patients with leptomeningeal hemangiomas and is secondary to maldevelopment and/or brain atrophy. Leptomeningeal angiomas are also associated with seizure disorders in approximately 83% percent of SWS patients.[144] The seizures are typically Jacksonian type on the side contralateral to the angiomas, and they frequently begin in infancy.[145] The seizures typically generalize with age, and patients may develop transient or permanent hemianopia or hemiparesis.[146]

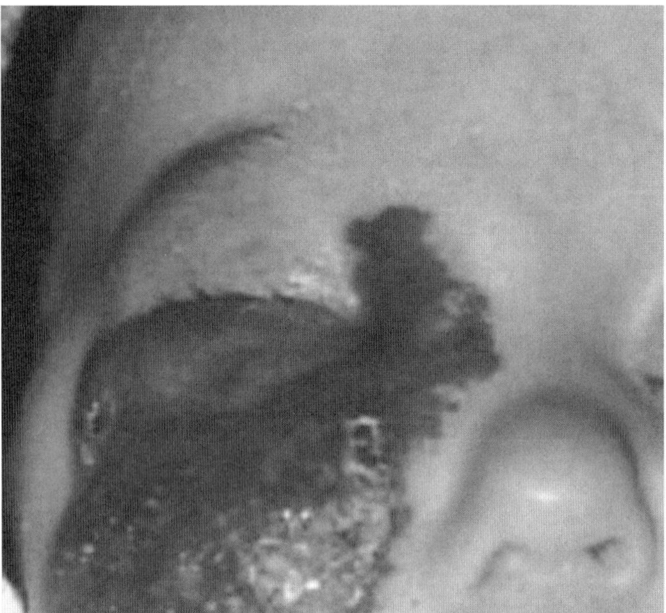

FIGURE 35.18. Port wine stain representing cavernous hemangioma involving the lower lid of a patient with Sturge–Weber syndrome.

Choroidal hemangiomas located ipsilaterally to the facial angioma are present in 40% to 50% of SWS patients. They consist of increased numbers of well-formed choroidal vessels yielding a deep red coloration to the retina, called a "tomato catsup" fundus.[147] Histologically, choroidal hemangiomas consist of numerous large, thin-walled vascular channels that are lined by a flat layer of endothelial cells and divided by thin intervascular septa (Figure 35.19). This choroidal angiomatosis is typically asymptomatic in childhood. However, the choroid can become quite thick as the lesion enlarges, producing visual symptoms in adulthood. There is frequently progressive hyperopia as the lesion enlarges. Longstanding lesions cause destruction of the overlying choriocapillaris, degeneration of the retinal pigment epithelium with loss of photoreceptors, and cystoid degeneration of the outer surface of the retina with gliosis. A serous retinal

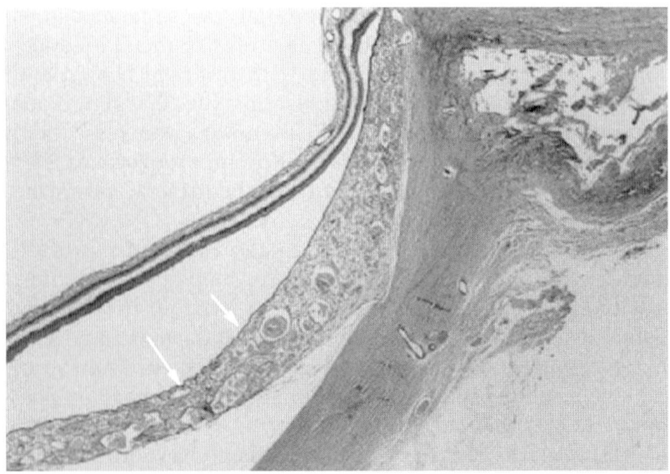

FIGURE 35.19. Choroidal hemangioma causing thickening of choroid (*arrows*) in a patient with Sturge–Weber syndrome. 10×.

detachment may occur and progress to total exudative retinal detachment, which can lead to severe secondary glaucoma.

Glaucoma occurs frequently, in 30% to 70% of cases, and is usually congenital, unilateral, and ipsilateral to facial angioma.[143,148] Patients whose hemangiomas affect the upper eyelid are particularly susceptible to the development of glaucoma.[149] Of the patients with glaucoma, 60% develop buphthalmos (ocular enlargement) as a result of increased intraocular pressure. Forty percent of patients do not develop glaucoma until later in childhood and therefore do not exhibit buphthalmos. The typical mechanisms for glaucoma development are (1) occlusion of the anterior chamber angle by peripheral anterior synechiae (PAS), which frequently develops secondary to iris neovascularization in patients with retinal detachment, or (2) malformation of the anterior chamber angle, which leads to obstruction of aqueous humor outflow.[101] Of note, some patients who develop glaucoma do not have either PAS or a malformed anterior chamber angle. Other ocular findings include a pinkish discoloration of the conjunctiva secondary to increased conjunctival vascularity, heterochromia iridis with the darker iris ipsilateral to facial angioma, and arteriovenous communications within the retina.

Treatment is generally symptomatic. Facial nevus flammus may be treated with laser therapy to improve cosmesis. Occasionally, intractable seizures are treated surgically with subtotal hemispherectomy.[150] Life expectancy is reduced in patients with SWS. Most early deaths occur in patients with severe forms of the disease, including profound mental retardation and intractable seizures.

Ataxia-Telangiectasia and Wyburn–Mason Syndrome

Ataxia-telangiectasia and Wyburn–Mason syndrome are frequently considered among the phakomatoses, although they do not fit the original description. Ataxia-telangiectasia (AT) is characterized by cerebellar ataxia, telangiectasias, immune deficiency, and propensity to develop neoplasms. Its inheritance is autosomal recessive. Homozygous patients present in early childhood with symptoms of cerebellar ataxia that are progressive.[149] Neoplasms associated with AT include lymphocytic leukemia,[151] medulloblastomas, and gliomas.[152] Of note, patients who are heterozygous for AT also have an increased risk of cancer.[153]

Wyburn–Mason syndrome (WMS) is characterized by arteriovenous malformations that are not distinct tumors, and the condition is therefore not a true phakomatosis. The retinal and ipsilateral CNS arteriovenous malformations (AVM) of WMS are congenital and progress with age.[154] There is no established hereditary pattern and no sex or racial predilection. No effective treatment is currently available for retinal AVMs. CNS AVMs can be managed with surgery or radiation.[95] Life expectancy is reduced secondary to intracranial bleeds from the AVMs and strokes related to their treatment.[111]

Systemic Malignancies

It is important for the oncologist to be familiar with potential ocular complications associated with systemic malignancies. Patients may be referred from the ophthalmologist for a systemic workup, or they may present to their oncologist with ocular symptoms that warrant a referral to an ophthalmologist. This section reviews the common and distinct ocular signs and symptoms associated with systemic malignancy.

There are two main mechanisms by which systemic malignancy can have ocular manifestations. (1) Certain genetic syndromes, such as Wilms' tumor, are associated with neoplasia and have eye findings. (2) Remote malignancies can produce paraneoplastic effects in the eye.

Aniridia

Although the term implies an absence of iris tissue, affected patients most commonly have some iris tissue. The amount of iris varies widely from minimal tissue present to minor defects in an otherwise normal iris. Aniridia is associated with Wilms' tumor in the "WAGR syndrome." Genitourinary abnormalities and mental retardation are the other components in the pneumonic WAGR. The syndrome is caused by an autosomal dominant mutation on chromosome 11p13,[155] the proximity of the WT-1 gene and the AN2 gene being responsible for the constellation of findings.[156] The AN2 gene is also responsible for other elements of ocular histogenesis, which explains the higher incidence of additional ocular findings such as peripheral corneal pannus, cataract, lens dislocation, foveal dysplasia, and optic nerve hypoplasia.[157,158] Photophobia and nystagmus can also occur in Wilms' tumor patients.[159,160] Glaucoma is present in 50% to 75% of patients with the autosomal dominant WAGR syndrome, but it does not normally appear until late childhood.[161] In patients with sporadic aniridia, 25% to 33% develop Wilms' tumor.[162–164]

Atypical Congenital Hypertrophy of the Retinal Pigment Epithelium (RPE)

Inclusion of the term *atypical* is used to distinguish this entity from the more common congenital hypertrophy of the retinal pigment epithelium (CHRPE). In contrast to the latter, atypical congenital hypertrophy is typically bilateral. Multiple lesions are present, with larger lesions in the periphery and smaller lesions near the posterior pole of the eye. These areas of hypertrophy are typically black, but they can be nonpigmented and their shape can be round, oval, kidney shaped, or pisiform. From 1 to 30 lesions are seen per fundus quadrant.[165,166] The areas of RPE hypertrophy are usually present at birth and are often the first manifestation of patients with the autosomal dominant syndromes familial adenomatous polyposis (FAP) and Gardner's syndrome.[167] These are syndromes in which thousands of precancerous colonic polyps develop at a young age. Please see elsewhere in this text for more details regarding these entities. There is a high concordance between the presence of these lesions and the development of Gardner's syndrome. Traboulsi and associates found atypical RPE hypertrophy in 90.2% of patients with Gardner's syndrome.[168] Further strengthening this connection is a study by Olea et al., which found that 100% of patients with a family history of FAP and five or more bilateral retinal lesions developed adenomatous polyposis.[169] For more information on FAP/Gardner's syndrome, please see the discussions elsewhere in this text.

Hyperplastic Corneal Nerves

Hyperplastic corneal nerves are observed with the biomicroscope as long, thin, linear opacities, running in various directions through the corneal stroma. They are a consistent finding in multiple endocrine neoplasias (MEN) type 2B;[170] however, they have also been described in 57% of patients with MEN type 2A.[171] MEN syndromes develop as the result of a mutation of the RET gene on chromosome 10.[172] The other ocular findings in MEN 2B include thickening and eversion of the upper eyelid margin and visible tarsal plates, large and prominent eyebrows, and neuromas of the eyelids and the conjunctiva.[170] MEN syndromes are discussed in detail elsewhere in this text.

Bilateral Diffuse Uveal Melanocytic Proliferation

Bilateral diffuse uveal melanocytic proliferation (BDUMP) is a rare paraneoplastic syndrome consisting of two striking findings in the eye: (1) multiple red patches in the posterior fundus that exhibit striking areas of hyperfluorescence on fluorescein angiography, and (2) multiple, slightly elevated uveal melanocytic tumors associated with diffuse thickening of the uveal tract.[173] These changes can produce vision loss, but when associated with retinal detachment or rapid cataract progression they produce a more swift and profound visual decline.

Machemer in 1966 reported the first case of a patient with bilateral uveal melanoma and pancreatic carcinoma.[174] The syndrome may occur slightly more frequently in females. Systemic tumors commonly associated with BDUMP are most commonly ovarian cancer in women and lung cancer in men. Multiple other malignancies, however, have also been associated with BDUMP, such as cancers of the colon, pancreas, gallbladder, breast, and esophagus.[175–182] No treatment has succeeded in arresting the visual field loss associated with BDUMP. Aggressive treatment of the underlying systemic malignancy offers the best hope for the patient's survival but may not prevent further visual loss.

Cancer-Associated Retinopathy

Cancer-associated retinopathy (CAR) is a retinal degeneration experienced by patients with systemic carcinomas. The visual decline can progress to complete blindness and may be rapid or prolonged over several years. Frequently, the visual symptoms of blurred vision, visual field defects, and impaired color vision are manifest before any cancer is diagnosed.

This syndrome has been most frequently recognized in association with small cell lung carcinoma, but it has also been observed with other types of cancer, including uterine cervical cancer, non-small cell carcinoma of the lung, infiltrating ductal adenocarcinoma of the breast, and undifferentiated endometrial carcinoma.[183,184]

Funduscopic examination typically reveals narrowing of the arterioles, changes in the retinal pigment epithelium, and inflammatory cells in the vitreous. The electroretinogram is markedly diminished in all cases.[183,184] Autoantibodies against recoverin, a 23-kDa calcium-binding protein expressed in rod and cone photoreceptors, are responsible for the changes seen in CAR. The gene for recoverin is located in close proximity to p53, and some tumors with elevated p53 expression might aberrantly express recoverin and induce the production of antirecoverin antibodies as well as the activation of antirecoverin-specific T cells.[185–187]

Melanoma-Associated Retinopathy

Melanoma-associated retinopathy (MAR) has been seen in 17 patients with cutaneous melanomas.[188–198] MAR is a retinal degenerative paraneoplastic syndrome that affects the bipolar cells of the retina, thus reducing the B wave on electroretinography.[199–203] The symptoms are normally less severe than those of CAR and include mild visual loss, night blindness, and shimmering or flickering light sensations.[188] Only one patient developed severe visual loss.[188] The B-wave reduction in the electroretinogram of MAR patients is most compatible with disorders in the neuronal transmission pathways beyond photoreceptor cells.

Ocular Flutter

Ocular flutter consists of episodic horizontal rapid eye movements without evidence of a slow phase. Each burst lasts only slightly longer than 1 second. It can coexist with saccadic dysmetria (inaccurate saccades) and opsoclonus (described in the next section). This eye movement abnormality, in the absence of known toxic-metabolic encephalopathy or encephalitis, should warrant workup, including cerebrospinal fluid analysis, MRI, and comprehensive search for occult malignancy.

Opsoclonus

Opsoclonus is defined as involuntary, arrhythmic, chaotic, irregular eye movements that are predominantly horizontal but can have vertical or oblique components. In children, opsoclonus can be related to neuroblastoma. In adults most commonly, opsoclonus is simply the sequela of a viral infection, but it has also been observed as part of a neoplastic process. Fourteen cases of adult opsoclonus associated with systemic carcinoma have been reported.[204]

Various types of cancer have been associated with opsoclonus, including undifferentiated lung carcinoma, oat cell carcinoma of the lung, uterine cancer, adenocarcinoma of the breast, and infiltrating ductal breast carcinoma.[204] There is no sex predilection, and generally there is no prodromal illness. Removal or treatment of the primary tumor has resulted in improvement.[205]

Histopathologic analysis of some cases at autopsy has demonstrated a loss of cerebellar Purkinje's cells, and blood samples from patients with this syndrome have contained anti-Purkinje cell antibodies. Although opsoclonus can be associated with a variety of disease processes, it can herald the onset of an occult malignant tumor, and an extensive evaluation (including anti-Ri and ANNA-2 antibodies) must be made when it is observed in an older individual.

Eyelid Malignancies and Other Malignancies

Basal Cell Carcinoma

Basal cell carcinomas (BCCs) are tumors derived from a pleuripotent stem cell within the basal epithelium that rests on the basement membrane separating the epidermis from

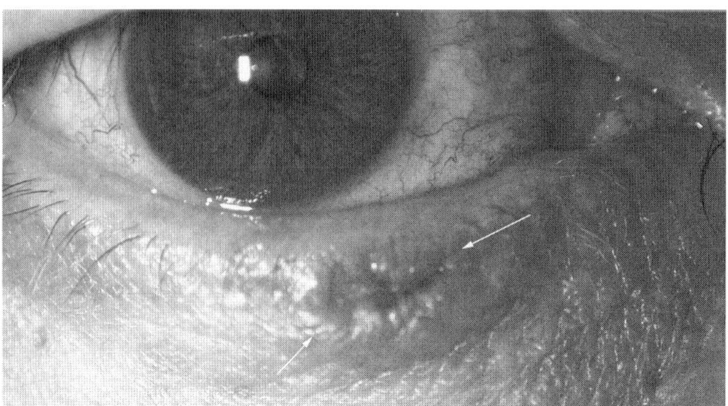

FIGURE 35.20. Basal cell carcinoma with typical pearly edges and excavated center occurring on lower lid.

the dermis. This type of tumor is also discussed in the chapter on skin disease. BCCs are the most common eyelid malignancy, accounting for 85% to 90% of malignant eyelid tumors.[206] These most often occur in fair-skinned individuals; more than 99% of those affected are Caucasian.[207] BCCs typically occur in older adults around the age of 60 but can occur in younger individuals as well. They have a predilection for males (2:1). BCCs arise in areas of sun-exposed skin, and the proposed etiology is actinic damage from ultraviolet light. In the area around the eye, they most commonly occur on the lower lid (50%–60%) followed by the medial canthus (25%–30%), upper lid (15%), and lateral canthus (5%).[208]

Their clinical appearance is that of a firm, raised, pink-pearly papule with a rolled translucent pearly border as the lesion increases in size. There are associated telangiectatic vessels, loss of lashes, and chronic conjunctivitis.

There are two major types of basal cell carcinomas: undifferentiated and differentiated. The subtypes of undifferentiated BCC include noduloulcerative, pigmented, morpheaform or fibrosing, superficial, and fibroepithelioma. The differentiated type of BCC includes adenoid (adenocystic) and basosquamous (metatypical). The most common form of BCC is the nodular type, accounting for 75% of all tumors. This type is the classic pink-pearly papule that has overlying telangiectasia and develops a translucent rolled border as it increases in size (Figure 35.20). The pigmented form is similar to the nodular form, but the pigment results in a bluish, black, or brown discoloration. The pigmented BCC may be confused clinically with malignant melanoma. The morpheaform or sclerosing type, accounting for 15% of all BCCs, is aggressive and can invade deep into the dermis, paranasal sinuses, and orbit. Clinically, it is a poorly defined, pale, yellowish-pink, flat plaque with induration. The superficial and fibroepithelioma forms arise more frequently on the trunk than on the eyelids. The superficial form has an erythematous, scaly patch with raised pearly borders. Fibroepithelioma BCC is a smooth, pink nodule that is pedunculated or sessile.

The basic pathology of undifferentiated BCC includes nests, lobules, and cords with peripheral palisading and stromal retraction (Figure 35.21). The tumor cells have small, hypochromatic cells of uniform size with scanty cytoplasm yielding a characteristically high nuclear-to-cytoplasm ratio. Unlike the other undifferentiated forms, the morpheaform BCC does not typically have peripheral palisading. This type is characterized by intense stromal fibrous proliferation with tumor cells in narrow cords that are only one to two cell layers thick (see Figure 35.21). The differentiated types have a glandular structure with mucinous stroma and a histopathologic appearance somewhere between basal cell carcinoma and squamous cell carcinoma.

Diagnosis is made based on the clinical appearance and is confirmed by histopathologic examination of a biopsy. The differential diagnosis includes malignant melanoma, sebaceous cell carcinoma, squamous cell carcinoma, squamous cell carcinoma in situ, actinic keratosis, keratoacanthoma, seborrheic keratosis, papillomatous lesions, and blepharitis.[209]

The most effective method of treatment is Mohs' micrographic surgery. With this method, the lesion is excised in layers and mapped three-dimensionally.[210] The margins are carefully examined for residual tumor using frozen sections.

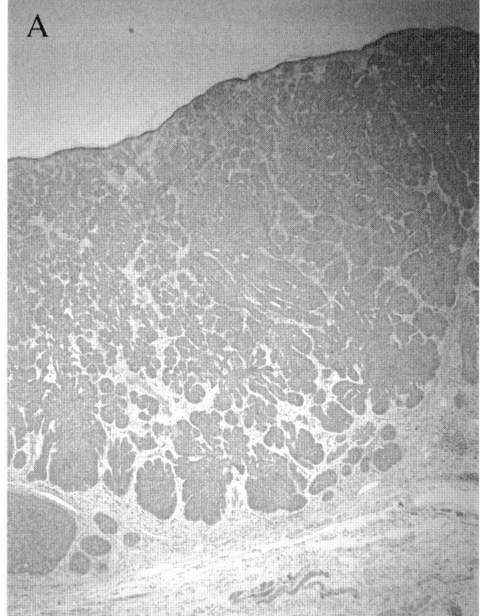

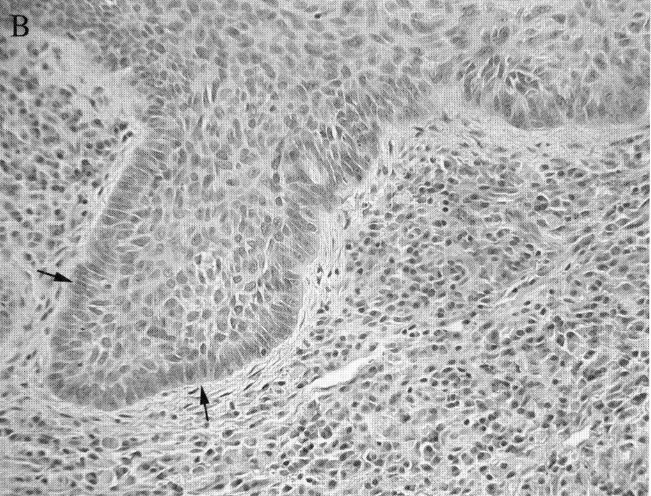

FIGURE 35.21. (A) Nodular basal cell carcinoma with characteristic dermal invasion. 2×. (B) Peripheral palisading of nuclei (*arrows*). 20×.

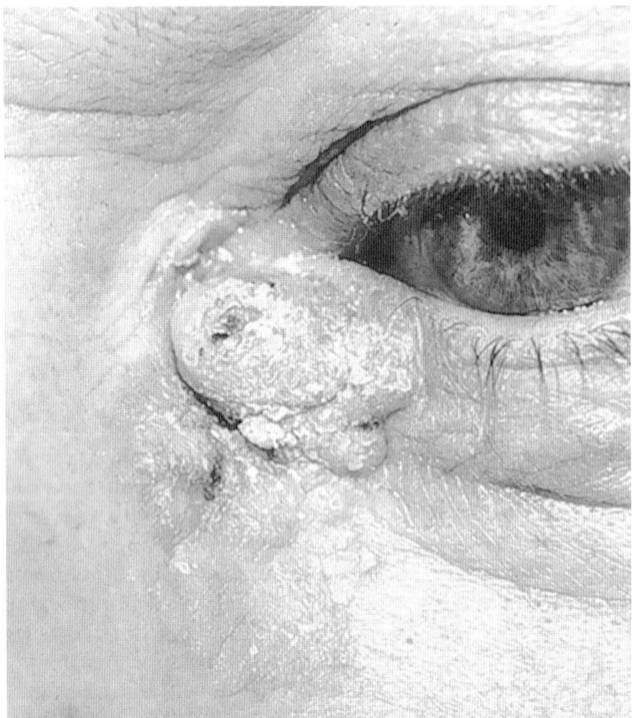

FIGURE 35.22. Hyperkeratotic plaque of squamous cell carcinoma involving the medial canthus. Note the erythema and irregular margins of the lesion.

Areas of residual tumor are identified, and the map is used to locate the areas for further excision until all the margins are free of tumor. One may also use a non-Mohs' technique of excision, also employing frozen section examination of margins to ensure that the tumor is completely excised. There are several other methods of treatment available, but they are generally not recommended for the periorbital region; these include radiation therapy, cryotherapy, chemotherapy, and photodynamic therapy.

Complete surgical excision of basal cell carcinoma is thought to be curative because the lesions rarely metastasize. Rates of metastasis vary from 0.028% to 0.55%,[211] and, in fact, many pathologists believe that if metastases occur, then the primary tumor was not basal cell. Death secondary to basal cell carcinoma is very rare, but it can occur with direct orbital and intracranial extension.

There are a few associated systemic syndromes. The most common syndrome, occurring in less than 1% of individuals with BCC, is basal cell nevus syndrome, also known as Gorlin–Goltz syndrome. This syndrome is characterized by multiple BCCs, jaw cysts, plantar/palmar pits, skeletal abnormalities, neurologic abnormalities, and endocrine disorders. Other rare syndromes include albinism and xeroderma pigmentosa, which are inherited autosomal recessive disorders, along with nevus sebaceous, Bazex's syndrome, linear unilateral basal cell nevus, and Rombo syndrome.[209]

Squamous Cell Carcinoma

Squamous cell carcinoma (SCC) is another malignant tumor that commonly affects the eyelids. Although SCC is approximately 40 times less common than BCC, it is more common on the upper eyelid and lateral canthus than basal cell carcinoma.[211] Unlike BCC, SCC has a greater potential for metastatic spread. SCCs typically arise from actinic damage, but they can arise de novo. Risk factors for developing SCC include ultraviolet light, ionizing radiation, human papillomavirus, and arsenic ingestion. Systemic conditions with a propensity to develop SCC include xeroderma pigmentosa and oculocutaneous albinism, both inherited autosomal recessive disorders.

Clinical presentation reveals an erythematous, indurated, hyperkeratotic plaque or nodule that has irregular margins (Figure 35.22). The lesions typically ulcerate. As noted, SCC commonly affects the upper and lower eyelid margins as well as the medial and lateral canthi.

Histopathologic examination of SCC reveals polygonal cells with abundant eosinophilic cytoplasm and hyperchromatic nuclei with mitotic figures (Figure 35.23A). There may also be evidence of dyskeratosis (Figure 35.23B), keratin pearls, and intercellular bridges.[212]

Diagnosis is made based on clinical appearance and confirmed by histopathologic examination of a biopsy. Differential diagnosis includes basal cell carcinoma, sebaceous cell carcinoma, squamous cell carcinoma in situ, actinic keratosis, keratoacanthoma, inverted follicular keratosis, seborrheic keratosis, verruca vulgaris, and papillomatous lesions.[209]

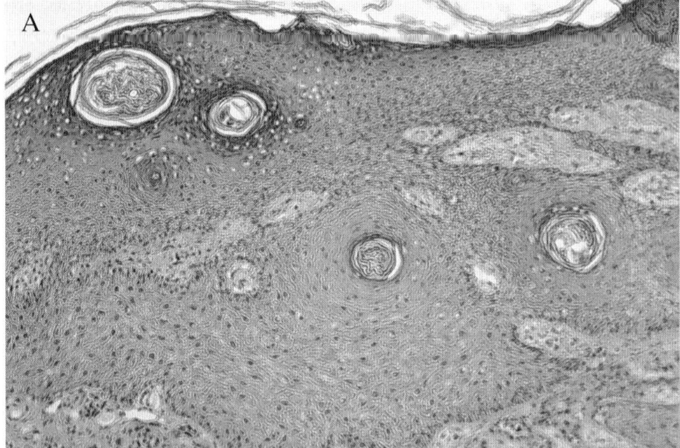

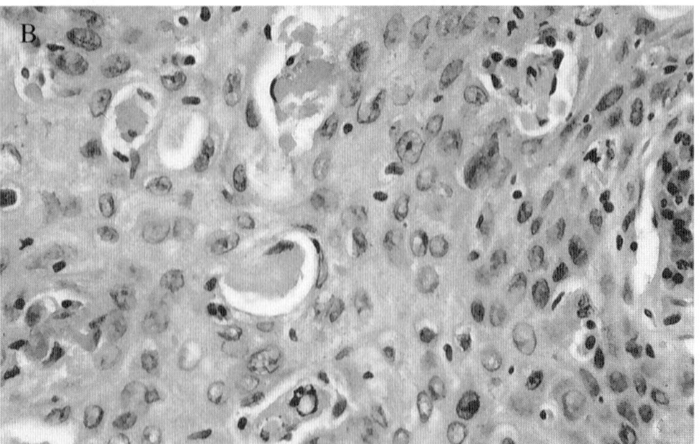

FIGURE 35.23. (A) Dermal invasion by squamous cell carcinoma. 4×. (B) Dyskeratosis in squamous cell carcinoma. 40×.

Treatment for SCC is similar to treatment for BCC. SCC is more aggressive and invasive, but SCC lesions of the eyelid rarely metastasize. Methods of treatment include Mohs' micrographic surgery, irradiation, and cryotherapy. More-extensive surgery may be needed for local control, such as orbital exenteration, if the tumor is deeply invasive.

As with BCC of the eyelid, SCC of the eyelid treated with wide local surgical excision is considered curative; however, metastasis can occur to the preauricular or submandibular lymph nodes, which would yield a guarded prognosis. For further discussion of SCC, including Broder's grading scale, see Chapter 60.

Sebaceous Gland Carcinoma

Sebaceous gland carcinoma (SGC) arises most commonly from the meibomian glands and less frequently from the glands of Zeis and the sebaceous glands of the caruncle and eyebrow. This is a highly malignant, aggressive tumor that has a high rate of metastasis, a high recurrence rate, and a relatively high mortality rate. It is the third most common eyelid malignancy after BCC and SCC but accounts for only 1% to 5.5% of all eyelid malignancies.[213–215] It occurs more frequently in women. Typically presenting in the sixth to seventh decade of life, it can also occur in younger individuals. The etiology is currently unknown. SGC most frequently affects the upper eyelid, with this being the site in approximately two-thirds of all cases. Nonetheless, it can occur in any periocular site. SGC invades overlying epithelium. In about 50% of cases, it may display pagetoid spread, forming nests of cancer cells. It may behave as an intraepithelial carcinoma with diffuse spreading and replacement of the conjunctiva.[209] The primary lesion may spread to other periocular structures, including the conjunctiva, cornea, lacrimal system, or nasal cavity.

The clinical appearance is often that of a firm, yellow nodule similar to a chalazion with possible thickening of the tarsal plate, destruction of meibomian gland orifices, and loss of eyelashes. It is considered to be one of the "masquerade syndromes" because it may mimic chalazion, meibomianitis, or chronic blepharoconjunctivitis, which are refractory to usual therapy.

Because it is uncommon and mimics many other conditions, SGC may be difficult to diagnose. A high index of suspicion is required when lesions do not respond to standard therapies. Diagnosis is confirmed by full-thickness wedge biopsy of the eyelid. Evaluation of the extent of spread may require a sampling of other local structures, given the propensity of this cancer for multicentric spread. Fresh tissue should be submitted for special lipid staining.[211]

Histologically, SGC has highly pleomorphic cells in irregular lobules or nests with hyperchromatic nuclei and a characteristic vacuolated (frothy) cytoplasm secondary to the high lipid content within the cell (Figure 35.24). There are four histologic variants: lobular, comedocarcinoma, papillary, and mixed. On staining for lipids, the cells are found to have fine lipid globules.[209] Given that SGC may exhibit pagetoid spread of malignant cells, the histologic differential diagnosis includes clear cell carcinoma, squamous cell carcinoma, malignant melanoma, and extramammary Paget's disease.[216]

Diagnosis is made on the basis of clinical suspicion confirmed by histopathologic examination of a biopsy. Differential diagnosis includes basal cell carcinoma, squamous cell carcinoma, papillomatous lesions, blepharitis, conjunctivitis, and superior limbic keratoconjunctivitis.[209]

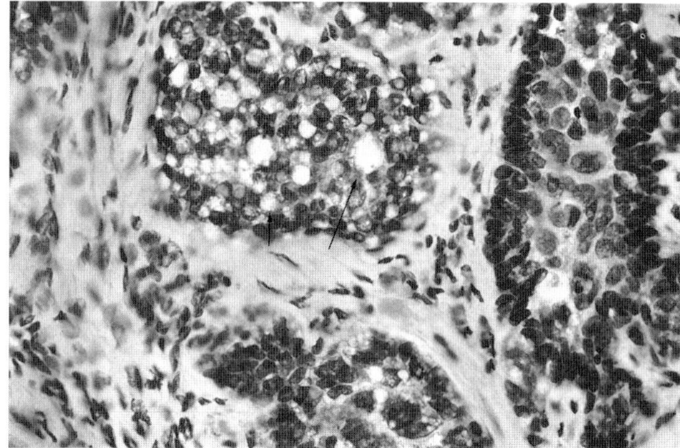

FIGURE 35.24. Sebaceous cell carcinoma with frothy cytoplasm (*arrows*) of tumor cells. 40×.

Treatment for SGC is similar to treatment for BCC and SCC with Mohs' micrographic surgery; this consists of wide excision with microscopic monitoring of the margins. However, given the likelihood of multicentric spread, this treatment is not always successful. If the tumor is large or involves deep orbital tissues, or if there is evidence of metastasis, a more-complex treatment plan is needed with possible orbital exenteration and radiation. The rate of mortality is 0% to 15% with no evidence of metastasis; with distant metastasis, the mortality rate rises to 50% to 67% at 5 years.[132] Although traditionally considered to be radioresistant with radiation reserved only for palliation, there has been some recent success reported with radiation therapy of greater than 55 Gy.[216,217]

Melanoma and Other Eyelid Malignancies

Briefly, malignant melanoma is more common in fair-skinned individuals. The major risk factor for developing malignant melanoma is a history of severe sunburns. Other risk factors include family history, Caucasian race, age over 20 years, congenital/dysplastic nevi, changing moles, or excessive sun exposure/sun sensitivity.[218] It causes only 1% of eyelid malignancies; however, it is responsible for two-thirds of all tumor-related deaths from skin cancers.[209] Pathology reveals diffuse hyperplasia of atypical melanocytes throughout the basal cell layer; there may be a mixture of epithelioid, spindle, and nevus-like cells. Treatment involves wide surgical excision leaving a 1-cm tumor-free margin. Metastatic evaluation should be performed if the tumor is greater than 1.5 mm in depth or shows evidence of lymphatic/vascular spread. For a more complete discussion, including staging, course, and outcome, see Chapter 59.

Other eyelid malignancies, which are quite uncommon, include Kaposi's sarcoma, Merkel cell tumor, mucinous sweat gland adenocarcinoma, adenocarcinoma of the gland of Moll, and metastasis.

References

1. Phillpotts BA, Sanders RJ, Shields JS, et al. Uveal melanomas in black patients: a case series and comparative review. J Natl Med Assoc 1995;87:709.
2. Cutler SJ, Young JL (eds) Third National Cancer Survey: incidence data. NCL Monogr 1975;41:1.
3. Robertson DM. Changing concepts in the management of choroidal melanoma. Am J Ophthalmol 2003;136:161–170.
4. Raivio I. Uveal melanoma in Finland: an epidemiological, clinical, histological and prognostic study. Acta Ophthalmol 1977;133(suppl):3.
5. Gialason I, Magnussen G, Tulinius H. Malignant melanoma of the uvea in Iceland. Acta Ophthalmol 1985;63:385–394.
6. Margo CE, Mulla Z, Billiris K. Incidence of surgically treated uveal melanoma by race and ethnicity. Ophthalmology 1998;105:1087.
7. Wilkes SR, Robertson DM, Kurland LT, et al. Incidence of uveal melanoma in the resident population of Rochester and Olmstead County, Minnesota. Am J Ophthalmol 1979;87: 639–674.
8. Scotto J, Fraumeni JF, Lee JAH. Melanoma of the eye and other noncutaneous sites. JNCI 1976;56:489.
9. Gass JDM, Gieser RG, Wilkinson CP, et al. Bilateral diffuse uveal melanocytic proliferation in patients with occult carcinoma. Arch Ophthalmol 1990;108:527–533.
10. Singh AD, De Potter P, Fijal BA, et al. Lifetime prevalence of uveal melanoma in white patients with oculo (dermal) melanocytosis. Ophthalmology 1998;105:195.
11. Yanoff M, Zimmerman LE. Histogenesis of malignant melanomas of the uvea. III. The relationship of congenital ocular melanocytosis and neurofibromatosis to uveal melanomas. Arch Ophthalmol 1967;77:331.
12. Van Hees CL, De Boer A, Jager MJ, et al. Are atypical nevi a risk factor for uveal melanoma? A case-control study. J Invest Dermatol 1994;103:202.
13. Egan KM, Gragoudas ES, Seddon JM, et al. Smoking and the risk of early metastases from uveal melanoma. Ophthalmology 1992;99:537.
14. Horn EP, Hartge P, Shields JA, et al. Sunlight and risk of uveal melanoma. J Natl Cancer Inst 1994;86:1476.
15. Wagoner MD, Albert DM. The incidence of metastases from untreated ciliary body and choroidal melanomas. Arch Opthalmol 1982;100(6):939–940.
16. Collaborative Ocular Melanoma Study Group. Assessment of metastatic disease status at death in 435 patients with large choroidal melanoma in the COMS: COMS report no. 15. Arch Opthalmol 2001;119(5):670–676.
17. Starr HJ, Zimmerman LE. Extrascleral extension and orbital recurrence of a malignant melanoma of the choroid and ciliary body. Int Opthalmol Clin 1962;2:369.
18. Folberg R, Pe'er J, Gruman LM, et al. The morphologic characteristics of tumor blood vessels as a marker of tumor progression in primary human uveal melanoma. Hum Pathol 1992;23:1298.
19. Folberg R, Rummelt V, Parys-Van Ginderdeuren R, et al. The prognostic value of tumor blood vessel morphology in primary uveal melanoma. Ophthalmology 1993;100:1389.
20. Sorensen FB, Gamel JW, McCurdy J. Stereologic estimation of nucleolar volume in ocular melanoma: a comparative study of size estimators with prognostic impact. Hum Pathol 1993;24:513.
21. Gamel JW, McCurdy JB, McLean IW. A comparison of prognostic covariates for uveal melanomas. Invest Ophthalmol Vis Sci 1992;33:1919.
22. Marcus DM, Minokovitz JB, Wardwell SD, et al. The value of nucleolar organizing regions in uveal melanoma. Am J Ophthalmol 1990;100:527.
23. Whelchel JC, Farah SE, McLean IW, et al. Immunohistochemistry of infiltrating lymphocytes in uveal malignant melanoma. Invest Ophthalmol Vis Sci 1993;34:2603–2606.
24. Gass JDM. Observation of suspected choroidal and ciliary body melanomas for evidence of growth prior to enucleation. Ophthalmology 1990;87:525.
25. Char DH, Kroll SM, Phillips TL. Uveal melanoma growth rate and prognosis. Arch Ophthalmol 1997;115:1014–1018.
26. Karlsson M, Boeryd B, Carstensen J, et al. DNA ploidy and S-phase fraction as prognostic factors in patients with uveal melanomas. Br J Cancer 1995;71:177.
27. Coleman K, Baak JP, van Diest PF, et al. DNA ploidy status in 84 ocular melanomas: a study of DNA quantitation in ocular melanomas by flow cytometry and automatic and interactive static image analysis. Hum Pathol 1995;26:99.
28. Mooy C, Vissers K, Luyton G. et al. DNA flow cytometry in uveal melanoma: the effect of pre-enucleation irradiation. Br J Ophthalmol 1995;79:174.
29. Collaborative Ocular Melanoma Study Group. Histopathologic characteristics of uveal melanomas in eyes enucleated from the Collaborative Ocular Melanoma Study. COMS report no. 6. Am J Opthalmol 1998;125(6):745–766.
30. Shields CL, Cater J, Shields JA, et al. Combination of clinical factors predictive of growth of small choroidal melanocytic tumors. Arch Ophthalmol 2000;118:360–364.
31. Meyer-Schwickerath G. The preservation of vision by treatment of the intraocular tumors with light coagulation. Arch Ophthalmol 1961;66:458.
32. Vogel MK. The application of photocoagulation in the treatment of the choroid. Ophthalmic Forum 1983;1:46.
33. Shields JA. The expanding role of laser photocoagulation for intraocular tumors. The 1993 H. Christian Zweng Memorial Lecture. Retina 1994;14:310.
34. Shields CL, Shields JA, Cater J, et al. Transpupillary thermotherapy for choroidal melanoma: tumor control and visual results in 100 consecutive cases. Ophthalmology 1998;105:581.
35. Finger PT, Berson A, Szechter A. Palladium-103 vs. iodine-125 for ophthalmic plaque radiotherapy. Int J Radiat Oncol Biol Phys 1993;27:849.
36. Finger PT, Berson A, Szechter A. Palladium-103 plaque therapy for choroidal melanoma. Ophthalmology 1999;106: 606.
37. Collaborative Ocular Melanoma Study Group. The COMS randomized trial of iodine 125 brachytherapy for choroidal melanoma. III: Initial mortality findings. COMS Report No. 18. Arch Opthalmol 2001;119(7):969–982.
38. Perez CA, Brady LW (eds) Principles and Practice of Radiation Oncology. Philadephia: Lippincott-Raven, 1998.
39. Wilson MW, Hungerford JL. Comparison of episcleral plaque and proton beam radiation therapy for the treatment of choroidal melanoma. Ophthalmology 1999;106:1579.
40. Collaborative Ocular Melanoma Study Group. COMS randomized trial of pre-enucleation radiation of large choroidal melanoma: I. Characteristics of patients enrolled and not enrolled. COMS Report No. 9. Am J Ophthalmol 1998; 125(6):767–778.
41. The Collaborative Ocular Melanoma Study–Quality of Life Study Group. Development and validation of disease specific measures for choroidal melanoma: COMS-QOL Report No. 2. Arch Opthalmol 2003;121(7):1010–1020.

42. Jampol LM, Moy CS, Murray TG. The COMS randomized trial of iodine-125 brachytherapy for choroidal melanoma: IV. Local treatment failure and enucleation in the first 5 years after brachytherapy. COMS Report No. 19. Ophthalmology 2002;109(12):2197–2206.
43. Anonymous. The Collaborative Ocular Melanoma Study (COMS) randomized trial of pre-enucleation radiation of large choroidal melanoma. III: Local complications and observations following enucleation. COMS Report No. 11. Am J Ophthalmol 1998;126(3):362–372.
44. Collaborative Ocular Melanoma Study Group. The Collaborative Ocular Melanoma Study (COMS) randomized trial of pre-enucleation radiation of large choroidal melanoma. II: Initial mortality findings. COMS Report No. 10. Am J Opthalmol 1998;125(6):779–796.
45. Peyman Ga, Apple DJ. Local excision of a choroidal malignant melanoma: full-thickness eyewall resection. Arch Ophthalmol 1974;92:216.
46. Damato BE, Paul J, Foulds WS. Risk factors for residual and recurrent uveal melanoma after trans-scleral local resection [comment]. Br J Ophthalmol 1996;80(2):102–108.
47. Sahel JA, Brini A, Albert DM. Pathology of the retina and vitreous. In: Albert DM, Jakobiec FA (eds). Principles and Practice of Ophthalmology, 2nd ed, vol 4. Philadelphia: Saunders, 2000:3750–3792.
48. Albert DM, Dryja TP. The eye. In: Cotran RS, Kumar V, Collins T (eds). Pathologic Basis of Disease, 6th ed. Philadelphia: Saunders, 1999:1359–1377.
49. McLean IW. Retinoblastomas, retinocytomas, and pseudoretinoblastomas. In: Ophthalmic Pathology: An Atlas and Textbook, 4th ed, vol 2. Philadelphia: Saunders, 1996:1332–1438.
50. Peterson RA, Friend SH, Albert DM. Prolonged survival of a child with metastatic retinoblastoma. J Pediatr Ophthalmol Strabismus 1987;24(5):247–248.
51. Abramson DH, Frnak CM, Susman M, et al. Presenting signs of retinoblastoma. J Pediatr 1998;132(3):505–508.
52. Friend SH, Bernards R, Rodlj S, et al. A human DNA segment with properties of the gene that predisposes to retinoblastoma and osteosarcoma. Nature (Lond) 1986;323: 643–646.
53. Cavenee WK, Dryja TP, Phillips RA, et al. Expression of recessive alleles by chromosomal mechanisms in retinoblastoma. Nature (Lond) 1983;305:779.
54. Dryja TP, Cavenee W, White R, et al. Homozygosity of chromosome 13 in retinoblastoma. N Engl J Med 1984;310: 550.
55. Wong FL, Boice JD Jr, Abramson DH, et al. Cancer incidence after retinoblastoma: radiation dose and sarcoma risk. JAMA 1997;278(15):1262–1266.
56. Eng C, Li FP, Abramson DH. Mortality from second tumors among long-term survivors of retinoblastoma. J Natl Cancer Inst 1993;85(14):1121–1128.
57. Shields JA, Stephens RT, Sarin LK. The differential diagnosis of retinoblastoma. In: Harley RD (ed). Pediatric Ophthalmology, 2nd ed. Philadelphia: Saunders, 1983:114.
58. Shields JA, Michelson JB, Leonard BC, et al. B-scan ultrasonography in the diagnosis of atypical retinoblastomas. Can J Ophthalmol 1976;11:42–51.
59. Hermsen VM. Echographic diagnosis. In: Blodi FC (ed). Retinoblastoma. New York: Churchill Livingstone, 1985: 111–127.
60. Donoso LA, Shields JA, Felber NT, et al. Intracranial malignancy in patients with bilateral retinoblastoma. Retina 1981;1:67–74.
61. Pratt CB, Meyer D, Chenaille P, et al. The use of bone marrow aspirates and lumbar puncture at the time of diagnosis of retinoblastoma. J Clin Oncol 1989;7:140–143.
62. Moll AC, Imhof AM, Schouten-Van Meeteren AYN, et al. At what age could screening for familial retinoblastoma be stopped? A register based study 1945–98. Br J Ophthalmol 2000;84:1170–1172.
63. Castillo BV Jr, Kaufman L. Pediatric tumors of the eye and orbit. Pediatr Clin N Am 2003;50(1):149–172.
64. Hungerford J, Toma N, Plowman P, et al. External beam radiotherapy for retinoblastoma: I. Whole eye technique. Br J Ophthalmol 1995;79:109–111.
65. Shields C, Shields J, Needle M, et al. Combined chemoreduction and adjuvant treatment for introcular retinoblastoma. Ophthalmology 1997;104(12):2101–2111.
66. Hall LS, Ceisler E, Abramson D. Visual outcomes in children with bilateral retinoblastoma. J Pediatr Ophthalmol Strabismus 1999;3:138–142.
67. Shields C, Shields J. Recent developments in the management of retinoblastoma. J Pediatr Ophthalmol Strabismus 1999;36:8–18.
68. Magramm I, Abramson D, Ellsworth R. Optic nerve involvement in retinoblastoma. Ophthalmology 1989;96: 217–222.
69. Shields CL, Shields JA, De Potter P. New treatment modalities for retinoblastoma. Curr Opin Ophthalmol 1996; 7(111):20–26.
70. De Potter P. Current treatment of retinoblastoma. Curr Opin Ophthalmol 2002;13:331–336.
71. Shields CL, Honavar SG, Meadows AT, et al. Chemoreduction plus focal therapy for retinoblastoma: factors predictive of need for treatment with external beam radiotherapy or enucleation. Am J Ophthalmol 2002;133:657–664.
72. Friedman DL, Limelstein B, Shields CL, et al. Chemoreduction and local ophthalmic therapy for intraocular retinoblastoma. J Clin Oncol 2000;18:12–17.
73. Shields CL, Shields JA, De Potter P, et al. The effect of chemoreduction on the retinoblastoma-induced retinal detachment. J Pediatr Ophthalmol Strabismus 1997;34: 165–169.
74. Shields CL, Santos MC, Diniz W, et al. Thermotherapy for retinoblastoma. Arch Ophthalmol 1999;117:885–893.
75. Shields CL, Shields JA, Minelli, et al. Regression of retinoblastoma after plaque radiotherapy. Am J Ophthalmol 1993;115:181–187.
76. Shields CL, Shields JA, De Potter P, et al. Plaque radiotherapy in the management of retinoblastoma: use as a primary and secondary treatment. Ophthalmology 1993;100:216–224.
77. Cassady J. Radiation therapy for retinoblastoma. In: Albert DM, Jakobiec FA (eds). Principles and Practice of Ophthalmology, 2nd ed, vol 5. Philadelphia: Saunders, 2000:3285–3297.
78. Grabowski EF, Abramson DH. Intraocular and extraocular retinoblastoma. Hematol Oncol Clinc N Am 1987;1: 721–735.
79. Pratt CB, Fontanesi J, Chenaille P, et al. Chemotherapy for extraocular retinoblastoma. Pediatr Hematol Oncol 1994; 11:301–309.
80. White L. Chemotherapy for retinoblastoma. Med Pediatr Oncol 1995;24:341–342.
81. Ferry AP, Font RL. Carcinoma metastatic to the eye and orbit. I: A clinicopathologic study of 227 cases. Arch Ophthalmol 1974;92:276.

82. Castro PA, Albert DM, Wang WJ, Ni C. Tumors metastatic to the eye and adnexa. Int Ophthalmol Clin 1982;22:189.
83. Bloch RS, Gartner S. The incidence of ocular metastatic carcinoma. Arch Ophthalmol 1971;85:673.
84. Stephens RF, Shields JA. Diagnosis and management of cancer metastatic to the uvea: a study of 70 cases. Ophthalmology 1979;86:1336–1349.
85. Albert DM, Rubenstein RA, Scheie HG: Tumor metastases to the eye. I: Incidence in 213 patients with generalized malignancy. Am J Ophthalmol 1967;63:723.
86. Shields CL, Shields JA, Gross NE, et al. Survey of 520 eyes with uveal metastases. Ophthalmology 1997;104:1265–1276.
87. Freedman MI, Folk JC. Metastatic tumors to the eye and orbit: patient survival and clinical characteristics. Arch Ophthalmol 1987;105:1215.
88. Shields JA. Diagnosis and Management of Intraocular Tumors. St. Louis: Mosby-Year Book, 1983.
89. Char DH. Clinical Ocular Oncology, 2nd ed. Philadelphia: Lippincott-Raven, 1997:89–165.
90. Merrill CF, Kaufman DI, Dimitrov NV. Breast cancer metastatic to the eye is a common entity. Cancer (Phila) 1991;68:623–627.
91. Mewis L, Young SF. Breast carcinoma metastatic to the choroids: analysis of 67 patients. Ophthalmology 1982;89: 147–151.
92. Thatcher N, Thomas PRM. Choroidal metastases from breast carcinoma: a survey of 42 patients and the use of radiation therapy. Clin Radiol 1975;26:549–553.
93. Chu FC, Huh SH, Nisce LZ, et al. Radiation therapy of choroidal metastasis from breast cancer. Int J Radiat Oncol Biol Phys 1977;2:273–279.
94. Albert DM, Volpe MJ. Metastases to the uvea. In: Albert DM, Jakobiec FA (eds). Principles and Practice of Ophthalmology, 2nd ed. Philadelphia: Saunders, 2000;5073–5084.
95. Ebert EM, Boger W, Albert DM. In: Albert DM, Jakobeic FA (eds). Principles and Practice of Ophthalmology, 2nd ed, vol 6. Philadelphia: Saunders, 2000:5117–5146.
96. Beauchamp GR. Neurofibromatosis type 1 in children. Trans Am Ophthalmol Soc 1995;93:445–472.
97. Sipple K. Ocular findings in neurofibromatosis type 1. Int Ophthalmol Clin 2001;41(1):25–40.
98. Fountain JW, Wallace MR, Bruce MA, et al. Physical mapping of a translocation breakbpoint in neurofibromatosis. Science 1989;244:1085–1087.
99. Jadayel D, Fain P, Upadhyaya M, et al. Paternal origin of new mutations in neurofibromatosis. Nature (Lomd) 1990;343: 558–559.
100. Neurofibromatosis. Conference Statement. National Institute of Health Consensus Development Conference. Arch Neurology 1988;45:575–580.
101. Font RL, Ferry AP. The phakomatoses. Int Ophthalmol Clin 1972;12:1–50.
102. Barbagallo JS, Kolodzieh MS, Silverberg NB, et al. Neurocutaneous disorders. Dermatol Clin 2002;20(3):547–560.
103. Hope DJ, Mulvihill JJ. Malignancy in neurofibromatosis. Adv Neurol 1981;29:33–56.
104. Riccardi VM. von Recklinghausen neurofibromatosis. N Engl J Med 1981;305:1617–1627.
105. Sipple K. Ocular findings in neurofibromatosis type 1. Int Ophthalmol Clin 2001;41(1):25–40.
106. Font RL, Ferry AP. The phakomatoses neurofibromatosis. Int Ophthalmol Clin 1972;12:1–50.
107. Benedict PH, Szabo G, Fitzpatrick TB, Sinesi SJ. Melanotic macules in Albright's syndrome and in neurofibromatosis. JAMA 1968;205:72–80.
108. Grant WM, Walton DS. Distinctive gonioscopic findings in glaucoma due to neurofibromatosis. Arch Ophthal 1968;79: 127–134.
109. Kandt RS. Tuberous sclerosis complex and neurofibromatosis type 1: the two most common neurocutaneous diseases. Neurol Clin 2002;20(4):941–964.
110. Dutton JJ. Gliomas of the anterior visual pathway. Surv Ophthalmol 1994;38:427–452.
111. Augsburger JJ, Bolling JP. Phakomatoses. In: Yanoff M, Duker JS (eds). Ophthalmology, 2nd ed, vol 158. Philadelphia: Saunders, 2004:1097–1102.
112. Lewis RA, Riccardi VM. Von Recklinghausen neurofiromatosis: incidence of iris hamartomata. Ophthalmology 1981;88:348–354.
113. Hudson S, Jones D, Beck L. Ophthalmic manifestations of neurofibromatosis. Br J Ophthalmol 1987;71:235–238.
114. Brownstein S, Little JM. Ocular neurofibromatosis. Ophthalmology 1983;91:1595–1599.
115. Kurosawa A, Kurosawa H. Ovoid bodies in choroidal neurofibromatosis. Arch Ophthalmol 1982;100:1939–1941.
116. Riccardi VM. Von Recklinghausen neurofibromatosis. N Engl J Med 1981;305:1617–1627.
117. Wiznia RA, Freedman JK, Mancini AD, Shields JA. Malignant melanoma of the choroid in neurofibromatosis. Am J Ophthalmol 1978;86:684–687.
118. Parry DM, Eldridge R, Kaiser-Kupfer MI, et al. Neurofibromatosis 2 (NF2): clinical characteristics of 63 affected individuals and clinical evidence for heterogeneity. Am J Med Gen 1994;52:450–461.
119. Richards SC, Bachynski BN. Ophthalmic manifestations of neurofibromatosis type 2. Int Pediatr 1990;5:270.
120. Rouleau BG, Wertelecki W, Haines JL, et al: Genetic linkage of bilateral aoustic neurofibromatosis to a DNA marker on chromosome 22. Nature (Lond) 1987;329:246.
121. Ragge NK, Baser ME, Klein J, et al. Ocular abnormalities in neruofibromatosis 2. Am J Ophthalmol 1995;120: 634.
122. Kaye LD, Rothner AD, Beauchamp GR, et al. Ocular findings associated with neurofibromatosis type II. Ophthalmology 1992;99:1424.
123. Landau K, Dossetor FM, Hoyt WF, et al. Retinal hamartoma in neurofibromatosis 2. Arch Ophthalmol 1990;108:328.
124. Good WV, Brodsky MC, Edwards MS, et al. Bilateral retinal hamartomas in neurofibromatosis type 2. Br J Ophthalmol 1991;75:190.
125. National Institute of Health Consensus Development Conferences Statement on Acoustic Neuroma, December 11–13, 1991. Consensus Development Panel. Arch Neurol 1994;51:201–207.
126. Crino PB, Henske EP. New developments in the neurobiology of tuberous sclerosis complex. Neurology 1999;53: 1384–1390.
127. Ebert EM, Boger W, Albert DM. In: Albert DM, Jakobeic FA (eds). Principles and Practice of Ophthalmology, 2nd ed, vol 6. Philadelphia: Saunders, 2000: 5117–5146.
128. Kandt RS. Tuberous sclerosis complex and neurofibromatosis type 1: the two most common neurocutaneous diseases. Neurol Clin 2002;20(4):941–964.
129. Roach ES, Gomez MR, Northrup H. Tuberous sclerosis complex consensus conference: revised clinical diagnostic criteria. J Child Neurol 1998;13:624–628.

130. Barbagallo JS, Kolodzieh MS, Silverberg NB, et al. Neurocutaneous disorders. Dermatol Clin 2002;20(3):547–560.
131. Font RL, Ferry AP. The phakomatoses. Int Ophthalmol Clin 1972;12:1–50.
132. Lagos JC, Gomez MR. Tuberous sclerosis: reappraisal of a clinical entity. Mayo Clin Proc 1967;42:26–49.
133. Melmon KL, Rosen SW. Lindau's disease: review of the literature and study of a large kindred. Am J Med 1964;36: 595–617.
134. Maher ER, Yates JRW, Harries R, et al. Clinical features and natural history of von Hippel–Lindau disease. Q J Med 1990;66:233.
135. Hardwig P, Robertson DM. von Hippel–Lindau disease: a familial, often lethal, multi-system phakomatosis. Ophthalmology 1984;91:263–270.
136. Oakes WJ. The natural history of patients with the Sturge–Weber syndrome. Pediatr Neurosurg 1992;18: 287–290.
137. Eisenhofer G, Walther MM, Huynh TT, et al. Pheochromocytomas in von Hippel–Lindau syndrome and multiple endocrine neoplasia type 2 display distinct biochemical and clinical phenotypes. J Clin Endocrinol Metab 2001;86(5): 1999–2008.
138. Font RL, Ferry AP. The phakomatoses. Int Ophthalmol Clin 1972;12:1–50.
139. Welch RB. Von Hippel-Lindau disease: the recognition and treatment of early angiomatosis retinae and the use of cryosurgery as an adjunct to therapy. Trans Am Ophthalmol Soc 1970;66:367.
140. Maher ER, Yates JRW, Harries R, et al. Clinical features and natural history of von Hippel-Lindau disease. Q J Med 1990;66:233.
141. Enjolras O, Riche MC, Merland JJ. Facial port-wine stains and Sturge-Weber syndrome. Pediatrics 1985;76:48–51.
142. Ebert EM, Boger W, Albert DM. In: Albert DM, Jakobeic FA (eds). Principles and Practice of Ophthalmology, 2nd ed, vol 6. Philadelphia: Saunders, 2000:5117–5146.
143. Sullivan TJ, Clarke MP, Morin JD. The ocular manifestations of the Sturge-Weber syndrome. J Pediatr Ophthalmol Strabismus 1992;29:349.
144. Kerrison B. Neuro-ophthalmology of the phacomatoses. Curr Opin Ophthalmol 2000;11:413–420.
145. Sujansky E, Conradi S. Sturge–Weber syndrome: age of onset of seizures and glaucoma and the prognosis for affected children. J Child Neurol 1995;10:49–58.
146. Font RL, Ferry AP. The phakomatoses. Int Ophthalmol Clin 1972;12:1–50.
147. Susac JO, Smith JL, Scelfo RJ. The "tomato-catsup" fundus in Sturge-Weber syndrome. Ophthalmology 1979;86: 1360.
148. Sujansky E, Conradi S. Outcome of Sturge-Weber syndrome in 52 adults. Am J Med Genet 1995;57:35–45.
149. Kerrison B. Neuro-ophthalmology of the phacomatoses. Curr Opin Ophthalmol 2000;11:413–420.
150. Ito M, Sato K, Ohnuki A, Uto A. Sturge-Weber disease: operative indications and surgical results. Brain Dev 1990;12: 473–477.
151. Hecht F, Koler RD, Rigas DA, et al. Leukemia and lymphoctes in ataxia telangiectasia. Lancet 1996;2:1193.
152. Gatti RA, Boder E, Vinters HV, et al. Ataxia-telangiectasia: an interdisciplinary approach to pathogenesis. Medicine (Baltim) 1991;70:99–117.
153. Swift M, Reitnauer PF, Morrell D, et al. Breast and other cancers in families with ataxia-telangiectasia. New Engl J Med 1987;316:1289–1294.
154. Willinsky RA, Lasjaunias P, Terbrugge K, et al. Multiple cerebral arteriovenous malformations (AVMs). Review of our experience from 203 patients with cerebral vascular lesions. Neuroradiology 1990;32:207–210.
155. Schmickel R. Chromosomal deletions and enzyme deficiencies. J Pediatr 1986;108:244–246.
156. Walther C, Gruss P. Pax-6, a murine paired box gene, is expressed in the developing CNS. Development (Camb) 1991;113:1435–1449.
157. Hanson I, Fletcher J, Jordon T, et al. Mutations at the PAX6 locus are found in heterogeneous anterior segment malformations including Peters' anomaly. Nat Genet 1994;6: 168–173.
158. Mirzayans F, Pearce W, MacDonald I, Walter M. Mutation of the PAX6 gene in patients with autosomal dominant keratitis. Am J Hum Genet 1995;57:539–548.
159. Harnois C, Boisjoly HM, Jotterand V. Sporadic aniridia and Wilms' tumor: visual function evaluation of three cases. Graefes Arch Clin Exp Ophthalmol 1989;227: 244–247.
160. Nelson LB, Spaeth GL, Nowinski TS, et al. Aniridia. A review. Surv Ophthalmol 1984;28:621–642.
161. Shields MB. Textbook of Glaucoma, 4th ed. Baltimore: Williams & Wilkins, 1998.
162. Shannon RS, Mann JR, Harper E, et al. Wilms' tumour and aniridia: clinical and cytogenetic features. Arch Dis Child 1982;57:685–690.
163. Mackintosh TF, Girdwood TG, Parker DJ, Strachan IM. Aniridia and Wilms' tumour (nephroblastoma). Br J Ophthalmol 1968;52:846–848.
164. Cotlier E, Rose M, Moel SA. Aniridia, cataracts, and Wilms' tumor in monozygous twins. Am J Ophthalmol 1978;86: 129–132.
165. Traboulsi EI, Maumenee IH, Krush AJ, et al. Pigmented ocular fundus lesions in the inherited gastrointestinal polyposis syndromes and in hereditary nonpolyposis colorectal cancer. Ophthalmology 1988;95:964–969.
166. Stein EA, Brady KD. Ophthalmologic and electro-oculographic findings in Gardner's syndrome. Am J Ophthalmol 1988;106:326–331.
167. Blair N, Trempe C. Hypertrophy of the retinal pigment epithelium associated with Gardner's syndrome. Am J Ophthalmol 1980;90:661–667.
168. Traboulsi EI, Krush AJ, Gardner EJ, et al. Prevalence and importance of pigmented ocular fundus lesions in Gardner's syndrome. N Engl J Med 1987;316:661–667.
169. Olea JL, Mateos JM, Llompart A, et al. Frequency of congenital hypertrophy of the retinal pigment epithelium in familial adenomatosis polyposis. Acta Ophthalmol Scand 1996;74:48–50.
170. Nasir M, Yee R, Piest K, et al. Multiple endocrine neoplasia type III. Cornea 1991;10:454–459.
171. Kinoshita S, Tanaka F, Ohashi Y, et al. Incidence of prominent corneal nerves in multiple endocrine neoplasia type 2A. Am J Ophthalmol 1991;111:311.
172. Morrison PJ, Nevin NC. Multiple endocrine neoplasia type 2B (mucosal neuroma syndrome, Wagenmann–Froboese syndrome). J Med Genet 1996;33:779–782.
173. Gass JDM, Gieser RG, Wilkinson CP, et al. Bilateral diffuse uveal melanocytic proliferation in patients with occult carcinoma. Arch Ophthalmol 1990;108:527–533.

174. Machemer R. Zur Pathogenese des flachenhaften malignen Melanoms. Klin Monatsbl Augenheilkd 1966;148:641–652.
175. Prusiner P, Butler A, Yavitz W, Stern W. Metastatic adenocarcinoma presenting as bilateral blindness. Ann Ophthalmol 1983;15:653–656.
176. Ryll D, Campbell R, Robertson D, Brubaker S. Pseudometas-tatic lesions of the choroid. Ophthalmology 1980;87:1181–1186.
177. Prause J, Jensen O, Eisgart F, et al. Bilateral diffuse malignant melanoma of the uvea associated with large cell carcinoma, giant cell type, of the lung. Case report of a newly described syndrome. Ophthalmologica 1984;189:221–228.
178. Mullaney J, Mooney D, O'Connor M, McDonald G. Bilateral ovarian carcinoma with bilateral uveal melanoma. Br J Ophthalmol 1984;68:261–267.
179. de Wolff-Rouendall D. Bilateral diffuse benign melanocytic tumors of the uveal tract. A clinicopathological study. Int Ophthalmol 1985;7:149–160.
180. Filipic M, Ambler J. Bilateral diffuse melanocytic uveal tumours associated with systemic malignant neoplasm. Aust N Z J Ophthalmol 1986;14:293–299.
181. Tsukahara S, Wakui K, Ohzeki S. Simultaneous bilateral primary diffuse malignant uveal melanoma: case report with pathological examination. Br J Ophthalmol 1986;70: 33–38.
182. Rohrbach JM, Roggendorf W, Thanos S, et al. Simultaneous bilateral diffuse melanocytic uveal hyperplasia. Am J Ophthalmol 1990;10:49–56.
183. Thirkill CE, Roth AM, Keltner J. Cancer-associated retinopathy. Arch Ophthalmol 1987;105:372–375.
184. Grofts JW, Bachynski BN, Odel JG. Visual paraneoplastic syndrome associated with undifferentiated endometrial carcinoma. Can J Ophthalmol 1988;23:128–132.
185. Polans A, Witkowska D, Haley T, et al. Recoverin, a photoreceptor-specific calcium binding protein, is expressed by the tumor of a patient with cancer associated retinopathy. Proc Natl Acad Sci USA 1995;92:9176–9180.
186. Wiechmann a, Akots G, Hammarback J, et al. Genetic and physical mapping of human recoverin: a gene expressed in retinal photoreceptors. Invest Ophthalmol Vis Sci 1994;35: 325–331.
187. Murakami A, Yajima T, Inana G. Isolation of human retinal genes: recoverin cDNA and gene. Biochem Biophys Res Commun 1992;187:234–244.
188. Kellner U, Bornfeld N, Foerster M. Severe course of cutaneous melanoma associated paraneoplastic retinopathy. Br J Ophthalmol 1995;79:746–752.
189. Ripps H, Carr R, Siegel I, Greenstein V. Functional abnormalities in vincristine-induced night blindness. Invest Ophthalmol Vis Sci 1984;25:787–794.
190. Berson E, Lessell S. Paraneoplastic night blindness with malignant melanoma. Am J Ophthalmol 1988;106:307–311.
191. DuBois L, Sadun A, Lawton T. Inner retinal layer loss in complicated migraine. Arch Ophthalmol 1988;106:1035–1037.
192. DuBois L, Sadun A, Lawton T. Inner retinal layer loss in complicated migraine. In reply. Arch Ophthalmol 1988;109: 175.
193. Alexander K, Fishman G, Peachey N, et al. "On" response defect in paraneoplastic night blindness with cutaneous malignant melanoma. Invest Ophthalmol Vis Sci 1992;33: 477–483.
194. Mackay C, Gouras P, Yamamoti S. S-cone and rod ERGs in paraneoplastic retinal degeneration. Invest Ophthalmol Vis Sci 1992;33:1074.
195. Andreasson S, Ponjavic V, Ehinger B. Full field electroretinogram in a patient with cutaneous melanoma-associated retinopathy. Acta Ophthalmol 1993;71:487–490.
196. Kim R, Retsas S, Fitzke F, et al. Cutaneous melanoma-associated retinopathy. Ophthalmology 1994;101:1837–1843.
197. Milam A, Saari J, Jacobson S, et al. Autoantibodies against retinal bipolar cells in cutaneous melanoma-associated retinopathy. Invest Ophthalmol Vis Sci 1993;34:91–100.
198. Rush J. Paraneoplastic retinopathy in malignant melanoma. Am J Ophthalmol 1993;115:390–391.
199. Weinstein J, Kelman S, Bresnick G, Korngluth S. Paraneoplastic retinopathy associated with antiretinal bipolar cell antibodies in cutaneous malignant melanoma. Ophthalmology 1994;101:1236–1243.
200. Cideciyan A, Jacobson S. Negative electroretinograms in retinitis pigmentosa. Invest Ophthalmol Vis Sci 1993;34: 3252–3263.
201. Kellner U, Brummer S, Foerster M, Wessing A. X-linked congenital retinoschisis. Graefes Arch Clin Exp Ophthalmol 1990;228:432–437.
202. Kellner U, Foerster M. Cone dystrophies with negative photopic electroretinogram. Br J Ophthalmol 1993;77:404–409.
203. Ripps H. Night blindness revisited; from man to molecules. Invest Ophthalmol Vis Sci 1982;23:588–609.
204. Digre EB. Opsoclonus in adults—report of three cases and review of the literature. Neurology 1986;43:1165.
205. Furman JMR, Eidelman BH, Fromm GH. Spontaneous remission of paraneoplastic ocular flutter and saccadic intrusions. Neurology 1988;38:499–501.
206. Margo CE, Waltz K. Basal cell carcinoma of the eyelid and periocular skin. Surv Ophthalmol 1993;38:169–192.
207. Haas AF, Kielty DW. Basal cell carcinoma. In: Mannis MJ, Macasai MS, Huntley AC (eds). Eye and Skin Disease. Philadelphia: Lippincott-Raven, 1996:395–403.
208. Doxanas MT, Green WR, Iliff CE. Factors in successful surgical management of basal cell carcinoma of the eyelids. Am J Ophthalmol 1981;215:1239–1241.
209. Vaughn GJ, Dortzbach RK, Gayre GS. Eyelid malig-nancies. In: Yanoff M, Duker JS (eds). Ophthal-mology, 2nd ed, vol 93. Philadelphia: Mosby, 2004:711–719.
210. Mohs FE. Micrographic surgery for microscopically controlled excision of eyelid tumors. Arch Ophthalmol 1986; 104:901–909.
211. Font RL. Eyelids and lacrimal drainage system. In: Spencer WH (ed). Ophthalmic Pathology: An Atlas and Textbook, 4th ed, vol 4. Philadephia: Saunders, 1996:2218–2443.
212. Kwitko ML, Bonuik M, Zimmerman LE. Eyelid tumors with reference to lesions confused with squamous cell carcinoma. I. Incidence and errors in diagnosis. Arch Ophthalmol 1963;69:693–697.
213. Rao NA, Hidayat AA, McLean IW, et al. Sebaceous gland carcinomas of the ocular adnexa: a clinicopathologic study of 104 cases, with five-year follow-up data. Hum Pathol 1982;13:113–122.
214. Doxanas MT, Green WR. Sebaceous gland carcinoma. Arch Ophthalmol 1984;102:245–249.
215. Kass LG, Hornblass A. Sebaceous carcinoma of the ocular adnexa. Surv Ophthalmol 1989;33:477–490.
216. Conill C, Toscas I, Morilla I, et al. Radiation therapy as a curative treatment in extraocular sebaceous carcinoma (Correspondence). Br J Ophthalmol 2003;149(2):441–442.

217. Yen MT, Tse DT, Wu X, et al. Radiation therapy for local control of eyelid sebaceous cell carcinoma: report of two cases and review of the literature. Ophthal Plast Reconstr Surg 2000;16(3):211–215.

218. Rhodes AR, Weinstock MA, Fitzpatrick TB, et al. Risk factors for cutaneous melanoma: a practical method of recognizing predisposed individuals. JAMA 1987;258:3146–3154.

36 Head and Neck Cancer

Ezra E.W. Cohen, Kerstin M. Stenson, Michael Milano, and Everett E. Vokes

Cancers of the head and neck include a variety of tumors of different histology and behavior. The different subtypes represented by these tumors include squamous cell cancers, paranasal sinus cancers, nasopharyngeal carcinomas, salivary gland cancers, thyroid gland malignancies, melanomas, sarcomas, small cell neuroendocrine carcinoma, and lymphomas. By far the most commonly encountered cancers in this group, accounting for more than 90% of tumors, are the squamous cell carcinomas of the oral cavity, oropharynx, hypopharynx, larynx, and paranasal sinuses. This chapter concentrates on squamous cell carcinoma of the head and neck (SCCHN), nasopharyngeal carcinoma (NPC), and cancers of the salivary glands.

The annual worldwide incidence of head and neck cancer is approximately 500,000, whereas, in the United States, approximately 40,000 new cases are diagnosed annually.[1,2] Cancer of the head and neck accounts for 3% of all cancers in incidence in the United States and is the eighth most prevalent and deadly malignancy worldwide.[1,3] SCCHN is more common in individuals over the age of 60, in males, and in lower socioeconomic groups. These differences likely parallel the most common environmental risk factors (see following). Despite progress in diagnosis, staging, and therapy of these cancers over the past several decades, the 5-year overall survival rate remains essentially unchanged at 50%. These mortality rates are influenced by competing causes such as cardiac and respiratory disease and second primary tumors to which these individuals can be susceptible.[4,5] Nevertheless, significant developments have occurred on many fronts in the management of head and neck cancer, driven by evidence from laboratory-based and clinical research.

Squamous Cell Carcinoma

Etiology and Epidemiology

Environmental Risk Factors

There are well-recognized risk factors for SCCHN (Table 36.1), with tobacco and alcohol being the two most significant. In fact the use of these agents parallels endemic areas of SCCHN incidence such as France, Southeast Asia, and the Indian subcontinent.[6] The form of tobacco use varies with culture, but all have been associated with a higher risk of developing SCCHN. The relative risk does increase with the quantity and time of tobacco exposure, with rough estimates of 10 to 20 times greater relative risk.[7–9] In addition, although SCCHN is associated with heavy alcohol consumption without concurrent tobacco use (approximately 5 times greater risk), the dual exposure seems to increase risk synergistically up to 100 times compared with nonexposed individuals.[10] It is unclear whether second-hand smoke increases risk, although some studies have reported a 2- to 3-fold increased risk.[11]

Betel quid or areca nut chewing is practiced in many parts of Asia, although the habit is becoming less common. There are several variations of the habit depending on region, but overall, it does appear to increase risk of SCCHN, especially of the oral cavity, although odds ratios vary widely with the population studied.[12] The combination of tobacco smoking, alcohol, and betel quid chewing is especially dangerous and can increase risk of oral cancer significantly.[12]

Field Cancerization

The concept of field cancerization is an important one in SCCHN as the foremost risk factor for the disease, tobacco, results in exposure of the entire upper aerodigestive tract. The hypothesis, first described in 1953,[13] contends that environmentally related malignancies develop in a tissue that is exposed to the implicating carcinogen. Because the entire tissue is exposed, metachronous or simultaneous cancers can develop in different parts of the tissue. The upper aerodigestive tract serves as a model for this hypothesis, as evidenced by molecular derangements found in normal-appearing mucosa of SCCHN patients, the high incidence of second SCCHN primary tumors, and the high incidence of lung and upper esophageal malignancies in these patients. In fact, investigators have been able to establish clonality between second lung or esophageal tumors and the original SCCHN.[14,15] The occurrence of second cancers in this patient population accounts for a significant cause of mortality, with annual incidence rates of approximately 5%.

Viral Agents

Despite the strong association of tobacco and alcohol consumption with SCCHN, approximately 25% of patients have had no significant exposure to these carcinogens. The human papillomavirus (HPV) has been implicated in cancer of other sites including the uterine cervix, and in the early 1980s pathologists began noting morphologic changes in SCCHN that were reminiscent of HPV exposure.[16] Thus, it was hypothesized that HPV may play an etiologic role in a subset

TABLE 36.1. Risk factors for squamous cell carcinoma of the head and neck (SCCHN).

Environmental	Tobacco (smoking, chewing) Alcohol Betel quid chewing
Infectious	Human papilloma virus (oropharynx) Epstein–Barr virus (nasopharynx) *Candida albicans*
Genetic (e.g., Fanconi anemia, Li–Fraumeni syndrome)	
Ultraviolet or ionizing radiation	
Poor oral health	

of SCCHN patients. Several reports have now confirmed the presence of HPV DNA in SCCHN tissue samples,[17] and a recent meta-analysis examining 94 studies including 4,680 specimens revealed that, compared to normal oral mucosa, HPV was 2 to 3 times more likely to be detected in precancerous mucosa and 4.7 times more likely to be detected in oral carcinoma.[18] Although there are more than 100 known types of the virus, HPV 16 has been most consistently linked with SCCHN.[19]

Studies have begun to define a subset of SCCHN patients in whom HPV may be the etiologic agent.[17,20] This subset is composed of oropharangeal cancers, specifically palatine and lingual tonsil and base of tongue, younger patients, nonsmokers, and nondrinkers. The molecular biology of these cancers appears also to be different in that they are less likely to contain inactivating mutations of p53[17,20,21]; this may be due to the ability of the HPV E6 gene to inactivate p53, a necessary step during infection and propagation of the virus. In addition, several reports have also suggested that HPV-positive tumors tend to have a better prognosis compared to their non-HPV-containing counterparts.[17] To date there are few data supporting an etiologic role of other viruses in SCCHN, with the exception of Epstein–Barr virus (EBV) and NPC (see following).

Molecular Biology

Studies have shown that SCCHN harbors common molecular derangements including chromosomal, epigenetic, and specific protein alterations. Deletion of specific chromosome arms is often found including loss of 3p, 5q, 8p, 9p, 17p, 18q, and 21q.[22,23] Chromosomal deletions that appear to be particularly common, especially in precancerous lesions, are 9p21, 3p21, and 17p13. Genes of interest in these areas include p16 (9p21), FHIT and RASSF1A (3p21), and p53 (17p13).[24–30] Meanwhile, by using comparative genomic hybridization investigators have commonly observed amplification of 3q, 5p, 11q13, and 19q.[31–33] Of these, 11q13 contains a number of oncogenes including cyclin D1, which has been shown to be overexpressed in 40% to 60% of SCCHN.[34,35]

High expression levels of the epidermal growth factor receptor (EGFR) and its primary ligand, transforming growth factor-alpha (TGF-α), have also been observed in SCCHN and form an autocrine loop spurring tumor growth and survival.[36,37] Expression of EGFR has been linked with poorer survival in patients undergoing surgery or radiation.[36,38] There is also evidence that the EGFR pathway contributes to angiogenesis and metastasis of SCCHN tumors.[39,40] Other oncogenes that have been linked with worse outcome in SCCHN include the eukaryotic initiation factor 4E (eIF4E),[41] cyclooxygenase 2,[42] and p63.[43] Hypermethylation, the addition of methyl groups to CpG islands in the promoter region of a gene, is commonly observed in the context of specific genes in SCCHN,[44] including p16,[29,45,46] E-cadherin,[47] *O*-6-methylguanine-DNA-methyltransferase (MGMT),[45,47] and death-associated protein (DAP) kinase,[45,47] resulting in their silencing.

By comparing the pattern of gene expression in normal, precancerous, and cancerous tissue, investigators have created an hypothetical model of SCCHN tumorigenesis.[48] It appears that deletion of 3p and 9p are relatively early events, followed by deletion of 17p, inactivation of p16, and overexpression of cyclin D1. Mutation of p53, deletion of 10q, 13q, and 18q, and other aberrations occur later in the progression model. It is important to note that the exact sequence of events is not universal or necessary and that any lesion causing genetic instability is more likely to progress to the malignant state.

Recent evidence highlights the significance of genetic instability in SCCHN development. DNA aneuploidy, even more than grade of dysplasia, appears to be a reliable predictor of subsequent development of carcinomas in lesions of the oral cavity including leukoplakias and erythroplakias.[49–51] In fact, lesions with aneuploid DNA predicted a higher recurrence rate and mortality rate from SCCHN.

Although not associated with a single molecular event, angiogenesis is implicated in the development of every solid tumor and SCCHN is not excepted. Several proangiogenic factors including interleukin 8,[52] basic fibroblast growth factor,[53] platelet-derived growth factor,[54] and vascular endothelial growth factor (VEGF)[55,56] are secreted in SCCHN. Angiogenesis has been shown to be essential to development of early lesions and is often associated with a higher recurrence rates, distant failure, and poor survival.

Diagnosis

The great majority of SCCHN patients are diagnosed with locoregional disease, whereas only 10% of patients present with metastatic disease, usually to the lungs or bone.[57] The initial spread of SCCHN is to regional lymph nodes and is usually predictable based on anatomic drainage patterns (Figure 36.1). Patients often present with local symptoms including pain, dysphagia, and odynophagia. Specific symptoms depend on the location of the primary tumor and lymph node metastases and can include otalgia, loose teeth, poor tongue mobility, speech impairment, and hoarseness. Cranial nerve deficits are uncommon in locoregionally advanced SCCHN, with the exception of NPC and salivary gland tumors.

Clinical suspicion is confirmed by pathologic examination, which includes grading of the tumor as well-, moderately, or poorly differentiated carcinoma. Although this descriptive system is applied to almost all cases of SCCHN, tumor grade has little influence on prognosis and management.

The diagnostic evaluation also includes radiologic imaging of the head and neck, usually by computed tomography (CT) scanning. Additional studies can include panoramic radiographs if mandibular invasion is suspected and magnetic resonance imaging if CT scanning is inadequate, although these studies are often complementary. A

Cervical lymphatics.

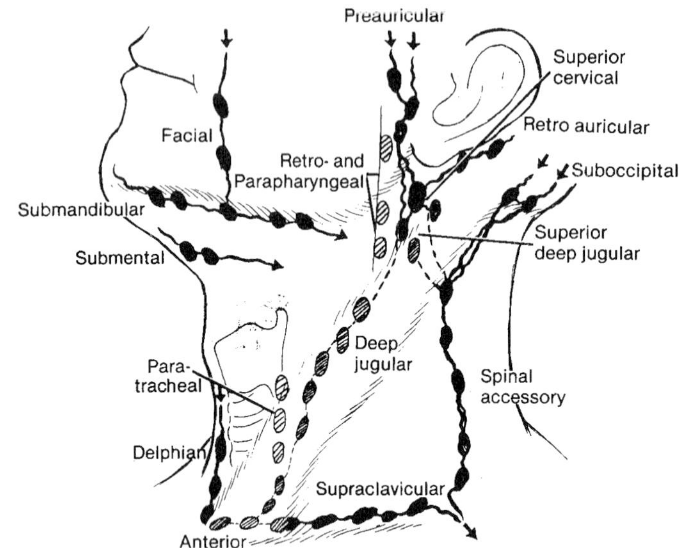

FIGURE 36.1. Cervical lymph node drainage of the head and neck. (Adapted from Cummings et al.,[172] by permission of *Otolaryngology—Head & Neck Surgery*.)

determination of baseline swallowing function is usually performed by videofluoroscopy.[58] CT scanning of the chest is often also performed, especially if advanced neck nodal spread is encountered. This practice, however, has not been tested in clinical trials, although it appears prudent to exclude metastatic disease in stage III, IVa, and IVb patients.

A subset of patients, approximately 2% to 9% of SCCHN cases, present with an expanding cervical lymph node metastasis without an obvious primary tumor.[59] When a primary site is found it is often of the oropharynx, especially the tonsil and base to tongue, likely secondary to the extensive lymphatic supply to this region, allowing early nodal spread. Often a careful clinical examination followed by radiographic tests reveals the location of the primary tumor. Occasionally patients require random biopsies of the base of tongue, pyriform sinus, and nasopharynx, or bilateral tonsillectomy depending on the location of cervical nodes. The availability of fluorodeoxyglucose positron emission tomography (FDG-PET) scanning does not appear to aid significantly in the diagnostic evaluation, allowing detection of the primary tumor in a small minority of cases.[60] For patients in whom the primary tumor is never found, the approach to treatment in these instances varies and randomized trials are lacking.[61] Neck dissection followed by extensive radiation including bilateral neck and mucosa appears to reduce local recurrence and improve survival, especially in advanced nodal disease (N2 or higher).[61]

Staging

Staging of SCCHN is based on the tumor-node-metastasis (TNM) system, which forms the single most important determinant of therapy and prognosis, making accuracy paramount. Specific staging varies with location of the primary tumor; however, some generalizations can be made across disease sites with NPC being the notable exception (see following). T4 implies that the primary tumor has invaded adjacent soft tissue or bony structures. Nodal staging is classified by the size and of involved lymph nodes, and N2 stage is further divided into N2a (one lymph node between 3 and 6cm in diameter), N2b (two or more ipsilateral lymph nodes less than 6cm in diameter), and N2c (contralateral lymph nodes less than 6cm in diameter). Of note in the staging system is that stage IV does not necessarily imply distant disease. In fact, stages IVa and IVb are still confined to locoregional involvement and only stage IVc indicates metastatic disease. Across tumor sites, T4 tumors tend to have higher local failure rates whereas N2 and N3 tumors are prone to distant failure.

Therapy

Modalities

Surgery

The Role of Endoscopy Patients with head and neck cancer are more likely to develop second primary cancers than any other group of patients with malignancies. In addition, the development of second primary tumors is the most common cause of posttreatment failure after 3 years, with an annual rate of development of 2.7% to 4 % per year.[5] Panendoscopy (laryngoscopy, esophagoscopy, bronchoscopy) is typically completed during primary site tumor staging and has been appraised by many surgeons in terms of its ability to detect second primaries. The overall second primary incidence ranges from 13.5% to 16.2% (2.6%–6.4% synchronous and 8%–9.8% metachronous).[62,63] Lung and head and neck were the most common sites of second primary tumor, followed by esophageal primary. The role of prospective panendoscopy, as a means to detect second primaries at an earlier stage, has also been studied.[64] A 2.5-fold-improved yield of metachronous tumors was seen for patients undergoing prospective panendoscopy. Routine panendoscopy remains controversial in terms of cost-effectiveness. Nonetheless, many head and neck surgeons view panendoscopy as a low-risk procedure that may greatly influence treatment decisions.

Control of Primary Site Control of the primary tumor site, regardless of modality or stage, is paramount. Local primary site failure is highly correlated with ultimate treatment failure and decreased survival. Complete wide surgical resection with adequate margins is critical when surgery is employed as primary therapy. Resected tumors with margins less than 5 mm are as likely to locally recur as a frankly positive margin.[63] Intraoperative methods to assess margin status have received attention recently. Portugal et al. prospectively studied 50 consecutive patients undergoing surgical resection of various head and neck primaries.[65] The authors applied toluidine blue, a dye that binds to nuclear material of early malignant lesions, to the remaining in situ mucosa. The toluidine blue identified a positive margin in 3 cases, which was confirmed by frozen and permanent pathologic analysis. In addition, three cases of second primary tumors were identified with this staining technique.

Postoperative techniques of assessing surgical margins have focused on application of immunostaining to paraffin-embedded mucosal margins. Ball et al. immunostained surgical margins from 24 patients with oral cavity/oropharyngeal carcinomas for abnormal p53 (tumor suppressor gene) protein.[66] There was a 5.33-fold-higher chance of local recurrence with at least one surgical margin p53 positive by sample odds ratio test. Nathan et al. evaluated the histologically free tumor margins of 52 tumor specimens for presence or absence of eIF4E, p53, and MMP-9.[67] The authors found that overexpression of eIF4E occurred in 98% of tumors and that eIF4E was a significant predictor of recurrence and disease-free interval.

The head and neck surgeon may find that the measured in situ margin differs from that reported by histopathologic measurement. Johnson et al. quantified the change in muscle and mucosal margins after resection, fixation, and slide preparation of simulated mucosal tumors in 10 mongrel dogs.[65] They found that mucosal and muscle margins shrunk significantly, 30% to 47%. The greatest proportion of shrinkage occurred immediately after resection. To obtain a 5-mm margin, the surgeon must have an in situ margin of at least 8 to 10 mm.

The Clinically Negative Neck

The hallmark of advanced (stage III or IV) head and neck cancer when associated with a small (T1 or T2) primary is the presence of a metastatic cervical node. Although there are several radiographic methods of detecting carcinoma in a cervical node, none can currently identify microscopic or occult nodal disease. The negative impact of nodal status on survival is well known and introduces the controversies surrounding the treatment of the N0 neck. The possibility of carcinoma in the cervical lymphatics, the uncertainty over who will develop clinical disease if left untreated, and the choice of modality to most effectively detect, prevent, and treat occult nodal disease are areas of fervent debate. Complete discussion of these issues extends beyond the scope of this section. However, several recent studies could help clarify the ongoing uncertainties.

Treatment recommendations for the N0 neck can be analyzed on a site-by-site basis.[68] There is a significant incidence of occult nodal disease in all but the earliest and most superficial carcinomas of the oral cavity, oropharynx, larynx, and hypopharynx. Expectant management of the neck is not recommended given the observation that neck failures after observation tend to be high stage and portend a poor prognosis.[68] Therefore, most surgeons support the following management philosophy: if the risk of occult metastatic disease exceeds 15%, the neck should be electively treated. If surgery is chosen for the primary tumor, elective selective neck dissection is advised. Alternatively, if the primary tumor is to be irradiated, the neck should be electively irradiated.

Functional neck surgery represents a shift in the surgical management of occult cervical metastatic disease. By saving important anatomic structures that were routinely sacrificed in the classic radical neck dissection, the selective neck dissection produces less functional morbidity and aesthetic defects than the radical neck dissection.

Several authors have studied the utility of selective neck dissection in patients with a clinically and radiographically N0 neck.[69] Selective neck dissection was found to be as effective as a comprehensive neck dissection, and recurrences outside the dissected levels in the selective neck dissection group were not significant. The authors strongly advocate elective neck dissection in patients with N0 disease, as this is the most accurate method available to diagnose occult metastatic disease. The prognostic information obtained from the pathologic specimen is invaluable in terms of staging accuracy and in identifying high-risk patients who would benefit from postoperative therapy.

Sentinel Lymph Node Biopsy

Sentinel lymph node mapping was originally developed as a means to stage the first-echelon lymphatics of cutaneous melanoma. Recent literature has supported its application in mucosal head and neck squamous cell carcinoma.[70] Researchers have found that the technique is minimally invasive, technically feasible, and predictive of cervical metastatic disease. This method is currently under investigation at several institutions and promises to further refine the assessment of occult regional metastases.

Radiotherapy

For early-stage cancer, surgery or radiotherapy alone is effective. Radiotherapy can be delivered via external beam and/or interstitial brachytherapy (where radioactive sources are inserted into needles that are placed into the tumor). For intermediate- and advanced-stage cancer, surgery and radiation or definitive radiation alone is effective. Unresectable cancers, particularly most early-stage nasopharyngeal cancers, can be cured by radiation alone.

Radiation Therapy Techniques Radiation is delivered to the primary site, including involved lymph nodes, as well as lymph nodes at risk for occult, microscopic disease. Hence, radiation planning requires a thorough understanding of the risk of clinical lymph node involvement, the risk of pathologic, occult lymph node involvement, and the patterns of nodal failure; these vary by the site of the primary and stage of disease.[71,72] Knowledge of subclinical spread at the primary site is also important.

Traditionally radiation has been delivered to the primary site and upper cervical lymph nodes with opposed lateral (OL) fields, with the dose prescribed to midplane. A supraclavicular is delivered with an anteroposterior (AP) field, matched to the opposed lateral field. A block on either the OL or AP field protects the spinal cord at the match line, although it is important that this block not traverse through gross tumor. Periodic field shifts at the match line (termed feathering) allow for any radiation hot spots to be better distributed. After spinal cord tolerance has been reached (~45 Gy), the opposed lateral fields are modified such that an anterior opposed lateral field is matched to a posterior electron field; because electrons are less penetrating, the spinal cord does not receive any further dose.

Three-dimensional (3-D) planning necessitates a CT scan during planning and provides detailed dose–volume information on the target as well as normal structures. Modification of the fields with either multiple segmented fields or variable weighting of fields can improve the homogeneity of the dose distribution. Intensity-modulated radiation therapy (IMRT) is a form of 3-D planning that allows more conformal radiation delivery by varying the radiation beams spatially and/or temporally.[72–74] Hence, IMRT allows for greater sparing of normal structures such as salivary glands, esophagus, optic nerves, brainstem, and spinal cord.[75,76] IMRT avoids the limitations of tumor boost doses, eliminates the need for posterior neck electron therapy, and enables simultaneous boosting, a technique that allows for higher doses to be delivered to regions at higher risk for failure (such as gross disease), with lower doses prescribed to areas of microscopic disease.[77]

IMRT is readily applied to head and neck cancer as the region is readily immobilized and gross disease will often be adjacent to critical normal tissue. Patients who are most likely to benefit, therefore, are those in whom the tumor volume may be compromised to spare normal tissue or where standard radiotherapy fields would encompass the salivary glands. Thus far randomized trials comparing IMRT with standard radiotherapy have not been completed. However, failures that have been observed on Phase I and II IMRT trials have been noted within high-dose regions, suggesting inherent tumor resistance rather than underdosing of subclinical disease.[78,79]

Postoperative Radiation Therapy Radiation is delivered post-operatively (PORT) to patients with locoregionally advanced disease. M.D. Anderson Cancer Center (MDACC) conducted a randomized trial comparing 57.6 Gy versus 63 Gy PORT in low-risk patients and 63.0 versus 68.4 Gy in high-risk patients, with patients stratified by stage, margin status, perineural invasion, extracapsular extension (ECE), number of lymph nodes, and size of lymph nodes.[80] The higher-dose arms did not afford any benefit in outcome. Performance status and radiation delay resulted in a worse prognosis. Adverse tumor-related factors included ECE and/or two or more of oral cavity primary site, positive margins, perineural invasion, more than two lymph nodes, and lymph nodes greater than 3 cm. In a follow-up study by MDACC, patients were stratified by risk factors.[81] Low-risk patients had no adverse tumor-related factors and therefore received no PORT. Intermediate-risk patients had one adverse risk factor, except ECE; these patients received 57.6 Gy PORT. High-risk patients were defined as having ECE and/or two or more other adverse risk factors. Five-year locoregional control in these groups was 90%, 94%, and 68%, respectively; 5-year overall survival was 83%, 66%, and 42%, respectively. The MDACC experience provides a guide to which patients may benefit from PORT and the doses to administer.

The Role of Edoscopy Conventional radiation fractionation (CF) implies daily radiation delivered 5 days a week. Altered fractionation is a variation of this. Important temporal variables include the repair of sublethal damage, reassortment of cells within the cell cycle, repopulation, and reoxygenation. Ideally, radiation is delivered in such a manner to maximize damage to cancerous cells while minimizing normal tissue damage. Altered fractionation schemes should be delivered such that they provide a biologically equivalent (or greater) dose than conventional fractionation. Hyperfractionation (HF) entails an increased number of fractions, with a decreased fraction dose, but unchanged overall treatment time. Accelerated fractionation (AF) implies the same number of fractions, same total dose, but delivered over shorter time duration.

Several randomized trials comparing CF to AF have shown no survival or tumor control benefit, and worse toxicity with AF.[82–84] The CHART trial compared 66 Gy in 2-Gy fractions to continuous delivery of 54 Gy in 1.5, three-times-daily fractions. Severe mucositis was worse in the CHART arm. Two randomized trials have shown improved outcomes with HF regimens delivering radiation in six or seven daily treatments per week.[85,86] Skladowski et al. showed improved overall survival and locoregional control with a 7-day-per-week versus a 5-day-per-week radiation regimen.[86] A Norwegian trial has shown improved locoregional control and disease-free survival with a 6-day-per-week versus 5-day-per-week radiation regimen, although overall survival was not significantly impacted.[85]

The RTOG conducted a randomized trial with four arms: (1) CF 70 Gy in 2-Gy daily fractions; (2) HF 81.6 Gy in 1.2-Gy twice-daily fractions; (3) AF split (2-week break) 67.2 Gy in 1.6-Gy twice-daily fractions; and (4) 32.4 Gy in 1.8-Gy daily fractions followed by twice-daily radiation, with 1.8 Gy to delivered to a large field and 1.5 Gy to the boost field (63 Gy total). The HF arm and simultaneous boost arm yielded the best locoregional control and disease-free survival, whereas overall survival was similar in all arms.

Chemotherapy

Traditionally, chemotherapy had been reserved for patients with incurable SCCHN, usually as a palliative measure. Several randomized trials have now clearly demonstrated that chemotherapy as part of a multimodality approach that includes surgery and radiotherapy does improve survival and allow for organ preservation in almost every setting (see following).[87] There are a number of chemotherapy agents that are active in SCCHN (Table 36.2), with platinum compounds being the mainstay of most chemotherapeutic regimens.[88] Cisplatin appears to be superior to carboplatin, as demonstrated by at least two randomized trials.[89,90] Antimetabolites are also active in SCCHN, with 5-fluorouracil commonly used in

TABLE 36.2. Active agents in SCCHN.

Agent	*Relative risk (RR)*	*Reference*
Methotrexate	6%–10%[a]	90, 187
5-Fluorouracil	13%[a]	188
Cisplatin	14%–17%[a]	187–189
Paclitaxel	40%	190
Docetaxel	20%–42%	191–193
Ifosfamide	4%–42%	194–197
Vinorelbine	8%–14%	198, 199
Gemcitabine	0%–13%	200, 201

[a] These response rates are based on Phase III randomized trials.

combination with cisplatin, and capecitabine more recently introduced. In addition, taxanes (paclitaxel and docetaxel), vinorelbine, gemcitabine, bleomycin, and mitomycin C also have single-agent activity in this disease.[88]

Stage-Specific Therapy

Early Stage

In general, patients with early-stage carcinomas of the upper aerodigestive tract enjoy an overall good prognosis when treated with a single curative-intent modality. Radiotherapeutic or surgical approaches are chosen based on anatomic location, surgical access, functional outcome, and long-term consequences of radiation. The following discussion focuses on operative management of early-stage head and neck cancer and highlights issues surrounding the choice of radiation versus surgery.

Oral Cavity The oral cavity includes the lip, anterior tongue, floor of mouth, hard palate, alveolar ridge, retromolar trigone, and buccal mucosa. Because of the permanent dry mouth that invariably develops from radiation to these areas, wide local excision is the preferred management of these early-stage patients. The resections are by nature both organ- and function preserving. Achieving negative margins is critical.[91,92] The lymphatics in the oral cavity are rich and often bilateral. In addition, occult cervical metastatic disease is highly correlated with tumor thickness.[93] Hence, the surgeon strongly considers selective neck dissection(s) for all but the most superficial carcinomas, as curative salvage neck surgery is associated with poor outcomes.[94] Rim mandibulectomy is performed for those tumors adjacent to or inseparable from the mandible, ascertaining that at least 10mm of inferior rim remains to prevent fracture.[95] Early-stage hard palate malignancies are resected en masse with palatal bone, preserving the underlying nasal mucosa if possible, or reconstruction with local flaps.[96]

There are many options for reconstruction of the surgical defect. Tongue, floor of mouth, and buccal defects can be left to granulate or grafted with split-thickness skin. The buccal myomucosal flap has been a very reliable and technically easy method to reconstruct a myriad of other oral cavity defects in many surgeons' hands.[97]

Oropharynx Carcinomas of the tongue base, soft palate, and tonsil areas have been historically and preferentially treated with radiotherapy because of difficult surgical access and reported poor functional outcomes with resection.[98] Currently, there are numerous acceptable treatments for carcinomas of the oropharynx, reflecting advances in imaging and operative and cytoreductive techniques.[99–101] Recent analyses of tongue base treatments have found that similar dysfunctions of the tongue remain after either surgical or nonoperative therapy.[102] More surgeons are performing a transhyoid pharyngotomy as a means for surgical access to the oropharynx.[100,103] This approach provides wide exposure and avoids the potential morbidity of lateral or paramedian mandibular osteotomy. Steiner et al. have popularized transoral laser microsurgery, which represents a recent innovation in the treatment of tongue base cancers.[104] This organ-preserving resection has exceptional functional and oncologic results for early-stage tongue base cancers. In addition, most surgeons would perform staging-selective neck dissection(s) for these lesions.

Hypopharynx Early-stage cancers of the piriform sinus, posterior pharyngeal wall, and postcricoid areas are fairly rare. Even small lesions often present with cervical and/or distant metastatic disease.[105] Although radiation offers similar survival rates for T1–T2 lesions, proponents of surgical therapy believe that salvage surgery for radiation failures yields dismal results. In addition, surgeons found that patients who underwent larger resections (laryngectomy or pharyngolaryngectomy) had significantly better survival than those who underwent partial pharyngectomy.[106] Fortunately, surgeons have pioneered resection and reconstructive techniques that permit organ and function preservation.

Lesions of the posterior pharyngeal wall can be accessed via a transhyoid pharyngotomy, resected with laryngeal preservation, and functionally reconstructed with free tissue transfer.[107] A technique called supracricoid hemilaryngopharyngectomy has gained recognition as a means to perform oncologically sound resection and tracheotomy decannulation while preserving phonation and swallowing.[108] Moreover, endoscopic laser microsurgery for piriform sinus carcinomas has resulted in preservation of function and high recurrence-free survival.[109] These state-of-art methods challenge the historical dogma of laryngopharyngectomy and may progress the standard of care for early-stage hypopharyngeal carcinoma.

Larynx Both radiation and surgery offer high survival rates for patients with early glottic and supraglottic carcinoma. Treatment recommendations are based upon careful radiologic and clinical staging, appropriate patient selection, methods available to the radiation oncologist, and expertise of the surgeon.

Glottis Endoscopic laser microresection has emerged as an oncologically sound, cost-effective, and voice-preserving modality for many patients with T1–T2 carcinoma of the vocal cords, including the anterior commissure.[110–114] The use of the operating microscope enhances the surgeon's detection of dysplastic versus normal wound architecture and ultimately enables simultaneous staging and definitive treatment in one setting. The neck is typically observed in early glottic cancers, due to the sparse lymphatics draining this region. Vertical hemilaryngectomy remains a viable option for selected patients, but unlike laser resection, requires laryngeal framework disassembly and reconstruction. More surgeons are reserving hemilaryngectomy for local radiation failures.

Supraglottis Supraglottic laryngectomy is the time-honored method for controlling early cancers of the supraglottic structures.[115,116] Temporary pulmonary aspiration frequently results from this voice-sparing surgery. Therefore, patients must preoperatively demonstrate adequate pulmonary reserve. Transoral laser resection limits much of the morbidity of open/transcervical surgery and is evolving into an important technique that provides oncologic, functional, and cost-effective results.[117] Unlike the glottic larynx, the supraglottic structures have rich, bilateral lymphatic drainage, which dictates bilateral selective neck dissections.

Intermediate Stage

Intermediate-stage tumors usually consist of stage III tumors and selected stage II malignancies, such as those arising from the base of the tongue or pyriform sinus. The term characterizes malignancies that are too advanced to be readily curable by a single-modality therapy such as surgery or radiation therapy yet carry a more-favorable prognosis than stage IV (M0) cancers, with cure rates ranging from 40% to 60%. Historically, treatment for this group of patients has consisted of surgery with postoperative radiation therapy.

The use of postoperative concurrent chemoradiotherapy has been of more interest. Initial pilot studies combining surgery with postoperative radiation and simultaneous cisplatin chemotherapy were promising. Recently, two large randomized trials investigating postoperative concurrent chemoradiotherapy have been reported. First was a trial conducted by the EORTC that compared postoperative radiation therapy with postoperative radiation (66 Gy) given with concurrent cisplatin administered 100 mg/m^2 on days 1, 22, and 43.[118] Eligible patients included "high-risk" resected patients defined by pathologic criteria such as positive surgical margins, involvement of two or more cervical lymph nodes, or extracapsular spread. The results of this trial were favorable and supported the administration of concomitant chemoradiotherapy. Progression-free survival (47% versus 36%; $P = 0.04$) and overall survival (53% versus 40%; $P = 0.02$) at 5 years were significantly in favor of the chemoradiotherapy arm. This result was attributed to the effect of combined treatment on locoregional control with 5-year locoregional relapse rates of 31% for radiotherapy and 18% for chemoradiotherapy ($P = 0.007$). A similar trial was conducted by the RTOG, comparing postoperative radiotherapy to 60 Gy with or without three doses of cisplatin on days 21, 42, and 63.[119] Again, locoregional control was improved with combination therapy (82% versus 72% at 2 years; $P = 0.01$). In addition, disease-free survival (hazard ratio, 0.78; $P = 0.04$), but not overall survival (hazard ratio, 0.84; $P = 0.19$), was also improved. With two positive trials showing similar findings, it can be argued that the combined evidence of these studies supports the administration of concomitant chemoradiotherapy in the postoperative setting.

Another recent randomized study with a focus on intermediate-state disease was the Larynx Intergroup Trial.[120] This trial followed up on the previous observations in the Veterans Administration laryngeal preservation trial that had compared surgery and postoperative radiotherapy with three cycles of induction chemotherapy followed by radiotherapy and surgical salvage.[121] That trial showed no difference in survival in patients treated on either arm of the study but confirmed a larynx preservation rate of 64% in patients receiving chemotherapy. Subsequently, the Intergroup conducted a three-arm trial comparing the induction chemotherapy arm as defined by the VA Larynx Trial with either radiation alone or radiotherapy with concomitant cisplatin.[120] Eligible patients included those with stage III and IV laryngeal cancer. However, patients with advanced T4 lesions characterized by invasion of the thyroid cartilage were excluded. Thus, this trial can be considered as applying to intermediate-stage patients. There was no difference in survival between the three arms. However, the larynx preservation rate was highest (85%) in patients receiving concurrent chemoradiotherapy. Similarly the proportion of patients alive with a functioning larynx was highest on the concurrent chemoradiotherapy arm (45% at 5 years versus 41% for patients treated with induction chemotherapy and 37% for the radiotherapy-alone group). Thus, concomitant chemoradiotherapy (with surgical salvage for patients with residual disease following completion of therapy or with later local recurrence) is the current standard therapy for patients with intermediate-stage larynx cancer.

Finally, pilot trials investigating concomitant chemoradiotherapy with surgical salvage for a broad group of patients with stages II and III head and neck cancer have been conducted. Haraf et al. from the University of Chicago reported on a Phase II trial in which patients received concurrent chemoradiotherapy utilizing fluorouracil (5-FU) and hydroxyurea administered with concurrent hyperfractionated radiation therapy every other week.[122] In this phase II trial, the 5-year disease-specific survival was 82%, with 86% of patients achieving long-term locoregional control, whereas the overall 3- and 5-year survival rates were 74% and 65%, respectively. These data suggested that concurrent chemoradiotherapy is a highly efficacious approach for intermediate-stage head and neck cancer and, similar to the aforementioned larynx Intergroup trial, suggest that most patients do not need to be exposed to a surgical approach as a first treatment option.

Locally Advanced Head and Neck Cancer

Patients with locoregionally advanced head and neck cancer have traditionally been treated with surgery and PORT or radiotherapy alone for patients with unresectable disease. As overall survival rates following this approach were low and significant functional and psychologic sequelae frequent, combined modality therapies have been investigated. Initially, strategies focused on the use of induction chemotherapy. Although regimens such as the combination of cisplatin and 5-FU were shown to be active, resulting in overall response rates exceeding 80% and complete response rates of approximately 50%,[121,123] most subsequent randomized trials demonstrated no significant effect on survival.[87] Meta-analyses evaluating the impact of chemotherapy on survival rates of advanced head and neck cancer also suggested no benefit from the use of induction chemotherapy.[124] Only an analysis of those trials specifically utilizing the combination of cisplatin and 5-FU suggested a small impact of approximately 5% on 5-year survival rates. However, despite the positive impact of induction therapy on distant failure, at this time there is no convincing evidence justifying the use of induction chemotherapy outside of a well-designed clinical trial in patients with SCCHN.

At the same time, several trials were initiated investigating the concurrent administration of chemotherapy and radiation. Because many patients with head and neck cancer fail locoregionally, the radiosensitizing effects of chemotherapy appear of particular importance. Early trials utilized single agents such as methotrexate,[125] bleomycin,[126] mitomycin-C,[127] or cisplatin[128] and were usually conducted in patients with unresectable disease. Many of these trials were in themselves inconclusive. However, a meta-analysis confirmed an 8% increase in absolute 5-year overall survival rate favoring concurrent chemoradiotherapy compared with radiotherapy alone.[124] This finding suggested that, for unresectable disease at least, concurrent chemoradiotherapy might be a more successful approach.

In recent years, several larger randomized trials comparing multiagent concurrent chemoradiotherapy (such as cisplatin and 5-FU) with radiation therapy alone have confirmed this prior observation.[87] Studies conducted both in the United States and Europe have demonstrated an increase of up to 20% in 3-year absolute survival rates for patients treated on the concurrent chemoradiotherapy arm.

Additional trials have utilized concurrent chemoradiotherapy as a definitive treatment strategy hoping for organ preservation in addition to increasing survival rates. Pilot trials conducted by the RTOG,[129] investigators at the University of Chicago,[130,131] and the Cleveland Clinic[132] have all suggested that high survival rates exceeding 50% can be achieved for patients with locoregionally advanced disease even when omitting surgery. For example, a study at the University of Chicago treating patients with a combination of paclitaxel, 5-fluorouracil, hydroxyurea, and twice-daily radiation therapy administered every other week, to a total radiation dose of 75 Gy, demonstrated a 3-year survival rate of 60% in patients with stage IV regionally advanced disease.[131]

Of note, when evaluating the pattern of failure in patients with regionally advanced disease treated with concurrent chemoradiotherapy alone, it became clear that a higher proportion of patients were failing distantly than were failing locally. This finding represents a reversal of the failure pattern observed in patients treated with surgery and/or radiotherapy and has led to recent interest in studies combining both induction chemotherapy (for better distant disease control) and concurrent chemoradiotherapy (for improved locoregional control). Pilot trials from the University of Chicago[133,134] as well as the University of Pennsylvania[135] have indicated that this approach is feasible and highly active. Randomized evaluation of the use of induction chemotherapy with concurrent chemoradiotherapy is planned for the near future.

Surgery and Reconstruction in the Patient Who Has Undergone Multimodality Therapy

The goals of multimodality strategies for patients with advanced head and neck cancer encompass organ preservation through less-radical surgery and improved survival. As multimodality organ preservation strategies are becoming more successful, the role of surgery is being redefined. Individualized treatment, with attention to important perioperative factors and utilization of vascularized tissue, is critical. These treatment approaches may help prevent surgical complications as well as help resolve the complications of multimodality therapy for these challenging patients. It is a general dogma held by most surgeons that performing surgery upon a patient who has previously undergone radiation or chemoradiation (CRT) is a challenging task. The surgery may not only be technically difficult but may be associated with a higher incidence of complications such as wound healing problems and infection.

Type of Neck Dissection The patient should undergo biopsy of the primary tumor site with frozen-section pathologic analysis. If the biopsy is negative for carcinoma, a selective neck dissection is completed at the same sitting as the biopsy. If the biopsy is indeterminate or positive, neck dissection is deferred until permanent pathology is available. In this manner, the primary tumor site and the neck may be operated at the same time if there is viable cancer at the primary site. The patient is consented to reflect these scenarios.

The selective type of dissection preserves the sternocleidomastoid muscle (SCM), internal jugular vein, and accessory nerve.[136] A supraomohyoid (levels 1–3) or lateral (levels 2–4) neck dissection is most often performed. If the SCM must be sacrificed (e.g., for gross tumor in SCM in salvage neck dissection), one should strongly consider placement of a pectoralis myofascial flap (PMMF) for vessel coverage and to provide the patient with a more aesthetic neck contour.[137] These flaps are straightforward, efficient to elevate, and can prevent the potentially catastrophic complication of carotid exposure and rupture.

Primary Site Recurrence In general, resection of primary site recurrences transgress the pharyngeal barrier and are prone to fistula and wound breakdown. Use of vascularized tissue and prolonged use of large suction drains has improved our wound management strategies.[138]

Larynx It is imperative that a patient requiring laryngectomy be evaluated by the Speech and Swallowing Pathologist before surgery. Patients who require laryngectomies for recurrence also undergo bilateral selective neck dissections if feasible and undergo G-tube placement before or at the same sitting as the laryngectomy. A Provox or other tracheoesophageal prosthesis is placed.[139] A "prophylactic" PMMF is placed over the suture line to prevent fistula and/or to hasten healing if a fistula should form. For laryngectomy defects that require resection of a large portion of pharynx (leaving 2 cm or less of pharyngeal wall), one should also consider use of free radial forearm. Large-bore drains are placed and remain for 10 days to 3 weeks to manage potential fistulas.

Tongue Hemitongue defects can be managed with radial forearm flap reconstruction.[140] The more-radical total glossectomy defects are better managed with the more bulky rectus free flap.[141] One should strongly consider laryngeal preservation in the young motivated patient with adequate pulmonary reserve. The bulk of the rectus flap allows control of oral secretions as well as understandable speech.

Composite Defects Patients who are edentulous and who have low-volume posterolateral jaw defects without significant soft tissue loss may heal and function well with PMMF. The bulk of the PMMF will prevent significant "drift" of this nonreconstructed edentulous mandible. Mandible–floor of mouth–tongue defects in the chemoradiated patient are best managed with vascularized bone flaps such as the fibula free flap with or without a radial forearm free flap. Often, external as well as internal coverage is provided with the fibula flap alone. A portion of the skin paddle is deepithelialized so that vascularized skin bridges both intraoral and skin defects.

Recurrent or Metastatic Disease

Patients who fail therapy or present with metastatic disease are usually treated with palliative intent to preserve comfort and quality of life. Notwithstanding, there are occasional patients with only local recurrence who can be offered surgical salvage (see foregoing discussion). Reports of case series have suggested 15% long-term survival in these selected patients. Nevertheless, for the majority of patients with recurrent disease or for those with metastatic foci, the mainstay of treatment is systemic chemotherapy. These patients

TABLE 36.3. Randomized trials in recurrent and/or metastatic SCCHN.

Regimens	*RR (%)*	*Reference*
CDDP/5-FU	11	187
CDDP/MTX	12	
MTX	6	
CDDP	14	
CDDP/5-FU	32	188
CDDP	17	
5-FU	13	
CDDP/5-FU	32	90
CBDCA/5-FU	21	
MTX	10	
CDDP/MTX/BLEO/VCR	34	189
CDDP/5-FU	31	
CDDP	15	
CDDP/5-FU/IFN-α2b	47	202
CDDP/5-FU	38	
CDDP/PAC (high dose)	35	203
CDDP/PAC (low dose)	36	
CDDP/5-FU	22	204
CDDP/PAC	28	

CDDP = cisplatin; CBDCA = carboplatin; IFN-α2b = interferon α2b; 5-FU = 5-fluorouracil; BLEO = bleomycin; PAC = paclitaxel; MTX = methotrexate; VCR = vincristine

have expected median survivals of 6 to 8 months and 1-year survival rates of 20% to 30%.[87]

Randomized clinical trials would suggest that combination chemotherapy with two agents, compared with single agents, yields superior response rates in the range of 30% to 40% (Table 36.3). However, combination chemotherapy has not proven superior with respect to overall survival compared to single agents and has never been tested against best supportive care. Despite this, it is common practice to treat patients in this setting with combination chemotherapy, usually consisting of cisplatin with 5-FU or a taxane. In the only randomized trials comparing cisplatin with carboplatin, the agents were combined with 5-FU, revealing an improved response rate in the cisplatin-treated patients.[89,90] The possible superiority of cisplatin, however, must be tempered by its toxicity, and carboplatin continues to be commonly administered, especially with a taxane.

The lack of a demonstrated survival advantage to cytotoxic chemotherapy and the poor survival of these patients have opened the door to testing targeted agents in this disease. The first class of agents to undergo testing in this setting is the EGFR inhibitors. The agents in clinical use include two small molecule inhibitors, gefitinib and erlotinib, and a monoclonal antibody, cetuximab. Both gefitinib and erlotinib have been tested in the Phase II setting, demonstrating 11%[142] and 4%[143] response rates, respectively. Cetuximab has undergone testing in a Phase III trial in combination with cisplatin compared to placebo.[144] This trial, enrolling 123 patients, revealed an improved response rate in the cisplatin/cetuximab arm, but no differences were observed in progression-free survival, the primary endpoint, or overall survival.

Chemoprevention

The concept of chemoprevention asserts that medical therapy has the ability to interrupt or delay the progression of premalignant lesions. The rationale behind chemoprevention strategies applied in SCCHN is based on knowledge of fundamental molecular derangements in its carcinogenesis (see foregoing), the ability to identify a group of patients at relatively high risk of developing cancer, and lesions that are clinically apparent (oral leukoplakia or erythroplakia). Although it is clear that the majority of leukoplastic and erythroplastic lesions do not progress to malignancy and that histology is a poor predictor of outcome,[145] this model has been the most commonly employed in early pilot trials. Recent work suggests that molecular markers such as aneuploidy are much better prognostic markers.[49–51]

The retinoic acid receptor (RAR) has been a subject of intensive research in chemoprevention as stimulation of the receptor is an integral part of mucosal differentiation and influences expression of several other key genes. Furthermore, RAR-β expression is reduced in premalignant lesions and can be restored by retinoic acid (RA) therapy (isotretinoin).[146] Early randomized trials employing high-dose 13-*cis* RA demonstrated efficacy in reversing premalignant lesions or fewer second malignancies[147,148]; however, this therapy was associated with unacceptable mucocutaneous toxicity and relapses once therapy was discontinued. Thus far, low-dose RA therapy, although tolerable, has not been efficacious.[149,150] A strategy of combination "bioadjuvant" therapy combining interferon-α, α-tocopherol, and 13-*cis* RA has shown promising results[151,152] and is currently being evaluated in a Phase III trial versus observation alone in stage III or IV patients with previously treated SCCHN.

More-recent chemopreventative approaches have employed virally delivered gene therapy,[153] cyclooxygenase 2 COX-2 inhibition,[154] and Bowan–Birk inhibitor concentrate.[155] Clearly, future success in this area will hinge on improved definition of high-risk molecular markers and an understanding of the molecular mechanism of action of any therapy. In addition, it will be necessary for any agent to either possess the ability to eliminate the genetically altered clones or be administered for prolonged periods of time to otherwise healthy individuals.

Nasopharyngeal Carcinoma

Nasopharyngeal carcinoma (NPC) is a well-defined subset of head and neck cancer that requires separate discussion with respect to its pathology, epidemiology, and treatment options. Etiologically, nasopharyngeal cancer is linked to Epstein–Barr virus (EBV) exposure. Evidence of persistent EBV latency in nasopharyngeal cancer cells is present in the majority of cases.[156] Patients with nasopharyngeal cancer are also known to have high EBV antibody titers, which appear to correlate with tumor burden.[157] Measurement of serum EBV DNA has been used to predict clinical treatment outcome.[158] Additional factors contributing to carcinogenesis in the nasopharynx have been implied, such as high-temperature indoor cooking, consumption of salted preserved fish,[159] or, in the United States and Western Europe, more traditional risk factors including smoking and alcohol exposure.

The epidemiology of NPC is highly distinct from that of other head and neck cancers. The disease occurs in

TABLE 36.4. Definition of nasopharyngeal cancer (NPC) TNM.

Tumor	
T1	Tumor confined to the nasopharynx
T2	Tumor extends to soft tissues
T2a	Tumor extends to the oropharynx and/or nasal cavity without parapharyngeal extension[a]
T2b	Any tumor with parapharyngeal extension[a]
T3	Tumor involves bony structures and/or paranasal sinuses
T4	Tumor with intracranial extension and/or involvement of cranial nerves, infratemporal fossa, hypopharynx, orbit, or masticator space
Regional lymph nodes	
NX	Regional lymph nodes cannot be assessed
N0	No regional lymph node metastasis
N1	Unilateral metastasis in lymph node(s), 6 cm or less in greatest dimension, above the supraclavicular fossa[b]
N2	Bilateral metastasis in lymph node(s), 6 cm or less in greatest dimension, above the supraclavicular fossa[b]
N3	Metastasis in a lymph node(s)[b] more than 6 cm and/or to supraclavicular fossa
N3a	Greater than 6 cm in dimension
N3b	Extension to the supraclavicular fossa[c]

[a] Parapharyngeal extension denotes posterolateral infiltration of tumor beyond the pharyngobasilar fascia.

[b] Midline nodes are considered ipsilateral nodes.

[c] Supraclavicular zone or fossa is relevant to the staging of nasopharyngeal carcinoma and is the triangular region originally described by Ho. It is defined by three points: (1) the superior margin of the sternal end of the clavicle, (2) the superior margin of the lateral end of the clavicle, and (3) the point where the neck meets the shoulder. Note that this would include caudal portions of levels IV and V. All cases with lymph nodes (whole or part) in the fossa are considered N3b.

Source: Used with the permission of the American Joint Committee on Cancer (AJCC), Chicago, Illinois. The original source for this material is the *AJCC Cancer Staging Manual*, sixth edition (2002), published by Springer-Verlag New York, www.springer-ny.com.

an endemic form in the Far East and the Mediterranean countries.[160] In addition, clustering in families has been observed.[161,162] These observations suggest the presence of genetic susceptibility as a cofactor with latent EBV infection as well as additional aforementioned factors.

The pathology of NPC has been defined by the World Health Organization.[163] Generally, three types of malignancy are identified; these include the most frequent undifferentiated form of NPC (type III) frequently also referred to as lymphoepithelioma. This is the form associated with the endemicity. Types I and II represent less-common forms of keratinizing (type I) and nonkeratinizing (type II) squamous cell cancers. Lymphomas and plasmacytomas are also observed.

Clinical Presentation

The clinical presentation of NPC can be quite succinct. Patients can present with epistaxis, stuffy nose, uni- or bilateral otitis media caused by blockage of the eustachian tube, or headaches and visual problems related to skull base invasion or cranial nerve involvement. Because of the rich perfusion of the nasopharynx by lymphatic and blood vessels, early spread to lymph nodes is frequently seen. As a consequence, patients can present with massive bilateral lymphadenopathy including lymph nodes in the posterior cervical chains.[164] Similarly, systemic dissemination to lungs, bones, and liver occurs more frequently and earlier than seen in other malignancies arising from head and neck mucosal tissues.[164]

The staging of NPC also differs from that of the other head and neck malignancies. Criteria for T stage are displayed in Tables 36.4 and 36.5. Similarly, the staging of lymph node involvement is different from that of other head and neck malignancies. In particular, the specific location of involved lymph nodes in the neck area plays a more important part. Involvement of low cervical or supraclavicular lymph nodes has clearly been identified as negative prognostic factors. The definition of lymph node staging and TNM classification for overall stage classification are shown in Table 36.5.

Therapy

The therapy of nasopharyngeal cancer has largely been defined by randomized trials conducted exclusively in patients with this disease. Many of these originate in Europe and the Far East, consistent with the higher incidence in those regions. As a rule, NPC is considered unresectable, and as a consequence the primary treatment modality has been radiotherapy. Single-modality radiotherapy can be curative, particularly when administered in high doses. Combined modality therapies have been evaluated.[165,166] In the United States, a randomized trial investigated the use of concomitant cisplatin followed by two cycles of adjuvant cisplatin and 5-FU.[165] It demonstrated a clear superiority in survival when compared with radiation therapy alone (3-year survival, 47% versus 78%; $P = 0.005$). This trial, Intergroup 0099, included a histologic mix of World Health Organization (WHO) types I, II, and III patients. In addition, the control arm of patients treated with radiotherapy alone did quite poorly. It has therefore been questioned whether these results could be applied to NPC in endemic areas. However, because NPC is rare in this country and the combined modality arm resulted in a significant survival advantage, it has been considered to provide sufficient evidence to adopt concurrent chemoradiotherapy as

TABLE 36.5. Stage grouping of NPC.

Stage	*T*	*N*	*M*
Stage 0	Tis	N0	M0
Stage I	T1	N0	M0
Stage IIA	T2a	N0	M0
Stage IIB	T1	N1	M0
	T2	N1	M0
	T2a	N1	M0
	T2b	N0	M0
	T2b	N1	M0
Stage III	T1	N2	M0
	T2a	N2	M0
	T2b	N2	M0
	T2b	N2	M0
	T3	N0	M0
	T3	N1	M0
	T3	N2	M0
Stage IVA	T4	N0	M0
	T4	N1	M0
	T4	N2	M0
Stage IVB	Any T	N3	M0
Stage IVC	Any T	Any N	M1

Source: Used with the permission of the American Joint Committee on Cancer (AJCC), Chicago, Illinois. The original source for this material is the *AJCC Cancer Staging Manual*, sixth edition (2002), published by Springer-Verlag New York, www.springer-ny.com.

a current standard. Concomitant chemoradiotherapy has also been shown to be of benefit in meta-analyses.[167]

Studies conducted in the Far East have been less conclusive. However, at least one study from Taiwan demonstrated an advantage for the concurrent administration of chemoradiotherapy with respect to progression-free and overall survival.[166] Another study, by Chan et al., showed a trend favoring concurrent chemoradiotherapy for progression-free survival that was statistically significant in patients with T3 and T4 disease.[168]

Investigations of sequential combined modality therapy (induction or adjuvant chemotherapy) have not succeeded at increasing survival rates in randomized settings,[169,170] although decreased systemic and local failure rates have been demonstrated.[171] It has been argued that induction chemotherapy can reasonably be offered to patients with very bulky primary tumors extending into the brain or in close proximity to the optic chiasm and/or brainstem. Given the sensitivity of these structures to high-dose radiation, such tumors would not be readily amenable to curative intent radiotherapy. Initial tumor shrinkage with chemotherapy thus might benefit overall treatment outcomes in these cases.

Parotid Malignancies

The majority of parotid neoplasms are benign, have a predictable clinical course, and are treated successfully with superficial or partial parotidectomy. Parotid malignancies, on the other hand, are variable in clinical behavior. Accurate pathologic diagnosis has critical implications for appropriate surgical and postoperative therapy.

Pathology

Pathologists have classified salivary gland malignancies into two groups, based on the historical correlation of histopathology with biologic/clinical behavior.[172] Low-grade malignancies include low-grade mucoepidermoid carcinoma and acinic cell carcinoma. High-grade malignancies consist of high-grade mucoepidermoid carcinoma, adenoid cystic carcinoma, adenocarcinoma, squamous cell carcinoma, carcinoma ex-pleomorphic adenoma, and the rare malignant mixed tumor. Mucoepidermoid carcinomas are the most common parotid gland malignancies.

Occult cervical nodal disease is frequently seen in high-grade malignancies. Other predictors of nodal involvement are facial nerve involvement, extraglandular tumor extension, T stage, and severe desmoplasia.[173–175] In fact, the absence of histopathologic adenopathy has been found to be the major predictor of disease-free survival.[174]

Diagnosis

Patients commonly present with an asymptomatic mass in the preauricular or mandibular angle regions. Rapid growth in a long-standing parotid mass is a classic sign of carcinoma ex-pleomorphic adenoma. Pain has been considered by some to be more frequently associated with malignancy.[172] Paresis or paralysis of facial nerve branches or palpable lymphadenopathy represent indisputable signs of malignancy. The clinician should perform a careful head and neck history and examination for these and other symptoms and signs. The parotid gland holds the first-echelon nodes for the surrounding scalp and auricular carcinomas. Therefore, a history of skin malignancy in the periparotid region dictates a thorough examination for detection of metastatic disease to the parotid gland.

TABLE 36.6. Staging of parotid gland.

TX	Primary tumor cannot be assessed
T0	No evidence of primary tumor
T1	Tumor 2 cm or less in greatest dimension without extraparenchymal extension
T2	Tumor more than 2 cm but not more than 4 cm without extraparenchymal extension
T3	Tumor more than 4 cm and/or having extraparenchymal extension
T4a	Tumor invades skin, mandible, ear canal, and/or facial nerve
T4b	Tumor invades skull base, pterygoid plates, or encases carotid artery

Source: Used with the permission of the American Joint Committee on Cancer (AJCC), Chicago, Illinois. The original source for this material is the *AJCC Cancer Staging Manual*, sixth edition (2002), published by Springer-Verlag New York, www.springer-ny.com.

Testing and Staging

Although not uniformly utilized, many surgeons have found that fine-needle aspiration of the parotid mass is a very useful diagnostic adjunct.[176] Preoperative recognition of malignancy facilitates therapeutic planning and helps prepare both the surgeon and patient for the planned procedures. CT scans are also useful in determining subclinical or metastatic disease.[177] Primary parotid malignancies are staged as shown in Table 36.6.[178]

Treatment

Low-grade T1–T2 malignancies (acinic cell and low-grade mucoepidermoid carcinoma) are sufficiently treated by performing nerve-sparing parotidectomy with clear margins. No adjuvant therapy is indicated because of the indolent biologic and clinical behavior of these neoplasms. All high-grade and larger low-grade malignancies are treated with total parotidectomy and dissection of node-positive necks. Surgeons should strongly consider performing selective posterior-lateral (levels II–V) neck dissection for high-grade tumors because of the high incidence of occult metastatic disease. Postoperative radiation and/or chemotherapy may improve survival.[174]

Electromyogram (EMG)-based continuous intraoperative facial nerve monitoring is utilized by many surgeons but is not considered the standard of care. Temporary nerve weakness was found to be decreased in monitored cases versus unmonitored parotid surgeries. However, the incidence of permanent paralysis (4% or less) is similar.[179,180] The facial nerve is preserved unless directly involved with tumor. Intentional or inadvertent transection of nerve branches dictates immediate intraoperative neurorrhaphy. There are numerous cervical sensory nerves that can be harvested individually or as a plexus. Composite facial nerve trunk grafting of cervical plexus to individual distal branches will provide tone and even voluntary facial movement over 12 to 18 months.[181]

Frey's syndrome (gustatory sweating) can be prevented by placing acellular dermis between the parotid defect and the external skin.[182] In addition, symptomatic postoperative Frey's syndrome is treated successfully with botulinum toxin.[183–186] Many patients with parotid malignancy receive postoperative radiotherapy, virtually eliminating the chance of gustatory sweating. If patients are expected to endure long-term paralysis, strong consideration should be given to surgical rehabilitation. Gold weight implantation, lower lid shortening, temporalis muscle transfer (to oral commissure), and lip-switch operations all provide cosmetic facial symmetry.

References

1. Jemal A, Tiwari RC, Murray T, et al. Cancer statistics, 2004. CA Cancer J Clin 2004;54:8–29.
2. Parkin DM, Pisani P, Ferlay J. Estimates of the worldwide incidence of 25 major cancers in 1990. Int J Cancer 1999;80:827–841.
3. Shibuya K, Mathers CD, Boschi-Pinto C, Lopez AD, Murray CJ. Global and regional estimates of cancer mortality and incidence by site: II. Results for the global burden of disease 2000. BMC Cancer 2002;2:37.
4. Argiris A, Brockstein BE, Haraf DJ, et al. Competing causes of death and second primary tumors in patients with locoregionally advanced head and neck cancer treated with chemoradiotherapy. Clin Cancer Res 2004;10:1956–1962.
5. Dhooge IJ, De Vos M, Van Cauwenberge PB. Multiple primary malignant tumors in patients with head and neck cancer: results of a prospective study and future perspectives. Laryngoscope 1998;108:250–256.
6. Reichart PA. Identification of risk groups for oral precancer and cancer and preventive measures. Clin Oral Invest 2001;5:207–213.
7. Rodriguez T, Altieri A, Chatenoud L, et al. Risk factors for oral and pharyngeal cancer in young adults. Oral Oncol 2004;40:207–213.
8. Znaor A, Brennan P, Gajalakshmi V, et al. Independent and combined effects of tobacco smoking, chewing and alcohol drinking on the risk of oral, pharyngeal and esophageal cancers in Indian men. Int J Cancer 2003;105:681–686.
9. Winn DM, Blot WJ, Shy CM, Pickle LW, Toledo A, Fraumeni JF Jr. Snuff dipping and oral cancer among women in the southern United States. N Engl J Med 1981;304:745–749.
10. Neville BW, Day TA. Oral cancer and precancerous lesions. CA Cancer J Clin 2002;52:195–215.
11. Zhang ZF, Morgenstern H, Spitz MR, et al. Environmental tobacco smoking, mutagen sensitivity, and head and neck squamous cell carcinoma. Cancer Epidemiol Biomarkers Prev 2000;9:1043–1049.
12. Ko YC, Huang YL, Lee CH, Chen MJ, Lin LM, Tsai CC. Betel quid chewing, cigarette smoking and alcohol consumption related to oral cancer in Taiwan. J Oral Pathol Med 1995;24:450–453.
13. Slaughter DP, Southwick HW, Smejkal W. Field cancerization in oral stratified squamous epithelium; clinical implications of multicentric origin. Cancer (Phila) 1953;6:963–968.
14. Califano J, Leong PL, Koch WM, Eisenberger CF, Sidransky D, Westra WH. Second esophageal tumors in patients with head and neck squamous cell carcinoma: an assessment of clonal relationships. Clin Cancer Res 1999;5:1862–1867.
15. Califano J, Westra WH, Koch W, et al. Unknown primary head and neck squamous cell carcinoma: molecular identification of the site of origin. J Natl Cancer Inst 1999;91:599–604.
16. Syrjanen K, Syrjanen S, Lamberg M, Pyrhonen S, Nuutinen J. Morphological and immunohistochemical evidence suggesting human papillomavirus (HPV) involvement in oral squamous cell carcinogenesis. Int J Oral Surg 1983;12:418–424.
17. Gillison ML, Koch WM, Capone RB, et al. Evidence for a causal association between human papillomavirus and a subset of head and neck cancers. J Natl Cancer Inst 2000;92:709–720.
18. Miller CS, Johnstone BM. Human papillomavirus as a risk factor for oral squamous cell carcinoma: a meta-analysis, 1982–1997. Oral Surg Oral Med Oral Pathol Oral Radiol Endod 2001;91:622–635.
19. Snijders PJ, Scholes AG, Hart CA, et al. Prevalence of mucosotropic human papillomaviruses in squamous-cell carcinoma of the head and neck. Int J Cancer 1996;66:464–469.
20. Koch WM, Lango M, Sewell D, Zahurak M, Sidransky D. Head and neck cancer in nonsmokers: a distinct clinical and molecular entity. Laryngoscope 1999;109:1544–1551.
21. Mork J, Lie AK, Glattre E, et al. Human papillomavirus infection as a risk factor for squamous-cell carcinoma of the head and neck. N Engl J Med 2001;344:1125–1131.
22. Van Dyke DL, Worsham MJ, Benninger MS, et al. Recurrent cytogenetic abnormalities in squamous cell carcinomas of the head and neck region. Genes Chromosomes Cancer 1994;9:192–206.
23. Jin Y, Mertens F, Mandahl N, et al. Chromosome abnormalities in eighty-three head and neck squamous cell carcinomas: influence of culture conditions on karyotypic pattern. Cancer Res 1993;53:2140–2146.
24. Mao L, Fan YH, Lotan R, Hong WK. Frequent abnormalities of FHIT, a candidate tumor suppressor gene, in head and neck cancer cell lines. Cancer Res 1996;56:5128–5131.
25. Nawroz H, van der Riet P, Hruban RH, Koch W, Ruppert JM, Sidransky D. Allelotype of head and neck squamous cell carcinoma. Cancer Res 1994;54:1152–1155.
26. Sartor M, Steingrimsdottir H, Elamin F, et al. Role of p16/MTS1, cyclin D1 and RB in primary oral cancer and oral cancer cell lines. Br J Cancer 1999;80:79–86.
27. Taylor D, Koch WM, Zahurak M, Shah K, Sidransky D, Westra WH. Immunohistochemical detection of p53 protein accumulation in head and neck cancer: correlation with p53 gene alterations. Hum Pathol 1999;30:1221–1225.
28. Mao L, Lee JS, Fan YH, et al. Frequent microsatellite alterations at chromosomes 9p21 and 3p14 in oral premalignant lesions and their value in cancer risk assessment. Nat Med 1996;2:682–685.
29. Reed AL, Califano J, Cairns P, et al. High frequency of p16 (CDKN2/MTS-1/INK4A) inactivation in head and neck squamous cell carcinoma. Cancer Res 1996;56:3630–3633.
30. Hogg RP, Honorio S, Martinez A, et al. Frequent 3p allele loss and epigenetic inactivation of the RASSF1A tumour suppressor gene from region 3p21.3 in head and neck squamous cell carcinoma. Eur J Cancer 2002;38:1585–1592.
31. Brzoska PM, Levin NA, Fu KK, et al. Frequent novel DNA copy number increase in squamous cell head and neck tumors. Cancer Res 1995;55:3055–3059.
32. Berenson JR, Yang J, Mickel RA. Frequent amplification of the bcl-1 locus in head and neck squamous cell carcinomas. Oncogene 1989;4:1111–1116.
33. Callender T, el-Naggar AK, Lee MS, Frankenthaler R, Luna MA, Batsakis JG. PRAD-1 (CCND1)/cyclin D1 oncogene amplification in primary head and neck squamous cell carcinoma. Cancer (Phila) 1994;74:152–158.
34. Jares P, Fernandez PL, Campo E, et al. PRAD-1/cyclin D1 gene amplification correlates with messenger RNA overexpression and tumor progression in human laryngeal carcinomas. Cancer Res 1994;54:4813–4817.
35. Izzo JG, Papadimitrakopoulou VA, Liu DD, et al. Cyclin D1 genotype, response to biochemoprevention, and progression rate to upper aerodigestive tract cancer. J Natl Cancer Inst 2003;95:198–205.

36. Grandis JR, Melhem MF, Gooding WE, et al. Levels of TGF-alpha and EGFR protein in head and neck squamous cell carcinoma and patient survival. J Natl Cancer Inst 1998;90:824–832.
37. Grandis JR, Melhem MF, Barnes EL, Tweardy DJ. Quantitative immunohistochemical analysis of transforming growth factor-alpha and epidermal growth factor receptor in patients with squamous cell carcinoma of the head and neck. Cancer (Phila) 1996;78:1284–1292.
38. Ang KK, Berkey BA, Tu X, et al. Impact of epidermal growth factor receptor expression on survival and pattern of relapse in patients with advanced head and neck carcinoma. Cancer Res 2002;62:7350–7356.
39. Barrandon Y, Green H. Cell migration is essential for sustained growth of keratinocyte colonies: the roles of transforming growth factor-alpha and epidermal growth factor. Cell 1987; 50:1131–1137.
40. Chen P, Xie H, Sekar MC, Gupta K, Wells A. Epidermal growth factor receptor-mediated cell motility: phospholipase C activity is required, but mitogen-activated protein kinase activity is not sufficient for induced cell movement. J Cell Biol 1994; 127:847–857.
41. Sorrells DL, Ghali GE, Meschonat C, et al. Competitive PCR to detect eIF4E gene amplification in head and neck cancer. Head Neck 1999;21:60–65.
42. Sudbo J, Ristimaki A, Sondresen JE, et al. Cyclooxygenase-2 (COX-2) expression in high-risk premalignant oral lesions. Oral Oncol 2003;39:497–505.
43. Patturajan M, Nomoto S, Sommer M, et al. DeltaNp63 induces beta-catenin nuclear accumulation and signaling. Cancer Cell 2002;1:369–379.
44. Hasegawa M, Nelson HH, Peters E, Ringstrom E, Posner M, Kelsey KT. Patterns of gene promoter methylation in squamous cell cancer of the head and neck. Oncogene 2002;21:4231–4236.
45. Sanchez-Cespedes M, Esteller M, Wu L, et al. Gene promoter hypermethylation in tumors and serum of head and neck cancer patients. Cancer Res 2000;60:892–895.
46. Rosas SL, Koch W, da Costa Carvalho MG, et al. Promoter hypermethylation patterns of p16, *O*-6-methylguanine-DNA-methyltransferase, and death-associated protein kinase in tumors and saliva of head and neck cancer patients. Cancer Res 2001;61:939–942.
47. Viswanathan M, Tsuchida N, Shanmugam G. Promoter hypermethylation profile of tumor-associated genes p16, p15, hMLH1, MGMT and E-cadherin in oral squamous cell carcinoma. Int J Cancer 2003;105:41–46.
48. Califano J, van der Riet P, Westra W, et al. Genetic progression model for head and neck cancer: implications for field cancerization. Cancer Res 1996;56:2488–2492.
49. Sudbo J, Lippman SM, Lee JJ, et al. The influence of resection and aneuploidy on mortality in oral leukoplakia. N Engl J Med 2004;350:1405–1413.
50. Sudbo J, Kildal W, Johannessen AC, et al. Gross genomic aberrations in precancers: clinical implications of a long-term follow-up study in oral erythroplakias. J Clin Oncol 2002;20:456–462.
51. Sudbo J, Kildal W, Risberg B, Koppang HS, Danielsen HE, Reith A. DNA content as a prognostic marker in patients with oral leukoplakia. N Engl J Med 2001;344:1270–1278.
52. Lingen MW, Polverini PJ, Bouck NP. Retinoic acid induces cells cultured from oral squamous cell carcinomas to become anti-angiogenic. Am J Pathol 1996;149:247–258.
53. Schultz-Hector S, Haghayegh S. Beta-fibroblast growth factor expression in human and murine squamous cell carcinomas and its relationship to regional endothelial cell proliferation. Cancer Res 1993;53:1444–1449.
54. Gleich LL, Srivastava L, Gluckman JL. Plasma platelet-derived growth factor: preliminary study of a potential marker in head and neck cancer. Ann Otol Rhinol Laryngol 1996;105:710–712.
55. Moriyama M, Kumagai S, Kawashiri S, Kojima K, Kakihara K, Yamamoto E. Immunohistochemical study of tumour angiogenesis in oral squamous cell carcinoma. Oral Oncol 1997; 33:369–374.
56. Petruzzelli GJ, Benefield J, Taitz AD, et al. Heparin-binding growth factor(s) derived from head and neck squamous cell carcinomas induce endothelial cell proliferations. Head Neck 1997;19:576–582.
57. Kotwall C, Sako K, Razack M, et al. Metastatic patterns in squamous cell cancer of the head and neck. Am J Surg 1987;154:439.
58. Pauloski BR, Rademaker AW, Logemann JA, et al. Pretreatment swallowing function in patients with head and neck cancer. Head Neck 2000;22:474–482.
59. Grau C, Johansen LV, Jakobsen J, Geertsen P, Andersen E, Jensen BB. Cervical lymph node metastases from unknown primary tumours. Results from a national survey by the Danish Society for Head and Neck Oncology. Radiother Oncol 2000;55:121–129.
60. Nieder C, Gregoire V, Ang KK. Cervical lymph node metastases from occult squamous cell carcinoma: cut down a tree to get an apple? Int J Radiat Oncol Biol Phys 2001;50:727–733.
61. Jereczek-Fossa BA, Jassem J, Orecchia R. Cervical lymph node metastases of squamous cell carcinoma from an unknown primary. Cancer Treat Rev 2004;30:153–164.
62. Stoeckli SJ, Zimmermann R, Schmid S. Role of routine panendoscopy in cancer of the upper aerodigestive tract. Otolaryngol Head Neck Surg 2001;124:208–212.
63. Jones AS, Morar P, Phillips DE, Field JK, Husband D, Helliwell TR. Second primary tumors in patients with head and neck squamous cell carcinoma. Cancer (Phila) 1995;75:1343–1353.
64. Haughey BH, Gates GA, Arfken CL, Harvey J. Meta-analysis of second malignant tumors in head and neck cancer: the case for an endoscopic screening protocol. Ann Otol Rhinol Laryngol 1992;101:105–112.
65. Johnson RE, Sigman JD, Funk GF, Robinson RA, Hoffman HT. Quantification of surgical margin shrinkage in the oral cavity. Head Neck 1997;19:281–286.
66. Ball VA, Righi PD, Tejada E, Radpour S, Pavelic ZP, Gluckman JL. p53 immunostaining of surgical margins as a predictor of local recurrence in squamous cell carcinoma of the oral cavity and oropharynx. Ear Nose Throat J 1997;76:818–823.
67. Nathan CA, Franklin S, Abreo FW, et al. Expression of eIF4E during head and neck tumorigenesis: possible role in angiogenesis. Laryngoscope 1999;109:1253–1258.
68. Robbins K. Neck dissection. In: Cummings C, Frederickson J, Harker L, Krause C, Schuller D (eds). Otolaryngology Head and Neck Surgery. St. Louis: Mosby-Year Book, 1998:1787.
69. Mira E, Benazzo M, Rossi V, Zanoletti E. Efficacy of selective lymph node dissection in clinically negative neck. Otolaryngol Head Neck Surg 2002;127:279–283.
70. Pitman KT, Johnson JT, Brown ML, Myers EN. Sentinel lymph node biopsy in head and neck squamous cell carcinoma. Laryngoscope 2002;112:2101–2113.
71. Mukherji SK, Armao D, Joshi VM. Cervical nodal metastases in squamous cell carcinoma of the head and neck: what to expect. Head Neck 2001;23:995–1005.
72. Chao KS, Wippold FJ, Ozyigit G, Tran BN, Dempsey JF. Determination and delineation of nodal target volumes for head-and-neck cancer based on patterns of failure in patients receiving definitive and postoperative IMRT. Int J Radiat Oncol Biol Phys 2002;53:1174–1184.
73. Eisbruch A, Lyden T, Bradford CR, et al. Objective assessment of swallowing dysfunction and aspiration after radiation concurrent with chemotherapy for head-and-neck cancer. Int J Radiat Oncol Biol Phys 2002;53:23–28.
74. Milano M, Vokes E, Witt M, et al. Retrospective comparison of intensity modulated radiation therapy (IMRT) and conventional

three-dimensional RT (3DCRT) in advanced head and neck patients treated with definitive chemoradiation. Proc Am Soc Clin Oncol 2003;22:499 (abstract 2007).
75. Chao KS, Deasy JO, Markman J, et al. A prospective study of salivary function sparing in patients with head-and-neck cancers receiving intensity-modulated or three-dimensional radiation therapy: initial results. Int J Radiat Oncol Biol Phys 2001; 49:907–916.
76. Eisbruch A, Kim HM, Terrell JE, Marsh LH, Dawson LA, Ship JA. Xerostomia and its predictors following parotid-sparing irradiation of head-and-neck cancer. Int J Radiat Oncol Biol Phys 2001;50:695–704.
77. Butler EB, Teh BS, Grant WH III, et al. Smart (simultaneous modulated accelerated radiation therapy) boost: a new accelerated fractionation schedule for the treatment of head and neck cancer with intensity modulated radiotherapy. Int J Radiat Oncol Biol Phys 1999;45:21–32.
78. Dawson LA, Anzai Y, Marsh L, et al. Patterns of local-regional recurrence following parotid-sparing conformal and segmental intensity-modulated radiotherapy for head and neck cancer. Int J Radiat Oncol Biol Phys 2000;46:1117–1126.
79. Lee N, Xia P, Fischbein NJ, Akazawa P, Akazawa C, Quivey JM. Intensity-modulated radiation therapy for head-and-neck cancer: the UCSF experience focusing on target volume delineation. Int J Radiat Oncol Biol Phys 2003;57:49–60.
80. Peters LJ, Goepfert H, Ang KK, et al. Evaluation of the dose for postoperative radiation therapy of head and neck cancer: first report of a prospective randomized trial. Int J Radiat Oncol Biol Phys 1993;26:3–11.
81. Ang KK, Trotti A, Brown BW, et al. Randomized trial addressing risk features and time factors of surgery plus radiotherapy in advanced head-and-neck cancer. Int J Radiat Oncol Biol Phys 2001;51:571–578.
82. Horiot JC, Bontemps P, van den Bogaert W, et al. Accelerated fractionation (AF) compared to conventional fractionation (CF) improves loco-regional control in the radiotherapy of advanced head and neck cancers: results of the EORTC 22851 randomized trial. Radiother Oncol 1997;44:111–121.
83. Jackson SM, Weir LM, Hay JH, Tsang VH, Durham JS. A randomised trial of accelerated versus conventional radiotherapy in head and neck cancer. Radiother Oncol 1997;43:39–46.
84. Dische S, Saunders M, Barrett A, Harvey A, Gibson D, Parmar M. A randomised multicentre trial of CHART versus conventional radiotherapy in head and neck cancer. Radiother Oncol 1997;44:123–136.
85. Overgaard J, Hansen HS, Specht L, et al. Five compared with six fractions per week of conventional radiotherapy of squamous-cell carcinoma of head and neck: DAHANCA 6 and 7 randomised controlled trial. Lancet 2003;362:933–940.
86. Skladowski K, Maciejewski B, Golen M, Pilecki B, Przeorek W, Tarnawski R. Randomized clinical trial on 7-day-continuous accelerated irradiation (CAIR) of head and neck cancer: report on 3-year tumour control and normal tissue toxicity. Radiother Oncol 2000;55:101–110.
87. Cohen EE, Lingen MW, Vokes EE. The expanding role of systemic therapy in head and neck cancer. J Clin Oncol 2004; 22:1743–1752.
88. Lamont EB, Vokes EE. Chemotherapy in the management of squamous-cell carcinoma of the head and neck. Lancet Oncol 2001;2:261–269.
89. De Andres L, Brunet J, Lopez-Pousa A, et al. Randomized trial of neoadjuvant cisplatin and fluorouracil versus carboplatin and fluorouracil in patients with stage IV-M0 head and neck cancer. J Clin Oncol 1995;13:1493–1500.
90. Forastiere AA, Metch B, Schuller DE, et al. Randomized comparison of cisplatin plus fluorouracil and carboplatin plus fluorouracil versus methotrexate in advanced squamous-cell carcinoma of the head and neck: a Southwest Oncology Group study. J Clin Oncol 1992;10:1245–1251.
91. Sessions DG, Spector GJ, Lenox J, et al. Analysis of treatment results for floor-of-mouth cancer. Laryngoscope 2000;110: 1764–1772.
92. Sessions DG, Spector GJ, Lenox J, Haughey B, Chao C, Marks J. Analysis of treatment results for oral tongue cancer. Laryngoscope 2002;112:616–625.
93. O'Brien CJ, Lauer CS, Fredricks S, et al. Tumor thickness influences prognosis of T1 and T2 oral cavity cancer—but what thickness? Head Neck 2003;25:937–945.
94. Kowalski LP. Results of salvage treatment of the neck in patients with oral cancer. Arch Otolaryngol Head Neck Surg 2002;128: 58–62.
95. Wax MK, Bascom DA, Myers LL. Marginal mandibulectomy vs. segmental mandibulectomy: indications and controversies. Arch Otolaryngol Head Neck Surg 2002;128:600–603.
96. Moore BA, Magdy E, Netterville JL, Burkey BB. Palatal reconstruction with the palatal island flap. Laryngoscope 2003;113: 946–951.
97. Landes CA, Kovacs AF. Nine-year experience with extended use of the commissure-based buccal musculomucosal flap. Plast Reconstr Surg 2003;111:1029–1039; discussion 1040–1042.
98. Harrison LB, Zelefsky MJ, Armstrong JG, Carper E, Gaynor JJ, Sessions RB. Performance status after treatment for squamous cell cancer of the base of tongue–a comparison of primary radiation therapy versus primary surgery. Int J Radiat Oncol Biol Phys 1994;30:953–957.
99. Robertson ML, Gleich LL, Barrett WL, Gluckman JL. Base-of-tongue cancer: survival, function, and quality of life after external-beam irradiation and brachytherapy. Laryngoscope 2001;111:1362–1365.
100. Azizzadeh B, Enayati P, Chhetri D, et al. Long-term survival outcome in transhyoid resection of base of tongue squamous cell carcinoma. Arch Otolaryngol Head Neck Surg 2002;128: 1067–1070.
101. Galati LT, Myers EN, Johnson JT. Primary surgery as treatment for early squamous cell carcinoma of the tonsil. Head Neck 2000;22:294–296.
102. Perlmutter MA, Johnson JT, Snyderman CH, Cano ER, Myers EN. Functional outcomes after treatment of squamous cell carcinoma of the base of the tongue. Arch Otolaryngol Head Neck Surg 2002;128:887–891.
103. Zeitels SM, Vaughan CW, Ruh S. Suprahyoid pharyngotomy for oropharynx cancer including the tongue base. Arch Otolaryngol Head Neck Surg 1991;117:757–760.
104. Steiner W, Fierek O, Ambrosch P, Hommerich CP, Kron M. Transoral laser microsurgery for squamous cell carcinoma of the base of the tongue. Arch Otolaryngol Head Neck Surg 2003; 129:36–43.
105. Eckel HE, Staar S, Volling P, Sittel C, Damm M, Jungehuelsing M. Surgical treatment for hypopharynx carcinoma: feasibility, mortality, and results. Otolaryngol Head Neck Surg 2001; 124:561–569.
106. Czaja JM, Gluckman JL. Surgical management of early-stage hypopharyngeal carcinoma. Ann Otol Rhinol Laryngol 1997; 106:909–913.
107. Julieron M, Kolb F, Schwaab G, et al. Surgical management of posterior pharyngeal wall carcinomas: functional and oncologic results. Head Neck 2001;23:80–86.
108. Laccourreye O, Merite-Drancy A, Brasnu D, et al. Supracricoid hemilaryngopharyngectomy in selected pyriform sinus carcinoma staged as T2. Laryngoscope 1993;103:1373–1379.
109. Steiner W, Ambrosch P, Hess CF, Kron M. Organ preservation by transoral laser microsurgery in piriform sinus carcinoma. Otolaryngol Head Neck Surg 2001;124:58–67.

110. Smith JC, Johnson JT, Myers EN. Management and outcome of early glottic carcinoma. Otolaryngol Head Neck Surg 2002;126: 356–364.
111. Gallo A, de Vincentiis M, Manciocco V, Simonelli M, Fiorella ML, Shah JP. CO2 laser cordectomy for early-stage glottic carcinoma: a long-term follow-up of 156 cases. Laryngoscope 2002; 112:370–374.
112. Pradhan SA, Pai PS, Neeli SI, D'Cruz AK. Transoral laser surgery for early glottic cancers. Arch Otolaryngol Head Neck Surg 2003;129:623–625.
113. Tamura E, Kitahara S, Ogura M, Kohno N. Voice quality after laser surgery or radiotherapy for T1a glottic carcinoma. Laryngoscope 2003;113:910–914.
114. Pearson BW, Salassa JR. Transoral laser microresection for cancer of the larynx involving the anterior commissure. Laryngoscope 2003;113:1104–1112.
115. Hartig G, Truelson J, Weinstein G. Supraglottic cancer. Head Neck 2000;22:426–434.
116. Scola B, Fernandez-Vega M, Martinez T, Fernandez-Vega S, Ramirez C. Management of cancer of the supraglottis. Otolaryngol Head Neck Surg 2001;124:195–198.
117. Iro H, Waldfahrer F, Altendorf-Hofmann A, Weidenbecher M, Sauer R, Steiner W. Transoral laser surgery of supraglottic cancer: follow-up of 141 patients. Arch Otolaryngol Head Neck Surg 1998;124:1245–1250.
118. Bernier J, Domenge C, Ozsahin M, et al. Postoperative irradiation with or without concomitant chemotherapy for locally advanced head and neck cancer. N Engl J Med 2004; 350:1945–1952.
119. Cooper JS, Pajak TF, Forastiere AA, et al. Postoperative concurrent radiotherapy and chemotherapy for high-risk squamous-cell carcinoma of the head and neck. N Engl J Med 2004; 350:1937–1944.
120. Forastiere AA, Goepfert H, Maor M, et al. Concurrent chemotherapy and radiotherapy for organ preservation in advanced laryngeal cancer. N Engl J Med 2003;349:2091–2098.
121. Induction chemotherapy plus radiation compared with surgery plus radiation in patients with advanced laryngeal cancer. The Department of Veterans Affairs Laryngeal Cancer Study Group. N Engl J Med 1991;324:1685–1690.
122. Haraf DJ, Kies M, Rademaker AW, et al. Radiation therapy with concomitant hydroxyurea and fluorouracil in stage II and III head and neck cancer. J Clin Oncol 1999;17:638–644.
123. Lefebvre JL, Chevalier D, Luboinski B, Kirkpatrick A, Collette L, Sahmoud T. Larynx preservation in pyriform sinus cancer: preliminary results of a European Organization for Research and Treatment of Cancer phase III trial. EORTC Head and Neck Cancer Cooperative Group. J Natl Cancer Inst 1996;88:890–899.
124. Pignon JP, Bourhis J, Domenge C, Designe L. Chemotherapy added to locoregional treatment for head and neck squamous-cell carcinoma: three meta-analyses of updated individual data. MACH-NC Collaborative Group. Meta-Analysis of Chemotherapy on Head and Neck Cancer. Lancet 2000;355:949–955.
125. Fu KK, Phillips TL, Silverberg IJ, et al. Combined radiotherapy and chemotherapy with bleomycin and methotrexate for advanced inoperable head and neck cancer: update of a Northern California Oncology Group randomized trial. J Clin Oncol 1987;5:1410–1418.
126. Shanta V, Krishnamurthi S. Combined bleomycin and radiotherapy in oral cancer. Clin Radiol 1980;31:617–620.
127. Haffty BG, Son YH, Papac R, et al. Chemotherapy as an adjunct to radiation in the treatment of squamous cell carcinoma of the head and neck: results of the Yale Mitomycin Randomized Trials. J Clin Oncol 1997;15:268–276.
128. Al-Sarraf M, Pajak TF, Marcial VA, et al. Concurrent radiotherapy and chemotherapy with cisplatin in inoperable squamous cell carcinoma of the head and neck. An RTOG Study. Cancer (Phila) 1987;59:259–265.
129. Garden AS, Harris J, Vokes EE, et al. Preliminary results of Radiation Therapy Oncology Group 97-03: a randomized phase II trial of concurrent radiation and chemotherapy for advanced squamous cell carcinomas of the head and neck. J Clin Oncol 2004;22(14):2856–2864.
130. Vokes EE, Kies MS, Haraf DJ, et al. Concomitant chemoradiotherapy as primary therapy for locoregionally advanced head and neck cancer. J Clin Oncol 2000;18:1652–1661.
131. Kies MS, Haraf DJ, Rosen F, et al. Concomitant infusional paclitaxel and fluorouracil, oral hydroxyurea, and hyperfractionated radiation for locally advanced squamous head and neck cancer. J Clin Oncol 2001;19:1961–1969.
132. Adelstein DJ, Saxton JP, Lavertu P, et al. Maximizing local control and organ preservation in stage IV squamous cell head and neck cancer with hyperfractionated radiation and concurrent chemotherapy. J Clin Oncol 2002;20:1405–1410.
133. Vokes EE, Stenson K, Rosen FR, et al. Weekly carboplatin and paclitaxel followed by concomitant paclitaxel, fluorouracil, and hydroxyurea chemoradiotherapy: curative and organ-preserving therapy for advanced head and neck cancer. J Clin Oncol 2003;21:320–326.
134. Haraf DJ, Rosen FR, Stenson K, et al. Induction chemotherapy followed by concomitant TFHX chemoradiotherapy with reduced dose radiation in advanced head and neck cancer. Clin Cancer Res 2003;9:5936–5943.
135. Machtay M, Rosenthal DI, Hershock D, et al. Organ preservation therapy using induction plus concurrent chemoradiation for advanced resectable oropharyngeal carcinoma: a University of Pennsylvania Phase II Trial. J Clin Oncol 2002;20:3964–3971.
136. Medina JE. A rational classification of neck dissections. Otolaryngol Head Neck Surg 1989;100:169–176.
137. Zbar RI, Funk GF, McCulloch TM, Graham SM, Hoffman HT. Pectoralis major myofascial flap: a valuable tool in contemporary head and neck reconstruction. Head Neck 1997;19:412–418.
138. Bastian RW, Park AH. Suction drain management of salivary fistulas. Laryngoscope 1995;105:1337–1341.
139. Ackerstaff AH, Hilgers FJ, Meeuwis CA, et al. Multi-institutional assessment of the Provox 2 voice prosthesis. Arch Otolaryngol Head Neck Surg 1999;125:167–173.
140. Urken ML, Biller HF. A new bilobed design for the sensate radial forearm flap to preserve tongue mobility following significant glossectomy. Arch Otolaryngol Head Neck Surg 1994;120:26–31.
141. Lyos AT, Evans GR, Perez D, Schusterman MA. Tongue reconstruction: outcomes with the rectus abdominis flap. Plast Reconstr Surg 1999;103:442–447; discussion 448–449.
142. Cohen EE, Rosen F, Stadler WM, et al. Phase II trial of ZD1839 in recurrent or metastatic squamous cell carcinoma of the head and neck. J Clin Oncol 2003;21:1980–1987.
143. Soulieres D, Senzer NN, Vokes EE, Hidalgo M, Agarwala SS, Siu LL. Multicenter phase II study of erlotinib, an oral epidermal growth factor receptor tyrosine kinase inhibitor, in patients with recurrent or metastatic squamous cell cancer of the head and neck. J Clin Oncol 2004;22:77–85.
144. Burtness B, Li Y, Flood W, Mattar B, Forastiere A. Phase III trial comparing cisplatin (C) + placebo (P) to C + anti-epidermal growth factor antibody (EGF-R) C225 in patients (pts) with metastatic/recurrent head & neck cancer (HNC). Proc Am Soc Clin Oncol 2002;21:226a (abstract 901).
145. Sudbo J, Reith A. Which putatively pre-malignant oral lesions become oral cancers? Clinical relevance of early targeting of high-risk individuals. J Oral Pathol Med 2003;32:63–70.
146. Lotan R, Xu XC, Lippman SM, et al. Suppression of retinoic acid receptor-beta in premalignant oral lesions and its up-regulation by isotretinoin. N Engl J Med 1995;332:1405–1410.
147. Hong WK, Endicott J, Itri LM, et al. 13-*cis*-Retinoic acid in the treatment of oral leukoplakia. N Engl J Med 1986;315: 1501–1505.

148. Hong WK, Lippman SM, Itri LM, et al. Prevention of second primary tumors with isotretinoin in squamous-cell carcinoma of the head and neck. N Engl J Med 1990;323:795–801.
149. Khuri FLJ, Lippman SM, Kim ES,et al. Isotretinoin effects on head and neck cancer recurrence and second primary tumors. In: American Society of Clinical Oncology Annual Meeting, Chicago, IL, 2003, vol 22.
150. Pinto HLY, Loprinzi C, Kardinal C, Adams G, Pandya K. Phase III trial of low-dose 13-*cis*-retinoic acid for prevention of second primary cancers in stage I–II head and neck cancer: an Eastern Cooperative Oncology Group Study. In: American Society of Clinical Oncology Annual Meeting, San Francisco, CA, 2001, vol 20.
151. Shin DM, Khuri FR, Murphy B, et al. Combined interferon-alfa, 13-*cis*-retinoic acid, and alpha-tocopherol in locally advanced head and neck squamous cell carcinoma: novel bioadjuvant phase II trial. J Clin Oncol 2001;19:3010–3017.
152. Papadimitrakopoulou VA, Clayman GL, Shin DM, et al. Biochemoprevention for dysplastic lesions of the upper aerodigestive tract. Arch Otolaryngol Head Neck Surg 1999;125: 1083–1089.
153. Rudin CM, Cohen EE, Papadimitrakopoulou VA, et al. An attenuated adenovirus, ONYX-015, as mouthwash therapy for premalignant oral dysplasia. J Clin Oncol 2003;21: 4546–4552.
154. Lin DT, Subbaramaiah K, Shah JP, Dannenberg AJ, Boyle JO. Cyclooxygenase-2: a novel molecular target for the prevention and treatment of head and neck cancer. Head Neck 2002; 24:792–799.
155. Armstrong WB, Kennedy AR, Wan XS, et al. Clinical modulation of oral leukoplakia and protease activity by Bowman-Birk inhibitor concentrate in a phase IIa chemoprevention trial. Clin Cancer Res 2000;6:4684–4691.
156. Chien YC, Chen JY, Liu MY, et al. Serologic markers of Epstein–Barr virus infection and nasopharyngeal carcinoma in Taiwanese men. N Engl J Med 2001;345:1877–1882.
157. Shotelersuk K, Khorprasert C, Sakdikul S, Pornthanakasem W, Voravud N, Mutirangura A. Epstein–Barr virus DNA in serum/plasma as a tumor marker for nasopharyngeal cancer. Clin Cancer Res 2000;6:1046–1051.
158. Lo YM, Chan LY, Chan AT, et al. Quantitative and temporal correlation between circulating cell-free Epstein–Barr virus DNA and tumor recurrence in nasopharyngeal carcinoma. Cancer Res 1999;59:5452–5455.
159. Yuan JM, Wang XL, Xiang YB, Gao YT, Ross RK, Yu MC. Preserved foods in relation to risk of nasopharyngeal carcinoma in Shanghai, China. Int J Cancer 2000;85:358–363.
160. Lee AW, Foo W, Mang O, et al. Changing epidemiology of nasopharyngeal carcinoma in Hong Kong over a 20-year period (1980–99): an encouraging reduction in both incidence and mortality. Int J Cancer 2003;103:680–685.
161. Zeng YX, Jia WH. Familial nasopharyngeal carcinoma. Semin Cancer Biol 2002;12:443–450.
162. Xiong W, Zeng ZY, Xia JH, et al. A susceptibility locus at chromosome 3p21 linked to familial nasopharyngeal carcinoma. Cancer Res 2004;64:1972–1974.
163. Vokes EE, Liebowitz DN, Weichselbaum RR. Nasopharyngeal carcinoma. Lancet 1997;350:1087–1091.
164. Altun M, Fandi A, Dupuis O, Cvitkovic E, Krajina Z, Eschwege F. Undifferentiated nasopharyngeal cancer (UCNT): current diagnostic and therapeutic aspects. Int J Radiat Oncol Biol Phys 1995;32:859–877.
165. Al-Sarraf M, LeBlanc M, Giri PG, et al. Chemoradiotherapy versus radiotherapy in patients with advanced nasopharyngeal cancer: phase III randomized Intergroup study 0099. J Clin Oncol 1998;16:1310–1317.
166. Lin JC, Jan JS, Hsu CY, Liang WM, Jiang RS, Wang WY. Phase III study of concurrent chemoradiotherapy versus radiotherapy alone for advanced nasopharyngeal carcinoma: positive effect on overall and progression-free survival. J Clin Oncol 2003;21: 631–637.
167. Huncharek M, Kupelnick B. Combined chemoradiation versus radiation therapy alone in locally advanced nasopharyngeal carcinoma: results of a meta-analysis of 1,528 patients from six randomized trials. Am J Clin Oncol 2002;25:219–223.
168. Chan AT, Teo PM, Ngan RK, et al. Concurrent chemotherapy-radiotherapy compared with radiotherapy alone in locoregionally advanced nasopharyngeal carcinoma: progression-free survival analysis of a phase III randomized trial. J Clin Oncol 2002;20:2038–2044.
169. Chi KH, Chang YC, Guo WY, et al. A phase III study of adjuvant chemotherapy in advanced nasopharyngeal carcinoma patients. Int J Radiat Oncol Biol Phys 2002;52:1238–1244.
170. Ma J, Mai HQ, Hong MH, et al. Results of a prospective randomized trial comparing neoadjuvant chemotherapy plus radiotherapy with radiotherapy alone in patients with locoregionally advanced nasopharyngeal carcinoma. J Clin Oncol 2001;19: 1350–1357.
171. Preliminary results of a randomized trial comparing neoadjuvant chemotherapy (cisplatin, epirubicin, bleomycin) plus radiotherapy vs. radiotherapy alone in stage IV(> or = N2, M0) undifferentiated nasopharyngeal carcinoma: a positive effect on progression-free survival. International Nasopharynx Cancer Study Group. VUMCA I trial. Int J Radiat Oncol Biol Phys 1996;35:463–469.
172. Cummings C, Frederickson J, Harker L, Krause C, Schuller D. Otolaryngology—Head & Neck Surgery, vol 4. St. Louis: Mosby, 1998:2908–2933.
173. Bhattacharyya N, Fried MP. Nodal metastasis in major salivary gland cancer: predictive factors and effects on survival. Arch Otolaryngol Head Neck Surg 2002;128:904–908.
174. Hocwald E, Korkmaz H, Yoo GH, et al. Prognostic factors in major salivary gland cancer. Laryngoscope 2001;111:1434–1439.
175. Regis De Brito Santos I, Kowalski LP, Cavalcante De Araujo V, Flavia Logullo A, Magrin J. Multivariate analysis of risk factors for neck metastases in surgically treated parotid carcinomas. Arch Otolaryngol Head Neck Surg 2001;127:56–60.
176. Zbaren P, Schar C, Hotz MA, Loosli H. Value of fine-needle aspiration cytology of parotid gland masses. Laryngoscope 2001;111:1989–1992.
177. Urquhart A, Hutchins LG, Berg RL. Preoperative computed tomography scans for parotid tumor evaluation. Laryngoscope 2001;111:1984–1988.
178. Greene F, Page D, Fleming I, et al. TNM Classification of Malignant Tumours. AJCC Cancer Staging Handbook. New York: Springer-Verlag, 2002:145–153.
179. Dulguerov P, Marchal F, Lehmann W. Postparotidectomy facial nerve paralysis: possible etiologic factors and results with routine facial nerve monitoring. Laryngoscope 1999;109: 754–762.
180. Terrell JE, Kileny PR, Yian C, et al. Clinical outcome of continuous facial nerve monitoring during primary parotidectomy. Arch Otolaryngol Head Neck Surg 1997;123:1081–1087.
181. Reddy PG, Arden RL, Mathog RH. Facial nerve rehabilitation after radical parotidectomy. Laryngoscope 1999;109:894–899.
182. Govindaraj S, Cohen M, Genden EM, Costantino PD, Urken ML. The use of acellular dermis in the prevention of Frey's syndrome. Laryngoscope 2001;111:1993–1998.
183. Guntinas-Lichius O. Increased botulinum toxin type A dosage is more effective in patients with Frey's syndrome. Laryngoscope 2002;112:746–749.
184. Arad-Cohen A, Blitzer A. Botulinum toxin treatment for symptomatic Frey's syndrome. Otolaryngol Head Neck Surg 2000; 122:237–240.

185. Laskawi R, Drobik C, Schonebeck C. Up-to-date report of botulinum toxin type A treatment in patients with gustatory sweating (Frey's syndrome). Laryngoscope 1998;108:381–384.
186. Blitzer A, Sulica L. Botulinum toxin: basic science and clinical uses in otolaryngology. Laryngoscope 2001;111:218–226.
187. A phase III randomised trial of cisplatinum, methotrexate, cisplatinum + methotrexate and cisplatinum + 5-FU in end stage squamous carcinoma of the head and neck. Liverpool Head and Neck Oncology Group. Br J Cancer 1990;61:311–315.
188. Jacobs C, Lyman G, Velez-Garcia E, et al. A phase III randomized study comparing cisplatin and fluorouracil as single agents and in combination for advanced squamous cell carcinoma of the head and neck. J Clin Oncol 1992;10:257–263.
189. Clavel M, Vermorken JB, Cognetti F, et al. Randomized comparison of cisplatin, methotrexate, bleomycin and vincristine (CABO) versus cisplatin and 5-fluorouracil (CF) versus cisplatin (C) in recurrent or metastatic squamous cell carcinoma of the head and neck. A phase III study of the EORTC Head and Neck Cancer Cooperative Group. Ann Oncol 1994;5:521–526.
190. Forastiere AA, Shank D, Neuberg D, Taylor SGt, DeConti RC, Adams G. Final report of a phase II evaluation of paclitaxel in patients with advanced squamous cell carcinoma of the head and neck: an Eastern Cooperative Oncology Group trial (PA390). Cancer (Phila) 1998;82:2270–2274.
191. Dreyfuss AI, Clark JR, Norris CM, et al. Docetaxel: an active drug for squamous cell carcinoma of the head and neck. J Clin Oncol 1996;14:1672–1678.
192. Couteau C, Chouaki N, Leyvraz S, et al. A phase II study of docetaxel in patients with metastatic squamous cell carcinoma of the head and neck. Br J Cancer 1999;81:457–462.
193. Catimel G, Verweij J, Mattijssen V, et al. Docetaxel (Taxotere): an active drug for the treatment of patients with advanced squamous cell carcinoma of the head and neck. EORTC Early Clinical Trials Group. Ann Oncol 1994;5:533–537.
194. Buesa JM, Fernandez R, Esteban E, et al. Phase II trial of ifosfamide in recurrent and metastatic head and neck cancer. Ann Oncol 1991;2:151–152.
195. Huber MH, Lippman SM, Benner SE, et al. A phase II study of ifosfamide in recurrent squamous cell carcinoma of the head and neck. Am J Clin Oncol 1996;19:379–382.
196. Sandler A, Saxman S, Bandealy M, et al. Ifosfamide in the treatment of advanced or recurrent squamous cell carcinoma of the head and neck: a phase II Hoosier Oncology Group trial. Am J Clin Oncol 1998;21:195–197.
197. Cervellino JC, Araujo CE, Pirisi C, Francia A, Cerruti R. Ifosfamide and mesna for the treatment of advanced squamous cell head and neck cancer. A GETLAC study. Oncology 1991;48:89–92.
198. Degardin M, Oliveira J, Geoffrois L, et al. An EORTC-ECSG phase II study of vinorelbine in patients with recurrent and/or metastatic squamous cell carcinoma of the head and neck. Ann Oncol 1998;9:1103–1107.
199. Saxman S, Mann B, Canfield V, Loehrer P, Vokes E. A phase II trial of vinorelbine in patients with recurrent or metastatic squamous cell carcinoma of the head and neck. Am J Clin Oncol 1998;21:398–400.
200. Catimel G, Vermorken JB, Clavel M, et al. A phase II study of Gemcitabine (LY 188011) in patients with advanced squamous cell carcinoma of the head and neck. EORTC Early Clinical Trials Group. Ann Oncol 1994;5:543–547.
201. Samlowski WE, Gundacker H, Kuebler JP, et al. Evaluation of gemcitabine in patients with recurrent or metastatic squamous cell carcinoma of the head and neck: a Southwest Oncology Group phase II study. Invest New Drugs 2001;19:311–315.
202. Schrijvers D, Johnson J, Jiminez U, et al. Phase III trial of modulation of cisplatin/fluorouracil chemotherapy by interferon alfa-2b in patients with recurrent or metastatic head and neck cancer. Head and Neck Interferon Cooperative Study Group. J Clin Oncol 1998;16:1054–1059.
203. Forastiere AA, Leong T, Rowinsky E, et al. Phase III comparison of high-dose paclitaxel + cisplatin + granulocyte colony-stimulating factor versus low-dose paclitaxel + cisplatin in advanced head and neck cancer: Eastern Cooperative Oncology Group Study E1393. J Clin Oncol 2001;19:1088–1095.
204. Gilson MK, Li Y, Murphy B, et al. Randomized phase III evaluation of cisplatin plus fluorouracil versus cisplatin plus paclitaxel in advanced head and neck cancer (E1395): an intergroup trial of the eastern cooperative oncology group. J Clin Oncol 2005;23:3562–3567.

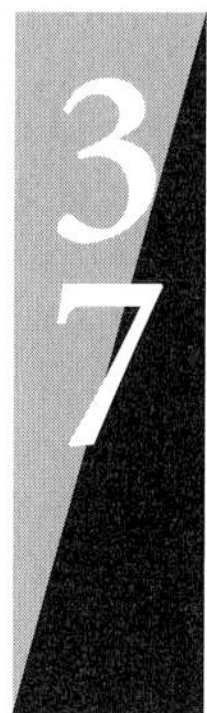

Lung Cancer

Hak Choy, Harvey I. Pass, Rafael Rosell, and Anne Traynor

Etiology

Lung cancer is the leading cause of cancer death in the United States and throughout the world.[1] In the United States, the manufactured cigarette emerged as the tobacco product of choice shortly after the turn of the 20th century. Lung cancer surfaced after years of inhalation of cigarette smoke, first among men and then among women. From 1995 to 1999, cigarette smoking and exposure to environmental tobacco smoke (ETS) accounted for approximately 160,000 annual deaths in the United States. Each year, 127,813 Americans die from smoking-attributable lung cancer deaths.

Smoking

Active Cigarette Smoking

Worldwide, approximately 4 million people die annually of tobacco-attributable diseases; the number of tobacco-attributable deaths is projected to rise to 8.4 million by 2020. China, with 20% of the world's population, smokes 30% of the world's cigarettes. Men smoke more than women, and the proportion of male deaths at ages 35 to 69 years attributable to tobacco has been predicted to rise over the next few decades from 13% (in 1988) to about 33%.[2] In Hong Kong, cigarette consumption reached its peak 20 years earlier than in mainland China. In the general population of Hong Kong, in 1988, tobacco caused about 33% of all male deaths at ages 35 to 69, plus 5% of all female deaths, and hence 25% of all deaths at these ages.[2]

A highly significant trend of increasing lung cancer mortality has been observed with increasing cigarette consumption. Smoking was considered causally related to cancers of the trachea, lung and bronchus, larynx, and lip by the first Surgeon General's Report in 1964.[3] In studies conducted through the 1960s, cigarette smoking was strongly associated with squamous and small cell cancers of the lung, but less so with adenocarcinoma. However, during the past two decades, there has been a noticeable shift in lung cancer histology patterns. The relative frequency of squamous cell carcinoma has decreased, whereas that of adenocarcinomas, often of peripheral origin, is clearly increasing. This shift has been attributed to changing cigarette design, in which filters removed much of the tar from inhaled tobacco smoke. The tar fraction contains most of the polycyclic aromatic hydrocarbons (PAH), including numerous carcinogens known to produce squamous cell lung cancer in animals. However, filters also retain some nicotine. As the use of filtered cigarettes has become predominant, smokers have inhaled more deeply and have retained smoke longer in the deep lung to satisfy nicotine craving.[4]

The mainstream smoke emerging from the mouthpiece of a cigarette is an aerosol containing about 1,010 particles/mL and 4,800 compounds. Experimentally, vapor-phase components of the smoke can be separated from the particulate phase by a glass fiber filter. The vapor-phase comprises more than 90% of the mainstream smoke weight. Potentially carcinogenic vapor-phase compounds include nitrogen oxides, isoprene, butadiene (BD), benzene, styrene, formaldehyde, acetaldehyde, acrolein, and furan. The particulate phase contains at least 3,500 compounds and many carcinogens including PAH, N-nitrosamines, aromatic amines, and metals.[5,6] A key aspect of the link between cigarette smoke and lung cancer is the chronic exposure of DNA to multiple metabolically activated carcinogens, leading to multiple DNA adducts and mutations (Figure 37.1).

PAH and other aromatics are also found in ambient and indoor air and in the diet. PAH, a major class of carcinogens present in ETS, leads to the formation of DNA adducts, which cause mutagenic events involving chromosomal aberrations, DNA strand breaks, oncogene activation, and tumor suppressor gene inactivation. Several epidemiologic and experimental studies have shown a good correlation between PAH and aromatic DNA adducts in blood and lung tissue from the same subjects. Genetic susceptibility plays an important role in the risk of developing lung cancer, and at present there are multiple biomarker assays to predict exposure risk[7] (Table 37.1).

Passive Smoking/Environmental Tobacco Smoke

Active cigarette smoking, passive smoking, various occupational exposures, and carcinogens in heavily polluted air are causally related to lung cancer. Environmental tobacco smoke (ETS) is a form of indoor air pollution resulting from the mixture of sidestream smoke, emitted from the smoldering of the distal part of the cigarette in between puff drawing, and the portion of mainstream smoke that is released into ambient air by actively smoking individuals. Most epidemiologic studies support the view that exposure to ETS involves a carcinogenic risk to humans. In rats treated with very high doses of a mixture of sidestream smoke and mainstream smoke, mimicking exposure to ETS, the formation of DNA adducts was observed in different organs and tissues.[8] The poor persistence of smoke-related adducts in the lung sug-

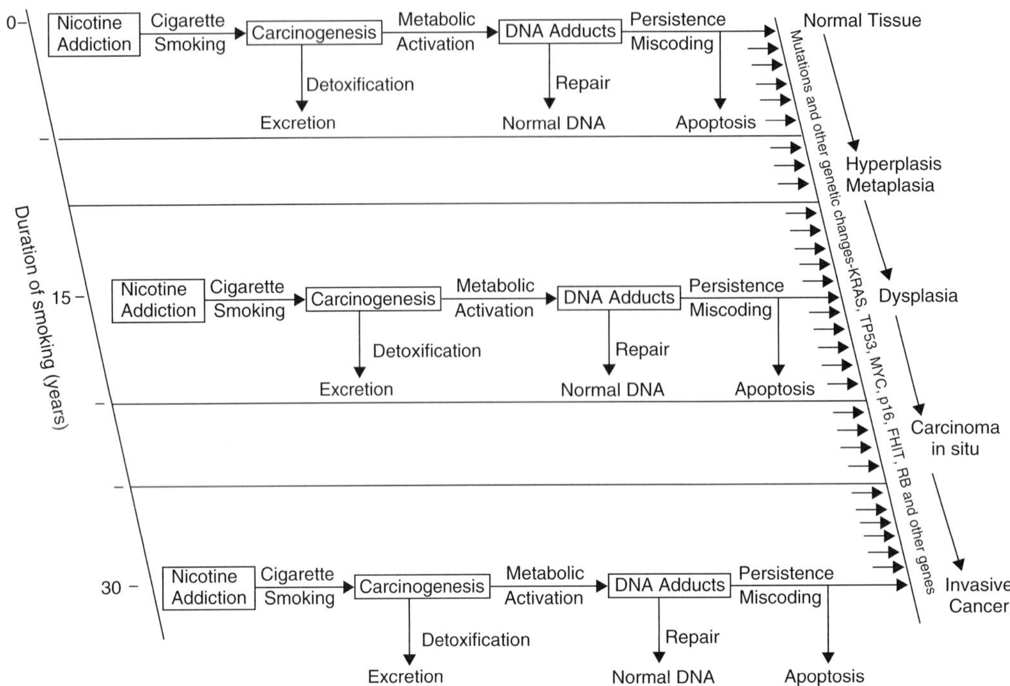

FIGURE 37.1. Genotoxicity of tobacco smoke.

gests that a continuative exposure is needed for fixation of DNA damage. It has been demonstrated that spending an average period of 3 hours in a smoky pub results in a considerably high exposure to carcinogenic ETS.

In one study, the mean ambient air concentration of benzo[*a*]pyrene, a widely known representative of carcinogenic PAH, was 6.3 ng/m3. The mean concentrations of this compound in smoking and nonsmoking homes were 1.0 and 0.4 ng/m^3, respectively. The values in commercial buildings were 1.07 ng/m3 for smoking zones and 0.39 ng/m3 for nonsmoking zones. In the ambient air of Silesia, Poland, a highly polluted industrial city, the mean concentrations of benzo[*a*]pyrene were 60 to 90 ng/m^3 in winter and 5 to 20 mg/m^3 in summer.[9]

Significantly, formation of DNA adducts was observed in the induced sputum of 3 of 15 healthy nonsmokers consequent to ETS exposure, establishing a plausible link between ETS and lung cancer.[9] The hypothesis that ETS is more potent than mainstream tobacco smoke as a lung carcinogen is supported by observations that cigarette sidestream smoke condensate is more carcinogenic in skin painting studies than full-smoke condensate. ETS-induced lung tumor risk in A/J mice occurs by a predominantly genotoxic mechanism of action, which may be suppressed partially by sustained high-level ETS exposure.

Trends in Lung Cancer Risk After Smoking Cessation

In both men and women, the age-related increase in lung cancer risk is lowest in people who have never smoked, intermediate in those who have quit at various ages, and highest in those who continue smoking. Among former smokers, the age-related increase is smaller the earlier the age of quitting.[3] Widespread cessation of smoking in the United Kingdom has

TABLE 37.1. Classification and examples of biomarkers for lung cancer.

Category	*Examples*
External exposure	Questionnaire data, Federal Trade Commission (FTC) yield
Biomarker of exposure	Polycyclic aromatic hydrocarbon in lung tissue Urinary measurement of tobacco constituent or metabolite, exhaled CO; carboxyhemoglobin, urinary mutagenicity
Biologically effective dose	Carcinogen–DNA adducts in human lung tissue Carcinogen–DNA hemoglobin adducts, chromosomal aberrations in cultured lymphocytes, lipid peroxidation
Biomarker of harm	Changes in RNA or protein expression, somatic mutations and LOH in normally or abnormally appearing tissue; change in methylation or gene control; mitochondrial mutations, mRNA expression arrays or proteomics Osteoporosis, hypertension, hyperplasia, dysplasia, lipids, blood coagulant pathways, mRNA expression arrays or proteomics Leukocytosis, hprt mutations, mRNA or protein expression via microarrays in cultured blood cells
Effect modifiers	Genetic polymorphisms for genes involved in disease pathways Enzyme induction of metabolizing enzymes

LOH, loss of heterozygosity.

approximately halved the lung cancer mortality that would have been expected if former smokers had continued to smoke.[10] However, for some individuals, such as those of advanced age and heavy smoking exposure, the risk of lung cancer may exceed 10% within 10 years even if they stop smoking.[11] The risk for lung cancer is increased for both current and former female smokers compared with female nonsmokers and declines for former smokers with increasing duration of abstinence.[12]

Occupational Exposure and Polluted Air

Workers in graphite-electrode manufacturing, as well as in coke-oven plants, are exposed to PAH by inhalation of volatile PAH and PAH bound to respiratory particulate matter. Mean 8-oxo-7,8-dihydro-2′-deoxyguanosine in white blood cells of exposed workers was between 1.38 and 2.15 times higher than levels found in control samples. An alkaline single-cell gel electrophoresis (Comet assay) was used to study DNA strand breaks that were found in exposed workers. These biomarkers may be appropriate for surveillance of workers exposed to PAH[13] (see Table 37.1).

Vehicles powered by diesel engines are a major source of suspended particulate matter, which is a suspected cause of lung cancer and allergic respiratory disease, including bronchial asthma. Diesel exhaust contains potent carcinogens and mutagens, such as PAH and nitrated PAH. PAH released from diesel exhaust particulates also generate DNA adducts that cause mutations in oncogenes and tumor suppressor genes and act as initiators of carcinogenesis. DNA adducts were identified in rats after both short-term (12 weeks) and long-term (30 months) exposure to diesel exhaust, and the level of DNA adducts was shown to be higher in lung tumor tissues than in normal tissues after chronic exposure.[14] Formation of DNA adducts is catalyzed by CYP1A1 and CYP1A2, which are inducible by PAH. CYPs oxidize PAH to reactive electrophilic metabolites, which bind to DNA bases to form DNA adducts. The level of cytochrome P-450 1A1 mRNA was shown by Northern blot analysis to be significantly increased in the lungs of rats exposed to 6 mg/m3 of diesel exhaust.[14]

1,3-BD is a major commodity chemical used in the manufacture of synthetic rubber and various plastics.[15] Global consumption of BD was 6.1 million metric tons in 1995, with consumption expected to rise to more than 7.5 million metric tons in the year 2000. BD is also a common air contaminant found in auto emissions and cigarette smoke. It is a component of automotive exhaust and of the vapor phase of environmental smoke (~400 mg/cigarette). BD is carcinogenic in rodent bioassays, and exposure of mice to BD at 20 parts per million for 4 days induced mutations in spleen lymphocytes at the hypoxanthine-guanine phosphoribosyl transferase (HPRT) locus.

Coexposure to cadmium, cobalt, lead, and other heavy metals occurs in many occupational settings, such as pigment and batteries production, galvanization, and recycling of electric tools.[16] The lifetime excess lung cancer risk for cadmium fumes of 100 mg/m^3 was estimated to be approximately 50 to 111 lung cancer deaths per 1,000 workers exposed to cadmium for 45 years. The principal mechanisms of cadmium genotoxicity, mutagenicity, and carcinogenicity are generation of reactive oxygen species, inhibition of DNA repair, depletion of glutathione, and possibly also suppression of apoptosis.

Diet and Lung Cancer Risk

Numerous epidemiologic studies have demonstrated a protective effect of vegetable or fruit consumption on cancer risk.[17–22] Statistically significant inverse associations were found with total vegetables and most vegetable groups in a Netherlands study.[17] The strongest effect was found for vegetables from the *Brassica* group (Brussels sprouts, cauliflower, cabbage, kale). Based on the results, it was calculated that a male current smoker who smoked 25 cigarettes per day for 40 years has a risk of lung cancer that is 18 times higher than that of a never-smoker. By eating 286 g vegetables per day, instead of 103 grams, he may reduce his risk by 29%.[17] The mechanisms underlying a cancer protection by fruit and vegetables are still uncertain. The possible protective compounds in vegetables and fruits include a wide variety of phytochemicals. Among them are the carotenoids, colorful compounds that are abundant as pigments in plants. The main carotenoids are α-carotene, β-carotene, lutein, zeaxanthin, β-cryptoxanthin, and lycopene. They are potent quenchers of free radicals, which are by-products of metabolic processes originating from environmental pollutants such as cigarette smoke.[23]

Blood levels of micronutrients and vitamins including beta-carotene have been inversely correlated with lung cancer risk.[24] However, large intervention studies with β-carotene supplementation found no clear protection against cancer or cardiovascular disease, and two studies were terminated because mortality or lung cancer incidence increased in the supplemented group.[25–27] Subsequent analyses suggested that the deleterious effect might occur primarily among heavy current smokers and/or alcohol drinkers and asbestos-exposed subjects.[28] It has been speculated that this represents a pro-oxidant interaction effect of β-carotene with such exposures or that it could be related to a high supplementation dose and unnaturally high serum levels.

Lung Cancer Susceptibility

Gender

It has been stated that females are more susceptible than males to tobacco carcinogenesis. Activation of gastrin-releasing peptide receptor (GRPR) in airways has been related to a proliferative response of bronchial cells to gastrin-releasing peptide and to long-term tobacco exposure. The GRPR gene is located on the X chromosome and escapes X-chromosome inactivation, which occurs in females. GRPR mRNA expression was detected in airway cells and tissues of more female than male nonsmokers and short-term smokers. Female smokers showed expression of GRPR mRNA at a lower mean pack-year (number of packs of cigarettes smoked per day multiplied by number of years of smoking) exposure than male smokers. These findings indicate that women may have a higher risk of developing lung cancer than men.[29] However, in a different study, the risk of lung cancer was comparable in women and men.[30]

Estrogen and progesterone receptors have been found to be present in resected lung cancers, regardless of the sex of the patient, although a female patient with squamous cell carcinoma showed an estrogen receptor level of 301 fmol/mg.[31] Catechol estrogens may act as carcinogens either by forming DNA adducts or by acting as oxidative intermediates. The CYP1B1*3 polymorphism, which can cause enhanced conversion of estradiol to 4-hydroxy-estrogen and its catechol estrogen metabolite, was found frequently among 203 lung cancer cases in comparison with 205 controls (odds ratio, 2.6). Gene–gene interactive associations were observed among females, but not among males, with the CYP1B1*3 allele, including increased adjusted odds ratios for coinheritance of at least one copy of the CYP1B1*3 allele and the DNA repair enzyme XPD exon 23 (Gln) allele (odds ratio, 5.7), or for coinheritance of CYP1B1*3 and the high or intermediate activity alleles of epoxide hydrolase (odds ratio, 9.1). The microsomal epoxide hydrolase enzyme could activate catechol estrogens to reactive intermediate.[32]

Lung cancer is the leading cause of cancer death in Taiwanese women, although less than 10% of female lung cancer patients are smokers. Half of the 141 lung tumors in these patients had human papillomavirus 16/18, compared with 26% of 60 noncancer control subjects. It is thought that the human papillomavirus infection is related to lung cancer development in nonsmoking females.[33]

An aggregation of lung cancer was seen in first-degree relatives of more than 800 lung cancer probands, and a significantly lower intake of dietary folate, critical for maintaining DNA integrity and synthesis, was observed in lung cancer cases compared with controls.[34]

Genetic

Alterations in Minisatellites and Variable Number of Tandem Repeats

Microsatellite instability, defined as changes in the number of short tandem DNA repeats in microsatellites, mainly associated with CA dinucleotides, has been reported in non-small cell lung cancer (NSCLC).[35] Genetic susceptibility to lung cancer is multifactorial, including alterations in minisatellites and variable number of tandem repeats (VNTR). The HRAS1 VNTR region, which maps 1 kb downstream from the canonical polyadenylation signal of the human proto-oncogene H-*ras*-1, consists of four common progenitor alleles, in addition to several rare variants that are thought to derive from germ-line mutations of the nearest common alleles. A higher percentage of rare HRAS1 VNTR alleles was found in lung cancer patients than in controls,[36] and a meta-analysis[37] showed suggestive but not statistically significant association for these alleles with lung cancer. Minisatellite alterations may cause dysregulation of gene expression. HRAS1 VNTR binds at members of the NF-kB family of transcriptional regulatory factors, and some HRAS1 VNTR alleles show a tendency to bind more avidly to transcriptional regulatory factors. Frequent allele loss for the marker HRAS on chromosome 11p (deleted region designated LOH11B) has been associated with cigarette consumption and gender. None of the nonsmokers had allele loss, as compared with 28% of the patients with low and 43% of those with high cigarette consumption. Allele loss was also more frequent in men (43%) than in women (11%). Median survival was lower for patients with allele loss.[38]

Adducts

DNA adducts are markers not only of exposure but also of risk for cancer development. Healthy current smokers who had elevated levels of DNA adducts in leukocytes were approximately three times more likely to be diagnosed with lung cancer 1 to 13 years later than current smokers with lower adduct concentrations.[39] A recent meta-analysis found an overall 83% excess of adducts in cases compared to controls in current smokers.[40]

DNA adducts have been found to be higher in women than in men with the same level of smoking.

S-Transferase

Glutathione *S*-transferase (GST) M1 is deleted in about half of Caucasians, and a GSTP1 polymorphism at codon 105 (Ile to Val) has been identified. The combined GSTM1 null/GSTP1 Val genotypes were associated with lung cancer before and after adjusting for adducts.[41] In addition, a meta-analysis of 43 published case-control studies including more than 18,000 subjects found a slight excess risk for lung cancer in individuals with the GSTM1 null genotype.[42]

Insulin-Like Growth Factor

A case-control analysis of plasma insulin-like growth factor (IGF) levels from lung cancer patients revealed that elevated plasma IGF-I was associated with an increased risk of lung cancer. An increased risk of lung cancer was also associated with reduced levels of IGF-binding protein (IGFBP)-3, which moderates the effect of IGF-I but also inhibits all growth and induces apoptosis.[43] Elevated levels of IGF-II are associated with a poor prognosis in human lung adenocarcinoma. Transgenic overexpression of IGF-II in lung epithelium induces lung tumors in mice. These tumors display morphologic characteristics of human pulmonary adenocarcinomas, such as expression of prosurfactant protein C, surfactant protein B, and thyroid transcription factor 1. Moreover, IGF-II induced proliferation and CREB phosphorylation in human lung cancer cell lines.[44]

Polymorphisms in DNA Repair Capacity (DRC) Genes

Host-specific factors modulate susceptibility to tobacco carcinogenesis, including variations in DNA repair, which may influence the rate of removal of DNA damage and of fixation of mutations. In a seminal study, DRC was measured in peripheral blood lymphocytes by means of the host-cell reactivation assay, which measured cellular reactivation of a reporter gene damaged by exposure to 75 mM benzo[*a*]pyrene diol epoxide. The mean level of DRC in lung cancer cases (3.3%) was significantly lower than in controls (5.1%). Younger cases (less than 65 years) and smokers were more likely than controls to have reduced DRC.[45] This finding was confirmed in a case-control study of 316 newly diagnosed lung cancer patients and 316 cancer-free controls. Case patients who were younger at diagnosis, female, or lighter smokers, or who reported a family history of cancer, exhibited the lowest DRC, suggesting that these subgroups may be especially susceptible to lung cancer.[46] Reduced DRC and increased DNA adduct levels are associated with increased risk of lung cancer.

Nucleotide excision repair (NER) is one of the principal pathways for repair of DNA adducts induced by smoking-related carcinogens. NER is also the main mechanism for removing cisplatin adducts.[47] The NER molecular machinery includes proteins that are mutated in xeroderma pigmentosum (XP) and Cockayne syndrome (CS) patients. In the global genome repair pathway, the protein complex XPC-HHR23B, which appears to be essential for the recruitment of all subsequent NER factors in the preincision complex, binds to damaged DNA. Then, the multicomponent transcription factor TFIIH, which is responsible for unwinding the damaged region of the DNA, is recruited. Next, XPG nuclease cleaves the DNA on the 3′-end. Following cleavage on the DNA, XPA/RPA proteins join the complex and recruit the ERCC1-XPF complex, which cleaves the 5′-end.[47,48]

Polymorphisms of a number of DNA repair genes involved in the NER pathway have the potential to affect protein function and subsequently DRC. In lung cancer patients, reduced expression levels of XPG and CSB have been observed in peripheral lymphocytes.[49] Moreover, ERCC1 and XPD mRNA levels in lymphocytes have been shown to correlate with DRC and could thus be useful surrogates of DRC.[50] A reduction in DRC was more significant in lung cancer patients who were homozygous for two XPD (also known as ERCC2) polymorphisms (Asp312Asn at exon 10 and Lys751Gln at exon 23) (−12.3% and −18.3%, respectively) than in controls (−3.3% and −5.4%, respectively). Lung cancer patients who were homozygous for XPD Asn312Asn or Gln751Gln had an increased risk of suboptimal DRC (odds ratios, 1.57 and 3.50, respectively), compared to those who were wild-type homozygous.[51] The intron 9 polymorphism of XPC [an 83-bp poly(AT) insertion] has also been correlated with DRC. XPC PAT+/+ homozygous subjects exhibited lower DRC than those with other XPC PAT genotypes, suggesting that XPC PAT+/+ is an adverse genotype.[52] A common single-nucleotide polymorphism (A to G) in the 5′-noncoding region of the XPA gene has been related to lung cancer. The presence of one or two copies of the G allele was associated with a reduced lung cancer risk. Control subjects with one or two copies of the G allele demonstrated more efficient DRC than those homozygous for the A allele.[48]

Polymorphisms in other pathways have been identified also. The XRCC3 (belonging to the homologous recombination repair pathway) Thr241Met at exon 7 and the XRCC1 (belonging to the base excision repair pathway) Arg399Gln at exon 10 have been related to lung cancer. The XRCC3 241Met allele was associated with higher DNA adduct levels, while the XRCC1 399Gln allele was associated with higher DNA adduct levels only in nonsmokers.[53] Gene–smoking interaction associations have been found for the XPD Asp312Asn and Lys751Gln and for the XRCC1 Arg399Gln polymorphisms. The odds ratios decreased as pack-years increased. For nonsmokers, the adjusted odds ratio was 2.4, whereas for heavy smokers (more than 55 pack-years), the odds ratio decreased to 0.5. When the three polymorphisms were evaluated together, the adjusted odds ratios for individuals with five or six variant alleles versus individuals with no variant alleles were 5.2 for nonsmokers and 0.3 for heavy smokers.[54]

Basic Science

Lung cancers are believed to arise after a series of progressive pathologic changes (preneoplastic lesions). Many of these preneoplastic changes are frequently detected in the respiratory mucosa of smokers. The molecular abnormalities involved in the multistep pathogenesis of lung carcinomas have been examined in lung cancer cell lines, microdissected primary lung tumors, respiratory epithelium from patients with lung cancer, and respiratory epithelium from nonsmokers[55] (Figure 37.2). Historically, the carcinogenesis sequence for squamous cell carcinomas shows that invasive lung cancer develops through a series of stages from mild, moderate, and severe atypia, carcinoma in situ, and then invasive cancer. The genetic changes of preneoplastic lesions can be analyzed in cytologic specimens, including sputum samples, bronchial brushes and bronchoalveolar lavage fluids (BAL) from smokers.

Atypical adenomatous hyperplasia (AAH) is considered to be the preinvasive lesion of adenocarcinoma. AAH is valued as a good target for delineating the timing and sequence of genetic alterations in the development of lung adenocarcinomas. Activation of the K-*ras* oncogene seems to be an early event involved in the initiation of AAH. Progression of AAH through increasing degrees of morphologic dysplasia requires the silencing of key tumor suppressor genes, such as p16. Ultimately, activation of telomerase and inactivation of the p53 tumor suppressor gene appear to be important in triggering invasive tumor growth.

Importantly, as discussed later, alterations of LKB1 function may represent one of the critical steps in the transition

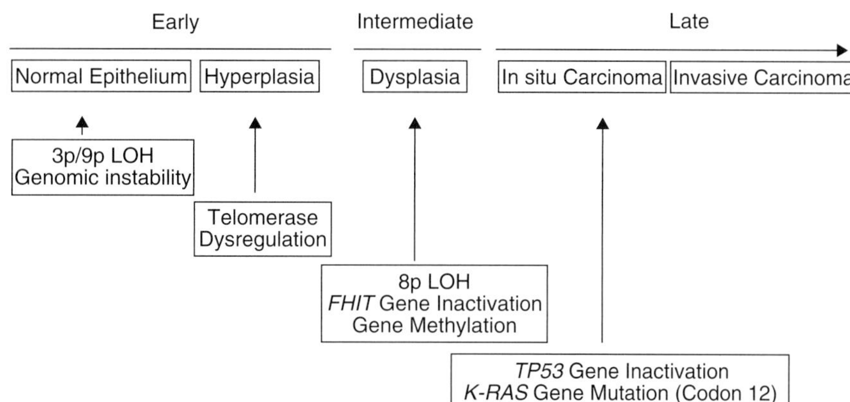

FIGURE 37.2. Sequential molecular changes during the multistage pathogenesis of squamous cell lung carcinoma.

from a benign to a potentially malignant proliferation of pneumocytes. Loss of LKB1 expression was more frequent (21%) in the high-grade AAH lesions (severe atypia) than in low-grade lesions (5%). Therefore, loss of LKB1 expression is associated with severe dysplasia.[56]

Genetic

Oncogenes and Tumor Suppressor Genes

In general, mutations follow a sequence. Allelic losses at chromosomes 3p, 9p, and 8p occur relatively early. Losses and inactivation of the retinoblastoma and p53 genes are intermediate, and losses at 5q are late events.[55] The losses at 3p are progressive, and advanced lesions and tumors have often lost most of the arm or the entire arm, whereas early lesions have more focal lesions.[57] In contrast, loss of heterozygosity (LOH) at 5q21 (APC-MMC region) and K-*ras* mutations are detected at the carcinoma in situ stage.[55] Some of the genetic changes involved in the pathogenesis of lung cancer are depicted in Table 37.2.

Mutations of the K-*ras* proto-oncogene are found in about 20% of the tumors with a mutation hot spot at codon 12. However, the mutation frequencies are significantly different among histologic subtypes of lung cancer. Most K-*ras* mutations are detected in lung adenocarcinoma.[58,59] *ras* mutations are not observed in small cell lung cancer (SCLC).[60] K-*ras* mutations are not correlated with sex of the patient, tumor extent, or prior therapy status.[60]

The p53 tumor suppressor gene is inactivated by mutations in more than 50% of NSCLC patients and in 90% of SCLC patients. p53 gene mutations in NSCLC cell lines with *ras* mutations tended to cluster at exon 8.[61]

Epidermal Growth Factor Pathway

Overexpression and/or hyperactivity of the epidermal growth factor receptor (EGFR) has been shown to play a causal role in the progression of lung tumors. EGFR is activated by the binding of ligands to its extracellular domain, which leads to receptor homodimerization or heterodimerization with any of the other three members of this family of transmembrane tyrosine kinases: HER2 (erbB2), HER3, and HER4. This results in the binding of adenosine triphosphate (ATP) to the receptor's catalytic site, activation of the receptor's tyrosine kinase, and autophosphorylation of C-terminal tyrosine residues, which in turn recruit several cytoplasmic signal transducers. These effector molecules include Ras-MEK-MAPK, phosphatidylinositol-3 kinase (PI3K) and its target Akt, p70S6 kinase, Src, and STATs, among others. Active Akt phosphorylates a number of substrates involved in apoptosis, cell-cycle regulation, protein synthesis, and glycogen metabolism, which include the Bcl-2 family member Bad, forkhead transcription factors, caspase 9, IKB kinase, p21, p27, mTOR, and nitric oxide synthase. Akt activity has been shown to be upregulated by loss of function of the phosphatase and tensin homologue (PTEN) phosphatase.[62] In addition, the activation of receptor tyrosine kinases and Src also leads to activation of the signal transducers and activators of the transcription (STAT) pathway.

Tyrosine kinase growth factor receptors are overexpressed in a large number of human lung cancers, with NSCLCs demonstrating overexpression of EGFR and its ligands EGF, amphiregulin, and tumor necrosis factor-alpha (TGF-α), whereas some SCLCs demonstrate c-Kit overexpression. STAT activation leads to increased transcription of cyclin, D1, and Myc. In NSCLC cells, Stat3 DNA-binding capacity is upregulated by EGF, interleukin 6 (IL-6), and the hepatocyte growth factor (HGF).[63] A model proposed in NSCLC is that either EGF, IL-6, or the HGF-Src-Stat3 signaling cascade may protect lung cancer cells from death signals through the upregulation of Stat3 activity. Interestingly, no constitutive Stat3 activity was found in a human lung carcinoma cell line that had constitutive Akt activity. Therefore, Stat3 signaling may be dispensable for tumors that have upregulated other survival signals such as Akt.[63] An increased understanding of molecular biology is necessary to piece together all the critical factors in lung cancer cell growth.

Angiogenesis

Angiogenesis is essential for tumor growth in vivo. Cytokines and growth factors, such as TGF-β, TGF-α, platelet-derived growth factor, basic fibroblast growth factor, and vascular endothelial growth factor (VEGF), are known to promote angiogenesis. VEGF expression is induced in cancer cells as a result of hypoxia and multiple genetic alterations, including p53 and PTEN loss-of-function, RAS and SRC gain-of-

TABLE 37.2. Summary of the histopathologic and molecular abnormalities of the major types of lung cancer.

Abnormality histopathology	*Small cell lung cancer (SCLC)*	*Squamous cell carcinoma*	*Adenocarcinoma*
Precursor	Unknown	Known	Probable
Lesion	Normal epithelium and hyperplasia	Squamous dysplasia and CIS	Adenomatous atypical hyperplasia (AAH)
Theory of development	Parallel	Sequential	Probably sequential
Molecular			
Gene abnormalities	*myc* overexpression TP53 LOH and mutation	TP53 LOH and mutation	K-*ras* mutation
LOH	High	Intermediate	Low
Frequency	90%	54%	10%
Chromosomal regions	5q21, 8p21–23, 9p21, 17p/TP53	8p21–23, 9p21, 17p/TP53	9p21, 17p/TP53
Genetic instability	High	Intermediate	Low
Frequency	68%	10%	13%

function and autocrine tyrosine kinase signaling pathways involving EGFR, HER-2/neu, and insulin growth factor 1 receptor (IGF-1R). In each case, VEGF expression is activated by hypoxia inducible factor 1 (HIF-1).[64] Cyclooxygenase (COX)-2, a catalyst in prostaglandin synthesis from arachidonic acid, also increases VEGF expression. Another angiogenesis modulator, nitric oxide synthase (NOS-2), stimulates VEGF as well. Immunohistochemical protein expression levels of COX-2, NOS-2, and VEGF correlated with microvessel density at the tumor-stromal interphase. NOS-2 and COX-2 levels correlated positively with VEGF status.[65]

Gene and Protein Expression Patterns

Comprehensive analysis of gene expression patterns could provide detailed molecular portraits including differences in gene expression profiles among lung adenocarcinomas. Thyroid transcription factor 1, as well as several surfactant-related genes, was identified as one of the genes whose expression is primarily restricted to lung adenocarcinomas.[66–69]

High-resolution two-dimensional polyacrylamide gel electrophoresis (2-D PAGE) analysis allows the simultaneous assessment of hundreds of known and unknown polypeptides. Protein expression profiles (proteomic analysis) of lung adenocarcinomas identified triosephosphate isomerase, a key component of the glycolytic pathway that converts dihydroxyacetone phosphate to glyceraldehyde 3-phosphate, to be significantly elevated in more advanced lung adenocarcinomas.[70] A glucose-regulated (GRP58) protein that was increased in tumors with K-*ras* mutations was also elevated.[70,71] Proteomic profiling of tumor tissue has the potential to uncover aberrantly expressed proteins resulting, in part, from numerous posttranslational modifications that may be altered in lung cancer.

Aberrant Methylation

To determine the extent of RASSF1A promoter methylation, sputum samples from lung cancer patients and from current and former smokers were examined using the common procedure of methylation-specific PCR. Fifty percent of SCLC and 21% of NSCLC patients had RASSF1A methylation, whereas 1 of 2 former smokers and 4 of 13 current smokers showed RASSF1A methylation in sputum. Furthermore, 2 of the 4 current smokers and 1 former smoker showing RASSF1A methylation in their sputum developed lung cancer within 12 to 14 months of bronchoscopy.[72]

Methylation status of p16, DAPK, and GSTP1 has been studied in bronchial brush samples from former smokers.[73] A total of 32% of the samples had methylation in at least one of the three genes tested.[73] Interestingly, in a study where DNA was isolated from sputum, bilateral BAL, and brushing taken at bronchoscopy, p16 promoter methylation and p53 mutations were observed in chronic smokers before any clinical evidence of neoplasia. However, K-*ras* mutations were exclusively seen in lung cancer patients.[74]

Genetic Alterations in Serum/Plasma

Elevated levels of free DNA in the serum of lung cancer patients were reported more than 25 years ago.[75] The cancer fingerprint in the form of microsatellite alterations in plasma DNA was found in 50% of SCLC patients. A microsatellite alteration was present in 76% of SCLC tumors and in 71% of plasma samples.[76] Microsatellite alterations, either as a shift (changes in the size of the microsatellite sequence), LOH, or both, have been found in tumor and serum/plasma DNA paired samples in NSCLC, using microsatellite markers at chromosome 3p.[77,78]

Intriguingly, plasma DNA abnormalities were found in 45% of tumors up to 2 cm in maximum diameter.[78] Similarly, findings indicate that quantification and molecular characterization of plasma DNA in lung cancer patients are valuable noninvasive tools for discriminating patients from unaffected individuals and for detecting early recurrence during follow-up.[79] LOH in plasma samples also predated a diagnosis of lung cancer by several months.[80] Other studies have reported p53 and K-*ras* mutations in serum DNA. Aberrant methylation of at least one of p16, DAPK, GSTP1, or MGMT was noted in 15 of 22 (68%) NSCLC tumors but not in any paired normal lung tissue. In these primary tumors with methylation, 11 of 15 (73%) samples also had abnormal methylated DNA in the matched serum samples.[81] Other genes are also methylated in primary tumors and paired preoperative serum samples from lung cancer patients.

Genetic and Molecular Alterations in Sputum

Sputum is the most commonly utilized biologic material to detect lung cancer cells in a noninvasive manner. Cancer cells harboring point mutations of oncogenes such as K-*ras*[82] and p53 might be detected in sputum of patients with early-stage lung cancer. Bronchoalveolar lavage has also been used as biologic material for the detection of lung cancer.[83] Microsatellite alterations might be detectable in cytologically negative sputum from patients with lung cancer.[82] In lung cancer, aberrant promoter methylation is frequently found in tumor suppressor genes.[84,85] Aberrant methylation of the p16 and/or *O*-6-methyl-guanine-DNA methyltransferase (MGMT) promoter can be found in 100% of patients with squamous cell lung carcinoma up to 3 years before clinical diagnosis.[86] Aberrant promoter methylation of p16 has also been seen in normal bronchial epithelium.[87]

Pathology

Premalignant Lesions

Bronchial preneoplastic lesions may be divided into three broad categories: reactive changes (histologically normal epithelium, hyperplasia, and metaplasia) having no increased risk other than smoke exposure; intermediate changes (mild and moderate dysplasia) having moderately increased risk; and high-risk lesions (severe dysplasia and carcinoma in situ) having considerably increased risk. The proportion of individuals with mild, moderate, or severe sputum cell atypia who will develop invasive lung cancer within 10 years was found to be 4%, 10%, and 40%, respectively.[88]

In a study of high-risk subjects enrolled because of a cigarette-smoking history of at least 30 pack-years, an airflow obstruction, and either an abnormal sputum cytology or a previous or suspected lung cancer, laser-induced fluorescence endoscopy (LIFE) was more sensitive than white-light bronchoscopy (WLB) in detecting preneoplastic bronchial changes.[89] LIFE was also better at identifying angiogenic squamous dysplasia (ASD) lesions than WLB. ASD is a unique lesion consisting of capillary blood vessels closely juxtaposed to and projecting into metaplastic or dysplastic squamous bronchial epithelium. ASD represents a qualitatively distinct from of angiogenesis in which there is architectural rearrangement of the capillary microvasculature. LOH at chromosome 3p was observed in 53% of ASD lesions. ASD was described in 34% of high-risk smokers without carcinoma and in 6 of 10 patients with squamous cell carcinoma who underwent LIFE.[90]

Atypical adenomatous hyperplasia (AAH) is considered to be the preinvasive lesion of adenocarcinoma. These lesions are usually less than 7 mm in diameter and are detected on computed tomography (CT) scan as small, ground-glass densities. In resected lungs, the incidence of AAH was estimated to be 9% to 21% in patients with primary lung cancer and 4% to 10% in patients without lung cancer.[88] The mere presence of AAH does not necessarily indicate sure and unremitting progression to adenocarcinoma.

Lung cancer is classified into two major clinicopathologic groups: small cell lung carcinoma (SCLC) and non-small cell lung carcinoma (NSCLC). Squamous cell carcinoma (SCC), adenocarcinoma, and large cell carcinoma are the major histologic types of NSCLC.

Non-Small Cell Lung Cancer (NSCLC)

Squamous Cell Carcinoma (SCC)

SCC (epidermoid carcinoma) of the lung is a malignant epithelial tumor with the differentiating features of squamous epithelium: keratinization, intercellular bridges, or both. SCC varies from small endobronchial obstructive tumors to large cavitated masses that can replace an entire lung. The masses are gray-white or yellowish, often with a dry flaky appearance that reflects the keratinization. Necrosis and hemorrhage are common; cavitation is seen in one-third of cases. Secondary infections may occur in cavitated masses. SCC of the lung may be divided into well-differentiated, moderately differentiated, and poorly differentiated subtypes depending on the degree of squamous differentiation present. Intercellular bridges and keratinization are most marked in well-differentiated tumors. SCCs tend to grow as nests of cells with surrounding stroma that may be desmoplastic and infiltrated by acute or chronic inflammatory cells. The nuclei are hyperchromatic, sometimes with prominent nucleoli and thick chromatin condensation along the nuclear membrane. SCC typically stains for both high and low molecular weight keratins. Other intermediate filaments may also be present, including vimentin and synaptophysin. SCC may also stain positively for epithelial membrane antigen (EMA), human milk fat globule (HMFG-2), S-100 protein, Leu-M1, and carcinoembryonic antigen (CEA).[91]

Adenocarcinoma

Adenocarcinoma of the lung is a glandular epithelial malignancy manifesting tubular, papillary, or acinar growth patterns or a solid growth pattern with mucin production. Unusual patterns include signet-ring adenocarcinoma, spindle cell adenocarcinoma, and adenocarcinoma showing hepatoid differentiation. Adenocarcinomas are generally peripheral, well-circumscribed masses often associated with overlying pleural fibrosis or puckering. On cut section, they are gray-white, sometimes lobulated, and often have central scarring that may contain anthracotic pigment. The cells comprising adenocarcinoma are large, cuboidal, columnar, or polygonal with large vesicular nuclei and prominent nucleoli. Solid adenocarcinomas may be virtually indistinguishable from large cell carcinomas except for the mucin production. Mucin stains (mucicarmine, periodic acid–Schiff diastase, Alcian blue) are required for diagnosis. Mucin production varies from occasional positive cells to large pools containing nests of tumor cells. Some pleomorphic adenocarcinomas have foci of spindle cells. Pulmonary adenocarcinomas may be positive for a number of neuroendocrine markers.[91]

Bronchoalveolar Carcinoma

Bronchoalveolar carcinoma (BAC), also called alveolar cell carcinoma or bronchoalveolar tumor, is a subset of pulmonary adenocarcinoma in which cylindrical tumor cells grow upon the walls of preexisting alveoli. The key feature is the preservation of the underlying architecture of the lung. BACs are separated into two major subtypes: nonmucinous, comprising two-thirds of cases, and mucinous, comprising most of the remainder. Nonmucinous BACs are composed of cells with Clara cell or type 2 cell differentiation or both. Mucinous BACs are composed of goblet or mucin-producing cells and are usually very well differentiated.[91]

Large Cell Carcinoma

Large cell carcinoma, also called large cell anaplastic carcinoma and large cell undifferentiated carcinoma, is defined as a malignant epithelial tumor with large nuclei, prominent nucleoli, and usually well-defined cell borders without the characteristic features of SCC, small cell, or adenocarcinoma. This definition is one of exclusion and is dependent on extensive sampling of a given tumor.[91]

Small Cell Lung Cancer

The International Association for the Study of Lung Cancer (IASLC) proposed that small cell carcinoma be divided into three categories: small cell carcinoma; mixed small cell/large cell carcinoma; and combined small cell carcinoma, which also has components of squamous cell and/or adenocarcinoma.[92] Small cell carcinoma is composed of small tumor cells with a round to fusiform shape, scant cytoplasm, finely granular nuclear chromatin, and absent or inconspicuous nucleoli. The tumor has a very hyperchromatic appearance because the cells have little cytoplasm and are situated very close to each other. Nuclear molding may be conspicuous but is more difficult to visualize in histologic sections than in cytologic preparations. Mitotic rates are characteristically high, sometimes exceeding 10 per single high-power field.[91]

Neuroendocrine Tumors

SCLC and large cell neuroendocrine (NE) carcinomas are high-grade NE tumors, whereas typical carcinoid and atypical carcinoid are low and intermediate grade, respectively. Large cell NE carcinoma is defined as a tumor with NE morphology, including organoid nesting, palisading, trabecular pattern, and rosette-like structures. A mitotic count of 11 or more mitoses per $2\,mm^2$ is the main criterion for separating large cell NE carcinoma and SCLC from atypical carcinoid. Large cell NE carcinoma and SCLC usually have very high mitotic rates, with an average of 70 to 80 per $2\,mm^2$. Large cell NE carcinoma and SCLC also generally have more extensive necrosis than atypical carcinoid. Large cell NE carcinoma is separated from SCLC using a constellation of criteria, which include larger cell size, abundant cytoplasm, prominent nucleoli, vesicular or coarse chromatin, polygonal rather than fusiform shape, less-prominent nuclear molding, and less-conspicuous DNA encrustation of blood vessel walls.[93]

Clinically, approximately 20% to 40% of patients with both typical and atypical carcinoids are nonsmokers, whereas virtually all patients with SCLC and large cell NE carcinoma are cigarette smokers. In contrast to SCLC and large cell NE carcinoma, both typical and atypical carcinoids can occur in patients with multiple endocrine neoplasia (MEN) type I. Histology heterogeneity with other major histologic types of lung carcinoma (squamous cell carcinoma, adenocarcinoma) occurs with both SCLC and large cell NE carcinoma but not with typical or atypical carcinoids. Furthermore, large cell NE carcinomas and SCLC have a high frequency of retinoblastoma direct inactivation related to retinoblastoma loss of protein expression. However, the typical carcinoids remain the only tumor type in the spectrum of neuroendocrine tumors that retain an intact retinoblastoma pathway. Moreover, p53 mutations leading to immunohistochemical aberrant overexpression of p53 protein are observed in 60% of large cell NE carcinomas and SCLC, in 20% of atypical carcinoids, and in no typical carcinoids. E2F1 regulated by p53-retinoblastoma pathways is overexpressed, as well as all its transcriptional target genes, in the majority of SCLC and large cell NE carcinomas, but not in carcinoids.[94]

Biologic Differences Between Histologic Subtypes

EGFR expression varies according to histologic subtypes. Squamous cell carcinoma expressed EGFR in 84% of tumors, adenocarcinoma in 65%, large cell carcinoma in 68%, and SCLC in 0%. Interestingly, a study of a small number of patients with bronchioloalveolar carcinoma (BAC) found that the large majority had either intermediate or high expression of EGFR by immunostaining. There was also a significant correlation between nonmucinous BAC and EGFR expression, while mucinous BAC histology was more frequently related to HER2 overexpression.[95]

In addition to differences in K-*ras* and p53 mutation frequencies between SCLC and NSCLC, there are other significant genetic distinctions. RASSF1A is inactivated by promoter methylation in more than 90% of SCLCs and in 40% of NSCLCs. Retinoblastoma is inactivated in more than 90% of SCLCs but only 15% of NSCLCs. p16 is almost never abnormal in SCLCs but is inactivated in more than 50% of NSCLCs. A study of hypermethylation in lung cancer for eight genes (p16, APC, CDH13, GSTP1, MGMT, RARb, CDH1, RASSF1A) revealed that the profile of methylated genes in SCLC was different from that of NSCLC.[84] Further details on methylation, including FHIT and DAPK, have been reviewed elsewhere.[85]

Prognostic Factors

Clinical

In a retrospective analysis of 2,531 NSCLC patients treated in the Southwest Oncology Group (SWOG) with extensive disease defined either as distant metastases or locoregional recurrence after definitive radiotherapy, a Cox modeling and recursive partitioning and amalgamation (RPA) was performed to determine independent predictive factors of outcome.[96] Patients were treated between 1974 and 1988. Performance status (PS) was defined as good (SWOG 0–1, no symptoms or with symptoms but fully ambulatory) or poor (SWOG 2–4, nonambulatory). Good performance status (PS), female sex, and age greater than 70 years were significant independent predictors. In a second Cox model for patients with good PS, hemoglobin levels above 11 g/dL, normal calcium, and a single metastatic site were significant favorable factors. The use of cisplatin was an additional independent predictor of improved outcome. An RPA performed in 904 patients from more-recent SWOG trials, almost all of whom were treated with cisplatin, revealed three distinct subsets based on PS, age, hemoglobin, and lactate dehydrogenase (LDH); 1-year survivals were 27%, 16%, and 6%, respectively. Until 1980, additional variables, such as weight loss (less than 10 or more than 10 pounds), were not included. In the multivariate survival analyses by prognostic variables and therapy discriminants, significant favorable SWOG factors were PS 0 to 1, female sex, age greater than 70 years, and then greater than 45 years in females, single metastatic lesion, less than 10 pounds of weight loss, normal LDH, normal alkaline phosphatase, and hemoglobin above 11 g/dL. Median survival was 1 to 3 months better for the good PS, female, single-lesion, and cisplatin-based therapy categories.[96] Intriguingly, LDH was important in the poor PS subset; patients with a normal LDH level and poor PS had a survival outcome similar to other subsets with a good PS.[96]

In the analysis of 1,052 patients included in clinical trials conducted by the European Lung Cancer Working Party (ELCWP), a Cox regression model found the following variables: Karnofsky PS (greater than 80 = SWOG 0–1; less than 70 = SWOG 2–4), neutrophil counts, metastatic involvement of skin, serum calcium level, age, and gender, as well as disease extent, because patients with stages I to III were included in the analysis. According to an RPA model, the best subgroup of patients was defined as female with limited disease and Karnofsky PS above 80.[97] In a third, smaller analysis including a homogenous group of stage III unresectable or inoperable patients receiving cisplatin $120\,mg/m^2$ plus vinca alkaloid combination chemotherapy, a multivariate analysis disclosed the following parameters associated with outcome: initial PS, with patients having a good PS displaying an increased objective response and survival; bone metastases, which were adversely predictive of response rate and survival; elevated LDH and male sex, both of which were associated with shortened survival; and the presence of two or more extrathoracic metastatic organ sites, which was associated with shortened survival.[98] When objective response with chemotherapy was included in the analysis, it was also strongly associated with longer survival.[98]

In a prospective Spanish Lung Cancer Group (SLCG) study[99] including 557 cisplatin combination-treated NSCLC patients, PS, gender, and weight loss were significant prognostic factors. Second, weight loss in lung cancer patients is associated with both impaired therapy outcome and reduced survival.[97]

In studies of multimodality treatment in stage IIIA (N2) and IIIB NSCLC, the SWOG study of concurrent cisplatin plus etoposide and chest radiotherapy followed by surgery observed that the strongest predictor of long-term survival after thoracotomy was absence of tumor in the mediastinal lymph nodes at surgery (median survivals, 30 versus 10 months and 3-year survival rates, 44% versus 18%).[100]

Some of these predictive markers of survival, such as PS, hemoglobin level, and bone, liver, or skin metastases, are understandable; however, why gender, LDH, or weight loss influence survival remains unclear. New pieces of information should shed light on these prognostic factors. First, there are interindividual differences in DRC that are accentuated according to age and gender, with females having a reduced DRC.[46] Based on this difference in DRC, females would have greater chemosensitivity than males. In vitro intrinsic cisplatin resistance was associated with elevated DRC in NSCLC cells.[101] DRC is a surrogate of the NER pathway, which eliminates cisplatin adducts,[47,50] and it has been demonstrated that NSCLC patients with effective systemic (host) DRC have poorer survival than patients with suboptimal DRC.[102] Patients who were in the top DRC quartile of the group (DRC greater than 9.2%) had a risk of death more than two times that of patients in the bottom quartile (DRC less than 5.8%). Median survival was 8.9 months for patients in the top DRC quartile, compared with 15.8 months for those in the bottom quartile ($P = 0.04$).[102]

Earlier findings suggest that the formation and persistence of cisplatin or carboplatin adducts in buccal cells or in leukocytes predict better response.[103,104] Cisplatin DNA adducts in nuclei of buccal cells were studied in a small group of patients who received radical radiotherapy and daily administration of low-dose cisplatin for inoperable NSCLC.[105] Nuclear staining was performed in buccal cells collected 1 hour after cisplatin on the fifth treatment day (after five daily doses of cisplatin 6 mg/m^2). Cisplatin DNA adduct staining remained a significant independent predictor of survival. Patients with low levels of induced DNA adducts in buccal cells showed a meager median survival of 5 months, in contrast with 30 months for patients with elevated DNA adduct levels.[106] Beyond the stratification for gender in future clinical trials, measuring DRC by functional assays or surrogates such as ERCC1 or XPD mRNA in peripheral lymphocytes[50] could help to predict responders.[98]

Metabolism

In contrast to normal mammalian cells, which use oxygen to generate energy, cancer cells rely on glycolysis for energy. Lung cancer patients with weight loss have elevated 3-phosphoglycerate and phosphoenolpyruvate, components of the glycolysis pathway[107] (Figure 37.3). Furthermore, c-Myc and HIF-1 overexpression deregulate glycolysis through the activation of the glucose metabolic pathway, which regulates lactate dehydrogenase and induces lactate overproduction[108] (Figure 37.3). Elevated serum LDH was associated with shortened survival and remission duration.[98] Elevated mRNA levels of phosphofructokinase, glyceraldehyde-3-phosphate dehydrogenase, phosphoglycerate kinase, and enolase were also reported.[108] Systematic identification of lung adenocarcinoma proteins using 2-D PAGE and mass spectrometry found that at least four proteins (phosphoglycerate kinase 1, phosphoglycerate mutase, alpha enolase, and pyruvate kinase M1), all of which are components of the glycolysis pathway (see Figure 37.3), were increased in expression and associated with poor survival in resected lung adenocarcinoma.[109] Expression of phosphoglycerate kinase 1, the sixth enzyme of the glycolytic pathway (Figure 37.3), reflects increased glycolysis in the tumor cells and is related to the induction of a multidrug resistant phenotype distinct from MDR1. The hypoxic nature of solid tumor triggers VEGF expression, which stimulates angiogenesis and glycolytic enzymes, including phosphoglycerate kinase, which facilitates anaerobic production of ATP.[110]

A surrogate of the cancer glycolytic pathway could be positron emission tomography (PET) reflecting the biochemical and physiologic processes occurring in the tissues being imaged. The most frequently used positron-emitting radiopharmaceutical is 18-fluor, labeled 2-deoxy-d-glucose (^{18}F-FDG), a radioactively labeled glucose analogue. The clinical use of ^{18}F-FDG-PET is based on the premise that cancer cells exhibit a higher glycolytic rate than do nonneoplastic cells. It is reasonable to speculate that a higher tumor uptake of the radiolabeled glucose analogue could be a surrogate of the glycolytic pathway. PET imaging has been used to assess changes in tumor glucose use during chemotherapy. In NSCLC, median time to progression and overall survival were significantly longer for ^{18}FDG-6-PET metabolic responders in the interval before and after the first chemotherapy cycle.[111]

Overexpression of ERCC1 mRNA and Other NER Genes

Moving toward a new prognostic classification, overexpression of ERCC1 mRNA and other NER genes has been associated with repair of cisplatin-induced DNA damage and clinical resistance to cisplatin. In a small study of cisplatin/gemcitabine-treated metastatic NSCLC patients, performance status, weight loss and low ERCC1 mRNA expression were independent prognostic factors. ERCC1 mRNA levels were even more significant than that of performance status.[112] Median survival for patients with low ERCC1 expression was 15 months in contrast to only 5 months for those harboring high expression.

M2 Subunit of Ribonucleotide Reductase

Also to be considered as a potential new predictive and prognostic marker is the ribonucleotide reductase activity, which is increased in cancer cells. The subunit M2 (or RRM2) is directly involved in a number of signaling pathways.[113] Among other drugs, gemcitabine decreases ribonucleotide reductase activity. In a retrospective analysis, better time to progression and survival were observed in gemcitabine/cisplatin-treated metastatic NSCLC patients who had low ribonucleotide reductase subunit M1 (or RRM1) mRNA expression.[114] Interestingly, retinoblastoma is sequentially phosphorylated by cyclin D-CDK4/6 and cyclin E/CDK2 during G_1/S cell-cycle transition. This modification leads to the dissociation of retinoblastoma from E2F/DP heterodimers, leaving them in a transcriptionally active state

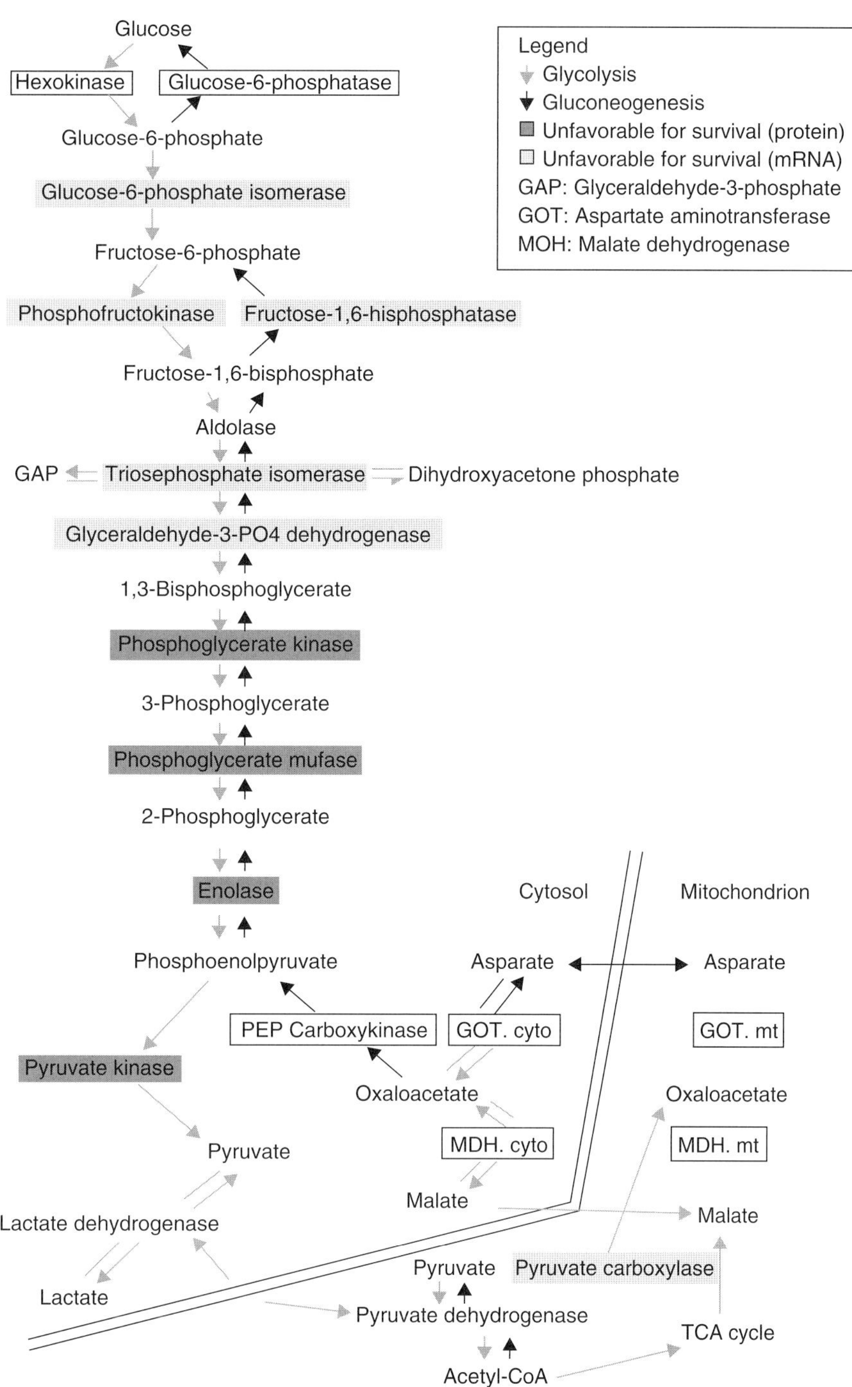

FIGURE 37.3. Glycolysis and gluconeogenesis pathway.

that regulates several DNA synthesis enzymes also involved in chemotherapy response, such as dihydrofolate reductase (DHFR), thymidylate synthase (TS), and ribonucleotide reductase.[115] In SCLC and NSCLC, p16/INK4A and retinoblastoma are reciprocally inactivated, resulting in the inactivation of the same p16/INK4A/RB pathway.[116] Therefore, in prospective studies the predictive and/or prognostic value of certain transcripts should be kept in mind. For example, in ribonucleotide-dependent chemotherapy combinations, the role of RRM1 and TS mRNA levels could influence response and survival, as proposed in the model in Figure 37.4.

Genetic

Since the first article describing K-*ras* mutations in lung adenocarcinomas,[51] a continual list of new genetic markers has been described, predicting disease-free survival and overall survival, mainly in surgically resected stage I NSCLC (Table 37.3). Tumors with K-*ras* mutations tend to be smaller and less differentiated than those without. The normal DNA sequence GGT at codon 12 is commonly switched to TGT.[52] K-*ras* mutations in NSCLC cell lines were related to poor survival in stage IIIB–IV.[117] Numerous reports have pointed out

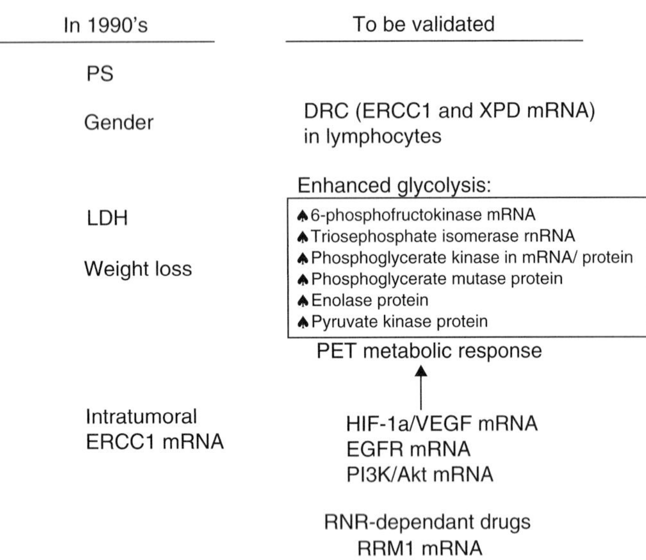

FIGURE 37.4. Factors associated with impaired therapy outcome and reduced survival.

the prognostic value of K-*ras* codon 12 mutations in stage I NSCLC.[52,118–120] However, in a recent report, neither K-*ras* nor p53 mutations influenced survival in all patients, although in patients receiving adjuvant chemotherapy, those without K-*ras* mutations had a median survival of almost 42 months, whereas for those with mutations, median survival bottomed out at nearly 25 months ($P = 0.09$; risk ratio = 0.59).[121] Such differences were not seen in patients who did not receive adjuvant chemotherapy. In a randomized neoadjuvant trial, K-*ras* mutations were more often found in the surgery-alone arm than in the neoadjuvant arm.[122] In a small neoadjuvant chemotherapy study of stage III NSCLC, the presence of K-*ras* mutations in the surgical specimens was a significant predictor of poor disease-free survival.[123]

Retinoic Acid Receptor and COX-2

In several retrospectively analyzed surgical series, high retinoic acid receptor-b mRNA levels by in situ hybridization correlated with poor survival in stage I NSCLC.[124] A significant relationship between elevated expression of cyclooxygenase 2 (COX-2) and worse survival has also been observed in stage I disease.[125,126]

Aberrant Methylation

Hypermethylation of death-associated protein kinase (DAPK) was found in 44% of tumors and linked to significantly poorer survival.[127] Similarly, hypermethylation of RASSF1A was linked to worse survival.[128] However, in a recent study, neither DAPK nor RASSF1A methylation in tumor or

TABLE 37.3. Genetic markers in resected non-small cell lung cancer (NSCLC).

Biomarker		*No. of patients*	*NSCLC*	*Survival*[a]	*P*
K-*ras* mutation[53]		19	Adenocarcinoma	≈18 months NR	0.002
wt		50			
RAR-β mRNA[124]	High	45	Stage I	Worse	0.045
	Low	115			
COX-2[125,126]	High	57	Stage I	66%	0.034
	Low	24		88%	
DAPK[127]	Methyl	59	Stage I	46%	0.007[b]
	Unmethyl	76		68%	
RASSF1A[128]	Methyl	32	Stage I	37 months	0.046[b]
	Unmethyl	75		49 months	
CRMP-1 mRNA[130]	Low	40	Stage I	28 months leveled off at 52%	0.016
	Normal	40			
IL-8 mRNA[131]	High	61	Stage I	Shorter	<0.001
	Normal	61		Longer	
IL-10[132]	Low	44	SCC	40.9%	0.080
	High	94		56%	
MIF mRNA[133]	Low	4	SCC	Longer	
	High	6		Shorter	
RANTES[134]	Low	36	Stage I	Shorter	0.002
	High	27		Longer	
IGFBP-3[135]	Methyl	51	Stage I	53%	0.006
	Unmethyl	32		86%	
11p15.5 LOH[136]	Present	26	Stage I	24.9 months	0.038
	Absent	50		36 months	
ERCC1 mRNA[137]	Low	NS	Stage I	35.5 months	0.010
	High			94.6 months	
128-gene set[138]	With	NS	Adenocarcinoma	Shorter	0.009

wt, wild-type; NS, not specified; SCC, squamous cell carcinoma; NR, not reached.

[a] Percentages indicate 5-year survival rates; months indicate median survival.

[b] Another study found no survival differences according to methylation patterns.

serum influenced survival in surgically resected NSCLC patients.[129]

Real-time (RT)-PCR of lung cancer specimens showed that reduced expression of collapsin response mediator protein 1 was statistically significantly associated with advanced disease, lymph node metastases, early postoperative relapse, and shorter survival.[130] Interleukin (IL)-8 mRNA overexpression was also associated with advanced disease, lymph node metastases, early relapse, and shorter survival.[131] Intriguingly, immunohistochemical analysis showed that patients whose tumors lacked IL-10 had worse survival than those whose tumors retained IL-10 expression.[132] Along the same lines, using RT-PCR, overexpression of macrophage migration inhibitory factor was associated with poor survival.[133] Regulated upon activation, normal T-cell-expressed and -secreted (RANTES) overexpression was a predictor of significantly better survival in stage I lung adenocarcinoma.[134] Also in stage I disease, patients with hypermethylated insulin-like growth factor-binding protein 3 (IGFBP-3) had a significantly lower disease-free and overall survival than those without IGFBP-3 methylation.[135] LOH on chromosome segment 11p15.5, which includes the gene for ribonucleotide reductase, confers poor survival in patients with stage I NSCLC.[136] Stage I patients with high ERCC1 mRNA expression also had significantly better survival than those with low ERCC1 expression, who could potentially benefit from adjuvant chemotherapy.[137] However, patients with efficient DNA repair mechanisms (high ERCC1 expression or without LOH on 11p15.5) could be chemoresistant and may not require adjuvant chemotherapy.

Proteomic and Gene Expression Signatures

Using microarray platforms, metastases-associated gene-expression signature has been identified. There were no survival differences in lung adenocarcinoma according to 9,248 highly varying genes; however, survival differences surfaced when using 128 metastases-associated genes.[138] Interestingly, these differences were also evident with the use of only 17 genes (8 upregulated and 9 downregulated genes). This signature, taken as a whole, seems to contain predictive information. Intriguingly, the gene-expression signature associated with metastases arises from both malignant and stromal elements in primary tumors, indicating that the large stromal component of the signature would have been missed had only malignant epithelial cells been isolated by laser capture microdissection.[138] Moreover, the use of mRNA-based gene expression profiles predicted survival in surgically resected NSCLC.[68,139] Interestingly, increased phosphoglycerate kinase 1 mRNA was significantly associated with poor survival in lung adenocarcinoma and mRNA levels correlated with the expression of the phosphoglycerate kinase 1 protein isoform.[109,139] Upregulation of genes in the pathway involving glycolysis and the Krebs cycle has been demonstrated in mesotheliomas with significant increases of glyceraldehyde-3-phosphate dehydrogenase, LDH, and phosphoglycerate kinase 1[140] (see Figure 37.3). Proteomic patterns could be used to accurately classify surgically resected NSCLC and identify individual protein isoforms that become tumor markers.[141] This knowledge opens the doors to the assessment of HIF-1 levels as a putative prognostic marker, because the upregulation of each HIF-1 in cancer functions as a key transcription factor that potentially regulates 9 of the 11 glycolytic enzymes (see Figure 37.3). Table 37.3 summarizes some genetic markers that have been identified as prognostic and predictive markers in stage I NSCLC.

Microvessel Density

A meta-analysis of more than 4,400 surgically resected NSCLC patients analyzed the microvessel count assessed on surgical samples by immunohistochemistry using factor VIII, CD34, and CD31. A high microvessel count in the primary lung tumor was a statistically significant poor prognostic factor for survival, regardless of the marker used.[142] A strong correlation between IL-8 mRNA expression and microvessel counts or macrophage counts has also been observed.[143] Higher IL-8 mRNA levels and higher macrophage counts were associated with lower survival. In addition, VEGF expression was positively related to microvessel density and negatively related to the degree of dendritic cell infiltration.[144] A multivariate analysis showed VEGF expression, microvessel density, and dendritic cell infiltration to be independent prognostic factors. The patient group with both high VEGF expression and low dendritic cell infiltration showed a worse prognosis. Angiopoietin 2 expression was significantly correlated with higher CD105-stained microvessel density in NSCLC.[145] CD105 is a proliferation-related endothelial antigen that is more selective than CD34, which is a pan-endothelial antigen reacting not only with newly forming vessels but also with stable vessels just trapped in tumors. Five-year survival for resected NSCLC patients was 71% when VEGF was low and angiopoietin was negative and 41% when angiopoietin was positive and VEGF was high.

Screening of Lung Cancer

Lung cancer screening is controversial. A number of studies have been performed using all three methods for the evaluation of screening tests, including randomized trials of screening, population-based studies of screening, and observation studies of screening in select cohorts. For lung cancer screening to be accepted as beneficial, it must unequivocably prolong life expectancy by detecting the disease at a time when its course will be altered with the institution of therapy. Moreover, the screening test should be specific enough not to create an inordinate number of false-positive exams that could do psychologic or physical harm to the participants through anxiety or through the advocacy of potentially harmful tests. Finally, the use of a screening test must be cost-effective and conform to an accepted standard for cost/lives saved.

To validate the utility of lung cancer screening, choices must be made that focus these efforts to enrich for those at highest risk. These choices include proper target (i.e., high-risk population), the choice of central or peripheral screening, the appropriate algorithm for patient follow-up once an abnormality has been detected, and the timing and magnitude of the intervention to prove that the detected abnormality is a life-threatening abnormality. Once confirmed as a life-threatening lung cancer, the management of the disease must conform to present standards of care until well-conducted studies prove that these treatment standards are excessive for these newly detected abnormalities.

Randomized Trials of Lung Cancer Screening

The earliest randomized trial for lung cancer screening started in 1960 with a randomization of 55,034 London men to either chest X-ray every 6 months for 3 years or to chest X-ray at the beginning and the end of the 3-year period. The detection rate and the number of respectable cancers was higher in the screened group, but there was no difference in lung cancer mortality.[146,147] In the 1970s and 1980s, the National Cancer Institute sponsored a study of 10,000 high-risk volunteers at Sloan Kettering,[148] Johns Hopkins,[149] and another 10,000 high-risk volunteers at the Mayo Clinic.[150–152] These trials, whose participants were all male smokers over 45 years of age who had a smoking history of at least 1 pack per day, were designed to investigate the efficacy of lung cancer screening using a combination of chest X-ray and conventional sputum cytology. A fourth study similar to the Mayo Clinic study was performed in Czechoslovakia.[153–155] In the Johns Hopkins and Memorial Sloan-Kettering trials, both experimental and control participants had annual screening chest radiography, and the experimental arm had sputum cytology every 4 months to address the incremental benefit of sputum cytology analysis rather than chest radiographs per se. Although they found that sputum analysis did not favorably influence outcome, these studies achieved survival rates among all groups three times higher than predicted by epidemiologic data.

A prevalence screening with chest X-ray and sputum cytology was performed in all individuals in the Mayo Lung Trial followed by randomization to radiographs and sputum cytology every 4 months or the recommendation to have these annually. The Czechoslovakian study, a 3-year study with 3-year follow-up, also began with a prevalence screen, then randomization to a screened or control group, and the control group was told not to get either radiograph or cytology during the 3-year study period. In both the Mayo and Czech studies, more lung cancers were found in the screened group, and there was a tendency toward earlier stage at diagnosis, resectability, and survival for the screened group. Five-year survival for the control group in the Mayo Study was 15% compared to 33% in the screened group.[151] Both studies demonstrated increases in cumulative lung cancer incidence in the experimental group above that of control groups, demonstrating significant improvements for the experimental groups in case fatality (number of cancer deaths/number of individuals with cancer) but not in significant reductions in lung cancer mortality (number of cancer deaths/number of individuals screened).

Lead-time bias, length bias, and overdiagnosis have been used to potentially explain the differences between lung cancer mortality and earlier stage at diagnosis, improved resectability, and survival of the screened.[156–159] Lead-time bias operates when the timing of diagnosis between screening and nonscreening cases is not adjusted; that is, earlier detection may result in longer survival from the time of diagnosis even if death is not delayed. Length bias occurs when conditions are not adjusted for the rate of cancer progression and the screening examination purportedly detects slow-growing cancers. In other words, the slower the growth of the neoplasm, the longer it is present without symptoms, and the greater the likelihood of detection. Overdiagnosis bias refers to the phenomenon of detecting a lung cancer that would otherwise have remained subclinical before death from other causes.

Supporters of the concept of lung cancer screening have argued that these original trials were flawed.[160] Arguments include the observations that (1) they did not include a "no-screening" study arm and thus no determination of true efficacy could be made; and (2) the sample size of these studies was inadequate, because both the Mayo Lung Project and the Czechoslovakian studies were powered to detect a 50% reduction in lung cancer mortality in the screened group compared with the control group, and the power to detect a smaller 10% reduction in mortality, which is still clinically significant, was much lower (only 0.21 and 0.16, respectively).[161,162]

High-Risk Populations: Smokers and Nonsmokers

The risk of lung cancer is influenced by duration of smoking, the number of cigarettes smoked per day, and the age at which a smoker stopped smoking; that is, the longer one lives after cessation of smoking, the greater the risk for developing lung cancer. The greater the consumption of tobacco as measured by pack-years, the greater the risk that one will develop lung cancer. Lung cancer prevalence is also influenced by the presence of airway obstruction. For individuals smoking 30 to 40 pack-years or more with airflow obstruction, defined by FEV_1/FVC less than 70% and an FEV_1 less than 70% predicted, the risk of lung cancer is three to four times higher than those individuals with normal airflow.[163] Individuals with previously surgically treated stage 1 NSCLC or head and neck primary neoplasms are also at increased risk for the development of a new lung primary cancer for up to 20 years, at an approximate rate of 1% to 2% per patient per year.[164] Occult lung cancers detected by sputum cytology also have an especially high rate of metachronous tumors, approaching 11% at 5 years with an incidence per patient-year of surveillance of 2.2%.[165] The incidence of a second primary tumor in patients treated for squamous cell carcinoma of the aerodigestive tract can be as high as 16.2%, with 6.4% being synchronous and 9.8% being metachronous.[166] Metachronous tumors are most likely in the lung (57%), placing these patients in one of the highest risk categories for the development of lung cancer.

Present Screening Efforts

There has been a realization by the medical community that the efficacy of lung cancer screening should now be investigated in a research setting using newer computed tomographic techniques. Moreover, individual centers as well as lung specialized program of research excellence (SPORES) have enrolled patients on either radiographic, sputum-based, or combination programs for lung cancer screening to develop potential molecular markers. All lung cancer screening programs are based on the premise that high-risk populations must be chosen to have any hope of cost-effectiveness, and, in addition to the technologic evolution alluded to above, there has been a greater refining of the demographics of the individual at high risk for lung cancer who may be a candidate for enrolling in lung cancer screening programs.

Chest X-Ray

The National Cancer Institute initiated a large randomized controlled screening trial using chest radiographs for lung cancer screening as part of the Prostate-Lung-Colorectal-Ovarian (PLCO) trial. One of the objectives of the trial, which is ongoing, was to determine whether screening reduces lung cancer-specific mortality by at least 10% relative to unscreened groups.[167] This trial remains under analysis at this writing.

Low-Dose Helical CT Scanning of the Chest

Nonrandomized Approaches

The Japanese Anti-Lung Cancer Association screened approximately 26,000 male smokers over 50 years of age from 1975 to 1993 with chest radiography and sputum cytology, and added spiral CT scanning to the regimen in 1993.[168] Significantly more cancers were detected in the CT era (36 over 5 years) compared to the pre-CT era (43 over 18 years), and 81% of the CT screened lung cancers were stage IA compared to 42% in the pre-CT era. There was a striking increase in the 5-year survival, from 48% to 82%. Single-spiral CT prevalence scanning was performed by another Japanese group in 3,967 of 5,483 persons aged 40 to 74 years, individuals who had previously been screened with yearly chest X-rays and sputum cytologic screening. Of the 223 individuals with abnormal findings, 19 cancers were detected, and 84% of these were found to be stage I;[169,170] the addition of CT scanning increased the rate of lung cancer diagnosis by approximately 12 fold.

The Early Lung Cancer Action Project (ELCAP) was initiated in the United States in 1993 to define the frequency with which malignancy was found in screen-detected nodules and the frequency with which malignant nodules were curable. A cohort of 1,000 high-risk persons was experimentally screened using a noncomparative design in which a single cohort was recruited for baseline and annual repeat CT screening.[170,171] The medically fit volunteers were aged 60 years or older, with at least 10 pack-years of cigarette smoking and no previous cancer.

Chest radiographs and low-dose CT were done for each participant, with the diagnostic/interventional investigation of screen-detected noncalcified pulmonary nodules by short-term high-resolution CT follow-up dictated primarily by size of the nodule. Noncalcified nodules were detected in 233 [23%; 95% confidence interval (CI), 21–26] participants by low-dose CT at baseline, compared with 68 (7%; 95% CI, 5–9) by chest radiography. Malignant disease was detected in 27 (2.7%; 95% CI, 1.8–3.8) by CT and 7 (0.7%; 95% CI, 0.3–1.3]) by chest radiography, and stage I malignant disease in 23 (2.3%; 95% CI, 1.5–3.3]) and 4 (0.4%; 95% CI, 0.1–0.9]), respectively. Of the 27 CT-detected cancers, 26 were respectable. Biopsies were done on 28 of the 233 participants with noncalcified nodules; 27 had malignant noncalcified nodules and 1 had a benign nodule. Another 3 individuals underwent biopsy against the ELCAP recommendations; all had benign noncalcified nodules. No participant had thoracotomy for a benign nodule.[171]

A follow-up report concentrating on 1,184 annual repeat screenings defined a positive result from the screening test as a newly detected nodule or one to six noncalcified pulmonary nodules with interim growth. Of the 1,184 repeat CT screenings, the test result was positive in 30 (2.5%). In 2 of these 30 cases, the individual died (of an unrelated cause) before diagnostic workup, and the nodule(s) resolved in another 12 individuals. In the remaining 16 individuals, the absence of further growth was documented by repeat CT in 8 individuals and further growth was documented in the remaining 8 individuals. All 8 individuals with further nodular growth underwent biopsy, and malignancy was diagnosed in 7. Six of these 7 malignancies were non-small cell carcinomas (5 of which were stage IA and 1 of which was stage IIIA), and the 1 small cell carcinoma was found to be of limited stage. The median size dimension of these malignancies was 8 mm. In another 2 subjects, symptoms prompted the interim diagnosis of lung carcinoma. Neither of these malignancies was nodule associated but rather was endobronchial; 1 was a stage IIB non-small cell carcinoma and the other was a small cell carcinoma of limited stage. The data from the ELCAP experience will be pooled with that of two initiatives, which are outgrowths of the original ELCAP, the New York ELCAP (NY-ELCAP) and the International Early Lung Cancer Action Program (I-ELCAP). These efforts share the same set of principles and protocol as well as the ELCAP web-based management and data-recording system and its associated teaching files.[172]

The Mayo Clinic also evaluated CT-based lung screening in a prospective cohort study of 1,520 individuals aged 50 years or older who had smoked 20 pack-years or more.[173] Participants underwent three annual low-dose CT examinations of the chest and upper abdomen. Two years after baseline CT scanning, 2,832 uncalcified pulmonary nodules were identified in 1,049 participants (69%). Forty cases of lung cancer were diagnosed: 26 at baseline (prevalence) CT examinations and 10 at subsequent annual (incidence) CT examinations. CT alone depicted 36 cases, and sputum cytologic examination alone, 2. There were 2 interval cancers. The mean size of the non-small cell cancers detected at CT was 15.0 mm. The stages were as follows: IA, 22; IB, 3; IIA, 4; IIB, 1; IIIA, 5; IV, 1; limited small cell tumor, 4. Twenty-one (60%) of the 35 non-small cell cancers detected at CT were stage IA at diagnosis.

Present Randomized Studies

The National Cancer Institute and the American College of Radiology Intervention Network is sponsoring a multicenter, randomized controlled trial of 88,000 individuals at high risk of developing lung cancer to see whether screening with low-dose helical CT can reduce lung cancer-specific mortality relative to chest radiographs. High risk is defined by age 55 to 74 years with a current or previous heavy smoking history equaling at least 30 pack-years; former smokers must have quit within the preceding 15 years. The experimental group will undergo screening with low-dose helical CT, and the control group will undergo screening with chest radiographs. Both groups will be screened annually for at least two incidence screens, and both groups will complete quality of life questionnaires. The primary endpoint of the trial is lung cancer-specific mortality. Intermediate endpoints include all-cause mortality; surgical stage at diagnosis; medical resource utilization; the impact of screening on quality of life and psychologic effects; and the economic consequences of helical CT screening.

Sputum Cytology Screening

Sputum cytology studies for lung cancer screening require huge numbers of subjects and are less attractive because of the low sensitivity (65%) of sputum analysis, as well as the inability to detect peripheral cancers with the same sensitivity as central tumors.[174] To be successful as a population-screening tool, sputum cytology sensitivity must be improved using such approaches as (1) immunostaining of abnormal epithelial cells, (2) computer-assisted image analysis of exfoliated sputum cells, (3) PCR-based assays to detect changes in dominant and recessive oncogenes, and (4) genetic epidemiology markers to more precisely define at-risk populations of current and former smokers.[175] Tockman has reported that an antibody to heterogeneous nuclear ribonucleoprotein (hnRNP) may improve the accuracy of preclinical lung cancer detection. HnRNP is overexpressed in exfoliated airway cells as a prelude to the development of lung cancer.[163,176,177] In a background of normal-appearing airway cells, abnormal staining for hnRNP with the antibody can be performed by quantitative densitometry of immunostained slides. In separate, ongoing prospective studies, sputum has been collected annually from stage I resected non-small cell lung cancer patients at high risk of developing a second primary lung cancer and Yunnan tin miners at high risk of primary lung cancer. These two prospective studies accurately predicted that 67% and 69% of those with hnRNP upregulation in their sputum would develop lung cancer in the first year of follow-up. Other investigators are quantitating malignancy-associated changes by computer-assisted image analysis to report nuclear distribution of DNA in histologically normal cells adjacent to preinvasive or invasive cancers. In a retrospective analysis, malignancy-associated changes in sputum cytology were able to correctly identify 74% of subjects who later developed lung cancer.[178] Other molecular markers that are being examined in sputum include microsatellite alterations,[179] methylation changes,[180] and point mutations in p53 and *ras* genes.[181–183]

The detection of sputum atypia and subsequent identification of the source of cells demands improvements in endoscopic visualization. Only 30% to 40% of carcinoma in situ are visible to an experienced endoscopist on conventional bronchoscopy. Autofluorescence bronchoscopy is now being used with greater frequency as a complementary technology to sputum screening to provide targeted biopsies of dysplastic lesions.[184] The technique is based on the observation that when the bronchial surface is illuminated by a blue light (405–442 nm), such as light from a helium-cadmium laser, there is a progressive reduction in the fluorescence intensity as the tissue becomes more abnormal, especially in the green wavelength band of the autofluorescence spectrum. The marked reduction in fluorescence intensity (up to 10-fold decrease in the green and about 5-fold in the red) in precancerous and cancerous tissue is thought to be caused by the combination of an increase in the thickness of the bronchial epithelium, a very slight increase in blood content in the area of the submucosa of the lesion, and a loss of fluorophore concentration or fluorescence quantum yield.[185] A multicenter clinical trial in 173 subjects with known or suspected lung cancer was performed in which conventional bronchoscopy was followed by fluorescence examination. The relative sensitivity of both examinations versus conventional bronchoscopy alone was 6.3 for intraepithelial neoplastic lesions and 2.71 when invasive carcinomas were also included.[186]

Staging

TNM Staging Classification

Staging of lung cancer (Table 37.4) uses the TNM staging system and was most recently revised in 1997.[187]

Mediastinal Staging

Staging of the mediastinum by either invasive or noninvasive techniques should efficiently and accurately determine whether patients are candidates for a potentially curative surgical resection, or for protocols involving multimodality approaches before or instead of attempted surgical resection. The most confounding aspect of the surgical staging of lung cancer involves accurate assessment of the mediastinum, which ideally should define (1) mediastinal lymph node status and (2) mediastinal invasion.

Mediastinal Involvement: Lymph Nodes

Approximately 26% to 44% of patients with newly diagnosed lung cancer have mediastinal lymph node involvement. Adverse prognostic factors associated with positive mediastinal nodes include extracapsular spread of tumor, multiple levels of involved lymph nodes, bulky enlarged nodes, and the size of the primary tumor.[188–191] Multiple studies have found that metastatic disease to the subcarinal lymph nodes adversely affected prognosis compared to other lymph nodes.[192–198] It is generally believed than multistation nodal disease has a somewhat worse prognosis than single-station disease, but the location of metastatic disease to a single nodal station probably has no significant effect.

The poor survival rates with surgery alone in N2 disease, without significant survival benefit for adjuvant postoperative radiotherapy,[199–201] has led to designing protocols that use nonsurgical (radiotherapy and/or chemotherapy) therapy first, often to convert the "unresectable" tumor to resectable, to improve long-term survival.[202] In general, patients with lymph nodes greater than 2 cm in short-axis diameter measured by CT, who have extranodal involvement, and multistation disease along with groups of multiple involved smaller lymph nodes, are considered to have bulky, unresectable disease. These patients are referred for protocols involving chemoradiation if they are functionally fit to tolerate the therapy. The heterogeneity of N2 prognostic categories can certainly confound ongoing prospective trials attempting to define good-risk candidates for multimodality therapy. The heterogeneity phenomenon of mediastinal lymph node involvement has been reviewed by Andre et al. in 702 consecutive patients having surgical resection of N2 non-small cell lung cancer.[203] A multivariable analysis using Cox regression identified four negative prognostic factors: clinically apparent N2 disease; the involvement of multiple lymph node stations; either pathologic stage T3 or T4 status; or no preoperative chemotherapy. For patients having primary

TABLE 37.4. Stage Grouping: TNM subsets.

Stage	*TNM subset*	*TNM descriptors*	
0	Carcinoma in situ		
IA	T1N0M0	T1	Tumor 3 cm or less in greatest dimension, surrounded by lung or visceral pleura, without bronchoscopic evidence of invasion more proximal than the lobar bronchus* (i.e., not in the main bronchus)
IB	T2N0M0	T2	Tumor with any of the following features of size or extent: More than 3 cm in greatest dimension; involves main bronchus, 2 cm or more distal to the carina; invades the visceral pleura; associated with atelectasis or obstructive pnuemonitis that extends to the hilar region but does not involve the entire lung.
IIA	T1N1M0	T3	Tumor of any size that directly invades any of the following: chest wall (including superior sulcus tumors), diaphragm, mediastinal pleura, parietal pericardium; or tumor in the main bronchus less than 2 cm distal to the carina, but without involvement of the carina; or associated atelectasis or obstructive pneumonitis of the entire lung.
IIB	T2N1M0 T3N0M0	T4	Tumor of any size that invades any of the following: mediastinum, heart, great vessels, trachea, esophagus, vertebral body, carina; or separate tumor nodules in the same lobe; or tumor with malignant pleural effusion.**
IIIA	T3N1M0 T1N2M0 T2N2M0 T3N2M0	N0 N1	No nodal involvement involving ipsilateral hilar or bronchial nodes
IIIB	T4 any N, M0 Any T, N3, M0	N2 N3	involving ipsilateral mediastinal nodes involving contralateral nodes or *scalene nodes*
IV	Any T, Any N M1	M0 M1	no distant metastases distant metastases present

*Note: The uncommon superficial tumor of any size with its invasive component limited to the bronchial wall, which may extend proximal to the main bronchus, is also classified T1.

**Note: Most pleural effusions associated with lung cancer are caused by tumor. However, there are a few patients in whom multiple cytopathologic examinations of pleural fluid are negative for tumor. In these cases, fluid is nonbloody and is not an exudate. Such patients may be further evaluated by video thoracoscopy and direct pleural biopsies. When these elements and clinical judgment dictate that the effusion is not related to the tumor, the effusion should be excluded as a staging element and the patient should be staged T1, T2, or T3.

Source: Used with the permission of the American Joint Committee on Cancer (AJCC), Chicago, Illinois. The original source for this material is the *AJCC Cancer Staging Manual*, Sixth Edition (2002), published by Springer-Verlag New York, www.springer-ny.com.

surgery, the 5-year survivals varied according to N2 characteristics: one-level involvement with microscopic disease (34%); multiple level lymph nodes with microscopic disease (11%); single-level clinically apparent disease (8%); and multilevel clinically apparent disease (3%). For patients with single-level microscopic disease, there was no difference in survival between different lymph node stations.

It is just as important to determine whether the extent of mediastinal involvement is T3 (nontransmural involvement of the pericardium, involvement of the phrenic nerve focally, or extrapericardial involvement of the pulmonary artery or veins) or T4 (involvement of the superior vena cava, aorta, main pulmonary artery, esophagus).[204] Extension of tumor into these structures radically alters the T status of the tumor and influences surgical decision making toward primary resection or protocol-directed induction therapy with later surgical consideration. The limited studies that deal with T3 involvement of the mediastinum report a 5-year survival approaching 25% if the mediastinal lymph nodes are not involved.[205] However, with T4 involvement of the superior vena cava, main pulmonary artery, or aorta, the 5-year survival rate in very limited series is approximately 15%, with the best survivals (30%) reported in patients with localized superior vena caval involvement.[205]

Noninvasive Staging Modalities

Computed Tomography

A recent review of 20 studies published since 1993 with a cohort of 3,438 patients evaluated the accuracy of CT scanning for the mediastinal staging of lung cancer.[204,206] There was marked heterogeneity for the sensitivity (pooled value = 0.57) and specificity (pooled value = 0.82), with positive predictive value of 0.56 and negative predictive value of 0.83. These data reinforce that findings on a CT scan cannot be used solely to determine mediastinal lymph node status and reveal that the accuracy of CT scanning of the mediastinum has not changed despite improvements in technology. Obstructive pneumonitis with resulting enlarged lymph nodes can account for the fact that 40% of lymph nodes thought, on CT scan, to be malignant were actually benign, and microscopic involvement of lymph nodes is encountered in up to 15% of patients having a complete mediastinal lymph node dissection for presumed stage I disease. The obvious conclusion for the standard of care in 2004 is that CT scanning findings of the mediastinum, when using the 1-cm cutoff limit, must be supplemented by other noninvasive and invasive techniques to have a higher confidence that abnormally enlarged lymph nodes truly represent IIIA or IIIB disease.

Magnetic Resonance Imaging

Magnetic resonance imaging (MRI) currently has a limited role in the noninvasive staging of bronchogenic carcinoma but may be used to evaluate for vascular or vertebral body invasion with suspected T4 tumors or to assess the integrity of the brachial plexus in patients with a Pancoast tumor.[207] Due to poorer spatial resolution and motion artifact, it is less sensitive in evaluation of the pulmonary parenchyma.

Noninvasive Staging Beyond CT: Positron Emission Tomography

Positron emission tomography (PET) scanning has become an ideal supplement to CT scanning because of its higher sensitivity and specificity for the evaluation of mediastinal lymph nodes. Toloza et al.[206] evaluated PET scanning for mediastinal staging in 1,111 patients from 29 reports in the literature, finding a pooled sensitivity of 0.85 and a pooled specificity of 0.88. The overall positive predictive value and negative predictive value were superior to CT scanning (0.78 and 0.93, respectively). Other reports have noted that the use of PET scanning can change decision strategies for patients in 10% to 20% of instances.[208] PET scanning, however, is limited in its anatomic interpretation and sensitivity when analyzing lesions less than 1.2 cm. Lymph node stations can be accurately identified when PET images and CT images are fused or interpreted simultaneously, but the volume or number of involved lymph nodes cannot be determined with present PET technology. The size limitations for sensitivity may not only have to do with spatial resolution software but with the type of lesion that is being visualized, as the PET intensity is known to be lower in bronchoalveolar lung cancer compared to other histologies.[209]

Surgical Staging

Minimally Invasive Techniques for Mediastinal Staging

Bronchoscopic Techniques Including Transbronchial Needle Aspiration Biopsy Bronchoscopy can play a key role in the staging of lung cancer. Carinal biopsy alone in the presence of an endobronchial tumor can have a yield as high as 5%,[210] and bronchoscopy may also detect other lesions unsuspected in the airway. Fluorescence bronchoscopy is being evaluated not only for finding occult lesions but also to define margins of resection of the bronchus that could influence stage, that is, proximity to the carina.[211] The yield for transbronchial needle aspiration (TBNA) varies widely in the literature (20% to 89%) and seems to be related to the size and location of the lesion as well as operator experience.[204] In a recent review regarding the accuracy of TBNA of the mediastinum in patients with lung cancer, the sensitivity was determined to be 76% with a specificity of 96%.[204] The problem with TBNA is that the false-negative rate can be as high as 30%, and the yield is reported to improve with at least seven passes with the TBNA needle.

Endobronchial Ultrasound Biopsy (EBUS) Endobronchial ultrasound allows visualization of the tracheobronchial and peribronchial lesions, mediastinal lymph nodes, and adjacent vascular structures as well as peripheral pulmonary tumors, but studies of its efficacy are limited because of its limited use by specialty centers. In 207 of 242 patients investigated using EBUS, the lymph nodes were successfully sampled (86%), and a diagnosis or cancer stage could be obtained in 172 patients (72%).[212]

Endoesophageal Ultrasound Fine-Needle Aspiration (EUS-FNA) Because the esophagus lies posteriorly and to the left of the trachea and is in proximity to the lymph nodes between these two structures, lymph node levels 5, 7, 8, and possibly 9 are accessible by endoesophageal ultrasound fine needle. Right-sided levels 2, 4, and the pretracheal space are not accessible with EUS-FNA. EUS-FNA is usually performed in the outpatient setting with conscious sedation. Wiersema et al.[213] reported that EUS-FNA was superior to TBNA in the diagnosis of mediastinal metastases in NSCLC. When performed in patients with enlarged lymph nodes, EUS-FNA has a high sensitivity and sensitivity (0.88 and 0.91, respectively), with an overall positive predictive value of 98% and negative predictive value of 77%.[214] EUS-FNA can also detect malignancy in normal-sized lymph nodes, and when successful has altered the staging of patients with normal-size lymph nodes from 18% to 42%. The sensitivity and specificity are low, however, with normal-sized lymph nodes due to the necessity to perform many aspirations of different sites to increase the yield.[214]

Transbronchial and Transesophageal Needle Biopsy: Recommendations These techniques are most useful for patients who have documented enlarged, nondiscrete lymph nodes with extensive mediastinal infiltration (clinical/radiographic evidence of N2/N3 disease). In this situation TBNA and EUS-NA provide the best chance for obtaining a diagnosis with the least morbidity. Multiple aspirates should be performed to avoid sampling error.

Invasive Surgical Staging of the Mediastinum

Based on the relationship between prognosis and the level of lymph node involvement, Naruke and colleagues developed a thoracic lymph node map that illustrates the location of various lymph nodes.[215] This map has been most recently revised in 1997 by Mountain and Dresler.[216] Each lymph node is assigned to a specific nodal station (N0, N1, N2, or N3) representing a prognostic subgroup or stage. In 1986 and subsequently in 1997, Mountain introduced and modified a new international staging system in which the extent of nodal spread serves as the principal prognostic determinant,[187,217] and multiple reports have validated the prognostic value of this staging system.

The method by which the mediastinum is explored depends on the site of the lesion. Cervical mediastinoscopy involves an initial digital exploration palpating suspicious nodes followed by placement of the scope to visualize and biopsy the appropriate lymph nodes. The N2 (levels 4, 7) and N3 nodal stations (2, scalenus/supraclavicular) with the exception of the aortic nodes (levels 5 and 6), the inferior pulmonary ligament nodes (level 9), and the paraesophageal nodes (level 8), are accessible for biopsy using this technique. Ginsberg has emphasized the importance of combining standard cervical mediastinoscopy with exploration of the scalenus fat pad[218] in patients with central nonsquamous tumors. Extended cervical mediastinoscopy is a technique that combines cervical mediastinoscopy with mediastinoscopic evaluation of the subaortic space as a single procedure.[219] More commonly, the subaortic space is approached using the Chamberlain procedure, which permits the surgeon to directly palpate the subaortic extrapleural space and biopsy the lymph nodes in this region.[220] Some surgeons prefer to use a mediastinoscope through a small anterior incision in the left chest and not remove the costal cartilage to perform a Chamberlain procedure.

Video-assisted thoracoscopic surgery (VATS), a minimally invasive surgical technique, is an alternative method to assess levels 5 and 6 as well as the paraesophageal (level 8) and pulmonary ligament (level 9) nodes.[221] Whether a surgeon surgically stages the ipsilateral and the contralateral mediastinal nodes in a lung cancer patient is being increasingly dictated by the use of PET scanning, although there are recommendations in the absence of PET scan findings (see following). In the absence of PET scanning availability, staging of the contralateral side usually is defined by nodal size on computerized tomography.

Mediastinoscopy or Mediastinotomy Mediastinal nodal enlargement by CT is an absolute indication for mediastinoscopy. For patients with mediastinal nodes of any size, the documentation of metabolic activity within single nodes or in multiple nodal basins in an individual with suspected lung cancer is also an indication for surgical staging of the suspicious mediastinum. For patients whose eligibility criteria require documentation of mediastinal disease, as in randomized or nonrandomized trials of induction therapy for locoregional lung cancer, mediastinal biopsy is mandated. A large mass or a lesion of any size located within the inner one-third of the lung field, especially if it is an adenocarcinoma or large cell carcinoma, correlates with an increased incidence of N2 nodal spread despite the finding of a normal mediastinum on CT scan.[222] Left-sided lung cancers also merit mediastinoscopy at certain centers. Because of the tendency for left lower lobe lesions to spread contralaterally, some centers recommend biopsy of bilateral mediastinal nodes, using mediastinoscopy to sample anterior 7, 2R, 4R, 2L, and 4L, and extended mediastinoscopy, mediastinotomy, or EUS-NA to sample 5L and 6L. Mediastinoscopy evaluation is also warranted for left upper lobe lesions to sample the level 4l nodes.[223]

In a review of more than 5,687 patients undergoing mediastinoscopy between 1983 and 1999, the overall sensitivity of standard cervical mediastinoscopy was 81%, with a negative predictive value of 91%.[204] Extended cervical mediastinoscopy used in combination with standard cervical mediastinoscopy will increase the overall sensitivity by 17% to 44% and improve negative predictive value by 10% to 20% when compared directly to standard mediastinoscopy.[219] The Chamberlain procedure or anterior mediastinotomy has a sensitivity of 63% to 86%, and its negative predictive value remains high whether it is performed alone (89% to 100%) or in combination with standard cervical mediastinoscopy (89% to 92%).[204]

Video-Assisted Thoracic Surgery and Mediastinal Staging Thoracoscopy has been used to not only assess left-sided lymph node stations not accessible by standard mediastinoscopy and for the inferior pulmonary ligament and paraesophageal lymph nodes, but also in very limited series to assess systematic nodal dissection for right-sided tumors. There are few series, however, describing the surgical technique in its entirety, and most operations involve the use of a 4.5- to 5-cm anterior incision that enhances visibility, yet in expert hands subcarinal lymph node dissection is possible.[224] It is generally concluded that VATS is used by a small group of surgeons in lung cancer mediastinal staging, and its chief use involves the assessment of pleural effusions associated with lung cancer adenopathy and the documentation of discontinuous pleural disease by direct visualization and roentgenographically negative pleural involvement.

Intraoperative Staging at the Time of Resection There is controversy whether complete ipsilateral mediastinal nodal dissection as opposed to minimal or more-extensive hilar and mediastinal lymph nodes sampling has greater efficacy in determining intraoperative stage and whether the degree of the dissection influences prognosis. A number of investigators have evaluated the extent of mediastinal biopsy necessary to obtain accurate staging information. Bollen et al. found that systematic sampling of mediastinal lymph nodes was as successful as mediastinal lymph node dissection in identifying N2 disease (discovery ratio, 2.7; CI, 1.04–4.2).[225] Bollen described more injuries to the recurrent nerve with lymph node dissection when compared to historic controls and that lymph node dissection lengthens the operation. Izbicki et al.[226] conducted a randomized prospective trial with 182 patients comparing systematic mediastinal lymph node sampling to mediastinal lymph node dissection, and found that the number of N2 positive levels was greater in the patients who underwent complete dissection, although the percentage of patients found to have N1 or N2 disease was not significantly different between the two study arms; there was no difference in blood loss or blood replacement.[226] A similar study was conducted by Sugi et al. in 115 patients with clinical T1N0 tumors that were less than 2 cm in diameter; mediastinal metastases were found in 13% of each group.[227] From these data, it appears that systematic lymph node dissection is no more accurate than mediastinal dissection for staging NSCLC.

Whether regional lymph node sampling or complete ipsilateral lymphadenectomy affects long-term survival is unclear. There has been no long-term study of the effects of a complete mediastinal lymphadenectomy. However, the retrospective study by Funatsu et al. has shown that 5-year survival was significantly better in 64 patients who underwent a lymph node sampling, when compared to 61 patients who underwent a radical mediastinal lymphadenectomy.[228] Conversely, in a series of 151 patients at Memorial Sloan-Kettering Cancer Center who had positive mediastinal lymph nodes, a 30% 5-year survival was observed as one of the highest in the literature today with mediastinal lymphadenectomy.[229] In Izbicki's randomized trial comparing mediastinal node sampling with mediastinal lymphadenectomy, no increase in morbidity or mortality was noted for lymphadenectomy, and there were no differences in survival. This trial, however, was underpowered to show differences in locoregional recurrence or survival.[226]

The Intergroup Trial 0115 of adjuvant therapy in patients with completely resected stages II and IIIA NSCLC had the patients stratified by the type of lymph node dissection before participation (dissection versus sampling). Of 373 eligible patients accrued to the study, 187 underwent sampling and 186 had dissection. Although no significant difference in stage distribution was observed between the two surgical procedures, complete dissection identified significantly more levels of N2 disease and was associated with improved survival with right-sided NSCLC compared to systematic sampling.[230]

Wu et al. recently presented the results of the largest randomized trial to date that compared the two techniques.[231] In this study of 471 eligible patients with stages I to IIIA NSCLC followed up for up to 10 years after resection, complete dissection was associated with significant improvement in survival: 59 months versus 34 months median survival. Significant differences in survival were present for all pathologic stages of disease and, on multivariate analysis, the type of lymph node dissection was found to be an independent predictor of survival.

Sentinel Lymph Node Mapping and Mediastinal Staging The first draining node from a primary lesion is known as the sentinel node, and determination of the sentinel node (SN) has been used to individualize lymph node dissection for melanoma and breast cancer, as well as to target those nodes for which thin-section immunohistochemical analysis of micrometastases is warranted. For patients with lung cancer with small tumors and clinically negative lymph nodes, SN mapping could be most beneficial because this group has a 15% and 20% incidence of occult nodal metastatic disease. The safety and efficacy of the SN technique have already been documented in patients with lung cancer. Liptay et al.[232,233] established the feasibility of this technique by defining the SN in 82% of patients with lung cancer intraoperatively with technetium colloid, reporting that upstaging from NO to N1 could occur in as high as 7% of patients. Schmidt,[234] Nomori,[235] and Sugi[236] achieved an identification rate for sentinel lymph nodes of more than 80%, 87%, and 63%, respectively. Although most of the SN were identified at station 12, the rate of mediastinal sentinel lymph nodes (skip metastases) was 20% to 35%. These detection rates had a false-negative rate of 2% to 5%, and may be influenced by the degree of the patient's chronic obstructive pulmonary disease with loss of lymphatic channels due to emphysema and/or the presence of large necrotic tumors.

The implications and utility of SN mapping will become more clear as greater experience with the technique is published to determine the appropriate isotope, timing, and intraoperative or preoperative injection, as well as the ability to intraoperatively determine nodal status using molecular techniques. By selecting only those lymph nodes with a high probability of metastases, molecular or protein identification of these occult metastases could radically stage shift these patients and have implications for therapy, either intraoperatively or postoperatively.

Restaging of the Mediastinum After Induction Therapy Patients with documented mediastinal lymph node disease will be found at surgery after multimodality therapy to be downstaged to N0 in approximately 45% of the cases,[237–239] and a recent report using docetaxel-cisplatinum induction therapy described mediastinal nodal sterilization in 65% of patients.[240] Mediastinal clearance and complete resection of disease in these patients has been associated with 3-year survival of 53% to 61%, compared to 11% to 18% for those without mediastinal clearance. These studies suggest that surgical resection should be avoided in patients after induction therapy who have definite, biopsy-proven residual tumor in the mediastinal nodes.

As mediastinal status after therapy appears to be a strong predictor of survival, the ability to restage the mediastinum in the least invasive fashion could guide therapeutic decisions with regard to (1) feasibility of surgical resection and (2) modification of nonsurgical strategies such as changing chemotherapy regimens if a response is not being achieved. Radiographic techniques are not reliable in the restaging of the mediastinum unless there is a complete disappearance of disease [potential complete response (CR)] or if the disease is obviously progressing.[202] Hence, one should histologically define the status of treated mediastinal adenopathy using less-invasive techniques than thoracotomy, with mediastinal lymph node dissection and intraoperative frozen section assessment of mediastinal disease clearance. There are controversial data to suggest that remediastinoscopy is feasible and may supply information in selected populations of patients. In a study by Mateu-Navarro et al.,[241] 24 patients underwent remediastinoscopy after receiving neoadjuvant chemotherapy with mitomycin, iphosphamide, and cisplatin or cisplatin and gemcitabine. In 12 (50%), remediastinoscopy was positive. The 12 remaining patients were operated on, and residual disease in mediastinal lymph nodes was detected in 5 patients (pN2) and hilar lymph nodes in 1 patient (pN1). The other 6 patients were free of nodal disease. The sensitivity, specificity, and accuracy of remediastinoscopy were 0.7%, 1%, and 0.8%, respectively. In a similar study by Van Schil et al., 27 of 31 identified candidates had remediastinoscopy without major technical difficulties after neoadjuvant therapy.[242] Remediastinoscopy was positive in 11 patients (40.7%) and negative in 16 (59.3%). Of these 16, 4 turned out to be false negatives, for a sensitivity of 71%, specificity of 100%, and accuracy of 84%. These data, although promising, do not establish remediastinoscopy as the gold standard for histologic verification of mediastinal restaging and do not address the issues that may occur with remediastinoscopy after induction chemoradiotherapy.

PET Scanning After Induction Chemo/Radiotherapy The role of PET scanning after both induction chemotherapy and chemoradiotherapy with regard to the status of the mediastinum has been reported by various groups with mixed degrees of enthusiasm, and there are recent reports that FDG-PET scanning can be performed as early as 4 to 12 weeks after radiotherapy with or without chemotherapy and is a better predictor of survival in these patients than CT.[243] In addition, survival and time to progression in Stage IIIb and IV are longer in patients who have a 46% to 60% reduction in standard uptake value (SUV) as early as 21 days after commencing therapy. Nevertheless, these studies do not involve surgical verification of the lymphadenopathy after therapy, and do not comment on nodal basin SUV as a separate region of interest.

One of the initial reports evaluating PET after induction therapy involved 15 surgically staged N2-NSCLC patients who underwent a first PET before three cycles of platinum-based induction chemotherapy.[244] After induction, a second PET was performed and locoregional therapy consolidated with surgery in 9 and radiotherapy in 6. Correlation with pathology of the 9 resection specimens revealed that the accuracy of PET in predicting mediastinal lymph node downstaging was 100% (6 true negatives; 3 true positives). Survival was significantly better in patients with mediastinal clearance ($P = 0.01$) or with a greater than 50% decrease in the SUV of the primary tumor ($P = 0.03$) after induction chemotherapy. A study from the Massachusetts General Hospital[245] investigated PET restaging in 26 patients with histologically confirmed stage III NSCLC [21 with stage IIIA (N2) NSCLC and 5 patients with a highly selected subset of stage IIIB] who were treated with preoperative chemoradiotherapy. All patients had an initial FDG-PET and another performed 2 weeks after completion of preoperative therapy. The FDG-PET images were evaluated qualitatively for uptake at the primary tumor sites and mediastinal lymph nodes. When a value of 3.0 was used as the SUV cutoff, sensitivity and specificity were 88% and 67%, respectively, for the primary tumor site restaging. The sensitivity and specificity of FDG-PET for mediastinal restaging were 58.0% and 93.0%. These results indicated that FDG-PET may be useful for monitoring the therapeutic effect of neoadjuvant chemoradiotherapy in patients with stage III NSCLC. For the primary lesions, SUV-based analysis has high sensitivity but limited specificity for detecting residual tumor. In contrast, for restaging of mediastinal lymph nodes, FDG-PET is highly specific but has limited sensitivity. In a study from Memorial Sloan Kettering Cancer Center,[246] FDG-PET was accurate in the detection of the presence or absence of disease in the primary site (positive and negative predictive values of the FDG scan were 98% and 29%, respectively) of 56 patients restaged postinduction therapy with FDG-PET. Most of the errors in tumor staging were related to understaging T4 disease. In predicting the presence of residual mediastinal nodal disease, however, the positive predictive value, the negative predictive value, sensitivity, and specificity for PET in all assessable patients were 46%, 79%, 67%, and 61%, respectively. This study, however, was limited by the absence of a majority of preinduction FDG-PET scans. More promising data for regional accuracy of lymph node prediction was reported by Cerfolio et al.[247] in a small group of 11 patients with N2 disease in whom repeat FDG-PET scans correctly predicted the absence or presence of cancer in all the N2 paratracheal lymph nodes in all patients. FDG-PET scanning was not as accurate in the other N2 stations, however, including levels 5, 6, and 7.

Future prospective trials of the utility of FDG-PET scanning to predict nodal clearance after induction therapy must be validated by histologic confirmation of disease either by intraoperative mediastinal dissection or by combining PET scanning with targeted positive nodes for remediastinoscopy[248] or EUS.[249]

Preoperative Evaluation

Based on the literature for more than 14,000 patients reported, the operative mortality rates for resection of lung cancer average 4% (lobectomy, 3%; pneumonectomy, 7%–9%), and the most common causes of death include pneumonia and respiratory failure (41%), myocardial infarction (14%), empyema and bronchopleural fistula (11%), hemorrhage (7%), and pulmonary embolus (6%).[250] Surgical selection should be defined by correlation of the functional cardiopulmonary reserve with the age of the patient instead of the chronologic age alone. In a recent review of the literature, the mortality of pulmonary resection for lung cancer in patients 70 to 79 years or more than 80 years was 6% and 8%, respectively.[250] For patients in their seventh decade or older, the mortality for lobectomy is 4% to 7%, and for pneumonectomy it is approximately 14% to 16%.[251] These rates may be more a function of comorbidity than age alone.

In a literature review of more than 9,000 patients, the overall operative morbidity for patients having lung cancer surgery is 34%, with the leading causes of major morbidity being pneumonia (6%), respiratory failure (5%), empyema/bronchopleural fistula (4%), cardiac failure (4%), hemorrhage (2%), myocardial infarction (1%), and pulmonary embolus (1%).[250] The most common minor morbidity is supraventricular tachyarrhythmia (12%).

Preoperative Pulmonary Assessment

The major parameters that have been used to predict postoperative mortality on preoperative studies include blood gas studies while breathing ambient air, and the forced expiratory volume in 1 second as an absolute number or as a percentage of predicted value. Preoperative arterial oxygen saturation less than 90% has been associated with an increased risk of postoperative complications.[252] Hypercapnea ($PaCO_2$ greater than 45 mmHg) cannot be used as an independent risk factor for increased complications but does call for further evaluation of pulmonary reserve.[253,254] The generally accepted guidelines for preoperative FEV_1 for lobectomy and pneumonectomy are values greater than 1.5 and 2 L, respectively, and in all cases the maximum voluntary ventilation (MVV) should be greater than 50% of predicted.[255] Preoperative diffusing capacity of the lung for carbon monoxide (DLCO) has also been linked to postresection morbidity and mortality. For pneumonectomy and lobectomy, a preoperative DLCO of greater than 60% and 50% are recommended for pneumonectomy and lobectomy, respectively. The risk of pulmonary complications also increases if the DLCO% is less than 80%.[256] In general, patients with an FEV_1 more than 80% predicted, a DLCO more than 80% predicted, and no significant cardiac history are suitable for pneumonectomy.[253]

Postoperative Prediction of Lung Function

The prediction of postoperative lung function after resection by using nuclear medicine perfusion scans and recently quantitative CT further defines pulmonary risk. A quantitative radionuclide perfusion scan measures the relative function of each lung.[257–259] In general, the threshold for postoperative FEV_1 for surgical resection is between 0.7 and 0.8 L.[260,261] It is difficult to predict the absolute cutoff for surgical resection and predicted postoperative FEV_1 by percent of normal, but a group of studies have suggested increased morbidity with a postoperative FEV_1 that is less than 40% of normal.[258,262] Moreover, a predicted postoperative DLCO less than 40% is also associated with increased morbidity.[258,263,264]

Exercise Testing

Stair climbing has been used historically to gauge an individual's cardiopulmonary conditioning. In general, lobectomy candidates were expected to climb three flights of stairs, and indeed this correlates with an FEV_1 greater than 1.7 L. Pneumonectomy patients who could climb five flights of stairs have an FEV_1 above 2 L.[265,266]

Formal cardiopulmonary exercise testing (CPET) with the measurement of oxygen consumption has also been used to stratify for the risk of perioperative complications. Patients with a preoperative oxygen consumption greater than 20 mL/kg/min are not at increased risk of complications or death,[255,267,268] whereas those with measurements less than 10 mL/kg/min are at high risk for postoperative complications.[267,269,270]

Specific Management of Lung Cancer Stages

Screen-Detected Central NSCLC

Occult lung cancers (those without radiographic or bronchoscopic findings) are usually detected in sputum screening programs of high-risk asymptomatic individuals and in patients who have had a previous aerodigestive malignancy. The majority of these sputum detected lesions are squamous cell carcinomas, and synchronous lung cancers occur in 7% to 10% and as high as 22% in some studies.[221] Occult lung cancers are usually carcinoma in situ or microinvasive cancer, and the "gold standard" for these lesions is pulmonary lobectomy. The use of autofluorescence bronchoscopic techniques has improved the detection of these occult lesions,[270,271] and 5-year survival with surgery approaches 90%.[272,273]

The depth of invasion of these lesions and the risk of lymphatic permeation can be derived from bronchoscopic evaluation of their size and shape (i.e., less than 10mm, superficial lesions have invasion in only 5% or less, whereas those that are polypoid lesions invade up to 27% of the time).[274] For the smaller lesions with less of a chance of invasion and for patients who will not tolerate a pulmonary resection, lung-preserving endobronchial therapies may be considered including photodynamic therapy, brachytherapy, electrocautery, cryotherapy, and neodymium-yttrium-garnet (Nd-Yag) laser therapy.[275,276,277] Photodynamic therapy of lesions less than 1 cm can ablate these lesions in 75% of the cases with a recurrence rate of approximately 30%.[276] Similar results are achieved with electrocautery,[278] endobronchial iridium-based brachytherapy,[277] and, most recently, cryotherapy.[279]

Stage I Lung Cancer (T1, T2N0M0)

Patients who are medically fit for surgery with lung cancers limited to the hemithorax without lymph node involvement, and with tumor extension no further than the visceral pleura (stage IA and B), should have complete surgical excision by a Board-certified general thoracic surgeon. In the event of positive pathologic margins, additional local therapies should be considered, including reoperation or radiation therapy. The use of adjuvant and induction therapies, specifically for the T2 subset, is discussed in another section of this chapter.

The 5-year survival rates of pathologic stage IA and IB disease after surgical resection are 70% and 55%, respectively, independent of the histology of the tumor.[280,281] The T status of the tumor is clearly important in the prognosis. A literature review of more than 1,600 cT1 tumors versus 1,800 cT2 tumors revealed a 5-year survival of 70% versus 47%,[282] while a review of more than 11,000 pT1 and pT1 tumors revealed survival differences of 71% and 55%, respectively. On average, about a third of the patients with stage I lung cancer will recur, with two-thirds of these recurrences being systemic and one-third local. Approximately 5% of patients with stage I lung cancer will develop a second primary at the rate of 2% per year.[282]

Primary Radiation Versus Surgery for Stage I NSCLC

There have been no randomized trials of surgery versus primary radiation therapy for stage I non-small cell lung cancer. In general, however, radiation therapy is only delivered to early-stage patients who refuse surgical management or who are deemed physiologically unable to undergo resection. A review of 978 patients from various studies of patients with poor performance statuses varying from 0% to 16% and radiation doses ranging from 50 to 80Gy reveals a cancer-specific survival of 23% for clinical stage I non-small cell lung cancer (versus the generally accepted 5-year survival of 51% for surgically resected clinical stage I lung cancer).[283–289] A meta-analysis evaluating the role of primary radiation therapy in stage I NSCLC patients receiving at least 40Gy in 20 fractions over 4 weeks revealed a cancer-specific survival of 13% to 39% at 5 years.[290]

Limited Resection and Early Lung Cancer

The controversies regarding the surgical management of stage IA and IB lung cancer include whether an anatomic resection should be preferred as opposed to wedge resection or less than a lobar anatomic resection, that is, segmentectomy, and the role of lymphadenectomy at the time of resection. Limited resection as a compromise procedure in patients with poor pulmonary reserve has a 5-year survival of 50%.[282] A 6% to 24% risk of local recurrence has been reported in earlier studies using wedge or segmental resection for stage I non-small cell lung cancer along with a 5-year survival of 55% to

TABLE 37.5. Lobectomy versus limited resection for lung cancer: nonrandomized trials.

Author	*Year*	*Lobectomies (n)*	*Limited resections (n)*	*Survival (5 year)*	*Recurrence rates*	*Comments*
Read[661]	1990	131	113	Same = 51%		
Pastorino[662]	1991	411	61	49% vs. 55%	38% vs. 36%	
Warren[663]	1994	68	105	Equal for tumors <3 cm	5% vs. 23%	Lobe for tumors >3 cm
Martini[291]	1995	511	62	77 vs. 59 vs. 35 (LSW)	50% for SW	
Landreneu[294]	1997	117	102	70% vs. 61%		Open or VATS wedge
Kodama[293]	1997	77	63	Same = 93%		
Okada[664]	2001	139	70	87% vs. 87%	No difference	All tumors <2 cm
Miller[295]	2002	75	25	71% vs. 33%	15% vs. 28%	All tumors <1 cm
Koike[666]	2003	159	74	90% vs. 89%	9/159 vs. 5/74	Tumors <2 cm

L, lobectomy; S, segmentectomy; W, wedge resection; VATS, video-assisted thoracic surgery.

TABLE 37.6. Lymph node involvement versus lesion size.

Author	*N*	*Node positive (%)*	*N1 positive (%)*	*N2 positive (%)*	*Size*
Konaka,[667] 1998	171	30 (14%)	10	20	<2 cm
Koike,[668] 1998	157	27 (17%)	11	16	<2 cm
Sugi,[227] 1998	115	22 (19%)	7	15	<2 cm
Kawahara,[669] 2000	49	14 (29%)	NA	NA	<2 cm
Watanabe,[670] 2001	225	38 (17%)	NA	NA	<2 cm (only adeno with positive nodes)
Miller,[665] 2002	100	7 (7%)	5	2	<1 cm

93% when performed in noncompromised individuals.[291–295] In more-recent studies that compare efficacy in single institutional series of lobectomy versus limited resection (Table 37.5), lobectomies were generally similar, especially for smaller lesions, yet the risk of recurrence was significantly increased for lesser resections. There has been one randomized prospective trial comparing limited resection to lobectomy for T1-2NO non-small cell lung cancer. The study, performed by the Lung Cancer Study Group with 247 patients assigned either lesser resection or lobectomy, revealed that the lung cancer recurrence rate was 75% greater in the limited resection due to a tripling of local tumor recurrence and that there was a 50% increase in cancer death.[296]

One must conclude at present that survival is better after lobectomy than after limited resection, and there is a two- to fourfold-higher local recurrence rate in limited resection. Nevertheless, the role of limited resection for lesions less than 1 cm and for lesions that are part solid or nonsolid (i.e., ground-glass opacities) remains under investigation.

The issues regarding mediastinal node dissection and nodal sampling have been described in the "staging" portion of this chapter. Table 37.6 reviews the issue of node positivity as a function of lesion size, showing that even small lesions less than 1 cm can have lymph node metastases if they are adenocarcinomas.

Stage II Lung Cancer

T1–T2N1M0

The majority of patients with pathologic stage II lung cancers (80%) have N1 disease involvement whereas the rest have T3N0 disease.[280,281] N1 nodal disease refers to involvement either by metastasis or direct extension to the subsegmental, segment, and lobar lymph nodes (stations 14, 13, 12) or to the interlobar (11) and hilar lymph nodes (10). The 5-year survival of patients with pathologic stage II (N1) disease is 40%, and the survival of T1N1 disease is approximately 15% higher than that for T2N1 patients.[189,297–300] Squamous stage II lung cancers have improved 5-year survival compared to adenocarcinoma,[298] and the site of recurrence in all N1 is usually systemic rather than local sites.[306] Although evaluated in few studies,[298,301,302] involvement of lobar lymph nodes has approximately a 15% survival advantage over the involvement of extralobar/hilar lymph nodes.

The major surgical issues regarding management of N1 disease involve whether sleeve resections (preservation of lung tissue using bronchoplastic reconstruction techniques) are as efficacious as pneumonectomies and the role of induction/neoadjuvant therapy. The risk of recurrence as well as the operative mortalities are equivalent for the two operations in the setting of sleeve lobectomy for NSCLC (Table 37.7). There are really no data that suggest that pneumonectomy for N1 disease is superior to sleeve resection in terms of survival.[303] The theoretic advantages of sleeve resection also include lung preservation in anticipation of a second primary lung cancer, as well as the increased risk of a cardiopulmonary death with pneumonectomy. The role of induction and postoperative adjuvant therapy for N1 involved patients is discussed elsewhere in this chapter.

Treatment of Stage II NSCLC: T3 Category

T3 tumors usually present without lymph node involvement, and this subset represents approximately 10% of all resected non-small cell lung cancers or 5% of all NSCLC.[281,282] T3 tumors invade the chest wall or diaphragm, the mediastinum (mediastinal pleura, pericardium, phrenic nerve, azygous vein, or right or left pulmonary artery), or have proximity (less than 2 cm) to the carina and involve the mainstem bronchus. Mediastinoscopy should be performed in patients with T3 central tumors before resection for reasons of occult N2 metastases, and the survival of T3N2 NSCLC with a primary surgical resection is low.

Chest Wall T3 Disease

Chest wall muscle, involvement of the parietal pleura, or rib invasion constitute 40% of T3 tumors, and with a complete

TABLE 37.7. Sleeve resections versus pneumonectomies.

Author	*Sleeve lobectomies vs. pneumonectomies (n)*	*Five-year survival*	*Recurrence*	*Operative mortality*
Gaissert[671]	72 vs. 72	42% vs. 44%	14% vs. NA	4% vs. 9%
Okada[318]	60 vs. 60	48% vs. 29%	8% vs. 10%	2%
Suen[672]	58 vs. 142	38% vs. 35%	NA	5.2 vs. 4.9

resection, the 5-year survival is approximately 50% to 60%. The prognosis of resected chest wall T3 disease depends on completeness of resection, nodal involvement, and depth of invasion.[304,305] If on exploration of the chest, the tumor is found to invade the parietal pleura or deeper, an en bloc resection of the tumor with chest wall with a minimum of 2 cm of normal chest wall in all directions beyond the tumor is the preferred surgical technique, and the morbidity of en bloc resection is similar to that of operations where an extrapleural resection is performed.[304,306,307] The decision to reconstruct the chest wall with prosthetic material will depend on the location of the tumor, the preoperative pulmonary status of the patient, and the extent of the resection. The few studies that address postoperative radiotherapy in patients who have undergone either a complete or an incomplete resection of T3 (chest wall) NSCLC have not identified a survival advantage.[305,308]

Pancoast (Superior Sulcus) Tumors

The symptoms arising from a tumor in the apex of the lung, with invasion of the first rib and associated involvement of the brachial plexus and stellate ganglion, create the classic Pancoast syndrome (rib erosion, shoulder pain radiating down the arm, Horner's syndrome). These are usually adenocarcinomas, and fine-needle aspiration has greater than 90% success rate in establishing a diagnosis. Poor prognostic factors for a superior sulcus tumor include mediastinal nodal involvement, the presence of a Horner's syndrome, vertebral body invasion, and great vessel involvement (T4 involvement). In the absence of mediastinal nodal involvement, the overwhelming problem with these tumors is local control. Preoperative radiation therapy of 3,000 to 4,500 cGy followed by en bloc resection of the involved lung, chest wall, and frequently the T1 nerve root has been the standard of care until recently, resulting in complete resection in approximately 66% of patients and a 5-year survival for completely resected patients of 40%. A minority of patients in the surgical series have mediastinal nodal involvement or have evidence of T4 disease.[309] Approximately 45% of resected patients recur locally, and another 25% recur systemically, chiefly in the brain.

The new standard of care for Pancoast tumors involves concurrent chemoradiation therapy followed by surgical resection. Initial results for 95 patients eligible for surgery in the Southwest Oncology Group Trial 9416 (Intergroup Trial 0160) using this approach revealed an operative mortality of 2.4% and a 92% complete resection rate. A pathologic complete response or minimal microscopic disease was seen in 65% of thoracotomy specimens. The 2-year survival was 55% for all eligible patients and 70% for patients who had a complete resection.[310] Presently a Phase II trial that evaluates the role of consolidation chemotherapy after this regimen is under way.

Mediastinal T3 Disease

If mediastinal invasion of the pleura, pericardium, or fat seen by an en bloc resection of the mediastinal tissue is over a small area and discovered only at the time of surgery, resection can usually be accomplished. The average 5-year survival of such patients is 25%.[205] The patients with mediastinal invasion usually have other major structures involved or concomitant mediastinal lymph node disease.[311,312]

Proximal Airway Involvement T3 Disease

Tumors within 2 cm of the carina can be resected by pneumonectomy, but in most of the series reported, especially with those tumors arising from the upper lobes and extending into the main bronchus, a sleeve resection is performed with preservation of the normal distal lung. In fact, patients with mainstem bronchial involvement are usually reported in series of sleeve resections, often mixed in with other stages (Table 37.7). The range of 5-year survival in reported series varies from 12% to 40%.[313–316] No randomized trials comparing sleeve lobectomy with pneumonectomy have been reported in the literature. In single-institution reports comparing pneumonectomy with sleeve resection, the complication rate and mortalities were increased in the pneumonectomy patients, but survival of the two techniques was equivalent. The survival of patients with proximal airway disease is influence by the ability to perform a complete resection (35% 5-year survival versus 18%, complete versus incomplete resection) and the presence of mediastinal nodal involvement (45% 5 year survival for N0 versus 37% for N1 and 0% for N2).[205,317,318] Although these studies are limited by their retrospective method and small numbers of patients, the authors agree with the conclusions of these articles that sleeve lobectomy is preferred over pneumonectomy whenever a complete pathologic resection can be obtained using bronchoplastic techniques.

Locally Advanced Lung Cancer: Stages IIIA and B

Stage IIIA (N2) Disease

Stage IIIA disease includes a T3N1 tumor or N2 nodal spread. The 5-year survival of T3N1 patients is approximately 22%, and the finding of T3N1 (4% of all lung cancers) disease is usually confirmed after resection of suspected T3N0 disease.

The role of surgery for N2 disease is much more complicated because of the heterogeneity of N2 scenarios in clinical presentation, treatment, and prognosis.

Surgery for Incidental N2 Disease

Despite careful preoperative staging including CT scan, PET, and mediastinoscopy, as many as 25% of patients will be found at thoracotomy to have metastases to mediastinal N2 lymph nodes, either intraoperatively or on the final pathologic examination of the surgical specimen. In others, metastases will be found intraoperatively at the time of a thoracotomy with frozen section examination of unsuspected, enlarged mediastinal nodes. In patients with an occult single-station mediastinal node metastasis that is recognized at thoracotomy and when a complete resection of the nodes and primary tumor is technically possible, most thoracic surgeons will proceed with the planned lung resection and a mediastinal lymphadenectomy. This is the best possible prognostic category for these patients because they are classified as clinical N0, microsopic N2, single station, and, according to Andre et al., have 5-year survivals of approximately 35%

to 40%.[203] If a complete resection is not possible or there is multistation or bulky, unresectable extracapsular nodal disease, then the planned lung resection should be aborted as the 5-year survival rate in this situation is only 5% to 10%. These patients can then be considered for induction therapies and potentially reexploration at the conclusion of their chemotherapy with or without radiation therapy. Although incomplete resection rarely results in long-term survival, collected results of surgery alone in stage IIIA (N2 disease) provides a 14% to 30% 5-year survival, with the best survival seen in cases with minimal N2 disease and complete resection.[191,192,194,195,215,319–321] However, if before thoracotomy metastatic disease is found in the N2 nodes at mediastinoscopy, further surgery at that time should be avoided.[322] If appropriate, induction therapy first is more advantageous (see later), followed later in selected patients by definitive surgical resection of the primary lung cancer along with as complete a mediastinal lymphadenectomy as possible.

Prognostic Factors Related to N2 Disease

Extracapsular tumor spread, multiple levels of involved lymph nodes, bulky enlarged nodes, and the size of the primary tumor have negative prognostic significance in stage III A disease.[188–192] Metastatic disease to the subcarinal lymph nodes adversely affects prognosis compared to other lymph nodes[192–198] and, as mentioned earlier, multistation nodal disease has a somewhat worse prognosis than single-station disease.

Potentially Resectable N2 Disease

The poor survival rate with surgery alone in N2 disease, even with adjuvant postoperative chemotherapy or radiotherapy, has led to efforts at giving initial nonsurgical (radiotherapy and/or chemotherapy) therapy first, often to convert the unresectable tumor to resectable and, as well, to improve long-term survival. Patients considered for such approaches include those with enlarged (more than 1.0-cm short-axis diameter) N2 nodes (IIIA) on chest CT. Tissue confirmation of nodal involvement must be performed in this setting to document that these nodes actually contain metastatic tumor, as approximately 40% of moderately enlarged nodes may be benign, especially if there is an associated recent pneumonitis.

Preoperative Chemotherapy in Early-Stage NSCLC

There remains a significant chance for recurrence in patients having surgery for Stage IB–IIB. Due to the feasibility and potential efficacy of induction therapy seen in a small series of randomized trial of IIIA disease, Phase II and III trials have explored the use of induction therapy before surgery in earlier-stage lung cancer patients. One of the first large studies to demonstrate data supporting the use of induction therapy (also discussed later in this chapter) came from a subset analysis of a trial that randomized over 300 patients with stages IB, II (188 patients), and IIIA to receive induction chemotherapy with mitomycin, ifosfamide, and cisplatin before surgery compared to surgery alone.[323] The survival benefit was primarily for patients with stages I and II, with an estimated 4-year survival of 44% for the induction group compared to 35% for the surgery-alone arm. There was a significant decrease in distant metastases and an increase in the length of disease-free survival for the patients treated with chemotherapy. Postoperative morbidity was increased in the combined modality treatment arm (6.7% versus 4.5% for surgery alone). There was no statistically significant benefit in the stage III subgroup.

A randomized study of 212 patients with stage I–IIIA from Shanghai, China, has been reported in abstract form only.[324] One hundred and three patients were randomized to one to two cycles of preoperative cisplatin based chemotherapy and 108 to immediate surgery. A response rate of 50% was seen following preoperative chemotherapy, but no survival benefit was found at 5 years (32% chemotherapy arm versus 37% surgery arm). In fact, the 5-year survival rates were significantly worse in stage II patients (20% versus 65%; $P = 0.042$). Further comments regarding this study will have to await the full publication.

The Phase II BLOT (Bimodality Lung Oncology Team) trial that evaluated preoperative paclitaxel and carboplatin established the feasibility and safety of this approach with encouraging survival.[325–327] Eligible patients had stage T2N0, T1N1, T2N1, and T3N0-1 NSCLC. This population was selected for study based on poor survival despite operability and resection (5-year survival rates, 38%–9%).[327] The study had two cohorts: 94 patients who received two induction and three postoperative paclitaxel/carboplatin cycles[327] and a second cohort of 39 patients who were treated with three induction and two postoperative cycles.[325] The response rate for the induction chemotherapy was 56%, and 94% of the patients underwent resection (86% had a complete resection). The pathologic CR rate was only 6% and the 5-year survival was 46%. An update on the BLOT trial that includes 40 additional patients reveals a 3-year survival of 63%. As seen with many adjuvant lung cancer studies, only 45% of the patients received the postoperative treatment. Forty-six percent of patients had relapsed at the time of the last analysis. The majority of these were distant (44%), with 13 (21%) occurring in the brain only. A combination of local and distant failure was seen in 18%, and 15% recurred locally only. This pattern of failure did not differ from historical controls.

The promising survival from this Phase II trial led to the development of the Phase III North American Intergroup trial S9900. This Southwest Oncology Group (SWOG)-led trial was a prospective, randomized trial that compared three cycles of induction chemotherapy with paclitaxel and carboplatin followed by surgery to surgical resection alone in patients with early-stage NSCLC. However, with the announcement of marked survival advantage to adjuvant chemotherapy as previously described in this chapter, the surgery-alone arm was no longer acceptable as the control, and S9900 was closed to accrual as of July 2004. Nevertheless, all the approximately 350 patients randomized to that point will be followed and the study will still yield valuable information.

The concern that induction chemotherapy given to patients with early-stage disease may increase operative morbidity and mortality[328] should be diminished by data from large surgical series as well as the trials already reviewed here. For example, at the M.D. Anderson Cancer Center, no significant increases in operative morbidity or mortality were found based on clinical stage, pathologic stage, extent of resection, or protocol enrollment. Investigators at Memorial Sloan-Kettering Cancer Center reported similar findings, with the exception that patients undergoing right pneumonectomy following induction therapy had increased operative risk.[329] Other international investigators also examined operative morbidity and mortality rates and found them acceptable following preoperative chemotherapy.[330,331]

Ongoing Early-Stage Induction Trials

Currently, there are randomized trials that compare preoperative chemotherapy to surgery alone in early-stage NSCLC ongoing in Europe. The NATCH trial in Spain is a three-arm study comparing three cycles of paclitaxel/carboplatin chemotherapy given before surgery or after surgery to surgery alone, and data should soon be available from this trial. In Italy, the CHEST study is comparing three cycles of gemcitabine/cisplatin chemotherapy before surgery to a surgery-alone control arm. The LU22 study in Great Britain compares three cycles of platin-based induction chemotherapy to a surgery-only control arm. Finally, the current French study administers chemotherapy to all early-stage NSCLC patients, with randomization to one of two different chemotherapy regimens (gemcitabine/cisplatin or paclitaxel/carboplatin).

Induction Chemotherapy and/or Radiotherapy in Stage IIIA

The modern era of induction regimens for higher-stage NSCLC began with a series of first-generation Phase II trials conducted utilizing cisplatin-based chemotherapy with or without radiotherapy as induction treatment before surgery.[332–336] Response rates from the induction therapy were 39% to 82%, resection rates (percent of original number accrued) were 14% to 88%, and the survival rates were highly variable. Staging and volume of tumor differences within these trials preclude conclusions about efficacy or comparisons across trials; however, these pivotal studies demonstrated the general safety of surgery after induction therapy and, in some instances, provided intriguing survival data and leading to a series of second-generation induction chemotherapy studies.[337–341] Although all second-generation studies required pathologic documentation of N2 disease, tumors with a wide range of disease bulk were accrued. Moreover, radiotherapy was variably given (intraoperative, postoperative, or not at all), and information on why radiotherapy was either given or withheld was not provided in detail for some of the studies. Thus, lack of concordance on the disease bulk and radiotherapy utilization variables makes comparison of results among the studies difficult. Resection rates for second-generation studies were 51% to 68%, and postoperative mortality, predominantly from pulmonary or cardiopulmonary toxicities, ranged from 0% to 18%.

The other major category of second-generation induction studies utilized concurrent chemoradiotherapy (chemoRT) induction therapy (Table 37.8.[237,342–345] The RT varied in schedule, all induction chemotherapy was cisplatin based, but the treatment prescribed after surgical resection was not uniform among these five studies. Biopsy documentation of N2 disease or T4 status (see later) was required only in the SWOG, Lung Cancer Study Group (LCSG), and Cancer and Leukemia Group B (CALGB) trials, and stage IIIA (N2) accounted for 47% to 87% of patients per trial. Two studies included T3N0 or T3N1 (21% and 20% in the Rush Presbyterian and CALGB studies, respectively), whereas all patients with stage IIIA disease in the SWOG 8805, LCSG 852, and Tufts trials had N2 nodal involvement. The stage IIIB subsets of T4 and/or N3 were allowed in all trials except the CALGB study and accounted for 6% to 53% of patients per trial.

Response or "response plus stable" (one study) rates were 56% to 92%, and 52% to 76% of the total number of patients accrued to each study had a complete resection at thoracotomy. The pathologic complete response (pCR) rates were 16%, 21%, and 27% in the LCSG, SWOG, and Rush Presby-

TABLE 37.8. Second-generation Phase II studies of induction chemoradiotherapy before surgery.

Investigators	*N*	*Disease burden*	*IIIA (N2) (%)*	*T3N0–1/T4 or N3 (%)*	*Treatment schema*	*Response rate (%)*[a]	*Complete resection rate (%)*[a]	*Treatment-related mortality (%)*[a]	*Operative Mortality (%)*[b]	*pCR (%)*[a]	*pCR in N2 (%)*[a]
SWOG 8805[237]	126	High volume	60	0/40	EP × 2 + 45 Gy → Surgery → EP × 2 + 14 Gy if persistent N2 /incomplete resection	59	71	10	8	15	38
LCSG 852[342]	85	High volume	85	0/13	PF × 2 + 30 Gy → Surgery	56	52	8	7	9	Not stated
Rush—Presbyterian[343]	85	Mixed volume	73	21/6	PF or PEF + 40 Gy (Split course) → Surgery	92[a]	71	3.5	5	20	26
CALGB I[344]	41	Mixed volume	80	20/0	PVF × 2 + 30 Gy → Surgery → PVF × 1 + 30 Gy	64+	61	15	10	17	Not stated
Tufts[345]	42	High volume	66	2/45	EP × 2 + 59.4 Gy→ surgery → PE × 4 or Carbo T × 4	69[a]	79	0	0	21	59

SWOG, Southwest Oncology Group; LCSG, Lung Cancer Study Group; CALGB, Cancer and Leukemia Group B; E, etoposide; P, cisplatin; F, 5-fluorouracil; V, vinblastine; Carbo, carboplatin; T, paclitaxel; Gy, gray.

[a] Percent of original number.

[b] Percent of patients subjected to surgery.

[c] Includes stable disease.

TABLE 37.9. Long-term survival in selected second-generation Phase II induction trials in NSCLC.

Investigators	*Disease burden*	*Included T3N0 or N1?*	*Biopsy proof of N2 status required?*	*Selected Stage IIIB included?*	*Long-term survival*
Memorial[338]	Mixed volume	No	Yes	No	28%, 3-year; 17%, 5-year
Toronto[339]	Mixed volume	No	Yes	No	26%, 3-year
SWOG 8805[237,346]	High volume	No	Yes	Yes	27%, 3-year, 20%, 6-year, stage IIIA (N2); 24%, 3-year, 22%, 6-year, stage IIIB
CALGB II[340]	High volume	Yes	No	No	28%, 3-year 22%, 7(+)-year
CALGB 8935[341]	High volume	No	Yes	No	23%, 3-year
Rush-Presbyterian[343]	Mixed volume	Yes	No	Yes	40%, 3-year
Tufts[345]	High volume	Yes	No	Yes	37%, 5-year

SWOG, Southwest Oncology Group: CALGB, Cancer and Leukemia Group B.

terian trials, respectively.[237,342,343] Postinduction assessment of nonresponse by CT scan was often misleading, because 46% of the 26 patients with resectable stable disease in the SWOG study had pCR or only rare microscopic foci.[237]

The operative mortalities were predominantly pulmonary related, as observed in the induction chemotherapy trials. The cause of death often resembled the adult respiratory distress syndrome (ARDS).

Long-term survival data were reported in several of the trials of induction chemotherapy and induction chemoRT (Table 37.9). Long-term follow-up of several of the trials suggested that a plateau emerged on the tails of the survival curves, and 5- to 7-year survivals of 17% to 34% were reported. Favorable outcome predictors included postinduction pCR, complete resection, T3N0 or T3N1 disease, T4N0 or N1 disease, and pathologic clearance of initial N2 or N3 involvement (nodal downstaging). The SWOG 8805 trial analysis showing that nodal downstaging was an independent favorable prognostic impact of intermediate (2- to 3-year) survival is of interest, and was the only significant factor in a multivariate model that included complete resection rate, pCR, and multiple other factors.[237] This variable was also the most important univariate discriminant of 6-year survival, although complete resection emerged as a long-term survival predictor as well.[346] The survival rates 3 and 6 years after thoracotomy for patients with uninvolved nodes at surgery were 41% and 33%, respectively, versus only 11% and 11% if there was persistent mediastinal disease.

Following on the aforementioned chemoRT trials came three Phase II induction trials [Massachusetts General Hospital (MGH), West German Cancer Center (WGCC), and the German Lung Cancer Cooperative Group (GLCCG)] using platinum-based chemotherapy and hyperfractionated radiotherapy either with a planned break (1) or with radiation intensification by delivering it in an accelerated fashion (2)[347–349] (Table 37.10). Treatment-related mortality was 7%, 6%, and 9% and postoperative mortality 5%, 7%, and 8% (of patients who underwent thoracotomy) in the MGH, WGCC, and GLCCG trials, respectively. The main perioperative complication seen in both WGCC and GLCCG trials was bronchial stump insufficiency, most often after right-sided resections. After both groups started reinforcing bronchial stumps with tissue later in each trial, the incidence of this problem dropped to zero. A complete resection with negative margins was accomplished in 81% of all patients in the MGH trial, and the median survival was 25 months with an overall survival of 66%, 37%, and 37% at 2, 3, and 5 years, respectively. Five-year survival was 79% if the nodes were downstaged to N0; 53% of the patients had complete resection with negative margins on the West German Cancer Center study and 26% had a complete pathologic response. Median survival was 20 and 18 months and 3-year survival rates were 36% and 31% for stages IIIA and IIIB, respectively (no statistical difference). A complete resection with negative margins was achieved in 63% of patients enrolled on the GLCCG trial, and over 50% of these exhibited a major histological response, defined as necrosis or fibrosis of more than 90% of tumor cells. Seven (13%) had pathologic complete response. The median survival for the whole group was 20 months, with 2- and 3-year survival of 40% and 30%, respectively. Median survivals for stages IIIA and IIIB (25 versus 17 months) showed no statistical significance, as did 2- and 3-year survivals (52% and 35% versus 30% and 26%).

Randomized Trials of Surgery Alone Versus Induction Therapy Followed by Surgery in Mixed-Stage, Resectable Disease

Several small randomized studies and one large Phase III trial of induction chemotherapy for NSCLC were conducted for patients with low-volume or "minimal" N2 disease and with a surgery-alone arm as the control (Table 37.11).[238,350–353] The NCI trial was the most homogeneous in the stage subsets accrued, whereas the treatment groups of the small M.D. Anderson and Spanish studies had heterogeneous stage subset distributions. The same stage mix issues existed in the large French Thoracic Cooperative Group (FTCG) trial, with some imbalance of stage subsets between the two arms ($P = 0.07$).[353]

TABLE 37.10. Third-generation Phase II trials of concurrent induction chemoradiotherapy with hyperfractionation in NSCLC.

Investigators	*Stage subsets(s)/ number of patients*	*Disease burden*	*Chemotherapy*	*Radiotherapy*	*Resection rate (%)*[a]	*Treatment -related mortality (%)*[a]	*Operative mortality (%)*	*Survival*	*Predictors of favorable outcome*
MGH[347]	Biopsy-proven stage IIIA (N2), $n = 42$	Mixed volume	PVF × 2 concurrent with RT → surgery → VF × 1 concurrent with RT	42 Gy split (1.5 bid × 7 → 10 day rest → 1.5 bid × 7); postoperative 12–18 Gy 1.5 bid)	93%	7	5	37%, 5-year	• Downstaging to N0 (79% 5-year survival) • Complete resection 4-year survival from registration: • complete resection, 46% vs. 11%, $P = 0.0001$
West German Cancer Center (WGCC)[348]	Mediastinoscopy required, 6; advanced T3 N0/1, 46; two or more N2 nodes, 42; IIIB (T4) or contralateral (N3) Total, $n = 94$	High volume	EP × 3 → reduced dose EP × 1 with RT → surgery	45 Gy (1.5 Gy bid over 3 weeks); PCI later in trial	53% (60% IIIA, 45% (IIIB)	6	7	28%, 4-year (31% IIIA 26% IIIB)	• N2/3 → N0 38% vs. 15%, $P = 0.11$ • LDH ≤240 or not, 37% vs. 0%, $P = 0.003$ • PCI Decrease **in first brain metastases,** $P = 0.005$ • >90% histologic regression (3-year survival, 48% vs.. 9%, $P = 0.007$) • Complete resection ($P = 0.009$)
German Lung Cancer Cooperative Group (GLCCG)[349]	N2, 25; (all biopsy-proven); T4 or N3, 29; Total, $n = 54$	High volume	ICE × 2 → PVd × 1 + RT → surgery	45 Gy (1.5 Gy bid over 3 weeks)	63% (R0)	9	8	30%, 3-year	

MGH, Massachusetts General Hospital; n, number of patients; P, cisplatin: V, vinblastine; F, 5-fluorouracil; E, etoposide; I, ifosfamide, C, carboplatin; Vd, vindesine; Gy, gray; PCI, prophylactic cranial irradiation.
p, pathologic.

TABLE 37.11. Randomized Phase III trials of surgery with or without induction therapy in resectable NSCLC.

Investigators	Stage subset(s)	Disease bulk	Chemotherapy	Radiotherapy	Patients (N)	Two- to 3-year survival		
						No. ChT	ChT	P value
NCI[238]	IIIA (N2) by biopsy	High volume	EP 2 cycles preoperative EP 4 cycles postoperative	Postoperative in no-ChT arm only (54–60 Gy)	28	21%	46%	0.12
M.D. Anderson[351,673]	IIIA (N2) not required; node biopsy not required; some IIIB	Low volume	CEP pre- and postoperative	Postoperative only if residual disease	60	15%	56%	<0.05
Spain[352,355]	IIIA (N2) not required; node biopsy not required	Low volume	PIM preoperative	Postoperative for both arms	60	0%	30%	<0.05
French Thoracic Cooperative Group[323]	Clinical T2N0, II, IIIA	Low volume	MIP × 2 preoperative; also postoperative, if objective response	Postoperative to 60 Gy, if pT3 or pN2 for both arms	355	41%*	52%*	$P = 0.15$**

E, etoposide; P, cisplatin; V, vinblastine; I, ifosfamide; Vd, vindesine; M, mitomycin C; C, cyclophosphamide; NS, not significant; NCI, National Cancer Institute; ChT, chemotherapy.

Furthermore, in the FTCG study, clinical staging alone was accepted and documentation of N2 status was not required. The induction chemotherapy regimens for the five trials were cisplatin based and were also variably given after surgery depending on the study design.

Three of the four trials closed before the target accrual goal was met. The National Cancer Institute (NCI) trial was halted due to slow accrual, whereas the M.D. Anderson and Spanish studies were stopped early because of large survival differences by data monitoring committees due to strongly positive results in favor of the induction chemotherapy arms.[354,355] With additional follow-up of the M.D. Anderson trial cohort (median follow-up, 81 months), 32% of patients were alive in the induction chemotherapy group versus 16% in the surgery-alone arm ($P = 0.06$).[351] The P value became significant if only deaths caused by cancer were considered. The update of the Spanish trial has revealed that no patients survived in the surgery group, whereas 16% were long-term survivors in the induction chemotherapy arm.[352]

These M.D. Anderson and Spanish trials generated extensive discussion and debate with a consensus that these results were provocative but not definitive. Suffice it to say that the major concerns were the marked substage heterogeneity within these two trials, and that the surgical control arms fared poorly, possibly because of substage imbalances.

The largest randomized Phase III trial of chemotherapy alone for induction was the French Thoracic Cooperative Group Trial, which enrolled patients with stage IB to IIIA disease.[323,353] The 1-, 2-, 3-, and 4-year survivals were 77%, 71%, 59%, and 44%, respectively, in the induction chemotherapy arm and 73%, 52%, 41%, and 35% in the surgery-alone arm. The difference did not reach statistical significance ($P = 0.15$). Stage-adjusted relative risk of death was 0.80 in the chemotherapy arm ($P = 0.089$). In a subset analysis, there was a benefit to induction for patients with N0-1 disease [relative risk (RR), 0.68; $P = 0.027$], but not for patients with N2 (RR, 1.04; $P = 0.85$). There was a nonsignificant excess of mortality (10% versus 5%) in the induction chemotherapy arm, consisting of pneumonia, emphysema, fistula, and pulmonary embolism.

The North American Intergroup trial 0139, chaired by RTOG, is the largest Phase III trial to date that addressed the potential value of surgery in stage IIIA(N2) NSCLC[356] (Table 37.12). The entry criteria for this study included T1-3 primary tumor, pathologically confirmed N2 disease, feasible resection from a surgical standpoint, and medical ability to undergo resection. The induction regimen was identical in both arms: 45 Gy of external radiotherapy given in once-daily fraction, concurrent with day 1 of induction chemotherapy, which was cisplatin, 50 mg/m^2 on days 1, 8, 29, and 36, and etoposide, 50 mg/m^2 days 1–5 and 29–33. Patients were reevaluated by a CT scan 2 to 4 weeks after completion of the induction regimen in the surgical arm, and in the RT arm, 1 week before completion of treatment. Those patients with no progression proceeded with their assigned treatment. In the surgical arm, the treatment consisted of resection of all known disease and mediastinal nodal sampling. In the RT arm, the radiotherapy continued to 61 Gy without a break. In both arms, consolidation chemotherapy (two cycles of cisplatin and etoposide) was given to all patients. At a median follow-up of 69 months, 392 patients were analyzable. Induction treatment was delivered as per the protocol equally in both arms. In the surgical arm, a thoracotomy was performed in 96%, and a complete resection was accomplished in 88% of patients for whom the data were available. There were 18% pathologic complete responses (T0N0) and 46% with pathologic nodal clearance. The chemoRT toxicity was similar in both arms, with the exception of esophagitis, which was more common in the chemoRT-alone arm. Consolidation chemotherapy was not administered to 42% of patients undergoing surgery, and 21% of those not having undergone surgery (P less than 0.001), reiterating the difficulty of deliv-

TABLE 37.12. Reported Phase III induction trials of chemoradiotherapy for NSCLC.

Investigators	*Stage subset*	*Question*	*Study design*	*No. of patients*	*Outcome comment*
NCI Canada[674]	Biopsy-proven stage IIIA (N2)	Postinduction surgery vs. RT	PV → surgery vs. RT	31	Closed early due to radiotherapy alone arm; survival curves superimposed at 2 years
RTOG 89-01[675]	Biopsy-proven stage IIIA (N2)	Postinduction surgery vs. RT	MVP or VP ↓ Surgery vs. RT ↓ MVP or VP	73	Closed early due to slow accrual; $P = 0.62$ for overall survival; 4-year: 22% for surgery vs. 22% for RT
CALGB[676]	Biopsy-proven stage IIIA (N2)	Induction RT or chemo	RT → surgery → RT vs. PV → surgery → PV → RT	57	Closed early due to slow accrual; median survival 24 months (RT/S/RT) and 18 months (CT/S/CT) ($P = 0.4$)
INT 0139[356]	Biopsy-proven IIIA (N2)	Postinduction surgery vs. chemoRT alone	PE/RT → surgery → PE vs. PE/RT → RT → PE	392	Preliminary results: CT/RT/S: 3-year OS, 38%; median OS, 22 months; 3-year PFS, 29%; $P = 0.51$; median PFS, 14 months CT/RT: 3-year OS, 33%; median OS, 21 months; 3-year PFS, 19%; $P = 0.02$; median PFS, 12 months

P, cisplatin; F, 5-fluorouracil; M, mitomycin C; V, vinblastine; E, etoposide; RTOG, Radiation Therapy Oncology Group; CALGB, Cancer and Leukemia Group B.

ering chemotherapy after "definitive" surgical treatment for lung cancer. Conversely, RT was delivered according to protocol in 81% on the chemoRT arm versus 97% on the surgery arm ($P = 0.002$). Three patients (1.6%) in the chemoRT arm and 14 (7%) patients in the chemoRT-surgery arm died of treatment-related toxicity. In the latter group, 10 of these deaths were caused by postoperative complications. Most of the deaths occurred in patients who underwent pneumonectomy (especially right-sided), and the most frequent cause of death was the adult respiratory distress syndrome (ARDS).

Median progression-free survival was 14.0 months and 11.7 months in the chemoRT-surgery arm and chemoRT arm, respectively. Three-year progression-free survival was 29% in the chemoRT-surgery arm versus 19% in the chemoRT arm (log rank, $P = 0.02$). The median overall survival was 22.1 months versus 21.7 months and the 3-year survival was 38% versus 33% in the chemoRT-surgery and chemoRT arms, respectively (log rank, $P = 0.51$). The overall survival curves cross over and begin to separate at 22 months. By 3 years, there was a 5% absolute survival benefit in the surgical arm, but the confidence intervals are wide and overlap. More patients died of treatment complications in the surgical arm, but more are alive without progression in the same treatment arm. Sites of relapse were also analyzed: 13% of patients in the chemoRT-surgery arm had locoregional relapse only versus 21% in the chemoRT arm ($P = 0.07$). Relapse in the primary site was three times more common in the nonsurgical arm. Brain was common site of first relapse in both arms (10% versus 18 % in the chemoRT and chemoRT-surgery arm, respectively; $P = 0.08$). Pretreatment factors predictive of favorable outcome were lower T stage, less than 5% weight loss, and younger age. Female sex and normal LDH did not reach statistical significance. After the induction treatment, patients who achieved complete response in the mediastinal nodes had median survival of 36.7 months and 3-year survival of about 50%, regardless of the response in the primary tumor.

The Stage IIIB Subgroup in Second-Generation (and Subsequent) Studies of ChemoRT Induction Trials

From a subset of these second-generation ChemoRT trials, data are available regarding the role of induction therapy followed by surgery in selected stage IIIB subsets. The SWOG 8805 trial was unique among the other chemoRT trials in that it included stage IIIB disease. Pathologic documentation of T4 or N3 disease was required and outcome was analyzed separately for this subset.[237,256] The median, 2-year, and 3-year survivals were identical for the IIIA(N2) versus the IIIB group in the SWOG 8805 study (27%, 24%).[237] Of note, in the SWOG 8805 study, the T4N0-1 subset had an outcome identical to the T1N2 substage and achieved a 2-year survival of 64%. This substage variable was the only independent predictor of favorable outcome from the time of registration to the study in a multivariate analysis.[237] Exploratory survival analyses were conducted within the N3 subset of the SWOG trial, of which 27 patients were accrued. The 2-year survival for the contralateral nodal N3 subgroup was zero, whereas it was 35% for the supraclavicular N3 subset. However, the resection rate in this latter group was only 39%. An update of SWOG 8805 provided 6-year survival statistics: IIIA (N2), 20%; T4N0-1, 49%; and N2 or N3, 18%.[357]

Subsequent studies have commented on the role of induction therapy for stage IIIB disease. Grunenwald et al. prospectively studied 40 patients with IIIB disease, of whom 30 had T4 disease and 18, N3.[358] Five patients had T4N0 tumors and 1 had T4N1. All patients underwent pretreatment surgical staging. Induction treatment consisted of 5-fluorouracil (5-FU), cisplatin, and vinblastine for two cycles. A total of 42 Gy of external radiotherapy was given split in two 21-Gy courses, 1.5 Gy bid, with 10 days of rest between the courses. Patients who responded to the induction regimen underwent thoracotomy. A clinical response was obtained in 73% of patients, and in 60% resection was performed. The resection was complete in all but 1 patient who underwent thoracotomy. Four patients (10%) had complete pathologic response and 30% had complete mediastinal clearance. There were 5 treatment-related deaths, and 7 additional patients suffered serious morbidity. Median survival was 15 months and 5-year overall survival was 19%. Thirty percent of the overall patient number had locoregional relapse and 50% had distant relapse. Pathologic mediastinal nodal downstaging was the only significant favorable prognostic factor in a multivariate analysis (5-year survival, 42% for postinduction N0/1 versus 12 % for postinduction N2/3 for resected patients). All long-term survivors had persistent viable tumor cells in the primary tumor but 6 of 7 were postinduction N0-1.

Pitz et al. treated patients with stage IIIB NSCLC with neoadjuvant gemcitabine and cisplatin without radiotherapy, followed by surgery in responding patients. There was a response rate of 66%, resection rate of 44%, and perioperative mortality of 2.4%. Median survival for all patients was 15.1 months and 3-year survival was 15%. The investigators found no difference in outcome between T4N0 and N2/N3 subsets. However, only patients with a response after induction chemotherapy were considered for surgical resection.[359] These trials highlight that the T4N0/1 substage as a group does particularly well with trimodality therapy.

Induction with Third-Generation Chemotherapy Agents

Third-generation chemotherapy agents have been tested in Phase II induction therapy protocols in stage III disease (Table 37.13). The Swiss Group for Clinical Cancer Research (SAKK) enrolled 90 potentially operable stage IIIA patients with biopsy-proven ipsilateral mediastinal nodal involvement.[240] The induction regimen consisted of cisplatin 40 mg/m^2 on days 1–2 plus docetaxel 85 mg/m^2 on day 1 for three cycles. All patients except those with progressive disease underwent thoracotomy. No postoperative chemotherapy was given, and postoperative RT to 60 Gy was reserved for patients found to have a positive resection margin and/or involvement of the uppermost mediastinal lymph node. There were 2 treatment-related deaths (3%). The overall clinical response was 66%, and complete resection was accomplished in only 48% of the entire patient group. An additional 43% underwent incomplete resection with positive margins and/or positive highest mediastinal lymph node, and their overall cisplatin dose intensity was less that that in patients with negative resection margins (80 versus 96 mg/m^2/cycle; P = 0.034). There were 14 patients (16%) with a complete pathologic response, and 45 (60%) had pathologic nodal clearance. The median survival was 27.6 months and 3-year survival was 33%. Mediastinal downstaging was the most powerful independent favorable prognostic factor (P = 0.0003), and patients with mediastinal downstaging had a 3-year survival rate of 61% as compared to 11% for those who did not. Complete resection was also predictive of favorable outcome (P = 0.006).

In another recent trial, three preoperative cycles of gemcitabine, paclitaxel, and cisplatin were delivered to 49 biopsy-documented N2 disease patients.[360] Patients with at least stable disease after the induction regimen underwent attempted surgical resection. Patients whose disease did not respond received RT alone, and the patients whose disease responded but did not undergo thoracotomy, received three more cycles of the same chemotherapy followed by RT. Postoperative RT was delivered for patients with persistent N2 disease or incomplete resection. There was 1 death during the induction. A response rate of 73.5% based on radiographic criteria was recorded, and a complete resection was performed in 55% of patients. Mediastinal nodal disease clearance occurred in 35% of cases and complete pathologic response in 16%. Median and progression-free survival were 23 and 18 months, respectively, and the brain was the most common metastatic site (16%). The Italian Lung Cancer Project completed a Phase II trial in 129 unresectable, locally advanced stage IIIA and IIIB NSCLC patients.[361] The induction regimen consisted of four cycles of gemcitabine 1,000 mg/m^2 on days 1 and 8 and cisplatin 70 mg/m^2 on day 2. The response rate was 80%, but the resectability rate was only 29%. There was no perioperative mortality and minimal morbidity. Postoperative RT was given for positive mediastinal lymph nodes and was continued to 60 Gy if the disease was unresectable. The median progression-free survival was 11 months and median survival was 20 months.

The European Organization for Research and Treatment of Cancer (EORTC) is conducting a Phase III trial (EORTC 08941) of induction chemotherapy followed by either radiotherapy or surgery for those patients with at least partial clinical response to induction (see discussion in section to follow).[362] The trial design allows a menu of induction combination chemotherapy so long as it includes cisplatin at 100 mg/m^2 or carboplatin at 400 mg/m^2. Two reports of feasibility and toxicity have been published to date of induction approaches, while the Phase III trial is ongoing.[363,364] The first

TABLE 37.13. Design and results of completed Phase II trials using third-generation chemotherapy drugs within the induction regimen.

Investigators	*Stage subset*	*Study design*	*No. of patients*	*Response rate (%)*	*Resection rate (RG)[a] (%)*	*pCR (%)*	*Survival*
SAKK[240]	IIIA (pN2), mixed bulk	PD × 3 → surgery → variable RT	90	66	48	16	3-year, 33%
De Marinis et al.[360]	IIIA (pN2), bulky	GTP × 3 → surgery → variable RT	49	74	55	16	Median, 23 months
ILCP[361]	IIIA, IIIB (clin), bulky	GP × 4 → surgery → variable RT	129	62	29	2	Median, 19 months
EORT[362,363,364]	IIIA (pN2), bulky	GC → surgery TC → Surgery	47 52	70 64	71 80	NR	NR

T, paclitaxel; C, carboplatin; P, cisplatin; D, docetaxel; G, gemcitabine; NR, not reported.

[a] Of the original number of patients.

TABLE 37.14. **Phase III trials of adjuvant radiotherapy in NSCLC.**

Study	N	Local recurrence rate (%)		Five year overall survival (%)		Statistical significance
		Observed	*Treated*	*Observed*	*Treated*	
Weisenbruger[366]	230	41	3*	38[a]	38[a]	NS
Stephens et al.[365]	308	47.4	37.7	19 months[b]	17.5 months[b]	NS
Lafitte et al.[367]	132	17	15	51.6	35.2	NS
Dautzenberg et al.[368]	728	34	28	43	30	$P = 0.002$
Granone et al.[369]	104	22	2*	70	83	NS

NS, not statistically significant.

[a] Obtained from data curves.

[b] Median survival in months.

* Statistically significant for local recurrence rate, $P < 0.025$.

pilot study was reported by Van Zandwijk et al. in which gemcitabine 1,000mg/m^2 and cisplatin 100mg/m^2 were used.[364] The dose of gemcitabine had to be reduced or omitted in more than half of the patients, mainly due to thrombocytopenia. Responses were observed in 70%. O'Brien et al. reported the use of induction paclitaxel, 200mg/m^2, and carboplatin, AUC of 6. Over 90% of patients were able to complete all induction treatment per protocol. The response rate was 64%. One patient died of postoperative complications.[363] In the two studies, resection rates of 71% and 80%, respectively, were reported.

Mortality After Induction Therapy

Although the use of neoadjuvant chemotherapy and/or radiotherapy appears to have potential advantages in the treatment of locally advanced lung cancer, concern has been raised in numerous publications about the perceived and real increase in morbidity and mortality of the subsequent lung resections. So far, there has been no difference in overall postoperative mortality rates compared to the surgery-alone control arms in trials with induction chemotherapy for early, more minimal bulk disease.[323,328,351] Pulmonary complications and deaths from pulmonary causes during the postoperative time period are the greatest concern after induction therapy, and collectively rates are probably greater than reported in the literature after surgery alone. In particular, events such as extensive pneumonitis, usually culture negative, ARDS, and bronchopleural fistula have a high mortality in the postoperative period. Pulmonary morbidity and mortality rates are often quoted to be greater after induction regimens with chemoRT than after induction chemotherapy alone. However, a careful review of all the literature available discloses great variability. Postoperative mortality rates from 3.1% to 17% were reported after mitomycin/vinblastine/cisplatin (MVP)- or VP16/cisplatin (VP)-containing induction chemotherapy (including some cases of ARDS), from 4% to 15% after second-generation induction chemoRT, and 5% to 7% after induction chemoRT with hyperfractionation. The specific type of mortal postoperative event may differ according to whether RT was included with induction chemotherapy or not, although this issue is not fully resolved. Moreover, the degree of pulmonary resection, that is, pneumonectomy, especially on the right, is associated with a higher morbidity and mortality.[329]

Adjuvant Radiotherapy

Randomized trials examining adjuvant radiotherapy for resected NSCLC are shown in Table 37.14, including four trials of greater than 100 patients that were incorporated into the 1998 PORT meta-analysis (see following).[365–369] None of these trials demonstrated a beneficial effect of postoperative radiotherapy on overall survival. However, findings from the LCSG 773 trial are notable for detecting a significant reduction in local recurrence (41% versus 3%) for patients receiving adjuvant radiotherapy.[366] Dautzenberg et al. detected inferior efficacy outcomes and an increased rate of intercurrent deaths in their large randomized trial; the intercurrent deaths were largely caused by cardiorespiratory failure and prompted concern regarding the utility of adjuvant radiotherapy in patients with resected stage I and II disease.[368]

The PORT meta-analysis encompassed updated data on 2,128 patients from nine randomized studies of adjuvant radiotherapy in resected NSCLC, approximately one-third of whom were enrolled in the trial of Dautzenberg et al.[368] The PORT meta-analysis found that radiation exerted a harmful effect, especially for N0-N1 patients, with a hazard ratio of death of 1.21. This translated to an absolute detriment of 7% at 2 years, reducing overall survival from 55% to 48%. Subgroup analyses revealed that adjuvant radiotherapy exerted no harmful effect on patients with N2 disease. Criticisms of this meta-analysis include its dependence on older studies that used outmoded radiation techniques such as lateral portals and the use of cobalt-60 units.[370] It is anticipated that modern radiotherapy procedures, relying on three-dimensional (3-D) conformal planning and using doses no greater than 45Gy in fraction sizes less than 2.0Gy, will reduce morbidity and mortality associated with adjuvant radiation, especially radiation pneumonitis.[371]

Interim analyses from a more recent investigation, incorporating modern radiotherapy techniques, did not detect deleterious effects of adjuvant radiation therapy.[369] Adjuvant radiation, administered using 50.4-Gy linear accelerator radiotherapy in 1.8-Gy fractions with 2-D and 3-D imaging support, was associated with a decline in local recurrence but exerted no effect on estimated 5-year overall survival. Preoperative and postradiation pulmonary function tests were not significantly different in this study population. Final results of this study are eagerly awaited as this trial tests the hypothesis that more modern radiation techniques will reduce the number of treatment-related, intercurrent deaths in the setting of adjuvant radiotherapy for NSCLC patients.

Published reports of adjuvant radiotherapy have failed to demonstrate improvements in overall survival in resected NSCLC patients, and have, in fact, raised the question of possible harmful effects for N0 and N1 treated patients. Although no survival benefit has been observed in patients with resected N2 disease, the preponderance of randomized evidence demonstrates improved local control in resected N2 patients who receive adjuvant radiotherapy. Off-study use of postoperative radiation cannot be recommended for completely resected NSCLC patients with N0 or N1 disease.

Adjuvant Chemotherapy

Table 37.15 demonstrates results from randomized trials investigating the role of adjuvant chemotherapy in resected NSCLC.[372–383] Until very recently, the clinical trial experience of adjuvant chemotherapy has been hampered by an inability to administer adequate dose intensity because of treatment-related toxicities. The Lung Cancer Study Group (LCGS) conducted three trials in the United States investigating the role of adjuvant cyclophosphamide, doxorubicin, and cisplatin (CAP) in patients with resected stage I–III disease.[372–374] Systemic adjuvant therapy did not improve overall survival in any of the three studies, or in two European trials (although treatment was associated with a positive impact when rates of pneumonectomy were controlled for in the trial of Niiranen et al.).[375,376]

Japanese investigators instituted a series of adjuvant trials with oral uracil-tegafur (UFT), an oral agent consisting of tegafur, a 5-fluorouracil derivative, and uracil at a 1:4 molar ratio. Tegafur is gradually converted to 5-fluorouracil in vivo. Treatment with UFT results in sustained concentrations of intratumoral 5-fluorouracil.[379] Results of these trials have been mixed (see Table 37.15), with only one trial conducted by the Japan Lung Cancer Research Group in patients with resected stage I (T1N0 or T1N1) adenocarcinomas being clearly positive.[383] However, subgroup analyses revealed that the survival benefit seen with UFT was restricted to the 269 patients with T2 lesions (improving 5-year survival from 73.5% to 84.9%; $P = 0.005$), and that no improvement was seen in the T1N0 subgroup. Other studies involving postoperative chemotherapy plus or minus UFT have been negative, although subgroup analysis[380,381] after controlling for baseline T or N stage,[381,382] or for baseline prognostic factors and the extent and completeness of surgery,[380] have suggested a possible role for UFT in very early stage disease. Confirmatory studies are certainly warranted.

In 1995, the Non-small Cell Lung Cancer Collaborative Group published a meta-analysis using updated data on individual patients from 52 randomized clinical trials.[384] One of their analyses examined randomized trials of adjuvant chemotherapy versus surgery alone in patients with resected NSCLC. Data were available from 14 trials, of which 5 used alkylating agents, 8 used cisplatin-based chemotherapy, and 3 used other combinations. Alkylating chemotherapy was associated with a hazard ratio of 1.15, or a 15% increase in the risk of death, translating into an absolute detriment of alkylating chemotherapy of 5% at 5 years. For regimens containing cisplatin, the overall hazard ratio was 0.87, or a 13% reduction in the risk of death, translating into an absolute benefit from chemotherapy of 5% at 5 years. This result was of borderline statistical significance ($P = 0.08$).

A number of randomized trials have examined the role of adjuvant chemotherapy in patients undergoing postoperative radiation for resected NSCLC (Table 37.16).[384–391] Investigators from the LCGS, Memorial Sloan Kettering, the Groupe d'Etude et de Traitement des Cancers Bronchiques, the U.S. Intergroup, and investigators from Germany did not detect

TABLE 37.15. Phase III trials of adjuvant chemotherapy in NSCLC.

Study	*N*	*Stage*	*Treatment*	*Five-year overall survival (%)*		*Statistical significance*
				Controls	*Treated*	
Feld et al.[372]	269	T1N1, T2N0	CAP vs. obs	58	54	NS
Holmes et al.[373]	141	T2N1, III	CAP vs. IP IT	15 months[a]	22 months[a]	NS
Figlin et al.[374]	188	II and III	CAP vs. obs	32.7 months[b]	32.7 months[b]	NS
Niiranen et al.[375]	110	T1–3N0	CAP vs. obs	63.7[c]	73.5[c]	NS
Waller et al.[376]	381	I–III	CDDP-based chemo vs. obs	NR	NR	HR = 1.00
Ohta et al.[377]	209	T3N0 and IIIA	CDDP + VND vs. obs	41	35	NS
Ichinose et al.[378]	119	IIIA (N2)	CDDP + VND vs. obs	35.2 months[a]	35.5 months[a]	NS
Wada et al.[379]	310	I–III	CDDP + VND + UFT vs. UFT vs. obs	49	64[d]	$P = 0.019$
Imaizumi[380]	309	I–III	CDDP + DOX + UFT vs. obs	58.1	61.8	NS
Wada et al.[381]	225	I and II	CDDP + VND + MMC + UFT vs. obs	71.1	76.8	NS
Tada et al.[382]	267	I–IIIA	UFT vs. obs (stage I) CDDP + VND + UFT vs. bs (stage II–IIIA)	57.6[e]	74.2[e]	$P = 0.045$
Kato et al.[383]	999	I adenocarcinoma	UFT vs. obs	85.4	87.9	$P = 0.036$

obs, observation; HR, hazard ratio; UFT, uracil-tegafur.

[a] Median survival, in months.

[b] Median survival in months, provided for study population as a whole.

[c] For resection less than pneumonectomy.

[d] UFT-only group.

[e] Overall survival at 8 years for patients with stage I disease.

TABLE 37.16. Phase III trials of adjuvant chemoradiation in NSCLC.

Study	N	Local recurrence rate (%)		Five-year overall survival (%)		Statistical significance
		RT alone	Chemo/RT	RT alone	Chemo/RT	
Lad et al.[386]	164	0.152[a]	0.093[a]	13 months[b]	20 months[b]	NS
Pisters et al.[387]	72	17	8	19 months[b]	16 months[b]	NS
Dautzenberg et al.[388]	267	26	34	19	18	NS
Keller et al.[389]	488	21	24	39	33	NS
Wolf et al.[390]	150	NR	NR	34 months[b]	34 months[b]	NS
Scagliotti et al.[391]	1,209	22	23	48 months[b]	55.2 months[b]	HR = 0.96[c]
Le Chevalier et al.[385]	1,867	NR	NR	40	45	$P < 0.03$

[a] Rate of local recurrence per person-years.
[b] Median survival in months.
[c] Hazard ratio for overall survival (95% CI, 0.79–1.12).

improvements in survival using cisplatin-based regimens in trials of adjuvant chemoradiation.[386–390]

The 1995 Non-small Cell Lung Cancer Collaborative Group meta-analysis examined seven trials randomizing patients to adjuvant chemoradiation versus radiation alone.[384] Radiation treatment doses ranged from 40 Gy in 10 fractions to 65 Gy in 33 fractions. They concluded that there was no benefit or adverse effects of adjuvant combined therapy for patients with resected NSCLC compared to postoperative radiotherapy alone.

Two large, recently completed international trials yielded conflicting results in terms of the efficacy of postoperative chemoradiation in patients with completely resected NSCLC. Results from the Adjuvant Lung Project Italy (ALPI)/EORTC study confirmed the lack of benefit in adding systemic cisplatin-based chemotherapy.[391] In this trial, 1,209 patients with stages I–IIIA NSCLC received postoperative radiotherapy (50–54 Gy over 5 to 6 weeks) at the investigator's discretion. As such, radiotherapy was planned in 4%, 60%, and 76% of stage I, II, and IIIA patients, respectively, and randomization was stratified accordingly. Patients were randomized to either three cycles of mitomycin, vindesine, and cisplatin adjuvant treatment or no chemotherapy. The study was designed to detect a 7% improvement in overall survival at 5 years, from 50% to 57% (or a 20% reduction in the relative risk of death). At over 5 years of follow-up, no statistically significant difference in progression-free or overall survival was detected between the two treatment arms. Comparison of the Kaplan–Meier curves for overall survival gave a hazard ratio of 0.96 (95% CI, 0.81–1.13; $P = 0.589$). This impact translated into an absolute increase in 5-year survival of 1%. There was an excess of early deaths (within 12 months after randomization) in the chemotherapy arm (90 patients), compared to the control arm (69 patients); this was attributable to cancer progression in 11 patients and to cardiopulmonary events in 7 patients. Rates of grade 4 neutropenia and nausea/vomiting for the patients receiving chemotherapy were 12% and 4%, respectively.

However, positive results were recently seen in the large randomized International Adjuvant Lung Trial (IALT) of adjuvant cisplatin-based chemotherapy.[385] Although patients were allowed to undergo postoperative radiotherapy at their physician's discretion, this study was primarily designed to assess the value of adjuvant chemotherapy in a large, heterogeneous sample of patients, and 1,867 patients were randomized in the late 1990s from 148 centers in 33 countries to observation or to undergo three or four cycles of cisplatin-based systemic treatment. The total dose of cisplatin was predetermined to be in the range of 300 to 400 mg/m^2. Most of the patients received etoposide as the second agent in the chemotherapy doublet (56%), while others received vinorelbine (27%), vinblastine (11%), or vindesine (6%). Patients were balanced in terms of pathologic stage, histology, and type of surgical procedure. At a median follow-up of 56 months, both disease-free and overall survival at 5 years was improved in patients treated with adjuvant chemotherapy (39.4% and 44.5% for the chemotherapy patients, and 34.3% and 40.4% for the control patients, respectively; P less than 0.03 for overall survival). No significant interaction between response to adjuvant chemotherapy was observed with respect to age, gender, performance status, type of surgery, pathologic stage, histology, cisplatin dose, choice of the second chemotherapy agent, and the addition of radiotherapy. Twenty-three percent of the chemotherapy-treated patients experienced at least one grade 4 toxicity, and the treatment-related mortality was 0.8%.

The authors of the IALT trial concluded that cisplatin-based adjuvant chemotherapy exerts a statistically significant positive impact on survival in resected patients, thereby potentially saving 7,000 lives worldwide annually. Why was the IALT trial positive in the face of so many prior negative studies of adjuvant chemotherapy? The IALT investigators were the first to design the statistical analyses of their outcomes to reflect the findings of the 1995 meta-analyses, in which an absolute survival advantage of 5% was seen with treatment. In contrast, earlier studies hypothesized a larger difference in the primary outcome of overall survival.[391] In addition, more than 70% of patients in the IALT trial received at least 240 mg/m^2 total of cisplatin during the course of their adjuvant treatment, a substantially higher dose intensity than had been delivered in most of the previous studies of postoperative chemotherapy.[372–374] Last, a lower percentage of patients in the ALPI/EORTC trial underwent pneumonectomy, in comparison to the IALT study (25% in ALPI/EORTC versus 35% in the IALT), possibly improving the survival of the control arm in the ALPI/EORTC sufficiently to mask a beneficial impact of chemotherapy, as was seen in the IALT.[385,391]

In conclusion, although the majority of trials of adjuvant therapy in resected NSCLC have been negative, recently published evidence points to the possible efficacy of UFT, particularly in early-stage disease, and cisplatin-based chemotherapy, especially when administered at doses of at least 240 mg/m^2.

Management of Locally Advanced Stage IIIB

The role of radiation therapy (RT) in management of patients with unresectable locally advanced NSCLC became accepted when the VA study in the late 1960s showed a survival benefit at 1 year (18.2% versus 13.9%) for those patients who received 35 Gy in 5 weeks of RT versus no RT.[392] This study's conclusions were confounded by inadequate dose of RT, inadequate techniques, and inclusion of patients with small cell histology. The role of RT was further refined by a randomized study by the Radiation Therapy Oncology Group (RTOG 73-01), which showed that response rate improved with higher dose of RT (60 Gy versus 40 and 50 Gy) and led to improved local tumor control and 3-year survival. Furthermore, inclusion of a split-course arm revealed that the standard fractionation led to a better outcome.[393] RR was 51% with 40 Gy, 66% with 50 Gy, and 61% with 60 Gy. Local control was inversely proportional to dose received: 77% at 3 years for the 60-Gy arm, 58% for the 50-Gy arm, and 48% for those treated with 40 Gy ($P = 0.02$).[393] However, although these trials indicate a role for high-dose thoracic RT in patients with NSCLC, the overall survival with this modality alone still left much to be desired [2-year overall survival (OS), 19%].[394] Meanwhile, the issue of whether thoracic RT was indicated as a single modality despite these studies continued to be a subject of debate. In the 1980s, a randomized trial designed to readdress this issue was reported by Johnson et al.[395] This trial randomized 319 patients to three arms: experimental chemotherapy (vindesine) arm, RT-alone arm (60 Gy/6 weeks), and vindesine and thoracic RT arm. The overall response rate was superior in the RT arms: 30% (RT alone), 34% (RT + chemo), and 10% (chemo alone) (P less than 0.001). However, there was no significant difference in median and overall survival. Median survival for vindesine arm was 10.1 months, for RT alone was 8.6 months, and 9.4 months for those receiving RT + vindesine ($P = 0.58$). It is important to note that 37% (36/98) of the vindesine-alone arm crossed over to the RT arm, and of these, 22% had response. Conversely, 25 patients crossed over to the vindesine arm from the RT arm, and of these patients, the response rate was 4%. The authors concluded that immediate radiation may not confer survival advantage to patients with locally advanced (LA) NSCLC, despite a statistically significant improvement in response rate. However, in retrospect, in view of our current knowledge that combined modality therapy improves survival compared to RT alone, and with up to one-third of the chemo-alone arm crossing over to RT in this study, it is possible that this arm, in reality, was partially a sequential chemo-RT arm. Regardless of the controversies, these and other studies clearly pointed to a need for improvement in the therapy of LA NSCLC patients.

Sequential Combined Modality Therapy (CMT) Defined for Locally Advanced NSCLC

Negative Studies

In the 1980s, several important Phase III studies conducted at various countries around the world helped to determine the role of combined modality therapy (CMT) for inoperable locally advanced NSCLC patients. Chemotherapy in these studies was administered mostly before (induction) or after (consolidation) the administration of thoracic RT.

The trial from Finland randomizing 238 patients to RT versus CMT, revealed no statistically significant difference in local and distant control and overall survival (Table 37.17).[396] In retrospect, their thoracic RT regimen was suboptimal in

TABLE 37.17. Sequential combined modality therapy (CMT) trials in the 1980s.

Study	*N*	*Median survival*	*Two-year survival*	*P*
Finnish Trial[396]				
CAP (induction, mid, consolidation) + split course RT 55 Gy/2.5–3 Gy/fx	119	11 months	19%	
RT alone	119	10.3 months	17%	P = ns
Italian Trial (Trovo et al.[397])				
RT 45 Gy/15 fx	62	11.74 months		
RT + CAMP × 12 cycles	49	10.03 months		P = ns
NCCTG (Morton et al.[398])				
MACC × 2 induction/consolidation + RT 60-Gy conventional fx	56	10.4 months	21%	
RT 60 Gy/2 Gy/fx	58	10.3 months	16%	$P = 0.69$
CALGB (Dillman et al.[399])				
PV × 2 cycles induction + RT 60 Gy/2 Gy/fx	78	13.7 months	26%	
RT alone	77	9.6 months	13%	$P = 0.012$
French Trial (Le Chevalier et al.[400]); included follow-up that showed statistical significance				
VCPC × 2 cycles + RT 65 Gy/26 fx	176	12	21%	
RT alone	177	10	14%	$P < 0.02$
Italian trial (Crino et al.[543])				
PE × 3 cycles + RT 56 Gy	33	14 months	30%	
RT alone	33	11 months	14%	$P = 0.056$

terms of total dose (55 Gy), fractionation (split course with 3-week break after 2 weeks, 30 Gy), nonstandard fractionations used [2.5 Gy/fraction (fx), 3 Gy/fx, and 4.5 Gy/fx], and technique (posterior cord block used during second course of RT). Therefore, the true value of combined modality was difficult to assess in this setting.

A group from Italy also published reports on CMT versus RT alone for locally advanced NSCLC.[397] In this study, chemotherapy was administered 4 weeks after completion of RT (sequential/consolidation) rather than as an induction phase. RT dose was 45 Gy in 15 fractions (fx) delivered in 3 weeks, which in retrospect is also a suboptimal dose; 111 patients were randomized to RT alone (n = 62) or RT + chemotherapy (n = 49). Response rate was 56.4% for RT alone versus 38.8% for RT + chemotherapy, which was not statistically significant (P = 0.9). Time to progression was 5.93 months for RT versus 7.02 months for RT/chemo (P = ns). Important to note was also the high cross-over rate: patients progressing on RT alone were allowed to be started on CAMP, and of the 54 patients who progressed in the RT-alone arm, 29 patients received CAMP. Median survival was 11.74 months in the RT arm versus 10.03 months in the RT/CAMP arm; however, there was a high cross-over rate (47%) in the RT arm, which makes this study difficult to analyze.

The North Central Cancer Treatment Group (NCCTG) also reported on their Phase III randomized study, which was also a negative trial for CMT.[398] Median survival times were equivalent between the chemo/RT arm versus the RT-alone arm (317 days versus 313 days, respectively), and 2-year survival showed a trend toward improved survival with CMT (16% versus 21%), but failed to reach statistical significance, and did not hold true on long-term follow-up at 5 years (7% for RT alone versus 5% for CMT). Unlike the Finnish study, their RT regimen was based on the RTOG 73-01 regimen, and patients received 60 Gy over 6 weeks. Furthermore, in both the Finnish and the NCCTG studies, patients with poor prognostic factors (poor performance status, liberal weight loss criteria, and presence of supraclavicular disease) were enrolled in the trials, which may have led to worse outcome.

Positive Studies

Meanwhile, two important randomized Phase III studies conducted by CALGB (Dillman et al.[399]) and the French group (Le Chevalier et al.[400]) both showed statistically significant improvement in OS with CMT (see Table 37.17).

In an attempt to clarify the issue of CMT versus RT alone, several groups performed meta-analysis and reported improvement of survival, albeit modestly so, favoring addition of chemotherapy to thoracic RT.[384,401,402] Marino et al. performed meta-analysis on 14 randomized trials from 1980–1994, comprising a total of 1,887 patients.[401] As expected, the studies involved used a variety of radiation regimen and a variety of chemotherapy regimen (10 of 14 were platinum based). This analysis reported a reduction in mortality of 18% at 2 years for the non-cisplatinum-based group, and 30% for the cisplatinum-based group. However, this improvement did not persist at 3 and 5 years.

Similarly, the Non-Small Cell Lung Cancer Collaborative Group also performed a meta-analysis, which was published in the *British Medical Journal* in 1995.[384] This was a larger meta-analysis comparing four treatment modalities including surgery versus surgery plus chemotherapy, and surgery plus radiotherapy with or without chemotherapy for early-stage disease, and RT versus RT + chemotherapy for locally advanced NSCLC. For the scope of this review, we briefly summarize their findings for unresectable locally advanced NSCLC. Altogether, data from 52 trials with 9,387 patients were used for analysis. For locally advanced NSCLC, data from 22 trials with 3,033 patients were available with varying CT regimens and various RT regimens. Results showed significant benefit of chemotherapy with a hazard ratio of 0.9 (P = 0.006), or a 10% reduction of risk of death, corresponding to a 2% benefit at 5 years (3% at 2 years). Cisplatin-based chemotherapy once again showed strongest benefit with a hazard ratio of 0.87 (P = 0.005), or a 13% reduction in risk of death, which equals a 4% benefit at 2 years and 2% at 5 years.

Finally, a similar meta-analysis by Pritchard et al. was published the next year in the *Annals of Internal Medicine*.[402] The main difference was that this group's analysis included trials by Sause and Jeremic and excluded trials by Wils and Crino.[402] They also had more updated data, as it was analyzed later, and the trials included were from 1987 to 1995. The main exclusion criteria difference was that they did not include any studies that have only been presented in abstract form or were in preliminary publications only. Fourteen studies were analyzed for total of 2,589 patients. In their analysis, they reported a reduction in risk of death up to 3 years using combined modality therapy of 10% to 20%. Mean gain in life expectancy was calculated to be approximately 2 months at the end of 3 years. Interestingly, cisplatin-based sequential chemotherapy had a RR of 0.77 (CI, 0.68–0.87), compared to 0.83 (CI, 0.77–0.9) for any chemotherapy. Median survival was improved from 10.3 months to 12.0 months with the addition of any chemotherapy.

As with all meta-analyses, one must be wary of the publication biases (i.e., negative trials tend not to be reported), but as the author interestingly points out in Pritchard's paper, 10 of 14 were initially published as negative trials. Furthermore, different agents were used for chemotherapy, different radiation regimens were also used, and sequencing of chemotherapy was not uniform in all studies. However, despite all these potentially confounding issues, these studies pointed toward a role for chemoradiation therapy. If anything, the meta-analysis may have underestimated the potential benefit of combined modality therapy in an appropriately selected patient population.

Therefore, these pivotal trials and the follow-up meta-analysis led to a new paradigm for therapy of unresectable NSCLC: that the addition of appropriate chemotherapy (particularly cisplatinum based) to the optimal RT regimen would improve survival. These studies led the way to investigation of some very important issues that pertain to optimizing combined modality therapy that include questions aimed at defining the optimal sequencing of the chemotherapy with radiation, the optimal agent or agents to be used with radiation, and the optimal dose and fractionation of RT that can be safely delivered with chemotherapy.

Concurrent Administration of Chemotherapy with RT for Locally Advanced NSCLC

As the trials in the 1980s indicated that addition of chemotherapy appears to confer significant survival benefit, likely secondary to decrease in metastasis rate, as alluded to by several studies,[400,401] sequential chemo/RT became the standard of care. However, local control was not always shown to be improved by this approach. Importance of local control in improving survival was first indicated by previous work by Perez et al.[393] This finding was further strengthened by the EORTC trial, which was the first randomized Phase III study comparing concurrent chemo/RT versus RT alone.[105] This study randomized 331 patients to three treatment arms: RT alone, RT + weekly cisplatin (30 mg/m^2), and RT + daily cisplatin (6 mg/m^2) during thoracic RT. RT was administered in split-course regimen: 3 Gy × 10 daily fractions, followed by 3 weeks of break, followed by 2 more weeks of 2.5 Gy × 10 fractions for a total of 55 Gy. Significant survival advantage and disease-free survival (DFS) were noted for patients treated with cisplatin, despite a split-course RT regimen. Local recurrence-free survival was also significantly improved with the addition of cisplatin. Interestingly, with the split-course regimen, the typical acute and late toxicities, including esophagitis and delayed lung injury (pneumonitis, fibrosis, and respiratory symptoms), were not significantly worsened by the addition of concurrent cisplatin.

The major trials addressing the efficacy of concurrent administration of chemotherapeutic agents with thoracic RT are outlined in Table 37.18 in chronologic order. The first reported trial that specifically compared head to head concurrent versus sequential chemo/RT was reported by the West Japan Lung Cancer Group.[403] This was a Phase III study randomizing 314 patients to concurrent versus sequential chemotherapy with RT. In the sequential arm, RT was delivered to 56 Gy and 2 Gy/fx without a break. Statistically significant improvement in response rate was achieved (84% versus 66.4%; $P = 0.002$). Overall median survival was 16.5 months versus 13.3 months ($P = 0.04$) favoring the concurrent arm, with 5-year OS at 15.8% versus 8.9%. On further analysis, local control was found to be directly impacted by the use of the concurrent approach, which found survival without local relapse was 30 months versus 11 months ($P = 0.0221$), which persisted on long-term follow-up of 5 years. Time to distant failure was not statistically different between the two arms ($P = 0.8$; log rank test), suggesting that local control was an important determinant of improved survival. Toxicity profile, in particular grade 3+ esophagitis, was not worse in the concurrent arm (4% concurrent versus 3% sequential), likely because of the split-course regimen employed in this study. This was the first published report of improvement of survival with concurrent chemoRT versus sequential chemoRT.

The GLOT-GFPC NPC 95-01 study was reported in ASCO 2001 by Pierre et al.[404] This randomized, multicenter, Phase III trial from France also addressed the issue of sequential versus concurrent administration of chemo/RT: 212 patients were randomized to sequential versus concurrent arms. Median survival was 13.8 months in the sequential and 15 months in the concurrent arm ($P = 0.41$), which was a trend for the concurrent arm. Two-year OS was 23% in the sequential and 35% in the concurrent arm, also indicating a trend toward increased survival for the concurrent regimen.

TABLE 37.18. Schema of major concurrent versus sequential CMT to date.

Trial	*Schema*	*Median survival*	*Grade 3+ esophagitis (acute)*
West Japan LC Group[403]	Sequential: MVP × 2 → Conventional RT Day 50 Concurrent: MVP × 2/Split course RT Day 1	13.3 months 16.5 months $P = 0.04$	3% 4%
RTOG 9410[409]	Sequential: Vinb/CisP × 2 → Stn RT day 50 Conc standard RT: Vinb/CisP × 2/Stn RT day 1 Conc hyperfractionated RT: CisP/Eto × 2/BID RT day 1	14.6 months 17 months ($P = 0.046$ vs. sequential) 15.2 months	4% 25% 46%
French Trial[404]	Sequential: CisP/Nav → Stn RT day 50 Concurrent: CisP/Etop × 2/RT → CisP/Etop	13.8 months 15 months $P = 0.41$	0% 26.1%
Czech Trial[405]	Sequential: Cisp/Nav × 4 → RT Concurrent: Cisp/Nav/RT → Cisp/Nav	13 months 20.2 months $P = 0.0216$	4.2% 17.6%
LAMP[406,407]	Sequential: Paclitaxel/Carbo → RT Induction → Conc: Paclitaxel/Carbo → p/c/RT Conc. → Consolidation: p/c/RT → Paclitaxel/Carbo	13 months 12.8 months 16.1 months P = ns	4% 20% 28%
BROCAT[408]	Sequential: Paclitaxel/Carbo × 2 → RT alone Concurrent: Paclitaxel/Carbo × 2 → weekly paclitaxel/RT	14.6 months 19.2 months	7.6% 15.8%

In ASCO 2002, two important trials addressing this same issue were highlighted. One study was presented by Zatloukal et al., for the Czech Lung Cancer Group.[405] This study employed vinorelbine and cisplatin, and 102 patients were enrolled and randomized to the two arms. Median survival time was 619 days in the concurrent arm and 396 days in the sequential arm ($P = 0.0216$). Time to progression was 366 days in the concurrent arm, and 288 days in the sequential arm ($P = 0.0506$). The concurrent arm had significantly higher grade 3/4 toxicities, including leukopenia (52.9% versus 18.8%), neutropenia (64.7% versus 39.6%), and esophagitis (17.6% versus 4.2%). Pulmonary toxicity was equivalent (3.9 % versus 2.1%) between the concurrent and sequential arms.

The locally advanced multimodality protocol (LAMP) trial is a randomized Phase II study whose preliminary results have been presented at ASCO 2001 and 2002.[406,407] One of the unique aspects of this trial was its liberal weight loss criterion, up to 10% before enrollment (most recent studies require less than 5% weight loss to be eligible). Three arms were as follows: arm 1 was a sequential arm where patients were administered two cycles of paclitaxel with carboplatin, followed by daily RT to 63 Gy. The second arm was the induction/concurrent arm, where patients were given induction chemo, as in arm 1, followed by weekly paclitaxel and carboplatin with RT for 7 weeks, also to 63 Gy. Finally, arm 3 consisted of a concurrent/consolidation mode in which patients were treated with concurrent RT as in arm 2, but followed by adjuvant chemo for two cycles (same as induction regimen). When all patients were considered, median survival was 13 months for sequential, 12.8 months for induction/concurrent, and 16.1 months for concurrent/adjuvant arm. When a subset analysis of patients with better weight criteria was conducted, the median survival and 2-year OS were 13 months/28%, 14.4 months/24%, and 17.2 months/35% for arms 1, 2, and 3 respectively. Both the total and subset analyses showed a trend toward the concurrent/consolidation arm but did not reach statistical significance on short-term follow-up. Toxicity profile showed grade 3/4 esophagitis to be 4%, 20%, and 28% on arms 1 to 3, respectively. The interesting result from this study was that delay of concurrent chemo/RT with induction chemotherapy appeared to have a negative impact on outcome; whether this was due to underpowering of this study ($n = 69$) or to the true impact of delaying initiation of concurrent chemo/RT is difficult to assess with certainty but is worth further investigation.

Most recently, in ASCO 2003, two trials were presented that gave further credence to concurrent chemo RT as the modality of choice over sequential CMT. One study was a long-term mature update of the RTOG 9410, which was first presented in ASCO in 2000. The other was a study from Germany reported by Huber for the BROCAT group.[408]

The BROCAT group schema involved initiation with two cycles of induction paclitaxel and carboplatin chemotherapy for 3 weeks.[408] After the induction, patients were analyzed, and if patients did not have progressive disease, they were randomized to the sequential arm (RT alone to 60 Gy), or the concurrent arm (weekly paclitaxel + RT as in sequential arm); 303 patients enrolled, and 262 patients were able to complete the induction chemotherapy. Median survival time was 14.6 months for sequential versus 19.2 months for concurrent arm. With this short follow-up, however, statistical significance was not reached.

RTOG 9410 is a Phase III randomized three-arm study ($n = 610$) that compared sequential chemotherapy followed by RT versus concurrent administration of hyperfractionated (69.9 Gy bid in 1.2 Gy/fx) or daily RT and chemotherapy.[409] Chemotherapeutic agents used were cisplatin and vinblastine; when given sequentially, two cycles were administered before RT (start on day 50), whereas in the concurrent arms, RT began on day 1 with the chemotherapy. In ASCO 2003, the long-term results of the trial were reported, with median survival for the sequential arm being 14.6 months, 17 months for the concurrent qd arm, and 15.2 months for the concurrent bid arm. This survival benefit was maintained on long-term follow-up with 4-year OS for the sequential arm being 12%, versus 21% for the concurrent qd arm and 17% for the concurrent bid arm. The difference between the sequential and concurrent qd arms reached a statistically significant difference with a P value of 0.046. There were significant acute toxicity issues with the concurrent and hyperfractionated arms. The concurrent arm had 25% grade 3 or 4 esophagitis and the hyperfractionated arm had 46% grade 3 or 4 esophagitis, whereas the sequential arm had 4% grade 3 or 4 esophagitis. There was no significant difference in acute grade 3 or 4 lung toxicity (within 90 days) of RT initiation, which was approximately 9% for the sequential arm, versus 4% for the concurrent arm and 4% for the hyperfractionated arm. There was no significant difference in late toxicities including esophagitis and pneumonitis.[409]

Optimal Sequencing for Combined Modality Therapy: Summary of Major Trials

In summary, when all these trials are evaluated together, a total of 709 patients were treated with one of the foregoing concurrent regimens and 716 on the sequential arm. Median survival of these studies summed together show a difference of 3 months: 17 months versus concurrent, and 14 months for sequential arms (P less than 0.05 Kruskal–Wallis test). Furthermore, these trials appear to validate the earlier sequential trials of the 1980s in that addition of chemotherapy appears to improve median survival. The most impressive and convincing data that are now beginning to emerge are that the benefits conferred by the concurrent regimen appear to be durable on long-term follow-up. Long-term follow-up of two important trials, WJLCG and RTOG 9410,[403,409] both show a significant long-term survival advantage to the concurrent arm. Similar data were seen on long-term follow-up of three sequential Phase II studies of concurrent chemo/RT by Choy et al., as reported in ASCO 2003.[410]

Toxicity of Concurrent Chemo/RT

Although the benefit of concurrent chemoRT appears to improve survival outcome in patients with LA NSCLC, the question of the cost or risks of this modality remained. The most apparent cost, however, is that of increased acute toxicities, mainly esophagitis and pneumonitis. A review of the data from multiple RTOG concurrent chemoRT trials (90-15, 91-06, 92-04, and 94-10), all involving cisplatin given concurrently with standard 60 Gy or hyperfractionated 69.6 Gy bid RT, was performed (personal communication, Werner et al.). Analysis included a total of 585 patients. Acute esophagitis of grade 3 or higher occurred in 37% of these patients, peaking and plateauing by 2 months after initiation of therapy.

When a similar analysis was performed to evaluate grade 3 or 4 esophagitis rates, the results showed that a 19.5% esophagitis rate was observed in the concurrent arm versus 4% in the sequential arm. Therefore, it appears that the concurrent arm does lead to superior survival at the expense of increased acute esophageal toxicity.

Similar to the foregoing analysis, Werner-Wasik et al. performed analysis on the same 585 patients from the various RTOG trials looking at late pneumonitis incidence.[411] Incidence of late pneumonitis of grade 3 or higher toxicity occurred in 20% of these patients. Time course of incidence showed that this could occur as late as 18 months after therapy, with 50% of these grade 3 or higher pneumonitis patients having symptoms at 6 months posttherapy. A majority of patients had pneumonitis occur between 6 and 12 months posttherapy.

In the RTOG 9410 trial, there appears to be no difference in the rate of pneumonitis in the three arms on long-term follow-up. For example, pneumonitis rate (grade 3 or 4) was 14% in the sequential arm, 12% in the concurrent arm, and 16% in the hyperfractionated arm (personal communications). Furthermore, although there was increased esophagitis acutely in the concurrent and the hyperfractionated arms as noted above, this appears to resolve on long-term follow-up, and the rate of esophagitis among the three arms became equivalent at 0.5%, 2.6%, and 4% for the sequential, concurrent, and hyperfractionated arms, respectively. It appears that the major disadvantage of concurrent arm, which is esophagitis, is not a sustained toxicity, and without significant evidence for undue late toxicity with this regimen, the survival advantage should convince us that concurrent strategy is superior to the sequential combined modality therapy. In lieu of a further confirmatory, larger randomized trial, the next important analysis would be to perform a meta-analysis of all studies comparing sequential versus concurrent therapy to improve the power to detect a significant difference in outcome and toxicities between these two approaches.

A variety of strategies for decreasing the toxicity of chemoRT treatment has been suggested. These include improvements in technology of RT delivery and utilization of pharmacocytoprotective strategies to decrease normal tissue toxicity. Technical innovations include usage of intensity modulated radiation therapy (IMRT) or 3-D conformal planning strategies, novel fractionation schemes, improved functional imaging to deliver therapy to a smaller target volume, and new strategies for RT delivery (i.e., determining for which patients mediastinal nodes could be omitted to decrease target volume). The more biologic approach includes suggestions of usage of agents such as keratinizing growth factor, tumor necrosis factor- beta (TGF-β, melatonin, glutamine, gene therapy (intratumoral injection of manganese superoxide dismutase plasmid/liposome, SOD2-PL), and use of amifostine, an organic thiophosphate compound that has been shown to protect normal tissue selectively against both radiation and chemotherapeutic agents.

Delivery of Radiotherapy: Hyperfractionation

Another brewing question in the field of treatment of unresectable NSCLC was regarding how RT should be administered. As previously mentioned, pioneering works by Perez et al. helped to clearly establish the appropriate dose and helped to establish that a split-course regimen was not as efficacious as the conventional continuous course RT. Investigation into hyperfractionated regimen dates back to the 1970s when RTOG 77-04 indicated that in treatment of squamous cell carcinoma of upper respiratory tract and esophagus, 1.5 Gy bid produced severe mucositis requiring treatment interruptions, where as with 1.25 Gy/fx bid, therapy could be carried to 60 Gy.

RTOG 81-08 was a feasibility study that helped to establish that 1.2 Gy bid fx to 69.6 Gy could be administered without significant acute toxicities in NSCLC.[412] RTOG 83-11 was performed as a randomized dose-escalation Phase I/II trial of hyperfractionated RT with total doses ranging from 60 to 79.2 Gy for stage III NSCLC patients.[413] The study had five arms, each involving 1.2 Gy bid to total doses of 60.0, 64.8, 69.6, 74.4, and 79.2 Gy. Their conclusion was that equal survival benefit was seen in the 69.6-Gy and above arms (median survival, 10 months versus 8.7 months versus 10.5 months for the 69.6-Gy, 74.4-Gy, and 79.2-Gy arms, respectively). However, significantly higher life-threatening pneumonitis occurred in the 79.2-Gy arm versus the 69.6-Gy arm (8.1% versus 5.7%). Median survival at 69.6 Gy was superior to the lower doses of 60 and 64.8 Gy, which was even more markedly pronounced when a subset of patients with the CALGB 84-33 good prognosis criteria were evaluated (median survival, 13 months in the 69.6-Gy arm versus 10 and 7.8 months for 60- and 64.8-Gy arms, respectively; $P = 0.07$). Furthermore, there was a dose–survival relationship in the CALGB group (i.e., dose received versus survival), with patients receiving 69.6 Gy surviving longer than those who received less [median survival for 69.6 Gy (±2.4 Gy) dose received was 13.7 months versus those who received 64.8 Gy (±2.4 Gy) was 12.7 months, and those who received 60 Gy (±2.4 Gy) was 8.9 months ($P = 0.02$)]. These results led to a Phase III trial (RTOG 88–08) investigating the role of hyperfractionated RT in this population of patients. The major hyperfractionation trials are listed and summarized in Table 37.19.

Negative Hyperfractionation Trials

A Phase III trial comparing (1) RT alone, (2) induction chemotherapy followed by RT, or (3) hyperfractionated RT (1.2 Gy bid to 69.6 Gy) was conducted by the U.S. intergroup.[414] In this trial, 452 patients were enrolled and eligible, with 149, 151, and 152 patients, respectively, in arms 1 to 3. Initial results showed median survival of 11.4 months, 13.8 months ($P = 0.03$ for chemoRT versus RT alone), and 12.3 months for arms 1 to 3 respectively, which validated the Dillman data.[399] Toxicity profile was reported as being acceptable, with similar grade 3 or 4 nonheme toxicity profile for the three patient groups who were followed to 18 months. Grade 4 toxicity related to RT was reported in 4 patients in the hyperfractionated arm, versus 1 on the standard and sequential arm; 2/4 grade 4 toxicity on the hyperfractionated arm was esophagitis. Updated reports published in 2000 reported similar findings with median survival of 11.4 months, 13.2 months, and 12 months, respectively, in arms 1 to 3.[415] The 5-year survival rates were 5%, 8%, and 6%, once again showing mild benefit to the sequential arm, but not in the hyperfractionated arm. There was an indication that in

TABLE 37.19. Comparison of hyperfractionated (tid, bid) versus conventional (qd) RT either with or without concurrent chemotherapy.

Study	*Median survival*	*Three-year OS*	*Five year OS*	*P value*	*Acute esophagitis (grade 3 or 4)*
RTOG 8808[415]					
Daily RT (no chemo)	11.4 months	9%	5%		Not available
BID RT	12 months	14%	6%	P = ns	Not available
RTOG 9410[416]		2-year OS	4-year OS		
Concurrent chemo + daily RT	17 months	35%	21%		25%
Concurrent chemo + bid RT	15.2 months	34%	17%	P = ns	46%
CHART[418,419]		2-year OS	4-year OS		
Daily RT	13 months	21%	12%		3%
TID RT	16.5 months	30%	7%	P = 0.008	19%
HART[420]					
Induction chemo + conventional RT	13.7 months	33%			16%
Induction chemo + tid RT	22.2 months	48%		P = NS	25%

squamous cell cancer histology, the hyperfractionated arm had a durable response of 5-year survival of 9% compared to 2% in the other two arms (P = ns).[414,415] However, as a whole, this was a negative trial for the hyperfractionated regimen, contrary to what was indicated by the RTOG 83–11 study. It did prove to be a confirmatory trial for the sequential arm with very similar median survival results as the Dillman study.

RTOG 94–10 also had a hyperfractionated arm as previously noted. The difference was that, in this study, chemotherapy was administered concurrently with the hyperfractionated regimen as described above, and as was the case in RTOG 88-08, the hyperfractionated arm failed to provide survival advantage over the concurrent or the sequential arm[416] (see Table 37.19). It is also quite clear that the acute toxicity was significantly higher in the hyperfractionated arm. Therefore, hyperfractionation using 1.2 Gy bid to 69.6 Gy does not appear to be a reasonable therapeutic option for this group of patients. However, this does not necessarily imply that hyperfractionation is not a good strategy in this setting.

Positive Hyperfractionated Trials

Continuous, Hyperfractionated, Accelerated Radiotherapy (CHART)

CHART was introduced in the mid-1980s and has a strong biologic rationale.[417] The goal for CHART is twofold: (1) to attempt to improve tumor control of cancer cells, which can proliferate and repopulate rapidly, by using more-frequent fractions, and (2) to minimize long-term normal tissue morbidity by using smaller fractions.[417] CHART employs a 1.5-Gy fx three times a day in 12 consecutive days. Saunders et al. reported on their trial, which randomized 563 patients to CHART (n = 338) versus conventional RT (n = 225) which was administered to 60 Gy in 30 daily fractions. Promising survival advantage with CHART, particularly in patients with SCCA histology, was demonstrated on short-term follow-up.[418] Results from long-term follow-up confirmed a significant reduction in death, with 2-year survival being 30% for CHART and 20% for the conventional arm (P = 0.008). This benefit was extended at 5 years, with OS being 12% for CHART and 7% for standard RT. There was also a 21% reduction in risk of local progression (P = 0.033). This benefit was more pronounced for patients with SCCA histology in terms of survival (20% versus 33%), and improvement in local control was substantial and statistically significant in this group.[419] Interestingly, there was also a significant 25% reduction in relative risk of metastasis (P = 0.043) and 27% reduction in risk of local progression (P = 0.0012) in the SCCA histology. Considering no chemotherapy was used in these patients, one could potentially argue that in the squamous histology, improvement of local control may be critically linked to inhibition of further metastatic progression. As one would expect, the rate of acute toxicity with CHART was higher than that of conventional, with the esophagitis rate being 19% in CHART versus 3% in the conventional arm (see Table 37.19). The late complications were not significantly different between the two groups, however. Interesting to note was that 81% of patients in the CHART trial were of squamous histology, and this trial included patients with stage IA, IB, and II disease (36% of enrolled patients), which may explain the significantly higher survival data even with conventional RT alone compared to historical controls. Is it also possible that CHART may have been more effective in patients with early-stage disease for whom ultimate local control has been the primary mode of therapy (i.e., surgery)? Despite these and other potential issues, the data from CHART are encouraging and worthy of further pursuit.

Hyperfractionated Accelerated Radiotherapy (HART)

Therefore, based on this, ECOG set forth to clarify this issue with a randomized Phase III multiinstitutional trial comparing standard thoracic RT to hyperfractionated accelerated radiotherapy (HART) (Table 37.19). The results of ECOG 2597 were recently presented at ASCO 2003.[420] They reported that

119 eligible patients were randomized to either standard RT or HART following two cycles of induction chemotherapy consisting of carboplatin (AUC = 6) and paclitaxel (225 mg/m^2) on day 1 of each 3-week cycle. The HART regimen was similar to CHART, consisting of 1.5 Gy tid over 2.5 weeks to a total of 57.6 Gy (no weekends). Standard RT involved 64 Gy in 2 Gy/day fractions. Only stage III patients were enrolled. The study was closed prematurely due to poor accrual. The results, nevertheless, are provocative. Median survival time for conventional RT is similar to historical control at 13.7 months. The HART regimen, meanwhile, conferred a trend toward survival benefit, with median survival at 22.2 months, and the 2-year survival was 33% for conventional and 48% for HART ($P = 0.20$). Grade 3 or 4 esophagitis was higher for the HART (14 patients, 25%) arm than the conventional arm (9 patients, 16%).

Role of Prophylactic Cranial Irradiation in Locally Advanced NSCLC

Chemotherapy combined with thoracic radiotherapy improves survival for patients with locally advanced NSCLC,[384,404,421] but the systemic relapse, including brain metastasis, remains a major problem (Table 37.20). Central nervous system (CNS) metastasis is a common and devastating problem for patients with NSCLC with reported incidence up to 54%.[100,422–430] The median survival of patients diagnosed with brain metastasis in NSCLC is less than a year.[431–433] Gaspar and colleagues reported a retrospective review of the SWOG database of stage IIIA/B NSCLC patients who underwent combined modality therapy on four SWOG protocols (S8805, S9019, S9416, and S9504).[434] There were a total of 422 patients enrolled on the SWOG trials, and 20% of the patients experienced isolated brain metastasis after primary therapy; 46% of the patients who had brain as the site of first relapse developed brain metastasis within 16 weeks of completion of therapy. The Radiation Therapy Oncology Group (RTOG) also showed that NSCLC patients with locally advanced disease with longest survival are at significant risk for developing CNS metastases.[435,436] The improvement in the treatment of locally advanced NSCLC with combination chemotherapy, radiotherapy, and surgery has shown that CNS metastases remains a major site of relapse with up to 33% of patients experiencing CNS as the first site of metastasis.[423,437] Similarly, the Lung Cancer Study Group (LCSG) reported that 21% of patients developed brain metastasis after undergoing neoadjuvant chemoradiotherapy followed by surgery for stage III NSCLC.[438] Martini et al. also reported that 28.5% of patients developed isolated brain metastasis after undergoing chemotherapy (cisplatin, vindesine or vinblastine, and mitomycin) followed by surgery.[439]

Three published prospective randomized trials investigated the role of prophylactic cranial irradiation (PCI) in patients with NSCLC. One of the early studies was from the Veterans Administration Lung Group (VALG) reported by Cox and colleagues in 1981.[425] The study reported the results of treatment for 281 inoperable NSCLC patients enrolled between 1975 and 1978. The treatment consisted of thoracic radiotherapy alone with dose up to 50 Gy in 25 daily fractions with or without PCI (20 Gy in 10 fractions); 6% of patients (7/136) who received PCI relapsed in the brain compared to 13% (16/145) of patients who did not receive PCI ($P = 0.38$). The reduction in brain relapse was not significant for squamous cell histology and addition of PCI did not alter the median survival of patients in the study. Umsawasdi and colleagues from the M.D. Anderson Cancer Center reported the results of a randomized trial testing the role of PCI in 1984.[427] The study included 100 patients with locally advanced NSCLC who were clinically free of lung cancer after combined modality therapy. Patients received two cycles of induction chemotherapy (cyclophasphamide, adriamycin, cisplatin) followed by thoracic radiotherapy administered concurrently with the same chemotherapy. Patients in the PCI group received 3,000 cGy in 10 daily fractions to the whole brain. PCI reduced the incidence of brain metastasis dramatically from 27% to 4% ($P = 0.002$). However, no survival benefit was seen with PCI because of the negative impact of frequent extracranial relapses. Finally, RTOG conducted a study that investigated the role of PCI in 187 patients with unresectable or inoperable adenocarcinoma or large cell carcinoma of the lung. Russell and colleagues reported the results of the randomized study that incorporated thoracic radiotherapy with or without PCI (30 Gy/10 daily fractions).[426] The dose to the chest was 60 Gy in 30 treatments for patients without prior surgery and 50 Gy in 25 treatments for those who had prior thoracotomy. Eighteen patients (19%) developed brain metastasis without PCI and 8 patients (9%) with PCI developed brain metastasis ($P = 0.10$). There was no survival difference seen due to the significant extracranial systemic (81%) and thoracic (61%) relapses (see Table 37.20).

Unresectable Locally Advanced NSCLC: Decades of Progress

Despite all the controversies that may persist in the field of locally advanced NSCLC therapy, the advancement of this field in the past 20 years has been substantial and noteworthy. The median survival, using standard of care therapy in the 1980s, was less than 10 months. In the 1980s, with the advent of sequential chemotherapy with improved RT techniques and conventional dosing, the survival was improved to the order of 14 months. Currently, utilizing concurrent

TABLE 37.20. Prophylactic cranial irradiation (PCI) for NSCLC: randomized trials.

			Median survival		*Brain metastasis*	
Study	*N*	*PCI dose (dose/fraction)*	*+PCI*	*–PCI*	*+PCI*	*–PCI*
VALG[425]	281	20 Gy/10	NA	NA	6%	13%
RTOG[426]	187	30 Gy/10	8.4	8.1	9%	19%
M.D. Anderson[427]	97	30 Gy/10	8.4	NA	4%	NA

VALG, Veterans Administration Lung Group; RTOG, Radiation Therapy Oncology Group.

chemoRT or CHART or sequential chemo-HART regimens, one can expect that patients with unresectable LA NSCLC would have median survival of the order of 17 to 18 months. Between 15% and 20% of patients with this disease may now expect to have survival of the order of 4 to 6 years (or more; longer follow-up not yet available) as seen in the WJLG, RTOG 9410, and Lun-27/56/63 studies. This prognosis is in contrast to 5-year survival of less than 5% in the 1980s, and translates to almost a threefold improvement in long-term survival for this cohort of patients. However, it is true that lung cancer is a disease that continues to humble us, as a majority of our patients with locally advanced NSCLC will succumb to this disease. Therefore, much more clinical, translational, and basic science research still needs to be devoted to this field.

Metastatic NSCLC

Cisplatin-Based Chemotherapy Versus Best Supportive Care

Through the 1980s, cisplatin formed the backbone of systemic treatment in metastatic NSCLC, demonstrating single-agent response rate activity of 10% to 17%.[440] Other active agents included mitomycin C, vinblastine, ifsofamide, and vindesine. However, the impact on patient survival using these agents remained in doubt, as multiple trials comparing cisplatin-based chemotherapy with best supportive care (BSC) drew conflicting conclusions (Table 37.21).[441–447,677]

Although conclusive prolongations in survival were not consistently seen with the use of chemotherapy in the advanced disease setting in the 8 studies compared to BSC, its use was frequently associated with symptom relief and improvements in quality of life.[448,449] For example, investigators in the Big Lung Trial found that the use of chemotherapy was associated with less grade 3 and 4 breathlessness and less pain, but worsened peripheral neuropathy, compared to patients receiving supportive care only.[450] In addition, quality of life as assessed by the EORTC QLC-LC13 questionnaire at 6 weeks confirmed an improvement for patients receiving cisplatin-based chemotherapy.[451] This randomized experience confirmed that seen in prior Phase II studies, in which rates of symptom relief often exceeded that of objective antitumor response, in that patients with stable disease experienced lessening of disease-related symptoms.[452,453]

Because of discrepant survival results in BSC trials, meta-analyses of chemotherapy versus BSC trials have been helpful in determining the role of systemic treatment in these patients. A 1993 analysis of 6 randomized trials concluded that the use of chemotherapy in this setting was associated with a statistically significant 24% reduction in the risk of death at 1 year, and that treatment was associated with a lengthening of overall survival from 16.7 weeks to 27.4 weeks.[454] A 1994 meta-analysis of published literature results and individual patient data confirmed the benefit of treatment, determining an odds ratio of death of 0.44 and an increase in estimated median survival from 3.9 months for BSC to 6.7 months for patients with advanced disease receiving chemotherapy.[455] The largest meta-analysis of individual patient data was compiled from 11 studies from 1965 to 1991 and was reported in 1995.[384] Findings from this analysis of more than 1,100 patients revealed that the use of cisplatin-based regimens was associated with a 27% reduction in the risk of death for patients with advanced NSCLC, translating into an absolute improvement in survival at 1 year of 10% (from 5% to 15%). The use of nonplatinum-containing regimens was not beneficial in the setting of advanced disease.

Newer Agents Versus Best Supportive Care

Clinical testing of newer, so-called "third-generation" chemotherapeutic agents in the treatment of NSCLC was active in the 1990s, with resultant improvements in the therapeutic index.[456–460] The antimicrotubule agent, paclitaxel, was administered over 1 hour, 3 hours, and 24 hours, at various doses and schedules, with response rates ranging from 21% to 56% in untreated patients.[461,462] Another taxane,

TABLE 37.21. Randomized trials of best supportive care versus cisplatin-based chemotherapy.

Study	*N*	*Therapy*	*Overall response rate (%)*	*Median survival (months)*	*One-year overall survival (%)*	*P value*
Rapp[441]	251	BSC		4.3	10	
		Cisplatin/vindesine	25.3	8.2	22	<0.01
		Cyclophosphamide/doxorubicin/cisplatin	15.3	6.2	21	<0.05
Ganz[442]		BSC		3.4		NS
		Cisplatin/vinblastine		5.1		
Woods[443]	201	BSC		4.3		NS
		Cisplatin/vindesine	28	6.8		
Cellerino[444]	128	BSC		5.3		NS
		Cyclophosphamide/epirubicin/cisplatin→ Methotrexate/etoposide/CCNU	21	8.6		
Cartei[445]	102	BSC		4		
		Cisplatin/cyclophosphamide/mitomycin		8.5		<0.0001
Thongprasert[446]	287	BSC		4.1	13	
		Ifosfamide/epirubicin/cisplatin, or	40	5.9	29.8	
		mitomycin/cisplatin/vinblastine	41.7	8.1	39.3	0.0003
Cullen[447]	351	BSC		4.8		
		Mitomycin/ifosfamide/cisplatin	32	6.7		0.03
Stephens[677]	725	BSC		5.7		HR = 0.77,
		Cisplatin-based		7.7		$P = 0.0015$

TABLE 37.22. Randomized trials of best supportive care (BSC) versus newer agents.

Study	*N*	*Therapy*	*Overall response rate (%)*	*Median survival (months)*	*One-year overall survival (%)*	*P value*
ELVIS[463]	161	BSC		5.3	14	HR = 0.65,
		Vinorelbine	19.7	7	32	*P* = 0.03
Roszkowski[464]	207	BSC		5.7	16	
		Docetaxel	13.1	6.0	25	<0.026
Ranson[465]	157	BSC		4.8	NR	
		Paclitaxel	16	6.8	NR	0.037
Anderson[466]	300	BSC		5.9	22	
		Gemcitabine	19	5.7	25	NS

docetaxel, demonstrated a 35% response rate in Phase II testing, while antitumor response rates of 25% and 32% were seen in early clinical trials of gemcitabine and irinotecan, respectively.[455,459,460]

The advent of these more-active agents prompted a renewal of BSC comparison trials, using these newer agents[463–466] (Table 37.22). These trials more consistently demonstrate statistically significant prolongations in survival (approximating 2 months), as well as frequently detecting improvements in quality of life due to symptom relief. No comparative study detected a detriment in quality of life associated with the use of palliative chemotherapy with these newer agents, and in the one study in which the survival was not lengthened with treatment, symptom improvement was statistically sustained with chemotherapy.[466] These trials provide the foundation for the use of palliative chemotherapy in metastatic NSCLC, with the expectation from single-agent therapy of an antitumor response seen in approximately one of five patients, and an average improvement in overall survival from 5 to 7 months, coincident with symptom improvement.

Combination Chemotherapies Versus Cisplatin Alone

The next challenge was to improve upon these single-agent results by combining chemotherapeutics, based upon the experience of combination chemotherapy in other disease settings. Prior combinations, using cisplatin with less-active drugs, yielded response rates similar to that seen with newer single-agent third-generation agents, namely in the 20% range, with median survivals of 5 to 6 months.[448,467] As such, no single combination could be recommended as first-line therapy for patients with advanced NSCLC.

Table 37.23 demonstrates the results from four randomized trials, comparing cisplatin alone versus cisplatin combinations using a newer, third-generation agent.[449,468–470] This table provides evidence that doublet, platinum-based chemotherapy combined with a newer active, third-generation agent positively impacts survival in most studies, without significantly worsening toxicity. Large cooperative groups, therefore, selected one of these doublets as their reference arm for treatment in subsequent comparative trials. Carboplatin appears to be able to inserted for cisplatin with no consistent loss in efficacy, and with an improvement in tolerability (please see following), such that it has often replaced cisplatin as the platinating agent of choice for treatment doublets.

Cisplatin Versus Carboplatin

Cisplatin, however, has been associated with a significant number of side effects, most notably nausea and vomiting. Although this toxicity has become much more manageable with the advent of the HT3 antiemetics, concerns remain regarding the renal toxicity, neuropathy, ototoxicity, and generalized fatigue and asthenia. To alleviate some of these side effects, clinicians have turned toward the platin analogue carboplatin. Although carboplatin has a relatively low single-agent response rate, data from most, but not all, randomized trials supports equivalent clinical benefit between cisplatin and carboplatin.[471] An EORTC study from the late 1980s demonstrated similar survival curves for cisplatin and carboplatin when each drug was combined with etoposide.[472]

TABLE 37.23. Randomized trials of cisplatin alone versus newer cisplatin-based combinations.

Study	*N*	*Therapy*	*Overall response rate (%)*	*Median survival (months)*	*One-year overall survival (%)*	*P value*
Wozniak[449]	432	Cisplatin	12	6	20	
		Cisplatin/vinorelbine	26	8	36	0.0018
Sandler[468]	522	Cisplatin	11.1	7.6	28	
		Cisplatin/gemcitabine	30.4	9.1	39	0.004
von Pawel[469]	446	Cisplatin	13.7	6.9	22.5	
		Cisplatin/tirapazamine	27.5	8.7	34	0.0078
Gatzemeier[470]	414	Cisplatin	17	8.6	36	
		Cisplatin/paclitaxel	26	8.1	30	NS

Another more-recent study compared carboplatin and gemcitabine to cisplatin and gemcitabine and showed similar survival from treatment with cisplatin- and carboplatin-based regimens.[473] In ECOG 1594, four different chemotherapy doublets were compared to each other; the comparator arm involved cisplatin and paclitaxel, while one of the experimental arms included carboplatin and paclitaxel.[474] Although the dose and infusion rate of the paclitaxel differed between the two arms (135 mg/m^2 over 24 hours in the cisplatin arm, and 225 mg/m^2 over 3 hours in the carboplatin arm), the overall response and median survival did not differ significantly (22% and 7.8 months in the cisplatin/paclitaxel arm, and 17% and 8.1 months in the carboplatin/paclitaxel arm, respectively). A Phase III trial by a Yugoslavian group found an improved survival by log rank analysis when carboplatin was substituted for cisplatin in combination with vindesine and mitomycin C, whereas a European trial comparing cisplatin/paclitaxel to carboplatin/paclitaxel, in which the dose and schedule of paclitaxel was identical between the two arms, found a statistically significant improvement in median survival (9.8 months) in the cisplatin arm, compared to 8.5 months in the carboplatin arm.[475,476] Another study reported by Fossella and colleagues compared docetaxel/cisplatin and docetaxel/carboplatin with vinorelbine/cisplatin, 75 mg/m^2 of docetaxel being given in both arms.[477] Although the study was not designed to compare the two docetaxel arms, the investigators reported a trend toward improved survival in the docetaxel/cisplatin arm (11.3 months) compared to the docetaxel/carboplatin arm (9.4 months). Essentially all these studies found decreased toxicity in the carboplatin arm. Thus, although it could be debated as to whether carboplatin produces exactly the same efficacy outcomes as cisplatin in advanced NSCLC, results appear to be roughly similar, and with improved tolerability seen with the use of carboplatin. Given the paramount importance of limiting toxicity and optimizing quality of life in the advanced disease setting, it certainly seems reasonable to incorporate carboplatin as the platinating agent of choice in first-line doublet therapy. However, in earlier-stage disease such as in the postoperative setting, where curability is defined as the treatment goal, the results of Rosell et al. and Fossella et al. raise the important question of whether cisplatin is superior to carboplatin in terms of disease activity.[476,477] Randomized trials comparing cisplatin and carboplatin in earlier-stage NSCLC are needed to address this question.

New Single Agents Versus New Combinations

Table 37.24 shows randomized trials comparing a newer single agent versus a newer platinum-based combination.[478–484] On the whole, these trials show that antitumor response is improved with doublet treatment, and that combination therapy potentially improves median survival by 2 months, although at higher rates of hematologic toxicity.

New Combinations Versus Older Combinations

Table 37.25 displays the results of nine randomized trials that compared an older cisplatin-based doublet with a platinum-based combination using a newer second agent.[478,484–491] In these trials, the newer agents, including palcitaxel, gemcitabine, docetaxel, and irinotecan, add the toxicities of myalgias/arthralgias/sensory neuropathy, nonclinically significant thrombocytopenia, edema, and diarrhea, respectively, without consistently exacerbating neutropenia. Statistically significant prolongations in overall survival are seen in nearly half of the trials.[478,488,489,491] Quality of life measures were improved for patients receiving the combinations with the newer agents, despite the absence of a corresponding survival benefit, in the trials of Giaccone et al. and Belani et al., revealing a clinically meaningful effect from the third-generation agents.[485,486] Although marked improvements in overall survival were not seen in all these trials, the bulk of evidence pointed to the fact that the newer combinations resulted in 1-year overall survival rates consistently exceeding 30% to 35%, and that an efficacious doublet could be individualized to match a patient's comorbidities contingent upon the newer

TABLE 37.24. Randomized trials of platinum-based doublets versus new single agents.[a]

Study	*N*	*Therapy*	*Overall response rate (%)*	*Median survival (months)*	*One-year overall survival (%)*	*P value*
Le Chevalier[478]	612	Cisplatin/vindesine	19	8.3	29	
		Vinorelbine	14	9.0	34	
		Cisplatin/vinorelbine	30	10.8	38	0.01-
ten Bokkel Huinink[479]	147	Gemcitabine	17.9	6.6	26	
		Cisplatin/etoposide	15.3	7.6	24	NS
Vansteenkiste[480]	169	Gemcitabine	20.2	6.7	22	
		Cisplatin/vindesine	20	5.5	19	NS
Lilenbaum[481]	584	Paclitaxel	17	6.7	33	
		Carboplatin/paclitaxel	29	8.8	37	<0.05[b]
Sederholm[482]	332	Gemcitabine	12	9	32	
		Carboplatin/gemcitabine	30	11	44	0.0024
Georgoulias[483]	307	Docetaxel	18	10	40	
		Cisplatin/docetaxel	35	13	45	NS
Negoro[484]	398	Irinotecan	20.5	11.5	41.8	
		Cisplatin/vindesine	31.7	11.4	38.3	
		Cisplatin/irinotecan	43.7	12.5	46.5	NS

[a] When adjusted for treatment centers.

[b] Wilcoxon analysis.

TABLE 37.25. Randomized trials of older cisplatin-based doublets versus newer platinum-based doublets.

Study	*N*	*Therapy*	*Overall response rate (%)*	*Median survival (months)*	*One-year overall survival (%)*	*P value*
Le Chevalier[478]	612	Cisplatin/vindesine	19	8.3	29	
		Cisplatin/vinorelbine	30	10.8	38	0.04[a]
Giaccone[485]	332	Cisplatin/teniposide	28	9.9	41	
		Cisplatin/paclitaxel	41	9.7	43	NS
Belani[486]	369	Cisplatin/etoposide	14	8.2	37	
		Carboplatin/paclitaxel	23	7.7	32	NS
Cardenal[487]	135	Cisplatin/etoposide	21.9	7.2	26	
		Cisplatin/gemcitabine	40.6	8.7	32	NS
Bonomi[488]	599	Cisplatin/etoposide	12.4	7.6	31.8	
		Cisplatin/paclitaxel (low)	25.3	9.5	37.4	
		Cisplatin/paclitaxel (high)	27.7	10	40.3	0.048[b]
Takiguchi[489]	210	Cisplatin/vindesine	22	11.6	48	
		Cisplatin/irinotecan	29	10.5	43	NS
Grigorescu[490]	198	Cisplatin/vinblastine	15	7.9	12	
		Carboplatin/gemcitabine	27	11.6	36	<0.05
Kubota[491]	302	Cisplatin/vindesine	21	9.6	43	
		Cisplatin/docetaxel	37	11.3	48	0.014
Negoro[484]	398	Cisplatin/vindesine	31.7	11.4	38.3	
		Cisplatin/irinotecan	43.7	12.5	46.5	NS

[a] When adjusted for treatment centers.

[b] When survival is combined for the low and high dose paclitaxel arms.

agent's toxicities. As such, practice has progressed from the "one size fits all" recipe for a platinum-based doublet for patients with advanced NSCLC, therefore expanding the number of patients eligible to receive therapy.

Doublet Combination Comparisons

Comparisons of platinum-based doublets incorporating third-generation agents have demonstrated improvements in treatment activity and overall survival in patients with a good performance status, but have yet to identify one clinically superior regimen.[473,474,476,477,492–495] Table 37.26 demonstrates that treatment with these combinations yields antitumor response rates of at least 30%, median survival times of 8 to 10 months, 1-year overall survival rates exceeding 30%, and, for the first time, 2-year survival rates exceeding 10%. These advances are measured against median survivals of 5.3 to 5.8 months and 1-year survival of less than 20% seen with platinum-based doublets combined with older, second-generation agents.[448,467] The therapeutic plateau achieved with the use of these newer doublets clearly speaks to the need to incorporate newer treatments, most notably the use of targeted agents, into clinical trials of new treatment combinations.

Selecting a regimen based upon comparisons across trials is fraught with potential error, given differences in sample populations and treatment plans (for example, ECOG 1594 enrolled patients with brain metastases and a lower percentage of patients with stage IIIB disease, compared to TAX 326, whereas the dosing of paclitaxel was lower in ECOG 1594, compared to the study of Rosell et al.).[474,476,477] Overall, clinical efficacy within trials appears to be roughly similar using platinum-based doublets that incorporate a newer, third-generation agent. In addition, toxicity with the newer combinations is manageable, and therefore, selection of a platinum-based doublet for therapy in advanced NSCLC may be individualized in terms of the toxicity profile of the particular doublet, as well as convenience and cost, as efficacies of the newer combinations are largely equivalent. The therapeutic plateau achieved with the use of these newer doublets clearly speaks to the need to incorporate newer treatments, most notably the use of targeted agents, into clinical trials.

Quality of life analyses were conducted in four of the trials from Table 37.26, with consistent, significant differences seen most strongly with the use of docetaxel in the Fossella trial.[476,477,493,495] Using the EuroQoL global health scale (EuroQoL) and the Lung Cancer Symptom Scale (LCSS), these investigators showed that treatment with docetaxel/cisplatin (DC) or docetaxel/carboplatin (DCb) was associated with significant improvements in quality of life, compared to treatment with vinorelbine/cisplatin (VC): [for DC versus VC, $P = 0.064$ (LCSS) and $P = 0.016$ (EuroQoL); for DCb versus VC, $P = 0.016$ (LCSS) and P less than 0.001 (EuroQoL)]. Declines in performance status and weight were mitigated with docetaxel therapy.[477] It has been noted in a discussion of these results that the cisplatin dose administered to patients in the vinorelbine arm was higher per treatment (at 100 mg/m^2, compared to 75 mg/m^2 in the docetaxel arms). Also, a higher dose of corticosteroids was given to patients receiving docetaxel. Both these factors may have contributed to an improvement in symptoms in patients in the docetaxel arms.[496] Regardless, in light of the efficacy plateau reached with the platinum-based doublets shown in Table 37.26, it remains paramount to incorporate quality of life and symptom management outcomes into the decision making of selecting treatments for patients in this palliative setting.

Two Versus Three Drugs

Table 37.27 shows the results of 13 trials randomizing patients with advanced NSCLC to treatment with two or three cytotoxic agents.[99,497–510] However, in 8 of the 13 trials, the comparison three-agent arm contains at least one single agent that is older and would not be used presently as a single agent for treatment (i.e., mitomycin C or ifosfamide).[497,500,501,503–507] In one of the remaining five trials, Sculier et al. combined the two platinating agents, cisplatin and carboplatin, in the three-drug arms, in an effort to maximize platinum exposure. The similar mechanisms of action of the two platinating agents confounds interpretation of the impact of these three-drug combinations.[505] The remaining 4 studies utilize newer, third-generation agents into their triplets; however, final results for 3 of the remaining 4 trials have yet to be published.[498,499,502] Although the three-agent combination of cisplatin/gemcitabine/navelbine was found by the Southern Italian Cooperative Oncology Group (SICOG) investigators to be superior to treatment with cisplatin/navelbine, the doublet arm in this study was surprisingly toxic, and was associated with two toxic deaths, and higher rates of chemotherapy discontinuation, severe neutropenia, and vomiting, compared to the other arms. This unexpected rate of toxicity with this doublet may have been related to the treatment schema of administering $120 mg/m^2$ of cisplatin on day 1 of each 4- to 6-week cycle.[498] The Spanish Lung Cancer Group 98-02 study detected higher rates of hematologic toxicity with no corresponding improvement in efficacy outcomes for treatment with their three-drug combination.[99] In contrast, preliminary results from a second SICOG study yielded improved survival with only a modest increase in toxicities with the use of either of two three-drug regimens.[499] Final results from this SICOG trial are anticipated.

In summary, the consensus of evidence and opinion, including the preliminary publication of two meta-analyses recently, conclude that treatment of good performance status patients with advanced NSCLC with two cytotoxic agents is better than with one (see Tables 37.23, 37.24), whereas the addition of a third agent likely only exacerbates toxicity.[508,509] However, the majority of these findings result from studies incorporating rather inactive, older agents into the three-agent arm. Favorable results with the use of three-drug regimens from the SICOG investigators and Paccagnella et al.

TABLE 37.26. Randomized trials of newer platinum-based doublets.

Study	*N*	*Therapy*	*Overall response rate (%)*	*Median survival (months)*	*One-year overall survival (%)*	*P value*
Kosmidis[492]	198	Carboplatin/paclitaxel (low)	25.6	9.5	37	
		Carboplatin/paclitaxel (high)	31.8	11.4	44	NS
Kelly[493]	408	Cisplatin/vinorelbine	28	8.1	36	
		Carboplatin/paclitaxel	25	8.6	38	NS
Fossella[477]	1220	Cisplatin/vinorelbine	25	10.1	41	
		Cisplatin/docetaxel	32	11.3	46	
		Carboplatin/docetaxel	24	9.4	38	0.044[a]
Schiller[474]	1207	Cisplatin/paclitaxel	21	7.8	31	
		Cisplatin/gemcitabine	22	8.1	36	
		Cisplatin/docetaxel	17	7.4	31	
		Carboplatin/paclitaxel	17	8.1	34	NS
Rosell[476]	618	Cisplatin/paclitaxel	26	9.8	38	
		Carboplatin/paclitaxel	23	8.2	33	0.019[b]
Zatloukal[473]	176	Cisplatin/gemcitabine	41	8.8	33	
		Carboplatin/gemcitabine	29	8.0	36	NS
Huang[494]	99	Carboplatin/paclitaxel	31	NR	NR	
		Carboplatin/docetaxel	22	NR	NR	NR
Scagliotti[495]	612	Cisplatin/gemcitabine	30	9.8	37	
		Carboplatin/paclitaxel	32	9.9	43	
		Cisplatin/vinorelbine	30	9.5	37	NS
Gebbia[678]	400	Cisplatin/vinorelbine	44	9.0	24	
		Cisplatin/gemcitabine	34	8.2	20	NS
Martoni[679]	276	Cisplatin/vinorelbine	30.5	9.0	NR	
		Cisplatin/gemcitabine	32.0	9.0	NR	NS
Ohe[680]	602	Cisplatin/irinotecan	30	NR	NR	
		Carboplatin/paclitaxel	31	NR	NR	
		Cisplatin/gemcitabine	28	NR	NR	
		Cisplatin/vinorelbine	31	NR	NR	NR

[a] Cisplatin/docetaxel versus cisplatin/vinorelbine.

[b] Intention-to-treat analysis, as of the survival update of September 2001.

TABLE 37.27. Randomized trials of two drugs versus three.

Study	*N*	*Therapie*	*Overall response rate (%)*	*Median survival (months)*	*One-year overall survival (%)*	*P value*
Crino[497]	307	Mitomycin/ifosfamide/cisplatin	26	9.6	34	
		Cisplatin/gemcitabine	38	8.6	33	NS
Comella[498]	180	Cisplatin/vinorelbine	25	8.8	34	
		Cisplatin/gemcitabine	30	10.5	40	
		Cisplatin/gemcitabine/vinorelbine	47	12.8	45	<0.01[a]
Alberola[99]	557	Cisplatin/gemcitabine	42	9.3	38	
		Cisplatin/gemcitabine/vinorelbine	41	8.2	33	
		Gemcitabine/vinorelbine→ ifosfamide/vinorelbine	27	8.1	34	NS
Comella[499]	343	Cisplatin/gemcitabine	28	9.5	39	
		Cisplatin/gemcitabine/vinorelbine	44	12.8	47	
		Cisplatin/gemcitabine/paclitaxel	48	12.8	46	<0.05[b]
Rudd[500]	422	Mitomycin/ifosfamide/cisplatin	40	6.5	28	
		Carboplatin/gemcitabine	37	10.0	38	0.028
Melo[501]	248	Mitomycin/vinblastine/cisplatin	27	6.4	NR	
		Cisplatin/vinorelbine	37.1	9.0	NR	
		Cisplatin/gemcitabine (early)	48.4	9.4	NR	
		Cisplatin/gemcitabine (late)	48.4	9.6	NR	0.05[c]
Paccagnella[502]	60	Carboplatin/paclitaxel/gemcitabine	33	NR	NR	
		Carboplatin/paclitaxel	15	NR	NR	NR
Gebbia[503]	247	Mitomycin/vindesine/cisplatin	42	8	14.7	
		Cisplatin/vinorelbine	39	7	15.2	NS
Kodani[504]	132	Vindesine/ifosfamide/cisplatin	49.3	12.4	49.3	
		Cisplatin/vindesine	44.6	9.3	35.3	NS
Sculier[505]	284	Cisplatin/carboplatin/ifosfamide	25	6.0	23	
		Cisplatin/Carboplatin/Gemcitabine	31	8.5	33	
		Ifosfamide/gemcitabine	26	7.5	35	NS
Souquet[506]	259	Cisplatin/ifosfamide/vinorelbine	35.7	8.2	33.7	
		Cisplatin/vinorelbine	34.6	10	38.4	NS
Danson[507]	372	Mitomycin/ifosfamide/cisplatin or mitomycin/vinblastine/cisplatin	33	8.3	32.5	
		Carboplatin/gemcitabine	30	7.9	33.2	NS
Williamson[510]	396	Carboplatin/paclitaxel/tirapazamine	18	7	NR	
		Carboplatin/paclitaxel	27	9	NR	0.74

[a] Cisplatin/vinorelbine versus the other two arms.

[b] Cisplatin/gemcitabine versus the other two arms.

[c] Mitomycin/vinblastine/cisplatin versus the other three arms.

require confirmation before their findings would impact practice patterns.[502] Nonetheless, incorporation of agents with novel, targeted mechanisms of action into new treatment regimens, administered to patients preselected based upon the molecular characteristics of their tumors, will likely bear better outcomes, rather than continuing to explore combinations of cytotoxic agents administered to patients without genomic preselection. The recently released results of SWOG 0003, revealing no improvement in efficacy outcomes for patients with advanced NSCLC receiving the three-drug regimen carboplatin, paclitaxel, and tirapazamine, confirms the need to consider incorporating molecular preselection criteria into study designs.[510]

Nonplatinum Combinations

Investigators have tested nonplatinum combinations in an effort to reduce treatment-related toxicity and extend therapy to more symptomatic patients. Table 37.28 illustrates nine recent studies comparing a platinum-based doublet with nonplatinum-containing regimens.[99,505,511–517] None of the trials detected a statistically significantly worse response activity or overall survival with use of the nonplatinum-containing regimens. However, in the seven trials for which there are data, median and/or overall survival at 1 year is numerically inferior when platinum is not employed.[99,505,511–516] Although the use of nonplatinum-containing regimens is sometimes associated with lower rates of grade 3 and 4 toxicities, especially related to nausea, vomiting, myelosuppression, and ototoxicity, consistent trends suggesting inferior efficacy have precluded widespread acceptance of these combinations as the treatment of choice for good performance status patients with metastatic NSCLC. Furthermore, a large study from Italy and Canada failed to identify a significant improvement in quality of life for patients treated with the nonplatinum regimen of gemcitabine plus vinorelbine, despite more frequent rates of severe myelosuppression, vomiting, alopecia, and ototoxicity seen in patients receiving either of the two platinum-containing regimens in this trial, cisplatin plus vinorelbine or cisplatin plus gemcitabine.[513] As such, first-line treatment of advanced NSCLC with a third-generation nonplatinum doublet remains the exception rather than the rule but may prove beneficial in patients less able to withstand platinum-related toxicities. Although no study has confirmed a statistically significant inferiority in terms of efficacy outcomes, reductions in treatment-related toxicities may not translate into meaningful improvements in quality of life.

Duration of Therapy

Three trials have examined the question of duration of first-line therapy in advanced NSCLC.[517–520] The investigators determined that optimal treatment outcomes, in terms of efficacy and quality of life, are achieved with three to four cycles of therapy, as opposed to prolonged treatment. These recent studies have guided practitioners in limiting the number of front-line cycles of chemotherapy, as nearly all patients who respond to treatment do so within the first three to four cycles (all in the Socinski trial and 48/58 patients in the Smith study), and administering additional cycles only serves to expose patients to additional toxicities.

Special Populations

Chemotherapy in the Elderly

Patients over the age of 65 comprise a large fraction of patients with advanced NSCLC. Their treatment tends to be complicated by increased medical comorbidities and multiple concurrent medications. Moreover, therapeutic treatment decisions in the elderly are complicated by their significant underrepresentation in clinical oncology trials.[521] However, a recent review from the National Cancer Institute in Naples found that elderly patients with lung cancer do not appear to have different characteristics at disease presentation, especially related to disease stage, performance status, and histology, compared to younger patients.[522] Moreover, when asked, elderly patients are as likely as their younger counterparts to accept chemotherapy for both curative and palliative purposes.[523]

Multiple retrospective reviews of cooperative group trials in advanced NSCLC that examined subsets of elderly patients (usually defined as 70 years of age) have shown that the "fit" elderly are as likely to benefit in terms of improvements in survival and quality of life as are younger patients, albeit at the expense of a slightly higher rate of the most severe toxicities.[524–528]

Prospective data regarding the experience of elderly patients with advanced NSCLC receiving chemotherapy were provided by Italian investigators who compared treatment with single-agent vinorelbine to best supportive care in patients over 70 years of age.[463] As shown in Table 37.29, vinorelbine-treated patients scored better than control patients on quality of life scales and had fewer lung cancer-related symptoms. Furthermore, there was a statistically significant survival advantage for elderly patients receiving vinorelbine, with median survival increasing from a baseline of 21 weeks to 28 weeks. Clinical research is active with this group of patients, as practitioners have come to accept that age alone should not preclude consideration of systemic treatment of advanced NSCLC. The combination of both gemcitabine with vinorelbine together appears only to increase toxicity without a corresponding improvement in efficacy or quality of life parameters.[529] The slightly lower response rates and survival in the study by Frasci et al. may point to the fact that this trial, in contrast to the MILES study, permitted patients with brain metastases.[530] Investigations of single-agent docetaxel or gemcitabine at varying doses and schedules for the treatment of the elderly with advanced NSCLC are ongoing.[531,532]

TABLE 37.28. Randomized trials of nonplatinum doublets.

Study	*N*	*Therapy*	*Overall response rate (%)*	*Median survival (months)*	*One-year overall survival (%)*	*P value*
Giaccone[511]	480	Cisplatin/paclitaxel	31	8.1	35.5	
		Cisplatin/gemcitabine	36	8.8	32.6	
		Paclitaxel/gemcitabine	27	6.9	26.5	0.09[a]
Alberola[99]	410	Cisplatin/gemcitabine	42	9.3	38	
		Gemcitabine/vinorelbine→ ifosfamide/vinorelbine	27	8.1	34	NS
Georgoulias[512]	441	Cisplatin/docetaxel	34.6	10	42	
		Gemcitabine/docetaxel	33.3	9.5	39	NS
Gridelli[513]	501	Cis/vinorelbine or Cis/gemcitabine	30	9.5	37	
		Gemcitabine/vinorelbine	25	8	31	NS
Kakolyris[514]	251	Cisplatin/vinorelbine	36	11.5	45.4	
		Gemcitabine/docetaxel	29	9.0	34.4	NS
Patel[515]	107	Gemcitabine/paclitaxel	26	NR	NR	
		Gemcitabine/docetaxel	33	NR	NR	NR
Kosmidis[516]	509	Carboplatin/paclitaxel	28	10.4	41.7	
		Gemcitabine/paclitaxel	35	9.8	41.4	NS
Sculier[505]	284	Cisplatin/carboplatin/ifosfamide	25	6.0	23	
		Cisplatin/carboplatin/gemcitabine	31	8.5	33	
		Ifosfamide/gemcitabine	26	7.5	35	NS
Treat[517]	474	Carboplatin/gemcitabine	32.4	NR	NR	
		Carboplatin/paclitaxel	34.7	NR	NR	
		Gemcitabine/paclitaxel	39.0	NR	NR	NR

[a]Paclitaxel/gemcitabine versus the other two arms.

TABLE 37.29. Randomized trials of chemotherapy treatment in the elderly.

Study	N	Therapy	Overall response rate (%)	Median survival (months)	One-year overall survival (%)	P value
ELVIS[463]	161	BSC		5.3	14	
		Vinorelbine	19.7	7	32	0.03
Frasci[530]	120	Vinorelbine	15	4.5	13	
		Gemcitabine/vinorelbine	22	7.3	30	<0.01
Gridelli[529]	698	Vinorelbine	18	9	38	
		Gemcitabine	16	7	28	
		Gemcitibine/vinorelbine	21	7.5	30	NS

Treatment of fit elderly patients with NSCLC should now include consideration of at least single-agent therapy, and possibly consideration of doublet therapy, in an attempt to improve quality of life, reduce symptoms, and prolong survival, as the studies in Table 37.29 demonstrate that age alone should not disqualify patients from consideration of treatment.[533,534] Further investigation of the pharmacokinetics and pharmacodynamics of chemotherapies in the elderly are needed to clarify the impact on chemotherapy-related toxicities of reduced renal function and hematopoietic reserve of the elderly.[535]

Chemotherapy for Patients with Performance Status 2

Advanced NSCLC tends to be a highly symptomatic disease, often impairing one's ability to perform activities of daily living. Poor functional capability, or poor performance status, consistently appears as a negative prognostic factor in treatment trials.[96,474] In a recent review of a large ECOG trial comparing platinum-based systemic therapies, Eton et al. determined baseline physical well-being, as assessed by the FACT-L scale, to be the strongest predictor of both response to therapy, as well as survival duration.[536] Most (although not all) clinical trials suggest that these patients do not derive substantial benefit from chemotherapy and thus should probably not be treated off a clinical protocol.[451] The increased number of deaths in the PS 2 population (7.35%) enrolled in ECOG 1594 was related to the worsened incidence of medical comorbidities in these patients, rather than being strictly a consequence of treatment-related toxicity.[452] Efficacy was poor in these patients, with response rate, median survival, and 1-year overall survival all worse in the PS 2 patients compared to the better performance status cohorts (14% versus 19%, 4.1 months versus 7.9 months, and 19% versus 33%, respectively). ECOG is actively enrolling patients onto a PS 2-dedicated trial to further assess the utility of systemic cytotoxic treatment in this symptomatic population. For now, chemotherapy cannot be recommended as a means to prolong survival for patients with advanced NSCLC who are PS 2. However, chemotherapy may improve quality of life in these symptomatic patients and, as such, may be a reasonable consideration.[451] This patient group appears especially appropriate for further investigation of novel, molecularly targeted therapy, as many of them have a reduced toxicity profile because of their inherent selectivity, compared to cytotoxic chemotherapy.

Second-Line Treatment

Approximately one-quarter to one-half of patients with advanced NSCLC go on to receive second-line therapy.[477,513,518] Cytotoxic chemotherapy with docetaxel has been shown in two large international trials to confer a survival and quality of life/symptom control benefit in this setting.[537,538] Based on these studies, patients receiving docetaxel for relapsed disease can expect about a 5% to 10% rate of antitumor response, about a 35% to 45% incidence of stable disease, and an improvement in survival, compared to best supportive care, of about 3 months. These findings extended to patients who had received prior first-line treatment with paclitaxel and were confirmed to be cost-effective.[539]

Clinical research of second-line treatment of advanced NSCLC is proceeding at a robust pace, comparing new cytotoxics, combinations, and administration schedules, and incorporating novel, targeted agents (please see next section). Hanna et al. recently presented preliminary findings comparing second-line docetaxel with pemetrexed, the novel multitargeted antifolate that inhibits thymidylate synthase, dihydrofolate reductase, and glycinamide ribonucleotide formyltransferase.[540] Response rates, time to progressive disease, and survival were similar in both treatment arms, but therapy with pemetrexed produced a significantly more favorable toxicity profile, with less myelosuppression and fewer hospitalizations from febrile neutropenia. Comparisons of weekly versus the standard every-3-week schedule of administration with second-line docetaxel have revealed slightly higher rates of grades 3 and 4 nonhematologic toxicities with the weekly schedule, in contrast to worsened hematologic toxicities with the standard schedule.[541,542] Docetaxel combinations have also been investigated, as have other cytotoxics, including weekly paclitaxel, gemcitabine, and irinotecan.[543,544] Although docetaxel represents standard second-line treatment for advanced NSCLC at the present time, this recommendation will likely revise repeatedly in the near future, with the expected U.S. Food and Drug Administration (FDA) approval of pemetrexed, as well as continued application of novel, targeted agents into clinic protocols.

Novel Targeted Agents in the Treatment of NSCLC

A very exciting and quickly paced field of lung cancer research is the continuing clinical application of novel, molecularly targeted therapies. By definition, these agents specifically interfere with the molecular and biochemical pathways that contribute to the malignant phenotype. The specificity of these agents, directed against pathways that are often abnormally activated or overexpressed in the malignant cell and not in the normal cell, should result in reduced toxicity.

Gefitinib is an oral small molecule that serves as the prototypic molecularly targeted agent, disrupting the tyrosine kinase activity of the epidermal growth factor receptor (EGFR), which is frequently overexpressed on the surface of lung cancer cells. Single-agent response rates of 11.8% to 18.4% and a median survival measuring 6.1 months resulted in international Phase II studies of heavily pretreated NSCLC patients, using the 250-mg daily dose.[545,546] Stable disease was observed in 31% to 36% of patients. Of critical importance was the finding that symptom improvement was achieved by more than 40% of patients, occurred promptly, and was often experienced by patients who lacked an objective radiographic response. Drug-related toxicities were limited in this large Phase II experience, consisting primarily of mild to moderate rash and diarrhea, such that less than 2% of patients discontinued treatment due to side effects. Based upon these Phase II findings, gefitinib was recently approved by the FDA for administration in patients who have previously received platinum and docetaxel chemotherapies. Somewhat surprisingly, concurrent administration of gefitinib with platinum-based doublets in patients with advanced NSCLC did not yield improved efficacy outcomes.[547,548] Toxicity was not worsened by administration of this novel agent with chemotherapy, but the reasons for an absence of clinical benefit are not clear, given the promising preclinical experience with the combination.[549] Questions regarding the impact of sequencing and scheduling of administration of gefitinib, which blocks cells in the G_1 phase, with cytotoxic agents, are of intense research interest, as are means to better preselect patients who may respond to these EGFR-blocking agents.[550] In contrast to the targeted therapy experience with anti-estrogen agents and the erbB-2 blocking monoclonal antibody, trastuzumab, the intensity of EGFR overexpression in tumor cells does not appear to correspond with clinical outcomes following treatment with EGFR inhibitors.[551] As such, further preclinical and clinical studies are needed to clarify pretreatment patient and/or tumor characteristics that may predispose a patient to respond to this well-tolerated agent. In that regard, work done by Clark et al. is of interest, in that in their Phase II study of the EGFR small molecule inhibitor, erlotinib, rash occurred more frequently in patients whose tumors responded to treatment, compared to nonresponders.[552] Although molecular characteristics obviously differ considerably between skin and tumor cells, further understanding of, and potential correlation with, the effects of EGFR blockade on surrogate tissue and corresponding tumor cells will hasten the clinical development of these targeted medications.

Erlotinib (Tarceva) is another oral tyrosine kinase inhibitor that targets EGF. Multiple Phase II trials have demonstrated striking responses in females, patients from Japan, never smokers, and patients with adenocarcinomas. In a randomized, double-blind, placebo-controlled trial, 731 patients were randomized 2:1 to receive either erlotinib, 150mg/day, or placebo. The primary endpoint showed that erlotinib did significantly prolong survival (median, 6.7 versus 4.7 months for erlotinib versus placebo). Patients receiving Erlotinib also exhibited a statistically significant tumor response (8.9% versus 0.9%). The IRESSA Survival Evaluation in lung cancer (ISEL) trial was a similar double-blinded, placebo-controlled, parallel group, multicenter, randomized Phase III survival study of 1,692 patients who were followed for a median of 7 months. The study compared survival data in patients receiving gefitinib, 250mg/day, plus best supportive care to placebo plus best supportive care in patients with advanced NSCLC who had received one or two prior chemotherapy regimens and were refractory or intolerant to the most recent regimen. The primary endpoint revealed that gefitinib did not significantly prolong survival in the overall population (median, 5.6 versus 5.1 months for gefitinib versus placebo), or for patients with adenocarcinoma (median, 6.3 versus 5.4 months for gefitinib versus placebo). Studies have found that the EGFR gene is mutated in a cohort of non-small cell lung cancers and that these mutations are associated with increased sensitivity to gefitinib or erlotinib.[553,554] Recent studies have found that EGFR gene mutations are more common among females, patients from Japan, never smokers, and patients with adenocarcinomas, the same groups that have the highest response rates to tyrosine kinase (TK) inhibitors. In lung cancer patients, mutations in the TK domain of the EGFR gene are more common in never smokers than in smokers (51% versus 10%), adenocarcinomas versus other types of lung cancer (40% versus 3%), in patients of East Asian ancestry than in other ethnicities (30% versus 8%), and in females versus males (42% versus 14%). Mutation status is not associated with age at diagnosis, clinical stage, the presence of certain histologic features, or overall survival, and mutations are not found in any normal tissue or tissue from other cancer types. EGFR TK domain mutations are the first known mutation to occur in never smokers. Moreover, KRAS mutations, which also are involved with the EGFR signaling pathways gene, is mutated in about 8% of lung cancers but not in any that had an EGFR gene mutation.[555]

Antiangiogenic treatment, as a means to inhibit tumor-related neovascularization, also represents an active area of clinic research. RhuMAb-VEGF (Bevacizumab; Avastin; Genentech, Inc.) is a recombinant human monoclonal antibody that targets the VEGF protein and sequesters VEGF-A inhibiting signal transduction. Both in vitro and in vivo data indicate that endothelial cell proliferation is inhibited and tumor growth is reduced with administration of this antibody.[556]

A Phase II, three-arm, multicenter trial randomized 99 patients with stage IIIB or IV NSCLC to standard therapy with carboplatin/paclitaxel or one of two experimental arms: carboplatin/paclitaxel with rhuMAb VEGF (7.5mg/kg) or carboplatin/paclitaxel with rhuMAb VEGF (15mg/kg).[556] Because the endpoints of the study were safety, response, and time-to-tumor progression, the control group was allowed to cross over to the antibody-alone arm if disease progression was witnessed. Addition of rhuMAb VEGF led to an increase in response rates by about 10% and prolongation of the time-to-tumor progression by about 3 months (4.5–7.5 months) in the high-dose antibody group. Six patients developed severe hemoptysis (four episodes were fatal). Assessment of the potential risk factors for this adverse event indicated that squamous histology and rhuMAb treatment were the only factors associated with hemoptysis. Trials with this drug were then limited to those patients with nonsquamous cell histology in NSCLC.[557] Given the positive impact on survival seen with this agent in patients with advanced colon cancer,[556] the results of an ECOG Phase III trial in which patients with advanced NSCLC were randomized to receive chemotherapy with or without bevacizumab were eagerly awaited. The data were presented at the ASCO 2005 meeting. In a recent elegant example of the potential ability to combine targeted, molecularly directed agents, which comes from investigators at Vanderbilt University, erlotinib and bevacizumab are combined.[558] This important work illustrates the capability to potentially disable multiple intracellular pathways that are interacting to stimulate tumor growth and spread; further studies of this type are needed to optimize the clinical application of these agents.

Other molecularly targeted agents undergoing clinical assessment in the treatment of NSCLC include treatment with inhibitors of cyclooxygenase (COX)-2,[559] adenovirus replication-deficient p53 gene replacement,[560] vaccination with the whole tumor cell vaccine GVAX,[561] the farnesyltransferase inhibitor R115777,[562] treatment with BAY 43-9006, an inhibitor of the raf kinase pathway,[563] use of the thrombospondin 1 mimetic peptide ABT-510,[564] the RXR selective retinoid bexarotene,[565] and treatment[559] with the ubiquitin proteasome pathway inhibitor, bortezomib.[566] Additionally, the emerging field of pharmacogenomics will enhance the ability to optimize treatment outcomes by individualizing chemotherapy to match a patient's pharmacodynamic makeup.[567] Rosell et al. recently used quantitative PCR to analyze the expression of beta-tubulin III, stathmin, RRM1, COX-2, and GSTP1 in mRNA isolated from paraffin-embedded tumor biopsies of 75 patients with advanced NSCLC who were treated as part of a large randomized trial.[114] Their findings showed that patients with low beta-tubulin III levels had a better response to carboplatin/paclitaxel, whereas patients with low RRM1 levels showed a tendency to respond better to treatment with cisplatin/gemcitabine. Similarly, low levels of gene expression of ERCC1, critical in the repair of cisplatin-related adducts, corresponded to longer survival in patients treated with cisplatin/gemcitabine.[112] These examples of integration of patient-specific molecular information and the corresponding individualization of therapy should result in improved treatment outcomes for patients with advanced NSCLC.

Small Cell Lung Cancer Therapy

Limited-Stage Small Cell Lung Cancer

Combined Modality Treatment of Small Cell Lung Cancer

Small cell lung cancer (SCLC) accounted for approximately 18% to 25% of the estimated 169,500 cases of lung cancer in 2001.[59,568] Most patients present with metastatic disease because of the aggressive nature of SCLC. Limited-stage disease (LD) accounts for approximately 40% of all SCLC cases. The VALG classified limited-stage disease as tumor limited to one hemithorax and its regional lymph nodes that can be encompassed by one radiation port. Extensive-stage disease (ED) is tumor spread beyond these boundaries.[569] Radiation therapy's main role is in the treatment of limited-stage disease. Because radiation only offers locoregional control, chemotherapy is necessary to destroy the micrometastatic disease that invariably is present. Multiple cooperative group trials have been performed to establish the role of radiation therapy in SCLC.[570–573]

In the early 1960s, surgery was the treatment of choice for patients with resectable SCLC. However, a trial performed in the United Kingdom that compared patients with limited disease treated with thoracic radiation alone versus surgery alone showed the 10-year survival for the surgery-alone arm was zero, but the 10-year survival for the radiation-alone arm was 5%.[574] In the 1970s and 1980s, multiple cooperative group trials were performed to test the role of adding thoracic radiation therapy to chemotherapy (Tables 37.30, 37.31). These trials randomized patients with LD-SCLC to chemotherapy

TABLE 37.30. **Studies of chemotherapy versus chemotherapy and radiation in patients with limited diseases-small cell lung cancer (LD-SCLC).**

					Median survival (months)		*Two-year survival*	
Study	*N*	*Chemotherapy regimen*	*Radiation dose*	*Radiation schedule*	*CT*	*CRT*	*CT*	*CRT*
SECSG[569]	369	CAV	30 Gy/15 fx/ weeks 1, 2, 7	Alternating	10.6	11.9	21%	29%
CALGB[570]	399	CEV/CAV	50 Gy/25 fx/ 5 weeks continuous	Concurrent starting on day 1 of cycle 1 through day 4 of cycle 3 No RT	7.7	11.2 11.8	8% 8%	15% 25%
ECOG[568,569]	310	CCM/EA	50 Gy/25 fx/ 5 weeks continuous	Sequential day 43	12.4	14.4	13%	19%
SWOG[571]	93	VMV/VAC	48 Gy/22 fx/ 6.5 week split	Sequential week 12	18.5		25%	35%
NCI[570,573]	96	CCM/VAP	40 Gy/15 fx/ 3 weeks bid continuous	Concurrent day 1	11.6	15	12%	28%
NCIC[568,572]	308	CAV/PE Alternating	40 Gy/15 fx Per week	Concurrent Day 22 (cycle 2) Day 106 (cycle 6)	15.4	21.2	40%	34%

CAV, cyclophosphamide/doxorubicin/vincristine; CEV, cyclophosphamide/epirubicin/vincristine; CCM, cyclophosphamide/lomustine/methotrexate; EA, etoposide/doxorubicin; VMV/VAC, vincristine, methotrexate, VP-16/vincristine, doxorubicin, cyclophosphamide; VAP, vincristine/doxorubicin/procarbazine; PE, cisplatin/etoposide.

alone versus chemotherapy with radiation. The schedule of radiation and type of chemotherapy used varied between trials, but all the trials used prophylactic cranial irradiation (PCI). The combination of radiation therapy and chemotherapy decreased the locoregional recurrence rates compared to the use of chemotherapy alone in the treatment of LD-SCLC (see Table 37.31). All the trials except the SWOG trial reported statistically significant improvements in survival. As a result of these studies, thoracic radiation therapy became a standard part of the therapy for patients with LD-SCLC.

Radiation Therapy

The optimal dose of radiation therapy for patients with limited-stage disease is unknown. Full-dose radiation therapy is critical to achieve the therapeutic gain of local tumor control.[575] Effective chemotherapy may allow a decrease in the radiation dose needed for local control. In the presence of chemotherapy, the radiation dose theoretically can be reduced 20% to control the tumor. Thus, the dose for complete response, approximately 70 Gy, can be decreased to 55 Gy.[575] Local recurrence is still about 40% to 50%.[576] Retrospective trials revealed that doses less than 40 Gy were not adequate for local control.[577]

Fractionation of radiation therapy is another important factor affects the biologically effects radiation dose. Pignon et al. performed a meta-analysis and included 13 randomized trials.[578] The fractionation dose varied between 2 and 4 Gy. The analysis revealed that as the fraction became larger, the toxicities increased.[578]

Hyperfractionated radiation decreases the fraction size but is repeated hours later. Theoretically, twice-daily radiation therapy decreases the repopulation of tumor cells. The CALGB trial by Choi et al. established the maximum tolerated dose of hyperfractionated radiation therapy given twice daily as 45 Gy in 30 fractions over 3 weeks, and the maximum tolerated conventional dose was 70 Gy in 35 fractions over 7 weeks.[579]

An intergroup randomized Phase III study compared daily versus hyperfractionated radiation therapy.[579] Patients were randomized to twice-daily radiation therapy (45 Gy over 3 weeks) or conventional radiation therapy (45 Gy over 5 weeks). Radiation therapy was started day 1, cycle 1, with four cycles of cisplatin and etoposide (CE). Local control trended better in the twice-daily arm. After a complete response, the recurrence rate was 75% in the daily radiation versus 42% in the twice-daily radiation arm. Local recurrence only rates were 52% versus 36%, respectively ($P = 0.058$). Median survival for the conventional radiation was 19 months and for the hyperfractionated radiation was 23 months. Five-year survival was 16% for conventional daily fractions and 26% for hyperfractionated radiation ($P = 0.04$). However, grade 3 or greater esophageal toxicity was higher for the twice-daily radiation (25.7% versus 10.9%, respectively).

Optimal radiation volume is still not well defined at this point. Several studies have tried to address the question of encompassing pre- versus postchemotherapy tumor volume.[569,571,580–582] Studies have been limited because of small patient numbers. The Mayo Clinic performed a retrospective analysis comparing radiation ports encompassing the prechemotherapy or the postchemotherapy tumor volume. No marginal failures occurred. Locoregional failures occurred in 10 of 31 patients treated with a prechemotherapy port versus 9 of 28 patients treated with a postchemotherapy radiation port.[580] Locoregional recurrences occurred within the radiation port. SWOG performed a randomized study evaluating this same question.[581] Patients were randomized per their tumor response to induction chemotherapy. Those patients who achieved a complete response after chemotherapy were randomized to either a wide-volume port followed by chemotherapy or chemotherapy alone. A wide-volume port was defined as the prechemotherapy tumor volume plus mediastinal adenopathy and a surrounding margin. Local recurrence rate of the patients treated with the wide volume was 50% versus chemotherapy alone was 72% ($P = 0.01$). The median survival of the group of complete responders was 18.5 months. Local recurrence rate of the group given wide-field radiation therapy was 32% versus 28% for the reduced-field radiation (not statistically different). In conclusion, there is no difference in locoregional recurrence when the volume of the port size is varied between pre- versus postchemotherapy tumor volume or margin size. Thus, larger volumes do not necessarily mean better control. If combined chemotherapy and radiation therapy is used, only postchemotherapy tumor volumes need to be included within the radiation port. However, prophylactic radiation of regional lymph nodes is still a subject to be evaluated.

TABLE 37.31. Local recurrence rates for chemotherapy alone versus chemotherapy and chest irradiation in patients with LD-SCLC.

		Local recurrence rates	
Study	*Radiation*	*CT*	*CRT*
SECSG[565,569]		79%	51%
CALGB[566,570]	Concurrent		74%
	No RT	32%	60%
ECOG[568,569]		NR	
SWOG[567,571]		72%	50%
NCI[570,573]		33%	70%
NCIC[568,572]	Day 22 (cycle 2)		59%
	Day 106 (cycle 4)		61%

RT, radiation; NR, not reported.

Combining Chemotherapy with Radiation Therapy

Several randomized studies have demonstrated that the combination of chemotherapy and radiation therapy improves overall survival compared to chemotherapy alone. The optimal timing and sequence of combining chemotherapy and radiation therapy is unknown for the treatment of limited-stage small cell lung cancer. Radiation can be combined with chemotherapy sequentially, alternating, or concurrently. When combined concurrently, radiation can be started early in the treatment or later during the treatment schedule.[582]

Three randomized Phase III studies have been performed evaluating sequential chemotherapy followed by radiation therapy versus chemotherapy alone in patients with LD-SCLC (Table 37.32). Carlson et al. randomized patients who responded to chemotherapy to chemotherapy only or radiation therapy.[583] No difference in overall survival was detected. A French group randomized 53 patients who achieved a complete response after chemotherapy to radiation of 46.5 Gy or no radiation therapy until disease relapse.[584] The median survival was 10.5 months for the radiation therapy group and

TABLE 37.32. Studies of chemotherapy versus sequential chemotherapy followed by radiation therapy in patients with LD-SCLC.

					Median survival (months)		Two-year survival	
Study	*N*	*Chemo*	*Radiation*	*Schedule*	*CT*	*CRT*	*CT*	*CRT*
Carlson[583]	48	CLVP/EAM	55 Gy/30 fx/7 weeks	Sequential after 6–9 months	18.9	20.3	42%	42%
Lebeau[585]	53	CCAE	46.5 Gy/ equivalent	Sequential after 8 cycles	16.5	10.5	38%	26%
SWOG[587]	93	VMV/VAC	48 Gy/22 fx 6.5 weeks Split	Sequential week 12	18.5		25%	35%

CLVP, cyclophosphamide/lomustine/vincristine/procarbazine; EAM, etoposide/doxorubicin/methotrexate; CCAE, cyclophosphamide/lomustine/doxorubicin/etoposide; VMV/VAC, vincristine, methotrexate, VP-16/vincristine, doxorubicin, cyclophosphamide.

16.5 months for the group who received radiation therapy at the time of relapse. The SWOG cooperative group randomized 93 patients who achieved complete responses after induction chemotherapy to split-course radiation therapy or chemotherapy alone.[571] The radiation therapy did improve local control compared to chemotherapy alone. The local recurrence rate was 50% versus 72%, respectively.

Two studies evaluated the alternating schedule, which is defined as chemotherapy given conventionally with radiation given in between the chemotherapy cycles for LD-SCLC. The Southeastern Cancer Study Group (SECSG) trial randomized patients to chemotherapy alone or chemotherapy alternating with radiation therapy.[569] The addition of radiation therapy improved local control and 2-year survival (64% versus 48% and 24% versus 16%, respectively).[569] A French trial randomized patients between alternating and concurrent schedules.[585] The median survival for the concurrent arm was 13.5 months and for the alternating arm was 14 months. The 3-year survival for the concurrent arm was 6% versus 11% for the alternating schedule arm. The differences were not statistically different.

A Japanese trial compared sequential delivery of chemotherapy and radiation therapy to concurrent delivery of chemotherapy and radiation.[586] Patients were randomized to receive concurrent hyperfractionated radiation therapy (day 2 of cycle 1 of chemotherapy) or to sequential chemotherapy followed after the fourth cycle by hyperfractionated radiation therapy. The radiation dose was 45 Gy given in 1.5-Gy fractions twice daily for a total of 30 fractions in 3 weeks. The chemotherapy given was cisplatin and etoposide. The median survival for the concurrent schedule was 29 months and for the sequential schedule was 19 months. The 2-year survival was 50% for the concurrent therapy and 40% for the sequential therapy.[587] These results favored concurrent therapy and are the best results to date for patients with LD-SCLC.

Other studies evaluated the question of whether early delivery of radiation concurrently with chemotherapy was better than late delivery. A study performed by the CALGB randomized patients to early (day 1, cycle 1), late (day 64, cycle 4), or no radiation therapy. The radiation therapy dose was 50 Gy over 6 weeks. Chemotherapy used in this trial was cyclophosphamide, etoposide, and vincristine. The local recurrence rate for the early, late, and no radiation therapy arms was 49%, 68%, and 82%, respectively. The 2-year progression-free survival rate was 15% for the early schedule arm versus 25% for the late schedule ($P = 0.078$). The 5-year survival rate for the early, late, and no radiation therapy arms was 6.6%, 12%, and 3%, respectively ($P = 0.007$). The poor 5-year survival rate for the early schedule was thought to be due to the significant decrease in chemotherapy dose needed for the early schedule group.[570,587]

The NCIC randomized patients to radiation therapy started either early or late with concurrent chemotherapy (cyclophosphamide, doxorubicin, and vincristine alternating with cisplatin and etoposide).[572] In the early arm, radiation was started on day 21 of cycle 2 (after the first cycle of cisplatin/etoposide). In the late arm, radiation was started on day 106 (cycle 6) with the third cycle of cisplatin and etoposide. The 5-year survival in the early delivery and late delivery arm was 20% and 11%, respectively ($P = 0.006$). The early delivery arm also had a decreased incidence of brain metastasis (18% versus 28%; $P = 0.042$), which could explain the improved 5-year survival.[572]

A Danish trial randomized 199 patients to either early radiation therapy or late radiation therapy given concurrently with chemotherapy.[588] The 5-year survival and local recurrence rate were not statistically different. The 5-year survival for the early arm was 10.8% versus 12% for the delayed radiation therapy arm. The local recurrence rate for the early radiation arm was 76.6% versus 72.8% for the delayed arm.[588]

The EORTC randomized patients to either start radiation therapy during week 6 (early) or after the chemotherapy during week 14 (late). No significant differences were noted for local recurrence (50.5% for early radiation versus 45.5% for late radiation) or 3-year survival (14% for both early and late radiation therapy).[589]

Another CALGB study randomized patients to early versus late delivery of hyperfractionated radiation given with carboplatin and etoposide chemotherapy.[590] In the early radiation arm, patients received radiation with chemotherapy during weeks 1 through 4. In the late radiation arm, patients received radiation with chemotherapy during weeks 6 through 9. The radiation dose for both arms was 54 Gy given in 36 fractions over 4 weeks. The radiation dose was also hyperfractionated, with 1.5 Gy given twice daily for 5 days per week. The locoregional recurrence rate for the early and late radiation was 42% and 65%, respectively. The median survival for the early radiation group was 34 months compared to 26 months in the late radiation group ($P = 0.052$). The 5-year survival for the early radiation group was 30% versus

15% for the late radiation group ($P = 0.027$). The results favored the early delivery of radiation therapy concurrently with platinum-based chemotherapy.[590]

Current data support the use of concurrent over sequential or alternating chemotherapy and radiation therapy. The optimal delivery of concurrent chemoradiation is still under study. Early delivery of radiation therapy may decrease dissemination by killing the chemoresistant tumor cells before their distant seeding. Late delivery of radiation therapy possibly reduces toxicities, and full chemotherapy doses can be delivered. However, even with increased toxicity, improved survival rates help establish as standard early delivery of concurrent radiation with platinum-based chemotherapy.

Prophylactic Cranial Irradiation for SCLC

Prophylactic cranial irradiation (PCI) use for SCLC began in the 1970s. The CNS is a sanctuary from most chemotherapy agents, and for patients with SCLC, relapse in the CNS is common. At diagnosis, 10% of patients with SCLC have brain metastasis, and 20% to 25% of patients with SCLC are diagnosed later with brain metastasis.[591] PCI is thought to decrease disease relapse in the CNS. Several studies have randomized patients after receiving definitive therapy for their systemic disease and achieving a complete remission to PCI versus no PCI. Of three randomized trials, PCI improved overall relapse rate and brain-only relapse rate (Table 37.33). A trend toward improved survival was also demonstrated.[592–594] A meta-analysis of PCI was performed including seven randomized trials.[594] A total of 847 patients with LD-SCLC and 140 patients with extensive disease SCLC were included in the meta-analysis. These patients were in complete remission and then randomized to PCI or observation. A 16% decrease in mortality was observed in those patients who received PCI. Also, a 5.4% increase in the 3-year survival was demonstrated (15.3% controls versus 20.7% PCI). From these data, PCI should be considered for patients who achieve a complete remission or near complete remission after initial therapy. The optimal dose and fractionation for PCI is unknown. The most commonly used dose for PCI is 25 Gy given over 10 fractions.

The randomized trials reported very few or no late neurologic complications from PCI for NSCLC. However, there are more data available regarding the late toxicity of PCI from SCLC patients who underwent PCI. In these trials of PCI for patients with SCLC, dementia was not commonly seen,[595–597] but attention deficit, memory changes, and changes in visual perception were noted.[595,598,599] Some investigators noted changes in the white matter in T_2-weighted MRI of the brain.[423,597,598] Most of the patients exhibiting these changes did not show significant deterioration in clinical status. In addition, the changes rarely affected daily life functions.[600] Recent data of prospective studies incorporating PCI in SCLC did not demonstrate a profound effect on neuropsychologic function.[592,593,600,601] In addition, recent studies have reported a significant portion of the patients with SCLC had cognitive dysfunction even before PCI,[600,601] and these patients did not have significant changes in their neuropsychologic status after PCI. This finding implied that neuropsychologic abnormalities seen with SCLC might have been the result of either systemic therapy or SCLC itself. Cecile Le Pechoux and colleagues reported follow-up data on 57 patients followed for more than 36 months in a randomized PCI trial.[602] There was no severe, late-onset neurotoxicity. However, memory loss and mood changes were believed to be more attributable to PCI. Memory loss was seen in 21% (7/33) of patients who received PCI versus 4% (1/24) of patients who did not receive PCI. Mood changes such as anxiety were seen in 18% (6/33) of the patients who received PCI versus 4% (1/24) of patients who did not receive PCI. Highest rates of toxicity have been seen when PCI was combined with concurrent chemotherapy or when high dose per fraction was used.[603]

TABLE 37.33. Summary of prophylactic cranial irradiation (PCI) for SCLC patients.

Study	PCI dose	Brain Metastasis +PCI	Brain Metastasis −PCI	P value
Arriagada[582]	24 Gy/8 Fx	41%	59%	$P < 0.0001$
Gregor[589]	36 Gy/18 Fx 30 Gy/10 Fx 24 Gy/12 Fx 8 Gy/1 Fx	29%	52%	$P = 0.0002$

+ Carboplatin.

Extensive-Stage Small Cell Lung Cancer

Cisplatin/Etoposide (EP) Versus Anthracycline-Based Chemotherapy

Cisplatin has been used frequently in the first-line treatment of patients with extensive SCLC in the United States and Japan since the 1980s, whereas anthracycline-based therapy cyclophosphamide, doxorubicin, vincristine (CAV), cyclophosphamide, epirubicin, vincristine (CEV) has been used more commonly in Europe.[604] In one of the few randomized clinical trials demonstrating the superiority of a combination regimen in patients with extensive SCLC, Evans et al. detected a statistically improved response rate (80% versus 63%), median survival (9.6 versus 8 months), and overall survival ($P = 0.03$) for patients receiving six cycles of the alternating regimen of cisplatin/etoposide (EP) and CAV, compared to patients receiving six cycles of CAV alone.[605] In contrast, no improvement in either antitumor response or survival was seen with either EP or CAV alternating with EP, compared to CAV, in a randomized trial of 437 patients with extensive disease published by the Southeastern Cancer Group Study.[606] A meta-analysis of nine trials comparing cisplatin-based treatment versus chemotherapy not containing cisplatin for all patients with SCLC yielded an odds ratio of 1.35 (95% CI, 1.18–1.55; P less than 0.00005) in favor of obtaining a response after receiving cisplatin. Patients treated with a cisplatin-containing regimen benefited from a significant reduction of risk of death at 12 months (odds ratio, 0.80, 95% CI, 0.69–0.93; $P = 0.002$), corresponding to a significant increase in the probability of survival of 4.4% at 1 year.[607] Additionally, a comprehensive meta-analysis of randomized chemotherapy treatment trials in patients with extensive disease only recently reported that the median survival time of patients receiving a cisplatin-based regimen was 9.5 months, compared to patients treated with a noncisplatin-containing combination (7.1 months).[608] Last, investigators from Norway recently published their 5-year results of a trial comparing five courses of EP to CEV for patients with both extensive and limited SCLC.[609] Median survival was improved for all patients who received EP (10.2 months), versus patients in the CEV arm (7.8 months; $P = 0.0004$). This trial was not powered to detect a statistical difference in survival for patients with extensive disease only, but the numerical superiority of the results with EP, combined with the findings from the above meta-analyses, confirms the clinical experience that treatment of patients with extensive SCLC is no worse than anthracycline-based treatment and may be better tolerated.

Refinement of EP: Replacing Etoposide with Irinotecan

In an effort to improve the stagnation in the treatment of extensive SCLC, Noda et al. replaced etoposide with irinotecan, in combination with cisplatin in a randomized Japan Clinical Oncology Group (JCOG) trial of 154 patients.[610] A survival advantage was experienced by patients receiving the investigational treatment (median survival, 12.8 months for the cisplatin/irinotecan group versus 9.4 months for patients receiving cisplatin/etoposide; $P = 0.002$). This survival advantage exceeded that seen in any of the 21 randomized trials reviewed by Chute et al. and prompted termination of accrual after two interim analyses (the first was planned and the second was early).[608] Use of irinotecan also yielded a significantly higher antitumor response rate (84.4 % versus 67.5% for patients receiving the standard EP). Treatment was fairly well tolerated in this study, with the exception of grade 3 and 4 diarrhea occurring more frequently in the irinotecan group.[610] Two multicenter randomized trials in the United States are attempting to confirm these impressive results.

Refining EP: Adding Agents Concurrently

Other investigators have attempted to improve upon the standard treatment of EP by adding concurrent additional active agents (Table 37.34).[611–613] In all three trials, toxicity was exacerbated with the addition of the third agent, such that platinum-based doublet therapy remains the standard of care for extensive SCLC.

Refining Cisplatin-Based Chemotherapy: Adding Maintenance Chemotherapy

Prior trials assessing the utility of maintenance chemotherapy added sequentially to induction treatment demonstrated a 2-month prolongation in time to progression, but no improvement in overall survival.[614,615] Two studies assessing the possible role for sequential maintenance treatment in nonprogressing patients with extensive SCLC have been published recently. The Eastern Cooperative Oncology Group trial 7593 attempted to exploit the potential synergistic antitumor effects of administering topoisomerase II and I inhibitors in sequence in randomizing patients to four cycles of topotecan or observation after their received cisplatin and etoposide.[616] Addition of the topotecan did not impact overall survival (8.9 months in the topotecan arm versus 9.3 months in the observation arm; $P = 0.53$), nor did it improve quality of life in the topotecan recipients per the FACT-L questionnaire. However, progression-free survival was statistically improved (3.7 months in the treated patients versus 2.3 months; P less than 0.001), confirming a trend seen in older studies of mixed populations.[614,616] Hanna et al. confirmed these findings after randomizing 144 patients to observation or three courses of oral daily etoposide following their initial treatment with etoposide, ifosfamide, and cisplatin.[617] Maintenance therapy again prolonged progression-free survival, from 6.5 to 8.23 months ($P = 0.0018$), but resulted in only a trend toward improving overall survival, from 11.2 to 12.2 months ($P = 0.0704$). Without a clear-cut improvement in overall survival from the addition of maintenance cytotoxic agents, it appears more prudent to investigate the utility of augmenting cytotoxic therapy with molecularly targeted agents, which often do not exacerbate toxicity to the same extent.

High-Dose Chemotherapy

The administration of high-dose chemotherapy, using late intensification chemotherapy with autologous bone marrow transplantation, did not improve overall survival in the single randomized trial to date that tested this paradigm.[618] Using higher doses of both cisplatin and etoposide in cycles 1 and 2 of a total of four cycles of treatment did not improve antitumor response or overall survival in a sample of 90 patients with extensive disease, despite increasing the dose intensity by 46%.[619] Investigators attempted to increase the dose intensity of cyclophosphaminde, 4′-epidoxorubicin, etoposide, and cisplatin by giving higher doses over a shorter number of cycles in a 1997 study from France.[620] Due to worsened toxicity in the high-dose arm, cumulative dose delivered was actually higher in the standard dose group. Use of the higher-dose treatment yielded a significantly shorter survival, suggesting that higher doses over fewer courses is not an advantageous route to dose intensity.[620] Last, the EORTC

TABLE 37.34. Adding a third cytotoxic agent to etoposide/cisplatin (EP).

Study	*N*	*Therapy*	*Overall response rate (%)*	*Time to progression (months)*	*Median survival (months)*	*One-year survival (%)*	*Comments*
Pujol et al.[611]	226	EP	61	6.3	9.3	29	PCDE with worsened myelosuppression, febrile neutropenia, cardiac toxicity.
		PCDE	76	7.2	10.5	40 ($P = 0.0067$)	
Mavroudis et al.[612]	133[a]	EP	48	9	10.5	37	Eight toxic deaths with TEP; none with EP. TEP with worsened myelosuppression, diarrhea, asthenia.
		TEP	50	11	9.5	38	
Niell et al.[613]	587	EP	NR	NR	9.8	35.7	TEP with 6.4% treatment related mortality, EP with 2.7%.
		TEP	NR	NR	10.3	36.2	

PCDE, cisplatin, cyclophosphamide, etoposide, 4′-epidoxorubicin; TEP, paclitaxel, etoposide, cisplatin.

[a] 74 patients had extensive disease; 59 patients had limited disease.

increased the dose intensity with accelerated CDE (cyclophosphamide, doxorubicin, and etoposide) by 70% with every-2-week administration (with growth factor support, for four cycles), compared to every-3-week treatment for five cycles.[621] Grade 3 and 4 anemia and thrombocytopenia, as well as stomatitis/mucositis, were not unexpectedly significantly worse with the accelerated treatment. Median survival times were equivalent (54 weeks on the standard arm and 52 weeks on the intensified arm; $P = 0.885$). These multiple negative results demonstrated that efforts to increase dose intensity that utilize fewer cycles of treatment should be abandoned.

Dose Density

In their recent review of dose-intensified chemotherapy in the treatment of SCLC, Tjan-Heijnen et al. point out that dose densification is the most effective means to improve efficacy outcomes with this paradigm, citing four studies (three with mixed populations of patients with extensive and limited disease) that, on average, yielded a prolongation of median survival of 2.7 months by reducing the treatment interval, but keeping the doses administered, the number of treatment cycles, and hence the cumulative dose, equivalent.[614] However, three recent negative studies argue against this method.[622–624] Weekly administration of the cisplatin, vincristine, doxorubicin, etoposide (CODE) regimen yielded a higher toxic death rate (8.2%) and no improvement in overall survival (0.98 years), compared to standard every-3-week alternating CAV/EP (0.9% and 0.91 years, respectively) in a Canadian/ SWOG trial of 220 patients with extensive SCLC.[624] The European Lung Cancer Working Party confirmed the absence of a survival benefit, despite an improved antitumor response rate, when accelerating chemotherapy from every 3 weeks to every 2 weeks, using epirubicin, vindesine, and ifosfamide.[622] Moreover, recently announced results from British investigators again detected no improvement in response rate or survival, despite nearly doubling the dose intensity of ICE (ifosfamide, carboplatin, and etoposide) for six cycles by administering it every 2 weeks [with granulocyte colony-stimulating factor (GCSF) support and transfusions of autologous blood], compared to every 4 weeks.[623] As such, despite the optimistic conclusions of Tjan-Heijnen et al., the use of dose-intensified treatment via treatment acceleration cannot be recommended.[614]

Experience with Cisplatin and Prolonged Oral Etoposide

Oral etoposide has been examined as a potentially less toxic regiment that might be suitable for patients with an impaired performance status. The CALGB combined oral etoposide for 21 days with intravenous cisplatin, while investigators from the Medical Research Council and the London Lung Cancer Group examined the use of 21 days of oral etoposide as a single agent (Table 37.35).[625–627] These results indicate that oral etoposide yields significant myelosuppression and, even when used as a single agent in untreated, symptomatic patients, inferior efficacy outcomes, compared to intravenous doublet therapy.

Treatment of the Elderly Patient with SCLC

Treatment of elderly patients with extensive SCLC is, again, complicated by their increased rate of medical comorbidities and relative underrepresentation in clinical oncology trials.[521,628] Nonetheless, multiple groups have retrospectively reviewed treatment outcomes with elderly patients and determined from subset analyses that survival is not limited by advanced age alone, despite the reduced dose intensity often administered to elderly patients.[629–631]

Prospective data reporting the experience of chemotherapy in the treatment of elderly patients with extensive SCLC is limited to small Phase II studies. Investigators from the British Columbia Cancer Agency in Vancouver treated 66 SCLC patients over the age of 65, 41 with extensive-stage disease, with four cycles of cisplatin ($30 mg/m^2$), doxorubicin ($40 mg/m^2$), vincristine ($1.0 mg/m^2$), and etoposide ($100 mg/m^2$), repeated every 3 weeks (PAVE).[632] All four cycles of PAVE were delivered to 64% of the patients treated with chemotherapy only; only 27% of such patients required dose reductions. Of the extensive-stage patients, 15% required hospitalization for supportive care of toxicities, namely, febrile neutropenia. Antitumor response with this regimen measured 87% (24% with a complete response), and median survival was 11.5 months. However, chemotherapy efficacy outcomes are confounded by the fact that half the patients with extensive-stage disease also received radiotherapy as a part of their treatment.[632]

Multiple groups have used the combination of carboplatin and etoposide in their treatment of elderly SCLC patients

TABLE 37.35. Experience with oral etoposide (E).

Study	*N*	*Therapy*	*Overall response rate (%)*	*Time to progression (months)*	*Median survival (months)*	*One-year survival (%)*	*Comments*
Miller et al.[625]	306	IV CDDP + IV E	57	7	9.5	NR	Worsened myelosuppression, deaths due to febrile neutropenia with oral etoposide.
		IV CDDP[a] + oral E[a]	61	7	9.9	NR	
Girling et al.[626]	339	IV EP or CAV	51	NR	6.1	13	Enrollment terminated early with inferior survival.
		Oral E[b]	45	NR	4.3 ($P = 0.03$)	11	
Souhami et al.[627]	155	IV EP alternating with CAV	46.3	5.6	5.9	19.3	Enrollment terminated early with inferior survival
		Oral E[c]	32.9	3.6	4.8	9.8 ($P < 0.05$)	

CDDP, cisplatin; CAV, cisplatin, adriamycin, vincristine.

[a] $50 mg/m^2$ orally daily for 21 days every 28 days.

[b] 50 mg orally twice daily for 10 days every 21 days.

[c] 100 mg orally twice daily for 5 days every 21 days.

TABLE 37.36. Carboplatin (Cb)/etoposide (E) in elderly patients with extensive SCLC.

Study	*N*	*Therapy*	*Overall response rate (%)*	*Median survival (months)*	*One-year overall survival (%)*
Evans et al.[681]	36	Cb: 150 mg/m^2 day 1 E: 100 mg/m^2 × 7 days po	67	11.3	NR
Matsui et al.[682]	22	Cb: Egorin's formula E: 760 mg/m^2 po over 14 days	71	8.6	NR
Okamoto et al.[683]	20	Cb: AUC 5 day 1 E: 100 mg/m^2 po days 1–3	85	10.1	47
Quoix et al.[684]	26	Cb: AUC 5 day 1 E: 100 mg/m^2 IV days 1–3	60.5	8.6	26.3
Larive et al.[685]	28	Cb: AUC 5 day 1 E: 100 mg/m^2 po days 1–5	59	9.3	21

(Table 37.36). The Phase II experience is certainly broadest using the combination of carboplatin and etoposide for the treatment of elderly patients with extensive SCLC. At present, it represents the most reasonable combination regimen to consider for this population; however, hematologic toxicity can be significant.[629] It is imperative that future clinical trials in this population incorporate improved methods to assess geriatric functional status and extent of comorbidities to assist in the selection of patients who may benefit from systemic treatment.[633]

Second-Line Treatment

Although the majority of patients with extensive SCLC respond to first-line chemotherapy, relapse is virtually inevitable, usually within 8 months.[610,611,624] Approximately 45% to 60% of patients who receive combination first-line treatment proceed to second-line therapy.[611,634] Patients who receive best supportive care at relapse typically survive 2 to 4 months. Although comparative data are lacking, treatment at relapse with chemotherapy appears to positively impact survival.[635] A critical predictive marker of antitumor response with second-line treatment is the duration of the time to relapse, in that patients with primary refractory disease or those who relapse within 2 to 3 months of completing their first-line treatment (refractory relapse) are less likely to respond to salvage chemotherapy than patients who recur later following initial therapy (sensitive relapse). For instance, response rates of 6.4% and 11% and a median survival of 5 months were seen in studies of patients with refractory relapse treated with topotecan.[636,637] In contrast, response rates of 15% to 38% and a median survival of up to 7 months resulted from the use of topotecan in patients with sensitive relapse.[636,638,639] Uncontrolled trials with small numbers of patients suggest that repeat treatment with the same regimen that was used in the patient's initial therapy may offer clinical benefit, given a sufficiently long progression-free interval.[640,641] Clinical investigators more recently have used the somewhat arbitrary time to relapse of 90 days to distinguish those patients with refractory versus sensitive relapse. Data regarding the impact of systemic treatment at relapse on quality of life are sparse.[638,642]

Table 37.37 demonstrates recent examples of clinical trials examining second-line systemic treatment in SCLC. von Pawel et al. compared intravenous topotecan, dosed at

TABLE 37.37. Second-line systemic treatment in SCLC.

Study	*N*	*Therapy*	*Overall response rate (%)*	*Time to progression (months)*	*Median survival (%)*	*One-year survival (%)*	*Comments*
von Pawel et al.[638]	211	CAV Topotecan 1.5 mg/m^2 IV qd × 5 days	18.3 24.3	3.1 3.3	6.2 6.3	14.4 14.2	Greater symptom improvement with topotecan
von Pawel[639]	304	Topotecan 1.5 mg/m^2 IV qd × 5 days Topotecan 2.3 mg/m^2 po qd × 5 days	21.9 18.3	NR NR	8.8 8.3	29 33	No differences in symptom control or QOL
Masters et al.[644]	46	Gemcitabine 1,000 mg/m^2 days 1, 8, 15	16.7 (s) 5.6 (r)	NR	7.3 (s) 6.9 (r)	NR	
Hoang et al.[643]	27	Gemcitabine 1,250 mg/m^2 days 1 and 8	0	1.5 (s) 1.4 (r)	8.8 (s) 4.2 (r)	33.3 (s) 16.7 (r)	
Ardizzoni et al.[649]	110	Cisplatin 60 mg/m^2 day 1 Topotecan 0.75 mg/m^2 days 1–5	29.4 (s) 23.8 (r)	4.7 (s) 3.0 (r)	6.4 (s) 6.1 (r)	19.7 (s) 15.2 (r)	
Naka et al.[647]	29	Cb: AUC 2 days 1, 8, 15 CPT-11: 50 mg/m^2 days 1, 8, 15	37.5 (s) 23.1 (r)	NR NR	6.1 (s) 5.7 (r)	NR NR	
Hirose et al.[648]	24	Cb: AUC 5 day 1 CPT-11: 50 mg/m^2 days 1,8	92.3 (s) 33.3 (r)	NR NR	8.2 (s) 8.2 (r)	NR NR	

(s), sensitive relapse; (r), refractory or resistant relapse; QOL, quality of life.

1.5 mg/m² daily times 5 days every 21 days, versus CAV in 107 patients with sensitive relapsed extensive SCLC.[638] Response rates (24.3% for topotecan and 18.3% for CAV), median times to progression (13.3 and 12.3 weeks, respectively, for topotecan and CAV), and median overall survivals (25 weeks for topotecan and 24.7 weeks for CAV) were virtually superimposable. Differences between the two salvage treatments were seen with respect to worsened myelotoxicity and improved symptom control in patients receiving topotecan.[638] Oral topotecan offers more convenient administration while maintaining similar efficacy in the relapsed setting.[639] Toxicity profiles and FACT-L quality of life measurements were comparable between the intravenous and oral forms of this agent.[642]

Median survivals between 6 and 7 months and acceptable toxicities were seen in two Phase II trials of salvage gemcitabine.[643,644] Additional cytotoxics that appear to exert antitumor activity as second-line single agents include irinotecan, vinorelbine, and docetaxel.[635,645,646] Compared to the single-agent experience, rates of moderate to severe hematologic toxicities, including febrile neutropenia, are higher in recent Phase II trials using combination regimens in the setting of relapsed SCLC, with no improvement in survival.[647–649] Clearly, systemic treatment of refractory and relapsed SCLC remains fertile ground for clinical investigation examining the incorporation of novel anticancer agents, in an effort to improve patient survival, symptom control, and quality of life.

Novel Agents in the Treatment of SCLC

As with NSCLC, incorporation of novel, molecularly targeted therapeutics for patients with SCLC attempts to disrupt overexpressed or inappropriately activated cellular pathways that may be stimulating tumor cell growth, proliferation, invasion, and protection from apoptosis. As an example, blocking the antiapoptotic activity of Bcl-2 with antisense technology is under active investigation in SCLC. Bcl-2, a prototypical antiapoptotic protein, is expressed frequently in SCLC samples and has been shown to correlate negatively with prognosis.[650] G3139, an 18-base antisense oligonucleotide complementary to the bcl-2 mRNA, is thought to inhibit Bcl-2 mRNA translation and result in Rnase H-mediated mRNA degradation, and thereby result in augmented chemosensitivity.[651] G3139 has been combined with carboplatin and etoposide in untreated patients with extensive SCLC in the Phase I setting, and a comparative randomized trial of this doublet, with or without G3139, will be conducted by the CALGB.[651,652]

Treatment of patients with SCLC using STI571 (Gleevec) is intended to inhibit the tyrosine kinase activity of the kit receptor, which is part of an autocrine growth loop in SCLC. Four of 19 patients (21%) with untreated or sensitive relapsed SCLC were found in a Phase II study of STI571 to have kit (CD117) positivity per IHC staining.[653] Treatment of all 19 patients with STI571 yielded no antitumor responses, although 1 patient had prolonged stabilization of disease. Future studies with this agent will incorporate kit (CD117) preselection, in an effort to target the patient population who may benefit from this agent.

Additional examples of molecularly targeted agents under investigation in the treatment of SCLC include adjuvant therapy with the BEC2 vaccine, which mimics the ganglioside GD3, use of the tyrosine kinase inhibitor SU11248, which is targeted at the platelet-derived growth factor receptor, kit, and FLT3 receptors, treatment with the ubitquitin proteasome pathway inhibitor bortezomib, and treatment with 2A11, a monoclonal antibody directed against gastrin-releasing peptide.[654–656]

References

1. Giovino G. Epidemiology of tobacco use in the United States. Oncogene 2002;21(48):7326–7340.
2. Lam T, Ho S, Hedley A, Mak K, Peto R. Mortality and smoking in Hong Kong: case-control study of all adult deaths in 1998. BMJ 2001;323(7309):s361.
3. Thun M, Henley S, Calle E. Tobacco use and cancer: an epidemiologic perspective for geneticists. Oncogene 2002;21: 7307–7325.
4. Bogen K, Witschi H. Lung tumors in A/J mice exposed to environmental tobacco smoke: estimated potency and implied human risk. Carcinogenesis (Oxf) 2002;23(3):511–519.
5. Pfeifer G, Denissenko M, Olivier M, Tretyakova N, Hecht S, Hainaut P. Tobacco smoke carcinogens, DNA damage and p53 mutations in smoking-associated cancers. Oncogene 2002; 21(48):7435–7451.
6. Arora A, Willhite C, Liebler D. Interactions of beta-carotene and cigarette smoke in human bronchial epithelial cells. Carcinogenesis (Oxf) 2001;22(8):1173–1178.
7. Shields P. Molecular epidemiology of smoking and lung cancer. Oncogene 2002;21(45):6870–6876.
8. Izzotti A, Bagnasco M, D'Agostini F, Cartiglia, Lubet R, Kelloff G, De Flora S. Formation and persistence of nucleotide alterations in rats exposed whole-body to environmental cigarette smoke. Carcinogenesis (Oxf) 1999;20(8):1499–1505.
9. Besaratinia A, Maas L, Brouwer E, et al. A molecular dosimetry approach to assess human exposure to environmental tobacco smoke in pubs. Carcinogenesis (Oxf) 2002;23(7):1171–1176.
10. Peto R, Darby S, Deo H, Silcocks P, Whitley E, Doll R. Smoking, smoking cessation, and lung cancer in the UK since 1950: combination of national statistics with two case-control studies. BMJ 2000;321(7257):323–329.
11. Bach P, Kattan M, Thornquist M, et al. Variations in lung cancer risk among smokers. J Natl Cancer Inst 2003;95(6):470–478.
12. Ebbert J, Yang P, Vachon C, et al. Lung cancer risk reduction after smoking cessation: observations from a prospective cohort of women. J Clin Oncol 2003;21(5):921–926.
13. Marczynski B, Rihs H, Rossbach B, et al. Analysis of 8-oxo-7,8-dihydro-2′-deoxyguanosine and DNA strand breaks in white blood cells of occupationally exposed workers: comparison with ambient monitoring, urinary metabolites and enzyme polymorphisms. Carcinogenesis (Oxf) 2002;23(2):273–281.
14. Sato H, Sone H, Sagai M, Suzuki K, Aoki Y Increase in mutation frequency in lung of Big Blue rat by exposure to diesel exhaust. Carcinogenesis (Oxf) 2000;21(4):653–661.
15. Abdel-Rahman S, Ammenheuser M, Ward J Jr. Human sensitivity to 1,3-butadiene: role of microsomal epoxide hydrolase polymorphisms. Carcinogenesis (Oxf) 2001;22(3):415–423.
16. Hengstler J, Bolm-Audorff U, Faldum A, et al. Occupational exposure to heavy metals: DNA damage induction and DNA repair inhibition prove co-exposures to cadmium, cobalt and lead as more dangerous than hitherto expected. Carcinogenesis (Oxf) 2003;24(1):63–73.
17. Voorrips L, Goldbohm R, Verhoeven D, et al. Vegetable and fruit consumption and lung cancer risk in the Netherlands Cohort Study on diet and cancer. Cancer Causes Control 2000;11(2): 101–115.

18. Feskanich D, Ziegler R, Michaud D, et al. Prospective study of fruit and vegetable consumption and risk of lung cancer among men and women. J Natl Cancer Inst 2000;92(22):1812–1823.
19. Breslow R, Graubard B, Sinha R, Subar A. Diet and lung cancer mortality: a 1987 National Health Interview Survey cohort study. Cancer Causes Control 2000;11(5):419–431.
20. Wright M, Mayne S, Swanson C, Sinha R, Alavanja M. Dietary carotenoids, vegetables, and lung cancer risk in women: the Missouri women's health study (United States). Cancer Causes Control 2003;14(1):85–96.
21. Darby S, Whitley E, Doll R, Key T, Silcocks P. Diet, smoking and lung cancer: a case-control study of 1000 cases and 1500 controls in South-West England. Br J Cancer 2001;84(5):728–735.
22. Takezaki T, Hirose K, Inoue M, et al. Dietary factors and lung cancer risk in Japanese: with special reference to fish consumption and adenocarcinomas. Br J Cancer 2001;84(9):1199–1206.
23. Voorrips L, Goldbohm R, Brants H, et al. A prospective cohort study on antioxidant and folate intake and male lung cancer risk. Cancer Epidemiol Biomarkers Prev 2000;9(4):357–365.
24. Nyberg F, Hou S, Pershagen G, Lambert B. Dietary fruit and vegetables protect against somatic mutation in vivo, but low or high intake of carotenoids does not. Carcinogenesis (Oxf) 2003;24(4): 689–696.
25. Hennekens C, Buring J, et al. Lack of effect of long-term supplementation with beta carotene on the incidence of malignant neoplasms and cardiovascular disease. N Engl Med 1996;3334: 1145–1149.
26. The Alpha-Tocopherol, B. C. C. P. S. G. The effect of vitamin E and beta carotene on the incidence of lung cancer and other cancers in male smokers. N Engl J Med 1994;330(15):1029–1035.
27. Omenn G, Goodman G, et al. Effects of a combination of beta carotene and vitamin A on lung cancer and cardiovascular disease. N Engl J Med 1996;334:1150–1155.
28. Djousse L, Dorgan J, Zhang Y, et al. Alcohol consumption and risk of lung cancer: the Framingham Study. J Natl Cancer Inst 2002;94(24):1877–1882.
29. Shriver S, Bourdeau H, Gubish C, et al. Sex-specific expression of gastrin-releasing peptide receptor: relationship to smoking history and risk of lung cancer. J Natl Cancer Inst 2000;92(1): 24–33.
30. Kreuzer M, Boffetta P, Whitley E, et al. Gender differences in lung cancer risk by smoking: a multicentre case-control study in Germany and Italy. Br J Cancer 2000;82(1):227–233.
31. Cagle P, Mody D, Schwartz M. Estrogen and progesterone receptors in bronchogenic carcinoma. Cancer Res 1990;50(20): 6632–6635.
32. Siegfried J, Stabile L, Lerdtragool S, Romkes M. Hormones: do they make a difference in lung cancer? Lung Cancer 2003; 41(suppl 3):S95.
33. Cheng Y-W, Chiou H-L, Sheu G-T, et al. The association of human papillomavirus 16/18 infection with lung cancer among nonsmoking Taiwanese women. Cancer Res 2001;61(7): 2799–2803.
34. Spitz M, Wu X, Wei Q. Identifying the high risk subject: assessment of DNA damage and repair. Lung Cancer 2003;41(suppl 3):S95.
35. Rosell R, Pifarre A, Monzo M, et al. Reduced survival in patients with stage-I non-small-cell lung cancer associated with DNA-replication errors. Int J Cancer 1997;74(3):330–334.
36. Rosell R, Calvo R, Sanchez J, et al. Genetic susceptibility associated with rare HRAS1 variable number of tandem repeats alleles in Spanish non-small cell lung cancer patients. Clin Cancer Res 1999;5(7):1849–1854.
37. Krontiris T, Devlin B, Karp D, Robert N, Risch N. An association between the risk of cancer and mutations in the HRAS1 minisatellite locus. N Engl J Med 1993;329(8):517–523.
38. Schreiber G, Fong K, Peterson B, Johnson B, O'Briant K, Bepler G. Smoking, gender, and survival association with allele loss for the LOH11B lung cancer region on chromosome 11. Cancer Epidemiol Biomarkers Prev 1997;6(5):315–319.
39. Tang D, Phillips D, Stampfer M, et al. Association between carcinogen-DNA adducts in white blood cells and lung cancer risk in the physicians health study. Cancer Res 2001;61(18): 6708–6712.
40. Veglia F, Matullo G, Vineis P. Bulky DNA adducts and risk of cancer: a meta-analysis. Cancer Epidemiol Biomarkers Prev 2003;12(2):157–160.
41. Perera F, Mooney L, Stampfer M, et al. Associations between carcinogen-DNA damage, glutathione S-transferase genotypes, and risk of lung cancer in the prospective Physicians' Health Cohort Study. Carcinogenesis (Oxf) 2002;23(10):1641–1646.
42. Benhamou S, Lee W, Alexandrie A, et al. Meta- and pooled analyses of the effects of glutathione S-transferase M1 polymorphisms and smoking on lung cancer risk. Carcinogenesis (Oxf) 2002; 23(8):1343–1350.
43. London S, Yuan J, Travlos G, Gao Y, Wilson R, Ross R, Yu M. Insulin-like growth factor I, IGF-binding protein 3, and lung cancer risk in a prospective study of men in China. J Natl Cancer Inst 2002;94(10):749–754.
44. Moorehead R, Sanchez O, Baldwin R, Khokha R. Transgenic overexpression of IGF-II induces spontaneous lung tumors: a model for human lung adenocarcinoma. Oncogene 2003;22(6): 853–857.
45. Wei Q, Cheng L, Hong W, Spitz M. Reduced DNA repair capacity in lung cancer patients. Cancer Res 1996;56(18):4103–4107.
46. Wei Q, Cheng L, Amos C, et al. Repair of tobacco carcinogen-induced DNA adducts and lung cancer risk: a molecular epidemiologic study. J Natl Cancer Inst 2000;92(21):1764–1772.
47. Furuta T, Ueda T, Aune G, Sarasin A, Kraemer K, Pommier Y. Transcription-coupled nucleotide excision repair as a determinant of cisplatin sensitivity of human cells. Cancer Res 2002; 62(17):4899–4902.
48. Wu X, Zhao H, Wei Q, et al. XPA polymorphism associated with reduced lung cancer risk and a modulating effect on nucleotide excision repair capacity. Carcinogenesis (Oxf) 2003;24(3): 505–509.
49. Cheng L, Spitz M, Hong W, Wei Q. Reduced expression levels of nucleotide excision repair genes in lung cancer: a case-control analysis. Carcinogenesis (Oxf) 2000;21(8):1527–1530.
50. Vogel U, Dybdahl M, Frentz G, Nexo B. DNA repair capacity: inconsistency between effect of over-expression of five NER genes and the correlation to mRNA levels in primary lymphocytes. Mutat Res 2000;461(3):197–210.
51. Spitz M, Wu X, Wang Y, et al. Modulation of nucleotide excision repair capacity by XPD polymorphisms in lung cancer patients. Cancer Res 2001;61(4):1354–1357.
52. Qiao Y, Spitz M, Shen H, et al. Modulation of repair of ultraviolet damage in the host-cell reactivation assay by polymorphic XPC and XPD/ERCC2 genotypes. Carcinogenesis (Oxf) 2002; 23(2):295–299.
53. Matullo G, Palli D, Peluso M, et al. XRCC1, XRCC3, XPD gene polymorphisms, smoking and (32)P-DNA adducts in a sample of healthy subjects. Carcinogenesis (Oxf) 2001;22(9):1437–1445.
54. Zhou W, Liu G, Miller D, et al. Polymorphisms in the DNA repair genes XRCC1 and ERCC2, smoking, and lung cancer risk. Cancer Epidemiol Biomarkers Prev 2003;12(4):359–365.
55. Wistuba I, Mao L, Gazdar A. Smoking molecular damage in bronchial epithelium. Oncogene 2002;21(48):7298–7306.
56. Ghaffar H, Sahin F, Sanchez-Cepedes M, et al. LKB1 protein expression in the evolution of glandular neoplasia of the lung. Clin Cancer Res 2003;9(8):2998–3003.
57. Wistuba I, Behrens C, Virmani A, et al. High resolution chromosome 3p allelotyping of human lung cancer and preneoplastic/preinvasive bronchial epithelium reveals multiple, discontinuous sites of 3p allele loss and three regions of frequent breakpoints. Cancer Res 2000;60(7):1949–1960.

58. Rodenhuis S, van de Wetering M, Mooi W, Evers S, van Zandwijk N, Bos J. Mutational activation of the K-ras oncogene. A possible pathogenetic factor in adenocarcinoma of the lung. N Engl J Med 1987;317(15):929–935.
59. Slebos R, Kibbelaar R, Dalesio O, et al. K-ras oncogene activation as a prognostic marker in adenocarcinoma of the lung. N Engl J Med 1990;323(9):561–565.
60. Mitsudomi T, Viallet J, Mulshine J, Linnoila R, Minna J, Gazdar A. Mutations of ras genes distinguish a subset of non-small-cell lung cancer cell lines from small-cell lung cancer cell lines. Oncogene 1991;6(8):1353–1362.
61. Mitsudomi T, Steinberg S, Nau M, et al. p53 gene mutations in non-small-cell lung cancer cell lines and their correlation with the presence of ras mutations and clinical features. Oncogene 1992;7(1):171–180.
62. Bianco R, Shin I, Ritter C, et al. Loss of PTEN/MMAC1/TEP in EGF receptor-expressing tumor cells counteracts the antitumor action of EGFR tyrosine kinase inhibitors. Oncogene 2003;22(18):2812–2822.
63. Song L, Turkson J, Karras J, Jove R, Haura E. Activation of Stat3 by receptor tyrosine kinases and cytokines regulates survival in human non-small cell carcinoma cells. Oncogene 2003;22(27):4150–4165.
64. Semenza G. Signal transduction to hypoxia-inducible factor 1. Biochem Pharmacol 2002;64(5–6):993–998.
65. Marrogi A, Travis W, Welsh J, et al. Nitric oxide synthase, cyclooxygenase 2, and vascular endothelial growth factor in the angiogenesis of non-small cell lung carcinoma. Clin Cancer Res 2000;6(12):4739–4744.
66. Jimenez A, Fernandez P, Dominguez O, Dopazo A, Sanchez-Cespedes M. Growth and molecular profile of lung cancer cells expressing ectopic LKB1: down-regulation of the phosphatidylinositol 3′-phosphate kinase/PTEN pathway. Cancer Res 2003;63(6):1382–1388.
67. Garber M, Troyanskaya O, Schluens K, et al. Diversity of gene expression in adenocarcinoma of the lung. Proc Natl Acad Sci USA 2001;98(24):13784–13789.
68. Bhattacharjee A, Richards W, Staunton J, et al. Classification of human lung carcinomas by mRNA expression profiling reveals distinct adenocarcinoma subclasses. Proc Natl Acad Sci USA 2001;98(24):13790–13795.
69. Giordano T, Shedden K, Schwartz D, et al. Organ-specific molecular classification of primary lung, colon, and ovarian adenocarcinomas using gene expression profiles. Am J Pathol 2001;159(4):1231–1238.
70. Chen G, Gharib T, Huang C, et al. Proteomic analysis of lung adenocarcinoma: identification of a highly expressed set of proteins in tumors. Clin Cancer Res 2002;8(7):2298–2305.
71. Chen G, Gharib T, Huang C, et al. Discordant protein and mRNA expression in lung adenocarcinomas. Mol Cell Proteomics 2002;1(4):304–313.
72. Honorio S, Agathanggelou A, Schuermann M, et al. Detection of RASSF1A aberrant promoter hypermethylation in sputum from chronic smokers and ductal carcinoma in situ from breast cancer patients. Oncogene 2003;22(1):147–150.
73. Soria J, Rodriguez M, Liu D, Lee J, Hong W, Mao L. Aberrant promoter methylation of multiple genes in bronchial brush samples from former cigarette smokers. Cancer Res 2002;62(2):351–355.
74. Kersting M, Friedl C, Kraus A, Behn M, Pankow W, Schuermann M. Differential frequencies of p16(INK4a) promoter hypermethylation, p53 mutation, and K-ras mutation in exfoliative material mark the development of lung cancer in symptomatic chronic smokers. J Clin Oncol 2000;18(18):3221–3229.
75. Leon S, Shapiro B, Sklaroff D, Yaros M. Free DNA in the serum of cancer patients and the effect of therapy. Cancer Res 1977;37(3):646–650.
76. Chen X, Stroun M, Magnenat J, et al. Microsatellite alterations in plasma DNA of small cell lung cancer patients. Nat Med,1996;2(9):1033–1035.
77. Sanchez-Cespedes M, Monzo M, Rosell R, et al. Detection of chromosome 3p alterations in serum DNA of non-small-cell lung cancer patients. Ann Oncol 1998;9(1):113–116.
78. Sozzi G, Musso K, Ratcliffe C, Goldstraw P, Pierotti M, Pastorino U. Detection of microsatellite alterations in plasma DNA of non-small cell lung cancer patients: a prospect for early diagnosis. Clin Cancer Res 1999;5(10):2689–2692.
79. Sozzi G, Conte D, Mariani L, et al. Analysis of circulating tumor DNA in plasma at diagnosis and during follow-up of lung cancer patients. Cancer Res 2001;61(12):4675–4678.
80. Allan J, Hardie L, Briggs J, et al. Genetic alterations in bronchial mucosa and plasma DNA from individuals at high risk of lung cancer. Int J Cancer 2001;91(3):359–365.
81. Esteller M, Sanchez-Cespedes M, Rosell D, Sidransky D, Baylin S, Herman J. Detection of aberrant promoter hypermethylation of tumor suppressor genes in serum DNA from non-small cell lung cancer patients. Cancer Res 1999;59(1):67–70.
82. Mao L. Recent advances in the molecular diagnosis of lung cancer. Oncogene 2002;21(45):6960–6969.
83. Scott F, Modali R, Lehman T, et al. High frequency of K-ras codon 12 mutations in bronchoalveolar lavage fluid of patients at high risk for second primary lung cancer. Clin Cancer Res 1997;3(3):479–482.
84. Toyooka S, Toyooka K, Maruyama R, et al. DNA methylation profiles of lung tumors. Mol Cancer Ther 2001;1(1):61–67.
85. Rosell R, Monzo M, O'Brate A, Taron M. Translational oncogenomics: toward rational therapeutic decision-making. Curr Opin Oncol 2002;14(2):171–179.
86. Palmisano W, Divine K, Saccomanno G, et al. Predicting lung cancer by detecting aberrant promoter methylation in sputum. Cancer Res 2000;60(21):5954–5958.
87. Belinsky S, Palmisano W, Gilliland L, et al. Aberrant promoter methylation in bronchial epithelium and sputum from current and former smokers. Cancer Res 2002;62(8):2370–2377.
88. McWilliams A, MacAulay C, Gazdar A, Lam S. Innovative molecular and imaging approaches for the detection of lung cancer and its precursor lesions. Oncogene 2002;21(45):6949–6959.
89. Hirsch F, Prindiville S, Miller Y, et al. Fluorescence versus white-light bronchoscopy for detection of preneoplastic lesions: a randomized study. J Natl Cancer Inst 2001;93(18):1385–1391.
90. Keith R, Miller Y, Gemmill R, et al. Angiogenic squamous dysplasia in bronchi of individuals at high risk for lung cancer. Clin Cancer Res 2000;6(5):1616–1625.
91. Colby T, Koss M, Travis W. Tumors of the lower respiratory tract. In: Rosai J, Sobin L (eds). Atlas of Tumor Pathology. Washington, DC: Armed Forces Institute of Pathology, 1995.
92. Hirsch F, Matthews M, Aisner S, et al. Histopathologic classification of small cell lung cancer. Changing concepts and terminology. Cancer (Phila) 1988;62(5):973–977.
93. Travis W. High-grade neuroendocrine (NE) tumors: what we know and important unanswered questions. Lung Cancer 2003;41(suppl 41):S101.
94. Brambilla E. Molecular pathology of neuroendocrine lung tumors. Lung Cancer 2003;41(suppl 41):S16–S17.
95. Hirsch F, Scagliotti G, Langer C, Varella-Garcia M, Franklin W. Epidermal growth factor family of receptors in preneoplasia and lung cancer: perspectives for targeted therapies. Lung Cancer 2003;41(suppl 41):S29–S42.
96. Albain K, Crowley J, LeBlanc M, Livingston R. Survival determinants in extensive-stage non-small-cell lung cancer: the Southwest Oncology Group experience. J Clin Oncol 1991;9(9):1618–1626.
97. Paesmans M, Sculier J, Libert P, et al. Prognostic factors for survival in advanced non-small-cell lung cancer: univariate and multivariate analyses including recursive partitioning and

amalgamation algorithms in 1,052 patients. The European Lung Cancer Working Party. J Clin Oncol 1995;13(5):1221–1230.
98. O'Connell J, Kris M, Gralla R, et al. Frequency and prognostic importance of pretreatment clinical characteristics in patients with advanced non-small-cell lung cancer treated with combination chemotherapy. J Clin Oncol 1986;4(11):1604–1614.
99. Alberola V, Camps C, Provencio M, et al. Cisplatin plus gemcitabine versus a cisplatin-based triplet versus nonplatinum sequential doublets in advanced non-small-cell lung cancer: a Spanish Lung Cancer Group phase III randomized trial. J Clin Oncol 2003;21(17):3207–3213.
100. Albain K, Rusch V, Crowley J, et al. Concurrent cisplatin/etoposide plus chest radiotherapy followed by surgery for stages IIIA (N2) and IIIB non-small-cell lung cancer: mature results of Southwest Oncology Group phase II study 8805. J Clin Oncol 1995;13(8):1880–1892.
101. Zeng-Rong N, Paterson J, Alpert L, Tsao M, Viallet J, Alaoui-Jamali M. Elevated DNA repair capacity is associated with intrinsic resistance of lung cancer to chemotherapy. Cancer Res 1995;55(21):4760–4764.
102. Bosken C, Wei Q, Amos C, Spitz M. An analysis of DNA repair as a determinant of survival in patients with non-small-cell lung cancer. J Natl Cancer Inst 2002;94(14):1091–1099.
103. Blommaert F, Michael C, Terheggen P, et al. Drug-induced DNA modification in buccal cells of cancer patients receiving carboplatin and cisplatin combination chemotherapy, as determined by an immunocytochemical method: interindividual variation and correlation with disease response. Cancer Res 1993;53(23):5669–5675.
104. Schellens J, Ma J, Planting A, et al. Relationship between the exposure to cisplatin, DNA-adduct formation in leuocytes and tumour response in patients with solid tumours. Br J Cancer 1996;73(12):1569–1575.
105. Schaake-Koning C, van den Bogaert W, Dalesio O, et al. Effects of concomitant cisplatin and radiotherapy on inoperable non-small-cell lung cancer. N Engl J Med 1992;326(8):524–530.
106. Van de Vaart P, Belderbos J, de Jong D, et al. DNA-adduct levels as a predictor of outcome for NSCLC patients receiving daily cisplatin and radiotherapy. Int J Cancer 2000;89(2):160–166.
107. Leij-Halfwerk S, van den Berg J, Sijens P, Wilson J, Oudkerk M, Dagnelie P. Altered hepatic gluconeogenesis during L-alanine infusion in weight-losing lung cancer patients as observed by phosphorus magnetic resonance spectroscopy and turnover measurements. Cancer Res 2000;60(3):618–623.
108. Osthus R, Shim H, Kim S, et al. Deregulation of glucose transporter 1 and glycolytic gene expression by c-Myc. J Biol Chem 2000;275(29):21797–21800.
109. Chen G, Gharib TG, Wang H, et al. Protein profiles associated with survival in lung adenocarcinoma. Proc Natl Acad Sci USA 2003;100(23):13537–13542.
110. Lay A, Jiang X, Kisker O, et al. Phosphoglycerate kinase acts in tumour angiogenesis as a disulphide reductase. Nature (Lond) 2000;408(6814):869–873.
111. Weber W, Petersen V, Schmidt B, et al. Positron emission tomography in non-small-cell lung cancer: prediction of response to chemotherapy by quantitative assessment of glucose use. J Clin Oncol 2003;21(14):2651–2657.
112. Lord R, Brabender J, Gandara D, et al. Low ERCC1 expression correlates with prolonged survival after cisplatin plus gemcitabine chemotherapy in non-small cell lung cancer. Clin Cancer Res 2002;8(7):2286–2291.
113. Lee Y, Vassilakos A, Feng N, et al. GTI-2040, an antisense agent targeting the small subunit component (R2) of human ribonucleotide reductase, shows potent antitumor activity against a variety of tumors. Cancer Res 2003;63(11):2802–2811.
114. Rosell R, Scagliotti G, Danenberg K, et al. Transcripts in pretreatment biopsies from a three-arm randomized trial in metastatic non-small-cell lung cancer. Oncogene 2003;22(23):3548–3553.
115. Sowers R, Toguchida J, Qin J, et al. mRNA expression levels of E2F transcription factors correlate with dihydrofolate reductase, reduced folate carrier, and thymidylate synthase mRNA expression in osteosarcoma. Mol Cancer Ther 2003;2(6):535–541.
116. Osada H, Takahashi T. Genetic alterations of multiple tumor suppressors and oncogenes in the carcinogenesis and progression of lung cancer. Oncogene 2002;21(48):7421–7434.
117. Mitsudomi T, Steinberg S, Oie H, et al. ras gene mutations in non-small cell lung cancers are associated with shortened survival irrespective of treatment intent. Cancer Res 1991;51(18):4999–5002.
118. Rosell R, Li S, Skacel Z, et al. Prognostic impact of mutated K-ras gene in surgically resected non-small cell lung cancer patients. Oncogene 1993;8(9):2407–2412.
119. Nelson H, Christiani D, Mark E, Wiencke J, Wain J, Kelsey K. Implications and prognostic value of K-ras mutation for early-stage lung cancer in women. J Natl Cancer Inst 1999;91(23):2032–2038.
120. Graziano S, Gamble G, Newman N, et al. Prognostic significance of K-ras codon 12 mutations in patients with resected stage I and II non-small-cell lung cancer. J Clin Oncol 1999;17(2):668–675.
121. Schiller J, Adak S, Feins R, et al. Lack of prognostic significance of p53 and K-ras mutations in primary resected non-small-cell lung cancer on E4592: a laboratory ancillary study on an Eastern Cooperative Oncology Group prospective randomized trial of postoperative adjuvant therapy. J Clin Oncol 2001;19(2):448–457.
122. Rosell R, Gomez-Codina J, Camps C, et al. A randomized trial comparing preoperative chemotherapy plus surgery with surgery alone in patients with non-small-cell lung cancer. N Engl J Med 1994;330(3):153–158.
123. Broermann P, Junker K, Brandt B, et al. Trimodality treatment in stage III nonsmall cell lung carcinoma: prognostic impact of K-ras mutations after neoadjuvant therapy. Cancer (Phila) 2002;94(7):2055–2062.
124. Khuri F, Lotan R, Kemp B, et al. Retinoic acid receptor-beta as a prognostic indicator in stage I non-small-cell lung cancer. J Clin Oncol 2000;18(15):2798–2804.
125. Achiwa H, Yatabe Y, Hida T, et al. Prognostic significance of elevated cyclooxygenase 2 expression in primary, resected lung adenocarcinomas. Clin Cancer Res 1999;5(5):1001–1005.
126. Khuri F, Wu H, Lee J, et al. Cyclooxygenase-2 overexpression is a marker of poor prognosis in stage I non-small cell lung cancer. Clin Cancer Res 2001;7(4):861–867.
127. Tang X, Khuri F, Lee J, et al. Hypermethylation of the death-associated protein (DAP) kinase promoter and aggressiveness in stage I non-small-cell lung cancer. J Natl Cancer Inst 2000;92(18):1511–1516.
128. Burbee D, Forgacs E, Zochbauer-Muller S, et al. Epigenetic inactivation of RASSF1A in lung and breast cancers and malignant phenotype suppression. J Natl Cancer Inst 2001;93(9):691–699.
129. Ramirez J, Sarries C, de Castro P, et al. Methylation patterns and K-ras mutations in tumor and paired serum of resected non-small-cell lung cancer patients. Cancer Lett 2003;193(2):207–216.
130. Shih J, Yang S, Hong T, et al. Collapsin response mediator protein-1 and the invasion and metastasis of cancer cells. J Natl Cancer Inst 2001;93(18):1392–1400.
131. Yuan A, Yang P, Yu C. Interleukin-8 messenger ribonucleic acid expression correlates with tumor progression, tumor angiogenesis, patient survival, and timing of relapse in non-small-cell lung cancer. Am J Respir Crit Care Med 2000;162(5):1957–1963.
132. Soria J, Moon C, Kemp B, et al. Lack of interleukin-10 expression could predict poor outcome in patients with stage I non-small cell lung cancer. Clin Cancer Res 2003;9(5):1785–1791.

133. Tomiyasu M, Yoshino I, Suemitsu R, Okamoto T, Sugimachi K. Quantification of macrophage migration inhibitory factor mRNA expression in non-small cell lung cancer tissues and its clinical significance. Clin Cancer Res 2002;8(12):3755–3760.
134. Moran C, Arenberg D, Huang C, et al. RANTES expression is a predictor of survival in stage I lung adenocarcinoma. Clin Cancer Res 2002;8(12):3803–3812.
135. Chang Y, Wang L, Liu D, et al. Correlation between insulin-like growth factor-binding protein-3 promoter methylation and prognosis of patients with stage I non-small cell lung cancer. Clin Cancer Res 2002;8(12):3669–3675.
136. Bepler G, Gautam A, McIntyre L, et al. Prognostic significance of molecular genetic aberrations on chromosome segment 11p15.5 in non-small-cell lung cancer. J Clin Oncol 2002;20(5): 1353–1360.
137. Simon G, Sharma S, Smith P, Bepler G. Increased ERCC1 expression predicts for improved survival in resected patients with non-small-cell lung cancer (NSCLC). Eur J Cancer 2002;38(suppl):S15.
138. Ramaswamy S, Ross K, Lander E, Golub T. A molecular signature of metastasis in primary solid tumors. Nat Genet 2003; 33(1):49–54.
139. Beer D, Kardia S, Huang C, et al. Gene-expression profiles predict survival of patients with lung adenocarcinoma. Nat Med 2002;8(8):816–824.
140. Singhal S, Wiewrodt R, Malden L, et al. Gene expression profiling of malignant mesothelioma. Clin Cancer Res 2003;9(8): 3080–3097.
141. Yanagisawa K, Shyr Y, Xu B, et al. Proteomic patterns of tumour subsets in non-small-cell lung cancer. Lancet 2003;362(9382): 433–439.
142. Meert A, Paesmans M, Martin B, et al. The role of microvessel density on the survival of patients with lung cancer: a systematic review of the literature with meta-analysis. Br J Cancer 2002;87(7):694–701.
143. Chen J, Yao P, Yuan A, et al. Up-regulation of tumor interleukin-8 expression by infiltrating macrophages: its correlation with tumor angiogenesis and patient survival in non-small cell lung cancer. Clin Cancer Res 2003;9(2):729–737.
144. Inoshima N, Nakanishi Y, Minami T, et al. The influence of dendritic cell infiltration and vascular endothelial growth factor expression on the prognosis of non-small cell lung cancer. Clin Cancer Res 2002;8(11):3480–3486.
145. Tanaka F, Ishikawa S, Yanagihara K, et al. Expression of angiopoietins and its clinical significance in non-small cell lung cancer. Cancer Res 2002;62(23):7124–7129.
146. Brett GZ. Earlier diagnosis and survival in lung cancer. Br Med J 1969;4:260–262.
147. Brett GZ. The value of lung cancer detection by six-monthly chest radiographs. Thorax 1968;23:414–420.
148. Melamed MR. Lung cancer screening results in the National Cancer Institute New York study. Cancer (Phila) 2000;89: 2356–2362.
149. Frost JK, Ball WCJ, Levin ML, et al. Early lung cancer detection: results of the initial (prevalence) radiologic and cytologic screening in the Johns Hopkins study. Am Rev Respir Dis 1984;130: 549–554.
150. Fontana RS, Sanderson DR, Taylor WF, et al. Early lung cancer detection: results of the initial (prevalence) radiologic and cytologic screening in the Mayo Clinic study. Am Rev Respir Dis 1984;130:561–565.
151. Fontana R.S. The Mayo Lung Project: a perspective, Cancer, 2000;89:2352–2355.
152. Fontana RS, Sanderson DR, Woolner LB, et al. Screening for lung cancer. A critique of the Mayo Lung Project. Cancer (Phila) 1991;67:1155–1164.
153. Kubik A, Parkin DM, Khlat M, Erban J, Polak J, Adamec M. Lack of benefit from semi-annual screening for cancer of the lung: follow-up report of a randomized controlled trial on a population of high-risk males in Czechoslovakia. Int J Cancer 1990;45: 26–33.
154. Kubik A, Polak J. Lung cancer detection. Results of a randomized prospective study in Czechoslovakia. Cancer (Phila) 1986; 57:2427–2437.
155. Kubik AK, Parkin DM, Zatloukal P. Czech Study on Lung Cancer Screening: post-trial follow-up of lung cancer deaths up to year 15 since enrollment. Cancer (Phila) 2000;89:2363–2368.
156. Black WC. Should this patient be screened for cancer? Effect Clin Pract 1999;2:86–95.
157. Marcus PM. Lung cancer screening: an update. J Clin Oncol 2001;19:83S–86S.
158. Marcus PM, Bergstralh EJ, Fagerstrom RM, et al. Lung cancer mortality in the Mayo Lung Project: impact of extended follow-up. J Natl Cancer Inst 2000;92:1308–1316.
159. Marcus PM, Prorok PC. Reanalysis of the Mayo Lung Project data: the impact of confounding and effect modification. J Med Screen 1999;6:47–49.
160. Strauss GM, Gleason RE, Sugarbaker DJ. Chest X-ray screening improves outcome in lung cancer. A reappraisal of randomized trials on lung cancer screening. Chest 1995;107:270S–279S.
161. Eddy DM. Screening for lung cancer. Ann Intern Med 1989;111: 232–237.
162. Patz EF Jr, Goodman PC, Bepler G. Screening for lung cancer. N Engl J Med 2000;343:1627–1633.
163. Tockman MS, Anthonisen NR, Wright EC, Donithan MG. Airways obstruction and the risk for lung cancer. Ann Intern Med 1987;106:512–518.
164. Johnson BE, Cortazar P, Chute JP. Second lung cancers in patients successfully treated for lung cancer. Semin Oncol 1997;24:492–499.
165. SaitoY, Nagamoto N, Ota S, et al. Results of surgical treatment for roentgenographically occult bronchogenic squamous cell carcinoma. J Thorac Cardiovasc Surg 1992;104:401–407.
166. Stoeckli SJ, Zimmermann R, Schmid S. Role of routine panendoscopy in cancer of the upper aerodigestive tract. Otolaryngol Head Neck Surg 2001;124:208–212.
167. Kramer BS, Gohagan J, Prorok PC, Smart C. A National Cancer Institute sponsored screening trial for prostatic, lung, colorectal, and ovarian cancers. Cancer (Phila) 1993;71:589–593.
168. Sone S, Li F, Yang ZG, et al. Results of three-year mass screening programme for lung cancer using mobile low-dose spiral computed tomography scanner. Br J Cancer 2001;84:25–32.
169. Sone S, Takashima S, Li F, et al. Mass screening for lung cancer with mobile spiral computed tomography scanner. Lancet 1998;351:1242–1245.
170. Henschke CI, Yankelevitz DF, Libby D, Kimmel M. CT screening for lung cancer: the first ten years. Cancer J 2002;8(suppl 1): S47–S54.
171. Henschke CI, McCauley DI, Yankelevitz DF, et al. Early Lung Cancer Action Project: overall design and findings from baseline screening. Lancet 1999;354:99–105.
172. Henschke CI, Yankelevitz DF, Smith JP, Miettinen OS. Screening for lung cancer: the early lung cancer action approach. Lung Cancer 2002;35:143–148.
173. Swensen SJ, Jett JR, Hartman TE, et al. Lung cancer screening with CT: Mayo Clinic experience. Radiology 2003;226:756–761.
174. Bocking A, Biesterfeld S, Chatelain R, Gien-Gerlach G, Esser E. Diagnosis of bronchial carcinoma on sections of paraffin-embedded sputum. Sensitivity and specificity of an alternative to routine cytology. Acta Cytol 1992;36:37–47.
175. Gazdar AF, Minna JD. Molecular detection of early lung cancer [editorial; comment]. J Natl Cancer Inst 1999;91:299–301.
176. Tockman MS, Mulshine JL. The early detection of occult lung cancer. Chest Surg Clin N Am 2000;10:737–749.
177. Tockman MS. Clinical detection of lung cancer progression markers. J Cell Biochem (Suppl) 1996;25:177–184.

178. Ikeda N, Macaulay C, Lam S, et al. Malignancy associated changes in bronchial epithelial cells and clinical application as a biomarker. Lung Cancer 1998;19:161–166.
179. Ahrendt SA, Chow JT, Xu LH, et al. Molecular detection of tumor cells in bronchoalveolar lavage fluid from patients with early stage lung cancer. J Natl Cancer Inst 1999;91:332–339.
180. Belinsky SA, Nikula KJ, Palmisano WA, et al. Aberrant methylation of p16(INK4a) is an early event in lung cancer and a potential biomarker for early diagnosis. Proc Natl Acad Sci U S A 1998;95:11891–11896.
181. Anderson M, Sladon S, Michels R, et al. Examination of p53 alterations and cytokeratin expression in sputa collected from patients prior to histological diagnosis of squamous cell carcinoma. J Cell Biochem (Suppl) 1996;25:185–190.
182. Dai Z, Lakshmanan RR, Zhu WG, et al. Global methylation profiling of lung cancer identifies novel methylated genes. Neoplasia 2001;3:314–323.
183. Mao L, Lee DJ, Tockman MS, Erozan YS, Askin F, Sidransky D. Microsatellite alterations as clonal markers for the detection of human cancer. Proc Natl Acad Sci U S A 1994;91:9871–9875.
184. Sato M, Sakurada A, Sagawa M, et al. Diagnostic results before and after introduction of autofluorescence bronchoscopy in patients suspected of having lung cancer detected by sputum cytology in lung cancer mass screening. Lung Cancer 2001;32: 247–253.
185. Lam S, Lam B, Petty TL. Early detection for lung cancer. New tools for case finding. Can Fam Physician 2001;47:537–544.
186. Lam S, Kennedy T, Unger M, et al. Localization of bronchial intraepithelial neoplastic lesions by fluorescence bronchoscopy. Chest 1998;113:696–702.
187. Mountain CF. Revisions in the International System for Staging Lung Cancer. Chest 1997;111:1710–1717.
188. Rusch VW. Surgery for stage III non-small cell lung cancer. Cancer Control 1994;1:455–466.
189. van Rens MT, de la Riviere AB, Elbers HR, van den Bosch JM. Prognostic assessment of 2,361 patients who underwent pulmonary resection for non-small cell lung cancer, stage I, II, and IIIA. Chest 2000;117:374–379.
190. Martini N, Flehinger BJ, Zaman MB, Beattie EJ Jr. Results of resection in non-oat cell carcinoma of the lung with mediastinal lymph node metastases. Ann Surg 1983;198:386–397.
191. Mountain CF. Surgery for stage IIIa-N2 non-small cell lung cancer. Cancer (Phila) 1994;73:2589–2598.
192. Vansteenkiste JF, De Leyn PR, Deneffe GJ, et al. Survival and prognostic factors in resected N2 non-small cell lung cancer: a study of 140 cases. Leuven Lung Cancer Group. Ann Thorac Surg 1997;63:1441–1450.
193. Miller DL, McManus KG, Allen MS, et al. Results of surgical resection in patients with N2 non-small cell lung cancer. Ann Thorac Surg 1994;57:1095–1100.
194. Watanabe Y, Hayashi Y, Shimizu J, Oda M, Iwa T. Mediastinal nodal involvement and the prognosis of non-small cell lung cancer. Chest 1991;100:422–428.
195. Goldstraw P, Mannam GC, Kaplan DK, Michail P. Surgical management of non-small-cell lung cancer with ipsilateral mediastinal node metastasis (N2 disease). J Thorac Cardiovasc Surg 1994;107:19–27.
196. Naruke T, Suemasu K, Ishikawa S. Lymph node mapping and curability at various levels of metastasis in resected lung cancer. J Thorac Cardiovasc Surg 1978;76:832–839.
197. Conill C, Astudillo J, Verger E. Prognostic significance of metastases to mediastinal lymph node levels in resected non-small cell lung carcinoma. Cancer (Phila) 1993;72:1199–1202.
198. Okada M, Tsubota N, Yoshimura M, Miyamoto Y, Matsuoka H. Prognosis of completely resected pN2 non-small cell lung carcinomas: what is the significant node that affects survival? J Thorac Cardiovasc Surg 1999;118:270–275.
199. Scagliotti GV, Novello S. Adjuvant therapy in completely resected non-small-cell lung cancer. Curr Oncol Rep 2003;5: 318–325.
200. Movsas B. Role of adjuvant therapy in resected stage II/IIIA non-small-cell lung cancer. Oncology (Huntingt) 2002;16:90–95, 100.
201. Keller SM, Adak S, Wagner H, et al. A randomized trial of postoperative adjuvant therapy in patients with completely resected stage II or IIIA non-small-cell lung cancer. Eastern Cooperative Oncology Group, N Engl J Med 2000;343:1217–1222.
202. Albain KS. Induction chemotherapy or chemoradiotherapy before surgery for non-small-cell lung cancer. Curr Oncol Rep 2000;2:54–63.
203. Andre F, Grunenwald D, Pignon JP, et al. Survival of patients with resected N2 non-small-cell lung cancer: evidence for a subclassification and implications. J Clin Oncol 2000;18:2981–2989.
204. Toloza EM, Harpole L, Detterbeck F, McCrory DC. Invasive staging of non-small cell lung cancer: a review of the current evidence. Chest 2003;123:157S–166S.
205. Detterbeck F, Kiser A, Detterbeck FC, Kiser AC. In: Detterbeck FC, Rivera MP, Socinski MA, Rosenman JG (eds). Anonymous Diagnosis and Treatment of Lung Cancer: An Evidence-Based Guide for the Practicing Clinician. Philadelphia: Saunders, 2001:223–232.
206. Toloza EM, Harpole L, McCrory DC. Noninvasive staging of non-small cell lung cancer: a review of the current evidence. Chest 2003;123:137S–146S.
207. Schaefer-Prokop C, Prokop M. New imaging techniques in the treatment guidelines for lung cancer. Eur Respir J (Suppl) 2002; 35:71s–83.
208. Margery J, Grahek D, Vaylet F, et al. Impact of FDG PET imaging on clinical management in patients with resectable NSCLC: a prospective multicentric French study. Lung Cancer 2003;41:s13 (abstract).
209. Yap CS, Schiepers C, Fishbein MC, Phelps ME, Czernin J. FDG-PET imaging in lung cancer: how sensitive is it for bronchioloalveolar carcinoma? Eur J Nucl Med Mol Imaging 2002;29:1166–1173.
210. Shure D, Fedullo PF. Transbronchial needle aspiration in the diagnosis of submucosal and peribronchial bronchogenic carcinoma. Chest 1985;88:49–51.
211. Sutedja TG, Venmans BJ, Smit EF, Postmus PE. Fluorescence bronchoscopy for early detection of lung cancer: a clinical perspective. Lung Cancer 2001;34:157–168.
212. Herth FJ, Becker HD, Ernst A. Ultrasound-guided transbronchial needle aspiration: an experience in 242 patients. Chest 2003;123: 604–607.
213. Wiersema M, Edell E, Midthun D. Prospective comparison of transbronchial needle aspirate (TBNA) and endosonography guided biopsy (EUS-FNA) of mediastinal lymph nodes in patients with known or suspected non small cell lung cancer. In: Anonymous 2002.
214. Devereaux B, Ciaccia D, Imperiale T. Clinical utility of endoscopic ultrasound guided FNA in the preoperative staging of non-small cell lung cancer in computerized tomography negative patients. In: Anonymous 2001.
215. Naruke T. Significance of lymph node metastases in lung cancer. Semin Thorac Cardiovasc Surg 1993;5:210–218.
216. Mountain CF, Dresler CM. Regional lymph node classification for lung cancer staging. Chest 1997;111:1718–1723.
217. Mountain CF. A new international staging system for lung cancer. Chest 1986;89:225S–233S.
218. Lee JD, Ginsberg RJ. Lung cancer staging: the value of ipsilateral scalene lymph node biopsy performed at mediastinoscopy. Ann Thorac Surg 1996;62:338–341.
219. Ginsberg RJ. Extended cervical mediastinoscopy. Chest Surg Clin N Am 1996;6:21–30.
220. Olak J. Parasternal mediastinotomy (Chamberlain procedure). Chest Surg Clin N Am 1996;6:31–40.

221. Landreneau RJ, Keenan RJ, Hazelrigg SR, Dowling RD, Mack MJ, Ferson PF. VATS wedge resection of the lung using the neodymium:yttrium-aluminum garnet laser. Ann Thorac Surg 1993;56:758–761.
222. Daly BD, Mueller JD, Faling LJ, et al. N2 lung cancer: outcome in patients with false-negative computed tomographic scans of the chest. J Thorac Cardiovasc Surg 1993;105:904–910.
223. Detterbeck F, Jones DR, Parker LA. Intrathoracic staging. In: Detterbeck F, Rivera M, Socinski MA, Rosenman JG (eds). Diagnosis and Treatment of Lung Cancer: An Evidence-Based Guide for the Practicing Physician. Philadelphia: Saunders: 2001:73–93.
224. Krasna MJ. Role of thoracoscopic lymph node staging for lung and esophageal cancer Oncology (Huntingt) 1996;10:793–802.
225. Bollen EC, van Duin CJ, Theunissen PH, vt Hof-Grootenboer BE, Blijham GH. Mediastinal lymph node dissection in resected lung cancer: morbidity and accuracy of staging. Ann Thorac Surg 1993;55:961–966.
226. Izbicki JR, Thetter O, Habekost M, et al. Radical systematic mediastinal lymphadenectomy in non-small cell lung cancer: a randomized controlled trial. Br J Surg 1994;81:229–235.
227. Sugi K, Nawata K, Fujita N, et al. Systematic lymph node dissection for clinically diagnosed peripheral non-small-cell lung cancer less than 2 cm in diameter, World J Surg 1998;22:290–294.
228. Funatsu T, Matsubara Y, Ikeda S, Hatakenaka R, Hanawa T, Ishida H. Preoperative mediastinoscopic assessment of N factors and the need for mediastinal lymph node dissection in T1 lung cancer. J Thorac Cardiovasc Surg 1994;108:321–328.
229. Martini N, Flehinger BJ. The role of surgery in N2 lung cancer. Surg Clin N Am 1987;67:1037–1049.
230. Keller SM, Adak S, Wagner H, Johnson DH. Mediastinal lymph node dissection improves survival in patients with stages II and IIIa non-small cell lung cancer. Eastern Cooperative Oncology Group. Ann Thorac Surg 2000;70:358–365.
231. Wu Y, Huang ZF, Wang SY, Yang XN, Ou W. A randomized trial of systematic nodal dissection in resectable non-small cell lung cancer. Lung Cancer 20002;36:1–6.
232. Liptay MJ, Grondin SC, Fry WA, et al. Intraoperative sentinel lymph node mapping in non-small-cell lung cancer improves detection of micrometastases. J Clin Oncol 2002;20:1984–1988.
233. Liptay MJ, Masters GA, Winchester DJ, et al. Intraoperative radioisotope sentinel lymph node mapping in non-small cell lung cancer. Ann Thorac Surg 2000;70:384–389.
234. Schmidt FE, Woltering EA, Webb WR, Garcia OM, Cohen JE, Rozans MH. Sentinel nodal assessment in patients with carcinoma of the lung. Ann Thorac Surg 2002;74:870–874.
235. Nomori H, Horio H, Naruke T, Orikasa H, Yamazaki K, Suemasu K. Use of technetium-99m tin colloid for sentinel lymph node identification in non-small cell lung cancer. J Thorac Cardiovasc Surg 2002;124:486–492.
236. Sugi K, Kaneda Y, Sudoh M, Sakano H, Hamano K. Effect of radioisotope sentinel node mapping in patients with cT1 N0 M0 lung cancer. J Thorac Cardiovasc Surg 2003;126:568–573.
237. Albain KS, Rusch VW, Crowley JJ, et al. Concurrent cisplatin/etoposide plus chest radiotherapy followed by surgery for stages IIIA (N2) and IIIB non-small-cell lung cancer: mature results of Southwest Oncology Group phase II study 8805. J Clin Oncol 1995;13:1880–1892.
238. Pass HI, Pogrebniak HW, Steinberg SM, Mulshine J, Minna J. Randomized trial of neoadjuvant therapy for lung cancer: interim analysis. Ann Thorac Surg 1992;53:992–998.
239. Bueno R, Richards WG, Swanson SJ, et al. Nodal stage after induction therapy for stage IIIA lung cancer determines patient survival. Ann Thorac Surg 2000;70:1826–1831.
240. Betticher DC, Hsu Schmitz SF, Totsch M, et al. Mediastinal lymph node clearance after docetaxel-cisplatin neoadjuvant chemotherapy is prognostic of survival in patients with stage IIIA pN2 non-small-cell lung cancer: a multicenter phase II trial. J Clin Oncol 2003;21:1752–1759.
241. Mateu-Navarro M, Rami-Porta R, Bastus-Piulats R, Cirera-Nogueras L, Gonzalez-Pont G. Remediastinoscopy after induction chemotherapy in non-small cell lung cancer. Ann Thorac Surg 2000;70:391–395.
242. Van Schil P, van der Schoot J, Poniewierski J, et al. Remediastinoscopy after neoadjuvant therapy for non-small cell lung cancer. Lung Cancer 2002;37:281–285.
243. MacManus MR, Hicks R, Fisher R, et al. FDG-PET-detected extracranial metastasis in patients with non-small cell lung cancer undergoing staging for surgery or radical radiotherapy: survival correlates with metastatic disease burden. Acta Oncol 2003;42:48–54.
244. Vansteenkiste JF, Stroobants SG, De Leyn PR, Dupont PJ, Verbeken EK. Potential use of FDG-PET scan after induction chemotherapy in surgically staged IIIa-N2 non-small-cell lung cancer: a prospective pilot study. The Leuven Lung Cancer Group. Ann Oncol 1998;9:1193–1198.
245. Ryu JS, Choi NC, Fischman AJ, Lynch TJ, Mathisen DJ. FDG-PET in staging and restaging non-small cell lung cancer after neoadjuvant chemoradiotherapy: correlation with histopathology. Lung Cancer 2002;35:179–187.
246. Akhurst T, Downey RJ, Ginsberg MS, et al. An initial experience with FDG-PET in the imaging of residual disease after induction therapy for lung cancer. Ann Thorac Surg 2002;73: 259–264.
247. Cerfolio RJ, Ojha B, Bryant AS, Bass CS, Bartalucci AA, Mountz JM. The role of FDG-PET scan in staging patients with nonsmall cell carcinoma. Ann Thorac Surg 2003;76:861–866.
248. Lardinois D, Schallberger A, Betticher D, Ris HB. Postinduction video-mediastinoscopy is as accurate and safe as video-mediastinoscopy in patients without pretreatment for potentially operable non-small cell lung cancer. Ann Thorac Surg 2003;75:1102–1106.
249. Kramer H, Douma WR, van Putten J, Post W, Groen H, Groen HJM. Endoscopic ultrasonography with fine needle aspiration in the staging of non-small cell lung cancer after a positive mediastinal PET. Lung Cancer 2003;41:S204 (abstract).
250. Kiser AC, Detterbeck FC. General aspects of surgical treatment. In: Detterbeck FC, Riverra MP, Sopcinski MA, Rosenman JG (eds). Diagnosis and Treatment of Lung Cancer: An Evidence-Based Guide for the Practicing Clinician. Philadelphia: Saunders, 2001:133–147.
251. Yellin A, Hill LR, Lieberman Y. Pulmonary resections in patients over 70 years of age. Isr J Med Sci 1985;21:833–840.
252. Ninan M, Sommers KE, Landreneau RJ, et al. Standardized exercise oximetry predicts postpneumonectomy outcome, Ann Thorac Surg 1997;64:328–332.
253. Wyser C, Stulz P, Soler M, et al. Prospective evaluation of an algorithm for the functional assessment of lung resection candidates. Am J Respir Crit Care Med 1999;159:1450–1456.
254. Celli BR. What is the value of preoperative pulmonary function testing? Med Clin N Am 1993;77:309–325.
255. Bolliger CT, Perruchoud AP. Functional evaluation of the lung resection candidate. Eur Respir J 1998;11:198–212.
256. Ferguson MK, Little L, Rizzo L, et al. Diffusing capacity predicts morbidity and mortality after pulmonary resection. J Thorac Cardiovasc Surg 1988;96:894–900.
257. Giordano A, Calcagni ML, MeduriG, Valente S, Galli G. Perfusion lung scintigraphy for the prediction of postlobectomy residual pulmonary function. Chest 1997;111:1542–1547.
258. Pierce RJ, Copland JM, Sharpe K, Barter CE. Preoperative risk evaluation for lung cancer resection: predicted postoperative product as a predictor of surgical mortality. Am J Respir Crit Care Med 1994;150:947–955.
259. Wu MT, Pan HB, Chiang AA, et al. Prediction of postoperative lung function in patients with lung cancer: comparison of quantitative CT with perfusion scintigraphy. AJR Am J Roentgenol 2002;178:667–672.

260. Pate P, Tenholder MF, Griffin JP, Eastridge CE, Weiman DS. Preoperative assessment of the high-risk patient for lung resection. Ann Thorac Surg 1996;61:1494–1500.
261. Olsen GN, Weiman DS, Bolton JW, et al. Submaximal invasive exercise testing and quantitative lung scanning in the evaluation for tolerance of lung resection. Chest 1989;95:267–273.
262. Bolliger CT, Wyser C, Roser H, Soler M, Perruchoud AP. Lung scanning and exercise testing for the prediction of postoperative performance in lung resection candidates at increased risk for complications. Chest 1995;108:341–348.
263. Wang J, Olak J, Ferguson MK. Diffusing capacity predicts operative mortality but not long-term survival after resection for lung cancer. J Thorac Cardiovasc Surg 1999;117:581–586.
264. Markos J, Mullan BP, Hillman DR, et al. Preoperative assessment as a predictor of mortality and morbidity after lung resection. Am Rev Respir Dis 1989;139:902–910.
265. Olsen GN, Bolton JW, Weiman DS, Hornung CA. Stair climbing as an exercise test to predict the postoperative complications of lung resection. Two years' experience. Chest 1991;99:587–590.
266. Bolton JW, Weiman DS, Haynes JL, Hornung CA, Olsen GN, Almond CH. Stair climbing as an indicator of pulmonary function. Chest 1987;92:783–788.
267. Bolliger CT, Jordan P, Soler M, et al. Exercise capacity as a predictor of postoperative complications in lung resection candidates. Am J Respir Crit Care Med 1995;151:1472–1480.
268. Walsh GL, Morice RC, Putnam JB Jr, et al. Resection of lung cancer is justified in high-risk patients selected by exercise oxygen consumption. Ann Thorac Surg 1994;58:704–710.
269. Brutsche MH, Spiliopoulos A, Bolliger CT, Licker M, Frey JG, Tschopp JM. Exercise capacity and extent of resection as predictors of surgical risk in lung cancer. Eur Respir J 2000;15:828–832.
270. Olsen GN, Weiman DS, Bolton JW, et al. Submaximal invasive exercise testing and quantitative lung scanning in the evaluation for tolerance of lung resection. Chest 1989;95:267–273.
271. Fujimura S, Sakurada A, Sagawa M, et al. A therapeutic approach to roentgenographically occult squamous cell carcinoma of the lung. Cancer (Phila) 2000;89:2445–2448.
272. Koike T, Terashima M, Takizawa T, et al. Surgical results for centrally-located early stage lung cancer. Ann Thorac Surg 2000;70:1176–1179.
273. Bechtel JJ, Kelley WR, Petty TL, Patz DS, Saccomanno G. Outcome of 51 patients with roentgenographically occult lung cancer detected by sputum cytoogic testing: a community hospital program. Arch Intern Med 1994;154:975–980.
274. Konaka C, Hirano T, Kato H, Furuse K, et al. Comparison of endoscopic features of early-stage squamous cell lung cancer and histological findings. Br J Cancer 1999;80:1435–1439.
275. Sheski FD, Mathur PN. Endoscopic treatment of early-stage lung cancer. Cancer Control 2000;7:35–44.
276. Mathur PN, Edell E, Sutedja T, Vergnon JM. Treatment of early stage non-small cell lung cancer. Chest 2003;123:176S–180S.
277. Perol M, Caliandro R, Pommier P, et al. Curative irradiation of limited endobronchial carcinomas with high-dose rate brachytherapy. Results of a pilot study. Chest 197;111:1417–1423.
278. van Boxem TJ, Venmans BJ, Schramel FM, et al. Radiographically occult lung cancer treated with fibreoptic bronchoscopic electrocautery: a pilot study of a simple and inexpensive technique. Eur Respir J 1998;11:169–172.
279. Deygas N, Froudarakis M, Ozenne G, Vergnon JM. Cryotherapy in early superficial bronchogenic carcinoma. Chest 2001;120:26–31.
280. Naruke T, Tsuchiya R, Kondo H, Asamura H. Prognosis and survival after resection for bronchogenic carcinoma based on the 1997 TNM-staging classification: the Japanese experience. Ann Thorac Surg 2001;71:1759–1764.
281. Mountain, C.F. Revision in the International System for Staging Lung Cancer, Chest, 111:1710–1717, 1997.
282. Jones D, Detterbeck F. Surgery for stage I non-small cell lung cancer. In: Detterbeck F, Rivera MP, Socinski MA, Rosenman JG (eds). Diagnosis and Treatment of Lung Cancer: An Evidence Based Guide for the Practicing Clinician. Philadelphia: Saunders, 2001:177–190.
283. Gauden S, Ramsay J, Tripcony L. The curative treatment by radiotherapy alone of stage I non-small cell carcinoma of the lung. Chest 1995;108:1278–1282.
284. Morita K, Fuwa N, Suzuki Y, et al. Radical radiotherapy for medically inoperable non-small cell lung cancer in clinical stage I: a retrospective analysis of 149 patients. Radiother Oncol 1997;42:31–36.
285. Sibley GS, Jamieson TA, Marks LB, Anscher MS, Prosnitz LR. Radiotherapy alone for medically inoperable stage I non-small-cell lung cancer: the Duke experience. Int J Radiat Oncol Biol Phys 1998;140:149–154.
286. Krol AD, Aussems P, Noordijk EM, Hermans J, Leer JW. Local irradiation alone for peripheral stage I lung cancer: could we omit the elective regional nodal irradiation? Int J Radiat Oncol Biol Phys 1996;34:297–302.
287. Graham PH, Gebski VJ, Langlands AO. Radical radiotherapy for early non-small cell lung cancer. Int J Radiat Oncol Biol Phys 1995;31:261–266.
288. Sandler HM, Curran WJ Jr, Turrisi AT III. The influence of tumor size and pre-treatment staging on outcome following radiation therapy alone for stage I non-small cell lung cancer. Int J Radiat Oncol Biol Phys 1990;19:9–13.
289. Kaskowitz L, Graham MV, Emami B, Halverson KJ, Rush C. Radiation therapy alone for stage I non-small cell lung cancer. Int J Radiat Oncol Biol Phys 1993;27:517–523.
290. Rowell NP, Williams CJ. Radical radiotherapy for stage I/II non-small cell lung cancer in patients not sufficiently fit for or declining surgery (medically inoperable): a systematic review. Thorax 2001;56:628–638.
291. Martini N, Bains MS, Burt ME, et al. Incidence of local recurrence and second primary tumors in resected stage I lung cancer. J Thorac Cardiovasc Surg 1995;109:120–129.
292. Jensik RJ, Faber LP, Kittle CF. Segmental resection for bronchogenic carcinoma. Ann Thorac Surg 1979;28:475–483.
293. Kodama K, Doi O, Higashiyama M, Yokouchi H. Intentional limited resection for selected patients with T1 N0 M0 non-small-cell lung cancer: a single-institution study. J Thorac Cardiovasc Surg 1997;114:347–353.
294. Landreneau RJ, Sugarbaker DJ, Mack MJ, et al. Wedge resection versus lobectomy for stage I (T1 N0 M0) non-small-cell lung cancer. J Thorac Cardiovasc Surg 1997;113:691–698.
295. Miller JI, Haticher CR. Limited resection of bronchogenic carcinoma in the patient with marked impairment of pulmonary function. Ann Thorac Surg 1987;44:340–343.
296. Ginsberg RJ, Rubinstein LV. Randomized trial of lobectomy versus limited resection for T1 N0 non-small cell lung cancer. Lung Cancer Study Group. Ann Thorac Surg 1995;60:615–622.
297. Inoue K, Sato M, Fujimura S, et al. Prognostic assessment of 1,310 patients with non-small-cell lung cancer who underwent complete resection from 1980 to 1993. J Thorac Cardiovasc Surg 1998l;116:407–411.
298. Yano T, Yokoyama H, Inoue T, Asoh H, Tayama K, Ichinose Y. Surgical results and prognostic factors of pathologic N1 disease in non-small-cell carcinoma of the lung. Significance of N1 level: lobar or hilar nodes. J Thorac Cardiovasc Surg 1994;107:1398–1402.
299. Adebonojo SA, Bowser AN, Moritz DM, Corcoran PC. Impact of revised stage classification of lung cancer on survival: a military experience. Chest 1999;115:1507–1513.

300. Martini N, Burt ME, Bains MS, et al. Survival after resection of stage II non-small cell lung cancer. Ann Thorac Surg 1992;54: 460–465.
301. Riquet M, Manac'h D, Le Pimpec-Barthes F, Dujon A, Chehab A. Prognostic significance of surgical-pathologic N1 disease in non-small cell carcinoma of the lung. Ann Thorac Surg 1999;67: 1572–1576.
302. van VE, de la Riviere AB, Elbers HJ, Lammers JW, van den Bosch JM. Type of lymph node involvement and survival in pathologic N1 stage III non-small cell lung carcinoma. Ann Thorac Surg 1999;67:903–907.
303. Fadel E, Yildizeli B, Chapelier AR, Dicenta I, Mussot S, Dartevelle PG. Sleeve lobectomy for bronchogenic cancers: factors affecting survival. Ann Thorac Surg 2002;74:851–858.
304. Harpole DH Jr, Healey EA, Decamp MM Jr, Mentzer SJ, Strauss GM, Sugarbaker DJ. Chest wall invasive non-small cell lung cancer: patterns of failure and implications for a revised staging system. Ann Surg Oncol 1996;3:261–269.
305. Ratto GB, Piacenza G, Frola C, et al. Chest wall involvement by lung cancer: computed tomographic detection and results of operation. Ann Thorac Surg 1991;51:182–188.
306. Downey RJ, Martini N, Rusch VW, Bains MS, Korst RJ, Ginsberg RJ. Extent of chest wall invasion and survival in patients with lung cancer. Ann Thorac Surg 1999;68:188–193.
307. Magdeleinat P, Alifano M, Benbrahem C, et al. Surgical treatment of lung cancer invading the chest wall: results and prognostic factors. Ann Thorac Surg 2001;71:1094–1099.
308. Patterson GA, Ilves R, Ginsberg RL, Cooper JD, Todd TRJ, Pearson FG. The value of adjuvant radiotherapy in pulmonary and chest wall resection for bronchogenic carcinoma. Ann Thorac Surg 1982;34:692–697.
309. Detterbeck F, Jones D, Rosenman JG. Pancoast tumors. In: Detterbeck F, Rivera MP, Socinski MA, Rosenman JG (eds). Diagnosis and Treatment of Lung Cancer: An Evidence Based Guide for the Practicing Clinician. Philadelphia: Saunders, 2001:233–243.
310. Rusch VW, Giroux DJ, Kraut MJ, et al. Induction chemoradiation and surgical resection for non-small cell lung carcinomas of the superior sulcus: initial results of Southwest Oncology Group Trial 9416 (Intergroup Trial 0160). J Thorac Cardiovasc Surg 2001;121:472–483.
311. Burt ME, Pomerantz AH, Bains MS, et al. Results of surgical treatment of stage III lung cancer invading the mediastinum. Surg Clin N Am 1987;67:987–1000.
312. Martini N, Yellin A, Ginsberg RJ, et al. Management of non-small cell lung cancer with direct mediastinal involvement. Ann Thorac Surg 1994;58:1447–1451.
313. Deslauriers J, Jacques LF. Sleeve pneumonectomy. Chest Surg Clin N Am 1995;5:297–313.
314. Deslauriers J, Ginsberg RJ, Dubois P, Beaulieu M, Goldberg M, Piraux M. Current operative morbidity associated with elective surgical resection for lung cancer. Can J Surg 1989;32:335–339.
315. Deslauriers J, Gaulin P, Beaulieu M, Piraux M, Bernier R, Cormier Y. Long-term clinical and functional results of sleeve lobectomy for primary lung cancer. J Thorac Cardiovasc Surg 1986;92:871–879.
316. Vogt-Moykopf I, Toomes H, Heinrich S. Sleeve resection of the bronchus and pulmonary artery for pulmonary lesions. Thorac Cardiovasc Surg 1983;31:193–198.
317. Pitz CC, de la Brutel RA, Elbers HR, Westermann CJ, van den Bosch JM. Results of resection of T3 non-small cell lung cancer invading the mediastinum or main bronchus. Ann Thorac Surg 1996;62:1016–1020.
318. Okada M, Tsubota N, Yoshimura M, et al. Extended sleeve lobectomy for lung cancer: the avoidance of pneumonectomy. J Thorac Cardiovasc Surg 1999;118:710–713.
319. Suzuki K, Nagai K, Yoshida J, et al. Conventional clinicopathologic prognostic factors in surgically resected nonsmall cell lung carcinoma: a comparison of prognostic factors for each pathologic TNM stage based on multivariate analyses. Cancer (Phila) 1999;86:1976–1984.
320. Wada H, Tanaka F, Yanagihara K, et al. Time trends and survival after operations for primary lung cancer from 1976 through 1990. J Thorac Cardiovasc Surg 1996;112:349–355.
321. Martini N, Flehinger BJ, Nagasaki F, Hart B. Prognostic significance of N1 disease in carcinoma of the lung. J Thorac Cardiovasc Surg 1983;86:646–653.
322. Pearson FG. Staging of the mediastinum Role of mediastinoscopy and computed tomography. Chest 1993;103:346S–348S.
323. Depierre A, Milleron B, Moro-Sibilot D, et al. Preoperative chemotherapy followed by surgery compared with primary surgery in resectable stage I (except T1N0), II, and IIIa non-small-cell lung cancer. J Clin Oncol 2002;20:247–253.
324. Liao ML, Zhou Y, Ding JA, et al. The study of peri-operative chemotherapy in stage I-IIIa NSCLC. Lung Cancer 2003;41: (abstract).
325. Pisters K, Ginsberg R, Giroux D, et al. Phase II bimodality lung oncology team trial of induction paclitaxel/carboplatin in early stage non-small cell lung cancer: long term followup of a phase II trial. Proc Am Soc Clin Oncol 2003;22:633a (abstract).
326. Pisters K, Ginsberg R, Giroux D, et al. Bimodality lung oncology team (BLOT) trial of induction paclitaxel/carboplatin in early stage non-small cell lung cancer (NSCLC): long-term follow-up of a phase II study. Proc Am Soc Clin Oncol 2003; (abstract).
327. Pisters KM, Ginsberg RJ, Giroux DJ, et al. Induction chemotherapy before surgery for early-stage lung cancer: a novel approach. Bimodality Lung Oncology Team. J Thorac Cardiovasc Surg 2000;119:429–439.
328. Siegenthaler MP, Pisters KM, Merriman KW, et al. Preoperative chemotherapy for lung cancer does not increase surgical morbidity. Ann Thorac Surg 2001;71:1105–1111.
329. Martin J, Abolhoda A, Bains MS. Long-term results of combined modality therapy in resectable non-small cell lung cancer. Proc Am Soc Clin Oncol 2001;20:311a (abstract).
330. Perrot E, Guibert B, Mulsant P, et al. Preoperative chemotherapy doesn't increase postoperative complications in patients undergoing resection for NSCLC: results of a retrospective study of 114 consecutive patients. Lung Cancer 2003;41: (abstract).
331. Toscana E, Roriz W, Biasi S, et al. Neoadjuvant chemotherapy in patients with operable NSCLC:Surgical results. Lung Cancer 2003;41: (abstract).
332. Skarin A, Jochelson M, Sheldon T, et al. Neoadjuvant chemotherapy in marginally resectable stage III M0 non-small cell lung cancer: long-term follow-up in 41 patients. J Surg Oncol 1989;40:266–274.
333. Eagan RT, Ruud C, Lee RE, Pairolero PC, Gail MH. Pilot study of induction therapy with cyclophosphamide, doxorubicin, and cisplatin (CAP) and chest irradiation prior to thoracotomy in initially inoperable stage III M0 non-small cell lung cancer. Cancer Treat Rep 1987;71:895–900.
334. Bitran JD, Golomb HM, Hoffman PC, et al. Protochemotherapy in non-small cell lung carcinoma: an attempt to increase surgical resectability and survival. A preliminary report. Cancer (Phila) 1986;57:44–53.
335. Elias AD, Skarin AT, Gonin R, et al. Neoadjuvant treatment of stage IIIA non-small cell lung cancer: long-term results. Am J Clin Oncol 1994;17:26–36.
336. Darwish S, Minotti V, Crino L, et al. Neoadjuvant cisplatin and etoposide for stage IIIA (clinical N2) non-small cell lung cancer. Am J Clin Oncol 1994;17:64–67.
337. Wagner H Jr, Lad T, Piantadosi S, Ruckdeschel JC. Randomized phase 2 evaluation of preoperative radiation therapy and preoperative chemotherapy with mitomycin, vinblastine, and cisplatin in patients with technically unresectable stage IIIA and

IIIB non-small cell cancer of the lung: LCSG 881. Chest 1994; 106:348S–354S.

338. Martini N, Kris MG, Flehinger BJ, et al. Preoperative chemotherapy for stage IIIa (N2) lung cancer: the Sloan-Kettering experience with 136 patients. Ann Thorac Surg 1993;55:1365–1373.
339. Pisters KM, Kris MG, Gralla RJ, Zaman MB, Heelan RT, Martini N. Pathologic complete response in advanced non-small-cell lung cancer following preoperative chemotherapy: implications for the design of future non-small-cell lung cancer combined modality trials. J Clin Oncol 1993;11:1757–1762.
340. Elias AD, Skarin AT, Leong T, et al. Neoadjuvant therapy for surgically staged IIIA N2 non-small cell lung cancer (NSCLC). Lung Cancer 1997;17:147–161.
341. Sugarbaker DJ, Herndon J, Kohman LJ, Krasna MJ, Green MR. Results of cancer and leukemia group B protocol 8935. A multiinstitutional phase II trimodality trial for stage IIIA (N2) non-small-cell lung cancer. Cancer and Leukemia Group B Thoracic Surgery Group. J Thorac Cardiovasc Surg 1995;109:473–483.
342. Weiden PL, Piantadosi S. Preoperative chemotherapy (cisplatin and fluorouracil) and radiation therapy in stage III non-small cell lung cancer. A phase 2 study of the LCSG. Chest 1994;106:344S–347S.
343. Faber LP, Kittle CF, Warren WH, et al. Preoperative chemotherapy and irradiation for stage III non-small cell lung cancer. Ann Thorac Surg 1989;47:669–675.
344. Strauss GM, Herndon JE, Sherman DD, et al. Neoadjuvant chemotherapy and radiotherapy followed by surgery in stage IIIA non-small-cell carcinoma of the lung: report of a Cancer and Leukemia Group B phase II study. J Clin Oncol 1992;10:1237–1244.
345. Law A, Karp DD, Dipetrillo T, Daly BT. Emergence of increased cerebral metastasis after high-dose preoperative radiotherapy with chemotherapy in patients with locally advanced non-small cell lung carcinoma. Cancer 2001;92:160–164.
346. Albain K, Rusch VR, Crowley J, et al. Long-term survival after concurrent cisplatin/etoposide plus chest radiotherapy followed by surgery in bulky, stages IIA(N2) and IIB non-small cell lung cancer: 6 year outcomes from Southwest Oncology Group Study 8805. Proc Am Soc Clin Oncol 1999;18:467a (abstract).
347. Choi NC, Carey RW, Daly W, et al. Potential impact on survival of improved tumor downstaging and resection rate by preoperative twice-daily radiation and concurrent chemotherapy in stage IIIA non-small-cell lung cancer. J Clin Oncol 1997;15:712–722.
348. Eberhardt WE, Albain KS, Pass H, et al. Induction treatment before surgery for non-small cell lung cancer. Lung Cancer 2003;42(suppl 1):S9–S14.
349. Stuschke M, Eberhardt W, Pottgen C, et al. Prophylactic cranial irradiation in locally advanced non-small-cell lung cancer after multimodality treatment: long-term follow-up and investigations of late neuropsychologic effects. J Clin Oncol 1999;17: 2700–2709.
350. Yoneda S, Hibino S, Gotoh I, et al. A comparative trial on induction chemoradiotherapy followed by surgery or immediate surgery for stage III NSCLC. Proc Am Soc Clin Oncol 1995;14: 367 (abstract).
351. Roth JA, Atkinson EN, Fossella F, et al. Long-term follow-up of patients enrolled in a randomized trial comparing perioperative chemotherapy and surgery with surgery alone in resectable stage IIIA non-small-cell lung cancer. Lung Cancer 1998;21:1–6.
352. Rosell R, Gomez-Codina J, Camps C, et al. Preresectional chemotherapy in stage IIIA non-small-cell lung cancer: a 7-year assessment of a randomized controlled trial. Lung Cancer 1999; 26:7–14.
353. Depierre A, Westeel V, Milleron B, et al. 5-year results of the French randomized study comparing preoperative chemotherapy followed by surgery and primary surgery in resectable stage I (except T1N0), II and IIIa non-small cell lung cancer. Lung Cancer 2003;41: (abstract).
354. Roth JA, Fossella F, Komaki R, et al. A randomized trial comparing perioperative chemotherapy and surgery with surgery alone in resectable stage IIIA non-small-cell lung cancer. J Natl Cancer Inst 1994;86:673–680.
355. Rosell R, Gomez-Codina J, Camps C, et al. A randomized trial comparing preoperative chemotherapy plus surgery with surgery alone in patients with non-small-cell lung cancer. N Engl J Med 1994;330:153–158.
356. Albain KS, Rusch VR, Turrisi A III, et al. Phase II comparison of concurrent chemotherapy and radiotherapy (CT/RT) and CT/RT followed by surgical resection for stage IIIA (pN2) NSCLC: initial results from North American Intergroup Trial 0139 (RTOG 9309). Proc Am Soc Clin Oncol 2003; (abstract).
357. Rusch VW, Albain KS, Crowley JJ, et al. Neoadjuvant therapy: a novel and effective treatment for stage IIIb non-small cell lung cancer. Southwest Oncology Group. Ann Thorac Surg 1994;58: 290–294.
358. Grunenwald DH, Andre F, Le PC, et al. Benefit of surgery after chemoradiotherapy in stage IIIB (T4 and/or N3) non-small cell lung cancer. J Thorac Cardiovasc Surg 2001;122:796–802.
359. Pitz CC, Maas KW, Van Swieten HA, de la Riviere AB, Hofman P, Schramel FM. Surgery as part of combined modality treatment in stage IIIB non-small cell lung cancer. Ann Thorac Surg 2002;74:164–169.
360. De Marinis MF, Nelli F, Migliorino MR, et al. Gemcitabine, paclitaxel, and cisplatin as induction chemotherapy for patients with biopsy-proven Stage IIIA (N2) non-small cell lung carcinoma: a Phase II multicenter study. Cancer (Phila) 2003;98: 1707–1715.
361. Cappuzzo F, Selvaggi G, Gregorc V, et al. Gemcitabine and cisplatin as induction chemotherapy for patients with unresectable Stage IIIA-bulky N2 and Stage IIIB non-small cell lung carcinoma: an Italian Lung Cancer Project Observational Study. Cancer (Phila) 2003;98:128–134.
362. Splinter TA, van Schil PE, Kramer GW, et al. Randomized trial of surgery versus radiotherapy in patients with stage IIIA (N2) non small-cell lung cancer after a response to induction chemotherapy. EORTC 08941. Clin Lung Cancer 2000;2:69–72.
363. O'Brien ME, Splinter T, Smit EF, et al. Carboplatin and paclitaxol (Taxol) as an induction regimen for patients with biopsy-proven stage IIIA N2 non-small cell lung cancer. an EORTC phase II study (EORTC 08958). Eur J Cancer 2003;39:1416–1422.
364. Van Zandwijk N, Smit EF, Kramer GWP, et al. Gemcitabine and cisplatin as induction regimen for patients with biopsy-proven stage IIIA N2 non-small-cell lung cancer: a phase II study of the European Organization for Research and Treatment of Cancer Lung Cancer Cooperative Group (EORTC 08955). J Clin Oncol 2000;18:2658–2664.
365. Stephens R, Girling D, Bleehen N, Moghissi K, Yosef H, Machin D. The role of post-operative radiotherapy in non-small-cell lung cancer: a multicentre randomised trial in patients with pathologically staged T1-2, N1-2, M0 disease. Medical Research Council Lung Cancer Working Party. Br J Cancer 1996;74(4): 632–639.
366. Weisenbruger T. Effects of postoperative mediastinal radiation on completely resected stage II and stage III epidermoid cancer of the lung. N Engl J Med 1986;315(22):1377–1381.
367. Lafitte J, Ribet M, Prevost B, Gosselin B, Copin M, Brichet A. Postresection irradiation for T2 N0 M0 non-small cell carcinoma: a prospective, randomized study. Ann Thorac Surg 1996; 62:830–834.
368. Dautzenberg B, Arriagada R, Chammard A, et al. A controlled study of postoperative radiotherapy for patients with completely resected nonsmall cell lung carcinoma. Groupe d'Etude et de Traitement des Cancers Bronchiques. Cancer (Phila) 1999;86(2): 265–273.
369. Granone P, Trodella L, Margaritora S, et al. Radiotherapy versus follow-up in the treatment of pathological stage Ia and Ib non-

small cell lung cancer. Early stopped analysis of a randomized controlled study. Eur J Cardiothorac Surg 2000;18(4):418–424.
370. Munro A. What now for postoperative radiotherapy for cancer? Lancet 1998;352:250–251.
371. Machtay M, Lee J, Shrager J, Kaiser L, Glatstein E. Risk of death from intercurrent disease is not excessively increased by modern postoperative radiotherapy for high-risk resected non-small-cell lung carcinoma. J Clin Oncol 2001;19(19):3912–3917.
372. Feld R, Rubenstein L, Thomas P, L.C.S. Group. Adjuvant chemotherapy with cyclophosphamide, doxorubicin, and cisplatin in patients with completely resected stage I non-small cell lung cancer. J Natl Cancer Inst 1993;85:299–306.
373. Holmes E, Gail M. Surgical adjuvant therapy for stage II and III adenocarcinoma and large-cell undifferentiated carcinoma. J Clin Oncol 1986;4:710–715.
374. Figlin R, Piantodosi S. A phase 3 randomized trial of immediate combination chemotherapy vs. delayed combination chemotherapy in patients with completely resected stage II and III non-small cell carcinoma of the lung. Chest 1994;106(suppl 6):310S–312S.
375. Niiranen A, Niitamo-Korhonen S, Kouri M, Assendelft A, Mattson K, Pyrhonen S. Adjuvant chemotherapy after radical surgery for non-small-cell lung cancer: a randomized study. J Clin Oncol 1992;10(12):1927–1932.
376. Waller D, Fairlamb D, Gower N, et al. The Big Lung Trial (BLT): determining the value of cisplatin-based chemotherapy for all patients with non-small cell lung cancer (NSCLC). Preliminary results in the surgical setting. Proc Am Soc Clin Oncol 2003.
377. Ohta M, Tsuchiya R, Shimoyama M, et al. Adjuvant chemotherapy for completely resected stage III non-small cell lung cancer. Results of a randomized prospective study. The Japan Clinical Oncology Group. J Thorac Cardiovasc Surg 1993;106(4):703–708.
378. Ichinose Y, Tada H, Koike T, et al. National Kyushu Cancer Center, Japan. A randomized phase III trial of postoperative adjuvant chemotherapy in patients with completely resected stage IIIA-N2 non-small cell lung cancer: Japan Clinical Oncology Group (JCOG 9304) trial. Proc Am Soc Clin Oncol 2001.
379. Wada H, Hitomi S, Teramatsu T. Adjuvant chemotherapy after complete resection in non-small-cell lung cancer. West Japan Study Group for Lung Cancer Surgery. J Clin Oncol 1996;14(4):1048–1054.
380. Imaizumi M. A randomized trial of postoperative adjuvant chemotherapy in non-small cell lung cancer (the second cooperative study). The Study Group of Adjuvant Chemotherapy for Lung Cancer (Chubu, Japan). Eur J Surg Oncol 1995;21(1):69–77.
381. Wada H, Miyahara R, Tanaka F, Hitomi S. Postoperative adjuvant chemotherapy with PVM (cisplatin + vindesine + mitomycin C) and UFT (uracil + tegaful) in resected stage I-II NSCLC (non-small cell lung cancer): a randomized clinical trial. West Japan Study Group for lung cancer surgery (WJSG). Eur J Cardiothorac Surg 1999;15(4):438–443.
382. Tada H, Yasumitu T, Iuchi K, Taki T, Kodama K, Mori T. Randomized study of adjuvant chemotherapy for completely resected non-small cell lung cancer: lack of prognostic significance in DNA ploidy pattern at adjuvant setting. 2002.
383. Kato H, Tsuboi M, Ohta M, et al. A randomized phase III trial of adjuvant chemotherapy with UFT for completely resected pathological stage I (T1NOMO, T2, NOMO) adenocarcinoma of the lung. Proc Am Soc Clin Oncol 2003.
384. Chemotherapy in non-small cell lung cancer: a meta-analysis using updated data on individual patients from 52 randomised clinical trials. Non-small Cell Lung Cancer Collaborative Group. BMJ 1995;311(7010):899–909.
385. Le Chevalier T. Results of the randomized international adjuvant lung cancer trial (IALT): cisplatin-based chemotherapy (CT) vs no CT in 1867 patients (pts) with resected non-small cell lung cancer (NSCLC). Proc Am Soc Clin Oncol 2003.
386. Lad T, Rubinstein L, Sadeghi A. The benefit of adjuvant treatment for resected locally advanced non-small-cell lung cancer. J Clin Oncol 1988;6(1):9–17.
387. Pisters K, Kris M, Gralla R, et al. Randomized trial comparing postoperative chemotherapy with vindesine and cisplatin plus thoracic irradiation with irradiation alone in stage III (N2) non-small cell lung cancer. J Surg Oncol 1994;56(4):236–241.
388. Dautzenberg B, Chastang C, Arriagada R, et al. Adjuvant radiotherapy versus combined sequential chemotherapy followed by radiotherapy in the treatment of resected nonsmall cell lung carcinoma. A randomized trial of 267 patients. GETCB (Groupe d'Etude et de Traitement des Cancers Bronchiques). Cancer (Phila) 1995;76(5):779–786.
389. Keller S, Adak S, Wagner H, et al. A randomized trial of postoperative adjuvant therapy in patients with completely resected stage II or IIIA non-small-cell lung cancer. Eastern Cooperative Oncology Group. N Engl J Med 2000;343(17):1217–1222.
390. Wolf M, Muller H, Seifart U, et al. Randomized phase III trial of adjuvant radiotherapy vs. adjuvant chemotherapy followed by radiotherapy in patients with N2 positive non small cell lung cancer (NSCLC). Proc Am Soc Clin Oncol 2001.
391. Scagliotti G, Fossati R, Torri V, et al. Randomized study of adjuvant chemotherapy for completely resected stage I, II, or IIIA non-small-cell lung cancer. J Natl Cancer Inst 2003;95(19):1453–1461.
392. Roswit B, Patno M, Rapp R, et al. The survival of patients with inoperable lung cancer: a large-scale randomized study of radiation therapy versus placebo. Radiology 1968;90(4):688–697.
393. Perez C, Bauer M, Edelstein S, Gillespie B, Birch R. Impact of tumor control on survival in carcinoma of the lung treated with irradiation. Int J Radiat Oncol Biol Phys 1986;12(4):539–547.
394. Perez C, Stanley K, Grundy G, et al. Impact of irradiation technique and tumor extent in tumor control and survival of patients with unresectable non-oat cell carcinoma of the lung: report by the Radiation Therapy Oncology Group. Cancer (Phila) 1982; 50(6):1091–1099.
395. Johnson D, Einhorn L, Bartolucci A, et al. Thoracic radiotherapy does not prolong survival in patients with locally advanced, unresectable non-small cell lung cancer. Ann Intern Med 1990;113(1):33–38.
396. Mattson K, Holsti L, Holsti P, et al. Inoperable non-small cell lung cancer: radiation with or without chemotherapy. Eur J Cancer Clin Oncol 1988;24(3):477–482.
397. Trovo M, Minatel E, Veronesi A, et al. Combined radiotherapy and chemotherapy versus radiotherapy alone in locally advanced epidermoid bronchogenic carcinoma. A randomized study. Cancer (Phila) 1990;65(3):400–404.
398. Morton R, Ett J, McGinnis W, et al. Thoracic radiation therapy alone compared with combined chemoradiotherapy for locally unresectable non-small cell lung cancer. A randomized, phase III trial. Ann Intern Med 1991;115(9):681–686.
399. Dillman R, Herndon J, Seagren S, Eaton W Jr, Green M. Improved survival in stage III non-small-cell lung cancer: seven-year follow-up of cancer and leukemia group B (CALGB) 8433 trial. J Natl Cancer Inst 1996;88(17):1210–1215.
400. Le Chevalier T, Arriagada R, Quoix E, et al. Radiotherapy alone versus combined chemotherapy and radiotherapy in nonresectable non-small-cell lung cancer: first analysis of a randomized trial in 353 patients. J Natl Cancer Inst 1991;83(6):417–423.
401. Marino P, Preatoni A, Cantoni A. Randomized trials of radiotherapy alone versus combined chemotherapy and radiotherapy in stages IIIa and IIIb nonsmall cell lung cancer. A meta-analysis. Cancer (Phila) 1995;76(4):593–601.
402. Pritchard R, Anthony S. Chemotherapy plus radiotherapy compared with radiotherapy alone in the treatment of locally advanced, unresectable, non-small-cell lung cancer. A meta-analysis. Ann Intern Med 1996;125(9):723–729.

403. Furuse K, Fukuoka M, Kawahara M, et al. Phase III study of concurrent versus sequential thoracic radiotherapy in combination with mitomycin, vindesine, and cisplatin in unresectable stage III non-small-cell lung cancer. J Clin Oncol 1999;17(9):2692–2699.
404. Pierre F, Maurice P, Gilles R, et al. A randomized phase III trial of sequential chemo-radiotherapy versus concurrent chemo-radiotherapy in locally advanced non small cell lung cancer (NSCLC) (GLOT-GFPC NPC 95-01 study). Proc Am Soc Clin Oncol 2001.
405. Zatloukal P, Petruzelka L, Zemanova M, et al. Concurrent versus sequential radiochemotherapy with vinorelbine plus cisplatin (V-P) in locally advanced non-small cell lung cancer. A randomized phase II study. Proc Am Soc Clin Oncol 2002.
406. Curran W Jr, Scott C, Bonomi P, et al. Initial report of locally advanced multimodality protocol (LAMP): ACR 427: a randomized 3-arm phase II study of paclitaxel (T), carboplatin (C), and thoracic radiation (RT) for patients with stage III non-small cell lung cancer (NSCLC). Proc Am Soc Clin Oncol 2001;20:312a (abstract 1244).
407. Choy H, Curran WJ Jr, Scott C, et al. Preliminary report of locally advanced multimodality protocol (LAMP): ACR 427: a randomized phase II study of three chemo-radiation regimens with paclitaxel, carboplatin, and thoracic radiation (RT) for patients with locally advanced non-small cell lung cancer (LA-NSCLC). Proc Am Soc Clin Oncol 2002;21:291A (abstract 1160).
408. Huber R, Schmidt M, Flentje M, et al. Induction chemotherapy and following simultaneous radio/chemotherapy versus induction chemotherapy and radiotherapy alone in inoperable NSCLC (stage IIIA/IIIB). Proc Am Soc Clin Oncol 2003;22:622 (abstract 2501).
409. Curran W Jr, Scott C, Langer C, et al. Long-term benefit is observed in a phase III comparison of sequential vs. concurrent chemo-radiation for patients with unresected stage III NSCLC: RTOG 9410. Proc Am Soc Clin Oncol 2003;22:621 (abstract 2499).
410. Choy H, Kim D, Akerley W, et al. Combined modality therapy (CMT) using concurrent radiation therapy (RT) with paclitaxel based chemotherapeutic regimen in unresectable locally advanced nonsmall cell lung cancer (LANSCLC): long term follow up on three sequential multi-institutional prospective phase III studies. Proc Am Soc Clin Oncol 2003.
411. Werner-Wasik M, Scott C, Movsas B, et al. Amifostine as mucosal protectant in patients with locally advanced non-small cell lung cancer (NSCLC) receiving intensive chemotherapy and thoracic radiotherapy (RT): results of the radiation therapy oncology group (RTOG) 98-01 study. Int J Radiat Oncol Biol Phys 2003;57:S216.
412. Seydel H, Diener-West M, Urtasun R, et al. Hyperfractionation in the radiation therapy of unresectable non-oat cell carcinoma of the lung: preliminary report of a RTOG Pilot Study. Int J Radiat Oncol Biol Phys 1985;11(10):1841–1847.
413. Cox J, Azarnia N, Byhardt R, Shin K, Emami B, Pajak T. A randomized phase I/II trial of hyperfractionated radiation therapy with total doses of 60.0 Gy to 79.2 Gy: possible survival benefit with greater than or equal to 69.6 Gy in favorable patients with Radiation Therapy Oncology Group stage III non-small-cell lung carcinoma: report of Radiation Therapy Oncology Group 83-11. J Clin Oncol 1990;8(9):1543–1555.
414. Sause W, Scott C, Taylor S, et al. Radiation Therapy Oncology Group (RTOG) 88-08 and Eastern Cooperative Oncology Group (ECOG) 4588: preliminary results of a phase III trial in regionally advanced, unresectable non-small-cell lung cancer. J Natl Cancer Inst 1995;87(3):198–205.
415. Sause W, Kolesar P, Taylor S IV, et al. Final results of phase III trial in regionally advanced unresectable non-small cell lung cancer: Radiation Therapy Oncology Group, Eastern Cooperative Oncology Group, and Southwest Oncology Group. Chest 2000;117(2):358–364.
416. Komaki R, Scott C, Sause W, et al. Induction cisplatin/vinblastine and irradiation vs. irradiation in unresectable squamous cell lung cancer: failure patterns by cell type in RTOG 88-08/ECOG 4588. Radiation Therapy Oncology Group. Eastern Cooperative Oncology Group. Int J Radiat Oncol Biol Phys 1997;39(3):537–544.
417. Dische S, Saunders M. The rationale for continuous, hyperfractionated, accelerated radiotherapy (CHART). Int J Radiat Oncol Biol Phys 1990;19(5):1317–1320.
418. Saunders M, Dische S, Barrett A, Harvey A, Gibson D, Parmar M. Continuous hyperfractionated accelerated radiotherapy (CHART) versus conventional radiotherapy in non-small-cell lung cancer: a randomised multicentre trial. CHART Steering Committee. Lancet 1997;350(9072):161–165.
419. Saunders M, Dische S, Barrett A, Harvey A, Griffiths G, Palmar M. Continuous, hyperfractionated, accelerated radiotherapy (CHART) versus conventional radiotherapy in non-small cell lung cancer: mature data from the randomised multicentre trial. CHART Steering committee. Radiother Oncol 1999;52(2):137–148.
420. Belani C, Wang W, Johnson D, et al. Induction chemotherapy followed by standard thoracic radiotherapy (Std. RT) vs. hyperfractionated accelerated radiotherapy (HART) for patients with unresectable stage III A & B non-small cell lung cancer (NSCLC): Phase III study of the Eastern Cooperative Oncology Group (ECOG 2597). Proc Am Soc Clin Oncol 2003;22:622 (abstract 2500).
421. Videtic G, Johnson B, Freidlin B, et al. The survival of patients treated for stage III non-small cell lung cancer in North America has increased during the past 25 years. Lung Cancer 2003; 41(suppl 2):S70 (abstract O-238).
422. Furuse K, Kubota K, Kawahara M, et al. Phase II study of concurrent radiotherapy and chemotherapy for unresectable stage III non-small-cell lung cancer. Southern Osaka Lung Cancer Study Group. J Clin Oncol 1995;13(4):869–875.
423. Stuschke M, Eberhardt W, Pottgen C, et al. Prophylactic cranial irradiation in locally advanced non-small-cell lung cancer after multimodality treatment: long-term follow-up and investigations of late neuropsychologic effects. J Clin Oncol 1999;17(9): 2700–2709.
424. Strauss G, Herndon J, Sherman D, et al. Neoadjuvant chemotherapy and radiotherapy followed by surgery in stage IIIA non-small-cell carcinoma of the lung: report of a Cancer and Leukemia Group B phase II study. J Clin Oncol 1992;10(8):1237–1244.
425. Cox J, Stanley K, Petrovich Z, Paig C, Yesner R. Cranial irradiation in cancer of the lung of all cell types. JAMA 1981;245(5): 469–472.
426. Russell A, Pajak T, Selim H, et al. Prophylactic cranial irradiation for lung cancer patients at high risk for development of cerebral metastasis: results of a prospective randomized trial conducted by the Radiation Therapy Oncology Group. Int J Radiat Oncol Biol Phys 1991;21(3):637–643.
427. Umsawasdi T, Valdivieso M, Chen T, et al. Role of elective brain irradiation during combined chemoradiotherapy for limited disease non-small cell lung cancer. J Neurooncol 1984;2(3):253–259.
428. Skarin A, Jochelson M, Sheldon T, et al. Neoadjuvant chemotherapy in marginally resectable stage III M0 non-small cell lung cancer: long-term follow-up in 41 patients. J Surg Oncol 1989; 40(4):266–274.
429. Robnett T, Machtay M, Stevenson J, Algazy K, Hahn S. Factors affecting the risk of brain metastases after definitive chemoradiation for locally advanced non-small-cell lung carcinoma. J Clin Oncol 2001;19(5):1344–1349.

430. Law A, Karp D, Dipetrillo T, Daly B. Emergence of increased cerebral metastasis after high-dose preoperative radiotherapy with chemotherapy in patients with locally advanced nonsmall cell lung carcinoma. Cancer (Phila) 2001;92(1):160–164.
431. Gaspar L, Scott C, Rotman M, et al. Recursive partitioning analysis (RPA) of prognostic factors in three Radiation Therapy Oncology Group (RTOG) brain metastases trials. Int J Radiat Oncol Biol Phys 1997;37(4):745–751.
432. Patchell R, Tibbs P, Walsh J, et al. A randomized trial of surgery in the treatment of single metastases to the brain. N Engl J Med 1990;322(8):494–500.
433. Vecht C, Haaxma-Reiche H, Noordijk E, et al. Treatment of single brain metastasis: radiotherapy alone or combined with neurosurgery? Ann Neurol 1993;33(6):583–590.
434. Gaspar L, Chansky K, Albain K, et al. Time from treatment to subsequent diagnosis of brain metastases in stage III non-small cell lung cancer (NSCLC): a retrospective review by the Southwest Oncology Group (SWOG). Proc Am Soc Clin Oncol 2003.
435. Komaki R, Scott C, Byhardt R, et al. Failure patterns by prognostic group determined by recursive partitioning analysis (RPA) of 1547 patients on four radiation therapy oncology group (RTOG) studies in inoperable non-small-cell lung cancer (NSCLC). Int J Radiat Oncol Biol Phys 1998;42(2):263–267.
436. Cox J, Scott C, Byhardt R, et al. Addition of chemotherapy to radiation therapy alters failure patterns by cell type within non-small cell carcinoma of lung (NSCCL): analysis of radiation therapy oncology group (RTOG) trials. Int J Radiat Oncol Biol Phys 1999;43(3):505–509.
437. Choi N, Carey R, Daly W, et al. Potential impact on survival of improved tumor downstaging and resection rate by preoperative twice-daily radiation and concurrent chemotherapy in stage IIIA non-small-cell lung cancer. J Clin Oncol 1997;15(2):712–722.
438. Eagan R, Ruud C, Lee R, Pairolero P, Gail M. Pilot study of induction therapy with cyclophosphamide, doxorubicin, and cisplatin (CAP) and chest irradiation prior to thoracotomy in initially inoperable stage III M0 non-small cell lung cancer. Cancer Treat Rep 1987;71(10):895–900.
439. Martini N, Kris M, Gralla R, et al. The effects of preoperative chemotherapy on the resectability of non-small cell lung carcinoma with mediastinal lymph node metastases (N2 M0). Ann Thorac Surg 1988;45(4):370–379.
440. Johnson D. Evolution of cisplatin-based chemotherapy in non-small cell lung cancer: a historical perspective and the Eastern Cooperative Oncology Group Experience. Chest 2000;117(4):133S–137S.
441. Rapp E, Pater J, Willan A, et al. Chemotherapy can prolong survival in patients with advanced non-small-cell lung cancer: report of a Canadian multicenter randomized trial. J Clin Oncol 1988;6:633–641.
442. Ganz P, Figlin R, Haskell C, La Soto N, Siau J. Supportive care versus supportive care and combination chemotherapy in metastatic non-small cell lung cancer. Does chemotherapy make a difference? Cancer (Phila) 1989;63(7):1271–1278.
443. Woods R, Williams C, Levi J, et al. A randomised trial of cisplatin and vindesine versus supportive care only in advanced non-small cell lung cancer. Br J Cancer 1990;61(4):608–611.
444. Cellerino R, Tummarello D, et al. Randomized trial of alternating chemotherapy versus best supportive care in advanced non-small-cell lung cancer. J Clin Oncol 1991;9(8):1453–1461.
445. Cartei G, Cartie F, Cantone A, et al. Cisplatin-cyclophosphamide-mitomycin combination chemotherapy with supportive care versus supportive care alone for treatment of metastatic non-small-cell lung cancer. J Natl Cancer Inst 1993;85:794–800.
446. Thongprasert S, Sanguanmitra P, Juthapan W, Clinch J. Relationship between quality of life and clinical outcomes in advanced non-small cell lung cancer: best supportive care (BSC) versus BSC plus chemotherapy. Lung Cancer 1999;24(1):17–24.
447. Cullen M, Billingham J, Woodroffe C, et al. Mitomycin, ifosfamide, and cisplatin in unresectable non-small-cell lung cancer: effects on survival and quality of life. J Clin Oncol 1999;17:3188–3194.
448. Weick J, Crowley J, Natale R, et al. A randomized trial of five cisplatin-containing treatments in patients with metastatic non-small cell lung cancer: a Southwest Oncology Group study. J Clin Oncol 1991;9:1157–1162.
449. Wozniak A, Crowley JJ, Balcerzak SP, et al. Randomized trial comparing cisplatin with cisplatin plus vinorelbine in the treatment of advanced non-small-cell lung cancer: a Southwest Oncology Group study. J Clin Oncol 1998;16(7):2459–2465.
450. Brown J, Thorpe H, Napp V, et al. The Big Lung Trial Quality of Life Study: determining the effect of cisplatin-based chemotherapy for supportive care in patients with non-small cell lung cancer (NSCLC). In: 10th World Conference on Lung Cancer, 2003, Vancouver, Canada.
451. Billingham L, Cullen M. The benefits of chemotherapy in patient subgroups with unresectable non-small-cell lung cancer. Ann Oncol 2001;12(12):1671–1675.
452. Tummarello D, Graziano F, Isidori P, Cellerino R. Symptomatic, stage IV, non-small-cell lung cancer (NSCLC): response, toxicity, performance status change and symptom relief in patients treated with cisplatin, vinblastine and mitomycin-C. Cancer Chemother Pharmacol 1995;35(3):249–253.
453. Ellis P, Smith I, Hardy J, et al. Symptom relief with MVP (mitomycin C, vinblastine and cisplatin) chemotherapy in advanced non-small-cell lung cancer. Br J Cancer 1995;71(2):366–370.
454. Grilli R, Oxman A, Julian J. Chemotherapy for advanced non-small-cell lung cancer: how much benefit is enough? J Clin Oncol 1993;11(10):1866–1872.
455. Marino P, Pampallona S, Preatoni A, Cantoni A, Inveinezzi F. Chemotherapy vs. supportive care in advanced non-small cell lung cancer: results of a meta-analysis of the literature. Chest 1994;106:861–865.
456. Depierre A, Lemarie E, Dabouis G, Garnier G, Jacoulet P, Dalphin J. A phase II study of navelbine (vinorelbine) in the treatment of non-small-cell lung cancer. Am J Clin Oncol 1991;14(2):115–119.
457. Fukuoka M, Niitani H, Suzuki A, et al. A phase II study of CPT-11, a new derivative of camptothecin, for previously untreated non-small-cell lung cancer. J Clin Oncol 1992;10:16–20.
458. Murphy W, Fossella F, Winn R, et al. Phase II study of taxol in patients with untreated advanced non-small-cell lung cancer. J Natl Cancer Inst 1993;85:384–388.
459. Francis P, Rigas J, Kris M, et al. Phase II trial of docetaxel in patients with stage III and IV non-small-cell lung cancer. J Clin Oncol 1994;12(6):1232–1237.
460. Fossella F, Lippman S, Shin D, et al. Maximum-tolerated dose defined for single-agent gemcitabine: a phase I dose-escalation study in chemotherapy-naive patients with advanced non-small-cell lung cancer. J Clin Oncol 1997;15(1):310–316.
461. Chang A, Kim K, Glick J, Anderson T, Karp D, Johnson D. Phase II study of taxol in patients with stage IV non-small cell lung cancer (NSCLC): the Eastern Cooperative Oncology Group (ECOG) results. Proc Am Soc Clin Oncol 1992;11:293 (abstract 981).
462. Akerley W III. Paclitaxel in advanced non-small cell lung cancer: an alternative high-dose weekly schedule. Chest 2000;117(4 suppl 1):152S–155S.
463. Anonymous. Effects of vinorelbine on quality of life and survival of elderly patients with advanced non-small cell lung cancer. The Elderly Lung Cancer Vinorelbine Italian Study Group. J Natl Cancer Inst 1999;91:66–72.
464. Roszkowski K, Pluzanska A, Krzakowski M, et al. A multicenter, randomized, phase III study of docetaxel plus best supportive care versus best supportive care in chemotherapy-naive

patients with metastatic or non-resectable localized non-small cell lung cancer (NSCLC). Lung Cancer 2000;27(3):145–157.

465. Ranson M, Davidson N, Nicolson M, et al. Randomized trial of paclitaxel plus supportive care versus supportive care for patients with advanced non-small-cell lung cancer. J Natl Cancer Inst 2000;92(13):1074–1080.
466. Anderson H, Hopwood P, Stephens R, et al. Gemcitabine plus best supportive care (BSC) vs BSC in inoperable non-small cell lung cancer: a randomized trial with quality of life as the primary outcome. UK NSCLC Gemcitabine Group. Non-Small Cell Lung Cancer. Br J Cancer 2000;83(4):447–453.
467. Ruckdeschel J, Finkelstein D, Ettinger D, et al. A randomized trial of the four most active regimens for metastatic non-small cell lung cancer. J Clin Oncol 1986;4:14–22.
468. Sandler A, Nemunaitis J, Denham C, et al. Phase III trial of gemcitabine plus cisplatin versus cisplatin alone in patients with locally advanced or metastatic non-small cell lung cancer. J Clin Oncol 2000;18:122–130.
469. von Pawel J, von Roemeling R, Gatzemeier U, et al. Tirapazamine plus cisplatin versus cisplatin in advanced non-small-cell lung cancer: a report of the international CATAPULT I study group. Cisplatin and tirapazamine in subjects with advanced previously untreated non-small-cell lung tumors. J Clin Oncol 2000;18(6):1351–1359.
470. Gatzemeier U, von Pawel J, Gottfried M, et al. Phase III comparative study of high-dose cisplatin versus a combination of paclitaxel and cisplatin in patients with advanced non-small-cell lung cancer. J Clin Oncol 2000;18(19):3390–3399.
471. Bonomi P, Finkelstein D, Ruckdeschel J, et al. Combination chemotherapy versus single agents followed by combination chemotherapy in stage IV non-small-cell lung cancer: a study of the Eastern Cooperative Oncology Group. J Clin Oncol 1989;7:1602–1613.
472. Klastersky J, Sculier J, Lacroix L, et al. A randomized study comparing cisplatin or carboplatin with etoposide in patients with advanced non-small-cell lung cancer: European Organization for Research and Treatment of Cancer, protocol 07861. J Clin Oncol 1990;8:1556–1562.
473. Zatloukal P, Petruzelka L, Zemanova M, et al. Gemcitabine plus cisplatin vs. gemcitabine plus carboplatin in stage IIIb and IV non-small cell lung cancer: a phase III randomized trial. Lung Cancer 2003;41(3):321–331.
474. Schiller J, Harrington D, Belani C, et al. Comparison of four chemotherapy regimens for advanced non-small cell lung cancer. N Engl J Med 2002;346(2):92–98.
475. Jelic S, Mitrovic L, Radosavljevic D, et al. Survival advantage for carboplatin substituting cisplatin in combination with vindesine and mitomycin C for stage IIIB and IV squamous-cell bronchogenic carcinoma: a randomized phase III study. Lung Cancer 2001;34(1):1–13.
476. Rosell R, Gatzemeier U, Betticher D, et al. Phase III randomized trial comparing paclitaxel/carboplatin with paclitaxel/cisplatin in patients with advanced non-small cell lung cancer: a cooperative multinational trial. Ann Oncol 2002;13(10):1539–1549.
477. Fossella F, Pereira J, von Pawel J, et al. Randomized, multinational, phase III study of docetaxel plus platinum combinations versus vinorelbine plus cisplatin for advanced non-small-cell lung cancer: the TAX 326 study group. J Clin Oncol 2003;21(16):3016–3024.
478. Le Chevalier T, Brisgand D, Douillard J, et al. Randomized study of vinorelbine and cisplatin versus vindesine and cisplatin versus vinorelbine alone in advanced non-small-cell lung cancer: results of a European multicenter trial including 612 patients. J Clin Oncol 1994;12:360–367.
479. ten Bokkel Huinink W, Bergman B, Chemaissani A, et al. Single-agent gemcitabine: an active and better tolerated alternative to standard cisplatin-based chemotherapy in locally advanced or metastatic non-small cell lung cancer. Lung Cancer 1999;26(2):85–94.
480. Vansteenkiste J, Vandebroek J, Nackaerts K, et al. Influence of cisplatin-use, age, performance status and duration of chemotherapy on symptom control in advanced non-small cell lung cancer: detailed symptom analysis of a randomised study comparing cisplatin-vindesine to gemcitabine. Lung Cancer 2003;40(2):191–199.
481. Lilenbaum R, Herndon J, List M. Single agent versus combination chemotherapy in advanced non-small cell lung cancer: a CALGB randomized trial of efficacy, quality of life, and cost effectiveness. Presented at the Amer Soc Clin Oncol, Orlando, Florida, 2002.
482. Sederholm C. Gemcitabine (G) compared with gemcitabine plus carboplatin (GC) in advanced non-small cell lung cancer (NSCLC): a phase III study by the Swedish Lung Cancer Study Group (SLUSG). Presented at the Amer Soc Clin Oncol, Orlando, Florida, 2002.
483. Georgoulias V, Ardavanis A, Agelidou M, et al. Preliminary analysis of a multicenter phase III trial comparing docetaxel (D) versus docetaxel/cisplatin (DC) in patients with inoperable advanced and metastatic non-small cell lung cancer (NSCLC). Presented at the Amer Soc Clin Oncol, Orlando, Florida, 2002.
484. Negoro S, Masuda N, Takada Y, et al. Randomised phase III trial of irinotecan combined with cisplatin for advanced non-small-cell lung cancer. Br J Cancer 2003;88(3):335–341.
485. Giaccone G, Splinter T, Debruyne C, et al. Randomized study of paclitaxel-cisplatin versus cisplatin-teniposide in patients with advanced non-small-cell lung cancer. The European Organization for Research and Treatment of Cancer Lung Cancer Cooperative Group. J Clin Oncol 1998;16(6):2133–2141.
486. Belani C, Natale R, Lee J, et al. Randomized phase III trial comparing cisplatin/etoposide versus carboplatin/paclitaxel in advanced and metastatic non-small cell lung cancer (NSCLC). Presented at the Amer Soc Clin Oncol, Los Angeles, California, 1998.
487. Cardenal F, Lopez-Cabrerizo M, Anton A, et al. Randomized phase III study of gemcitabine-cisplatin versus etoposide-cisplatin in the treatment of locally advanced or metastatic non-small-cell lung cancer. J Clin Oncol 1999;17(1):12–18.
488. Bonomi P, Kim K, Fairclough D, et al. Comparison of survival and quality of life in advanced non-small cell lung cancer patients treated with two dose levels of paclitaxel combined with cisplatin versus etoposide with cisplatin: results of an Eastern Cooperative Oncology Group trial. J Clin Oncol 2000;18(3):623–631.
489. Takiguchi Y, Nagao K, Nishiwaki A. The final results of a randomized phase III trial comparing irinotecan (CPT-11) and cisplatin (CDDP) with vindesine (VDS) and CDDP in advanced non-small-cell lung cancer (NSCLC). In: 9th World Conference on Lung Cancer, 2000.
490. Grigorescu A, Draghici I, Nitipir C, Gutulescu N, Corlan E. Gemcitabine (GEM) and carboplatin (CBDCA) versus cisplatin (CDDP) and vinblastine (VLB) in advanced non-small-cell lung cancer (NSCLC) stages III and IV: a phase III randomised trial. Lung Cancer 2002;37(1):9–14.
491. Kubota K, Watanabe K, Kunitoh H. Final results of a randomized phase III trial of docetaxel and cisplatin versus vindesine and cisplatin in stage IV non-small cell lung cancer (NSCLC). Presented at the Amer Soc Clin Oncol, Orlando, Florida, 2002.
492. Kosmidis P, Mylonakis N, Skarlos D, et al. Paclitaxel ($175 mg/m^2$) plus carboplatin (6 AUC) versus paclitaxel ($225 mg/m^2$) plus carboplatin (6 AUC) in advanced non-small-cell lung cancer (NSCLC): a multicenter randomized trial. Hellenic Cooperative Oncology Group (HeCOG). Ann Oncol 2000;11(7): 799–805.

493. Kelly K, Crowley J, Bunn P, et al. Randomized phase III trial of paclitaxel plus carboplatin versus vinorelbine plus cisplatin in the treatment of patients with advanced non-small-cell lung cancer: a Southwest Oncology Group trial. J Clin Oncol 2001; 19(13):3210–3218.
494. Huang C, Langer C, Minniti C, et al. Phase III toxicity trial of carboplatin (Cb) plus either docetaxel (D) or paclitaxel (P) in advanced non-small cell lung cancer (NSCLC): preliminary findings of OPN-001. Presented at the Amer Soc Clin Oncol, Orlando, Florida, 2002.
495. Scagliotti G, De Marinis F, Rinaldi M, et al. Phase III randomized trial comparing three platinum-based doublets in advanced non-small-cell lung cancer. J Clin Oncol 2002;20(21):4285–4291.
496. Harper P, Plunkett T, Khayat D. Quality trials and quality of life in non-small-cell lung cancer. J Clin Oncol 2003;21(16):3007–3008.
497. Crino L, Scagliotti G, Ricci S, et al. Gemcitabine and cisplatin versus mitomycin, ifosfamide, and cisplatin in advanced non-small-cell lung cancer: a randomized phase III study of the Italian Lung Cancer Project. J Clin Oncol 1999;17(11):3522–3530.
498. Comella P, Frasci G, Panza N, et al. Randomized trial comparing cisplatin, gemcitabine, and vinorelbine with either cisplatin and gemcitabine or cisplatin and vinorelbine in advanced non-small-cell lung cancer: interim analysis of a phase III trial of the Southern Italy Cooperative Oncology Group. J Clin Oncol 2000;18(7):1451–1457.
499. Comella P. Phase III trial of cisplatin/gemcitabine with or without vinorelbine or paclitaxel in advanced non-small cell lung cancer. Semin Oncol 2001;28(2 suppl 7):7–10.
500. Rudd R, Gower N, James L. Phase III randomised comparison of gemcitabine and carboplatin (GC) with mitomycin, ifosfamide and cisplatin (MIP) in advanced non-small cell lung cancer (NSCLC). Presented at the Amer Soc Clin Oncol, Orlando, Florida, 2002.
501. Melo M, Barradas P, Costa A, Cristovao M, Alves P. Results of a randomized phase III trial comparing 4 cisplatin (P)-based regimens in the treatment of locally advanced and metastatic non-small cell lung cancer (NSCLC): mitomycin/vinblastine/cisplatin (MVP) is no longer a therapeutic option. Presented at the Amer Soc Clin Oncol, Orlando, Florida, 2002.
502. Paccagnella A, Favaretto A, Bearz A, et al. Carboplatin/paclitaxel (CP) vs carboplatin/paclitaxel/gemcitabine (CPG) in advanced NSCLC: a phase II-III multicentric study. Presented at the Amer Soc Clin Oncol, Orlando, Florida, 2002.
503. Gebbia V, Galetta D, Riccardi F, et al. Vinorelbine plus cisplatin versus cisplatin plus vindesine and mitomycin C in stage IIIB-IV non-small cell lung carcinoma: a prospective randomized study. Lung Cancer 2002;37(2):179 S. Frustaci, F. Barbieri, F. Oniga, M. Ghi, R. Biason, M. Clerici, G. Ceresoli, A. 187.
504. Kodani T, Ueoka H, Kiura K, et al. A phase III randomized trial comparing vindesine and cisplatin with or without ifosfamide in patients with advanced non-small-cell lung cancer: long-term follow-up results and analysis of prognostic factors. Lung Cancer 2002;36(3):313–319.
505. Sculier J, Lafitte J, Lecomte J, et al. A three-arm phase III randomised trial comparing combinations of platinum derivatives, ifosfamide and/or gemcitabine in stage IV non-small-cell lung cancer. Ann Oncol 2002;13(6):874–882.
506. Souquet P, Tan E, Rodrigues Pereira J, et al. GLOB-1: a prospective randomised clinical phase III trial comparing vinorelbine-cisplatin with vinorelbine-ifosfamide-cisplatin in metastatic non-small-cell lung cancer patients. Ann Oncol 2002;13(12): 1853–1861.
507. Danson S, Middleton M, O'Byrne K, et al. Phase III trial of gemcitabine and carboplatin versus mitomycin, ifosfamide, and cisplatin or mitomycin, vinblastine, and cisplatin in patients with advanced non-small cell lung carcinoma. Cancer (Phila) 2003; 98(3):542–553.
508. Delbaldo C, Syz N, Michiels S, Le Chevalier T, Pignon J-P. Adding a second or a third drug to a chemotherapy regimen in patients with advanced non-small-cell lung carcinoma (NSCLC): a meta-analysis of the literature. Presented at the Amer Soc Clin Oncol, Chicago, Illinois, 2003.
509. Baggstrom M, Socinski M, Hensing T, Poole C. Addressing the optimal number of cytotoxic agents in stage IIIB/IV non-small cell lung cancer (NSCLC): a meta-analysis of the published literature. Presented at the Amer Soc Clin Oncol, Chicago, Illinois, 2003.
510. Williamson S, Crowley J, Lara P, et al. S0003: paclitaxel/carboplatin (PC) v PC + tirapazamine (PCT) in advanced non-small cell lung cancer (NSCLC). A Southwest Oncology Group (SWOG) trial. Presented at the Amer Soc Clin Oncol, Chicago, Illinois, 2003.
511. Giaccone G. Early results of a randomized phase III trial of platinum-containing doublets versus a nonplatinum doublet in the treatment of advanced non-small cell lung cancer: European Organization for Research and Treatment of Cancer 08975. Semin Oncol 2002;29(3 suppl 9):47–49.
512. Georgoulias V, Papadakis E, Alexopoulos A, et al. Cancer platinum-based and non-platinum-based chemotherapy in advanced non-small-cell lung cancer: a randomised multicentre trial. Lancet 2001;357(9267):1478–1484.
513. Gridelli C, Gallo C, Shepherd F, et al. Gemcitabine plus vinorelbine compared with cisplatin plus vinorelbine or cisplatin plus gemcitabine for advanced non-small-cell lung cancer: a phase III trial of the Italian GEMVIN Investigators and the National Cancer Institute of Canada Clinical Trials Group. J Clin Oncol 2003;21(16):3025–3034.
514. Kakolyris S, Tsiafaki X, Agelidou A, et al. Preliminary results of a multicenter randomized phase III trial of docetaxel plus gemcitabine (DG) versus vinorelbine plus cisplatin (VC) in patients with advanced non-small cell lung cancer. Presented at the Amer Soc Clin Oncol, Orlando, Florida, 2002.
515. Patel R, Keiser L, Justice G, et al. ACORN 9901: a multicenter randomized trial of docetaxel plus gemcitabine versus weekly paclitaxel plus gemcitabine in patients (pts) with non-small-cell lung cancer. Presented at the Amer Soc Clin Oncol, Orlando, Florida, 2002.
516. Kosmidis P, Mylonakis N, Nicolaides C, et al. Paclitaxel plus carboplatin versus gemcitabine plus paclitaxel in advanced non-small-cell lung cancer: a phase III randomized trial. J Clin Oncol 2002;20(17):3578–3585.
517. Treat J, Belani C, Edelman M, et al. A randomized phase III trial of gemcitabine (G) in combination with carboplatin (C) or paclitaxel (P) versus paclitaxel plus carboplatin in advanced (stage IIIB, IV) non-small cell lung cancer (NSCLC). Presented at the Amer Soc Clin Oncol, Chicago, Illinois, 2003.
518. Socinski M, Schell M, Peterman A, et al. Phase III trial comparing a defined duration of therapy versus continuous therapy followed by second-line therapy in advanced-stage IIIB/IV non-small-cell lung cancer. J Clin Oncol 2002;20(5):1335–1343.
519. Smith I, O'Brien M, Talbot D, et al. Duration of chemotherapy in advanced non-small-cell lung cancer: a randomized trial of three versus six courses of mitomycin, vinblastine, and cisplatin. J Clin Oncol 2001;19(5):1336–1343.
520. Depierre A, Quoix E, Mercier M. Maintenance chemotherapy in advanced non-small cell lung cancer (NSCLC): a randomized study of vinorelbine (V) versus observation (OB) in patients (Pts) responding to induction therapy (French Cooperative Oncology Group). Presented at the Amer Soc Clin Oncol, New Orleans, Louisiana, 2001.
521. Hutchins L, Unger J, Crowley J, Coltman C Jr, Albain K. Underrepresentation of patients 65 years of age or older in cancer-treatment trials. N Engl J Med 1999;341(27):2061–2067.

522. Montella M, Gridelli C, Crispo A, et al. Has lung cancer in the elderly different characteristics at presentation? Oncol Rep 2002;9(5):1093–1096.
523. Yellen S, Cella D, Leslie W. Age and clinical decision making in oncology patients. J Natl Cancer Inst 1994;86(23):1766–1770.
524. Kelly K, Giarritta S, Hayes S, et al. Should older patients (pts) receive combination chemotherapy for advanced stage non-small cell lung cancer (NSCLC)? An analysis of Southwest Oncology Trials 9509 and 9308. Presented at the Amer Soc Clin Oncol, New Orleans, Louisiana, 2001.
525. Langer C, Vangel M, Schiller J, et al. Age-specific subanalysis of ECOG 1594: fit elderly patients (70–80 yrs) with NSCLC do as well as younger pts (<70). Presented at the Amer Soc Clin Oncol, Chicago, Illinois, 2003.
526. Rocha Lima C, Herndon J II, Kosty M, Clamon G, Green M. Therapy choices among older patients with lung carcinoma: an evaluation of two trials of the Cancer and Leukemia Group B. Cancer (Phila) 2002;94(1):181–187.
527. Langer C, Manola J, Bernardo P, et al. Cisplatin-based therapy for elderly patients with advanced non-small-cell lung cancer: implications of Eastern Cooperative Oncology Group 5592, a randomized trial. J Natl Cancer Inst 2002;94(3):173–181.
528. Hensing T, Peterman A, Schell M, Lee J, Socinski M. The impact of age on toxicity, response rate, quality of life, and survival in patients with advanced, Stage IIIB or IV non-small cell lung carcinoma treated with carboplatin and paclitaxel. Cancer (Phila) 2003;98(4):779–788.
529. Gridelli C, Perrone F, Gallo C, et al. Chemotherapy for elderly patients with advanced non-small-cell lung cancer: the Multicenter Italian Lung Cancer in the Elderly Study (MILES) phase III randomized trial. J Natl Cancer Inst 2003;95(5):362–372.
530. Frasci G, Lorusso V, Panza N, et al. Gemcitabine plus vinorelbine versus vinorelbine alone in elderly patients with advanced non-small-cell lung cancer. J Clin Oncol 2000;18(13):2529–2536.
531. Quoix E, Breton J, Ducolone A, et al. First-line 4-weeks (4W) versus 3-weeks (3W) single agent gemcitabine (Gem) in elderly patients (pts) with NSCLC: A randomized multicentre phase II study. Presented at the Amer Soc Clin Oncol, Chicago, Illinois, 2003.
532. Hainsworth J, Burris H III, Litchy S, et al. Weekly docetaxel in the treatment of elderly patients with advanced nonsmall cell lung carcinoma. A Minnie Pearl Cancer Research Network phase II trial. Cancer (Phila) 2000;89(2):328–333.
533. Peake M, Thompson S, Lowe D, Pearson M. Ageism in the management of lung cancer. Age Ageing 2003;32(2):171–177.
534. Earle C, Tsai J, Gelber R, Weinstein M, Neumann P, Weeks J. Effectiveness of chemotherapy for advanced lung cancer in the elderly: instrumental variable and propensity analysis. J Clin Oncol 2001;19(4):1064–1070.
535. Gridelli C, Maione P, Barletta E. Individualized chemotherapy for elderly patients with non-small cell lung cancer. Curr Opin Oncol 2002;14(2):199–203.
536. Eton D, Fairclough D, Cella D, Yount S, Bonomi P, Johnson D. Early change in patient-reported health during lung cancer chemotherapy predicts clinical outcomes beyond those predicted by baseline report: results from Eastern Cooperative Oncology Group Study 5592. J Clin Oncol 2003;21(8):1536–1543.
537. Fossella F, Devore R, Crawford J, et al. Randomized phase III trial of docetaxel versus vinorelbine or ifosfamide in patients with advanced non-small-cell lung cancer previously treated with plantinum-containing chemotherapy regimens. The TAX 320 Non-Small Cell Lung Cancer Study Group. J Clin Oncol 2000;18(12):2354–2362.
538. Shepard F, Dancey J, Ramlau R, et al. Prospective randomized trial of docetaxel versus best supportive care in patients with non-small-cell lung cancer previously treated with platinum-based chemotherapy. J Clin Oncol 2000;18:2095–2103.
539. Leighl N, Shepherd R, Burkes R, Goodwin P. Economic analysis of the TAX 317 trial: Docetaxel versus best supportive care as second-line therapy of advanced non-small-cell lung cancer. J Clin Oncol 2002;20:1344–1352.
540. Hanna N, Shepherd F, Rosell R, et al. A phase III study of pemetrexed vs docetaxel in patients with recurrent non-small cell lung cancer (NSCLC) who were previously treated with chemotherapy. Presented at the Amer Soc Clin Oncol, Chicago, Illinois, 2003.
541. Gridelli C, Illiano A, Salvagni S, et al. Effect on quality-of-life (QOL) of weekly vs. 3-weekly docetaxel (D) in second-line treatment of advanced non-small-cell lung cancer. The DISTAL randomized phase 3 trial. Presented at the Amer Soc Clin Oncol, Chicago, Illinois, 2003.
542. Camps C, Massuti B, Jimenez A, et al. Second-line docetaxel adminstered every 3 weeks versus weekly in advanced non-small-cell lung cancer (NSCLC): a Spanish Lung Cancer Group (SLCG) phase III trial. Presented at the Amer Soc Clin Oncol, Chicago, Illinois, 2003.
543. Crino L, Mosconi A, Scagliotti G, et al. Gemcitabine as second-line treatment for relapsing or refractory advanced non-small cell lung cancer: a phase II trial. Semin Oncol 1998;25(4 suppl 9):23–26.
544. Socinski M, Schell M, Bakri K, et al. Second-line, low-dose, weekly paclitaxel in patients with stage IIIB/IV nonsmall cell lung carcinoma who fail first-line chemotherapy with carboplatin plus paclitaxel. Cancer (Phila) 2002;95(6):1265–1273.
545. Kris M, Natale R, Herbst R, et al. Efficacy of gefitinib, an inhibitor of the epidermal growth factor receptor tyrosine kinase, in symptomatic patients with non-small cell lung cancer: a randomized trial. JAMA 2003;290(16):2149–2158.
546. Fukuoka M, Yano S, Giaccone G, et al. Multi-institutional randomized phase II trial of gefitinib for previously treated patients with advanced non-small-cell lung cancer. J Clin Oncol 2003; 21(12):2237–2246.
547. Giaccone G, Johnson D, Manegold C, et al. Phase III clinical trial of ZD1839 ('Iressa') in combination with gemcitabine and cisplatin in chemotherapy-naive patients with advanced non-small-cell lung cancer (INTACT 1). Ann Oncol 2002;13(suppl 5):2.
548. Johnson D, Herbst R, Giaconne G, et al. ZD1839 ("Iressa") in combination with paclitaxel and carboplatin in chemotherapy-naive patients with advanced non-small-cell lung cancer: results from a phase III clinical trial (INTACT2). Ann Oncol 2002; 13(suppl 5):127–128.
549. Sirotnak F, Zakowiski M, Miller V, Scher H, Kris M. Efficacy of cytotoxic agents against human tumor xenografts is markedly enhanced by coadministration of ZD1839 (Iressa), an inhibitor of EGFR tyrosine kinase. Clin Cancer Res 2000;6:4885–4892.
550. Natale R, Shak S, Aronson N, et al. Quantitative gene expression in non-small cell lung cancer from paraffin-embedded tissue specimens: predicting response to gefitinib, an EGFR kinase inhibitor. Presented at the Amer Soc Clin Oncol, Chicago, Illinois, 2003.
551. Saltz L, Rubin M, Hochster H, et al. Cetuximab (IMC-C225) plus irinotecan (CPT-11) is active in CPT-11-refractory colorectal cancer (CRC) that expresses epidermal growth factor receptor (EGFR). Presented at the Amer Soc Clin Oncol, New Orleans, Louisiana, 2001.
552. Clark G, Perez-Soler R, Siu L, Gordon A, Santabarbara P. Rash severity is predictive of increased survival with erlotinib HCl. Presented at the Amer Soc Clin Oncol, Chicago, Illinois, 2003.
553. Lynch TJ, Bell DW, Sordella R, et al. Activating mutations in the epidermal growth factor receptor underlying responsiveness of non-small-cell lung cancer to gefitinib. N Engl J Med 2004; 350;2129–2139.

554. Paez JG, Janne PA, Lee JC, et al. EGFR mutations in lung cancer: correlation with clinical response to gefitinib therapy. Science 2004;304:1497–1500.
555. Shigematsu H, Lin L, Takahashi T, et al. Clinical and biological features associated with epidermal growth factor receptor gene mutations in lung cancers. J Natl Cancer Inst 2005;97(5):339–346.
556. Johnson DH, Fehrenbacher L, Novotny WF, et al. Randomized phase II trial comparing bevacizumab plus carboplatin and paclitaxel with carboplatin and paclitaxel alone in previously untreated locally advanced or metastatic non-small-cell lung cancer. J Clin Oncol. 2004;22(11):2184–2191.
557. Johnson D, DeVore R, Kabbinavar F, Herbst R, Holmgren E, Novotny W. Carboplatin (C) + paclitaxel (T) + RhuMab-VEGF (AVF) may prolong survival in advanced non-squamous lung cancer. Presented at the Amer Soc Clin Oncol, New Orleans, Louisiana, 2001.
558. Mininberg E, Herbst R, Henderson T, et al. Phase I/II study of the recombinant humanized monoclonal anti-VEGF antibody bevacizumab and the EGFR-TK inhibitor erlotinib in patients with recurrent non-small cell lung cancer (NSCLC). Presented at the Amer Soc Clin Oncol, Chicago, Illinois, 2003.
559. Johnson D, Csiki I, Gonzalez A, et al. Cyclooxygenase-2 (COX-2) inhibition in non-small cell lung cancer (NSCLC): preliminary results of a phase II trial. Presented at the Amer Soc Clin Oncol, Chicago, Illinois, 2003.
560. Schuler M, Herrmann R, De Greve J, et al. Adenovirus-mediated wild-type p53 gene transfer in patients receiving chemotherapy for advanced non-small cell lung cancer: results of a multicenter phase II study. J Clin Oncol 2001;19(6):1750–1758.
561. Nemunaitis J, Smith J, Sterman D, et al. A phase I/II trial of bystander GVAX cancer vaccine in non-small cell lung cancer (NSCLC). Presented at the Amer Soc Clin Oncol, Orlando, Florida, 2002.
562. Adjei A, Mauer A, Marks R. A phase II study of the farnesyltransferase inhibitor R115777 in patients with advanced non-small cell lung cancer. Proc Am Soc Clin Oncol 2002;21:290a (abstract 1156).
563. Strumberg D, Awada A, Piccart M, et al. Final report of the phase I clinical program of the novel raf kinase inhibitor BAY 43-9006 in patients with refractory solid tumors. Presented at the Amer Soc Clin Oncol, Chicago, Illinois, 2003.
564. Gordon M, Mendelson D, Guirguis M, Knight R, Humerickhouse R. ABT-510, an anti-angiogenic, thrombospondin-1 (TSP-1) mimetic peptide, exhibits favorable safety profile and early signals of activity in a randomized phase IB trial. Presented at the Amer Soc Clin Oncol, Chicago, Illinois, 2003.
565. Khuri F, Rigas J, Figlin R, et al. Multi-institutional phase I/II trial of oral bexarotene in combination with cisplatin and vinorelbine in previously untreated patients with advanced non-small-cell lung cancer. J Clin Oncol 2001;19(10):2626–2637.
566. Stevenson J, Nho C, Schick J, et al. Phase II clinical/pharmacodynamic trial of the proteasome inhibitor PS-341 in advanced non-small cell lung cancer. Presented at the Amer Soc Clin Oncol, Chicago, Illinois, 2003.
567. Danesi R, de Braud F, Fogli S, et al. Pharmacogenetics of anticancer drug sensitivity in non-small cell lung cancer. Pharmacol Rev 2003;55(1):57–103.
568. Murran J, Glatstein E, Pass H. Small cell lung cancer. In: Devita V Jr, Hellman S, Rosenberg S (eds). Cancer: Principles and Practice of Oncology. Philadephia: Lippincott, 2001:983–1018.
569. Birch R, Omura G, Greco F, Perez C. Patterns of failure in combined chemotherapy and radiotherapy for limited small cell lung cancer: Southeastern Cancer Study Group experience. Natl Cancer Inst Monogr 1988;6:265–270.
570. Perry M, Eaton W, Propert K, et al. Chemotherapy with or without radiation therapy in limited small-cell carcinoma of the lung. N Engl J Med 1987;316(15):912–918.
571. Kies M, Mira J, Crowley J, et al. Multimodal therapy for limited small-cell lung cancer: a randomized study of induction combination chemotherapy with or without thoracic radiation in complete responders; and with wide-field versus reduced-field radiation in partial responders: a Southwest Oncology Group Study. J Clin Oncol 1987;5(4):592–600.
572. Murray N, Coy P, Pater J, et al. Importance of timing for thoracic irradiation in the combined modality treatment of limited-stage small-cell lung cancer. The National Cancer Institute of Canada Clinical Trials Group. J Clin Oncol 1993;11(2):336–344.
573. Creech R, Richter M, Finkelstein D. Combination chemotherapy with or without consolidation radiation therapy (RT) for regional small cell carcinoma of the lung. Proc Am Soc Clin Oncol 1988.
574. Fox W, Scadding J. Medical Research Council comparative trial of surgery and radiotherapy for primary treatment of small-celled or oat-celled carcinoma of bronchus. Ten-year follow-up. Lancet 1973;2(7820):63–65.
575. Jenkin D, Chan H, Freedman M, et al. Hodgkin's disease in children: treatment results with MOPP and low-dose, extended-field irradiation. Cancer Treat Rep 1982;66(4):949–959.
576. Bergsagel D, Jenkin R, Pringle J, et al. Lung cancer: clinical trial of radiotherapy alone vs. radiotherapy plus cyclophosphamide. Cancer (Phila) 1972;30(3):621–627.
577. Turrisi A III, Glover D. Thoracic radiotherapy variables: influence on local control in small cell lung cancer limited disease. Int J Radiat Oncol Biol Phys 1990;19(6):1473–1479.
578. Pignon J, Arriagada R, Ihde D, et al. A meta-analysis of thoracic radiotherapy for small-cell lung cancer. N Engl J Med 1992; 327(23):1618–1624.
579. Choi N, Herndon J II, Rosenman J, et al. Phase I study to determine the maximum-tolerated dose of radiation in standard daily and hyperfractionated-accelerated twice-daily radiation schedules with concurrent chemotherapy for limited-stage small-cell lung cancer. J Clin Oncol 1998;16(11): 3528–3536.
580. Liengswangwong V, Bonner J, Shaw E, et al. Limited-stage small-cell lung cancer: patterns of intrathoracic recurrence and the implications for thoracic radiotherapy. J Clin Oncol 1994;12(3): 496–502.
581. Brodin O, Rikner G, Steinholtz L, Nou E. Local failure in patients treated with radiotherapy and multidrug chemotherapy for small cell lung cancer. Acta Oncol 1990;29(6):739–746.
582. Arriagada R, Pellae-Cosset B, Ladron de Guevara J, et al. Alternating radiotherapy and chemotherapy schedules in limited small cell lung cancer: analysis of local chest recurrences. Radiother Oncol 1991;20(2):91–98.
583. Carlson R, Sikic B, Gandara D, et al. Late consolidative radiation therapy in the treatment of limited-stage small cell lung cancer. Cancer (Phila) 1991;68(5):948–958.
584. Lebeau B, Chastang C, Brechot J, Capron F. A randomized trial of delayed thoracic radiotherapy in complete responder patients with small-cell lung cancer. Petites Cellules Group. Chest 1993;104(3):726–733.
585. Lebeau B, Urban T, Brechot J, et al. A randomized clinical trial comparing concurrent and alternating thoracic irradiation for patients with limited small cell lung carcinoma. "Petites Cellules" Group. Cancer (Phila) 1999;86(8):1480–1487.
586. Takada M, Fukuoka M, Furuse K, et al. Phase III study of concurrent versus sequential thoracic radiotherapy (RT) in combination with cisplatin (C) and etoposide (E) for limited-stage (LS) small cell lung cancer (SCLC): preliminary results of the Japan Clinical Oncology Group (JCOG). Proc Am Soc Clin Oncol 1996.
587. Perry M, Herndon J III, Eaton W, Green M. Thoracic radiation therapy added to chemotherapy for small-cell lung cancer: an update of Cancer and Leukemia Group B Study 8083. J Clin Oncol 1998;16(7):2466–2467.

588. Work E, Nielsen O, Bentzen S, Fode K, Palshof T. Randomized study of initial versus late chest irradiation combined with chemotherapy in limited-stage small-cell lung cancer. Aarhus Lung Cancer Group. J Clin Oncol 1997;15(9):3030–3037.
589. Gregor A, Drings P, Burghouts J, et al. Randomized trial of alternating versus sequential radiotherapy/chemotherapy in limited-disease patients with small-cell lung cancer: a European Organization for Research and Treatment of Cancer Lung Cancer Cooperative Group Study. J Clin Oncol 1997;15(8):2840–2849.
590. Jeremic B, Shibamoto Y, Acimovic L, Milisavljevic S. Initial versus delayed accelerated hyperfractionated radiation therapy and concurrent chemotherapy in limited small-cell lung cancer: a randomized study. J Clin Oncol 1997;15(3):893–900.
591. Gregor A. Prophylactic cranial irradiation in small-cell lung cancer: is it ever indicated? Oncology (Huntingt) 1998;12(1 suppl 2):19–24.
592. Arriagada R, Le Chevalier T, Borie F, et al. Prophylactic cranial irradiation for patients with small-cell lung cancer in complete remission. J Natl Cancer Inst 1995;87(3):183–190.
593. Gregor A, Cull A, Stephens R, et al. Prophylactic cranial irradiation is indicated following complete response to induction therapy in small cell lung cancer: results of a multicentre randomised trial. United Kingdom Coordinating Committee for Cancer Research (UKCCCR) and the European Organization for Research and Treatment of Cancer (EORTC). Eur J Cancer 1997;33(11):1752–1758.
594. Auperin A, Arriagada R, Pignon J, et al. Prophylactic cranial irradiation for patients with small-cell lung cancer in complete remission. Prophylactic Cranial Irradiation Overview Collaborative Group. N Engl J Med 1999;341(7):476–484.
595. Laukkanen E, Klonoff H, Allan B, Graeb D, Murray N. The role of prophylactic brain irradiation in limited stage small cell lung cancer: clinical, neuropsychologic, and CT sequelae. Int J Radiat Oncol Biol Phys 1988;14(6):1109–1117.
596. Lishner M, Feld R, Payne D, et al. Late neurological complications after prophylactic cranial irradiation in patients with small-cell lung cancer: the Toronto experience. J Clin Oncol 1990;8(2):215–221.
597. Twijnstra A, Boon P, Lormans A, ten Velde G. Neurotoxicity of prophylactic cranial irradiation in patients with small cell carcinoma of the lung. Eur J Cancer Clin Oncol 1987;23(7):983–986.
598. Van Oosterhout A, Ganzevles P, Wilmink J, De Geus B, Van Vonderen R, Twijnstra A. Sequelae in long-term survivors of small cell lung cancer. Int J Radiat Oncol Biol Phys 1996;34(5): 1037– 1044.
599. Johnson B, Patronas N, Hayes W, et al. Neurologic, computed cranial tomographic, and magnetic resonance imaging abnormalities in patients with small-cell lung cancer: further follow-up of 6- to 13-year survivors. J Clin Oncol 1990;8(1):48–56.
600. Komaki R, Meyers C, Shin D, et al. Evaluation of cognitive function in patients with limited small cell lung cancer prior to and shortly following prophylactic cranial irradiation. Int J Radiat Oncol Biol Phys 1995;33(1):179–182.
601. Van Oosterhout A, Boon P, Houx P, ten Velde G, Twijnstra A. Follow-up of cognitive functioning in patients with small cell lung cancer. Int J Radiat Oncol Biol Phys 1995;31(4):911–914.
602. Le Pechoux C, Laplache A, Borie F, et al. Long term results in terms of neurotoxicity among patients with limited small cell lung cancer included in a trial evaluating prophylactic cranial irradiation. Lung Cancer 2003;41(suppl 2):S21 (abstract O-64).
603. Surveillance, Epidemiology, and End Results (SEER) Program, Division of Cancer Control and Population Sciences, National Center for Health Statistics, Centers for Disease Control and Prevention. Stat 3.0. 1992–1997.
604. Johnson D. "The guard dies, it does not surrender!" progress in the management of small-cell lung cancer? J Clin Oncol 2002; 20(24):4618–4620.
605. Evans W, Feld R, Murray N, et al. Superiority of alternating non-cross-resistant chemotherapy in extensive small cell lung cancer. A multicenter, randomized clinical trial by the National Cancer Institute of Canada. Ann Intern Med 1987;107(4):451–458.
606. Roth B, Johnson D, Einhorn L, et al. Randomized study of cyclophosphamide, doxorubicin, and vincristine versus etoposide and cisplatin versus alternation of these two regimens in extensive small-cell lung cancer: a phase III trial of the Southeastern Cancer Study Group. J Clin Oncol 1992;10(2):282–291.
607. Pujol J, Carestia L, Daures J. Is there a case for cisplatin in the treatment of small-cell lung cancer? A meta-analysis of randomized trials of a cisplatin-containing regimen versus a regimen without this alkylating agent. Br J Cancer 2000;83(1): 8–15.
608. Chute J, Chen T, Feigal E, Simon R, Johnson B. Twenty years of phase III trials for patients with extensive-stage small-cell lung cancer: perceptible progress. J Clin Oncol 1999;17(6):1794–1801.
609. Sundstrom S, Bremnes R, Kaasa S, et al. Cisplatin and etoposide regimen is superior to cyclophosphamide, epirubicin, and vincristine regimen in small-cell lung cancer: results from a randomized phase III trial with 5 years' follow-up. J Clin Oncol 2002;20(24):4665–4672.
610. Noda K, Nishiwaki Y, Kawahara M, et al., J.C.O. Group. Irinotecan plus cisplatin compared with etoposide plus cisplatin for extensive small-cell lung cancer. N Engl J Med 2002;346(2): 85–91.
611. Pujol J, Daures J, Riviere A, et al. Etoposide plus cisplatin with or without the combination of 4'-epidoxorubicin plus cyclophosphamide in treatment of extensive small-cell lung cancer: a French Federation of Cancer Institutes multicenter phase III randomized study. J Natl Cancer Inst 2001;93(4):300–308.
612. Mavroudis D, Papadakis E, Veslemes M, et al. A multicenter randomized clinical trial comparing paclitaxel-cisplatin-etoposide versus cisplatin-etoposide as first-line treatment in patients with small-cell lung cancer. Ann Oncol 2001;12(4):463–470.
613. Niell H, Herndon J, Miller A, et al. Randomized phase III intergroup trial (CALGB 9732) of etoposide (VP-16) and cisplatin (DDP) with or without paclitaxel (TAX) and G-CSF in patients with extensive stage small cell lung cancer (ED-SCLC). Presented at the Amer Soc Clin Oncol, Orlando, Florida, 2002.
614. Tjan-Heijnen V, Wagener D, Postmus P. An analysis of chemotherapy dose and dose-intensity in small-cell lung cancer: lessons to be drawn. Ann Oncol 2002;13(10):1519–1530.
615. Giaccone G, Dalesio O, McVie G, et al. Maintenance chemotherapy in small-cell lung cancer: long-term results of a randomized trial. J Clin Oncol 1993;11(7):1230–1240.
616. Schiller J, Adak S, Cella D, DeVore R, Johnson D. Topotecan versus observation after cisplatin plus etoposide in extensive-stage small-cell lung cancer: E7593—a phase III trial of the Eastern Cooperative Oncology Group. J Clin Oncol 2001;19(8): 2114–2122.
617. Hanna N, Sandler A, Loehrer P, et al. Maintenance daily oral etoposide versus no further therapy following induction chemotherapy with etoposide plus ifosfamide plus cisplatin in extensive small-cell lung cancer: a Hoosier Oncology Group randomized study. Ann Oncol 2002;13:95–102.
618. Humblet Y, Symann M, Bosly A, et al. Late intensification chemotherapy with autologous bone marrow transplantation in selected small-cell carcinoma of the lung: a randomized study. J Clin Oncol 1987;5:1864–1873.
619. Ihde D, Mulshine J, Kramer B, et al. Prospective randomized comparison of high-dose and standard-dose etoposide and cisplatin chemotherapy in patients with extensive-stage small-cell lung cancer. J Clin Oncol 1994;12:2022–2034.
620. Pujol J, Douillard J, Riviere A, et al. Dose-intensity of a four-drug chemotherapy regimen with or without recombinant human granulocyte-macrophage colony-stimulating factor in

extensive-stage small-cell lung cancer: a multicenter randomized phase III study. J Clin Oncol 1997;15(5):2082–2089.
621. Ardizzoni A, Tjan-Heijnen V, Postmus P, et al. Standard versus intensified chemotherapy with granulocyte colony-stimulating factor support in small-cell lung cancer: a prospective European Organization for Research and Treatment of Cancer-Lung Cancer Group Phase III Trial-08923. J Clin Oncol 2002;20(19):3947–3955.
622. Sculier J, Paesmans M, Lecomte J, et al. A three-arm phase III randomised trial assessing, in patients with extensive-disease small-cell lung cancer, accelerated chemotherapy with support of haematological growth factor or oral antibiotics. Br J Cancer 2001;85(10):1444–1451.
623. Lorigan P, Woll P, O'Brien M, et al. Randomised phase 3 trial of dose dense ICE chemotherapy versus standard ICE in good prognosis small cell lung cancer (SCLC). Presented at the Amer Soc Clin Oncol, Chicago, Illinois, 2003.
624. Murray N, Livingston R, Shepherd F, et al. Randomized study of CODE versus alternating CAV/EP for extensive-stage small-cell lung cancer: an Intergroup Study of the National Cancer Institute of Canada Clinical Trials Group and the Southwest Oncology Group. J Clin Oncol 1999;17(8):2300–2308.
625. Miller A, Herndon J II, Hollis D, et al. Schedule dependency of 21-day oral versus 3-day intravenous etooside in combination with intravenous cisplatin in extensive-stage small-cell lung cancer: a randomized phase III study of the Cancer and Leukemia Group B. J Clin Oncol 1995;13(8):1871–1879.
626. Girling D. Comparison of oral etoposide and standard intravenous multidrug chemotherapy for small-cell lung cancer: a stopped multicentre randomised trial. Medical Research Council Lung Cancer Working Party. Lancet 1996;348(9027):563–566.
627. Souhami R, Spiro S, Rudd R, et al. Five-day oral etoposide treatment for advanced small-cell lung cancer: randomized comparison with intravenous chemotherapy. J Natl Cancer Inst 1997;89(8):577–580.
628. Weinmann M, Jeremic B, Bamberg M, Bokemeyer C. Treatment of lung cancer in elderly part II: small cell lung cancer. Lung Cancer 2003;40(1):1–16.
629. Kelly P, O'Brien A, Daly P, Clancy L. Small-cell lung cancer in elderly patients: the case for chemotherapy. Age Ageing 1991;20(1):19–22.
630. Nou E. Full chemotherapy in elderly patients with small cell bronchial carcinoma. Acta Oncol 1996;35(4):399–406.
631. Jara C, Gomez-Aldaravi J, Tirado R, Meseguer V, Alonso C, Fernandez A. Small-cell lung cancer in the elderly: is age of patient a relevant factor? Acta Oncol 1999;38(6):781–786.
632. Westeel V, Murray N, Gelmon K, et al. New combination of the old drugs for elderly patients with small-cell lung cancer: a phase II study of the PAVE regimen. J Clin Oncol 1998;16(5):1940–1947.
633. Gridelli C, Rossi A, Barletta E, et al. Carboplatin plus vinorelbine plus G-CSF in elderly patients with extensive-stage small-cell lung cancer: a poorly tolerated regimen. Results of a multicentre phase II study. Lung Cancer 2002;36(3):327–332.
634. Ettinger D, Finkelstein D, Ritch P, Lincoln S, Blum R. Study of either ifosfamide or teniposide compared to a standard chemotherapy for extensive disease small cell lung cancer: an Eastern Cooperative Oncology Group randomized study (E1588). Lung Cancer 2002;37(3):311–318.
635. Eckardt J. Second-line treatment of small-cell lung cancer. The case for systemic chemotherapy. Oncology (Huntingt) 2003;17(2):181–188, 191; discussion 191–192, passim.
636. Ardizzoni A, Hansen H, Dombernowsky P, et al. Topotecan, a new active drug in the second-line treatment of small-cell lung cancer: a phase II study in patients with refractory and sensitive disease. The European Organization for Research and Treatment of Cancer Early Clinical Studies Group and New Drug Development Office, and the Lung Cancer Cooperative Group. J Clin Oncol 1997;15(5):2090–2096.
637. Perez-Soler R, Glisson B, Lee J, et al. Treatment of patients with small-cell lung cancer refractory to etoside and cisplatin with the topoisomerase I poison topotecan. J Clin Oncol 1996;14(10):2785–2790.
638. von Pawel J, Schiller J, Shepherd F, et al. Topotecan versus cyclophosphamide, doxorubicin, and vincristine for the treatment of recurrent small-cell lung cancer. J Clin Oncol 1999;17(2):658–667.
639. von Pawel J, Gatzemeier U, Pujol J, et al. Phase ii comparator study of oral versus intravenous topotecan in patients with chemosensitive small-cell lung cancer. J Clin Oncol 2001;19(6):1743–1749.
640. Postmus P, Berendsen H, van Zandwijk N, Splinter T, Burghouts J, Bakker W. Retreatment with the induction regimen in small cell lung cancer relapsing after an initial response to short term chemotherapy. Eur J Cancer Clin Oncol 1987;23(9):1409–1411.
641. Giaccone G, Ferrati P, Donadio M, Testore F, Calciati A. Reinduction chemotherapy in small cell lung cancer. Eur J Cancer Clin Oncol 1987;23(11):1697–1699.
642. Gralla R, Eckardt J, von Pawel J, Grotzinger K, Ross G. Quality of life with single agent oral topotecan vs. intravenous topotecan in patients with chemosensitive small cell lung cancer (SCLC). An international phase III study. Presented at the 10th World Conference on Lung Cancer, Vancouver, British Columbia, 2003.
643. Hoang T, Kim K, Jaslowski A, et al. Phase II study of second-line gemcitabine in sensitive or refractory small cell lung cancer. Lung Cancer 2003;42(1):97–102.
644. Masters G, Declerck L, Blanke C, et al. Phase II trial of gemcitabine in refractory or relapsed small-cell lung cancer: Eastern Cooperative Oncology Group Trial 1597. J Clin Oncol 2003;21(8):1550–1555.
645. Sandler A. Irinotecan in small-cell lung cancer: the US experience. Oncology (Huntingt) 2001;15(1 suppl 1):11–12.
646. Furuse K, Kubota K, Kawahara M, et al. Phase II study of vinorelbine in heavily previously treated small cell lung cancer. Japan Lung Cancer Vinorelbine Study Group. Oncology 1996;53(2):169–172.
647. Naka N, Kawahara M, Okishio K, et al. Phase II study of weekly irinotecan and carboplatin for refractory or relapsed small-cell lung cancer. Lung Cancer 2002;37(3):319–323.
648. Hirose T, Horichi N, Ohmori T, et al. Phase II study of irinotecan and carboplatin in patients with the refractory or relapsed small cell lung cancer. Lung Cancer 2003;40(3):333–338.
649. Ardizzoni A, Manegold C, Debruyne C, et al. European organization for research and treatment of cancer (EORTC) 08957 phase II study of topotecan in combination with cisplatin as second-line treatment of refractory and sensitive small cell lung cancer. Clin Cancer Res 2003;9(1):143–150.
650. Fennell D. Bcl-2 as a target for overcoming chemoresistance in small-cell lung cancer. Clin Lung Cancer 2003;4(5):307–313.
651. Rudin C, Otterson G, Mauer A, et al. A pilot trial of G3139, a bcl-2 antisense oligonucleotide, and paclitaxel in patients with chemorefractory small-cell lung cancer. Ann Oncol 2002;13(4):539–545.
652. Rudin C, Kosloff M, Edelman M, Hoffman P, Szeto L, Vokes E. Phase I study of G3139 (oblimersen sodium), carboplatin, and etoposide in previously untreated extensive stage small cell lung cancer (SCLC). Presented at the Amer Soc Clin Oncol, Chicago, Illinois, 2003.
653. Soria J, Johnson B, Chevalier T. Imatinib in small cell lung cancer. Lung Cancer 2003;41(suppl 1):S49–S53.
654. Chaudhry A, Carrasquillo J, Avis I, et al. Phase I and imaging trial of a monoclonal antibody directed against gastrin-releasing

peptide in patients with lung cancer. Clin Cancer Res 1999;5(11): 3385–3393.
655. Abrams T, Lee L, Murray L, Pryer N, Cherrington J. SU11248 inhibits KIT and platelet-derived growth factor receptor beta in preclinical models of human small cell lung cancer. Mol Cancer Ther 2003;2:471–478.
656. Grant S, Kris M, Houghton A, Chapman P. Long survival of patients with small cell lung cancer after adjuvant treatment with the anti-idiotypic antibody BEC2 plus bacillus Calmette-Guerin. Clin Cancer Res 1999;5:1319–1323.
657. Lu H, Forbes R, Verma A. Hypoxia-inducible factor 1 activation by aerobic glycolysis implicates the Warburg effect in carcinogenesis. J Biol Chem 2002;277(26):23111–23115.
658. Durany N, Joseph J, Campo E, Molina R, Carreras J. Phosphoglycerate mutase, 2,3-bisphosphoglycerate phosphatase and enolase activity and isoenzymes in lung, colon and liver carcinomas. Br J Cancer 1997;75(7):969–977.
659. Giatromanolaki A, Koukourakis M, Sivridis E, et al. Relation of hypoxia inducible factor 1 alpha and 2 alpha in operable non-small cell lung cancer to angiogenic/molecular profile of tumours and survival. Br J Cancer 2001;85(6):881–890.
660. Laughner E, Taghavi P, Chiles K, Mahon P, Semenza G. HER2 (neu) signaling increases the rate of hypoxia-inducible factor 1alpha (HIF-1alpha) synthesis: novel mechanism for HIF-1-mediated vascular endothelial growth factor expression. Mol Cell Biol 2001;21(12):3995–4004.
661. Read RC, Yoder G, Schaeffer RC. Survival after conservative resection for T_1, N_0, M_0 nonsmall cell lung cancer. Ann Thorac Surg 1990;49:391–400.
662. Pastorino U, Valente M, Bedini V, Infante M, Tavecchio L, Ravasi G. Limited resection for Stage I lung cancer. Eur J Surg Oncol 1991;17:42–46.
663. Warren WH, Faber LP. Segmentectomy versus lobectomy in patients with stage I pulmonary carcinoma. Five-year survival and patterns of intrathoracic recurrence. J Thorac Cardiovasc Surg 1994;107:1087–1093.
664. Okada M, Yoshikawa K, Hatta T, Tsubota N. Is segmentectomy with lymph node assessment an alternative to lobectomy for non-small cell lung cancer of 2 cm or smaller? Ann Thorac Surg 2001;71:956–960.
665. Miller DL. Management of the subcentimeter pulmonary nodule. Semin Thorac Cardiovasc Surg 2002;14:281–285.
666. Koike T, Yamato Y, Yoshiya K, Shimoyama T, Suzuki R. Intentional limited pulmonary resection for peripheral T1 N0 M0 small-sized lung cancer. J Thorac Cardiovasc Surg 2003;125:924–928.
667. Konaka C, Ikeda N, Hiyoshi T, et al. Peripheral non-small cell lung cancers 2.0 cm or less in diameter: proposed criteria for limited pulmonary resection based upon clinicopathological presentation. Lung Cancer 1998;21:185–191.
668. Koike T, Terashima M, Takizawa T, Watanabe T. Intentional limited resection for primary lung cancer. Jpn J Thorac Cardiovasc Surg 1998;46(suppl):120–123.
669. Kawahara K, Iwasaki A, Yoshinaga Y, et al. Lymph node metastasis and prognosis in small peripheral non-small-cell lung cancers. Jpn J Thorac Cardiovasc Surg 2000;48:618–624.
670. Watanabe S, Oda M, Go T, et al. Should mediastinal nodal dissection be routinely undertaken in patients with peripheral small-sized (2 cm or less) lung cancer? Retrospective analysis of 225 patients. Eur J Cardiothorac Surg 2001;20:1007–1011.
671. Gaissert HA, Mathisen DJ, Moncure AC, Hilgenberg AD, Grillo HC, Wain JC. Survival and function after sleeve lobectomy for lung cancer, J Thorac Cardiovasc Surg 1996;111:948–953.
672. Suen HC, Meyers BF, Guthrie T, et al. Favorable results after sleeve lobectomy or bronchoplasty for bronchial malignancies. Ann Thorac Surg 1999;67:1557–1562.
673. Roth JA, Fossella F, Komaki R, et al. A randomized trial comparing perioperative chemotherapy and surgery with surgery alone in resectable stage IIIA non-small-cell lung cancer. J Natl Cancer Inst 1994;86:673–680.
674. Shepherd FA, Johnston MR, Payne D, et al. Randomized study of chemotherapy and surgery versus radiotherapy for stage IIIA non-small-cell lung cancer: a National Cancer Institute of Canada Clinical Trials Group Study. Br J Cancer 1998;78:683–685.
675. Johnstone DW, Byhardt RW, Ettinger D, Scott CB. Phase III study comparing chemotherapy and radiotherapy with preoperative chemotherapy and surgical resection in patients with non-small-cell lung cancer with spread to mediastinal lymph nodes (N2); final report of RTOG 89-01. Radiation Therapy Oncology Group. Int J Radiat Oncol Biol Phys 2002;54:365–369.
676. Elias AD, Kumar P, Herndon J III, Skarin AT, Sugarbaker DJ, Green MR. Radiotherapy versus chemotherapy plus radiotherapy in surgically treated IIIA N2 non-small-cell lung cancer. Clin Lung Cancer 2002;4:95–103.
677. Stephens R, Fairlamb D, Gower N, et al. The big lung trial (BLT): Determining the value of cisplatin-based chemotherapy for all patients with non-small cell lung cancer (NSCLC). Preliminary results in the supportive care setting. Presented at the Amer Soc Clin Oncol, Orlando, Florida, 2002.
678. Gebbia V, Galetta D, Caruso M, et al. Gemcitabine and cisplatin versus vinorelbine and cisplatin versus ifosfamide + gemcitabine followed by vinorelbine and cisplatin versus vinorelbine and cisplatin followed by ifosfamide and gemcitabine in stage IIIB-IV non small cell lung carcinoma: a prospective randomized phase III trial of the Gruppo Oncologico Italia Meridionale. Lung Cancer 2003;39(2):179–189.
679. Martoni A, Marino A, Sperandi F, et al. Multicenter randomized clinical trial of cisplatin (CP) + vinorelbine (VNR) vs. CP + gemcitabine (GEM) in advanced NSCLC: Results of the first analysis. Presented at the Amer Soc Clin Oncol, Chicago, Illinois, 2003.
680. Ohe Y, Saijo N, Ohashi Y, et al. Preliminary results of the Four-Arm Cooperative Study (FACS) for advanced non-small cell lung cancer (NSCLC) in Japan. Presented at the Amer Soc Clin Oncol, Chicago, Illinois, 2003.
681. Evans WK, Radwi A, Tomiak E, et al. Oral etoposide and carboplatin. Effective therapy for elderly patients with small cell lung cancer. Am J Clin Oncol 1995;18(2):149–155.
682. Matsui K, Masuda N, Fukuoka M, et al. Phase II trial of carboplatin plus oral etoposide for elderly patients with small-cell lung cancer. Br J Cancer 1998;77(11):1961–1965.
683. Okamoto H, Watanabe K, Nishiwaki Y, et al. Phase II study of area under the plasma-concentration-versus-time curve-based carboplatin plus standard-dose intravenous etoposide in elderly patients with small-cell lung cancer. J Clin Oncol 1999;17(11): 3540–3545.
684. Quoix E, Breton J, Daniel C, et al. Etoposide phosphate with carboplatin in the treatment of elderly patients with small-cell lung cancer: a phase II study. Ann Oncol 2001;12(7):957–962.
685. Larive S, Bombaron P, Riou R, et al. Carboplatin-etoposide combination in small cell lung cancer patients older than 70 years: a phase II trial. Lung Cancer 2002;35(1):1–7.
686. Eckardt JR. Topotecan in relapsed small-cell lung cancer: can good things come in small packages? Clin Lung Cancer 2003; 4(4):229–230.

38

Therapy for Malignant Pleural Mesothelioma

Harvey I. Pass, Nicholas Vogelzang, Steven Hahn, and Michele Carbone

Malignant mesotheliomas, highly aggressive neoplasms arising primarily from the surface serosal cells of the pleural, peritoneal, and pericardial cavities, are caused primarily from exposure to asbestos fibers.[1,2] Recent investigations have also implicated simian virus 40 (SV40) and genetic predisposition in the etiology of some malignant mesothelioma.[1–3] The disease is characterized by a long latency from the time of exposure to asbestos to the onset of disease. Early evidence provided by karyotypic analysis supports the theory that multiple somatic genetic events are required for tumorigenic conversion of a normal mesothelial cell. Although a specific chromosomal change is not shared by all malignant mesotheliomas, several prominent sites of chromosomal loss have been identified in this malignancy. Tumor suppressor genes (TSGs) residing in these deleted chromosomal regions may be responsible for the tumorigenic conversion of mesothelial cells, and recent studies have begun to identify the specific TSGs that contribute to the development and progression of malignant mesothelioma. Here we review the clinical aspects of this malignancy, focusing on etiology, pathology, epidemiology, symptoms, diagnosis, imaging methods, and treatment.

Genetic Predisposition to Mesothelioma

Recent evidence indicates that genetic predisposition plays an important role in determining individual susceptibility to mineral fibers carcinogenesis and to the development of mesothelioma. In the 1970s, asbestos was the only known causative agent for mesothelioma. In three small villages in Turkey, Karain (population ~600), Tuzkoy (population ~1,400), and Sarihidir (this village was abandoned) in Cappadocia, 50% or more of deaths are caused by malignant mesothelioma.[4–8] These villages, similar to most other villages in the region, were built with stones mined from the nearby natural caves. Studies in Cappadocia concluded that in this region, asbestos is almost everywhere, as it is a natural component of the volcanic terrain, and asbestos-tremolite-based stucco was widely used in building construction in all Cappadocian villages.[5–9] However, it was concluded that asbestos could not account for the unique high incidence of mesotheliomas in these three villages.[5–9] Another type of mineral fiber, erionite, a type of fibrous zeolite commonly found in the stones of the houses of Karain, Sarihidir, and Tuzkoy,[2,8–10] had been detected in the lungs of several villagers and was suspected as a possible causative agent.[5–9] Erionite was injected intrapleurally into animals, causing mesothelioma,[11] and it was concluded that erionite was the cause of mesothelioma in these villages.[8,9,12] Erionite, therefore, appeared much more potent than asbestos in causing mesothelioma.[10] Studies tried to link erionite to other human tumors. With the exception of mesotheliomas, there is no significant difference in the incidence of any other tumor types in these two villages compared with the rest of Turkey.[2]

Homes in these areas of Turkey are inhabited by multiple generations and passed down. Closer observation revealed that mesotheliomas only occurred in certain homes and not in others, although all homes contained similar amounts of erionite according to recent mineralogic analysis.[2,13] Furthermore, in the nearby village of Karlik, where homes are built from the same materials and contain the same types of erionite fibers, only one mesothelioma had been known to occur, which was in a woman who had migrated from Karain.[2,13] Further analysis of pedigrees of families who lived in homes where mesotheliomas occurred showed that these mesotheliomas appeared to be inherited in an autosomal dominant pattern. About 50% of descendents of affected parents developed mesotheliomas. When members of unaffected families married into affected families, 50% of their descendents also developed mesotheliomas.[2,13] Whether genetics alone or in conjunction with erionite are responsible for these mesotheliomas remains unknown, but clearly genetics is a key factor, because mesotheliomas do not develop in nonaffected families regardless of environmental exposure.

Familial malignant mesothelioma has been occasionally described in the United States and in Europe.[2,14] These families, however, were too small to prove genetic transmission. Furthermore, in these families, mesothelioma may also have been linked to asbestos exposure or/and SV40 infection.[2] It is hoped that isolation of this putative mesothelioma susceptibility gene will lead to future preventative and therapeutic approaches.

Pathology of Mesothelioma

Benign Mesotheliomas

True malignant mesothelioma is an aggressive malignancy with a dismal prognosis. There are, however, a number of benign mesothelial proliferations that must be distinguished from malignant mesothelioma, such as multicystic mesothelioma, also called multilocular peritoneal inclusion cyst. Multicystic mesothelioma is a benign mesothelial lesion, characteristically formed by multiple cysts arranged in grape-like clusters. Adenomatoid mesotheliomas are benign mesothelial lesions of the genital system. Mesothelioma of the atrioventricular node is neither a mesothelioma nor a tumor but a congenital heterotopia of the endodermal sinus in the atrioventricular node.

Well-differentiated papillary mesothelioma (WDPM) is found more often in the abdominal cavity of young women. Histologically, it is formed by multiple papillary structures covered by cytologically benign mesothelial cells. The lesion is benign, but there have been occasional cases in which several years after diagnosis the patient developed a true mesothelioma. Consultation with a pathologist who sees numerous mesothelial lesions and malignant mesothelioma is highly recommended to rule out a well-differentiated epithelial malignant mesothelioma, based mostly on the absence of invasion in these benign lesions. Patients with WDPM may be more likely to die of the complication of therapy for a misdiagnosed malignant mesothelioma compared to the risk of dying of WDPM if left untreated.[15]

Localized fibrous tumor of the pleura (FTP), often referred to as localized mesothelioma, is thought to originate from the submesothelial cells, but it is unclear what submesothelial cells are. More than 700 FTPs have been reported in the literature and, on presentation, are frequently confused with pleural mesothelioma. These tumors are similar to other fibrous tumors found elsewhere in the body; the cells have a benign appearance, and are usually immersed in a fibrous and characteristically vascular stroma. FTP is characteristically negative for cytokeratin, a mesothelial cell marker, and positive for CD34, suggesting that these cells are not of mesothelial origin. Occasionally, localized FTPs are histologically and cytologically malignant and until recently were called hemangiopericytomas. These tumors are the more cellular and histologically aggressive tumors; however, they are still FTPs and should be called fibrous tumors (of the pleura if in the pleura). They are characterized by multiple recurrences after resection and, often, a poor prognosis. The most important predictive factor in the prognosis of FTP is whether the tumor can be completely resected. Thus pedunculated tumors have a much better prognosis than tumors that grow over a broad pleural area. Tumor array studies may in the future provide us with tools to identify rare "benign malignant mesothelioma" from classical epithelial malignant mesothelioma; however, the majority of the markers that have been found to be significant in the expression arrays are already used as part of the standard immunohistochemical panel.[16]

Malignant Mesothelioma

The diagnosis of malignant mesothelioma, in contrast to common belief, is usually straightforward, provided that the pathologist has extensive experience with this malignancy. Histologically malignant mesothelioma can show an epithelial morphology (malignant mesothelioma epithelial type), the most common, about 50% to 60% of cases; a fibrous morphology (malignant mesothelioma fibrous type, also called sarcomatoid type), 10% of cases; or a combination of both (mixed type or biphasic malignant mesothelioma), about 30% to 40% of cases. Tumors with a prevalently sarcomatous morphology are quite resistant to therapy and have median survivals less than 1 year from diagnosis. They are difficult to diagnose because they show a morphology that can be essentially identical to other primary or metastatic pleural sarcomas. Immunohistochemistry showing positive staining for pankeratin may be considered confirmatory. Only a fraction, which varies depending on the study, of sarcomatoid malignant mesothelioma stain positive for calretinin, and some of them are positive for WT-1. Thus, negative staining for these two mesothelial markers does not rule out the diagnosis of malignant mesothelioma, but should prompt the pathologist to consider other differentials. Electron microscopy (EM) has a limited role in diagnosing sarcomatoid malignant mesothelioma because these cells do not have the diagnostic long branching microvilli of the epithelial type. However, EM can identify characteristics of other sarcomatoid tumors besides microvilli that can help to rule out the diagnosis of sarcomatoid malignant mesothelioma.

Mostly epithelial-type tumors, especially well-differentiated variants, are associated with prolonged survivals up to 2 years from diagnosis. Epithelial malignant mesothelioma typically shows large and well-differentiated epithelioid cells, with centrally placed nuclei, lack of atypia, abundant cytoplasm, and often form glandlike spaces or tubular-like spaces, although some epithelial mesotheliomas instead grow forming sheets of epithelioid cells. To be classified as biphasic, assume that at least 10% of the tumor must have a fibrous (or epithelial) component for the malignant mesothelioma. In fact, most malignant mesothelioma could be considered biphasic, as most mesothelioma show both morphologies if in a very tiny fraction, which is the characteristic histologic feature of this malignancy. Unusual morphologic variants exist, but are rare. In addition, some malignant mesotheliomas cannot be subcategorized histologically and should be called poorly differentiated malignant mesothelioma.[15]

The experienced pathologist will recognize these tumors as mesothelial in origin; however, occasionally a carcinoma with a typically more aggressive and atypical histology can look very much like a malignant mesothelioma, or a malignant mesothelioma can look so atypical that it resembles a metastatic carcinoma. Therefore, to rule out these rare mimics, confirmatory immunohistochemistry should be completed. Epithelial-type mesothelioma tumor cells are positive for pankeratin, keratin 5/6, calretinin, and WT-1 and negative for the epithelial markers carcinoembryonic antigen (CEA), LeuM1, B72.3, Ber-EP4, Moc-1, TTF-1, etc. Positive staining for pankeratin and calretinin and negative staining for three epithelial markers is considered sufficient for diagnosis; however, some carcinomas may stain positive for calretinin or negative for some of the epithelial markers and therefore additional testing may be required. In these difficult cases, EM showing the classic long branching microvilli of human mesothelial cells compared to the short nonbranching microvilli of carcinomas can still be considered the gold standard for a correct diagnosis.

Clinical Presentation of Malignant Pleural Mesothelioma

Classically, mesothelioma affects older men in their fifties, sixties, and seventies because of the aforementioned 25- to 40-year latency period between occupational asbestos exposure and the development of the tumor. Latency periods between first exposure to asbestos and a diagnosis of mesothelioma vary by occupation, intensity, and duration of exposure, with shorter latencies for insulators and dock workers and longer intervals for shipyard and maritime workers, as well as for domestic exposures. Table 38.1 lists the most common industries identified in 1,048 cases of histologically confirmed mesothelioma cases reviewed by Roggli et al.[17]

Women and children can have the disease but the male to female ratio is approximately 3–5 : 1.[18] There are many reports of childhood mesothelioma; however, on review of the pathology, the diagnosis is erroneous in as many as 50% of the cases, and there does not seem to be a relationship in these pediatric cases with asbestos, radiation, or isoniazid.[19]

Symptoms

The majority of patients (~60%) present with nonpleuritic chest pain, classically located posterolaterally and low in the thorax. The pain typically has increased over time and may be severe enough to warrant narcotics for pain management. Intractable chest pain often indicates chest wall invasion beyond the endothoracic fascia. Approximately 5% of patients also have metastatic disease at presentation, usually to the lungs. The right side is affected more than the left side (60% versus 40%), most likely due to its greater volume. Dyspnea is present in 50% to 70% of the cases, and some 80% of the patients present with dyspnea and effusion. In some series the symptoms of shortness of breath and chest pain are seen either singly or in combination in 90% of the cases.[20] The presence of a pleural effusion will be documented at some time in the course of the disease in 95% of patients with malignant pleural mesothelioma. Cough, fever, fatigue, and weight loss occur in approximately 30% of the patients, and a minority of cases present with hoarseness, hemoptysis, Horner's syndrome, superior vena caval syndrome, or paralysis from invasion of the spinal canal.

The duration of symptoms varies; however, the range can extend from 2 weeks to 2 years, with most series having a median time to diagnosis from symptoms of 2 to 3 months. Unfortunately, as many as 25% of patients with the disease have symptoms for 6 months or more before seeking medical attention.

TABLE 38.1. Occupational exposure and mesothelioma.

	Single exposure	*Multiple exposures*	*% of total*
Shipbuilding[a]	203	86	30
U.S. Navy[b]	91	84	18
Construction[c]	99	35	13
Insulation[d]	92	11	10
Oil and chemical	78	10	8
Power plant	50	10	5
Railroad	37	16	4
Automotive[e]	24	27	4
Steel/metal[f]	33	10	3
Asbestos manufacturing[g]	34	5	3
Paper mill	7	0	1
Ceramics/glass	6	0	1

[a] Includes joiner, shipwright, rigger, sandblaster, shipfitter, electrician, painter, and welder.

[b] Includes merchant marine seamen.

[c] Includes construction worker, laborer, carpenter, painter, drywall/plasterer.

[d] Includes pipe coverer, insulator, asbestos sawyer, asbestos sprayer.

[e] Includes auto mechanic, brake repair worker, brakeline worker.

[f] Includes steel, aluminium, and iron foundry workers; furnace worker; potroom worker.

[g] Includes asbestos textile, asbestos manufacture, asbestos plant worker.

Source: Maggi et al.,[103] by permission of *European Journal of Cardiothoracic Surgery*.

Physical Examination

Physical examination usually reveals signs associated with a pleural effusion with decreased breath sounds, dullness to percussion, or decreased motion of the involved chest wall. In patients with severe dyspnea, the effusion may occupy the entire chest, resulting in mediastinal shift and compromise of the opposite lung volumes. Dyspnea continuing after thoracentesis may be an indication of fixation of a nonexpanding, contracted, and trapped lung (i.e., failure to expand after fluid removal). In the late stages of the disease there is often dramatic cachexia, marked contraction of the involved chest with narrowed interspaces, and hypertrophy of the contralateral hemithorax. A chest wall mass occurs in up to 25% of patients, often at the site(s) of prior thoracentesis, thoracotomy, or thoracoscopy wounds. Lymph node examination should concentrate on the cervical, supraclavicular, and axillary basins, and any externally palpated asymmetrically enlarged nodes should be biopsied. The abdomen must be inspected for signs of ascites.

Laboratory Examination

The most striking laboratory abnormality is thrombocytosis (more than 400,000), which is seen in 60% to 90% of patients,[21] and elevated platelet counts (more than 1,000,000) in approximately 15% of patients. In addition, nonspecific laboratory findings including hypergammaglobulinemia, eosinophilia, and/or anemia of chronic disease may be seen. It has been recently noted that 14% to 15% of patients have elevated homocysteine levels reflecting folic acid deficiency, 17% have biochemical evidence of B_{12} deficiency and 32% have biochemical signs of B_6 deficiency.[22]

At present, validated serum markers that are both sensitive and specific for mesothelioma do not exist. Hyaluronic acid is elevated in the mesothelioma pleural effusions in approximately 60% of the patients[23,24]; however, this is only seen in the serum in advanced cases and has not proven to be a reliable marker. Measurement of low molecular weight cytokeratins has been reported to aid in the diagnosis of mesothelioma when combined with other pleural effusion markers including CEA but prospective validation studies are lacking.[25] Serum CEA should be less than 5 ng/mL in more than 95% of cases. Recently, a dual monoclonal forward sandwich enzyme-linked immunosorbent assay (ELISA) for the measurement of soluble members of the mesothelin/megakaryocyte potentiating factor (MPF) family of proteins expressed by mesothelial cells has been reported to predict the development of mesothelioma in high-risk individuals as well as to reflect the influence of therapeutic efficacy in mesothelioma.[26]

Radiologic Examination/Imaging Studies

Malignant mesothelioma can have a diverse radiographic appearance. Many of the early changes are associated with a previous exposure to asbestos, consisting of both pleural and parenchymal changes, including pleural plaques or parenchymal pulmonary fibrosis.

Chest Radiography

The presence of a pleural effusion, diffuse pleural thickening, and nodularity are the most common features associated with progression and symptoms. The involved hemithorax can eventually have smooth, lobular pleural masses that infiltrate the pleural space and fissures[27–29] in 45% to 60% of patients with contraction and fixation of the chest. The lung becomes encased, and the mediastinum shifts because of volume loss. The apex may appear to have minimal pleural thickening on the chest radiograph, which may be better visualized with computerized tomography (CT). The effusion can completely obscure a view of the diaphragm, lower lobes, and pericardium indicative of complete collapse. One must assess the contralateral chest for effusion, which could raise the possibility of two-cavity involvement, or reveal worrisome nodularity or evidence of asbestos involvement that may impact on the functional ability of the patient to undergo diagnostic or therapeutic interventions.

Usually the chest radiograph adds little to the staging of mesothelioma; however, it may guide the workup toward a thoracoscopy if fluid is present.

Computerized Tomography

CT imaging allows for density resolution that is not available with chest radiography, and these characteristics are useful not only in the evaluation of the patient with mesothelioma but also with asbestos-related diseases.[30] Such asbestos-induced parenchymal changes on CT frequently include subpleural lines and parenchymal bands, prominent pulmonary arcades, subpleural dependent densities, reticulation, and parenchymal honeycomb patterns. Pleural changes seen on CT include pleural plaques, diffuse pleural thickening, and pleural effusion. Up to 10% of pleural plaques are calcified, and they appear characteristically on the posterolateral aspect of the lower parietal pleura or diaphragm.

The patient with mesothelioma may have all the previously mentioned findings in addition to the aborementioned circumferentially lobulated, soft tissue mass with lower-zone predominance. Additional CT features of mesothelioma include localized nodular or plaquelike pleural thickening possibly associated with pleural effusion. The lobulated pleural encasement frequently causes lower lobe collapse. Intrapulmonary nodules can occur in 60% of patients, and infiltration into fissures along with enlarged hilar and mediastinal lymph nodes may be seen. CT allows a better view of the involved pericardium, which is irregularly thickened and associated with infiltration to the pericardial fat pad. Chest wall involvement is still difficult to assess with CT and, unfortunately, this finding is an important aspect in the staging of the disease. Occasionally CT will demonstrate focal chest wall invasion at a previous biopsy site, surgical scar, or chest tube tract.[31] CT signs of chest wall invasion include distortion of the intercostal spaces, infiltration of extrapleural soft tissue and ribs, and undefined densities infiltrating the chest wall musculature. A clear fat plane between the inferior diaphragmatic surface and the adjacent abdominal organs as well as a smooth inferior diaphragmatic contour may imply resectability.[32] CT may reveal a hemidiaphragm encased by a mass or poor definition between the liver, stomach, and inferior diaphragmatic surface.

Volumetric estimates of tumor volume using three-dimensional reconstruction have also been investigated for the staging of mesothelioma.[33] Tumor volumes associated with mesothelioma patients who are found to have no spread to lymph nodes are significantly smaller than in those patients with positive nodes. Moreover, progressively higher stage is associated with higher median preoperative solid volume of tumor in these patients.

Magnetic Resonance Imaging

Magnetic resonance imaging (MRI) is appealing because of the differential signal intensity, depending upon the sequence used, and the ability to image in the coronal, sagittal, and transverse planes. Tumors are found to have intermediate signal intensity on the T_1-weighted image, whereas on T_2-weighted images there is an increase in signal intensity, fluid is clearly seen as high signal intensity and there are focal areas of very high signal intensity. More recent studies have suggested gadolinium contrast enhancement MRI can improve tumor detection and extension. Detection of diaphragm invasion and invasion of endothoracic fascia or a single chest wall focus may be better with MRI compared to CT.[31]

Positron Emission Tomography

There are a number of studies of positron emission tomography (PET) and the radionuclide imaging agent [^{18}F]fluorodeoxyglucose (FDG) in mesothelioma. Four studies have reported that FDG-PET is accurate in the diagnosis of pleural malignancies, specifically mesothelioma , and that it may be superior to CT for defining mediastinal lymph node involvement.[34–37] Moreover, the ability to define extrathoracic, otherwise occult disease in newly diagnosed patients can be as high as 10% to 11% and 45% in those followed after therapy. One of the more intriguing aspects of the technology is quantitational prognostication using the standardized uptake value (SUV). The data suggest that patients with higher SUVs have tumors that are more metabolically active and have a shortened median survival compared with those with a lower SUV. In the most recent report, the SUV of the tumor before resection was significant in discriminating longer- from shorter-surviving patients and was able to stratify very good risk versus very bad risk patients: those with low SUV and epithelial histology had the best prognosis whereas those with high SUV and nonepithelial histology did the worst.[38]

Follow-Up Radiologic Assessment

After thoracoscopy or thoracentesis, a postprocedure X-ray can be done to determine whether the patient has trapped lung. The failure of the lung to expand should alert the clinician that the lung may require decortication in addition to parietal pleurectomy if surgical therapy is required. Such a situation implies that the lung has been trapped for a considerable amount of time and may point to the use of a ventilation perfusion scan to assess functional contribution of that lung. The discovery of a trapped lung rules out the ability to successfully palliate the effusion with a talc pleurodesis, although the patient may still be a candidate for insertion of a Pleurex catheter (see Supportive Care section).

The standards for postoperative radiographic follow-up for patients having mesothelioma surgery are undefined; however, CT should be performed at regular intervals after extrapleural pneumonectomy (EPP) or pleurectomy decortication to monitor for progressive disease. After EPP, CT scanning of the resected hemithorax will reveal a smooth-walled, well-defined postoperative membrane lining the pneumonectomy space that is usually concentrically smooth, but as the interval from operation to follow-up lengthens, the membrane may actually get thicker. Unexplained irregular focal thickening at the base of the chest should alert the clinician to a recurrence of disease. This finding is especially pronounced in the pleurectomy patient in whom the recurrent mesothelioma may start to thicken rapidly and infiltrate the underlying lung. Other presentations of recurrence include the development of new mediastinal adenopathy or ascites otherwise undetectable by physical examination. The development of asymptomatic abdominal fluid after EPP is an ominous sign and calls for paracentesis. CT will usually reveal diaphragmatic thickening or diffuse mesenteric infiltration in these cases.

Without recurrence, however, the space is smooth walled, especially on the parietal pleura and mediastinal surfaces. The prosthetic Goretex diaphragm eventually becomes radiopaque and the diaphragmatic surface requires close inspection, for at the lower sulci the initial appearance may not be smoothly contoured.

Another important role of follow-up or sequential CT scanning is in the assessment of the response of mesothelioma to chemotherapy. Multicenter protocols now require measuring the thickness of the pleural rind at one to three locations on the rind on three separate slices of the CT every 6 to 9 weeks. If the total thickness has decreased by 30% or more, the patient has shown a response to treatment whereas 20% or greater increase in thickness equals progressive disease.[39] This method of response assessment correlated with outcome in Phase II trials and in an international trial, which showed that cisplatin plus pemetrexed was superior to cisplatin alone. Research is still needed to validate the three-step process: (1) selection of the CT sections in which the disease is most prominent, (2) identification of specific sites within these sections that demonstrate the greatest extent of tumor, and (3) the actual measurement of tumor thickness at these sites that generate these measurements.

The role of PET imaging to follow response or progression to chemotherapy is also under evaluation.

Diagnosis

Thoracentesis and Closed Pleural Biopsy

Patients who present with a large, unexplained pleural effusion and minimal or moderate evidence of pleural thickening should have initial thoracentesis and pleural biopsy. Multiple closed pleural biopsies to avoid sampling error are able to aid in the diagnosis in 30% to 50% of cases.[40] Using both histochemical and immunohistochemical staining techniques along with EM analysis of a preserved pleural fluid cell block, the diagnosis of mesothelioma can be obtained from pleural effusion in as high as 84% of suspected cases.[41,42]

Thoracoscopy

Patients at risk for mesothelioma who develop a large effusion and who do not have malignant cells on thoracentesis and pleural biopsy or who recur with effusion after initial thoracentesis should have a video-assisted thoracoscopy[43–45]; this allows evaluation of specific areas for guided biopsy and assessing the ability of the lung to expand. Thoracoscopy can be invaluable for estimating extent of disease with regard to the diaphragm, pericardium, chest wall, and nodes. The compulsive use of thoracoscopy led to the finding that exclusive involvement of the diaphragmatic pleura and parietal pleura (stage IA) has a median survival of 31.2 months whereas involvement into visceral pleura led to a median survival of 6.75 months.[46] There is a 10% chance of later development of chest wall masses from seeding of the biopsy site or surgical scar from any diagnostic procedure, but this can usually be avoided by radiotherapy to the scar if appropriate,[47] although this is controversial (see Radiation Therapy section).

Open Pleural Biopsy

Open biopsy is indicated when there is no free pleural space as a result of previous treatment and the bulk of the disease in the hemithorax is solid. Such a biopsy should be infrequent and carefully planned such that the scar could be incorporated into the incision if a major resection is planned after definitive diagnosis. Bronchoscopy may be necessary to rule out carcinoma of the lung until unequivocal pathologic confirmation is reported. Mediastinoscopy should generally be performed when enlarged mediastinal lymph nodes are detected by imaging and to rule out contralateral disease.[48] This step may, however, underestimate the extent of nodal involvement because the majority of mediastinal nodal involvement in mesothelioma is below the subcarinal level.[49]

Natural History

Most patients with pleural mesothelioma will die of complications of their local disease; these include increasing tumor bulk causing progressive respiratory compromise, pneumonia or myocardial dysfunction with arrhythmias, narcotic usage leading to pulmonary complications and cachexia, and/or occasionally dysphagia from tumor compression of the esophagus. Small bowel obstruction from direct extension through the diaphragm develops in approximately one-third, and 10% die of pericardial or myocardial involvement.[50] Extrathoracic metastases occur late in the course of disease and are not usually the direct cause of the patient's death.

Prognostic Indicators

Although the overall prognosis for patients with mesothelioma is poor, there are some patients who do not conform to the norm and live with their disease for a considerable period of time. Retrospective analysis of prognostic variables to define these outliers is difficult for reasons of nonuniformity of pathologic staging and reporting criteria. Recently, however, larger studies have been published that give insight into potential prognostic variables in mesothelioma.

The most important predictor of survival in nonsurgical studies of mesothelioma is performance status. The Cancer and Leukemia Group B conducted 10 clinical trials in which patients were required to have a performance status of 0–2 at entry. Analysis of survival of 337 patients in these studies showed that overall median survival was 7 months; however, in the subgroup of patients with a performance status of 0, median survival was 13 to 14 months.[51] In addition, chest pain, dyspnea, platelet count greater than 400,000/μL, weight loss, serum lactate dehydrogenase level greater than 500 IU/L, pleural involvement, low hemoglobin level, high white blood cell count, and increasing age over 75 years predicted shorter survival.[51]

The European Organization for Research and Treatment of Cancer (EORTC) studied 204 adults with malignant pleural mesothelioma. The median survival was 13 months from diagnosis and 8 months from trial entry. Poor prognosis was again associated with a poor performance status as well as a high white blood cell count, male gender, and the sarcomatous histologic subtype[52] in the multivariate analysis.

The molecular prognostication of mesothelioma has been explored by two groups. These data require further validation in larger prospective analyses but imply that gene expression data in mesothelioma at the time of initial biopsy may predict clinical outcome.[53,54]

Staging

The commonly used American Joint Committee on Cancer (AJCC) staging system for mesothelioma (Table 38.2) was adopted from that proposed by the International Mesothelioma Interest Group (IMIG) in 1995 and has been validated in a number of surgical-based trials.[55–58] There was a redefinition of the T categories from the original Butchart system dividing T1 lesions into involvement of the parietal pleura only (T1a) and involvement of the visceral pleura (T1b), creating stage IA and IB from stage I. T3 is defined as a locally advanced but potentially resectable tumor and T4 is defined as a locally advanced, technically unresectable tumor. The AJCC system classifies any nodal involvement, either intrapleural or extrapleural, as stage III disease. The Brigham and Women's Staging System has also been proposed for pleural mesothelioma and differs from the AJCC by defining intrapleural adenopathy as stage II disease and extrapleural adenopathy as stage III disease.[59–62]

Treatment

Overview

No standards exist for the management of resectable pleural mesothelioma, and treatment decisions are influenced by the functional evaluation of these often-elderly individuals and the philosophy of the treating physician. Treatment of mesothelioma can consist of supportive care only, surgery, radiotherapy, chemotherapy, and/or combinations of these modalities. Geographic locale can dictate the type of treatment given. In the United Kingdom, less than half of mesotheliomas are treated by radical resection (E.G. Butchart, personal communication). Currently however, a randomized trial of EPP compared with nonsurgical treatment is under way.[62] In the United States, a cohort of cancer centers using Phase I/II protocols are defining the use of surgery in mesothelioma with or without intraoperative and/or postoperative innovative adjuvant therapies and, in general, innovative, multimodality protocols that incorporate surgery as part of the package are being explored in larger numbers of patients.

Supportive Care

The median survival of patients who select active symptom control only for mesothelioma ranges from 4 months[63] to 13 months[50] because of variations in tumor biology, host response to tumor, detection bias, lead time bias, and the use of ad hoc or unreported treatments by some patients and physicians. Factors predictive of survival were poorly defined when many of the "natural history" series were published; therefore, survival data can only be used for historical comparisons if the prognostic factors of that group are taken into account.

Control of pleural effusion can be accomplished with repeated thoracenteses, talc pleurodesis, pleuroperitoneal shunting, or placement of a Pleurex catheter. Success rates in effusion control with talc, used either via thoracoscopy or via slurry, approach 90%.[64,65] Failure of these techniques is usually associated with the standard reasons for poor prognosis. In such cases, the Pleurex catheter can be implanted under local anesthesia into the fluid collection and the patients can drain themselves at home,[66] or internal drainage from the pleura to the abdomen may be accomplished using the Denver pleuroperitoneal shunt.

Pain management frequently requires narcotics and consultation by a dedicated pain management team to optimize the patient's quality of life. Insertion of subcutaneous epidural catheters for long-term outpatient use has also been used in selective cases.

In 2002, the British Thoracic Society (BTS) proposed a Phase III clinical trial to compare the use of ACS with ACS plus two different chemotherapeutic regimens to measure overall survival, symptom palliation, performance, quality of life, and other endpoints.[67] The chemotherapeutic regimens mitomycin, vinblastine, cisplatin (MVP) and vinorelbine (N) were chosen because of their record of symptom control. More recently, in 2004, a study was conducted to determine if this study was feasible and it was concluded to be.[68] This study is now under way and will be the first to indicate if ACS alone or ACS plus chemotherapy is more effective in symptom control in mesothelioma patients.

Surgery

Aggressive therapy of pleural mesothelioma often entails a multimodality approach of which surgery is only a part. Surgical procedures include pleurectomy/decortication or EPP, and the indication for each of these operations depends on the extent of disease, performance, and functional status of the patient and the philosophy and experience of the treating

TABLE 38.2. International staging system for diffuse malignant pleural mesothelioma.

Stage	*T*	*N*	*M*
Stage I	T1	N–Lymph nodes	M–Metastases
Ia	T1a	NX Regional lymph nodes cannot be assessed	MX Distant metastases cannot be assessed
T1aN0 M0	Tumor involves ipsilateral parietal (mediastinal, diaphragmatic) pleura **No involvement of the visceral pleura**	N0 No regional lymph node metastases	
Ib	T1b		M0 No distant metastasis
T1bN0 M0	Tumor involves ipsilateral parietal (mediastinal, diaphragmatic) pleura, **with focal involvement of visceral pleura**		
Stage II	T2		
T2 N0 M0	Tumor involves any of the ipsilateral pleural surfaces (parietal, mediastinal, diaphragmatic, and visceral pleura) with at least one of the following features: —confluent visceral pleural tumor (including fissure) • invasion of diaphragmatic muscle • invasion of lung parenchyma		
Stage III	T3		
Any T3 M0	Describes locally advanced but **potentially resectable** tumor. Tumor involves any of the ipsilateral pleural surfaces (parietal, mediastinal, diaphragmatic, and visceral pleura), with at least one of the following: • invasion of the endothoracic fascia • invasion into the mediastinal fat • solitary focus of tumor invading the soft tissues of the chest wall • nontransmural involvement of the pericardium		
Any N1 M0		N1 Metastases in the ipsilateral bronchopulmonary and/or hilar node(s)	
Any N2 M0		N2 Metastases in the subcarinal and/or the ipsilateral internal mammary or mediastinal lymph node(s)	
Stage IV	T4		
Any T4	Describes locally advanced **technically unresectable** tumor Tumor involving all the ipsilateral pleural surfaces (parietal, mediastinal, diaphragmatic, and visceral pleura) with at least one of the following: • diffuse extension or multifocal invasion of soft tissues in the chest wall —any involvement of rib • invasion of the diaphragm to the peritoneum • invasion of any mediastinal organ • direct extension of the contralateral pleura —invasion into the spine • extension to the internal surface of the pericardium —pericardial effusion with positive cytology —invasion of the brachial plexus		
Any N3		N3 Metastases in the contralateral mediastinal, internal mammary, or hilar lymph nodes, and/or ipsilateral, or contralateral supraclavicular or scalene lymph nodes	
Any M1			M1 Distant metastasis present

Source: Used with the permission of the American Joint Committee on Cancer (AJCC), Chicago, Illinois. The original source for this material is the *AJCC Cancer Staging Manual*, sixth edition (2002), published by Springer-Verlag New York, www.springer-ny.com.

institution. Operative intervention in mesothelioma fall into one of three categories: (1) primary effusion control as described for supportive care purposes, (2) cytoreduction before to multimodal therapy, or (3) to deliver and monitor innovative intrapleural therapies. Currently studies are under way to determine the benefits of aggressive therapy using surgery as part of a multimodality approach.

Most mesothelioma patients are older individuals with a long latency period between asbestos exposure and tumor development. A detailed physiologic and functional evaluation assessing cardiac and pulmonary status must be performed before any surgical intervention. The degree of asbestos exposure, smoking history, trapped lung, and patient age all influence pulmonary function. Fiber-related fibrosis and reduced CO_2 diffusion capacity increases dyspnea in these patients, and abnormal chest wall motion resulting in reduced lung volumes on the affected side will influence the patient's respiratory functional reserve and the extent of surgery.

Patients without objective evidence of cardiac injury require nuclear medicine studies to rule out reversible perfusion defects indicative of myocardium at risk. Patients with a left ventricular ejection fraction (LVEF) less than 45% or who have sustained a myocardial infarction within the past 3 months are not candidates for EPP. Patients who undergo angioplasty before operative intervention for their disease may be better candidates after such interventions if a multimodality approach is being contemplated.

In addition, before surgery, any drugs that could impact platelet function or anticoagulant therapies must be halted. If a multimodality program utilizing drugs with potential renal toxicity (i.e., cisplatin) is planned, a preoperative creatinine clearance should be performed.

Staging and Operative Therapy

The goal of a surgical resection in mesothelioma is to leave only microscopic residual disease, that is, a near-complete cytoreduction. Eligibility includes all patients who are clinically IMIG stages I–III, although there is increasing skepticism whether patients with stage III mesothelioma are benefited by surgery. No guidelines exist that can assure the patient preoperatively which operation will be necessary to accomplish tumor removal. A large effusion with minimal bulk disease may call for pleurectomy decortication, whereas the presence on CT of irregular, bulky disease that infiltrates into the fissures probably dictates that an EPP should be performed. Hence, stage II mesothelioma may indeed be an absolute indication for EPP as opposed to pleurectomy. Moreover, some surgeons reserve EPP for those patients with bulk disease that prevents simple pleurectomy, whereas others believe that the greatest chance for complete gross excision is via EPP performed in the patient with minimal disease. This important factor, preoperative quantitative bulk of disease, may not only influence the choice or resection but may be an important preoperative prognostic factor in any patient with mesothelioma. The final decision as to whether pleurectomy and decortication or EPP is to be performed, given these caveats, becomes an intraoperative decision unless a protocol calls specifically for one operation or the other.

The influence of nodal status and eligibility for surgery is not well defined because only 30% to 40% of nodes involved from resected mesothelioma patients are accessible to routine mediastinoscopy.[56] The involvement of any nodes, making the patient Stage III, is an ominous prognostic sign; however, it is unclear whether the prognostic importance of mediastinal nodal involvement in mesothelioma is equivalent to the prognostic importance of the nodes within the visceral envelope of the lung which may reflect disease at a later time point. It is possible that FDG PET scanning as previously discussed will help to at least define those patients with node involved mesothelioma in the future. Until then, without routine thoracoscopic sampling of multiple nodal stations in mesothelioma before definitive resection, mediastinoscopy may be justified in those patients with obvious (i.e., larger than 1.5 cm) nodal involvement in levels 7, 4R, 4L, 5L, or 6L, or in patients with a suspicion for contralateral nodal involvement on presentation.[48]

Pleurectomy

Most diffuse malignant mesotheliomas cannot be surgically removed en bloc with truly negative histologic margins. A minority of patients have a margin-free resection, and because those patients who have margin-free resections usually have less-bulky disease, it may be justifiable to spare functioning lung if the visceral pleura is minimally involved; this can be accomplished by performing a radical parietal pleurectomy instead of EPP. "Minimal visceral pleural disease" is an undefined entity and there are no criteria for how many sites should be involved, the size of these involved sites, or whether involvement of the fissure is worse than nonfissural involvement. In general, patients who have pleurectomy decortications for mesothelioma have lesser disease and live longer.

Pleurectomy and decortication are very effective in controlling malignant pleural effusion. Effusion control has been reported in 88% of patients having decortication, 98% of patients having pleurectomy,[69] and 86% of patients having partial decortication and pleurectomy.[70] When performed routinely, pleurectomy for mesothelioma has few major complications, the most common of which is prolonged air leak lasting longer than 7 days occurring in 10% of the patients. The modern-day mortality for pleurectomy for mesothelioma is generally considered to be 1.5% to 2% with death from either respiratory insufficiency or hemorrhage.[71,72]

Many of the published series using pleurectomy for palliative management have added therapies postoperatively in an uncontrolled, institution-related fashion (Table 38.3). The overall median survival for patients having pleurectomy alone is approximately 13 months. The patients who receive pleurectomy and decortication usually have early effusive disease with minimal bulk tumor. If these patients have epithelial mesothelioma, and are not found to have nodal involvement, survival rates can be significantly longer than that quoted above. For additional discussion of pleurectomy and multitherapy, see the Multimodality section.

Extrapleural Pneumectomy

Although a minority of patients have margin-free resections, in one of the largest series of EPPs performed for mesothelioma, 66 of 183 patients were defined as having negative resection margins after surgery. Patients with negative margins at resection, without nodal involvement, and epithe-

TABLE 38.3. Results for pleurectomy.

Year	Author	N	Survival: Median (months)	Survival: Two-year (%)
2003(a)	Sugarbaker et al.	44	10–20	—
2002	Aziz et al.	47	14	—
2002	Lee at al.	26	18.1	—
2001	Martin-Ucar et al.	51	7.2	—
2001	Takagi et al.	73	—	26.1
1997(a)	Pass et al.	39	14.5	—
1996	Rusch and Venkataraman	51	18.3	—
1994	Allen et al.	56	9	8.9
1991	Brancatisano et al.	45	16	21
1990	Harvey et al.	9	11.9	—
1989	Ruffie et al.	63	9.8	—
1988	Faber	33	10	12
1986	DaValle et al.	23	11.2	—
1984	Law et al.	28	20	32
1982	Brenner et al.	69	15	—
1982	Chahinian et al.	30	13	27
1976	Wanebo et al.	33	16.1	—

[a]All patients received intrapleural hyperthermic chemotherapy.

Source: Modified from Singhal S, Kaiser LR. *Surg Clin N Am* 2002;82:797–831.

lial histology were found to have 2- and 5-year survival rates of 68% and 46%, respectively.[60]

EPP is a more-extensive dissection and a more-complete resection than a pleurectomy, chiefly in the diaphragmatic and visceral pleural surfaces. For EPP, pericardiotomy and partial pericardiectomy are performed during the resection because this maneuver aids in the exposure of the vessels and allows intrapericardial control to prevent a surgical catastrophe. Some surgeons include diaphragmatic resection and pericardial resection with their pleurectomies also to accomplish removal of all gross disease.

EPP should only be performed at those centers that have specialized expertise in the surgical management of mesothelioma, loosely defined as having a caseload of 20 or more EPPs per year. Moreover, expansion of surgical eligibility criteria should occur only at those institutions that are conducting institution-based, human investigation committee-approved physician-initiated surgical protocols for the disease or who are participating in consortium-based surgical mesothelioma protocols through cooperative groups or other mechanisms.

Often, during exploration, a cohort of patients planned for EPP are found to be unresectable at the time of the operation. Eligibility for EPP ranged from 50% to 63% at three different instutions,[60,73,74] and in a study in the 1980s it was reported to be as low as 24%.[71]

EPP has significantly greater risk than pleurectomy, and major complication rates range from 20% to 40% with arrhythmia requiring medical management being the most common complication. Morbidity of some type has been reported to be as high as 60.4%.[75] In addition, rates for some morbidities such as bronchopleural fistula is greater with right-sided EPPs, with an overall fistula rate of 3% to 20%. The bronchopleural fistula can be handled for the most part with open thoracostomy drainage with or without muscle flap interposition.

Median survival ranges from 9.3 to 17 months, with longer survival shown in a series heavily weighted in stage I patients (see Table 38.4).[56,60,72,75–78] Mortality rates have declined over the last 30 years and range from 3.8 to 8%, death occurring chiefly in older patients from respiratory failure, myocardial infarction, or pulmonary embolus.[75,77,78] The pattern of recurrence following surgery has been reported as chiefly local progression after pleurectomy and systemic failures after EPP.[72]

Currently, a unique multimodality pilot study is underway in the UK (Treasure, unpublished data) to determine if EPP is useful in the management of mesothelioma; this is described in detail in the Induction Chemotherapy followed by Surgery Section.

TABLE 38.4. Photodynamic therapy for mesothelioma.

Group	N	Mortality (%)	Sensitizer	Operations	Median survival (months)
Pass et al. 1997b, NCI (Phase III)	25	0	Photofrin	11 P; 14 EPP	14.4
Takita and Dougherty 1995, Roswell Park	40	7.5	Photofrin	28 P; 7 EPP; 5 other	15
Schouwink et al. 2001, Rotterdam	28	10	mTHPC	28 EPP	10
Friedberg et al. 2003, Jefferson	26	10	mTHPC	7 P; 19 EPP	12.4

P, pleurectomy; EPP, extrapleural pneumonectomy; mTHPC, *m*-tetrahydroxyphenylchlorin.

Radiotherapy for Mesothelioma

Palliation Using Radiation Therapy

Palliation with radiotherapy in mesothelioma involves the management of dyspnea and chest pain and is most commonly used to palliate pain in patients with advanced mesothelioma and to treat painful chest wall metastases. Palliation was improved with the use of 400-cGy fractions compared with 300-cGy fractions (50% to 72% rate of symptom improvement); however, pain recurrence within the treated field remained a significant problem.[79,80] These investigators reported that short courses of radiation (2,000 cGy in 5 fractions) were as efficacious for symptom relief as more protracted courses of radiation (3,000–4,000 cGy in 10–15 fractions). There is some evidence that total doses greater than 4,500 cGy are the most efficacious,[70] as reported in the results of palliative radiation therapy in 85 patients with mesothelioma.[81] However, in a study with 1,100 patients, 71 of 1,100 patients were treated with radiation for symptoms and more than 60% of patients had some symptomatic benefit from radiation therapy with no dose response.[82] Therefore, the standard approach is to offer patients short courses of treatment (2,000 cGy in 5 fractions) rather than longer courses of radiotherapy.

Curative Radiation Therapy as a Single Modality

Administration of "curative" radiotherapy for malignant pleural mesothelioma adds the risk of severe toxicity to surrounding normal tissue from the large treatment volumes, typically in the 5,000 to 5,500 cGy range. Survival in patients receiving 5,000 to 5,500 cGy to the pleural space using a rotational technique[83] ranged from 3 to 10 months, with one patient who was alive and well 4 years after the completion of treatment. In additional studies, median survival ranged from 9.8 to 17 months.[70,80,84] Patients receiving palliative therapy only had a median survival of 7 months. Selection bias may explain these differences, with those fit enough to undergo a full course of radiation likely to have a greater survival regardless of treatment given. The median survival is 4 to 5 months[79,83] when only local radiotherapy has been delivered solely for chest wall pain or chest wall nodules.

Radiotherapy to Prevent Malignant Seeding

As noted in the thoracoscopy section, there is a 10% chance of later development of chest wall masses from seeding of the biopsy site or surgical scar from any diagnostic procedure. In a recent study designed to determine if a single 9-MeV electron treatment following invasive thoracic procedures would eliminate tract metastasis, 58 patients were randomized to single-dose treatment or no treatment. No significant differences were seen between the two treatments.[85,86]

The best evidence for prevention of malignant seeding by the use of radiotherapy following invasive diagnostic procedures comes from a 1996 study in France.[47] Investigators enrolled 40 patients with histologically proven malignant pleural mesothelioma who had undergone thoracoscopy. Half of the subjects (20) were given 2,100 cGy over 3 days in 700-cGy fractions within 10 to 15 days of the procedure. The other 20 patients were given no additional treatment to the thoracoscopy site. In the radiotherapy arm of the study, not 1 patient developed metastasis at the entry tract, compared with 8 of 20 (40%) who did in the other study arm. These findings support the use of early local radiation therapy at appropriate doses following procedures such as thoracoscopy, needle biopsy, and chest tube placements in eliminating malignant seeding.

Combined Surgical Resection and Definitive Radiotherapy

Surgical resection, when feasible, is the desired treatment for patients with malignant pleural mesothelioma. After an EPP, radical radiotherapy can be administered without concern for damage to the underlying ipsilateral lung because it has been removed surgically. However, radical radiotherapy after a pleurectomy continues to place the ipsilateral lung at risk for substantial loss of function.

No difference in survival was reported in two series when decortication or EPP was followed by radiation therapy for a total dose of 5,000 to 5,500 cGy in 12 and 8 patients, respectively, with pleural mesothelioma.[70,83] Toxicities from this regimen were minimal and included nausea, malaise, transient radiation hepatitis, and mild esophagitis.

Some investigators have used brachytherapy or intraoperative external-beam radiation in combination with surgery. In a study of 41 patients with pleural mesothelioma, parietal pleurectomy resulted in residual disease being left in the majority of patients. Either brachytherapy or radioisotopes were used to eradicate gross residual disease.[87] Measurable gross residual disease was treated with permanent ^{125}I brachytherapy implants, for diffuse residual disease, temporary ^{192}Ir implants were placed 3 to 5 days after the pleurectomy, and for gross disease on the lung surface, a ^{32}P solution was instilled into the pleural cavity 5 to 7 days after thoracotomy. External-beam radiation to a dose of 4,500 cGy was delivered to the pleural surface 4 to 6 weeks after surgery via a combination of photons and electron. There was no mortality and minimal toxicity from this treatment strategy. Six patients (15%) developed complications from treatment: subcutaneous emphysema ($n = 2$), pneumonitis ($n = 1$), pulmonary fibrosis ($n = 1$), pericardial effusion ($n = 1$), and esophagitis ($n = 1$). The median survival was 21 months, with 1-year and 2-year survivals of 65% and 40%, respectively. Local failure occurred in 17% of the patients, perhaps because of the aggressive local therapy. It was concluded that although aggressive surgical resection is an essential portion of treatment, it is often very difficult to remove all sites of disease. The results of this study showed that intraoperative brachytherapy followed by external-beam radiation therapy was effective in controlling local recurrence.

In a Phase II trial at Memorial Sloan Kettering Cancer Center, 67 subjects with malignant pleural mesothelioma received postoperative radiotherapy.[77] Most patients ($n = 62$) underwent an EPP, followed by 5,400 cGy given through anterior and posterior fields in 30 fractions of 180 cGy. Five patients were treated with a pleurectomy, during which 1,500 cGy was given intraoperatively using a high-dose iridium applicator; this was followed by 5,400 cGy to the hemithorax via anterior and posterior fields, in the same fractionation schedule as those who underwent EPP. Not all patients were able to complete the radiation therapy. There were 7 postoperative deaths from pulmonary complications in patients who had undergone an EPP. A total of 33 patients had some complications, the most common being atrial arrythmias (n = 17), respiratory failure (n = 6), pneumonia (n = 5), and empyema (n = 5). In general, radiation was well tolerated, with grade 3 toxicities mainly related to fatigue, nausea, and esophagitis. There were five grade 4 toxicities, the most serious being an esophagopleural fistula. Survival analysis was completed for the 62 EPP patients. Median survival was 17 months, with an overall survival of 27% at 3 years. Locoregional recurrence was 13%, primarily the result of distant metastases. The results of the study showed aggressive surgery with EPP followed by high-dose radiation to the entire hemithorax provided a favorable outcome for those patients who were able to complete the therapy compared with historical data. It should be noted that almost 25% of the enrolled patients were unresectable and were not included in the survival analysis, perhaps introducing a bias in the reported results.

In a recent retrospective review of the efficacy and toxicity of surgery with intraoperative radiotherapy followed by chemotherapy, 24 patients underwent pleurectomy/decortication and intraoperative radiotherapy consisting of 4 to 9 MeV electrons for a median dose of 1,500 cGy (range, 500 to 1,500 cGy).[88] Following surgery, external-beam conformal radiation was given to 14 patients and intensity-modulated radiation therapy (IMRT) was completed in 10 patients. The goal of this radiation therapy was to treat the affected tissue while sparing the underlying normal tissue. The median dose of radiation delivered was 4,140 cGy (range, 3,010–4,880 cGy). Chemotherapy consisting of cisplatin, doxorubicin, and cyclophosphamide was administered to selected patients beginning 1 to 2 months after radiation was completed. There were no deaths, and postoperative complications consisted of atrial fibrillation (n = 3) and a persistent air leak (n = 1). Radiation was also well tolerated; pneumonitis occurred in 4 patients and pericarditis in 1 patient. All symptoms resolved with conservative management. The median overall survival was 18.1 months and the median progression-free interval was 12.2 months. Locoregional relapse was the most common site of failure. It was concluded that this approach was a potential treatment option for adjuvant radiotherapy in patients who were unable to tolerate an EPP.

IMRT offers the potential for administering higher doses of radiotherapy to the hemithorax while minimizing normal tissue toxicities. In a study of 28 patients given IMRT after EPP, the hemithorax was treated with doses totaling 4,500 to 5,000 cGy in most cases, with some regions getting boosted to a total dose of 6,000 cGy.[89,90] Radiation dose homogeneity to the entire hemithorax was excellent. Side effects included nausea, vomiting, dyspnea, and esophagitis. The median follow-up was 9 months, the local control rate was 100%, and 1-year survival was 65%. These early results are encouraging and are worthy of additional study.

Adjuvant Therapy For Surgically Cytoreduced Mesothelioma Patients

Although there are no published Phase III trials of adjuvant therapy in mesothelioma, patients treated with surgery followed by postoperative adjuvant therapy have an apparent improved survival compared with palliative therapy alone in consecutively treated patients from single institutions. These results may be explained by selection bias or by a number of other factors, yet the possibility remains that surgery and adjuvant therapy changes the course of the disease. Mesothelioma is characterized by chemotherapy resistance and infrequent surgical cure, yet an EPP dramatically reduces the amount of visible cancer. The importance of the cytoreduction has been quantified by Pass et al.,[33] and in patients who have a more complete cytoreduction, the time to progression as documented by CT and survival time is longer. In a comparison of patients treated at the National Cancer Institute (NCI), Bethesda, from 1990 to 1993 who did not receive adjuvant therapy and patients treated from 1993 to 1996 and who received cytoreduction followed by adjuvant immunochemotherapy with cisplatin, interferon, and tamoxifen, the addition of postoperative adjuvant therapy influenced postoperative survival.[91,92] These data have been corroborated by Rusch et al.[93] Strong consideration should be given to treating patients with postoperative chemotherapy (if pleurectomy was performed) and/or radiotherapy (if EPP was performed)[94] as Phase III trials are rare and unlikely in this disease.

Multimodality Treatment

Pleurectomy/Intraoperative Brachytherapy and Postoperative Radiation

The Memorial Sloan Kettering Cancer Center has been the leading proponent of this technique, which includes as complete debulking by parietal pleurectomy as possible followed by permanent (^{125}I) or temporary (^{192}Ir) implantation to deliver 3,000 rads in 3 days to a 1-cm distance from the implant plane. Radioactive ^{32}P is selectively instilled intrapleurally 5 to 7 days after thoracotomy, and external-beam radiation therapy commences 4 to 6 weeks postoperatively using electrons and photons to deliver 4,500 rads in 4.5 weeks. In a series from 1984 there was minimum morbidity in 41 patients, and median survival was 21 months at the time of their report.[95] Most patients (54%) recurred at distant sites with or without local recurrence. There have been no subsequent publications on this novel approach; however, the use of intraoperative radiotherapy has been explored recently. Radical pleurectomy/decortication has been combined with intraoperative radiotherapy and postoperative three-dimensional conformal radiation therapy or with IMRT. The study resulted in a median survival of 18 months and median time to progression of 12 months but requires greater maturation. Moreover, the adjuvant therapy did not seem to have an impact on patterns of recurrence after pleurectomy.[96]

Pleurectomy/Intrapleural Chemotherapy and Postoperative Chemotherapy

There has been interest in combining debulking surgery with intracavitary treatment of pleural mesothelioma since the first reports of intrapleural chemotherapy alone for malignant mesothelioma. Rusch et al. used intrapleural chemotherapy with cisplatin and cytarabine after surgical debulking followed by systemic chemotherapy in 10 patients.[97] A subsequent report used an even more aggressive regimen of pleurectomy, immediate intracavitary cisplatin, and mitomycin C with two cycles of systemic cisplatin and mitomycin C.[98] In the initial trial there was one postoperative death and the chemotherapy complications were reversible, making such an approach feasible. The most recent trial revealed an overall survival rate of 68% at 2 years and 44% at 2 years in the 27 patients who received the therapy, with a median survival of 17 months.[97,98] Recurrences, however, were chiefly locoregional. A very similar regimen combining pleurectomy or EPP with cisplatin and mitomycin C resulted in a disappointing median survival of 13 months, and only 50% of the chemotherapy treatments were delivered adjuvantly. In an Italian study of 20 patients, pleurectomy and diaphragmatic or pericardial resection, combined with intrapleural chemotherapy with cisplatin and cytarabine for 4 hours immediately after pleurectomy, followed by systemic chemotherapy with epirubicin and mitomycin C, revealed a median time to disease progression of 7.4 months and median survival of only 11.5 months.[99]

The intrapleural route with standard agents or radiation therapy remains intriguing but unanswered with regard to its efficacy. Phase II studies with the following design principles continue to be needed: (1) a tolerable regimen without chronic side effects, (2) a standard debulking approach with definition of the extent of residual disease, and (3) careful documentation of recurrence patterns.

Extrapleural Pneumonectomy/Intravenous Chemotherapy and Postoperative Radiotherapy

A multimodal approach to malignant mesothelioma using EPP, postoperative chemotherapy, and targeted postoperative radiotherapy has been ongoing since 1980 at the Brigham and Women's Hospital in Boston.[100] The adjuvant therapy presently includes two cycles of paclitaxel and carboplatin with concurrent radiation to a dose of 4,050cGy. Over a 19-year period, 183 patients have been treated with a perioperative mortality of 3.8%. The median survival in this group of patients is approximately 17 months, which is a significant improvement over other trials. Favorable subgroups include those with no mediastinal nodal involvement and epithelial histology.[100]

A large nonrandomized series from Germany has also demonstrated apparent increased survival with multimodal treatment compared to best supportive care.[101] The treated patients, however, were younger, had a better performance status at presentation, and had no medical contraindications to surgery. These 93 patients chose either best supportive care or multimodal treatment. Surgery consisted of pleurectomy decortication or EPP followed by systemic chemotherapy with doxorubicin, cyclophosphamide, and vindesine. Patients in remission at the end of the chemotherapy (16 of the 57 accrued) received 4,500 to 6,000cGy of radiation therapy to the hemithorax. Median survival was 13 months compared to 7 months for those receiving best supportive care.

In a series of 32 patients from Italy, Maggi et al.[102–104] used the Brigham and Women's protocol of EPP followed by adjuvant chemotherapy and concurrent hemithoracic radiation up to a total dose of 5,500cGy. The results were encouraging with only a 6.25% operative mortality rate. However, a median survival of only 9.5 months was reported as 50% of the patients were found to be in stage III after the procedure.

Induction Chemotherapy Followed by Surgery

Induction or neoadjuvant therapy for pleural mesothelioma followed by surgery has been patterned after such therapy with non-small cell lung cancer. Results have been disappointing due to the inability of the patients to tolerate both the cytotoxic chemotherapy and the surgery. There also appeared to be difficulty in performing the surgical dissection after induction chemotherapy with doxorubicin because of the dense adhesions, perhaps caused by fibrosis following cancer kill by chemotherapy. With the improved efficacy of doublet chemotherapy (gemcitabine/cisplatin or pemetrexed/cisplatin), there is renewed interest in investigating a neoadjuvant approach for mesothelioma. A Swiss neoadjuvant study used three cycles of cisplatin 80mg/m^2 on day 1 and gemcitabine 1,000mg/m^2 on days 1, 8, and 15 every 28 days followed by surgery. Radiation therapy was considered after EPP to areas at risk. In all, 30 patients entered thus far have been reported. After chemotherapy, 22 (73%) underwent EPP. Histology after surgery revealed epithelioid (10) , mixed (11), and sarcomatoid disease (3). There was 1 postoperative fatality. The median overall survival was 20 months and the 1-year survival rate was 77%.[105] A similar trial performed by de Perrot et al. involved induction chemotherapy, surgery, and postoperative hemithorax radiation therapy with a 6% operative mortality and 74% 1-year survival.[106] A neoadjuvant approach is presently being investigated in the United States as a multicenter trial of four cycles of pemetrexed and cisplatin followed by EPP and postoperative hemithorax radiation therapy.

Currently, a pilot feasibility study of neoadjuvant chemotherapy followed by EPP and postoperative radiotherapy is under way in the United Kingdom (unpublished). The mesothelioma and radical surgery (MARS, unpublished) trial is intended to help determine the usefulness of EPP in the management of mesothelioma. In this clinical trial, 670 patients will be enrolled over 3 years. Before randomization, the patients will have histologically proven mesothelioma with no distant metastases, with resectable disease, and have undergone three cycles of cisplatin-based chemotherapy. Following their chemotherapy, each patient will be randomized to the EPP + radiotherapy arm or the no further intervention arm of the study. Follow-up for the patient is expected to be 5 years.

Novel Intrapleural Approaches: New Techniques with New/Old Agents

Intrapleural Photodynamic Therapy

Photodynamic therapy involves the light-activated sensitization of malignant cells[92] using a photosensitizer such as Photofrin II that is retained by malignant tissue in vivo in comparison to normal tissue. The sensitizer is activated by 630-nm light and then interacts with molecular oxygen to produce an excited reactive oxygen species. After a series of Phase I and II trials, a group of 63 patients with localized mesothelioma were randomized to surgery, with or without

TABLE 38.5. Pleural perfusion for mesothelioma.

Group	*N*	*Mortality/morbidity (%)*	*Treatment*	*Surgeries*	*Median survival (months)*
Ratto et al. 1999	7	0/28	Cisplatin 40°–42°C	4 EPP; 3 P	N/A
Yellin et al. 2001	7	0/33	Cisplatin 41.5°C	4 EPP; 3 other	15
Carrey et al. 1993	3	0/33	Mitomycin C 40°C	3 P	N/A
Van Ruth et al. 2003	20	0/65	Adriamycin, cisplatin 40°–41°C + postoperative RT	8 EPP; 6 P; 5 incomplete	11
Sugarbaker et al. 2003	44	11/44	Cisplatin 42°C	44 P	13

N/A, not available; P, pleurectomy; EPP, extrapleural pneumonectomy; RT, radiation therapy.

intraoperative photodynamic therapy (PDT). All patients received postoperative immunochemotherapy with cisplatin, tamoxifen, and interferon. There were no differences in median survival (14.4 versus 14.1 months) or median progression-free time (8.5 versus 7.7 months), and sites of first recurrence were similar. Thus, aggressive multimodal therapy incorporating PDT can be delivered for patients with higher-stage mesothelioma, but first-generation PDT does not prolong survival or increase local control for mesothelioma. Other Phase II trials of photodynamic therapy and mesothelioma have not demonstrated therapeutic efficacy,[107–109] and most recently preliminary results using intrapleural PDT with meta-tetrahydroxy-phenylchlorin after EPP have revealed significant toxicities without survival benefit[110] (Table 38.5).

Pleural Perfusion

Hyperthermic chemoperfusion of the pleura after resection of mesothelioma is based on the hypothesis that the treatment will provide increased local control and avoid systemic chemotherapy toxicity. Ratto et al. delivered cisplatin to the pleural space after pleurectomy or EPP in 10 patients[111] and recorded the pharmacokinetics but did not comment on survival or recurrences. Other small Phase II studies using cisplatin or doxorubicin with cisplatin have recorded morbidity rates of 33% to 65% using temperatures of 40°a to 42°C without impacting on survival[112,113] (Table 38.6). Sugarbaker et al. presented a Phase I/II trial using hyperthermic cisplatin (42°C) to perfuse both the abdomen and the pleura after pleurectomy/decortication. Operative mortality was 11%, and survival of all patients was 10.5 months; however, in the group of patients surviving surgery who received 225 mg/m^2 of cisplatin, the median survival was 22 months and disease-free survival was 20 months.[114]

Novel Gene and Cytokine-Related Therapies

By transferring the herpes simplex virus (HSV-tk) thymidine kinase gene to a tumor by infecting it with an adenovirus construct containing the TK gene (AdHSVtk), one essentially kills the tumor with the addition of gancyclovir. A Phase I trial of intrapleural suicide gene therapy has been reported that delivered a replication-deficient adenovirus encoding HSV-tk (Ad.HSV-tk) which, in preclinical studies, was found to transduce mesothelioma cells and treat human mesothe-

TABLE 38.6. Results for extrapleural pneumonectomy.

Year	*Author*	*N*	*Median survival (months)*	*Two-year survival (%)*
2001	Rusch et al. 2001[a]	61	17	—
2001	Schouwink et al. 2001[b]	28	10	—
2000	Takagi et al. 2001	116	—	29.7
1999	Sugarbaker et al. 1999[c]	183	19	38
1997	Pass et al. 1997a[d]	39	9.4	—
1996	Rusch and Venkatraman 1996	50	9.9	—
1994	Allen et al. 1994	40	13.3	22.5
1990	Harvey et al. 1990	7	5.4	28.5
1989	Ruffie et al. 1989	23	9.3	17
1988	Faber 1988	33	13.5	24
1986	DaValle et al. 1986		17.8	24
1982	Chahinian et al. 1982	6	18	33
1978	DeLaria et al. 1978	11	18	—
1976	Butchart et al. 1976	29	4.5	10.3

[a] Postoperative hemithorax radiation therapy; all patients; stages I/II, 33.8; Stages III/IV, 10.

[b] Intraoperative photodynamic therapy.

[c] Postoperative multimodal therapy.

[d] Phase I trials of photodynamic therapy or immunochemotherapy.

Source: Modified from Singhal S, Kaiser LR. *Surg Clin N Am* 2002;82:797–831.

lioma xenografts in SCID mice.[115] Gene transfer was demonstrated in 17 of 25 evaluable patients and was dose dependent. There was 1 partial response, 3 of the first 18 patients remained stable for up to 2 years following treatment, and 1 early-stage patient was tumor free for more than 31 months. The median survival of all patients was 11 months.

Immunomodulatory gene therapy is also being investigated for mesothelioma by transfecting tumors with cytokine genes that can activate CD4 T cells or stimulate CD8 T cells. The IL-2 gene has been inserted into a replication-deficient vaccinia virus, and six patients have been, treated with one to three weekly injections of vaccinia virus-IL-2 (VV-IL-2) intratumorally. No clinical responses were seen, although expression of VV-IL-2 mRNA was detected in tumor biopsies and a T-cell infiltrate was detected in 50% of tumor biopsies at the site of injection.[116–118] Preclinical trials of the transfection of interferon-β,[119,120] interleukin 4, and p14[121,122] into mesothelioma are ongoing. An approach that combines suicide gene therapy and vaccination strategies uses genetically modified allogeneic irradiated ovarian cancer cells transduced with the HSV-tk gene followed with systemic gancyclovir treatment.[118–120,123–125] In in vitro mixing experiments, gene-modified ovarian tumor cells killed both mouse and human mesothelioma cells in a dose-dependent manner. Use of the ovarian HSV-TK ovarian cells also prolonged survival of mice with mesothelioma in a dose-dependent fashion. These data have served as the basis for an ongoing Phase I clinical gene therapy trial to determine the maximum tolerated dose of HSV-TK-transduced ovarian cancer cells infused into the pleural cavities of mesothelioma patients followed by systemic gancyclovir.

Intrapleural and Systemic Cytokine Therapy

The use of intrapleural cytokine therapy by infusional techniques has chiefly been investigated in earlier-stage mesothelioma, and the effectiveness of interferon-γ by this route has been documented by Boutin et al.[126,127] Interferon was administered at a dose of 40 million units twice a week for 8 weeks intrapleurally via a catheter or an implantable port for 89 patients over 46 months. Thoracoscopic or surgical biopsy was performed if CT scan 2 weeks after the end of treatment demonstrated a reduction in tumor size. Eight histologically confirmed complete responses and 9 partial responses with at least a 50% reduction in tumor size were obtained. The overall response rate was 20%. The response rate for patients with stage I disease was 45% with the main side effects being hyperthermia, liver toxicity, neutropenia, and catheter-related infection.

Intrapleural interleukin-2-based regimens have also been exploited in mesothelioma.[128] Intrapleural IL-2 (21 × 10^6 IU/m^2/day for 5 days) was given to 22 patients with mesothelioma. Patients had stage IA ($n = 3$), stage IB ($n = 1$), stage II ($n = 16$), stage III ($n = 1$), or stage IV ($n = 1$) disease (Butchart classification). Histology comprised epithelial ($n = 19$), mixed ($n = 2$), and fibrosarcomatous ($n = 1$) mesothelioma. Patients were evaluated for response 36 days after treatment by CT scan and thoracoscopy with biopsies. There were 11 partial responses and 1 complete response. Stable disease occurred in 3 patients and disease progression in 7 patients. The overall median survival time was 18 months, and the 24-month and 36-month survival rates for responders were 58% and 41%, respectively. Surprisingly, no confirmatory trials of this promising approach have been published.

Chemotherapy And Newer Agents

The rarity and dismal survival of pleural mesothelioma has precluded, until recently, Phase III trials. It was not surprising, therefore, that early studies with single-agent chemotherapeutics were tested in 20 to 40 patients[21,129–133] with the hope that a major therapeutic advance would be discovered with limited numbers of patients. The most common single-agent drugs used for mesothelioma have been the anthracyclines, platinum agents, and antimetabolites.[134] The anthracyclines have had response rates of 0% to 15%, with median survivals of 4.4 to 9.5 months. Cisplatinum or carboplatinum have had response rates of 7% to 16%, with median survivals of 5 to 8 months. Antimetabolites as single agents have had response rates from 0% to 37%, the highest observed in methotrexate (37%) and gemcitabine (31%).[134] Typically, tumor regression of short duration associated with symptomatic improvement occurred in 15% of patients treated with chemotherapy but the median survival remained at about 7 to 9 months. Recently, however, a clinical benefit in up to 40% to 50% of patients was seen with single-agent vinorelbine.[135]

In general, combination regimens have had higher response rates and longer median survival times. Anthracycline-based combinations had response rates from 11% to 32% and median survivals from 5.5 to 13.8 months, and those with platinum have had response rates of 6% to 48% with median survivals of 5.8 to 16 months.[134]

A 1998 report from the U.K. suggested that clinical benefit as measured by reduction in pain and dyspnea occurred in up to 40% to 50% of patients treated with a regimen of mitomycin C, vinblastine, and cisplatin (MVC).[136] Therefore, a study is under way that will randomize more than 800 patients with mesothelioma to single-agent vinorelbine, the MVC combination, or supportive care to determine whether chemotherapy improves either quality of life or length of life in this disease.[137]

A role for the antifolates has been suggested since it was reported that methotrexate induced regressions in 37% of patients.[138] Other antifolates had consistent but low activity as well[139–143] (Table 38.7). A novel antifolate, pemetrexed, binds with high affinity to folate transport proteins,[144] is extensively polyglutamated, inhibits dihydrofolate reductase (DHFR), thymidylate synthase (TS), and glycinamide ribonucleotide formyltransferase (GARFT), and demonstrated broad antitumor activity in Phase I and II trials.[145] In Phase I studies, the combination of cisplatin and pemetrexed induced regressions in 5 of 12 (38%) of pleural mesothelioma patients in one study[146] and significant radiologic improvements in approximately 40% of patients in another.[147] These two trials led to a Phase II trial of pemetrexed as a single agent in the treatment of mesothelioma[148] in which 14% of patients responded. A comprehensive multivariate analysis of ongoing Phase II and III trials revealed that elevated serum homocysteine and methylmalonic acid (MMA) levels indicated folic acid and vitamin B_{12} deficiency states were the major contributors to grade 3 and 4 toxicity of pemetrexed.[149] Subsequently, the enforced initiation of folic acid therapy (400–1,000 μg/day) and B_{12} injections every 9 weeks reduced myelosuppression and

TABLE 38.7. Single-agent antifolate studies.

Drug	Author and year of report	No. of patients	Response rate
Methotrexate	Solheim et al. 1992	63	37%
CB-3717	Calvert et al. 1987; Cantwell et al. 1986	18	5%
Trimetrexate	Vogelzang et al. 1994	52	12%
Edatrexate	Kindler et al. 1999	60	25%
Pemetrexed	Scagliotti and Novello 2003	64	15%

gastrointestinal toxicity while preserving and possibly enhancing efficacy.

Encouraging results in Phase I and II trials prompted a Phase III trial with 448 evaluable patients comparing every-3-week single-agent cisplatin (75mg/m^2) versus pemetrexed (500mg/m^2 IV bolus over 10 minutes) plus cisplatin (75mg/m^2). Median survival time was clearly superior with combination therapy (12.1 months versus 9.3 months, respectively). An average 30% reduction in the thickness of the pleural rind measured by CT scan was 41.3% in the combination arm versus 16.7% in the cisplatin-alone arm. Time to disease progression, pulmonary function, and quality of life also improved in a statistically significant manner in the pemetrexed/cisplatin-treated patients.

Treatment with the combination regimen had resulted in more serious adverse events including drug-related death, grades 3 and 4 neutropenia, thrombocytopenia, and nausea and vomiting compared with cisplatin alone; however, supplementation with folic acid and vitamin B_{12} significantly reduced the incidence of these toxicities and was associated with longer survival (P less than 0.01) in the pemetrexed/cisplatin arm only. Sustained improvement in quality of life and symptom relief (including pain, dyspnea, fatigue, anorexia, and cough) were also seen in the combination arm when compared with cisplatin alone.[150] These results suggest treatment with pemetrexed and cisplatin, supplemented with folic acid and vitamin B_{12}, provides an improved risk-to-benefit ratio in the treatment of mesothelioma.

Powerful predictors of increased survival and decreased survival were consistent with those reported previously in this chapter. Pulmonary function tests (PFTs) before each cycle of therapy in both treatment arms were improved in both the responder and stable-disease patients.[151] Changes in slow vital capacity (SVC), forced vital capacity (FVC), or forced expiratory volume in 1 second (FEV_1) all correlated significantly with tumor response status. Therefore, the commonly used objective measurement with PFTs may be helpful and more sensitive than CT scanning in detecting treatment efficacy for patients with a response.

An additional two drug regimens containing a platinating agent (cisplatin, carboplatin, and oxaliplatin) have been studied in Phase II trials and appear to be associated with response rates and median survivals similar to that of the pemetrexed/cisplatin-treated patients. The combination of the older chemotherapeutic agent cisplatin combined with the antimetabolite gemcitabine showed a 30% or greater reduction in the thickness of the pleural rind and improvement in symptoms in 10 of 21 (47%) of patients in one study[152]; in another, a 26% rate of activity was seen but median survival was only 7.5 months.[153] Other multicenter Phase II studies have shown promising activity with combination chemotherapy using gemcitabine/carboplatin, leading to widespread use of this regimen.[154–156]

Following an encouraging Phase II experience with ranpirase, a ribonuclease derived from frogs' eggs,[157] a Phase III trial compared the median survival of 154 patients randomized to treatment with either single-agent doxorubicin or ranpirnase (Onconase). No difference in the median survivals of 7 to 8 months in each group was seen. Poor-risk patients were heavily weighted in the ranpirnase arm, and elimination of those patients from the analysis showed median survival for rapirnase was 11 months. The trial has now been extended to compare doxorubicin to doxorubicin plus ranpirnase and will accrue a total of up to 300 patients. Ranpirnase has recently been granted orphan drug status for the treatment of mesothelioma by the European Union.

In a 3-year period from November 1999 to January 2003, 250 patients were randomized into a Phase III study of cisplatin alone or cisplatin plus raltitrexed, a thymidine synthase inhibitor. Previously, Phase I and Phase II studies had shown an overall response rate of 20% to 35% in the combination arm and 21% with cisplatin alone. Patients must have had histologically confirmed mesothelioma that was unresectable, had not been pretreated with chemotherapy, and a performance status of 0 to 2. Cisplatin (80mg/m^2) or cisplatin (80mg/m^2) plus raltitrexed (3mg/m^2) was given every 3 weeks until progression, unacceptable toxicity, or patient refusal occurred. The population was 80% male, median age 58 years, and mostly histological subtype epithelial (68%). Most patients had a performance status of 1 (62%). Grade 3 and 4 toxicities were roughly double in the combination arm for neutropenia, thrombocytopenia, fatigue, nausea, and emesis. Interestingly, more patients with greater pleuritic pain were in the cisplatin-alone arm when compared with combination therapy ($n = 10$ versus 6, respectively), and dyspnea was equivalent in the two treatment arms. There were 207 patients with measurable disease who were followed by RECIST criteria during the study. Partial response was seen in 14 cisplatin-alone patients compared with 24 in the combination arm. In addition, 1 patient in the combination arm achieved completed response. Overall response rates and median and 1-year survivals were better for the combination therapy compared with cisplatin alone, showing a trend toward improved survival in combination (23% versus 14 %, 11.2 versus 8.8 months, and 45% versus 40%, respectively); however, these results were not statistically significant.

In spite of these modestly heartening results, chemotherapeutic agents have historically had little effectiveness against mesothelioma. Most of the larger studies require unresectable patients; therefore, the benefit of these drug regimens in early-stage mesothelioma is not well studied. However, in the studies reported, newer agents seem to be somewhat more effective and the pemetrexed and cisplatin combination alters the natural history of mesothelioma. Second-line chemotherapy may also alter the natural history of mesothelioma, but Phase III trials using a placebo-control population are needed. Effective agents with unique mechanisms of action against mesothelioma are still desperately needed. Vascular endothelial growth factor (VEGF) signal transduction inhibitors are being tested and have clinical activity. To optimally test the many newer agents, referral of fit patients with no prior exposure to systemic therapy to clinical trials is strongly encouraged.

Malignant Peritoneal Mesothelioma

Presentation

Peritoneal mesotheliomas account for 25% to 33% of all mesotheliomas. Similar to pleural mesothelioma, it is diagnosed later in life (median age, 60 years), and there is a male to female ratio of 3:1. The relationship between mesothelioma and heavy exposure to airborne asbestos fibers is statistically proven, and pleural plaques are seen in approximately 50% of patients with peritoneal primaries.[158]

Presentation commonly includes increased abdominal girth from ascites (49%), pain (43%), and weight loss (22%) and includes a pain-predominant or ascites-predominant clinical type,[159] with concomitant abdominal distension and abdominal pain in 14% of the patients. A tumor mass is seen in 6% of patients with localized abdominal pain with little or no ascites, and the abdominal mass is usually represents omental caking.[160] Most patients have had symptoms for 6 months to 2 years before diagnosis. Men can present with an inguinal or umbilical hernia, and women can present with a pelvic mass. Some patients present with a new-onset hernia. Other signs of advanced disease include fever, leukocytosis, and thrombocytosis, and are associated with poor prognostic signs.[161]

Diagnosis

Radiography and Tissue Procurement

The workup of the patient with a peritoneal mesothelioma usually includes abdominal ultrasonography,[162] CT of the abdomen,[163–165] MRI,[166,167] and most recently PET scanning.[168] On routine endoscopy, the appearance of mesothelioma is consistent with metastatic tumors with nodules, plaques, and masses that will involve the parietal and visceral peritoneum. The absence of hepatic parenchymal metastases should alert the physician to the possibility that the pathology is mesothelioma. Patients may present with massive ascites without demonstrable solid disease, ascites with infiltration of the mesentery leading to mesenteric thickening, peritoneal studding with masses of varying sizes, and/or hemorrhage within a dominant tumor mass.[169,170] Peritoneal fluid from malignant ascites may be a watery transudate or a viscous fluid rich in mucopolysaccharides. Cytology establishes the diagnosis in only 5% to 10% of cases; however, viscous ascites with high fluid hyaluronidase levels may suggest the diagnosis. Definitive diagnosis requires CT-guided core biopsy of tumor masses or infiltrated omentum,[171] paracentesis with cell block for immunohistochemical staining, or preferably adequate tissue sampling from a laparoscopy with biopsy[172,173] or an open directed biopsy. Laparoscopy, in addition to evaluating the extent of disease, should carefully examine the ovaries and the bowel to rule out nonmesothelioma neoplasms. Sufficient tissue must be obtained to perform immunohistochemical staining to differentiate an abdominal mesothelioma from other more-common causes of peritoneal carcinomatosis.

Peritoneal mesotheliomas must be differentiated from papillary tumors of the peritoneum (WDPM) because these tumors have a completely different natural history (see Benign Mesotheliomas). Although the ability to diagnose cystic mesotheliomas of the peritoneum before or at the time of exploratory laparotomy is limited, there has been advocacy for the avoidance of treatment unless there is evidence of progressive disease.[174] Differential diagnosis from ovarian cancer or true mesothelioma, however, may be possible only after the surgically resected ovaries and tumor are examined pathologically to document that there is no minimal or superficial invasion of the ovarian cortex or through immunohistochemical methods.[175] Because the amount of residual disease may be a prognostic factor, all such patients should be debulked to no macroscopic disease. Nevertheless, despite initial surgical resection, approximately one-half recur locally, and outcome is not associated with lesion size or proliferation.[176] There are recent anecdotal reports of an aggressive approach to these tumors either by adding adjuvant platinum-based chemotherapy after resection or primary treatment with cytoreductive surgery, and heated chemoperfusion may prove worthwhile.[177]

Staging and Natural History of Malignant Peritoneal Mesothelioma

There is no staging system for peritoneal mesothelioma. The tumor is typically confined to the abdomen until late in the course and usually spreads to one or both pleural cavities rather than disseminating hematogenously. Most patients die without metastases or involvement of the chest. Involvement of the serosa overlying the small and large bowel, the liver, the spleen, and other organs leads to encasement of these organs in tumor tissue and repeated bowel obstructions. The median survival of untreated patients is 5 to 12 months.[178,179]

Treatment

A multidisciplinary aggressive approach has evolved at specialized centers for treating peritoneal mesothelioma. Complete surgical resection is rarely, if ever, feasible and has not shown a survival benefit in the absence of additional therapy. Nevertheless, in the absence of clear evidence-based data, it may be that effective local therapy has a substantial effect on the survival of patients with this disease, and peritoniectomy and cytoreduction is an integral part of multimodality therapy for the disease. Because of the low response rates of systemic chemotherapy, novel approaches involving either induction therapy followed by surgery, or postoperative intraperitoneal drug delivery after surgical debulking, were explored. Intraperitoneal chemotherapy with a variety of agents including cisplatinum, mitomycin C, doxorubicin, epidoxorubicin, etoposide, and cytarabine used either singly or in combination has been reported with responses up to 50% in small Phase II studies.[180–184] Whole abdominal radiotherapy as an adjunct to intraperitoneal chemotherapy and surgery was first described in 10 patients with peritoneal mesothelioma in which 6 of the 10 patients received the multimodality approach between 1968 and 1985. The 6 patients remained free of disease at 19+ to 78+ months after diagnosis whereas the 4 patients not treated with this multimodality approach died of the disease.[185] The intraperitoneal infusion of radioisotopes for peritoneal mesothelioma remains of historical interest only[186,187]; however, intraperitoneal chemotherapy is of continued interest.

Intraperitoneal Chemotherapy

Intravenous chemotherapy results in patients with malignant mesothelioma have been disappointing. Given the tendency of the disease to remain confined to the peritoneum, interest has focused on the use of intraperitoneal chemotherapy. The primary theoretical obstacle to this form of treatment is the shallow depth of drug penetration into tumor nodules. Advantages include greatly enhanced drug concentrations in the peritoneal cavity and decreased systemic toxicity. In addition, substantial intravenous drug concentrations are obtained from peritoneal absorption of some drugs such as cisplatin. Thus, the combination of free surface diffusion and intracapillary drug flow may be potentially more efficacious than intravenous treatment alone.

The use of intraperitoneal chemotherapy for mesothelioma has been extensively reviewed.[188,189] Intraperitoneal cisplatin and intravenous thiosulfate protection have resulted in a 59% complete response rate. However, many patients in this study relapsed quickly after treatment, implying incomplete eradication of tumor using cisplatin alone.[190] Intraperitoneal cisplatin was given to 18 of 19 patients and cisplatin alone was given to 1, resulting in 2 patients (10.5%) being disease free more than 5 years after therapy.[191] The combination of cisplatin and etoposide resulted in 1 complete response in 5 patients with measurable disease.

Another study showed a response for two of four patients receiving cisplatin-based intraperitoneal therapy, one of which was a complete response. A 2-year follow-up laparotomy revealed only adhesions.[192] Additionally, a case report noted continuing complete response at 53 months in a patient treated with intraperitoneal cisplatin and cytarabine.[193]

Combined Modality Approaches

Several institutions have researched combined modality, which typically involves surgery with cytoreduction, intraperitoneal intraoperative treatment with cytotoxic chemotherapy, and postoperative chemotherapy and/or radiation therapy,[194,195] and many of these reviews are reported next in this section. In a retrospective review of 15 women with peritoneal mesothelioma, it was reported that the response rate to first-line chemotherapy regimens was 30% overall but 67% to paclitaxel and cisplatin.[196] The median survival of all patients was 12 months; however, survival was longer for patients who underwent cytoreductive surgery versus biopsy only (14 versus 6 months, $P = 0.24$) and chemotherapy versus none (29 versus 1 month, $P = 0.03$).

Three sequential series of patients reported by Taub et al.[195] (1980 to 1982, 1982 to 1985, 1986 to 1988) were treated at the Dana Farber Cancer Institute and Joint Center for Radiation Therapy. In the initial trial, 1 of 9 patients treated with surgery and intravenous cyclophosphamide, doxorubicin, and dimethyltriazenoimidazole carboxamide (DTIC), before and after whole abdominal radiotherapy, survived more than 10 years after diagnosis. In the second Phase I trial between 1982 and 1985, 6 of 13 patients having a debulking resection of all lesions of more than 1 cm in size were treated with intraperitoneal doxorubicin (6 to 50 mg/m^2) and cisplatin (60 to 100 mg/m^2) for a total of 8 to 12 treatments. At the time of the second laparotomy for removal of the access device, all 6 patients had a minimum decrease of 50% in the size of the tumor. The complete treatment package of surgical resection and chemotherapy followed by whole abdominal irradiation was completed in 4 patients. Four of the 6 patients, including 3 of the 4 who received irradiation, remained disease free for at least 36, 48, 60, and 61 months after diagnosis. In the third Phase II series, patients were treated with surgical debulking and intraperitoneal cisplatin and doxorubicin every 2 weeks for 20 weeks. Patients with no visible disease at second-look laparotomy received whole abdominal external-beam radiotherapy, and patients with macroscopic residual disease were treated with intravenous cyclophosphamide and doxorubicin and then radiation therapy. Thirteen patients had responded to therapy (partial response, $n = 7$; complete response, $n = 6$; although random biopsies were positive in all patients). Three patients with partial responses relapsed at 8, 24, and 25 months. At the time of reporting, all 6 patients with complete responses had remained in remission from 9 to 30 months (median, 25 months). Toxicity was generally mild, including nausea, vomiting, transient elevation in creatinine, and mild to moderate hematologic toxicity, and there were no discontinuations due to toxicity. Two episodes of small bowel obstructions in responding patients resolved without surgical intervention.

In a series of 17 early-stage patients between 1984 and 1999[195] who underwent cytoreductive surgery followed by five cycles of intraperitoneal doxorubicin (25 mg/m^2) and cisplatin (75 mg/m^2), 11 patients responded (65%) as assessed by second-look laparotomy or CT scan and received total abdominal radiation (3,000 cGy, $n = 3$), intravenous chemotherapy ($n = 3$), or both ($n = 4$). Ten patients completed all planned treatment. Toxicity included nausea, fatigue, and myelosuppression. Median survival for this group was 27.6 months (range, 3.6–66 months), and 8 patients were alive at the 24-month median follow-up (range, 3–49 months).

Taub et al.[197] also pioneered the use of surgery, intraperitoneal chemotherapy, and postoperative radiotherapy for peritoneal mesothelioma. Ten symptomatic patients were registered to be surgically debulked and receive five courses of intraperitoneal cisplatin and doxorubicin postoperatively, weekly over 10 weeks via the laparotomy-placed catheter. After reexploration to document disease status and to resect residual disease, patients were to receive 3,080 cGy to the abdomen and pelvis. Of the 10, 5 patients underwent surgical debulking and intraperitoneal chemotherapy but did not receive planned radiotherapy and 4 completed all three modalities of treatment. Three patients died of disease progression. The remaining 7 patients survived longer than 9 months; 4 had minimal or undetectable stable disease, and 3 had detectable intraabdominal disease.

Other investigators have combined hyperthermia to 42°C with the chemotherapy at the time of the cytoreduction.[198–200] As part of three consecutive Phase I trials conducted at the National Cancer Institute, 18 patients (13 had associated ascites) underwent tumor debulking followed by a 90-minute continuous hyperthermic peritoneal profusion with cisplatin. Results showed symptomatic, multiply recurrent, benign, cystic peritoneal mesothelioma (n = 1), reperfusion due to recurrence after 6 months or more, a progression-free interval following continuous hyperthermic peritoneal profusion (n = 3), superficial wound infections (n = 2), and atrial fibrillation, pancreatitis, fascial dehiscence, ileus, line sepsis, and *Clostridium difficile* colitis (n = 1 for each). No toxic deaths occurred. Renal toxicity occurred at cisplatin doses above the recommended Phase II dose. Postoperative resolution of ascites occurred in 9 of 10 patients. Three patients with recurrent ascites at 10, 22, and 27 months after initial treatment had resolution of their ascites with ongoing responses at 4, 6, and 24 months after reperfusion. The median progression-free survival was 26 months, and the overall 2-year survival was 80% at early follow-up.

In the series of Loggie,[198] 12 patients underwent exploratory laparotomy with cytoreduction followed by a 2-hour hyperthermic chemoperfusion using mitomycin C. One patient died 50 days postoperatively from complications relating to small bowel perforation. Hematologic toxicity of the procedure was minimal. Ascites was controlled in all patients and permanently in 86% of patients presenting with ascites. To date, median survival is 34.2 months with median follow-up of 45.2 months; however, long-term follow-up is lacking, and whether any of these patients had cystic mesothelioma must be determined. The Sugarbaker et al. series of 51 patients reports an encouraging median survival of 50 to 60 months using cytoreduction and heated chemotherapy with adriamycin and cisplatinum followed by paclitaxel[201]; however, further delineation of the histology of the patients is needed.

Malignant Mesothelioma of the Tunica Vaginalis Testis

Fewer than 100 cases of gonadal mesothelioma have been reported in the literature, and although most patients are 50 years of age or older, approximately 10% of the patients are younger than 25 years.[202] Asbestos exposure is documented in approximately one-half of the more recently reported cases.[203] Patients generally present with a hydrocele or hernia. An accurate preoperative diagnosis has been reported in only two cases.[204]

All patients with a suspected testicular malignancy should undergo a radical or high inguinal orchiectomy. Local resection of the tumor or hydrocelectomy is associated with a high recurrence rate compared with high inguinal orchiectomy. Because preoperative diagnosis of gonadal mesothelioma is difficult, management should be as for any testicular tumor. The inguinal approach avoids interruption of the scrotal lymphatics, which would alter the metastatic pathway of the tumor, and also allows complete removal of the spermatic cord up to the internal ring. Patients with evidence of disease extending into the retroperitoneal nodes should undergo a retroperitoneal lymphadenectomy.

The overall recurrence rate (local and disseminated) for gonadal mesothelioma can be as high as 52%, with 38% of patients dying of disease progression.[205] Local recurrence is seen in 36% of patients who undergo local resection of the hydrocele wall, 10% after scrotal orchiectomy, and 12% after inguinal orchiectomy.[205] More than 60% of recurrences developed within the first 2 years of the follow-up. The overall median survival is 23 months. There are few data regarding the use of adjuvant therapy after resection of gonadal mesothelioma.

Malignant Mesothelioma of the Pericardium

A recent review of the primary pericardial mesothelioma has been published.[206] It is a rare neoplasm with a reported incidence of 0.0022% in an autopsy series of 5,000,000 case studies[207] and a calculated annual incidence of 1 in 40 million in a Canadian epidemiologic survey.[208] An antemortem diagnosis was made in less than one-third of 150 reported cases in the literature. Pericardial mesotheliomas can occur at any age, but people in the fourth to seventh decades of life are most likely to be afflicted, and there is a 2:1 male to female ratio.[209,210] Patients generally present with a pericardial effusion,[211] congestive heart failure, an anterior mediastinal mass, or tamponade.[212] Presentation is usually nonspecific, and chest radiography may demonstrate only an enlarged cardiac silhouette, making diagnosis difficult. Echocardiography can reveal evidence of an effusion, thickening of the pericardium, or mass involvement of the myocardium.[213] CT scanning or MRI can show a thickened pericardium and may help determine invasion into myocardium.[214,215] Currently, surgical excision is the treatment for primary pericardial mesothelioma primarily to palliate symptoms of constriction or tamponade.

References

1. Price B. Analysis of current trends in United States mesothelioma incidence. Am J Epidemiol 1997;145:211–218.
2. Carbone M, Kratzke RA, Testa JR. The pathogenesis of mesothelioma. Semin Oncol 2002;29:2–17.
3. Gazdar AF, Butel JS, Carbone M. SV40 and human tumours: myth, association or causality? Nat Rev Cancer 2002;2:957–964.
4. Baris YI, Sahin AA, Ozesmi M, et al. An outbreak of pleural mesothelioma and chronic fibrosing pleurisy in the village of Karain/Urgup in Anatolia. Thorax 1978;33:181–192.
5. Artvinli M, Baris YI. Malignant mesotheliomas in a small village in the Anatolian region of Turkey: an epidemiologic study. J Natl Cancer Inst 1979;63:17–22.
6. Baris YI, Artvinli M, Sahin AA. Environmental mesothelioma in Turkey. Ann N Y Acad Sci 1979;330:423–432.
7. Baris YI, Saracci R, Simonato L, Skidmore JW, Artvinli M. Malignant mesothelioma and radiological chest abnormalities in two villages in Central Turkey. An epidemiological and environmental investigation. Lancet 1981;1:984–987.
8. Baris I, Simonato L, Artvinli M, et al. Epidemiological and environmental evidence of the health effects of exposure to erionite fibres: a four-year study in the Cappadocian region of Turkey. Int J Cancer 1987;39:10–17.
9. Baris B, Demir AU, Shehu V, Karakoca Y, Kisacik G, Baris YI. Environmental fibrous zeolite (erionite) exposure and malignant tumors other than mesothelioma. J Environ Pathol Toxicol Oncol 1996;15:183–189.

10. Baris YI. Asbestos and Erionite Related Chest Diseases. Ankara, Turkey: Semih Ofset Matbaacilik, 1987.
11. Wagner JC, Skidmore JW, Hill RJ, Griffiths DM. Erionite exposure and mesotheliomas in rats. Br J Cancer 1985;51:727–730.
12. Emri S, Demir A, Dogan M, et al. Lung diseases due to environmental exposures to erionite and asbestos in Turkey. Toxicol Lett 2002;127:251–257.
13. Roushdy-Hammady I, Siegel J, Emri S, Testa JR, Carbone M. Genetic-susceptibility factor and malignant mesothelioma in the Cappadocian region of Turkey. Lancet 2001;357:444–445.
14. Ascoli V, Mecucci C, Knuutila S. Genetic susceptibility and familial malignant mesothelioma. Lancet 2001;357:1804.
15. Battifora H, McCaughey WTE. Atlas of Tumor Pathology, vol 3, fascicle 15. Washington, DC: Armed Forces Institute of Pathology, 2003.
16. Gordon GJ, Jensen RV, Hsiao LL, et al. Translation of microarray data into clinically relevant cancer diagnostic tests using gene expression ratios in lung cancer and mesothelioma. Cancer Res 2002;62:4963–4967.
17. Roggli VL, Sharma A, Butnor KJ, Sporn T, Vollmer RT. Malignant mesothelioma and occupational exposure to asbestos: a clinicopathological correlation of 1445 cases. Ultrastruct Pathol 2002;26:55–65.
18. Connelly RR, Spirtas R, Myers MH, Percy CL, Fraumeni JF Jr. Demographic patterns for mesothelioma in the United States. J Natl Cancer Inst 1987;78:1053–1060.
19. Fraire AE, Cooper S, Greenberg SD, Buffler P, Langston C. Mesothelioma of childhood. Cancer (Phila) 1988;2:838–847.
20. Kannerstein M, Churg J, McCaughey WT. Asbestos and mesothelioma: a review. Pathol Annu 1978;13(pt 1):81–129.
21. Herndon JE, Green MR, Chahinian AP, Corson JM, Suzuki Y, Vogelzang NJ. Factors predictive of survival among 337 patients with mesothelioma treated between 1984 and 1994 by the Cancer and Leukemia Group B. Chest 1998;113:723–731.
22. Vogelzang NJ, Emri S, Boyer M, et al. Effect of folic acid and vitamin b12 supplementation on risk-benefit ratio from phase III study of pemetrexed + cisplatin versus cisplatin in malignant pleural mesothelioma. Proc Am Soc Clin Oncol 2003;22:657 (abstract).
23. Hedman M, Arnberg H, Wernlund J, Riska H, Brodin O. Tissue polypeptide antigen (TPA), hyaluronan and CA 125 as serum markers in malignant mesothelioma. Anticancer Res 2003;23:531–536.
24. Thylen A, Hjerpe A, Martensson G. Hyaluronan content in pleural fluid as a prognostic factor in patients with malignant pleural mesothelioma. Cancer (Phila) 2001;92:1224–1230.
25. Paganuzzi M, Onetto M, Marroni P, et al. Diagnostic value of CYFRA 21-1 tumor marker and CEA in pleural effusion due to mesothelioma. Chest 2001;119:1138–1142.
26. Pass HI, Bones J, Hellstrom KE, et al. A sensitive serum test for monitoring of malignant pleural mesothelioma. Proc 2003;8:30 (abstract).
27. Wechsler RJ, Rao VM, Steiner RM. The radiology of thoracic malignant mesothelioma. Crit Rev Diagn Imaging 1984;20:283–310.
28. Heller RM, Janower ML, Weber AL. The radiological manifestations of malignant pleural mesothelioma. Am J Roentgenol Radium Ther Nucl Med 1979;108:53–59.
29. Solomon A. Radiological features of diffuse mesothelioma. Environ Res 1970;3:330–338.
30. Gamsu G, Aberle DR, Lynch D. Computed tomography in the diagnosis of asbestos-related thoracic disease. J Thorac Imaging 1989;4:61–67.
31. Miller BH, Rosado-de-Christenson ML, Mason AC, Fleming MV, White CC, Krasna MJ. From the archives of the AFIP. Malignant pleural mesothelioma: radiologic-pathologic correlation. Radiographics 1996;16:613–644.
32. Patz EF Jr, Shaffer K, Piwnica-Worms DR, et al. Malignant pleural mesothelioma: value of CT and MR imaging in predicting resectability. AJR Am J Roentgenol 1992;159:961–966.
33. Pass HI, Temeck BK, Kranda K, Steinberg SM, Feuerstein IR. Preoperative tumor volume is associated with outcome in malignant pleural mesothelioma. J Thorac Cardiovasc Surg 1998;115:310–317.
34. Flores RM, Akhurst T, Gonen M, Larson SM, Rusch VW. Positron emission tomography defines metastatic disease but not locoregional disease in patients with malignant pleural mesothelioma. J Thorac Cardiovasc Surg 2003;126:11–16.
35. Schneider DB, Clary-Macy C, Challa S, et al. Positron emission tomography with F18-fluorodeoxyglucose in the staging and preoperative evaluation of malignant pleural mesothelioma. J Thorac Cardiovasc Surg 2000;120:128–133.
36. Benard F, Sterman D, Smith RJ, Kaiser LR, Albelda SM, Alavi A. Metabolic imaging of malignant pleural mesothelioma with fluorodeoxyglucose positron emission tomography. Chest 1998;114:713–722.
37. Gerbaudo VH, Sugarbaker DJ, Britz-Cunningham S, Di Carli MF, Mauceri C, Treves ST. Assessment of malignant pleural mesothelioma with (18)F-FDG dual-head gamma-camera coincidence imaging: comparison with histopathology. J Nucl Med 2002;43:1144–1149.
38. Flores R, Akhurst T, Gonen M, Larson SM, Rusch VW. FDG-PET predicts survival in patients with malignant pleural mesothelioma. Proc Am Soc Clin Oncol 2003;22:620 (abstract).
39. Therasse P, Arbuck SG, Eisenhauer EA, et al. New guidelines to evaluate the response to treatment in solid tumors. European Organization for Research and Treatment of Cancer, National Cancer Institute of the United States, National Cancer Institute of Canada. J Natl Cancer Inst 2000;92:205–216.
40. Herbert A, Gallagher PJ. Pleural biopsy in the diagnosis of malignant mesothelioma. Thorax 1982;37:816–821.
41. Whitaker D, Shilkin KB, Sterrett GF. Cytological appearances of malignant mesothelioma. In: Henderson DW, Shilkin KB, Langlois SL, Whitaker D (eds). Malignant Mesothelioma. New York: Hemisphere, 1992:167–182.
42. Whitaker D. The cytology of malignant mesothelioma. Cytopathology 2000;11:139–151.
43. Blanc FX, Atassi K, Bignon J, Housset, B. Diagnostic value of medical thoracoscopy in pleural disease: a 6-year retrospective study. Chest 2002;121:1677–1683.
44. Kendall SW, Bryan AJ, Large SR, Wells FC. Pleural effusions: is thoracoscopy a reliable investigation? A retrospective review. Respir Med 1992;86:437–440.
45. Boutin C. Thoracoscopy in malignant mesothelioma. Pneumologie 1989;43:61–65.
46. Boutin C, Schlesser M, Frenay C, Astoul P. Malignant pleural mesothelioma. Eur Respir J 1998;12:972–981.
47. Boutin C, Rey F, Viallat JR. Prevention of malignant seeding after invasive diagnostic procedures in patients with pleural mesothelioma. A randomized trial of local radiotherapy. Chest 1995;108:754–758.
48. Schouwink JH, Kool LS, Rutgers EJ, et al. The value of chest computer tomography and cervical mediastinoscopy in the preoperative assessment of patients with malignant pleural mesothelioma. Ann Thorac Surg 2003;75:1715–1718.
49. Rusch VW, Venkatraman ES. Important prognostic factors in patients with malignant pleural mesothelioma, managed surgically. Ann Thorac Surg 1999;68:1799–1804.
50. Antman KH, Blum RH, Greenberger JS, Flowerdew G, Skarin AR, Canellos GP. Multimodality therapy for malignant mesothelioma based on a study of natural history. Am J Med 1980;68:356–362.
51. Herndon JE, Green MR, Chahinian AP, Corson JM, Suzuki Y, Vogelzang NJ. Factors predictive of survival among 337 patients

with mesothelioma treated between 1984 and 1994 by the Cancer and Leukemia Group B. Chest 1998;113:723–731.
52. Curran DT, Sahmoud P, van Therasse MJ, Postmus PE, Giaccone G. Prognostic factors in patients with pleural mesothelioma: the European Organization for Research and Treatment of Cancer experience. J Clin Oncol 1998;16:145–152.
53. Gordon GJ, Jensen RFV, Hsiao LL, et al. Using gene expression ratios to predict outcome among patients with mesothelioma. J Natl Cancer Inst 2003;95:598–605.
54. Pass HI, Liu Z, Wali A, et al. Gene expression profiles predict survival and progression of pleural mesothelioma. Clin Cancer Res 2004;10:849–859.
55. Rusch VW. A proposed new international TNM staging system for malignant pleural mesothelioma from the International Mesothelioma Interest Group. Lung Cancer 1996;14:1–12.
56. Rusch VW, Venkatraman ES. Important prognostic factors in patients with malignant pleural mesothelioma, managed surgically. Ann Thorac Surg 1999;68:1799–1804.
57. Pass HI, Temeck BK, Kranda K, Steinberg SM, Feuerstein IR. Preoperative tumor volume is associated with outcome in malignant pleural mesothelioma. J Thorac Cardiovasc Surg 1998;115:310–317.
58. Pass HI, Temeck BK, Kranda K, et al. Phase III randomized trial of surgery with or without intraoperative photodynamic therapy and postoperative immunochemotherapy for malignant pleural mesothelioma. Ann Surg Oncol 1997;4:628–633.
59. Zellos LS, Sugarbaker DJ. Diffuse malignant mesothelioma of the pleural space and its management. Oncology 2002;16:907–913.
60. Sugarbaker DJ, Flores RM, Jaklitsch MT, et al. Resection margins, extrapleural nodal status, and cell type determine postoperative long-term survival in trimodality therapy of malignant pleural mesothelioma: results in 183 patients. J Thorac Cardiovasc Surg 1999;117:54–63.
61. Sugarbaker DJ, Garcia JP. Multimodality therapy for malignant pleural mesothelioma. Chest 1997;112:272S–275S.
62. Waller DA. Malignant mesothelioma: British surgical strategies. Lung Cancer 2004;45(suppl 1):S81–S84.
63. Edwards JG, Abrams KR, Leverment JN, Spyt TJ, Waller DA, O'Byrne KJ. Prognostic factors for malignant mesothelioma in 142 patients: validation of CALGB and EORTC prognostic scoring systems. Thorax 2000;55:731–735.
64. Canto A, Guijarro R, Arnau A, Galbis J, Martorell M, Garcia AR. Videothoracoscopy in the diagnosis and treatment of malignant pleural mesothelioma with associated pleural effusions. Thorac Cardiovasc Surg 1997;45:16–19.
65. Viallat JR, Rey F, Astoul P, Boutin C. Thoracoscopic talc poudrage pleurodesis for malignant effusions. A review of 360 cases. Chest 1996;110:1387–1393.
66. Pien GW, Gant MJ, Washam CL, Sterman DH. Use of an implantable pleural catheter for trapped lung syndrome in patients with malignant pleural effusion. Chest 2001;119:1641–1646.
67. Girling DJ, Muers MF, Qian W, Lobban D. Multicenter randomized controlled trial of the management of unresectable malignant meothelioma porposed by the British Thoracic Society and the British Medical Research Council. Semin Oncol 2002;29(1):97–101.
68. Muers M F, Rudd RM, O'Brien ME, et al. A randomised trial of single-dose radiotherapy to prevent procedure tract metastasis by malignant mesothelioma. Br J Cancer 2004;91(1):9–10.
69. Brancatisano RP, Joseph MG, McCaughan BC. Pleurectomy for mesothelioma. Med J Aust 1991;154:455–457, 460.
70. Ruffie P, Feld R, Minkin S, et al. Diffuse malignant mesothelioma of the pleura in Ontario and Quebec: a retrospective study of 332 patients. J Clin Oncol 1989;7:1157–1168.
71. Rusch VW. Pleurectomy/decortication in the setting of multimodality treatment for diffuse malignant pleural mesothelioma. Semin Thorac Cardiovasc Surg 1997;9:367–372.
72. Pass HI, Kranda K, Temeck BK, Feuerstein I, Steinberg SM. Surgically debulked malignant pleural mesothelioma: results and prognostic factors. Ann Surg Oncol 1997;4:215–222.
73. Butchart EG, Ashcroft T, Barnsley WC, Holden MP. Pleuropneumonectomy in the management of diffuse malignant mesothelioma of the pleura. Experience with 29 patients. Thorax 1976;31:15–24.
74. Faber LP. 1986: Extrapleural pneumonectomy for diffuse, malignant mesothelioma. Updated in 1994. Ann Thorac Surg 1994;58:1782–1783.
75. Sugarbaker DJ, Jaklitsch MT, Bueno R, et al. Prevention, early detection, and management of complications after 328 consecutive extrapleural pneumonectomies. J Thorac Cardiovasc Surg 2002;128:138–146.
76. Rusch VW, Figlin R, Godwin D, Piantadosi S. Intrapleural cisplatin and cytarabine in the management of malignant pleural effusions: a Lung Cancer Study Group trial. J Clin Oncol 1991;9:313–319.
77. Rusch VW, Rosenzweig K, Venkatraman E, et al. A phase II trial of surgical resection and adjuvant high-dose hemithoracic radiation for malignant pleural mesothelioma. J Thorac Cardiovasc Surg 2001;122:788–795.
78. Rusch VW. Indications for pneumonectomy. Extrapleural pneumonectomy. Chest Surg Clin N Am 1999;9:327–338.
79. de Graaf-Strukowska L, et al. Factors influencing the outcome of radiotherapy in malignant mesothelioma of the pleura: a single-institution experience with 189 patients. Int J Radiat Oncol Biol Phys 1999;43:511–516.
80. Ball DL, Cruickshank DG. The treatment of malignant mesothelioma of the pleura: review of a 5-year experience, with special reference to radiotherapy. Am J Clin Oncol 1990;13:4–9.
81. Gordon W Jr, Antman KH, Greenberger JS, Weichselbaum RR, Chaffey JT. Radiation therapy in the management of patients with mesothelioma. Int J Radiat Oncol Biol Phys 1982;8:19–25.
82. Davis SR, Tan L, Ball DL. Radiotherapy in the treatment of malignant mesothelioma of the pleura, with special reference to its use in palliation. Australas Radiol 1994;38:212–214.
83. Alberts AS, Falkson G, Goedhals L, Vorobiof DA, Van der Merwe CA. Malignant pleural mesothelioma: a disease unaffected by current therapeutic maneuvers. J Clin Oncol 1988;6:527–535.
84. Law MR, Gregor A, Hodson ME, Bloom HJ, Turner-Warwick M. Malignant mesothelioma of the pleura: a study of 52 treated and 64 untreated patients. Thorax 1984;39:255–259.
85. Bissett D, Macbeth FR, Cram I. The role of palliative radiotherapy in malignant mesothelioma. Clin Oncol (R Coll Radiol) 1991;3:315–317.
86. Bydder S, Phillips M, Joseph DJ, A randomised trial of single-dose radiotherapy to prevent procedure tract metastasis by malignant mesothelioma. Br J Cancer 2004;91:9–10.
87. Hilaris BS, Nori D, Kwong E, Kutcher GJ, Martini N. Pleurectomy and intraoperative brachytherapy and postoperative radiation in the treatment of malignant pleural mesothelioma. Int J Radiat Oncol Biol Phys 1984;10:325–331.
88. Lee TT, Everett DL, Shu HK, et al. Radical pleurectomy/decortication and intraoperative radiotherapy followed by conformal radiation with or without chemotherapy for malignant pleural mesothelioma. J Thorac Cardiovasc Surg 2002;124:1183–1189.
89. Ahamad A, Stevens CW, Smythe WR, et al. Intensity-modulated radiation therapy: a novel approach to the management of malignant pleural mesothelioma. Int J Radiat Oncol Biol Phys 2003;55:768–775.
90. Forster KM, Smythe WR, Starkschall G, et al. Intensity-modulated radiotherapy following extrapleural pneumonectomy for the treatment of malignant mesothelioma: clinical implementation. Int J Radiat Oncol Biol Phys 2003;55:606–616.

91. Pass HI, Kranda K, Temeck BK, Feuerstein I, Steinberg SM. Surgically debulked malignant pleural mesothelioma: results and prognostic factors. Ann Surg Oncol 1997;4:215–222.
92. Pass HI, Temeck BK, Kranda K, et al. Phase III randomized trial of surgery with or without intraoperative photodynamic therapy and postoperative immunochemotherapy for malignant pleural mesothelioma. Ann Surg Oncol 1997;4:628–633.
93. Rusch VW, Venkatraman ES. Important prognostic factors in patients with malignant pleural mesothelioma, managed surgically. Ann Thorac Surg 1999;68:1799–1804.
94. Rusch VW, Rosenzweig K, Venkatraman E, et al. A phase II trial of surgical resection and adjuvant high-dose hemithoracic radiation for malignant pleural mesothelioma. J Thorac Cardiovasc Surg 2001;122:788–795.
95. Hilaris BS, Nori D, Kwong E, Kutcher GJ, Martini N. Pleurectomy and intraoperative brachytherapy and postoperative radiation in the treatment of malignant pleural mesothelioma. IntJ Radiat Oncol Biol Phys 1984;10:325–331.
96. Lee TT, Everett DL, Shu HK, et al. Radical pleurectomy/decortication and intraoperative radiotherapy followed by conformal radiation with or without chemotherapy for malignant pleural mesothelioma. J Thorac Cardiovasc Surg 2002;124:1183–1189.
97. Rusch V, Saltz L, Venkatraman E, et al. A phase II trial of pleurectomy/decortication followed by intrapleural and systemic chemotherapy for malignant pleural mesothelioma. J Clin Oncol 1994;12:1156–1163.
98. Rusch VW, Niedzwiecki D, Tao Y, et al. Intrapleural cisplatin and mitomycin for malignant mesothelioma following pleurectomy: pharmacokinetic studies. J Clin Oncol 1992;10:1001–1006.
99. Colleoni M, Sartori F, Calabro F, et al. Surgery followed by intracavitary plus systemic chemotherapy in malignant pleural mesothelioma. Tumori 1996;82:53–56.
100. Zellos LS, Sugarbaker DJ. Diffuse malignant mesothelioma of the pleural space and its management. Oncology (Huntingt) 2002;16:907–913.
101. Calavrezos A, Koschel G, Husselmann H, et al. Malignant mesothelioma of the pleura. A prospective therapeutic study of 132 patients from 1981–1985. KlinWochenschr 1988;66:607–613.
102. Maggi G, Casadio C, Giobbe R, Ruffini E. The management of malignant pleural mesothelioma. Eur J Cardiothorac Surg 2003;23:255–256.
103. Maggi G, Giobbe R, Casadio C, Rena O. Palliative surgery for malignant pleural mesothelioma. Eur J Cardiothorac Surg 2002;21:1128–1129.
104. Maggi G, Casadio C, Cianci R, Rena O, Ruffini E. Trimodality management of malignant pleural mesothelioma. Eur J Cardiothorac Surg 2001;19:346–350.
105. Stahel R, Weder W, Ballabio P, et al. Neoadjuvant chemotherpay followed by pleuropneumonectomy for pleural mesothelioma: a multicenter phase II trial of the SAKK. Lung Cancer 2003;41(suppl 2):S59 (abstract).
106. de Perrot M, Ginsberg R, Payne D, et al. A phase II trial of induction chemotherapy followed by extrapleural pneumonectomy and high-dose hemiothoracic radiation for malignant pleural mesothelioma. Lung Cancer 2003;41(suppl 2):S59.
107. Bonnette P, Heckly GB, Villette S, Fragola A. Intraoperative photodynamic therapy after pleuropneumonectomy for malignant pleural mesothelioma. Chest 2002;122:1866–1867.
108. Schouwink H, Rutgers ET, et al. Intraoperative photodynamic therapy after pleuropneumonectomy in patients with malignant pleural mesothelioma: dose finding and toxicity results. Chest 2001;120:1167–1174.
109. Baas P, Murrer L, Zoetmulder FA, et al. Photodynamic therapy as adjuvant therapy in surgically treated pleural malignancies. Br J Cancer 1997;76:819–826.
110. Friedberg JS, Mick R, Stevenson J, et al. A phase I study of Foscan-mediated photodynamic therapy and surgery in patients with mesothelioma. Ann Thorac Surg 2003;75:952–959.
111. Ratto GB, Civalleri D, Esposito M, et al. Pleural space perfusion with cisplatin in the multimodality treatment of malignant mesothelioma: a feasibility and pharmacokinetic study. J Thorac Cardiovasc Surg 1999;117:759–765.
112. Yellin A, Simansky DA, Paley M, Refaely Y. Hyperthermic pleural perfusion with cisplatin: early clinical experience. Cancer (Phila) 2001;92:2197–2203.
113. van Ruth S, Baas P, Haas RL, Rutgers EJ, Verwaal VJ, Zoetmulder FA. Cytoreductive surgery combined with intraoperative hyperthermic intrathoracic chemotherapy for stage I malignant pleural mesothelioma. Ann Surg Oncol 2003;10:176–182.
114. Sugarbaker DJ, Richards W, Zellos L, et al. Feasibility of pleurectomy and intraoperative bicavitary hyperthermic cisplatin lavage for mesothelioma: a phase I–II study. Proc Am Soc Clin Oncol 2003:22 (abstract).
115. Sterman DH, Kaiser LR, Albelda SM. Gene therapy for malignant pleural mesothelioma. Hematol Oncol Clin N Am 1998;12:553–568.
116. Mukherjee S, Nelson D, Loh S, et al. The immune anti-tumor effects of GM-CSF and B7–1 gene transfection are enhanced by surgical debulking of tumor. Cancer Gene Ther 2991;8:580–588.
117. Mukherjee S, Haenel T, Himbeck R, et al. Replication-restricted vaccinia as a cytokine gene therapy vector in cancer: persistent transgene expression despite antibody generation. Cancer Gene Ther 2000;7:663–670.
118. Nowak AK, Lake RA, Kindler HL, Robinson BW. New approaches for mesothelioma: biologics, vaccines, gene therapy, and other novel agents. Semin Oncol 2002;29:82–96.
119. Odaka M, Wiewrodt R, DeLong P, et al. Analysis of the immunologic response generated by Ad.IFN-beta during successful intraperitoneal tumor gene therapy. Mol Ther 2002;6:210–218.
120. Odaka M, Sterman DH, Wiewrodt R, et al. Eradication of intraperitoneal and distant tumor by adenovirus-mediated interferon-beta gene therapy is attributable to induction of systemic immunity. Cancer Res 2001;61:6201–6212.
121. Yang CT, You L, Lin YC, Lin CL, McCormick F, Jablons DM. A comparison analysis of anti-tumor efficacy of adenoviral gene replacement therapy (p14ARF and p16INK4A) in human mesothelioma cells. Anticancer Res 2003;23:33s–38s.
122. Yang CT, You L, Uematsu K, Yeh CC, McCormick F, Jablons DM. p14(ARF) modulates the cytolytic effect of ONYX-015 in mesothelioma cells with wild-type p53. Cancer Res 2001;61:5959–5963.
123. Harrison LH Jr, Schwarzenberger PO, Byrne PS, Marrogi AJ, Kolls JK, McCarthy KE. Gene-modified PA1-STK cells home to tumor sites in patients with malignant pleural mesothelioma. Ann Thorac Surg 2000;70:407–411.
124. Schwarzenberger P, Byrne P, Kolls JK. Immunotherapy-based treatment strategies for malignant mesothelioma. Curr Opin Mol Ther 1999;1:104–111.
125. Schwarzenberger P, Lei D, Freeman SM, et al. Antitumor activity with the HSV-tk-gene-modified cell line PA-1-STK in malignant mesothelioma. Am J Respir Cell Mol Biol 1998;19:333–337.
126. Boutin C, Nussbaum E, Monnet I, et al. Intrapleural treatment with recombinant gamma-interferon in early stage malignant pleural mesothelioma. Cancer (Phila) 1994;74:2460–2467.
127. Driesen P, Boutin C, Viallat JR, Astoul PH, Vialette JP, Pasquier J. Implantable access system for prolonged intrapleural immunotherapy. Eur Respir J 194;7:1889–1892.
128. Astoul P, Picat-Joossen D, Viallat JR, Boutin C. Intrapleural administration of interleukin-2 for the treatment of patients with malignant pleural mesothelioma: a Phase II study [see comments]. Cancer (Phila) 1998;83:2099–2104.
129. Antman K, Shemin R, Ryan L, et al. Malignant mesothelioma: prognostic variables in a registry of 180 patients, the Dana-

Farber Cancer Institute and Brigham and Women's Hospital experience over two decades, 1965–1985. J Clin Oncol 1988; 6:147–153.
130. Curran D, Sahmoud T, Therasse P, van Meerbeeck J, Postmus PE, Giaccone G. Prognostic factors in patients with pleural mesothelioma: the European Organization for Research and Treatment of Cancer experience. J Clin Oncol 1998;16:145–152.
131. Chahinian AP, Pajak TF, Holland JF, Norton L, Ambinder RM, Mandel EM. Diffuse malignant mesothelioma. Prospective evaluation of 69 patients. Ann Intern Med 1982;96:746–755.
132. Vogelzang NJ, Schultz SM, Iannucci AM, Kennedy BJ. Malignant mesothelioma. The University of Minnesota experience. Cancer (Phila) 1984;53:377–383.
133. Samuels BL, Herndon JE, Harmon DC, et al. Dihydro-5-azacytidine and cisplatin in the treatment of malignant mesothelioma: a phase II study by the Cancer and Leukemia Group B. Cancer (Phila) 1998;82:1578–1584.
134. Janne PA. Chemotherapy for malignant pleural mesothelioma. Clin Lung Cancer 2003;5(2):98–106.
135. Steele JP, Shamash J, Evans MT, Gower NH, Tischkowitz MD, Rudd RM. Phase II study of vinorelbine in patients with malignant pleural mesothelioma. J Clin Oncol 2000;18:3912–3917.
136. Middleton GW, Smith IE, O'Brien ME, et al. Good symptom relief with palliative MVP (mitomycin-C, vinblastine and cisplatin) chemotherapy in malignant mesothelioma. Ann Oncol 1998;9:269–273.
137. Girling DJ, Muers MF, Qian W, Lobban D. Multicenter randomized controlled trial of the management of unresectable malignant mesothelioma proposed by the British Thoracic Society and the British Medical Research Council. Semin Oncol 2002; 29:97–101.
138. Solheim OP, Saeter G, Finnanger AM, Stenwig AE. High-dose methotrexate in the treatment of malignant mesothelioma of the pleura. A phase II study. Br J Cancer 1992;65:956–960.
139. Calvert AH, Alison DL, Harland SJ, et al. A phase I evaluation of the quinazoline antifolate thymidylate synthase inhibitor, N10-propargyl-5,8-dideazafolic acid, CB3717. J Clin Oncol 1986; 4:1245–1252.
140. Cantwell BM, Earnshaw M, Harris AL. Phase II study of a novel antifolate, N10-propargyl-5,8 dideazafolic acid (CB3717), in malignant mesothelioma. Cancer Treat Rep 1986;70:1335–1336.
141. Vogelzang NJ, Weissman LB, Herndon JE, et al. Trimetrexate in malignant mesothelioma: a Cancer and Leukemia Group B Phase II study. J Clin Oncol 1994;12:1436–1442.
142. Kindler HL, Belani CP, Herndon JE, Vogelzang NJ, Suzuki Y, Green MR. Edatrexate (10-ethyl-deaza-aminopterin) (NSC #626715) with or without leucovorin rescue for malignant mesothelioma. Sequential phase II trials by the cancer and leukemia group B. Cancer (Phila) 1999;86:1985–1991.
143. Scagliotti GV, Shin DM, Kindler HL, et al. Phase II study of pemetrexed with and without folic acid and vitamin B12 as front-line therapy in malignant pleural mesothelioma. J Clin Oncol 2003;21:1556–1561.
144. Westerhof GR, Schornagel JH, Kathmann I, et al. Carrier- and receptor-mediated transport of folate antagonists targeting folate-dependent enzymes: correlates of molecular-structure and biological activity. Mol Pharmacol 1995;48:459–471.
145. Rusthoven JJ, Eisenhauer E, Butts C, et al. Multitargeted antifolate LY231514 as first-line chemotherapy for patients with advanced non-small-cell lung cancer: a phase II study. National Cancer Institute of Canada Clinical Trials Group. J Clin Oncol 1999;17:1194.
146. Thodtmann R, Depenbrock H, Dumez H, et al. Clinical and pharmacokinetic phase I study of multitargeted antifolate (LY231514) in combination with cisplatin. J Clin Oncol 1999;17:3009–3016.
147. Hughes A, Calvert P, Azzabi A, et al. Phase I clinical and pharmacokinetic study of pemetrexed and carboplatin in patients with malignant pleural mesothelioma. J Clin Oncol 2002,20: 3533–3544.
148. Shin DM, Scagliotti G, Kindler HL, et al. A phase II trial of pemetrexed in malignant pleural mesothelioma patients: clinical outcome, role of vitamin supplementation, respiratory symptoms and lung function. Proc Am Soc Clin Oncol 2003;21: (abstract).
149. Niyikiza C, Baker SD, Seitz DE, et al. Homocysteine and methylmalonic acid: markers to predict and avoid toxicity from pemetrexed therapy. Mol Cancer Ther 2002;1:545–552.
150. Gralla R, Hollen PJ, Liepa AM, et al. Improving quality of life in patients with malignant pleural mesothelioma: results of the randomized pemetrexed + cisplatin vs. cisplatin trial using the LCSS-meso instrument. Proc Am Soc Clin Oncol 2003;22:621 (abstract).
151. Paoletti P, Pistolesi M, Rusthoven J, et al. Correlation of pulmonary function tests with best tumor response status: results from the phase III study of pemetrexed + cisplatin vs. cisplatin in malignant pleural mesothelioma. Proc Am Soc Clin Oncol 2003;22:659 (abstract).
152. Byrne MJ, Davidson JA, Musk AW, et al. Cisplatin and gemcitabine treatment for malignant mesothelioma: a phase II study. J Clin Oncol 1999;17:25–30.
153. Nowak AK, Byrne MJ, Williamson R, et al. A multicentre phase II study of cisplatin and gemcitabine for malignant mesothelioma. Br J Cancer 2002;87:491–496.
154. van Haarst JM, Baas P, Manegold C, et al. Multicentre phase II study of gemcitabine and cisplatin in malignant pleural mesothelioma. Br J Cancer 2002;86:342–345.
155. Vogelzang NJ. Gemcitabine and cisplatin: second-line chemotherapy for malignant mesothelioma? J Clin Oncol 1999;17: 2626–2627.
156. Favaretto AG, Aversa SM, Paccagnella A, et al. Gemcitabine combined with carboplatin in patients with malignant pleural mesothelioma: a multicentric phase II study. Cancer (Phila) 2003;97:2791–2797.
157. Mikulski SM, Costanzi JJ, Vogelzang NJ, et al. Phase II trial of a single weekly intravenous dose of ranpirnase in patients with unresectable malignant mesothelioma. J Clin Oncol 2002; 20:274–281.
158. Antman KH. Clinical presentation and natural history of benign and malignant mesothelioma. Semin Oncol 1981;8:313–320.
159. Mohamed F, Sugarbaker PH. Peritoneal mesothelioma. Curr Treat Options Oncol 2002;3:375–386.
160. Mohamed F, Sugarbaker PH. Peritoneal mesothelioma. Curr Treat Options Oncol 2002;3:375–386.
161. Antman K, Shemin R, Ryan L, et al. Malignant mesothelioma: prognostic variables in a registry of 180 patients, the Dana-Farber Cancer Institute and Brigham and Women's Hospital experience over two decades, 1965–1985. J Clin Oncol 1988; 6:147–153.
162. Latief KH, Somers JM, Hewitt M. High-resolution ultrasound in the diagnosis of childhood malignant peritoneal mesothelioma. Pediatr Radiol 1998;28:173.
163. Puvaneswary M, Chen S, Proietto T. Peritoneal mesothelioma: CT and MRI findings. Australas Radiol 2002;46:91–96.
164. Sugarbaker PH, Acherman YI, Gonzalez-Moreno S, et al. Diagnosis and treatment of peritoneal mesothelioma: the Washington Cancer Institute experience. Semin Oncol 2002;29: 51–61.
165. Guest PJ, Reznek RH, Selleslag D, Geraghty R, Slevin M. Peritoneal mesothelioma: the role of computed tomography in diagnosis and follow up. Clin Radiol 1992;45:79–84.
166. Puvaneswary M, Chen S, Proietto T. Peritoneal mesothelioma: CT and MRI findings. Australas Radiol 2002;46:91–96.
167. Ozgen A, Akata D, Akhan O, Tez M, Gedikoglu G, Ozmen MN. Giant benign cystic peritoneal mesothelioma: US, CT, and MRI findings. Abdom Imaging 1998;23:502–504.

168. Eade TN, Fulham MJ, Constable CJ. Primary malignant peritoneal mesothelioma: appearance on F-18 FDG positron emission tomographic images. Clin Nucl Med 2002;27:924–925.
169. Whitley NO, Brenner DE, Antman KH, Grant D, Aisner J. CT of peritoneal mesothelioma: analysis of eight cases. AJR Am J Roentgenol 1982;138:531–535.
170. Raptopoulos V, Gourtsoyiannis N. Peritoneal carcinomatosis. Eur Radiol 2001;11:2195–2206.
171. Pombo F, Rodriguez E, Martin R, Lago M. CT-guided core-needle biopsy in omental pathology. Acta Radiol 1997;38:978–981.
172. Stamat JC, Chekan EG, Ali A, Ko A, Sporn TA, Eubanks WS. Laparoscopy and mesothelioma. J Laparoendosc Adv Surg Tech A 1999;9:433–437.
173. Piccigallo E, Jeffers LJ, Reddy KR, Caldironi MW, Parenti A, Schiff ER. Malignant peritoneal mesothelioma. A clinical and laparoscopic study of ten cases. Dig Dis Sci 1988;33:633–639.
174. Hoekman K, Tognon G, Risse EK, Bloemsma CA, Vermorken JB. Well-differentiated papillary mesothelioma of the peritoneum: a separate entity. Eur J Cancer 1996;32A:255–258.
175. Ordonez NG. Role of immunohistochemistry in distinguishing epithelial peritoneal mesotheliomas from peritoneal and ovarian serous carcinomas. Am J Surg Pathol 1998;22:1203–1214.
176. Datta RV, Paty PB. Cystic mesothelioma of the peritoneum. Eur J Surg Oncol 1997;23:461–462.
177. Sethna K, Mohamed F, Marchettini P, Elias D, Sugarbaker PH. Peritoneal cystic mesothelioma: a case series. Tumori 2003;89: 31–35.
178. Antman KH, Osteen RT, Klegar KL, et al. Early peritoneal mesothelioma: a treatable malignancy. Lancet 1985;2:977–981.
179. Loggie BW, Fleming RA, McQuellon RP, Russell GB, Geisinger KR, Levine EA. Prospective trial for the treatment of malignant peritoneal mesothelioma. Am Surg 2001;67:999–1003.
180. Markman M. Intraperitoneal chemotherapy. Crit Rev Oncol Hematol 1999;31:239–246.
181. Markman M. Intracavitary chemotherapy. Crit Rev Oncol Hematol 1985;3:205–233.
182. Langer CJ, Rosenblum N, Hogan M, et al. Intraperitoneal cisplatin and etoposide in peritoneal mesothelioma: favorable outcome with a multimodality approach. Cancer Chemother Pharmacol 1993;32:204–208.
183. Howell SB, Pfeifle CE. Peritoneal access for intracavitary chemotherapy. Cancer Drug Deliv 1986;3:157–161.
184. Howell SB, Pfeifle CL, Wung WE, et al. Intraperitoneal cisplatin with systemic thiosulfate protection. Ann Intern Med 1982; 97:845–851.
185. Lederman GS, Recht A, Herman T, Osteen R, Corson J, Antman KH. Long-term survival in peritoneal mesothelioma. The role of radiotherapy and combined modality treatment. Cancer (Phila) 1987;59:1882–1886.
186. Brady LW. Mesothelioma: the role for radiation therapy. Semin Oncol 1981;8:329–334.
187. Legha SS, Muggia FM. Therapeutic approaches in malignant mesothelioma. Cancer Treat Rev 1977;4:13–23.
188. Antman KH, Pass HI, Schiff PB. Benign and malignant mesothelioma. In: DeVita VT Jr, Hellman S, Rosenberg SA (eds). Cancer: Principles and Practice of Oncology, 6th ed. Philadelphia: Lippincott-Raven, 2001:1943–1970.
189. Markman M. Intraperitoneal chemotherapy. Crit Rev Oncol Hematol 1999;31:239–246.
190. Howell SB, Pfeifle CL, Wung WE, et al. Intraperitoneal cisplatin with systemic thiosulfate protection. Ann Intern Med 1982; 97:845–851.
191. Markman M, Kelsen D. Efficacy of cisplatin-based intraperitoneal chemotherapy as treatment of malignant peritoneal mesothelioma. J Cancer Res Clin Oncol 1992;118:547–550.
192. Vlasveld LT, Taal BG, Kroon BB, Gallee MP, Rodenhuis S. Intestinal obstruction due to diffuse peritoneal fibrosis at 2 years after the successful treatment of malignant peritoneal mesothelioma with intraperitoneal mitoxantrone. Cancer Chemother Pharmacol 1992;29:405–408.
193. Garcia Moore ML, Savaraj N, Feun LG, Donnelly E. Successful therapy of peritoneal mesothelioma with intraperitoneal chemotherapy alone. A case report. Am J Clin Oncol 1992;15: 528–530.
194. Taylor RA, Johnson LP. Mesothelioma: current perspectives. West J Med 1981;134:379–383.
195. Taub RN, Keohan ML, Chabot JC, Fountain KS, Plitsas M. Peritoneal mesothelioma. Curr Treat Options Oncol 2000; 1:303–312.
196. Eltabbakh GH, Piver MS, Hempling RE, Recio FO, Intengen ME. Clinical picture, response to therapy, and survival of women with diffuse malignant peritoneal mesothelioma. J Surg Oncol 1999;70:6–12.
197. Taub RN, Keohan ML, Chabot JC, Fountain KS, Plitsas M. Peritoneal mesothelioma. Curr Treat Options Oncol 2000; 1:303–312.
198. Loggie BW. Malignant peritoneal mesothelioma. Curr Treat Options Oncol 2001;2:395–399.
199. Mohamed F, Sugarbaker PH. Peritoneal mesothelioma. Curr Treat Options Oncol 2002;3:375–386.
200. Park BJ, Alexander HR, Libutti SK, et al. Treatment of primary peritoneal mesothelioma by continuous hyperthermic peritoneal perfusion (CHPP). Ann Surg Oncol 1999;6:582–590.
201. Sugarbaker PH, Acherman YI, Gonzalez-Moreno S, et al. Diagnosis and treatment of peritoneal mesothelioma: the Washington Cancer Institute experience. Semin Oncol 2002;29:51–61.
202. Khan MA, Puri P, Devaney D. Mesothelioma of tunica vaginalis testis in a child. J Urol 1997;158:198–199.
203. Antman K, Cohen S, Dimitrov NV, Green M, Muggia F. Malignant mesothelioma of the tunica vaginalis testis. J Clin Oncol 1984;2:447–451.
204. Gupta SC, Gupta AK, Misra V, Singh PA. Pre-operative diagnosis of malignant mesothelioma of tunica vaginalis testis by hydrocele fluid cytology. Eur J Surg Oncol 1998;24:153–154.
205. Plas E, Riedl CR, Pfluger H. Malignant mesothelioma of the tunica vaginalis testis: review of the literature and assessment of prognostic parameters. Cancer (Phila) 1998;83:2437–2446.
206. Vigneswaran WT, Stefanacci PR. Pericardial mesothelioma. Curr Treat Options Oncol 2000;1:299–302.
207. Cohen JL. Neoplastic pericarditis. Cardiovasc Clin 1976;7: 257–269.
208. McDonald AD, Harper A, McDonald JC, el Attar OA. Epidemiology of primary malignant mesothelial tumors in Canada. Cancer (Phila) 1970;26:914–919.
209. Kahn EI, Rohl A, Barrett EW, Suzuki Y. Primary pericardial mesothelioma following exposure to asbestos. Environ Res 1980; 23:270–281.
210. Churg A, Warnock ML, Bensch KG. Malignant mesothelioma arising after direct application of asbestos and fiber glass to the pericardium. Am Rev Respir Dis 1978;118:419–424.
211. Eker R, Cantez T, Dogan O, Demiryent M, Celik A, Karabocuoglu M. Pericardial mesothelioma. A pediatric case report. Turk J Pediatr 1989;31:305–309.
212. Aggarwal P, Wali JP, Agarwal J. Pericardial mesothelioma presenting as a mediastinal mass. Singapore Med J 1991;32:185–186.
213. Agatston AS, Robinson MJ, Trigo L, Machado R, Samet P. Echocardiographic findings in primary pericardial mesothelioma. Am Heart J 1986;111:986–988.
214. Thomason R, Schlegel W, Lucca M, Cummings S, Lee S. Primary malignant mesothelioma of the pericardium. Case report and literature review. Tex Heart Inst J 1994;21:170–174.
215. Gossinger HD, Siostrzonek P, Zangeneh M, et al. Magnetic resonance imaging findings in a patient with pericardial mesothelioma. Am Heart J 1988;115:1321–1322.

Mediastinum

Alexander S. Krupnick
and Joseph B. Shrager

Because tumors of the mediastinum make up only a small portion of thoracic oncology and the cases are relatively few, treatment-based outcomes of only a few mediastinal diseases processes have been evaluated by powerful level I data consisting of randomized, controlled trials.[1,2] The majority of the data guiding treatment of mediastinal tumors, therefore, come from level II data.

Anatomy and Embryology

The mediastinum comprises an anatomic space located between the thoracic inlet and the diaphragm and bordered on the left and right sides by the pleural cavities. This central anatomic location houses or borders upon vital structures of almost every major organ system: the thymus of the immune system, the heart and great vessels of the circulatory system, the esophagus and major airways of the aerodigestive tract, and important nerves such as the phrenic and vagus. The oncologist or operating surgeon treating mediastinal disease must be familiar, therefore, with both the anatomic configuration and the pathophysiologic derangements that may occur in each of these systems.

By the fourth week of gestation, the intraembryonic coelom, or primordial body cavity, is separated into several body cavities that will ultimately form the boundaries of the mediastinum. These cavities are the pericardial cavity, the peritoneal cavity, and two pericardioperitoneal canals that connect the two cavities. Growth of the lung buds as well as mesenchymal tissue into the pericardioperitoneal canals further divides these cavities and creates the mesothelial lining, which will ultimately form the pleura and serve as the lateral borders of the mediastinum. The primitive mediastinum, consisting of solid mesenchymal tissue, becomes a true entity by the seventh week of gestation as the pericardioperitoneal membranes fuse with the mesoderm ventral to the esophagus. At approximately the same time, the primitive bilobed thymus, derived from the third pharyngeal pouch epithelium, descends into the mediastinum. By this time in gestation, all adult structures are present in the primitive mediastinum, but they begin to function only at different points in development or even at birth.[3]

Despite the complex developmental relationships between what are to become the mediastinal structures, postnatal anatomic divisions can be organized on the basis of simple radiographic anatomy. The most anatomically appropriate model for organization of the mediastinum is a modification of the three-compartment model as refined by Shields.[4] According to this system, the mediastinum is divided into what are essentially anterior, middle, and posterior compartments based on the borders of anatomic structures as seen on a lateral radiograph (Figure 39.1). The anterior compartment that Shields terms the *prevascular zone* is bordered anteriorly by the sternum and posteriorly by the pericardium and the great vessels. It contains the thymus, variable amounts of fat and lymphatic tissue, and the internal mammary arteries and veins. The middle mediastinum (Shield's *visceral compartment*) extends from the anterior to the posterior pericardium and contains the heart, great vessels, trachea, main bronchi, and esophagus, along with all associated lymph nodes. It is bordered by the main segments of the phrenic nerves. The posterior mediastinum or *paravertebral sulci* is bounded anteriorly by the posterior pericardium and extends posteriorly to the chest wall. It contains the descending thoracic aorta, inferior vena cava, and sympathetic chain and is variably deemed to include the esophagus with associated vagi. One of the main advantages of this system is the ability it confers to generate a differential diagnosis for a mediastinal mass based on the structures naturally contained within the compartment in which it arises (Table 39.1). Such a classification thus allows the thoracic surgeon or oncologist to proceed systematically to the appropriate diagnostic or therapeutic approach depending on this differential diagnosis.

Signs and symptoms of mediastinal tumors can vary widely at presentation and usually offer only nonspecific clues to the nature of the underlying disease process. Although more than 60% of patients do present with symptoms, it is not uncommon for an asymptomatic mass to be detected on a routine screening examination.[5] As a rule, two-thirds of all mediastinal masses are benign, and more than three-fourths of asymptomatic patients with mediastinal lesions have a benign lesion. The majority of patients who present with symptoms, however, have an underlying malignant process.[5] The presenting symptoms vary widely based on anatomic location. Although anterior mediastinal masses can present with symptoms of anatomic impingement such as cough, chest pain, or dyspnea, the presence of systemic symptoms such as fevers and night sweats heightens the suspicion for lymphoma whereas new-onset myasthenic symptoms are suggestive of thymoma. Posterior mediastinal tumors, which are most commonly benign and neurogenic in nature, are usually asymptomatic at presentation.[6]

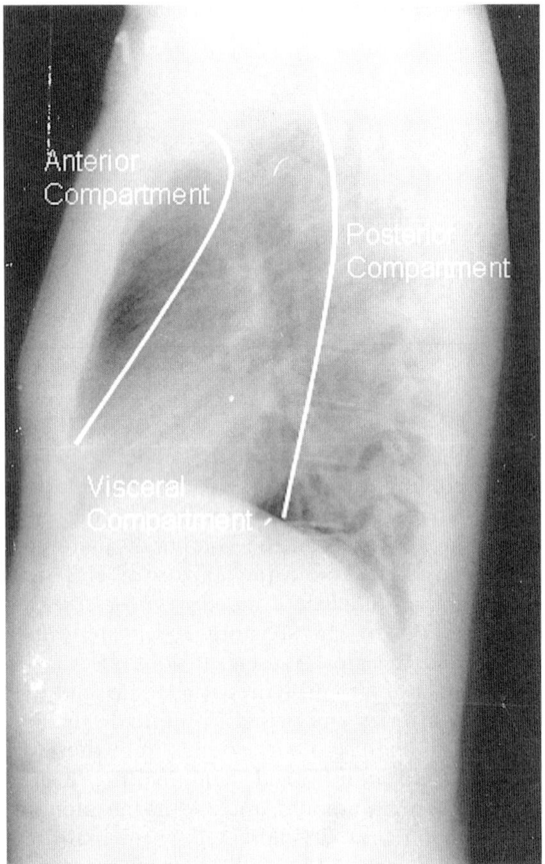

FIGURE 39.1. Traditionally, the mediastinum has been divided into anterior, middle, and posterior compartments based on the lateral radiograph.

Anterior Mediastinal Masses

Differential Diagnosis

Fifty percent of all mediastinal masses are located in the anterior mediastinum, and the majority of all malignant mediastinal lesions occur in this compartment.[5,7] In descending order of frequency, the common malignant lesions here consist of thymic tumors, lymphoma, and germ cell tumors (see Table 39.1).

History and Physical Examination

After the initial chest radiograph, a history and physical examination focusing on factors that suggest one of these diagnoses is performed. Lymphomas and germ cell tumors should be high on the differential diagnosis in patients under 40 years of age. Symptoms such as fevers, night sweats, and weight loss can further enhance the suspicion for lymphoma. Lymphoma symptoms are classified as A, if there are no systemic symptoms, and as B, if fevers are above 38°C, drenching night sweats occur, and weight loss is greater than 10% body weight. The presence of remote, palpable lymphadenopathy also raises the likelihood of lymphoma and may simplify tissue diagnosis via superficial lymph node excisional biopsy.

Thymoma usually affects adults over 40 years of age.[7,8] Nearly one-half of patients with thymoma suffer from one or more of the paraneoplastic symptoms associated with this disease.[8–10] Myasthenia gravis is the most common such parathymic syndrome, and 30% to 50% of patients with thymoma concurrently have this disease. A careful history focusing on weakness and fatigability with repeated activity and a detailed neuromuscular examination may suggest this diagnosis and the diagnosis of thymoma.

Germ cell tumors account for only 1% to 4% of mediastinal tumors.[11] The majority of patients present with symptoms caused by the mass lesion of the anterior mediastinum, including chest pain, dyspnea, and cough. A small portion of patients presents with constitutional symptoms such as fever, night sweats, and malaise similar to patients with systemic lymphoma. Asymptomatic cervical lymphadenopathy has also been reported as the initial presenting sign of both lymphoma and malignant germ cell tumor.[12] Finally, germ cell tumors can rarely be associated with testicular masses in men, so a thorough testicular examination is important in this population.

Serum Studies

Serologic evaluation plays an important role in the diagnosis of mediastinal tumors and is the next step after history and physical examination. It is now widely accepted that the neuromuscular abnormalities of myasthenia gravis are caused by an antibody-mediated process, and 90% of patients with myasthenia have detectable serum levels of antibodies to the acetylcholine receptor (anti-Achr Ab), even if asymptomatic.[13] Although serum titers do not necessarily correlate

TABLE 39.1. Normal anatomic and pathologic content of the mediastinum.

Anterior mediastinum	*Middle mediastinum*	*Posterior mediastinum*
Thymus	Heart	Sympathetic chain
Thyroid (if ectopic)	Ascending and transverse aortic arch	Esophagus
Parathyroid (if ectopic)	Superior and inferior vena cava	Descending aorta
Lymphatic tissue	Pulmonary arteries and veins	Inferior vena cava
Internal mammary artery and vein	Lymph nodes	
Thymic neoplasms	Pericardial cyst	Neurogenic tumor
Lymphoma	Bronchogenic cyst	Esophageal disease
Germ cell tumors	Enteric cyst	
	Metastatic cancer	

with the magnitude of the disease,[14] the presence of such antibodies is diagnostic of the disease. Detectable anti-Achr Ab combined with radiographic features of thymic enlargement or a discrete thymic mass render the diagnosis of thymoma likely and allow the clinician to proceed directly to surgical therapy. As only 40% to 50% of thymomas are associated with myasthenia, however, the absence of detectable anti-Achr Ab does little to eliminate thymoma from the differential diagnosis of an anterior mediastinal mass.

Serum tumor markers play a critical role in the diagnosis, treatment, and follow-up of patients with mediastinal tumors. β-Human chorionic gonadotropin (β-HCG) and alpha fetoprotein (AFP) are two of the most common markers used in this diagnosis, and all patients with anterior mediastinal masses should undergo serum evaluation for these proteins. Alpha fetoprotein is synthesized by the fetal liver with structural and functional similarities to albumin, whereas β-HCG is normally produced by the placenta and most likely functions to maintain uterine integrity during pregnancy. In adults, both AFP and β-HCG levels remain exceptionally low except in pregnancy and certain disease states such as cirrhosis, hepatic and gastrointestinal cancers, and malignant germ cell tumors.

An elevation in AFP is diagnostic of a nonseminomatous component of a malignant germ cell tumor and is elevated in 80% to 90% of patients. β-HCG is also elevated in the majority of nonseminomatous germ cell tumors. Primary mediastinal seminoma, on the other hand, does not result in an elevation of AFP, but 10% of tumors may show a slight elevation (less than 100ng/mL) of β-HCG.[15] This small amount of protein does not originate within the seminomatous tumor itself but rather from the syncytiotrophoblasts scattered throughout the tumor. Thus, the presence of elevated AFP and β-HCG in patients with a known mediastinal mass is suggestive of a germ cell tumor, and pure AFP elevation is most likely the result of a mediastinal seminoma whereas a pure elevation of β-HCG makes the discrimination slightly more difficult. High levels of AFP and β-HCG (more than 600 ng/mL) are virtually diagnostic of a malignant nonseminomatous germ cell tumor. Although no definitive data exist, a large number of thoracic oncologists would initiate therapy for nonseminomatous germ cell tumor without tissue diagnosis in this scenario. In addition to the initial diagnostic value of these markers, they also play a critical role in assessing the response to therapy and detection of recurrence of malignant germ cell tumors. Benign germ cell tumors such as mature teratoma do not elaborate AFP or β-HCG.

Imaging

The plain chest radiogram provides only limited information necessary to tailor diagnostic options. It is therefore important to proceed to either computerized tomography (CT) or magnetic resonance imaging (MRI) for cross-sectional imaging.[16–18] With few exceptions, CT can provide all the data necessary to either diagnose or select the appropriate further diagnostic workup for a mediastinal mass. The initial question that must be answered by cross-sectioning imaging is whether the mass truly arises from the mediastinum or may be involving the mediastinum secondarily from the contiguous lung, pleura, or chest wall. The lungs must be examined for pathology, as mediastinal lymphadenopathy secondary to metastatic disease, most commonly from primary lung cancer, is more common than primary neoplasms of the mediastinum.[19] A primary pulmonary malignancy itself, however, can be confused with a mediastinal mass if it arises adjacent to the mediastinal pleura. A mass with its broadest base in the mediastinum and a smooth edge, however, is usually mediastinal in origin. Masses with irregular or spiculated edges rarely arise in the mediastinum.[16] If clinical suspicion is high for lymphoma, support for this diagnosis is often obtained by a CT showing lymphadenopathy within the chest that is remote from the main anterior mediastinal mass.

After determination that the mediastinal mass does not arise from a contiguous structure, the location within the three-compartment model is confirmed by CT. The mass is next evaluated for its major components—fat, calcium, and higher-density soft tissue—and it is classified as solid or cystic. Fat can be recognized due to its low Hounsfield units (70–130), whereas calcification is best seen in the unenhanced series of images. For the most part, the discovery that the mass has a large fatty component suggests that it is benign. A caudad, anterior mediastinal mass could represent omental fat in a foramen of Morgagni hernia, and mediastinal lipomatosis has been reported in Cushing's disease or steroid therapy.[20] Lipomas or liposarcomas can present in the mediastinum, but they are very rare, and fat may no longer be present in undifferentiated tumors.[21]

Most mediastinal masses in the adult consist primarily of nonfatty soft tissue. Spontaneous hyperattenuation, or a CT finding of tissue that is brighter than muscle on unenhanced CT, is uncommon. This finding usually restricts the differential diagnosis to intrathoracic thyroid goiters, which are bright as a result of the high iodine content, or fresh hematoma, reflecting the high hemoglobin content of fresh blood. Masses that strongly enhance with intravenous contrast are usually vascular tumors such as hemangiomas, thymic carcinoids, medullary cancers of the thyroid, or metastatic tumors. Such tumors, however, are rare, and most tumors of the thymus mimic the CT density of normal young thymus. The intensity is slightly lower than that of muscle because of the presence of some fat, and enhancement does increase with administration of contrast.

Noninvasive thymomas can appear as round or oval masses growing either within or adjacent to the thymus. These tumors can also present as diffuse enlargement of the thymus rather than as a discrete mass.[17,21,22] An invasive thymoma may appear as an irregularly shaped mass growing to or through the pleural surface or invading adjacent great vessels. *Drop* metastases separate from the main mass, usually on the parietal or visceral pleural surface of the adjacent hemithorax, may be seen in 15% of the cases. Diagnostic criteria for aggressiveness of thymic tumors have classically been based on gross evidence of invasion at the time of surgical resection (see following section on Masaoka staging system, under Histology and Classification Systems). CT diagnosis of an aggressive thymoma or thymic carcinoma according to these traditional criteria must thus rely on the demonstration of direct invasion into adjacent structures or obliteration of peritumoral fat planes and direct apposition of tumor to mediastinal structures. However, caution should be exercised in both overdiagnosing and underdiagnosing aggressive behavior based on radiographic findings, as absence of cleavage planes is not a strictly reliable criteria of invasion.

The differentiation between noninvasive and invasive thymoma is a pathologic diagnosis. Although thymic carcinoma behaves more aggressively than thymoma and frequently invades the pleura or other mediastinal structures, distinguishing the two disease processes on CT scan is unreliable.[23,24]

The CT features of malignant germ cell tumors are similar to those of other malignant tumors of the anterior mediastinum. As for thymic malignancies, invasion of adjacent structures is difficult to determine radiographically. The benign germ cell tumor, mature teratoma, contains a mixture of solid, fatty, and calcified components. Occasionally, diagnostic features such as the presence of fat–fluid level or spherical calcifications of dental material may render the diagnosis of benign teratoma nearly certain. None of these features, however, is entirely specific for benignity.[25,26] These benign radiographic features, along with normal AFP and β-HCG, however, only very rarely turn up anything other than a benign teratoma.

Although MRI does offer some advantages over CT, including lack of iodinated intravenous contrast, multiplanar imaging, and excellent soft tissue and tissue–vessel contrast, in clinical practice MRI provides little beyond CT in the diagnosis and workup of mediastinal tumors.[18,21] Compared with CT, MRI offers less spatial resolution and does not show calcification, both of which can be critical to the diagnostic workup of mediastinal masses. MRI characteristics of malignant mediastinal tumors such as thymoma and germ cell tumors are similar to skeletal muscle, with intermediate to low signal intensity on T_1-weighted images and high signal intensity on T_2-weighted images. The multiplanar imaging capability and high-contrast resolution of MRI may facilitate staging by demonstrating local invasion of a mediastinal tumor not apparent on CT, but the clinical value of this finding is still uncertain.[27] The finding of a fat–fluid level by MRI in a mediastinal mass has been reported to be diagnostic of teratoma, but these benign tumors possess classic CT characteristics as well, so MRI adds little to the diagnosis.[25] Similar limitations are encountered when imaging both mediastinal lymphomas and lymphadenopathy, as there is a significant overlap in both T_1-weighted and T_2-weighted images of benign and malignant lymphadenopathy.[28] It is more common for MRI to be used as a problem-solving study further evaluating abnormalities detected by CT, such as suspected great vessel or chest wall invasion, rather than as a primary imaging modality during the workup of an anterior mediastinal mass.

Positron emission tomography using the 2-deoxy-2-fluoro[^{18}F]-D-glucose analogue of glucose (FDG-PET) has a developing role in the diagnosis and staging of many malignancies.[29] Several groups have attempted to apply this imaging modality for a similar purpose to tumors of the mediastinum. Kubota and colleagues[30] performed both preoperative FDG-PET and CT scans on 22 patients with primary mediastinal tumors, and FDG-PET added little diagnostic information to the CT scan. Although biopsy-proven malignant lesions such as invasive thymoma and thymic carcinoma did show higher levels of FDG uptake than benign lesions, the relatively wide distribution of radioisotope uptake and the inability to differentiate lymphoma from primary thymic malignancy put the clinical utility of this imaging modality in question. Some benign inflammatory masses such as mediastinal sarcoidosis demonstrated FDG uptake similar to malignant lesions, further hampering the diagnostic value of FDG-PET. Further evaluation of this imaging modality by other groups, including larger studies as well as case reports, reached nearly the same conclusions.[31–33] The rapid advancement of this technology does hold future diagnostic potential, but its current role in diagnostic evaluation of a mediastinal mass is not established.

Diagnostic Biopsy Versus Resection

A preresectional tissue diagnosis is often not indicated in the management algorithm of anterior mediastinal masses. In a patient over 40 years of age, with negative tumor markers, absence of systemic *B* symptoms or remote lymphadenopathy, and a well-circumscribed anterior mediastinal mass, most surgeons would proceed with surgical resection for both diagnosis and cure. The presumed diagnosis for such a clinical scenario is thymoma, and resection without prior biopsy avoids violation of the capsule and potential seeding of surrounding tissues with thymic tumor cells that are known to have a propensity for local dissemination. Myasthenic symptoms or serum antiacetylcholine antibodies increase the suspicion of this diagnosis further.

This direct excisional approach is also recommended if the presumed diagnosis is benign, mature teratoma with typical appearance on imaging and normal serum AFP and β-HCG. Most oncologists would also be willing to initiate treatment with cisplatinum-based multidrug chemotherapy for presumed malignant, nonseminomatous germ cell tumors based on extreme elevation of AFP and β-HCG and a typical CT appearance.

A perhaps equally large group of patients, however, requires tissue diagnosis before initiation of therapy. This group includes those in which lymphoma is the leading diagnosis, metastatic lung or esophageal cancer is thought to be a possibility, or a germ cell tumor is suspected but serum markers are not sufficiently high to be pathognomonic. Tissue diagnosis is also useful in cases of unresectable-appearing mediastinal tumors by imaging studies with negative serum tumor markers, as such a neoplasm could represent lymphoma, aggressive thymoma that might benefit from neoadjuvant treatment, or germ cell tumor. Tissue diagnosis is necessary in such a case because of the differing treatment of these tumors.

Techniques of Diagnostic Biopsy

A tissue diagnosis from an anterior mediastinal mass may be best obtained by either open surgical or percutaneous techniques, depending upon the circumstances.

Percutaneous Needle Biopsy

CT-guided percutaneous fine-needle biopsy or aspiration (FNA) represents the least invasive modality that may be used to diagnose a mediastinal mass. Several anatomic approaches have been used for CT-guided FNA. The transpulmonary approach requires that the needle transverse the lung as well as both the visceral and mediastinal pleura. The risk of pneumothorax with this technique is 11% to 19%.[34,35] The parasternal, extrapleural approach has been reported as a useful modality to sample a mediastinal mass and can be performed under either CT or ultrasound (US) guidance avoiding violation of the pleural space.[35,36] Although this approach minimizes the risk of pneumothorax, the potential risk of accidental injury to the mammary vessels is high and has been reported to result in life-threatening hemorrhage.[37,38] The transsternal approach for needle access to mediastinal masses has been described in several series with a low reported complication rate. Although this technique has been used to sample lesions in all areas of the mediastinum, it is most appropriate for anterior mediastinal masses, which are located in the prevascular space immediately beneath the sternum.[39] Aside from the transthoracic approach for biopsy, the recent introduction of endoscopic ultrasound (EUS) in the diagnosis and staging of esophageal cancer has resulted in numerous reports describing the success of transesophageal EUS-FNA in the diagnosis of mediastinal masses.[40] Other studies report similar success rates of FNA in the diagnosis and treatment stratification of mediastinal masses.

Not all investigators, however, have had equally positive experience with FNA in the evaluation of mediastinal masses, and its appropriate application remains controversial. In a series from the Memorial Sloan-Kettering Cancer Center, 48 patients with operatively proven thymoma were evaluated by a preoperative biopsy: 26 patients underwent an open biopsy and 22 an FNA. The FNA diagnosis was accurate in only 59% of patients compared with an 81% accuracy by open biopsy. This issue is even more controversial due to reports describing the shedding of tumor cells into the mediastinum after capsule violation by preoperative biopsy.[41,42] Based on such reports, it is currently our policy to proceed with surgical excision in good surgical candidates in whom thymoma is thought to be the likely diagnosis, without a preoperative biopsy, either percutaneous or open.

The role of FNA in the clinical management of presumed mediastinal lymphoma is even more unclear. While FNA combined with immediate cytologic analysis may sometimes provide a rapid and cost-effective diagnosis, cytology alone plays only a small role in the initial diagnosis of mediastinal lymphoma. As stratification and proper clinical treatment usually involves subtyping lymphoma by flow cytometry and architectural pattern, FNA can rarely provide enough tissue for this entire workup. A large multiinstitutional study evaluated the role of FNA in the diagnosis and management of anterior mediastinal masses; over half the lymphomas identified by FNA required more tissue for further subclassification and confirmation of the diagnosis. A portion of the lymphomas were also misclassified as thymoma or metastatic melanoma based on FNA diagnosis.[43] As such mistakes can have disastrous consequences in proper patient management, it is rare in our practice to base the diagnosis and therapy of mediastinal lymphoma on FNA, and we most often perform a chamberlain procedure (anterior mediastinotomy; see following) in patients with anterior mediastinal masses thought to be most suspicious for lymphoma. FNA may, on the other hand, be appropriate as the sole diagnostic modality in identifying a relapse of mediastinal lymphoma when surgical tissue is available from the initial diagnosis to confirm FNA-based cytology.

Lymphoblastic lymphoma may represent the sole exception to the otherwise limited role of FNA in the initial diagnosis of lymphomas. This tumor has a characteristic cytologic appearance and lacks the architectural organization and extracellular fibrosis common to other mediastinal lymphomas. As this high-grade malignancy can present with rapidly progressing obstructive symptoms in the anterior mediastinum, the rapidity of FNA with immediate cytologic analysis can allow earlier initiation of therapy. Some small series have documented the success of FNA as the sole diagnostic modality for initiation of treatment for lymphoblastic lymphoma.[44]

TABLE 39.2. Representative studies evaluating fine-needle aspiration (FNA) in diagnosis of mediastinal masses.

Representative sample of studies reporting success of FNA in the diagnosis of a mediastinal mass	vanSonnenberg et al.[175] Morrissey et al.[176] Catalano et al.[40] Wakely et al.[44]
Representative sample of studies reporting failure or misdiagnosis of FNA for mediastinal masses	Gossot et al.[48] Blumberg et al.[41] Powers et al.[43]

Core needle biopsy or aspiration using a large 14- or 18-gauge needle may overcome some of the limitations of percutaneous biopsy for lymphoma by providing a larger volume of tissue with preserved architectural integrity for diagnosis. While large studies evaluating the value to core needle biopsy in patients with systemic lymphoma report a high rate of success in diagnosis, these results do not necessarily apply to isolated mediastinal lymphoma.[45,46] Because of the large size of the needle and high risk of pneumothorax, the transpulmonary approach is rarely chosen.[34,47] The direct mediastinal parasternal approach is favored for core needle biopsy but is limited by the potential damage to and bleeding from the mammary vessels.[37,38] Based on these inherent difficulties, only limited data are available regarding the success of this diagnostic modality for mediastinal lymphoma (Table 39.2).

Video-Assisted Thoracoscopic Biopsy

Video-assisted thoracoscopy (VATS) can be a cumbersome means for accessing the mediastinum and is potentially associated with a higher morbidity than other methods of mediastinal sampling.[48] Most importantly, there is a real concern that biopsy of a thymoma, in particular, is not prudent from this approach given the propensity of loose thymic cells to seed the pleural space even in cases in which transpleural biopsy has not been done.

Chamberlain Procedure

Anterior mediastinotomy, also known as the Chamberlain procedure, is in our opinion the optimal approach to the biopsy of most anterior mediastinal masses for which biopsy is indicated. This procedure is carried out through a 5-cm transverse skin incision made directly over the second costal cartilage.

Mediastinoscopy

Cervical mediastinoscopy in trained hands is a safe procedure, but as originally described and most widely applied, it allows access to the middle mediastinum and not the anterior mediastinum.

Extended Mediastinoscopy

The *extended* cervical mediastinoscopy allows for full staging of these areas through a single cervical incision by creating a tunnel to the aorticopulmonary window between the origins of the innominate and carotid arteries.[49] This technique requires considerable experience and carries a significant risk of bleeding due to the proximity to the great vessels. Few are trained in its use.

Transcervical, Sternum-Lifting Approach

A final approach to the anterior mediastinum that can be of use in certain circumstances is the transcervical, sternum-lifting approach that is used for transcervical thymectomy. Cooper described a device that, by lifting the sternum, allows an extended transcervical thymectomy to be performed with excellent visualization of the entire anterior mediastinum.[50] This technique has been adopted by the authors' group to biopsy of a wide variety of anterior mediastinal masses.[51]

Thymoma

A variety of tumors can arise from the thymus, but thymoma, derived from the thymic epithelial cells, is the most common neoplasm. Interest in thymomas developed secondarily to early investigations into autoimmune disease. Several independent investigators in the late 19th and early 20th centuries described the association of myasthenia gravis with thymic neoplasms.[52] Based on this evidence, Blalock pioneered the use of thymectomy as a therapy.[53,54] Advances in the use of positive-pressure ventilation increased the acceptability of thymectomy.[55] A major barrier to the diagnosis and treatment of thymic neoplasms throughout the 1900s was the lack of a standardized system for subclassification of these tumors. In 1999 the World Health Organization recognized this problem and developed a standardized system of nomenclature derived from the cellular origin of thymic neoplasms[56] (Table 39.3).

TABLE 39.3. Classification of thymic tumors.

Epithelial tumors: thymoma, thymic carcinoma
Neuroendocrine tumors: carcinoid, small cell carcinoma, large cell neuroendocrine carcinoma
Germ cell tumors
Lymphomas
Stromal tumors: thymolipoma, thymoliposarcoma, solitary fibrous tumor
Tumor like lesions: thymic hyperplasia, lymphoid hyperplasia, thymic cyst
Neck tumors of thymic or related branchial pouch derivation: ectopic hamartomatous thymoma, ectopic cervical thymoma, spindle epithelial tumor with thymus-like differentiation, carcinoma showing thymus-like differentiation
Metastatic tumors
Unclassified tumors

Source: From Rosai and Sobin,*56* by permission of Springer.

Histology and Classification Systems

Histologically, a thymoma is composed of a mixture of thymic epithelial cells with bland, benign-appearing histologic features as well as lymphocytes. Unlike other solid tumors that contain mature lymphocytes derived from the peripheral immune system, the majority of lymphocytes in a thymoma are immature and can be found in various stages of development, thus mirroring lymphocytes found in the normal thymus. Despite this histologic appearance, it has become accepted that the neoplastic cell of origin is the thymic epithelial cell and not the lymphocyte[57] (Figure 39.2A,B).

Determining the aggressive potential of a thymoma is of critical importance for proper therapy, becuase early-stage "noninvasive" tumors are associated with an excellent prognosis after surgical resection alone, whereas "malignant" tumors may benefit from neoadjuvant and/or adjuvant

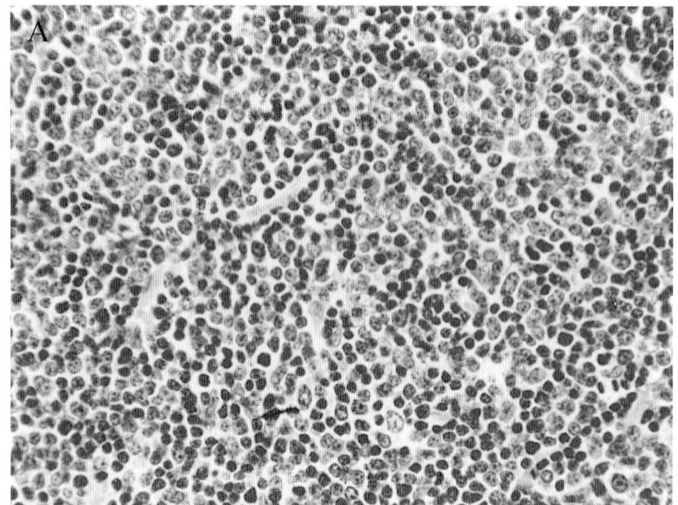

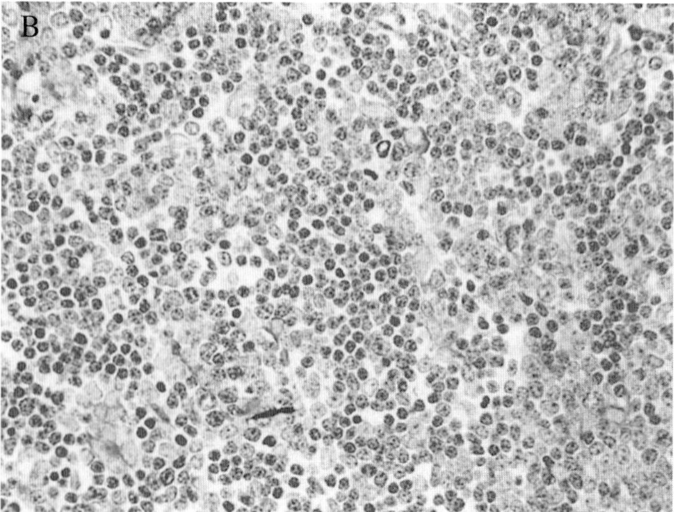

FIGURE 39.2. (A) Histologically thymoma is composed of various combinations of thymic epithelial cells and immature lymphocytes. (B) Immunohistochemical staining for cytokeratin can be used to differentiate lymphocytes from thymic epithelial cells. (Courtesy of Dr. Leslie A. Litzky, Department of Pathology, Hospital of the University of Pennsylvania.)

TABLE 39.4. Clinical staging of thymoma according to Masaoka et al.[61]

Stage I	Macroscopically completely encapsulated and microscopically no capsular invasion
Stage II	Macroscopic invasion into surrounding fatty tissue or mediastinal pleura, or microscopic invasion into the capsule
Stage III	Macroscopic invasion into neighboring organ, i.e., pericardium, great vessels, or lung
Stage IVa	Pleural or pericardial dissemination
Stage IVb	Lymphogenous or hematogenous metastasis

Source: From Masaoka et al.,[61] by permission of *Cancer*.

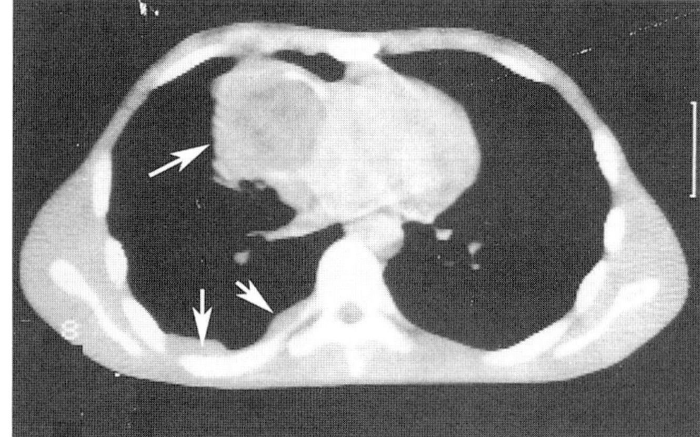

FIGURE 39.4. CT scan showing a malignant thymoma with radiographic evidence of pleural metastasis (*arrows*). (Courtesy of Dr. Wallace Miller, Department of Radiology, Hospital of the University of Pennsylvania.)

therapy. A 1961 paper from the Mayo Clinic proposed a histologic grading system classifying thymoma based on the lymphocyte to epithelial cell ratio[58]: lymphocytic, mixed, epithelial, and spindle. Predominantly epithelial cell tumors were considered more aggressive and carried a worse prognosis.[8,59] Not all investigations, however, supported this view.[60]

In 1981 Masaoka and colleagues, recognizing the difficulty of pure histologic criteria for stratification, developed clinical staging criteria.[61] After excluding other tumors of thymic origin, they staged epithelial thymomas based on their local invasiveness. Stage 1 tumors were completely encapsulated without gross or microscopic capsular invasion, stage 2 tumors showed microscopic invasion into the capsule or macroscopic invasion into surrounding fat or mediastinal pleura, stage 3 tumors showed gross local invasion into neighboring organs, and stage 4 tumors had evidence of pleural, pericardial or hematogenous dissemination (Table 39.4). The clinical stage both was prognostic[62] and allowed stratification for adjuvant therapy. A difficulty with this system is that staging is based on findings at surgical resection, thus preventing its use for triage to neoadjuvant therapies (Figures 39.3, 39.4).

Histologic classification of thymoma was revisited in 1985 by Marino and Müller-Hermelink,[63] who proposed a novel classification system dividing thymomas into different categories based on the histologic appearance of the neoplastic epithelial cells. Tumors composed of large, round, or polygonal epithelial cells were classified as cortical thymomas due to similarity of such cells to normal cortical epithelium. Medullary thymomas, on the other hand, contain smaller, spindle-shaped epithelial cells with irregular nuclei. All thymomas could thus be classified as cortical, medullary, or mixed histology. Subsequent studies indeed found that the Marino and Müller-Hermelink histologic classification reliably predicts tumor behavior and prognosis. In a large series, Pescarmona and colleagues[60] found that this histologic classification could be used to predict prognosis, with cortical thymomas exhibiting a more-malignant behavior. Of the 80 patients studied, those with medullary thymomas had essentially benign disease while patients with cortical thymomas showed evidence of invasive and malignant disease. Later studies found that both the Masaoka staging and the Müller-Hermelink grading classifications are strong and independent prognostic indicators of both overall and disease-free survival.[62,64,65] It has now become accepted that the Müller-Hermelink classification used in combination with the Masaoka staging system provides perhaps the most accurate prognostic information for recurrence. The recently adopted World Health Organization classification system represents an effort to combine the Masaoka and Müller-Hermelink criteria[56] (see Table 39.3).

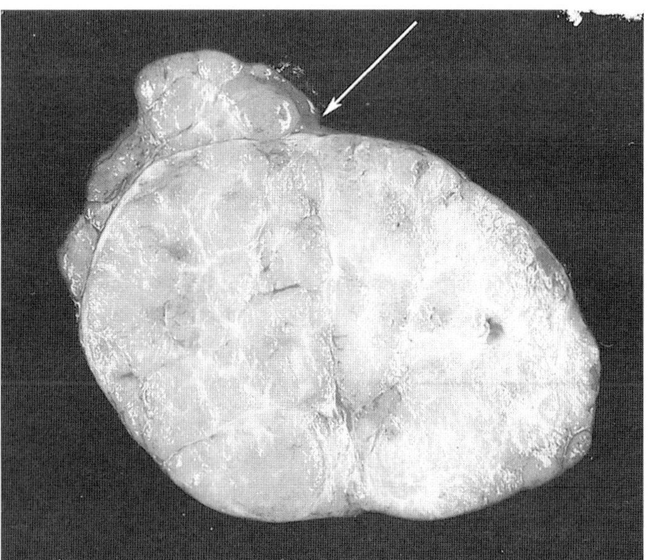

FIGURE 39.3. Stage 2 thymoma showing gross invasion past the thymic capsule (*arrow*). (Courtesy of Dr. Leslie A. Litzky, Department of Pathology, Hospital of the University of Pennsylvania.)

Presentation and Evaluation

Thymomas typically occur in adults over 40 years of age and are uncommon in children. They are slow-growing tumors with little propensity for hematogenous metastasis and are usually discovered incidentally on an imaging modality obtained for another purpose. Those patients who are symptomatic, with more-aggressive tumors, can present with symptoms of local obstruction or invasion, such as chest pain, cough, or even superior vena cava syndrome, or the symptoms of one of the autoimmune-related paraneoplastic syndromes associated with thymoma (Table 39.5). A standard chest radiograph is typically the initial diagnostic study, and it usually reveals an anterior mediastinal mass. Cross-sectional imaging

TABLE 39.5. Symptoms caused by or associated with thymoma.

Compressive/obstructive symptoms: cough, dysphagia, superior vena cava syndrome
Neuromuscular disorders: myasthenia gravis, myotonic dystrophy, Eaton–Lambert syndrome, myositis
Collagen vascular autoimmune disorders: rheumatoid arthritis, lupus, polymyositis
Hematologic disorders: red cell aplasia, megakaryocytopenia, pancytopenia

Source: Modified from Graeber and Tamim,[10] by permission of *Seminars in Thoracic and Cardiovascular Surgery.*

such as the CT scan is the best study following the chest radiography. There are no pathognomonic imaging features identifying thymoma from other mediastinal solid tumors, but the diagnosis may be strongly suggested by CT. Although it can be difficult to be certain preoperatively that one is dealing with a thymoma (see previous sections on Differential Diagnosis), ideally a noninvasive thymoma is resected directly, without preoperative biopsy (see previous section on Diagnostic Biopsy Versus Resection).

Neoadjuvant and Surgical Therapy

Although no prospective randomized trials exist, numerous groups have evaluated neoadjuvant and multimodality therapy for invasive or locally metastatic thymoma.[66–68] The overwhelming majority of the studies have supported the effectiveness of this approach. Neoadjuvant therapy for unresectable tumors was used initially in the early 1990s. Several groups demonstrated the efficacy of combining cisplatin-based preoperative chemotherapy with or without radiation therapy in downstaging unresectable tumors. All 23 patients in two of these early studies demonstrated a response, and complete resection was possible in 8 patients who had been considered unresectable before treatment. Those with an incomplete resection received additional postoperative therapy. Median survival was longer than that of historical control series without neoadjuvant treatment.[67,69] Several larger studies performed in the late 1990s confirmed these results.[70,71] Recent data suggest that chemotherapy alone might be as effective as radiation as a neoadjuvant agent. Delaying radiation until the postoperative period eliminates the concerns that some raise about operating in a radiated field. One study showed that preoperative chemotherapy alone with cisplatinum, doxorubicin, prednisone, and cyclophosphamide for stage III and IV tumors, followed by resection and adjuvant therapy, can result in 100% survival after 3.5 years.[72] Stratification of patients with aggressive tumors to neoadjuvant therapy based on the Muller-Hermelink grade combined with the Masaoka staging system resulted in a similar increase in survival versus historical controls.[66]

Despite the impressive results with neoadjuvant chemotherapy and radiation therapy, surgical resection remains the cornerstone therapy for thymoma. The accepted approach to the surgical management of thymoma has been complete resection of the mass along with all thymic tissue and the en bloc resection of adjacent structures involved by tumor. These structures most commonly include portions of lung and/or the great vessels (which, other than the innominate vein, require reconstruction if resected). This approach has been supported by several large studies showing that complete resection of all tumor is the most important prognostic factor for survival, even more important than Masaoka staging.[73] Simple tumor debulking, even when followed by radiation therapy, provides no survival advantage over biopsy alone.[74]

Approach through a median sternotomy provides the broadest and most generally accepted access for resection of thymoma. It is generally accepted that sacrifice of one phrenic nerve can be performed in a patient with otherwise adequate pulmonary function if this maneuver will result in a complete resection. Certainly, both phrenic nerves cannot be resected, and even one should not be divided if one would still be unable to achieve complete resection.

Surgical management of vascular structures involved by tumor is also controversial.[75,76] It is the authors' policy to resect and reconstruct involved vascular structures if this results in a complete resection.

Maximal exposure via median sternotomy for resection of thymoma is currently considered the standard of care, but a more minimally invasive approach for resection of suspected thymoma has been reported, including the transcervical approach.[51,77,78] The use of minimally invasive techniques such as video thoracoscopy for resection of thymoma has also been described,[79–81] but in our opinion this approach is less likely to provide a *clean* resection.

Adjuvant Radiation

Because thymomas are sensitive to radiation, radiation has become widely accepted for unresectable stage III and IV tumors. Several small retrospective studies suggest that survival of patients with either unresectable or residual invasive thymoma after attempted surgical resection may be improved by postoperative radiation therapy.[82,83] One study even noted that survival of stage III patients who underwent a complete resection without irradiation was identical to those who underwent incomplete resection with postoperative radiation therapy.[59] This finding, however, is controversial.[74]

Although the benefits of postoperative radiation in unresectable or residual stage III–IV thymoma have been accepted, the role of postoperative radiation therapy in stage II disease, which is highly likely to have been completely resected at surgery, is still debated. Survival is no higher in those who receive postoperative radiation, and radiation also did not influence disease-free survival. Local recurrence is as prevalent in patients who receive radiation as in those who did not.[84,85] Based on these data, we recommend that patients with completely resected stage II thymomas may be safely followed by serial radiographic examination and do not warrant postoperative radiation therapy. The role of adjuvant radiation for completely resected stage III disease, although generally accepted, is also supported by only some of the data available.

Similar to data for noninvasive and stage II disease, complete resection of invasive thymoma is the most important prognostic factor affecting survival, and postoperative radiation played no role in recurrence or survival if complete surgical resection was obtainable.[73] However, Curran and colleagues found a 38% local recurrence rate in patients who did not receive adjuvant radiation versus 0% for those who did.[86] The differences between these and other studies are difficult to understand; nevertheless, most clinicians continue to "recommend postoperative radiotherapy" for invasive disease, even after complete resection.[73]

Adjuvant Chemotherapy

Similar to preoperative neoadjuvant therapy, postoperative chemotherapy has been shown to improve survival in both retrospective and prospective studies. In a large retrospective series of patients across several French cancer centers, Cowen and colleagues reviewed the impact of platinum-based postoperative chemotherapy on survival. Multivariate analysis revealed that postoperative chemotherapy was one of the factors influencing disease-free survival. This finding was most pronounced in patients with stage III and IV disease who presented with symptoms of mediastinal compression.[87]

The European Organization for Research and Treatment of Cancer Lung Cancer Cooperative group reported a prospective phase II trial of cisplatinum- and etoposide-based chemotherapy for recurrent or metastatic malignant thymoma.[88] Although the trial was small and consisted of only 16 patients, the authors were able to document complete remission in 5 patients, a partial remission in 4, and no progression of disease in any of the patients while on treatment. The median survival time increased over historical controls with survival rates of 69%, 50%, and 42% at 3, 5, and 7 years, respectively. Other prospective studies support these conclusions and have shown that adjuvant chemotherapy can extend progression-free survival for patients with recurrent or unresectable disease, especially if combined with radiation therapy.[89] Based on these data, postresection adjuvant therapy is now considered the standard treatment for recurrent or unresectable disease.

Reresection

The overwhelming evidence supporting the role of complete surgical resection for curative treatment of thymoma has brought the issue of reresection for recurrent disease to the forefront. In the same study mentioned previously, Regnard and colleagues found a survival benefit for reresection of recurrent tumor. Similar to primary disease, complete reresection offered a survival advantage over incomplete reresection (53% versus 11% at 10-year survival).[73] Other slightly larger studies support this conclusion.[41,84]

Prognosis

Venuta and colleagues evaluated the survival benefit of aggressive multimodality therapy.[66] These authors retrospectively evaluated 83 patients who underwent surgical resection for thymoma between 1965 and 1988, before the advent of multimodality treatment beyond surgery. Starting in 1989, all patients with newly diagnosed thymoma were preoperative stratified as having benign, invasive, and malignant disease. This stratification was based on the Masaoka staging protocols as well as biopsy-proven histology, with cortical thymomas considered more aggressive. Patients with benign disease underwent radical resection only, those with invasive disease received adjuvant chemotherapy and radiotherapy, even in cases of complete resection, and those with malignant disease received both neoadjuvant as well as postoperative cisplatin-based adjuvant chemotherapy and radiation. All patients were able to complete the multimodality treatment, and only 1 patient with stage IV thymoma had a delayed recovery because of myelosuppression. Long-term survival of patients treated by multimodality therapy after 1989 improved significantly over those in the pre-1989 era who were treated by surgery alone (Figure 39.5A,B). Improvement

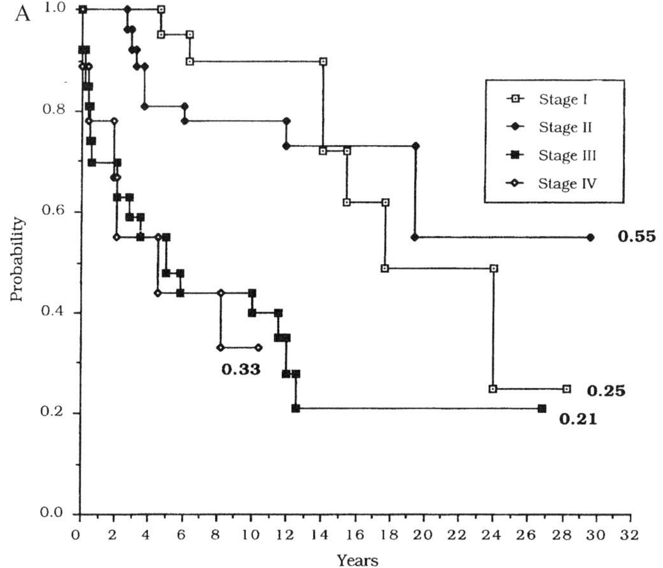

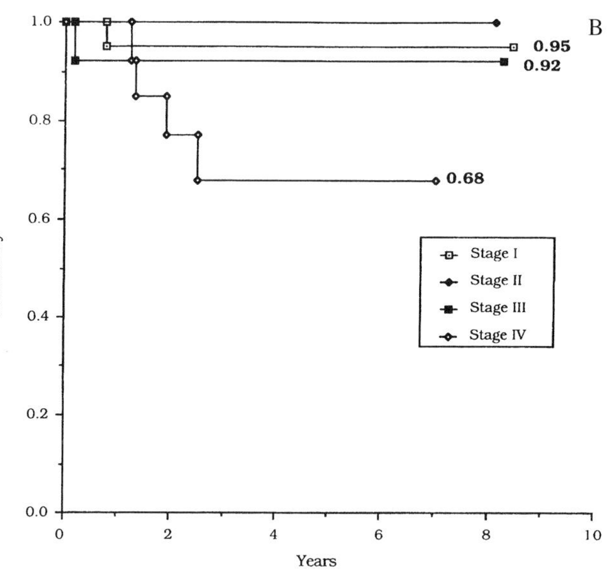

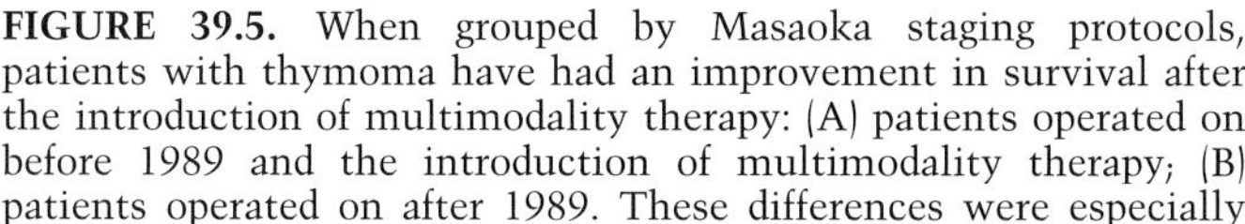
FIGURE 39.5. When grouped by Masaoka staging protocols, patients with thymoma have had an improvement in survival after the introduction of multimodality therapy: (A) patients operated on before 1989 and the introduction of multimodality therapy; (B) patients operated on after 1989. These differences were especially prevalent for advanced disease and survival of stage III patients after the introduction of multimodality therapy approximates that of stage I and II before 1989. (From Venuta et al.,[66] by permission of *Annals of Thoracic Surgery*.)

was seen across all stages of disease but was especially pronounced for invasive disease. Survival of patients with stage III disease after multimodality therapy approached that of stages I and II in the earlier series. Further improvements in chemotherapy and radiation therapy offer the possibility of increasing survival still further.

Thymic Carcinoma

Thymic carcinoma is a highly aggressive neoplasm of thymic epithelial origin, with less than 50% of patients surviving 5 years after diagnosis.[90–92] These tumors account for only a small portion of thymic neoplasms, estimated as 20% of epithelial malignancies. The true incidence is difficult to determine as only recently have these tumors become recognized as a separate entity from aggressive thymoma, and several studies have reported treatment outcomes for thymic carcinoma along with thymoma.[62,89] Histologically, thymic carcinomas are distinct from thymomas because of malignant cytologic features such as anaplasia, nuclear and cellular atypia, and a high number of mitosis. Whether thymic carcinoma arises from malignant degeneration of benign thymoma or is a separate entity is still undetermined. The reported finding of concomitant thymoma within specimens of thymic carcinoma as well as thymic carcinoma developing in patients with a past medical history of thymoma favors the malignant degeneration hypothesis. The possibility of a common cause for both disease processes, however, cannot be excluded.[90,91] Unlike the classic thymoma, the infiltrating leukocytes of thymic carcinoma are usually mature.

The majority of patients with thymic carcinoma present with symptoms of local invasion or compression such as cough, chest pain, or superior vena cava syndrome.[90,93] Traditionally, it has been thought that concominant paraneoplastic syndromes favor the diagnosis of thymoma over thymic carcinoma, but the data supporting this are thin, only a few patients in two studies, and controversial.[90,94]

Staging of thymic carcinoma has traditionally relied on the Masaoka staging system, similar to thymoma. The validity of this system for predicting survival in thymic carcinoma and thus establishing therapeutic options, however, has never been validated. Because thymic carcinomas, unlike thymomas, not infrequently metastasize by hematogenous as well as lymphatic routes, the use of the TNM staging system may be more appropriate.[95] In a large series, Suster and Rosai proposed a morphologic grading system for thymic carcinoma that could be used to predict clinical behavior. They discovered that patients with thymic carcinoma could be subdivided into two distinct clinical groups. Eighty-five percent of patients in group one, with aggressive tumors with high-grade histology, died of their disease, whereas all patients in group two, with low-grade histology, survived (Table 39.6). Other histologic markers such as the number of mitotic counts per high power field, lobular growth pattern, and circumscribed versus infiltrating morphology were also predictive of survival.[90] Such histologic grading criteria along with staging could be reliably used to triage patients into various treatment options.

Due to the rarity of this disease, most therapy has been based on the experience with treatment of thymoma. Thus, resection of both local and extensive disease, if possible, has been the guiding principle. Ogawa and colleagues determined that complete resection was a significant prognostic factor for survival on multivariate analysis.[96] Seventy-five percent of patients treated by complete resection versus 4% of those with incomplete resection were alive at follow-up. Surgical resection is currently proposed as the primary therapy for thymic carcinoma. However, the role of complete surgical resection, especially with sacrifice of vital structures, is not as strong as that for thymoma.[93,97,98]

TABLE 39.6. Histologic classification of thymic carcinoma.

Low-grade histology: well-differentiated (keratinizing) squamous cell carcinoma, well-differentiated mucoepidermoid carcinoma, basaloid carcinoma
High-grade histology: lymphoepithelioma-like carcinoma, small cell/neuroendocrine carcinoma, sarcomatoid carcinoma, clear cell carcinoma

Source: From Suster and Rosai,[90] by permission of *Cancer*.

Due to the aggressive nature of this tumor, more than half of patients may present with locally advanced, potentially unresectable disease.[90] The utility of both radiation and chemotherapy for neoadjuvant and adjuvant therapy has been addressed in several small studies, but standardization of treatment has been difficult to achieve because of the rarity of the disease. Yano and colleagues reported a series of patients, the majority of whom had unresectable disease, treated with both chemotherapy as well as radiation.[99] The role of chemotherapy was limited, but radiation resulted in a high response rate (seven of eight patients) and a prolonged survival over previous series. Other investigators report a similar improvement in survival in patients who received radiation therapy after complete or partial surgical resection compared to those who did not.[97,100] Using multivariate analysis, several investigators found that the routine use of chemotherapy with or without surgical resection or radiation therapy had no impact on survival.[94,96] Although both these groups report a relatively large number of patients, the variety of chemotherapeutic regimens used as well as combination of chemotherapy with surgery and radiation in some patients makes it difficult to reach definitive conclusions from these series alone. The reported success of multimodality therapy in the treatment of thymoma and the reported sensitivity of thymic carcinoma to radiation make it difficult to justify chemotherapy alone as the sole modality for the treatment of thymic carcinoma. One small series published in 1993 did evaluate the impact of chemotherapy alone on progression of disease after biopsy or incomplete resection of thymic carcinoma.[101] The authors' findings were similar to those for thymoma; patients treated with the single agent of cisplatin showed a poor response whereas those treated with a multiagent regimen in addition to cisplatin demonstrated partial and even some complete responses.

The role of aggressive multimodality therapy in the treatment of thymic carcinoma has been evaluated by several groups. Lucchi and colleagues reported a series of seven patients with biopsy-proven thymic carcinoma who took part in multimodality treatment consisting of cisplatin-based multiagent neoadjuvant chemotherapy followed by surgical resection after hematologic recovery and postoperative radiation therapy to the tumor bed.[102] All seven patients reported showed at least a partial response to chemotherapy, and complete surgical resection was possible in four patients. Those with complete resection received 45 Gy to the mediastinum while those with incomplete resection received 60 Gy to the mediastinum and residual tumor areas. During the follow up period, ranging from 16 to 136 months, one patient died of metastatic disease, one patient died in a motor vehicle accident without evidence of disease at autopsy, three patients are disease free, and two patients are alive but with recurrent tumor. Both the patients with recurrence as well as the patient who died of metastatic tumor had high-grade lymphoepithelioma-like tumor. Other slightly larger retrospective series have found a similar survival advantage to multimodality treatment of neoadjuvant chemotherapy, surgical resection, and postoperative radiotherapy.[94,96,103] Although it is unlikely that much larger series or prospective, randomized trials will be possible in the treatment of thymic carcinoma due to the rarity of this disease, these small series have made it possible to identify therapeutic regimens that can offer maximal benefit.

Other Thymic Neoplasms

Thymic carcinoid is a rare neoplasm of the thymus that has a strong association with multiple endocrine neoplasia type I[104,105] (see Chapter 55). Unlike other carcinoids, they rarely present with carcinoid syndrome but can secrete ectopic adrenocorticotropic hormone (ACTH), leading to Cushing's syndrome. This tumor is more frequently found in men and can present either with endocrinopathy or with a mass effect such as cough, chest pain, or superior vena cava (SVC) syndrome.[106] The majority of thymic carcinoids are locally invasive at presentation, and close to half of all patients have metastatic disease on presentation.[107]

Surgery has been considered the cornerstone of therapy. As most tumors are locally invasive on presentation, complete resection is often impossible. Despite this, several small series suggest that complete resection does offer a survival advantage and propose aggressive therapy of complete resection followed by adjuvant chemotherapy and radiation therapy and reresection of recurrent and metastatic disease.[108,109] Because of the aggressive nature of this disease, radiation therapy is almost always administered, either as primary therapy for unresectable disease or even after complete resection. Numerous authors have reported good control and amelioration of paraneoplastic symptoms.[110–113] Chemotherapy has been based on experience with carcinoids of the intestine; however, no standardized regimen has been established. Despite these efforts, prognosis of thymic carcinoids is overall poor, with few long-term survivors and median survival of 2 to 5 years after diagnosis.[108,109]

Thymolipoma is a benign tumor of the thymus that consists of mature fat intermixed with normal thymic epithelium.[114] These can reach a relatively large size, and tumors occupying the whole mediastinum and one hemithorax have been reported.[115] Although a large number of patients are diagnosed with this tumor incidentally by an unrelated imaging study, they can present with obstructive symptoms such as shortness of breath and cough.[114] Surgical resection is curative, and even asymptomatic thymolipoma should be resected as they can grow in size and result in obstructive symptoms.

Thymic hyperplasia is a benign condition describing a histologically normal thymus that is enlarged for the patient's age. This condition can present as a spectrum of disease ranging from respiratory compromise to an incidental finding on an unrelated imaging study. This condition has most frequently been described as a rebound thymic hyperplasia after chronic illness or stress-related atrophy of the gland.[116,117] The main diagnostic dilemma for the chest physician is to differentiate benign thymic hyperplasia from malignant disease.

Germ Cell Tumors

Mediastinal germ cell tumors include benign and malignant teratoma and malignant seminomatous and nonseminomatous tumors. They are a heterogeneous group of neoplasms resulting from malignant change in primordial germ cells.[115] Collectively, they account for approximately 20% of all anterior mediastinal tumors, and this location is the most common extragonadal site for germ cell malignancies. Their origin in sites heterotopic to the gonads may result from aberrant migration of germ cells during embryonic development or as a part of normal embryogenesis.[118,119] Based on the need for standard classification, investigators from the Armed Forces Institute of Pathology developed a reproducible histologic system of classification based on review of more than 300 cases. They concurrently proposed a clinical staging system that could help in planning therapy and defining prognosis[120] (Table 39.7).

Teratomatous Tumors

Teratomas are defined by the presence of tissue from more than one of the three primitive germinal layers.[121] They are the most common of the mediastinal germ cell tumors.[122] Mature (benign) teratomas are composed of well-differentiated mature elements such as mesodermally derived fat and cartilage, endodermal intestinal tissue, and ectodermal hair and skin with occasional formation of well-developed teeth. Immature (malignant) teratomas consist of mature elements derived from one or two embryonic layers combined with immature fetal tissue composing the remaining layer. Ter-

TABLE 39.7. Classification of germ cell tumors of the mediastinum.

Teratomatous tumors
Mature teratomas (composed of well-differentiated, mature elements)
Immature teratomas (with the presence of immature mesenchymal or neuroepithelial tissue)
Teratomas with additional malignant components:
Type I: with another germ cell tumor (seminoma, embryonal carcinoma, yolk-sac tumor)
Type II: with a nongerm cell epithelial component (squamous carcinoma, adenocarcinoma)
Type III: with a malignant mesenchymal component (rhabdomyosarcoma, chondrosarcoma)
Type IV: with any combination of the above
Nonteratomatous tumors
Seminomas
Yolk-sac tumors
Embryonal carcinomas
Choriocarcinomas
Combined nonteratomatous tumors (a combination of any of the above)

Source: From Moran and Suster,[120] by permission of *Cancer*.

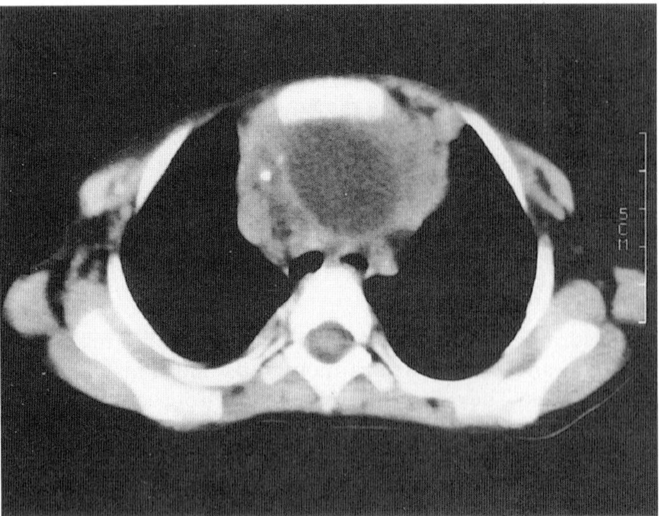

FIGURE 39.6. A benign cystic teratoma can be identified by the presence of a variety of tissues in an anterior mediastinal mass such as soft tissue, fluid, and calcium. (Courtesy of Dr. Wallace Miller, Department of Radiology, Hospital of the University of Pennsylvania.)

atomas may also be mixed tumors with additional malignant components derived from other germ cell tumors or nongerm cell epithelial or mesenchymal components (see Table 39.7).

Most mature teratomas are asymptomatic on presentation but may in a minority of patients present with symptoms resulting from impingement on mediastinal structures. In one of the larger series reported to date, some patients presented with nonspecific symptoms such as chest, back, or shoulder pain as well as cough and dyspnea.[123] Infection of a cystic component of a teratoma may result in signs of systemic infection, and erosion into the airway may lead to trichoptysis, the expectoration of hair and oily secretions, a presentation that is pathognomonic of a ruptured mediastinal teratoma.[7,124]

Radiographic characteristics of mature teratomas have been described previously in this chapter. Chest CT provides a firm diagnosis with identifying characteristics such as the combination of calcium, fat, and fluid in a soft tissue mass in the anterior mediastinum[125] (Figure 39.6). Serum tumor markers are not elevated unless a concurrent nonseminomatous component is present.

The accepted treatment for benign mediastinal teratoma is complete surgical excision, which is curative for the disease. Radiation and chemotherapy play no therapeutic role unless concurrent malignant disease is present.[15,123]

Seminoma

Unlike teratomas, which are equally distributed in men and women, malignant germ cell tumors, both seminomas and nonseminomatous tumors, are almost exclusively diseases of men. Seminoma is the most common malignant mediastinal germ cell tumor of single histology and usually presents in relatively young men during the third to fourth decade of life.[15,123,126] Most patients are symptomatic on presentation, with chest pain and dyspnea present in 40% to 50% and as many as one-third of all patients showing evidence of superior vena cava obstruction.[123] More than 60% of patients have metastatic disease on presentation, with intrathoracic organs being the most common site of metastasis. Widely metastatic disease to bone, brain, liver, and lymph nodes mimicking lymphoma is not uncommon.[12] As with other mediastinal masses, a chest radiograph and chest CT scan are the initial imaging studies of choice. As most seminomas reach a relatively large size before presentation, they can usually be seen on chest radiography. On CT scanning these tumors have the appearance of a bulky homogeneous anterior mediastinal mass that may obscure tissue planes or invade adjacent structures.[127] Calcification may rarely be seen in the mass, and the tumor is often surrounded by bulky lymphadenopathy. Serum tumor markers can be positive for low levels of β-HCG in about 10% of patients. Elevation of AFP is never evident in pure seminoma and indicates a nonseminomatous tumor component. Although a staging system has been proposed by some authors, it has been difficult to establish a reliable system for staging and predicting prognosis due to the rarity of this disease.[121,128] A biopsy is usually necessary to define the diagnosis. Although it has been proposed that the diagnosis of mediastinal seminoma necessitates abdominal CT scan and testicular imaging to rule out metastatic disease from an occult gonadal primary tumor,[15] one of the largest series detailing the clinical course of 120 patients with mediastinal seminoma found no evidence that mediastinal seminoma was a part of metastatic gonadal primary.[126]

This tumor is highly sensitive to both radiation and chemotherapy, and successful outcomes have been achieved with both regimens. Similar to primary testicular seminoma, mediastinal seminoma responds to cisplatin-based therapy, and because most patients present with metastatic disease, chemotherapy should be considered first-line treatment. Successful therapeutic regimens reported in the literature consist of cisplatin, dactinomycin, cyclophosphamide, bleomycin and vinblastine, or cisplatin and etoposide, with an 88% remission rate and a 85% long-term survival with chemotherapy alone.[129] Most recent reports are even more encouraging and describe 100% long-term survival after cisplatin-based chemotherapy[130] (Table 39.8).

The addition of radiation therapy for locoregional control can increase the response rate even further, with 100% 5-year actuarial survival reported in one study.[131] Radiation therapy alone has also been reported as a successful modality for treating patients with local mediastinal disease without extrathoracic metastasis. This approach led to a 75% 5-year rate of survival.[15] The role of surgical resection in this disease is controversial. Some authors have suggested resection as primary therapy for small mediastinal seminomas,[132] and others have proposed resection for residual masses larger than 3cm after chemotherapy.[133,134] None of these series showed a survival or local control advantage over radiation or salvage chemotherapy, and we do not favor surgical intervention for mediastinal seminoma.

Nonseminomatous Germ Cell Tumors

The group of malignant, nonseminomatous germ cell tumors consists of embryonal cell carcinoma, yolk cell tumor, choriocarcinoma, and mixed germ cell tumors. Some have classified teratomas with a malignant, immature component within this category as well (see Table 39.7). These tumors are rare and represent only 1% to 2% of all germ cell tumors

TABLE 39.8. Representative survival of patients with mediastinal seminoma based on therapy.

Author	*No. of patients reported*	*Primary form of therapy*	*Survival*
Sterchi et al.[177]	105	Radiation	58% at 5 years
Polansky et al.[178]	107	Radiation	75% at 5 years
Takeda et al.[123]	13	Multimodality therapy	83% survival ranging from 8 months to 19 years posttreatment
Bokemeyer et al.[145]	51	Chemotherapy alone, 74% of patients Radiotherapy alone, 9% of patients Chemo and radiation, 17%	88% at 5 years
Gholam et al.[130]	12	Chemotherapy only	100% at 7 years

in men,[135] with a particularly high incidence in men with Klinefelter's syndrome.[136] A primary mediastinal location of nonseminomatous germ cell tumors is considered by the International Germ Cell Collaborative Group (IGCCG) to be an independent adverse prognostic risk factor separate from tumor markers or sites of metastasis. In general, these tumors carry a worse prognosis and are more resistant to therapy than their histologic counterparts elsewhere in the body[137]. Nonseminomatous malignant germ cell tumors, especially those with yolk-sac histology, are also associated with a variety of hematologic malignancies, which occur independently of the chemotherapy used to treat the tumor.[138] Similar to seminoma, the majority of patients have metastatic disease on presentation and are symptomatic due to tumor burden.[12] Reported symptoms range from chest pain, the most common, to dyspnea, hoarseness, and superior vena cava syndrome.[123,139] Similar to seminoma, common metastatic sites include lung, liver, and regional lymph nodes.

Imaging studies typically reveal a large, irregular anterior mediastinal mass with poorly defined margins and multiple areas of central necrosis and hemorrhage.[127] In contrast to seminoma, more than 90% of patients with a nonseminomatous germ cell tumor have an elevation of either β-HCG or AFP[15,140,141] (Figure 39.7). Although no definitive data exist, the finding that AFP is elevated only in nonseminomatous germ cell tumors has motivated some oncologists to initiate therapy based on imaging studies and serology alone, without a tissue diagnosis.

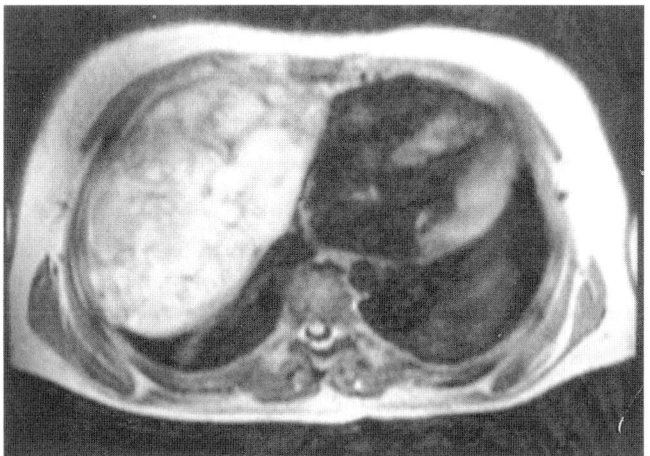

FIGURE 39.7. Magnetic resonance imaging (MRI) of embryonal carcinoma reveals a large heterogeneous mass displacing the mediastinum and replacing a large portion of the right pleural cavity. (Courtesy of Dr. Wallace Miller, Department of Radiology, Hospital of the University of Pennsylvania.)

Because most patients present with extremely bulky or metastatic disease, surgical resection is not the usual first-line treatment. Radiation therapy alone has also been unsuccessful for management of nonseminomatous germ cell tumors.[131] Historically, patients diagnosed with nonseminomatous germ cell tumors had an exceptionally poor median survival of 4.0 months after diagnosis[141]; this has improved dramatically with the advent of cisplatin-based multiagent chemotherapy. One of the earlier series from Indiana University reported the results of aggressive multimodality cisplatin-, etoposide-, and bleomycin-based chemotherapy combined with salvage chemotherapy for initial failures as well as surgical resection for postchemotherapy radiographic residual masses.[142] Of the 31 patients enrolled in the study, 18 (58%) obtained disease-free status after therapy, with 3 recurrences of the malignant germ cell tumors and 15 long-term disease-free survivors. These results represented a significant improvement from the 18% disease-free survival reported in the early 1980s.[141] A follow-up series from the same Indiana University group reported an even higher 61% survival with a broader variety of multimodality therapy, including autologous peripheral stem cell transplantation after high-dose chemotherapy.[143] Similar results have been replicated by others.[12]

Current attempts to improve survival in nonseminomatous germ cell tumors (NSGCT) have involved high-dose chemotherapy combined with autologous peripheral blood stem cell transplantation. One recently published prospective trial from Germany reported the results of high-dose cisplatin, etoposide, and ifosfamide chemotherapy followed by autologous peripheral blood stem cell transplantation and granulocyte colony-stimulating factor (G-CSF) support.[144] Nineteen of the 28 (68%) patients enrolled obtained disease-free status after three or four cycles of therapy, with 1 patient succumbing to a relapse of nonseminomatous germ cell tumor. Two patients died of concurrent hematologic malignancies. Overall progression-free survival rates were reported as 64% at 2 years and 56% at 5 years, which compare favorably with the 46% and 42% progression-free survival rates reported with standard cisplatin-based therapy from 1979 to 1996 by the International Extragonadal Germ Cell Tumor Study Group.[145,146]

TABLE 39.9. Survival of patients with mediastinal nonseminomatous germ cell tumors based on therapy.

Author	*No. of patients*	*Therapy*	*Survival*
Kersh et al.[131]	14	Radiation	8.8% at 5 years
Kesler et al.[143]	91	Chemotherapy and surgical resection	61% at 4 years
Bokemeyer et al.[144]	28	High-dose chemotherapy and autologous peripheral blood stem cell transplantation	68% at 2 years

Although surgery plays at most a diagnostic role in the initial management of NSGCT, it is a critical component of treatment after completion of chemotherapy. The M.D. Anderson Cancer Center recently reported a series of 20 patients who underwent surgical resection after completion of chemotherapy.[12] Eleven patients received no additional treatment beyond initial chemotherapy and 9 others received salvage chemotherapy after failure of the initial regimen. Of the 11 patients in the initial treatment only group, 9 survived the course of chemotherapy and all patients normalized levels of serum tumor markers after completion of chemotherapy. One patient demonstrated a complete radiographic response and did not undergo an operation, whereas 8 patients had evidence of residual mediastinal mass and underwent surgical resection. Of the 9 patients in the salvage group, there were 5 deaths during chemotherapy and 4 patients survived the course of treatment. One patient in this group had both a serologic and radiographic response and did not undergo mediastinal exploration. Three patients in the salvage group underwent surgical resection for residual mediastinal mass. Of all 11 resected tumors, 3 demonstrated complete tumor necrosis, 1 showed necrosis with mature teratoma, 3 showed mature teratoma only, and 2 showed near-complete necrosis and small microscopic rests of viable tumor. Two patients in this series had grossly viable tumor despite chemotherapy. One of these patients was the only patient in the series who had persistently elevated tumor markers after chemotherapy and succumbed to recurrent tumor, whereas the other patient with residual disease developed acute leukemia and died before restarting postresection savage chemotherapy. At 2-year follow-up, the survival of patients treated by this aggressive multimodality therapy was 72%, with 9 of 11 patients surviving without evidence of disease. These results are the highest rates ever reported for mediastinal NSGT. Survival of the "salvage group," or patients who had failed an initial course of chemotherapy at another institution before treatment at M.D. Anderson Cancer Center, was worse, with 4 of 9 patients (39%) alive 2 years after the initiation of treatment; 1 patient is alive with disease and 3 are free of disease.

Although this study supports previous series suggesting that resection should be undertaken in patients who have postchemotherapy residual mediastinal masses with tumor marker normalization,[135,147] the role of surgery in the face of persistently elevated tumor markers is more controversial. Some favor salvage chemotherapy in patients with persistently elevated tumor markers and a residual mediastinal mass, but others have presented data supporting the idea that survival may be improved by postchemotherapy resection of residual masses. A retrospective 17-year review of 91 patients treated at Indiana University showed that surgical resection after initial chemotherapy could lead to tumor marker normalization and improve survival in a subgroup of patients.[143] This finding combined with the overall poor long-term survival of patients requiring salvage chemotherapy has increased the acceptance of surgical resection for residual mediastinal NSGCT despite elevation of tumor markers (Table 39.9). Larger series will be necessary to convincingly demonstrate the efficacy of this form of treatment.

Middle Mediastinum

Although the middle mediastinum contains numerous vital structures of the aerodigestive tract, lymphoma and benign mediastinal cysts remain the most common primary middle mediastinal masses. Because the middle mediastinal lymph nodes are a frequent site of metastasis from bronchogenic carcinoma, however, metastatic carcinoma is probably the most common cause for middle mediastinal masses overall.

The diagnosis and treatment of lymphoma in the middle mediastinum does not differ from disease located primarily in the anterior mediastinum other than the fact that the diagnosis is typically made by mediastinoscopy rather than Chamberlain procedure (mediastinotomy). Congenital foregut cysts are the most common middle mediastinal cysts and represent benign, aberrant development of foregut structures. They almost never undergo malignant degeneration, but familiarity with these entities is important to distinguish them from malignant tumors of the mediastinum. Bronchogenic cysts recapitulate the structure of the tracheobronchial tree and can contain all histologic structures found in the normal airway such as respiratory epithelium, cartilage, and bronchial glands.[148,149] Enterogenous cysts recapitulate alimentary tract structures of the foregut, although they may contain gastric mucosa or pancreatic tissue. Because many of these patients eventually develop symptoms of obstruction or cyst infection, resection of these structures is generally recommended on discovery[150] (Figure 39.8). Minimally invasive techniques that allow resection of these cysts with little morbidity have made resection all the more attractive.[151] However, it is certainly reasonable to follow a simple, thin-walled, asymptomatic cyst that has all the radiologic characteristics of a benign process.

Pericardial cysts represent aberrant fusion of the anterior pericardial recess and can be located attached to the diaphragm or the pericardium. These are usually unilocular cysts filled with clear fluid, with no malignant potential, and they are resected only if symptomatic or if the diagnosis is in doubt.[150,152]

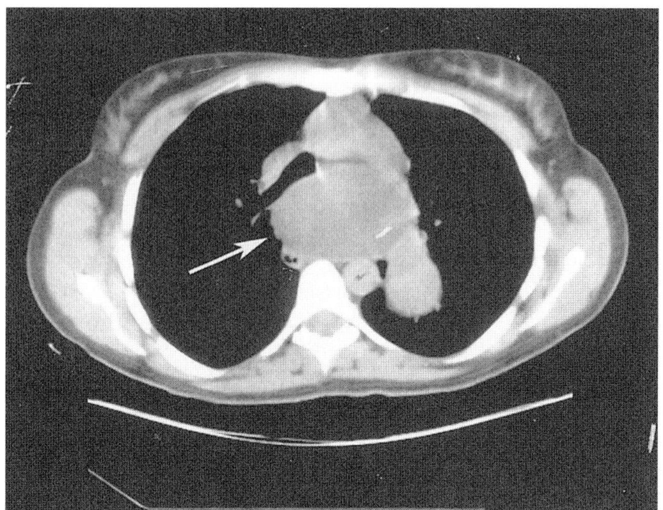

FIGURE 39.8. Large foregut duplication cyst (*arrow*) can present with signs and symptoms of dysphagia as well as airway obstruction as a result of impingement on the aerodigestive tract. (Courtesy of Dr. Wallace Miller, Department of Radiology, Hospital of the University of Pennsylvania.)

Posterior Mediastinum

Neurogenic tumors are the most common posterior mediastinal masses. Collectively, they represent approximately 14% of all mediastinal masses in the adult.[5] The overwhelming majority of these tumors are benign, and most patients are asymptomatic. These neoplasms are generally grouped into three categories based on the neurogenic tissue of origin. Tumors arising from the nerve sheath include schwannoma, neurofibroma, and malignant nerve sheath tumor. They are the most common neurogenic tumors in the adult. Sympathetic ganglion tumors include ganglioneuroma, ganglioneuroblastoma, and neuroblastoma. Parasympathetic ganglion tumors such as chemodectoma and pheochromocytoma have been reported to occur in the posterior mediastinum but are exceedingly rare in that location.

Esophageal duplication cysts and bronchogenic cysts also occur with some frequency in the posterior mediastinum. The approach to their management is as described previously for simple middle mediastinal cysts, but the surgical approach often involves thoracoscopic resection.

Schwannoma and neurofibroma are the most common mediastinal neurogenic tumors.[153] These are benign and slow-growing tumors. They appear as well-marginated, encapsulated masses, most commonly in the costovertebral sulci. Both tumors behave in a benign manner and most patients are asymptomatic on presentation, although symptoms of plexopathy, neurologic symptoms from the involved intercostals nerve(s) or intraspinal extension, or airway irritation are not unusual.[150,154,155] More than one-third of patients with neurofibromas have von Recklinghausen's disease or neurofibromatosis. These patients usually have with multiple neurofibromas and tend to present at an earlier age.[150,156] The definitive treatment of these tumors is surgical resection, although as for benign-appearing cysts, observation is not unreasonable in some patients due to the slow growth and low malignant potential. Some of the larger series have shown that complete resection by a thoracotomy can be achieved in more than 90% of the patients, and of those with complete resection, only 5% present with local recurrence.[154] Thoracoscopic resection of such tumors has also been reported with favorable results,[157,158] and this is now commonly performed. Combined thoracic and neurosurgical resection of dumbbell tumors with intraspinal extension can also be achieved with low morbidity.[159]

The malignant version of the nerve sheath tumor, neurofibrosarcoma, is a rare malignancy arising most likely from malignant degeneration of neurofibroma.[160] Although it is a rare malignancy in the population as a whole, this cancer can affect as many as 29% of patients with neurofibromatosis.[161] Unlike benign tumors, most of these malignancies are symptomatic, with pain and symptoms of nerve impingement being common at presentation.[160] On CT these tumors typically present as rounded masses with areas of central hemorrhage and necrosis.[150] Radical surgical excision is the procedure of choice. However, 5-year survival is as low as 16% in patients with neurofibromatosis, with no survival benefit derived from adjuvant therapy.[160,162]

Sympathetic ganglion tumors represent malignant degeneration of the nerve cell, rather than the nerve sheath. These tumors tend to occur in the sympathetic ganglia and adrenal gland and probably represent a spectrum of the same tumor, with ganglioneuroma representing the most benign version of the disease. Ganglioneuromas are the most common of the thoracic sympathetic chain tumors and are composed of well-differentiated ganglion cells.[163] Most patients are asymptomatic at presentation, but symptoms related to secretory activity of catecholamines has been reported.[164] Complete resection is the definitive and highly successful treatment.[165] Ganglioneuroblastoma is a tumor that is histologically composed of ganglioneuroma-like elements as well as neuroblastoma-like features. The degree of malignant behavior is generally related to the degree of neuroblastic differentiation. Overall, these tumors have a high 5-year survival after resection.[166]

Neuroblastoma represents the most malignant of the sympathetic ganglion tumors. This disease is almost exclusively limited to children, and 90% of the cases are reported in children less then 5 years of age.[167] The majority of the patients are symptomatic on presentation, and distant metastases are common. Symptoms may include chest pain, dyspnea, myelopathy from spinal canal involvement, and symptoms related to excess catecholamine production.[168] The International Neuroblastoma Staging System, reflecting factors such as the primary tumor size, lymph node involvement, and extent of unresectable disease, can be used to predict survival.[169] Amplification of the oncogene, N-*myc*, has also been shown to correlate with poor prognosis.[167]

Localized neuroblastoma, both abdominal and thoracic, has a favorable 89% to 96% survival rate with surgery alone.[170,171] Survival can be improved in patients with residual disease after resection and in those with positive lymph node involvement by combining chemotherapy and radiation therapy.[172] Traditionally, thoracic neuroblastoma has been considered a positive prognostic factor, less likely to have N-*myc* amplification or DNA ploidy, and thus conferring a better survival rate.[173] More recent studies, however, have shown that patients with early-stage thoracic and abdominal neuroblastomas have a similar survival.[174]

References

1. Fishman A, Martinez F, Naunheim K, et al. A randomized trial comparing lung-volume-reduction surgery with medical therapy for severe emphysema. N Engl J Med 2003;348:2059–2073.
2. Chemotherapy in non-small cell lung cancer: a meta-analysis using updated data on individual patients from 52 randomised clinical trials. Non-small Cell Lung Cancer Collaborative Group. BMJ 1995;311:899–909.
3. Moore K, Persaud T. The Developing Human: Clinically Oriented Embryology, 6th ed. Philadelphia: Saunders, 1998.
4. Shields T. Mediastinal Surgery. Philadelphia: Lea & Febiger, 1991.
5. Davis RD Jr, Oldham HN Jr, Sabiston DC Jr. Primary cysts and neoplasms of the mediastinum: recent changes in clinical presentation, methods of diagnosis, management, and results. Ann Thorac Surg 1987;44:229–237.
6. Reeder LB. Neurogenic tumors of the mediastinum. Semin Thorac Cardiovasc Surg 2000;12:261–267.
7. Strollo DC, Rosado de Christenson ML, Jett JR. Primary mediastinal tumors. Part 1: Tumors of the anterior mediastinum. Chest 1997;112:511–522.
8. Lewis JE, Wick MR, Scheithauer BW, Bernatz PE, Taylor WF. Thymoma. A clinicopathologic review. Cancer (Phila) 1987;60: 2727–2743.
9. Beard ME, Krantz SB, Johnson SA, Bateman CJ, Whitehouse JM. Pure red cell aplasia. Q J Med 1978;47:339–348.
10. Graeber GM, Tamim W. Current status of the diagnosis and treatment of thymoma. Semin Thorac Cardiovasc Surg 2000;12: 268–277.
11. Clamon GH. Management of primary mediastinal seminoma. Chest 1983;83:263–267.
12. Walsh GL, Taylor GD, Nesbitt JC, Amato RJ. Intensive chemotherapy and radical resections for primary nonseminomatous mediastinal germ cell tumors. Ann Thorac Surg 2000;69: 337–343.
13. Drachman DB. Myasthenia gravis. N Engl J Med 1994;330:1797–1810.
14. Drachman DB, Adams RN, Josifek LF, Self SG. Functional activities of autoantibodies to acetylcholine receptors and the clinical severity of myasthenia gravis. N Engl J Med 1982;307: 769–775.
15. Wood DE. Mediastinal germ cell tumors. Semin Thorac Cardiovasc Surg 2000;12:278–289.
16. Woodring JH, Johnson PJ. Computed tomography distinction of central thoracic masses. J Thorac Imaging 1991;6:32–39.
17. Chen JL, Weisbrod GL, Herman SJ. Computed tomography and pathologic correlations of thymic lesions. J Thorac Imaging 1988; 3:61–65.
18. Erasmus JJ, McAdams HP, Donnelly LF, Spritzer CE. MR imaging of mediastinal masses. Magn Reson Imaging Clin N Am 2000;8:59–89.
19. Cameron R, Loehrer P, Thomas C. Neoplasms of the mediastinum. In: DeVita V, Hellman S, Rosenberg S (eds). Cancer: Principles and Practice of Oncology. Philadelphia: Lippincott Williams & Wilkins, 2001 pp. 1019–1036.
20. Rodriguez E, Soler R, Gayol A, Freire R. Massive mediastinal and cardiac fatty infiltration in a young patient. J Thorac Imaging 1995;10:225–226.
21. Laurent F, Latrabe V, Lecesne R, et al. Mediastinal masses: diagnostic approach. Eur Radiol 1998;8:1148–1159.
22. Rosado-de-Christenson ML, Galobardes J, Moran CA. Thymoma: radiologic-pathologic correlation. Radiographics 1992; 12:151–168.
23. Quagliano PV. Thymic carcinoma: case reports and review. J Thorac Imaging 1996;11:66–74.
24. Lee JD, Choe KO, Kim SJ, Kim GE, Im JG, Lee JT. CT findings in primary thymic carcinoma. J Comput Assist Tomogr 1991;15: 429–433.
25. Fulcher AS, Proto AV, Jolles H. Cystic teratoma of the mediastinum: demonstration of fat/fluid level. AJR Am J Roentgenol 1990;154:259–260.
26. Quillin SP, Siegel MJ. CT features of benign and malignant teratomas in children. J Comput Assist Tomogr 1992;16:722–726.
27. Verstandig AG, Epstein DM, Miller WT Jr, Aronchik JA, Gefter WB, Miller WT. Thymoma: report of 71 cases and a review. Crit Rev Diagn Imaging 1992;33:201–230.
28. Gefter WB. Magnetic resonance imaging in the evaluation of lung cancer. Semin Roentgenol 1990;25:73–84.
29. Jerusalem G, Hustinx R, Beguin Y, Fillet G. PET scan imaging in oncology. Eur J Cancer 2003;39:1525–1534.
30. Kubota K, Yamada S, Kondo T, et al. PET imaging of primary mediastinal tumours. Br J Cancer 1996;73:882–886.
31. Sasaki M, Kuwabara Y, Ichiya Y, et al. Differential diagnosis of thymic tumors using a combination of ^{11}C-methionine PET and FDG PET. J Nucl Med 1999;40:1595–1601.
32. Naumann R, Beuthien-Baumann B, Fischer R, et al. Simultaneous occurrence of Hodgkin's lymphoma and eosinophilic granuloma: a potential pitfall in positron emission tomography imaging. Clin Lymphoma 2002;3:121–124.
33. Naumann R, Beuthien-Baumann B. Positron emission tomography in the management of patients with indolent non-Hodgkin's lymphoma. Clin Lymphoma 2003;4:50–51.
34. Herman SJ, Holub RV, Weisbrod GL, Chamberlain DW. Anterior mediastinal masses: utility of transthoracic needle biopsy. Radiology 1991;180:167–170.
35. Weisbrod GL. Percutaneous fine-needle aspiration biopsy of the mediastinum. Clin Chest Med 1987;8:27–41.
36. Bressler EL, Kirkham JA. Mediastinal masses: alternative approaches to CT-guided needle biopsy. Radiology 1994;191: 391–396.
37. Glassberg RM, Sussman SK, Glickstein MF. CT anatomy of the internal mammary vessels: importance in planning percutaneous transthoracic procedures. AJR Am J Roentgenol 1990;155: 397–400.
38. Glassberg RM, Sussman SK. Life-threatening hemorrhage due to percutaneous transthoracic intervention: importance of the internal mammary artery. AJR Am J Roentgenol 1990;154: 47–49.
39. Gupta S, Wallace MJ, Morello FA, Jr., Ahrar K, Hicks ME. CT-guided percutaneous needle biopsy of intrathoracic lesions by using the transsternal approach: experience in 37 patients. Radiology 2002;222:57–62.
40. Catalano MF, Rosenblatt ML, Chak A, Sivak MV, Jr., Scheiman J, Gress F. Endoscopic ultrasound-guided fine needle aspiration in the diagnosis of mediastinal masses of unknown origin. Am J Gastroenterol 2002;97:2559–2565.
41. Blumberg D, Port JL, Weksler B, et al. Thymoma: a multivariate analysis of factors predicting survival. Ann Thorac Surg 1995;60:908–913; discussion 914.
42. Weissberg D, Goldberg M, Pearson FG. Thymoma. Ann Thorac Surg 1973;16:141–147.
43. Powers CN, Silverman JF, Geisinger KR, Frable WJ. Fine-needle aspiration biopsy of the mediastinum. A multi-institutional analysis. Am J Clin Pathol 1996;105:168–173.
44. Wakely PE Jr, Kornstein MJ. Aspiration cytopathology of lymphoblastic lymphoma and leukemia: the MCV experience. Pediatr Pathol Lab Med 1996;16:243–252.
45. Pappa VI, Hussain HK, Reznek RH, et al. Role of image-guided core-needle biopsy in the management of patients with lymphoma. J Clin Oncol 1996;14:2427–2430.
46. Ben-Yehuda D, Polliack A, Okon E, et al. Image-guided core-needle biopsy in malignant lymphoma: experience with 100

patients that suggests the technique is reliable. J Clin Oncol 1996;14:2431–2434.
47. Protopapas Z, Westcott JL. Transthoracic hilar and mediastinal biopsy. J Thorac Imaging 1997;12:250–258.
48. Gossot D, Toledo L, Fritsch S, Celerier M. Mediastinoscopy vs. thoracoscopy for mediastinal biopsy. Results of a prospective nonrandomized study. Chest 1996;110:1328–1331.
49. Ginsberg RJ, Rice TW, Goldberg M, Waters PF, Schmocker BJ. Extended cervical mediastinoscopy. A single staging procedure for bronchogenic carcinoma of the left upper lobe. J Thorac Cardiovasc Surg 1987;94:673–678.
50. Cooper JD, Al-Jilaihawa AN, Pearson FG, Humphrey JG, Humphrey HE. An improved technique to facilitate transcervical thymectomy for myasthenia gravis. Ann Thorac Surg 1988; 45:242–247.
51. Deeb ME, Brinster CJ, Kucharzuk J, Shrager JB, Kaiser LR. Expanded indications for transcervical thymectomy in the management of anterior mediastinal masses. Ann Thorac Surg 2001; 72:208–211.
52. Bell ET. Tumors of the thymus in myasthenia gravis. J Nerv Mental Dis 1917;45:130.
53. Blalock A, Mason M, Morgan H. Myasthenia gravis and tumors of the thymic region: Report of a case in which the tumor was removed. Ann Surg 1939;110:544.
54. Blalock A. Thymectomy in the treatment of myesthenia gravis: report of twenty cases. J Thorac Cardiovasc Surg 1944;13:316.
55. Andrus WD, Foot NC. Report of a large thymic tumor successfully removed by operation. J Thorac Surg 1937;6:648.
56. Rosai J, Sobin LH. Histological typing of tumours of the thymus. World Health Organization: International Histological Classification of Tumours, vol 2. Berlin: Springer, 1999.
57. Lauriola L, Maggiano N, Marino M, Carbone A, Piantelli M, Musiani P. Human thymoma: immunologic characteristics of the lymphocytic component. Cancer (Phila) 1981;48:1992–1995.
58. Bernatz PE, Harrison EG, Clagett OT. Thymoma: a clinicopathologic study. J Thorac Cardiovasc Surg 1961;42:424–444.
59. Gripp S, Hilgers K, Wurm R, Schmitt G. Thymoma: prognostic factors and treatment outcomes. Cancer (Phila) 1998;83:1495–1503.
60. Pescarmona E, Rendina EA, Venuta F, Ricci C, Ruco LP, Baroni CD. The prognostic implication of thymoma histologic subtyping. A study of 80 consecutive cases. Am J Clin Pathol 1990; 93:190–195.
61. Masaoka A, Monden Y, Nakahara K, Tanioka T. Follow-up study of thymomas with special reference to their clinical stages. Cancer (Phila) 1981;48:2485–2492.
62. Lardinois D, Rechsteiner R, Lang RH, et al. Prognostic relevance of Masaoka and Muller–Hermelink classification in patients with thymic tumors. Ann Thorac Surg 2000;69:1550–1555.
63. Marino M, Muller-Hermelink HK. Thymoma and thymic carcinoma. Relation of thymoma epithelial cells to the cortical and medullary differentiation of thymus. Virchows Arch A Pathol Anat Histopathol 1985;407:119–149.
64. Quintanilla-Martinez L, Wilkins EW Jr, Choi N, Efird J, Hug E, Harris NL. Thymoma. Histologic subclassification is an independent prognostic factor. Cancer (Phila) 1994;74:606–617.
65. Ricci C, Rendina EA, Pescarmona EO, et al. Correlations between histological type, clinical behaviour, and prognosis in thymoma. Thorax 1989;44:455–460.
66. Venuta F, Rendina EA, Pescarmona EO, et al. Multimodality treatment of thymoma: a prospective study. Ann Thorac Surg 1997;64:1585–1591; discussion 1591–1582.
67. Macchiarini P, Chella A, Ducci F, et al. Neoadjuvant chemotherapy, surgery, and postoperative radiation therapy for invasive thymoma. Cancer (Phila) 1991;68:706–713.
68. Hejna M, Haberl I, Raderer M. Nonsurgical management of malignant thymoma. Cancer (Phila) 1999;85:1871–1884.
69. Rea F, Sartori F, Loy M, et al. Chemotherapy and operation for invasive thymoma. J Thorac Cardiovasc Surg 1993;106:543–549.
70. Akaogi E, Ohara K, Mitsui K, et al. Preoperative radiotherapy and surgery for advanced thymoma with invasion to the great vessels. J Surg Oncol 1996;63:17–22.
71. Tomiak EM, Evans WK. The role of chemotherapy in invasive thymoma: a review of the literature and considerations for future clinical trials. Crit Rev Oncol Hematol 1993;15:113–124.
72. Shin DM, Walsh GL, Komaki R, et al. A multidisciplinary approach to therapy for unresectable malignant thymoma. Ann Intern Med 1998;129:100–104.
73. Regnard JF, Magdeleinat P, Dromer C, et al. Prognostic factors and long-term results after thymoma resection: a series of 307 patients. J Thorac Cardiovasc Surg 1996;112:376–384.
74. Ciernik IF, Meier U, Lutolf UM. Prognostic factors and outcome of incompletely resected invasive thymoma following radiation therapy. J Clin Oncol 1994;12:1484–1490.
75. Nakahara K, Ohno K, Hashimoto J, et al. Thymoma: results with complete resection and adjuvant postoperative irradiation in 141 consecutive patients. J Thorac Cardiovasc Surg 1988;95:1041–1047.
76. Okumura M, Miyoshi S, Takeuchi Y, et al. Results of surgical treatment of thymomas with special reference to the involved organs. J Thorac Cardiovasc Surg 1999;117:605–613.
77. Kark AE, Kirschner PA. Total thymectomy by the transcervical approach. Br J Surg 1971;58:321–326.
78. Kark AE, Papatestas AE. Some anatomic features of the transcervical approach for thymectomy. Mt Sinai J Med 1971;38: 580–585.
79. Kaiser LR. Video-assisted thoracic surgery. Current state of the art. Ann Surg 1994;220:720–734.
80. Kaiser LR. Thymoma. The use of minimally invasive resection techniques. Chest Surg Clin N Am 1994;4:185–194.
81. Takeo S, Sakada T, Yano T. Video-assisted extended thymectomy in patients with thymoma by lifting the sternum. Ann Thorac Surg 2001;71:1721–1723.
82. Wang LS, Huang MH, Lin TS, Huang BS, Chien KY. Malignant thymoma. Cancer (Phila) 1992;70:443–450.
83. Mornex F, Resbeut M, Richaud P, et al. Radiotherapy and chemotherapy for invasive thymomas: a multicentric retrospective review of 90 cases. The FNCLCC trialists. Federation Nationale des Centres de Lutte Contre le Cancer. Int J Radiat Oncol Biol Phys 1995;32:651–659.
84. Singhal S, Shrager JB, Rosenthal DI, LiVolsi VA, Kaiser LR. Comparison of stage I–II thymoma treated by complete resection with or without adjuvant radiation. Ann Thorac Surg 2003;76(5): 1635–1641; discussion 1641–1642.
85. Mangi AA, Wright CD, Allan JS, et al. Adjuvant radiation therapy for stage II thymoma. Ann Thorac Surg 2002;74:1033–1037.
86. Curran WJ Jr, Kornstein MJ, Brooks JJ, Turrisi AT III. Invasive thymoma: the role of mediastinal irradiation following complete or incomplete surgical resection. J Clin Oncol 1988;6:1722–1727.
87. Cowen D, Richaud P, Mornex F, et al. Thymoma: results of a multicentric retrospective series of 149 non-metastatic irradiated patients and review of the literature. FNCLCC trialists. Federation Nationale des Centres de Lutte Contre le Cancer. Radiother Oncol 1995;34:9–16.
88. Giaccone G, Ardizzoni A, Kirkpatrick A, Clerico M, Sahmoud T, van Zandwijk N. Cisplatin and etoposide combination chemotherapy for locally advanced or metastatic thymoma. A phase II study of the European Organization for Research and Treatment of Cancer Lung Cancer Cooperative Group. J Clin Oncol 1996;14:814–820.
89. Loehrer PJ Sr, Chen M, Kim K, et al. Cisplatin, doxorubicin, and cyclophosphamide plus thoracic radiation therapy for limited-

stage unresectable thymoma: an intergroup trial. J Clin Oncol 1997;15:3093–3099.
90. Suster S, Rosai J. Thymic carcinoma. A clinicopathologic study of 60 cases. Cancer (Phila) 1991;67:1025–1032.
91. Suster S, Moran CA. Thymoma, atypical thymoma, and thymic carcinoma. A novel conceptual approach to the classification of thymic epithelial neoplasms. Am J Clin Pathol 1999;111:826–833.
92. Suster S, Moran CA. Primary thymic epithelial neoplasms: spectrum of differentiation and histological features. Semin Diagn Pathol 1999;16:2–17.
93. Truong LD, Mody DR, Cagle PT, Jackson-York GL, Schwartz MR, Wheeler TM. Thymic carcinoma. A clinicopathologic study of 13 cases. Am J Surg Pathol 1990;14:151–166.
94. Blumberg D, Burt ME, Bains MS, et al. Thymic carcinoma: current staging does not predict prognosis. J Thorac Cardiovasc Surg 1998;115:303–308; discussion 308–309.
95. Tsuchiya R, Koga K, Matsuno Y, Mukai K, Shimosato Y. Thymic carcinoma: proposal for pathological TNM and staging. Pathol Int 1994;44:505–512.
96. Ogawa K, Toita T, Uno T, et al. Treatment and prognosis of thymic carcinoma: a retrospective analysis of 40 cases. Cancer (Phila) 2002;94:3115–3119.
97. Hsu CP, Chen CY, Chen CL, et al. Thymic carcinoma. Ten years' experience in twenty patients. J Thorac Cardiovasc Surg 1994; 107:615–620.
98. Shimizu J, Hayashi Y, Morita K, et al. Primary thymic carcinoma: a clinicopathological and immunohistochemical study. J Surg Oncol 1994;56:159–164.
99. Yano T, Hara N, Ichinose Y, Asoh H, Yokoyama H, Ohta M. Treatment and prognosis of primary thymic carcinoma. J Surg Oncol 1993;52:255–258.
100. Hasserjian RP, Klimstra DS, Rosai J. Carcinoma of the thymus with clear-cell features. Report of eight cases and review of the literature. Am J Surg Pathol 1995;19:835–841.
101. Weide LG, Ulbright TM, Loehrer PJ Sr, Williams SD. Thymic carcinoma. A distinct clinical entity responsive to chemotherapy. Cancer (Phila) 1993;71:1219–1223.
102. Lucchi M, Mussi A, Basolo F, Ambrogi MC, Fontanini G, Angeletti CA. The multimodality treatment of thymic carcinoma. Eur J Cardiothorac Surg 2001;19:566–569.
103. Lucchi M, Mussi A, Ambrogi M, et al. Thymic carcinoma: a report of 13 cases. Eur J Surg Oncol 2001;27:636–640.
104. Rosai J, Higa E, Davie J. Mediastinal endocrine neoplasm in patients with multiple endocrine adenomatosis. A previously unrecognized association. Cancer (Phila) 1972;29:1075–1083.
105. Rosai J, Higa E. Mediastinal endocrine neoplasm, of probable thymic origin, related to carcinoid tumor. Clinicopathologic study of 8 cases. Cancer (Phila) 1972;29:1061–1074.
106. Wick MR, Carney JA, Bernatz PE, Brown LR. Primary mediastinal carcinoid tumors. Am J Surg Pathol 1982;6:195–205.
107. Wang DY, Chang DB, Kuo SH, et al. Carcinoid tumours of the thymus. Thorax 1994;49:357–360.
108. de Montpreville VT, Macchiarini P, Dulmet E. Thymic neuroendocrine carcinoma (carcinoid): a clinicopathologic study of fourteen cases. J Thorac Cardiovasc Surg 1996;111:134–141.
109. Economopoulos GC, Lewis JW Jr, Lee MW, Silverman NA. Carcinoid tumors of the thymus. Ann Thorac Surg 1990;50:58–61.
110. Chakravarthy A, Abrams RA. Radiation therapy in the management of patients with malignant carcinoid tumors. Cancer (Phila) 1995;75:1386–1390.
111. Kondo K, Monden Y. Therapy for thymic epithelial tumors: a clinical study of 1,320 patients from Japan. Ann Thorac Surg 2003;76:878–884; discussion 884–875.
112. Asbun HJ, Calabria RP, Calmes S, Lang AG, Bloch JH. Thymic carcinoid. Am Surg 1991;57:442–445.
113. Caceres W, Baldizon C, Sanchez J. Carcinoid tumor of the thymus: a unique neoplasm of the mediastinum. Am J Clin Oncol 1998;21:82–83.
114. Moran CA, Rosado-de-Christenson M, Suster S. Thymolipoma: clinicopathologic review of 33 cases. Mod Pathol 1995;8:741–744.
115. Rosado-de-Christenson ML, Pugatch RD, Moran CA, Galobardes J. Thymolipoma: analysis of 27 cases. Radiology 1994;193:121–126.
116. Mishra SK, Melinkeri SR, Dabadghao S. Benign thymic hyperplasia after chemotherapy for acute myeloid leukemia. Eur J Haematol 2001;67:252–254.
117. Cohen M, Hill CA, Cangir A, Sullivan MP. Thymic rebound after treatment of childhood tumors. AJR Am J Roentgenol 1980;135:151–156.
118. Schlumberger H. Teratoma of the anterior mediastinum. Arch Pathol 1946;41:398–444.
119. Friedman NB. The function of the primordial germ cell in extragonadal tissues. Int J Androl 1987;10:43–49.
120. Moran CA, Suster S. Primary germ cell tumors of the mediastinum: I. Analysis of 322 cases with special emphasis on teratomatous lesions and a proposal for histopathologic classification and clinical staging. Cancer (Phila) 1997;80:681–690.
121. Moran CA. Germ cell tumors of the mediastinum. Pathol Res Pract 1999;195:583–587.
122. Nichols CR. Mediastinal germ cell tumors. Clinical features and biologic correlates. Chest 1991;99:472–479.
123. Takeda S, Miyoshi S, Ohta M, Minami M, Masaoka A, Matsuda H. Primary germ cell tumors in the mediastinum: a 50-year experience at a single Japanese institution. Cancer (Phila) 2003; 97:367–376.
124. Lewis BD, Hurt RD, Payne WS, Farrow GM, Knapp RH, Muhm JR. Benign teratomas of the mediastinum. J Thorac Cardiovasc Surg 1983;86:727–731.
125. Brown LR, Muhm JR, Aughenbaugh GL, Lewis BD, Hurt RD. Computed tomography of benign mature teratomas of the mediastinum. J Thorac Imaging 1987;2:66–71.
126. Moran CA, Suster S, Przygodzki RM, Koss MN. Primary germ cell tumors of the mediastinum: II. Mediastinal seminomas: a clinicopathologic and immunohistochemical study of 120 cases. Cancer (Phila) 1997;80:691–698.
127. Strollo DC, Rosado-de-Christenson ML. Primary mediastinal malignant germ cell neoplasms: imaging features. Chest Surg Clin N Am 2002;12:645–658.
128. Cefaro GA, Luzi S, Turriziani A, Salvi G, Marmiroli L. Primary mediastinal seminoma. Br J Urol 1988;62:461–464.
129. Motzer RJ, Bosl GJ, Geller NL, et al. Advanced seminoma: the role of chemotherapy and adjunctive surgery. Ann Intern Med 1988;108:513–518.
130. Gholam D, Fizazi K, Terrier-Lacombe MJ, Jan P, Culine S, Theodore C. Advanced seminoma: treatment results and prognostic factors for survival after first-line, cisplatin-based chemotherapy and for patients with recurrent disease: a single-institution experience in 145 patients. Cancer (Phila) 2003;98: 745–752.
131. Kersh CR, Eisert DR, Constable WC, et al. Primary malignant mediastinal germ-cell tumors and the contribution of radiotherapy: a southeastern multi-institutional study. Am J Clin Oncol 1987;10:302–306.
132. Aygun C, Slawson RG, Bajaj K, Salazar OM. Primary mediastinal seminoma. Urology 1984;23:109–117.
133. Puc HS, Heelan R, Mazumdar M, et al. Management of residual mass in advanced seminoma: results and recommendations from the Memorial Sloan-Kettering Cancer Center. J Clin Oncol 1996;14:454–460.
134. Osada H, Kojima K, Yamate N. Primary mediastinal seminoma. Efficacy of chemo-radiotherapy alone. Jpn J Thorac Cardiovasc Surg 1998;46:810–814.

135. Wright CD, Kesler KA, Nichols CR, et al. Primary mediastinal nonseminomatous germ cell tumors. Results of a multimodality approach. J Thorac Cardiovasc Surg 1990;99:210–217.
136. Dexeus FH, Logothetis CJ, Chong C, Sella A, Ogden S. Genetic abnormalities in men with germ cell tumors. J Urol 1988;140: 80–84.
137. International Germ Cell Consensus Classification: a prognostic factor-based staging system for metastatic germ cell cancers. International Germ Cell Cancer Collaborative Group. J Clin Oncol 1997;15:594–603.
138. Nichols CR, Roth BJ, Heerema N, Griep J, Tricot G. Hematologic neoplasia associated with primary mediastinal germ-cell tumors. N Engl J Med 1990;322:1425–1429.
139. Moran CA, Suster S, Koss MN. Primary germ cell tumors of the mediastinum: III. Yolk sac tumor, embryonal carcinoma, choriocarcinoma, and combined nonteratomatous germ cell tumors of the mediastinum: a clinicopathologic and immunohistochemical study of 64 cases. Cancer (Phila) 1997;80:699–707.
140. Bukowski RM, Wolf M, Kulander BG, Montie J, Crawford ED, Blumenstein B. Alternating combination chemotherapy in patients with extragonadal germ cell tumors. A Southwest Oncology Group study. Cancer (Phila) 1993;71:2631–2638.
141. Economou JS, Trump DL, Holmes EC, Eggleston JE. Management of primary germ cell tumors of the mediastinum. J Thorac Cardiovasc Surg 1982;83:643–649.
142. Nichols CR, Saxman S, Williams SD, et al. Primary mediastinal nonseminomatous germ cell tumors. A modern single institution experience. Cancer (Phila) 1990;65:1641–1646.
143. Kesler KA, Rieger KM, Ganjoo KN, et al. Primary mediastinal nonseminomatous germ cell tumors: the influence of post-chemotherapy pathology on long-term survival after surgery. J Thorac Cardiovasc Surg 1999;118:692–700.
144. Bokemeyer C, Schleucher N, Metzner B, et al. First-line sequential high-dose VIP chemotherapy with autologous transplantation for patients with primary mediastinal nonseminomatous germ cell tumours: a prospective trial. Br J Cancer 2003;89: 29–35.
145. Bokemeyer C, Nichols CR, Droz JP, et al. Extragonadal germ cell tumors of the mediastinum and retroperitoneum: results from an international analysis. J Clin Oncol 2002;20:1864–1873.
146. Hartmann JT, Nichols CR, Droz JP, et al. Prognostic variables for response and outcome in patients with extragonadal germ-cell tumors. Ann Oncol 2002;13:1017–1028.
147. Fizazi K, Culine S, Droz JP, et al. Primary mediastinal nonseminomatous germ cell tumors: results of modern therapy including cisplatin-based chemotherapy. J Clin Oncol 1998;16: 725–732.
148. Reed JC, Sobonya RE. Morphologic analysis of foregut cysts in the thorax. Am J Roentgenol Radium Ther Nucl Med 1974;120: 851–860.
149. Zambudio AR, Lanzas JT, Calvo MJ, Fernandez PJ, Paricio PP. Non-neoplastic mediastinal cysts. Eur J Cardiothorac Surg 2002; 22:712–716.
150. Strollo DC, Rosado-de-Christenson ML, Jett JR. Primary mediastinal tumors: part II. Tumors of the middle and posterior mediastinum. Chest 1997;112:1344–1357.
151. Smythe WR, Bavaria JE, Kaiser LR. Mediastinoscopic subtotal removal of mediastinal cysts. Chest 1998;114:614–617.
152. Dernellis J, Theodosiou P, Fois L. An asymptomatic giant pericardial cyst. Int J Cardiol 2001;78:185–187.
153. Davidson KG, Walbaum PR, McCormack RJ. Intrathoracic neural tumours. Thorax 1978;33:359–367.
154. Topcu S, Alper A, Gulhan E, Kocyigit O, Tastepe I, Cetin G. Neurogenic tumours of the mediastinum: a report of 60 cases. Can Respir J 2000;7:261–265.
155. Akwari OE, Payne WS, Onofrio BM, Dines DE, Muhm JR. Dumbbell neurogenic tumors of the mediastinum. Diagnosis and management. Mayo Clin Proc 1978;53:353–358.
156. Ribet ME, Cardot GR. Neurogenic tumors of the thorax. Ann Thorac Surg 1994;58:1091–1095.
157. Divisi D, Battaglia C, Crisci R, et al. Diagnostic and therapeutic approaches for masses in the posterior mediastinum. Acta Biomed Ateneo Parmense 1998;69:123–128.
158. Canvasser DA, Naunheim KS. Thoracoscopic management of posterior mediastinal tumors. Chest Surg Clin N Am 1996;6: 53–67.
159. Vallieres E, Findlay JM, Fraser RE. Combined microneurosurgical and thoracoscopic removal of neurogenic dumbbell tumors. Ann Thorac Surg 1995;59:469–472.
160. Ducatman BS, Scheithauer BW, Piepgras DG, Reiman HM, Ilstrup DM. Malignant peripheral nerve sheath tumors. A clinicopathologic study of 120 cases. Cancer (Phila) 1986;57:2006–2021.
161. McComb EN, McComb RD, DeBoer JM, Neff JR, Bridge JA. Cytogenetic analysis of a malignant triton tumor and a malignant peripheral nerve sheath tumor and a review of the literature. Cancer Genet Cytogenet 1996;91:8–12.
162. Ghosh BC, Ghosh L, Huvos AG, Fortner JG. Malignant schwannoma. A clinicopathologic study. Cancer (Phila) 1973;31:184–190.
163. Shimada H, Chatten J, Newton WA Jr, et al. Histopathologic prognostic factors in neuroblastic tumors: definition of subtypes of ganglioneuroblastoma and an age-linked classification of neuroblastomas. J Natl Cancer Inst 1984;73:405–416.
164. Geoerger B, Hero B, Harms D, Grebe J, Scheidhauer K, Berthold F. Metabolic activity and clinical features of primary ganglioneuromas. Cancer (Phila) 2001;91:1905–1913.
165. Gale AW, Jelihovsky T, Grant AF, Leckie BD, Nicks R. Neurogenic tumors of the mediastinum. Ann Thorac Surg 1974;17: 434–443.
166. Adam A, Hochholzer L. Ganglioneuroblastoma of the posterior mediastinum: a clinicopathologic review of 80 cases. Cancer (Phila) 1981;47:373–381.
167. Castleberry RP. Neuroblastoma. Eur J Cancer 1997;33:1430–1437; discussion 1437–1438.
168. Schwab M, Westermann F, Hero B, Berthold F. Neuroblastoma: biology and molecular and chromosomal pathology. Lancet Oncol 2003;4:472–480.
169. Brodeur GM, Seeger RC, Barrett A, et al. International criteria for diagnosis, staging, and response to treatment in patients with neuroblastoma. J Clin Oncol 1988;6:1874–1881.
170. Alvarado CS, London WB, Look AT, et al. Natural history and biology of stage A neuroblastoma: a Pediatric Oncology Group Study. J Pediatr Hematol Oncol 2000;22:197–205.
171. Nitschke R, Smith EI, Shochat S, et al. Localized neuroblastoma treated by surgery: a Pediatric Oncology Group Study. J Clin Oncol 1988;6:1271–1279.
172. Castleberry RP, Kun LE, Shuster JJ, et al. Radiotherapy improves the outlook for patients older than 1 year with Pediatric Oncology Group stage C neuroblastoma. J Clin Oncol 1991;9:789–795.
173. Morris JA, Shcochat SJ, Smith EI, et al. Biological variables in thoracic neuroblastoma: a Pediatric Oncology Group study. J Pediatr Surg 1995;30:296–302.
174. Haberle B, Hero B, Berthold F, von Schweinitz D. Characteristics and outcome of thoracic neuroblastoma. Eur J Pediatr Surg 2002;12:145–150.
175. vanSonnenberg E, Casola G, Ho M, et al. Difficult thoracic lesions: CT-guided biopsy experience in 150 cases. Radiology 1988;167:457–461.
176. Morrissey B, Adams H, Gibbs AR, Crane MD. Percutaneous needle biopsy of the mediastinum: review of 94 procedures. Thorax 1993;48:632–637.
177. Sterchi M, Cordell AR. Seminoma of the anterior mediastinum. Ann Thorac Surg 1975;19:371–377.
178. Polansky SM, Barwick KW, Ravin CE. Primary mediastinal seminoma. AJR Am J Roentgenol 1979;132:17–21.

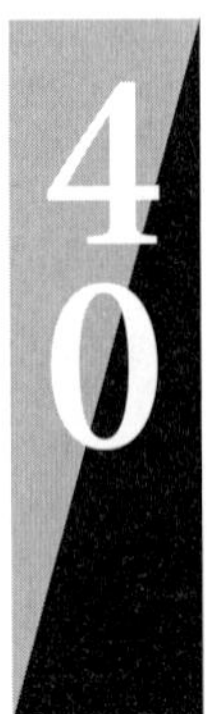

Esophageal Cancer

John D. Urschel

Esophageal cancer is a notoriously difficult cancer to treat. Locoregional therapies, such as surgery and radiotherapy, are hampered by the anatomic proximity of the esophagus to vital structures, its rich and multidirectional lymphatic plexus, and, typically, by the late stage of symptomatic disease. Currently available systemic therapies, such as chemotherapy, are effective but they leave much to be desired. Chemotherapy's effectiveness, perhaps surprisingly, relates in large measure to its synergism with radiotherapy at the locoregional level. All the major treatment modalities are hampered by the typical patient's inability to easily tolerate aggressive therapy, but this is especially so for surgical therapy. One only has to contrast the rigors of esophagectomy, especially after chemoradiation, with the tolerability of breast cancer surgery or right hemicolectomy, to see this point. Taking these factors together, esophageal cancer remains one of the most difficult cancers for an oncologist of any discipline to treat and one of the most difficult malignant illnesses that a patient can face. Sadly, it is also a cancer that is rapidly increasing in incidence, at least in the Western world.

Despite the gloomy introductory remarks to this chapter, there is some reason for optimism. Progress, albeit modest, has been made in the past several decades.[1] The stage-specific effectiveness of the major therapies—surgery, radiotherapy, and chemotherapy—has improved markedly. This change relates, in part, to real progress in each field, but better patient selection and stage migration have also played a role. Population-based statistics from several countries now show 5-year survivals in excess of 10%, instead of the consistently single-digit figures from previous eras.[2] Although these data largely confirm that true progress has been made, a cynic might still take exception. The disease itself has changed, at least in the Western world, and the new disease, with its predilection for the distal esophagus, is in some ways easier to treat.

Not all improvements in oncology can be measured with endpoints such as 5-year survival. Progress in the areas of imaging and staging has been particularly striking, and patients have benefited greatly from these advances. Many have been spared the exploratory operations and incomplete "palliative" resections that were so common in the past. Advances have also been made in the palliation of malignant symptoms, especially dysphagia. Endoscopic techniques have replaced surgical interventions for dysphagia, and the endoscopic methods themselves have become less morbid. Although these advances cannot be captured in survival data, they are nevertheless very important. Progress in esophageal cancer treatment has been made, and practitioners should be excited and hopeful about the future.

This chapter is not a uniform overview of all aspects of esophageal cancer. Following the theme of this textbook, emphasis is placed on subject areas that have been studied by randomized controlled trials. The randomized controlled trials, in aggregate, provide the evidence upon which we base our clinical practices. The chapter also emphasizes the questions in clinical practice that are characterized by hard choice constraints, where we must decide between two alternatives (for example, primary surgery versus definitive chemoradiation), as opposed to soft choice constraints, where we decide if an additional intervention may be valuable [for example, computed tomography (CT) scanning versus CT and positron emission tomography (PET)]. This is not to say that soft constraints, which involve issues of cost, feasibility, and efficiency, are not important; they are. For clinicians (and by extension, patients), however, it is the choice between mutually exclusive treatment options that weigh most heavily on the mind. Finally, the chapter seeks to clarify topics that are prone to confusion, such as those relating to surgery, while avoiding duplication of topics covered elsewhere in the textbook, such as diagnostic imaging.

Problems of Data Aggregation

One of the purposes of this textbook is to help clinicians make sense of the huge body of published data on any given malignancy. In the process of aggregating data we, by necessity, ignore certain types of information in each original data source or, stated differently, we abstract the critical information from the less-important detail. It is easy to lose sight of the simplifying assumptions that we make during data aggregation, and this is especially the case for the esophageal cancer literature. The major problems in aggregating esophageal cancer data that distinguish this subject of study from others in this textbook are the following: (i) different histologies, that is, squamous carcinoma and adenocarcinoma; (ii) different classification and staging schemes for adenocarcinomas involving the esophagogastric junction; and (iii) East versus West dichotomy.[3,4]

Squamous carcinomas and adenocarcinomas are arguably very similar in their very general features of lethality and response to treatment. However, even if this is assumed to be the case, the two histologies diverge in other important ways.

The typical patient suffering from squamous cancer of the esophagus differs from one with adenocarcinoma and poses different treatment challenges. The profile of the former includes a history of smoking and consuming alcohol, poor nutrition, a tumor in proximity to the tracheobronchial tree, involvement of lymphatics adjacent to the recurrent laryngeal nerves, difficult surgical resections that usually require a thoracotomy approach, radial resection margins that are commonly positive, and a propensity to postoperative pulmonary complications. In contrast, a typical patient suffering from adenocarcinoma is often a heavy-set nonsmoker, with a more readily resectable distal esophageal tumor (often not requiring a thoracotomy), but with lymphatic involvement of both the mediastinal and abdominal lymphatics. These generalizations, as simplistic as they are, should be kept in mind as we review aggregated patient data.

Turning to the second issue, adenocarcinomas that involve the esophagogastric junction present a major problem for the classification and staging of foregut cancers and the interpretation of published literature. These adenocarcinomas of the esophagogastric junction, or AEGs, frustrate our attempts to develop valid treatment concepts in both esophageal and gastric disease sites. Controversy abounds as how to best classify these tumors. Are they all variants of the same malignant condition, or are they very different? That question has bearing on their classification. Siewert's classification organizes tumors that involve the esophagogastric junction into three types.[5] AEG I tumors arise in the distal esophagus from malignant transformation of Barrett's esophagus (which in turn is caused by gastroesophageal reflux), and extend to the esophagogastric junction. They are primarily esophageal tumors and should be treated as such. The surgical therapy is esophagectomy. AEG type III tumors arise in the proximal stomach and extend upward into the junction. They share a common etiology with other gastric tumors (*Helicobacter pylori* infection and nutritional risk factors) and should be treated as gastric tumors. The surgical therapy is total gastrectomy and abdominal lymph node dissection. AEG type II tumors, or true tumors of the cardia, arise at the esophagogastric junction. Their origin is hotly debated, and their optimal treatment is unclear. Siewert makes a case for treating these tumors as gastric cancers, with the surgical treatment being total gastrectomy and limited resection of the distal esophagus. Others favor operations that place the cancer at the epicenter of the resection (esophagogastrectomy).

Readers may be forgiven for thinking that the AEG classification is primarily of interest to surgeons, but they will nevertheless be mistaken. Two virtually identical AEG tumors may be classified, staged, treated, and reported in completely different fashions, depending on the point of view of the treating physicians. This practice causes tremendous confusion in the data aggregation process. For example, one center might classify an AEG tumor as an esophageal cancer, treat with chemoradiation followed by transhiatal or transthoracic total esophagectomy (based on a published randomized controlled trial), stage involved celiac nodes as stage IVA–M_{1a} (distant lymph nodes; Table 40.1) disease, and report the results accordingly. Another center may classify the same AEG tumor as a gastric cancer, proceed with staging laparoscopy followed by total gastrectomy and D2 lymph node dissection, give postoperative chemoradiation (based on a published randomized controlled trial), stage the involved celiac axis nodes according to the total number of involved nodes (versus location), assign a final stage that is much more favorable than stage IV, and report the results accordingly. Both centers, arguably, have proceeded correctly. This problem frustrates rational attempts at data aggregation.

TABLE 40.1. Definition of TNM and stage grouping for esophageal carcinoma.

Primary tumor (T)			
TX	Primary tumor cannot be assessed		
T0	No evidence of primary tumor		
Tis	Carcinoma in situ		
T1	Tumor invades lamina propria or submucosa		
T2	Tumor invades muscularis propria		
T3	Tumor invades adventitia		
T4	Tumor invades adjacent structures		
Regional lymph nodes (N)			
NX	Regional lymph nodes cannot be assessed		
N0	No regional lymph node metastasis		
N1	Regional lymph node metastasis		
Distant metastasis (M)			
MX	Distant metastasis cannot be assessed		
M0	No distant metastasis		
M1	Distant metastasis		
Stage grouping			
Stage 0	Tis	N0	M0
Stage I	T1	N0	M0
Stage IIA	T2	N0	M0
	T3	N0	M0
Stage IIB	T1	N1	M0
	T2	N1	M0
Stage III	T3	N1	M0
	T4	Any N	M0
Stage IV	Any T	Any N	M1
Stage IVA	Any T	Any N	M1a
Stage IVB	Any T	Any N	M1b

Source: Used with the permission of the American Joint Committee on Cancer (AJCC), Chicago, Illinois. The original source for this material is the *AJCC Cancer Staging Manual*, sixth edition (2002), published by Springer-Verlag New York, www.springer-ny.com.

The third problem, East–West dichotomy, at first glance seems a redundant restatement of the differential histology problem. Admittedly, that is partly the case. Its importance, however, relates to the assessment of trials across time. The East–West dichotomy shows a widening trend, so as more trials are done it will be increasingly difficult to justify the inclusion of both East and West experience in a single meta-analysis or review.[4]

Epidemiology and Screening

At one time esophageal cancer was considered a single disease, squamous cancer, with its incidence varying across the world in accordance with known risk factors.[6] Risk factors for squamous cancer include smoking, alcohol consumption, nutritional deficiencies, and low socioeconomic status. In the United States, poor black males were commonly affected. Since the 1970s adenocarcinoma of the esophagus has increased in incidence in the West while the incidence of squamous cancer has decreased.[7] Adenocarcinoma is now the dominant form of esophageal cancer in the West whereas squamous cancer continues to dominate in the East. Risk factors for adenocarcinoma of the esophagus include gastroesophageal reflux, obesity, and, to a lesser extent, cigarette smoking. Almost all esophageal adenocarcinomas arise in specialized intestinal metaplastic epithelium (Barrett's esophagus) and pass through a metaplasia–dysplasia–cancer sequence.[8] Barrett's esophagus, in turn, is caused by chronic reflux. Although obesity and reflux affect males and females almost equally, adenocarcinoma typically affects males (white males). Our understanding of this disease is obviously incomplete.

Preventive strategies for squamous cancer include avoidance of smoking and excess alcohol consumption and eating a balanced diet that includes fresh vegetables. The decline in squamous cancer incidence in the West is probably (at least in part) the result of these types of behavioral change. Prevention of adenocarcinoma is more controversial. Few would take exception with recommendations to avoid obesity and cigarette smoking (although cigarette smoking is much less important in the etiology of adenocarcinoma than it is in squamous cancer). Dealing with reflux, however, is problematic. Symptoms can be controlled with medications, but the underlying reflux of harmful, usually alkaline, gastroduodenal material continues. Some have suggested a role for antireflux surgery to eliminate reflux and thereby reduce the risk of adenocarcinoma. Large-scale population-based antireflux surgery programs, while perhaps a dream in certain surgical circles, are simply not practical or warranted. Importantly, antireflux surgery has not been proven to reduce the risk of adenocarcinoma, and the surgery itself is not innocuous.[9,10] Other areas of preventive interest include the role of *H. pylori* infection, or rather the lack thereof, and the possible protective effect of cyclooxygenase 2 (COX-2) inhibitors. There is some suggestion that *H. pylori* infection, although central to the genesis of gastric cancer, may somehow protect against esophageal adenocarcinoma. This, however, is far from clear. Interest in COX-2 inhibitors follows from their use as chemopreventive agents in other gastrointestinal sites, notably the colon.

Clinicians are very aware that the prospective for cure is greatest among patients whose esophageal cancer is detected by screening, either formal or ad hoc. However, that does not mean that screening for esophageal cancer is effective as a population-level health strategy.[11] The issues are not simple, as this textbook's two chapters on screening make clear. Salient problems (in the West) include the uncertainty of diagnosis of high-grade dysplasia, inability to predict progression from dysplasia to invasive cancer, and the operative mortality of esophagectomy. Readers familiar with the (apparent) success of cervical cancer screening programs should ask themselves what might have happened if cone biopsies were not really reliable and hysterectomy carried an operable mortality of 15% in nonspecialized centers. Finally, clinicians embarking on the screening of elderly or frail patients might want to reconsider. The unfortunate combination of postesophagectomy death and a "negative" pathology report is not unknown.

Staging and Patient Assessment

Advances in the staging of esophageal cancer have greatly influenced the contemporary management of this disease.[1,12] Many of these advances belong to the field of diagnostic imaging, and readers are referred to the chapters on thoracic and gastrointestinal imaging for detailed treatment of these subjects. The benefits of accurate staging are difficult to overstate. Once common, but futile, surgical interventions are now less frequent than in previous eras. The modern staging exercise can be stratified into three salient questions: (i) is metastatic disease present? (ii) if not, what is the precise locoregional stage? and (iii) how fit is the patient for aggressive treatments, especially surgery?

The first question is best answered with a combination of CT scanning and PET scanning. PET scanning identifies metastatic disease in approximately 20% of patients who appear to be free of metastases on other imaging studies.[13] This accuracy in the detection of metastatic disease, along with PET's promising role in assessing response to treatment, makes PET scanning a major advance in esophageal cancer management.[14] Once metastatic disease is confirmed, further detailed staging investigations are generally not needed.

Precise locoregional staging is best accomplished with endoscopic ultrasonography (EUS) and, to a lesser extent, multislice CT scanning. EUS provides the most accurate assessment of T stage, with its accuracy being especially sharp (near 90%) if clinically relevant and relatively simple discriminations, such as T1–T2 versus T3–T4 assessments are made (as opposed to T-specific measures). Newer, slimmer instruments have partly solved the problem of a tight stricture, which has previously precluded passage of the endoscopic probe. Arguably, however, failure to pass the standard EUS instrument is itself an indicator of advanced T stage. EUS also provides valuable staging information about regional lymph node involvement. Unlike CT determinations, which are mostly based on node size, EUS gives an image of both size and character (central necrosis, for example). Endoscopic transesophageal fine-needle aspiration biopsy techniques have extended the usefulness of EUS in regional lymph node staging.

The place of invasive staging, namely thoracoscopy and laparoscopy, is not well defined.[12,15] Proponents of invasive staging hope to duplicate the success of mediastinoscopy in non-small cell lung cancer staging (one of the few established examples of surgical staging). Mediastinoscopy in lung cancer, however, provides a fairly simple outpatient assessment of the lymph nodes of interest, answers a focused and specific question, and is relatively accurate. Proficient operators can sample the relevant nodes in approximately 20 minutes. Thoracoscopy, in contrast, is much more involved, and the question or questions of interest are not as focused. One lung anesthesia is required. Dissection of relevant nodes takes time. As a rule, postoperative hospitalization and a chest tube are needed. Hospitalization can extend to several days.[15] Although thoracoscopy incisions are small, the associated pain is often out of proportion to size because of intercostal nerve trauma.

Laparoscopy is better tolerated than thoracoscopy. In gastric cancer, a malignancy known for its propensity for intraperitoneal dissemination, laparoscopy makes sense; imaging studies often miss peritoneal seeding. However, the rationale for routine laparoscopy in esophageal cancer staging is less compelling. Peritoneal metastases are not frequent. One of the alleged advantages of laparoscopy, obtaining information on celiac axis node involvement, is suspect. In many reported series the celiac nodes are simply visually inspected; fully dissecting the celiac nodes, while at the same time preserving the vessels, is not a minor undertaking. In summary, the case for routine invasive staging of esophageal malignancies is tenuous.

Assessment of fitness is an important aspect of a patient's workup, especially if surgery is considered. The preoperative assessment process has been formalized in several specialized esophageal surgery centers. Composite scoring systems have been developed that accurately stratify patients according to operative risk. One system emphasizes general status, cardiac, hepatic, and pulmonary function, while another uses age, FEV_1 (forced expiratory volume in 1 second), and performance status.[16,17] Unfortunately, composite scoring systems do not enjoy widespread use.

Treatment: General Concepts

The treatment of esophageal cancer, similar to that of other solid tumors, is dictated by cancer stage and patient fitness.[1,4,18,19] Although it is possible to think of treatment and develop algorithms in terms of each specific cancer stage, the process of data aggregation across clinical trials does not lend itself to this degree of precision. Rather, crude stage groupings must be used. A useful stage grouping categorizes patients into three groups: (1) early-stage disease (T1–2N0), (2) locoregional disease (more advanced than early-stage disease but no metastatic disease), and (3) metastatic disease. A few additional qualifications to this simplified scheme are helpful. Within the second category of locoregional disease, a practical subdivision can be made based on surgical considerations. The group can be divided into those patients who have a reasonable expectation of undergoing a complete, or R0, resection if primary surgery is performed and those who do not. This distinction is not always easy; considerable experience and good judgment are needed. The third category, metastatic disease, can be expanded to include frail patients who cannot tolerate aggressive, curative-intent, treatment. These patients are often treated along the same lines as those with metastatic disease, but for different reasons.

Treatment: Early-Stage Esophageal Cancer

Patients with early-stage esophageal cancer cannot be approached in an evidence-based fashion, at least not in the usual sense of the term. Large-scale randomized trials have not been conducted in this group of patients, nor are they likely to be done in the near future. Treatment is instead based on what might be called a reason-based approach.[18,19] Surgical resection is effective in this group of patients, so it is reasonable to deem this the standard by which other treatments are compared. Five-year survivals in excess of 50% are reported, and operative mortality is lower than that of unselected surgical patients (well below 5%). Nevertheless, it is very possible that the same results, or perhaps better, could be obtained with other treatments such as chemoradiation. Because patients with unfavorable comorbidities tend to be treated nonoperatively, fair comparisons are hard to come by.

Patients with very early disease (subgroups of T1a) may be treated with various endoscopic approaches, such as endoscopic mucosal resection, and in this way esophagectomy is avoided. However, these endoscopic treatments may have a higher cancer recurrence rate than traditional esophageal resection. Recurrence can result from underestimation of the true stage of disease (staging imprecision), inherent limitation of endoscopic treatment methods, or a combination of the two. The techniques are probably best suited for patients too frail to safely undergo esophageal resection.

Treatment: Locoregional Esophageal Cancer

This stage of esophageal cancer has generated the greatest controversy in management and, appropriately, the largest number of randomized controlled trials (RCTs). As a result of RCTs there is now broad agreement on several points: concurrent chemoradiation is superior to radiotherapy as a nonoperative treatment, preoperative radiotherapy is not effective, and the routine administration of postoperative radiotherapy is not warranted. Nevertheless, many controversies exist. One seemingly basic problem is the choice of a standard treatment (control arm) for comparison purposes. One approach is to start with treatments that have history on their side, such as surgery. This rationale is used by those who proclaim surgery as the "gold" standard. Not only does the term gold seem excessive (5-year survival is typically 20% to 25%), but the logic of using history as a criterion is questionable. Surgery is standard through precedent; other treatments require compelling evidence to become standard. The failure of a notable American intergroup trial, which tried to compare chemoradiation and surgery to surgery alone, to accrue patients suggests that, in the United States, at least, clinicians are uncomfortable with the historical surgical standard. An alternative approach is to use frequency of use as a basis for the standard. Using this argument, chemoradiation is a standard treatment for locoregional esophageal cancer in the United States.[18] In this chapter two treatments, surgery alone and definitive chemoradiation (not to be confused with neoadjuvant chemoradiation), are discussed as standard treatments, and then other treatment options are measured against them. These other treatments are grouped into three categories: (1) investigational treatments of current interest, (2) investigational treatments of some interest, and (3) treatments shown to be inferior (of no current interest) (Table 40.2).

TABLE 40.2. Treatment options for locoregional stage esophageal cancer (curative intent).

I. Standard treatments, against which other treatments are compared:
  1. Surgery alone
  2. Definitive chemoradiation

II. Investigational treatments of current interest:
  1. Neoadjuvant chemotherapy and surgery
  2. Neoadjuvant chemoradiation and surgery
  3. Definitive chemoradiation with possible salvage esophagectomy

III. Investigational treatments of some interest:
  1. Surgery and adjuvant chemotherapy
  2. Surgery and adjuvant chemoradiation

IV. Inferior treatments (of no interest):
  1. Radiation alone
  2. Neoadjuvant radiation and surgery
  3. Surgery and adjuvant radiation

Standard Treatments

Surgery Alone

Esophagectomy for locoregional stage cancer typically cures 20% to 25% of patients (a higher percentage if patients are very carefully selected), but approximately 5% to 10% of patients succumb to postoperative complications (a lower percentage if patients are carefully selected or statistical liberties are taken).[20] Unlike chemotherapy and radiotherapy, surgery is difficult to standardize. The innumerable ways to remove an esophagus, and then put something in its place, provide surgeons with an endless list of topics to debate at meetings and frustrate the nonsurgeon who wishes to abstract the essential surgical concepts from the trivia. In what follows, an abstraction of the essential surgical concepts and controversies is presented (Table 40.3).

Generally Accepted Surgical Concepts

The central concept of surgery for cancer of the esophagus has changed over the past several decades.[19] Surgeons once performed esophagectomy because it effectively palliated dysphagia and because a few fortunate, and largely a priori unidentifiable, patients were cured. There are now less-morbid methods to palliate dysphagia, so palliative intent esophagectomy is no longer a valid concept. The goal of modern esophageal cancer resection is to perform a complete (R0) cancer resection. Microscopically (R1) and macroscopically (R2) incomplete resections provide little benefit. In fact, these incomplete resections are often harmful. Not only is perioperative mortality high in this group, but potentially curative alternatives such as definitive chemoradiation are foregone. Primary surgery should therefore only be offered to patients in whom there is a reasonable expectation of achieving a complete resection. Patients with bulky tumors that are closely apposed to vital structures (for example, the tracheobronchial tree and aorta) should be viewed with caution, as should those with obvious lymph node metastases. It is difficult to perform a complete resection in these patients.

TABLE 40.3. Surgical concepts: agreement and controversies.

Agreement:
1. A complete (R0) resection is the overriding goal of surgical therapy
2. Incomplete resections are of little, if any, benefit
3. There is no place for palliative-intent surgery
4. Primary surgery should be restricted to those patients in whom there is a reasonable expectation of an R0 resection
5. There is a relationship between surgical volumes and outcomes

Controversies:
1. Operative approach (transthoracic, transhiatal, other)
2. Extent of resection (axial, radial, lymphatic)
3. Methods of reconstruction
4. Surgery as a component of multimodality therapy
5. Validity of the salvage esophagectomy concept

How can we tell, after the fact, if a resection was complete? The pathology report is obviously critical, but so is a thoughtfully dictated operative report. The pathologist can only comment on the submitted specimens, not the tissues and lymph nodes remaining in situ; it is up to the surgeon to describe these things. We usually think in terms of resection margins, but physicians often unduly emphasize one margin (the easiest to quantify and conceptualize) while paying less attention to the other margins (the more difficult to quantify and conceptualize). There are three resection margins: axial (proximal and distal), radial, and lymphatic.[4,19] The axial margins tend to receive the greatest attention. They are the easiest for the pathologist to measure and report and the easiest for physicians to understand. Positive proximal or distal margins indicate an incomplete resection and portend a future anastomotic recurrence. Not surprisingly, generous (many centimeters in the fixed specimen) margins give a lower risk of anastomotic recurrence than close margins (a centimeter or two).[21] Remarkably, microscopically involved margins do not seem to increase the risk of postoperative anastomotic leakage.[22] The radial margins, in contrast to the axial margins, are difficult for the pathologist to assess. Ideally, the esophagus is resected in such a way that normal mediastinal soft tissues completely envelope the area of tumor. By inking the radial margins, the pathologist can state whether the radial margin is clear and by how many millimeters (note the different scale of measurement for axial and radial margins). Often, however, the radial margin is almost nonexistent; this is the rule for a T3 tumor adjacent to the trachea. Here it is difficult for the pathologist, and the surgeon, to tell if a R0 resection has been done. Involved radial margins raise the possibility of recurrence in the tumor bed.

Finally, the lymphatic margin or, more specifically, the lymph node ratio, is often completely ignored. This concept is best described by way of an example. Imagine two seemingly similar pathology reports, each reporting an identical T-stage primary, negative axial and radial resection margins, and cancer in three lymph nodes. The postoperative TNM stage will be the same, and some might imagine a similar prognosis for the two patients. But, what if one specimen shows 3 of 30 nodes positive (lymph node ratio of 0.1) while the other shows 3 of 4 positive (lymph node ratio of 0.75)? One patient has a clear lymphatic margin and a favorable prognosis (lymph node ratio less than 0.2) while the other's R0 status is suspect, along with the prognosis.[23]

Surgical treatment of esophageal cancer, as measured by survival and operative mortality, has improved markedly over the past few decades. Surgery, per se, is not more effective as a cancer treatment than in the past. Progress in esophageal cancer surgery is instead attributable to improved patient selection (better staging), better postoperative care, and surgical experience.[1,24] The experience factor cannot be underestimated. There is now overwhelming evidence that the results of esophageal cancer surgery are better when surgery is done at high-volume hospitals and by experienced surgeons.[25–27] Specialized esophageal surgery centers consistently achieve operative mortalities of less than 5% while the comparable figure for low-volume hospitals and surgeons is closer to 15%. A final factor that may contribute to improved results, at least in the West, is the epidemiologic shift from squamous to adenocarcinomas. Infracarinal esophageal tumors are generally easier to resect, and easier to resect completely, than equivalent stage supracarinal tumors.

Controversies in Esophageal Cancer Surgery

There are five main areas of controversy in esophageal cancer surgery, but most of these controversies are linked in some way to at least one of the other controversies (see Table 40.3).[4] For example, proponents of very radical surgery (extent of resection controversy) usually favor a transthoracic operation (operative approach controversy), and they often view surgery alone as an effective curative treatment strategy (multimodality therapy controversy). Nevertheless, this bundling of the controversies is often overstated and assumed to be present when in fact it is not. Nonsurgeons (and less-experienced surgeons), for example, often mistakenly believe that a transthoracic esophagectomy is, by definition, a more-radical operation than a transhiatal esophagectomy. This is simply not true. The clinics of the world are replete with (unsuspecting) patients who possess the unfortunate combination of a large thoracotomy scar and a pithy pathology report. Conversely, very radical infracarinal en bloc resections of distal esophageal tumors can be done through a transhiatal route.[19]

Operative approaches include (i) laparotomy and right thoracotomy (Ivor Lewis, or Lewis–Tanner), (ii) laparotomy, right thoracotomy, and cervicotomy (McKeown, or three-incision), (iii) left thoracoabdominal, (iv) transhiatal (laparotomy and cervicotomy), and (v) minimally invasive versions of these operations (especially iv and ii).[4] Worldwide, the Lewis transthoracic approach is popular and broadly applicable. It offers generous exposure for dissection, but has the disadvantage of postthoracotomy morbidity, and its intrathoracic anastomosis occasionally gives rise to catastrophic complications.

The McKeown adaptation (properly called three incision, not three field) adds a cervicotomy for fashioning of a cervical anastomosis and gives a little longer proximal resection margin. The cervical anastomosis is a mixed blessing; leaks are less lethal and easier to manage, but most surgeons (not all) have noted an increased tendency for these anastomoses to leak (incidence of 10%–15% versus 5% for intrathoracic anastomoses).[22] The left thoracoabdominal approach gives excellent exposure of the gastric cardia and is one valid option for treatment of type II AEG cancers but otherwise has little to recommend it. Inexperienced operators are easily seduced by its quickness and simplicity, but they often shortchange the proximal margin (the aortic arch is in the way), and the low intrathoracic esophagogastric anastomosis can produce severe reflux. Variations of this operation that take the dissection and the anastomosis above the aortic arch are perfectly acceptable but not popular.

The transhiatal esophagectomy is best suited to infracarinal tumors. Not coincidentally, its surge in popularity mirrors the rise of adenocarcinoma as the dominant cancer in the Western world. The main advantages of the operation are avoidance of thoracotomy (less pain and fewer pulmonary complications) and the mixed blessing of a cervical anastomosis. A radical infracarinal resection can be done (more or less under direct vision), but aggressive dissection cephalad to the carina can create unwanted surprises. In the United States, at least, some surgeons have mistakenly assumed that the lack of a thoracotomy somehow excuses the operator from having a basic familiarity with intrathoracic dissection.

Minimally invasive adaptations of the transhiatal and McKeown esophagectomies have been successfully performed at selected centers throughout the world with good results.[28] There is no reason to condemn these innovations. However, the operations require extraordinary skill, if they are to be done well, and this may limit their use.

Is there any evidence that one operative approach is superior to another? Many comparisons of transhiatal and transthoracic (various types) approaches have been done. Two systematic quantitative reviews of multiple nonrandomized and several underpowered randomized controlled trials (RCTs) failed to show a convincing difference between these approaches.[29,30] However, the most recent RCT, and the only one that was adequately powered, showed lower pulmonary morbidity with the transhiatal approach;[31] this confirms what advocates of the approach have always maintained. Nevertheless, other important outcomes, such as operative mortality and cancer survival, were not shown to be different. Proponents of the transhiatal operation point out that operative mortality was slightly lower (not significant) in the transhiatal group, whereas advocates of transthoracic operations instead dwell on the nonsignificant trend toward better cancer survival with the transthoracic approach. The RCT, as well designed and conducted as it was, still leaves room for debate.

Surgeons agree that a complete (R0) resection is needed, but they differ on how far one must go to achieve this. Both the extent of tumor resection and the extent of lymph node dissection are debated, but these two questions are virtually always bundled together into a single surgical philosophy.[32,33] Tumor resections range from those that simply remove the involved esophagus (little attention to the radial margin), to those that remove the tumor en bloc within a sheath of normal surrounding tissues (for example, the mediastinal fat, posterior pericardium, mediastinal pleura bilaterally, and thoracic duct). En bloc resections of infracarinal tumors are easier to perform than those done for supracarinal tumors; the trachea gets in the way of an anatomically satisfying en bloc resection.

The extent of lymph node dissection ranges from a cursory sampling of regional nodes to a formal anatomic dissection across multiple body sites (abdomen, chest, neck). The term two-field suggests a formal dissection of abdominal and mediastinal nodes, while a three-field dissection adds a neck dissection (the terms two-field and three-field should be used to denote lymph node dissections, not the number of operative incisions). Is there any good evidence that the extent of tumor resection and lymph node dissection make a difference? The aforementioned RCT of transthoracic versus transhiatal esophagectomy is helpful.[31] The transthoracic group received aggressive resections and two-field lymph node dissections; there was a nonsignificant trend toward longer survival. Aggressive resections, although strictly of unproven benefit, may confer some modest benefit.[32–34] The benefit, if it exists, is probably the result of better locoregional control, as opposed to a direct Halstedian impact on cure. One note of caution is in order. Skilled surgeons can perform radical esophageal operations, including a two-field node dissection, with acceptable morbidity. An analogy to the case of D2 dissections for gastric cancer is appropriate. The three-field dissection, however, is another matter. Complications, most commonly related to recurrent laryngeal nerve injury, are very frequent. Without proof of effectiveness, it is difficult to justify routine neck (three-field) dissection for esophageal cancer, especially distal adenocarcinomas.[35]

Controversies surrounding methods of esophageal reconstruction center on the quality of neoforegut function after esophagectomy.[36] The issues include postreconstruction swallowing, conduit emptying, reflux, early satiety, anastomotic and conduit recurrence, and reconstruction-related postoperative mortality. Many of these issues have been studied in RCTs, but because these questions are primarily surgical in nature, interested readers are referred to other sources.[37–40] In brief, most surgeons favor reconstruction with a gastric conduit (versus colon) placed in the posterior mediastinum (versus anterior), and a high thoracic (versus low thoracic) or cervical esophagogastric anastomosis, which can be fashioned by hand or with a stapling instrument (equivalent). A pyloric drainage procedure (pyloroplasty or pyloromyotomy) may be omitted if a narrow gastric tube is used, and care is taken to avoid kinking or twisting of the conduit. Otherwise, a drainage procedure is wise. The final two surgical controversies featured in Table 40.3, surgery as a component of multimodality therapy and salvage esophagectomy, are discussed later in this chapter.

Definitive Chemoradiation

Definitive chemoradiation is the standard nonoperative treatment of locoregional esophageal cancer and rivals surgery as the current treatment of choice.[18,41,42] Many RCTs have compared chemoradiation to radiation alone, the nonoperative standard treatment of the past (Tables 40.4, 40.5).[43–57] Although many of these trials have been negative, most featured suboptimal doses of radiation or chemotherapy. Additionally, many delivered chemotherapy and radiation sequentially (versus concurrently), an approach that is now recognized as inferior. The American RTOG 8501 trial is the only major RCT to feature adequate doses of radiation (50 Gy, 2 Gy per day) and adequate doses of concurrent chemotherapy [5-fluorouracil (5-FU) and cisplatin].[51,52] Its impressive survival results (median survival, 14 versus 9 months; 5-year survival, 27% versus 0%; $P = 0.001$) have made chemoradiation the standard nonoperative treatment throughout the world. Nevertheless, a local failure rate (persistent and recurrent disease) of approximately 45% leaves much room for improvement. Many (innumerable) modifications have since been made to both the radiation and chemotherapy protocols, but many of these apparent improvements have not been assessed in RCTs. One important modification, radiation dose escalation, has been studied in a RCT. High-dose radiation (64.8 Gy) was compared to the previous standard of 50.4 Gy; no survival or local control benefit was seen.[58] A nonrandomized study that added brachytherapy, in the hope of improving local control, was also disappointing. There was a high incidence of treatment-related esophagorespiratory fistulae.[59]

TABLE 40.4. Chemoradiation (concomitant) versus radiation alone: RCTs.

Author	Year	Histology	Study arms, number of patients	Chemotherapy	RT (Gy)	Median survival, months	Five-year survival (%)	Other survival (%)
Earle[43]	1980	Squamous	RT, 44		~55	6		2 years (11%)
			CTRT, 47	Bleomycin	~55	6		2 years (9%)
Zhang[44]	1984	Squamous, adeno	RT, 51		~60	9		2 years (20%)
			CTRT, 48	Bleomycin	~60	15		2 years (42%) ($P < 0.05$)
Andersen[45]	1984	Squamous	RT, 42		63			2 years (12%)
			CTRT, 40	Bleomycin	55			2 years (12.5%)
Araujo[46]	1991	Squamous	RT, 31		50	15	6	
			CTRT, 28	5-FU, MMC, bleomycin	50	17	16	
Roussel[47]	1994	Squamous	RT, 111		40	8		2 years (16%)
			CTRT, 110	Cisplatin	40	10		2 years (20%)
Kaneta[48]	1997	Squamous	RT, 12		~70	7		1 year (24%)
			CTRT, 12	Cisplatin	~70	9		1 year (40%)
Slabber[49]	1998	Squamous	RT, 36		40	5		1 year (20%)
			CTRT, 34	Cisplatin, 5-FU	40	6		1 year (28%)
Smith[50a]	1998	Squamous	RT, 60		40–60	9		2 years (12%)
			CTRT, 59	5-FU, MMC	40–60	15		2 years (27%)
Herskovic[51]	1992	Squamous, adeno	RT, 62		64	9	0	($P = 0.04$)
Cooper[52]	1999		CTRT, 61	5-FU, cisplatin	50	14 ($P < 0.001$)	26	

RCTs, randomized controlled trials; RT, radiation therapy; CTRT, chemoradiation; adeno, adenocarcinoma; MMC, mitomycin C; 5-FU, 5-fluorouracil.

[a] Trial permitted surgery, so its place within this table is not clear.

Only P values less than 0.05 are shown.

TABLE 40.5. Chemoradiation (sequential) versus radiation alone: RCTs.

Author	*Year*	*Histology*	*Study arms, number of patients*	*Chemotherapy*	*RT (Gy)*	*Median survival, months*	*Five-year survival (%)*	*Other survival (%)*
Roussel[53]	1989	Squamous	RT, 86		56	8	4	
			CTRT, 84	Methotrexate	56	9	7	
Zhou[54]	1991	Squamous	RT, 32		~70			2 years (35%)
			CTRT, 32	Cisplatin, 5-FU	~70			2 years (56%)
Hishikawa[55]	1991	Squamous	RT, 25		60–70	8.8		2 years (13%)
			CTRT, 24	Futrafur	60–70	11		2 years (20%)
Hatlevoll[56]	1992	Squamous	RT, 51		63	5.5		2 years (11%)
			CTRT, 46	Cisplatin, 5-FU	63	5.5		2 years (5%)
Lu (57)	1995	Squamous	RT, 30		~65			1 year (37%)
			CTRT, 30	Adriamycin, 5-FU, cisplatin	50			1 year (64%)

RCTs, randomized controlled trials; Chemo; chemotherapy; RT, radiation therapy; CTRT, chemoradiation; adeno, adenocarcinoma; 5-FU, 5-fluorouracil.
Only P values less than 0.05 are shown.

Comparisons of the Two Standards: Surgery Alone and Definitive Chemoradiation

Direct comparisons of the two standard treatments for locoregional esophageal cancer, in the form of RCTs, have not been done. However, the outcomes of the two standard treatments, when compared in a very crude and unscientific way, seem roughly equivalent. Surgery typically provides median survivals of 15 to 18 months and 5-year survival rates of 20% to 25%; treatment mortality is 5% to 10%. Chemoradiation typically provides median survivals of 12 to 18 months and 5-year survivals of 15% to 20%; Treatment mortality is about 2%. Fair comparisons are difficult to find, because patients with poorer prognoses tend to be treated nonoperatively. Two nonrandomized comparative studies of surgery versus chemoradiation, as weak as this form of clinical research is, showed no difference in survival.[60,61]

It is easy to call for a RCT comparing surgery alone to definitive chemoradiation but difficult to actually do it. Clinicians and patients often have strong preferences, even if the equipoise condition seems to be satisfied. Rather than address the question directly, it is probably more practical to pose related questions about the role of surgery, such as (i) is chemoradiation-surgery superior to chemoradiation without surgery or (ii) can we treat with definitive chemoradiation and reserve surgery for selected patients who show persistent or recurrent local disease, or patients who early during chemoradiation show a lack of response (as assessed by PET scan, or some yet to be developed discriminating test)? Some of the more interesting investigational treatments are discussed next.

Investigational Treatments of Current Interest

Neoadjuvant Chemotherapy and Surgery

Given the generally poor results of surgery alone in patients with locoregional esophageal cancer, the interest in induction or neoadjuvant therapy is not surprising. In theory, neoadjuvant chemotherapy offers early treatment of micrometastatic disease, and it can facilitate surgical resection by "downstaging" cancers. In addition, esophageal cancer patients generally tolerate preoperative (neoadjuvant) chemotherapy better than postoperative (adjuvant) chemotherapy. However, induction therapy is not without morbidity (both independently, and after surgery), and it may cause harm by delaying definitive, albeit modestly effective, treatment with surgery.

Several RCTs have compared neoadjuvant chemotherapy and surgery to surgery alone (Table 40.6).[62–70] Three trials are very notable. The Hong Kong study showed that there was no survival benefit to the combination of chemotherapy and surgery but that chemotherapy responders did better than nonresponders. Nonresponders actually fared worse than those treated with surgery alone.[66] In effect, the responders benefited at the expense of the nonresponders. This observation, although not sufficient to justify combined modality therapy, is nevertheless important, especially in the era of PET scanning. PET can discriminate between the two groups with impressive accuracy.[14]

The two largest RCTs, the U.S. and U.K. trials, are similar in many respects but markedly different in outcome. The American intergroup study showed no difference in survival for the two treatments and no difference in treatment mortality.[68] The pathologic complete response rate (no viable tumor in resected specimen) was disappointingly low (less than 10%). In contrast, the Medical Research Council (MRC) trial from the U.K. showed a significant survival advantage for the combination of chemotherapy and surgery [hazard ratio, 0.79; 95% confidence interval (CI) 0.67–0.93; $P = 0.004$).[70] This discrepancy between trials is a puzzle. One popular explanation is that the U.K. trial featured a shorter period of preoperative treatment than the American trial (two cycles of chemotherapy versus three), so nonresponders (a conceptual subgroup) in the combined therapy group moved to surgery quickly. In other words, the responders no longer benefited at the expense of the nonresponders.

Meta-analysis can be useful when individual trials show different results, but the meta-analysis process is not without difficulty and the conclusions should be considered accordingly. One meta-analysis showed no overall survival benefit for neoadjuvant chemotherapy and no difference in treatment-related mortality.[71] Interestingly, the chemotherapy plus surgery patients were less likely to undergo resection but

TABLE 40.6. Neoadjuvant chemotherapy and surgery versus surgery alone: RCTs.

Author	*Year*	*Histology*	*Study arms, number of patients*	*Chemotherapy*	*Median survival, months*	*Survival (%)*
Roth[62]	1988	Squamous	CTS, 19 S, 20	Cisplatin, vindesine, bleomycin	9 9	3 years (25%) 3 years (5%)
Nygaard[63]	1992	Squamous	CTS, 56 S, 50	Cisplatin, bleomycin		2 years (6%) 2 years (12%)
Schlag[64]	1992	Squamous	CTS, 22 S, 24	Cisplatin, 5-FU	10 10	
Maipang[65]	1994	Squamous	CTS, 24 S, 22	Cisplatin, vinblastine, bleomycin	17 17	3 years (31%) 3 years (36%)
Law[66]	1997	Squamous	CTS, 74 S, 73	Cisplatin, 5-FU	17 13	2 years (44%) 2 years (31%)
Kok[67]	1997	Squamous	CTS, 74 S, 74	Cisplatin, etoposide	18 11 ($P = 0.002$)	
Kelsen[68]	1998	Squamous, adeno	CTS, 233 S, 234	Cisplatin, 5-FU	15 16	2 years (35%) 2 years (37%)
Ancona[69]	2001	Squamous	CTS, 47 S, 47	Cisplatin, 5-FU	25 24	3 years (44%) 3 years (42%)
MRC[70]	2002	Squamous, adeno	CTS, 400 S, 402	Cisplatin, 5-FU	17 13	2 years (43%) 2 years (34%) ($P = 0.004$)

RCTs, randomized controlled trials; Chemo, chemotherapy; CTS, chemotherapy followed by surgery; S, surgery alone; adeno, adenocarcinoma; 5-FU, 5-fluorouracil. Only P values less than 0.05 are shown.

more likely to undergo a complete (R0) resection. We can explain this observation in two ways: chemotherapy may act as a selection tool (patients with poor cancer prognoses never make it to surgery), and it may also "downstage" (this term is not without problems) tumors and make complete resection more likely. Both mechanisms are probably operational.

The interpretation of RCT evidence seems to vary according to geography. In the U.K., the MRC trial has made neoadjuvant chemotherapy and surgery a standard treatment for locoregional esophageal cancer. In the United States, however, the American intergroup trial has largely eliminated enthusiasm for neoadjuvant chemotherapy followed by surgery. The prevailing American notion is that currently available chemotherapy regimens are simply ineffective as (single-modality) induction treatments.

Neoadjuvant Chemoradiation and Surgery Compared to the Standard of Surgery Alone

Neoadjuvant chemoradiation followed by surgery is a strategy that has been formerly compared to both standard treatments, surgery alone (Table 40.7)[63,72–81] and definitive chemoradiation (Table 40.8).[82,83] The former implies the question: Does chemoradiation add anything to surgery? The latter asks: Does surgery add anything to chemoradiation?

Many of the concepts discussed in the previous section are transposable to the question of neoadjuvant chemoradiation and surgery versus surgery alone. The theoretical foundations, early treatment of micrometastatic disease, facilitating complete resection, and tolerance of preoperative therapy, are the same. Additionally, chemotherapy and radiation act synergistically on locoregional disease; pathologic complete response rates of 25%, as opposed to 10% with induction chemotherapy, are typically encountered. However, the issue of treatment-related toxicity looms larger with neoadjuvant chemoradiation than it does for neoadjuvant chemotherapy. For example, few who argue against neoadjuvant chemotherapy justify their position with morbidity concepts; instead, they point to a simple lack of treatment effect. In contrast, it is possible to argue against neoadjuvant chemoradiation on two fronts: lack of effect and morbidity. In fact, one can even argue in favor of a positive treatment effect, but one that is offset by a negative morbidity effect. Interesting theoretical arguments aside, we now turn to the evidence.

Of the many RCTs done on this question (see Table 40.7), only one showed a benefit for chemoradiation plus surgery. Many of the other trials showed an effect directionally in favor of the combined treatment but not significantly so. The lone unequivocally positive trial, reported by Walsh, has therefore come under intense scrutiny;[74,75] it seems that no review of this subject is complete without a few disparaging comments about the trial. The major criticisms relate to less than optimal preoperative staging and an unusually poor survival in the surgery-alone arm (less than 10% at 3 years). The first criticism cannot be completely dismissed, but the poor surgery-alone survival is partly explainable. The RCT was done at a single general hospital (a remarkable feat) and more than 70% of patients referred to the hospital unit were enrolled in the trial. Therefore, the patient selection forces at work in most RCTs involving cancer surgery, especially multicenter trials, were not present. Given that the study's population was unusually unselected ("all comers") and that 80% of the patients in the surgery-alone arm were lymph node positive, the dismal survival rate with surgery alone is not all that surprising.

Many of the negative trials show a treatment effect that is directionally, but nonsignificantly, in favor of chemoradiation and surgery. A beneficial treatment effect, if it exists, may be too modest to detect in relatively small (underpow-

TABLE 40.7. Neoadjuvant chemoradiation and surgery versus surgery alone: RCTs.

Author	*Year*	*Histology*	*Study arms, number of patients*	*Chemotherapy*	*RT (Gy)*	*Median survival, months*	*Three-year survival (%)*
Nygaard[63]	1992	Squamous	CTRTS, 53 S, 50	Cisplatin, bleomycin	35	7 7	15 8
Le Prise[72]	1994	Squamous	CTRTS, 41 S, 45	Cisplatin, 5-FU	20	10 11	19 14
Apinop[73]	1994	Squamous	CTRTS, 35 S, 34	Cisplatin, 5-FU	40	10 7	26 20
Walsh[74,75]	1996	Adeno	CTRTS, 58 S, 55	Cisplatin, 5-FU	40	16 11 ($P = 0.01$)	32 6 ($P = 0.01$)
Bosset[76]	1997	Squamous	CTRTS, 143 S, 139	Cisplatin	37	19 19	39 37
Law[77]	1998	Squamous	CTRTS, 30 S, 30	Cisplatin, 5-FU	40	26 27	
Walsh[78]	2000	Squamous	CTRTS, 46 S, 52	Cisplatin, 5-FU	40	12 8 ($P = 0.02$)	
Urba[79]	2001	Adeno, squamous	CTRTS, 50 S, 50	Cisplatin, vinblastine, 5-FU	45	17 18	30 16
Burmeister[80]	2002	Adeno, squamous	CTRTS, 128 S, 128	Cisplatin, 5-FU	35	22 18	
Lee[81]	2003	Squamous	CTRTS, 52 S, 50	Cisplatin, 5-FU	46	28 27	

RCTs, randomized controlled trials; Chemo, chemotherapy; RT, radiation therapy; CTRTS, chemoradiation followed by surgery; S, surgery alone; adeno, adenocarcinoma; 5-FU, 5-fluorouracil.

Only P values less than 0.05 are shown.

ered) RCTs. Meta-analysis can be useful here, but once again, it is not without problems. A meta-analysis showed improved 3-year survival [odds ratio (OR), 0.66; 95% CI, 0.47, 0.92; $P = 0.016$], and reduced locoregional recurrence (OR, 0.38, 95% CI, 0.23, 0.63; $P = 0.0002$), in the chemoradiation/surgery-treated patients.[84] Subgroup analysis showed that concurrent chemoradiation was beneficial but sequential chemoradiation was not. In common with the neoadjuvant chemotherapy data, there was a lower rate of esophageal resection with induction treatment, but a higher rate of complete resection. Treatment-related mortality was higher in the combined modality treatment patients, but this did not quite reach statistical significance (OR, 1.63, 95% CI, 0.99, 2.68; $P = 0.053$).

Because only one RCT shows a significant benefit for neoadjuvant chemoradiation and surgery, we cannot proclaim this treatment as proven, or standard, even if a meta-analysis is "positive." Nevertheless, there is probably a modest survival benefit for neoadjuvant chemoradiation and surgery over surgery alone. A cancer survival benefit may be partly negated by treatment-related mortality. This possibility was apparent in the French trial; disease-free survival was longer in the experimental arm but treatment-related mortality was higher.[76] Further RCTs are needed. However, investigative interest around the world is shifting somewhat to related clinical research questions, such as does surgery add benefit over chemoradiation?

Neoadjuvant Chemoradiation and Surgery: Compared to the Standard of Definitive Chemoradiation

Two recently completed RCTs have compared neoadjuvant chemoradiation to definitive chemoradiation, and the results are more or less consistent (Table 40.8).[82,83] The French FFCD 9102 RCT compared chemoradiation without surgery (defin-

TABLE 40.8. Definitive chemoradiation versus neoadjuvant chemoradiation and surgery: RCTs.

Author	*Year*	*Pts*	*Histology*	*Study arms*	*Chemotherapy*	*RT (Gy)*	*Median survival, months*	*Survival (%)*	*Treatment mortality (%)*
Bedenne[82]	2002	259	Squamous, adeno	CTRT CTRTS	Cisplatin, 5-FU Cisplatin, 5-FU	66 46	19 18	2 years (40%) 2 years (34%) ($P = 0.56$)	1 9 ($P = 0.002$)
Stahl[83]	2003	177	Squamous	CTRT	Cisplatin, 5-FU, leucovorin, etoposide	More than 60	15	3 years (20%)	3.5
				CTRTS	Cisplatin, 5-FU, leucovorin, etoposide	40	16	3 years (28%) ($P = 0.22$)	10

RCTs, randomized controlled trials; PTs, number of patients; Chemo, chemotherapy; RT, radiation therapy; adeno, adenocarcinoma; CTRT, definitive chemoradiation; CTRTS, chemoradiation followed by surgery; 5-FU, 5-fluorouracil.

itive chemoradiation) to neoadjuvant chemoradiation followed by planned surgery.[82] Four hundred fifty-five patients with T3–T4, N0–N1 squamous carcinoma or adenocarcinoma were treated with two cycles of 5-fluorouracil and cisplatin, plus radiotherapy (46 Gy). Patients showing at least a partial response, and fit for surgery (259 patients), were randomized to surgery or further chemoradiation (three cycles of chemotherapy and 15–20 Gy radiotherapy). Median survival was 17.7 months in the chemoradiation plus surgery group and 19.3 months in the chemoradiation group. Two-year survival was 34% in the chemoradiation-surgery group and 40% in the chemoradiation group ($P = 0.56$). Ninety-day treatment mortality was 9% in the patients treated surgically and 1% in patients treated with definitive chemoradiation ($P = 0.002$). After completion of treatment, 78% of patients treated with chemoradiation plus surgery, and 87% of those treated with definitive chemoradiation, had a World Health Organization performance status of 0 or 1 ($P = 0.08$). Surgically treated patients were less likely to need palliative endoscopic interventions for dysphagia (P values for stenting and dilatation, 0.005 and 0.07, respectively).

The German Oesophageal Cancer Study Group performed a similar trial.[83] One hundred seventy-seven patients with locally advanced squamous cancer were randomized to treatment with either (i) three cycles of chemotherapy (5-fluorouracil, cisplatin, etoposide, leucovorin) followed by chemoradiation (cisplatin, etoposide, and 40 Gy) and then surgery, or (ii) chemotherapy (same), followed by definitive chemoradiation (cisplatin, etoposide, and more than 60 Gy). Median and 3-year survival were 16 months and 28% in the chemoradiation-surgery group versus 15 months and 20% in the definitive chemoradiation group ($P = 0.22$). There was a trend toward better local control in the chemoradiation-surgery group ($P = 0.08$) but also a higher overall treatment mortality (10% versus 3.5%). Not surprisingly, responders in both treatment arms fared better than nonresponders. Although the nonresponders in the chemoradiation-surgery arm had a dismal 3-year survival, 18%, a small subgroup that could still undergo a complete resection did better (35% 3-year survival). The denominator of this group is small, and overemphasis on this point may be unwarranted.

Taken together, the French and German trials show that definitive chemoradiation, and neoadjuvant chemoradiation followed by surgery, provide equivalent overall survival in patients with locoregional esophageal cancer. The inclusion of surgery in treatment provides modest benefit in terms of local control and palliation of dysphagia, but at the cost of higher treatment-related mortality.

Definitive Chemoradiation with Possible Salvage Esophagectomy

Because definitive chemoradiation provides survival that is equivalent (or perhaps better) to that observed with chemoradiation plus surgery, but has a high local failure rate, it is logical to ask the question: Is there a role for esophagectomy as a selective salvage strategy in patients with local failures after definitive chemoradiation? This question has been implicit in much of the foregoing discussion, especially in the comparisons of definitive chemoradiation and chemoradiation-surgery; herein it is addressed explicitly. In part the question of salvage esophagectomy is one of feasibility, and in part it is one of effectiveness. RCTs have not been done, but the U.S. Radiation Therapy Oncology Group, along with other groups, is keenly interested in this question.

The feasibility of salvage esophagectomy for local failures (persistent or recurrent disease) of definitive chemoradiation relates to two major issues: properly identifying patients for salvage surgery (true local failure, and lack of disseminated disease), and performing salvage esophagectomy with acceptable operative mortality.[85,86] In contrast to the primary diagnosis of esophageal cancer, which is exceptionally simple, the diagnosis of persistent or recurrent local disease can be very difficult. Endoscopic biopsies can be "negative" despite the presence of viable tumor in deeper layers of the posttreatment esophagus. A persistent stricture is often the clue that malignant disease is present, but this is hardly a specific diagnostic criterion. EUS and CT scanning are also less accurate in the posttreatment setting. An apparent paradox in relation to diagnostic accuracy is noteworthy. In the context of neoadjuvant chemoradiation and planned surgery, little effort is expended in assessing the exact status of the tumor before surgery, and an absence of viable tumor in the resected specimen brings cheers from all concerned. However, in the context of salvage esophagectomy, an inherently selective approach, the lack of tumor in the resected specimen is a diagnostic failure, and a particularly difficult one should the patient die (disease free) after surgery.

Although experience with salvage esophagectomy is limited, there is little doubt that it is a more morbid operation than both esophagectomy alone and planned esophagectomy after neoadjuvant chemoradiation.[85,87] Within the salvage esophagectomy framework there are two patient subgroups, each with different, but negative, implications. One group has persistent local disease that is apparent at the completion of definitive chemoradiation, and they promptly undergo salvage esophagectomy. This situation is very similar to planned surgery after neoadjuvant chemoradiation (although the radiation dose may be a bit higher), but being nonresponders, the anticipated survival is poor. The second group manifests local disease months after treatment. They may have a better cancer prognosis (initially responding), but the salvage esophagectomy can be technically difficult (later in the evolution of radiation tissue injury). It is not surprising that taken together these two groups of patients have a propensity for poor outcomes, but for different reasons.

Finally, a third group of patients can be considered for a slightly different form of surgical salvage. These are patients who are treated with definitive chemoradiation but early in the course of treatment show features of nonresponse. The lack of response usually portends a poor outcome irrespective of treatment, but promptly offering an operation is sensible. PET scanning holds tremendous promise as a response discriminator.[14]

Investigational Treatments of Some Interest

Surgery and Adjuvant Chemotherapy

Postoperative chemotherapy is an accepted therapeutic strategy for several solid tumor sites (breast, colon), but it is not very practical in postoperative esophageal cancer patients. It

TABLE 40.9. Surgery and adjuvant chemotherapy versus surgery alone: RCTs.

Author	*Year*	*Histology*	*Study arms, number of patients*	*Chemotherapy*	*Median survival (months)*	*Five-year survival (%)*
Pouliquen[88]	1996	Squamous	SCT, 52 S, 68	Cisplatin, 5-FU	13 14	12 14
Ando[89]	1997	Squamous	SCT, 105 S, 100	Cisplatin, vindesine		48 45
Ando[90]	2003	Squamous	SCT, 120 S, 122	Cisplatin, 5-FU		52 61

RCTs, randomized controlled trials; Chemo, chemotherapy; SCT, surgery and postoperative chemotherapy; S, surgery alone; 5-FU, 5-fluorouracil.

takes weeks or sometimes months for a patient to recover after an esophagectomy; temporary nutritional compromise and postoperative weight loss are the rule. Patients with squamous cancer, in particular, are often malnourished before esophagectomy, and they are especially frail after surgery. Predictably, trials of adjuvant chemotherapy after surgery for squamous cancer have been characterized by a high rate of incomplete treatments. Even patients undergoing esophagectomy for adenocarcinoma have difficulty completing postoperative chemotherapy treatment.[68]

Several RCTs have studied the question of adjuvant chemotherapy, but none has shown a benefit (Table 40.9).[88–90] Admittedly, the most recent Japanese trial showed a significant improvement in disease-free survival.[90] Although a modest beneficial effect is plausible, the current evidence does not support the routine use of postoperative chemotherapy after esophageal cancer resection.

Surgery and Adjuvant Chemoradiation

The question of chemoradiation after esophagectomy for esophageal cancer has not been studied in RCTs. Several nonrandomized studies have been encouraging, but selection bias probably plays a role in these studies;[91] being fit enough to be considered for postoperative chemoradiation could, in itself, be a favorable prognostic factor. Postoperative chemoradiation is even more taxing than postoperative chemotherapy, and this feasibility problem has dampened interest. However, postoperative chemoradiation was shown to be effective after gastric cancer resection in the U.S. intergroup trial (problems of inadequate surgery aside).[92] That trial included patients who had tumors of the cardia (patients often included in esophageal cancer trials). Although adjuvant chemoradiation after esophagectomy is an interesting question for study, current investigational interest generally focuses on neoadjuvant treatment.

Treatments Shown to Be Inferior

Radiation Alone

RCTs of concurrent chemoradiation versus radiation alone are summarized in Table 40.4.[43–52] Most researchers and clinicians have been convinced by the RTOG trial, and radiation alone is no longer a standard treatment for locoregional esophageal cancer.[42] Critics could point to the many negative trials on this subject, or suggest that very modern radiation techniques have not been compared to chemoradiation in proper trials, but the general oncology community is not receptive to these arguments. If a patient is fit for chemoradiation, chemoradiation is preferable to radiation alone.

Neoadjuvant Radiation and Surgery

Eight RCTs of preoperative radiation and surgery versus surgery alone have been performed (some included additional postoperative treatment).[63,93–99] The trials are of historic interest; they are not deemed important enough to summarize in a table. The radiation regimens varied considerably, with doses ranging from 20 to 53 Gy. None of them showed a survival advantage for preoperative radiation. A published meta-analysis, based on updated individual data (1,147 patients), reported a hazard ratio of death of 0.89 (95% CI, 0.78–1.01; $P = 0.06$) for the preoperative radiation patients.[100] This result could be interpreted as being consistent with a very modest benefit. However, another meta-analysis that included an additional published trial found a relative risk of 1.01 (95% CI, 0.88–1.16; $P = 0.90$).[101] The combination of neoadjuvant radiation and surgery is no longer a valid treatment.

Surgery and Adjuvant Radiation

Four RCTs of surgery and postoperative radiation versus surgery alone have been conducted (not summarized in table form).[99,102–104] None showed a survival benefit for postoperative radiation, and in one trial the survival was actually significantly shorter.[103] Postoperative treatment impaired quality of life in another trial.[104] Postoperative radiation is not indicated after complete resection of esophageal cancer. Most oncologists are tempted to offer some further therapy after an incomplete resection, but not necessarily radiation alone. There is little evidence to guide therapy in this situation.

Treatment: Metastatic Disease, and Palliation of Dysphagia

The primary goal of treatment in metastatic disease is palliation of symptoms. Prolongation of life is a second objective. Chemotherapy has some palliative benefit, but it has not been shown to increase survival over supportive care, at least not in RCTs.[105,106] Few RCTs have specifically addressed this issue in esophageal cancer. In gastric cancer, a related malignancy, some (but not all) RCTs have shown a modest survival benefit for chemotherapy (refer to Chapter 41).

Many different strategies can be used to palliate dysphagia, and there is no single best treatment. External-beam radiation is the traditional standard, but brachytherapy, chemotherapy, and a host of endoscopic treatments are also effective. Endoscopic treatments include laser (thermal ablation) therapies, stents (plastic, expandable metal, covered expandable metal), photodynamic therapy (PDT), and ethanol (and other chemical agents) injections into the tumor. These endoscopic treatments have been compared in RCTs;[107–117] these are briefly summarized next.

Endoscopic PDT palliates dysphagia with fewer treatments than Nd:YAG laser treatment, but cost and photosensitivity are drawbacks.[107] Newer expandable metal stents have justifiably replaced older plastic stents, despite their higher per unit cost and the lack of conclusive (randomized) supporting evidence.[108] Higher per unit costs are usually favorably offset by reduced costs of treating complications. The slimmer introducer of the metal expandable stents minimizes the need for preliminary dilatation (so often the source of complications with plastic stents), and success rates for placement approach 100%. The multiple brands of stent are broadly equivalent.[109] Covered stents prevent tumor ingrowth, but they are more expensive than uncovered stents and more prone to migration.[110]

RCTs comparing laser treatment to metal expandable stenting are inconsistent.[111,112] Because a major drawback of laser therapy, compared to stenting, is the need for repetitive treatments, combinations of laser therapy and radiotherapies (external beam or brachytherapy) have been investigated. These combinations reduce the need for repetitive laser interventions[113,114] but they still seem inferior to stenting.[115] Brachytherapy also effectively palliates dysphagia, but it should be used cautiously in the setting of previous chemoradiation as fistulae may result.[59,116] Overall, brachytherapy is as effective as stenting.[117] Stenting palliates dysphagia immediately, but the palliative effect of brachytherapy is more durable.

What should clinicians, especially those not active in endoscopy, think of this maze of RCTs on endoscopic palliative interventions? Although broad treatment themes are properly shaped by RCTs, individual patient circumstances and institutional expertise often (correctly) determine the specifics of endoscopic palliation. Proficiency with a given method is probably more important than the choice of method itself.

Future Directions

It is always difficult to predict the future direction of cancer care, but certain general themes deserve mention. Chemopreventative approaches for adenocarcinoma are interesting, as are developments in the therapy of reflux. Modern RCTs are needed to address the impact of antireflux surgery on cancer risk. An accurate way to determine cancer risk in patients with Barrett's esophagus and dysplasia is needed. In the area of treatment, a more individualized approach is desirable. Surgery, it can be argued, should be used more selectively. Perhaps its main value is in early disease, as a sole therapy, and in more-advanced disease as salvage therapy. The trend toward regionalization of surgery to specialized centers should be encouraged. PET scanning shows great promise in assessing response to treatment, predicting outcome, and generally guiding treatment decisions. Newer chemotherapeutic agents and targeted therapies, it is hoped, will also improve the prospects for cure in the future. Finally, if we consider obesity to be an important causal (versus confounding) factor in the rise of adenocarcinoma, then the epidemic of obesity in the West, especially in the United States, desperately needs a solution, and preferably not one that surgically inflicts a new disease.

References

1. Stein HJ, Siewert JR. Improved prognosis of resected esophageal cancer. World J Surg 2004;28:520–525.
2. Sihvo EI, Luostarinen ME, Salo JA. Fate of patients with adenocarcinoma of the esophagus and the esophagogastric junction: a population-based analysis. Am J Gastroenterol 2004;99:419–424.
3. Rusch VW. Are cancers of the esophagus, gastroesophageal junction, and cardia one disease, two, or several? Semin Oncol 2004; 31:444–449.
4. Law S, Wong J. What is appropriate treatment for carcinoma of the thoracic esophagus? World J Surg 2001;25:189–195.
5. Siewert JR, Feith M, Werner M, et al. Adenocarcinoma of the esophagogastric junction: results of surgical therapy based on anatomical/topographic classification in 1,002 consecutive patients. Ann Surg 2000;232:353–361.
6. Crew KD, Neugut AI. Epidemiology of upper gastrointestinal malignancies. Semin Oncol 2004;31:450–464.
7. Blot WJ, Devesa SS, Kneller RW, et al. Rising incidence of adenocarcinoma of the esophagus and gastric cardia. JAMA 1991; 265:1287–1289.
8. Theisen J, Nigro JJ, DeMeester TR, et al. Chronology of the Barrett's metaplasia-dysplasia-carcinoma sequence. Dis Esophagus 2004;17:67–70.
9. Spechler SJ, Lee E, Ahnen D, et al. Long-term outcome of medical and surgical therapies for gastroesophageal reflux disease: follow-up of a randomized controlled trial. JAMA 2001; 285:2331–2338.
10. Parrilla P, Martinez de Haro LF, Ortiz A, et al. Long-term results of a randomized prospective study comparing medical and surgical treatment of Barrett's esophagus. Ann Surg 2003;237: 291–298.
11. Gerson LB, Triadafilopoulos G. Screening for esophageal adenocarcinoma: an evidence-based approach. Am J Med 2002; 113:499–505.
12. Wallace MB, Nietert PJ, Earle C, et al. An analysis of multiple staging management strategies for carcinoma of the esophagus: computed tomography, endoscopic ultrasound, positron emission tomography, and thoracoscopy/laparoscopy. Ann Thorac Surg 2002;74:1026–1032.
13. Flamen P, Lerut A, Van Cutsem E, et al. Utility of positron emission tomography for the staging of patients with potentially operable esophageal carcinoma. J Clin Oncol 2000;18: 3202–3210.
14. Brucher BL, Weber W, Bauer M, et al. Neoadjuvant therapy of esophageal squamous cell carcinoma: response evaluation by positron emission tomography. Ann Surg 2001;233:300–309.
15. Krasna MJ, Reed CE, Nedzwiecki D, et al. CALGB 9380: a prospective trial of the feasibility of thoracoscopy/laparoscopy in staging esophageal cancer. Ann Thorac Surg 2001;71: 1073–1079.
16. Bartels H, Stein HJ, Siewert JR. Preoperative risk analysis and postoperative mortality of oesophagectomy for resectable oesophageal cancer. Br J Surg 1998;85:840–844.
17. Ferguson MK, Durkin AE. Preoperative prediction of the risk of pulmonary complications after esophagectomy for cancer. J Thorac Cardiovasc Surg 2002;123:661–669.
18. Suntharalingam M, Moughan J, Coia LR, et al. The national practice for patients receiving radiation therapy for carcinoma

of the esophagus: results of the 1996–1999 Patterns of Care Study. Int J Radiat Oncol Biol Phys 2003;56:981–987.
19. Siewert JR, Stein HJ, Feith M, et al. Histologic tumor type is an independent prognostic parameter in esophageal cancer: lessons from more than 1,000 consecutive resections at a single center in the Western world. Ann Surg 2001;234:360–369.
20. Muller JM, Erasmi H, Stelzner M, et al. Surgical therapy of oesophageal carcinoma. Br J Surg 1990;77:845–857.
21. Law S, Arcilla C, Chu KM, et al. The significance of histologically infiltrated resection margin after esophagectomy for esophageal cancer. Am J Surg 1998;176:286–290.
22. Urschel JD. Esophagogastrostomy anastomotic leaks complicating esophagectomy: a review. Am J Surg 1995;169:634–640.
23. Roder JD, Busch R, Stein HJ, et al. Ratio of invaded to removed lymph nodes as a predictor of survival in squamous cell carcinoma of the oesophagus. Br J Surg 1994;81:410–413.
24. Whooley BP, Law S, Murthy SC, et al. Analysis of reduced death and complication rates after esophageal resection. Ann Surg 2001;233:338–344.
25. Begg CB, Cramer LD, Hoskins WJ, et al. Impact of hospital volume on operative mortality for major cancer surgery. JAMA 1998;280:1747–1751.
26. Birkmeyer JD, Stukel TA, Siewers AE, Goodney PP, et al. Surgeon volume and operative mortality in the United States. N Engl J Med 2003;349:2117–2127.
27. Miller JD, Jain MK, de Gara CJ, et al. The effect of surgical experience on results of esophagectomy for esophageal carcinoma. J Surg Oncol 1997;65:20–21.
28. Luketich JD, Alvelo-Rivera M, Buenaventura PO, et al. Minimally invasive esophagectomy: outcomes in 222 patients. Ann Surg 2003;238:486–495.
29. Hulscher JB, Tijssen JG, Obertop H, et al. Transthoracic versus transhiatal resection for carcinoma of the esophagus: a meta-analysis. Ann Thorac Surg 2001;72:306–313.
30. Rindani R, Martin CJ, Cox MR. Transhiatal versus Ivor-Lewis oesophagectomy: is there a difference? Aust NZ J Surg 1999; 69:187–194.
31. Hulscher JB, van Sandick JW, de Boer AG, et al. Extended transthoracic resection compared with limited transhiatal resection for adenocarcinoma of the esophagus. N Engl J Med 2002; 347:1662–1669.
32. Altorki N, Skinner D. Should en bloc esophagectomy be the standard of care for esophageal carcinoma? Ann Surg 2001;234: 581–587.
33. Orringer MB, Marshall B, Iannettoni MD. Transhiatal esophagectomy: clinical experience and refinements. Ann Surg 1999;230:392–403.
34. Hagen JA, DeMeester SR, Peters JH, et al. Curative resection for esophageal adenocarcinoma: analysis of 100 en bloc esophagectomies. Ann Surg 2001;234:520–531.
35. Law S, Wong J. Two-field dissection is enough for esophageal cancer. Dis Esophagus 2001;14:98–103.
36. Urschel JD. Does the interponat affect outcome after esophagectomy for cancer? Dis Esophagus 2001;14:124–130.
37. Urschel JD, Urschel DM, Miller JD, et al. A meta-analysis of randomized controlled trials of route of reconstruction after esophagectomy for cancer. Am J Surg 2001;128:470–475.
38. Urschel JD, Blewett CJ, Bennett WF, et al. Handsewn or stapled esophagogastric anastomosis after esophagectomy for cancer. A meta-analysis of randomized controlled trials. Dis Esophagus 2001;14:212–217.
39. Urschel JD, Blewett CJ, Young JEM, et al. Pyloric drainage (pyloroplasty) or no drainage in gastric reconstruction after esophagectomy. A meta-analysis of randomized controlled trials. Dig Surg 2002;19:160–164.
40. Ferguson MK. Reconstructive Surgery of the Esophagus. New York: Futura, 2002.
41. Brenner B, Ilson DH, Minsky BD. Treatment of localized esophageal cancer. Semin Oncol 2004;31:554–565.
42. Wong RK, Malthaner RA, Zuraw L, et al. Combined modality radiotherapy and chemotherapy in nonsurgical management of localized carcinoma of the esophagus: a practice guideline. Int J Radiat Oncol Biol Phys 2003;55:930–942.
43. Earle JD, Gelber RD, Moertel CG, et al. A controlled evaluation of combined radiation and bleomycin therapy for squamous cell carcinoma of the esophagus. Int J Radiat Oncol Biol Phys 1980; 6:821–826.
44. Zhang Z. Radiation combined with bleomycin for esophageal carcinoma: a randomized study of 99 patients. Clin J Oncol 1984; 6:372–374.
45. Andersen AP, Berdal P, Edsmyears F, et al. Irradiation, chemotherapy and surgery in esophageal cancer: a randomized clinical study. The first Scandinavian trial in esophageal cancer. Radiother Oncol 1984;2:179–188.
46. Araujo CM, Souhami L, Gil RA, et al. A randomized trial comparing radiation therapy versus concomitant radiation therapy and chemotherapy in carcinoma of the thoracic esophagus. Cancer (Phila) 1991;67:2258–2261.
47. Roussel A, Haegele P, Paillot B, et al. Results of the EORTC-GTCCG phase III trial of irradiation vs. irradiation and CDDP in inoperable esophageal cancer. Proc Am Soc Clin Oncol 1994; 13:199 (abstract).
48. Kaneta T, Takai Y, Nemoto K, et al. Effect of combination chemotherapy with daily low-dose CDDP for esophageal cancer: results of a randomized trial. Jpn J Cancer Chemother 1997; 24:2099–2104.
49. Slabber CF, Nel JS, Schoeman L, et al. A randomized study of radiotherapy alone versus radiotherapy plus 5-fluorouracil and platinum in patients with inoperable, locally advanced squamous cancer of the esophagus. Am J Clin Oncol 1998; 21:462–465.
50. Smith TJ, Ryan LM, Douglass HO Jr, et al. Combined chemoradiotherapy vs. radiotherapy alone for early stage squamous cell carcinoma of the esophagus: a study of the Eastern Cooperative Oncology Group. Int J Radiat Oncol Biol Phys 1998;42:269–276.
51. Herskovic A, Martz K, al-Sarraf M, et al. Combined chemotherapy and radiotherapy compared with radiotherapy alone in patients with cancer of the esophagus. N Engl J Med 1992; 326:1593–1598.
52. Cooper JS, Guo MD, Herskovic A, et al. Chemoradiotherapy of locally advanced esophageal cancer: long-term follow-up of a prospective randomized trial (RTOG 85-01). JAMA 1999;281: 1623–1627.
53. Roussel A, Bleiberg H, Dalesio O, et al. Palliative therapy of inoperable oesophageal carcinoma with radiotherapy and methotrexate: Final results of a controlled clinical trial. Int J Radiat Oncol Biol Phys 1989;16:67–72.
54. Zhou JC. [Randomized trial of combined chemotherapy including high dose cisplatin, and radiotherapy for esophageal cancer (in Chinese).] Chung Hua Chung Liu Tsa Chih 1991;13:291–294.
55. Hishikawa Y, Miura T, Oshitani T, et al. A randomized prospective study of adjuvant chemotherapy after radiotherapy in unresectable esophageal carcinoma. Dis Esophagus 1991;4:85–90.
56. Hatlevoll R, Hagen S, Hansen HS, et al. Bleomycin/cis-platin as neoadjuvant chemotherapy before radical radiotherapy in localized, inoperable carcinoma of the esophagus: a prospective randomized multicentre study. The second Scandinavian trial in esophageal cancer. Radiother Oncol 1992;24:114–116.
57. Lu XJ, Miao RH, Li XQ. [Combination of selective arterial infusion chemotherapy with radiotherapy in the treatment of advanced esophogeal carcinoma (in Chinese).] Chin J Clin Oncol 1995;22:262–265.
58. Minsky BD, Pajak TF, Ginsberg RJ, et al. INT 0123 (Radiation Therapy Oncology Group 94-05) phase III trial of combined-modality therapy for esophageal cancer: high-dose versus

standard-dose radiation therapy. J Clin Oncol 2002;20:1167–1174.
59. Gaspar LE, Winter K, Kocha WI, et al. Swallowing function and weight change observed in a phase I/II study of external-beam radiation, brachytherapy and concurrent chemotherapy in localized cancer of the esophagus (RTOG 9207). Cancer J 2001;7:388–394.
60. Chan A, Wong A. Is combined chemotherapy and radiation therapy equally effective as surgical resection in localized esophageal carcinoma? Int J Radiat Oncol Biol Phys 1999;45:265–270.
61. Murakami M, Kuroda Y, Nakajima T, et al. Comparison between chemoradiation protocol intended for organ preservation and conventional surgery for clinical T1–T2 esophageal carcinoma. Int J Radiat Oncol Biol Phys 1999;45:277–284.
62. Roth JA, Pass HI, Flanagan MM, et al. Randomized clinical trial of preoperative and postoperative adjuvant chemotherapy with cisplatin, vindesine, and bleomycin for carcinoma of the esophagus. J Thorac Cardiovasc Surg 1988;96:242–248.
63. Nygaard K, Hagen S, Hansen HS, et al. Pre-operative radiotherapy prolongs survival in operable esophageal carcinoma: a randomized, multicenter study of pre-operative radiotherapy and chemotherapy. The second Scandinavian trial in esophageal cancer. World J Surg 1992;16:1104–1110.
64. Schlag PM. Randomized trial of preoperative chemotherapy for squamous cell cancer of the esophagus. Arch Surg 1992;127:1446–1450.
65. Maipang T, Vasinanukorn P, Petpichetchian C, et al. Induction chemotherapy in the treatment of patients with carcinoma of the esophagus. J Surg Oncol 1994;56:191–197.
66. Law S, Fok M, Chow S, et al. Preoperative chemotherapy versus surgical therapy alone for squamous cell carcinoma of the esophagus: a prospective randomized trial. J Thorac Cardiovasc Surg 1997;114:210–217.
67. Kok TC, van Lanschot J, Siersema PD, et al. Neoadjuvant chemotherapy in operable esophageal squamous cell cancer: final report of a phase III multicenter randomized controlled trial. Proc Am Soc Clin Oncol 1997;16:277 (abstract).
68. Kelsen DP, Ginsberg R, Pajak TF, et al. Chemotherapy followed by surgery compared with surgery alone for localized esophageal cancer. N Engl J Med 1998;339:1979–1984.
69. Ancona E, Ruol A, Santi S, et al. Only pathologic complete response to neoadjuvant chemotherapy improves significantly the long term survival of patients with resectable esophageal squamous cell carcinoma: final report of a randomized, controlled trial of preoperative chemotherapy versus surgery alone. Cancer (Phila) 2001;91:2165–2174.
70. Medical Research Council Oesophageal Cancer Working Group. Surgical resection with or without preoperative chemotherapy in oesophageal cancer: a randomised controlled trial. Lancet 2002;359:1727–1733.
71. Urschel JD, Vasan H, Blewett CJ. Meta-analysis of randomized controlled trials that compared neoadjuvant chemotherapy and surgery to surgery alone for resectable esophageal cancer. Am J Surg 2002;183:274–279.
72. Le Prise E, Etienne PL, Meunier B, et al. A randomized study of chemotherapy, radiation therapy, and surgery versus surgery for localized squamous cell carcinoma of the esophagus. Cancer (Phila) 1994;73:1779–1784.
73. Apinop C, Puttisak P, Preecha N. A prospective study of combined therapy in esophageal cancer. Hepatogastroenterology 1994;41:391–393.
74. Walsh TN, Noonan N, Hollywood D, et al. A comparison of multi-modality therapy and surgery for esophageal adenocarcinoma. N Engl J Med 1996;335:462–467.
75. Walsh TN, Grennell M, Mansoor S, et al. Neoadjuvant treatment of advanced stage esophageal adenocarcinoma increases survival. Dis Esophagus 2002;15:121–124.
76. Bosset JF, Gignoux M, Triboulet JP, et al. Chemoradiotherapy followed by surgery compared with surgery alone in squamous-cell cancer of the esophagus. N Engl J Med 1997;337:161–167.
77. Law S, Kwong DLW, Tung HM, et al. Preoperative chemoradiation for squamous cell esophageal cancer: a prospective randomized trial. Can J Gastroenterol 1998;12(suppl B):161 (abstract).
78. Walsh TN, McDonnell CO, Mulligan ED, et al. Multimodal therapy versus surgery alone for squamous cell carcinoma of the esophagus: a prospective randomized trial. Gastroenterology 2000;118(suppl 2):1008 (abstract).
79. Urba SG, Orringer MB, Turrisi A, et al. Randomized trial of preoperative chemoradiation versus surgery alone in patients with locoregional esophageal carcinoma. J Clin Oncol 2001;19:305–313.
80. Burmeister BH, Smithers BM, Fitzgerald L, et al. A randomized phase III trial of preoperative chemoradiation followed by surgery (CR-S) versus surgery alone (S) for localized resectable cancer of the esophagus. Proc Am Soc Clin Oncol 2002;21:518 (abstract).
81. Lee J-L, Kim S-B, Jung H-Y, et al. A single institutional phase III trial of preoperative chemotherapy with hyperfractionation radiotherapy plus surgery (CRT-S) versus surgery (S) alone for stage II, III resectable esophageal squamous cell carcinoma (SCC): an interim analysis. Proc Am Soc Clin Oncol 2003;22:1043 (abstract).
82. Bedenne L, Michel P, Bouche O, et al. Randomized phase III trial in locally advanced esophageal cancer: radiochemotherapy followed by surgery versus radiochemotherapy alone (FFCD 9102). Proc Am Soc Clin Oncol 2002;21:519 (abstract).
83. Stahl M, Wilke H, Walz MK, et al. Randomized phase III trial in locally advanced squamous cell carcinoma (SCC) of the esophagus: chemoradiation with and without surgery. Proc Am Soc Clin Oncol 2003;22:1001 (abstract).
84. Urschel JD, Vasan H. A meta-analysis of randomized controlled trials that compared neoadjuvant chemoradiation and surgery to surgery alone for resectable esophageal cancer. Am J Surg 2003;185:538–543.
85. Swisher SG, Wynn P, Putnam JB, et al. Salvage esophagectomy for recurrent tumors after definitive chemotherapy and radiotherapy. J Thorac Cardiovasc Surg 2002;123:175–183.
86. Urschel JD, Ashiku S, Thurer R, Sellke FW. Salvage or planned esophagectomy after chemoradiation therapy for locally advanced esophageal cancer: a review. Dis Esophagus 2003;16:60–65.
87. Urschel JD, Sellke FW. Complications of salvage esophagectomy. Med Sci Monit 2003;9:173–180.
88. Pouliquen X, Levard H, Hay JM, et al. 5-Fluorouracil and cisplatin therapy after palliative surgical resection of squamous cell carcinoma of the esophagus. A multicenter randomized trial. French Associations for Surgical Research. Ann Surg 1996;223:127–133.
89. Ando N, Iizuka T, Kakegawa T, et al. A randomized trial of surgery with and without chemotherapy for localized squamous carcinoma of the thoracic esophagus: the Japan Clinical Oncology Group Study. J Thorac Cardiovasc Surg 1997;114:205–209.
90. Ando N, Iizuka T, Ide H, et al. Surgery plus chemotherapy compared with surgery alone for localized squamous cell carcinoma of the thoracic esophagus: a Japan Clinical Oncology Group study, JCOG 9204. J Clin Oncol 2003;21:4592–4596.
91. Bedard EL, Inculet RI, Malthaner RA, et al. The role of surgery and postoperative chemoradiation therapy in patients with lymph node positive esophageal carcinoma. Cancer (Phila) 2001;91:2423–2430.
92. Macdonald JS, Smalley SR, Benedetti J, et al. Chemoradiotherapy after surgery compared with surgery alone for adenocarcinoma of the stomach or gastroesophageal junction. N Engl J Med 2001;345:725–730.

93. Launois B, Delarue D, Campion JP, et al. Preoperative radiotherapy for carcinoma of the esophagus. Surg Gynecol Obstet 1981;153:690–692.
94. Gignoux M, Roussel A, Paillot B, et al. The value of preoperative radiotherapy in esophageal cancer: results of a study of the E.O.R.T.C. World J Surg 1987;11:426–432.
95. Wang M, Gu XZ, Yin W, et al. Randomized clinical trial on the combination of preoperative irradiation and surgery in the treatment of esophageal carcinoma: report on 206 patients. Int J Radiat Oncol Biol Phys 1989;16:325–327.
96. Iizuka T, Ide H, Kakegawa T, et al. Preoperative radioactive therapy for esophageal carcinoma. Randomized evaluation trial in eight institutions. Chest 1988;93:1054–1058.
97. Huang GJ, Gu XZ, Wang LJ, et al. Combined preoperative irradiation and surgery versus surgery alone for squamous cell carcinoma of the midthoracic esophagus: a prospective randomized study in 360 patients. In: Ferguson MK, Little AG, Skinner DB (eds). Diseases of the Esophagus. New York: Futura, 1990; 275–281.
98. Arnott SJ, Duncan W, Kerr GR, et al. Low dose preoperative radiotherapy for carcinoma of the oesophagus: results of a randomized clinical trial. Radiother Oncol 1992;24:108–113.
99. Fok M, McShane J, Law SYK, et al. Prospective randomised study in the treatment of oesophageal carcinoma. Asian J Surg 1994;17:223–229.
100. Arnott SJ, Duncan W, Gignoux M, et al. Preoperative radiotherapy in esophageal carcinoma: a meta-analysis using individual patient data (Oesophageal Cancer Collaborative Group). Int J Radiat Oncol Biol Phys 1998;41:579–583.
101. Malthaner R, Wong RKS, Rumble RB, et al. Neoadjuvant or adjuvant therapy for resectable esophageal cancer. 2002; http://www.cancercare.on.ca/pdf/pebc2-11f.pdf.
102. Teniere P, Hay JM, Fingerhut A, et al. Postoperative radiation therapy does not increase survival after curative resection for squamous cell carcinoma of the middle and lower esophagus as shown by a multicenter controlled trial. Surg Gynecol Obstet 1991;173:123–130.
103. Fok M, Sham JS, Choy D, et al. Postoperative radiotherapy for carcinoma of the esophagus: a prospective, randomized controlled study. Surgery (St. Louis) 1993;113:138–147.
104. Zieren HU, Muller JM, Jacobi CA, et al. Adjuvant postoperative radiation therapy after curative resection of squamous cell carcinoma of the thoracic esophagus: a prospective randomized study. World J Surg 1995;19:444–449.
105. Shah MA, Schwartz GK. Treatment of metastatic esophagus and gastric cancer. Semin Oncol 2004;31:574–587.
106. Levard H, Pouliquen X, Hay JM, et al. 5-Fluorouracil and cisplatin as palliative treatment of advanced oesophageal squamous cell carcinoma. A multicentre randomised controlled trial. The French Associations for Surgical Research. Eur J Surg 1998;164: 849–857.
107. Lightdale CJ, Heier SK, Marcon NE, et al. Photodynamic therapy with porfimer sodium versus thermal ablation therapy with Nd:YAG laser for palliation of esophageal cancer: a multicenter randomized trial. Gastrointest Endosc 1995;42:507–512.
108. O'Donnell CA, Fullarton GM, Watt E, et al. Randomized clinical trial comparing self-expanding metallic stents with plastic endoprostheses in the palliation of oesophageal cancer. Br J Surg 2002;89:985–992.
109. Siersema PD, Hop WC, van Blankenstein M, et al. A comparison of 3 types of covered metal stents for the palliation of patients with dysphagia caused by esophagogastric carcinoma: a prospective, randomized study. Gastrointest Endosc 2001; 54:145–153.
110. Vakil N, Morris AI, Marcon N, et al. A prospective, randomized, controlled trial of covered expandable metal stents in the palliation of malignant esophageal obstruction at the gastroesophageal junction. Am J Gastroenterol 2001;96:1791–1796.
111. Dallal HJ, Smith GD, Grieve DC, et al. A randomized trial of thermal ablative therapy versus expandable metal stents in the palliative treatment of patients with esophageal carcinoma. Gastrointest Endosc 2001;54:549–557.
112. Adam A, Ellul J, Watkinson AF, et al. Palliation of inoperable esophageal carcinoma: a prospective randomized trial of laser therapy and stent placement. Radiology 1997;202:344–348.
113. Sargeant IR, Tobias JS, Blackman G, et al. Radiotherapy enhances laser palliation of malignant dysphagia: a randomised study. Gut 1997;40:362–369.
114. Spencer GM, Thorpe SM, Blackman GM, et al. Laser augmented by brachytherapy versus laser alone in the palliation of adenocarcinoma of the oesophagus and cardia: a randomised study. Gut 2002;50:224–227.
115. Konigsrainer A, Riedmann B, De Vries A, et al. Expandable metal stents versus laser combined with radiotherapy for palliation of unresectable esophageal cancer: a prospective randomized trial. Hepatogastroenterology 2000;47:724–727.
116. Sur RK, Levin CV, Donde B, et al. Prospective randomized trial of HDR brachytherapy as a sole modality in palliation of advanced esophageal carcinoma: an International Atomic Energy Agency study. Int J Radiat Oncol Biol Phys 2002;53: 127–133.
117. Homs MY, Essink-Bot ML, Borsboom GJ, Steyerberg EW, Siersema PD; the Dutch SIREC Study Group. Quality of life after palliative treatment for oesophageal carcinoma: a prospective comparison between stent placement and single dose brachytherapy. Eur J Cancer 2004;40:1862–1871.

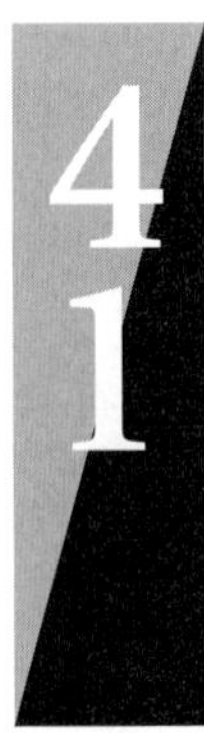

Stomach

Scott A. Hundahl, John S. Macdonald, and Stephen R. Smalley

Neoplasms of the stomach encompass both benign and malignant tumors, with more than 95% of the latter consisting of adenocarcinomas. Until approximately 1980, gastric cancer was the most common solid organ tumor in the world, and today it is eclipsed only by lung cancer in incidence and mortality.[1]

This chapter addresses the classification, epidemiology, staging, and evidence-based treatment of gastric adenocarcinoma. Less-common gastric neoplasms, such as gastrointestinal stromal sarcomas (GIST), carcinoid tumors, and gastric lymphomas, are comprehensively reviewed in other chapters. Despite the necessary emphasis on new findings and improved treatments, background items of historical significance are also mentioned, lest we underappreciate previous work and the difficulty of progress.

Gastric Adenocarcinoma

Classification

Borrmann first characterized gastric carcinoma on the basis of gross characteristics in 1926, based on a review of 5,000 European cases.[2] He described four macroscopic tumor growth patterns: (1) type I, nodular polypoid tumor without ulceration and usually with a broad base; (2) type II, a fungating, exophytic, circumscribed tumor with defined sharp margins, devoid of ulceration except at its dome; (3) type III, an ulcerating tumor with a penetrating, infiltrating ulcer base; (4) type IV, a diffuse thickening of the gastric wall without a discretely marginated mass or ulceration, corresponding to the "leather bottle," nondistensible stomach termed linitis plastica. Still used today, the Borrmann classification has proved useful in guiding surgical treatment, especially the extent of gross tumor clearance necessary for reliable negative margin resection.

The histology of gastric adenocarcinoma falls into two distinct subtypes, first identified by the Finnish authors Jarvi and Lauren in 1951 and refined in 1965[3,4]: (1) intestinal type and (2) diffuse type. Intestinal-type cancers (Figure 41.1), often found in association with chronic atrophic gastritis and intestinal metaplasia, demonstrate gland formation and locally/progressively invade the gastric wall. Diffuse-type cancers (Figure 41.2) present as a sheet of discohesive individual cells that diffusely spread within the gastric wall, often spreading considerable distances from the site of origin. Diffuse tumors elicit a particularly brisk scirrhous proliferation of fibroblasts.

Histoepidemiologically, gastric adenocarcinomas generally sort into three broad patterns, based on simple combinations of Lauren type and location within the stomach.[5]

1. Intestinal-type tumors arising in the antrum or antral–corpus junction (*Helicobacter pylori* associated)
2. Diffuse-type cancers involving the corpus (*H. pylori* associated)
3. Intestinal-type cancers of the gastroesophageal junction

In regions of high gastric cancer incidence, approximately two-thirds of the incident cancers are of the intestinal-antral type associated with chronic *Helicobacter pylori* infection, multifocal atrophic gastritis, and intestinal metaplasia. This process usually begins at the lesser curve and the antral–corpus junction, and this is the most frequent site of cancer in high-incidence regions of the world. In such areas, most of the remaining cancers are also associated with *H. pylori* infection, but not intestinal metaplasia, and afflict younger age groups (usually those under 50 years). In this presentation, the cancer is of the diffuse type involving the body of the stomach and is associated with a brisk mucosal inflammatory infiltrate related to the *H. pylori* infection. *Helicobacter pylori* (see below) is therefore associated with both the antral-intestinal and the corpus-diffuse patterns.[6,7] Gastroesophageal junction (GE junction) tumors, on the other hand, tend to be associated with Barrett's metaplasia of the esophagus and are proportionately far less common in high-incidence regions but are an increasingly frequent subtype in low-incidence areas.

For the sake of completeness, a somewhat less common fourth subset of gastric cancer is also seen: intestinal-type cancers of the corpus associated with chronic autoimmune gastritis, G-cell hyperplasia, and achlorhidria. This less-common subtype is usually seen in Northern Europeans.[5]

Before the development of antral–intestinal-type adenocarcinoma, antecedent histologic changes occur that can be viewed as tissue markers along the multistep path to frank neoplasia. Multifocal atrophic gastritis, literally a thinning, chronic inflammation of the gastric mucosa, is generally thought to be the result of decades of superficial gastritis associated with *H. pylori* infection (Figure 41.3) and other factors. So-called intestinal metaplasia (Figure 41.4) is the characteristic histologic feature of atophic gastritis, and it occurs in two forms: (1) complete type intestinal metaplasia and (2) incomplete type intestinal metaplasia. Complete type intestinal metaplasia (Figure 41.4) closely duplicates the mucosa of the small intestine, with small intestine-like mucin-negative

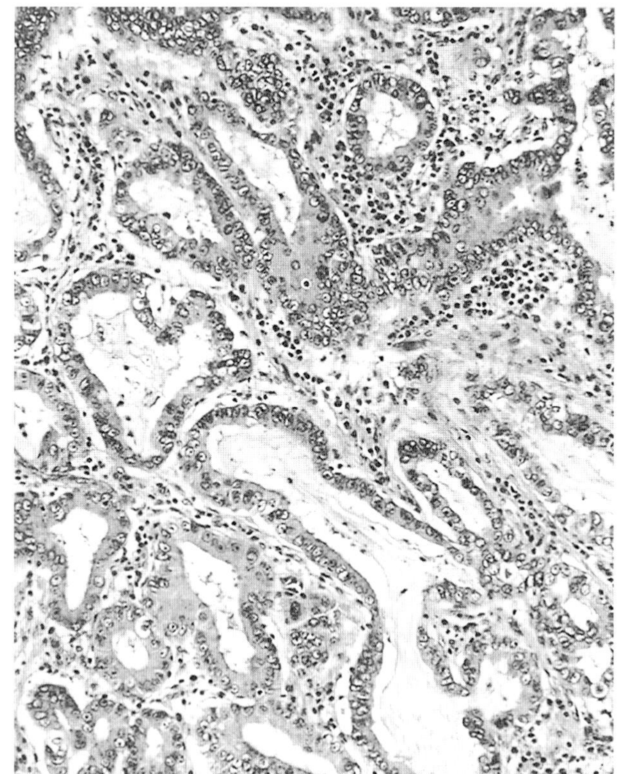

FIGURE 41.1. Intestinal-type cancer. Hematoxylin and eosin (H&E). (Courtesy of Alfredo Asuncion, M.D.)

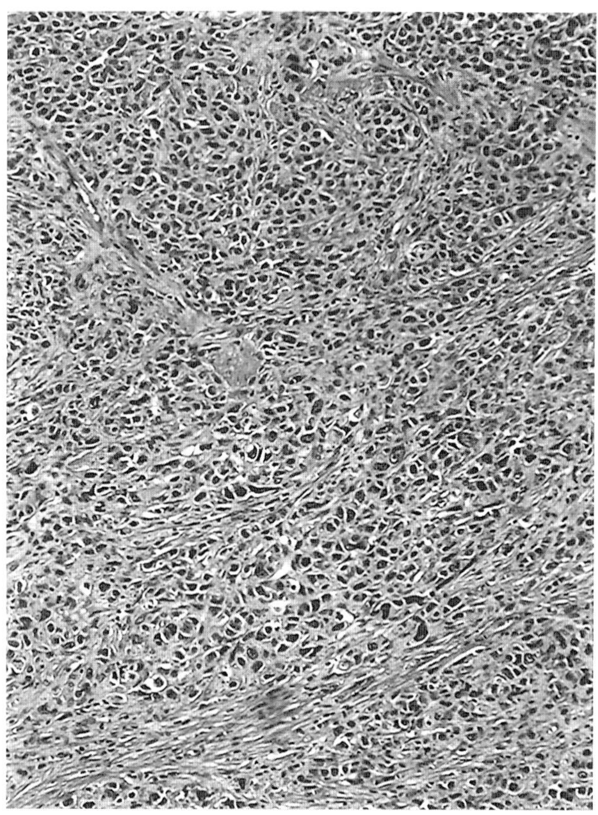

FIGURE 41.2. Diffuse-type cancer. H&E. (Courtesy of Alfredo Asuncion, M.D.)

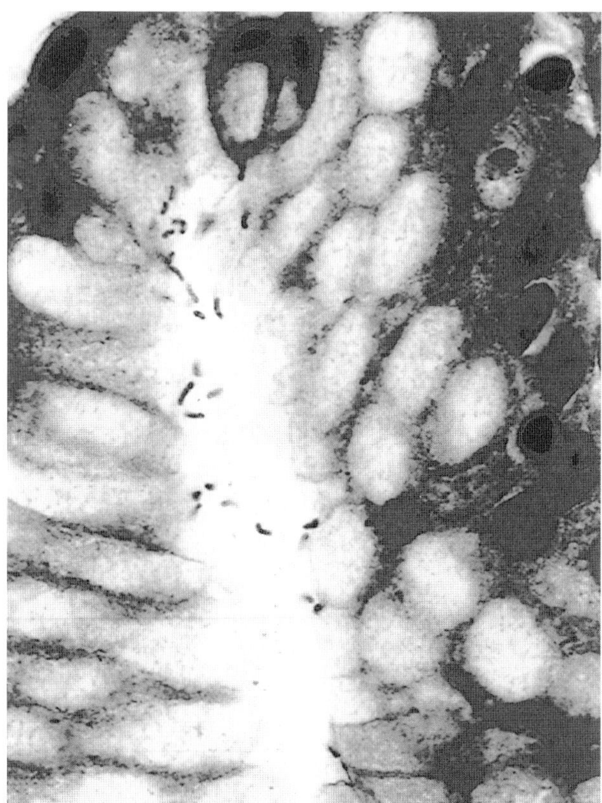

FIGURE 41.3. *Helicobacter pylori* (small rodlike organisms in crypt), Warthin–Starry stain. 100×. (Courtesy of Alfredo Asuncion, M.D.)

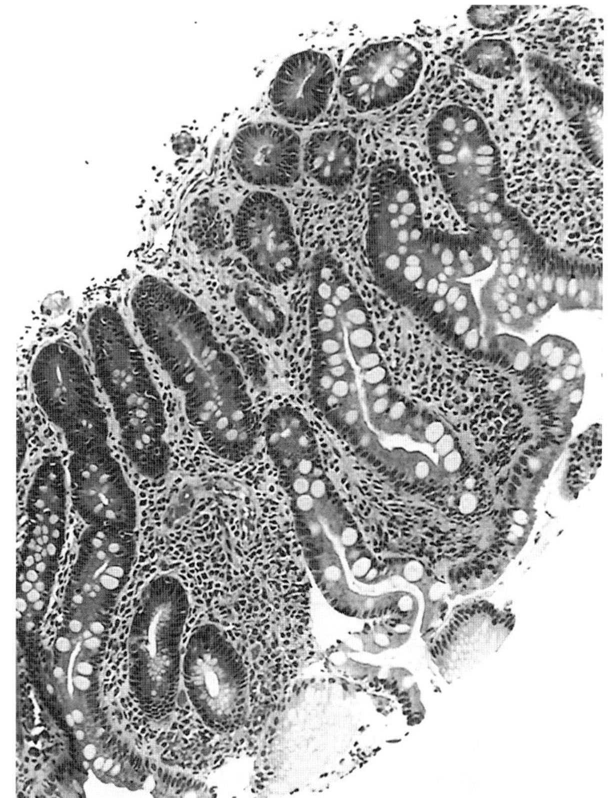

FIGURE 41.4. Intestinal metaplasia. H&E. Goblet cells, not normally seen in gastric mucosa, are numerous. (Courtesy of Alfredo Asuncion, M.D.)

absorptive cells and Alcian blue-positive, sialomucin-positive goblet cells. This process usually begins at the antral–corpus interface, especially along the lesser curve near the incisura.[8] When antral-intestinal metaplasia is still of limited area and spotty, and the remaining oxyntic gastric mucosa is still pumping out acid normally, peptic ulceration of affected areas is frequent, hence explaining the historical association between gastric ulcer and gastric cancer. Incomplete intestinal metaplasia represents a more-advanced process in which absorptive enterocytes disappear in favor of columnar, brush-border-free, colon-like cells with prominent mucous droplets and sulfomucins. Additionally, in incomplete intestinal metaplasia, Paneth cells are absent.[8] In both types of intestinal metaplasia, cells produce enzymes not normally present in the stomach, including sucrase, aminopeptidase, disaccharidases, and, most-importantly, alkaline phosphatase.[9] The latter enzyme may be used to grossly stain and map the distribution of intestinal metaplasia within the stomach ex vivo.[8]

Of the many alternative histologic gastric cancer classification schemes based on morphology, such as the World Health Organization Classification,[10] or histogenesis-based classifications such as that of Mulligan and Rember,[11] degree of differentiation such as Broder's classification[12] and the Nagayo–Komagome classification,[13] or classifications that include growth pattern such as the Ming classification,[14] none has proven of more "beyond-TNM" prognostic value than the Goseki classification.[15,16] In the Goseki scheme, degree of tubular differentiation (well versus poor) is combined with mucin staining pattern (mucin rich versus mucin poor) to divide gastric adenocarcinomas into four groups. Although of apparent prognostic value, it has yet to find widespread use.

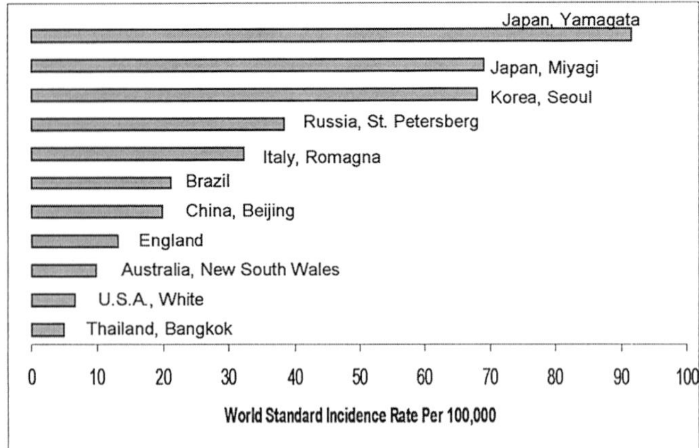

FIGURE 41.5. World Standard incidence of gastric adenocarcinoma (rate per 100,000 World Standard population, males). (Data from Cancer in Five Continents,[19] vol VIII.)

Epidemiology

In incidence and mortality, gastric cancer ranks as the second in the world.[1] In raw numbers, it ranks third.[1,17] Of the estimated global cancer burden of 10 million cases in the year 2000, 876,000 are stomach cancers.[1,17] An estimated 38% of incident cases in the world occurs in China, where it is the most common cancer in both males and females.[18] In almost all registries, gastric cancer incidence for males is approximately twice that of females.[19]

Figure 41.5 depicts widespread variation in gastric cancer incidence in various population-based registries around the world. The registries selected for this figure reflect those with both high numbers of incident cases and relatively low death-certificate-only cases, which suggests good case-finding. The highest world standard incidence rate (91.3 cases per age-standardized 100,000) is reported from Yamagata, Japan. The lowest rates are reported from Bangkok, Thailand, as well as from England, Australia, and the United States.

Age-adjusted gastric cancer incidence rates are declining in most countries throughout the world.[18] The age adjustment of such rates tends to obscure the fact that, as a result of population growth and aging, the numerical burden of gastric cancer cases is actually expected to increase by 30% in 2010, to approximately 1 million cases.[18]

Unifying a vast body of epidemiologic, pathologic, and biologic research, Correa in 1975 proposed a multistep, multicausal model of gastric carcinogenesis, which he refined in 1988 and again in 1992.[20–22] Chronic gastric mucosal irritation, particularly that associated with the gastric mucosal bacterium *Helicobacter pylori*,[23–25] initiates a superficial gastritis, which, especially in a setting of a diet rich in salt-preserved foods and high NaCl intake,[26] progresses to atrophic gastritis and intestinal metaplasia (first the complete type and subsequently the higher-risk incomplete type). This transformation, and the subsequent march to dysplasia and cancer, is facilitated by diminished oxyntic acid output, increasing gastric pH, bacterial growth, and high-nitrate-containing diet. In such an intragastric environment, dietary nitrates are converted to carcinogenic *N*-nitroso compounds.[27–33] Many other carcinogenic compounds, such as polycyclic aromatic hydrocarbons, are also implicated. Certain ingested compounds, such as vitamin C, can interrupt this process.[34–36] Additional risk factors for epidemic gastric cancer include smoking and a diet deficient in fresh fruits, vegetables, and antioxidants.[26,37,38] Blood group A,[39] gastric ulcer,[40] ionizing radiation,[41,42] family history,[39,43–52] and previous gastric resection[53] are also associated risk factors.

A vast body of data now supports *Helicobacter pylori* as a key factor in epidemic gastric cancer,[23–25] and the International Agency for Research on Cancer (IARC) has recognized it as a human carcinogen with both direct and indirect effects.[54] Strains containing the cagA gene appear more dangerous.[55–57] Summarizing a large body of surveillance data, Parkin and colleagues observe that more than 80% of individuals in developing countries are infected with *H. pylori*. The figure for developed countries is approximately 50%.[18,58] An odds ratio for *H. pylor*i and gastric cancer of 2.1 has been estimated.[18,58] Based on this, Parkin and colleagues estimate that 42% of the world total gastric cancer cases can be attributed to the impact of infection with this bacterium.[18]

Decades-long *H. pylori* infection, usually starting in childhood, begets superficial gastritis and chronic atrophic gastritis and intestinal metaplasia, which, once established, usually persists even after the *H. pylori* infection has disappeared because of the resulting achlohydric gastric luminal environment (the bacterium requires an acid environment to live). Atrophic gastritis and intestinal metaplasia were once believed to be irreversible. This does not appear to be entirely true, however. The pharmacologic elimination of *H. pylori*

TABLE 41.1. Hereditary Syndromes in Gastric Cancer.

Well-recognized association:
Hereditary diffuse gastric cancer syndrome
E-cadherin germ-line mutation syndrome
Hereditary non-polyposis colon cancer (HNPCC)
Li–Fraumeni syndrome (p53 mutations)
Possible, weak association:
Familial adenomatous polyposis (FAP) syndrome

along with favorable dietary intervention has led to documented regression of atrophic gastritis and intestinal metaplasia.[34,59–65] Unfortunately for the purpose of cancer prevention, however, a (somewhat underpowered) Chinese *H. pylori* elimination trial in Fujian Province has recently documented a significant decrease in gastric cancer incidence only in participants without preexisting intestinal metaplasia and no significant decrease when such metaplasia was already established.[66] Ongoing *Helicobacter* eradication trials include one in Venezuela,[64] and one in Japan, the Japanese Intervention Trial on *H. pylori*.[67]

Molecular Biology

The genetics and molecular biology of gastric cancer continue to be elucidated. With each clue to understanding the biology of gastric neoplasia, both targeted prevention and targeted therapy seem more and more feasible.

Between 8% and 10% of gastric cancer cases appear to be associated with a hereditary component, and these cases provide significant clues.[68] Dominant inheritance patterns and familial clusters have certainly been documented.[69–71] Notably, Napoleon Bonaparte's family was afflicted by hereditary gastric cancer, and this (rather than arsenic poisoning) appears to have caused his death.[72]

Table 41.1 summarizes recognized hereditary conditions associated with gastric cancer.[73] Perry Guilford and colleagues were among the first to describe germline E-cadherin mutations in a Maori kindred afflicted with diffuse-type gastric cancer,[52,74] and such mutations have also been described in African-American and European kindreds.[52,75] Gastric cancer is one of the neoplasms associated with the hereditary nonpolyposis colon cancer (HNPCC) syndrome, and such HNPCC-associated cancers are almost exclusively of the intestinal type.[43,76] It is also overrepresented in those afflicted with germline p53 mutations, Li–Fraumeni syndrome.[50,77] Asian reports of association of gastric cancer with familial polyposis coli (FAP) syndrome[78] have not been reported for other populations,[79] and the relationship remains controversial.

Table 41.2 summarizes genetic and molecular abnormalities frequently described in sporadic cases of gastric carcinoma. Immortalizing telomerase activity is commonly noted in advanced gastric cancers, but not in surrounding normal gastric mucosa,[80] and is associated with a poor prognosis.[81] Inactivation of the p53 gene and abnormal expression has been detected in more than 60% of gastric cancers.[82] In diffuse-type tumors, E-cadherin expression is reduced in as many as 92% of tumors, compared to adjacent normal tissue.[83] Reduced expression of alpha-catenin, which forms intracytoplasmic complexes with the cadherins, is noted in 56% of tumors.[84] Overexpression of the MET gene that encodes a tyrosine kinase receptor for hepatocyte growth factor (HGF) is seen in approximately half of gastric cancers and tends to be associated with poor prognosis.[85–87] Loss of trefoil peptide, the isomerization of which relates to repair of gut mucosa,[88] occurs in approximately half of gastric carcinomas, especially the intestinal type.[89–92] Proliferation of gastric cancer cell lines is decreased by this peptide.[93] Expression tends to be decreased in intestinal metaplasia.[94] This family of peptides appears to play a key role in the multistep progression to gastric cancer.[95] Epidermal growth factor (EGF) is detected in more than 50% of gastric cancers and epidermal growth factor receptor in approximately a third, and these have been associated with invasiveness and poor prognosis.[96–99] Subtypes c-erb-B1 and -B2 (HER-2/neu) have also been detected[100] in up to a third of cases, and the latter has similarly been associated with poor prognosis.[100–102] Similarly, fibroblast growth factor is expressed in 54% to 70% of gastric cancers.[103,104] Cyclin D is another protein variably overexpressed in gastric cancer, with incidence of overexpression approximately 20% to 30% in sporadic cases,[105–108] and possibly more in familial tumors.[109] COX-2 is not normally expressed in gastric mucosa but is in tumors,[110,111] precancerous lesions,[112] and inflammatory states (especially those induced by *H. pylori*).[113,114] In tumors, its presence seems to correlate with angiogenesis and invasiveness, and it tends to inhibit apoptosis.[115–117] For these reasons, and observational evidence of possible chemoprevention by aspirin,[118–121] COX-2 inhibitors have been proposed as chemopreventive agents in gastric cancer.[122]

Differences among molecular and genetic patterns for gastrointestinal cancers can also provide clues to etiology and therapy. Ras proto-oncogene mutations, which are frequent in colon cancer, are infrequent in gastric cancer.[123]

Paracrine-like interactions between gastric cancer and fibroblasts have also been reported, particularly those involv-

TABLE 41.2. Frequent genetic and molecular abnormalities in sporadic gastric cancer.

Telomerase expression	85% of advanced tumors, poor prognosis
E-cadherin	In 92%, downregulation or mutation
p53 mutations	More than 60% of tumors
Trefoil peptide, TFF-1 (sP2)	Loss in 50% of gastric tumors, and decrease in intestinal metaplasia
MET, c-*met*	Overexpression in approximately 50%, a marker for poor prognosis
Epidermal growth factor (EGF)	Expression in more than 50% of advanced cancers
Fibroblast growth factor	70% expression, especially undifferentiated tumors
Cyclooxygenase 2 (COX-2)	Expressed frequently in tumors and precancerous lesions, but not in normal mucosa

ing transforming growth factor-beta (TGF-β) and hepatocyte growth factor (HGF),[80,124] as well as other factors.[125] Such tissue interactions appear to impact on the proliferation of neoplastic and preneoplastic cells.

Diagnosis

Data from a registry-based American College of Surgeons Patient Care Evaluation Study nicely documents the presenting symptoms of patients with gastric cancer: weight loss in 62%, abdominal or epigastric pain in 52%, nausea in 34%, anorexia or early satiety in 32%, frank dysphagia in 26%, and melena in 18%.[126] Specific signs of gastric cancer are generally associated with more-advanced disease; these include palpable epigastric mass, ascites, left supraclavicular adenopathy, and Blummer's shelf palpable on rectal examination.

In low-incidence countries, fecal occult blood testing, when positive, triggers endoscopic investigation of both upper and lower gastrointestinal (GI) tract; this can lead to a diagnosis of early disease. Patients in defined higher-risk groups (e.g., positive family history or previously documented intestinal metaplasia) are increasingly being screened by surveillance endoscopy, and this, too, leads to diagnosis of more-localized disease. Overall in the United States and most low-incidence regions, stage IB or less (see following for staging) disease is detected in fewer than 23% of cases.[127]

In high-incidence countries, such as Japan, mass screening with upper GI contrast studies and endoscopy have proven successful in shifting stage distribution to lower stages, with measurable improvement in overall survival rates (level of evidence, II-1).[128–133] Pepsinogen I/II ratio of less than 2.0 (a marker of loss of oxyntic mucosa and the extent of intestinal metaplasia) has also been used as a mass screening tool.[134] In Japan, where mass screening has been established as national policy, the percentage of early gastric cancer cases among screening program participants is a staggering 74%.[135] Unfortunately, such mass screening is far less feasible in the poorer, less-developed nations of the world where gastric cancer tends to occur more frequently.[136]

Extent-of-Disease Evaluation

Most patients undergo upper endoscopy as part of their initial evaluation. Key information gleaned from this examination includes tumor location and extent of mucosal involvement, distance from the esophagogastric junction, and Borrmann type.

Endoscopic ultrasound examination (EUS), using a 7.5- to 12-MHz transducer at the end of an endoscope, offers a reliable means of preoperatively assessing the depth of tumor penetration of the wall and a fairly reliable means of assessing for gross lymph node enlargement.[137–139] Concordance of EUS and pathologic T stage in most series is 85% or better.[137,140] Endoscopic ultrasound examination appears more accurate than even helical computed tomography.[137,141]

CT scanning of the abdomen and chest should be performed in most cases. It is very helpful in detecting distant metastatic disease, extraregional adenopathy, and signs of locally-advanced disease unlikely to be removed to negative margins with up-front surgery. Helical CT, particularly if enhanced by the triphasic water-filling scanning technique, appears to be more sensitive than conventional CT.[142]

Positron emission tomography (PET) with [^{18}F]fluorodeoxyglucose (FDG) and PET-CT fusion scanning have enhanced detection of distant metastases in a variety of cancers. Unfortunately, gastric adenocarcinoma is not as suited for PET scanning as other tumors.[143] Primary tumor uptake is seen in only approximately 75% of cases, and the technique is less sensitive than CT for detecting nodal disease.[144] Neither mucus-containing tumors nor diffuse-type scirrhous tumors image well.[145] Furthermore, different regions of the normal stomach have different uptake of FDG,[146] thus complicating image interpretation. PET does appear to be somewhat helpful in detecting certain distant organ metastases, however.[147,148]

Laparoscopy and minilaparotomy represent invasive procedures, but can accurately detect serosal spread and small peritoneal implants, as well as extraregional nodal disease and small hepatic metastases.[149–151] In a recent large series, laparoscopy outperformed EUS and CT in detecting signs of unresectability and/or extraregional metastases.[152] It consistently outperforms CT.[153] In a recent series, laparoscopy proved more accurate than peritoneal fluid cytology in detecting peritoneal implants.[154] Lack of a prospective randomized trial showing resultant outcome differences makes inclusion of laparoscopy in pretreatment staging a level II-1 recommendation, however.[155]

Staging and Prognosis

Since 1987, the American Joint Committee on Cancer (AJCC) and the Union Internationale Contra le Cancer (UICC) systems for the staging of cancer have been identical.[156] Fifth and sixth edition UICC/AJCC TNM staging for adenocarcinoma of the stomach is summarized in Table 41.3.[157] This TNM staging system differs from previous versions with respect to nodal classification. Formerly, nodal classification was based on anatomic location of lymph nodes. In the current fifth–sixth edition system, nodal staging is based on the number of pathologically involved nodes, thus (at least partially) addressing the thorny issue of stage migration related to extent of lymphadenectomy.

The staging of tumor depth, or T staging, for this site has not changed since 1988. The reader should be aware that T staging for this site differs from that of colorectal cancer. Invasion of the lamina propria or submucosa, but not the muscularis propria of the gastric wall, is deemed T1 disease. Invasion of the muscularis propria or a breach of the muscularis propria without a serosal breach is deemed T2 disease. A tumor may extend into the lesser omentum or the greater omentum adjoining the stomach and, provided the serosa (i.e., visceral peritoneum) is not breached, the tumor is deemed T2. A T3 tumor breaches the serosa, thus placing the patient at increased risk of peritoneal dissemination. Microscopic breach of the serosa can be difficult for the pathologist to detect, but prognostically, presence or absence of such penetration has great impact (e.g., one recent study from Hong Kong reports 5-year survival of 64% versus 10% based on this feature alone).[158] A T4 tumor invades adjacent structures such as spleen, transverse colon, liver, diaphragm, pancreas, abdominal wall, adrenal gland, kidney, small intestine, or retroperitoneum. Intramural extension to the duodenum or the esophagus is not considered invasion of an adjacent structure, and a tumor exhibiting such intramural extension is

TABLE 41.3. UICC/AJCC Staging for Gastric Adenocarcinoma, 6th ed.

Primary tumor (T)	
Tx	Primary tumor cannot be assessed
T0	No evidence of primary tumor
Tis	Carcinoma in situ: intraepithelial tumor without invasion of the lamina propria
T1	Tumor invades lamina propria or submucosa
T2	Invades muscularis propria or subserosa[a]
T2a	Tumor invades mucularis propria
T2b	Tumor invades subserosa
T3	Tumor penetrates serosa (visceral peritoneum) without invasion of adjacent structures[b,c]
T4	Tumor invades adjacent structures[b,c]
Regional lymph nodes (N)	
NX	*Regional lymph nodes* cannot be assessed
N0	No regional node metastasis[d]
N1	Metastasis in 1 to 6 regional lymph nodes
N2	Metastasis in 7 to 15 regional lymph nodes
N3	Metastasis in more than 15 regional lymph nodes
Distant metastasis (M)	
Mx	*Distant metastasis* cannot be assessed
M0	No distant metastasis
M1	Distant metastasis

[a] A tumor may penetrate the muscularis propria with extension into the gastrocolic or gastrohepatic ligaments, or into the greater or lesser omentum, without perforation of the visceral peritoneum covering these structures. In this case, the tumor is classified T2. If there is perforation of the visceral peritoneum covering the gastric ligaments or the omentum, the tumor should be classified T3.

[b] The adjacent structures of the stomach include the spleen, transverse colon, liver, diaphragm, pancreas, abdominal wall, adrenal gland, kidney, small intestine, and retroperitoneum.

[c] Intramural extension to the duodenum or esophagus is classified by the depth of the greatest invasion in any of these sites, including the stomach.

[d] A designation of pN0 should be used if all examined lymph nodes are negative, regardless of the total number removed and examined.

Stage grouping	
0	TisN0M0
IA	T1N0M0
IB	T1N1M0 T2a/bN0M0
II	T1N2M0 T2a/bN1M0 T3N0M0
IIIA	T2a/bN2M0 T3N1M0 T4N0M0
IIIB	T3N2M0
IV	T4N1-3M0 T1-3N3M0 Any T/Any N/M1

Source: Used with the permission of the American Joint Committee on Cancer (AJCC), Chicago, Illinois. The original source for this material is the *AJCC Cancer Staging Manual*, sixth edition (2002), published by Springer-Verlag New York, www.springer-ny.com.

staged based on the depth of greatest invasion, as described above.[157]

Nodal staging in the fifth and sixth edition UICC/AJCC system is by number of involved nodes. Absence of nodal metastasis is considered N0 disease. Nodal metastasis in 1 to 6 nodes is considered N1 disease and metastasis in 7 to 15 nodes is considered N2 disease. Metastasis to more than 15 lymph nodes is considered N3 disease, and most regard this extent of nodal disease as incompatible with survival following surgery treatment alone; hence, any N3 case is classified as stage IV.

Nodal data for prognostic estimates in large databases encompass hematoxylin and eosin (H&E) staining of nodes. Methods of nodal analysis such as immunohistochemistry or polymerase chain reaction analysis enhance sensitivity to a degree far beyond H&E analysis. Prognostic implications for nodes positive only by such methods are likely different, and to a degree that remains controversial.

Distant metastasis is scored as M1 disease and all such cases are deemed stage IV. Common sites of M1 disease include the peritoneal cavity, extraregional lymph nodes (e.g., paraaortic, retropancreatic, portal, retroperitoneal, and mesenteric lymph nodes), liver, ovaries, and, less commonly, lung and bone.[157]

The TNM staging matrix for stomach cancer is summarized in Table 41.3. If one creates a 2×2 table with T stages representing rows and N stages representing columns, stage categories generally map to the diagonals (i.e., if the sum of T and N is 1, stage IA; if the sum is 2, then stage IB; if the sum is 3, then stage II; if the sum is 4, then stage IIIA). Stage IIIB is reserved for stage T3N2M0 tumors. All cases with N3 disease, and all cases with a sum of T and N greater than 5, are considered stage IV.

Five-year and 10-year relative survival rates for U.S. cases treated by gastrectomy and pathologically staged according to the fifth–sixth edition UICC/AJCC system are depicted in Table 41.4.[127] Comparison of these rates suggests that 10-year relative survival (versus 5-year relative survival) should probably be considered as the preferred outcome standard for this cancer; in modern series, survival curves tend to plateau not at 5 years, but rather between 7 and 8 years.[127]

Clinicians in Japan and elsewhere often use an alternate staging system derived from a set of "General Rules for Gastric Cancer Study," first published in 1963 and revised many times since.[159] A complete version of the 12th edition of this staging system, usually referred to as the "General Rules," has been published in English, complete with color tables and diagrams.[159,160] The T stages in this system are similar to those in the UICC/AJCC system, but it is otherwise different. Nodal staging differs considerably, with node-level definitions ranging from (regional) N1 and N2 nodal levels to (generally considered extraregional) N3 and N4 levels. The specific definitions for such levels vary according to location of tumor within the stomach (e.g., proximal third, middle third, distal third). The system includes macroscopic

TABLE 41.4. TNM staging and relative survival for U.S. cases treated by gastrectomy, 1985–1996 (n = 50, 169).

6th edition UICC/AJCC stage	*Five-year relative survival*	*Ten-year relative survival*
IA	78%	65%
IB	58%	42%
II	34%	26%
IIIA	20%	14%
IIIB	8%	3%
IV	7%	5%

Source: Data from Hundahl et al.[127]

description of the tumor (e.g., early gastric carcinoma type or, if more advanced, Borrmann type), but such description does not directly impact on final stage assignment. Peritoneal metastases are described separately (e.g., P0–P3), as are liver metastases (e.g., H0–H3). Other sites are described conventionally (i.e., M0, M1). In the overall "General Rules" staging matrix, limited peritoneal or hepatic disease is lumped in stage IVA, and other distant metastatic disease is classified as stage IVB. In this Japanese system, nodal disease that one might term extraregional in the UICC/AJCC classification (e.g., General Rules N3 disease), is incorporated into stage IIIA or IIIB if the depth of invasion is T1 or T2. Fortunately, it is fairly easy to translate from the General Rules staging to UICC/AJCC staging, provided accurate node counts are also available.[159]

The Japanese General Rules system is of interest primarily because the extent of surgical lymphadenectomy in stomach cancer has been historically defined according to this system's lymph node classification. Before the mid-1990s, the Japanese described as an "R-level" the extent of lymphadenectomy according to the highest echelon of lymph node stations completely dissected by the surgeon. To avoid confusion with the UICC R-factor, which described completeness of resection, extent of lymphadenectomy was described as a "D-factor" after the 12th edition of the General Rules.[159,160] In reviewing earlier literature in gastric cancer, one should be aware of the dual use of "R" terminology. Also, one should remember that the D-level description for level of lymphadenectomy is based on the Japanese nodal classification system (e.g., a lymphadenectomy is classified as D4 if all Japanese General Rules N1–N4 nodes are surgically removed, D3 if all N1–N3 but not all N4 nodes are cleared, etc.).[159,160]

In the current AJCC/UICC staging system, the choice of numerical thresholds for nodal categories represents a point of ongoing controversy. A number of investigators have observed progressive decrease in survival with increasing number of involved nodes,[161–168] with an apparent dropoff in survival when more than 3 nodes are involved.[162–167,169] Another dropoff when more than 6 nodes are involved has been reported.[163,165,167,168,170,171] Involvement beyond 15 or 16 nodes has been observed to be largely incompatible with long-term survival.[161,169,171] UICC/AJCC cutoffs are based on these observations, but it must be recognized that differences in the pathologic analysis of surgical specimens and differences in the extent of surgical lymphadenectomy can alter thresholds. A National Cancer Data Base (NCDB) report of 50,169 cases, all treated by gastrectomy, from 1985 through 1995, has documented that only 18% of U.S. gastric cancer cases have more than 15 nodes analyzed by the pathologist,[127] as recommended by the AJCC for accurate nodal staging.[157] The study further documented that stage migration related to nodal analysis persists in the United States despite the move to the fifth edition AJCC staging system based on based on number of nodes positive. Inadequate nodal analysis generated observed survival differences within assigned stage levels of up to 20%, and this was clearly related to the number of nodes analyzed. Nodal analysis beyond 15 nodes failed to generate any measurable enhancement in stage-stratified survival rates. Overall, 5-year relative survival was 28% and 10-year relative survival was 20%. Of the 10-year survivors in this series, 67% were node negative and 98% had 8 or fewer nodes involved.[127] Despite documented variation in nodal sampling and analysis, however, assigning nodal stage categories based on the number of involved lymph nodes does appear to generate better prognostic estimates compared to previous versions of the UICC/AJCC system[172–174] and the Japanese General Rules.[173]

Recently, Kattan and colleagues at Memorial Sloan-Kettering Cancer Center in the United States have published a prognostic normogram based on multivariate analysis of 1,039 completely resected cases that somewhat corrects for inadequate nodal analysis in gastric cancer cases. Higher relapse risk is assigned when number of nodes analyzed is suboptimal.[175] This potentially useful prognostic tool awaits validation in a separate cohort.

Residual disease after surgical treatment is not included in the UICC/AJCC TNM stage grouping matrix. It nonetheless represents a powerful, significant, independent prognostic factor.[176] The UICC and AJCC code residual disease as R0 for none, R1 for microscopic residual, and R2 for macroscopic residual tumor.[157] The completeness of resection R-factor should be specifically assigned and recorded for all patients undergoing surgical treatment.

Surgical Treatment

Historical Overview

In the United States, increasingly radical surgical approaches for gastric cancer during the 1940s and 1950s[177–180] fell into disfavor in the late 1960s and 1970s with recognition of the sometimes considerable mortality such procedures entail, at least when performed on U.S. or European patients, given the level of patient selection and the level of postoperative care possible in that era.[181]

Encouraged by generally lower surgical mortality rates and favorable 5-year survival rates, Japanese surgeons, led principally by Kajitani and colleagues, adopted a related, but distinct, approach: negative-margin gastrectomy (with initial gross margins guided by the Borrmann type of the tumor: 2cm for exophytic nodular tumors and 5+cm for ulcerated infiltrating tumors or linitis plastica) combined with aggressive removal of regional/extraregional lymph nodes, omentum, and en bloc removal of the peritoneum lining of the floor of the omental bursa along with the pancreatic capsule and associated fatty nodal tissue (i.e., omentobursectomy). Also, depending on tumor location, resection of contiguous organs such as tail of pancreas and spleen were advocated in an effort to better clear lymph node stations along the splenic artery and the splenic hilum.[182–185] Reports from large cancer hospitals in Japan emphasized increasingly favorable stage-stratified results with such techniques, multiplied by screening-driven trends to earlier-stage diagnosis and improvement in overall survival.[186–189]

Genuinely increased overall survival as a result of early diagnosis in Japan has been generally accepted as valid.[190–193] However, claims by Japanese surgeons that more-radical surgical treatment was simultaneously generating better stage-for-stage results[189,194–198] failed to uniformly win international acceptance, given the previous observation of high perioperative mortality accompanying U.S.-style radical surgery.[181] By the late 1980s, however, remarkably low 30-day postoperative mortality rates reported from major Japanese institutions (e.g., 0.6% for expert institutions such as the National Cancer

TABLE 41.5. Prospective, randomized surgical trials.

Lymphadenectomy trials	*Inclusion criteria*	*N*	*Mortality/survival*	*Mortality/ survival*	*P value (survival)*	*General comments*
			D1	**D2**		
Cape Town[209,210]	T1–3; N0–1; M0, age <75	43	0%/78% (3-year survival)	0%/76% (3-year survival)	n.s.	Solid design. Early closure due to poor accrual & inadequate power to detect.
British MRC[216–218]	Stage I–III, age >20	400	6%/35% (5-year survival)	13%/33% (5-year survival)	n.s.	Unique definition of "D1" and "D2". Skimpy quality control.
Dutch[219–220,222]	Stage I–II, age <85	711	4%/45% (5-year survival)	10%/47% (5-year survival)	n.s.	Solid design. Despite superb quality control efforts, substantial protocol noncompliance. Trial question confounded by adverse effect of pancreaticosplenectomy.
			D2	**D4**		
Japanese D2 vs. D4 Trial[226]	Deep T2–T4		0.8%/–	0.8%/–	ongoing	Ongoing trial. Immature with respect to survival.
			Subtotal	**Total**		
French[211]	Antral tumor, M0		3%/48% (5-year survival)	1%/48% (5-year survival)	n.s.	Pioneering trial. Straightforward design.
Italian[213,214]	>6 cm proximal margin possible all, but not mandated M0		1%/65% (5-year survival)	2%/62% (5-year survival)	n.s.	D2 recommended all, but not mandated. Straightforward design.
			Subtotal + D1	**Total + D3**		
Hong Kong[215]	Antral >6 cm margin, M0, age <75		0%/1,511 median survival	3%/922 days median survival	0.04 days 0.07	Dual *P* values reported. Transfusion issue.

Center Hospital in Tokyo)[194] stimulated renewed interest in Japanese surgical methods. The much higher proportion of low-stage (early gastric cancer) patients in Japanese series, combined with marked differences between the Japanese staging system (see earlier) and the UICC/AJCC staging system, confounded direct international comparison of survival rates. The UICC and AJCC successfully standardized staging worldwide in 1987,[199,200] thus facilitating stage-stratified comparisons between Japanese and non-Japanese gastric cancer cohorts. Such comparisons revealed substantial stage-stratified survival differences,[126,201] prompting some to question whether gastric cancer in Japan was a "different disease" from that seen in Western industrial countries.[202] Several retrospective analyses from Japan and elsewhere suggested that Japanese-style surgical treatment generated higher stage-stratified survival.[203–207] With seemingly uniform UICC/AJCC staging, large apparent differences in stage-stratified survival rates were noted, with 5-year survival rates for each stage routinely much higher in the more radically treated Japanese cohorts.[126,208] Such observations set the stage for prospective, randomized clinical trials addressing the following two surgical questions: (1) What is the optimal extent of lymphadenectomy (i.e., Japanese D1 versus Japanese D2) in the treatment of gastric cancer? and (2) Is routine total gastrectomy with or without extended node dissection more effective than simple subtotal gastrectomy? Results of these trials are summarized next and in Table 41.5.

Prospective, Randomized Trials of Surgical Treatment

The Cape Town South Africa Trial (1982–1986)[209,210] of D1 Versus D2 Lymphadenectomy (termed Japanese R1 versus R2 at that time) was conducted between January 1982 and November 1986 by Dent and colleagues. Inclusion criteria included T1–T3, N0–N1 disease, no distant metastases, absence of significant comorbidity, and age less than 75 years. Patients from "remote areas" were excluded. For accurate staging, biopsies of celiac, common hepatic, hepatic nodes, and "any abnormal nodes" were taken for all patients. D2 (aka R2 dissection in the nomenclature of the time) was performed according to the Japanese methods described by Kajitani and Nakajima (i.e., removal of omentum, superior leaf of peritoneum on the transverse mesocolon, removal of the capsule of the pancreas, aka omentobursectomy, and celiac-based lymph node dissection).[182,185] For the gastric resection itself, gross proximal clearance of 5 cm was required in both arms, and reconstructive techniques were specified. Over the period of study, 608 cases were reportedly evaluated; 403 were deemed surgical candidates, but only 43 (7% overall and 11% at laparotomy) were deemed to meet all eligibility criteria. Following treatment and discharge, patients were followed by examination at 3-month intervals. No attempt was made to screen for recurrence.[209,210] No survival differences were noted. In-hospital mortality was zero for both groups. The trial did document increased operative time (*P* less than 0.005), increased blood transfusions (*P* less than 0.005), and longer hospital stay (*P* less than 0.05) for the D2 group. This single-institution trial was halted when single-institution accrual to adequate statistical power for the question was deemed unlikely.[209,210]

The French Subtotal Versus Total Gastrectomy Trial,[211] by the French Association for Surgical Research, was conducted between 1980 and 1985 to address the potential value of routine total gastrectomy versus the higher mortality and morbidity associated with this procedure, as documented by

McNeer and others.[180,212] Eligibility criteria included presence of an adenocarcinoma located in the distal half of the stomach, good organ function, and no evidence of nodal involvement higher than the gastroesophageal junction or in the splenopancreatic region. Cases of superficial carcinoma (in situ or early T1) were to be excluded, as were cases of obvious linitis plastica type extensive infiltration within the gastric wall. Extensive lymph node dissection was not mandated, but proximal ligation/resection of the left gastric artery was. A Billroth II gastrojejeunostomy reconstruction was used for all subtotal gastrectomy cases, reconstruction for all total gastrectomy cases consisted of Roux-en-Y esophagojejeunostomy, and 169 patients were randomized. Somewhat paradoxically, postoperative mortality was observed to be lower in the total gastrectomy group (1.3% versus 3.2%). Five-year survival rate for both groups was identical at 48%.[211]

The Italian Subtotal Versus Total Gastrectomy Trial[213,214] was conducted from April 1982 through December 1993. Six hundred eighteen patients with localized gastric adenocarcinoma of the antrum were randomized to subtotal gastrectomy versus total gastrectomy. A D2 lymphadenectomy and omentobursectomy was recommended for all patients but not mandated. Inclusion criteria included histologic confirmation of adenocarcinoma, age less than 75, absence of serious comorbid conditions, and no history of previous malignancy, gastric surgery, or chemotherapy. Additionally, during laparotomy, all patients were required to have a tumor-free proximal margin of 6 cm and absence of any extraregional nodes, hepatic metastases, peritoneal metastases, or unresectable infiltration of contiguous organs. Over this 1982–1993 period, 1,372 patients from 31 Italian institutions were evaluated and 648 randomized; after exclusions, 311 were left in the subtotal gastrectomy group and 296 in the total gastrectomy group.[213,214] With median 72-month follow-up, 5-year Kaplan–Meier survival was 65.3% for the subtotal gastrectomy group and 62.4% for the total gastrectomy group (P = n.s.).[213,214]

The Hong Kong Trial of D1 Subtotal Versus D3 Total Gastrectomy[215] was conducted between October 1987 and December 1991 by Robertson and colleagues at the Prince of Wales Hospital in Hong Kong. The trial was open to patients undergoing laparotomy for grossly localized antral tumors that could be cleared to a 6-cm proximal margin with subtotal gastrectomy. Additional entry criteria included negative distal margin, absence of liver metastases, absence of peritoneal metastases, age less than 75 years, and absence of serious comorbid conditions. Neither intraoperative cytologic nor histologic analyses were performed. In the D3 group, distal pancreatectomy and splenectomy and D3 lymph node dissection were routinely performed, but without omentobursectomy. The R1 subtotal group underwent simple distal gastrectomy with a 6-cm proximal margin, high ligation of the right and left gastric arteries, and simple omentectomy, but no other node dissection. Over the study period, 55 cases were randomized, 25 in the D1 subtotal group and 30 in the D3 total group.[215] In this trial, survival was actually better for the more simply treated D1 subtotal group (median survival, 1511 versus 922 days; P less than 0.05). The D3 total group had longer operative time (260 versus 140 minutes; P less than 0.05), more transfusions (P less than 0.05), and much longer hospital stay (16 versus 8 days; P less than 0.05). No patient in the D1 subtotal group died postoperatively in hospital, in contrast to 1 patient in the D3 total group (P = n.s.).[215]

The Medical Research Council (MRC) Trial of Modified "D1" Versus Modified "D2" Lymphadenectomy[216–218] was conducted in 1986 through 1995, by Cushieri, Fielding, Craven, Joypaul, and colleagues of the Surgical Co-operative Group. In this trial, a D1 procedure was defined in a manner at variance with the definition used by the JRSGC. For this trial, a D1 lymph node dissection was one in which only those lymph nodes within 3 cm of the tumor were removed (consistent with pre-1997 TNM definitions of N1 nodes). The D2 procedure was defined as one in which TNM N2 nodes (i.e., "celiac, hepatoduodenal, retroduodenal, splenic, and retropancreatic nodes, depending on location of the tumor," as well as perigastric nodes more than 3 cm from the tumor) were removed and the omental bursa resected (omentobursectomy). Distal pancreaticosplenectomy was performed almost exclusively in the D2 group, and splenectomy in both groups, but more frequently in the D2 group. Eligibility was assessed at staging laparotomy. Prelaparotomy exclusions included age less than 20 and those with serious comorbid disease. All patients were assessed, at laparotomy, for the presence of peritoneal implants, liver metastases, and extraregional/periaortic adenopathy, particularly in the area of the left renal vein. Those with disease in these sites were excluded. Intraoperative peritoneal cytology was not used. Eligible cases were deemed to have TNM stage I–III disease with negative margins of resection and a proximal margin of at least 2.5 cm free of gross disease. Of 737 cases registered, 337 were deemed ineligible at staging laparotomy because of advanced disease, leaving 400 cases for intraoperative randomization.[216–218] With median follow-up of 6.5 years, 5-year overall survival for the D1 group was 35% versus 33% for the D2 group (P = n.s.). Recurrence-free survival and disease-specific survival did not differ significantly. Unfortunately, splenic resection, performed more frequently in the D2 group, and pancreatic resection, performed almost exclusively in the D2 group, seriously impacted survival and proved to be independent predictors of poor survival. Complications and mortality were higher in the D2 group, and pancreaticosplenectomy appeared to be a powerful influence. The adverse impact of pancreaticosplenectomy, particularly pancreatectomy, somewhat confounded this trial with respect to the lymphadenectomy question.[216–218]

The Dutch Trial of D1 Versus D2 Lymphadenectomy[219,220] was conducted between August 1989 and July 1993 by surgeons participating in the Dutch Gastric Cancer Group. Eligibility criteria included age less than 85 years, adequate physical condition with no serious comorbid diseases, no previous cancer, no previous gastric surgery, and histologically confirmed gastric adenocarcinoma without evidence of distant metastases. Patients in both groups underwent distal or total gastrectomy according to the location of the tumor, with subtotal gastrectomy allowed if a proximal tumor-free margin of 5 cm could be achieved. At the onset of the trial, surgeons from 80 centers and 8 expert consulting surgeons were extensively instructed concerning Japanese-type surgical treatment according to Japan Research Society for Gastric Cancer (JRSGC) definitions and guidelines.[160,182,221] Patients were randomized preoperatively to arrange for the intraoperative presence of an expert consultant surgeon for all D2 cases. A Japanese expert surgeon attended every case during the first 4 months of the trial. The D1 procedure involved removal of all JRSGC-defined N1 nodes, generally the perigastric nodes at stations 1–6 along the greater and lesser curvatures of the stomach, along with removal of the lesser and greater omentum. The D2 procedure involved omentobursectomy (i.e., removal of greater and lesser omentum, the superior leaf of the transverse mesocolon and the capsule of the pancreas), frequent distal pancreatectomy and splenectomy (depending on tumor location), and removal of all JRSGC-defined N2 nodes at stations 7–12 (i.e., left gastric, celiac, common hepatic, proper hepatic, and splenic arteries and splenic hilar nodes). Reconstruction following completion of the D2 node dissection was left to the local institutional surgeon, as was the postoperative care of the patient[219,220]. Of the 1,078 cases randomized preoperatively, 82 (8%) were excluded for various reasons, most commonly, unavailability of a consultant reference surgeon (35 cases), poor physical condition, or lack of histologic confirmation of the diagnosis. Of the remaining 996 patients randomized and entered into the study, 285 had evidence of incurable/extraregional disease and were excluded; 711 deemed potentially curable underwent the randomly assigned treatment (i.e., D1 or D2 resection) with curative intent. The 380 cases in the D1 group and the 331 cases in the D2 group were well balanced with respect to age, gender, tumor location, and tumor depth. Eighty-nine percent of the cases in each group underwent apparent, pathologically confirmed, negative-margin resection. A slightly higher proportion of cases in the D2 group underwent total gastrectomy (38% versus 30% in the D1 group).[219,220]

Among randomized cases, morbidity (25% versus 43%; P less than 0.001) and in-hospital mortality (4% versus 10%; $P = 0.004$) were higher for the D2 group. With a median follow-up of 72 months, 5-year survival was 45% for the D1 group and 47% for the D2 group (P = n.s.). Pancreatic and splenic resection, performed mostly in the D2 group (and mandated for particular tumor subsites) were associated with significantly higher morbidity and mortality in this study. Restricting the analysis to patients who did not undergo pancreatic or splenic resection (a post hoc, selected analysis), survival was higher for the D2 group (59% for the D1 group versus 71% for the D2 group; $P = 0.02$).[222] Overall, however, for those who indeed had a negative-margin resection deemed potentially curative, risk of relapse at 5 years was 43% for the D1 group versus 37% for the D2 group (difference between relapse rates was not significant). An 11-year follow-on report for this trial indicates that of the 89 cases with pathologic N2 disease, there were nine 10-year survivors, and 8 of the 9 were in the D2 group ($P = 0.01$ for this post hoc analysis of the N2 subgroup).[222] Overall survival at the 11-year mark is 31% versus 35% for D1 and D2, respectively ($P = 0.53$). Post hoc subset analysis notwithstanding, overall, this trial fails to support routine D2 lymphadenectomy.[219,220]

At the time, both the MRC trial and the Dutch Trial were initiated, pancreaticosplenectomy was still deemed a standard part of a Japanese-type operation for cancers involving the cardia. By the mid-1990s, Japanese recommendations with respect to pancreaticosplenectomy had shifted[223–225]; however, both trials were already well under way. Perhaps in response to MRC and Dutch Trial findings, pancreas-preserving D2 (or D2+) operations are now favored by the Japanese and others, unless resection of these organs is required to achieve negative margins.[223–225]

A multicenter Japanese Trial of D2 Versus D4 Lymphadenectomy,[226] initiated by Sasako, Sano, and colleagues, dwells on the potential value of paraaortic lymph node dissection for deep T2 (i.e., serosal invasion suspected) and T3–T4 proximal tumors. In both Japan and Italy, microscopic disease in such nodes is not infrequent, and resection of such diseased nodes can generate approximately 15% 5-year survival.[227–231] This trial has now completed accrual of 523 eligible cases. Thirty-day operative mortality for both D2 and D4 groups in this trial is 0.8%.[226] The trial remains immature with respect to survival.[226]

Summarizing results from all these surgical trials, neither routine D2 (or greater) lymphadenectomy with pancreatic-splenic resection nor routine total gastrectomy can be routinely recommended (level of evidence, I). Overall, the somewhat arbitrary D-level system for guiding lymphadenectomy has not proven helpful in increasing survival. However, the potential value of pancreas/spleen-preserving lymphadenectomy, particularly if performed in low-mortality centers (e.g., those in Japan and certain other expert centers) remains an open question.

In-Hospital Mortality Rates Associated with Gastrectomy for Cancer

In both the MRC trial (6.5% versus 13%, $P = 0.04$)[217] and the Dutch Trial (4% versus 10%, $P = 0.004$).[219,232] in-hospital mortality was significantly associated with pancreatic-splenic resection,[217,232] which, in turn, was far more frequent in the D2 group (mandated component of D2 for most nonantral tumors). Viewed critically, in-hospital mortality was also very high for the D1 groups. In the aforementioned Japanese multicenter D2 versus D4 trial, surgical mortality was only 0.8% for both groups.[226] Certainly, comorbid cardiovascular disease probably differs among international patient populations, but other factors such as surgical experience, technique, and variation in morbidity management can also play a role.[233] In U.S. studies, surgeon volume and hospital volume persistently impact on in-hospital mortality.[234–236] The mechanisms for the volume–mortality relationship have yet to be fully elucidated. Specialists, well-equipped and well-staffed operating rooms, and specialized services, including sophisticated ICU care, tend to be more available in larger hospitals.[237,238] Additionally, when surgeons have open access to various hospitals, high-volume surgeons might preferentially prefer to practice in such environments.[237,238] For a major procedure such as gastrectomy for cancer, there is evidence of both a learning curve[239] and value to volume. Referral to specialist centers has been proposed.[240,241]

Maruyama Index of Unresected Disease and Computer-Guided Lymphadenectomy

In the late 1980s, Keiichi Maruyama and colleagues at the National Cancer Center Hospital in Tokyo created a computer program (known as the Maruyama Program) that searched a meticulously-maintained 3,843-patient database of gastric cancer cases treated by extensive lymphadenectomy, matching cases with similar characteristics to a given case. With seven demographic and clinical inputs (all identifiable preoperatively or intraoperatively), the program predicts the statistical likelihood of nodal disease for each of 16 (JRSGC-defined) nodal stations around the stomach (note that current JRSGC General Rules identify 33 nodal stations, substations,

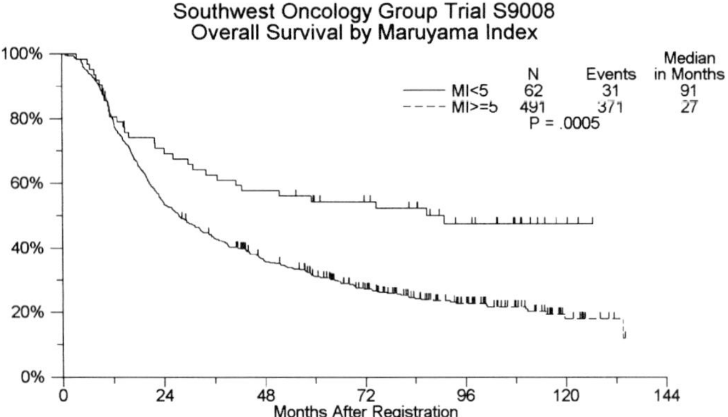

FIGURE 41.6. Impact of a surgical factor, Maruyama Index of Unresected Disease (MI), on overall survival for cases enrolled in SWOG 9008/INT 0116, a large U.S. adjuvant trial. (Updated data courtesy of Southwest Oncology Group.[246])

and optional sites). Maruyama Program predictions have been assessed in Japanese, German, and Italian populations and found to be highly accurate.[242–244] The tool is designed to be used by surgeons preoperatively or intraoperatively as a convenient means of rationally planning the optimal extent of lymphadenectomy for a given patient. Since the late 1980s, the program has been used in exactly this way by surgeons at the National Cancer Institute Hospital in Tokyo and by many gastric cancer surgeons around the world. In an effort to expand use of this computerized tool, a CD-ROM with expanded case volume has been prepared.[245]

In a prospectively planned surgical analysis of a large multicenter U.S. trial of adjuvant postoperative chemoradiation in gastric cancer (SWOG 9008/Intergroup 0116; see following), the extent of surgical treatment was specifically assessed and prospectively coded through both detailed reporting forms and review of records (e.g., operative reports). The prospectively planned surgical analysis of survival in Intergroup 0116 made use of a novel means of quantifying the adequacy of lymphadenectomy relative to likely extent of nodal disease: the "Maruyama Index of Unresected Diease" (MI). The Maruyama Index of Unresected Diease was defined (by the author, S.H.) as the sum of Maruyama Program predictions for those Japanese-defined regional node stations (stations 1–12) left in situ by the surgeon.[246] Based on the Intergroup trial's entry criteria, and the definition of MI, every case registered to INT-0116 could have had an MI of 0; this variable was under the surgeon's control. Before any survival analysis in this trial, it was speculated that patients with MI less than 5 would have measurably superior survival. As shown in Figure 41.6, this indeed proved to be the case, with median overall survival for the MI less than 5 subgroup 91 months versus 27 months ($P = 0.005$). By multivariate analysis, adjusting for treatment, T stage, and number of nodes positive, MI proved an independent predictor of survival ($P = 0.0049$). Data for disease-free survival are similar.[246,247] The overall median Maruyama Index of Unresected Diease in this chemoradiation trial was 70 (range, 0–429), suggesting undertreatment. An effect for "dose of surgery," as measured by MI, was also evident: median survival was 20 months for the highest MI quartile and 46 months for the lowest MI quartile (treatment-adjusted $P = 0.002$).[246] In summary, by univariate analysis and by multivariate analysis, MI proved to be a strong and significant predictor of prognosis.[246,248]

To further assess of the utility of MI as a prognostic tool, the Dutch Trial has recently been reanalyzed. Blinded to survival, and eliminating cases with incomplete information, 648 of the 711 patients treated with curative intent had MI assigned. Median MI was 26 and varied according to UICC stage, nodal stratum, T stage, D level, and tumor involvement of overlapping sites, in that order. In contrast to D level, MI less than 5 proved an independent predictor of both overall [$P = 0.016$, hazard ratio (HR) = 1.45, 95% confidence interval (CI) = 1.07–1.95] and relapse risk ($P = 0.010$, HR = 1.72, 95% CI = 1.14–2.60).[249] As shown in Figures 41.7 and 41.8, a dose–response effect was also evident.[249] This blinded

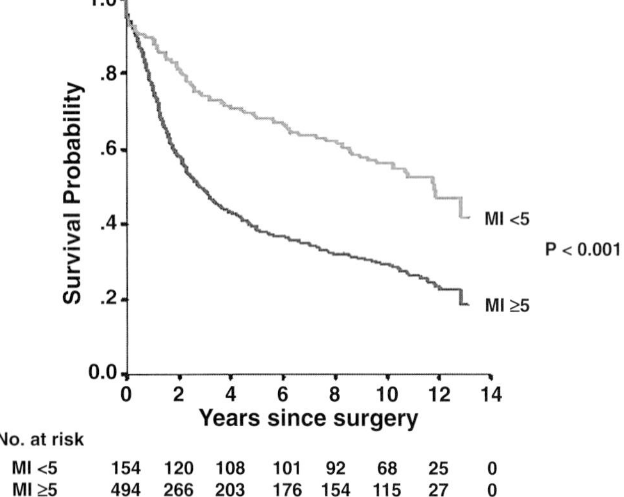

FIGURE 41.7. Reanalysis of the Dutch D1–D2 Trial. Maruyama Index of Unresected Disease (MI) is a major independent prognostic factor. Low MI is associated with superior survival. (From Peeters et al.,[249] by permission of *World Journal of Surgery*.)

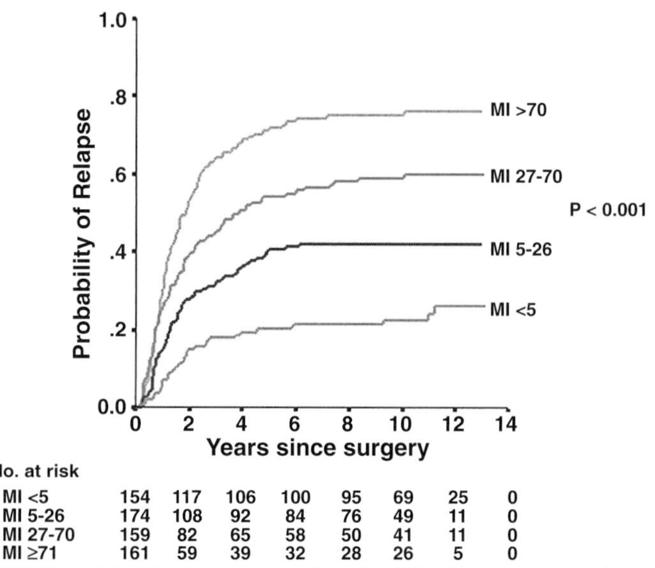

FIGURE 41.8. Dose–response effect for MI with respect to relapse in the Dutch D1–D2 Trial (data for survival similar, not shown). (From Peeters et al.,[249] by permission of *World Journal of Surgery*.)

reanalysis further supports the utility of the Maruyama computer program in customizing the extent of lymphadenectomy in individual gastric cancer cases according to the predicted extent of nodal disease. "Low Maruyama Index" surgery, which can easily be accomplished by using the Maruyama Program to prospectively plan lymphadenectomy for a given patient, appears to enhance survival (level II-1 evidence). This conclusion has yet to be validated in a prospective, randomized trial.

Endoscopic Mucosal Resection of Selected T1 Cancers

In countries such as Japan, where the incidence of early gastric cancer (i.e., T1 tumor) is high, endoscopic mucosal resection (EMR) has emerged as a reasonable option for selected cases.[250–255] In the traditional technique of endoscopic mucosal resection, submucosal injection of saline floats the small area of tumor-bearing mucosa off the underlying muscularis propria and the lesion is resected with a special cautery snare with hooks to preserve specimen orientation for margin analysis. The procedure can be technically challenging, but innovations such as use of incision endo-forceps,[256] aspiration mucosectomy,[257] use of a stabilizing distal magnetic anchor,[258] or use of the double endoscope resection technique[259] can facilitate its proper execution. Percutaneous traction assist techniques using small percutaneous ports and instrumentation can also facilitate the procedure,[260] but percutaneous violation of the gastric lumen in such cases can risk unnecessary intraabdominal or port site tumor implantation. For this reason, laparoscopic resection for superficial T1 tumors suitable for EMR has been viewed with caution.[255]

Selection of cases suitable for EMR hinges on the absence of disease in the regional lymphatics. A combined series of 5,265 surgically treated T1 cases from the National Cancer Center Hospital and the Cancer Institute Hospital in Tokyo offers unsurpassed level II guidance.[261] For *intramucosal tumors*, none of 1,230 well-differentiated cancers of less than 30mm diameter, regardless of ulceration findings, were associated with metastases (95% CI, 0%–0.3%). Regardless of tumor size, none of 929 cancers without ulceration were associated with nodal metastases (95% CI, 0%–0.4%). For *submucosal cancers*, there was a significant correlation between tumor size larger than 30mm and lymphatic-vascular involvement with an increased risk of nodal involvement. None of the 145 well-differentiated adenocarcinomas of less than 30mm diameter without lymphatic or venous permeation were associated with nodal involvement, provided that the lesion had invaded less than 500μm into the submucosa (95% CI, 0%–2.5%).[261]

In an 11-year, 445 case series by Ono and colleagues from the National Cancer Center Hospital in Tokyo, there were no gastric cancer related deaths during a median follow up period of 38 months (3–120 months).[250] Although bleeding and perforation occurred in 5%, there were no treatment-related deaths.[250] For selected superficial T1 cancers, endoscopic mucosal resection performed by experienced personnel can generate superb results and can certainly be recommended, especially because local recurrences can be addressed with salvage gastrectomy (level II-2 evidence).

Adjuvant Treatments

Radiation and Chemoradiation

For locally advanced tumors deemed unresectable to negative margins, radiation and concomitant chemoradiation appear to make long-term disease-free survival possible for a small, but significant, subset of patients.[262] In a Mayo Clinic series published in 1969, Moertel and colleagues documented rare long-term survivals with regional chemoradiation.[263] In a follow-up prospective, randomized trial of radiation alone ($n = 23$) versus concomitant bolus 5-fluorouracil (5-FU) plus radiation ($n = 25$), mean survival was 13 months versus 6 months, favoring combined therapy (P less than 0.05) and 5-year survival was 12% versus 0%.[264] In a follow-up study, the Gastrointestinal Tumor Study Group randomized 90 eligible cases to receive either combination chemotherapy alone or concomitant chemoradiation with further, follow-on chemotherapy. Early nutritional and myelosuppressive complications rendered initial survival of the chemoradiation arm inferior, but with minimum 5-year follow-up, survival was significantly higher for the chemoradiation arm, with 16% alive disease free compared to 7% among those treated with chemotherapy alone (P less than 0.05).[265]

For cases treated surgically, historical pattern-of-failure data from clinical, operative second look, and autopsy sources document that approximately 60% of node-positive and/or transserosal cancers (T3 or more) recur in regional nodes, tumor bed, or anastomosis, with 20% of tumors recurring only locoregionally (Table 41.6).[262,266–270] Such data compellingly invited application of locoregional radiation or chemoradiation as an adjuvant to surgical treatment. Figure 41.9 depicts a early proposal by Gunderson and Sosin for a radiation treatment field encompassing frequent locoregional areas of failure, based on Wangensteen's University of Minnesota reoperative series.[271]

Between 1991 and 1998, the Southwest Oncology Group and the Gastric Intergroup conducted SWOG 9008/INT 0116, a two-armed prospective randomized trial of postoperative adjuvant chemoradiation versus surgery alone in patients with completely resected adenocarcinoma of the stomach and esophagogastric junction. Eligibility criteria for this trial specified complete negative-margin resection, registration 20–41 days postoperatively, adequate organ function, good performance status (i.e., Zubrod 1 or 2), postoperative caloric intake of more than 1,500kcal per day, and fourth edition TNM stage IB or higher, distant-metastasis-negative, disease.[272] Of 603 cases accrued to the study, 46 (8%) were ineligible, leaving

TABLE 41.6. Patterns of failure after "curative" resection of gastric cancer.

Incidence in total patient group (%)			
Pattern of Failure	*Clinical*	*Reoperation*	*Autopsy*
A. Locoregional	38	67	80–93
B. Peritoneal seeding	23	41	30–50
—Localized		–19	
—Diffuse		–22	
C. Distant metastases	52	22	49

Modified from Smalley et al.,[262] by permission of *International Journal of Radiation Biology Oncology Physics.*

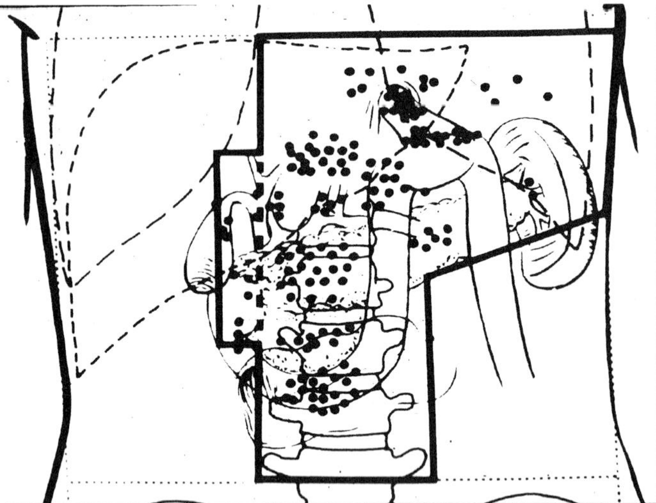

FIGURE 41.9. Early proposal by Gunderson and Sosin for a radiation treatment field encompassing frequent locoregional areas of failure, based on Wangensteen's University of Minnesota reoperative series. (From Gunderson and Sosin,[267] by permission of *International Journal of Radiation Oncology Biology Physics*.)

556 cases; 20% of eligible cases registered had disease of the cardia/gastroesophageal junction, and advanced-stage cases were overrepresented. Eighty-five percent of cases were node positive. Using AJCC/UICC fifth edition criteria, fully 69% of the cases had AJCC IIIA or IIIB disease (46% and 23%, respectively) and only 8% had stage IB disease.[272] Of the cases in this trial, 54% underwent D0 (i.e., less than D1 lymphadenectomy), a source of subsequent criticism. The treatment consisted of one cycle of 5-FU (425 mg/m^2) and leucovorin (LV, 20 mg/m^2) in a daily × 5 regimen followed by 4,500 cGy (180 cGy/day, M–F) given with 5-FU/LV (400 mg/m^2 and 20 mg/m^2) on days 1 through 4 and on the last 3 days of radiation. On completion of the radiation, two additional cycles of daily × 5% FU/LV were given at the original dose levels at monthly intervals.[272] Results for this trial were recently updated with more than 6 years of median follow-up (Figure 41.10).[273] Overall survival was 35 months median for chemoradiation versus 26 months for surgery alone [$P = 0.006$; hazard ratio, 1.31 (1.08–1.61)]. Disease-free survival was also significantly different at 30 months median for chemoradiation and 19 months for surgery alone [P less than 0.001; hazard ratio, 1.52 (1.75–1.85)].[273]

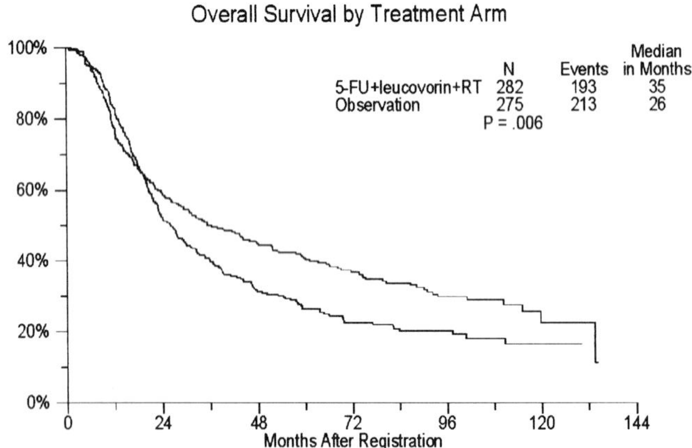

FIGURE 41.10. Updated survival with more than 6 years median follow-up for INT-0116, a trial of postoperative adjuvant chemoradiation (*upper curve*) versus postoperative observation (see text). (Updated data courtesy of Southwest Oncology Group.[272,273])

Exploratory subgroup analyses for INT-0116 were recently performed for six variables: gender, T stage, N stage, gastric subsite, D level of dissection, and diffuse versus intestinal histology. Positive treatment effects were seen in all subsets. A possible treatment interaction was seen, with diffuse-type histology cases doing poorly with therapy, but after adjusting for multiple testing, this result was not significant.[273]

The likely burden of unresected locoregional disease in this trial is problematic.[274] Less than D1 lymphadenectomy, considered suboptimal in the opinion of most experts, was performed in 54% of the cases.[246,272] As noted in the previous section, cases with Maruyama Index of Unresected Disease (MI) less than 5 enjoyed significantly greater survival (median overall survival for the MI less than 5 subgroup, 91 months versus 27 months; $P = 0.005$), and this was an independent predictor of survival.[246] By D level, median survival was 27 months for D0 lymphadenectomy and 48 months for D2 lymphadenectomy, but only 10% of cases registered to this trial underwent D2, and this difference was not significant.[246] Surgical undertreatment may have played a role in making this a positive trial.[274]

On the basis of INT 0116, adjuvant chemoradiation has been recommended in the United States for all patients with stage IB or greater, M0 disease (i.e., locoregional disease), *provided* they meet criteria for adequate caloric intake (more than 1,500 cal/day), good organ function, and good performance status.[272] Do all patient subgroups really benefit? The power to detect differing treatment effect in various subgroups in this trial (especially the stage IB subset) is low. Statistical tests of treatment interaction with pathology and surgical variables have been negative, however.[272] A cautionary note concerning the lower-risk, stage IB subgroup (i.e., patients with T2N0 or T1N1 disease) has been voiced.[274]

On the basis of this study, a new U.S. Intergroup trial, examining postoperative etoposide, cisplatin, and 5-FU (ECF) chemotherapy before and after radiation with continuous infusion 5-FU versus adjuvant treatment according to the INT-0116 protocol, is now under way, as well as other, similar trials in Europe.

Early Postoperative Intraperitoneal Chemotherapy

Japanese investigators have advocated intraperitoneal and intralymphatic installation of mitomycin C bound to microcarbon particles for some time.[275] This treatment has been tested in an Austrian prospective randomized trial with negative results.[276] Another Austrian prospective randomized trial of perioperative cisplatin has also been reported as negative.[277] A Japanese trial of intraperitoneal OK-432 in addition to systemic therapy has also been negative.[278] Phase II investigations of intraperitoneal therapy have also been conducted in the United States and elsewhere,[279,280] with some investigators enthusiastic[281] and some advising caution because of the associated morbidity.[282]

One positive prospective randomized clinical trial of perioperative intraperitoneal has been reported.[283] Between 1990 and 1995, 248 Korean patients with biopsy-proven gastric

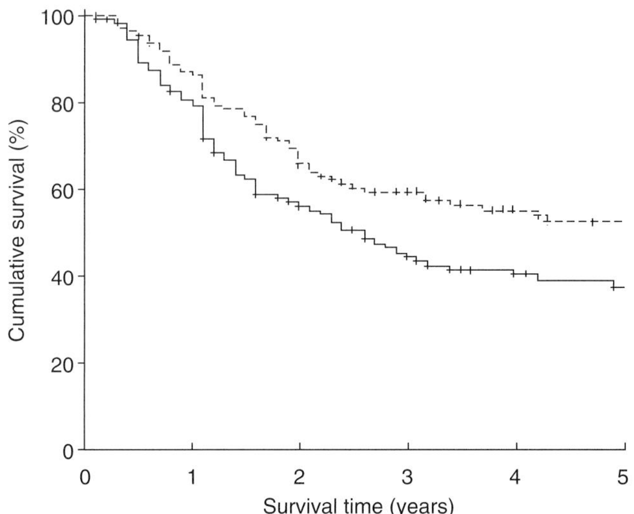

FIGURE 41.11. Kaplan–Meier overall survival for group treated with early postoperative intraperitoneal chemotherapy (mitomycin C on postoperative day 1 and 5-fluorouracil (5-FU) daily on postoperative days 2–5; *upper curve*) versus controls receiving surgery alone (*lower curve*). With mean follow-up of 36 months, survival difference is significant ($P = 0.0278$). (From Yu et al.,[283] by permission of *World Journal of Surgery*.)

cancer without intraoperatively detected distant organ metastases were randomized intraoperatively following complete resection and minimum D2 lymphadenectomy to receive postoperative intraperitoneal mitomycin C and 5-FU versus surgery alone (Figure 41.11). Stage I cases and those more than 70 years of age were excluded. Postoperative adjuvant treatment, delivered intraperitoneally through a Tenckhoff catheter, consisted of 10 mg/m^2 mitomycin C delivered at body temperature in 1 L dialysis solution on the first postoperative day, followed by 700 mg/m^2 5-FU plus 50 mEq sodium bicarbonate in 1 L dialysis solution daily on days 2 through 5. No further antitumor treatment was administered during the disease-free interval. In-hospital mortality was 6.4% in the treated group versus 1.6% in the surgery-only group (P = n.s.). Among morbidities, intraabdominal bleeding (10% versus 1%; $P = 0.002$) and intraabdominal abscess/peritonitis (14% versus 4%; $P = 0.008$) were more frequent among treated cases. Follow-up consisted of regular physical examinations, but CT scans, paracentesis, etc., were initiated only at the discretion of the surgeon to confirm clinical findings. The initial report of this trial in 1998 reported a significant positive effect on survival only for stage III cases.[284] A subsequent follow-up in 2001 reported significantly improved overall survival for the treatment group (54% versus 38%; $P = 0.0278$).[283] Subset analysis revealed the benefit was enjoyed predominantly by those with fifth–sixth edition UICC TNM stage III (57% versus 23%; $P = 0.0024$) and stage IV (28% versus 5%; $P = 0.0098$) disease.[283] Further subset analysis showed benefit for those with involved lymph nodes (46% versus 22%; $P = 0.0027$) and those with serosal invasion (52% versus 25%; $P = 0.0004$).[283] Although this trial has yet to be duplicated, and there are some methodological criticisms, it has encouraged continued investigation of both perioperative intraperitoneal therapy and methods to decrease the associated morbidity. In the view of advocates, this trial constitutes level I evidence in favor of such intraperitoneal therapy.[281]

Chemotherapy Without Radiation

A succession of meta-analyses concerning the value (or nonvalue) of systemic chemotherapy for gastric cancer have been conducted over the past decade. In 1993, Hermans et al. published a meta-analysis of 11 randomized trials of adjuvant chemotherapy, mostly involving treatment with 5-FU-based regimens, conducted over the previous decade. The odds ratio of 0.88 among treated patients was not significant.[285] A year later, in response to a journal letter,[286] two additional trials were added, and the addition of 318 cases from the two erroneously omitted trials lowered the odds ratio to 0.82; this was of borderline significance (CI, 0.68–0.98).[287] In 1999, Earle and Maroun published a 13-trial meta-analysis of non-Asian trials published between 1980 and 1996, with a similar odds ratio for death in the treated group of 0.80 (95% CI, 0.66–0.97).[288] In 2000, Mari et al. published a 20-article, 3,658 patient meta-analysis with an odds ratio for the treated group of 0.82; with the additional trials and patients, this was significant (95% CI, 0.75–0.89; P less than 0.001).[289] Nonetheless, even including subgroup analyses, only a few trials showed significant results favoring chemotherapy,[290–295] and the authors still considered adjuvant chemotherapy as investigational.[289] In 2002, Panzini et al., from Italy, restricted meta-analysis to those trials where all patients were treated with "radical" surgical techniques. Of the 17 papers eligible for inclusion, 3,118 patients were available for analysis. Odds ratio for death among the treated cases was 0.72 (95% CI, 0.62–0.84),[296] and on the basis of this, a large confirmatory randomized controlled trial of cisplatin-based chemotherapy was recommended.[296] In 2001, a less-selective, but more-comprehensive, meta-analysis was conducted by the Swedish Council of Technology Assessment in Health Care (SBU),[297] based on 153 scientific papers, 18 reviews, 60 randomized studies, and 57 prospective studies encompassing 12,367 patients. The authors' meta-analysis of 21 randomized adjuvant studies revealed a statistically significant survival benefit with odds ratio 0.84 (95% CI, 0.74–0.96); however, analyzing Western world and Asian studies separately, a statistically significant difference was noticed: Western world studies showed an odds ratio of 0.96 (95% CI, 0.83–1.12) and the Asian studies an odds ratio of 0.58 (95% CI, 0.44–0.76).[297] The authors concluded that adjuvant chemotherapy could not be recommended in Western patients, but that benefit in Japanese series was evident.[297] Overall, the benefit of adjuvant therapy in all these meta-analyses equates to an odds ratio of approximately 0.80 at best. The extent of surgical resection for patients entered into these adjuvant studies, and the consequent burden of residual locoregional microscopic disease, may, as Panzini et al. suggest, be the key confounding variable.[296] Nakajima et al., in a meta-analysis of 10 Japanese trials conducted at the Cancer Institute Hospital in Tokyo on radically treated surgical cases from 1959 to 1982 (n = 1,177 cases), noted a much better odds ratio of 0.63 favoring the treatment groups (P less than 0.01).[298]

As depicted in Table 41.7, most trials of adjuvant systemic chemotherapy versus surgery alone have been negative.[291,294,295,299–311] For the positive trials, unusually low control group survival,[295] or findings at odds with other trials,[294] undermine general applicability.

Following the aforementioned INT-0116 adjuvant chemoradiation trial, for patients with disease resectable to

TABLE 41.7. Prospective randomized trials of adjuvant systemic chemotherapy.

Author	Year	Treatment group	N	Five-year survival	Survival Median survival	P value
Nakajima et al.[299]	1984	MMC + 5-FU+araC →F	81	68%	>60 months	0.09
		MMC + ftorafur + araC→ftora	83	63%	>60 months	
		Surgery alone	79	51%	>60 months	
Engstrom et al.[300]	1985	5-FU + MeCCNU	91	—	36.6 months	0.73
		Surgery alone	89	—	32.7 months	
Coombes et al.[301]	1990	FAM (5-FU + Adria+MMC)	148	35%	36 months	0.17
		Surgery alone	133	46%	36 months	
Krook et al.[302]	1991	5-FU + Adria	64	33%	34 months	0.88
		Surgery alone	61	32%	36 months	
Grau et al.[291]	1993	MMC	68	41%	—	0.025*
		Surgery alone	66	26%	—	
Hallissey et al.[303]	1994	FAM	138	19%	17.3 months	0.14
		Postoperative radiotherapy alone	153	12%	12.9 months	
		Surgery alone	145	20%	14.7 months	
Macdonald et al.[304]	1995	FAM	93	—	32 months	0.57
		Surgery alone	100	—	28 months	
Tsavaris et al.[305]	1996	5-FU-epirub-MMC (FEM)	42	—	64 months	ns
		Surgery alone	42	—	81 months	
Neri et al.[295]	1996	5-FU-LV-epirub	48	25%	20.4 months	0.01*
		Surgery alone	55	13%	13.6 months	
Grau et al.[329]	1998	MMC-ftorafur	43	67%	—	0.04
		MMC	42	44%	—	
Nakajima et al.[306]	1999	MMC-5-FU-UFT	285	85.8%	>5 years	0.17
		Surgery alone	288	82.9%	>5 years	
Cirera et al.[294]	1999	MMC-tegafur	76	56%	74	0.04*
		Surgery alone	72	36%	29	
Langman et al.[307]	1999	Cimetidine	221	21%	13	0.42
		Surgery alone	221	18%	11	
Nashimoto et al.[308]	2003	MMC-5-FU-araC	126	91.2%	—	0.13
		Surgery alone	126	86.1%	—	
Chipponi et al.[309]	2004	5-FU-LV-CDDP	101	39%	—	ns
		Surgery alone	104	39%	—	
Sato et al.[310]	2004	5-DFUR	143	62.9%	—	0.79
		5-DFUR + OKT-432	144	63.8%		
Hartgrink et al.[311]	2004	Preop (neoadjuvant) FAMTX	29	—	18 months	0.17
		Surgery alone	30	—	30 months	

negative margins, clinical trials involving arms with only surgery or only postoperative adjuvant chemotherapy have become less feasible in the United States.[272,273]

To date, no neoadjuvant preoperative chemotherapy regimen has been shown superior to postoperative therapy or surgery alone in a Phase III prospective randomized trial, despite promising Phase II results.[312] Further, a recently reported trial of neoadjuvant FAMTX versus surgery alone showed median survival of 18 months for the treated group versus 30 months for the surgery-alone group ($P = 0.17$). On the basis of this result, the risk that neoadjuvant treatment with insufficiently effective chemotherapy might jeopardize survival must be considered.[311]

Advanced and Metastatic Disease

A variety of combination chemotherapy regimens have been used in the palliative management of patients with gastric cancer.[313–319] Although the EAP type regimens pioneered by Preusser, Wilke, and colleagues[317] led to a new era in combination chemotherapy, in which expectations of response rates in excess of 30%, and some complete tumor regressions, were possible, the EAP regimen is now utilized only rarely because of its significant toxicity.[320] There are now other regimens that are widely used. The major regimens of current interest include methotrexate-directed 5-FU combinations,[321] infusional 5-FU regimens,[37,314,322] and combinations containing taxanes[316] and irinotecan-based regimens.[315,323]

Over the past decade, there has been interest in the use of prolonged infusion of 5-FU as a part of the combination chemotherapy treatment for stomach cancer. Crookes and colleagues[314] used continuous infusion 5-FU as a major component of a neoadjuvant program described below. Webb and colleagues reported important results with a combination regimen designated ECF (epirubicin, cisplatin, and 5-FU).[322] Of note, ECF uses protracted infusion of 5-FU at a daily rate of 200 mg/m^2 with intermittent epirubicin and cisplatinum. Epirubicin is an anthracycline analogue available in Western Europe for several years and now commercially available in the United States (although its approval indication is for breast cancer, not gastrointestinal cancer, in the United States). ECF was tested in a major Phase III randomized trial reported in 1997.[322] This study compared ECF with FAMTX in patients with gastroesophageal adenocarcinoma. In this study, 274 patients with adenocarcinoma or undifferentiated cancer were randomized between FAMTX and ECF. The FAMTX regimen caused significant hematologic toxicity and was inferior in regard to response rate and survival when compared to ECF. The overall response rate for ECF was 45% versus 21% for FAMTX ($P = 0.002$). The median survival for ECF was 8.9 versus 5.7 months ($P = 0.0009$). At 1 year, 36% of ECF and 21% of FAMTX patients were alive. Webb and colleagues also assessed global quality of life scores in their study. The global quality of life was superior for ECF at 24 weeks. This advantage in quality of life, however, did not persist as patients were followed further on the study.[322] Of interest, Ross and colleagues performed a Phase III study of ECF versus a very similar regimen, MCF, that substituted mitomycin C (7 mg/m^2 every 6 weeks) for epirubicin and uses somewhat different doses of 5-FU (300 mg/m^2/day × 24 weeks) and cisplatin (50 mg/m^2 every 3 weeks).[324] The overall rates of survival were no different between the ECF and MCF regimens. This trial supports the use of MCF if either epirubicin is not available or a clinician would prefer not to use an anthracycline.[320]

Other, more-recent, regimens include the combination of docetaxel–cisplatin[316] and the regimen of irinotecan–cisplatin.[315] The irinotecan and cisplatin combination has been evaluated and shown to have good activity in gastroesophageal cancers. The response rate for adenocarcinoma with the regimen was 12 of 23 (57%), with excellent palliation of tumor-related symptoms.[315] Another regimen of interest recently is the combination of docetaxel and cisplatin.[316] In a European study of 85 patients with advanced gastric cancer, the overall response rate was 36%, and 7 of 85 (8%) had complete responses. The median survival in this study was 10 months, and grade IV toxicity was seen in only 4% of cases.[316]

Data on therapy of advanced gastric cancer allow one to draw some conclusions in regard to the standard recommendations for patients with metastatic stomach cancer. It is reasonable to assume that several approaches can be considered appropriate chemotherapeutic management for patients with advanced gastric cancer. FAMTX is well tolerated and can certainly result in some complete responses in patients with gastric cancer, but it is no longer considered a front-line regimen for advanced gastric cancer (level I evidence). More promising approaches entail the use of continuous infusions of fluorinated pyrimidines, such as 5-FU. The ECF regimen, along with similar regimens using alternate anthracyclines, continue to be investigated. Finally, taxane- and iritonecan-based regimens are also of interest and appropriate for use in patients with advanced gastric cancer (level IIc data). However, it is important to stress that none of these regimens results in long-term control of metastatic adenocarcinoma of the stomach.

For a subset of cases with advanced locoregional disease followed by major response to chemotherapy, eventual R0 surgical resection is sometimes possible, and occasional long-term disease-free survival can result.[325–327] It should also be noted that surgical resection of isolated hepatic metastases, before or after chemotherapy, can also result in occasional long-term disease-free survival.[328] In general, however, although some chemotherapy regimens produce major partial responses and complete response rates as high as 15%, such responses are usually not durable.

References

1. Parkin DM, Bray FI, Devesa SS. Cancer burden in the year 2000. The global picture. Eur J Cancer 2001;37(suppl 8:S4–S66.
2. Borrmann R. Geschweulste des Magens und Duodenums, vol 4. Berlin: Springer Verlag, 1926.
3. Jarvi O, Lauren P. On the role of heterotopias of the intestinal epithelium in the pathogenesis of gastric cancer. Acta Pathol Microbiol Scand 1951;29(1):26–44.
4. Lauren T. The two histologic main types of gastric carcinoma. Acta Pathol Microbiol Scand 1965;64:31–49.
5. Stemmermann G, Fenoglio-Preiser C. Gastric cancer: epidemiology. In: Kelsen D, Daly J, Kern S, Levin B, Tepper J (eds). Gastrointestinal Oncology: Principles and Practice. Philadelphia: Lippincott Williams & Wilkins, 2002:311–324.
6. Fenoglio-Preiser CM, Noffsinger AE, Belli J, Stemmermann GN. Pathologic and phenotypic features of gastric cancer. Semin Oncol 1996;23(3):292–306.
7. Stemmermann GN, Fenoglio-Preiser C. Gastric carcinoma distal to the cardia: a review of the epidemiological pathology of the precursors to a preventable cancer. Pathology 2002;34(6): 494–503.
8. Stemmermann GN, Hayashi T. Intestinal metaplasia of the gastric mucosa: a gross and microscopic study of its distribution in various disease states. J Natl Cancer Inst 1968;41(3):627–634.
9. Matsukura N, Suzuki K, Kawachi T, et al. Distribution of marker enzymes and mucin in intestinal metaplasia in human stomach and relation to complete and incomplete types of intestinal metaplasia to minute gastric carcinomas. J Natl Cancer Inst 1980;65(2):231–240.
10. Watanabe H, Jass J, Sobin L. Histological typing of gastric and oesophageal tumors. In: Organization WH (ed). International Histologic Classification of Tumors, 2nd ed. Berlin: Springer, 1990.
11. Mulligan RM, Rember RR. Histogenesis and biologic behavior of gastric carcinoma: study of one hundred thirty-eight cases. AMA Arch Pathol 1954;58(1):1–25.
12. Broders A. Carcinoma and other malignant lesions of the stomach: pathologic considerations. In: Waltman W, Gray H, Priestley J (eds). Carcinoma and Other Malignant Lesions of the Stomach. Philadelphia: Sanders, 1942:127.
13. Nagayo T, Komagome T. Histological studies of gastric mucosal cancer with special reference to relationship of histological pictures between the mucosal cancer and the cancer-bearing gastric mucosa. Gann Monogr 1961;56:101.
14. Ming SC. Gastric carcinoma. A pathobiological classification. Cancer. Jun 1977;39(6):2475–2485.
15. Goseki N, Takizawa T, Koike M. Differences in the mode of the extension of gastric cancer classified by histological type: new histological classification of gastric carcinoma. Gut 1992;33(5): 606–612.
16. Songun I, van de Velde CJ, Arends JW, et al. Classification of gastric carcinoma using the Goseki system provides prognostic information additional to TNM staging. Cancer (Phila) 1999; 85(10):2114–2118.
17. Parkin DM. Global cancer statistics in the year 2000. Lancet Oncol 2001;2(9):533–543.
18. Parkin DM, Pisani P, Ferlay J. Global cancer statistics. CA Cancer J Clin 1999;49(1):33–64, 31.
19. Cancer Incidence in Five Continents, vol VIII. Lyon: IARCPress, 2002.
20. Correa P. A human model of gastric carcinogenesis. Cancer Res 1988;48(13):3554–3560.

21. Correa P, Haenszel W, Cuello C, Tannenbaum S, Archer M. A model for gastric cancer epidemiology. Lancet 1975;2(7924):58–60.
22. Correa P. Human gastric carcinogenesis: a multistep and multifactorial process: First American Cancer Society Award Lecture on Cancer Epidemiology and Prevention. Cancer Res 1992;52(24):6735–6740.
23. Parsonnet J, Friedman GD, Vandersteen DP, et al. *Helicobacter pylori* infection and the risk of gastric carcinoma. N Engl J Med 1991;325(16):1127–1131.
24. Parsonnet J, Vandersteen D, Goates J, Sibley RK, Pritikin J, Chang Y. *Helicobacter pylori* infection in intestinal- and diffuse-type gastric adenocarcinomas. J Natl Cancer Inst 1991;83(9):640–643.
25. Nomura A, Stemmermann GN, Chyou PH, Kato I, Perez-Perez GI, Blaser MJ. *Helicobacter pylori* infection and gastric carcinoma among Japanese Americans in Hawaii. N Engl J Med 1991;325(16):1132–1136.
26. Kono S, Ikeda M, Ogata M. Salt and geographical mortality of gastric cancer and stroke in Japan. J Epidemiol Community Health 1983;37(1):43–46.
27. Leach SD, Cook A, Challis B. Bacterially Mediated *N*-Nitrosation Reactions and Endogenous Formation of *N*-Nitroso Compounds, vol 84. Lyon: IARC, 1987.
28. Tannenbaum SR, Moran D, Rand W, Cuello C, Correa P. Gastric cancer in Colombia. IV. Nitrite and other ions in gastric contents of residents from a high-risk region. J Natl Cancer Inst 1979;62(1):9–12.
29. De Bernardinis G, Guadagni S, Pistoia MA, et al. Gastric juice nitrite and bacteria in gastroduodenal disease and resected stomach. Tumori 1983;69(3):231–237.
30. Wogan GN. Diet and nutrition as risk factors for cancer. Princess Takamatsu Symp 1985;16:3–10.
31. Tannenbaum SR. Diet and exposure to N-nitroso compounds. Princess Takamatsu Symp 1985;16:67–75.
32. Choi NW, Miller AB, Fodor JG, et al. Consumption of precursors of N-nitroso compounds and human gastric cancer. IARC Sci Publ 1987(84):492–496.
33. Leach SA, Thompson M, Hill M. Bacterially catalysed N-nitrosation reactions and their relative importance in the human stomach. Carcinogenesis (Oxf) 1987;8(12):1907–1912.
34. Sasazuki S, Sasaki S, Tsubono Y, et al. The effect of 5-year vitamin C supplementation on serum pepsinogen level and *Helicobacter pylori* infection. Cancer Sci 2003;94(4):378–382.
35. Bartsch H, Ohshima H, Pignatelli B. Inhibitors of endogenous nitrosation. Mechanisms and implications in human cancer prevention. Mutat Res 1988;202(2):307–324.
36. Bartsch H, Pignatelli B, Calmels S, Ohshima H. Inhibition of nitrosation. Basic Life Sci 1993;61:27–44.
37. Webb PM, Bates CJ, Palli D, Forman D. Gastric cancer, gastritis and plasma vitamin C: results from an international correlation and cross-sectional study. The Eurogast Study Group. Int J Cancer 1997;73(5):684–689.
38. Kono S, Ikeda M, Tokudome S, Kuratsune M. A case-control study of gastric cancer and diet in northern Kyushu, Japan. Jpn J Cancer Res 1988;79(10):1067–1074.
39. McConnell R. The Genetics of Gastro-intestinal disorders. London: Oxford University Press, 1966.
40. Nagayo T. Microscopical cancer of the stomach: a study on histogenesis of gastric carcinoma. Int J Cancer 1975;16(1):52–60.
41. Brown WM, Doll R. Mortality from cancer and other causes after radiotherapy for ankylosing spondylitis. Br Med J 1965;5474:1327–1332.
42. Tarbell NJ, Gelber RD, Weinstein HJ, Mauch P. Sex differences in risk of second malignant tumours after Hodgkin's disease in childhood. Lancet 1993;341(8858):1428–1432.
43. Lynch HT, Smyrk T, Lynch J. An update of HNPCC (Lynch syndrome). Cancer Genet Cytogenet 1997;93(1):84–99.
44. Lehtola J. Family study of gastric carcinoma, with special reference to histological types. Scand J Gastroenterol Suppl 1978;50:3–54.
45. Lehtola J. Family behaviour of gastric carcinoma. Ann Clin Res 1981;13(3):144–148.
46. Ihamaki T, Sipponen P. Family characteristics of gastric carcinoma. Ann Clin Res 1981;13(3):149–150.
47. Bonney GE, Elston RC, Correa P, et al. Genetic etiology of gastric carcinoma: I. Chronic atrophic gastritis. Genet Epidemiol 1986;3(4):213–224.
48. Mecklin JP, Jarvinen HJ. Tumor spectrum in cancer family syndrome (hereditary nonpolyposis colorectal cancer). Cancer (Phila) 1991;68(5):1109–1112.
49. Keller G, Rotter M, Vogelsang H, et al. Microsatellite instability in adenocarcinomas of the upper gastrointestinal tract. Relation to clinicopathological data and family history. Am J Pathol 1995;147(3):593–600.
50. Varley JM, McGown G, Thorncroft M, et al. An extended Li-Fraumeni kindred with gastric carcinoma and a codon 175 mutation in TP53. J Med Genet 1995;32(12):942–945.
51. Aarnio M, Mecklin JP, Aaltonen LA, Nystrom-Lahti M, Jarvinen HJ. Life-time risk of different cancers in hereditary nonpolyposis colorectal cancer (HNPCC) syndrome. Int J Cancer 1995;64(6):430–433.
52. Guilford PJ, Hopkins JB, Grady WM, et al. E-cadherin germline mutations define an inherited cancer syndrome dominated by diffuse gastric cancer. Hum Mutat 1999;14(3):249–255.
53. Tersmette AC, Offerhaus GJ, Tersmette KW, et al. Meta-analysis of the risk of gastric stump cancer: detection of high risk patient subsets for stomach cancer after remote partial gastrectomy for benign conditions. Cancer Res 1990;50(20):6486–6489.
54. Schistosomes, Liver Flukes, and *Helicobacter pylori*, vol 61. Lyon: IARC, 1994.
55. Huang JQ, Zheng GF, Sumanac K, Irvine EJ, Hunt RH. Meta-analysis of the relationship between cagA seropositivity and gastric cancer. Gastroenterology 2003;125(6):1636–1644.
56. Queiroz DM, Mendes EN, Rocha GA, et al. cagA-positive *Helicobacter pylori* and risk for developing gastric carcinoma in Brazil. Int J Cancer 1998;78(2):135–139.
57. Grimley CE, Holder RL, Loft DE, Morris A, Nwokolo CU. *Helicobacter pylori*-associated antibodies in patients with duodenal ulcer, gastric and oesophageal adenocarcinoma. Eur J Gastroenterol Hepatol 1999;11(5):503–509.
58. Pisani P, Parkin DM, Munoz N, Ferlay J. Cancer and infection: estimates of the attributable fraction in 1990. Cancer Epidemiol Biomarkers Prev 1997;6(6):387–400.
59. Zhou L, Sung JJ, Lin S, et al. A five-year follow-up study on the pathological changes of gastric mucosa after *H. pylori* eradication. Chin Med J (Engl) 2003;116(1):11–14.
60. Walker MM. Is intestinal metaplasia of the stomach reversible? Gut 2003;52(1):1–4.
61. Ito M, Haruma K, Kamada T, et al. *Helicobacter pylori* eradication therapy improves atrophic gastritis and intestinal metaplasia: a 5-year prospective study of patients with atrophic gastritis. Aliment Pharmacol Ther 2002;16(8):1449–1456.
62. van Grieken NC, Meijer GA, Kale I, et al. Quantitative assessment of gastric antrum atrophy shows restitution to normal histology after *Helicobacter pylori* eradication. Digestion 2004;69(1):27–33.
63. Yamada T, Miwa H, Fujino T, Hirai S, Yokoyama T, Sato N. Improvement of gastric atrophy after *Helicobacter pylori* eradication therapy. J Clin Gastroenterol 2003;36(5):405–410.
64. Munoz N, Kato I, Peraza S, et al. Prevalence of precancerous lesions of the stomach in Venezuela. Cancer Epidemiol Biomarkers Prev 1996;5(1):41–46.
65. Gammon MD, Terry MB, Arber N, et al. Nonsteroidal anti-inflammatory drug use associated with reduced incidence of adenocarcinomas of the esophagus and gastric cardia that over-

express cyclin D1: a population-based study. Cancer Epidemiol Biomarkers Prev 2004;13(1):34–39.

66. Wong BC, Lam SK, Wong WM, et al. *Helicobacter pylori* eradication to prevent gastric cancer in a high-risk region of China: a randomized controlled trial. JAMA 2004;291(2):187–194.
67. Takahashi S. Long-term *Helicobacter pylori* infection and the development of atrophic gastritis and gastric cancer in Japan. J Gastroenterol 2002;37(suppl 13:24–27.
68. La Vecchia C, Negri E, Franceschi S, Gentile A. Family history and the risk of stomach and colorectal cancer. Cancer (Phila) 1992;70(1):50–55.
69. Palli D, Galli M, Caporaso NE, et al. Family history and risk of stomach cancer in Italy. Cancer Epidemiol Biomarkers Prev 1994;3(1):15–18.
70. Goldgar DE, Easton DF, Cannon-Albright LA, Skolnick MH. Systematic population-based assessment of cancer risk in first-degree relatives of cancer probands. J Natl Cancer Inst 1994; 86(21):1600–1608.
71. Videback A, Mosbeck J. The etiology of gastric carcinoma elucidated by a study of 302 pedigrees. Acta Med Scand 1954; 149:159–173.
72. Powell SM, Smith MF. Gastric cancer: molecular biology and genetics. In: Kelsen DP, Daly JM, Kern SE, Levin B, Tepper JE (eds). Gastrointestinal Oncology: Principles and Practice. Philadelphia: Lippincott Williams & Wilkins, 2002:325–340.
73. El-Rifai W, Powell SM. Molecular biology of gastric cancer. Semin Radiat Oncol 2002;12(2):128–140.
74. Guilford P, Hopkins J, Harraway J, et al. E-cadherin germline mutations in familial gastric cancer. Nature (Lond) 1998; 392(6674):402–405.
75. Gayther SA, Gorringe KL, Ramus SJ, et al. Identification of germ-line E-cadherin mutations in gastric cancer families of European origin. Cancer Res 1998;58(18):4086–4089.
76. Lynch HT, Smyrk TC, Lanspa SJ, et al. Upper gastrointestinal manifestations in families with hereditary flat adenoma syndrome. Cancer (Phila) 1993;71(9):2709–2714.
77. Sugano K, Taniguchi T, Saeki M, Tsunematsu Y, Tomaru U, Shimoda T. Germline p53 mutation in a case of Li-Fraumeni syndrome presenting gastric cancer. Jpn J Clin Oncol 1999; 29(10):513–516.
78. Utsunomiya J. The concept of hereditary colorectal cancer adn the implications of its study. In: Utsunomiya J, Lynch HT (eds). Hereditary Colorectal Cancer: Proceedings of the Fourth International Symposium of Colorectal Cancer (ISCC-4), November 9–11, 1989, Kobe, Japan. New York: Springer-Verlag, 1990:3–16.
79. Offerhaus GJ, Giardiello FM, Krush AJ, et al. The risk of upper gastrointestinal cancer in familial adenomatous polyposis. Gastroenterology 1992;102(6):1980–1982.
80. Tahara E. Molecular biology of gastric cancer. World J Surg 1995; 19(4):484–488; discussion 489–490.
81. Hiyama E, Yokoyama T, Tatsumoto N, et al. Telomerase activity in gastric cancer. Cancer Res 1995;55(15):3258–3262.
82. Hollstein M, Shomer B, Greenblatt M, et al. Somatic point mutations in the p53 gene of human tumors and cell lines: updated compilation. Nucleic Acids Res 1996;24(1):141–146.
83. Mayer B, Johnson JP, Leitl F, et al. E-cadherin expression in primary and metastatic gastric cancer: down-regulation correlates with cellular dedifferentiation and glandular disintegration. Cancer Res 1993;53(7):1690–1695.
84. Gofuku J, Shiozaki H, Tsujinaka T, et al. Expression of E-cadherin and alpha-catenin in patients with colorectal carcinoma. Correlation with cancer invasion and metastasis. Am J Clin Pathol 1999;111(1):29–37.
85. Nakajima M, Sawada H, Yamada Y, et al. The prognostic significance of amplification and overexpression of c-*met* and c-*erb* B-2 in human gastric carcinomas. Cancer (Phila) 1999; 85(9):1894–1902.
86. Taniguchi K, Yonemura Y, Nojima N, et al. The relation between the growth patterns of gastric carcinoma and the expression of hepatocyte growth factor receptor (c-*met*), autocrine motility factor receptor, and urokinase-type plasminogen activator receptor. Cancer (Phila) 1998;82(11): 2112–2122.
87. Yokozaki H, Kuniyasu H, Yasui W, Tahara E. [Genetic characteristics of scirrhous gastric carcinomas.] Gan To Kagaku Ryoho 1994;21(14):2371–2377.
88. Marchbank T, Westley BR, May FE, Calnan DP, Playford RJ. Dimerization of human pS2 (TFF1) plays a key role in its protective/healing effects. J Pathol 1998;185(2):153–158.
89. Luqmani Y, Bennett C, Paterson I, et al. Expression of the pS2 gene in normal, benign and neoplastic human stomach. Int J Cancer 1989;44(5):806–812.
90. Muller W, Borchard F. pS2 protein in gastric carcinoma and normal gastric mucosa: association with clinicopathological parameters and patient survival. J Pathol 1993;171(4):263–269.
91. Machado JC, Carneiro F, Ribeiro P, Blin N, Sobrinho-Simoes M. pS2 protein expression in gastric carcinoma. An immunohistochemical and immunoradiometric study. Eur J Cancer 1996; 32A(9):1585–1590.
92. Wu MS, Shun CT, Wang HP, Lee WJ, Wang TH, Lin JT. Loss of pS2 protein expression is an early event of intestinal-type gastric cancer. Jpn J Cancer Res 1998;89(3):278–282.
93. Calnan DP, Westley BR, May FE, Floyd DN, Marchbank T, Playford RJ. The trefoil peptide TFF1 inhibits the growth of the human gastric adenocarcinoma cell line AGS. J Pathol 1999; 188(3):312–317.
94. Fujimoto J, Yasui W, Tahara H, Tahara E, Kudo Y, Yokozaki H. DNA hypermethylation at the pS2 promoter region is associated with early stage of stomach carcinogenesis. Cancer Lett 2000; 149(1-2):125–134.
95. Katoh M. Trefoil factors and human gastric cancer (review). Int J Mol Med 2003;12(1):3–9.
96. Onda M, Tokunaga A, Nishi K, et al. The correlation of epidermal growth factor with invasion and metastasis in human gastric cancer. Jpn J Surg 1990;20(3):269–274.
97. Yasui W, Sumiyoshi H, Hata J, et al. Expression of epidermal growth factor receptor in human gastric and colonic carcinomas. Cancer Res 1988;48(1):137–141.
98. Yoshiyuki T, Shimizu Y, Onda M, et al. Immunohistochemical demonstration of epidermal growth factor in human gastric cancer xenografts of nude mice. Cancer (Phila) 1990;65(4): 953–957.
99. Gamboa-Dominguez A, Dominguez-Fonseca C, Quintanilla-Martinez L, et al. Epidermal growth factor receptor expression correlates with poor survival in gastric adenocarcinoma from Mexican patients: a multivariate analysis using a standardized immunohistochemical detection system. Mod Pathol 2004; 17(5):579–587.
100. Pinto-de-Sousa J, David L, Almeida R, et al. c-erb B-2 expression is associated with tumor location and venous invasion and influences survival of patients with gastric carcinoma. Int J Surg Pathol 2002;10(4):247–256.
101. Aoyagi K, Kohfuji K, Yano S, et al. Evaluation of the epidermal growth factor receptor (EGFR) and c-erbB-2 in superspreading-type and penetrating-type gastric carcinoma. Kurume Med J 2001;48(3):197–200.
102. Ghaderi A, Vasei M, Maleck-Hosseini SA, et al. The expression of c-erbB-1 and c-erbB-2 in Iranian patients with gastric carcinoma. Pathol Oncol Res 2002;8(4):252–256.
103. el-Hariry I, Pignatelli M, Lemoine N. Fibroblast growth factor 1 and fibroblast growth factor 2 immunoreactivity in gastrointestinal tumours. J Pathol 1997;181(1):39–45.
104. Ueki T, Koji T, Tamiya S, Nakane PK, Tsuneyoshi M. Expression of basic fibroblast growth factor and fibroblast growth factor

receptor in advanced gastric carcinoma. J Pathol 1995;177(4):353–361.
105. Yu J, Leung WK, Ebert MP, et al. Absence of cyclin D2 expression is associated with promoter hypermethylation in gastric cancer. Br J Cancer 2003;88(10):1560–1565.
106. Oshimo Y, Nakayama H, Ito R, et al. Promoter methylation of cyclin D2 gene in gastric carcinoma. Int J Oncol 2003;23(6):1663–1670.
107. Takano Y, Kato Y, Masuda M, Ohshima Y, Okayasu I. Cyclin D2, but not cyclin D1, overexpression closely correlates with gastric cancer progression and prognosis. J Pathol 1999;189(2):194–200.
108. Muller W, Noguchi T, Wirtz HC, Hommel G, Gabbert HE. Expression of cell-cycle regulatory proteins cyclin D1, cyclin E, and their inhibitor p21 WAF1/CIP1 in gastric cancer. J Pathol 1999;189(2):186–193.
109. Yu J, Miehlke S, Ebert MP, et al. Expression of cyclin genes in human gastric cancer and in first degree relatives. Chin Med J (Engl) 2002;115(5):710–715.
110. Uefuji K, Ichikura T, Mochizuki H, Shinomiya N. Expression of cyclooxygenase-2 protein in gastric adenocarcinoma. J Surg Oncol 1998;69(3):168–172.
111. Ristimaki A, Honkanen N, Jankala H, Sipponen P, Harkonen M. Expression of cyclooxygenase-2 in human gastric carcinoma. Cancer Res 1997;57(7):1276–1280.
112. Sheu BS, Yang HB, Sheu SM, Huang AH, Wu JJ. Higher gastric cycloxygenase-2 expression and precancerous change in *Helicobacter pylori*-infected relatives of gastric cancer patients. Clin Cancer Res 2003;9(14):5245–5251.
113. Buskens CJ, Ristimaki A, Offerhaus GJ, Richel DJ, van Lanschot JJ. Role of cyclooxygenase-2 in the development and treatment of oesophageal adenocarcinoma. Scand J Gastroenterol Suppl 2003(239):87–93.
114. Sakamoto C. Roles of COX-1 and COX-2 in gastrointestinal pathophysiology. J Gastroenterol 1998;33(5):618–624.
115. Yu LZ, Gao HJ, Bai JF, et al. Expression of COX-2 proteins in gastric mucosal lesions. World J Gastroenterol 2004;10(2):292–294.
116. Xue YW, Zhang QF, Zhu ZB, Wang Q, Fu SB. Expression of cyclooxygenase-2 and clinicopathologic features in human gastric adenocarcinoma. World J Gastroenterol 2003;9(2):250–253.
117. Tatsuguchi A, Matsui K, Shinji Y, et al. Cyclooxygenase-2 expression correlates with angiogenesis and apoptosis in gastric cancer tissue. Hum Pathol 2004;35(4):488–495.
118. Jolly K, Cheng KK, Langman MJ. NSAIDs and gastrointestinal cancer prevention. Drugs 2002;62(6):945–956.
119. Gonzalez-Perez A, Garcia Rodriguez LA, Lopez-Ridaura R. Effects of non-steroidal anti-inflammatory drugs on cancer sites other than the colon and rectum: a meta-analysis. BMC Cancer 2003;3(1):28.
120. Zaridze D, Borisova E, Maximovitch D, Chkhikvadze V. Aspirin protects against gastric cancer: results of a case-control study from Moscow, Russia. Int J Cancer 1999;82(4):473–476.
121. Wong BC, Zhu GH, Lam SK. Aspirin induced apoptosis in gastric cancer cells. Biomed Pharmacother 1999;53(7):315–318.
122. Jiang XH, Wong BC. Cyclooxygenase-2 inhibition and gastric cancer. Curr Pharm Res 2003;9(27):2281–2288.
123. Koshiba M, Ogawa O, Habuchi T, et al. Infrequent *ras* mutation in human stomach cancers. Jpn J Cancer Res 1993;84(2):163–167.
124. Inoue T, Chung YS, Yashiro M, et al. Transforming growth factor-beta and hepatocyte growth factor produced by gastric fibroblasts stimulate the invasiveness of scirrhous gastric cancer cells. Jpn J Cancer Res 1997;88(2):152–159.
125. La Rosa S, Uccella S, Erba S, Capella C, Sessa F. Immunohistochemical detection of fibroblast growth factor receptors in normal endocrine cells and related tumors of the digestive system. Appl Immunohistochem Mol Morphol 2001;9(4):319–328.
126. Wanebo HJ, Kennedy BJ, Chmiel J, Steele G Jr, Winchester D, Osteen R. Cancer of the stomach. A patient care study by the American College of Surgeons. Ann Surg 1993;218(5):583–592.
127. Hundahl SA, Phillips JL, Menck HR. The National Cancer Data Base Report on poor survival of U.S. gastric carcinoma patients treated with gastrectomy: fifth edition American Joint Committee on Cancer staging, proximal disease, and the "different disease" hypothesis. Cancer (Phila) 2000;88(4):921–932.
128. Fujii M. [Results of mass gastric examination in Fukuoka prefecture, with special reference to the comparison with detection of stomach diseases among out-patients.] Igaku Kenkyu 1970;40(5):459–476.
129. Okui K, Tejima H. Evaluation of gastric mass survey. Acta Chir Scand 1980;146(3):185–187.
130. Takagi K. [Japanese cancer: retrospective and prospective views, gastric cancer.] Gan To Kagaku Ryoho 1984;11(3 pt 2):716–726.
131. Fukutomi H, Sakita T. Analysis of early gastric cancer cases collected from major hospitals and institutes in Japan. Jpn J Clin Oncol 1984;14(2):169–179.
132. Hisamichi S, Sugawara N. Mass screening for gastric cancer by X-ray examination. Jpn J Clin Oncol 1984;14(2):211–223.
133. Kampschoer GH, Fujii A, Masuda Y. Gastric cancer detected by mass survey. Comparison between mass survey and outpatient detection. Scand J Gastroenterol 1989;24(7):813–817.
134. Yoshihara M, Sumii K, Haruma K, et al. The usefulness of gastric mass screening using serum pepsinogen levels compared with photofluorography. Hiroshima J Med Sci 1997;46(2):81–86.
135. Sasamori N, Hinohara S, Tamura M, et al. Results of screening for cancer in Japanese in the prime of life: an analysis of nationwide MHTS and human dry dock statistics. Preventive Medicine Committee of the Japan Hospital Association. Jpn Hosp 1999(18):71–78.
136. Rozen P. Cancer of the gastrointestinal tract: early detection or early prevention? Eur J Cancer Prev 2004;13(1):71–75.
137. Habermann CR, Weiss F, Riecken R, et al. Preoperative staging of gastric adenocarcinoma: comparison of helical CT and endoscopic US. Radiology 2004;230(2):465–471.
138. Botet JF, Lightdale C. Endoscopic sonography of the upper gastrointestinal tract. AJR Am J Roentgenol 1991;156(1):63–68.
139. Botet JF, Lightdale CJ, Zauber AG, et al. Preoperative staging of gastric cancer: comparison of endoscopic US and dynamic CT. Radiology 1991;181(2):426–432.
140. Smith JW, Brennan MF, Botet JF, Gerdes H, Lightdale CJ. Preoperative endoscopic ultrasound can predict the risk of recurrence after operation for gastric carcinoma. J Clin Oncol 1993;11(12):2380–2385.
141. Kienle P, Buhl K, Kuntz C, et al. Prospective comparison of endoscopy, endosonography and computed tomography for staging of tumours of the oesophagus and gastric cardia. Digestion 2002;66(4):230–236.
142. Takao M, Fukuda T, Iwanaga S, Hayashi K, Kusano H, Okudaira S. Gastric cancer: evaluation of triphasic spiral CT and radiologic-pathologic correlation. J Comput Assist Tomogr 1998;22(2):288–294.
143. Ho CL. Clinical PET imaging: an Asian perspective. Ann Acad Med Singapore 2004;33(2):155–165.
144. Mochiki E, Kuwano H, Katoh H, Asao T, Oriuchi N, Endo K. Evaluation of ^{18}F-2-deoxy-2-fluoro-D-glucose positron emission tomography for gastric cancer. World J Surg 2004;28(3):247–253.
145. Stahl A, Ott K, Weber WA, et al. FDG PET imaging of locally advanced gastric carcinomas: correlation with endoscopic and histopathological findings. Eur J Nucl Med Mol Imaging 2003;30(2):288–295.
146. Koga H, Sasaki M, Kuwabara Y, et al. An analysis of the physiological FDG uptake pattern in the stomach. Ann Nucl Med 2003;17(8):733–738.

147. Yeung HW, Macapinlac H, Karpeh M, Finn RD, Larson SM. Accuracy of FDG-PET in gastric cancer. Preliminary experience. Clin Positron Imaging 1998;1(4):213–221.
148. Yoshioka T, Yamaguchi K, Kubota K, et al. Evaluation of ^{18}F-FDG PET in patients with a metastatic or recurrent gastric cancer. J Nucl Med 2003;44(5):690–699.
149. Giger U, Schafer M, Krahenbuhl L. Technique and value of staging laparoscopy. Dig Surg 2002;19(6):473–478.
150. Ozmen MM, Zulfikaroglu B, Ozalp N, Ziraman I, Hengirmen S, Sahin B. Staging laparoscopy for gastric cancer. Surg Laparosc Endosc Percutan Tech 2003;13(4):241–244.
151. Lavonius MI, Gullichsen R, Salo S, Sonninen P, Ovaska J. Staging of gastric cancer: a study with spiral computed tomography, ultrasonography, laparoscopy, and laparoscopic ultrasonography. Surg Laparosc Endosc Percutan Tech 2002;12(2):77–81.
152. Clements DM, Bowrey DJ, Havard TJ. The role of staging investigations for oesophago-gastric carcinoma. Eur J Surg Oncol 2004;30(3):309–312.
153. Blackshaw GR, Barry JD, Edwards P, Allison MC, Thomas GV, Lewis WG. Laparoscopy significantly improves the perceived preoperative stage of gastric cancer. Gastric Cancer 2003;6(4): 225–229.
154. Wilkiemeyer MB, Bieligk SC, Ashfaq R, Jones DB, Rege RV, Fleming JB. Laparoscopy alone is superior to peritoneal cytology in staging gastric and esophageal carcinoma. Surg Endosc 2004; 18(5):852–856.
155. Rau B, Hunerbein M. Diagnostic laparoscopy: indications and benefits. Langenbecks Arch Surg 2005;390:187–196.
156. Sobin LH, Hermanek P, Hutter RV. TNM classification of malignant tumors. A comparison between the new (1987) and the old editions. Cancer (Phila) 1988;61(11):2310–2314.
157. Fleming ID, Cooper JS, Henson DE, et al. AJCC Cancer Staging Manual, 5th ed. Philadelphia: Lippincott-Raven, 1997.
158. Hayes N, Ng EK, Raimes SA, et al. Total gastrectomy with extended lymphadenectomy for "curable" stomach cancer: experience in a non-Japanese Asian center. J Am Coll Surg 1999;188(1):27–32.
159. Japanese Gastric Cancer A. Japanese Classification of Gastric Carcinoma, 2nd English ed. Gastric Cancer 1998;1(1):10–24.
160. Japanese Classification of Gastric Carcinoma, 1st English ed. Tokyo: Kanehara, 1995.
161. Ichikura T, Fujino K, Ikawa H, Tomimatsu S, Uefuji K, Tamakuma S. Proposal of a risk score for recurrence in patients with curatively resected gastric cancer. Surg Today 1993;23(9): 759–764.
162. Shiu MH, Perrotti M, Brennan MF. Adenocarcinoma of the stomach: a multivariate analysis of clinical, pathologic and treatment factors. Hepatogastroenterology 1989;36(1):7–12.
163. Okusa T, Nakane Y, Boku T, et al. Quantitative analysis of nodal involvement with respect to survival rate after curative gastrectomy for carcinoma. Surg Gynecol Obstet 1990;170(6):488–494.
164. de Manzoni G, Verlato G, Guglielmi A, Laterza E, Genna M, Cordiano C. Prognostic significance of lymph node dissection in gastric cancer. Br J Surg 1996;83(11):1604–1607.
165. Jatzko GR, Lisborg PH, Denk H, Klimpfinger M, Stettner HM. A 10-year experience with Japanese-type radical lymph node dissection for gastric cancer outside of Japan. Cancer (Phila) 1995;76(8):1302–1312.
166. Bottcher K, Becker K, Busch R, Roder JD, Siewert JR. [Prognostic factors in stomach cancer. Results of a uni- and multivariate analysis.] Chirurg 1992;63(8):656–661.
167. Makino M, Moriwaki S, Yonekawa M, Oota M, Kimura O, Kaibara N. Prognostic significance of the number of metastatic lymph nodes in patients with gastric cancer. J Surg Oncol 1991;47(1):12–16.
168. Adachi Y, Kamakura T, Mori M, Baba H, Maehara Y, Sugimachi K. Prognostic significance of the number of positive lymph nodes in gastric carcinoma. Br J Surg 1994;81(3):414–416.
169. Ichikura T, Tomimatsu S, Okusa Y, Uefuji K, Tamakuma S. Comparison of the prognostic significance between the number of metastatic lymph nodes and nodal stage based on their location in patients with gastric cancer. J Clin Oncol 1993;11(10): 1894–1900.
170. Jaehne J, Meyer HJ, Maschek H, Geerlings H, Burns E, Pichlmayr R. Lymphadenectomy in gastric carcinoma. A prospective and prognostic study. Arch Surg 1992;127(3):290–294.
171. Roder JD, Bottcher K, Busch R, Wittekind C, Hermanek P, Siewert JR. Classification of regional lymph node metastasis from gastric carcinoma. German Gastric Cancer Study Group. Cancer (Phila) 1998;82(4):621–631.
172. Karpeh MS, Leon L, Klimstra D, Brennan MF. Lymph node staging in gastric cancer: is location more important than Number? An analysis of 1,038 patients. Ann Surg 2000; 232(3):362–371.
173. Ichikura T, Tomimatsu S, Uefuji K, et al. Evaluation of the New American Joint Committee on Cancer/International Union against cancer classification of lymph node metastasis from gastric carcinoma in comparison with the Japanese classification. Cancer (Phila) 1999;86(4):553–558.
174. Yoo CH, Noh SH, Kim YI, Min JS. Comparison of prognostic significance of nodal staging between old (4th edition) and new (5th edition) UICC TNM classification for gastric carcinoma. International Union Against Cancer. World J Surg 1999;23(5): 492–497; discussion 497–498.
175. Kattan MW, Karpeh MS, Mazumdar M, Brennan MF. Postoperative nomogram for disease-specific survival after an R0 resection for gastric carcinoma. J Clin Oncol 2003;21(19): 3647–3650.
176. Siewert JR, Bottcher K, Stein HJ, Roder JD. Relevant prognostic factors in gastric cancer: ten-year results of the German Gastric Cancer Study. Ann Surg 1998;228(4):449–461.
177. McNeer G, Sunderland D, McInnes G. A more thorough operation for gastric cancer: anatomical basis and description of technique. Cancer (Phila) 1951;4:957–967.
178. Lewis F, Wangensteen O. Exploration following resection of the colon, rectum, or stomach for carcinoma with lymph node metastases. Surg Forum 1950;1950:535–540.
179. Remine W, Priestley L. Late results after total gastrectomy. Surg Gynecol Obstet 1952;94:519–525.
180. McNeer G, Pack G. Neoplasms of the Stomach. Philadelphia: Lippincott, 1967.
181. Gilbertson V. Results of treatment of stomach cancer: an appraisal of efforts for more extensive surgery and a report of 1,983 cases. Cancer (Phila) 1969;23:1305–1308.
182. Kajitani T. The general rules for the gastric cancer study in surgery and pathology. Part I. Clinical classification. Jpn J Surg 1981;11(2):127–139.
183. Kajitani T, Hoshino T. Studies on five-year survivals after surgery for gastric carcinoma. Rev Surg 1965;22(6):398–399.
184. Kajitani T, Nishi M. [Surgical treatment of gastric cancer: pyloric gastrectomy.] Gan No Rinsho 1972;Suppl:269–274.
185. Nakajima T, Kajitani T. Surgical treatment of gastric cancer with special reference to lymph node dissection. In: Friedman M, Ogawa M, Kisner D (eds). Diagnosis and Treatment of Upper Gastrointestinal Tumors. Amsterdam: Excerpta Medica, 1981: 207–223.
186. Takagi K, Nishi M, Kajitani T. Surgical treatment of gastric cancer today. Wien Klin Wochenschr 1987;99(12):410–415.
187. Nakajima T, Fukami A, Ohashi I, Kajitani T. Long-term follow-up study of gastric cancer patients treated with surgery and adjuvant chemotherapy with mitomycin C. Int J Clin Pharmacol Biopharm 1978;16(5):209–216.
188. Ohta K, Nishi M, Nakajima T, Kajitani T. [Indications for total gastrectomy combined with pancreaticosplenectomy in the treatment of middle gastric cancer.] Nippon Geka Gakkai Zasshi 1989;90(9):1326–1330.

189. Maruyama K, Okabayashi K, Kinoshita T. Progress in gastric cancer surgery in Japan and its limits of radicality. World J Surg 1987;11(4):418–425.
190. Watanabe S, Arimoto H. Standardized mortality rates of cancer by prefecture in 1979–1981 and 1984–1986 in Japan. Jpn J Clin Oncol 1990;20(3):316–337.
191. Davis DL, Hoel D, Fox J, Lopez A. International trends in cancer mortality in France, West Germany, Italy, Japan, England and Wales, and the USA. Lancet 1990;336(8713):474–481.
192. The Third Japan-US Conference on Biostatistics in the Study of Human Cancer. November 11–13, 1988, Hiroshima, Japan. Proceedings. Environ Health Perspect 1990;87:1–178.
193. Nagata T, Ikeda M, Nakayama F. Changing state of gastric cancer in Japan. Histologic perspective of the past 76 years. Am J Surg 1983;145(2):226–233.
194. Maruyama K, Gunven P, Okabayashi K, Sasako M, Kinoshita T. Lymph node metastases of gastric cancer. General pattern in 1931 patients. Ann Surg 1989;210(5):596–602.
195. Maruyama K, Sasako M, Kinoshita T. Wert der systematischen erweiterten Lymphknotendissektion: Ergebnisse in Japan. [Value of systematic extended lymph node dissection: results in Japan.] Langenbecks Arch Chir Suppl Kongressbd 1992:130–135.
196. Sakakibara N, Asakura A. [Evaluation of 5-year survival after extensive radical surgery for gastric carcinoma.] Geka Chiryo 1966;15(2):156–161.
197. Kodama Y, Kano T, Tamada R, Kumashiro R, Okamura T, Inokuchi K. Combined effect of prophylactic lymphadenectomy and long term combination chemotherapy for curatively resected carcinoma of the stomach. Jpn J Surg 1982;12(4):244–248.
198. Kaibara N, Okamoto T, Kimura O, et al. Possible role of lymph node dissection in the surgical treatment of gastric cancer with disseminating peritoneal metastasis. Jpn J Surg 1983;13(5): 404–408.
199. Manual for Staging of Cancer, 3rd ed. Philadelphia: Lippincott, 1988.
200. Hutter RV. At last: worldwide agreement on the staging of cancer. Arch Surg 1987;122(11):1235–1239.
201. Bollschweiler E, Boettcher K, Hoelscher AH, et al. Is the prognosis for Japanese and German patients with gastric cancer really different? Cancer (Phila) 1993;71(10):2918–2925.
202. Fielding JW. Gastric cancer: different diseases. Br J Surg 1989; 76(12):1227.
203. Kodama Y, Sugimachi K, Soejima K, Matsusaka T, Inokuchi K. Evaluation of extensive lymph node dissection for carcinoma of the stomach. World J Surg 1981;5(2):241–248.
204. de Aretxabala X, Konishi K, Yonemura Y, et al. Node dissection in gastric cancer. Br J Surg 1987;74(9):770–773.
205. Csendes A, Caracci M, Parr G, Pavez J, Venturelli A. [Clinical and therapeutic aspects of gastric cancer (1973–1979). A cooperative interhospital study.] Rev Med Chil 1983;111(3):262–267.
206. Shiu MH, Moore E, Sanders M, et al. Influence of the extent of resection on survival after curative treatment of gastric carcinoma. A retrospective multivariate analysis. Arch Surg 1987;122(11):1347–1351.
207. Hundahl SA, Stemmermann GN, Oishi A. Racial factors cannot explain superior Japanese outcomes in stomach cancer. Arch Surg 1996;131(2):170–175.
208. Miwa K. Evolution of the TNM classification of stomach cancer and proposal for its rational stage grouping. Jpn J Clin Oncol 1984;14(3):385–410.
209. Dent DM. Radical surgery for curable gastric carcinoma. S Afr Med J 1994;84(2):56–57.
210. Dent DM, Madden MV, Price SK. Randomized comparison of R1 and R2 gastrectomy for gastric carcinoma. Br J Surg 1988; 75(2):110–112.
211. Gouzi JL, Huguier M, Fagniez PL, et al. Total versus subtotal gastrectomy for adenocarcinoma of the gastric antrum. A French prospective controlled study. Ann Surg 1989;209(2):162–166.
212. McNeer G, Bowden L, Booner RJ, McPeak CJ. Elective total gastrectomy for cancer of the stomach: end results. Ann Surg 1974;180(2):252–256.
213. Bozzetti F, Marubini E, Bonfanti G, et al. Total versus subtotal gastrectomy: surgical morbidity and mortality rates in a multicenter Italian randomized trial. The Italian Gastrointestinal Tumor Study Group. Ann Surg 1997;226(5):613–620.
214. Bozzetti F, Marubini E, Bonfanti G, Miceli R, Piano C, Gennari L. Subtotal versus total gastrectomy for gastric cancer: five-year survival rates in a multicenter randomized Italian trial. Italian Gastrointestinal Tumor Study Group. Ann Surg 1999;230(2): 170–178.
215. Robertson CS, Chung SC, Woods SD, et al. A prospective randomized trial comparing R1 subtotal gastrectomy with R3 total gastrectomy for antral cancer. Ann Surg 1994;220(2):176–182.
216. Cunha P, Cunha JF, Burnay MO, Galhordas A, Fernandes R, Calinas F. [Gastric adenocarcinoma and carcinoid.] Acta Med Port 1998;11(6):577–580.
217. Cuschieri A, Fayers P, Fielding J, et al. Postoperative morbidity and mortality after D1 and D2 resections for gastric cancer: preliminary results of the MRC randomised controlled surgical trial. The Surgical Cooperative Group. Lancet 1996;347(9007): 995–999.
218. Cuschieri A, Weeden S, Fielding J, et al. Patient survival after D1 and D2 resections for gastric cancer: long- term results of the MRC randomized surgical trial. Surgical Co- operative Group. Br J Cancer 1999;79(9-10):1522–1530.
219. Bonenkamp JJ, Hermans J, Sasako M, van de Velde CJ. Extended lymph-node dissection for gastric cancer. Dutch Gastric Cancer Group. N Engl J Med 1999;340(12):908–914.
220. Bonenkamp JJ, Songun I, Hermans J, et al. Randomised comparison of morbidity after D1 and D2 dissection for gastric cancer in 996 Dutch patients. Lancet 1995;345(8952):745–748.
221. The general rules for gastric cancer study in surgery. Jpn J Surg 1973;3(1):61–71.
222. Hartgrink HH, van de Velde CJ, Putter H, et al. Extended lymph node dissection for gastric cancer: who may benefit? Final results of the randomized Dutch gastric cancer group trial. J Clin Oncol 2004;22(11):2069–2077.
223. Maruyama K, Sasako M, Kinoshita T, Sano T, Katai H, Okajima K. Pancreas-preserving total gastrectomy for proximal gastric cancer. World J Surg 1995;19(4):532–536.
224. Uyama I, Ogiwara H, Takahara T, et al. Spleen- and pancreas-preserving total gastrectomy with superextended lymphadenectomy including dissection of the para-aortic lymph nodes for gastric cancer. J Surg Oncol 1996;63(4):268–270.
225. Kaminishi M, Shimoyama S, Yamaguchi H, et al. Results of subtotal gastrectomy with complete dissection of the N2 lymph nodes preserving the spleen and pancreas in surgery for gastric cancer. Hepatogastroenterology 1994;41(4):384–387.
226. Sano T. Update on D2 versus D4 trial. Presented at: 4th International Gastric Cancer Congress, 2001; New York.
227. Baba M, Hokita S, Natsugoe S, et al. Paraaortic lymphadenectomy in patients with advanced carcinoma of the upper-third of the stomach. Hepatogastroenterology 2000;47(33):893–896.
228. De Manzoni G, Di Leo A, Guglielmi A, et al. [Abdominal metastasis of cardiac adenocarcinoma.] Minerva Chir 2000;55(3): 105–111.
229. Kunisaki C, Shimada H, Yamaoka H, et al. Indications for paraaortic lymph node dissection in gastric cancer patients with paraaortic lymph node involvement. Hepatogastroenterology 2000;47(32):586–589.
230. Kunisaki C, Shimada H, Yamaoka H, et al. Significance of para-aortic lymph node dissection in advanced gastric cancer. Hepatogastroenterology 1999;46(28):2635–2642.
231. De Manzoni G, Di Leo A, Borzellino G, et al. [Para-aortic lymph node involvement in gastric adenocarcinoma.] Ann Chir 2001; 126(4):302–306; discussion 306–307.

232. Hartgrink HH, Van De Velde CJ, Putter H, et al. Extended lymph node dissection for gastric cancer: who may benefit? Final results of the Randomized Dutch Gastric Cancer Group Trial. J Clin Oncol 2004;22:2069–2077.
233. Sasako M, Katai H, Sano T, Maruyama K. Management of complications after gastrectomy with extended lymphadenectomy. Surg Oncol 2000;9(1):31–34.
234. Maerki SC, Luft HS, Hunt SS. Selecting categories of patients for regionalization. Implications of the relationship between volume and outcome. Med Care 1986;24(2):148–158.
235. Romano PS, Roos LL, Jollis JG. Adapting a clinical comorbidity index for use with ICD-9-CM administrative data: differing perspectives. J Clin Epidemiol 1993;46(10):1075–1079; discussion 1081–1090.
236. Hannan EL, Radzyner M, Rubin D, Dougherty J, Brennan MF. The influence of hospital and surgeon volume on in-hospital mortality for colectomy, gastrectomy, and lung lobectomy in patients with cancer. Surgery (St. Louis) 2002;131(1):6–15.
237. Kizer KW. The volume-outcome conundrum. N Engl J Med 2003;349(22):2159–2161.
238. Birkmeyer JD, Stukel TA, Siewers AE, Goodney PP, Wennberg DE, Lucas FL. Surgeon volume and operative mortality in the United States. N Engl J Med 2003;349(22):2117–2127.
239. Irvin TT, Bridger JE. Gastric cancer: an audit of 122 consecutive cases and the results of R1 gastrectomy. Br J Surg 1988;75(2): 106–109.
240. Luft HS. Hospital Volume, Physician Volume, and Patient Outcomes: Assessing the Evidence. Ann Arbor: Health Administration Press Perspectives, 1990.
241. Parikh D, Johnson M, Chagla L, Lowe D, McCulloch P. D2 gastrectomy: lessons from a prospective audit of the learning curve. Br J Surg 1996;83(11):1595–1599.
242. Kampschoer GH, Maruyama K, van de Velde CJ, Sasako M, Kinoshita T, Okabayashi K. Computer analysis in making preoperative decisions: a rational approach to lymph node dissection in gastric cancer patients. Br J Surg 1989;76(9):905–908.
243. Bollschweiler E, Boettcher K, Hoelscher AH, et al. Preoperative assessment of lymph node metastases in patients with gastric cancer: evaluation of the Maruyama computer program. Br J Surg 1992;79(2):156–160.
244. Guadagni S, de Manzoni G, Catarci M, et al. Evaluation of the Maruyama computer program accuracy for preoperative estimation of lymph node metastases from gastric cancer. World J Surg 2000;24(12):1550–1558.
245. Siewert JR, Kelsen D, Maruyama K, et al. Gastric cancer diagnosis and treatment: an interactive training program. Spinger Electronic Media [CD-ROM]. New York: Springer, 2000.
246. Hundahl SA, Macdonald JS, Benedetti J, Fitzsimmons T. Surgical treatment variation in a prospective, randomized trial of chemoradiotherapy in gastric cancer: the effect of undertreatment. Ann Surg Oncol 2002;9(3):278–286.
247. Hundahl SA, Macdonald JS, Benedetti J. Durable survival impact of "Low Maruyama Index Surgery" in a trial of adjuvant chemoradiation for gastric cancer. 2004 ASCO GI Symposium, San Francisco, January 22, 2004, p 48.
248. Hundahl SA, Macdonald JS, Benedetti J. Durable survival impact of "Low Maruyama Index Surgery" in a trial of adjuvant chemoradiation for gastric cancer. San Francisco: 2004 ASCO GI Symposium; January 22, 2004 (abstract #48).
249. Peeters KCMJ, Hundahl SA, Kranenbarg EK, Hartgrink H, vandeVelde CJH. "Low-Maruyama-Index" surgery for gastric cancer—a blinded re-analysis of the Dutch D1-D2 Trial. World Journal of Surgery. 2005; in press.
250. Ono H, Kondo H, Gotoda T, et al. Endoscopic mucosal resection for treatment of early gastric cancer. Gut 2001;48(2):225–229.
251. Pathirana A, Poston GJ. Lessons from Japan: endoscopic management of early gastric and oesophageal cancer. Eur J Surg Oncol 2001;27(1):9–16.
252. Sano T, Katai H, Sasako M, Maruyama K. The management of early gastric cancer. Surg Oncol 2000;9(1):17–22.
253. Sasako M. Treatment of early gastric cancer. Chir Ital 1997; 49(3):9–13.
254. Hiki Y. [Endoscopic mucosal resection (EMR) for early gastric cancer.] Nippon Geka Gakkai Zasshi 1996;97(4):273–278.
255. Kobayashi T, Kazui T, Kimura T. Surgical local resection for early gastric cancer. Surg Laparosc Endosc Percutan Tech 2003; 13(5):299–303.
256. Yamamoto H, Sekine Y, Higashizawa T, et al. Successful en bloc resection of a large superficial gastric cancer by using sodium hyaluronate and electrocautery incision forceps. Gastrointest Endosc 2001;54(5):629–632.
257. Yoshikane H, Sakakibara A, Hidano H, Niwa Y, Goto H, Yokoi T. Piecemeal endoscopic aspiration mucosectomy for large superficial intramucosal tumors of the stomach. Endoscopy 2001;33(9):795–799.
258. Kobayashi T, Gotohda T, Tamakawa K, Ueda H, Kakizoe T. Magnetic anchor for more effective endoscopic mucosal resection. Jpn J Clin Oncol 2004;34(3):118–123.
259. Kuwano H, Mochiki E, Asao T, Kato H, Shimura T, Tsutsumi S. Double endoscopic intraluminal operation for upper digestive tract diseases: proposal of a novel procedure. Ann Surg 2004; 239(1):22–27.
260. Kondo H, Gotoda T, Ono H, et al. Percutaneous traction-assisted EMR by using an insulation-tipped electrosurgical knife for early stage gastric cancer. Gastrointest Endosc 2004;59(2): 284–288.
261. Gotoda T, Yanagisawa A, Sasako M, et al. Incidence of lymph node metastasis from early gastric cancer: estimation with a large number of cases at two large centers. Gastric Cancer 2000;3(4):219–225.
262. Smalley SR, Gunderson L, Tepper J, et al. Gastric surgical adjuvant radiotherapy consensus report: rationale and treatment implementation. Int J Radiat Oncol Biol Phys 2002;52(2): 283–293.
263. Moertel CG, Childs DS Jr, Reitemeier RJ, Colby MY Jr, Holbrook MA. Combined 5-fluorouracil and supervoltage radiation therapy of locally unresectable gastrointestinal cancer. Lancet 1969;2(7626):865–867.
264. Holbrook MA. Cancer of the gastrointestinal tract. Radiation therapy. JaAMA 1974;228(10):1289–1290.
265. Schein PS, Smith FP, Woolley PV, Ahlgren JD. Current management of advanced and locally unresectable gastric carcinoma. Cancer (Phila) 1982;50(suppl 11):2590–2596.
266. Smalley S, Gunderson LL. Stomach. In: Perez C, Brady LW (eds). Principles and Practice of Radiation Oncology. Philadelphia: Lippincott-Raven, 1997.
267. Gunderson LL, Sosin H. Adenocarcinoma of the stomach: areas of failure in a re-operation series (second or symptomatic look) clinicopathologic correlation and implications for adjuvant therapy. Int J Radiat Oncol Biol Phys 1982;8(1):1–11.
268. Landry J, Tepper JE, Wood WC, Moulton EO, Koerner F, Sullinger J. Patterns of failure following curative resection of gastric carcinoma. Int J Radiat Oncol Biol Phys 1990;19(6):1357–1362.
269. McNeer G, Vandenberg H Jr, Donn FY, Bowden L. A critical evaluation of subtotal gastrectomy for the cure of cancer of the stomach. Ann Surg 1951;134(1):2–7.
270. Thompson FB, Robbins RE. Local recurrence following subtotal resection for gastric carcinoma. Surg Gynecol Obstet 1952;95: 341–344.
271. Gunderson LL, Sosin H. Areas of failure found at reoperation (second or symptomatic look) following "curative surgery" for adenocarcinoma of the rectum. Clinicopathologic correlation and implications for adjuvant therapy. Cancer (Phila) 1974; 34(4):1278–1292.
272. Macdonald JS, Smalley SR, Benedetti J, Hundahl SA et al. Chemoradiotherapy after surgery compared with surgery alone

for adenocarcinoma of the stomach or gastroesophageal junction. N Engl J Med 2001;345(10):725–730.
273. Macdonald JS. Postoperative combined radiation and chemotherapy improves disease-free survival (DFS) and overall survival (OS) in resected adenocarcinoma of the stomach and gastroesophageal junction: update of the results of Intergroup Study INT-0116 (SWOG 9008). Presented at: 2004 Gastrointestinal Cancers Symposium, 2004, San Francisco.
274. Kelsen DP. Postoperative adjuvant chemoradiation therapy for patients with resected gastric cancer: intergroup 116. J Clin Oncol 2000;18(suppl 21):32S–34S.
275. Takahashi T, Sawai K, Hagiwara A, Takahashi S, Seiki K, Tokuda H. Type-oriented therapy for gastric cancer effective for lymph node metastasis: management of lymph node metastasis using activated carbon particles adsorbing an anticancer agent. Semin Surg Oncol 1991;7(6):378–383.
276. Rosen HR, Jatzko G, Repse S, et al. Adjuvant intraperitoneal chemotherapy with carbon-adsorbed mitomycin in patients with gastric cancer: results of a randomized multicenter trial of the Austrian Working Group for Surgical Oncology. J Clin Oncol 1998;16(8):2733–2738.
277. Schiessel R, Funovics J, Schick B, et al. Adjuvant intraperitoneal cisplatin therapy in patients with operated gastric carcinoma: results of a randomized trial. Acta Med Aust 1989;16(3-4):68–69.
278. Sugimachi K, Maehara Y, Akazawa K, et al. Postoperative chemotherapy including intraperitoneal and intradermal administration of the streptococcal preparation OK-432 for patients with gastric cancer and peritoneal dissemination: a prospective randomized study. Cancer Chemother Pharmacol 1994;33(5):366–370.
279. Leichman L, Silberman H, Leichman CG, et al. Preoperative systemic chemotherapy followed by adjuvant postoperative intraperitoneal therapy for gastric cancer: a University of Southern California pilot program. J Clin Oncol 1992;10(12):1933–1942.
280. Glehen O, Mohamed F, Gilly FN. Peritoneal carcinomatosis from digestive tract cancer: new management by cytoreductive surgery and intraperitoneal chemohyperthermia. Lancet Oncol 2004;5(4):219–228.
281. Sugarbaker PH, Yu W, Yonemura Y. Gastrectomy, peritonectomy, and perioperative intraperitoneal chemotherapy: the evolution of treatment strategies for advanced gastric cancer. Semin Surg Oncol 2003;21(4):233–248.
282. Hall JJ, Loggie BW, Shen P, et al. Cytoreductive surgery with intraperitoneal hyperthermic chemotherapy for advanced gastric cancer. J Gastrointest Surg 2004;8(4):454–463.
283. Yu W, Whang I, Chung HY, Averbach A, Sugarbaker PH. Indications for early postoperative intraperitoneal chemotherapy of advanced gastric cancer: results of a prospective randomized trial. World J Surg 2001;25(8):985–990.
284. Yu W, Whang I, Suh I, Averbach A, Chang D, Sugarbaker PH. Prospective randomized trial of early postoperative intraperitoneal chemotherapy as an adjuvant to resectable gastric cancer. Ann Surg 1998;228(3):347–354.
285. Hermans J, Bonenkamp JJ, Boon MC, et al. Adjuvant therapy after curative resection for gastric cancer: meta-analysis of randomized trials. J Clin Oncol 1993;11(8):1441–1447.
286. Pignon JP, Ducreux M, Rougier P. Meta-analysis of adjuvant chemotherapy in gastric cancer: a critical reappraisal. J Clin Oncol 1994;12(4):877–878.
287. Hermans S, Benekamp K. In reply. J Clin Oncol 1994;12:879–880.
288. Earle CC, Maroun JA. Adjuvant chemotherapy after curative resection for gastric cancer in non-Asian patients: revisiting a meta-analysis of randomised trials. Eur J Cancer 1999;35(7):1059–1064.
289. Mari E, Floriani I, Tinazzi A, et al. Efficacy of adjuvant chemotherapy after curative resection for gastric cancer: a meta-analysis of published randomised trials. A study of the GISCAD (Gruppo Italiano per lo Studio dei Carcinomi dell'Apparato Digerente). Ann Oncol 2000;11(7):837–843.
290. Estape J, Grau JJ, Lcobendas F, et al. Mitomycin C as an adjuvant treatment to resected gastric cancer. A 10- year follow-up. Ann Surg 1991;213(3):219–221.
291. Grau JJ, Estape J, Alcobendas F, Pera C, Daniels M, Teres J. Positive results of adjuvant mitomycin-C in resected gastric cancer: a randomised trial on 134 patients. Eur J Cancer 1993;3:340–342.
292. Chou FF, Sheen-Chen SM, Liu PP, Chen FC. Adjuvant chemotherapy for resectable gastric cancer: a preliminary report. J Surg Oncol 1994;57(4):239–242.
293. Douglas HO, Stablein DM. A comparison of combination chemotherapy and combined modality therapy for locally advanced gastric carcinoma. Gastrointestinal Tumor Study Group. Cancer (Phila) 1982;49(9):1771–1777.
294. Cirera L, Balil A, Batiste-Alentorn E, et al. Randomized clinical trial of adjuvant mitomycin plus tegafur in patients with resected stage III gastric cancer. J Clin Oncol 1999;17(12):3810–3815.
295. Neri B, de Leonardis V, Romano S, et al. Adjuvant chemotherapy after gastric resection in node-positive cancer patients: a multicentre randomised study. Br J Cancer 1996;73(4):549–552.
296. Panzini I, Gianni L, Fattori PP, et al. Adjuvant chemotherapy in gastric cancer: a meta-analysis of randomized trials and a comparison with previous meta-analyses. Tumori 2002;88(1):21–27.
297. Janunger KG, Hafstrom L, Nygren P, Glimelius B. A systematic overview of chemotherapy effects in gastric cancer. Acta Oncol 2001;40(2-3):309–326.
298. Nakajima T, Ota K, Ishihara S, Oyama S, Nishi M, Hamashima N. [Meta-analysis of 10 postoperative adjuvant chemotherapies for gastric cancer in CIH.] Gan To Kagaku Ryoho 1994;21(11):1800–1805.
299. Nakajima T, Takahashi T, Takagi K, Kuno K, Kajitani T. Comparison of 5-fluorouracil with ftorafur in adjuvant chemotherapies with combined inductive and maintenance therapies for gastric cancer. J Clin Oncol 1984;2(12):1366–1371.
300. Engstrom PF, Lavin PT, Douglass HO Jr, Brunner KW. Postoperative adjuvant 5-fluorouracil plus methyl-CCNU therapy for gastric cancer patients. Eastern Cooperative Oncology Group study (EST 3275). Cancer (Phila) 1985;55(9):1868–1873.
301. Coombes RC, Schein PS, Chilvers CE, et al. A randomized trial comparing adjuvant fluorouracil, doxorubicin, and mitomycin with no treatment in operable gastric cancer. International Collaborative Cancer Group. J Clin Oncol 1990;8(8):1362–1369.
302. Krook JE, O'Connell MJ, Wieand HS, et al. A prospective, randomized evaluation of intensive-course 5-fluorouracil plus doxorubicin as surgical adjuvant chemotherapy for resected gastric cancer. Cancer (Phila) 1991;67(10):2454–2458.
303. Hallissey MT, Dunn JA, Ward LC, Allum WH. The second British Stomach Cancer Group trial of adjuvant radiotherapy or chemotherapy in resectable gastric cancer: five-year follow-up. Lancet 1994;343(8909):1309–1312.
304. Macdonald JS, Fleming TR, Peterson RF, et al. Adjuvant chemotherapy with 5-FU, adriamycin, and mitomycin-C (FAM) versus surgery alone for patients with locally advanced gastric adenocarcinoma: A Southwest Oncology Group study. Ann Surg Oncol 1995;2(6):488–494.
305. Tsavaris N, Tentas K, Kosmidis P, et al. A randomized trial comparing adjuvant fluorouracil, epirubicin, and mitomycin with no treatment in operable gastric cancer. Chemotherapy 1996;42(3):220–226.
306. Nakajima T, Nashimoto A, Kitamura M, et al. Adjuvant mitomycin and fluorouracil followed by oral uracil plus tegafur in serosa-negative gastric cancer: a randomised trial. Gastric Cancer Surgical Study Group. Lancet 1999;354(9175):273–277.

307. Langman MJ, Dunn JA, Whiting JL, et al. Prospective, double-blind, placebo-controlled randomized trial of cimetidine in gastric cancer. British Stomach Cancer Group. Br J Cancer 1999;81(8):1356–1362.
308. Nashimoto A, Nakajima T, Furukawa H, et al. Randomized trial of adjuvant chemotherapy with mitomycin, fluorouracil, and cytosine arabinoside followed by oral fluorouracil in serosa-negative gastric cancer: Japan Clinical Oncology Group 9206-1. J Clin Oncol 2003;21(12):2282–2287.
309. Chipponi J, Huguier M, Pezet D, et al. Randomized trial of adjuvant chemotherapy after curative resection for gastric cancer. Am J Surg 2004;187(3):440–445.
310. Sato Y, Kondo M, Kohashi S, et al. A randomized controlled study of immunochemotherapy with OK-432 after curative surgery for gastric cancer. J Immunother 2004;27(5):394–397.
311. Hartgrink HH, van de Velde CJ, Putter H, et al. Neo-adjuvant chemotherapy for operable gastric cancer: long term results of the Dutch randomised FAMTX trial. Eur J Surg Oncol 2004;30(6):643–649.
312. VanCutsem E. Neoadjuvant and adjuvant treatment of gastric cancer. Presented at 2004 Gastrointestinal Cancers Symposium, Jan. 22–24, 2004, San Francisco.
313. Cascinu S, Labianca R, Alessandroni P, et al. Intensive weekly chemotherapy for advanced gastric cancer using fluorouracil, cisplatin, epi-doxorubicin, 6S-leucovorin, glutathione, and filgrastim: a report from the Italian Group for the Study of Digestive Tract Cancer. J Clin Oncol 1997;15(11):3313–3319.
314. Crookes P, Leichman CG, Leichman L, et al. Systemic chemotherapy for gastric carcinoma followed by postoperative intraperitoneal therapy: a final report. Cancer (Phila) 1997;79(9):1767–1775.
315. Ilson DH, Saltz L, Enzinger P, et al. Phase II trial of weekly irinotecan plus cisplatin in advanced esophageal cancer. J Clin Oncol 1999;17(10):3270–3275.
316. Ridwelski K, Gebauer T, Fahlke J, et al. Combination chemotherapy with docetaxel and cisplatin for locally advanced and metastatic gastric cancer. Ann Oncol 2001;12(1):47–51.
317. Preusser P, Wilke H, Achterrath W, et al. Phase II study with the combination etoposide, doxorubicin, and cisplatin in advanced measurable gastric cancer. J Clin Oncol 1989;7(9):1310–1317.
318. Wils J, Bleiberg H, Dalesio O, et al. An EORTC Gastrointestinal Group evaluation of the combination of sequential methotrexate and 5-fluorouracil, combined with adriamycin in advanced measurable gastric cancer. J Clin Oncol 1986;4(12):1799–1803.
319. Wils JA, Klein HO, Wagener DJ, et al. Sequential high-dose methotrexate and fluorouracil combined with doxorubicin: a step ahead in the treatment of advanced gastric cancer. A trial of the European Organization for Research and Treatment of Cancer Gastrointestinal Tract Cooperative Group. J Clin Oncol 1991;9(5):827–831.
320. Macdonald JS. Chemotherapy in the management of gastric cancer. J Clin Oncol 2003;21(suppl 23):276s–279s.
321. Kelsen D, Atiq OT, Saltz L, et al. FAMTX versus etoposide, doxorubicin, and cisplatin: a random assignment trial in gastric cancer. J Clin Oncol 1992;10(4):541–548.
322. Webb A, Cunningham D, Scarffe JH, et al. Randomized trial comparing epirubicin, cisplatin, and fluorouracil versus fluorouracil, doxorubicin, and methotrexate in advanced esophagogastric cancer. J Clin Oncol 1997;15(1):261–267.
323. Ajani JA. Irinotecan and other agents in upper gastrointestinal and colorectal carcinomas. The University of Texas M.D. Anderson Cancer Center Investigators' Workshop, vol 3. Introduction. Oncology (Huntingt) 2003;17(9 suppl 8):10–12.
324. Ross P, Nicolson M, Cunningham D, et al. Prospective randomized trial comparing mitomycin, cisplatin, and protracted venous-infusion fluorouracil (PVI 5-FU) with epirubicin, cisplatin, and PVI 5-FU in advanced esophagogastric cancer. J Clin Oncol 2002;20(8):1996–2004.
325. Fink U, Stein HJ, Schuhmacher C, Wilke HJ. Neoadjuvant chemotherapy for gastric cancer: update. World J Surg 1995;19(4):509–516.
326. Fink U, Schuhmacher C, Stein HJ, et al. Preoperative chemotherapy for stage III-IV gastric carcinoma: feasibility, response and outcome after complete resection. Br J Surg 1995;82(9):1248–1252.
327. Ajani JA, Mansfield PF, Ota DM. Potentially resectable gastric carcinoma: current approaches to staging and preoperative therapy. World J Surg 1995;19(2):216–220.
328. Ochiai T, Sasako M, Mizuno S, et al. Hepatic resection for metastatic tumours from gastric cancer: analysis of prognostic factors. Br J Surg 1994;81(8):1175–1178.
329. Grau JJ, Estape J, Fuster J, et al. Randomized trial of adjuvant chemotherapy with mitomycin plus ftorafur versus mitomycin alone in resected locally advanced gastric cancer. J Clin Oncol 1998;16(3):1036–1039.

42

Colon, Rectal, and Anal Cancer Management

John M. Skibber and Cathy Eng

Treatment of Precancerous Conditions

Neoplastic Polyps (Adenomas)

Adenomas are the most common neoplasms in the large bowel. They are classified into three types—tubular, tubulovillous, and villous—according to the histologic appearance. Tubular adenomas account for 75% of polyps found, tubulovillous adenomas account for 25%, and villous adenomas account for 10%.[1] The malignancy rate of tubular adenomas is about 5%, but it rises to about 40% in villous adenomas. The entire colon should be examined if a histologically proven adenoma has been removed from the colon or is found on endoscopic biopsy.[2,3] Endoscopic removal of polyps should be performed to confirm the diagnosis of a benign or malignant polyp.[4] Polyps with a stalk can be removed by endoscopic snare polypectomy. Judgment must be used to assess the practicality of attempting endoscopic removal of sessile polyps, especially in the relatively thin-walled abdominal colon.[5]

Further management and timing of surveillance depends on the characteristics of the adenomas removed initially, as well as on their number and the clinical risk status of the patient. Follow-up of small adenomas containing in situ carcinoma or severe dysplasia that have been completely removed is the same as that for benign adenomas: routine follow-up colonoscopy at 3-year intervals once the colon is cleared.[6] Patients having multiple adenomas are at higher risk for oversight of synchronous adenomas, and therefore these patients should be examined at 1 year. Small polyps (less than 1 cm) carry a low likelihood of malignancy and are adequately treated with excisional biopsy.[7]

Villous adenomas (i.e., more than 2 cm in diameter) have a malignant potential that is significantly greater than that for other adenomatous polyps. Villous adenomas require complete excision for adequate histologic examination. Large sessile polyps with villous features have a significant rate of local recurrence.[8] Even if endoscopic excision of a large sessile polyp is done, the patients should be reexamined 3 months later to evaluate the completeness of resection.[9] Ultimately, surgery can be required, as these polyps are highly likely to harbor invasive cancer. For rectal polyps, local excision techniques may be an acceptable form of excisional biopsy. Submucosal techniques of transanal excision are appropriate in the excision of rectal villous adenomas.[10]

Management of Malignant Polyps

A malignant polyp is one where cancer cells have extended into the submucosal layer. Theoretically, this results from the cancer cells gaining access to lymphatics and blood vessels in this layer and thereby having the potential for regional and systemic spread.[11,12] In a pedunculated malignant polyp, there is an opportunity for complete excision because of the stalk. Sessile tumors often cannot be endoscopically completely excised in a manner that allows for an accurate examination of the margin and the completeness of excision.[13]

Essentially, the risk of local recurrence of a malignant polyp or undetected regional lymph node spread must be weighed against the patient's operative risk.[14] The risk of local recurrence is related to the completeness of excision and resection margin. The definition of an adequate resection margin varies from 3 to 1 mm or simply the absence of malignant cells at the cut edge.[15–17] In one study, simply the assessment of the adequacy of the resection by the endoscopist was an adequate criteria for a low risk of recurrence.[18] Piecemeal excision or improper retrieval or processing of the polyp makes assessment of the margin indeterminate.

The risk of regional lymphatic spread appears to be increased in cases in which the malignant component has poor differentiation or lymphatic/vascular invasion. Poor differentiation appears to be a factor correlated with lymph node metastases in endoscopically removed polyps.[18] Vascular and lymphatic or perineural invasion increases the risk of lymphatic metastases.[19–22]

Haggitt et al.[23] (1985) have described various levels of invasion of carcinoma into pedunculated polyps (Table 42.1). They noted that, in a pedunculated polyp, an invasive component in the head of the polyp may be a substantial distance from the submucosa and therefore may be resected endoscopically with a significant margin. In a sessile polyp, the invasive component has early access to the submucosa and therefore has an earlier opportunity for dissemination. Sessile polyps have a higher incidence of lymph node metastasis than pedunculated polyps with invasive cancer.[24] When the invasive cancer is limited to the head of a pedunculated polyp, lymph node metastasis rates appear to be approximately 3%, in contrast to 10% to 25% for sessile polyps (Table 42.2).

The operative mortality for elective colon resection scores from 0.2% to 2%.[25,26] For low-risk malignant polyps, the incidence of residual disease appears to be less than this.[25,27,28] The criteria of incomplete excision or poor histologic appearances

TABLE 42.1. AJCC/UICC TNM staging of colon and rectal cancer.

Primary tumor (T)	
TX	Primary tumor cannot be assessed
T0	No evidence of primary tumor
Tis	Carcinoma in situ: intraepithelial or invasion of lamina propria[a]
T1	Tumor invades submucosa
T2	Tumor invades muscularis propria
T3	Tumor invades through muscularis propria into subserosa, or into nonperitonealized pericolic or perirectal tissues
T4	Tumor directly invades other organs or structures, and/or perforates visceral peritoneum[b,c]
Regional lymph nodes (N)	
NX	Regional lymph nodes cannot be assessed
N0	No regional lymph node metastasis
N1	Metastasis in 1 to 3 regional lymph nodes
N2	Metastasis in 4 or more regional lymph nodes
Distant metastasis (M)	
MX	Distant metastasis cannot be assessed
M0	No distant metastasis
M1	Distant metastasis

[a] This includes cancer cells confined within the glandular basement membrane (intraepithelial) or lamina propria (intramucosal) with no extension through the muscularis mucosae into the submucosa.

[b] Direct invasion in T4 includes invasion of other segments of the colorectum by way of the serosa, for example, invasion of the sigmoid colon by a carcinoma of the cecum.

[c] Tumor that is adherent to other organs or structures, macroscopically, is classified R4. However, if no tumor is present in the adhesion, microscopically, the classification should be pT3. The V and L substaging should be used to identify the presence or absence of vascular or lymphatic invasion.

Source: Used with the permission of the American Joint Committee On Cancer (AJCC), Chicago, Illinois. The original source for this material is the AJCC Cancer Staging Manual, sixth edition (2002), published by Springer-Verlag New York, www.springer-ny.com.

or identifiers for a high risk of an adverse outcome has been confirmed on long-term follow-up.[29,30] Patients with poor prognostic factors can have local, regional, or systemic spread in 8.5% to 14.4% of cases.[31] In cases where operative risk is higher (in the elderly), the mortality associated with resection may exceed the risk of residual disease.[32,33] As laparoscopic techniques for colon resection become more common, it will be important to include the tattooing of suspected malignant polyp sites for identification of the polypectomy site.[34] Intraoperative colonoscopy may be an important aid in the identification of the polyp site.[35] Most commonly, the issue dictating surgical resection will be an inadequate or questionable margin.[36]

After colonoscopic removal of the malignant polyp, it is important to document carefully the site of polypectomy in the event that surgical resection is warranted. We commonly perform this procedure using endoscopically placed clips, which are both palpable and evident on abdominal radiographs. Follow-up colonoscopy is generally performed 3 to 6 months after removal of a malignant polyp to assess the polypectomy site for any residual mass. Presence of a mass is an indication for surgical resection. In patients in whom there is no further evidence of residual carcinoma, colonoscopic follow-up can be carried out at 1 year.[37]

Management of Potentially Curable Colon Cancer

Pretreatment Evaluation

Surgical management is required for most patients with a diagnosis of colon carcinoma. The appropriateness of a surgi-

TABLE 42.2. Cancer in polyps: risk of lymph node metastases.

	Patients resected	*Lymph node metastases*
Sessile polyps with invasive cancer:		
Grinnelle and Lane[359]	13	3
Waye and Frankel[360]	9	1
Wolff and Shyna[361]	5	2
Lock et al.[362]	12	4
Kodaira et al.[363]	34	2
Nivatvongs[364]	25	3
	Lymph nodes with metastases = 15%	
Pedunculated polyps with invasive cancer:		
Grinnell and Lane[359]	39	3
Waye and Frankel[360]	8	0
Wolff and Shinya[361]	11	0
Shatney et al.[365]	23	1
Lock et al.[362]	15	1
Coutsoftides et al.[366]	13	0
Colachio et al.[367]	24	6
Kodaira et al.[363]	64	3
Shatney et al.[365]	16	3
	Lymph nodes with metastases = 8%	
Pedunculated polyps with invasive cancer limited to head of polyp:		
Grinnell and Lane[359]	28	0
Shatney et al.[365]	14	0
Nivatvongs[364]	12	0
Colachio et al.[367]	11	2
	Lymph nodes with metastases = 3%	

Source: Used by permission of Nivatvongs S. Management of polyps containing invasive carcinoma. In: Codner IJ, Fry RD, Roe JP (eds.). Colon, Rectal, and Anal Surgery. St. Louis: Mosby, 1985:183.

cal resection will be determined by the extent of disease and comorbidities. In cases of metastatic colorectal carcinoma, surgery may be required for palliation. Some authors have documented an ability to manage colon cancer patients nonoperatively in the presence of metastatic disease without significant complications from bleeding, perforation, or obstruction.[38]

A well-conducted history and physical examination will provide a great deal of information about the patient's extent of disease and suitability for treatment. Specific aspects of the history taking should focus on a personal history of cancer or polyps and family history of colorectal cancer or polyps.

Complete colonic examination not only allows a biopsy of the index lesion but also provides information about the exact location of the lesion. Additionally, it provides information on the presence or absence of synchronous colon cancers, which are present in 1.5% to 7.6% of cases. In addition, significant synchronous polyps can occur in 25% to 40% of patients.[39–41] The colon should be endoscopically cleared of these lesions. If polyps cannot be removed endoscopically, they should be included in the planned resection. Preoperative colonoscopy can change the nature of the planned surgical procedures in about 10% to 13% of cases.[42–44]

Computed tomography (CT) scanning is used to reveal clinically unapparent liver metastases or local extension to adjacent organs. The negative predictive value of CT scan for synchronous liver metastases has been estimated at 90%.[45] The argument has been made that a CT scan often does not change management compared to the findings at operation alone.[46]

The value of a chest X-ray for the primary workup of a patient may be in evaluating the patient for comorbid diseases that would have an effect on planning for surgery, as well as to indicate the presence of pulmonary metastases. It is interesting to note that even in patients with liver metastases, when the initial chest X-ray is negative, chest CT is positive in about 30% of patients. However, Kronawitter and associates found that only 5% of high-risk patients had malignant lesions identified.[47]

In those who are curatively treated, there is little prognostic value to preoperative carcinoembryonic antigen (CEA) levels.[48,49] Preoperative CEA levels have been demonstrated to have prognostic value and to be correlated with stage. CEA levels are increased in 65% to 85% of patients with Dukes' D colorectal cancers.[50] Among patients with high-risk (i.e., C1 and C2 disease) cancers, high (greater than 5 mg/ml) CEA levels preoperatively correlated with significantly shorter survival. In this retrospective study of 218 patients, CEA was not useful to predict survival in Dukes' A or B patients.[51]

The value of preoperative ^{18}F-fluorodeoxyglucose positron emission tomography (FDG-PET) scanning in the primary evaluation of patients with colorectal cancer has only recently been addressed. In a study of 38 consecutive patients with colorectal primary cancers, PET was compared to CT and sonography. Its accuracy for liver metastases was about 91%, which was similar to CT. In this study, PET is said to have changed the treatment modality in 8% of patients and the extent of surgery in 13%. The studies demonstrated extrahepatic lesions in 4 of 38 patients that could be identified as malignant. Overall, most of the change in therapy (3 of 6 cases) was to avoid operation at all in cases of "generalized malignancy." In 2 of 6 cases, the patient underwent surgery anyway, and in 1 of 6 of the patients the nature of the surgery was changed to a smaller palliative procedure.[52] In other single institutional studies, the predictive accuracy in the detection of liver metastases in those with primary colon and rectal cancer is greater than with CT.[53] It has yet to be demonstrated in long-term follow-up that clinical management decisions made on the basis of PET scanning will produce either survival or quality of life benefits.

Surgical Management of Carcinoma of the Colon

Radical resection with curative intent is appropriate for 80% to 90% of patients with colon carcinoma.[54] Surgical resection is the mainstay of treatment for curable colorectal cancer. It is the only treatment required for tumors limited to the bowel wall. Although this is commonly accomplished by palpation and inspection, intraoperative ultrasonography of the liver has increased the rate of detection of small metastases.[55,56] The findings of exploration in regard to the fixation or extent of the primary tumor, local or regional adenopathy, involvement of adjacent structures, and sites of metastases should be documented in the surgical report.[57]

Extent of Resection

The extent of colonic resection is determined by the blood vessels that must be divided to remove the lymphatic drainage of the tumor-bearing portion of the colon with tumor-free margins.[58] This is the primary treatment approach in patients with colon carcinoma.[59] Resection of intermediate and principal nodes requires ligation and division of the main vascular trunks to the affected colon segment.[60] Tumor-free margins usually are accomplished by resection of at least 5 cm of normal bowel proximal and distal to the tumor.[61] Uncontrolled data exist to demonstrate improvement in outcomes from extending this resection.[62]

Extent of Lymph Node Resection

Adequate lymphadenectomy is crucial. In addition to its therapeutic benefits of preventing local progression and subsequent development of symptoms caused by mesenteric recurrence, lymphadenectomy is critical in the staging of patients with colon carcinoma.[63] In colon cancer, recovery of cancer-bearing lymph nodes is the parameter most often used for adjuvant therapy recommendations in the United States.[64] Mesenteric resection should be extensive enough to harvest at least 12 lymph nodes for examination to allow for accurate staging.[65]

Controversy exists over the curative efficacy of extensive lymphadenectomy in patients with colon carcinoma. Excellent results have been obtained with wide mesenteric resection.[66,67] Other studies have found patients with principal node involvement to be incurable.[68] Slanetz and Grimson[69] reviewed 2,409 cases of curative resections. They found that specific groups of patients benefited from high ligation of the vascular pedicle; these were the patients with transmural node-negative tumors and those with limited nodal spread. Those in whom the highest nodes were involved did not appear to benefit. A prospective multicenter study was unable to confirm a survival benefit confined by wider mesenteric resection in left colon cancer.[70]

TABLE 42.3. Sentinel lymph node biopsy in colon cancer.

Study	*N*	*IHC Used*	*Upstage (H&E or IHC)*	*SCN detected*	*True positive*	*SN false (–)*
Prospective consecutive cases: Wood et al.[326]	100	Yes	24%	97%	95%	5%
Prospective consecutive cases: Trocha et al.[327]	50	Yes	Gy IHC 20.5%	98%	93.8%	6%
Not stated: Paramo et al.[328]	45	Yes	11%	82%	98%	3%
Multicenter prospective: Saha et al.[329]	203	Yes	14%	98%	—	—
Multicenter prospective: Bilchick et al.[330]	40	Yes	10%	100%	100%	0
Not stated: Joosten et al.[331]	50	Yes	N/A	70%	NS	24%
Prospective: Merrie et al.[332]	26	No	N/A	88%	55%	45%

N, number of patients; IHC, immunohistochemical staining; H&E, hemotoxylin and eosin staining; SN, sentinel node; NS, not significant.

Sentinel Lymph Node Biopsy for Colon Cancer

In an effort to increase the detection of lymphatic metastases in patients undergoing the resection of a colon cancer, sentinel lymph node biopsy has been used. In colon cancer, it is used to stage the patient in a more-sensitive way as opposed to eliminating or minimizing the extent of the lymphatic resection (Table 42.3).

Among patients with node-positive cancers, survival can be affected by the number of positive nodes. Patients with one positive node may have survival rates in the 69% to 75% range whereas 5-year survival for those with four or more positive nodes or metastases along a named vascular trunk are in the 27% to 40% range.[71] Overall, survival rates for patients with node-positive cancers appear to be approximately 40% to 50%. The analysis by Cohen et al.[72] of node-positive colon cancer patients treated with resection alone showed a significant difference in survival for patients having one to three positive nodes (66% 5-year survival) and those with four or more positive nodes (37% 5-year survival). It has been demonstrated, however, that up to 75% of all positive nodes in resectable colon cancer may be under 2mm in size and therefore gross dissection alone may underestimate nodal status.[73]

Contiguous Organ Involvement

For tumors that are adherent to adjacent organs, adhesions should not be divided. In one-half of cases, the adherence may be caused by malignant invasion of these adjacent organs.[74] Separation of sites of adherence can disrupt the tumor, increase recurrence, and reduce survival rates. Adjacent organ involvement should be resected in continuity with the colon and primary tumor. Radical resection may still be curative in 20% to 50% of patients, even if adjacent tissues are invaded by malignant infiltration.[74] In a review of 25 patients with locally advanced colon cancer requiring en bloc resection, median survival was 38.2 months and 5-year survival was 49%. External-beam and intraoperative therapy was used to obtain these results.[75]

Surgical Technique

Molecular techniques have enhanced the ability to detect cancer cells released into the circulation during operative manipulation.[76] A prospective, randomized trial by Wiggers et al.[77] showed that in patients who underwent preliminary ligation of vessels liver metastases appeared later than in patients who did not undergo this procedure. However, no overall survival benefit was demonstrated.

Possibly because the local recurrence rate for colon cancer approximates 4%, surgical technique for colon resection may be seen as less critical in many cases.[78,79] Hospital volume seemed to have a greater effect on patient outcome than did individual surgeon volume in a review of a large administrative database.[80]

Laparoscopic Colectomy

Laparoscopic techniques have become widely used in the management of benign and malignant colorectal conditions.[81] With laparoscopic colectomies, there is a theoretical advantage of a shortened hospital stay and a more rapid recovery.[82]

The overall complications of laparoscopic colorectal surgery were comparable to those of open resection in a large randomized trial of laparoscopic and open colectomy in the United States.[83] Data that are available on the extent of lymphadenectomy and resection margins suggest that oncologic laparoscopic resection is comparable to open colectomy for cancer.[84] Studies have documented estimated recurrence rates in port sites of 1.08% to 3.8% after laparoscopic resection. These recurrence rates are similar to those associated with laparotomy wounds in patients treated by open resection.[83]

Two prospective, randomized trials have been done to compare the efficacy of laparoscopic colectomy with open colectomy for carcinoma.[85,86] The COST study involves patients with right, left, or sigmoid colon adenocarcinoma, and patients are randomly assigned to laparoscopically assisted or open colectomy. The primary endpoints of the study are disease-free and overall survival. The secondary endpoints are examinations of morbidity, cost-effectiveness, and quality of life (Table 42.4).

The COST trial demonstrated, in a multiinstitutional trial, that rates of recurrence and overall survival rates were equivalent for open and laparoscopic colectomy.[85] Wound recurrence rates were less than 1% in both groups. Complication rates were similar in both groups. It is important to recognize that this trial excluded rectal cancer and transverse

TABLE 42.4. Laparoscopic versus open resection for colon cancer.

	Open recurrence rate	*Laparoscopic recurrence rate*	*Open survival*	*Laparoscopic survival*
COST[85] (*n* = 872)	18	16	85	86
Lacy et al.[86] (*n* = 219)	27	18	~75	~85

colon cancer. The authors also had strict controls over the quality of the surgery and the experience of the surgeons before enrolling patients in the study.

In the study by Lacy et al., the criteria for entry were similar; however, it was conducted in a single hospital unit.[86] This study favors laparoscopic resection in terms of survival and recurrence rates. Lower rates of wound infection and ileus were noted in the laparoscopic resection group, and this was responsible for an overall lower morbidity rate for this group. The cancer-related probability of survival was significantly higher in the laparoscopic resection group.

Prophylactic Oophorectomy

Ovarian metastases and colorectal cancer can occur at the time of presentation in 2% to 8% of patients and as a subsequent site of metastases in 1% to 7% of curatively resected patients. Survival from ovarian metastases is poor in both settings, being 9% with synchronous metastases and 20% with metachronous metastases.[87]

Prophylactic removal of the ovaries at the time of colorectal cancer resection has been considered to reduce the risks of poor survival from metachronous metastases; this is pertinent only for the 1% to 7% of women who develop metachronous metastases, of whom only 6% to 20% have disease confined to the ovaries.

In a study of prophylactic oophorectomy in postmenopausal women by Sielezneff et al.,[88] the incidence of occult ovarian metastases was 2.4%. The 5-year survival rates in this study were equal, whether or not a prophylactic oophorectomy was performed.[89] In a preliminary report of a randomized trial of prophylactic oophorectomy in patients with Dukes' stage B and C colorectal cancer treated at the Mayo Clinic, no incidence of gross or microscopic ovarian metastases was found in 77 patients randomized to oophorectomy. No differences were seen in overall survival, whether or not patients were randomized to oophorectomy. A trend was noted toward an improved recurrence-free survival with prophylactic oophorectomy. No selection criteria based on tumor size, grade, or other characteristics exist at this time.[90]

Oncologic Results of Surgical Management

For node-negative patients, survival with surgery alone varies between 75% and 90%.[71] Even in these cancers, such factors as depth of penetration, contiguous organ involvement, lymphatic and vascular invasion, differentiation and perineural invasion, as well as molecular and cellular characteristics, will affect survival.[91]

Important issues in surgically resected, apparently node-negative colon cancer are the methods of lymph node evaluation and the detection of occult metastatic disease. Studies have indicated that 12 to 15 lymph nodes should be examined to indicate true nodal negativity.[65,92,93] Standardizing node evaluation and using immunohistochemical techniques can identify occult nodal metastases in up to 26% of those whose nodes test negatively by routine techniques.[94] There is a high likelihood that standard dissection will identify node-negative patients if an adequate number of nodes are examined.[73] Some have questioned the relevance of occult micrometastatic disease in patients who have undergone curative resection.[95] In a group of surgically resected patients with micrometastases in resected nodes and original Dukes' stage A or B colorectal cancer, survival time was 48 months, which equaled the survival time for patients without micrometastases. In a review of 243 cases from NSABP trials that were node negative by standard techniques, immunohistochemical demonstration of nodal micrometastases did not correlate with overall or recurrence-free survival in node-negative patients.[96]

Specific Management Problems

Synchronous Cancer

Synchronous cancers are relatively uncommon, having an incidence of 3.4%, as described by Finan et al.[97] In addition to the presence of another malignancy, there can be up to 30% to 40% incidence of synchronous neoplastic polyps in the colon of a patient with a large bowel carcinoma.[98]

If removal of all polyps cannot be accomplished owing to obstructive lesions or an emergency operation for perforation, the index lesion should be addressed at the time of surgery and subsequent complete colonoscopic examination should be carried out in the early postoperative period.[99]

Passman et al.[100] conducted an 18-year multiinstitutional database study of 4,878 patients with colon cancer. They found a 3.3% incidence of synchronous tumors; they also found that patients with synchronous colon cancers have the same survival rate as patients with solitary colon tumors when the highest stage of the synchronous tumor is considered.[100]

Obstructing Cancers

Intestinal obstruction is the most common emergency presentation of colorectal carcinoma.[101] Poor prognosis is associated with this presentation, even when analyzed stage for stage, with an overall survival rate of 31% at 5 years. Patients who present with this problem are frequently elderly or in poor condition because of dehydration, and operative mortality can approach 28%.[101]

Staged resection is most useful in elderly persons with multiple comorbidities.[101] Further alternatives for obstruction lesions distal to the splenic flexure have been studied. The first is subtotal colectomy, the second is an extended right colectomy to include the obstruction lesion without colonic decompression, and a third is the use of intraoperative colonic lavage and segmental resection. Nyam et al.[89] reported on a series of 103 patients with obstructing left-side colon carcinomas undergoing an extended right colectomy without colonic decompression or a segmental left colectomy with intraoperative lavage. They found that both procedures had an acceptably low anastomotic leak rate and mortality. Poon et al.[102] studied emergency primary resection and anastomosis with intraoperative colonic lavage for left-sided obstruction. Hospital mortality rate was 5% to 9%; the anastomotic leak rate with this approach was 4%.

The alternative approach of subtotal colectomy with ileorectal anastomosis has been compared with intraoperative lavage in primary colonic anastomosis in a randomized trial.[103] This trial showed no difference in mortality or morbidity rates. However, patients with subtotal colectomy had a higher postoperative frequency of bowel movements.[103]

Perforating Cancers

Perforation of the colon due to carcinoma can occur either at the site of the colon tumor itself (in approximately 65% to 82% of patients with perforation) or in the bowel proximal to an obstructing tumor (in 18% to 35% of patients).[104] Overall 5-year survival for patients with localized perforation is approximately 44%. This complication occurs in 2% to 8% of all patients with colorectal cancer.

The presence of a perforation or fistula increases cancer recurrence rates. Local recurrence rates of 23% have been reported by Carraro et al.[104] in a study of 83 patients with large bowel perforation and colorectal cancer; this compares with figures of 28% to 44% reported in the literature. Peritoneal seeding is a particularly common failure in patients with perforated colorectal cancers, with carcinomatosis rates of 17% to 18%.

Radiation Therapy for Colon Cancer

The overall component that local failure contributes to the recurrence of resected colon cancer is low. However, it has been possible to demonstrate that those with obstruction or perforation have higher local recurrence rates compared to those without these complications of colon cancer. In a retrooperative study of 77 patients with obstruction and 34 patients with perforated colon cancers, the local failure rates were 42% and 44%, respectively, compared with a local failure rate of 14% in other resected patients without these features.[105] From subset analysis of colon cancer adjuvant trials it has been implied that local recurrences can occur in 20% to 27% of resected node-positive patients and that this is not changed by 5-fluorouracil-based chemotherapy. This analysis further concluded that the addition of whole abdominal irradiation reduced local relapse rates to 12% for these high-risk colon cancers.[106]

Postoperative irradiation alone was demonstrated to reduce local failure rates compared to historical control rates where doses of 4,300 to 6,300 cGy were delivered to the tumor bed.[107] In another study of postoperative radiation therapy in Astler–Coller stage B2, B3, and C patients, local failure rates were reduced to 8%, 21%, and 31%, respectively, in those receiving radiotherapy compared to 31%, 36%, and 53%, respectively, in those treated with surgery alone.[108] A later follow-up of this series after 5-fluorouracil-based therapy was added to node-positive patients identified Astler–Coller stage B3 and C3 patients. Tumors associated with abscess or fistula formation and a subset of those with residual gross disease after resection are potential candidates for this approach.[109] Similar results were obtained in B2 and C colon cancer patients when doses of 50 to 55 cGy were given along with fluorouracil. In this study, local control rates dropped from 96% with doses of radiation of 50 to 55 Gy to 76% when less than 45 Gy was given.[110] A 10-year retrospective analysis of this approach also confirmed this management in reducing local failure in this group of patients.[111]

Two studies looked at the effect of whole abdominal radiation after the resection of high-risk colon cancer with 5-fluorouracil. In an analysis of 18 patients, local failure was seen in 17%, whereas 28% of patients required treatment breaks of 2 weeks or more and 11% had grade 3 or 4 toxicity.[112] In another pilot study, 41 transmural node-negative patients were treated with postoperative 5-fluorouracil, whole abdominal irradiation to 30 Gy, and a boost to the tumor bed. Local control rates compared favorably with similar patients treated with chemotherapy alone. However, 17% of patients had severe toxicity and 7% had life-threatening toxicity. These studies demonstrate positive results with this approach but confirm substantial toxicity for whole abdominal irradiation.[113]

On an examination of the role of intraoperative radiation therapy (IORT) in advanced colon cancer where postoperative radiation and chemotherapy were also used, it was found that IORT reduced local failure rate in these with residual disease from 82% to 1%. This result was associated with a 5-year survival improvement for those with residual disease who were treated with IORT compared with external-beam treatment alone.[114] For patients with recurrent colon cancer who undergo resection, IORT and external-beam radiation can produce long term survival.[115]

Chemotherapy for Colon Carcinoma

The treatment of colon carcinoma with curative intent is best achieved in the earliest stages of diagnosis. The estimated 5-year survival of a patient with American Joint Committee on Cancer (AJCC) stage I is approximately 90% with surgery alone. However, the majority of patients present with AJCC stage II/III disease; more than 80% will be rendered disease free following surgical resection but approximately 50% of these patients will develop recurrent disease.[116] It is presumed the etiology for the resurgence of colon carcinoma is attributed to microscopic disease that is not self-evident on surgical or radiologic assessment. Therefore, adjuvant chemotherapy is often considered to prevent the manifestation of recurrent tumor that may not be amenable to treatment. Existing heterogeneity in stage II/III patients including surgical technique, the number of lymph nodes involved, colonic obstruction, visceral perforation, histology, age at presentation, coexisting morbidities, and molecular makeup confound the medical oncologist's perspective of what is deemed a simple categorical AJCC stage II or III that can be further subdivided into AJCC subgroups of A, B, or C. For the purposes of this chapter, the discussion of adjuvant chemotherapy is only in reference to surgically resected AJCC stage II (Duke's B2) and III (Dukes' C) patients.

A meta-analysis of 17 randomized adjuvant chemotherapy trials involving 6,791 patients was conducted and published

TABLE 42.5. INT-0035: Adjuvant chemotherapy in Dukes' C colon patients ($n = 929$).

	Observation	*Levamisole*	*5-Fluorouracil (5-FU)/levamisole*
Reduction in recurrence	—	NS	41% ($P < 0.0001$)
Decrease in mortality	—	NS	33% ($P = 0.006$)
Overall survival	55%	NS	71% ($P = 0.0064$)

NS, not statistically significant.

in 1988.[117] When evaluating all clinical trials published in the English periodical literature through the year 1987, the benefits of adjuvant chemotherapy could not be determined. However, when evaluating 5-fluorouracil (5-FU)-only-containing regimens ($n = 4{,}700$), the odds of death were 10% lower in comparison to the control arm, and the estimated benefit in 5-year survival was 2.3% to 5.7% higher relative to the control arm, although not statistically significant. If the treatment provided was prolonged for 1 year or more, the absolute 5-year survival benefit was disappointingly less than 5%. Such a small risk-to-benefit ratio in the setting of a patient population that has been surgically cured could not support the use of adjuvant chemotherapy in this setting.

The National Surgical Adjuvant Breast and Bowel Project (NSABP) cooperative group conducted the first large-scale study to evaluate the potential benefits of adjuvant chemotherapy, NSABP C-01.[118,119] More than 1,100 patients with AJCC stage II and stage III colon cancer were randomized to (a) observation alone, (b) 5-FU, semustine, and vincristine (MOF), or (c) inoculation with the bacillus Calmette–Guerin (BCG) vaccine. The initial use of MOF relative to the control arm indicated a benefit in disease-free survival (DFS) ($P = 0.02$) and overall survival ($P = 0.05$); these findings were not supported after a median follow-up of 8 years ($P = 0.10$ and $P = 0.12$, respectively).[120] A considerable drawback to the use of the MOF regimen was the development of chemotherapy-related leukemia. There was no survival benefit with the use of BCG.

5-FU/Levamisole

Immunomodulation of 5-FU with levamisole has been extensively investigated in several randomized trials. Traditionally, levamisole was used as an antihelminthic agent in animals and humans. Its mechanism of action relative to 5-FU is poorly understood but may result in selective stabilization of mRNA.[121] The North Central Cancer Treatment Group (NCCTG) completed the first study to examine the potential immunomodulatory effects of levamisole on 5-FU.[122] Four hundred eleven Dukes' B2 or C patients following surgical resection were randomized to (a) observation, (b) single-agent levamisole (50 mg t.i.d., days 1–3 every 14 days × 1 year), or (c) 5-FU (450 mg/m^2/day × 5 days every 28 days × 1 year)/levamisole (same schedule and dose as single-agent arm). Patients were followed closely for more than 5 years. It should be noted that two-thirds of patients were Dukes' C colon carcinoma patients; a minority of rectal carcinoma patients were represented. After a median follow-up of 7 years, 5-FU/levamisole versus observation resulted in superiority of disease-free survival (DFS) ($P = 0.02$) and overall survival (OS) ($P = 0.03$) in Dukes' C patients only; no benefit could be derived in Dukes' B2 patients. The levamisole-alone arm demonstrated a trend in improved DFS and OS but this finding was not statistically significant ($P = 0.06$).

To verify the findings reported in the NCCTG study, Intergroup study, INT-0035, involving members of the NCCTG, Southwest Oncology Group (SWOG) and the Eastern Cooperative Group (ECOG) was completed.[123] A total of 1,296 patients were enrolled in this study; three-fourths of the patients were Dukes' C patients. Eligibility criteria were identical to that of the original NCCTG study but rectal carcinoma patients were not included. Preliminary results after a median follow-up of 3.5 years concluded that 5-FU/levamisole provided a significant reduction in recurrence and OS (Table 42.5). Toxicities associated with 5-FU and levamisole were considered to be tolerable. Results of the Dukes' B2 colon carcinoma patients ($n = 318$) were premature and were reported at a later date. This pivotal trial culminated in the Consensus Panel of the National Institute of Health (NIH) recommending 5-FU/levamisole as adjuvant therapy for all node-positive (AJCC stage III/Dukes' C) colon carcinoma patients and became widely accepted as the standard of care in the United States.[64] The NIH Consensus Panel concluded that Dukes' B2 (AJCC stage II) colon cancer patients are at high risk for recurrence and warrant further evaluation. After a median follow-up of 7 years, the superior benefits of 5-FU/levamisole were confirmed in Dukes' C patients.[124] Single-agent levamisole failed to provide any clinical benefit in the adjuvant setting.

Altering the Paradigm of Adjuvant Chemotherapy to 5-FU/Leucovorin

Whether levamisole provided any true benefit to 5-FU is questionable and may in part be attributed to the large number of patients accrued. An oversight in initial trial design of INT-0035 was to not include an 5-FU-only arm to determine the actual additive benefit of levamisole in this setting.

During the next 5 years, levamisole shortly became replaced by leucovorin (folinic acid), an immunomodulatory agent whose mechanism of action is clearly defined. Leucovorin (LV) biochemically modifies 5-FU by stabilizing the metabolite 5-FdUMP (5-fluorodeoxyuridine monophosphate) to thymidylate synthase (TS), enhancing inhibition of 5-FU on TS. Initial interest in LV in the adjuvant setting developed after a meta-analysis of 18 randomized trials determined superiority in response rate and 1-year overall-survival.[125] Hence, the adjuvant setting appeared to be the most appropriate for evaluating a survival benefit.

TABLE 42.6. Adjuvant chemotherapy trials of 5-fluorouracil (5-FU)/leucovorin (LV) following surgical resection.

	Adjuvant treatment	*N*	*Three-year DFS*	*Three-year OS*	*Reduction in mortality*
NSABP C-03[358]	MOF × 5	524	64% (95% CI, 60%–68%)	77%	—
	5-FU/LV × 6 cycles	521	73% (95% CI, 69%–77%)	84% ($P = 0.003$)	32%
IMPACT[126]	Observation	772	62%	78%	—
	5-FU (370–400 mg/m^2)/ LV (200 mg/m^2) daily × 5 days, every 28 days	754	71%	83%	22%

MOF, 5-FU, semustine, and vincristine; DFS, disease-free survival; OS, overall survival.

Multiple trials have since been conducted examining 5-FU/LV in the adjuvant setting (Table 42.6). NSABP C-03 randomized 1,081 patients with Dukes' B2 and C colon cancer between the years of 1987 and 1989 to MOF or 5-FU /LV on the basis of the promising results of NSABP C-01 using MOF as the control arm.[120] Results from this study clearly designated 5-FU/LV as superior to MOF with an advantage in both DFS (13%) and OS (12%).

Despite the earlier recommendations by the NIH Consensus Panel, doubt in the international community existed regarding the use of adjuvant chemotherapy. A pooled analysis of three cooperative groups, the International Multicentre Pooled Analysis of Colon Cancer Trials (IMPACT), was created randomizing 1,526 patients to 5-FU/LV versus observation only following a surgical resection.[126] The IMPACT study concluded that the use of 5-FU/LV is an effective adjuvant chemotherapy regimen for Dukes' C colon carcinoma patients (Table 42.7). A subset analysis of Dukes' B2 patients failed to demonstrate any benefit in DFS or OS for patients receiving 5-FU/LV. With the advent of adjuvant chemotherapy in the setting of Dukes' C patients, the optimal schedule and use of levamisole, leucovorin, or the combination of levamisole/leucovorin, with 5-FU remained undefined.

These concerns were addressed by O'Connell and colleagues who conducted an intergroup trial led by the NCCTG with the National Cancer Institute of Canada Clinical Trials Group assessing appropriate duration of treatment.[127] After a median follow-up of 5.1 years, it was concluded that the doublet 5-FU/levamisole for 1 year was inferior to the triplet combination of 5-FU/levamisole/leucovorin for 6 months (P less than 0.01). Greater grade 3–4 gastrointestinal toxicities were observed in the three-drug combination arm (P less than 0.0005). This study failed to directly compare 5-FU/LV to 5-FU/levamisole.

Two landmark trials, NSABP C-04 and INT-0089, provided the impetus for the extinction of levamisole in the treatment of colon carcinoma.[128] NSABP C-04 accrued 2,151 patients in less than 2 years to the doublet regimens of 5-FU/levamisole or LV versus that of the triplet combination of 5-FU/LV/levamisole (see Table 42.7). At the conclusion of this study, a survival advantage was not detected in any arm. However, superior DFS ($P = 0.04$) was achieved with 5-FU/LV relative to 5-FU/levamisole. The addition of levamisole to 5-FU/LV did not confer any additional benefit in DFS or OS.

TABLE 42.7. NSABP C-04.

Chemotherapy regimen	*N*	*Five-year DFS*	*Five-year OS*
5-FU/LV	691	65% ($P = 0.04$)	74% ($P = 0.07$)
5-FU/levamisole	691	60%	70%
5-FU/levamisole/LV	696	65% ($P = 0.67$)	74% ($P = 0.99$)

DFS, disease-free survival; OS, overall survival.

INT-0089 is the single largest study created to examine the benefits of adjuvant chemotherapy in Dukes' B2 and C colon carcinoma patients.[129] Dukes' B2 patients represented 20% of all patients accrued. Patients were randomized to one of four arms: (1) 5-FU/levamisole × 1 year, (2) 8 months of 5-FU/LV (Roswell Park), (3) six cycles of 5-FU/LV (Mayo Clinic), or (4) six cycles of the Mayo regimen of 5-FU/LV + levamisole. Initial results were presented in 1996 and updated in 1998. Final evaluation of the Dukes' B2 patients was reported in a separate study. A subset analysis determined the triplet combination of Mayo Clinic regimen of 5-FU/LV + levamisole was superior in OS relative to 5-FU/levamisole but equivalent to that of the Mayo Clinic regimen alone. The benefits of levamisole were determined to be negligible, and its use could not be advocated. Furthermore, the Roswell Park schedule was equivalent in response and 5-year overall survival to that of the Mayo Clinic regimen (Table 42.8). At the conclusion of the study, 5-FU/LV scheduled in either fashion was recommended as the standard of care in patients with high-risk colon cancer (AJCC stage III/Dukes' C). Remarkably, the final publication regarding this breakthrough study has yet to be published.

Novel Chemotherapeutics in Adjuvant Chemotherapy

Irinotecan (CPT-11)

For the past four decades, 5-FU has been the sole chemotherapy agent for both the adjuvant and metastatic settings. Other than biomodulation with levamisole or leucovorin, few modifications in this regimen had occurred. The topoisomerase I inhibitor, irinotecan, and the third-generation platinum analogue, oxaliplatin, were to shortly alter the approach to chemotherapy.

Two large Phase III clinical trials conducted both in the United States and Europe provided the foundation for combined chemotherapy with 5-FU/LV in advanced colorectal cancer. Both clinical trials randomized AJCC stage IV advanced colorectal cancer patients to a regimen of weekly bolus irinotecan/5-FU/LV (IFL) versus bolus 5-FU/LV or irinotecan/infusional 5-FU/LV (FOLFIRI) versus infusional 5-FU/LV, respectively (Table 42.9). In short, the combined irinotecan/5-FU/LV arms demonstrated exceptional time to progression, response rate, and OS relative to the 5-FU/LV arms.[130,131]

The use of infusional 5-FU/LV is commonplace in the European community rather than the bolus 5-FU/LV as in the Mayo Clinic or Roswell Park regimens. Of interest is that pre-

TABLE 42.8. Variable schedules in 5-fluorouracil (5-FU)/leucovorin (LV) administration as adjuvant chemotherapy.

Regimen	*Dose and schedule*	*Five-year OS*	*Common toxicities*
Mayo	5-FU (425 mg/m^2)/LV (20 mg/m^2) daily × 5 days, repeat every 28 days	66%	Stomatitis, leukopenia
Roswell	5-FU (500 mg/m^2)/LV (500 mg/m^2) daily × 5 days, repeat every 28 days	65%	Diarrhea

5-FU, 5-fluorouracil; LV, leucovorin.

vious studies had determined infusional 5-FU/LV resulted in a higher response rate (32.6% versus 14.4%) and progression-free survival (27.6 versus 22 months) when compared to the Mayo Clinic 5-FU/LV but no statistical benefit in overall survival ($P = 0.067$).[132]

The irinotecan/infusional 5-FU/LV regimen reported by Douillard and colleagues[131] was found to be superior in OS, but the positive results of the IFL regimen reported by Saltz and colleagues[130] led the U.S. Food and Drug Administration (FDA) to approve weekly bolus irinotecan/5-FU/LV (IFL) as front-line therapy in advanced colorectal cancer. Subsequently, in the year 2000, the weekly bolus IFL regimen became the standard of care for all patients in the United States with advanced stage IV disease unless clinically contraindicated.

Hence, interest in the use of irinotecan/5-FU/LV in the adjuvant setting arose. The largest study to examine the impact of IFL as adjuvant treatment was created by the Cancer and Leukemia Group B (CALGB). CALGB 89803 randomized 1,263 patients with stage III colon carcinoma to either the Roswell Park regimen of 5-FU/LV or to weekly bolus IFL.[133,134] Paradoxically, a recent interim analysis after a median follow-up of 2.1 years found no difference in time to progression (TTP) or OS between the treatment arms. Thus, the use of weekly bolus IFL cannot be advocated as adjuvant treatment for stage III colon cancer. Whether irinotecan/infusional 5-FU/LV will also be of negative benefit in stage II or III colon cancer is unclear at this time; two Phase III European trials (PETAC 3 and ACCORD02) have completed patient accrual ($N = 1{,}250$), with final results to be reported at a later date.

Oxaliplatin

For the past decade, the diaminocyclohexane platinum analogue oxaliplatin (Eloxatin) has been extensively investigated as a single agent and in combination with other chemotherapy agents. Oxaliplatin is the first platinum agent that has demonstrated activity in colorectal cancer and lacks cross-reactivity with other platinum agents. Potential adverse toxicities unique to oxaliplatin compared to other platinum agents may include cold pharyngeal dysesthesia and cumulative reversible peripheral neuropathy. Its activity as a single agent is rather disappointing and is reported 10% at best.[135] However, when combined with infusional 5-FU/LV synergistic cytotoxic activity is evident.[136–138]

De Gramont and colleagues proceeded to evaluate oxaliplatin in combination with infusional 5-FU/LV. [136] Despite a superior difference in relative risk (RR) and TTP, this study was not powered to establish a benefit in OS. Consequently, the Oncologic Drugs Advisory Committee (ODAC) and the FDA did not approve the first-line indication of oxaliplatin in advanced colorectal cancer. Clinical investigators continued to explore its role.

A large, pivotal intergroup study headed by the North Central Cancer Treatment Group, NCCTG 9741, accrued 741 chemotherapy-naïve patients with advanced stage IV colorectal cancer, randomizing them to (a) weekly bolus IFL, (b) oxaliplatin/infusional 5-FU/LV (FOLFOX 4), or (c) oxaliplatin/irinotecan.[139] The infusional 5-FU/LV (FOLFOX 4) regimen prevailed after a median follow-up of 20.4 months with an impressive median OS of 19.8 months, the longest median overall survival reported to date with standard chemotherapy agents. This study was fraught with questions regarding its clinical trial design for second-line therapy. Sixty percent of patients with progression of disease (PD) while on FOLFOX4 were allowed to receive irinotecan as second-line therapy versus only 24% of patients on the IFL arm who were able to receive oxaliplatin because it was not FDA approved at the time of the study. Regardless, this trial established oxaliplatin as a valuable agent in the armamentarium against advanced colorectal cancer. Its effectiveness as second-line therapy after irinotecan is less than 10% but clearly demonstrates a clinical benefit.[138] In September 2002, the FDA advocated the use of oxaliplatin/infusional 5-FU/LV as second-line therapy after irinotecan-treated failures. Worldwide, it is accepted as front-line therapy in the treatment of advanced colorectal cancer.

The role of oxaliplatin may not be limited to the advanced disease setting. The multicenter international study of oxaliplatin/5-FU/LV in the adjuvant treatment of colon cancer "MOSAIC" trial has recently reported promising preliminary results from a large randomized Phase III study of FOLFOX4

TABLE 42.9. Efficacy of bolus and infusional irinotecan/5-FU/LV in advanced colorectal cancer.

	N	*RR*	*TTP*	*Median OS*
Saltz et al.[130]				
Bolus irinotecan/5-FU/LV (IFL), weekly × 4 of every 6 weeks	231	21%	4.3 M	12.6
Mayo Clinic 5-FU/LV	226	39%	7.0 M	14.8
Douillard et al.[131]				
Infusional 5-FU/LV	187	22%	4.4 M	14.1 M
Irinotecan/infusional 5-FU/LV	198	41%	6.7 M	17.4 M

RR, relative risk; TTP, time to progression; M, months.

TABLE 42.10. The Phase III MOSAIC Trial.

	Infusional 5-FU/LV	*FOLFOX4*	*Risk reduction*
Stage II (Dukes' B2)	83.9%	86.6%	18%
Stage III (Dukes' C)	65.5%	71.8%	24%
Overall 3-year DFS	72.8%	77.9%	23% ($P < 0.01$)

FOLFOX4, oxaliplatin/infusional 5-FU/LV; DFS, disease-free survival.

versus infusional 5-FU/LV as adjuvant therapy. This impressive study accrued 2,246 patients diagnosed with Dukes' B2/Dukes' C colon carcinoma who were subsequently treated for a 6-month duration (Table 42.10).[140] Although the final analysis of this study will be reported at a later date, these encouraging findings may permanently alter the approach to adjuvant therapy. Furthermore, this may be the first study to indicate additional benefit for adjuvant chemotherapy in Dukes' B2 colon carcinoma.

The Controversy of Stage II/Dukes' B2 Patients

Although a patient with stage II colon cancer has a more favorable prognosis than that of a stage III patient, poor prognostic markers may place the stage II patient at increased risk for local or metastatic disease recurrence.[105,141–144] Of the four largest clinical studies conducted over the past decade to evaluate this subpopulation of patients, the overwhelming majority of studies have reported no added benefit in OS when adjuvant chemotherapy is administered.

After a median follow-up of 7 years, investigators of INT-0035 substratified the stage II/Dukes' B2 patients ($n = 318$), reporting a trend in reduced recurrence with the use 5-FU/levamisole versus that of observation only (32% decline; $P = 0.10$).[145] The investigators of the International Multicentre Pooled Analysis of Colon Cancer Trials (IMPACT) created a pooled analysis of five separate clinical trials, IMPACT B2, involving 1,016 patients. Patients had been randomized to six adjuvant cycles of 5-FU/LV versus that of observation alone.[146] After a median follow-up of 5.75 years, patients who had received chemotherapy did not experience an improvement in event-free survival (EFS) (76% versus 73%) or OS (82% versus 80%). After a median follow-up of 5 years, Intergroup Study 0089 failed to validate a benefit in OS for Dukes' B2 patients with the use of either leucovorin and/or levamisole when combined with 5-FU, in doublet or triplet combination.[129] Likely, this study was inadequately powered to evaluate this subgroup with only 20% of all patients accrued with Dukes' B2 disease. Hence, the consideration of adjuvant chemotherapy for a stage II patient was not recommended.

The only positive pooled analysis before to the MOSAIC study[134] was conducted by the NSABP in Dukes' B2 and C patients. Patients of four separate trials, C-01, C-02, C-03, and C-04, addressed the plausible benefit of not one particular regimen but simply the benefit of 5-FU-based chemotherapy overall. Of the 4,006 patients enrolled, 41% of patients ($n = 1,565$) were diagnosed with a Dukes' B2 carcinoma. In brief, C-01 and C-02 compared 5-FU/LV to observation only, and Studies C-03 and C-04 compared 5-FU/LV with either MOF or the combination of 5-FU/LV/levamisole. When the data of all four studies were combined, a 30% reduction in mortality was determined in Dukes' B2 patients and an 18% reduction was noted in Dukes' C patients. Despite these positive findings, this study was heavily criticized and not advocated to alter the standard of care at the time the study was conducted as a result of the lack of uniformity among the chemotherapy regimens. In contrast, the recent findings supported by the MOSAIC study may result in a paradigm shift in the consideration of treatment for all Dukes' B2/stage II patients unless contraindicated.[147]

Microsatellite Instability (MSI) on the Decision of Adjuvant Therapy

Significant discussion has recently risen when considering adjuvant chemotherapy for high-frequency microsatellite instability (MSI) patients. MSI results in a defect in DNA mismatch repair as a result of frame-shift mutations and base-pair substitutions found in short, tandemly repeated nucleotide sequences. MSI is associated with familial inherited malignancies as the hereditary nonpolyposis colorectal cancer (HNPCC, or Lynch syndrome) but may be found in approximately 15% of sporadic colorectal carcinomas also as a result of hypermethylation of the promoter region on MLH1.[148,149] High-frequency MSI has been determined to be an independent prognostic factor and is a positive predictive survival factor.[148] Whether adjuvant chemotherapy provides additional benefit in these patients is unclear. Conflicting results have been reported in both stage II and stage III patients.[148,150] Ribic and colleagues confirmed that patients with high-frequency MSI had longer OS and DFS but concluded that adjuvant 5-FU/LV was of no benefit in OS ($P = 0.12$) or DFS ($P = 0.06$) for stage II/III patients exhibiting MSI.[150] Elsaleh and colleagues have suggested that sex, location, and MSI status may have a bearing on survival following adjuvant 5-FU/LV.[151] It is not the intent of this chapter to elaborate in full detail regarding MSI status and outcome but to note that additional clinical studies are warranted to clarify this issue further.

Management Options for Rectal Carcinoma

Improving the management of resectable rectal cancer involves the optimization of patient outcomes through (1) a detailed understanding of the pathology of rectal cancer and its relation to surgical techniques; (2) multidisciplinary management; and (3) organ and function conservation. The goal of the treatment of rectal carcinoma is cure or local control of disease with maintenance of quality of life. The biology of a particular patient's tumor is the most important factor in overall outcome. Adequate surgical removal of the tumor is the major treatment factor affecting local control and cure.[152] Appropriate adjuvant therapies can enhance local control, reduce systemic recurrence, and increase organ preservation.[153–155]

The chief reason for this difference between colon cancer and rectal cancer outcomes is related to a difference in local recurrence.[156] Abdominoperineal resection (APR) has been used for management with excellent results. However, APR requires a permanent colostomy, which adversely affects the patient's quality of life.[157] Advances in rectal cancer management and surgical techniques have improved our ability to achieve oncologic control and optimal patient function without APR, even in patients with low rectal cancers.[158] Even in the absence of adjuvant therapy, 79 of 95 patients with T3 N0 rectal cancer had sphincter-preserving procedures with local recurrence rates less than 10%.[159] This study as well as others have continued to demonstrate that there is no difference in local recurrence rates between sphincter-preserving surgery for rectal cancer and APR.[160]

Surgical Approaches and Techniques

Local Excision

Full-thickness local excision can be effective in the treatment of selected early low rectal cancers. Local excision can be used as curative therapy for patients who have superficial tumors (Table 42.11).

Transanal excision is the most common method of local excision. Selection factors based on tumor size and degree of circumferential involvement predict the potential for a successful transanal excision. The local excision is performed in a full-thickness manner.

Transanal endoscopic microsurgery can be done with success and low complication rates.[161–163] Whichever method is selected, the full-thickness excision must have at least 1-cm margins of normal tissue surrounding the tumor. An inadequate margin is a predictor of failure.[164] Piecemeal submucosal excision is not considered adequate surgical treatment of invasive rectal cancer. Fragmentation of the tumor is associated with an increased incidence of local recurrence.[165] If the lesion cannot be adequately resected by local excision, then a more standard surgical approach should be used. In a curative case, the patient should be counseled to consider local excision as a form of definitive biopsy, especially when transmural penetration or adverse histologic characteristics are found in the local excision specimen. In a retrospective review of 155 patients it was found that disease-free survival was 94.1% for the group undergoing immediate surgery for adverse findings after local excision, compared to 55% for the delayed salvage group.[165]

The criteria used to select patients for local excision are intended to make a negative-margin, full-thickness local excision technically feasible and to ensure a low risk of lymph node metastasis (Table 42.12). The most useful test in this regard has been found to be endorectal ultrasound.[166] Factors that can help identify patients who are at low risk for lymphatic metastasis include small tumors, absence of lymphatic and vascular invasion, well- or moderately differentiated tumor, and absence of clinical or radiologic evidence of enlarged lymph nodes. The assumed low risk in patients treated with local excision alone is accepted because such procedures do not involve resection of the mesorectal lymph nodes.

TABLE 42.11. Local excision without adjuvant radiotherapy.

	N	*Local recurrence*
Mellgren et al.[333]	108	28%
Balani et al.[334]	20	0%
Garcia-Aguilar et al.[335]	82	24%
Paty et al.[280]	97	17%

TABLE 42.12. Indications for the local excision of rectal cancer.

Tumor less than 3 cm in greatest dimension.
Invades only the submucosa or superficial muscularis.
Favorable pathologic grade.

Source: From Nivatvongs and Wolff,[336] by permission of *World Journal of Surgery*.

The major factor predicting patient survival and perirectal lymph node metastasis is the depth of penetration of the primary tumor. In 1966, Morson[167] reported that lymphatic metastasis arose from 10% of tumors confined to the submucosa, 12% of tumors invading the muscularis propria, and 58% of tumors extending beyond the bowel wall. In a study of tumors treated by radical resection, the incidence of lymphatic metastasis was 12% for T1 tumors and 22% for T2 tumors.[168]

The incidence of lymph node metastasis in patients with T1 tumors approximates the recurrence rate for T1 cancers treated by local excision alone. Studies describe a 3% to 10% rate of local recurrence after excision alone.[169] Survival rates in patients with T1 rectal carcinomas treated with local excision alone or radical resection are 90% to 100%.[170] Local excision alone is a reasonable treatment for T1 carcinoma of the rectum if the tumor meets the previous selection criteria. A caveat is that blood vessel or lymphatic invasion is a significant predictor of lymph node involvement and poor survival. In such cases, either a standard surgical therapy involving total mesorectal excision or, if the patient refuses or cannot tolerate standard surgical therapy, the use of adjuvant therapy after local excision should be considered.

In patients with T2 rectal carcinomas, the risk of lymph node metastasis is 10% to 30%.[167,168] Recurrence rates range from 17% to 24% in patients with T2 tumors. Survival rates are 78% to 82% with excision alone.

Many studies, mostly retrospective and single-institution, have examined the results of local excision alone in the management of T1/T2 rectal cancer. Graham et al.[169] found the combined local recurrence rate for T1 lesions to be 5% (range, 0%–12%) and for T2 lesions, 18% (range, 8%–27%). The clinically significant rate of local recurrence, especially compared with lower rates of local recurrence in historical series of similar patients treated with APR (0%–10%),[170–172] has driven multiple studies examining the use of both postoperative radiotherapy and postoperative chemoradiation after local excision in selected patients.

In one of the first series with an adequately long follow-up, Bailey et al.[173] reported their experience with local excision between 1978 and 1988. Of the 65 study patients, 34 (54%) received postoperative radiotherapy, and 2 of those (5.9%) had local recurrences. The crude 5-year survival rate in this series was 74.3% and the 5-year disease-specific survival rate was 90.3%. This study provided some of the first indirect evidence regarding the long-term efficacy of adjuvant radiotherapy.

In a similar report from the Massachusetts General and Emory University Hospitals, 52 patients were treated with local excision alone while 47 patients were given postoperative adjuvant radiotherapy.[174] Although the patients chosen to receive postoperative radiotherapy were at higher risk of local failure because they had higher-stage lesions than the patients treated with local excision alone (70% T2 versus 15% T2, respectively), 5-year local recurrence-free survival (LRFS) and disease-free survival (DFS) rates were significantly better in the patients who received adjuvant therapy (LRFS, 10% versus 28%; DFS, 74% versus 66%). The authors concluded that adjuvant chemoradiation should be offered to all T2 patients undergoing local excision as well as all T1 patients with high-risk histologic features (advanced grade or lymphatic/vascular invasion).

A prospective series from The University of Texas M.D. Anderson Cancer Center reported excellent local control rates for 46 patients treated with local excision and postoperative chemotherapy or radiation therapy.[175] T3 tumors were also treated in this way in patients who were medically compromised or refused standard therapy. All patients underwent negative-margin, full-thickness excisions. The overall survival rate at 3 years was 93%. Table 42.13 shows the pattern of treatment failure by the American Joint Committee on Cancer (AJCC) T stage. Local recurrence-free survival at 3 years was 90%. None of the patients with T1 tumors demonstrated treatment failure. An update of the M.D. Anderson Cancer Center experience with local excision seems to support these findings, with 4-year LRFS rates of 9%, 80%, and 73% for T1, T2, and T3 tumors, respectively.[164]

Perhaps the best data regarding the modern-day approach to local excision for T1/T2 rectal cancer come from the initial results of a Cancer and Leukemia Group (CALG) prospective Phase II trial.[176] This study enrolled patients who met the usual criteria for the local excision of distant rectal cancer: mobile tumors confirmed up to the rectal wall (T1/T2), less than 4 cm in size, less than 40% of the bowel wall circumference in size, and with no evidence of lymph node involvement. Patients were registered after a negative-margin, full-thickness local excision. Patients with T1 tumors received no further treatment whereas patients with T2 tumors received adjuvant chemoradiation therapy.

A total of 110 eligible patients completed the study protocol, 59 with T1 tumors and 51 with T2 tumors. The 6-year overall disease-free survival rates were 85% and 78%. Overall, 9 patients (2 with T1 tumors, 7 with T2 tumors) had local recurrence of disease, and 4 of them died of the disease.

Table 42.14 shows the timing of local recurrence in selected large series of patients who did or did not receive postoperative radiotherapy. As the data suggest, postoperative radiotherapy seems to result in a shift toward later local failure when compared with local excision alone. In the combined experience of Massachusetts General and Emory University Hospitals, the median time to local recurrence was 13.5 months for patients treated with local excision alone and 55 months for patients treated with postoperative radiotherapy.[174]

TABLE 42.13. Patterns of failure by AJCC T stage of disease after local excision and adjuvant therapy.

	T1 (n = 16)	*T2 (n = 15)*	*T3 (n = 15)*	*Total (n = 46)*
Local recurrence only	0	0	2	2 (4%)
Distant recurrence only	0	0	4	4 (7%)
Combined recurrence	0	1	1	2 (4%)

Source: From Ota et al.,[175] by permission of *Surgical Clinics of North America*.

TABLE 42.14. Patterns of local recurrence (LR) following local excision with and without the use of postoperative radiotherapy.

Series	*N*	*LR (n)*	*LR (n) more than 2 years postoperative*
Local excision alone:			
Chakravarti et al.[174]	52	10	2 (20%)
Bailey et al.[173]	28	2	1 (50%)
Willett et al.[337]	40	6	1 (17%)
Biggers et al.[338]	141	36	4 (11%)
Local excision + postoperative radiotherapy:			
Chakravarti et al.[174]	47	8	6 (75%)
Bailey et al.[173]	34	2	1 (50%)
Willett et al.[337]	26	4	2 (50%)

Results of attempted surgical salvage in patients with local recurrence after local excision (with or without adjuvant therapy) are summarized in Table 42.15. In these combined series comprising 493 patients, 73 patients suffered local failure either alone or in combination with distant disease. In 44 (60%) of these patients, a potentially curative, margin-negative salvage procedure had been performed, most often by APR. Of these 44 patients, 21 (48%) had no evidence of disease at varying lengths of follow-up. Salvage seems to be possible in more than half of patients with isolated local failure after local excision; however, more than 50% of those patients will eventually die of their disease. Therefore, it appears that the argument for a liberal approach to selecting patients for local excision based on good salvage potential in patients whose disease recurs is not supported by the literature.

Baron et al.[177] examined the issue of salvage after local excision at the Memorial Sloan-Kettering Cancer Center. They compared the outcome in 21 patients who had undergone local excision followed by immediate APR or low anterior resection (LAR) for tumors with adverse histologic features with the outcome in 21 patients who underwent local excision followed by LAR or APR at the time of clinical local recurrence. Disease-free survival was significantly improved in the patients undergoing immediate LAR or APR (94.1% versus 55.5%; P less than 0.05), a finding that again emphasizes that salvage after local excision does not seem to be an optimal strategy.

Alternative forms of local therapy for T1 and T2 rectal cancer have been reported, including endocavitary irradiation, fulguration, cryosurgery, and Nd:YAG laser therapy.[178] Of these modalities, endocavity irradiation has received the most attention. In Papillon's[179] initial experience with this technique in 1972, the local recurrence rate was 7% and the 5-year overall survival rate was 72% among a selected low-risk group of patients. The potential advantage of endocavitary irradiation over external-beam radiotherapy is the ability to deliver a higher dose of radiation in a more concentrated fashion to the tumor. Both Papillon and others have subse-

TABLE 42.15. Surgical salvage of locoregional recurrence following local excision of T1/T2 rectal carcinoma.

Series	*N*	*LR (n)*[a]	*Salvaged (n)*[b]	*Salvage procedure*	*Outcome*
Chakravarti et al.[174]	99	18	10 (56%)	9 APR 1, exenteration	5, DOD 3, DOC 2, NED
Wong et al.[245]	25	6	5 (83%)	4, APR 1, exenteration	3, DOD 2, NED
Steele et al.[176]	59 (T1)	3	2 (67%)	All APR	1, DOD 1, NED
	51 (T2)	7	7 (100%)	All APR	3, DOD 4, NED
Bailey et al.[173]	53	4	3 (75%)	2, APR 1, LE	1, DOD 2, NED
Bleday et al.[339c]	48	4	3 (75%)	All APR	1, DOD 1, AWD 1, NED
Valentini et al.[340]	21	3	2 (67%)	All APR	1, DOD 1, NED
Taylor et al.[341]	47	17	7 (50%)	5, APR 2, LE	3, DOD 1, AWD 3, NED
Bouvet et al.[164]	90	11	5 (45%)	All APR	5, NED

APR, abdominoperineal resection; LE, local excision; DOD, dead of disease; DOC, dead of other causes; AWD, alive with disease; NED, no evidence of disease.

[a] Local recurrences alone and combined with distant recurrences.

[b] Number of potentially curative (margin-negative) salvage procedures.

[c] Five patients had T3 tumors.

quently reported similar results, again among highly selected low-risk patients.[180–182] Birnbaum et al.[183] identified "ideal" characteristics of rectal lesions for treatment by combination endocavitary and external beam irradiation (Table 42.16). Among 72 patients, they found that recurrence was significantly less likely in those patients with "ideal" tumors than in those with nonideal tumors (15% versus 48%,;$P = 0.01$). These authors stressed the importance of careful clinical and endorectal ultrasound staging to identify patients ideally suited to this treatment approach.

Transanal endoscopic microsurgery (TEM), in which either submucosal excision (for adenomas) or full-thickness excision (for invasive carcinomas) is performed through an operating rectoscope, has recently emerged as an option for the local treatment of rectal cancer.[184,185] In a recent series, local recurrence occurred in 2 of 16 patients (12.5%) with T1 lesions undergoing TEM.[184] However, the authors of this series thought that TEM alone was not appropriate treatment for T2 lesions.

TABLE 42.16. Ideal characteristic of rectal cancer lesions for combination endocavitary and external-beam radiation.

- Well or moderately differentiated
- Mobile
- Not ulcerated
- Less than 3 cm in diameter
- Less than 12 cm from the anal verge

Source: From Birnbaum et al.,[183] by permission of *Diseases of the Colon andRectum*.

Despretz et al.[186] reported results in 25 patients with rectal cancer treated with preoperative external radiation therapy (35 Gy) followed by local excision and brachytherapy. Local recurrence developed in 5 of the 25 patients. Mohiuddin et al.[187] reported results in 14 patients who underwent preoperative radiation (45 Gy) followed by a full-thickness excision; local recurrence developed in 3 patients. The preoperative use of chemotherapy and radiation therapy to downstage the disease and permit a more satisfactory local excision may be feasible.[188] In a series of 10 patients with T2/T3 primary tumors, such an approach demonstrated an absence of local recurrence and a 78% 2 year survival.[189]

Pretreatment Locoregional Staging for Rectal Cancer

Two factors can make pretreatment locoregional staging important in the evaluation of patients with resectable rectal cancer. First is the use of local excision, which could be considered in tumors confined to the bowel wall. Second, and much more common, is the use of preoperative radiation or chemoradiation, which is used in tumors considered to be high risk. This approach has been favored in decision analysis.[190] These are usually tumors that are transmural or those with evidence of metastatic perirectal lymph nodes.

The modalities used for determining the depth of penetration of the primary tumor and enlargement of perirectal lymph nodes are CT, magnetic resonance imaging (MRI), and endorectal ultrasound (EUS) Digital rectal exam (DRE) has been estimated to be a poor selector of patients for preoperative treatment.[191] Table 42.17 shows the accuracy of EUS,

Table 42.17. Accuracy of locoregional staging for rectal cancer.

		EUS, %		*MRI, %*		*CT, %*	
	DRE, %	*T*	*N*	*T*	*N*	*T*	*N*
Harewood et al.[166]		91	82			71	76
Brown et al.[191]	40	48		88			
Panzironi et al.[342]		100	72	92	76	75	88
Shami et al.[343]		89	85			45	68
Mathur et al.[344]				76		41	
Fuchsjager et al.[345]		64	70	64	62		
Nesbakken et al.[346]		74	65				
Marusch et al.[347]		63					
Tobaruela et al.[348]		72					
Gagliardi et al.[349]				86	69		
Kim et al.[350]		81	64				
Garcia-Aguilar et al.[351]		69	64				
Gualdi et al.[352]		77		84			
Beets-Tan et al.[353]				83			
Hunerbein et al.[354]		86	86				
Chiesura-Corona et al.[355]						82	79
Civelli et al.[356]						86	73
Akasu et al.[357]		96	72				

DRE, digital rectal examination; EUS, endorectal ultrasound; MRI, magnetic resonance imaging; CT, computed tomography.

MRI, and CT for the T and N staging of rectal cancer preoperatively. Overall, it appears EUS is the most accurate way to stage the depth of penetration.

MRI has been shown to predict the potential for a positive circumferential margin better than DRE or EUS.[191] In a treatment algorithm where preoperative treatment was used for those with deep mesorectal invasion or extension of the mesorectal fascia, MRI was the dominant strategy over DRE or EUS in terms of cost-effectiveness.[191] In another study of cost-effectiveness, a strategy of CT and EUS dominated CT- and MRI-only approaches when the demonstration of transmural rectal cancer was the prompt for preoperative radiotherapy.[192]

In the staging of patients after neoadjuvant therapy, the dominant component of the lesion seen on EUS is fibrosis. Thus, the technique really stages the extent of fibrosis and not the true residual tumor, which may be microscopic only.[193] Overall accuracy for pathologic T stage may drop to 48% in preoperatively treated patients who are restaged with EUS. From these data, it appears that EUS is unreliable in evaluating the degree of residual disease after neoadjuvant therapy.[194] CT and MRI suffer from similar limitations in the restaging of irradiated rectal cancers.[195,196]

When PET scanning is used to stage primary rectal cancer, in a preoperative study where EUS or MRI/CT was also used, 78% of cases had no change in management and in an additional 4% there were changes in treatment independent of the PET results. The management changes appear to result chiefly from the detection or confirmation of metastatic disease.[51] After neoadjuvant chemoradiation, PET has been used to identify tumor response.[197] In a preoperative study of restaging with PET scanning, the degree of rectal cancer response was not able to be differentiated between macroscopic residual disease versus microscopic residual disease after chemoradiation.[198] A prospective study of PET restaging in 15 resectable high-risk rectal cancer patients found that visual assessment of the response in PET correlated with pathologic response in 60% of cases.[199] Lymph node staging by PET scanning appears to be limited even before changes induced by chemoradiation with a sensitivity of 22% to 29%.[52]

Locoregional Resection for Rectal Cancer

Patients with stage II or III rectal cancer have tumors that are large and biologically aggressive. Disease at this stage carries a higher risk of local and systemic recurrence after surgical treatment. Accordingly, strategies have been developed to address these issues through locoregional resection and multimodality therapy.[200] However, adequate surgical resection and choice of technique are the most critical treatment factors determining patient outcome.[201,202]

The risk of spread to local lymph nodes and the risk of local recurrence increase as tumor penetration of the rectal wall increases. This understanding has led to the development of operations such as the APR that achieve tumor-free proximal and distal tissue margins and remove the upward pathways of lymphatic spread from rectal cancer.[203] The distal margin has been shown to be adequate when it is 2 cm from the edge of the tumor in unirradiated patients.[204,205] However, more recently the work of Quirke and others has dramatically demonstrated the importance of lateral tumor spread in the local recurrence of resected rectal cancers.[206,207]

Among patients with local recurrence, tumor involvement at the circumferential margin of resection has been found in 85% of cases.[206] Because of problems in obtaining adequate exposure in the low pelvis and surrounding structures, circumferential margins around rectal cancers can be highly variable and minimal. In this regard, surgeon experience and surgical technique play key roles in the prevention

TABLE 42.18. Importance of distal mesorectal spread in producing an involved radial margin.

Curative resection specimens (n = 20)	*Distal mesorectal spread*	*Involvement of radial margin*
16	Negative	2 (13%)
4	Positive	2 (50%)

Source: From Adam et al.,[207] by permission of *Lancet*.

of local recurrence.[208] Involvement of the circumferential margins can result from direct spread, mesenteric implants, vascular or lymphatic invasion, or cancer-bearing lymph nodes.[209] Tumor involvement of the circumferential margins of resection is frequently due to spread in the mesorectum distal to the tumor (Table 42.18).[207] The long-term outcome is poor in the presence of a positive circumferential margin.[207] Total mesorectal excision has been demonstrated to be effective in the surgical management of rectal cancer.[210]

McAnena and coworkers described the long-term outcome of 57 patients treated by this approach.[210] The mean follow-up was 4.8 years. Local recurrence was seen in only 3.5% of the patients, and overall 5-year survival rate was 81%. It should also be noted that "serious" postoperative complications occurred in 17% of patients. This effect of the adaptation of total mesorectal excision on complication rates has been confirmed by others.[211] In a subsequent larger review of their experience with total mesorectal excision for rectal cancer, MacFarlane and colleagues[212] studied 135 patients with Dukes' B and C rectal cancers who were treated with surgery only, by one surgeon over a 13-year period with a mean follow-up of 7.5 years. None of these patients received adjuvant radiation or chemotherapy, yet there was only a 5% local recurrence rate. Further long-term follow-up of a larger group of patients confirmed these findings by finding a 10-year local recurrence rate of 4% and a 10-year disease-free survival rate of 78%.[213] These results compare favorably with the results from the North Central Cancer Treatment Group study that form the basis for current recommendations for adjuvant therapy in the United States.[214]

In North America, similar results have been obtained with high rates of local recurrence-free survival when a total mesorectal excision is done by meticulous sharp dissection along the pelvic sidewalls. Enker's report[215] on this subject called for full rectal mobilization along anatomic planes to obtain complete mesorectal excision. In a series of 42 men who underwent sphincter-preserving surgery for low rectal cancer with this technique, only 1 had local recurrence (median follow-up, 20 months). Moreover, potency was preserved in 88% of the patients.

Wide pelvic lymphadenectomy has been proposed for the treatment of rectal cancer. Although there is little doubt that the presence of metastasis in such lymph nodes is a highly significant negative prognostic factor, there is no evidence to support a therapeutic benefit of the routine addition of extensive lymphadenectomy to standard locoregional procedures.[216–218]

To address the effect of training and experience in rectal cancer surgery in a region of Sweden where all rectal cancer surgery has been concentrated in one colorectal unit, survival seems to have improved and local recurrence rates have dropped.[219] Over the past 5 years, several studies have suggested that the surgeon's experience is an important prognostic factor in rectal cancer. In a population-based study of 683 patients, Porter and colleagues[220] found a significant local recurrence and survival advantage among the patients of surgeons with colorectal surgery fellowship training or surgeons with a higher caseload. In addition, a greater rate of sphincter preservation for low rectal cancer was also found to be associated with these surgeon groups. Other studies suggest that hospital volume, hospital type (university versus community), and surgeon experience influence survival and recurrence outcomes.[221–223]

In general, three operative procedures can be performed for resectable rectal cancer, all of which conform to the principles of total mesorectal excision: LAR, APR, and total proctectomy with coloanal anastamosis (CAA).[157,160,224]

Low anterior resection involves the transabdominal resection of the rectum and mesorectum above the level of the levator ani complex. After complete mobilization of the rectum *en bloc* with the mesorectum, the rectum is divided at least 2 cm below the distal edge of the tumor. There is evidence that total mesorectal excision is not required for upper rectal cancers.[225] Reconstruction of the rectum is then carried out between the completely mobilized left colon and the remaining rectal stump. The double-stapled technique has permitted an easier and lower anastomosis, with leak rates (clinical or radiographic) similar to or better than those obtained with hand-sewn techniques.[226–228] Second, although 5 cm was previously thought to be the minimum acceptable distal margin, acceptance of a 2-cm distal margin has allowed lower tumors to be resected by LAR.[155,205]

Abdominoperineal resection involves a combined transabdominal and perineal approach to complete resection of the rectum, mesorectum, levator muscles, and anus with formation of a permanent colostomy. The rectum and mesorectum are mobilized via an abdominal approach. A perineal approach is used to widely resect the levator complex and anus along with an appropriate margin of perianal skin. A permanent end colostomy is carried out. As sphincter preservation has increased, the overall proportion of rectal cancer patients undergoing APR has decreased.[219]

Proctectomy with CAA has emerged as a well-accepted surgical option in carefully selected patients. This approach can spare patients a permanent colostomy while still producing good functional and cancer-related outcomes. A recent review of 117 patients from the Mayo and Cleveland Clinics provides a perspective on the utility of proctectomy and CAA for patients with low rectal cancer.[229] The patients were treated over a 10-year period (1981–1991). The median distance of the tumor from the anal verge was 6 to 7 cm. The technique that was used required complete mobilization of the rectum to the levators, transanal transaction of the rectum, complete mobilization of the left colon, and endanal anastomosis. The authors recommended loop ileostomy for most patients. The effectiveness of this procedure in preventing local recurrence was demonstrated by the low local recurrence rate of 7%. Fecal continence was satisfactory in 78% of the cases. There were no surgery-related deaths. Early and late complications were related mainly to the anastomosis leaking (10%) and healing with a stricture (21%).

Several groups have reported on patients who had a 6- to 10-cm colonic J-pouch reservoir constructed with no additional risk or compromise of the anastomosis.[230] The formation of the colon pouch has been compared with the straight CAA in randomized clinical trials.[231] Physiologic measures and short-term outcomes seem to be improved with the pouch, although these findings are disputed by some.[232,233] However, these differences in function may disappear with time.

Major long-term postoperative problems after CAA are related to rectal capacitance and compliance and manifest as urgency and frequency of bowel movements. In a series from the Mayo Clinic described by Drake and colleagues,[234] patients who had a CAA for malignancies had a stool frequency of 2.6 per 24 hours, and only 1 of 19 patients was incontinent. Results from the Mayo and Cleveland Clinics Study are similar to those of others describing proctectomy and CAA for rectal cancer.[235] Even when combined with preoperative irradiation, coloanal anastomosis can result in good to excellent bowel function in 77% of patients. The median number of bowel movements per day was 2 in a Phase I/II trial.[236]

In a randomized clinical trial by the Gastrointestinal Tumor Study Group intended to examine the benefit of adjuvant therapy in rectal cancer, patients who underwent APR had a higher recurrence rate than did patients undergoing LAR (P less than 0.05),[237] and this has been seen in other studies.[238] However, this probably reflected the presence of larger, more-advanced tumors in the patients undergoing APR. Several other studies involving large numbers of rectal cancer patients have shown no significant differences in local recurrence or survival rates between patients undergoing APR and those undergoing sphincter preservation.[239–242] In summary, there is no evidence that, in appropriately selected patients, sphincter-preserving locoregional procedures compromise oncologic outcome.

Adjuvant Radiation and Chemoradiation for Resectable Rectal Cancer

The first adjuvant therapy in rectal cancer to be assessed for efficacy was postoperative radiotherapy. Both the Gastrointestinal Tumor Study Group and the National Adjuvant Breast and Bowel Project performed randomized clinical trials and found decreased local recurrence rates, but not improved survival, in stage II and III rectal cancer patients receiving postoperative radiotherapy compared with patients undergoing surgery alone.[204,237]

The addition of chemotherapy to postoperative radiotherapy seemed logical in an effort to influence the development of systemic disease and increase the therapeutic effect of radiation. A study conducted by the North Central Cancer Treatment Group was reported in 1991 by Krook and colleagues. This large, randomized trial for high-risk (stage II and III) rectal cancer patients compared postoperative fluorouracil and radiation with postoperative radiation alone.[214] Reduced local recurrence, systemic recurrence, and cancer-related death as well as improved overall survival were seen in patients randomly assigned to receive chemotherapy in addition to postoperative radiotherapy.

Another major step in adjuvant therapy for rectal cancer came from a report from an Intergroup trial testing the role of protracted or continuous intravenous infusion of fluorouracil combined with radiation therapy as postoperative therapy. The rationale for this protocol was based on in vitro studies indicating that optimal cytotoxicity was obtained by continuous exposure of tumor cells to fluorouracil after irradiation.[243] A study by Rich and coworkers[244] showed the regimen to be well tolerated during radiation therapy. In a trial of 680 patients, significant reductions were seen in overall rates of tumor relapse and distant metastasis.[245] Survival was significantly increased in those who received the protracted infusion of fluorouracil during irradiation. The National Institutes of Health Consensus Conference has recommended a standard approach widely used in North America for postoperative chemoradiation.[64]

Neoadjuvant Therapy

Although there have been many randomized clinical trials comparing preoperative radiation with surgery alone, most of these trials did not use radiotherapy dosing strategies currently considered appropriate.[246–248] Local recurrence seemed to be reproducibly reduced with preoperative radiotherapy compared to surgery alone.[249,250] However, more recently, the Swedish Rectal Cancer Study showed a significant improvement in local recurrence and survival with the use of a short course of radiotherapy versus surgery alone.[251] Notably, patients in this trial did not receive chemotherapy, and the delivery of radiotherapy (25 Gy, given over 5 days beginning 1 week preoperatively) differed substantially from the delivery strategy traditionally used in North America (45–50 Gy, given over 25–30 days beginning 4–6 weeks preoperatively). A French study that examined the issue of interval between completion of radiotherapy and surgery found that a longer period was beneficial in terms of response and sphincter preservation.[252]

In a meta-analysis of the results of 19 randomized trials of preoperative radiotherapy and 9 trials of postoperative radiation therapy by the Colorectal Cancer Collaborative Group, the absolute risks of any recurrence and local recurrence were reduced significantly by the use of radiotherapy either preoperatively or postoperatively. Trials of preoperative radiation therapy appeared to have a greater effect on the reduction of local recurrence at lower radiation doses than did postoperative radiation regimens. Early deaths for noncancer cases appeared to increase when radiation was carried out.[253] The effect of short-course preoperative radiation alone seen in the randomized Swedish Rectal Cancer Trial was to reduce local recurrence rates from 27% to 12% in the group receiving surgery and radiation[254]; this result indicated that this approach did not result in greater late-term morbidity.[255]

The improvement in local recurrence rate with preoperative short-course radiation therapy is still seen when modern rectal cancer surgery techniques of total mesorectal excision and quality control of the circumferential margin are carried out.[256] The randomized Dutch trial indicates that radiotherapy is helpful along with this technique.[257,258]

Minsky and colleagues[235] reported on the efficacy and toxicity of preoperative radiation with proctectomy and CAA for low rectal cancer in patients who otherwise would have required an APR. Twenty-two patients with a diagnosis of invasive resectable T2 or T3 primary adenocarcinoma of the distal rectum (median distance from anal verge, 4 cm) were treated. External-beam radiation therapy was given to a total dose of 50.4 Gy. Four to 5 weeks later, resection was performed in 21 of those 22 patients, and 10% of patients had a complete response. Therapy was well tolerated, and the anastomotic leak rate was only 6%. Eighty-nine percent had a good or excellent functional result. Local failure alone occurred in 5%. These data reveal acceptable local control, survival, and functional results in selected patients treated with preoperative radiation therapy and proctectomy with CAA as an alternative to APR. Outstanding sphincter-preserving results in the treatment of low rectal cancers after preoperative radiation have been described by Marks and coworkers[258a] at Thomas Jefferson University. They demonstrated long-term adequate sphincter function in 91% of patients, with local recurrence rates of less than 13%. The addition of preoperative endocavitary boost dose to low rectal cancers treated with external-beam radiation improved sphincter preservation rates over external-beam treatment alone.[259]

Prolonging the interval between radiation and surgery did not appear to significantly change the ability to do sphincter preservation in a randomized trial despite greater tumor response with a longer interval.[260] Similar results were seen when chemoradiation was used preoperatively.[261] Radiation alone has produced complete pathologic response rates of 10% to 17%.[247,248,262] Concurrent preoperative chemoradiation has produced complete response rates of 20% to 30%.[263] Among patients who had tumors less than 7 cm from the anal verge and who underwent preoperative chemoradiation, Janjan and coworkers[264] found a high rate of sphincter preservation in patients who had a complete response compared to those who did not (53% versus 38%).

However, the meaning of a pathologic complete response for a patient in long-term follow-up is unclear, although preliminary evidence suggests that it may be a prognostic factor for improved survival.[265] Moreover, the absence of mucosal tumor clearly does not assure a complete response because residual tumor may be found within or beyond the rectal wall or within lymph nodes in the absence of residual mucosal tumor.[263,265] Among 41 patients with partial or complete primary tumor response to preoperative chemoradiation, 9 (16%) were found to have metastatic disease in mesorectal lymph nodes.[265] In a larger series of patients, similar results were seen despite an overall decrease in the number of patients with positive mesorectal nodes.[266] Obviously, shrinking the tumor may allow achievement of acceptable negative margins and may facilitate sphincter preservation. In a review of 94 patients from a preoperative database where preoperative chemoradiation was given for low rectal cancers, distal margins of 1 cm or more did not compromise local control rates.[267] Although overall these effects tend to produce the ability to perform more sophisticated low rectal cancer operations that preserve sphincter function, they do not appear to support local excision in all but highly selected patients.[268,269]

Preoperative chemoradiation therapy has been demonstrated to be less toxic than postoperative chemoradiation.[270] Minsky et al. reported that when identical chemoradiation regiments were given preoperatively or postoperatively, significantly fewer patients experienced grade 3 or 4 toxic effects when the adjuvant treatment was given preoperatively. In this study,[270] 13% of patients treated preoperatively experienced gastrointestinal toxicity, whereas 48% of patients treated postoperatively had grade 3 or 5 gastrointestinal or genitourinary toxic effects.

The addition of chemotherapy to preoperative irradiation for rectal cancer was studied across two different institutions. In a multivariate analysis of 403 patients, the use of concomitant 5-FU resulted in an increase in sphincter preservation rates for patients with tumors less than 6 cm from the anal verge.[271] Similar to the results of an endocavitary boost with radiotherapy alone, the use of an external-beam boost dose to the tumor bed increased sphincter preservation for low rectal tumors.[272] Even among patients thought to require APR or initial assessment, up to 85% can be treated with sphincter preservation after such regimens.[273]

Rich and colleagues[274] reported on the outcome of 77 patients treated with preoperative chemoradiation therapy who then underwent resection of low rectal T3 cancers staged by ultrasonography.[274] The preoperative treatment given was continuous-infusion fluorouracil (300 mg/m^2/day) given with daily irradiation (45 Gy in 25 fractions over 5 weeks). Sphincter preservation was accomplished in 67% of these patients, in whom the mean distance of the tumor from the anal verge was 5 cm. A complete pathologic response was found in 29% and local recurrence in 4% of cases.

There are data comparing preoperative chemoradiation versus postoperative chemoradiation in resectable rectal cancer. This type of regimen given preoperatively can result in high sphincter preservation rates without compromising local recurrence rates, as previously mentioned. A preliminary report of the NSABP R-03 randomized trial of 5-fluorouracil and levocorin and 50.4 Gy given pre- or postoperatively indicated that sphincter preservation was increased from 33% to 50% in the preoperatively treated group. Complications of surgery were similar in both groups.[275] In a recently reported trial of a preoperative versus postoperative chemoradiation with continuous infusion 5-FU and standardized surgery with total mesorectal excision (TME), 628 patients with high risks (pT3/4 or N+) cancer were randomized. The trial showed postoperative complications were 12% to 13% in both arms. This result confirmed that neoadjuvant therapy did not carry a higher risk of perioperative morbidity.[276] In a later report of this trial with 825 patients randomized and with a median follow-up of 43 months, pelvic and distant recurrence rates were reduced in the preoperative treatment while overall survival rates were similar. Fewer patients were found to have anastomotic stenosis in the preoperative group whereas overall postoperative morbidity was equivalent between the two groups. In a subgroup of patients with low-lying tumors who were randomized, sphincter preservation rates were significantly increased to 39% in the preoperatively treated group, compared to 19% in the other group. This is a major step forward in confirming the value of preoperative conventional dose chemoradiation in the management of high-risk rectal cancer.[277]

If function is poor after sphincter-preserving surgery, then the patient's quality of life may be impaired more than if a permanent colostomy is present.[278] Kollmorgen and coworkers[279] studied the long-term effects of chemoradiation therapy on bowel function when this adjuvant therapy was given postoperatively. One hundred patients were studied after extensive exclusions were made to minimize confounding variables affecting outcomes. The group of patients who did not receive postoperative treatment uniformly had fewer problems with bowel function. In contrast, clustering of bowel movements, stool frequency, and fecal soiling were all increased when the reconstructed rectum was postoperatively irradiated (Table 42.19). As is clear from this study, long-term

TABLE 42.19. Long-term effect of postoperative chemoradiation therapy on bowel function in rectal cancer patients.

			Percent of patients			
Postoperative therapy	*Median bowel movement per day*	*Clustering of bowel movements*	*Fecal incontinence Occasional*	*Fecal incontinence Frequent*	*Urgency*
None	2	3%	7%	0%	19%
Chemoradiation	7	42%	39%	17%	17%

Source: From Kollmorgen et al.,[279] by permission of *Annals of Surgery*.

detrimental effects on bowel function can result from postoperative chemoradiation. Further support for this conclusion can be drawn from the results of a study by Paty and colleagues on the outcomes of CAA for rectal cancer.[280]

Sphincter preservation during multivisceral resections for locally advanced rectal cancer can be performed in patients who have involvement of adjacent pelvic organs. Selected patients may benefit from intraoperative radiation therapy or brachytherapy.[281]

Anal Cancer

Anal cancer is an uncommon malignancy in the digestive tract and will be found in about 4,000 patients each year.[282] Although a variety of histologic types of cancer can be located in the anal canal, the most common type is squamous cell carcinoma.[283,284] Basiloid and cloacogenic subtypes of anal cancer have the same survival and treatment responses as squamous cell cancer (SCC).[284,285] This discussion is limited to the treatment of invasive epidermoid or squamous cell cancer of the anal canal.

The lining of the upper anal canal is the anal transition zone and the lower portion is lined by the nonkeratinized anodermis.[286] The dentate line divides these. The lymphatic drainage above the dentate line is primarily to the perirectal and inferior mesenteric nodes and secondary to the internal iliac nodes. Below the dentate line the drainage is primarily to the inguinal lymph nodes and secondarily to the internal iliac nodes.[287]

Prognosis

The staging of anal cancer is based on tumor size and the presence of nodal and distant metastases.[288] Failures of therapy occur more commonly in T3 and T4 tumors than in T1 and T2 cases.[289,290] Multiple studies have identified positive inguinal or perirectal lymph nodes as a factor that predicts higher rates of cancer death, local failure, and the need for colostomy formation and salvage surgery.[291–293] Sentinel lymph node biopsy is feasible in these patients and may help to tailor radiation treatment fields.[294]

Surgery

In an analysis of local excision alone for small and superficially invasive cancers, Boman et al. found that it was successful in 12 of 13 patients so selected. However, in a larger group of patients treated by APR, the recurrence rate was 40% with survival of only 71%. This finding was probably due to the larger size of tumors selected for APR as a treatment along with the higher likelihood of nodal metastases in such patients. Even in patients undergoing APR, the predominant site of failure was still in the pelvis in 80%.[295] This failure pattern has been noted by others and is believed to be attributable to residual pelvic nodal disease after surgical approaches, with positive nodes being seen in surgical specimens in 30% to 60% of patients.[296]

Radiation Alone

Treatment with external-beam radiation alone can result in high rates of local control for early-stage tumors. When this approach was used for T1 and T2 cancers, local control rates were 100% but the doses were up to 67 Gy.[297] When radiation alone was delivered to doses of 60 to 62 Gy, the 5-year survival was noted to be 84% for T1 and T2 tumors but only 58% to 74% for T3 and T4 tumors. Although local control rates were 76%, the overall anal conservation rate was only 62% and normal anal function was maintained in only 55% of patients. The results are indicative of the local toxicity of high-dose external beam irradiation alone for SCC of the anus.[298] Total radiation dose was the factor that correlated best with late severe complications of radiation resulting in the need for colostomy formation.[289] In an additional series, primary radiation alone resulted in 5-year survivals of 57% with local recurrence rates of 14%.[299]

Definitive Treatment with Chemoradiation

The initial report of the potential success of definitive chemoradiation was from Nigro et al., who reported complete responses to a preoperative complete responses to a preoperative combination of 30 Gy external-beam radiotherapy and 5-fluorouracil and mitomycin-C in patients then treated with APR.[300] A later report by the same group revealed an even more limited role for surgery. Twenty-eight patients were given this combined chemoradiation treatment preoperatively and, of the 12 who underwent APR, 7 had no residual cancer in the specimen while 1 patient had only microscopic disease 4 to 6 weeks after completion of chemoradiation. The reliability of the clinical evaluation of the response to treatment was verified in 14 patients from this series who had a clinical complete response. They had excision of the scar, and none were found to have residual disease. Two additional patients with complete response on clinical examination were followed without biopsy and remained free of disease.[300]

Single-institution studies showed control of SCC of the anus was improved by the addition of chemotherapy; this was especially true for larger tumors with moderate doses of radiation. Sischy demonstrated a control rate of 89% for SCC of the anus in 29 patients with 5-FU and mitomycin-C.[301] Leichman et al. reported a complete response rate of 84% in patients treated with this regimen with no recurrence among these patients with a complete response.[302] Flam et al. reported even 5- and 10-year treatment with 41.4 Gy and 5-FU with mitomycin-C resulted in survival of 92% and 85%, respectively. Grade 3 or 4 late toxicity in this study was limited to 15% of patients, mainly in the form of chronic diarrhea. These excellent results were confirmed in T3–T4 and node-positive patients.[303] Local control rates of 84% with preservation of sphincter function in 80% of patients have been demonstrated with such regimens.[304]

A retrospective comparison of radiation therapy alone (using a brachytherapy boost) and chemoradiation for anal cancer failed to show a local control, survival, or sphincter preservation advantage to the combined approach.[305] However, in a much larger study of 191 patients treated according to sequential protocols of radiation, radiation with 5-FU and mitomycin-C, and radiation with 5-FU, it was found that radiation with both 5-FU and mitomycin-C was superior to the other approaches. The control with 5-FU and mitomycin-C was 86% versus 56% to 60% for the other regimens.[291] In a comparison of the quality of life in anal cancer survivors treated with or without chemotherapy, there did not appear to be a difference on long-term follow-up.[306]

The definitive advantage of chemoradiation over radiation alone has been demonstrated in two randomized prospective trials. In the UKCCCR trial involving 585 randomized patients, results were compared between radiation alone and radiation with 5-FU and mitomycin-C. The chief endpoint was local failure. Treatment with chemoradiation reduced local failure rates from 59% to 36%. The risk of death from anal cancer was also significantly reduced, but overall survival was not different in the groups.[307] In another trial with 110 randomized patients, the addition of 5-FU and mitomycin-C to 45 Gy radiation over 5 weeks with an external beam boost of 15 to 20 Gy was studied. In this EORTC study, the addition of chemotherapy increased complete remission rates to 80% from 54%. In this study, significant improvements in local control and colostomy-free survival were found for combined treatment.[308]

In a Phase III randomized trial, the role of mitomycin-C in addition to 5-FU during chemoradiation was studied in a cooperative group setting. Treatment groups were randomized to radiation and 5-FU or radiation with 5-FU and mitomycin-C. Patients who achieved less than a complete response 4 to 6 weeks after treatment underwent biopsy. If the biopsy revealed residual cancer, an additional 9 Gy radiation and cisplatin was given with concurrent 5-FU. Persistence of disease beyond 4 to 6 weeks after treatment was evaluated by biopsy and if confirmed was treated with APR. Patients receiving mitomycin-C had a higher rate of complete response with a corresponding increase in colostomy-free survival. The colostomy rate was lowered from 22% to 9% by the addition of the mitomycin-C. However, the group treated with mitomycin-C had a higher rate of complete response with a corresponding increase in colostomy-free survival. The colostomy rate was lowered from 22% to 9% by the addition of the mitomycin-C. However the group treated with mitomycin-C had a higher rate of grade 4 toxicity and two deaths due to neutropenic sepsis.[293] Because of concerns over this toxicity, the alternative use of cisplatin has been advocated. The use of 5-FU and cisplatin with radiation has been shown in a retrospective study of 92 patients to produce 5-year survival rates of 85% with colostomy-free survival rates of 82%; this was accomplished with few grade 4 toxicities and moderate (55 Gy) doses of radiation.[309] Others have demonstrated high complete response rates for this regimen when induction chemotherapy is used followed by chemoradiation with 5-FU and cisplatin. In a Phase II study of this approach, complete response rates of 93% were seen even in poor prognosis tumors.[310]

Management of Persistent or Recurrent Disease

In 8% to 10% of patients, there will be residual disease 4 to 6 weeks after the completion of initial therapy,[307] which may be a residual ulcer or a mass. Despite this, regression has been documented more than 3 to 12 months after therapy.[291] In addition to having concern over being misled by the biopsy of a regressing lesion, there can be concern over poor healing and fibrosis of the anal canal from biopsy in a heavily irradiated field. Excisional biopsy has been correlated with grade 4 long-term morbidity in irradiated patients.[311]

Most authors have defined persistent disease as the diagnosis of persistent tumor or recurrent tumor within the first 6 months after multimodality treatment. Recurrent disease has been considered the diagnosis of recurrent tumor at least 6 months after a complete clinical response. The largest series on salvage APR consist of 35 and 38 patients, respectively.[312,313] The prognosis after failure of primary chemoradiation therapy is dire. Table 42.20 illustrates the selected series that have been published after salvage APR for failure of primary treatment, mainly radiation combined with chemoradiation. The overall 5-year survival has been reported to be between 0% and 60%, and the overall recurrence rate is between 42% and 62%.[284,312–318]

After salvage APR, the major morbidity is related to the perineal wounds. Perineal wound problems, including infection and nonhealing wounds, have been reported to occur in at least 30% to 60% of the patients after salvage APR.[312,317] The use of musculocutaneous flaps offers tissue both to obliterate the pelvic defect and for vaginal reconstruction. Tei et al. reported on 14 patients who underwent vertical rectus abdominis musculocutaneous flap reconstruction to cover the perineal defect after salvage APR.[319]

Management of Lymph Node Metastasis

Studies of surgical lymphadenectomy alone can have local failure rates of 20% to 40%.[295,320] There are reports of a long-term disease-free interval in 60% of patients with inguinal lymph node metastasis managed by limited groin dissection following 45-Gy radiation therapy.[321] Others have reported control of clinically abnormal nodes in 71% of patients with high-dose radiation alone. In a review of 270 patients with inguinal lymph node metastases, treatment of synchronous metastases with irradiation and 5-FU with cisplatin resulted in a 5-year survival rate of 54%.[322]

Clinically evident metachronous lymph node metastases will be isolated treatment failures after radiation in approximately 8% of patients. Metachronous lymph node metastasis can be resected with a 5-year survival rate as high as 55%

TABLE 42.20. Results of salvage surgery for persistent or recurrent cancer.

Author	*Year*	*Prior therapy*	*No. of patients*	*Procedure*	*Overall recurrence (%)*	*Local recurrence (%)*	*Overall survival (%), 3 years*	*Overall survival (%), 5 years*
Longo[314]	1994	LE, LE + RT, LE + CRT	17	APR		NS		57
Ellenhorn[312]	1994	CRT	38	APR	61	66[a]	72[b]	44
Pocard[315]	1998	RT	21	APR	61	NS	29[c]	60[c] 0
Klas[284]	1999	CRT	13	APR			62[d]	
Allal[316]	1999	RT only, CRT	23/3	APR/LE	58	73[e]	44.5	
van der Wal[317]	2001	CRT	17 (13 "curative")	APR/PPE	62	100[f]	47	
Smith[318]	2001	CRT	22	APR		81	72	
Nilsson[313]	2002	RT only, CRT	35	APR	42	93	52	

CRT, chemoradiation; LE, local excision; APR, abdominoperineal resection; PPE, posterior pelvic exenteration; RT, radiotherapy; NS, not significant.

[a] Pelvis.

[b] Persistent disease.

[c] Recurrent disease.

[d] Alive and disease free, mean follow-up of 32 months.

[e] Local and regional.

[f] Five patients pelvis or groin and three patients pelvis and distant.

following lymphadenectomy.[323] The lymphadenectomy can be accompanied by significant morbidity in terms of wound problems related to seromas or infections.[324] In patients who have received no prior inguinal irradiation for initial therapy, a program of chemoradiation after inguinal dissection achieved a 5-year survival rate of 41%.[322] Ilioinguinal lymph node dissections can be carried out with a higher rate of morbidity from lymphedema, but again with some degree of success.[325]

References

1. Konishi F, Morson BC. Pathology of colorectal adenomas: a colonoscopic survey. J Clin Pathol 1982;35(8):830–841.
2. Winawer SJ, Zauber AG, O'Brien MJ, et al. Randomized comparison of surveillance intervals after colonoscopic removal of newly diagnosed adenomatous polyps. The National Polyp Study Workgroup. N Engl J Med 1993;328(13):901–906.
3. Morson BC, Konishi F. Contribution of the pathologist to the radiology and management of colorectal polyps. Gastrointest Radiol 1982;7(3):275–281.
4. Gillespie PE, Chambers TJ, Chan KW, Doronzo F, Morson BC, Williams CB. Colonic adenomas—a colonoscopy survey. Gut 1979;3:240–245.
5. Shirai M, Nakamura T, Matsuura A, Ito Y, Kobayashi S. Safer colonoscopic polypectomy with local submucosal injection of hypertonic saline-epinephrine solution. Am J Gastroenterol 1994;89(3):334–338.
6. Winawer SJ, Zauber AG, Ho MN, et al. Prevention of colorectal cancer by colonoscopic polypectomy. The National Polyp Study Workgroup. N Engl J Med 1993;329(27):1977–1981.
7. Waye JD, Lewis BS, Frankel A, Geller SA. Small colon polyps. Am J Gastroenterol 1988;83(2):120–122.
8. Binmoeller KF, Bohnacker S, Seifert H, Thonke F, Valdeyar H, Soehendra N. Endoscopic snare excision of "giant" colorectal polyps. Gastrointest Endosc 1996;43(3):183–188.
9. Cohen LB, Waye JD. Treatment of colonic polyps—practical considerations. Clin Gastroenterol 1986;15(2):359–376.
10. Pello MJ. Transanal excision of large sessile villous adenomas using an endorectal traction flap. Surg Gynecol Obstet 1987;164(3):280–282.
11. Fenoglio CM, Kaye GI, Lane N. Distribution of human colonic lymphatics in normal, hyperplastic, and adenomatous tissue. Its relationship to metastasis from small carcinomas in pedunculated adenomas, with two case reports. Gastroenterology 1973;64(1):51–66.
12. Cooper HS. Surgical pathology of endoscopically removed malignant polyps of the colon and rectum. Am J Surg Pathol 1983;7(7):613–623.
13. Bond JH. Polyp guideline: diagnosis, treatment, and surveillance for patients with colorectal polyps. Practice Parameters Committee of the American College of Gastroenterology. Am J Gastroenterol 2000;95(11):3053–3063.
14. Gordon MS, Cohen AM. Management of invasive carcinoma in pedunculated colorectal polyps. Oncology (Huntingt) 1989;3(7):99–104; discussion 104–105.
15. Fucini C, Wolff BG, Spencer RJ. An appraisal of endoscopic removal of malignant colonic polyps. Mayo Clin Proc 1986;61(2):123–126.
16. Williams CB, Whiteway JE, Jass JR. Practical aspects of endoscopic management of malignant polyps. Endoscopy 1987;19(suppl 1):31–37.
17. Lipper S, Kahn LB, Ackerman LV. The significance of microscopic invasive cancer in endoscopically removed polyps of the large bowel. A clinicopathologic study of 51 cases. Cancer (Phila) 1983;52(9):1691–1699.
18. Morson BC, Whiteway JE, Jones EA, Macrae FA, Williams CB. Histopathology and prognosis of malignant colorectal polyps treated by endoscopic polypectomy. Gut 1984;25(5):437–444.
19. Minsky BD, Mies C, Rich TA, Recht A, Chaffey JT. Potentially curative surgery of colon cancer: the influence of blood vessel invasion. J Clin Oncol 1988;6(1):119–127.
20. Minsky B, Mies C. The clinical significance of vascular invasion in colorectal cancer. Dis Colon Rectum 1989;32(9):794–803.
21. Shirouzu K, Isomoto H, Kakegawa T, Morimatsu M. A prospective clinicopathologic study of venous invasion in colorectal cancer. Am J Surg 1991;162(3):216–222.

22. Muller S, Chesner IM, Egan MJ, et al. Significance of venous and lymphatic invasion in malignant polyps of the colon and rectum. Gut 1989;30(10):1385–1391.
23. Haggitt RC, Glotzbach RE, Soffer EE, Wruble LD. Prognostic factors in colorectal carcinomas arising in adenomas: implications for lesions removed by endoscopic polypectomy. Gastroenterology 1985;89(2):328–336.
24. Netzer P, Forster C, Biral R, et al. Risk factor assessment of endoscopically removed malignant colorectal polyps. Gut 1998;43(5):669–674.
25. Wilcox GM, Beck JR. Early invasive cancer in adenomatous colonic polyps ("malignant polyps"). Evaluation of the therapeutic options by decision analysis. Gastroenterology 1987;92(5 pt 1):1159–1168.
26. Fitzgerald SD, Longo WE, Daniel GL, Vernava AM III. Advanced colorectal neoplasia in the high-risk elderly patient: is surgical resection justified? Dis Colon Rectum 1993;36(2):161–166.
27. Christie JP. Polypectomy or colectomy? Management of 106 consecutively encountered colorectal polyps. Am Surg 1988; 54(2):93–99.
28. Eckardt VF, Fuchs M, Kanzler G, Remmele W, Stienen U. Follow-up of patients with colonic polyps containing severe atypia and invasive carcinoma. Compliance, recurrence, and survival. Cancer (Phila) 1988;61(12):2552–2557.
29. Coutsoftides T, Sivak MV Jr, Benjamin SP, Jagelman D. Colonoscopy and the management of polyps containing invasive carcinoma. Ann Surg 1978;188(5):638–641.
30. Volk EE, Goldblum JR, Petras RE, Carey WD, Fazio VW. Management and outcome of patients with invasive carcinoma arising in colorectal polyps. Gastroenterology 1995;109(6):1801–1807.
31. Coverlizza S, Risio M, Ferrari A, Fenoglio-Preiser CM, Rossini FP. Colorectal adenomas containing invasive carcinoma. Pathologic assessment of lymph node metastatic potential. Cancer (Phila) 1989;64(9):1937–1947.
32. Greenburg AG, Saik RP, Coyle JJ, Peskin GW. Mortality and gastrointestinal surgery in the aged: elective vs. emergency procedures. Arch Surg 1981;116(6):788–791.
33. Limpert P, Longo WE, Kelemen PR, et al. Colon and rectal cancer in the elderly. High incidence of asymptomatic disease, less surgical emergencies, and a favorable short-term outcome. Crit Rev Oncol Hematol 2003;48(2):159–163.
34. Shatz BA, Weinstock LB, Swanson PE, Thyssen EP. Long-term safety of India ink tattoos in the colon. Gastrointest Endosc 1997;45(2):153–156.
35. Kuramoto S, Ihara O, Sakai S, Tsuchiya T, Oohara T. Intraoperative colonoscopy in the detection of nonpalpable colonic lesions: how to identify the affected bowel segment. Surg Endosc 1988;2(2):76–80.
36. Whitlow C, Gathright JB Jr, Hebert SJ, et al. Long-term survival after treatment of malignant colonic polyps. Dis Colon Rectum 1997;40(8):929–934.
37. Markowitz AJ, Winawer SJ. Management of colorectal polyps. CA Cancer J Clin 1997;47(2):93–112.
38. Scoggins CR, Meszoely IM, Blanke CD, Beauchamp RD, Leach SD. Nonoperative management of primary colorectal cancer in patients with stage IV disease. Ann Surg Oncol 1999;6(7):651–657.
39. Winawer SJ, Zauber AG, Gerdes H, et al. Risk of colorectal cancer in the families of patients with adenomatous polyps. National Polyp Study Workgroup. N Engl J Med 1996;334(2): 82–87.
40. Ekelund GR, Pihl B. Multiple carcinomas of the colon and rectum. Cancer (Phila) 1974;33(6):1630–1634.
41. Pagana TJ, Ledesma EJ, Mittelman A, Nava HR. The use of colonoscopy in the study of synchronous colorectal neoplasms. Cancer (Phila) 1984;53(2):356–359.
42. Askew A, Ward M, Cowen A. The influence of colonoscopy on the operative management of colorectal cancer. Med J Aust 1986;145(6):254–255.
43. Arenas RB, Fichera A, Mhoon D, Michelassi F. Incidence and therapeutic implications of synchronous colonic pathology in colorectal adenocarcinoma. Surgery (St. Louis) 1997;122(4):706–709; discussion 709–710.
44. Barrier A, Houry S, Huguier M. The appropriate use of colonoscopy in the curative management of colorectal cancer. Int J Colorectal Dis 1998;13(2):93–98.
45. Chapuis P, Kos S, Bokey L, Dent O, Newland R, Hinder J. How useful is pre-operative computerized tomography scanning in staging rectal cancer? Aust N Z J Surg 1989;59(1):31–34.
46. Isbister WH, al-Sanea O. The utility of pre-operative abdominal computerized tomography scanning in colorectal surgery. J R Coll Surg (Edinb) 1996;41(4):232–234.
47. Kronawitter U, Kemeny NE, Heelan R, Fata F, Fong Y. Evaluation of chest computed tomography in the staging of patients with potentially resectable liver metastases from colorectal carcinoma. Cancer (Phila) 1999;86(2):229–235.
48. Lewi H, Blumgart LH, Carter DC, et al. Pre-operative carcinoembryonic antigen and survival in patients with colorectal cancer. Br J Surg 1984;71(3):206–208.
49. Lunde OC, Havig O. Clinical significance of carcinoembryonic antigen (CEA) in patients with adenocarcinoma in colon and rectum. Acta Chir Scand 1982;148(2):189–193.
50. Wanebo HJ, Rao B, Pinsky CM, et al. Preoperative carcinoembryonic antigen level as a prognostic indicator in colorectal cancer. N Engl J Med 1978;299(9):448–451.
51. Wang WS, Lin JK, Chiou TJ, et al. Preoperative carcinoembryonic antigen level as an independent prognostic factor in colorectal cancer: Taiwan experience. Jpn J Clin Oncol 2000; 30(1):12–16.
52. Heriot AG, Hicks RJ, Drummond EG, et al. Does positron emission tomography change management in primary rectal cancer? A prospective assessment. Dis Colon Rectum 2004;47(4):451–458.
53. Abdel-Nabi H, Doerr RJ, Lamonica DM, et al. Staging of primary colorectal carcinomas with fluorine-18 fluorodeoxyglucose whole-body PET: correlation with histopathologic and CT findings. Radiology 1998;206(3):755–760.
54. Beart RW, Steele GD Jr, Menck HR, Chmiel JS, Ocwieja KE, Winchester DP. Management and survival of patients with adenocarcinoma of the colon and rectum: a national survey of the Commission on Cancer. J Am Coll Surg 1995;181(3):225–236.
55. Charnley RM, Morris DL, Dennison AR, Amar SS, Hardcastle JD. Detection of colorectal liver metastases using intraoperative ultrasonography. Br J Surg 1991;78(1):45–48.
56. Rafaelsen SR, Kronborg O, Larsen C, Fenger C. Intraoperative ultrasonography in detection of hepatic metastases from colorectal cancer. Dis Colon Rectum 1995;38(4):355–360.
57. Nelson H, Petrelli N, Carlin A, et al. Guidelines 2000 for colon and rectal cancer surgery. J Natl Cancer Inst 2001;93(8):583–596.
58. Bruch HP, Schwandner O, Schiedeck TH, Roblick UJ. Actual standards and controversies on operative technique and lymph-node dissection in colorectal cancer. Langenbecks Arch Surg 1999;384(2):167–175.
59. Fazio VW, Tjandra JJ. Primary therapy of carcinoma of the large bowel. World J Surg 1991;15(5):568–575.
60. Morikawa E, Yasutomi M, Shindou K, et al. Distribution of metastatic lymph nodes in colorectal cancer by the modified clearing method. Dis Colon Rectum 1994;37(3):219–223.
61. Devereux DF, Deckers PJ. Contributions of pathologic margins and Dukes' stage to local recurrence in colorectal carcinoma. Am J Surg 1985;149(3):323–326.
62. Tagliacozzo S, Tocchi A. Extended mesenteric excision in right hemicolectomy for carcinoma of the colon. Int J Colorectal Dis 1997;12(5):272–275.
63. Wu JS, Paul P, McGannon EA, Church JM. APC genotype, polyp number, and surgical options in familial adenomatous polyposis. Ann Surg 1998;227(1):57–62.

64. NIH Consensus Conference. Adjuvant therapy for patients with colon and rectal cancer. JAMA 1990;264(11):1444–1450.
65. Scott KW, Grace RH. Detection of lymph node metastases in colorectal carcinoma before and after fat clearance. Br J Surg 1989;76(11):1165–1167.
66. Enker WE, Laffer UT, Block GE. Enhanced survival of patients with colon and rectal cancer is based upon wide anatomic resection. Ann Surg 1979;190(3):350–360.
67. Toyota S, Ohta H, Anazawa S. Rationale for extent of lymph node dissection for right colon cancer. Dis Colon Rectum 1995; 38(7):705–711.
68. Malassagne B, Valleur P, Serra J, et al. Relationship of apical lymph node involvement to survival in resected colon carcinoma. Dis Colon Rectum 1993;36(7):645–653.
69. Slanetz CA Jr, Grimson R. Effect of high and intermediate ligation on survival and recurrence rates following curative resection of colorectal cancer. Dis Colon Rectum 1997;40(10): 1205–1218; discussion 1218–1219.
70. Rouffet F, Hay JM, Vacher B, et al. Curative resection for left colonic carcinoma: hemicolectomy vs. segmental colectomy. A prospective, controlled, multicenter trial. French Association for Surgical Research. Dis Colon Rectum 1994;37(7):651–659.
71. Laurie J, Moertel C, Flemming T, et al. Surgical adjuvant therapy of poor prognosis colorectal cancer with levamisole alone or combined levamisol and 5-fluorouracil: a North Central Cancer Treatment Group and Mayo Clinic Study. Proc Am Soc Clin Oncol 1986;5(81):81 (abstract).
72. Cohen AM, Tremiterra S, Candela F, Thaler HT, Sigurdson ER. Prognosis of node-positive colon cancer. Cancer (Phila) 1991; 67(7):1859–1861.
73. Brown HG, Luckasevic TM, Medich DS, Celebrezze JP, Jones SM. Efficacy of manual dissection of lymph nodes in colon cancer resections. Mod Pathol 2004;17(4):402–406.
74. Gall FP, Tonak J, Altendorf A. Multivisceral resections in colorectal cancer. Dis Colon Rectum 1987;30(5):337–341.
75. Taylor WE, Donohue JH, Gunderson LL, et al. The Mayo Clinic experience with multimodality treatment of locally advanced or recurrent colon cancer. Ann Surg Oncol 2002;9(2):177–185.
76. Sales JP, Wind P, Douard R, Cugnenc PH, Loric S. Blood dissemination of colonic epithelial cells during no-touch surgery for rectosigmoid cancer. Lancet 1999;354(9176):392.
77. Wiggers T, Jeekel J, Arends JW, et al. No-touch isolation technique in colon cancer: a controlled prospective trial. Br J Surg 1988;75(5):409–415.
78. Gordon NL, Dawson AA, Bennett B, Innes G, Eremin O, Jones PF. Outcome in colorectal adenocarcinoma: two seven-year studies of a population. BMJ 1993;307(6906):707–710.
79. Read TE, Mutch MG, Chang BW, et al. Locoregional recurrence and survival after curative resection of adenocarcinoma of the colon. J Am Coll Surg 2002;195(1):33–40.
80. Schrag D, Panageas KS, Riedel E, et al. Surgeon volume compared to hospital volume as a predictor of outcome following primary colon cancer resection. J Surg Oncol 2003;83(2):68–78; discussion 78–79.
81. Ota DM. Laparoscopic resection for colon cancer: a favorable view. Important Adv Oncol 1996:227–229.
82. Schwenk W, Bohm B, Witt C, Junghans T, Grundel K, Muller JM. Pulmonary function following laparoscopic or conventional colorectal resection: a randomized controlled evaluation. Arch Surg 1999;134(1):6–12; discussion 13.
83. Fleshman JW, Nelson H, Peters WR, et al. Early results of laparoscopic surgery for colorectal cancer. Retrospective analysis of 372 patients treated by Clinical Outcomes of Surgical Therapy (COST) Study Group. Dis Colon Rectum 1996;39(suppl 10): S53–S58.
84. Kockerling F, Reymond MA, Schneider C, et al. Prospective multicenter study of the quality of oncologic resections in patients undergoing laparoscopic colorectal surgery for cancer. The Laparoscopic Colorectal Surgery Study Group. Dis Colon Rectum 1998;41(8):963–970.
85. A comparison of laparoscopically assisted and open colectomy for colon cancer. N Engl J Med 2004;350(20):2050–2059.
86. Lacy AM, Garcia-Valdecasas JC, Delgado S, et al. Laparoscopy-assisted colectomy versus open colectomy for treatment of non-metastatic colon cancer: a randomised trial. Lancet 2002; 359(9325):2224–2229.
87. Huang PP, Weber TK, Mendoza C, Rodriguez-Bigas MA, Petrelli NJ. Long-term survival in patients with ovarian metastases from colorectal carcinoma. Ann Surg Oncol 1998;5(8):695–698.
88. Sielezneff I, Salle E, Antoine K, Thirion X, Brunet C, Sastre B. Simultaneous bilateral oophorectomy does not improve prognosis of postmenopausal women undergoing colorectal resection for cancer. Dis Colon Rectum 1997;40(11):1299–1302.
89. Nyam DC, Leong AF, Ho YH, Seow-Choen F. Comparison between segmental left and extended right colectomies for obstructing left-sided colonic carcinomas. Dis Colon Rectum 1996;39(9):1000–1003.
90. Young-Fadok TM, Wolff BG, Nivatvongs S, Metzger PP, Ilstrup DM. Prophylactic oophorectomy in colorectal carcinoma: preliminary results of a randomized, prospective trial. Dis Colon Rectum 1998;41(3):277–283; discussion 283–285.
91. Mulcahy HE, Toner M, Patchett SE, Daly L, O'Donoghue DP. Identifying stage B colorectal cancer patients at high risk of tumor recurrence and death. Dis Colon Rectum 1997;40(3): 326–331.
92. Joseph NE, Sigurdson ER, Hanlon AL, et al. Accuracy of determining nodal negativity in colorectal cancer on the basis of the number of nodes retrieved on resection. Ann Surg Oncol 2003; 10(3):213–218.
93. Tepper JE, O'Connell MJ, Niedzwiecki D, et al. Impact of number of nodes retrieved on outcome in patients with rectal cancer. J Clin Oncol 2001;19(1):157–163.
94. Mainprize KS, Kulacoglu H, Hewavisinthe J, Savage A, Mortensen N, Warren BF. How many lymph nodes to stage colorectal carcinoma? J Clin Pathol 1998;51(2):165–166.
95. Oberg A, Stenling R, Tavelin B, Lindmark G. Are lymph node micrometastases of any clinical significance in Dukes Stages A and B colorectal cancer? Dis Colon Rectum 1998;41(10): 1244–1249.
96. Yasuda K, Adachi Y, Shiraishi N, Yamaguchi K, Hirabayashi Y, Kitano S. Pattern of lymph node micrometastasis and prognosis of patients with colorectal cancer. Ann Surg Oncol 2001; 8(4):300–304.
97. Finan PJ, Ritchie JK, Hawley PR. Synchronous and "early" metachronous carcinomas of the colon and rectum. Br J Surg 1987;74(10):945–947.
98. Isler JT, Brown PC, Lewis FG, Billingham RP. The role of preoperative colonoscopy in colorectal cancer. Dis Colon Rectum 1987;30(6):435–439.
99. Tate JJ, Rawlinson J, Royle GT, Brunton FJ, Taylor I. Pre-operative or postoperative colonic examination for synchronous lesions in colorectal cancer. Br J Surg 1988;75(10):1016–1018.
100. Passman MA, Pommier RF, Vetto JT. Synchronous colon primaries have the same prognosis as solitary colon cancers. Dis Colon Rectum 1996;39(3):329–334.
101. Koperna T, Kisser M, Schulz F. Emergency surgery for colon cancer in the aged. Arch Surg 1997;132(9):1032–1037.
102. Poon RT, Law WL, Chu KW, Wong J. Emergency resection and primary anastomosis for left-sided obstructing colorectal carcinoma in the elderly. Br J Surg 1998;85(11):1539–1542.
103. Single-stage treatment for malignant left-sided colonic obstruction: a prospective randomized clinical trial comparing subtotal colectomy with segmental resection following intraoperative irrigation. The SCOTIA Study Group. Subtotal Colectomy versus On-table Irrigation and Anastomosis. Br J Surg 1995; 82(12):1622–1627.

104. Carraro PG, Segala M, Orlotti C, Tiberio G. Outcome of large-bowel perforation in patients with colorectal cancer. Dis Colon Rectum 1998;41(11):1421–1426.
105. Willett C, Tepper JE, Cohen A, Orlow E, Welch C. Obstructive and perforative colonic carcinoma: patterns of failure. J Clin Oncol 1985;3(3):379–384.
106. Estes NC, Giri S, Fabian C. Patterns of recurrence for advanced colon cancer modified by whole abdominal radiation and chemotherapy. Am Surg 1996;62(7):546–549; discussion 549–550.
107. Duttenhaver JR, Hoskins RB, Gunderson LL, Tepper JE. Adjuvant postoperative radiation therapy in the management of adenocarcinoma of the colon. Cancer (Phila) 1986;57(5):955–963.
108. Willett CG, Tepper JE, Skates SJ, Wood WC, Orlow EC, Duttenhaver JR. Adjuvant postoperative radiation therapy for colonic carcinoma. Ann Surg 1987;206(6):694–698.
109. Willett CG, Fung CY, Kaufman DS, Efird J, Shellito PC. Postoperative radiation therapy for high-risk colon carcinoma. J Clin Oncol 1993;11(6):1112–1117.
110. Amos EH, Mendenhall WM, McCarty PJ, et al. Postoperative radiotherapy for locally advanced colon cancer. Ann Surg Oncol 1996;3(5):431–436.
111. Willett CG, Goldberg S, Shellito PC, et al. Does postoperative irradiation play a role in the adjuvant therapy of stage T4 colon cancer? Cancer J Sci Am 1999;5(4):242–247.
112. Ben-Josef E, Court WS. Whole abdominal radiotherapy and concomitant 5-fluorouracil as adjuvant therapy in advanced colon cancer. Dis Colon Rectum 1995;38(10):1088–1092.
113. Fabian C, Giri S, Estes N, et al. Adjuvant continuous infusion 5-FU, whole-abdominal radiation, and tumor bed boost in high-risk stage III colon carcinoma: a Southwest Oncology Group Pilot study. Int J Radiat Oncol Biol Phys 1995;32(2):457–464.
114. Schild SE, Gunderson LL, Haddock MG, Wong WW, Nelson H. The treatment of locally advanced colon cancer. Int J Radiat Oncol Biol Phys 1997;37(1):51–58.
115. Pezner RD, Chu DZ, Wagman LD, Vora N, Wong JY, Shibata SI. Resection with external beam and intraoperative radiotherapy for recurrent colon cancer. Arch Surg 1999;134(1):63–67.
116. Midgley R, Kerr D. Colorectal cancer. Lancet 1999;353(9150):391–399.
117. Buyse M, Zeleniuch-Jacquotte A, Chalmers TC. Adjuvant therapy of colorectal cancer. Why we still don't know. JAMA 1988;259(24):3571–3578.
118. Wolmark N, Fisher B, Rockette H, et al. Postoperative adjuvant chemotherapy or BCG for colon cancer: results from NSABP protocol C-01. J Natl Cancer Inst 1988;80(1):30–36.
119. Saltz LB, Minsky B. Adjuvant therapy of cancers of the colon and rectum. Surg Clin N Am 2002;82(5):1035–1058.
120. Wolmark N, Rockette H, Fisher B, et al. The benefit of leucovorin-modulated fluorouracil as postoperative adjuvant therapy for primary colon cancer: results from National Surgical Adjuvant Breast and Bowel Project protocol C-03. J Clin Oncol 1993;11(10):1879–1887.
121. AbdAlla EE, Blair GE, Jones RA, Sue-Ling HM, Johnston D. Mechanism of synergy of levamisole and fluorouracil: induction of human leukocyte antigen class I in a colorectal cancer cell line. J Natl Cancer Inst 1995;87(7):489–496.
122. Laurie JA, Moertel CG, Fleming TR, et al. Surgical adjuvant therapy of large-bowel carcinoma: an evaluation of levamisole and the combination of levamisole and fluorouracil. The North Central Cancer Treatment Group and the Mayo Clinic. J Clin Oncol 1989;7(10):1447–1456.
123. Moertel CG, Fleming TR, Macdonald JS, et al. Levamisole and fluorouracil for adjuvant therapy of resected colon carcinoma. N Engl J Med 1990;322(6):352–358.
124. Moertel CG, Fleming TR, Macdonald JS, et al. Intergroup study of fluorouracil plus levamisole as adjuvant therapy for stage II/Dukes' B2 colon cancer. J Clin Oncol 1995;13(12):2936–2943.
125. Piedbois P. Survival benefit of 5-FU/LV over 5-FU bolus in patients with advanced colorectal cancer: an updated meta-analysis based on 2,751 patients. Proc Annu Meet Am Soc Clin Oncol 2003;22:a1180.
126. Efficacy of adjuvant fluorouracil and folinic acid in colon cancer. International Multicentre Pooled Analysis of Colon Cancer Trials (IMPACT) investigators. Lancet 1995;345(8955):939–944.
127. O'Connell MJ, Laurie JA, Kahn M, et al. Prospectively randomized trial of postoperative adjuvant chemotherapy in patients with high-risk colon cancer. J Clin Oncol 1998;16(1):295–300.
128. Wolmark N, Rockette H, Mamounas E, et al. Clinical trial to assess the relative efficacy of fluorouracil and leucovorin, fluorouracil and levamisole, and fluorouracil, leucovorin, and levamisole in patients with Dukes' B and C carcinoma of the colon: results from National Surgical Adjuvant Breast and Bowel Project C-04. J Clin Oncol 1999;17(11):3553–3559.
129. Haller D, Catalano P, Macdonald J. Fluorouracil (FU), leucovorin (LV), and levamisole (LeV) adjuvant therapy for colon cancer: 5-year final report of INT-0089. Proc Annu Meet Am Soc Clin Oncol 1998;17:a982.
130. Saltz LB, Cox JV, Blanke C, et al. Irinotecan plus fluorouracil and leucovorin for metastatic colorectal cancer. Irinotecan Study Group. N Engl J Med 28 2000;343(13):905–914.
131. Douillard JY, Cunningham D, Roth AD, et al. Irinotecan combined with fluorouracil compared with fluorouracil alone as first-line treatment for metastatic colorectal cancer: a multicentre randomised trial. Lancet 2000;355(9209):1041–1047.
132. de Gramont A, Bosset JF, Milan C, et al. Randomized trial comparing monthly low-dose leucovorin and fluorouracil bolus with bimonthly high-dose leucovorin and fluorouracil bolus plus continuous infusion for advanced colorectal cancer: a French intergroup study. J Clin Oncol 1997;15(2):808–815.
133. Pflzer U.S. Medical Information, Camptosar as adjuvant therapy in colorectal cancer, Sept. 8, 2003.
134. Degramont A, Banzi M, Navarro M. Oxaliplatin/5-FU/LV in adjuvant colon cancer: results of the international MOSAIC trial. Proc Annu Meet Am Soc Clin Oncol 2003;22:a1015.
135. Becouarn Y, Rougier P. Clinical efficacy of oxaliplatin monotherapy: phase II trials in advanced colorectal cancer. Semin Oncol 1998;25(2 suppl 5):23–31.
136. de Gramont A, Figer A, Seymour M, et al. Leucovorin and fluorouracil with or without oxaliplatin as first-line treatment in advanced colorectal cancer. J Clin Oncol 2000;18(16):2938–2947.
137. Becouarn Y, Gamelin E, Coudert B, et al. Randomized multicenter phase II study comparing a combination of fluorouracil and folinic acid and alternating irinotecan and oxaliplatin with oxaliplatin and irinotecan in fluorouracil-pretreated metastatic colorectal cancer patients. J Clin Oncol 15 2001;19(22):4195–4201.
138. Rothenberg ML, Oza AM, Bigelow RH, et al. Superiority of oxaliplatin and fluorouracil-leucovorin compared with either therapy alone in patients with progressive colorectal cancer after irinotecan and fluorouracil-leucovorin: interim results of a phase III trial. J Clin Oncol 2003;21(11):2059–2069.
139. Goldberg R, Morton R, Sargent D. N9741: oxaliplatin or CPT-11+5-FU/LV or oxaliplatin + CPT-11 in advanced colorectal cancer: updated efficacy and quality of life data from an Intergroup study. Proc Annu Meet Am Soc Clin Oncol 2003;22:a1009.
140. Gramont Ad, Banzi M, Navarro M. Oxaliplatin/5-FU/LV in adjuvant colon cancer: results of the international randomized phase III "MOSAIC" trial. Proc Annu Meet Am Soc Clin Oncol 2003;22:a1015.
141. Willett C, Tepper JE, Cohen A, Orlow E, Welch C, Donaldson G. Local failure following curative resection of colonic adenocarcinoma. Int J Radiat Oncol Biol Phys 1984;10(5):645–651.
142. Cascinu S, Georgoulias V, Kerr D, Maughan T, Labianca R, Ychou M. Colorectal cancer in the adjuvant setting: perspectives

on treatment and the role of prognostic factors. Ann Oncol 2003;14(suppl 2):ii25–ii29.
143. Watanabe T, Wu TT, Catalano PJ, et al. Molecular predictors of survival after adjuvant chemotherapy for colon cancer. N Engl J Med 2001;344(16):1196–1206.
144. Ogunbiyi OA, Goodfellow PJ, Herfarth K, et al. Confirmation that chromosome 18q allelic loss in colon cancer is a prognostic indicator. J Clin Oncol 1998;16(2):427–433.
145. Moertel CG, Fleming TR, Macdonald JS, et al. Fluorouracil plus levamisole as effective adjuvant therapy after resection of stage III colon carcinoma: a final report. Ann Intern Med 1995;122(5):321–326.
146. Efficacy of adjuvant fluorouracil and folinic acid in B2 colon cancer. International Multicentre Pooled Analysis of B2 Colon Cancer Trials (IMPACT B2) Investigators. J Clin Oncol 1999; 17(5):1356–1363.
147. Mamounas E, Wieand S, Wolmark N, et al. Comparative efficacy of adjuvant chemotherapy in patients with Dukes' B versus Dukes' C colon cancer: results from four National Surgical Adjuvant Breast and Bowel Project adjuvant studies (C-01, C-02, C-03, and C-04). J Clin Oncol 1999;17(5):1349–1355.
148. Gryfe R, Kim H, Hsieh ET, et al. Tumor microsatellite instability and clinical outcome in young patients with colorectal cancer. N Engl J Med 2000;342(2):69–77.
149. Lynch HT, Drouhard T, Vasen HF, et al. Genetic counseling in a Navajo hereditary nonpolyposis colorectal cancer kindred. Cancer (Phila) 1996;77(1):30–35.
150. Ribic CM, Sargent DJ, Moore MJ, et al. Tumor microsatellite-instability status as a predictor of benefit from fluorouracil-based adjuvant chemotherapy for colon cancer. N Engl J Med 2003;349(3):247–257.
151. Elsaleh H, Joseph D, Grieu F, Zeps N, Spry N, Iacopetta B. Association of tumour site and sex with survival benefit from adjuvant chemotherapy in colorectal cancer. Lancet 2000; 355(9217):1745–1750.
152. Compton CC, Fielding LP, Burgart LJ, et al. Prognostic factors in colorectal cancer. College of American Pathologists Consensus Statement 1999. Arch Pathol Lab Med 2000;124(7):979–994.
153. Lipshultz SE, Colan SD, Gelber RD, Perez-Atayde AR, Sallan SE, Sanders SP. Late cardiac effects of doxorubicin therapy for acute lymphoblastic leukemia in childhood. N Engl J Med 1991;324(12):808–815.
154. Tveit KM, Guldvog I, Hagen S, et al. Randomized controlled trial of postoperative radiotherapy and short-term time-scheduled 5-fluorouracil against surgery alone in the treatment of Dukes B and C rectal cancer. Norwegian Adjuvant Rectal Cancer Project Group. Br J Surg 1997;84(8):1130–1135.
155. Wolmark N, Wieand HS, Hyams DM, et al. Randomized trial of postoperative adjuvant chemotherapy with or without radiotherapy for carcinoma of the rectum: National Surgical Adjuvant Breast and Bowel Project Protocol R-02. J Natl Cancer Inst 2000; 92(5):388–396.
156. Olson RM, Perencevich NP, Malcolm AW, Chaffey JT, Wilson RE. Patterns of recurrence following curative resection of adenocarcinoma of the colon and rectum. Cancer (Phila) 1980; 45(12):2969–2974.
157. Dehni N, McFadden N, McNamara DA, Guiguet M, Tiret E, Parc R. Oncologic results following abdominoperineal resection for adenocarcinoma of the low rectum. Dis Colon Rectum 2003;46(7):867–874; discussion 874.
158. Tocchi A, Mazzoni G, Lepre L, et al. Total mesorectal excision and low rectal anastomosis for the treatment of rectal cancer and prevention of pelvic recurrences. Arch Surg 2001;136(2): 216–220.
159. Merchant NB, Guillem JG, Paty PB, et al. T3N0 rectal cancer: results following sharp mesorectal excision and no adjuvant therapy. J Gastrointest Surg 1999;3(6):642–647.
160. Nakagoe T, Ishikawa H, Sawai T, et al. Survival and recurrence after a sphincter-saving resection and abdominoperineal resection for adenocarcinoma of the rectum at or below the peritoneal reflection: a multivariate analysis. Surg Today 2004;34(1):32–39.
161. Nakagoe T, Sawai T, Tsuji T, et al. Local rectal tumor resection results: gasless, video-endoscopic transanal excision versus the conventional posterior approach. World J Surg 2003;27(2): 197–202.
162. Neary P, Makin GB, White TJ, et al. Transanal endoscopic microsurgery: a viable operative alternative in selected patients with rectal lesions. Ann Surg Oncol 2003;10(9):1106–1111.
163. Sutton CD, Marshall LJ, White SA, Flint N, Berry DP, Kelly MJ. Ten-year experience of endoscopic transanal resection. Ann Surg 2002;235(3):355–362.
164. Bouvet M, Milas M, Giacco GG, Cleary KR, Janjan NA, Skibber JM. Predictors of recurrence after local excision and postoperative chemoradiation therapy of adenocarcinoma of the rectum. Ann Surg Oncol 1999;6(1):26–32.
165. Willett CG, Tepper JE, Donnelly S, et al. Patterns of failure following local excision and local excision and postoperative radiation therapy for invasive rectal adenocarcinoma. J Clin Oncol 1989;7(8):1003–1008.
166. Harewood GC, Wiersema MJ, Nelson H, et al. A prospective, blinded assessment of the impact of preoperative staging on the management of rectal cancer. Gastroenterology 2002;123(1): 24–32.
167. Morson BC. Factors influencing the prognosis of early cancer of the rectum. Proc R Soc Med 1966;59(7):607–608.
168. Minsky BD, Rich T, Recht A, Harvey W, Mies C. Selection criteria for local excision with or without adjuvant radiation therapy for rectal cancer. Cancer (Phila) 1989;63(7):1421–1429.
169. Graham RA, Garnsey L, Jessup JM. Local excision of rectal carcinoma. Am J Surg 1990;160(3):306–312.
170. McDermott FT, Hughes ES, Pihl E, Johnson WR, Price AB. Local recurrence after potentially curative resection for rectal cancer in a series of 1008 patients. Br J Surg 1985;72(1):34–37.
171. Sticca RP, Rodriguez-Bigas M, Penetrante RB, Petrelli NJ. Curative resection for stage I rectal cancer: natural history, prognostic factors, and recurrence patterns. Cancer Invest 1996; 14(5):491–497.
172. Wilson SM, Beahrs OH. The curative treatment of carcinoma of the sigmoid, rectosigmoid, and rectum. Ann Surg 1976; 183(5):556–565.
173. Bailey HR, Huval WV, Max E, Smith KW, Butts DR, Zamora LF. Local excision of carcinoma of the rectum for cure. Surgery (St. Louis) 1992;111(5):555–561.
174. Chakravarti A, Compton CC, Shellito PC, et al. Long-term follow-up of patients with rectal cancer managed by local excision with and without adjuvant irradiation. Ann Surg 1999; 230(1):49–54.
175. Ota DM, Skibber J, Rich T. M.D. Anderson Cancer Center experience with local excision and multimodality therapy for rectal cancer. Surg Clin N Am 1992;1:147–152.
176. Steele GD, Jr., Herndon JE, Bleday R, et al. Sphincter-sparing treatment for distal rectal adenocarcinoma. Ann Surg Oncol 1999;6(5):433–441.
177. Baron PL, Enker WE, Zakowski MF, Urmacher C. Immediate vs. salvage resection after local treatment for early rectal cancer. Dis Colon Rectum 1995;38(2):177–181.
178. Crile G Jr, Turnbull RB Jr. The role of electrocoagulation in the treatment of carcinoma of the rectum. Surg Gynecol Obstet 1972;135(3):391–396.
179. Papillon J. Endocavity irradiation of early rectal cancers for cure: a series of 123 cases. Proc R Soc Med 1973;66(12):1179–1181.
180. Hull TL, Lavery IC, Saxton JP. Endocavitary irradiation. An option in select patients with rectal cancer. Dis Colon Rectum 1994;37(12):1266–1270.

181. Myerson RJ, Ualz BJ, Kodner IJ, Fleshman J, Fri RD, Konefal JB. Endocavitary radiation therapy for rectal cancer: results with and without external beam. Endocurie Hypertherm Oncol 1989; 5:195–199.
182. Papillon J, Berard P. Endocavitary irradiation in the conservative treatment of adenocarcinoma of the low rectum. World J Surg 1992;16(3):451–457.
183. Birnbaum EH, Ogunbiyi OA, Gagliardi G, et al. Selection criteria for treatment of rectal cancer with combined external and endocavitary radiation. Dis Colon Rectum 1999;42(6):727–733; discussion 733–725.
184. Saclarides TJ. Transanal endoscopic microsurgery: a single surgeon's experience. Arch Surg 1998;133(6):595–598; discussion 598–599.
185. Buess G, Kipfmuller K, Hack D, Grussner R, Heintz A, Junginger T. Technique of transanal endoscopic microsurgery. Surg Endosc 1988;2(2):71–75.
186. Despretz J, Otmezguine Y, Grimard L, Calitchi E, Julien M. Conservative management of tumors of the rectum by radiotherapy and local excision. Dis Colon Rectum 1990;33(2):113–116.
187. Mohiuddin M, Marks G, Bannon J. High-dose preoperative radiation and full thickness local excision: a new option for selected T3 distal rectal cancers. Int J Radiat Oncol Biol Phys 1994;30(4):845–849.
188. Habr-Gama A, de Souza PM, Ribeiro U Jr, et al. Low rectal cancer: impact of radiation and chemotherapy on surgical treatment. Dis Colon Rectum 1998;41(9):1087–1096.
189. Ruo L, Guillem JG, Minsky BD, Quan SH, Paty PB, Cohen AM. Preoperative radiation with or without chemotherapy and full-thickness transanal excision for selected T2 and T3 distal rectal cancers. Int J Colorectal Dis 2002;17(1):54–58.
190. Telford JJ, Saltzman JR, Kuntz KM, Syngal S. Impact of preoperative staging and chemoradiation versus postoperative chemoradiation on outcome in patients with rectal cancer: a decision analysis. J Natl Cancer Inst 2004;96(3):191–201.
191. Brown G, Davies S, Williams GT, et al. Effectiveness of preoperative staging in rectal cancer: digital rectal examination, endoluminal ultrasound or magnetic resonance imaging? Br J Cancer 2004;91(1):23–29.
192. Harewood GC, Wiersema MJ. Cost-effectiveness of endoscopic ultrasonography in the evaluation of proximal rectal cancer. Am J Gastroenterol 2002;97(4):874–882.
193. Gavioli M, Bagni A, Piccagli I, Fundaro S, Natalini G. Usefulness of endorectal ultrasound after preoperative radiotherapy in rectal cancer: comparison between sonographic and histopathologic changes. Dis Colon Rectum 2000;43(8):1075–1083.
194. Vanagunas A, Lin DE, Stryker SJ. Accuracy of endoscopic ultrasound for restaging rectal cancer following neoadjuvant chemoradiation therapy. Am J Gastroenterol 2004;99(1):109–112.
195. Watanabe M, Sugimura K, Kuroda S, Okizuka H, Ishida T. CT assessment of postirradiation changes in the rectum and perirectal region. Clin Imaging 1995;19(3):182–187.
196. Sugimura K, Carrington BM, Quivey JM, Hricak H. Postirradiation changes in the pelvis: assessment with MR imaging. Radiology 1990;175(3):805–813.
197. Delrio P, Lastoria S, Avallone A, et al. [Early evaluation using PET-FDG of the efficiency of neoadjuvant radiochemotherapy treatment in locally advanced neoplasia of the lower rectum.] Tumori 2003;89(suppl 4):50–53.
198. Calvo FA, Domper M, Matute R, et al. ^{18}F-FDG positron emission tomography staging and restaging in rectal cancer treated with preoperative chemoradiation. Int J Radiat Oncol Biol Phys 2004;58(2):528–535.
199. Guillem JG, Puig-La Calle J Jr, Akhurst T, et al. Prospective assessment of primary rectal cancer response to preoperative radiation and chemotherapy using 18-fluorodeoxyglucose positron emission tomography. Dis Colon Rectum 2000;43(1): 18–24.
200. Gunderson LL, Sargent DJ, Tepper JE, et al. Impact of T and N stage and treatment on survival and relapse in adjuvant rectal cancer: a pooled analysis. J Clin Oncol 2004;22(10):1785–1796.
201. Fernandez-Represa JA, Mayol JM, Garcia-Aguilar J. Total mesorectal excision for rectal cancer: the truth lies underneath. World J Surg 2004;28(2):113–116.
202. Martijn H, Voogd AC, van de Poll-Franse LV, Repelaer van Driel OJ, Rutten HJ, Coebergh JW. Improved survival of patients with rectal cancer since 1980: a population-based study. Eur J Cancer 2003;39(14):2073–2079.
203. Miles WE. A method of performing abdomino-perineal excision for carcinoma of the rectum and of the terminal portion of the pelvic colon (1908). CA Cancer J Clin 1971;21(6):361–364.
204. Fisher B, Wolmark N, Rockette H, et al. Postoperative adjuvant chemotherapy or radiation therapy for rectal cancer: results from NSABP protocol R-01. J Natl Cancer Inst 1988;80(1):21–29.
205. Pollett WG, Nicholls RJ. The relationship between the extent of distal clearance and survival and local recurrence rates after curative anterior resection for carcinoma of the rectum. Ann Surg 1983;198(2):159–163.
206. Quirke P, Durdey P, Dixon MF, Williams NS. Local recurrence of rectal adenocarcinoma due to inadequate surgical resection. Histopathological study of lateral tumour spread and surgical excision. Lancet 1986;2(8514):996–999.
207. Adam IJ, Mohamdee MO, Martin IG, et al. Role of circumferential margin involvement in the local recurrence of rectal cancer. Lancet 1994;344(8924):707–711.
208. Stocchi L, Nelson H, Sargent DJ, et al. Impact of surgical and pathologic variables in rectal cancer: a United States community and cooperative group report. J Clin Oncol 2001;19(18): 3895–3902.
209. Quirke P, Scott N. The pathologist's role in the assessment of loal recurrence in rectal carcinoma. Surg Oncol Clin N Am 1992;1:1–17.
210. McAnena OJ, Heald RJ, Lockhart-Mummery HE. Operative and functional results of total mesorectal excision with ultra-low anterior resection in the management of carcinoma of the lower one-third of the rectum. Surg Gynecol Obstet 1990; 170(6):517–521.
211. Nesbakken A, Nygaard K, Westerheim O, Lunde OC, Mala T. Audit of intraoperative and early postoperative complications after introduction of mesorectal excision for rectal cancer. Eur J Surg 2002;168(4):229–235.
212. MacFarlane JK, Ryall RD, Heald RJ. Mesorectal excision for rectal cancer. Lancet 1993;341(8843):457–460.
213. Heald RJ, Moran BJ, Ryall RD, Sexton R, MacFarlane JK. Rectal cancer: the Basingstoke experience of total mesorectal excision, 1978–1997. Arch Surg 1998;133(8):894–899.
214. Krook JE, Moertel CG, Gunderson LL, et al. Effective surgical adjuvant therapy for high-risk rectal carcinoma. N Engl J Med 1991;324(11):709–715.
215. Enker WE. Potency, cure, and local control in the operative treatment of rectal cancer. Arch Surg 1992;127(12):1396–1401; discussion 1402.
216. Moreira LF, Hizuta A, Iwagaki H, Tanaka N, Orita K. Lateral lymph node dissection for rectal carcinoma below the peritoneal reflection. Br J Surg 1994;81(2):293–296.
217. Hojo K, Koyama Y, Moriya Y. Lymphatic spread and its prognostic value in patients with rectal cancer. Am J Surg 1982; 144(3):350–354.
218. Glass RE, Ritchie JK, Thompson HR, Mann CV. The results of surgical treatment of cancer of the rectum by radical resection and extended abdomino-iliac lymphadenectomy. Br J Surg 1985; 72(8):599–601.
219. Dahlberg M, Glimelius B, Pahlman L. Changing strategy for rectal cancer is associated with improved outcome. Br J Surg 1999;86(3):379–384.

220. Porter GA, Soskolne CL, Yakimets WW, Newman SC. Surgeon-related factors and outcome in rectal cancer. Ann Surg 1998; 227(2):157–167.
221. Holm T, Johansson H, Cedermark B, Ekelund G, Rutqvist LE. Influence of hospital- and surgeon-related factors on outcome after treatment of rectal cancer with or without preoperative radiotherapy. Br J Surg 1997;84(5):657–663.
222. Hermanek P, Wiebelt H, Staimmer D, Riedl S. Prognostic factors of rectum carcinoma–experience of the German Multicentre Study SGCRC. German Study Group Colo-Rectal Carcinoma. Tumori 1995;81(suppl 3):60–64.
223. Simons AJ, Ker R, Groshen S, et al. Variations in treatment of rectal cancer: the influence of hospital type and caseload. Dis Colon Rectum 1997;40(6):641–646.
224. Tiret E, Poupardin B, McNamara D, Dehni N, Parc R. Ultralow anterior resection with intersphincteric dissection—what is the limit of safe sphincter preservation? Colorectal Dis 2003; 5(5):454–457.
225. Lopez-Kostner F, Lavery IC, Hool GR, Rybicki LA, Fazio VW. Total mesorectal excision is not necessary for cancers of the upper rectum. Surgery (St. Louis) 1998;124(4):612–617; discussion 617–618.
226. Steichen FM, Ravitch MM. History of mechanical devices and instruments for suturing. Curr Probl Surg 1982;19(1):1–52.
227. Beart RW Jr, Kelly KA. Randomized prospective evaluation of the EEA stapler for colorectal anastomoses. Am J Surg 1981; 141(1):143–147.
228. Docherty JG, McGregor JR, Akyol AM, Murray GD, Galloway DJ. Comparison of manually constructed and stapled anastomoses in colorectal surgery. West of Scotland and Highland Anastomosis Study Group. Ann Surg 1995;221(2):176–184.
229. Cavaliere F, Pemberton JH, Cosimelli M, Fazio VW, Beart RW Jr. Coloanal anastomosis for rectal cancer. Long-term results at the Mayo and Cleveland Clinics. Dis Colon Rectum 1995; 38(8):807–812.
230. Lazorthes F, Fages P, Chiotasso P, Lemozy J, Bloom E. Resection of the rectum with construction of a colonic reservoir and colo-anal anastomosis for carcinoma of the rectum. Br J Surg 1986;73(2):136–138.
231. Sailer M, Fuchs KH, Fein M, Thiede A. Randomized clinical trial comparing quality of life after straight and pouch coloanal reconstruction. Br J Surg 2002;89(9):1108–1117.
232. Hallbook O, Pahlman L, Krog M, Wexner SD, Sjodahl R. Randomized comparison of straight and colonic J pouch anastomosis after low anterior resection. Ann Surg 1996;224(1):58–65.
233. Hida J, Yasutomi M, Maruyama T, et al. Indications for colonic J-pouch reconstruction after anterior resection for rectal cancer: determining the optimum level of anastomosis. Dis Colon Rectum 1998;41(5):558–563.
234. Drake DB, Pemberton JH, Beart RW Jr, Dozois RR, Wolff BG. Coloanal anastomosis in the management of benign and malignant rectal disease. Ann Surg 1987;206(5):600–605.
235. Minsky BD, Cohen AM, Enker WE, Sigurdson E. Phase I/II trial of pre-operative radiation therapy and coloanal anastomosis in distal invasive resectable rectal cancer. Int J Radiat Oncol Biol Phys 1992;23(2):387–392.
236. Minsky BD, Cohen AM, Enker WE, Paty P. Sphincter preservation with preoperative radiation therapy and coloanal anastomosis. Int J Radiat Oncol Biol Phys 1995;31(3):553–559.
237. Prolongation of the disease-free interval in surgically treated rectal carcinoma. Gastrointestinal Tumor Study Group. N Engl J Med 1985;312(23):1465–1472.
238. Law WL, Chu KW. Impact of total mesorectal excision on the results of surgery of distal rectal cancer. Br J Surg 2001; 88(12):1607–1612.
239. Nissan A, Guillem JG, Paty PB, et al. Abdominoperineal resection for rectal cancer at a specialty center. Dis Colon Rectum 2001;44(1):27–35; discussion 35–36.
240. Paty PB, Enker WE, Cohen AM, Lauwers GY. Treatment of rectal cancer by low anterior resection with coloanal anastomosis. Ann Surg 1994;219(4):365–373.
241. Zaheer S, Pemberton JH, Farouk R, Dozois RR, Wolff BG, Ilstrup D. Surgical treatment of adenocarcinoma of the rectum. Ann Surg 1998;227(6):800–811.
242. Williams NS, Johnston D. Survival and recurrence after sphincter saving resection and abdominoperineal resection for carcinoma of the middle third of the rectum. Br J Surg 1984; 71(4):278–282.
243. Byfield JE, Calabro-Jones P, Klisak I, Kulhanian F. Pharmacologic requirements for obtaining sensitization of human tumor cells in vitro to combined 5-fluorouracil or ftorafur and X rays. Int J Radiat Oncol Biol Phys 1982;8(11):1923–1933.
244. Rich TA, Lokich JJ, Chaffey JT. A pilot study of protracted venous infusion of 5-fluorouracil and concomitant radiation therapy. J Clin Oncol 1985;3(3):402–406.
245. Wong CS, Stern H, Cummings BJ. Local excision and post-operative radiation therapy for rectal carcinoma. Int J Radiat Oncol Biol Phys 1993;25(4):669–675.
246. Ghanem AN, Perry KC. Malignant lymphoma as a complication of ureterosigmoidostomy. Br J Surg 1985;72(7):559–560.
247. Rider WD, Palmer JA, Mahoney LJ, Robertson CT. Preoperative irradiation in operable cancer of the rectum: report of the Toronto trial. Can J Surg 1977;20(4):335–338.
248. Roswit B, Higgins GA, Keehn RJ. Preoperative irradiation for carcinoma of the rectum and rectosigmoid colon: report of a National Veterans Administration randomized study. Cancer (Phila) 1975;35(6):1597–1602.
249. Gerard A, Buyse M, Nordlinger B, et al. Preoperative radiotherapy as adjuvant treatment in rectal cancer. Final results of a randomized study of the European Organization for Research and Treatment of Cancer (EORTC). Ann Surg 1988;208(5):606–614.
250. Martling A, Holm T, Johansson H, Rutqvist LE, Cedermark B. The Stockholm II trial on preoperative radiotherapy in rectal carcinoma: long-term follow-up of a population-based study. Cancer (Phila) 2001;92(4):896–902.
251. Improved survival with preoperative radiotherapy in resectable rectal cancer. Swedish Rectal Cancer Trial. N Engl J Med 1997; 336(14):980–987.
252. Gerard JP. The use of radiotherapy for patients with low rectal cancer: an overview of the Lyon experience. Aust N Z J Surg 1994;64(7):457–463.
253. Adjuvant radiotherapy for rectal cancer: a systematic overview of 8,507 patients from 22 randomised trials. Lancet 2001; 358(9290):1291–1304.
254. Initial report from a Swedish multicentre study examining the role of preoperative irradiation in the treatment of patients with resectable rectal carcinoma. Swedish Rectal Cancer Trial. Br J Surg 1993;80(10):1333–1336.
255. Frykholm GJ, Glimelius B, Pahlman L. Preoperative or post-operative irradiation in adenocarcinoma of the rectum: final treatment results of a randomized trial and an evaluation of late secondary effects. Dis Colon Rectum 1993;36(6):564–572.
256. Kapiteijn E, Marijnen CA, Nagtegaal ID, et al. Preoperative radiotherapy combined with total mesorectal excision for resectable rectal cancer. N Engl J Med 2001;345(9):638–646.
257. McCall JL, Cox MR, Wattchow DA. Analysis of local recurrence rates after surgery alone for rectal cancer. Int J Colorectal Dis 1995;10(3):126–132.
258. Hill GL, Rafique M. Extrafascial excision of the rectum for rectal cancer. Br J Surg 1998;85(6):809–812.
258a. Marks G, Modiuddin M, Eitan A, Masoni L, Rakinic J. High-dose preoperative radiation and radical sphincter-preserving surgery for rectal cancer. Arch Surg 1991;126(12):1534–1540.
259. Gerard JP, Chapet O, Nemoz C, et al. Improved sphincter preservation in low rectal cancer with high-dose preoperative

radiotherapy: the Lyon R96–02 randomized trial. J Clin Oncol 2004;22(12):2404–2409.
260. Francois Y, Nemoz CJ, Baulieux J, et al. Influence of the interval between preoperative radiation therapy and surgery on downstaging and on the rate of sphincter-sparing surgery for rectal cancer: the Lyon R90–01 randomized trial. J Clin Oncol 1999;17(8):2396.
261. Moore HG, Gittleman AE, Minsky BD, et al. Rate of pathologic complete response with increased interval between preoperative combined modality therapy and rectal cancer resection. Dis Colon Rectum 2004;47(3):279–286.
262. Cohen A, Minsky B, Schildky R. Cancer of the rectum. In: De Vita V, Hellman S, Rosenberg S (eds). Cancer: Principles and Practice of Oncology, 5th ed. Philadelphia: Lippincott Raven, 1997:1197–1234.
263. Meterissian S, Skibber J, Rich T, et al. Patterns of residual disease after preoperative chemoradiation in ultrasound T3 rectal carcinoma. Ann Surg Oncol 1994;1(2):111–116.
264. Janjan NA, Khoo VS, Abbruzzese J, et al. Tumor downstaging and sphincter preservation with preoperative chemoradiation in locally advanced rectal cancer: the M.D. Anderson Cancer Center experience. Int J Radiat Oncol Biol Phys 1999; 44(5):1027–1038.
265. Fleming J, Hunt K, Feig BW, et al. Primary tumor response to preoperative chemoradiation does not ensure the absence of regional lymph node metastases in patients with locally advanced rectal cancer. Presented at the 40th Meeting of the Society of Surgery of the Alimentary Tract, May 16–19, 1999, Orlando, FL.
266. Stipa F, Zernecke A, Moore HG, et al. Residual mesorectal lymph node involvement following neoadjuvant combined-modality therapy: rationale for radical resection? Ann Surg Oncol 2004;11(2):187–191.
267. Moore HG, Riedel E, Minsky BD, et al. Adequacy of 1-cm distal margin after restorative rectal cancer resection with sharp mesorectal excision and preoperative combined-modality therapy. Ann Surg Oncol 2003;10(1):80–85.
268. Pigot F, Dernaoui M, Castinel A, Juguet F, Chaume JC, Faivre J. [Local excision with postoperative radiotherapy for T2 or T3 distal rectal cancer. Long-term results.] Ann Chir 2001; 126(7):639–643.
269. Kim CJ, Yeatman TJ, Coppola D, et al. Local excision of T2 and T3 rectal cancers after downstaging chemoradiation. Ann Surg 2001;234(3):352–358; discussion 358–359.
270. Minsky BD, Cohen AM, Kemeny N, et al. Combined modality therapy of rectal cancer: decreased acute toxicity with the preoperative approach. J Clin Oncol 1992;10(8):1218–1224.
271. Crane CH, Skibber JM, Birnbaum EH, et al. The addition of continuous infusion 5-FU to preoperative radiation therapy increases tumor response, leading to increased sphincter preservation in locally advanced rectal cancer. Int J Radiat Oncol Biol Phys 2003;57(1):84–89.
272. Janjan NA, Crane CN, Feig BW, et al. Prospective trial of preoperative concomitant boost radiotherapy with continuous infusion 5-fluorouracil for locally advanced rectal cancer. Int J Radiat Oncol Biol Phys 2000;47(3):713–718.
273. Grann A, Minsky BD, Cohen AM, et al. Preliminary results of preoperative 5-fluorouracil, low-dose leucovorin, and concurrent radiation therapy for clinically resectable T3 rectal cancer. Dis Colon Rectum 1997;40(5):515–522.
274. Rich TA, Skibber JM, Ajani JA, et al. Preoperative infusional chemoradiation therapy for stage T3 rectal cancer. Int J Radiat Oncol Biol Phys 1995;32(4):1025–1029.
275. Hyams DM, Mamounas EP, Petrelli N, et al. A clinical trial to evaluate the worth of preoperative multimodality therapy in patients with operable carcinoma of the rectum: a progress report of National Surgical Breast and Bowel Project Protocol R-03. Dis Colon Rectum 1997;40(2):131–139.
276. Sauer R, Fietkau R, Wittekind C, et al. Adjuvant versus neo adjuvant radiochemotherapy for locally advanced rectal cancer. A progress report of a phase-III randomized trial (protocol CAO/ARO/AIO-94). Strahlenther Onkol 2001;177(4):173–181.
277. Sauer R. Adjuvant versus neoadjuvant combined modality treatment for locally advanced rectal cancer: first results of the German rectal cancer study (CAO/ARO/AIO-94). Int J Radiat Oncol Biol Phys 2003;57(suppl 2):S124–S125.
278. Sprangers MA, Taal BG, Aaronson NK, te Velde A. Quality of life in colorectal cancer. Stoma vs. nonstoma patients. Dis Colon Rectum 1995;38(4):361–369.
279. Kollmorgen CF, Meagher AP, Wolff BG, Pemberton JH, Martenson JA, Illstrup DM. The long-term effect of adjuvant postoperative chemoradiotherapy for rectal carcinoma on bowel function. Ann Surg 1994;220(5):676–682.
280. Paty PB, Enker WE, Cohen AM, Minsky BD, Friedlander-Klar H. Long-term functional results of coloanal anastomosis for rectal cancer. Am J Surg 1994;167(1):90–94; discussion 94–95.
281. Weinstein GD, Rich TA, Shumate CR, et al. Preoperative infusional chemoradiation and surgery with or without an electron beam intraoperative boost for advanced primary rectal cancer. Int J Radiat Oncol Biol Phys 1995;32(1):197–204.
282. Jemal A, Thomas A, Murray T, Thun M. Cancer statistics, 2002. CA Cancer J Clin 2002;52(1):23–47.
283. Bendell JC, Ryan DP. Current perspectives on anal cancer. Oncology (Huntingt) 2003;17(4):492–497, 502–503; discussion 503, 507–509
284. Klas JV, Rothenberger DA, Wong WD, Madoff RD. Malignant tumors of the anal canal: the spectrum of disease, treatment, and outcomes. Cancer (Phila) 1999;85(8):1686–1693.
285. Olofinlade O, Adeonigbagbe O, Gualtieri N, et al. Anal carcinoma: a 15-year retrospective analysis. Scand J Gastroenterol 2000;35(11):1194–1199.
286. Moore HG, Guillem JG. Anal neoplasms. Surg Clin N Am 2002;82(6):1233–1251.
287. Dujovny N, Quiros RM, Saclarides TJ. Anorectal anatomy and embryology. Surg Oncol Clin N Am 2004;13(2):277–293.
288. AJCC Cancer Staging Handbook, 6th ed. New York: Springer, 2002.
289. Peiffert D, Bey P, Pernot M, et al. Conservative treatment by irradiation of epidermoid cancers of the anal canal: prognostic factors of tumoral control and complications. Int J Radiat Oncol Biol Phys 1997;37(2):313–324.
290. Gerard JP, Ayzac L, Hun D, et al. Treatment of anal canal carcinoma with high dose radiation therapy and concomitant fluorouracil-cisplatinum. Long-term results in 95 patients. Radiother Oncol 1998;46(3):249–256.
291. Cummings BJ, Keane TJ, O'Sullivan B, Wong CS, Catton CN. Epidermoid anal cancer: treatment by radiation alone or by radiation and 5-fluorouracil with and without mitomycin C. Int J Radiat Oncol Biol Phys 1991;21(5):1115–1125.
292. Allal AS, Mermillod B, Roth AD, Marti MC, Kurtz JM. The impact of treatment factors on local control in T2-T3 anal carcinomas treated by radiotherapy with or without chemotherapy. Cancer (Phila) 15 1997;79(12):2329–2335.
293. Flam M, John M, Pajak TF, et al. Role of mitomycin in combination with fluorouracil and radiotherapy, and of salvage chemoradiation in the definitive nonsurgical treatment of epidermoid carcinoma of the anal canal: results of a phase III randomized intergroup study. J Clin Oncol 1996;14(9):2527–2539.
294. Perera D, Pathma-Nathan N, Rabbitt P, Hewett P, Rieger N. Sentinel node biopsy for squamous-cell carcinoma of the anus and anal margin. Dis Colon Rectum 2003;46(8):1027–1029; discussion 1030–1031.
295. Boman BM, Moertel CG, O'Connell MJ, et al. Carcinoma of the anal canal. A clinical and pathologic study of 188 cases. Cancer (Phila) 1984;54(1):114–125.

296. Frost DB, Richards PC, Montague ED, Giacco GG, Martin RG. Epidermoid cancer of the anorectum. Cancer (Phila) 1984; 53(6):1285–1293.
297. Martenson JA Jr, Gunderson LL. External radiation therapy without chemotherapy in the management of anal cancer. Cancer (Phila) 1993;71(5):1736–1740.
298. Schlienger M, Krzisch C, Pene F, et al. Epidermoid carcinoma of the anal canal treatment results and prognostic variables in a series of 242 cases. Int J Radiat Oncol Biol Phys 1989;17(6): 1141–1151.
299. Dobrowsky W. Radiotherapy of epidermoid anal canal cancer. Br J Radiol 1989;62(733):53–58.
300. Nigro ND, Vaitkevicius VK, Considine B Jr. Combined therapy for cancer of the anal canal: a preliminary report. Dis Colon Rectum 1974;17(3):354–356.
301. Sischy B. The use of radiation therapy combined with chemotherapy in the management of squamous cell carcinoma of the anus and marginally resectable adenocarcinoma of the rectum. Int J Radiat Oncol Biol Phys 1985;11(9):1587–1593.
302. Leichman L, Nigro N, Vaitkevicius VK, et al. Cancer of the anal canal. Model for preoperative adjuvant combined modality therapy. Am J Med 1985;78(2):211–215.
303. Flam MS, John MJ, Mowry PA, Lovalvo LJ, Ramalho LD, Wade J. Definitive combined modality therapy of carcinoma of the anus. A report of 30 cases including results of salvage therapy in patients with residual disease. Dis Colon Rectum 1987; 30(7):495–502.
304. Grabenbauer GG, Schneider IH, Gall FP, Sauer R. Epidermoid carcinoma of the anal canal: treatment by combined radiation and chemotherapy. Radiother Oncol 1993;27(1):59–62.
305. Allal A, Kurtz JM, Pipard G, et al. Chemoradiotherapy versus radiotherapy alone for anal cancer: a retrospective comparison. Int J Radiat Oncol Biol Phys 1993;27(1):59–66.
306. Allal AS, Sprangers MA, Laurencet F, Reymond MA, Kurtz JM. Assessment of long-term quality of life in patients with anal carcinomas treated by radiotherapy with or without chemotherapy. Br J Cancer 1999;80(10):1588–1594.
307. Epidermoid anal cancer: results from the UKCCCR randomised trial of radiotherapy alone versus radiotherapy, 5-fluorouracil, and mitomycin. UKCCCR Anal Cancer Trial Working Party. UK Co-ordinating Committee on Cancer Research. Lancet 1996; 348(9034):1049–1054.
308. Bartelink H, Roelofsen F, Eschwege F, et al. Concomitant radiotherapy and chemotherapy is superior to radiotherapy alone in the treatment of locally advanced anal cancer: results of a phase III randomized trial of the European Organization for Research and Treatment of Cancer Radiotherapy and Gastrointestinal Cooperative Groups. J Clin Oncol 1997;15(5):2040–2049.
309. Hung A, Crane C, Delclos M, et al. Cisplatin-based combined modality therapy for anal carcinoma: a wider therapeutic index. Cancer (Phila) 2003;97(5):1195–1202.
310. Peiffert D, Giovannini M, Ducreux M, et al. High-dose radiation therapy and neoadjuvant plus concomitant chemotherapy with 5-fluorouracil and cisplatin in patients with locally advanced squamous-cell anal canal cancer: final results of a phase II study. Ann Oncol 2001;12(3):397–404.
311. Allal AS, Mermillod B, Roth AD, Marti MC, Kurtz JM. Impact of clinical and therapeutic factors on major late complications after radiotherapy with or without concomitant chemotherapy for anal carcinoma. Int J Radiat Oncol Biol Phys 1997; 39(5):1099–1105.
312. Ellenhorn JD, Enker WE, Quan SH. Salvage abdominoperineal resection following combined chemotherapy and radiotherapy for epidermoid carcinoma of the anus. Ann Surg Oncol 1994; 1(2):105–110.
313. Nilsson PJ, Svensson C, Goldman S, Glimelius B. Salvage abdominoperineal resection in anal epidermoid cancer. Br J Surg 2002;89(11):1425–1429.
314. Longo WE, Vernava AM III, Wade TP, Coplin MA, Virgo KS, Johnson FE. Recurrent squamous cell carcinoma of the anal canal. Predictors of initial treatment failure and results of salvage therapy. Ann Surg 1994;220(1):40–49.
315. Pocard M, Tiret E, Nugent K, Dehni N, Parc R. Results of salvage abdominoperineal resection for anal cancer after radiotherapy. Dis Colon Rectum 1998;41(12):1488–1493.
316. Allal AS, Laurencet FM, Reymond MA, Kurtz JM, Marti MC. Effectiveness of surgical salvage therapy for patients with locally uncontrolled anal carcinoma after sphincter-conserving treatment. Cancer (Phila) 1999;86(3):405–409.
317. van der Wal BC, Cleffken BI, Gulec B, Kaufman HS, Choti MA. Results of salvage abdominoperineal resection for recurrent anal carcinoma following combined chemoradiation therapy. J Gastrointest Surg 2001;5(4):383–387.
318. Smith AJ, Whelan P, Cummings BJ, Stern HS. Management of persistent or locally recurrent epidermoid cancer of the anal canal with abdominoperineal resection. Acta Oncol 2001; 40(1):34–36.
319. Tei TM, Stolzenburg T, Buntzen S, Laurberg S, Kjeldsen H. Use of transpelvic rectus abdominis musculocutaneous flap for anal cancer salvage surgery. Br J Surg 2003;90(5):575–580.
320. Stearns MW Jr, Urmacher C, Sternberg SS, Woodruff J, Attiyeh F. Cancer of the anal canal. Curr Probl Cancer 1980;4(12):1–44.
321. Papillon J, Montbarbon JF. Epidermoid carcinoma of the anal canal. A series of 276 cases. Dis Colon Rectum 1987;30(5): 324–333.
322. Gerard JP, Chapet O, Samiei F, et al. Management of inguinal lymph node metastases in patients with carcinoma of the anal canal: experience in a series of 270 patients treated in Lyon and review of the literature. Cancer (Phila) 2001;92(1):77–84.
323. Greenall MJ, Magill GB, Quan SH, DeCosse JJ. Recurrent epidermoid cancer of the anus. Cancer (Phila) 1986;57(7): 1437–1441.
324. Humphrey LJ. Reducing leg edema after groin dissection. J Surg Oncol 1992;50(1):19.
325. Spratt J. Groin dissection. J Surg Oncol 2000;73(4):243–262.
326. Wood TF, Nora DT, Morton DL, et al. One hundred consecutive cases of sentinel lymph node mapping in early colorectal carcinoma: detection of missed micrometastases. J Gastrointest Surg 2002;6(3):322–329; discussion 229–330.
327. Trocha SD, Nora DT, Saha SS, Morton DL, Wiese D, Bilchik AJ. Combination probe and dye-directed lymphatic mapping detects micrometastases in early colorectal cancer. J Gastrointest Surg 2003;7(3):340–345; discussion 345–346.
328. Paramo JC, Summerall J, Poppiti R, Mesko TW. Validation of sentinel node mapping in patients with colon cancer. Ann Surg Oncol 2002;9(6):550–554.
329. Saha S, Bilchik A, Wiese D, et al. Ultrastaging of colorectal cancer by sentinel lymph node mapping technique—a multicenter trial. Ann Surg Oncol 2001;8(suppl 9):94S–98S.
330. Bilchik AJ, Saha S, Wiese D, et al. Molecular staging of early colon cancer on the basis of sentinel node analysis: a multicenter phase II trial. J Clin Oncol 2001;19(4):1128–1136.
331. Joosten JJ, Strobbe LJ, Wauters CA, Pruszczynski M, Wobbes T, Ruers TJ. Intraoperative lymphatic mapping and the sentinel node concept in colorectal carcinoma. Br J Surg 1999;86(4): 482–486.
332. Merrie AE, van Rij AM, Phillips LV, Rossaak JI, Yun K, McCall JL. Diagnostic use of the sentinel node in colon cancer. Dis Colon Rectum 2001;44(3):410–417.
333. Mellgren A, Sirivongs P, Rothenberger DA, Madoff RD, Garcia-Aguilar J. Is local excision adequate therapy for early rectal cancer? Dis Colon Rectum 2000;43(8):1064–1071; discussion 1071–1074.
334. Balani A, Turoldo A, Braini A, Scaramucci M, Roseano M, Leggeri A. Local excision for rectal cancer. J Surg Oncol 2000; 74(2):158–162.

335. Garcia-Aguilar J, Mellgren A, Sirivongs P, Buic D, Madoff RD, Rothenberger DA. Local excision of rectal cancer without adjuvant therapy: a word of caution. Ann Surg 2000;231(3):345–351.
336. Nivatvongs S, Wolff BG. Technique of per anal excision for carcinoma of the low rectum. World J Surg 1992;16(3):447–450.
337. Willett CG, Tepper JE, Donnelly S, et al. Patterns of failure following local excision and local excision and postoperative radiation therapy for invasive rectal adenocarcinoma. J Clin Oncol 1989;7(8):1003–1008.
338. Biggers OR, Beart RW Jr, Ilstrup DM. Local excision of rectal cancer. Dis Colon Rectum 1986;29(6):374–377.
339. Bleday R, Breen E, Jessup JM, Burgess A, Sentovich SM, Steele G Jr. Prospective evaluation of local excision for small rectal cancers. Dis Colon Rectum 1997;40(4):388–392.
340. Valentini V, Morganti AG, De Santis M, et al. Local excision and external beam radiotherapy in early rectal cancer. Int J Radiat Oncol Biol Phys 1996;35(4):759–764.
341. Taylor RH, Hay JH, Larsson SN. Transanal local excision of selected low rectal cancers. Am J Surg 1998;175(5):360–363.
342. Panzironi G, De Vargas Macciucca M, Manganaro L, et al. Preoperative locoregional staging of rectal carcinoma: comparison of MR, TRUS and multislice CT. Personal experience. Radiol Med (Torino) 2004;107(4):344–355.
343. Shami VM, Parmar KS, Waxman I. Clinical impact of endoscopic ultrasound and endoscopic ultrasound-guided fine-needle aspiration in the management of rectal carcinoma. Dis Colon Rectum 2004;47(1):59–65.
344. Mathur P, Smith JJ, Ramsey C, et al. Comparison of CT and MRI in the pre-operative staging of rectal adenocarcinoma and prediction of circumferential resection margin involvement by MRI. Colorectal Dis 2003;5(5):396–401.
345. Fuchsjager MH, Maier AG, Schima W, et al. Comparison of transrectal sonography and double-contrast MR imaging when staging rectal cancer. AJR Am J Roentgenol 2003;181(2):421–427.
346. Nesbakken A, Lovig T, Lunde OC, Nygaard K. Staging of rectal carcinoma with transrectal ultrasonography. Scand J Surg 2003;92(2):125–129.
347. Marusch F, Koch A, Schmidt U, et al. Routine use of transrectal ultrasound in rectal carcinoma: results of a prospective multicenter study. Endoscopy 2002;34(5):385–390.
348. Tobaruela E, Arribas D, Mortensen N. Is endosonography useful to select patients for endoscopic treatment of rectal cancer? Rev Esp Enferm Dig 1999;91(9):614–621.
349. Gagliardi G, Bayar S, Smith R, Salem RR. Preoperative staging of rectal cancer using magnetic resonance imaging with external phase-arrayed coils. Arch Surg 2002;137(4):447–451.
350. Kim NK, Kim MJ, Yun SH, Sohn SK, Min JS. Comparative study of transrectal ultrasonography, pelvic computerized tomography, and magnetic resonance imaging in preoperative staging of rectal cancer. Dis Colon Rectum 1999;42(6):770–775.
351. Garcia-Aguilar J, Pollack J, Lee SH, et al. Accuracy of endorectal ultrasonography in preoperative staging of rectal tumors. Dis Colon Rectum 2002;45(1):10–15.
352. Gualdi GF, Casciani E, Guadalaxara A, d'Orta C, Polettini E, Pappalardo G. Local staging of rectal cancer with transrectal ultrasound and endorectal magnetic resonance imaging: comparison with histologic findings. Dis Colon Rectum 2000;43(3):338–345.
353. Beets-Tan RG, Beets GL, Vliegen RF, et al. Accuracy of magnetic resonance imaging in prediction of tumour-free resection margin in rectal cancer surgery. Lancet 2001;357(9255):497–504.
354. Hunerbein M, Totkas S, Ghadimi BM, Schlag PM. Preoperative evaluation of colorectal neoplasms by colonoscopic miniprobe ultrasonography. Ann Surg 2000;232(1):46–50.
355. Chiesura-Corona M, Muzzio PC, Giust G, Zuliani M, Pucciarelli S, Toppan P. Rectal cancer: CT local staging with histopathologic correlation. Abdom Imaging 2001;26(2):134–138.
356. Civelli EM, Gallino G, Mariani L, et al. Double-contrast barium enema and computerised tomography in the pre-operative evaluation of rectal carcinoma: are they still useful diagnostic procedures? Tumori 2000;86(5):389–392.
357. Akasu T, Kondo H, Moriya Y, et al. Endorectal ultrasonography and treatment of early stage rectal cancer. World J Surg 2000;24(9):1061–1068.
358. Wolmark N, Rockette H, Fisher B, et al. The benefit of leucovorin-modulated fluorouracil as postoperative adjuvant therapy for primary colon cancer: results from National Surgical Adjuvant Breast and Bowel Project protocol C-03. J Clin Oncol 1993;11(10):1879–1887.
359. Grinnell RS, Lane N. Benign and malignant adenomatous polyps and papillary adenomas of the colon and rectum: an analysis of 1,856 tumors in 1,335 patients. Surg Gynecol Obstet 1958;106(6):519–538.
360. Waye JD, Frankel A. Treatment of early colon cancer. Gastroenterology 1974;66:796.
361. Wolff WI, Shinya H. Definitive treatment of "malignant" polyps of the colon. Ann Surg 1975;182(4):516–525.
362. Lock MR, Cairns DW, Ritchie JK, Lockhart-Mummery HE. The treatment of early colorectal cancer by local excision. Br J Surg 1978;65(5):346–349.
363. Kodaira S, Teramoto T, Ono S, Takizawa K, Katsumata T, Abe O. Lymph node metastases from carcinomas developing in pedunculated and semipedunculated colorectal adenomas. Aust N Z J Surg 1981;51(5):429–433.
364. Nivatvongs S. Management of polyps containing invasive carcinoma. In: Codner I, Fry R, Roe J (eds). Colon, Rectal, and Anal Surgery. St. Louis: CV Mosby; 1985:183.
365. Shatney CH, Lober PH, Gilbertson V, Sosin H. Management of focally malignant pedunculated adenomatous colorectal polyps. Dis Colon Rectum 1976;19(4):334–341.
366. Coutsoftides T, Lavery I, Benjamin SP, Sivak MV, Jr. Malignant polyps of the colon and rectum: a clinicopathologic study. Dis Colon Rectum 1979;22(2):82–86.
367. Colachio TA, Forde KA, Scantlebury VP. Endoscopic polypectomy: inadequate treatment for invasive colorectal carcinoma. Ann Surg 1981;194(6):704–707.

43

Adenocarcinoma and Other Small Intestinal Malignancies

John H. Donohue

Despite the enormous surface area of the small intestinal mucosa and the rapid turnover of the enterocytes, malignancies of the small bowel are uncommon. Of the more than 250,000 digestive system cancers projected for diagnosis in the United States in 2003, only an estimated 5,300 were small intestinal malignancies.[1] There is a slight predominance of men diagnosed with these tumors. An estimated 1,100 Americans died of small intestinal malignancies in 2003.[1] Because of the low incidence of small bowel cancers and the common occurrence of four distinct histologic types, namely adenocarcinoma, lymphoma, gastrointestinal stromal tumor (GIST), and carcinoid tumor, even major clinical centers have limited experience in treating patients with these diseases. As a result, controlled data evaluating treatment variables and other aspects of small intestinal malignancies are virtually nonexistent.

This chapter reviews what is known about the etiology, diagnosis, treatment, and outcomes for adenocarcinoma, lymphoma, and GIST of the small intestine. Carcinoid tumors are reviewed in Chapter 60.

Etiology

A number of protective factors have been proposed to explain the low incidence of malignant transformation in the small intestinal mucosa, especially when compared to the large bowel. First of all, the liquid chyme is less irritating to the mucosa than solid fecal matter. Both the rapid transit of digesting food through the small intestine and the rapid turnover of enterocytes limit the exposure time of ingested carcinogens to individual mucosal cells. The alkaline pH of the small bowel contents, mucosal hydroxylases, and a several-log-lower concentration of bacteria than that present in the colon all lead to lower rates of carcinogen formation in the small intestine. Last, secretory IgA levels are significantly higher in the small bowel and may provide additional protection against malignant transformation.[2]

Most patients diagnosed with small bowel malignancies have no apparent underlying predisposition. Evidence for an adenoma–carcinoma sequence similar to that well-documented progression in colon cancers has been reported in the small intestine.[3] Facts supporting this theory include these: (1) a third of all small bowel adenomas contain cancer, (2) the distributions of benign and malignant growths within the small intestine are the same, and (3) the mean age of patients with benign adenomas is lower than that for adenocarcinomas, whereas the gender ratios are identical for both types of tumor.[3]

Among patients with inherited causes for colorectal cancer, both those with familial adenomatous polyposis (FAP is the result of a mutation of the APC gene)[4,5] and hereditary nonpolyposis colorectal carcinoma [HNPCC is due mostly to mutations of the mismatch repair (MMR) enzyme genes hMLH1 and hMSH2][6,7] are known to have increased risk of small intestinal adenocarcinoma. In FAP patients, the majority of small bowel cancers are duodenal adenocarcinomas, most of which arise in the periampullary area subsequent to total proctocolectomy.[5] In sharp contrast, small intestinal adenocarcinomas in HNPCC families are more evenly distributed throughout the small bowel and at least half may be the first tumor diagnosed in these kindreds.[8] In both FAP and HNPCC patients, the lifetime risk of small intestinal adenocarcinoma has been estimated to be more than 100 times that of the normal population.[8]

Peutz–Jeghers syndrome (PJS; the result of a mutation of the LKB1 gene that encodes a serine threonine kinase, STK11) results in the development of multiple hamartomatous polyps of the small intestine.[9] Although the nonneoplastic nature of the PJS polyps was long believed not to put these patients at increased risk of gastrointestinal malignancy, this hypothesis is now known to be false.[10,11] PJS patients are estimated to have an 18-fold-increased risk of intestinal cancer.[11] Most of the small bowel cancers in PJS appear to arise from hamartomas that transform into adenomas which then follow the usual adenoma–carcinoma sequence.[12] Given the wide distribution of hamartomatous polyps, small intestinal adenocarcinomas in PJS patients appear to be distributed differently than sporadic tumors, although the documentation of this pattern is incomplete.[13]

Several inflammatory conditions of the intestinal tract are also well recognized as risk factors for cancers of the small intestine. Crohn's disease is an idiopathic transmural inflammatory disease that may involve any part of the gastrointestinal tract but most commonly affects the terminal ileum. Although sporadic small bowel carcinomas are most common in the duodenum and rarest in the ileum, approximately two-thirds of adenocarcinomas in patients with Crohn's disease occur in the ileum, 30% in the jejunum, and rarely in the duodenum.[14] The estimated risk of adenocarcinoma in Crohn's disease has varied significantly because of small sample sizes but is likely more than 100 times that of the normal population.[15] Factors that especially increase the risk of cancer in Crohn's disease include male gender, excluded loops of diseased bowel, long duration of disease, fistula tracts, and multiple strictures.[16] Approximately 10 patients with small intestinal lymphoma in the setting of chronic Crohn's disease have been reported.[17] Although a causal link between these conditions may exist, the rare combination of Crohn's disease and small bowel lymphoma has prevented a quantitative analysis of risk.

Celiac disease, or celiac sprue, is a chronic inflammatory disease of the small intestine caused by exposure to dietary glutens. Patients with celiac disease are at increased risk for both intestinal and extraintestinal malignancies, a predisposition that a gluten-free diet seems to reverse. In a study of 235 celiac disease patients with more than 250 cancers, more than half were malignant lymphomas, incredibly with 80% of these tumors occurring in the small intestine.[18] These tumors are most commonly T-cell lymphomas of the jejunum, whereas sporadic small intestinal lymphomas are predominantly of B-cell origin and occur most often in the ileum. These so-called enteropathy-associated T-cell lymphomas (EATL) presumably arise from intraepithelial-infiltrating lymphocytes, a routine finding in celiac disease patients. Because many patients with mild celiac disease symptoms are not diagnosed, the true prevalence of small intestinal lymphoma in celiac disease is unknown, but risk estimates range from 25 to 120 times that for the general population.[17] The next most common type of malignancy in celiac disease patients is small intestinal adenocarcinoma, occurring at a prevalence 83 times greater than in unaffected patients.[18] The majority of these cancers occur in the jejunum.[17]

A small number of patients have been reported with ileal adenocarcinomas after a long-standing Brooke ileostomy,[19] Kock pouch,[20] or ileal pouch–anal anastomosis[21] following total proctocolectomy. Most of these patients had chronic ulcerative colitis as the reason for their proctocolectomy. The patients with both pouch reconstructions had chronic, severe inflammation of the pouch mucosa.[20,21] In Brooke ileostomy patients, colonic metaplasia and dysplasia have been described as histologic precursors of adenocarcinoma.[19] In patients with FAP and an ileal pouch–anal anastomosis, the probability of an adenomatous polyp in the pouch increases from 7% at 5 years to 75% at 15 years after the operation.[22] Because most of these reports have been published in the last 15 years, ileal cancers following proctocolectomy will likely become a more common problem in the future.

Patients with both inherited forms of immunosuppression (e.g., Wiskott–Aldrich syndrome and ataxia telangiectasia) and acquired immunocompromise, including immunosuppressive treatment for solid organ transplantation and human immunodeficiency virus (HIV) infection, are at significantly higher risk of non-Hodgkin's lymphoma. Extranodal sites, including the gastrointestinal tract, are more common than in patients without immunosuppression. Only a small number of these lymphomas, however, originate in the small intestine.[23]

Basic Science and Pathology

Adenocarcinoma

Although the duodenum makes up only 4% of the total length of the small intestine, 50% of small bowel adenocarcinomas occur there, and more than half of duodenal carcinomas occur in the periampullary region. Bile exposure has been hypothesized as an explanation for this distribution, but this speculation about bile as a carcinogen has not been proven. The proximal duodenum originates from the foregut, whereas the remainder of the small intestine arises from the midgut. This distinction has been hypothesized as another possible cause for the significant difference in cancer prevalence between these parts of the small bowel.[24] Jejunal adenocarcinomas are more common than ileal tumors, but because of similarities between cancers at these two sites and the small numbers at both locations, these malignancies are usually combined in discussions of small bowel carcinoma.

In the colon cancer adenoma–carcinoma sequence, early mutations usually occur in the APC and cyclooxygenase (COX-2) genes, with subsequent mutations in K-*ras*, SMAD4, DCC, and P53 genes being commonplace. Another pathway, seen in patients with HNPCC, involves DNA mismatch repair enzyme gene mutations (mismatch repair or MMR phenotype). Many of the later genetic alterations seen in the first pathway also occur in HNPCC patients. The published data on genetic mutations in small bowel carcinomas are sparse because of the rarity of these tumors. A recent summary of published data showed no one mutation present in more than 45% of tumors and some possible differences in the genetic mutation pathways leading to malignant transformation in duodenal and jejunuoileal carcinomas[24] (Table 43.1). One small study analyzing 12 duodenal cancers found a clear distinction in gene mutations between tumors following the classic adenoma–carcinoma pathway and those with an MMR phenotype,[25] but this has not been a consistent finding. In a recent study of 35 small bowel cancers (12 duodenal, 23 jejunal or ileal), 40% overexpressed P53 protein whereas only 9% of tumors had a mutation at codon 12 in

TABLE 43.1. Prevalence of genetic mutations in small bowel adenocarcinomas.

	Gene mutation (n)				
Tumor location	*APC*	*K-ras*	*p53*	*DCC*	*MMR*
Duodenum	18% (32)	34% (38)	32% (41)	9% (32)	15% (20)
Jejunum/ileum	6% (35)	25% (43)	44% (36)	6% (35)	37% (8)

APC, adenomatous polyposis coli; DCC, detected in colon cancer; MMR, mismatch repair.
Source: Data from Hutchins et al.[24]

the K-*ras* gene. The latter finding led the authors to conclude that the adenoma–carcinoma sequence was not of great importance in the development of most small bowel tumors.[26] Other reports have shown strong COX-2 expression and high levels of other eicosanoid production enzymes in most small bowel cancers[27] and frequent 18q chromosomal deletions that result in SMAD4 mutations.[28] These findings support a molecular pathway similar to that noted in large bowel tumor development. In another report,[29] among 89 small intestine adenocarcinomas studied, 16 (18%) showed microsatellite instability, an indicator of MMR phenotype. MLH1 mutations were the cause of these abnormalities in about half the patients, with MSH2 mutations accounting for most of the remaining MMR mutations in younger patients.[29] This prevalence of MMR abnormalities is similar to that found in colorectal cancer patients. We have recently found replication errors to be significantly more common in small bowel adenocarcinomas arising in patients with celiac disease compared to sporadic small intestinal cancers.[29a] More genetic analyses on larger numbers of tumors are needed to better clarify the prevalence and types of genetic alterations that occur in small intestinal adenocarcinomas.

Lymphoma

The gastrointestinal tract is the most common site of extranodal lymphomas, with the stomach being involved most commonly (approximately two-thirds of primary gastrointestinal lymphomas) and the small intestine and colon having similar numbers of tumors.[30] Although many advanced-stage nodal lymphomas involve the gastrointestinal tract, primary intestinal lymphomas can be distinguished by the absence of peripheral or mediastinal adenopathy, a normal peripheral blood smear and bone marrow biopsy, and a primary tumor of the bowel with or without mesenteric nodal involvement.[31] The majority of intestinal lymphomas in the United States are non-Hodgkin's lymphomas of B-cell origin and occur most commonly in the ileum, less frequently in the jejunum, and least often in the duodenum. This distribution correlates with the amount of mucosal-associated lymphoid tissue (MALT) in the different parts of the small intestine. Table 43.2 outlines the classification system for gastrointestinal non-Hodgkin's lymphomas.[32]

The predominant type of small bowel lymphoma differs significantly from one part of the world to another. In the Western world, high-grade MALT lymphomas are the most common histologic type of lymphoma in adults. Although gastric low-grade MALT lymphomas usually occur with *Helicobacter pylori* infestation and regress with treatment that eliminates this bacterium, no link with *H. pylori* infection has been determined for small intestinal lymphoma. In children in both the West and parts of the Middle East, Burkitt's-like lymphomas of the ileocecal region are the most common form of intestinal lymphoma.[32] Around the Mediterranean Sea and, less commonly, in the rest of Africa, Eastern Asia, and Latin America, a very different MALT-type lymphoma is the most common intestinal lymphoma. Immunoproliferative small intestinal disease (IPSID) is a disease of younger persons (peak incidences in the second and third decades), usually in poorer socioeconomic classes, that involves the jejunum most often but in later stages causes diffuse disease of the small intestine. Because of the epicenter of the disease

TABLE 43.2. Classification of primary gastrointestinal non-Hodgkin's lymphomas.

B-cell
Mucosa-associated lymphoid tissue (MALT) type
Low-grade
High-grade ± low-grade component
Immunoproliferative small intestinal disease (IPSID)
Low-grade
High-grade ± low-grade component
Mantel-cell (lymphomatous polyposis)
Burkitt's-like and Burkitt's
Other lymphomas corresponding to lymph node equivalents
T-cell
Enteropathy-associated T-cell lymphoma (EATL)
Non-EATL

Source: Data from Isaacson.[32]

and the usual detection of an alpha heavy-chain protein, IPSID has also been termed Mediterranean lymphoma or alpha heavy-chain disease. In the earliest stage of IPSID, the tumor often responds to treatment with broad-spectrum antibiotics, consistent with a benign immunoproliferative disorder arising in response to bacterial flora antigen(s). Over time, the malignant centrocytic-like cells that are initially confined to the bowel and regional lymph nodes spread to distant sites. Progression of IPSID carries a poorer prognosis and requires chemotherapy for treatment.[33] In countries where celiac disease is common (e.g., the United Kingdom), up to a third of small intestinal lymphomas are of T-cell origin, so-called enteropathy-associated T-cell lymphomas (EATL).[34] The link between celiac disease and EATL has long been suspected, but only recently have molecular studies clearly shown these conditions to be related. Patients with celiac disease have a chronic inflammatory infiltration of the small bowel mucosa that generally improves with a gluten-free diet. Patients who no longer respond to a gluten-free diet have refractory sprue, and their involved mucosa contains a monoclonal T-cell population, a finding that is also present in ulcerative jejunitis, another complication of celiac disease. These monoclonal T-cell populations have been shown to be clonally identical to those found in subsequent EATLs.[35] Patients with refractory sprue and ulcerative jejunitis require chemotherapy for their neoplastic T-cell disease.

Multiple lymphomatous polyposis (MLP) of the gastrointestinal tract is a rare lymphoma that presents with multiple polyps located anywhere from the stomach to the rectum, with small bowel involvement in almost all patients. A bulky tumor mass is often present and occurs most commonly in the ileocecal region. Given the histologic, immunohistochemical, and molecular characteristics of MLP, it is considered the gastrointestinal form of mantle cell lymphoma, a more indolent form of lymphoma.[36] Follicular lymphoma, a common type of non-Hodgkin's nodal lymphoma (NHL), rarely occurs in the small intestine. The distal ileum is the most common site within the bowel. The histologic appearance, surface markers, and molecular changes [increased BCL-2 expression caused by a t(14:18) involving the BCL-2 and immunoglobulin heavy-chain loci] are comparable to nodal follicular lymphomas. The intestinal form of follicular lymphoma rarely spreads to sites away from the gastrointestinal tract. These lymphomas appear to arise from a mucosal population of B cells.[37,38] Hodgkin's disease is also a common form of nodal lymphoma and the bowel is often involved in advanced stages of disease; however, primary gastrointestinal Hodgkin's disease is very uncommon. Many intestinal Hodgkin's disease cases have arisen in patients with chronic inflammatory bowel disease treated with immunosuppressive medications. The tumor cells demonstrate infection with Epstein–Barr virus, the likely stimulus for lymphoproliferation in this unusual disease.[39]

Gastrointestinal Stromal Tumors

Gastrointestinal stromal tumor (GIST) is the most common type of mesenchymal tumor of the small intestine. The prevalence of this neoplasm in the different parts of the small bowel is proportional to the length of these segments, with most occurring in the jejunum, the next largest number in the ileum, and the fewest in the duodenum.[40] Once classified as smooth muscle tumors and called leiomyomas or leiomyosarcomas depending on whether they histologically appeared benign or malignant, GIST are now thought to arise from the interstitial cell of Cajal (pacemaker cell of the gut) or a pluripotential stem cell.[41] GIST generally express CD117 (KIT, a tyrosine kinase receptor for stem cell factor) and have either a spindle cell or epithelioid histologic pattern. Mutations in exon 11 (and rarely either exon 9 or exon 13) of the c-*kit* gene are common in GIST. These mutations are generally activation mutations and are thought to be the molecular cause for tumorigenesis in GIST.[41] A recent evaluation of nearly 300 GIST revealed differences in surface marker expression between sites in the gastrointestinal tract. CD34 (a hematopoietic progenitor cell antigen) is present in only half of small intestinal GIST but approximately 90% of gastric GIST. Small bowel GIST are slightly more likely to stain for smooth muscle actin and S100 protein than gastric GIST, but tumor cells at both sites rarely express desmin.[42] GIST with benign and malignant behavior both have similar DNA losses, including deletions in chromosomes 14q and 22q, but DNA copy gains are seen predominantly in malignant GIST. Specific tumor suppressor gene loss and oncogene activation mutations responsible for GIST development, and different biologic behaviors have as yet not been identified.[41]

Prognostic Factors

As with most adult cancers, stage is the strongest predictor of survival for small bowel adenocarcinomas. The most recent American Joint Commission on Cancer Staging System for Small Bowel Carcinomas (sixth edition) is shown in Table 43.3.[43] The largest reported series of almost 5,000 small bowel adenocarcinomas treated between 1985 and 1995 in the United States was retrieved from the National Cancer Data Base.[44] In this publication, higher tumor stage, patient age greater than 75 years, and duodenal origin were adverse predictors of disease-specific survival using multivariate analysis. Figure 43.1 shows the survival curves of patients by tumor stage with 5-year disease-specific survivals of 65%, 48%, 35% and 4% for stages I, II, III, and IV, respectively. In Figure 43.2, the outcomes of jejunal and ileal adenocarcinoma patients are seen as essentially identical (both 38% 5-year disease-specific survival) and significantly better than duodenal adenocarcinomas (28% 5-year disease-specific survival; *P* less than 0.0001).[44] Tumor grade, when comparing poorly dif-

TABLE 43.3. American Joint Committee on Cancer (AJCC) staging for small intestinal cancers.

Primary tumor (T)	
TX	Primary tumor cannot be assessed
T0	No evidence of primary tumor
Tis	Carcinoma in situ
T1	Tumor invades lamina propria or submucosa
T2	Tumor invades muscularis propria
T3	Tumor invades through muscularis propria into the subserosa or into the nonperitonealized perimuscular tissue (mesentery or retroperitoneum) with extension 2 cm or less[a]
T4	Tumor perforates visceral peritoneum or directly invades other organs or structures (includes other loops of small intestine, mesentery, or retroperitoneum more than 2 cm, and abdominal wall by way of serosa; for duodenum only, invasion of pancreas)
Regional lymph nodes (N)	
NX	Regional lymph nodes cannot be assessed
N0	No regional lymph node metastasis
N1	Regional lymph node metastasis
Distant metastases (M)	
MX	Distant metastasis cannot be assessed
M0	No distant metastasis
M1	Distant metastasis

[a] The nonperitonealized perimuscular tissue is, for jejunum and ileum, part of the mesentery and, for duodenum in areas where serosa is lacking, part of the retroperitoneum.

Stage grouping			
0	Tis	N0	M0
I	T1/2	N0	M0
II	T3/4	N0	M0
III	Any T	N1	M0
IV	Any T	Any N	M1

Used with the permission of the American Joint Committee on Cancer (AJCC), Chicago, Illinois. The original source for this material is the *AJCC Cancer Staging Manual*, sixth edition (2002), published by Springer-Verlag New York, www.springer-ny.com.

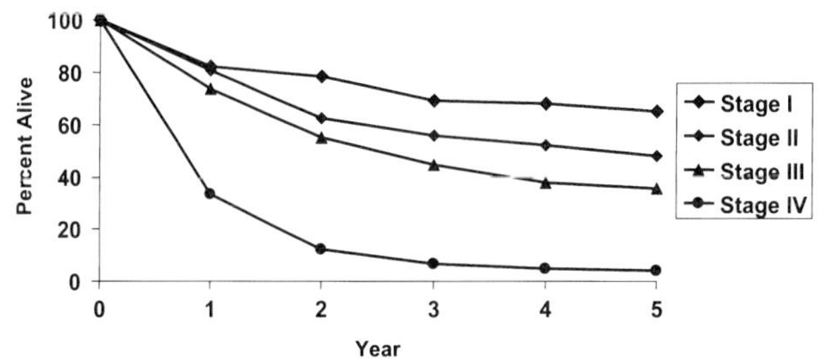

AJCC Stage	1	2	3	4	5	95% CI s	Median	Cases
Stage I	82.4	78.7	69.4	68.0	65.1	54.7-75.5	> 60	96
Stage II	80.9	62.7	56.1	52.2	48.1	38.8-57.4	54.5	138
Stage III	73.7	55.1	44.7	37.8	35.4	26.0-44.7	29.8	129
Stage IV	33.5	12.2	6.7	5.0	4.2	0.8-7.6	9.0	188

FIGURE 43.1. Patient survival for small bowel adenocarcinoma by tumor stage. Data from the National Cancer Data Base (NCDB). (From Howe et al.,[44] by permission of *Cancer*.)

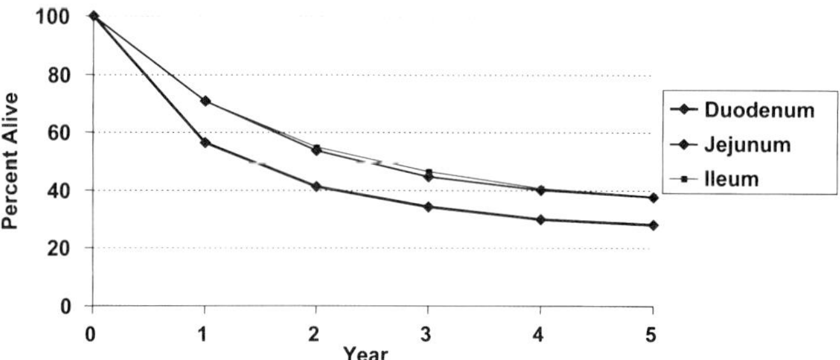

Site	1	2	3	4	5	95% CI s	Median	Cases
Duodenum	56.3	41.1	34.0	29.9	28.2	25.1-31.2	16.9	1006
Jejunum	70.6	53.8	44.4	40.0	37.6	32.0-43.1	28.9	335
Ileum	70.6	54.9	46.2	40.5	37.8	31.0-44.6	30.8	246

FIGURE 43.2. Patient survival for adenocarcinomas of the duodenum, jejunum, and ileum. The difference in outcome for duodenal cancer patients compared to the other two sites was highly significant ($P < 0.0001$). Data from the NCDB. (From Howe et al.,[44] by permission of *Cancer*.)

ferentiated tumors with either moderately or well-differentiated adenocarcinomas, revealed a significant survival difference, whereas the latter two tumor grades had similar survivals.[44] Other much smaller patient series[45,46] have also found grade to be a significant predictor of patient outcome, but only in univariate analysis. Vascular invasion and incomplete excision have also been reported as adverse prognostic indicators,[46,47] but these studies lack multivariate analysis and significant patient numbers. No molecular markers have been reported as prognostic indicators for patients with small intestinal adenocarcinomas.

Extranodal lymphomas have traditionally been staged using a modification of the Ann Arbor system.[48] As reformulated by Musshoff in 1977, this nomenclature included designations for extranodal origin (E) and subcategories of regional nodal involvement for mesenteric and paraaortic locations (stages IIE1 and IIE2, respectively).[49] Within the past decade, a new staging system has been proposed.[50] These three systems for staging gastrointestinal lymphomas are displayed in Table 43.4.[48–50] In the latest staging system, the E designation has returned to the original meaning within the Ann Arbor classification, namely, extension to an adjacent structure, rather than extranodal disease in general. Stage III has been eliminated and is included with stage IV. The stage of disease at presentation has routinely been found to be a significant prognostic factor for small intestinal lymphomas.[30,34,51–54]

Other adverse prognostic factors have been described for small intestinal lymphomas. In general, T-cell lymphomas have a worse prognosis than B-cell phenotypes.[34,49,54] Older patient age,[52,54] B symptoms,[54] perforation,[34,52] and multifocal disease[34,52] have all been reported as adverse prognostic indicators. Higher-grade lesions have been found to have poorer outcome in some studies,[34,50] but stage and other variables have not always been accounted for in these analyses.

There is currently no formal staging system for GIST. Because lymph node metastases are very uncommon, GIST presents with either localized disease or distant metastases (most commonly liver, lung, or bone). Not surprisingly, patients with localized GIST have better survival than those who present with metastatic disease. In an effort to classify primary GIST by their risk of metastasis, pathologists sepa-

TABLE 43.4. Gastrointestinal lymphoma staging systems.

Modified Ann Arbor[48]		*Musshoff*[49]		*Rohatiner*[50]	
IE	Single GI focus only	IE	GI tumor alone	I	GI tumor alone
IIE	GI focus, nodal involvement on one side diaphragm	IIE_1	GI tumor and regional nodal involvement (i.e. mesentery celiac)	II	Tumor involving other abdominal structures
IIIE	GI focus, nodal involvement on both sides of diaphragm involvement (paraaortic)	IIE_2	GI tumor and extraregional subdiaphragmatic nodal	II_1 II_2	Local nodes (i.e., para-intestinal) Distant nodes (i.e. mesenteric paraaortic)
IIIES	Spleen involved	IIIE	GI tumor and nodal involvement on both sides of the diaphragm	IIE	Penetration of serosa with adjacent organ involvement [If both nodes and organ involved, each is noted (i.e., II_1E pancreas)]
IVE	GI focus, disseminated extranodal site(s) involvement (e.g. bone marrow, liver)	IVE	GI tumor with other extranodal site(s) of involvement (i.e., bone marrow, liver)	IV	GI tumor with supradiaphragmatic nodal or disseminated extranodal involvement
GI, gastrointestinal; E, extranodal.		GI, gastrointestinal; E, extranodal.		GI, gastrointestinal; E, extension to adjacent structures.	

rate them into low-risk and high-risk categories. The criteria used for this distinction include tumor diameter (less than 5 cm versus 5 cm and more), mitotic rate [fewer than 2 mitoses/10 high-power fields (hpf) versus 2 or more mitoses/hpf], and the proliferation index (10% or less versus more than 10%). Low-risk tumors include those that are less than 5 cm with fewer than 2 mitoses/hpf and tumors that are either 5 cm or more in diameter or have 2 or more mitoses/hpf with a proliferation index of 10% or less. High-risk GIST have both larger size and higher mitotic index, or either of these factors plus a proliferation index greater than 10%.[55] Tumor size has consistently been a predictor of patient outcome both when evaluating smooth muscle tumors of the gastrointestinal tract[40,56] and with analysis of only GIST.[57,58]

Some low-risk GIST do metastasize. Recent findings of activation mutations in the KIT gene seem to correlate with malignant behavior in GIST. About 40% to 50% of GIST, most with a malignant phenotype, have a missense mutation in the juxtamembrane portion of the KIT molecule (exon 11), and the presence of this mutation correlates with poor prognosis.[59,60] New mutational hot spots have recently been detected in tumors lacking a mutation in exon 11. These mutations localized to exons 9 and 13 of KIT have occurred uncommonly (less than 10%) in the GIST screened and correlate with malignant tumor behavior.[61] Mutations in exon 9 were seen mostly in small bowel GIST in one report,[61] whereas this correlation did not occur in a second study.[62] The number of DNA sequence copy number changes[57] and loss of $p16^{INK4}$ protein expression in GIST have also been correlated with poorer patient outcome. Other still undiscovered mutations activating KIT or having another effect on GIST behavior are likely to exist and will impact on tumor biology.

Diagnosis

Small intestinal malignancies do not produce any specific symptoms or signs, with the exception of carcinoid tumors. Because of their insidious presentation and the inability to directly visualize most tumors, the diagnosis of small bowel cancer is often delayed. Compounding this problem is the frequent cessation of the diagnostic evaluation of the gastrointestinal tract once the large bowel, esophagus, and stomach have been deemed normal. In patients with evidence of gastrointestinal blood loss, partial bowel obstruction, or both, the workup is never complete until the small intestine has also been fully evaluated for a source of these abnormalities. The presence of a genetic mutation or inflammatory bowel disease that places a patient at higher risk for these rare tumors (see section on Etiology) should only heighten the clinician's level of suspicion. In FAP patients, the duodenum should be routinely screened for polyps to prevent malignant degeneration and to detect duodenal cancers at an earlier stage.

Abdominal pain, ranging from a vague, dull discomfort to diffuse, acute signs of peritonitis, when a bowel perforation has occurred, is the most common symptom of small bowel malignancy. Up to 30% of small bowel lymphomas present with a surgical emergency. Progressive cramping pain with nausea, vomiting, and change in bowel habits caused by a partial luminal obstruction occurs frequently. Blood loss is usually occult and chronic in nature, but may be clinically apparent and massive, especially in a patient with a GIST. Symptoms of malabsorption, especially in a patient with celiac disease, may be a sign of lymphoma. Periampullary duodenal cancers, especially adenocarcinomas, may initially present as obstructive jaundice. Jaundice can also occur with extensive hepatic involvement from small intestinal adenocarcinoma or GIST. As with any other primary cancer, weight loss, evidence of malnourishment, and decreased performance status are commonly the result of advanced disease.[63]

Most duodenal adenocarcinomas occur within the first two portions of the duodenum and are detected during the course of a routine upper endoscopy. All duodenal neoplasms and some proximal jejunal cancers can be visualized with an extended upper endoscopy using a standard endoscope or colonoscope. More extensive direct visualization of the small intestinal mucosa can be accomplished with push or Sonde enteroscopy.[64,65] Intraoperative or laparoscopic enteroscopy are also options, but most small bowel malignancies are apparent with visual inspection and palpation at laparoscopy or laparotomy, making these diagnostic tools of less value than with benign small bowel pathology. Compared to radiographic studies of the small bowel, endoscopy offers the advantage of pathologic sampling of any abnormality that can be visualized.

A plain film of the abdomen will rarely provide a diagnosis, but findings that may lead to the diagnosis of a small bowel malignancy include air–fluid levels indicative of a partial bowel obstruction plus a proximal or distal location, a mass effect from a large lymphoma or GIST, and calcifications within a GIST. Because many small bowel tumors are inaccessible to endoscopy, contrast radiography continues to have a role in their diagnosis. Standard barium upper gastrointestinal series with small bowel follow-through will detect an abnormality in one-half to three-quarters of malignant tumors, but only 30% to 40% will show direct evidence of the cancer.[66] Enteroclysis has been shown to have a higher detection rate for several small bowel pathologies, including malignancies. In one comparison of enteroclysis and small bowel follow-through, enteroclysis had a sensitivity of 95% and detection rate of 90% compared to a sensitivity of 61% and tumor detection of 33% for small bowel follow-through.[67]

If a patient has a palpable tumor or evidence of a small bowel malignancy is detected on a contrast study, two-dimensional imaging is usually obtained to better define the site, local extent of the primary neoplasm, and evidence of regional or distant metastases. Although computerized tomography (CT) is more commonly utilized, magnetic resonance imaging (MRI) can be more accurate, especially in patients with a high-grade bowel obstruction where luminal contrast cannot be used. A recent study comparing MRI and helical CT scans in patients with bowel obstruction showed the sensitivity, specificity, and accuracy of MRI (95%, 100%, and 96%, respectively) to be superior to helical CT scan (71%, 71%, and 71%, respectively).[68]

Although not all small intestinal malignancies can be differentiated by their radiographic characteristics, many can be distinguished from one another based on the radiologic findings. Adenocarcinomas most commonly cause a discrete "apple core" lesion on both contrast and cross-sectional imaging studies (Figure 43.3). This stricture is usually rigid, whereas strictures from lymphoma and GIST may alter on

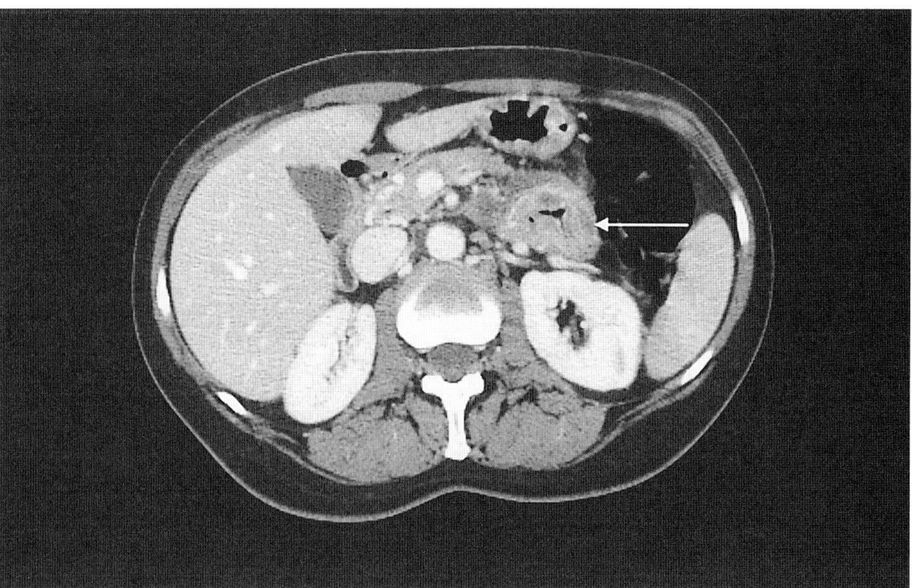

FIGURE 43.3. Computed tomography (CT) image showing tumor mass and luminal narrowing (apple-core lesion) of an adenocarcinoma of the fourth portion of the duodenum.

fluoroscopic imaging with compression. A polypoid intraluminal mass most commonly occurs with a duodenal adenocarcinoma, although more distal polypoid small bowel cancers can present with intussusception. Large high-grade carcinomas may ulcerate and be difficult to distinguish from other small intestinal cancer, especially lymphomas. The cross-sectional images should be assessed for growth into adjacent structures, regional adenopathy, peritoneal seeding, and hepatic metastases. Small bowel lymphomas can be multicentric, but most commonly they present as a segmental infiltrating mass that markedly thickens the bowel wall and often has aneurysmal dilatation of the intestinal lumen (Figure 43.4). Regional lymph nodes are commonly enlarged in lymphoma patients and may form a bulky mass of matted nodes with secondary involvement of small intestinal loops. Small intestinal GIST are generally discrete, round or lobulated, solitary tumors. Larger GIST often have heterogeneous contrast uptake and may display central necrosis, sometimes with calcifications (Figure 43.5). Large GIST show a predominant exenteric growth pattern, but some GIST have predominantly an endoenteric location. The latter growth pattern causes an eccentric stricture of the bowel lumen with or without ulceration that can frequently be demonstrated on either contrast or cross-sectional images.[66,69]

Recently, use of a miniature video capsule for diagnosing occult small bowel pathology has been reported.[70] This technology provides frequent, but not continuous, imaging of the entire bowel. The capsule cannot control its orientation during passage through the gastrointestinal tract. Although this technology will continue to improve and provide a diagnosis in subtle and early-stage small intestinal neoplasms, because most small bowel cancers present at a size amenable to detection with standard imaging, its role may remain a limited one for these tumors.

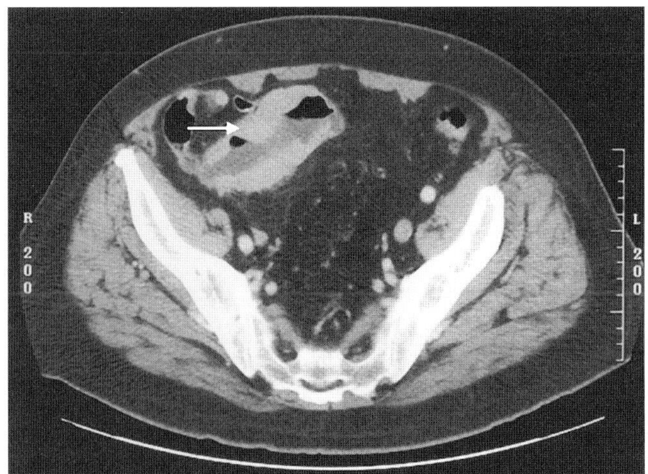

FIGURE 43.4. CT image of an ileal B-cell lymphoma with segmental thickening of bowel wall and aneurysmal dilatation of the bowel lumen.

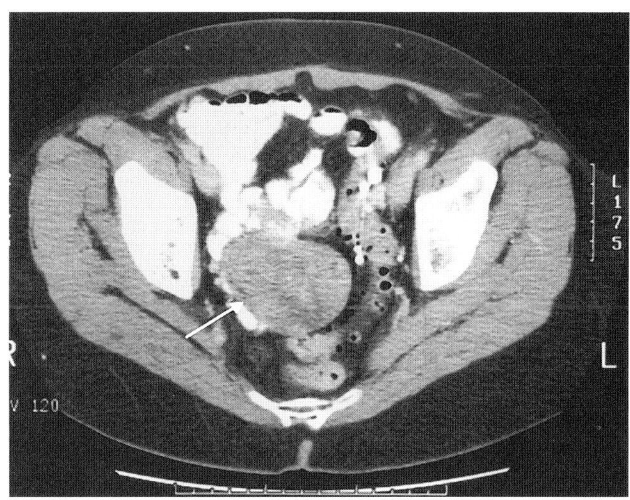

FIGURE 43.5. CT image of jejunal gastrointestinal stromal tumor (GIST) with predominant exenteric growth pattern and heterogeneous vascularity of tumor mass.

Treatment

Adenocarcinoma

Small bowel adenocarcinomas are best treated surgically with a segmental bowel resection and removal of the regional lymph nodes most likely to be involved by metastases (Table 43.5). In the jejunum and all but the terminal ileum, the optimal operative procedure consists of removal of a wide margin (more than 10 cm proximally and distally) of adjacent bowel and mesentery with a primary anastomosis. All clinically involved mesenteric lymph nodes should be removed with the cancer, but the proximal mesenteric resection is limited by the superior mesenteric vessels. Any structure adherent to the primary cancer should be resected en bloc when a curative operation is possible. For cancers of the terminal ileum, a right colectomy should be performed to remove the draining lymph nodes along the ileocolic vessels. Among 779 jejunal and 602 ileal carcinomas included in the National Cancer Data Base review, approximately 90% underwent some type of resection (curative operations were not distinguished from noncurative procedures).[44]

Invasive duodenal adenocarcinomas of the periampullary region can only be cured by a pancreaticoduodenectomy. Villous adenomas of the duodenum, especially those presenting with jaundice or other signs of malignancy, are more prone to contain malignancy. The sensitivity of endoscopic biopsy for malignancy in these polyps can be as low as 50%, making a pancreaticoduodenectomy, especially for periampullary tumors, the best operative choice.[71,72] For distal duodenal tumors, the lymphatic drainage includes lymph nodes along the superior mesenteric vessels that are not included in a standard pancreaticoduodenectomy. Although several older papers[73,74] advocated pancreaticoduodenectomy for all duodenal adenocarcinomas, more-recent publications[75–78] have found equally good outcomes with segmental duodenectomy for distal duodenal adenocarcinomas. In individual institutional reports of duodenal carcinomas,[75,76,79–81] the resectability rates of patients surgically explored range from 53% to 87%, and 5-year survivals for curatively resected patients are between 45% and 60%. Data from the National Cancer Data Base for 1,425 duodenal carcinomas indicated only 52% of patients had some type of cancer resection.[44]

At the present time, no adjuvant therapy can be recommended based on objective data for small intestinal adenocarcinomas. Similarities between small and large bowel adenocarcinomas have led some investigators to treat small bowel cancers with chemotherapy regimens of benefit in colon carcinoma, such as 5-fluorouracil and leucovorin. No controlled data exist showing an impact of these treatments in small intestinal cancers. Similarly, patients with duodenal cancers requiring pancreaticoduodenectomy are commonly recommended for adjuvant chemoradiation therapy,[82] although no significant survival benefit has been apparent in retrospective reports.[76,81] No major clinical trials looking at adjuvant or palliative treatment in small bowel adenocarci-

TABLE 43.5. Summary of small intestinal cancers.

Small intestinal cancers are rare.	
Etiology	
Inherited:	Familial adenomatous polyposis (FAP), hereditary nonpolyposis colorectal carcinoma (HNPCC), Peutz–Jeghers— adenocarcinoma
Inflammation:	Crohn's disease—adenocarcinoma (lymphoma)
	Celiac disease—T-cell lymphoma (adenocarcinoma)
Immunosuppression:	Wiskcott–Aldrich syndrome, organ transplantation, human immunodeficiency (HIV) lymphoma
Basic science/pathology	
Adenocarcinoma:	Most common in duodenum, least frequent in ileum
	Adenoma–carcinoma sequence and mismatch repair (MMR) pathways
Lymphoma:	Most common in ileum, least common in duodenum
	Most B-cell non-Hodgkin's lymphoma (NHL) of mucosal-associated lymphoid tissue (MALT) origin
	T-cell lymphoma in celiac disease
GIST:	Most common in jejunum, less in ileum, least frequent in duodenum
	Express CD117 (KIT) and most have c-kit activation mutations
Prognosis	
Tumor stage most important	
Adenocarcinoma:	TNM staging, duodenal tumors poorer outcome
Lymphoma:	Modified Ann Arbor and other staging systems
	T-cell lymphoma poor outcome
GIST:	No definite staging system
	Metastasis implies poor outcome
Diagnosis	
GI source of pathology not excluded without evaluating small bowel	
Duodenum, proximal jejunum–extended upper endoscopy	
Most jejunum, ileum–enteroclysis, enteroscopy, video capsule	
CT/MR scan to stage disease	
Treatment	
Adenocarcinoma:	Segmental resection of bowel and adjacent lymph nodes
	(Whipple for periampullary duodenal cancers)
	Colon carcinoma chemotherapy
Lymphoma:	Resection of primary tumor to prevent complications
	Combination chemotherapy dependent on histology
GIST:	Resection primary tumor (lymphadenectomy unnecessary)
	Imitinab for metastatic tumors that express KIT

noma are currently under way, in large part because of the rarity of this condition.

Lymphoma

Because patients with gastrointestinal lymphomas amenable to complete gross resection more often survive than those with unresected lymphoma,[83,84] many surgeons continue to recommend operative intervention for all early-stage lymphomas.[85] Experience with gastric lymphomas treated with primary chemotherapy and consolidation radiation therapy, when indicated, provides comparable survival to patients initially treated with resection and later with chemotherapy. Despite concerns about hemorrhage and perforation with primary chemotherapy in gastrointestinal lymphomas, very few patients with gastric lymphoma need any surgical treatment.[86,87] Because small intestinal lymphomas are even rarer than gastric lymphomas, no controlled or even large-scale uncontrolled data exist comparing primary surgical and neoadjuvant therapy of these cancers. Most recent reports on small intestinal lymphoma[88–90] have recommended combination therapy with surgical removal of all disease when feasible and multidrug chemotherapy dependent on the tumor histology. Some data indicate a trend toward treatment without operative intervention. In one study,[89] a complete remission rate of nearly 50% was noted with chemotherapy in advanced-stage (stage IV) small bowel lymphoma patients, irrespective of whether initial debulking was performed. In another study,[88] early-stage (stages I and II) patients had similar complete rates of response, survival, and disease-free survival regardless of whether complete resection, limited tumor removal, or no resection was performed.

At present, most clinicians still recommend complete tumor removal in early-stage disease when feasible, to avoid tumor perforation or obstruction, and selective surgical intervention for advanced-stage small intestinal lymphomas. All patients except those with low-grade lymphomas limited to the submucosa should be considered for postoperative combination chemotherapy.[89] For intermediate- and high-grade lymphomas, CHOP (cyclophosphamide, doxorubicin, vincristine, and prednisone) remains the treatment of choice. For indolent lymphomas, such as mantle cell and follicular lymphomas, the anti-CD20 antibody rituximab has shown excellent promise in enhancing the response to chemotherapy.[85] Intestinal T-cell lymphomas are generally unresponsive to traditional combination chemotherapy and have a significantly worse prognosis compared to B-cell non-Hodgkin's lymphomas.[91] Lymphomas associated with HIV infection generally have a poor prognosis due to treatment- and underlying disease-related complications plus low complete response rates with standard chemotherapy.[92] Although radiation therapy has been recommended for bulky and advanced-stage lymphomas, the incidence of complications is high for gastrointestinal lymphomas,[85] and many advanced-stage patients do not survive long enough to receive treatment.[91] In general, 5-year disease-free survival for small intestinal lymphomas is approximately 50% to 70% following combination therapy.[85]

Gastrointestinal Stromal Tumors

Complete surgical excision of GIST is the treatment of choice. In most portions of the small intestine, this involves a segmental bowel resection with en bloc excision of any adherent structures, but not extensive removal of the mesentery, because nodal metastases are uncommon. Duodenal GIST, especially of the proximal duodenum, may require pancreaticoduodenectomy to achieve complete removal, although segmental resection may be feasible if the GIST does not involve the periampullary region and clear margins can be achieved with a less-extensive excision. If all tumor is removed, the 5-year survival rate ranges from 50% to 65%.[93] Palliative tumor resection is indicated in metastatic GIST, especially with hemorrhage or perforation.

Following complete tumor removal, local recurrence and peritoneal and hepatic metastases are the most common types of tumor recurrence,[94] at a median time of 20 months.[95] Up to one-third of patients with recurrent GIST are amenable to total removal of recurrent tumor, but the median survival following a second operation is only 15 months with no further treatment. Patients with isolated hepatic metastases have the longest survival.[95] Postoperative intraperitoneal mitoxantrone appears to reduce the prevalence of peritoneal recurrence but has no impact on the development of hepatic metastases following recurrent GIST excision.[96]

GIST have been notoriously resistant to conventional chemotherapy and radiation therapy. In the recent past, imatinib mesylate, a competitive inhibitor of several tyrosine kinases, including c-*kit*, c-ABL, and platelet-derived growth factor receptor, has been shown to be an effective treatment for metastatic and unresectable GIST. In a Phase II trial of 147 patients, 38% had a partial tumor response (greater than 50% tumor volume reduction), and the U.S. Food and Drug Administration approved imatinib mesylate for use in the treatment of patients with advanced GIST.[97] From data presented in two recent publications,[98,99] it appears that GIST with activating mutations of KIT at exon 11 respond best to imatinib mesylate (83.5% partial response rate, compared to 48% with KIT mutations in exon 9). No responses were seen in 9 patients without detectable KIT or platelet-derived growth factor receptor alpha mutations.[99] Two Phase III trials evaluating the impact of imitinab in metastatic GIST have been completed, but the results have not been published yet. A third prospective, randomized study of the effect of adjuvant imitinab in high-risk primary GIST following complete resection is currently under way.

References

1. Jemal A, Murray T, Samuels A, et al. Cancer statistics, 2003. Ca Cancer J Clin 2003;53:5–26.
2. Cooper MJ, Williamson RC. Enteric adenoma and adenocarcinoma. World J Surg 1985;9:914–920.
3. Sellner F. Investigations on the significance of the adenoma-carcinoma sequence in the small bowel. Cancer (Phila) 1990; 66:701–715.
4. Jones TR, Nance FC. Periampullary malignancy in Gardner's syndrome. Ann Surg 1977;185:565–573.
5. Jagelman DG, DeCosse JJ, Bussey HJ. Upper gastrointestinal cancer in familial adenomatous polyposis. Lancet 1988; 1:1149–1151.
6. Lynch HT, Smyrk TC, Lynch PM, et al. Adenocarcinoma of the small bowel in lynch syndrome II. Cancer (Phila) 1989;64: 2178–2183.
7. Vasen HF, den Hartog Jager FC, Menko FH, Nagengast FM. Screening for hereditary non-polyposis colorectal cancer: a study of 22 kindreds in The Netherlands. Am J Med 1989;86:278–281.

8. Rodriguez-Bigas MA, Vasen HF, Lynch HT, et al. Characteristics of small bowel carcinoma in hereditary nonpolyposis colorectal carcinoma. International Collaborative Group on HNPCC. Cancer (Phila) 1998;83:240–244.
9. Westerman AM, Entius MM, de Baar E, et al. Peutz–Jeghers syndrome: 78-year follow-up of the original family. Lancet 1999; 353:1211s–1215s.
10. Dozois RR, Judd ES, Dahlin DC, Bartholomew LG. The Peutz–Jeghers syndrome: is there a predisposition to the development of intestinal malignancy? Arch Surg 1969;98:509–517.
11. Giardiello FM, Welsh SB, Hamilton SR, et al. Increased risk of cancer in the Peutz–Jeghers syndrome. N Engl J Med 1987; 316:1511–1514.
12. Perzin KH, Bridge MF. Adenomatous and carcinomatous changes in hamartomatous polyps of the small intestine (Peutz–Jeghers syndrome): report of a case and review of the literature. Cancer (Phila) 1982;49:971–983.
13. Hemminki A. The molecular basis and clinical aspects of Peutz–Jeghers syndrome. Cell Mol Life Sci 1999;55:735–750.
14. Hawker PC, Gyde SN, Thompson H, Allan RN. Adenocarcinoma of the small intestine complicating Crohn's disease. Gut 1982;23:188–193.
15. Senay E, Sachar DB, Keohane M, Greenstein AJ. Small bowel carcinoma in Crohn's disease. Distinguishing features and risk factors. Cancer (Phila) 1989;63:360–363.
16. Ribeiro MB, Greenstein AJ, Heimann TM, et al. Adenocarcinoma of the small intestine in Crohn's disease. Surg Gynecol Obstet 1991;173:343–349.
17. Green PH, Jabri B. Celiac disase and other precursors to small-bowel malignancy. Gastroenterol Clin N Am 2002;31:625–639.
18. Swinson CM, Slavin G, Coles EC, Booth CC. Coeliac disease and malignancy. Lancet 1983;1:111–115.
19. Gadacz TR, McFadden DW, Gabrielson EW, et al. Adenocarcinoma of the ileostomy: the latent risk of cancer after colectomy for ulcerative colitis and familial polyposis. Surgery (St. Louis) 1990;107:698–703.
20. Cox CL, Butts DR, Roberts MP, et al. Development of invasive adenocarcinoma in a long-standing Kock continent ileostomy: report of a case. Dis Colon Rectum 1997;40:500–503.
21. Heuschen UA, Heuschen G, Autschbach F, et al. Adenocarcinoma in the ileal pouch: late risk of cancer after restorative proctocolectomy. Int J Colorectal Dis 2001;16:126–130.
22. Parc YR, Olschwang S, Desaint B, et al. Familial adenomatous polyposis: prevalence of adenomas in the ileal pouch after restorative proctocolectomy. Ann Surg 2001;233:360–364.
23. Karp JE, Broder S. Acquired immunodeficiency syndrome and non-Hodgkin's lymphomas. Cancer Res 1991;51:4743–4756.
24. Hutchins RR, Bani Hani A, Kojodjojo P, et al. Adenocarcinoma of the small bowel. Aust N Z J Surg 2001;71:428–437.
25. Achille A, Baron A, Zamboni G, et al. Molecular pathogenesis of sporadic duodenal cancer. Br J Cancer 1998;77:760–765.
26. Nishiyama K, Yao T, Yonemasu H, et al. Overexpression of p53 protein and point mutation of K-ras genes in primary carcinoma of the small intestine. Oncol Rep 2002;9:293–300.
27. Wendum D, Svrcek M, Rigau V, et al. COX-2 inflammatory secretory secreted PLA2, and cytoplasmic PLA2 protein expression in small bowel adenocarcinomas compared with colorectal adenocarcinomas. Mod Pathol 2003;16:130–136.
27a. Potter DD, Murray JA, Donohue JH, et al. The role of defective mismatch repair in small bowel adenocarcinoma in celiac disease. Cancer Res 2004;64:7073–7077.
28. Blaker H, von Herbay A, Penzel R, et al. Genetics of adenocarcinomas of the small intestine: frequent deletions at chromosome 18q and mutations of the SMAD4 gene. Oncogene 2002; 21:158–164.
29. Planck M, Ericson K, Piotrowska Z, et al. Microsatellite instability and expression of MLH1 and MSH2 in carcinomas of the small intestine. Cancer (Phila) 2003;97:1551–1557.
30. Weingrad DN, DeCosse JJ, Sherlock P, et al. Primary gastrointestinal lymphoma: a 30-year review. Cancer (Phila) 1982; 49:1258–1265.
31. Dawson IMP, Cornes JS, Morson BC. Primary malignant lymphoid tumours of the intestinal tract: report of 37 cases with a study of factors influencing prognosis. Br J Surg 1961;49:80–89.
32. Isaacson PG. Gastrointestinal lymphoma. Hum Pathol 1994; 25:1020–1029.
33. Fine KD, Stone MJ. Alpha-heavy chain disease, Mediterranean lymphoma, and immunoproliferative small intestinal disease: a review of clinicopathological features, pathogenesis, and differential diagnosis. Am J Gastroenterol 1999;94:1139–1152.
34. Domizio P, Owen RA, Shepherd NA, et al. Primary lymphoma of the small intestine. A clinicopathological study of 199 cases. Am J Surg Pathol 1993;17:429–442.
35. Bagdi E, Diss TC, Munson P, Isaacson PG. Mucosal intra-epithelial lymphocytes in enteropathy-associated T-cell lymphoma, ulcerative jejunitis, and refractory celiac disease constitute a neoplastic population. Blood 1999;94:260–264.
36. Ruskone-Fourmestraux A, Delmer A, Lavergne A, et al. Multiple lymphomatous polyposis of the gastrointestinal tract: prospective clinicopathologic study of 31 cases. Group D'etude des Lymphomes Digestifs. Gastroenterology 1997;112: 7–16.
37. LeBrun DP, Kamel OW, Cleary ML, et al. Follicular lymphomas of the gastrointestinal tract. Pathologic features in 31 cases and bcl-2 oncogenic protein expression. Am J Pathol 1992;140: 1327–1335.
38. Bende RJ, Smit LA, Bossenbroek JG, et al. Primary follicular lymphoma of the small intestine: alpha4beta7 expression and immunoglobulin configuration suggest an origin from local antigen-experienced B cells. Am J Pathol 2003;162:105–113.
39. Kumar S, Fend F, Quintanilla-Martinez L, et al. Epstein–Barr virus-positive primary gastrointestinal Hodgkin's disease: association with inflammatory bowel disease and immunosuppression. Am J Surg Pathol 2000;24:66–73.
40. Blanchard DK, Budde JM, Hatch GF III, et al. Tumors of the small intestine. World J Surg 2000;24:421–429.
41. Miettinen M, Lasota J. Gastrointestinal stromal tumors: definition, clinical, histological, immunohistochemical, and molecular genetic features and differential diagnosis. Virchows Arch 2001;438:1–12.
42. Miettinen M, Sobin LH, Sarlomo-Rikala M. Immunohistochemical spectrum of GISTs at different sites and their differential diagnosis with a reference to CD117 (KIT). Mod Pathol 2002;13:1134–1142.
43. Small intestine. In: Greene FL, Page DL, Fleming ID, et al. (eds). AJCC Cancer Staging Manual, 6th ed. New York: Springer Verlag, 2002:107–112.
44. Howe JR, Karnell LH, Mench HR, Scott-Conner C. The American College of Surgeons Commission on Cancer and the American Cancer Society. Adenocarcinoma of the small bowel: review of the National Cancer Data Base, 1989–1995. Cancer (Phila) 1999;86:2693–2706.
45. Veyrieres M, Baillet P, Hay J, et al. Factors influencing long-term survival in 100 cases of small intestine primary adenocarcinoma. Am J Surg 1997;173:237–239.
46. Abrahams NA, Halverson A, Fazio VW, et al. Adenocarcinoma of the small bowel: a study of 37 cases with emphasis on histologic prognostic factors. Dis Colon Rectum 2002;45:1496–1502.
47. Brucher BL, Stein HJ, Roder JD, et al. New aspects of prognostic factors in adenocarcinomas of the small bowel. Hepatogastroenterology 2001;48:727–732.
48. Carbone PP, Kaplan HS, Musshoff K, et al. Report of the Committee on Hodgkin's Disease Staging Classification. Cancer Res 1971;31:1860–1861.
49. Musshoff K. Klinische stadienne inteilung der Niebt-Hodgkin lymphoma. Stahlertherapie 1977;153:218–221.

50. Rohatiner A, d'Amore F, Coiffier B, et al. Report on a workshop convened to discuss the pathological and staging classifications of gastrointestinal tract lymphomas. Ann Oncol 1994;5:397–400.
51. Rosenfelt F, Rosenberg SA. Diffuse histiocytic lymphoma presenting with gastrointestinal tract lesions: the Stanford experience. Cancer (Phila) 1980;45:2188–2193.
52. Amer MH, El-Akkad S. Gastrointestinal lymphoma in adults: clinical features and management of 300 cases. Gastroenterology 1994;106:846–858.
53. Krugmann J, Dirnhofer S, Gschwendtner A, et al. Primary gastrointestinal B-cell lymphoma: a clinicopathological and immunohistochemical study of 61 cases with an evaluation of prognostic parameters. Pathol Res Pract 2001;197:385–393.
54. Nakamura S, Matsumoto T, Iida M, et al. Primary gastrointestinal lymphoma in Japan: a clinicopathologic analysis of 455 patients with special reference to its time trends. Cancer (Phila) 2003;97:2462–2473.
55. Franguemont DW. Differentiation and risk assessment of gastrointestinal stromal tumors. Am J Clin Pathol 1995;103:41–47.
56. Howe JR, Karnell LH, Scott-Conner C. Small bowel sarcoma: analysis of survival from the National Cancer Data Base. Ann Surg Oncol 2001;8:496–508.
57. Langer C, Gunawan B, Schuler P, et al. Prognostic factors influencing surgical management and outcome of gastrointestinal stromal tumors. Br J Surg 2003;90:332–339.
58. Schneider-Stock R, Boltze C, Lasota J, et al. High prognostic value of p16[INK4] alterations in gastrointestinal stroma tumors. J Clin Oncol 2003;21:1688–1697.
59. Lasota J, Jasinski M, Sarlomo-Rikala M, Miettinen M. Mutations in exon 11 of c-kit occur preferentially in malignant versus benign gastrointestinal stromal tumors and do not occur in leiomyomas or leiomyosarcomas. Am J Pathol 1999;154:53–60.
60. Taniguchi M, Nishida T, Hirota S, et al. Effect of c-kit mutation on prognosis of gastrointestinal stromal tumors. Cancer Res 1999;59:4297–4300.
61. Lasota J, Wozniak A, Sarlomo-Rikala M, et al. Mutations in exons 9 and 13 of KIT gene are rare events in gastrointestinal stromal tumors: a study of 200 cases. Am J Pathol 2000;157:1091–1095.
62. Sakurai S, Oguni S, Hironaka M, et al. Mutations in c-kit gene exons 9 and 13 in gastrointestinal stromal tumors among Japanese. Jpn J Cancer Res 2001;92:494–498.
63. Donohue JH, Kelly KA. Cancers of the small intestine. In: Moossa AR, Schimpff SC, Robson MC, Doyle LA, Kaplan RS, Green MR (eds). Comprehensive Textbook of Oncology. Baltimore: Williams & Wilkins, 1991:892–903.
64. Lewis BS. Radiology versus endoscopy of the small bowel. Gastrointest Endosc Clin N Am 1999;9:13–27.
65. Forouzandeh B, Wright R. Diagnostic yield of push-type enteroscopy in relation to indication. Gastrointest Endosc 1998;48:645–647.
66. Korman MU. Radiologic evaluation and staging of small intestine neoplasms. Eur J Radiol 2002;42:193–205.
67. Bessette JR, Maglinte DD, Kelvin FM, Chernish SM. Primary malignant tumors in the small bowel: a comparison of the small bowel enema and conventional follow-through examination. AJR Am J Roentgenol 1989;153:741–744.
68. Beall DP, Fortman BJ, Lawler BC, Regan F. Imaging bowel obstruction: a comparison between fast magnetic resonance imaging and helical computed tomography. Clin Radiol 2002;57:719–724.
69. Buckley JA, Fishman EK. CT evaluation of small bowel neoplasms: spectrum of disease. Radiographics 1998;18:379–392.
70. Gong F, Swain P, Mills T. Wireless endoscopy. Gastrointest Endosc 2000;51:725–729.
71. Pezet D, Rotman N, Slim K, et al. Villous tumors of the duodenum: a retrospective study of 47 cases by the French Association for Surgical Research. J Am Coll Surg 1995;180:541–544.
72. Farnell MB, Sakorafas GH, Sarr MG, et al. Villous tumors of the duodenum: reappraisal of local vs. extended resection. J Gastrointest Surg 2000;4:13–23.
73. Cortese AF, Cornell GN. Carcinoma of the duodenum. Cancer (Phila) 1972;29:1010–1015.
74. Spira IA, Ghazi A, Wolff WI. Primary adenocarcinoma of the duodenum. Cancer (Phila) 1977;39:1721–1726.
75. Barnes G Jr, Romero L, Hess KR, Curley SA. Primary adenocarcinoma of the duodenum: management and survival in 67 patients. Ann Surg Oncol 1994;1:73–78.
76. Bakaeen FG, Murr MM, Sarr MG, et al. What prognostic factors are important in duodenal adenocarcinoma? Arch Surg 2000;135:635–642.
77. Kaklamanos IG, Bathe OF, Franceschi D, et al. Extent of resection in the management of duodenal adenocarcinoma. Am J Surg 2000;179:37–41.
78. Tocchi A, Mazzoni G, Puma F, et al. Adenocarcinoma of the third and fourth portions of the duodenum. Arch Surg 2003;138:80–85.
79. Rotman N, Pezet D, Fagniez P-L, et al. Adenocarcinoma of the duodenum: factors influencing survival. Br J Surg 1994;81:83–85.
80. Rose DM, Hochwald SN, Klimstra DS, Brennan MF. Primary duodenal adenocarcinoma: a ten-year experience with 79 patients. J Am Coll Surg 1996;183:89–96.
81. Sohn TA, Lillemoe KD, Cameron JL, et al. Adenocarcinoma of the duodenum: factors influencing long-term survival. J Gastrointest Surg 1998;2:79–87.
82. Chakravarthy A, Abrams RA, Yeo CJ, et al. Intensified adjuvant combined modality therapy for resected periampullary adenocarcinoma: acceptable toxicity and suggestion of improved 1-year disease-free survival. Int J Radiat Oncol Biol Phys 2000;48:1089–1096.
83. Dragosics B, Bauer P, Radaszkiewicz T. Primary gastrointestinal non-Hodgkin's lymphomas: a retrospective clinicopathologic study of 150 cases. Cancer (Phila) 1985;55:1060–1073.
84. Radaszkiewicz T, Dragosics B, Bauer P. Gastrointestinal malignant lymphomas of the mucosa-associated lymphoid tissue: factors relevant to prognosis. Gastroenterology 1992;102:1628–1638.
85. Koniaris LG, Drugas G, Katzman PJ, Salloum R. Management of gastrointestinal lymphoma. J Am Coll Surg 2003;197:127–141.
86. Maor MH, Velasquez WS, Fuller LM, Silvermintz KB. Stomach conservation in stage IE and IIE gastric non-Hodgkin's lymphoma. J Clin Oncol 1990;8:266–271.
87. Gobbi PG, Dionigi P, Barieri F, et al. The role of surgery in the multimodal treatment of primary gastric non-Hodgkin's lymphoma: a report of 76 cases and review of the literature. Cancer (Phila) 1990;65:2528–2536.
88. Salles G, Herbrecht R, Tilly H, et al. Aggressive primary gastrointestinal lymphomas: review of 91 patients treated with the LNH-84 regimen. A study of the Groupe d'Etude des Lymphomes Agressifs. Am J Med 1991;90:77–84.
89. Tondini C, Giardini R, Bozzetti F, et al. Combined modality treatment for primary gastrointestinal non-Hodgkin's lymphoma: The Milan Cancer Institute experience. Ann Oncol 1993;4:831–837.
90. Ruskone-Fourmestraux A, Aegerter P, Delmer A, et al. Primary digestive tract lymphoma: a prospective multicentric study of 91 patients. Gastroenterology 1993;105:1662–1671.
91. Daum S, Ullrich R, Heise W, et al. Intestinal non-Hodgkin's lymphoma: a multicenter prospective clinical study from the German Study Group on Intestinal Non-Hodgkin's Lymphoma. J Clin Oncol 2003;21:2740–2746.

92. Wang C-Y, Snow JL, Su WPD. Lymphoma associated with human immunodeficiency virus infection. Mayo Clin Proc 1995;70:665–672.
93. Connolly EM, Gaffney E, Reynolds JV. Gastrointestinal stromal tumours. Br J Surg 2003;90:1178–1186.
94. DeMatteo RP, Lewis JJ, Leung D, et al. Two-hundred gastrointestinal stromal tumors: recurrence patterns and prognostic factors for survival. Ann Surg 2000;231:51–58.
95. Mudan SS, Conlon KS, Woodruff JM, et al. Salvage surgery for patients with recurrent gastrointestinal sarcoma: prognostic factors in guide patient selection. Cancer (Phila) 2000;88:66–74.
96. Eilber FC, Rosen G, Forscher C, et al. Surgical resection and intraperitoneal chemotherapy for recurrent abdominal sarcomas. Ann Surg Oncol 1999;6:645–650.
97. Dagher R, Cohen M, Williams G, et al. Approval summary: imatinib mesylate in the treatment of metastatic and/or unresectable malignant gastrointestinal stromal tumors. Clin Cancer Res 2002;8:3034–3038.
98. Bumming P, Andersson J, Meis-Kinidblom JM, et al. Neoadjuvant, adjuvant and palliative treatment of gastrointestinal stromal tumors (GIST) with imatinib: a centre-based study of 17 patients. Br J Cancer 2003;89:460–464.
99. Heinrich MC, Corless CL, Demetri GD, et al. Kinase mutations and imatinib response in patients with metastatic gastrointestinal stromal tumor. J Clin Oncol 2003;21:4342–4349.

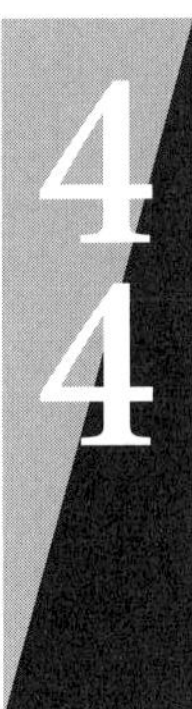

Cancer of the Liver and Bile Ducts

Michael L. Kendrick, Annette Grambihler, Gregory J. Gores, Steven Alberts, and David M. Nagorney

Hepatocellular Carcinoma

Hepatocellular carcinoma (HCC) is the fifth most common neoplasm in the world and the third most common cause of cancer death worldwide.[1] More than 500,000 deaths per year are attributed to HCC, representing 10% of all deaths from cancer. In select areas of Asia and Africa, HCC is the most common cause of death due to cancer. The incidence in Europe and the United States is relatively low but is increasing. In Europe, HCC is now the leading cause of death among patients with cirrhosis.[2] In the United States, epidemiologic studies have demonstrated a doubling of HCC incidence over the past two decades.[3] This increase, which has been attributed to the increasing prevalence of chronic hepatitis C virus (HCV) infection, is expected to continue over the next two decades, given the lag time between the onset of chronic hepatitis and development of HCC.

Etiology

Unique among many other cancers, HCC has well-defined major risk factors. Cirrhosis is the strongest predisposing factor for development of HCC, present in 80% of patients. Chronic viral infection is the most frequent major risk factor for development of HCC. In Asia and Africa, hepatitis B viral (HBV) infection is common, whereas in the West and Japan, hepatitis C virus (HCV) is the main risk factor. The association of HCC and HBV infection is one of the most well recognized etiologic relationships in cancer biology.[4] In epidemiologic studies, the prevalence of HBV carriers correlates with incidence of HCC. Chronic HBV carriers have a 100-fold relative risk of developing HCC compared with noncarriers.[5] Up to 40% of HBV carriers who develop HCC do not have evidence of cirrhosis, demonstrating the direct carcinogenic potential of HBV infection.[6] Prevention of HBV infection reduces the incidence of HCC, as demonstrated in Taiwan, where vaccination of infants reduced the incidence of HBV carriers and simultaneously decreased the incidence of HCC by 60% compared with nonimmunized children.[7,8] In developed countries, HCC arises in cirrhotic livers as a result of HCV infection or excessive alcohol intake. Approximately 170 million people are infected with HCV.[9] Vaccination for prevention of HCV infection is currently not available. Prevention is focused on preventing transmission by transfusion of blood products and in halting the progression of infected individuals to cirrhosis by antiviral regimens such as pegylated interferon and ribavirin. Cirrhosis independent of the etiology is thought in most instances to increase the risk of HCC. The degree of association between cirrhosis and HCC, however, is dependent on the primary condition. Cirrhosis from HCV, HBV, alcohol abuse, and hemochromatosis portends a greater risk for HCC than other conditions such as autoimmune hepatitis, primary biliary cirrhosis, α_1-antitrypsin deficiency, and Wilson's disease, where HCC is uncommon.[10]

The environmental carcinogen aflatoxin B_1 (produced by *Aspergillus flavus*) is a contaminant found in corn, peanuts, and rice that increases the risk of HCC threefold due to a specific mutation on codon 249 of the p53 tumor suppressor gene, leading to unregulated cell growth.[11] Aflatoxins do not cause chronic hepatitis, but metabolite intermediates bind selectively to guanine residues in hepatocyte DNA, resulting in mutations of the p53 tumor suppressor gene that lead to unregulated cell proliferation.[12] Clinically, aflatoxins likely act as cocarcinogens in the pathogenesis of HCC in patients with underlying cirrhosis or hepatitis.

Clinical Evaluation

Patients with HCC typically present with either constitutional symptoms or abdominal complaints due to advanced disease. Abdominal pain is present in nearly one-half of patients; anorexia, nausea, weight loss, and fatigue also occur commonly. Presentation may also be related to the degree of cirrhosis and hepatic decompensation manifested by ascites, gastrointestinal hemorrhage, or encephalopathy. Physical examination may be significant only for signs of cirrhosis; however, a discrete mass may be palpable in large tumors.

Serum α-fetoprotein levels are increased in more than 80% of patients with HCC, and this marker provides a sensitivity of 85% and specificity of 90% for detecting the presence of HCC. The presence of a liver mass with an α-fetoprotein level of 500 ng/mL or more is virtually diagnostic of HCC. Serum des-γ-carboxyprothrombin, a precursor of prothrombin, has a sensitivity and specificity similar to α-fetoprotein but is less commonly used.

An accurate assessment of the number, size, and location of HCC is best obtained by using multiple complementary imaging studies. The goals of imaging are to define the number and location of lesions and the relationship of the HCC to major hepatic and portal veins and hepatic ducts and to delineate cirrhosis, splenomegaly, ascites, regional adenopathy, and presence of metastatic disease. Abdominal ultrasonography is a useful initial study in suspected patients based on its noninvasive and cost-effective profile. After the basic characteristics of HCC are defined with ultrasonography, additional imaging with rapid contrast-enhanced computed tomography (CT) is recommended. In addition to confirming ultrasonographic findings, CT further defines evidence for local invasion, vascular invasion, regional and distant metastases, and portal hypertension. It also provides the ability to calculate the resection volume and the expected remnant volume in resection planning, which are essential in determining the functional resectability of HCC, particularly in patients with cirrhosis. Magnetic resonance imaging (MRI) is an accurate method for imaging HCC. It is the single best imaging method to simultaneously evaluate the liver, tumor vascularity, vascular structural relationships, and bile duct anatomy but lacks the clarity of CT for assessment of extrahepatic disease. MRI has largely supplanted the need for angiography in most patients and is the study of choice for patients with impaired renal function. Hepatic angiography in our practice has a decreasing role in diagnostic evaluation, and its primary use is directed in therapy. Hepatic angiography with the contrast agent lipiodol is particularly accurate for the diagnosis of small HCC when CT and MRI are indeterminate. Hepatic angiography with chemoembolization is used to reduce the size of HCC to enhance resectability, as neoadjuvant therapy in patients before transplantation, or as palliative treatment for patients with unresectable disease. Portal vein embolization can be used to increase resectability by inducing hypertrophy of the contralateral lobe when the predicted postresection remnant is small and the risk of hepatic failure is increased.[13–15]

Staging and Prognosis

Prognostic modeling in HCC is complex, because survival is determined not only by the tumor characteristics and metastases but also by the underlying liver function, which in turn affects the applicability of treatment options. HCC is staged according to the tumor, node, and metastases classification of the American Joint Committee on Cancer or the International Union Against Cancer (AJCC-UICC) scheme (Table 44.1). Although improvements in the prognostic value of this staging system have been realized with modifications, accuracy is still limited because of its predominant histopathologic focus and neglect of accounting for underlying liver function. The Okuda classification includes variables related to pathologic staging and liver function and has been used extensively, but it is unable to distinguish between early and advanced stages.[16] Multiple other classifications have been proposed but have not been fully validated or have not received universal acceptance.

TABLE 44.1. American Joint Committee on Cancer (AJCC) staging of hepatocellular carcinoma (HCC) and intrahepatic cholangiocarcinoma.

Stage	*Tumor*	*Node*	*Metastasis*
I	T1	N0	M0
II	T2	N0	M0
IIIA	T3	N0	M0
IIIB	T4	N0	M0
IIIC	Any T	N1	M0
IV	Any T	Any N	M1

T_1, solitary tumor without vascular invasion; T_2, solitary with vascular invasion or multiple tumors less than 5 cm; T_3, multiple tumors greater than 5 cm or tumor involving a major branch of the portal or hepatic vein(s); T_4, tumors(s) with direct invasion of adjacent organs other than the gallbladder or with perforation of visceral peritoneum; N_1, regional lymph node metastases; M_1, distant metastases.

Source: Used with the permission of the American Joint Committee on Cancer (AJCC), Chicago, Illinois. The original source for this material is the *AJCC Cancer Staging Manual, 6th Edition* (2002), published by Springer-Verlag New York, www.springer-ny.com.

Management

The treatment of HCC is broadly divided into curative and palliative. Curative treatments include resection, liver transplantation, and percutaneous ablation and induce complete responses in a high proportion of patients. Palliative treatments are not aimed at cure but may exhibit partial response rates and even improve survival. In the West, only 30% to 40% of patients undergo curative treatments. In Japan, this percentage is increased to 60% to 90%, which is largely attributed to implementation of surveillance. No level I evidence is currently available evaluating the different methods of curative treatment.

Resection

Hepatic resection aimed at complete extirpation of the tumor is the treatment of choice for HCC in noncirrhotic patients. The treatment of patients with underlying cirrhosis may involve either hepatic resection or transplantation, depending on hepatic function and organ availability. Despite the enthusiasm and theoretical advantages of liver transplantation for HCC patients with cirrhosis, hepatic resection plays a predominant role in the treatment of select patients with well-preserved liver function (Child–Pugh class A) as a result of the lack of organ availability for liver transplantation. There are currently no well-designed controlled trials comparing hepatic resection with transplantation for patients with HCC and cirrhosis.

Hepatic resection is reserved for those patients with HCC grossly limited to the liver and is primarily dependent on the intrahepatic extent of the HCC and the hepatic function. Criteria for resectability are exclusion of extrahepatic metastases, anatomic intrahepatic accessibility of the tumor, and adequate hepatic functional reserve. Major resections in experienced centers can be performed with minimal mortality and excellent outcome. Table 44.2 lists the large contemporary series of hepatic resection in patients with HCC. Overall mortality of hepatic resection is 1% to 15% with an overall 5-year survival of 25% to 50%. Perioperative morbidity and mortality is adversely affected by the presence of cirrhosis,

TABLE 44.2. Hepatic resection for hepatocellular carcinoma.

Reference	*Year*	*N*	*Level of evidence*	*Median follow-up (months)*	*Mortality (%)*	*5-year disease-free survival (%)*	*5-year actuarial survival (%)*
Wayne[162]	2002	249	III	42	6	N/A	41
Poon[163]	2001	203	III	102	N/A	20[a]	37[a]
Fong[164]	1999	154	III	27	4.5	44[b]	37
Lise[165]	1998	100	III	29	7	26	38
Mazziotti[166]	1998	229	III	40	5	N/A	41
Takenaka[167]	1996	280	III	N/A	2	29	50
Vauthey[168]	1995	106	III	52	6	N/A	41
Kawasaki[169]	1995	112	III	N/A	2	33[c]	79[c]

N/A, not available.
[a]Actual survival data.
[b]For tumors less than 5 cm.
[c]3-year survival data.

which is present in up to 80% of patients. The most frequent serious complications after liver resection in patients with HCC remain perioperative bleeding and liver failure. Several important considerations should be understood when interpreting reports on hepatic resection in patients with HCC. First, each series of patients is highly selected, and overall resectability rate is only 10% of all patients with HCC. Second, the definition of resectability varies widely, with some series excluding patients on the basis of tumor size, vascular invasion, lymph node metastases, and degree of portal hypertension. Third, 75% to 80% of patients who undergo resection have underlying cirrhosis. The degree of hepatic dysfunction, although progressive, may fluctuate and influence perioperative hepatic decompensation and mortality. Moreover, the cause of cirrhosis varies, and the natural history of the underlying liver disease also varies widely. Clearly, there is substantial heterogeneity among patients with resected HCC, and overall comparison of patients frequently neglects these differences.

Tumor recurrence complicates 70% of patients at 5 years, including both true recurrence and de novo tumor.[17] Several predictors of recurrence that have been established include microvascular invasion, poor histologic differentiation, and satellite tumors.[18,19]

Liver Transplantation

Liver transplantation is a well-established treatment option in cirrhotic patients with HCC. Theoretical advantages include simultaneous cure of the tumor and the underlying cirrhosis. Early reports of transplantation for patients with HCC described poor results, with tumor recurrence rates of 32% to 54% and 5-year survival of less than 40%.[20] Careful scrutiny of these reports, however, has enabled identification of optimal candidates for transplantation. With highly selected patients, transplantation has been shown to provide excellent 5-year survival and decreased recurrence rates. Established criteria include patients with one HCC smaller than 5 cm or up to three nodules smaller than 3 cm. With these criteria, 5-year survival of up to 70% and recurrence rates less than 15% have been reported.[17,21–24] Expansion of these criteria has been proposed but remains to be validated.

A crucial consideration in the role of transplantation for treatment of HCC is organ availability, and thus the waiting time, which can exceed 12 months in many centers, results in a dropout rate of 20% to 50%.[18,25] However, because of the disparate number of patients with HCC needing liver transplantation compared to the number of available donors, the United Network of Organ Sharing (UNOS) has adapted the model for end-stage liver disease (MELD) to prioritize the waiting list. This model provides consideration for patients with HCC and underlying liver disease. Living donor liver transplantation is emerging as the most feasible alternative to deceased donor liver transplantation. The theoretical unlimited availability of donors is encouraging but is presently unrealized.

Percutaneous Ablation

For patients with HCC who are not operative candidates, percutaneous approaches are the best option for potential curative treatment. Multiple destructive techniques have been described including both chemical (alcohol, acetic acid) and temperature modification (radiofrequency, microwave, and cryoablation). Percutaneous ethanol injection has been extensively evaluated. Advantages are its procedural simplicity, low cost, and minimal adverse effects. Response rates of 90% to 100% in HCC smaller than 2 cm, 70% in those up to 3 cm, and 50% in those up to 5 cm in diameter have been reported.[26,27] Selected patients with a complete response have been reported to achieve a 5-year survival of 50%.[26,28] Radiofrequency ablation (RFA) represents an alternative percutaneous treatment option for patients with unresectable HCC. Potential advantages over ethanol injection include fewer treatment sessions and better local tumor control. In one randomized controlled trial comparing percutaneous ethanol injection and radiofrequency ablation, RFA-treated patients were associated with better local tumor control; however, there was no difference in overall survival.[29]

Arterial Embolization

Arterial embolization is frequently used for treatment for patients with unresectable HCC. Embolization agents, typically gelatin, may be administered alone or in combination with selective intraarterial chemotherapy (chemoembolization). Arterial embolization achieves partial responses in 15% to 55% of patients and substantially delays tumor progression and vascular invasion.[30–33] A meta-analysis of randomized controlled trials comparing arterial embolization or chemoembolization with conservative management demonstrated a survival benefit for chemoembolization.[34]

Systemic Treatment

The majority of patients presenting with HCC have advanced disease at the time of presentation. It is estimated that only 15% to 30% of patients have potentially resectable disease. However, on further evaluation only about one-half of these patients truly have tumors that are resectable. For patients with unresectable disease confined to the liver, several options of therapy are available, including chemoembolization and alcohol ablation. For patients with disease that has spread beyond the liver, few effective options are available. Despite multiple prior studies of chemotherapy, either as single agents or in combination, only limited benefit for patients with unresectable or metastatic HCC has been observed (Table 44.3).

A variety of studies have assessed single-agent chemotherapy. Anthracyclines, particularly doxorubicin, have often served as the chemotherapy drug of reference. Only level II and III evidence exists for the efficacy of doxorubicin. Objective responses to doxorubicin have generally been about 10% with an associated short median survival.[35–40] Limited data from trials with epirubicin suggest better response rates but not necessarily longer survival.[41,42] A variety of phase II studies with an anthracycline combined with another agent have not led to a consistent improvement in outcome compared to single-agent studies. However, no phase III trials have been performed.

Fluorouracil (5-FU)- and platinum (CDDP)-based regimens have been evaluated in a large number of clinical trials. All these trials provide level II or III evidence of activity. A combination of 5-FU, CDDP, doxorubicin, and interferon (PIAF) has frequently been cited as an active regimen. Following a complete response to this regimen in a case report,[43] a subsequent phase II clinical trial in 50 patients reported a 26% partial response rate and median overall survival rate of 8.9 months.[44] Although the proportion of patients responding to this regimen was not notably different from that in other platinum-based regimens, 9 of the 13 responding patients were able to undergo surgical resection of previously unresectable tumors. The use of regimens such as PIAF has been limited by the toxicity of the regimens and frequently by the advanced stage of liver dysfunction in most patients with HCC.

Several meta-analyses of published trials have concluded that systemic chemotherapy offers little benefit to patients with HCC.[45–47] Given the apparent limited benefit of chemotherapy, other agents have been evaluated, including hormonal therapy.

Preclinical studies have shown varying levels of sex hormone receptors in HCC, leading to an evaluation of hormonal agents in HCC.[48,49] Several older underpowered phase II trials showed potential benefit with tamoxifen compared to a placebo.[50,51] Subsequently, a number of randomized multicenter trials of tamoxifen, compared to best supportive care, have shown no benefit for tamoxifen.[52–55] Phase II trials of other hormonal-based therapies have not clearly shown a benefit,[56–59] although several small clinical trials have suggested potential activity that has yet to be confirmed.[60,61]

Several clinical trials have evaluated the role of adjuvant therapy for patients undergoing surgical resection of HCC. In one of these trials, 49 patients were randomized to receive chemotherapy with epirubicin and mitomycin or observation.[62] A lower rate of recurrence and better overall survival were observed in patients receiving chemotherapy. The small size of this trial provides only level II evidence of benefit. Most trials have evaluated liver-directed therapy rather than systemic chemotherapy.[63] To date, the various approaches assessed have not shown any clear improvement in overall survival or disease-free survival compared to surgery alone.

Cholangiocarcinoma

Cholangiocarcinoma is the second most common primary liver cancer in the world, after the more common hepatocellular carcinoma. The tumor usually occurs over the age of 50 to 60 years and is slightly more frequent in men than in women. In the United States, the annual incidence of cholangiocarcinoma is approximately 7 per million.[64] Recently, several epidemiologic studies have been published demonstrating an increase in the incidence and mortality of intrahepatic cholangiocarcinoma over the past 30 years in the United States,[64] as well as in numerous other countries.[65,66] According to these analyses, the age-adjusted death rates in the United States increased from 0.15 per 100,000 in the 1970s to 0.66 per 100,000 in the 1990s; similar data were reported for many other Western countries, especially England, Wales, and Australia. The reason for the rising incidence and mortality of cholangiocarcinoma is as yet unclear; it may in part be better recognition of the intrahepatic form of this disease, and some authors have suggested that new and not yet defined environmental factors might contribute to a more frequent development of this disease.

Etiology and Pathogenesis

In contrast to hepatocellular carcinoma, cholangiocarcinoma does not develop preferentially in the cirrhotic liver; in some studies only 4% to 7% of cholangiocarcinomas originated from cirrhotic livers.[67] A number of risk factors have been established, including primary sclerosing cholangitis, liver fluke infestation, Caroli's disease, congenital choledochal cysts, chronic hepatolithiasis, and Thorotrast deposition. However, many patients who are diagnosed with cholangiocarcinoma have none of these factors in their history.

In the United States and Europe, primary sclerosing cholangitis (PSC) is one of the most important risk factors. The estimated risk of a patient with PSC for cholangiocarcinoma is approximately 0.5% to 1.5% per year after diagnosis, and about 10% to 20% of patients with PSC eventually develop cholangiocarcinoma.[68,69]

Other established risk factors for cholangiocarcinoma include liver flukes (infection with *Clonorchos sinensis* or *Opisthorchis viverrini*), Caroli's disease, congenital choledochal cysts, and chronic hepatolithiasis.[70] In Japan, hepatitis

TABLE 44.3. Review of clinical trials of systemic therapy for hepatocellular carcinoma.

Regimen	*No. of patients*	*Response (95% CI)*	*Overall survival*	*Reference*	*Level of evidence*
Gemcitabine-based					
Gemcitabine 1250mg/m² weekly × 3 over 30min	28	PR—17.8% (2.7–32.9%)	4.8 months	Yang[170]	II
Gemcitabine 1000mg/m² weekly × 3 over 30min	20	PR—5%	7.5 months	Kubicka[134]	II
Gemcitabine 1000mg/m² weekly × 3 over 30min	30	No responses	6.9 months	Fuchs[171]	II
Gemcitabine 1. 1250mg/m² weekly × 2 over 30min 2. 1250mg/m² weekly × 2 at 10mg/m²/min	1. 25 2. 23	1. PR—4% (0.1–20.4%) 2. No responses	3.2 months	Guan[172]	II
Gemcitabine 2200mg/m² every 2 weeks over 30min	17	No responses	8.5 months	Ulrich-Pur[173]	II
Gemcitabine 1250mg/m² over 30min days 1,8 + doxorubicin 30mg/m² day 1	34	PR—11.8% (0.8–22.8%)	4.6 months	Yang[174]	II
1. Gemcitabine 1000mg/m² at 10mg/m²/min day 1 + oxaliplatin 100mg/m² day 2 2. Gemcitabine 1500mg/m² over 30min + oxaliplatin 85mg/m², day 1	1. 11 2. 10	1. PR—10% 2. PR—10%	5 months	Taieb[175]	III
Fluorouracil-based					
5-FU 370mg/m² + LV 200mg/m² × 5 days	14	No responses	3.2 months	Zaniboni[176]	III
5-FU 425mg/m² + LV 20mg/m² × 5 days	29	PR—10%	5.5 months	van Eeden[177]	II
5-FU 250–450mg/m², days 1–5 + LV 500mg/m²/d CI days 1–5	15	PR—7%	3.8 months	Tetef[178]	II
5-FU 370mg/m²/d + LV 200mg/m²/d, days 1–5	25	1 CR + 6 PR: 28% (10.1–45.9%)	Not stated	Porta[179]	II
5-FU + LV + Hydrea				Gebbia[180]	
5-FU 750mg/m² weekly + IFN 9MU TIW	10	No responses	10 months	Stuart[181]	III
5-FU 200mg/m²/d × 21 days + IFN 4MU/m² TIW	36	PR—14.3% (4–32.7%)	15.5 months	Patt[182]	II
UFT 300mg/m²/d + LV 90mg/d PO TID × 28 days	14	No responses	>10 months	Mani[183]	II
Eniluracil 10mg/m² + 5-FU 1mg/m² PO BID × 28 days	45	No responses	11.5 months	Llovet[184]	II
Eniluracil 10mg/m² + 5-FU 1mg/m² PO BID × 28 days	36	No responses	8 months	Benson[185]	II
Platinum-based					
CDDP 90mg/m²	9	PR—11%	2.3 months	Ravry[143]	III
CDDP 75mg/m²	35	PR—6% (0–17%)	3.5 months	Falkson[186]	II
CDDP 80mg/m²	26	PR—15.4% (4.4–34.9%)	Not stated	Okada[187]	II
5-FU 170mg/m²/d CI × 7 days + CDDP 3mg/m²/d × 5 days, weekly × 3	37	PR—47%	6.1 months	Tanioka[188]	II
5-FU 250mg/m² × 5 days + CDDP 10mg/m² × 5 days + IFN 2.5MU TIW	6	PR—33%	Not stated	Komorizono[189]	III
5-FU 400mg/m² days 1–4 + doxoubicin 40mg/m² day 1 + CDDP 20mg/m² days 1–4 + IFN 5MU/m² days 1–4	50	PR—26%	8.9 months	Leung[44]	II
5-FU 200mg/m²/d × 21 days + epirubicin 50mg/m² day 1 + CDDP 60mg/m² day 1	7	PR—29%	8 months	Ellis[151]	III
5-FU 200mg/m²/d × 21 days + epirubicin 60mg/m² day 2 + CDDP 50mg/m² day 2	21	PR—14.5% (1–28%)	10 months	Boucher[190]	III
Oxaliplatin 85–110mg/m² day 1 + topotecan 0.5–1.5mg/m²/d × 5 days	13	PR—8%	8 months	Alexandre[191]	III
CDDP 20mg/m² + topotecan 1.25mg/m² × 5 days	10	PR—10%	Not stated	Lee[192]	III
Anthracycline-based					
Doxorubicin 60mg/m²	109	No responses	Not stated	Sciarrino[37]	III
Doxorubicin 75mg/m²	46	PR—11%	4.2 months	Chlebowski[35]	III
1. Doxorubicin 60–75mg/m² 2. Observation	1. 60 2. 46	PR—3.3%	1. 2.5 months 2. 1.8 months	Lai[36]	II
Liposomal doxorubicin 30mg/m²	16	No responses	4.6 months	Halm[38]	II
Liposomal doxorubicin 30–45mg/m²	40	PR—13% (2–24%)	3 months	Hong[39]	II
Liposomal doxorubicin 40mg/m²	17	CR—7%	12 months	Schmidinger[40]	II
Epirubicin varying doses	18	PR—17% (0–34%)	3 months	Hochster[41]	III
Epirubicin 20mg/m² days 1, 8, 15	44	1 CR + 3 PR: 36%	13.7 months	Pohl[42]	II
Doxorubicin 20mg/m² + IFN 20MU/m²	21	PR—10%	Not stated	Feun[193]	II
Doxorubicin 20mg/m², weekly + 5-FUDR 80mg/kg, weekly + IFN 6MU/m², TIW	30	PR—7%	3 months	Feun[194]	II
Epirubicin 25mg/m², weekly + IFN 3MU/m², days 1–5	30	PR—3%	9.5 months	Bokemeyer[195]	II
Epirubicin 40mg/m² day 1 + VP-16 120mg/m² days 1,3,5	36	1 CR + 13 PR: 39% (23–55%)	10 months	Bobbio[196]	II

(continued)

TABLE 44.3. **Review of clinical trials of systemic therapy for hepatocellular carcinoma.** (continued)

Regimen	*No. of patients*	*Response (95% CI)*	*Overall survival*	*Reference*	*Level of evidence*
Epirubicin 40–60 mg/m² day 1 + 5-FU 800 mg/m² days 1	22	14	11.7 months	Kajanti[197]	II
Hormonal-based					
Flutamide 750 mg QD	32	No responses	2.5 months	Chao[56]	II
Megestrol 160 mg QD	11	No responses	3 months	Colleoni[57]	III
Megestrol 160 mg QD	46	No responses	4 months	Chao[58]	II
Octreotide 30 mg IM	21	PR—5%	4.2 months	Raderer[59]	II
Tamoxifen 20 mg BID	33	No responses	6 months	Engstrom[198]	II
1. Tamoxifen 60 mg QD 2. Placebo	44	Not stated	1. 17 months 2. 12 months	Elba[50]	II
1. Tamoxifen 10 mg BID 2. Placebo	36	Not stated	1. 8.6 months 2. 5.7 months	Martinez[51]	II
1. Tamoxifen 20 mg QD 2. Placebo	120	No responses	1. 20 months 2. 17 months	Castells[52]	I
1. Tamoxifen 40 mg QD 2. Placebo	77	Not stated	1-year survival 1. 30% 2. 37.8%	Riestra[199]	II
1. Tamoxifen 40 mg QD 2. No treatment	480	Not stated	1. 15 months 2. 16 months	Perrone[53,200]	I
1. Tamoxifen 30 mg QD 2. Placebo	119	Not stated	1. 1.5 months 2. 1.5 months	Liu[54]	I
1. Tamoxifen 120 mg QD 2. Tamoxifen 60 mg QD 3. Placebo	1. 130 2. 74 3. 120	Not assessed	1. 2.2 months 2. 2.1 months 3. 2.7 months	Chow[55]	I
Tamoxifen 40 mg/day + VP-16 50 mg/m² days 1–21	33	PR—24.2% (11–42%)	Not stated	Cheng[201]	II
Tamoxifen 40 mg QID, days 1–7 + doxorubicin 60 mg/m² day 4	36	PR—33.3% (17–51%)	Not stated	Cheng[202]	II
1. Doxorubicin 60 mg/m² 2. Tamoxifen 10 mg BID, daily + doxorubicin 60 mg/m², day 1	59	1. PR—11% 2. PR—16%	1. 2 months 2. 2.5 months	Melia[203]	II
1. Tamoxifen 30 mg BID 2. Tamoxifen 30 mg BID, daily + doxorubicin 50 mg/m², day 1	1. 16 2. 16	Not stated	1. 3.2 months 2. 4.9 months	Schachschal[204]	III
1. Octreotide 250 mcg SQ BID 2. Observation	1. 28 2. 30	Not stated	1. 13 months 2. 4 months	Kouroumalis[60]	II
1. Octreotide 30 mg IM 2. Observation	1. 35 2. 35	No responses	1. 1.9 months 2. 2 months	Yuen[205]	II
1. Tamoxifen + Octreotide 2. 5-FU + MMC	1. 24 2. 15	1. 4 CR + 7 PR 2. No responses	1. 12.8 months 2. 5.5 months	Pan[61]	II
Other agents					
CPT-11 125 mg/m²	14	PR—7% (0–20%)	8.2 months	O'Reilly[206]	II
Ifosfamide 2.5 gm/m²/d CI × 5 days	10	No responses	3 months	Lin[207]	III
MMC varying doses	30	PR—48%	7 months	Cheirsilpa[208]	III
Mitoxantrone 12 mg/m²	18	PR—23% (10–47%)	5 months	Colleoni[209]	II
Mitoxantrone 12 mg/m², day 1 + IFN varying doses	38	PR—23% (11–40%)	8 months	Colleoni[210]	II
Paclitaxel 175 mg/m²	20	No responses	3 months	Chao[211]	II
Thalidomide 200–600 mg QD	63	1 CR + 3 PR: 6.3% (0–12.5%)	4.5 months	Hsu[212]	II
Topotecan		PR—13.9% (4.7–29.5%)	8 months	Wall[213]	II
Vindesine 3 mg/m²	16	No responses	5 months	Falkson[214]	II

PR, partial response; CR, complete response.

C virus infection is frequently found in patients with cholangiocarcinoma,[71] and Kobayashi et al. found that 3.5% of HCV-infected patients developed cholangiocarcinoma within a 10-year observation period.[72] Moreover, dietary habits have been suggested to contribute to the regional variability in incidence, especially the regular intake of certain salted fish products in Asia, which can contain the bacterial product dimethylnitrosamine.[73,74]

Most of these risk factors have in common that they are causes of chronic inflammation and/or cholestasis. Thus, as is the case in many other gastrointestinal tumors, chronic inflammation of the biliary tree appears to be an important factor in the development of cholangiocarcinoma.

A large number of molecular alterations have been found in human cholangiocarcinoma (Table 44.4). However, it must be noted that the most of these alterations have been described in intrahepatic mass-forming cholangiocarcinomas, and their relevance to the ductal-infiltrating and intraductal growth forms as well as extrahepatic tumors is unclear.

TABLE 44.4. **Molecular alterations in cholangiocarcinoma.**

Molecular finding	*Biologic effect*
Chronic inflammation/growth factors	
INOS overexpression	DNA damage and mutation Inhibition of DNA repair COX-2 and IL-6 overexpression Inhibition of apoptosis Angiogenesis
COX-2 overexpression	Inhibition of apoptosis Angiogenesis
IL-6/gp130 overexpression	iNOS induction Proliferation
HGF/c-met overexpression	Proliferation
c-erbB-2 overexpression	Proliferation
Tumor suppressors/oncogenes	
K-*ras* mutation/activation	Proliferation
Retinoblastoma/p16/CDK4 inactivation	Loss of cell-cycle control
p14/MDM/p53 inactivation	Loss of cell-cycle control Apoptosis resistance
p53 mutation/overexpression	Loss of cell-cycle control Apoptosis resistance
Apoptosis resistance and immune escape	
Mcl-1 overexpression	Inhibition of apoptosis
Bcl-2 overexpression	Inhibition of apoptosis
Disruption of TGF-beta signaling	Inhibition of apoptosis Loss of cell-cycle control
FasL expression	T-cell apoptosis
Other	
Telomerase reverse transcriptase	Immortalization

As some of the molecular and genetic changes of cholangiocarcinoma can already be detected in preneoplastic inflammatory bile duct lesions, it is generally presumed that chronic inflammation or cholestasis or both cause a sequence of events leading first to hyperplasia and dysplasia of the biliary epithelia, and eventually to the development of carcinoma. Figure 44.1 gives an overview of this hypothesis.

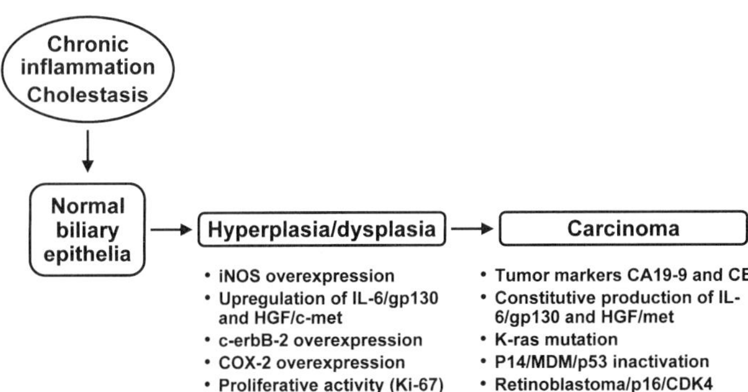

FIGURE 44.1. Molecular alterations in reactive hyper- and dysplasia and in cholangiocarcinoma. Chronic inflammation and cholestasis cause premalignant hyper- and dysplasia of biliary epithelia with distinct molecular alterations such as inducible nitric oxide synthase (iNOS) overexpression, upregulation of growth factors and their receptors, cyclooxygenase (COX)-2 overexpression, increased proliferation, and telomerase activity. With the development of cholangiocarcinoma, malignant cells constitutively express growth factors, mutation of tumor suppressor genes occurs, and oncogenes are observed. There is also dysregulation of antiapoptotic proteins along with expression of classic tumor markers.

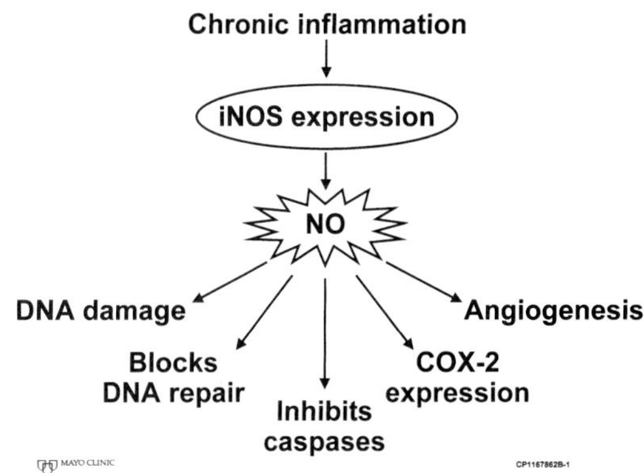

FIGURE 44.2. Nitric oxide in cholangiocarcinogenesis. In chronic inflammation of the bile ducts [e.g., in sclerosing cholangitis (PSC)], cytokines cause biliary epithelia to express iNOS, which in turn generates nitric oxide (NO); NO contributes to carcinogenesis by damaging DNA and inhibiting DNA repair proteins leading to mutation, by inactivating caspases and thus inhibiting apoptosis, by promoting angiogenesis, and by inducing COX-2 expression, which also inhibits apoptosis and triggers angiogenesis.

Chronic Inflammation: DNA Damage

Chronic inflammation is associated with generation of cytokines both by inflammatory cells and by cholangiocytes. A key proinflammatory cytokine is interleukin 6, a strong mitogen for cholangiocytes and cholangiocarcinoma cells. Proinflammatory cytokines including interleukin 6, interleukin 1, interferon-γ, and tumor necrosis factor-α cause cholangiocytes to express the inducible form of nitric oxide synthase (iNOS), a potent generator of nitric oxide (NO). NO itself or NO derivatives (Figure 44.2) can modify or alter DNA bases, resulting in direct DNA damage.[75] NO may also nitrosylate and inactivate DNA repair proteins, leading to an accumulation of damaged DNA bases, thereby further promoting mutagenesis [76]. In addition, NO has been shown to also disable proapoptotic proteins such as caspases.[77]

Consistent with these data, iNOS expression and generation of NO can often be detected in diseases that predispose to cholangiocarcinoma; for example, cholangiocytes in PSC and cholangiocarcinoma cells have been shown to express iNOS,[78] and elevated serum nitrate values as a result of iNOS activity can be observed in patients with fluke infections.[79] Therefore, it has been proposed that iNOS expression and NO generation play an important role in the pathogenesis of cholangiocarcinoma, and that iNOS inhibitors may be chemopreventive in diseases predisposing to the development of cholangiocarcinoma such as PSC, especially because in animal models of intestinal and lung cancer, deletion or inhibition of iNOS can be chemopreventive.[80,81]

Bile Acids: Regulation of Proliferation and Apoptosis

Cholangiocarcinomas often grow within or along the bile duct lumen, suggesting that they may not only have developed mechanisms to survive the toxic constituents in bile but actually use bile to promote growth and survival. Indeed, cholangiocytes and cholangiocarcinoma cells are resistant to apoptosis when exposed to bile acids in vitro, in contrast to hepatocytes and hepatoma cells, for which most bile acids are toxic. Furthermore, bile acids have been shown to transactivate the epidermal growth factor receptor in cholangiocarcinoma cells and induce expression of cyclooxygenase (COX)-2,[82] an enzyme that generates prostanoids and can inhibit apoptosis, facilitate growth, and promote angiogenesis in a variety of malignancies.[83] In addition to inducing COX-2 expression, bile acids also enhance the cellular protein levels of myeloid cell leukemia protein 1 (Mcl-1), a potent antiapoptotic protein, in vitro.[84] Mcl-1 protein levels are also frequently elevated in human cholangiocarcinoma in vivo.[85]

Thus, chronic inflammation as well as the ability to survive and proliferate in the toxic bile milieu appears to contribute to the development of cholangiocarcinoma. It remains to be elucidated whether cholestasis alone, or alterations in bile composition caused by chronic inflammation, or both are responsible for the antiapoptotic and growth-promoting effects of bile on cholangiocarcinoma.

Histology

Histologically, most cholangiocarcinomas are well to moderately differentiated tubular adenocarcinomas, with formation of glands and an abundance of dense desmoplastic stroma; calcification may be present. Mucus, but not bile secretion, is observed in the majority of tumors. The glandular lumens are lined by well-differentiated columnar or cuboidal cells with uniform nuclei and small nucleoli. In poorly differentiated adenocarcinoma, a definite tubular formation is rarely found, and the cells are pleomorphic with irregular nuclei.

In addition to the most common tubular form of cholangiocellular adenocarcinoma, other variants have been described, such as papillary adenocarcinoma, signet-ring carcinoma, squamous cell or mucoepidermoid carcinoma, a spindle cell variant, and a lymphoepithelioma-like form.

Classification

Cholangiocarcinoma is broadly classified as intrahepatic or extrahepatic. Extrahepatic cholangiocarcinoma is further classified as perihilar, midduct, and distal. Major differences in presentation, evaluation, staging, and operative management warrant separate discussion of intrahepatic and extrahepatic cholangiocarcinoma.

Intrahepatic Cholangiocarcinoma

Intrahepatic cholangiocarcinoma (ICC) is the second most common primary liver cancer after HCC, with a prevalence of 10% to 30%.[86,87] Cholangiocarcinoma of the intrahepatic ducts is far less common than that of the extrahepatic ducts, typically accounting for less than 10% of all cholangiocarcinoma.

Clinical Evaluation

In a review of 61 patients with ICC surgically treated at the Mayo Clinic over a 31-year period, the most common presenting symptom was abdominal pain, followed by signs of weight loss and anorexia. Jaundice is an unusual finding in ICC that is present in only 15%.[88] The physical examination is frequently nonspecific for ICC; an abdominal mass is the most common finding but is present in only one-third of patients. Other signs such as ascites, cachexia, and splenomegaly are infrequent and nonspecific. Typically, when patients with ICC present with symptoms, the disease is frequently advanced and the likelihood of a curative resection is low.

Other than mild increases in alkaline phosphatase and aminotransferases, laboratory findings are typically normal in patients with ICC. Tumor markers such as the carcinoembryonic antigen (CEA) and α-fetoprotein are infrequently increased, whereas the carbohydrate antigen 19-9 is more frequently elevated in patients with ICC.

The imaging of ICC is similar to that of HCC. Frequently ultrasonography is the initial diagnostic evaluation that is useful to identify the tumor location and characteristics. As for HCC, CT is an excellent imaging modality to assess the tumor location, extent of invasion, and evidence of extrahepatic disease. Because of the intense fibrosis associated with cholangiocarcinoma, a decreased tumoral vascularity of ICC is frequently noted compared to that of HCC.

Pathology and Staging

The gross appearance of intrahepatic cholangiocarcinomas is of a gray-white scirrhous mass, with an abundance of stroma and mucin secretion, but little vascularization. The masses may be solitary or multinodular and can be relatively well demarcated or infiltrating, growing along the intrahepatic bile ducts.

The Liver Cancer Study Group of Japan has further classified intrahepatic cholangiocarcinoma into three principal types: a mass-forming type that is usually localized with a round shape and distinct borders, a periductal-infiltrating type with diffuse infiltration along the bile ducts, and an intraductal growth type showing intraductal papillary or granular growth.[89] Among these, the mass-forming type is the most frequent and the intraductal growth type the rarest; overlap, especially between the mass-forming and the periductal-infiltrating type, is very common. This new classification appears to be useful, because the three forms have been shown to differ not only in gross appearance but also in their genetic alterations and prognosis.[90,91] ICC is staged using the same AJCC tumor, node, and metastases classification as for HCC (see Table 44.1).

Operative Management

Resection remains the only curative treatment in the management of ICC. In our experience, patients with resected ICC are the only long-term survivors, with a 3-year survival of 60% with resection compared to 7% without resection.[88] Operative mortality and morbidity for resection in patients with ICC are typically less than 2% and 15%, respectively.

Hepatic resection is the standard for intrahepatic cholangiocarcinoma. The extent of resection is determined by the anatomic location of the tumor and by the objective of achieving a complete macroscopic and microscopic (R0) resection. Recent series of outcomes after resection of ICC are shown in Table 44.5. Factors associated with decreased survival are stage, vascular invasion, intrahepatic metastases, and positive lymph nodes. Intrahepatic cholangiocarcinoma spreads along

TABLE 44.5. Hepatic resection for perihepatic cholangiocarcinoma.

Reference	*Year*	*N*	*Level of evidence*	*Mortality (%)*	*Hepatectomy (%)*	*Negative margin (%)*	*5-year survival (%)*
Rea[122]	2004	46	III	9	100	80	26
Jarnagin[101]	2001	80	III	10	78	78	27
Kitagawa[215]	2001	110	III	10	95	N/A	31[a]
Nimura[102]	2000	142	III	9[b]	90	76	26
Gazzaniga[111]	2000	75	III	10	67	61	18
Lee[119]	2000	128	III	6	87	70	22[c]
Launois[216]	1999	40	III	13	63	80	13
Neuhaus[120]	1999	80	III	8	83	44	22
Burke[97]	1998	30	III	7	73	83	45
Iwatsuki[217]	1998	34	III	15	100	59	9
Miyazaki[218]	1998	76	III	15	86	71	26

N/A, not available.
[a]For node-negative patients
[b]For patients with curative resection.
[c]For patients with hepatic resection.

Glisson's sheath by way of lymphatics to metastasize to regional lymph nodes. The incidence of lymph node metastases for ICC ranges from 6% to 46%.[92,93] In an autopsy series of ICC, lymph node metastases were present in up to 72%.[94] Patients with lymph node metastases have an extremely poor prognosis. Inohue and colleagues evaluated 52 patients with intrahepatic cholangiocarcinoma and reported an overall 5-year survival rate of 36%, but no long-term survivors among 21 patients with lymph node metastases.[95] Routine lymph node dissection in patients with ICC remains controversial. Currently, there is no strong evidence to suggest that lymph node dissection offers a survival benefit, and no randomized trials have been performed. Additionally, hilar lymphadenectomy does not ensure removal of lymph node metastases because the lymphatic drainage of the liver is not exclusively via the hepatoduodenal ligament but also through the coronary, falciform, and triangular ligaments. The presence of lymph node metastases, however, is an ominous finding and should preclude hepatic resection.[95,96] Routine lymphadenectomy with frozen section analysis before proceeding to hepatic resection has been advocated.[96]

Extrahepatic Cholangiocarcinoma

Perihilar cholangiocarcinoma (PCC) accounts for approximately 60% of extrahepatic cholangiocarcinomas. Midduct (15%) and distal (20%) cholangiocarcinomas comprise the remainder.

Clinical Evaluation

The majority of patients with extrahepatic cholangiocarcinoma present with progressive, painless jaundice. Biochemical confirmation typically prompts diagnostic ultrasonography. Albeit operator dependent, ultrasonography can demonstrate several salient features of PCC such as tumor morphology, portal vein or hepatic artery obstruction, intrahepatic metastases, and regional lymph node metastases. Because distant disease precludes curative resection and evidence of unresectability will prompt palliative stenting, CT should precede cholangiographic evaluation. CT provides an excellent overall assessment and can characterize local tumor extension, hepatic lobar atrophy, portal vein compression in invasion, and lymph node and other metastases. The presence of lobar atrophy is frequently associated with ipsilateral portal vein involvement, is a major harbinger of unresectable disease, and should prompt a thorough vascular evaluation.

Cholangiography provides the best evaluation of ductal involvement and extension. Critical in the ductal evaluation is the proximal extent of the disease. Clear delineation of the confluence and proximal biliary system is imperative to correctly classify the tumor and plan surgical resection and reconstruction. Endoscopic retrograde cholangiography (ERC) may not provide sufficient evaluation of the proximal extent of the disease, and percutaneous transhepatic cholangiography may be necessary. The Bismuth–Corlette classification, although not intended to stage PCC, provides a useful conceptualization based on preoperative imaging when considering the extent of resection necessary for a curative intent and communication in reporting (Figure 44.3).

Magnetic resonance imaging (MRI) provides several advantages in the evaluation of cholangiocarcinoma. It provides a noninvasive assessment of the liver, bile ducts, and vessels. Unlike direct cholangiography, however, MRI does not provide equivalent cholangiographic image resolution,

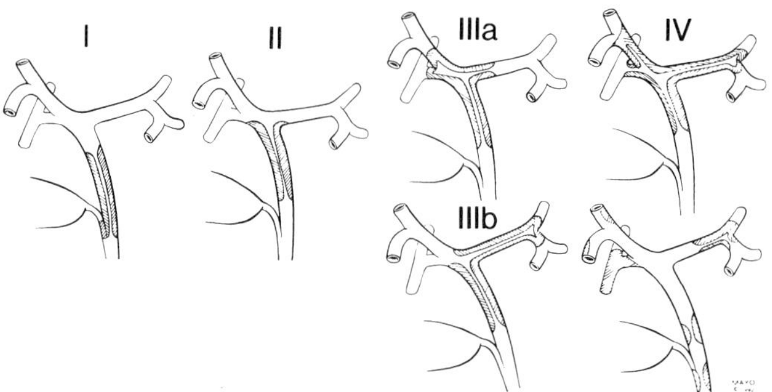

FIGURE 44.3. Bismuth–Corlette classification of perihilar cholangiocarcinoma. (Reprinted by permission of Mayo Foundation for Medical Education and Research.)

access for brush cytology, or the ability of biliary ductal drainage for relief of obstruction and palliation.

A thorough clinical evaluation of the patient's functional status and coexisting medical comorbidities is important before extensive radiographic evaluation. Patients deemed unfit for operative intervention do not need such extensive evaluations, and alternate palliative goals should be considered.

In determining the resectability of PCC, four key issues must be addressed: extent of biliary involvement, vascular (hepatic artery or portal vein) invasion, hepatic atrophy, and metastatic disease. Specific criteria of unresectability have been suggested[97]: these include (1) bilateral ductal extension to the secondary or segmental biliary radicals; (2) encasement or occlusion of the main portal vein proximal to its bifurcation; (3) lobar atrophy with encasement of the contralateral portal vein branch or hepatic artery; (4) lobar atrophy with contralateral involvement of secondary biliary radicals; (5) unilateral segmental ductal extension with contralateral vascular encasement; and (6) distant metastases.

Pathology and Staging

Extrahepatic cholangiocarcinomas have also been subclassified based on their gross appearance as either papillary, nodular, or sclerosing.[98,99] Sclerosing tumors comprise approximately 70% of hilar cholangiocarcinomas and cause an annular thickening of the bile duct wall with longitudinal and radial tumor infiltration as well as infiltration and fibrosis of the periductal tissue. Nodular tumors are characterized by a firm nodule projecting into the bile duct lumen. Tumors featuring characteristics of both nodular and sclerosing forms are relatively frequent. The papillary variant only accounts for approximately 10% and is most commonly seen in the distal bile duct; its prognosis is generally more favorable than that of the two other forms.[98,100] Extrahepatic cholangiocarcinoma is staged according to the AJCC-UICC tumor, node, and metastases classification (Table 44.6). Unlike intrahepatic cholangiocarcinoma where staging is combined with other primary liver tumors, the extrahepatic cholangiocarcinoma staging system is unique to cholangiocarcinoma and has undergone significant revisions. Previous editions of the AJCC staging were criticized for neglect of vascular invasion or hepatic atrophy, which are thought to affect resectability and outcome. Jarnagin and colleagues, in a review of 225 patients with hilar cholangiocarcinoma, proposed a modification of the T staging to include these two factors.[101] On univariate analysis, both vascular invasion and hepatic lobar atrophy were prognostic indicators; however, on multivariate analysis they failed to demonstrate prognostic validity. Although both these factors are clinically useful for evaluating resectability and planning resection, the staging system proposed by Jarnagin and colleagues does not appear to have been adapted by others, albeit the *AJCC Cancer Staging Manual, 6th Edition* now includes vascular invasion as part of the tumoral staging.

TABLE 44.6. American Joint Committee on Cancer (AJCC) staging for extrahepatic cholangiocarcinoma.

Stage	*Tumor*	*Node*	*Metastasis*
0	Tis	N0	M0
IA	T1	N0	M0
IB	T2	N0	M0
IIA	T3	N0	M0
IIB	T1–3	N1	M0
III	T4	Any N	M0
IV	Any T	Any N	M1

T_{is}, carcinoma in situ; T_1, tumor confined to the bile duct histologically; T_2, tumor invades beyond the wall of the bile duct; T_3, tumor invades the liver, gallbladder, pancreas, and/or unilateral branches of the portal vein (right or left) or hepatic artery (right or left); T_4, tumor invades any of the following: main portal vein or its branches bilaterally, common hepatic artery, or other adjacent structures, such as colon, stomach, duodenum, or abdominal wall; N_1, regional lymph node metastases; M_1, distant metastases.

Source: Used with the permission of the American Joint Committee on Cancer (AJCC), Chicago, Illinois. The original source for this material is the *AJCC Cancer Staging Manual, 6th Edition* (2002), published by Springer-Verlag New York, www.springer-ny.com.

Operative Management

Complete tumor resection currently offers the only opportunity for cure. As such, all patients with cholangiocarcinoma should be offered an attempt at resection unless specific contraindications exist. Both patient-related factors and tumor-related factors must be considered when assessing patients for potential operative intervention. Clearly, the patient's functional status must be sufficient to tolerate a major operation, and the preoperative tumor assessment must suggest that a curative resection is possible with opportunity for prolonged survival.

The role of preoperative percutaneous or endoscopic biliary drainage in patients with PCC remains an area of controversy. Proponents argue that the improved hepatic function, reduction of cholangitis, and assistance with hilar dissection afforded by biliary drainage warrant its use.[102,103] Opponents claim that the increased rate of wound infection, bacterobilia, and potential for tumor seeding contraindicate preoperative biliary drainage.[104] Outcome comparisons regarding regeneration after portal vein embolization, hepatic function, and liver failure with or without drainage for hepatic resection in patients with PCC are lacking, and practice guidelines are based on institutional preference.

Patients in whom resection of up to 70% to 75% of the functional liver volume is expected are candidates for portal vein embolization (PVE). The rationale for PVE is to induce hypertrophy and hyperplasia in the anticipated hepatic remnant before resection, theoretically increasing functional capacity and decreasing the risk of postoperative liver failure. In a prospective nonrandomized trial of patients undergoing right hepatectomy for either primary or metastatic liver disease, Farges and colleagues demonstrated a decreased incidence of postoperative complications including liver dysfunction or failure among patients with chronic liver disease who had preoperative PVE.[13] Similar findings of reduced postoperative liver dysfunction or failure were reported by Hemming and colleagues in patients undergoing extended hepatectomy with PVE compared to those without PVE.[14] No randomized controlled trials have been performed assessing the role and utility of PVE in patients undergoing major hepatic resection. The authors have not employed PVE to treat PCC. Although the potential use of PVE has merit, extended hepatic resections are generally well tolerated if the planned liver remnant is well drained preoperatively and if evidence for adequate hepatic function exists.

Intraoperative assessment of patients undergoing exploration for potential curative resection includes exclusion of metastases and assessment of the extent of local invasion. Overall resectability among patients undergoing exploration is nearly 65%. The pendulum of operative management of extrahepatic cholangiocarcinoma has swung from a bile-duct-only resection to that of a combined bile duct and hepatic resection. This change is attributed to the recognition of the propensity for intrahepatic ductal extension and hepatic parenchymal invasion as well as the ability to perform hepatic resection with lower morbidity and mortality. With bile duct resection alone, resectability rates of 15% to 20% were reported.[105–107] Multiple reports have confirmed that increases in hepatic resection for PCC correlate with increases in negative margin resections (R0 resection).[108,109] With hepatic resection rates of 20% to 29%, negative margin rates were achieved in only 15%, compared to a negative margin rate of 60% to 88% with hepatic resection rates of 60% to 89%. Multiple other series have demonstrated that resectability rates parallel hepatic resection rates.[110–112] Level I data are currently unavailable comparing outcomes of bile-duct-only resection versus that combined with hepatic resection. Outcomes of aggressive hepatic resection for management of PCC are shown in Table 44.5.

Significant consideration has been given to the caudate lobe in the operative management of PCC. Caudate biliary ductal tributaries frequently drain into the posterior aspect of the right or left hepatic ducts near the confluence.[113,114] Careful histopathologic examination of resected specimens has demonstrated caudate lobe involvement in 42% to 100% of patients.[114–117] The impact of caudate lobe resection for treatment of PCC is evident by a 20% local recurrence in the caudate lobe when it is not resected.[110] In contrast, when the caudate lobe was incorporated into the hepatic resection, local recurrence decreased and 5-year survival increased from 8% to 25%.[111]

Resection of PCC mandates removal of the gallbladder, the extrahepatic duct from the hepatic hilus to the pancreas, regional lymphadenectomy, and Roux-en-Y hepaticojejunostomy. Hepatic resection is generally not required for Bismuth–Corlette type I PCC. Type II and III require resection of caudate and additional segments, dependent on local invasion or ductal extension.

Perioperative mortality and 5-year survival for patients with hepatic resection are shown in Table 44.5. The most frequent serious complications after hepatic resection for PCC are hepatic failure, infection, hemorrhage, and renal or cardiorespiratory failure.

Although no level I data are available comparing outcomes of patients with resected versus nonresected PCC, survival of patients with unresected or advanced-stage PCC has ranged from 6 to 12 months.[118] Before acceptance of hepatic resection, 5-year survival was infrequent and only marginally better than patients without resection.[105] In contrast, the 5-year survival in series utilizing hepatic resection ranges from 9% to 45% (see Table 44.5).

Clearly, the major predictor of long-term survival is complete resection with negative margins (R0 resection).[102,119,120] Existing data suggest that patients with positive margins at resection demonstrate no consistent survival advantage compared to patients without resection.[101,121] In a recent review of our experience with 46 patients undergoing major hepatic resection for PCC, an R0 resection was achieved in 80% with an operative mortality rate of 9%. Actual 1-, 3-, and 5-year survival rates were 80%, 39%, and 26%, respectively.[122] On multivariate analysis, the only predictor of recurrence was tumor grade 3 or 4, whereas negative predictors of survival were history of hepatitis, direct bilirubin at presentation greater than 6.4 mg/dL, blood transfusion requirement greater than 4 units, and male sex. Factors demonstrated to be adversely associated with survival include distant lymph node metastases, vascular invasion, and lobar atrophy.[102,119,120]

Systemic Treatment

The role of palliative chemotherapy in patients with unresectable hepatobiliary cancer has been assessed in a number of clinical trials. The potential benefit of chemotherapy for this group of cancers is derived primarily from trials providing level II and III evidence (Table 44.7), consisting primarily of phase II and insufficiently powered phase III clinical trials. As such, the standards of therapy for unresectable disease remain uncertain. Even less evidence exists on the potential benefit of either adjuvant or neoadjuvant therapy.

For patients with metastatic disease, chemotherapy remains the primary form of therapy, principally for palliation of symptoms. A randomized trial of chemotherapy [5-fluorouracil (5-FU) and leucovorin (LV) or 5-FU, LV, and etoposide] and best supportive care compared to best supportive care alone in patients with metastatic pancreatic or biliary tract cancers demonstrated improved quality of life and overall survival in those receiving chemotherapy.[123]

A variety of chemotherapy agents have been evaluated, but in general the response to these agents has been limited (see Table 44.7). Several older studies evaluated 5-FU alone or in combination with other forms of chemotherapy and showed mixed results. Many of these studies were statistically underpowered and combined biliary cancers with pancreatic cancer or hepatocellular carcinoma, making their interpretation difficult. In general, 5-FU as a single agent produces few responses and an overall survival of less than 6 months.[124,125] However, several recent small trials have suggested high-dose 5-FU or 5-FU in combination with other agents may produce partial responses in up to one-third of patients.[126–130] Despite improved response rates, the duration of response is generally short and little increase in overall survival with 5-FU is seen. Only one phase III study has been performed to assess the added benefit of 5-FU combined with other agents to 5-FU alone.[124] That trial indicated that 5-FU, used alone, was equivalent to or superior to combination therapy. However, this trial provided only level II evidence based on the inadequate sample size.

More recently, trials have focused on gemcitabine as well as other newer agents. Several recent case reports have suggested that gemcitabine may have activity in biliary tract and gallbladder carcinoma.[131,132] A variety of phase II trials have now been published providing level II evidence for the use of gemcitabine.[127,133–139] The appropriate dose and schedule of gemcitabine continue to be evaluated. In a phase II trial of gemcitabine in patients with biliary tract or gallbladder carcinoma, two different schedules were evaluated.[139] Gemcitabine at 1,200 mg/m^2 given weekly for 3 weeks, followed by a 2-week rest period, resulted in 4 of 24 patients (17%) achieving a partial response. The median survival was

TABLE 44.7. Review of clinical trials of systemic therapy for biliary tract and gallbladder cancer.

Regimen	*No. of patients*	*Response (95% CI)*	*Overall survival*	*Reference*	*Level of evidence*
Gemcitabine-based					
Gemcitabine 800 mg/m^2 weekly over 30 min	Gallbladder—14 Biliary tract—14	PR—30%	14 months	Tsavaris[133]	II
Gemcitabine 1000 mg/m^2 weekly × 3 over 30 min	Biliary tract—23	PR—30%	9.3 months	Kubicka[134]	II
Gemcitabine 1000 mg/m^2 weekly × 3 over 30 min	Gallbladder—26	PR—36% (17.1–57.9%)	7.5 months	Gallardo[135]	II
Gemcitabine 1200 mg/m^2 weekly × 3 over 30 min	Gallbladder—5 Biliary tract—14	PR—16%	6.5 months	Raderer[127]	II
Gemcitabine 2200 mg/m^2 every 2 weeks over 30 min	Gallbladder—10 Biliary tract—22	PR—21.9% (9.3–40%)	11.5 months	Penz[136]	II
Gemcitabine 1000 mg/m^2 weekly × 3 over 30 min	Gallbladder—5	PR—60%	9.8 months	Teufel[137]	III
Gemcitabine 1000 mg/m^2 weekly × 3 over 30 min	Biliary tract—13	PR—8%	16 months	Metzger[138]	III
Gemcitabine 1. 1200 mg/m^2 weekly × 3 over 30 min 2. 2200 mg/m^2 every 2 weeks over 30 min	1. Gallbladder—8 Biliary tract—16 2. Gallbladder—5 Biliary tract—9	1. PR—16.7% (5–37%) 2. PR—28.6% (8–58%)	1. 6.8 months 2. 10.5 months	Valencak[139]	III
Gemcitabine 24-h infusion weekly × 3 1. 150 mg/m^2 (no prior therapy) 2. 100 mg/m^2 (prior therapy)	Biliary tract—9 Pancreas—15 Unknown—1	1. PR—8% 2. 0%	Not stated	Eckel[219]	III
Gemcitabine 1000 mg/m^2 weekly × 3 over 30 min	Gallbladder—case report	PR	Not stated	Castro[131]	IV
Gemcitabine 1000 mg/m^2 weekly × 3 over 30 min	Gallbladder—case report	PR	Not stated	Gallardo[132]	IV
Gemcitabine 1000 mg/m^2 over 30 min + 5-FU 500 mg/m^2 over 3 h, weekly × 3	Biliary tract—9	PR—33%	Not stated	Murad[140]	III
Gemcitabine 1000 mg/m^2 over 30 min + 5-FU variable doses, weekly × 3	Gallbladder—1 Biliary tract—3	PR—25%	14.8 months	Boxberger[141]	IV
Gemcitabine 1000 mg/m^2 over 30 min, days 1,8 + CDDP 70 mg/m^2 day 1	Gallbladder—11	CR—9% PR—55%	10.5 months	Malik[220]	III
Gemcitabine 1000 mg/m^2 over 30 min + CPT-11,100 mg/m^2, day 1, 8	Gallbladder—10 Biliary tract—6	PR—14% (interim report)	Not stated	Bhargava[221]	II
Gemcitabine 1000 mg/m^2 over 30 min + docetaxel 35 mg/m^2 over 3 h, weekly × 3	Gallbladder—26 Biliary tract—15	PR—9.3%	11 months	Kuhn[222]	II
Fluorouracil-based					
5-FU 375 mg/m^2/d + LV 25 mg/m^2/d, days 1–5	Gallbladder—9 Biliary tract—19	CR—2% PR—25%	6 months	Choi[223]	II
5-FU 2600 mg/m^2 + LV 150 mg/m^2 over 24 h, weekly × 6	Gallbladder—6 Biliary tract—13	PR—33% (14–57%)	7.0 months	Chen[126]	II
UFT 300 mg/m^2/d + LV 90 mg/d daily for 28 days	Gallbladder + Biliary tract—13	No responses	7 months	Mani[224]	II
1. 5-FU 600 mg/m^2/d × 5 2. 5-FU 600 mg/m^2/d + STZ 500 mg/m^2/d, days 1–5 3. 5-FU 500 mg/m^2/d, days 1–5 + MeCCNU 150 mg/m^2, day 1	1. 30 patients 2. 26 patients 3. 31 patients	GB / Biliary 1. 11% / 8% 2. 13% / 0 3. 5% / 17%	GB / Biliary 1. 5.25 / 5.25 2. 3.5 / 3.0 3. 2.5 / 2.0	Falkson[124]	II
5-FU 750 mg/m^2/d days 1–5 + IFN_2b 5 MU/m^2, days 1, 3, 5	Gallbladder—25 Biliary tract—10	PR—34% (18.6–53.2%)	12 months	Patt[182]	II
5-FU 2000 mg/m^2 + LV 500 mg/m^2 over 24 h, weekly × 6 + CTX 300 mg/m^2 monthly + tamoxifen 20 mg BID	Gallbladder—7 Biliary tract—23	No responses	7.3 months	Eckel[225]	II
5-FU 400 mg/m^2 + LV 200 mg/m^2, days 1–4 + mito C 8 mg/m^2, day 1	Gallbladder—7 Biliary tract—13	PR—25%	9.5 months	Raderer[127]	II
5-FU 2600 mg/m^2 + LV 150 mg/m^2 over 24 hours, weekly × 6 + MMC 10 mg/m^2 day 1, every 8 weeks	Gallbladder—3 Biliary tract—22	PR—26% (14–57%)	6 months	Chen[128]	II
5-FU 350 mg/m^2 + LV 350 mg/m^2, days 1–4 + MMC 10 mg/m^2, day 1	Gallbladder—4 Biliary tract—9	PR—23% (5–54%)	4.5 months	Polyzos[129]	II
5-FU 600 mg/m^2, days 1, 8, 29, 36 + ADR 30 mg/m^2, days 1, 29 + MMC 10 mg/m^2, day 1	Biliary tract—17	PR—31%	Not stated for entire group	Harvey[130]	II
1. 5-FU 310 mg/m^2, days 1–5, 22–26 2. 5-FU 310 mg/m^2, days 1–5, 22–26 + ADR 12 mg/m^2, day 8 + MMC 6 mg/m^2, day 1	1. Gallbladder—10 Biliary tract—8 2. Gallbladder—10 Biliary tract—8	No responses in either arm	Not stated	Takada[125]	II
5-FU 600 mg/m^2 + epirubicin 20 mg/m^2 + MTX 150 mg/m^2, weekly × 3	Gallbladder—6 Biliary tract—16	No responses	9 months	Kajanti[226]	II

TABLE 44.7. (continued)

Regimen	*No. of patients*	*Response (95% CI)*	*Overall survival*	*Reference*	*Level of evidence*
Platinum-based					
CDDP 90 mg/m² every 3 weeks	Biliary tract—9	No responses	Not stated	Ravry[143]	III
CDDP 80 mg/m² every 4 weeks	Gallbladder—1 Biliary tract—12	PR—7.7% (0.2–36%)	5.5 months	Okada[144]	II
5-FU 1000 mg/m²/d × 5 days + CDDP 100 mg/m² day 2	Gallbladder—11 Biliary tract—14	PR—25% (6–42%)	10 months	Ducreux[145]	II
LV 200 mg/m² days 1, 2 + 5-FU 400 mg/m² bolus followed by 2200 mg/m² over 22 h, days 1, 2 + CDDP 50 mg/m² day 2	Gallbladder—6 Biliary tract—23	CR 1 + PR 9: 34% (23–45%)	9.5 months	Taieb[146]	II
LV 500 mg/m² + 5-FU 2–2.6 g/m² weekly × 6 + CDDP 50 mg/m² every other week	Biliary tract—4	No responses	3.9 months	Caroli-Bosc[147]	III
5-FU 500 mg/m²/d × 5 days + epirubicin 50 mg/m² day 1 + CDDP 80 mg/m² day 1	Gallbladder—32 Biliary tract—5	PR—19% (6–32%)	6 months	Morizane[150]	II
5-FU 200 mg/m²/d × 21 days + epirubicin 50 mg/m² day 1 + CDDP 60 mg/m² day 1	Gallbladder—9 Biliary tract—12	PR—40% (19–64%)	11 months	Ellis[151]	II
5-FU 500 mg/m²/d × 3 days + doxoubicin 40 mg/m² day 1 + CDDP 80 mg/m² day 1 + IFN	Gallbladder—19 Biliary tract—22	1 CR + 7 PR 21% (10–37%)	14 months	Patt[152]	II
5-FU 400 mg/m² + LV 25 mg/m², days 1–4 + CBDCA 300 mg/m² day 1	Gallbladder—4 Biliary tract—10	1 CR + 2 PR 21.4%	5 months	Sanz-Altamira[148]	II
LV 500 mg/m² days 1, 2 + 5-FU 1.5–2 g/m² over 22 h, days 1, 2 + oxaliplatin 85 mg/m² day 1	Gallbladder—7 Biliary tract—9	PR—19% (0–41%)	9.5 months	Nehls[149]	II
Other agents					
CPT-11 100–125 mg/m² weekly × 4	Gallbladder—24 Biliary tract—15	1 CR + 2 PR: 8% (2–23%)	6.1 months	Alberts[153]	II
CPT-11 125 mg/m² weekly × 4	Gallbladder—10 Biliary tract—15	PR—8% (0–18%)	10 months	Sanz-Altamira[154]	II
Docetaxel 100 mg/m² every 3 weeks	Gallbladder—16 Biliary tract—9	2 CR + 3 PR—20% (4–36%)	8 months	Papakostas[155]	II
MMC 15 mg/m² every 6 weeks	Gallbladder—13 Biliary tract—17	PR—10% (2–27%)	4.5 months	Taal[227]	II
Paclitaxel 170–240 mg/m² every 21 days	Gallbladder—4 Biliary tract—11	No responses	Not stated	Jones[156]	II

6.8 months and the time to progression was 3.5 months. In the second arm of this study, gemcitabine 2,200 mg/m² was given every 2 weeks, and 4 of 14 patients (29%) achieved a partial response. The median survival with this schedule was 10.5 months and the median time to progression was 4.8 months. In 2002, on review of the available data, the FDA approved a diagnosis of cholangiocarcinoma as an indicator for the use of gemcitabine. Phase III studies to establish the efficacy of gemcitabine have yet to be performed.

Gemcitabine combined with other agents have produced responses ranging from 25% to 64% with median survivals of 10 to 15 months.[140–142] However, this finding is based on level III and IV evidence and as such is of uncertain value. No phase III trials or appropriately powered phase II trials have been published. It therefore remains unclear if multiagent therapy, using gemcitabine, has any benefit over gemcitabine alone. The potential added toxicity of a second agent has also not been assessed in comparison to gemcitabine.

In addition to 5-FU and gemcitabine, platinum compounds represent the other most commonly evaluated chemotherapy drugs. Most studies have evaluated cisplatin (CDDP) alone or in combination with 5-FU and LV and provide level II or III evidence of activity.[143–147] There appears to be no justification for the use of single-agent CDDP, with less than 10% of patients having a response and overall survival under 6 months.[143,144] An improved response rate is seen with the addition of 5-FU and LV. Prolonged infusion of 5-FU appears to increase the response rate to approximately one-third of patients.[146] However, overall survival does not appear to differ between infusional and bolus regimens of 5-FU.[145,146] The use of other platinum drugs, such as carboplatin (CBDCA) or oxaliplatin, also does not appear to change response rates or overall survival.[148,149] Finally, the addition of an anthracycline (doxorubicin or epirubicin) to CDDP and 5-FU does not improve its activity.[150–152] No level I evidence is currently available to establish the activity of platinum-based regimens in comparison to other regimens or single agents such as gemcitabine.

The activity of several newer chemotherapy drugs has been assessed in phase II trials. These trials have shown no obvious improvement in outcome, based on level II evidence, when the drugs CPT-11, docetaxel, or paclitaxel were used.[153–156] Clinical trials with novel or targeted agents have not yet been published.

Until recently, no randomized trials had assessed the potential benefit of chemotherapy following resection of gallbladder or biliary tract carcinoma. In a study of resected pancreatic (n = 173), bile duct (n = 135), gallbladder (n = 140), or ampulla of Vater (n = 56), patients were randomized to either surgery alone or to adjuvant chemotherapy following surgery.[157] For those randomized to adjuvant chemotherapy, patients were given mitomycin C (MMC) and 5-FU for two cycles followed by oral 5-FU until the time of recurrence. Patients with resected gallbladder cancer who received adjuvant chemotherapy had a significantly better 5-year survival rate if they received chemotherapy (26% versus 14%; P =

0.0367). No benefit of adjuvant chemotherapy was seen in patients with resected bile duct cancers. Although this study provides level I evidence for use of adjuvant chemotherapy, at least for resected gallbladder cancer, further studies are needed to confirm the findings of this study and to evaluate the potentially more active chemotherapy drugs including gemcitabine.

The role of adjuvant radiotherapy with or without chemotherapy in combination with hepatic resection for extrahepatic cholangiocarcinoma remains controversial. Although some institutions have demonstrated improved local control and improved overall survival,[158,159] others have reported no benefit.[160,161]

References

1. Parkin DM, Bray F, Ferlay J, et al. Estimating the world cancer burden: GLOBOCAN 2000. Int J Cancer (Phila) 2001;94:153–156.
2. Fattovich G, Giustina G, Degos F, et al. Morbidity and mortality in compensated cirrhosis type C: a retrospective follow-up study of 384 patients. Gastroenterology 1997;112:463–472.
3. El-Serag HB, Mason AC. Rising incidence of hepatocellular carcinoma in the United States. N Engl J Med 1999;340:745–750.
4. Alberti A, Pontisso P. Hepatitis viruses as aetiological agents of hepatocellular carcinoma. Ital J Gastroenterol 1991;23:452–456.
5. Beasley RP, Hwang LY, Lin CC, et al. Hepatocellular carcinoma and hepatitis B virus; a prospective study of 22,707 men in Taiwan. Lancet 1981;2:1129–1133.
6. Zhou XD, Tang ZY, Yang BH, et al. Experience of 1000 patients who underwent hepatectomy for small hepatocellular carcinoma. Cancer (Phila) 2001;91:1479–1486.
7. Chang MH, Chen CJ, Lai MS, et al. Universal hepatitis B vaccination in children. N Engl J Med 1997;336:1855–1859.
8. Change MH, Shau WY, Chen CJ, et al. The Taiwan Childhood Hepatoma Study Group: hepatitis B vaccination and hepatocellular carcinoma rates in boys and girls. JAMA 2000;284:3040–3042.
9. WHO. Hepatitis C: global prevalence. Wkly Epidemiol Rec 1997;72:341–344.
10. Niederau C, Fischer R, Sonnenberg A, et al. Survival and causes of death in cirrhotic and in noncirrhotic patients with primary hemochromatosis. N Engl J Med 1985;313:1256–62.
11. Sun Z, Lu P, Gail MH. Increased risk of hepatocellular carcinoma in male hepatitis B surface antigen carriers with chronic hepatitis who have detectable aflatoxin metabolite M1. Hepatology 1999;30:379–383.
12. Ozturk M. p53 mutation in hepatocellular carcinoma after aflatoxin exposure. Lancet 1991;338:1356–1359.
13. Farges O, Belghiti J, Kianmanesh R, et al. Portal vein embolization before right hepatectomy: prospective clinical trial. Ann Surg 2003;237:208–217.
14. Hemming AW, Reed AI, Howard RJ, et al. Preoperative portal vein embolization for extended hepatectomy. Ann Surg 2003;237:686–691.
15. Abdalla EK, Barnett CC, Doherty D, et al. Extended hepatectomy in patients with hepatobiliary malignancies with and without preoperative portal vein embolization. Arch Surg 2002;137:675–681.
16. Okuda K, Ohtsuki T, Obata H, et al. Natural history of hepatocellular carcinoma and prognosis in relation to treatment. Study of 850 patients. Cancer (Phila) 1985;56:918–928.
17. Bismuth H, Majno P. Hepatobiliary surgery. J Hepatol 2000;32:208–224.
18. Llovet JM, Fuster J, Bruix J. Intention-to-treat analysis of surgical treatment for early hepatocellular carcinoma: resection versus transplantation. Hepatology 1999;39:1434–1440.
19. Nagasue N, Uchida M, Makino Y, et al. Incidence and factors associated with intrahepatic recurrence following resection of hepatocellular carcinoma. Gastroenterology 1993;105:488–494.
20. Ringe B, Pichlmayr R, Wittekind C, et al. Surgical treatment of hepatocellular carcinoma: experience with liver resection and transplantation in 198 patients. World J Surg 1991;15:270–285.
21. Mazzaferro V, Regalia E, Doci R, et al. Liver transplantation for the treatment of small hepatocellular carcinomas in patients with cirrhosis. N Engl J Med 1996;334:693–699.
22. Bismuth H, Majno PE, Adam R. Liver transplantation for hepatocellular carcinoma. Semin Liver Dis 1999;19:311–322.
23. Jonas S, Bechstein WO, Steinmuller T, et al. Vascular invasion and histopathologic grading determine outcome after liver transplantation for hepatocellular carcinoma in cirrhosis. Hepatology 2001;33:1080–1086.
24. Yao FY, Ferrell L, Bass NM, et al. Liver transplantation for hepatocellular carcinoma: expansion of the tumor size limits does not adversely impact survival. Hepatology 2001;33:1394–1403.
25. Yao FY, Bass NM, Nikolai B, et al. Liver transplantation for hepatocellular carcinoma: analysis of survival according to the intention-to-treat principle and dropout from the waiting list. Liver Transplant 2002;8:873–883.
26. Livraghi T, Giorgio A, Marin G, et al. Hepatocellular carcinoma and cirrhosis in 746 patients: long term results of percutaneous ethanol injection. Radiology 1995;197:101–108.
27. Lencioni R, Pinto F, Armillotta N, et al. Long-term results of percutaneous ethanol injection therapy for hepatocellular carcinoma in cirrhosis: a European experience. Eur Radiol 1997;7:514–519.
28. Arri S, Yamaoka Y, Futagawa S, et al. Results of surgical and nonsurgical treatment for small-sized hepatocellular carcinomas: a retrospective and nationwide survey in Japan. Hepatology 2000;32:1224–1229.
29. Lencioni RA, Allgaier HP, Cioni D, et al. Small hepatocellular carcinoma in cirrhosis: randomized comparison of radio-frequency thermal ablation versus percutaneous ethanol injection. Radiology 2003;228:235–240.
30. Bruix J, Llovet JM. Prognostic prediction and treatment strategy in hepatocellular carcinoma. Hepatology 2002;35:519–524.
31. Bruix J, Llovet JM Castells A, et al. Transarterial embolization versus symptomatic treatment in patient with advanced hepatocellular carcinoma: results of a randomized, controlled trial in a single institution. Hepatology 1998;27:1578–1583.
32. Lo CM, Ngan H, Tso WK, et al. Randomized controlled trial of transarterial lipiodol chemoembolization for unresectable hepatocellular carcinoma. Hepatology 2002;35:1164–1171.
33. Llovet JM, Real MI, Montana X, et al. Arterial embolisation or chemoembolisation versus symptomatic treatment in patients with unresectable hepatocellular carcinoma: a randomised controlled trial. Lancet 2002;359:1734–1739.
34. Llovet JM, Bruix J. Systematic review of randomized trials for unresectable hepatocellular carcinoma: chemoembolization improves survival. Hepatology 2003;37:429–442.
35. Chlebowski RT, Brzechwa-Adjukiewicz A, Cowden A, et al. Doxorubicin ($75\,mg/m^2$) for hepatocellular carcinoma: clinical and pharmacokinetic results. Cancer Treat Rev 1984;68:487–491.
36. Lai CL, Wu PC, Chan GC, et al. Doxorubicin versus no antitumor therapy in inoperable hepatocellular carcinoma. A prospective randomized trial. Cancer (Phila) 1988;62:479–483.
37. Sciarrino E, Simonetti RG, Le Moli S, et al. Adriamycin treatment for hepatocellular carcinoma. Experience with 109 patients. Cancer (Phila) 1985;56:2751–2755.

38. Halm U, Etzrodt G, Schiefke I, et al. A phase II study of pegylated liposomal doxorubicin for treatment of advanced hepatocellular carcinoma. Ann Oncol 2000;11(1):113–114.
39. Hong RL, Tseng YL. A phase II and pharmacokinetic study of pegylated liposomal doxorubicin in patients with advanced hepatocellular carcinoma. Cancer Chemother Pharmacol 2003;51:433–438.
40. Schmidinger M, Wenzel C, Locker GJ, et al. Pilot study with pegylated liposomal doxorubicin for advanced or unresectable hepatocellular carcinoma. Br J Cancer 2001;85:1850–1852.
41. Hochster HS, Green MD, Speyer J, et al. 4′-Epidoxorubicin (epirubicin): activity in hepatocellular carcinoma. J Clin Oncol 1985;3:1535–1540.
42. Pohl J, Zuna I, Stremmel W, et al. Systemic chemotherapy with epirubicin for treatment of advanced or multifocal hepatocellular carcinoma. Chemotherapy 2001;47:359–365.
43. Patt YZ, Hoque A, Roh M, et al. Durable clinical and pathologic response of hepatocellular carcinoma to systemic and hepatic arterial administration of platinol, recombinant interferon alpha 2B, doxorubicin, and 5-fluorouracil: a communication. Am J Clin Oncol 1999;22:209–213.
44. Leung TW, Patt YZ, Lau WY, et al. Complete pathological remission is possible with systemic combination chemotherapy for inoperable hepatocellular carcinoma. Clin Cancer Res 1999;5:1676–1681.
45. Malaguarnera M, Trovato G, Restuccia S, et al. Treatment of nonresectable hepatocellular carcinoma: review of the literature and meta-analysis. Adv Ther 1994;11:303–319.
46. Simonetti RG, Liberati A, Angiolini C, et al. Treatment of hepatocellular carcinoma: a systematic review of randomized controlled trials. Ann Oncol 1997;8:117–136.
47. Mathurin P, Rixe O, Carbonell N, et al. Review article: Overview of medical treatments in unresectable hepatocellular carcinoma—an impossible meta-analysis? Aliment Pharmacol Ther 1998;12:111–126.
48. Jiang SY, Shyu RY, Yeh MY, et al. Tamoxifen inhibits hepatoma cell growth through an estrogen receptor independent mechanism. J Hepatol 1995;23:712–719.
49. Boix L, Bruix J, Castells A, et al. Sex hormone receptors in hepatocellular carcinoma. Is there a rationale for hormonal treatment? J Hepatol 1993;17:187–191.
50. Elba S, Giannuzzi V, Misciagna G, et al. Randomized controlled trial of tamoxifen versus placebo in inoperable hepatocellular carcinoma. Ital J Gastroenterol 1994;26:66–68.
51. Martinez Cerezo FJ, Tomas A, Donoso L, et al. Controlled trial of tamoxifen in patients with advanced hepatocellular carcinoma. J Hepatol 1994;20:702–706.
52. Castells A, Bruix J, Bru C, et al. Treatment of hepatocellular carcinoma with tamoxifen: a double-blind placebo-controlled trial in 120 patients. Gastroenterology 1995;109:917–922.
53. Perrone F, Gallo C, Daniele B, et al. Tamoxifen in the treatment of hepatocellular carcinoma: 5-year results of the CLIP-1 multicentre randomised controlled trial. Curr Pharm Des 2002;8:1013–1019.
54. Liu CL, Fan ST, Ng IO, et al. Treatment of advanced hepatocellular carcinoma with tamoxifen and the correlation with expression of hormone receptors: a prospective randomized study. Am J Gastroenterol 2000;95:218–222.
55. Chow PK, Tai BC, Tan CK, et al. High-dose tamoxifen in the treatment of inoperable hepatocellular carcinoma: a multicenter randomized controlled trial. Hepatology 2002;36(5):1221–1226.
56. Chao Y, Chan WK, Huang YS, et al. Phase II study of flutamide in the treatment of hepatocellular carcinoma. Cancer (Phila) 1996;77:635–639.
57. Colleoni M, Nelli P, Vicario G, et al. Megestrol acetate in unresectable hepatocellular carcinoma. Tumori 1995;81(5):351–353.
58. Chao Y, Chan WK, Wang SS, et al. Phase II study of megestrol acetate in the treatment of hepatocellular carcinoma. J Gastroenterol Hepatol 1997;12:277–281.
59. Raderer M, Hejna MH, Muller C, et al. Treatment of hepatocellular cancer with the long acting somatostatin analog lanreotide in vitro and in vivo. Int J Oncol 2000;16:1197–1201.
60. Kouroumalis E, Skordilis P, Thermos K, et al. Treatment of hepatocellular carcinoma with octreotide: a randomised controlled study. Gut 1998;42:442–447.
61. Pan DY, Qiao JG, Chen JW, et al. Tamoxifen combined with octreotide or regular chemotherapeutic agents in treatment of primary liver cancer: a randomized controlled trial. Hepatobiliary Pancreat Dis Int 2003;2:211–215.
62. Huang YH, Wu JC, Lui WY, et al. Prospective case-controlled trial of adjuvant chemotherapy after resection of hepatocellular carcinoma. World J Surg 2000;24:551–555.
63. Schwartz JD, Schwartz M, Mandeli J, et al. Neoadjuvant and adjuvant therapy for resectable hepatocellular carcinoma: review of the randomised clinical trials. Lancet Oncol 2002;3:593–603.
64. Patel T. Increasing incidence and mortality of primary intrahepatic cholangiocarcinoma in the United States. Hepatology 2001;33:1353–1357.
65. Patel T. Worldwide trends in mortality from biliary tract malignancies. BMC Cancer 2002;2:10.
66. Khan SA, Taylor-Robinson SD, Toledano MB, et al. Changing international trends in mortality rates for liver, biliary and pancreatic tumours. J Hepatol 2002;37:806–813.
67. Terada T, Kida T, Nakanuma Y, et al. Intrahepatic cholangiocarcinomas associated with nonbiliary cirrhosis. A clinicopathologic study. J Clin Gastroenterol 1994;18:335–342.
68. Bergquist A, Glaumann H, Persson B, et al. Risk factors and clinical presentation of hepatobiliary carcinoma in patients with primary sclerosing cholangitis: a case-control study. Hepatology 1998;27:311–316.
69. Bergquist A, Ekbom A, Olsson R, et al. Hepatic and extrahepatic malignancies in primary sclerosing cholangitis. J Hepatol 2002;36:321–327.
70. Khan SA, Davidson BR, Goldin R, et al. Guidelines for the diagnosis and treatment of cholangiocarcinoma: consensus document. Gut 2002;51(suppl 6):VI1–VI9.
71. Okuda K, Nakanuma Y, Miyazaki M. Cholangiocarcinoma: recent progress. Part 1: epidemiology and etiology. J Gastroenterol Hepatol 2002;17:1049–1055.
72. Kobayashi M, Ikeda K, Saitoh S, et al. Incidence of primary cholangiocellular carcinoma of the liver in Japanese patients with hepatitis C virus-related cirrhosis. Cancer (Phila) 2000;88:2471–2477.
73. Fong YY, Chan WC. Bacterial production of di-methyl nitrosamine in salted fish. Nature (Lond) 1973;243:421–422.
74. Herrold KM. Histogenesis of malignant liver tumors induced by dimethylnitrosamine. An experimental study in Syrian hamsters. J Natl Cancer Inst 1967;39:1099–1111.
75. Jaiswal M, LaRusso NF, Gores GJ. Nitric oxide in gastrointestinal epithelial cell carcinogenesis: linking inflammation to oncogenesis. Am J Physiol Gastrointest Liver Physiol 2001;281:G626–G634.
76. Jaiswal M, LaRusso NF, Shapiro RA, et al. Nitric oxide-mediated inhibition of DNA repair potentiates oxidative DNA damage in cholangiocytes. Gastroenterology 2001;120:190–199.
77. Mannick JB, Hausladen A, Liu L, et al. Fas-induced caspase denitrosylation. Science 1999;284:651–654.
78. Jaiswal M, LaRusso NF, Burgart LJ, et al. Inflammatory cytokines induce DNA damage and inhibit DNA repair in cholangiocarcinoma cells by a nitric oxide-dependent mechanism. Cancer Res 2000;60:184–190.
79. Parkin DM, Srivatanakul P, Khlat M, et al. Liver cancer in Thailand. I. A case-control study of cholangiocarcinoma. Int J Cancer 1991;48:323–328.

80. Rao CV, Indranie C, Simi B, et al. Chemopreventive properties of a selective inducible nitric oxide synthase inhibitor in colon carcinogenesis, administered alone or in combination with celecoxib, a selective cyclooxygenase-2 inhibitor. Cancer Res 2002;62:165–170.
81. Kisley LR, Barrett BS, Bauer AK, et al. Genetic ablation of inducible nitric oxide synthase decreases mouse lung tumorigenesis. Cancer Res 2002;62:6850–6856.
82. Yoon JH, Higuchi H, Werneburg NW, et al. Bile acids induce cyclooxygenase-2 expression via the epidermal growth factor receptor in a human cholangiocarcinoma cell line. Gastroenterology 2002;122:985–993.
83. Gupta RA, Dubois RN. Colorectal cancer prevention and treatment by inhibition of cyclooxygenase-2. Nat Rev Cancer 2001;1:11–21.
84. Yoon JH, Werneburg NW, Higuchi H, et al. Bile acids inhibit Mcl-1 protein turnover via an epidermal growth factor receptor/Raf-1-dependent mechanism. Cancer Res 2002; 62:6500–6505.
85. Okaro AC, Deery AR, Hutchins RR, et al. The expression of antiapoptotic proteins Bcl-2, Bcl-X(L), and Mcl-1 in benign, dysplastic, and malignant biliary epithelium. J Clin Pathol 2001;54:927–932.
86. Pichlmayr R, Lamesch P, Weimann A, et al. Surgical treatment of cholangiocellular carcinoma. World J Surg 1995;19:83–88.
87. Colombari R, Tsui WM. Biliary tumors of the liver. Semin Liver Dis 1995;15:402–413.
88. Lieser MJ, Barry MK, Rowland C, et al. Surgical management of intrahepatic cholangiocarcinoma: a 31-year experience. J Hepatobiliary Pancreat Surg 1998;5:41–47.
89. Liver Cancer Study Group of Japan. Classification of primary liver cancer. Tokyo: Kanehara-Shuppan, 1997.
90. Kang YK, Kim WH, Lee HW, et al. Mutation of p53 and K-ras, and loss of heterozygosity of APC in intraphepatic cholangiocarcinoma. Lab Invest 1999;79(4):477–483.
91. Ohashi K, Nakajima Y, Kanehiro H, et al. Ki-ras mutations and p53 protein expressions in intrahepatic cholangiocarcinomas: relation to gross tumor morphology. Gastroenterology 1995; 109:1612–1617.
92. Roayaie S, Guarrera JV, Ye MQ, et al. Aggressive surgical treatment of intrahepatic cholangiocarcinoma: predictors of outcomes. J Am Coll Surg 1998;187:365–372.
93. Chou FF, Sheen-Chen SM, Chen YS, et al. Surgical treatment of cholangiocarcinoma. Hepatogastroenterology 1997;44:760–765.
94. Nakajima T, Kondo Y, Miyazaki M, et al. A histopathologic study of 102 cases of intrahepatic cholangiocarcinoma: histologic classification and modes of spreading. Hum Pathol 1988; 19:1228–1234.
95. Inohue K, Makuuchi M, Takayama T, et al. Long-term survival and prognostic factors in the surgical treatment of mass-forming type cholangiocarcinoma. Surgery (St. Louis) 2000;127:498–505.
96. Chu KM, Lai ECS, Al-Hadeedi S, et al. Intrahepatic cholangiocarcinoma. World J Surg 1997;21:301–306.
97. Burke EC, Jarnagin WR, Hochwald SN, et al. Hilar cholangiocarcinoma: patterns of spread, the importance of hepatic resection for curative operation, and a presurgical clinical staging system. Ann Surg 1998;228:385–394.
98. Weinbren K, Mutum SS. Pathological aspects of cholangiocarcinoma. J Pathol 1983;139:217–238.
99. Sako K, Seitzinger GL, Garside E. Carcinoma of the extrahepatic bile ducts: review of the literature and report of six cases. Surgery(St. Louis) 1957;41:416–437.
100. Pitt HA, Dooley WC, Yeo CJ, et al. Malignancies of the biliary tree. Curr Probl Surg 1995;32:1–90.
101. Jarnagin WR, Fong Y, DeMatteo RP, et al. Staging, resectability, and outcome in 225 patients with hilar cholangiocarcinoma. Ann Surg 2001;234:507–519.
102. Nimura Y Kamiya J, Kondo S, et al. Aggressive preoperative management and extended surgery for hilar cholangiocarcinoma: Nagoya experience. J Hepatobiliary Pancreat Surg 2000; 7:155–162.
103. Kawasaki S, Makuuchi M, Miyagawa S, et al. Radical operation after portal embolization for tumor of the hilar bile duct. J Am Coll Surg 1994;178:480–486.
104. Hochwald SN, Burke EC, Jarnagin WR, et al. Association of preoperative biliary stenting with increased postoperative infectious complications in proximal cholangiocarcinoma. Arch Surg 1999;134:261–266.
105. Gallinger S, Gluckman D, Langer B. Proximal bile duct cancer. Adv Surg 1990;23:89–118.
106. Cameron JL, Pitt HA, Zinner MJ, et al. Management of proximal cholangiocarcinomas by surgical resection and radiotherapy. Am J Surg 1990;159:91–97.
107. Gerhards MF, van Gulik TM, de Wit LT, et al. Evaluation of morbidity and mortality after resection for hilar cholangiocarcinoma – a single center experience. Surgery (St. Louis 2000;127:395–404.
108. Mulholland MW, Yahanda A, Yeo CJ. Multidisciplinary management of perihilar bile duct cancer. J Am Coll Surg 2001; 193:440–447.
109. Tabata M, Kawarada Y, Yokoi H, et al. Surgical treatment for hilar cholangiocarcinoma. J Hepatobiliary Pancreat Surg 2000; 7:148–154.
110. Gazzaniga GM, Ciferri E, Bagarolo C, et al. Primitive hepatic hilum neoplasm. J Surg Oncol 1993;3:140–146.
111. Gazzaniga GM, Filauro M, Bagarolo C, et al. Surgery for hilar cholangiocarcinoma: an Italian experience. J Hepatobiliary Pancreat Surg 2000;7:122–127.
112. Tsao JI, Nimura Y, Kamiya J, et al. Management of hilar cholangiocarcinoma: comparison of an American and a Japanese experience. Ann Surg 2000;232:166–174.
113. Nimura Y, Haykawa N, Kamiya J, et al. Hilar cholangiocarcinoma: surgical anatomy and curative resection. J Hepatobiliary Pancreat Surg 1995;2:239–248.
114. Kawarada Y, Suzuki H, Mizumoto R. Surgical treatment of hilar carcinoma of the bile duct, with special reference to anatomy of the hepatic hilum and caudate lobe. Jpn J Gastroenterol Surg 1984;17:1684–1688.
115. Nimura Y, Hayakawa N, Kamiya J, et al. Hepatic segmentectomy with caudate lobe resection for bile duct carcinoma of the hepatic hilus. World J Surg 1990;14:535–543.
116. Ogura Y, Mizumoto R, Tabata M. Surgical treatment of carcinoma of the hepatic duct confluence: analysis of 55 resected carcinomas. World J Surg 1993;17:85–92.
117. Sugiura Y, Nakamura S, Iisda S, et al. Extensive resection of the bile ducts combined with liver resection for cancer of the main hepatic duct junction: a cooperative study of the Keio Bile Duct Cancer Study Group. Surgery (St/Louis) 1994;115:445–451.
118. Farley DR, Weaver AL, Nagorney DM. Natural history of unresected cholangiocarcinoma: patient outcome after noncurative intervention. Mayo Clin Proc 1995;70:425–429.
119. Lee SG, Lee YJ, Park KM. One hundred and eleven liver resections for hilar bile duct cancer. J Hepatobiliary Pancreat Surg 2000;7:135–141.
120. Neuhaus P, Jonas S, Bechstein WO, et al. Extended resections for hilar cholangiocarcinoma. Ann Surg 1999;230:808–818.
121. Launois B, Reding R, Lebeau G. Surgery for hilar cholangiocarcinoma: French experience in a collective survey of 552 extrahepatic bile duct cancers. J Hepatobiliary Pancreat Surg 2000;7:128–134.
122. Rea DJ, Munoz-Juarez M, Farnell MB, et al. Major hepatic resection for hilar cholangiocarcinoma: analysis of 46 patients. Arch Surg 2004;139:514–525.

123. Glimelius B, Hoffman K, Sjoden PO, et al. Chemotherapy improves survival and quality of life in advanced pancreatic and biliary cancer. Ann Oncol 1996;7:593–600.
124. Falkson G, MacIntyre JM, Moertel CG. Eastern Cooperative Oncology Group experience with chemotherapy for inoperable gallbladder and bile duct cancer. Cancer (Phila) 1984;54:965–969.
125. Takada T, Kato H, Matsushiro T, et al. Comparison of 5-fluorouracil, doxorubicin and mitomycin C with 5-fluorouracil alone in the treatment of pancreatic-biliary carcinomas. Oncology 1994;51:396–400.
126. Chen JS, Jan YY, Lin YC, et al. Weekly 24h infusion of high-dose 5-fluorouracil and leucovorin in patients with biliary tract carcinomas. Anti-Cancer Drugs 1998;9:393–397.
127. Raderer M, Hejna MH, Valencak JB, et al. Two consecutive phase II studies of 5-fluorouracil/leucovorin/mitomycin C and of gemcitabine in patients with advanced biliary cancer. Oncology 1999;56:177–180.
128. Chen JS, Lin YC, Jan YY, et al. Mitomycin C with weekly 24-h infusion of high-dose 5-fluorouracil and leucovorin in patients with biliary tract and periampullar carcinomas. Anticancer Drugs 2001;12(4):339–343.
129. Polyzos A, Nikou G, Giannopoulos A, et al. Chemotherapy of biliary tract cancer with mitomycin-C and 5-fluorouracil biologically modulated by folinic acid. A phase II study. Ann Oncol 1996;7:644–645.
130. Harvey JH, Smith FP, Schein PS. 5-Fluorouracil, mitomycin, and doxorubicin (FAM) in carcinoma of the biliary tract. J Clin Oncol 1984;2:1245–1248.
131. Castro MP. Efficacy of gemcitabine in the treatment of patients with gallbladder carcinoma: a case report. Cancer (Phila) 1998; 82:639–641.
132. Gallardo J, Fodor M, Gamargo C, et al. Efficacy of gemcitabine in the treatment of patients with gallbladder carcinoma: a case report. Cancer (Phila) 1998;83:2419–2421.
133. Tsavaris N, Kosmas C, Gouveris P, et al. Weekly gemcitabine for the treatment of biliary tract and gallbladder cancer. Invest New Drugs 2004;22:193–198.
134. Kubicka S, Rudolph KL, Tietze MK, et al. Phase II study of systemic gemcitabine chemotherapy for advanced unresectable hepatobiliary carcinomas. Hepato-Gastroenterology 2001;48: 783–789.
135. Gallardo JO, Rubio B, Fodor M, et al. A phase II study of gemcitabine in gallbladder carcinoma. Ann Oncol 2001;12: 1403–1406.
136. Penz M, Kornek GV, Raderer M, et al. Phase II trial of two-weekly gemcitabine in patients with advanced biliary tract cancer. Ann Oncol 2001;12:183–186.
137. Teufel A, Lehnert T, Stremmel W, et al. Chemotherapy with gemcitabine in patients with advanced gallbladder carcinoma. Z Gastroenterol 2000;38:909–912.
138. Metzger J, Sauerbruch T, Ko Y, et al. Phase II trial of gemcitabine in gallbladder and biliary tract carcinomas. Onkologie 1998; 21:232–234.
139. Valencak J, Kornek GV, Raderer M, et al. Gemcitabine for the treatment of advanced biliary tract carcinomas: evaluation of two different dose regimens. Onkologie 1999;22:498–501.
140. Murad AM, Guimaraes RC, Aragao BC, et al. Phase II trial of the use of gemcitabine and 5-fluorouracil in the treatment of advanced pancreatic and biliary tract cancer. Am J Clin Oncol 2003;26:151–154.
141. Boxberger F, Jungert B, Brueckl V, et al. Palliative chemotherapy with gemcitabine and weekly high-dose 5-fluorouracil as 24-h infusion in metastatic biliary tract and gall bladder adenocarcinomas. Anticancer Drugs 2003;14:87–90.
142. Malik IA, Aziz Z, Zaidi SH, et al. Gemcitabine and cisplatin is a highly effective combination chemotherapy in patients with advanced cancer of the gallbladder. Am J Clin Oncol 2003; 26:174–177.
143. Ravry MJR, Omura GA, Bartolucci AA, et al. Phase II evaluation of cisplatin in advanced hepatocellular carcinoma and cholangiocarcinoma: a Southeastern Cancer Study Group Trial. Cancer Treat Rep 1986;70:311–312.
144. Okada S, Ishii H, Nose H, et al. A phase II study of cisplatin in patients with biliary tract carcinoma. Oncology 1994;51:515–517.
145. Ducreux M, Rougier P, Fandi A, et al. Effective treatment of advanced biliary tract carcinoma using 5-fluorouracil continuous infusion with cisplatin. Ann Oncol 1998;9:653–656.
146. Taieb J, Mitry E, Boige V, et al. Optimization of 5-fluorouracil (5-FU)/cisplatin combination chemotherapy with a new schedule of leucovorin, 5-FU and cisplatin (LV5FU2-P regimen) in patients with biliary tract carcinoma. Ann Oncol 2002;13: 1192–1196.
147. Caroli-Bosc FX, Van Laethem JL, Michel P, et al. A weekly 24-h infusion of high-dose 5-fluorouracil (5-FU) + leucovorin and bi-weekly cisplatin (CDDP) was active and well tolerated in patients with non-colon digestive carcinomas. Eur J Cancer 2001;37:1828–1832.
148. Sanz-Altamira PM, Ferrante K, Jenkins RL, et al. A phase II trial of 5-fluorouracil, leucovorin, and carboplatin in patients with unresectable biliary tree carcinoma. Cancer (Phila) 1998; 82:2321–2325.
149. Nehls O, Klump B, Arkenau HT, et al. Oxaliplatin, fluorouracil and leucovorin for advanced biliary system adenocarcinomas: a prospective phase II trial. Br J Cancer 2002;87:702–704.
150. Morizane C, Okada S, Okusaka T, et al. Phase II study of cisplatin, epirubicin, and continuous-infusion 5-fluorouracil for advanced biliary tract cancer. Oncology 2003;64:475–476.
151. Ellis PA, Norman A, Hill A, et al. Epirubicin, cisplatin and infusional 5-fluorouracil (5-FU) (ECF) in hepatobiliary tumours. Eur J Cancer 1995;31A:1594–1598.
152. Patt YZ, Hassan MM, Lozano RD, et al. Phase II trial of cisplatin, interferon alpha-2b, doxorubicin, and 5-fluorouracil for biliary tract cancer. Clin Cancer Res 2001;7:3375–3380.
153. Alberts SR, Fishkin PA, Burgart LJ, et al. CPT-11 for bile-duct and gallbladder carcinoma: a phase II North Central Cancer Treatment Group (NCCTG) study. Int J Gastrointest Cancer 2002;32:107–114.
154. Sanz-Altamira PM, O'Reilly E, Stuart KE, et al. A phase II trial of irinotecan (CPT-11) for unresectable biliary tree carcinoma. Ann Oncol 2001;12:501–504.
155. Papakostas P, Kouroussis C, Androulakis N, et al. First-line chemotherapy with docetaxel for unresectable or metastatic carcinoma of the biliary tract. A multicentre phase II study. Eur J Cancer 2001;37:1833–1838.
156. Jones DV Jr, Lozano R, Hoque A, Markowitz A, Patt YZ. Phase II study of paclitaxel therapy for unresectable biliary tree carcinomas. J Clin Oncol 1996;14:2306–2310.
157. Takada T, Amano H, Yasuda H, et al. Is postoperative adjuvant chemotherapy useful for gallbladder carcinoma? A phase III multicenter prospective randomized controlled trial in patients with resected pancreaticobiliary carcinoma. Cancer (Phila) 2002;95(8):1685–1689.
158. Todoroki T, Ohara K, Kawamoto T, et al. Benefits of adjuvant radiotherapy after radical resection of locally advanced main hepatic duct carcinoma. Int J Radiat Oncol Biol Phys 2000; 46:581–587.
159. Gonzalez D, Gerard JP, Maners AW, et al. Results of radiation therapy in carcinoma of the proximal bile ducts (Klatskin tumor). Semin Liver Dis 1990;10:131–141.
160. Cameron JL, Pitt HA, Zinner MJ, et al. Management of proximal cholangiocarcinomas by surgical resection and radiotherapy. Am J Surg 1990;159:91–98.
161. Pitt HA, Nakeeb A, Abrams RA, et al. Perihilar cholangiocarcinoma: postoperative radiotherapy does not improve survival. Ann Surg 1995;221:778–798.

162. Wayne JD, Lauwers GY, Ikai I, et al. Perioperative predictors of survival after resection of small hepatocellular carcinomas. Ann Surg 2002;235:722–731.
163. Poon RTP, Ng IOL, Fan ST, et al. Clinicopathologic features of long-term survivors and disease-free survivors after resection of hepatocellular carcinoma: a study of a prospective cohort. J Clin Oncol 2001;19:3037–3044.
164. Fong Y, Sun RL, Jarnagin W, et al. An analysis of 412 cases of hepatocellular carcinoma at a western center. Ann Surg 1999;229:790–800.
165. Lise M, Bacchetti S, Da Pian, P, et al. Prognostic factors affecting long term outcome after liver resection for hepatocellular carcinoma: results in a series of 100 Italian patients. Cancer (Phila) 1998;82:1028–1036.
166. Mazziotti A, Frazi GL, Cavallari A. Surgical treatment of hepatocellular carcinoma on cirrhosis: a western experience. Hepatogastroenterology 1998;45:1281–1287.
167. Takenaka K, Kawahara N, Yamamoto K, et al. Results of 280 liver resections for hepatocellular carcinoma. Arch Surg 1996; 131:71–76.
168. Vauthey JN, Klimstra D, Franceschi D, et al. Factors affecting long-term outcome after hepatic resection for hepatocellular carcinoma. Am J Surg 1995;169:28–34.
169. Kawasaki S, Makuuchi M, Miyagawa S, et al. Results of hepatic resection for hepatocellular carcinoma. World J Surg 1995; 19:31–34.
170. Yang TS, Lin YC, Chen JS, et al. Phase II study of gemcitabine in patients with advanced hepatocellular carcinoma. Cancer (Phila) 2000;89:750–756.
171. Fuchs CS, Clark JW, Ryan DP, et al. A phase II trial of gemcitabine in patients with advanced hepatocellular carcinoma. Cancer (Phila) 2002;94:3186–3191.
172. Guan Z, Wang Y, Maoleekoonpairoj S, et al. Prospective randomised phase II study of gemcitabine at standard or fixed dose rate schedule in unresectable hepatocellular carcinoma. Br J Cancer 2003;89:1865–1869.
173. Ulrich-Pur H, Kornek GV, Fiebiger W, et al. Treatment of advanced hepatocellular carcinoma with biweekly high-dose gemcitabine. Oncology 2001;60:313–315.
174. Yang TS, Wang CH, Hsieh RK, et al. Gemcitabine and doxorubicin for the treatment of patients with advanced hepatocellular carcinoma: a phase I-II trial. Ann Oncol 2002;13:1771–1778.
175. Taieb J, Bonyhay L, Golli L, et al. Gemcitabine plus oxaliplatin for patients with advanced hepatocellular carcinoma using two different schedules. Cancer (Phila) 2003;98:2664–2670.
176. Zaniboni A, Simoncini E, Marpicati P, et al. Phase II study of 5-fluorouracil (5-FU) and high dose folinic acid (HDFA) in hepatocellular carcinoma. Br J Cancer 1988;57:319.
177. van Eeden H, Falkson G, Burger W, et al. 5-Fluorouracil and leucovorin in hepatocellular carcinoma. Ann Oncol 1992; 3:404–405.
178. Tetef M, Doroshow J, Akman S, et al. 5-Fluorouracil and high-dose calcium leucovorin for hepatocellular carcinoma: a phase II trial. Cancer Invest 1995;13:460–463.
179. Porta C, Moroni M, Nastasi G, et al. 5-Fluorouracil and *d,l*-leucovorin calcium are active to treat unresectable hepatocellular carcinoma patients: preliminary results of a phase II study. Oncology 1995;52:487–491.
180. Gebbia V, Maiello E, Serravezza G, et al. 5-Fluorouracil plus high dose levofolinic acid and oral hydroxyurea for the treatment of primary hepatocellular carcinomas: results of a phase II multicenter study of the Southern Italy Oncology Group (G.O.I.M.). Anticancer Res. 1999;19:1407–1410.
181. Stuart K, Tessitore J, Huberman M. 5-Fluorouracil and alpha-interferon in hepatocellular carcinoma. Am J Clin Oncol 1996; 19:136–139.
182. Patt YZ, Jones DV, Hoque A, et al. Phase II trial of intravenous fluorouracil and subcutaneous interferon alfa-2b for biliary tract cancer. J Clin Oncol 1996;14:2311–2315.
183. Mani S, Schiano T, Garcia JC, et al. Phase II trial of uracil/tegafur (UFT) plus leucovorin in patients with advanced hepatocellular carcinoma. Invest New Drugs 1998;16:279–283.
184. Llovet JM, Ruff P, Tassopoulos N, et al. A phase II trial of oral eniluracil/5-fluorouracil in patients with inoperable hepatocellular carcinoma. Eur J Cancer 2001;37:1352–1358.
185. Benson AB III, Mitchell E, Abramson N, et al. Oral eniluracil/5-fluorouracil in patients with inoperable hepatocellular carcinoma. Ann Oncol 2002;13:576–581.
186. Falkson G, Ryan LM, Johnson LA, et al. A random phase II study of mitoxantrone and cisplatin in patients with hepatocellular carcinoma. An ECOG study. Cancer (Phila) 1987;60:2141–2145.
187. Okada S, Okazaki N, Nose H, et al. A phase 2 study of cisplatin in patients with hepatocellular carcinoma. Oncology 1993; 50:22–26.
188. Tanioka H, Tsuji A, Morita S, et al. Combination chemotherapy with continuous 5-fluorouracil and low-dose cisplatin infusion for advanced hepatocellular carcinoma. Anticancer Res 2003; 23:1891–1897.
189. Komorizono Y, Kohara K, Oketani M, et al. Systemic combined chemotherapy with low dose of 5-fluorouracil, cisplatin, and interferon-alpha for advanced hepatocellular carcinoma: a pilot study. Dig Dis Sci 2003;48:877–881.
190. Boucher E, Corbinais S, Brissot P, et al. Treatment of hepatocellular carcinoma (HCC) with systemic chemotherapy combining epirubicin, cisplatinum and infusional 5-fluorouracil (ECF regimen). Cancer Chemother Pharmacol 2002;50:305–308.
191. Alexandre J, Tigaud JM, Gross-Goupil M, et al. Combination of topotecan and oxaliplatin in inoperable hepatocellular cancer patients. Am J Clin Oncol 2002;25:198–203.
192. Lee GY, Kim BS, Seo YT, et al. Phase II study to topotecan and cisplatin in advanced hepatocellular carcinoma. Korean J Int Med 2003;18:104–108.
193. Feun LG, Savaraj N, Hung S, et al. A phase II trial of recombinant leukocyte interferon plus doxorubicin in patients with hepatocellular carcinoma. Am J Clin Oncol 1994;17:393–395.
194. Feun LG, O'Brien C, Molina E, et al. Recombinant leukocyte interferon, doxorubicin, and 5FUDR in patients with hepatocellular carcinoma: a phase II trial. J Cancer Res Clin Oncol 2003; 129:17–20.
195. Bokemeyer C, Kynast B, Harstrick A, et al. No synergistic activity of epirubicin and interferon-alpha 2b in the treatment of hepatocellular carcinoma. Cancer Chemother Pharmacol 1995;35:334–338.
196. Bobbio-Pallavicini E, Porta C, Moroni M, et al. Epirubicin and etoposide combination chemotherapy to treat hepatocellular carcinoma patients: a phase II study. Eur J Cancer 1997; 33:1784–1788.
197. Kajanti MJ, Pyrhonen SO. Phase II intravenous study of epirubicin with 5-fluorouracil in patients with advanced hepatocellular carcinoma. Eur J Cancer 1991;27:1620–1622.
198. Engstrom PF, Levin B, Moertel CG, et al. A phase II trial of tamoxifen in hepatocellular carcinoma. Cancer (Phila) 1990; 65:2641–2643.
199. Riestra S, Rodriguez M, Delgado M, et al. Tamoxifen does not improve survival of patients with advanced hepatocellular carcinoma. J Clin Gastroenterol 1998;26:200–203.
200. Anonymous. Tamoxifen in treatment of hepatocellular carcinoma: a randomised controlled trial. CLIP Group (Cancer of the Liver Italian Programme) [see comment]. Lancet 1998; 352:17–20.
201. Cheng AL, Chen YC, Yeh KH, et al. Chronic oral etoposide and tamoxifen in the treatment of far-advanced hepatocellular carcinoma. Cancer (Phila) 1996;77:872–877.

202. Cheng AL, Yeh KH, Fine RL, et al. Biochemical modulation of doxorubicin by high-dose tamoxifen in the treatment of advanced hepatocellular carcinoma. Hepatogastroenterology 1998;45:1955–1960.
203. Melia WM, Johnson PJ, Williams R. Controlled clinical trial of doxorubicin and tamoxifen versus doxorubicin alone in hepatocellular carcinoma. Cancer Treat Rep 1987;71:1213–1216.
204. Schachschal G, Lochs H, Plauth M. Controlled clinical trial of doxorubicin and tamoxifen versus tamoxifen monotherapy in hepatocellular carcinoma. Eur J Gastroenterol Hepatol 2000;12:281–284.
205. Yuen MF, Poon RT, Lai CL, et al. A randomized placebo-controlled study of long-acting octreotide for the treatment of advanced hepatocellular carcinoma. [see comment] [erratum appears in Hepatology 2003;37:489]. Hepatology 2002;36: 687–691.
206. O'Reilly EM, Stuart KE, Sanz-Altamira PM, et al. A phase II study of irinotecan in patients with advanced hepatocellular carcinoma. Cancer (Phila) 2001;91:101–105.
207. Lin J, Shiu W, Leung WT, et al. Phase II study of high-dose ifosfamide in hepatocellular carcinoma. Cancer Chemother Pharmacol 1993;31:338–339.
208. Cheirsilpa A, Leelasethakul S, Auethaveekiat V, et al. High-dose mitomycin C: activity in hepatocellular carcinoma. Cancer Chemother Pharmacol 1989;24:50–53.
209. Colleoni M, Nole F, Di Bartolomeo M, et al. Mitoxantrone in patients affected by hepatocellular carcinoma with unfavorable prognostic factors. Oncology 1992;49:139–142.
210. Colleoni M, Buzzoni R, Bajetta E, et al. A phase II study of mitoxantrone combined with beta-interferon in unresectable hepatocellular carcinoma. Cancer (Phila) 1993;72(11):3196–3201.
211. Chao Y, Chan WK, Birkhofer MJ, et al. Phase II and pharmacokinetic study of paclitaxel therapy for unresectable hepatocellular carcinoma patients. Br J Cancer 1998;78:34–39.
212. Hsu C, Chen CN, Chen LT, et al. Low-dose thalidomide treatment for advanced hepatocellular carcinoma. Oncology 2003; 65:242–249.
213. Wall JG, Benedetti JK, O'Rourke MA, et al. Phase II trial to topotecan in hepatocellular carcinoma: a Southwest Oncology Group study. Invest New Drugs 1997;15:257–260.
214. Falkson G, Burger W. A phase II trial of vindesine in hepatocellular cancer. Oncology 1995;52:86–87.
215. Kitagawa Y, Nagino M, Kamiya J, et al. Lymph node metastases from hilar cholangiocarcinoma: audit of 110 patients who underwent regional and paraaortic node dissection. Ann Surg 2001; 233:385–392.
216. Launois B, Terblanche J, Lakehal M, et al. Proximal bile duct cancer: high resectability rate and 5-year survival. Ann Surg 1999;230:266–275.
217. Iwatsuki S, Todo S, Marsh JW, et al. Treatment of hilar cholangiocarcinoma (Klatskin tumors) with hepatic resection or transplantation. J Am Coll Surg 1998;187:358–364.
218. Miyazaki H, Ito H, Nakagawa K, et al. Aggressive surgical approaches to hilar cholangiocarcinoma: hepatic or local resection? Surgery (St. Louis) 1998;123:131–136.
219. Eckel F, Lersch C, Assmann G, et al. Toxicity of a 24-hour infusion of gemcitabine in biliary tract and pancreatic cancer: a pilot study. Cancer Invest 2002;20:180–185.
220. Malik IA, Aziz Z. Prospective evaluation of efficacy and toxicity of 5-FU and folinic acid (Mayo Clinic regimen) in patients with advanced cancer of the gallbladder. Am J Clin Oncol 2003; 26:124–126.
221. Bhargava P, Jani CR, Savarese DM, et al. Gemcitabine and irinotecan in locally advanced or metastatic biliary cancer: preliminary report. Oncology (Huntingt) 2003;17:23–26.
222. Kuhn R, Hribaschek A, Eichelmann K, et al. Outpatient therapy with gemcitabine and docetaxel for gallbladder, biliary, and cholangio-carcinomas. Invest New Drugs 2002;20:351–356.
223. Choi CW, Choi IK, Seo JH, et al. Effects of 5-fluorouracil and leucovorin in the treatment of pancreatic-biliary tract adenocarcinomas. Am J Clin Oncol 2000;23:425–428.
224. Mani S, Sciortino D, Samuels B, et al. Phase II trial of uracil/tegafur (UFT) plus leucovorin in patients with advanced biliary carcinoma. Invest New Drugs 1999;17:97–101.
225. Eckel F, Lersch C, Assmann G, et al. Phase II trial of low-dose cyclophosphamide, leucovorin, high-dose 5-fluorouracil 24-hour continuous infusion and tamoxifen in advanced biliary tract cancer. Ann Oncol 2000;11:762–763.
226. Kajanti M, Pyrhonen S. Epirubicin-sequential methotrexate-5-fluorouracil-leucovorin treatment in advanced cancer of the extrahepatic biliary system. A phase II study. Am J Clin Oncol 1994;17:223–226.
227. Taal BG, Audisio RA, Bleiberg H, et al. Phase II trial of mitomycin C (MMC) in advanced gallbladder and biliary tree carcinoma. An EORTC Gastrointestinal Tract Cancer Cooperative Group Study. Ann Oncol 1993;4:607–609.

45

An Evidence-Based Approach to the Management of Pancreatic Cancer

Dan Laheru

In 2001, a number of prominent pancreas cancer specialists from the medical community met with industry and pancreatic cancer advocacy partners to make comprehensive formal recommendations for the National Cancer Institute's pancreatic cancer research agenda. They published an executive summary identifying barriers to progress and highlighted research priorities that could lead to real progress for this cancer.[1] As we approach the end of 2004, much has changed, yet much has remained the same for the management of pancreatic cancer. We now have an understanding of how normal duct epithelium progresses to infiltrating cancer at the molecular level.[2] We finally have available reliable mouse models of early pancreatic ductal lesions[3] that will provide unprecedented potential to identify early pancreatic lesions and allow testing of new drugs for prevention and treatment. The technology for pancreatic tumor animal xenografting exists that will allow more efficient testing of new drugs and identifying mechanisms of drug resistance.

Despite reason for optimism that meaningful progress is on the horizon, the current reality is that 5-year survival remains approximately 15% to 20% for resectable disease and 3% for all stages combined.[4] There remains no current universal standard of care for adjuvant therapy. Gemcitabine still remains the standard of care for metastatic disease.

Therapy for Adjuvant Disease

The current standard of 5-fluorouracil (5-FU)-based combined modality chemoradiotherapy is based on in vitro data, animal studies, and a series of human studies, most notable from the Gastrointestinal Tumor Study Group (GITSG). This study utilized split-course irradiation in modest doses with concurrent bolus 5-FU followed by maintenance 5-FU. The study reported a survival advantage for adjuvant chemoradiotherapy in comparison to surgery alone.[5] While criticized for slow and limited accrual, the GITSG study was the first and only study to document that adjuvant therapy following surgical resection for pancreatic surgery prolonged survival. Additional studies by the GITSG demonstrated the benefit of combined chemoradiotherapy versus chemotherapy alone or radiation therapy alone for patients with resectable disease.[6]

Subsequently, additional groups have further developed this approach[4–21] (Table 45.1). The Johns Hopkins Hospital published results of two single-institution prospective but nonrandomized trials that were designed to evaluate survival benefit in patients with pancreatic cancer following surgical resection.[10] This report, involving 174 patients, demonstrated that patients receiving GITSG-style chemoradiotherapy with maintenance 5-FU truncated at 6 months (rather than 2 years), or a more-intensive regimen involving higher doses of irradiation as well as hepatic irradiation administered without interruption and with continuous-infusion 5-FU chemotherapy augmented with leukovorin, did better than patients receiving no postsurgical therapy. The median survival for the more-standard regimen was 21 months, with 1- and 2-year survival at 80% and 44%, respectively. For the intensive regimen, the median survival was 17.5 months with 1- and 2-year survival at 70% and 22%, respectively. For the control arm, the median survival was 13.5 months with 1- and 2-year survival at 54% and 30%, respectively. The intensive therapy had no survival advantage when compared to the standard therapy group, but there was a statistically significant difference between the standard arm versus control with P less than 0.002. Multivariate analysis confirmed prognostic factors for disease recurrence including margin and lymph node status, tumor size, and degree of differentiation. This approach, showing the importance of multiple prognostic factors in addition to adjuvant therapy on postsurgical outcomes, has been further refined by Sohn et al.[4] and Abrams et al.[12] The critical factors appear to be the histologic status of resection margins, lymph node involvement (especially more than three lymph nodes involved), tumor size greater than 3 cm, and the presence of a poorly differentiated component within the tumor. Using these factors, patients can be segregated into high-risk and low-risk groups, with median survival after standard adjuvant therapy being 30.5 months for low-risk patients and 14.0 months for high-risk patients.

In an effort to enhance the activity of chemotherapy in pancreatic cancer, other agents have been examined in combination with 5-FU. Mitomycin-C (MMC) is an antitumor antibiotic with activity in several gastrointestinal cancers including pancreatic cancer. The UCLA group has published

TABLE 45.1. Adjuvant studies in pancreatic cancer.

Adjuvant study	*No. of patients*	*EBRT dose (Gy)*	*Chemotherapy*	*MS, months*	*One-year survival*	*Two-year survival*	*Five-year survival*
GITSG (1985)	22 pts surgery alone	None	None	11	49%	15%	NR
	21 pts to chemorad	40 split course	5-FU bolus	20 $P = 0.01$	63%	42%	NR
GITSG (1987)	30	40 split course	5-FU bolus	18	67%	46%	NR
Whittington (1991)	33 pts surgery alone	None	None	15	70% (est)	30% (est)	8% (3 years)
	10 pts rad alone	45–63	None	15	72% (est)	40% (est)	5% (3 years)
	28 pts chemorad	45–63	5-FU bolus and MMC	16	75% (est)	55% (est)	34% (3 years)
Foo (1993)	29	35.1–60	5-FU bolus	22.8	NR	48%	12%
Spitz (1997)	19	50.4	5-FU CI	22	70% (est)	42% (est)	40% (est)
Yeo (1997)	53 pts surgery alone	None	None	13.5	54%	30%	NR
	99 pts "standard"	40–45 split course	5-FU bolus	21 $P = 0.002$	80%	44%	NR
	21 pts "intensive"	50.4–57.6 + liver 23–27	5-FU CI	17.5 $P = 0.252$	70%	22%	NR
Demeure (1998) (stage I, 29 pts)	30 pts surgery alone	None	None	16.9	90% (est)	20% (est)	0%
	31 pts chemorad	50.4–54	5-FU bolus or CI	24.2 $P < 0.05$	100% (est)	50% (est)	50% (est)
Pendurthi (1998)	23	50.4	5-FU bolus or CI	25			
Abrams (1999)	23	50.4–57.6 + liver 23–27	5-FU CI	15.9	62% (est)	25% (est)	NR
EORTC (1999)	54 pts surgery alone	None	None	12.6	40% (est)	23%	10%
	60 pts chemorad	40	5-FU bolus	17.1 $P = 0.099$	65% (est)	37%	20%
Paulino (1999)	30 pts chemorad	30.6–64.8	5-FU bolus or CI	26 $P = 0.004$	84%	52%	NR
	8 pts rad alone	30.6–64.8	None	5.5	0%	0%	0%
Mehta (2000)	52	54	5-FU CI	32	80%	62%	39%
Nukui (2000)	16 pts	45–54	5-FU bolus or CI	18.5	92% (est)	84%	Not reached
	17 pts	45–54	5-FU CI/cisplatin/IFN-alpha	Not reached	80% (est)	50% (est)	25% (est)
Chakravarthy (2000)	29	50 split course	5-FU CI with MMC/ DPM	16	84%	60%	NR
Sohn (2000) (retrospective study)	119 pts surgery alone	None	None	11	48%	22% (est)	9%
	333 pts adjuvant tx	40–50	5-FU ± MMC, DPM	19 $P < 0.0001$	71%	38% (est)	20%
ESPAC1 (2001)	200 pts surgery alone	None	None	16.1	N/A	N/A	NR
	103 pts chemorad	40 split course	None	15.5	N/A	N/A	NR
	166 pts chemo alone	None	5-FU bolus	19.7	60% (est)	39% (est)	16% (est)
	72 pts chemorad/chemo	40 split course	5-FU bolus	N/A	N/A	N/A	NR
Picozzi (2003)	53	45–50	5-FU CI/cisplatin/IFN-alpha	46	88%	53%	49%
Van Laethem (2003)	22	40 split course	Gemcitabine	15	50% (est)	15% (est)	NR
ESPAC 1 (2004)	73	40 split course	5-FU bolus	13.9 15.9			7
	72	40 split course	5-FU bolus + 6 cycles	19.9			13
	69	None	None	16.9 17.9			11
	75	None	5-FU × 6 cycles	21.6			29

pts, patients; EBRT, external-beam radiation therapy; chemorad, chemoradiation therapy; rad, radiation therapy; 5-FU, 5-fluorouracil; MMC, mitomycin-C; DPM, dipyridamole; IFN, interferon; CI, continuous infusion; MS, mean survival; NR, no response; est, estimated; N/A, not applicable.

their experience using MMC (10 mg/m^2 IV q 6 weeks) and 5-FU (200 mg/m^2/day administered via continuous infusion), in combination with leukovorin (30 mg/m^2 weekly) and dipyridamole (75 mg po daily) in 38 patients with locally advanced pancreatic carcinoma.[11] There were 14 partial responders with 1 complete response. The median survival for all patients was 15.5 months, which is an improvement over historical data for locoregional advanced disease. This regimen has subsequently been applied to pancreatic cancer in combination with radiotherapy. The Hopkins group recently presented data of 39 patients with pancreatic cancer following surgical resection treated with combined radiotherapy (50 Gy in 25 fractions with planned 2-week break after 25 Gy) and chemotherapy consisting of 5-FU 400 mg/m^2 days 1–3, MMC 10 mg/m^2 day 1, leukovorin 20 mg/m^2 days 1–3, and dipyridamole 75 mg po qid days 0–4 administered on weeks 1 and 4. One month following combined chemoradiotherapy, patients received four additional cycles (4 months) of the same chemotherapy alone. At 12.6 months median follow-up, median survival was 16 months.[12]

Subsequently, the Stanford group published their experience of 52 patients with pancreatic cancer following definitive surgical resection to combined radiotherapy (45 Gy to tumor bed and nodes in 1.8-Gy fractions with boost to total of 54 Gy if surgical margins were positive) and chemotherapy (5-FU 200–250 mg/m^2/day administered without break throughout radiation therapy). All patients were able to complete therapy without grade IV toxicities. With median follow-up of 24 months, the median survival was reported at 32 months.[15]

The Virginia Mason Medical Center published their experience of 33 patients with resected pancreatic adenocarcinoma who received combined radiotherapy (external beam at a dose of 45–54 Gy in standard fractions, days 1–35) and chemotherapy (5-FU 200 mg/m^2/day as continuous infusion, weekly cisplatin 30 mg/m^2 IV bolus, interferon-α 3 million units SQ every other day) during radiation or GITSG-type chemotherapy with radiation therapy. Following combined modality chemoradiotherapy, chemotherapy alone was administered (5-FU 200 mg/m^2/day as continuous infusion) in two 6-week courses during weeks 9–14 and 17–22. Of note, 13 of 17 patients randomized to the interferon-based chemoradiotherapy had positive lymph nodes compared to 7 of 16 patients randomized to the GITSG-based chemoradiotherapy. There were significant grade III/IV gastrointestinal (GI) toxicities including vomiting, mucositis, diarrhea, and GI bleeding in the interferon-based chemotherapy, requiring hospitalization in 35% of patients. However, the majority of patients were still able to receive more than 80% of planned therapy. The median overall survival and 2-year actuarial survival rate were 18.5 months and 54% for patients receiving GITSG-based chemoradiotherapy. In contrast, the median survival and 2-year survival were more than 24 months and 84% for the interferon-based chemoradiotherapy.[16] The Virginia Mason Group has recently presented a follow-up study of 53 patients with resected pancreas cancer treated with similar interferon-based chemoradiotherapy. Toxicities including anorexia, dehydration, diarrhea, mucositis, nausea, and vomiting necessitated hospitalization in 23 of 53 patients. However, the clinical efficacy remains very encouraging, with median survival of 46 months and 2-year survival of 53%.[19] As such, The American College of Surgery Oncology Group (ACOSOG) has opened a multiinstitutional Phase II study in patients with pancreatic adenocarcinoma who are candidates for resection.

In July 2002, the Radiation Therapy Oncology Group (RTOG) closed R97-04. This Phase III study of 518 pancreatic cancer patients randomized between 5-FU continuous infusion (250 mg/m^2/day for 3 weeks), followed by 5-FU continuous infusion (250 mg/m^2/day) during radiation therapy (50.4 Gy in 1.8-Gy fractions), followed by two cycles 5-FU continuous infusion, versus gemcitabine 1,000 mg/m^2 weekly $\times$ 3, followed by 5-FU continuous infusion during radiation therapy, followed by three cycles gemcitabine alone. The experimental question being asked was whether gemcitabine before and after 5-FU-based chemoradiotherapy would be more efficacious than continuous infusion 5-FU before and after the same 5-FU-based chemoradiotherapy. In 1997, when this study was designed, there was inadequate knowledge regarding how to safely administer gemcitabine concurrently with irradiation to allow for concurrent gemcitabine and radiotherapy. This study was the first North American Co-Operative group trial since the GITSG trial. Although the survival results for this trial will not be known until possibly late 2004, a number of important observations have already been made: neither arm was associated with unacceptable acute toxicity during the trial, accrual was quite rapid (12–14 patients per month), reflecting the support of both the Eastern Co-Operative Oncology Group and the Southwest Oncology Group, and the willingness of patients and their physicians to participate in adjuvant trials for pancreatic cancer.

Despite a growing body of literature supporting the benefit of adjuvant combined modality therapy following potentially definitive resection in patients with high risk for recurrence, adjuvant chemoradiation has not been universally accepted as a standard of care. One of the criticisms has been that none of these studies included an observation-only arm. There have been three studies that have demonstrated contrasting conclusions.

A European Organization for Research and Treatment of Cancer (EORTC) trial randomized 218 patients with pancreatic and nonpancreatic periampullary adenocarcinoma 2 to 8 weeks following potentially curative resection to either observation or to combined radiotherapy (40 Gy using a three- or four-field technique in 2-Gy fractions with 2-week break at midtreatment) and chemotherapy (5-FU administered as a continuous infusion 25 mg/kg/day during the first week of each 2-week radiation therapy module only). No postradiation chemotherapy was administered. Median progression-free survival was 16 months in the observation arm versus 17.4 months in the treatment arm ($P = 0.643$). Median survival was 19 months in the observation group versus 24.5 months in the treatment group, but this was not statistically significant ($P = 0.737$). For the subgroup of patients with pancreatic adenocarcinoma ($n = 114$), the median survival was 12.6 months in the observation group versus 17.1 months in the treatment arm, but this was not statistically significant ($P = 0.099$). Of note, 21 of 104 patients randomized to the treatment arm were not treated. In addition, although the original dose of 5-FU was already modest, 35 patients in the treatment arm received only 3 days of 5-FU during the second module of radiotherapy secondary to grade I/II toxicities. Therefore, this study could be better described as an underpowered positive study.[13]

TABLE 45.2. Active or planned adjuvant or neoadjuvant studies.

Study	*Regimen*	*Study phase*
EORTC	Arm I: Gemcitabine weekly × 3 every 4 weeks × 2 cycles followed by Gem/EBRT Arm II: Observation	II/III
ACOSOG	EBRT (50 Gy/5-FU CI/cisplatin/IFN, 5-FU CI) × 2 cycles	II
Johns Hopkins	GM-CSF allo vaccine, 5-FU CI, 5-FU CI/XRT, 5-FU CI × 2 cycles followed by GM-CSF allogeneic vaccine X 4	II
ECOG 1200	Arm A: Gem 500 mg/m² over 50 min weekly × 6 with EBRT 50.4 followed by surgery, gem 1,000 mg/m² over 100 min × 5 cycles Arm B: Gem 175 mg/m² over 30 min days 1, 5, 29, 33/cisplatin 20 mg/m² days 1–4, 29–33, 5-FU 600 mg/m² over 21 hours days 1–4, 29–32 followed by EBRT 50.4, surgery, gemcitabine × 3 cycles	II
ESPAC-3	Arm I: Observation Arm II: 5-Fluorouracil/LV days 1–5 × 6 cycles Arm III: Gemcitabine weekly ×3 every 4 weeks × 6 cycles	III

gem, gemcitabine; IFN, interferon-alpha; RTOG, Radiation Therapy Oncology Group; CI, continuous infusion; ACOSOG, American College of Surgery Oncology Group; ECOG, Eastern Cooperative Oncology Group.

The European Study Group for Pancreatic Cancer (ESPAC) randomized 541 patients with pancreatic adenocarcinoma in a four-arm design based on a two-by-two factorial design: (a) observation; (b) concomitant chemoradiotherapy alone (20 Gy in 10 fractions over 2 weeks with 500 mg/m² 5-FU IV bolus during the first 3 days of radiation therapy; the module is repeated after a planned 2-week break) followed by no additional chemotherapy; (c) chemotherapy alone (leukovorin 20 mg/m² bolus followed by 5-FU 425 mg/m² administered for 5 consecutive days repeated every 28 days for six cycles); and (d) chemoradiotherapy followed by chemotherapy.[18] The data set for 289 patients randomized just through the two-by-two design was recently reported.[21] The four arms were subsequently uniquely combined to make additional comparisons (no chemoradiotherapy versus chemoradiotherapy and no chemotherapy versus chemotherapy). There appeared to be a survival advantage for patients receiving no chemoradiotherapy (17.9 months) versus chemoradiotherapy (15.9 months, $P = 0.05$). In addition, there was a survival advantage for those who received chemotherapy (20.1 months) versus those who did not receive chemotherapy (15.5 months, $P = 0.009$). When the four arms were analyzed individually, there appeared to be a survival benefit for chemotherapy alone (median survival, 21.6 months) versus observation alone (16.9 months), chemoradiotherapy alone (13.9 months), or chemoradiotherapy followed by chemotherapy (19.9 months). However, the study was not powered to examine these arms separately. Multivariate analysis for known prognostic factors including margin status, lymph node involvement, and tumor grade and size did not alter the effect for chemoradiotherapy treatment. The study authors concluded that there was no survival benefit for adjuvant chemoradiotherapy. In addition, the authors concluded that a potential benefit existed for adjuvant chemotherapy alone following surgical resection. Based on these results, the follow-up ESPAC study (ESPAC-3) does not include radiation therapy and is designed as a randomized study of three different chemotherapy schedules (5-FU and leukovorin versus gemcitabine versus observation) following surgery.

Although this was a randomized study consisting of more than 500 patients with a smaller subset of 289 patients included in the two-by-two design, the conclusions of the study should be carefully measured. To encourage maximal patient recruitment, the study was modified in that 68 patients were assigned separately and randomized to either chemoradiotherapy or observation. In addition, 188 patients were subsequently assigned separately and randomized to either chemotherapy alone or observation. In a sense, three randomizations were possible for inclusion into the same original study design. Also, patients in the additional two randomizations could have received "background chemotherapy or chemotherapy," which was not specifically defined. The background treatment was not known in 82 eligible patients. Of note, these patients were still assigned into an arm of the study despite lack of definitive knowledge of prior therapy. Finally, 25 of the eligible 541 patients refused to accept their randomization and an additional 25 patients withdrew secondary to treatment toxicities.

Although the smaller subset of 289 patients does not include these additional "randomized" patients, other fundamental issues concerning these are patients worthy of comment. First, the absence of a central review of radiotherapy fields and quality control/assurance is essential in such a study design and alone could explain the results of the study. Equally important, the radiation as well as the chemotherapy used in the ESPAC-1 study are not considered contemporary therapy. Doses of radiation therapy integrated with chemotherapy are currently in the range of 45 to 54 Gy. The lower doses of radiation used in ESPAC-1 might explain the high incidence of local recurrence in 109 of 158 patients (62%) with recurrent disease.

As the debate continues, several studies have recently opened or have been proposed by either the cooperative groups or through single institutions. Table 45.2 summarizes open or planned studies in the adjuvant setting. These future studies will be characterized by the addition of multiagent chemotherapy to irradiation at the cooperative group level by the addition of Gemcitabine to the period of chemoradiation and by the use of conformal, three-dimensional (3-D) irradiation planned to patient-specific anatomic and surgical pathologic data.

Future Concepts for Adjuvant Therapy

The identification of overexpressed/underexpressed genes, tumor-dependent growth pathways, and the search for tumor-specific proteins or antigens have for many years been the triple holy grail for oncologists. The impact from such discoveries would potentially not only revolutionize the management of disease but would also have implications for early detection and for monitoring disease. A number of these molecular targeted drugs (Cetuximab and Bevacizumab) have been approved by the U.S. Food and Drug Administration (FDA) for other malignancies and are currently being tested in combination with Gemcitabine in patients with metastatic pancreatic cancer. To date, no molecular targeted agents have been tested in the adjuvant setting.

Immune-based therapy is a novel therapeutic approach that has the ability to recruit and activate tumor-specific T cells and induce a cytotoxic response. The potential of this approach is attractive for many reasons.[22] First, tumor killing by activated tumor-specific T cells occurs via a mechanism that is distinct from chemotherapy or radiation therapy and would represent a noncross-resistant treatment with an entirely different spectrum of toxicities. Second, the immune system is capable of recognizing a broad diversity of potential antigens with selective and specific cytotoxic responses. These features may be essential in recognizing and eliminating a heterogeneous tumor population while avoiding normal tissue toxicity. Third, preclinical animal models using active immunotherapy (vaccines) have been able to eliminate small burdens of established tumors, a situation that corresponds to the state of minimal residual disease commonly found after resection of human tumors. Fourth, there are data to suggest that human tumor-specific antigens can be manipulated to be effectively recognized by the immune system and that these antigens may be shared broadly among tumors of similar histologies.[23] Finally, vaccine cells do not need to be HLA compatible with host immune cells to effectively prime both the $CD4^+$ T-cell (regulatory) arm and the $CD8^+$ T-cell (cytolytic) arm of the immune response.[24,25]

Although the use of autologous tumor cells may preserve unique antigens expressed by each patient's cancer, the development of an autologous vaccine has limitations that preclude the use of autologous cellular vaccine for most cancers including pancreatic adenocarcinoma. Recent data support the immunologic rationale for using allogeneic tumor cells rather than autologous cells as the source of antigen used for the vaccination.[24] Taken together, the data suggest that relevant tumor antigens can be delivered by an allogeneic tumor and still sufficiently mount an effective immune response.

The Johns Hopkins group has developed allogeneic cell lines from neoplastic tissue harvested from the surgical specimens of patients undergoing pancreaticoduodenectomy at the Johns Hopkins Hospital. All these cell lines have been characterized as 100% epithelial by cytokeratin staining. In addition, all these cell lines carry the same k-*ras* mutation as the original tumor specimen, which supports the conclusion that these lines are derived from malignant pancreatic tumor cells. Two cell lines had been chosen for further testing because they contain the most common k-*ras* mutation at codon 12 found in greater than 90% of pancreatic cancer. These lines were genetically modified to secrete granulocyte-macrophage colony-stimulating factor (GM-CSF). These lines were previously tested for safety in 14 patients with stage 1, 2, or 3 pancreatic adenocarcinoma.[26]

This study was the first clinical trial to test the hypothesis that allogeneic GM-CSF-secreting pancreatic tumor cell lines can prime a systemic immune response in patients with resected pancreatic adenocarcinoma. Fourteen patients with stage 2 or 3 disease received an initial vaccination 8 weeks following resection; this was a dose escalation study in which 3 patients each received 1×10^7, 5×10^7, and 1×10^8 tumor cells. An additional 5 patients received 5×10^8 vaccine cells. Study patients were jointly enrolled in an adjuvant chemoradiation protocol for 6 months. Following the completion of adjuvant chemoradiation, patients were reassessed, and those who were still in remission were treated with three additional vaccinations given 1 month apart at the same original dose that they received for the first vaccination. Toxicities were limited to grade I/II local reactions at the vaccine site. Postvaccination delayed-type hypersensitivity (DTH) responses to autologous tumor cells have been used in previously reported vaccine studies as a surrogate to identify and characterize specific immune responses that are associated with vaccination. In the pancreatic cancer vaccine trial, postvaccination DTH responses to autologous tumor cells were observed in 1 of 3 patients receiving 1×10^8 and in 2 of 4 patients receiving 5×10^8 vaccine cells.

The major limitation of defined antigen-based vaccines has been the lack of identified pancreatic tumor antigens that are the known targets of the immune response. Thus, current immune-based approaches either target a small group of candidate antigens expressed by the tumor or rely on whole tumor cells as the immunogen. In addition, postvaccination DTH response to autologous tumor provided only indirect evidence of vaccine-derived antitumor immune response. However, with the recent sequencing of the human genome and the development of rapid methods for identifying genes that are differentially expressed by tumor cells,[2] potential candidate immune targets were expected to be discovered that may serve as immunogens for treatment as well as prevention. Recently, mesothelin, a transmembrane glycoprotein member of the mesothelin/megakaryocyte potentiating factor (MPF) family, was identified by differential gene expression to be overexpressed by most pancreatic adenocarcinomas.[27] Mesothelin has been shown to be recognized by vaccinated uncultured $CD8^+$ T cells isolated from the three patients who are long-term survivors from the previously described phase I GM-CSF pancreatic cancer vaccine study but not in the other patients who received the vaccine but subsequently relapsed.[28] These data suggest that mesothelin may be used as an in vitro marker of vaccine-specific T-cell responses to correlate with in vivo DTH response to autologous tumors and to clinical responses.

Based on the phase I study, the Johns Hopkins Hospital initiated a 60-patient study, administering a total of five vaccinations integrated around chemoradiotherapy for patients with resected pancreatic adenocarcinoma. The study is planned to complete accrual by the end of 2004.

Role of Neoadjuvant Therapy

Neoadjuvant therapy is a potentially attractive alternative to current standard adjuvant chemoradiation for several reasons: (1) radiation is more effective on well-oxygenated cells that have not been devascularized by surgery, (2) contamination and subsequent seeding of the peritoneum with tumor cells secondary to surgery could theoretically be reduced, (3) patients with metastatic disease on restaging following adjuvant therapy would not need to undergo definitive resection and might benefit from palliative intervention, and (4) the risk of delaying adjuvant therapy would be eliminated because it would be delivered in the neoadjuvant setting. A number of groups have further developed this approach[9,29–41] (Table 45.3).

TABLE 45.3. Neoadjuvant studies in patients with resectable pancreatic cancer.

Study	*Evaluable pts*	*% resected*	*EBRT (Gy)*	*Chemotherapy*	*MS (all pts, months)*	*MS (resected pts, months)*	*One-year survival*	*Two-year survival*	*Five-year survival*
Evans (1992)	28	17 (61%)	50.4 + IORT	5-FU CI	Not available (N/A)	Not available	N/A	N/A	N/A
Hoffman (1995)	34	11 (32%)	50.4	5-FU bolus and MMC	N/A	45	70% (est)	60% (est)	40% (est)
Staley (1996)	39	39 (100%)	30 or 50.4 and IORT	5-FU CI	19	19	75% (est)	35% (est)	N/A
Spitz (1997)	91	52 (57%)	30 or 50.4	5-FU CI	20.2	19.2	76% (est)	38% (est)	28% (est)
Pendurthi (1998)	70	25 (36%)	50.4	5-FU bolus and MMC	N/A	20	75% (est)	40% (est)	8% (est)
Hoffman (1998)	53	24 (45%)	50.4	5-FU bolus and MMC	9.7	15.7	72%	27%	8%
Pisters (1998)	35	20 (74%)	30 + IORT	5-FU CI	7	25	84%	56% (est)	N/A
Todd (1998)	38	4 (10%)	none	5-FU CI/MMC/DPM	15.5				
White (2001)	111	39 (35%)	45	5-FU CI and MMC/CDDP	Not reached				
Breslin (2001)	132	132 (100%)	30–50.4 and/or IORT	5-FU CI or Gem or Taxol	21	21	78% (est)	50% (est)	23%
Moutardier (2002)	19	15 (79%)	30 or 45	5-FU bolus and CDDP	20	30	N/A	52%	N/A
Arnoletti (2002)	26	14 (54%)	50.4	5-FU and/or MMC or Gem	N/A	34	75% (est)	68%	45%
Pisters (2002)	35	20 (57%)	30 and IORT	Paclitaxel	12	19	75% (est)	35% (est)	10% (est)
Magnin (2003)	32	19 (59%)	30 or 45	5-FU CI + cisplatin	16	30	82% (est)	59%	N/A

The Fox Chase Cancer Center published their experience of 53 patients with localized resectable pancreatic cancer who were treated preoperatively with radiation therapy (5,040 cGy in 180-cGy fractions) and chemotherapy (MMC 10 mg/m^2 on day 2 with 5-FU 1,000 mg/m^2/day by continuous infusion on days 2–5 and 29–32). Forty-one patients subsequently underwent exploratory laparotomy at the conclusion of preoperative chemoradiation. From this group of patients, 17 were not resectable (including 11 patients with hepatic or peritoneal metastases and 6 patients with local extension that precluded resection). Twenty-four patients eventually underwent potentially curative resection. Significant treatment-related hematologic and nonhematologic toxicities were identified, including 1 patient with treatment-related toxicities that precluded reexploration. Median survival for the entire group was 9.7 months and 15.7 months for the group that underwent surgical resection.[31]

The MD Anderson Cancer Center (MDACC) published their experience of 132 patients with localized resectable pancreatic adenocarcinoma were treated preoperatively with radiation therapy (45–50.4 Gy in standard 1.8-Gy fractions or consisting of 30-Gy rapid fractionation in 3 Gy/fraction) combined with chemotherapy (5-FU continuous infusion 300 mg/m^2/day or gemcitabine 400 mg/m^2/week or paclitaxel 60 mg/m^2/week), followed by surgical resection. There were no surgical delays in the neoadjuvant group but there were noted to be delays in 6 of 25 patients who underwent surgical resection first. At median follow-up of 19 months, no significant differences in survival were noted between treatment groups, with overall median survival of 21 months.[37]

The Fox Chase group has since published a follow-up study of 30 patients with localized resectable pancreatic cancer of whom 26 received preoperative radiation therapy (50.4 Gy) with 5-FU continuous infusion. Fourteen patients who received preoperative therapy subsequently underwent resection. Median survival was 34 months for the resected group compared to 8 months in the group that could not be resected.[39]

The MDACC have also used paclitaxel 60 mg/m^2 over 3 hours weekly with 30-Gy radiation therapy rapid fractionation. Of note, if patients could undergo surgical resection, they could also have received external-beam intraoperative radiation therapy (EB-IORT). Grade III hematologic and nonhematologic toxicities were identified in 16 patients. No delays in surgery were attributable to preoperative therapy. Twenty of 25 patients who underwent exploratory laparotomy underwent surgical resection. There were no histologic complete responders. With median follow-up of 45 months, 3-year survival for those patients following potentially curative resection was 28% with overall median survival of 19 months.[41]

Currently, the Eastern Co-operative Oncology Group (ECOG) is planning to open a prospective randomized trial randomizing patients to intensified gemcitabine-based or gemcitabine/5-FU/platinum-based chemoradiotherapy. This trial makes an important distinction between clearly unresectable disease and potentially resectable disease, especially around the issues of partial versus complete encasement of the superior mesenteric artery and length of superior mesenteric vein involved by tumor at initial presentation. To date, the current data demonstrate that although neoadjuvant chemoradiotherapy can be administered safely, there is no clear advantage to this strategy compared to postoperative therapy. In the realm of marginally resectable patients, it remains to be seen whether there is a meaningful cohort of patients for whom this approach may represent an important therapeutic advantage based on "downstaging" and improved surgical outcomes.

Treatment of Locally Advanced Disease

Pancreatic tumors frequently invade adjacent structures such as superior mesenteric and celiac vascular structures, making curative resection difficult if not impossible. The Memorial Sloan Kettering group recently reviewed their experience of 163 patients with locally advanced pancreas cancer. A number of chemotherapy regimens were integrated with radiation therapy and administered to 87 patients. Only 3 patients had sufficient radiographic response to justify surgical exploration. Of these selected patients, one-third underwent resection for curative intent.[42] For the approximately 30% to 40% of pancreatic cancer patients who present with such locally advanced, nonmetastatic disease, optimal management is controversial. Palliative surgery, chemoradiation, chemotherapy alone, and locally directed therapies have all been employed in this setting.

Chemoradiation Approaches

Although external-beam radiation therapy (EBRT) alone can improve symptoms associated with locally advanced disease, the high local failure rate and synergy observed when EBRT is combined with chemotherapy have led to trials using both modalities. Chemoradiation approaches have shown improved survival compared to either modality alone, but the improvements are modest, and local control remains a significant challenge. There have been no randomized comparisons of radiation and/or chemotherapy versus supportive care (aside from subset analyses in trials for metastatic disease).

Several prospective randomized trials have shown a benefit with chemoradiation compared to either radiation or chemotherapy alone in the management of locally advanced disease.[43–49] The first trial was published in 1969 and included patients with different types of gastrointestinal (GI) cancers, 64 of whom had locally unresectable pancreatic cancer randomized to either 5-FU or placebo combined with 35–40 Gy radiation. Median survival in the combined modality arm was significantly higher than in the radiation therapy-only arm (10.4 versus 6.3 months).[43] The Gastrointestinal Tumor Study Group (GITSG) randomized 194 locally advanced pancreatic cancer patients to receive split-course EBRT, either alone (60 Gy) or combined (either 40 or 60 Gy) with 5-FU 500 mg/m^2 on the first 3 days of each 20 Gy of radiation.[44] The EBRT-alone arm was discontinued after an interim analysis showed improved median time to progression (TTP) and overall survival (OS) in the combined modality arms. There were no significant differences between the high- and low-dose EBRT in the chemoradiation arms, although there were trends favoring the higher-dose arm in time to progression and survival. A second GITSG study compared SMF (streptozotocin, mitomycin, and 5-FU) chemotherapy alone versus SMF combined with EBRT (54 Gy), and showed a significant improvement in median survival (9.7 versus 7.4 months) for the chemoradiation arm.[46] In contradistinction to the GITSG studies, a randomized ECOG study of 91 patients comparing 5-FU 600 mg/m² weekly with or without EBRT (40 Gy, which has been criticized as an insufficient dose) did not find a significant benefit to combined modality therapy over chemotherapy alone.[45] Thus, three randomized studies have demonstrated a modest survival benefit of combined modality therapy over chemotherapy or EBRT alone, and one ECOG study with a possibly suboptimal dose of EBRT (40 Gy) did not show benefit over 5-FU alone.

Several trials have examined the use of different chemotherapy agents with radiation therapy in the locally advanced setting. The first was a Southwest Oncology Group (SWOG) study published in 1980 randomizing 69 patients to mCCNU (methyl lomustine) and 5-FU with or without testolactone, combined with 60 Gy of radiation.[47] There was no significant difference in overall survival, and myelosuppression (87%) and GI toxicity (23%) were common. A GITSG study randomized 143 patients to EBRT with either weekly 5-FU or doxorubicin.[48] Median survival was similar in both arms (approximately 8 months), but the doxorubicin arm had more frequent severe toxicity. Finally, a randomized Phase II study of 87 patients compared the radiation sensitizer hycanthone to 5-FU, both given with 60 Gy of split-course radiation, and found no difference in survival.[49] Thus, three trials failed to demonstrate a survival advantage of different chemotherapy regimens given with radiation therapy compared to 5-FU, which tended to have less toxicity.

Chemoradiation Using Gemcitabine

There has been considerable interest in combining EBRT with gemcitabine because of its clinical benefit in the metastatic setting and potent radiosensitizing properties. Studies combining radiotherapy with gemcitabine have proceeded cautiously because of this synergy. Early trials were designed to determine the maximal tolerated dose of gemcitabine when delivered weekly and integrated with radiation therapy consisting of 50.4 Gy in standard 1.8-Gy fractions. A margin of 3 cm around the gross target volume was required for the initial field of 39.6 Gy. The margin was subsequently reduced to 2 cm for the final 10.8-Gy boost. The starting dose of gemcitabine was 300 mg/m². Hematologic and gastrointestinal toxicities were identified as dose limiting at 700 mg/m².[50] Blackstock and colleagues examined, in a Phase I study, gemcitabine (starting at 20 mg/m²) twice weekly in combination with radiation therapy (total dose, 50.4 Gy in 1.8-Gy fractions) in 19 patients with locally advanced pancreatic adenocarcinoma. Thrombocytopenia, neutropenia, and nausea/vomiting were dose-limiting toxicities. Of the 15 patients assessable for response, 3 partial responses were identified.[51] A dose of 40 mg/m² twice weekly in combination with radiotherapy to a total dose of 50.4 Gy was subsequently examined by the Cancer and Leukemia Group B (CALGB) in a Phase II study of 38 patients with locally advanced pancreatic cancer. Following chemoradiotherapy, patients without disease progression received Gemcitabine alone at 1,000 mg/m² weekly × 3 every 4 weeks for five additional cycles. Grade III/IV hematologic toxicity was significant and identified in 60% of patients; in addition, grade III/IV GI toxicity was identified in 42% of patients. With median follow-up of 10 months, median survival was 7.9 months.[52]

The MD Anderson Cancer Center (MDACC) has since published a corollary phase I study of 18 patients with locally advanced disease using rapid fractionation external-beam radiation. Patients received dose escalation gemcitabine from 350 mg/m² to 500 mg/m² weekly × 7 with concurrent rapid fractionation 3,000-cGy external-beam radiation therapy during the first 2 weeks of therapy. Hematologic and nonhematologic toxicities were significant in all three patient cohorts. There were 8 responses (4 minor and 4 partial). One of 2 patients who were subsequently explored had a curative resection. The recommended Phase II testing dose of gemcitabine was 350 mg/m².[53]

These dose-finding studies would suggest that the maximal tolerated dose of gemcitabine when combined with radiation therapy is dependent on the radiation therapy field size. Planned confirmatory studies will follow up on these observations.

The University of Michigan has described an alternative approach by using standard doses of gemcitabine at 1,000 mg/m² weekly × 3 every 4 weeks and administering radiation therapy as dose escalation beginning at 24 Gy (1.6-Gy fractions in 15 fractions) in 34 patients with locally advanced disease. The majority of patients received chemotherapy after combined modality treatment at the discretion of the treating physician; 75% of patients received at least 85% of planned gemcitabine. Two of 6 assessable patients experienced dose-limiting toxicity at the final planned radiation dose of 42 Gy in 2.8-Gy fractions. An additional 2 patients developed late GI toxicities at this dose level. Six patients were documented to have a partial response, with a complete radiographic response in 2 patients. In addition, 4 patients with documented stable disease at time of study entry experienced objective responses (2 partial and 2 complete responses). Definitive resection was achieved for 1 of 3 surgically explored patients. With median follow-up of 22 months, median survival for the entire group was 11.6 months. The recommended Phase II radiation dose was 36 Gy in 2.4-Gy fractions.[54]

Other chemotherapy agents have been added to Gemcitabine combined with radiation therapy. The Eastern Cooperative Oncology Group (ECOG) published a Phase I study of seven patients with locally advanced disease using 5-FU/Gemzar combined with radiation therapy to a maximum 59.4 Gy in 1.8-Gy fractions. 5-FU (200 mg/m²/day as continuous infusion throughout radiation therapy) was administered with weekly gemcitabine dose escalation beginning at 100 mg/m². Because of dose-limiting toxicities seen in two of the first three patients, the study was amended to lower the initial dose of gemcitabine to 50 mg/m². However, dose-limiting toxicities were subsequently seen in three of four patients at the 50 mg/m² dose. Three of the five dose-limiting toxicities occurred at radiation doses less than 36 Gy. The study was subsequently closed.[55]

Gemcitabine has also been combined with cisplatin and radiation in published Phase I trials, following up on promising preclinical synergistic data. A study based at the Mayo clinic gave twice-weekly gemcitabine and cisplatin for 3 weeks during radiation (50.4 Gy in 28 fractions). Dose-limiting toxicities consisted of grade 4 nausea and vomiting, and the recommended phase II dose was gemcitabine 30 mg/m² and cisplatin 10 mg/m².[56] Another trial used strictly time-scheduled gemcitabine (days 2, 5, 26, and 33 after a weekly regimen was too toxic) and cisplatin (days 1–5 and 29–33) combined with radiation, with a recommended Phase II dose of 20 mg/m^2 for cisplatin and 300 mg/m^2 for gemcitabine.[57] The response to chemoradiation allowed 10 of 30 initially unresectable patients to undergo surgery, with a R0 resection in 9 cases and a complete response (CR) in 2 cases.

Given the current published data, would 5-FU or gemcitabine be better suited to be used concurrently with radiation therapy for either resected or locally advanced disease? The MDACC retrospectively examined their database of 114 patients with locally advanced disease treated with combination radiation therapy (rapid fractionation 30 Gy in 10 fractions) with either 5-FU by continuous infusion 200–300 mg/m^2 (61 patients) or gemcitabine 250–500 mg/m^2 weekly × 7 (53 patients). Patients receiving gemcitabine developed a significantly higher incidence of severe acute toxicity, defined as toxicity requiring a hospital stay of more than 5 days, mucosal ulceration with bleeding, more than three dose deletions of gemcitabine or discontinuation of 5-FU, or toxicity resulting in surgical intervention or death, compared with those patients receiving 5-FU (23% versus 2%; P less than 0.0001). Five of 53 patients treated with gemcitabine/radiation therapy subsequently underwent surgical resection compared to 1 of 61 patients treated with 5-FU/radiation therapy. However, with short median follow-up, median survival was similar (11 months versus 9 months ($P = 0.19$).[58]

Chemotherapeutic Approaches

Because the benefit of chemoradiation is relatively modest, and the aforementioned randomized ECOG study showed no benefit to radiation added to 5-FU alone, some oncologists recommend chemotherapy alone for locally advanced disease. Gemcitabine is the most commonly used agent, extrapolating from the metastatic disease setting; this is based on the randomized trial by Burris et al. in which 26% of the study subjects had locally advanced disease. Gemcitabine ameliorated symptoms and modestly improved survival compared to 5-FU, but the results for patients with locally advanced disease were not reported separately.[59] An ECOG Phase III trial (E4201) comparing gemcitabine (600 mg/m^2 weekly)/radiation (50.4 Gy in 28 fractions) followed by weekly gemcitabine (1,000 mg/m^2 weekly, 3 of 4 weeks) versus gemcitabine alone, which opened in April 2003, is examining this issue.

Locally Directed Therapy

Both brachytherapy and intraoperative radiotherapy (IORT) have been employed in the setting of locally advanced disease. Both modalities are aimed at improving locoregional control. Given the propensity of this disease to disseminate, especially into the liver and adjacent peritoneum, what can be achieved overall for patients by the addition of either modality to external-beam irradiation and chemotherapy is not completely clear. Mohiuddin et al. reported on 81 patients with localized unresectable carcinoma of the pancreas managed at Thomas Jefferson using intraoperative iodine-125 implants, external-beam irradiation, and perioperative systemic chemotherapy.[60] The radioactive iodine implant was designed to deliver a minimum peripheral dose up to 1,200 cGy over 1 year. Patients were also treated with 50 to 55 Gy of external-beam irradiation with systemic chemotherapy consisting of 5-FU, mitomycin, and occasionally CCNU. Implants were performed at laparotomy. There was a 5% mortality rate, and a 34% acute morbidity rate with cholangitis, upper GI bleeding, and gastric outlet obstruction being the most common. In addition, there was a 32% late morbidity rate, with GI bleeding, cholangitis, and radiation enteritis being the most common late developments. Local control was obtained in 39 of 53 (71%) of evaluable patients. Of 14 patients undergoing reexploration more than 6 months following implantation, 86% showed extensive fibrosis and had negative biopsies from the region of the tumor. In 8 patients undergoing autopsy, 5 (63%) were without evidence of locoregional tumor. Nevertheless, 52 of these 81 patients (62%) failed with intraabdominal disease, primarily hepatic and peritoneal. With a minimum follow-up of 2 years at the time of publication, the median survival for the total group was 12 months, the 2-year survival was 21%, and the 5-year survival was 7%. Despite satisfactory local control in several patients, many centers would not be willing to accept this level of therapeutic intensity in a group of patients for whom management is ultimately primarily noncurative.

Nori et al. have reported on a series of 15 patients undergoing similar management but using palladium-103 instead of iodine-125.[61] The implant was designed to provide a matched peripheral dose of 1,100 cGy. Patients also received external-beam irradiation of 4,500 cGy over 4.5 weeks and chemotherapy with 5-FU and MMC. Median survival was 10 months. The authors concluded that palladium-103 is an alternative to iodine-125 for interstitial brachytherapy for unresectable patients, and that symptom relief appeared to occur somewhat faster. The study did not show any improvement in the median survival as compared to ^{125}I. Finally, a note of caution was raised by Raben et al. on the use of palladium brachytherapy for locally unresectable carcinoma of the pancreas. In their series of 11 patients, they found an unacceptably high complication rate including gastric outlet obstruction, duodenal perforation, and sepsis.[62] They did not find an improvement in median survival over other modalities and did not recommend this approach for further study.

The use of intraoperative radiation therapy (IORT) using single-fraction electron beam treatment has also been extensively studied. In experienced hands, IORT can be given with acceptable morbidity. However, there are occasional reports of unacceptably high complication rates. Generally, IORT has been given in combination with external-beam radiation therapy (EBRT) in the range of 45 to 50.4 Gy with 5-FU alone or 5-FU-based combination chemotherapy. The RTOG reported on 51 patients with locally unresected nonmetastatic pancreatic cancer treated with IORT and EBRT/5-FU and found a major postoperative complication rate of 12%. Two patients had major morbidity leading to death.[63] A neoadjuvant approach was taken by Garton et al. at the Mayo Clinic, where EBRT (50–54 Gy) with or without 5-FU was given preoperatively, followed by IORT (20 Gy).[64] In 27 patients with unresectable disease because of locoregional considerations, local control was achieved in 78%, although 70% of patients developed distant metastases, including peritoneum and liver. Median survival from diagnosis was 14.9 months. Zerbi et al. have suggested that the use of IORT as an adjuvant to resection decreases the risk of local recurrence.[65] Mohiuddin et al. have also reported excellent results with IORT in the management of unresectable pancreatic cancer when combined with postoperative EBRT.[66] As reviewed by Willett and Warshaw, the dose of intraoperative radiation therapy is generally in the range of 10 to 20 Gy, with some investigators prescribing to the 90% line and others prescribing to the 100% line.[67]

In addition to local radiation delivery, a variety of other techniques and agents are under development for the treatment of locally advanced pancreatic cancer. One example is intratumoral injection via endoscopic ultrasound of ONYX-015, an engineered adenovirus that selective replicates in tumor cells. A Phase I/II trial of this agent combined with gemcitabine in 21 patients showed that the technique was feasible with transgastric injections (2 duodenal perforations occurred early in the trial), and 2 partial responses were seen.[68] Another novel biologic agent in development is TNFerade, a replication-deficient adenovector carrying a transgene encoding for human tumor necrosis factor-alpha regulated by a radiation-inducible promoter. Weekly intratumoral injections have been given in combination with chemoradiation (50.4 Gy with continuous infusion 5-FU 200 mg/m^2 daily).[69] Two of 17 patients in a Phase I trial converted from unresectable to resectable, and 1 of these had a pathologic CR.

Treatment Recommendation for Locally Advanced Disease

The optimal treatment for locally advanced pancreatic cancer remains controversial. There have been no randomized trials comparing chemoradiation strategies versus best supportive care, or chemotherapy alone (aside from the GITSG trial in which both 5-FU and radiation were added to SMF chemotherapy), and the survival benefit from combined modality therapy for locally advanced disease has been modest in various trials. Nonetheless, most practitioners in the United States employ radiation therapy (typically 54 Gy in 1.8-Gy fractions) with simultaneous chemotherapy, the standard being 5-FU. Although several chemotherapy regimens have been compared to 5-FU in randomized trials, none have proven more efficacious, and these are typically more toxic. Various ways of giving 5-FU have been used in these trials, but most practitioners choose either continuous infusion at 200 mg/m^2/day during radiation therapy, or a 500 mg/m^2 bolus given on the first 3 days and last 3 days of radiation. Studies are under way that will examine the role of gemcitabine (both alone, and combined with radiation) for locally advanced disease. In addition, given the limited success of current treatments, several novel approaches are being actively explored with the aim of allowing patients who present with unresectable disease to undergo curative surgery.

Therapy for Metastatic Disease

Historically, 5-fluorouracil (5-FU)-based chemotherapy has been the most widely studied chemotherapeutic agent for all stages of pancreatic cancer. Despite more recent attempts to modify the delivery of 5-FU, response rates have remained unchanged in the 10% to 20% range, with median survival of 4 to 5 months for patients with stage IV disease.[70–74]

The Role of Gemcitabine in Metastatic Pancreatic Cancer

Gemcitabine is a prodrug deoxycytidine (2′-deoxy-2′,2′-difluorocytidine monohydrochloride) analogue that is metabolized by deoxycytidine kinase to active diphosphate (dFdCDP) and triphosphate (dFdCTP) nucleosides. These metabolites inhibit ribonucleotide reductase with the effect of decreasing intracellular levels of required deoxynucleotide triphosphates for continued DNA synthesis. In addition, gemcitabine triphosphate directly competes with dCTP for incorporation into DNA. Recently, gemcitabine has demonstrated promise as an active agent in treating pancreatic cancer. Casper and colleagues reported the results of a Phase II trial using weekly gemcitabine at 800–1,250 mg/m^2 in 44 patients with unresectable pancreatic cancer. The response rate was noted to be 11% but with median survival of 5.6 months and a 1-year actuarial survival of 23%.[75] Subsequently, Burris and colleagues randomized 126 patients with unresectable pancreatic cancer to either gemcitabine (1,000 mg/m^2 weekly over a 30-minute infusion X 7 followed by 1 week rest then weekly × 3 every 4 weeks) or 5-FU (600 mg/m^2 weekly). Although the primary endpoints were issues related to quality of life, median survival was 5.7 months in the gemcitabine arm compared to 4.4 months in the 5-FU arm. In addition, 1-year survival was 18% in the gemcitabine arm compared to 2% in the 5-FU arm (P = 0.0025), with median time to progression also favoring gemcitabine (9 weeks compared to 4 weeks in the 5-FU arm; P = 0.0002). Gemcitabine was well tolerated, with the majority of side effects related to grade 3 or 4 neutropenia (26%) without associated infections, low-grade fevers (30%), and nausea and vomiting (9.5% and 3.2%). Gemcitabine has since been approved by the FDA in 1996 as a first-line therapy in metastatic pancreatic cancer.[59] In addition, Rothenberg and colleagues evaluated gemcitabine (1,000 mg/m^2 weekly × 7 with 1 week off then weekly × 3 with 1 week off) in 63 patients with unresectable disease who had been previously treated with 5-FU. The overall salvage response was 10.5% with median time to progression at 2.5 months and median survival at 3.85 months, with a toxicity profile similar to first-line therapy.[76] Recent strategies include identifying alternative dosing schedules of gemcitabine that might both enhance drug delivery to tumor cells as well as identifying synergistic combinations with other chemotherapeutic agents. Tempero and colleagues randomized 93 patients to either gemcitabine (2,200 mg/m^2) over the standard 30-minute infusion or gemcitabine (1,500 mg/m^2) at a rate of 10 mg/m^2/min. With analysis completed on 67 patients, the response rate was 17% versus 3% in favor of the longer infusion rate. In addition, median survival (6.1 months versus 4.7 months) and 1-year survival (23% versus 0%) favored the longer infusion rate.[77]

Combination Chemotherapy

Recent efforts have focused on developing strategies that would enhance the efficacy of gemcitabine and ultimately improve median survival. Table 45.4 summarizes the most recent studies[59,75–108]

Gemcitabine with 5-Fluorouracil

Preclinical data have also demonstrated a synergistic and non-cross-resistant effect of 5-FU when given with gemcitabine.[73]

TABLE 45.4. Recent studies in advanced pancreatic cancer.

Study	*Patient no.*	*Chemotherapy*	*PR/CR rate*	*Median survival (months)*	*One-year survival*
Casper (1994)	44	Gemcitabine	5 (11%)	5.6	23%
Burris (1997)	63 63	5-FU bolus Gemcitabine	0 (0%) 3 (5.4%)	4.4 5.7 $P = 0.0025$	2% 18%
Rothenberg (1996)	63 (2nd line)	Gemcitabine	6 (10.5%)	3.8	4%
Hidalgo (1999)	26	Gem + 5-FU CI	5 (19.2%)	10.3	40%
Berlin (2000)	36	Gem + 5-FU bolus	5 (14%)	4.4	9%
Miller (2000)	42	Pemetrexed	2 (5.7%)	6.5	28%
Heinemann (2000)	41	Gem + cisplatin	4 (11%)	8.2	27%
Marantz (2001)	29	Gem + 5-FU bolus	6 (21%)	8.4	36%
Louvet (2001)	62	Gem + LV5FU2	16 (25.9%)	9	32%
Philip (2001)	42	Gem + cisplatin	11 (26%)	7.1	19%
Colucci (2001)	54 53	Gemcitabine Gem + cisplatin	5 (9.2%) 14 (26.4%)	5 7.5 $P = 0.43$	11% 11%
Kozuch (2001)	34 (2nd line)	Gem + 5-FU + LV Irinotecan/cisplatin	8 (24%)	10.3	20%
Konstadoulakis (2001)	19	Rubitecan	4 (21%)	5.2	17%
Tomao (2002)	27	Gem + tamoxifen	3 (11%)	8	31%
Cartwright (2002)	42	Xeloda	3 (7.3%)	6.1	NR
Rothenberg (2002)	58 (1st line) 48 (2nd line)	5-FU bolus + Eniluracil	3 total (2%)	3.6 3.4	16% 10%
Feliu (2002)	43	Gem + UFT	14 (33%)	11	32%
Ducreux (2002)	103 104	5-FU bolus 5-FU + cisplatin	0 (0%) 10 (10%)	3.4 3.7 $P = 0.1$	9% 17%
Ryan (2002)	34	Gem + Taxol	6 (18%)	8.9	29%
Rocha Lima (2002)	45	Gem + Irinotecan	9 (20%)	5.7	27%
Fine (2002)	33	Gem/Taxol/Xeloda	20 (66%)	Not reached	NR
Louvet (2002)	30 LR 34 metastatic	Gem + Oxaliplatin Gem + Oxaliplatin	9 (31%) 10 (30%)	11.5 8.7	47% 26%
Kindler (2002)	42	Gem + pemetrexed	6 (15%)	6.5	29%
Hess (2003)	36	Gem + Xeloda	5 (14%)	6.4	33%
Scheithauer (2003)	42 43	Biweekly Gem Gem + Xeloda	6 (14%) 7 (17%)	8.2 9.5 (P = ns)	37% 32%
Kralidis (2003)	25	Gem + Tomudex	3 (12%)	6.2	12%
Cascinu (2003)	45	Gem + cisplatin	5 (9%)	5.6	NR
Alberts (2003)	47	Gem + Oxaliplatin	5 (11%)	6.2	18%
Heinemann (2003)	96 99	Gem Gem + cisplatin	NR NR	6 8.3 $P = 0.12$	NR NR
Rocha Lima (2003)	173 169	Gem Gem + Irinotecan	8 (4.4%) 27 (16%)	6.6 6.3 P = ns	21% 22%
Louvet (2003)	156 152	Gem Gem + Oxaliplatin	25 (16%) 39 (26%)	NR NR	NR NR
Tempero (2003)	49 43	Gem Fixed dose Gem	2/22 (9%) 1/17 (5%)	5 8 ($P = 0.013$)	9% 29%
Kindler (2004)	45	Gem + Avastin	9 (21%)	9	37%
O'Reilly (2004)	340	Gem ± Exatecan	6.3 vs. 8.2	6.3 months vs. 6.7 ($P = 0.52$)	21% vs. 23%
Richards (2004)	565	Gem ± Pemetrexed	9.1 vs. 18.3	6.3 months vs. 6.2 ($P = 0.85$)	21% vs. 20%
Louvet (2004)	313	Gem vs. Gem (FDR) + Oxaliplatin	17.3 vs. 26.8	7.1 vs. P ($P = 0.13$)	28% vs. 35%
Abbruzzese (2004)	41	Gem + Cetuximab	5 (12.2%)	7.1	31.7%

CR, complete response; PR, partial response; NR, no response.

However, the combination of 5-FU and gemcitabine has not consistently resulted in significant improvement over gemcitabine alone.[79,80,83,84,100] Early studies had designed the use of gemcitabine with bolus infusion of 5-FU with no significant improvement when compared to single-agent gemcitabine.[79] However, subsequent studies focusing on infusional schedules of 5-FU with gemcitabine suggested a clinical parallel to the data using infusional 5-FU in the therapy of metastatic colorectal cancer. Hidalgo et al. examined the combination of 5-FU administered as a continuous infusion (200 mg/m^2 throughout the study) with gemcitabine 700–900 mg/m^2 weekly × 3 repeated every 4 weeks. The reported median survival was 10.3 months.[80] In addition, Louvet et al. reported a Phase II study of infusional 5-FU and leukovorin (leukovorin 400 mg/m^2 in a 2-hour infusion followed by 5-FU 400 mg/m^2 bolus followed by 2–3 g/m^2 continuous-infusion 5-FU, in a schedule known as LV5FU2) with gemcitabine 1,000 mg/m^2 on day 3, repeating the cycle every 2 weeks. The reported median survival was 9 months.[84] However, in a recent study by Hess et al. using gemcitabine (1,000 mg/m^2, days 1 and 8) and capecitabine (starting 500 mg/m^2 divided bid × 14 days) in 36 patients with advanced pancreas cancer repeated every 21 days, the median survival was 6.4 months.[85] A number of modulators of 5-FU have been previously examined, including interferon-alpha and *N*-(phosphonoacteyl)-L-aspartate disodium (PALA), and all have been of no additional benefit. There has been interest in examining other 5-FU formulations, either alone or with gemcitabine, including the multitargeted folate inhibitor pemetrexed that has activity against thymidylate synthase (TS), dihyrofolate reductase (DHFR), and glyncinamide ribonucleotide formyltransferase (GARFT).[81,84]

Gemcitabine with Platinum Chemotherapy

Another potentially synergistic agent that has been used with gemcitabine is cisplatin. This combination is thought to be synergistic either by enhancing dFdCTP incorporation into DNA or via increasing DNA adduct formation.[78] Early studies identified median survival from 5.6 to 8.2 months.[82,86,102] This combination has recently been examined in two Phase III studies. Colucci and colleagues treated 107 patients with advanced pancreas cancer with either gemcitabine alone at standard dose and schedule or gemcitabine and cisplatin (25 mg/m^2 weekly × 3 every 4 weeks). The combination of gemcitabine and cisplatin improved median time to disease progression (2.7 months for gemcitabine alone versus 5 months for combination gemcitabine and cisplatin; $P = 0.048$) with no significant differences in toxicities. However, although the median survival for the gemcitabine group was 5 months compared to 7.5 months for the combination chemotherapy, the P value of 0.43 was not statistically significant.[87] More recently, Heinemann et al. presented the Phase III data of 195 patients randomized to either gemcitabine alone at standard dose and schedule versus gemcitabine and cisplatin (50 mg/m^2 weekly × 3 repeated every 4 weeks). Although a difference in median survival was noted (6 months for gemcitabine alone versus 8.3 months for the combination), this result was not statistically significant.[104]

Gemcitabine with Oxaliplatin

Oxaliplatin is a diaminocyclohexane (DACH) platinum compound that received FDA approval in August 2002 for use in combination with infusional 5-FU) and leucovorin for the treatment of patients with colorectal cancer whose disease has recurred or become worse following initial therapy with a combination of irinotecan with bolus 5-FU and leucovorin. Based on preclinical data that identified synergistic antitumor activity, oxaliplatin has since also been evaluated in combination with gemcitabine in patients with advanced pancreatic cancer. The French Cooperative group GERCOR examined gemcitabine 1,000 mg/m^2 as a 10 mg/m^2/min prolonged infusion administered on day 1 in combination with oxaliplatin 100 mg/m^2 as a 2-hour infusion administered on day 2, repeated every 2 weeks, in 64 patients with chemonaive metastatic pancreas cancer. Response rate was noted to be 30.6 % with a clinical benefit response of 40%. Median progression-free survival and overall survival were 5.3 months and 9.2 months, respectively, with 36% 1-year survival. The combination was safe, with reported side effects including grade 3 or 4 neutropenia/thrombocytopenia of 11%, nausea and vomiting of 14%, diarrhea of 6.2%, and peripheral neuropathy of 11%.[98]

The North Central Cancer Treatment Group (NCCTG) completed a Phase I study of gemcitabine and oxaliplatin in 18 patients with metastatic pancreas cancer. Dose-limiting toxicities (DLT) of neutropenia and severe infection were identified at the maximum tolerated dose of gemcitabine, 1,250 mg/m^2 (day 1 and day 8 every 21 days) and oxaliplatin, 130 mg/m^2 (day 1 every 21 days).[103]

Louvet et al. recently presented a Phase III study of 308 patients randomized to either gemcitabine or to gemcitabine with oxaliplatin (gemcitabine 1,000 mg/m^2 as a 10 mg/m^2/min prolonged infusion administered on day 1 in combination with oxaliplatin 100 mg/m^2 as a 2-hour infusion administered on day 2 repeated every 2 weeks) versus gemcitabine alone. Although there was a difference in progression-free survival (4 months for gemcitabine alone versus 6.25 months for combination chemotherapy; $P = 0.05$), the median survival was statistically significant.[106]

Gemcitabine with Irinotecan

Rocha Lima et al. completed a Phase II study of 45 patients treated with gemcitabine at 1,000 mg/m^2 over 30 minutes and irinotecan at 100 mg/m^2, both weekly × 2 repeated every 3 weeks. Median survival was 5.7 months.[96] Rocha Lima et al. also presented the follow-up Phase III study recently of 342 patients randomized to either gemcitabine alone or gemcitabine + irinotecan. Although there was a higher response rate for combination gemcitabine and irinotecan (16% versus 4%), the median survival was no different (6.6 months for gemcitabine alone versus 6.3 months for the combination).[105]

Gemcitabine with Other Chemotherapy

There has been additional interest based on preclinical data to synergistically combine multiple chemotherapy agents with gemcitabine. Early data suggest that such combinations have similar safety profiles with some of the gemcitabine combinations and are active schedules. Fine and colleagues have published preliminary data with a schedule known as GTX (gemcitabine 750 mg/m^2 over 2 hours days 4 and 11, Taxotere 30 mg/m^2 over 30 minutes days 4 and 11, and Xeloda 1,500 mg/m^2 po divided doses bid days 1–14 repeated every 21 days) in patients with locally advanced and metastatic disease. Patients without metastatic disease received gemcitabine 200 mg/m^2 weekly × 6 concurrent with EBRT to 45 to 50 Gy followed by surgery if indicated. Toxicities included 25% grade 3 leukopenia, 20% grade 3 asthenia, 20% grade 3 diarrhea, and 15% erythrodyesthesia. In 9 patients who presented with locally advanced but nonmetastatic disease, 8 patients were resected, with complete response in 6 patients. In patients who presented with metastatic disease, there were partial responses in 12 patients. Median survival for both groups has not been reported.[97]

Kozuch and colleagues treated 34 patients who had been previously treated with gemcitabine either alone or in combination with a schedule known as G-FLIP (day 1: gemcitabine 500 mg/m^2 over 50 minutes, leukovorin 300 mg over 30 minutes, irinotecan 80 mg/m^2 over 80 minutes, 5-FU bolus 400 mg/m^2 over 10 minutes, then 600 mg/m^2 over 8 hours; day 2: leukovorin 300 mg over 30 minutes, 5-FU bolus 400 mg/m^2 over 10 minutes, cisplatin 50–75 mg/m^2 with mannitol over 45 minutes and 5-FU 600 mg/m^2 over 8 hours). Toxicities were largely hematologic. Median survival for this pretreated group was 10.3 months.[88]

New Drugs in Pancreatic Cancer

During the last few years, an increasing number of new drugs, many of them targeted to specific alterations in malignant cells, have been tested in pancreatic cancer as well as in other tumors. The rationale to develop these drugs in pancreatic cancer comes from the better understanding of the biologic basis of the disease, which has made possible the identification and validation of some of these targets in pancreatic cancer. In addition, the poor prognosis of patients with this disease and the evidence from clinical trials discussed previously that conventional chemotherapy may have reached a plateau in improving outcome have also motivated an aggressive evaluation of new drugs in pancreatic cancer.

Matrix Metalloproteinase Inhibitors

The matrix metalloproteinases (MMPs) are a group of closely related proteases that are dysregulated in the majority of human neoplasms, including pancreatic cancer. The increased activity of these enzymes has been related to the tumor growth, progression, invasion, generation of blood vessels, and metastasis. Several inhibitors of the MMP have been developed as anticancer agents, and two of them, marimastat and BAY12-9566, have been more extensively studied in pancreatic cancer.[109]

Marimastat is a hydroxamate peptidomimetic broad-spectrum inhibitor of the MMP family including MMPs 1, 2, and 9. In Phase I studies in pancreatic cancer, doses from 10 to 25 mg orally twice a day were well tolerated. A large Phase II study that enrolled 113 patients, 90% of whom were treated with 25 mg in a once a day dose, reported a 30% decline or stabilization in the tumor marker CA-19-9 and a median survival of 3.8 months. and 51% of the patients had improvement in symptoms. Twenty-nine percent of the patients developed arthralgias, the most common toxicity encountered with marimastat.[110] The efficacy and toxicity of marimastat at doses of 5, 10, and 25 mg twice a day was compared to gemcitabine in a Phase III study. Patients treated with gemcitabine had a longer progression-free survival of 3.8 months versus 1.9 to 2 months for the marimastat-treated group (P = 0.001). Overall survival was also better for gemcitabine and significantly worse for patients treated with marimastat at doses of 5 and 10 mg, while no statistically significant differences were observed in overall survival with the 25 mg twice a day dose. A subset analysis in this study showed that the benefit of gemcitabine was restricted to patients with advanced disease and that patients with locally advanced tumors benefited from marimastat, supporting the hypothesis that these drugs may be more active in the situation of early disease.[111] Finally, the combination of gemcitabine with marimastat was tested against gemcitabine in a randomized Phase III study with no improvement in any parameter of outcome in the combined treatment group.[112]

The second MMP inhibitor extensively studied in pancreatic cancer is BAY12-9566, a peptidomimetic inhibitor specific for MMP-2 and MMP-9. The drug was compared in a Phase III study to single-agent gemcitabine in which 270 patients of a planned sample of 350 were enrolled after an interim analysis demonstrated that patients treated with gemcitabine had a significantly better time to tumor progression (3.5 versus 1.6 months; P less than 0.001) and overall survival (6.59 versus 3.74; P less than 0.001). Quality of life analysis also favored gemcitabine.[113] In summary, these studies suggest that current MMP inhibitors do not have relevant antitumor activity in patients with advanced pancreatic cancer. Whether or not these drugs or newer generation analogs would be effective in earlier stages of pancreatic cancer remains to be determined.

Angiogenesis Inhibitors

Pancreatic cancer is not an exception to the rule that tumors require the generation of blood vessels to grow, invade, and metastasize. The drug of this class that appears more promising is pancreatic cancer is bevacizumab, a recombinant human monoclonal antibody against vascular endothelial growth factor (VEGF), a growth factor that has been implicated in pancreatic cancer progression in several preclinical studies. Bevacizumab has been studied in combination with gemcitabine in a Phase II study in patients with pancreatic cancer.[114] Patients with advanced or locally advanced pancreatic cancer received gemcitabine 1,000 mg/m^2 on days 1, 8, and 15 every 28 days and bevacizumab 10 mg/kg intravenously on days 1 and 15. Results on the first 45 evaluable patients have been reported with a response rate of 21%, median survival of 9 months, and an estimated 1-year survival of 37%. Correlative studies suggest that patients with higher baseline levels of VEGF tend to do worse.[115] The Cancer and Leukemia Group B (CALGB) is currently leading a phase III study of gemcitabine ± bevacizumab.

Inhibitors of the Oncogene Ras

Mutation in the oncogene Ras is the most frequent genetic abnormality in pancreatic cancer. Because Ras requires to be farnesylated to be active, a posttranslational modification mediated by the enzyme farnesyl transferase, inhibitors of this enzyme have been developed as potential Ras inhibitors.[116] Two of these agents, tipifarnib and lonafarnib, have been studied in disease-oriented studies in pancreatic cancer. Tipifarnib was tested in a single-agent Phase II study in patients with advanced pancreatic cancer administered at a dose of 300 mg orally twice a day. Twenty patients were treated with no objective responses and a median survival of less than 5 months. Correlative studies conducted in peripheral blood mononuclear cells demonstrated partial inhibition of the target farnesyl transferase enzyme.[117] In parallel to this study, a randomized Phase III study compared the combination of R115777 with gemcitabine against gemcitabine plus placebo in patients with advanced pancreatic cancer. Treatment of 688 patients did not demonstrate any improvement in outcome in patients treated with R115777 and gemcitabine.[118] Lonafarnib was evaluated in a randomized Phase II study in comparison to gemcitabine. The 3-month progression-free survival rate for patients treated with lonafarnib was 23% and 31% for gemcitabine, and the median overall survival was 3.3 and 4.4 months, respectively. There were two partial responses in patients treated with lonafarnib and one partial response observed in 1 patient treated with gemcitabine. Overall, lonafarnib was better tolerated than gemcitabine in that study.[119]

Inhibitors of the EGFR Family of Receptors

The epidermal growth factor receptor (EGFR) family of receptors is formed by four related transmembrane receptors that are composed of an external ligand binding domain, a transmembrane domain, and an intracellular domain with tyrosine kinase (TK) activity. These receptors are frequently dysregulated in cancer and have been associated with the process of tumor growth, invasion, and metastasis, exciting considerable interest in developing these drugs for cancer treatment. Pharmacologically, the inhibitors of the EGFR belong to two broad classes of drugs including monoclonal antibodies against the extracellular domain of the receptor and small molecules inhibitors of the intracellular TK domain.[120] The studies conducted in pancreatic cancer have mainly tested the combination of these drugs with gemcitabine. Safran and collaborators reported a Phase II study of trastuzumab, a monoclonal antibody that targets the Her-2 receptor, in combination with gemcitabine in patients with pancreatic cancer.[120] Up to 21% of pancreatic cancers are Her-2 positive, and preclinical studies have shown that inhibition of Her-2 signaling with trastuzumab is associated with antitumor effects in pancreatic cancer models. Patients with Her-2-positive (2 or 3 + as determined by immunohistochemistry) pancreatic cancer received gemcitabine, 1,000 mg/m^2 weekly for 7 consecutive weeks followed by 1 week of rest and then weekly for 3 weeks every 4 weeks, and trastuzumab, 2 mg/kg/week following an initial loading dose of 4 mg/kg. Data on 23 patients have been reported thus far. Five patients had a partial response (response rate, 24%), and the median survival and 1-year survival were 7.5 months and 24%, respectively. Nine of 18 evaluable patients (50%) have had greater than 50% reduction in CA 19-9. A Phase II study of gemcitabine and cetuximab, a monoclonal antibody against EGFR, in EGFR-positive pancreatic cancer patients was conducted. Forty-one patients were treated in the study. The overall response rate was 12.5% with a median survival of 7.1 months and 1-year survival of 32%.[121] The Southwest Oncology Group (SWOG) is currently leading a Phase III study of gemcitabine ± cetuximab.

The second clinically relevant classes of agents that inhibit the EGFR are small molecule inhibitors of the receptor TK. Several of these agents are currently in clinical development. Two of these compounds, EKB-569 and erlotinib, have been specifically developed in pancreatic cancer. EKB-569, an irreversible inhibitor of EGFR and the Her-2 receptors, has completed a Phase I study in combination with gemcitabine, and a randomized Phase III study through NCI–Canada of gemcitabine plus erlotinib or placebo has completed enrollment.

Future Directions and Conclusions

The principal need to identify more effective therapies to supplement surgical gains in resected patients is unchallenged. What remain unresolved and controversial are the means to this end. Progress in the context of adjuvant trials has been slow. Current controversies may result in part from trial design issues, inadequate consideration of factors other than therapy that may impact on outcomes, and the limited efficacy of single chemotherapeutic agents for pancreatic cancer.

Current efforts are aimed at refining our understanding of the impact of nontherapeutic factors on outcomes (stratification factors for future trials), proceeding to multiagent chemotherapy alone or in combination with irradiation, identifying pancreatic tumor-specific antigens that provide an opportunity for molecular target-based drugs or immunotherapy, and identifying accurate predictors of microscopic disease and of response to therapy.

For metastatic disease, understanding of the molecular pathways that are thought to drive cellular growth is at the heart of the new paradigm of drug development. The utilization of xenografts to rapidly and efficiently screen drugs as well as improved collaboration with industry provide some promise that better therapies are on the horizon.

References

1. Kern S, Tempero M, et al. Pancreatic Cancer: An Agenda for Action Report of the Pancreatic Cancer Progress Review Group. http://prg.cancer.gov/pdfprgreports/2001pancreatic.pdf.
2. Iacobuzio-Donahue CA, Maitra A, Sheng-Ong GL, et al: Discovery of novel tumor markers of pancreatic cancer using global gene expression technology. Am J Pathol 2002;60:1239–1249.
3. Hingorani SR, Petricoin EF, Maitra A, et al. Preinvasive and invasive ductal pancreatic canecr and its early detection in the mouse. Cancer Cell 2003;4:437–450.
4. Sohn TA, Yeo CJ, Cameron JL, et al. Resected adenocarcinoma of the pancreas-616 patients: results, outcomes, and prognostic indicators. J Gastrointest Surg 2000;4:567–579.
5. Kalser MH, Ellenberg SS. Pancreatic cancer: adjuvant combined radiation and chemotherapy following curative resection. Arch Surg 1985;120:899–903.
6. Gastrointestinal tumor study group. Further evidence of effective adjuvant combined radiation and chemotherapy following curative resection of pancreatic cancer. Cancer (Phila) 1987;59: 2006–2010.
7. Whittington R, Bryer MP, Haller DG, et al. Adjuvant therapy of resected adenocarcinoma of the pancreas. Int J Radiat Oncol Biol Phys 1991;21:1137–1143.
8. Foo ML, Gunderson LL, Nagorney DM, et al. Patterns of failure in grossly resected pancreatic ductal adenocarcinoma treated with adjuvant irradiation ± 5-fluorouracil. Int J Radiat Oncol Biol Phys 1993;26:483–489.

9. Spitz FR, Abbruzzese JL, Lee JE, et al. Preoperative and postoperative chemoradiation strategies in patients treated with pancreaticoduodenectomy for adenocarcinoma of the pancreas. J Clin Oncol 1997;15:928–937.
10. Yeo CJ, Abrams RA, Grochow LB, et al. Pancreaticoduodenectomy for pancreatic adenocarcinoma: Postoperative adjuvant chemoradiation improves survival. Ann Surg 1997;225(5): 621–636.
11. Todd KE, Gloor B, Lane JS, et al. Resection of locally advanced pancreatic cancer after downstaging with continuous infusion 5-fluorouracil, mitomycin-C, leukovorin and dipyridamole. J Gastrointest Surg 1998;2:159–166.
12. Abrams RA, Grochow LB, Chakravarthy A, et al: Intensified adjuvant therapy for pancreatic and periampullary adenocarcinoma: survival results and observations regarding patterns of failure, radiotherapy dose and CA19-9 levels. Int J Radiat Oncol Biol Phys 1999;44(5):1039–1046.
13. Klinkenbijl JH, Jeekel J, Sahmoud T, et al. Adjuvant radiotherapy and 5-fluorouracil after curative resection of cancer of the pancreas and periampullary region. Ann Surg 1999;230(6):776–784.
14. Paulino AC. Resected pancreatic cancer treated with adjuvant radiotherapy with or without 5-fluorouracil: treatment results and patterns of failure. Am J Clin Oncol 1999;22(5):489–498.
15. Mehta VK, Fisher GA, Ford JM, et al. Adjuvant radiotherapy and concomitant 5-fluorouracil by protracted venous infusion for resected pancreatic cancer. Int J Radiat Oncol Biol Phys 2000; 48(5):1483–1487.
16. Nukui Y, Picozzi VJ, Travesro LW. Interferon based adjuvant chemoradiation therapy improves survival after pancreaticoduodenectomy for pancreatic adenocarcinoma. Am J Surg 2000; 179(5):367–371.
17. Chakravarthy A, Abrams RA, Yeo CJ. Intensified adjuvant combined modality therapy for resected periampullary adenocarcinoma: acceptable toxicity and suggestion of improved 1 year survival. Int J Radiat Oncol Biol Phys 2000;48(4):1089–1096.
18. Neoptolemos JP, Dunn JA, Stocken DD, et al. Adjuvant chemoradiotherapy and chemotherapy in resectable pancreatic cancer: a randomized controlled trial. Lancet 2001;358:1576–1585.
19. Picozzi VJ, Kozarek RE, Jacobs AD, et al. Adjuvant therapy for resected pancreas cancer (PC) using alpha-interferon (IFN)-based chemoradiation: completion of a phase II trial. Proc ASCO 2003; 22:265 (abstract 1061).
20. Van-Laethem JL, Demols A, Gay F, et al. Postoperative adjuvant gemcitabine and concurrent radiation after curative resection of pancreatic head carcinoma: a phase II study. Int J Radiat Oncol Biol Phys 2003;56(4):974–980.
21. Neoptolemos JP, Stocken DD, Friess H, et al. A randomized trial of chemoradiotherapy and chemotherapy after resection of pancreatic cancer. N Engl J Med 2004;350:1200–1210.
22. Greten TF, Jaffee EM. Cancer vaccines. J Clin Oncol 1999;17(3): 1047–1060.
23. Cox AL, Skipper J, Chen Y, et al. Identification of a peptide recognized by five melanoma specific human cytotoxic T cell lines. Science 1994;264:716–719.
24. Dranoff G, Jaffee EM, Golumbek P, et al. Vaccination with irradiated tumor cells engineered to secrete murine GM-CSF stimulates potent, specific and long lasting anti tumor immunity. Proc Natl Acad Sci USA 1993;90:3539–3543.
25. Huang AY, Golumbek PT, Ahmadzadeh M, et al. Role of bone marrow derived cells in presenting MHC class I restricted tumor antigens. Science 1994;264:961–965.
26. Jaffee EM, Hruban R, Biedrzycki B, et al. A novel allogeneic GM-CSF secreting tumor vaccine for pancreatic cancer: a Phase I trial of safety and immune activation. J Clin Oncol 2001;19(1): 145–156.
27. Argani P, Iacobuzio-Donahue C, Ryu B, et al. Mesothelin is overexpressed in the vast majority of ductal adenocarcinomas of the pancreas: identification of a new pancreatic cancer marker by serial analysis of gene expression (SAGE). Clin Cancer Res 2001; 3862(7):3862–3868.
28. Thomas AM, Santarsiero LM, Armstrong T, et al. A functional genomic approach identifies mesothelin as an immune target in human pancreatic cancer. J Exp Med 2004;200:297–306.
29. Todd KE, Gloor B, Lane JS, et al. Resection of locally advanced pancreatic cancer after downstaging with continuous infusion 5-fluorouracil, mitomycin-c, leukovorin and dipyridamole. J Gastrointest Surg 1998;2(2):159–166.
30. Evans DB, Rich TA, Byrd DR, et al. Pre-operative chemoradiation and pancreaticoduodenectomy for adenocarcinoma of the pancreas. Arch Surg 1992;127:1335–1339.
31. Hoffman JP, Weese JL, Solin LJ, et al. A pilot study of preoperative chemoradiation for patients with localized adenocarcinoma of the pancreas. Am J Surg 1995;169:71–78.
32. Staley CA, Lee JE, Cleary KR, et al. Preoperative chemoradiation, pancreaticoduodenectomy, and intraoperative radiation therapy for adenocarcinoma of the pancreatic head. Am J Surg 1996;171:118–125.
33. Pendurthi TK, Hoffman JP. Pre-operative versus postoperative chemoradiation for patients with resected pancreatic adenocarcinoma. Am Surg 1998;64(7):686–695.
34. Hoffman JP, Lipsitz S, Pisansky T, et al. Phase II trial of preoperative radiation therapy and chemotherapy for patients with localized, resectable adenocarcinoma of the pancreas: an Eastern Cooperative Oncology Group study. J Clin Oncol 1998;16(1): 317–323.
35. Pisters PW, Abbruzzese JL, Janjan NA, et al. Rapid fractionation pre-operative chemoradiation, pancreaticoduodenectomy, and intraoperative radiation therapy for resectable pancreatic adenocarcinoma. J Clin Oncol 1998;16:3843–3850.
36. White RR, Hurwitz HI, Morse MA, et al. Neoadjuvant chemoradiation for localized adenocarcinoma of the pancreas. Ann Surg Oncol 2001;8(10):758–765.
37. Breslin TM, Hess KR, Harbison DB, et al. Neoadjuvant chemoradiotherapy for adenocarcinoma of the pancreas: treatment variables and survival duration. Ann Surg Oncol 2001;8(2):123–132.
38. Moutardier V, Giovanni M, Lelong B, et al. A phase II single institutional experience with pre-operative radiochemotherapy in pancreatic adenocarcinoma. Eur J Surg Oncol 2002;28: 531–539.
39. Arnoletti JP, Hoffman JP, Ross EA, et al. Pre-operative chemoradiation in the management of adenocarcinoma of the body of the pancreas. Am Surg 2002;68(4):330–335.
40. Magnin V, Moutardier V, Giovannini MH, et al. Neoadjuvant pre-operative chemoradiation in patients with pancreatic cancer. Int J Radiat Oncol Biol Phys 2003;55(5):1300–1304.
41. Pisters PWT, Wolff RA, Janjan NA, et al. Preoperative paclitaxel and concurrent rapid fractionation radiation for resectable pancreatic adenocarcinoma: toxicities, histologic response rates and event-free outcome. J Clin Oncol 2002;20(10):2537–2544.
42. Kim HJ, Kzischke K, Brennan MF, et al. Does neoadjuvant chemoradiation downstage locally advanced pancreatic cancer? J Gastrointest Surg 2002;6:763–769.
43. Moertel CG, Childs DS Jr, Reitemeier RJ, et al. Combined 5-fluorouracil and supervoltage radiation therapy of locally unresectable gastrointestinal cancer. Lancet 1969;2(7626):865–867.
44. Moertel CG, Frytak S, Hahn RG, et al. Therapy of locally unresectable pancreatic carcinoma: a randomized comparison of high dose (6000 rads) radiation alone, moderate dose radiation (4000 rads + 5-fluorouracil), and high dose radiation + 5-fluorouracil. The Gastrointestinal Tumor Study Group. Cancer (Phila) 1981; 48:1705–1710.
45. Klaassen DJ, MacIntyre JM, Catton GE, et al. Treatment of locally unresectable cancer of the stomach and pancreas: a randomized comparison of 5-fluorouracil alone with radiation plus concurrent and maintenance 5-fluorouracil: an Eastern Cooperative Oncology Group Study. J Clin Oncol 1985;3:373–378.

46. Gastrointestinal Tumor Study Group. Treatment of locally unresectable carcinoma of the pancreas: comparison of combined-modality therapy (chemotherapy plus radiotherapy) to chemotherapy alone. J Natl Cancer Inst 1988;80:751–755.
47. McCracken JD, Ray P, Heilbrun LK, et al. 5-Fluorouracil, methyl-CCNU, and radiotherapy with or without testolectone for localized adenocarcinoma of the exocrine pancreas. A Southwest Oncology Group Study. Cancer (Phila) 1980;46:1518–1522.
48. Gastrointestinal Tumor Study Group. Radiation therapy combined with adriamycin or 5-fluorouracil for the treatment of locally unresectable pancreatic carcinoma. Cancer (Phila) 1985; 56:2563–2568.
49. Earle JD, Foley JF, Wieand HS, et al. Evaluation of external-beam radiation therapy plus 5-fluorouracil (5-FU) versus external-beam radiation therapy plus hycanthone (HYC) in confined, unresectable pancreatic cancer. Int J Radiat Oncol Biol Phys 1994;28:207–211.
50. McGinn CJ, Zalupski MM. Radiation therapy with once-weekly gemcitabine in pancreatic cancer: current status of clinical trials. Int J Radiat Oncol Biol Phys 2003;56(suppl 4):10–15.
51. Blackstock AW, Bernard SA, Richards F, et al. Phase I trial of twice-weekly gemcitabine and concurrent radiation in patients with advanced pancreatic cancer. J Clin Oncol 1999;17(7): 2208–2212.
52. Blackstock AW, Tempero MA, Niedwiecki D, et al. Phase II chemoradiation trial using gemcitabine in patients with locoregional adenocarcinoma of the pancreas. Proc ASCO 2001;20: 158a (abstract 627).
53. Wolff RA, Evans DB, Gravel DM, et al. Phase I trial of gemcitabine combined with radiation for the treatment of locally advanced pancreatic adenocarcinoma. Clin Cancer Res 2001; 2246(7):2246–2253.
54. McGinn CJ, Zalupski MM, Shureiqi I, et al. Phase I trial of radiation dose escalation with concurrent weekly full-dose gemcitabine in patients with advanced pancreatic cancer. J Clin Oncol 2001;19(22):4202–4208.
55. Talamonti MS, Catalano PJ, Vaughn DJ, et al. Eastern Cooperative Oncology Group phase I trial of protracted venous infusion fluorouracil plus weekly gemcitabine with concurrent radiation therapy in patients with locally advanced pancreas cancer: a regimen with unexpected early toxicity. J Clin Oncol 2000;18: 3384–3389.
56. Martenson JA, Vigliotti APG, Pitot HC, et al. A phase I study of radiation therapy and twice-weekly gemcitabine and cisplatin in patients with locally advanced pancreatic cancer. Int J Radiat Oncol Biol Phys 2003;55(5):1305–1310.
57. Brunner TB, Grabenbauer GG, Klein P, et al. Phase I trial of strictly time-scheduled gemcitabine and cisplatin with concurrent radiotherapy in patients with locally advanced pancreatic cancer. Int J Radiat Oncol Biol Phys 2003;55(1):144–153.
58. Crane CH, Abbruzzese JL, Evans DB, et al. Is the therapeutic index better with gemcitabine based chemoradiation than with 5-fluorouracil based chemoradiation in locally advanced pancreatic cancer? Int J Radiat Oncol Biol Phys 2002;52(5): 1293–1302.
59. Burris HA 3rd, Moore MJ, Andersen J, et al. Improvements in survival and clinical benefit with gemcitabine as first-line therapy for patients with advanced pancreas cancer: a randomized trial. J Clin Oncol 1997;15(6):2403–2413.
60. Mohiuddin M, Rosato F, Barbot D, et al. Long-term results of combined modality treatment with I-125 implantation for carcinoma of the pancreas. Int J Radiat Oncol Biol Phys 1992;23: 305–311.
61. Nori D, Merimsky O, Osian AD, et al. Palladium-103: a new radioactive source in the treatment of unresectable carcinoma of the pancreas: a phase I–II study. J Surg Oncol 1996;61:300–305.
62. Raben A, Mychalczak B, Brennan MF, et al. Feasibility study of the treatment of primary unresectable carcinoma of the pancreas with ^{103}PD brachytherapy. Int J Radiat Oncol Biol Phys 1996; 35(2):351–356.
63. Tepper JE, Noyes D, Krall JM, et al. Intraoperative radiation therapy of pancreas carcinoma: a report of RTOG-8505. Radiation Therapy Oncology Group. Int J Radiat Oncol Biol Phys 1991;21(5):1145–1149.
64. Garton GR, Gunderson LL, Nagorney DM, et al. High-dose preoperative external beam and intraoperative irradiation for locally advanced pancreatic cancer. Int J Radiat Oncol Biol Phys 1993;27:1153–1157.
65. Zerbi A, Fossati V, Parolini D, et al. Intraoperative radiation therapy adjuvant to resection in the treatment of pancreatic cancer. Cancer (Phila) 1994;73:2930–2935.
66. Mohiuddin M, Regine WF, Stevens J, et al. Combined intraoperative radiation and perioperative chemotherapy for unresectable cancers of the pancreas. J Clin Oncol 1995;13(11): 2764–2768.
67. Willett CG, Warshaw AL. Intraoperative electron beam irradiation in pancreatic cancer. Front Biosci 1998;3:e207–e213.
68. Hecht JR, Bedford R, Abbruzzese JL, et al. A phase I/II trial of intratumoral endoscopic ultrasound injection of ONYX-015 with intravenous gemcitabine in unresectable pancreatic carcinoma. Clin Cancer Res 2003;9:555–561.
69. Hanna N, Chung T, Hecht R, et al. TNFerade in pancreatic cancer: results of a run-in phase of a major randomized study in patients with locally advanced pancreatic cancer. Proc ASCO 2003;22:271 (abstract 1086).
70. Ahlgren JD. Chemotherapy for pancreatic carcinoma. Cancer (Phila) 1996;78:653–663.
71. DeCaprio JA, Mayer RJ, Gonin R, et al. Fluorouracil and high dose leukovorin in previously untreated patients with advanced pancreatic adenocarcinoma: results of a phase II trial. J Clin Oncol 1991;9:2128–2133.
72. Crown J, Casper ES, Botet J, et al. Lack of efficacy of high dose leukovorin and fluorouracil in patients with advanced pancreatic adenocarcinoma. J Clin Oncol 1991;9:1682–1686.
73. Peters GJ, van der Wilt CL, van Moorsel CJ, et al. Basis for effective combination cancer chemotherapy with antimetabolites. Pharmacol Ther 2000;87:227–253.
74. DiMagno E, Reber HA, Tempero MA. AGA technical review on the epidemiology, diagnosis, and treatment of pancreatic ductal adenocarcinoma. Gastroenterology 1999;117(6):1463–1484.
75. Casper E, Green MR, Kelson DP, et al. Phase II trial of gemcitabine in patients with pancreatic adenocarcinoma. Invest New Drugs 1994;12:29–34.
76. Rothenberg ML, Moore MJ, Cripps MC, et al. A phase II trial of gemcitabine in patients with 5-FU refractory pancreas cancer. Ann Oncol 1996;7:347–353.
77. Tempero M, Plunkett W, van Haperen V, et al. Randomized phase II comparison of dose intense gemcitabine: thirty minute infusion and fixed dose infusion in patients with pancreatic adenocarcinoma. J Clin Oncol 2003;21:3402–3408.
78. Peters GJ, van der Wilt CL, van Moorsel CJ, et al. Basis for effective combination cancer chemotherapy with antimetabolites. Pharmacol Ther 2000;87:227–253.
79. Berlin JD, Adak S, Vaughn DJ, et al. A phase II study of gemcitabine and 5-fluorouracil in metastatic pancreatic cancer: an Eastern Cooperative Oncology Group Study. Oncology 2000;58(3):215–218.
80. Hidalgo M, Castellano D, Paz-Ares, L, et al. Phase I–II study of gemcitabine and fluorouracil as a continuous infusion in patients with pancreatic cancer. J Clin Oncol 1999;17(2): 585–592.
81. Miller KD, Picus J, Blanke C, et al. Phase II study of the multitargeted antifolate LY231514 (ALIMTA, MTA, pemetrexed disodium) in patients with advanced pancreatic cancer. Ann Oncol 2000;11:101–103.

82. Heinemann V, Wilke H, Mergenthaler HG, et al. Gemcitabine and cisplatin in the treatment of advanced or metastatic pancreatic cancer. Ann Oncol 2000;11:1399–1403.
83. Marantz A, Jovtis S, Almira E, et al. Phase II study of gemcitabine,5-fluorouracil and leukovorin in patients with pancreatic cancer. Semin Oncol 2001;28(3S10):44–49.
84. Louvet C, Andre T, Hammel P, et al. Phase II trial of bimonthly leukovorin, 5-fluorouracil and gemcitabine for advanced pancreatic adenocarcinoma (FOLFUGEM). Ann Oncol 2001;12: 675–679.
85. Hess V, Salzberg M, Borner M, et al. Combining capecitabine and gemcitabine in patients with advanced pancreatic carcinoma: a phase I/II trial. J Clin Oncol 2003;21(1):66–68.
86. Philip PA, Zalupski MM, Vaitkevicius VK, et al. Phase II study of gemcitabine and cisplatin in the treatment of patients with advanced pancreatic cancer. Cancer (Phila) 2001;92:569–577.
87. Colucci G, Giuliani F, Gebbia V, et al. Gemcitabine alone or with cisplatin for the treatment of patients with locally advanced and/or metastatic pancreatic carcinoma. Cancer (Phila) 2002;94: 902–910.
88. Kozuch P, Grossbard ML, Barzdins A, et al. Irinotecan combined with gemcitabine, 5-fluorouracil, leukovorin and cisplatin (G-FLIP) is an effective and non-cross resistant treatment for chemotherapy refractory metastatic pancreatic cancer. Oncologist 2001;6:488–495.
89. Konstadoulakis MM, Antonakis PT, Tsibloulis BG, et al. A phase II study of 9-nitrocamptothecin in patients with advanced pancreatic adenocarcinoma. Cancer Chemother Pharmacol 2001;48:417–420.
90. Tomao S, Romiti A, Massidda B, et al. A phase II study of gemcitabine and tamoxifen in advanced pancreatic cancer. Anticancer Res 2002;22:2361–2364.
91. Cartwright TH, Cohn A, Varkey JA, et al. Phase II study of oral capecitabine in patients with advanced or metastatic pancreatic cancer. J Clin Oncol 2002;20(1):160–164.
92. Rothenberg ML, Benedetti JK, Macdonald JS, et al. phase II trial of 5-fluorouracil plus eniluracil in patients with advanced pancreatic cancer: a Southwest Oncology Group study. Ann Oncol 2002;13:1576–1582.
93. Feliu J, Mel R, Borrega P, et al. Phase II study of a fixed dose-rate infusion of gemcitabine associated with uracil/tegafur in advanced carcinoma of the pancreas. Ann Oncol 2002;13: 1756–1762.
94. Ducreux M, Rougier P, Pignon JP, et al. A randomized trial comparing 5-FU with 5-FU plus cisplatin in advanced pancreatic carcinoma. Ann Oncol 2002;13:1185–1191.
95. Ryan DP, Kulke MH, Fuchs CS, et al. A phase II study of gemcitabine and docetaxel in patients with metastatic pancreatic carcinoma. Cancer (Phila) 2002;94:97–103.
96. Rocha Lima C, Savarese D, Bruckner H, et al. Irinotecan plus gemcitabine induces both radiographic and CA19-9 tumor marker responses in patients with previously untreated advanced pancreatic cancer. J Clin Oncol 2002;20:1182–1191.
97. Fine RL, Sherman W, Chabot J, et al. Biochemically synergistic chemotherapy for advanced pancreatic cancer. Proc ASCO 2002;21:144a (abstract 575).
98. Louvet C, Andre T, Lledo G, et al. Gemcitabine combined with oxaliplatin in advanced pancreatic adenocarcinoma: final results of a GERCOR multicenter phase II study. J Clin Oncol 2002; 20(6):1512–1518.
99. Kindler H, Dugan W, Hochster H, et al. Clinical outcome in patients with advanced pancreatic cancer treated with pemetrexed/gemcitabine. Proc ASCO 2002;21:125a (abstract 499).
100. Scheithauer W, Schull B, Ulrich-Pur H, et al. Biweekly high dose gemcitabine alone or in combination with capecitabine in patients with metastatic pancreatic adenocarcinoma: a randomized phase II trial. Ann Oncol 2003;14:97–104.
101. Kralidis E, Aebi S, Friess H, et al. Activity of raltitrexed and gemcitabine in advanced pancreatic cancer. Ann Oncol 2003; 14:574–579.
102. Cascinu S, Labianca R, Catalano V, et al. Weekly gemcitabine and cisplatin chemotherapy: a well tolerated but ineffective chemotherapeutic regimen in advanced pancreatic cancer patients. A report from the Italian Group for the Study of Digestive Tract Cancer (GISCAD). Ann Oncol 2003;14:205–208.
103. Alberts SR, Townley PM, Goldberg RM, et al. Gemcitabine and oxaliplatin for metastatic pancreatic adenocarcinoma: a North Central Cancer Treatment Group phase II study. Ann Oncol 2003;14:580–585.
104. Heinemann V, Quietzsch D, Gieseler F, et al. A phase III trial comparing gemcitabine plus cisplatin vs. gemcitabine alone in advanced pancreatic cancer. Proc ASCO 2003;22:250 (abstract 1003).
105. Rocha Lima CMS, Rotche R, Jeffrey M, et al. A randomized phase III study comparing efficacy and safety of gemcitabine and Irinotecan to gemcitabine alone in patients with locally advanced or metastatic pancreatic cancer who have not received prior systemic therapy. Proc ASCO 2003;22:250 (abstract 1005).
106. Louvet C, Labianca R, Hammel G, et al. GEMOX (gemcitabine + oxaliplatin) versus gem (Gemcitabine) in nonresectable pancreatic adenocarcinoma: final results of the GERCOR/GISCAD Intergroup Phase III. Proc ASCO 2004;23: (abstract 4008).
107. Cheverton P, et al. Phase III results of exatecan (DX-8951f) versus gemcitabine (Gem) in chemotherapy-naïve patients with advanced pancreatic cancer. Proc ASCO 2004;23: (abstract 4005).
108. Richards DA, Kindler HL, Oettle H, et al. A randomized phase II study comparing gemcitabine + pemetrexed versus gemcitabine in patients with locally advanced and metastatic pancreas cancer. Proc ASCO 2004;23: (abstract 4007).
109. Hidalgo M, Eckhardt SG. Development of matrix metalloproteinase inhibitors in cancer therapy. J Natl Cancer Inst 2001; 93(3):178–193.
110. Evans JD, et al. A phase II trial of marimastat in advanced pancreatic cancer. Br J Cancer 2001;85(12):1865–1870.
111. Bramhall SR, et al. Marimastat as first-line therapy for patients with unresectable pancreatic cancer: a randomized trial. J Clin Oncol 2001;19(15):3447–3455.
112. Bramhall SR, et al. A double-blind placebo-controlled, randomised study comparing gemcitabine and marimastat with gemcitabine and placebo as first line therapy in patients with advanced pancreatic cancer. Br J Cancer 2002;87(2):161–167.
113. Moore MJ, et al. Comparison of gemcitabine versus the matrix metalloproteinase inhibitor BAY 12-9566 in patients with advanced or metastatic adenocarcinoma of the pancreas: a Phase III trial of the National Cancer Institute of Canada Clinical Trials Group. J Clin Oncol 2003;21(17):3296–3302.
114. Kindler HL, Friberg G, Stadler WM, et al. Bevacizumab plus gemcitabine is an active combination in patients with advanced pancreatic cancer: interim results of an ongoing phase II trial from the University of Chicago Phase II consortium. Proc GI ASCO 2004; (abstract 86).
115. Adjei AA. Blocking oncogenic Ras signaling for cancer therapy. J Natl Cancer Inst 2001;93(14):1062–1074.
116. Cohen SJ, et al. Phase II and pharmacodynamic study of the farnesyltransferase inhibitor R115777 as initial therapy in patients with metastatic pancreatic adenocarcinoma. J Clin Oncol 2003; 21(7):1301–1306.
117. Van Cutsem E, van de Velde H, Karasek P, et al. Phase III trial of gemcitabine + tipifarnib compared to gemcitabine + placebo in advanced pancreatic cancer. J Clin Oncol 2004;22:1430–1438.
118. Lersch C, Amado R, Ehninger G, et al. Randomized phase II study of SCH 66336 and gemcitabine in the treatment of metastatic adenocarcinoma of the pancreas. Proc Am Soc Clin Oncol 2001; (abstract 608).

119. Grunwald V, Hidalgo M. Developing inhibitors of the epidermal growth factor receptor for cancer treatment. J Natl Cancer Inst 2003;95(12):851–867.
120. Safran H, et al. Herceptin and gemcitabine for metastatic pancreatic cancer. Eur J Cancer 2001;37(suppl 6):S310.
121. Xiong HQ, Rosenberg A, LoBuglio A, et al. Cetuximab, a monoclonal antibody targerting the epidermal growth factor receptor, in combination with gemcitabine for advanced pancreatic cancer: a multicenter phase II trial. J Clin Oncol 2004;22:2610–2616.

Renal Cell Cancer

Joseph I. Clark, Craig Hofmeister,
Vicki Keedy, and Jeffrey A. Sosman

More than 80% of tumors originating in the kidney are renal cell carcinomas. Tumors of the renal pelvis make up another 10%, and the remaining tumors include a variety of rare lesions such as collecting duct carcinomas, renal sarcomas, or other rare epithelial tumors. This chapter presents evidence-based literature only for renal cell carcinoma and its histologic subtypes.

Epidemiology

Renal cell cancer (RCC) is responsible for approximately 2% of the total incidence and mortality caused by cancer in the United States in 2004.[1] During the past 30 years, based on the Surveillance, Epidemiology, and End Results (SEER) program of the National Cancer Institute (NCI), which covers about 10% of the U.S. population, there has been a rising incidence of renal cell carcinoma.[2] There will be an estimated 35,700 newly diagnosed cases of renal cancer and another 12,800 deaths during 2004, compared with an incidence of 27,000 and mortality of 10,900 in 1993. The increases over the 20 years in the SEER database (1975–1995) were observed in both genders and in both black and white populations. The upward incidence of advanced RCC with increased mortality is certainly not simply the result of detection of tumors in the presymptomatic stage. The reasons for this rise in RCC are not obvious and are likely multifactorial. The main risk factor for RCC, tobacco abuse, actually decreased in incidence during this time frame. Whether there are other identifiable environmental factors is unknown, but this is significant as understanding may lead to prevention (primary and secondary) strategies for RCC. Last, it is well known that the incidence of RCC in male subjects is twofold that of female subjects. The median age of diagnosis is around 64 years for Caucasians and 58 years for African-Americans. It is unusual to see the occurrence of RCC in individuals below the age of 40 years. The 5-year survival for all RCC is between 50% and 60%. This rate is lowest among African-American men, based on SEER data from 1985 to 1996. Although 5-year survival has improved for Caucasians, this has not been true for African-Americans. The increase in cancer-related mortality due to RCC has been most apparent in the African-American populations.

A number of studies have examined the association of environmental factors and renal cancer. The largest cohort trial involved 363,000 adult men enrolled from 1971 to 1992 in Sweden. The increased risk of RCC has appeared to meet the required level of significance only for three risk factors: cigarette smoking, obesity, and hypertension (Tables 46.1, 46.2, 46.3).[3,4] In general, cigarette smoking is a more significant factor in men whereas obesity is more of an important factor for women. Even though there is an increase in risk associated to all three factors, the relative risks are small compared with other cancers (see Table 46.1) (1.2–2.5). For example, cigarette smoking has a greater relative risk in transitional cell cancer of the renal pelvis (greater than 3.5). Smoking has been calculated to account for 20% to 30% of RCC in men but only 10% to 15% of the incidence in women.

Genetic Association

There is a distinct familial or hereditary component in only around 4% of renal cancers (Table 46.4). In general, these renal cancers are distinguishable by their early age of onset, multiplicity, bilaterality, and their equivalent male: female distribution.[5] The other distinguishing factors include an association with distinct syndromes involving other cancers or other organ abnormalities. The syndromes include von Hippel–Lindau, tuberous sclerosis, and Birt–Hogg–Dube syndrome. All three are autosomal dominant in their transmission.[5–8] Additionally, familial RCC can manifest itself more restrictively in the kidneys alone, such as hereditary papillary RCC (type I), familial renal oncocytoma, and finally hereditary and familial clear cell RCC (with or without chromosome 3 translocation).[5,9–11]

von Hippel–Lindau disease (VHL) is an autosomal dominant disease with prevalence in North America or Europe of 1 in 36,000 to 40,000.[6,12,13] Although clear cell carcinoma of the kidneys is a prominent manifestation in 28% to 45% of the cases, there are a large number of associated characteristics including retinal angiomas, cerebellar and spinal hemangioblastomas, pheochromocytomas, pancreatic cystic disease (serous cystadenomas), pancreatic neuroendocrine cancers, endolymphatic sac tumors of the labrinyth of the inner ears, epididymal cystadenoma, and renal cystic disease. The VHL gene, mutated in the germ-line VHL patient on chromosome 3p25, is accompanied by the loss of the other allele in the tumor consistent with VHL being a tumor suppressor gene (TSG).[14,15] This same gene is mutated, deleted, or not expressed in 55% to 85% of sporadic RCC of the clear cell type, emphasizing its importance to the general pathogenesis of clear cell RCC.[14] The protein product of the gene, pVHL, binds to a complex of proteins including elongin B, C, and Cul2 to form an ubiquitin ligase that facilitates ubiquitin-

TABLE 46.1. Cigarette smoking and renal carcinoma.

Reference	*Type of study*	*Number of patients [renal cell carcinoma (RCC)/control]*	*Relative risk*	*Association with exposure*	*Summary*	*Importance*
210	Case-control/ population based	1,732/2,309	1.4 current smokers 1.1–2.1 for <10 to >20 cigarettes/day	Yes	Adjusted for age, gender, body mass index (BMI)	Smoking is responsible for attributable for 24% in men and 9% in women
211	Case-control/ population based	495/697	1.6 ever smoked 1.2–2.3 for <20 to >50 pack-years, men 1.9 ever smoked, women	Yes	More significant risk for men and women	30% in men and 24% in women, attributable risk due to smoking
212	Case control/ population based	518/1,381	2.0 and 2.3 for ever and current smokers, men 1.9 and 2.2 for ever smoked and current smoker, women	No; no trends with amount of smoking	Risk increase after 20 years and decline after stopping for 20 years	No trend with amount of smoking is concerning

TABLE 46.2. Obesity and renal carcinoma.

Reference	*Type of study*	*No. of patients (RCC/control)*	*Relative risk*	*Summary*	*Importance*
210	Case-control/ population based	1,732/2,309	1.6 BMI highest quarter, men 2.0 BMI highest quarter, women	Significant trend in women; rate of weight change in women	Important primarily in women; no effect of height or physical activity
212	Case-control/ population based	518/1,381	2.2 BMI highest quarter	Effect in both women and men, with trend; recent weight in women; earlier weight in men	Importance in both genders
3	Cohort study based	102 RCC from 46,827 hospital-discharged patients, 1977–1987, Denmark	2.67 risk obesity in women 1.52 risk obesity in men	Cohort trial: but diagnosis-only based on hospital discharged	Prospective: effect greatest in women

TABLE 46.3. High blood pressure (hypertension) and renal carcinoma.

Reference	*Type of study*	*No. of patients (RCC/control)*	*Relative risk (RR)*	*Summary*	*Importance*
210	Case-control/ population based	1,732/2,309	1.7 Hypertension	Antihypertensive effects adjusted for; then 1.4 risk	Diuretics not a risk factor; possible role for beta-blockers
4	Cohort	759 from 363,992 men Sweden	RR approximately 2.0 Almost 70% on diuretics	Cohort trial, significant risk for RCC with hypertension (HTN) Role of drugs to treat	Important based on prospective nature of study; difficult to adjust for other factors
213	Case-control nested in cohort	206/206	RR 2.0 men RR 1.9 women	Diuretic use and beta-blocker use appear to play major role	RR of HTN without anti-HTN agents-only 0.8 Role of drugs more pronounced in women

TABLE 46.4. Genetics and syndrome associated with RCC.

Disease	*Locus*	*Gene*	*Protein*	*Renal manifestations*
VHL	3p25	VHL	VHL	Clear cell carcinoma, simple and complex cysts
HPRCC (papillary type I)	7q31	MET	Tyrosine kinase	Type I papillary carcinoma
Tuberous sclerosis	9q34 16p13.3	TSC1 TSC2	Hamartin Tuberin	Angiomyelolipoma (most common), renal cysts, clear cell carcinoma, papillary carcinoma, chromophobe carcinoma
HLRCC (papillary type II)	1q42-q44	FH	Fumarate hydratase	Type II papillary carcinoma
BHD	17p11.2	BHD	Folliculin	Chromophobe (34%), chromophobe/oncocytoma (50%), clear cell carcinoma (9%), papillary carcinoma (2%)
FRO[214]	Unknown	Unknown	Unknown	Oncocytoma
Familial clear cell renal cell carcinoma with balanced translocation	3p14:8q24[a]	Fragile histidine triad	Unknown	Clear cell carcinoma
Familial clear renal cell carcinoma with intact VHL	Unknown	Unknown	Unknown	Clear cell carcinoma (typically solitary and unilateral and occurs later in life)
FPTC-PRN[215]	1q21[b]	Unknown	Unknown	Papillary tumors
HPT-JT[216]	2p16 3p31.3	mutS homologue mutL homologue[c]	DNA mismatch Repair genes	Transitional cell carcinoma of the renal pelvis and ureter

VHL, von Hippel–Lindau syndrome; HPRCC, hereditary papillary renal cell cancer; HLRCC, hereditary leiomyoma renal cell cancer; BHD, Birt–Hogg–Dube; FRO, familial renal oncocytoma; HPT-JT, familial renal hamartomas associated with hyperparathyroidism-jaw tumor; HNPCC, hereditary non-polyposis colon cancer; FPTC-PRN, papillary thyroid cancer with papillary renal neoplasia.

[a] In addition, balanced translocations between chromosome 3 and other chromosomes have been reported in some families.

[b] Derived from linkage analysis of one family with FPTC-PRN.

[c] These two genes account for 70% of cases.

mediated degradation of cellular protein through the proteosome.[16,17] A key protein that requires this complex for its breakdown and rapid turnover is hypoxia-inducing factor-1α (HIF-1α).[18–20] When the pVHL is not present or not functioning correctly, the presence of HIF-1α builds up within the cell, binds to its partner HIF-1β, crosses into the nucleus, and then as a transcription factor activates a number of downstream genes important to the cellular response to hypoxia. The downstream genes appear critical to mechanisms of oncogenesis in clear cell RCC, including VEGF (vascular endothelial growth factor), EGF (epidermal growth factor), TGF-α (transforming growth factor-α), EGFR (epidermal growth factor receptor), PDGF-α/β (platelet-derived growth factor-α/β), erythropoietin (EPO), GLUT1, and carbonic anhydrase IX (CAIX).[21–23] HIF-1α and its activated downstream genes are critical to the pathophysiology of RCC and offer therapeutic targets (discussed later).

Tuberous sclerosis complex (TSC) is an autosomal dominant neurocutaneous syndrome with a high degree of variability in clinical manifestations.[7,24] The incidence is estimated at 1 in 10,000 based on wide screening. There are a number of cases that are sporadic without a definite family history. Two genes, TSC1 and TSC2, are responsible for the manifestations of the complex.[25] These are both considered TSG, with TSC1 located on 9q34 coding for a protein, hamartin, and TSC2 located on 16p13.3 and coding for a protein tuberin. In the kidney, the predominant manifestation of TSC is the development of multiple angiomyolipomas (AML). These *benign* tumors can displace all the functioning kidney and lead to renal failure or cause catastrophic hemorrhage. Additionally, TSC patients also manifest large renal cysts and finally an increase in renal cell cancers. The histology of these RCC covers a wide spectrum including clear cell, papillary, chromophobe, and even oncocytomas. Renal cell cancer is found in 2.5% to 4.0% of patients with TSC.

Birt–Hogg–Dube (BHD) is an autosomal dominant syndrome associated with inherited internal cancer, primarily renal cancers.[8,26] The most prominent features of the BHD syndrome are the skin and skin appendage triad of fibrofolliculomas (hair follicle tumors), trichodiscomas, and acrochordons. The renal tumors may vary from chromophobe or mixed chromophobe-oncocytomas, papillary, and clear cell. The mutation has been identified on 17p11.2, and the gene product is known as folliculun. Renal cysts, colonic cancers and polyps, and multiple lipomas have also been associated with BHD.

Hereditary papillary RCC (HPRCC) is a familial cancer syndrome characterized by papillary RCC (type I).[27] There are two types of papillary RCC,[28,29] which are differentiated by their different histologies. Type I contains basophilic, small cells and, in the core of the papillae, foamy macrophages and psammoma bodies. Type II has large, eosinophilic cells lining the papillae. The type I lesions are seen in hereditary papillary RCC. In sporadic cases of papillary RCC, those cancers with type I histology appear less aggressive than those with type II histology. HPRCC is also associated with a number of other cancers including breast, pancreas, lung, skin, and stomach. It has been characterized primarily as showing a gain of function mutation in the oncogene c-*met*.[9,27] The gene product is a tyrosine kinase-associated cell-surface receptor for hepatocyte growth factor or scatter factor.

Familial non-VHL clear cell RCC ± chromosomal 3 translocation is a well-recognized syndrome characterized more than 20 years ago.[9,30] We now know the translocation involves the 3p14, and in one family the FHIT gene is directly involved in the translocation.[5] The familial CCRCC without chromosomal 3 translocation fails to present at an early age and is rarely bilateral or multiple.

More recently, rare syndromes have been described and genetically mapped. Familial renal hamartomas associated with hyperparathyroidism-jaw tumor (HPT-JT) (1q21–32) is associated with papillary RCC (type I); hereditary leiomyomatosis and renal cell cancer (HLRCC) (1q42–44) are associated with papillary RCC (type 2) and uterine leiomyomas and leiomyosarcomas, breast cancer, and bladder cancer.[10]

Pathology

International agreement has been reached on the histologic classification of renal cortical epithelial neoplasms based on light microscopy.[31] Histologic classifications have subsequently been consistent with the molecular genetics of renal cancer.[12,31,32] Renal tumor classifications segregate with their observed genetic abnormalities. Some terms previously used to describe certain morphologic features such as granular or cystic have been eliminated, and most are now classified within the major histologic subtypes: clear cell, papillary, and chromophobe. Sarcomatoid remains, not as a separate identity, but instead as a high-grade variant of any histologic subtype.

Oncocytomas represent about 5% of renal cortical neoplasms[33]; they are typically large and have a central stellate scar. The histology of these benign tumors includes cells arranged in islands, solid sheets, tubules, or cysts. The tumor cells show a prominent eosinophilic cytoplasm due to the abundance of mitochondria. They are not graded by their benign behavior but must be differentiated from the chromophobe and clear cell renal cancers when providing a differential diagnosis.

Clear cell carcinoma is the conventional neoplasm associated with the renal cortex in adults[34] and represents at least 70% of renal cortical neoplasm. Most have a clear cytoplasm but some are either eosinophilic or granular. Some cases have an abundance of cystic structures lined by small clear cells. The *cystic* clear cell renal cancer must be 75% composed of cystic structures to meet the definition; these are usually both low grade and low stage with a generally good prognosis. As stated elsewhere in this chapter, the loss of genes on the 3p chromosome is a frequent finding in sporadic clear cell cancer. The predominant lesions include the loss of the VHL gene, VHL gene mutation, or even VHL gene inactivation through regulatory CpG islands that are hypermethylated.[35] One of these processes leads to the loss of functional VHL protein in most (more than 75%) of clear cell renal cancers. A small (5%) number of cases may have sarcomatoid change in areas of the tumor. This feature in itself represents a very high grade tumor with a poor prognosis.

Papillary renal cell carcinoma (PRCC) accounts for 15% of renal cortical cancers and includes those lesions that in the past would have been called chromophilic.[28,29] These neoplasms are highly associated with certain cytogenetic changes whether or not papillary architecture is observed. Genetic abnormalities not only include trisomies of 7 and 17 but also abnormalities of 3q, 12, 16, and 20 and loss of Y chromosome.[11,36] Delahunt and Eble have proposed the existence of two PRCC subtypes, type 1 with papillae covered by a single or double layer of small basophilic cells with scanty cytoplasm and type 2 with papillae covered by cells with abundant eosinophilic cytoplasm, arranged in a pseudostratified or irregularly stratified manner.[37] Studies show the tumor stage at diagnosis is significantly higher in type 2 than in type 1 PRCCs, suggesting these subtypes could be clinicopathologic entities with a different prognosis.[29] Also, it has been found that the more-common type I variant of papillary renal adenocarcinoma was less vascular on computed tomography (CT) scan, larger in size, and had a lower amount of nuclear pleomorphism as well as decreased expression of cytokeratin 7. The more-aggressive biologic variant, type II, presents in the earlier decades of life, with a smaller but more-vascular cancer with greater nuclear pleomorphism.

Chromophobe renal carcinoma accounts for 5% of the renal cell carcinomas.[38,39] The cytoplasm is full of a number of microvesicles and stains blue with a colloidal iron stain. Around the nucleus there is a halo caused by cytoplasmic condensation. The major dilemma is differentiating this neoplasm from oncocytoma. Oncocytomas may also stain with the iron stains, but their staining pattern is membranous, not cytoplasmic.

Collecting duct carcinoma is a rare and high-grade neoplasm that represents less than 1% of primary renal cortical neoplasms.[40] It can be difficult to recognize but usually demonstrates very irregular epithelial-lined channels in the background of extensive fibrosis and stroma. The cells have a hobnail appearance. These tumors can be accompanied by areas of renal parenchyma with dysplastic collecting duct epithelium, the tissue of origin.

Grading of Renal Cell Carcinoma

It has been known for a number of decades that grading of renal cell carcinoma is of great importance to the prognosis and outcome of disease.[2,34,41] The Fuhrman grading system is the predominant approach to grading done in the United States. Grades I through IV are based on size (10–20 μm) and shape of nuclei, prominence of nucleoli, and admixture of bizarre pleomorphic cells. Grade IV cytology can frequently include polylobulated and spindle-shaped nuclei. There have been difficulties in separating outcome for each individual grade, especially grade II–III. Grade I tumors do quite well whereas grade IV tumors present at an advanced stage and have a very dismal prognosis. The main issues relate to grade I versus II and grade II and III. Survival advantages have been seen with multiple cutoff points; between I and II; between III and IV; or between II and III in various studies. Grading has also been difficult to reproduce even among expert pathologists. It is likely refinement and use of molecular markers will have to occur in the future to make this system more practical and improve our ability to define the significance of each grade.[42] Other histologic characteristics that have been suggested as helpful in staging include mitotic rate, microvasculature presence, and microvessel density.

In the future, it is likely that pathologists will characterize RCC not by histologic appearance or even by cytogenetic or specific chromosomal changes, but instead by utilizing gene expression patterns of thousands of genes or even complex arrays of protein expression patterns. The group at the National Cancer Institute (NCI) led by Marston Lineham examined 58 fresh specimens from renal cancers.[42] They found a set of 45 genes could predict survival outcome as an independent factor. Of this set of genes, only a few genes or gene products appeared critical. VCAM-1 appeared to be the most important gene in predicted outcome.[42] Upregulation of VCAM-1 was associated with a better prognosis whereas downregulation was associated with a poor prognosis. Other data obtained in a set of clear cell RCC-VHL-expressing cell lines suggest that CXCR4 downregulation was associated with a poor prognosis and regulated by VHL expression.[43] Finally, others have shown that global gene expression patterns could accurately predict the histologic subtype of renal cancer.[44] This approach may ultimately direct us to genes and proteins that may be ideal for molecularly targeted treatment.

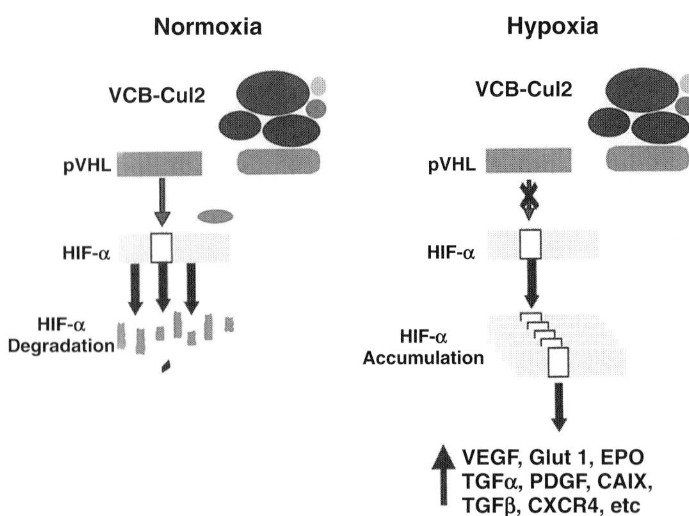

FIGURE 46.1. Von Hippel–Lindau disease (VHL) regulation of hypoxia-inducible factor (HIF)-1α and the downstream expression of HIF-1α-controlled genes.

Molecular Pathogenesis

Clear Cell Carcinoma

A major breakthrough in renal cancer biology came when the von Hippel–Lindau (VHL) gene was cloned in 1993.[13] This tumor suppressor gene (TSG) was cloned by positional cloning knowing that the gene had to be within the 3p25–p26 region of the chromosome. Loss of the gene was demonstrated among translocations and deletions, as well as mutations, all consistent with its possible role as a TSG. Even at this early point intragenic mutations were found in cell lines derived from sporadic renal cancer in addition to the cell lines from VHL patients.[13] Initially, there was little understanding of biology gained from the pVHL structure. It was a gene that was definitely evolutionarily conserved. It was also known that in CCRCC with VHL defects a number of growth factors and their receptors were highly expressed. A critical molecule regulating the expression of these genes or the genes induced by hypoxia was hypoxia-inducing-factor-1α (HIF-1 α).[23,45,46] Furthermore, it was known that HIF-1α was increased in hypoxic situations and in renal cancer cell lines because of an increase in its protein stability. Although in normal cells this increased stability was known to occur only in hypoxic situations, in RCC cells it occurred under normoxic conditions. HIF-1α was a key component of a very widespread oxygen cellular response mechanism.[45,46] Ultimately, it was demonstrated that native pVHL binds to HIF-1α as part of a complex, which led to the ubiquination of the HIF-1α protein to allow trafficking to and subsequent destruction by the proteosome. In normal cells with adequate oxygen, the hydroxylation of pVHL allowed for its binding to HIF-1α, again allowing for rapid degradation of HIF-1α. This oxygen-sensing and -regulating system is disturbed and dysfunctional in tumors from VHL patients, as well as in a large number of sporadic RCC. The implications are obvious (Figure 46.1): the induction of gene expression for a large number of genes regulated by HIF-1α including VEGF, EPO, Glut-1, PDGFα/β, TGFα, TGFb, CRCX4, and CAIX, plus many others. The overexpression of these factors and their receptors leads to many manifestations of clear cell carcinoma of the kidney (CCRCC), including its intense vascularity. The frequency of VHL gene mutation, deletion, or suppression by epigenetic mechanisms in sporadic RCC has been debated but has been estimated to be as high as 85% to 95% and as low as 55%. There may even be prognostic implications to the status of the VHL gene (mutated, deleted, or not expressed through epigenetic changes).[47]

It has been known that, besides VHL, there were other regions in chromosome 3p lost in RCC. A gene deleted (3p21.3) in a number of both clear cell and papillary renal cancer is the RASSF1a (Ras association family 1A gene).[48] This RASSF1A gene is frequently silenced because of the hypermethylation of its promoter region. RASSF1A has been shown to interact with Ras in its mutated form, potentially mediating some of the downstream effects.[49]

Finally, sporadic papillary renal cancer only rarely has mutations in the c-*met* gene, which is frequently mutated in familial papillary RCC. c-*met* has even been shown to be overexpressed in some of the papillary RCC cases. Therefore, only the RASSF1A gene has been identified consistently in sporadic papillary renal cancer.

Clinical and Laboratory Features

Renal cell cancer is an unpredictable tumor. The minority of patients present with the classic triad of flank pain, hematuria, and a palpable abdominal mass. Paraneoplastic syndromes are well described and some may be secondary to the loss of a functional VHL protein increasing levels of HIF-1α. Further discoveries in the basic biology of RCC may help explain the myriad of signs and symptoms from which other patients suffer.

Local Symptoms from Primary

The principal presenting complaints of renal cell cancer are hematuria, abdominal pain and mass, and/or symptoms and signs related to invasion of adjacent blood vessels or distant metastases. The classic triad of flank pain, hematuria, and a palpable abdominal mass occurred together in only 9% of patients in a 1971 review of 309 patients[50] and is likely even less frequent at present. With an increase in incidental diagnoses, it might be better termed the *radiologist's tumor*.

Metastatic Disease

Older series report that approximately 25% of patients present with either distant metastases or advanced locoregional disease. Historically, metastatic disease often presented with a wide array of symptoms and laboratory abnormalities such that renal cell carcinoma was termed "the internist's tumor."

Frequent sites of metastases include the lung, bone, lymph nodes, pleura, brain, ipsilateral adrenal gland, and liver.

Paraneoplastic Syndromes

A large amount has been written about paraneoplastic syndromes despite little knowledge of these syndromes or their etiologies.[51] Still, a minority of patients with renal cell carcinoma develop paraneoplastic syndromes.

Without bony metastases, hypercalcemia is one of the most common of the paraneoplastic syndromes, affecting up to 20% of patients via increased production of parathyroid hormone-related peptide, osteoclast-activating factor, transforming growth factor-α, and/or tumor necrosis factor.[52] The main hypercalcemic factor identified in patients with solid malignancies and hypercalcemia has been parathyroid hormone-related protein. Metastatic renal cell carcinoma complicated by hypercalcemia has been found to shorten survival, and it represents one of the five poor prognostic factors incorporated into Motzer's model (see following).[53,54]

Renal cell carcinoma can be associated with increased production of inflammatory cytokines,[55] and the subsequent inflammation leads to a number of signs and symptoms. Fever is usually intermittent and is frequently accompanied by night sweats, anorexia, weight loss, fatigue, and cachexia. Anemia of chronic inflammatory disease can frequently precede the diagnosis of renal cell carcinoma by a number of months.

An often-discussed but not very often seen paraneoplastic manifestation is erythrocytosis. The loss of the protein product of the VHL gene, pVHL, is common in sporadic clear-cell renal carcinomas. Therefore HIF-1α accumulates and activates the transcription of hypoxia-inducible genes, including erythropoietin. The overproduction of erythropoietin accounts for the association of paraneoplastic erythrocytosis with kidney cancer and hemangioblastoma.[56] The much less frequent overproduction of a soluble VEGF receptor may lead to the paraneoplastic hypertension and proteinuria.[56,57]

A recognized syndrome of hepatic dysfunction in the absence of liver metastases (Stauffer's syndrome)[58] has been reported to occur in up to 20% of patients with renal carcinoma. Hepatosplenomegaly, fever, elevated alkaline phosphatase levels, prolonged partial thromboplastin time, and elevated serum haptoglobin levels characterize this idiopathic syndrome. As an example among 365 patients in one report, 77 (21%) had a paraneoplastic elevation in the serum level of alkaline phosphatase. When present, it is frequently observed in association with fever, weight loss, and fatigue.[59]

Staging

Computed tomography (CT) scan of the abdomen is generally the first noninvasive staging tool used in renal cell carcinoma. The urologist in planning the surgical approach often uses magnetic resonance imaging (MRI) to evaluate renal vein and inferior vena cava (IVC) involvement.[60] For staging, it is required to evaluate the extent of vascular invasion from the tumor when present. Preoperative staging may or may not include a CT of the chest. A bone scan should only be considered in patients with bone pain or an elevated serum alkaline phosphatase.[61]

Systems

Tumor stage, which reflects the anatomic spread and involvement of disease, is recognized as the most important prognostic factor for the clinical behavior and outcome of RCC.[62] The Robson's classification, which includes consideration of vascular involvement, is often cited in the literature and can be compared with the tumor, nodes, and metastasis (TNM) staging system proposed by the International Union Against Cancer in Table 46.5.[63]

Initially, the Robson staging system was widely used; however, it was subsequently demonstrated to correlate poorly with prognosis.[64] Patients with renal vein involvement (Robson stage IIIa) but with cancer confined to the kidney had similar survival rates when compared with patients whose disease were confined to the renal capsule (stage I) or Gerota's fascia (stage II). In contrast, the TNM system emphasized local growth, nodal spread, and distant metastasis and therefore more accurately classifies the extent of tumor involvement.[64] The 2002 TNM classification system[65] is summarized in Table 46.6.

TABLE 46.5. Robson staging compared to the 1997 TNM staging: tumor stage for renal cell carcinoma.

Robson stage	*TNM (1997)*	*Disease extent*
I	T1-2N0M0	Organ confined
II	T3aN0M0	Perinephric fat or adrenal involvement
IIIA	T3b-cN0M0	Venous involvement
IIIB	TxN+M0	Lymphatic involvement
IVA	T4N0M0	Locally advanced
IVB	TxNxM+	Systemic metastases

Source: Bostwick and Eble,[31] by permission of *Urology Clinics of North America*.

TABLE 46.6. American Joint Committee on Cancer (AJCC) Cancer Staging for Cancer of the Kidney, sixth edition.

Primary tumor (T)	
TX	Primary tumor cannot be assessed
T0	No evidence of primary tumor
T1	Tumor 7 cm or less in greatest dimension, limited to the kidney
T1a	Tumor 4 cm or less in greatest dimension, limited to the kidney
T1b	Tumor more than 4 cm but not more than 7 cm in greatest dimension, limited to the kidney
T2	Tumor more than 7 cm in greatest dimension, limited to the kidney
T3	Tumor extends into major veins or invades adrenal gland or perinephric tissue but not beyond Gerota's fascia
T3a	Tumor directly invades adrenal gland or perirenal and/or renal sinus fat but not beyond Gerota's fascia
T3b	Tumor grossly extends into the renal vein or its segmental (muscle-containing) branches, or vena cava below the diaphragm.
T3c	Tumor grossly extends into vena cava above diaphragm or invades the wall of the vena cava
T4	Tumor invades beyond Gerota's fascia
Regional lymph nodes (N)	
NX	Regional lymph nodes cannot be assessed
N0	No regional lymph node metastases
N1	Metastasis in a single regional lymph node
N2	Metastasis in more than one regional lymph node
Distant metastasis (M)	
MX	Distant metastasis cannot be assessed
M0	No distant metastasis
M1	Distant metastasis

Stage grouping			
Stage I	T1	N0	M0
Stage II	T2	N0	M0
Stage III	T1-3	N0-1	M0
		Not including T1N0 or T2N0	
Stage IV	T4	N0-1	M0
	Any T	N2	M0
	Any T	Any N	M1

Source: Used with the permission of the American Joint Committee on Cancer (AJCC), Chicago, Illinois. The original source for this material is the *AJCC Cancer Staging Manual*, sixth edition (2002), published by Springer-Verlag New York, www.springer-ny.com.

Nephrectomy for Primary Therapy

Renal cell carcinoma is not the only malignant lesion in the kidney. In addition, any number of benign cysts, adenomas, and lipomas can arise from the renal parenchyma and are frequently seen incidentally on radiographic imaging. Malignant renal tumors in children include Wilms' tumors, neuroblastomas, and rhabdomyosarcomas, whereas sarcomas, lymphomas, metastatic lesions, renal pelvis transitional cell cancer, and renal cell carcinomas account for most adult kidney cancers.

The surgical approach and the extent of resection should be based primarily on the size of the primary tumor. Patients with T1 tumors should be considered for partial nephrectomy. Any tumor T2 or above by preoperative staging should undergo a radical nephrectomy, if feasible by the least invasive method possible. Those with radiologic evidence of abdominal lymphadenopathy should still be offered a radical nephrectomy as suspicious nodes are often enlarged because of reactive inflammation.

Radical Nephrectomy

The results from a retrospective study by Robson et al.[63] of 88 cases operated on from 1949 to 1964 set the standard for oncologic care from simple to radical nephrectomy. Simple nephrectomy is performed through the lumbar approach. Perinephric tissue is removed only if the tumor extends visually beyond the renal capsule and the adrenal gland is removed only if there was an upper pole lesion. Radical nephrectomy begins with a thoracoabdominal, extrapleural supracostal, or anterior transabdominal approach to the medial border of the tumor, followed by dissection of the renal vein and artery. These vessels are then ligated early to prevent putative tumor emboli, the kidney is removed without incising Gerota's fascia to theoretically reduce the risk of tumor seeding, the ipsilateral adrenal gland is removed, and the paraaortic and paracaval nodes are dissected. Dr. Robson reported tumors isolated to the kidney in 33 patients, to the perirenal fat in 15, and spread to the vessels or lymphatics in 27, and distant metastases present in 12 patients, with 5-year survivals at 66%, 64%, 42%, and 11%, respectively. Dr. Robson reported the superiority of the overall 52% 5-year survival compared with the 40% to 50% survival of simple nephrectomy in four other published reports from 1939 to 1966. His retrospective study was later supported[66] and disputed[50,67] by other retrospective studies, a prospective randomized study was never published, and radical nephrectomy became the standard of care mostly for theoretical reasons.

Since the publication by Robson et al. in 1969, the procedure for radical nephrectomy has been significantly refined with regard to removing the adrenal gland, dissecting regional lymph nodes, and in evaluating and removing tumor thrombus. Adrenalectomy is now limited to patients with large upper pole tumors, those with solitary metastasis identified by preoperative staging to the ipsilateral adrenal gland, or when the adrenal gland is displaced or not identified on preoperative imaging. A normal-appearing adrenal gland visualized preoperatively by CT essentially rules out neoplastic adrenal involvement.[68] Renal cell carcinoma that has spread to local lymph nodes not only defines a higher stage but also may be indicative of a tumor that is less likely to respond to therapy. In fact, there is some evidence that patients with regional nodal metastases have a shorter survival than those with distant metastases without regional node disease.[69] Lymphadenectomy at the time of nephrectomy may improve response to subsequent immunotherapy[70] but is rarely a part of a curative procedure.[71] Finally, renal cell carcinoma is complicated by tumor thrombus involving the inferior vena cava or right atrium in 5% to 10% of cases.[72] Small studies support the use of MRI to evaluate the presence and extent of associated tumor thrombi.[60] Simple thrombectomy may suffice for patients with thrombus extending below the major hepatic veins, whereas for thrombi located above the major hepatic veins, cardiopulmonary bypass and hypothermic circulatory arrest may be required for complete resection.[73]

Partial Nephrectomy

Since Robson et al. published their landmark papers[74,75] proposing radical nephrectomy as the new standard for renal cell carcinoma, the incidence of incidentally discovered tumors has increased,[76] along with technologic advances allowing partial nephrectomies with less risk of renal insufficiency[77] and laparoscopic surgeries with shorter hospital stays and less pain than standard laparotomies.[78]

Partial nephrectomy is performed with a close eye on reducing damage to the uninvolved kidney while performing an oncologically sound procedure. Generally an extraperitoneal flank incision through the bed of the 11th or 12th rib is performed, the kidney is mobilized within Gerota's fascia while leaving the perirenal fat intact, and the renal artery is interrupted. The renal vein remains patent to reduce ischemic damage. The kidney is then cooled with ice slush for 10 to 15 minutes and the tumor is excised. Campbell et al.[79] have previously shown that intraoperative ultrasound can assist in delineating the limit of intrarenal tumors, show collecting system structures, and overall help avoid inadvertent entry into the renal sinus. In patients with sarcomatoid histology on frozen section or with renal vessel invasion, surgery should be extended when possible to a radical nephrectomy as these patients have a higher risk of recurrence and incomplete resection. Although not supported by any prospective studies, retrospective reviews support the notion that the width of the targeted resection margin should be greater than or equal to 3 mm with negative microscopic margins.[80,81]

The performance of a partial nephrectomy has been the standard of care for select patients with renal cell carcinoma involving an isolated kidney or in patients at high risk of cancer involving the contralateral kidney. However, concerns that such a procedure might put the patient at higher risk for recurrence have hindered its widespread use.

Partial nephrectomy should be considered in the following clinical situations:

1. Renal masses less than 4 cm (T1) or those located within the cortex where up to 23% have been reported to be benign.[82] Several groups have recommended that tumors less than 4 cm be considered for partial nephrectomy as the chance for disease-free survival is greater than 95%.[82,83]
2. Mass in a patient with a single kidney or with compromised renal function.[84]
3. Synchronous bilateral renal tumors or patients with von Hippel–Lindau syndrome at high risk of renal cell cancer in the contralateral kidney.[85] One prospective study in 96 patients with von Hippel–Lindau disease or hereditary papillary renal cancer recommended a maximum size of 3 cm by preoperative staging for patients sent for partial nephrectomy to minimize the need for more-frequent surgery.

Partial nephrectomy is not without potential complications: one study reported urinary fistula, acute tubular necrosis, need for temporary dialysis, and the requirement of permanent dialysis in 7.4%, 6.3%, 4.9%, and 1.9%, respectively. The risk of worsened renal insufficiency or failure is approximately 5% in an elective partial nephrectomy and may increase to 15% to 20% or more in symptomatic tumors, T2 or larger lesions, lesions that involve excision of more than 50% of the parenchyma, and when the ischemia time is greater than 1 hour.[86]

The risk of urinary fistula has been reported to range from 2% to 21%. The risk is decreased among subjects undergoing elective surgery after 1988 when the routine injection of methylene blue was initiated to identify anastomotic leaks and for smaller lesions. There is an increased risk in those with tumors larger than 4 cm, central or hilar lesions, and surgery involving reconstruction of the collecting system.[87]

Overall partial nephrectomies should be performed on patients with small tumors, those with impaired renal function, or those with an inherited risk of subsequent renal carcinomas such as von Hippel–Lindau. The approach should be via a standard laparotomy until the laparoscopic technique is proven to be safe.

Laparoscopic Nephrectomy

Laparoscopic nephrectomy, first performed in 1990, represents a reasonable alternative to open radical nephrectomy for patients with renal cell cancers less than 10 cm.[88] The three laparoscopic approaches to radical nephrectomy are transperitoneal, retroperitoneal, and hand-assisted. The transperitoneal approach provides ample working space, and multiple landmarks are available to guide the surgeon, but it does require reflection of multiple abdominal structures to gain access to the kidney, intracorporeal placement of the specimen in a bag is required, and removing large renal specimens is cumbersome. The retroperitoneal approach is generally a shorter procedure but is technically more difficult and is generally not suited for large renal tumors.[89] There is no difference in blood loss, complications, pain, or length of stay when compared with the transperitoneal approach[90] (Table 46.7). The hand-assisted approach involves placing the nondominant hand into the abdomen via an incision below the umbilicus; this may be technically easier than a transperitoneal approach, with an associated shorter operative time,[91] but still requires reflection of multiple abdominal structures and is ill suited for small, thin patients.

Destroying the renal tumor, termed morcellation, before removal allows for a smaller incision, improves cosmesis, and is thought to result in less pain. Meticulous care must be taken to avoid tumor contamination during morcellation; at least one patient with a T3 lesion developed a port site recurrence at 25 months.[92] One of the disadvantages of morcellation is that the tumor size cannot be determined pathologically although the histology, grade, and stage are still accurate.[93] Because of the prolonged operative times, increased expense, risk of tumor contamination, and no proven benefits beyond a smaller incision, intact specimen removal is the more-prudent route.

Laparoscopic nephrectomy has demonstrated similar recurrence rates in retrospective reviews,[78,94] but no prospective trials have been published. This technique is becoming more popular as the advantages of decreased postoperative analgesia and pain, shorter hospital stays, and improved cosmesis are published and more technical experience is gained with this method.

The maximum tumor size limit for laparoscopic nephrectomy has not been specifically studied, although the maximum tumor diameter generally ranges from 12 to 14 cm in published reports.[78,95,96] Laparoscopy was initially reserved

TABLE 46.7. Complications of laparoscopic nephrectomy.

Reference	No. (years), indication	Major operative complications
Gill[97]	185 (1990–1993): 153 benign 32 malignant	6 (3%): 4 bleeding, 1 pneumothorax, 1 small bowel cutaneous fistula Conversion to open in 3 patients due to complications and in 7 because of difficult dissection
Rassweiler[88]	482 (1992–1996): 444 benign 38 malignant	29 (6%): 22 bleeding, 3 bowel injury, 2 hypercarbia, pleural injury in 1, pulmonary embolism in 1 Conversion to open in 26 patients due to complications and in 20 because of difficult dissection
Ono[202]	60 (1992–1998): All malignant	6 (10%): duodenal injury was treated by open duodenojejunostomy Left renal artery injury, splenic injury, adrenal injury, and periureteral injury were treated laparoscopically One pulmonary embolism
Dunn[209]	61 (1990–1999): 46 malignant 15 benign	2 (3%): superior mesenteric artery ligation, renal vein incomplete ligation leading to conversion to open procedure
Chan[96]	67 (1991–1999) All malignant	3 (4%): bowel injury during morcellation, small bowel obstruction due to an incisional hernia, pulmonary embolus
Kim[203]	114 (1998–2002): 35 radical (LRN) 79 partial (LPN) All malignant	LRN: 4 (11%): 1 mesenteric injury, 1 liver injury, and 2 serosal tear LPN: 3 (4%): 1 lumbar vein tear, 1 splenic capsule tear, 1 ureteral injury

LRN, laparoscopic radical nephrectomy; LPN, laparoscopic partial nephrectomy.

for clinical stage T1–T2 tumors, but pathologic T3 tumors have also been removed laparoscopically.[78]

Tumor Ablation

Cryoablation, radiofrequency ablation, and high-intensity focused ultrasound are three newer, less-invasive strategies that have been developed for small tumors in patients who are not operative candidates. The goal of energy-based tissue ablative procedures is to achieve targeted destruction of a predetermined volume of tissue that would otherwise be excised during a traditional partial nephrectomy, that is, the tumor itself and a surrounding margin of healthy parenchyma.

Cryotherapy-induced cytonecrosis is a sequential two-step process involving the rapid intracellular formation of ice followed by delayed microcirculatory failure, rendering the area necrotic due to ischemia. The most commonly used reagents include liquid nitrogen or argon. Limited experience with cryoablation suggests that it is effective in more than 90% of T1 renal cell cancers, but only limited follow-up data are available.[97,98]

Radiofrequency ablation utilizes a high-frequency electrical current to create molecular friction, denaturation of cellular protein, and cell membrane disintegration. The threshold temperature necessary for tissue thermal destruction ranges from 40° to 70°C. The use of radiofrequency ablation for kidney tumors is emerging as a viable technique,[99,100] but this procedure can often be complicated by perinephric hematomas, and viable tumor unfortunately was shown to remain in every patient in one trial.[101]

High-intensity focused ultrasound is the least invasive ablative technique. Ultrasound frequency beams are generated by a cylindrical piezoelectric element, then focused by a paraboloid reflector. Similar to extracorporeal shockwave lithotripsy, this beam is focused on a lesion to cause localized hemorrhage, coagulative necrosis, and chronic inflammatory infiltration. The size and configuration of the radiolesion are related to ablation time, the amount of delivered energy, the electrolyte content of the targeted tissue, and the surface area of the electrode. High-intensity focused ultrasound may become an effective technique once the technical problems of protecting against superficial skin burns and incomplete ablation have been solved.[102]

Adjuvant Therapy for High-Risk Renal Cell Cancer

Adjuvant therapy in solid tumors is based on the concept that chemotherapy after a cytoreductive surgery will serve to eliminate micrometastatic disease at a time when the tumor is growing rapidly and is therefore most susceptible to incorporating chemotherapeutic toxins. Unfortunately, no proven adjuvant therapy exists for renal cell carcinoma; in fact, trials using immunotherapy have shown distant metastasis as the most common site of relapse, suggesting that nonselective immune stimulators such as interferons or interleukins are ineffective in micrometastatic disease. Recent trials using autologous tumor cell vaccines provide hope that reeducating the body's immune system to attack this cancer is possible.

Characteristics of High-Risk Tumors

Tumors at high risk of recurrence are generally thought to be ideal candidates for adjuvant therapy. Unfortunately, a number of trials performed to date in renal cell carcinoma have shown no benefit to adjuvant chemotherapy or immunotherapy despite well-done studies on populations at high risk of recurrence (Table 46.8).

Characteristics of high-risk disease are based generally on tumor size and Fuhrman histologic grade, extent of local invasion, ipsilateral adrenal gland involvement, or nodal positivity. Three centers have reviewed their large retrospective database of patients who have undergone nephrectomy as primary curative therapy: Mayo Clinic, Memorial Sloan Kettering Cancer Center (MSKCC), and UCLA (University of

California at Los Angles).[103–105] The largest experience reported is that of the Mayo Clinic based on surgery performed from 1970 to 2000.[103] Their 1,671 clear cell carcinoma patients presented with symptomatic primary disease in more than 70% of the cases. The factors of greatest importance were tumor stage, lymph node status, tumor size (cutoff of 5 or 10cm), nuclear grade (1–4), and histologic tumor necrosis. All were very significant in a multivariate analysis. By assigning points from 0 to 4 for these characteristics, a prognostic model was developed. Ten-year metastases-free survival could be predicted for three cohorts with low (0–2 points), intermediate (3–5 points), and high (6 points or more) at 92%, 64%, and 24%, respectively. These factors in this model were called the SSIGN score. For T1 lesions alone, both size (0–5 or 5–7cm) and histologic grade were predictive of recurrence. The MSKCC group reviewed 601 patients who had undergone a nephrectomy from 1989 to 1998 for primary RCC.[104] A normogram was constructed with the factors that were significant by multivariate analysis. The entire groups were generally at an earlier stage than the Mayo study. More than two-thirds of the patients had disease found incidentally without even local symptoms. The normogram included symptoms (none, local, or systemic), histology (chromophobe, papillary, or clear cell), tumor size, and tumor stage including T1, T2, T3a, and T3b/c. Only 66 of the 601 patients had recurred at this time of the analysis, compared with the Mayo database in which 479 of 1,671 patients had recurred. Finally, the UCLA Urology Group has created a prognostic model called UISS.[105] This model has been made applicable for any patient undergoing nephrectomy, whether metastatic or only primary disease. The factors of most significance were included in a multivariate model based on 661 patients undergoing nephrectomy from 1989 to 1999. The overall model included nuclear grade, tumor stage, number of symptoms, nodes involved, and immunotherapy received. However, for primary disease alone, only nuclear grade (0–4) and performance status (0 versus 1 or more) were predictive of survival.

Although trials to detect the benefits of adjuvant therapy for resected renal cell carcinoma have traditionally based their eligibility criteria on tumor size, T3–T4, and the presence of nodal involvement, better indicators for patients who will respond to adjuvant therapy are being developed.

Role for Postoperative Radiation

In the past 20 years, only two poorly designed studies of postoperative radiation therapy after nephrectomy have been published, both describing treatment failures similar to previously reported data.[106] Although the more-recent trial[107] suggests that modern radiation therapy is likely safe, no trials have been published to detect its possible benefit, if any, in an adjuvant setting. In addition, studies have shown that patients who relapse after nephrectomy rarely have isolated renal bed lesions and that disseminated disease is the predominant problem.

Adjuvant Immunotherapy

Two adjuvant studies with interferon[108,109] and one with high-dose interleukin-2 (IL-2)[110] have all failed to show any benefit. The most recent controlled trial was conducted by the Cytokine Working Group[110] comparing observation to the treatment arm using high-dose IL-2, usually in an intensive care unit to monitor and treat for IL-2-induced capillary leak syndrome. Unfortunately, this trial's statistical power to detect a benefit from adjuvant therapy was hindered by slow accrual and an ambitious predicted clinical benefit using high-dose IL-2. When the study was designed, it was estimated that the 2-year disease-free survival (DFS) after resection of locally advanced RCCa was 40%.[111] With an estimated accrual of 68 patients with locally advanced RCCa, the goal was to detect an absolute increase in DFS from 40% to 70%. Between September 1997 and June 2002, 69 patients were accrued. At a predefined interim analysis, 16 of 21 patients with locally advanced disease receiving IL-2 experienced relapse, compared with 15 of 23 patients in the observation arm ($P = 0.73$) (Figure 46.2). The study was therefore closed early when the Data Safety and Monitoring Board concluded that the anticipated improvement in 2-year DFS was unattainable even if full accrual occurred.

The largest and most well designed trial to date tested lymphoblastoid interferon in patients who had undergone radical nephrectomy and were found to have unilateral, locally advanced (pathologic stage T3–T4), and/or node-positive renal cell carcinoma conducted under the Eastern Cooperative Oncology Group (ECOG) from May 1987 to April 1992.[109] Two hundred ninety-four patients were randomly assigned to receive up to 12 cycles of interferon-α (IFN-α)-NL or observation until recurrence or progression. Only 70% in the treatment group received completed normal lymphoblastoid therapy, with the remainder withdrawing because of grade 3–4 toxicities. No benefit was seen for disease-free or overall survival. At a median follow-up of 10.4 years, median survival was 5.1 years in the treatment arm and

TABLE 46.8. **Patterns of recurrence for resected node-negative pT1–T3 renal cell carcinomas.**

Reference	*N*	*Surgery*	*TNM*	*Lung*	*Bone*	*Abdomen*	*Average. time to relapse (years)*	*Asymptomatic relapse (%)*
Sandock[117]	137	RN	1992	19	10	13	2.5	19
Levy[115]	286	RN	1997	31	12	14	1.9	23
Ljungberg[118]	187	RN	1997	30	15	9	1.2	NR
Gofrit[116]	200	RN/NS	1997	11	6	10	NR	54
Fergany[86]	327	NS	1992	NR	NR	NR	2.0	37

RN, radical nephrectomy; NS, nephron-sparing surgery; NR, not reported.

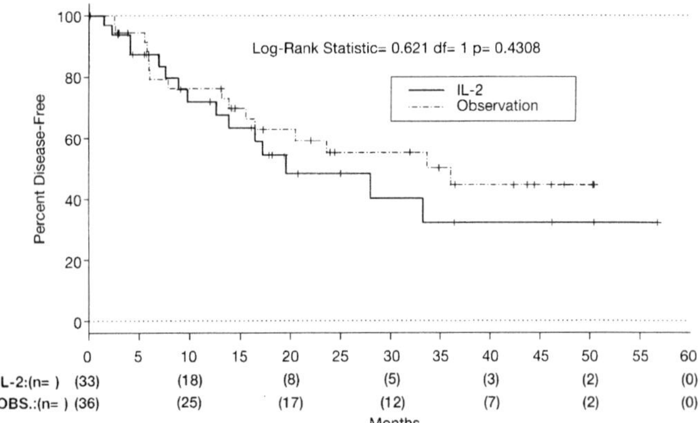

FIGURE 46.2. Disease-free survival by treatment group for all patients. Interleukin-2 (IL-2) median, 19.5 months; observation (OBS.) median, 36 months. (From Clark et al.[110] by permission of J Clin Oncol.)

7.4 years in the observation arm. In patients who recurred, 71% had distant metastases alone, arguing against a significant antitumor effect against micrometastatic disease.

The second trial with interferon, a multicenter Italian trial, began in February 1990 and enrolled 247 patients who had undergone a radical nephrectomy finding pathologic staged T3a/bN0M0 or T2/3N1–M0.[108] One hundred twenty-three patients were treated with 6 million IU IFN α-2b intramuscularly three times per week for 6 months starting within 1 month of surgery. After a median follow-up period of 62 months, relapses occurred in 38 (31%) of the 124 controls and in 51 (41%) of the 123 treated patients. The overall survival probability at 5 years was 67% for controls and 66% for treated patients.

Adjuvant Vaccine Therapy

There are three published large clinical trials using autologous tumor lysate vaccines[112–114] after nephrectomy. In a randomized placebo-controlled trial of 120 patients with stage I–III renal cell carcinoma from January 1987 to December 1991,[112] 4 weeks after complete resection, patients were randomized to receive three intradermal injections of 10^7 autologous irradiated tumor cells or placebo. The first two injections were mixed with 10^7 viable bacillus Calmette–Guèrin organisms in hopes of boosting the host's immune response. Delayed cutaneous hypersensitivity reactions to autologous tumor cells were demonstrated in 70% of treated patients: 25 of 44 patients at 6 months and 16 of 28 patients at 12 months. Unfortunately, with a median follow-up of 61 months, the probability of 5-year disease-free survival was 63% for treated patients and 72% for control patients, with an overall survival of 69% and 78%, respectively.

From data presented in January 2002 at the 11th International Hamburg Symposium on Tumor Markers, Dr. Rüdiger Repmann[113] reported on a nonrandomized prospective controlled study of 360 patients accrued between 1990 and 1995 who underwent a radical nephrectomy. The study was limited to the 236 patients who were found to have T2N0M0 or T3N0M0 renal cell carcinoma. Of this group, 148 received a median of 13 adjuvant injections of autologous tumor cell lysates every 4 weeks. The 5-year overall survival was 71.4% in the control group compared with 86% in the vaccine group ($P = 0.0059$). A prospective randomized multicenter Phase III trial was started in 1997 to confirm these results is described next.[114]

A recent trial of an autologous cancer vaccine was published in 2004 in *Lancet*[114]; this was a randomized non-placebo-controlled trial of patients with T2 or T3 RCC with endpoints of progression-free survival (PFS). The randomization took place preoperatively for which the rationale was unclear. There was a very large loss of patients following surgery because of incorrect stage, incorrect diagnosis, and a number of other factors. Therefore, of the 558 patients enrolled only 379 were analyzed and continued therapy. The trial did seem to offer an improved PFS at 5 years and 70 months. The effect was predominantly seen in those patients with T2 disease RCC. The overall survival is not discussed in the article.

In summary, there is little evidence to support adjuvant immunotherapy up to the present time. There is good evidence to support withholding adjuvant interferon interleukin-2 for high-risk renal cell carcinoma, and there is a suggestion that tumor lysate vaccine therapy may have a future role.

Follow-Up

Any recommendations for follow-up after nephrectomy for RCCa should bear in mind the patterns of relapse and whether any follow-up protocol has led to a survival benefit in a disease where recurrence is notoriously difficult to treat. Unfortunately, there are only a handful of studies documenting sites of recurrence, no prospective trials that used a uniform follow-up protocol, and no trials to show that any type of follow-up improves survival.[115–118]

Overview of Therapy of Metastatic Renal Cell Cancer

Prognostic Factors in Metastatic Renal Cell Cancer

Although therapy of metastatic disease has progressed at a painfully slow pace, the development of models to accurately predict prognosis and survival have allowed for much better counseling of patients regarding their prognosis. These studies are summarized in Table 46.9.[119–123] It is critical that these prognostic factors be used to better understand the meaning of Phase II trials and better cohort balance through stratification with these factors in large Phase III trials. Overall time from diagnosis to metastases, poor performance status or number of symptoms, lack of nephrectomy, and elevated serum lactic dehydrogenase (LDH) have been poor prognostic factors in a number of clinical databases and must be taken into consideration when discussing prognosis and designing and evaluating outcomes from clinical trials.

TABLE 46.9. Independent prognostic factors identified in previous studies including different populations of patients with metastatic renal cell carcinoma.

Reference	*No. of patients*	*Identified independent factors*
Elson et al.[119]	610	PS, time from diagnosis to treatment Number of metastatic sites Prior chemotherapy Weight loss
Motzer[53]	670	Absence of nephrectomy Karnofsky PS less than 80 Serum LDH > 1.5 × ULN Corrected serum Ca^{2+} elevation Anemia
Zisman[105]	477	ECOG PS Fuhrman nuclear grade TNM stage for M1 disease Number of symptoms Regional LN involvement Immunotherapy given
Negrier[153]	782	CRP or ESR elevation Interval from diagnosis to metastases Neutrophil count (>7.5) PS Number of metastatic sites, liver, bone Anemia Elevated serum alkaline phosphatase
Atzpodien[204]	425	Neutrophil count (>6.5) Time from diagnosis to metastases Serum LDH > 1.5 ULN Elevated serum CRP Number of metastatic sites Bone metastases

PS, performance score; LDH, lactic dehydrogenase; CRP, C-reactive protein; ESR, erythrocyte sedimentation rate; ULN, upper limit of normal.

Surgery in the Metastatic Setting

Debulking Nephrectomy

There are several accepted reasons to excise the primary renal cell carcinoma in the presence of metastatic disease. Palliative nephrectomy for severe pain, hemorrhage, and endocrinopathy appears to be justified in the patient who is expected to live at least 6 months. Angioinfarction is another option in patients with intractable pain or hematuria from inoperable local disease.

The role of debulking nephrectomy in the presence of metastatic disease stems from the unique biology of renal cell carcinoma. There is a rare phenomenon of spontaneous regression of metastatic disease following nephrectomy. Although single centers have published extensively on the benefits of cytoreductive nephrectomy before immune therapy,[124–128] two prospective studies provide the only randomized data.[129,130] The European Organization for Research and Treatment of Cancer (EORTC) Genitourinary Group trial 30–947 was a Phase III study of 85 patients with metastatic renal cell carcinoma who were randomized to either IFN-α-2b alone or nephrectomy followed by interferon.[129] Nephrectomy was performed on 42 patients with only 6 perioperative complications requiring that 1 patient not receive immunotherapy. They reported no significant difference in the response rates to systemic therapy between the two groups (19% versus 12%; $P = 0.38$) but did note a prolonged time to progression (5 months versus 3 months; $P = 0.04$) and overall survival benefit (17 months versus 7 months, respectively; $P = 0.03$).

The Southwest Oncology Group (SWOG) trial 8949 examined the role of cytoreductive nephrectomy in combination with IFN-α-2b therapy in 241 patients with metastatic renal cell carcinoma as part of a multicenter randomized phase III trial performed in the United States.[130] There were 121 patients in the interferon-alone arm and 120 patients in the nephrectomy-plus-interferon arm. In this clinical trial, there was 1 perioperative death, 5 major surgical complications, and 16 mild to moderate surgical complications. Despite the complications, 98% of the patients in the surgery arm were able to receive interferon. Again, this study reported no difference in response rates to systemic interferon therapy in the two groups, 3.3% in the nephrectomy arm versus 3.6% in the immunotherapy-alone arm. Despite the low overall response rates, the study demonstrated a significant survival advantage for patients who underwent cytoreductive nephrectomy and immunotherapy when compared with patients who received immunotherapy alone (12.5 months versus 8.1 months, respectively; $P = 0.012$).

Table 46.10 summarizes results from the SWOG and EORTC trials as well as the largest single-institution retrospective from the NCI describing their 11-year experience with 195 patients who underwent nephrectomy with an overall 13% surgical complication rate.[98,99] One hundred twenty-one (62%) patients who underwent nephrectomy in the NCI series went on to receive immunotherapy. Only 18 (9%) patients missed systemic treatment because of surgical complications. The NCI's 37.9% failure to receive immunotherapy likely indicates the rate of off-protocol adjuvant therapy rather than the 2% seen in the SWOG and EORTC trials.

Based on these results from these two randomized studies, debulking nephrectomy in those patients with distant metastatic disease is indicated in those patients with a good performance status deemed capable of proceeding on to systemic immunotherapy.

Metastatectomy

Approximately 25% to 59% of patients with renal cell carcinoma already have multiple distant metastases at tumor diagnosis, including the lungs (55%), lymph nodes (38%), liver (35%), or bones (33%). Moreover, metachronous metastatic disease may develop in approximately 50% of patients who have undergone seemingly curative radical nephrectomy.[131] In the rare patient with a solitary synchronous metastasis, radical nephrectomy and excision of the solitary metastasis provide a 5-year survival rate of 23 to 35%.[132]

TABLE 46.10. Trials of nephrectomy in metastatic disease followed by immunotherapy.

Trial	*N*	*Mortality (%)*	*% that missed immunotherapy*	*Immunotherapy response rate (%)*
NCI[2]	195	1.0	37.9	17.8
SWOG[130]	120	0.8	2.0	3.3
EORTC[129]	42	0	2.4	19.0

n, number of patients enrolled on trial.

Memorial Sloan Kettering[133] retrospectively reviewed 278 patients with recurrent renal cell carcinoma from 1980 to 1993. They stated that 141 patients underwent a curative resection for their first recurrence with an overall 44% 5-year survival. Those who underwent noncurative surgery or who were treated nonsurgically had 14% and 11% 5-year survival rates, respectively. Favorable features included a disease-free interval greater than 12 months, solitary metastasis, and age less than 60 years. Of the 94 patients with solitary metastasis, 50 patients had a single pulmonary lesion resected, leading to a 54% 5-year survival rate compared with 11 patients with a solitary brain metastasis with an 18% 5-year survival rate. Their conclusion was that patients with a single site of recurrence and/or a long disease-free interval will have a good chance at long-term survival with curative resection of disease. Surgical resection of solitary metastases should be considered standard of care when feasible.

Chemotherapy-Based Treatment of Renal Cell Cancer

Many single-agent chemotherapeutic agents have been studied in metastatic RCC. These trials have not shown any single chemotherapeutic agent to have significant efficacy in renal cell carcinoma. In 1988, Bergerat et al. found a 42% response rate in patients treated with combination interferon and vinblastine, leading to hopes that vinblastine would prove to be an effective agent.[134] Unfortunately, subsequent randomized trials have been less promising.[135] In a study of 160 patients treated with IFN-2α plus vinblastine versus vinblastine alone, the vinblastine arm showed only a 2.5% response rate.[135] Similarly, early Phase II studies also showed promising results for 5-fluorouracil (5-FU)[136,137]; however, Negrier et al., comparing IFN-α plus IL-2 with or without 5-FU, showed no added benefit from chemotherapy in survival and a very poor response rate in both arms.[138]

Similarly, combination therapies have not been proven effective in randomized controlled trials. Many studies have concentrated on platinum- fluorouracil-, and gemcitabine-based therapies, all in Phase II trials of various size populations.[139,140] A single-arm Phase II trial by Rini et al. of gemcitabine with continuous 5-FU showed a 17% objective response rate.[141]

In the past few years, newer chemotherapeutic drugs have been studied. A large number of Phase II studies of newer chemotherapeutic drugs have shown no improvement in survival or significant response rates but have occasionally suggested a prolonged stable disease.[142–149] Therapies that have been studied include bryostatin-1, a protein kinase C inhibitor; flavopiridol, a cyclin-dependent kinase inhibitor; troxacitabine, a nucleoside analogue; irofulvin, which covalently binds to DNA, inhibits DNA synthesis, and induces apoptosis; the 5-fluorouracil, folinic acid, and oxaliplatin (FOLFOX-4 regimen); arsenic trioxide (As_2O_3); razoxane, an antiangiogenic topoisomerase II inhibitor; and most recently, PS-341, a proteosome inhibitor, to name a few. In general, chemotherapy has failed to improve or even match the objective responses seen with cytokine therapy, and none has shown improvement in survival.

TABLE 46.11. Hormone therapy in advanced renal cell carcinoma.

Therapy	*Patients (n)*	*% response (range)*
Progestational agents	695	5 (0–17)
Androgenic agents	190	3 (0–14)
Hormonal responses by year of reporting		
1967–1971	228	17
1971–1976	415	2

Hormonal Therapy of Advanced Renal Cell Cancer

Numerous trials have explored the role of hormonal therapy in treatment of patients with metastatic renal cell carcinoma (Table 46.11). These studies were prompted by preclinical studies in which progesterone was shown to be effective in inhibiting both tumor development and tumor growth.[150,151] Progestins have been the most actively studied clinically as well and have produced response rates ranging from 0% up to 20%. More recent studies using standard defined response criteria have produced response rates of only 1% to 5%.[152] In reviewing the data on medroxyprogesterone,[150] it was concluded that irrespective of dose or schedule, human renal cell carcinoma is neither hormone dependent nor hormone responsive. Nonetheless, patients with severe anorexia and weight loss may occasionally derive significant symptomatic relief from the administration of medroxyprogesterone, even in the absence of any direct antitumor effect.

Cytokine-Based Therapy of Renal Cell Cancer

Although there have been innumerable trials examining a number of biologic agents in treatment of advanced RCC, few have provided strong evidence for the clear benefit of one treatment over another. The majority of studies have been focused on the clinical effects of two cytokines: interleukin (IL)-2 and interferon-alpha. These have been extensively studied alone and in combination in Phase I and II trials; surprisingly few trials have compared the two treatments in a randomized Phase III design.[138,153–155] Other cytokines have been tested in numerous phase I and II settings including IL-4, IL-6, IL-12, Flt3L, and others without any real suggestion of significant activity in trials of small cohorts of patients.[156–161] The cytokine therapy of RCC suffers greatly from an abundance of relatively small unconfirmed Phase II trials and very few properly sized and statistically sound Phase III trials.

Interferon-Alpha (IFN-α)

There is an extensive literature examining single agent IFN-α in the treatment of advanced RCC.[162–166] In the early studies, a number of different and noncloned interferons were utilized and RCC was chosen as a target disease. In numerous trials, antitumor activity in terms of tumor regression and disease stabilization was observed. Additionally, it has been suggested that the objective rules we use to evaluate complete and partial responses do not capture the ability of IFN-α to extend survival without objective disease regression. Meta-analyses encompassing a large number of trials and patients with RCC in the 1980s supported the following results.

1. The various interferons, that is, lymphoblastoid, leukocyte, IFN-α2a, and IFN-α2b, all demonstrated similar results with complete responses between 1% and 4% and partial responses as high as 10% and 15% and as low as 5% in other trials.[164]

2. Doses between 3 and 10 MIU/day appear as active as and less toxic than higher doses.[164–167]

3. SC or IM was the most effective route, and other IFNs such as IFN-β and IFN-γ had lower activity than IFN-α.[168–172]

Several important Phase III trials have tried to determine whether the combination of other agents with IFN-α could improve therapy in RCC. Several Phase I and II trials combining IFN-α with vinblastine, an agent initially approved for advanced RCC but rarely applied to the disease, reported promising results with objective response rates exceeding 20% to 25% and median survivals up to 70 weeks (16+ months).[173] This finding led to a Phase III trial that selected vinblastine (Vbl) as control and IFN-α plus Vbl as the experimental arm,[134] with a total of 160 patients enrolled. For those in the Vbl arm alone, the median survival was only 37.8 weeks, with an objective response rate of 2.5% (2 patients). This result compared poorly to Vbl plus IFN-α patients,[174] who demonstrated a 16.5% response rate (P = 0.0025) and median survival of 67.6 weeks (P = 0.0049). One obvious conclusion is that Vbl alone has no value as a single agent in advanced RCC. The benefit of the combined arm was likely totally the result of the contribution of IFN-α.

Another attempt to improve the effects of IFNa in RCC was led by Motzer at MSKCC. Based upon a Phase II trial combining IFN-α with 13-*cis*-retinoic acid (CRA),[175] a Phase III trial was then conducted at multiple centers through ECOG and MSKCC and enrolled 284 patients with advanced RCC in slightly more than 2 years.[169] In the 139 patients on IFN-α plus CRA, there were 16 responses [5 complete responses (CRs) and 11 partial responses (PRs)] for a response rate of 12%, compared with 9 (1 CR and 8 PRs) (6%) among the 145 patients receiving only IFN-α (P = 0.14) The duration of the responses was long in both cohorts but longer (P = 0.03) in those receiving IFN-α plus CRA (33 versus 22 months). The median survival for all patients, 15 months, was not significantly different between the groups (P = 0.26). The quality of life of patients receiving both IFN-α and CRA was decreased.

Smaller but definitive studies have shown that IFN-γ, when added to IFN-α, did not increase the response rate.[171] In fact, among the 102 patients enrolled, 7 of 53 responded to IFN-α alone, whereas only 2 of 45 responded to IFN-α plus IFN-γ. Finally, two randomized control trials examined the role of nephrectomy in patients with advanced RCC who followed surgical intervention with systemic therapy such as IFN-α.[170] An EORTC trial of 85 patients and a SWOG Intergroup trial both showed an improved outcome for both survival and progression-free survival when patients treated with IFN-α had nephrectomy before surgery,[129,130] although the objective response rate to IFN-α in the 85-patient EORTC trial was 19% and 12% (P = 0.38), respectively, for patients with and without nephrectomy. On the other hand, among the 246 patients enrolled on the SWOG trial, of those with measurable disease only 3% to 4% of patients had evidence for objective responses whether or not they had undergone prior nephrectomy. This finding implied that the statistically significant improvement in overall survival was not completely dependent on improving the number and quality of tumor regressions induced by IFN-α.[130]

Interleukin-2 (IL-2)

Since its rapid translation from animal models to clinical trials back in the mid-1980s, IL-2 has been the focus of both great excitement and great disappointment[176,177] (Table 46.12). Initially, trials of a high-dose bolus regimen administered at 600,000–720,000 units/kg intravenously (IV) every 8 hours for 14 doses (maximum) on days 1–5 and 15–19 of every 8–12 weeks with ex vivo IL-2-activated peripheral blood mononuclear cells (LAK cells) demonstrated response rates as high as 30% to 40% in patients with advanced RCC.[176] These trial included highly selected groups of patients.[176,178] Later, it became clear that ex vivo LAK cells were not essential and very costly.[179,180] Additionally, it became apparent that the response rate was lower (15%–25%); however, the durability of the responses persisted as the most impressive finding. These findings culminated in the 1995 publication by Fyfe et al. of 255 patients with advanced RCC who had been entered on seven Phase II clinical trials from 21 different institutions.[181] This database included all patients with advanced RCC treated with high-dose bolus IL-2 as a single agent. As in many high-dose IL-2 trials that were subsequently reported, the patients were selected for excellent organ function (cardiac, respiratory, renal, hematologic), no evidence of brain metastases, and excellent performance score (PS) of 0–1 or Karnofsky 70–100. Eighty-five percent had prior nephrectomy, 65% had a PS = 0 or certainly Karnofsky PS above 80, whereas 44% had initial diagnosis with 12 months of IL-2 therapy. No data were available on the number of patients with elevated serum LDH, elevated serum calcium, or anemia (Motzer prognostic factors). Of the 255 patients, 36 (14%) demonstrated objective evidence of response, 12 CRs and 24 PRs.[181] Most impressive was the duration of the responses, 19 months for PRs and 8 of 12 ongoing responses in the CR patients (5+ to 62+). Responses were observed in patients with bulky disease (larger than 25 cm^2). As expected, toxicity was quite impressive, with grade 3–4 hypotension in nearly 75% of patients and grade 3–4 mental status changes in nearly 30% of patients. Oliguria/anuria and symptoms such as nausea, vomiting, diarrhea, and fever were severe (grade 3–4) in 24% to 46% of patients. In this group of patients, many were treated before a full understanding of toxicity management, and therefore treatment-related mortality was 4% (11 patients). An additional follow-up report more than 12 months later on the same cohort of 255 RCC patients showed even better durability, with very rare if any late relapses among any of the objective responders.[182]

The year 2003 saw a completed Phase III trial (actually two Phase III trials combined) published in the *Journal of Clinical Oncology*.[154,155] From 1991 to 2001, 306 patients were randomized between high-dose bolus IL-2 (720,000 U/kg/dose) versus low-dose bolus IL-2 (72,000 U/kg/dose). Another 94 patients were randomized to outpatient subcutaneous IL-2 from 1993 to 2001. The trial began as a two-arm trial, and after the initial 117 patients were accrued, the trial was modified into a three-arm Phase III with an additional

TABLE 46.12. Trials with interleukin-2 in renal cell cancer.

Author	*Regimen*	*Dose of IL-2*	*No. of patients*	*No. of responses*	*% response*	*95% CI for RR*	*CR*	*PR*	*Response duration, months*	*P value*
Sleijfer[205] Phase II	SC IL-2, 5 days for 6 weeks of 9	18 MIU/day 9 MIU/day	26	6	23	9%–44%	2	4	CR: 19+, 21+ PR: 13+, 15+, 16+, 20	NA
Atzpodien[204] Phase II	SC IL-2 + IFN, 5 days for 6 weeks	20 MIU 10 MIU	152	38	25	19%–32%	9	29	CR: median 16 + PR: median 9	
Figlin[206] Phase II	CI IL-2–4 days + IFN SC 4 weeks of 6	2 MIU/m²/day	30	9	30	15%–49%	0	9 (→2 sCR)	PR: median 12+	
Fyfe[181] Phase II	Bolus IL-2, 14 doses q 8 h	600–720 KIU/kg	255	36	14	10%–19%	12	24	PR: median 19 CR: median not reached	
Negrier[138] Phase III	SC IL-2 + SC IFN QOW 1, 3, 5, 7	IL-2 9 MIU/day, IFN 6 MIU TIW	70	1	1.4	NA	0	1	NA	0.1
	Same + 5-FU CI, week 1, 5	Same + 5-FU at 600/m²/day	61	5	8.2	NA	0	5	NA	
Negrier[153] Phase III	IL-2 CI IFN SC	18 MIU/m² 18 MIU	138 147	9 11	7.7 7.8	NA NA	NA NA	NA NA	NA NA	$P < 0.01$ EFS at 12 months, $P = 0.01$
	IL-2 CI + IFN SC	18 MIU IL-2 6 MIU IFN	140	26	21.3	NA	NA	NA	NA	OS, $p = 0.55$
Yang[154]	HD IL-2 bolus	720 K/kg	156	33	21	NA	11	22	Not reached, 8/11 ongoing CR 3/6	RR HD vs. LD, $P = 0.048$
Phase III	IL-2 LD bolus	72 K/kg	150	19	13	NA	6	13	remain in CR 1/2 remain in CR	Not significant for OS
	IL-2 SC	250 K/kg 125 K/kg	94	9	10	NA	2	7		
McDermott[155] Phase III	HD bolus IL-2	600 kIU/kg	97	22	23	NA	8	14	Response duration 14 months median	$P = 0.035$ for RR
	IL-2 + IFN SC 4 of 6 weeks	IL-2 5 MIU/m²/day IFN 5 MIU/m²/day	96	9	9	NA	3	6	Response duration 7 months median	$P = 0.08$ for 3 years for PFS $P = 0.069$ for OS

MIU, million international units; IL-2, interleukin 2; IFN, interferon; CI, continuous infusion; 5-FU, fluorouracil; HD, high dose; LD, low dose; CR, complete response; PR, partial response; QOW, every other week; CI, confidence interval; RR, relative risk; EFS, event-free survival; PFS, progression-free survival; OS, overall survival.

TABLE 46.13. Thalidomide in renal cell carcinoma.

Single-agent thalidomide studies	*Maximum daily dose allowed (mg)*	*Total no. of patients*	*No. of assessable patients*	*Partial response*	*% of patients*	*Stable disease for 3–6 months*	*% of patients*
Stebbing et al.[184]	100	18	18	3	17	13	72
Minor et al.[186]	1,200	15	12	1	8	3	25
Stebbing et al.[184]	600	25	22	2	9	7	32
Li et al.[9]	1,200	36	29	2	7	9	31
Escudier et al.[185]	1,200	40	33	2	6	9	27
Motzer et al.[183]	800	26	25	0	0	16	64
Daliani et al.[187]	1,200	20	19	2	11	9	47
Total	207	185	12	6	73	39	

IFN, interferon.

283 patients then randomized. When all results were combined, high-dose bolus IL-2 was associated with a 21% response rate among 155 evaluable patients (11 CRs and 22 PRs) versus 13% for low-dose bolus IL-2 (6 CRs and 13 PRs) ($P = 0.048$ by chi-square test). The patients receiving subcutaneous IL-2 as outpatients had a response rate of 10%, with 2 CRs and 7 PRs among the 93 patients. Compared with the IL-2 high-dose bolus randomized simultaneously, the statistical difference favored high-dose IL-2 ($P = 0.033$ by χ^2 testing), although the study did not show a definitive overall survival advantage for those receiving high-dose IL-2. Overall, the responses to high-dose IL-2 were more durable; in fact, the responding patients getting high-dose IL-2 had a better survival than responders in the low-dose IL-2 bolus arm ($P = 0.04$). Responses were more frequent and the responses were apparently more durable.

In another trial conducted by the Cytokine Working Group, 193 patients with advanced RCC were randomized between high-dose bolus IL-2 and outpatient subcutaneous IL-2 plus IFN-α based on the Atzpodien regimen.[155] This trial accrued patients from 1997 through 2000 with 96 patients accrued to each arm and eligible. Similar to the NCI randomized trial, high-dose IL-2 had a significantly better response rate versus IL-2/IFN-α outpatients (23 versus 9%; $P = 0.018$). Again, the response duration was greater with high-dose IL-2 (14 versus 7 months). Finally, only 2 of the 9 IL-2/IFN-α responders were progression free at 17+ and 35+ months, whereas 9 of 22 high-dose IL-2 responders remained progression free at 22+ to 44+ months. Together, these trials support high-dose bolus IL-2 as the preferred treatment of metastatic RCC at centers where experience and clinical support exist. On the other hand, only approximately 10% of patients ultimately obtain very meaningful benefit with high-dose IL-2 and far more do not get a major benefit.

Thalidomide

Based on the in vitro antiangiogenic activity of thalidomide, it has attracted much interest for the treatment of RCC.[183–187] A number of Phase II studies have been performed demonstrating partial responses ranging from 0% to 8% and stable disease at 6 months of 23% to 30% (Table 46.13).[183–187] A randomized ECOG Phase III study was recently reported in abstract form[188]; it compared treatment with IFN-α alone to IFN-α in combination with thalidomide and enrolled 353 patients, of whom 342 were eligible, with a median age of 59 years (range, 24–84), including 227 men and 115 females with a median ECOG PS 1. Of these, 254 patients had undergone a prior nephrectomy and 236 had a disease-free interval of 1 year or less. Treatment consisted of IFN-α, 1 million IU SC bid alone or in combination with thalidomide (intrapatient dose escalation from 200 mg/day to 1,000 mg/day maximum). The study was designed to detect an improvement in progression-free survival (PFS) at 6 months of 35% compared with 20% in the "standard IFN-α" arm and a 50% improvement in median overall survival (OS) from 12 to 18 months. Fatigue, myelosuppression, and thrombotic events (12 versus 4) were greater in the thalidomide + IFN-α arm. There was no difference in response rates or overall survival, although PFS was longer, and the difference was significant statistically, in the IFN + thalidomide arm (Table 46.14). Quality of life and fatigue scores were worse on the IFN + thalidomide arm. The addition of thalidomide to this IFN regimen modestly improves PFS but not OS and worsens quality of life in RCC patients.

Other Therapies Applied to Renal Cell Cancer

Adoptive Cellular Therapy

Transfer of immune cells for the treatment of renal cancer has been an integral component of research over the years in RCC. There was an interest in the role of LAK cells in the setting of high-dose interleukin-2, and this was presumed to be a critical component of the IL-2 therapy. However, a randomized trial revealed that it added little in terms of response rate and overall survival. The results may have trended toward an advantage with cellular therapy, but it was certainly not worth the labor, cost, and added toxicity.[179,180]

TABLE 46.14. Thalidomide contribution to RCC treatment.

	CR (%)	*PR (%)*	*RR (%)*	*6-month PFS*	*Median PFS*	*Median OS*
IFN alone	0	2	2.2	26%	2.8 months	12.2 months
IFN + T	2	4	6.5	29.3%	3.8 months $P = 0.04$	10.8 months $P = 0.93$

T, thalidomide 100 mg/day po escalating to 1,000 mg; IFN, interferon 1 mm/BID sq daily.

Probably the most ambitious effort was led by the investigators at UCLA. Over a number of years the group treated 55 patients with autologous CD8 selected tumor-infiltrating (TIL) cells from prior resection specimens; an additional 7 patients could not undergo the therapy. There were 5 complete responses and 14 partial remissions for an overall response rate of 35%. The patients also received IL-2 but at doses that rarely induced a response rate greater than 10%. The responses were durable, with a median of 14 months. These data were the impetus for a Phase III trial of the same schedule and dose of IL-2 with or without CD8+ selected TIL cells in which 178 patients were enrolled and 160 patients were randomized.[189] Twenty additional patients did not receive any therapy because of postoperative complications, mortality, or simply inability to tolerate the IL-2 therapy. Of 72 patients designated to receive CD8+ TIL cells, 33 did not have adequate cells generated. In the end, with intent to treat, the responses in both groups were around 10% and 1-year survival was similar at approximately 50%. This experience showed the difficulty in exporting highly technical cellular approaches into a large multicenter trial. The need for a single-institution commitment cannot easily be recreated in a multicenter trial.

Vaccination strategies in RCC have differed from melanoma primarily because of the lack of obvious tumor antigens that appeared to be recognized by T cells.[190,191] This finding may have changed recently as a result of the expression pattern of some enzymes associated with VHL mutations such as CAIX,[192] which has lead to efforts using the antigens from tumor cells without specific knowledge of what they are or having to isolate them. The first approach explored the use of tumor cell-autologous tumor hybrids. An initial report from Kugler et al. in Germany included 17 patients with advanced renal cancer.[191] Of the 17 patients, 7 had objective responses with 4 CRs, 2 PRs, and 1 mixed response. Two other patients had prolonged stable disease for more than 12 months each. Although this report was quite promising, it was retracted later with a great deal of suspicion about the validity of any of the findings. Others have not reported this approach in RCC, primarily because of technical difficulties with the fusion and growth culturing procedures.[193] More recently, the group at Duke led by Vieweg and Gilboa have attempted a slightly different strategy of isolating RNA from the RCC specimens and then transfecting the RNA into autologous dendritic cells (DC).[194] This approach appeared to be successful at inducing CTL activity by ELISPOT assays in most patients of the 10 treated. These immune responses included those directed to specific antigens, telomerase, G250, RNA tumor-loaded DC, and oncofetal antigens. None of the 10 patients had obvious tumor regression; however, 7 of the 10 remain alive with a median follow-up of almost 20 months. This result could represent a significant effect of the treatment or simply a matter of patient selection and the presence of only good prognosis patients.

Nonmyeloablative HLA-Matched Sibling Stem Cell Transplants as a Form of Immunotherapy

A new paradigm for treating renal cancer appeared in 1998–2000 when Childs and his colleagues at the NCI and National Institutes of Health (NIH) reported on the use of allogeneic stem cells transplants utilizing nonmyeloablative chemotherapy regimens in the treatment of RCC.[111] The approach was based on the well-known association of graft-versus-host disease with improved clinical outcome and even clinical regressions in hematologic malignancies. The hope was for a graft-versus-tumor (GVT) effect. Ten of the first 19 patients with RCC who underwent the procedure had a clinical remission after failing cytokine therapy.[111] Three complete responses remained ongoing at 16+ to 27+ months. Regression of disease was frequently delayed up to 4 to 6 months after the allogeneic stem cell therapy. In a number of cases the patient did not demonstration chimerism, a sign of the engraftment of donor cells. In these cases, frequently additional donor lymphocytes were infused to enhance the potential for a GVT effect. The risk and importance of graft-versus-host disease (GVHD) was emphasized. GVHD occurred in 10 of the patients at grade II–IV, being associated with transplant mortality in 2 patients (Table 46.15).

Although overall this approach to RCC therapy is exciting and scientifically of great interest,[195–197] it is far from established, is associated with great toxicity, and should only be performed as part of a clinical trial. The center where it is performed must be truly committed to optimally studying these patients and understanding how to improve the efficacy and diminishing the toxicity.

Novel Therapy of Advanced Clear Cell RCC Based on Its Cancer Biology

As reviewed, the cloning of the VHL gene, the understanding of its role in HIF-1α stability and activity, and the large number of HIF-1α-regulated genes that are expressed in RCC. These genes appear to have uncovered numerous molecular targets for therapeutic intervention, which include VEGF, PDGF, TGF-α, EGFR, and carbonic anhydrase IX, and appear important to the behavior of this malignancy.[198] Small molecule kinase inhibitors and/or antibodies have been developed to either selectively block many of these pathways or inhibit a number of pathways on their own. These agents have now entering clinical trials at the Phase I/II/III stage (Table 46.16).

The data as published in peer-reviewed journals so far are most compelling for a humanized antibody to VEGF (anti-VEGF; Avastin, Bevicizamab). In a randomized, double-blinded Phase II trial of placebo versus anti-VEGF at 3 mg/kg/2 weeks versus 10 mg/kg/2 weeks in which 50 patients were to be enrolled into each arm, RCC patients were followed for the primary endpoint of time to progression (TTP), as well as objective clinical responses and overall survival.[199] All patients either had prior interleukin-2 or were unable to receive it. Most patients had previously undergone nephrectomy. The trial was terminated at the enrollment of the 116th patient because "the difference in outcome in the three arms mandated closure by the DSMB." There were only 4 responses (all PR) among 39 [confidence interval (CI) at 95%, 2.9%–24.2% relative risk (RR)] patients treated with the high dose of anti-VEGF (10 mg/kg). There were no other responses among the other 74 patients. At the time of unblinding, the median TTP was 4.8 months for the high-dose anti-VEGF versus 2.5 months for placebo [P less than 0.001; hazard ratio (HR) = 2.55]. The difference in median TTP for those receiv-

TABLE 46.15. Results of nonmyeloablative transplant regimens reported for metastatic renal cell carcinoma.

Investigators	*Conditioning agents*	*GVHD prophylaxis*	*Comment*	*Median time to response*	*Response in other solid tumors*
Childs et al.[111]	Cyclophosphamide 120 mg/kg, fludarabine 125 mg/m^2	CSA +/– MMF	Immunosuppression tapered and DLI given based on T cell	5 months	Currently being evaluated
Rini et al.[207]	Cyclophosphamide 2,000 mg/m^2, fludarabine 90 mg/m^2	FK506 + MMF	High incidence of graft rejection (3/4 patients treated); cyclophosphamide increased to 4 g/m^2 and fludarabine increased to 150 mg/m^2	>100 days	Not evaluated
Bregni et al.[208]	Thiotepa 5 mg/kg, fludarabine 60 mg/m^2, cyclophosphamide 60 mg/kg	CSA + methotrexate	CSA tapering based on disease status; delayed response observed in 3/3 treated RCC patients	>100 days	Yes (response seen in breast cancer and ovarian cancer patient)

GVHD, graft-versus-host disease; RCC, renal cell carcinoma; CSA, cyclosporine; MMF, mycophenolate mofetil; DLI, donor lymphocyte infusions; NA, not available.

ing low-dose anti-VEGF versus placebo nearly reached statistical significance ($P = 0.053$; HR = 1.26). The percent that were progression free on each of the arms at 4 and 8 months are shown in Table 46.17.

There was crossover allowed for those progressing patients to receive the anti-VEGF at the high dose (10 mg/kg) if they were initially in the placebo or 3 mg/kg arm of anti-VEGF. This choice likely made the overall survival evaluation impossible. Nevertheless, the excitement generated by these results has led to a number of other trials including a large multicenter trial of IFN-α versus IFN-α plus anti-VEGF, Phase II trials of combination blockade with anti-VEGF and EGFR tyrosine kinase inhibitors. The later trial of anti-VEGF and an EGFR inhibitor was very promising. The combination produced a 21% objective response rate in a group of 58 evaluable patients with advanced RCC. An additional 45% of patients had stable disease/minor response for 6 months or more.[200] More recently, Phase II and III trials of a number of agents look especially promising via inhibition of VEGF, PDGF, Raf, and mTOR signaling.[217–220]

TABLE 46.16. Clinical trials of novel therapies for clear cell RCC.

Therapeutic agent	*Mechanism of action*	*Target molecule(s)*	*Advantages*	*Disadvantages*	*Clinical status*
Anti-VEGF	Humanized antibody to VEGF	VEGF	Specificity	Intravenous	Phase II/III
SU5416	Tyrosine kinase inhibitor	VEGFR1 and VEGFR2		Toxicities	Program closed
PTK787	Tyrosine kinase inhibitor	VEGFR2 and PDGFR	Oral		Phase II/III
VEGF Trap	Cytokine trap (FcIg-receptor)	VEGFR1 and VEGFR2	Prolong t1/2	Intravenous	Phase I/II
STI-571 (Gleevec)	Tyrosine kinase inhibitor	Bcr/Abl, c-*kit*, PDGFR	Oral	Non-specificity	Phase II/III
C225 (Imclone)	Humanized antibody to EGFR	EGFR	ADCC	Intravenous	Phase II/III
ABX (Abgenix)	Human antibody to EGFR	EGFR	ADCC	Intravenous	Phase II
ZD1839 (Iressa)	Tyrosine kinase inhibitor	EGFR	Oral		Phase II/III
OSI-774 (Tarceva)	Tyrosine kinase inhibitor	EGFR	Oral		Phase II/III
SU011248	Tyrosine kinase inhibitor	VEGFR2, PDGFR, Flt 3, c-*kit*	Oral		Phase II
ZD6474	Tyrosine kinase inhibitor	VEGFR2, EGFR	Oral		Phase I/II
Bay 43-9006 (Sorafenib)	Kinase inhibitor	VEGFR2, PDGFR, Raf	Oral		Phase II, III
AG013736	Tyrosine kinase inhibitor	VEGFR2, PDGFR, Flt 3, c-, c-*kit*	Oral		Phase II
CCI-779 (Temsirolumas)	mTOR inhibitor	mTOR, PTEN/Akt pathway		Intravenous weekly	Phase III

VEGF, vascular endothelial growth factor; EGFR, epithelial growth factor receptor; PDGFR, platelet-derived growth factor receptor; ADCC, antibody dependent cellular cytotoxicity.

TABLE 46.17. **Antivascular epithelial growth factor (anti-VEGF) prolongs progression-free survival (PFS).**

	Anti-VEGF at 10 mg/kg	*Anti-VEGF at 3 mg/kg*	*Placebo*
PFS at 4 months	64%	39%	20%
PFS at 8 months	30%	14%	5%

References

1. Jemal A, Tiwari RC, Murray T, et al. Cancer statistics, 2004. CA Cancer J Clin 2004;54:8–29.
2. Chow WH, Devesa SS, Warren JL, Fraumeni JF, Jr. Rising incidence of renal cell cancer in the United States. JAMA 1999;281:1628–1631.
3. Mellemgaard A, Moller H, Olsen JH, Jensen OM. Increased risk of renal cell carcinoma among obese women. J Natl Cancer Inst 1991;83:1581–1582.
4. Chow WH, Gridley G, Fraumeni JF, Jr., Jarvholm B. Obesity, hypertension, and the risk of kidney cancer in men. N Engl J Med 2000;343:1305–1311.
5. Hwang JJ, Uchio EM, Linehan WM, Walther MM. Hereditary kidney cancer. Urol Clin North Am 2003;30:831–842.
6. Lamiell JM, Salazar FG, Hsia YE. von Hippel-Lindau disease affecting 43 members of a single kindred. Medicine (Baltimore) 1989;68:1–29.
7. Lendvay TS, Marshall FF. The tuberous sclerosis complex and its highly variable manifestations. J Urol 2003;169:1635–1642.
8. Pavlovich CP, Walther MM, Eyler RA, et al. Renal tumors in the Birt-Hogg-Dube syndrome. Am J Surg Pathol 2002;26:1542–1552.
9. Cohen AJ, Li FP, Berg S, et al. Hereditary renal-cell carcinoma associated with a chromosomal translocation. N Engl J Med 1979;301:592–595.
10. Takahashi M, Kahnoski R, Gross D, Nicol D, Teh BT. Familial adult renal neoplasia. J Med Genet 2002;39:1–5.
11. Schmidt L, Duh FM, Chen F, et al. Germline and somatic mutations in the tyrosine kinase domain of the MET proto-oncogene in papillary renal carcinomas. Nat Genet 1997;16:68–73.
12. Pavlovich CP, Schmidt LS, Phillips JL. The genetic basis of renal cell carcinoma. Urol Clin North Am 2003;30:437–454, vii.
13. Nelson JB, Oyasu R, Dalton DP. The clinical and pathological manifestations of renal tumors in von Hippel-Lindau disease. J Urol 1994;152:2221–2226.
14. Zbar B, Brauch H, Talmadge C, Linehan M. Loss of alleles of loci on the short arm of chromosome 3 in renal cell carcinoma. Nature 1987;327:721–724.
15. Iliopoulos O, Kibel A, Gray S, Kaelin WG, Jr. Tumour suppression by the human von Hippel-Lindau gene product. Nat Med 1995;1:822–826.
16. Stebbins CE, Kaelin WG, Jr., Pavletich NP. Structure of the VHL-ElonginC-ElonginB complex: implications for VHL tumor suppressor function. Science 1999;284:455–461.
17. Pause A, Lee S, Worrell RA, et al. The von Hippel-Lindau tumor-suppressor gene product forms a stable complex with human CUL-2, a member of the Cdc53 family of proteins. Proc Natl Acad Sci U S A 1997;94:2156–2161.
18. Ohh M, Park CW, Ivan M, et al. Ubiquitination of hypoxia-inducible factor requires direct binding to the beta-domain of the von Hippel-Lindau protein. Nat Cell Biol 2000;2:423–427.
19. Kamura T, Sato S, Iwai K, Czyzyk-Krzeska M, Conaway RC, Conaway JW. Activation of HIF1alpha ubiquitination by a reconstituted von Hippel-Lindau (VHL) tumor suppressor complex. Proc Natl Acad Sci U S A 2000;97:10430–10435.
20. Cockman ME, Masson N, Mole DR, et al. Hypoxia inducible factor-alpha binding and ubiquitylation by the von Hippel-Lindau tumor suppressor protein. J Biol Chem 2000;275:25733–25741.
21. Sargent ER, Gomella LG, Belldegrun A, Linehan WM, Kasid A. Epidermal growth factor receptor gene expression in normal human kidney and renal cell carcinoma. J Urol 1989;142:1364–1368.
22. de Paulsen N, Brychzy A, Fournier MC, et al. Role of transforming growth factor-alpha in von Hippel–Lindau (VHL)(–/–) clear cell renal carcinoma cell proliferation: a possible mechanism coupling VHL tumor suppressor inactivation and tumorigenesis. Proc Natl Acad Sci U S A 2001;98:1387–1392.
23. Lonergan KM, Iliopoulos O, Ohh M, et al. Regulation of hypoxia-inducible mRNAs by the von Hippel-Lindau tumor suppressor protein requires binding to complexes containing elongins B/C and Cul2. Mol Cell Biol 1998;18:732–741.
24. Kandt RS. Tuberous sclerosis complex and neurofibromatosis type 1: the two most common neurocutaneous diseases. Neurol Clin 2002;20:941–964.
25. Yeung RS. Multiple roles of the tuberous sclerosis complex genes. Genes Chromosom Cancer 2003;38:368–375.
26. Toro JR, Glenn G, Duray P, et al. Birt-Hogg-Dube syndrome: a novel marker of kidney neoplasia. Arch Dermatol 1999;135:1195–1202.
27. Schmidt L, Junker K, Nakaigawa N, et al. Novel mutations of the MET proto-oncogene in papillary renal carcinomas. Oncogene 1999;18:2343–2350.
28. Mydlo JH, Weinstein R, Misseri R, Axiotis C, Thelmo W. Radiologic, pathologic and molecular attributes of two types of papillary renal adenocarcinomas. Scand J Urol Nephrol 2001;35:262–269.
29. Mejean A, Hopirtean V, Bazin JP, et al. Prognostic factors for the survival of patients with papillary renal cell carcinoma: meaning of histological typing and multifocality. J Urol 2003;170:764–767.
30. Pathak S, Strong LC, Ferrell RE, Trindade A. Familial renal cell carcinoma with a 3;11 chromosome translocation limited to tumor cells. Science 1982;217:939–941.
31. Bostwick DG, Eble JN. Diagnosis and classification of renal cell carcinoma. Urol Clin North Am 1999;26:627–635.
32. Zambrano NR, Lubensky IA, Merino MJ, Linehan WM, Walther MM. Histopathology and molecular genetics of renal tumors toward unification of a classification system. J Urol 1999;162:1246–1258.
33. Morra MN, Das S. Renal oncocytoma: a review of histogenesis, histopathology, diagnosis and treatment. J Urol 1993;150:295–302.
34. Moch H, Gasser T, Amin MB, Torhorst J, Sauter G, Mihatsch MJ. Prognostic utility of the recently recommended histologic classification and revised TNM staging system of renal cell carcinoma: a Swiss experience with 588 tumors. Cancer 2000;89:604–614.
35. Kondo K, Kaelin WG, Jr. The von Hippel-Lindau tumor suppressor gene. Exp Cell Res 2001;264:117–125.
36. Kovacs G, Fuzesi L, Emanual A, Kung HF. Cytogenetics of papillary renal cell tumors. Genes Chromosom Cancer 1991;3:249–255.
37. Delahunt B, Eble JN. Papillary renal cell carcinoma: a clinicopathologic and immunohistochemical study of 105 tumors. Mod Pathol 1997;10:537–544.
38. Thoenes W, Storkel S, Rumpelt HJ, Moll R, Baum HP, Werner S. Chromophobe cell renal carcinoma and its variants—a report on 32 cases. J Pathol 1988;155:277–287.
39. Speicher MR, Schoell B, du Manoir S, et al. Specific loss of chromosomes 1, 2, 6, 10, 13, 17, and 21 in chromophobe renal cell carcinomas revealed by comparative genomic hybridization. Am J Pathol 1994;145:356–364.

40. Kennedy SM, Merino MJ, Linehan WM, Roberts JR, Robertson CN, Neumann RD. Collecting duct carcinoma of the kidney. Hum Pathol 1990;21:449–456.
41. Mejean A, Oudard S, Thiounn N. Prognostic factors of renal cell carcinoma. J Urol 2003;169:821–827.
42. Vasselli JR, Shih JH, Iyengar SR, et al. Predicting survival in patients with metastatic kidney cancer by gene-expression profiling in the primary tumor. Proc Natl Acad Sci U S A 2003;100:6958–6963.
43. Staller P, Sulitkova J, Lisztwan J, Moch H, Oakeley EJ, Krek W. Chemokine receptor CXCR4 downregulated by von Hippel-Lindau tumour suppressor pVHL. Nature 2003;425:307–311.
44. Takahashi M, Yang XJ, Sugimura J, et al. Molecular subclassification of kidney tumors and the discovery of new diagnostic markers. Oncogene 2003;22:6810–6818.
45. Yu F, White SB, Zhao Q, Lee FS. HIF-1alpha binding to VHL is regulated by stimulus-sensitive proline hydroxylation. Proc Natl Acad Sci U S A 2001;98:9630–9635.
46. Jaakkola P, Mole DR, Tian YM, et al. Targeting of HIF-alpha to the von Hippel-Lindau ubiquitylation complex by O2-regulated prolyl hydroxylation. Science 2001;292:468–472.
47. Yao M, Yoshida M, Kishida T, et al. VHL tumor suppressor gene alterations associated with good prognosis in sporadic clear-cell renal carcinoma. J Natl Cancer Inst 2002;94:1569–1575.
48. Dreijerink K, Braga E, Kuzmin I, et al. The candidate tumor suppressor gene, RASSF1A, from human chromosome 3p21.3 is involved in kidney tumorigenesis. Proc Natl Acad Sci U S A 2001;98:7504–7509.
49. Morrissey C, Martinez A, Zatyka M, et al. Epigenetic inactivation of the RASSF1A 3p21.3 tumor suppressor gene in both clear cell and papillary renal cell carcinoma. Cancer Res 2001;61: 7277–7281.
50. Skinner DG, Colvin RB, Vermillion CD, Pfister RC, Leadbetter WF. Diagnosis and management of renal cell carcinoma. A clinical and pathologic study of 309 cases. Cancer 1971;28:1165–1177.
51. Gold PJ, Fefer A, Thompson JA. Paraneoplastic manifestations of renal cell carcinoma. Semin Urol Oncol 1996;14:216–222.
52. Fahn HJ, Lee YH, Chen MT, Huang JK, Chen KK, Chang LS. The incidence and prognostic significance of humoral hypercalcemia in renal cell carcinoma. J Urol 1991;145:248–250.
53. Motzer RJ, Bacik J, Schwartz LH, et al. Prognostic factors for survival in previously treated patients with metastatic renal cell carcinoma. J Clin Oncol 2004;22:454–463.
54. Motzer RJ, Mazumdar M, Bacik J, Berg W, Amsterdam A, Ferrara J. Survival and prognostic stratification of 670 patients with advanced renal cell carcinoma. J Clin Oncol 1999;17:2530–2540.
55. Blay JY, Rossi JF, Wijdenes J, et al. Role of interleukin-6 in the paraneoplastic inflammatory syndrome associated with renal-cell carcinoma. Int J Cancer 1997;72:424–430.
56. Janik JE, Sznol M, Urba WJ, et al. Erythropoietin production. A potential marker for interleukin-2/interferon-responsive tumors. Cancer 1993;72:2656–2659.
57. Maynard SE, Min JY, Merchan J, et al. Excess placental soluble fms-like tyrosine kinase 1 (sFlt1) may contribute to endothelial dysfunction, hypertension, and proteinuria in preeclampsia. J Clin Invest 2003;111:649–658.
58. Stauffer MH. Nephrogenic hepatosplenomegaly. Gastroenterology 1961;40:694.
59. Chuang YC, Lin AT, Chen KK, Chang YH, Chen MT, Chang LS. Paraneoplastic elevation of serum alkaline phosphatase in renal cell carcinoma: incidence and implication on prognosis. J Urol 1997;158:1684–1687.
60. Aslam Sohaib SA, Teh J, Nargund VH, Lumley JS, Hendry WF, Reznek RH. Assessment of tumor invasion of the vena caval wall in renal cell carcinoma cases by magnetic resonance imaging. J Urol 2002;167:1271–1275.
61. Koga S, Tsuda S, Nishikido M, et al. The diagnostic value of bone scan in patients with renal cell carcinoma. J Urol 2001;166: 2126–2128.
62. Thrasher JB, Paulson DF. Prognostic factors in renal cancer. Urol Clin North Am 1993;20:247–262.
63. Robson CJ, Churchill BM, Anderson W. The results of radical nephrectomy for renal cell carcinoma. 1969. J Urol 2002;167: 873–875; discussion 876–877.
64. Bassil B, Dosoretz DE, Prout GR, Jr. Validation of the tumor, nodes and metastasis classification of renal cell carcinoma. J Urol 1985;134:450–454.
65. Sobin LH, Wittekind C. TNM classification of malignant tumours, 6th edition. New York: Wiley-Liss, 2002.
66. Patel NP, Lavengood RW. Renal cell carcinoma: natural history and results of treatment. J Urol 1978;119:722–726.
67. Ramon J, Goldwasser B, Raviv G, Jonas P, Many M. Long-term results of simple and radical nephrectomy for renal cell carcinoma. Cancer 1991;67:2506–2511.
68. Gill IS, McClennan BL, Kerbl K, Carbone JM, Wick M, Clayman RV. Adrenal involvement from renal cell carcinoma: predictive value of computerized tomography. J Urol 1994;152:1082–1085.
69. Pantuck AJ, Zisman A, Dorey F, et al. Renal cell carcinoma with retroperitoneal lymph nodes. Impact on survival and benefits of immunotherapy. Cancer 2003;97:2995–3002.
70. Pantuck AJ, Zisman A, Dorey F, et al. Renal cell carcinoma with retroperitoneal lymph nodes: role of lymph node dissection. J Urol 2003;169:2076–2083.
71. Giuliani L, Giberti C, Martorana G, Rovida S. Radical extensive surgery for renal cell carcinoma: long-term results and prognostic factors. J Urol 1990;143:468–473; discussion 473–464.
72. Hatcher PA, Anderson EE, Paulson DF, Carson CC, Robertson JE. Surgical management and prognosis of renal cell carcinoma invading the vena cava. J Urol 1991;145:20–23; discussion 23–24.
73. Chiappini B, Savini C, Marinelli G, et al. Cavoatrial tumor thrombus: single-stage surgical approach with profound hypothermia and circulatory arrest, including a review of the literature. J Thorac Cardiovasc Surg 2002;124:684–688.
74. Robson CJ, Churchill BM, Anderson W. The results of radical nephrectomy for renal cell carcinoma. J Urol 1969;101:297–301.
75. Robson CJ. Radical nephrectomy for renal cell carcinoma. J Urol 1963;89:37.
76. Mevorach RA, Segal AJ, Tersegno ME, Frank IN. Renal cell carcinoma: incidental diagnosis and natural history: review of 235 cases. Urology 1992;39:519–522.
77. McKiernan J, Simmons R, Katz J, Russo P. Natural history of chronic renal insufficiency after partial and radical nephrectomy. Urology 2002;59:816–820.
78. Stifelman MD, Handler T, Nieder AM, et al. Hand-assisted laparoscopy for large renal specimens: a multi-institutional study. Urology 2003;61:78–82.
79. Campbell SC, Fichtner J, Novick AC, et al. Intraoperative evaluation of renal cell carcinoma: a prospective study of the role of ultrasonography and histopathological frozen sections. J Urol 1996;155:1191–1195.
80. Sutherland SE, Resnick MI, Maclennan GT, Goldman HB. Does the size of the surgical margin in partial nephrectomy for renal cell cancer really matter? J Urol 2002;167:61–64.
81. Castilla EA, Liou LS, Abrahams NA, et al. Prognostic importance of resection margin width after nephron-sparing surgery for renal cell carcinoma. Urology 2002;60:993–997.
82. Belldegrun A, Tsui KH, deKernion JB, Smith RB. Efficacy of nephron-sparing surgery for renal cell carcinoma: analysis based on the new 1997 tumor-node-metastasis staging system. J Clin Oncol 1999;17:2868–2875.
83. Thrasher JB, Robertson JE, Paulson DF. Expanding indications for conservative renal surgery in renal cell carcinoma. Urology 1994;43:160–168.

84. Adkins KL, Chang SS, Cookson MS, Smith JA, Jr. Partial nephrectomy safely preserves renal function in patients with a solitary kidney. J Urol 2003;169:79–81.
85. Frydenberg M, Malek RS, Zincke H. Conservative renal surgery for renal cell carcinoma in von Hippel-Lindau's disease. J Urol 1993;149:461–464.
86. Fergany AF, Hafez KS, Novick AC. Long-term results of nephron sparing surgery for localized renal cell carcinoma: 10-year followup. J Urol 2000;163:442–445.
87. Campbell SC, Novick AC, Streem SB, Klein E, Licht M. Complications of nephron sparing surgery for renal tumors. J Urol 1994;151:1177–1180.
88. Rassweiler J, Tsivian A, Kumar AV, et al. Oncological safety of laparoscopic surgery for urological malignancy: experience with more than 1,000 operations. J Urol 2003;169:2072–2075.
89. Abbou CC, Cicco A, Gasman D, et al. Retroperitoneal laparoscopic versus open radical nephrectomy. J Urol 1999;161:1776–1780.
90. Gill IS, Matin SF, Desai MM, et al. Comparative analysis of laparoscopic versus open partial nephrectomy for renal tumors in 200 patients. J Urol 2003;170:64–68.
91. Nelson CP, Wolf JS, Jr. Comparison of hand assisted versus standard laparoscopic radical nephrectomy for suspected renal cell carcinoma. J Urol 2002;167:1989–1994.
92. Fentie DD, Barrett PH, Taranger LA. Metastatic renal cell cancer after laparoscopic radical nephrectomy: long-term follow-up. J Endourol 2000;14:407–411.
93. Landman J, Lento P, Hassen W, Unger P, Waterhouse R. Feasibility of pathological evaluation of morcellated kidneys after radical nephrectomy. J Urol 2000;164:2086–2089.
94. Cadeddu JA, Ono Y, Clayman RV, et al. Laparoscopic nephrectomy for renal cell cancer: evaluation of efficacy and safety: a multicenter experience. Urology 1998;52:773–777.
95. Gill IS, Schweizer D, Hobart MG, Sung GT, Klein EA, Novick AC. Retroperitoneal laparoscopic radical nephrectomy: the Cleveland clinic experience. J Urol 2000;163:1665–1670.
96. Chan DY, Cadeddu JA, Jarrett TW, Marshall FF, Kavoussi LR. Laparoscopic radical nephrectomy: cancer control for renal cell carcinoma. [comment]. J Urol 2001;166:2095–2099; discussion 2099–2100.
97. Gill IS, Novick AC, Meraney AM, et al. Laparoscopic renal cryoablation in 32 patients. Urology 2000;56:748–753.
98. Rukstalis DB, Khorsandi M, Garcia FU, Hoenig DM, Cohen JK. Clinical experience with open renal cryoablation. Urology 2001;57:34–39.
99. Farrell MA, Charboneau WJ, DiMarco DS, et al. Imaging-guided radiofrequency ablation of solid renal tumors. AJR Am J Roentgenol 2003;180:1509–1513.
100. Gervais DA, McGovern FJ, Arellano RS, McDougal WS, Mueller PR. Renal cell carcinoma: clinical experience and technical success with radio-frequency ablation of 42 tumors. Radiology 2003;226:417–424.
101. Rendon RA, Kachura JR, Sweet JM, et al. The uncertainty of radio frequency treatment of renal cell carcinoma: findings at immediate and delayed nephrectomy. [comment]. J Urol 2002;167:1587–1592.
102. Kohrmann KU, Michel MS, Gaa J, Marlinghaus E, Alken P. High intensity focused ultrasound as noninvasive therapy for multilocal renal cell carcinoma: case study and review of the literature. J Urol 2002;167:2397–2403.
103. Leibovich BC, Blute ML, Cheville JC, et al. Prediction of progression after radical nephrectomy for patients with clear cell renal cell carcinoma: a stratification tool for prospective clinical trials. Cancer 2003;97:1663–1671.
104. Kattan MW, Reuter V, Motzer RJ, Katz J, Russo P. A postoperative prognostic nomogram for renal cell carcinoma. J Urol 2001;166:63–67.
105. Zisman A, Pantuck AJ, Dorey F, et al. Mathematical model to predict individual survival for patients with renal cell carcinoma. J Clin Oncol 2002;20:1368–1374.
106. Finney R. The value of radiotherapy in the treatment of hypernephroma—a clinical trial. British J Urol 1973;45:258–269.
107. Gez E, Libes M, Bar-Deroma R, Rubinov R, Stein M, Kuten A. Postoperative irradiation in localized renal cell carcinoma: the Rambam Medical Center experience. Tumori 2002;88:500–502.
108. Pizzocaro G, Piva L, Colavita M, et al. Interferon adjuvant to radical nephrectomy in Robson stages II and III renal cell carcinoma: a multicentric randomized study. J Clin Oncol 2001;19: 425–431.
109. Messing EM, Manola J, Wilding G, et al. Phase III study of interferon alfa-NL as adjuvant treatment for resectable renal cell carcinoma: an Eastern Cooperative Oncology Group/Intergroup trial. [comment]. J Clin Oncol 2003;21:1214–1222.
110. Clark JI, Atkins MB, Urba WJ, et al. Adjuvant high-dose bolus interleukin-2 for patients with high-risk renal cell carcinoma: a cytokine working group randomized trial. J Clin Oncol 2003;21:3133–3140.
111. Childs R, Chernoff A, Contentin N, et al. Regression of metastatic renal-cell carcinoma after nonmyeloablative allogeneic peripheral-blood stem-cell transplantation. N Engl J Med 2000;343:750–758.
112. Galligioni E, Quaia M, Merlo A, et al. Adjuvant immunotherapy treatment of renal carcinoma patients with autologous tumor cells and bacillus Calmette-Guerin: five-year results of a prospective randomized study. Cancer 1996;77:2560–2566.
113. Repmann R, Goldschmidt AJ, Richter A. Adjuvant therapy of renal cell carcinoma patients with an autologous tumor cell lysate vaccine: a 5-year follow-up analysis. Anticancer Research 2003;23:969–974.
114. Jocham D, Richter A, Hoffmann L, et al. Adjuvant autologous renal tumour cell vaccine and risk of tumour progression in patients with renal-cell carcinoma after radical nephrectomy: phase III, randomised controlled trial. Lancet 2004;363:594–599.
115. Levy DA, Slaton JW, Swanson DA, Dinney CP. Stage specific guidelines for surveillance after radical nephrectomy for local renal cell carcinoma. J Urol 1998;159:1163–1167.
116. Gofrit ON, Shapiro A, Kovalski N, Landau EH, Shenfeld OZ, Pode D. Renal cell carcinoma: evaluation of the 1997 TNM system and recommendations for follow-up after surgery. Eur Urol 2001;39:669–674; discussion 675.
117. Sandock DS, Seftel AD, Resnick MI. A new protocol for the followup of renal cell carcinoma based on pathological stage. J Urol 1995;154:28–31.
118. Ljungberg B, Alamdari FI, Rasmuson T, Roos G. Follow-up guidelines for nonmetastatic renal cell carcinoma based on the occurrence of metastases after radical nephrectomy. BJU International 1999;84:405–411.
119. Elson PJ, Witte RS, Trump DL. Prognostic factors for survival in patients with recurrent or metastatic renal cell carcinoma. Cancer Res 1988;48:7310–7313.
120. Negrier S, Escudier B, Gomez F, et al. Prognostic factors of survival and rapid progression in 782 patients with metastatic renal carcinomas treated by cytokines: a report from the Groupe Francais d'Immunotherapie. Ann Oncol 2002;13:1460–1468.
121. Atzpodien J, Kuchler T, Wandert T, Reitz M. Rapid deterioration in quality of life during interleukin-2- and alpha-interferon-based home therapy of renal cell carcinoma is associated with a good outcome. Br J Cancer 2003;89:50–54.
122. Blay JY, Negrier S, Combaret V, et al. Serum level of interleukin 6 as a prognosis factor in metastatic renal cell carcinoma. Cancer Res 1992;52:3317–3322.
123. Bui MH, Seligson D, Han KR, et al. Carbonic anhydrase IX is an independent predictor of survival in advanced renal clear cell carcinoma: implications for prognosis and therapy. Clin Cancer Res 2003;9:802–811.

124. Rackley R, Novick A, Klein E, Bukowski R, McLain D, Goldfarb D. The impact of adjuvant nephrectomy on multimodality treatment of metastatic renal cell carcinoma. J Urol 1994;152:1399–1403.
125. Wolf JS, Jr., Aronson FR, Small EJ, Carroll PR. Nephrectomy for metastatic renal cell carcinoma: a component of systemic treatment regimens. [see comment]. J Surg Oncol 1994;55:7–13.
126. Fallick ML, McDermott DF, LaRock D, Long JP, Atkins MB. Nephrectomy before interleukin-2 therapy for patients with metastatic renal cell carcinoma. J Urol 1997;158:1691–1695.
127. Walther MM, Yang JC, Pass HI, Linehan WM, Rosenberg SA. Cytoreductive surgery before high dose interleukin-2 based therapy in patients with metastatic renal cell carcinoma. J Urol 1997;158:1675–1678.
128. Franklin JR, Figlin R, Rauch J, Gitlitz B, Belldegrun A. Cytoreductive surgery in the management of metastatic renal cell carcinoma: the UCLA experience. Semin Urol Oncol 1996;14:230–236.
129. Mickisch GH, Garin A, van Poppel H, et al. Radical nephrectomy plus interferon-alfa-based immunotherapy compared with interferon alfa alone in metastatic renal-cell carcinoma: a randomised trial. [comment]. Lancet 2001;358:966–970.
130. Flanigan RC, Salmon SE, Blumenstein BA, et al. Nephrectomy followed by interferon alfa-2b compared with interferon alfa-2b alone for metastatic renal-cell cancer. [comment]. N Engl J Med 2001;345:1655–1659.
131. Kozlowski JM. Management of distant solitary recurrence in the patient with renal cancer. Contralateral kidney and other sites. Urol Clin North Am 1994;21:601–624.
132. Tolia BM, Whitmore WF, Jr. Solitary metastasis from renal cell carcinoma. J Urol 1975;114:836–838.
133. Kavolius JP, Mastorakos DP, Pavlovich C, Russo P, Burt ME, Brady MS. Resection of metastatic renal cell carcinoma. J Clin Oncol 1998;16:2261–2266.
134. Bergerat JP, Herbrecht R, Dufour P, et al. Combination of recombinant interferon alpha-2a and vinblastine in advanced renal cell cancer. Cancer 1988;62:2320–2324.
135. Pyrhonen S, Salminen E, Ruutu M, et al. Prospective randomized trial of interferon alfa-2a plus vinblastine versus vinblastine alone in patients with advanced renal cell cancer. J Clin Oncol 1999;17:2859–2867.
136. Hofmockel G, Langer W, Theiss M, Gruss A, Frohmuller HG. Immunochemotherapy for metastatic renal cell carcinoma using a regimen of interleukin-2, interferon-alpha and 5-fluorouracil. J Urol 1996;156:18–21.
137. Ellerhorst JA, Sella A, Amato RJ, et al. Phase II trial of 5-fluorouracil, interferon-alpha and continuous infusion interleukin-2 for patients with metastatic renal cell carcinoma. Cancer 1997;80:2128–2132.
138. Negrier S, Caty A, Lesimple T, et al. Treatment of patients with metastatic renal carcinoma with a combination of subcutaneous interleukin-2 and interferon alfa with or without fluorouracil. Groupe Francais d'Immunotherapie, Federation Nationale des Centres de Lutte Contre le Cancer. J Clin Oncol 2000;18:4009–4015.
139. Mertens WC, Eisenhauer EA, Moore M, et al. Gemcitabine in advanced renal cell carcinoma. A phase II study of the National Cancer Institute of Canada Clinical Trials Group. Ann Oncol 1993;4:331–332.
140. De Mulder PH, Weissbach L, Jakse G, Osieka R, Blatter J. Gemcitabine: a phase II study in patients with advanced renal cancer. Cancer Chemother Pharmacol 1996;37:491–495.
141. Rini BI, Vogelzang NJ, Dumas MC, Wade JL, 3rd, Taber DA, Stadler WM. Phase II trial of weekly intravenous gemcitabine with continuous infusion fluorouracil in patients with metastatic renal cell cancer. J Clin Oncol 2000;18:2419–2426.
142. Haas NB, Smith M, Lewis N, et al. Weekly bryostatin-1 in metastatic renal cell carcinoma: a phase II study. Clin Cancer Res 2003;9:109–114.
143. Stadler WM, Vogelzang NJ, Amato R, et al. Flavopiridol, a novel cyclin-dependent kinase inhibitor, in metastatic renal cancer: a University of Chicago Phase II Consortium study. J Clin Oncol 2000;18:371–375.
144. Townsley CA, Chi K, Ernst DS, et al. Phase II study of troxacitabine (BCH-4556) in patients with advanced and/or metastatic renal cell carcinoma: a trial of the National Cancer Institute of Canada-Clinical Trials Group. J Clin Oncol 2003;21:1524–1529.
145. Stadler WM, Kuzel T, Shapiro C, Sosman J, Clark J, Vogelzang NJ. Multi-institutional study of the angiogenesis inhibitor TNP-470 in metastatic renal carcinoma. J Clin Oncol 1999;17:2541–2545.
146. Braybrooke JP, O'Byrne KJ, Propper DJ, et al. A phase II study of razoxane, an antiangiogenic topoisomerase II inhibitor, in renal cell cancer with assessment of potential surrogate markers of angiogenesis. Clin Cancer Res 2000;6:4697–4704.
147. Bennouna J, Delva R, Gomez F, et al. A phase II study with 5-fluorouracil, folinic acid and oxaliplatin (FOLFOX-4 regimen) in patients with metastatic renal cell carcinoma. Oncology 2003;64:25–27.
148. Vuky J, Yu R, Schwartz L, Motzer RJ. Phase II trial of arsenic trioxide in patients with metastatic renal cell carcinoma. Invest New Drugs 2002;20:327–330.
149. Davis NB, Taber DA, Ansari RH, et al. Phase II trial of PS-341 in patients with renal cell cancer: a University of Chicago phase II consortium study. J Clin Oncol 2004;22:115–119.
150. Kjaer M. The role of medroxyprogesterone acetate (MPA) in the treatment of renal adenocarcinoma. Cancer Treat Rev 1988;15:195–209.
151. Cummings KB, Wheelis RF, Nelson FW. Role of hormones in growth kinetics of renal cell carcinoma in vitro. J Urol 1977;117:269–271.
152. Kriegmair M, Oberneder R, Hofstetter A. Interferon alfa and vinblastine versus medroxyprogesterone acetate in the treatment of metastatic renal cell carcinoma. Urology 1995;45:758–762.
153. Negrier S, Escudier B, Lasset C, et al. Recombinant human interleukin-2, recombinant human interferon alfa-2a, or both in metastatic renal-cell carcinoma. Groupe Francais d'Immunotherapie. N Engl J Med 1998;338:1272–1278.
154. Yang JC, Sherry RM, Steinberg SM, et al. Randomized study of high-dose and low-dose interleukin-2 in patients with metastatic renal cancer. J Clin Oncol 2003;21:3127–3132.
155. McDermott D, Flaherty L, Clark J, et al. A randomized phase III trial of high dose interleukin-2 (HD IL2) versus subcutaneous (SC) IL-2/interferon (IFN) in patients with metastatic renal cell carcinoma (RCC). J Clin Oncol 2005;23:133–141.
156. Margolin K, Aronson FR, Sznol M, et al. Phase II studies of recombinant human interleukin-4 in advanced renal cancer and malignant melanoma. J Immunother Emphasis Tumor Immunol 1994;15:147–153.
157. Weiss GR, Margolin KA, Sznol M, et al. A phase II study of the continuous intravenous infusion of interleukin-6 for metastatic renal cell carcinoma. J Immunother Emphasis Tumor Immunol 1995;18:52–56.
158. Atkins MB, Robertson MJ, Gordon M, et al. Phase I evaluation of intravenous recombinant human interleukin 12 in patients with advanced malignancies. Clin Cancer Res 1997;3:409–417.
159. Motzer RJ, Rakhit A, Schwartz LH, et al. Phase I trial of subcutaneous recombinant human interleukin-12 in patients with advanced renal cell carcinoma. Clin Cancer Res 1998;4:1183–1191.
160. Motzer RJ, Rakhit A, Thompson JA, et al. Randomized multicenter phase II trial of subcutaneous recombinant human interleukin-12 versus interferon-alpha 2a for patients with advanced renal cell carcinoma. J Interferon Cytokine Res 2001;21:257–263.

161. Rini BI, Paintal A, Vogelzang NJ, Gajewski TF, Stadler WM. Flt-3 ligand and sequential FL/interleukin-2 in patients with metastatic renal carcinoma: clinical and biologic activity. J Immunother 2002;25:269–277.
162. Nathan PD, Eisen TG. The biological treatment of renal-cell carcinoma and melanoma. Lancet Oncol 2002;3:89–96.
163. Minasian LM, Motzer RJ, Gluck L, Mazumdar M, Vlamis V, Krown SE. Interferon alfa-2a in advanced renal cell carcinoma: treatment results and survival in 159 patients with long-term follow-up. J Clin Oncol 1993;11:1368–1375.
164. Motzer RJ, Bacik J, Murphy BA, Russo P, Mazumdar M. Interferon-alfa as a comparative treatment for clinical trials of new therapies against advanced renal cell carcinoma. J Clin Oncol 2002;20:289–296.
165. Fossa S, Jones M, Johnson P, et al. Interferon-alpha and survival in renal cell cancer. Br J Urol 1995;76:286–290.
166. Muss HB, Costanzi JJ, Leavitt R, et al. Recombinant alfa interferon in renal cell carcinoma: a randomized trial of two routes of administration. J Clin Oncol 1987;5:286–291.
167. Fossa SD, Martinelli G, Otto U, et al. Recombinant interferon alfa-2a with or without vinblastine in metastatic renal cell carcinoma: results of a European multi-center phase III study. Ann Oncol 1992;3:301–305.
168. Garnick MB, Reich SD, Maxwell B, Coval-Goldsmith S, Richie JP, Rudnick SA. Phase I/II study of recombinant interferon gamma in advanced renal cell carcinoma. J Urol 1988;139:251–255.
169. Motzer RJ, Murphy BA, Bacik J, et al. Phase III trial of interferon alfa-2a with or without 13-cis-retinoic acid for patients with advanced renal cell carcinoma. J Clin Oncol 2000;18:2972–2980.
170. Wagstaff J, Smith D, Nelmes P, Loynds P, Crowther D. A phase I study of recombinant interferon gamma administered by s.c. injection three times per week in patients with solid tumours. Cancer Immunol Immunother 1987;25:54–58.
171. De Mulder PH, Oosterhof G, Bouffioux C, van Oosterom AT, Vermeylen K, Sylvester R. EORTC (30885) randomised phase III study with recombinant interferon alpha and recombinant interferon alpha and gamma in patients with advanced renal cell carcinoma. The EORTC Genitourinary Group. Br J Cancer 1995;71:371–375.
172. Sagaster P, Micksche M, Flamm J, Ludwig H. Randomised study using IFN-alpha versus IFN-alpha plus coumarin and cimetidine for treatment of advanced renal cell cancer. Ann Oncol 1995;6:999–1003.
173. Sertoli MR, Brunetti I, Ardizzoni A, et al. Recombinant alpha-2a interferon plus vinblastine in the treatment of metastatic renal cell carcinoma. Am J Clin Oncol 1989;12:43–45.
174. Shih SC, Claffey KP. Role of AP-1 and HIF-1 transcription factors in TGF-beta activation of VEGF expression. Growth Factors 2001;19:19–34.
175. Motzer RJ, Schwartz L, Law TM, et al. Interferon alfa-2a and 13-cis-retinoic acid in renal cell carcinoma: antitumor activity in a phase II trial and interactions in vitro. J Clin Oncol 1995;13:1950–1957.
176. Rosenberg SA, Lotze MT, Muul LM, et al. A progress report on the treatment of 157 patients with advanced cancer using lymphokine-activated killer cells and interleukin-2 or high-dose interleukin-2 alone. N Engl J Med 1987;316:889–897.
177. West WH, Tauer KW, Yannelli JR, et al. Constant-infusion recombinant interleukin-2 in adoptive immunotherapy of advanced cancer. N Engl J Med 1987;316:898–905.
178. Rosenberg SA, Yang JC, Topalian SL, et al. Treatment of 283 consecutive patients with metastatic melanoma or renal cell cancer using high-dose bolus interleukin 2. JAMA 1994;271:907–913.
179. Rosenberg SA, Lotze MT, Yang JC, et al. Prospective randomized trial of high-dose interleukin-2 alone or in conjunction with lymphokine-activated killer cells for the treatment of patients with advanced cancer. J Natl Cancer Inst 1993;85:622–632.
180. Law TM, Motzer RJ, Mazumdar M, et al. Phase III randomized trial of interleukin-2 with or without lymphokine-activated killer cells in the treatment of patients with advanced renal cell carcinoma. Cancer 1995;76:824–832.
181. Fyfe G, Fisher RI, Rosenberg SA, Sznol M, Parkinson DR, Louie AC. Results of treatment of 255 patients with metastatic renal cell carcinoma who received high-dose recombinant interleukin-2 therapy. J Clin Oncol 1995;13:688–696.
182. Fisher RI, Rosenberg SA, Sznol M, Parkinson DR, Fyfe G. High-dose aldesleukin in renal cell carcinoma: long-term survival update. Cancer J Sci Am 1997;3 Suppl 1:S70–72.
183. Motzer RJ, Berg W, Ginsberg M, et al. Phase II trial of thalidomide for patients with advanced renal cell carcinoma. J Clin Oncol 2002;20:302–306.
184. Stebbing J, Benson C, Eisen T, et al. The treatment of advanced renal cell cancer with high-dose oral thalidomide. Br J Cancer 2001;85:953–958.
185. Escudier B, Lassau N, Couanet D, et al. Phase II trial of thalidomide in renal-cell carcinoma. Ann Oncol 2002;13:1029–1035.
186. Minor DR, Monroe D, Damico LA, Meng G, Suryadevara U, Elias L. A phase II study of thalidomide in advanced metastatic renal cell carcinoma. Invest New Drugs 2002;20:389–393.
187. Daliani DD, Papandreou CN, Thall PF, et al. A pilot study of thalidomide in patients with progressive metastatic renal cell carcinoma. Cancer 2002;95:758–765.
188. Gordon MS, Manola J, Fairclough DL, et al. Low dose interferon-α2b (IFN) + thalidomide (T) in patients (pts) with previously untreated renal cell cancer (RCC). Improvement in progression-free survival (PFS) but not quality of life (QoL) or overall survival (OS). A phase III study of the Eastern Cooperative Oncology Group (E2898). Proc Am Soc Clin Oncol 2004;22: 4516, 386s.
189. Figlin RA, Thompson JA, Bukowski RM, et al. Multicenter, randomized, phase III trial of CD8(+) tumor-infiltrating lymphocytes in combination with recombinant interleukin-2 in metastatic renal cell carcinoma. J Clin Oncol 1999;17:2521–2529.
190. Holtl L, Rieser C, Papesh C, et al. Cellular and humoral immune responses in patients with metastatic renal cell carcinoma after vaccination with antigen pulsed dendritic cells. J Urol 1999;161:777–782.
191. Kugler A, Stuhler G, Walden P, et al. Regression of human metastatic renal cell carcinoma after vaccination with tumor cell-dendritic cell hybrids. Nat Med 2000;6:332–336.
192. Hernandez JM, Bui MH, Han KR, et al. Novel kidney cancer immunotherapy based on the granulocyte-macrophage colony-stimulating factor and carbonic anhydrase IX fusion gene. Clin Cancer Res 2003;9:1906–1916.
193. Marten A, Renoth S, Heinicke T, et al. Allogeneic dendritic cells fused with tumor cells: preclinical results and outcome of a clinical phase I/II trial in patients with metastatic renal cell carcinoma. Hum Gene Ther 2003;14:483–494.
194. Su Z, Dannull J, Heiser A, et al. Immunological and clinical responses in metastatic renal cancer patients vaccinated with tumor RNA-transfected dendritic cells. Cancer Res 2003;63: 2127–2133.
195. Slavin S, Nagler A, Naparstek E, et al. Nonmyeloablative stem cell transplantation and cell therapy as an alternative to conventional bone marrow transplantation with lethal cytoreduction for the treatment of malignant and nonmalignant hematologic diseases. Blood 1998;91:756–763.
196. Hentschke P, Barkholt L, Uzunel M, et al. Low-intensity conditioning and hematopoietic stem cell transplantation in patients with renal and colon carcinoma. Bone Marrow Transplant 2003;31:253–261.
197. Khouri IF, Keating M, Korbling M, et al. Transplant-lite: induction of graft-versus-malignancy using fludarabine-based nonablative chemotherapy and allogeneic blood progenitor-cell

transplantation as treatment for lymphoid malignancies. J Clin Oncol 1998;16:2817–2824.
198. George DJ, Kaelin WG, Jr. The von Hippel-Lindau protein, vascular endothelial growth factor, and kidney cancer. N Engl J Med 2003;349:419–421.
199. Yang JC, Haworth L, Sherry RM, et al. A randomized trial of bevacizumab, an anti-vascular endothelial growth factor antibody, for metastatic renal cancer. N Engl J Med 2003;349:427–434.
200. Hainsworth JD, Sosman J, Spigel DR, et al. Phase II trial of bevacizumab and erlotinib in patients with metastatic renal carcinoma (RCC). Proc Am Soc Clin Oncol 2004;22:4502, 382s.
201. Mandel JS, McLaughlin JK, Schlehofer B, et al. International renal-cell cancer study. IV. Occupation. Int J Cancer 1995;61:601–605.
202. Ono Y, Kinukawa T, Hattori R, et al. Laparoscopic radical nephrectomy for renal cell carcinoma: a five-year experience. Urology 1999;53:280–286.
203. Kim FJ, Rha KH, Hernandez F, Jarrett TW, Pinto PA, Kavoussi LR. Laparoscopic radical versus partial nephrectomy: assessment of complications. J Urol 2003;170:408–411.
204. Atzpodien J, Lopez Hanninen E, Kirchner H, et al. Multiinstitutional home-therapy trial of recombinant human interleukin-2 and interferon alfa-2 in progressive metastatic renal cell carcinoma. J Clin Oncol 1995;13:497–501.
205. Sleijfer DT, Janssen RA, Buter J, de Vries EG, Willemse PH, Mulder NH. Phase II study of subcutaneous interleukin-2 in unselected patients with advanced renal cell cancer on an outpatient basis. J Clin Oncol 1992;10:1119–1123.
206. Figlin RA, Belldegrun A, Moldawer N, Zeffren J, deKernion J. Concomitant administration of recombinant human interleukin-2 and recombinant interferon alfa-2A: an active outpatient regimen in metastatic renal cell carcinoma. J Clin Oncol 1992;10:414–421.
207. Rini BI, Zimmerman T, Stadler WM, Gajewski TF, Vogelzang NJ. Allogeneic stem-cell transplantation of renal cell cancer after nonmyeloablative chemotherapy: feasibility, engraftment, and clinical results. J Clin Oncol 2002;20:2017–2024.
208. Bregni M, Dodero A, Peccatori J, et al. Nonmyeloablative conditioning followed by hematopoietic cell allografting and donor lymphocyte infusions for patients with metastatic renal and breast cancer. Blood 2002;99:4234–4236.
209. Dunn MD, Portis AJ, Shalhav AL, et al. Laparoscopic versus open radical nephrectomy: a 9-year experience. J Urol 2000;164(4):1153–1159.
210. McLaughlin JK, Lindblad P, Mellemgaard A, et al. International renal-cell cancer study. I. Tobacco use. Int J Cancer 1995;60(2):194–198.
211. Hunt JD, van der Hel OI, McMillan GP, Boffetta P, Brennan P. Renal cell carcinoma in relation to cigarette smoking: meta-analysis of 24 studies. Int J Cancer 2005;11:101–108.
212. Kreiger N, Marrett LD, Dodds L, Hilditch S, Darlington GA. Risk factors for renal cell carcinoma: results of a population-based case-control study. Cancer Causes Control 1993;4(2):101–110.
213. Weinmann S, Glass AG, Weiss NS, Psaty BM, Siscovick DS, White E. Use of diuretics and other antihypertensive medications in relation to the risk of renal cell cancer. Am J Epidemiol 1994;140(9):792–804.
214. Weirich G, Glenn G, Junker K, et al. Familial renal oncocytoma: clinicopathological study of 5 families. J Urol 1998;160:335–340.
215. Malchoff CD, Sarfarazi M, Tendler B, et al. Papillary thyroid carcinoma associated with papillary renal neoplasia: genetic linkage analysis of a distinct heritable tumor syndrome. J Clin Endocrinol Metab 2000;85(5):1758–1764.
216. Aarnio M, Mecklin JP, Aaltonen LA, Nystrom-Lahti M, Jarvinen HJ. Life-time risk of different cancers in hereditary non-polyposis colorectal cancer (HNPCC) syndrome. Int J Cancer 1995;64:430–433.
217. Motzer RJ, Rini BI, Michaelson MD, et al. Phase 2 trials of SU11248 show antitumor activity in second-line therapy for patients with metastatic renal cell carcinoma (RCC). J Clin Oncol 2005;23:4508 (abstract), 380s.
218. Rini B, Rixe O, Bukowski R, et al. AG-013736, a multi-target tyrosine kinase receptor inhibitor, demonstrates anti-tumor activity in a Phase 2 study of cytokine-refractory, metastatic renal cell cancer (RCC). J Clin Oncol 2005;23:4509 (abstract), 380s.
219. Escudier B, Szezylik C, Eisen T, et al. Randomized phase III trial of the Raf kinase and VEGFR inhibitor sorafenib (BAY 43-9006) in patients with advanced renal cell carcinoma (RCC). J Clin Oncol 2005;23:4510 (abstract), 380s.
220. Atkins MB, Hidalgo M, Stadler WM, et al. Randomized phase II study of multiple dose levels of CCI-779, a novel mammalian target of rapamycin kinase inhibitor, in patients with advanced refractory renal cell carcinoma. J Clin Oncol 2004;22(5):909–918.

47

Ureter, Bladder, Penis, and Urethra

Cheryl T. Lee, Brent Hollenbeck, and David P. Wood, Jr.

Evidence-based clinical medicine has been proven to produce the best outcomes.[1] Unfortunately, many tumor sites do not have adequate randomized clinical trials to provide the necessary data to reach treatment and diagnostic consensus. The ureter, bladder, penis, and urethra fall into this category. There are several reasons for a lack of randomized clinical trials in these sites, but the primary reason is the relatively low incidence of each tumor. Of these tumors, bladder cancer has the highest incidence (16 per 100,000 people), followed by ureteral cancer (10 per 100,000) and subsequently penis and urethra (less than 2 per 100,000)[2]; this is in contrast to prostate cancer, which has an incidence of 75 per 100,000 men.[2] Despite the limited randomized clinical trials in these sites, there are excellent Phase II clinical and historical trials that can shed light on management of these rare tumors.

In this chapter we describe the etiology, basic science, pathology, prognostic factors, screening tests, diagnostic tests, and treatment for cancer of the ureter, bladder, penis, and urethra. The ureter, bladder, and urethra are discussed as one tumor type as they are all components of transitional cell carcinoma (TCCa). Penile cancer is considered separately.

Ureter, Bladder, and Urethra

Etiology

Many data suggest that bladder cancers are carcinogen induced.[3] Factors reported to be causally related to bladder cancer include occupational chemicals, tobacco, coffee, analgesic abuse, artificial sweeteners, bladder calculi, pelvic irradiation, and certain types of chemotherapeutic agents. Inhaled or ingested carcinogens are filtered by the kidney and concentrated in the urine where they are stored in the bladder for prolonged periods of time before excretion. Repeated exposure of the urothelium to these carcinogens can lead to genetic alteration and tumor formation. Multiple lesions or genetic mutations are likely required to cause malignant transformation of the urothelium, as evidenced by the multitude of chromosomal abnormalities recorded in TCCa.[4,5]

The most common environmental exposure that promotes bladder cancer is tobacco.[6] Cigarette smokers have a fourfold higher incidence of bladder cancer than nonsmokers do. The risk correlates with the number of cigarettes smoked, the duration of smoking, and the degree of inhalation. Although males are more commonly affected with TCCa than females (3 to 1 ratio), this ratio has decreased as women have increased their tobacco use. An estimated one-third of bladder cancer cases may be caused by cigarette smoking. The specific chemical carcinogen is unknown; however, nitrosamine has been implicated. Occupational exposures also increase the risk of urothelial malignancies. Aniline dyes containing xenylamine and benzidine, for example, are known urothelial carcinogens in humans and in animals.[7]

Genetic mutations appear to play an important role in formation of TCCa.[4] Figure 47.1 illustrates consensus genetic changes that occur in bladder cancer.[4,8] Bladder cancer is typically stratified into superficial and invasive tumors. Superficial tumors have a high recurrence rate but invade and metastasize in a minority of cases. Conversely, invasive TCCa has a highly metastatic potential. Genetic mutations appear different in the two tumor types. Superficial bladder cancers are typically associated with loss of 9q, ink4A, and p16; invasive tumors have loss of p53, Rb, p14, and p16. Several monoclonal tests have been developed to detect these markers in urine, but the reproducibility is unclear.

Pathology

As with many tumors, pathologic evaluation of TCCa is critical in determining appropriate therapy. The pathology description for TCCa is divided into grade (1 to 3) and stage (Tis to T4).[9] Grade is associated with the aggressiveness of the disease, whereas stage is a reflection of the time the tumor has been present and its ability to metastasis. Tumor staging is generally based on the TNM system (Table 47.1). The T stage is defined by the depth of invasion into the bladder, ureteral, or urethral wall. Nodal disease is based on number as well as location of metastatic lymph nodes. Metastatic sites most commonly involve lung, bone, and liver. *Clinically, the precise TNM stage is used rather than the overall stage.* Recently, the World Health Organization (WHO) has reclassified superficial bladder cancer from grades 1 to 3 to low malignant potential tumors to high malignant tumors.[10] Low malignant potential TCCa has a high recurrence rate (60% to 80%) but a low rate of invasion (less than 10%). Conversely, high malignant potential superficial bladder cancer has a high risk of recurrence and invasion (70%). Treatment decisions are highly predicated on the pathology.

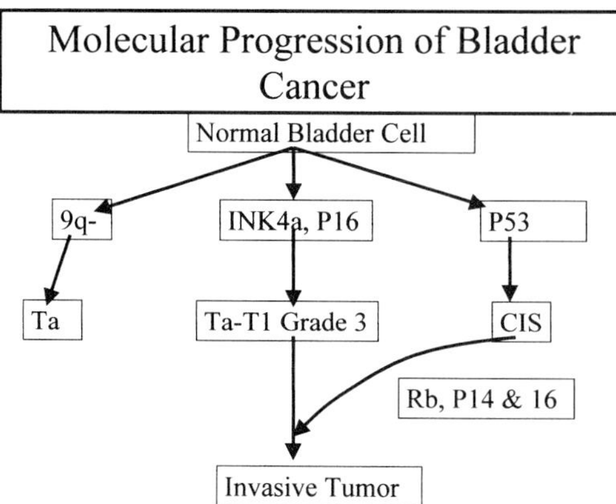

FIGURE 47.1. Bladder cancer progression.

Prognostic Factors

Multiple factors may influence the prognosis of bladder cancer. Pathologic parameters have been studied in great depth and have traditionally been the primary means of predicting prognosis. More recently, an increased study of molecular alterations and disease outcome has led to novel approaches to therapy and methods for patient stratification.

Pathologic Factors

Although grade and presence of vascular invasion have been proposed as predictors of adverse outcome,[11] pathologic stage is the most powerful predictor of survival outcome. Increased stage, particularly extravesical disease and nodal or visceral involvement, results in diminished survival when compared to organ-confined disease.[12–14] Despite the excellent 87% to 97% local control provided by radical cystectomy, metastatic recurrence in patients with extravesical disease is common.[12,15] The respective 10-year overall survival (OS) of 54%, 22%, 22%, and 23% for organ-confined, pT3, pT4a, and N+ disease has been demonstrated in a large retrospective series of 1,054 patients.[12] Pretreatment clinical predictors of extravesical disease include hydronephrosis and a palpable mass on bimanual examination. Unilateral and bilateral hydronephrosis are associated with T3–T4, N– disease in 33% and 36%, and metastatic disease in 34% and 55%, respectively.[16] Although bimanual examination is believed to correlate with extravesical or unresectable tumors, there remains a paucity of data confirming its sensitivity and specificity apart from other clinical staging.[17,18]

For earlier-stage cT1 disease, the depth of penetration is also an important predictor of progression and death from bladder cancer. In a prospective, nonrandomized study of 121 patients with cT1 disease, tumor penetration of the muscularis mucosa (T1b) was associated with a 53% risk of

TABLE 47.1. The 2002 American Joint Committee on Cancer (AJCC) staging of bladder cancer: TNM definitions.

Primary tumor (T)	
TX	Primary tumor cannot be assessed
T0	No evidence of primary tumor
Ta	Noninvasive papillary carcinoma
Tis	Carcinoma in situ: "flat tumor"
T1	Tumor invades subepithelial connective tissue
T2	Tumor invades muscle
pT2a	Tumor invades superficial muscle (inner half)
pT2b	Tumor invades deep muscle (outer half)
T3	Tumor invades perivesical tissue
pT3a	Microscopically
pT3b	Macroscopically (extravesical mass)
T4	Tumor invades any of the following: prostate, uterus, vagina, pelvic wall, or abdominal wall
T4a	Tumor invades the prostate, uterus, vagina
T4b	Tumor invades the pelvic wall, abdominal wall
Regional lymph nodes (N)	
NX	Regional lymph nodes cannot be assessed
N0	No regional lymph node metastasis
N1	Metastasis in a single lymph node, 2 cm or less in greatest dimension
N2	Metastasis in a single lymph node, more than 2 cm but not more than 5 cm in greatest dimension; or multiple lymph nodes, none more than 5 cm in greatest dimension
N3	Metastasis in a lymph node, more than 5 cm in greatest dimension
Distant metastasis (M)	
MX	Distant metastasis cannot be assessed
M0	No distant metastasis
M1	Distant metastasis

Source: Used with the permission of the American Joint Committee on Cancer (AJCC), Chicago, Illinois. The original source for this material is the *AJCC Cancer Staging Manual*, sixth Edition (2002), published by Springer-Verlag New York, www.springer-ny.com.

progression compared with a 31% risk with superficial penetration (T1a) of the lamina propria (P less than 0.05).[19] At a minimum of 5 years of follow-up, death from bladder cancer occurred in 44% of T1a and 23% of T1b patients (P less than 0.05).

Molecular Markers

p53

In an effort to complement prognostic information obtained from pathologic and imaging criteria, several molecules important in cancer biology have been explored. The most extensively studied marker in bladder cancer is the tumor suppressor gene p53. Upregulation of p53 protein induces cell-cycle arrest, which allows repair of damaged DNA. Mutations result in accumulation of abnormal protein in the cell nucleus. The suspected importance of this gene began with observations of p53 mutations in a high proportion of bladder cancers.[20] Detection of nuclear p53 staining by immunohistochemistry has been independently associated with diminished survival after cystectomy or systemic chemotherapy.[21–23] Other studies have demonstrated a correlation between nuclear accumulation of p53 protein and bladder cancer progression and an increased risk of disease recurrence and decreased overall survival (OS).[24,25] These findings have provided the rationale for a randomized study from the University of Southern California for patients with organ-confined bladder cancer (stage pT1–pT2) and p53 mutations. Patients with p53-positive tumors are randomized to three cycles of MVAC (methotrexate, vinblastine, doxorubicin, cisplatin) or observation after radical cystectomy.

Epidermal Growth Factor Receptor

Epidermal growth factor receptor (EGFR) is a transmembrane receptor tyrosine kinase that is overexpressed in bladder cancer. EGFR activation influences cellular proliferation and the cell cycle, and affects other cellular processes, including angiogenesis, apoptosis, motility, adhesion, invasion, and metastasis.[26] Bladder tumors that overexpress EGFR are more likely to recur, progress to muscle-invasion, and have diminished survival.[27,28] In other reports, however, EGFR expression has not been associated with tumor progression or survival.[29]

HER2-Neu

The HER-2/neu proto-oncogene encodes a transmembrane receptor kinase. Overexpression of HER2, seen in 30% of bladder tumors,[30] has been correlated with increased tumor grade and is an independent prognostic factor of tumor-specific survival.[31] Further, overexpression of HER2 in primary tumors is predictive of increased HER2 expression in metastases.[30] Currently, however, it is unclear whether HER2 expression levels provide any additional prognostic information over tumor stage and grade for bladder cancer.[32,33] The availability of therapeutic antibodies to the HER2 protein has resulted in several ongoing clinical trials to determine the efficacy of these agents in advanced bladder cancer patients.

Other markers outlined in Table 47.2 may have potential prognostic benefit in bladder cancer. A great deal of preclinical investigation continues to delineate the impact of alteration of these markers and the resultant clinical implication. Unfortunately, none of these molecular prognostic markers has been confirmed to be useful for clinical decision making at this time.[34] With the continued development of relevant therapeutics, patient benefit will be assessed through neoadjuvant studies in surgical patients and treatment trials in the advanced disease state.

TABLE 47.2. Prognostic markers of bladder cancer.

Marker	*Biological function*	*Potential prognostic value*
T138	Tumor-associated antigen	Association with progression and metastasis, diagnostic marker
ABO	Blood group antigens	Diagnostic marker, association with progression in secretory individuals
c-H-*ras*, c-*myc*, c-*erb*-B2, mdm-2	Oncogenes	Prognosticators of disease recurrence (ras) or survival (erb), correlation with tumor grade (erb, myc) or metastasis (erb)
Rb, p53, p21, p27	Cell-cycle regulators	Correlation with progression/survival (Rb), markers of progression (p53) or recurrence and survival (p21, p53), association with tumor grade and survival (p27)
Ki-67, PCNA, MCM	Proliferation-associated antigens	Markers of recurrence, progression, and survival (Ki-67), correlation with recurrence (PCNA) and grade (MCM)
Vessel density, thrombspondin-1	Angiogenesis and inhibitors of angiogenesis	Markers of progression (V.d.), recurrence (Thromb-1) and survival (V.d., Thromb-1)
Cadherins, integrins, Ig-super family	Cell adhesion molecules	Association with metastasis, tumor grade and stage (E-cadherin) and survival (E-cadherin, integrins)
Laminin-P1, cathepsin D, U-PA, matrix-metalloproteases and -inhibitors	Extracellular matrix proteases	Correlation with tumor size and number (laminin), association with survival (Cathepsin D) or metastasis (u-PA), correlation with tumor stage, grade, and survival (MMPs)
EGFR	Growth factor receptors	Correlation with recurrence and progression
EGF, FGF, TGF-α, TGF-β, VEGF	Peptide growth factors	Correlation with survival (EGF, TGF-α), or tumor stage, grade and recurrence (FGF, VEGF)
Bcl2, Bax, Fas, Fas-L, survivin	Markers of apoptosis	Correlation with recurrence (survivin, bcl-2/bax) or survival (Fas)
CD44	Cell–cell/matrix interactions	Correlation with survival, diagnostic value

Source: Adapted from Kausch and Böhle,[34] by permission of *European Urology*.

TABLE 47.3. Selected diagnostic urinary tests.

	Sensitivity (%)	*Specificity (%)*
BTA	41–83	72–95
BTA trak	54–78	95–97
BTA stat	75–90	72–95
BTF	80	75
FDP	82	86–96
FISH	81	>95
HA/HAase	86–92	84–92
ImmunoCyt	86–95	90
Microsatellite DNA (ex. MAUS)	89	100
NMP-22	47–100	60–90
TRAP (telomerase)	50–100	80–90
Urine cytology	20–58	>95

BTA, bladder tumor antigen; BTF, bladder tumor fibronectin; FDP, fibrin degradation product; FISH, fluorescent in situ hybridization; HA, hyaluronic acid; HAase, hyaluronidase; MAUS, microsatellite analysis of urinary sediment; NMP22, nuclear matrix protein 22; TRAP, telomeric repeat amplification protocol.

Screening

Although cystoscopy remains the "gold standard" for diagnosis, it is not a good tool for general bladder cancer screening because it is invasive and expensive. Urine cytology uses a morphologic assessment to evaluate cells shed in the urine. The very favorable 97% to 99% specificity is offset by its lack of sensitivity, particularly suboptimal for low-grade tumors, and also limits its use as a general screening tool. Several noninvasive tests have been developed to augment the sensitivity of urine cytology while maintaining the specificity (Table 47.3). Although several of these tests have been investigated for general screening, the use has primarily been in screening for tumor recurrence in patients with a prior diagnosis of bladder cancer. Currently, there is not a clear consensus on the clinical utility of many of these markers.

Fluorescent In Situ Hybridization

Fluorescent in situ hybridization (FISH) uses fluorescently labeled centromeric and locus-specific DNA probes to detect chromosomal abnormalities in exfoliated cells in the urine, specifically looking at chromosomes 17, 3, 7, and 9p21. The specificity rivals urine cytology at 96%.[35] The sensitivity for Ta tumors is 65%, for Tis is 100%, and for T1–T4 is 95%. This technique is much more sensitive at picking up invasive disease as nearly all tumors of T1 or above have multiple chromosomal alterations. FISH may also allow earlier detection of tumors than urine cytology.

BTA Stat

The BTA Stat test is a qualitative test performed on voided urine. It measures "bladder tumor antigen" complement factor H-related proteins and is relatively easy to interpret, although weak positive results can be difficult. BTA has a higher sensitivity than urine cytology and a similar specificity.[1]

Fibrin/Fibrinogen Degradation Product (FDP)

Fibrin/fibrinogen degradation product (FDP) was introduced for the detection of occult and rapidly recurring disease after transurethral resection of bladder tumor (TURBT). FDP assesses fibronectin fragments excreted in urine.[37] These fibrin products are widely distributed on cells involved in the mechanism of human bladder cancer cell invasion.

Nuclear Matrix Protein (NMP)

Nuclear matrix protein (NMP) is a quantitative test that measures tumor-related proteins in urine. Nuclear matrix proteins make up portions of the nuclear structure, organize chromatin, regulate critical aspects of mitosis, and are elevated in patients with active TCCa of bladder.[38]

Microsatellite Analysis of Urinary Sediment (MAUS)

Although not currently approved for surveillance in bladder cancer, microsatellite analysis of urinary sediment (MAUS) markers may be useful as clonal markers for the detection of human cancer. Microsatellite analysis can detect loss of heterozygosity and may reveal genetic instability marked by areas of increased repetition of DNA sequences. The test is based on the detection of exfoliated urothelial cells with genetic alterations consistent with specifically identified microsatellite regions common in TCCa.[39] It, too, may provide early tumor detection by examining the DNA of urinary sediment.

Telomeric Repeat Amplification Protocol (TRAP)

Telomeric repeat amplification protocol (TRAP) detects telomerase activity. Telomerase plays an important role in cellular immortalization and oncogenesis, is a marker for carcinogenesis, and has increased expression in bladder cancer patients. It has a higher sensitivity in bladder washings than in voided urines[40] and is a promising tool.

Diagnosis

The majority of patients diagnosed with bladder cancer have signs or symptoms. Typically, gross painless hematuria is present but may be associated with urgency, frequency, and dysuria, all signs of bladder cancer, particularly carcinoma in situ (CIS). The signs associated with advanced TCCa are a palpable mass in the abdomen, a urethral mass, urethral spotting, or bone pain. The tumor site may be suggested by the timing of gross hematuria. Initial gross hematuria is likely associated with a urethral abnormality, whereas midstream hematuria is associated with a bladder abnormality, and finally late or terminal hematuria may be associated with a ureteral lesion.

The evaluation required to make the diagnosis of TCCa is a combination of endoscopic and radiologic techniques. For patients with gross or microscopic hematuria, imaging of the upper urinary tracts and the bladder is required. The American Urological Association recently published a summary of the best practice policies for the evaluation of symptomatic microscopic hematuria.[41] Upper tract imaging with an intravenous pyelogram (IVP) or computerized tomography (CT) scan is recommended. An office cystoscopy to evaluate the bladder mucosa and a urine cytology to detect malignant cells complete the evaluation. For patients with invasive tumors, appropriate metastatic evaluation consists of a chest X-ray,

CT scan of abdomen and pelvis, and a bone scan, if the serum alkaline phosphatase is elevated or bone symptoms exist.

Upper tract abnormalities on imaging studies should prompt retrograde pyelography and ureteroscopic evaluation with ureteral cytology and washings as well as biopsy of suspicious areas. The endoscopic evaluation may provide valuable clarification of tumor histology, grade, and, potentially, stage; however, ureteroscopic biopsy can be hampered by small fragments that leave one relying on visual inspection. Transurethral resection of bladder tumor (TURBT), performed under general or regional anesthesia, is mandatory to obtain pathologic diagnosis and staging of any bladder lesion identified on cystoscopy. It should include an examination under anesthesia (EUA) and sampling of the bladder muscular wall to fully assess depth of invasion. It may also be appropriate to biopsy multiple areas of mucosa to identify multifocal CIS.

Treatment of Bladder Cancer

The treatment of bladder cancer can be complex and frequently involves a combination of surgery and chemotherapy/immunotherapy or radiation. Treatment approach is essentially a reflection of tumor behavior patterns, which are commonly stage specific. For nonmetastatic disease, the goals of therapy include complete tumor resection followed by adjuvant treatments, when appropriate, that will diminish the risk of tumor recurrence and progression.

Early-Stage Disease: Ta/Tis/T1

Transurethral Resection

The initial treatment of all bladder tumors generally begins with TURBT. Resection of all visible tumor, when possible, is performed, with care taken to assess detrusor muscle below the lesion. For extensive but clearly well-differentiated papillary tumors, staged endoscopic resections may be necessary for complete tumor excision. Large or bulky tumors may not be feasible to remove with TURBT, and thus deep biopsies are taken for purposes of staging.

Restaging TURBT within 2 to 6 weeks is recommended in the patient with incomplete, undersampled, or uncertain resection. This repeat is especially important in the patient with Tis, Ta, or T1 disease, as well as the patient with suspected T2 disease who is being considered for a bladder preservation treatment strategy. Up to 29% of patients thought to have superficial or early-stage disease may be upstaged and 22% of individuals believed to have muscle-invasive disease may be downstaged, ultimately altering treatment in 33% of patients.[42] Rates of residual tumor detected by the second TURBT are 55% to 76% for all stages sampled.[43] For cT1 disease, a 33% to 78% residual tumor rate is detected if muscle is present in the sample for evaluation; up to 28% of these patients are upstaged to muscle-invasive disease. If muscle is absent, up to 83% will be upstaged on the restaging TURBT when muscle is ultimately sampled.

Disease recurrence rates of superficial and early invasive bladder cancer after TURBT range from 50% to 70%, and progression rates range from 5% to 40%.[44] Thus, TURBT is limited as the sole treatment for early-stage disease. Patients at increased risk of both disease recurrence and progression include those with (1) invasion into the lamina propria (cT1), (2) high-grade disease, (3) multifocal tumors, and (4) associated CIS. Adjuvant treatments are generally applied to high-risk patients or low-risk patients with recurrent disease.

Intravesical Therapy

Intravesical treatments are the primary adjunctive strategies aimed at reducing recurrence and possibly progression after TURBT (Table 47.4). Intravesical treatment is desirable as the risk of systemic absorption is generally low; however, local side effects can result in significant irritative symptoms. Intravesical chemotherapy used in conjunction with TURBT can reduce the risk of recurrence by 44% to 73% in patients with primary Ta and T1 tumors and by 38% to 65% in patients with recurrent Ta, T1, and Tis tumors when compared to TURBT alone.[45,46]

Bacillus Calmette–Guérin (BCG) is an attenuated strain of *Mycobacterium bovis* that has stimulatory effects on immune responses.[47] Intravesical immunotherapy using BCG provides a significant reduction in recurrence that is greater than 50% in patients with superficial and early invasive disease and may also improve progression.[48,49] Several randomized Phase III studies support the use of BCG as a first-line intravesical agent (see Table 47.4). The Southwest Oncology Group studied intravesical and percutaneous BCG versus intravesical doxorubicin in patients with rapidly recurrent Ta, Tis, and T1 disease.[50] This study demonstrated a significantly improved 5-year disease-free survival (DFS) for patients treated with BCG as compared to doxorubicin. The 45% DFS in patients with CIS was quite encouraging and was confirmed in another prospective randomized study in which BCG was found to be superior to doxorubicin and thiotepa in DFS and progression-free survival for superficial tumors.[51] A subsequent randomized Phase III study by the EORTC demonstrated the superiority of intravesical BCG over epirubicin.[52] The addition of percutaneous BCG to intravesical therapy does not increase treatment efficacy, and its use has been abandoned.[53]

Despite improved rates of DFS, standard induction courses of intravesical chemotherapy and immunotherapy do not improve disease-specific survival (DSS) and therefore may not have long-term impact on the evolution of early-stage bladder cancer.[54,55] However, when an induction course of BCG is followed by a series of maintenance doses consisting of weekly BCG given for 3 weeks at 3, 6, 12, 18, 24, 30, and 36 months after induction, DFS can be prolonged.[56] Median DFS for the maintenance group was 76.8 months, whereas DFS for the induction therapy alone was 35.7 months (P less than 0.0001). Overall 5-year survival was 78% in the no-maintenance arm compared with 83% in the maintenance arm. For patients who fail an initial or maintenance course of intravesical therapy, it may be reasonable to try another agent, such as MMC, doxyrubicin, interferon-alpha, or gemcitabine as these agents may salvage 20% to 50% of patients with early-stage disease who fail to respond to BCG.[57–59]

Mitomycin C is an antitumor antibiotic that has been used in the treatment of patients with superficial bladder cancer intravesically since the early 1960s.[60] Although mitomycin C is inferior to BCG in patients with Ta/T1 and Tis tumors,[61] its use in the immediate perioperative period provides a unique clinical application. A single dose of MMC administered immediately after TURBT can improve the rate of tumor recurrence of low-grade superficial tumors.[62] In this study of 452 eligible patients, 1 dose of perioperative MMC

TABLE 47.4. Randomized trials of intravesical treatments for superficial and early-invasive bladder cancer.

Trial	*Reference*	*Accrual years*	*Patient no.*	*Stage*	*Intervention/ design*	*Median follow-up (F/U), months*	*DFS*	*Result*
SWOG	50	1983–1985	262	Ta, T1 or CIS	BCG vs. Doxorubicin	65	5-year Ta/T1: 37% vs. 17% ($P = 0.015$) CIS: 45% vs. 18%	BCG superior to Doxorubicin
Martinez-Pineiro	51	1980–1988	176	Ta/T1	BCG vs. Doxorubicin vs. Thiotepa	36	3-year: 87% vs. 57% ($P = 0.002$) vs. 64% ($P = 0.004$)	BCG superior to both drugs Doxorubicin similar to Thiotepa
EORTC	52	1992–1997	837	Int-high risk Ta/T1	Epirubicin vs. BCG vs. BCG + INH	41	3-year: 49% vs. 65% vs. 64%; ($P = 0.0001$)	BCG better than Epirubicin INH offers no benefit
SWOG	56	1985–1988	384	Ta/T1 + CIS	BCG vs. BCG + maintenance BCG	120	Median DFS: 36 vs. 77 months ($P < 0.0001$) 5-year: 41% vs. 60%	Maintenance BCG improves DFS
SWOG	61	1988–1992	447	Ta/T1	BCG vs. MMC	30	Median DFS: 44 vs. 22 months ($P = 0.017$)	BCG superior to mitomycin
MRC	62	1984–1986	452	Ta/T1	TUR vs. TUR ± MMC × 1 vs. TUR ± MMC × 5	84	40% vs. 55% ($P = 0.010$) vs. 63% ($P = 0.0001$)	TURBT + MMC × 1 is superior No benefit to MMC × 5 vs. × 1

DFS, disease-free survival; INH, Isoniazid; TUR, transurethral resection; MMC, mitomycin C; BCG, bacillus Calmette–Guérin.

(40mg/40mL) given within 24 hours of TURBT decreased the risk of recurrence by 34% when compared to TURBT alone.

Muscle-Invasive Disease: T2

Transurethral Resection

TURBT is generally not effective in the treatment of cT2 disease; however, this modality may be of benefit in selected patients. Herr reported 10-year outcome of TURBT in 151 patients with cT2 bladder cancer who were downstaged to T0 or T1 after a restaging TURBT.[63] Of these 151 patients, 99 received definitive TURBT and 52 had immediate cystectomy. The 10-year DSS was 76% in the 99 patients treated with TURBT; 57% had their bladder preserved. The 52 treated with immediate cystectomy had a 71% DSS ($P = 0.3$). Thirty-four patients (34%) treated with definitive TURBT relapsed in the bladder; 18 were salvaged with cystectomy, but 16 died of disease. Radical TURBT may thus be of benefit, particularly in those ineligible for radical surgery or chemotherapy. However, this technique is best augmented with radiotherapy.

Partial Cystectomy

Because of the risk of recurrent tumors, indications for partial cystectomy are limited and generally apply to isolated tumors or those within diverticula. The 5-year survival rates range from 25% to 50%, with local recurrence ranging from 40% to 80%. Candidates should have unifocal lesions amenable to a resection with a 2-cm margin, and still have a reasonable remaining bladder capacity. Classic teaching suggests that patients with CIS should not be candidates, although the use of intravesical BCG to treat CIS may broaden this teaching.

Radical Cystectomy

Radical cystectomy remains the standard of care for patients with muscle-invasive disease and is the most effective means of cancer control of nonmetastatic TCCa of the bladder, with a 10-year DFS rate of 66%. The broad indication for cystectomy is a superficial, early-stage, or invasive tumor that is refractory to or unlikely to be controlled by transurethral resection and intravesical therapy. Local control in the pelvis is achieved in 93% of cases.[12]

The standard technique of radical cystectomy in men requires resection of the bladder and surrounding prostate and seminal vesicles because of the risk of prostatic urethral invasion and incidental prostate cancer.[64] In women, anterior pelvic exenteration may be required for high-volume disease, necessitating removal of portions of neighboring reproductive and sex organs at risk for direct extension. A complete total pelvic lymphadenectomy provides staging information and also treatment benefit. Although node-positive patients have a significantly shortened survival when compared to node-negative patients, 30% DFS at 5 and 10 years is still achievable despite extravesical disease in the primary specimen.[12] Recently, extended node dissection has been advocated because a 27% improved 5-year survival has been observed in patients who receive a standard node dissection when compared to those who have no dissection.[65] At least 11 to 14 nodes are necessary to define node-negative status accurately and to optimize cure by surgery in node-positive cases.

Patients with muscle-invasive bladder cancer are at risk for distant relapse after cystectomy; recurrence typically occurs within 2 years after treatment. This finding partly relates to the 30% to 40% understaging rate of preoperative assessment. Modern pelvic imaging tools such as CT and magnetic resonance imaging (MRI) are often unable to detect low-volume perivesical invasion; thus, many patients are upstaged at the time of cystectomy.

Bladder Preservation

A feasible alternative to radical surgery for selected patients with limited cT2 disease is radical radiotherapy. This modality has been of benefit for patients who are ineligible for or refuse radical surgery or those who desire organ preservation. Aggressive TURBT is followed by radiotherapy, which offers an improved rate of survival when performed in conjunction with chemotherapy.[66] A 5-year DSS rate of 20% to 40% is expected in patients with preserved bladders, with the best overall survival outcome in younger patients with lower-stage tumors without lymphovascular or nodal invasion.[66,67] Superficial or early-stage recurrence approaches 50%, but it can be managed with TURBT with or without intravesical chemotherapy, although salvage cystectomy must be heavily considered. Because of the high local recurrence rate and low survival rate, it is accepted that radical cystectomy provides superior local control and more-efficacious survival for muscle-invasive disease and is therefore the preferred local therapy. A competing treatment strategy for those patients desiring bladder preservation has been early cystectomy and orthotopic neobladder diversion, which is able to simulate a natural voiding pattern, has very acceptable rates of continence, and avoids an external appliance.[68]

To improve the efficacy of radical radiotherapy, neoadjuvant and concomitant chemotherapy has been applied. The Radiation Therapy Oncology Group (RTOG) performed a series of Phase II studies and ultimately a randomized Phase III study that examined the efficacy of peritreatment chemotherapy. In RTOG 85-12, aggressive TURBT was followed by concurrent radiotherapy and cisplatin, a treatment regimen that offered a 64% 4-year survival rate for patients with cT2 disease and 24% for patients with cT3–T4 disease.[69] RTOG 89-03, a Phase III study, assessed the effect of cisplatin/methotrexate/vinblastine (CMV) as a neoadjuvant to concurrent radiotherapy and cisplatin.[70] The primary objective was survival, although secondary objectives included bladder preservation, tolerance, and toxicity. Poor patient tolerance to the CMV regimen was demonstrated despite a 5-year survival of 49% in the 123 patients who were entered into the trial.[71] Toxicity resulted in 3 treatment-related deaths, primarily due to neutropenia and severe sepsis. No difference in survival or bladder preservation was observed in patients who did or did not receive neoadjuvant CMV. Radiation sensitizers, such as gemcitabine and taxol, are currently being investigated.[70]

Extravesical Disease: T3/T4/N+

Patients with clinical evidence of extravesical tumor have a 5-year overall survival (OS) rate as high as 30% to 40% after cystectomy.[12,15] As tumor recurrence is common in this population, perioperative systemic chemotherapy has been advocated. Both neoadjuvant and adjuvant chemotherapy offer advantages and disadvantages to the patient. Adjuvant therapy has several benefits: (1) pathologic staging is the best prognostic indicator and will be known after surgical treatment; (2) low-risk patients are spared unnecessary treatment and toxicity if their staging is favorable; (3) no delay in surgery exists; (4) chance of cure for patients with chemoresistant disease is maximized; and (5) the lower toxicity of newer combination chemotherapy is likely to improve tolerance of and compliance with postoperative therapy. Neoadjuvant therapy also has several benefits: (1) prognostic information can be obtained from response to therapy of the primary lesion; (2) chemotherapy is not delayed, thus treating chemosensitive microscopic metastases immediately; (3) bladder preservation may be considered in complete responders, (4) patients may be downstaged increasing the opportunity for complete surgical resection; and (5) the presurgical patient is more likely to tolerate and be compliant with treatment.

Neoadjuvant Chemotherapy

Neoadjuvant chemotherapy is increasingly being advocated for patients with muscle-invasive disease who will undergo radical cystectomy. Table 47.5 outlines several randomized trials that examined the survival effect of neoadjuvant chemotherapy.[72–78] Most recently, an Intergroup study initiated by the SWOG lent further support for the use of neoadjuvant chemotherapy before radical cystectomy in patients with muscle-invasive disease.[78] In this study, 307 patients were randomized to receive three cycles of methotrexate, vinblastine, adriamycin, and cisplatin (MVAC) chemotherapy before cystectomy or cystectomy alone. With a median follow-up over 8 years, survival in the MVAC arm was significantly superior to survival in the no-MVAC arm, with a hazard ratio of 0.74 and estimated median survival times of 6.2 and 3.8 years, respectively. The improved median DSS and decreased total number of deaths was most pronounced in the patients with T3 and T4 disease. An added benefit in the chemotherapy arm was the downstaging of patients to pT0, confirmed at cystectomy. Criticisms regarding the study's methodology and lengthy accrual period of 11 years have led to some controversy.[79] Although a statistically significant improvement in DFS and median survival was appreciated, the overall survival benefit of the neoadjuvant cohort was relatively modest (less than 6%), and the toxicity from the treatment was significant.

The results of the SWOG-led study have contrasted those of the largest trial of neoadjuvant chemotherapy. The international intergroup trial initiated by the MRC and EORTC of CMV before cystectomy or radiotherapy enrolled 976 patients from 106 institutions in 5.5 years.[80] The trial, powered to detect a 10% improvement in survival, observed a 15% reduction in the risk of death in the chemotherapy arm, which translated into a 3-year survival benefit of 5.5% (50% in the no-chemotherapy arm and 55% in the chemotherapy arm.) The median length of follow-up for patients who were still alive was 4 years. The significance of these results have been debated, and follow-up analyses at 7 years suggest a possible significant survival benefit for the chemotherapy arm. Although interpretation of these randomized trials (see Table 47.5) has been difficult, it is clear that long term survival rates after cystectomy alone are poor for cT3 and T4 disease, and so a perioperative chemotherapy strategy makes sense.

TABLE 47.5. Randomized trials of neoadjuvant chemotherapy for invasive bladder cancer.

Trial	*Reference*	*Accrual years*	*Patient no./ evaluable Patients*	*Stage*	*Neoadjuvant regimen*	*Median F/U (years)*	*Survival (chemo + Cx) vs. (Cx alone)*	*Chemo benefit*
Cortesi	72	1988–1992	171/153	T2–4 N0	MVEC 3 cycles	2.8	NR	No
Martinez-Pineiro	73	1984–1989	122/121	T2–4a Nx–N2	Cisplatin 3 cycles	6.5	OS: 35.5% (Cis) vs. 37.3% (Cx); $P = 0.95$	No
Abol-Eneim	74	1984–1996	196/196	T2–4a Nx	CMV 2 cycles	2.7	5-year DFS: 62% (CMV) vs. 42% (Cx) $P = 0.01$	Yes
Mamstrom (Nordic I)	75	1985–1989	325/311	G3 T1–T4a NxM0	Cisplatin + Doxorubicin 2 cycles	Min. 5	5-year OS: 59% (CA) vs. 51% (Cx) $P = 0.1$	No
Sherif (Nordic II)	76	1990–1997	317/309	T2–4a NxM0	Cisplatin + MTX 3 cycles	5.3	5-year OS: 53% (CM) vs. 46% (Cx); $P = 0.24$	No
Grossman (Intergroup)	78	1987–1998	317/307	T2–4a N0M0	MVAC 3 cycles	8.4	5-year OS: 57% (MVAC) vs. 43% (Cx); $P = 0.06$	Yes
MRC/ EORTC	80	1989–1995	976/976	T2–4a N0/NxM0	CMV 3 cycles	4.0 (living patients)	3-year OS 55.5% (CMV) vs. 50% (Cx); $P = 0.075$	No

CMV, cisplatin or carboplatin, methotrexate, vinblastine; MVAC, methotrexate, vinblastine, doxorubicin, cisplatin; MVEC, methotrexate, vinblastine, epirubicin, cisplatin; DFS, disease-free survival; G3, grade 3; MTX, methotrexate; Cx, cystectomy alone; OS, overall survival; NR, not reported.

Adjuvant Chemotherapy

Four randomized studies have evaluated the benefit of adjuvant chemotherapy after cystectomy (Table 47.6).[81–85] Two of these trials did not show a benefit when adjuvant treatment was compared with observation.[83,84] The study by Studer[83] and colleagues has been criticized for using an inferior regimen, single-agent cisplatin, when a cisplatin-based multidrug regimen such as MVAC was known to be more efficacious at that time.[86] The study by Freiha et al.[84] has been criticized for being underpowered.

In the Skinner study,[81] patients with stage T3–T4 or node-positive disease were randomized to observation or four cycles of adjuvant CAP (cyclophophamide, adriamycin, cisplatin). A significant delay in recurrence was observed in the adjuvant chemotherapy group when compared to those treated with cystectomy alone (70% versus 46% 3-year-DFS, respectively). A significant improvement in OS (4.3 versus 2.4 years) was also observed. This study was criticized for the small number of patients (91), flawed statistical methods, premature termination, and the use of nonstandardized chemotherapy. Moreover, chemotherapy compliance was poor; only 70% of patients in the chemotherapy group received any treatment and only 62% received the planned number of cycles.

In the study by Stockle et al.,[82] 49 patients with stage pT3a–pT4a or node-positive TCCa were randomized to MVAC, MVEC, or observation. Patients in the observation group did not receive chemotherapy at relapse. A significant reduction in the risk of tumor recurrence was observed in the chemotherapy arm: 3 (17%) of 18 patients who received chemotherapy relapsed compared with 18 (82%) of 23 untreated patients. This study also faced poor chemotherapy compliance, with only 75% of patients in the chemotherapy group receiving any treatment and only 48% receiving the planned number of cycles. Unfortunately, both the Skinner and Stockle trials ended prematurely based on interim analyses favoring adjuvant chemotherapy.

TABLE 47.6. Randomized trials of adjuvant chemotherapy for invasive bladder cancer.

Trial	*Reference*	*Accrual period*	*No. of patients*	*Stage*	*Adjuvant regimen*	*Median F/U, months*	*Survival*	*Chemo benefit*
Skinner	81	1980–1988	91	T3 Nx	CISCA	32	3-year DFS: 70% (Cx/CISCA) vs. 46% (Cx); $P = 0.01$; 3-year OS: 66% (Cx/CISCA) vs. 50% (Cx); ($P = 0.099$)	Yes for DFS; No for OS
Stockle	82	1987–1990	49	pT3, pT4 N+	MVAC/MVEC	>12	DFS in 73% (Cx/chemo) vs. 18% (Cx); $P = 0.0012$	Yes for DFS
Studer	83	1984–1989	77	pT1–4 N0–2	Cisplatin	69	5-year OS: 57% (Cx/Cis) vs. 54% (Cx); ($P = 0.65$)	No for OS
Freiha	84	1986–1993	50	pT3b, pT4 N0–1	CMV	62	Median OS: 63 (Cx/CMV) vs. 36 months (Cx); ($P = 0.32$)	No for OS

CISCA, cisplatin, methotrexate, vinblastine; CMV, cisplatin or carboplatin, methotrexate, vinblastine; MVAC, methotrexate, vinblastine, doxorubicin, cisplatin; MVEC, methotrexate, vinblastine, epirubicin, cisplatin; DFS, disease-free survival; OS, overall survival; Cx, cystectomy alone.

Despite criticisms of adjuvant treatment trials, there is a suggested survival benefit for patients with extravesical or nodal extension or extension to neighboring viscera. Currently, a large international Intergroup study is under way to determine whether adjuvant chemotherapy is effective.[87] This randomized study will compare delayed versus immediate chemotherapy (gemcitabine plus cisplatin, MVAC or high-dose MVAC plus granulocyte colony-stimulating factor) after radical cystectomy for pT3–pT4 or node-positive, but M0 TCCa, of the bladder.

Distant Urothelial Metastases: M+

There have been several randomized clinical trials evaluating chemotherapeutic regimens for the treatment of metastatic TCCA (Table 47.7).[88–98] Although chemotherapeutic regimens can result in response rates as high as 65%, the median survival is at best 12 to 15 months. The most active chemotherapeutic regimen for TCCa is MVAC.[93,94] Its use has been limited by its significant toxicity, including an associated 3% to 4% treatment mortality rate.[94,96,97] Gemcitabine/cisplatin has similar survival but an improved toxicity profile, and in many respects it has become the standard therapy for metastatic TCCa.[96] Variants of the traditional MVAC dosing may also make the regimen more tolerable while maintaining survival rates.[97]

Newer Phase I and Phase II studies using a combination of monoclonal antibodies and chemotherapy are under way at single institutions. Some of these studies have shown promise, particularly the use of Herceptin in the treatment of patients with tumors that express Her-2/neu. Although TCCa appears to be responsive to chemotherapy, the number of complete long-term responders is low, and the development of additional chemotherapeutic regimens will be necessary to make an advance in this disease.

Treatment of Ureteral Cancer

When the diagnosis of upper tract urothelial cancer is well established, it is critical to consider multiple tumor and patient factors when making a treatment decision. Tumor size, grade, stage, and location all guide treatment strategy, but tumor stage remains the most important prognostic factor for recurrence and DSS.[99] Apart from stage, one must also weigh the value of renal preservation against the reality of tumor threat. Organ preservation is entertained if a patient has a solitary functioning kidney, multifocal urothelial tumors, or an abnormal or threatened contralateral kidney. This strategy is considered in view of the significant mortality of dialysis, with a 5-year survival rate of 19% in patients between 65 and 74 years of age.[100] Modern endoscopic strategies have also permitted a wider application of conservative treatment options.

Endoscopic Options

Endoscopic treatment of low-grade, low-volume, noninvasive renal pelvic and ureteral tumors is now possible with improved instrumentation in ureteroscopy and enhanced experience with percutaneous techniques. Figure 47.2 demonstrates a typical papillary ureteral tumor visualized during ureteral imaging (Figure 47.2A) and through a ureteroscope (Figure 47.2B). Retrograde ureteroscopic tumor biopsy and treatment may be accomplished using flexible instrumentation of an accessible ureteral orifice. Electrocautery and the holmium and neodymium YAG lasers have all been used

TABLE 47.7. Randomized trials of chemotherapeutic intervention for metastatic bladder cancer.

Trial	*Reference*	*Accrual*	*No. of evaluable patients*	*Chemotherapy regimen*	*RR (%)*	*CR (%)*	*Median survival*	*Treatment mortality (%)*	*Outcome*
Soloway	88	1978–1982	109	Cisplatin vs. cisplatin + cyclophosphamide	20 12	10 5	NR	0 0	No survival difference
Khandekar	89	1978–1981	130	Cisplatin vs. CAP	17 33	2 22	6 7.3	0 1.6	No survival difference
Troner	90	NR	91	Cisplatin vs. CAP	15 21	0 5	5.2 7.2	3.5 1.9	No survival difference
Gagliano	91	1976–1979	92	Doxorubicin vs. Doxorubicin + cisplatin	19 43	0 3	4 7.8	0 2.7	No survival difference
Hillcoat	92	1982–1986	108	Cisplatin vs. cisplatin + MTX	31 45	9 9	7.2 8.7	2 3.8	No survival difference
Logothetis	93	1985–1989	110	CISCA vs. MVAC	46 65	25 35	9 12	1.8 0	MVAC better
Loehrer	94	1984–1989	246	Cisplatin vs. MVAC	12 39	3 13	8.2 12.5	0 4	MVAC better
Mead	95	1991–1995	214	MTX + vinblastine vs. CMV	19 46	7 10	4.5 7	0 4	CMV better
von der Maase	96	1996–1998	405	MVAC vs. Gemcitabine + cisplatin	46 49	12 12	14.8 13.8	3 1	No survival difference
Sternberg	97	1993–1998	263	MVAC vs. HD-MVAC/ G-CSF	50 62	9 21	14.1 15.5	4 3	No survival difference

CAP, cyclophosphomide, doxorubicin, cisplatin; CMV, cisplatin or carboplatin, methotrexate, vinblastine; MVAC, methotrexate, vinblastine, doxorubicin, cisplatin; CISCA, cisplatin, methotrexate, vinblastine; G-CSF, granulocyte colony-stimulating factor; HD-MVAC, high-dose MVAC; MTX, methotrexate; NR, not reported; RR, response rate; CR, complete response.

Source: Adapted from Juffs et al.,[98] by permission of *Lancet Oncology*.

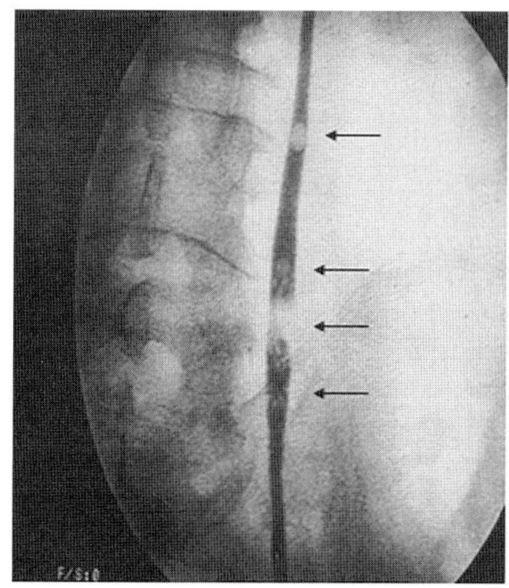

A

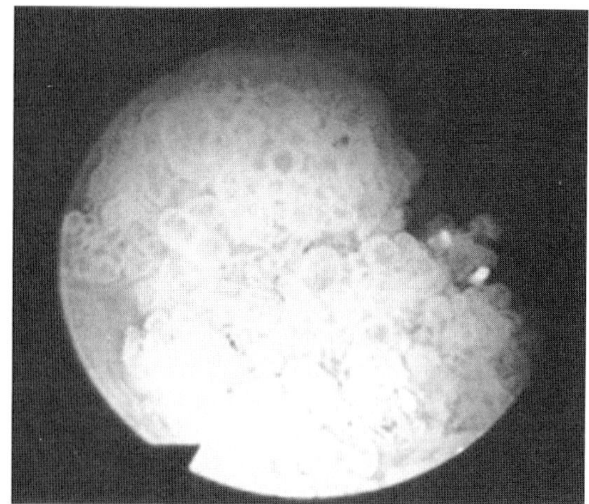

B

FIGURE 47.2. Identification of a papillary urothelial tumor. (A) Tumors are detected during ureteral imaging as filling defect (*black arrows*). (B) Tumors are readily visualized using ureteroscopy.

successfully for primary upper tract tumor ablation. Small working endoscopic channels with decreased irrigant flow can compromise the visual field, however, and can limit the therapeutic applications. Percutaneous management, a better approach to selected renal pelvic tumors, has the benefit of larger working channels that can accommodate resections and cautery instruments, permitting more complete biopsy, fulguration, and staging. However, percutaneous management has the potential risk of extravasation of cancer cells when obtaining renal access and dilating the nephrostomy tract. The authors do not recommend elective endoscopic or percutaneous management of T1 disease in the patient with a normal contralateral kidney in view of the 20% to 55% progression rates experienced for grade II/III primary tumors.[101]

Tumor recurrence remains the most serious consequence of conservative treatments. With any conservative approach, one must ensure that salvage therapy is available for failures. When surveyed closely, most patients are still candidates for open resection if they fail endoscopic approaches. Recurrence rates of renal pelvic and ureteral tumors treated with ureteroscopy are 33% to 35% and 31% to 32%, respectively. Tumor grade and size do impact recurrence, with a rate of 26% for grade I, 44% for grade II, and 25% for lesions less than 1.5cm compared with 50% for tumors larger than 1.5cm.[101,102] A reasonable initial approach to the small (less than 1.5cm) low-grade ureteral or renal pelvic tumor would be ureteroscopic ablation. Multiple or large low-grade renal pelvic tumors in the patient who is a poor candidate for nephroureterectomy would likely benefit from initial percutaneous management.

Upper Tract Chemotherapy or Immunotherapy

Carcinoma in situ presents a much greater treatment challenge than low-grade superficial disease, in part because of its often multifocal nature; this is reflected in the higher recurrence and progression rates of high-grade superficial disease treated endoscopically or percutaneously.[101] Upper tract immunotherapy and chemotherapy have been used as adjuvant strategies for Ta and CIS. Logistic problems often arise relative to delivering adequate drug dosage whether by antegrade or retrograde techniques. There is limited experience with all agents, with only few reports describing the use of BCG, thiotepa, and mitomycin C; the efficacy of these agents remains unclear.[101,102] Although BCG delivery can be cumbersome, a recent study of 41 renal units treated in 37 patients with primary Ta or Tis disease demonstrated that percutaneous BCG can be delivered without seeding the nephrostomy tract and without undue morbidity; acceptable 3% and 5% rates of BCG inflammation and septicemia, respectively, were observed.[103] The median recurrence free and progression free survival was 21 and 34 months at 42 months of follow-up.

Segmental or Distal Ureterectomy

The best results with preservative procedures for upper tract urothelial tumors are seen in the treatment of isolated tumors of the lower third of the ureter. Complete distal ureterectomy with reimplantation of the ureter can yield results very similar to those obtained with a nephroureterectomy if appropriate cases are chosen, particularly for low-grade noninvasive tumors. The proximal margin of the ureter must be examined intraoperatively. Using this approach in the patient with high-grade and invasive disease must be done with caution as a significant number of these patients will die of recurrent disease.[99] The temptation of segmental ureterectomy for midureteral lesions should be avoided in the patient without renal compromise in view of the 30% recurrence rate within the ureter distal to the initial lesion.[104]

Nephroureterectomy

Nephroureterectomy with bladder cuff excision continues to be the standard treatment for organ-confined invasive or recurrent superficial upper tract TCCa, particularly in the mid- to upper ureter and renal pelvis. Partial nephrectomy and pyelotomy with tumor excision are undesirable but are considered in the presence of a solitary kidney, diminished renal function, or bilateral disease. The major concern after conservative procedures is tumor spillage and local recurrence, which can approach 62% for open renal pelvic procedures.[105] Excision of the entire ureter with a small cuff of bladder ensures total removal of the intramural ureter and avoids unnecessary recurrence. Historically, recurrence of 48% was reported after nephrectomy alone, 32% after nephrectomy and partial ureterectomy, 24% with nephrectomy and subtotal ureterectomy, and only 12% after total nephroureterectomy, illustrating the importance of total ureterectomy.[104] An incomplete ureterectomy also leaves an ipsilateral ureteral stump that is difficult to survey for recurrent disease. Laparoscopic nephroureterectomy has several benefits over open nephroureterectomy for primary upper tract tumors including more rapid recovery, shorter hospital stay, and less requirement of pain medication. Rates of recurrence, local control, and disease-specific survival are comparable to open nephroureterectomy, and consequently laparoscopic nephroureterectomy has become standard treatment in many centers.[106] Success of upper tract treatments is heavily reliant on tumor stage. Five-year DSS is 100% for Ta/CIS, 92% for T1, 73% for T2, 41% for T3, and 0% for T4.[99] Median DSS for T4 patients is 6 months.

Treatment of Urethral Cancer

Treatment of urethral cancer is complex and often requires a multidisciplinary approach. Patients often present at a later stage requiring radical surgery with adjuvant chemotherapy or radiation.[107] Because of the uncommon nature of the disease, there is a lack of uniform treatment. In women, because of the short urethra, fewer conservative treatment strategies exist. Therapy for superficial low-grade tumors may be treated endoscopically; however, one risks disrupting the continence sphincteric mechanism. For invasive disease, total urethrectomy is performed along with cystectomy and, depending on the tumor bulk and age of the patient, partial resection of neighboring sexual and reproductive organs. Urinary diversion is then required.

Urethral Cancer in Women

In a retrospective case series from Memorial Sloan Kettering, 72 women with urethral cancer were followed for a median of 84 months; 68% presented with cT2–cT4 tumors.[107] Forty (56%) underwent major or radical surgery including anterior or total pelvic exenteration, urethrectomy, cystectomy, or diverticulectomy; 10 of those undergoing anterior pelvic exenteration received preoperative radiotherapy. A total of 25 patients (35%) were treated with external-beam radiotherapy with or without brachytherapy. The 5-year DFS and DSS were 46% for the entire cohort, 83% to 89% for low-stage women, and 33% for high-stage patients. In a multivariate analysis, primary stage, nodal status, and site of disease were independent predictors of survival. Primary treatment with either surgery or radiation resulted in similar DFS and DSS; however, preoperative radiotherapy significantly improved DFS.

Organ preservation may be achieved with the use of brachytherapy and radiotherapy.[108] In a retrospective case series of 34 women treated with external-beam radiotherapy with or without brachytherapy, brachytherapy reduced the risk of local recurrence by a factor of 4.2. Its effect was most prominently seen in patients with bulky primary disease. Large tumor size was the only independent adverse predictor of DFS and DSS. The 7-year DSS was 45%.

Urethral Cancer in Men

In men, the location and stage of the tumor dictates the treatment. Small or low-grade superficial tumors may be treated endoscopically throughout the urethra. However, bulkier tumors require surgical resection and often adjuvant chemoradiation. Tumors in the distal or anterior male urethra may be treated with subtotal urethrectomy with or without partial penectomy depending upon tumor extension. More proximal disease in the prostatic or pendulous urethra may require cystoprostatectomy with urethrectomy and urinary diversion.

Dalbagni et al. retrospectively reviewed the Memorial Sloan Kettering experience over a 38-year period during which 46 men were treated for primary urethral cancer.[109] The majority (70%) presented with locally advanced or nodal disease, with a median interval of 7.5 months from the onset of symptoms to diagnosis. The infrequent nature of the disease led to nonstandard treatment with conservative (endoscopy, partial urethrectomy, partial penectomy) and radical (total urethrectomy, total penectomy, cystectomy, pelvic exenteration) surgery. Six patients received preoperative radiation, although no benefit in local recurrence-free survival was observed in this group. At a median follow-up of 125 months, the 5-year DSS and OS were 50% and 42%, respectively. Tumors in the bulbar (proximal) urethra had a worse prognosis when compared to those in the anterior (distal) urethra (26% versus 69% OS, respectively). In view of the low disease incidence, evidence-based treatments will only be realized through national cooperative group studies.

Penis

Etiology

Carcinoma of the penis is an uncommon malignancy, with an estimated 1,400 new cases in 2003.[110] Epidemiologic evidence suggests that penile cancer has several similarities with other anogenital malignancies. Specifically, these tumors occur more commonly among those of lower social class and those who are separated or divorced. Furthermore, these cancers occur infrequently in Jewish populations.[111] Although potential risk factors of penile cancer have been studied extensively, a true etiology remains unclear.

Human papilloma virus (HPV) is a sexually transmitted virus that has been associated with anogenital infections in men and women.[112] The prevalence of HPV infection in penile cancers is variable (22%–71%),[113–115] and less prevalent than in genital warts,[113] suggesting distinct pathogenesis of these conditions. Historically, penile carcinomas were thought to arise from cellular atypia or intraepithelial neoplasia[116] associated with HPV infection.[117] Two case-control studies detected an increased risk (4.5 to 5.9 times) of penile cancer in men with genital warts, implicating HPV as a potential causal agent.[114,118] Because of the variable association of HPV with carcinoma of the penis, however, its oncogenicity is likely additive to other causal factors.

Other risk factors commonly associated with invasive or in situ carcinoma of the penis include tobacco use/exposure, phimosis, penile injury, poor hygiene, physical inactivity, and history of genital rash.[114,118,119] Men with prolonged exposure to ultraviolet A and B radiation in the treatment of psoriasis, prospectively followed for 12 years, demonstrated a 59-fold-

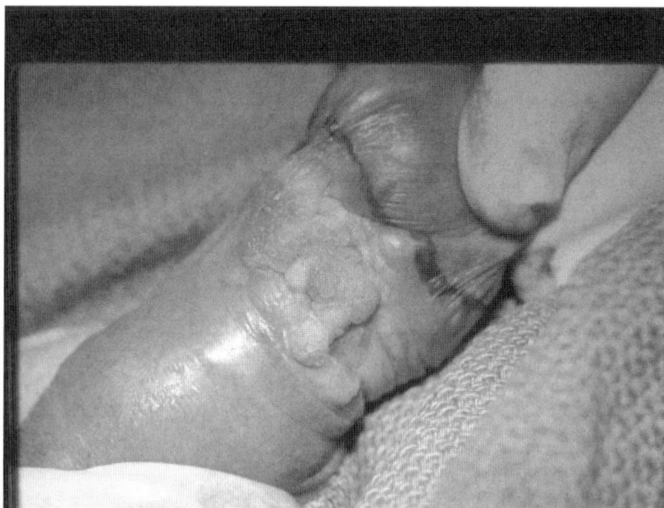

FIGURE 47.3. Photograph of a penile cancer on the shaft of the penis.

increased risk of developing invasive or in situ penile cancer when compared to unexposed men.[120] This risk was strongly dose dependent, suggesting a high susceptibility of the genitalia to the carcinogenic effects of ultraviolet radiation.

Although newborn circumcision is not routinely recommended by the American Academy of Pediatrics or the American College of Obstetrics and Gynecology,[121] there is some evidence to suggest that newborn circumcision may prevent the development of penile cancer.[114] It is unclear whether this effect is mediated by improved hygiene[119] or prevention of complications related to phimosis.[118,119] However, the incidence of penile cancer among American circumcised men is essentially nonexistent, with a lifetime risk of developing penile cancer of 1 in 600.[122]

Pathology

Most penile cancers are of squamous cell origin, resembling those malignancies that develop in nongenital skin (Figure 47.3). Because of the implications of pathogenesis and morphology on prognosis, squamous cell carcinoma (SCCa) of the penis has been classified into three histologic subtypes.[113,123,124] The most common subtype is typical SCCa. Other subtypes—warty and basaloid—correspond to those found in vulvar malignancies. Warty SCCa of the penis morphologically resembles other verruciform lesions of the penis such as giant condyloma and verrucous carcinoma.[124] Unlike the latter two lesions, warty carcinoma is uniformly associated with HPV infection[114] and has the ability to metastasize.[124,125] The association of basaloid carcinomas with HPV infection (80% of cases)[5] is similar to that of the warty subtype, whereas the most common variant, typical SCCa, is infrequently associated with this viral infection (35% of cases).[113] In contradistinction to the warty subtype, the basaloid variant is commonly associated with deeper invasion and diminished survival.[123] Collectively, these data suggest that these subtypes of penile carcinoma may have distinct pathogenesis and pathophysiology. The frequent association of basaloid and warty subtypes with HPV DNA may also provide a molecular basis for a viral etiology in their development. Staging of penile cancers is based on that of the American Joint Committee on Cancer TNM staging system (Table 47.8).[126] *Clinically, the precise TNM stage is used rather than the overall stage.*

Prognostic Factors

Clinical variables (e.g., palpable adenopathy) and primary tumor factors (e.g., vascular invasion) associated with regional lymph node metastasis have been described as prognostic factors (Table 47.9). To date, there have been no randomized clinical trials in the management of inguinal lymph nodes in patients with or without palpable adenopathy. Consequently, the current evidence is based on multiple, single-institutional case series. Despite these limitations, these data, in conjunction with the pathologic stage of the regional lymph nodes, have been useful in defining various measures of survival (see Table 47.9).

Regional Lymph Nodes

The morbidity of a modified inguinal lymph node dissection (ILND), including lymphedema, flap necrosis, deep venous thrombosis, and wound infection, precludes its routine use in the treatment of patients with penile cancer.[127,128] Consequently, factors predictive of lymph node involvement have been sought.

Lymphatic and Vascular Invasion

Multiple studies[129–131] have demonstrated the importance of vascular invasion in the penile specimen as an independent predictor of subsequent lymph node metastasis. Among 82 patients treated with penectomy and bilateral ILND between 1953 and 1992, those with lymphatic embolization of tumor cells in the penile specimen were nine times more likely to have positive lymph nodes compared to those without lymphatic invasion.

TABLE 47.8. The TNM staging system for carcinoma of the penis.

Primary tumor (T)	
TX	Primary tumor cannot be assessed
T0	No evidence of primary tumor
Tis	Carcinoma in situ
Ta	Noninvasive verrucous carcinoma
T1	Tumor invades subepithelial connective tissue
T2	Tumor invades corpus spongiosum or cavernosum
T3	Tumor invades urethra or prostate
T4	Tumor invades other adjacent structures
Regional lymph nodes (N)	
NX	Regional lymph nodes cannot be assessed
N0	No regional lymph node metastasis
N1	Metastasis in single superficial, inguinal lymph node involvement
N2	Metastasis in multiple or bilateral inguinal lymph nodes
N3	Metastasis in deep inguinal or pelvic lymph node(s) unilateral of bilateral
Distant metastasis (M)	
MX	Distant metastasis cannot be assessed
M0	No distant metastasis
M1	Distant metastasis

Source: Used with the permission of the American Joint Committee on Cancer (AJCC), Chicago, Illinois. The original source for this material is the *AJCC Cancer Staging Manual*, sixth edition (2002), published by Springer-Verlag New York, www.springer-ny.com.

TABLE 47.9. Factors that are associated with regional lymph node involvement and/or survival.

Reference	No. of patients	Years	Design	Stage (%)	Median follow-up (months)	Survival	Prognostic factors
Lopes[130]	145	1953–1985	Case series	T1 1 N0 40 T2 28 N1 18 T3 59 N2 28 T4 5 N3 3	33	5-year DFS 45% 5-year OS 54%	**LN status**: lymphatic/venous embolization **DFS**: + nodes, N stage **OS**: + nodes, N stage, age, eosinophilic infiltrate
Soria[140]	102	1973–1993	Case series	T1 67 N0 76 T2 25 N1 12 T3 6 N2 8 N3 1	111	5-year DFS 56% 10-year DFS 42% 5-year DSS 72% 10-year DSS 66%	**OS**: corporal involvement, palpable node
Emerson[139]	22	1989–1998	Case series	T1 77 T2 9 T3 14	21		**PFS**: vascular invasion, depth, stage, grade
McDougal[163]*	76	1960–1980	Case series	1 7 2A 25 2B 36 3 32	>36	3-year DFS Immediate ILND 75%–92% Delayed ILND 33%	Early ILND better than delayed
Sarin[134]	101	1960–1990	Case series	T1 79 N0 82 T2 13 N1 6 T3 3 N2 5 T4 5 N3 7	562.4 (mean)	5-year DSS 66% 10-year DSS 57%	**DSS**: poorly differentiated, age > 60, ulcerative, + nodes
Lopes[129]	82	1953–1992	Case series	T2 26 N0 40 T3/4 74 N1 13 N2 34 N3 13	89 (mean)	OS 5-year 10-year T2 53 53 T3/4 47 37 N0 56 50 N1 27 13 N2 63 53 N3 18 18	**LN status**: lymphatic embolization, p53 + **OS**: + nodes, age > 50
Martins[132]	50	1978–1995	Case series	pT1NO 36 pT2–4N0 36 pT2–4N+ 20 pT1N+ 8	108		**LN status**: grade, pT stage, p53 +
Slaton[131]	48	1980–1992	Case series		59		**LN status**: vascular invasion, >50% poorly differentiated, tumor stage
Bezerra[135]	85	1953–1993	Case series		89	DSS 10 years HPV+ 68–69 LN+ 45–89	**DSS**: + nodes
Horenblas[133]	118	1956–1989	Case series	T1 33 T2 51 T3 14 T4 2	48	DSS 5 years T1 94 N0 93 T2 59 N1 57 T3 52 N2 50 N3 17	**OS**: grade, N stage
Srinivas[136]	119	1950–1980	Case series			5-year OS N+ 28%	**OS**: unilateral LN involvement better than bilateral involvement

DFS, disease-free survival; OS, overall survival; DSS, disease-specific survival; PFS, progression-free survival; ILND, inguinal lymph node dissection; LN, lymph node; *, modified Jackson Staging System.

Accumulation of p53

Inactivation of the tumor suppressor gene, p53, has been associated with pathogenesis and progression of multiple malignancies. In penile cancer, lymph node metastasis has been associated with nuclear accumulation of dysfunctional p53 protein.[129,132]

Pathologic Stage/Grade of Primary Tumor

Pathologic stage of the primary tumor is also associated with lymph node involvement.[131,132] Invasion of the corpus spongiosum or cavernosum (pT2 or greater) independently portends increased risk for nodal involvement.[131] Poorly differentiated primary tumors also offer increased risk of lymph node metastasis.[131] These data highlight the importance of careful pathologic analysis of the primary tumor.

Disease Progression and Survival

Nodal Status

The presence of inguinal lymph node metastasis at the time of ILND is the single greatest predictor of overall[129,130,133] and disease-specific[134,135] survival among patients with penile cancer. In one series, patients with lymph node involvement were 8.3 times more likely to die of penile cancer than those patients without nodal disease. Moreover, bilateral lymph node metastasis portends a worse prognosis than unilateral disease, with 5-year DSS decreasing to 9% from 56%, respectively.[36] Involvement of the deep inguinal or pelvic lymph nodes heralds aggressive disease with 5-year survival of less than 18%.[29,33,36] The number of lymph nodes involved at the time of ILND is also associated with survival. Specifically, the presence of metastasis in more than two lymph nodes results in significant declines in 5-year survival.[136] Moreover, the likelihood of pelvic metastasis rises as the number of involved inguinal lymph nodes increases.[136,137]

Age

Not surprisingly, older age (classified as more than 50 to 60 years of age) has been associated with a decline in overall survival among patients with penile cancer.[129,130] However, advanced age has also been shown to be independently associated with lower DSS.[134] In fact, men over the age of 60 were 3.4 times more likely to die of penile cancer than younger men.

Tumor Grade

Patients with high-grade or poorly differentiated cancers are more likely to succumb to their disease or have progressive disease than those with low-grade tumors.[134,138,139] Multiple other factors have been associated with diminished OS (eosinophilic infiltrate on pathologic examination,[130] corporal involvement,[140] and p53 immunoreactivity[132]), DSS (ulcerative tumors),[134] and tumor progression (pathologic stage, depth of invasion, and vascular invasion).[139]

Diagnosis

The diagnosis of penile cancer is made by excisional, incisional, or punch or needle biopsy methods depending on the location of the tumor. Once the diagnosis is confirmed, subsequent local treatment (e.g., partial or total penectomy, laser surgery, or Moh's micrographic surgery) can be undertaken based on biopsy results and extent of the primary tumor (see Treatment: Local). Additional staging may be performed with a chest radiograph, an abdominal-pelvic CT scan (to assess for pelvic adenopathy), and a bone scan (in patients with extensive disease, bone pain, or abnormal serum chemistries, such as alkaline phosphatase, calcium).

Evaluation of the regional (superficial and deep inguinal) lymph nodes poses a greater problem because of the lack of sensitivity of various imaging modalities and the potential for significant morbidity associated with ILND.[128,141] Multiple attempts have been made to clarify the accuracy of the various staging modalities. Horenblas and colleagues[138] described their experience with staging techniques among 118 patients with cancer of the penis. The investigators noted that the sensitivities for physical examination, lymphangiography, computed tomography, and fine-needle aspiration were 90%, 31%, 36%, and 71%, respectively. The respective specificities for these tests were 21%, 100%, 100%, and 100%. The authors concluded that imaging is useful in determining the management of the regional lymph nodes: negative findings are essentially meaningless. Rather, imaging may be helpful in the context of evaluating the pelvic lymph nodes and in determining the extent of disease.

Invasive techniques for assessing the inguinal lymph nodes include modified ILND, dynamic sentinel lymph node biopsy, and fine-needle aspiration. Some investigators have demonstrated improved postoperative recovery following the saphenous vein-sparing modified ILND with transient lymphedema and scrotal edema in 20% of patients and no long-term complications.[127,142] Morbidity with this procedure appears to be greater when performed as a palliative procedure rather than prophylactically in the setting of clinically negative nodes.[128] Although the modified dissection is perhaps the most popular form of lymphadenectomy currently utilized, some investigators advocate a more-extensive dissection because of its worrisome local recurrence rates (up to 15%).[141]

The use of fine-needle aspirations has also proven problematic because of false-negative rates of at least 10%.[143] Among 20 patients who underwent extensive fine-needle biopsy using lypmhangiographic and fluoroscopic guidance, 2 patients (10%) were found to have false-negative results at the time of ILND. Attempts to improve upon the sensitivity of needle biopsy and morbidity of ILND resulted in the use of dynamic sentinel lymph node biopsy.[144,145] Initial findings of high false-negative rates as manifested by subsequent progression or the presence of metastasis at the time of ILND1[46–148] have prompted technique modification. Recent efforts employing preoperative lymphoscintigraphy, vital blue dye, and gamma-ray detection probes have made considerable inroads into improving technique sensitivity. However, current results reiterate that sentinel node sampling continues to be imperfect[149] and results in false-negative rates of at least 20%.[150] Despite this, recent evidence suggests that universal application of this technique in cT2–cT3 patients can improve DSS at 3 years when compared to surveillance. These findings highlight the importance of early treatment of the inguinal lymph nodes in those with nodal involvement.[151]

Therapy

Carcinoma of the penis typically follows a stepwise progression in which the disease proceeds from the penis to regional inguinal lymph nodes to distant sites. Because of this predictable pattern of spread, the extent of radical surgery is often measured against the high probability of surgical-related morbidity. Consequently, less-deforming modalities of therapy have been utilized to strike a balance between therapy and morbidity.

Local

Excisional biopsy encompassing normal neighboring skin is the initial local treatment for small superficial penile cancers. Lesions confined to the preputial skin can successfully be managed with circumcision alone.[152] For more-extensive cancers involving the glans, the shaft, and other local structures (e.g., prostate), the standard treatment includes either partial or total penectomy, depending on the extent of the primary tumor.[137,153] Partial penectomy is indicated when an adequate 2-cm tumor margin[154] can be achieved while maintaining sufficient penile length for upright micturition. Margins less than 2 cm may also provide adequate local control, because penile cancers are focal and do not spread in a discontinuous fashion.[153] Several studies have documented the efficacy of margins less than 1 cm when performing partial penectomy, thus increasing the eligible patient population for the procedure.[153,155]

Because of the morbidity of total or partial penectomy, less-disfiguring treatments have been implemented in select patients including laser therapy,[156] Moh's micrographic surgery,[157] and multimodality regimens that incorporate conservative surgery, radiation (external beam or brachytherapy), and systemic chemotherapy.[158–162] The aggregate of data suggest that responses to these modalities are highly variable and that local recurrence rates for these less-invasive treatments is higher than for extirpative surgery. Consequently, these conservative modalities should be reserved for selected patients with smaller, well-differentiated disease.[162]

Regional

Standard treatment for documented inguinal lymph node metastasis is ILND. Certainly, despite its modifications,[142] the ILND is commonly associated with postoperative morbidity,[128] excluding its routine use in all patients with carcinoma of the penis. Historically, patients with palpable inguinal lymph nodes at the time of primary treatment were initially managed with a 6-week course of antibiotics to treat adenopathy related to infection or inflammation.[152] Persistent adenopathy following antimicrobial therapy was associated with tumor invasion in at least 70% of patients.[136,137] Likewise, development of palpable inguinal nodes after treatment of the primary tumor generally represents tumor extension rather than inflammation.[152]

Early or prophylactic ILND provides improved cancer control[131,136,163] and less morbidity than lymphadenectomy performed in the presence of known lymph node metastasis (therapeutic) or for palliation.[128] Selected patients eligible for observation instead of ILND include those with low grade (grades 1–2), low stage (Ta, Tis, T1) tumors without vascular invasion. In this setting, close surveillance is critical as delayed ILND may result in increased tumor burden manifested by extranodal disease, pelvic lymph node metastasis or contralateral inguinal spread.[151]

Controversial issues in the management of the regional lymph nodes include whether or not to perform a bilateral dissection and the utility of a pelvic lymphadenectomy in the setting of positive inguinal lymph nodes. The lymphatic drainage of the penis to both the right and left inguinal lymph nodes is well documented.[150,164] Hence, bilateral ILND would seem warranted in the setting of prophylactic dissection. This methodology is further substantiated by the aforementioned benefits of an early ILND. The indication for pelvic lymphadenectomy is less clear because the presence of pelvic nodal metastases portends a poor prognosis with a 5-year survival of 10%.[152] Consequently, pelvic lymphadenectomy is rarely curative, and patients with demonstrable pelvic nodes may receive more benefit from neoadjuvant systemic therapy.

Distant

Patients uncommonly present with distant disease (less than 3%).[165] Table 47.10 summarizes the efficacy of single-agent and combination chemotherapy in the setting of advanced penile cancer.

TABLE 47.10. Selected chemotherapeutic studies directed at the treatment of advanced penile carcinoma.

Reference	*Year of study*	*No. of patients*	*Design*	*Stages*	*Treatment regimen*	*Median survival (months)*	*Conclusions*
Hussein[171]	—	5	Phase II	Regional, bone metastasis	Cisplatin + 5-fluorouracil	15	All had clinical PR, all received subsequent XRT
Haas[170]	1986–1994	40	Phase II	Locally advanced or metastatic disease	Cisplatin + methotrexate + bleomycin	28 (progression-free survival, 14 weeks)	CR 12.5% PR 20% Treatment-related death in 12.5% 15% life-threatening toxicities
Sklaroff[166]	1970s	11	Phase II	Regional	Cisplatin Prior treatments: 50% ILND 63% XRT 88% chemo		OR 33% 1 patient had CR of 7 months
Ahmed[167]	—	39	Phase II	Advanced disease	Methotrexate 13 Bleomycin 14 Cisplatin 12	2 to 8 (nonresponders vs. responders)	Median response (in months): Methotrexate 3 Bleomycin 3 Cisplatin 8
Dexeus[173]	1987–1989	12	Phase II	Advanced; 93% nodal disease	Cisplatin + methotrexate + bleomycin	10	OR 72% CR 14% PR 57%
Sklaroff[168]	1970s	8	Phase I	Advanced 88% nodal, 38% liver, 50% pulmonary	Methotrexate Prior treatments: 75% ILND 38% XRT 25% chemo		OR 38% lasting 2–11 months
Shammas[172]	1985–1990	8	Phase II	Metastatic disease/ inoperable	Cisplatin + 5-fluorouracil	12	PR 25% Response facilitated subsequent surgery
Edsmyr[159]	1971–1984	42	Case series	T1 36 T2 45 T3 19	Group 1 45 Gy + bleomycin Group II 58 Gy + bleomycin	77% 5-year survival	Group I CR 86% Group II CR 94% Local recurrence 10%

Large, multiinstitutional trials are uncommon in penile cancer, largely because of its low incidence. Single-agent cisplatin,[166,167] methotrexate,[167,168] and bleomycin[159,167] have all demonstrated treatment efficacy, with partial responses occurring in 14% to 53% of patients. However, complete and durable responses following single-agent chemotherapy are rare, occurring in 7% to 8% of patients.[167] A multiinstitutional SWOG study treated 26 chemotherapy-naïve patients with cisplatin. The investigators noted a modest response of 15% with 1 to 3 months durability.[169]

Suboptimal responses with single-agent chemotherapy prompted the use of multidrug regimens. A Phase II intergroup study, SWOG 8520, treated 40 patients with locally advanced or metastatic disease with cisplatin, bleomycin, and methotrexate. The median overall and progression-free survival in this population was 28 months and 14 weeks, respectively.[170] The overall response rate in this cohort of patients was 33%. However, the toxicity of the regimen was prohibitive, with treatment-related deaths occurring in 13% and life-threatening grade 4 toxicity in 15%.

Because of its squamous cell origin, established regimens utilized in the management of head and neck cancers have been tested in advanced penile cancer. The combination of cisplatin and 5-fluorouracil has demonstrated promising results, with median survival of 15 to 57 months in responders.[171,172] Moreover, this regimen has documented efficacy in improving the feasibility of salvage surgery. Its use may be limited by toxicity because only 38% of patients received more than two cycles. Other regimens have provided modest responses in advanced disease.[173]

In summary, combination chemotherapy appears to offer the best efficacy in the treatment of advanced/nonsurgical carcinoma of the penis. Current regimens offer a modest response rate and may facilitate subsequent surgery, although the role of this methodology is evolving and the effectiveness is uncertain. Certainly, the use of novel agents and drug combinations is warranted in this disease.

References

1. Diringer MN. Evidence-based medicine: what do you do when there's no evidence? Crit Care Med 2003;31(2):659–660.
2. Jemal A, Murray T, et al. Cancer statistics, 2003. CA Cancer J Clin 53(1):5–26. Summary of the AUA best practice policy recommendations. Am Fam Physician 2003;63(6):1145–1154.
3. Cole P, Hoover R, et al. Occupation and cancer of the lower urinary tract. Cancer (Phila) 1972;29(5):1250–1260.
4. Sandberg AA. Cytogenetics and molecular genetics of bladder cancer: a personal view. Am J Med Genet 2002;115(3):173–182.
5. Obermann EC, Junker K, et al. Frequent genetic alterations in flat urothelial hyperplasias and concomitant papillary bladder cancer as detected by CGH, LOH, and FISH analyses. J Pathol 2003;199(1):50–57.
6. Burch JD, Rohan TE, et al. Risk of bladder cancer by source and type of tobacco exposure: a case-control study. Int J Cancer 1989;44(4):622–628.
7. Morrison AS, Cole P. Epidemiology of bladder cancer. Urol Clin N Am 1976;3(1):13–29.
8. Berger CS, Sandberg AA, et al. Chromosomes in kidney, ureter, and bladder cancer. Cancer Genet Cytogenet 1986;23:1–24.
9. Millar J. Review on bladder cancer. New rather than old TNM staging system should have been used. BMJ 1999; 318(7187):875–876.
10. Busch C, Algaba F. The WHO/ISUP 1998 and WHO 1999 systems for malignancy grading of bladder cancer. Scientific foundation and translation to one another and previous systems. Virchows Arch 2002;441(2):105–108.
11. Lopez JI, Angulo JC. The prognostic significance of vascular invasion in stage T1 bladder cancer. Histopathology (Oxf) 1995; 27(1):27–33.
12. Stein JP, Lieskovsky G, Cote R, et al. Radical cystectomy in the treatment of invasive bladder cancer: long-term results in 1,054 patients. J Clin Oncol 2001;19:666–675.
13. Van Der Meijden A, Sylvester R, Collette L, Bono A, Ten Kate F. The role and impact of pathology review on stage and grade assessment of stages Ta and T1 bladder tumors: a combined analysis of 5 European Organization for Research and Treatment of Cancer Trials. J Urol 2000;164,1533–1537.
14. Schultz PK, Herr HW, Zhang ZF, et al. Neoadjuvant chemotherapy for invasive bladder cancer: prognostic factors for survival of patients treated with M-VAC with 5-year follow-up. J Clin Oncol 1994;12(7):1394–1401.
15. Madersbacher S, Hochreiter W, Burkhard F, et al. Radical cystectomy for bladder cancer today—a homogeneous series without neoadjuvant therapy. J Clin Oncol 2003;21(4):690–696.
16. Haleblian GE, Skinner EC, Dickinson MG, et al. Hydronephrosis as a prognostic indicator in bladder cancer patients. J Urol 1998;160(6 pt 1):2011–2014.
17. Fossa SD, Ous S, Berner A. Clinical significance of the "palpable mass" in patients with muscle-infiltrating bladder cancer undergoing cystectomy after pre-operative radiotherapy. Br J Urol 1991;67(1):54–60.
18. See WA, Fuller JR. Staging of advanced bladder cancer. Current concepts and pitfalls. Urol Clin N Am 1992;19(4):663–683.
19. Holmang S, Hedelin H, Anderstrom C, et al. The importance of the depth of invasion in stage T1 bladder carcinoma: a prospective cohort study. J Urol 1997;157(3):800–803.
20. Sidransky D, Von Eschenbach A, Tsai YC, et al. Identification of p53 gene mutations in bladder cancers and urine samples. Science 1991;252(5006):706–709.
21. Esrig D, Elmajian D, Groshen S, et al. Accumulation of nuclear p53 and tumor progression in bladder cancer. N Engl J Med 1994; 331(19):1259–1264.
22. Sarkis AS, Dalbagni G, Cordon-Cardo C, et al. Nuclear overexpression of p53 protein in transitional cell bladder carcinoma: a marker for disease progression. J Natl Cancer Inst 1993; 85(1):53–59.
23. Sarkis AS, Bajorin DF, Reuter VE, et al. Prognostic value of p53 nuclear overexpression in patients with invasive bladder cancer treated with neoadjuvant MVAC. J Clin Oncol 1995;13(6): 1384–1390.
24. Esrig D, Elmajian D, Groshen S, Freeman JA, Stein JP. Accumulation of nuclear p53 and tumor progression in bladder cancer. N Engl J Med 1994;33:1259–1264.
25. Llopis J, Alcaraz A, Ribal MJ, et al. p53 expression predicts progression and poor survival in T1 bladder tumours. Eur Urol 2000;37:644–653.
26. Woodburn JR. The epidermal growth factor receptor and its inhibition in cancer therapy. Pharmacol Ther 1999;82(2–3):241–250.
27. Small EJ, Halabi S, Dalbagni G, et al. Cancer and Leukemia Group B. Overview of bladder cancer trials in the Cancer and Leukemia Group B. Cancer (Phila) 2003;97(8):2090–2098.
28. Lipponen P, Eskelinen M. Expression of epidermal growth factor receptor in bladder cancer as related to established prognostic factors, oncoprotein (c-erbB-2, p53) expression and long-term prognosis. Br J Cancer 1994;69(6):1120–1125.
29. Ravery V, Grignon D, Angulo J, et al. Evaluation of epidermal growth factor receptor, transforming growth factor alpha, epidermal growth factor and c-erbB2 in the progression of invasive bladder cancer, epidermal growth factor and c-erbB2 in the progression of invasive bladder cancer. Urol Res 1997;25:9–17.

30. Jimenez RE, Hussain M, Bianco FJ Jr, et al. Her-2/neu overexpression in muscle-invasive urothelial carcinoma of the bladder: prognostic significance and comparative analysis in primary and metastatic tumors. Clin Cancer Res 2001;7(8):2440–2447.
31. Sato K, Moriyama M, Mori S, et al. An immunohistologic evaluation of c-erb-B2 gene product in patients with urinary bladder carcinoma. Cancer (Phila) 1992;70:2493–2498.
32. Mellon JK, Lunec J, Wright C, Horne CH, Kelly P, Neal DE. C-erbB-2 in bladder cancer: molecular biology, correlation with epidermal growth factor receptors and prognostic value. J Urol 1996;155:321.
33. Underwood M, Bartlett J, Reeves J, Gardiner DS, Scott R, Cooke T. C-erb-B2 gene amplification: a molecular marker in recurrent bladder tumors? Cancer Res 1995;55:2422–2430.
34. Kausch I, Böhle A. Molecular aspects of bladder cancer: III. Prognostic markers of bladder cancer. Eur Urol 2002;41:15–29.
35. Halling KC, King W, Sokolova IA, et al. A comparison of cytology and fluorescence in situ hybridization for the detection of urothelial carcinoma. J Urol 2000;164(5):1768–1775.
36. Sarosdy MF, DeVere White RW, Soloway MS, et al. Results of a multicenter trial using the BTA test to monitor for and diagnose recurrent bladder cancer. J Urol 1995;154:379–384.
37. Schmetter BS, Habicht KK, Lamm DL, et al. A multicenter trial evaluation of the fibrin/fibrinogen degradation products test for detection and monitoring of bladder cancer. J Urol 1997;158: 801–805.
38. Shelfo SW, Soloway MS. The role of nuclear matrix protein 22 in the detection of persistent or recurrent transitional-cell cancer of the bladder. World J Urol 1997;15(2):107 111.
39. Steiner G, Schoenberg MP, Linn JF, Mao L, Sidransky D. Detection of bladder cancer recurrence by microsatellite analysis of urine. Nat Med 1997;3(6):621–624.
40. Yoshida K, Sugino T, Tahara H, et al. Telomerase activity in bladder carcinoma and its implication for noninvasive diagnosis by detection of exfoliated cancer cells in urine. Cancer (Phila) 1997;79:362.
41. Grossfeld GD, Wolf JS Jr, et al. Asymptomatic microscopic hematuria in adults: summary of the AUA best practice policy recommendations. Am Fam Physician 2001;63(6):1145–1154.
42. Herr HW. The value of a second transurethral resection in evaluating patients with bladder tumors. J Urol 1999;162:74–76.
43. Miladi M, Peyromaure M, Zerbib M, Saighi D, Debre B. The value of a second transurethral resection in evaluating patients with bladder tumours. Eur Urol 2003;43:241–245.
44. Herr HW, Badalament RA, Amato DA, Laudone VP, Fair WR, Whitmore WF Jr. Superficial bladder cancer treated with bacillus Calmette-Guerin: a multivariate analysis of factors affecting tumor progression. J Urol 1989;141(1):22–29.
45. Huncharek M, Geschwind JF, Witherspoon B, McGarry R, Adcock D. Intravesical chemotherapy prophylaxis in primary superficial bladder cancer: a meta-analysis of 3703 patients from 11 randomized trials. J Clin Epidemiol 2000;53:676–680.
46. Huncharek M, McGarry R, Kupelnick B. Impact of intravesical chemotherapy on recurrence rate of recurrent superficial transitional cell carcinoma of the bladder: results of a meta-analysis. Anticancer Res 2001;21:765–770.
47. Alexandroff AB, Jackson AM, O'Donnell MA, James K. BCG immunotherapy of bladder cancer: 20 years on. Lancet 1999;353: 1689–1694.
48. Shelley MD, Kynaston H, Court J, et al. A systematic review of intravesical bacillus Calmette-Guérin plus transurethral resection vs. transurethral resection alone in Ta and T1 bladder cancer. BJU Int 2001;88:209–216.
49. Sylvester RJ, van der Meijden AP, Lamm DL. Intravesical bacillus Calmette-Guerin reduces the risk of progression in patients with superficial bladder cancer: a meta-analysis of the published results of randomized clinical trials. J Urol 2002;168(5): 1964–1970.
50. Lamm DL, Blumenstein BA, Crawford ED, et al. A randomized trial of intravesical doxorubicin and immunotherapy with bacille Calmette-Guerin for transitional-cell carcinoma of the bladder. N Engl J Med 1991;325(17):1205–1209.
51. Martinez-Pineiro JA, Jimenez LJ, Martinez-Pineiro L Jr, et al. Bacillus Calmette-Guerin versus doxorubicin versus thiotepa: a randomized prospective study in 202 patients with superficial bladder cancer. J Urol 1990;143(3):502–506.
52. van der Meijden AP, Brausi M, Zambon V, Kirkels W, de Balincourt C, Sylvester R. Members of the EORTC Genito-Urinary Group. Intravesical instillation of epirubicin, bacillus Calmette-Guerin and bacillus Calmette-Guerin plus isoniazid for intermediate and high risk Ta, T1 papillary carcinoma of the bladder: a European Organization for Research and Treatment of Cancer genitourinary group randomized phase III trial. J Urol 2001;166(2):476–481.
53. Lamm DL, DeHaven JI, Shriver J, Sarosdy MF. Prospective randomized comparison of intravesical with percutaneous bacillus Calmette-Guerin versus intravesical bacillus Calmette-Guerin in superficial bladder cancer. J Urol 1991;145(4):738–740.
54. Pawinski A, Sylvester R, Kurth KH, et al. A combined analysis of European organization for research and treatment of cancer, and medical research council randomized clinical trials for the prophylactic treatment of stage TaT1 bladder cancer. J Urol 1996;156:1934–1941.
55. Herr H. Tumor progression and survival of patients with high grade, noninvasive papillary (TaG3) bladder tumors: 15-year outcome. J Urol 2000;163:60–62.
56. Lamm DL, Blumenstein BA, Crissman JD, et al. Maintenance bacillus Calmette-Guérin immunotherapy for recurrent Ta, T1 and carcinoma in situ transitional cell carcinoma of the bladder: a randomized Southwest Oncology Group study. J Urol 2000; 163:1124–1129.
57. O'Donnell MA, Krohn J, DeWolf WC. Salvage intravesical therapy with interferon-alpha 2b plus low dose bacillus Calmette-Guerin is effective in patients with superficial bladder cancer in whom bacillus Calmette-Guerin alone previously failed. J Urol 2001;166(4):1300–1304.
58. Dalbagni G, Russo P, Sheinfeld J, et al. Phase I trial of intravesical gemcitabine in bacillus Calmette-Guerin-refractory transitional-cell carcinoma of the bladder. J Clin Oncol 2002; 20(15):3193–3198.
59. Steinberg G, Bahnson R, Brosman S, et al. Efficacy and safety of valrubicin for the treatment of bacillus Calmette-Guerin refractory carcinoma in situ of the bladder: The Valrubicin Study Group. J Urol 2000;163:761–767.
60. Richie JP. Intravesical chemotherapy. Treatment selection, techniques, and results. Urol Clin N Am 1992;19(3):521–527.
61. Lamm DL, Blumenstein BA, Crawford ED, et al. Randomized Intergroup comparison of bacillus Calmette-Guerin immunotherapy and mitomycin C chemotherapy prophylaxis in superficial transitional cell carcinoma of the bladder. Urol Oncol 1995;1:119–126.
62. Tolley DA, Parmar MK, Grigor KM, et al. The effect of intravesical mitomycin C on recurrence of newly diagnosed superficial bladder cancer: a further report with 7 years of follow up. J Urol 1996;155(4):1233–1238.
63. Herr HW. Transurethral resection of muscle-invasive bladder cancer: 10-year outcome. J Clin Oncol 2001;19(1):89–93.
64. Revelo MP, Cookson MS, Chang SS, Shook MF, Smith JA Jr, Shappell SB. Incidence and location of prostate and urothelial carcinoma in prostates from cystoprostatectomies: implications for possible apical sparing surgery. J Urol 2004;171:646–651.
65. Herr HW. Surgical factors in bladder cancer: more (nodes) + more (pathology) = less (mortality). BJU Int 2003;92(3):187–188.
66. Rodel C, Grabenbauer GG, Kuhn R, et al. Combined-modality treatment and selective organ preservation in invasive bladder cancer: long-term results. J Clin Oncol 2002;20:3061–3071.

67. Fossa SD, Waehre H, Aass N, Jacobsen AB, Olsen DR, Ous S. Bladder cancer definitive radiation therapy of muscle-invasive bladder cancer. A retrospective analysis of 317 patients. Cancer (Phila) 1993;72:3036–3043.
68. Hautmann RE, Petriconi RD, Gottrried H-W. The ileal neobladder: complications and functional results in 363 patients after 11 years of followup. J Urol 1999;161:422–428.
69. Shipley WU, Prout GR Jr, Einstein AB, et al. Treatment of invasive bladder cancer by cisplatin and radiation in patients unsuited for surgery. JAMA 1987;258(7):931–935.
70. Shipley WU, Kaufman DS, Tester WJ, Pilepich MV, Sandler HM. Radiation Therapy Oncology Group. Overview of bladder cancer trials in the Radiation Therapy Oncology Group. Cancer (Phila) 2003;97(8):2115–2119.
71. Shipley WU, Winter KA, Kaufman DS, et al. Phase III trial of neoadjuvant chemotherapy in patients with invasive bladder cancer treated with selective bladder preservation by combined radiation therapy and chemotherapy: initial results of Radiation Therapy Oncology Group 89-03. J Clin Oncol 1998;16(11): 3576–3583.
72. Cortesi E. Neoadjuvant treatment for locally advanced bladder cancer: a randomized prospective clinical trial. Proc Am Soc Clin Oncol 1995;14:237a (abstract).
73. Martinez-Pineiro JA, Gonzalez Martin M, Arocena F, et al. Neoadjuvant cisplatin chemotherapy before radical cystectomy in invasive transitional cell carcinoma of the bladder: a prospective randomized phase III study. J Urol 1995;153:964–973.
74. Abol-Eneim H, El-Mekresh M, El-Baz M, Ghoneim MA. Neoadjuvant chemotherapy in the treatment of invasive transitional bladder cancer: a controlled, prospective randomized study. Br J Urol 1997;79(suppl 4):43.
75. Malmstrom PU, Rintala E, Wahlqvist R, Hellsten S, Sander S. Five-year followup of a prospective trial of radical cystectomy and neoadjuvant chemotherapy: Nordic Cystectomy Trial I. The Nordic Cooperative Bladder Cancer Study Group. J Urol 1996; 155(6):1903–1906.
76. Sherif A, Rintala E, Mestad O, et al. Neoadjuvant cisplatin-methotrexate chemotherapy for invasive bladder cancer: Nordic cystectomy trial 2. Scand J Urol Nephrol 2002;36(6):419–425.
77. Advanced Bladder Cancer Meta-analysis Collaboration. Neoadjuvant chemotherapy in invasive bladder cancer: a systematic review and meta-analysis. Lancet 2003;361:1927–1934.
78. Grossman HB, Natale RB, Tangen CM, et al. Neoadjuvant chemotherapy plus cystectomy compared with cystectomy alone for locally advanced bladder cancer N Engl J Med 2003; 349(9):859–866.
79. Sternberg CN, Parmar M. Neoadjuvant chemotherapy is not (yet) standard treatment for muscle-invasive bladder cancer. J Clin Oncol 2001;19(18S):21s–26s.
80. Neoadjuvant cisplatin, methotrexate, and vinblastine chemotherapy for muscle-invasive bladder cancer: a randomised controlled trial. International collaboration of trialists. Lancet 1999;354(9178):533–540.
81. Skinner DG, Daniels JR, Russell CA, et al. The role of adjuvant chemotherapy following cystectomy for invasive bladder cancer: a prospective comparative trial. J Urol 1991;145(3):459–464.
82. Stockle M, Meyenburg W, Wellek S, et al. Advanced bladder cancer (stages pT3b, pT4a, pN1 and pN2): improved survival after radical cystectomy and 3 adjuvant cycles of chemotherapy. Results of a controlled prospective study. J Urol 1992;148: 302–307.
83. Studer UE, Bacchi M, Biedermann C, et al. Adjuvant cisplatin chemotherapy following cystectomy for bladder cancer: results of a prospective randomized trial. J Urol 1994;152(1):81–84.
84. Freiha F, Reese J, Torti FM. A randomized trial of radical cystectomy versus radical cystectomy plus cisplatin, vinblastine and methotrexate chemotherapy for muscle invasive bladder cancer. J Urol 1996;155(2):495–500.
85. Bono AV, Benvenuti C, Reali L, et al. Adjuvant chemotherapy in advanced bladder cancer. Italian Uro-Oncologic Cooperative Group. Prog Clin Biol Res 1989;303:533–540.
86. Loehrer PJ Sr, Einhorn LH, Elson PJ, et al. A randomized comparison of cisplatin alone or in combination with methotrexate, vinblastine, and doxorubicin in patients with metastatic urothelial carcinoma: a cooperative group study. J Clin Oncol 1992; 10(7):1066–1073.
87. de Wit R. European Organization for Research and Treatment. Overview of bladder cancer trials in the European Organization for Research and Treatment. Cancer (Phila) 2003;97:2120–2126.
88. Soloway MS, Einstein A, Corder MP, et al. A comparison of cisplatin and the combination of cisplatin and cyclophosphamide in advanced urothelial cancer. A National Bladder Cancer Collaborative Group A Study. Cancer (Phila) 1983;52(5):767–772.
89. Khandekar JD, Elson PJ, DeWys WD, et al. Comparative activity and toxicity of cis-diamminedichloroplatinum (DDP) and a combination of doxorubicin, cyclophosphamide, and DDP in disseminated transitional cell carcinomas of the urinary tract. J Clin Oncol 1985;3(4):539–545.
90. Troner M, Birch R, Omura GA, et al. Phase III comparison of cisplatin alone versus cisplatin, doxorubicin and cyclophosphamide in the treatment of bladder (urothelial) cancer: a Southeastern Cancer Study Group trial. J Urol 1987;137(4): 660–662.
91. Gagliano R, Levin H, El-Bolkainy MN, et al. Adriamycin versus adriamycin plus cis-diamminedichloroplatinum (DDP) in advanced transitional cell bladder carcinoma. A Southwest Oncology Group study. Am J Clin Oncol 1983;6(2):215–218.
92. Hillcoat BL, Raghavan D, Matthews J, et al. A randomized trial of cisplatin versus cisplatin plus methotrexate in advanced cancer of the urothelial tract. J Clin Oncol 1989;7(6):706–709.
93. Logothetis CJ, Dexeus FH, Finn L, et al. A prospective randomized trial comparing MVAC and CISCA chemotherapy for patients with metastatic urothelial tumors. J Clin Oncol 1990; 8(6):1050–1055.
94. Loehrer PJ Sr, Einhorn LH, Elson PJ, et al. A randomized comparison of cisplatin alone or in combination with methotrexate, vinblastine, and doxorubicin in patients with metastatic urothelial carcinoma: a cooperative group study. J Clin Oncol 1992; 10(7):1066–1073.
95. Mead GM, Russell M, Clark P, et al. A randomized trial comparing methotrexate and vinblastine (MV) with cisplatin, methotrexate and vinblastine (CMV) in advanced transitional cell carcinoma: results and a report on prognostic factors in a Medical Research Council study. MRC Advanced Bladder Cancer Working Party. Br J Cancer 1998;78(8):1067–1075.
96. von der Maase H, Hansen SW, Roberts JT, et al. Gemcitabine and cisplatin versus methotrexate, vinblastine, doxorubicin, and cisplatin in advanced or metastatic bladder cancer: results of a large, randomized, multinational, multicenter, phase III study. J Clin Oncol 2000;18(17):3068–3077.
97. Sternberg CN, de Mulder PH, Schornagel JH, et al. Randomized phase III trial of high-dose-intensity methotrexate, vinblastine, doxorubicin, and cisplatin (MVAC) chemotherapy and recombinant human granulocyte colony-stimulating factor versus classic MVAC in advanced urothelial tract tumors: European Organization for Research and Treatment of Cancer Protocol no. 30924. J Clin Oncol 2001;19(10):2638–2646.
98. Juffs HG, Moore MJ, Tannock IF. The role of systemic chemotherapy in the management of muscle-invasive bladder cancer. Lancet Oncol 2002;3(12):738–747.
99. Hall MC, Womack S, Sagalowsky AI, Carmody T, Erickstad MD, Roehrborn CG. Prognostic factors, recurrence, and survival in transitional cell carcinoma of the upper urinary tract: a 30-year experience in 252 patients. Urology 1998;52:594–601.

100. Held PJ, Brunner F, Odaka M, et al. Five-year survival for end-stage renal disease patients in the United States, Europe, and Japan: 1982 to 1987. Am J Kidney Dis 1990;15:451.
101. Jabbour ME, Smith AD. Primary percutaneous approach to upper urinary tract transitional cell carcinoma. Urol Clin N Am 2000;27(4):739–750.
102. Assimos DG, Hall MC, Martin JH. Ureteroscopic management of patients with upper tract transitional cell carcinoma. Urol Clin N Am 2000;27(4):751–760.
103. Thalmann GN, Markwalder R, Walter B, Studer UE. Long-term experience with bacillus Calmette-Guerin therapy of upper urinary tract transitional cell carcinoma in patients not eligible for surgery. J Urol 2002;168:1381–1385.
104. Tawfiek ER, Bagley DH. Upper-tract transitional cell carcinoma. Urology 1997;50(3):321–329.
105. Zincke H, Neves RJ. Feasibility of conservative surgery for transitional cell carcinoma of the upper urinary tract. Urol Clin N Am 1984;11:717.
106. Gill IS, Sung GT, Hobart MG, et al. Laparoscopic radical nephroureterectomy for upper tract transitional cell carcinoma: The Cleveland Clinic experience. J Urol 2000;164:1513–1522.
107. Dalbagni G, Zhang ZF, Lacombe L, Herr HW. Female urethral carcinoma: an analysis of treatment outcome and a plea for a standardized management strategy. Br J Urol 1998;82:835–841.
108. Milosevic MF, Warde PR, Banerjee D, et al. Urethral carcinoma in women: results of treatment with primary radiotherapy. Radiother Oncol 2000;56(1):29–35.
109. Dalbagni G, Zhang ZF, Lacombe L, Herr HW. Male urethral carcinoma: analysis of treatment outcome, Urology 1999;53(6):1126–1132.
110. American Cancer Society. Cancer Facts and Figures 2003. Washington, DC: American Cancer Society, 2003.
111. Peters RK, Mack TM, Bernstein L. Parallels in the epidemiology of selected anogenital carcinomas. J Natl Cancer Inst 1984;72(3):609–615.
112. Barrasso R, De Brux J, Croissant O, Orth G. High prevalence of papillomavirus-associated penile intraepithelial neoplasia in sexual partners of women with cervical intraepithelial neoplasia. N Engl J Med 1987;317(15):916–923.
113. Rubin MA, Kleter B, Zhou M, et al. Detection and typing of human papillomavirus DNA in penile carcinoma: evidence for multiple independent pathways of penile carcinogenesis. Am J Pathol 2001;159:1211.
114. Maden C, Sherman KJ, Beckmann AM, et al. History of circumcision, medical conditions, and sexual activity and risk of penile cancer [comment]. J Natl Cancer Inst 1993;85:19.
115. Gregoire L, Cubilla AL, Reuter VE, Haas GP, Lancaster WD. Preferential association of human papillomavirus with high-grade histologic variants of penile-invasive squamous cell carcinoma. J Natl Cancer Inst 1995;87:1705.
116. Cubilla AL. Carcinoma of the penis. Mod Pathol 1995;8:116.
117. Aynaud O, Ionesco M, Barrasso R. Penile intraepithelial neoplasia. Specific clinical features correlate with histologic and virologic findings. Cancer (Phila) 1994;74:1762.
118. Tsen HF, Morgenstern H, Mack T, Peters RK. Risk factors for penile cancer: results of a population-based case-control study in Los Angeles County (United States). Cancer Causes Control 2001;12:267.
119. Brinton LA, Li JY, Rong SD, et al. Risk factors for penile cancer: results from a case-control study in China. Int J Cancer 1991;47:504.
120. Stern RS. Genital tumors among men with psoriasis exposed to psoralens and ultraviolet A radiation (PUVA) and ultraviolet B radiation. The Photochemotherapy Follow-up Study. N Engl J Med 1990;322:1093.
121. American College of Obstetricians and Gynecologists. Committee on Obstetric Practice: ACOG Committee Opinion. Circumcision. Number 260, October 2001. Obstet Gynecol 2001;98:707.
122. Kochen M, McCurdy S. Circumcision and the risk of cancer of the penis. A life-table analysis. Am J Dis Child 1980;134:484.
123. Cubilla AL, Reuter VE, Gregoire L, et al. Basaloid squamous cell carcinoma: a distinctive human papilloma virus-related penile neoplasm: a report of 20 cases. Am J Surg Pathol 1998;22(6):755–761.
124. Cubilla AL, Velazques EF, Reuter VE, et al. Warty (condylomatous) squamous cell carcinoma of the penis: a report of 11 cases and proposed classification of 'verruciform' penile tumors. J Surg Pathol 2000;24:505.
125. Kraus FT, Perezmesa C. Verrucous carcinoma. Clinical and pathologic study of 105 cases involving oral cavity, larynx and genitalia. Cancer (Phila) 1966;19:26.
126. American Joint Committee on Cancer. Penis. In: Greene FL, Page DL, Fleming ID, et al (eds). Cancer Staging Manual, 6th ed. New York: Springer, 2002:303.
127. Jacobellis U. Modified radical inguinal lymphadenectomy for carcinoma of the penis: technique and results. J Urol 2003;169(4):1349–1352.
128. Bevan-Thomas R, Slaton JW, Pettaway CA. Contemporary morbidity from lymphadenectomy for penile squamous cell carcinoma: the M.D. Anderson Cancer Center Experience. J Urol 2002;167:1638.
129. Lopes A, Bezerra AL, Pinto CA, Serrano SV, de Mello CA, Villa LL. p53 as a new prognostic factor for lymph node metastasis in penile carcinoma: analysis of 82 patients treated with amputation and bilateral lymphadenectomy. J Urol 2002;168:81.
130. Lopes A, Hidalgo GS, Kowalski LP, Torloni H, Rossi BM, Fonseca FP. Prognostic factors in carcinoma of the penis: multivariate analysis of 145 patients treated with amputation and lymphadenectomy. J Urol 1996;156(5):1637–1642.
131. Slaton JW, Morgenstern N, Levy DA, et al. Tumor stage, vascular invasion and the percentage of poorly differentiated cancer: independent prognosticators for inguinal lymph node metastasis in penile squamous cancer. J Urol 2001;165:1138.
132. Martins AC, Faria SM, Cologna AJ, Suaid HJ, Tucci S Jr. Immunoexpression of p53 protein and proliferating cell nuclear antigen in penile carcinoma. J Urol 2002;167:89.
133. Horenblas S, van Tinteren H. Squamous cell carcinoma of the penis. IV. Prognostic factors of survival: analysis of tumor, nodes and metastasis classification system. J Urol 1994;151:1239.
134. Sarin R, Norman AR, Steel GG, Horwich A. Treatment results and prognostic factors in 101 men treated for squamous carcinoma of the penis. Int J Radiat Oncol Biol Phys 1997;38(4):713–722.
135. Bezerra AL, Lopes A, Santiago GH, Ribeiro KC, Latorre MR, Villa LL. Human papillomavirus as a prognostic factor in carcinoma of the penis: analysis of 82 patients treated with amputation and bilateral lymphadenectomy. Cancer (Phila) 2001;91:2315.
136. Srinivas V, Morse MJ, Herr HW, Sogani PC, Whitmore WF Jr. Penile cancer: relation of extent of nodal metastasis to survival. J Urol 1987;137(5):880–882.
137. Ornellas AA, Seixas AL, Marota A, Wisnescky A, Campos F, de Moraes JR. Surgical treatment of invasive squamous cell carcinoma of the penis: retrospective analysis of 350 cases. J Urol 1994;151:1244.
138. Horenblas S, van Tinteren H, Delemarre JF, Moonen LM, Lustig V, Kroger R. Squamous cell carcinoma of the penis: accuracy of tumor, nodes and metastasis classification system, and role of lymphangiography, computerized tomography scan and fine needle aspiration cytology. J Urol 1991;146:1279.
139. Emerson RE, Ulbright TM, Eble JN, Geary WA, Eckert GJ, Cheng L. Predicting cancer progression in patients with penile squamous cell carcinoma: the importance of depth of invasion and vascular invasion. Mod Pathol 2001;14:963.

140. Soria JC, Fizazi K, Piron D, et al. Squamous cell carcinoma of the penis: multivariate analysis of prognostic factors and natural history in monocentric study with a conservative policy. Ann Oncol 1997;8(11):1089–1098.
141. Lopes A, Rossi BM, Fonseca FP, Morini S. Unreliability of modified inguinal lymphadenectomy for clinical staging of penile carcinoma. Cancer (Phila) 1996;77(10):2099–2102.
142. Catalona WJ. Modified inguinal lymphadenectomy for carcinoma of the penis with preservation of saphenous veins: technique and preliminary results. J Urol 1988;140(2):306–310.
143. Scappini P, Piscioli F, Pusiol T, Hofstetter A, Rothenberger K, Luciani L. Penile cancer. Aspiration biopsy cytology for staging. Cancer (Phila) 1986;58(7):1526–1533.
144. Cabanas RM. Anatomy and biopsy of sentinel lymph nodes. Urol Clin N Am 1992;19:267.
145. Cabanas RM. An approach for the treatment of penile carcinoma. Cancer (Phila) 1977;39:456.
146. Pettaway CA, Pisters LL, Dinney CP, et al. Sentinel lymph node dissection for penile carcinoma: the M.D. Anderson Cancer Center experience. J Urol 1995;154:1999.
147. Perinetti E, Crane DB, Catalona WJ. Unreliability of sentinel lymph node biopsy for staging penile carcinoma. J Urol 1980; 124:734.
148. Valdes Olmos RA, Tanis PJ, Hoefnagel CA, et al. Penile lymphoscintigraphy for sentinel node identification. Eur J Nuclear Med 2001;28:581.
149. Wespes E, Simon J, Schulman CC. Cabanas approach: is sentinel node biopsy reliable for staging penile carcinoma? Urology 1986;28(4):278–279.
150. Tanis PJ, Lont AP, Meinhardt W, Olmos RA, Nieweg OE, Horenblas S. Dynamic sentinel node biopsy for penile cancer: reliability of a staging technique. J Urol 2002;168:76.
151. Lont AP, Horenblas S, Tanis PJ, Gallee MP, Tinteren H, Nieweg OE. Management of clinically node negative penile carcinoma: Improved survival after the introduction of dynamic sentinel lymph node biopsy. J Urol 2003;170:783.
152. Lynch DF Jr, Pettaway CA. Tumors of the penis. In: Walsh PC, Retik AB, Vaughn ED Jr, et al (eds). Campbell's Urology, 8th ed. Philadelphia: Saunders, 2002:2945.
153. Agrawal A, Pai D, Ananthakrishnan N, Smile SR, Ratnakar C. The histological extent of the local spread of carcinoma of the penis and its therapeutic implications. BJU Int 2000;85: 299.
154. Donat SM, Cozzi PJ, Herr HW. Surgery of penile and urethral carcinoma. In: Walsh PC, Retik AB, Vaughn ED Jr, et al (eds). Campbell's Urology, 8th ed. Philadelphia: Saunders, 2001:2983.
155. Hoffman MA, Renshaw AA, Loughlin KR. Squamous cell carcinoma of the penis and microscopic pathologic margins: how much margin is needed for local cure? Cancer (Phila) 1999;85: 1565.
156. van Bezooijen BP, Horenblas S, Meinhardt W, Newling DW. Laser therapy for carcinoma in situ of the penis. J Urol 2001;166: 1670.
157. Mohs FE, Snow SN, Larson PO. Mohs micrographic surgery for penile tumors. Urol Clin N Am 1992;19:291.
158. Ravi R, Chaturvedi HK, Sastry DV. Role of radiation therapy in the treatment of carcinoma of the penis. Br J Urol 1994;74:646.
159. Edsmyr F, Andersson L, Esposti PL. Combined bleomycin and radiation therapy in carcinoma of the penis. Cancer (Phila) 1985;56(6):1257–1263.
160. Bissada NK, Yakout HH, Fahmy WE, et al. Multi-institutional long-term experience with conservative surgery for invasive penile carcinoma. J Urol 2003;169(2):500–502.
161. Mitropoulos D, Dimopoulos MA, Kiroudi-Voulgari A, Zervas A, Dimopoulos C, Logothetis CJ. Neoadjuvant cisplatin and interferon-alpha 2B in the treatment and organ preservation of penile carcinoma. J Urol 1994;152:1124.
162. Gotsadze D, Matveev B, Zak B, Mamaladze V. Is conservative organ-sparing treatment of penile carcinoma justified? Eur Urol 2000;38:306.
163. McDougal WS. Carcinoma of the penis: improved survival by early regional lymphadenectomy based on the histological grade and depth of invasion of the primary lesion. J Urol 1995;154: 1364.
164. Horenblas S, Jansen L, Meinhardt W, Hoefnagel CA, de Jong D, Nieweg OE. Detection of occult metastasis in squamous cell carcinoma of the penis using a dynamic sentinel node procedure. J Urol 2000;163:100.
165. el Demiry MI, Oliver RT, Hope-Stone HF, Blandy JP. Reappraisal of the role of radiotherapy and surgery in the management of carcinoma of the penis. Br J Urol 1984;56:724.
166. Sklaroff RB, Yagoda A. cis-Diamminedichloride platinum II (DDP) in the treatment of penile carcinoma. Cancer (Phila) 1979; 44:1563.
167. Ahmed T, Sklaroff R, Yagoda A. Sequential trials of methotrexate, cisplatin and bleomycin for penile cancer. J Urol 1984; 132(3):465–468.
168. Sklaroff RB, Yagoda A. Methotrexate in the treatment of penile carcinoma. Cancer (Phila) 1980;45:214.
169. Gagliano RG, Blumenstein BA, Crawford ED, Stephens RL, Coltman CA Jr, Costanzi JJ. cis-Diamminedichloroplatinum in the treatment of advanced epidermoid carcinoma of the penis: a Southwest Oncology Group Study. J Urol 1989;141:66.
170. Haas GP, Blumenstein BA, Gagliano RG, et al. Cisplatin, methotrexate and bleomycin for the treatment of carcinoma of the penis: a Southwest Oncology Group study. J Urol 1999;161: 1823.
171. Hussein AM, Benedetto P, Sridhar KS. Chemotherapy with cisplatin and 5-fluorouracil for penile and urethral squamous cell carcinomas. Cancer (Phila) 1990;65:433.
172. Shammas FV, Ous S, Fossa SD. Cisplatin and 5-fluorouracil in advanced cancer of the penis. J Urol 1992;147:630.
173. Dexeus FH, Logothetis CJ, Sella A, et al. Combination chemotherapy with methotrexate, bleomycin and cisplatin for advanced squamous cell carcinoma of the male genital tract. J Urol 1991;146:1284.

48

Prostate Cancer

Richard Whittington and David J. Vaughn

Prostate cancer presents one of the most controversial challenges to clinicians today. Where controversies may exist as to how best to treat many diseases, the controversies in prostate cancer start with the question, "Should we even try to diagnose this disease before it becomes clinically evident?" When the disease is found, the next question is whether the disease should be treated and whether the cure is worse than the disease. The next set of controversies revolve around how to most effectively treat the tumor. If a decision is made to proceed with radiation, the final controversies revolve around radiation fields and techniques. Each of these decision points can provoke heated discussions among recognized authorities in the field. This chapter attempts to discuss the controversies with the data supporting each point. It is likely that partisans of any argument will find support for their position, but it is also likely that a disinterested observer will see logic in each position. Before reviewing the controversies, it is necessary to develop a common foundation for the discussion.

Prostate cancer is the second leading cause of cancer death in the United States, second only to lung cancer, with an estimated 221,000 new cases in 2003 with an expected 28,900 deaths. It represents nearly one-third of all cancers diagnosed in men but only 10% of the deaths. The age-adjusted incidence of prostate cancer has increased by 70% in the past 25 years but is still 25% lower than values from 1993. There is a disequilibrium in the racial distribution of prostate cancer, with a very high incidence in African-Americans and a lower incidence in Asian-Americans (Table 48.1).[1]

The staging of prostate cancer has also been modified twice in recent years, which confuses staging. Initially, stage B tumors (palpable nodule) were divided into B1(n), a nodule smaller than 1 cm entirely surrounded by normal prostate stroma; B1, which was a larger or peripheral unilateral nodule; and B2, representing a bilateral nodule. This scheme was modified shortly after prostate-specific antigen (PSA) screening became available to describe B1 as a nodule encompassing half of one lobe and B2 as a unilateral nodule encompassing more than one-half of a lobe. B3 tumors were palpable bilaterally. This system also introduced the T1c tumor, which is not palpable but is diagnosed based on a biopsy for an elevated PSA or ultrasound abnormality. In 2001, this system was again revised to classify B1 tumors as unilateral and B2 as bilateral nodules. In the current system, T1 tumors are nonpalpable and T2 tumors are palpable and organ confined, whereas T3 tumors have palpable extraprostatic disease and T4 tumors invade adjacent structures.

The problem with this system is that T1a tumors represent incidental tumors found at transurethral resection (TUR) of the prostate for obstructive symptoms. The patient has less than 5% of the chips involved and a Gleason score less than 7. T1b tumors represent more-extensive disease or poorly differentiated tumors found at TUR, and T1c tumors are tumors discovered through PSA screening. T1b tumors may involve 6% or 90% of the chips or be very aggressive; this includes a wide range of tumors, as a T1c tumor may have one positive screening biopsy up to all biopsies involved. These more-extensive T1b and T1c tumors actually are more similar to T2b or T3 tumors and are more likely to have nodal metastases whereas the T1c tumor with 1 positive core of 12 to 24 is more similar to T1a tumors. This approach makes any conclusions based on an analysis of results based on stage highly uncertain. Nodal staging is based on the absence (N0) or presence (N1) of pelvic nodal metastases. Stage classification sets stage I as T1a N0 tumors, T2 includes any T1b/c N0 or T2 N0 tumor, stage III includes all T3 N0 tumors, and stage IV includes all T4 or N1 or M1 tumors.

Utility of Prostate-Specific Antigen as a Screening Tool

The availability of serum PSA determination has dramatically increased the number of cases of prostate cancer diagnosed in the United States. Although the American Urologic Association and the American Society of Therapeutic Radiology and Oncology argue that this finding supports the widespread availability of screening, the American College of Physicians–American Society of Internal Medicine argues that the tumors identified are not clinically significant and that they are less likely to alter the quantitative or qualitative survival. The incidence of subclinical prostate cancer in a contemporary autopsy series in an unscreened population is shown in Table 48.2.[2] Older publications have reported a higher incidence of subclinical cancers, as high as 50% at age 60 and 80% at age 80, although many of these studies date from the 1950s when PIN was not a defined entity and many of these lesions may have been interpreted as carcinoma. The incidence, mortality, and age distribution of prostate cancer and breast cancer are similar and yet there is controversy over the need to screen men for prostate cancer and little discussion of the need for screening mammography.[3] The difference is largely due to the perceived effect of both tumor and treatment on lifestyle and the effectiveness of available treat-

TABLE 48.1. Incidence and mortality caused by prostate cancer in the United States, 2003.

Ethnic group	*Incidence*[a]	*Mortality*[a]
Caucasian	172.9	32.9
African-American	275.3	75.1
Asian/Pacific Islander	107.2	15.1
Native American	60.7	18.8
Hispanic	127.6	22.6

[a] Rates per 100,000 population.
Source: Some data from Jemal et al.[1]

ments. Whether this distinction is justified is beyond the scope of this chapter.

Several studies have reviewed large screened populations for the incidence of occult prostate cancer. PSA is a serine protease inhibitor produced by both normal and malignant prostate. The malignant prostate will leak more of this protein into the circulation than normal prostate. The malignant prostate also allows a larger protein, a serine protease inhibitor, into the blood as well. These two proteins circulate in the blood as a complex that is detected by the PSA assay along with the free PSA. The picture is complicated by the fact that the infected, inflamed, and traumatized prostate gland also leaks increased quantities of PSA into the blood. Kane also reported that increased prostate volume will produce higher serum PSA levels. Using the accepted cutoff of 4.0, 95% of men with prostates smaller than 35 cm^3 have a normal PSA whereas only 75% of men with prostates larger than 45 cc^3 will have a normal value.

The normal value of 4.0 was established in studies reported by Catalona et al. and Brawer et al. of men undergoing digital rectal exam, transrectal ultrasound, and biopsy.[4,5] They found that this value found prostate cancer in 2.2% and 2.6% of asymptomatic men, respectively. In Catalona's series, the sensitivity of the PSA cutoff of 4.0 was 79% with a specificity of 59%; the predictive value of a positive test was 40% and the predictive value of a negative test was 89% for an overall accuracy of 64%. Subsequent investigations have tried to use PSA density (serum PSA/prostate volume), PSA velocity (dPSA/dt), and free PSA level to improve the specificity of the test and reduce the number of negative biopsies, without notable success.[6] The current sensitivity and specificity data would suggest that only 15% to 25% of men with PSAs between 4.0 and 7.0 have prostate cancer on biopsy.

TABLE 48.2. Incidence of prostate cancer in an autopsy series of unscreened patients.

Age (years)	*Incidence of cancer (%)*	*Incidence of high-grade (PIN)*
20–30	3.6	7.1
31–40	8.9	12
41–50	14	36
51–60	24	38
61–70	31	45
71–80	33	48

Source: Data from Sanchez-Chapado et al.[2]

Natural History of Untreated Prostate Cancer

There are a number of reviews of patients managed expectantly with localized prostate cancer with conflicting results. There are a number of reasons for this. Some series include men with incidental disease found at TUR, which has a low risk of progression to clinically significant disease, whereas other series allow men and their physicians to select treatment if they believe the risks of tumor progression outweigh the risks of treatment. Some studies observed men and selected men who did not show progression over an interval but excluded men with progression during that interval. The unknown value is the annual probability that a clinically occult tumor will progress to become clinically evident with either local tumor manifesting as a palpable nodule, bladder invasion, or outlet obstruction. This is the key value that must be applied to decisions regarding screening. As in other issues in prostate cancer, the value probably depends upon the Gleason score and other tumor characteristics.

The Veterans Administration trials in prostate cancer during the 1950s provide the basis for the Gleason scoring system for prostate cancer.[7] This was the first and is still the most important factor used to estimate the risk of metastatic disease and death. This study was confined to men with clinical stage T2–T4 Nx M0 so that it is not strictly applicable to patients seen today with T1c prostate cancers due to the lead time bias caused by the application of PSA screening. Table 48.3 shows the annual cancer-specific mortality reported in their review and the projected 15-year survival based on the mortality observed. In evaluating a patient with a newly diagnosed prostate cancer, it is necessary to balance an estimate of the cancer-specific morbidity and mortality against the mortality of competing conditions. In making these considerations, it is necessary to factor in life expectancy. The most useful estimate may come from the Internal Revenue Service, given the relationship between death and taxes. They calculate the median survival at age 60 is 24.2 years, at age 70, 16 years, and at age 80, 9.5 years.

A number of series have reviewed the survival of men electing a course of watchful waiting instead of potentially curative treatment. The most famous of these series is the series reported and updated by Johansson et al. from Uppsala.[8–10] This study is not strictly applicable, because among men with T1–T2 tumors 72 of the 223 patients appear to have had T1a tumors. They report a progression-free

TABLE 48.3. Annual mortality in men with localized prostate cancer.

Gleason score	*Annual cancer-specific mortality (%)*	*Anticipated 15-year cancer-specific survival*
2	0	100
3	1	86
4	2	74
5	2	74
6	5	54
7	7	34
8	11	17
9	11	17
10	21	2

TABLE 48.4. Complications observed in Johansson's series of men treated expectantly for T1–T2 prostate cancer.

Event	*Frequency (%)*
Moderate to severe outlet obstruction	30
Surgery required	16
Catheter dependent	11
Local problem (edema/pain)	12
Hospitalization	19

Source: Data from references 8 through 10.

survival at 5 years of 72% and a cancer-specific survival of 94%; the figures were 53% and 87% at 10 years and 31% and 81% at 15 years, respectively. Of concern in this series, however, is that there is substantial morbidity in this population. Specific complications reported at 10 years are listed in Table 48.4. Fifty-three percent of the men had a major complication in the first 10 years, and it must be remembered that 32% of the men had T1a tumors that would not have been treated with any therapy and had only a 14% risk of progression. This finding would indicate that 72% of the men experienced a significant cancer-related effect on quality of life as well as the reported 13% mortality. Adolfsson reported a similar series from Stockholm restricted to men with well or moderately differentiated tumors and T1 or T2 tumors. At 10 years, it was found that 55% of the patients had progressed to T3 tumors, 28% had developed metastatic disease, and 16% had died.

In the United States, Whitmore et al. reported a series of 75 patients that has been cited extensively.[11] The concern with this study is that it included only men with clinical T2 tumors who were evaluated on two occasions more than one year apart without any evidence of clinical progression. The progression-free survival is then back-dated to the date of the first evaluation. There are no data available on how many men were lost to follow-up or treated for progressive disease before the second evaluation.

The concept of early diagnosis and treatment is supported by the work of Hugosson and Aus, who reviewed the results of expectant management in 490 men in Goteborg.[12] They included deaths caused by underlying conditions exacerbated by prostate cancer as well as those men dying of conditions caused by prostate cancer as cancer-related deaths. They did not include deaths due to cardiac events in men on estrogen therapy. They reported that the cause-specific survival was 43% at 15 years in T2 lesions, 23% in grade 2 and 3 tumors, and 60% in grade I lesions. They found that prostate cancer comprised 4 of 11 deaths in the first 5 years but increased to 15 of 28 deaths between 5 and 10 years and 24 of 32 deaths occurring after the 10th year.[13]

It is clear that the only solution is a randomized clinical trial, although these are difficult to construct and complete. There are questions as to whether to include patients with very early stage tumors (T1c) and those with advanced tumors (T3), because the one group may have tumors that would not be discovered in other settings and the latter group has a tumor that has already demonstrated biologic aggressiveness by extending beyond the prostate. Similarly, the study must stratify patients by tumor grade and must be able to estimate the global state of patient health to estimate the anticipated survival, which is necessary to estimate the anticipated benefit. Any study also needs to include a quality of life assessment because both tumor and treatment may affect bowel and bladder function as well as performance status. Finally, it is necessary to decide whether to study expectant management or noncurative treatment, as many men will insist on androgen deprivation at some time due to changes in PSA or prostate palpation. As well, there are differential effects of hormones and no therapy on tumor and quality of life.

Holmberg et al. reported a comparison of expectant management versus radical prostatectomy.[14] Although the early follow-up demonstrates no improvement in 8-year survival with a relative risk of death in the prostatectomy group of 0.83 [95% confidence interval (CI), 0.57–1.2; $P = 0.31$], there was a significant reduction in prostate cancer deaths with a relative risk of 0.50 (95% CI, 0.27–0.91; $P = 0.02$). Similarly, there was a reduction in the relative risk of metastatic disease with a relative risk of 0.63 (95% CI, 0.41–0.96; $P = 0.03$). This study needs longer follow-up to determine if there is a significant difference in outcome between the two groups.

A second randomized trial has been completed by Moon et al. randomizing men to radical prostatectomy or conservative therapy including early hormonal therapy in asymptomatic men.[15] This study will likely require an additional 10 to 12 years to mature. Until we have a definitive answer from these trials, the clinician is left to estimate the prostate cancer mortality and competing mortalities, factoring in the tumor stage and grade as well as the extent of prostate involvement, and balance that against the patient's coexistent medical problems to determine whether the risks of treatment outweigh the risk of tumor progression and the probability of tumor-related death.

Local Therapy: Radical Prostatectomy Versus Radiation Therapy

Although the decision to treat or observe is controversial, the question of best therapy of limited disease is perhaps more controversial. This problem reflects the fact that there are two specialties that can effectively treat prostate cancer, although time required, the side effects, and quality-of-life effects are distinctly different. The controversy is accentuated by the fact that the patients who are not treated successfully are frequently referred to the other specialty for palliative care. Patients initially treated with surgery may develop metastatic disease and are referred for palliative radiation, where a radiation oncologist is more likely to note incontinence and pelvic pain while being less cognizant of the rectal effects of radiation. Similarly, the management of local recurrences after surgery is generally left to the radiation oncologist, who may be inclined to question the wisdom of surgery in high-risk patients.

Radiation oncologists do not consider the problems with subsequent pelvic surgery for vascular disease, diverticulitis, and colon polyps or neoplasms to be complications of treatment. Bladder neck contracture, urethral stricture, and hematuria all subsequent to radiation are urologic problems managed by urology. Radiation oncologists also generally lose track of patients with local recurrences and bladder invasion after radiation, as their problems are managed by urologists. Each specialty sees more of its own successes and the failures

TABLE 48.5. Results of radical prostatectomy in selected series.

Author	*Institution*	*No. of patients*	*Follow-up (years)*	*Prostate-specific antigen (PSA) 10.0 or less (%)*	*Gleason score 6 or less (%)*
Partin	Johns Hopkins	1,955	10	78	64
D'Amico	Penn-Harvard		8	73	73
Bauer	Walter Reed	378	5	69	60
Iselin	Duke	1,242	10	Not specified	53

Source: Data from references 27 through 30.

of the other specialty. The resultant competitive atmosphere in many institutions reflects the biblical observation that it is easier to note the sliver in our brother's eye while being oblivious to the board in our own eye.

Radical Prostatectomy

Radical prostatectomy has been a widely practiced effective approach to men with organ-confined prostate cancer since the perineal approach was described by Young in 1905.[16] Millen first reported the retropubic approach in 1945 in a paper republished as a classic paper in urology.[17] Both these papers describe the complete anatomic removal of the prostate and its capsule with urethral–vesical anastomosis to control the tumor. Retropubic prostatectomy will also try to remove portions of the proximal seminal vesicle that cannot always be achieved with the perineal approach. Neither treatment gained widespread popularity because of the problems with bleeding, incontinence, and impotence and a relatively low cure rate. This latter was largely related to the frequent diagnosis of the tumor after extracapsular extension had occurred. Relapse rates were high, and there was not a clear advantage over expectant management because of the long natural history of the disease. Two advances have made radical prostatectomy a safe, effective, and attractive treatment option for prostate cancer. The first is the description by Walsh of the nerve-sparing anatomic radical prostatectomy that preserved potency in a high percentage of men without incontinence.[18] A better understanding of the pelvic anatomy with an improved understanding of the patterns of tumor extension and spread has led to better surgical planning and more complete tumor excision. The second advance was the development of a radioimmunoassay for serum prostate-specific antigen (PSA) for screening large populations of men at risk for prostate cancer[19]; this has changed the spectrum of disease presenting to the clinician. The prevalent wisdom in 1970 was the rule of four; one-fourth of patients presented with metastatic disease, one-fourth with extraprostatic disease confined to the pelvis (T3 or N+), one-fourth with organ-confined disease, and one-fourth with subclinical disease (T1a–T1b). Today, in regions of the country where PSA screening is prevalent, more than 50% of the patients present with nonpalpable disease detected by screening PSA (T1c). A review of the technique for radical retropubic and perineal prostatectomy is beyond the scope of this chapter. For a full description and illustration of the procedure, the reader is referred to *Campbell's Textbook of Urology*.[21,22]

As large numbers of men have undergone radical prostatectomy and been followed, a number of factors have been identified that will predict the risk of biochemical recurrence. Initially it was noted that extracapsular extension, positive surgical margins and seminal vesicle involvement are associated with local recurrence after surgery. Roach developed formulae to predict the risk of occult nodal involvement and seminal vesicle involvement.[23] Many series have reported the results of treatment in large numbers of men with reasonably long follow-up.[24–26] Four large recently reported series are reported by Partin and Walsh from Johns Hopkins,[27] D'Amico from the University of Pennsylvania and Harvard,[28] Bauer, et al. from Walter Reed Army Medical Center,[29] and Iselin and Paulson from Duke.[30] In the first three series patients underwent retropubic prostatectomy and the Duke patients underwent perineal prostatectomy. The characteristics of the four series are reported in Table 48.5.

The groups are not comparable due to differences in the distribution of PSA and Gleason scores in the different populations, with Iselin's group having a higher Gleason score and not reporting PSA values in a number of patients operated on in the pre-PSA era.[30] Two-thirds of the patients from Duke University had PSA follow-up, and their data demonstrate that nearly all biochemical recurrences occur in the first 5 years after surgery. Median time to recurrence was less than 2 years in men with Gleason score 8–10 tumors and was more than 3 years in men with Gleason score 7 tumors. Men with Gleason scores of 6 or lower had a lower recurrence rate and a median time to recurrence that was longer still (Table 48.6). They do show that patients with extracapsular extension have a higher recurrence rate and among men dying of prostate cancer the survival is shorter, confirming that histologic factors correlate with biologic aggressiveness of the tumors.

Bauer et al. reviewed a group of 378 men undergoing radical prostatectomy at Walter Reed Army Medical Center between 1985 and 1995 and identified race, PSA, surgical Gleason score, and capsular transgression as critical parameters affecting recurrence risk.[29] The model required a sigmoid transformation of the PSA value and assigned a value of 1 for race = African-American and 0 for race = other. The value was 0 for organ-confined tumors and 1 for extracapsular extension or positive surgical margins. The formula was relative risk (RR) = exp[(0.51 × race) + (0.12 × PSA_{ST}) + (0.25 × postopera-

TABLE 48.6. Results of radical perineal prostatectomy (Duke University).

Group	*Five-year bNED survival*	*Median survival (years)*	*Fifteen-year cancer-specific survival*
Organ confined	92%	Not reached	86%
Specimen confined	65%	16.3	77%
Positive margins	35%	14.2	38%
Node positive	Not specified	7.2	38%

bNED, no biochemical evidence of disease.

TABLE 48.7. Risk of recurrence following radical prostatectomy according to Partin.

Risk group	*Low*	*Moderate*	*High*	*Very high*
Characteristics	Organ confined or extracapsular extension Gleason 2–6 Margins negative	Organ confined or extracapsular extension Gleason 7 Margins negative OR Gleason 2–6 and margins Positive	Organ confined or extracapsular extension Gleason 8–10 Margins positive or negative OR Gleason 7 Margins positive OR Seminal vesicle involvement	All node-positive patients
Ten-year bNED survival	95%	72%	41%	13%

Source: Data from Khan et al.[27]

tive Gleason sum) + (0.89 × organ confinement)]. Using this method, it was possible to separate the population into three groups with low (less than 10%) risk of recurrence versus intermediate (10% to 30%) versus high risk (more than 30%). The utility is limited because it does not lend itself to easy grouping of clinical risk.

Partin reported that there were four prognostic groups identified based on Gleason score, pathologic stage, and surgical margins.[27] He was able to derive a similar equation based on a multivariate analysis of the patients undergoing radical prostatectomy at Johns Hopkins and was then able to separate the population into four groups with different risk of recurrence (Table 48.7). This is the first effort to quantitate the risk of recurrence and separate patients into risk groups based on easily identified pathologic characteristics.

The preferred method of evaluation would be to predict the risk of local recurrence based on preoperative tumor characteristics. D'Amico identified clinical tumor characteristics associated with biochemical recurrence including Gleason score, preoperative PSA, and findings on magnetic resonance imaging (MRI) with an endorectal coil.[24] Partin at the same time created a series of tables predicting the risk of organ-confined and specimen-confined tumors based on the clinical stage and Gleason score.[25] Both Partin and D'Amico have shown that the factors associated with the risk of biochemical recurrence include Gleason score.

D'Amico has developed a prognostic system based on the preoperative clinical and pathologic findings. He identified a low-risk group based on a Gleason score of 6 or less and a preoperative PSA 10.0 or less. The high-risk population included men with Gleason score of 8 or more and PSA of 20.0 or more. The intermediate-risk group with Gleason score of 7 and PSA between 10.0 and 20.0 were further divided by D'Amico based on the percentage of biopsies containing tumor, showing that men with 17% or less of the biopsies containing cancer had a lower risk of biochemical recurrence and those with more than 50% positive biopsies had a high risk of recurrence. For the intermediate-risk patients, MRI was useful in identifying clinically significant extracapsular extension and seminal vesicle involvement.[26] The risk of biochemical recurrence in the low-risk population was less than 20% at 3 years, whereas the risk of biochemical recurrence was greater than 50% in the high-risk population. A description of the three populations is shown in Table 48.8.

The morbidity of radical prostatectomy is difficult to define and will vary according to the experience of individual surgeons. Begg et al.[31] reviewed the results from six metropolitan areas in five states using the Surveillance, Epidemiology, and End Results (SEER)–Medicare database using a consistent assessment method. They demonstrated that the risk of incontinence rises with increasing age. They also demonstrated that increasing the annual number of procedures per surgeon reduced the risk of postoperative complications, late urinary complications, corrective procedures, and incontinence. The most common late urinary complication was anastomotic stricture, which comprised 70% of the complications. The frequency of complications based on age and surgical volume is shown in Table 48.9. Although no relationship was found between age and mortality or urinary complications, there was a strong association with the severity of comorbidities (P less than 0.002). The study clearly shows that the risk of stricture, incontinence, and other morbidities is lower in younger patients who are undergoing surgery by surgeons who perform more procedures.

Radiation Therapy

Paralleling the development of surgery was the development of radiation therapy as a specialty with the ability to effectively treat prostate cancer. Because the prostate is situated deep within the pelvis, treatment developed slowly because of difficulty delivering an effective dose of radiation to the tumor without injuring the adjacent bladder and rectum. Localization of the prostate gland was also difficult until the development of cross-sectional imaging, first with computed tomography (CT) and later MRI. The earliest use of megavoltage radiation to treat prostate cancer in a substantial number of men was reported in 1965 by Bagshaw et al.[20] Tech-

TABLE 48.8. Risk of recurrence following radical prostatectomy according to D'Amico.

Low Risk (<20%)	*Intermediate risk (20%–50%)*	*High risk (more than 50%)*
Gleason score ≤6 AND PSA < 10.0 AND ≤50% positive Bx OR Gleason score = 7 and PSA < 20.0 OR Gleason score ≤6 and 10.0 < PSA < 20.0 AND <17% positive Bx	Gleason Score ≤6 AND PSA ≤ 10.0 AND >50% positive Bx OR Gleason score 7 OR 10.0 < PSA ≤ 20.0 AND 17% < positive Bx < 50%	Gleason score ≥8 OR PSA >20.0 OR Gleason score 7 OR 10.0 < PSA ≤ 20 AND ≥50% positive Bx

TABLE 48.9. Incidence of operative complications.

Complications based on patient age				
Age	*60-day mortality (%)*	*Postoperative complications (%)*	*Urinary age complications*	*Incontinence*
≤69	0.5	28	25	18
70–74	0.6	31	25	19
≥75	0.9	35	28	24
P value	0.12	<0.001	0.34	<0.001
Complications based on surgical caseload				
Caseload (patients/year)	*Mortality (%)*	*Postoperative complications (%)*	*Late urinary complications (%)*	*Incontinence (%)*
≤10	0.5	32	28	20
11–19	0.5	31	26	20
20–32	0.6	30	27	19
≥33	0.6	26	20	16
*P** value*	0.59	<0.001	0.001	0.04

*Adjusted for clustering and case mix.

Source: From Begg et al.,[31] by permission of *N Engl J Med.*

niques have been improved since that time with the development of CT-based computerized treatment planning, three-dimensional conformal radiation, and intensity-modulated radiation therapy to allow the delivery of higher doses of radiation to the prostate with better sparing of the adjacent normal tissues, which produces higher control rates with less morbidity. Brachytherapy has also been shown to be an effective treatment option. There are still a number of major questions that produce controversy. What is the optimal dose of radiation? Is there any benefit to treating the lymph nodes? Is there any benefit to adding external radiation to brachytherapy? Who benefits from adjuvant hormonal therapy? How long should hormonal therapy last? Is androgen deprivation as effective as combined androgen blockade?

The definition of the target in prostate radiation depends on the stage and grade of the tumor. It is easiest to think in terms of expanding and infiltrating tumors. Low-grade and early-stage tumors are generally assumed to be confined to the prostate and limited by the prostate capsule. As the tumor proliferates, these tumors with limited invasive potential are more likely to remain confined within the prostate, so as the tumor proliferates the prostate expands. In these cases the clinical target volume (CTV) includes only the prostate. Advanced-stage and high-grade tumors may extend grossly or subclinically beyond the capsule to invade adjacent structures. In this situation of infiltrating tumor the CTV will extend further beyond the prostate to encompass these areas at risk for subclinical infiltration.

How much radiation is enough?

To answer this question is difficult because prostate cancer is more difficult to assess on follow-up than many tumors because the low proliferative activity of many tumors causes nodules to regress slowly, and postradiation fibrosis may make it difficult to assess the local control status of many tumors. Bone scans are sensitive, but lack specificity as a follow-up tool, and the utility of acid phosphatase is limited by its lack of both sensitivity and specificity. The development of PSA testing has improved the follow-up of patients treated in the last 10 years, but the incidence of late clinical failures complicates the follow-up because there is no accurate correlation of biochemical recurrence with clinical failure and progression to metastatic disease and death.

The largest series of men with clinically localized tumors treated with conventional radiation techniques with consistent long-term follow-up is the group reported by Bagshaw et al. from Stanford.[32] These patients were treated to doses of 70 Gy using multiple shaped fields and in most cases received adjuvant radiation to the pelvic lymph nodes.

To try to achieve an earlier indication of local control, many institutions have biopsied men following radiation with the idea that a negative biopsy may predict local control and cure. This is difficult to accomplish because postradiation atypia may mimic prostate cancer. Similarly, because radiation causes a lethal injury that is expressed at mitosis, well-differentiated tumors that have low growth fractions and prolonged doubling times may regress slowly, although ultimately are controlled. Crook et al.[33] performed serial biopsies every 6 months and demonstrated that a minimum follow-up of 24 to 30 months is necessary to assess the histologic local control.

A group of institutions reported the biochemical disease-free survival in a group of patients with a minimum biochemical follow-up of 2 years (median, 4 years) and found four groups with distinct survival curves.[34] Patients with PSA values of 9.2 or less had a 5-year biochemical disease-free survival of 81%, whereas patients with PSA values higher than 9.2 but less than 19.7 had a bNED (no evidence of biochemical disease) survival of 69%. Patients with PSAs higher than 19.7 were divided into those with Gleason score of 6 or less, who had a 47% 5-year bNED survival, whereas those with Gleason scores of 7 or more had a 29% bNED survival. A substantial number of patients were followed for up to 8 years, and the biochemical relapse rate after 5 years was 5%.[34] They used strict criteria for diagnosing recurrences that included all patients with three consecutive rises in PSA at least 1 month apart with failure back-dated to the date halfway between the last nonincreasing PSA and the first increasing PSA. The institutions used a number of dose levels in this

TABLE 48.10. Prostate cancer-specific survival (%) following radiation therapy.

Clinical stage					
Stage/follow-up	***5 years***	***10 years***	***15 years***	***20 years***	***25 years***
Stage T0	99	84	78	78	78
Stage T1	89	78	68	59	58
Stage T2	88	67	47	38	38
Stage T3	72	49	33	24	24
Stage T4	35	27	27	n.s.	n.s.
Prostate cancer-specific survival (%) Gleason score					
Gleason score/follow-up	***5 years***	***10 years***	***15 years***	***20 years***	***25 years***
2–5	97	84	82	75	75
6	86	67	52	47	40
7	77	58	30	15	n.s.
8–10	61	38	26	23	13
Clinical relapse-free survival (%)					
Stage/follow-up	***5 years***	***10 years***	***15 years***	***20 years***	***25 years***
Stage T0	86	75	75	70	70
Stage T1	74	60	47	37	32
Stage T2	64	40	29	27	27
Stage T3	45	28	20	17	12
Stage T4	23	18	18	0	0
Clinical local control (%)					
Stage/follow-up	***5 years***	***10 years***	***15 years***	***20 years***	***25 years***
Stage T0	98	94	94	88	88
Stage T1	90	79	70	57	54
Stage T2	84	64	53	53	53
Stage T3	78	63	50	50	40
Stage T4	64	64	64	0	0

study, so one cannot use the bNED survival rates as reflecting the results of radiation; they do, however, suggest that early PSA results may be a useful marker of cure rate (Table 48.10).

Because of the higher local recurrence rate in patients treated with conventional radiation therapy, many institutions have investigated the utility of increased radiation dose. In a recursive partitioning analysis, Horowitz et al.[35] identified four risk groups and studied the effect of dose on bNED survival (Table 48.11). While the results are complicated, they demonstrate that higher T stage and higher PSA require higher doses of radiation to produce local control.

Investigators at M.D. Anderson began a randomized trial in 1993 to assess the value of dose-escalated radiation in managing prostate cancer.[36] Patients with stage T1 to T3 prostate cancer were randomly assigned to doses of 70 or 78 Gy over 7 to 8 weeks. There was a longer time to treatment failure in the group treated by 78 Gy, but on subset analysis, the group that benefited from the higher dose were men with pretreatment PSA values greater than 10.0.

Many clinicians are concerned about the tolerance of the adjacent bladder and rectum and worry that doses of 75 to 80 Gy may not be safely delivered. A number of trials have been reported in men at risk for occult metastatic disease

TABLE 48.11. Recursive partition analysis of results of radiation for prostate cancer.

Risk	*T stage*	*Gleason score*	*Pretreatment PSA*	*Dose*
Low	T1–T2a	Any	<10.0	<7,179
	T1–T2a	Any	<20.0	>7,235
	T2b–T3	Any	<20.0	>7,629
Intermediate	T2b–T3	Any	<10.0	<7,179
	Any	Any	<10.0	7,179–7,235
	Any	Any	10.0–19.9	<7,235
	T2b–T3	Any	<20.0	7,235–7,629
	T2b–T3	2–6	≥20.0	>7,482
	Any	7–10	≥20.0	>7,742
High	Any	Any	≥20.0	≤7,482
	Any	7–10	≥20.0	7,482–7,742
Very high	T1–T2a	2–6	≥20.0	>7,462

Source: From Horowitz et al.,[35] by permission of *Cancer*.

treated with radiation and hormones. Some have questioned whether hormones could be combined with lower doses of radiation to achieve the same effect as higher doses of radiation with reduced morbidity and comparable local control. It would appear logical that hormonal therapy would reduce the intraprostatic tumor burden by two to three logs, which would lower the tumor control dose. Nguyen et al.[37] reported the results of a comparison of two cohorts from the Fox Chase series. Men with high-risk prostate cancer (PSA greater than 20.0, Gleason 8–10 or T3–T4) treated with doses less than 75 Gy (62–75 Gy;-median, 71.8 Gy) and 2 to 6 months of androgen deprivation were compared with those who received doses greater than 75 Gy (75–80 Gy; median, 75.8 Gy) without hormones. Median follow-up was 52 months in the high-dose radiotherapy (RT) group and 69 months in the androgen deprivation group. The 5-year bNED survival was 36% in the adjuvant hormone group and 55% in the high-dose RT group. In a multivariate analysis, there was no evidence that short-term androgen deprivation reduced the risk of local recurrence or distant metastases.[37] There was also no survival benefit noted.

The major current controversy in external-beam radiation concerns the safest method of delivering an effective dose of radiation with the least morbidity. Before 1990, most patients were treated with conventional radiation with shaped fields or rotational techniques. Patients underwent simulation to the prostate region as defined by bony landmarks with or without contrast. It was known that the prostate lay posterior to the symphysis pubis, inferior to the bladder, anterior to the rectum, and superior to the urogenital diaphragm. The structures were located using the lateral pelvic film with contrast in the bladder and rectum. The inferior margin could be located by performing a urethrogram to find the cone-shaped tapering of the urethra as it passed through the diaphragm or by using a Foley catheter, because the posteriormost extension of the urethra is where it passes through the urogenital diaphragm and this can be seen on a lateral radiograph. The lateral margins were arbitrarily assigned based on the clinician's perception of the prostate width on palpation, although some centers would include data from the ultrasound or CT scan. Lymph nodes may or may not have been treated, although the benefit of lymph node irradiation may have been related to the dose of radiation delivered to the periprostatic structures and perhaps even to more complete coverage of the prostate. Lymph nodes routinely included in the target volume included the obturator and external and internal (hypogastric) lymph nodes, and may also have included the common iliac lymph nodes. Lymph nodes were generally treated with two or four fixed shaped fields.

Since 1990, three-dimensional conformal radiation (3-D CRT) has been developed as CT data became more routinely available in radiation oncology departments and computer programs were developed to use the images from the CT scan to create digitally reconstructed radiographs. The target size and location was defined in three dimensions from a treatment planning study and transferred to the treatment planning computer to develop a plan using shaped fields to treat the target volume defined by the clinician. The locations of the rectum and bladder were also defined, and the treatment plan was developed to deliver the maximum dose of radiation to the target while minimizing the dose to the bladder, rectum, and femoral heads. In general, four to six treatment

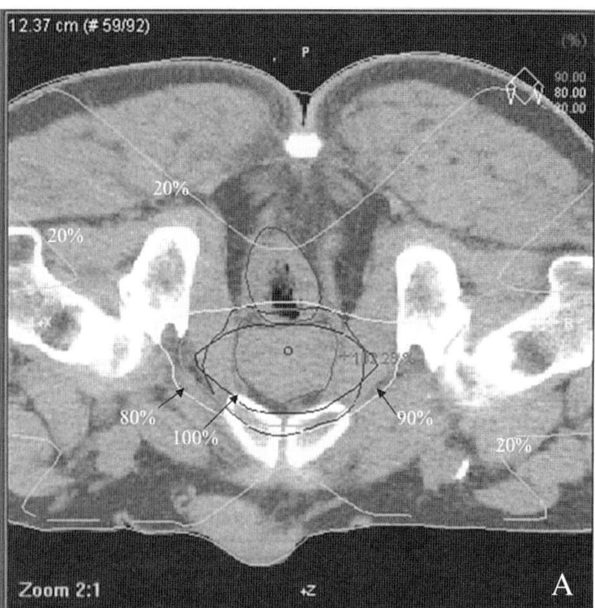

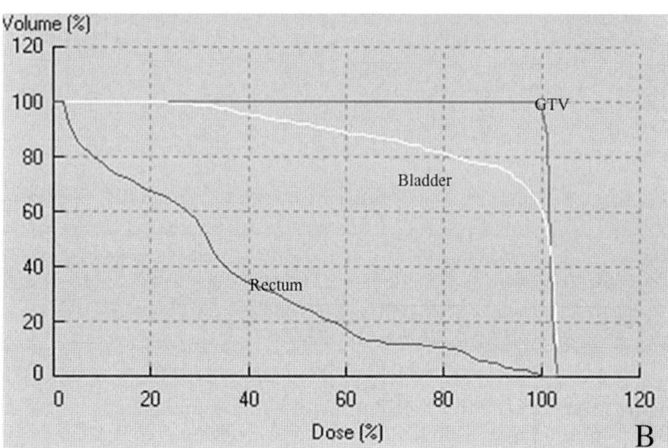

Figure 48.1. (A) Distribution of typical six-field technique on prone patient: 50% of dose delivered with two lateral fields and 50% delivered with four oblique fields. (B) Dose–volume histogram for six-field prone technique: dose to tumor, 78 Gy with inhomogeneity of +2% to –4% (95% volume ± 2%); dose to rectum, median 35 Gy with 82% less than 50 Gy and 90% less than 65 Gy; dose to bladder, median 78 Gy with 20% less than 65 Gy and maximum dose of 78 Gy.

fields are used, although arc techniques with variable collimation have been explored and are used in some institutions. A sample treatment plan using a six-field technique is shown in Figure 48.1.

Within the last 5 to 6 years, intensity-modulated radiation therapy (IMRT) has been used for prostate cancer. Intensity-modulated radiation therapy uses an inverse treatment planning methodology to define the desired dose to the target volume and the tolerable dose to normal structures. IMRT uses more fields, frequently five to nine, to treat the target, and the shape of each field is changed several times during each treatment. The treatment is optimized to minimize the radiation dose to the surrounding normal tissue, which is done by treating individual segments of each field so that each segment treats a portion of the tumor and maximizes the shielding of the normal tissue. The total number of segments is usually between 50 and 90 with each segment receiving a

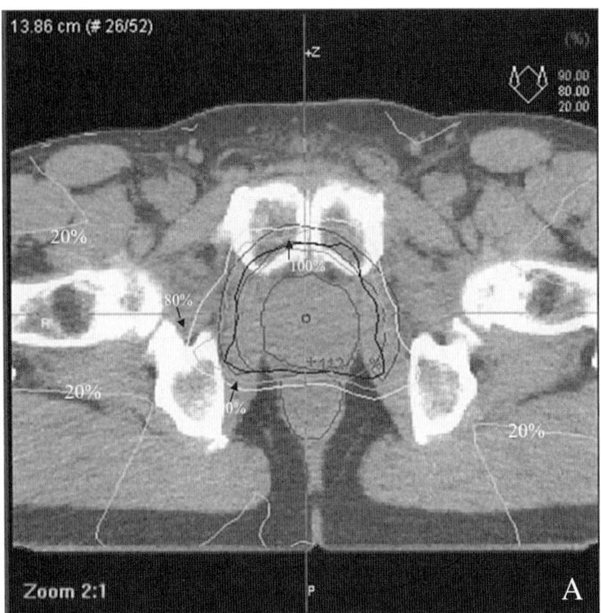

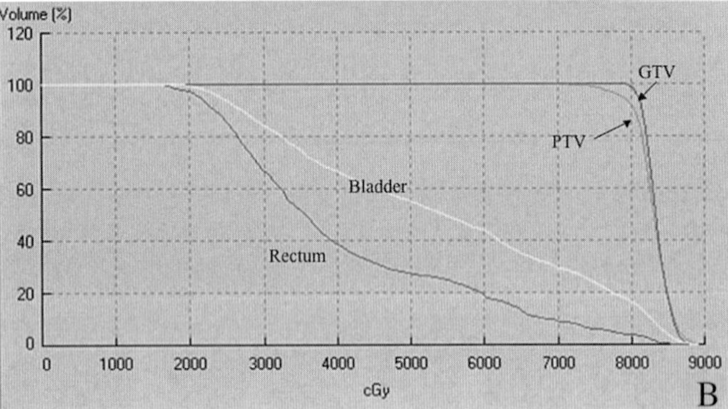

Figure 48.2. (A) Dose distribution of typical intensity-modulated radiation therapy (IMRT) plan on same volume. Note that 70% volume is somewhat smaller whereas 10% and 20% lines cover more of the volume; this is the additional region receiving 8–16 Gy. (B) Dose–volume histogram for plan shown in (A). Prostate dose, 78 Gy with inhomogeneity of +10% to 10% (95% volume +8% to −4%); dose to rectum, median 32 Gy with 68% less than 50 Gy and 90% less than 71 Gy; dose to Bladder, median 52 Gy with 65% less than 65 Gy and maximum dose of 87 Gy.

very small dose of radiation. When the cumulative dose is calculated, the tumor has received the prescribed daily dose, usually 1.80 to 2.0 Gy, but the maximum dose to the adjacent normal tissue is reduced. A sample treatment plan for prostate cancer using IMRT techniques is shown in Figure 48.2.

The difference in dose distribution between 3-D CRT and IMRT is that the dose homogeneity is somewhat better with 3-DCRT but the maximum dose to the adjacent normal tissue, especially the bladder, is higher. With IMRT, the maximum tumor dose is higher but the minimum target dose may be lower, and the maximum dose to adjacent normal tissues is lower, although a somewhat larger volume of tissue is treated to a low or moderate dose. Whether one technique is superior is unknown as there have been no randomized trials to compare the methods. Although some institutions have reported that higher doses can be delivered to the prostate with reduced morbidity, it is not clear that the long-term control will be similar. Because multiple segments are used and it is necessary to interrupt the treatment many times to change the collimator settings to alter the field shape, the treatment takes longer. A significant proportion of the damage caused to the tumor is through the accumulation of short-lived intermediate compounds, DNA strand breaks, and free radicals. Because the effective dose rate with IMRT is frequently 20% to 25% of the dose rate with 3-D conformal radiation, it is not clear whether there is reduced efficacy. Many authors claim that the complication rate is reduced with the use of IMRT, although comparisons may not be possible due to advances in target localization. Daily localization of the prostate with ultrasound, CT, or electronic portal imaging has allowed treatment planners to reduce the margin around the target that must be added for organ motion and uncertainty of target location. These reduced margins also allow higher doses to be delivered with reduced dose to bladder and rectum.

Brachytherapy

Prostate brachytherapy is the method that delivers the maximum dose of radiation to the prostate and minimizes the radiation exposure of the bladder and rectum. There is an extensive literature on two different techniques. The most common method is low dose rate brachytherapy initially developed by Hilaris and colleagues at Memorial Sloan-Kettering Cancer Center.[38] Men initially underwent retropubic exposure of the prostate and needles were placed into the prostate through the incision. This treatment required a 4-day hospitalization, and although an attempt was made to distribute the seeds evenly though the gland, dose inhomogeneity was a frequent problem.

For these reasons, the procedure was subsequently superseded by the transperineal ultrasound-guided implant developed by Blasko and colleagues.[39] Computer programs have been developed to use parallel ultrasound images obtained at the time of implant to produce three-dimensional reconstructions of the prostate and rapidly produce plans that provide a homogeneous radiation distribution through the prostate and minimize radiation dose to the urethra and the periprostatic structures. Needles can be loaded to complete the implant quickly and allow the patient to be discharged to home with self-care the same day. If a preplan is used and needles are preloaded, the procedure takes between 30 and 45 minutes. If real-time planning is done in the operating room, the procedure can be completed in 45 to 90 minutes.

Two isotopes have been used for low dose rate prostate brachytherapy, iodine-125 and palladium-103. Both isotopes produce low-energy photons that travel short distances in tissue. The two processes that determine the dose are energy absorption by tissue and inverse square falloff as distance from the source increases. Because the sources are placed inside the prostate, all normal tissue is further from the seeds than the tumor, and the inverse square law stipulates that the dose falls off in proportion to the square of the distance from the source, that is, doubling the distance reduces the dose by 75%. The tissue absorption of energy by both isotopes is approximately 50% for every 2 cm of tissue. Combining these two factors means that increasing the distance form the source from 2 to 4 cm will reduce the dose by 87.5% (50% attenuation by absorption × 75% reduction due to inverse square falloff).

One advantage of low dose rate low-energy brachytherapy is that the radiation may have a greater biologic effect on a slow-growing tumor cell that may be hypoxic than on an exponentially growing cell such as is found in the rectal mucosa. Freeman et al.[40] investigated this by exposing Chinese hamster ovary fibroblasts to radiation at various dose rates from both iodine-125 (average energy, 27 keV) and cesium-137 (average energy, 662 keV). They showed there was greater effect on slowly growing or plateau-phase cultures, similar to well to moderately differentiated prostate cancer, than there was on the exponentially growing cells, similar to rectal mucosa. This effect was also more pronounced at dose rates seen in low-dose permanent implants such as are used in prostate brachytherapy than they are in high dose rates as are used in temporary implants.

The largest reported series of men treated with brachytherapy and external radiation is the series from the Seattle group.[41] They report that 10-year biochemical disease-free survival is 86% in patients with Gleason score of 6 or less and PSA less than 10.0 and 90% among men with tumors of Gleason score of 7 or more and a PSA of 10.0 to 20.0. Among men with Gleason score of 8 or more or PSA of 20.0 or more, the 10-year bNED survival was 49%. In a second report of men treated with brachytherapy alone, they report the 5-year bNED survival is 88% among men treated with brachytherapy alone and 79% among patients with intermediate-risk disease.[42] Because of patient selection issues, it remains to be determined whether there is any benefit to the addition of external radiation to brachytherapy.

Dosoretz et al. have reported the results of a nonrandomized patient series of 130 high-risk patients with Gleason scores of 8 to 10 or PSA of 20.0 or more or clinical stage T2c or T3 treated with 45-Gy external radiation and hormones with implant (130 patients) and found that the 5-year bNED survival was 90% compared with 78% in 82 high-risk patients treated with hormones and brachytherapy and with 62% in 37 high-risk patients treated with brachytherapy alone. These results suggest that external-beam radiation and hormones may serve complementary effects in men with aggressive prostate cancer.[43]

The effects of the treatment with brachytherapy are similar to those reported with external radiation. Both procedures cause bladder irritative symptoms with frequency, urgency, and nocturia usually lasting 8 to 16 weeks. The reported risk of rectal ulcer with tenesmus, pain, or bleeding is 2% to 4% in series reporting either interstitial or external radiation. Some series report that an additional 10% of men may have intermittent painless rectal bleeding. Perineal discomfort is common after transperineal brachytherapy but is usually controlled with nonsteroidal antiinflammatory analgesics with small doses of codeine-like medication used intermittently during the first 2 to 4 days. There is a small risk of urinary retention lasting 2 to 4 days that is caused by edema of the gland due to the multiple punctures, similar to the risk reported after prostate biopsy. The severity of the edema and the risk of retention is also affected by the skill of the brachytherapist in placing the needles, as multiple punctures to reposition the needles increase the risk of retention.

The duration of postoperative catheter drainage of the bladder can also affect the risk of retention as the catheter will stabilize the urethra during the period that the edema develops. Most institutions use 6 to 24 hours of drainage, and we have reported that the risk is 5% after 24 hours of drainage.[44] The major putative advantage of brachytherapy is a lower risk of impotence associated with interstitial therapy. Sanchez-Ortiz et al. reported the results of a survey following brachytherapy or external-beam radiation with a strict definition of impotence, erection sufficient for intromission, and ability to achieve orgasm without mechanical or pharmacologic assistance[45]; 49% of men undergoing brachytherapy were potent and an additional 26% had partial erections or were fully potent with sildenafil. Talcott et al.[46] reported that only 30% of men treated with external radiation were fully potent following external radiation. The effects of combinations of external radiation and brachytherapy have not been studied to know whether this would lead to increased effect on sexual function or rectal or bladder effects.

Selection of patients for brachytherapy is critical for a successful brachytherapy program. For mechanical reasons it is technically difficult to implant prostates larger than 55 cm^3 due to interference from the ischium. Patients with larger prostates may be candidates if they undergo androgen deprivation for 3 to 6 months. We have treated men and carried out serial ultrasounds.[47] Among men in the largest quartile, that is, glands greater than 56 cm^3, the median reduction in volume was 60%, which would suggest that men with glands as large as 80 cm^3 may undergo the procedure. The reduction in volume appears to be related to the extent of benign prostatic hyperplasia (BPH) as the volume reduction was only 10% among men with glands smaller than 24 cm^3. Men with PSA greater than 20 or Gleason score of 8 to 10 do not do well with androgen deprivation and subsequent prostate brachytherapy; this is likely related to the shorter doubling times of a poorly differentiated tumor. Also, the highly conformal nature of the dose distribution of prostate brachytherapy is a disadvantage in these patients because they are at higher risk for occult extracapsular tumor or distant metastatic disease. Other contraindications to brachytherapy include men with recurrent prostate infections, as the placement of foreign bodies within the prostate increases the risk of recurrent infection and possibly abscess, and men with moderate to severe bladder outlet obstruction do not tolerate brachytherapy well as these symptoms frequently worsen in these men. Additionally, men with prior transurethral resection of the prostate are not good candidates for the procedure if these is a substantial central defect, as this prostate tissue is necessary to hold sources and there is a greater risk of stricture or bladder neck contracture due to fibrosis from two procedures.

High dose rate brachytherapy using temporary implants has also been studied in men with locally advanced prostate cancer to increase the dose of radiation to the tumor while limiting the dose to the bladder and rectum. Guerriero et al.[48] reported a series of men treated with external radiation and radioactive gold-198 implant. In this procedure only three to four seeds were used, which made the dosimetry much more sensitive to source position. There is a theoretical advantage to the high dose rate implant as there is less attenuation of the energy by tissue so that the dose to tissues immediately adjacent to the prostate is higher, which may treat microscopic extracapsular disease more effectively. Similarly, it may deliver a higher dose to T3 tumors with a lower dose to the rectum.

Guerriero et al. delivered 46 Gy to the prostate with external radiation and carried out two implants to deliver a total dose of approximately 80 Gy. They report a 5-year bNED survival among high-risk patients with poorly differentiated Gleason of 7 or more or PSA of 10.0 or more or locally advanced tumors (T2b or greater) as 74% without the addition of adjuvant hormonal therapy.

A similar experience has been reported by physicians at the Swedish hospital in Seattle.[50] They have treated a similar number of patients, with a large percentage falling into the high-risk population, with a median follow-up of 45 months. No patient received adjuvant hormonal therapy. They combined 50.4-Gy external radiation with four implants delivering 3.0 to 4.0 Gy each time to the prostate. They report a 5-year bNED survival of 84%.[49]

To Treat the Nodes or Not to Treat the Nodes?

This is a controversial issue among radiation oncologists because the data can be interpreted to support both positions. Many institutions have routinely delivered radiation to the lymph nodes to treat high-risk patients for occult nodal involvement, whereas others have insisted that nodal involvement in patients with clinically limited disease is invariably associated with occult distant metastatic disease, arguing that the effect on survival and disease-free survival is greater than that observed in node-positive breast cancer.

Two early reports supported the application of prophylactic nodal radiation based on retrospective reviews of single-institution data.[50,51] McGowan reported a review of 342 patients treated between 1970 and 1978 with doses of 60 Gy in 6 weeks to the prostate or a dose of 32.5 Gy to the pelvic lymph nodes with a 27.5-Gy boost dose to the prostate.[50] Treatment policy changed during this time to treat the nodes as well as the prostate instead of the prostate only. The 5-year clinical disease-free survival among 36 patients treated to the prostate only was 35% compared to 62% for 91 patients treated to the pelvis and prostate.[50]

Results from Stanford supported this finding after they went through a similar evolution in treatment policy.[51] The dose delivered was 70 Gy. The 10-year clinical disease-free survival was 70% for patients treated to the prostate and nodes versus 40% for patients treated to the prostate only. In the same report, Bagshaw describes the results in 58 patients undergoing node sampling and treated with prostate only radiation at Memorial Sloan-Kettering Cancer Center with iodine-125 implant only versus 86 patients treated to the prostate and pelvic nodes at Stanford. There was no significant difference in survival between the two groups.

The Radiation Therapy Oncology Group (RTOG) conducted a randomized prospective trial determine the benefit of prophylactic lymph node radiation in patients with node-negative prostate cancer.[52] Patients were accepted after either a negative lymph node sampling or lymphangiogram or CT scan. However, both CT scan and lymphangiogram are relatively insensitive in detecting nodal metastases because CT scans require that nodes be enlarged to at least 1.0 cm in greatest dimension before they are called radiographically positive and the lymphangiogram does not evaluate the first two echelons of lymph nodes, that is, the obturator and internal iliac lymph nodes, so they only detect the common iliac nodes if they are involved. Both studies have sensitivities that are less than 50%. In a final analysis of this trial (RTOG 77-06) in stage T1b and T2 patients, there was no difference in disease-free survival between prostate-only radiation and pelvis-plus-prostate radiation at 12 years, although the survival was 26% in patients undergoing lymphangiographic or CT staging compared to 38% among surgically staged patients (P = 0.003).[52] At the same time, RTOG 75-06 accrued patients with pathologically involved lymph nodes and randomized them to pelvis and prostate radiation versus paraaortic, pelvic, and prostate radiation. There was no difference in survival between the two groups and, more importantly, there were only 2 bNED survivors at 10 years among 90 patients.

All these studies were developed and reported before the availability of PSA studies and the development of three-dimensional conformal radiation and intensity-modulated radiation. The radiation doses were lower than are commonly used today, and target volumes were smaller than are used today. The observations from these older RTOG trials still ask the clinician to explain why it seems that if the nodes are not involved there is no need to treat the lymph nodes, and if the nodes are involved there is no benefit to treating the nodes, yet if the nodal status is not known there is a benefit to prophylactic nodal radiation. Possible explanations include the following: (1) a benefit to patients with truly limited disease that may not be detected pathologically because the extremely limited microscopic involvement of the nodes may have been missed; (2) pelvic radiation may have compensated for the difficulty in defining the prostate target volume and better treated the peripheral portions of the gland and the adjacent soft tissues; or (3) there may have been a volume effect because of the greater tissue effects due to the vascular and lymphatic effects of pelvic radiation, which may have enhanced the cytocidal effects of the prostate radiation or may have impaired tumor progression.

A recent RTOG study (94-13) included patients with locally advanced tumor but radiographically node-negative patients in whom there is an estimated risk of occult lymph node involvement greater than 15% based on the equation (2/3)*PSA + [(Gleason score–6)*10] greater than 15.[53] Patients in this trial were randomized to whole pelvis + prostate radiation versus prostate-only radiation and were also randomized to neoadjuvant and concurrent combined androgen blockade (2 months before and during radiation; total, 4 months) versus adjuvant combined androgen blockade (beginning after the completion of radiation). They found an improvement in 4-year biochemical disease-free survival from 47% to 54% with the addition of pelvic radiation independent or hormonal effects. These patients again did not undergo CT-based treatment planning or three-dimensional conformal radiation or intensity-modulated radiation. Because these patients were selected for the increased risk of occult nodal involvement, the treatment effect may reflect the effect of nodal radiation, or it may reflect the better coverage of periprostatic soft tissues in patients who also had a high risk of capsular transgression. It is unlikely that another randomized trial can be justified, and it remains for the individual clinician to decide on the treatment volume in this patient group. It is clear that there is a benefit to larger fields in these poor-risk patients, but the exact target is not clear.

Treatment Selection Issues

Based on the data reported by all the previously mentioned studies, the question arises as to the optimal treatment. There is unfortunately only one small randomized trial reported that randomized men to surgery or radiation for localized prostate cancer. Paulson et al. reported the results of a small series of 97 patients randomized to radiation versus radical prostatectomy.[54] Their analysis did purport to show a higher 5-year disease-free survival in patients undergoing surgery, 86% versus 59%. However, the conclusions from this trial have been called into question by some of the coauthors.[55] Unfortunately, the group was disbanded before the completion of the study and some of the coauthors complained that they did not have the opportunity to review the data or the manuscript before publication. A number of problems in data analysis were raised in the second publication,[55] including the issue that 12% of the radiation patients and 19% of the surgery patients did not receive the assigned treatment and that they were analyzed by treatment group and not intention to treat. They also point out that 48% of the radiated patients and 66% of the surgery patients did not complete follow-up. Additionally, nearly all the recurrences were documented by bone scan, which has a high probability of false-positive studies due to the multiple causes of bone scan abnormalities. Finally, there was also no central review of studies documenting recurrent disease. It should also be noted that the dose of radiation used (66 Gy) is significantly lower than is used today. The results of this study[54] and the ensuing controversy[55] have precluded any potential for completing a full randomized study of this question. A subsequent attempt by the Southwest Oncology Group in concert with all the other major oncology research groups in the United States failed because of poor accrual. Two large nonrandomized patient series have also attempted to address this question.[56,57]

D'Amico et al. compared the results of patients at the University of Pennsylvania treated with radical prostatectomy or palladium-103 brachytherapy with patients treated with external-beam radiation to a dose of 66 Gy at the Joint Center for Radiation Therapy. In low-risk patients, the 8-year biochemical disease-free survival was 88% for radical prostatectomy and 78% for radiation therapy. In intermediate-risk patients the bNED survival was 79% for surgery and 65% for radiation.[57] More recently, Kupelian et al.[56] compared the results of external-beam radiation therapy, brachytherapy, and radical retropubic prostatectomy of a single-institution retrospective study. They found that in the group of patients with stage T1–T3 disease treated with radiation alone the 7-year bNED survival was significantly better if patients were treated with a dose greater than 72 Gy (81% versus 48%). These results were independent of treatment Gleason score or PSA. The treatment results with radiation to doses of 72 Gy or more were comparable to the results with radical prostatectomy.

Overall, in selecting treatment for a specific cohort of patients with localized prostate cancer, it is necessary to evaluate the institutional treatment results including the risks of morbidity and the available resources including 3-D CRT and IMRT. It is also necessary to allow each patient to understand the relative risks of potential rectal complications of radiation and the risk of postsurgical incontinence as well as the effects of each treatment on potency. External-beam radiation therapy will not relieve obstructive symptoms, and brachytherapy may make obstructive symptoms worse, at least transiently, whereas surgery will relieve them. Some patients may prefer surgery because of the reassurance that they receive from an undetectable PSA and may be less satisfied with a low, but stable, PSA as found following radiation therapy. Others may take comfort from the potential effect of salvage radiation. Younger patients have a longer anticipated survival, and radiation or brachytherapy may complicate the management of subsequent pelvic problems including diverticular disease and bladder and rectal neoplasms. This possibility must be balanced against the higher risk of surgical incontinence and impotence with increasing age, whereas a similar trend has not been demonstrated with radiation therapy.

Locally Advanced Prostate Cancer: Combined Radiation and Hormones

Early results with radiation for T3 prostate cancer showed a high risk of recurrence and metastatic disease following radiation therapy. One of the earliest efforts to improve the results in these high-risk patients was reported from M.D. Anderson in 82 patients using diethylstilbestrol (DES) with radiation in a randomized trial compared to radiation alone, recently updated by Zagars et al. with a median follow-up of 14.5 years.[58] Fifteen-year relapse-free survival was 57% for radiation + DES versus 37% for radiation alone. The overall survival was 33% for radiation alone and 25% for radiation + DES. The major reason for the difference between disease-free survival and overall survival was the excess mortality in the DES group resulting from cardiovascular events. Since this trial was completed, other studies have examined the same question but have used luteinizing hormone-releasing hormone (LHRH) agonists with or without antiandrogens. RTOG 86-10 randomized men with T3–T4 or bulky T2 prostate cancer to radiation alone or radiation with 2 months of combined androgen blockade (CAB) before radiation and 2 months during radiation versus radiation alone.[59] With 8 years follow-up, the overall and disease-specific survival are not significantly different, 47% and 55% with radiation and CAB versus 44% and 56% with radiation alone. The study did show an improved bNED survival with neoadjuvant and concurrent hormones, 63% versus 45% (P less than 0.001). Some bias may be introduced into the interpretation of these data by the inclusion of men with T2 tumors and extensive BPH and limited tumors. An important finding from this study was that the quality and duration of subsequent hormonal response among men who suffered relapses was not adversely affected by the short-course hormonal therapy.

RTOG 85-31 is a Phase III clinical trial that included men with clinical T3 prostate cancer as well as men with any T stage node-positive prostate cancer, and men undergoing radical prostatectomy for stage T1–T2 disease with pathologically documented extracapsular disease or seminal vesicle involvement.[60] These men were randomized to treatment with radiation with or without lifelong androgen deprivation. Local recurrence rates were improved with hormonal therapy, 16% versus 29% (P less than 0.001). Additionally, the 5-year clinical NED survival was improved, 60% versus 44% (P less than 0.001), as was bNED survival, 53% versus 20% (P less than 0.001), but there was no difference in 5-year absolute survival, 75% versus 71% ($P = 0.52$). Patients were stratified for Gleason score (7 or less versus 8–10) and for surgery and nodal status.

The only group showing a survival benefit thus far is men with Gleason score 8 to 10 not undergoing surgery, 66% with hormones versus 48% without hormone after 5 years ($P = 0.01$).

The first report that showed a clear survival advantage with the addition of hormonal therapy was reported by Bolla et al. for the EORTC,[61] in which 415 men with high-grade T1–T2 or any grade T3 tumors were randomized to conventional dose radiation to the lymph nodes and prostate to a dose of 50Gy, followed by a boost to the prostate to a dose of 70Gy with or without 3 years of LHRH agonist therapy. With a 66-month median follow-up, the incidence of clinical locoregional failure was 16% in the radiation-alone group and 2% in the combined therapy group (P less than 0.0001). The risk of distant metastases was reduced from 29% to 10% (P less than 0.0001), and the 5-year clinical disease-free survival was increased from 40% to 74% by the addition of hormones. Overall 5-year survival was also increased by the addition of hormonal therapy from 60% to 78% (P less than 0.0001). Importantly, the addition of LHRH agonist therapy did not increase the risk of cardiovascular events as was observed with estrogen therapy.

The RTOG 92-02 study was a randomized trial in high-risk T2b and T3–T4 prostate cancer that randomized men to neoadjuvant and concurrent androgen deprivation therapy during external-beam radiation therapy with or without 2 years of maintenance androgen deprivation.[62] Regional nodes were treated to 44 to 46Gy and the prostate was treated to 65 to 70Gy. A small number of node-positive patients were also included, and very few patients had pathologic nodal involvement. The median PSA was 20, and most patients had Gleason scores of 7 or more. With the use of 2 years of postradiation androgen deprivation, local recurrences were reduced from 12% to 6% (P less than 0.0001); the risk of distant metastases was reduced from 17% to 11% ($P = 0.03$), and the 5-year disease-free survival was increased from 28% to 46% (P less than 0.0001). However, the overall survival was not significantly improved, being 78% for short-term androgen deprivation and 80% for the longer course of treatment.

Although the survival curves published in the RTOG 92-02 study were not analyzed, it appears that the extended disease-free survival was approximately 2 years, reflecting the longer course of treatment in this population.[62] The disease-free survival curve does not appear to plateau through 7 years. This result would suggest that the 2 years of postradiation androgen deprivation treatment may delay rather than prevent recurrences, and further follow-up is needed to determine whether there is a survival advantage. Indeed, the EORTC study[61] has been criticized because serum testosterone levels were not followed, and some have suggested that 3 years of androgen deprivation may have induced lifelong gonadal failure, and that the survival benefit seen in this trial may reflect a prolonged effect on gonadal dysfunction. The disease-free survival appears poorer in the RTOG report,[62] although the Gleason score of the RTOG patients was generally higher than in the EORTC study.[61] There may also be a better overall survival in the RTOG population because of the generally earlier application of palliative hormonal therapy in the United States than in Europe. Patients in both studies were stratified based on Gleason score, PSA, and clinical stage.[61,62] Future subset analyses may clarify which patients benefit from prolonged hormones.

Management of Node-Positive Prostate Cancer

When prostate cancer metastasizes to lymph nodes, the implications for therapy are not dissimilar to those in breast cancer. When men with node-positive prostate cancer are followed, the results with any monotherapy are poor. Early reports showed that the risk of recurrence is high with surgery and radiation and that the major sites of recurrence were distant.[63–66] Patients treated with hormonal therapy alone have similarly poor results but more problems with symptomatic local progression.[10] Table 48.4 has previously shown that men with localized tumors treated expectantly with palliative hormonal therapy when symptoms develop have a greater than 50% risk of symptomatic local progression. The results with local therapy are shown in Table 48.12. The dominant pattern of clinical recurrence in each of these series is distant metastasis.

There is only one randomized trial of combined modality therapy in men with node-positive nonmetastatic tumors. Messing et al. reported a randomized trial of men undergoing radical prostatectomy who were randomized to either observation or androgen ablation therapy with either orchiectomy or lifelong goserelin[67] in which 98 men were randomized and the median follow-up was more than 7 years. In this patient series, there was a high incidence of seminal vesicle involvement, 60%, and positive surgical margins, 65%. Half had Gleason score 7 tumors and 15% had Gleason score 8–10 tumors, although 80% had an undetectable PSA after surgery. The 7-year overall survival was 84% with adjuvant hormones and 57% for surgery alone ($P = 0.02$), and the prostate cancer-specific survival was 97% versus 63% (P less than 0.01). The 7-year disease-free survival was improved to 83% using immediate postsurgical hormonal therapy versus 34% with surgery alone.

There are no randomized trials in men treated with radiation for node-positive prostate cancer. Two attempts at randomized trials have failed due to poor accrual. There are two sizable series of men treated with combined hormonal and radiation therapy that have shown substantially better disease-free and overall survival compared to series of radiation alone.[68,69] These patients are not comparable to the surgical trial[67] as there is a higher percentage of patients with T3 disease and more patients have gross nodal disease before treatment. Sands et al. reported a series of 208 men with node-positive prostate cancer treated at M.D. Anderson with hormones alone (181 patients) or hormones plus local radiation (27 patients).[68] Both groups received lifelong androgen ablation and the prostate was treated to 66Gy. They report that

TABLE 48.12. Result with local therapy alone in node-positive prostate cancer.

Author	*Reference*	*Follow-up*	*Cancer-specific survival*	*Clinical NED survival*	*bNED survival*
Surgery					
Sgrignoli	63	10 years	NR	47%	12%
Myers	64	10 years	65%	0%	NR
Hanks	65	10 years	29%	7%	NR
Gervasi	66	10 years	43%	7%	NR

NR, not reported.

TABLE 48.13. Results of combined modality therapy in node-positive prostate cancer.

Author	*Treatment*	*T3*	*Gleason score 8–10*	*No. of patients*	*bNED survival*	*Overall survival*
Messing[67]	S + H	0%	30%	47	84% at 7 years	83% at 7 years
Sands[68]	RT + H	59%	15%	27	100% 4 years	100% at 4 years
Robnett[69]	RT + H	70%	51%	79	61% at 12 years	81% at 12 years

S, surgery; RT, radiation therapy; H, hormone therapy.

the 4-year bNED survival was 47% with hormones alone and the incidence of local progression was 22%. Only 10% of patients had distant metastatic disease without clinical local progression. Men treated with combined hormonal-radiation therapy were all biochemically NED at 4 years. Robnett et al.[69] recently updated the results from the University of Pennsylvania in a similar group of 79 patients treated with combined hormonal-radiation therapy. Clinically uninvolved pelvic lymph nodes were treated to 45 Gy and involved nodes were treated to 50 Gy. The prostate was treated to 66 to 72 Gy. The median follow-up was 7.2 years with more than 25% of the patients followed for more than 10 years. The 12-year actuarial clinical disease-free survival was 81% and the bNED survival was 61%. This series showed no difference between androgen ablation therapy and combined androgen blockade. They did note that all 5 patients with residual gross nodal disease at the start of radiation did recur and that more than 50% of recurrences after 5 years were prostate only without distant metastases. A comparison of the combined therapies in the three series including the randomized surgical trail and two single-institution radiation therapy series are shown in Table 48.13. The evidence from each report strongly suggests that combined therapy is superior to monotherapy as these patients are at extremely high risk for occult distant disease but hormones alone cannot reliably produce durable local control.

Management of Advanced Disease

Hormonal therapy has been the mainstay in the management of advanced disease since the observations of Huggins et al. in 1943 demonstrated the high rate of symptomatic response to orchiectomy in advanced prostate cancer.[70] The initial results were encouraging, but the advantage was partially offset by the increased risk of cardiovascular events in men treated with estrogen therapy.[71] In this study of stage III and IV prostate cancer patients, they found that the prostate cancer mortality was 31% among 485 men treated with placebo, 28% among 469 men treated with orchiectomy, and 21% among 476 men treated with DES.[70,71] Cardiovascular mortality among this group was 29% in men treated with placebo, 31% in men treated with orchiectomy, and 39% among men treated with DES.

Since 1985, the use of LHRH agonists has largely supplanted the use of DES and orchiectomy. In a large meta-analysis, Seidenfeld et al. reported that the results with LHRH agonists were comparable and equivalent to the results achieved with orchiectomy.[72]

During this same time, the antiandrogens have also been developed, and there have been a large number of investigations comparing androgen ablation therapy with either orchiectomy or LHRH agonist with or without antiandrogen. These results were recently reviewed using a meta-analysis.[73] Antiandrogens have the disadvantage of causing gynecomastia as well as a small risk of liver injury. Antiandrogens also substantially increase the cost of treatment. In a meta-analysis of androgen deprivation therapy versus combined with androgen blockade, no significant difference was found in survival between the two treatments when antiandrogens were reserved for a time when patients progressed on antiandrogen therapy.[73]

There is a spectrum of endocrine sensitivity in patients with prostate cancer that extends from the very sensitive cells that need testosterone to survive and undergo apoptosis as a result of androgen deprivation to cells whose growth characteristics are unaffected by hormones. There also appears to be a population that needs androgen stimulation to proliferate, but not to survive. For this reason, many oncologists will continue androgen ablation therapy even when refractory tumor emerges, although there are no randomized trials to support this treatment approach. Many clinicians also add cytotoxic therapy to the androgen ablation therapy. Whether the cytostatic effects of hormones affect the sensitivity to cytotoxics is also unknown.

There are two common effects of androgen deprivation therapy that patients find disturbing, vasomotor instability (hot flashes) and osteoporosis. There are a number of anecdotal reports that some drugs may reduce or eliminate the symptoms of hot flashes. Selective serotonin reuptake inhibitor (SSRI) antidepressants have been approved for women with menopausal symptoms, but similar trials have not been carried out in men undergoing androgen deprivation, although 80% of men treated with androgen deprivation, either orchiectomy or LHRH agonist, report symptoms. Quella et al. reported the results of a survey of men and women treated with megesterol for symptoms.[74] These patients continued therapy for up to 3 years, and 88% reported a benefit with doses as low as 10 mg twice daily. Townsend et al. reviewed a single-institution experience with androgen deprivation therapy and found that the cumulative risk of bone fracture unrelated to metastasis was 9% at 6 years.[75] Smith reviewed bone mineral density data in a small group of men with M0 prostate cancer and found that the annual decrease in bone mineral density was 5%, comparable to that observed in postmenopausal women. This risk was the same with orchiectomy or LHRH agonist, although a small group of men treated with DES had only a 1% annual loss in bone mineral density.[76] Diamond et al. carried out a randomized prospective double-blind cross-over study of pamidronate infusion, 90 mg given monthly, versus placebo in men treated with combined androgen blockade and found that pamidronate produced a 2% increase in femoral neck density compared to a 2.3% loss with placebo.[77] These data suggest that bisphosphonate therapy merits consideration in men beginning androgen ablation therapy.

The greatest question in the use of hormonal therapy is when to initiate therapy. There is only one large prospective randomized trial of immediate versus delayed therapy in men with prostate cancer not undergoing curative therapy.[78] This study accrued asymptomatic men with prostate cancer including T2–T4 tumors, N0 or N+ and M0 or M1. Patients were treated with either orchiectomy or LHRH agonists and the patients randomized to delayed treatment began hormonal therapy when the patient and physician identified a symptom likely to benefit from hormonal therapy; 938 men were registered to this trial, with 53% of the men having metastatic disease, and 19% were not evaluated for metastasis. With a median follow-up of more than 5 years, patients assigned to initial deferred treatment required treatment after a median time on study of 18 months, 10 months for M1 patients and 30 months for M0 and Mx patients. Patients treated with early hormonal therapy had fewer bone fractures, 21 versus 11; myelopathy, 23 versus 9; and ureteric obstruction, 55 versus 33. There were fewer overall deaths (328 versus 361) and deaths due to prostate cancer (203 versus 257) in the early therapy group. The group receiving early therapy also has a longer interval to the development of hormone refractory disease, 4.0 versus 6.5 years. These data suggest that presymptomatic hormonal therapy will improve the quality of life and may improve overall survival.

There is a wealth of data reporting the results of screening, staging, and treating prostate cancer, including patients with subclinical, localized, and metastatic disease. The practicing clinician needs to make decisions at several levels. It is first necessary to estimate the probability that prostate cancer is present. If cancer is present, it is then necessary to determine the extent and biologic aggressiveness of the tumor. The patient and clinician must then weigh the institutional capabilities and lifestyle preferences of the patient in making a treatment decision. Some would argue that the high incidence of subclinical or nonaggressive prostate cancer would mitigate against screening, while others argue that it is wise to know the characteristics of the tumor to determine whether treatment is desirable. Pending the results of the large VA trial of observation versus radical prostatectomy, each patient and clinician need to evaluate the issue and jointly make a decision.

Cytotoxic Chemotherapy

Recent developments in cytotoxic chemotherapy have offered prostate cancer patients another therapeutic option. In general, chemotherapy is used in the setting of the development of metastatic androgen-independent disease. Many controversies surround the utilization of chemotherapy in prostate cancer. How do we define androgen independence with respect to eligibility for clinical trials? What therapeutic endpoints are most useful in assessing effectiveness of chemotherapy? Which chemotherapy regimen is most effective? Is there a role for chemotherapy in earlier stages of the disease, including hormone-naïve disease?

Until recently, prostate cancer has been viewed as a chemotherapy-resistant neoplasm without a standard role in the management of the disease.[79] However, early chemotherapy trials were difficult to compare and interpret because of diverse entry criteria and response assessment. To address these and other issues, the Prostate-Specific Antigen Working Group published in 1999 consensus guidelines for phase II clinical trials in androgen-independent disease.[80] These guidelines define specific patient groups as they relate to eligibility for a trial. In addition, criteria for objective assessment of response including PSA response endpoints were defined. This landmark achievement stands as an important step forward in the more recent evolution of chemotherapy in prostate cancer. In 2004, all clinical trials assessing cytotoxic chemotherapy should incorporate this important work into trial design.

Mitoxantrone is an anthracenedione with documented single-agent activity in prostate cancer.[81] Tannock et al. reported a Phase III trial in which 161 patients with symptomatic (pain) androgen-independent prostate cancer were randomized to mitoxantrone plus prednisone (MP) versus prednisone (P) alone.[82] A unique aspect of this study was that the primary endpoint was pain relief. A favorable palliative response was noted in 23 of 80 patients who received MP (29%; 95% CI, 19%–40%) as opposed to only 10 of 81 who received P alone (12%; 95% CI, 6%–22%). In addition, the duration of palliative benefit was improved in the MP group (43 weeks versus 18 weeks; *P* less than 0.001). There was no statistically significant difference in either the PSA response rate or overall survival between the two groups. A correlative study demonstrated that treatment with MP was associated with improvement in several health-related quality of life domains compared to P alone.[83]

The Cancer and Leukemia Group B also studied the combination of mitoxantrone plus hydrocortisone (MH) versus hydrocortisone (H) alone in androgen-independent patients.[84] The primary endpoint of this trial was not pain relief but overall survival. In this trial, 242 patients were randomized to either MH or H alone. There was no difference in survival between the two groups (12.3 months versus 12.6 months). A post hoc analysis demonstrated that 42 of 112 patients (38%) treated with MH demonstrated a 50% PSA response compared to 25 of 116 patients (22%) treated with H alone (P = 0.008). In addition, there was a trend toward improved quality of life in the MH group. Based upon these studies, the U.S. Food and Drug Administration approved mitoxantrone in combination with a steroid as a palliative treatment for men with androgen-independent prostate cancer.

Estramustine phosphate (EMP) is a nornitrogen mustard–estrogen conjugate. Preclinical studies have demonstrated synergy of estramustine with M-phase-specific cytotoxic drugs.[85] Based upon Phase II trials combining EMP with agents such as vinblastine, Hudes et al. performed a Phase III trial of vinblastine (V) versus V plus EMP in 201 patients with androgen-independent prostate cancer. The median survival of the two groups trended toward the V/EMP arm (11.9 months versus 9.2 months; P = 0.08).[86] The V/EMP arm was statistically superior in terms of time to progression and 50% PSA response rate.

More recent trials have focused upon combinations of EMP with a taxane. An exhaustive review of the Phase II trials of EMP/docetaxel and EMP/paclitaxel is well beyond the scope of this review. CALGB 9780 is examined as an example of these trials. In this trial, Savarese et al. treated 47 men with androgen-independent disease with a combination of EMP, docetaxel, and hydrocortisone.[87] In the 44 patients with an elevated pretreatment PSA, the 50% PSA response rate was 68%. In 24 patients with measurable disease, the objective response rate was 50% (95% CI, 27%–73%). The median survival demonstrated in this trial was 20 months.

It is of interest that the median survival noted in CALGB 9780 is superior to those noted in the MP trials. Obviously, patient selection and other biases could result in this difference. SWOG 9916 is a randomized trial comparing MP to EMP/docetaxel in patients with androgen-independent prostate cancer. The primary endpoint of this trial is to detect a 33% increase in median survival in the EMP/docetaxel arm. The trial has completed accrual of 770 patients and the results are eagerly awaited. A second randomized trial that deserves mention is the industry-sponsored TAX 327, a three-arm randomized trial comparing MP to docetaxel/prednisone without EMP (arms 2 and 3 represent an every-3-week docetaxel schedule and a weekly docetaxel schedule, respectively). This trial is also closed to accrual, and the results are forthcoming.

Given the recent advances in chemotherapy development for patients with metastatic androgen-independent prostate cancer, the next obvious step is to move chemotherapy to earlier stages of the disease. A number of investigator-initiated, industry-sponsored, and cooperative group trials are addressing this issue, and two are described here. In RTOG 9902, patients with poor-risk localized prostate cancer are randomized to radiation therapy plus androgen ablation (the standard arm) versus a combination of radiation therapy plus androgen ablation plus cytotoxic chemotherapy (paclitaxel, etoposide, EMP). This ongoing trial hopes to accrue 1,440 patients, with the primary endpoint being survival. ECOG 1899 addresses the role of cytotoxic chemotherapy in patients with androgen-independent prostate cancer but no metastases. In this trial, EMP/docetaxel is being compared to a standard "salvage" hormone regimen, ketoconazole plus hydrocortisone. The primary endpoint of this ongoing trial is progression-free survival. These two trials and others will further define the role of chemotherapy in the management of prostate cancer. As always, clinicians are encouraged to offer patients access to well-designed clinical trials.

References

1. Jemal A, Murray T, Samuels A, Ghafoor A, Ward E, Thun M. Cancer statistics, 2003. CA Cancer J Clin 2003;53:5–26.
2. Sanchez-Chapado M, Olmedilla G, Cabeza M, Donat E, Ruiz A. Prevalence of prostate cancer and prostatic intraepithelial neoplasia in Caucasian Mediterranean males: an autopsy study. Prostate 2003;54(3):238–247.
3. Pienta KJ. Etiology, epidemiology, and prevention of carcinoma of the prostate. In: Walsh P, Retik AB, Vaughan ED, Wein AJ (eds) Campbell's Urology. Philadephia: Saunders, 1998:2191.
4. Catalona WJ, Smith DS, Ratliff TL, Coplen DE, Yuan JJ, Petros JA, Andriole GL. Measurement of prostate-specific antigen in serum as a screening test for prostate cancer. N Engl J Med 1991; 324(17):1156–1161.
5. Brawer MK, Chetner MP, Beatie J, Buchner DM, Vessela RL. Screening for prostatic carcinoma with prostate-specific antigen. J Urol 1992;147:841–845.
6. Mettlin C, Littrup PJ, Kane RA, et al. Relative sensitivity and specificity of serum prostate specific antigen (PSA) level compared with age-referenced PSA, PSA density, and PSA change. Data from the American Cancer Society National Prostate Cancer Detection Project. Cancer (Phila) 1994;74(5):1615–1620.
7. Gleason DF, Mellinger GT, and The Veterans Administration Cooperative Urologic Group. Prediction of prognosis for prostatic adenocarcinoma by combined histological grading and clinical staging. J Urol 1974;111(1):58–64.
8. Johansson J-E, Andersson S-O, Krusemo UB, Adami H-O, Bergstrom R, Kraaz W. Natural history of localised prostatic cancer: A population-based study in 223 untreated patients. Lancet 1989;1:799–803.
9. Johansson J-E, Adami H-O, Andersson S-O, Bergstrom R, Holmberg L, Krusemo UB. High 10-year survival rate in patients with early, untreated prostatic cancer. JAMA 1992;267:2191–2196.
10. Johansson J-E, Holmberg L, Johansson S, Andersson S-O, Bergstrom R, Adami H-O. Fifteen year survival in prostate cancer: a prospective, population based study. JAMA 1997;277: 467–471.
11. Whitmore WF, Warner JA, Thompson IM. Expectant management of localized prostate cancer. Cancer (Phila) 1991;67: 1091–1096.
12. Hugosson J, Aus G, Norlen L. Surveillance is not a viable and appropriate treatment option in the management of localized prostate cancer. Urol Clin N Am 1996;23:557–573.
13. Hugosson J, Aus G, Bergdahl C, Bergdahl S. Prostate cancer mortality in patients surviving more than 10 years after diagnosis. J Urol 1995;154:2115–2117.
14. Holmberg L, Bill-Axelson A, Helgesen F, et al. A randomized trial comparing radical prostatectomy with watchful waiting in early prostate cancer. N Engl J Med 2002;347:781–789.
15. Moon TD, Brawer MK, Wilt TJ. Prostate Intervention Versus Observation Trial (PIVOT): a randomized trial comparing radical prostatectomy with palliative expectant management for treatment of clinically localized prostate cancer. PIVOT Planning Committee. J Natl Cancer Inst Monogr 1995;19:69–71.
16. Young HH. The early diagnosis and radical cure of carcinoma of the prostate: being a study of 40 cases and presentation of a radical operation which was carried out in four cases. Johns Hopkins Hosp Bull 1905;16:315–321.
17. Millen T. Retropubic prostatectomy: a new extravesical technique report on 20 cases. J Urol 2002;167(2 pt 2):976–979.
18. Walsh PC, Donker PJ. Impotence following radical prostatectomy: insight into etiology and prevention. J Urol 1982;182: 482–497.
19. Liedtke RJ. Batjer JD. Measurement of prostate-specific antigen by radioimmunoassay. Clin Chem 1984;30:649–652.
20. Bagshaw MA, Kaplan HS, Sagerman RH. Linear accelerator supervoltage radiotherapy. VII. Carcinoma of the prostate. Radiology 1965;85:121–129.
21. Walsh PC. Anatomical radical retropubic prostatectomy. In: Walsh P, Retik AB, Vaughan ED, Wein AJ (eds) Campbell's Urology. Philadelphia: Saunders, 1998:2565–2588.
22. Gibbons RP. Radical perineal prostatectomy. In: Walsh P, Retik AB, Vaughan ED, Wein AJ (eds) Campbell's Urology. Philadelphia: Saunders, 1998:2589–2604.
23. Roach M III, Chen A, Song J, Diaz A, Presti J Jr, Carroll P. Pretreatment prostate-specific antigen and Gleason score predict the risk of extracapsular extension and the risk of failure following radiotherapy in patients with clinically localized prostate cancer. Semin Urol Oncol 2000;18(2):108–114.
24. D'Amico AV, Altschuler MD, Whittington R, Kao G, Malkowicz SB, Wein AJ. The use of clinical parameters in an interactive statistical package to predict pathologic features associated with local failure after radical prostatectomy. Clin Perf Qual Health Care 1993;1:219–222.
25. Partin AW, Yoo J, Carter HB, et al. The use of prostate specific antigen, clinical stage and Gleason score to predict pathological stage in men with localized prostate cancer. J Urol 1993;150(1): 110–114.

26. Lieberfarb ME, Schultz D, Whittington R, et al. Using PSA, biopsy Gleason score, clinical stage, and the percentage of positive biopsies to identify optimal candidates for prostate-only radiation therapy. Int J Radiat Oncol Biol Phys 2002;53:898–903.
27. Khan MA, Partin AW, Mangold LA, Epstein JI, Walsh PC. Probability of biochemical recurrence by analysis of pathologic stage, Gleason score, and margin status for localized prostate cancer. Urology 2003;62:866–871.
28. D'Amico AV, Whittington R, Malkowicz SB, et al. Biochemical outcome after radical prostatectomy or radiation therapy for clinically localized prostate carcinoma in the prostate specific antigen era. Cancer (Phila) 2002;95:281–286.
29. Bauer JJ, Conelly RR, Seterhenn IA, et al. Biostatistical modeling using traditional preoperative and pathological prognostic variables in the selection of men at high risk for disease recurrence after radical prostatectomy for prostate cancer. J Urol 1998;159:929–933.
30. Iselin CE, Robertson JE, Paulson DF. Radical perineal prostatectomy: Oncologic outcome during a 20-year period. J Urol 1999; 161:163–168.
31. Begg CB, Reidel ER, Bach PB, et al. Variations in morbidity after radical prostatectomy. N Engl J Med 2002;346:1138–1144.
32. Bagshaw MA, Kaplan ID, Cox RC. Radiation therapy for localized disease. Cancer (Phila) 71:939–952.
33. Crook JM, Perry GA, Tobertson S, Esche BA. Routine prostate biopsies following radiotherapy for prostate cancer: results for 226 patients. Urology 1995;445:624–632.
34. Shipley WU, Thames HD, Sandler HM, et al. Radiation therapy for clinically localized prostate cancer: a multi-institutional pooled analysis. JAMA 1999;281:1598–1604.
35. Horowitz EM, Hanlon AL, Pinover WH, Anderson PR, Hanks GE. Defining the optimal radiation dose with three dimensional conformal radiation therapy for patients with nonmetastatic prostate cancer by using recursive partitioning techniques. Cancer (Phila) 2001;92:1281–1287.
36. Pollack A, Zagars GK, Starkschall G, et al. Prostate cancer radiation dose response: results of the M.D. Anderson phase III randomized clinical trial. Int J Radiat Oncol Biol Phys 2002;53:1097–1105.
37. Nguyen KH, Horwitz EM, Hanlon AL, Uzzo RG, Pollack A. Does short-term androgen deprivation substitute for radiation dose in the treatment of high risk prostate cancer. Int J Radiat Oncol Biol Phys 2003;52:377–383.
38. Whitmore WF, Hilaris BS, Grabstald H, Batata MA. Implantation of 125-I in prostate cancer. Surg Clin N Am 1974;54: 887–895.
39. Blasko JC, Ragde H, Schumacher D. Transperineal percutaneous iodine-125 implantation for prostate carcinoma using transrectal ultrasound and template guidance. Endocuriether Hypertherm Oncol 1987;3:131–139.
40. Freeman ML, Goldhagen P, Sierra E, Hall EJ. Studies with encapsulated ^{125}I sources. II. Determination of the relative biological effectiveness using cultured mammalian cells. Int J Radiat Oncol Biol Phys 1982;8:1355–1361.
41. Sylvester JE, Blasko JC, Grimm PD, Meier R, Malmgren JA. Ten-year biochemical relapse-free survival after external beam radiation and brachytherapy for localized prostate cancer: the Seattle experience. Int J Radiat Oncol Biol Phys 2003;57(4):944–952.
42. Vicini FA, Martinez A, Hanks G, et al. An interinstitutional and interspecialty comparison of treatment outcome data for patients with prostate carcinoma based on predefined prognostic categories and minimum follow-up. Cancer (Phila) 2002; 95:2126–2135.
43. Dosoretz AM, Stock RG, Cesaretti JA, Stone NN. Role of external radiation and hormonal therapy in low, intermediate, and high risk patients treated with permanent radioactive seed implantation. Int J Radiat Oncol Biol Phys 57(suppl 2):S227.
44. Blank KR, Whittington R, Arjomandy B, et al. Neoadjuvant androgen deprivation prior to transperineal prostate brachytherapy: smaller volumes, less morbidity. Cancer J Sci Am 1999; 5:70–73.
45. Sánchez-Ortiz RF, Broderick GA, Rovner ES, Whittington R, Wein AJ, Malkowicz SB. Erectile function and health-related quality of life after interstitial radiation therapy for prostate cancer. Int J Impot Res 2000;12:S18–S24.
46. Talcott JA, Manola J, Clark JA, et al. Time course and predictors of symptoms after primary prostate cancer therapy. J Clin Oncol 2003;21:3979–3986.
47. Whittington R, Broderick GA, Arger P, Malkowicz SB, Epperson RD, Arjormandy B, Kassaee A. The effect of androgen deprivation on the early changes in prostate volume following transperineal ultrasound guided interstitial therapy for localized carcinoma of the prostate. Int J Radiat Oncol Biol Phys 1999; 44:1107–1110.
48. Guerriero WG, Carlton CE Jr, Hudgins PT. Combined interstitial and external radiotherapy in the definitive management of carcinoma of the prostate. Cancer (Phila) 1980;15:1922–1923.
49. Mate TP, Gottesman JE, Hatton J, Gribble M, Van Hollebeke L. High dose-rate after loading ^{192}iridium prostate brachytherapy: feasibility report. Int J Radiat Oncol Biol Phys 1998;41:525–533.
50. McGowan DG. The value of extended field radiation therapy in carcinoma of the prostate. Int J Radiat Oncol Biol Phys 1981; 7:1333–1339.
51. Bagshaw MA. Current conflicts in the management of prostatic cancer. Int J Radiat Oncol Biol Phys 1986;12:1721–1727.
52. Asbell SO, Martz KL, Shin KH, et al. Impact of surgical staging in evaluating the radiotherapeutic outcome in RTOG 77-06, a phase III study for T1BN0M0 and T2N0M0 prostate carcinoma. Int J Radiat Oncol Biol Phys 1998;40:769–782.
53. Roach M, Desilvio M, Lawton C, et al. Phase III trial comparing whole-pelvic versus prostate-only radiotherapy and neoadjuvant versus adjuvant combined androgen suppression: Radiation Therapy Oncology Group 9413. J Clin Oncol 2003;21: 1904–1911.
54. Paulson DF, Lin GH, Hinshaw W, Stephani S, of the Uro-oncology Research Group. Radical surgery versus radiotherapy for adenocarcinoma of the prostate. J Urol 1982;128:502–504.
55. Byhardt RW, Greenlaw RH, Jensen R, et al. Re: Radical surgery versus radiotherapy for adenocarcinoma of the prostate. J Urol 1983;130:1205–1206.
56. Kupelian PA, Potters L, Khnutia D, et al. Radical prostatectomy, external beam radiation therapy < 72 Gy, external beam radiotherapy > 72 Gy, permanent seed implantation, or combined seeds/external radiotherapy for stage T1-T2 prostate cancer. Int J Radiat Oncol Biol Phys 2004;58:25–33.
57. D'Amico AV, Whittington R, Malkowicz SB, et al. Biochemical outcome after radical prostatectomy or external beam radiation therapy for patients with clinically localized prostate carcinoma in the prostate specific antigen era. Cancer (Phila) 2002;95: 281–286.
58. Zagars GK, Johnson DE, von Eschenbach AC, Hussey DH. Adjuvant estrogen following radiation therapy for stage C adenocarcinoma of the prostate: long-term results of a prospective randomized study. Int J Radiat Oncol Biol Phys 1988;14(6): 1085–1091.
59. Shipley WU, Lu JD, Pilepich MV, et al. Effect of short course neoadjuvant hormonal therapy on the response to subsequent androgen suppression in prostate cancer patients with relapse after radiotherapy: a secondary analysis of the randomized protocol RTOG 86-10. Int J Radiat Oncol Biol Phys 2002;54: 1302–1310.
60. Pilepich MV, Caplan R, Byhardt RW, et al. Phase III trial of androgen suppression using goserelin in unfavorable-prognosis carcinoma of the prostate treated with definitive radiotherapy: report

of Radiation Therapy Oncology Group protocol 85-31. J Clin Oncol 1997;15:1013–1021.
61. Bolla M, Collette L, Blank L, et al. Long-term results with immediate androgen suppression and external radiation in patients with locally advanced prostate cancer (an EORTC study): a phase III randomised trial. Lancet 2002;360:105–108.
62. Hanks GE, Pajak TF, Porter A, et al. Phase III trial of long- term adjuvant androgen deprivation after neoadjuvant hormonal cytoreduction and radiotherapy in locally advanced carcinoma of the prostate: the Radiation Therapy Oncology Group protocol 92-02. J Clin Oncol 2002;21:3972–3978.
63. Sgrignoli AR, Walsh PC, Steinberg GD, Steiner MS, Epstein JI. Prognostic factors in men with stage D1 prostate cancer: identification of patients less likely to have prolonged survival after radical prostatectomy. J Urol 1994;152:1077–1081.
64. Myers RP, Zincke H, Fleming TR, Farrow GM, Furlow WL, Utz DC. Hormonal treatment at time of radical retropubic prostatectomy for stage D1 prostate cancer. J Urol 1983;130:99–101.
65. Hanks GE, Buzydlowski J, Sause WT, et al. Ten-year outcomes for pathologic node-positive patients treated in RTOG 75-06. Int J Radiat Oncol Biol Phys 1998;40(4):765–768.
66. Gervasi LA, Mata J, Easley JD, et al. Prognostic significance of lymph nodal metastases in prostate cancer. J Urol 1989;142: 332–336.
67. Messing EM, Manola J, Sarosdy M, Wilsing G, Crawford ED, Trump D. Immediate hormonal therapy compared with observation after radical prostatectomy and pelvic lymphadenectomy in men with node-positive prostate cancer. N Engl J Med 1999; 341:1781–1788.
68. Sands ME, Pollack A, Zagars GK. Influence of radiotherapy on node-positive prostate cancer treated with androgen ablation. Int J Radiat Oncol Biol Phys 1995;31:13–19.
69. Robnett TJ, Whittington R, Malkowicz SB, et al. Long term use of combined radiation therapy and hormonal therapy in the management of stage D1 prostate cancer. Int J Radiat Oncol Biol Phys 2002;53:1146–1151.
70. Huggins C, Stevens RE, Hodges CV. Studies on prostatic cancer. II: The effects of castration on advanced carcinoma of the prostate. Arch Surg 1943;43:209–223.
71. Blackard CE, Byar DP, Jordan WP. Orchiectomy for advanced prostate cancer: a reevaluation. Urology 1973;1:553–560.
72. Seidenfeld J, Samson DJ, Hasselblad V, et al. Single-therapy androgen suppression in men with advanced prostate cancer: a systematic review and meta-analysis. Ann Intern Med 2000;132: 566–577.
73. Samson DJ, Seidenfeld J, Schmitt B, et al. Systematic review and meta-analysis of monotherapy compared with combined androgen blockade for patients with advanced prostate carcinoma. Cancer (Phila) 2002;95:361–376.
74. Quella SK, Loprinzi CL, Sloan JA, et al. Long term use of megesterol acetate by cancer survivors for the treatment of hot flashes. Cancer (Phila) 1998;82:1784–1788.
75. Townsend MF, Sanders WH, Northway RO, Graham SD. Bone fractures associated with luteinizing hormone-releasing hormone agonists used in the treatment of prostate carcinoma. Cancer (Phila) 1997;79:545–550.
76. Smith MR. Diagnosis and management of treatment-related osteoporosis in men with prostate cancer. Cancer 2003;97(suppl 3):789–795.
77. Diamond TH, Winters J, Smith A, et al. The antiosteoporotic efficacy of intravenous pamidronate in men with prostate carcinoma receiving combined androgen blockade: a double blind, randomized, placebo-controlled crossover study. Cancer (Phila) 2001;92:1444–1450.
78. The Medical Research Council Prostate Cancer Working Party Investigators Group. Immediate versus deferred treatment for advanced prostatic cancer: initial results of the Medical Research Council trial. Br J Urol 1997;79:235–246.
79. Yagoda A, Petrylak D. Cytotoxic chemotherapy for advanced hormone-resistant prostate cancer. Cancer (Phila) 1993;71: 1098.
80. The Prostate-Specific Antigen Working Group. Eligibility and response guidelines for phase II clinical trials in androgen-independent prostate cancer: recommendations from the Prostate-Specific Antigen Working Group. J Clin Oncol 1999;17: 3461–3467.
81. Kantoff PW, Block C, Letvak, et al. 14-day continuous infusion of mitoxantrone in hormone-refractory metastatic adenocarcinoma of the prostate. Am J Clin Oncol 1993;6:489–491.
82. Tannock IF, Osaba D, Stockler MR, et al. Chemotherapy with mitoxantrone plus prednisone or prednisone alone for symptomatic hormone-resistant prostate cancer: a Canadian randomized trial with palliative endpoints. J Clin Oncol 1996;14: 1756–1764.
83. Osoba D, Tannock IF, Ernst DS, et al. Health-related quality of life in men with metastatic prostate cancer treated with prednisone alone or mitoxantrone and prednisione. J Clin Oncol 1999;17:1654–1663.
84. Kantoff PW, Halabi S, Conaway M, et al. Hydrocortisone with or without mitoxantrone in men with hormone-refractory prostate cancer: results of the Cancer and Leukemia Group B 9182 study. J Clin Oncol 1999;17:2506–2513.
85. Kreis W, Budman D, Calabro A. Unique synergism or antagonism of combinations of chemotherapeutic and hormonal therapy in human prostate cancer cell lines. Br J Urol 1997;79: 196–202.
86. Hudes G, Einhorn L, Ross E, et al. Vinblastine versus vinblastine plus oral estramustine phosphate for patients with hormone-refractory prostate cancer: a Hoosier Oncology Group and Fox Chase Network trial. J Clin Oncol 1999;17: 3160–3166.
87. Savarese DM, Halabi S, Hars V, et al. Phase II study of docetaxel, estramustine, and low dose hydrocortisone in men with hormone-refractory prostate cancer: a final report of CALGB 9780.

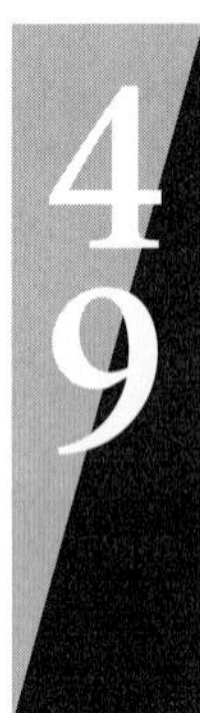

Testis Cancer

Timothy Gilligan and Phillip W. Kantoff

The treatment of testicular cancer is one of the great success stories of Western medical science. More than 90% of patients are now cured, and essentially all patients, regardless of how advanced their disease is at the time of diagnosis, have a real chance of cure. In contrast, 50 years ago, metastatic testicular cancer was almost always fatal. Testicular cancer represents an example of what can be learned from a systematic and determined clinical trials effort. The current standard chemotherapeutic regimens are based on a long series of randomized controlled trials, despite the fact that this is a relatively rare disease. Because there is almost always the possibility of achieving a cure and because current standard therapies have been based on a solid scientific foundation, mistakes in the management of testicular cancer patients can be particularly costly and difficult to justify. Patients with testicular cancer should be treated by physicians familiar with the disease and with the germ cell tumor literature.[1]

The vast majority of testicular cancers are germ cell tumors (GCT), and most GCTs occur in the testicles. It is worth noting that there are important biologic and therapeutic differences between GCTs in adult or adolescent males, which are discussed in this chapter, and other GCTs, which include dermoid cysts, gestational trophoblastic neoplasia, intracranial GCTs of childhood and adolescence, and neonatal yolk-sac tumors and teratomas. Ovarian GCTs have many similarities to testicular GCTs, but these are discussed in a different chapter.

Epidemiology

Testicular cancer is rare, with about 7,600 cases diagnosed and 400 deaths reported annually in the United States.[2] Worldwide, an estimated 49,000 cases are diagnosed and 9,000 men die of the disease annually.[3] It is the most common malignancy among U.S. males 20 to 34 years of age and the second most common malignancy among white males in the United States between the ages of 15 to 19 and 35 to 39.[4] Testicular cancers represent up to 60% of malignancies diagnosed in men aged 20 to 40 years in Western countries. The incidence of nonseminomatous GCTs peaks between the ages of 20 and 35, whereas seminomas are most common between the ages of 30 and 45. Nearly 95% of all testicular cancers are diagnosed between the ages of 15 and 54, and the median age of diagnosis is 34 years.[2,5]

The incidence of testicular cancer has increased in the United States and worldwide, but with substantial regional variation between the years 1950 and 2000.[6] During that period, the U.S. incidence of testicular cancer increased 168% while mortality declined 73% and relative 5-year survival improved from 57% to 96%.[2] Between 1975 and 2000, the incidence increased 54%, to 5.7 cases per 100,000 males.[2] During the same period, mortality declined by 71%. Most of the decline in mortality occurred between 1973 and 1983, when cisplatin-based chemotherapy became widely used, but a slower downward mortality trend has continued.[7] For unknown reasons, testicular cancer is especially rare in black men. White males in the United States have a 0.42% lifetime risk of being diagnosed with testicular cancer compared to a 0.10% risk among African-Americans.[2]

The major risk factors for testicular cancer are cryptorchidism, an affected first-degree relative, and a personal history of contralateral testicular cancer. Male infertility and subfertility have also been strongly associated with an increased incidence of testicular cancer.[8–10] Cryptorchidism confers a relative risk of testicular cancer that has been reported to range from 2 to 18, and a meta-analysis reported a relative risk of 7.8.[11,12] The increased risk of cancer is seen in both the nondescended testicle and, to a lesser degree, the contralateral testicle. Although different studies have reached different conclusions, it appears that orchiopexy before age 10 either reduces or eliminates the increased risk of cancer.[11,13,14] Men with a father or son with testicular cancer have a relative risk of testicular cancer of 2.0 to 5.7,[15–19] whereas men with a brother with testicular cancer have a relative risk of 8.3 to 13 and a lifetime risk of testicular cancer of about 2% to 3%, suggesting that maternal factors may be important. Men with testicular cancer have a 1% to 4% risk of developing a second primary GCT in the contralateral testicle.[20–24] Among men with bilateral cancers, the median time interval between the diagnoses of the two tumors is about 5 years, and as many as 25% of metachronous tumors are diagnosed more than 10 years after the first cancer.[22,24] Men with gonadal dysgenesis and testicular atrophy also manifest an increased incidence of testicular GCTs.[25]

Basic Science

Cell of Origin

Testicular GCTs, with the exception of spermatocytic seminomas, are thought to develop from primordial germ cells or slightly later gonocytes that have transformed into the premalignant cells that constitute carcinoma in situ of the testis, also referred to as intratubular germ cell neoplasia (ITGCN).[26] This transformation is believed to occur in utero, because an increased risk of testicular cancer has been associated with (1) severe maternal nausea, (2) neonatal jaundice, (3) parity, (4) advanced maternal age, and (5) both low and high birth weights.[27–29] In addition, men with a fraternal twin with testicular cancer have a higher relative risk of being diagnosed with the disease than do men with an identical twin with testicular cancer.[30] These findings support the hypothesis that high estrogen levels and other factors during pregnancy stimulate the transformation of primordial germ cells into premalignant tissue.[27] Similarly, the association of testicular atrophy and abnormal sperm counts with testicular cancer, as well as the finding that the incidence of testicular cancer rises sharply shortly after puberty, suggest that increased gonadotropin levels may drive the transformation of ITGCN into GCTs. Increased follicle-stimulating hormone (FSH), estrogen, and testosterone have been documented in patients with newly diagnosed testicular cancer.

The biologic relationship between pure seminomas and nonseminomatous or mixed GCTs remains poorly defined. It is currently believed that the default pathway from ITGCN is to seminoma and that additional genetic events are needed for the development of nonseminomatous tumors. An alternative hypothesis is that seminomas and nonseminomas represent different development pathways from ITGCN.

Cytogenetics

The specific genetic events involved in the malignant transformation of germ cells remain to be defined. Most GCTs are associated with an isochromosome of the short arm of chromosome 12 (i(12p)). Germ cell tumors without an i(12p) uniformly show increased 12p sequences.[31,32] The short arm of chromosome 12 is thought to encode about 120 genes, including SOX5, JAW1, and K-*ras*, but the identity of the critical genes on 12p has not been established. Overrepresentation of the long arm of chromosome 17 has been reported in more than 50% of testicular cancers.[26]

Basis of Chemosensitivity

The unique sensitivity of testicular germ cell cancer to cisplatin-based chemotherapy represents one of the most striking attributes of this disease. The derivation of these tumors from germ cell precursors, which are highly prone toward apoptosis, makes this sensitivity less surprising. Several factors have been identified that likely contribute to these tumors' chemosensitivity. Wild-type p53 protein is overexpressed in most GCTs, and p53 mutations are only rarely seen.[33] Although the role of P53 in inducing apoptosis makes these findings provocative, it has not been clearly demonstrated that p53 status is central to GCT chemosensitivity. Indeed, most chemoresistant GCTs have no p53 mutations, and Burger et al. have demonstrated, in cell line studies, that functional p53 is not necessary for cisplatin-induced apoptosis.[34,35] Similarly, the antiapoptotic protein BCL2 has been shown to be either absent from or expressed at very low levels in most GCTs, but BCL2 expression has not been consistently linked to chemotherapy resistance or other clinical outcomes. In reviewing the literature in this area, Mayer and Bokemeyer and colleagues have proposed that GCT chemosensitivity may result from a low expression of chemotherapy export pumps, impairment of both cisplatin detoxification and DNA repair pathways, a relatively high sensitivity to DNA damage, and corresponding low threshold for activation of apoptosis, as well as an intact apoptotic cascade.[36,37] Currently, there are not adequate data to validate this model. Zurita et al. have reported that expression of the lung resistance-related protein in testicular cancers was associated with shorter overall survival and may be associated with chemoresistance.[38] Although it is clear that GCTs show a greater propensity for undergoing apoptosis, both spontaneously and in response to chemotherapy, the specific apoptotic pathway(s) involved are unknown and the specific basis of chemosensitivity remains to be clearly defined.

Teratomas, in contrast to seminomas, choriocarcinomas, embryonal carcinomas, and yolk-sac tumors, are highly resistant to chemotherapy. Although the reason for this resistance is not well defined, several differences have been noted. Teratomas more often express p21 and the retinoblastoma protein, both of which mediate G_1/S cell-cycle arrest.[37] In addition, teratomas show a higher expression of the antiapototic protein Bcl-2 and lower expression of the proapoptotic Bax protein.[37] Collectively, these findings suggest that although the other GCT subtypes are prone toward apoptosis and have an impaired ability to arrest the cell cycle and repair chemotherapy-damaged DNA, teratomas are more resistant to apoptosis and instead respond to DNA damage by stopping the cell cycle.[36]

Serum Tumor Markers

The serum tumor markers alpha fetoprotein (AFP), human chorionic gonadotropin (HCG), and lactate dehydrogenase (LDH) play a major role in the management of GCTs. They can help to confirm the diagnosis, estimate the prognosis, determine appropriate therapy, and monitor for progression, regression, and relapse. In cases of metastatic carcinoma of unknown primary, a highly elevated AFP or HCG may suggest a diagnosis of a poorly differentiated GCT, but elevated serum tumor markers in this setting have not been shown to predict a response to platinum-based chemotherapy, and therefore the utility of measuring the markers in such tumors remains debatable.[39] In men with disseminated GCTs, a very high AFP, HCG, or LDH is associated with a poorer prognosis and generally leads to more-aggressive therapy.[40] Similarly, in men with no radiologic evidence of disseminated disease, a persistent elevation of serum tumor markers is generally interpreted as evidence of occult metastases. During treatment, a decline in serum tumor markers in accordance with their predicted biologic half-lives has been associated with a more-favorable prognosis, whereas a sluggish decline suggests chemoresistance and rising markers imply refractory disease. Men whose markers fail to normalize with chemotherapy are at higher risk of relapse, and when men with nonseminomatous GCTs relapse, the most common initial manifestation is rising tumor markers.

An unresolved issue is whether sluggishly declining tumor markers during chemotherapy are an indication that the chemotherapy regimen should be changed.[41] Among men receiving second-line chemotherapy, an HCG half-life greater than 3.5 days or an AFP half-life greater than 7 days is associated with shorter event-free and overall survival.[42] A follow-up study reported that among men receiving first-line chemotherapy, overall survival was 95% in men with a normal rate of decline of HCG and AFP compared to 72% among men with a slow rate of decline.[43] However, it has never been demonstrated that switching therapy based on the rate of marker decline yields improved outcomes, and this remains a question for clinical trials.

Although tumor markers help monitor the response to therapy, they must be interpreted with care.[44] Initiation of chemotherapy can result in tumor lysis that leads to a rise in markers during the first 10 days of therapy, and such a rise should not be interpreted as indicative of resistance to chemotherapy.[45] The baseline marker levels to be used for monitoring response to chemotherapy should thus be drawn at the end of the first week of treatment. Similarly, chemotherapy can result in hepatotoxicity that results in rising serum AFP levels in the absence of viable germ cell cancer.[46] HCG assays may cross-react with luteinizing hormone, and hypogonadal men with elevated gonadotropins may thus test as having a mildly elevated HCG. Administration of testosterone lowers gonadotropin secretion from the pituitary and can thus help identify false-positive results.[47] Heterophile antibodies can also result in false-positive HCG results.[48] Mild, stable elevations in markers do not always indicate the presence of residual malignancy; the entire clinical picture must be considered.[44,45]

Alpha Fetoprotein

Serum AFP is elevated in 40% to 60% of patients with testicular nonseminomatous germ cell tumors (NSGCT). AFP is a single-chain polypeptide with a serum half-life of 5 to 7 days.[49] It is produced by the fetal yolk sac, liver, and intestines and, except during pregnancy, an AFP level above 15 ng/mL is abnormal.[45] AFP is elevated not only in NSGCTs but also in pregnancy, hepatitis, hepatocellular carcinoma, and, less often, carcinomas of the stomach,[50–52] colon and rectum,[53] and other gastrointestinal sites.[54] Within the context of GCTs, AFP is most strongly associated with yolk-sac tumors but can also be produced by embryonal carcinomas. Seminomas do not produce AFP. *The presence of an elevated serum AFP in a patient with a histologic diagnosis of pure seminoma is interpreted as a sign of occult nonseminomatous elements, and such patients are treated as having mixed GCTs.* Men with a clinical stage I NSGCT who have a persistently elevated serum AFP following orchiectomy are at high risk of having distant metastases and are typically treated with chemotherapy. As noted previously, a rising AFP can result not only from relapsed disease but also from chemotherapy-related liver toxicity.

Human Chorionic Gonadotropin

Serum HCG is elevated in 25% to 50% of men with disseminated seminomas and in 2% to 12% of men with stage I disease. In contrast, in men with nonseminomatous testicular GCTs, HCG is elevated in 45% to 60% of metastatic cases and in 25% to 50% of stage I cases. HCG is a glycoprotein consisting of an α-chain and a β-chain. The serum half-life of HCG is about 24 to 36 hours, and the upper limit of normal serum HCG in men ranges from 0.1 to 5 IU/L, depending on the assay. Different assays can produce widely varying results, and when false-positive results are suspected, repeating the test using a different assay may be helpful.[55–57] The α-chain in HCG has a polypeptide sequence identical to the α-chain found in the other glycoprotein hormones: thyroid-stimulating hormone, luteinizing hormone (LH), and follicle-stimulating hormone (FSH). The β-chain of each of these hormones is unique and gives the hormone its specificity. Assays for HCG typically test for both the beta-subunit (β-HCG) and for intact HCG, but cross-reactivity with other glycoprotein hormones sometimes occurs, particularly with LH.[58,59]

In healthy individuals, HCG is produced by placental trophoblasts and pituitary gonadotrophs. Elevated HCG levels occur in pregnancy as well as in gestational trophoblastic disease, hydatidiform moles, choriocarcinoma, and other GCTs. Elevated levels of β-HCG are found in 45% to 60% of patients with biliary and pancreatic cancer and 10% to 30% of most other cancers, but more than a mild elevation of intact HCG is rare in non-germ cell tumors.[59,60]

In the context of GCTs, elevated serum HCG is most strongly associated with choriocarcinomas, which can result in HCG levels in the hundreds of thousands or even millions (IU/L). Less-extreme elevations of serum HCG are seen in other GCTs. Many experts consider serum HCG levels higher than 200 to 300 IU/L incompatible with pure seminoma and advocate treating patients with such results as having mixed germ cell tumors, but there are few data to support these opinions.[59,61,62] Pure seminomas have been reported in which the serum HCG was highly elevated, but it is possible such cases represent mixed GCTs misdiagnosed as pure seminomas. The International Germ Cell Cancer Collaborative Group's pooled analysis reported that, among men with disseminated seminoma receiving first-line chemotherapy, 3% of the subjects had a serum HCG above 1,000 IU/L. It does not appear that an elevated HCG in seminoma is associated with a poorer prognosis, but the data are mixed.[63]

Lactate Dehydrogenase

Lactate dehydrogenase (LDH) is an enzyme that catalyzes the conversion between lactate and pyruvate. LDH is elevated in about 50% to 75% of patients with disseminated seminoma.[64–67] An elevated LDH can be seen in many settings of cell death and rapid cellular turnover, including lymphomas, myocardial infarction, and liver disease. An elevated LDH is not specific, and LDH level is not helpful in establishing or ruling out a diagnosis of germ cell cancer. Serum LDH levels do carry prognostic information once the diagnosis has been made, particularly in seminomas, which are less likely than nonseminomas to have other elevated serum tumor markers.[66] An elevation of serum LDH at diagnosis and a sluggish decay of elevated serum LDH are each associated with a higher relapse rate in seminomas.[63] Assays for LDH measure enzymatic activity, and the normal range is therefore assay dependent and varies widely among different tests. Knowing the LDH level without knowing the specific assay's normal range is thus meaningless.

Pathology

Most testicular cancers are GCTs, which are divided into two broad categories, seminomas and nonseminomas, by differences in natural history and treatment. Nonseminomatous germ cell tumors (NSGCTs) include embryonal carcinomas, yolk-sac tumors, teratomas, and choriocarcinomas. Most NSGCTs are mixed tumors that are composed of two or more GCT subtypes. Mixed GCTs that include both nonseminomatous and seminomatous histology are considered NSGCTs for treatment and prognostic purposes. Testicular malignancies that are not GCTs include Leydig cell tumors, Sertoli cell tumors, gonadoblastomas, granuloma-thecal cell tumors, and carcinoma of the rete testis. Pathologic staging of the primary tumor is based on the presence or absence of (a) lymphatic or vascular invasion (henceforth referred to as lymphovascular invasion, LVI), (b) invasion beyond the tunica albuginea into the tunica vaginalis, (c) invasion of the spermatic cord, and (d) invasion of the scrotum. In seminomas, the size of the primary tumor and the presence or absence of invasion of the rete testis are also of prognostic significance.[68]

Intratubular Germ Cell Neoplasia

Testicular GCTs in adults, with the exception of spermatocytic seminomas, develop from the testicular form of carcinoma in situ, also referred to as intratubular germ cell neoplasia (ITGCN). ITGCN consists of noninvasive malignant-appearing cells within the seminiferous tubules. The presence of ITGCN in an orchiectomy specimen in men with testicular cancer does not carry any prognostic implications with regard to the risk of relapse of the cancer.[69] However, in men with unilateral testicular GCTs, contralateral testicular biopsies reveal ITGCN in about 5% of cases, and half of these men develop invasive testicular cancers over the subsequent 5 years.[70] In some countries, men with testicular cancer are subjected to a biopsy of the contralateral testicle to evaluate for ITGCN.[71] Men with positive biopsies are then typically treated with low-dose radiotherapy (14–20 Gy) to the testis, which kills the neoplastic cells and preserves testosterone production but sacrifices fertility.[72] Screening biopsies for ITGCN in testis cancer patients is controversial because half the men treated are treated unnecessarily and because screening has not been shown to result in improved survival or quality of life. Testis biopsies are rare in the United States.

Seminoma

The most common type of testicular GCT, seminomas occur at an older average age than nonseminomatous tumors, with most cases diagnosed in the fourth or fifth decade of life.[73] Syncytiotrophoblasts, which stain positive for HCG, can be identified in up to 24% of cases of pure seminoma but are of no clear prognostic significance.[73] Lymphocytic infiltrates and granulomatous reactions are often seen, and seminomas appear to be associated with an increased incidence of sarcoidosis.[74,75] Seminomas can produce moderately elevated serum levels of HCG but they do not produce AFP. Even if histopathology shows a pure seminoma, an elevated serum AFP should be interpreted as indicating the presence of yolk-sac tumor elements, and the tumor should be treated as a mixed GCT.

Spermatocytic Seminomas

Although they share a similar name, spermatocytic seminomas are biologically distinct from classic seminomas. These are very rare tumors and occur at a mean age of 54 to 67 years.[76,77] These tumors are almost always cured with orchiectomy alone, although many patients have received prophylactic paraaortic radiation. Metastatic disease has only been reported once.[77] Unlike other testicular GCTs, spermatocytic seminoma is not associated with a history of cryptorchidism.

Embryonal Carcinoma

Embryonal carcinomas consist of undifferentiated malignant cells resembling cells from early-stage embryos. The microscopic appearance of these tumors varies considerably, and they may grow in solid sheets or in papillary, glandular, or tubular patterns. Hemorrhagic and necrotic areas are often present. In some cases, syncytiotrophoblasts are identified. Embryonal carcinomas are aggressive tumors associated with a high rate of metastasis, often in the context of normal serum tumor markers. As discussed next, the presence and proportion of embryonal carcinoma has been associated with the likelihood of postorchiectomy relapse in clinical stage I tumors.

Choriocarcinoma

Choriocarcinomas of the testicles are rare and very aggressive tumors that typically present with very highly elevated serum HCG and disseminated disease. Common sites of metastases include the lungs and brain, but reports have also been made of metastases to the skin and eye.[78,79] Microscopically, the tumors are composed of syncytiotrophoblasts and cytotrophoblasts, and the former stain positively for HCG. As noted previously, syncytiotrophoblasts can also be present in seminomas and embryonal carcinoma. Choriocarcinoma is distinguished by the presence of these cells together with cytotrophoblasts.[73] Areas of hemorrhage and necrosis are prominent. As in gestational trophoblastic disease, testicular choriocarcinoma is prone to hemorrhage, sometimes both spontaneously and immediately after chemotherapy is initiated, and such bleeding can be catastrophic.[80]

Yolk-Sac Tumors

In adults, pure yolk-sac tumors (sometimes called endodermal sinus tumors) represent a very small fraction of testicular cancers but are common among mediastinal GCTs. Nonetheless, mixed GCTs of the testis often include elements of yolk-sac tumor. Yolk-sac tumors almost always produce AFP but not HCG. Among men with clinical stage

I testicular GCTs with normal serum tumor markers, finding elements of yolk-sac tumor is associated with a lower risk of relapse, but this finding may simply be a result of serum tumor markers (i.e., AFP) having a higher sensitivity for detecting micrometastatic disease in this type of GCT.[81]

Teratoma

Teratomas are tumors that contain well- or incompletely differentiated elements of endoderm, mesoderm, and ectoderm. Well-differentiated tumors are labeled mature teratomas whereas those that are incompletely differentiated are called immature teratomas. Mature teratomas may include elements of mature bone, cartilage, teeth, hair, and squamous epithelium, a fact that most likely explains the name teratoma, which roughly means "monster tumor" in Greek. In adults, both mature and immature testicular teratomas have the potential to metastasize, and the distinction carries no clear prognostic significance.[82] Teratomas are generally associated with normal serum tumor markers, but they may cause mildly elevated serum AFP levels.

Diagnosis and Staging

Presentation

Testicular cancers typically present as testicular nodules or enlargement, but testicular atrophy can also be a sign of cancer. Although testicular cancers are classically described as painless masses, half of all patients complain of testicular pain or tenderness at the time of presentation. Such symptoms can lead practitioners to mistake cancers for orchitis or epididymitis and to delays in diagnosis. GCTs are also associated with gynecomastia, and men with this condition should be evaluated for testicular cancer. The most common site of metastatic disease is the retroperitoneum and men with disease in this region may present with back pain. Palpable supraclavicular adenopathy can also be a presenting sign.

Diagnostic and Staging Studies

Physical examination of a man suspected of having testicular cancer should include a careful testicular palpation for induration or nodules. Any firm or fixed areas within the tunica albuginea should be considered suspicious for cancer until proven otherwise. Examination should also include lymph node evaluation, particularly in the supraclavicular region, and the abdomen should be palpated for retroperitoneal masses.

Men with suspicious or ambiguous findings on testicular palpation should be referred for testicular ultrasound, and measurement of serum AFP, HCG, and LDH should be considered. With high-frequency (7.5-MHz) transducers, lesions as small as 1 to 2 mm can be identified with very high sensitivity and specificity.[83] Testicular cancers are typically heterogeneous, hypoechoic intratesticular masses, and such a finding on ultrasound should lead to an inguinal orchiectomy to make a definitive diagnosis. *Transscrotal biopsy and scrotal orchiectomy are contraindicated because of the risk of seeding the scrotum with tumor and complicating subsequent management.* Serum tumor markers should always be measured before orchiectomy; this is particularly important with regard to AFP, because an elevated AFP precludes a diagnosis of pure seminoma regardless of the results of histopathologic evaluation. In rare cases where transscrotal ultrasound results are ambiguous, testicular magnetic resonance imaging (MRI) may be helpful.

Men who are found to have testicular cancer in their orchiectomy specimen should be staged with a computed tomography (CT) scan of the abdomen and pelvis and a plain chest radiograph. Chest CT scans in men with normal chest radiographs and normal abdominopelvic CT scans is extremely low yield. Only 4% of men with normal abdominal CT scans have thoracic disease, and a prospective study of 120 patients undergoing both plain radiographs and chest CT scans identified only a single case in which the CT identified disease that had not been detected on the radiograph.[84,85] However, because up to 40% of men with abnormal abdominal CT scans have chest metastases, a chest CT is appropriate in this subpopulation. CT or MRI scans of the brain are not routinely indicated in testicular cancer patients who do not have neurologic symptoms but should be obtained in men with choriocarcinoma and/or highly elevated postorchiectomy serum HCG (greater than 10,000 IU/L) or AFP (greater than 1,000 ng/mL). Positron emission tomography (PET) scanning has not proven useful thus far in staging testicular cancers but may be of aid in evaluating residual masses in men with pure seminoma following radiation or chemotherapy. Because teratoma does not show increased activity on PET, this modality is of limited utility with NSGCTs.

Although many staging systems for testicular cancer have been used historically, current staging follows the American Joint Committee on Cancer (Tables 49.1, 49.2).[86] For patients with disseminated disease, low-risk, intermediate-risk, and high-risk patients can be identified using the International Germ Cell Consensus Classification (Table 49.3).[40] According to this system, the prognosis of disseminated seminomas is based solely on the presence (intermediate risk) or absence (good risk) of nonpulmonary visceral metastases. For NSGCTs, prognosis depends on the level of postorchiectomy serum tumor markers, the presence of nonpulmonary visceral metastases, and the primary site of the tumor.

Treatment of Stage I Disease

Stage I Seminoma

Stage I testicular seminoma has a 5-year cause-specific survival of more than 99%.[68] Because the risk of dying of the disease is so low, minimizing treatment-related toxicity represents a priority. Standard management historically was external-beam radiation, but, due to concern about secondary malignancies and other radiation toxicities, close surveillance has become a widely accepted alternative. More recently, near-perfect results have been achieved with single-agent carboplatin chemotherapy, which has produced the lowest relapse rate of any treatment thus far. All three approaches produce comparable overall and disease-specific survival to

TABLE 49.1. American Joint Committee on Cancer (AJCC) staging of testicular germ cell tumors.

Definition of TNM

Primary tumor (pT)

pTX	Primary tumor cannot be assessed
pTO	Primary tumor cannot be assessed (e.g., histologic scar in testis)
pTis	Intratubular germ cell neoplasia (carcinoma in situ)
pT1	Tumor limited to the testis and epididymis without vascular/lymphatic invasion; tumor may invade into the tunica albuginea but not the tunica vaginalis
pT2	Tumor limited to the testis and epididymis with vascular/lymphatic invasion, or tumor extending through the tunica albuginea with involvement of the tunica vaginalis
pT3	Tumor invades the spermatic cord with or without vascular/lymphatic invasion
pT4	Tumor invades the scrotum with or without vascular/lymphatic invasion

Regional lymph nodes (N)

Clinical

NX	Regional lymph nodes cannot be assessed
NO	No regional lymph node metastasis
N1	Metastasis with a lymph node mass 2 cm or less in greatest dimension; or multiple lymph nodes, none more than 2 cm in greatest dimension
N2	Metastasis with a lymph node mass, more than 2 cm but not more than 5 cm in greatest dimension; or multiple lymph nodes, any one mass greater than 2 cm but not more than 5 cm in greatest dimension
N3	Metastasis with a lymph node mass more than 5 cm in greatest dimension

Pathologic (pn)

pNX	Regional lymph nodes cannot be assessed
pN0	No regional lymph node metastasis
pN1	Metastasis with a lymph node mass, 2 cm or less in greatest dimension and less than or equal to 5 nodes positive, none more than 2 cm in greatest dimension
pN2	Metastasis with a lymph node mass, more than 2 cm but not more than 5 cm in greatest dimension; or more than 5 nodes positive, none more than 5 cm; or evidence of extranodal extension of tumor
pN3	Metastasis with a lymph node mass more than 5 cm in greatest dimension

Distant metastasis (M)

MX	Distant metastasis cannot be assessed
M0	No distant metastasis
M1	Distant metastasis M1a Nonregional nodal or pulmonary metastasis M1b Distant metastasis other than to nonregional lymph nodes and lungs

Serum tumor markers (S)

SX	Marker studies not available or not performed
S0	Marker study levels within normal limits
S1	LDH less than 1.5 × N **AND**
	hCG (mIu/mL) less than 5000 **AND**
	AFP (ng/mL) less than 1000
S2	LDH 1.5–10 × N **OR**
	HCG = 5,000–50,000 mIu/mL **OR**
	AFP = 1,000–10,000 ng/mL
S3	LDH greater than 10 × N **OR**
	hCG > 50,000 mIu/mL **OR**
	AFP > 10,000 ng/mL

N, upper limit of normal for the lactate dehydrogenase (LDH) assay.

Source: Used with the permission of the American Joint Committee on Cancer (AJCC), Chicago, Illinois. The original source for this material is the *AJCC Cancer Staging Manual*, sixth edition (2002), published by Springer-Verlag New York, www.springer-ny.com.

TABLE 49.2. American Joint Committee on Cancer (AJCC) staging of testicular germ cell tumors.

Stage 0	pTis, N0, M0, S0	Stage IIC	Any pT/Tx, N3, M0, S0
Stage I	pT1–4, N0, M0, SX		Any pT/Tx, N3, M0, S1
Stage IA	pT1 , N0, M0, S0	Stage III	Any pT/Tx, any N, M1, SX
Stage IB	pT2, N0, M0, S0 pT3, N0, M0, S0 pT4, N0, M0, S0	Stage IIIA Stage IIIB	Any pT/Tx, any N, M1a, S0 Any pT/Tx, any N, M1a, S1 Any pT/Tx, N1–3, M0, S2
Stage IS	Any pT/Tx, N0, M0, S1–3		Any pT/Tx, any N, M1a, S2
Stage II	Any pT/Tx, N1–3, M0, SX	Stage IIIC	Any pT/Tx, N1–3, M0, S3
Stage IIA	Any pT/Tx, N1 , M0, S0 Any pT/Tx, N1, M0, S1		Any pT/Tx, any N, M1a, S3 Any pT/Tx, any N, M1b, any S
Stage IIB	Any pT/Tx, N2, M0, S0 Any pT/Tx, N2, M0, S1		

Source: Used with the permission of the American Joint Committee on Cancer (AJCC), Chicago, Illinois. The original source for this material is the *AJCC Cancer Staging Manual*, sixth edition (2002), published by Springer-Verlag New York, www.springer-ny.com.

TABLE 49.3. International germ cell consensus classification for disseminated tumors.

GOOD PROGNOSIS	
Non-seminoma	***Seminoma***
Testis/retroperitoneal primary	Any primary site
AND	AND
No nonpulmonary visceral metastases	No nonpulmonary visceral metastases
AND	AND
All of the following:	Normal AFP, any HCG, any LDH
AFP less than 1,000 ng/mL	
HCG less than 5,000 mIu/mL	
LDH less than 1.5 × upper limit of normal (ULN)	
5-year progression-free survival = 89%	5-year progression-free survival = 82%
5-year overall survival = 92%	5-year overall survival = 86%
INTERMEDIATE PROGNOSIS	
Non-seminoma	***Seminoma***
Testis/retroperitoneal primary	Any primary site
AND	AND
No nonpulmonary visceral metastases	Nonpulmonary visceral metastases
AND	AND
Any of the following:	Normal AFP, any HCG, any LDH
AFP 1,000 or more and 10,000 ng/mL or less	
HCG 5,000 or more and 50,000 mIu/mL or less	
LDH 1.5 or more × ULN and 10 × ULN or less	
5-year progression-free survival = 75%	5-year progression-free survival = 67%
5-year overall survival = 80%	5-year overall survival = 72%
POOR PROGNOSIS	
Non-seminoma	***Seminoma***
Mediastinal primary	
AND/OR	
Nonpulmonary visceral metastases	No seminoma patients classified as poor prognosis
AND/OR	
Any of the following:	
AFP more than 10,000 ng/mL	
HCG more than 50,000 mIu/mL	
LDH more than 10 × ULN	
5-year progression-free survival = 41%	
5-year overall survival = 48%	

Source: From International Germ Cell Consensus Classification,[40] by permission of *Journal of Clinical Oncology*.

TABLE 49.4. Results of carboplatin, radiation, and surveillance for stage I Seminoma.

Study	*N*	*Median follow-up*	*Relapses*	*% relapsed*	*Five-year OS (%)*	*Five-year DFS (%)*	*Five-year RFS (%)*
Surveillance:							
Warde[b] 2002[68]	638	84	121	19.0	97.7	99.3	82.3
Daugaard 2003[155]	394	60	69	17.5	98.6	100	83
Totals	1,032		190	18.4			
Carboplatin (2 cycles):							
Oliver 2001[96]	57	128	1	1.8	100.0	100	98.2
Krege 1997[97]	43	28	0	0		100[c]	100[c]
Dieckmann 2000[101]	32	45	0	0	100.0	100	100
Aparicio 2003[88]	60	52	2	3.3	96.7	100	96.6
Steiner 2002[99]	108	60	2	1.9	100.0	100	
Reiter 2001[95]	107	74	0	0	94.4	100	100
Kratzik 1993[100]	39	20	1	2.6	N/A	N/A	N/A
Aparicio 2004[90]	204	20	5	2.5	100.0[a]	100[a]	96.4[a]
Totals	650		11	1.7			
Radiation:							
Warde 1995[91]	194	97	11	5.7	97.0	100.0	94.5
Logue 2003[113]	431	62	15	3.5	98.0	99.8	96.3
Bamberg 1999[114]	483	55	18	3.7		99.8	95.8
Bauman 1998[118]	169	90	5	3.0		100.0	95.0
Giacchetti 1993[121]	184	216	4	2.2	96.0	97.0	
Fossa 1999[116]	478	54	18	3.8	99.6		96.0
Santoni 2003[115]	487	105	21	4.3	97[d]		
Classen 2004[306]	675	61	26	3.9		99.6	95.8
Oliver 2004[102]	904	36	36	4.0	99.4[e]	99.9[e]	96.6[a]
Totals	4,005		154	3.8			

OS, overall survival; DFS, disease-free survival; RFS, relapse-free survival.
[a] Three-year survival.
[b] Pooled international analysis.
[c] Results at 28-month median follow-up.
[d] Ten-year survival.
[e] Results at 36-month median follow-up.

the extent that data are available (Table 49.4). Mature randomized trials are lacking.

Overall, about 15% to 20% of men with clinical stage I testicular seminomas who receive no postorchiectomy treatment will relapse within 5 years of diagnosis and a few percent more will relapse in later years.[68,87,88] If all men are treated with radiation or chemotherapy, then roughly 80% receive unneeded treatment. Efforts have been made to find risk factors for relapse that would allow clinicians to identify low-risk patients for whom surveillance would be particularly attractive and high-risk patients for whom the side effects of active treatment would be more justifiable. The most consistently identified risk factor for relapse has been tumor size. von der Maase and colleagues reported that 4-year relapse-free survival was 94%, 82%, and 64% for men with tumor diameters less than 3 cm, 3 to 6 cm, and greater than or equal to 6 cm, respectively.[89] Other identified risk factors include invasion of the rete testis, younger age at diagnosis, and lymphovascular invasion. A pooled international analysis of 638 men with clinical stage I seminoma undergoing surveillance reported that, in multivariate analysis, only larger tumor size and rete testis invasion were associated with relapse, but this prognostic model was unable to identify a group of patients with a risk of relapse either greater than 32% or less than 12%.[68] These risk criteria have now been prospectively validated by the Spanish Germ Cell Cancer Group, which studied risk-adapted management of stage I seminoma.[90] Among 300 patients with stage I seminoma, those with tumors 4 cm or smaller and no invasion of the rete testis underwent surveillance whereas those who had rete testis invasion and/or tumors larger than 4 cm were treated with two cycles of carboplatin. With a median follow-up of 20 months, 4 of 96 (4.2%) low-risk patients put on surveillance had relapsed whereas 5 of the 204 (2.4%) high-risk patients receiving carboplatin relapsed. Although this strategy effectively identified a very low risk group and spared up to 92 men unnecessary treatment, overtreatment was a problem: 208 men received chemotherapy while only 60 would have been expected to relapse without therapy.

Surveillance

Surveillance offers patients the obvious advantage of avoiding postorchiectomy therapy unless it becomes necessary because of relapsed disease. Given the well-documented increased late mortality associated with radiation therapy as a result of excess cardiac events and secondary cancers, as well as the possibility of long-term side effects from carboplatin chemotherapy, the opportunity to avoid treating at least 80 of 100 men is attractive. Almost all relapsing patients are salvaged, and 5-year disease-specific survival ranges from 99% to 100%.[88,89,91,92] In an international pooled analysis of 638 patients, 5-year overall and disease-specific survival were 97.7% and 99.3%, respectively.[68] There is no evidence that surveillance compromises or improves long-term survival so long as patients comply with the surveillance schedule.

Different centers have used difference surveillance schedules, and no randomized trials comparing surveillance schedules have been published. The National Cooperative Cancer Network and the Princess Margaret Hospital both have proposed evaluations every 4 months for the first 3 years, every 6 months for years 4 to 7, and every 12 months during years 8 through 10.[68,93] At each visit serum LDH, AFP, and HCG are measured, a physical examination is performed (including a testicular examination), and an abdominopelvic CT scan in obtained. A chest radiograph is recommended at alternate visits, although the three largest published surveillance series have reported thoracic relapses in only 3 of 576 men (0.52%).[89,91,92]

The success of surveillance results from the relatively low relapse rate and the success of salvage therapy. In large published series, 74% to 83% of relapses are limited to the retroperitoneal lymph nodes, with most of the remainder involving the pelvis.[89,91] Most postorchiectomy relapses are stage IIA or IIB and can be treated with paraaortic radiation at doses ranging from 25 to 37 Gy.[91] The Princess Margaret Hospital in Toronto reported a median retroperitoneal lymph node size of 3 cm with a range of 1.5 to 9 cm, whereas the Spanish Germ Cell Cancer Cooperative Group reported a median relapsed tumor size of 3.3 cm with a range of 0 to 6 cm.[88,91] In published surveillance series from Toronto, Denmark, and the Royal Marsden Hospital, 74% to 76% of relapsing patients have received radiation therapy, with most of the remainder receiving systemic chemotherapy as a result of bulky or disseminated disease.[89,91,92] Combining the data from these reports, 11 of 70 (16%) patients receiving radiation therapy for relapsed disease subsequently required chemotherapy for a second relapse, and only 1 death from seminoma was reported. Of all the men entered on these surveillance protocols, 6% ultimately required chemotherapy as part of their salvage therapy, which is comparable to the proportion of men requiring salvage chemotherapy for relapse following postorchiectomy radiation.

Adjuvant Carboplatin Chemotherapy

Adjuvant chemotherapy using single-agent carboplatin represents the newest postorchiectomy treatment for clinical stage I seminoma and has produced the lowest relapse rates. Judging from numerous phase II trials, carboplatin appears to offer patients a way to dramatically lower their risk of relapse without exposing themselves to the long-term toxicities of radiation therapy. Most of these trials have given two doses of carboplatin 21 to 28 days apart at a dose of 400 mg/m^2, although the Anglian Germ Cell Cancer Group doses carboplatin at an AUC (area under the curve) of 7.[94] A phase III trial comparing a single dose of carboplatin to radiation therapy has been completed and early results presented, but mature data have not been published.

Results from eight phase II trials of two cycles of single-agent carboplatin are available, including data from 650 men[88,90,95–101] (see Table 49.4). Only 11 (1.7%) had relapsed and all were successfully salvaged with additional therapy. None died of seminoma or acute treatment toxicity; disease-specific survival was 100%. Looking only at studies with a mean follow-up of at least 5 years, only 3 of 272 men (1.1%) have relapsed and all have relapsed within 2 years of receiving carboplatin.[95,96,99] Although a risk of late relapses has been posited as a theoretical concern, no late relapses have been documented thus far. The European Oncology Research and Treatment Group and Medical Research Council randomized phase III trial comparing radiation to a single dose of carboplatin dosed at an AUC of 7 reported its preliminary results in abstract form in 2004.[102] With 1,447 men enrolled and a median follow-up of 3 years, relapse-free survival was 96.6% in the radiation arm and 95.4% in the carboplatin arm, and the 95% confidence intervals excluded an increased risk in the carboplatin arm of more than 4%. No disease- or treatment-related deaths were reported in the carboplatin arm and only 1 was reported in the radiation arm. Seven patients receiving radiation developed second germ cell cancers compared to only 1 patient receiving carboplatin. This trial appears to establish equivalency between a single dose of carboplatin and radiation for stage I seminoma, but mature results are needed. This is the second study, however, to suggest that a single cycle of carboplatin is inferior to two cycles.[101]

Carboplatin also looks favorable from a toxicity perspective. No cases of febrile neutropenia have been reported, and carboplatin at these doses has not been associated with secondary malignancies. Two patients in the published seminoma series developed severe thrombocytopenia and received platelet transfusions, but no bleeding complications have been reported. In a randomized phase II trial, Oliver et al. reported that chemotherapy resulted in greater myelosuppression and altered taste than radiation but that radiation resulted in greater nausea, diarrhea, and fatigue.[96] Assessing the impact of testicular cancer chemotherapy on fertility represents a challenge, because most men have abnormal sperm counts at the time of diagnosis and testicular cancer is associated with infertility both before diagnosis and following treatment with orchiectomy alone.[9,10,103–105] After treatment, sperm counts typically improve. Reassuring data were published by Reiter et al., who found that normospermia increased from 35% following orchiectomy to 68% following chemotherapy.[106] Similarly, no renal or neurologic toxicity has been documented. Multiagent platinum-based chemotherapy for testicular cancer has been associated with dyslipidemia, hypertension, and an increased long-term risk of cardiovascular events in some studies, but no increase in mortality has been reported.[107–111] Most of the patients in these studies received cisplatin, rather than carboplatin, but one study that evaluated both agents found no evidence that carboplatin was safer in the context of a multidrug regimen.[107] There are inadequate long-term follow-up data to assess whether two cycles of single-agent carboplatin have any impact on vascular health, but this is an issue that clearly warrants future monitoring.

Radiation Therapy

Previously, radiation therapy was considered the preferred therapy for stage I seminomas.[112] It is highly effective, producing a 5-year relapse-free survival of 95% to 97% and a disease-specific survival of 99% to 100% in almost all published series.[63,91,113–121] Interest in developing alternative therapies stems from concern not about radiation therapy's effectiveness at disease control but rather its side effects. Because the 5-year relapse-free survival rate is about 15% to 20% with surveillance and about 5% with radiation, only 10 to 15 men for every 100 treated appear to benefit from radiation. There is no evidence of a survival benefit from radiation compared to surveillance. Given the outstanding prognosis of men who receive no postorchiectomy treatment and are followed on a surveillance protocol, treatments for stage I disease with significant long-term toxicity are difficult to tolerate. Radiation therapy has been associated with a variety of secondary cancers as well as with cardiovascular disease and peptic ulcers. Largely in response to these concerns, the radiation dose and field have diminished substantially over time. However, these changes in treatment have occurred too recently for there to be follow-up data clarifying whether, and if so, to what extent, they reduce long-term toxicities.

Radiation Field and Dose

Although the radiation field previously extended to include the mediastinum, supraclavicular region, paraaortic region, and ipsilateral hemipelvis, radiation above the diaphragm is now considered inappropriate, with the risks of additional toxicity outweighing any small benefit in disease control. Multiple retrospective studies have reported a twofold or greater excess cardiac mortality among patients receiving mediastinal radiation,[122–124] and it does not appear that mediastinal radiation significantly improves cancer control outcomes.[125] Prophylactic mediastinal radiation is therefore currently contraindicated.

Many centers omit treatment of the pelvis, using a paraaortic field only that typically extends from the 10th vertebral body down to the L4–L5 or L5–S1 disk space.[114,116] The lateral margins vary, sometimes extending to the renal hilum on the same side as the involved testicle and to the *processus transversus* on the contralateral side.[116] Others treat to the *processus transversus* bilaterally. Alternatively, a lymphangiogram may be obtained to visualize the lymphatic anatomy and then the lateral margins can be tailored to these radiographic findings. The other commonly used field is the "dog-leg" or "hockey-stick" field, which uses the same superior margins as the paraaortic field but extends more inferolaterally to the ipsilateral pelvis. A randomized controlled trial conducted by the Medical Research Council assigned 478 men with clinical stage I seminoma to either paraaortic or dog-leg irradiation with a dose of 30 Gy.[116] With a median follow-up of 4.5 years, 9 patients had relapsed in each arm, yielding a 3-year relapse-free survival of 96.0% in the paraaortic field arm and 96.6% in the dog-leg field arm. Nausea, vomiting, diarrhea, and leukopenia occurred less often in the paraaortic arm, and recovery of sperm counts was delayed in the dog-leg arm. However, 4 relapsing patients in the paraaortic arm relapsed in the pelvis whereas there were no pelvic relapses in the dog-leg arm. Use of a paraaortic field was thus associated with equivalent efficacy and less toxicity and was therefore advanced as a new standard of care, but some still use a dog-leg field because of concern about pelvic relapses.

Radiation Dose

The radiation dose used to treat seminomas has declined over time. Although 30 Gy or higher was often used for clinical stage I disease in older trials, recent studies have reported equally favorable results with lower doses, and many consider 25 Gy to be the standard dose today.[126] Medical Research Council study TE18 randomized 625 patients to either 20 Gy in 10 fractions or 30 Gy in 15 fractions.[127,128] With 37 months median follow-up, the relapse-free survival was 97% in each arm. A separate multicenter study of 431 men in the United Kingdom reported that treatment with 20 Gy resulted in a 5-year relapse-free survival rate of 96.3% and a disease-specific survival of 99.8%, figures entirely comparable to studies of higher doses.[113]

Patterns of Failure

The few men who relapse following radiation therapy for stage I seminoma tend to relapse outside the field that was irradiated.[63,91,113–118] Slightly over half relapse above the diaphragm, typically in the lungs, the mediastinum, or supraclavicular lymph nodes. Most of the remaining relapses occur in the pelvis, while about 15% are in the retroperitoneum. Paraaortic field radiation is associated with about a 2% pelvic relapse rate compared to a 0.6% rate in those treated with a dog-leg field.[91,113–118] Late relapses are unusual, with the median time to relapse in most studies ranging from 13 to 17 months, and relapses beyond 36 months are unusual. Postradiation surveillance should include a chest radiograph, physical examination, and serum tumor marker measurement (LDH, AFP, and HCG) every 3 months for the first year, every 4 months the second year, every 6 months the third year, and then annually for at least 3 years. A CT scan of the abdomen and pelvis is obtained annually by many but not all centers, even though only about 1% of men treated with a dog-leg field and 2% of those treated with a paraaortic field will relapse in the abdomen or pelvis. Some advocate pelvic CTs without including the abdomen for those patients who are treated using a paraaortic field and no CT scan for those treated with a dog-leg field. Randomized trials comparing different surveillance strategies have not been conducted.

Secondary Malignancies and Other Radiation Toxicities

Toxicity from radiation therapy includes acute side effects such as fatigue, nausea and vomiting, diarrhea and mild leukopenia.[129] These side effects are milder and less common with smaller fields (paraaortic rather than dog-leg)[116] and lower doses (20 Gy versus 30 Gy).[128,130] Late and long-term side effects include secondary non-germ cell malignancies, peptic ulcer disease, cardiovascular toxicity, and compromised fertility. Numerous papers have documented an elevated relative risk of secondary non-germ cell malignancies in men receiving radiation therapy for testicular seminoma.[120,131–136] For instance, Travis and colleagues reported an analysis of 16 population-based tumor registries including more than 15,000 men with testicular seminomas.[132] Men who had received radiation therapy had a relative risk of 1.45 for developing secondary non-germ cell cancers ($P = 0.05$), with increased risks of cancers of the colon, kidneys, stomach, pancreas, and urinary bladder. Chemotherapy, by contrast, was not associated with an overall increased risk of cancer [relative risk (RR) = 0.90; P more than 0.05], although men receiving etoposide chemotherapy are known to be at a low but increased risk of developing leukemia. Similarly, a review of the M.D. Anderson Cancer Center's experience with radiation therapy for testicular seminoma reported that there were 91% more cancer deaths than expected [95% confidence interval (CI); RR, 1.30–2.71], but this increase only appeared 15 years after treatment.[120] Others have reported relative risks from 1.6 to 3.4 for second cancers.[123,137,138] Because it takes 15 to 20 years for secondary cancers to develop, studies with short follow-up periods are uninformative, and the meaningful data on secondary malignancies are unavoidably based on older radiation therapy planning and dosing. It is unknown whether modern radiotherapy with smaller doses and treatment fields will result in significantly fewer secondary malignancies, and there is no guarantee that this will be the case.

A second major concern with radiation therapy is cardiovascular toxicity. The M.D. Anderson Cancer Center reported a 61% increase in cardiac deaths among men receiving radiation therapy, and the increased risk was seen even among patients who received no mediastinal radiation. Others have reported relative risk of cardiac deaths as high as 2.3,[123] and other reports have confirmed that an increased risk of cardiac events is seen among men receiving radiation therapy limited to a paraaortic field.[107–109,123] Similar findings of excess cardiac events (but not mortality) have been reported for men receiving chemotherapy for testicular cancer but not among men being followed on a postorchiectomy surveillance schedule.[107,108]

Radiation for seminoma has also been associated with peptic ulcer disease and infertility. Reported rates of peptic ulcers have ranged from 0% to 16%.[91,116,139–143] The MRC TE10 phase III study comparing paraaortic to dog-leg radiation fields collected toxicity data systematically and reported that, with a median follow-up of 4.5 years, 33 of 478 men (7%) were diagnosed with a peptic ulcer.[116] Regarding fertility, a series of 451 men with GCTs who had undergone orchiectomy followed by surveillance, retroperitoneal lymph node dissection, chemotherapy, or radiation reported that patients who had received radiation therapy had an odds ratio for achieving conception of 0.35 compared to men who had received chemotherapy ($P = 0.017$) despite the use of testicular shielding.[144] In contrast, modern studies of stage I seminoma have reported that 60% to 90% of men who try to father children following radiation therapy are successful.[115,144]

Conclusion

Current data do not permit a definitive recommendation for the treatment of stage I seminoma.[112] Surveillance, carboplatin, and radiation are each associated with disease-specific survival exceeding 99%, although the long-term toxicity of radiation is concerning and the long-term toxicity of carboplatin is unknown (see Table 49.4). Men should be informed of the three treatment options and the associated side effects so that they can participate in choosing the treatment that is best for them.[112]

Stage I Nonseminomatous Germ Cell Tumors

Clinical stage I testicular NSGCTs have an excellent prognosis, with a 5-year survival rate of 98% to 99% with any of the following three postorchiectomy therapies: close surveillance, two cycles of bleomycin, etoposide, and cisplatin (BEP) chemotherapy, or retroperitoneal lymph node dissection (RPLND) (Table 49.5). As a result of the near-perfect survival rate with any of these approaches, decisions about treatment often hinge on provider bias and patient preference as well as on the side effects of the different treatment options and the availability of the appropriate technology and surgical expertise. Patients with clinical stage I disease but persistently elevated serum tumor markers following orchiectomy, however, are presumed to have disseminated disease and are generally treated with chemotherapy for advanced disease (see later section).

Risk Classification

Men with clinical stage I testicular NSGCTs and serum tumor markers that are either normal or that are falling at a pace consistent with the markers' predicted biologic half-life face a 25% to 30% risk of relapsing without additional treatment. With the aim of treating only those men who are most likely to relapse while sparing low-risk men unnecessary treatment, many centers have attempted to identify criteria that predict relapse. The Medical Research Council (MRC) identified and then prospectively validated four independent risk factors for relapse: vascular invasion, lymphatic invasion, the presence of embryonal carcinoma elements, and the absence of yolk-sac tumor.[81,145] However, even among men with three or four of the risk factors, fewer than half (47%) relapsed. With regard to identifying low-risk patients, 24 of 141 (17%) men with zero or one risk factors relapsed, and these low-risk men represented 39% of the study participants; 21% of men with two risk factors relapsed, and this group represented 39% of the participants, which is similar to the average relapse rate of stage I nonseminoma patients in general. The MRC approach was thus of limited utility in identifying appropriate patients for surveillance and for treatment: more than half those identified as high risk would be treated unnecessarily whereas 4 of 10 men could not be classified as either high or low risk.

Subsequent efforts at risk classification have identified lymphovascular invasion (LVI) and embryonal carcinoma (EC) as the two elements most predictive of relapse.[146–155] However, prospective validation of models other than that of the MRC is lacking. Taking into account the proportion of the tumor that is EC rather than simply the presence or absence of this tissue type has led to models with greater predictive power.[147] Moul and colleagues reported, in a sample of 149 patients with clinical stage I disease who underwent RPLND, that they could accurately identify the pathologic stage in 88% using a combination of LVI and percent EC.[148] They reported that occult retroperitoneal lymph node metastases can be demonstrated in 89% of clinical stage I patients whose tumor showed either more that 80% EC or the combination of LVI and more than 45% EC. Similarly, Indiana University reported that 62% of men whose tumors showed LVI and a predominance of EC were found to have metastatic disease subsequently,[153] whereas Memorial Sloan-Kettering Cancer Center reported that 73% of men with pure EC had metastases detected at RPLND.[151] Other studies have suggested that

TABLE 49.5. Results of primary chemotherapy, retroperitoneal lymph node dissection (RPLND, and surveillance for stage I testicular nonseminomatous germ cell tumors.

Study	*N*	*Median follow-up*	*Relapses*	*% relapsed*	*OS (%)*	*DSS (%)*	*GCT-related deaths*
Surveillance							
Freedman 1987[145]	259	30	70	27.0	98.0	98.0	1.2%
Read 1992[81]	396	60	100	25.3	98.0	99.0	1.3%
Sogani 1998[150]	105	135.6	27	25.7		97.1	2.9%
Colls 1999[149]	248	53	70	28.2	97.6	98.0	1.2%
Spermon 2002[307]	90	92.4	23	25.6		98.5	1.1%
Daugaard 2003[155]	301	60	86	28.6	98.6	100.0	0.0%
Gels 1995[154]	154	84	42	27.3	98.7	98.7	1.3%
Alexandre 2001[157]	88	51.6	24	27.3		98.9%	1.1%
Total	**1,641**		**442**				**1.1%**
Chemotherapy[a]							
Pont 1996[308]	29	79	2	6.9%	93.0	96.5	3.45%
Cullen 1996[188]	114	48	2	1.8%	98.0	98.0	1.75%
Bohlen 1999[189]	58	93	2	3.4%	100.0	100.0	0.00%
Abratt 1994[309]	20	31	0	0.0%	N/A	100.0	0.00%
Ondrus 1998[194]	18	36	0	0.0%	100.0	100.0	0.00%
Mourey 2003[191]	64	51	1	1.6%	100.0	100.0	0.00%
Oliver 2004[192]	148	33	6	4.1%	97.3	97.3	1.35%
Amato 2004[193]	68	38	1	1.5%	100.0	100.0	0.00%
Hendry 2000[195]	60	60	2	3.3%	98.3%	98.3%	1.67%
Total	**579**		**16**	**2.8%**			**1.04%**

Study	*N*	*N, PSI*	*Median follow-up (months)*	*Relapses among PSI*	*Relapses among CSI*	*Relapse rate among PSI*	*Relapse rate among CSI*	*OS*	*DSS*	*Deaths related to GCT*
RPLND										
Spermon 2002[307]	101	70	82.8	7	7	10.0%	6.9%	98%	98%	1.0%
Hermans 2000[310]	292	226	46	23	30	10.2%	10.3%	NR	NR	NR
McLeod 1991[209]	264	264	63	27	27	10.2%	N/A	96.6%	98.1%	1.9%
Klepp 1997[184]	99	85	40	13	13	15.3%	13.1%	100.0%	100	0%
Donohue 1993[172]	378	266	75	31	53	11.7%	14.0%	99.2%	99.2%	0.8%
Total	**1,134**	**911**		**101**	**130**	**11.1%**	**11.5%**			**0.7%**

OS, overall survival; DSS, disease-specific survival; PSI, pathologic stage I; CSI, clinical stage I; GCT, germ cell tumor.

[a]Patients selected for primary chemotherapy trials had above-average risk of postorchiectomy relapse based on the histopathology of their primary tumor.

immunohistochemical staining with the MIB-1 antibody against the Ki-67 receptor is associated with metastatic disease, but such staining has not been incorporated into common practice.[156]

Men with low risk of occult metastatic disease have also been identified. In the Indiana series, 84% of men with clinical stage I disease and neither LVI nor a predominance of EC remained relapse free with at least 2 years follow-up.[153] In Moul's model, men with either less than 45% EC or the combination of no LVI and less than 80% EC had only a 13% risk of having metastases detected at RPLND.[148] The presence of mature teratoma has also been associated with low risk of occult metastases,[157] but in multivariate analyses mature teratoma has generally been eclipsed by LVI and the proportion of EC. Even men with clinical stage I pure mature teratomas of the testicle have a 19% risk of occult metastatic disease to the retroperitoneal lymph nodes.[158]

Retroperitoneal Lymph Node Dissection (RPLND)

Retroperitoneal lymph node dissection (RPLND) involves the removal of the lymph nodes that constitute the primary draining site of the testicles. This procedure is well tolerated and has both diagnostic and therapeutic benefits by helping to define the stage of the cancer while also reducing the subsequent relapse rate. The major benefit of RPLND is to reduce the proportion of patients who require treatment with chemotherapy. It is a major operation but is extremely well tolerated in patients who have received no prior chemotherapy.

Surgical Technique

Historically, a bilateral dissection of all retroperitoneal nodal material was performed, extending from the crus of the diaphragm to the bifurcation of the common iliac arteries and laterally to the ureters.[159] In addition, a complete and wide excision of the spermatic cord and surrounding lymphatic tissues was and is recommended.[160] The field of resection was subsequently reduced, first with the superior margin coming down to the renal vessels (infrahilar dissection) and then with the development of distinct right and left modified templates.[161–164] Studies carefully mapping the location of microscopic lymph node metastases in testicular cancer revealed that bilateral dissections in clinical stage I disease were unnecessary, as contralateral metastases were very rare, with the exception that right-sided tumors showed the potential to spread to preaortic lymph nodes between the renal vessels and the inferior mesenteric artery (IMA).[165] Just as the venous drainage from the testicles is asymmetric, with the right gonadal vein moving toward midline and draining into the inferior vena cava while the left gonadal vein remains more lateral and drains into the left renal vein, so too is the lymphatic drainage. Therefore, the right-sided template extends to the left of midline above the IMA while the left sided template remains unilateral.[166]

Complications

Loss of antegrade ejaculatory function is the most common long-term side effect of RPLND; this should not be confused with erectile dysfunction, which is **not** associated with RPLND. The use of the unilateral modified templates reduced the incidence of dry ejaculation from nearly 100% to less than 50%.[167] The next development was the introduction of nerve-sparing RPLND, which involved prospectively identifying the sympathetic fibers in the field of dissection before the dissection of the nodal tissue.[168] In the hands of an experienced surgeon, nerve-sparing RPLND has resulted in preservation of ejaculation in 93% to 100% of patients.[168–170] Other complications are rare.[167] Wound infections in less than 5% and small bowel obstruction in less than 2% are well-established risks, whereas some centers have reported a rare incidence of a prolonged ileus, incisional hernia, and urethral strictures.[171] RPLNDs performed to remove residual masses following chemotherapy for advanced-stage GCTs are associated with a higher rate of complications than RPLNDs performed on men with clinical stage I disease.

Outcomes

Among clinical stage I patients undergoing RPLND, 25% to 30% have retroperitoneal nodal metastases (pathologic stage II disease), and overall survival is 98% to 99%.[172,173] Pathologic stage I patients with normal or normalizing serum tumor markers before RPLND have about a 10% risk of relapsing, but a recent single-institution study reported that that rate had dropped from 10% before 1999 to 3% in subsequent years.[172–174] The risk of relapse among patients with pathologic stage N1 disease and normal pre-RPLND tumor markers has been reported at 8% to 16%.[166,175] Patients with elevated serum tumor markers before RPLND face a high risk of relapsing following RPLND. Studies of RPLND that have not excluded patients with elevated markers have reported less-favorable relapse-free survival figures than those just cited.[166,176] Indiana University has reported that 5 of 6 men (83%) with persistently elevated AFP relapsed following RPLND, as did 6 of 24 (25%) with a persistently elevated HCG, whereas Memorial Sloan-Kettering reported that persistently elevated markers were associated with a relative risk for relapse of 8.0 (95% CI, 2.3–27.8).[166,177] RPLND is therefore **not** recommended for men with persistently elevated or sluggishly declining serum tumor markers following orchiectomy: such men should receive chemotherapy for disseminated disease.

Patients with tumors with lymphovascular invasion (LVI) and/or a predominance of embryonal carcinoma (EC) have a higher risk of having occult stage II disease, as discussed previously, and RPLND is less likely to be curative without subsequent chemotherapy.[147,151,153] In the Memorial Sloan-Kettering experience, half of all clinical stage I patients with pure EC treated with RPLND subsequently received chemotherapy. Indiana University reported that men with predominantly EC have a 32% risk of having retroperitoneal lymph node metastases and that 35% of these men will relapse without adjuvant chemotherapy.[152,153] Of the 68% of these men with no disease found at RPLND, 20% will relapse without adjuvant chemotherapy. If LVI and a predominance of EC are both present, the risk of lymph node metastases rises to 47%, of whom 36% will relapse without chemotherapy while 29% of those without lymph node metastases relapse without chemotherapy. These figures indicate that at least a third of men with predominant EC and LVI require chemotherapy following RPLND, whereas additional men may be advised to undergo chemotherapy to lower their risk of relapse. Because of the high risk of receiving chemotherapy following RPLND, some have questioned the appropriateness of surgery for men with predominantly EC and LVI.

Laparoscopy

Laparascopic RPLND has been investigated.[178–182] The results thus far are favorable, with a relapse rate in pathologic stage I patients of 5% to 13% reported with median follow-up times of at least 40 months and loss of antegrade ejaculation reported in 0% to 3.5%.[178,180–183] Complications have included injury to the bowel, renal artery, and ureter, and the procedure is associated with a steep learning curve. In experienced hands, the results appear favorable but there are few centers with experience.

Surveillance

Postorchiectomy surveillance for clinical stage I testicular NSGCTs and normal or normalizing serum AFP, HCG, and LDH is a well-accepted option that results in disease-specific survival ranging from 97% to 100% in published series.[81,145,149,150,154,155,157,184,185] This approach has the benefit of sparing 71% to 74% of men any postorchiectomy treatment. The disadvantage of surveillance is mainly that the 26% to 29% of men who relapse then require three to four cycles of chemotherapy, which carries a higher toxicity profile than either RPLND or the two cycles of chemotherapy offered to men as primary chemotherapy for stage I disease. Men with persistently elevated tumor markers are not appropriate candidates for surveillance but instead should be treated for presumed disseminated disease with chemotherapy (three to four cycles depending on the degree of marker elevation and the choice of regimen), unless a nonmalignant source for marker elevation can be established. Similarly, men who would be unable to comply with the schedule of clinic visits and medical tests involved in surveillance and men who live in an area where such services are unavailable should be advised to undergo active treatment to reduce the risk of relapse.

Overall, 26% to 29% of men on surveillance schedules will relapse, but almost all can be successfully salvaged with therapy at the time of relapse, and the long-term outcome for men on surveillance is similar to that of men undergoing RPLND or primary chemotherapy, although no randomized trials have been published. Surveillance schedules vary considerably among institution. Most relapses occur within the first 6 months, 76% to 90% occur in the first year, and 87% to 100% occur within 2 years. Relapses later than 5 years are highly unusual, affecting fewer than 1% of patients (in contrast, second primary tumors involving the contralateral testis are more common, affecting about 3% of patients). The most common site of relapse is the abdomen, with 60% to 80% manifesting retroperitoneal adenopathy, while a similar proportion will have elevated tumor markers. Marker elevation is the sole indication of relapse in 7% to 30% of patients. Marker-negative relapses limited to the thorax occur in less than 10% of relapsing patients.

A typical schedule includes visits every month for year 1, every 2 months for year 2, every 3 months for year 3, every 6 months for year 4, and annually thereafter. A history and physical as well as blood tests of AFP, HCG, and LDH should be performed at each visit. Some advocate obtaining a chest radiograph at every visit or every other visit, but chest imaging leads to earlier detection of relapse in only 0% to 2.6% of men undergoing surveillance. CT scans of the abdomen or abdomen and pelvis are typically obtained every 3 months during year 1, every 4 months during years 2 and 3, every 6 months during year 4, and annually thereafter. The Medical Research Council reported a multicenter surveillance trial in which different centers used different schedules, finding no difference in disease burden at relapse among men undergoing CT scans annually compared to those undergoing scans three to five times per year.[81,186] No consensus exists regarding how long surveillance should be continued beyond year 5, and some have advocated indefinite annual surveillance, whereas the National Cooperative Cancer Network has recommended that surveillance continue for a minimum of 7 years.[187]

Primary Chemotherapy

After cisplatin-based chemotherapy was shown to be highly effective against disseminated disease, a number of European cancer centers studied an abbreviated course of chemotherapy following orchiectomy as treatment for men with clinical stage I disease and normal serum tumor markers. This approach has resulted in the lowest relapse rate of any approach to stage I disease and is associated with similar near-perfect long-term survival rates as those seen with RPLND and surveillance. However, limited long-term follow-up data are available, and thus it is impossible to currently assess the risks of long-term chemotherapy toxicity and of late relapses resulting from undertreatment of occult disseminated disease.

At least nine studies of primary chemotherapy have been published, with most patients receiving two cycles of cisplatin and bleomycin plus either vinblastine (PVB) or etoposide (BEP)[188–195] (see Table 49.5). With almost 600 cases reported, the relapse rate is 2.8% with a disease-specific survival rate of 98.8%. In studies with at least 4 years of follow-up, 265 cases have been reported, and the relapse rate is 2.6% whereas the survival rate is 98.9%. These figures are all the more impressive in that most studies of primary chemotherapy have restricted enrollment to stage I patients at high risk of relapse.

Toxicity from two cycles of BEP is less than that seen with three to four cycles but is not negligible. Acute bleomycin pulmonary toxicity has not been reported. No treatment-related deaths have been reported, except for one patient who died of a thromboembolic stroke during chemotherapy. The Medical Research Council study has conducted the most detailed evaluation of toxicity from primary chemotherapy. They reported that pre- and postchemotherapy testing revealed that 15 of 16 tested patients suffered a decline in pulmonary diffusion capacity (average decline was 15%) and that 4 of 32 tested patients (12%) showed high-pitch hearing loss, but the clinical relevance of these changes was unclear.[188] They found no evidence of a negative impact on sperm count or motility.

Conclusion

As all three treatment options of RPLND, surveillance, and chemotherapy offer similar, near-perfect long-term survival, decisions about treatment are often based on provider bias, on patient preference, and on side effects and convenience. In parts of the world where regular surveillance is not feasible, chemotherapy may seem the best option as it is associated with the lowest relapse rate. The optimal strategy would be to surveil those patients who are not destined to relapse while treating patients with lymph-node-only metastases with RPLND and those with occult distant metastases with chemotherapy. However, our ability to identify these subgroups prospectively remains crude. Risk-adapted treatment strategies in which low-risk patients are assigned to surveillance have reported relapse rates of 12% to 27%.[184,192,194] And, although most patients with LVI and tumors consisting mostly of EC have been shown to have occult metastases in retrospective series, this risk stratification approach has yet to be prospectively validated. An additional consideration concerns the presence of teratoma in the orchiectomy specimen. Patients with teratoma in the primary tumor are more likely to have teratoma in their retroperitoneal lymph nodes.[196] Because teratoma generally does not respond to chemotherapy, some have argued that these patients should be treated with RPLND rather than chemotherapy. By the same token, the finding that pathologic stage I patients with lymphovascular invasion and a predominance of EC have a 29% chance of relapsing following RPLND has led some to advocate chemotherapy for this high-risk population.[197] Given the near-perfect long-term survival seen with any of the three approaches, it is reasonable to present patients with all three options (see Table 49.5).

Treatment of Stage II Disease

Stage II Seminoma

Treatment of stage II seminomas is less controversial than treatment of stage I disease. The current standard of care is to administer external-beam radiation therapy for nonbulky disease while treating bulky stage II disease with the same chemotherapy used for disseminated disease. Bulky disease has been defined inconsistently among studies but typically refers to tumors greater than 5 cm in transverse dimension. The rationale for this treatment strategy is that radiation is generally considered to have less acute toxicity than cisplatin-based chemotherapy and thus is preferable for early-stage disease, but postradiation relapse rates are substantially higher for bulky disease. However, there are no randomized trials comparing radiation to chemotherapy to definitively address this issue and how the acute toxicity of chemotherapy (e.g., febrile neutropenia and bleomycin lung injury) and the late risk of secondary cancers from radiation balance out with regard to long-term survival is unknown. Patients with stage IIA or IIB seminomas who have contraindications for radiation therapy should receive chemotherapy for advanced-stage disease. These patients include those with either a horseshoe or pelvic kidney or patients with disease sufficiently lateral in location to necessitate significant radiation exposure by one of the kidneys or the liver.[198]

Smalley and Van Veldhuizen reviewed the radiation experience with stage II seminomas and reported that, among 340 men treated for nonbulky disease, 30 (9%) relapsed and 322 (95%) survived their disease.[199] In contrast, among 356 men treated for bulky stage II disease, 124 (35%) relapsed. The Princess Margaret Hospital has recently reported similar results, with 5-year disease-free survival rates of 92% for stage IIA and 90% for stage IIB disease following radiation.[200] However, 9 of 16 (56%) stage IIC patients treated with radiation subsequently relapsed compared to only 1 of 23 (4.3%) IIC patients treated with chemotherapy ($P = 0.0004$).

Modern radiation therapy for stage II disease uses a dog-leg field as described for stage I seminoma. Historically, an inverted-Y field was often used such that the pelvis was treated bilaterally, but contralateral pelvic relapses are uncommon, and this is no longer considered necessary. Similarly, as discussed for stage I disease, supradiaphragmatic radiation has been abandoned by most centers. The radiation dose is similar to that used for stage I disease (25 Gy), with the enlarged lymph nodes receiving a boost to a total dose of 35 Gy. Chemotherapy for bulky disease is identical to treatment of favorable-risk disseminated disease: three cycles of bleomycin, etoposide, and cisplatin (BEP) or four cycles of etoposide and cisplatin (EP).[66,67,201] Five-year overall and disease-free survival in stage IIC patients following chemotherapy are 85% and 78%, respectively.[67]

Stage II Nonseminomas

Stage II nonseminomas with persistently elevated serum tumor markers are managed with chemotherapy for disseminated disease. If the markers normalize following orchiectomy, the option of performing a retroperitoneal lymph node dissection also exists. Five-year survival is 95% to 98% with either approach in the setting of normal markers.[202–204] There is no consensus regarding how best to chose between the two approaches. No randomized trials have compared chemotherapy to RPLND in this setting. One goal is to limit the toxicity of treatment by trying to avoid having to use both modalities. However, if both modalities are to be used, it appears to be safer to perform surgery first, because prechemotherapy RPLND is associated with fewer complications than postchemotherapy RPLND and because only two cycles of chemotherapy are given in the adjuvant, post-RPLND setting compared to three to four cycles given as primary therapy.[167,205,206] An additional concern, however, is that delaying chemotherapy to perform RPLND presents an opportunity for any occult distant metastatic disease to progress. A common practice is to perform RPLND for stage IIA patients and to give chemotherapy to patients with IIB or IIC disease based on the finding that post-RPLND relapse rates rise as disease bulk rises.[176,204]

The following issues must be taken into account when deciding between RPLND and chemotherapy. About 12% to 24% of clinical stage II patients are found to have no nodal involvement at RPLND, and surgery spares them unneeded chemotherapy.[203,205] In contrast, men who are found to have pathologic stage IIB or higher disease at RPLND are generally advised to subsequently undergo two cycles of chemotherapy because their risk of relapse is about 50%.[176] Treating such men with chemotherapy instead of RPLND is usually curative in itself, but about one-third will have less than a complete radiologic response and will require postchemotherapy RPLND for resection of residual masses.[205] The risk of having a residual mass following chemotherapy is higher in men with teratoma in the primary tumor, and thus some have advocated primary RPLND for men with such histology.[207] In contrast, embryonal carcinomas, particularly if lymphovascular invasion is seen in the primary tumor, are likely to spread hematogenously and have a high relapse rate following RPLND.[153] Moreover, it has been reported that embryonal carcinomas are more likely to respond completely to chemotherapy than other histologies.[204,208] RPLND for stage II disease typically involves a bilateral dissection rather than the unilateral templates used in stage I. As a result, ejaculatory dysfunction occurs more often in this setting along with other surgical complications, but nerve-sparing surgery, where feasible, can reduce this risk.[205]

Adjuvant Chemotherapy for Pathologic Stage II Disease

When RPLND reveals pathologic stage II disease, adjuvant chemotherapy should be considered. Among patients with five or fewer nodes involved and none larger than 2 cm, the relapse rate of 6% to 15% is similar to the 6% to 10% rate seen among those with no involved nodes.[166,175,209] However, relapse rates are about 50% for bulkier lymph node involvement.[176] Therefore, it has become standard practice to give two cycles of bleomycin, etoposide, and cisplatin (BEP) for patients with pathologic stage IIB or IIC disease. An alternative regimen is to give two cycles of etoposide and cisplatin. A randomized intergroup study, however, demonstrated that although BEP dramatically lowered the relapse rate, survival was not compromised by surveilling stage II patients after RPLND.[176] After undergoing RPLND, 195 men were randomized to surveillance or two cycles of BEP. Of the 98 who were surveilled, 49 relapsed but almost all were salvaged, with only 3 dying of testicular cancer. In the BEP arm, 6 relapsed (6%) and 1 man died of testis cancer, but of the 6 relapses, only 1 had in fact received adjuvant chemotherapy. Subsequently, a study of 82 men who received two cycles of BEP for pathologic stage (PS) II disease reported a single relapse,[210] while a separate report of two cycles of EP reported a similar 1.1% relapse rate.[211]

Treatment of Disseminated Disease

The development of effective systemic therapy for disseminated germ cell cancers represents one of the greatest success stories of cancer research, and the key step was the implementation of cisplatin in the 1970s. A major breakthrough was the 1977 study by Einhorn and Donohue in which they reported that 35 of 50 men (70%) achieved a complete remission to cisplatin, vinblastine, and bleomycin (PVB), while disease-free survival was 64%.[212] This report was followed 10 years later by an intergroup study showing that, compared to PVB, the combination of bleomycin (30 units on days 2, 9, and 15), etoposide (100 mg/m^2, days 1–5), and cisplatin (20 mg/m^2, days 1–5) (BEP) resulted in lower toxicity and similar efficacy, with 80% 2-year survival. Retrospective subgroup analysis revealed that patients with bulky disease had better outcomes with BEP with regard to complete responses (77% versus 61%; P less than 0.05) and survival ($P = 0.048$). The toxic death rate in the study was 4.7%, half of which was due to neutropenic sepsis. Five men (2.0%) died of bleomycin-induced pulmonary fibrosis. Four cycles of BEP was thus established as the new standard of care.

It had become clear that different prognostic groups of patients could be identified who had different probabilities of being cured. After four cycles of BEP was established as the standard treatment, most subsequent trials focused either on good-prognosis or poor-prognosis patients, with an aim toward reducing the toxicity of treatment for the former while increasing the efficacy of treatment for the latter. A variety of prognostic systems were developed at different centers, most of which were focused on the location and bulk of metastatic disease, but it subsequently became clear that the serum tumor marker levels also carried important prognostic implications. In 1997, collaborative groups from 10 countries pooled their data on 5,862 patients with disseminated GCTs and developed the International Germ Cell Consensus Classification system, which categorizes patients as good risk, intermediate risk, or poor risk (see Table 49.3).[40] This multivariate analysis reported that disease bulk was not important. Rather, in seminomas the only poor prognostic factor was nonpulmonary visceral metastases, whereas in NSGCTs, risk factors included highly elevated serum tumor markers, nonpulmonary visceral metastases, and a mediastinal primary tumor.

Special Considerations Regarding Chemotherapy

Chemotherapy for disseminated testicular GCTs represents an unusually high-stakes situation for the oncologist: the disease is almost uniformly fatal without chemotherapy, but chemotherapy can cure a large majority of patients. There are few such moments in oncology where chemotherapy can grant many decades of life. Unnecessary treatment failures resulting from substandard treatment can have tragic consequences. Testicular cancer is a rare disease, and most oncologists see no more than a few cases annually. Those without substantial experience treating testicular cancer should consider consulting a cancer center with appropriate expertise because specialist centers produce superior outcomes.[1,213]

The major chemotherapy issues are not simply which regimen to use and how many cycles to give but also how to monitor for toxicity and under what circumstances to delay treatment, reduce doses, or change the treatment plan. Regarding dose adjustments, the practice in most modern first-line chemotherapy trials has been to treat at full dose, on schedule regardless of day 1 cell counts. Patients who are neutropenic on day 1 should have blood counts checked every 1 to 2 days and etoposide should be held on day 5 if counts have not recovered. If the prior cycle was complicated by febrile neutropenia or thrombocytopenic bleeding, then etoposide and ifosfamide doses are reduced by 25%. Cisplatin is given on schedule at full dose unless serum creatinine rises above 3 mg/dL. In *good-risk patients*, several trials have adjusted doses or delayed treatment up to 7 days in patients with day 1 neutropenia or thrombocytopenia without any evidence of compromising results,[214,215] but there are no randomized data to indicate whether such a policy has an impact on survival.

Bleomycin should be discontinued if there is evidence of pulmonary toxicity, *but if bleomycin is discontinued, additional adjustments are required.* In patients with favorable-risk disease who were scheduled to receive three cycles of BEP, discontinuing the bleomycin can be accommodated by switching to etoposide and cisplatin (EP) and giving a fourth cycle, because four cycles of EP appears to be nearly equivalent to three cycles of BEP.[216] In intermediate- and poor-risk patients scheduled to receive four cycles of BEP, ifosfamide can be substituted for bleomycin with no loss in efficacy (if ifosfamide is substituted for bleomycin, then the daily etoposide dose is reduced to 75 mg/m^2).[217,218] Monitoring for bleomycin pulmonary toxicity involves a careful history and physical examination before each bleomycin administration. Symptoms and signs of pulmonary toxicity include dyspnea, a persistent nonproductive cough, inspiratory rales, and an inspiratory lag. Pulmonary toxicity is also associated with a decline in pulmonary diffusion capacity. Some centers obtain pulmonary function tests every 3 weeks during chemotherapy, particularly in patients scheduled to receive four cycles of bleomycin, although the utility of pulmonary function tests in reducing the incidence or severity of bleomycin-induced pulmonary fibrosis has never been demonstrated. A low threshold for discontinuing bleomycin if pulmonary toxicity is suspected can be justified by the availability of ifosfamide, an equally efficacious drug, albeit one associated with greater myelosuppression.

Chemotherapy for Good-Risk Disease

Strategies for reducing the toxicity of treatment for good-risk patients have included reducing the number of cycles, eliminating bleomycin, and substituting carboplatin for cisplatin (Table 49.6). Only the first goal has been unambiguously accomplished.

Reducing the Number of Cycles

In 1989, the Southeastern Cancer Study Group reported a study of 184 good- to moderate-risk patients randomized to either three or four cycles of BEP.[219] No significant difference was seen between three and four cycles with regard to either complete response rate (98% versus 97%) or the relapse rate (5% in each arm). No bleomycin deaths were reported. Long-term follow-up of the 188 patients who had been treated at Indiana University reported that 7 patients (6%) had died of either germ cell cancer or treatment-related toxicities, with 4 deaths in the three-cycle arm and 3 deaths in the four-cycle arm.[220] When this trial was conducted, the importance of

TABLE 49.6. Randomized controlled trials for good-risk disseminated germ cell tumors.

Regimen	*N*	*Median follow-up (months)*	*Complete response*	*Relapses*	*Deaths*	*Conclusion*
Number of cycles:						
BEP × 3[219,220]	88	NR	98%	5	6	Equivalent
BEP × 4	96		97%	5	3	
BEP × 3[215]	406	25	73%	24	12	Equivalent
BEP × 3 + EP × 1	406		75%	23	12	
BEP × 3[214]	83	33		6	3	Standard BEP superior to modified BEP
$B_{30}E_{360}P$ × 4	83			12	13	
Is bleomycin necessary?						
VAB-6 × 3[311]	82		96%	7		Equivalent
EP × 4	82		93%	7		
BEP × 3[222]	86	49.2	92%	8	4	BEP superior
EP × 3	85		79%	17	14	
$BE_{360}P$ × 4[223]	200	87.6	95%	8	7	Modified BEP superior to modified EP
$E_{360}P$ × 4	195		87%	8	12	
BEP × 3[216]	131	51	81%	9	5	Trend favoring BEP (p = 0.07)
EP × 4	127		69%	17	10	
Can carboplatin replace cisplatin?						
BEP × 3[226]	29	33	81%	4	1	BEP superior
$CE_{360}B$ × 4	25		76%	8	4	
EP × 4[312]	134	22.4	90%	4	NR	EP superior
EC × 4	131		88%	16	NR	
BEP[225]	268	36	94%	15	10	BEP superior
CEB	260		87%	46	27	

NR, no response; BEP, bleomycin, etoposide, cisplatin; EP, etoposide and cisplatin; CEB, carboplatin, etoposide, and bleomycin; EC, etoposide and carboplatin B_{30}, reduced bleomycin dose of 30 units per cycle; E_{360}, reduced etoposide dose of 360 mg/m^2 per cycle.

serum tumor marker levels was not appreciated, and men with highly elevated HCG levels were included. Among men with HCG levels below 1,000 IU/L, 98% were alive with no evidence of disease with a median follow-up of 10 years, whereas 5 of 14 (36%) with HCG levels above 1,000 IU/L died disease-related deaths. Such patients are now considered intermediate risk and should receive four cycles of BEP or VIP. A larger European study randomized 812 men to either three cycles of BEP or three cycles of BEP followed by a fourth cycle of etoposide and cisplatin (EP).[215] With 2 years follow-up, 2-year progression-free survival was 90% and 89%, respectively, and a 5% difference could be excluded. These two trials established three cycles of BEP as a standard treatment option for men with good-risk disseminated germ cell cancers.

Attempting to Eliminate Bleomycin

Bleomycin is associated with potentially fatal pulmonary fibrosis as well as a more-common occurrence of Raynaud's phenomenon and mucositis. People who have received bleomycin also have an elevated incidence of sometimes fatal postoperative pulmonary complications. Fortunately, dropping the fourth cycle of BEP in good-risk patients has almost eliminated fatal pulmonary complications. Six trials administering three cycles of BEP to 1,142 patients reported 2 (0.18%) fatalities.[111,214,215,219,221,222] However, nonfatal pulmonary complications have been reported in 12% to 17% in studies that have reported detailed toxicity data.[214,215] Numerous randomized controlled trials have studied whether eliminating bleomycin compromises efficacy. Based on the existent evidence, a number of centers have adopted four cycles of EP as an alternative to three cycles of BEP, and the two regimens are considered equivalent by many in the field. However, the equivalence of these regimens has never been established by comparative trials, and BEP is better supported by the available data.[216]

Prospective randomized trials have demonstrated that three cycles of BEP produced superior overall survival than three cycles of EP (95% versus 86%; $P = 0.01$),[222] that three cycles of BEP produce a higher complete response rate than four cycles of EP (95% versus 87%; $P = 0.0075$) when using the lower European etoposide dose (360 mg/m^2/cycle instead of 500 mg/m^2/cycle),[223] and that PBV results in superior disease control compared to a cisplatin and vinblastine doublet.[224] A randomized trial comparing four cycles of EP to three cycles of a historical regimen referred to as VAB-6 showed no difference in efficacy, but VAB-6 has never been compared to BEP, so the relevance of this trial to current practice is ambiguous. After retrospective data suggested that three cycles of BEP may produce disease control superior to that of four cycles of EP,[221] a randomized trial was completed that assigned 131 men to the BEP × 3 arm and 127 to the EP × 4 arm.[216] With a median follow-up of 51 months, the 4-year event-free survival with BEP was 89% compared to 84% with EP ($P = 0.09$). When the 6 men with nonpulmonary visceral metastases (poor-risk patients) were excluded from the analysis, this difference became significant (91% versus 84%; $P = 0.037$). Overall survival showed a nonsignificant trend in favor of BEP (96% versus 92%; $P = 0.1$). Grade 3 to 4 neutropenia was more common with EP (90%) than BEP (73%), but cutaneous toxicity and neurotoxicity were more common with BEP. This trial was unable to exclude clinically relevant inferiority concerning disease control with EP. However, because the intent-to-treat analysis did not show a statistically significant difference between the two regimens, four cycles of EP is still accepted by many as a standard treatment option for good-risk disseminated NSGCTs.

Carboplatin

Cisplatin is associated with much higher rates of renal, neurologic, gastrointestinal, and vascular toxicity than is carboplatin. In addition, large volumes of intravenous fluid are given with cisplatin to avoid renal toxicity by maintaining a brisk urine output, and the infusion of fluids substantially increases the time necessary to administer treatment. Multiple attempts have been made to substitute carboplatin for cisplatin in favorable-risk disease, and these randomized controlled trials have clearly established that cisplatin is more effective and is associated with higher survival rates (see Table 49.6).[225–227] Nonetheless, carboplatin is a highly active agent and, in patients with renal failure or extremely severe cisplatin neurotoxicity, the question of substituting carboplatin for cisplatin arises; treatment decisions in such extraordinary cases must weigh the risks and benefits associated with the available regimens.

Conclusion

Standard chemotherapy for good-risk disseminated testicular GCTs is three cycles of BEP or four cycles of EP, but there is evidence that the BEP regimen may be more effective.

Intermediate- and Poor-Risk Disease

Despite two decades of trials, *four cycles of BEP remains the standard of care for intermediate- and poor-risk disease*, and this regimen is associated with overall survival rates of about 80% and 60%, respectively, for these two risk groups.[112,217] The search for a more-effective regimen continues but has thus far been unsuccessful. A randomized Eastern Cooperative Oncology Group trial compared BEP to etoposide, ifosfamide, and cisplatin (VIP) and reported no significant differences in complete response (31% versus 37%; $P = 0.26$), failure-free survival (60% versus 64%; $P = 0.29$), or overall survival (71% versus 74%; $P = 0.78$).[217,218] Although the trends in this trial favored VIP, a multicenter European trial also reported no difference between the two regimens, with the trend favoring BEP.[215] Both studies reported greater leukopenia and thrombocytopenia in the VIP arm. BEP was therefore concluded to be the preferred regimen, except in patients with compromised pulmonary status at baseline, for whom VIP represents a good alternative.

Efforts to improve results through increased dose density or dose intensity have similarly failed. Rapid cycling of three courses of bleomycin, vincristine, and cisplatin followed by three cycles of VIP proved no better than BEP in a randomized trial.[228] Similarly, a randomized multicenter U.S. trial comparing standard BEP to BEP using double-dose cisplatin (200 mg/m² per cycle) reported the same 74% survival and almost identical disease-free survival in the two arms.[229] Although numerous other regimens have been studied, using up to seven different chemotherapeutic agents and many using alternating cycles of different regimens, none has been shown to produce superior results to BEP.[230–234]

High-Dose Chemotherapy as First-Line Treatment

The use of high-dose chemotherapy with stem cell support has been investigated in Europe and the United States, with promising phase II trial results but no informative phase III studies yet available. The largest series using this approach come from the German Testicular Cancer Study Group and Memorial Sloan-Kettering Cancer Center. A recent update of the German experience with dose escalation describes 182 patients with poor-prognosis disseminated germ cell cancers.[235] Treatment consisted of one cycle of standard-dose VIP with subsequent stem cell collection of stem cells, followed by three to four cycles of high-dose VIP. With a median follow-up of 4 years, progression-free and disease-specific survival were 69% and 79%, respectively, at 2 years and 68% and 73% at 5 years. Severe toxicity included toxic deaths (4%), leukemia (1%), chronic renal insufficiency (3%), chronic renal failure (1%), and persistent neuropathy (5%). This regimen is being compared to four cycles of standard BEP in a randomized phase III trial by the EORTC. In the United States, a multicenter phase III trial comparing four cycles of BEP to two cycles of BEP followed by two cycles of high-dose CEC (carboplatin, etoposide, and cyclophosphamide) completed accrual in 2003, and results are expected to be presented soon.

Management of Residual Masses

Pure Seminomas

Men with stage II or III seminomas commonly have residual radiographic lesions following radiation or chemotherapy. Roughly 60% of men have residual masses after chemotherapy.[66,236] Unlike nonseminomas, where surgical resection of any residual masses represents an important part of standard care, resecting residual seminomas following radiation or chemotherapy is often technically difficult or impossible and is associated with a higher rate of major surgical complications than RPLND in nonseminomas. Indiana University reported that 37 of 97 men (38%) undergoing postchemotherapy RPLND for residual tumors that contained seminomatous elements (including 88 with pure seminoma primary tumors) required a total of 47 additional intraoperative procedures, including 25 nephrectomies, 9 inferior vena cava resections, 5 arterial grafts, 5 bowel resections, and 3 hepatic resections or biopsies.[237] In contrast, additional procedures were required in only 340 of 1,269 men (26.8%) without seminomatous elements ($P = 0.02$). Relative to nonseminomas and mixed GCTs, residual viable neoplastic disease is less likely to be present when the primary tumor was a pure seminoma. For these reasons, surgery is used more selectively in seminomas,[238] but it must be remembered that resection of residual disease is curative for most patients and remains an important treatment modality for patients at high risk of having residual neoplasm.[238–240] Moreover, only 7% to 14% of poorly defined, difficult-to-resect masses harbor cancer, compared to 46% to 55% of well-defined, more easily resected masses.[239,241] In one series of 55 men with residual masses following treatment of pure seminomas, a complete resection was possible in 78% of those whose masses were well defined on CT scan compared to only 44% of those whose masses were not well defined.[239] Extensive biopsies were taken when resection was impossible. Residual seminoma or teratoma was found in 8 of 27 (30%) men with masses at least 3cm in diameter compared to 0 of 28 with masses less than 3cm. Three series with a total of 202 men with residual masses reported that 22 of 74 (30%) with masses that were 3cm or larger had viable cancer, compared to 5 of 128 (4%) with smaller masses.[238,241,242]

Treating residual postchemotherapy masses with radiation therapy has fallen out of favor based on several retrospective analyses showing that routinely irradiating residual masses had a low radiographic response rate[243] and had no appreciable effect on subsequent relapse rates.[236] Although there is no clear consensus on the management of these patients, low-risk patients (masses smaller than 3cm) are generally surveilled whereas high-risk patients (masses 3cm or greater) undergo surgical exploration with either resection of residual masses or, where resection is impossible, extensive biopsies. Patients who have unresectable pathologically confirmed residual seminoma should undergo salvage chemotherapy.

The seminoma patient with residual masses represents one of the only settings in testicular cancer care where PET scans show some promise. A multiinstitutional series of 56 scans of 51 patients reported a sensitivity of 80% and specificity of 100%.[238] Among 37 scans of men with lesions less than 3cm, increased uptake was present in 1 of the 3 men who were subsequently found to have residual cancer. In contrast, PET was 100% accurate with lesions larger than 3cm, correctly identifying the 7 with residual disease and the 12 without. An earlier study was less promising, however, and the utility of PET scans needs to be confirmed.[244]

Nonseminomatous Germ Cell Tumors

Residual masses are detected in an estimated 20% to 25% of men following chemotherapy for metastatic NSGCTs.[245] *The current standard of care is to resect any residual masses if the serum tumor markers have normalized and if technically feasible.* As discussed next, some centers have advocated retroperitoneal exploration and lymphadenectomy in all patients with prechemotherapy retroperitoneal adenopathy or masses, regardless of the findings on postchemotherapy radiologic imaging, but this practice is not widespread.[245] Resections of postchemotherapy masses in GCT patients are generally complex and, given the rarity of the disease, extensive experience is limited to a small fraction of practicing surgeons. Referral to a center of excellence is strongly encouraged.

The rationale for resection of residual masses derives from the finding that roughly 35% to 45% of residual masses contain teratoma, 10% to 20% contain residual seminoma, yolk-sac tumor, choriocarcinoma, and/or embryonal carcinoma, while the remaining 45% to 50% contain only necrotic tissue and fibrosis.[246–248] Following salvage (as opposed to primary) chemotherapy, up to 50% of patients have viable nonteratomatous germ cell cancer.[249] Interpreting these figures is not entirely straightforward, because the observed relapse rates in men who do not undergo postchemotherapy RPLND are lower than these numbers would predict.[250] Although it thus appears that some residual teratomas are not destined to progress, this issue is poorly characterized and poorly understood.

Surgically removing residual teratoma is generally curative in itself, and men who have only teratoma or necrosis/fibrosis discovered at surgery share an excellent prognosis, with a roughly 90% 2-year progression-free survival.[251] Men with residual cancer, however, have a poorer prognosis and are generally advised to undergo additional chemotherapy following surgery.[249] Resection of residual masses is thus both therapeutic and diagnostic. However, half of these masses are purely necrotic/fibrotic, and resection of fibrosis and necrosis is unlikely to confer any benefit upon the patient. Numerous attempts have thus been made to develop a model that would predict the histology of residual masses with the goal of reducing unnecessary operations.[245–247,252,253] Indiana University reported that, based on an analysis of 295 men with disseminated NSGCTs who had undergone primary chemotherapy, 92% of men who achieved a radiologic and serologic complete remission were continuously disease free with a median follow-up of 5 years.[253] However, no other group could be identified with less than a 25% risk of relapse without undergoing postchemotherapy RPLND.

A more-sophisticated model has been developed by Steyerberg and colleagues, taking into account the following variables that were associated with the absence of viable teratoma or cancer in residual masses: absence of teratoma elements in the primary tumor, normal prechemotherapy HCG, normal prechemotherapy AFP, elevated prechemotherapy LDH, smaller postchemotherapy residual disease bulk, and a large percent decline in disease bulk during chemotherapy.[247] The model was developed using a pooled international data set of 544 patients and later validated on 172 subsequent patients. In the validation study, no tumor was found at RPLND in the 15 patients predicted to have less than a 10% chance of having residual cancer or teratoma. However, in a second validation study limited to 105 good-risk patients, only 4 patients were predicted to have less than a 30% chance of having residual viable tumor. Three of these 4 (75%) had benign histology found at RPLND. The prediction rule was accurate but affected the management of only 4% of the patients. More-recent attempts to develop a clinically useful model have similarly failed.[254] Further complicating decision making, the Norwegian Radium Hospital has reported an analysis of 87 patients with disseminated NSGCTs undergoing RPLND for postchemotherapy masses smaller than 20mm. Of the 87 total patients, 29 (33%) had residual tumor, including 23 (26%) with residual teratoma and 6 (7%) with residual cancer. Of the 54 with masses no larger than 10mm, 5 (9%) had residual cancer and 11 (20%) had teratoma. Thus, 29% of patients with normal postchemotherapy CT scans had residual tumor. Nonetheless, chemotherapy trials have reported that fewer than 8% of patients with radiologic and serologic complete responses subsequently relapse.[208,215,253] The low relapse rate seen in men with complete responses to chemotherapy as well as the complications seen in postchemotherapy RPLNDs have led most centers to avoid RPLND unless there are residual masses greater than 10mm.[245]

Managing Residual Masses in Men with Persistently Elevated Serum Tumor Markers

Men with rising or persistently elevated serum tumor markers are at high risk for having progressive disseminated cancer and have typically been treated with salvage chemotherapy. However, no randomized trials exist to support this practice, and data clarifying the best management of these patients remain sparse. Published series have reported that resection of residual disease is curative for most men with a persistently elevated or rising serum AFP following chemotherapy, but relapse and mortality rates range from 70% to 100% when serum HCG remains elevated in most series.[255–257] It has also been reported that patients with rising markers have a poorer postoperative prognosis than those with stable elevated markers.[258] A persistently elevated AFP is thus not a contraindication to resecting residual disease, but operating in the setting of a significantly elevated HCG or rising AFP is usually futile. Any decision to operate in the setting of elevated markers should be carefully considered. As previously discussed, it is essential to exclude nonneoplastic etiologies for elevated serum tumor markers following chemotherapy.

Complications and Extent of Resection

Historically, postchemotherapy RPLND has been associated with a substantially higher complication rate than primary RPLND, but the surgical template for the postchemotherapy operation has diminished over time and the complication rate has declined.[259,260] Nonetheless, Indiana University reported that among 150 men undergoing postchemotherapy RPLND between 2000 and 2002, 29% had intraoperative complications requiring additional procedures such as nephrectomy or inferior vena cava resection and 6.7% experienced postoperative complications such as ascites, wound infections, or prolonged ileus.[260] Although no patients in this report suffered fatal complications, others have reported a perioperative mortality rate of nearly 1%.[206,261] The higher complication rate following chemotherapy derives from the greater bulk of disease, the higher frequency of invasion of or adherence to vital structures, the effect of chemotherapy on the patient's overall condition, and the increased rate of postoperative pulmonary complications seen in patients with prior bleomycin exposure. However, the rate of pulmonary complications appears to have declined with the implementation of anesthesia precautions, which include limiting the partial pressure of oxygen and the volume of intravenous fluids delivered to the patient during surgery and the perioperative period. Several recent studies have reported no fatal pulmonary complications.[206,260]

A major change in the template of postchemotherapy RPLNDs has occurred during the past two decades. Historically, an extensive bilateral dissection was performed in addition to removing any visible residual disease. More recently, favorable results have been reported following a more-limited resection in which all visible residual masses are removed and a more-limited template dissection is performed, with nerve sparing when possible, if no residual tumor is found on frozen section.[262–264] In cases where frozen section shows viable tumor, most reporting centers have performed an extensive bilateral dissection. Memorial Sloan-Kettering Cancer Center reported, in 62 patients undergoing such an approach, that 37 showed only necrosis on frozen section (and thus underwent a limited dissection), and only 1 of these 37 relapsed in the retroperitoneum. Among the total 62 patients, only 3 had teratoma or cancer outside the palpable disease and only 2 relapsed within the retroperitoneum.[265] In patients with residual masses in the lungs, liver, or other sites, standard practice has been to resect these lesions as well, either in a single operation sequentially, if all residual disease can be resected. Whether a finding of necrosis only in the retroperitoneum justifies aborting any attempt to resect other sites of residual disease remains controversial.[266,267] Most reports have advocated a resection of all residual masses because up to 23% of men with necrosis in the retroperitoneum have teratoma or cancer in the thorax. In cases in which a complete resection is impossible, a resection of those masses that are resectable is not generally recommended because the benefit of a partial resection has not been established.

Treatment of Men with Viable Cancer in Postchemotherapy Masses

Men with viable cancer discovered at postchemotherapy surgery have a poor prognosis compared to those with necrosis or teratoma.[249,268–270] Hannover University reported, among 27 patients undergoing resection of residual masses, that overall survival was 87% among those found to have necrosis or residual teratoma versus 22% among those found to have viable cancer.[271] EORTC reported that 23 of 26 (88%) men with residual teratoma were alive without evidence of disease compared to 13 of 22 (59%) of those with residual cancer.[270] Some have therefore recommended chemotherapy for these patients following surgery, and the standard practice among those giving chemotherapy has been to administer two cycles of cisplatin-based chemotherapy, typically either EP, VIP, or VeIP. An international multivariate analysis of 146 patients with viable cancer in residual masses reported a progression-free survival advantage favoring chemotherapy (69% versus 52%; P less than 0.001) but no overall survival difference when comparing those who received adjuvant chemotherapy to those who did not.[272] The three factors independently associated with overall survival were complete versus incomplete resection, less than 10% viable malignant cells, and a good-risk international germ cell consensus classification (IGCCC).

Treatment of Relapsed and Refractory Disease

Progressive disease during or following first-line chemotherapy carries a distinctly poorer prognosis than metastatic chemonaive disease. Although ifosfamide and etoposide have activity in patients with cisplatin-resistant disease, they have produced disappointing long-term survival. Subsequently, paclitaxel and gemcitabine were shown to have activity in cisplatin-resistant disease, but whether regimens incorporating these drugs can improve survival remains unproven, favorable phase II trial results notwithstanding. Great interest has developed in high-dose chemotherapy as salvage treatment, but data showing a survival advantage are lacking.

Standard-Dose Salvage Chemotherapy

The most widely used salvage chemotherapy regimens for relapsed or refractory GCTs have been cisplatin, ifosfamide, and either etoposide (VIP) or vinblastine (VeIP), and these remain the standard of care. Because most patients now receive etoposide as part of their first-line chemotherapy, VeIP, which offers two new agents to men who have previously been treated with either EP or BEP, is the most commonly used salvage regimen. In patients with relapsed NSGCTs, VIP and VeIP have resulted in long-term survival of 20% to 30%.[273–277] Men with relapsing seminoma fare better, with VeIP and other ifosfamide-cisplatin-based regimens producing long-term survival of 53% to 54%.[65,278] These results led to the investigation of alternative regimens and the use of high-dose chemotherapy with stem cell rescue. Gemcitabine and paclitaxel both have activity against cisplatin-resistant GCTs, with response rates in the 11% to 30% range and reports of rare durable remissions.[279–282] Using these agents in multidrug regimens has produced more-favorable results. Motzer et al. reported 30 relapsing GCT patients with favorable prognostic features in whom paclitaxel, ifosfamide, and cisplatin (TIP) produced an overall and progression-free survival of 80% and 73%, respectively, at a median follow-up of 33 months.[283] Because this study involved a favorable subset of relapsed patients, comparing the results to other regimens is problematic, but a multicenter U.S. randomized phase III trial comparing TIP to VeIP is under way. The combination of gemcitabine and paclitaxel has been investigated in relapsing patients with adverse prognostic features.[284] Six of 28 (21.4%) responded, including 3 complete responses and 2 durable responses at 15 and 25 months. Oxaliplatin, alone or combined with gemcitabine, has also shown modest levels of activity in heavily pretreated patients.[285,286]

High-Dose Salvage Chemotherapy

High-dose chemotherapy with stem cell support for patients with relapsing or refractory GCTs has been investigated since the early 1980s as salvage therapy, but early results in heavily pretreated patients were disappointing, with more than 20% of patients suffering toxic deaths and few long-term survivors. More recently, high-dose salvage chemotherapy has been used on less heavily pretreated patients and the results, as discussed next, have been more promising. Whether high-dose salvage chemotherapy results in better long-term outcomes than standard-dose chemotherapy remains unresolved. Prognostic criteria have been identified that help predict the likelihood of a successful outcome with high-dose salvage chemotherapy. Analyzing 310 patients treated at four centers between 1984 and 1993, Beyer et al. reported that five factors were associated with treatment failure: progressive disease immediately before high-dose chemotherapy, HCG level above 1,000U/L, mediastinal primary tumor, and disease that was relatively refractory (progression within 4 weeks of treatment) or absolutely refractory (progression during treatment) to cisplatin.[287] Using a scoring system that gave each prognostic factor one point, except for mediastinal primary or absolutely refractory disease, which each were worth two points, the study identified a good-risk category (no points), an intermediate-risk category (one or two points), and a poor risk category (more than two points). Failure-free survival was 51%, 27%, and 5%, respectively. Indiana University, however, reported that among the 23 poor-risk patients transplanted using a tandem transplant strategy, failure-free survival was 30% (95% CI, 11%–49%) and the most important adverse prognostic factor was a mediastinal primary tumor (0% survival in the Indiana series compared to 12% survival in Beyer's study). In contrast, recent European studies using a single cycle of high-dose chemotherapy have reported no survivors among 18 poor-risk patients.[288–290] Whether these results indicate that poor-risk patients are poor candidates for transplant or that they require at least two cycles of high-dose chemotherapy is controversial.[291]

Different institutions have used different regimens and have targeted different prognostic groups, with the result that comparing results among different institutions is challenging. Recent studies, however, have reported that about 50% of relapsing or refractory patients can be successfully salvaged with high-dose chemotherapy when it is used at first or second relapse.[290,292–294] Although many centers have evaluated multiple cycles of high-dose chemotherapy, the benefit of this approach relative to a single cycle remains untested; the high-dose results appear favorable compared to historical results with standard-dose regimens, but the patients undergoing high-dose therapy have been more carefully selected. A European trial randomized 280 men to either four cycles of standard salvage therapy (VeIP or VIP) or three cycles of standard therapy followed by one cycle of high-dose carboplatin, etoposide, and cyclophosphamide.[295] Men who were relatively or absolutely refractory to cisplatin were excluded, but men with mediastinal primary tumors were permitted. Three-year overall survival was 53% in each arm, indicating no advantage to high-dose chemotherapy, but mature results have not been published. A retrospective matched-pair analysis has been published comparing the outcomes of men who relapsed after first-line cisplatin-based chemotherapy and received either high-dose or standard-dose salvage chemotherapy.[296] This analysis reported a statistically significant 10% 2-year survival advantage with high-dose chemotherapy, but it is subject to all the limitations of a retrospective, nonrandomized investigation.

Men who relapse following high-dose salvage chemotherapy relapse early and have a poor prognosis. Indiana University reported 101 relapsing patients, all of whom relapsed within 17 months of high-dose therapy.[297] After relapse, 47 underwent chemotherapy, either with (n = 35) or without (n = 12) surgery, and 7 underwent surgery alone. The response rate to chemotherapy was 18% and only 5 patients (5%) were disease free at the time of the report, all of whom had received surgery as part of their treatment. A French study of 32 relapsing patients reported similarly poor chemotherapy results: 6 patients were successfully salvaged, all of whom had had surgical resection of residual masses as part of their treatment.[298]

Conclusion

Currently, high-dose salvage chemotherapy represents a standard treatment option at most centers treating a large volume of germ cell cancers. Choosing between standard- and high-dose chemotherapy presents a challenge in the absence of mature randomized trials. The only setting in which high-dose chemotherapy appears to be almost completely ineffectual is relapsed mediastinal GCTs.

Extragonadal Germ Cell Tumors

Germ cell tumors in adolescent and adult men also occur in the retroperitoneum and mediastinum. Primary mediastinal GCTs almost always occur in the anterior mediastinum, which is a rare site of metastasis for testicular or retroperitoneal GCTs.[299] As part of the diagnostic workup, it is standard practice to obtain a scrotal ultrasound to exclude a testicular primary. Although retroperitoneal GCTs carry the same prognosis as testicular GCTs after correcting for stage, mediastinal NSGCTs carry a worse prognosis and are considered poor-risk GCTs unless they are composed of mature teratoma.[40,300] Mediastinal seminomas have an excellent prognosis that is no different from that of disseminated testicular seminomas. They are treated with the same systemic chemotherapy protocols as disseminated testicular seminomas and carry the same good or intermediate prognosis, depending on whether nonpulmonary visceral metastases are present. Residual masses are handled in the same fashion as in gonadal seminomas. The treatment of retroperitoneal GCTs is similar to that of testicular tumors with respect to the choice of chemotherapy and the practice of rapid diagnostic workup and treatment, including, in nonseminomatous tumors, the resection of all residual masses. Retroperitoneal seminomas are considered favorable risk unless nonpulmonary visceral metastases are present and are generally treated with chemotherapy using the same chemotherapy protocols used for disseminated testicular seminoma. Although radiation therapy may be an acceptable alternative for low-volume disease, retrospective analysis has suggested better progression-free survival with chemotherapy (87% versus 33%; $P = 0.01$).[301] Retroperitoneal NSGCTs are also staged and treated in the same fashion as testicular NSGCTs. Patients with retroperitoneal GCTs typically present either with abdominal or back pain or with symptoms of advanced disease such as weight loss, fevers, night sweats, or venous thrombosis. Most patients are found to have a significant disease burden at the time of diagnosis. Median primary tumor size is 7 cm and 8 cm for seminomas and NSGCTs, respectively. Metastases are present at diagnosis in 46% of patients with seminomas and 76% of those with NSGCTs, and most patients have elevated tumor markers.[301]

Mediastinal NSGCTs differ from testicular NSGCTs in several respects. The distinction of pure teratomas from other histologies and the distinction of mature versus immature teratoma carries a prognostic significance in mediastinal tumors that does not apply to testicular cancers. Mature teratomas of the mediastinum are benign tumors that can be cured with surgical resection alone in almost all patients. In three series reporting a total of 157 patients, the only 2 deaths were due to surgical complications.[299,302,303] Immature teratomas, in contrast, often behave more malignantly in individuals over 15 years of age (in children, teratomas of the mediastinum are benign regardless of whether there are immature elements). Dulmet et al. reported that among 6 adult patients with immature teratoma, 4 died of the disease.[302] In contrast, Hiroshima et al. found that 5 of 6 men with immature teratomas survived when treated with chemotherapy followed by complete surgical resection.[303]

Nonseminomas of the mediastinum have a poorer prognosis than other GCTs and are considered poor risk regardless of the extent of disease. The pooled analysis by Bokemeyer et al. of 287 cases from around the world reported that 49% were alive at a median follow-up of 19 months. Standard treatment is four cycles of BEP chemotherapy followed by a resection of any residual masses. An aggressive postchemotherapy surgical approach resecting all residual disease when possible is standard, partly because relapses are extremely difficult to cure. A representative study reported that among 79 patients receiving second-line chemotherapy for recurrent disease, only 9 (8%) were alive at a median follow-up of 45 months.[300] High-dose salvage chemotherapy has been similarly ineffective in this population. Indiana University reported that all 28 patients receiving high-dose salvage chemotherapy subsequently relapsed.[220] An international pooled analysis reported that failure-free survival following high-dose salvage che-motherapy was only 12%.[287] In contrast, 2-year progression-free and overall survival were 64% and 68%, respectively, following *first-line* treatment with high-dose chemotherapy, but whether first-line high-dose chemotherapy results in superior results compared with standard BEP has not been addressed in prospective trials.[304]

Mediastinal NSGCTs are associated with an increased risk of hematologic malignancies, particularly disorders of the megakaryocyte lineage. Analysis by Hartmann et al. of 287 patients treated in the United States and Europe reported 17 individuals (5.9%) with fatal hematologic malignancies.[305] The median time from diagnosis of the mediastinal tumor to the diagnosis of the hematologic neoplasm was 6 months. These tumors appear to share their origin with that of the mediastinal tumor, as they often share the isochromosome 12p seen in GCTs. They are highly resistant to treatment and are almost universally fatal, with a median survival of 5 months.

References

1. Collette L, Sylvester RJ, Stenning SP, et al. Impact of the treating institution on survival of patients with "poor-prognosis" metastatic nonseminoma. European Organization for Research and Treatment of Cancer Genito-Urinary Tract Cancer Collaborative Group and the Medical Research Council Testicular Cancer Working Party. J Natl Cancer Inst 1999;91(10):839–846.
2. Ries LAG, Eisner MP, Kosary CL, et al. SEER Cancer Statistics Review, 1975–2000. Bethesda: National Cancer Institute, 2003.
3. Parkin DM, Bray FI, Devesa SS. Cancer burden in the year 2000. The global picture. Eur J Cancer 2001;37(suppl 8):S4–S66.
4. Brown LM. Testis. In: Harras A (ed) Cancer: Rates and Risks. Bethesda: National Cancer Institute, 1996:194–196.
5. Bernstein L, Smith MA, Liu L, et al. Germ cell, trophoblastic and other gonadal neoplasms. In: Ries LAG, et al. (eds). Cancer Incidence and Survival among Children and Adolescents: United States SEER Program 1975–1995 (NIH Pub. No. 99-4649). Bethesda, MD: National Cancer Institute, 1999.
6. Huyghe E, Matsuda T, Thonneau P. Increasing incidence of testicular cancer worldwide: a review. J Urol 2003;170(1): 5–11.

7. Ries LAG, Eisner MP, Kosary CL, et al. In: Ries LAG, et al. (eds). SEER Cancer Statistics Review, 1973–1998. Bethesda, MD: National Cancer Institute. 2001.
8. Moller H, Skakkebaek NE. Risk of testicular cancer in subfertile men: case-control study. BMJ 1999;318(7183):559–562.
9. Jacobsen R, Bostofte E, Engholm G, et al. Risk of testicular cancer in men with abnormal semen characteristics: cohort study. BMJ 2000;321(7264):789–792.
10. Jacobsen R, Bostofte E, Engholm G, et al. Fertility and offspring sex ratio of men who develop testicular cancer: a record linkage study. Hum Reprod 2000;15(9):1958–1961.
11. Herrinton LJ, Zhao W, Husson G. Management of cryptorchism and risk of testicular cancer. Am J Epidemiol 2003;157(7): 602–605.
12. Castejon Casado J, Jimenez Alvarez C, Alaminos Mingorance M, et al. [Cancer: cryptorchism meta-analysis.] Cir Pediatr 2000;13(3):92–96.
13. Moller H, Prener A, Skakkebaek NE. Testicular cancer, cryptorchidism, inguinal hernia, testicular atrophy, and genital malformations: case-control studies in Denmark. Cancer Causes Control 1996;7(2):264–274.
14. Aetiology of testicular cancer: association with congenital abnormalities, age at puberty, infertility, and exercise. United Kingdom Testicular Cancer Study Group. Bmj 1994;308(6941): 1393–1399.
15. Forman D, Oliver RT, Brett AR, et al. Familial testicular cancer: a report of the UK family register, estimation of risk and an HLA class 1 sib-pair analysis. Br J Cancer 1992;65(2):255–262.
16. Dong C, Lonnstedt I, Hemminki K. Familial testicular cancer and second primary cancers in testicular cancer patients by histological type. Eur J Cancer 2001;37(15):1878–1885.
17. Sonneveld DJ, Sleijfer DT, Schrafford Koops H, et al. Familial testicular cancer in a single-centre population. Eur J Cancer 1999;35(9):1368–1373.
18. Heimdal K, Olsson H, Tretli S, et al. Familial testicular cancer in Norway and southern Sweden. Br J Cancer 1996;73(7): 964–969.
19. Westergaard T, Olsen JH, Frisch M, et al. Cancer risk in fathers and brothers of testicular cancer patients in Denmark. A population-based study. Int J Cancer 1996;66(5):627–631.
20. Pamenter B, De Bono JS, Brown IL, et al. Bilateral testicular cancer: a preventable problem? Experience from a large cancer centre. BJU Int 2003;92(1):43–46.
21. Geczi L, Gomez F, Bak M, et al. The incidence, prognosis, clinical and histological characteristics, treatment, and outcome of patients with bilateral germ cell testicular cancer in Hungary. J Cancer Res Clin Oncol 2003;129(5):309–315.
22. Holzbeierlein JM, Sogani PC, Sheinfeld J. Histology and clinical outcomes in patients with bilateral testicular germ cell tumors: the Memorial Sloan Kettering Cancer Center experience 1950 to 2001. J Urol 2003;169(6):2122–2125.
23. Ondrus D, Hornak M, Mat'oska J. Bilateral testicular germ-cell tumors—a single centre long-term experience. Int Urol Nephrol 2001;33(3):521–524.
24. Wanderas EH, Fossa SD, Tretli S. Risk of a second germ cell cancer after treatment of a primary germ cell cancer in 2201 Norwegian male patients. Eur J Cancer 1997;33(2):244–252.
25. Skakkebaek NE, Holm M, Hoei-Hansen C, et al. Association between testicular dysgenesis syndrome (TDS) and testicular neoplasia: evidence from 20 adult patients with signs of maldevelopment of the testis. APMIS 2003;111(1):1–9; discussion 9–11.
26. Oosterhuis JW, Looijenga LH. Current views on the pathogenesis of testicular germ cell tumours and perspectives for future research: highlights of the 5th Copenhagen Workshop on Carcinoma in situ and Cancer of the Testis. APMIS 2003;111(1): 280–289.
27. Oliver RT. Germ cell cancer. Curr Opin Oncol 1999;11(3): 236–241.
28. Wanderas EH, Grotmol T, Fossa SD, et al. Maternal health and pre- and perinatal characteristics in the etiology of testicular cancer: a prospective population- and register-based study on Norwegian males born between 1967 and 1995. Cancer Causes Control 1998;9(5):475–486.
29. Moller H, Skakkebaek NE. Testicular cancer and cryptorchidism in relation to prenatal factors: case-control studies in Denmark. Cancer Causes Control 1997;8(6):904–912.
30. Swerdlow AJ, De Stavola BL, Swanwick MA, et al. Risks of breast and testicular cancers in young adult twins in England and Wales: evidence on prenatal and genetic aetiology. Lancet 1997;350(9093):1723–1728.
31. Suijkerbuijk RF, Sinke RJ, Meloni AM, et al. Overrepresentation of chromosome 12p sequences and karyotypic evolution in i(12p)-negative testicular germ-cell tumors revealed by fluorescence in situ hybridization. Cancer Genet Cytogenet 1993;70(2):85–93.
32. Atkin NB, Fox MF, Baker MC, et al. Chromosome 12-containing markers, including two dicentrics, in three i(12p)-negative testicular germ cell tumors. Genes Chromosomes Cancer 1993;6(4):218–221.
33. Heidenreich A, Schenkman NS, Sesterhenn IA, et al. Immuno histochemical and mutational analysis of the p53 tumour suppressor gene and the bcl-2 oncogene in primary testicular germ cell tumours. APMIS 1998;106(1):90–99; discussion 99–100.
34. Burger H, Nooter K, Boersma AW, et al. Distinct p53-independent apoptotic cell death signalling pathways in testicular germ cell tumour cell lines. Int J Cancer 1999;81(4):620–628.
35. Burger H, Nooter K, Boersma AW, et al. Lack of correlation between cisplatin-induced apoptosis, p53 status and expression of Bcl-2 family proteins in testicular germ cell tumour cell lines. Int J Cancer 1997;73(4):592–599.
36. Mayer F, Honecker F, Looijenga LH, et al. Towards an understanding of the biological basis of response to cisplatin-based chemotherapy in germ-cell tumors. Ann Oncol 2003;14(6):825–832.
37. Mayer F, Stoop H, Scheffer GL, et al. Molecular determinants of treatment response in human germ cell tumors. Clin Cancer Res 2003;9(2):767–773.
38. Zurita AJ, Diestra JE, Condom E, et al. Lung resistance-related protein as a predictor of clinical outcome in advanced testicular germ-cell tumours. Br J Cancer 2003;88(6):879–886.
39. Currow DC, Findlay M, Cox K, et al. Elevated germ cell markers in carcinoma of uncertain primary site do not predict response to platinum based chemotherapy. Eur J Cancer 1996;32A(13): 2357–2359.
40. International Germ Cell Consensus Classification: a prognostic factor-based staging system for metastatic germ cell cancers. International Germ Cell Cancer Collaborative Group. J Clin Oncol 1997;15(2):594–603.
41. Bidart JM, Thuillier F, Augereau C, et al. Kinetics of serum tumor marker concentrations and usefulness in clinical monitoring. Clin Chem 1999;45(10): 1695–1707.
42. Murphy BA, Motzer RJ, Mazumdar M, et al. Serum tumor marker decline is an early predictor of treatment outcome in germ cell tumor patients treated with cisplatin and ifosfamide salvage chemotherapy. Cancer (Phila) 1994;73(10):2520–2526.
43. Mazumdar M, Bajorin DF, Bacik J, et al. Predicting outcome to chemotherapy in patients with germ cell tumors: the value of the rate of decline of human chorionic gonadotrophin and alphafetoprotein during therapy. J Clin Oncol 2001;19(9):2534–2541.
44. Morris MJ, Bosl GJ. Recognizing abnormal marker results that do not reflect disease in patients with germ cell tumors. J Urol 2000;163(3):796–801.
45. Bower M, Rustin GJ. Serum tumor markers and their role in monitoring germ cell cancers of the testis. In: Vogelzang NJ, et

al. (eds) Comprehensive Textbook of Genitourinary Oncology. New York: Lippincott Williams & Wilkins, 2000:927–938.

46. Germa JR, Llanos M, Tabernero JM, et al. False elevations of alpha-fetoprotein associated with liver dysfunction in germ cell tumors. Cancer (Phila) 1993;72(8):2491–2494.
47. Hoshi S, Suzuki K, Ishidoya S, et al. Significance of simultaneous determination of serum human chorionic gonadotropin (hCG) and hCG-beta in testicular tumor patients. Int J Urol 2000;7(6):218–223.
48. Mills JN, Nguyen TT, Williams RD. Falsely increased beta-human chorionic gonadotropin with a testicular epidermoid cyst. J Urol 2001;166(6):2314.
49. Gillespie JR, Uversky VN. Structure and function of alpha-fetoprotein: a biophysical overview. Biochim Biophys Acta 2000;1480(1-2):41–56.
50. Marx GM, Boyce A, Goldstein D. Elevated alpha-foetoprotein and hepatic metastases—it's not always what it seems! Ann Oncol 2002;13(1):167–169.
51. Adachi Y, Tsuchihashi J, Shiraishi N, et al. AFP-producing gastric carcinoma: multivariate analysis of prognostic factors in 270 patients. Oncology 2003;65(2):95–101.
52. Chen J, Rocken C, Treiber G, et al. Clinical implications of alpha-fetoprotein expression in gastric adenocarcinoma. Dig Dis 2003;21(4):357–362.
53. Yachida S, Fukushima N, Nakanishi Y, et al. Alpha-fetoprotein-producing carcinoma of the colon: report of a case and review of the literature. Dis Colon Rectum 2003;46(6):826–831.
54. Mcintire KR, Waldmann TA, Moertel CG, et al. Serum alpha-fetoprotein in patients with neoplasms of the gastrointestinal tract. Cancer Res 1975;35(4): 991–996.
55. Cole LA. Immunoassay of human chorionic gonadotropin, its free subunits, and metabolites. Clin Chem 1997;43(12): 2233–2243.
56. Butler SA, Cole LA. Use of heterophilic antibody blocking agent (HBT) in reducing false-positive hCG results. Clin Chem 2001; 47(7):1332–1333.
57. Butler SA, Cole LA. Falsely elevated human chorionic gonadotropin leading to unnecessary therapy. Obstet Gynecol 2002;99(3):516–517.
58. Porakishvili N, Jackson AM, De Souza JB, et al. Epitopes of human chorionic gonadotropin and their relationship to immunogenicity and cross-reactivity of beta-chain mutants. Am J Reprod Immunol 1998;40(3):210– 214.
59. Stenman UH, Alfthan H, Hotakainen K. Human chorionic gonadotropin in cancer. Clin Biochem 2004;37(7):549–561.
60. Marcillac I, Troalen F, Bidart JM, et al. Free human chorionic gonadotropin beta subunit in gonadal and nongonadal neoplasms. Cancer Res 1992;52(14):3901–3907.
61. Ruther U, Rothe B, Grunert K, et al. Role of human chorionic gonadotropin in patients with pure seminoma. Eur Urol 1994;26(2):129–133.
62. Thomas G, Jones W, Vanoosterom A, et al. Consensus statement on the investigation and management of testicular seminoma 1989. Prog Clin Biol Res 1990;357:285–294.
63. Weissbach L, Bussar-Maatz R, Lohrs U, et al. Prognostic factors in seminomas with special respect to HCG: results of a prospective multicenter study. Seminoma Study Group. Eur Urol 1999;36(6):601–608.
64. Mencel PJ, Motzer RJ, Mazumdar M, et al. Advanced seminoma: treatment results, survival, and prognostic factors in 142 patients. J Clin Oncol 1994;12(1):120–126.
65. Miller KD, Loehrer PJ, Gonin R, et al. Salvage chemotherapy with vinblastine, ifosfamide, and cisplatin in recurrent seminoma. J Clin Oncol 1997;15(4):1427–1431.
66. Fossa SD, Oliver RT, Stenning SP, et al. Prognostic factors for patients with advanced seminoma treated with platinum-based chemotherapy. Eur J Cancer 1997;33(9):1380–1387.
67. Gholam D, Fizazi K, Terrier-Lacombe MJ, et al. Advanced seminoma: treatment results and prognostic factors for survival after first-line, cisplatin-based chemotherapy and for patients with recurrent disease: a single-institution experience in 145 patients. Cancer (Phila) 2003;98(4):745–752.
68. Warde P, Specht L, Horwich A, et al. Prognostic factors for relapse in stage I seminoma managed by surveillance: a pooled analysis. J Clin Oncol 2002;20(22):4448–4452.
69. Von Eyben FE, Jacobsen GK, Rorth M, et al. Microinvasive germ cell tumour (MGCT) adjacent to testicular germ cell tumours. Histopathology (Oxf) 2004;44(6):547–554.
70. Von Der Maase H, Rorth M, Walbom-Jorgensen S, et al. Carcinoma in situ of contralateral testis in patients with testicular germ cell cancer: study of 27 cases in 500 patients. Br Med J (Clin Res Ed) 1986;293(6559):1398–1401.
71. Dieckmann KP, Skakkebaek NE. Carcinoma in situ of the testis: review of biological and clinical features. Int J Cancer 1999;83(6): 815–822.
72. Petersen PM, Giwercman A, Daugaard G, et al. Effect of graded testicular doses of radiotherapy in patients treated for carcinoma-in-situ in the testis. J Clin Oncol 2002;20(6):1537–1543.
73. Cheville JC. Classification and pathology of testicular germ cell and sex cord-stromal tumors. Urol Clin N Am 1999;26(3): 595–609.
74. Rayson D, Burch PA, Richardson RL. Sarcoidosis and testicular carcinoma. Cancer (Phila) 1998;83(2):337–343.
75. Tjan-Heijnen VC, Vlasveld LT, Pernet FP, et al. Coincidence of seminoma and sarcoidosis: a myth or fact? Ann Oncol 1998;9(3):321–325.
76. Eble JN. Spermatocytic seminoma. Hum Pathol 1994;25(10): 1035–1042.
77. Chung PW, Bayley AJ, Sweet J, et al. Spermatocytic seminoma: a review. Eur Urol 2004;45(4):495–498.
78. Osada K, Iijima H, Imasawa M, et al. Metastatic uveal tumor secondary to testicular choriocarcinoma. Jpn J Ophthalmol 2004;48(1):85–87.
79. Tinkle LL, Graham BS, Spillane TJ, et al. Testicular choriocarcinoma metastatic to the skin: an additional case and literature review. Cutis 2001;67(2):117–120.
80. Motzer RJ, Bosl GJ. Hemorrhage: a complication of metastatic testicular choriocarcinoma. Urology 1987;30(2):119–122.
81. Read G, Stenning SP, Cullen MH, et al. Medical Research Council prospective study of surveillance for stage I testicular teratoma. Medical Research Council Testicular Tumors Working Party. J Clin Oncol 1992; 10(11):1762–1768.
82. Leibovitch I, Foster RS, Ulbright TM, et al. Adult primary pure teratoma of the testis. The Indiana experience. Cancer (Phila) 1995;75(9):2244–2250.
83. Benson CB. The role of ultrasound in diagnosis and staging of testicular cancer. Semin Urol 1988;6(3):189–202.
84. Jochelson MS, Garnick MB, Balikian JP, et al. The efficacy of routine whole lung tomography in germ cell tumors. Cancer (Phila) 1984;54(6): 1007–1009.
85. See WA, Hoxie L. Chest staging in testis cancer patients: imaging modality selection based upon risk assessment as determined by abdominal computerized tomography scan results. J Urol 1993;150(3):874–878.
86. American Joint Committee on Cancer, Testis. In: Cancer Staging Manual. Philadelphia: Lippincott-Raven, 1997:225–230.
87. Chung P, Parker C, Panzarella T, et al. Surveillance in stage I testicular seminoma: risk of late relapse. Can J Urol 2002;9(5):1637–1640.
88. Aparicio J, Garcia Del Muro X, Maroto P, et al. Multicenter study evaluating a dual policy of postorchidectomy surveillance and selective adjuvant single-agent carboplatin for patients with clinical stage I seminoma. Ann Oncol 2003;14(6):867–872.
89. Von Der Maase H, Specht L, Jacobsen GK, et al. Surveillance following orchidectomy for stage I seminoma of the testis. Eur J Cancer 1993;29A(14): 1931–1934.

90. Aparicio J, Germa JR, Garcia Del Muro X, et al. Risk-adapted management of stage I seminoma: the second Spanish Germ Cell Cancer Group study. Proc Am Soc Clin Oncol 2004;23:385 (abstract 4518).
91. Warde P, Gospodarowicz MK, Panzarella T, et al. Stage I testicular seminoma: results of adjuvant irradiation and surveillance. J Clin Oncol 1995;13(9):2255–2262.
92. Horwich A, Alsanjari N, A'hern R, et al. Surveillance following orchidectomy for stage I testicular seminoma. Br J Cancer 1992;65(5):775–778.
93. Motzer RJ, Bhanson RR, Carducci MA, et al. Clinical Practice Guidelines in Oncology: Testicular Cancer. TEST-3. Jenkintown, PA: National Cooperative Cancer Network, 2003.
94. Oliver RT, Edmonds PM, Ong JY, et al. Pilot studies of 2 and 1 course carboplatin as adjuvant for stage I seminoma: should it be tested in a randomized trial against radiotherapy? Int J Radiat Oncol Biol Phys 1994;29(1):3–8.
95. Reiter WJ, Brodowicz T, Alavi S, et al. Twelve-year experience with two courses of adjuvant single-agent carboplatin therapy for clinical stage I seminoma. J Clin Oncol 2001;19(1):101–104.
96. Oliver T, Boublikova L, Ong J. Fifteen year follow up of the Anglian Germ Cell Cancer Group adjuvant studies of carboplatin as an alternative to radiation or surveillance for stage I seminoma. Proc Am Soc Clin Oncol 2001;20: abstract 780.
97. Krege S, Kalund G, Otto T, et al. Phase II study: adjuvant single-agent carboplatin therapy for clinical stage I seminoma. Eur Urol 1997;31(4):405–407.
98. Dieckmann KP, Krain J, Kuster J, et al. Adjuvant carboplatin treatment for seminoma clinical stage I. J Cancer Res Clin Oncol 1996;122(1):63–66.
99. Steiner H, Holtl L, Wirtenberger W, et al. Long-term experience with carboplatin monotherapy for clinical stage I seminoma: a retrospective single-center study. Urology 2002;60(2):324–328.
100. Kratzik C, Kuhrer I, Wiltschke C. Carboplatin-monotherapie bei seminomen in stadium I. Acta Chir Aust 1993;25:27–28.
101. Dieckmann KP, Bruggeboes B, Pichlmeier U, et al. Adjuvant treatment of clinical stage I seminoma: is a single course of carboplatin sufficient? Urology 2000;55(1):102–106.
102. Oliver RT, Mason M, Von Der Maase H, et al. A randomised comparison of single agent carboplatin with radiotherapy in the adjuvant treatment of stage I seminoma of the testis, following orchidectomy: MRC TE19/EORTC 30982. Proc Am Soc Clin Oncol 2004;23:385 (abstract 4517).
103. Herr HW, Bar-Chama N, O'sullivan M, et al. Paternity in men with stage I testis tumors on surveillance. J Clin Oncol 1998;16(2):733–734.
104. United Kingdom Testicular Cancer Study Group, Aetiology of testicular cancer: association with congenital abnormalities, age at puberty, infertility, and exercise. BMJ 1994;308(6941):1393–1399.
105. Richiardi L, Akre O, Montgomery SM, et al. Fecundity and twinning rates as measures of fertility before diagnosis of germ-cell testicular cancer. J Natl Cancer Inst 2004;96(2):145–147.
106. Reiter WJ, Kratzik C, Brodowicz T, et al. Sperm analysis and serum follicle-stimulating hormone levels before and after adjuvant single-agent carboplatin therapy for clinical stage I seminoma. Urology 1998;52(1):117–119.
107. Huddart RA, Norman A, Shahidi M, et al. Cardiovascular disease as a long-term complication of treatment for testicular cancer. J Clin Oncol 2003;21(8):1513–1523.
108. Meinardi MT, Gietema JA, Van Der Graaf WT, et al. Cardiovascular morbidity in long-term survivors of metastatic testicular cancer. J Clin Oncol 2000;18(8):1725–1732.
109. Gietema JA, Sleijfer DT, Willemse PH, et al. Long-term follow-up of cardiovascular risk factors in patients given chemotherapy for disseminated nonseminomatous testicular cancer. Ann Intern Med 1992;116(9):709–715.
110. Kollmannsberger C, Kuzcyk M, Mayer F, et al. Late toxicity following curative treatment of testicular cancer. Semin Surg Oncol 1999;17(4):275–281.
111. Bokemeyer C, Berger CC, Kuczyk MA, et al. Evaluation of long-term toxicity after chemotherapy for testicular cancer. J Clin Oncol 1996;14(11):2923–2932.
112. Schmoll HJ, Souchon R, Krege S, et al. European consensus on diagnosis and treatment of germ cell cancer: a report of the European Germ Cell Cancer Consensus Group (EGCCCG). Ann Oncol 2004;15(9):1377–1399.
113. Logue JP, Harris MA, Livsey JE, et al. Short course para-aortic radiation for stage I seminoma of the testis. Int J Radiat Oncol Biol Phys 2003;57(5):1304–1309.
114. Bamberg M, Schmidberger H, Meisner C, et al. Radiotherapy for stages I and IIA/B testicular seminoma. Int J Cancer 1999;83(6):823–827.
115. Santoni R, Barbera F, Bertoni F, et al. Stage I seminoma of the testis: a bi-institutional retrospective analysis of patients treated with radiation therapy only. BJU Int 2003;92(1):47–52; discussion 52.
116. Fossa SD, Horwich A, Russell JM, et al. Optimal planning target volume for stage I testicular seminoma: a Medical Research Council randomized trial. Medical Research Council Testicular Tumor Working Group. J Clin Oncol 1999;17(4):1146.
117. Lederman GS, Herman TS, Jochelson M, et al. Radiation therapy of seminoma: 17-year experience at the Joint Center for Radiation Therapy. Radiother Oncol 1989;14(3):203–208.
118. Bauman GS, Venkatesan VM, Ago CT, et al. Postoperative radiotherapy for Stage I/II seminoma: results for 212 patients. Int J Radiat Oncol Biol Phys 1998;42(2):313–317.
119. Epstein BE, Order SE, Zinreich ES. Staging, treatment, and results in testicular seminoma. A 12-year report. Cancer (Phila) 1990;65(3):405–411.
120. Zagars GK, Ballo MT, Lee AK, et al. Mortality after cure of testicular seminoma. J Clin Oncol 2004;22(4):640–647.
121. Giacchetti S, Raoul Y, Wibault P, et al. Treatment of stage I testis seminoma by radiotherapy. Long-term results: a 30-year experience. Int J Radiat Oncol Biol Phys 1993;27(1):3–9.
122. Lederman GS, Sheldon TA, Chaffey JT, et al. Cardiac disease after mediastinal irradiation for seminoma. Cancer (Phila) 1987;60(4):772–776.
123. Hanks GE, Peters T, Owen J. Seminoma of the testis: long-term beneficial and deleterious results of radiation. Int J Radiat Oncol Biol Phys 1992;24(5):913–919.
124. Peckham MJ, Mcelwain Tj. Radiotherapy of testicular tumours. Proc R Soc Med 1974;67(4):300–303.
125. Sommer K, Brockmann WP, Hubener KH. Treatment results and acute and late toxicity of radiation therapy for testicular seminoma. Cancer (Phila) 1990;66(2):259–263.
126. Thomas GM. Over 20 years of progress in radiation oncology: seminoma. Semin Radiat Oncol 1997;7(2):135–145.
127. Jones WG, Fossa SD, Mead GM, et al. A randomised trial of two radiotherapy schedules in the adjuvant treatment of stage I seminoma (MRC TE18). Eur J Cancer 2001;37(suppl 6):S157.
128. Fossa SD, Jones WG, Stenning SP. Quality of life (QL) after radiotherapy (RT) for stage I seminoma: results from a randomised trial of two RT schedules (MRC TE18). Proc Am Soc Clin Oncol 2002;21(1):188a (abstract 750).
129. Khoo VS, Rainford K, Horwich A, et al. The effect of antiemetics and reduced radiation fields on acute gastrointestinal morbidity of adjuvant radiotherapy in stage I seminoma of the testis: a randomized pilot study. Clin Oncol (R Coll Radiol) 1997;9(4):252–257.
130. Melchior D, Hammer P, Fimmers R, et al. Long term results and morbidity of paraaortic compared with paraaortic and iliac adjuvant radiation in clinical stage I seminoma. Anticancer Res 2001;21(4B):2989–2993.
131. Travis LB, Curtis RE, Hankey BF. Second malignancies after testicular cancer. J Clin Oncol 1995;13(2):533–534.

132. Travis LB, Curtis RE, Storm H, et al. Risk of second malignant neoplasms among long-term survivors of testicular cancer. J Natl Cancer Inst 1997;89(19):1429–1439.
133. Horwich A, Bell J. Mortality and cancer incidence following radiotherapy for seminoma of the testis. Radiother Oncol 1994; 30(3):193–198.
134. Oliver RT. Second tumors after radiation treatment of testicular germ cell tumors. J Clin Oncol 1993;11(11):2286–2287.
135. Stein ME, Steiner M, Lachter J, et al. Second primary cancer in irradiated stage I testicular seminoma. Strahlenther Onkol 1993;169(11):672–677.
136. Ruther U. Second malignancies following pure seminoma. Oncology 2000;58(1):75–82.
137. Van Leeuwen FE, Stiggelbout AM, Van Den Belt-Dusebout AW, et al. Second cancer risk following testicular cancer: a follow-up study of 1,909 patients. J Clin Oncol 1993;11(3):415–424.
138. Hughes MA, Wang A, Deweese TL. Two secondary malignancies after radiotherapy for seminoma: case report and review of the literature. Urology 2003;62(4):748.
139. Glanzmann C, Schultz G, Lutolf UM. Long-term morbidity of adjuvant infradiaphragmatic irradiation in patients with testicular cancer and implications for the treatment of stage I seminoma. Radiother Oncol 1991;22(1):12–18.
140. Vallis KA, Howard GC, Duncan W, et al. Radiotherapy for stages I and II testicular seminoma: results and morbidity in 238 patients. Br J Radiol 1995;68(808):400–405.
141. Akimoto T, Takahashi I, Takahashi M, et al. Long-term outcome of postorchiectomy radiation therapy for stage I and II testicular seminoma. Anticancer Res 1997;17(5B):3781–3785.
142. Stein M, Steiner M, Moshkowitz B, et al. Testicular seminoma: 20-year experience at the Northern Israel Oncology Center (1968–1988). Int Urol Nephrol 1994;26(4):461–469.
143. Fossa SD, Aass N, Kaalhus O. Radiotherapy for testicular seminoma stage I: treatment results and long-term post-irradiation morbidity in 365 patients. Int J Radiat Oncol Biol Phys 1989; 16(2):383–388.
144. Huyghe E, Matsuda T, Daudin M, et al. Fertility after testicular cancer treatments: results of a large multicenter study. Cancer (Phila) 2004;100(4):732–737.
145. Freedman LS, Parkinson MC, Jones WG, et al. Histopathology in the prediction of relapse of patients with stage I testicular teratoma treated by orchidectomy alone. Lancet 1987;2(8554): 294–298.
146. Heidenreich A, Sesterhenn IA, Mostofi FK, et al. Prognostic risk factors that identify patients with clinical stage I nonseminomatous germ cell tumors at low risk and high risk for metastasis. Cancer (Phila) 1998;83(5):1002–1011.
147. Moul JW. Percentage of embryonal carcinoma and of vascular invasion predicts pathological stage in clinical stage I nonseminomatous testicular cancer. Cancer Res 1994;54(2):362–364.
148. Moul JW, Heidenreich A. Prognostic factors in low-stage nonseminomatous testicular cancer. Oncology (Huntingt) 1996; 10(9):1359–1368, 1374; discussion 1377–1378.
149. Colls BM, Harvey VJ, Skelton L, et al. Late results of surveillance of clinical stage I nonseminoma germ cell testicular tumours: 17 years experience in a national study in New Zealand. BJU Int 1999;83(1):76–82.
150. Sogani PC, Perrotti M, Herr HW, et al. Clinical stage I testis cancer: long-term outcome of patients on surveillance. J Urol 1998;159(3):855–858.
151. Pohar KS, Rabbani F, Bosl GJ, et al. Results of retroperitoneal lymph node dissection for clinical stage I and II pure embryonal carcinoma of the testis [comment]. J Urol 2003;170(4 pt 1):1155–1158.
152. Hermans BP, Sweeney CJ, Foster RS, et al. Risk of systemic metastases in clinical stage I nonseminoma germ cell testis tumor managed by retroperitoneal lymph node dissection. J Urol 2000;163(6):1721– 1724.
153. Sweeney CJ, Hermans BP, Heilman DK, et al. Results and outcome of retroperitoneal lymph node dissection for clinical stage I embryonal carcinoma: predominant testis cancer. J Clin Oncol 2000;18(2):358–362.
154. Gels ME, Hoekstra HJ, Sleijfer DT, et al. Detection of recurrence in patients with clinical stage I nonseminomatous testicular germ cell tumors and consequences for further follow-up: a single-center 10-year experience. J Clin Oncol 1995;13(5):1188–1194.
155. Daugaard G, Petersen PM, Rorth M. Surveillance in stage I testicular cancer. APMIS 2003;111(1):76–85.
156. Albers P, Siener R, Kliesch S, et al. Risk factors for relapse in clinical stage I nonseminomatous testicular germ cell tumors: results of the German Testicular Cancer Study Group Trial. J Clin Oncol 2003;21(8):1505–1512.
157. Alexandre J, Fizazi K, Mahe C, et al. Stage I non-seminomatous germ-cell tumours of the testis: identification of a subgroup of patients with a very low risk of relapse. Eur J Cancer 2001;37(5):576–582.
158. Heidenreich A, Moul JW, Mcleod DG, et al. The role of retroperitoneal lymphadenectomy in mature teratoma of the testis. J Urol 1997;157(1):160–163.
159. Donohue JP. Retroperitoneal lymphadenectomy: the anterior approach including bilateral suprarenal-hilar dissection. Urol Clin N Am 1977;4(3):509–521.
160. Chang SS, Mohseni HJ, Leon A, et al. Paracolic recurrence: the importance of wide excision of the spermatic cord at retroperitoneal lymph node dissection. J Urol 2002;167(1):94–96.
161. Donohue JP, Foster RS. Retroperitoneal lymphadenectomy in staging and treatment. The development of nerve-sparing techniques. Urol Clin N Am 1998;25(3):461–468.
162. Richie JP. Modified retroperitoneal lymphadenectomy for patients with clinical stage I testicular cancer. Semin Urol 1988; 6(3):216–222.
163. Richie JP. Clinical stage 1 testicular cancer: the role of modified retroperitoneal lymphadenectomy. J Urol 1990;144(5):1160–1163.
164. Fossa SD, Klepp O, Ous S, et al. Unilateral retroperitoneal lymph node dissection in patients with non-seminomatous testicular tumor in clinical stage I. Eur Urol 1984;10(1):17–23.
165. Donohue JP, Zachary JM, Maynard BR. Distribution of nodal metastases in nonseminomatous testis cancer. J Urol 1982; 128:315–320.
166. Rabbani F. Low-volume nodal metastases detected at retroperitoneal lymphadenectomy for testicular cancer: pattern and prognostic factors for relapse. J Clin Oncol 2001;19(7):2020–2025.
167. Baniel J, Sella A. Complications of retroperitoneal lymph node dissection in testicular cancer: primary and post-chemotherapy. Semin Surg Oncol 1999;17:263–267.
168. Donohue JP, Foster RS, Rowland RG, et al. Nerve-sparing retroperitoneal lymphadenectomy with preservation of ejaculation. J Urol 1990;144(2 pt 1): 287–291; discussion 291–292.
169. Donohue JP, Thornhill JA, Foster RS, et al. Retroperitoneal lymphadenectomy for clinical stage A testis cancer (1965 to 1989): modifications of technique and impact on ejaculation. J Urol 1993;149(2):237–243.
170. Heidenreich A, Albers P, Hartmann M, et al. Complications of primary nerve sparing retroperitoneal lymph node dissection for clinical stage I nonseminomatous germ cell tumors of the testis: experience of the German Testicular Cancer Study Group. J Urol 2003;169(5):1710–1714.
171. Jewett MA, Wesley-James T. Early and late complications of retroperitoneal lymphadenectomy in testis cancer. Can J Surg 1991;34(4):368–373.
172. Donohue JP, Thornhill JA, Foster RS, et al. Primary retroperitoneal lymph node dissection in clinical stage A non-seminomatous germ cell testis cancer. Review of the Indiana University experience 1965–1989. Br J Urol 1993;71(3):326–335.
173. Sonneveld DJ, Koops HS, Sleijfer DT, et al. Surgery versus surveillance in stage I non-seminoma testicular cancer. Semin Surg Oncol 1999;17(4):230–239.

174. Stephenson AJ, Bosl GJ, Motzer RJ, et al. Primary retroperitoneal lymph node dissection (RPLND) for non-seminomatous germ-cell tumor (NSGCT): impact of trends in patient selection on retroperitoneal pathology and outcome. Proc Am Soc Clin Oncol 2004;22(14S):4523.
175. Richie JP. Is adjuvant chemotherapy necessary for patients with stage B1 testicular cancer? J Clin Oncol 1991;9(8):1393–1396.
176. Williams SD, Stablein DM, Einhorn LH, et al. Immediate adjuvant chemotherapy versus observation with treatment at relapse in pathological stage II testicular cancer. N Engl J Med 1987;317(23):1433–1438.
177. Saxman SB. The management of patients with clinical stage I nonseminomatous testicular tumors and persistently elevated serologic markers [see comments]. J Urol 1996;155(2):587–589.
178. Steiner H, Peschel R, Janetschek G, et al. Long-term results of laparoscopic retroperitoneal lymph node dissection: a single-center 10-year experience. Urology 2004;63(3):550–555.
179. Corvin S, Kuczyk M, Anastasiadis A, et al. Laparoscopic retroperitoneal lymph node dissection for nonseminomatous testicular carcinoma. World J Urol 2004;22(1):33–36.
180. Bhayani SB, Allaf ME, Kavoussi LR. Laparoscopic RPLND for clinical stage I nonseminomatous germ cell testicular cancer: current status. Urol Oncol 2004;22(2):145–148.
181. Bhayani SB, Ong A, Oh Wk, et al. Laparoscopic retroperitoneal lymph node dissection for clinical stage I nonseminomatous germ cell testicular cancer: a long-term update. Urology 2003;62(2):324–327.
182. Rassweiler JJ, Frede T, Lenz E, et al. Long-term experience with laparoscopic retroperitoneal lymph node dissection in the management of low-stage testis cancer. Eur Urol 2000;37(3):251–260.
183. Janetschek G, Hobisch A, Peschel R, et al. Laparoscopic retroperitoneal lymph node dissection for clinical stage I nonseminomatous testicular carcinoma: long-term outcome. J Urol 2000;163(6):1793–1796.
184. Klepp O, Dahl O, Flodgren P, et al. Risk-adapted treatment of clinical stage 1 non-seminoma testis cancer. Eur J Cancer 1997;33(7):1038–1044.
185. Roeleveld TA, Horenblas S, Meinhardt W, et al. Surveillance can be the standard of care for stage I nonseminomatous testicular tumors and even high risk patients. J Urol 2001;166(6): 2166–2170.
186. Mead GM, Stenning SP, Parkinson MC, et al. The Second Medical Research Council study of prognostic factors in nonseminomatous germ cell tumors. Medical Research Council Testicular Tumour Working Party. J Clin Oncol 1992;10(1): 85–94.
187. Motzer RJ, Bahnson RR, Carducci MA, et al. National Comprehensive Cancer Network Practice Guidelines in Oncology: Testicular Cancer, Version 1. Rockledge, PA: National Comprehensive Cancer Network, 2001.
188. Cullen MH, Stenning SP, Parkinson MC, et al. Short-course adjuvant chemotherapy in high-risk stage I nonseminomatous germ cell tumors of the testis: a Medical Research Council report. J Clin Oncol 1996;14(4):1106–1113.
189. Bohlen D, Borner M, Sonntag RW, et al. Long-term results following adjuvant chemotherapy in patients with clinical stage I testicular nonseminomatous malignant germ cell tumors with high risk factors. J Urol 1999;161(4):1148–1152.
190. Abratt RP, Pontin AR, Barnes RD, et al. Adjuvant chemotherapy for stage I non-seminomatous testicular cancer. S Afr Med J 1994;84(9):605–607.
191. Mourey L, Flechon A, Droz JP, et al. Cohort study of surveillance (S) and adjuvant chemotherapy (CT) in high risk stage I non seminomatous germ cell testicular tumors (NSGCTT I). Proc Am Soc Clin Oncol 2003;22:389 (abstract 1562).
192. Oliver RT, Ong J, Shamash J, et al. Long-term follow-up of Anglian Germ Cell Cancer Group surveillance versus patients with Stage 1 nonseminoma treated with adjuvant chemotherapy. Urology 2004;63(3):556–561.
193. Amato RJ, Ro JY, Ayala AG, et al. Risk-adapted treatment for patients with clinical stage I nonseminomatous germ cell tumor of the testis. Urology 2004;63(1):144–148; discussion 148–149.
194. Ondrus D, Matoska J, Belan V, et al. Prognostic factors in clinical stage I nonseminomatous germ cell testicular tumors: rationale for different risk-adapted treatment. Eur Urol 1998;33(6):562–566.
195. Hendry WF, Norman A, Nicholls J, et al. Abdominal relapse in stage 1 nonseminomatous germ cell tumours of the testis managed by surveillance or with adjuvant chemotherapy. BJU Int 2000;86(1):89–93.
196. Foster RS, Baniel J, Leibovitch I, et al. Teratoma in the orchiectomy specimen and volume of metastasis are predictors of retroperitoneal teratoma in low stage nonseminomatous testis cancer. J Urol 1996;155(6):1943–1945.
197. Studer UE, Burkhard FC, Sonntag RW. Risk adapted management with adjuvant chemotherapy in patients with high risk clinical stage i nonseminomatous germ cell tumor. J Urol 2000; 163(6):1785–1787.
198. Milosevic MF, Gospodarowicz M, Warde P. Management of testicular seminoma. Semin Surg Oncol 1999;17(4):240–249.
199. Smalley SR, Earle JD, Evans RG, et al. Modern radiotherapy results with bulky stages II and III seminoma. J Urol 1990;144(3):685–689.
200. Chung PW, Gospodarowicz MK, Panzarella T, et al. Stage II testicular seminoma: patterns of recurrence and outcome of treatment. Eur Urol 2004;45(6):754–760.
201. Loehrer PJ, Sr., Birch R, Williams SD, et al. Chemotherapy of metastatic seminoma: the Southeastern Cancer Study Group experience. J Clin Oncol 1987;5(8):1212–1220.
202. Horwich A, Norman A, Fisher C, et al. Primary chemotherapy for stage II nonseminomatous germ cell tumors of the testis. J Urol 1994;151(1):72–77; discussion 77–78.
203. Donohue JP, Thornhill JA, Foster RS, et al. Clinical stage B nonseminomatous germ cell testis cancer: the Indiana University experience (1965–1989) using routine primary retroperitoneal lymph node dissection. Eur J Cancer 1995;31A(10):1599–1604.
204. Logothetis CJ, Swanson DA, Dexeus F, et al. Primary chemotherapy for clinical stage II nonseminomatous germ cell tumors of the testis: a follow-up of 50 patients. J Clin Oncol 1987;5(6):906–911.
205. Weissbach L, Bussar-Maatz R, Flechtner H, et al. RPLND or primary chemotherapy in clinical stage IIA/B nonseminomatous germ cell tumors? Results of a prospective multicenter trial including quality of life assessment. Eur Urol 2000;37(5): 582–594.
206. Gels ME, Nijboer AP, Hoekstra HJ, et al. Complications of the post-chemotherapy resection of retroperitoneal residual tumour mass in patients with non-seminomatous testicular germ cell tumours. Br J Urol 1997;79(2):263–268.
207. Rabbani F, Gleave ME, Coppin CM, et al. Teratoma in primary testis tumor reduces complete response rates in the retroperitoneum after primary chemotherapy. The case for primary retroperitoneal lymph node dissection of stage IIb germ cell tumors with teratomatous elements. Cancer (Phila) 1996;78(3): 480–486.
208. Williams S, Birch R, Einhorn L, et al. Treatment of disseminated germ-cell tumors with cisplatin, bleomycin, and either vinblastine or etoposide. N Engl J Med 1987;316(23):1435–1440.
209. Mcleod DG, Weiss RB, Stablein DM, et al. Staging relationships and outcome in early stage testicular cancer: a report from the Testicular Cancer Intergroup Study. J Urol 1991;145(6): 1178–1183; discussion 1182–1183.
210. Behnia M. Adjuvant bleomycin, etoposide and cisplatin in pathological stage II non-seminomatous testicular cancer. the

Indiana University experience [see comments]. Eur J Cancer 2000;36(4):472–475.
211. Kondagunta GV, Sheinfeld J, Mazumdar M, et al. Relapse-free and overall survival in patients with pathologic stage II nonseminomatous germ cell cancer treated with etoposide and cisplatin adjuvant chemotherapy. J Clin Oncol 2004;22(3):464–467.
212. Einhorn LH, Donohue J. *cis*-Diamminedichloroplatinum, vinblastine, and bleomycin combination chemotherapy in disseminated testicular cancer. Ann Intern Med 1977;87(3):293–298.
213. Harding MJ, Paul J, Gillis CR, et al. Management of malignant teratoma: does referral to a specialist unit matter? Lancet 1993;341(8851):999–1002.
214. Toner GC, Stockler MR, Boyer MJ, et al. Comparison of two standard chemotherapy regimens for good-prognosis germ-cell tumours: a randomised trial. Australian and New Zealand Germ Cell Trial Group. Lancet 2001;357(9258):739–745.
215. De Wit R, Roberts JT, Wilkinson PM, et al. Equivalence of three or four cycles of bleomycin, etoposide, and cisplatin chemotherapy and of a 3- or 5-day schedule in good-prognosis germ cell cancer: a randomized study of the European Organization for Research and Treatment of Cancer Genitourinary Tract Cancer Cooperative Group and the Medical Research Council. J Clin Oncol 2001;19(6):1629–1640.
216. Culine S, Kerbrat P, Bouzy J, et al. The optimal chemotherapy regimen for good-risk metastatic non seminomatous germ cell tumors (MNSGCT) is 3 cycles of bleomycin, etoposide and cisplatin: mature results of a randomized trial. Proc Am Soc Clin Oncol 2003;22: abstract 1536.
217. Hinton S, Catalano PJ, Einhorn LH, et al. Cisplatin, etoposide and either bleomycin or ifosfamide in the treatment of disseminated germ cell tumors: final analysis of an intergroup trial. Cancer (Phila) 2003;97(8):1869–1875.
218. Nichols CR, Catalano PJ, Crawford ED, et al. Randomized comparison of cisplatin and etoposide and either bleomycin or ifosfamide in treatment of advanced disseminated germ cell tumors: an Eastern Cooperative Oncology Group, Southwest Oncology Group, and Cancer and Leukemia Group B Study [see comment]. J Clin Oncol 1998;16(4):1287–1293.
219. Einhorn LH, Williams SD, Loehrer PJ, et al. Evaluation of optimal duration of chemotherapy in favorable-prognosis disseminated germ cell tumors: a Southeastern Cancer Study Group protocol. J Clin Oncol 1989;7(3):387–391.
220. Saxman SB, Finch D, Gonin R, et al. Long-term follow-up of a phase III study of three versus four cycles of bleomycin, etoposide, and cisplatin in favorable-prognosis germ-cell tumors: the Indian University experience. J Clin Oncol 1998;16(2):702–706.
221. Culine S, Theodore C, Terrier-Lacombe Mj, et al. Are 3 cycles of bleomycin, etoposide and cisplatin or 4 cycles of etoposide and cisplatin equivalent optimal regimens for patients with good risk metastatic germ cell tumors of the testis? The need for a randomized trial. J Urol 1997;157(3):855–858; discussion 858–859.
222. Loehrer PJ, Sr., Johnson D, Elson P, et al. Importance of bleomycin in favorable-prognosis disseminated germ cell tumors: an Eastern Cooperative Oncology Group trial. J Clin Oncol 1995;13(2):470–476.
223. De Wit R, Stoter G, Kaye SB, et al. Importance of bleomycin in combination chemotherapy for good-prognosis testicular nonseminoma: a randomized study of the European Organization for Research and Treatment of Cancer Genitourinary Tract Cancer Cooperative Group. J Clin Oncol 1997;15(5):1837–1843.
224. Levi JA, Raghavan D, Harvey V, et al. The importance of bleomycin in combination chemotherapy for good-prognosis germ cell carcinoma. Australasian Germ Cell Trial Group. J Clin Oncol 1993;11(7):1300–1305.
225. Horwich A, Sleijfer DT, Fossa SD, et al. Randomized trial of bleomycin, etoposide, and cisplatin compared with bleomycin, etoposide, and carboplatin in good-prognosis metastatic nonseminomatous germ cell cancer: a Multiinstitutional Medical Research Council/European Organization for Research and Treatment of Cancer Trial. J Clin Oncol 1997;15(5):1844–1852.
226. Bokemeyer C, Kohrmann O, Tischler J, et al. A randomized trial of cisplatin, etoposide and bleomycin (PEB) versus carboplatin, etoposide and bleomycin (CEB) for patients with 'good-risk' metastatic non-seminomatous germ cell tumors. Ann Oncol 1996;7(10):1015–1021.
227. Bajorin DF, Sarosdy MF, Pfister DG, et al. Randomized trial of etoposide and cisplatin versus etoposide and carboplatin in patients with good-risk germ cell tumors: a multiinstitutional study. J Clin Oncol 1993;11(4):598–606.
228. Kaye SB, Mead GM, Fossa S, et al. Intensive induction-sequential chemotherapy with BOP/VIP-B compared with treatment with BEP/EP for poor-prognosis metastatic nonseminomatous germ cell tumor: a Randomized Medical Research Council/European Organization for Research and Treatment of Cancer study. J Clin Oncol 1998;16(2):692–701.
229. Nichols C, Williams S, Loehrer P, et al. Randomized study of cisplatin dose intensity in advanced germ cell tumors: a Southeastern Cancer Study Group and Southwest Oncology Group protocol. J Clin Oncol 1991;1991(9):1163–1172.
230. Bower M, Newlands ES, Holden L, et al. Treatment of men with metastatic non-seminomatous germ cell tumours with cyclical POMB/ACE chemotherapy. Ann Oncol 1997;8(5):477–483.
231. Culine S, Theodore C, Bekradda M, et al. Experience with bleomycin, etoposide, cisplatin (BEP) and alternating cisplatin, cyclophosphamide, doxorubicin (CISCA(II))/vinblastine, bleomycin (VB(IV)) regimens of che-motherapy in poor-risk nonseminomatous germ cell tumors. Am J Clin Oncol 1997;20(2):184–188.
232. Gerl A, Clemm C, Hentrich M, et al. Etoposide, cisplatin, bleomycin, and cyclophosphamide (ECBC) as first-line chemotherapy for poor-risk non-seminomatous germ cell tumors. Acta Oncol 1993;32(5):541–546.
233. De Wit R, Stoter G, Sleijfer DT, et al. Four cycles of BEP versus an alternating regime of PVB and BEP in patients with poor-prognosis metastatic testicular non-seminoma; a randomised study of the EORTC Genitourinary Tract Cancer Cooperative Group. Br J Cancer 1995;71(6):1311–1314.
234. Bhala N, Coleman JM, Radstone CR, et al. The management and survival of patients with advanced germ-cell tumours: improving outcome in intermediate and poor prognosis patients. Clin Oncol (R Coll Radiol) 2004;16(1):40–47.
235. Schmoll HJ, Kollmannsberger C, Metzner B, et al. Long-term results of first-line sequential high-dose etoposide, ifosfamide, and cisplatin chemotherapy plus autologous stem cell support for patients with advanced metastatic germ cell cancer: an extended phase I/II study of the German Testicular Cancer Study Group. J Clin Oncol 2003;21(22):4083–4091.
236. Duchesne GM, Stenning SP, Aass N, et al. Radiotherapy after chemotherapy for metastatic seminoma: a diminishing role. MRC Testicular Tumour Working Party. Eur J Cancer 1997;33(6):829–835.
237. Mosharafa AA, Foster RS, Bihrle R, et al. Does retroperitoneal lymph node dissection have a curative role for patients with sex cord-stromal testicular tumors? Cancer (Phila) 2003;98(4):753–757.
238. De Santis M, Becherer A, Bokemeyer C, et al. 2-^{18}Fluoro-deoxy-D-glucose positron emission tomography is a reliable predictor for viable tumor in post-chemotherapy seminoma: an update of the prospective multicentric SEMPET trial. J Clin Oncol 2004;22(6):1034–1039.
239. Herr HW, Sheinfeld J, Puc HS, et al. Surgery for a post-chemotherapy residual mass in seminoma. J Urol 1997;157(3):860–862.

240. Hofmockel G, Gruss A, Theiss M. Chemotherapy in advanced seminoma and the role of postcytostatic retroperitoneal lymph node dissection. Urol Int 1996;57(1):38–42.
241. Ravi R, Ong J, Oliver RT, et al. The management of residual masses after chemotherapy in metastatic seminoma. BJU Int 1999;83(6):649–653.
242. Puc HS, Heelan R, Mazumdar M, et al. Management of residual mass in advanced seminoma: results and recommendations from the Memorial Sloan-Kettering Cancer Center. J Clin Oncol 1996;14(2):454–460.
243. Crawford ED, Goodman P, Nabors WL, et al. Treatment of stages B3 and C seminoma with chemotherapy followed by irradiation therapy. Southwest Oncology Group Study. Urology 1992;39(5): 457–460.
244. Stephens AW, Gonin R, Hutchins GD, et al. Positron emission tomography evaluation of residual radiographic abnormalities in postchemotherapy germ cell tumor patients. J Clin Oncol 1996;14(5):1637–1641.
245. Kuczyk M, Machtens S, Stief C, et al. Management of the post-chemotherapy residual mass in patients with advanced stage non-seminomatous germ cell tumors (NSGCT). Int J Cancer 1999;83(6):852–855.
246. Steyerberg EW, Gerl A, Fossa SD, et al. Validity of predictions of residual retroperitoneal mass histology in nonseminomatous testicular cancer. J Clin Oncol 1998;16(1):269–274.
247. Steyerberg EW, Keizer HJ, Fossa SD, et al. Prediction of residual retroperitoneal mass histology after chemotherapy for metastatic nonseminomatous germ cell tumor: multivariate analysis of individual patient data from six study groups. J Clin Oncol 1995;13(5):1177–1187.
248. Fossa SD, Qvist H, Stenwig AE, et al. Is postchemotherapy retroperitoneal surgery necessary in patients with nonseminomatous testicular cancer and minimal residual tumor masses? J Clin Oncol 1992;10(4):569–573.
249. Fox EP, Weathers TD, Williams SD, et al. Outcome analysis for patients with persistent nonteratomatous germ cell tumor in postchemotherapy retroperitoneal lymph node dissections. J Clin Oncol 1993;11(7):1294–1299.
250. Oldenburg J, Alfsen GC, Lien HH, et al. Postchemotherapy retroperitoneal surgery remains necessary in patients with nonseminomatous testicular cancer and minimal residual tumor masses. J Clin Oncol 2003;21(17):3310–3317.
251. Stenning SP, Parkinson MC, Fisher C, et al. Postchemotherapy residual masses in germ cell tumor patients: content, clinical features, and prognosis. Medical Research Council Testicular Tumour Working Party. Cancer (Phila) 1998;83(7):1409–1419.
252. Vergouwe Y, Steyerberg EW, De Wit R, et al. External validity of a prediction rule for residual mass histology in testicular cancer: an evaluation for good prognosis patients. Br J Cancer 2003;88(6):843–847.
253. Debono DJ, Heilman DK, Einhorn LH, et al. Decision analysis for avoiding postchemotherapy surgery in patients with disseminated nonseminomatous germ cell tumors. J Clin Oncol 1997;15(4):1455–1464.
254. Albers P, Weissbach L, Krege S, et al. Prediction of necrosis after chemotherapy of advanced germ cell tumors: results of a prospective multicenter trial of the German Testicular Cancer Study Group. J Urol 2004;171(5):1835–1838.
255. Kisbenedek L, Bodrogi I, Szeldeli P, et al. Results of salvage retroperitoneal lymphadenectomy (RLA) in the treatment of patients with nonseminomatous germ cell tumours remaining marker positive after inductive chemotherapy. Int Urol Nephrol 1995;27(3): 325–329.
256. Habuchi T, Kamoto T, Hara I, et al. Factors that influence the results of salvage surgery in patients with chemorefractory germ cell carcinomas with elevated tumor markers. Cancer (Phila) 2003;98(8): 1635–1642.
257. Wood DP, Jr., Herr HW, Motzer RJ, et al. Surgical resection of solitary metastases after chemotherapy in patients with nonseminomatous germ cell tumors and elevated serum tumor markers. Cancer (Phila) 1992;70(9):2354–2357.
258. Coogan CL, Foster RS, Rowland RG, et al. Postchemotherapy retroperitoneal lymph node dissection is effective therapy in selected patients with elevated tumor markers after primary chemotherapy alone. Urology 1997;50(6):957–962.
259. Chang SS, Smith JA, Jr., Girasole C, et al. Beneficial impact of a clinical care pathway in patients with testicular cancer undergoing retroperitoneal lymph node dissection. J Urol 2002;168(1): 87–92.
260. Mosharafa AA, Foster RS, Koch MO, et al. Complications of post-chemotherapy retroperitoneal lymph node dissection for testis cancer. J Urol 2004;171(5):1839–1841.
261. Baniel J, Sella A. Complications of retroperitoneal lymph node dissection in testicular cancer: primary and post-chemotherapy. Semin Surg Oncol 1999;17(4):263–267.
262. Rabbani F. Retroperitoneal lymphadenectomy for post-chemotherapy residual masses: is a modified dissection and resection of residual masses sufficient? Br J Urol 1998;81(2): 295–300.
263. Aprikian AG, Herr HW, Bajorin DF, et al. Resection of postchemotherapy residual masses and limited retroperitoneal lymphadenectomy in patients with metastatic testicular nonseminomatous germ cell tumors. Cancer (Phila) 1994;74(4): 1329–1334.
264. Coogan CL, Hejase MJ, Wahle GR, et al. Nerve sparing post-chemotherapy retroperitoneal lymph node dissection for advanced testicular cancer. J Urol 1996;156(5):1656–1658.
265. Herr HW. Does necrosis on frozen-section analysis of a mass after chemotherapy justify a limited retroperitoneal resection in patients with advanced testis cancer? Br J Urol 1997;80(4): 653–657.
266. Brenner PC, Herr HW, Morse MJ, et al. Simultaneous retroperitoneal, thoracic, and cervical resection of postchemotherapy residual masses in patients with metastatic nonseminomatous germ cell tumors of the testis. J Clin Oncol 1996;14(6): 1765–1769.
267. Einhorn LH. Do all germ cell tumor patients with residual masses in multiple sites require postchemotherapy resections? J Clin Oncol 1997;15(1):409–410.
268. Hollender A, Stenwig EA, Ous S, et al. Survival of patients with viable malignant non-seminomatous germ cell tumour persistent after cisplatin-based induction chemotherapy. Eur Urol 1997;31(2):141–147.
269. Hartmann JT, Candelaria M, Kuczyk MA, et al. Comparison of histological results from the resection of residual masses at different sites after chemotherapy for metastatic non-seminomatous germ cell tumours. Eur J Cancer 1997;33(6): 843–847.
270. Jansen RL, Sylvester R, Sleyfer DT, et al. Long-term follow-up of non-seminomatous testicular cancer patients with mature teratoma or carcinoma at postchemotherapy surgery. EORTC Genitourinary Tract Cancer Cooperative Group (EORTC GU Group). Eur J Cancer 1991;27(6):695–698.
271. Hartmann JT, Schmoll HJ, Kuczyk MA, et al. Postchemotherapy resections of residual masses from metastatic non-seminomatous testicular germ cell tumors. Ann Oncol 1997;8(6):531–538.
272. Fizazi K, Tjulandin S, Salvioni R, et al. Viable malignant cells after primary chemotherapy for disseminated nonseminomatous germ cell tumors: prognostic factors and role of postsurgery chemotherapy: results from an international study group. J Clin Oncol 2001;19(10):2647–2657.
273. Mccaffrey JA, Mazumdar M, Bajorin DF, et al. Ifosfamide- and cisplatin-containing chemotherapy as first-line salvage therapy in germ cell tumors: response and survival. J Clin Oncol 1997;15(7):2559–2563.
274. Gerl A, Clemm C, Schmeller N, et al. Prognosis after salvage treatment for unselected male patients with germ cell tumours. Br J Cancer 1995;72(4):1026–1032.

275. Loehrer PJ, Sr, Gonin R, Nichols CR, et al. Vinblastine plus ifosfamide plus cisplatin as initial salvage therapy in recurrent germ cell tumor. J Clin Oncol 1998;16(7):2500–2504.
276. Loehrer PJ, Sr, Einhorn LH, Williams SD. VP-16 plus ifosfamide plus cisplatin as salvage therapy in refractory germ cell cancer. J Clin Oncol 1986;4(4):528–536.
277. Motzer RJ, Bajorin DF, Vlamis V, et al. Ifosfamide-based chemotherapy for patients with resistant germ cell tumors: the Memorial Sloan-Kettering Cancer Center experience. Semin Oncol 1992;19(6 suppl 12): 8–11.
278. Vuky J, Tickoo SK, Sheinfeld J, et al. Salvage chemotherapy for patients with advanced pure seminoma. J Clin Oncol 2002;20(1): 297–301.
279. Motzer RJ, Bajorin DF, Schwartz LJ, et al. Phase II trial of paclitaxel shows antitumor activity in patients with previously treated germ cell tumors. J Clin Oncol 1994;12(11):2277–2283.
280. Sandler AB, Cristou A, Fox S, et al. A phase II trial of paclitaxel in refractory germ cell tumors. Cancer (Phila) 1998;82(7): 1381–1386.
281. Einhorn LH, Stender MJj, Williams SD. Phase II trial of gemcitabine in refractory germ cell tumors. J Clin Oncol 1999;17(2): 509–511.
282. Bokemeyer C, Gerl A, Schoffski P, et al. Gemcitabine in patients with relapsed or cisplatin-refractory testicular cancer. J Clin Oncol 1999;17(2):512–556.
283. Motzer RJ, Sheinfeld J, Mazumdar M, et al. Paclitaxel, ifosfamide, and cisplatin second-line therapy for patients with relapsed testicular germ cell cancer. J Clin Oncol 2000;18(12): 2413–2418.
284. Hinton S, Catalano P, Einhorn LH, et al. Phase II study of paclitaxel plus gemcitabine in refractory germ cell tumors (E9897): a trial of the Eastern Cooperative Oncology Group. J Clin Oncol 2002;20(7):1859–1863.
285. Kollmannsberger C, Rick O, Derigs HG, et al. Activity of oxaliplatin in patients with relapsed or cisplatin-refractory germ cell cancer: a study of the German Testicular Cancer Study Group. J Clin Oncol 2002;20(8):2031–2037.
286. Kollmannsberger C, Beyer J, Liersch R, et al. Combination chemotherapy with gemcitabine plus oxaliplatin in patients with intensively pretreated or refractory germ cell cancer: a study of the German Testicular Cancer Study Group. J Clin Oncol 2004;22(1):108–114.
287. Beyer J, Kramar A, Mandanas R, et al. High-dose chemotherapy as salvage treatment in germ cell tumors: a multivariate analysis of prognostic variables. J Clin Oncol 1996;14(10):2638–2645.
288. Rick O, Beyer J, Kingreen D, et al. High-dose chemotherapy in germ cell tumours: a large single centre experience. Eur J Cancer 1998;34(12):1883–1888.
289. Rick O, Bokemeyer C, Beyer J, et al. Salvage treatment with paclitaxel, ifosfamide, and cisplatin plus high-dose carboplatin, etoposide, and thiotepa followed by autologous stem-cell rescue in patients with relapsed or refractory germ cell cancer. J Clin Oncol 2001;19(1):81–88.
290. Mcneish IA, Kanfer EJ, Haynes R, et al. Paclitaxel-containing high-dose chemotherapy for relapsed or refractory testicular germ cell tumours. Br J Cancer 2004;90(6):1169–1175.
291. Vaena DA, Abonour R, Einhorn LH. Long-term survival after high-dose salvage chemotherapy for germ cell malignancies with adverse prognostic variables. J Clin Oncol 2003;21(22): 4100–4104.
292. Bhatia S, Abonour R, Porcu P, et al. High-dose chemotherapy as initial salvage chemotherapy in patients with relapsed testicular cancer. J Clin Oncol 2000;18(19):3346–3351.
293. Motzer RJ, Mazumdar M, Sheinfeld J, et al. Sequential dose-intensive paclitaxel, ifosfamide, carboplatin, and etoposide salvage therapy for germ cell tumor patients. J Clin Oncol 2000;18(6):1173–1180.
294. Rodenhuis S, De Wit R, De Mulder PH, et al. A multi-center prospective phase II study of high-dose chemotherapy in germ-cell cancer patients relapsing from complete remission. Ann Oncol 1999;10(12):1467–1473.
295. Rosti G, Pico J-L, Wandt H, et al. High-dose chemotherapy (HDC) in the salvage treatment of patients failing first-line platinum chemotherapy for advanced germ cell tumors (GCT); first results of a prospective randomised trial of the European Group for Blood and Marrow Transplantation (EBMT): IT-94 study. Proc Am Soc Clin Oncol 2002;21: abstract 716.
296. Beyer J, Stenning S, Gerl A, et al. High-dose versus conventional-dose chemotherapy as first-salvage treatment in patients with non-seminomatous germ-cell tumors: a matched-pair analysis. Ann Oncol 2002;13(4):599–605.
297. Porcu P, Bhatia S, Sharma M, et al. Results of treatment after relapse from high-dose chemotherapy in germ cell tumors. J Clin Oncol 2000;18(6):1181–1186.
298. Flechon A, Rivoire M, Biron P, et al. Importance of surgery as salvage treatment after high dose chemotherapy failure in germ cell tumors. J Urol 2001;165(6 pt 1):1920–1926.
299. Takeda S, Miyoshi S, Ohta M, et al. Primary germ cell tumors in the mediastinum: a 50-year experience at a single Japanese institution. Cancer (Phila) 2003;97(2):367–376.
300. Bokemeyer C, Nichols CR, Droz JP, et al. Extragonadal germ cell tumors of the mediastinum and retroperitoneum: results from an international analysis. J Clin Oncol 2002;20(7):1864–1873.
301. Bokemeyer C, Droz JP, Horwich A, et al. Extragonadal seminoma: an international multicenter analysis of prognostic factors and long term treatment outcome. Cancer (Phila) 2001;91(7):1394–1401.
302. Dulmet EM, Macchiarini P, Suc B, et al. Germ cell tumors of the mediastinum. A 30-year experience. Cancer (Phila) 1993; 72(6):1894–1901.
303. Hiroshima K, Toyozaki T, Iyoda A, et al. Apoptosis and proliferative activity in mature and immature teratomas of the mediastinum. Cancer (Phila) 2001;92(7):1798–1806.
304. Bokemeyer C, Schleucher N, Metzner B, et al. First-line sequential high-dose VIP chemotherapy with autologous transplantation for patients with primary mediastinal nonseminomatous germ cell tumours: a prospective trial. Br J Cancer 2003;89(1): 29–35.
305. Hartmann JT, Nichols CR, Droz JP, et al. Hematologic disorders associated with primary mediastinal nonseminomatous germ cell tumors. J Natl Cancer Inst 2000;92(1):54–61.
306. Classen J, Schmidberger H, Meisner C, et al. Para-aortic irradiation for stage I testicular seminoma: results of a prospective study in 675 patients. A trial of the German testicular cancer study group (GTCSG). Br J Cancer 2004;90(12):2305–2311.
307. Spermon JR, Roeleveld TA, Van Der Poel HG, et al. Comparison of surveillance and retroperitoneal lymph node dissection in Stage I nonseminomatous germ cell tumors. Urology 2002; 59(6):923–929.
308. Pont J, Albrecht W, Postner G, et al. Adjuvant chemotherapy for high-risk clinical stage I nonseminomatous testicular germ cell cancer: long-term results of a prospective trial. J Clin Oncol 1996;14(2):441–448.
309. Abratt RP, Pontin AR, Barnes RD, et al. Adjuvant chemotherapy for stage I non-seminomatous testicular cancer. S Afr Med J 1994;84(9):605–607.
310. Hermans BP, Sweeney CJ, Foster RS, et al. Risk of systemic metastases in clinical stage I nonseminoma germ cell testis tumor managed by retroperitoneal lymph node dissection. J Urol 2000;163(6):1721–1724.
311. Bosl GJ, Geller NL, Bajorin D, et al. A randomized trial of etoposide + cisplatin versus vinblastine + bleomycin + cisplatin + cyclophosphamide + dactinomycin in patients with good-prognosis germ cell tumors. J Clin Oncol 1988;6(8):1231–1238.
312. Bajorin DF. Randomized trial of etoposide and cisplatin versus etoposide and carboplatin in patients with good-risk germ cell tumors: a multiinstitutional study [see comments]. J Clin Oncol 1993;11(4):598–606.

50

Cervix, Vulva, and Vagina

Julian C. Schink

In the United States and other developed countries, remarkable progress has been made in the prevention and treatment of cancer of the female lower genital track. Cervical cancer is still the most prevalent of the lower genital tract cancers, followed by vulvar cancer and finally vaginal cancer, which is quite rare. Unfortunately, invasive cervical carcinoma remains one of the most common causes of cancer death for women in the developing world. On a global basis, cervical cancer remains a significant health problem, with 500,000 new cases occurring each year and an annual death rate of 230,000 worldwide.[1] In the United States, approximately 13,000 new cases of cervical cancer are diagnosed each year and only 4,500 deaths due to cervical cancer. This stark contrast between the low number of cases in the United States and tragic number of cases in the developing world is primarily a reflection of the effectiveness of screening for and treating preinvasive cervical disease.

Cervical, vaginal, and vulvar cancer are usually squamous cell carcinomas arising from a preinvasive lesion. The relatively slow progression from an in situ lesion to invasive cancer, which may take anywhere from 5 to 20 years, offers an important opportunity for screening interventions to prevent invasive cancer from developing in these women. Cervical cytology screening lowers the mortality from cervical cancer, as evidenced by both population-based and case-controlled studies.[2] Women having cervical cytology screening at least every 3 years have a 10-fold decrease in their risk of cervical cancer when compared with women who have never been screened.[3] The focus of this chapter is primarily on the evaluation and treatment of squamous cell carcinoma of the cervix, vagina, and vulva because the principles of treating squamous cell carcinoma in these tissues are applicable to the other histologies. Cervical cancer is clearly the most common of the lower genital tract malignancies in women, accounting for approximately 16% of all gynecologic cancers. Vulvar cancer is quite uncommon and represents only 4% of malignancies in the female genital tract and, in contrast to cervical cancer, occurs most commonly in elderly women, compared to cervical cancer where the mean age is 51 years old. Vaginal cancer is even more rare, accounting for only 1% of gynecologic malignancies. In this chapter, we concentrate first on cervical cancer, then vulvar cancer, and finish with the diagnosis and management of vaginal cancer.

Cervical Cancer

Background and Prevalence

Cervical cancer remains a common event in the developing countries, with annual incidence rates ranging from a high of 83 cases per 100,000 women per year in Brazil to as low as 3 per 100,000 in developed countries such as Israel and the United States. The highest risk areas around the world are in Central and South America, the Caribbean, and southern and eastern Africa.[4] The marked contrast in these incidence rates has been attributed primarily to the success of screening programs in the United States and other developed countries. Other explanations for the high incidence in underdeveloped countries, which are lacking consistent evidence, include the higher rate of cigarette smoking and the more frequent early age of initiating sexual intercourse.

The prevention of cervical cancer is attributed to screening asymptomatic women on a regular basis with cervical cytology. The identification of preinvasive cervical dysplasia, which can be successfully treated with a number of modalities including cryotherapy, surgical excision, or laser ablation, has resulted in a marked decrease in the number of women developing cervical cancer. In countries where cervical cytology screening is commonly performed, such as the United States, at least half the cases of cervical cancer occur in women who have not had regular Papanicolaou (Pap) smear screening. The cases that do occur in women who have had regular Pap smear screening tend to be unusual tumors, such as adenocarcinoma arising within the glands of the cervix, or in women who have been incompletely or previously treated for preinvasive disease and then develop a lesion high in the cervical canal.

The risk factors for developing cervical cancer are tied closely to the commonly identified etiologic agent human papillomavirus (HPV).[5] This HPV is considered to be a necessary and critical factor in the development of cervical intraepithelial neoplasia and the subsequent progression to cervical cancer. Cervical carcinoma usually arises in metaplastic squamous epithelium at the junction of the ectocervix and endocervical canal. This squamous epithelium, which has undergone metaplasia during adolescence, appears to be particularly susceptible to the tumor suppressor effects of

HPV. The preinvasive lesions of cervical dysplasia, also called cervical intraepithelial neoplasia, will progress to invasive cervical cancer in 30% to 70% of women if left untreated. Fortunately, this progression usually takes between 10 to 20 years, allowing many opportunities to prevent the development of invasive cancer. The HPV is easily transmitted by sexual intercourse, so many of the risk factors for cervical cancer relate to sexual activity. Risk factors associated with the development of cervical cancer include early age of first intercourse, lower socioeconomic status, number of sexual partners, and a smoking history.[6] Smoking is associated with both cervical dysplasia and invasive cancer, suggesting that cigarette by-products may affect the early evolution of HPV-related lesions, possibly by increasing the rate of cell turnover or by the presence of carcinogens in cervical mucus combined with the immunosuppressive effects of HPV.[7] In 2002, results of the first controlled trial of an HPV vaccine were published, documenting an HPV-16 vaccine's efficacy in reducing the incidence of HPV-16-related cervical dysplasia.[8] The editorial response to this vaccine breakthrough was "The Beginning of the End for Cervical Cancer?," emphasizing the importance of preventing HPV infection and thus decreasing the incidence of both cervical dysplasia and cervical cancer.[9]

Although vaccination to prevent HPV infection worldwide carries great promise, there are several short-term barriers to the success of this strategy. First, there are numerous oncogenic strains of HPV, with HPV-16 only accounting for half the cases of cervical cancer. A multivalent vaccine is currently in clinical trials; if effective it will be a next critical step in vaccine development. Second, vaccination does not appear to reduce the incidence of cervical cancer or dysplasia in women already infected with HPV. Therefore, the benefits of an HPV vaccination program will be confined to women who are not yet infected by HPV, and will take several decades before a marked reduction in cervical cancer results. Unfortunately, despite the possible long-term benefits of an HPV vaccine, in our lifetime we will continue to see women with cervical, vaginal, and vulvar cancer.

Diagnosis

The diagnosis of cervical cancer segregates into two groups of patients. The asymptomatic patient identified on cervical cytology screening often has an early stage 1 cancer. In contrast, women who have not had regular cervical cytology screening usually present with signs and symptoms of advanced disease, including pelvic pain and vaginal bleeding.

The Asymptomatic Patient

Most asymptomatic patients will be diagnosed with a Pap smear showing either malignant cells or a preinvasive lesion, possibly even atypical squamous cells of undetermined significance (ASC). The evaluation of an abnormal Pap smear includes the use of colposcopic inspection of the cervix followed by colposcopically directed biopsies. If the colposcopy, or the biopsies, suggest an invasive malignancy, then a cone biopsy will confirm both the presence of invasion, the size of the tumor, and the depth of invasion. Occasionally, a patient with a more-advanced cervical cancer remains asymptomatic and has false-negative cervical cytology. These false-negative cytology tests usually occur because the tumor originated high in the endocervical canal or did not shed malignant cells.

Symptoms of Cervical Cancer

The most common symptom of cervical cancer is abnormal vaginal bleeding, often presenting as postcoital bleeding. Women with cervical cancer also frequently complain of a watery and malodorous discharge. As cervical cancer becomes more progressive, patients may note urinary frequency, bladder pressure, or back pain. In the most advanced cases, patients can present with inguinal lymph node metastasis, lower extremity edema secondary to pelvic sidewall invasion or tumor replacing the pelvic lymph nodes, or in stage IV cases vesicovaginal or rectovaginal fistula.

Physical Findings of Cervical Cancer

The physical examination findings of cervical cancer are an essential component to the clinical staging of this cancer. The examination focuses on defining the extent of local invasion, primarily by pelvic examination. This examination includes visual inspection of the cervix and vagina, bimanual pelvic/abdominal examination, and rectovaginal examination. Evidence of vaginal mucosal involvement, parametrial tumor invasion, uterosacral tumor invasion, rectovaginal septum involvement, and fixation of one or both of the pelvic sidewalls are important considerations. An observational study by Hoffman and colleagues demonstrated only 50% accuracy in predicting tumor diameter when pelvic exam findings were compared with pathology specimens,[10] but clinicians are accurate in predicting other prognostic factors, including outer third invasion (80%) and vaginal involvement (90%). Determining the extent of local and distant metastasis is critical in selecting between surgical and radiotherapy treatment options. Because physical examination findings are not very reliable, especially for tumors larger than 4 cm, most clinicians rely on magnetic resonance imaging (MRI), computed tomography (CT), and positron emission tomography (PET) imaging, when available, to better define the extent of disease. The most common patterns of spread of cervical cancer are direct extension and lymphatic metastasis. Examination of the groin and supraclavicular nodes for evidence of extensive nodal spread is critically important. Although hematogenous metastasis is less likely, especially with early cervical cancer, chest radiography at a minimum is indicated in the initial evaluation of all patients.

Histologic Diagnosis of Cervical Cancer

A clinical diagnosis or cytology diagnosis of cervical cancer must be confirmed by biopsy-proven histology. A cytologic evaluation is not definitive evidence of invasive disease in these patients and is rarely adequate evidence to proceed with treatment. A colposcopically directed biopsy for a patient with a visual lesion is generally adequate for establishing the diagnosis, and these patients can usually be spared the risks and treatment delay that may result from a surgical biopsy known as cold knife conization. The pathologic diagnosis of invasive disease is sometimes difficult in women with a small lesion and only minimal invasion. The histologic features of early invasion of squamous cancer of the cervix include differentiation of the invading squamous cells and a brisk adjacent inflammatory response. Involvement of the endocervical glands by carcinoma in-situ is a common finding in preinvasive disease, and any question of invasion versus glandular involvement deserves thorough pathology review. For patients with a microinvasive lesion, complete excision of the lesion by cervical conization with negative margins is mandatory to determine the extent of disease and the risk of metastatic disease.

Pathology

Squamous cell carcinoma and adenocarcinoma are the most frequent histopathologic types of cervical carcinoma. Squamous cell carcinoma has been subcategorized into keratinizing, nonkeratinizing, and small cell carcinomas. Adenocarcinoma has been subcategorized to include endometrioid adenocarcinoma, endocervical adenocarcinoma, and clear cell adenocarcinoma. Other much less common histologies seen with cervical cancer include adenosquamous carcinoma, small cell carcinoma, adenoid cystic carcinoma, and undifferentiated carcinoma.

Squamous Cell Carcinoma

The majority of squamous cell carcinomas are exophytic or ulcerative lesions that arise within the transformation zone of the cervix. These lesions are generally visible on the ectocervix and are easily biopsied. The current classification scheme for squamous cell carcinomas was developed by the World Health Organization and divides these tumors into large cell keratinizing, large cell nonkeratinizing, and small cell nonkeratinizing types. The presence of keratin pearls is required for the tumor to be classified as keratinizing.[11] Small cell squamous carcinomas are as common as the keratinizing large cell carcinomas and are characterized by focal squamous differentiation without keratin pearl formation. It is important to distinguish small cell squamous carcinoma from small cell undifferentiated carcinoma, which may have neuroendocrine features and a significantly more-aggressive behavior.

Verrucous carcinoma is a variant of squamous cell carcinoma that is characterized by its exophytic growth resembling a giant condyloma. Verrucous carcinomas tend to be locally aggressive and may spread to adjacent organs including the vagina and the endometrium. The malignant behavior of this tumor is unpredictable, although some have suggested that the risk of nodal metastasis is considerably lower. Nodal metastases have been reported with this tumor, as has aggressive dedifferentiation when treated with radiotherapy.

Invasive Adenocarcinoma

In the United States and other developed countries where cervical cancer screening is common, there has been a relative increase in the incidence of adenocarcinomas of the cervix. In some studies adenocarcinomas now comprise between 15% and 25% of invasive cervical carcinomas. Adenocarcinomas are most commonly mucinous adenocarcinoma arising from endocervical glands, usually developing within the endocervical canal. These tumors are likely to be endophytic and may expand the cervix before becoming clinically apparent. Although the prognosis associated with adenocarcinomas has remained controversial, most studies have demonstrated that prognosis is similar to squamous lesions size for size and stage for stage. In one recently published Italian randomized clinical trial of radical surgery versus radiation therapy for stage 1B and 2A cervical cancer, 46 of the 343 patients had adenocarcinomas. In that study, there is a suggestion that adenocarcinomas were more radiation resistant as the overall survival for adenocarcinoma patients treated with surgery was 79% versus 59% for patients treated with radiotherapy. This difference was statistically significant for the adenocarcinoma group, but in the squamous cell carcinoma group there was no difference in survival.[12] Intestinal-type mucinous adenocarcinomas of the cervical canal have the histologic appearance of cells that would ordinarily arise as intestinal adenocarcinomas but in this case arise within the endocervical canal. Endometrioid adenocarcinoma has a histologic appearance of its endometrial counterpart. It is important to distinguish the primary location of this tumor as it may represent endocervical extension of an endometrial carcinoma.

Well-differentiated villoglandular adenocarcinomas are a variant of adenocarcinoma typically seen in young women and may be associated with oral contraceptive use. Initial reports of this tumor included no recurrences or deaths among 37 patients, suggesting that metastasis was unlikely. Unfortunately, subsequent cases of metastatic disease, especially nodal metastasis, have been reported and are typically associated with deep cervical invasion; this is an important distinction that has lead to the recommendation that these patients be treated in the same fashion as any other adenocarcinoma of the cervix.[13]

Clear cell carcinoma of the cervix can be seen in patients with a history of diethylstilbesterol (DES) exposure or as an extremely rare variant of adenocarcinoma. These tumors frequently present at an advanced stage and as a high-grade lesion and have a relatively poor prognosis.[14]

Adenosquamous carcinoma is a cervical cancer with both squamous and glandular features. These tumors can have a wide range of presentations, including atypical squamous cell carcinoma with small areas of mucin to an endometrioid-appearing carcinoma with squamous differentiation, to a single carcinoma of endocervical type with both squamous and glandular differentiation. Some controversy is expressed within the literature as to whether the prognosis associated with this malignancy is unfavorable, and it likely depends on which of these different types of adenosquamous carcinoma is involved.[11]

Neuroendocrine small cell undifferentiated carcinoma is a very aggressive malignancy that is characterized by the presence of neuroendocrine granules. This highly aggressive tumor has been identified as having a very poor prognosis, with a 5-year survival as low as 14%.[15]

Adenoid cystic carcinoma is a malignant lesion with poor prognosis that resembles its more-common counterpart within the salivary glands. It is very important to distinguish adenoid cystic carcinomas from adenoid basal carcinoma, which is typically a small lesion associated with cervical dysplasia or early invasive squamous cancer and carrying with it a very good prognosis.

Although a wide range of histologies can arise within the uterine cervix, the treatment principles for these lesions are generally quite similar. The exceptions are neuroendocrine small cell carcinomas, which have an extremely aggressive behavior, and villoglandular and verrucous carcinomas, which are not particularly aggressive. With neuroendocrine tumors, many clinicians have advocated using lung cancer chemotherapy regimens in addition to chemoradiation; however, there are no prospective trial data for this rare histology that support or confirm the benefit of this management.

Staging and Pretreatment Evaluation

Cervical cancer is staged clinically because the majority of patients are treated with a nonsurgical therapy. The commonly accepted staging system for cervical cancer was adopted by the International Federation of Gynecology and Obstetrics (FIGO) in 1994 (Table 50.1; 2002 staging).[16] The clinical staging rules are based on clinical evaluation and basic radiographic studies. The only examinations of the patient allowed for staging include palpation, inspection, colposcopy with biopsy and endocervical curettage, cervical conization, hysteroscopy, proctoscopy, intravenous pyelogram, and plain film radiographs of the chest and bones. Suspected bladder or rectal involvement must be confirmed by biopsy, with histologic evidence of invasion into the mucosa of either the bladder or rectum required for a diagnosis of involvement of those organs. If there is any doubt between two stages, the lower stage must be chosen. Because the majority of patients with cervical cancer are treated in the underdeveloped world where CT scans and MRI are not available, the use of those studies has not been adopted for the clinical staging of cervical cancer. Patients undergoing surgical assessment or further radiographic assessment with newer imaging modalities should have these findings noted and treatment directed based on the results of these studies, even though they are not allowed to change the clinical staging for these patients. Fine-needle aspiration of scan-detected suspicious lymph nodes may be helpful in treatment planning but is not allowed as part of the staging.

TABLE 50.1. International Federation of Gynecology and Obstetrics (FIGO) staging of cervical cancer, 2002.

Carcinoma of the cervix uteri	
Stage 0	Carcinoma in situ.
Stage I	Cervical carcinoma confined to uterus (extension to corpus should be disregarded).
Stage IA	Invasive carcinoma diagnosed only by microscopy. All macroscopically visible lesions, even with superficial invasion, are IB. Stromal invasion with a maximal depth of 5.0mm measured from the base of the epithelium and a horizontal spread of 7.0mm or less. Vascular space involvement, venous or lymphatic, does not affect classification. IA1—Measured stromal invasion of 3.0mm or less in depth and 7.0mm or less in horizontal spread. IA2—Measured stromal invasion more than 3.0mm and not more than 5.0mm with a horizontal spread 7.0mm or less.
Stage IB	Clinically visible lesions confined to the cervix or microscopic lesion greater than IA2. IB1—Clinically visible lesion 4cm or less in greatest dimension. IB2—Clinically visible lesion more than 4cm in greatest dimension.
Stage II	Cervical carcinoma invades beyond the uterus, but not to the pelvic wall or to the lower third of the vagina. IIA—Tumor without parametrial invasion. IIB—Tumor with parametrial invasion.
Stage III	Tumor extends to pelvic wall and/or involves lower third of the vagina and/or hydronephrosis or nonfunctioning kidney. IIIA—Tumor involves lower third of vagina, no extension to pelvic wall. IIIB—Tumor extends to pelvic wall and/or hydronephrosis or nonfunctioning kidney.
Stage IVA	Tumor invades mucosa of the bladder or rectum and/or extends beyond true pelvis (bullous edema is not sufficient evidence to classify a tumor as T4).

Source: Used with the permission of the American Joint Committee on Cancer (AJCC), Chicago, Illinois. The original source for this material is the *AJCC Cancer Staging Manual*, sixth edition (2002), published by Springer-Verlag New York, www.springer-ny.com.

Although the rules for clinical staging are very clear that only plain film radiographs and routine available examination techniques may be considered in the assignment of the clinical stage, most patients in the United States are further investigated either by surgical staging or with noninvasive diagnostic studies ranging from lymphangiography to PET scanning. The goal of more-extensive imaging evaluation is to better define the radiation treatment fields and doses. The risk of paraaortic lymph node metastasis is 16% for stage II disease and 29% for stage III cervical cancer.[17] The added toxicity of including the paraaortic lymph nodes in the radiation field has motivated investigators to look for better ways to identify nodal disease.

For many years, bipedal lymphangiography was considered to be one of the more-sensitive techniques for identifying nodal metastasis in cervical cancer patients. The difficulty in reading lymphangiograms as well as the technical challenges of performing this study combined with the side effects and high false-positive rate have led to lymphangiography falling out of favor. CT and MRI remain popular tools for better defining nodal metastasis and evaluating tumor size and parametrial infiltration.

Magnetic resonance imaging may be particularly important in evaluating patients as possible candidates for surgical therapy because it is useful in identifying parametrial invasion, a relative contraindication to primary surgical therapy in cervical cancer. Pakkal and colleagues evaluated the accuracy of MRI for the assessment of parametrial and lymph node involvement in cervical cancer patients undergoing surgical therapy. They compared the surgical staging and pathology findings with the MRI results and found accuracy in detecting parametrial and lymph node involvement in patients with cervical carcinoma to be 71% and 86%, respectively. Their conclusion was that MRI helps decide operability and the type of operation and aids in the selection of patients who need to be considered for specialist referral to a gynecologic oncologist.[18] A recent retrospective analysis of 106 consecutive cervical cancer patients treated in the United Kingdom showed that pretreatment tumor volume measured using MRI with both an endovaginal and an external coil provides a more-accurate prediction of prognosis and defines a population at high risk of recurrence and death. Their results suggest that a tumor volume of 13 cm^3 or greater is associated with poor prognosis and is more important in determining outcome than depth of invasion or invasion beyond the cervix.[19]

Recent studies of strategies to detect cervical cancer metastasis have focused on ^{18}F-fluorodeoxyglucose positron emission tomography (FDG-PET scanning) and on surgical staging with or without sentinel node biopsies. These studies have shown the utility of both surgical staging and PET scanning in detecting occult nodal disease and in treatment planning. A study by Grigsby and colleagues at Washington University demonstrated excellent lymph node control in a group of 208 women with cervical cancer evaluated by both PET and CT scan. They accomplished control of PET-positive pelvic and paraaortic lymph nodes in most patients using radiation doses tailored to the size of the lymph nodes and the PET status of the nodal disease. They found no nodal failures in the 76 patients with PET-negative pelvic lymph nodes less than or equal to 1 cm when treated with a nodal radiation mean dose of 66.8 Gy. They also showed remarkably good regional control for patients with PET-positive pelvic nodes as follows: only 3 of 89 failures for nodes less than or equal to 1 cm treated with 66.8 Gy, and for nodes ranging from 3.1 to 4.0 cm treated with 74.1 Gy, there were no failures in the 5 patients. There were no failures for the 33 women with PET-positive paraaortic lymph nodes ranging up to 3 cm in diameter when treated with a mean paraaortic lymph node dose of 43.3 Gy. The most common site of failure in this study was distant metastasis, which was best predicted by PET-positive lymph nodes of any size.[20]

Surgical staging with laparoscopic lymphadenectomy has been markedly refined over the past decade. Thorough evaluation of the pelvic and paraaortic lymph nodes can now be accomplished with minimal morbidity for these women. Although minimally invasive surgery (MIS) using laparoscopy is thorough and safe, the survival benefit of this surgical staging has not been established in a clinical trial and is unlikely to be so in the future. It is difficult to justify the need to identify occult positive lymph nodes by surgical resection considering the nodal control rates demonstrated by Grigsby using PET and CT imaging and with the improved regional control now seen with the combination of chemotherapy and radiotherapy.[20]

The use of sentinel lymph node biopsies has been studied as a strategy to plan radiation treatment fields and minimize the complications of complete lymphadenectomy, most notably lymphedema. Although some of these trials have reported an excellent correlation between the sentinel node and subsequent lymphadenectomy results, others have failed to demonstrate the excellent results seen in breast cancer and melanoma. A prospective clinical study from France in particular raises concern about the use of sentinel lymph node biopsy as a strategy for further improving on surgical staging. In this study of 28 patients, multilevel sectioning followed by cytokeratin immunohistochemistry was used to identify micrometastasis within lymph nodes. Five of the 28 patients had metastasis; in 2 patients these metastases were in the sentinel lymph node, but in the other 3 patients the sentinel lymph node was negative and the metastases were in nonsentinel pelvic lymph nodes.[21]

Currently, in the United States most women with cervical cancer undergo thorough pretreatment staging with chest radiograph and either CT scan or MRI. PET scanning is also rapidly being integrated into the treatment planning, especially for patients being treated with chemoradiation. Pretreatment cystoscopy and proctosigmoidoscopy are generally reserved for patients with radiographic or clinical evidence of bladder or rectal invasion. Prospective randomized trials showing improved outcomes, in particular improved survival, with either surgical or PET staging have not been published.[22]

Treatment

Stage I Cervical Cancer

The treatment of cervical cancer is divided into two groups of patients, those with early disease, stage I, and those with advanced disease, stage II and beyond. In early local disease, the decision is between surgical therapy and chemoradiation therapy. For cervical cancer patients, surgery and radiation therapy are equally effective in stage 1 disease, and the decision on which treatment modality to use is based primarily on patient preference and the respective side effects. Stage 1a cervical carcinoma represents microscopic disease and is broken down into two subgroups; stage 1a1 is microinvasive disease with stromal invasion of 3 mm or less, squamous histology, and less than or equal to 7 mm of horizontal spread of the lesion. Ostor et al. reported on more than 3,000 women who met the criteria for stage 1a1 disease and found the incidence of lymph node metastasis is about 1%.[23] The recurrence rate is about 1% and the death rate is 0.2% for stage 1a1 cervical carcinoma. The treatment options range from cervical conization, which is adequate treatment so long as all margins are free of disease, to extrafascial hysterectomy.

For patients with lymphovascular space invasion, there may be an increased risk of nodal metastasis or recurrence, but this is controversial. In DiSaia and Creasman's *Clinical Gynecologic Oncology*, it is stated: " . . . the role of vascular space involvement in this group of patients does not predict lymph node metastasis nor recurrence."[24] However, Benedette et al. showed, in these stage 1a1 patients with lymphovascular space invasion, an increased risk of recurrence in the range of 3% to 4%.[25,26] Based on these findings, the presence of lymphovascular invasion suggests the need for more-radical treatment with particular attention paid to the regional lymph nodes.

Patients with 1a2 cervical carcinoma have a significantly greater risk of lymph node metastasis, in the range of 6%.[27] Stage 1a2 is characterized as having more than 3 mm but not more than 5 mm of invasion and still less than 7 mm of horizontal spread. As invasion into the cervical stromal increases, so does the risk of lymph node metastasis. This higher risk of nodal metastasis precludes conservative therapy with cervical conization or extrafascial hysterectomy. Management of these early cervical carcinomas must include evaluation or treatment of the regional lymph nodes. Surgical therapy with radical hysterectomy and pelvic lymphadenectomy results in a 95% 5-year survival.

A fertility-sparing variation avoiding radical hysterectomy is radical trachelectomy with pelvic lymphadenectomy. The published results of this procedure using a vaginal and laparoscopic approach have outcomes that are comparable to radical pelvic surgery.[28–30] The best candidates for radical trachelectomy have tumor less than 2 cm, no lymphovascular space involvement, stage IA2 or IB1, and either adenocarcinoma or squamous carcinoma (Table 50.2). Pelvic radiotherapy is an acceptable approach for these stage I patients but is generally confined to those women who are not candidates for surgical therapy, because the late side effects of radiotherapy are generally more troublesome than the minimal late effects of surgery. These consequences of pelvic radio-

TABLE 50.2. Radical trachelectomy: a fertility-sparing treatment alternative for early-stage cervical cancer.

Trial	*Reference*	*Year*	*No. of patients*	*Study design*	*Median follow-up*	*Procedures aborted*	*Recurrence rate*	*Survival*
Plante	28	2004	82	Prospective serial	60 months	10	4.2%	2.8%
Covens	29	2002	93	Prospective	30 months	0	7.3%	4.2%

The patients with recurrent disease generally have tumors more than 2cm or high-risk histology. The best candidates for radical trachelectomy have tumor less than 2cm, no lymphovascular space involvement, stage IA2 or IB1 disease, and either adenocarcinoma or squamous carcinoma.[30]

therapy include radiation cystitis, proctitis, and ovarian failure in premenopausal patients.

Microinvasive Adenocarcinoma

The concept of microinvasive adenocarcinoma is controversial because of a lack of extensive data on prognosis for these patients and a lack of a clear definition of microinvasion for glandular lesions. The definition of microinvasion is challenging because these tumors tend to arise within endocervical glands, making the point of measurement difficult. It is debated whether invasion should be from the base of the surface epithelium or from the endocervical gland. The volume of involved stroma and the risk of lymphovascular space invasion by these tumors vary considerably depending on where in the endocervical canal the lesion arises. Glandular lesions also tend to be multifocal as evidenced by a study by Ostor et al. in which 27% of the 77 patients had multicentric lesions.[31] In patients with adenocarcinoma lesions invading from 2 to 5mm, Berek et al. identified positive lymph nodes in 2 of 18 women.[32] Both Ostor and Berek report no lymph node metastasis in women with less than 2mm of invasion.

Successful treatment of microinvasive cervical carcinoma requires a strict adherence to the staging definitions. The diagnosis of microinvasive disease is based on complete surgical resection of the lesion by cone biopsy with negative surgical margins. When these criteria are met and other factors such as lymphovascular space invasion are taken into account, we can expect a death rate of much less than 1% for stage 1a1 lesions and a death rate of approximately 2.4% for stage 1a2 lesions.

Stage 1B

When the tumor exceeds 5mm of invasion or 7mm of lateral extent or is visible but confined to the uterine cervix, it is stage 1b. Tumor size is the most important prognostic factor in stage 1 lesions and therefore stage 1b has been further categorized into stage 1b1, where the tumor is less than or equal to 4cm in size, and stage 1b2, which is greater than 4cm. The overall survival for patients with stage 1b cervical carcinoma is comparable whether they are treated with radical hysterectomy and pelvic lymphadenectomy or primary radiotherapy. An Italian prospective randomized clinical trial in stage 1b cervical cancer compared radical hysterectomy with primary radiotherapy.[12] In this study, patients undergoing radical hysterectomy who had high-risk features identified in the pathology specimen then received adjuvant radiotherapy also. The two treatment groups had identical 5-year survival (83%), comparing the radiation group with the surgery plus tailored postoperative radiotherapy group. Severe toxicity was noted in 28% of patients in the surgery group and only in 12% of patients in the radiotherapy group. In this study, 54% of the stage 1b1 patients (those with tumors 4cm or less) received adjuvant radiotherapy, and 84% of the stage 1b2 patients received adjuvant radiotherapy. This study clearly served to highlight the added toxicity that results from combining surgery and radiotherapy in this patient population. In the current era of treating all radiotherapy patients with concurrent chemotherapy, the rationale of including a treatment group that receives both surgery and radiation is increasingly difficult to support. A justification voiced for combining surgery and radiotherapy is the concept that large tumors may have poor oxygenation, compromising the radiation effectiveness and therefore hampering the central pelvic control. To date there are no controlled trials supporting that concern, and with the increasing effectiveness of the chemoradiation schema's central pelvic control it is unlikely to be a critical issue in stage I disease treated with chemoradiotherapy.

Although radical hysterectomy clearly has the option of preserving ovarian function and minimizing the late effects of radiation therapy, there remains a role for postoperative adjuvant therapy in radical hysterectomy patients with specific risk factors. The addition of pelvic radiotherapy with concurrent cisplatin chemotherapy significantly improves the overall survival rate when compared to radiation therapy alone for patients with metastatic disease in the form of pelvic nodal metastasis, positive margins, or extension into the parametrial tissues.[33] Radical hysterectomy patients with negative lymph nodes but with large tumors, deep cervical stromal invasion, and lymphovascular space involvement also benefit from adjuvant radiotherapy. A Gynecologic Oncology Group (GOG) study of 277 women with stage 1b1 cervical cancer and negative lymph nodes identified that those with risk factors including tumor size greater than 4 cm, stromal invasion greater than one-third of the cervical stroma, or presence of lymphovascular space involvement benefited from adjuvant pelvic radiotherapy.[34] In this study, the recurrence rates were 15% for those patients who received radiotherapy and 28% for those who received no further therapy. In that study, the grade 3 and 4 toxicity rates were 9.3% for the radiotherapy group and only 2.1% for the no further therapy arm, but considering the significant improvement in recurrence-free survival, those toxicities were considered acceptable (Table 50.3).

Stage II–IVA

Chemoradiation

Radiotherapy to the cervix, parametria, and nodal areas at risk for metastatic disease, using external-beam irradiation combined with brachytherapy inserted directly into the cervix, provides a reasonable chance of cure even in advanced disease. The 5-year survival rates are 50% to 80% for stage IIB and 25% to 50% for stage III.[35] There are several different strategies for brachytherapy, ranging from high dose rate (HDR) to low dose rate techniques to interstitial therapy, all with fairly comparable outcomes. Surgery alone is not effective in controlling advanced-stage cervical cancer.

TABLE 50.3. Adjuvant radiotherapy in stage 1 cervical cancer.

Trial	*Year*	*Stage*	*No. of patients*	*Study design*	*Median follow-up*	*Intervention*	*Disease-free survival*	*Conclusions*
Sedlis (GOG 92)[34]	1998	IB	277	Randomized Cooperative Group Trial	5 years	No further therapy versus pelvic radiotherapy	72% versus 85%	For women with at least two risk factors: more than one-third invasion, CLS, or tumor more than 4–5 cm, the addition of pelvic radiotherapy significantly improves disease-free survival RR 0.53, $P = 0.008$
Peters[33]	2000	IA2, IB, IIA	268	Randomized Intergroup Trial	42 months	Radiotherapy alone versus radiotherapy plus chemotherapy: cisplatin 70 mg/m^2, days 1, 22 5-FU 1,000 mg/m^2/day, for 96 hours		The addition of chemotherapy to adjuvant pelvic radiotherapy significantly improves disease-free survival for women with node-positive early-stage disease $P = 0.03$

These two cooperative group trials established the benefit of adjuvant radiotherapy in high-risk early-stage cervical cancer, and that the addition of chemotherapy to adjuvant radiotherapy is beneficial.

The combination of cytotoxic chemotherapy given as a radiation-sensitizing agent has markedly improved outcomes in the last decade. Cisplatin is the most effective single agent and has been shown in cell lines to be synergistic with radiotherapy. The interaction between chemotherapy and radiation inhibits DNA repair after sublethal damage, especially increasing the sensitivity of hypoxic cells.[36] The early side effects of the combination of chemotherapy and radiotherapy are now well known and appear quite safe. The late chronic effects of radiotherapy on the rectum, urinary tract, and vagina may increase with combined therapy, but long-term data are still pending.

In the 1990s, several Phase II studies established the relative safety of combining chemotherapy with radiotherapy for cervical cancer. Although most of the studies were small, two larger series served to demonstrate that combining chemotherapy and radiation in women with cervical cancer was feasible.[37,38] These prospective Phase II studies paved the way for several Phase III trials that ultimately demonstrated the significantly improved outcomes of combination chemotherapy and radiotherapy[39–41] (Table 50.4). This table details the improved disease control and survival and compare the toxicity data from the three pivotal studies. Although the incidence of grade III and IV toxicity is quite variable, one study reported acute grade III and IV toxicity in 49% of patients. As the widespread use of chemoradiation for cervical cancer is still relatively new, the incidence of grade III and IV late toxicity is not yet well defined.

In 1999, with several large randomized trials demonstrating benefit for concomitant cytotoxic chemotherapy with radiation (chemoradiotherapy), the National Cancer Institute issued a clinical alert stating that chemoradiation should be considered for all patients with advanced cervical cancer.[42] These compelling results prompted a recent meta-analysis from the Cochrane Review of data available from 11 trials to directly, or indirectly, estimate a hazard ratio (HR) for overall survival.[43] They found a highly significant overall survival benefit for chemoradiation. The HR of 0.71 across all trials [95% confidence interval (CI) = 0.63–0.81; P less than 0.0001] represents a 29% reduction in the risk of death and an absolute improvement in survival of 12% (95% CI = 8%–16%) from 40% to 52%. For progression-free survival, the overall results also support the use of chemoradiotherapy, with a HR of 0.61 (95% CI = 0.55–0.68) and an absolute improvement in progression-free survival of 16% (95% CI = 13%–19%) from 47% to 63%. The significant toxicities (grade III and IV) for these chemoradiation trials are shown in Table 50.4. As expected, the hematologic toxicity occurred in a significantly greater proportion of patients in the chemoradiotherapy group compared to the control group (white cell count, 16% versus 8%; platelets, 1.5% versus 0.2%; hematologic, 29% versus 1.3%). Grade III or IV gastrointestinal toxicity is also more common in the combined arm (9% versus 4%). Other toxicities including neurologic, skin, and urinary are essentially comparable for the two groups. Late toxicity is only available for one of the large Phase III studies.[40] There is no evidence to date of a difference in the late side effects, but follow-up is still relatively early.

In view of the marked survival benefit of combining chemotherapy with radiation therapy and the relatively minimal impact on toxicity, chemoradiation has emerged as the treatment standard for large or advanced cervical cancer, usually beginning with stage IB2 (lesion greater than 4 cm). The combination of chemotherapy and radiation therapy appears to improve the therapeutic ratio and results in improved local control. The majority of the improvement for these patients is in local control, implying that radiation sensitization is the most important factor in improving outcomes for these patients. However, in the Phase III Gynecologic Oncology Group (GOG) trial the frequency of lung metastasis was 3% and 4% for the two cisplatin arms and 10% for the less-active hydroxyurea arm.[41] These data certainly suggest that some patients may also derive improved distant control when treated with a cisplatin-based regimen.

Initial studies of chemoradiation considered drugs such as hydroxyurea and 5-fluorouracil (5-FU). In the 1980s, with chemoradiation proliferating for the treatment of head and neck malignancies, the promising combination of cisplatin

TABLE 50.4. Radiotherapy with or without chemotherapy as the primary treatment of cervical cancer.

Trial	*Year*	*Stage*	*No. of patients*	*Study design*	*Median follow-up*	*Intervention*	*Progression-free survival*	*Toxicity*	*Conclusions*
Keys (GOG)[39]	1999	IB Tumor > or = to 4 cm	369	Randomized Cooperative Group Trial	36 months	Radiotherapy alone versus radiotherapy combined with cisplatin 40 mg/m^2 weekly for 6 weeks	63% vs. 79% favoring the combined therapy arm	Grade 3–4 Hematologic: 2% vs. 21% GI: 5% vs. 14%	Adding weekly cisplatin to pelvic radiotherapy significantly improves survival, while increasing transient toxicities but not long term toxicity HR 0.51 for combined therapy $P < 0.001$
Morris (RTOG)[40]	1999	IB2-IVA	403	Randomized Cooperative Group Trial	43 months	Radiotherapy alone versus radiotherapy combined with 2 cycles of 5-FU and cisplatin	40% vs. 67% favoring combined therapy	No significant difference in the late side effects	The rates of both local and distant metastasis were significantly higher for the radiotherapy-only arm $P < 0.001$
Rose (GOG)[41]	1999	IIB,III, IVA	526	Randomized Cooperative Group Trial	35 months	Radiotherapy combined with either: weekly cisplatin, vs. 2 cycles of cisplatin, 5-FU and hydroxyurea vs. hydroxurea alone	67% vs. 64% vs. 47%, respectively, at 24 months	There were no treatment related deaths; the three-drug regimen had the highest frequency of adverse events	Regimens that combine cisplatin with radiotherapy improve survival in locally advanced cervical cancer $P < 0.001$

Randomized cooperative group trials have clearly demonstrated the benefit of combining cisplatin with radiotherapy in the treatment of cervical cancer.

and 96-hour 5-FU was tested in several Phase II trials. In the GOG trial that compared cisplatin alone or in combination, the rate of progression-free survival was significantly better in the group given radiotherapy combined with cisplatin therapy (109 of 176; P less than 0.001) and for patients given radiotherapy combined with treatment with cisplatin, fluorouracil, and hydroxyurea (106 of 173; P less than 0.001) than among patients in the group given radiotherapy combined with hydroxyurea therapy (73 of 177).[41] The progression-free survival and the overall survival for the group receiving cisplatin 40 mg/m^2 weekly 4 hours before radiotherapy were almost identical to the group receiving cisplatin 50 mg/m^2 days 1 and 29 combined with two 96-hour infusions of 5-FU and hydroxyurea. The frequencies of both grade 3 and grade 4 leukopenia in the group given radiotherapy combined with treatment with cisplatin, fluorouracil, and hydroxyurea were more than double the frequencies in the other two groups (P less than 0.001). Based on comparable efficacy, and less toxicity, the weekly cisplatin 40 mg/m^2 regimen has emerged as the preferred combination chemoradiation treatment.

Neoadjuvant Chemotherapy

The concept of neoadjuvant chemotherapy before surgery or radiotherapy to reduce tumor burden and facilitate local treatment is popular in some parts of the world.[44–46] In a randomized prospective trial of 205 women with stage IB cervical cancer with lesions more than 2 cm in diameter, patients were randomly assigned to either surgery followed by radiotherapy or neoadjuvant chemotherapy followed by surgery and adjuvant radiotherapy.[44] The neoadjuvant chemotherapy regimen for this study was three courses of cisplatin 50 mg/m^2, vincristine 1 mg/m^2, and bleomycin 25 mg/m^2 on days 1 to 3, at 10-day intervals. The neoadjuvant chemotherapy arm of this trial had a higher rate of negative margins (100% versus 85%) and significantly fewer pelvic failures. However, there was no significant difference in the overall survival for the study. For the women with larger lesions (stage IB2), there was an improvement in long-term survival with neoadjuvant chemotherapy of 80% versus 61%. A critique of this study is that no chemoradiation was used in the control arm, despite data showing the significant improvement that occurs when chemotherapy is added to adjuvant radiotherapy.[33] A meta-analysis of randomized controlled trials of neoadjuvant chemotherapy before radiotherapy found insufficient evidence of a survival benefit, despite showing a significant reduction in disease volume by chemotherapy.[47]

Radiation Therapy Techniques

The two radiation therapy modalities used in treating cervical cancer are external-beam radiotherapy and brachytherapy. The brachytherapy is usually placed intracavitary, through the cervix into the uterus, using any of a variety of afterloading or high dose rate applicators. Interstitial brachytherapy is used for women with advanced disease involving the lower vagina or extensive parametrial involvement that cannot be adequately treated with an intracavitary insertion.

The American Brachytherapy Society (ABS) has recently published guidelines for the use of either high dose rate or low dose rate brachytherapy as a component of cervical cancer treatment.[48,49] The treatment dose and technique depend on many variables including disease volume, ability to displace the bladder and rectum, and institutional practices. Low-dose brachytherapy, usually with ^{137}Cs, is more common; however, the number of institutions using high dose rate (HDR) applicators with ^{192}Ir is rapidly increasing. The radiation safety and patient convenience factors have made the HDR approach attractive. In several randomized trials of women with cervical cancer, HDR was comparable to low dose rate (LDR) brachytherapy in terms of survival and complication rates. It is now accepted by the GOG as comparable to low dose rate therapy for their clinical trials.[50–52]

Improved regional control of the paraaortic lymph nodes can be accomplished with extended-field radiation. The RTOG conducted a Phase III trial evaluating the effect of prophylactic paraaortic radiation to 45 Gy in patients with tumors greater than 4 cm but confined to IB2 and Stage II cervical cancers. In this trial of patients who were without clinical evidence of paraaortic nodal disease, there was a significantly better 5-year survival rate of 66% versus 55% favoring the paraaortic extended-field arm.[53] In this trial, severe gastrointestinal toxicity, especially in patients with a history of prior abdominal surgery, was more common in the extended-field group. Future clinical trials will need to address whether pretreatment evaluation using newer modalities such as PET scan can eliminate the role of empiric extended-field radiation for patients with poor prognostic factors such as tumor size greater than 4 cm or high-risk histology.

Primary and Recurrent Distant Metastatic Disease

For patients presenting with stage IVB disease, or recurring with distant metastatic disease, the prognosis is quite poor, with only 20% surviving for 1 year. For these women the role of chemotherapy is palliative; a complete response to chemotherapy is quite rare. The single-agent response rates to various agents typically range from 25% for cisplatin to 17% for paclitaxel. Studies of multiagent regimens have shown improved response rates but no improvement in survival. Compared with cisplatin alone, cisplatin plus ifosfamide had a significantly higher response rate (33% versus 19%) and progression-free survival (PFS) (4.6 versus 3.2 months), but no significant improvement in survival. As expected, the adverse side effects of neutropenia, nephrotoxicity, and neurotoxicity were increased in the ifosfamide-containing arm.[54] Additional evidence of the lack of benefit comes from another GOG trial that compared cisplatin 50 mg/m^2 every 3 weeks versus paclitaxel 135 mg/m^2 and cisplatin 50 mg/m^2. This study, GOG 169, demonstrated response rates of 19% and 36% for the single- versus two-drug regimens, respectively. In this trial again the median PFS was improved for the two-drug regimen, but there was no difference in the overall survival or quality of life between single-agent cisplatin and the two-drug regimen.[55] Recently, Long et al. reported on a GOG Phase III study comparing cisplatin alone with cisplatin and 3-day topotecan that demonstrated a significant improvement in survival for the women receiving the cisplatin and topotecan combination. This regimen of cisplatin 50 mg/m^2 on day 1 and topotecan 0.75 mg/m^2 on days 1 to 3 had a progression-free survival of 4.6 months and an overall survival of 9.4 months. The authors suggest, based on these results, which are superior to any Phase III results reported to date, that the cisplatin/topotecan doublet should be the new standard therapy[56] (Table 50.5).

TABLE 50.5. Chemotherapy for cervical cancer.

Trial	*Year*	*Stage*	*No. of patients*	*Study design*	*Intervention*	*Response rate*	*Progression-free survival (PFS)*	*Survival*	*Toxicity*	*Conclusions*
Moore (GOG)[55]	2004	IVB, recurrent or persistent	280	Randomized Cooperative Group Trial	Cisplatin with or without paclitaxel	19% for cisplatin alone, 36% for cisplatin and paclitaxel.	2.8 months vs. 4.8 months $P < 0.001$	8.8 vs. 9.7 months not significant	Grade 3 & 4 anemia, 13% vs. 28%	Adding paclitaxel to cisplatin improves the response rate and PFI but did not significantly improve survival
Omura (GOG)[54]	1997	IVB, recurrent or persistent	454	Randomized Cooperative Group Trial	Cisplatin versus cisplatin plus mitolactol versus cisplatin and ifosfamide	18% for cisplatin alone, and 31% for cisplatin and ifosfamide; mitolactol showed no benefit	3.2 months vs. 4.6 months $P = 0.003$	8.0 vs. 8.3 months Not significant	CNS toxicity was greater with addition of ifosfamide	The addition of ifosfamide improved the response rate and PFS compared with cisplatin given alone, but is more toxic and does not improve survival
Long[56]	2004	IVB, recurrent or persistent	356	Randomized Cooperative Group Trial	Cisplatin versus topotecan and cisplatin versus methotrexate, vinblastine, adriamycin, cisplatin (MVAC)	19% for cisplatin alone, and 27% with the addition of topotecan (including 10% CR)	2.9 months vs. 4.6 months $P = 0.014$	6.5 months vs. 9.4 months $P = 0.017$	MVAC arm discontinued because of excessive toxicity	The improved overall survival and best reported duration of survival make topotecan 0.75 mg/m^2 days 1–3 and cisplatin 50 mg/m^2 the most active regimen reported to date

The addition of a second active drug to the chemotherapy regimen for women with recurrent or metastatic cervical cancer improves PFI and response rate. Before the cisplatin and topotecan doublet, there was no improvement in overall survival with the addition of a second drug.

SALVAGE SURGICAL THERAPY

RADICAL SURGERY AND EXENTERATION

In selected patients with central pelvic recurrence after radiation therapy, it is possible to completely resect this disease with either a radical hysterectomy or a total pelvic exenteration. Total pelvic exenteration involves the surgical removal of the bladder, uterus, cervix, parametria, vagina, and rectum. In most cases, this is accompanied by reconstruction of the vagina, formation of a urinary conduit, and reanastamosis of the rectal stump. The place of pelvic exenteration as salvage therapy continues to decrease as radiotherapy treatments and chemoradiation have markedly improved the central pelvic control for women with cervical cancer. For the rare patient with an isolated distant recurrence, such as a single pulmonary lesion, consideration should be given to surgical resection or local radiotherapy, acknowledging that there are no data demonstrating a large group of such survivors.

Posttreatment Surveillance

After completing treatment, cervical cancer patients are typically evaluated every 3 to 4 months for 2 years, then every 6 months until 5 years, and annually therafter.[57] The role of the Papanicolaou (Pap) smear as posttreatment surveillance is controversial. The National Comprehensive Cancer Network (NCCN) Clinical Practice Guidelines recommend obtaining a cytology specimen at each visit. However, in a retrospective evaluation of 1,096 Stage Ib cervical cancer patients treated at the M.D. Anderson Cancer Center between 1983 and 1993, all asymptomatic pelvic recurrences were diagnosed by pelvic examination. In this study, there were 114 symptomatic and 19 asymptomatic recurrences, and Pap smears did not detect a single asymptomatic recurrence.[58] Furthermore, there are no data to suggest that additional surveillance strategies with CT scan, MRI, or blood tests for squamous cell carcinoma antigen levels are of any survival benefit.

Vulvar Cancer

Vulvar cancer remains a relatively uncommon gynecologic malignancy, with an estimate of 4,000 new cases in the United States in 2004 and only 850 estimated deaths.[59] The 5-year survival for this cancer ranges from 98% for stage I disease to 31% for women with stage IV disease.[60] This cancer occurs primarily in elderly women with a mean age at diagnosis of 65 years old, and a significant fraction of these cases occur in women over the age of 80. Because of the socially awkward location of vulvar cancer and the associated symptoms, there is often a delay in the diagnosis of this relatively slow-growing malignancy. In addition to the patient's reluctance to complain about a vulvar lesion, a component of physician delay in the diagnosis of vulvar cancer is also common. Many of these patients report symptoms of vulvar cancer lasting for more than a year before the definitive diagnosis. Since 1960 when Dr. Stanley Wei first described the radical surgical resection of vulvar cancer, we have made remarkable progress in the treatment of this disease and in our ability to preserve structure and function of the lower genital tract, bladder, and rectum.[61]

Background and Etiology

There is no clear etiology to the development of vulvar cancer. There is an association between human papillomavirus (HPV) and the development of vulvar intraepithelial neoplasia, which is a preinvasive precursor to some but not all vulvar carcinoma. In contrast to cervical cancer, only a fraction of patients with vulvar carcinoma have tumors positive for the human papillomavirus. This group of patients tends to be younger, often uses tobacco products, and is more likely to have multifocal disease. HPV-positive patients also include women who are chronically immunosuppressed, either because of steroid use for connective tissue diseases, asthma, or organ transplantation or from human immunodeficiency virus (HIV) infection. Because of this causal association with human papillomavirus, the risk factors for vulvar cancer also include sexual activity and a history of genital warts.

For elderly women, the association with human papillomavirus is usually absent. A significant fraction of these women, however, do have an associated vulvar dystrophy. The most common of the associated vulvar dystrophies is lichen sclerosis. It has estimated that as many as 50% of elderly women with vulvar cancer have associated lichen sclerosis. For women with lichen sclerosis, however, the likelihood of developing vulvar carcinoma may be as high as 21%, with overexpression of p53 identified as a potential factor in the etiology of this cancer.[62]

Symptoms of Vulvar Cancer

The most common symptom of vulvar cancer is pruritus. Because itching and discomfort are often associated with lichen sclerosis, those symptoms are frequently dismissed by elderly women and/or their physicians. Other symptoms include vulvar bleeding, a painful mass, malodorous discharge, or enlarged inguinal lymph nodes.

Signs of Vulvar Cancer

Vulvar cancer generally presents as an ulcerated red lesion that is slightly raised and friable. Occasionally the patient has a wartlike thick plaque with what appears to be intact epithelium. These lesions, particularly ulcerated lesions, can be quite tender to palpation.

HISTOLOGIC DIAGNOSIS

Vulvar cancer is diagnosed by histologic biopsy, typically accomplished by using either a Keyes or Baker punch biopsy. Ideally, the biopsy should be obtained from the center of the lesion and should be deep enough to include the underlying tissue to establish the presence of invasion and the depth of invasion. An excisional biopsy is not warranted unless needed to distinguish between a noninvasive lesion and early invasion. If there is a suggestion of a large raised lesion being noninvasive, then wide local excision of that lesion

TABLE 50.6. Vulvar cancer: tumor size as a risk factor for lymph node metastasis.

Study	Year	No. of patients	Trial design	<2.1 cm	2.1–3.0 m	3.1–4 cm	>4 cm
Homesley et al.[60] (GOG)	1991	381	Prospective Cooperative Group Surgicopathology Study	36 of 190 19%	55 of 175 31%	44 of 81 54%	64 of 134 48%

In one of the only prospective vulvar cancer trials, size greater than 2 cm was established as an important prognostic indicator of risk for nodal metastasis.

should be preformed to establish the presence or absence of invasion.

Patterns of Spread

Vulvar cancer spreads primarily by direct extension to the adjacent vagina, urethra, perineum, and rectum. As the depth of invasion increases and the lateral extent of this disease increases, so does the risk of metastatic spread to the inguinal/femoral lymph nodes. Fortunately, hematogenous spread is generally a late occurrence associated with either advanced nodal involvement, or recurrent cancer. The lymphatic spread of vulvar cancer is in an orderly fashion, starting in the inguinal femoral region and then, as those lymph nodes become involved, spreading to the pelvic lymph nodes. Isolated pelvic lymph node metastasis, without inguinal femoral node involvement, is quite rare. The incidence of inguinal lymph node metastasis ranges from 10% for stage 1 disease up to 89% for patients with stage 4 disease. The most important predictors of lymph node metastasis are stage, tumor size (Table 50.6), and depth of invasion. Only 20% of patients with positive groin nodes have positive pelvic lymph nodes.

Hematogenous Metastasis

Hematogenous metastasis of vulvar cancer is a rare late occurrence. Most patients with hematogenous spread of their disease have advanced-stage vulvar cancer and in most cases have positive pelvic lymph nodes. A small fraction of these patients with widely metastatic disease develop a paraneoplastic hypercalcemia, either as a direct consequence of their squamous cell carcinoma or secondary to their lung metastasis.

Pathology

Squamous cell carcinoma is the most common histology causing vulvar cancer. Vulvar melanomas are quite rare in comparison to squamous cell carcinoma of the vulva and account for less than 5% of vulvar cancers. Basal cell carcinomas may also occur on the vulva and represent only about 2% of vulvar cancers. Extramammary Paget's disease of the vulva is generally an adenocarcinoma in situ, but in 10% to 12% of patients there is an underlying invasive component of Paget's disease and in 4% to 8% of patients there is an underlying gastrointestinal (GI) tract adenocarcinoma.[63] Adenocarcinoma of the vulva may also arise within the Bartholin's gland and simulate a vulvar primary cancer. Bartholin's gland cancer is generally managed as a vulvar cancer; half the cancers arising within the Bartholin's gland are squamous malignancies and the other half are adenocarcinoma.

Verrucous carcinoma is an uncommon variant of squamous cell carcinoma of the vulva that is associated with exophytic growth which may result in a very large warty tumor of the vulva. Verrucous carcinomas tend to be slow growing and locally invasive with a relatively low likelihood of lymph node metastasis.[64] Some reports have suggested that radiation therapy may induce a highly malignant transformation of verrucous carcinomas, resulting in subsequent aggressive behavior and regional or distant metastasis. Although that concept was originally reported in 1973, subsequent studies have had difficulty confirming this aggressive behavior associated with radiotherapy.[65]

Melanoma

Vulvar melanomas are a relatively rare malignancy that occurs most commonly in postmenopausal women. The areas of the vulva most commonly affected are the labia minora and the clitoris. Any pigmented lesion of the vulva must be biopsied to rule out melanoma. The other pigmented lesion of the vulva is squamous carcinoma in situ, so careful histologic evaluation of these pigmented lesions is essential in treatment planning. The staging and management of vulvar melanoma follow the treatment guidelines for melanoma rather than squamous malignancies of the vulva.

Staging

The FIGO surgical staging system was most recently revised in 2000 (Table 50.7); within the staging system, depth of invasion is used in stage 1 to distinguish between stage 1a and 1b disease.[66] Depth of invasion is defined as the measurement of tumor from the epithelial–stromal junction of the adjacent most superficial dermal papilla to the deepest point of invasion. Depth of invasion is an important prognostic factor for lymph node metastasis, noting that in many large series tumors with less than 1 mm invasion have no lymph node metastasis, whereas tumors with 1 to 3 mm of invasion have an approximately 8% to 10% risk of nodal metastasis and tumors that invade more than 5 mm have an approximately 35% risk of nodal metastasis.

Pretreatment Evaluation

Radiographic evaluation with chest X-ray and a complete laboratory study are essential in any patient diagnosed with vulvar carcinoma. In addition to the routine cancer staging studies, colposcopy of the vulva, vagina, and cervix is essential to define the extent of preinvasive disease, especially in younger patients where associated preinvasive lesions of the vagina or cervix may be present. A CT scan of the inguinal femoral lymph nodes and pelvis can be helpful in identifying enlarged lymph nodes in the groin or pelvis. This identification is particularly important if nodal disease is suspected as the extent of inguinal femoral lymphadenectomy may be

TABLE 50.7. Staging of vulvar cancer.

Categories	
TX	Primary tumor cannot be assessed
TO	No evidence of primary tumor
Tis	Carcinoma in situ (preinvasive carcinoma)
T1	Tumor confined to vulva or vulva and perineum, 2 cm or less in greatest dimension T1A Tumor confined to vulva or vulva and perineum, 2 cm or less in greatest dimension and with stromal invasion no greater than 1.0 mm* T1B Tumor confined to vulva or vulva and perineum, 2 cm or less in greatest dimension and with stromal invasion greater than 1.0 mm[a]
T2	Tumor confined to the vulva or vulva and perineum, more than 2 cm in greatest dimension
T3	Tumor of any size with contiguous spread to the lower urethra, and/or vagina or anus
T4	Tumor invades any of the following: upper urethra, bladder mucosa, rectal mucosa, or is fixed to the pubic bone

Regional lymph nodes *(N)*:
- NX—Regional lymph nodes cannot be assessed;
- N0—No regional lymph node metastasis;
- N1—Unilateral regional lymph node metastasis;
- N2—bilateral regional lymph node metastases.

Distant metastasis *(M)*.
- MX—Distant metastasis cannot be assessed;
- M0—No distant metastasis;
- M1—Distant metastasis.

Carcinoma of the Vulva: Stage Grouping.

FIGO stage	*Union Internationale Conta la Cancrum (UICC)*		
	T	*N*	*M*
0	Tis	N0	M0
I	T1	N0	M0
IA	T1A	N0	M0
IB	T1B	N0	M0
II	T2	N0	M0
III	T1	N1	M0
	T2	N1	M0
	T3	N1	M0
IVA	T1	N2	M0
	T2	N2	M0
	T3	N2	M0
	T4	Any N	M0
IVB	Any T	Any N	M1

[a]The depth of invasion is defined as the measurement of the tumor from the epithelial–stromal junction of the adjacent most superficial dermal papilla, to the deepest point of invasion.

Histopathologic types:
Squamous cell carcinoma is the most frequent form of cancer of the vulva. Malignant melanoma is the second most common tumor and should be reported separately. Other histopathologic types are adenocarcinoma underlying Paget's disease of vulva, verrucous carcinoma, Bartholin gland carcinoma, adenocarcinoma not otherwise specified (NOS), basal cell carcinoma.

- Histopathologic grades (G):
- Gx—Grade cannot be assessed;
- G1—Well-differentiated;
- G2—Moderately differentiated;
- G3—Poorly or undifferentiated.

Source: Used with the permission of the American Joint Committee on Cancer (AJCC), Chicago, Illinois. The original source for this material is the *AJCC Cancer Staging Manual*, sixth edition (2002), published by Springer-Verlag New York, www.springer-ny.com.

tailored to remove only the involved nodes if it is known that radiotherapy will be administered postoperatively.

Treatment

The surgical management of vulvar carcinoma requires the experience and additional training provided by a Gynecologic Oncology Fellowship. The treatment strategy must focus on adequate radical excision of the local lesion without disrupting the physiologic function of the adjacent bladder, urethra, or rectum. This excision should be designed to consider and preserve sexual functioning if possible. Management of the regional lymph nodes is based on the concept that nodal metastasis occurs by embolization of tumor cells from the primary tumor to the regional lymph nodes. This concept has allowed for surgical management to evolve from an ultraradical massive resection of the inguinal femoral lymph nodes en bloc with the vulva to the use of separate groin incision and a vulvar incision. The ultraradical en bloc excision of groin and vulva was complicated by a 50% to 75% wound breakdown rate and fairly devastating psychosexual morbidity. The transition to less radical surgery and individualized surgical resection has resulted in significantly less operative morbidity without compromising the cure rate. A contemporary radical vulvectomy is now a surgical procedure with a goal of resecting the tumor with a 1.0- to 2.0-cm margin and dissection down to the underlying fascia. A review by Heaps and colleagues from University of California at Los Angeles (UCLA) of 135 vulvar cancer patients with all stages of disease revealed that a 1-cm tumor-free surgical margin resulted in excellent local control.[67] Although the term radical vulvectomy implies that the entire vulva is removed, in fact most vulvar cancers can be managed with a modified procedure that spares the uninvolved vulva. Because many of the lesions only involve the posterior vulva, preservation of the anterior vulva and clitoris is often possible for these patients.

Surgical Management of the Inguinal Femoral Lymph Nodes

The risk of lymph node metastasis ranges from 8% for lesions 2 mm thick to almost 80% for large, deeply invasive lesions. The spread to regional lymph nodes is relatively orderly, beginning with the inguinal lymph nodes before spreading to the pelvic nodes.[68] Lymph node metastases are also reasonably lateralized so that lesions more than 1 to 2 cm from the midline can be managed with unilateral lymphadenectomy. The contralateral nodes are at risk, however, if the ipsilateral groin nodes are positive, and this must be considered in planning any postoperative adjuvant therapy. Involvement of the regional lymph nodes is the most important prognostic indicator in squamous cell carcinoma of the vulva.[60]

Control rates as high as 70% have been reported for patients with positive groin nodes treated by surgical resection and radiation therapy at the time of initial diagnosis. If, however, vulvar cancer recurs in a previously undissected groin, the salvage prospects are very poor.[69] Because of the poor prognosis associated with groin node recurrence, exquisite attention is paid to the thoroughness of the inguinal femoral lymphadenectomy, and an inguinal femoral lymphadenectomy is required in any patient with more than 1 mm of stromal invasion or a lesion more than 2 mm thick.

The serious toxicity associated with inguinal femoral lymphadenectomy includes lymphedema in 15% to 30% of patients and is most common in those women receiving postoperative radiotherapy or those with chronic lymphangitis. This toxicity has prompted investigators to look at modifications to complete lymphadenectomy, many of which have been proposed but not yet verified in a prospective clinical trial. Replacing lymphadenectomy by groin irradiation was studied by the GOG in a randomized trial that was closed early because of excessive number of groin recurrences in the radiotherapy arm. In this study 5 of 26 patients in the radiation-only treatment arm had recurrence in the groin. In the surgical arm of this study, 5 of 23 patients had positive groin nodes and, when they received postoperative radiotherapy, none recurred.[70] This study was later criticized because the target depth dose for the radiation was deemed to be too superficial, at 3 cm, when a quality evaluation of the patients by CT scan revealed the average depth of the groin nodes to be 6 cm.[71]

In a small, 48-patient, retrospective study Petereit and colleagues demonstrated adequate nodal control using groin irradiation and found less morbidity.[72] In view of the poor GOG study outcome, however, it is unlikely that groin irradiation will ever gain a significant place in the primary management of vulvar cancer. Another proposed treatment modification was to perform only a superficial lymphadenectomy, noting that this cancer rarely bypasses the superficial nodes and that if these are positive the patient would receive adjuvant radiotherapy.[73] When this was studied by the GOG, however, there were 6 recurrences in 121 women with negative superficial lymph nodes and early-stage lesions.[74] This disturbingly high recurrence rate suggests that a complete superficial and deep lymphadenectomy should be performed until a proven alternative is found. The most recent proposed treatment modification is sentinel lymph node biopsy, which may allow a much more limited lymph node dissection and consequently a decrease in the associated morbidity such as lymphedema and lymphangitis. In a recent study of 52 patients undergoing primary surgery for vulvar cancer, using isosulfan blue dye a sentinel lymph node was identified in 57 of 76 groins examined (75%) and in 46 of 52 patients (88%).[75] An ongoing GOG trial using both isosulfan blue and lymphoscintigraphy is expected to define the sensitivity and utility of sentinel lymph node biopsies in the management of vulvar cancer.

Advanced Vulvar Cancer

Patients with advanced vulvar cancer comprise three groups with a wide range of prognoses. First, women with evidence of occult nodal metastasis, with one or two positive nodes at the time of radical vulvectomy and inguinal femoral lymphadenectomy, who are then treated with radiotherapy, have a 75% disease-free survival.[60] Women with locally advanced disease involving either the urethra, bladder, rectum, or bilateral enlarged lymph nodes have a 55% to 75% complete response with a combination of surgery, radiation, and in some cases chemotherapy as a radiation-sensitizing agent. Finally, for women with distant metastatic disease, whether it be primary or recurrent, the prognosis is quite poor and these patients are treated with palliative intent.

Patients with more than one microscopic positive groin node metastasis, or occult macroscopically positive nodes, should receive radiation to the bilateral pelvis and groins. This strategy grew out of a GOG randomized trial in which patients with positive groin nodes received either ipsilateral pelvic lymph node dissection or radiotherapy to 45 to 50 Gy. In this trial, the 2-year survival for the radiation group was 68% versus 54% for the surgery group. Recurrence in the groin was rare (5%) in the radiotherapy arm, and occurred in 24% of those women treated with lymphadenectomy alone.[76]

Treating women with large vulvar tumors involving critical structures such as the rectum or urethra with a combination of chemotherapy and radiotherapy can frequently avoid an ultraradical resection of the vulva in combination with the bladder or rectum. This concept was first proposed by Boronow in the early 1970s as an alternative to pelvic exenteration.[77] Boronow later described 37 of his patients, noting a 5-year survival of 75% for locally advanced disease treated with radiotherapy followed by surgery.[78] In the 1980s and 1990s, with radiation-sensitizing chemotherapy emerging for cervical cancer treatment, it was logical to add chemotherapy to the management of these women with locally advanced vulvar cancers. Several studies have considered various combinations of chemotherapy using 5-FU, cisplatin, and mitomycin C either alone or in combination, with 5-year survival as high as 54%.[79–83] The role of surgical resection of the primary tumor site after completion of radiotherapy has been controversial. This procedure is usually complicated by slow and poor wound healing and has not been shown to improve outcomes. Our current recommendation is to reserve surgical resection for the patient with persistent disease and then to anticipate the need to reconstruct the area with a myocutaneous flap to improve to prospects for healing.

Locally Recurrent Disease

Local recurrence of vulvar cancer occurs most commonly in patients with a large primary tumor, a close margin (less than 1 cm),[67] or chronic immunosuppression. For patients with large tumors or close margins, the disease recurrence is usually adjacent to the urethra or rectum, which explains the compromised margin. These lesions are often best managed with local radiotherapy, with or without sensitizing chemotherapy. If surgical resection can be accomplished with adequate margins, then plastic reconstruction is usually required as a component of this procedure. Hoffman and colleagues from the Moffat Cancer Center reported on excellent salvage results using aggressive radiotherapy techniques including interstitial brachytherapy.[84] They report survival of 9 of 10 patients treated with locally aggressive radiotherapy, but also noted severe radiation morbidity in 6 of the 10 women.

Vaginal Cancer

Background

The rarest of the lower genital tract gynecologic malignancies is vaginal cancer; 80% are squamous cell carcinomas, and the remainder are adenocarcinoma, melanoma, and sarcoma. This malignancy mostly occurs in elderly women with a median age of 60 years.[85] Similar to vulvar carcinoma, human papillomavirus appears to be an etiologic agent in some but

TABLE 50.8. FIGO staging of vaginal cancer.

Stage	*Description*
0	Carcinoma in situ
I	Tumor confined to the vagina
II	Tumor invades paravaginal tissues but not to pelvic wall
III	Tumor extends to pelvic wall
IVA	Tumor invades mucosa of the bladder or rectum and/or extends beyond the true pelvis (bullous edema is not sufficient evidence to classify a tumor as T4)

Source: Used with the permission of the American Joint Committee on Cancer (AJCC), Chicago, Illinois. The original source for this material is the *AJCC Cancer Staging Manual*, sixth edition (2002), published by Springer-Verlag New York, www.springer-ny.com.

not all cases of vaginal carcinoma. The presence of vaginal intraepithelial neoplasia, an HPV-related precursor lesion comparable to cervical intraepithelial neoplasia, is present in some patients with squamous cell carcinoma of the vagina. The incidence of precursor lesions and the time to progression from vaginal intraepithelial neoplasia to invasive cancer is not nearly as well defined for vaginal cancer as compared with cervical cancer.[86]

Staging

Vaginal carcinoma is staged according to the criteria of FIGO shown in Table 50.8. The staging of vaginal cancer follows the clinical staging rules for cervical carcinoma. In particular, the stage is assigned on the basis of clinical examination and may include cystoscopy and proctosigmoidoscopy as well as routine laboratory studies and chest X-ray. Further radiographic or other imaging techniques such as CT scan, PET scan, and MRI, although they may be useful in treatment planning, are not allowed as a component of the staging examination.

The FIGO staging of vaginal cancer identifies any vaginal lesion that also involves the cervix as being a cervical cancer. Similarly, any vaginal lesion that also involves the vulva is defined as vulvar carcinoma. In a patient who has a prior history of cervical carcinoma and develops a lesion within the vagina less than 5 years after treatment for cervical cancer, it is considered to be a recurrence of cervical carcinoma, but after 5 years is considered to be a new vaginal carcinoma.

Signs and Symptoms

Irregular vaginal bleeding or profuse watery discharge are the most common symptoms of vaginal carcinoma. Pelvic or back pain, lower extremity swelling, urinary frequency, change in the caliber of stool, or hematochezia are all symptoms of advanced-stage disease.

Diagnosis

Occult vaginal cancer may be diagnosed by Pap smear or colposcopic examination. For patients with a grossly visible lesion, a punch biopsy using a cervical biopsy instrument or Keys punch can be used to provide adequate histologic evidence of this cancer. For patients in whom histology reveals an adenocarcinoma, consideration should be given to other primary sites of disease such as colorectal cancer, metastatic endometrial carcinoma, or a Bartholin's gland cancer. In rare patients adenocarcinoma of the rectovaginal septum may arise in a remnant of residual endometriosis; this is particularly true in patients who may have undergone hysterectomy for endometriosis treatment and then been treated with unopposed estrogen therapy.

Patterns of Spread

Vaginal carcinoma is similar to both vulvar cancer and cervical cancer in its propensity for direct invasion into surrounding tissues and lymphatic metastasis. Although the most common site of vaginal carcinoma is the upper third of the vagina, these generally spread directly to the pelvic lymphatics in a fashion similar to cervical carcinoma. Lesions in the lower one third of the vagina may spread to either the inguinal femoral lymph nodes or the pelvic lymph nodes, so particular care must be taken to ensure that treatment consideration is given to both these sites of lymph nodes.

Treatment

Surgical therapy plays a minor role in the management of vaginal cancer because of the difficulty in obtaining adequate surgical margins. For lesions involving the posterior vagina, the presence of the rectum immediately adjacent to the posterior vaginal wall precludes obtaining an adequate margin for anything but the earliest microinvasive lesion; this is also true for anterior vaginal lesions where the immediately adjacent bladder precludes adequate tissue margin to effect cure by surgery alone. For patients with advanced local disease involving the bladder or rectum, a pelvic exenteration may be required to adequately control this disease.

Radiotherapy

Because a majority of patients with vaginal carcinoma are treated with radiation therapy, it should be noted that if the lesion is in the upper two thirds of the vagina the treatment plans generally parallel those that would be used for cervical carcinoma. If the lesion involves the lower one third of the vagina, then consideration must be given to treating the inguinal femoral lymph nodes as well as the pelvic lymph nodes. For lower vaginal lesions as well as bulky vaginal lesions, the use of interstitial brachytherapy is often required to effect adequate radiation dose to the tumor.

There is no evidence confirming the beneficial affects of adding chemotherapy to the radiation treatment plan for vaginal carcinoma. Given the significant improvement in outcomes for patients with cervical carcinoma when treated with combined therapy, most academic centers now treat these patients with chemoradiation using cervical carcinoma treatment schemes.

Treatment-Related Complications

The immediately adjacent bladder and rectum often receive very high doses of radiation therapy as a component of treatment for vaginal carcinoma, and therefore the patients may have significant radiation cystitis or proctitis. In the worst cases, patients may develop a fistula between either the bladder or rectum, depending on the location of the lesion and the dose of radiation required to control that lesion. Vaginal function is often disrupted by these treatments, with fibrosis, stenosis, and significantly decreased lubrication resulting from the local radiation therapy. The use of a vaginal dilator and personal lubricants may help preclude some of this loss of function.

Prognosis

The prognosis for vaginal cancer is worse than that seen with cervical or vulvar carcinoma. In a compilation of several studies, Berek et al. identified a 5-year survival of 69% for stage 1 vaginal cancer, 46% for stage 2, 30% for stage 3, and 18% for stage 4 diseases.[87] They note that most recurrences of this disease are within the pelvis, either from lack of regional control of involved lymph nodes or from inability to control the primary tumor. For those patients with an isolated central pelvic failure, consideration may be given to salvage treatment with pelvic exenteration.

Pathology

Although the majority of vaginal cancers are squamous cell carcinomas, other histologic types occur rarely.

Clear Cell Carcinoma Arising After Diethylstilbestrol Exposure

In 1971, Herbst et al. reported on seven women who developed clear cell adenocarcinoma of the vagina.[88] They linked this unusual preponderance of clear cell carcinoma in young women to in utero exposure to diethylstilbestrol (DES). In the late 1940s and particularly in the early 1950s, DES was prescribed to women with a history of pregnancy loss. It was believed that DES decreased the likelihood of spontaneous abortion and early pregnancy loss. A randomized clinical trial in 1954 by Dieckmann and colleagues at the University of Chicago showed that DES was not effective in preventing pregnancy loss.[89] Despite early evidence that DES was not effective, it was still commonly prescribed in many parts of the country throughout the 1950s and into the 1960s.

Women who were DES exposed have several other associated complications of that exposure, including adenosis of the upper vagina, an increased risk of cervical dysplasia, and increased risk of preterm delivery, ectopic pregnancy, and uterine malformations. Although those gynecologic consequences are relatively common after DES exposure, the risk of developing a clear cell adenocarcinoma in the exposed young women is estimated to be 1 in 1,000. The mean age of clear cell carcinoma of the vagina occurring in DES-exposed women is 19 years old. As this cohort of women has aged, the incidence of these DES-exposed clear cell carcinomas has clearly decreased. There is no evidence to date of other DES-induced malignancies in the lower genital tract, but continued surveillance is indicated to detect a second peak incidence of in utero exposure-related malignancy.

Sarcoma

Vaginal sarcomas are extremely rare and are generally managed by a combination of surgical resection followed by adjuvant chemotherapy or radiation therapy. Embryonal rhabdomyosarcoma is a pediatric variant of vaginal sarcoma that is treated by the combined modality approach involving neoadjuvant chemotherapy followed by radiation therapy and in some cases surgery. This multimodality approach has led to significant improvements in survival during the past 20 years.

Melanoma

Malignant melanoma involving the vagina is also exceedingly rare and in many cases has a very poor prognosis. The median age of this disease is 58 years old, with most patients presenting with a Clark's level 4 lesion at the time of detection. Because of the deep invasion at the time of diagnosis, it is quite common for patients to develop hematogenous metastasis from this disease, and the 5-year survival is only 10%. For women with melanoma involving the vagina, it is often necessary to perform anterior, posterior, or total pelvic exenteration to obtain adequate surgical margins around the melanoma.[90]

References

1. Parkin DM, Pisani P, Ferlay J. Global cancer statistics. CA Cancer J Clin 1999;49:33–64.
2. Miller AB, Lindsay J, Hill GB. Mortality from cancer of the uterus in Canada and its relationship to screening for cancer of the cervix. Int J Cancer 1976;17:602–612.
3. La Vecchia C, Franceschi S, Decarli A, Fasoli M, Gentile A, Tognoni G. Pap smear and the risk of cervical neoplasia: quantitative estimates from a case-control study. Lancet 1984;2:779–782.
4. Fanco EL, Duarte-Franco E, Ferenczy A. Cervical cancer: epidemiology, prevention and the role of human papillomavirus infection. Can Med Assoc J 2001;164:1017–1025.
5. Wlboomers JM, Jacobs MV, Manos MM, et al. Human papillomavirus is a necessary cause of invasive cervical cancer worldwide. Pathology 1999;189:12–19.
6. Schiffman MH, Bauer HM, Hoover RN, et al. Epidemiologic evidence showing that human papillomavirus infection causes most cervical intraepithelial neoplasia. J Natl Cancer Inst 1993; 85:958–964.
7. Haverkos HW. Viruses, chemicals and co-carcinogenesis. Oncogene 2004;23:6492–6499.
8. Koutsky LA, Ault KA, Wheeler CM, et al. A controlled trial of a human papillomavirus type 16 vaccine. N Engl J Med 2002; 347:1645–1651.
9. Crum CP. The beginning of the end for cervical cancer? N Engl J Med 2002;347:1703–1705.
10. Hoffman MS, Cardosi RJ, Roberts WS, Fiorica JV, Grendys EC Jr, Griffin D. Accuracy of pelvic examination in the assessment of patients with operable cervical cancer. Am J Obstet Gynecol 2004; 190:986–993.
11. Silverberg SG. Pathology of cervical cancer. Cancer J 2003;9: 335–337.
12. Landoni F, Maneo A, Colomb A, et al. Randomized study of radical surgery versus radiotherapy for stage Ib-IIA cervical cancer. Lancet 1997;350:535.
13. Kamura T, Shigmatsu T, et al. Adenocarcinoma of the uterine cervix with predominantly villoglandular papillary growth pattern. Gynecol Oncol 1964;64:147–152.
14. Hanselaar A, van Loosbroek M, Schuurdiers O, et al. Clear cell adenocarcinoma of the vagina and cervix an update of the central Netherlands registry showing twin average incidence peaks. Cancer (Phila) 1997;79:2229–2236.
15. Abeler VM, Holm R, Nesland JM, et al. Small cell carcinoma of the cervix: a clinical pathologic study of 26 patients. Cancer (Phila) 1994;73:672–677.

16. Creasman WT. New gynecologic cancer staging. Gynecol Oncol 1995;58:157–158.
17. Berek JS, Hacker NF. Practical Gynecologic Oncology, 3rd ed. Philadelphia: Lippincott Williams & Wilkins, 2000:354.
18. Pakkal MV, Rudralingam V, McCluggage WG, Kelly BE. MR staging in carcinoma of the endometrium and carcinoma of the cervix. Ulster Med J 2004;73:20–24.
19. Soutter WP, Hanoch J, D'Arcy T, Dina R, McIndoe GA, DeSouza NM. Pretreatment tumour volume measurement on high-resolution magnetic resonance imaging as a predictor of survival in cervical cancer. Br J Obstet Gynecol 2004;111:741–747.
20. Grigsby PW, Siegel BA, Dehdashti F. Lymph node staging by positron emission tomography in patients with carcinoma of the cervix. J Clin Oncol 2001;19:3745–3749.
21. Marchiole P, Buenerd A, Scoazec JY, Dargent D, Mathevet P. Sentinel lymph node biopsy is not accurate in predicting lymph node status for patients with cervical carcinoma. Cancer (Phila) 2004;100:2154–2159.
22. Schneider A, Hertel H. Surgical and radiographic staging in patients with cervical cancer. Curr Opin Obstet Gynecol 2004;16:11–18.
23. Ostor AG. Pandora's box or Ariadne's thread? Definition and prognostic significance of microinvasion into uterine cervix. Ann Pathol 1995;30(2):103–136.
24. DiSaia PJ, Creasman WT. Clinical Gynecologic Oncology, 6th ed. St. Louis: Mosby.
25. Benedette J, Odicino F, Maisonneuve P, et al. Carcinoma of the cervix uteri. J Epidemiol Biostat 1998;3:5–34.
26. Benedette JL, Anderson GH. Stage 1a carcinoma of the cervix revisited. Obstet Gynecol 1996;87:1052–1059.
27. Ostor AG, Rome RM. Microinvasive squamous cell carcinoma of the cervix: a clinical pathologic study of 200 cases with long term follow up. Int J Gynecol Cancer 1994;4:257.
28. Plante M, Renaud M-C, François H, Roy M. Vaginal radical trachelectomy: an oncologically safe fertility-preserving surgery. An updated series of 72 cases and review of the literature. Gynecol Oncol 2004;94:614–623.
29. Covens A, Shaw P, Murphy J, et al. Is radical trachelectomy a safe alternative to radical hysterectomy for patients with stage IA-B carcinoma of the cervix? Cancer (Phila) 1999;86(11):2273–2279.
30. Ramirez PT, Levenback C. Radical trachelectomy: is it here to stay? Gynecol Oncol 2004;94:611–613.
31. Ostor A, Rome R, Quinn M. Microinvasive adenocarcinoma of the cervix: a clinicopathologic study of 77 women. Obstet Gynecol 1997;89:88–93.
32. Berek JS, Hacker NF, Fu Y-S, Sokale JR, Leuchter RC, Lagasse LD. Adenocarcinoma of the uterine cervix: histologic variables associated with lymph node metastasis and survival. Obstet Gynecol 1985;65:46–52.
33. Peters WA, Liu PY, Barrett RJ, et al. Concurrent chemotherapy and pelvic radiotherapy compared with pelvic radiotherapy alone as adjuvant therapy after radical surgery in high risk early stage cancer of the cervix. J Clin Oncol 2000;18:1608–1613.
34. Sedlis A, Bundy BN, Rjotman MZ, Lentz SS, Muderspach LI, Zaino RJ. A randomized trial of pelvic radiation therapy versus no further therapy in selected patients with stage IB carcinoma of the cervix after radical hysterectomy and pelvic lymphadenectomy: a Gynecologic Oncology Group study. Gynecol Oncol 1999;73:177–183.
35. Coia L, Won M, Lanciano R, et al. The Patterns of Care Outcome Study for cancer of the uterine cervix. Results of the Second National Practice Survey. Cancer (Phila) 1990;66:2451.
36. Britten RA, Evans AJ, Allalunis-Turner MJ, Pearcey RG. Effect of cisplatin on the clinically relevant radiosensitivity of human cervical carcinoma cell lines. Int J Radiat Oncol Biol Phys 1996;34:367–374.
37. Stehman FB, Bundy BN, Kucera PR, Deppe G, Reddy S, O'Connor DM. Hydroxyurea, 5-fluorouracil infusion, and cisplatin adjunct to radiation therapy in cervical carcinoma: a phase I-II trial of the Gynecologic Oncology Group. Gynecol Oncol 1997;66:262–267.
38. Malfetano J, Keys H, Kredentser D, Cunningham M, Kotlove D, Weiss L. Weekly cisplatin and radical radiation therapy for advanced, recurrent, and poor prognosis cervical carcinoma. Cancer (Phila) 1993;71:3703–3706.
39. Keys HM, Bundy BN, Stehman FB, et al. Cisplatin, radiation, and adjuvant hysterectomy compared with radiation and adjuvant hysterectomy for bulky stage IB cervical carcinoma. N Engl J Med 1999;340:1154–1161.
40. Morris M, Eifel PJ, Lu J, et al. Pelvic radiation with concurrent chemotherapy compared with pelvic and para-aortic radiation for high-risk cervical cancer. N Engl J Med 1999;340:1137–1143.
41. Rose PG, Bundy BN, Watkins EB, et al. Concurrent cisplatin-based radiotherapy and chemotherapy for locally advanced cervical cancer. N Engl J Med 1999;340:1144–1153.
42. National Cancer Institute. Concurrent chemoradiation for cervical cancer. Clinical announcement. Bethesda: NCI, February 22, 1999.
43. Green J, Kirwan J, Tierney J, et al. Concomitant chemotherapy and radiation therapy for cancer of the uterine cervix. The Cochrane Database of Systematic Reviews, 18 November, 2003.
44. Sardi JE, Giaroli A, Sananes C, et al. Long-term follow-up of the first randomized trial using neoadjuvant chemotherapy in stage IB squamous carcinoma of the cervix: the final results. Gynecol Oncol 1997;67:61.
45. Serur E, Mathews RP, Gates J, et al. Neoadjuvant chemotherapy in stage IB2 squamous cell carcinoma of the cervix. Gynecol Oncol 1997;65:348.
46. Park DC, Kim JH, Lew YO, et al. Phase II trial of neoadjuvant paclitaxel and cisplatin in uterine cervical cancer. Gynecol Oncol 2004;92:59.
47. Tierney JF, Stewart LA, Parmar MKB. MRC Clinical Trials Unit, Cambridge, England. Can the published data tell us about the effectiveness of neoadjuvant chemotherapy for locally advanced cancer of the uterine cervix? Eur J Cancer 1999;35:406–409.
48. Nag S, Erickson B, Thomadsen B, et al. The American Brachytherapy Society recommendations for high-dose-rate brachytherapy for carcinoma of the cervix. Int J Radiat Oncol Biol Phys 2000;48:201.
49. Nag S, Chao C, Erickson B, et al. The American Brachytherapy Society recommendations for low-dose-rate brachytherapy for carcinoma of the cervix. Int J Radiat Oncol Biol Phys 2002;52:33.
50. Patel FD, Sharma SC, Negi PS, et al. Low dose rate vs. high dose rate brachytherapy in the treatment of carcinoma of the uterine cervix: a clinical trial. Int J Radiat Oncol Biol Phys 1994;28:335.
51. Lertsanguansinchai P, Lertbutsayanukul C, Shotelersuk K, et al. Phase III randomized trial comparing LDR and HDR brachytherapy in treatment of cervical carcinoma. Int J Radiat Oncol Biol Phys 2004;59:1424.
52. Hareyama M, Sakata K, Oouchi A, et al. High-dose-rate versus low-dose-rate intracavitary therapy for carcinoma of the uterine cervix: a randomized trial. Cancer (Phila) 2002;94:117.
53. Rotman M, Pajak TF, Choi K, et al. Prophylactic extended-field irradiation of para-aortic lymph nodes in stages IIB and bulky IB and IIA cervical carcinomas: ten-year treatment results of RTOG 79-20. JAMA 1995;274:387–393.
54. Omura GA, Blessing JA, Vaccarello L, et al. A randomized trial of cisplatin versus cisplatin plus mitolactol versus cisplatin plus ifosfamide in advanced squamous carcinoma of the cervix: a Gynecologic Oncology Group study. J Clin Oncol 1997;15:165–171.

55. Moore DH, Blessing JA, McQuellon RP, et al. Phase III study of cisplatin with or without paclitaxel in stage IVB, recurrent, or persistent squamous cell carcinoma of the cervix: a gynecologic oncology group study. J Clin Oncol 2004;22:3113–3119.
56. Long HJ, Bundy BN, Grendys ED, et al. Randomized phase III trial of cisplatin (P) vs. cisplatin plus topotecan (T), vs. MVAC in stage IVB, recurrent or persistent carcinoma of the uterine cervix: a Gynecologic Oncology Group study. Gynecol Oncol 2004;92:(abstract).
57. National Comprehensive Cancer Network (NCCN). Clinical Practice Guidelines in Oncology. http://www.nccn.org/professionals/physician, June 2004 version.
58. Bodurka-Bevers D, Morris M, Eifel PJ, et al. Posttherapy surveillance of women with cervical cancer: an outcomes analysis. Gynecol Oncol 2000;78:187–193.
59. Jemal A, Tiwari RC, Murray T, et al. Cancer Statistics, 2004. CA Cancer J Clin 2004;54:8–29.
60. Homesley HD, Bundy BN, Sedlis A, et al. Assessment of current International Federation of Gynecology and Obstetrics staging of vulvar carcinoma relative to prognostic factors for survival (a Gynecologic Oncology Group Study). Am J Obstet Gynecol 1991;164:997–1004.
61. Wei S. Carcinoma of the vulva. Am J Obstet Gynecol 1960;79: 692–699.
62. Carlson JA, Ambros R, Malfetano J, et al. Vulvar lichen sclerosus and squamous cell carcinoma: a cohort, case control, and investigational study with historical perspective; implications for chronic inflammation and sclerosis in the development of neoplasia. Hum Pathol 1998;29:932–948.
63. Fanning J, Lambert L, Hale TM, Morris PC, Schuerch C. Paget's disease of the vulva: prevalence of associated vulvar adenocarcinoma, invasive Paget's disease and recurrence after surgical excision. Am J Obstet Gynecol 1999;180:24–27.
64. Gallousis S. Verrucous carcinoma: report of three vulvar cases and a review of the literature. Obstet Gynecol 1972;40:502–508.
65. Demian SDE, Bushkin FL, Echevarria RA. Perineural invasion and anaplastic transformation of verrucous carcinoma. Cancer (Phila) 1973;32:395–399.
66. Benedet JL, Bender H, Jones H III, Ngan HYS, Pecorelli S. Staging classifications and clinical practice guidelines of gynaecologic cancers. Int J Gynecol Obstet 2000;70:207–312.
67. Heaps JM, Fu YS, Montz FJ, Hacker NF, Berek JS. Surgical-pathologic variables predictive of local recurrence in squamous cell carcinoma of the vulva. Gynecol Oncol 1990;38:309–314.
68. Way S. The anatomy of the lymphatic drainage of the vulva and its influence on the radical operation for carcinoma. Ann R Coll Surg Engl 1948;3:187.
69. Hacker NF. Current treatment of small vulvar cancers. Oncology 1990;4:21.
70. Stehman F, Bundy B, Thomas G, et al. Groin dissection versus groin radiation in carcinoma of the vulva: a Gynecologic Oncology Group study. Int J Radiat Oncol Biol Phys 1992;24: 389–396.
71. Koh W-J, Chin M, Stelzer K, et al. Femoral vessel depth and the implication for groin node radiation. Int J Radiat Oncol Biol Phys 1993;27:969–974.
72. Petereit DG, Mehta MP, Buchler DA, Kinsella TJ. Inguinofemoral radiation of N0,N1 vulvar cancer may be equivalent to lymphadenectomy if proper radiation technique is used. Int J Radiat Oncol Biol Phys 1993;27:963.
73. DiSaia PJ, Creasman WT, Rich WM. An alternate approach to early cancer of the vulva. Am J Obstet Gynecol 1979;133:825.
74. Stehman FB, Bundy BN, Droretsky PM, Creasman WT. Early stage 1 carcinoma of the vulva treated with ipsilateral superficial inguinal lymphadenectomy and modified radical hemivulvectomy: a prospective study of the Gynecologic Oncology Group. Obstet Gynecol 1992;79:490–496.
75. Levenback C, Coleman RL, Burke TW, et al. Intraoperative lymphatic mapping and sentinel node identification with blue dye in patients with vulvar cancer. Gynecol Oncol 2001;83:276.
76. Homesley HD, Bundy BN, Sedlis A, Adcock L. Radiation therapy versus pelvic node resection for carcinoma of the vulva with positive groin nodes. Obstet Gynecol 1986;68:733–738.
77. Boronow RC. Therapeutic alternative to primary exenteration for advanced vulvovaginal cancer. Gynecol Oncol 1973;1:223–229.
78. Boronow RC, Hickman BT, Reagan MT, Smith RA, Steadham RE. Combined therapy as an alternative to exenteration for locally advanced vulvovaginal cancer: II. Results, complications and dosimetric and surgical considerations. Am J Clin Oncol 1987;10:171–181.
79. Landoni F, Maneo A, Zanetta G, et al. Concurrent preoperative chemotherapy with 5-fluoruracil and mitomycin-C and radiotherapy (FUMIR) followed by limited surgery in locally advanced and recurrent vulvar carcinoma. Gynecol Oncol 1996;61: 321–327.
80. Lupi G, Raspagliesi F, Zucali R, et al. Combined preoperative chemoradiotherapy followed by radical surgery in locally advanced vulvar carcinoma. Cancer (Phila) 1996;77:1472–1478.
81. Cunningham MJ, Goyer RP, Bibbons SK, Kredentser DC, Malfetano JH, Keys H. Primary radiation, cisplatin and 5-fluourouracil for advanced squamous cell carcinoma of the vulva. Gynecol Oncol 1997;66:258–261.
82. Leiserowitz GS, Russell AH, Kinney WK, Smith LH, Taylor HM, Scudder SA. Prophylactic chemoradiation of inguinal femoral lymph nodes in patients with locally extensive vulvar cancer. Gynecol Oncol 1997;66:509–514.
83. Thomas G, Dembo A, DePetrillo A, et al. Concurrent radiation and chemotherapy in vulvar carcinoma. Gynecol Oncol 1989;34: 263–267.
84. Hoffman M, Greenberg S, Greenberg H, et al. Interstitial radiotherapy for the treatment of advanced or recurrent vulvar and distal vaginal malignancy. Am J Obstet Gynecol 1990;162: 1278–1282.
85. Rutledge F. Cancer of the vagina. Am J Obstet Gynecol 1967;97; 635–655.
86. Benedet JL, Saunders DH. Carcinoma in situ of the vagina. Am J Obstet Gynecol 1984;148:695–700.
87. Berek JS, Hacker NF. Practical Gynecologic Oncology, 3rd ed. Philadelphia: Lippincott Williams & Wilkins, 2000:604–605.
88. Herbst AL, Ulfelder H, Poskanzer DC. Adenocarcinoma of the vagina: association of maternal stilbestrol therapy with tumor appearance in young women. N Engl J Med 1971;284:878–882.
89. Dieckmann WJ, Davis ME, Rynkiewicz LM, Pottinger RE. Does the administration of diethylstilbestrol during pregnancy have therapeutic value? Am J Obstet Gynecol 1953;66:1962.
90. Morrow CP, DiSaia PJ. Malignant melanoma of the female genitalia: a clinical analysis. Obstet Gynecol Surv 1976;31:233–241.

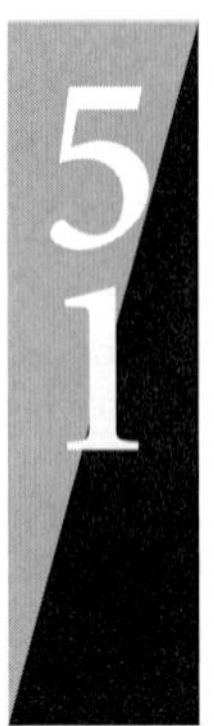

Gestational Trophoblastic Neoplasia

John R. Lurain

Gestational trophoblastic neoplasia includes invasive mole, choriocarcinoma, and placental site trophoblastic tumor. The overall care rate in the treatment of these tumors currently exceeds 90%. This success is the result of the inherent chemotherapy sensitivity of trophoblastic neoplasms, the effective use of the tumor marker human chorionic gonadotropin (hCG) for diagnosis of disease and monitoring of therapy, the referral of patients to or consultation with specialized treatment centers, the identification of prognostic factors that enhance individualization of therapy, and the development of active combinations of chemotherapy agents used in conjunction with irradiation and surgery to treat patients with the most advanced disease.[1]

Diagnosis and Classification

Gestational trophoblastic neoplasia is diagnosed by rising or plateauing hCG levels following evacuation of a hydatidiform mole, a histopathologic diagnosis of invasive mole, choriocarcinoma or placental site trophoblastic tumor, or persistent elevation of hCG usually in conjunction with demonstrated metastases following any pregnancy event. Once the diagnosis of a gestational trophoblastic neoplasm has been made, it is necessary to determine the extent of disease. After a thorough history and physical examination, the following clinical studies should be obtained: chest X-ray, computed tomography (CT) scans of the chest, abdomen, and pelvis, CT or magnetic resonance imaging (MRI) of the brain, complete blood and platelet counts, serum chemistries including liver and renal function studies, and quantitative serum hCG.

After these initial studies, patients are categorized as having nonmetastatic, metastatic low-risk, or metastatic high-risk gestational trophoblastic neoplasia. Patients with metastatic tumors were originally classified as being at higher risk for treatment failure based on one or more of the following poor prognostic factors described by investigators at the National Cancer Institute (NCI): (1) more than 4 months from antecedent pregnancy to diagnosis; (2) pretreatment hCG level more than 100,000 IU/24-hour urine or more than 40,000 mIU/mL serum; (3) metastases to sites other than the lung and vagina; (4) antecedent term pregnancy; and (5) previous failed therapy.[2] In 1983, the World Health Organization (WHO) adopted a prognostic scoring system, initially proposed by Bagshawe and subsequently modified, based on the patient's age, parity, and type of antecedent pregnancy, the interval between antecedent pregnancy and trophoblastic tumor event, hCG level, number and sites of metastases, largest tumor mass, and previous chemotherapy. A weighted numerical value is applied to each prognostic factor and then added together; the resultant score is used to divide patients into low-risk (less than 7) and high-risk (7 or more) groups (Table 51.1). An anatomic staging system was adopted by the International Federation of Gynecology and Obstetrics (FIGO) Cancer Committee in 1982 (Table 51.2) and changed to include the modified WHO score in 2000.[3] In this system, the modified WHO score is depicted by an Arabic numeral following and separated by a colon from the stage, which is depicted by a Roman numeral.

Patients with nonmetastatic (FIGO stage I) and low-risk metastatic (FIGO stages II and III, WHO score less than 7) gestational trophoblastic neoplasia can be treated with single-agent chemotherapy resulting in a survival rate approaching 100%. Patients with high-risk metastatic disease (FIGO stage IV or WHO score 7 or higher) should be treated more aggressively with initial combination chemotherapy with or without adjuvant radiotherapy or surgery to achieve a cure rate of 80% to 90%. Patients with gestational trophoblastic neoplasia must be chosen for single-agent or multiagent chemotherapy based on careful attention to selection criteria to ensure the best outcome with the least morbidity.

Development of Chemotherapy for Gestational Trophoblastic Neoplasia

Investigators at the National Cancer Institute (NCI) in the United States first demonstrated the efficacy of chemotherapy in the treatment of metastatic gestational trophoblastic disease in the late 1950s and early 1960s. In 1948, Hertz[4] presented data demonstrating that fetal tissues required large amounts of folic acid to support trophoblastic growth in experimental animals and that this growth could be inhibited by the folic acid antagonist methotrexate. In 1956, Li et al.[5] first reported complete regression of metastatic gestational trophoblastic disease in women treated with methotrexate. During the decade that followed, the group at the NCI systematically studied the effects of chemotherapy on gestational trophoblastic disease.[6–8] In patients with metastatic disease, they obtained complete sustained remissions in 47% using methotrexate alone and in 74% using methotrexate and actinomycin D (an antitumor antibiotic that intercalates DNA), sequentially. In patients with nonmetastatic disease, they achieved complete remissions in 93% using methotrex-

TABLE 51.1. Modified World Health Organization (WHO) scoring system for gestational trophoblastic neoplasia.

	SCORE			
Risk factors	0	1	2	4
Age factors	<39	>39		
Antecedent pregnancy	Hydatidiform mole	Abortion	Term	
Pregnancy event to treatment interval (months)	<4	4–6	7–12	>12
Pretreatment human chorionic gonadotropin(hCG) (mIU/mL) < 10^3	<10^3	10^3–10^4	10^4–10^5	>10^5
Largest tumor mass, including uterus (cm)		3–4	>5	
Site of metastases		Spleen kidney	Gastrointestinal tract	Brain Liver
Number of metastases		1–4	4–8	>8
Previous failed chemotherapy			1 drug	>2 drugs

The total score for a patient is obtained by adding the individual scores for each prognostic factor: <7 = low risk; ≥7 = high risk.

ate without hysterectomy and an overall cure rate of 98%.

The NCI investigators made many important contributions to the treatment of trophoblastic disease and to cancer chemotherapy in general. First, they proved that metastatic, as well as nonmetastatic, cancer could be cured by drug therapy. Second, they established that higher-dose intermittent chemotherapy was more effective than a lower daily dose. Third, they demonstrated that chemotherapy response could be effectively monitored by accurately measuring hCG. They also recognized that the outcome of therapy depended largely on duration of disease, height of the pretreatment hCG level, presence or absence of brain or liver metastases, and expertise in the use of chemotherapy drugs. More than 95% of patients who were diagnosed early and treated vigorously were cured, whereas patients in whom there was a delay in diagnosis or inappropriate therapy resulting in more-extensive disease had only a 36% remission rate.

Chemotherapeutic agents other than methotrexate and actinomycin D were subsequently found to be effective in gestational trophoblastic disease. Sung et al.[9] and Bagshawe[10] reported on the use of 6-mercaptopurine (6-MP), an antimetabolite purine analogue. There seemed to be no advantage of 6-MP over methotrexate or actinomycin D, and toxicity was significantly greater. The alkylating agents cyclophosphamide and chlorambucil were combined with methotrexate and actinomycin D (MAC) to produce some cures in patients resistant to single-agent chemotherapy.[11]

Sung et al.[12] reported excellent results with 5-fluorouracil (5-FU), an antimetabolite fluoropyrimidine. Yim et al.[13] were able to demonstrate a good response to bleomycin, an antitumor antibiotic that induces single-strand breaks in DNA. They suggested that bleomycin should not replace methotrexate or actinomycin D as first-line therapy because of pulmonary and cutaneous toxicity, but should be used in combination chemotherapy regimens for patients who become resistant to more-conventional drugs. The vinca alkaloids vincristine and vinblastine, which inhibit microtubular polymerization, thereby arresting function of the mitotic spindle, have known activity in gestational trophoblastic disease and have been used in combination therapy.[14,15]

In the 1970s, Newlands et al.[16–18] identified etoposide (VP16-213), an epipodophyllotoxin that binds to the microtubules and interferes with the normal functioning of the topoisomerase II enzyme, as a very active agent in the treatment of resistant gestational trophoblastic neoplasia and suggested that it be incorporated into initial chemotherapy for high-risk disease. Ifosfamide, an alkylating agent similar to cyclophosphamide, has been used successfully alone or in combination for the treatment of resistant gestational trophoblastic tumors.[19] Cisplatin and carboplatin, alkylating-type drugs that form platinum adducts with DNA, have been employed in combination with other drugs, most commonly etoposide, bleomycin, and ifosfamide, for the treatment of resistant trophoblastic disease.[14,15,20–23] Most recently, paclitaxel, an extract from the bark of the Western yew tree *Taxus brevifolia* that binds to and stabilizes the intracellular microtubules disrupting normal mitotic spindle function, has been shown to inhibit growth of choriocarcinoma in vitro,[24,25] and a few remissions using paclitaxel in patients with resistant gestational trophoblastic neoplasia have been reported.[26–28]

TABLE 51.2. International Federation of Gynecology and Obstetrics (FIGO) staging for gestational trophoblastic neoplasia.

Stage I	Disease confined to the uterus
Stage II	Disease extends outside the uterus but is limited to genital structures (adnexa, vagina, broad ligament)
Stage III	Disease extends to lungs with or without genital tract involvement
Stage IV	Disease involves other metastatic sites

Nonmetastatic Disease

Patients with nonmetastatic gestational trophoblastic neoplasia (FIGO stage I) should be treated with single-agent methotrexate (MTX) or actinomycin D (Act D) chemotherapy. Several different outpatient chemotherapy protocols have been used, all yielding excellent and fairly comparable results (Table 51.3). Hysterectomy is used as part of primary therapy in patients who no longer wish to preserve fertility and when the diagnosis is placental site trophoblastic tumor or as secondary therapy for resistant uterine disease.

Methotrexate given IM or IV for 5 days every 2 weeks has been the traditional treatment. In 1995, we reviewed nearly 30 years of experience in treating nonmetastatic gestational trophoblastic neoplasia at the Brewer Trophoblastic Disease Center to determine effectiveness of therapy, evaluate toxicity, and assess factors associated with chemotherapy resis-

TABLE 51.3. Chemotherapy for nonmetastatic and low-risk metastatic gestational trophoblastic neoplasia.

Drug	*Dosing regimen*
Methotrexate (MTX)	0.4 mg/kg/day i.v. or i.m. (max. 25 mg) for 5 days Repeat every 14 days (9-day window)
Actinomycin D	10–12 mg/kg/day i.v. for 5 days Repeat every 14 days (9-day window)
Methotrexate	1.0–1.5 mg/kg i.m. every other day for 4 doses (days 1, 3, 5, 7) Folinic acid (FA) 0.1–0.15 mg/kg i.m. every other day for 4 doses (days 2, 4, 6, 8) Repeat every 15–18 days (7- to 10-day window)
Methotrexate	100 mg/m^2 i.v. push, then 200 mg/m^2 in 500 mL D 5W over 12 h Folinic acid 15 mg i.m. or p.o. every 12 h for 4 doses beginning 24 h after the start of MTX Repeat every 18 days, as needed
Methotrexate[a]	30–50 mg/m^2 i.m. weekly
Actinomycin D[a]	1.25 mg/m^2 i.v. every 2 weeks

[a] Should not be used for patients with metastatic or resistant disease.

tance using the 5-day MTX regimen.[29] Of 337 patients treated between 1962 and 1990, 253 were initially treated with single-agent MTX 0.4 mg/kg (maximum, 25 mg) IV daily for 5 days every other week (9-day window). Primary remission was achieved in 226 (89.3%). Of the 27 patients (10.9%) resistant to methotrexate, 22 (8.7%) were placed into remission with a second agent, Act D. Multiagent chemotherapy or surgery was required in only 5 patients (2.0%). Relapse from remission occurred in 6 patients (2.4%) from 1 to 9 months after completing initial therapy. All 253 patients were eventually placed into permanent remission. Factors found to be significantly associated with the development of MTX resistance were pretreatment hCG levels greater than 50,000 mIU/mL, nonmolar antecedent pregnancy, and clinicopathologic diagnosis of choriocarcinoma. Significant toxicity to MTX necessitating a change to another chemotherapeutic agent occurred in only 12 patients (4.7%); no life-threatening toxicity occurred. There was no alopecia related to MTX, and nausea was not a common side effect. The most common toxic reaction to MTX was oropharyngeal ulcerations (stomatitis), which were managed symptomatically with "cocktails" including antacids, sulcralfate, viscous lidocaine, and antifungals. These manifestations usually persisted for only a short time but must have been resolved before another course of chemotherapy was initiated. Other less common or minor toxic side effects were conjunctivitis, pleuritic or peritoneal pain, and skin rash. Our results of approximately 90% complete response and 100% overall survival confirmed earlier reports from our center and others that single-agent methotrexate in a 5-day outpatient course every 2 weeks is a highly effective and well-tolerated treatment for nonmetastatic gestational trophoblastic neoplasia.

In an attempt to reduce toxicity to methotrexate, Bagshawe and Wilde[30] introduced folinic acid rescue. Methotrexate with folinic acid (MTX-FA) has been applied to the treatment of nonmetastatic gestational trophoblastic neoplasia. This regimen uses slightly high doses of MTX, 1.0–1.5 mg/kg IM every other day for 4 doses, plus FA 0.1–0.15 mg/kg IM 24 hours after each MTX dose, repeated as needed after a minimum rest period of 7 days. Berkowitz et al.[31] from the New England Trophoblastic Disease Center reported that MTX-FA induced primary remission in 147 (90.2%) of 163 patients with nonmetastatic disease. Complete remission was subsequently achieved in all patients, but 7.1% required multiagent chemotherapy or surgery. Bagshawe et al.,[32] from Charing Cross Hospital in London, reported that they were able to cure 99.7% of 348 low-risk patients (most with nonmetastatic disease) with the use of MTX-FA. They noted that 26% of patients had to switch treatment because of drug resistance (20%) or drug-induced toxicity (6%). Similarly, Wong et al.[33] from Hong Kong treated 68 low-risk patients with MTX-FA. Sustained remission was achieved in 76% with MTX-FA alone; 11.8% developed drug resistance requiring multiagent chemotherapy to achieve cure, and 8.8% had a treatment change because of MTX toxicity.

Rotmensch et al.[34] suggested that the reduced toxicity of the MTX-FA regimen compared with MTX alone was due to the every-other-day scheduling of MTX and not to FA. They measured plasma methotrexate levels in patients being treated with MTX-FA and noted that MTX levels at the time of FA administration were below levels necessitating FA rescue.

Single, weekly dose scheduling of methotrexate has been devised in an attempt to develop a more-efficient and less costly, yet safe and effective, chemotherapy for patients with nonmetastatic gestational trophoblastic neoplasia. The Gynecologic Oncology Group used single, weekly IM doses of MTX 30–50 mg/m^2 to treat patients with nonmetastatic postmolar disease. Homesley et al.[35] reported a primary remission rate of 74% in 62 patients using this regimen; 4.8% required multiagent chemotherapy, 3.2% required surgery, and 1 patient eventually died. Hoffman et al.[36] subsequently reported on a single-institution experience using weekly IM MTX to treat 20 similar patients. The primary remission rate was 60%; 5% required multiagent chemotherapy for cure.

High-dose methotrexate IV infusion with folinic acid rescue (HDMTX-FA) has been used to treat patients with nonmetastatic gestational trophoblastic disease. Berkowitz and colleagues[37,38] reported on the use of a 100 mg/m^2 IV bolus and then a 200 mg/m^2 12-hour IV infusion of MTX followed by FA 15 mg IM or PO every 12 hours for 4 doses starting 24 hours after beginning MTX. The primary control rate was only 69%, and 18.8% of patients required multiagent chemotherapy to attain remission. Elit et al.[39] treated 65 patients with a 1,000 mg, 6-hour MTX infusion followed by FA rescue at 24 hours, resulting in a remission rate of 86%. Wong et al.,[40] using a similar MTX infusion protocol in 51 patients, obtained a 90% remission rate.

Different MTX chemotherapy regimens for treatment of nonmetastatic disease have been compared. At the Southeastern Regional Trophoblastic Disease Center, Smith et al.[41] compared 29 patients treated with MTX-FA with 39 historical controls treated with a 5-day course of MTX. A change in chemotherapy because of MTX resistance was required in 27.5% of patients receiving MTX-FA compared with 7.7% of patients receiving MTX alone. Gleeson et al.[42] reported primary remission rates of 69% in 13 patients treated with weekly IM MTX and 75% in 12 patients treated with MTX-FA.

The lower primary remission rates achieved with the MTX-FA, weekly MTX, and MTX infusion protocols compared with 5-day MTX regimen may be attributable to shorter overall duration of chemotherapy exposure of trophoblastic cells to inhibiting levels of the drug during the S phase of the cell cycle, where MTX exerts its cytotoxic effect by interrupting thymidylic acid biosynthesis.[43] Methotrexate administrated at set intervals over 5 days affords increased drug exposure compared to other MTX regimens. Another reason for increased failure to achieve remission with various MTX protocols is that some patients may actually have metastatic disease. Mutch et al.[44] reported that at least 40% of patients with negative chest X-rays, who presumably had nonmetastatic disease, actually had micropulmonary metastases on CT of the lungs, and that 50% of these patients developed resistance to treatment with MTX-FA. Therefore, one must take into consideration toxicity, patient convenience, and cost, as well as the chance of requiring a change in chemotherapy, including multiagent chemotherapy, to achieve cure when choosing a MTX regimen for treatment of nonmetastatic disease.

Actinomycin D 10–12 μg/kg IV daily for 5 days or as a single 1.25 mg/m² IV dose every 2 weeks is an acceptable alternative to MTX for treatment of nonmetastatic gestational trophoblastic neoplasia. Act D generally causes more nausea and alopecia than MTX and produces local tissue injury if IV extravasation occurs. Therefore, Act D is most often used as secondary therapy in the presence of MTX resistance rather than as primary therapy. However, Act D is the appropriate primary therapy for patients with hepatic or renal disease or effusions contraindicating the use of MTX.

The New England Trophoblastic Disease Center first reported on the use of the 5-day Act D regimen to treat 31 patients with nonmetastatic gestational trophoblastic neoplasia, yielding a primary remission rate of 94%.[45] Subsequently, Petrilli and Morrow[46] and Kohorn[47] reported 77% and 88% primary remission rates in 13 and 43 patients, respectively. In our series from the Brewer Center, 78% of 13 patients initially treated with Act D achieved primary remission.[29] Pulsed Act D (1.25 mg/m² every 2 weeks) has been used to treat nonmetastatic postmolar disease.[48–50] Complete response rates of 75% to 100% have been reported in a small number of patients meeting these limited criteria.

Alternating 5-day regimens of MTX and Act D every other week for treatment of nonmetastatic trophoblastic neoplasia have been suggested to decrease drug resistance and cumulative toxicity. Smith[51] first reported a 100% primary remission rate using this scheme. Rose and Piver[52] and Lurain and Elfstrand[29] subsequently confirmed the excellent results with this treatment plan. The tendency, however, has been to use MTX as primary therapy and avoid Act D if possible because of the greater hair loss and nausea as well as local IV infiltration tissue damage associated with Act D.

In summary, single-agent chemotherapy with MTX or Act D by a variety of regimens is the appropriate treatment for

TABLE 51.4. Results of chemotherapy for nonmetastatic gestational trophoblastic neoplasia.

Chemotherapy regimen	*Primary remissions, %*	*Multiagent chemotherapy, %*	*Surgery for resistance, %*
MTX 5-day	91	1	1
MTX-FA	75	5	2
MTX weekly	70	5	3
MTX high-dose infusion with FA	69	19	—
Act D 5-day	92	—	—
Act D pulse	80	—	—

Modified from Lurain,[1] by permission of *Current Treatment Options in Oncology*.

nonmetastatic gestational trophoblastic neoplasia (Table 51.4). Overall, cure is anticipated in essentially all patients with nonmetastatic disease. Approximately 85% to 90% of patients can be cured by the initial chemotherapy regimen. Most of the remaining patients will be placed into permanent remission with additional single-agent chemotherapy. Rarely do patients require multiagent chemotherapy or surgery for cure.

Low-Risk Metastatic Disease

Patients categorized into the low-risk metastatic disease group (FIGO stages II and III, WHO score less than 7) should be treated with single-agent chemotherapy using 5-day dosage schedules of MTX or Act D or the 8-day MTX-FA protocol. The weekly MTX or biweekly Act D single-dose protocols currently in use for nonmetastatic postmolar disease should not be employed for treatment of metastatic disease. If resistance to the initial drug occurs, the alternate single agent in a 5-day dosage schedule is begun. Patients who develop resistance to sequential single-agent MTX and Act D chemotherapy are then treated with combination chemotherapy, as for high-risk disease. Hysterectomy may be performed as adjuvant treatment coincident with the institution of chemotherapy to shorten the duration of therapy or to eradicate persistent, chemotherapy-resistant disease in the uterus. Several studies have demonstrated the high curability of low-risk metastatic disease using this approach.[53–55]

DuBeshter et al.[53] at the New England Trophoblastic Disease Center treated 48 patients with low-risk metastatic gestational trophoblastic neoplasia with single-agent MTX with or without FA or Act D between 1965 and 1990. All patients achieved sustained remission, although 50% required a second single agent, 14% needed multiagent chemotherapy, and 12% underwent surgical resection of resistant tumor foci. Multiagent chemotherapy was more often required after the use of MTX-FA protocols (30%) than single-agent MTX or Act D (4%).

Soper et al.[54] at the Southeastern Regional Trophoblastic Disease Center retrospectively analyzed 52 patients with low-risk metastatic gestational trophoblastic disease treated with 5-day cycles of IM MTX repeated every 14 days. Primary remission was achieved in 60%. Therapy was changed because of drug-resistance in 19% and toxicity in 21%. Only 2 patients (4%) required multiagent chemotherapy, 1 of whom also underwent hysterectomy. Pretherapy hCG at

TABLE 51.5. Single-agent chemotherapy for low-risk metastatic gestational trophoblastic neoplasia.

Series	*No. of patients*	*Primary remission, %*	*Multiagent chemotherapy, %*	*Surgery for resistance, %*	*Survival, %*
DuBeshter et al.[53]	48	48	15	12	100
Soper et al.[54]	52	60	4	2	100
Roberts and Lurain[55]	92	67	1	0	100

Source: Modified from Roberts and Lurain,[55] by permission of *American Journal of Obstetrics and Gynecology*.

more than 10,000 mIU/mL was associated with the development of drug resistance. Sustained remission was achieved in all patients.

At the Brewer Center, we treated 92 low-risk metastatic disease patients between 1962 and 1992.[55] Initial treatment consisted of 5-day cycles of IV MTX (61), Act D (4), alternating MTX/ACT D (5), and hysterectomy with single-agent chemotherapy (22). All patients were cured. Remission was achieved in 98.9% of patients with MTX and Act D used alone or sequentially with or without hysterectomy; only one patient (1.1%) needed multiagent chemotherapy. Toxicity was relatively mild and easily remedied, necessitating a change in chemotherapeutic agents in 10.7% of patients. Patients in whom initial therapy failed tended to be older and had higher pretreatment hCG levels and WHO scores than those successfully treated; however, the only statistically significant finding was that patients with large vaginal metastases were more likely to require secondary therapy.

In summary, single-agent chemotherapy with MTX or Act D, each given for 5 consecutive days every other week, is the preferred treatment for patients with low-risk metastatic gestational trophoblastic neoplasia (Table 51.5). With appropriate selection of patients as well as proper administration of treatment, cure should approach 100%, and the greater morbidity associated with the use of multiagent chemotherapy can usually be avoided. Approximately 30% to 50% of patients in this category develop resistance to the first chemotherapeutic agent and require alternate treatment. Eventually, 5% to 15% of patients treated with sequential single-agent chemotherapy will require multiagent chemotherapy with or without surgery to achieve remission.

High-Risk Metastatic Disease

Patients with high-risk metastatic gestational trophoblastic neoplasia (FIGO stage IV or WHO score 7 or more) should be treated with initial multiagent rather than single-agent chemotherapy with or without adjuvant radiotherapy or surgery.[56] During most of the 1970s and 1980s, the primary multidrug regimen used was MAC: methotrexate, actinomycin D, and cyclophosphamide or chlorambucil. Reported cure rates ranged from 63% to 71%.[57] In the late 1970s, Bagshawe and colleagues at Charing Cross Hospital in London introduced the seven-drug CHAMOCA protocol, using cyclophosphamide, hydroxyurea, actinomycin D, methotrexate with folinic acid, vincristine and doxorubicin, for treatment of high-risk patients and reported a primary remission rate of 82%.[58] However, in a randomized clinical trial comparing MAC and CHAMOCA for primary treatment of high-risk patients, the Gynecologic Oncology Group found that the MAC regimen was more effective (cure rates, 95% versus 70%, respectively) and less toxic than the CHAMOCA regimen.[59] After the discovery in the late 1970s that etoposide (VP16-213) was a very effective chemotherapeutic agent for gestational trophoblastic neoplasia, Newlands et al.[60] formulated the EMA-CO regimen, employing etoposide, high-dose methotrexate with folinic acid, actinomycin D, cyclophosphamide, and vincristine (Table 51.6). They originally reported an 80% complete clinical response rate and 82% survival with minimal toxicity in 76 high-risk patients who had not received any prior chemotherapy. Since then, complete response rates and long-term survival rates of more than 80% have been reported by several groups, making the EMA-CO protocol, or some variation of it, the initial multiagent chemotherapy of choice for treatment of patients with high-risk metastatic gestational trophoblastic neoplasia (Table 51.7).

Bolis et al.[61] reported an initial complete response rate of 94% and survival in 88% of 17 patients with high-risk disease treated primarily with EMA-CO. Only 1 patient failed to achieve an initial complete response, and 3 patients (19%) relapsed from remission. In 1992 we reported our preliminary results with EMA-CO for primary treatment of patients with high-risk metastatic gestational neoplasia at the Brewer Trophoblastic Disease Center between 1986 and 1991. Ten

TABLE 51.6. EMA-CO chemotherapy regimen for high-risk gestational trophoblastic neoplasia.

Day	*Drug*	*Dosing*
1	Etoposide	100 mg/m^2 i.v. infusion over 30 min
	Actinomycin D	0.5 mg i.v. push
	Methotrexate	100 mg/m^2 i.v. push, then 200 mg/m^2 in 500 mL D5W over 12 h
2	Etoposide	100 mg/m^2 i.v. infusion over 30 min
	Actinomycin D	0.5 mg i.v. push
	Folinic acid	15 mg i.m. or p.o. every 12 h for 4 doses beginning 24 h after the start of methotrexate
8	Cyclophosphamide	600 mg/m^2 i.v. infusion
	Vincristine	1.0 mg/m^2 i.v. push

EMA-CO: etoposide, high-dose methotrexate with folinic acid, actinomycin D, cyclophosphamide, and vincristine.

Repeat cycle on days 15, 16, and 22 (every 2 weeks).

TABLE 51.7. Results of EMA ± CO chemotherapy for high-risk gestational trophoblastic neoplasia.

Series	*Primary therapy No. of patients*	*Complete response, %*	*Survival, %*	*Secondary therapy No. of patients*	*Complete response, %*	*Survival, %*
Bower et al.[65]	151	78	85	121	79	90
Kim et al.[66]	96	—	91	69	—	74
Escobar et al.[67]	25	—	94	20	—	90
Soto-Wright et al.[a,68]	7	71	100	22	95	100
Matsui et al.[a,69]	27	78	89	12	67	83

[a] EMA only.

Source: Modified from Lurain,[1] by permission of *Current Treatment Options in Oncology.*

of 12 patients (83%) had lasting complete clinical responses to EMA-CO.[62] Soper and colleagues[63] treated 22 high-risk patients with EMA-CO. Four (67%) of six patients receiving primary therapy and 13 (81%) of 16 patients receiving secondary therapy had complete responses; 6 (35%) of 17 complete responders developed recurrences within 6 months of therapy. Overall, 68% of patients remained without evidence of disease. Quinn et al.[64] from Australia treated 35 patients with metastatic disease with EMA-CO. Most of the patients had high-risk features and all had WHO scores above 4. The survival rate was 89%. All four deaths occurred in patients who had hepatic and/or central nervous system metastases.

More recently, Bower et al.[65] updated the Charing Cross-London experience using EMA-CO to treat 272 women with high-risk disease. There were 11 (4%) early deaths, 214 (78%) complete remissions to EMA-CO, and an additional 33 (12%) complete responses to subsequent cisplatin-based chemotherapy and surgery, yielding an overall survival rate of 88%. Kim et al.[66] from Korea treated 165 high-risk patients with the EMA-CO regimen. Of 96 patients who received EMA-CO as first-line treatment, 87 (91%) had complete remissions, whereas only 51 (74%) of the 69 patients who received EMA-CO as second- or third-line therapy entered into remission. The overall survival rate was 84%. Factors that predicted poor prognosis were tumor age greater than 12 months, metastases to more than two organ systems, and previous inadequate chemotherapy or unplanned surgery. In patients with two or three of these factors, death rates were 18% and 57%, respectively. We recently updated our experience with EMA-CO for treatment of high-risk disease at the Brewer Center from 1986 to 2001.[67] Of the 45 patients treated with EMA-CO (25 as primary therapy and 20 as secondary therapy), 32 (71%) had a complete response, 9 (20%) developed resistance but were subsequently placed into remission with platinum-based chemotherapy, and 4 (9%) died of widespread metastatic disease, resulting in an overall survival rate of 91%.

Two groups have reported on the use of an EMA protocol without CO for treatment of high-risk disease, yielding similar results. Soto-Wright et al.[68] from the New England Trophoblastic Disease Center were able to achieve remissions in 5 (71%) of 7 patients treated primarily with EMA and in 21 (95%) of 22 patients treated secondarily with EMA, eventually placing all 29 patients into remission. Matsui et al.[69] from Japan reported obtaining complete remissions in 21 (78%) of 27 patients treated primarily with EMA and in 8 (67%) of 12 patients who had received chemotherapy prior to EMA. The overall survival rate was 87%. Of note, grade 4 neutropenia and thrombocytopenia occurred in 5.3% and 6.4% of treatment cycles, respectively, resulting in one chemotherapy-related death.

In almost all the reports, treatment with EMA ± CO was generally well tolerated and toxicity was mild. In our series, there were no treatment-related deaths or life-threatening toxicity.[67] Neutropenia necessitating a 1-week delay of treatment occurred in 13.5% of 257 treatment cycles. We have been using granulocyte colony-stimulating factor (G-CSF, 300 μg SC days 9–14 of each subsequent treatment cycle) if any neutropenia-associated treatment delay is encountered. Anemia requiring blood transfusions and grade 3–4 neutropenia without thrombocytopenia were associated with only 5.8% and 1.9% of treatment cycles, respectively.

Primary treatment of high-risk gestational trophoblastic disease using cisplatin/etoposide-containing combinations has also been reported. Theodore et al.[70] treated 8 patients with high-risk disease primarily with cisplatin/etoposide/actinomycin D combination chemotherapy. All eight patients had complete responses to this chemotherapy and were apparently cured. Although all patients had WHO scores above 7, several had nonmetastatic disease and none had metastases to more than one organ site, usually the lungs. Bakri and associates[71,72] reported using a similar regimen as primary therapy for patients presenting with brain or liver metastases. Eight (67%) of 12 patients survived. Surwit and Childers[73] substituted etoposide (100 mg/m^2) and cisplatin (80 mg/m^2) (EP) for cyclophosphamide and vincristine (CO) on day 8 in the EMA-CO regimen, as suggested by Newlands et al.,[74] for primary treatment of high-risk patients. They reported remission in the four patients treated with this EMA-EP protocol. In general, primary treatment of high-risk patients using cisplatin/etoposide combinations results in significant cumulative toxicity, often before a complete response is accomplished, and may compromise the ability to deliver adequate salvage chemotherapy.

When central nervous system metastases are present, whole-brain irradiation (3,000 cGy in 200-cGy fractions) is usually given simultaneously with the initiation of chemotherapy.[75–77] Brain irradiation has the dual purpose of being both tumoricidal and hemostatic. Yordan et al.[75] reported that death due to brain involvement occurred in 11 of 25 patients (44%) treated with chemotherapy alone but in none of 18 patients treated with brain irradiation and chemotherapy. During radiotherapy, the methotrexate infusion dose in the EMA-CO protocol is increased to 1 g/m^2, and 30 mg folinic acid is given every 12 hours for 3 days starting 32 hours after the infusion begins. Overall, 50% to 80% of patients with brain metastases can be cured, depending on patient symptoms as well as number, size, and location of the brain lesions.

Evans et al.,[76] at the Southeastern Regional Trophoblastic Disease Center, treated 42 patients with brain metastases with brain irradiation and chemotherapy. Twelve of 16 patients (75%) who presented initially with evidence of brain lesions and no prior therapy were successfully treated. Five of 23 patients (22%) survived who had received prior treatment (5 of 13) or developed brain lesions while undergoing systemic chemotherapy (0 of 10). At the Brewer Trophoblastic Disease Center, 26 (4.1%) of 631 patients who underwent treatment for trophoblastic neoplasia between 1962 and 1994 had or developed evidence of brain metastases. Patients were treated with chemotherapy and whole-brain irradiation. The overall 5-year actuarial survival rate was 51%:100% (6 of 6) for patients with asymptomatic or minimally symptomatic brain disease at presentation, 39% (5 of 14) for patients with symptomatic brain metastases at presentation, and 17% (1 of 6) for patients who developed brain metastases during chemotherapy.[77]

As an alternative to whole-brain irradiation, the Charing Cross Hospital group has recommended the addition of intrathecal methotrexate or surgical excision with steriotactic irradiation in selected patients. Eighty-six percent of their patients with brain lesions achieved complete remission using this approach.[78] Bakri and associates,[71] at the New England Trophoblastic Disease Center, reported achieving sustained remissions in four of eight patients (50%) with brain metastases who were treated with systemic chemotherapy combined with intrathecal methotrexate without brain irradiation.

Resistant High-Risk Disease

Approximately 30% of high-risk patients have an incomplete response to first-line chemotherapy or relapse from remission and require secondary chemotherapy. Salvage chemotherapy with drug regimens employing etoposide and platinum agents, often combined with surgical resection of sites of persistent tumor (usually in the uterus or lungs), will result in cure of most of these high-risk patients with resistant disease.[56]

The EMA-EP regimen, substituting etoposide and cisplatin for cyclophosphamide and vincristine in the EMA-CO protocol, seems to be the most appropriate therapy for patients who have responded to EMA-CO but have plateauing low hCG levels or who have developed reelevation of hCG levels after having had a complete response to EMA-CO. Newlands et al.[74] reported curing 30 (88%) of 34 patients with disease refractory to EMA-CO by treating them with the EMA-EP regimen. The majority of these patients had only low-level hCG plateaus and also underwent surgical procedures; however, 9 of 11 patients treated with EMA-EP without adjuvant surgery were cured.

High-risk patients who have clearly developed resistance to methotrexate-containing treatment protocols should be treated with platinum–etoposide drug combinations. Theodore and associates[70] used a cisplatin–etoposide + actinomycin D regimen to treat 14 patients with drug-resistant trophoblastic disease. Eleven (78%) achieved remission; however, all but 2 had failed only a single- or double-agent methotrexate or actinomycin D chemotherapy regimen. Soper et al.[79] treated 7 patients who demonstrated resistance to multiagent chemotherapy with the combination of etoposide 100 mg/m^2 and cisplatin 20 mg/m^2 each, given IV daily for 5 consecutive days every 21 days. Six patients (86%) had return of their hCGs to normal, but only 3 (43%) had sustained remissions. Hematologic and renal toxicity were significant.

The combination of cisplatin, vinblastine, and bleomycin (PVB) has been used in the past to induce remissions in some patients with resistant high-risk gestational trophoblastic neoplasia.[14,15,20] More recently, etoposide has replaced vinblastine in this regimen.[18,21] The BEP protocol (cisplatin 20 mg/m^2 IV and etoposide 100 mg/m^2 IV on days 1–4 repeated every 21 days, as well as bleomycin 30 U IV weekly starting on day 1) is currently our first chemotherapy choice for patients with resistance to EMA-CO/EMA-EP. Ifosfamide has also been combined with etoposide and cisplatin to treat patients with refractory gestational trophoblastic disease, resulting in some cures.[19] The VIP protocol that we have used is etoposide 75 mg/m^2 IV, ifosfamide 1.2 g/m^2 IV, and cisplatin 20 mg/m^2 IV every day for 4 days. Mesna is given as a 120 mg/m^2 IV bolus just before the first dose of ifosfamide, followed by a 1.2 g/m^2 12-hour IV infusion daily after each ifosfamide dose.[22] If significant cisplatin-induced renal or neurologic toxicity occurs, carboplatin can be substituted for cisplatin in the ICE protocol: ifosfamide 1.2 g/m^2 on days 1–3 with mesna as noted above, carboplatin 300 mg/m^2 IV on day 1, and etoposide 75 mg/m^2 IV on days 1–3.[23] Both regimens are repeated every 21 days. To decrease the incidence of severe neutropenia, which occurs almost universally with these protocols, and to avoid treatment delays, G-CSF is administered on days 6–14 of each treatment cycle, and a complete blood count is obtained on days 8 and 15.[80]

Another approach to improving response to secondary therapy for high-risk disease is to administer chemotherapy agents with known activity at doses much higher than usual. Collins et al.[81] treated a patient with refractory disease in the lung and brain after both EMA-CO and PVB chemotherapy with very high dose etoposide, 4,200 mg/m^2 at 60 hours IV infusion and cyclophosphamide 50 mg/kg IV daily, for 4 days without bone marrow support. Although severe mucositis and pancytopenia occurred, the hCG level returned to normal within 14 days of therapy and the patient was disease free 15 months later. We treated two patients similarly; both achieved normal hCG levels immediately after treatment, but disease recurred in both, 4 and 6 months later.[82] Lotz et al.[83] treated five patients with gestational trophoblastic tumors who were refractory to standard therapy with high-dose chemotherapy, consisting of ifosfamide 1,500 mg/m^2 and carboplatin 200 mg/m^2, both given IV daily for 5 days, followed by autologous bone marrow transplantation. Only two of the patients had normalization of their hCG levels, for 68 and 2 months, respectively, and 1 patient died of therapy-related complications. Giacolone et al.[84] and van Besian et al.[85] each reported on one patient with refractory gestational trophoblastic disease who had a complete response to high-dose chemotherapy. Further data on the use of high-dose chemotherapy with autologous bone marrow transplantation or peripheral stem cell support are necessary before this form of treatment can be recommended as initial salvage therapy for patients failing EMA-CO.

Newer anticancer agents have been developed that may also have a role in the treatment of gestational trophoblastic neoplasia. Paclitaxel has been shown to inhibit growth of choriocarcinoma in tissue culture.[24,25] Jones et al.,[26] Termrungruanglert et al.,[27] and Gershon et al.[28] each reported remissions using paclitaxel in patients with resistant gestational choriocarcinoma. Obsorne et al.[86] recently reported achieving remission in patients with resistant high-risk disease using a doublet of paclitaxel/etoposide and paclitaxel/cisplatin alternating every 2 weeks. The topoisomerase I inhibitor campthecins, topotecan and irinotecan, and new antimetabolites, such as gemcitabine, have been shown to have significant antitumor activity against a wide range of cancers and need to be evaluated in resistant gestational trophoblastic neoplasia.

Adjuvant surgical procedures, especially hysterectomy and thoracotomy, may be of use in removing known foci of chemotherapy-resistant disease in selected patients with persistent or recurrent high-risk gestational trophoblastic neoplasia.[87–89] Chemotherapy is usually administered at the time of surgery to (1) eradicate any occult metastases that may also be present, (2) reduce the likelihood of tumor dissemination at surgery, and (3) maintain cytotoxic levels of chemotherapy in tissues and plasma in the event that viable tumor cells are disseminated at the time of surgery.

Patients with evidence of uterine disease but no or very little extrauterine disease may benefit from hysterectomy. Mutch et al.[90] reported curing 10 (71%) of 14 patients who had hysterectomy as part of their treatment for recurrent disease. Resection of pulmonary nodules in highly selected patients with drug-resistant disease (solitary pulmonary nodule, no evidence of other metastatic sites or uterine disease, hCG level less than 1,000 mIU/mL) may also be successful in inducing remission. Tomoda et al.[91] were able to cure 14 (93%) of 15 patients who satisfied their criteria by resection of resistant pulmonary disease. Mutch et al.[90] reported that 4 (44%) of 9 patients who underwent thoracotomy with pulmonary wedge resection of resistant choriocarcinoma survived. Prompt hCG regression within 1 to 2 weeks of surgical resection predicts a favorable outcome.[90–92]

Surgery may also have a role in the therapy of high-risk disease as a means of controlling tumor hemorrhage, relieving bowel or urinary obstruction, treating infection, or dealing with other life-threatening complications. Selective angiographic embolization of the uterine arteries may be used to control uterine or pelvic tumor bleeding in lieu of surgical intervention.[93]

In summary, intensive multimodality therapy with EMA-CO or some variation of it, along with adjuvant radiotherapy and surgery when indicated, has resulted in cure rates of 80% to 90% in patients with high-risk metastatic gestational trophoblastic neoplasia. Approximately 30% of high-risk patients will fail first-line therapy or relapse from remission. Most of these patients have a clinicopathologic diagnosis of choriocarcinoma, multiple metastases to sites other than the lungs and vagina, and inadequate previous chemotherapy. Salvage chemotherapy with drug regimens combining platinum agents, etoposide, and bleomycin, ifosfamide, or paclitaxel, often in conjunction with surgical resection of sites of persistent tumor, will result in cure of most of these high-risk patients. Colony-stimulating factors should be used to prevent treatment delays and dose reductions. Newer anticancer drugs, such as paclitaxel and gemcitabine, or high-dose chemotherapy may have a role in the future management of selected patients.

Placental-Site Trophoblastic Tumor

Placental-site trophoblastic tumor (PSTT) is an uncommon variant of gestational trophoblastic neoplasia. Pathologically, it consists predominantly of intermediate trophoblasts that secrete human placental lactogen (hPL), is associated with less vascular invasion, necrosis, and hemorrhage than typical choriocarcinoma, and has a propensity for lymphatic spread. The most common presentation is irregular vaginal bleeding, often distant from a preceding nonmolar gestation. Placental-site tumors tend to remain within the uterus, disseminate late, and produce low levels of hCG relative to their tumor mass. The clinical classification schemes and scoring systems used for other gestational trophoblastic neoplasms do not apply to PSTT. These tumors are relatively resistant to chemotherapy.

Hysterectomy is the treatment of choice for PSTT. Patients with metastatic disease should be treated with EMA-EP chemotherapy. Newlands et al.[74] managed 17 patients with PSTT: 8 nonmetastatic and 9 metastatic to lungs (5), pelvis (3), and lymph nodes (1). All but 1 patient had a hysterectomy, and 14 had chemotherapy. The overall survival rate was 76% : 100% for nonmetastatic disease and 56% for metastatic disease. The most significant adverse prognostic variable was an interval of more than 2 years from antecedent pregnancy event to treatment. Cure was achieved in all 12 patients whose interval was less than 2 years compared with only 1 of 5 whose interval was more than 2 years.

Follow-Up After Treatment for Gestational Trophoblastic Neoplasia

Disease Surveillance

After completion of chemotherapy, serum quantitative hCG levels should be obtained at 1-month intervals for 12 months. The risk of recurrence is exceedingly low after 1 year. Physical examinations are performed at 6- to 12-month intervals; other examinations such as chest X-rays are rarely indicated. Contraception should be maintained during treatment, preferably with oral contraceptives, and for 1 year after completion of chemotherapy. During a subsequent pregnancy, pelvic ultrasound is recommended in the first trimester to confirm a normal gestation, because these patients are at increased risk for another gestational trophoblastic disease event. The products of conception or placentas from future pregnancies should be carefully examined histopathologically, and an hCG level should be obtained 6 weeks after any pregnancy event.

Reproductive Performance

The successful treatment of gestational trophoblastic neoplasia with chemotherapy has resulted in a large number of women whose reproductive potential has been retained despite exposure to drugs that have ovarian toxicity and teratogenic potential. Most women resume normal ovarian function following chemotherapy and exhibit no increase in infertility. Many successful pregnancies have been reported.[94] In general, these women experience no increase in incidences of abortions, stillbirths, congenital anomalies, prematurity, or major obstetric complications. There is no evidence for reactivation of disease because of a subsequent pregnancy, although patients who have had one trophoblastic disease episode (hydatidiform mole or choriocarcinoma) are at greater risk for developing a second episode in a subsequent pregnancy, unrelated to whether they had previously received chemotherapy.

Secondary Malignancies

Because many anticancer drugs are known carcinogens, there is concern that the chemotherapy used to induce long-term remissions or cures of one cancer may induce second malignancies. Until recently, there were no reports of increased susceptibility to the development of other malignancies after successful chemotherapy for gestational trophoblastic tumors[95]; this was probably due to the relatively short exposure of patients to intermittent schedules of methotrexate and actinomycin D and the infrequent use of alkylating agents. However, after the introduction of etoposide-containing drug combinations for treatment of gestational trophoblastic tumors in the 1980s, an increased risk of secondary malignancies, including acute myelogenous leukemia, colon cancer, melanoma, and breast cancer, was identified.[96]

References

1. Lurain JR. Treatment of gestational trophoblastic tumors. Curr Treat Options Oncol 2002;3:113–124.
2. Lurain JR, Casanova LA, Miller DS, Rademaker AW. Prognostic factors in gestational trophoblastic tumors. Am J Obstet Gynecol 1991;164:611–616.
3. Kohorn EI. The new FIGO 2000 staging and risk factor scoring system for gestational trophoblastic disease: description and critical assessment. Int J Gynecol Cancer 2001;11:73–77.
4. Hertz R. Interference with estrogen-induced tissue growth in the chick genital tract by a folic acid antagonist. Science 1948; 107:300–302.
5. Li MD, Hertz R, Spencer DB. Effects of methotrexate therapy upon choriocarcinoma and chorioadenoma. Proc Soc Exp Biol Med 1956;93:361–366.
6. Hertz R, Lewis J Jr, Lipsett MD. Five years experience with chemotherapy of metastatic choriocarcinoma and related tumors in women. Am J Obstet Gynecol 1961;82:631–640.
7. Ross GT, Goldstein DP, Hertz R, et al. Sequential use of methotrexate and actinomycin D in the treatment of metastatic choriocarcinoma and related trophoblastic diseases in women. Am J Obstet Gynecol 1965;93:223–229.
8. Hammond CB, Hertz R, Ross GT, Lipsett MD, Odell WD. Primary chemotherapy for nonmetastatic gestational trophoblastic neoplasms. Am J Obstet Gynecol 1967;98:71–78.
9. Sung HC, Wu PC, Ho TH. Treatment of choriocarcinoma and chorioadenoma destruens with 6-mercaptopurine and surgery. Chin Med J (Engl) 1963;82:24–28.
10. Bagshawe KD. Trophoblastic tumors. Chemotherapy and developments. Br Med J 1963;2:1303–1310.
11. Brewer JI, Gerbie AB, Dolkart RE, Skom JH, Nalge RG, Torok EE. Chemotherapy of trophoblastic diseases. Am J Obstet Gynecol 1964;90:566–570.
12. Sung HC, Wu PC, Yang HY. Re-evaluation of 5-fluorouracil as a single therapeutic agent for gestational trophoblastic neoplasms. Am J Obstet Gynecol 1984;150:69–73.
13. Yim CM, Wong LC, Ma HK. Clinical trial of bleomycin in the treatment of gestational trophoblastic disease. Gynecol Oncol 1979;8:296–299.
14. Gordon AN, Kavanagh JJ, Gershenson DM, et al. Cisplatin, vinblastine, and bleomycin combination therapy in resistant gestational trophoblastic disease. Cancer (Phila) 1986;58:1407–1410.
15. DuBeshter B, Berkowitz RS, Goldstein DP. Vinblastine, cisplatin, and bleomycin as salvage therapy for refractory high-risk metastatic gestational trophoblastic disease. J Reprod Med 1989;34:189–192.
16. Newlands ES, Bagshawe KD. Anti-tumor activity of the epipodophyllin derivative VP16-213 (Etoposide: NSC-141540) in gestational choriocarcinoma. Eur J Cancer 1980;16:401–405.
17. Newlands ES. New chemotherapeutic agents in the management of gestational trophoblastic disease. Semin Oncol 1885; 12:37–43.
18. Newlands ES. VP 16 in combinations in first-line treatment of malignant germ cell tumors and gestational choriocarcinoma. Semin Oncol 1982;9:239–244.
19. Sutton GP, Soper JT, Blessing JA, et al. Ifosfamide alone and in combination in the treatment of refractory malignant gestational trophoblastic disease. Am J Obstet Gynecol 1992;167: 489–493.
20. Azab M, Droz JP, Theodore C, et al. Cisplatin, vinblastine, and bleomycin combination in the treatment of resistant high-risk gestational trophoblastic tumors. Cancer (Phila) 1989;64:1829–1832.
21. Willemse PHB, Aalders JG, Bouma J, et al. Chemotherapy-resistant gestational trophoblastic neoplasia successfully treated with cisplatin, etoposide, ifosfamide and bleomycin. Obstet Gynecol 1988;71:438–440.
22. Garris PD, Gallup DG, Melton K. Long-term remission of previously resistant choriocarcinoma with a combination of etoposide, ifosfamide, and cisplatin. Gynecol Oncol 1995;57: 254–256.
23. Piamsomboon S, Kudelka AP, Termangruanglert W, et al. Remission of refractory gestational trophoblastic disease in the brain with ifosfamide, carboplatin, and etoposide (ICE): first report and literature review. Eur J Gynecol Oncol 1997;18:453–456.
24. Koechli OR, Schaer GN, Sevin BU, et al. In vitro chemosensitivity of paclitaxel and other chemotherapeutic agents in malignant gestational trophoblastic neoplasms. Anti-Cancer Drugs 1995;6:94–100.
25. Marth C, Lang T, Widschwendter M, et al. Effects of Taxol on choriocarcinoma cells. Am J Obstet Gynecol 1995;173:1835–1842.
26. Jones WB, Schneider J, Shapiro F, et al. Treatment of resistant gestational choriocarcinoma with Taxol: a report of two cases. Gynecol Oncol 1996;61:126–130.
27. Termrungruanglert W, Kudelka AP, Piamsomboon S, et al.: Remission of refractory gestational trophoblastic disease with high-dose paclitaxel. Anti-Cancer Drugs 1996;7:503–506.
28. Gershon R, Serrano A, Delcarmen Bello M, et al. Response of choriocarcinoma to paclitaxel. Case report and review of resistance. Eur J Gynecol Oncol 1997;18:108–110.
29. Lurain JR, Elfstrand EP. Single-agent methotrexate chemotherapy for the treatment of nonmetastatic gestational trophoblastic tumors. Am J Obstet Gynecol 1995;172:574–579.
30. Bagshawe KD, Wilde CE. Infusion therapy for pelvic trophoblastic tumors. Br J Obstet Gynecol 1964;71:565–570.
31. Berkowitz RS, Goldstein DP, Bernstein MR. Ten years' experience with methotrexate and folinic acid as primary therapy for gestational trophoblastic disease. Gynecol Oncol 1986;23: 111–118.

32. Bagshawe KD, Dent J, Newlands ES, et al. The role of low-dose methotrexate and folinic acid in gestational trophoblastic tumors. Br J Obstet Gynecol 1989;96:795–802.
33. Wong LC, Choo YC, Ma HK. Methotrexate with citrovorum factor rescue in gestational trophoblastic disease. Am J Obstet Gynecol 1985;152:59–62.
34. Rotmensch J, Rosenshein N, Donehower R, Dillon M, Villar J. Plasma methotrexate levels in patients with gestational trophoblastic neoplasia treated by two methotrexate regimens. Am J Obstet Gynecol 1984;178:730–734.
35. Homesley HD, Blessing JA, Schlaerth J, et al. Rapid escalation of weekly intramuscular methotrexate for nonmetastatic gestational trophoblastic disease. Obstet Gynecol 1988;72:413–418.
36. Hoffman MS, Fiorica JV, Gleeson NC, et al. A single institution experience with weekly intramuscular methotrexate for nonmetastatic gestational trophoblastic disease. Gynecol Oncol 1996;60:292–294.
37. Berkowitz RS, Goldstein DP, Bernstein MR. Methotrexate infusion with folinic acid in primary therapy of nonmetastatic trophoblastic tumors. Gynecol Oncol 1990;36:56–59.
38. Garrett AP, Garner EO, Goldstein DP, Berkowitz RS. Methotrexate infusion and folinic acid as primary therapy for nonmetastatic and low-risk metastatic gestational trophoblastic tumors. J Reprod Med 2002;47:355–362.
39. Elit L, Covens A, Osborne R, et al. High-dose methotrexate for gestational trophoblastic disease. Gynecol Oncol 1994;54:282–287.
40. Wong LC, Ngan HYS, Cheng DKL, et al. Methotrexate infusion in low-risk gestational trophoblastic disease. Am J Obstet Gynecol 2000;183:1579–1582.
41. Smith EB, Weed JC Jr, Tyrey L, et al. Treatment of nonmetastatic gestational trophoblastic disease: results of methotrexate alone versus methotrexate folinic acid. Am J Obstet Gynecol 1982;144:88–92.
42. Gleeson NC, Finan MA, Fiorica JV, et al. Nonmetastatic gestational trophoblastic disease. Weekly methotrexate compared with 8-day methotrexate-folinic acid. Eur J Gynecol Oncol 1993; XIV:461–465.
43. Hilgers RD, Hermann JJ, Sandefer JC. Failure of single-dose methotrexate followed by citrovorum factor in nonmetastatic gestational trophoblastic neoplasia. Gynecol Oncol 1990;37: 412–416.
44. Mutch DG, Soper JT, Baker ME, et al. Role of computed axial tomography of the chest in staging patients with nonmetastatic trophoblastic disease. Obstet Gynecol 1986;68:348–352.
45. Osathanondh R, Goldstein DP, Pastorfide GB. Actinomycin D as the primary agent for gestational trophoblastic disease. Cancer (Phila) 1975;36:863–866.
46. Petrilli ES, Morrow CP. Actinomycin D toxicity in the treatment of trophoblastic disease. A comparison of the 5-day course to single-dose administration. Gynecol Oncol 1980;9:18–22.
47. Kohorn EI. Decision making for chemotherapy administration in patients with low-risk gestational trophoblastic neoplasia. Int J Gynecol Cancer 1996;6:279–285.
48. Twiggs LB. Pulse actinomycin D scheduling in nonmetastatic gestational trophoblastic neoplasia: cost-effective chemotherapy. Gynecol Oncol 1982;16:190–195.
49. Schlaerth JB, Morrow CP, Nalick RH, et al. Single-dose actinomycin D in the treatment of postmolar trophoblastic disease. Gynecol Oncol 1984;19:53–56.
50. Petrilli ES, Twiggs LB, Blessing JA, et al. Single-dose actinomycin D treatment for nonmetastatic gestational trophoblastic disease. Cancer (Phila) 1987;60:2173–2176.
51. Smith JP. Chemotherapy in gynecologic cancer. Clin Obstet Gynecol 1975;18:113–116.
52. Rose PG, Piver MS. Alternating methotrexate and dactinomycin in nonmetastatic gestational trophoblastic disease. J Surg Oncol 1989;41:148–152.
53. DuBeshter B, Berkowitz RS, Goldstein DP, et al. Management of low-risk gestational tumors. J Reprod Med 1991;36:36–39.
54. Soper JT, Clarke-Pearson DL, Berchuck A, et al. Five-day methotrexate for women with metastatic gestational trophoblastic disease. Gynecol Oncol 1994;54:76–79.
55. Roberts JP, Lurain JR. Treatment of low-risk metastatic gestational trophoblastic tumors with single-agent chemotherapy. Am J Obstet Gynecol 1996;174:1917–1924.
56. Lurain JR. Advances in management of high-risk gestational trophoblastic tumors. J Reprod Med 2002;47:451–459.
57. Lurain JR, Brewer JI. Treatment of high-risk gestational trophoblastic disease with methotrexate, actinomycin D and cyclophosphamide chemotherapy. Obstet Gynecol 1985;65: 830–834.
58. Begent RHJ, Bagshawe KD. The management of high-risk choriocarcinoma. Semin Oncol 1982;9:198–203.
59. Curry SL, Blessing JA, Disaia PJ, et al. A prospective randomized comparison of methotrexate, actinomycin D and chlorambucil (MAC) versus modified Bagshawe regimen in "poor-prognosis" gestational trophoblastic disease. Obstet Gynecol 1989;73:357–362.
60. Newlands ES, Bagshawe KD, Begent RJH, et al. Results with EMA/CO (etoposide, methotrexate, actinomycin D, cyclophosphamide, vincristine) regimen in high-risk gestational trophoblastic tumors (1979–1989). Br J Obstet Gynecol 1991; 98:550–557.
61. Bolis G, Bonazzi C, Landoni F, et al. EMA/CO regimen in high-risk gestational trophoblastic tumor. Gynecol Oncol 1988;31:439–444.
62. Schink JC, Singh DK, Rademaker AW, Miller DS, Lurain JR. Etoposide, methotrexate, actinomycin D, cyclophosphamide, and vincristine for the treatment of metastatic, high-risk gestational trophoblastic disease. Obstet Gynecol 1992;80: 817–820.
63. Soper JT, Evans AC, Clarke-Pearson DL, et al. Alternating weekly chemotherapy with etoposide, methotrexate, dactinomycin/cyclophosphamide-vincristine for high-risk gestational trophoblastic disease. Obstet Gynecol 1994;83:113–117.
64. Quinn M, Murray J, Friedlander M, et al. EMA/CO in high-risk gestational trophoblastic disease; the Australian experience Aust NZ J Obstet Gynecol 1994;34:90–92.
65. Bower M, Newlands ES, Holden L, et al. EMA/CO for high-risk gestational trophoblastic disease results; from a cohort of 272 patients. J Clin Oncol 1997;15:2636–2643.
66. Kim SJ, Bae SN, Kim JH, et al. Risk factors for the prediction of treatment failure in gestational trophoblastic tumors treated with EMA/CO regimen. Gynecol Oncol 1998;71:247–253.
67. Escobar PF, Lurain JR, Singh DK, Bozorgi K, Fishman DA. Treatment of high-risk gestational trophoblastic neoplasia with etoposide, methotrexate, actinomycin D, cyclophosphamide, and vincristine chemotherapy. Gynecol Oncol 2003; 91:552–557.
68. Soto-Wright V, Goldstein DP, Bernstein MR, et al. The management of gestational trophoblastic tumors with etoposide, methotrexate, and actinomycin D. Gynecol Oncol 1997;64: 156–159.
69. Matsui H, Suzuka K, Iitsuka Y, et al. Combination chemotherapy with methotrexate, etoposide, and actinomycin D for high-risk gestational trophoblastic tumors. Gynecol Oncol 2000;78: 28–31.
70. Theodore C, Azab M, Droz J-P, et al. Treatment of high-risk gestational trophoblastic disease with chemotherapy combinations containing cisplatin and etoposide. Cancer (Phila) 1989;64: 1824–1829.
71. Bakri Y, Berkowitz RS, Goldstein DP, et al. Brain metastases of gestational trophoblastic tumor. J Reprod Med 1994;39:179–182.
72. Bakri YN, Subhi J, Amer M, et al. Liver metastases of gestational trophoblastic tumor. Gynecol Oncol 1993;48:110–113.

73. Surwit EA, Childers JM. High-risk metastatic gestational trophoblastic disease. A new dose-intensive, multi-agent chemotherapeutic regimen. J Reprod Med 1991;36:45–48.
74. Newlands ES, Mulholland PJ, Holden L, et al. Etoposide and cisplatin/etoposide, methotrexate and actinomycin D (EMA) chemotherapy for patients with high-risk gestational trophoblastic tumors refractory to EMA/cyclophosphamide and vincristine and patients presenting with metastatic placental site trophoblastic tumors. J Clin Oncol 2000;18:854–859.
75. Yordan EL, Schlaerth J, Gaddis O, et al. Radiation therapy in the management of gestational choriocarcinoma metastatic to the central nervous system. Obstet Gynecol 1987;69:627–630.
76. Evans AC Jr, Soper JT, Clarke-Pearson DL, et al. Gestational trophoblastic disease metastatic to the central nervous system. Gynecol Oncol 1995;59:226–230.
77. Small W Jr, Lurain JR, Shetty RM, et al. Gestational trophoblastic disease metastatic to the brain. Radiology 1996;200: 277–280.
78. Rustin GJ, Newlands ES, Begent RH, et al. Weekly alternating etoposide, methotrexate, and actinomycin D/vincristine and cyclophosphamide chemotherapy for the treatment of CNS metastases of choriocarcinoma. J Clin Oncol 1989;7:900–904.
79. Soper JT, Evans AC, Rodriguez G, et al. Etoposide-platin combination therapy for chemorefractory gestational trophoblastic disease. Gynecol Oncol 1995;56:421–424.
80. Okomato T, Nawa A, Nakanishi T, et al. Usefulness of colony-stimulating factor on neutropenia in patients with invasive mole and choriocarcinoma. Oncology 1995;52:159–162.
81. Collins RH Jr, White CS, Stringer CA, et al. Successful treatment of refractory gestational trophoblastic neoplasm with high-dose etoposide and cyclophosphamide. Gynecol Oncol 1991;43:317–319.
82. Bozorgi K, Fishman DA, Lurain JR. High-dose etoposide for resistant gestational choriocarcinoma. Presented at XIth World Congress on Gestational Trophoblastic Disease, Santa Fe, NM, October 30, 2001.
83. Lotz JP, Andre T, Donsimoni R, et al. High-dose chemotherapy with ifosfamide, carboplatin, and etoposide combined with autologous bone marrow transplantation for the treatment of poor-prognosis germ cell tumors and metastatic trophoblastic disease in adults. Cancer (Phila) 1995;75:874–885.
84. Giacolone PL, Benos P, Donnadio D, et al. High-dose chemotherapy with autologous bone marrow transplantation for refractory metastatic gestational trophoblastic disease. Gynecol Oncol 1995;58:383–385.
85. Van Besian K, Verschraegen C, Mehra R, et al. Complete remission of refractory gestational trophoblastic disease with brain metastases treated with multicycle ifosfamide, carboplatin, and etoposide (ICE) and stem cell rescue. Gynecol Oncol 1997;65: 366–369.
86. Osborne R, Dodge J, Covens A, Gerulath A. Use of a paclitaxel-containing doublet (TE/TP) as salvage therapy for EP/EMA failures. Presented at XIIth World Congress on Gestational Trophoblastic Disease, Boston, MA, September 28–October 1, 2003.
87. Hammond CB, Weed JC Jr, Currie JL. The role of operation in the current therapy of gestational trophoblastic disease. Am J Obstet Gynecol 1980;136:844–856.
88. Soper JT. Surgical therapy of gestational trophoblastic disease. J Reprod Med 1994;39:168–174.
89. Jones WB, Wolchok J, Lewis JL Jr. The role of surgery in the management of gestational trophoblastic disease. Int J Gynecol Cancer 1996;6:261–266.
90. Mutch DG, Soper JT, Babcock CJ. Recurrent gestational trophoblastic disease. Cancer (Phila) 1990;66:978–982.
91. Tomoda Y, Arii Y, Kaseki S, et al. Surgical indications for resection in pulmonary metastases of choriocarcinoma. Cancer (Phila) 1980;46:2723–2730.
92. Saitoh K, Harado K, Nakayama H, et al. Role of thoracotomy in pulmonary metastases from gestational choriocarcinoma. J Thorac Cardiovasc Surg 1983;85:815–820.
93. Vogelzang RL, Nemeck AA, Skrtic Z, et al. Uterine arteriovenous malformations: primary treatment with therapeutic embolization. J Vasc Intervent Radiol 1991;2:517–522.
94. Matsui H, Iitsuka Y, Suzuka K, et al. Early pregnancy outcomes after chemotherapy for gestational trophoblastic tumor. J Reprod Med 2004;49:531–534.
95. Sarwar N, Newlands ES, Seckl MJ. Gestational trophobalstic-neoplasia: The managemetn of relapsing patients and other recent advances. Curr Oncol Rep 2004;6:476–482.
96. Osborne R, Covens A, Merchandani DE, et al. Successful salvage of relapsed high-risk gestational trophoblastic neoplasia patients using a novel paclitaxel-containing doublet. J Reprod Med 2004; 49:655–661.

52

Ovarian Cancer

Yukio Sonoda and David Spriggs

Ovarian cancer consistently ranks as the most common cause of death among the gynecologic malignancies. There will be an estimated 16,090 deaths attributable to this illness in the year 2004,[1] and with 25,580 annual new cases of ovarian cancer, it ranks as the fifth most common cancer among females in the United States. The incidence rates for this particular malignancy are higher in white compared to black women.[2] The lifetime risk in the general population is 1.4%, with incidence increasing with age up to age 80.

The management of ovarian cancer, fallopian tube cancer, and primary peritoneal cancer are generally indistinguishable. The number of fallopian tube cancers is far too small to constitute an independent literature whereas the diagnosis of primary peritoneal cancer is often presumptive, based on the distribution of tumor deposits or prior oophorectomy. The surgical and chemotherapy management principles described here for ovarian cancer can be generally applied to fallopian tube cancers or peritoneal cancers unless otherwise specified. For purposes of conceptualization, it is useful to imagine ovarian cancer as a series of networked *disease states* or groups of patients with similar outcomes. The material is organized within this framework.

Screening and Prevention

Epidemiology of Ovarian Cancer

Multiple risk factors have been associated with an increased risk of ovarian cancer. Race and country of origin have been associated with increased risk for this disease. Industrialized countries, with the exception of Japan, have the highest rates of ovarian cancer and the nonindustrialized countries the lowest. The incidence in the United States among the white population is 14.2 per 100,000. In Japan, the incidence is 2.7 per 100,000 and in India it is 4.6 per 100,000. However, when immigrants from Japan move to the United States, after one or two generations, their risk is similar to that of a native-born American.[3]. Race may also play a role in the development of this disease because the risk of developing ovarian cancer is 46% greater in Caucasians compared to African-Americans.[4]

Diet

Dietary factors such as dietary fat intake, milk product consumption, and antioxidant intake all have been investigated as potential risk factors. Although epidemiology and case-control studies have suggested increased risk associated with each of these factors, none has been confirmed in the large, prospective Nurses Health Study cohort. In that study, subjects' dietary intake was assessed using a self-administered food frequency questionnaire.[5–7] There were 301 cases of invasive epithelial ovarian cancer confirmed among 80,258 participants. None of the dietary features studied were found to increase ovarian cancer risk. For dietary fat, those women in the highest quintile of fat intake had a relative risk of 1.03 [confidence interval (CI) 0.72, 1.45; $P = 0.97$] of developing ovarian cancer when compared to women in the lowest quintile.

Lactose and its metabolic product galactose have also been implicated in retrospective analysis.[8] Using the Nurses' Health Study data, Fairfield et al. observed a 40% increase in risk of all types of ovarian cancer for subjects in the highest category of lactose consumption compared to those in the lowest.[9] This increase of risk did not achieve statistical significance. In the same study, Fairfield et al. prospectively assessed the consumption of vitamins A, C, and E, and specific carotenoids as well as fruit and vegetable intake among 80,326 women in the Nurses' Health Study. A high consumption of these antioxidant vitamins or intake of fruits did not translate into a decreased risk of ovarian cancer.[10] In summary, diet has not been convincingly shown to contribute to ovarian cancer incidence.

Reproductive Factors

There have been multiple studies examining the effect of parity on the incidence of ovarian cancer. Whittemore et al., reporting for the Collaborative Ovarian Cancer Group, summarized the results of 12 case-controlled studies from the United States and demonstrated a significant protective effect from pregnancy.[11] A single term pregnancy resulted in a significant reduction in risk of ovarian cancer [odds ratio (OR), 0.47; 95% CI, 0.40–0.56]. This risk reduction continued with future pregnancies; after six term pregnancies, the OR was 0.29 (95% CI, 0.20–0.42).

Reproductive factors were prospectively studied in the Nurses Cohort study, which followed 121,700 women since 1976.[12] The authors found that each parity reduced the risk of ovarian cancer (OR, 0.84; 95% CI, 0.77–0.91 for each pregnancy). This protective effect of parity supports the "incessant ovulation" hypothesis, which is based on the premise that ovarian cancer develops from an aberrant repair process of the surface epithelium that is ruptured and repaired during each ovulatory cycle.[13] By reducing the number of ovulatory cycles by pregnancy, there theoretically is a reduction in the probability that a cancer would develop.

Genetic Predisposition

This strongest risk factor for the development of ovarian cancer is genetic predisposition. Family history of ovarian cancer has long been known to be a strong risk factor for ovarian cancer. Case-controlled studies have demonstrated that relatives of patients with ovarian cancer had an increased risk themselves of developing ovarian cancer.[14] The odds ratios for patients with first- or second- degree relatives with ovarian cancer were 3.6 (95% CI, 1.8–7.1) and 2.9 (95% CI, 1.6–5.3) when compared to subjects without a family history of this disease.

It has been estimated that approximately 10% of all epithelial ovarian carcinomas result from a hereditary predisposition, and two distinct syndromes have been currently identified.[15] The most common is the hereditary breast-ovarian cancer syndrome, which accounts for 75% to 90% of all hereditary ovarian cancers. It is linked to mutations of the BRCA 1and BRCA 2 genes, which were both identified in the early 1990s. These genes are inherited in an autosomal dominant manner, which leads to increased susceptibility to ovarian cancer with variable penetrance. Linkage studies have demonstrated that the lifetime risk for the development of ovarian cancer for carriers of the BRCA 1 gene is in the range of 16% to 63%.[15] Similar studies have estimated the risk in BRCA 2 carriers to be 16% to 27%. These genes clearly place one at significantly higher risk than the 1.4% risk of the general population.[16,17]

The second recognized ovarian cancer syndrome is the hereditary nonpolyposis colorectal cancer syndrome (HNPCC). Mutations in the DNA mismatch-repair (MMR) genes are responsible for this syndrome. Specifically, mutations in MLH1 and MSH2 account for 90% of subjects with HNPCC.[18] In a study of 50 HNPCC families, Aarnio et al. determined the average lifetime risk of ovarian cancer in patients belonging to the HNPCC kindred is 12%.[19] Although this syndrome accounts for only a small fraction of hereditary ovarian cancer, these patients clearly have a lifetime risk significantly higher than the general population and should be considered for prophylactic surgery or screening.

Risk Reduction

Oral Contraceptive Pills

Oral contraceptive pills are one of the established findings to be associated with risk reduction for ovarian cancer. They have been shown to provide a protective effect for the development of ovarian cancer in many case-controlled trials. The World Health Organization (WHO) conducted a review of 368 patients with ovarian cancer compared to 2,397 matched controls.[20] The relative risk for women who had ever used oral contraceptives was 0.75. The risk decreased with increasing time since cessation of use and with longer duration of use.

Although the early studies that demonstrated the protective effect of oral contraceptives were based on formulations containing 50µg or more estrogen, recent case-controlled studies have demonstrated that the lower-dose formulations also provide a similar degree of risk reduction. In a case-controlled study, Ness et al. demonstrated that ovarian cancer risk reduction was similar when on oral contraceptives independent of low-dose and high-dose formulations.[21] Similar findings were reported in a study from Norway and Sweden consisting of 103,551 patients. Any use of oral contraceptives was associated with a decreased relative risk of 0.6 (95% CI, 0.5–0.8), and longer duration of use appeared to have an increasing protective effect.[22] The obvious benefits observed with oral contraceptive use in the general population are also evident in those patients who are members of a hereditary ovarian cancer syndrome.[23]

Prophylactic Surgery

The high mortality associated with ovarian cancer has prompted physicians to recommend that patients who are at risk for developing this deadly malignancy may opt to undergo prophylactic surgery to remove the source before it can develop. This concept of removing the ovaries to prevent a potential ovarian cancer is not new, as gynecologists have been performing this for many years at the time of surgery for benign disease. It has also been used in premenopausal patients as a hormonal adjuvant treatment for metastatic breast cancer. Patients with a germline mutation in *BRCA1/2* or the MMR genes or those with a clinical diagnosis of hereditary breast-ovarian cancer (HBOC) or HNPCC syndrome are typically candidates for this procedure. In the majority of cases, prophylactic oophorectomy can be performed by laparoscopy as an outpatient procedure with an acceptable complication rate.[24]

Because the majority of these patients have a genetic predisposition for cancer, occasionally an unrecognized ovarian cancer is found in patients undergoing prophylactic oophorectomy. Rebbeck et al. identified 6 (2.3%) stage I ovarian cancers in 259 patients with germline *BRCA* mutations at time of prophylactic oophorectomy.[25] There were also 2 cases of primary peritoneal cancer diagnosed 3.8 and 8.6 years, respectively, after the procedure. This result was compared to a control group of 292 patients who did not undergo prophylactic oophorectomy. After a mean follow up of 8.8 years, 58 (19.9%) women in the control group were diagnosed with ovarian cancer; thus, there was a 96% risk reduction for coelomic epithelial cancer in those patients undergoing a prophylactic oophorectomy. The risk of breast cancer was also decreased by 53% in those patients who had a prophylactic oophorectomy. Kauff et al. reported such a finding in 98 women who underwent a prophylactic bilateral salpingo-oophorectomy.[24] One primary peritoneal cancer was diagnosed, whereas in the control group there were 5 ovarian or primary peritoneal cancers, resulting in a risk reduction of 85%. A reduction in the risk of breast cancer by almost 70% was also reported.

Patients at high risk for ovarian cancer are likely at increased risk for carcinoma of fallopian tube cancer.[26] Thus, a complete bilateral salpingo-oophorectomy is warranted, with emphasis on removing as much of the tube as is technically possible. It is likely that a small interstitial portion of the tube will remain within the cornu of the uterus. Some may recommend a hysterectomy to remove this, but fallopian tube cancers tend to arise at the fimbria or in the isthmus portion and not within the interstitial portion. There have been no reports of fallopian tube cancer arising subsequent to a prophylactic bilateral salpingo-oophorectomy. Some may contemplate a hysterectomy at the time of prophylactic oophorectomy for the prevention of endometrial cancer; however, there are no good data to support that germline *BRCA* mutations increase the risk of endometrial cancer. In contrast, patients belonging to the hereditary nonpolyposis colorectal cancer syndrome group are at significant risk of developing ovarian and endometrial cancer. Such patients should be offered prophylactic hysterectomy and bilateral salpingo-oophorectomy.

Prophylactic surgery is not 100% effective. Patients undergoing prophylactic surgery should be made aware of the risk of primary peritoneal cancer. Previous estimates of this risk after prophylactic surgery are in the range of 0.5% to 2.0%.[24,25,27] In a retrospective review of 22 Jewish patients with primary peritoneal cancer, Levine et al. predicted the lifetime risk for BRCA mutation carriers to be 1.3%.[26]

Extensive counseling before prophylactic surgery, whether bilateral salpingo-oophorectomy with or without a hysterectomy, requires a detailed discussion of the risks and benefits with the patient. The after-effects of such surgery should be addressed before the procedure because some of these patients will experience symptoms such as vaginal dryness and pain with sex, which can significantly contribute to dissatisfaction with surgery.[28]

Screening and Early Detection

Who Should Be Screened?

Although the majority of patients with ovarian cancer present with advanced disease and have a poor prognosis, those patients fortunate enough to have their cancer detected when it is still limited to the ovaries have an associated 5-year survival between 80% and 90%.[29] Because the majority of patients are found to have ovarian cancer at an advanced stage, an effective screening program for this disease would clearly be beneficial. Unfortunately, such a program has yet to be determined. Although the average lifetime risk of developing ovarian cancer is 1 in 70, only 1 in 2,500 women will develop the disease in any given year. This low incidence necessitates that any test used for ovarian cancer screening be both highly sensitive and highly specific. To date, however, the sensitivity and specificity of available screening technologies (i.e., transvaginal ultrasound and serum CA 125) are not adequate to be used in women at average risk.[30]

Because of the low prevalence of disease in the general population, research in screening for this disease has begun to focus on populations at increased risk. As mentioned, epidemiologic studies have identified a number of risk factors for ovarian cancer. Although both reproductive and environmental influences may modify risk to a small degree, family history of early-onset breast cancer and ovarian cancer is clearly the most important risk factor identified to date. It is believed that approximately 10% of all ovarian cancers are the result of an inherited mutation in either the *BRCA1* or *BRCA2* genes. A much smaller proportion of inherited ovarian cancer is caused by mutations in the genes associated with the hereditary nonpolyposis colon cancer (HNPCC) syndrome. These women are at significantly higher risk and are recommended to participate in ovarian cancer screening with transvaginal ultrasound and CA 125 starting no later than the mid-thirties. Risk-reducing salpingo-oophorectomy after child bearing has also been shown to reduce the risk of subsequent breast and gynecologic cancer in *BRCA* mutation carriers and should be discussed.[24]

Efficacy of Screening

Serum Markers

Screening modalities that have drawn the most attention over the past two decades have been serum markers and radiologic imaging. Bast et al. initially reported on the CA 125 assay in 1983.[31] CA 125 is a high molecular weight glycoprotein that is recognized by the murine OC 125 monoclonal antibody. Since that time, CA 125 has been the most extensively studied tumor marker for ovarian cancer screening.

Several large prospective studies have investigated the use of CA 125 levels as an initial test to screen for ovarian cancer. Einhorn et al. screened 5,500 healthy Swedish women at least 40 years of age with CA 125.[32] One hundred seventy-five women with elevated CA 125 levels and an age-matched control group were followed with pelvic examination and sonography every 6 months and serial CA 125 levels every 3 months. Six ovarian cancers were found in the study population, 2 stage IA, 2 stage IIB, and 2 stage IIIC. In each of these 6 cases, CA 125 either doubled or reached 95U/ml during a median follow-up of 32 months. Three women in the control group developed an ovarian cancer. CA 125 levels greater than 35U/mL exhibited a specificity of 98.5% in women age 50 or older.

Jacobs et al. conducted a randomized control trial on 22,000 healthy postmenopausal women who were screened with CA 125.[33] Patients with a value of 30U/mL or greater were examined with a pelvic ultrasound (transabdominal in the first year of study, then transvaginal in the subsequent enrollees), and those with an abnormal ultrasound were surgically explored. Twenty-nine patients underwent surgical exploration that identified 6 (3 stage I) ovarian cancers during the first 3 years of screening. Ten additional women developed ovarian cancer in the 8 years following their screening. Twenty women in the no-screening group developed ovarian cancer. The positive predictive value of this screening protocol was 20.7%. There was a higher percentage of early-stage ovarian cancers in the screened group (31.3% with stage I/II disease versus 10% in the nonscreened group), but this difference was not significant ($P = 0.17$). Ovarian cancer patients in the screened group did have a longer median survival than those in the control group (72 versus 42 months; $P = 0.011$), but this may be due to a lead-time bias rather than a true benefit from screening.

Ultrasound

Transabdominal ultrasound has been studied as a screening modality for ovarian cancer. In a prospective study, 5,479 asymptomatic women were subjected to three annual sonographic evaluations. Patients with abnormal findings were referred for surgical evaluation. An abnormal sonogram was found in 326 patients (5.9%), and 5 patients with ovarian cancer (all stage I) were identified. More than 25% of the false-positive sonograms had no ovarian pathology at exploration, and 74.3% had benign ovarian abnormalities. This screening method resulted in 51 surgical procedures for each cancer found.[34]

In an attempt to improve on this, transvaginal ultrasound has been studied as an alternative modality. van Nagell et al. reported on 1,300 asymptomatic postmenopausal women who were screened with transvaginal ultrasound.[35] Ovarian abnormalities were found in 33 women (2.5%). Of these, 27 went on to have laparotomy, and 2 were found to have stage IA ovarian cancer. The same group subsequently reported on 3,220 postmenopausal women using both transvaginal ultrasound and a specific morphologic index. Morphologic index was abnormal in 44 of the women, and 3 were found to have ovarian cancer (2 stage IA and 1 stage IIIB).

The same authors undertook a more targeted approach directing screening to patients who were classified as at risk for ovarian cancer.[36] The group included women older than age 50 and women older than age 25 with a family history of ovarian cancer. Annual transvaginal sonogram was performed on 14,469 women. Patients with an abnormal scan had a repeat in 4 to 6 weeks, and those with a second abnormal scan had a CA 125, tumor morphology indexing, Doppler flow, and surgical evaluation. Of 180 patients who underwent surgical evaluation, 17 ovarian cancers were detected (11 stage I, 3 stage II, and 3 stage III). Among patients with normal screening sonograms, 4 were considered to have false-negative screening tests (development of ovarian cancer or peritoneal cancer within 12 months of a normal sonogram). The sensitivity for ovarian cancer was 81%, specificity was 98.9%, and the positive predictive value was 9.4%. The sensitivity for detecting stage I ovarian cancer (excluding borderline and granulosa tumors) was 31%.

Summary of Screening for Ovarian Cancer

Although screening for ovarian cancer using CA 125 and ultrasound can detect disease in its earliest stage (Table 52.1), the low prevalence of this disease makes the positive predictive value (PPV) too low for use in the general population. CA 125 alone lacks specificity, especially in the premenopausal population, and may lack sensitivity for early-stage disease. Ultrasound screening still is considered experimental in the general population.[37] Combining CA 125 and ultrasound may sacrifice sensitivity and only achieves a high PPV in the postmenopausal population.

To be effective, a screening test should result in a decrease in mortality. There has yet to be a well-designed clinical study that has been able to demonstrate this. Currently, there are three large ongoing randomized trials that, it is hoped, will provide more information on the role of CA 125 and ultrasound in the screening for ovarian cancer in the general population. The Prostate, Lung, Colon, and Ovarian trial is being conducted by the National Institutes of Health and is a randomized trial of screening versus no screening for these cancers. Approximately 74,000 women over age 60 years will be randomized to CA 125 testing, ultrasound, and physical examination or to a no-screening control group. This sample size will require 16 years of follow-up to have an 80% power to detect a 30% decrease in mortality.

Two European groups are also conducting large randomized screening trials. The St. Bartholomew's group will randomize 120,000 postmenopausal women over 50 years to annual CA 125 screening or to a no-screening control group. Women with an abnormal CA 125 will have follow-up with a sonogram, which may lead to surgical evaluation. This study is designed to have an 80% power to detect a 30% reduction in mortality. Third, the European Multicentre Study group will randomize 120,000 postmenopausal women to screening with transvaginal sonography or no screening.

These large randomized studies will provide more information on the role of CA 125 and ultrasound for the screening of ovarian cancer in the general population. Until such results are available, screening in the general population remains unproven. Participation in screening clinical trials is an option for these people. For patients belonging to a hereditary ovarian cancer syndrome group who have a higher risk of developing ovarian cancer, screening with CA 125, clinical examination, and transvaginal sonography can be recommended, and eventually these patients may consider prophylactic surgery when childbearing is completed.

Primary Surgery for Ovarian Cancer

Surgery is essential for the diagnosis and treatment of ovarian cancer. Not only does it provide a pathologic diagnosis in cases of suspected ovarian cancer, it provides an opportunity

TABLE 52.1. Large screening trials.

Trial	*Reference*	*Year*	*No. of patients*	*No. of invasive cancers*	*No. with stage I*	*Initial intervention*	*No. of positive screens*	*No. of positive screens/cancer*
Einhorn	32	1992	5,550	6	2	CA125	175	29
Jacobs	167	1993	22,000	11	4	CA125[a]	41	3.7
Grover	168	1995	2,550	1	0	CA125[a]	16	16
Adonakis	169	1996	2,000	1	1	CA125[a]	15	15
Jacobs	33	1999	10,958[b]	6	3	CA125[a]	29	4.8
Van Nagell	35	1995	8,500	8	6	TVS[c]	121	15
Campbell	34	1989	5,479	5	5	TAS	326	65
Sato	170	2000	51,550	22	17	TVS[c]	324	15
DePriest	171	1997	6,470	6	5	TVS[c]	90	15
Van Nagell	36	2000	14,169	17	11	TVS[c]	180	10.6

[a] Followed by pelvic sonogram if CA125 abnormal.
[b] Randomized controlled trial with 10,977 controls.
[c] Followed by additional testing if abnormal.

TABLE 52.2. Comprehensive staging for ovarian cancer.

Peritoneal cytology
Intact tumor removal
Complete abdominal exploration
Removal of the remaining ovary, uterus, and tubes (may be preserved in select cases)
Infracolic omentectomy
Pelvic and paraaortic lymph node sampling
Multiple biopsies from areas at risk for spread (i.e., diaphragm, paracolic gutters, pelvis)

for the cytoreduction of advanced-stage disease or the staging of apparent early-stage disease. The International Federation of Gynecology and Obstetrics (FIGO) staging system involves a comprehensive surgical staging system based on the known patterns of spread. Essential elements of this are given in Table 52.2.

Impact of "Maximal Surgical Effort" on Outcome

The term *maximal surgical effort* was first introduced for patients with ovarian cancer in 1968 by Munnell when he reported an improved survival in patients who underwent a "definitive surgery" compared to those who had "partial removal" or "biopsy only."[38] Similar reports illustrating improved survival in patients who underwent surgical cytoreduction followed.[39]

Quantification of residual disease was first described by Griffiths in 1975,[40] who reported on 102 patients with stage II or III ovarian cancer who were treated with single-agent melphalan after primary surgical cytoreduction. The patients were stratified based on the largest diameter of residual disease after primary debulking surgery. Median survival was 39 months for patients with no gross residual disease, 29 months for those with residual tumor less than 0.5 cm, 18 months for patients with 0.6 to 1.5 cm residual tumor, and 11 months for patients with residual tumor greater than 1.5 cm. Others have demonstrated the benefit of primarily cytoreductive surgery in the management of patients with ovarian cancer in retrospective series.

There have been several studies that have demonstrated that the number of residual lesions may have an effect on outcome. Gall et al. demonstrated that, in patients with less than 3 cm of residual disease, those with 1 lesion had improved survival compared to those with more than 1 lesion.[41] Hoskins et al. reported on the re-review of another stage III (optimal) Gynecologic Oncology Group study and found a significant difference in progression-free interval and survival based on the number of residual lesions.[42] Patients had an increase in relative risk for greater than 20 residual lesions.

Although diameter of residual disease may be only one of the factors that may influence prognosis, it remains the most widely used method to quantify the effects of cytoreductive surgery. Typically, the patients are reported using the terminology of "optimal" and "suboptimal"; however, the precise cutoff and the measure of outcome may vary between studies. Typically, the reported cutoffs have been between 0.5 and 3.0 cm, and currently, the Gynecologic Oncology Group (GOG) employs a cutoff of largest residual nodule 1 cm or less as being "optimal." Outcome measurements that have been employed include response to chemotherapy, likelihood of achieving a negative second look, and survival, but in all parameters, a clear benefit exists to patients in whom "optimal" cytoreduction is achieved.

Recently the benefits of maximal cytoreductive surgery have been illustrated in a large meta-analysis. Bristow et al. identified 53 studies on patients who predominantly had stage III or IV epithelial ovarian cancer and who underwent initial cytoreductive surgery followed by chemotherapy that included either cisplatin or carboplatin.[43] Maximal cytoreduction was considered to have occurred if the residual disease measured 3 cm or less in largest diameter. Ninety-five percent of studies used either 1 or 2 cm as the cutoff for defining maximum cytoreduction. There was a statistically significant positive correlation between percent maximal cytoreduction and log median survival time. Each 10% increase in maximal cytoreduction was associated with a 5.5% increase in median survival time. When survival was compared between a cohort who had 25% or less maximal cytoreductive surgery to one with greater than 75%, there was a 50% increase in median survival time in the group with the higher percent of maximum cytoreductive surgery. The authors concluded that maximal cytoreduction was one of the most powerful determinants of cohort survival among patients with stage III and IV ovarian cancer, and consistent referral of patients with suspected advanced ovarian cancer to expert centers for primary surgery may be the best means available for improving overall survival.

Value and Extent of Retroperitoneal Lymph Node Dissection

Ovarian cancer can disseminate by several proposed methods: direct extension, exfoliation of cells into the peritoneal cavity, lymphatic spread, or hematogenous dissemination. The role of retroperitoneal lymph node dissection is another topic of debate in the surgical management of ovarian cancer. Lymphatic spread to the retroperitoneal lymph nodes is believed to follow the vascular drainage of the ovary; thus, lymphatic tissue up to the level of the left renal vein is at risk for disease spread.

The diagnostic value of retroperitoneal node dissection cannot be questioned in apparent clinical stage I disease. Because adjuvant chemotherapy is prescribed in all but the earliest cases of ovarian cancer, determining node status is imperative for the management of early-stage disease. In patients with clinically apparent early-stage disease, approximately 10% will have pathologic evidence of nodal metastasis.[44]

Patients with advanced-stage (III and IV) disease require chemotherapy as part of their management, and lymph node dissection has a lesser impact on management plan. The therapeutic benefits of systemic lymph node dissection are not clear. Burghardt et al. retrospectively reviewed the 5-year actuarial survival rate for stage III ovarian cancer patients who had and had not undergone pelvic lymphadenectomy.[45] The patients who had undergone lymphadenectomy had a 5-year actuarial survival rate of 53% compared to 13% in those patients who did not. Obviously, the no-lymphadenectomy group may well have been more advanced, based on selection bias.

In a comparative study of stage IIIC–IV optimally (gross residual disease less than 2 cm) cytoreduced patients with epithelial ovarian cancer, Scarabelli et al. demonstrated that systemic pelvic and paraaortic lymphadenectomy significantly improved survival in previously untreated patients.[46] With a median follow up of 26 months (range, 9–60), the estimated 4-year survival for patients who had undergone lymphadenectomy was 22% compared to those who had not, 0% (P less than 0.001). Twenty-three of the 30 patients (76.6%) who had undergone a systematic lymphadenectomy had positive pelvic and/or paraaortic nodes. There was a significant difference in survival based on nodal status, with an estimated 2-year survival of 46% for the node-positive patients compared to 100% in the node-negative patients. As in untreated patients who were optimally reduced at primary surgery, a similar survival benefit has also been shown in untreated patients with advanced-stage ovarian cancer who underwent complete resection of disease in the peritoneal cavity and who undergo systemic pelvic and paraaortic lymphadenectomy. The use of systematic lymphadenectomy does not affect survival if patients are left with suboptimally debulked disease.[47]

In an attempt to better define the impact of aortic and pelvic lymphadenectomy in patients with advanced-stage ovarian cancer, Spirtos et al. conducted a prospective study of 77 consecutive patients with advanced-stage epithelial ovarian cancer who were undergoing exploratory laparotomy.[48] Complete pelvic and paraaortic lymphadenectomy was attempted whenever maximal cytoreduction was obtained to residual tumor nodules less than 1 cm. Fifty-six of the 77 patients (73%) enrolled underwent systematic lymphadenectomy. Twenty-one patients (27%) did not undergo the procedure because it would not have impacted the cytoreductive status or because intraoperative conditions precluded it. Positive lymph nodes were found in 36 of the 56 (64%) patients who had a lymphadenectomy, and of these 23 (64%) were macroscopically positive. With a median follow-up of 30 months, 10 of 20 (50%) of patients with negative lymph nodes, 6 of 13 (46%) with microscopically positive lymph nodes, 10 of 23 (43%) with resected macroscopically positive nodes, and 2 of 21 (10%) with residual disease at least 1 cm in diameter were alive without evidence of disease. The authors concluded that lymphadenectomy offers little benefit if the nodes are macroscopically negative. However, removal of macroscopically positive nodes was advocated because survival in this group was similar to that of patients with microscopically positive nodes.

Although it appears that systematic pelvic and paraaortic lymphadenectomy may have a role in the primary surgical management of advanced ovarian cancer if patients can be maximally cytoreduced, one explanation may be that a portion of patients who have undergone maximal cytoreduction may have macroscopically enlarged nodal disease greater than 1 cm, 14.3% of patients in one prospective series.[49] The results of an internationally randomized trial to evaluate the role of systematic lymphadenectomy versus resection of any bulky nodes in optimally debulked patients may provide more information to help formulate surgical algorithms.

Role of Neoadjuvant Therapy

The traditional sequence of management for ovarian cancer is composed of initial surgery followed by chemotherapy. This sequence seems to be the optimal approach in most women because it provides an opportunity to confirm a suspected diagnosis of ovarian cancer, remove large tumor masses that may have poor blood supply, and theoretically increase the chemosensitivity of remaining tumor nodules by causing a greater number of tumor cells to enter the dividing phase.

However, the traditional approach of surgery followed by adjuvant chemotherapy may not be the best sequence to treat all patients who present with advanced ovarian cancer. In particular, patients who are too ill to tolerate a large debulking procedure or patients with tumor that cannot be reduced to remaining disease with a greatest diameter less than 2 cm may be better served by receiving chemotherapy first. This approach has the advantage of avoiding aggressive surgery in patients with chemoresistant disease.

Neoadjuvant chemotherapy, which is given to patients with advanced ovarian cancer before cytoreductive surgery, has several theoretical advantages over primary cytoreduction: (1) improvement of performance status, especially in elderly patients and those with pleural effusions and ascites; (2) decrease in the extent and morbidity of surgery by reducing tumor volume preoperatively; and (3) increase in the percentage of patients undergoing optimal cytoreduction.

Several retrospective studies have evaluated this approach in the management of advanced ovarian cancer. Vergote et al. reported on 285 patients with advanced ovarian cancer treated between 1980 and 1997.[50] Between 1980 and 1988, all patients underwent primary debulking surgery. Between 1989 and 1997, patients were surgically evaluated to determine if they should receive chemotherapy first (43%) or cytoreductive surgery (57%). Crude 3-year survival when the neoadjuvant approach was applied in the latter part of the study was 42%, compared to 26% during the early time period when all patients underwent primary debulking surgery.

Ansquer et al. reported the French multicenter experience with neoadjuvant chemotherapy for ovarian cancer deemed unresectable by either laparoscopy (61%) or laparotomy (39%).[51] Patients received a median of four cycles of chemotherapy preoperatively. Eighty percent responded to chemotherapy and underwent subsequent debulking, which was optimal in 91% of patients. The authors concluded that neoadjuvant chemotherapy in unresectable ovarian cancer led to a selection of chemosensitive patients who could subsequently undergo optimal cytoreduction in the majority of cases. In addition, aggressive cytoreduction was avoided in patients with initial chemoresistance. The absence of any prospective evaluation of the neoadjuvant approach make its routine application inappropriate at this time.

A concept that has been combined with neoadjuvant chemotherapy is interval cytoreduction. In spite of the fact that employing more-aggressive surgical procedures can increase the "optimal" debulking rate, a portion of patients will undoubtedly be left with "suboptimal' residual disease. Because these patients have a substantially worse prognosis than those who are optimally cytoreduced, some have evaluated the benefit of a brief course of chemotherapy followed by a second attempt at cytoreduction ("interval cytoreduction") before completing a prescribed chemotherapy regimen. Lawton and coworkers attempted cytoreduction of 28 patients after three cycles of platinum-based chemotherapy and were successful in debulking 25 patients to residual disease of less than 2 cm.[52] Ng and associates described 38 patients who underwent interval cytoreduction after two intensive courses of platinum-based chemotherapy and reported that 30 of these patients could be cytoreduced to less than 1 cm of residual disease.[53] Thus, it appears that interval cytoreduction can be quite successful in allowing patients a second opportunity for optimal cytoreduction. The effect of this interval cytoreduction on long-term prognosis, however, is less clear. Neijt and coauthors did not find the survival rate of a small group of patients who underwent interval cytoreduction to be as high as that of those who underwent successful cytoreduction at the initial operation.[54]

Although it appears feasible to improve the percentage of patients who can be reduced to optimal disease by presurgical treatment with chemotherapy, existing data are insufficient to determine whether this approach results in improved median survival. Comparison to patients who were cytoreduced initially may bias this because of the potential "favorable biology" of those who could be cytoreduced initially. A true comparison would be with those patients who could not be cytoreduced and not undergo interval cytoreduction.

The use of interval debulking for ovarian cancer has been studied in a large prospective randomized fashion by the European Organization for the Research and Treatment of Cancer (EORTC).[55] Patients with FIGO IIb-IV ovarian cancer who had been suboptimally debulked were included in this study. Four hundred twenty-five patients were initially treated with three courses of chemotherapy consisting of cisplatin and cyclophosphamide after which they were randomized to undergo either an interval laparotomy followed by another three courses of chemotherapy or another three courses of chemotherapy alone. One hundred six women were not eligible for randomization because of progression of disease, uncompleted chemotherapy, contraindication to surgery, or other reasons. Patients undergoing interval surgery had a significantly improved 2-year overall survival and progression-free survival compared to those patients treated with chemotherapy alone: 56% versus 46% and 38% versus 26%, respectively. Median survival in the interval laparotomy group was 26 months compared to 20 months in the control group.

The Gynecologic Oncology Group (GOG) undertook a similar study to evaluate the role of interval cytoreduction on progression-free and overall survival in patients with suboptimally debulked ovarian cancer. Patients who had suboptimal disease after initial therapy were clinically reassessed. Those who were responding or those with stable disease were randomized to interval cytoreduction or no surgery. All patients received an additional three courses of chemotherapy. Median overall survival and progression-free survival were not significantly different between those who underwent interval cytoreduction and the control group: 32 months versus 33 months and 10.5 months versus 10.8 months, respectively. Based on these results, the authors concluded that interval secondary cytoreductive surgery is not beneficial in regard to overall survival and progression-free survival for patients with advanced-stage suboptimal disease who had previously undergone maximal primary cytoreductive surgery. An explanation for the conflicting results of these two large randomized trials may rest in the extent of initial suboptimal surgery in that all patients in the GOG trial were initially operated on by surgeons specifically trained in ovarian cancer surgery whereas the surgical expertise level in the EORTC trial was not as consistent. Based on these findings, interval cytoreduction does not appear to have a role in patients who have undergone an aggressive initial attempt at cytoreduction by a gynecologic oncologist and are left with suboptimal disease. Neoadjuvant chemotherapy with interval cytoreduction may have a role in patients who, at initial diagnosis, are truly deemed unresectable via CT scan or laparoscopy or those who are initially felt to be medically unfit to undergo surgery.

Impact of Spillage in Stage IC Disease

Several controversial issues surround the surgical staging of early-stage disease. The significance of intraoperative rupture in cases with disease otherwise confined to the ovaries is a situation that has attracted much attention. Dembo et al. examined the prognostic factors in stage I epithelial ovarian cancer (EOC).[56] This study was a two-part study in which data from 252 Canadian patients were used to generate a hypothesis and the result was applied to a separate group of 267 Norwegian patients. The presence of tumor rupture was not a poor prognostic factor in the relapse-free rate. Ahmed et al. reported on a series of 194 patients with stage I epithelial ovarian cancer who were entered into a trial of observation only after surgery.[57] Patients who had rupture at time of surgery did not have a significantly worse survival. Similar conclusions were reached by Sevelda et al., who performed a case-controlled analytical study on 60 patients who had tumor confined to one or both ovaries.[58] Half the patients had their tumors removed intact and the others had intraoperative rupture. All patients underwent a staging procedure consisting of bilateral salpingo-oophorectomy, hysterectomy, omentectomy, and pelvic lymphadenectomy. All patients except 10 received whole abdominal radiation therapy. Tumors were of significantly higher grade and there were more bilateral tumors in the group who had intraoperative rupture. On multivariate analysis, tumor grade, stage, and intraoperative rupture did not have a prognostic influence on 5-year survival. The authors concluded that prognosis of patients with stage I tumors does not depend on intraoperative rupture. Other studies examining the effect of intraoperative rupture on recurrence-free survival in untreated patients have also demonstrated similar findings.[59]

Intraoperative rupture has been reported to be a poor prognostic factor in other series. In a large retrospective study of 1,545 patients with FIGO stage I invasive epithelial ovarian cancers from the Netherlands, Vergote et al. correlated disease-free survival with various clinical and pathologic variables.[60] All patients underwent laparotomy, hysterectomy, bilateral salpingo-oophorectomy, and infracolic omentectomy. Peritoneal washings, diaphragmatic scrapings, and retroperitoneal lymphadenectomy were not routinely done. Tumor rupture and timing of such was recorded. On multivariate analysis, degree of differentiation (moderate and poor), preoperative and intraoperative rupture, and age at diagnosis were predictive of recurrence.

The issue of intraoperative rupture remains controversial. However, capsular rupture whether preoperative or intraoperative does result in upstaging according to FIGO criteria, and adjuvant treatment should be prescribed accordingly.

Second-Look Surgery

Second-look surgery was first introduced as a diagnostic and therapeutic intervention for patients with gastrointestinal malignancies. In the management of ovarian cancer, it can be defined as a comprehensive surgical exploration in an asymptomatic patient who has completed initial surgery and a planned program of chemotherapy. After initial surgery, patients may not have measurable disease; thus, second-look surgery was initially used as a means of determining when a patient's chemotherapy could be discontinued.[61] The procedure was widely used in the 1970s and 1980s, but its enthusiasm has waned, and it remains a topic of controversy.

Second-look surgery has been evaluated in patients with early-stage disease. Reporting the Ovarian Cancer Study Group and the GOG patients, Walton et al. reported on 112 patients with FIGO stage I or II ovarian carcinomas who underwent second-look surgery after completion of adjuvant therapy.[62] Of the 95 patients who were asymptomatic at 18 months, only 5% had positive findings, compared to the 17 patients who were symptomatic (bowel obstruction, abdominal or pelvic complaints, weight loss, or other symptoms suspicious for recurrent disease). Of these patients, 53% had disease at second-look surgery.

In a smaller series, Rubin et al. reported on 54 stage I patients who underwent second-look surgery following complete surgical staging and adjuvant chemotherapy.[63] They found, as did Walton et al., that only 5.5% of patients had disease. None of the patients with grade 1 tumors had disease. Tumor grade was a significant predictor of recurrence following a negative second look, with grade 1 and 2 having a 0% risk of recurrence compared to 52% in the grade 3 tumors. Substage, histologic type, and chemotherapy type or duration did not predict recurrence. Given the small positive yield of second-look surgery in early-stage patients who have been initially comprehensively staged, it is not routinely recommended.

In patients with advanced ovarian cancer, the issues of second-look surgery are not as clearly defined. Surgical evaluation remains the most accurate method to date of evaluating patients with small-volume disease. In a prospective study of patients with ovarian cancer, Meier et al. demonstrated a 50% false-negative rate when correlating CA 125 levels with surgical findings.[64] Of those patients with stage III/IV disease and found to be disease free at second-look surgery, more than half have a recurrence of their disease with continued follow-up.[65] This finding brings the utility of second look into question. Experience from a large GOG randomized trial illustrates these issues. In a comparison of progression-free survival and overall survival in patients from GOG Protocol 158, Ozols and Greer compared 393 subjects preselected to undergo second look to 399 patients who did not. Second-line chemotherapy was not standardized in the study.[66] Two hundred ninety-four (75%) of the second-look group went on to have the procedure. The adjusted relative risk was 0.88 (95% CI, 0.73, 1.06), and the difference in median progression free survival was 2.1 months for the second-look group (25.0 versus 22.9 months). There was no difference in survival between the groups, and they concluded second-look surgery combined with various second-line therapies improved progression-free survival or overall survival in primarily positive patients.

Although a true benefit to second-look surgery alone has yet to be proven, the procedure does allow an opportunity for secondary cytoreduction if feasible. Several retrospective series have shown a benefit to secondary cytoreduction at time of second look. In a retrospective review of 150 patients with ovarian cancer from the Mayo Clinic who underwent second-look surgery, Dowdy et al. demonstrated that patients with macroscopic disease of 1 cm or more and who were able to be cytoreduced to microscopic disease had a better survival compared to those subjects who had residual macroscopic disease and those with disease of 1 cm or more who were secondarily cytoreduced to microscopic disease.[67] Other studies in the literature have also demonstrated such a benefit.[68,69]

Second-look surgery does not appear to have a role in the management of patients with early-stage ovarian cancers. Its role in patients with advanced-stage disease still is controversial, although it can be justified in the clinical trial setting when response to therapy must be accurately determined. Certain situations such as placement of an intraperitoneal catheter may justify its routine use in patients with advanced-stage disease. If gross residual disease is found, strong consideration should be given to secondary cytoreduction if microscopic residual can be obtained.

Primary Chemotherapy for Ovarian Cancer

In the clinical management of ovarian cancer, management has traditionally been divided into low-stage (FIGO stage I and stage 2) cancer and advanced disease, based on the results of surgical staging. The clinical outcome for low-stage cancers is far superior to that of more-advanced disease. The clinical trials and analyses are routinely divided into these two groups, which allows the most clear-cut evaluation of the clinical data.

Low-Stage Disease

Adjuvant Treatment for Stage 1 and Stage 2 Epithelial Ovarian Cancer

The benefit of immediate adjuvant therapy for low-stage ovarian cancer is a key question when surgical therapy alone can lead to a long-term disease-free survival in excess of 80%. In the early 1980s, the Gynecologic Oncology Group conducted a pair of randomized adjuvant therapy trials for comprehensively staged patients with stage I tumors.[70] In the first, eligible patients had FIGO stage IA or IB tumors that were of well- or moderately differentiated grade. Patients either were observed or treated with adjuvant melphalan. After a median follow-up of more than 6 years, there was no significant difference between the two groups. The 5-year disease-free survival was 91% versus 98% ($P = 0.041$) and the overall survival was 94% versus 98% ($P = 0.43$) in the observation and melphalan group, respectively. Three (38%) of 8 patients who had clear cell histology relapsed as compared to only 2 (3%) of 63 patients with other histologic types. This finding led the authors to define a low-risk group that included patients with disease confined to one or both ovaries, intact capsule, no adhesions or extracystic tumor, no ascites, negative peritoneal washings, and well- or moderately differentiated histology. A prospective, observational study of 194 patients

TABLE 52.3. Adjuvant chemotherapy for early-stage ovarian cancer.

Author	*Reference*	*Year*	*Stage*	*No. of patients*	*Treatment*	*Median follow-up (F/U)*	*Outcome (%)*	*P value*
Young	70	1990	IA–B grade 1, 2	43 38	Melphalan No treatment	>6 years	98 (5-year DFS) 91	0.41
Bolis	72	1995	IA–B, grade 2–3	41 42	CDDP No treatment	76 months	83 (5-year DFS) 65	0.095
Trope	73	2000	I	81 81	Carboplatin No treatment	46 months	70 (5-year DFS) 71	0.9
Trimbos (ACTION)	74	2003	I–IIA	224 224	Platinum-based No treatment	5.5 years	76 (5-year DFS) 68	0.02[¥]
Colombo (ICON1)	75	2003	I–III[a]	241 236	Platinum-based No treatment	51 months	73 (5-year DFS) 62	0.01
Trimbos (ICON1 and ACTION)	74	2003	I–III[a]	465 460	Platinum-based No treatment	>4 years	76 (5-year DFS) 65	0.001

DFS, disease-free survival.

[a] Majority of patients are stage I/II.

[¥] No difference in disease-free survival for optimally staged patients.

with stage I disease reported similar survivals from stage 1A and 1B disease.[71] It appears that well-staged patients with disease limited to the ovaries and who have well-differentiated tumors have high enough survival rates that they do not derive benefit from adjuvant therapy. The recommendation for patients with stage IA or IB, grade 2 disease still remains controversial, with some recommending adjuvant therapy while others do not. The importance of comprehensive staging before withholding adjuvant therapy cannot be stressed enough, given that as many as 31% of patients will have subclinical metastasis, which should be treated.[70]

In contrast to the low-risk patients, patients with grade 3 cancers, stage 1C disease or stage 2 disease, are generally considered to be at high risk, and adjuvant treatment is more likely to be beneficial. Chemotherapy use as adjuvant treatment has also been studied in prospective fashion (Table 52.3). The Italian collaborative group, Gruppo Interregionale Collaborativo in Ginecologia Oncologica (GICOG), conducted two simultaneous randomized trials.[72] The first trial included patients with stage IA and IB, grade 2 and 3 tumors who were randomized to adjuvant therapy with cisplatin (50mg/m^2 every 28 days for six cycles) or no further treatment. The second trial randomized stage IC patients of any grade to cisplatin (50mg/m^2 every 28 days for six cycles) or intraperitoneal phosphorus-32 (^{32}P) (15mCi). With a median follow-up of 76 months, the 5-year disease-free survival was 83% (cisplatin) compared to 65% (no treatment) in the first trial ($P = 0.09$) and 85% (cisplatin) compared to 65% (^{32}P arm) in the second trial ($P = 0.008$). In both trials, the difference was primarily due to a reduction of relapses in the pelvis only. In neither of the two trials was there a significant difference in 5-year overall survival due to the initiation of platinum-based chemotherapy at time of relapse for the no-treatment group. The authors also suggested the lack of difference in overall survival may be due to the limited impact of adjuvant therapy, low doses at which the cisplatin was administered, impact of salvage therapy, or that the study was underpowered. Trope et al. reported on their randomized study of adjuvant chemotherapy in stage I high-risk ovarian cancers.[73] They defined high risk as FIGO grade 1 aneuploid, grade 2 or 3, or clear cell carcinomas. One hundred sixty-two patients were randomized to receive either adjuvant carboplatin [area under the curve (AUC) 7] every 28 days for six courses or no adjuvant treatment. With a median follow-up of 46 months, estimated 5-year disease-free survivals were similar, at 70% and 71% in the treatment group and control group, respectively. Five-year disease-specific survival was 86% and 85% in the treatment and control groups, respectively. The authors believed the results were inconclusive because of the small size of the study.

More recently, the results of two large prospective randomized European trials of chemotherapy treatment have been published. These trials attempted to address the issue of adjuvant chemotherapy use in high-risk early-stage ovarian cancer. Unfortunately, the patient populations from these studies were flawed by an absence of consistent, comprehensive staging. In an EORTC trial, patients were accrued from 40 centers in nine European countries. Eligibility criteria for this trial included patients with FIGO stage IA–IB (grade 2 or 3)–IIA tumors or patients with stage I–IIA clear cell carcinomas who underwent surgical treatment that consisted of total abdominal hysterectomy and bilateral salpingo-oophorectomy in most cases, in addition to surgical staging. The surgical staging consisted of at least careful inspection of the peritoneal surfaces, with biopsy of any suspicious lesion. Surgical staging had four classifications ranging from optimal, if a comprehensive staging procedure as previously described was performed, to inadequate, if peritoneal surfaces were carefully inspected. Four hundred forty-eight patients were randomized to receive either adjuvant platinum-based chemotherapy or observation, with the endpoints being overall survival and recurrence-free survival. The overall survival was similar comparing adjuvant therapy to observation with a hazard ratio of 1.45 (CI, 0.93–2.27; $P = 0.10$). The recurrence-free survival was improved in the patients who had adjuvant therapy, with a hazard ratio of 1.59 (CI, 1.09–2.31; $P = 0.02$). Because comprehensive staging was not mandated, only approximately one-third of patients qualified as being optimally staged. When the patients were analyzed based on thoroughness of staging, the patients who were not optimally staged had improved disease-free and overall survival rates if treated with adjuvant chemotherapy; however, no difference was identified among the optimally staged patients, a much smaller group. The authors concluded that adjuvant chemotherapy was associated with improved recurrence-free survival. However, the benefits of chemotherapy appear limited to those patients who do not undergo optimal staging and thus are at risk for having subclinical disease.

Over a similar time period, the International Collaborative Ovarian Neoplasm Collaborators group conducted their own adjuvant chemotherapy trial for early-stage ovarian cancer (ICON 1).[74,75] The eligibility criteria were even less stringent in that entry into the trial was based on the clinician's judgment, which probably resulted in some occult advanced stage patients being included in the trial. If the clinician was uncertain if the patient required adjuvant chemotherapy, the patient was eligible for the ICON 1 trial, so long as she had all visible disease removed. Hysterectomy, bilateral salpingo-oophorectomy, and omentectomy were the minimum surgical requirements. Patients were randomized to a platinum-containing regimen or observation. With a median follow-up of 51 months, the 5-year overall survival was 79% in the adjuvant therapy group, which was significantly better than the 70% in the observation arm. The disease-free survival was also significantly better in the adjuvant treatment arm (73% versus 62%). The authors concluded that platinum-based adjuvant therapy improves survival and delays recurrence in patients with early-stage epithelial ovarian cancer.

In a preplanned combined analysis of the ACTION and ICON1 trials, the authors published the results of all 925 patients. With a median follow-up of more than 4 years, 5-year overall survival was 82% in the chemotherapy arm and 74% in the observation arm ($P = 0.008$). Five-year recurrence-free survival was also improved in the chemotherapy arm compared to the observation arm (76% versus 65%, respectively; $P = 0.001$). However, because the majority of patients in this joint study were not optimally staged, the argument still remains as to whether the presence of unappreciated residual disease could account for the apparent beneficial effect of adjuvant chemotherapy in this joint analysis. Although platinum-based adjuvant therapy appears to have a role in the incompletely staged population, its role in the comprehensively staged, early-stage patient remains unanswered by this trial.[76]

The drugs to be used in this setting have never been directly tested. In advanced disease, platinum-based therapy has been shown to be superior to nonplatinum therapy and combination therapy is superior to single-agent treatment.[77] That information has been extrapolated to low-stage disease, and all recent trials employ platinum-based therapy. The American approach, dictated by the Gynecologic Oncology Group (GOG), is to employ paclitaxel and carboplatin in the chemotherapy approach, although the contribution of paclitaxel in this setting has not been established. The issue of duration of adjuvant therapy has been addressed. The GOG recently reported the results of its randomized trial of adjuvant treatment for poor prognosis, early-stage ovarian cancer. The objective of this study was to determine if adding an additional three cycles of chemotherapy would significantly lower the rate of cancer recurrence. They compared adjuvant therapy with six cycles of paclitaxel (175 mg/m^2 over 3 hours) and carboplatin (7.5 AUC over 30 minutes) to the standard arm of three cycles of the same.[78] All patients were required to have undergone a comprehensive staging laparotomy including retroperitoneal lymph node sampling, and of the 457 accrued patients, 107 were deemed ineligible due to incomplete surgical staging. Of the 321 eligible patients, 241 (75%) were alive without recurrence with a median follow-up of 4.5 years. The risk of recurrence was 33% lower (27% in the three-cycle arm versus 19% in the six-cycle arm); however, this number did not reach statistical significance. When the analysis was performed to include incompletely staged patients, the recurrence rate was 24% less on the six-cycle regimen, which was not statistically significant. Toxicity was significantly greater in the six-cycle arm. The authors concluded that the additional three cycles of carboplatin and paclitaxel did not significantly improve the rate of recurrence in these early-stage patients but that it did result in more toxicity.

Value of Radiation-Based Therapy

Two types of radiation have been studied as adjuvant therapy for early-stage disease. Both external-beam radiation and intraperitoneal radiation have been evaluated, but some of the studies have included patients with advanced-stage disease who have been optimally debulked, and this must be kept in mind when interpreting these studies.

Because ovarian cancer tends to disseminate throughout the entire peritoneal cavity, adjuvant external-beam radiation therapy should be directed to encompass both the abdomen and pelvis. There have been two prospective randomized trials comparing the role of pelvic radiation to observation. A GOG study randomized 168 stage I patients between observation, pelvic radiation, and melphalan.[79] Of the entire group, only 86 were eligible for analysis; thus, the treatment arms were not equally matched for prognostic variables. Neither pelvic radiation nor melphalan reduced the recurrence rates when compared to observation. Similar results were found by Dembo et al., who randomized 41 stage IA patients to pelvic radiation therapy or observation. There were four relapses in the radiation arm and one in the observation arm.[80] They concluded that there was no benefit in survival or prevention of relapse from pelvic radiation because the entire peritoneal cavity was at risk for failure.

The lack of effective control with pelvic radiation therapy led to studies using whole abdominal radiation (WAR). Several randomized trials comparing WAR to chemotherapy as adjuvant treatment for early-stage ovarian cancer have been reported in the literature (Table 52.4). Of these, only one demonstrated a significant benefit.

Dembo et al. reported their experience with 147 patients with stage I–III ovarian cancer. Patients were treated with either abdominopelvic radiation or pelvic radiation with or without chlorambucil.[80] The benefit was seen only in patients with less than 2 cm or no residual disease, whose 10-year survival was 64% compared to 40% in the pelvic radiation group ($P = 0.0007$). Patients with residual disease greater than 2 cm did not show any benefit. In a randomized trial of WAR (2,600–2,800 cGy) with a 2,000-cGy pelvic boost versus melphalan (12 cycles of 0.2 mg/kg/day for 5 days), Smith et al. reported a 2-year disease-free survival of 85% versus 90% in the stage I patients treated with WAR and chemotherapy, respectively.[81] For stage II patients, disease-free survival was 55% and 58%, respectively. No statistical significance information was reported in the study. Klaassen et al. evaluated 257 patients with ovarian cancers ranging from stage I to III optimally debulked patients who were randomized to intraperitoneal ^{32}P (10–15 mCi), melphalan (8 mg/m^2/day for 4

TABLE 52.4. Randomized trials of adjuvant whole abdominal radiation (WAR) for early-stage ovarian cancer.

Author	*Reference*	*Year*	*Stage*	*No. of patients*	*Treatment arms*	*Outcome (%)*	*P value*
Klaassen	82	1988	IA, B	107	WAR	62 (5-year OS)	NS
			(grade 3)	106	Melphalan	61	
			IC-III OD	44	P32	66	
Smith	81	1975	I	14	WAR	85 (2-year DFS)	NR
				28	Melphalan	90	
Smith	81	1975	II	37	WAR	55 (2-year DFS)	NR
				29	Melphalan	58	
Sell	172	1990	I	60	WAR	63 (4-year OS)	NS
				58	Pelvic RT and cytoxan	55	
Chiara	83	1994	I–II	44	Cisplatin/Cytoxan	74 (5-year DFS)	0.07
				25	WAR	50	
Dembo	173	1984	I–III OD	76	WAR	64 (10-year OS)	0.0007
				71	Pelvic RT ± chlorambucil	40	

OD, optimally debulked; NS, not significant; DFS, disease-free survival; OS, overall survival; NR, not reported; RT, radiation therapy; WAR, whole abdominal radiation.

Source: Adapted from Rubin SC, Sutton GP (eds) Ovarian Cancer, 2nd ed. Philadelphia: Lippincott Williams & Wilkins, 2001.

days every 4 weeks for 18 cycles), or WAR (2,250 cGy over 20 fractions using moving strip technique).[82] Comprehensive staging was not mandatory. All patients were initially treated with pelvic radiation (2,250 cGy before WAR or 4,500 cGy before melphalan or ^{32}P). With a median follow-up of 8 years, 5-year disease-free survivals were similar at 66%, 61%, and 62% for the three arms, respectively, but the authors also noted that protocol violations in the whole abdominal target volume were associated with reduced survival.

Although earlier randomized trials have compared WAR to nonplatinum-based forms of chemotherapy, the Northwest Oncologic Cooperative Group of Italy attempted to compare WAR (4,330 cGy/24 fractions of pelvic radiation plus 3,020 cGy to the upper abdomen) to six cycles of adjuvant cisplatin (50 mg/m^2) and cytoxan (600 mg/m^2) chemotherapy in patients with stage I and II disease.[83] The study was closed early due to poor protocol compliance and low accrual. With a median follow-up of 60 months, 5-year survival was 71% and 53 % ($P = 0.16$), and relapse-free survival was 74% and 50% ($P = 0.07$) for the chemotherapy and WAR arms, respectively. When the data were analyzed according to treatment received rather than treatment assigned, no significant difference could be detected in relapse-free survival (73% versus 60%) or overall survival (73% versus 68%) for patients receiving chemotherapy and WAR, respectively.

The role of external-beam radiation as adjuvant therapy for the treatment of early-stage ovarian cancer remains unclear. It is apparent that adjuvant radiation therapy should encompass the entire abdomen because these patients are at risk for relapse in the entire peritoneal cavity. Although the older studies have seemed to demonstrate that WAR may be as effective as chemotherapy, these results have yet to be adequately demonstrated in patients with early-stage disease who have been treated with modern chemotherapy. The evolution of modern-day chemotherapy for ovarian cancer may make further efforts to study adjuvant radiation therapy difficult.

Intraperitoneal Radioactive Isotopes

Radioactive isotopes have been used as adjuvant therapy for the treatment of early-stage ovarian cancer. The isotope most commonly used has been ^{32}P. It is an emitter of beta radiation only, which avoids the toxicity associated with gamma radiation. It has a half-life of 14.3 days and an average tissue penetration of 1.4–3.0 mm. After it is instilled into the abdomen, the patient is placed in several positions to assure adequate distribution throughout the peritoneal cavity. As one might suspect, distribution of the radioactive colloid may be a potential problem. The intraperitoneal distribution can be tested before ^{32}P instillation with radioactive technetium sulfur colloid or after radiocolloid instillation with scintigraphic imaging of Bremsstrahlung photons.

Distribution patterns of intraperitoneal ^{32}P have been studied by Vergote et al.[84] They used a gamma camera to detect Bremsstrahlung photons in 297 patients. Images were obtained 2 to 24 hours and 3 to 7 days following administration of P32. They demonstrated that there was an uneven distribution in 165 patients, loculation in 2%, leakage in 3%, and uptake in the thoracic lymph nodes in 54%. There was uneven accumulation of isotope in the pelvis (60%) and right flank (33%). Forty-six percent of patients were noted to initially have even distribution but later were found to have major accumulation at 3 to 7 days. No relationship was noted between uneven distribution, loculation, or leakage of ^{32}P and relapse or bowel obstruction.

Several studies have compared the use of intraperitoneal ^{32}P as adjuvant treatment for early-stage disease (Table 52.5). As previously mentioned, the National Cancer Institute of Canada examined the use of intraperitoneal ^{32}P compared to whole abdominal radiation and melphalan in patients with high-risk stage I–II disease or optimally debulked stage III disease.[83] Comprehensive staging was not mandatory, and with a median follow-up of 8 years, 5-year survival was similar. The authors noted a high incidence of bowel complications in the ^{32}P and pelvic radiation arm, and this trial was closed prematurely.

The GOG studied adjuvant treatment use in 141 patients with stage I poorly differentiated or stage II tumors.[70] Patients were randomly assigned to treatment with either melphalan (0.2 mg/kg/day) for 5 days every 4 to 6 weeks for 12 cycles or one dose (15 mCi) of intraperitoneal ^{32}P at time of surgery. With a median follow-up of greater than 6 years, the disease-

TABLE 52.5. Adjuvant intraperitoneal ^{32}P for early-stage ovarian cancer.

Author	*Reference*	*Year*	*Stage*	*No. of patients*	*Treatment*	*Outcome (%)*	*P value*
Young	70	1990	IA–B (grade 3), stage II	68 73	Melphalan P32	80 (5-year DFS) 80	0.87
Young	79	2003	IA–B (grade 3), stage II	107 98	CDDP/CTX P32	77 (5-year DFS) 66	0.08
Vergote	84	1993	I, II, III OD	171 169	CDDP P32	75 (5-year DFS) 81	0.57
Bolis	72	1995	IC	82 79	CDDP P32	85 (5-year DFS) 65	0.008
Klaassen	82	1988	IA, B (grade 3) IC-III OD	107 106 44	WAR Melphalan P32	62 (5-year OS) 61 66	NS

DFS, disease-free survival; CDDP, cisplatin; CTX, cyclophosphamide; OD, optimally debulked; OS, overall survival; NS, not significant.
Source: Adapted from Rubin SC, Sutton GP (eds) Ovarian Cancer, 2nd ed. Philadelphia: Lippincott Williams & Wilkins, 2001.

free survival was 80% in both arms, and the overall survival was 81% and 78% with melphalan and ^{32}P, respectively (P = 0.48). Twenty-four of the patients were reclassified as borderline tumors but were evenly distributed among the two groups. Excluding these patients reduced the 5-year survival to 76%. When comparing the two treatment regimens, the GOG decide to label ^{32}P as the standard, given its lower cost, ease of administration, and lack of leukemia risk.

The GOG subsequently compared adjuvant ^{32}P to three cycles of cyclophosphamide and cisplatin in patients with stage IC and II with no macroscopic residual disease and stage IA and stage IB poorly differentiated tumors.[79] There were 205 patients randomized, and median follow-up was 6 years. The 5-year recurrence-free survival was 77% for the chemotherapy arm and 66% for the ^{32}P arm. After adjusting for stage and histologic grade, the estimated recurrence rate was 31% lower for the chemotherapy arm; however, this was not statistically significant (P = 0.075). Overall 5-year survival was 84% for the chemotherapy arm and 76% for the ^{32}P arm. Although there was no significant difference between the two arms, the better progression-free interval with the cyclophosphamide and cisplatin and the associated problems with ^{32}P distribution and bowel toxicities made platinum-based combinations the standard adjuvant therapy for patients with early-stage, high-risk ovarian cancer.

Vergote et al. reported their experience with 347 patients with stage I–III epithelial ovarian cancer without residual disease.[84] Comprehensive staging was not required in this series. Patients were randomized to receive intraperitoneal ^{32}P (7–10mCi) or six cycles of cisplatin (50mg/m^2). Patients randomized to the ^{32}P arm and who were found to have intraperitoneal adhesions were treated with WAR. With a median follow-up of 62 months, the estimated 5-year rates of crude survival and disease-free survival were similar. In the ^{32}P arm, these were 83% and 81%, respectively, compared to the cisplatin arm, 81% and 75%. Bowel obstruction occurred with a significantly higher frequency in the ^{32}P or WAR groups compared to the cisplatin group. The authors recommended that cisplatin be used for adjuvant therapy in future studies.

The Italian collaborative group, Gruppo Interregionale Collaborativo in Ginecologia Oncologica (GICOG), simultaneously reported on two randomized trials for adjuvant therapy for early-stage ovarian cancer.[72] In these trials. patients underwent surgical staging without routine nodal assessment, which was done by presurgical lymphangiogram or optional surgical biopsy. The first trial included patients with stage IA and IB, grade 2 and 3 tumors, who were randomized to adjuvant therapy with cisplatin (50mg/m^2 every 28 days for six cycles) or no further treatment. The second of the trials randomized stage IC patients of any grade to cisplatin (50mg/m^2 every 28 days for six cycles) or intraperitoneal ^{32}P (15mCi). With a median follow-up of 76 months, the 5-year disease-free survival was 83% (cisplatin) versus 65% (no treatment) (P = 0.09) in the first trial and 85% (cisplatin) compared to 65% (^{32}P arm) (P = 0.008) in the second trial. In both trials the difference was primarily due to a reduction of relapses in the pelvis only. In neither of the two trials was there a significant difference in 5-year overall survival, which the authors suggested may result from the limited impact of adjuvant therapy, low doses at which the cisplatin was administered, impact of salvage therapy, or that the study was underpowered.

In summary, the literature on treatment of low-stage ovarian cancer is limited by poor staging and low frequency of relapse. Randomized data suggest that low-risk patients (stage 1A, 1B with grade 1 and grade 2 histology) have an excellent prognosis and cannot be shown to benefit from adjuvant therapy. Although the randomized trial results are discordant, meta-analysis and the largest clinical trials agree that platinum-based chemotherapy appears to decrease recurrence and increase survival in high-risk patients.[85] The duration of platinum-based therapy is still uncertain, although the benefit at least three cycles is not in dispute. The contribution of paclitaxel in this setting is unknown. Randomized trials suggest that radiation therapy is probably similar to chemotherapy in survival benefit.

Primary Chemotherapy for Advanced-Stage (IIc–1V) Disease

Platinum-Based Therapy

The evolution of chemotherapy for advanced ovarian cancer began with single alkylating agents and evolved into combination therapy by the early 1980s. Cyclophosphamide, doxorubicin, altretamine, and 5-fluorouracil were all employed with limited success. This evolution culminated with the widespread implementation of platinum complex (cisplatin)-

TABLE 52.6. Platinum-based primary therapy of advanced-stage ovarian cancer: selected studies.

Author	Reference	Year	Residual disease	No. of patients	Treatment	Response	DFS (%)	Survival	P value
Swenerton	87	1992	Macroscopic	Total 447	Cisplatin + CTX Carboplatin + CTX	57% 59%	56 weeks 58 weeks	100 weeks 110 weeks	NS
Alberts	88	1992	Suboptimal	Total 342	Cisplatin + CTX Carboplatin + CTX	52% 61%		17.4 months 20.0 months	NS
ICON 2	89	1998	Stage I–IV	766 760	CAP Carboplatin	NR	70 (5-year DFS) 71	33 months 33 months	HR 1.0
Ozols	66	2003	Optimal	Total 792	Cisplatin/paclitaxel Carboplatin/paclitaxel	NA	19.4 months 20.7 months	48.7 months 57.4 months	HR 0.84 (0.7–1.02)[b]
du Bois	90	2003	I–III[a]	Total 798	Cisplatin/paclitaxel Carboplatin/paclitaxel	NR	19.1 months 17.2 months	44 months 43 months	NS

HR, hazard ratio; CAP, cyclophosphamide, doxorubicin, and cisplatin.
[a]CAP + cyclophosphamide, doxorubicin, cisplatin.
[b]95% confidence interval.

based treatment by the end of that decade. That question has been definitively resolved with level 1 evidence and is not revisited here. The interested reader is referred to comprehensive meta-analyses for discussion of this point.[77,86] However, the question of which platinum complex is best has been more recently resolved (Table 52.6). In a series of comparison, either alone or in combination with cyclophosphamide and doxorubicin, carboplatin has been consistently equivalent to cisplatin treatment.[87–89] More recently, two large studies of cisplatin/paclitaxel versus carboplatin/paclitaxel have been reported.[66,90] As was seen in cyclophosphamide combinations a decade earlier, there is not a statistically significant difference between the two paclitaxel-containing regimens. Equivalence between carboplatin and cisplatin has also been confirmed in meta-analysis.[77] Because carboplatin is generally better tolerated with substantially less toxicity, the current treatment depends on carboplatin therapy. The value of oxaliplatin in ovarian cancer treatment is uncertain. Cyclophosphamide and oxaliplatin were compared to cisplatin and cyclophosphamide in a small randomized trial with similar efficacy in previously treated patients.[91]

Anthracyclines have been proposed to improve outcome in ovarian cancer. Omura and colleagues compared cyclophosphamide–doxorubicin–cisplatin to cyclophosphamide and cisplatin.[92] Although there was no statistical difference, there was a trend toward improved survival. A meta-analysis confirmed a modest advantage to doxorubicin-containing regimens.[93] However, following the advent of paclitaxel, doxorubicin therapy has generally fallen from favor. Two large randomized trials of paclitaxel and carboplatin plus or minus epirubicin have been reported in abstract form, and neither survival or overall survival have been improved in these studies. Toxicity was clearly increased.

Paclitaxel-Based Therapy

With the initial report of the GOG 111 study by McGuire et al., chemotherapy of ovarian cancer entered the taxane era.[94] The randomized studies examining the value of paclitaxel in ovarian cancer are listed in Table 52.7. Two of these trials (GOG 111 and OV 10) are clearly positive whereas two later trials (GOG 132 and ICON 3) suggest that therapy with taxane adds little to the effect of platinum complex therapy.

TABLE 52.7. Paclitaxel-based treatment of advanced ovarian cancer.

Author	Reference	Year	Residual disease	No. of patients	Treatment	Response	DFS (%)	Survival	P value
McGuire	94	1996	Suboptimal	Total 410	Cisplatin + CTX Cisplatin + paclitaxel	60% 73%	13 months 18 months	24 months 38 months	$P < 0.001$
Piccart	95	2000	Stage II–IV	Total 680	Cisplatin + CTX Cisplatin + paclitaxel	45% 59%	11.5 months 15.5 months	25.8 months 35.6 months	$P < 0.0016$
ICON 3	96	2002	Stage I–IV	Total 2,074	Paclitaxel + cisplatin or carboplatin CAP Carboplatin	NR	17.3 months 16.1 months	36.1 months 35.4 months	HR = 0.98 NS
Muggia	174	2000	Suboptimal	Total 648	Cisplatin Paclitaxel Cisplatin + paclitaxel	67% 42% 67%	16.3 months 11.2 months 14.0 months	30.2 26.0 26.6	— HR = 1.15 HR = 0.99
Ozols	66	2003	Optimal	Total 792	Cisplatin/paclitaxel Carboplatin/paclitaxel	NA	19.4 months 20.7 months	48.7 months 57.4 months	HR 0.84 (0.7–1.02)[b]
du Bois	90	2003	I–III[a]	Total 798	Cisplatin/paclitaxel Carboplatin/paclitaxel	NR	19.1 months 17.2 months	44 months 43 months	NS

[a]CAP + cyclophosphamide, doxorubicin, cisplatin.
[b]95% confidence interval.

GOG 111 was the first trial of paclitaxel that compared paclitaxel/cisplatin to cyclophosphamide/cisplatin in patients with suboptimally debulked ovarian cancer.[94] The paclitaxel arm showed a distinct advantage for both progressive-free survival (18 versus 13 months) and overall survival (38 versus 24 months). These results were essentially duplicated by a confirmatory trial performed by the EORTC and the National Cancer Institute of Canada, which found that a paclitaxel/cisplatin arm was superior for both progression-free survival (16 versus 12 months) and overall survival (35 versus 25 months).[95] Unfortunately, the issue was reopened when a subsequent GOG study, GOG 132, found that the same experimental arm of cisplatin/paclitaxel was not significantly better than cisplatin alone at 100mg/m^2. In this study, the progression-free survival for the taxane arm and the cisplatin arms were similar (14 versus 16 months) and survival was not different (26 versus 30 months). Another very large study, ICON 3, was also initiated as a confirmatory study and, similar to GOG 132, could not confirm the superiority of taxane-based therapy. In the ICON 3 study, the time to treatment failure was 17.3 months for the paclitaxel-containing arm and 16.1 for the nontaxane treatment. The survival of the paclitaxel arm was similar to that seen with the control arm of either carboplatin or cisplatin, doxorubicin, and cyclophosphamide (36.1 versus 35.4 months).[96]

The explanation for the discordance remains uncertain. In a meta-analysis, Sandercock and colleagues examined the potential design differences that might lead to the disagreement.[97] They make several points of interest. The time to progression is remarkably similar for the paclitaxel/platinum arms (16–18 months) in the four studies but both GOG 11 and OV 10 have a surprisingly poor outcome for the cyclophosphamide / cisplatin control groups and a negative effect of cyclophosphamide has been postulated. Results from randomized trials that compared cyclophosphamide/doxorubicin/cisplatin, a control arm in ICON 3, to cyclophosphamide/cisplatin have been inconclusive, but meta-analysis has suggested that cyclophosphamide/cisplatin may be inferior.[92,98,99] It is also noted that paclitaxel was not available for recurrent disease patients whereas late treatment of control arm patients in the other trials might blunt the survival differences compared to GOG 111. The issue remains unresolved. In the United States, the National Comprehensive Cancer Network (NCCN) has supported paclitaxel and platinum as the standard of therapy; this standard is generally accepted around the world, and it is unlikely that additional studies of this issue will be initiated.

Dose and Schedule

The dose, frequency, and duration of primary chemotherapy have also been subjects of intensive investigation. Dose intensity/schedule studies for platinum complex therapy are summarized in Table 52.8. The doses of cisplatin and carboplatin have both been carefully investigated without any evidence that either agent has a significant dose response within the clinically useful range.[100–103] The analysis by Egorin and colleagues suggested that a carboplatin dose above an AUC of 5–6 is fruitless and even a carboplatin AUC 4 maybe sufficient.[104,105] Although a small study by Kaye et al. suggested a modest survival advantage, they also recommended a maximum dose of 75mg/m^2 for toxicity reasons.[106] Duration of platinum-based treatment has not been as well examined. Two small randomized trials in the prepaclitaxel era have failed to show an advantage to prolonged therapy. A study of 5 cycles versus 10 cycles of cyclophosphamide, doxorubicin, and cisplatin showed no difference.[107] Another study of the same three-drug regimen showed no advantage for 12 cycles of therapy compared to a more standard 6 cycles.[108] No randomized examination of duration of therapy for carboplatin plus paclitaxel has been performed.

The number of paclitaxel schedule/dose intensity studies is smaller but the results are similar. A two by two factorial study of infusion time and dose compared 135mg/m^2 with 175mg/m^2 and 3-hour infusions with 24-hour infusions.[109] No statistical difference was identified. A GOG study comparing 135mg/m^2, 175mg/m^2, and 250mg/m^2 was similarly negative for survival advantage, although the 250mg/m^2 dose arm had a modest increase in response rate to paclitaxel therapy.[110] In a carboplatin combination study, Bolis and colleagues randomized 504 patients between carboplatin and paclitaxel at 175mg/m^2 and carboplatin and paclitaxel at 225mg/m^2.[111] Although the higher dose was more toxic, there was no improvement in survival. In a single randomized study of weekly paclitaxel, a weekly dose of 67mg/m^2 was nearly identical to a 200mg/m^2 dose of paclitaxel given once every 3 weeks.[112]

Intraperitoneal Therapy

Because ovarian cancer is primarily a disease of the peritoneal cavity, regional therapy has been an area of considerable interest. Models of intraperitoneal (IP) chemotherapy show distinct theoretical advantages, especially for small-volume disease.[113,114] The use of intraperitoneal chemotherapy has been carefully explored in several large randomized clinical trials conducted by the GOG. Although each appears to favor the arm containing intraperitoneal therapy, quirks in trial design and treatment toxicity have prevented intraperitoneal therapy from becoming the single standard of care.[115,116] The first randomized compared cyclophosphamide plus 100mg/m^2 of cisplatin, given either by the intravenous or intraperitoneal route.[115] The study showed a survival advantage (HR = 0.76) but was overtaken by the introduction of carboplatin and paclitaxel in the primary treatment paradigm. The next study included a preparative regimen of two cycles of carboplatin (AUC = 9) and then six cycles of cisplatin and paclitaxel.[116] As in the first study, the survival difference was statistically significant in favor of the IP arm (HR = 0.81), even though a substantial fraction of the IP arm received little or no IP therapy because of toxicity. A third large randomized trial using IP cisplatin and IP paclitaxel has also been completed. The IP arm had a superior progressive-free survival, but overall survival analysis is not yet complete.[117]

The failure of IP therapy to assume a position of therapeutic prominence is a complicated problem. Certainly, 100mg/m^2 of cisplatin is toxic, and the renal, gastrointestinal, and neurologic toxicities are all daunting. The technical aspects of IP administration are also a factor. Without experienced surgeons, nurses, and medical oncologists, the frequency of complications including catheter failure, infection, and renal damage is unacceptably high.[118] Despite the pres-

TABLE 52.8. Platinum dose intensity, duration of therapy, and paclitaxel dose intensity.

Author	*Reference*	*Year*	*Residual disease*	*No. of patients*	*Treatment*	*Response*	*DFS (%)*	*Survival*	*P value*
Conte	101	1996	Suboptimal	Total 145	Cyclo + doxorubicin Cisplatin 50 mg/m^2 Cisplatin 100 mg/m^2	61% 57%	18 months 13 months	29 months 24 months	NS
McGuire	102	1995	Suboptimal	Total 485 223 235	Cyclophosphamide + cisplatin 100 mg/m^2 cisplatin 50 mg/m^2	55% 60%	14.3 months 12.1 months	21.3 months 19.5 months	$P = 0.18$
Jakobsen	100	1997	II–IV	Total 222	Carboplatin AUC 4 Carboplatin AUC 8				NS
Gore	103	1998	II–IV	Total 227 117 110	Carboplatin AUC 6 Carboplatin AUC 12	64% 55%	12 months 11 months	29months 36 months	NS
Colombo	175	1992	NR	Total 296	Cisplatin 50 mg/m^2/week Cisplatin 75 mg/m^2 every 3 weeks	66% 61%		36 months 33 months	NS
Kaye	106	1996	II–IV	Total 159	Cyclophosphamide 750 mg/m^2 + cisplatin 100 mg/m^2 Cisplatin 50 mg/m^2	61% 34%		5 years 32% 26%	$P = 0.043$
Duration:									
Hakes	107	1992	II–IV	Total 78 41 37	Cyclophosphamide Doxorubicin Cisplatin × 5 cycles Cyclophosphamide Doxorubicin Cisplatin × 10 cycles	CR 34% CR 35%		24 months 27 months	NS $P = 0.34$
Bertelsen	108	1993	III–IV	Total 202 66 136	Cyclophosphamide Doxorubicin Cisplatin × 6 cycles Cyclophosphamide Doxorubicin Cisplatin × 12 cycles	NR	NR	23 months 27 months	NS $P = 0.45$
Paclitaxel Intensity:									
Eisenhauer	109	1994	Relapsed disease	Total 382 199 192	Paclitaxel 135 mg/m^2 × 3 h Paclitaxel 135 mg/m^2 × 24 h Paclitaxel 175 mg/m^2 × 3 h Paclitaxel 175 × 24 h	15% 20%	14 weeks 19 weeks	48 weeks 50 weeks	PFS $P < 0.02$
Omura	110	2003	Relapsed disease	Total 330 164 166	Paclitaxel at 175 mg/m^2 250 mg/m^2 + G-CSF	27% 36%	4.8 months 5.5 months	13.1 months 12.3 months	Survival NS
Bolis	111	2004	IIB–IV	Total 502 244 250	Carbo AUC 6 + paclitaxel 175 mg/m^2 Carbo AUC 6 + paclitaxel 225 mg/m^2	Pathologic CR 63.8% 55.7%	4-year PFS 41% 39%	4-year survival 46% 47%	NS
Rosenberg	112	2002	Taxane naïve	Total 208 105 mg/m^2 200 mg/m^2	Paclitaxel 67 mg/m^2/week Paclitaxel 200 mg/m^2/ 3 weeks	37% 38%	6.1 months 8.1 months	13.6 months 14.7 months	$P = 0.98$

AUC, area under the curve; G-CSF, granulocyte colony-stimulating factor; Carbo, carboplatin; CR, complete response; NR, no response; PFS, progression-free survival.

ence of a survival advantage, it seems likely that IP cisplatin therapy never become widely accepted, and studies of IP carboplatin are being initiated.

Consolidation Therapy

Paclitaxel Based Therapy

One of the most controversial areas in ovarian cancer treatment is the use of "consolidation therapy," defined as additional therapy for patients in clinical complete response at the end of primary treatment (Table 52.9).[119] Intraperitoneal therapy, immune-based treatments, and extended cytotoxic therapies have all been examined in Phase II and occasional Phase III trials. No consensus has yet emerged, and the state of the art is based on comparison to no treatment rather than direct therapeutic comparisons. The only trial to show a modest advantage was GOG 178, a randomized comparison of 12 months of paclitaxel to a shorter, 3-month paclitaxel treatment.[120] This trial showed a progression-free survival advantage that was highly significant in favor of 12 months of treatment, but the trial was closed by the data safety monitoring committee and survival data will not be available. Unfortunately, without the survival analysis, this trial has

TABLE 52.9. Consolidation strategies.

Author	*Reference*	*Phase*	*Year*	*Assessment*	*No. of patients*	*Treatment*	*Median DFS (%)*	*Median survival*	*P value*
Intraperitoneal (IP) therapy:									
Barakat	121	II	1998	PCR	36 46	IP Etoposide 200 mg/m² IP Cisplatin 100 mg/m² Observation (not randomized)	Not reached 28.5 months	Not reached	$P < 0.03$
Piccart	123	III	2003	PCR	Total 153 76 76	IP Cisplatin 90 mg/m² Observation	HR = 0.89 (0.6–1.3)	HR = 0.82 (0.5–1.3)	
Tournigand	122	Retrospective analysis	2003	PCR	68	IP Cisplatin, mitoxantrone, and etopisde	34 months	74 months	Not comparative
Radiation therapy:									
Sorbe	176	III	2003	PCR or micro +	Total 172	Observation Whole-abdominal RT 6 cycles cisplatin 50 mg/m² IV Doxorubicin 50 mg/m² IV	32 months 37 months 116 months $P - 0.034$	5-year survival 64.5% 68.8% 57.1%	
IV Chemotherapy:									
Markman	120	III	2003	Clinical CR	Total 262	Paclitaxel 175 mg/m² monthly × 3 months Paclitaxel 175 mg/m² monthly × 12 months	21 months 28 months (p = 0.0023)	NR (closed early)	NR
De Placido	125	III	2004	Clinical responders	Total 273	Observation Toptoecan 1.5 mg/m² for 4 cycles	28.4 months 18.2 months HR = 1.18 (0.86–1.63)	NR $P = 0.30$	NR
Immune Interventions:									
Hall	128	III	2004	Ic-IV End of chemotherapy	Total 300 149 149	Observation Interfereon-alpha	10.3 months 10.4 months	32 months 27 months	NS
Seiden	126	III	2004	Ic-IV Clinical CR 345	Total 702 357	Observation	HR = 0.90 (0.68–1.19)	HR = 1.15 (0.82–1.63)	
Berek	127	2004	2004	Clinical CR	345	Placebo Oregovomab IV			NS

PCR, pathologic complete response.

been unable to change the standard of care, although it clearly has sparked new investigations in this area.

Intraperitoneal Therapy

As noted previously, intraperitoneal chemotherapy has never achieved common usage. Although many agents (cisplatin, floxuridine, mitoxantrone, paclitaxel, and others) have had Phase I/II testing, few Phase III data exist. Although a very large IP experience reported by investigators at Memorial showed that patients receiving IP therapy had very long median survivals compared to historical controls, the lack of prospective randomized controls is a major limitation.[121] These investigators have reported a prospective Phase II trial of IP cisplatin and etoposide.[121] More than 65% of the patients remained disease free with a median follow-up of 3.5 years. These results are similar to those reported by Tourigand et al. in a similar study of negative second-look patients.[122] A randomized trial of this concept comparing intraperitoneal cisplatin with a no-treatment control arm was recently reported by the EORTC.[123] The study was terminated for poor accrual and only reached one-half of the planned enrollment. Although no statistical difference could be discerned, the progression-free survival (5.4 versus 3.6 years), the overall survival (9.7 versus 7.3 years), and the fraction alive at 5 years (70% versus 60.5%) all favored the IP treatment arm.

Cytotoxic Chemotherapy

Because many optimally debulked patients begin chemotherapy with no evidence of clinical disease, all primary therapy can be considered to be "consolidation." Extension of therapy beyond the consensus six cycles of platinum complex therapy might also be a form of consolidation, proven to be an unsuccessful strategy as already noted. More recently, extended treatment with paclitaxel was also proposed as a form of consolidation, based on the toxicity profile and possible vascular targeting of paclitaxel. In a randomized trial, 277 patients were randomized between 3 months of paclitaxel and 12 months of paclitaxel at 175/m^2.[124] At a planned interim analysis, the progression-free survival was found to strongly favor the 12-month arm (21 versus 28 months; P less than 0.0023), and the study was terminated early. No survival data are expected from this study because it was terminated early and many patients crossed over to the 12-month arm. The survival value of this intervention remains controversial, and future trials planned by the Gynecologic Oncology Group will continue both a no-treatment control arm and a paclitaxel treatment arm to confirm this finding. However, not all chemotherapy appears to have this function. In a study of noncross-resistant chemotherapy, four cycles of topotecan were tested in 273 patients in patients completing six cycles of carboplatin and paclitaxel.[125] No difference in progression-free survival was noted, and the study was not designed to analyze for survival. In summary, consolidation therapy remains an area of active investigation, and to date no intervention has shown a definitive survival advantage.

Immunotherapy

Although immunotherapy has been proposed as a logical strategy for ovarian cancer consolidation, the results so far have been disappointing. Two different monoclonal antibody agents, Oregovomab and a yttrium-labeled anti-HMG1 antibody, have failed to show significant effects in randomized trials.[126,127] A study of alpha interferon has also been negative.[128]

Chemotherapy for Recurrent Disease

In the majority of ovarian cancer patients, the cancer will recur and, with few exceptions, those patients who have recurrences die of their disease. Although surgery is sometimes employed, chemotherapy forms the bulwark of therapy for recurrent disease. Based on retrospective studies, at least two clinical subgroups have been identified. By convention, patients with progression while receiving platinum-based therapy, patients who fail to achieve a complete clinical response, and those who relapse within 6 months of the end of therapy are classified as platinum resistant. Beyond 6 months, the response to platinum retreatment appears to increase with the duration of the so-called platinum-free interval. Although this dichotomy may be an oversimplification, it is a useful intellectual construct to understand principles of management.

Potentially Platinum-Sensitive Disease

In the group of patients whose disease recurs after at least 6 months, platinum-based chemotherapy is generally preferred over nonplatinum agent therapy (Table 52.10). This practice is based on informal comparison of response rates between platinum-based therapy and nonplatinum agents. The number of randomized trials for this question is small. Cantu and coworkers compared paclitaxel to cyclophosphamide, doxorubicin, and cisplatin.[129] Certainly, the group of patients with a platinum-free interval in excess of 12 months are almost always treated with carboplatin, building on primary treatment data comparing carboplatin and cisplatin. The other issue in ovarian cancer treatment is the utility of combination therapy compared with single-agent treatment. A summary of the largest randomized studies for platinum sensitive patients is shown in Table 52.10. From this summary, it is apparent that both time to progression and overall survival appear to favor combinations of carboplatin and a second agent. The choice of the best second agent is not known, but the overall survival data imply that crossover to other agents occurs frequently and probably blunts the effect of initial choice in this group of patients. A second consistent finding is that combination therapy certainly results in more toxicity than sequential single-agent treatment. The failure of epidoxorubicin to improve on carboplatin alone may be a reflection of the lower activity of epidoxirubicin compared to paclitaxel and gemcitabine.[130] It can be seen that nonplatinum therapy with single-agent paclitaxel, topotecan, or liposomal doxorubicin appears to be inferior to platinum-based therapy in response rate and, to a lesser extent, in overall survival.[131–133] It is also of note that retrospective analysis suggests that a patient's time to progression following second-line treatment is almost always shorter than that patient's time to progression following primary therapy. The use of single-agent topotecan or liposomal doxorubicin in the patients with a relapse within 6 to 12 months appears to have a better response rate and overall survival, compared to the resistant population, possibly based on subsequent platinum-based therapy.[134]

Duration of therapy for recurrent disease is controversial. Many authorities recommend treatment to best response and then a chemotherapy holiday. It should be noted that the large randomized trials have generally encouraged treatment for up to 12 months in those patients without evidence of progression.[131–133] No comparative trials are available for duration of therapy.

Platinum-Refractory Disease

The management of platinum-refractory disease is an area with limited high-quality data. Only one combination of nonplatinum agents has been tested in randomized Phase III settings (Table 52.11).[135] No advantage was observed for a combination of anthracycline with paclitaxel to paclitaxel alone. Several of the randomized trials in platinum-resistant disease were performed during the prepaclitaxel era. From the data in hand, it can be seen that oxaliplatin, paclitaxel,

TABLE 52.10. Recurrent disease treatment: platinum-sensitive disease.

Author	*Reference*	*Year*	*Disease-free interval*	*No. of patients*	*Treatment*	*Response*	*Median DFS*	*Median survival*	*P value*
Cantu	129	2002	>12 months	Total 97					
				47	Paclitaxel 175 mg/m^2	45%	9.7 months	25.8 months	
							15.9 months	34.7%	
				47	Cyclophosphamide 500 mg/m^2 Doxorubicin 50 mg/m^2	55%			
					Cisplatin 50 mg/m^2		$P = 0.08$	$P = 0.16$	
Bolis	130	2001	>6 months	Total 190	Carboplatin	55%	14 months	NR	
				95	Carboplatin + epidoxorubicin	58%	17 months		
				95					
							NS		
Parmar	177	2003	>6 months	Total 802					
				410	Platinum-based therapy	NR	9 months	24 months	$P < 0.02$ (survival)
				392	Paclitaxel and platinum		12 months HR = 0.76	29 months HR = 0.82	$P < 0.0004$ (DFS)
Pfisterer	178	2004	>6 months	Total 365					
				178	Carboplatin AUC 5 day 1	30.9%	5.8 months		DFS $P < 0.0031$
				178	Carboplatin AUC 4 day 1 + Gemcitabine 1000 mg/m^2 Days 1 and 8	47.2%	8.6 months HR = 0.72	NR	
Gordon	133	2001	>6 months	Total 220					
				109	Liposomal Doxorubicin	31%	28.9 weeks	108 weeks	
				111	Topotecan	32%	23.3 weeks $P = 0.037$	71 weeks $P = 0.008$	

topotecan, and liposomal doxorubicin have very modest response rates and median survival of less than 1 year.[131,133,136,137] Randomized studies of these agents against supportive care have not been performed, although the superiority of intravenous topotecan to oral topotecan for overall survival implies a modest survival advantage for intravenous topotecan therapy.[136] A number of agents have been also examined in Phase II single-agent studies. In this setting, etoposide and gemcitabine stand out as two agents with modest activity.[138–143] Gemcitabine is often favored over etoposide, based on the small incidence of acute leukemia associated with etoposide treatment. Special mention should

TABLE 52.11. Recurrent disease: platinum-resistant disease.

Author	*Reference*	*Year*	*No. of patients*	*Treatment*	*Response*	*Median DFS*	*Median survival*	*P value*
ten Bokkel Huinink	131	1997	Total 226					
			112	Topotecan 1.5 mg/m^2 daily × 5	20.5%	23 weeks	61 weeks	$P = 0.002$ for DFS
			114	Paclitaxel 175 mg/m^2 over 3 h	13.2%	20 weeks	43 weeks	
Bolis	179	1998	Total 81				Two-year survival	$P = 0.10$ for response
			40	Paclitaxel 175 mg/m^2	17.1%	NR	18%	
			41	Paclitaxel 150 mg/m^2 + epidoxorubicn 120 mg/m^2	34.1%		10%	
Piccart	137	2000	Total 87					
			41	Paclitaxel 175 mg/m^2	17%	14 weeks	37 weeks	NS for all
			45	Oxaliplatin 130 mg/m^2	16%	12 weeks	42 weeks	
Gordon	133	2001	Total 254	Liposomal	16%	9.1 weeks	35 weeks	NS for all
			130	Doxorubicin 50 mg/m^2				
			124	Topotecan 1.5 mg/m^2 × 5 days	8%	13.6 weeks	41 weeks	
Gore	136	2002	Total 266	Total 266 Oral topotecan				
			135	2.3 mg/m^2 × 5 days	13%	13 weeks	51 weeks	$P = 0.033$ for survival
			131	Topotecan 1.5 mg/m^2 × 5 days	20%	17 weeks	58 weeks	

be made of the taxanes in this setting. Weekly paclitaxel has a response rate in excess of 20% for patients previously resistant to an every-3-week cycle, and this schedule enjoys an excellent side effect profile.[138,144] There is also some suggestion that docetaxel is not completely cross reistant with paclitaxel in ovarian cancer treatment.[145–147] The choice among these agents can be based on toxicity preferences. No data exist for a preferred sequence, and it appears that there is little cross-resistance among agents.[132,148]

It is also of note that a "platinum-resistant" cohort will contain some patients who may respond to additional platinum-based therapy. The GINECO investigators reviewed their experience with platinum-based chemotherapy for patients classified as "platinum resistant" by the standard definition. In that presentation, there was still a modest (but statistically significant) survival advantage to platinum-based chemotherapy.[149] In the Memorial Sloan Kettering experience, most of the platinum responders in "platinum-resistant" cohort are patients with early relapse following platinum-based therapy.[150]

Appropriate Follow-Up Interventions

Interval

The ideal follow-up of asymptomatic patients who have completed primary surgery and chemotherapy has yet to be determined. Typically, patients are followed at 3- to 4-month intervals for the first 2 years. Using a 15-question survey, Barnhill et al. illustrated the practice patterns for patient follow up after primary treatment of gynecologic cancers among 94 gynecologic oncologists.[151] The majority of the physicians surveyed recommended visits every 3 months for the first year, every 3 to 4 months for the second year, every 6 months for years 3 to 5, and annually thereafter.

The National Comprehensive Cancer Network (www.NCCN.org) has published their guidelines for monitoring patients with epithelial ovarian cancer who have had a complete response. Visits are every 2 to 4 months for the first 2 years, then every 6 months for the third year, followed by annual visits. Physical examination with pelvic exam and CA 125 (if initially elevated) is performed at each visit, and a complete blood count is obtained annually. Other testing is performed only if indicated.

Olaitan et al. recently reviewed their follow up protocols for 81 patients with gynecologic cancers at a tertiary referral center.[152] This regimen was similar to the one previously mentioned in that patients have visits with the specialists every 3 months for the first 2 years, every 6 months for the next 2 years, and then annually. There was a total of 14 recurrences, of which 8 (57.1%) were diagnosed at the scheduled appointments, and the remainder were diagnosed by either unscheduled visits to the general practitioner or emergency room. There were 10 cases of recurrent ovarian cancer of which 7 were diagnosed at scheduled clinic visits. Four of the 7 had symptoms of recurrence for at least 1 month before their scheduled visit, and 1 patient had symptoms for 4 months. Two recurrences were detected by CA 125 elevations, 2 patients presented to the general practitioners with several days of symptoms of recurrence, and 1 patient presented to the emergency room with a bowel obstruction. In total, 354 visits were required to diagnose 8 recurrences. The authors identified that patients with scheduled visits may delay reporting symptoms until the visit. They suggested an open-access system according to patient need may be a more cost-effective model and are currently performing a prospective randomized trial for follow-up.[153]

Appropriate Examinations

In Barnhill's survey, examination of the breasts, pelvis, lymph nodes, and abdomen were performed by the majority of physicians at each exam.[151] Physical examination by itself is limited in its ability to detect subclinical or persistent disease, but on occasion, a pelvic mass may be detected. The other test that is routinely performed in the follow-up of patients with ovarian cancer is CA 125. According to a survey of gynecologic oncologists, the median recommended number of times the CA 125 level was checked in patients with epithelial ovarian cancer was four during the first 2 years, two over the next 3 years, and either none, one, or two times annually after the fifth year.

The accuracy of CA 125 for determining recurrence was illustrated by Niloff et al.[154] Serum levels of CA 125 were obtained from 55 women with epithelial ovarian cancer both before and after second-look surgery. Patients were clinically and radiologically disease free and were followed until clinical recurrence. Patients with an elevated CA 125 at time of second look had a 60% chance of recurring within 4 months compared to only a 5% chance in patients with a normal CA 125. Elevation in serial CA 125 during the monitoring period was associated with recurrence in 94% of cases with a median lead time of 3 months. The accuracy of CA 125 in determining relapse illustrates its importance for ovarian cancer follow-up. However, given that there may be a lead time before detectable recurrence, ideal treatment for an elevated CA 125 alone raises a new question that is being addressed in a multicenter Medical Research Council/European Organization for Research and Treatment of Cancer (MRC/EORTC) prospective trial. The primary endpoint for this trial is overall survival, with quality of life and health economics designated as secondary endpoints.

Surgery in Relapse

Secondary Debulking

The value of primary cytoreductive surgery is well recognized. Removal of large tumors reduces the tumor load, and thus the number of chemotherapy cycles needed to eradicate residual tumor is also reduced. This concept of reducing tumor burden has also been applied to patients who have already undergone a primary cytoreductive surgery followed by chemotherapy. The data on this remain retrospective in nature and include a mixed population of patients.

Secondary operations for ovarian cancer can be grouped into four different clinical situations:

1. Recurrent disease: those patients with at least a 6-month disease-free interval.
2. Second-look laparotomy: patients who are clinically without evidence of disease and are found to have gross disease at second-look surgery.
3. Interval debulking: patients with bulky, unresectable disease at initial surgery who undergo neoadjuvant chemotherapy.

4. Progressive disease: patients with disease progression on primary chemotherapy.

Secondary surgery for recurrent disease is addressed in this section.

Because the majority of patients with advanced-stage ovarian cancer will eventually have a recurrence of their disease in spite of a period of clinical remission, the question of whether cytoreductive surgery is of therapeutic benefit at time of relapse remains. A number of retrospective studies have addressed this question of secondary cytoreduction at time of relapse.

Berek et al. described their experience with secondary cytoreductive surgery for ovarian cancer,[155] which included 32 patients who underwent secondary cytoreduction at the time of second-look laparotomy, at surgery for clinically detected disease, or at the time of bowel obstruction surgery. The median interval between primary and secondary surgery was 12 months, and optimal resection (defined as residual disease less than 1.5 cm) was accomplished in 38% of patients. When patients undergoing second-look surgery were excepted, 6 (29%) underwent optimal cytoreduction and had a median survival of 18 months compared to the 15 suboptimally debulked patients who had a median survival of 5 months. Although this series contained a heterogeneous group of patients, several poor prognostic variables were identified, including greater residual disease after primary surgery, disease-free interval less than 1 year, large tumor size at recurrence, ascites, and greater residual disease after secondary surgery. Several other series have reviewed the impact of residual disease on survival, and most have shown a benefit if residual disease is of small volume.

Although the majority of studies regarding the utility of secondary cytoreduction are retrospective, a prospective study was conducted by Eisenkop et al. that evaluated the feasibility and benefit of secondary cytoreduction.[156] Thirty-six patients who had undergone primary cytoreduction followed by platinum-based chemotherapy and who had relapsed at least 6 months after primary therapy were enrolled for secondary cytoreduction. All patients had disease greater than 1 cm at recurrence, and complete cytoreduction was achieved in 30 (83%) of patients using an aggressive surgical approach. Morbidity occurred in 30.1% of patients, and there was 1 (2.8%) postoperative mortality. Although there was not a control group who did not undergo secondary cytoreductive surgery, median survival in the group was significantly better in the patients completely resected before salvage therapy compared to those with macroscopic residual disease (43 versus 5 months; $P = 0.03$, respectively). Based on these retrospective series, secondary cytoreduction appears to be beneficial in patients with resectable recurrent disease and a reasonable disease-free interval.

It should be kept in mind that the retrospective series published on secondary cytoreduction included heterogeneous groups of patients and surgeons, involved tumors with different biologic behavior, and had strong selection bias in the authors' criteria for surgical interventions. The GOG (Protocol 213) is currently conducting a prospective bifactorial randomized trial addressing the use of sequence-dependent chemotherapy and secondary cytoreductive surgery in platinum-sensitive, recurrent ovarian and primary peritoneal cancers. Patients will be randomized to either treatment with topotecan or carboplatin or secondary cytoreduction followed by treatment with topotecan or carboplatin.

Value and Impact of Surgery for Obstruction

Progression of ovarian cancer results in symptoms of diffuse intraabdominal spread and can lead to progressive encasement of the bowel and its mesentery, resulting in symptoms of mechanical obstruction. This is a common finding among patients with recurrent ovarian cancer, and many will eventually succumb to this problem. In a study to determine the incidence of bowel obstruction in patients with ovarian cancer, Lund et al.[139] followed the clinical courses of 310 consecutive patients with ovarian cancer. With a median observation time of 46 months, the estimated incidence of intestinal obstruction was 26% at 5 years. The complication rate associated with surgery for obstruction was high, and only 32% of patients had a survival of greater than 60 days with palliation of symptoms. The most commonly associated variables included initial stage III or IV disease, suboptimal (larger than 2 cm tumor nodules) tumor debulking at initial surgery, and the presence of intestinal carcinomatosis at initial surgical exploration.

Initial management of patients with obstruction is typically a trial of conservative management with nasogastric drainage. However, Krebs and Goplerud reported that such an approach results in sufficient improvement for discharge in only about one-third of cases, and the majority of these patients return with a subsequent obstruction within a mean of 5.5 weeks.[157] In cases that do not resolve with conservative management, surgical correction may be considered. This option is associated with a high rate of morbidity and mortality, and the chances of successful palliation, risk of reobstruction, and quality of life after the surgery must be taken into consideration.

A number of retrospective studies have examined the role of surgery for obstruction in patients with ovarian cancer. Pothuri et al. reported. from Memorial Sloan-Kettering Cancer Center 64 patients who underwent 68 operations.[158] The obstruction was surgically corrected in 57 (84%) of the 68 procedures. Of this group, 71% were able to tolerate a regular or low-residue diet at least 60 days postoperatively, and 79% were able to receive more chemotherapy. The surgical morbidity was 22% and the perioperative mortality was 6%. Median survival was significantly longer in the patients who had successful palliation compared to those who did not, 11.6 months and 3.9 months, respectively (P less than 0.01). A number of other studies have demonstrated that surgical correction is possible; however, these studies include a patient pool that is heavily preselected. Successful palliation, defined as survival greater than 60 days from surgery, was achieved for 51% to 80% of patients; however, perioperative mortality (4%–32%) and morbidity (7%–64%) can be significant.

In an attempt to better define patients who may benefit from a surgical procedure, Krebs and Goplerud used age, nutritional status, tumor spread, ascites, previous chemotherapy, and previous radiation to formulate a prognostic index.[159] Using a scoring system of 0–2 for each variable, they reported that 84% of patients with a score of 6 or less survived at least 60 days postsurgery compared to 0% of patients with a score of 7 or more. It would be beneficial to identify patients who would not benefit from surgery, and other series have confirmed the validity of using a prognostic index.[160] Not all reports, however, have been able to demonstrate that such variables are predictive of successful palliation or improved survival.[161]

Supportive Care

Total Parenteral Nutrition

The role of total parenteral nutrition is a question that may arise in patients with malignant intestinal obstruction. Due to the predilection for intraabdominal spread, intestinal obstruction in patients with advanced ovarian cancer is not an uncommon situation. Many patients may present with or develop bowel obstruction related to unresectable disease. In such cases which do not appear amenable to surgical correction, supportive care should be the focus of treatment. The extent of supportive efforts can be a difficult topic to address.

Many patients or families suffering from altered gastrointestinal function from unresectable ovarian cancer may raise the possibility of using total parenteral nutrition (TPN). In spite of decreased oral intake, more than 60% of terminally ill cancer patients experience no hunger or thirst.[162] Thus, the value of TPN in patients with end-stage ovarian cancer remains questionable. The potential risks associated with TPN and the training required for home administration may justify its use in patients with expected survivals of more than 3 months.[163] With the exception of certain situations, such as patients who are undergoing surgical correction for obstruction or being administered TPN in conjunction with systemic chemotherapy for newly diagnosed ovarian cancer, TPN is not routinely recommended.

A review of patients with small bowel obstruction and advanced ovarian cancer demonstrated some of the rare indications for the use of TPN in advanced ovarian cancer patients. Abu-Rustum et al. identified 21 patients (3 newly diagnosed and 18 heavily treated for persistent or recurrent disease) who received chemotherapy in an attempt to restore bowel function.[164] All patients had a drainage gastrostomy placed. Eleven patients also received TPN (all newly diagnosed and 8 recurrent/persistent). Two of the 3 chemotherapy-naïve patients had relief of their bowel obstruction, compared to none of the patients with recurrent or persistent disease. Median survival for patients who received TPN with chemotherapy was 89 days compared to 71 days in patients who received chemotherapy alone ($P = 0.031$). However, the authors did not believe that the additional 18 days justified the routine administration of TPN and discouraged its use.

Percutaneous Endoscopic Gastrostomy Tube Drainage

Patients with malignant obstruction who either choose not to undergo a surgical procedure or who are poor candidates for surgical correction can be managed with percutaneous endoscopic gastrostomy (PEG) drainage of the stomach and small bowel. PEG has many advantages over a nasogastric tube, including patient comfort, lack of damage to the gastric mucosa, more efficient drainage due to a wide tube, and providing the satisfaction of oral liquids in spite of obstruction. PEG can be placed without necessitating a surgical procedure that may be associated with increased morbidity. Retrospective studies have demonstrated that PEG tubes can be placed in the majority of patients with success rates of 89% to 100%.[165,166]

Complications rates are typically low, with the major risks being leakage of gastric contents, intestinal perforation, and peritonitis. After successful placement of the PEG tube, patients can resume a liquid or soft diet in 84% to 100% of cases.[165,166] Because improvement in comfort of the terminally ill cancer patient should be the major goal, PEG drainage should be considered in patients with malignant bowel obstruction.

References

1. Jemal A, Tiwari RC, Murray T, et al. Cancer statistics, 2004. CA Cancer J Clin 2004;54(1):8–29.
2. Mink PJ, Sherman ME, Devesa SS. Incidence patterns of invasive and borderline ovarian tumors among white women and black women in the United States. Results from the SEER Program, 1978–1998. Cancer (Phila) 2002;95(11): 2380–2389.
3. Buell P, Dunn JE, Jr. Cancer mortality among Japanese Issei and Nisei of California. Cancer (Phila) 1965;18:656–664.
4. Goodman MT, Tung KH, McDuffie K, Wilkens LR, Donlon TA. Association of caffeine intake and CYP1A2 genotype with ovarian cancer. Nutr Cancer 2003;46(1):23–29.
5. Zhang M, Yang ZY, Binns CW, Lee AH. Diet and ovarian cancer risk: a case-control study in China. Br J Cancer 2002;86(5):712–717.
6. Bertone ER, Rosner BA, Hunter DJ, et al. Dietary fat intake and ovarian cancer in a cohort of US women. Am J Epidemiol 2002;156(1):22–31.
7. Bosetti C, Negri E, Franceschi S, et al. Diet and ovarian cancer risk: a case-control study in Italy. Int J Cancer 2001;93(6):911–915.
8. Cramer DW, Harlow BL, Willett WC, et al. Galactose consumption and metabolism in relation to the risk of ovarian cancer. Lancet 1989;2(8654):66–71.
9. Fairfield KM, Hunter DJ, Colditz GA, et al. A prospective study of dietary lactose and ovarian cancer. Int J Cancer 2004;110(2):271–277.
10. Fairfield KM, Hankinson SE, Rosner BA, Hunter DJ, Colditz GA, Willett WC. Risk of ovarian carcinoma and consumption of vitamins A, C, and E and specific carotenoids: a prospective analysis. Cancer (Phila) 2001;92(9):2318–2326.
11. Whittemore AS, Harris R, Itnyre J. Characteristics relating to ovarian cancer risk: collaborative analysis of 12 US case-control studies. IV. The pathogenesis of epithelial ovarian cancer. Collaborative Ovarian Cancer Group. Am J Epidemiol 1992;136(10):1212–1220.
12. Hankinson SE, Colditz GA, Hunter DJ, et al. A prospective study of reproductive factors and risk of epithelial ovarian cancer. Cancer (Phila) 1995;76(2):284–290.
13. Purdie DM, Bain CJ, Siskind V, Webb PM, Green AC. Ovulation and risk of epithelial ovarian cancer. Int J Cancer 2003;104(2):228–232.
14. Hildreth NG, Kelsey JL, LiVolsi VA, et al. An epidemiologic study of epithelial carcinoma of the ovary. Am J Epidemiol 1981;114(3):398–405.
15. Boyd J. Molecular genetics of hereditary ovarian cancer. Oncology (Huntingt) 1998;12(3):399–406; discussion 409–410, 413.

16. Ford D, Easton DF, Stratton M, et al. Genetic heterogeneity and penetrance analysis of the BRCA1 and BRCA2 genes in breast cancer families. The Breast Cancer Linkage Consortium. Am J Hum Genet 1998;62(3):676–689.
17. Struewing JP, Hartge P, Wacholder S, et al. The risk of cancer associated with specific mutations of BRCA1 and BRCA2 among Ashkenazi Jews. N Engl J Med 1997;336(20):1401–1408.
18. Lynch HT, Snyder CL, Lynch JF, Riley BD, Rubinstein WS. Hereditary breast-ovarian cancer at the bedside: role of the medical oncologist. J Clin Oncol 2003;21(4):740–753.
19. Aarnio M, Sankila R, Pukkala E, et al. Cancer risk in mutation carriers of DNA-mismatch-repair genes. Int J Cancer 1999; 81(2):214–218.
20. Epithelial ovarian cancer and combined oral contraceptives. The WHO Collaborative Study of Neoplasia and Steroid Contraceptives. Int J Epidemiol 1989;18(3):538-545.
21. Ness RB, Grisso JA, Klapper J, et al. Risk of ovarian cancer in relation to estrogen and progestin dose and use characteristics of oral contraceptives. SHARE Study Group. Steroid Hormones and Reproductions. Am J Epidemiol 2000;152(3):233–241.
22. Kumle M, Weiderpass E, Braaten T, Adami HO, Lund E. Risk for invasive and borderline epithelial ovarian neoplasias following use of hormonal contraceptives: the Norwegian-Swedish Women's Lifestyle and Health Cohort Study. Br J Cancer 2004;90(7):1386–1391.
23. Narod SA, Dube MP, Klijn J, et al. Oral contraceptives and the risk of breast cancer in BRCA1 and BRCA2 mutation carriers. J Natl Cancer Inst 2002;94(23):1773–1779.
24. Kauff ND, Satagopan JM, Robson ME, et al. Risk-reducing salpingo-oophorectomy in women with a BRCA1 or BRCA2 mutation. N Engl J Med 2002;346(21):1609–1615.
25. Rebbeck TR, Lynch HT, Neuhausen SL, et al. Prophylactic oophorectomy in carriers of BRCA1 or BRCA2 mutations. N Engl J Med 2002;346(21):1616–1622.
26. Levine DA, Argenta PA, Yee CJ, et al. Fallopian tube and primary peritoneal carcinomas associated with BRCA mutations. J Clin Oncol 2003;21(22):4222–4227.
27. Piver MS, Jishi MF, Tsukada Y, Nava G. Primary peritoneal carcinoma after prophylactic oophorectomy in women with a family history of ovarian cancer. A report of the Gilda Radner Familial Ovarian Cancer Registry. Cancer (Phila) 1993;71(9):2751–2755.
28. Robson M, Hensley M, Barakat R, et al. Quality of life in women at risk for ovarian cancer who have undergone risk-reducing oophorectomy. Gynecol Oncol 2003;89(2): 281–287.
29. Benedet JL, Bender H, Jones H, 3rd, Ngan HY, Pecorelli S. FIGO staging classifications and clinical practice guidelines in the management of gynecologic cancers. FIGO Committee on Gynecologic Oncology. Int J Gynaecol Obstet 2000; 70(2):209–262.
30. Burke W, Daly M, Garber J, et al. Recommendations for follow-up care of individuals with an inherited predisposition to cancer. II. BRCA1 and BRCA2. Cancer Genetics Studies Consortium. JAMA 1997;277(12):997–1003.
31. Bast RC, Jr., Klug TL, St John E, et al. A radioimmunoassay using a monoclonal antibody to monitor the course of epithelial ovarian cancer. N Engl J Med 1983;309(15):883–887.
32. Einhorn N, Sjovall K, Knapp RC, et al. Prospective evaluation of serum CA 125 levels for early detection of ovarian cancer. Obstet Gynecol 1992;80(1):14–18.
33. Jacobs IJ, Skates SJ, MacDonald N, et al. Screening for ovarian cancer: a pilot randomised controlled trial. Lancet 1999;353(9160):1207–1210.
34. Campbell S, Bhan V, Royston P, Whitehead MI, Collins WP. Transabdominal ultrasound screening for early ovarian cancer. Br Med J 1989;299(6712):1363–1367.
35. van Nagell JR, Jr., Gallion HH, Pavlik EJ, DePriest PD. Ovarian cancer screening. Cancer (Phila) 1995;76(suppl 10):2086–2091.
36. van Nagell JR, Jr., DePriest PD, Reedy MB, et al. The efficacy of transvaginal sonographic screening in asymptomatic women at risk for ovarian cancer. Gynecol Oncol 2000;77(3):350–356.
37. DePriest PD, DeSimone CP. Ultrasound screening for the early detection of ovarian cancer. J Clin Oncol 2003; 21(suppl 10): 194–199.
38. Munnell E. The changing prognosis and treatment in cancer of the ovary. A report of 235 patients with primary ovarian carcinoma 1952–1961. Am J Obstet Gynecol 1961;100(6): 790–805.
39. Elclos L, Quinlan EJ. Malignant tumors of the ovary managed with postoperative megavoltage irradiation. Radiology 1969;93(3):659–663.
40. Griffiths CT. Surgical resection of tumor bulk in the primary treatment of ovarian carcinoma. Natl Cancer Inst Monogr 1975;42:101–104.
41. Gall S, Bundy B, Beecham J, et al. Therapy of stage III (optimal) epithelial carci-noma of the ovary with melphalan or melphalan plus *Corynebacterium parvum* (a Gynecologic Oncology Group Study). Gynecol Oncol 1986;25(1): 26–36.
42. Hoskins WJ, Bundy BN, Thigpen JT, Omura GA. The influence of cytoreductive surgery on recurrence-free interval and survival in small-volume stage III epithelial ovarian cancer: a Gynecologic Oncology Group study. Gynecol Oncol 1992;47(2):159–166.
43. Bristow RE, Tomacruz RS, Armstrong DK, Trimble EL, Montz FJ. Survival effect of maximal cytoreductive surgery for advanced ovarian carcinoma during the platinum era: a meta-analysis. J Clin Oncol 2002;20(5):1248–1259.
44. Suzuki M, Ohwada M, Yamada T, Kohno T, Sekiguchi I, Sato I. Lymph node metastasis in stage I epithelial ovarian cancer. Gynecol Oncol 2000;79(2):305–308.
45. Burghardt E, Pickel H, Lahousen M, Stettner H. Pelvic lymphadenectomy in operative treatment of ovarian cancer. Am J Obstet Gynecol 1986;155(2):315–319.
46. Scarabelli C, Gallo A, Visentin MC, Canzonieri V, Carbone A, Zarrelli A. Systematic pelvic and para-aortic lymphadenectomy in advanced ovarian cancer patients with no residual intraperitoneal disease. Int J Gynecol Cancer 1997; 7(1):18–26.
47. Saygili U, Guclu S, Uslu T, Erten O, Ture S, Demir N. Does systematic lymphadenectomy have a benefit on survival of suboptimally debulked patients with stage III ovarian carcinoma? A DEGOG* Study. J Surg Oncol 2002;81(3): 132–137.
48. Spirtos NM, Gross GM, Freddo JL, Ballon SC. Cytoreductive surgery in advanced epithelial cancer of the ovary: the impact of aortic and pelvic lymphadenectomy. Gynecol Oncol 1995;56(3):345–352.
49. Eisenkop SM, Spirtos NM. The clinical significance of occult macroscopically positive retroperitoneal nodes in patients with epithelial ovarian cancer. Gynecol Oncol 2001;82(1):143–149.

50. Vergote I, De Wever I, Tjalma W, Van Gramberen M, Decloedt J, van Dam P. Neoadjuvant chemotherapy or primary debulking surgery in advanced ovarian carcinoma: a retrospective analysis of 285 patients. Gynecol Oncol 1998;71(3):431–436.
51. Ansquer Y, Leblanc E, Clough K, et al. Neoadjuvant chemotherapy for unresectable ovarian carcinoma: a French multicenter study. Cancer (Phila) 2001;91(12):2329–2334.
52. Lawton FG, Redman CW, Luesley DM, Chan KK, Blackledge G. Neoadjuvant (cytoreductive) chemotherapy combined with intervention debulking surgery in advanced, unresected epithelial ovarian cancer. Obstet Gynecol 1989;73(1):61–65.
53. Ng LW, Rubin SC, Hoskins WJ, et al. Aggressive chemosurgical debulking in patients with advanced ovarian cancer. Gynecol Oncol 1990;38(3):358–363.
54. Neijt JP, ten Bokkel Huinink WW, van der Burg ME, et al. Randomised trial comparing two combination chemotherapy regimens (Hexa-CAF vs CHAP-5) in advanced ovarian carcinoma. Lancet 1984;2(8403):594–600.
55. van der Burg ME, van Lent M, Buyse M, et al. Gynecological Cancer Group of the EORTC. The role of interval debulking surgery in ovarian cancer. Curr Oncol Rep 2003;5:473–481.
56. Dembo AJ, Davy M, Stenwig AE, Berle EJ, Bush RS, Kjorstad K. Prognostic factors in patients with stage I epithelial ovarian cancer. Obstet Gynecol 1990;75(2):263–273.
57. Ahmed FY, Wiltshaw E, A'Hern RP, et al. Natural history and prognosis of untreated stage I epithelial ovarian carcinoma. J Clin Oncol 1996;14(11):2968–2975.
58. Sevelda P, Vavra N, Schemper M, Salzer H. Prognostic factors for survival in stage I epithelial ovarian carcinoma. Cancer (Phila) 1990;65(10):2349–2352.
59. Monga M, Carmichael JA, Shelley WE, et al. Surgery without adjuvant chemotherapy for early epithelial ovarian carcinoma after comprehensive surgical staging. Gynecol Oncol 1991;43(3):195–197.
60. Vergote I, De Brabanter J, Fyles A, et al. Prognostic importance of degree of differentiation and cyst rupture in stage I invasive epithelial ovarian carcinoma. Lancet 2001; 357(9251):176–182.
61. Rutledge F, Burns BC. Chemotherapy for advanced ovarian cancer. Am J Obstet Gynecol 1966;96(6):761–772.
62. Walton L, Ellenberg SS, Major F, Jr, Miller A, Park R, Young RC. Results of second-look laparotomy in patients with early-stage ovarian carcinoma. Obstet Gynecol 1987;70(5): 770–773.
63. Rubin SC, Jones WB, Curtin JP, Barakat RR, Hakes TB, Hoskins WJ. Second-look laparotomy in stage I ovarian cancer following comprehensive surgical staging. Obstet Gynecol 1993;82(1):139–142.
64. Meier W, Stieber P, Eiermann W, Schneider A, Fateh-Moghadam A, Hepp H. Serum levels of CA 125 and histological findings at second-look laparotomy in ovarian carcinoma. Gynecol Oncol 1989;35(1):44–46.
65. Rubin SC, Randall TC, Armstrong KA, Chi DS, Hoskins WJ. Ten-year follow-up of ovarian cancer patients after second-look laparotomy with negative findings. Obstet Gynecol 1999;93(1):21–24.
66. Ozols RF, Bundy BN, Greer BE, et al. Phase III trial of carboplatin and paclitaxel compared with cisplatin and paclitaxel in patients with optimally resected stage III ovarian cancer: a Gynecologic Oncology Group study. J Clin Oncol 2003;21(17):3194–3200.
67. Dowdy SC, Constantinou CL, Hartmann LC, et al. Long-term follow-up of women with ovarian cancer after positive second-look laparotomy. Gynecol Oncol 2003;91(3):563–568.
68. Williams L, Brunetto VL, Yordan E, DiSaia PJ, Creasman WT. Secondary cytoreductive surgery at second-look laparotomy in advanced ovarian cancer: a Gynecologic Oncology Group Study. Gynecol Oncol 1997;66(2):171–178.
69. Hoskins WJ, Rubin SC, Dulaney E, et al. Influence of secondary cytoreduction at the time of second-look laparotomy on the survival of patients with epithelial ovarian carcinoma. Gynecol Oncol 1989;34(3):365–371.
70. Young RC, Walton LA, Ellenberg SS, et al. Adjuvant therapy in stage I and stage II epithelial ovarian cancer. Results of two prospective randomized trials. N Engl J Med 1990; 322(15):1021–1027.
71. Ahmed FY, Wiltshaw E, A'Hern RP, et al. Natural history and prognosis of untreated stage I epithelial ovarian carcinoma. J Clin Oncol 1996;14:2968–2975.
72. Bolis G, Colombo N, Pecorelli S, et al. Adjuvant treatment for early epithelial ovarian cancer: results of two randomised clinical trials comparing cisplatin to no further treatment or chromic phosphate (^{32}P). G.I.C.O.G.: Gruppo Interregionale Collaborativo in Ginecologia Oncologica. Ann Oncol 1995;(9):887–893.
73. Trope C, Kaern J, Hogberg T, et al. Randomized study on adjuvant chemotherapy in stage I high-risk ovarian cancer with evaluation of DNA-ploidy as prognostic instrument. Ann Oncol 2000;11(3):281–288.
74. Trimbos JB, Parmar M, Vergote I, et al. International Collaborative Ovarian Neoplasm trial 1 and Adjuvant ChemoTherapy in Ovarian Neoplasm trial: two parallel randomized phase III trials of adjuvant chemotherapy in patients with early-stage ovarian carcinoma. J Natl Cancer Inst 2003;95(2):105–112.
75. Colombo N, Guthrie D, Chiari S, et al. International Collaborative Ovarian Neoplasm trial 1: a randomized trial of adjuvant chemotherapy in women with early-stage ovarian cancer. J Natl Cancer Inst 2003;95(2):125–132.
76. Trimbos JB, Vergote I, Bolis G, et al. Impact of adjuvant chemotherapy and surgical staging in early-stage ovarian carcinoma: European Organisation for Research and Treatment of Cancer-Adjuvant ChemoTherapy in Ovarian Neoplasm trial. J Natl Cancer Inst 2003;95(2):113 125.
77. Aabo K, Adams M, Adnitt P, et al. Chemotherapy in advanced ovarian cancer: four systematic meta-analyses of individual patient data from 37 randomized trials. Advanced Ovarian Cancer Trialists' Group. Br J Cancer 1998;78(11): 1479–1487.
78. Bell J, Brady M, Lage J, et al. A randomized trial of three versus six cycles of carboplatin and paclitaxel as adjuvant treatment in early stage ovarian epithelial carcinoma: a GOG study. Proc Soc Gynecol Oncol 2003;34 (abstract 1).
79. Young RC, Brady MF, Nieberg RK, et al. Adjuvant treatment for early ovarian cancer: a randomized phase III trial of intraperitoneal ^{32}P or intravenous cyclophosphamide and cisplatin: a gynecologic oncology group study. J Clin Oncol 2003;21(23):4350–4355.
80. Dembo AJ, Bush RS, Beale FA, Bean HA, Pringle JF, Sturgeon JF. The Princess Margaret Hospital study of ovarian cancer: stages I, II, and asymptomatic III presentations. Cancer Treat Rep 1979;63(2):249–254.
81. Smith JP, Rutledge FN, Delclos L. Postoperative treatment of early cancer of the ovary: a random trial between post-

operative irradiation and chemotherapy. Natl Cancer Inst Monogr 1975; 42:149–153.
82. Klaassen D, Shelley W, Starreveld A, et al. Early stage ovarian cancer: a randomized clinical trial comparing whole abdominal radiotherapy, melphalan, and intraperitoneal chromic phosphate: a National Cancer Institute of Canada Clinical Trials Group report. J Clin Oncol 1988;6(8):1254–1263.
83. Chiara S, Conte P, Franzone P, et al. High-risk early-stage ovarian cancer. Randomized clinical trial comparing cisplatin plus cyclophosphamide versus whole abdominal radiotherapy. Am J Clin Oncol 1994;17(1):72–76.
84. Vergote IB, Winderen M, De Vos LN, Trope CG. Intraperitoneal radioactive phosphorus therapy in ovarian carcinoma. Analysis of 313 patients treated primarily or at second-look laparotomy. Cancer (Phila) 1993;71(7):2250–2260.
85. Winter-Roach B, Hooper L, Kitchener H. Systematic review of adjuvant therapy for early stage (epithelial) ovarian cancer. Int J Gynecol Cancer 2003;13(4):395–404.
86. Stewart A. Chemotherapy in advanced ovarian cancer: an overview of randomised clinical trials. Advanced Ovarian Cancer Trialists Group. B Med J 1991;303(6807):884–893.
87. Swenerton K, Jeffrey J, Stuart G, et al. Cisplatin-cyclophosphamide versus carboplatin-cyclophosphamide in advanced ovarian cancer: a randomized phase III study of the National Cancer Institute of Canada Clinical Trials Group. J Clin Oncol 1992;10(5):718–726.
88. Alberts DS, Green S, Hannigan EV, et al. Improved therapeutic index of carboplatin plus cyclophosphamide versus cisplatin plus cyclophosphamide: final report by the Southwest Oncology Group of a phase III randomized trial in stages III and IV ovarian cancer. J Clin Oncol 1992;10(5):706–717.
89. ICON2: randomised trial of single-agent carboplatin against three-drug combination of CAP (cyclophosphamide, doxorubicin, and cisplatin) in women with ovarian cancer. ICON Collaborators. International Collaborative Ovarian Neoplasm Study. Lancet 1998;352(9140):1571–1576.
90. du Bois A, Luck HJ, Meier W, et al. A randomized clinical trial of cisplatin/paclitaxel versus carboplatin/paclitaxel as first-line treatment of ovarian cancer. J Natl Cancer Inst 2003;95(17):1320–1329.
91. Misset JL, Vennin P, Chollet PH, et al. Multicenter phase II–III study of oxaliplatin plus cyclophosphamide vs. cisplatin plus cyclophosphamide in chemonaive advanced ovarian cancer patients. Ann Oncol 2001;12(10):1411–1415.
92. Omura GA, Bundy BN, Berek JS, Curry S, Delgado G, Mortel R. Randomized trial of cyclophosphamide plus cisplatin with or without doxorubicin in ovarian carcinoma: a Gynecologic Oncology Group Study. J Clin Oncol 1989;7(4):457–465.
93. A'Hern RP, Gore ME. Impact of doxorubicin on survival in advanced ovarian cancer. J Clin Oncol 1995;13(3):726–732.
94. McGuire WP, Hoskins WJ, Brady MF, et al. Cyclophosphamide and cisplatin compared with paclitaxel and cisplatin in patients with stage III and stage IV ovarian cancer. N Engl J Med 1996;334(1):1–6.
95. Piccart MJ, Bertelsen K, James K, et al. Randomized intergroup trial of cisplatin-paclitaxel versus cisplatin-cyclophosphamide in women with advanced epithelial ovarian cancer: three-year results. J Natl Cancer Inst 2000;92(9):699–708.
96. ICON3Investigators. Paclitaxel plus carboplatin versus standard chemotherapy with either single-agent carboplatin or cyclophosphamide, doxorubicin, and cisplatin in women with ovarian cancer: the ICON3 randomised trial. Lancet 2002;360(9332):505–515.
97. Sandercock J, Parmar MK, Torri V, Qian W. First-line treatment for advanced ovarian cancer: paclitaxel, platinum and the evidence. Br J Cancer 2002;87(8):815–824.
98. Conte PF, Bruzzone M, Chiara S, et al. A randomized trial comparing cisplatin plus cyclophosphamide versus cisplatin, doxorubicin, and cyclophosphamide in advanced ovarian cancer. J Clin Oncol 1986;4(6):965–971.
99. Omura GA, Brady MF, Homesley HD, et al. Long-term follow-up and prognostic factor analysis in advanced ovarian carcinoma: the Gynecologic Oncology Group experience. J Clin Oncol 1991;9(7):1138–1150.
100. Jakobsen A, Bertelsen K, Andersen JE, et al. Dose-effect study of carboplatin in ovarian cancer: a Danish Ovarian Cancer Group study. J Clin Oncol 1997;15(1):193–198.
101. Conte PF, Bruzzone M, Carnino F, et al. High-dose versus low-dose cisplatin in combination with cyclophosphamide and epidoxorubicin in suboptimal ovarian cancer: a randomized study of the Gruppo Oncologico Nord-Ovest. J Clin Oncol 1996;14(2):351–356.
102. McGuire WP, Hoskins WJ, Brady MF, et al. Assessment of dose-intensive therapy in suboptimally debulked ovarian cancer: a Gynecologic Oncology Group study. J Clin Oncol 1995;13(7):1589–1599.
103. Gore M, Mainwaring P, A'Hern R, et al. Randomized trial of dose-intensity with single-agent carboplatin in patients with epithelial ovarian cancer. London Gynaecological Oncology Group. J Clin Oncol 1998;16(7):2426–2434.
104. Jodrell DI, Egorin MJ, Canetta RM, et al. Relationships between carboplatin exposure and tumor response and toxicity in patients with ovarian cancer. J Clin Oncol 1992;10(4):520–528.
105. Egorin MJ, Reyno LM, Canetta RM, et al. Modeling toxicity and response in carboplatin-based combination chemotherapy. Semin Oncol 1994;21(5 suppl 12):7–19.
106. Kaye SB, Paul J, Cassidy J, et al. Mature results of a randomized trial of two doses of cisplatin for the treatment of ovarian cancer. Scottish Gynecology Cancer Trials Group. J Clin Oncol 1996;14(7):2113–2119.
107. Hakes TB, Chalas E, Hoskins WJ, et al. Randomized prospective trial of 5 versus 10 cycles of cyclophosphamide, doxorubicin, and cisplatin in advanced ovarian carcinoma. Gynecol Oncol 1992;45(3):284–289.
108. Bertelsen K, Jakobsen A, Stroyer J, et al. A prospective randomized comparison of 6 and 12 cycles of cyclophosphamide, adriamycin, and cisplatin in advanced epithelial ovarian cancer: a Danish Ovarian Study Group trial (DACOVA). Gynecol Oncol 1993;49(1):30–36.
109. Eisenhauer EA, ten Bokkel Huinink WW, Swenerton KD, et al. European-Canadian randomized trial of paclitaxel in relapsed ovarian cancer: high-dose versus low-dose and long versus short infusion. J Clin Oncol 1994;12(12):2654–2666.
110. Omura GA, Brady MF, Look KY, et al. Phase III trial of paclitaxel at two dose levels, the higher dose accompanied by filgrastim at two dose levels in platinum-pretreated epithelial ovarian cancer: an intergroup study. J Clin Oncol 2003;21(15):2843–2848.
111. Bolis G, Scarfone G, Polverino G, et al. Paclitaxel 175 or 225 mg per meters squared with carboplatin in advanced ovarian cancer: a randomized trial. J Clin Oncol 2004;22(4):686–690.

112. Rosenberg P, Andersson H, Boman K, et al. Randomized trial of single agent paclitaxel given weekly versus every three weeks and with peroral versus intravenous steroid premedication to patients with ovarian cancer previously treated with platinum. Acta Oncol 2002;41(5):418–424.
113. Dedrick RL, Myers CE, Bungay PM, DeVita VT, Jr. Pharmacokinetic rationale for peritoneal drug administration in the treatment of ovarian cancer. Cancer Treat Rep 1978;62(1):1–11.
114. Dedrick RL, Flessner MF. Pharmacokinetic problems in peritoneal drug administration: tissue penetration and surface exposure. J Natl Cancer Inst 1997;89(7):480–487.
115. Alberts DS, Liu PY, Hannigan EV, et al. Intraperitoneal cisplatin plus intravenous cyclophosphamide versus intravenous cisplatin plus intravenous cyclophosphamide for stage III ovarian cancer. N Engl J Med 1996;335(26):1950–1955.
116. Markman M, Bundy BN, Alberts DS, et al. Phase III trial of standard-dose intravenous cisplatin plus paclitaxel versus moderately high-dose carboplatin followed by intravenous paclitaxel and intraperitoneal cisplatin in small-volume stage III ovarian carcinoma: an intergroup study of the Gynecologic Oncology Group, South-western Oncology Group, and Eastern Cooperative Oncology Group. J Clin Oncol 2001;19(4):1001–1007.
117. Armstrong D. Preliminary Results GOG 172. Proc ASCO 2002; (abstract 803).
118. Makhija S, Leitao M, Sabbatini P, et al. Complications associated with intraperitoneal chemotherapy catheters. Gynecol Oncol 2001;81(1):77–81.
119. Chi DS, Sabbatini P. Advanced ovarian cancer. Curr Treat Options Oncol 2000;1(2):139–146.
120. Markman M, Liu PY, Wilczynski S, et al. Phase III randomized trial of 12 versus 3 months of maintenance paclitaxel in patients with advanced ovarian cancer after complete response to platinum and paclitaxel-based chemotherapy: a Southwest Oncology Group and Gynecologic Oncology Group trial. J Clin Oncol 2003;21(13):2460–2465.
121. Barakat RR, Almadrones L, Venkatraman ES, et al. A phase II trial of intraperitoneal cisplatin and etoposide as consolidation therapy in patients with Stage II–IV epithelial ovarian cancer following negative surgical assessment. Gynecol Oncol 1998;69(1):17–22.
122. Tournigand C, Louvet C, Molitor JL, et al. Long-term survival with consolidation intraperitoneal chemotherapy for patients with advanced ovarian cancer with pathological complete remission. Gynecol Oncol 2003;91(2):341–345.
123. Piccart MJ, Floquet A, Scarfone G, et al. Intraperitoneal cisplatin versus no further treatment: 8-year results of EORTC 55875, a randomized phase III study in ovarian cancer patients with a pathologically complete remission after platinum-based intravenous chemotherapy. Int J Gynecol Cancer 2003;13(suppl 2):196–203.
124. Markman M, Markman J, Webster K, et al. Duration of response to second line platinum-based chemotherapy for ovarian cancer: implications for patient management and clinical trial design. J Clin Oncol 2004;22(22):3120–3125.
125. De Placido S, Scambia G, Di Vagno G, et al. Topotecan compared with no therapy after response to surgery and carboplatin/paclitaxel in patients with ovarian cancer: Multicenter Italian Trials in Ovarian Cancer (MITO-1) randomized study. J Clin Oncol 2004;22(13):2635–2642.
126. Seiden M, Benigno B, Verheijen R, et al. A pivotal phase III trial to evaluate the efficacy of adjuvant treatment with R1549 (ytterium-90-labeled HMFG1 murine monoclonal antibody) in epithelial ovarian cancer (EOC). Proc ASCO 2004;23 (abstract 5008).
127. Berek J, Taylor P, Gordon A, et al. Randomized placebo controlled study of oregovomab for consolidation of clinical remission in patients with advanced ovarian cancer. J Clin Oncol 2004;22(15):3120–3125.
128. Hall GD, Brown JM, Coleman RE, et al. Maintenance treatment with interferon for advanced ovarian cancer: results of the Northern and Yorkshire gynaecology group randomised phase III study. Br J Cancer 2004;91(4):621–626.
129. Cantu MG, Buda A, Parma G, et al. Randomized controlled trial of single-agent paclitaxel versus cyclophosphamide, doxorubicin, and cisplatin in patients with recurrent ovarian cancer who responded to first-line platinum-based regimens. J Clin Oncol 2002;20(5):1232–1237.
130. Bolis G, Scarfone G, Giardina G, et al. Carboplatin alone vs carboplatin plus epidoxorubicin as second-line therapy for cisplatin- or carboplatin-sensitive ovarian cancer. Gynecol Oncol 2001;81(1):3–9.
131. ten Bokkel Huinink W, Gore M, Carmichael J, et al. Topotecan versus paclitaxel for the treatment of recurrent epithelial ovarian cancer [see comments]. J Clin Oncol 1997;15(6):2183–2193.
132. Gore M, ten Bokkel Huinink W, Carmichael J, et al. Clinical evidence for topotecan-paclitaxel non-cross-resistance in ovarian cancer. J Clin Oncol 2001;19(7):1893–1900.
133. Gordon AN, Fleagle JT, Guthrie D, Parkin DE, Gore ME, Lacave AJ. Recurrent epithelial ovarian carcinoma: a randomized phase III study of pegylated liposomal doxorubicin versus topotecan. J Clin Oncol 2001;19(14):3312–3322.
134. Markman M, Markman J, Webster K, et al. Duration of response to second line platinum-based chemotherapy for ovarian cancer: implications for patient management and clinical trial design. J Clin Oncol 2004;22(15):3120–3125.
135. Buda A, Floriani I, Rossi R, et al. Randomised controlled trial comparing single agent paclitaxel vs epidoxorubicin plus paclitaxel in patients with advanced ovarian cancer in early progression after platinum-based chemotherapy: an Italian Collaborative Study from the Mario Negri Institute, Milan, G.O.N.O. (Gruppo Oncologico Nord Ovest) group and I.O.R. (Istituto Oncologico Romagnolo) group. Br J Cancer 2004;90(11):2112–2117.
136. Gore M, Oza A, Rustin G, et al. A randomised trial of oral versus intravenous topotecan in patients with relapsed epithelial ovarian cancer. Eur J Cancer 2002;38(1):57–63.
137. Piccart MJ, Green JA, Lacave AJ, et al. Oxaliplatin or paclitaxel in patients with platinum-pretreated advanced ovarian cancer: a randomized phase II study of the European Organization for Research and Treatment of Cancer Gynecology Group. J Clin Oncol 2000;18(6):1193–1202.
138. Markman M. Second-line treatment of ovarian cancer with single-agent gemcitabine. Semin Oncol 2002;29(suppl 1):9–10.
139. Lund B, Hansen OP, Neijt JP, Theilade K, Hansen M. Phase II study of gemcitabine in previously platinum-treated ovarian cancer patients. Anticancer Drugs 1995;6(suppl 6):61–62.
140. D'Agostino G, Amant F, Berteloot P, Scambia G, Vergote I. Phase II study of gemcitabine in recurrent platinum-and paclitaxel-resistant ovarian cancer. Gynecol Oncol 2003;88(3):266–269.

141. Alici S, Saip P, Eralp Y, Aydiner A, Topuz E. Oral etoposide (VP16) in platinum-resistant epithelial ovarian cancer (EOC). Am J Clin Oncol 2003;26(4):358–362.
142. Kavanagh JJ, Tresukosol D, De Leon CG, et al. Phase II study of prolonged oral etoposide in refractory ovarian cancer. Int J Gynecol Cancer 1995;5(5):351–354.
143. de Wit R, van der Burg ME, van den Gaast A, Logmans A, Stoter G, Verweij J. Phase II study of prolonged oral etoposide in patients with ovarian cancer refractory to or relapsing within 12 months after platinum-containing chemotherapy. Ann Oncol 1994;5(7):656–657.
144. Fennelly D, Aghajanian C, Shapiro F, et al. Phase I and pharmacologic study of paclitaxel administered weekly in patients with relapsed ovarian cancer. J Clin Oncol 1997; 15(1):187–192.
145. Kavanagh JJ, Kudelka AP, de Leon CG, et al. Phase II study of docetaxel in patients with epithelial ovarian carcinoma refractory to platinum. Clin Cancer Res 1996;2(5):837–842.
146. Kaye SB, Piccart M, Aapro M, Kavanagh J. Docetaxel in advanced ovarian cancer: preliminary results from three phase II trials. EORTC Early Clinical Trials Group and Clinical Screening Group, and the MD Anderson Cancer Center. Eur J Cancer 1995;31A(suppl 4):S14–S17.
147. Verschraegen CF, Sittisomwong T, Kudelka AP, et al. Docetaxel for patients with paclitaxel-resistant Mullerian carcinoma. J Clin Oncol 2000;18(14):2733– 2739.
148. Eisenhauer EA, Vermorken JB, van Glabbeke M. Predictors of response to subsequent chemotherapy in platinum pretreated ovarian cancer: a multivariate analysis of 704 patients [see comments]. Ann Oncol 1997;8(10):963–968.
149. Pujade-Lauraine E, Paraiso D, Joly F, provencal J, Goupil A, et al. Is there a role of platinum in the treatment of patients with "platinum resistant" relapsed advanced ovarian cancer. Proc ASCO 2002;22:451 (abstract 1811).
150. Leitao MM, Jr., Hummer A, Dizon DS, et al. Platinum retreatment of platinum-resistant ovarian cancer after non-platinum therapy. Gynecol Oncol 2003;91(1):123–129.
151. Barnhill D, O'Connor D, Farley J, Teneriello M, Armstrong D, Park R. Clinical surveillance of gynecologic cancer patients. Gynecol Oncol 1992;46(3):275–280.
152. Olaitan A, Weeks J, Mocroft A, Smith J, Howe K, Murdoch J. The surgical management of women with ovarian cancer in the south west of England. Br J Cancer 2001;85(12): 1824–1830.
153. Moses S, Olaitan A, Murdoch J, Goodwin A. Pilot study and randomized controlled study of three models of follow-up of patients treated for gynaecological cancer: attitudes in general practice and feasibility of randomization. J Obstet Gynecol 2004;24(2):165.
154. Niloff JM, Knapp RC, Lavin PT, et al. The CA 125 assay as a predictor of clinical recurrence in epithelial ovarian cancer. Am J Obstet Gynecol 1986; 155(1):56–60.
155. Berek JS, Hacker NF, Lagasse LD, Nieberg RK, Elashoff RM. Survival of patients following secondary cytoreductive surgery in ovarian cancer. Obstet Gynecol 1983;61(2): 189–193.
156. Eisenkop SM, Friedman RL, Spirtos NM. The role of secondary cytoreductive surgery in the treatment of patients with recurrent epithelial ovarian carcinoma. Cancer (Phila) 2000;88(1):144–153.
157. Krebs HB, Goplerud DR. Surgical management of bowel obstruction in advanced ovarian carcinoma. Obstet Gynecol 1983;61(3):327–330.
158. Pothuri B, Vaidya A, Aghajanian C, Venkatraman E, Barakat RR, Chi DS. Palliative surgery for bowel obstruction in recurrent ovarian cancer: an updated series. Gynecol Oncol 2003;89(2):306–313.
159. Krebs HB, Goplerud DR. The role of intestinal intubation in obstruction of the small intestine due to carcinoma of the ovary. Surg Gynecol Obstet 1984;158(5):467–471.
160. Larson JE, Podczaski ES, Manetta A, Whitney CW, Mortel R. Bowel obstruction in patients with ovarian carcinoma: analysis of prognostic factors. Gynecol Oncol 1989;35(1):61–65.
161. Rubin SC, Hoskins WJ, Benjamin I, Lewis JL, Jr. Palliative surgery for intestinal obstruction in advanced ovarian cancer. Gynecol Oncol 1989;34(1):16–19.
162. McCann RM, Hall WJ, Groth-Juncker A. Comfort care for terminally ill patients. The appropriate use of nutrition and hydration. JAMA 1994;272(16):1263–1266.
163. Cozzaglio L, Balzola F, Cosentino F, et al. Outcome of cancer patients receiving home parenteral nutrition. Italian Society of Parenteral and Enteral Nutrition (S.I.N.P.E.). JPEN J Parenter Enteral Nutr 1997;21(6):339–342.
164. Abu-Rustum NR, Barakat RR, Venkatraman E, Spriggs D. Chemotherapy and total parenteral nutrition for advanced ovarian cancer with bowel obstruction. Gynecol Oncol 1997;64(3):493–495.
165. Herman LL, Hoskins WJ, Shike M. Percutaneous endoscopic gastrostomy for decompression of the stomach and small bowel. Gastrointest Endosc 1992;38(3):314–318.
166. Cunningham MJ, Bromberg C, Kredentser DC, Collins MB, Malfetano JH. Percutaneous gastrostomy for decompression in patients with advanced gynecologic malignancies. Gynecol Oncol 1995;59(2):273–276.
167. Jacobs I, Davies AP, Bridges J, et al. Prevalence screening for ovarian cancer in postmenopausal women by CA 125 measurement and ultrasonography. Br Med J 1993;306(6884): 1030–1034.
168. Grover S, Quinn MA, Weideman P, et al. Screening for ovarian cancer using serum CA 125 and vaginal examination: report on 2550 females. Int J Gynecol Cancer 1995;5(4): 291–295.
169. Adonakis GL, Paraskevaidis E, Tsiga S, Seferiadis K, Lolis DE. A combined approach for the early detection of ovarian cancer in asymptomatic women. Eur J Obstet Gynecol Reprod Biol 1996;65(2):221–225.
170. Sato S, Yokoyama Y, Sakamoto T, Futagami M, Saito Y. Usefulness of mass screening for ovarian carcinoma using transvaginal ultrasonography. Cancer (Phila) 2000;89(3): 582–588.
171. DePriest PD, Gallion HH, Pavlik EJ, Kryscio RJ, van Nagell JR, Jr. Transvaginal sonography as a screening method for the detection of early ovarian cancer. Gynecol Oncol 1997;65(3):408–414.
172. Sell A, Bertelsen K, Andersen JE, Stroyer I, Panduro J. Randomized study of whole-abdomen irradiation versus pelvic irradiation plus cyclophosphamide in treatment of early ovarian cancer. Gynecol Oncol 1990;37(3):367–373.
173. Dembo AJ. Radiotherapeutic management of ovarian cancer. Semin Oncol 1984;11(3):238–250.
174. Muggia FM, Braly PS, Brady MF, et al. Phase III randomized study of cisplatin versus paclitaxel versus cisplatin and paclitaxel in patients with suboptimal stage III or IV ovarian cancer: a gynecologic oncology group study. J Clin Oncol 2000;18(1):106–115.
175. Colombo N, Maggioni A, Vignali M, Parma G, Mangioni C. Options for primary chemotherapy in advanced ovarian cancer: the European perspective. Gynecol Oncol 1994;55(3 pt 2):S108–S113.

176. Sorbe B. Consolidation treatment of advanced (FIGO stage III) ovarian carcinoma in complete surgical remission after induction chemotherapy: a randomized, controlled, clinical trial comparing whole abdominal radiotherapy, chemotherapy, and no further treatment. Int J Gynecol Cancer 2003; 13(3):278–286.
177. Parmar MK, Ledermann JA, Colombo N, et al. Paclitaxel plus platinum-based chemotherapy versus conventional platinum-based chemotherapy in women with relapsed ovarian cancer: the ICON4/AGO-OVAR-2.2 trial. Lancet 2003;361(9375):2099–2106.
178. Pfisterer J, Plante M, du Bois A, Wagner U, Hirte H, al E. Gemcitabine/carboplatin vs. carboplatin in platinum sensitive disease. Proc ASCO 2004;23:450s (abstract 5005).
179. Bolis G, Parazzini F, Scarfone G, et al. Paclitaxel vs epidoxorubicin plus paclitaxel as second-line therapy for platinum-refractory and -resistant ovarian cancer. Gynecol Oncol 1999;72(1):60–64.

53

Uterine Malignancies

Gini F. Fleming, Anthony C. Montag,
Arno J. Mundt, and S.D. Yamada

Etiology, Epidemiology, and Risk Factors

The American Cancer Society estimates that, in 2004, endometrial cancer will be the most common gynecologic malignancy in North America, accounting for 40,320 new cases and 7,090 deaths. Endometrial cancer is primarily a disease of postmenopausal women, with the incidence peaking between the ages of 55 and 65 years. Among Caucasian women, the incidence of uterine cancer is about twice that of African-American women; however, African-American women are less likely to survive this disease. Between 1992 and 1999, the 5-year survival for Caucasian women was 86% as compared to 60% for African-American women.[1] This disparity in survival has persisted over the past 25 years and may reflect the preponderance of tumors in African-Americans with unfavorable histology, higher grade and, possibly, more-advanced stage at diagnosis.

It is believed that there are two types of endometrial cancer: estrogen related and non-estrogen related. More than 80% of early-stage endometrial cancers are endometrioid and, most likely, estrogen related.[2] The majority of these cases develop from preexisting endometrial hyperplasia and reflect the effect of endogenous or exogenous estrogen stimulation. The risk and rate of progression to cancer are not well defined, although it has been estimated that endometrial hyperplasia with nuclear atypia has a 25% risk of progression to endometrial carcinoma, in contrast to hyperplasia without cytologic atypia, which has an exceedingly low rate of progression.[3]

Numerous factors, many related to estrogen stimulation, have been associated with the development of endometrial hyperplasia and, subsequently, endometrial cancer. Estrogen without concurrent progestin use increases the risk of endometrial carcinoma by four- to eightfold. This risk increases with both duration and amount of estrogen exposure.[4] In the PEPI trial (Postmenopausal Estrogen and Progesterone Intervention Trial), 75 of 119 (62%) women who used unopposed estrogen 0.625 mg/day (conjugated equine estrogen) over the course of 3 years developed endometrial hyperplasia. Atypical endometrial hyperplasia occurred in a statistically higher percentage of women taking unopposed estrogen as opposed to placebo: 11.8% versus 0% (*P* less than 0.001).[5] Progestins used in conjunction with estrogen reduce the risk of endometrial cancer and should be prescribed to all women with an intact uterus receiving hormone replacement therapy. In the HOPE trial (Women's Health, Osteoporosis, Estrogen, Progestin Trial), doses of 0.625 mg conjugated equine estrogen (CEE) or 0.45 mg CEE with medroxyprogesterone 2.5 mg daily did not produce any cases of hyperplasia.[6]

As a result of prolonged exposure of the endometrium to estrogen stimulation, obesity, nulliparity, and late menopause increase the risk of endometrial cancer development, as do feminizing ovarian tumors (granulosa cell tumors) and polycystic ovarian syndrome. Diabetes and hypertension are also associated with increased risk of disease development but may be surrogates for other risk factors such as obesity.

Tamoxifen use in women with breast cancer also increases the relative risk of endometrial cancer six- to sevenfold, with the risk being most pronounced after 2 years of use.[7] Tamoxifen inhibits the action of estradiol by competitively binding to the estrogen receptor, but it inherently also has a weak estrogenic effect. In the NSABP B-14 study, the use of tamoxifen was associated with a rate of 1.6 cases of endometrial cancer in 1,000 women as compared to 0.2 cases per 1,000 women in the placebo group. The relative risk for the development of endometrial cancer increases with prolonged use: the relative risk is 2.0 [95% confidence interval (CI) 1.2–3.2) with 2 to 5 years of use and 6.9 (95% CI, 2.4–19.4) for 5 years or more of use as compared to nonusers. Although the vast majority of uterine cancers found in association with tamoxifen use are low-grade endometrial carcinomas, the long-term use of tamoxifen has been associated with the development of poor prognostic subtypes such as carcinosarcomas.[8]

Although the majority of uterine cancer cases develop in an environment of estrogen stimulation, some cases develop in the absence of hyperplasia or significant risk factors such as obesity. These endometrial cancers are often found to be of higher grade and may contain poorer prognostic histologic subtypes than their estrogen-related counterparts.

Endometrial cancer is infrequently associated with a genetic component; however, members of families with the Lynch II syndrome or hereditary nonpolyposis cancer syndromes, where there are mutations in the DNA mismatch repair genes *hMSH2* and *hMLH1*, have a lifetime risk of 25% to 50%[9] of developing endometrial cancer in addition to colon, breast, and ovarian cancer. Finally, pelvic radiation has also been associated with the development of certain poor prognostic cancers such as sarcomas.

Diagnosis and Screening

The diagnosis of uterine cancer is most frequently established through an office endometrial biopsy, usually instituted as a result of postmenopausal vaginal bleeding. In the absence of bleeding, endometrial cancer occasionally presents with abdominal pain as a result of an obstructed, blood-filled uterus, or, rarely, with abnormal endometrial cells on routine Pap smear screening. When atypical endometrial cells are seen on a Pap smear, the risk that an endometrial adenocarcinoma will be found is approximately 20%. This risk increases to approximately 41% in women who are at least 60 years old. Grossly normal endometrial cells in a Pap smear of a postmenopausal woman should also raise suspicion for malignancy. Approximately 10% of postmenopausal women less than 60 years old and up to 20% of those who are older with endometrial cells on Pap smear have an underlying adenocarcinoma, the majority of which are grade 1 or 2 endometrioid adenocarcinomas.[10]

An office endometrial biopsy will diagnose endometrial cancer with certainty in nearly 95% of cases. With small tissue samples it is sometimes difficult to distinguish complex hyperplasia from adenocarcinoma. In this case, a dilatation and curettage (D&C) may be necessary. In fact, in women with complex hyperplasia with atypia found on biopsy, up to 43% of patients in a prospective Gynecologic Oncology Group study correlating findings on biopsy with final hysterectomy diagnosis were found to have endometrial carcinoma.[11]

Once a uterine cancer is found, a careful pelvic examination is performed to determine if there is clinically apparent extension of the tumor beyond the confines of the uterus. In more than 75% of patients there will be no clinical evidence of extrauterine disease, and preoperative studies would then include a chest X-ray and routine blood tests. In patients with evidence of extrauterine spread or in patients with known aggressive histologic subtypes of tumor (see following), a computed tomography (CT) scan or magnetic resonance imaging (MRI) may delineate other areas of disease extension.

For the general population, there is no benefit to routine screening (transvaginal ultrasound and/or endometrial sampling) for endometrial cancer in asymptomatic women, even those on hormone replacement therapy.[12] Screening for women who have an increased risk for the development of endometrial cancer, such as patients on tamoxifen, has been studied extensively using a variety of techniques including transvaginal ultrasound (TVUS), sonohysterography, and hysteroscopy. The results of key prospective studies including studies of breast cancer patients on tamoxifen and controls not on tamoxifen are shown in Table 53.1. The majority of patients with abnormalities on ultrasound have benign disease in the form of atrophy, polyps, or simple hyperplasia. Tamoxifen has also been shown to cause stromal condensation that may be misinterpreted as a thickened endometrial lining on ultrasound. It is not cost-effective to screen asymptomatic breast cancer patients on tamoxifen. Most patients with significant abnormalities will manifest their disease with signs of vaginal bleeding. Only patients who experience vaginal bleeding on tamoxifen, therefore, should be further evaluated by endometrial tissue sampling. Screening even in patients with higher risk of development of endometrial cancer, such as members of hereditary nonpolyposis colon cancer syndrome (HNPCC) families, has been shown to be of limited value. Forty-one women in an HNPCC cohort, the majority of whom were postmenopausal, underwent annual TVUS exams with a median follow-up of 5 years. A total of 179 TVUSs led to 17 endometrial biopsies in which 3 patients with complex hyperplasia and 1 patient with endometrial cancers were identified.[13]

Pathology of Neoplasia of the Uterine Corpus: Carcinomas

Uterine lesions can be broadly divided into lesions that take their origin from the epithelium, from the stroma (whether endometrial stroma or myometrial smooth muscle), or mixed tumors containing both epithelial and stromal elements. Mixed tumors may contain a benign epithelial and malignant stromal component (adenosarcoma), the converse (carcinofibroma), or two malignant components (carcinosarcoma).

Endometrioid Adenocarcinoma

Most endometrial carcinomas are adenocarcinomas, displaying glandular differentiation mimicking one of the Mullerian-derived epithelia: endometrial, tubal, or cervical (Figure 53.1). Endometrioid carcinoma is the most common histology, comprising approximately 60% of endometrial carcinomas. Endometrioid tumors mimic normal endometrial glands to varying degrees; well-differentiated tumors form glands with several layers of cells that retain some of the normal polarity of proliferative endometrium. More poorly differentiated tumors lose the tendency to form glands, taking on a more-solid architecture, with loss of nuclear polarity and increasing cytologic atypia. The endometrioid histology and its subtypes are estrogen related, frequently accompanied by adenomatous hyperplasia, express estrogen and progesterone receptors, and tend to present at a lower stage and grade. Grading is according to the International Federation of Gynecology and Obstetrics (FIGO) system, based on the amount of solid growth pattern (excluding squamous areas): grade I is 5% or less solid, grade II is 6% to 50% solid, and grade III is more than 50% solid. If significant nuclear atypia is present, the grade should be increased by one degree. Diffuse nuclear atypia may indicate serous or clear cell histology.

Serous and Clear Cell Adenocarcinoma

In the early 1980s Bokhman[14] proposed two clinically and histologically distinct forms of endometrial carcinoma: type I or endometrioid and its variants, and type II, including serous and clear cell histologies. The latter frequently arise in a background of relative atrophy, are not associated with estrogen-related risk factors, occur in an older population, and are clinically more aggressive lesions. Hendrickson et al.[15] presented similar clinicopathologic support for two forms of endometrial carcinoma in their description of papillary serous carcinoma of the endometrium and its delineation from the villoglandular variant of endometrioid carcinoma. Patients with papillary serous carcinoma were on average 5 years older, had more-advanced tumors, more-frequent lymphatic involvement, and a tendency to recur in the upper abdomen. Serous tumors of the endometrium are considered to be high-grade lesions by definition and are not further graded by histology.

TABLE 53.1. Prospective studies of screening for endometrial cancer in women on tamoxifen.

Study	*Reference*	*Year*	*No. of patients*	*Tamoxifen dose*	*Screening method*	*Classification*	*Screening interval*	*Duration of tamoxifen use (median)*	*Primary uterine cancers detected*	*Cases detected with abnormal vaginal bleeding*	*Positive predictive value for uterine abnormality*
Fung	160	2003	304 (T)	20 mg/day	TVUS with CFDI, EMB	Normal <10 mm Abnormal ≥10 mm Bleeding	6–12 months	48 months	6	6	43.3%
Gerber	161	2000	247 (T) 98 (C)	20–30 mg/day	TVUS	Abnormal ≥10 mm	6 months	2–5 years	3	2	
Vosse	162	2002	317 (T) 823 (C)	Not noted	TVUS, EMB	Abnormal ≥8 mm	12 months	Not noted	5 (72 of 133 abnormal TVUS underwent EMB) 0	2	64%
Fong	163	2001	138 (T)	20 mg/day	TVUS (138), hysterosonography (133), hysteroscopy (117)	All	N/A				
Strauss	164	2000	70 (T)		TVUS	Abnormal ≥10 mm or bleeding			0	0	
Barakat	165	2000	159 (T)	20 mg/day	EMB on entry	All	6 months	36 months	0	0	
Seoud	166	1999	80 (T)	Not noted	TVUS, EMB	Baseline biopsy, TVUS, EMB q 6 months	6 months	30 months	1	1	
Love	167	1999	357 (T) 130 (C)	20 mg/day	TVUS, hysteroscopy if abnormal	Abnormal ≥5 mm (postmenopausal)	Not stated	62 months	0 145/357 required hysteroscopy: 46% false positive, atrophy	0	
Timmer-man	168	1998	53 (T)	20 or 40 mg/day	TVUS, hysteroscopy	Abnormal >4 mm			1 metastatic breast cancer	0	
Cecchini	169	1996	737 (T)	20 mg/day	TVUS, EMB	Abnormal >6 mm	12 months	50 months	1 (but 209 abnormal US, 108 with EMB)	0	

T, tamoxifen; C, control; TVUS, transvaginal ultrasound; EMB, endometrial biopsy; CFDI, color flow Doppler.

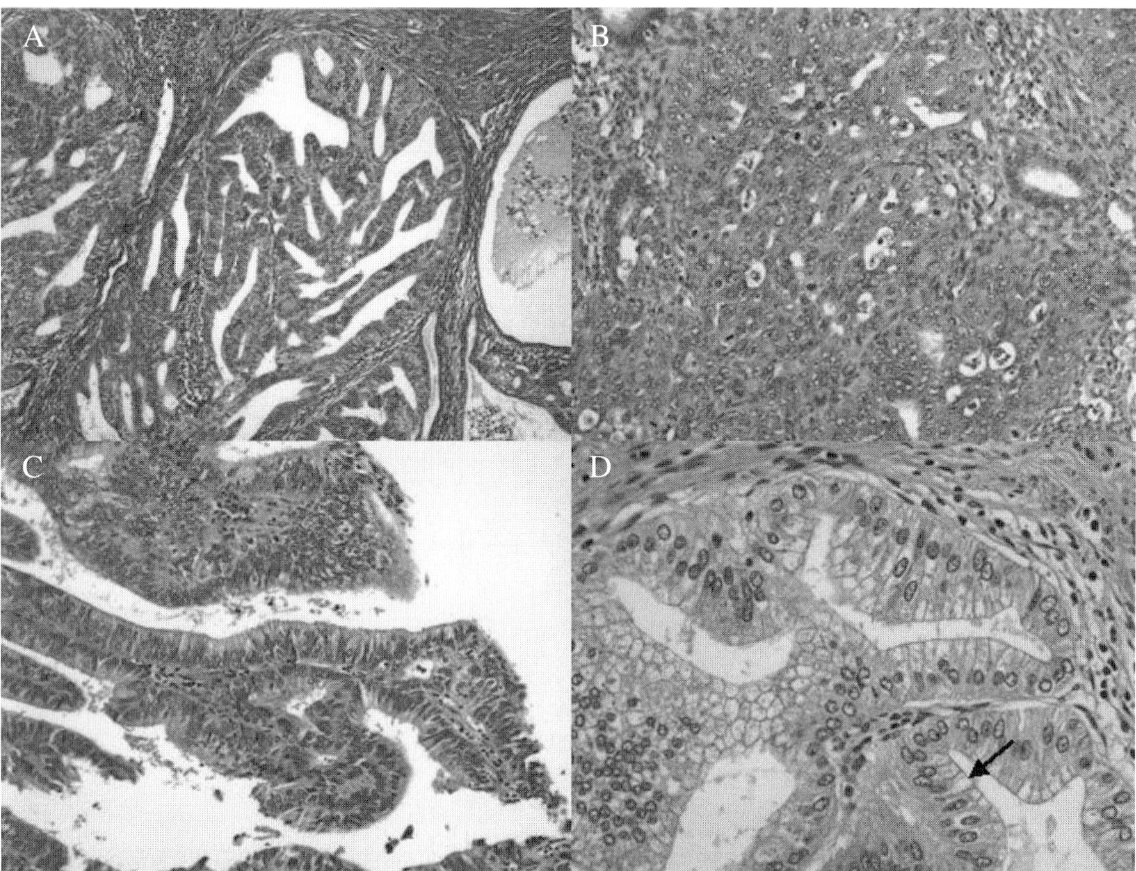

FIGURE 53.1. Endometrioid adenocarcinoma and its variants. (A) Grade I endometrioid carcinoma with cribriforming architecture. (B) Grade III endometrioid carcinoma with predominantly solid architecture. (C) Villoglandular variant with long slender villous projections but with bland cytology. (D) Secretory variant with supranuclear vacuoles (*arrow*).

Clear cell carcinoma is characterized by an architecture that ranges from papillary to tubulocystic or solid and a cytologic appearance that includes clear cells, eosinophilic cells, and hobnail cells. In contrast to vaginal and cervical clear cell tumors, endometrial clear cell carcinoma has no association with maternal diethylstilbestrol (DES) exposure. Clear cell carcinoma is regarded as a high-grade histology and is not further graded.

Carcinosarcoma

Carcinosarcoma, or malignant mixed Mullerian tumor, usually occurs in older, postmenopausal women and frequently presents as a polypoid uterine mass (Figure 53.2). Histologically carcinosarcomas have both epithelial and mesenchymal differentiation, frequently including elements of endometrial stromal sarcoma and leiomyosarcoma, but also heterologous elements not native to the endometrium such as cartilaginous and rhabdomyoblastic differentiation as well. In the past, heterologous elements were believed to correlate with poor prognosis; however, recent studies have shown the mesenchymal component to have no prognostic significance. Clinically, nearly all metastatic foci are either carcinoma or contain both carcinoma and sarcoma, suggesting that the lesion is more likely a metaplastic carcinoma than a collision tumor with separate epithelial and mesenchymal elements. By analysis of X chromosome inactivation and mutations of p53 and K-*ras*, more than 85% of cases have identical findings in the epithelial and mesenchymal components.[16] Similarly, analysis of microsatellite markers supports a monoclonal origin as an epithelial tumor with genetic progression to mesenchymal differentiation.[17]

Precursor Lesions

Endometrioid carcinoma and its variants are associated with endometrial hyperplasia and increased estrogenic effect. Patients with complex atypical hyperplasia have a significant risk of developing endometrial adenocarcinoma, 29%, as opposed to 1% for simple hyperplasia and 3% for complex hyperplasia without atypia.[3]

The precursor lesion of serous carcinoma of the endometrium has been called serous endometrial intraepithelial carcinoma, endometrial carcinoma in situ, or surface serous carcinoma,[18] and has been found in up to 89% of hysterectomy specimens with serous carcinoma (Figure 53.3). The lesion frequently arises in atrophic endometrium, replacing the surface endometrium with highly atypical cells resembling invasive serous carcinoma, displaying increased nuclear/cytoplasmic ratio, irregular nuclear membranes, abnormal chromatin texture, and atypical mitotic figures.

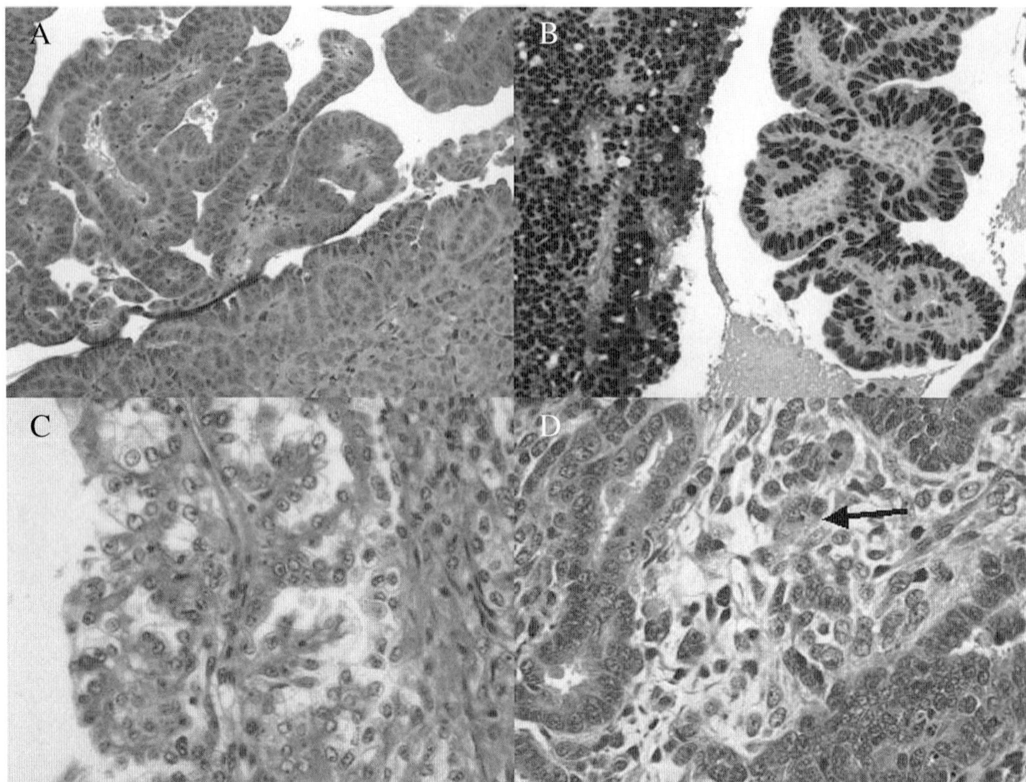

FIGURE 53.2. Type II endometrial carcinoma and carcinosarcoma. (A) Papillary serous carcinoma with fine papillae and marked cytologic atypia. (B) Immunohistochemical stain for p53 protein in papillary serous carcinoma showing uniform nuclear staining in tumor cells. (C) Clear cell carcinoma with nuclear atypia and clear cytoplasm. (D) Carcinosarcoma (malignant mixed Mullerian tumor) with malignant epithelial and stromal (*arrow*) components.

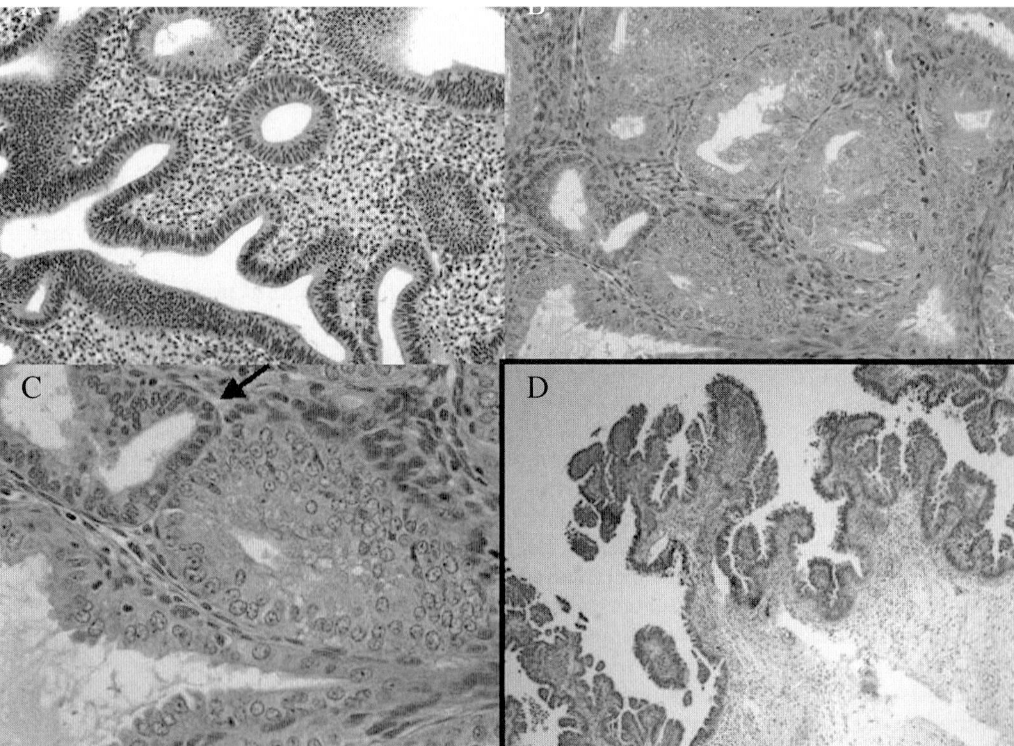

FIGURE 53.3. Precursor lesions of endometrial carcinoma. (A) Simple hyperplasia with architectural budding and branching but minimal increase in the ratio of glands to stroma. (B) Complex atypical hyperplasia with architectural crowding and increased gland to stroma ratio. (C) Complex atypical hyperplasia. Note the loss of nuclear polarity as compared to simple hyperplasia, nuclear enlargement, and abnormal chromatin texture as compared to adjacent normal gland (*arrow*). (D) Endometrial intraepithelial neoplasia (serous carcinoma in situ) arising on the surface of an atrophic endometrial polyp.

Molecular Pathogenesis

Recent molecular studies have confirmed the concept of two pathways of carcinogenesis in endometrial carcinoma. The details of the two pathways involve numerous classes of receptors, cell-cycle regulators, and genes involved in DNA maintenance.

In endometrioid, or type I, carcinoma, the earliest molecular finding appears to be inactivation of DNA mismatch-repair genes (MMR), leading to an accumulation of other mutations that result in cellular dysregulation. Germ-line mutations in the MMR genes MLH-1 and MSH-2 are responsible for the hereditary nonpolyposis colon cancer syndrome (HNPCC), and endometrial carcinoma is the second most common malignancy found in that disorder.[19] Sporadic endometrial carcinomas of endometrioid histology, in contrast, more frequently have methylation of the promoter region of an MMR gene. Goodfellow et al. recently reported the analysis of 127 cases of endometrial carcinomas for abnormalities in DNA mismatch-repair genes[20]: 115 of 127 cases had an abnormality in mismatch-repair genes involving either promoter methylation or somatic or germline mutation.

Microsatellite instability (MSI), the tendency of short repetitive segments of DNA to mutate, is a measure of an overall increased tendency of the cell to mutation. MSI is correlated with abnormalities of DNA mismatch-repair genes and is seen in endometrioid carcinoma and its precursors. Cohn et al.[21] found MI in 51 of 210 cases of endometrioid carcinoma, and of 21 of those cases with accompanying hyperplasia, 20 had MSI in the hyperplastic foci. Conversely, absence of MSI is highly correlated with normal expression of DNA mismatch-repair genes. MSI is almost never seen in serous carcinomas or their in situ precursor endometrial intraepithelial carcinoma (EIC). Tashiro et al. found that none of 34 cases of serous carcinoma had MSI.[22]

The key gatekeeper in endometrioid carcinoma appears to be lipid phosphatase and tensin homologue deleted on chromosome 10 (PTEN), an inositol phospholipid phosphatase that acts as a tumor suppressor by negatively regulating the Akt (phosphatidylinositol protein kinase B) pathway, promoting apoptosis.[23] Human germ-line PTEN mutations are found in Cowden's syndrome, an autosomal dominant multiple hamartoma syndrome that carries an increased risk of carcinoma of the breast, thyroid, and endometrium. Deletion of 10q23, the region that includes the PTEN gene, is seen in sporadic melanomas and glioblastoma, whereas sporadic endometrioid carcinomas may have either deletion or mutation of the PTEN gene.[24] Loss of the expression of PTEN protein by immunohistochemistry (IHC) or evidence of mutation or deletion by molecular analysis is seen in the majority of endometrioid carcinomas in most studies, while serous carcinomas rarely display an abnormality of PTEN. The combination of estrogen-driven proliferation, abnormal DNA repair mechanisms, and decreased apoptosis and cell-cycle dysregulation caused by loss of PTEN function sets the stage for uncontrolled growth and the acquisition of additional mutations.

K-*ras* mutations are seen in 10% to 35% of endometrioid carcinomas, but rarely in serous carcinoma.[21,25] Only a few cases of clear cell carcinoma have been examined for K-*ras* mutations, but mutations were present in two of three cases examined.[26]

Abnormalities of p53 expression appear to play little role in the evolution of endometrioid carcinoma, whereas the majority of serous and clear cell lesions have abnormalities in p53 expression. p53 abnormalities were found in none of 117 cases of endometrial hyperplasia by molecular methods.[27] Indeed, in cases of mixed serous and endometrioid histology, it appears that an area of the endometrioid carcinoma develops a mutation of p53, resulting in a serous component with a different phenotype. Serous carcinomas rarely have microsatellite instability, loss of PTEN expression, or K-*ras* mutations. As in invasive serous carcinoma, serous intraepithelial carcinoma is associated with p53 mutation, indicating that this is an early change in the carcinogenesis of serous tumors.[28]

Clear cell carcinoma has a rate of p53 mutation midway between that seen in clear cell and endometrioid carcinoma.[29] Cases with intermixture of serous elements have a higher rate of p53 mutation and frequently have coexisting serous intraepithelial carcinoma. Cases associated with endometrioid histology tend not to have abnormalities of p53, suggesting that there may be two pathways for the development of the clear cell histology.

Abnormalities in the adenomatous polyposis coli (APC)-beta catenin pathway are also found in type I endometrial carcinoma. In normal epithelial cells, the APC gene product binds to beta catenin, targeting the latter's degradation. Although mutations in the APC gene have not been reported in endometrial carcinoma, 47% of type I endometrial carcinomas have hypermethylation of the APC gene promoter, indicating a loss of APC function.[30] Nuclear beta-catenin accumulation has been documented in several studies ranging from 10% to 55%[31] and is almost exclusively limited to type I histology, having been reported in only 1 of 85 serous carcinomas examined.[30] When compared to other type I endometrial carcinomas, nuclear beta-catenin accumulation is associated with grade I histology, premenopausal status, and expression of estrogen and progesterone receptors.[32]

Stage and Prognosis

The International Federation of Gynecology and Obstetrics (FIGO) introduced a surgical staging classification system for endometrial carcinoma in 1988 (Table 53.2) because clinical

TABLE 53.2. International Federation of Gynecology and Obstetrics (FIGO) staging for carcinoma of the corpus uteri.

Stage	*Description*
IA Grades 1, 2, 3	Tumor confined to the endometrium
IB Grades 1, 2, 3	Invasion to less than one-half of myometrium
IC Grades 1, 2, 3	Invasion to more than one-half of myometrium
IIA Grades 1, 2, 3	Endocervical glandular involvement
IIB Grades 1, 2, 3	Cervical stromal involvement
IIIA Grades 1, 2, 3	Tumor invades the serosa and/or adnexae, and/or positive peritoneal cytology
IIIB Grades 1, 2, 3	Vaginal metastases
IIIC Grades 1, 2, 3	Metastases to pelvic and/or paraaortic lymph nodes
IVA Grades 1, 2, 3	Tumor invasion of bladder or bowel mucosa
IVB	Distant metastases including intraabdominal involvement or inguinal lymph node involvement

TABLE 53.3. Clinical staging for carcinoma of the corpus uteri.

Stage	*Description*
I	Confined to the corpus
IA	Uterine cavity 8 cm or less
IB	Uterine cavity more than 8 cm
II	Involvement of corpus and cervix
III	Extension outside the uterus but not outside the true pelvis May not involve mucosa of the bladder or rectum
IV	Extension beyond the true pelvis or involves mucosa of the bladder or rectum
IVA	Spread to adjacent organs: bladder, rectum, sigmoid, small bowel
IVB	Spread to distant organs

assessment was found to be inaccurate in approximately 40% of cases.[33] At this time, clinical staging (Table 53.3) is relevant only for patients treated with primary radiation therapy. Although there is no specific staging system for uterine sarcomas, some clinicians utilize the surgical staging system for endometrial corpus cancers to classify sarcomas. Surgical staging encompasses a total abdominal hysterectomy with bilateral salpingo-oophorectomy, peritoneal washings for cytology, and, if deemed necessary, pelvic and paraaortic lymph node assessment. Suspicious lymph nodes should be resected or biopsied if unresectable. Relative depth of myometrial invasion (none, inner half, outer half) and the presence or absence of cervical involvement can be determined by gross examination or, if necessary, a frozen section, to determine pathologic factors for which lymphadenectomy would be warranted. For patients with known uterine papillary serous carcinoma, clear cell carcinoma, or carcinosarcoma, where there is risk of omental involvement, some surgeons incorporate an omentectomy into the staging procedure. A lymph node assessment should be performed in these patients with poor prognostic histologic subtypes.

Tumor stage is a well-recognized prognostic factor for uterine cancer. Overall, 5-year survival for endometrial cancers between 1992 and 1999 was 84.4%, which is primarily due to the early stage of presentation in the majority of cases. For patients who are staged, the 5-year survivals are stage I and II, 96.2%, stage III, 64.7%, and stage IV, 26%.[1] In contrast, the prognosis for uterine sarcomas is significantly poorer, with only 20% to 35% of patients surviving 5 years.[34] Clinical factors including patient age, race, and medical comorbidities also significantly impact on outcome. Although incorporated into the surgical staging system, individual pathologic risk factors also act as prognostic factors. These are grouped into uterine and extrauterine factors. Uterine factors include histologic cell type, tumor grade, depth of myometrial invasion, tumor size, capillary or lymphatic vessel involvement, and extension to the cervix. Extrauterine factors include adnexal metastasis, intraperitoneal involvement, lymph node involvement, and positive peritoneal cytology. Risk of extrauterine disease is most strongly related to depth of uterine invasion, followed by tumor grade (Table 53.4).[35] The risk of pelvic lymph node involvement is less than 1% for patients whose tumor is confined to the endometrium. In contrast, if the outer half of the myometrium is involved, the risk of pelvic lymph node involvement increases to about 10% and 20% for grade 1 and grade 2 tumors, respectively, and 34% for grade 3 tumors. Corresponding percentages for paraaortic lymph node involvement in deeply invasive cancers are 6% and 14% for grade 1 and 2 tumors, respectively, and 23% for grade 3 tumors.[33] In patients with a combination of deep myometrial invasion and grade 3 tumor, 30% of patients in a cohort followed prospectively by PORTEC (Post-Operative Radiation Therapy in Endometrial Carcinoma) trialists experienced distant metastases despite the use of adjuvant radiation therapy.[36] Positive peritoneal cytology has also been identified as a factor that can influence prognosis in early-stage endometrial cancer patients; however, its role as an independent prognostic factor remains controversial because cytologic findings frequently correlate with increasing tumor grade and depth of invasion.[37]

As mentioned earlier, histologic cell types such as the papillary serous carcinomas and clear cell carcinomas carry a poorer prognosis than the endometrioid cancers. Much of this difference in outcome is due to the presence of occult disseminated disease.[38] Sarcomas and carcinosarcomas are also particularly aggressive, with more than 50% of apparent stage I carcinosarcomas showing evidence of extrauterine spread when surgically staged.[39]

Therapeutic Modalities

Surgery

Surgery for uterine cancers including the endometrial cancers, papillary serous cancers, and carcinosarcomas consists of a total abdominal hysterectomy, bilateral salpingo-oophorectomy, pelvic and paraaortic lymph node assessment, and cytologic washings. Surgery provides both prognostic information in the form of staging and, in stage IV disease, may be of therapeutic value. Improved survival has been demonstrated in those patients who were optimally surgically cytoreduced to less than 1 cm of disease.[40] In patients with stage IVB endometrioid, serous, and mixed cell types who were optimally debulked, survival was 34.3 months in comparison to 11 months ($P = 0.0001$) in suboptimally debulked patients.

Radical hysterectomy, an extended hysterectomy in which additional parametrial tissue is removed with the surgical specimen, has been used for patients with known cervical involvement and has been associated with an

TABLE 53.4. Frequency of nodal metastasis with individual risk factors.

Risk factor	No. of patients (Creasman)	Pelvic number (%) (Creasman)	Aortic number (%) (Creasman)	No. of patients (Grigsby)	Five-year DFS (%) (Grigsby)
Histology					
Adenocarcinoma	459	40 (9%)	21 (5%)	768	88.6%
Others	99	2 (9%)	4 (18%)	71	80.5%–88.9%
Grade					
1 Well	180	5 (3%)	3 (2%)	340	94.7%
2 Moderate	288	25 (9%)	14 (5%)	255	88.4%
3 Poor	153	28 (18%)	17 (11%)	161	73.2%
Myometrial invasion					
Endometrial only	87	1 (1%)	1 (1%)	199	93.4%
Superficial	279	15 (5%)	8 (3%)	250	89.6%
Middle	116	7 (6%)	1 (1%)	112	89.8%
Deep	139	25 (25%)	24 (17%)	88	67.8%
Peritoneal cytology					
Negative	537	38 (7%)	20 (4%)	240	91.5%
Positive	75	19 (25%)	14 (19%)	21	56.1%
Tumor location					
Fundus	524	42 (8%)	20 (4%)	447	88.8%
Isthmus-cervix	97	16 (16%)	14 (14%)	23	73.1%
Adnexal involvement					
Negative	587	47 (8%)	27 (5%)		
Positive	34	11 (32%)	7 (20%)		
Capillary space involvement					
Negative	528	37 (7%)	19 (9%)	549	88.9%
Positive	93	21 (27%)	15 (19%)	65	75.0%

Source: Adapted from Creasman et al. Surgical pathologic spread patterns of endometrial cancer. Cancer (Phila) 1987;60:2035–2041 (columns 2–4).

Source: Adapted from Grigsby et al. Stage I endometrial cancer: prognostic factors for local control and distant metastasis and implications of the new FIGO surgical staging system. Int J Radiat Oncol Biol Phys 1992;22:905–911 (columns 5, 6).

improvement in survival.[41] However, whether more-extensive surgery is of benefit in stage II disease remains controversial.

Debate also exists as to which patients with disease presumptively confined to the uterus should undergo lymph node assessment and how extensive a lymph node assessment is required as a component of the surgical staging. Proponents of lymph node sampling or lymphadenectomy in *all* patients with endometrial cancer note that relying on a staging algorithm based on intraoperative identification of high-risk factors (grade 3, papillary serous, clear cell, deep myometrial invasion, or cervical involvement) will miss 5% to 7% of patients with these risk factors.[42] In addition, reliance on palpably enlarged nodes during surgery has been shown to identify positive nodes less than 10% of the time in prospective studies.[33] The question of whether there is a therapeutic value to the removal of lymph nodes in endometrial cancer is also a matter of controversy. An analysis of the SEER (Surveillance, Epidemiology, and End Results) data to determine whether pelvic lymph node sampling impacted on survival did not show a correlation with survival. Information on use of adjuvant therapy was not available for this analysis.[43] No randomized studies have been performed to elicit the specific value of a lymphadenectomy in the removal of microscopic or macroscopic nodal metastases. Overall survival appears to be better, however, for patients with positive nodes if they undergo a paraaortic lymphadenectomy than if they do not (77% versus 42%; $P = 0.05$).[44]

Radiation Therapy

Radiation therapy (RT) has long occupied a role in the management of patients with endometrial carcinoma. For much of the past century, RT was commonplace in the treatment of these patients, particularly preoperative RT. By the 1980s, however, the use of preoperative RT declined, replaced by primary surgical approaches. Currently, RT is delivered almost exclusively following surgery in women with adverse pathologic features.

Today, the most common external-beam RT approach in endometrial cancer is pelvic RT, delivered at most centers with a four-field approach to a total dose of 45–50.4 Gy. Select patients receive extended-field or whole abdominal RT, delivered with opposed anteroposterior fields. Prescribed doses are 45 to 50 Gy (extended field) and 25 to 30 Gy (whole abdominal). In the latter case, the pelvis is boosted to 45–50 Gy.

The most common brachytherapy approach is intracavitary vaginal brachytherapy, delivered with either low dose rate (LDR) or high dose rate (HDR) techniques. With LDR, 60–70 Gy is prescribed to the vaginal surface (25–35 Gy if combined with pelvic RT). Various HDR schedules are recommended, including 7 Gy × 3, 5.5 Gy × 4, and 4.7 Gy × 5 (at 0.5-cm depth) and 10.5 Gy × 3, 8.8 Gy × 4, and 7.5 Gy × 5 (at the vaginal surface). When combined with pelvic RT, 5.5 Gy × 2 or 4 Gy × 3 (at 0.5 cm) or 8 Gy × 2 or 6 Gy × 3 (at the surface) is used.[45]

Recently, intensity-modulated radiation therapy (IMRT) has received increasing attention in gynecologic tumors. Unlike conventional techniques, IMRT conforms the prescription dose to the shape of the target in three dimensions, thereby sparing nearby normal tissues. Multiple investigators have compared IMRT and conventional planning, noting significant reductions in the volume of all normal tissues irradiated (small bowel, bladder, rectum, and bone marrow) with IMRT. In a series of reports, investigators at the University of Chicago have reported fewer acute and chronic sequelae in gynecology patients treated with IMRT compared to conventional pelvic RT.[25] Recently, these investigators reported no pelvic failures in a cohort of 31 stage I–IV endometrial cancer patients treated with IMRT at a median follow-up of 24 months.[46]

Therapy for Stage I/II Disease

Therapy for stage I/II disease usually consists of surgery with or without RT. Patients with surgically staged IA and IB grade 1 cancers with low-volume tumor (less than 2 cm) can be successfully managed with observation, as the cancer-related and recurrence-free survivals are 97% and 96%, respectively.[47] Surgically staged patients who have stage IB grade 2 disease with low-volume tumor (less than 2 cm) can also be successfully observed without adjuvant RT, although some investigators would administer vaginal brachytherapy.

Radiotherapy

Preoperative Radiotherapy

Radiotherapy was commonplace for many years in the treatment of early-stage endometrial cancer. However, its benefit in clinical stage I disease is unclear and today it is performed at only a few centers. A stronger rationale exists for its use in clinical stage II disease, particularly in patients with gross cervical involvement.

Adjuvant Radiotherapy

The role of adjuvant RT in early-stage endometrial cancer is controversial (Table 53.5). At some centers, nearly all patients receive postoperative RT, even those with minimally invasive, low-grade tumors. At others, it is rarely administered, even in women with deeply invasive, high-grade disease. Even when it is used, controversy exists over *how* it should be performed.

The decision to administer adjuvant RT in early-stage patients is typically based on pathologic features in the hysterectomy specimen including depth of myometrial invasion, grade, and cervical involvement. Other factors cited include tumor size, lymphovascular invasion, and lower uterine segment involvement. However, the significance of lower uterine segment involvement in the absence of other high-risk factors remains unclear.[48]

To date, three prospective randomized trials have been published evaluating postoperative RT in early-stage disease (Table 53.6). The first was performed in Norway and published in 1980.[49] All patients had clinical stage I disease and underwent primary surgery without lymph node sampling. Excluding those found to have extrauterine disease, 540 women were treated with vaginal brachytherapy and then randomized to observation versus pelvic RT. Overall, no difference was seen in the 5-year survival between the two groups (91% observation, 89% pelvic RT). However, pelvic RT was associated with a significantly lower incidence of vagina/pelvic recurrences in women with deep myometrial invasion (14.7% observation, 6.6% pelvic RT) and high-grade disease (14.1% observation, 3.2% pelvic RT). Chronic toxicities were seen in 1.2% and 0.8%, respectively, of patients treated with and without pelvic RT.

Gynecologic Oncology Group trial 99 (GOG 99) was initially presented in 1998 and ultimately published in 2004.[50] Four hundred forty-eight stage IB, IC, and occult II patients were enrolled. Patients underwent primary surgery with pelvic and paraaortic lymph node sampling and were randomized to pelvic RT or no further therapy. Overall, irradiated patients had a superior 2-year recurrence-free survival (97% versus 88%; $P = 0.007$) compared to surgery-alone patients. Two-year rates of isolated vaginal failure in the surgery-alone and irradiated patients were 7.4% and 1.6%, respectively. The benefit of RT was most evident in the subset of 132 patients with "high" intermediate risk features (94% versus 74%), defined as (1) grade 2–3 with lymphovascular

TABLE 53.5. Surgery and postoperative radiation therapy stage I–II endometrial carcinoma (series after 1998).

Author	*Reference*	*Year*	*N*	*Stage*	*Radiation therapy*	*Vaginal recurrence*	*Pelvic recurrence*	*Five-year survival*	*Comments*
Boz	170	1998	125	IAg3-IC	P		4%	94%	All patients underwent pelvic and paraaortic lymph node sampling
Irwin	171	1998	314	IA–C	VB, P ± VB		5%–6%	79%–82%	
Calvin	172	1999	44	IIA–B	P ± VB, VB	2%	4%	85.2% (DFS)	Select stage IIA patients received VB alone
Chadha	53	1999	124	IBg3-IC	VB		0%	93%	
Weiss	173	1999	159	I–II	P ± VB		0%	77%–92% (DFS)	
Weiss	54	1999	61	IC	P	0%	1.6%	86.7% (DFS)	Included unfavorable histology patients
Alektiar	174	2002	233	IBg1–2	VB		4%	94%	High dose-rate VB
Horowitz	175	2002	164	IB-II	VB	1.2%	1.2%	87%	High dose-rate VB
Ng	56	2001	77	IBg3–IC	VB	9%	1.3%	94%	

VB, vaginal brachytherapy; P, pelvic radiotherapy; g, grade; DFS, disease-free survival.

TABLE 53.6. Surgery and postoperative radiation therapy: randomized trials.

Author	*Reference*	*Year*	*Eligible patients*	*Randomization*	*N*	*Recurrence*	*Five-year survival*	*Comments*
Aalders	49	1980	Clinical stage I	TAH-BSO + VB TAH-BSO + VB + pelvic RT	264 254	14.7% (pelvic)[a] 6.6% (pelvic)*	91% 89%	Chronic toxicities: pelvic RT (1.8%) versus. no pelvic RT (0.8%)
Creutzberg	51	2000	Pathologic stage I (grade 1 > 50% MI, grade 2 any MI, grade 3 < 50% MI)	TAH-BSO TAH-BSO + pelvic RT	360 354	14% (pelvic) 4% (pelvic)	81% 85%	$P < 0.001$ (pelvic recurrence); $P = 0.31$ (survival)
Keys	50	2004	Pathologic stage IB, IC, occult II	TAH-BSO/LNS TAH-BSO/LNS + pelvic RT	202 190	12% (2-year) 3% (2-year)	86% (4- year) 92% (4- year)	$P = 0.007$ (recurrence); $P = 0.56$ (survival)

TAH-BSO, total abdominal hysterectomy and bilateral salpingo-oophorectomy; VB, vaginal brachytherapy; RT, radiation therapy; MI, myometrial invasion.
[a]Deep myometrial invasion patients only.

invasion and more than 1–3 myometrial invasion, (2) at least 50 years of age with any two of the above factors, or (3) at least 70 years of age with any one of the above factors. Overall, irradiated patients had a better 4-year overall survival (92% versus 86%); however, this difference failed to reach significance ($P = 0.56$). Significantly higher rates of hematologic, gastrointestinal, genitourinary, and cutaneous toxicities were seen in the irradiated group; however, acute and chronic toxicities were combined in the analysis.

Creutzberg and coworkers reported the results of the PORTEC trial.[51] All patients underwent primary surgery without nodal sampling. Eligible women had grade 1 tumors with more than 50% myometrial invasion, grade 2 tumors, or grade 3 tumors with less than 50% invasion. Seven hundred fifteen women were randomized to receive either pelvic RT or no further therapy. At a median follow-up of 52 months, irradiated patients had a superior 5-year pelvic control (96% versus 86%; P less than 0.001). However, no difference was noted in overall survival (81% RT group, 85% control group). As in the GOG trial, treatment sequelae were more common in irradiated patients (25% versus 6%; P less than 0.001).

Although these trials consistently demonstrate that RT reduces the risk of pelvic failure in patients with adverse pathologic features, it is unclear whether survival is improved. This is far from being an academic issue, for the lack of a survival benefit has led some to withhold RT. However, none of these trials is well suited to answer this question. First, their follow-up is limited. Longer observational times are needed to assess outcomes of patients who relapse following surgery. Second, only two include a no-RT control arm, for all women in the Norwegian trial received brachytherapy. Finally, the GOG *included* many low-risk patients (58% IB, 82% grades 1–2), whereas PORTEC *excluded* high-risk women (stage IC grade 3, stage II). The former thus included women the least likely to benefit whereas the latter excluded those the most likely to benefit. Although the GOG analyzed "high"-risk patients separately, the small number of such patients significantly limited the power of the analysis.

The optimal approach in early-stage patients who do receive postoperative RT is unclear. It is noteworthy that most pelvic recurrences in the GOG surgery-alone arm were in the vagina.[50] Such a failure pattern suggests that, at least in surgically staged patients, vaginal brachytherapy may be as efficacious as pelvic RT. The more-favorable toxicity profile of vaginal brachytherapy is certainly appealing. The ongoing PORTEC-2 study randomizes between external-beam radiotherapy and vaginal brachytherapy.

The decision whether to irradiate an individual patient rests on a careful assessment of the benefits and risk of treating (and of not treating). The likelihood of cure and toxicity following adjuvant RT needs to be weighed against the likelihood of salvage and toxicity if treatment is withheld. If administered, the approach that maximizes tumor control while minimizing toxicity should be selected. The least aggressive approach should always be used if outcome is not compromised, for example, vaginal brachytherapy instead of pelvic RT in surgically staged patients.

It is difficult to give clear guidelines regarding the use of adjuvant RT in early-stage endometrial cancer, given the lack of consensus between investigators. In general, most investigators do not administer adjuvant RT in women with stage IA grade 1–2 or stage IB grade 1 disease. Stage IA grade 3 patients usually receive either vaginal brachytherapy or pelvic RT.

Patients with stage IB grade 2 tumors undergo pelvic RT or vaginal brachytherapy. Given the excellent pelvic control and low toxicity associated with brachytherapy alone, it is the preferred approach, particularly in surgically staged patients. Women with stage IB grade 3 tumors typically undergo *both* pelvic RT and brachytherapy. However, pelvic RT alone is associated with excellent control rates and less toxicity.[52] In surgically staged patients, brachytherapy alone appears to results in equally favorable outcomes with low rates of toxicity.[53]

At most centers, patients with stage IC tumors receive pelvic RT. At others, they undergo both pelvic RT and vaginal brachytherapy. However, this practice should be discouraged. In a review of 541 stage I patients with deep myometrial invasion from 12 published studies, Weiss et al. noted vaginal recurrences in 1.04% of patients undergoing pelvic RT alone versus 0.97% of patients receiving pelvic RT and vaginal brachytherapy.[54] Moreover, toxicity is more common with the combined approach.[52] In surgically staged patients, brachytherapy alone results in an excellent pelvic control rate with a low risk of sequelae.[53] Interest has emerged recently in whether surgically staged patients with stage IC disease can be observed without adjuvant radiation. One study comparing two cohorts of patients with stage IC (all grades) disease with and without RT demonstrated a 6% chance of recurrence in the RT cohort and 12% in the observation cohort but with similar 5-year overall survivals in both groups (92% versus 90%, respectively; $P = 0.717$). Five-year disease-free survival was improved only in the grade 1 tumor group receiving RT (100% versus 80%; $P = 0.036$). However, studies such as these have been retrospective in nature with observation groups chosen by physician preference.[55]

Patients with stage II disease typically receive both pelvic RT and brachytherapy. However, stage IIA tumors can be treated with pelvic RT alone or, if surgically staged, vaginal brachytherapy.[56] Patients with stage IIB disease should receive both pelvic RT and vaginal brachytherapy.

Definitive Radiotherapy

Although most endometrial cancer patients are treated with surgery, a subset of patients with multiple medical comorbidities and/or advanced age are considered medically inoperable. Such patients are often treated with RT, with curative intent. In addition, patients with locally advanced disease may undergo RT alone.

The most favorable outcomes following RT alone are seen in clinical stage I patients, with 5-year survival rates ranging from 48% to 66%.[57,58] After correcting for intercurrent deaths, 5-year *cause-specific* survivals in these women range from 72% to 87%, with survivals in many series exceeding 80%. Less-favorable outcomes have been reported in clinical stage II and III patients.[57] Pelvic/uterine control rates are high in most patients treated with definitive RT, particularly in those with stage I disease (more than 80%).[59]

Systemic Therapy

There are currently no data supporting the addition of systemic therapy to adjuvant RT in early-stage endometrial cancer. Older randomized trials of adjuvant progestins showed no benefit.[60] The highest risk group are those with high-grade, deep myometrial invasion and no lymph node sampling. A recent registration trial from the PORTEC group followed 99 women with stage IC grade 3 tumors who did not undergo pelvic/paraaortic node dissection. All received postoperative pelvic radiotherapy. There were 13 vaginal/pelvic relapses and 31 distant relapses, with 30 deaths due to endometrial cancer.[36] The Radiation Therapy Oncology Group (RTOG) recently completed a Phase II trial evaluating chemoradiotherapy in high-risk patients (grade 2–3 tumors with more than 50% invasion, cervical stromal invasion, or pelvic-only extrauterine disease).[61] All patients received pelvic RT with cisplatin (50 mg/m^2, days 1 and 28), vaginal brachytherapy, and then four cycles of cisplatin (50 mg/m^2) and paclitaxel (175 mg/m^2). Although the regimen was thought to be feasible, severe (grade 3–4) acute and chronic toxicities were noted in 29% and 18% of patients, respectively. At 24 months, the pelvic recurrence, distant recurrence, disease-free survival, and overall survival of the entire group were 2%, 17%, 83%, and 90%, respectively. A recent randomized trial launched by the RTOG using this cisplatin/paclitaxel chemotherapy in stage I/II disease failed to accrue. Patients with high-risk tumors who have lymph node staging performed, and are known to be node negative, have a lower risk of recurrence than those in whom lymph node assessment is not performed, and it is not likely that adequately powered randomized trials in this subgroup will be feasible. Patients with stage I/II serous/clear cell tumors do merit consideration for adjuvant chemotherapy, as discussed next. In the future, molecular markers may aid in the selection of patients for adjuvant chemotherapy trials.

Therapy for Stage III and "Optimally Debulked" Stage IV Disease

Radiation Therapy

Adjuvant RT has been used in the postoperative treatment of stage III–IV endometrial cancer patients for many years. Patients with disease limited to the pelvis received pelvic RT with and without vaginal brachytherapy, analogous to stage I–II disease. Those with more-extensive disease were treated with more comprehensive fields, such as extended-field and whole abdominal RT.

Table 53.7 summarizes representative recent adjuvant RT series in stage III–IV disease.[62–68] Unsurprisingly, outcomes

TABLE 53.7. Surgery and postoperative radiotherapy: stage III–IV endometrial carcinoma (series after 1997).

Author	*Reference*	*Year*	*N*	*Stage*	*Site(s)*	*Radiation therapy*	*Five-year survival*	*Comments*
Onda	62	1997	30	IIIC	Pelvic/PA nodes	P/E	84%	
Connell	63	1999	12	IIIA	Adnexa only	P ± VB	70.9% (DFS)	
Nelson	64	1999	17	IIIC	Pelvic nodes	P/WA ± VB	72%	
Nicklin	65	2000	14	IIIB	Vagina	P ± VB	13%	Includes some nonirradiated patients
Smith	66	2000	22	III-IV	Various	WA ± VB	89% (3-year)	
Ashman	67	2001	15	IIIA	Serosa	P ± VB	41.5% (DFS)	
Mundt	68	2001	30	IIIC	Pelvic/PA nodes	P/E/W ± VB	55.8% (DFS)	

DFS, disease-free survival; PA, paraaortic; P, pelvic RT; E, extended-field RT; WA, whole abdominal RT; VB, vaginal brachytherapy.

vary widely, with the best results seen in stage IIIA disease, particularly in patients with isolated adnexal or peritoneal fluid involvement. In contrast, less-favorable outcomes are seen in stage III–IV patients with involvement of multiple extrauterine sites and residual upper abdominal disease.

Considerable interest formerly existed for intraperitoneal ^{32}P in patients with isolated involvement of the peritoneal cytology. Today, interest has waned in light of reports questioning the prognostic significance of positive cytology in the absence of other adverse features.[69] Moreover, significant gastrointestinal toxicities may occur in patients receiving both ^{32}P and external-beam RT.

In the past, stage IIIA patients with isolated adnexal involvement received aggressive therapy, including whole abdominal RT. However, pelvic RT is most likely sufficient. Similarly, recent data have called into questions the role of whole abdominal RT in stage IIIA patients with isolated serosal involvement.[67] Stage IIIB disease is rare. These patients are usually clinically staged and undergo preoperative (or definitive) irradiation. Limited data are available to guide therapeutic decisions.[65]

Adjuvant irradiation in stage IIIC disease has received considerable attention. Numerous authors have reported long-term cures in women with positive paraaortic nodes following extended-field RT, with 5-year survivals ranging from 36% to 84%.[62,68] Patients with pelvic nodal involvement alone represent a favorable group. Nelson and coworkers treated 17 stage IIIC patients with positive pelvic (and negative paraortic) nodes with pelvic ($n = 13$) or whole abdominal ($n = 4$) RT. The 5-year disease-free and overall survivals of the entire group were 81% and 72%, respectively.[64]

Patients with involvement of multiple extrauterine sites pose a therapeutic challenge. In a review of stage III patients, Greven et al. noted abdominal failures in 10% and 25% of women with involvement of one versus three or more extrauterine sites ($P = 0.03$), providing a rationale for whole abdominal RT in the latter group.[70] Promising results have been reported using whole abdominal RT in these as well as in stage IV patients. A GOG phase II trial (GOG 94) of whole abdominal RT included 77 optimally debulked stage III–IV patients. The 3-year progression-free and overall survival of this group was 35% and 31%, respectively.[71]

No prospective Phase III trial has been performed comparing surgery versus surgery plus postoperative RT in any subgroup of stage III–IV disease. Thus, the benefit of *any* form of adjuvant RT in these patients remains unclear. Today, interest is shifting increasingly away from postoperative RT toward systemic chemotherapy. Recently, the GOG completed a randomized trial (GOG 122) comparing adjuvant whole abdominal RT versus chemotherapy (doxorubicin/cisplatin) in optimally (less than 2 cm residual disease) debulked stage III/IV patients. This trial has not yet been published in full; at a median follow-up of 52 months, chemotherapy patients had a superior 2-year disease-free (59% versus 46%) and overall (70% versus 59%) survival. Recurrences were frequent, predominantly in the pelvis and abdomen, in both groups.[72] A concern was the high rate of vaginal cuff recurrences in the RT group because vaginal brachytherapy was not routinely delivered.

Little interest today remains for whole abdominal RT *alone* except at select centers.[66] However, whole abdominal RT is currently being evaluated combined with either concomitant (GOG 9907) or sequential (GOG 9908) chemotherapy. An earlier phase I trial (GOG 9001) demonstrated the feasibility of concomitant chemoradiotherapy in this setting.[73] Given the heterogeneity of stage III–IV disease, it is unlikely that a single approach is appropriate in all patients. Unfortunately, the limited numbers of locally advanced patients preclude the ability to define the optimal approach in every subgroup.

Systemic Therapy

As discussed above, the only randomized trial evaluating chemotherapy in stage III disease is GOG 122, which compared whole abdominal radiotherapy to cisplatin/doxorubicin chemotherapy. About 73% of the patients had stage III disease. Survival benefit with chemotherapy was seen for both the stage III patients [hazard ratio (HR) 0.67, 0.47–0.95] and the stage IV patients (HR 0.64, 0.42–0.99). A small number (about 15%) of these "optimally debulked" stage IV patients appear to be disease free at 5 years. Fifty percent to 60% of stage III patients were disease free at 5 years.[72]

Although select stage III patients may benefit from RT alone, current interest focuses on combined chemoradiotherapy approaches. The addition of radiotherapy to chemotherapy is supported by the high rate of locoregional failure both in GOG 122 and in retrospective series of patients treated with chemotherapy alone.[74] A subsequent GOG stage III trial, GOG 184, prescribed "involved field" (pelvic ± para-aortic ± intravaginal) radiotherapy to all patients; this was followed by either cisplatin/doxorubicin or paclitaxel/doxorubicin/cisplatin chemotherapy. Results of this trial are not yet available. Growth factor (granulocyte colony-stimulating factor, G-CSF) is required for most patients when pelvic radiotherapy precedes chemotherapy to maintain reasonable dose intensity.

Cisplatin/doxorubicin is the only chemotherapy combination for which any positive randomized trial data exist for use in the adjuvant setting. However, based on preliminary results in metastatic disease and ongoing adjuvant clinical trials, other regimens, such as paclitaxel/doxorubicin/cisplatin or carboplatin/paclitaxel, may be used in the future.[75]

Advanced/Recurrent Disease

With the exception of isolated vaginal recurrences or the occasional solitary, resectable pulmonary nodule, therapy for metastatic or recurrent endometrial carcinoma remains palliative.

Salvage Surgery

After radiation therapy, patients with localized central recurrences have been treated surgically with a complete pelvic exenteration for curative intent. Although the complication rate is high, 5-year disease-free survival in this small group of patients was 45%.[76]

Salvage Radiotherapy

Approximately 50% of endometrial cancer patients who relapse following surgery fail in the pelvis, of whom 50%

recur in the vaginal vault. Patients with recurrent disease limited to the pelvis often undergo salvage, particularly those with isolated vaginal recurrences.

Numerous investigators have reported the outcome of patients with recurrent endometrial cancer following salvage RT.[77–79] Survival rates vary considerably between the published reports, ranging from 18% to 71%. Patients with isolated vaginal recurrences represent a favorable group. Pai and coworkers evaluated the outcome of 20 patients with isolated vaginal involvement treated with salvage RT. The 10-year actuarial local control and cause-specific survival of the entire group were 74% and 71%, respectively.[79] In contrast, others have reported poor survivals (24%–33%) in patients with isolated vaginal recurrences.[77] Additional favorable prognostic factors include long disease-free intervals, low-grade disease, adenocarcinoma histology, and no prior RT.

Local control is achieved in 35% to 92% of patients treated with salvage RT, with most series reporting control rates between 40% and 70%.[78] A major determinant of local control is tumor size. Wylie and coworkers reported 5-year local control rates of 80% and 54% in tumors of 2 cm or less and more than 2 cm, respectively ($P = 0.02$).[80] Others have reported similar results.

Hormonal Therapy

Endometrial cancers frequently express both estrogen (ER) and progesterone (PR) receptors, and high levels of PR expression have been shown to correlate inversely with stage and grade, as well as being an independently favorable prognostic indicator in some series of early-stage disease.[81] About 20% of unselected patients with metastatic endometrial carcinoma will respond to therapy with progestins. Other hormonal agents may also have some activity.

Factors that have been found to predict for response to progestins and, to a limited extent, to other hormonal therapies include well-differentiated tumors, a long interval between diagnosis and tumor recurrence, and high levels of estrogen receptors (ER) and progesterone receptors (PR).[82] However, these criteria are imperfect; for example, high-grade tumors sometimes respond to hormonal therapy. Attempts have been made to standardize definitions of ER and PR positivity so that endometrial cancer patients could be selected for hormonal therapy in a manner similar to breast cancer patients, but this has not occurred. Concern exists over the fact that some patients defined as "receptor negative" by various cutoff criteria nonetheless respond to hormones, that there can be heterogeneity between the hormone receptor status of the primary tumor and the metastatic sites, and that various metastatic sites can be discordant.[83,84] Moreover, PR-specific antibodies may fail to detect PRB in formalin-fixed, wax-embedded tissue despite their ability to do so by immunoblot analysis,[85] and PRB may be important in response to hormonal therapy.[86]

Cytotoxic Chemotherapy

Taxanes, anthracyclines, and platinum agents have shown the most activity as single agents to date. It should be kept in mind that dose intensity in some single-agent trials is limited by the older age and prior pelvic radiotherapy of many patients. For example, the Eastern Cooperative Oncology Group (ECOG) trial of topotecan in chemotherapy-naïve women with metastatic/recurrent disease found 0.8 mg/m²/day × 5 (versus the FDA-approved dose of 1.5 mg/m²/day × 5 for second-line therapy for ovarian cancer) to be the tolerable dose in women with prior pelvic radiotherapy for endometrial cancer.[87]

Table 53.8 shows randomized trials of combination therapy. In general, combinations have been shown to produce higher response rates than single-agent therapy and have therefore become standard for healthy patients. Most recently, the three-drug combination of paclitaxel, doxorubicin, and cisplatin showed a survival advantage over the two-drug combination of doxorubicin and cisplatin, but it produced more neurotoxicity[88] and required growth factor support. As treatment in the setting of metastatic disease is generally palliative, decisions about choice of regimen should be based on individual needs and wishes of the patient. The median survival from time of entry onto a chemotherapy protocol for measurable recurrent disease is about a year.

Unfavorable Histology

Papillary Serous/Clear Cell

Because of the rarity of these subtypes, many publications represent small retrospective single-institution series that include patients diagnosed over several decades with a conglomerate of stages and treatments. Often uterine papillary serous carcinomas (UPSC) and clear cell carcinomas (CCC) are analyzed together.

Surgery

Because of the propensity for lymphatic and hematogenous spread, patients with papillary serous and clear cell carcinomas should be surgically staged. This procedure should include a total abdominal hysterectomy, bilateral salpingo-oophorectomy, cytologic washings, pelvic and paraaortic lymph node assessment, and an omentectomy, as 37% to 50% of patients believed to have cancer confined to the uterus will have extrauterine involvement found upon surgical staging.[89,90] Twenty-six of 34 (76%) patients from selected retrospective studies who were surgically staged and shown to have disease confined to the endometrium (stage IA) were observed without adjuvant radiation or chemotherapy. Five of these 26 patients (19%) developed a recurrence in either the pelvis or abdomen. The majority, however, remain disease free.[89–92] Other retrospective studies of presumptive stage IA patients have shown higher recurrence rates (30%) but are difficult to interpret given the lack of surgical staging.[93]

Radiotherapy

The role of RT in patients with unfavorable histologies (papillary serous, clear cell) is controversial. Because papillary serous tumors have a propensity to relapse in the upper abdomen, attention has focused primarily on whole abdominal RT. In a study of 26 patients (80% papillary serous) treated with abdominopelvic radiotherapy, Smith et al. noted a 3-year disease-free and overall survival of 87% and 87% in stage I–II and 32% and 61% in stage III–IV patients, respectively.[66] A Phase II study of whole abdominal RT conducted by the GOG (GOG 94) enrolled 88 papillary serous/clear cell patients, 49

TABLE 53.8. Randomized chemotherapy trials (first-line).

Author	*Reference*	*Year*	*Regimen*	*N*	*RR%*	*Median OS (months)*	*Comments*
Ayoub	176	1988	CAF[a]	20	15%	11	OS difference not significant
			CAF + MPA/tamoxifen[b]	23	43%	14	
Aapro	177	2003	Doxorubicin 60 mg/m² q 4 weeks	87	17%	7	$P = 0.06$ for OS
			Doxorubicin 60 mg/m² + Cisplatin 50 mg/m² q 4 weeks	90	43%	9	
Thigpen	178	2004	Doxorubicin 60 mg/m² q 3 weeks (dox 45 mg/m² if prior RT or age >65)	122	25%	9.2	$P = 0.004$ for RR
			Doxorubicin 60 mg/m² + cisplatin 50 mg/m² q 3 weeks (dox 45 mg/m² if prior RT or age >65)	101	42%	9.0	
Thigpen	179	1994	Doxorubicin 60 mg/m² q 3 weeks	132	22%	6.7	No significant difference in unadjusted RR or OS
			Doxorubicin 60 mg/m² + cyclophosphamide 500 mg/m² q 3 weeks (25% dose reduction if prior RT or age >65)	144	30%	7.3	
Gallion	180	2003	Doxorubicin 60 mg/m² + cisplatin 60 mg/m² q 3 weeks (dox 45 mg/m² if prior RT or age >65)	169	46%	11.2	No difference between standard and "circadian-timed" chemotherapy
			Doxorubicin 60 mg/m² (6 AM) + cisplatin 60 mg/m² (6 PM) q 3 weeks (dox 45 mg/m² if prior RT or age >65)	173	49%	13.2	
Fleming	181	2004	Doxorubicin 60 mg/m² + cisplatin 50 mg/m² q 3 weeks (dox 45 mg/m² + cis 40 mg/m² if prior RT or age >65)	157	40%	12.6	No difference between arms
			Doxorubicin 50 mg/m² + Paclitaxel 150 mg/m²/24 h + G-CSF (dox 40 mg/m² + paclitaxel 120 mg/m² if prior RT or age >65)	160	43%	13.6	
Fleming	88	2004	Doxorubicin 60 mg/m² + cisplatin 50 mg/m² q 3 weeks (Dox 45 mg/m² if prior RT or age >65)	132	34%	12.3	Significant difference in RR and OS. No initial dose reduction in three-drug arm
			Dox 45 mg/m² + cisplatin 50 mg/m² + paclitaxel 160 mg/m² + G-CSF	134	57%	15.3	
Weber	75	2003	Doxorubicin 60 mg/m² + cisplatin 50 mg/m²	29	28%	—	Preliminary report
			Paclitaxel 175 mg/m² + carboplatin AUC 5	34	35%	—	

[a] CAF = Dox 30 mg/m² on day 1, plus Ctx 400 mg/m² on days 1 and 8, plus 5-FU 400 mg/m² on days 1 and 8, q 4 weeks.

[b] MPA/TAM = medroxyprogesterone acetate 200 mg/day × 3 weeks, alternating with tamoxifen 20 mg/day × 3 weeks.

of whom were pathologic stage I/II. The 5-year disease-free survival of stage I–II papillary serous ($n = 31$) and clear cell ($n = 18$) patients were 35% and 61%, respectively.[71] Some others have also reported less-favorable results with whole abdominal RT.[71]

No prospective Phase III trial evaluating whole abdominal RT in papillary serous tumors has been conducted. Its benefit thus remains unclear, particularly in pathologic stage I–II patients. In a review of 193 stage I–II patients from nine studies, Mehta et al. noted abdominal failures in 6 of 68 patients (9%) treated with versus 10 of 125 patients (8%) treated without whole abdominal RT. A benefit in pelvic control was seen, however, with the use of pelvic and/or vaginal irradiation (11% irradiated, 73% nonirradiated patients).[94] Given the high risk of distant failure, a reasonable approach may be chemotherapy combined with pelvic and/or vaginal RT.[95]

Fewer data are available evaluating the role of RT in clear cell carcinoma. These tumors are often grouped with papillary serous tumors and treated with whole abdominal RT, even when confined to the uterus.[66] However, it remains unclear whether whole abdominal RT is beneficial. Murphy and colleagues reviewed the outcome of 38 clear cell patients treated with primary surgery.[96] Pelvic recurrence was seen in 0 of 22 patients treated with versus 8 of 16 (50%) without adjuvant RT (P less than 0.0001). Although no patient received whole abdominal RT, only 1 (2%) failed in the upper abdomen.

Systemic Therapy: Recurrent/Metastatic Disease

The worse prognosis associated with USPC and CCC appears to be related to the very high rates of advanced stage at presentation. Once a tumor has spread outside the uterus, there is no evidence that the chemotherapeutic treatment for women with UPSC or CCC should be different from that for women with high-grade endometrioid carcinomas, despite the different molecular pathways involved. UPSC and CCC do not usually express hormone receptors[97] and should not generally be treated with hormonal therapies such as progestins. Response rates and overall survival for UPSC did not differ from that for all other histologies in two large randomized trials of patients with advanced or recurrent endometrial cancer using cisplatin, paclitaxel, and doxorubicin (GOG 163 and GOG 177).

Clear cell carcinoma is less common than UPSC, and it is difficult to arrive at meaningful conclusions about how well it responds to chemotherapy. Abeler et al. reported that four of six patients treated with platinum-containing chemotherapy showed a response.[98] Three of 10 and 3 of 8 patients with clear cell carcinoma treated on GOG 163 and GOG 177, respectively, had a major response.

Adjuvant Systemic Therapy

Twenty-one percent of patients on GOG 122 had UPSC and 4% had CCC.[72] As discussed earlier, this trial demonstrated an overall superiority for chemotherapy; this was true regardless of histology, and chemotherapy therefore appears to be appropriate therapy for women with stage III and debulked stage IV endometrial cancer of all histologic subtypes, UPSC and CCC included.

The particular dilemmas in the systemic treatment of CCC and UPSC arise in the stage I and II patients. First, was the patient adequately staged? What criteria should be used to determine if the patient had an adequate surgical procedure to exclude more-advanced disease? Second, what is the prognosis of a true extensively surgically staged stage I UPSC or CCC patient? Given the rarity of these histologic subtypes, adequately powered randomized trials testing adjuvant treatment strategies are not feasible. Decisions about adjuvant chemotherapy must be made on a best estimate of risk of recurrence in the absence of systemic treatment and the assumption that if chemotherapy can reduce the risk of recurrence in stage III disease, it can also do so in high-risk stage I/II disease.

GOG 94 prospectively treated patients with clinical stage I/II UPSC/CCC with whole abdominal radiotherapy.[99] A preliminary report noted only a 35% 5-year progression-free survival (PFS) for stage I/II UPSC patients ($n = 31$) and a 61% PFS for stage I/II CCC patients ($n = 18$). On the other hand, as already discussed, a number of small single-institutional series using very extensive surgical staging have reported 85% to 100% 5-year survivals using no adjuvant therapy for patients with stage Ia disease.[91,100,101]

Patients with UPSC who have disease limited to a polyp or the endometrium and who have no further disease found in the hysterectomy specimen or by surgical staging probably have excellent survival and would not benefit from chemotherapy. This is a fairly rare situation. Those who have stage Ia disease based on extensive surgical staging, with a reasonable number of nodes dissected, the omentum and peritoneum sampled, and washings taken, probably also have survivals of 80% or more and will have limited benefit from adjuvant chemotherapy. Most series suggest that the remainder of stage I patients have a risk of recurrence of at least 20%, and they may benefit from chemotherapy.

UPSC and CCC have been suggested to have a higher frequency of HER2 amplification than endometrioid endometrial cancers.[102] The GOG reported results of HER2/neu evaluation on patients from GOG 177. A 3+ level of immunohistochemical staining was detected in 46 of 236 (20%) of cases overall; 10 of 38 USPC (26%), and 36/198 for all others (18%).[103] One complete response to trastuzumab was reported in a 2003 ASCO abstract.[104] However, a GOG trial of single-agent trastuzumab in patients with endometrial cancers staining 2+ or 3+ by immunohistochemical analysis noted no responses in the first stage of accrual.[105] That trial was amended to include only patients with HER2/neu gene amplification [i.e., fluorescence in situ hybridization (FISH) positive] patients of any histologic subtype, and accrual is ongoing.

Carcinosarcomas

Carcinosarcomas, similary to uterine papillary serous carcinomas, have a high rate (75%) of unsuspected metastatic disease.[106] These patients should be surgically staged, if possible, for counseling with regard to prognosis and for recommendations with regard to adjuvant therapy. Survival is directly related to stage of disease. In patients with disease truly confined to the uterus based upon staging, 5-year survival is as high as 74%, in contrast to patients who have known extrauterine disease where survival is only 24% ($P = 0.0013$).[107] However, even in patients left with no gross residual disease, 44% of patients have been shown to develop recurrent disease.[108]

Radiotherapy

Controversy exists regarding the role of RT in carcinosarcoma. Unfortunately, the available outcome data are difficult to interpret because many older reports fail to distinguish between carcinosarcomas and other uterine sarcomas (leiomyosarcoma, endometrial stromal sarcoma) in their analyses. Of note, most,[109] but not all, studies that group the various sarcoma histologies together report improved pelvic control with adjuvant RT. Moreover, most [109–111] but not all[112] note improved survival as well.

Hornback and coworkers evaluated the impact of pelvic RT in uterine sarcoma patients enrolled on GOG-20 (a randomized trial of adjuvant doxorubicin). In this study, pelvic RT was optional. Of 109 stage I–II patients (87% carcinosarcoma), the pelvis was the first site of failure in 10% and 23% of irradiated and nonirradiated patients, respectively.[113] In a separate GOG study, irradiated clinical stage I–II patients had a lower rate of first relapse in the pelvis (17%) than nonirradiated patients (24%).[114] Most studies focusing *solely* on carcinosarcoma have reported better pelvic control rates in irradiated patients, particularly in stage I–II disease.[115–117] Impact on survival has been mixed, with a benefit seen in some but not all reports.

Based on studies that noted a predominance of failures in the upper abdomen,[118] increasing attention has been focused on the use of whole abdominal RT in carcinosarcomas. Currently, the GOG is conducting a randomized trial (GOG 150) of adjuvant whole abdominal RT versus chemotherapy in optimally debulked stage I–IV carcinosarcoma patients. The results of this trial may help define the optimal approach to these patients.

Adjuvant Systemic Therapy

The effects of adjuvant chemotherapy have not been well studied. The only randomized trial performed (GOG 20) tested single-agent doxorubicin versus no chemotherapy after surgery, and demonstrated no difference between the arms in recurrence rate, progression-free survival, or overall survival.[119] This trial included stage I/II uterine carcinosarcomas, leiomyosarcomas, and sarcomas of other histologies, and the numbers in each histologic subset were too small for definitive analysis. Moreover, as discussed, use of pelvic irradiation was at the discretion of the investigator. Forty-five percent of the patients with carcinosarcoma treated on GOG 20 recurred. The current GOG adjuvant trial (GOG 150) randomizes women with optimally debulked stages I–IV carcinosarcoma to whole abdominal radiotherapy versus combination ifosfamide/cisplatin chemotherapy.

Systemic Therapy in Advanced/Recurrent Disease

In advanced or recurrent disease, the number of agents studied is limited, and older trials tended to study carcinosarcomas along with leiomyosarcomas and other sarcomas. Paclitaxel, ifosfamide, and cisplatin clearly produce response rates above 10%, with the highest response rates documented for ifosfamide, although these have also been the most dose-intense and toxic regimens. No randomized trials (Table 53.9) have proven any survival benefit for chemotherapy with advanced/recurrent disease, and median survival for this group of patients remains less than 1 year.

Uterine Mesenchymal Tumors (Sarcomas)

Uterine sarcomas, in general, are rare. However, leiomyosarcomas are responsible for a disproportionate number of deaths from uterine malignancy (40%–50% of stage I–II cancers will recur). As is the case for other soft tissue sarcomas, grade is prognostically very important.[120–122] The overall incidence of uterine malignancies including endometrial carcinomas is lower in black patients (15.31 per 100,000 woman-years; 95% CI, 14.61–16.04) than in white non-Hispanic patients (23.43 per 100,000 woman-years; 95% CI, 23.06–23.81). However, based on SEER (Surveillance, Epidemiology, and End Results) data from 1992–1998, blacks had significantly higher incidence rates of the poorer prognostic histologic types such as carcinosarcoma and sarcoma as compared to white non-Hispanics. The comparison rate ratios for blacks were 2.33 (95% CI, 1.99–2.72) for carcinosarcomas and 1.56 (95% CI, 1.31–1.86) for sarcomas. Mortality attributable to these rare aggressive tumor types accounted for 53% of mortality among black patients as compared to 36% among white patients.[123] Although there is no specific staging system for uterine sarcomas, some clinicians utilize the surgical staging system for endometrial corpus cancers to classify sarcomas.

Pathology

Uterine mesenchymal neoplasms can be broadly classified into those associated with endometrial stroma and those arising from the smooth muscle of the myometrium.

Endometrial Stromal Tumors

Endometrial stromal tumors are characterized by an appearance similar to the stroma of proliferative endometrium, being

TABLE 53.9. Randomized chemotherapy trials in advanced uterine carcinosarcoma.

Author	*Reference*	*Year*	*Prior chemotherapy*	*Regimen*	*N evaluable*	*RR% (n)*	*Median OS*	*Comments*
Sutton	182	2000	N	Ifosfamide 1.5 g/m^2 d × 5 d q 21 d vs. Ifosfamide 1.5 g/m^2 d × 4–5 d + CDDP 20 mg/m^2/d × 4–5 d q 21 d	102	36% (37)	7.6 months	$P = 0.07$ for survival, 17% gr 3–4 CNS toxicity Doses reduced to 4 days in combination arm because of toxicity; 6 deaths before dose reduction
				Ifosfamide 1.2 g/m^2 if prior RT both arms	92	54% (50)	9.4 months	
Muss	183	1985	N	Doxorubicin 60 mg/m^2 q 21 days vs. doxorubicin 60 mg/m^2 + cyclophosphamide 500 mg/m^2 q 21 days Doxorubicin dose 45 mg/m^2 in patients with prior RT, age >65 years, or PS 2–3, both arms	20	25% (5)	—	Part of a trial including uterine leiomyosarcoma Response rates given for patients with measurable disease, both arms combined
Omura	184	1983	Mixed	Doxorubicin 60 mg/m^2 q 21 days vs. doxorubicin 60 mg/m^2 + DTIC 250 mg/m^2/day × 5 q 21 days	41	10% (4)	—	Part of a trial including uterine leiomyosarcomas
				Chemotherapy doses reduced 25% for prior RT, both arms	31	23% (7)	—	

DTIC, dacarbazine; PS, performance status; CNS, central nervous system; gr, grade.

composed of short blue spindle cells and small arterioles. Based on the pattern of growth, they are separated into benign stromal nodules, low-grade endometrial stromal sarcoma, and undifferentiated endometrial sarcoma. The latter was formerly classified as high-grade endometrial stromal sarcoma, but as it is histologically, immunophenotypically, and cytogenetically distinct and has a dismal prognosis by comparison, it is best considered as a different entity rather than a less-differentiated example of stromal sarcoma.[124]

Endometrial stromal nodules are uncommon lesions, usually presenting as an intramural or polypoid well-circumscribed round or oval lesion less than 5 cm in diameter. They are most often discovered as incidental findings on hysterectomy. Microscopically they have an expansile, noninfiltrative growth pattern and are composed of bland stromal cells with variable mitotic activity. Stromal nodules are benign, and tend not to recur even if treated with simple excision.[125]

Low-grade endometrial stromal sarcoma may appear circumscribed or infiltrative on gross examination, but classically presents with a worm-ridden appearance to the myometrium. Areas of cystic degeneration and necrosis may be present. Microscopically, most cases have broad tongues of infiltrating tumor peculating through the myometrium and involving lymphatic spaces. Cells are uniform, nuclear atypia is minimal, and mitotic activity is usually low, although the latter is no longer a diagnostic criterion.[126] Stromal sarcoma typically expresses estrogen and progesterone receptors, CD10, and smooth muscle actin, but lacks expression of desmin.[127,128] Most endometrial stromal sarcomas have at (7: 17) translocation involving JAZF1 and JJAZ1.[129] Survival data from many studies are biased by the inclusion of cases of undifferentiated endometrial sarcoma; however, nearly half of stromal sarcoma patients will experience recurrence, often more than 5 years from initial diagnosis. Hormonal therapy has been effective in treating metastatic disease.[130]

Undifferentiated endometrial sarcoma, formerly known as high-grade endometrial stromal sarcoma, occurs in an older population than low-grade endometrial stromal sarcoma and has a dismal prognosis: most patients present with advanced stage and the median survival is less than 2 years. The tumor is composed of spindle or polygonal pleomorphic mesenchymal cells that bear little resemblance to endometrial stromal cells. Mitotic activity is typically brisk and necrosis is often present. Undifferentiated endometrial sarcoma rarely expresses estrogen or progesterone receptors, lack CD10 expression, and has a complex karyotype.[131] Because of the marked difference in behavior, histology, and immunoprofile, it is recommended that the term high-grade endometrial stromal sarcoma be replaced by undifferentiated endometrial sarcoma.[132]

Smooth Muscle Tumors

Leiomyomas are the most common uterine neoplasm, present in as many as 25% of women over 30. Grossly they are usually well circumscribed, white, and firm to rubbery, although when degenerative changes are present they may range from deep red to yellow and have a soft consistency. Microscopically, they are composed of fascicles of smooth muscle cells with bland cytology. Mitotic activity is usually low, although in reproductive years an otherwise typical leiomyoma may have up to 20 mitoses per 10 high-power fields (mitotically active leiomyoma) and still be benign. Although areas of hyalinization, red or carneous degeneration, or even necrosis may be present, they are different form the geographic coagulative tumor necrosis associated with leiomyosarcoma. Variants of leiomyoma include symplastic leiomyoma, with markedly atypical bizarre cells; epithelioid leiomyoma, with polygonal cells rather than spindled cells; and cellular leiomyoma, composed of cells with scant cytoplasm. Leiomyomas that have undergone treatment with gonadotropin-releasing hormone analogues may display coagulative necrosis or apoptosis.[133]

Leiomyosarcoma is the most common uterine sarcoma, with an incidence of approximately 1 per 10^5 population. Grossly the tumors are more likely to be poorly circumscribed, soft, fleshy, and necrotic or hemorrhagic. Microscopically, compared to leiomyomas, they are more cellular, more mitotically active, and frequently have coagulative necrosis. The histologic spectrum ranges from lesions that have recognizable smooth muscle differentiation to high-grade tumors that bear little resemblance to their cell of origin. The separation of low-grade leiomyosarcoma from leiomyoma is problematic. Taylor and Norris in 1966,[134] reporting on 63 highly cellular smooth muscle tumors, found that cases with fewer than 10 mitoses per 10 high-power fields (hpf) did not metastasize. They also noted that 74% of sarcomas had necrosis, as compared to 12% of leiomyomas. Kempson and Bari[135] studied 29 cases of problematic smooth muscle tumors and found that 6 of 7 cases with 5 to 9 mitoses/hpf recurred when associated with atypia. The malignant criteria of greater than 10 mitoses/10 hpf without atypia and greater than 5 mitoses/hpf with atypia were used for decades based on these studies. In 1988 Perrone and Dehner[136] found that mitotic index did not predict poor prognosis in cases that otherwise lacked atypia. They also noted that infiltrative margins and coagulative necrosis were seen in tumors with malignant behavior. Bell et al.[137] reported their experience with 213 "problematic" smooth muscle tumors in 1994, finding in a multivariant analysis that coagulative tumor necrosis, atypia, and mitotic activity were the important predictors of malignant behavior. When some but not all of these criteria are present, the diagnosis of atypical leiomyoma is made, which carries a small risk of malignant behavior. This expansion of malignant criteria to include coagulative necrosis is especially important in two circumstances: women with mitotically active smooth muscle tumors that lack atypia and necrosis, and tumors with necrosis and atypia that lack significant mitotic activity. The former, mitotically active leiomyomas, occur in women in the reproductive years, particularly under the influence of progesterone, and are benign even if mitotic activity is greater than 10 mitoses/10 hpf. The latter are sarcomas or atypical leiomyomas with some risk of recurrence, even if the mitotic index is low.

Although a clear sequence of neoplastic progression from precursor lesion to fully malignant tumor is seen in other organs, such as colonic adenocarcinoma, there are only anecdotal examples of leiomyosarcoma developing from preexisting leiomyomas. Indeed, the presence of multiple leiomyomas does not increase the risk of sarcoma, and the tumors have different cytogenetic and molecular characteristics.[138]

Surgery

The standard surgical procedure for patients with sarcomas of the uterus is a total abdominal hysterectomy and bilateral salpingo-oophorectomy. Often, the diagnosis will be made incidentally in a patient believed to have a benign leiomyoma. The incidence of ovarian metastasis is relatively low (5%), even in patients with high-grade sarcomas. In patients with low-grade sarcomas, there were no patients with ovarian metastases in a cohort of 108 patients. The role of lymphadenectomy and surgical staging is not of proven benefit in leiomyosarcomas of the uterus. The only patients ($n = 3$ of 37) with positive nodes (8%) in one study from Memorial Sloan Kettering had grossly enlarged lymph nodes. No patients with disease confined to the uterus or cervix had positive nodes.[139] Therefore, there is no documented benefit to taking a patient back to surgery for extended surgical staging. A young patient who underwent a myomectomy only, however, may benefit from undergoing a completion hysterectomy if high-grade leiomyosarcoma was found as there may be residual sarcoma remaining in the uterus.[140]

Radiation Therapy

Limited data are available regarding the role of RT in uterine leiomyosarcomas and endometrial stromal sarcomas. Although some investigators have reported a benefit to adjuvant RT in endometrial stromal sarcoma,[118] others have not.[141] Weitman et al. evaluated 15 endometrial stromal sarcoma patients (80% stage I–II) treated with surgery and adjuvant RT. The 5-year pelvic control and overall survivals were 93% and 79%, respectively.[142] Results have been mixed in leiomyosarcomas, with a benefit seen in terms of pelvic control[143,144] and survival[144] in some reports. Others have noted no benefit to adjuvant irradiation.[121]

Systemic Therapy

Uterine Leiomyosarcomas: Adjuvant Therapy

Neither adjuvant chemotherapy nor adjuvant radiotherapy has been proven to produce a survival benefit, but adequately powered randomized trials do not exist. Results for those patients with leiomyosarcoma entered on the one published randomized trial (doxorubicin versus no chemotherapy) suggest a possible modest benefit from adjuvant deoxorubicin.[119]

Uterine Leiomyosarcomas: Advanced/Recurrent Disease

As is the case for other leiomyosarcomas, ifosfamide and doxorubicin have single-agent activity in metastatic disease. The combination of these two agents has been reported to produce a response rate of 29%[145] but is toxic, and the median survival of 9.5 months observed is similar to that seen in a variety of single-agent studies. Cisplatin, which has reproducible activity in uterine carcinosarcomas, is not effective in the treatment of leiomyosarcomas. Interestingly, the GOG has recently reported a response rate of 19% to single-agent gemcitabine,[146] which has not demonstrated activity against advanced sarcomas or leiomyosarcomas in general.[147] A study by Hensley et al.[148] used the combination of docetaxel and gemcitabine and reported an overall response rate of 53% with a median overall survival of 17.9 months in a group of patients with leiomyosarcoma (85% had uterine leiomyosarcoma, and half had prior chemotherapy). A confirmatory trial is underway in the GOG.

Low Grade Endometrial Stromal Sarcoma (ESS): Systemic Therapy

Although low-grade ESS (previously known as endolymphatic stromal myosis) has a relatively good prognosis, it may recur late. It has been reported that 30% to 50% of tumors localized to the uterus at the time of diagnosis eventually recur.[149] Aubry et al. described 16 patients with lung metastases from metastatic low-grade ESS. In that series, the diagnosis of ESS had been made an average of 9.8 years previously.[150] Low-grade ESS frequently expresses ER and PR. It has been suggested that the ovaries should be removed in premenopausal women with low-grade ESS and/or that adjuvant progestins should be given,[149] but data to support these recommendations are insufficient.

There are, however, multiple case reports documenting responses of low-grade ESS to various hormonal manipulations, including aromatase inhibitors such as aminoglutethimide[130] and letrozole,[151] progestins such as megestrol acetate,[152,153] and, preoperatively, to gonadotropin-releasing hormone (GnRH) agonists such as leuprolide.[154] Because the tumor is indolent, resection of metastases is also an option. Among the 16 patients with lung metastases described by Aubry et al.,[150] 14 were alive and 7 were without evidence of disease at a median follow-up of 4.1 years after diagnosis of lung metastases. The interventions used consisted primarily of resection of lung nodules and hormonal therapy.

Undifferentiated Endometrial Sarcoma

Undifferentiated endometrial sarcoma (high grade) is less common than uterine leiomyosarcoma but has a similar prognosis.[122,155,156] In recurrent undifferentiated endometrial sarcoma, chemotherapy is generally tried. A prospective trial of ifosfamide in 22 patients with recurrent or disease yielded a response rate of 32%.[157] Multiple case reports have documented responses to doxorubicin,[158] and a complete response to paclitaxel and carboplatin has also been reported.[159]

References

1. http://www.cancer.org/downloads/STT/CAFF finalPWSecured.pdf. Accessed 4/8/04.
2. Pecorelli S. FIGO annual report on the results of treatment in gynaecological cancer. J Epidemiol Biostat 1998;3:41.
3. Kurman RJ, Kaminski PF, Norris HJ. The behavior of endometrial hyperplasia. A long-term study of "untreated" hyperplasia in 170 patients. Cancer (Phila) 1985;56:403–412.
4. Grady D, Gebretsadik T, Kerlikowske K, Ernster V, Petitti D. Hormone replacement therapy and endometrial cancer risk: a meta-analysis. Obstet Gynecol 1995;85:304–313.
5. Writing Group for the PEPI Trial. Effects of hormone replacement therapy on endometrial histology in postmenopausal women: the Postmenopausal Estrogen/Progestin Interventions (PEPI) Trial. JAMA 1996;275:370–375.
6. Weiderpass E, Adami HO, Baron JA, et al. Risk of endometrial cancer following estrogen replacement with and without progestins. J Natl Cancer Inst 1999;91:1131–1137.
7. Fisher B, Costantino JP, Redmond CK, Fisher ER, Wickerham DL, Cronin WM. Endometrial cancer in tamoxifen-treated breast cancer patients: findings from the National Surgical

Adjuvant Breast and Bowel Project (NSABP) B-14. J Natl Cancer Inst 1994;86:527–537.
8. Curtis RE, Freedman DM, Sherman ME, Fraumeni JF Jr. Risk of malignant mixed mullerian tumors after tamoxifen therapy for breast cancer. J Natl Cancer Inst 2004;96:70–74.
9. Vasen HF, Stormorken A, Menko FH, et al. MSH2 mutation carriers are at higher risk of cancer than MLH1 mutation carriers: a study of hereditary nonpolyposis colorectal cancer families. J Clin Oncol 2001;19:4074–4080.
10. Cherkis RC, Patten SF Jr, Andrews TJ, Dickinson JC, Patten FW. Significance of normal endometrial cells detected by cervical cytology. Obstet Gynecol 1988;71:242–244.
11. Trimble CL, Kauderer J, Silverberg S, et al. Concurrent endometrial carcinoma (ED) in women with biopsy diagnosis of atypical endometrial hyperplasia: a GOG study. Gynecol Oncol 2004;92:393.
12. Fleischer AC, Wheeler JE, Lindsay I, et al. An assessment of the value of ultrasonographic screening for endometrial disease in postmenopausal women without symptoms. Am J Obstet Gynecol 2001;184:70–75.
13. Rijcken FE, Mourits MJ, Kleibeuker JH, Hollema H, van der Zee AG. Gynecologic screening in hereditary nonpolyposis colorectal cancer. Gynecol Oncol 2003;91:74–80.
14. Bokhman KH. Two pathogenetic types of endometrial carcinoma. Gynecol Oncol 1983;15:10–17.
15. Hendrickson M, Ross J, Eifel P, Martinez A, Kempson R. Uterine papillary serous carcinoma: a highly malignant form of endometrial adenocarcinoma. Am J Surg Pathol 1982;6:93–108.
16. Wada H, Enomoto T, Fujita M, et al. Molecular evidence that most but not all carcinosarcomas of the uterus are combination tumors. Cancer Res 1997;57:5379–5385.
17. Fujii H, Yoshida M, Gong ZX, et al. Frequent genetic heterogeneity in the clonal evolution of gynecological carcinosarcoma and its influence on phenotypic diversity. Cancer Res 2000;60: 114–120.
18. Ambros RA, Sherman ME, Zahn CM, Bitterman P, Kurman RJ. Endometrial intraepithelial carcinoma: a distinctive lesion specifically associated with tumors displaying serous differentiation. Hum Pathol 1995;26:1260–1267.
19. Millar AL, Pal T, Madlensky L, et al. Mismatch repair gene defects contribute to the genetic basis of double primary cancers of the colorectum and endometrium. Hum Mol Genet 1999;8: 823–829.
20. Goodfellow PJ, Buttin BM, Herzog TJ, et al. Prevalence of defective DNA mismatch repair and MSH6 mutation in an unselected series of endometrial cancers. Proc Natl Acad Sci USA 2003;100:5908–5913.
21. Cohn DE, Mutch DG, Herzog TJ, et al. Genotypic and phenotypic progression in endometrial tumorigenesis: determining when defects in DNA mismatch repair and KRAS2 occur. Genes Chromosomes Cancer 2001;32:295–301.
22. Tashiro H, Lax SF, Gaudin PB, Isacson C, Cho KR, Hedrick L. Microsatellite instability is uncommon in uterine serous carcinoma. Am J Pathol 1997;150:75–79.
23. Ali IU. Gatekeeper for endometrium: the PTEN tumor suppressor gene. J Natl Cancer Inst 2000;92:861–863.
24. Waite KA, Eng C. Protean PTEN: form and function. Am J Hum Genet 2002;70:829–844.
25. Lax SF, Kendall B, Tashiro H, Slebos RJ, Hedrick L. The frequency of p53, K-ras mutations, and microsatellite instability differs in uterine endometrioid and serous carcinoma: evidence of distinct molecular genetic pathways. Cancer (Phila) 2000; 88:814–824.
26. Semczuk A, Berbec H, Kostuch M, Cybulski M, Wojcierowski J, Baranowski W. K-ras gene point mutations in human endometrial carcinomas: correlation with clinicopathological features and patients' outcome. J Cancer Res Clin Oncol 1998;124: 695–700.
27. Kohler MF, Nishii H, Humphrey PA, et al. Mutation of the p53 tumor-suppressor gene is not a feature of endometrial hyperplasias. Am J Obstet Gynecol 1993;169:690–694.
28. Zheng W, Khurana R, Farahmand S, Wang Y, Zhang ZF, Felix JC. p53 immunostaining as a significant adjunct diagnostic method for uterine surface carcinoma: precursor of uterine papillary serous carcinoma. Am J Surg Pathol 1998;22:1463–1473.
29. Lax SF, Pizer ES, Ronnett BM, Kurman RJ. Clear cell carcinoma of the endometrium is characterized by a distinctive profile of p53, Ki-67, estrogen, and progesterone receptor expression. Hum Pathol 1998;29:551–558.
30. Moreno-Bueno G, Hardisson D, Sanchez C, et al. Abnormalities of the APC/beta-catenin pathway in endometrial cancer. Oncogene 2002;21:7981–7990.
31. Schlosshauer PW, Ellenson LH, Soslow RA. Beta-catenin and E-cadherin expression patterns in high-grade endometrial carcinoma are associated with histological subtype. Mod Pathol 2002;15:1032–1037.
32. Scholten AN, Creutzberg CL, van den Broek LJ, Noordijk EM, Smit VT. Nuclear beta-catenin is a molecular feature of type I endometrial carcinoma. J Pathol 2003;201:460–465.
33. Creasman WT, Morrow CP, Bundy BN, Homesley HD, Graham JE, Heller PB. Surgical pathologic spread patterns of endometrial cancer. A Gynecologic Oncology Group Study. Cancer (Phila) 1987;60:2035–2041.
34. Dinh TV, Slavin RE, Bhagavan BS, Hannigan EV, Tiamson EM, Yandell RB. Mixed mullerian tumors of the uterus: a clinicopathologic study. Obstet Gynecol 1989;74:388–392.
35. Morrow CP, Bundy B, Kurman RJ. Relationship between surgical-pathological risk factors and outcome in clinical stage I and II carcinoma of the endometrium: a Gynecologic Oncology Group study. Gynecol Oncol 1991;40:55.
36. Creutzberg CL, van Putten WL, Warlam-Rodenhuis CC, et al. Outcome of high-risk stage IC, grade 3, compared with stage I endometrial carcinoma patients: the Postoperative Radiation Therapy in Endometrial Carcinoma Trial. J Clin Oncol 2004;22: 1234–1241.
37. Kadar N, Homesley HD, Malfetano JH. Positive peritoneal cytology is an adverse factor in endometrial carcinoma only if there is other evidence of extrauterine disease. Gynecol Oncol 1992; 46:145–149.
38. Goff BA, Kato D, Schmidt RA, et al. Uterine papillary serous carcinoma: patterns of metastatic spread. Gynecol Oncol 1994; 54:264–268.
39. Uterine carcinosarcomas: incidence and trends in management and survival. Gynecol Oncol 1998;65:153–163.
40. Bristow RE, Zerbe MJ, Rosenshein NB, Grumbine FC. Stage IVB endometrial carcinoma: the role of cytoreductive surgery and determinants of survival. Gynecol Oncol 2000;78:83–84.
41. Cornelison TL, Trimble EL, Kosary CL. SEER data, corpus uteri cancer: treatment trends versus survival for FIGO stage II, 1988–1994. Gynecol Oncol 1999;74:350–355.
42. Malviya VK, Deppe G, Malone JM Jr, Sundareson AS, Lawrence WD. Reliability of frozen section examination in identifying poor prognostic indicators in stage I endometrial adenocarcinoma. Gynecol Oncol 1989;34:299–304.
43. Trimble EL, Kosary C, Park RC. Lymph node sampling and survival in endometrial cancer. Gynecol Oncol 1998;71:340–343.
44. Mariani A, Webb MJ, Galli L, Podratz KC. Potential therapeutic role of para-aortic lymphadenectomy in node-positive endometrial cancer. Gynecol Oncol 2000;76:348–356.
45. Nag S, Erickson B, Parikh S, Gupta N, Varia M, Glasgow G. The American Brachytherapy Society recommendations for high-dose-rate brachytherapy for carcinoma of the endometrium. Int J Radiat Oncol Biol Phys 2000;48:779–790.
46. Knab B, Mehta N, Roeske JC, et al. Outcome of endometrial cancer patients treated with adjuvant intensity modulated pelvic radiation therapy. Presented at the 46th Annual Meeting of the

American Soceity for Therapeutic Radiology and Oncology, Atlanta, GA, October 3–7, 2004.
47. Mariani A, Webb MJ, Keeney GL, Haddock MG, Calori G, Podratz KC. Low-risk corpus cancer: is lymphadenectomy or radiotherapy necessary? Am J Obstet Gynecol 2000;182:1506–1519.
48. Phelan C, Montag AG, Rotmensch J, Waggoner SE, Yamada SD, Mundt AJ. Outcome and management of pathological stage I endometrial carcinoma patients with involvement of the lower uterine segment. Gynecol Oncol 2001;83:513–517.
49. Aalders J, Abeler V, Kolstad P, Onsrud M. Postoperative external irradiation and prognostic parameters in stage I endometrial carcinoma: clinical and histopathologic study of 540 patients. Obstet Gynecol 1980;56:419–427.
50. Keys HM, Roberts JA, Brunetto VL, et al. A phase III trial of surgery with or without adjunctive external pelvic radiation therapy in intermediate risk endometrial adenocarcinoma: a Gynecologic Oncology Group study. Gynecol Oncol 2004;92: 744–751.
51. Creutzberg CL, van Putten WL, Koper PC, et al. Surgery and postoperative radiotherapy versus surgery alone for patients with stage-1 endometrial carcinoma: multicentre randomised trial. PORTEC Study Group: Post Operative Radiation Therapy in Endometrial Carcinoma. Lancet 2000;355:1404–1411.
52. Randall ME, Wilder J, Greven K, Raben M. Role of intracavitary cuff boost after adjuvant external irradiation in early endometrial carcinoma. Int J Radiat Oncol Biol Phys 1990;19:49–54.
53. Chadha M, Nanavati PJ, Liu P, Fanning J, Jacobs A. Patterns of failure in endometrial carcinoma stage IB grade 3 and IC patients treated with postoperative vaginal vault brachytherapy. Gynecol Oncol 1999;75:103–107.
54. Weiss MF, Connell PP, Waggoner S, Rotmensch J, Mundt AJ. External pelvic radiation therapy in stage IC endometrial carcinoma. Obstet Gynecol 1999;93:599–602.
55. Straughn JM, Huh WK, Orr JW, Jr., et al. Stage IC adenocarcinoma of the endometrium: survival comparisons of surgically staged patients with and without adjuvant radiation therapy. Gynecol Oncol 2003;89:295–300.
56. Ng TY, Nicklin JL, Perrin LC, Cheuk R, Crandon AJ. Postoperative vaginal vault brachytherapy for node-negative Stage II (occult) endometrial carcinoma. Gynecol Oncol 2001;81:193–195.
57. Patanaphan V, Salazar OM, Chougule P. What can be expected when radiation therapy becomes the only curative alternative for endometrial cancer? Cancer (Phila) 1985;55:1462–1467.
58. Sorbe B, Frankendal B, Risberg B. Intracavitary irradiation of endometrial carcinoma stage I by a high dose-rate afterloading technique. Gynecol Oncol 1989;33:135–145.
59. Abayomi O, Tak W, Emami B, Anderson B. Treatment of endometrial carcinoma with radiation therapy alone. Cancer (Phila) 1982;49:2466–2469.
60. Macdonald RR, Thorogood J, Mason MK. A randomized trial of progestogens in the primary treatment of endometrial carcinoma. Br J Obstet Gynaecol 1988;95:166–174.
61. Greven K, Winter K, Underhill K, Fontenesci J, Cooper J, Burke T. Preliminary analysis of RTOG 9708: adjuvant postoperative radiotherapy combined with cisplatin/paclitaxel chemotherapy after surgery for patients with high-risk endometrial cancer. Int J Radiat Oncol Biol Phys 2004;59:168–173.
62. Onda T, Yoshikawa H, Mizutani K, et al. Treatment of node-positive endometrial cancer with complete node dissection, chemotherapy and radiation therapy. Br J Cancer 1997;75:1836–1841.
63. Connell PP, Rotmensch J, Waggoner S, Mundt AJ. The significance of adnexal involvement in endometrial carcinoma. Gynecol Oncol 1999;74:74–79.
64. Nelson G, Randall M, Sutton G, Moore D, Hurteau J, Look K. FIGO stage IIIC endometrial carcinoma with metastases confined to pelvic lymph nodes: analysis of treatment outcomes, prognostic variables, and failure patterns following adjuvant radiation therapy. Gynecol Oncol 1999;75:211–214.
65. Nicklin JL, Petersen RW. Stage 3B adenocarcinoma of the endometrium: a clinicopathologic study. Gynecol Oncol 2000; 78:203–207.
66. Smith RS, Kapp DS, Chen Q. Treatment of high-risk uterine cancer with whole abdominopelvic radiation therapy. Int J Gynecol Cancer 2000;48:767.
67. Ashman JB, Connell PP, Yamada D, Rotmensch J, Waggoner SE, Mundt AJ. Outcome of endometrial carcinoma patients with involvement of the uterine serosa. Gynecol Oncol 2001;82:338–343.
68. Mundt AJ, Murphy KT, Rotmensch J, Waggoner SE, Yamada SD, Connell PP. Surgery and postoperative radiation therapy in FIGO Stage IIIC endometrial carcinoma. Int J Radiat Oncol Biol Phys 2001;50:1154–1160.
69. Naumann RW, Higgins RV, Hall JB. The use of adjuvant radiation therapy by members of the Society of Gynecologic Oncologists. Gynecol Oncol 1999;75:4–9.
70. Greven KM, Lanciano RM, Corn B, Case D, Randall ME. Pathologic stage III endometrial carcinoma. Prognostic factors and patterns of recurrence. Cancer (Phila) 1993;71:3697–3702.
71. Axelrod J, Bundy J, Roy T. Advanced endometrial carcinoma (EC) treated with whole abdominal irradiation (WAI): a Gynecologic Oncology Group (GOG) study. Gynecol Oncol 1995;56: 135.
72. Randall ME, Brunetto G, Muss HB, Mannel R, Spirtos N. Whole abdominal radiotherapy versus combination doxorubicin-cisplatin chemotherapy in advanced endometrial carcinoma: a randomized phase III trial of the Gynecologic Oncology Group. Proc Am Soc Clin Oncol 2003;22:2.
73. Reisinger SA, Asbury R, Liao SY, Homesley HD. A phase I study of weekly cisplatin and whole abdominal radiation for the treatment of stage III and IV endometrial carcinoma: a Gynecologic Oncology Group pilot study. Gynecol Oncol 1996;63:299–303.
74. Mundt AJ, McBride R, Rotmensch J, Waggoner SE, Yamada SD, Connell PP. Significant pelvic recurrence in high-risk pathologic stage I–IV endometrial carcinoma patients after adjuvant chemotherapy alone: implications for adjuvant radiation therapy. Int J Radiat Oncol Biol Phys 2001;50:1145–1153.
75. Weber B, Mayer F, Bougnoux P, et al. What is the best chemotherapy regimen in recurrent or advanced endometrial carcinoma? Proc Am Soc Clin Oncol 2003;22:453.
76. Morris M, Alvarez RD, Kinney WK, Wilson TO. Treatment of recurrent adenocarcinoma of the endometrium with pelvic exenteration. Gynecol Oncol 1996;60:288–291.
77. Aalders JG, Abeler V, Kolstad P. Recurrent adenocarcinoma of the endometrium: a clinical and histopathological study of 379 patients. Gynecol Oncol 1984;17:85–103.
78. Nag S, Yacoub S, Copeland LJ, Fowler JM. Interstitial brachytherapy for salvage treatment of vaginal recurrences in previously unirradiated endometrial cancer patients. Int J Radiat Oncol Biol Phys 2002;54:1153–1159.
79. Pai HH, Souhami L, Clark BG, Roman T. Isolated vaginal recurrences in endometrial carcinoma: treatment results using high-dose-rate intracavitary brachytherapy and external beam radiotherapy. Gynecol Oncol 1997;66:300–307.
80. Wylie J, Irwin C, Pintilie M, et al. Results of radical radiotherapy for recurrent endometrial cancer. Gynecol Oncol 2000;77: 66–72.
81. Fukuda K, Mori M, Uchiyama M, Iwai K, Iwasaka T, Sugimori H. Prognostic significance of progesterone receptor immunohistochemistry in endometrial carcinoma. Gynecol Oncol 1998; 69:220–225.
82. Creasman WT. Prognostic significance of hormone receptors in endometrial cancer. Cancer (Phila) 1993;71:1467–1470.

83. Runowicz CD, Nuchtern LM, Braunstein JD, Jones JG. Heterogeneity in hormone receptor status in primary and metastatic endometrial cancer. Gynecol Oncol 1990;38:437–441.
84. Niemann TH, Maymind M, Fowler J. Expression of estrogen receptor and progesterone receptor in advanced stage endometrial cancer. Gynecol Oncol 1999;72.
85. Mote PA, Johnston JF, Manninen T, Tuohimaa P, Clarke CL. Detection of progesterone receptor forms A and B by immunohistochemical analysis. J Clin Pathol 2001;54:624–630.
86. Dai D, Wolf DM, Litman ES, White MJ, Leslie KK. Progesterone inhibits human endometrial cancer cell growth and invasiveness: down-regulation of cellular adhesion molecules through progesterone B receptors. Cancer Res 2002;62:881–886.
87. Wadler S, Levy DE, Lincoln ST, Soori GS, Schink JC, Goldberg G. Topotecan is an active agent in the first-line treatment of metastatic or recurrent endometrial carcinoma: Eastern Cooperative Oncology Group Study E3E93. J Clin Oncol 2003;21: 2110–2114.
88. Fleming GF, Brunetto VL, Cella D, et al. Phase III trial of doxorubicin plus cisplatin with or without paclitaxel plus filgrastim in advanced endometrial carcinoma: a Gynecologic Oncology Group Study. J Clin Oncol 2004;22:2159–2166.
89. Chan JK, Loizzi V, Youssef M, et al. Significance of comprehensive surgical staging in noninvasive papillary serous carcinoma of the endometrium. Gynecol Oncol 2003;90:181–185.
90. Slomovitz BM, Burke TW, Eifel PJ, et al. Uterine papillary serous carcinoma (UPSC): a single institution review of 129 cases. Gynecol Oncol 2003;91:463–469.
91. Grice J, Ek M, Greer B, et al. Uterine papillary serous carcinoma: evaluation of long-term survival in surgically staged patients. Gynecol Oncol 1998;69:69–73.
92. Bristow RE, Asrari F, Trimble EL, Montz FJ. Extended surgical staging for uterine papillary serous carcinoma: survival outcome of locoregional (Stage I–III) disease. Gynecol Oncol 2001;81: 279–286.
93. Lim P, Al Kushi A, Gilks B, Wong F, Aquino-Parsons C. Early stage uterine papillary serous carcinoma of the endometrium: effect of adjuvant whole abdominal radiotherapy and pathologic parameters on outcome. Cancer (Phila) 2001;91:752–757.
94. Mehta N, Yamada SD, Rotmensch J, Mundt AJ. Outcome and pattern of failure in pathologic stage I–II papillary serous carcinoma of the endometrium: implications for adjuvant radiation therapy. Int J Radiat Oncol Biol Phys 2003;57:1004–1009.
95. Turner BC, Knisely JP, Kacinski BM, et al. Effective treatment of stage I uterine papillary serous carcinoma with high dose-rate vaginal apex radiation (192Ir) and chemotherapy. Int J Radiat Oncol Biol Phys 1998;40:77–84.
96. Murphy KT, Rotmensch J, Yamada SD, Mundt AJ. Outcome and patterns of failure in pathologic stages I–IV clear-cell carcinoma of the endometrium: implications for adjuvant radiation therapy. Int J Radiat Oncol Biol Phys 2003;55:1272–1276.
97. Carcangiu ML, Chambers JT, Voynick IM, Pirro M, Schwartz PE. Immunohistochemical evaluation of estrogen and progesterone receptor content in 183 patients with endometrial carcinoma. Part I: Clinical and histologic correlations. Am J Clin Pathol 1990;94:247–254.
98. Abeler VM, Vergote IB, Kjorstad KE, Trope CG. Clear cell carcinoma of the endometrium. Prognosis and metastatic pattern. Cancer (Phila) 1996;78:1740–1747.
99. Sutton G, Bundy B, Axelrod J. Whole-abdominal radiotherapy in Stage I and II papillary serous (PS) or clear-cell cancers of the uterus (a GOG study). Gynecol Oncol 2002;84:535.
100. Gitsch G, Friedlander ML, Wain GV, Hacker NF. Uterine papillary serous carcinoma. A clinical study. Cancer (Phila) 1995;75: 2239–2243.
101. Gehtrig PA, Groben PA, Fowler J. Noninvasive papillary serous carcinoma of the endometrium. Obstet Gynecol 2001;97: 153–157.
102. Rolitsky CD, Theil KS, McGaughy VR, Copeland LJ, Niemann TH. HER-2/neu amplification and overexpression in endometrial carcinoma. Int J Gynecol Pathol 1999;18:138–143.
103. Grushko TA, Ridderstrale K, Olopade OI. Identification of HER-2/neu oncogene amplification by fluorescence in situ hybridization in endometrial carcinoma from patients included in Gynecologic Oncology Group trial 177. Proc Am Soc Clin Oncol 2003;22:468.
104. Villela JA, Cohen S, Tiersten A, Smith DH. HER-2/neu expression in uterine papillary serous cancers. Proc Am Soc Clin Oncol 2003;22:465.
105. Fleming GF, Sill MA, Thigpen JT. Phase II evaluation of trastuzumab in patients with advanced or recurrent endometrial carcinoma: a report of GOG 181b. Proc Am Soc Clin Oncol 2003; 22:453.
106. Macasaet MA, Waxman M, Fruchter RG, et al. Prognostic factors in malignant mesodermal (mullerian) mixed tumors of the uterus. Gynecol Oncol 1985;20:32–42.
107. Yamada SD, Burger RA, Brewster WR, Anton D, Kohler MF, Monk BJ. Pathologic variables and adjuvant therapy as predictors of recurrence and survival for patients with surgically evaluated carcinosarcoma of the uterus. Cancer (Phila) 2000; 88:2782–2786.
108. Inthasorn P, Carter J, Valmadre S, Beale P, Russell P, Dalrymple C. Analysis of clinicopathologic factors in malignant mixed Mullerian tumors of the uterine corpus. Int J Gynecol Cancer (Phila) 2002;12:348–353.
109. Ferrer F, Sabater S, Farrus B, et al. Impact of radiotherapy on local control and survival in uterine sarcomas: a retrospective study from the Grup Oncologic Catala-Occita. Int J Radiat Oncol Biol Phys 1999;44:47–52.
110. Sorbe B. Radiotherapy and/or chemotherapy as adjuvant treatment of uterine sarcomas. Gynecol Oncol 1985;20:281–289.
111. Moskovic E, MacSweeney E, Law M, Price A. Survival, patterns of spread and prognostic factors in uterine sarcoma: a study of 76 patients. Br J Radiol 1993;66:1009–1015.
112. Vongtama V, Karlen JR, Piver SM, Tsukada Y, Moore RH. Treatment, results and prognostic factors in stage I and II sarcomas of the corpus uteri. Am J Roentgenol 1976;126:139–147.
113. Hornback NB, Omura G, Major FJ. Observations on the use of adjuvant radiation therapy in patients with stage I and II uterine sarcoma. Int J Radiat Oncol Biol Phys 1986;12:2127–2130.
114. Majors FJ, Blessing JA, Silverberg S. Prognostic factors in early-stage uterine sarcoma. A Gynecologic Oncology Group Study 1993;71:1702.
115. Echt G, Jepson J, Steel J, et al. Treatment of uterine sarcomas. Cancer (Phila) 1990;66:35–39.
116. Perez CA, Askin F, Baglan RJ, et al. Effects of irradiation on mixed mullerian tumors of the uterus. Cancer (Phila) 1979;43: 1274–1284.
117. Kohern EI, Schwartz PE, Chambers JT. Adjuvant therapy in mixed mullerian tumors of the uterus. Gynecol Oncol 1986;23: 212.
118. Rose PG, Boutselis JG, Sachs L. Adjuvant therapy for stage I uterine sarcoma. Am J Obstet Gynecol 1987;156:660–662.
119. Omura GA, Blessing JA, Major F, et al. A randomized clinical trial of adjuvant adriamycin in uterine sarcomas: a Gynecologic Oncology Group Study. J Clin Oncol 1985;3:1240–1245.
120. Gadducci A, Landoni F, Sartori E, et al. Uterine leiomyosarcoma: analysis of treatment failures and survival. Gynecol Oncol 1996; 62:25–32.
121. Mayerhofer K, Obermair A, Windbichler G, et al. Leiomyosarcoma of the uterus: a clinicopathologic multicenter study of 71 cases. Gynecol Oncol 1999;74:196–201.
122. Gadducci A, Sartori E, Landoni F, et al. The prognostic relevance of histological type in uterine sarcomas: a Cooperation Task Force (CTF) multivariate analysis of 249 cases. Eur J Gynaecol Oncol 2002;23:295–299.

123. Sherman ME, Devesa SS. Analysis of racial differences in incidence, survival, and mortality for malignant tumors of the uterine corpus. Cancer (Phila) 2003;98:176–186.
124. Chang KL, Crabtree GS, Lim-Tan SK, Kempson RL, Hendrickson MR. Primary uterine endometrial stromal neoplasms. Am J Surg Pathol 1990;14:415–438.
125. Tavassoli FA, Nottis HJ. Mesenchymal tumours of the uterus. VII. A clinicopathological study of 60 endomterial stromal nodules. Histopathology (Oxf) 1981;5:1–10.
126. Chuang JT, Van Velden DJ, Graham JB. Carcinosarcoma and mixed mesodermal tumor of the uterine corpus. Review of 49 cases. Obstet Gynecol 1970;35:769–780.
127. Toki T, Shimizu M, Takagi Y, Ashida T, Konishi I. CD10 is a marker for normal and neoplastic endometrial stroma cells. Int J Gynecol Pathol 2002;21:41–47.
128. Blom R, Malmstrom H, Guerrieri C. Endometrial stromal sarcoma of the uterus: a clinicopathologic, DNA flow cytometric, p53, and mdm-2 analysis of 49 cases. Int J Gynecol Cancer 1999;9:98–104.
129. Koontz JI, Soreng AL, Nucci M, et al. Frequent fusion of the JAZF1 and JJAZ1 genes in endometrial stromal tumors. Proc Natl Acad Sci USA 2001;98:6348–6353.
130. Spano JP, Soria JC, Kambouchner M, et al. Long-term survival of patients given hormonal therapy for metastatic endometrial stromal sarcoma. Med Oncol 2003;20:87–93.
131. Gil-Benso R, Lopez-Gines C, Navarro S, Carda C, Llombart-Bosch A. Endometrial stromal sarcomas: immunohistochemical, electron microscopical and cytogenetic findings. Virchows Arch 1999;434:307–314.
132. Evans HL. Endometrial stromal sarcoma and poorly differentiated endometrial sarcoma. Cancer (Phila) 1982;50:2170–2182.
133. Sreenan JJ, Prayson RA, Biscotti CV, Thornton MH, Easly KA, Hart WR. Histopathologic findings in 107 uterine leiomyomas treated with leuprolide acetate compared with 126 controls. Am J Surg Pathol 1996;20:427–432.
134. Taylor HB, Norris HJ. Mesenchymal tumors of the uterus IV. Diagnosis and prognosis of leiomyosarcoma. Arch Pathol 1966; 82:40–44.
135. Kempson RL, Bari W. Uterine sarcomas. Classification, diagnosis, and prognosis. Hum Pathol 1970;1:331–339.
136. Perrone T, Dehner LP. Prognostically favorable "mitotically active" smooth muscle tumors of the uterus. A clinicopathologic study of ten cases. Am J Surg Pathol 1988;12:1–8.
137. Bell SW, Kempson RL, Hendrickson MR. Problematic uterine smooth muscle neoplasms. A clinicopathologic study of 213 cases. Am J Surg Pathol 1994;18:535–558.
138. Nibert M, Heim S. Uterine leiomyoma cytogenetics. Genes Chromosomes Cancer 1990;2:3–13.
139. Leitao MM, Sonoda Y, Brennan MF, Barakat RR, Chi DS. Incidence of lymph node and ovarian metastases in leiomyosarcoma of the uterus. Gynecol Oncol 2003;91:209–212.
140. Berchuck A, Rubin SC, Hoskins WJ, Saigo PE, Pierce VK, Lewis JL Jr. Treatment of uterine leiomyosarcoma. Obstet Gynecol 1988;71:845–850.
141. DeFusco PA, Gaffey TA, Malkasian GD. Endometrial stromal sarcoma: review of Mayo Clinic experience. Gynecol Oncol 1989;35:8.
142. Weitman HD, Kucera H, Knocke TH. Surgery and adjuvant radiation therapy of endometrial stromal sarcoma. Wien Klin Wochenschr 2002;114:44.
143. Wheelock JB, Krebs HB, Schneider V, Goplerud DR. Uterine sarcoma: analysis of prognostic variables in 71 cases. Am J Obstet Gynecol 1985;151:1016–1022.
144. Giuntoli RL II, Metzinger DS, DiMarco CS, et al. Retrospective review of 208 patients with leiomyosarcoma of the uterus: prognostic indicators, surgical management, and adjuvant therapy. Gynecol Oncol 2003;89:460–469.
145. Sutton G, Blessing JA, Malfetano JH. Ifosfamide and doxorubicin in the treatment of advanced leiomyosarcomas of the uterus: a Gynecologic Oncology Group study. Gynecol Oncol 1996;62: 226–229.
146. Look KY, Sandler A, Blessing JA, Lucci JA III, Rose PG. Phase II trial of gemcitabine as second-line chemotherapy of uterine leiomyosarcoma: a Gynecologic Oncology Group (GOG) Study. Gynecol Oncol 2004;92:644–647.
147. Okuno S, Ryan LM, Edmonson JH, Priebat DA, Blum RH. Phase II trial of gemcitabine in patients with advanced sarcomas (E1797): a trial of the Eastern Cooperative Oncology Group. Cancer (Phila) 2003;97:1969–1973.
148. Hensley ML, Maki R, Venkatraman E, et al. Gemcitabine and docetaxel in patients with unresectable leiomyosarcoma: results of a phase II trial. J Clin Oncol 2002;20:2824–2831.
149. Chu MC, Mor G, Lim C, Zheng W, Parkash V, Schwartz PE. Low-grade endometrial stromal sarcoma: hormonal aspects. Gynecol Oncol 2003;90:170–176.
150. Aubry MC, Myers JL, Colby TV, Leslie KO, Tazelaar HD. Endometrial stromal sarcoma metastatic to the lung: a detailed analysis of 16 patients. Am J Surg Pathol 2002;26:440–449.
151. Maluf FC, Sabbatini P, Schwartz L, Xia J, Aghajanian C. Endometrial stromal sarcoma: objective response to letrozole. Gynecol Oncol 2001;82:384–388.
152. Sabini G, Chumas JC, Mann WJ. Steroid hormone receptors in endometrial stromal sarcomas. A biochemical and immunohistochemical study. Am J Clin Pathol 1992;97:381–386.
153. Wade K, Quinn MA, Hammond I, Williams K, Cauchi M. Uterine sarcoma: steroid receptors and response to hormonal therapy. Gynecol Oncol 1990;39:364–367.
154. Schilder JM, Hurd WW, Roth LM, Sutton GP. Hormonal treatment of an endometrial stromal nodule followed by local excision. Obstet Gynecol 1999;93:805–807.
155. Nordal RR, Thoresen SO. Uterine sarcomas in Norway 1956–1992: incidence, survival and mortality. Eur J Cancer 1997;33:907–911.
156. Brooks SE, Zhan M, Cote T, Baquet CR. Surveillance, Epidemiology, and End Results analysis of 2677 cases of uterine sarcoma 1989–1999. Gynecol Oncol 2004;93:204–208.
157. Sutton G, Blessing JA, Park R, DiSaia PJ, Rosenshein N. Ifosfamide treatment of recurrent or metastatic endometrial stromal sarcomas previously unexposed to chemotherapy: a study of the Gynecologic Oncology Group. Obstet Gynecol 1996;87:747–750.
158. Berchuck A, Rubin SC, Hoskins WJ, Saigo PE, Pierce VK, Lewis JL Jr. Treatment of endometrial stromal tumors. Gynecol Oncol 1990;36:60–65.
159. Szlosarek PW, Lofts FJ, Pettengell R, Carter P, Young M, Harmer C. Effective treatment of a patient with a high-grade endometrial stromal sarcoma with an accelerated regimen of carboplatin and paclitaxel. Anticancer Drugs 2000;11:275–278.
160. Fung MF, Reid A, Faught W, et al. Prospective longitudinal study of ultrasound screening for endometrial abnormalities in women with breast cancer receiving tamoxifen. Gynecol Oncol 2003;91:154–159.
161. Gerber B, Krause A, Muller H, et al. Effects of adjuvant tamoxifen on the endometrium in postmenopausal women with breast cancer: a prospective long-term study using transvaginal ultrasound. J Clin Oncol 2000;18:3464–3470.
162. Vosse M, Renard F, Coibion M, Neven P, Nogaret JM, Hertens D. Endometrial disorders in 406 breast cancer patients on tamoxifen: the case for less intensive monitoring. Eur J Obstet Gynecol Reprod Biol 2002;101:58–63.
163. Fong K, Kung R, Lytwyn A, et al. Endometrial evaluation with transvaginal US and hysterosonography in asymptomatic postmenopausal women with breast cancer receiving tamoxifen. Radiology 2001;220:765–773.
164. Strauss HG, Wolters M, Methfessel G, Buchmann J, Koelbl H. Significance of endovaginal ultrasonography in assessing tamox-

ifen-associated changes of the endometrium. A prospective study. Acta Obstet Gynecol Scand 2000;79:697–701.

165. Barakat RR, Gilewski TA, Almadrones L, et al. Effect of adjuvant tamoxifen on the endometrium in women with breast cancer: a prospective study using office endometrial biopsy. J Clin Oncol 2000;18:3459–3463.
166. Seoud M, Shamseddine A, Khalil A, et al. Tamoxifen and endometrial pathologies: a prospective study. Gynecol Oncol 1999;75:15–19.
167. Love CD, Muir BB, Scrimgeour JB, Leonard RC, Dillon P, Dixon JM. Investigation of endometrial abnormalities in asymptomatic women treated with tamoxifen and an evaluation of the role of endometrial screening. J Clin Oncol 1999;17:2050–2054.
168. Timmerman D, Deprest J, Bourne T, Van den Berghe I, Collins WP, Vergote I. A randomized trial on the use of ultrasonography or office hysteroscopy for endometrial assessment in postmenopausal patients with breast cancer who were treated with tamoxifen. Am J Obstet Gynecol 1998;179:62–70.
169. Cecchini S, Ciatto S, Bonardi R, et al. Screening by ultrasonography for endometrial carcinoma in postmenopausal breast cancer patients under adjuvant tamoxifen. Gynecol Oncol 1996;60:409–411.
170. Boz G, De Paoli A, Innocente R, et al. Postoperative radiotherapy and surgery in stage I endometrial carcinoma: a 10-year experience. Tumori 1998;84:52–56.
171. Irwin C, Levin W, Fyles A, Pintilie M, Manchul L, Kirkbride P. The role of adjuvant radiotherapy in carcinoma of the endometrium-results in 550 patients with pathologic stage I disease. Gynecol Oncol 1998;70:247–254.
172. Calvin DP, Connell PP, Rotmensch J, Waggoner S, Mundt AJ. Surgery and postoperative radiation therapy in stage II endometrial carcinoma. Am J Clin Oncol 1999;22:338–343.
173. Weiss E, Hirnle P, Arnold-Bofinger H, Hess CF, Bamberg M. Therapeutic outcome and relation of acute and late side effects in the adjuvant radiotherapy of endometrial carcinoma stage I and II. Radiother Oncol 1999;53:37–44.
174. Alektiar KM, McKee A, Venkatraman E, et al. Intravaginal high-dose-rate brachytherapy for Stage IB (FIGO Grade 1, 2) endometrial cancer. Int J Radiat Oncol Biol Phys 2002;53:707–713.
175. Horowitz NS, Peters WA III, Smith MR, Drescher CW, Atwood M, Mate TP. Adjuvant high dose rate vaginal brachytherapy as treatment of stage I and II endometrial carcinoma. Obstet Gynecol 2002;99:235–240.
176. Ayoub J, Audet-Lapointe P, Methot Y, et al. Efficacy of sequential cyclical hormonal therapy in endometrial cancer and its correlation with steroid hormone receptor status. Gynecol Oncol 1988;31:327–337.
177. Aapro MS, van Wijk FH, Bolis G, et al. Doxorubicin versus doxorubicin and cisplatin in endometrial carcinoma: definitive results of a randomised study (55872) by the EORTC Gynaecological Cancer Group. Ann Oncol 2003;14:441–448.
178. Thigpen JT, Brady MF, Homesley HD, et al. Phase III trial of doxorubicin with or without cisplatin in advanced endometrial carcinoma: a gynecologic oncology group study. J Clin Oncol 2004;22:3902–3908.
179. Thigpen JT, Blessing JA, DiSaia PJ, Yordan E, Carson LF, Evers C. A randomized comparison of doxorubicin alone versus doxorubicin plus cyclophosphamide in the management of advanced or recurrent endometrial carcinoma: a Gynecologic Oncology Group study. J Clin Oncol 1994;12:1408–1414.
180. Gallion HH, Brunetto VL, Cibull M, et al. Randomized phase III trial of standard timed doxorubicin plus cisplatin versus circadian timed doxorubicin plus cisplatin in stage III and IV or recurrent endometrial carcinoma: a Gynecologic Oncology Group Study. J Clin Oncol 2003;21:3808–3813.
181. Fleming GF, Filiaci VL, Bentley RC, et al. Phase III randomized trial of doxorubicin + cisplatin versus doxorubicin + 24-h paclitaxel + filgrastim in endometrial carcinoma: a Gynecologic Oncology Group study. Ann Oncol 2004;15:1173–1178.
182. Sutton G, Brunetto VL, Kilgore L, et al. A phase III trial of ifosfamide with or without cisplatin in carcinosarcoma of the uterus: A Gynecologic Oncology Group Study. Gynecol Oncol 2000;79:147–153.
183. Muss HB, Bundy B, DiSaia PJ, et al. Treatment of recurrent or advanced uterine sarcoma. A randomized trial of doxorubicin versus doxorubicin and cyclophosphamide (a phase III trial of the Gynecologic Oncology Group). Cancer (Phila) 1985;55:1648–1653.
184. Omura GA, Major FJ, Blessing JA, et al. A randomized study of adriamycin with and without dimethyl triazenoimidazole carboxamide in advanced uterine sarcomas. Cancer (Phila) 1983; 52:626–632.

54

Evidence-Based Management of Breast Cancer

Lisa A. Newman and Daniel F. Hayes

The magnitude of the worldwide breast cancer burden is substantial and is increasing. Known to be a disease of greatest prevalence in heavily industrialized nations, its incidence and mortality rates are rising internationally as the populations of relatively less developed countries adopt the lifestyle and commercialism that characterize Western communities. Breast cancer has therefore been the subject of numerous clinical trials designed to improve our ability to screen for, to treat, and even to prevent the disease. This chapter reviews the highest levels of evidence that have been published for the major categories of interest in the contemporary management of breast cancer:

1. Screening/early detection
2. Primary surgery
3. Medical/systemic therapy
4. Radiation issues
5. Primary medical management (neoadjuvant chemotherapy)
6. Management of ductal carcinoma in situ (DCIS)
7. Risk reduction/prevention
8. Evaluation and treatment of metastatic disease

Breast Cancer Screening

The most commonly-accepted age-specific breast cancer screening recommendations regarding breast self-examination (BSE), clinical breast examination (CBE), and mammography are as follows:

20–40 years old: monthly BSE (optional); CBE every 1–3 years
40 years old and older: monthly BSE (optional); CBE annually; mammogram annually

BSE is generally perceived as a cost-efficient means of promoting breast health awareness, but data to document its efficacy in reducing breast cancer mortality are lacking.[1–3] Some clinicians have even criticized this approach because of concerns that it creates excessive cancerphobia in some women, and one meta-analysis revealed that it tended to result in an excess of unnecessary biopsies for benign fibrocystic changes.[2] On the other hand, it may represent the only viable alternative for women who do not meet screening eligibility requirements or for whom mammography services are simply unavailable.[4,5] Furthermore, Shen and Zelen[6] analyzed data from selected mammography screening trials and found the sensitivity of BSE (39%–59%) to be appreciable.

Utilization of annual mammographic screening in women beginning at age 40 is promoted by the majority of medical societies and advocacy organizations, such as the American Cancer Society, the American College of Surgeons, the American Society of Clinical Oncology, and the Susan G. Komen Breast Cancer Foundation. One issue that has generated substantial controversy involves the role of screening mammography in women 40 to 49 years old. In contrast to the annual mammography recommendation espoused by the majority of societies, the American Academy of Family Physicians and the American College of Preventive Medicine recommend that annual surveillance mammography should not begin until age 50. The U.S. Preventive Services Task Force[7] has compiled a comprehensive evidence-based analysis of published screening trials and concluded that mammographic surveillance (with or without clinical breast examination) is appropriate at 1- to 2-year intervals for women beginning at age 40, and they also reported that data are inadequate to fully assess the value of BSE.

The history of breast imaging dates back to the early 1900s, and it has evolved into the sophisticated technology of contemporary mammographic screening. Between 1963 and 1990, eight different prospective randomized studies were conducted worldwide in an attempt to define the optimal standards for breast cancer surveillance with screening mammography. Breast cancer mortality was the endpoint for all these studies, and participants were randomized to receive either periodic mammographic imaging or "routine" health care. The design of the various studies is shown in Table 54.1,[7–14] demonstrating notable differences between them regarding patient populations, screening intervals, and type of mammogram offered. Most of the studies were designed to be population based, and the women in the study arm were "invited" to undergo mammography, but the only trials with 100% uptake on initial screen were the two national programs coordinated in Canada. Uptake in the other six trials averaged approximately 80%. Furthermore, compliance with return for the second screen in the mammography arms ranged from only 54% to 90%, and many studies had significant contamination (13%–25%) of the control arms by patients who received mammography despite their random-

TABLE 54.1. Phase III studies of screening mammography.

		No. randomized			Mammography	
Trial	*Screening period*	*Mammography screening*	*No mammography*	*Age at accrual (years)*	*interval (months)*	*No. of views*
HIP[7,8]	1963–1969	30,239	30,256	40–64	12	2
Malmo[7,9]	1976–1990	21,088	21,195	45–70	18–24	1–2
Swedish Two-County[7,9–11]	1977–1985	77,080	55,985	40–74	24–33	1
Edinburgh[7,12]	1979–1988	28,628	26,015	45–64	24	1–2
CNBSS-1[7,13]	1980–1987	25,214	25,216	40–49	12	2
CNBSS-2[14]	1980–1987	19,711	19,694	50–59	12	2
Stockholm[7,9]	1981–1985	40,318	19,943	40–64	24–28	1
Gothenberg[7,9]	1982–1988	20,724	28,809	39–59	18	1–2

HIP, Health Insurance Plan of Greater New York; CNBSS, Canadian National Breast Screening Study.

ization assignment. The "intent-to-treat" statistical design of these studies mandated that all participants were analyzed according to their randomization assignment, regardless of whether the assignment was fulfilled. Nonetheless, a 21% to 26% lower breast cancer mortality rate was seen among the women randomized to receive screening mammography in these studies (Table 54.2). It is likely that the survival benefit associated with mammography is underestimated by these studies as a consequence of the suboptimal compliance and contamination issues.

Subset analysis based on age from these trials has revealed that most of the mammography-associated reduction in breast cancer mortality was seen among patients age 50 and older, where the magnitude of protection was 23%. To some extent this is an expected finding: breast cancer incidence is substantially lower for women aged 40 to 49 years, and the relatively greater breast density of younger women can complicate the interpretation of mammographic images. The Canadian National Breast Screening Study (CNBSS) represented an attempt to specifically address the question of mammography efficacy in younger women. In this study, 50,000 Canadian women aged 40 to 49 years were randomized to annual mammography versus routine health care and, with an average follow-up of 13 years, breast cancer mortality was unaffected by screening (rate ratio, 1.06; 95% confidence interval, 0.80–1.40).[13] A parallel study conducted in Canadian women aged 50 to 59 years yielded similar 13-year results (rate ratio, 1.02; 95% confidence interval, 0.78–1.33).[14] However, the validity of these results has been questioned because of criticisms regarding trial conduct. A fourfold excess of advanced disease was seen in the screened cohort, leading to allegations of bias in the CNBSS patient selection and randomization process.[15,16]

Additional screening-related controversy has been generated by investigators Gotzsche and Olsen, from the Cochrane Collaboration. Their interpretations that the methods

TABLE 54.2. Mammography screening trials: outcome and results.

	All participants			Participants <50 years old			Participants ≥50 years old		
Trial	*Median follow-up (months)*	*N*	*Mortality relative risk (95% CI)*	*N*	*Age range (years)*	*Mortality relative risk (95% CI)*	*N*	*Age range (years)*	*Mortality relative risk (95% CI)*
HIP[7,8]	18	60,490	0.77 (0.61–0.98)	27,480	40–49	0.78 (0.56–1.08)	33,010	50–64	0.79 (0.58–1.06)
Malmo[7,9]	17.1	42,283	0.82 (0.67–1.00)	8,054	45–49	0.73 (0.51–1.04)	16,873	55–64	0.80 (0.57–1.12)
Swedish Two-County[7,9–11]	17.3	133,065	0.68 (0.59–0.80)	35,448	40–49	0.87 (0.54–1.41)	40,290	50–59	0.66 (0.46–0.93)
Edinburgh[7,12]	13	54,643	0.79[a] (0.60–1.02)	22,746	45–49	0.75[a] (0.48–1.18)	21,746	50–54	0.99[a] (0.62–1.58)
								55–59	0.65[a] (0.43–0.99)
								60–64	0.80[a] (0.51–1.25)
CNBSS-1[7,13]	13	NA		50,430	40–49	0.97 (0.74–1.27)	NA		
CNBSS-2[14]	13	NA					39,405	50–59	1.02 (0.78–1.33)
Stockholm[7,9]	13.8	60,117	0.91 (0.65–1.27)	22,324	40–49	1.52 (0.80–2.88)	24,367	50–59	0.56 (0.32–0.97)
Gothenberg[7,9]	12.8	50,200	0.76 (0.56–1.04)	24,091	40–49	0.58 (0.35–0.96)	26,109	50–59	0.94 (0.62–1.43)

[a]Adjusted for socioeconomic factors.

employed in the various mammography trials were substantially flawed led them to conclude that mammographic surveillance yields no longevity benefit.[17,18] A counterargument, however, is that any retrospective critical review of the mammography trials is irrelevant to contemporary screening practices. Current mammography techniques and equipment are substantially more advanced in comparison to the methods of the screening trials. In fact, screening was not implemented on an annual basis in many of these trials, nor did it uniformly involve two-view imaging.

In the United States, the practices and performance of mammography centers are now regulated by the federally mandated Mammography Quality Standards Act, implemented in 1992 and reauthorized by Congress in 1998. This program has established benchmarks regarding the necessary equipment utilized in imaging centers as well as for minimum mammogram volume requirements for individual radiologists to maintain adequate expertise in evaluating these studies. Furthermore, in an era of chemoprevention availability, mammography represents the primary means of identifying high-risk women harboring lesions that contain atypical hyperplasia. Although it would likely be impossible to replicate a Phase 3 mammography screening trial today, it appears logical to assume that widespread mammographic surveillance over the past 10 to 20 years is largely responsible for the recent declines in breast cancer mortality that have been observed in the United States as well as abroad in the United Kingdom[19] and in Sweden.[20,21]

When an abnormal breast lesion is detected on routine, surveillance mammography, comprehensive imaging maneuvers should be promptly pursued, including comparisons with prior studies whenever possible. Diagnostic mammographic views (compression, magnification, etc.) should be obtained, and ultrasound imaging should be obtained for evaluation of densities as necessary. The abnormality should be characterized as per the American College of Radiology standardized Breast Imaging Reporting and Data Systems (BIRADS)[22]:

0: Additional imaging required.

1: Negative; no architectural disturbances identified.

2: Benign finding; negative mammogram, but some benign-appearing lesion identified.

3: Probably benign finding; short-interval follow-up suggested; some lesion identified that has a high probability of being benign, but establishing its stability is preferred.

4: Suspicious abnormality; biopsy should be considered; lesion detected that is not necessarily typical of cancer, but risk of malignancy is sufficiently high that a biopsy is warranted. The radiologist may comment specifically on the likelihood of cancer based on the type of lesion detected (calcifications, mass, etc).

5: Highly suggestive of malignancy; appropriate action should be taken; these lesions have a high probability of being cancer, and histopathologic confirmation should be sought accordingly.

The limitations of conventional screening mammography are well known. A subset of palpable breast tumors will be mammographically occult, and the overall false-negative rate of mammography averages 10% to 15%. Imaging of the dense breast can be particularly challenging, leading to difficulties in evaluating the fibrocystic changes seen in young women, and in women with a history of prolonged hormone replacement therapy. These issues may result in a patient "call-back" for additional diagnostic views to assess overlapping densities. This step in turn is the source of significant anxiety among patients, especially in those cases where a biopsy is ultimately necessary to definitively establish the benign versus malignant nature of a mammographically indeterminate lesion. Also, the burden of storing millions of screening mammograms has become an increasingly formidable task over time. The ability to compare a current mammogram with prior images is essential for optimal, accurate interpretations, but maintaining and archiving the growing volume of these studies is a difficult task.

In response to these acknowledged limitations, several alternative imaging modalities are being explored for their potential value in breast cancer screenings. Digital mammography is an advanced form of screening that offers electronic archiving of breast studies, with improved contrast resolution over a larger dynamic range. These advantages may obviate the need for many "call-backs" and eliminate the film storage problem. Furthermore, electronic studies can be transmitted to radiologists at any distance from the patient, thus facilitating second-opinion interpretations via telemammography, and they offer the potential value of computer-aided interpretations.

The major hindrances preventing widespread conversion to digital mammography programs include the considerable expenses of purchasing the advanced equipment and training staff in its use as well as maintenance. Another complexity is the difficulty inherent in comparing serial mammograms performed during the transition period and accurately distinguishing true interval changes from simple differences in tissue imaging related to technique. Prospective trials evaluating these two forms of mammography are currently under way.

Alternative methods for breast cancer screening, such as whole-breast ultrasound, magnetic resonance imaging (MRI), and positron emission tomography (PET) scanning, are also being actively investigated. Ultrasound evaluation of the breast was initially utilized to distinguish cystic versus solid lesions detected on either mammogram or physical examination. It has evolved into a highly specialized imaging modality that is useful in targeted breast studies to characterize the nature of solid mass lesions and frequently guides percutaneous needle biopsies (discussed further below). It is also possible that ultrasound may expand into the screening area. Unfortunately, whole-breast ultrasound is fairly labor intensive and is always operator dependent. Nonetheless, promising data have emerged indicating that screening with whole-breast ultrasound may be useful, particularly for women with mammographically dense tissue. Kolb et al.[23] reported a 97% sensitivity rate for the combination of whole-breast ultrasound and mammography in screening 4,897 BI-RADS category II–IV cases compared to 74% for the combination of mammography and physical examination. Kaplan et al.[24] reported a 0.3% cancer detection rate among women previously found to have a normal mammogram and clinical breast exam.

Breast imaging with magnetic resonance imaging (MRI) is of well-documented benefit in the evaluation of occult breast cancer in patients presenting with palpable axillary nodal metastases, where it reliably identifies those patients who may be safely treated with breast conservation (i.e., axillary surgery and breast irradiation).[25] It is also useful in detecting leakage from silicone implant rupture. In screening the otherwise normal and clinically negative breast of a normal-risk adult female, the indications for MRI are less clear. A recently completed prospective observational clinical trial conducted in women with hereditary susceptibility for breast cancer (as determined by either BRCA sequencing or Claus model calculations) demonstrated promising results regarding the efficacy of breast MRI in screening high-risk patients.[26] This study followed 1,909 high-risk women for a median of 2.9 years, with independently read annual mammography and breast MRI. Mammography was inferior to MRI in overall sensitivity (33% versus 80%), and MRI detected cancers at earlier stages, but mammography was slightly more specific (95% versus 90%). A total of 45 evaluable cancers were identified in this cohort; 32 were visible on MRI (including 22 that were mammographically occult) and 18 were visible on mammography (including 8 that were occult on MRI). One cancer was detected by clinical exam only, and four interval cancers developed. As noted by Liberman,[27] these results must be interpreted with caution, because the participating centers all had substantial expertise in MR imaging.

The potential advantages and limitations of breast MRI are summarized by Morris.[28] MRI can detect invasive breast cancer with a sensitivity rate approaching 100% and a negative study can therefore confidently clear the breast. Falsely negative MRIs can occur in the presence of ductal carcinoma in situ, and this modality may therefore be somewhat less reliable in evaluating microcalcifications. Invasive lobular cancer may also be missed, although MRI has been reported to be more sensitive in detecting this histopathology than other imaging modalities. Any hypervascular lesion may show enhancement on breast MRI, and even benign fibroadenomas may therefore occasionally result in a falsely positive study. These patterns contribute to the unreliable MRI specificities, ranging from 37% to 97%.[29] Nonetheless, these limitations may be acceptable in the effort to aggressively screen women at risk for the early-onset disease associated with mutations in the BRCA-1 and -2 breast cancer susceptibility genes.[26,30,31]

Use of breast MRI has also been suggested as a means of screening newly diagnosed breast cancer patients for the presence of multicentric disease, thereby refining the identification of candidates for breast-conserving therapy, especially in women with mammographically dense breasts[32,33] However, the sensitivity of breast MRI may actually be so high that occult foci of disease would be detected that might otherwise have been eradicated by breast radiotherapy. Whether a breast cancer diagnosis has been established or not, a final limitation of breast MRI is that few institutions have the capability to directly biopsy MRI-detected lesions.

Primary Surgical Management of Breast Cancer

Breast Conservation Therapy

The dawn of the 20th century marked a critical landmark in the management of breast cancer. Before this time the disease was widely considered untreatable and therefore universally fatal. It was not until Sir William Stuart Halsted popularized the radical mastectomy as surgical management for breast cancer that some degree of locoregional control of disease was achieved, and in a few cases long-term disease-free survival was observed. Early reports of this surgical approach appeared in the medical literature in the 1890s[34]; over the next three-quarters of a century, the radical mastectomy was established as the standard of care and sole treatment option for all stages of operable breast cancer.

In 1974, the National Surgical Adjuvant Breast Project (NSABP) published the initial outcome findings from their B-04 trial evaluating the safety of departing from the radical mastectomy as definitive treatment for breast cancer.[35] This study was designed to prove that variations in the locoregional management of breast cancer would not affect survival, thereby demonstrating that the major risk from this disease is related to the presence of micrometastases as opposed to whether the disease can be completely extirpated surgically. The B-04 study actually consisted of two clinical trials conducted in parallel. One trial involved randomization of 1,079 patients with clinically node-negative, operable breast cancer to one of three treatment arms: (i) radical mastectomy; (ii) total mastectomy followed by axillary nodal irradiation; and (iii) total mastectomy alone. The companion trial randomized 586 women with resectable, but clinically node-positive, disease to either radical mastectomy or total mastectomy and locoregional irradiation. Twenty-five-year follow-up from this study has recently been reported,[36] with survival equivalence continuing to be seen for the three arms of the clinically node-negative patients (25%, 19%, and 26%, respectively), and the two arms of the node-positive patients (14% for both arms).[36]

Once the concept was established that breast cancer outcome is primarily determined by early detection and the related risk of micrometastatic disease, it was a natural progression to explore treatment options involving breast preservation within the context of clinical trials. Six such studies (and one combined analysis of two trials) and one meta-analysis[37] have now reported long-term outcome revealing survival equivalence for stage-matched breast cancer patients randomized to mastectomy versus breast conservation (Table 54.3). The addition of breast irradiation to lumpectomy results in a statistically significant decrease in risk of local recurrence, as demonstrated by the NSABP B-06 trial,[38] where 1,851 stage I/II breast cancer patients were randomized to either radical mastectomy, lumpectomy and axillary lymph node dissection (ALND), or lumpectomy, ALND, and breast irradiation. Twenty-year follow-up confirms that mastectomy does not confer any survival advantage over breast preservation; however, breast irradiation lowers the risk of in-breast tumor recurrence from 39.2% to 14.3%.[38] As demonstrated by the Guy's Hospital experience, however, locoregional control should be optimized with delivery of appropriate radiotherapy doses. The potential contribution of locoregional irradiation to breast cancer outcome is discussed further next.

Management of the Axilla

The NSABP B-04 trials have also provided the basis for ongoing controversy regarding elective management of the axilla in newly diagnosed breast cancer patients. The B-04 trial that randomized patients with palpable, suspicious axillary disease to either radical mastectomy or total mastectomy

TABLE 54.3. Randomized trials comparing mastectomy and breast conservation therapy (BCT).

Trial	Accrual years	No. of patients	Maximum tumor size (cm)	Minimum lumpectomy margin	XRT (with BCT)	Median follow-up (years)	OS		LR/IBTR	
							Mastectomy	BCT	BCT	Mastectomy
NSABP B-06[38]	1976–84	1,851	4	Microscopically free at inked edge	50 Gy	20	47%	Lump only Lump + XRT 47%	39.2% 46% 14.3%	10.2%
Milan Cancer Institute[183]	1973–80	701	2		50 Gy + 10 Gy boost	20	58.8%	58.3%	8.8%	2.3%
NCI[184]	1979–87	237	5	Grossly negative	45–50.4 Gy + 15–20 Gy boost	18.4	58%	54%	22%[a]	0%[a]
EORTC[185,186]	1980–86	868	5	Grossly negative	50 Gy + 25 Gy boost	13.4	66%	65%	20%	12%
Institut Gustav Roussy[187]	1970–82	179	2	Grossly negative		10	79%	78%	4%	NR
DBCCG[188]	1983–89	905	5	Grossly negative	50 Gy + 10–25 Gy boost	6	82%	79%	NR	NR
EORTC and DBCCG (pooled results)[189]	1980–89	1,772	5	Grossly negative	50 bGy + 10–25 Gy boost	9.8	67%	67%	9%	10%
Guy's Hospital[67]	1961–71	374	5**	Grossly 3 cm	Regional nodes:[b] 25–27 Gy Breast: 35–38 Gy	10	N0: 80% N1: 60%	N0: 80% N1: 30%	N0: 0% N1: 2%	N0: 0% N1: 0%
	1971–75	255	5**	Grossly 3 cm	Regional nodes:[b] 25–27 Gy Breast: 35–38 Gy	9	82%	60%	30%	8%
	1961–75 (combined trial results)	629	5**	Grossly 3 cm	Regional nodes:[b] 25–27 Gy Breast: 35–38 Gy	24.7	56%[c]	43%[c]	50%	26%

OS, overall survival; BCT, breast conservation therapy; Lump, lumpectomy; XRT, irradiation; NSABP, National Surgical Adjuvant Breast Project; EORTC, European Organization for the Research and Treatment of Cancer; DBCCG, Danish Breast Cancer Cooperative Group; NCI, National Cancer Institute; LR, local recurrence; IBTR, in-breast tumor recurrence; Gy, gray.

[a] There were no isolated chest wall events/recurrences in the mastectomy arm, but 8 patients experienced a local failure with a regional and/or distant event; and 3 patients experienced a regional-only recurrence. In the BCT arm, 27 patients (22%) experienced an isolated local recurrence; there were 4 local with regional and/or distant failure; and there were no isolated regional recurrences.

[b] The initial Guy's Hospital trial randomized women with operable breast cancers and clinically node-negative as well as node-positive disease; patients randomized to lumpectomy arm had no surgical treatment to the axilla. After 1971 patients with clinically node-positive disease were excluded because of the high regional and distant failure rates. Regional XRT fields included supraclavicular, internal mammary, and axillary nodes; radical mastectomy arm also received 25–27 Gy regional XRT.

[c] Survival rates reported for the combined Guy's Hospital trial are 25-year rates of breast cancer-specific survival.

and locoregional breast irradiation (XRT) did demonstrate the superiority of surgery for durable control of bulky, symptomatic nodal disease. The regional failure rate of the patients randomized to radiation was 11%, compared to 8% for the patients randomized to ALND via the radical mastectomy procedure. The inaccuracy of clinical assessment for the axillary status was also apparent in this trial; of the nearly 300 patients whose axillae were assessed as being positive, 25% were found to be pathologically node negative by results of the radical mastectomy ALND.

On the other hand, numerous questions have arisen regarding management of the clinically axillary node-negative patients, and the long-term study results have been the subject of several different interpretations. It is assumed that nearly 40% of those in the two study arms randomized to nonsurgical management of the axilla (total mastectomy alone or total mastectomy plus axillary irradiation) had nonpalpable axillary metastases, because all three study arms were clinically matched and 39% of the radical mastectomy patients were found to be node positive. Nonetheless, clinically evident axillary relapse requiring delayed ALND developed in only 19% of the total mastectomy-only patients, suggesting that approximately half of untreated, occult axillary metastases will remain indolent. Only 4% of the total mastectomy plus axillary XRT arm required a delayed, therapeutic ALND (equivalent to the proportion of regional failures occurring in the radical mastectomy arm), and this finding suggests that axillary irradiation is an acceptable alternative for regional control of nonpalpable disease.

On critical reappraisal of the B-04 trial results, several concerns emerge. Pathology review of the mastectomy specimens revealed that nearly one-quarter of the total mastectomy cases actually included the incidental resection of some axillary lymph nodes, and the risk of axillary failure was inversely proportional to the number of lymph nodes retrieved. Also, this trial was not powered to address the outcome benefits of ALND, and because 22% of the long-term survivors from this study were patients found to be node positive based on pathology from the radical mastectomy procedure, the possibility of a survival contribution from the ALND cannot be definitively ruled out.

During the 1980s and 1990s, debate regarding a survival benefit from the ALND became irrelevant because of the identification of effective systemic therapy for breast cancer in the form of both endocrine and chemotherapeutic agents. Pathologic confirmation of the axillary nodal status then became a critical component of surgical breast cancer management as a means of determining which patients would be most likely to benefit from systemic treatment. Unfortunately, this is at the expense of committing breast cancer patients to the lifelong risk of lymphedema, reported to occur in 10% to 49% of ALND cases.[39–42] Features that increase the risk of lymphedema following ALND include obesity, regional irradiation, and a level III/apical axillary dissection.

Development of lymphatic mapping and the sentinel lymph node biopsy technology for breast cancer patients in the mid-1990s revolutionized the surgical care of breast cancer patients. This therapy, initially described by Krag et al. in 1993 with single-agent radioisotope and by Giuliano et al. in 1994 using single-agent blue dye, launched an era of minimally invasive surgery for the identification of node-negative patients who could be spared the morbidity of a standard level I/II ALND. The procedure involves injection of the mapping agent into the breast to replicate the pathway that cancer cells would traverse through the intramammary lymphatics en route to the primary nodal basin (which is the ipsilateral axilla for more than 90% of cases). The sentinel nodes represent the initial nodes likely to have been seeded by metastases, and they are distinguished by visual inspection to identify the blue-stained node(s), and/or detection of the radioactive nodes with an intraoperative gamma detector probe. Documentation of the accuracy of the sentinel lymph node biopsy was obtained by performing a concomitant level I/II ALND. This strategy permits calculation of the identification rate (number of cases where the sentinel node is found versus the number of cases where the procedure is attempted) and the false-negative rate (number of cases where the sentinel lymph node is negative but metastases are detected in nonsentinel nodes versus the total number of cases where any axillary metastases are detected).

Two meta-analyses have been conducted with reported pooled accuracy rates for the lymphatic mapping technology. General findings have included improved identification rates when dual- versus single-agent mapping is performed, and both the false negativity and identification rates are optimized when the learning curve has been passed. The 1999 meta-analysis[43] involved eleven studies involving 912 patients; the overall identification rate was 97% and the false negative rate was 5%. Another meta-analysis was presented at the 2002 American Society of Clinical Oncology meeting,[44] and this more recent study reported the pooled results of 69 published studies in the worldwide literature (37% from institutions within the United States), with data contributed by lymphatic mapping and completion ALND procedures performed on 10,454 breast cancer patients. The overall identification rate was 74%, but nearly half of the studies reported identification rates of 90% or greater. The pooled analysis revealed a false-negative rate of 8.4% (range, 0%–29%) but studies that performed more than 100 cases had a lower false-negative rate of 6.7%. An additional finding from the early studies of lymphatic mapping performed in conjunction with the ALND is that metastases will be limited to the sentinel node(s) in from one-third to two-thirds of cases, and this supports the biologic validity of the mapping concept.

The future results from two multicenter, prospective clinical trials coordinated by the NSABP and the American College of Surgeons Oncology Group (ACOSOG) will provide the most definitive long-term data on locoregional control of disease achieved after a sentinel lymph node biopsy performed for early-stage breast cancer.[45] The NSABP trial randomized clinically node-negative patients to undergo sentinel lymph node biopsy with completion ALND versus sentinel lymph node biopsy with ALND only if the sentinel node was positive for metastasis. The ACOSOG trial is prospectively following more than 5,000 breast cancer patients after sentinel node biopsy for breast cancer, and patients with a positive sentinel node are eligible for the companion trial that randomizes these node-positive cases to either completion ALND or axillary observation. The primary aim of the NSABP trial is therefore to compare the impact of sentinel node biopsy alone versus ALND on recurrence-free survival in women who are node negative. The primary aim of the ACOSOG randomized trial is to determine the impact of a standard ALND on survival in patients with node-positive breast cancer. Both cooperative groups will be evaluating the prognostic value of micrometastases identified in sentinel nodes via immunohistochemical staining for cytokeratin. There is extensive variability in the techniques utilized to perform the lymphatic mapping[46] in terms of injection site for the labeling agent (peritumoral versus overlying skin versus subareolar) and timing of the radioisotope label (same-day versus 1 day preoperatively). Thus far, excellent results have been observed with all the various strategies, and the randomized trials will include outcome data on the complete spectrum of mapping techniques.

Adjuvant Systemic Therapy for Breast Cancer

The benefits of adjuvant systemic therapy for breast cancer in eliminating micrometastases and thereby reducing risk of distant relapse have been recognized for several decades. Although breast cancer staging based on tumor size and nodal status carries strong prognostic value, 15% to 20% of patients diagnosed with stage I disease ultimately experience treatment failure, despite having been diagnosed with small, node-negative lesions. The necessity to address systemic manifestations of breast cancer before they are clinically apparent therefore became quite clear to the oncology community during the latter half of the 20th century. Success in achieving this goal, however, was dependent on identifying medical therapies that were cytotoxic and/or cytostatic against occult breast cancer metastases in distant organs.

The hormonally active, nonsteroidal estrogen receptor modulator tamoxifen became recognized as a valuable strategy in the endocrine regulation of this hormonally driven disease during the 1970s.[47] The ability to reliably assess for the presence of estrogen and progesterone receptors via widely reproducible immunohistochemical assays confirmed the validity of this approach, particularly for tumors selected on the basis of hormone receptor expression. Investigations of chemotherapeutic agents with activity against breast tumor biology strengthened these adjuvant therapy efforts and offered promise to women with hormone receptor-negative disease. In an effort to add clarity and balance to the discussion of benefit conferred by hormonal therapy and/or chemotherapy to breast cancer outcome, the Early Breast Cancer Trialists Collaborative Group (EBCTCG) was established. These distinguished international experts have convened periodically to review and statistically analyze the pooled results of various approaches for the adjuvant systemic therapy of breast cancer. Findings from these meta-analyses (commonly called the Overview Analyses), involving phase III trials of tamoxifen, chemotherapy, ovarian ablation, and radiation as adjuvant therapy, are summarized in Table 54.4.

The Overview Analyses have essentially documented a proportional odds reduction in the risk of breast cancer relapse in conjunction with the delivery of adjuvant systemic therapy. The magnitude of absolute benefit is therefore dependent on the baseline risk of relapse, defined by the stage of disease at diagnosis. Although the heterogeneity of individual breast tumor biology allows for the potential existence of life-threatening distant micrometastases associated with even the earliest stage lesions, the potential life-threatening adverse events associated with any adjuvant systemic therapy mandates that patients cautiously appraise the risks and benefits of these treatments. Guidelines promoted by the National Cancer Institute[48,49] include recommendations that

TABLE 54.4. Summary of worldwide overview analyses.

Treatment analyzed	*No. of trials analyzed*	*No. of women analyzed*	*Proportional reduction*			*Comments*
			Relapse	*Mortality*	*Contralateral breast cancer*	
Tamoxifen for early-stage breast cancer[190,191]	55	37,000	1 year: 21% 2 years: 29% 5 years: 47%	1 year: 12% 2 years: 17% 5 years: 26%	1 year: 13% 2 years: 26% 5 years: 47%	Risk of endometrial cancer doubled in trials of 1 or 2 years and quadrupled in trials of 5 years. Approximately 8,000 women had tumors with low/zero ER content; these patients had negligible benefit from tamoxifen for relapse and mortality. They are excluded from relapse and mortality data, but are included in contralateral risk data.
Multi-agent CTX for early breast cancer[192,193]	47	18,000[a]	<50 years old: 35% 50–69 years old: 20%	<50 years old: 27% 50–69 years old: 11%	NR NR	No significant survival advantage for more than approximately 3 months of polychemotherapy. Anthracycline-containing regimens better than CMF alone.
Ovarian ablation for early breast cancer[59,60]	12	2,102	18.5%	6.3%	NS	Benefit of ovarian ablation strongest in women not receiving CTX.
Radiotherapy for early breast cancer[69,94]	40	20,000	32.4%[b]	NS	NS	XRT reduced the annual breast cancer mortality rates by 13.2%, but increased the annual mortality rates from other causes (primarily vascular) by 21.2%. XRT reduced the annual breast cancer

CTX, chemotherapy; NR, not reported; NS, not significantly different.

[a] Including 6,000 women in 11 trials of longer versus shorter CTX, and 6,000 women in 11 trials of doxorubicin-containing CTX versus CMF (cyclophosphamide/methotrexate/fluorouracil).

[b] Local recurrence.

adjuvant systemic therapy be considered for all invasive breast cancers measuring at least 1 cm in size, and/or tumors of any size when associated with nodal metastases. In practice, endocrine therapy with tamoxifen tends to be the first-line approach for hormone receptor-positive disease, and polychemotherapy is delivered for hormone receptor-negative disease and/or patients with node-positive breast cancer.

Endocrine Therapy for Breast Cancer

Tamoxifen was originally developed as an antifertility medication, and alternative uses in the oncology field were sought because of its dismal failure in this area because of tamoxifen's ovulatory effects. As a very effective antagonist of estrogen receptors on mammary tissue, however, it has remained extremely powerful as first-line adjuvant systemic therapy in breast cancer management. Tamoxifen's selective estrogen receptor activity also yields estrogen agonist activity on the uterus, cardiovascular, cerebrovascular, and osseous tissues; this results in the mixed benefits and risks of uterine cancer, lowered cholesterol levels, vasomotor symptoms, and protection against osteoporosis. Tamoxifen was also found to decrease the incidence of contralateral new primary tumors, motivating extension of its applications to the chemoprevention arena.

Several other endocrine therapies have been studied recently as alternatives to tamoxifen (Table 54.5), with the hope that side effects can be minimized and protection from relapse prolonged.[50] All have proven efficacy in the setting of metastatic disease and are now used in the adjuvant setting as well. One category of endocrine agents includes other selective estrogen receptor modulators and another category includes the aromatase inhibitors (AIs). The AIs exert anticancer activity via inhibition of the nonovarian hormone production that occurs in postmenopausal women and is mediated through peripheral conversion of adrenal substances.

The ATAC Trial[51] was an international study that randomized 9,366 postmenopausal women to receive 5 years of the AI anastrozole, versus tamoxifen, versus a combination of these two therapies. At 33 months follow-up, the anastrozole-alone arm fared significantly better with regard to risk of relapse and new breast events; unfortunately, this improved outcome came at the expense of higher rates of osteoporotic complications.

The NSABP B-14 trial[52] randomized early-stage breast cancer patients to receive 5 versus 10 years of tamoxifen postoperatively, and found that extended therapy resulted in higher rates of adverse events that were not outweighed by added protection. Unfortunately, substantial numbers of estrogen receptor-positive breast cancer patients continue to relapse after 5 years of tamoxifen, and this pattern motivated implementation of the MA-17 trial,[53,54] where 5,187 postmenopausal breast cancer patients who had already completed 5 years of adjuvant tamoxifen therapy were randomized to receive 5 years of the AI letrozole versus placebo. This trial has revealed improved disease-free outcome in favor of prolonged endocrine therapy with letrozole.

Another recent trial, the Intergroup Exemestane Study,[55] randomized nearly 5,000 postmenopausal breast cancer patients to receive the AI exemestane for 2 to 3 years following tamoxifen, to a total adjuvant therapy course of 5 years, versus receiving tamoxifen for the entire 5-year course. At 31 months follow-up, the patients receiving exemestane had fewer relapses, suggesting superiority of AI therapy.

The selective estrogen receptor modulator (SERM) fulvestrant is a tamoxifen alternative that has no estrogen receptor agonist effects. Preliminary studies of application after tamoxifen failure in the setting of metastatic disease have been promising because fulvestrant does not appear to be cross-resistant with tamoxifen.[56] Evaluations of this therapy in the adjuvant setting are therefore likely to be forthcoming.

Removal or suppression of functional, estrogen-producing ovaries to control the progression of hormonally responsive

TABLE 54.5. Table of selected Phase III trials evaluating adjuvant endocrine therapy.

Trial	Accrual years	Median follow-up (months)	No. of patients	Randomization arms	Outcome: DFS	Outcome: OS	Outcome: Contralateral cancer
NSABP B-14[52a]	1982–1988	81	1,172	Adjuvant tamoxifen 5 years	82%	94%	2.9%
				Adjuvant tamoxifen 10 years	78%	91%	3.5%
ATAC[51,195b]	1996–1000	33	9,366	Anastrozole	89%	NR	0.4%
				Tamoxifen	87%	NR	1.1%
				Anastrozole + tamoxifen	87%	NR	0.9%
NCIC MA17[53,54c]	1998–2002	30	5,187	Tamoxifen × 5 years alone	90%	NR	1%
				Tamoxifen × 5 years followed by letrozole × 5 years	95%	NR	0.5%
Intergroup Exemestane Study[55d]	1998–2003	31	4,742	Tamoxifen × 5 years alone	87%	NR	0.8%
				Tamoxifen × 2–3 years followed by exemestane to the completion of 5 years adjuvant therapy	92%	NR	0.4%

[a] Improved survival in tamoxifen 5 years arm was statistically significant; difference in rate of contralateral cancer was not significant; there were more endometrial cancers in the tamoxifen 10 years arm (12, 2.1% versus 6, 1.1%; RR 2, 95% CI 0.7–6.6).

[b] Significantly fewer endometrial cancers, cardiovascular events, and thromboembolic complications in anastrazole arm; fewer osteoporotic complications in tamoxifen arm; 47-month median follow-up report demonstrated a statistically-significant 18% reduction in risk of relapse for estrogen receptor-positive patients receiving anastrozole, and a 44% reduction in risk of contralateral new cancers.

[c] Difference in disease-free outcome statistically significant in favor of letrozole following tamoxifen arm.

[d] Differences in disease-free outcome and contralateral new primary cancers statistically significant in favor of exemestane arm; Kaplan–Meier estimates for overall survival not reported, but the 93 all-cause deaths in the exemestane group was not statistically different from the 106 all-cause deaths in the tamoxifen-only arm.

breast cancer has a long history associated with several lines of evidence suggesting that this should be a successful therapeutic strategy. Unfortunately, the Phase III studies addressing this issue have usually been flawed by limited data on the estrogen expression levels of the participating patients, or by the fact that they were actually designed to answer a different question and have been interpreted retrospectively to evaluate the role of ovarian ablation and/or ovarian suppression. The benefits of this strategy must be balanced against the morbid osteoporotic and cardiovascular artherosclerotic sequelae of premature menopause.

Bilateral oophorectomy represents one of the oldest forms of systemic therapy for breast cancer, dating back to reports by Beatson[57] and Lett[58] from approximately 100 years ago. Although surgical removal of the ovaries remains a viable and certainly effective means of eliminating ovarian estrogen, the past several decades have seen the implementation of pelvic irradiation to obliterate the ovaries, as well as the development of medical therapy to suppress function. The overview analysis[59,60] reported an 18.5% reduction in the odds of disease relapse and a 6.3% reduction in the odds of death associated with either surgical or radiotherapeutic ablation of the ovaries. These benefits are comparable in magnitude to those achieved with adjuvant chemotherapy.

Surgical oophorectomy can be performed with relatively low morbidity as a laparoscopic procedure, although it requires general anesthesia. It also provides immediate, complete, and irreversible elimination of ovarian function. Another advantage of oophorectomy is that it can be offered in medically underserved parts of the world as straightforward and fairly cost-efficient endocrine management of breast cancer.

Pelvic irradiation also results in an irreversible blockade of ovarian function, but the extent of gonadal tissue effected and the interval to achieve this ablation can be variable. Furthermore, long-term effects on the pelvic contents may include adhesions, radiation enteritis, and/or colorectal stricture.

Medical therapies for ovarian suppression include chemotherapy-induced amenorrhea and luteinizing hormone-releasing hormone (LHRH) agonists. Chemotherapy will cause ovarian failure in 30% to 80% of cases,[61,62] with likelihood and duration of amenorrhea varying by age of patient (older premenopausal patients at increased risk compared to younger patients), type of chemotherapy [cyclophosphamide, methotrexate, and 5-fluorouracil (CMF) causing more amenorrhea than adjuvant chemotherapy (AC), and the addition of a taxane further increasing rates], and number of chemotherapy cycles. Some studies have reported that patients experiencing amenorrhea from chemotherapy have an improved outcome related to this diminished circulating estrogen.[63–65] Although these effects are provocative in supporting a role for ovarian suppression to manage premenopausal breast cancer, chemotherapy-induced amenorrhea is an unreliable strategy because of its unpredictability and uncertain duration.

Use of LHRH agonists to disrupt the physiologic hypothalamic–pituitary–gonadal axis is becoming increasingly accepted as a reasonable alternative for achieving ovarian suppression. Normal estrogen production by the ovaries is regulated by the pulsatile production of LHRH by the hypothalamus. LHRH stimulates gonadotropin-releasing hormone (GnRH) production by the pituitary, and this induces estrogen production from the ovaries of a premenopausal woman. LHRH agonists such as goserelin bind to the GnRH receptors with strong affinity, causing an initial surge in estrogen production (which can cause the so-called tumor flare that may occur clinically), followed by a blockade of the physiologic pulsatile and ongoing effects of natural LHRH. The patient is therefore rendered medically menopausal, but the suppressed ovarian function is reversible. This potential for restoring fertility is attractive, but the impact on cancer control is uncertain. The evidence from several prospective randomized trials evaluating ovarian ablation/ovarian suppression is summarized in Table 54.6.

Chemotherapy for Breast Cancer

The earliest studies of chemotherapy for breast cancer involved perioperative administration of medications that are considered inferior to the effective agents currently available, and the goal of these early investigations was to eliminate dissemination of cancer cells that might have occurred in conjunction with surgical manipulation of tumors. The NSABP B-01[66] trial (conducted nearly 40 years ago) therefore involved intravenous thiotepa versus placebo administered at the time of radical mastectomy and over the first 2 days postoperatively. Not surprisingly, this regimen failed to produce any improvements in outcome for the entire group of treated patients, but the subset of highest risk women (those with four or more metastatic nodes) did experience some overall survival advantages. Subsequent trials conducted during the 1970s and 1980s revealed the power of cyclophosphamide and combination chemotherapy (CTX) regimens in reducing breast cancer relapse rates as well as mortality risks.

Until fairly recently, the two regimens of cyclophosphamide/methotrexate/fluorouracil and cyclophosphamide/doxorubicin/fluorouracil, delivered in every-3-week cycles, have been the most commonly employed regimens for adjuvant therapy of breast cancer. During the late 1990s, the taxanes emerged as an alternative and highly effective agent against breast cancer. Furthermore, the development of active and tolerable bone marrow supportive therapy in the form of granulocyte colony-stimulating factors has opened the door to dose-dense regimens allowing safe delivery of higher cumulative CTX doses within shorter time frames. Selecting the appropriate cases for the various regimens has been challenging, but as shown in Table 54.7, several Phase III studies have successfully addressed many of the pertinent issues.

Collectively, these studies suggest that adjuvant CTX regimens that include a taxane as well as doxorubicin appear to be most reasonable for node-positive breast cancer patients. This conclusion is supported by findings from the CALGB 9344, NSABP B-28, and BCIRG 001 Phase III studies. These three trials all randomized node-positive patients to receive doxorubicin-based combinations versus doxorubicin CTX plus a taxane, and all three demonstrated an outcome advantage for the taxane arms. The CALGB 9741 and 9344 trials also revealed superiority of dose-dense therapy (9741), but no outcome advantage for increased doses of doxorubicin (9344). Questions regarding superiority of one taxane versus the other (paclitaxel versus docetaxol) remain unanswered.

TABLE 54.6. Prospective randomized trials of ovarian ablation/ovarian suppression.

Study	*N*	*Eligibility profile*	*Median follow-up (years)*	*Treatment arms*	*Outcome*
Scottish Trial 1993[196]	332	Premenopausal Node-positive Any ER status	Maximum 12	CMF OA	No significant difference in 8-year OS (hazard ratio 1.12; 95% CI 0.76–1.63) but ovarian ablation better in cases with ER >20 fmol/mg
Roche 1996[197a]	162	Premenopausal Node-positive ER and PR-positive	7	Surgical or radiotherapeutic OA FAC × 6	7-year DFS 83% for OA vs. 55% for FAC (significant on univariate,but not multivariate analysis after accounting for number of metastatic nodes) 7-year OS 84% for OA vs. 74% for FAC (not significant)
Ejlertsen 1999[198]	732	Premenopausal ER-positive Node-positive and/or tumor >5 cm	5.7	OA CMF × 9	5-year DFS 67%; OS 78% 5-year DFS 66%; OS 82% (no significant difference in DFS or OS)
Rutqvist 1999[199b]	2,631	Premenopausal	4.3	Goserelin × 2 years alone Tamoxifen × 2 years alone Goserelin and tamoxifen × 2 years No adjuvant endocrine therapy	Event-free hazard benefit in favor of goserelin use (relative risk, 0.77; 95% CI, 0.66–0.90)
Boccardo 2000[200]	244	Premenopausal ER-positive	6.3	CMF OA/OS[c] + tamoxifen	No significant difference in DFS or OS
Schmid 2002[201]	589[d]	Premenopausal Node-positive ER-positive		CMF Leuprolin	No significant difference in DFS or OS
IBCSG 2001[202]	174	Premenopausal Node-positive ER-positive s/p therapeutic ovarian ablation	4.1	Tamoxifen × 5 years AC × 4, then tamoxifen × 5 years	No significant difference in DFS or OS
Jonat 2002[203] and Kauffmann 2003[204] (ZEBRA Study)	1,614	Premenopausal Node-positive (any ER status[e])	7.3	CMF × 6 Goserelin × 2 years	No significant difference in DFS or OS for ER-positive disease; CMF better for ER-negative disease

Jakesz 2002[205]	1,034	Premenopausal ER-positive	5	CMF × 6 Goserelin × 3 years + tamoxifen × 5 years	5-year DFS 76% 5-year DFS 81% ($P = 0.37$; significant in favor of endocrine therapy)
Love 2002[206]	709	Premenopausal Operable breast cancer (node positive or tumor >2 cm size)	3.6	Oophorectomy + tamoxifen × 5 years Observation	5-year DFS 75%; 5-year OS 78% 5-year DFS 58%; 5-year OS 70% ($P < 0.05$; significant for DFS and OS in favor of adjuvant therapy)
Castiglione-Gertsch 2003[207]	1,063	Premenopausal Node-negative (any ER status[f])	7	Goserelin × 2 years CMF × 6 CMF × 6 + goserelin × 1.5 years	DFS significantly superior in favor of CMF for ER-negative tumors (5-year DFS 84% for CMF alone and 88% for CMF + goserelin vs. 73% for goserelin alone) DFS similar for all three arms in ER-positive tumors (5-year DFS 81% for either goserelin or CMF alone; and 86% for CMF + goserelin)
Arriagada 2003[208]	926	Premenopausal Operable breast cancer (Any ER status[g])	9.5	OA/OS + CTX[g] CTX[g]	10-year DFS 48%; 10-year OS 65% 10-year DFS 49%; 10-year OS 68% (no significant differences in DFS or OS)
Davidson 2003[209]	1,504	Premenopausal Node-positive ER-positive	9.6	FAC × 6 FAC × 6 + goserelin × 5 years FAC × 6 + goserelin + tamoxifen × 5 years	9-year DFS 57%; 9-year OS 70% 9-year DFS 60%; 9-year OS 73% 9-year DFS 68%; 9-year OS 76%[h]

OA, ovarian ablation; CMF, cyclophosphamide, methotrexate, 5-fluorouracil; ER, estrogen receptor; PR, progesterone receptor; FAC, 5-fluorouracil, doxorubicin, cyclophosphamide; CTX, chemotherapy; DFS, disease-free survival; OS, overall survival; CI, confidence interval.

[a] Trial closed in 1989 because of poor accrual, with 153 evaluable patients.

[b] Pooled results from similar trials conducted by the Cancer Research Campaign; the Breast Cancer Trials Group; the Stockholm Breast Cancer Study Group; the South-East Sweden Breast Cancer Group; and the Gruppo Interdisciplinare Valutazione Interventi in Oncologia (GIVIO); adjuvant chemotherapy use varied by individual protocols and participating centers.

[c] Surgical oophorectomy, 6 patients; radiotherapeutic oophorectomy, 31 patients; goserelin, 87 patients.

[d] Reported data on 227 evaluable patients from interim analysis.

[e] Approximately 20% of participants were ER negative; these were evenly distributed between the two trial arms.

[f] Approximately 30% of participants were ER negative; these were evenly distributed between the two trial arms.

[g] Approximately 24% of participants were ER negative; these were evenly distributed between the two trial arms; the adjuvant CTX delivered included an anthracycline in 77%; OA/OS was via irradiation or LHRH agonists.

[h] Outcome differences not significantly different, but trends favoring OS in women who did not become amenorrheic with CTX, and favoring tamoxifen in women who did become amenorrheic.

TABLE 54.7. Table of selected Phase III trials evaluating adjuvant chemotherapy.

Study	*Eligibility*	*N*	*Median follow-up*	*Randomization*	*DFS*	*OS*
CALGB 9344[210]	Node-positive	3,121	69 months	AC	65%	77%
				AC + paclitaxel	70%	80%
				Significance	*P* = 0.0023	*P* = 0.0064
NSABP B-28[211]	Node-positive	3,060	64 months	AC	72%	85%
				AC + paclitaxel	76%	85%
				Significance	*P* = 0.008	*P* = 0.46
BCIRG 001[212]	Node-positive	1,491	55 months	TAC	75%	87%
				FAC	68%	81%
				Significance	*P* = 0.001	*P* = 0.008
CALGB[a] 9741[213]	Node-positive	2,005	36 months	Conventional (q 3 weeks) ACP	75%	90%
				Dose-dense (q 2 weeks) ACP + G-CSF	82%	92%
				Significance	*P* = 0.010	*P* = 0.013

CALGB, Cancer and Leukemia Group B; NSABP, National Surgical Adjuvant Breast Project; BCIRG, Breast Cancer International Research Group; TAC, taxol (paclitaxel), adriamycin (doxorubicin), cytoxin (cyclophosphamide); AC, adriamycin (doxorubicin), cytoxin (cyclophosphamide); FAC, fluorouracil, adriamycin (doxorubicin), cytoxin (cyclophosphamide); ACP, adriamycin (doxorubicin), cytoxin (cyclophosphamide), paclitaxel (taxol).

[a] The CALGB Trial 9741 also evaluated sequential adriamycin × 4 followed by paclitaxel × 4 followed by cytoxin × 4 versus concurrent adriamycin and cytoxin × 4 followed by paclitaxel × 4 and found no significant effect on outcome based on these schedule variations.

Radiation Therapy for Breast Cancer

Radiation therapy and surgery are the primary modalities for treatment of locoregional manifestations of breast cancer. Radiation therapy alone can sterilize some breast tumors, but at the expense of excessively toxic doses. The standard rationale is therefore to rely on surgery to control grossly apparent breast lesions and to utilize irradiation to eliminate residual microscopic disease. Results from the Phase III studies of BCT summarized in Table 54.3 demonstrate the success of this approach. Adjuvant breast radiation delivered after surgical lumpectomy will effectively decrease the incidence of in-breast tumor recurrences. Most trials, however, have demonstrated equivalent overall survival rates following lumpectomy regardless of whether radiation was delivered. This finding suggested that breast cancer outcome was largely determined by ability to control progression of micrometastases and that irradiation would make a marginal or negligible contribution to survival. In contrast, the Guy's Hospital BCT Trials[67] used a breast XRT regimen that would be considered inferior to contemporary radiation schedules, and this resulted in significantly inferior survival rates. Level I evidence therefore supports the inclusion of appropriate radiation therapy (5,000–6,000 rads) into the management of conservatively treated breast cancer patients.

A recent meta-analysis[68] of Phase III clinical trials involving breast irradiation has motivated additional consideration of the survival benefits associated with radiation therapy in BCT patients. Vinh-Hung and Verschraegen pooled the outcomes of 13 trials involving more than 8,000 patients. The mortality hazard for patients treated by lumpectomy without radiation therapy was 1.086 (95% confidence interval, 1.003–1.175). This corresponds to a possible 8% survival benefit conferred by radiation.

The issue of postmastectomy chest wall irradiation (PMRT) has generated extensive controversy over the past few decades. Clinical trials conducted thus far have failed to render a consistent answer to the question of whether sterilization of microscopic disease on the chest wall of a mastectomized patient yields a worthwhile outcome advantage to all breast cancer patients. The EBCTCG studied this question indirectly in their meta-analysis of radiation for early-stage breast cancer patients.[69,70] Although this study revealed a reduced breast cancer mortality risk associated with adjuvant XRT (by 13%), it was at the expense of a 21% increase in nonbreast cancer-related mortality. This pooled analysis, however, involved studies whose primary design involved mastectomy versus BCT, systemic therapy versus no systemic therapy, and variable axillary management strategies. This heterogeneity precludes the ability to draw well-defined conclusions.

Table 54.8 summarizes the results from Phase III prospective randomized trials conducted internationally that have contributed data regarding PMRT in women whose management has also included ALND as well as adjuvant systemic therapy. The results of these trials suggest that patients with four or more metastatic axillary lymph nodes represent the subset most likely to derive a benefit from PMRT, primarily because of their inherently increased risk for chest wall recurrence (range, 20%–40%). The ability to reduce locoregional relapses (to rates of 6%–14%) in these patients with the delivery of PMRT appears to improve the overall survival as well. The National Cancer Institute, the American Society of Clinical Oncology, and the American Society of Therapeutic Radiation Oncology have all issued position statements recommending PMRT for breast cancer patients with four or more metastatic nodes.

The Danish Breast Cancer Group[71,72] reported survival benefits from PMRT in women with one to three metastatic axillary nodes as well; however, this trial has been criticized because of the surgical treatment rendered. The average number of nodes retrieved from the ALND specimens (six) was somewhat lower than would be expected in a standard level I and II dissection. This finding prompts the concern that inadequate regional surgery may have contributed to the increased incidence of locoregional failures. Unfortunately, a clinical trial designed by the Radiation Therapy Oncology Group designed to address the question of PMRT in patients with one to three metastatic axillary lymph nodes was recently closed because of poor accrual, and this question therefore remains unanswered.

TABLE 54.8. Randomized trials of postmastectomy irradiation in patients treated with axillary lymph node dissection and adjuvant systemic therapy, including subset analyses based on extent of nodal metastases (where available) and randomized trials of postmastectomy irradiation in patients treated with axillary lymph node dissection and adjuvant systemic therapy, including subset analyses based on extent of nodal metastases (where available).

Study		Year	No. of patients	Median follow-up (months)	LRF		OS (%)	
					No PMRT	PMRT	No PMRT	PMRT
DBCG 82b[71]	All	1997	1,708	114	32%	9%	45%	54%
	1–3 Nodes Positive		1,061	114	30%	7*	54%	62%
	≥4 Nodes Positive		510	114	42%	14%	20%	32%
DBCG 82c[72]	All	1999	1,375	123	35%	8%	36%	45%
	1–3 Nodes Positive		794	123	31%	6%	44%	55%
	≥4 Nodes Positive		448	123	46%	11%	17%	24%
Glasgow[214]	All	1986	219	63	25%	11%	57%	61%
	1–3 Nodes Positive		141	63	NR	NR	68%	76%
	≥4 Nodes Positive		72	63	NR	NR	46%	54%
BC[215]	All	1997	318	150	33%	13%	46%	54%
	1–3 Nodes Positive		183	150	33%	13%	NR	NR
	≥4 Nodes Positive		112	150	46%	21%	NR	NR
DFCI[216a]	1–3 Nodes Positive	1987	83	53	5%	2%	85%	77%
	≥4 Nodes Positive		123	45	20%	6%	63%	59%
SECSG[217b]	≥4 Nodes Positive	1992	295	120	23%	13%	44%	55%
South Sweden (Tamoxifen)[218]		1993	483	96	18%	6%	NR	NR
South Sweden (Cyclophosphamide)[218]		1993	287	96	17%	6%	NR	NR
ECOG[219]		1997	312	109	24%	15%	47%	46%
Mayo[220–223]		1984	217	48 (min)	30%	10%	66%	68%
German BCG[224]		2000	71	36 (mean)	NR	NR	84%	96%
Israel[222,223,225]		2000	112	NR	24%	4%	71%	61%
Portugal[223,226]		1998	112	NR	NR	NR	35%	33%
M.D. Anderson[222,223]		2001	97	NR	NR	NR	56%	35%
Helsinki[227]		1987	79	NR	60%	13%	69%	94%
Piedmont[228]		1991	76	132 (min)	35%	18%	48%	61%
Köln (Germany)[223,229]		1982	71	36 (mean)	NR	NR	84%	96%

DFCI, Dana Farber Cancer Institute; DBCG, Danish Breast Cancer Group; BC, British Columbia; SECSG, Southeast Cancer Study Group; NR, not reported; ECOG, Eastern Cooperative Oncology Group; German BCG, German Breast Cancer Group.

[a] DFCI Trial patients with 1–3 nodes positive received CMF adjuvant chemotherapy; patients with four or more positive nodes received AC adjuvant chemotherapy.

[b] All SECSG Trial patients had at least 4 positive nodes.

Primary Chemotherapy for Breast Cancer

Implementation of preoperative chemotherapy protocols (also commonly referred to as neoadjuvant or induction chemotherapy) revolutionized the management of locally advanced breast cancer (LABC) cases, and this approach is now considered the standard of care for patients with bulky breast and/or axillary disease. Early skepticism regarding this treatment sequence was based on concerns that preoperative chemotherapy would exert an adverse effect on (i) surgical complication rates, (ii) the prognostic value of the axillary nodal status, and (iii) overall survival as a consequence of delayed surgery. Nonetheless, the generally dismal results of treating LABC with primary surgery, radiation alone, or chemotherapy alone motivated investigations of multimodality therapy, and the benefits as well as the safety of preoperative downstaging of disease to improve respectability became apparent.

Broadwater et al.[73] demonstrated comparable operative morbidity among nearly 200 LABC patients treated with mastectomy, approximately half of whom received preoperative doxorubicin-based chemotherapy. The induction chemotherapy patients in fact had a lower rate of postoperative seroma formation. Danforth et al.[74] similarly reported that preoperative chemotherapy had no adverse effect on surgical complication rates and did not result in delayed delivery of any postoperative cancer care. Most patients will be ready to undergo surgery approximately 3 weeks after the last chemotherapy treatment, when the absolute neutrophil and platelet counts have normalized (greater than 1,500 and 100,000, respectively).

McCready et al.[75] confirmed that the axillary nodal status retains its prognostic value in the neoadjuvant chemotherapy setting. Their study of 136 LABC undergoing modified radical mastectomy following induction chemotherapy revealed that patients with no axillary metastases in the postchemotherapy mastectomy specimen had an excellent outcome, with nearly 80% surviving 5 years. In contrast, less than 10% of patients with 10 or more positive nodes survived 5 years, and patients with an intermediate number of residual metastatic nodes had an intermediate survival rate.

The third issue, regarding induction chemotherapy and its relative impact on breast cancer survival in comparison to conventional postoperative adjuvant therapy, remains controversial. It is clear, however, that preoperative treatment and deferral of surgery do not increase rates of unresectability. On the contrary, approximately 80% of patients will have at least 50% shrinkage of the primary tumor mass, and only 2% to 3% will have signs of progressive disease.[76–78] Fears that the surgeon will lose a "window of opportunity" to resect chest wall disease are therefore unfounded, and preoperatively treated patients are likely to be rendered improved operative candidates. A surgical resection is essential in accurately documenting chemotherapy response and in achieving durable locoregional control of disease, as the clinical assessment of response will overestimate the actual pathologic extent by two- to threefold.[79,80]

The induction CTX benefits of tumor downstaging and the ability to rapidly identify chemoresistant disease by in vivo observation motivated expanded applications of this treatment to the setting of early-stage disease. Accordingly, outcomes from prospective clinical trials have now been reported in which preoperative chemotherapy has been compared directly to postoperative chemotherapy in women with LABC as well as early-stage disease. Some of these Phase III clinical trial results are shown in Table 54.9.[81–88] All have demonstrated overall survival equivalence for the two treatment sequences, confirming the oncologic safety of the neoadjuvant approach.

Subset analyses of the Phase III studies, however, reveal that patients found to have a complete pathologic response (pCR) do have a statistically significant survival benefit, substantiating the concept that primary breast tumor response is a reliable surrogate for chemoeffect on micrometastases. In the NSABP B-18 trial,[88] patients with stage I–III breast cancer who were randomized to receive four cycles of doxorubicin and cytoxin preoperatively and who experienced a pCR had a 5-year overall survival of 86%, which was statistically superior to the outcome seen in all other study participants. Similarly, the University of Texas M.D. Anderson Cancer Center[89] reported an overall survival rate of 89% for pCR patients treated on preoperative chemotherapy protocols designed specifically for LABC, and this outcome also represented a statistically significant benefit compared to patients with a lesser response. Unfortunately, both studies found that only 12% to 13% of patients experience a pCR when treated with a doxorubicin-based regimen, and this proportion is simply insufficient in yielding a survival benefit for the entire pool of preoperatively treated patients. Predictors of a pCR include relatively smaller size primary breast tumors, estrogen receptor negativity, and high-grade lesions.[89] The latter two features probably characterize rapidly cycling tumors that may be particularly sensitive to chemotherapy effects.

The ability to downsize the primary breast tumor, thereby facilitating attainment of a margin-negative lumpectomy with a smaller-volume lumpectomy, is a major advantage of the neoadjuvant CTX sequence. A feasibility study reported by Singletary et al.[90] addressed many of the concerns that induction CTX might leave a field of microscopic satellite lesions, with a resulting increased risk of margin failure and/or excessive local recurrence rates. The Singletary study involved a pathology review of the mastectomy specimens in 143 LABC cases that had been treated with preoperative CTX; approximately one-quarter had adequate shrinkage of tumor and adequate eradication of disease in surrounding breast tissue as well as skin, such that they would have been candidates for successful lumpectomy. Table 54.9 demonstrates the overall comparability of local recurrence rates in subsequent clinical trials of women receiving BCT with versus without neoadjuvant CTX.

The NSABP B-18 trial[87,88,91] randomized more than 1,500 women with stages I–IIIA breast cancer to receive preoperative versus postoperative chemotherapy. This study demonstrated a statistically significant increase in breast conservation therapy utilization for the preoperative chemotherapy arm (68% versus 60%). With a median follow-up of 72 months, the local recurrence rates were 7.9% and 5.8% (no statistically significant difference) following BCT in the preoperative and postoperative chemotherapy arms, respectively. The conversion rate to BCT eligibility was greatest in the patients with T3 tumors at diagnosis. The NSABP also reported that local recurrence was somewhat higher in the subset of lumpectomy patients who were downstaged to become BCT eligible in comparison to the BCT patients who were BCT candidates at presentation.[88] However, this subset of downstaged BCT cases was predominantly composed of T3 tumors, and because local recurrence is one manifestation of underlying tumor biology, it would be expected that the more advanced stage lesions might have increased local recurrence rates regardless of surgery type and treatment sequence. Also, radiation boost doses were not consistently used in the lumpectomy patients, and tamoxifen therapy was only used in patients over 50 years of age. Both these interventions, if implemented uniformly, might have influenced local recurrence rates in downstaged tumors. Last, the NSABP requires that margin-negative lumpectomies be free of any tumor cells at an inked margin; a more-aggressive approach to margin control might be necessary for lumpectomies in tumors that have been downsized by preoperative CTX.

Newman et al.[92] analyzed a series of 100 patients treated at the M.D. Anderson Cancer Center on a prospective protocol of preoperative sequential taxotere and adriamycin-based chemotherapy in patients with stage I–III breast cancer. These investigators reported that 34% of patients initially ineligible for BCT were converted to lumpectomy candidates with this preoperative chemotherapy regimen. Final pathology review of all surgical specimens revealed that clinical assessment of BCT eligibility following induction chemotherapy was inaccurate for invasive lobular cancers, multicentric disease, and diffuse microcalcifications. Difficulties with assessment of chemoresponse in lobular cancers have also been noted by Mathieu et al.[93]

Induction chemotherapy is a reasonable and safe treatment approach for patients with breast cancer of any stage if the clinician is certain that chemotherapy would be recommended in the postoperative setting. The risk of overtreatment can be minimized by obtaining multiple diagnostic core biopsy specimens to confirm that a lesion is predominantly invasive, as it would clearly be inappropriate to treat large-volume or palpable DCIS tumors (with or without microinvasion) with CTX in any setting. Patients presenting with multiple tumors or extensive calcifications on initial mammogram should be counseled that preoperative chemotherapy will not convert them to BCT eligibility, regardless of extent of their primary tumor shrinkage. If the tumor is not associated with any microcalcifications, then a radiopaque clip should be inserted (preferably under ultrasound guidance) either before delivery of the neoadjuvant CTX or within the first couple of cycles. In the event that the patient should have a complete clinical response to the preoperative chemotherapy, this clip will serve

TABLE 54.9. Randomized trials of neoadjuvant versus adjuvant chemotherapy for breast cancer.

Study	Accrual years	N	Stages	Median follow-up (months)	BCT rate		Local recurrence after BCT		Overall survival at median follow-up	
					Preoperative CTX	Postoperative CTX	Preoperative CTX	Postoperative CTX	Preoperative CTX	Postoperative CTX
Institut Bergonie[81,82]	1985–1989	272	II-IIIA (T > 3 cm)	124	63.1%	0%	XRT: 34% L/ALND/XRT: 23%	NA	55%[a]	55%[a]
Institut Curie[230–232]	1983–1990	414	IIA-IIIA	66	82%	77%	24%	18%	86%	78%
Royal Marsden[85,86,233]	1990–1995	309	I-IIIB	48	89%	78%	3%[b]	4%[b]	80%[a]	80%[a]
NSABP[87,88,91]	1988–1993	1,523	I-IIIA	108	60%	68%	10.7%	7.6%	69%[c]	70%[c]
EORTC[234]	1991–1999	698	I-IIIA	56	37%	21%	NR	NR	NR	NR
ECTO[235]	2001	892	I-IIIA	23	71%	35%	NR	NR	NR	NR
ABCSG[236]	1991–1996	423	I-IIIB	NR	67%	60%	NR[d]	NR[d]	NR[d]	NR[d]

XRT, radiation; L, lumpectomy; ALND, axillary lymph node dissection; NA, not applicable; NR, not reported.

NSABP, National Surgical Adjuvant Breast Project; EORTC, European Organization for Research and Treatment of Cancer; ECTO, European Cooperative Trial in Breast Cancer; ABCS, Austrian Breast and Colorectal Study Group.

[a] Rate estimated from graph.

[b] Local recurrence rates reported for lumpectomy and mastectomy patients combined.

[c] Overall survival rate at 9 years.

[d] Recurrence and survival rates not reported, but relapse-free survival noted to be lower in neoadjuvant CTX arm, while overall survival similar for the two study arms.

as the target for subsequent mammography-assisted wire localization lumpectomy when the patient is ready for surgery. Lesions associated with microcalcifications have an inherent target for subsequent localization.

There is ongoing debate regarding the optimal method for integrating sentinel node staging of the axilla into induction CTX protocols. The standard treatment sequence for neoadjuvant CTX patients involves a percutaneous needle biopsy for establishment of the cancer diagnosis, delivery of chemotherapy, breast/axillary surgery, followed by irradiation in selected cases, and endocrine therapy for hormone receptor-positive disease. It was therefore logical for initial investigations to evaluate the results of sentinel lymph node biopsy performed after the delivery of preoperative CTX and concomitantly with the breast surgery. Concerns arose early in these discussions that the lymphatic mapping concept might be compromised by the following:

i. Lymphatic obstruction by tumor emboli from the relatively larger tumors that are more likely to be managed with neoadjuvant CTX;
ii. CTX effect on axillary metastases might not be uniform; and/or
iii. CTX might obliterate intramammary lymphatic channels.

Any combination of these factors could result in higher rates of sentinel node nonidentification or false negativity. Studies reported by Bedrosian et al.[94] and Chung et al.[95] documented the accuracy of lymphatic mapping for T2 and T3 breast cancers. Breslin et al.[96] reported the first series of patients undergoing sentinel lymph node biopsy and completion ALND after neoadjuvant CTX in a 2000 study from the M.D. Anderson Cancer Center, and these investigators demonstrated that the lymphatic mapping technology is indeed feasible in these cases, but accuracy rates are optimized when the surgical team has progressed through the learning curve of mapping in the setting of CTX-treated axillary tissue.

As shown in Table 54.10, several other investigators have now reported varying success rates with lymphatic mapping performed after delivery of neoadjuvant CTX. Identification rates range from 85% to 97%, and false-negative sentinel nodes are identified in 0% to 33% of cases. One feature supporting the biologic rationale for this approach is the persistent observation that even after neoadjuvant CTX, the sentinel node is frequently the isolated site of axillary metastases. A meta-analysis of reported studies conducted by Xing et al.[97] revealed an overall accuracy of 95% for sentinel node biopsy in this setting.

Nonetheless, the suboptimal false-negative results have prompted many surgeons to perform sentinel node biopsy for axillary staging before delivery of neoadjuvant CTX. The disadvantage to this approach is that some women will be subjected to unnecessary ALNDs, because the node-positive patients identified at presentation will be committed to a completion ALND after induction CTX, despite the fact that the sentinel node(s) may have been the only sites of disease for some cases, and for others the CTX may have eliminated any residual axillary metastases.

TABLE 54.10. Studies of sentinel lymph node biopsy performed after neoadjuvant chemotherapy.

Study	*T status*	*Sample size*	*Sentinel node identification rate*	*False-negative rate*	*Metastases limited to sentinel node(s)*
Breslin[96] (2000)	2, 3	51	85% (42/51)	12% (3/25)	40% (10/25)
Nason[237] (2000)	2, 3	15	87% (13/15)	33% (3/9)	≥11%* (≥1/9)
Haid[238] (2001)	1–3	33	88% (29/33)	0% (0/22)	50% (11/22)
Fernandez[239] (2001)	1–4	40	90% (36/40)	20% (4/20)	20% (4/20)
Tafra[240] (2001)	1, 2	29	93% (27/29)	0% (0/15)	NR
Stearns[241] (2002)	3, 4	T4d (inflammatory) 8	75% (6/8)	40% (2/5)	24% (5/21)
		Noninflammatory 26	88% (23/26)	6% (1/16)	
Julian[242] (2002)	1–3	34	91% (31/34)	0% (0/12)	42% (5/12)
Miller[243] (2002)	1–3	35	86% (30/35)	0% (0/9)	44% (4/9)
Brady[244] (2002)	1–3	14	93% (13/14)	0% (0/10)	60% (6/10)
Piato[245] (2003)	1, 2	42	98% (41/42)	17% (3/18)	0% (0/18)
Balch[246] (2003)	2–4	32	97% (31/32)	5% (1/19)	56% (10/18)
Schwartz[247] (2003)	1–3	21	100% (21/21)	9% (1/11)	64% (7/11)
Reitsamer[248] (2003)	2, 3	30	87% (26/30)	7% (1/15)	53% (8/15)
Mamounas[249] (2002)	1–3	428	85% (363/428)	11% (15/140)	50% (70/140)

Management of Ductal Carcinoma In Situ

Because DCIS is largely a disease whose manifestations are confined to in-breast pathology, management strategies focus on various combinations of local therapy: mastectomy, lumpectomy, and breast irradiation. Axillary metastases are sufficiently rare with DCIS that nodal staging with the conventional level I/II lymph node dissection and its associated risk of lymphedema is generally considered unnecessary. However, in cases of extensive DCIS, where the risk of coexisting invasive disease is significant, information regarding the axillary nodal status becomes more relevant. The advent of lymphatic mapping and sentinel lymph node biopsy has greatly facilitated the handling of this dilemma. Adjuvant systemic therapy provides no survival benefit for pure DCIS because of the exceedingly low risk of micrometastases. However, hormonally active medical therapies such as selective estrogen receptor modulators and aromatase inhibitors exert a suppressive effect on abnormal proliferative activity in the breast, and these agents can therefore be useful in contributing to local control of disease as well as prevention of new breast primary cancerous events. Table 54.11[98–103] summarizes the results reported by Phase III studies designed to compare DCIS treatment options.

Local Therapy

Mastectomy was the standard management approach for DCIS until approximately 25 years ago. During the 1980s, two developments provided the impetus for expanded surgical options in the treatment of this condition: (i) publication of prospective, randomized clinical trials from the United States and from Europe confirming the safety of breast conservation therapy as management for early-stage invasive breast cancer; and (ii) implementation of widespread screening mammography programs and the resulting increased rates of detection for localized foci of DCIS. Despite concerns that DCIS represented a diffuse pattern of disease in the breast, it became increasingly difficult for clinicians to support the paradox of offering breast-sparing treatment to women with invasive palpable breast cancer while women with mammographically detected DCIS were penalized with a routine recommendation for mastectomy. Hence, breast conservation strategies were explored and have been proven to be oncologically safe for appropriately selected DCIS cases.

Nonetheless, mastectomy remains a reasonable treatment option for DCIS, resulting in prolonged disease-free survival. Advances in plastic surgery techniques for immediate or delayed breast reconstruction have further improved the results achieved by mastectomy for DCIS. In certain clinical scenarios, mastectomy remains the preferred approach:

1. Patients with diffuse, suspicious-appearing microcalcifications in the breast
2. Inability to obtain margin control by lumpectomy and/or reexcision(s)
3. Patients with a contraindication to chest wall irradiation (XRT) or who lack access to an XRT facility, in cases in which it has been determined that breast XRT would be a necessary adjunct to lumpectomy
4. Patients with a primary personal preference for mastectomy
5. Patients with multiple, clinically apparent foci of DCIS that are not amenable to resection within a single margin-negative lumpectomy
6. Suboptimal tumor-to-breast size ratio, where a margin-negative lumpectomy will yield an unacceptable cosmetic result (as defined by the patient)

Mastectomy and lumpectomy have never been directly compared in a prospective, randomized trial designed for DCIS patients. However comparable survival has been confirmed by indirect comparisons from retrospective studies and from DCIS patients who were incidentally included in the NSABP B-06 trial.[98] The B-06 trial was designed to evaluate the outcome of approximately 1,800 stage I and II breast cancer patients randomized to treatment by breast conservation therapy (with versus without breast irradiation) or by mastectomy. Centralized pathology review subsequently identified 78 cases of DCIS that were randomized as well[98] and equally divided between the three study arms. The overall survival for all three arms was similar (approximately 96% at 6 years), but the addition of breast irradiation to lumpectomy decreased local recurrence (LR) from 43% to 7% (see Table 54.11).

As shown by Table 54.11, lumpectomy alone results in consistently higher rates of LR (range, 20%–43%) in comparison to patients treated by lumpectomy and breast radiation (range, 7%–12%). Commonly cited risk factors for LR have included suboptimal margin control, young age at diagnosis, and high-grade tumors with comedo-necrosis. Although margin status is frequently implicated in risk for developing LR, there is no consensus regarding the optimal extent of a negative margin. Furthermore, as noted in a meta-analysis of BCT for DCIS by Boyages et al.,[104] studies published before 1998 often neglected to include margin status in their analyses. In the more-recent studies, a negative margin was variously defined as a minimum of 1, 2, or 3mm of microscopically normal tissue at the inked lumpectomy borders.

Another consistent finding between studies was that approximately half of all locally recurrent lesions are in the form of invasive disease. The decision to be treated by breast preservation therefore involves a different category of risk that is assumed by the DCIS patient compared to the patient undergoing lumpectomy for invasive cancer. In the latter case, the risk for distant micrometastases is present from the time of diagnosis, and decisions regarding the need for adjuvant systemic therapy are addressed at that time. In the former case, however, there would be no need to consider treatment of micrometastases, because DCIS biologically would not be expected have the ability to extend beyond the local tissue environment of the breast. The development of a local recurrence alters this prognostically favorable situation, and affected patients then face the risk of breast cancer mortality from distant spread. The proportion of invasive LR was similar for the patients treated by lumpectomy alone versus lumpectomy and XRT. Because the risk of LR is lower for the radiated patients, however, the assumption would be that radiation reduces the incidence of a potentially life-threatening pattern of disease progression. One could further postulate that mastectomy is the safest treatment for DCIS patients because of the exceptionally low rate of LR. Although low, this risk is not nonexistent,[105,106] indicating

TABLE 54.11. Phase III studies of management strategies for ductal carcinoma in situ (DCIS).

Study	*NSABP B-06*[98a]			*EORTC*[99,103]		*NSABP B-17*[100,102]		*NSABP B-24*[101]		*UK*			
Eligibility requirements	• Designed to evaluate the safety of breast conservation for Stage I/II breast cancer • Inked margin tumor-free			• Designed to evaluate lumpectomy with versus without breast XRT • Mammographically detected DCIS ≤5 cm • No margin specification		• Designed to evaluate lumpectomy with versus without breast XRT • DCIS detected by mammogram or physical exam • Inked margin tumor-free		• Designed to evaluate the added benefit of tamoxifen as adjuvant therapy for DCIS patients treated with lumpectomy and breast XRT • DCIS detected by mammogram or physical exam • Inked margin tumor-free		• Screen-detected DCIS • Inked margin tumor-free			
Average follow-up (months)	83			65		90		74		53			
Randomization arms	Lump	Lump + XRT	Mastectomy	Lump	Lump + XRT	Lump	Lump + XRT	Lump + XRT	Lump + XRT + Tam	Lump	Lump + XRT	Lump + Tam	Lump + XRT + Tam
Number of patients	21	27	28	426	437	403	411	902	902	544	267	567	316
Number of local recurrences (%)	9 (42.8%)	2 (7.4%)	0 (0%)	83 (19.5%)	54 (12.4%)	104 (25.8%)	47 (11.4%)	87 (9.6%)	63 (7.0%)	119 (22%)	22 (8%)	101 (18%)	21 (6%)
Number of invasive local recurrences (%)	5/9 (45%)	1/2 (50%)	NA	37/83 (44%)	23/54 (45%)	53/104 (51%)	17/47 (36%)	40/87 (46%)	23/63 (37%)	39 (33%)	12 (55%)	43 (43%)	14 (67%)
Overall survival	96%	96%	96%	97%	97%	97%	96%	97%	97%	98%	97%	98%	95%
Risk factors for local recurrence	Lack of XRT following lumpectomy Comedonecrosis			Lack of XRT Age ≤40 years Symptomatic DCIS Involved margins Solid/cribriform/comedo patterns		Lack of XRT Calcifications on mammogram		Lack of tamoxifen Age <50 years Involved margins Comedonecrosis Symptomatic DCIS		Lack of XRT			

Lump, lumpectomy; XRT, breast irradiation; Tam, tamoxifen; Symptomatic DCIS, palpable mass,; nipple discharge.

[a] There were 76 cases randomized in NSABP B-06 that were found to be pure DCIS on retrospective pathology review.

that rare forms of DCIS do possess a biologically aggressive nature (or that an occult focus of invasion was present in the breast). Despite this concern, the Phase III clinical trials summarized in Table 54.11 reveal similarly high overall survival rates for DCIS patients treated by lumpectomy with or without breast irradiation.

Because of the expense, inconvenience, and potential adverse effects of XRT, several investigators have attempted to identify subsets of DCIS patients with sufficiently low-risk lesions that they could routinely be treated by lumpectomy alone. The obvious candidates would be small-volume, low-grade DCIS with widely negative margins on lumpectomy. Some groups have developed grading systems that stratify DCIS patients based on the risk of developing LR. The most popular of these is the Van Nuys Prognostic Index (VNPI), developed by Silverstein et al.[107] and based on the detailed pathology analyses and follow-up of several hundred DCIS patients. This index utilizes a point system to categorize patients on the basis of nuclear grade (with versus without necrosis); extent of DCIS (15mm or less versus 16–40mm versus more than 40mm); and margin width (10mm or more versus 1–9mm versus less than 1mm). Cumulative points resulting in scores of 3 or 4 identify patients who should be safely managed by lumpectomy only, whereas scores of 8 or 9 would be indications for mastectomy. Intermediate scores would be consistent with safe treatment by lumpectomy and XRT. This index was recently modified to include age (less than 40 versus 40–60 versus more than 60 years).[108] Several studies have been unable to validate the accuracy of the VNPI in predicting LR. A major disadvantage to the VNPI is that it was developed by retrospective review of treated patients and therefore has some inherent biases. Despite the difficulties in developing a reproducible and accurate scoring system for DCIS, an international and multidisciplinary panel of DCIS experts convened a consensus panel several years ago, and collectively decreed that all pathology reports on DCIS should include a description of morphology, nuclear grade, and necrosis.[109]

Several investigative groups have implemented prospective clinical trials designed to evaluate the long-term results of treating highly selected subsets of DCIS patients by lumpectomy alone. One such study, conducted by the Dana-Farber/Harvard Cancer Center, utilized DCIS grade 1 or 2, size up to 2.5cm, and final margins of at least 1cm as eligibility criteria. After accrual of 157 patients (of an accrual goal of 200), the early closure of this study was recently reported[110] because of an excessive LR rate. At a median follow-up of 40 months, 13 patients experienced a LR (9 were invasive recurrences), corresponding to a 5-year rate of 12.5% and a per annum rate of 2.5% per patient-year. A Phase 3 clinical trial implemented by the Radiation Therapy Oncology Group (RTOG), which randomizes small, low-grade DCIS to lumpectomy with versus without XRT and with versus without tamoxifen, is currently under way.

Regional Treatment and Management of the Axilla

Past studies of mastectomy performed for DCIS revealed axillary metastases in approximately 2% of DCIS cases. It is commonly assumed that these are related to a focus of invasive disease in the breast that was overlooked on pathologic tissue sampling. This low risk of detecting nodal disease and the wish to minimize risk of lymphedema prompted most surgeons to abandon the routine practice of performing a conventional level I/II ALND in DCIS patients. For those patients requiring a mastectomy because of diffuse DCIS, the need for axillary staging becomes more relevant because of the associated increased risk of coexisting microinvasion. In these cases the standard approach was to include a level I ALND with the mastectomy.

Integration of the lymphatic mapping technology into breast cancer surgery during the past decade presented a novel and minimally invasive method for detecting axillary metastases. Several investigators have now reported their findings from series of DCIS patients undergoing sentinel lymph node biopsy, with interesting results. Intra et al.[111] found axillary metastases in 7 of 223 (3.1%) DCIS patients, and Pendas et al.[112] reported a 6% rate of sentinel node positivity in 87 DCIS cases. These increased rates of upstaging patients previously thought to have preinvasive DCIS are inconsistent with established overall long-term survival rates of 98% for DCIS patients. It must be noted, however, that in both these series the majority of sentinel node disease was micrometastatic, detected by immunohistochemistry, and completion ALNDs rarely demonstrated additional metastases in nonsentinel nodes. The biologic significance of axillary metastases in this setting is therefore questionable. Given this uncertainty, the current standard of care is to defer axillary staging by lymphatic mapping in DCIS cases managed with breast preservation unless invasion is detected in the lumpectomy specimen, in which case the patient can be returned to the operating room for a subsequent sentinel lymph node biopsy. In contrast, it is not technically feasible to perform a lymphatic mapping procedure after the breast has been removed, and a different approach must be used for DCIS patients undergoing mastectomy. If there is a significant likelihood of a coexisting invasive focus, based on prior biopsy findings, or based on extent of DCIS, it is therefore reasonable to perform the lymphatic mapping procedure concomitantly with the mastectomy. Immunohistochemistry should not be routinely performed for these cases outside of a clinical trial.

Medical Therapy for DCIS

Because of the known prevalence of ER expression in DCIS lesions, and because of tamoxifen's known ability to suppress breast ductal proliferative activity, it has been reasonable to explore utilization of this selective ER receptor modulator as adjuvant therapy for DCIS. As shown in Table 54.11, the NSABP's B-24 study[101] randomized 1,800 DCIS cases to treatment by lumpectomy and XRT followed 5 years of tamoxifen versus placebo. At a median follow-up of 74 months, tamoxifen was found to result in a significantly lower risk of both ipsilateral and contralateral breast cancer events. There were 130 breast cancer events in the placebo arm versus 84 in the placebo arm, consistent with a 37% reduction for the tamoxifen patients (P = 0.0009). There was no requirement for margin control in this trial and, interestingly, there were fewer ipsilateral breast cancer events in the tamoxifen-treated arm even among those patients with involved margins. The pattern of benefit conferred by tamoxifen in NSABP B-24 was also notable, with most of the risk reduction occurring in contralateral breast events. Tamoxifen reduced the risk of contralateral invasive and noninvasive disease by 52% ($P = 0.01$).

For the ipsilateral breast there was a significant reduction in invasive recurrences, by 44% ($P = 0.03$), but the reduction in recurrent DCIS was only by 18% ($P = 0.43$).

Another prospective randomized trial conducted in the United Kingdom[113] (commonly called the UK Trial) had a two-by-two factorial design and evaluated the relative contributions of breast irradiation and tamoxifen therapy to the outcome of DCIS patients treated with lumpectomy. This study found that although both approaches are effective in decreasing risk of local recurrence, tamoxifen had only marginal benefit in patients receiving breast XRT. The UK Trial has been criticized because of its design, which allowed for some bias because patients were allowed to self-select regarding adjuvant therapy to some extent.

Allred et al. conducted a meticulous study of the ER expression in DCIS lesions from the NSABP tamoxifen-treated arm and reported a close association between the pattern of hormone receptor positivity and likelihood benefit from tamoxifen.[114] With a median follow-up of 104 months, the rate of LR for ER-positive DCIS was 10%, compared to 23% for the ER-negative lesions. It should be noted, however, that Allred et al. utilized a very specific grading and interpretation of ER staining by immunohistochemistry. Their findings with regard to DCIS and tamoxifen are biologically plausible; however, whether their methods can be widely replicated for standardized clinical practice warrants further study.

The ATAC Trial yielded provocative results regarding the activity of the aromatase inhibitor anastrozole for adjuvant management ER-positive postmenopausal breast cancer. This trial randomized more than 9,000 early-stage breast cancer patients to receive anastrozole, tamoxifen, or the combination of anastrozole with tamoxifen, as systemic adjuvant therapy. The risk of contralateral new breast cancers was reduced to a significantly greater degree in the anastrozole compared to the tamoxifen arm (odds ratio, 0.42; $P = 0.007$).[51] These findings prompted the design and implementation of NSABP B-35, a Phase 3 trial that randomizes postmenopausal DCIS patients treated by breast conservation therapy to receive adjuvant tamoxifen versus anastrozole for the prevention of additional breast cancer events.[115]

Breast Cancer Risk Reduction

Until recently, the primary message of breast health awareness programs has been that "early detection is a woman's best protection" against breast cancer because there was no way to prevent the disease. Currently, however, tamoxifen is U.S. Food and Drug Administration (FDA) approved for chemoprevention of breast cancer in high-risk women, and numerous investigators are evaluating other medications that may decrease the risk of breast cancer. Data have also become available regarding the efficacy of surgical strategies to reduce breast cancer risk.

The ability to hormonally manipulate breast tissue and thereby reduce proliferative changes that would otherwise evolve into cancer has been recognized over the past several decades. Women using tamoxifen for a unilateral breast cancer were seen to have a 40% lower risk of second primary/contralateral breast cancer compared to breast cancer patients not treated with tamoxifen. These data motivated implementation of the first large-scale chemoprevention trial conducted in the United States, the National Surgical Adjuvant Breast Project (NSABP) P-1 study,[116] a prospective, placebo-controlled randomized study of tamoxifen in 13,880 high-risk women. Eligibility criteria to participate in the P-1 Study included age at least 60 years; a 5-year Gail model breast cancer risk estimate of more than 1.66%; and history of lobular carcinoma in situ (LCIS). After 54 months median follow-up, the trial was unblinded early because of the magnitude of difference in breast cancer incidence between the treated and control arms of the study, revealing that tamoxifen lowered breast cancer risk by 49%. It therefore now considered the standard of care to evaluate breast cancer risk factor information in women and to counsel high-risk women about the options of chemoprevention.

Unfortunately, however, making a commitment to 5 years of tamoxifen is not easy, as several potentially severe adverse reactions can be associated with this therapy. Tamoxifen effects on estrogen receptors in the uterus, vascular system, and central nervous system increase risks of uterine cancer, thromboembolic phenomena (deep vein thrombosis and pulmonary emboli), and vasomotor symptoms (e.g., hot flashes, night sweats), respectively. Partially offsetting these risks are tamoxifen's estrogen agonist effects on the skeletal system and lipid profile, resulting in a reduced incidence of osteoporosis and lower serum cholesterol levels. NSABP P-1 study participants in the premenopausal age range appeared to be relatively protected from adverse tamoxifen effects;[116] however, the safety of tamoxifen during fetal development has not been established, and chemoprevention with this agent is therefore contraindicated in women who are contemplating pregnancy.

Complicating the chemoprevention decision process further is the fact that tamoxifen will only reduce the incidence of estrogen receptor-positive tumors. Tamoxifen has no impact on the occurrence of estrogen receptor-negative disease, a potentially significant issue in counseling women who harbor mutations in one of the breast cancer susceptibility genes. Subset analysis of genetically tested NSABP P-1 participants demonstrated that tamoxifen does not reduce breast cancer risk in BRCA-1 mutation carriers; however, it does appear to offer some chemoprevention benefit in BRCA-2 mutation carriers.[117] This finding is consistent with prior studies revealing that BRCA-2 mutation-associated tumors are similar in histopathology to sporadic breast cancer, whereas BRCA-1 cancers are more likely to be estrogen receptor negative and aneuploid.

The ideal SERM would retain antiproliferative activity in the breast, but without subjecting the patient to the negative risks. Toward this end, the (NSABP) is currently accruing to the second chemoprevention trial, the Study of Tamoxifen and Raloxifene (STAR). STAR randomizes high-risk postmenopausal women to receive either tamoxifen or raloxifen, a SERM that is presently FDA approved for treatment of osteoporosis. Preliminary evidence indicates that raloxifen has similar breast cancer risk reduction activity compared to tamoxifen, but with a lower incidence of uterine neoplasia. Premenopausal women are ineligible for STAR participation because of the absence of data on raloxifen effects in young, ovulating women.

One theory of breast carcinogenesis proposes that risk of malignant transformation is related to lifetime exposure of breast tissue to cyclic extremes in the levels of circulating hormones. Accordingly, it is postulated that stabilization of estrogen levels will decrease the incidence of mammary neoplasia. Studies of gonadotropin-releasing hormone agonists in conjunction with low-dose hormone replacement therapy are therefore under way as a means of testing this hypothesis, and preliminary results have shown that this approach can successfully decrease mammographic density;[118] however, longer follow-up is needed to evaluate actual chemoprevention efficacy.

Recent data on the efficacy of aromatase inhibitors for adjuvant therapy in breast cancer have revealed that these agents also possess significant chemoprevention activity.[119] Table 54.12[116,119–128] summarizes reported data on the risk-reducing strength of various medical therapies.

Premenopausal prophylactic oophorectomy and prophylactic mastectomy are additional options as surgical strategies for breast cancer risk reduction. Surgical menopause before age 35 years is an established protective factor against breast cancer risk. Availability of BRCA testing has resulted in the identification of women from hereditary breast-ovarian cancer families, and these women are especially motivated to consider prophylactic removal of the ovaries. Published case-control data (level II evidence) by Rebbeck et al.[129] and Kauff et al.[130] have confirmed that prophylactic oophorectomy in this setting can decrease breast cancer incidence by approximately 50%. Premature menopause, however, is associated with an increased risk of osteoporosis and atherosclerotic cardiovascular disease. Interestingly, the breast cancer protection afforded by prophylactic oophorectomy was not diminished by hormone replacement therapy in the Rebbeck et al. study.

Prophylactic mastectomy is a dramatic and extreme maneuver to decrease breast cancer risk, yet only recently has its efficacy in high-risk women been documented. Early reports of prophylactic mastectomy in humans[131,132] demonstrated a 1% to 2% failure rate, but these studies were flawed by limited follow-up and by the inclusion of many women who were probably at low risk for developing breast cancer. Women at risk for hereditary breast cancer would potentially be most susceptible to a failed prophylactic mastectomy, as in these cases any microscopic amount of residual breast tissue would harbor the germ-line predisposition for malignant transformation.

Hartmann et al.[133] have made valuable contributions to our understanding of the efficacy of prophylactic mastectomy through their meticulous scrutiny of the Mayo clinic database. This analysis yielded 639 prophylactic mastectomy patients with documented increased risk on the basis of family history of breast and/or ovarian cancer. These high-risk patients were further stratified into very-high (214 patients) and moderately-high risk (425 patients) subsets based on extent of family history. Outcome regarding number of subsequent breast cancers occurring among the very high risk subset was compared to the number of breast cancers developing among the female siblings of these patients. For the moderate-risk patients, efficacy of the prophylactic surgery was evaluated by calculating the number of expected cancers based on summing of the individual Gail model risk estimates for the entire group. Survival analyses were performed by projecting anticipated longevity based on population-based data. With a median follow-up of approximately 14 years, 7 breast cancers were detected in the prophylactic mastectomy patients (3 in the very high risk subset and 4 in the moderate-risk subset), consistent with a 90% reduction in breast cancer risk and mortality in both categories of high-risk patients.

Subsequent study of the Hartmann database[134] reported results of prophylactic mastectomy in women who were also found to be BRCA mutation carriers and confirmed an equivalent magnitude of breast cancer risk reduction. Similarly, Meijers-Heijboer et al.[135] reported outcome for 76 BRCA mutation carriers followed prospectively after having undergone prophylactic mastectomy and found no tumors developing with an average follow-up of nearly 3 years. Hence, reliable evidence does indicate that prophylactic mastectomy will effectively and substantially reduce the incidence of breast cancer in high-risk women, although the protection conferred is not complete.

Metastatic Breast Cancer

Goals of Therapy

Although few if any patients with metastatic breast cancer are cured by treatment, many will remain in remission for prolonged periods and enjoy acceptable quality of life. Treatment modestly prolongs survival, perhaps by 20% to 30% proportionally, and palliation is achieved for many if not all patients.[136–140]

Taken together, these considerations suggest that judicious, serial application of available therapies should result in the main goals of treatment of metastatic disease: palliation and modest survival prolongation. To achieve these goals, the clinician needs to first assess the patient's status in regard to diagnosis, prognosis, and prediction.

Diagnosis

Certain constellations of abnormalities may be so compelling that tissue confirmation of a new finding suggestive of metastatic disease is not required. However, it is strongly recommended that a biopsy of a suspicious lesion be performed to document that one is, in fact, dealing with metastatic breast cancer and not a benign lesion or a second, primary cancer. Such biopsies can be performed by fine-needle aspiration, core needle biopsy, or excision, depending on the circumstances. Biopsy of a metastatic lesion also permits reanalysis of the patient's tumor for predictive factors.

Prognosis

Chemotherapy is more likely to induce a clinical response than endocrine therapy or trastuzumab. However, chemotherapy is also usually more likely to have more toxicity, and so either endocrine or trastuzumab treatment is preferred as first therapy for estrogen receptor- or HER2-positive metastatic disease, respectively. However, chemotherapy is indicated as first-line therapy for patients with evidence of rapidly progressive visceral metastases, especially if there is evidence of substantial end-organ dysfunction, such as elevated liver function tests (especially bilirubin) and/or pulmonary symptoms, regardless of predictive factors.

TABLE 54.12. Phase III trials of breast cancer chemoprevention.

Study	Primary chemoprevention study?	N	Eligibility criteria	Age range (years)	Randomization	Intended treatment duration (years)	Median follow-up	Breast cancer hazard
Royal Marsden[120,121]	Yes	2,471	High risk, family history	30–70	Tam vs. placebo	5–8	70 months	1.06 (0.7–1.7) Tam. vs. placebo
NSABP P-01[116,120]	Yes	13,388	≥1.67% 5-year risk LCIS Age >60 years	35	Tam vs. placebo	5	54.6 months	0.51 (0.39–0.66)
Italian Tamoxifen Study Group[120,122–124]	Yes	5,408	S/p hysterectomy	35–70	Tam vs. placebo	5	81.2 months	All: 0.75 (0.48–1.18) No HRT: 0.99 (0.59–1.68) HRT: 0.36 (0.14–0.91)
IBIS[120,125]	Yes	7,139	RR *0.132	35–70	Tam vs. placebo	5	50 months	0.68 (0.50–0.92)
Tamoxifen Chemoprevention Overview Analysis[120]	Yes, collective review	28,406	NA	NA	Tam vs. placebo	NA	70.6×10^3 women-years	0.62 (0.54–0.72)
MORE[120,126]	No	7,705	Postmenopausal; osteoporosis	Median, 66.5	Raloxifene vs. placebo	4	3 years	0.28 (0.17–0.46)
STAR[250]	Yes	Accrual goal 19,000	Postmenopausal; ≥1.67% 5-year risk LCIS	Accrual not yet completed	Tam vs. raloxifene	5	Accrual not yet completed	NA
Fenritimide/4-HPR[127]	Yes	1,574	Early-stage unilateral breast cancer	28–67	4-HPR vs. placebo	7	97 months	Premenopausal: 0.66 (0.41–1.07) Postmenopausal: 1.32 (0.82–2.15)
Tamoxifen Adjuvant Therapy Overview Analysis[120,190]	No	14,170	Operable breast cancer	NA	Tam vs. no adjuvant therapy	≥5 (average, 5)	5 years	0.54 (0.43–0.69)
ATAC[119]	No	9,366	Postmenopausal, early-stage breast cancer	Mean, 64 years	Arimidex vs. Tam vs. Tam + arimidex	5	33.3 months	0.42 (0.22–0.79)

Prediction

For most patients, careful selection of the optimal therapy can result in considerable and often relatively long-lasting palliation. Expression of estrogen and progesterone receptors (ER, PgR) is highly predictive of response to endocrine treatments.[141,142] HER-2 is the protein product of the erbB-2 gene, a member of the epidermal growth factor receptor family that consists of four members: epidermal growth factor receptor (EGFR, also called HER1), HER2 (also called erbB-2 and c-neu), HER3, and HER4. HER2 is amplified and/or overexpressed in 25% to 40% of breast cancers, and the humanized monoclonal anti-HER2 antibody, trastuzumab, appears to be effective only in patients with HER2-positive breast cancer.[143–145]

There are no good predictive factors for individual chemotherapy agents. Chemotherapy resistance assays have been studied for more than two decades, but none of these technologies has been shown in rigorous studies to be sufficiently accurate for routine clinical use.[146–148] Therefore, selection of specific chemotherapy is empiric. For example, patients who relapse within 1 year of adjuvant therapy are very unlikely to respond to the same agents again. Moreover, cumulative toxicities, especially cardiac failure with the anthracyclines, may preclude additional treatment even if the agent is likely to be effective.

Selection of Therapy: Local Versus Systemic

Local therapies (surgery, radiation, hyperthermia) often preclude concurrent systemic therapy and therefore are most appropriate for patients who have isolated metastases and/or who have impending crises, such as long bone fracture, spinal cord metastases, or intracranial metastases.

Systemic Therapy: Endocrine Therapy

For most patients with metastatic disease, selection of systemic therapy is preferable. Patients with ER- and/or PgR-positive tumors should receive endocrine therapy. There is no role for combined endocrine and chemotherapy; there are some preclinical and adjuvant data suggesting that they may be antagonistic.[149,150] Regardless, because palliation is the goal, if endocrine treatment alone is appropriate it is more likely to induce palliation. If not, then there is no reason to use it, and chemotherapy should be initiated alone.

For the past 20 years, tamoxifen has been the first-line endocrine treatment of choice, because it is equally or more effective and has fewer side effects than previously available therapies. However, because most hormone receptor-positive patients receive tamoxifen in the adjuvant setting, second-line endocrine therapy, in fact, becomes "first line" if patients recur on tamoxifen. Several prospective randomized trials have demonstrated that for postmenopausal women with ER-positive metastatic breast cancer, the selective aromatase inhibitors are more effective with fewer side effects than older second-line therapies, such as megestrol acetate or aminoglutethimide[151–154] (Table 54.13). Recently, similar studies have demonstrated that survival is superior for women treated with AIs compared to tamoxifen as first line therapy for metastatic disease[136,155,156] (Table 54.13). Because they do not inhibit ovarian estrogen production, aromatase inhibitors should not be used in premenopausal women.

Fulvestrant, similar to tamoxifen, binds to the ER. However, instead of modulating ER dimerization and binding to estrogen response elements in the nucleus, fulvestrant prevents dimerization and induces downregulation of the receptor. Prospective randomized trials have demonstrated that fulvestrant is as effective as anastrozole as second-line therapy and, recently, more effective than tamoxifen as first-line therapy[157–159] (see Table 54.13).

Premenopausal women with hormone receptor-positive metastatic breast cancer are probably best treated with ovarian function cessation, either by surgical oophorectomy or by chemical cessation of ovary function with the use of luteinizing hormone-releasing hormone antagonists such as goserelin. Addition of either tamoxifen, an aromatase inhibitor, or fulvestrant to ovarian cessation appears to improve outcome, but the side effects are greater. However, because the aromatase inhibitors appear more effective than tamoxifen in postmenopausal women, it is not unreasonable to combine ovarian ablation with an aromatase inhibitor.[160,161]

Side effects of endocrine treatments are generally related to antiestrogenic effects, including hot flashes, moodiness, and vaginal dryness and dysparunia. The aromatase inhibitors all seem to have a small rate of arthralgias and of gastrointestinal upset. Because tamoxifen has estrogenic properties in the liver, it increases thrombogenesis, with consequent increased risk of deep venous thrombosis and cerebral vascular accident. Long-term use of aromatase inhibitors is associated with increased risk of osteoporosis and fracture, whereas tamoxifen has estrogenic effects in bone and is therefore protective from this effect. However, in women with metastatic disease, this is rarely an issue because they rarely remain on the agent for more than a few months due to progression, and they are frequently treated with bisphosphonates (see following).

Systemic Therapy: Chemotherapy

Of the common solid tumor malignancies, breast cancer is one of the most sensitive to chemotherapy, although, as noted, metastatic breast cancer exhibits a fundamental pattern of resistance that ultimately, and nearly universally, leads to death. Nonetheless, responses, and one therefore hopes improvement in symptoms, occur in 20% to 60% of patients when treated with single-agent alkylating agents, antimetabolites (purine and pyrimidine analogues), anthracyclines and anthraquinones, and taxanes. Of these, the anthracyclines (doxorubicin, epirubicin) and taxanes (paclitaxel, docetaxel) appear to have the highest single-agent activity.

Through the 1980s, combination chemotherapy was widely applied in metastatic breast cancer, cyclophosphamide, methotrexate, and 5-fluorouracil (CMF) and cyclophosphamide, doxorubicin (adriamycin), and 5-fluorouracil (CAF).[162,163] In the 1990s, use of sequential single-agent therapy was more widely applied to avoid overlapping toxicities of combination therapy.[164–169] Results of two recently published studies have suggested a modest survival advantage for combination therapy using either docetaxel and capecitabine or paclitaxel and gemcitabine.[138,170] These two studies notwithstanding, in the absence of rapidly progressive visceral disease, it seems just as reasonable to treat patients with single-agent chemotherapy, offering the next therapy if the first is either ineffective or intolerable.

TABLE 54.13. Prospective randomized trials of endocrine therapy for metastatic breast cancer.

Comparison	*Reference*	*Clinical benefit**	*TTP (HR for progression)*	*Overall survival (HR for death)*
Selective aromatase inhibitors versus aminoglutethimide				
Letrozole vs. aminoglutethimide	153	36.3% 28.9% (NS)	0.72 (P = 0.008)	0.64 (P = 0.002)
Selective aromatase inhibitors versus megestrol acetate				
Anastrozole vs. megestrol acetate	151	42.2% 40.3% (NA)	0.94 (NS)	0.78 (P = 0.025)
Letrozole vs. megestrol acetate	152	34.5% 31.7% (NS)	0.80 (P = 0.07)	0.82 (P = 0.15)
Letrozole vs. megestrol acetate	251	26.7% 23.4% (NA)	0.99 (NS)	0.92 (P = 0.49)
Exemestane vs. megestrol acetate	252	37.4% 34.6% (NS)	0.82 (P = 0.04)	NA (P = 0.04)
One selective aromatase inhibitor versus another				
Letrozole vs. anastrozole	253	27% 23%	1.0 (P = 0.92)	0.95 (P = 0.62)
Selective estrogen receptor downregulator versus selective aromatase inhibitor				
Fulvestrant vs. anastrozole	158	42.2% 36.1% (P = 0.26)	0.92 (P = 0.43)	NA
Fulvestrant vs. anastrozole	157	44.6% 45% (NS)	0.98 (P = 0.84)	NA
Selective aromatase inhibitors versus tamoxifen (selective estrogen receptor modulator)				
Anastrozole vs. tamoxifen	254	56.2% 55.5% (NS)	0.99 (P = 0.94)	NA
Anastrozole vs. tamoxifen	255	59% 46% (P = 0.01)	0.69 (P = 0.005)	NA
Letrozole vs. tamoxifen	155	49% 38% (P = 0.001)	0.70 (P = 0.0001)	NA
Exemestane vs. tamoxifen	156	57% 42% (P = NA)	NA	NA

In summary, chemotherapy can induce quite satisfactory palliation, in spite of its side effects, if applied judiciously. There does not appear to be an optimal regimen, schedule, or dose, although general guidelines can be drawn from a number of well-performed prospective randomized trials.

Novel Targeted Therapies

Trastuzumab is a humanized monoclonal antibody that selectively binds HER2. Phase II trials have shown it to induce responses in 10% to 25% of patients with HER2-positive breast cancers.[144,171,172] Perhaps more importantly, a single prospective randomized clinical trial has demonstrated that response rates, progression-free survival, and even overall survival are improved by chemotherapy (either CAF or paclitaxel) plus trastuzumab versus chemotherapy alone.[139] These exciting findings have led to combination studies of trastuzumab with several chemotherapeutic agents, with the suggestion of increased response rates than might be expected from historical controls.[173–175]

There are two important caveats regarding trastuzumab therapy. First, in the pivotal metastatic trial, congestive heart failure was observed in more than 25% of patients treated with combination doxorubicin and trastuzumab and in more than 10% of those who received paclitaxel and trastuzumab.[139] Currently combination therapy with trastuzumab and an anthracycline should be considered contraindicated. Second, HER2 is most commonly evaluated in breast cancer tissue by immunohistochemistry (IHC). The only IHC test for HER2 testing that is approved by the FDA is the so-called Herceptest. Substantial data suggest that, using the recommended readout scale of 0–3+, only those patients whose tumors are read as "3+" are likely to benefit from trastuzumab.[176] Likewise, it also appears that HER2 amplification, which is evaluated by fluorescent in situ hybridization (FISH), is also an accurate predictor of benefit from trastuzumab.[176] A reasonable algorithm is to perform IHC first. Patients with tumor HER2 scores of 0–1+ are unlikely to benefit, whereas those who are 3+ are good candidates for trastuzumab. For patients whose tumors are 2+, FISH should be performed to distinguish those who should receive trastuzumab from those who should not.

Other novel therapies that appear to have some benefit include bevacizumab, a monoclonal antibody directed against vascular endothelial growth factor (VEGF) and the orally available inhibitors of the EGFR-family tyrosine kinases.[177–179] However, none of these has been studied in a sufficiently rigorous manner to determine if it has a role in routine clinical care.

Monitoring Patients with Metastatic Breast Cancer

Palliative therapy should be continued so long as it appears to be successful and tolerated, as determined by history, physical examination, radiographs, and serologic/blood testing. Commonly a patient is followed for several cycles of therapy, lasting weeks to months, until progression is obvious and therapy should be changed. During this period of time, the patient may have been exposed to the toxicities of the therapy needlessly, if it was of little or no value in reducing the cancer burden.

Serial plain radiographs, computerized tomography, magnetic resonance imaging, and bone scintigraphy can provide evidence of response or, more importantly, progression. It is critical that the clinician be aware of causes of false-positive evidence of progression, in particular the so-called scintigraphic healing flare associated with response of bone metastases and conversion from lytic to sclerotic lesions. Because more than 50% of patients with metastases may have bone-predominant or bone-only metastases, monitoring may be quite difficult.

The value of positron emission tomography for monitoring metastatic breast cancer has not been shown in prospective, well-designed clinical trials, although this technology appears to have substantial promise. Serial circulating tumor markers, in particular carcinoembryonic antigen (CEA) and products of the MUC1 gene (identified by the commercially available assays CA 15-3 or CA 27.29), appear reasonably accurate for monitoring patients with metastatic disease.[180] However, approximately 25% of patients may experience a false-positive increase, or "tumor marker spike," during the first 30 to 60 days of therapy, and the clinician also needs to be aware of other reasons for nonmalignant tumor marker elevation, for example, as observed with acute hepatic dysfunction. Recently, results of a prospective clinical trial have suggested that circulating tumor cell (CTC) levels, as evaluated by an automated immunomagnetic technique, may be strongly associated with clinical outcome of patients with metastatic breast cancer.[181,182] These data, and the potential benefits of changing therapy very early for patients with elevated CTC, require validation in future studies.

In summary, high levels of evidence support the benefits of careful application of systemic therapies for patients with metastatic disease. Prospective randomized clinical trials have demonstrated the benefits of various endocrine treatments for those with hormone receptor-positive disease, for specific chemotherapeutic regimens for patients with very poor prognosis or those with hormone-refractory metastases, and for the use of trastuzumab alone or in combination with chemotherapy for patients with HER2-positive breast cancer. Ongoing research offers promise to further improve quality of life and even survival for patients who suffer with distant disease, and it is hoped that future investigations may even result in cure rates approaching those of Hodgkins' disease, non-Hodgkins' lymphoma, and testicular cancer.

References

1. Baxter N. Preventive health care, 2001 update: should women be routinely taught breast self-examination to screen for breast cancer? Cam Med Assoc J 2001;164:1837–1846.
2. Hackshaw AK, Paul EA. Breast self-examination and death from breast cancer: a meta-analysis. Br J Cancer 2003;88:1047–1053.
3. Thomas DB, Gao DL, Ray RM, et al. Randomized trial of breast self-examination in Shanghai: final results. J Natl Cancer Inst 2002;94:1445–1457.
4. Liberman L. The breast imaging reporting and data system: positive predictive value of mammographic features and final assessment categories. AJR Am J Roengtenol 1998;171:35–40.
5. Warner E. Breast self-examination. C Med Assoc J 2002;166:163; author reply 166, 168.
6. Shen Y, Zelen M. Screening sensitivity and sojourn time from breast cancer early detection clinical trials: mammograms and physical examinations. J Clin Oncol 2001;19:3490–3499.
7. Humphrey L, Helfand M, Chan B, Woolf S. Breast Cancer Screening: A Summary of the Evidence, vol 2003. Washington, DC: U.S. Preventive Services Task Force, 2002.
8. Shapiro S. Periodic screening for breast cancer: the HIP randomized controlled trial. J Natl Cancer Inst Monogr 1997;22: 27–30.
9. Nystrom L, Andersson I, Bjurstam N, Frisell J, Nordenskjold B, Rutqvist LE. Long-term effects of mammography screening: updated overview of the Swedish randomised trials. Lancet 2002;359:909–919.
10. Tabar L, Vitak B, Chen HH, et al. The Swedish Two-County Trial twenty years later. Updated mortality results and new insights from long-term follow-up. Radiol Clin N Am 2000;38:625–651.
11. Tabar L, Fagerberg G, Chen HH, et al. Efficacy of breast cancer screening by age. New results from the Swedish Two-County Trial. Cancer (Phila) 1995;75:2507–2517.
12. Alexander FE, Anderson TJ, Brown HK, et al. 14 years of follow-up from the Edinburgh randomised trial of breast-cancer screening. Lancet 1999;353:1903–1908.
13. Miller AB, To T, Baines CJ, Wall C. The Canadian National Breast Screening Study 1: breast cancer mortality after 11 to 16 years of follow-up. A randomized screening trial of mammography in women age 40 to 49 years. Ann Intern Med 2002;137: 305–312.
14. Tran NV, Evans GR, Kroll SS, et al. Postoperative adjuvant irradiation: effects on tranverse rectus abdominis muscle flap breast reconstruction. Plast Reconstr Surg 2000;106:313–317; discussion 318–320.
15. Kopans DB, Feig SA. The Canadian National Breast Screening Study: a critical review. AJR Am J Roentgenol 1993;161:755–760.
16. Tarone RE. The excess of patients with advanced breast cancer in young women screened with mammography in the Canadian National Breast Screening Study. Cancer (Phila) 1995;75: 997–1003.
17. Gotzsche PC, Olsen O. Is screening for breast cancer with mammography justifiable? Lancet 2000;355:129–134.

18. Olsen O, Gotzsche PC. Cochrane review on screening for breast cancer with mammography. Lancet 2001;358:1340–1342.
19. Feig SA. Effect of service screening mammography on population mortality from breast carcinoma. Cancer (Phila) 2002;95:451–457.
20. Tabar L, Vitak B, Chen HH, Yen MF, Duffy SW, Smith RA. Beyond randomized controlled trials: organized mammographic screening substantially reduces breast carcinoma mortality. Cancer (Phila) 2001;91:1724–1731.
21. Duffy SW, Tabar L, Chen HH, et al. The impact of organized mammography service screening on breast carcinoma mortality in seven Swedish counties. Cancer (Phila) 2002;95:458–469.
22. Radiology ACo. Breast Imaging-Reporting and Data System (BI-RADS). Reston, VA: American College of Radiology, 1998.
23. Kolb TM, Lichy J, Newhouse JH. Comparison of the performance of screening mammography, physical examination, and breast US and evaluation of factors that influence them: an analysis of 27,825 patient evaluations. Radiology 2002;225:165–175.
24. Kaplan SS. Clinical utility of bilateral whole-breast US in the evaluation of women with dense breast tissue. Radiology 2001;221:641–649.
25. Olson JA Jr, Morris EA, Van Zee KJ, Linehan DC, Borgen PI. Magnetic resonance imaging facilitates breast conservation for occult breast cancer. Ann Surg Oncol 2000;7:411–415.
26. Kriege M, Brekelmans CT, Boetes C, et al. Efficacy of MRI and mammography for breast-cancer screening in women with a familial or genetic predisposition. N Engl J Med 2004;351:427–437.
27. Liberman L. Breast cancer screening with MRI: what are the data for patients at high risk? N Engl J Med 2004;351:497–500.
28. Morris EA. Illustrated breast MR lexicon. Semin Roentgenol 2001;36:238–249.
29. Klimberg VS, Harms SE, Henry-Tillman RS. Not all MRI techniques are created equal. Ann Surg Oncol 2000;7:404–405.
30. Warner E, Plewes DB, Shumak RS, et al. Comparison of breast magnetic resonance imaging, mammography, and ultrasound for surveillance of women at high risk for hereditary breast cancer. J Clin Oncol 2001;19:3524–3531.
31. Stoutjesdijk MJ, Boetes C, Jager GJ, et al. Magnetic resonance imaging and mammography in women with a hereditary risk of breast cancer. J Natl Cancer Inst 2001;93:1095–1102.
32. Tillman GF, Orel SG, Schnall MD, Schultz DJ, Tan JE, Solin LJ. Effect of breast magnetic resonance imaging on the clinical management of women with early-stage breast carcinoma. J Clin Oncol 2002;20:3413–3423.
33. Hlawatsch A, Teifke A, Schmidt M, Thelen M. Preoperative assessment of breast cancer: sonography versus MR imaging. AJR Am J Roentgenol 2002;179:1493–1501.
34. Halsted W. The effects of adduction and abduction on the length of the limb in fractures of the neck of the femur. 1884. Clin Orthop Relat Res 1998;3(348):4–9.
35. Fisher B, Montague E, Redmond C, et al. Comparison of radical mastectomy with alternative treatments for primary breast cancer. A first report of results from a prospective randomized clinical trial. Cancer (Phila) 1977;39:2827–2839.
36. Fisher B, Jeong JH, Anderson S, Bryant J, Fisher ER, Wolmark N. Twenty-five-year follow-up of a randomized trial comparing radical mastectomy, total mastectomy, and total mastectomy followed by irradiation. N Engl J Med 2002;347:567–575.
37. Morris AD, Morris RD, Wilson JF, et al. Breast-conserving therapy vs. mastectomy in early-stage breast cancer: a meta-analysis of 10-year survival. Cancer J Sci Am 1997;3:6–12.
38. Fisher B, Anderson S, Bryant J, et al. Twenty-year follow-up of a randomized trial comparing total mastectomy, lumpectomy, and lumpectomy plus irradiation for the treatment of invasive breast cancer. N Engl J Med 2002;347:1233–1241.
39. Beaulac SM, McNair LA, Scott TE, LaMorte WW, Kavanah MT. Lymphedema and quality of life in survivors of early-stage breast cancer. Arch Surg 2002;137:1253–1257.
40. Coen JJ, Taghian AG, Kachnic LA, Assaad SI, Powell SN. Risk of lymphedema after regional nodal irradiation with breast conservation therapy. Int J Radiat Oncol Biol Phys 2003;55:1209–1215.
41. Petrek JA, Senie RT, Peters M, Rosen PP. Lymphedema in a cohort of breast carcinoma survivors 20 years after diagnosis. Cancer (Phila) 2001;92:1368–1377.
42. Erickson VS, Pearson ML, Ganz PA, Adams J, Kahn KL. Arm edema in breast cancer patients. J Natl Cancer Inst 2001;93:96–111.
43. Miltenburg DM, Miller C, Karamlou TB, Brunicardi FC. Meta-analysis of sentinel lymph node biopsy in breast cancer. J Surg Res 1999;84:138–142.
44. Kim T, Agboola O, Lyman G. Lymphatic mapping and sentinel lymph node sampling in breast cancer. In: Proceedings of the American Society of Clinical Oncology 2002 Annual Symposium, Orlando, FL, 2002. Chicago: American Society of Clinical Oncology, 2002.
45. Wilke LG, Giuliano A. Sentinel lymph node biopsy in patients with early-stage breast cancer: status of the National Clinical Trials. Surg Clin N Am 2003;83:901–910.
46. Newman L. Lymphatic mapping and sentinel lymph node biopsy in breast cancer patients: a comprehensive review of variations in performance and technique. J Am Coll Surg 2004;199(5):804–816.
47. Jordan VC. Third Annual William L. McGuire Memorial Lecture. Studies on the estrogen receptor in breast cancer: 20 years as a target for the treatment and prevention of cancer. Breast Cancer Res Treat 1995;36:267–285.
48. NCI. Breast Cancer (PDQ®): Treatment Health Professional Version, vol 2004. Washington, DC: National Cancer Institute, 2004.
49. NIH. Adjuvant therapy for breast cancer: NIH Consensus Statement. NIH 2000;17(4):1–35.
50. Gradishar WJ. Tamoxifen—what next? Oncologist 2004;9:378–384.
51. Anastrozole alone or in combination with tamoxifen versus tamoxifen alone for adjuvant treatment of postmenopausal women with early breast cancer: first results of the ATAC randomised trial. Lancet 2002;359:2131–2139.
52. Fisher B, Dignam J, Bryant J, Wolmark N. Five versus more than five years of tamoxifen for lymph node-negative breast cancer: updated findings from the National Surgical Adjuvant Breast and Bowel Project B-14 randomized trial. J Natl Cancer Inst 2001;93:684–690.
53. Goss P, Ingle J, Martino S, et al. Updated analysis of the NCIC CTG MA.17 randomized placebo-controlled trial of letrozole after five years of tamoxifen in postmenopausal women with early stage breast cancer. In: American Society of Clinical Oncology 2003 Annual Meeting, New Orleans, LA. Chicago: American Society of Clinical Oncology, 2003.
54. Goss PE, Ingle JN, Martino S, et al. A randomized trial of letrozole in postmenopausal women after five years of tamoxifen therapy for early-stage breast cancer. N Engl J Med 2003;349:1793–1802.
55. Coombes RC, Hall E, Gibson LJ, et al. A randomized trial of exemestane after two to three years of tamoxifen therapy in postmenopausal women with primary breast cancer. N Engl J Med 2004;350:1081–1092.
56. Gradishar WJ, Morrow M. Advances in endocrine therapy of metastatic breast cancer. Br J Surg 2002;89:1489–1492.
57. Beatson G. On the treatment of inoperable cases of carcinoma of the mamma: suggestions for a new method of treatment with illustrative cases. Lancet 1896;2:104–107, 162–165.
58. Lett H. An analysis of 99 cases of inoperable carcinoma of the breast treated by oophorectomy. Lancet 1905:227–228.

59. Ovarian ablation in early breast cancer: overview of the randomised trials. Early Breast Cancer Trialists' Collaborative Group. Lancet 1996;348:1189–1196.
60. Ovarian ablation for early breast cancer. Cochrane Database Syst Rev 2000:CD000485.
61. Prowell TM, Davidson NE. What is the role of ovarian ablation in the management of primary and metastatic breast cancer today? Oncologist 2004;9:507–517.
62. Sainsbury R. Ovarian ablation as a treatment for breast cancer. Surg Oncol 2003;12:241–250.
63. Poikonen P, Saarto T, Elomaa I, Joensuu H, Blomqvist C. Prognostic effect of amenorrhoea and elevated serum gonadotropin levels induced by adjuvant chemotherapy in premenopausal node-positive breast cancer patients. Eur J Cancer 2000;36: 43–48.
64. Del Mastro L, Venturini M, Sertoli MR, Rosso R. Amenorrhea induced by adjuvant chemotherapy in early breast cancer patients: prognostic role and clinical implications. Breast Cancer Res Treat 1997;43:183–190.
65. Pagani O, O'Neill A, Castiglione M, et al. Prognostic impact of amenorrhoea after adjuvant chemotherapy in premenopausal breast cancer patients with axillary node involvement: results of the International Breast Cancer Study Group (IBCSG) Trial VI. Eur J Cancer 1998;34:632–640.
66. Fisher B, Ravdin RG, Ausman RK, Slack NH, Moore GE, Noer RJ. Surgical adjuvant chemotherapy in cancer of the breast: results of a decade of cooperative investigation. Ann Surg 1968; 168:337–356.
67. Fentiman IS. Long-term follow-up of the first breast conservation trial: Guy' wide excision study. Breast 2000;9:5–8.
68. Vinh-Hung V, Verschraegen C. Breast-conserving surgery with or without radiotherapy: Pooled-analysis for risks of ipsilateral breast tumor recurrence and mortality. J Natl Cancer Inst 2004;96:115–121.
69. Effects of radiotherapy and surgery in early breast cancer. An overview of the randomized trials. Early Breast Cancer Trialists' Collaborative Group. N Engl J Med 1995;333:1444–1455.
70. Favourable and unfavourable effects on long-term survival of radiotherapy for early breast cancer: an overview of the randomised trials. Early Breast Cancer Trialists' Collaborative Group. Lancet 2000;355:1757–1770.
71. Overgaard M, Hansen PS, Overgaard J, et al. Postoperative radiotherapy in high-risk premenopausal women with breast cancer who receive adjuvant chemotherapy. Danish Breast Cancer Cooperative Group 82b Trial. N Engl J Med 1997;337:949–955.
72. Overgaard M, Jensen MB, Overgaard J, et al. Postoperative radiotherapy in high-risk postmenopausal breast-cancer patients given adjuvant tamoxifen: Danish Breast Cancer Cooperative Group DBCG 82c randomised trial. Lancet 1999;353:1641–1648.
73. Broadwater JR, Edwards MJ, Kuglen C, Hortobagyi GN, Ames FC, Balch CM. Mastectomy following preoperative chemotherapy. Strict operative criteria control operative morbidity. Ann Surg 1991;213:126–129.
74. Danforth DN Jr., Lippman ME, McDonald H, et al. Effect of preoperative chemotherapy on mastectomy for locally advanced breast cancer. Am Surg 1990;56:6–11.
75. McCready DR, Hortobagyi GN, Kau SW, Smith TL, Buzdar AU, Balch CM. The prognostic significance of lymph node metastases after preoperative chemotherapy for locally advanced breast cancer. Arch Surg 1989;124:21–25.
76. De Lena M, Varini M, Zucali R, et al. Multimodal treatment for locally advanced breast cancer. Result of chemotherapy-radiotherapy versus chemotherapy-surgery. Cancer Clin Trials 1981;4:229–236.
77. Perloff M, Lesnick GJ, Korzun A, et al. Combination chemotherapy with mastectomy or radiotherapy for stage III breast carcinoma: a Cancer and Leukemia Group B study. J Clin Oncol 1988;6:261–269.
78. Papaioannou A, Lissaios B, Vasilaros S, et al. Pre and postoperative chemoendocrine treatment with or without postoperative radiotherapy for locally advanced breast cancer. Cancer (Phila) 1983;51:1284–1290.
79. Hortobagyi GN, Ames FC, Buzdar AU, et al. Management of stage III primary breast cancer with primary chemotherapy, surgery, and radiation therapy. Cancer (Phila) 1988;62:2507–2516.
80. Lippman ME, Sorace RA, Bagley CS, Danforth DW Jr, Lichter A, Wesley MN. Treatment of locally advanced breast cancer using primary induction chemotherapy with hormonal synchronization followed by radiation therapy with or without debulking surgery. Natl Cancer Inst Monogr 1986;1986:153–159.
81. Mauriac L, Durand M, Avril A, Dilhuydy JM. Effects of primary chemotherapy in conservative treatment of breast cancer patients with operable tumors larger than 3 cm. Results of a randomized trial in a single centre. Ann Oncol 1991;2:347–354.
82. Mauriac L, MacGrogan G, Avril A, et al. Neoadjuvant chemotherapy for operable breast carcinoma larger than 3 cm: a unicentre randomized trial with a 124-month median follow-up. Institut Bergonie Bordeaux Groupe Sein (IBBGS). Ann Oncol 1999;10:47–52.
83. Schwartz GF, Birchansky CA, Komarnicky LT, et al. Induction chemotherapy followed by breast conservation for locally advanced carcinoma of the breast. Cancer (Phila) 1994;73:362–369.
84. Schwartz GF, Lange AK, Topham AK. Breast conservation following induction chemotherapy for locally advanced carcinoma of the breast (stages IIB and III). A surgical perspective. Surg Oncol Clin N Am 1995;4:657–669.
85. Powles TJ, Hickish TF, Makris A, et al. Randomized trial of chemoendocrine therapy started before or after surgery for treatment of primary breast cancer. J Clin Oncol 1995;13:547–552.
86. Makris A, Powles TJ, Ashley SE, et al. A reduction in the requirements for mastectomy in a randomized trial of neoadjuvant chemoendocrine therapy in primary breast cancer. Ann Oncol 1998;9:1179–1184.
87. Fisher B, Brown A, Mamounas E, et al. Effect of preoperative chemotherapy on local-regional disease in women with operable breast cancer: findings from National Surgical Adjuvant Breast and Bowel Project B-18. J Clin Oncol 1997;15:2483–2493.
88. Fisher B, Bryant J, Wolmark N, et al. Effect of preoperative chemotherapy on the outcome of women with operable breast cancer. J Clin Oncol 1998;16:2672–2685.
89. Kuerer HM, Newman LA, Smith TL, et al. Clinical course of breast cancer patients with complete pathologic primary tumor and axillary lymph node response to doxorubicin-based neoadjuvant chemotherapy. J Clin Oncol 1999;17:460–469.
90. Singletary SE, McNeese MD, Hortobagyi GN. Feasibility of breast-conservation surgery after induction chemotherapy for locally advanced breast carcinoma. Cancer (Phila) 1992;69:2849–2852.
91. Wolmark N, Wang J, Mamounas E, Bryant J, Fisher B. Preoperative chemotherapy in patients with operable breast cancer: nine-year results from National Surgical Adjuvant Breast and Bowel Project B-18. J Natl Cancer Inst Monogr 2001;2001:96–102.
92. Newman LA, Buzdar AU, Singletary SE, et al. A prospective trial of preoperative chemotherapy in resectable breast cancer: predictors of breast-conservation therapy feasibility. Ann Surg Oncol 2002;9:228–234.
93. Mathieu MC, Rouzier R, Llombart-Cussac A, et al. The poor responsiveness of infiltrating lobular breast carcinomas to neoadjuvant chemotherapy can be explained by their biological profile. Eur J Cancer 2004;40:342–351.
94. Bedrosian I, Reynolds C, Mick R, et al. Accuracy of sentinel lymph node biopsy in patients with large primary breast tumors. Cancer (Phila) 2000;88:2540–2545.

95. Chung M, Ye W, Giuliano A. Role for sentinel lymph node dissection in the management of large (> or +5 cm) invasive breast cancer. Ann Surg Oncol 2001;8:688–692.
96. Breslin TM, Cohen L, Sahin A, et al. Sentinel lymph node biopsy is accurate after neoadjuvant chemotherapy for breast cancer. J Clin Oncol 2000;18:3480–3486.
97. Xing Y, Ding M, Cox D, Ross M, Hunt K, Cormier J. Meta-analysis of sentinel lymph node biopsy following preoperative chemotherapy in patients with operable breast cancer. ASCO Ann Meet 2004, (abstract 561).
98. Fisher ER, Leeming R, Anderson S, Redmond C, Fisher B. Conservative management of intraductal carcinoma (DCIS) of the breast. Collaborating NSABP investigators. J Surg Oncol 1991;47:139–147.
99. Julien JP, Bijker N, Fentiman IS, et al. Radiotherapy in breast-conserving treatment for ductal carcinoma in situ: first results of the EORTC randomised phase III trial 10853. EORTC Breast Cancer Cooperative Group and EORTC Radiotherapy Group. Lancet 2000;355:528–533.
100. Fisher ER, Dignam J, Tan-Chiu E, et al. Pathologic findings from the National Surgical Adjuvant Breast Project (NSABP) eight-year update of Protocol B-17: intraductal carcinoma. Cancer (Phila) 1999;86:429–438.
101. Fisher B, Dignam J, Wolmark N, et al. Tamoxifen in treatment of intraductal breast cancer: National Surgical Adjuvant Breast and Bowel Project B-24 randomised controlled trial. Lancet 1999;353:1993–2000.
102. Fisher B, Dignam J, Wolmark N, et al. Lumpectomy and radiation therapy for the treatment of intraductal breast cancer: findings from National Surgical Adjuvant Breast and Bowel Project B-17. J Clin Oncol 1998;16:441–452.
103. Bijker N, Peterse JL, Duchateau L, et al. Risk factors for recurrence and metastasis after breast-conserving therapy for ductal carcinoma-in-situ: analysis of European Organization for Research and Treatment of Cancer Trial 10853. J Clin Oncol 2001;19:2263–2271.
104. Boyages J, Delaney G, Taylor R. Predictors of local recurrence after treatment of ductal carcinoma in situ: a meta-analysis. Cancer (Phila) 1999;85:616–628.
105. Clark L, Ritter E, Glazebrook K, Tyler D. Recurrent ductal carcinoma in situ after total mastectomy. J Surg Oncol 1999;71:182–185.
106. Montgomery R, Goldstein L, Hoffman J, et al. Local recurrence after mastectomy for ductal carcinoma in situ. Breast J 1998;4:430–436.
107. Silverstein MJ, Lagios MD, Craig PH, et al. A prognostic index for ductal carcinoma in situ of the breast. Cancer (Phila) 1996;77:2267–2274.
108. Silverstein MJ. The University of Southern California/Van Nuys prognostic index for ductal carcinoma in situ of the breast. Am J Surg 2003;186:337–343.
109. Consensus conference of the classification of ductal carcinoma in situ. Cancer (Phila) 1997;1997:1798–1802.
110. Wong J, Gadd M, Gelman R, et al. Wide excision alone for ductal carcinoma in situ of the breast. In: Proceedings of the 26th Annual San Antonio Breast Cancer Symposium, Breast Cancer Research and Treatment, San Antonio, TX, 2003, vol 82 (suppl 1).
111. Intra M, Veronesi P, Mazzarol G, et al. Axillary sentinel lymph node biopsy in patients with pure ductal carcinoma in situ of the breast. Arch Surg 2003;138:309–313.
112. Pendas S, Dauway E, Giuliano R, Ku N, Cox CE, Reintgen DS. Sentinel node biopsy in ductal carcinoma in situ patients. Ann Surg Oncol 2000;7:15–20.
113. Houghton J, George WD, Cuzick J, Duggan C, Fentiman IS, Spittle M. Radiotherapy and tamoxifen in women with completely excised ductal carcinoma in situ of the breast in the UK, Australia, and New Zealand: randomised controlled trial. Lancet 2003;362:95–102.
114. Allred C. 25th Annual San Antonio Breast Cancer Symposium, San Antonio, Texas, 2002.
115. Julian T, Land S, Wolmark N. NSABP B-35: A clinical trial to compare anastrazole and tamoxifen for postmenopausal patients with ductal carcinoma in situ undergoing lumpectomy with radiation therapy. Breast Diseases: A Yearbook Quarterly 2003;14:121–122.
116. Fisher B, Costantino JP, Wickerham DL, et al. Tamoxifen for prevention of breast cancer: report of the National Surgical Adjuvant Breast and Bowel Project P-1 Study. J Natl Cancer Inst 1998;90:1371–1388.
117. King MC, Wieand S, Hale K, et al. Tamoxifen and breast cancer incidence among women with inherited mutations in BRCA1 and BRCA2: National Surgical Adjuvant Breast and Bowel Project (NSABP-P1) Breast Cancer Prevention Trial. JAMA 2001;286:2251–2256.
118. Gram IT, Ursin G, Spicer DV, Pike MC. Reversal of gonadotropin-releasing hormone agonist induced reductions in mammographic densities on stopping treatment. Cancer Epidemiol Biomarkers Prev 2001;10:1117–1120.
119. Baum M, Budzar AU, Cuzick J, et al. Anastrozole alone or in combination with tamoxifen versus tamoxifen alone for adjuvant treatment of postmenopausal women with early breast cancer: first results of the ATAC randomised trial. Lancet 2002;359:213–219.
120. Cuzick J, Powles T, Veronesi U, et al. Overview of the main outcomes in breast-cancer prevention trials. Lancet 2003;361:296–300.
121. Powles T, Eeles R, Ashley S, et al. Interim analysis of the incidence of breast cancer in the Royal Marsden Hospital tamoxifen randomised chemoprevention trial. Lancet 1998;352:98–101.
122. Veronesi U, Maisonneuve P, Rotmensz N, et al. Italian randomized trial among women with hysterectomy: tamoxifen and hormone-dependent breast cancer in high-risk women. J Natl Cancer Inst 2003;95:160–165.
123. Veronesi U, Maisonneuve P, Sacchini V, Rotmensz N, Boyle P. Tamoxifen for breast cancer among hysterectomised women. Lancet 2002;359:1122–1124.
124. Veronesi U, Maisonneuve P, Costa A, et al. Prevention of breast cancer with tamoxifen: preliminary findings from the Italian randomised trial among hysterectomised women. Italian Tamoxifen Prevention Study. Lancet 1998;352:93–97.
125. First results from the International Breast Cancer Intervention Study (IBIS-I): a randomised prevention trial. Lancet 2002;360:817–824.
126. Cauley JA, Norton L, Lippman ME, et al. Continued breast cancer risk reduction in postmenopausal women treated with raloxifene: 4-year results from the MORE trial. Multiple outcomes of raloxifene evaluation. Breast Cancer Res Treat 2001;65:125–134.
127. Veronesi U, De Palo G, Marubini E, et al. Randomized trial of fenretinide to prevent second breast malignancy in women with early breast cancer. J Natl Cancer Inst 1999;91:1847–1856.
128. Nagata C, Takatsuka N, Inaba S, Kawakami N, Shimizu H. Effect of soymilk consumption on serum estrogen concentrations in premenopausal Japanese women. J Natl Cancer Inst 1998;90:1830–1835.
129. Rebbeck TR, Levin AM, Eisen A, et al. Breast cancer risk after bilateral prophylactic oophorectomy in BRCA1 mutation carriers. J Natl Cancer Inst 1999;91:1475–1479.
130. Kauff ND, Satagopan JM, Robson ME, et al. Risk-reducing salpingo-oophorectomy in women with a BRCA1 or BRCA2 mutation. N Engl J Med 2002;346:1609–1615.
131. Pennisi VR, Capozzi A. Subcutaneous mastectomy data: a final statistical analysis of 1500 patients. Aesthetic Plast Surg 1989;13:15–21.

132. Woods JE, Meland NB. Conservative management in full-thickness nipple-areolar necrosis after subcutaneous mastectomy. Plast Reconstr Surg 1989;84:258–264; discussion 265–266.
133. Hartmann LC, Schaid DJ, Woods JE, et al. Efficacy of bilateral prophylactic mastectomy in women with a family history of breast cancer. N Engl J Med 1999;340:77–84.
134. Hartmann LC, Sellers TA, Schaid DJ, et al. Efficacy of bilateral prophylactic mastectomy in BRCA1 and BRCA2 gene mutation carriers. J Natl Cancer Inst 2001;93:1633–1637.
135. Meijers-Heijboer H, van Geel B, van Putten WL, et al. Breast cancer after prophylactic bilateral mastectomy in women with a BRCA1 or BRCA2 mutation. N Engl J Med 2001;345:159–164.
136. Ingle JN, Suman VJ. Aromatase inhibitors versus tamoxifen for management of postmenopausal breast cancer in the advanced disease and neoadjuvant settings. J Steroid Biochem Mol Biol 2003;86:313–319.
137. Ahmann DL, Schaid DJ, Bisel HF, Hahn RG, Edmonson JH, Ingle JN. The effect on survival of initial chemotherapy in advanced breast cancer: polychemotherapy versus single drug. J Clin Oncol 1987;5:1928–1932.
138. O'Shaughnessy J, Miles D, Vukelja S, et al. Superior survival with capecitabine plus docetaxel combination therapy in anthracycline-pretreated patients with advanced breast cancer: phase III trial results. J Clin Oncol 2002;20:2812–2823.
139. Slamon DJ, Leyland-Jones B, Shak S, et al. Use of chemotherapy plus a monoclonal antibody against HER2 for metastatic breast cancer that overexpresses HER2. N Engl J Med 2001;344:783–792.
140. Chia S, Speers C, Kang A, et al. The impact of new chemotherapeutic and hormonal agents on the survival of women with metastatic beast cancer in a population based cohort. Proc Am Soc Clin Oncol 2003;22:6a.
141. Osborne CK. Tamoxifen in the treatment of breast cancer. N Engl J Med 1998;339:1609–1618.
142. Early Breast Cancer Trialist's Collaborative Group. Tamoxifen for early breast cancer: an overview of the randomised trials. Lancet 1998;351:1451–1467.
143. Mass R. The role of HER-2 expression in predicting response to therapy in breast cancer. Semin Oncol 2000;27:46–52; discussion 92–100.
144. Vogel CL, Cobleigh MA, Tripathy D, et al. Efficacy and safety of trastuzumab as a single agent in first-line treatment of HER2-overexpressing metastatic breast cancer. J Clin Oncol 2002;20:719–726.
145. Seidman A, Berry D, Cirrincione C, et al. CALGB 9840: Phase III study of weekly paclitaxel via 1-hour infusion versus standard 3h infusion every third week in the treatment of metastatic breast cancer with trasuzumab for HER2 positive MBC and randomized for trastuzumab in HER2 normal MBC. Proc Am Soc Clin Oncol 2004;23:6s (abstract 512).
146. Schrag D, Garewal HS, Burstein HJ, Samson DJ, Von Hoff DD, Somerfield MR. American Society of Clinical Oncology Technology Assessment: chemotherapy sensitivity and resistance assays. J Clin Oncol 2004;22:3631–3638.
147. Samson DJ, Seidenfeld J, Ziegler K, Aronson N. Chemotherapy sensitivity and resistance assays: a systematic review. J Clin Oncol 2004;22:3618–3630.
148. Styczynski J, Wysocki M. Is the in vitro drug resistance profile the strongest prognostic factor in childhood acute lymphoblastic leukemia? J Clin Oncol 2004;22:963–964.
149. Osborne CK, Kitten L, Arteaga CL. Antagonism of chemotherapy-induced cytotoxicity for human breast cancer cells by antiestrogens. J Clin Oncol 1989;7:710–717.
150. Albain KS, Green S, Ravdin P, et al. Adjuvant chemohormonal therapy for primary breast cancer should be sequential instead of concurrent: Initial results from intergroup trial 0100. Proc Am Soc Clin Oncol 2002;21:37a (abstract 143).
151. Buzdar AU, Jonat W, Howell A, et al. Anastrozole versus megestrol acetate in the treatment of postmenopausal women with advanced breast carcinoma: results of a survival update based on a combined analysis of data from two mature phase III trials. Arimidex Study Group. Cancer (Phila) 1998;83:1142–1152.
152. Dombernowsky P, Smith I, Falkson G, et al. Letrozole, a new oral aromatase inhibitor for advanced breast cancer: double-blind randomized trial showing a dose effect and improved efficacy and tolerability compared with megestrol acetate. J Clin Oncol 1998;16:453–461.
153. Gershanovich M, Chaudri HA, Campos D, et al. Letrozole, a new oral aromatase inhibitor: randomised trial comparing 2.5 mg daily, 0.5 mg daily and aminoglutethimide in postmenopausal women with advanced breast cancer. Letrozole International Trial Group (AR/BC3). Ann Oncol 1998;9:639–645.
154. Marty M, Gershanovich M, Campos B, et al. Letrozole, a new potent, selective aromatase inhibitor (AI) superior to aminoglutethimide in postmenopausal women with advanced breast cancer previously treated with antiestrogens. Proc Am Soc Clin Oncol 1997;16: abstract 544.
155. Mouridsen H, Gershanovich M, Sun Y, et al. Superior efficacy of letrozole versus tamoxifen as first-line therapy for postmenopausal women with advanced breast cancer: results of a phase III study of the International Letrozole Breast Cancer Group. J Clin Oncol 2001;19:2596–2606.
156. Paridaens R, Dirix L, Lohrisch C, et al. Mature results of a randomized phase II multicenter study of exemestane versus tamoxifen as first-line hormone therapy for postmenopausal women with metastatic breast cancer. Ann Oncol 2003;14:1391–1398.
157. Howell A, Robertson JF, Quaresma Albano J, et al. Fulvestrant, formerly ICI 182,780, is as effective as anastrozole in postmenopausal women with advanced breast cancer progressing after prior endocrine treatment. J Clin Oncol 2002;20:3396–3403.
158. Osborne CK, Pippen J, Jones SE, et al. Double-blind, randomized trial comparing the efficacy and tolerability of fulvestrant versus anastrozole in postmenopausal women with advanced breast cancer progressing on prior endocrine therapy: results of a North American trial. J Clin Oncol 2002;20:3386–3395.
159. Howell A, Robertson JF, Abram P, et al. Comparison of fulvestrant versus tamoxifen for the treatment of advanced breast cancer in postmenopausal women previously untreated with endocrine therapy: a multinational, double-blind, randomized trial. J Clin Oncol 2004;22:1605–1613.
160. Klijn JG, Blamey RW, Boccardo F, Tominaga T, Duchateau L, Sylvester R. Combined tamoxifen and luteinizing hormone-releasing hormone (LHRH) agonist versus LHRH agonist alone in premenopausal advanced breast cancer: a meta-analysis of four randomized trials. J Clin Oncol 2001;19:343–353.
161. Taylor CW, Green S, Dalton WS, et al. Multicenter randomized clinical trial of goserelin versus surgical ovariectomy in premenopausal patients with receptor-positive metastatic breast cancer: an intergroup study. J Clin Oncol 1998;16:994–999.
162. Aisner J, Weinberg V, Perloff M, et al. Chemotherapy versus chemoimmunotherapy (CAF v CAFVP v CMF each ± MER) for metastatic carcinoma of the breast: a CALGB study. J Clin Oncol 1987;5:1523–1533.
163. Hayes DF, Henderson IC. CAF in metastatic breast cancer: standard therapy or another effective regimen. J Clin Oncol 1987;5:1497–1499.
164. Heidemann E, Stoeger H, Souchon R, et al. Is first-line single-agent mitoxantrone in the treatment of high-risk metastatic breast cancer patients as effective as combination chemotherapy? No difference in survival but higher quality of life were found in a multicenter randomized trial. Ann Oncol 2002;13:1717–1729.

165. Cocconi G, Bisagni G, Bella M, et al. Comparison of CMF (cyclophosphamide, methotrexate, and 5-fluorouracil) with a rotational crossing and a sequential intensification regimen in advanced breast cancer: a prospective randomized study. Am J Clin Oncol 1999;22:593–600.
166. Miles D, von Minckwitz G, Seidman AD. Combination versus sequential single-agent therapy in metastatic breast cancer. Oncologist 2002;7(suppl 6):13–19.
167. Bishop JF, Dewar J, Toner GC, et al. Initial paclitaxel improves outcome compared with CMFP combination chemotherapy as front-line therapy in untreated metastatic breast cancer. J Clin Oncol 1999;17:2355–2364.
168. Sledge GW, Neuberg D, Bernardo P, et al. Phase III trial of doxorubicin, paclitaxel, and the combination of doxorubicin and paclitaxel as front-line chemotherapy for metastatic breast cancer: an intergroup trial (E1193). J Clin Oncol 2003;21:588–592.
169. Sparano JA. Taxanes for breast cancer: an evidence-based review of randomized phase II and phase III trials. Clin Breast Cancer 2000;1:32–40; discussion 41–42.
170. Albain KS, Nag S, Calderillo-ruiz G, et al. Global phase III study of gemcitabine plus paclitaxel vs. paclitaxel as frontline therapy for metastatic breast cancer: first report of overall survival. Proc Am Soc Clin Oncol 2004;23:5 (abstract 510).
171. Baselga J, Tripathy D, Mendelsohn J, et al. Phase II study of weekly intravenous recombinant humanized anti-p185HER2 monoclonal antibody in patients with HER2/neu-overexpressing metastatic breast cancer. J Clin Oncol 1996;14: 737–744.
172. Cobleigh MA, Vogel CL, Tripathy D, et al. Multinational study of the efficacy and safety of humanized anti-HER2 monoclonal antibody in women who have HER2-overexpressing metastatic breast cancer that has progressed after chemotherapy for metastatic disease. J Clin Oncol 1999;17:2639–2648.
173. Burstein HJ, Kuter I, Campos SM, et al. Clinical activity of trastuzumab and vinorelbine in women with HER2-overexpressing metastatic breast cancer. J Clin Oncol 2001;19:2722–2730.
174. Miller KD, Sisk J, Ansari R, et al. Gemcitabine, paclitaxel, and trastuzumab in metastatic breast cancer. Oncology (Huntingt) 2001;15:38–40.
175. O'Shaughnessy J, Vukelja SJ, Marsland T, Kimmel G, Ratnam S, Pippen J. Phase II trial of gemcitabine plus trastuzumab in metastatic breast cancer patients previously treated with chemotherapy: preliminary results. Clin Breast Cancer 2002; 3(suppl 1):17–20.
176. Hayes DF, Thor AD. c-erbB-2 in breast cancer: development of a clinically useful marker. Semin Oncol 2002;29:231–245.
177. Cobleigh MA, Langmuir VK, Sledge GW, et al. A phase I/II dose-escalation trial of bevacizumab in previously treated metastatic breast cancer. Semin Oncol 2003;30:117–124.
178. Albain K, Elledge RM, Gradishar WJ, et al. Open-label, phase II, multicenter trial of ZD1839 ('Iressa') in patients with advanced breast cancer. Breast Cancer Res Treat 2002;76:S33.
179. Baselga J, Albanell J, Ruiz A, et al. Phase II and tumor pharmacodynamic study of gefitinib in patients with advanced breast cancer. Proc Am Soc Clin Oncol 2003;22:7 (abstract 24).
180. Stearns V, Yamauchi H, Hayes DF. Circulating tumor markers in breast cancer: accepted utilities and novel prospects. Breast Cancer Res Treat 1998;52:239–259.
181. Cristofanilli M, Budd GT, Ellis MJ, et al. Circulating tumor cells, disease progression, and survival in metastatic breast cancer. N Engl J Med 2004;351:781–791.
182. Allard WJ, Matera J, Miller MC, et al. Tumor cells circulate in the peripheral blood of all major carcinomas but not in healthy subjects or patients with nonmalignant diseases. Clin Cancer Res 2004;10:6897–6904.
183. Veronesi U, Cascinelli N, Mariani L, et al. Twenty-year follow-up of a randomized study comparing breast-conserving surgery with radical mastectomy for early breast cancer. N Engl J Med 2002;347:1227–1232.
184. Poggi MM, Danforth DN, Sciuto LC, et al. Eighteen-year results in the treatment of early breast carcinoma with mastectomy versus breast conservation therapy: the National Cancer Institute Randomized Trial. Cancer (Phila) 2003;98:697–702.
185. Van Dongen J, Bartelink H, Fentiman I. Factors influencing local relapse and survival and results of salvage treatment after breast-conserving therapy in operable breast cancer: EORTC trial 10801, breast conservation compared with mastectomy in TNM stage I and II breast cancer. Eur J Cancer 1992;28A:801–805.
186. van Dongen JA, Voogd AC, Fentiman IS, et al. Long-term results of a randomized trial comparing breast-conserving therapy with mastectomy: European Organization for Research and Treatment of Cancer 10801 trial. J Natl Cancer Inst 2000;92: 1143–1150.
187. Sarrazin D, Le MG, Arriagada R, et al. Ten-year results of a randomized trial comparing a conservative treatment to mastectomy in early breast cancer. Radiother Oncol 1989;14:177–184.
188. Blichert-Toft M, Rose CA, Anderson J. Danish randomized trial comparing breast conservation therapy with mastectomy: six years of life-table analysis, Danish Breast Cancer Cooperative Group. J Natl Cancer Inst Monogr 1992;11:19–25.
189. Voogd AC, Nielsen M, Peterse JL, et al. Differences in risk factors for local and distant recurrence after breast-conserving therapy or mastectomy for stage I and II breast cancer: pooled results of two large European randomized trials. J Clin Oncol 2001;19:1688–1697.
190. Tamoxifen for early breast cancer: an overview of the randomised trials. Early Breast Cancer Trialists' Collaborative Group. Lancet 1998;351:1451–1467.
191. Tamoxifen for early breast cancer. Cochrane Database Syst Rev 2001:CD000486.
192. Multi-agent chemotherapy for early breast cancer. Cochrane Database Syst Rev 2002:CD000487.
193. Polychemotherapy for early breast cancer: an overview of the randomised trials. Early Breast Cancer Trialists' Collaborative Group. Lancet 1998;352:930–942.
194. Radiotherapy for early breast cancer. Cochrane Database Syst Rev 2002:CD003647.
195. Klijn J, Group AT. The ATAC trial: An efficacy update, focusing on breast cancer events, based on a median follow-up of 47 months. Proc Am Soc Clin Oncol 2003;22: abstract 338.
196. Adjuvant ovarian ablation versus CMF chemotherapy in premenopausal women with pathological stage II breast carcinoma: the Scottish trial. Scottish Cancer Trials Breast Group and ICRF Breast Unit, Guy's Hospital, London. Lancet 1993;341:1293–1298.
197. Roche H, Mihura J, de Lafontan B, et al. Castration and tamoxifen versus chemotherapy (FAC) for premenopausal, node and receptor-positive breast cancer patients: a randomized trial with a 7 years median follow-up. Proc Am Soc Clin Oncol 1996;15:117 (abstract 134).
198. Ejlertsen B, Dombernowsky P, Mouridsen H, et al. Comparable effect of ovarian ablation and CMF chemotherapy on premenopausal hormone receptor positive breast cancer patients, abstract no. 248. Proc Am Soc Clin Oncol 1999;18:66a.
199. Rutqvist L. Zoladex [trade] and tamoxifen as adjuvant therapy in premenopausal breast cancer: a randomised trial by the Cancer Research Campaign (C.R.C.) Breast Cancer Trials Group, the Stockholm Breast Cancer Study Group, the South-East Sweden Breast Cancer Group, & the Gruppo Interdisciplinare Valutazione Interventi in Oncologia (G.I.V.I.O). Proc Am Soc Clin Oncol 1999, (abstract 251).
200. Boccardo F, Rubagotti A, Amoroso D, et al. Cyclophosphamide, methotrexate, and fluorouracil versus tamoxifen plus ovarian

suppression as adjuvant treatment of estrogen receptor-positive pre-/perimenopausal breast cancer patients: results of the Italian Breast Cancer Adjuvant Study Group 02 randomized trial. boccardo@hp380.ist.unige.it. J Clin Oncol 2000;18:2718–2727.

201. Schmid P, Untch M, Wallwiener D, et al. Cyclophosphamide, methotrexate and fluorouracil (CMF) versus hormonal ablation with leuprorelin acetate as adjuvant treatment of node-positive, premenopausal breast cancer patients: preliminary results of the TABLE-study (Takeda Adjuvant Breast cancer study with Leuprorelin Acetate). Anticancer Res 2002;22:2325–2332.
202. International Breast Cancer Study Group. Randomized controlled trial of ovarian function suppression plus tamoxifen versus the same endocrine therapy plus chemotherapy: Is chemotherapy necessary for premenopausal women with node-positive, endocrine-responsive breast cancer? First results of International Study Group Trial 11–93. Breast 2001;10:130–138.
203. Jonat W, Kaufmann M, Sauerbrei W, et al. Goserelin versus cyclophosphamide, methotrexate, and fluorouracil as adjuvant therapy in premenopausal patients with node-positive breast cancer: The Zoladex Early Breast Cancer Research Association Study. J Clin Oncol 2002;20:4628–4635.
204. Kaufmann M, Jonat W, Blamey R, et al. Survival analyses from the ZEBRA study. Goserelin (Zoladex) versus CMF in premenopausal women with node-positive breast cancer. Eur J Cancer 2003;39:1711–1717.
205. Jakesz R, Hausmaninger H, Kubista E, et al. Randomized adjuvant trial of tamoxifen and goserelin versus cyclophosphamide, methotrexate, and fluorouracil: evidence for the superiority of treatment with endocrine blockade in premenopausal patients with hormone-responsive breast cancer: Austrian Breast and Colorectal Cancer Study Group Trial 5. J Clin Oncol 2002;20:4621–4627.
206. Love RR, Duc NB, Allred DC, et al. Oophorectomy and tamoxifen adjuvant therapy in premenopausal Vietnamese and Chinese women with operable breast cancer. J Clin Oncol 2002;20:2559–2566.
207. Castiglione-Gertsch M, O'Neill A, Price KN, et al. Adjuvant chemotherapy followed by goserelin versus either modality alone for premenopausal lymph node-negative breast cancer: a randomized trial. J Natl Cancer Inst 2003;95:1833–1846.
208. Arriagada R, Le M, Spielmann M, et al. Randomized trial of adjuvant ovarian suppression in 926 premenopausal patients with early breast cancer treated with adjuvant chemotherapy. Proc Am Soc Clin Oncol 2003;22:14a (abstract 14).
209. Davidson NE, O'Neill A, Vukov A. Chemohormonal therapy in premenopausal node-positive, receptor-positive breast cancer: an Eastern Cooperative Oncology Group phase III intergroup trial (E5188, INT-0101). Proc Am Soc Clin Oncol 2003;22:15a (abstract 15).
210. Henderson IC, Berry DA, Demetri GD, et al. Improved outcomes from adding sequential Paclitaxel but not from escalating Doxorubicin dose in an adjuvant chemotherapy regimen for patients with node-positive primary breast cancer. J Clin Oncol 2003;21:976–983.
211. Mamounas E, Bryant J, Lembersky B, et al. Paclitaxel following doxorubicin/cyclophosphamide as adjuvant chemotherapy for node-positive breast cancer: Results from NSABP B-28. Proc Am Soc Clin Oncol 2003;22: abstract 12.
212. Martin M, Pienkowski T, Mackey J, et al. TAC improves disease-free survival and overall survival over FAC in node-positive early breast cancer patients, BCIRG 001:55 months follow-up. In: San Antonio Breast Cancer Symposium 2003, San Antonio, TX, 2003, abstract 43.
213. Citron ML, Berry DA, Cirrincione C, et al. Randomized trial of dose-dense versus conventionally scheduled and sequential versus concurrent combination chemotherapy as postoperative adjuvant treatment of node-positive primary breast cancer: first report of Intergroup Trial C9741/Cancer and Leukemia Group B Trial 9741. J Clin Oncol 2003;21:1431–1439.
214. McArdle CS, Crawford D, Dykes EH, et al. Adjuvant radiotherapy and chemotherapy in breast cancer. Br J Surg 1986;73:264–266.
215. Ragaz J, Jackson SM, Le N, et al. Adjuvant radiotherapy and chemotherapy in node-positive premenopausal women with breast cancer. N Engl J Med 1997;337:956–962.
216. Griem KL, Henderson IC, Gelman R, et al. The 5-year results of a randomized trial of adjuvant radiation therapy after chemotherapy in breast cancer patients treated with mastectomy. J Clin Oncol 1987;5:1546–1555.
217. Velez-Garcia E, Carpenter JT, Jr., Moore M, et al. Postsurgical adjuvant chemotherapy with or without radiotherapy in women with breast cancer and positive axillary nodes: a South-Eastern Cancer Study Group (SEG) Trial. Eur J Cancer 1992;28A:1833–1837.
218. Tennvall-Nittby L, Tengrup I, Landberg T. The total incidence of loco-regional recurrence in a randomized trial of breast cancer TNM stage II. The South Sweden Breast Cancer Trial. Acta Oncol 1993;32:641–646.
219. Olson JE, Neuberg D, Pandya KJ, et al. The role of radiotherapy in the management of operable locally advanced breast carcinoma: results of a randomized trial by the Eastern Cooperative Oncology Group. Cancer (Phila) 1997;79:1138–1149.
220. Ahmann DL, O'Fallon JR, Scanlon PW, et al. A preliminary assessment of factors associated with recurrent disease in a surgical adjuvant clinical trial for patients with breast cancer with special emphasis on the aggressiveness of therapy. Am J Clin Oncol 1982;5:371–381.
221. Martinez A, Ahmann DL, O'Fallon J. An interim analysis of the randomized surgical adjuvant trial for patients with unfavorable breast cancer. Int J Radiat Oncol Biol Phys 1984;10(suppl 2):106.
222. Recht A, Edge SB, Solin LJ, et al. Postmastectomy radiotherapy: clinical practice guidelines of the American Society of Clinical Oncology. J Clin Oncol 2001;19:1539–1569.
223. Recht A, Edge SB. Evidence-based indications for postmastectomy irradiation. Surg Clin N Am 2003;83:995–1013.
224. Schmoor C, Bastert G, Dunst J, et al. Randomized trial on the effect of radiotherapy in addition to 6 cycles CMF in node-positive breast-cancer patients. The German Breast-Cancer Study Group. Int J Cancer 2000;86:408–415.
225. Hayat H, Brufman G, Borovik R. Adjuvant chemotherapy and radiation therapy vs. chemotherapy alone for Stage II breast cancer patients. Ann Oncol 1990;1S:21.
226. Gervasio H, Alves H, Rito A. Phase III study: adjuvant chemotherapy versus adjuvant radiotherapy plus chemotherapy in women with node-positive breast cancer. Breast J 1998;4(suppl 1):S88.
227. Klefstrom P, Grohn P, Heinonen E, Holsti L, Holsti P. Adjuvant postoperative radiotherapy, chemotherapy, and immunotherapy in stage III breast cancer. II. 5-year results and influence of levamisole. Cancer (Phila) 1987;60:936–942.
228. Muss HB, Cooper MR, Brockschmidt JK, et al. A randomized trial of chemotherapy (L-PAM vs. CMF) and irradiation for node positive breast cancer. Eleven year follow-up of a Piedmont Oncology Association trial. Breast Cancer Res Treat 1991;19:77–84.
229. Schulz KD, Reusch K, Schmidt-Rhode P. Consecutive radiation and chemotherapy in the adjuvant treatment of operable breast cancer. In: Salmon S, Jones S (eds) Adjuvant Therapy of Cancer, vol III. New York: Grune & Stratton, 1982:411–418.
230. Scholl SM, Asselain B, Palangie T, et al. Neoadjuvant chemotherapy in operable breast cancer. Eur J Cancer 1991;27:1668–1671.
231. Scholl SM, Fourquet A, Asselain B, et al. Neoadjuvant versus adjuvant chemotherapy in premenopausal patients with tumours considered too large for breast conserving surgery:

preliminary results of a randomised trial: S6. Eur J Cancer 1994;30A:645–652.
232. Scholl SM, Pierga JY, Asselain B, et al. Breast tumour response to primary chemotherapy predicts local and distant control as well as survival. Eur J Cancer 1995;31A:1969–1975.
233. Makris A, Powles TJ, Dowsett M, et al. Prediction of response to neoadjuvant chemoendocrine therapy in primary breast carcinomas. Clin Cancer Res 1997;3:593–600.
234. van der Hage JA, van de Velde CJ, Julien JP, Tubiana-Hulin M, Vandervelden C, Duchateau L. Preoperative chemotherapy in primary operable breast cancer: results from the European Organization for Research and Treatment of Cancer trial 10902. J Clin Oncol 2001;19:4224–4237.
235. Gianni L, Baselga J, Eiermann W, et al. First report of the European Cooperative Trial in Operable Breast Cancer (ECTO): effects of primary systemic therapy (PST) on local-regional disease. Proc Am Soc Clin Oncol 2002;2002: abstract 132.
236. Jakesz R, Group ABCCS. Comparison of pre- vs. postoperative chemotherapy in breast cancer patients: four-year results of Austrian Breast and Colorectal Study Group (ABCSG) Trial 7. Proc Am Soc Clin Oncol 2001;2001: abstract 125.
237. Nason KS, Anderson BO, Byrd DR, et al. Increased false negative sentinel node biopsy rates after preoperative chemotherapy for invasive breast carcinoma. Cancer (Phila) 2000;89: 2187–2194.
238. Haid A, Tausch C, Lang A, et al. Is sentinel lymph node biopsy reliable and indicated after preoperative chemotherapy in patients with breast carcinoma? Cancer (Phila) 2001;92:1080–1084.
239. Fernandez A, Cortes M, Benito E, et al. Gamma probe sentinel node localization and biopsy in breast cancer patients treated with a neoadjuvant chemotherapy scheme. Nucl Med Commun 2001;22:361–366.
240. Tafra L, Verbanac KM, Lannin DR. Preoperative chemotherapy and sentinel lymphadenectomy for breast cancer. Am J Surg 2001;182:312–315.
241. Stearns V, Ewing CA, Slack R, Penannen MF, Hayes DF, Tsangaris TN. Sentinel lymphadenectomy after neoadjuvant chemotherapy for breast cancer may reliably represent the axilla except for inflammatory breast cancer. Ann Surg Oncol 2002; 9:235–242.
242. Julian TB, Dusi D, Wolmark N. Sentinel node biopsy after neoadjuvant chemotherapy for breast cancer. Am J Surg 2002; 184:315–317.
243. Miller AR, Thomason VE, Yeh IT, et al. Analysis of sentinel lymph node mapping with immediate pathologic review in patients receiving preoperative chemotherapy for breast carcinoma. Ann Surg Oncol 2002;9:243–247.
244. Brady EW. Sentinel lymph node mapping following neoadjuvant chemotherapy for breast cancer. Breast J 2002;8:97–100.
245. Piato JR, Barros AC, Pincerato KM, Sampaio AP, Pinotti JA. Sentinel lymph node biopsy in breast cancer after neoadjuvant chemotherapy. A pilot study. Eur J Surg Oncol 2003;29:118–120.
246. Balch GC, Mithani SK, Richards KR, Beauchamp RD, Kelley MC. Lymphatic mapping and sentinel lymphadenectomy after preoperative therapy for stage II and III breast cancer. Ann Surg Oncol 2003;10:616–621.
247. Grunwald Z, Moore JH, Schwartz GF. Bilateral brachial plexus palsy after a right-side modified radical mastectomy with immediate TRAM flap reconstruction. Breast J 2003;9:41–43.
248. Reitsamer R, Peintinger F, Rettenbacher L, Prokop E. Sentinel lymph node biopsy in breast cancer patients after neoadjuvant chemotherapy. J Surg Oncol 2003;84:63–67.
249. Mamounas E, Brown A, Smith R, et al. Accuracy of sentinel lymph node biopsy after neoadjuvant chemotherapy in breast cancer: Updated results from NSABP B-27. Proc Am Soc Clin Oncol 2002;21: abstract 140.
250. Vogel VG, Costantino JP, Wickerham DL, Cronin WM, Wolmark N. The study of tamoxifen and raloxifene: preliminary enrollment data from a randomized breast cancer risk reduction trial. Clin Breast Cancer 2002;3:153–159.
251. Buzdar A, Douma J, Davidson N, et al. Phase III, multicenter, double-blind, randomized study of letrozole, an aromatase inhibitor, for advanced breast cancer versus megestrol acetate. J Clin Oncol 2001;19:3357–3366.
252. Kaufmann M, Bajetta E, Dirix LY, et al. Exemestane is superior to megestrol acetate after tamoxifen failure in postmenopausal women with advanced breast cancer: results of a phase III randomized double-blind trial. The Exemestane Study Group. J Clin Oncol 2000;18:1399–1411.
253. Rose C, Vtoraya O, Pluzanska A, et al. An open randomised trial of second-line endocrine therapy in advanced breast cancer. Comparison of the aromatase inhibitors letrozole and anastrozole. Eur J Cancer 2003;39:2318–2327.
254. Bonneterre J, Thurlimann B, Robertson JF, et al. Anastrozole versus tamoxifen as first-line therapy for advanced breast cancer in 668 postmenopausal women: results of the Tamoxifen or Arimidex Randomized Group Efficacy and Tolerability study. J Clin Oncol 2000;18:3748–3757.
255. Nabholtz JM, Buzdar A, Pollak M, et al. Anastrozole is superior to tamoxifen as first-line therapy for advanced breast cancer in postmenopausal women: results of a North American multicenter randomized trial. Arimidex Study Group. J Clin Oncol 2000;18:3758–3767.

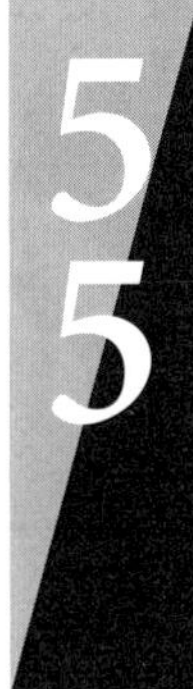

Thyroid and Parathyroid

Gerard M. Doherty

Thyroid and parathyroid diseases combine the focuses of endocrinology and oncology, as one must consider both the hormonal function effects of the tumor and its treatment and the management of the malignancy, or potential malignancy. This chapter addresses the malignant forms of thyroid and parathyroid diseases and their epidemiology, diagnosis, treatment, and follow-up.

Thyroid Nodule

A palpable solitary nodule caused by a carcinoma in the neck is often impossible to distinguish from a benign nodule. However, a hard and firm consistency in especially a relatively fast growing nodule indicates a higher risk for malignancy than a soft slowly growing nodule, and multinodular disease is associated with lower risk of malignancy compared with a solitary nodule.[1] A solitary nodule is best investigated by fine-needle aspiration (FNA), as well as ultrasound (Figure 55.1). FNA, however, is limited in its ability to differentiate benign from malignant disease for follicular tumors, because the diagnostic criteria rely on thorough examination of capsular invasion. Ultrasound-guided FNA may improve the diagnostic yield of FNA, but interpretation problems of the aspirate remain.

FNA biopsy has a sensitivity and specificity of 95% and 97.5%, respectively, in the diagnosis of thyroid cancer. The diagnostic accuracy of FNA cytology is more than 95% for papillary thyroid cancer (PTC). FNA cytology in patients with PTC commonly shows psammoma bodies, papillary structure, and the nuclear features of PTC (Figure 55.2). The FNA cytology may be suspicious or indeterminate, including follicular and Hürthle cell neoplasms, and in such cases patients should undergo thyroidectomy because about 20% prove to be thyroid cancer. In cases in which the FNA biopsy is nondiagnostic the FNA should be repeated; this is important because about 10% of these neoplasms are malignant.

Diagnostic ^{131}I- or technetium-thallium scintigraphy was used in the past to identify hypofunctional areas in the thyroid corresponding to a palpable lesion—*cold* nodules. However, this method has very low specificity and should only be used for patients with suppressed thyroid-stimulating hormone (TSH). There is no indication for scintigraphy in a euthyroid patient with a thyroid nodule.

There are no available diagnostic approaches that can distinguish follicular carcinoma from follicular adenoma, other than diagnostic lobectomy and histologic evaluation. Therefore, for follicular thyroid neoplasms by cytology, diagnostic lobectomy is generally indicated. If the thyroid nodule is large or otherwise suspicious for a carcinoma, the patient should have a total thyroidectomy, at the discretion of the surgeon and the patient.

Thyroid Cancer

Epidemiology

Thyroid cancer is the most common endocrine malignancy; it also has the highest mortality among endocrine neoplasms. According to estimates by the American Cancer Society, about 23,600 new cases of thyroid cancer will occur in 2004 in the United States and about 1,460 people will die of thyroid cancer. In addition, although thyroid cancer is more common in women than in men (M:F ratio, 5,960:17,640), death from thyroid cancer occurs in a higher proportion of the men (M:F, 620:840).[2] The lifetime risk of developing thyroid carcinoma is 0.33% for men and 0.9% for women, according to U.S. Surveillance, Epidemiology and End Results (SEER) data estimates.[3] Thyroid cancers have a wide range of aggressiveness, from relative indolence for most papillary thyroid cancer (PTC) to near-uniform lethality for anaplastic thyroid cancer. Fortunately, PTC accounts for about 80% of all thyroid cancer cases in iodine-sufficient areas and is associated with a relatively good prognosis.

Significant advances in our knowledge of the molecular biology, diagnosis, and prognosis of thyroid cancer have been made over the past three decades. The treatment of differentiated thyroid cancer remains controversial, with debates among experts regarding the most appropriate extent of thyroidectomy, the use of postoperative radioactive iodine ablation, and the need for thyroid hormone for TSH suppression. In addition, the understanding of the molecular changes leading to papillary thyroid cancer and medullary thyroid cancer have created optimism that specific therapies will be developed.

Follicular Cell-Derived Thyroid Cancer

The normal thyroid gland consists mainly of follicular cells. These specialized cells concentrate iodide from circulating blood through the sodium iodide symporter (NIS), synthesize thyroid hormone and thyroglobulin, and respond to thyroid-stimulating hormone (TSH) by both growth and hormone

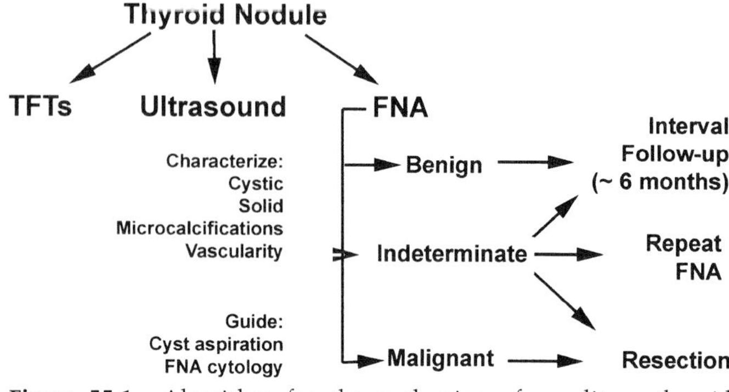

Figure 55.1. Algorithm for the evaluation of a solitary thyroid nodule. All patients should have thyroid function tests. Ultrasound is extremely helpful in the characterization of the nodule, and in the guidance of percutaneous interventions. Fine-needle aspiration cytology is the mainstay of thyroid nodule assessment and is very reliable. Thyroid scintigraphy does not have a place in the routine evaluation of a thyroid nodule unless the patient is hyperthyroid.

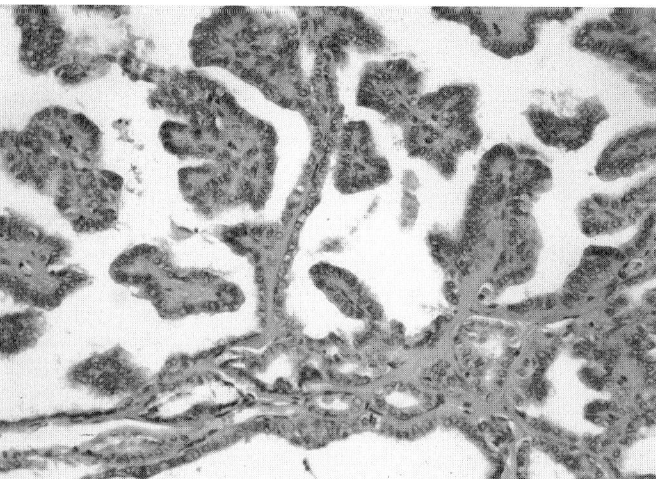

Figure 55.2. Papillary thyroid cancer histology. The classic papillary thyroid cancer has thin vascularized stalks lined by follicular cell-derived thyroid cancer (FCDTC) cells with typical nuclear changes. These can be diagnosed on cytology by the nuclear changes and by the fragments of papillary architecture that are sometimes identifiable.

release. Follicular cell-derived thyroid cancer (FCDTC) cells lose some of the normal signals that control cell growth and division, but often maintain some of the functions of normal thyroid follicular cells. The function that is most frequently lost is the ability to synthesize thyroid hormone. Very few thyroid carcinomas make thyroid hormone or cause hyperthyroidism. However, the NIS is present and functional in most FCDTC, and forms the basis for the use of radioiodine therapy in its management. Most FCDTC also retain the ability to synthesize thyroglobulin, which allows the use of serum levels of thyroglobulin after treatment as a tumor marker for follow-up. Finally, most FCDTC continue to express the TSH receptor and to respond to TSH with growth and increased thyroglobulin release. This understanding is important in the treatment of FCDTC, as suppression of TSH with thyroid hormone can decrease the recurrence rate. In addition, during follow-up, administration of TSH can increase the sensitivity of thyroglobulin tumor marker measurement.

FCDTC includes several related histologic and clinical subtypes. The main types are papillary thyroid cancer (about 80%), follicular thyroid cancer (about 15%), and Hürthle cell cancer. A variety of subcategories also exist, some of which have prognostic implications (Table 55.1).

Papillary Thyroid Carcinoma

Clinical Features

Almost all patients (98% or more) who present with clinical evidence of PTC present with a mass located in the thyroid gland (67%), a mass associated with cervical lymphadenopathy (13%), and only with cervical lymphadenopathy (20%).[4] Children and young adults more frequently present with palpable nodal metastases.[5] The peak incidence of PTC is in the third and fourth decade of life, and there is a female-to-male ratio of 3:1. Depending on the series and whether prophylactic neck node dissection was performed, the rate of cervical node metastases is 11% to 80%. Most studies from the United States report a rate of 30% to 40% cervical node metastases when therapeutic neck node dissections are done.[6] Distant metastasis is less common (2%–14%). The most common sites of distant metastases are to the lung and bone, and less commonly to the soft tissue, central nervous system, and liver.

Papillary thyroid cancer is the most common tumor that occurs in patients with Graves' disease, accounting for about 75% of the thyroid cancers associated with Graves' disease.[7] Some investigators report more-aggressive thyroid cancers in patients with Graves' disease whereas others do not.[7,8] Confounding factors that cloud the debate regarding whether patients with Graves' disease have more-aggressive tumors are (1) whether the thyroid cancer was diagnosed clinically or on histologic evaluation, (2) whether surgical or medical treatment was used, (3) history of radiation to the head and neck, and (4) level of microscopic histologic evaluation for the presence of thyroid cancer. The similarity of the thyroid-stimulating antibodies, present in Graves' patients, and TSH

TABLE 55.1. Histologic variants of follicular cell-derived thyroid carcinoma.

Variants with similar clinical behavior	*Variants with more aggressive behavior*
Follicular variant of papillary	Tall cell
Minimally invasive follicular thyroid carcinoma (FTC)	Diffuse sclerosing
Encapsulated	Columnar
Solid/trabecular	Oxyphil (Hürthle) Oncocytic papillary thyroid cancer (PTC) (similar to Hürthle) Clear cell FTC InsularMixed MTC/FTC (behaves like medullary thyroid carcinoma, MTC)

is clearly documented. The fact that TSH promotes tumor growth, invasion, angiogenesis, and inhibits apoptosis in vitro supports the possibility that thyroid cancer may be more aggressive in these patients. It appears that patients who present with clinical evidence of thyroid cancer and who have Graves' disease have more-aggressive tumors, whereas patients with occult thyroid cancers who are treated for Graves' disease have an excellent prognosis.

Pathologic Features

PTC is typically firm with an irregular border, has a whitish color, and may contain microcalcifications. However, there is variation in the tumor gross characteristics related to the different morphologic variants of PTC. For example, the encapsulated follicular variant of PTC may have a well-defined margin with a fleshy appearance similar to a follicular adenoma. Depending on the evaluation of the entire thyroid gland, a microscopic examination, and the thickness of histologic section, up to 80% tumor multicentricity is reported for PTC. Carcangiu and associates found 22% of PTC were multifocal on routine histologic examination whereas Katoh et al., on thin (0.5-µm) microscopic section evaluation, found 78% of PTC were multifocal.[4,9] Overall, most studies report 20% to 30% of PTC are multicentric. Vascular invasion by PTC is uncommon compared with follicular thyroid cancer, occurring rarely.

The presence of papillae and unique nuclear features are the defining characteristic of PTC. The papillae appear as fibrovascular stalks lined by the neoplastic epithelial follicular cells. The nuclear features are hyperchromatic nuclei, absent nucleoli, nuclear grooves, and intranuclear inclusions. Several variants of PTC exist, and their diagnosis is established by the presence of these distinct nuclear features of PTC. Some variants behave similar to typical PTC whereas others have a more-aggressive behavior. In 1960, Lindsay made the initial observation that some "follicular carcinoma" had papillae and a less-aggressive clinical course than typical follicular carcinoma.[10] Subsequent studies confirmed these observations, and the follicular variant of PTC is now regarded as a variant of PTC. This variant is characterized by the presence of ground-glass (clear nucleoli) nuclei and may have some or no papillary elements on histology. The micropapillary, "occult," or "minimal" variant of PTC is smaller than 10mm by definition and is commonly found incidentally. Patients with occult PTC (less than 1cm) have a near-normal life expectancy. The encapsulated variant of PTC accounts for about 10% of all PTC and is characterized by a total surrounding fibrous capsule that may have focal invasion but has the nuclear features consistent with PTC. In the solid/trabecular variant of PTC are foci of solid and/or trabecular growth pattern in most (more than 50%) or all of the tumor with the typical nuclear features of PTC. The presence of this morphologic variant is important to recognize to avoid misclassification as a poorly differentiated thyroid cancer.

The tall cell variant of PTC has a typical appearance with the height of the follicular cells greater than twice the width with an intense eosinophilic cytoplasm lining the glandular and papillary structures.[11] In this variant, nuclear grooves and intranuclear invaginations are commonly present. Hazard and Hawk observed that these tumors occurred in older patients and were larger in size (greater than 5cm), with frequent extrathyroid extension and a higher incidence of vascular invasion.[12] Studies by Johnson et al. and Moreno-Egea et al. comparing patients with the tall cell variants to patients with typical PTC, which matched patients for age and gender, found a higher recurrence rate and mortality in patients with the tall cell variant of PTC.[11,14] Vickery and associates were the first to describe the diffuse sclerosing variant of PTC, which is characterized by dense intrathyroidal lymphocytic invasion, severe fibrosis, squamous metaplasia, and numerous psammoma bodies involving one or both thyroid lobes.[15,16] Importantly, this morphologic variant was associated with a slightly worse prognosis and occurred more frequently in children. Compared with typical PTC, most subsequent studies have shown a higher rate of nodal and distant metastases, and also a higher recurrence rate for the diffuse sclerosing variant, but not a significant difference in mortality. According to the World Health Organization thyroid histologic classification, oxyphil or Hürthle cell carcinomas that display classic papillary architecture on histology are considered a variant of PTC. Herrera and associates have reported that this morphologic variant compared with typical PTC is associated with a higher recurrence rate and mortality.[17]

Risk Factors and Associated Hereditary Conditions

Several hereditary conditions and environmental factors increase the risk of developing thyroid cancer. A history of radiation exposure increases the risk of developing differentiated thyroid cancer. Most of the external radiation exposure was used in children to treat them for tinea capitus, hypertrophic thymus, tonsillitis, acne, and external otitis in the 1940s and 1950s. Large case-control retrospective studies by Shore et al. and Ron et al. confirmed the increased risk of thyroid cancers and benign thyroid nodules in children exposed to low-dose therapeutic radiation.[18–21] Shore and colleagues reported among 2,650 children exposed to therapeutic low-dose radiation, there is an increased relative risk of 45 for malignant thyroid tumors and a relative risk of 15 for benign thyroid tumors. Ron and associates found a relative risk of 4 for malignant thyroid tumors and 2 for benign thyroid tumors in a cohort of 10,834 children exposed to therapeutic radiation for tinea capitus. A linearly increased risk of thyroid cancer to dose of radiation exposure has been observed with an even higher risk among those exposed at a young age. A minimum 3- to 5-year latency period has been observed between radiation exposure and tumor development. The number of cases continues to increase for at least three decades after exposure and then decreases. About 90% of the radiation-associated thyroid cancers reported have been PTC. Today, radiation-induced thyroid cancer accounts for about 9% of all thyroid cancers. In addition to age and dose of radiation exposure, other environmental or genetic factors may play a role in which individuals develop thyroid neoplasm. Perkel and associates, in a study of 286 sib pairs, reported a significant ($P = 0.05$) familial concordance for thyroid neoplasms (benign and malignant) but not for thyroid cancer.[22] Schneider et al. have followed 2,634 children in Chicago and 40% have developed thyroid neoplasms (all types) and 12% thyroid cancer.[23] The use of low-dose radiation treatment in patients with benign conditions has been abandoned in the past 40 years because of the recognized increased risk for thyroid cancer.

Radiation exposure from diagnostic radiation or therapeutic high-dose external-beam radiation accounts for the medical-related exposure in patients today. Investigations in children exposed to nuclear fallout accidents in the Marshall Islands, Nevada test sites, and Chernobyl clearly document an increased risk of thyroid cancer among patients exposed to acute ionized radiation.[24–26] As in the studies of patients exposed to low-dose therapeutic radiation, age at exposure and dose of radiation exposure were significant factors in the increased relative risk. Other risk factors such as dietary, sex hormones, goitrogens, and environmental factors have also been identified but not all studies show an increased risk of thyroid cancer (Table 55.2). Epidemiologic studies show that both high-iodine and low-iodine diets can increase the risk of thyroid cancer.

Patients with familial adenomatous polyposis (FAP) have an increased risk of benign and malignant thyroid neoplasms[27,28]; they can develop either papillary or follicular tumors.

Diagnosis of Papillary Thyroid Cancer

The majority of patients with PTC present with a neck mass originating from the thyroid gland or from a cervical node metastasis. When there is significant local tumor invasion, patients may have local symptoms such as hoarseness, changes to the singing voice, or difficulty swallowing. A careful history and physical examination with emphasis on a history of head and neck radiation or familial thyroid disorders is important. If a patient has had previous neck surgery or has had any change in his or her voice, indirect or direct laryngoscopy can evaluate the status of the vocal cords. Although hyperfunctioning PTC are rare, careful evaluation for symptoms or signs of hypothyroidism with serum TSH level determination should be done.

A diagnosis of PTC is usually established by fine-needle aspiration (FNA). FNA cytology is highly accurate for diagnosing PTC. Simultaneous thyroid ultrasonography may be used during FNA biopsy, especially if the thyroid nodule is cystic, to obtain cellular element from the solid component (Figure 55.3).

Intraoperative frozen section in patients with PTC is not necessary for patients with PTC by cytologic examination. In patients who have enlarged lymph nodes or when there is a question of lymph node metastases, a frozen section can be helpful in confirming nodal metastases and for confirming the diagnosis intraoperatively.

TABLE 55.2. Risk classification systems for patients with papillary follicular cell-derived thyroid cancer (FCDTC).

System	*Prognostic factors included*
AGES	Age, tumor grade, extrathyroidal invasion, distant metastases, tumor size
AMES	Age, extrathyroidal invasion, distant metastases, tumor size
EORTC	Gender, tumor histology type, extrathyroidal invasion, distant metastases
MACIS	Age, extrathyroidal invasion, distant metastases, completeness of resection, tumor size

EORTC, European Organization for Research and Treatment of Cancer.

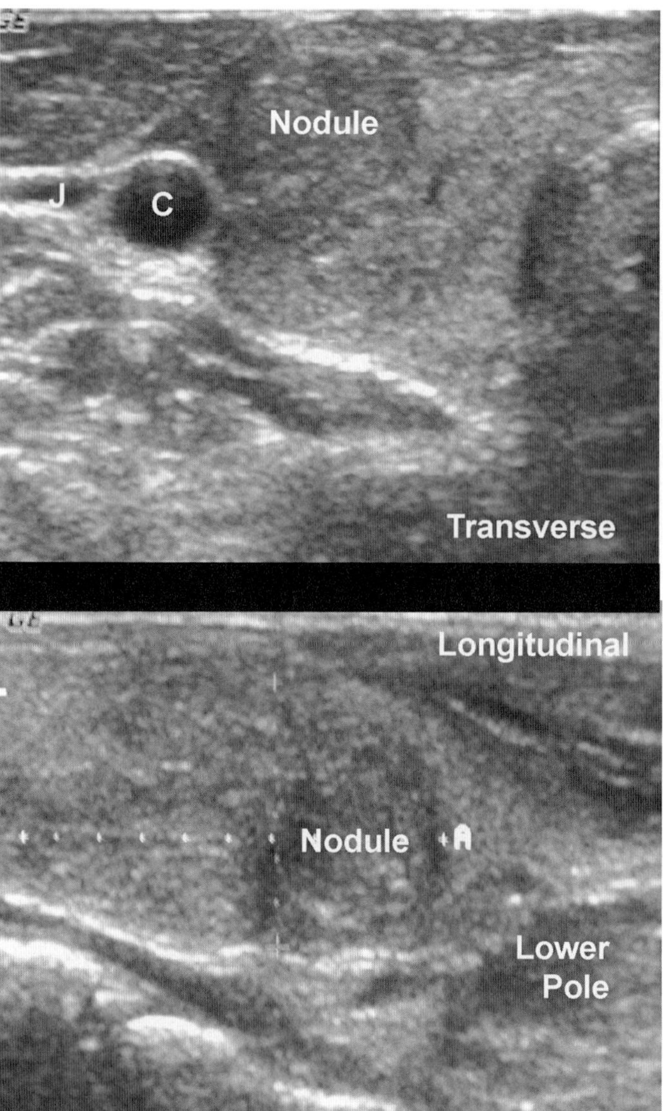

Figure 55.3. Thyroid ultrasound. Ultrasound is extremely useful for the characterization of cervical anatomy and thyroid nodules. This nodule in the lower pole of the right lobe of the thyroid gland is well circumscribed, slightly hypoechoic, and deforms the surface of the thyroid gland. Upon resection, this was a tall cell carcinoma of the thyroid. *J*, jugular vein; *C*, carotid artery.

Treatment of Papillary Thyroid Cancer

Controversy remains regarding optimal treatment of patients with differentiated thyroid cancer. The controversy persists because there are no prospective randomized control studies evaluating the merit of extent of thyroidectomy, postoperative radioactive iodine therapy, and TSH suppressive therapy. Such a trial would require a large multicenter trial with a long follow-up time required because of the relatively good prognosis and low incidence of thyroid cancer.

Extent of Thyroidectomy

Thyroidectomy is safe and effective and it is the primary treatment in patients with PTC. In patients who have bilateral lobe tumors, extrathyroidal tumor extension, and/or high-risk PTC, there is a general consensus that total thyroidectomy is warranted. However, in low-risk patients conflicting points of view by experts persist. Generally, three surgical approaches have been advocated among experts: (1) thyroid lobectomy or hemithyroidectomy (total removal of one lobe and isthmus), (2) near-total (total lobectomy and subtotal resection on the contralateral side leaving less than 1g thyroid tissue), and (3) total thyroidectomy. The most important reasons for performing a total or near-total thyroidectomy in patients with PTC are (1) a lower dose of radioactive iodine can be used to identify and ablate residual thyroid cancer, and (2) the serum thyroglobulin level following total thyroidectomy is a more accurate marker of recurrent/persistent PTC. Up to 80% of PTC are multicentric and tumor foci may occur in the contralateral lobe, thus representing a potential site of recurrence. There is about a 1% risk of a differentiated thyroid cancer progressing to anaplastic thyroid cancer, which is uniformly lethal. Hay et al. from the Mayo clinic also specifically studied local recurrence and nodal and distant metastases in patients with low-risk PTC based on the AMES prognostic classification system, finding those patients who had unilateral procedure (lobectomy only) had a higher local recurrence rate (14%) and nodal metastases (19%) than those patients treated with bilateral procedures.[29] However, there was no significant difference in survival rate and distant metastases.

Although advocates of lesser procedures contend that there is a higher risk of complications after total thyroidectomy, numerous surgeons with experience in total thyroidectomy report complication rates of less than 2%. The risk of complication from thyroidectomy depends primarily on the extent of thyroid disease, the experience of the surgeon, and anatomic variation of the parathyroid glands, recurrent laryngeal nerves, and external laryngeal nerves. The most common and serious complications of thyroidectomy are injury to the recurrent laryngeal nerves or parathyroid glands. It seems obvious that the risk of complication is higher with total thyroidectomy because of dissection on the side contralateral to the tumor. However, comparable complication rates for total thyroidectomy, near-total thyroidectomy, and lesser procedures are achieved by many surgeons.[30,31] Even among the less than 2% of patients who had complications, these patients were more likely to have more-invasive tumors involving the recurrent laryngeal nerve. Although the evidence suggests that total thyroidectomy should be associated with little or no higher complication rate than lesser procedures, these data are based upon the outcomes of experienced surgeons. The public policy issue of whether it is preferable to advocate a less-effective approach (lobectomy) that is more applicable by the occasional thyroid surgeon is made moot if patients are cared for by those with experience performing these operations.

Total thyroidectomy is the treatment of choice for virtually all patients with PTC when postoperative radioactive iodine is considered. This group includes virtually all patients except those with the very best prognosis, that is, small tumor (less than 1cm), confined to the thyroid without evident metastases, in an otherwise healthy woman under 45 years. Even in patients with low-risk PTC, total or near-total thyroidectomy is associated with a lower recurrence rate and mortality.[6,29] Serum thyroglobulin levels after total thyroidectomy are a more accurate marker for follow-up of patients with PTC, and postoperative radioactive iodine scanning and ablation is more effective. If a total thyroidectomy cannot be performed without injury to the recurrent laryngeal nerve or parathyroid glands, a near-total thyroidectomy can be done with a small amount of thyroid tissue left behind that can subsequently be ablated with radioactive iodine.

Lymph Node Dissection

Up to 80% of patients with PTC have cervical lymph node metastases; however, the prognostic significance of lymph node metastases is controversial. Patients with PTC and matted lymph nodes or tumor extending through the lymph node capsule have a worse prognosis.[6,32,33] When patients are matched for age and sex, lymph node metastases also appears to be associated with a higher recurrence rate. Patients with PTC treated with prophylactic node dissection compared with only therapeutic node dissection (removal of palpable enlarged lymph nodes) have essentially the same survival rate. Even though up to 80% of patients with PTC have occult cervical lymph node metastases, most of these metastases can be ablated with radioactive iodine treatment postoperatively and some do not appear to grow. Lymph node dissection during thyroidectomy has a higher complication rate, probably because it is associated with more tumor, especially around the parathyroid glands. Therapeutic lymph node dissection with removal of the ipsilateral central neck nodes and perithyroid lymph nodes (Delphian node and lymph nodes medial to the carotid sheath) is important for clinically involved nodes. If there are clinically involved lateral neck nodes, then a compartment-based resection, rather than a "node-plucking" operation, has a better rate of control of the nodal disease. A functional modified radical neck dissection removing all fibrofatty tissue with lymph nodes but preserving all motor (phrenic, vagus, and spinal accessory nerves) and sensory nerves as well as the sternocleidomastoid muscle and internal jugular vein unless invaded by tumor is the best approach. Contralateral lymph node dissection should also be performed for gross evidence of lymph node metastases. The superior mediastinal lower nodes and periesophageal nodes are often involved, and can often be removed through the cervical excision.

Recurrent and Persistent PTC

Most patients with PTC are diagnosed with persistent or recurrent disease by an elevated serum Tg level and/or by a positive radioactive iodine scan. Some patients with recurrent PTC may have an elevated Tg with a negative radioactive iodine scan. In this situation, a therapeutic dose of ^{131}I (100–200mCi) may help some patients by showing uptake (diagnostic benefit) or by response to this therapy (therapeutic benefit).[34] Local recurrences are often associated or precede distant metastases in patients with PTC; an evaluation for metastatic disease is important to define the extent of the recurrence. When recurrent PTC is identified in the neck by radioiodine scan, computed tomography (CT) scan, magnetic resonance imaging (MRI), or ultrasound with a positive FNA biopsy, a neck dissection can eliminate disease. Patients with solitary metastases (usually to the bone and rarely to the lung, which tend to be multiple) can benefit from operative resection. About two-thirds of patients with lung or bone metastases from differentiated thyroid cancer respond to ^{131}I therapy. In patients who are not operative candidates, and for most patients after resection of isolated metastasis to bone, external-beam radiation can be helpful in local tumor control or for symptomatic relief. In those patients with PTC that fail ^{131}I ablation or external-beam radiotherapy and who are not surgical candidates, cytotoxic chemotherapy may be useful in patients with progressive PTC.[35]

Follicular Thyroid Carcinoma

Clinical Features

The clinical presentation of follicular thyroid carcinoma (FTC) is very similar to PTC. Most patients present with a mass in the thyroid. However, FTC is less likely to be associated with cervical lymph node metastases than is PTC, so it is unusual to have a lateral neck mass as the presenting sign. FTC can be associated with distant metastases, particularly in older patients. In contrast to patients with follicular adenoma, patients with follicular thyroid cancers are more likely to have local symptoms; these can include difficulty swallowing, dysphonia, stridor, or pain. Patients can also present with evidence of distant metastases, most typically metastases in the bone, lung, brain, or liver. Apparently because of its propensity for vascular invasion, follicular tumors often metastasize via hematogenous pathways, and only rarely via cervical lymph nodes as would be more typical of papillary cancer. Biopsy at these distant sites may demonstrate relatively benign-appearing follicular tumor; however, by its behavior it has defined itself as an invasive malignant variety. Thus, follicular cancers typically present as a slowly growing solitary thyroid mass in a middle-aged to older person. About 25% of the patients have extrathyroidal invasion at the time of presentation. Between 10% and 33% of patients have distant metastasis at the time of initial diagnosis.

Most follicular cancers are nonfunctional ("cold") by radioiodine thyroid scan. Occasionally, a follicular cancer retains the ability to concentrate iodine to a degree similar to adjacent thyroid tissue ("warm") or even to a greater degree then the normal thyroid ("hot"). The rare "functional" thyroid cancer is nearly always a follicular carcinoma rather than a papillary tumor.

Follicular thyroid cancers can occur in any age group, but the median age of groups with follicular cancers is typically higher than groups with papillary cancers. The median age at presentation is in the sixth decade of life. Similar to papillary cancer, the female to male ratio is between 2:1 and 5:1.[36]

Pathologic Features

The important features that distinguish FTC from follicular adenomas are vascular and capsular invasion.[37] Follicular carcinomas can appear very similar to follicular adenoma on cytology and gross examination and therefore impossible to identify by either the cytologist, surgeon, or pathologist before complete pathologic assessment. The well-differentiated follicular carcinomas are identified by signs of minimal invasion such as microscopic evidence of capsule discontinuity. Other follicular tumors may be less differentiated, widely invading surrounding thyroid or even extrathyroidal tissues. The tumor cells vary in their histologic differentiation, but are generally bland, monomorphic cells lacking nuclear changes typical of PTC. Thus, follicular carcinoma cells can appear differentiated and may resemble normal thyroid tissue even when recurrent or metastatic; this can be misinterpreted as a "thyroid remnant" and not treated properly. The precise histologic pattern may be described as follicular, trabecular, or solid or display combinations of these. In the widely invasive forms, the tumor demonstrates areas of solid growth, frequent mitoses, and atypical cells. Signs of dedifferentiation are frequent as the disease proceeds.

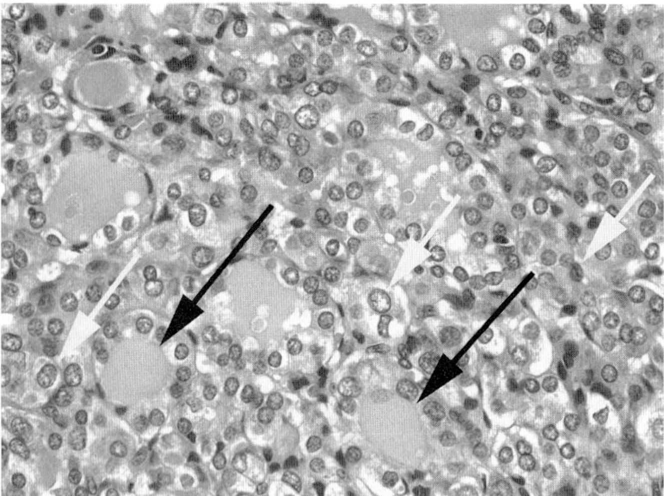

Figure 55.4. Follicular variant of papillary thyroid cancer. This variant has the follicular architecture of follicular thyroid carcinoma (FTC) (*black arrows*) without papillary structures, but has the nuclear features of papillary thyroid cancer (PTC) (*white arrows*) with nuclear grooves, clearing, and clumped chromatin.

Tumors with a mix of papillary and follicular features often show follicular differentiation, expressing follicular structures, but have nuclear features of papillary carcinoma (for example, psammoma bodies, or nuclear grooves or pseudoinclusions) (Figure 55.4). They can be difficult to diagnose on cytology, but once recognized they have the clinical course and prognosis of PTC rather than FTC.

Risk Factors and Associated Hereditary Conditions

In areas with sufficient intake of iodine, most of the differentiated thyroid carcinomas are papillary. In areas with iodine deficiency and endemic goiter, the total incidence of thyroid carcinoma is similar, with a relative increase in follicular thyroid carcinoma that are sometimes even more frequent than papillary carcinomas. A substantial intake of vegetables from the cruciferous family that block iodine uptake (goitrogenic food) can contribute to these findings. The stimulatory factor in the low-iodine areas leading to thyroid tumors appears to be TSH, although no clear correlation has been documented. Nevertheless, iodine supplementation coincides with an increase in the incidence of papillary carcinomas, with reduction in follicular and especially poorly differentiated and anaplastic carcinomas.[38] External radiation has not been associated with follicular carcinoma. Investigations after the Chernobyl accident generally support these earlier findings, although there are occasional reports of follicular thyroid carcinomas.[39] Nearly all follicular thyroid carcinomas are sporadic, but may in rare cases also be associated with familial colon polyposis or Gardner's syndrome, as well as Cowden's syndrome.

Treatment of Follicular Thyroid Cancer

Surgical resection is the only available method for FTC in the thyroid. As for PTC, the choice of hemithyroidectomy or total thyroidectomy as the procedure of choice for FTC has been debated. Hemithyroidectomy or total thyroidectomy with extirpation of central lymph nodes without radioiodine are both adequate for survival outcomes in patients with invasive follicular carcinoma confined to the thyroid, that is, T1–T2N0M0.

However, for larger tumors (above T2), total thyroidectomy with at least central lymph node dissection is appropriate for a number of reasons. This treatment allows postoperative ^{131}I ablation, as well as diagnostic scintigrams for follow-up. Arguments against total thyroidectomy have been increased risk for surgical complications such as injury to the recurrent laryngeal nerve or permanent hypoparathyroidism. However, for experienced surgeons, total thyroidectomy is a safe procedure, with minor complication rates. Therefore, in T3–4 tumors, a more-extensive treatment is mandatory. Although follicular tumors metastasize to lymph nodes in the neck less frequently than papillary tumors (approximately 35% versus 67%), therapeutic modified neck dissection should be performed when clinically apparent disease is present, followed by postoperative ^{131}I diagnostic procedures and radioiodine ablation therapy.

Hürthle Cell Carcinoma

Hürthle cell carcinoma is a variant of follicular carcinoma, which is sometimes called an oxyphilic or oncocytic carcinoma. These tumors may be remarkably similar on gross examination but are microscopically characterized by an acidophilic cytoplasm with small pyknotic central nuclei. It is important to distinguish these tumors from each other, because the oncocytic carcinomas have a much lower capacity for uptake of iodine, which makes postoperative diagnostic and therapeutic ^{131}I scintigrams difficult. They have a natural history and prognosis similar to FTC, which supports similar treatment.[40]

Postoperative Management of Differentiated Thyroid Carcinoma

Prognosis

FCDTC is the direct cause of death of more patients than all other endocrine malignancies combined. Nevertheless, with a crude mortality rate of only around 7%, the vast majority of patients with FCDTC are either cured, or lives with cancer, often for many years.

Overall recurrence rates after apparent surgical cure of the primary tumor range from 10% to 35%,[41,42] depending on histologic subtype and stage at diagnosis.[41–45] Recurrence may sometimes occur many years after the initial, apparently successful, treatment.[46] Thyroid carcinomas exhibit among the widest range of malignant potential of any human cancer. They range from the almost benign, incidentally discovered, papillary microcarcinoma, which probably has no impact on long-term survival, to extremely aggressive poorly differentiated carcinomas with a median life expectancy of only a few months. Within the FCDTC group, life expectancy and the likelihood of cure vary widely.

There have been many attempts to identify prognostic factors for patients with FCDTC. Unfortunately, there are no randomized, prospective trials of any aspect of thyroid cancer management, largely because of the relative rarity of the tumor, its generally slow clinical course with long survivorship, and the difficulty and expense of mounting large multicenter studies over prolonged periods. Nevertheless, a great deal of information is available from large retrospective reviews from a number of centers that can be used to influence all aspects of management of the patient with differentiated thyroid cancer (DTC). To select appropriate therapy and follow-up, and to provide prognostic information to the patient, the initial step in the postoperative care of the patient with FCDTC is to categorize the patient's risk of recurrence and death from disease.

American Joint Committee on Cancer (AJCC) Staging

Pathologists apply the pTNM classification system to tumors of all types, providing a convenient shorthand method to describe the tumor extent (Table 55.3).[47] Using this system, the tumor is assessed according to the size of the primary tumor mass, with T1 representing tumors of 1 cm or less, T2 those between 1 and 4 cm in maximum diameter, T3 those greater than 4 cm, and T4 represents tumors of any size exhibiting local extrathyroidal invasion. The presence (N1) or absence (N0) of lymph node spread, and the presence (M1) or absence (M0) of distant metastases are similarly easily defined at the time of the original diagnosis, and the pTNM classification is generally straightforward to determine within a few hours of operation. Although the prognosis for many tumor types is determined largely or exclusively by the extent of disease, described efficiently by the pTNM classification, FCDTC are unique, in that the strongest influence on prognosis is patient age at diagnosis. As a result, the AJCC staging system uses patient age in defining stage for follicular cell-derived thyroid carcinoma.

In this staging system, all patients under the age of 45 with FCDTC have stage I disease unless they have evidence of distant metastases, which makes them stage II. More-advanced stages are restricted to patients over the age of 45, with locally invasive tumors (stage III), or with evidence of nodal (stage III) or distant (stage IV) metastases. The pTNM system is the most widely accepted tool to describe the extent of disease for staging in thyroid carcinoma. The AJCC stage correlates well with outcome of FCDTC, in both retrospective and prospectively collected data, with stage I and II disease exhibiting a less than 1% overall mortality at 5 years.[48] In contrast, more-advanced stages of disease, limited to those patients over the age of 45 with locally invasive or metastatic disease, carry a less-favorable prognosis. For stage III disease, the 5-year mortality was 6% for PTC and 18% for FTC, whereas stage IV disease had a 5-year mortality in excess of 50% in both tumor types.

Despite its simplicity and utility, however, the AJCC staging does not provide all the information a clinician may need to adequately classify a patient with DTC and to assist in making therapeutic decisions. It does not use several additional independent prognostic variables and may therefore risk misclassification of a significant number of patients. For this reason, several other classification schemes remain in clinical use that may permit more accurate decision making, at least for patients with FCDTC.

TABLE 55.3. American Joint Committee on Cancer (AJCC) thyroid cancer staging.

Primary tumor (T)	
TX	Primary tumor cannot be assessed
T0	No evidence of primary tumor
T1	Tumor 2 cm or less in greatest dimension limited to the thyroid
T2	Tumor more than 2 cm but not more than 4 cm in greatest dimension limited to the thyroid
T3	Tumor more than 4 cm in greatest dimension limited to the thyroid or any tumor with minimal extrathyroid extension (e.g, extension to sternothyroid muscle or perithyroid soft tissues)
T4a	Tumor of any size extending beyond the thyroid capsule to invade subcutaneous soft tissues, larynx, trachea, esophagus, or recurrent laryngeal nerve
T4b	Tumor invades prevertebral fascia or encases carotid artery or mediastinal vessels
All anaplastic carcinomas are considered T4 tumors.	
T4a	Intrathyroidal anaplastic carcinoma—surgically resectable
T4b	Extrathyroidal anaplastic carcinoma—surgically unresectable
Regional lymph nodes (N)	
NX	Regional lymph nodes cannot be assessed.
N0	No regional lymph node metastasis
N1	Regional lymph node metastasis
N1a	Metastasis to Level VI (pretracheal, paratracheal, and prelaryngeal/Delphian lymph nodes)
N1b	Metastasis to unilateral, bilateral, or contralateral cervical of superior mediastinal lymph nodes
Distant metastasis (M)	
MX	Distant metastasis cannot be assessed
M0	No distant metastasis
M1	Distant metastasis

Stage grouping[a]

Papillary or Follicular				**Medullary Carcinoma**			
Under 45 years							
Stage I	Any T	Any N	M0	Stage I	T1	N0	M0
Stage II	Any T	Any N	M1	Stage II	T2	N0	M0
				Stage III	T3	N0	M0
					T1	N1a	M0
					T2	N1a	M0
					T3	N1a	M0
				Stage IVA	T4a	N0	M0
					T4a	N1a	M0
					T1	N1b	M0
					T2	N1b	M0
					T3	N1b	M0
					T4a	N1b	M0
				Stage IVB	T4b	Any N	M0
				Stage IVC	Any T	Any N	M1
Papillary or Folicular				**Anaplastic Carcinoma**			
45 years and older				All anaplastic carcinomas are considered			
Stage I	T1	N0	M0	Stage IV			
Stage II	T2	N0	M0				
Stage III	T3	N0	M0				
	T1	N1a	M0				
	T2	N1a	M0				
	T3	N1a	M0				
Stage IVA	T4a	N0	M0	Stage IVA	T4a	Any N	M0
	T4a	N1a	M0				
	T1	N1b	M0				
	T2	N1b	M0				
	T3	N1b	M0				
	T4a	N1b	M0				
Stage IVB	T4b	Any N	M0	Stage IVB	T4b	Any N	M0
Stage IVC	Any T	Any N	M1	Stage IVC	Any T	Any N	M1

[a]Separate stage groupings are recommended for papillary or follicular, medullary, and anaplastic (undifferentiated) carcinoma.

Source: Used with the permission of the American Joint Committee on Cancer (AJCC), Chicago, Illinois. The original source for this material is the *AJCC Cancer Staging Manual*, sixth edition (2002), published by Springer-Verlag New York, www.springer-ny.com.

Clinicopathologic Prognostic Schemes for FCDTC

For patients with FCDTC, age at initial treatment, tumor size, the presence of extrathyroidal invasion, and the presence of distant metastases at diagnosis are the most important risk factors for recurrence and for cause-specific mortality. However, unlike almost any other cancer type, the presence of lymph node metastases in PTC has little influence on cause-specific mortality from this disease, although it increases the risk of locoregional recurrence.

Several other factors, not included in the AJCC staging scheme, are also independent prognostic variables in rigorous multivariate analyses, including tumor grade in PTC, which is rarely assessed in routine histologic examination; extent of microinvasion of capsule or of blood vessels in FTC; DNA aneuploidy in Hürthle cell cancer and PTC, but not in nonoxyphilic FTC; delay to initial surgical intervention; and completeness of surgical resection of the primary tumor. These prognostic factors are not of equal importance in predicting mortality or recurrence, with the most predictive factors generally being regarded as the presence of distant metastases, the age of the patient, and the extent of the tumor.[49]

Several prognostic systems have been developed that include a number of these variables, weighted according to their importance in predicting outcomes, in multivariate analyses, of retrospectively analyzed large cohorts of patients (see Table 55.2). Each of these schemes permits classification of patients with FCDTC (particularly PTC, the most common type) into low-, medium-, and high-risk groups, accurately predicting long term outcome for these patients. Each of the prognostic schemes includes a slightly different group of variables, weighted in slightly different ways. However, all have certain features in common, and all include both tumor and patient variables, emphasizing the likely importance of host–tumor interaction in the behavior of this group of cancers.

Almost all the schemes, except the Ohio State University system, include the patient's age as an important variable predicting outcome. The size of the primary tumor, its histologic type, the presence of extrathyroidal invasion, and the presence of distant metastases are almost universally included. Controversy remains about the importance of nodal metastases and of patient gender. Tumor grade (and DNA ploidy in certain tumor types) is almost certainly an important independent prognostic variable but is rarely assessed.

The MACIS score (named for its predictive variables of *M*etastases, *A*ge, *C*ompleteness of surgical excision, local *I*nvasion, and tumor *S*ize) was derived from a retrospective review of almost 1,800 patients with PTC treated at one institution over a period of up to 50 years (median, 17 years follow-up).[50] Approximately half of the patients (from 1940 to 1964) were selected to represent the "training" group, and a formal multivariate analysis was performed on this group to identify the independently predictive prognostic variables from the data set. Each of these variables had a significant predictive value on outcomes in univariate analysis, but also remained significantly correlated with outcome in multivariate analysis.

The MACIS equation was generated to weight the importance of each of the predictive variables, generating a single score for patient classification (Table 55.4). This equation was tested on the remaining 1,015 patients in the original data set (the "test group"), and on the group as a whole, and proved to be a reliable predictor of outcome over a 20-year period in these patients.[50]

TABLE 55.4. The MACIS score.

Metastasis
Age
Completeness of resection
Invasion (local)
Size (primary tumor)

MACIS = 3.0 (for distant metastases at presentation)
+ 3.1 (for age less than 40 years) *or* (0.08 × age)
+ 1.0 (for incomplete tumor resection)
+ 1.0 (if locally invasive)
+ 0.3 × tumor size (in centimeters)

MACIS score	*20-year cause-specific mortality*
<6.0	<2%
6–6.99	11%
7–7.99	44%
>8	76%

Source: From Hay et al.,[50] by permission of *Surgery*.

A MACIS score of less than 6.0, representing the lowest risk group, carries a less than 1% cause-specific 20-year mortality risk from PTC and encompasses more than 80% of all patients presenting with PTC. A score between 6.0 and 6.9 has an 11% 20-year mortality; scores between 7.0 and 7.9 have a mortality rate of 44%; and scores of 8.0 and over (fortunately, a rare occurrence, affecting less than 5% of this group of patients) have a predicted disease-specific mortality of 76% at 20 years. This broad range of outcomes is predicted rapidly and easily at the bedside on the day after primary surgery, using data that should be available in every case from the operative and pathology reports, and from simple, universally available preoperative screening tests.

The other prognostic systems provide a similar rapid, accurate assignment of risk group category. The choice of prognostic scheme remains a matter more of preference than of science; however, it appears rational to use some system, in addition to the AJCC classification, to assign prognosis and guide therapeutic decisions for patients. Such classification allows accurate identification of the majority (80%–85%) of patients with FCDTC at low risk of cause-specific mortality. These patients can be reassured and managed with less-intensive intervention. More-intensive follow-up, and perhaps more-aggressive adjuvant therapy, can then be targeted to the higher-risk patients, the minority who are most likely to benefit from a more-aggressive management strategy.

Predicting Disease Recurrence

Recurrence of FCDTC is considerably more likely than death. The recurrences carry significant physical and psychologic morbidity and increase the likelihood of subsequent mortality. Recurrent disease is often predictable, and follows the patterns of spread observed at diagnosis. These vary with the type of FCDTC; PTC exhibits early spread to (and frequent recurrence in) regional lymph nodes, and less frequently distant spread, principally to the lungs and later to skeleton. Hürthle cell cancer follows a similar pattern, although perhaps more frequently exhibiting distant metastases.

Typical nonoxyphilic FTC, however, less often involves lymph nodes, spreading preferentially by a hematogenous route to lungs, bones, and brain. Metastatic spread to other organs has also been reported.

Local recurrence occurs mainly within the thyroid bed, ipsilateral to the primary tumor site, as a result of incomplete surgical resection, local invasiveness of the primary tumor, or failure of adjunctive therapy to destroy persistent microscopic tumor deposits. Local recurrence at sites other than the thyroid bed may result from unrecognized local spread of the tumor within the thyroid remnant or multifocal tumor that has been incompletely removed or ablated.

Regional recurrence also occurs frequently in the central compartment lymph nodes, often as a result of incomplete initial surgical exploration. These nodes are involved in up to 25% of patients with PTC at the time of diagnosis, and adequate primary surgery should include their resection, at least ipsilateral to the tumor. Jugular chain lymph nodes may also commonly be the site of regional recurrence, presumably as a result of unrecognized micrometastases present at the time of the original diagnosis. Adequate assessment of the jugular chain nodes is essential before and during the primary surgery. Preoperative ultrasound before the initial operation may provide the most sensitive method of detection of affected nodes, to enable therapeutic node dissection to potentially decrease the recurrence rate.[51]

The development of distant metastases, fortunately, is rare in FCDTC but heralds a poor prognosis, particularly for older patients, with cause-specific mortality rates of up to 60% at 10 years for stage IV disease.[45] By contrast, the presence of distant metastases, particularly micrometastases in the lungs, in young patients need not signal an imminent demise, with long-term survivorship being the norm, justifying their classification as stage II disease.

The risk factors for the development of distant metastatic disease in PTC mirror those established for mortality.[52,53] The age of the patient, the size of the tumor, and the presence of local invasion or incomplete surgical resection dominate the models. In addition, however, the involvement of lymph nodes with PTC, particularly those in the jugular chains, at the time of diagnosis, substantially increases the risk of future regional recurrences. The role of lymph node metastases in the prediction of distant spread remains controversial. For FTC, the presence of vascular invasion within the primary tumor, and possibly extensive capsular invasion, substantially increases the subsequent risk of developing distant metastases.

Postoperative Adjuvant Therapy

Two major forms of adjuvant therapy are commonly used following surgical treatment of FCDTC: radioactive iodine and thyroid hormone suppression of TSH. The availability of radioactive iodine (in the form of ^{131}I) as an effective adjuvant, its ease of use, and perhaps misconceptions regarding its efficacy, have resulted occasionally in complacency regarding the initial surgical treatment of these tumors. The importance of the primary surgical procedure cannot be overstated. Although the adjuvant therapies do have important impacts and roles, the long-term outcome for the patient depends largely on the adequacy of resection, particularly for patients at higher-than-average risk of death or recurrence.

Thyroid Hormone

The suppression of TSH by administration of supraphysiologic doses of thyroid hormone is probably the most widely used adjuvant therapy for FCDTC. In use for more than 40 years, this treatment is based on the belief that suppression of TSH removes an essential growth factor for cells of thyroid follicular origin, thus delaying or preventing the regrowth of the cancer. However, firm evidence that TSH-suppressive therapy is truly effective in the postoperative management of DTC is hard to obtain, in the absence of any randomized prospective trials.

Initially, the goal of TSH suppression therapy was to attain an absent response to intravenous TRH administration, assessed on a first-generation TSH radioimmunoassay, consistent with essentially complete suppression of the pituitary thyrotrope. With the development of more-sensitive TSH assays in the 1980s, it became possible simply to maintain an undetectable TSH, measured using a sensitive (second-generation) immunometric TSH assay, with a lower limit of detection of around 0.1 mU/L. Since the advent of "ultrasensitive" TSH assays (third- and fourth-generation), with lower limits of detection of 0.01 mU/L, 0.001 mU/L, or less, it has become possible to titrate the dose of thyroid hormone in the majority of patients to achieve levels of TSH within prespecified ranges. Unfortunately, there are not good data to help with decision making, so that the "desirable range" for TSH is speculative at the present time.

The contemporary data to support TSH suppression are limited. A recent retrospective, multicenter study of 683 patients, stratified by the National Thyroid Cancer Treatment Cooperative Study (NTCTCS) stage, who had been treated and followed at 14 institutions over a 10-year period, showed a significantly reduced risk of disease progression (defined as cause-specific mortality or recurrence) in stage III and IV patients with FCDTC treated with suppressive doses of thyroid hormone.[54] No such difference in outcome was observed in stage I and II patients.

The use of supraphysiologic doses of thyroid hormone may, however, carry some risk of adverse consequences.[55,56] A small proportion of patients experience hyperthyroid symptoms of tremor, anxiety, sleep disturbance, heat intolerance, and palpitations. which can be intolerable and can sometimes require reductions in thyroid hormone dosage. The impact of TSH suppression on bone turnover is also a concern, particularly in postmenopausal women, who have an increased risk of osteoporosis. The danger of this is probably negligible in premenopausal women, although it remains unclear whether estrogen replacement after menopause is equally protective. The possible impact of TSH suppression on bone health in men remains unknown.

A suppressed TSH is also a risk factor for the development of atrial fibrillation (AF), with its consequent increased risk of cerebrovascular events.[56] TSH suppression increases the odds ratio for the development of AF by threefold over baseline. This finding was based on prospectively collected data from the Framingham cohort and did not distinguish between endogenous and exogenous sources of thyroid hormone as the cause of the suppressed TSH. Because triiodothyronine (T_3) is the active hormone at the cardiac level, and because T_3 concentrations are somewhat lower for any given concentration of TSH when exogenous thyroxine is the source of thyroid hormone excess, the actual risk may be somewhat lower than indicated from the Framingham data. Nevertheless, the potential for significant morbidity exists, and may not be balanced by an improvement in outcome of the FCDTC, at least for stage I and II patients.

The recent guidelines of the National Comprehensive Cancer Network (Version 1.2003 available at *http://www.nccn.org/physician_gls/f_guidelines.html*) make no distinction regarding the level of TSH suppression between patients with cancers of varying risk. However, the joint recommendations of the American Association of Clinical Endocrinologists (AACE) and the American Association of Endocrine Surgeons (AAES) suggest a stratified approach, according to either AJCC stage or patient risk as assessed by one of the clinical prognostic schemes.[57] One approach, then, is for patients at low-risk (MACIS score less than 6.0, or AJCC stage 1 PTC), whose life expectancy is essentially normal, and whose lifetime risk of recurrence is less than 5%, the serum TSH is maintained at or just below the lower limit of the normal range. Because the risk of tumor recurrence in these low-risk patients falls to less than 1% in the 20 years beyond the first 5 postoperative years, the thyroid replacement can be adjusted to allow the TSH to rise into the lower third of the normal range after 5 recurrence-free years. This strategy avoids the potential morbidity associated with long-term TSH suppression. Lifelong monitoring of thyroid hormone status, by annual measurement of serum TSH concentration, is recommended.

Patients at intermediate risk of tumor recurrence include those patients with PTC whose MACIS score lies between 6.0 and 6.9, AJCC stages I and II, or stage III with only lymph node metastases, and patients with minimally invasive FTC. These groups almost certainly warrant rather more aggressive management than the low-risk patients. The TSH should be maintained in the subnormal range, without achieving frank hyperthyroidism. The target TSH concentration is below 0.1 mU/L, ideally in the range between 0.05 and 0.1 mU/L.

High-risk patients, including those with widely invasive FTC or Hürthle cell cancer, or PTC with MACIS scores over 7.0, stage IV disease, or stage III disease with local (extrathyroidal) invasion, should maintain virtually complete TSH suppression (TSH less than 0.05 mU/L). These patients may experience hyperthyroid symptoms when TSH suppression is achieved, although this may be transient. The potential for morbidity must be recognized, and these patients should have screening and monitoring of bone density, at least in postmenopausal women, with appropriate prophylactic and therapeutic management of bone disease.

Radioactive Iodine Therapy

The majority (75% or more) of FCDTC retain the capacity to take up and concentrate iodine, although frequently rather less efficiently than normal thyroid tissue, as is evident from the fact that most thyroid carcinomas are "cold" nodules on preoperative thyroid scintigraphy. This residual differentiated function permits radioactive isotopes of iodine to be used for both the detection and treatment of residual thyroid follicular cells.[43]

Administered orally, iodine isotopes are absorbed rapidly and reliably from the upper gastrointestinal (GI) tract, circulate transiently in the bloodstream, and are concentrated in tissues that express a functional sodium iodide transporter (NIS); these include normal and cancerous thyroid tissue, salivary gland, breast, stomach, and colon. The NIS is also expressed in the kidney, which transports as well as filters iodine, and circulating iodine is excreted rapidly through the urine and stool. The uptake of iodine into both normal and cancerous thyroid tissue is dependent on TSH, which causes upregulation of expression, and possibly increased function, of NIS.

Radioactive isotopes of iodine (^{131}I, ^{129}I) emit gamma rays, which can be detected using an appropriate detection apparatus (a gamma-camera), thus permitting imaging of iodine-concentrating tissues, and thereby the detection of residual or metastatic thyroid tissue, provided there has been sufficient prior stimulation with TSH. Although γ-rays are high energy, their tissue absorption is low, and the majority of these particles pass through the cell and surrounding tissue. Although ideal for imaging purposes, treatment of residual thyroid carcinoma with radioactive iodine depends on β-particle emission, the major emitted particle released by the decay of ^{131}I β-particles have moderately high energy travel and only short distances, less than 1 cm, before interacting with surrounding tissue. The resulting ionization and generation of superoxide radicals causes DNA damage, including double-strand DNA breaks; this activates the p53 pathway (commonly intact in differentiated thyroid carcinoma) and leads to apoptosis of the affected cell.

Radioiodine Remnant Ablation

Postoperative ablation of any remnant thyroid by treatment with 30 to 100 mCi of ^{131}I is often used to "complete" the initial surgical treatment in FCDTC.[43] Controversy remains about the optimal dose required to achieve this. A typical dose is between 30 and 75 mCi. Most often, radioactive iodine is administered 4 to 6 weeks after surgery, with the patient in a hypothyroid state, to maximize TSH-stimulated iodine uptake and whole-body iodine retention. Some authorities advocate a low-iodine diet during preparation for ^{131}I treatment and scanning. Hypothyroidism may be achieved by avoiding thyroid hormone replacement therapy postoperatively, and waiting for at least 4 weeks for endogenous hormone concentrations to fall. Alternatively, initial substitution for 4 weeks with triiodothyronine (Cytomel) followed by 2 weeks of withdrawal can be used and may shorten the duration of symptomatic hypothyroidism. After confirmation of a serum TSH elevated to at least 30 mIU/L, and a negative serum pregnancy test in women of childbearing potential, oral ^{131}I is administered, most often in an outpatient setting.

There is little doubt that even quite substantial remnants of normal thyroid tissue can be eliminated by this approach. Whether small amounts of residual thyroid carcinoma are also eliminated by these remnant ablative doses is uncertain, because carcinoma cells may be several orders of magnitude less efficient than normal follicular cells in the accumulation of iodine.[52] Many groups regard remnant ablation as a necessary first step before proceeding, at a later date, to higher-dose treatment of known residual (or recurrent) disease.

Elimination of a postsurgical remnant has three goals. First, this may destroy residual normal thyroid tissue, making subsequent neck and whole-body scans easier to interpret, because areas of more subtle uptake (for example, in metastatic tumor within regional lymph nodes) might otherwise be overshadowed. Second, it may simplify interpretation of serum thyroglobulin (Tg) concentrations, because residual normal thyroid tissue otherwise contributes, to some degree, to the production of Tg, particularly in the stimulated state (i.e., with elevated TSH). Third, it may make subsequent therapeutic doses of radioiodine more effective, as there will be no competition for the dose from normal thyroid tissue.

There are few data to ascertain whether remnant ablation with ^{131}I improves the outcome of patients with thyroid carcinoma. No randomized trials have been reported of radioactive iodine therapy, and none are in progress. The understanding of the risks and benefits of this widely used therapeutic approach is based entirely on observational, retrospectively analyzed, nonrandomized studies.

In low-risk patients who have had adequate primary operations, with small intrathyroidal papillary tumors (pT1–2, stage I disease), ^{131}I ablation provides no detectable benefit with respect to either cause-specific survival or the risk of recurrent disease.[58] Even in those patients with regional nodal involvement, ^{131}I does not further improve the already very low-risk of either death or recurrence in these otherwise low-risk patients. It is also extremely difficult to detect improvements in survival rates that approach 100%.

The possible benefit of such ablation in higher-risk patients, without evidence of residual disease, continues to stimulate heated debate. These arguments are fueled by apparently contradictory data from a few major centers. On the one hand are data from Mazzaferri, showing that 30-year recurrence rates, in patients with tumors larger than 1.5 cm, were halved (from 38% to 16%) in the 350 patients who received ablation with ^{131}I, compared with the 802 who did not.[59] Similarly, cause-specific 30-year mortality rates fell from 8% to 3%, with no deaths observed in patients who received ^{131}I in whom there was no evidence of residual disease. This view is shared by DeGroot and by the M.D. Anderson group.[60,61]

Contradicting this view are data reported by Hay, which have failed to show any significant benefit of ^{131}I ablation in patients with adequate primary surgery, including selective node dissection, in whom no evidence of residual disease was detected.[45] Analysis of a total of 1,542 patients with PTC, treated at Mayo Clinic, of similar stage to those reported by Mazzaferri, showed recurrence rates (16.6% versus 19.1%; $P = 0.89$) and mortality rates (5.9% versus 7.8%; $P = 0.43$) that were no different with or without ^{131}I remnant ablation.

The recurrence rates reported in this Mayo Clinic study are considerably lower than other reports, even in the absence of routine ^{131}I ablation. This finding may reflect the completeness of surgical excision of the primary tumor and emphasizes the importance of the primary operation in determining outcome. It may be that ^{131}I ablation has proven useful in other studies because of the presence of unrecognized residual disease, almost certainly within regional lymph nodes, the site of the majority of recurrences in several studies. With adequate preoperative assessment (using ultrasound), and careful intraoperative exploration of these affected nodes, the rate of later recurrence may be reduced to the level of the Mayo data and may obviate the need for the radioiodine.

Long-term data show that ablative doses of ^{131}I are safe and are not associated with significant side effects or carcinogenic risk.[62,63] The financial cost and inconvenience to the patient may outweigh any potential benefit, however, at least in low-risk patients who had undergone adequate primary operation. These data support the highly selective use of ^{131}I remnant ablation as adjunctive therapy following adequate primary surgery. In contrast, those patients at moderate or high risk of tumor recurrence based on postoperative risk assessment may benefit more, because they require follow-up by isotope scans and by stimulated Tg concentrations, and may need treatment for residual or recurrent disease. FTC, and particularly its Hürthle cell variant, carry somewhat higher risks for recurrent and metastatic disease than PTC, and these patients may be likely to benefit from ^{131}I ablation and treatment.

Radioiodine Therapy for Locally Residual Disease

Microscopic residual disease is likely to remain after resection of locally invasive (pT4) tumors, even if adequate clearance of gross residual disease is achieved surgically; this may be detected histologically as tumor presence at the surgical margin at the time of the initial resection, even in some tumors initially thought to be contained within the thyroid. Such microscopic disease increases the risk of true PTC thyroid-bed recurrence, and of cause-specific mortality, at least in older (stage III) patients.[64] Similarly, invasive Hürthle cell variant FTC is more likely to recur within the thyroid bed and can prove difficult or impossible to eradicate. Treatment with ^{131}I can be effective for the elimination or control of residual disease in some patients. Approximately 75% to 85% of FCDTC concentrate iodine appreciably when sufficiently stimulated by TSH, and adequate doses of orally administered ^{131}I can induce apoptosis in these cells and in surrounding tissue in a radius of up to 2 mm.

Either ^{131}I or external-beam irradiation improved local recurrence and 20-year cause-specific survival rates in patients with microscopic residual disease.[65,66] Traditionally, treatment of residual disease is a two-step process, with a relatively low dose (30–75 mCi) administered for ablation, and a higher treatment dose (100–200 mCi) given, at a later date, for treatment. There is no empirical evidence that this approach is superior to administration of therapeutic doses on the first occasion. From a diagnostic view, however, a significant thyroid remnant may overshadow the presence of subtler uptake in extrathyroidal tissues, and so the presence of residual disease can be masked on a posttherapy scan.

A few patients present with locally advanced disease, which makes complete surgical resection difficult or impossible, and a small number of these patients have gross residual disease in the neck despite an optimal surgical procedure. An aggressive primary surgical approach for these patients, including partial resection of trachea or esophagus, if necessary, to achieve local control is reasonable, with careful preservation of function. When this is not possible, the presence of gross residual disease is an independent risk factor for both recurrence and cause-specific mortality. Radioactive iodine provides a therapeutic option in this setting, and divided doses of up to 500 mCi may be necessary in an attempt to achieve local control. Some groups advocate even higher total doses of ^{131}I, guided by dosimetry studies, to achieve the maximum dose possible, to a point just short of bone marrow toxicity. Consequences of very high dose ^{131}I therapy include significant permanent xerostomia, dysphagia, bone marrow suppression, and risk of secondary malignancy, including leukemia, lymphoma, transitional cell bladder carcinoma, and colon carcinoma.

Dosimetry has a number of significant potential errors in predicting the radiation dose received by tumor tissue in response to a dose of ^{131}I. The estimated volume of the residual or recurrent tumor to be treated is, at best, only an approximation. The uptake of iodine may vary from one area of residual tumor to another, and may be heterogeneous within a single focus of recurrence. Additionally, the effective half-life of ^{131}I may vary substantially between patients, and even within a single patient, between the tracer and the therapeutic dose. Finally, the use of a prior tracer dose of ^{131}I, necessary to calculate dosimetry, may result in "stunning" of the tumor tissue, and so decrease the uptake of a subsequent therapeutic dose.[67] This stunning effect, if it truly exists, may be minimized by using a low (less than 5 mCi) scanning dose of ^{131}I, or ^{123}I (a gamma-emitter), as the tracer. Nevertheless, dosimetry remains a controversial tool in the administration of therapeutic ^{131}I and is used by a minority of practitioners.

Residual or recurrent FCDTC, even in the presence of gross disease, is often slow growing, may be alternatively treated by external-beam irradiation, and may be amenable to local control by intermittent repeat surgical neck exploration. Very high dose ^{131}I therapy (more than 500 mCi) is of unproven efficacy and has significant associated morbidity. External-beam radiotherapy may be a more-effective alternative.

Radioiodine Therapy for Metastatic Disease

Metastatic FCDTC may concentrate iodine in up to 80% of cases, and TSH can stimulate this uptake. Treatment with ^{131}I is therefore used widely to treat distant metastases, whether they are present at the time of the original diagnosis or appear at a later time. In the treatment of microscopic pulmonary metastases, ^{131}I appears effectively to minimize further growth, and possibly induce regression, at least in children and young adults.[5] This approach may lower the serum Tg concentration and reduce or eliminate iodine trapping, although the chest X-ray may never return entirely to normal and later recurrences remain a possibility. Whether ^{131}I improves survival in these cases remains unproven, but seems likely, and certainly long-term survival is expected in younger patients with PTC, treated with adequate surgery and ^{131}I, even when pulmonary metastatic disease exists at presentation.

There are also numerous anecdotal reports and case series that show significant shrinkage of pulmonary and other distant metastases in older patients after effective ^{131}I treatment.[68] There are no prospective data to show an improvement in survival with this treatment. Larger metastases (greater than ~1 cm in maximum diameter) are significantly less responsive to ^{131}I. Hypoxia within these larger tumor masses induces relative radioresistance, possibly by limiting the production of superoxide radicals, thus reducing the impact of radioactivity on tissue injury.

Initial enlargement of treated metastases occurs commonly, presumably some variable combination of a response to the trophic effect of the elevation of TSH necessary to induce iodine trapping and the edema that occurs in response to effective tumor tissue injury. Such enlargement can cause significant problems from space-occupying lesions in critical locations such as within the brain or adjacent to the spinal cord. Prophylactic steroid administration may be helpful.

The effective ^{131}I dose is lower after the use of recombinant human thyrotropin (rhTSH) than after thyroid hormone withdrawal, however, because hypothyroidism decreases renal ^{131}I clearance, increasing its effective biologic half-life. This effect does not occur after rhTSH therapy and therefore more attention to dosimetry may be necessary when treating after rhTSH use. The efficacy of ^{131}I therapy after rhTSH stimulation has not been evaluated and currently represents an unlicensed use of this product, except for compassionate use in selected patients.

Alternative therapeutic modalities, including resection and localized external-beam irradiation, may also play a role in the management of metastases from FCDTC, and ^{131}I should be viewed as merely one component of a multimodal therapeutic approach.

Postoperative Surveillance and Follow-Up

Recurrence rates for FCDTC range from 10% to 35%.[41–45] The majority of recurrences occur within the first 5 to 10 postoperative years; however, recurrences can occur as long as 25 years after apparently successful primary treatment. Many of the recurrences are easily amenable to treatment, particularly if detected early, before vital structures are compromised. Some form of sensitive surveillance is desirable to detect recurrences before they become clinically apparent.

The vast majority of patients with PTC are at low risk of recurrence, and these patients are unlikely to succumb to their disease. Follow-up surveillance must involve negligible risk, minimal morbidity or discomfort, and must be financially rational. The follow-up should be tailored to the patient's level of risk, with high-risk patients receiving more-intensive assessment, directed to the likely sites of recurrence, whereas low-risk patients should be reassured, and have much less intensive (and less-expensive) follow-up. The clinical staging and risk assessment schemes such as MACIS provide a logical and accurate basis to determine an appropriate follow-up strategy.

Anatomic Evaluation

The majority of recurrences of FCDTC occur in the thyroid bed or within regional lymph nodes in the neck. Ultrasound examination, using high-resolution transducers, permits accurate evaluation of the postoperative neck and is the imaging modality of choice for postoperative surveillance. Recurrent PTC, in particular, has sonographic features that are highly characteristic, with calcifications which result in multiple tiny bright echogenic foci within the tumor deposit. Lymph node architecture by ultrasound is also distinctive for nodal metastases, with enlargement, rounding, and loss of the normally visible, hyperechoic hilar structures. Ultrasound has a major added advantage over other imaging modalities in that ultrasound-guided FNAB can provide cytologic confirmation of the presence of metastatic cancer.

MRI and CT scanning are also widely used to assess the postoperative neck. CT scanning is usually performed without contrast, because the iodine loading from the contrast material otherwise obviates the subsequent use of radioactive iodine therapy. Although either of these techniques can be used to detect recurrences in the neck, their resolution is less good than ultrasound, in part because thyroid carcinoma exhibits similar spin-decay kinetics and similar X-ray density to other soft tissue structures in the neck. The minimum detectable size of recurrent tumor deposits within the neck using these techniques is about 0.5 to 1.0 cm. These techniques are also substantially more expensive than ultrasound. For these reasons, they are used as specialized tests to answer specific issues with regard to a recurrence, rather than as a surveillance tool, for most patients.

Spiral CT scanning (without contrast) may be useful to detect the pulmonary metastases that can occur in FCDTC. However, although the lung and mediastinum represent the most frequent distant metastatic sites for FCDTC of all types, the majority of patients are at very low risk of this event, and a chest X-ray may be sufficient on a routine basis, to exclude pulmonary metastases, in the majority of low-risk patients. In higher-risk patients, radioactive iodine scanning may prove even more useful than CT scanning because it also provides information regarding the possible future treatment of the detected disease with ^{131}I.

Functional Evaluation

Isotope Scanning Functional scanning with radioactive iodine (^{131}I or ^{123}I) remains the most widespread, and often the only, postoperative surveillance undertaken. Although less efficient than normal thyroid, the majority of (~80%), but not all, FCDTCs retain the capacity to concentrate iodine and its isotopes. A gamma-camera permits imaging of the neck within 24 hours of ingestion of oral ^{131}I or ^{123}I, whereas whole-body scanning requires clearance of the physiologically accumulated gastrointestinal and renal iodine and therefore requires 48 to 72 hours between administration of the isotope and imaging. Positive imaging demonstrates functional thyroid tissue and implies that it may be amenable to destruction with the beta-emitter ^{131}I.

Whole-body scanning is commonly performed using doses of 1 to 5 mCi ^{131}I. Follicular cell iodide uptake is a TSH-dependent process, in both normal and malignant tissue. Preparation for scanning has traditionally required withdrawal of thyroid hormone therapy for several weeks, to allow high levels of endogenous TSH to develop, thus stimulating uptake.[69] Serum TSH concentrations of more than 30 mU/L are recommended for scanning and treatment purposes. During the withdrawal of thyroid hormone, which lasts 4 weeks or more, patients develop hypothyroidism, with all its attendant morbidity, and efforts to limit this, by conversion to T_3 (Cytomel) before thyroid hormone withdrawal, are incompletely effective. In addition, a small number of patients are unable to mount an adequate endogenous TSH response because of hypopituitarism, or may be particularly sensitive to the effects of hypothyroidism because of various nonthyroidal illnesses.

Genetic engineering has permitted the large-scale production of recombinant human thyrotropin (rhTSH), and this is now approved for human diagnostic, but not therapeutic, use. Several large studies have been completed, comparing withdrawal scans with rhTSH-stimulated scans.[69,70] Clearly, patients experience considerably fewer hypothyroid symptoms during rhTSH stimulation, when compared with withdrawal scanning, and patients report higher quality of life scores during the days before the scan. rhTSH, which is administered by intramuscular injection, has limited side effects that are relatively minor for most patients.

The usual dose of rhTSH is two injections on consecutive days, with the second injection administered 24 hours before ingestion of the iodine isotope.[57] This approach requires some logistic commitment because the whole process of rhTSH administration followed by scanning requires approximately 5 days to complete. rhTSH fails to trigger urinary iodine retention, and the effective biological half-life of ^{131}I is therefore somewhat lower for rhTSH than for withdrawal scans. This results in rather lower whole-body iodide retention and so marginally poorer quality scans. This problem may be compensated by using higher tracer isotope doses (raising concerns about stunning), or by prolonging the acquisition time in "count-poor" scans, and under these circumstances the detection rate of metastatic disease approaches that of the withdrawal scan.[57] In carefully controlled, blinded studies of hormone withdrawal versus rhTSH-stimulated scans, a small number of "discordant" scans have been reported, with rather more areas of uptake missed following rhTSH stimulation than after withdrawal scanning in the same patients. The addition of stimulated Tg measurements to the scan itself improves the identification rate of patients with residual or recurrent disease to levels similar to withdrawal scanning. Very few treatment decisions would be altered by this minimal difference in sensitivity, but the approach remains a trade-off of sensitivity for symptom minimization.

Except in a compassionate use setting, rhTSH is not currently approved for treatment with radioiodine, because the difference in renal iodide clearance may make such treatment less effective. Studies of the use of rhTSH for ^{131}I therapy are under way. It has been used in a small number of patients with hypopituitarism, who are unable to mount an endogenous TSH rise with conventional hormone withdrawal.

The precise role for rhTSH-stimulated radioiodine scanning in the routine postoperative follow-up of patients with DTC remains unclear. Although the small difference in sensitivity may have minimal clinical impact, the current inability to follow a positive scan immediately by administration of therapeutic radioiodine remains a significant hurdle to its widespread use. For high-risk patients, in whom therapy with ^{131}I is believed likely to be required, withdrawal scanning seems more appropriate, to allow treatment to follow immediately. In low-risk patients, isotope scanning may not be necessary. Those intermediate-risk patients who might best benefit from this new approach remain to be clearly defined.

Other Functional Scans A variety of other isotopic scanning approaches have been assessed in thyroid cancer detection. The most promising of these is positron emission tomography (PET) scanning, which depends on the tumor uptake and sequestration of fluorodeoxyglucose (FDG) tracer.[71,72] It provides a combination of functional and anatomic imaging. The precise sensitivity and specificity of this technique for the detection of recurrent thyroid carcinoma remains to be adequately assessed. The initial experiences show that the less well differentiated FCDTC, which are less likely to image with radioiodine scans, are more likely to image with FDG-PET scan. Thus, the thyroglobulin-positive/radioiodine-negative patient in whom a recurrence is suspected may be best imaged with the FGD-PET technique.

Octreotide scanning, using isotope-labeled octreotide and traditional gamma-camera imaging or SPECT (gamma-camera tomography) imaging, can identify tumors expressing the appropriate receptor (type 2 somatostatin receptors). This may be a useful adjunctive method for the detection of some unusual FCDTC that express the somatostatin receptor. At present, however, it has no role in the routine management of FCDTC.

Tumor Marker

Serum thyroglobulin (Tg) is a highly specific product of the thyroid follicular cell and is detectable in the circulation of patients with residual normal or abnormal thyroid tissue.[57] After total thyroidectomy and remnant ablation, an elevated or rising Tg concentration is a highly specific and sensitive marker of recurrent FCDTC. Tg may be produced by residual normal thyroid tissue following surgery, and even after ^{131}I thyroid remnant ablation, so a low stable level of Tg might not indicate residual disease. A few tumors, particularly those that are high grade and less well differentiated, may not produce large amounts of Tg, making a recurrence without elevated Tg a possibility. Nevertheless, measurement of serum Tg is an important component of a comprehensive surveillance program, allowing detection of early recurrent disease in the majority of such patients, and identifying some patients who might benefit from more-aggressive anatomic imaging.

Tg production and secretion into the circulation are TSH dependent, and Tg concentrations increase following withdrawal of thyroxine therapy, or following stimulation with rhTSH. However, the majority of patients with clinically significant recurrent disease have an elevated Tg level even when on suppressive thyroxine therapy.[57] It is not clear that TSH-stimulated Tg measurement is worthwhile in the majority of patients at low risk of recurrent disease. Radioactive iodine remnant ablation, discussed previously, lowers basal and stimulated Tg concentrations by ablating a postsurgical thyroid remnant. However, this ablation is often incomplete, even with relatively high doses of ^{131}I, and the Tg concentration may remain detectable even in this setting. A serum Tg concentration greater than 5ng/mL (while on suppressive thyroxine therapy) is a useful trigger for further investigation; however, it is not uncommon for patients with Tg concentrations of 5 to 20ng/mL to have no anatomic or functional evidence of disease and to have stable, nonprogressive Tg levels.

The measurement of serum Tg is complicated, in as many as 20% of patients, by the presence of circulating anti-Tg antibodies as a result of autoimmune thyroiditis.[57] Depending on the assay, these antibodies may artificially raise or lower the measured Tg concentration and significantly complicate its interpretation. All assays should include screening for anti-Tg antibodies, and their presence should lead to caution in interpretation of the result. Autoantibody titers can wax and wane; even long-term trends in Tg concentrations may not reliably reflect the underlying growth of thyroid tissue in these patients.

Anaplastic Thyroid Carcinoma

Anaplastic thyroid carcinoma (ATC) is extraordinarily aggressive, relentless, and resistant to treatment. Its typical course stands in stark contrast to that observed for FCDTC. Few therapies have discernible value, and those affected typically suffer rapid tumor progression and death.

Epidemiology

ATC consistently has a median age of onset in the seventh decade of life and is characterized by a female preponderance ranging from 55% to 77%. In the comprehensive 1997 SEER report, which did not reexamine histology but which was conducted entirely in the modern immunohistochemical era, ATC accounted for 1.6% of all thyroid carcinomas.[73]

Clinical Features

Patients with ATC typically present with a suddenly enlarging neck mass. Local compressive symptoms are frequent and can include stridor, dysphagia, dyspnea, hoarseness, weight loss, and superior vena cava syndrome. Patients often have distant metastases at presentation that are usually pulmonary but can also involve bone, brain, and soft tissues. Preexistent thyroid conditions are frequent and can include prior benign thyroid nodules, differentiated thyroid carcinoma, goiter, and Graves' disease.[73–75]

Multiple retrospective clinical series on ATC document its demographic profile and lethality.[73–75] Gender is not a prognostic factor reliably impacting upon survival, nor is the use of radiation therapy. The presence of distant metastases at diagnosis predicts earlier demise from ATC. Small tumor size, defined as less than 5–6cm, is associated with improved survival compared with larger tumors. In a careful multivariate analysis, small tumor size (less than T3) was one of only three identified independent prognostic factors; the others were distant metastasis and the use of thyroxine, while surgical resection, radiation therapy (XRT), and radioiodine ablation had no influence on survival.

Treatment of Anaplastic Thyroid Cancer

Local Therapy

Surgical resection of ATC does not reliably improve local control or survival. A modern-era large series from M.D. Anderson Cancer Center, after reviewing histology to exclude lymphomas, observed no benefit to radical operation for ATC compared with less-radical resection.[76] Similarly, a large multivariate analysis also found no survival benefit to operation for ATC.[77] Resection of ATC may occur in association with better survival, whereas small tumor size is associated with better survival whether ATC is resected or not. Large tumors are impossible to resect, but it does not follow that it is the resection that improves survival.

The significance of focal anaplastic change observed histologically in a differentiated thyroid carcinoma is an occasional observation that may be quite important. In a small recent series, 8 of 65 patients with tall cell or insular carcinoma were found on histologic review to have focal anaplastic carcinoma, defined as a microscopic area or areas of anaplastic dedifferentiation within the primary tumor or nodal metastasis seen only on one slide.[78] All patients were treated by thyroidectomy, half received subsequent radioiodine ablation, and 4 of 8 patients had distant metastases at presentation. The group with foci of anaplastic change experienced increased mortality compared with patients with tall cell or insular carcinoma by both univariate and multivariate analysis, and 7 of 8 died of disease a mean of 11 months later. The authors concluded that even small anaplastic foci predict a fatal outcome. Another report of 17 patients with ATC noted that complete surgical excision of small ATC foci was the only factor associated with survival longer than 12 months. In ATC, the variables of tumor size and anaplastic foci require further study. Patients noted to have foci of ATC within FCDTC may have a prognosis dictated by the ATC focus. Although the data for this are limited, they are compelling. Unfortunately, there are few treatment options to offer patients with this disease.

Given the poor prognosis observed when microscopic foci of ATC are identified incidentally at thyroidectomy for FCDTC, it appears even more difficult to make a case for routine surgical resection of preoperatively identified ATC lesions. After the possibility of ATC is entertained based on history and physical examination, a core needle biopsy establishes the diagnosis in most patients. The role of surgery is limited to open biopsy when needle biopsy fails to obtain enough tissue to differentiate ATC from thyroid lymphoma and securing the airway via tracheostomy when necessary in individual patients. Emergent management of tracheal compression by tumor is occasionally necessary; if the airway is tenuous (less than 4mm in diameter) on CT imaging, before induction of radiation therapy, a tracheostomy is prudent.

Treatment after diagnosis focuses upon local tumor control in the neck. Conventional local therapy is based upon the reports that once-weekly low-dose doxorubicin ($10 mg/m^2$) given as a radiosensitizer with hyperfractionated radiotherapy can produce local tumor regression.[79] The radiation therapy is carried out at a fractional dose of 1.6Gy per treatment twice a day for 3 days per week with a total tumor dose of 5.76Gy. The initial report appeared to offer a modest survival benefit compared with historical controls that has not been borne out in subsequent studies. Use of radiotherapy in combination with a variety of systemic therapies has also failed to demonstrate a survival advantage. The efficacy of radiotherapy at local control has not yet been tested formally in a trial, but numerous studies have reported substantial rates, with local control typically achieved in more than two-thirds of patients (16%–84%), allowing death from distant metastases.[79,80] Use of radiation also potentially facilitates the use of an effective systemic therapy should such an agent be identified.

Systemic Therapy

There are no known systemic therapies that reduce mortality from ATC. ATC has poor concentration of radioiodine, and this modality has no role in therapy. Some reports have suggested a possible role for paclitaxel.[81,82] However, the benefit appears limited and the response durations short.

In summary, ATC is a rare rapidly fatal disease for which there is no known effective therapy, in contrast to FCDTC. There are few data to support a role for resection in patients diagnosed preoperatively with large ATC tumors. However, there may be a benefit to resection of small ATC (less than 5 cm). Anaplastic foci noted within well-differentiated thyroid cancer portend a poor prognosis. Local irradiation may sometimes provide palliative control of disease in the neck.

Medullary Thyroid Carcinoma

Clinical Features

Medullary thyroid carcinomas (MTCs) are 5% to 9% of all thyroid cancers seen in the United States. The cells of origin are the C cells, also called parafollicular cells, derived from the neural crest. C cells are about 1% of the total thyroid mass and are dispersed throughout the gland, with the highest concentration in the upper poles. The C cells have the unique ability to synthesize and secrete calcitonin. Although calcitonin is integral in calcium homeostasis in other vertebrate species, its role in humans is unclear. Calcitonin is used as a specific tumor marker for MTC. It is extremely useful in the screening of individuals predisposed to the hereditary forms of the disease and in the follow-up of patients who have been treated. C cells are also capable of secreting other hormones, including carcinoembryonic antigen (CEA), histaminase, neuron-specific enolase, calcitonin gene-related peptide, somatostatin, thyroglobulin, thyrotropin-stimulating hormone, adrenocortical-stimulating hormone, gastrin-related peptide, serotonin, chromogranin, and substance P.

The clinical presentation of patients with sporadic MTC is similar to patients with FCDTC, in that they usually have a mass in the thyroid gland, and may also have palpable cervical lymph node metastases. Sporadic MTC presents in the third through fifth decades of life, with a roughly equal proportion of men and women. Patients with very large tumor burdens may also have diarrhea as a manifestation of the hormonal function of the tumor. The diagnosis is often suspected based upon cytologic assessment, and the suspicion may be strengthened by an elevated basal serum calcitonin level. However, the presence of an elevated calcitonin level alone is not diagnostic of MTC, even in the presence of a palpable thyroid mass.[83]

Patients from multiple endocrine neoplasia kindreds (MEN-2a, MEN-2b, and familial medullary thyroid carcinoma) often now present without any thyroid mass or discernable thyroid abnormality. Optimally, they are discovered based on direct genetic testing of the RET protooncogene, leading to presymptomatic therapy.

Pathologic Features

MTC was recognized as a unique entity by Hazard, Hawk, and Creile in 1959.[84] Before 1959, MTC was classified as a variant of anaplastic thyroid carcinoma with amyloid stroma. MTCs are well-demarcated, firm, gray-white tumors that may have a gritty consistency. Calcifications may be present on imaging studies. Histologically, the tumors contain uniform polygonal cells with finely granular eosinophilic cytoplasm and central nuclei. The presence of amyloid is a distinctive feature of MTC, although it is not found in all cases. The amyloid is thought to be formed from calcitonin or procalcitonin molecules. In patients with sporadic disease, approximately 70% are solitary and unilateral and 30% are bilateral or multifocal. In patients with RET mutations, 95% are bilateral or multifocal, and only 5% are solitary.[85] C-cell hyperplasia is associated with MTC, particularly in the familial forms. It is presumed that C-cell hyperplasia is a precursor lesion to MTC.

Tumors that exhibit mixed features of MTC and FTC, or, more rarely, MTC and PTC, are unusual, but do occur.[86,87] The WHO recognizes the mixed MTC/FTC as a distinct histologic entity, but the clinical implications of this diagnosis are unclear. They should probably be managed in the same way as more-typical MTC. The possibility of successful treatment of such mixed tumors with radioactive iodine has been entertained, but no data exist.

Risk Factors and Associated Hereditary Conditions

There are no known risk factors for MTC, other than the hereditary syndromes that predispose to it (Table 55.5). The multiple endocrine neoplasia (MEN) type 2 syndromes include MEN 2A, MEN 2B, and familial, non-MEN medullary

TABLE 55.5. **Clinical features of sporadic MTC, multiple endocrine neoplasia (MEN) 2A, MEN 2B, and familial, non-MEN medullary thyroid carcinoma (FMTC).**

Clinical setting	*Features of MTC*	*Inheritance pattern*	*Associated abnormalities*	*Genetic defect*
Sporadic MTC	Unifocal	None	None	No germ-line defect
MEN 2A	Multifocal, bilateral	Autosomal dominant	Pheochromocytoma Hyperparathyroidism	Germ-line misssense mutations in extracellular cysteine codons of RET
MEN 2B	Multifocal, bilateral	Autosomal dominant	Pheochromocytoma Mucosal neuroma Megacolon Skeletal abnormalities	Germ-line misssense mutation in tyrosine kinase domain of RET
FMTC	Multifocal, bilateral	Autosomal dominant	none	Germ-line misssense mutations in extracellular or intracellular cysteine codons of RET

thyroid carcinoma (FMTC).[88] These are autosomal dominant inherited syndromes caused by germ-line mutations in the RET proto-oncogene. The cellular growth and malignant transformation are caused by a gain-of-function mutation, with enhanced intrinsic tyrosine kinase activity (codons 609, 611, 618, 620 of exon 10; codon 634 of exon 11; codon 768 of exon 13; codon 844 of exon 14), or an alteration of substrate recognition (codon 883 of exon 15; codon 918 of exon 16). Medullary thyroid carcinoma (MTC) is the hallmark of these syndromes, with tumors that are multifocal, bilateral, and usually occur at a young age. There is almost complete penetrance of MTC in patients affected by these syndromes; all persons who inherit the disease allele develop MTC. Other features of the syndromes are variably expressed, with incomplete penetrance.

In MEN 2A, patients develop multifocal, bilateral MTC associated with C-cell hyperplasia. Approximately 40% of gene carriers develop adrenal pheochromocytomas, which may also be multifocal and bilateral but not extraadrenal, which are usually associated with adrenal medullary hyperplasia. Hyperparathyroidism develops in 25% to 35% of patients, and is due to hyperplasia, which may be asymmetric, with one or more glands becoming enlarged. The hyperparathyroidism is generally relatively mild compared with MEN 1. Parathyroid carcinoma has been reported in one patient with MEN 2A. Hirschsprung's disease, characterized by the absence of autonomic ganglion cells within the distal colonic parasympathetic plexus, resulting in obstruction and megacolon, is infrequently associated with MEN 2A.

In MEN 2B, 40% to 50% of patients develop pheochromocytomas, and all individuals develop neural gangliomas, particularly in the mucosa of the digestive tract, conjunctiva, lips, and tongue. MEN 2B patients also have megacolon, skeletal abnormalities, and markedly enlarged peripheral nerves. MEN 2B patients do not develop hyperparathyroidism. MTC develops at a very young age (infancy) and appears to be the most aggressive form of hereditary MTC, although its aggressiveness may be more related to the extremely early age of onset, rather than the biologic virulence of the tumor. MTC in patients with MEN 2B is rarely curable once it develops, although it may be preventable by prophylactic thyroidectomy.

Familial, non-MEN medullary thyroid carcinoma (FMTC) is characterized by the development of MTC without any other endocrinopathies. MTC in these patients has a later age of onset and a more-indolent clinical course than MTC in patients with MEN 2A and MEN 2B. These patients do not develop any of the extrathyroidal manifestations of MEN 2A or 2B.

Prognosis of Medullary Thyroid Cancer

Although the prognosis of sporadic MTC is considered to be favorable, long-term studies report a 5- and 10-year-survival rate of only 80% to 90 % and 60% to 80 %, respectively.[89,90] More than 50% of all patients with sporadic MTC eventually die of their disease. TNM tumor stage is the most powerful predictor of prognosis in sporadic MTC. Most patients die of distant metastases (stage IV), which have the single greatest influence on outcome. In addition, patients with lymph node metastases (stage III) have a worse outcome compared with those patients without lymph node metastases. The impact of lymph node metastases on survival is greater than primary tumor size. The often-reported better prognosis of hereditary MTC is most likely biased by those hereditary cases that are diagnosed at an early tumor stage by screening procedures, notably by calcitonin measurement or mutation analysis of the RET proto-oncogene.

Treatment of Medullary Thyroid Cancer

Resection is the treatment of choice in MTC. This offers the only prospect of definitive cure, both in primary and in locally recurrent MTC. Whenever feasible, all efforts should be directed at eradicating the tumor.

Primary Operation

Localized or Regional Disease Because of the frequent multicentricity of sporadic MTC (20%), total thyroidectomy is appropriate for all cases of sporadic MTC, regardless of primary tumor size. Controversy exists, however, regarding the indication for and the extent of lymph node surgery. The central neck lymph node compartment is involved in at least 33% of patients with tumors of 10mm or less (pT1) in size (Table 55.6).[91,92] With this frequent involvement of the central neck compartment with small cancers, a dissection of the central neck should be performed for all patients for accurate staging and therapy for micrometastases. In the presence of

TABLE 55.6. Medullary carcinoma of the thyroid: frequency and distribution of nodal metastases.

Tumor size	No. of patients	Central node metastases (patients)	Ipsilateral level II–V metastases (patients)	Contralateral level II–V metastases (patients)
Unilateral tumor				
0–0.9 cm	4	3/4	3/4	1/4
1–1.9 cm	9	8/9	8/9	3/9
2– 2.9 cm	5	4/5	3/5	3/5
3–3.9 cm	5	2/5	4/5	3/5
4 cm or larger	9	9/9	8/9	4/9
Total	32	26/32 (81%)	26/32 (81%)	14/32 (44%)
Bilateral tumors (largest size)				
0–0.9	12	8/12	9/12	4/12
1–1.9	7	5/7	6/7	4/7
2–2.9	8	7/8	4/8	5/8
3–3.9	7	7/7	6/7	5/7
4 cm or larger	7	5/7	4/7	2/7
Total	41	32/41 (78%)	29/41 (71%)	20/41 (49%)

Central nodes refer to right and left level VI and VII nodes.
Source: Data from Moley and DeBenedetti.[92]

central neck lymph node metastases, demonstrated preoperatively by ultrasonography or intraoperatively, dissection of at least the ipsilateral neck compartments (levels 2–5) with curative intent is advocated because of the frequent occurrence of lateral neck lymph node metastases (Table 55.6). Contralateral metastases are present in at least 40% of patients, and these compartments may also require dissection, either under the same anesthetic, or subsequently if the calcitonin levels fail to normalize after thyroidectomy with central and ipsilateral dissection.

MTC with Distant Metastases Patients with distant metastases at presentation usually have an unfavorable course that does not warrant extended surgery apart from total thyroidectomy, central lymphadenectomy, and selective removal of symptomatic lymph nodes or tumor masses. Even with widespread disease, patients often have a prolonged survival despite their debilitating symptoms from tumor persistence or progression. Selected procedures may be indicated for symptomatic control. Judicious palliative reoperative resection of discrete symptomatic lesions may provide significant long-term control of symptoms, improving quality of life for patients with metastatic MTC.

Reoperation

Hypercalcitoninemia after primary surgery is a frequent phenomenon. For patients with locoregional recurrence without detectable distant metastases after inadequate primary surgery, reoperation to try to achieve local control and possibly cure is appropriate. Inadequate primary procedures should not be allowed to eliminate the chance for the patient to be cured, if the remaining disease can be excised. The indication for and the extent of surgery in patients with postoperative hypercalcitoninemia depends on the extent of locoregional recurrence or tumor persistence. Despite the persistence of hypercalcitoninemia, a substantial proportion of patients exhibit neither locoregional nor distant tumor foci by noninvasive imaging techniques.

Locoregional reoperation with curative intent is indicated in patients without demonstrable distant metastases.[93] Due to the frequency of bilateral lymph node metastases at reoperation, reoperative procedures should be designed to remove residual disease from the central neck, as well as to accomplish adequate bilateral neck dissection.

Locoregional recurrence after adequate primary surgery can be caused by either local recurrence within the former thyroid bed or locoregional lymph node metastases. It is important to localize the site of recurrence carefully in these patients who have had previous neck clearance. Central neck recurrence should be eradicated because tumor-related complications affecting the tracheoesophageal axis are difficult to manage and cannot be treated effectively by external-beam radiation. Solitary locoregional lymph node recurrence after adequate primary surgery is best treated by selective lymphadenectomy.

Preventative Resection for MEN 2A, 2B, or FMTC Gene Carriers

Individuals with MEN 2A, 2B, and FMTC are virtually certain to develop MTC at some point in their lives (usually before age 30). Therefore, at-risk family members who are found to have inherited a RET gene mutation should have thyroidectomy, regardless of their plasma calcitonin levels.

In a report of preventative thyroidectomy for RET mutation carriers, Wells and colleagues reported a series of 49 children with MEN 2A and MEN 2B.[94] In this series, 14 children had a prophylactic thyroidectomy based on genetic testing. The average age of the children at the time of surgery was 10.5 years. Postoperative calcitonin levels were all undetectable, and there was no evidence of recurrent MTC with a mean follow-up of 1.3 years. In an interim report of 3-year follow-up of the earliest group of 18 patients, no recurrence of disease was noted.[95]

The finding of carcinoma in the glands of many of these young patients with normal stimulated calcitonin testing indicates that the operation was therapeutic, not prophylactic. The ideal age for performance of thyroidectomy in those patients found to be genetically positive has not been determined unequivocally. Six years of age is accepted as a reasonable time for thyroidectomy in patients with MEN 2A and FMTC. Patients with MEN2B should undergo thyroidectomy during infancy, because of the aggressiveness and earlier age of onset of MTC in these patients. Follow-up over the next decades will determine whether there is a significant rate of recurrence following preventative thyroidectomy. At present, it is advisable to follow these patients with plasma calcitonin levels every 1 to 2 years. These patients must also continue to be followed for the development of pheochromocytoma and hyperparathyroidism.

External Irradiation

MTC is not very sensitive to external irradiation. Some retrospective studies report a reduced risk of local recurrence after radiation; however, operative removal of all tumor should be performed whenever feasible.[96] External irradiation may have distressing long-term side effects, notably cough and mucous membrane dryness. Scarring in the neck hampers future assessment of local recurrences and renders reoperation more difficult or impossible. When operative treatment has been successful in normalizing the calcitonin level, there is no need for radiation. In the event of locoregional recurrence, reoperation is the preferred treatment. Radiation therapy should be avoided unless local disease is either symptomatic or rapidly progressing and is not amenable to resection. Radiation may be useful in the treatment of symptomatic distant metastases, especially in bone metastases.

Chemotherapy

Experience with chemotherapy is limited to advanced or metastatic MTC, and no consistent benefit has been shown.[88] Drugs investigated include cisplatin, cyclophosphamide, dacarbazine (DTIC), doxorubicin, 5-fluorouracil (5-FU), streptozocin, vincristine, and vindesine.

Follow-Up of Medullary Thyroid Cancer

The postoperative follow-up for patients with sporadic MTC primarily consists in monitoring serum calcitonin levels. When an elevated or rising serum calcitonin is identified, further diagnostic workup or therapeutic intervention is indicated, including additional imaging and possibly surgery. The diagnostic workup must differentiate between local and systemic recurrence.

Parathyroid Carcinoma

Parathyroid carcinoma can be difficult to diagnose. At the time of the initial cervical exploration, it may be overlooked due to lack of overt malignant tumor characteristics such as adherence to the trachea, thyroid, recurrent laryngeal nerve, or esophageal wall and/or the presence of lymph node metastases. On microscopic evaluation, unless there is evidence of capsular or vascular invasion, the diagnosis may remain ambiguous. The combined intraoperative findings provided by an experienced surgeon and a meticulous microscopic evaluation are often required to confirm the suspicious diagnosis of malignancy. Because the first operation offers the best chance of local tumor control, it is imperative that the surgeon is aware of the clinical course of parathyroid cancer and participates in the management and follow-up.

Clinical Features of Parathyroid Carcinoma

In contrast to benign hyperparathyroidism, patients with parathyroid cancer are younger at diagnosis (44 to 53 years) with equal sex distribution.[97,98] Clinical symptoms are usually conspicuous in patients with a parathyroid malignancy. The general symptoms are fatigue, both muscular and mental, depression, nausea, vomiting, dehydration, polydipsia, and polyuria. Each of these can be attributed to the marked hypercalcemia usually found in these patients. Skeletal changes occur in approximately 40% to 70% of the patients. Elevated serum alkaline phosphatase levels are common. Nephrolithiasis occurs in about 70%, and nephrocalcinosis with severe renal dysfunction is found in 20% to 50%. Pancreatitis and peptic ulcerations are reported to occur in 10% to 15%. Among 95 patients with the diagnosis of parathyroid cancer, the median serum calcium level was 3.6 mmol/L (range, 2.5–6.1), and 20% had a palpable cervical mass.[98]

The combination of both renal and bone disease is frequently encountered in parathyroid cancer patients in contrast to those with benign hyperparathyroidism (HPT); this should raise the suspicion of cancer. A palpable, usually firm, cervical tumor is present in 30% to 50% of the patients. Thus, a diagnosis of parathyroid cancer should be strongly considered in a patient with a relative rapid onset of symptoms, with laboratory findings consistent with severe primary hyperparathyroidism (pHPT), an elevated serum alkaline phosphatase, and a palpable neck mass.

Treatment of Parathyroid Carcinoma

The most characteristic intraoperative findings are a firm grayish white tumor, grossly adherent to adjacent structures.[99] Most malignant tumors are larger (more than 2 cm, median weight 4 g), but size or glandular weight alone is not sufficient for diagnosis. The same operative strategy applies to benign and malignant parathyroid neoplasms in making every effort to preserve the capsule of the tumor. When the tumor invades a neighboring structure such as the thyroid gland, the strap muscles, or the esophageal wall, these structures should be removed in continuity with the tumor. When adherent to the recurrent laryngeal nerve that is known to function, an attempt to shave the tumor from the nerve is justifiable and indicated when the diagnosis of carcinoma is questionable. Most functioning nerves can be dissected free from contiguous malignant tumors. If this cannot be accomplished, the nerve may have to be sacrificed, which is preferable to cutting into tumor.

Breaking the tumor capsule can cause tumor seeding and puts the patient at risk for developing local recurrence even if the tumor is benign. Seeding of tumor cells or parathyromatosis can be extremely hard to differentiate from invasive carcinoma. Resection en bloc with the ipsilateral thyroid lobe is frequently required. Several authors and results from the collected international series of parathyroid carcinomas showed that a more extensive procedure including lymph node dissection did not affect prognosis.[97,98] Lymph node metastases were a rare finding. Reliance on intraoperative microscopic diagnosis should be avoided because of the difficulties in applying the diagnostic criteria of malignancy in a frozen section. Bilateral exploration for an evaluation of the other glands to rule out a concomitant benign neoplasm or multiglandular disease is recommended.

Parathyroid cancer can follow a variably aggressive course. Even at initial exploration, the macroscopic appearance of the tumor can be misleading. Hypercalcemia from parathyroid carcinoma may have a slow or a rapid onset, although the average time to recurrence is 3 years after initial diagnosis.[100] When signs of acute hypercalcemic crisis are evident, urgent treatment is indicated; this includes rehydration with intravenous saline, restoration of electrolyte balance, loop diuretics, and bisphosphonates.[101] Intravenous bisphosphonates (pamidronate) usually have an effect within 48 to 72 hours that may be sustained for up to 3 weeks. The mechanism of action is inhibition of osteoclastic bone resorption. The drug is well tolerated and not associated with any major complications.

Surgical removal of metastatic or recurrent disease is appropriate whenever feasible. The most common locations for recurrent or metastatic disease are the neck and the lungs, followed by the liver and the skeleton. Cervical recurrences may require repeated neck explorations. A lateral approach (anterior to the sternocleidomastoid, and lateral to the strap muscles) is preferred and may prevent damage to a recurrent laryngeal nerve.[102] Patients with lung metastases have been successfully treated or palliated by limited resection.

Prognosis and Follow-Up

Comparative studies have shown that parathyroid cancer can sometimes be controlled by aggressive surgical interventions; when that is not possible, the best palliative drug treatment for maintaining eucalcemia is intravenous bisphosphonate. There is a significant difference in survival in the collected international series of parathyroid carcinomas when comparing the survival of patients with metastatic disease to those without metastases (30% versus 85% after 5 years).[98] These findings stress the importance of early diagnosis, appropriate initial surgical procedure, and the variability in tumor biology.

References

1. Kumar H, Daykin J, Holder R, Watkinson JC, Sheppard MC, Franklyn JA. Gender, clinical findings, and serum thyrotropin measurements in the prediction of thyroid neoplasia in 1005 patients presenting with thyroid enlargement and investigated by fine-needle aspiration cytology. Thyroid 1999;9:1105–1109.
2. Cancer Facts and Figures 2004. Atlanta: American Cancer Society, 2004.
3. Ries LAG, Eisner MP, Kosary CL, et al (eds). SEER Cancer Statistics Review, 1975–2001. Bethesda, MD: National Cancer Institute, 2004.
4. Carcangiu ML, Zampi G, Pupi A, Castagnoli A, Rosai J. Papillary carcinoma of the thyroid. A clinicopathologic study of 241 cases treated at the University of Florence, Italy. Cancer (Phila) 1985;55:805–828.
5. Grigsby PW, Gal-or A, Michalski JM, Doherty GM. Childhood and adolescent thyroid carcinoma. Cancer (Phila) 2002;95:724–729.
6. DeGroot LJ, Kaplan EL, McCormick M, Straus FH. Natural history, treatment, and course of papillary thyroid carcinoma. J Clin Endocrinol Metab 1990;71:414–424.
7. Ozaki O, Ito K, Kobayashi K, Toshima K, Iwasaki H, Yashiro T. Thyroid carcinoma in Graves' disease. World J Surg 1990;14:437–440; discussion 440–441.
8. Mazzaferri EL. Thyroid cancer and Graves' disease. J Clin Endocrinol Metab 1990;70:826–829.
9. Katoh R, Sasaki J, Kurihara H, Suzuki K, Iida Y, Kawaoi A. Multiple thyroid involvement (intraglandular metastasis) in papillary thyroid carcinoma. A clinicopathologic study of 105 consecutive patients. Cancer (Phila) 1992;70:1585–1590.
10. Lindsay S. Carcinoma of the Thyroid Gland. Springfield: Thomas, 1960.
11. Johnson TL, Lloyd RV, Thompson NW, Beierwaltes WH, Sisson JC. Prognostic implications of the tall cell variant of papillary thyroid carcinoma. Am J Surg Pathol 1988;12:22–27.
12. Hawk WA, Hazard JB. The many appearances of papillary carcinoma of the thyroid. Cleve Clin Q. 1976;43(4):207–215.
13. Moreno-Egea A, Rodriguez-Gonzalez JM, Sola-Perez J, Soria-Cogollos T, Parrilla-Paricio P. Multivariate analysis of histopathological features as prognostic factors in patients with papillary thyroid carcinoma. Br J Surg 1995;82:1092–1094.
14. Moreno Egea A, Rodriguez Gonzalez JM, Sola Perez J, Soria Cogollos T, Parrilla Paricio P. Prognostic value of the tall cell variety of papillary cancer of the thyroid. Eur J Surg Oncol 1993;19:517–521.
15. Vickery AL Jr. Thyroid papillary carcinoma. Pathological and philosophical controversies. Am J Surg Pathol 1983;7:797–807.
16. Moreno Egea A, Rodriguez Gonzalez JM, Sola Perez J, Soria T, Parrilla Paricio P. Clinicopathological study of the diffuse sclerosing variety of papillary cancer of the thyroid. Presentation of 4 new cases and review of the literature. Eur J Surg Oncol 1994;20:7–11.
17. Herrera MF, Hay ID, Wu PS, et al. Hurthle cell (oxyphilic) papillary thyroid carcinoma: a variant with more aggressive biologic behavior. World J Surg 1992:16:669–674; discussion 674–685.
18. Shore RE. Issues and epidemiological evidence regarding radiation-induced thyroid cancer. Radiat Res 1992;131:98–111.
19. Shore RE, Hildreth N, Dvoretsky P, Andresen E, Moseson M, Pasternack B. Thyroid cancer among persons given x-ray treatment in infancy for an enlarged thymus gland. Am J Epidemiol 1993;137:1068–1080.
20. Ron E, Lubin JH, Shore RE, et al. Thyroid cancer after exposure to external radiation: a pooled analysis of seven studies. Radiat Res 1995;141:259–277.
21. Ron E, Modan B. Benign and malignant thyroid neoplasms after childhood irradiation for tinea capitis. J Natl Cancer Inst 1980;65:7–11.
22. Perkel VS, Gail MH, Lubin J, et al. Radiation-induced thyroid neoplasms: evidence for familial susceptibility factors. J Clin Endocrinol Metab 1988;66:1316–1322.
23. Schneider AB, Ron E, Lubin J, Stovall M, Gierlowski TC. Dose-response relationships for radiation-induced thyroid cancer and thyroid nodules: evidence for the prolonged effects of radiation on the thyroid. J Clin Endocrinol Metab 1993;77:362–369.
24. Kerber RA, Till JE, Simon SL, et al. A cohort study of thyroid disease in relation to fallout from nuclear weapons testing [see comment]. JAMA 1993;270:2076–2082.
25. Hamilton TE, van Belle G, LoGerfo JP. Thyroid neoplasia in Marshall islanders exposed to nuclear fallout. JAMA 1987;258:629–636.
26. Nikiforov Y, Gnepp DR. Pediatric thyroid cancer after the Chernobyl disaster. Cancer (Phila) 1994;74:748–766.
27. Cetta F, Montalto G, Gori M, Curia MC, Cama A, Olschwang S. Germline mutations of the APC gene in patients with familial adenomatous polyposis-associated thyroid carcinoma: results

from a European cooperative study. J Clin Endocrinol Metab 2000; 85:286–292.

28. Cetta F, Curia MC, Montalto G, et al. Thyroid carcinoma usually occurs in patients with familial adenomatous polyposis in the absence of biallelic inactivation of the adenomatous polyposis coli gene. J Clin Endocrinol Metabol 2001;86:427–432.
29. Hay ID, Grant CS, Bergstralh EJ, Thompson GB, van Heerden JA, Goellner JR. Unilateral total lobectomy: is it sufficient surgical treatment for patients with AMES low-risk papillary thyroid carcinoma? Surgery (St. Louis) 1998;124:958–964; discussion 964–966.
30. Reeve T, Thompson NW. Complications of thyroid surgery: how to avoid them, how to manage them, and observations on their possible effect on the whole patient. World J Surg 2000;24:971–975.
31. Ley PB, Roberts JW, Symmonds J, et al. Safety and efficacy of total thyroidectomy for differentiated thyroid carcinoma: a 20-year review. Am Surg 1993;59:110–114.
32. Akslen LA. Prognostic importance of histologic grading in papillary thyroid carcinoma. Cancer (Phila) 1993;72:2680–2685.
33. Akslen LA, Haldorsen T, Thoresen SO, Glattre A. Survival and causes of death in thyroid cancer: a population-based study of 2479 cases from Norway. Cancer Res 1991;51:1234–1241.
34. Pineda JD, Lee T, Ain K, Reynolds JC, Robbins J. Iodine-131 therapy for thyroid cancer patients with elevated thyroglobulin and negative diagnostic scan [see comment]. J Clin Endocrinol Metab 1995;80:1488–1492.
35. Ain KB. Papillary thyroid carcinoma. Etiology, assessment, and therapy. Endocrinol Metabol Clin N Am 1995;24:711–760.
36. Correa P, Chen VW. Endocrine gland cancer. Cancer (Phila) 1995; 75:338–352.
37. Rosai J, Carcangiu ML, DeLellis RA. Tumors of the Thyroid Gland, Series 3, Fascicle 5. Washington, DC: Armed Forces Institute of Pathology, 1992.
38. Bacher-Stier C, Riccabona G, Totsch M, Kemmler G, Oberaigner W, Moncayo R. Incidence and clinical characteristics of thyroid carcinoma after iodine prophylaxis in an endemic goiter country. Thyroid 1997;7:733–741.
39. Pacini F, Vorontsova T, Demidchik EP, et al. Post-Chernobyl thyroid carcinoma in Belarus children and adolescents: comparison with naturally occurring thyroid carcinoma in Italy and France. J Clin Endocrinol Metab 1997;82:3563–3569.
40. Cooper DS, Schneyer CR. Follicular and Hurthle cell carcinoma of the thyroid. Endocrinol Metab Clin N Am 1990;19:577–591.
41. Hay ID. Papillary thyroid carcinoma. Endocrinol Metab Clin N Am 1990;19:545–576.
42. Grebe SK, Hay ID. Follicular thyroid cancer. Endocrinol Metab Clin N Am 1995;24:761–801.
43. Mazzaferri EL. An overview of the management of papillary and follicular thyroid carcinoma. Thyroid 1999;9:421–427.
44. Mazzaferi FL. Papillary thyroid carcinoma: factors influencing prognosis and current therapy. Semin Oncol 1987;14:315–332.
45. Grebe SK, Hay ID. Follicular cell-derived thyroid carcinomas. Cancer Treat Res 1997;89:91–140.
46. Robbins J, Merino MJ, Boice JD Jr, et al. Thyroid cancer: a lethal endocrine neoplasm. Ann Intern Med 1991;115:133–147.
47. Greene F. AJCC Cancer Staging Manual, 6th ed. New York: Springer-Verlag, 2002.
48. Hundahl SA, Fleming ID, Fremgen AM, Menck HR. A National Cancer Data Base report on 53,856 cases of thyroid carcinoma treated in the U.S., 1985–1995 [see comments]. Cancer (Phila) 1998;83:2638–2648.
49. Dean DS, Hay ID. Prognostic indicators in differentiated thyroid carcinoma. Cancer Control 2000;7:229–239.
50. Hay ID, Bergstralh EJ, Goellner JR, Ebersold JR, Grant CS. Predicting outcome in papillary thyroid carcinoma: development of a reliable prognostic scoring system in a cohort of 1779 patients surgically treated at one institution during 1940 through 1989. Surgery (St. Louis) 1993;114:1050–1057; discussion 1057–1058.
51. Kouvaraki MA, Shapiro SE, Fornage BD, et al. Role of preoperative ultrasonography in the surgical management of patients with thyroid cancer. Surgery (St. Louis) 2003;134:946–954; discussion 954–955.
52. Grebe SK, Hay ID. Thyroid cancer nodal metastases: biologic significance and therapeutic considerations. Surg Oncol Clin N Am 1996;5:43–63.
53. Jorda M, Gonzalez-Campora R, Mora J, Herrero-Zapatero A, Otal C, Galera H. Prognostic factors in follicular carcinoma of the thyroid. Arch Pathol Lab Med 1993;117:631–635.
54. Cooper DS, Specker B, Ho M, et al. Thyrotropin suppression and disease progression in patients with differentiated thyroid cancer: results from the National Thyroid Cancer Treatment Cooperative Registry. Thyroid 1998;8:737–744.
55. Toivonen J, Tahtela R, Laitinen K, Risteli J, Valimaki MJ. Markers of bone turnover in patients with differentiated thyroid cancer with and following withdrawal of thyroxine suppressive therapy. Eur J Endocrinol 1998;138:667–673.
56. Sawin CT, Geller A, Wolf PA, et al. Low serum thyrotropin concentrations as a risk factor for atrial fibrillation in older persons [see comment]. N Engl J Med 1994;331:1249–1252.
57. Thyroid Carcinoma Task Force. AACE/AAES medical/surgical guidelines for clinical practice: management of thyroid carcinoma. American Association of Clinical Endocrinologists. American College of Endocrinology. Endocr Pract 2001;7:202–220.
58. Hay ID, Grant CS, van Heerden JA, Goellner JR, Ebersold JR, Bergstralh EJ. Papillary thyroid microcarcinoma: a study of 535 cases observed in a 50-year period. Surgery (St. Louis) 1992;112: 1139–1146; discussion 1146–1147.
59. Mazzaferri EL, Young RL. Papillary thyroid carcinoma: a 10 year follow-up report of the impact of therapy in 576 patients. Am J Med 1981;70:511–518.
60. DeGroot LJ, Kaplan EL, Straus FH, Shukla MS. Does the method of management of papillary thyroid carcinoma make a difference in outcome? World J Surg 1994;18:123–130.
61. Samaan NA, Schultz PN, Hickey RC, et al. The results of various modalities of treatment of well differentiated thyroid carcinomas: a retrospective review of 1599 patients. J Clin Endocrinol Metab 1992;75:714–720.
62. Franklyn JA, Maisonneuve P, Sheppard M, Betteridge J, Boyle P. Cancer incidence and mortality after radioiodine treatment for hyperthyroidism: a population-based cohort study [see comment]. Lancet 1999;353:2111–2115.
63. Franklyn JA. Thyroid disease and its treatment: short- and long-term consequences. J R Coll Phys Lond 1999;33:564–567.
64. Hay ID, Bergstralh EJ, Grant CS, et al. Impact of primary surgery on outcome in 300 patients with pathologic tumor-node-metastasis stage III papillary thyroid carcinoma treated at one institution from 1940 through 1989. Surgery (St. Louis) 1999;126: 1173–1181; discussion 1181–1182.
65. Taylor T, Specker B, Robbins J, et al. Outcome after treatment of high-risk papillary and non-Hurthle-cell follicular thyroid carcinoma. Ann Intern Med 1998;129:622–627.
66. Sherman SI, Brierley JD, Sperling M, et al. Prospective multicenter study of thyroid carcinoma treatment: initial analysis of staging and outcome. National Thyroid Cancer Treatment Cooperative Study Registry Group [see comment]. Cancer (Phila) 1998;83:1012–1021.
67. Park HM, Park YH, Zhou XH. Detection of thyroid remnant/metastasis without stunning: an ongoing dilemma. Thyroid 1997; 7:277–280.
68. Maxon MR, Smith HS. Radioactive ^{131}I in the diagnosis and treatment of metastatic well differentiated thyroid cancer. Endocrinol Metab Clin N Am 1990;19:685–718.

69. Ladenson PW, Braverman LE, Mazzaferri EL, et al. Comparison of administration of recombinant human thyrotropin with withdrawal of thyroid hormone for radioactive iodine scanning in patients with thyroid carcinoma [see comment]. N Engl J Med 1997;337:888–896.
70. Haugen BR, Pacini F, Reiners C, et al. A comparison of recombinant human thyrotropin and thyroid hormone withdrawal for the detection of thyroid remnant or cancer. J Clin Endocrinol Metab 1999;84:3877–3885.
71. Hooft L, Hoekstra OS, Deville W, et al. Diagnostic accuracy of 18F-fluorodeoxyglucose positron emission tomography in the follow-up of papillary or follicular thyroid cancer. J Clin Endocrinol Metab 2001;86:3779–3786.
72. Wang W, Macapinlac H, Larson SM, et al. [^{18}F]-2-Fluoro-2-deoxy-D-glucose positron emission tomography localizes residual thyroid cancer in patients with negative diagnostic [^{131}]I whole body scans and elevated serum thyroglobulin levels. J Clin Endocrinol Metab 1999;84:2291–2302.
73. Gilliland FD, Hunt WC, Morris DM, Key CR. Prognostic factors for thyroid carcinoma. A population-based study of 15,698 cases from the Surveillance, Epidemiology and End Results (SEER) program 1973–1991. Cancer (Phila) 1997;79:564–573.
74. McIver B, Hay ID, Giuffrida DF, et al. Anaplastic thyroid carcinoma: a 50-year experience at a single institution. Surgery (St. Louis) 2001;130:1028–1034.
75. Kobayashi T, Asakawa H, Umeshita K, et al. Treatment of 37 patients with anaplastic carcinoma of the thyroid. Head Neck 1996;18:36–41.
76. Venkatesh YSS, Ordonez NG, Schultz PN, Hickey RC, Goepfert H, Samoan NA. Anaplastic carcinoma of the thyroid. Cancer (Phila) 1990;66:321–330.
77. Staunton MD. Thyroid cancer: a multivariate analysis on influence of treatment on long-term survival. Eur J Surg Oncol 1994;20:613–621.
78. van den Brekel MW, Hekkenberg RJ, Asa SL, Tomlinson G, Rosen IB, Freeman JL. Prognostic features in tall cell papillary carcinoma and insular thyroid carcinoma. Laryngoscope 1997; 107:254–259.
79. Kim JH, Leeper RD. Treatment of locally advanced thyroid carcinoma with combination doxorubicin and radiation therapy. Cancer (Phila) 1987;60:2372–2375.
80. Schlumberger M, Parmentier C, Delisle MJ, Couette JE, Droz JP, Sarrazin D. Combination therapy for anaplastic giant cell thyroid carcinoma. Cancer (Phila) 1991;67:564–566.
81. Sweeney PJ, Haraf DJ, Recant W, Kaplan EL, Vokes EE. Anaplastic carcinoma of the thyroid. Ann Oncol 1996;7:739–744.
82. Ain KB, Tofiq S, Taylor KD. Antineoplastic activity of taxol against human anaplastic thyroid carcinoma cell lines in vitro and in vivo. J Clin Endocrinol Metab 1996;81:3650–3653.
83. Niccoli P, Wion-Barbot N, Caron P, et al. Interest of routine measurement of serum calcitonin: study in a large series of thyroidectomized patients. The French Medullary Study Group [see comment]. J Clin Endocrinol Metab 1997;82:338–341.
84. Hazard JB, Hawk WH, Creile GJ. Medullary (solid) carcinoma of the thyroid-clinicopathologic entity. J Clin Endocrinol Metab 1959;19:704.
85. Block MA, Jackson CE, Greenawald KA, et al. Clinical characteristics distinguishing hereditary from sporadic medullary thyroid carcinoma. Arch Surg 1980;115:142.
86. Apel RL, Alpert LC, Rizzo A, LiVolsi VA, Asa SL. A metastasizing composite carcinoma of the thyroid with distinct medullary and papillary components. Arch Pathol Lab Med 1994;118:1143–1147.
87. Lax SF, Beham A, Kronberger-Schonecker D, Langsteger W, Denk H. Coexistence of papillary and medullary carcinoma of the thyroid gland-mixed or collision tumour? Clinicopathological analysis of three cases. Virchows Arch 1994;424:441–447.
88. Moley JF. Medullary thyroid carcinoma. Curr Treat Options Oncol 2003;4:339–347.
89. Modigliani E, Cohen R, Campos JM, et al. Prognostic factors for survival and for biochemical cure in medullary thyroid carcinoma: results in 899 patients. The GETC Study Group. Groupe d'etude des tumeurs a calcitonine. Clin Endocrinol 1998;48: 265–273.
90. Bergholm U, Bergstrom R, Ekbom A. Long-term follow-up of patients with medullary carcinoma of the thyroid. Cancer (Phila) 1997;79:132–138.
91. Gimm O, Ukkat J, Dralle H. Determinative factors of biochemical cure after primary and reoperative surgery for sporadic medullary thyroid carcinoma. World J Surg 1998;22:562–567; discussion 567–568.
92. Moley JF, DeBenedetti MK. Patterns of nodal metastases in palpable medullary thyroid carcinoma: recommendations for extent of node dissection. Ann Surg 1999;229:880–887; discussion 887–888.
93. Moley JF, Debenedetti MK, Dilley WG, Tisell LE, Wells SA. Surgical management of patients with persistent or recurrent medullary thyroid cancer. J Intern Med 1998;243:521–526.
94. Skinner MA, DeBenedetti MK, Moley JF, Norton JA, Wells SA Jr. Medullary thyroid carcinoma in children with multiple endocrine neoplasia types 2A and 2B. J Pediatr Surg 1996;31: 177–181; discussion 181–182.
95. Wells SA Jr, Skinner MA. Prophylactic thyroidectomy, based on direct genetic testing, in patients at risk for the multiple endocrine neoplasia type 2 syndromes. Exp Clin Endocrinol Diabetes 1998;106:29–34.
96. Steinfeld AD. The role of radiation therapy in medullary carcinoma of the thyroid. Radiology 1977;123:745.
97. Sandelin K. Parathyroid carcinoma. Cancer Treat Res 1997;89: 183–192.
98. Sandelin K, Auer G, Bondeson L, Grimelius L, Farnebo LO. Prognostic factors in parathyroid cancer: a review of 95 cases. World J Surg 1992;16:724–731.
99. Bondeson L, Sandelin K, Grimelius L. Histopathological variables and DNA cytometry in parathyroid carcinoma. Am J Surg Pathol 1993;17:820–829.
100. Shane E, Bilezikian JP. Parathyroid carcinoma: a review of 62 patients. Endocr Rev 1982;3:218.
101. Bilezikian JP. Management of acute hypercalcemia. N Engl J Med 1992;326:1196–1203.
102. Moley JF, Lairmore TC, Doherty GM, Brunt LM, DeBenedetti MK. Preservation of the recurrent laryngeal nerves in thyroid and parathyroid reoperations. Surgery (St. Louis) 1999;126:673–677; discussion 677–679.

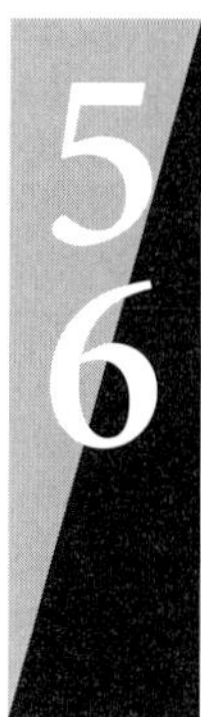

Tumors of the Endocrine System

Jeffrey A. Norton

Endocrine cancer includes the thyroid, parathyroid, endocrine gastrointestinal tract, and the adrenal. Cancer of the endocrine system is uncommon. The overall incidence is 11.2 and 4.5 per 100,000 woman and men, respectively.[1] Because ovary and breast are not included under endocrine cancer, thyroid cancer is the most common type, and it is covered in depth in Chapter 55. The remaining types are even less common, with an annual incidence of 1 to 20 per million. This chapter informs the reader about these rare tumors. Further, we characterize the multiple endocrine neoplasia syndromes, several autosomal dominant familial endocrine cancer syndromes that simultaneously affect multiple endocrine glands.

Adrenal Tumors

Adrenal adenoma is a benign neoplasm of adrenal cortical cells. It is not greater than 5 cm in diameter or 100 g in weight. Cellular pleomorphism and necrosis are rare. It may be hormonally functional. Adenomas produce syndromes of hypercortisolism and hyperaldosteronism and not virilization or feminization. Tumors larger than 6 cm that produce sex hormones are usually carcinoma. Pleomorphism, tumor necrosis, and mitotic activity are more common in carcinoma. The prognosis of adrenal cortical adenoma secreting cortisol is excellent, and surgical resection is curative. However, resection of aldosteronomas does not cure hypertension in some patients. Resection is followed by a favorable response in blood pressure and serum level of potassium; however, 30% of patients may develop recurrent hypertension.

Adrenal cortical carcinoma is a malignant neoplasm of adrenal cortical cells. It is rare and is less than 0.2% of all cancer. It occurs at a rate of only 2 per million. Women develop functional adrenal cancer more often than men. Men have nonfunctioning malignant adrenal tumors more often than women. There is a bimodal occurrence by age, with a peak incidence at less than 5 years and a second peak in the fourth and fifth decade. Adrenal cortical carcinomas are greater than 6 cm in size and weigh between 100 and 5,000 g. Areas of necrosis and hemorrhage are common. Invasion and metastases also occur. Microscopically, the appearance is variable. Cells with big nuclei, hyperchromatism, and enlarged nucleoli are all consistent with malignancy. Nuclear pleomorphism is more common in tumors larger than 500 g. Vascular invasion and many mitoses are diagnostic of malignancy.

Adrenal cortical carcinoma is part of Li–Fraumeni, a hereditary syndrome, including sarcoma, breast, and lung cancer. Mutations in the p53 gene occur in these families. Genetic changes are more common in malignant adrenal tumors. The most frequent DNA copy number changes include losses of 1p, 2q, 3p, 3q, 6q, 9p, and 11q. There are also gains and amplifications of 5q, 9q, 9q, 12q, and 20q.[2] Adrenal cortical cancer is associated with rearrangements at the 11p15 locus and IGF-II gene overexpression.[3] Insulin-like growth factor (IGF)-II may be a major determinant of progression and a target for future therapies. Predictors of survival include distant metastases, venous, capsular, and adjacent organ invasion, tumor necrosis, mitotic rate, atypical mitosis, and mdm-2 expression.[4]

Adrenal cancers may have tumor-specific mutations in p53 that serve as a marker for the tumor.[5] Mutations in the p53 gene have been used to diagnose malignancy.[6] Quantitative nuclear analysis demonstrates that nuclei from adrenal cancers are larger than those in adenomas, and DNA density is diploid in adenomas and aneuploid in carcinomas. Adrenal cancer cells in culture can spontaneously transition between two subtypes by switching expression of two genes, BRG1 and Brm, at the posttranscriptional level. This mechanism allows the cell to adapt to environmental factors that may suppress growth or cause death.[7] Finally, in general carcinomas produce abnormal amounts of androgens and 11-deoxysteroids. However, this is merely suggestive of malignancy, because only 10% of malignant tumors produce masculinization whereas the rest secrete cortisol, aldosterone, or nothing.

Cushing's Syndrome

Cushing's syndrome, or endogenous hypercortisolism, is caused by (in order of frequency) (a) excessive secretion of adrenocorticotropic hormone (ACTH) by a pituitary tumor, (b) cortisol by an adrenal tumor, or (c) ACTH by an ectopic tumor. Cushing's syndrome is potentially lethal and, if untreated, is associated with excessive mortality.[8] Determining the cause of the hypercortisolism involves sophisticated testing.

The signs and symptoms of hypercortisolism are ubiquitous and diverse; nearly every organ in the body is affected (Table 56.1). Progressive weight gain is the most common symptom. Obesity is usually truncal. Patients have thin extremities due to muscle wasting. Increased fat in the dorsal neck region combined with kyphosis secondary to osteo-

TABLE 56.1. Signs and Symptoms of hypercorticolism (Cushing's syndrome).

Weight gain
Truncal obesity
Muscle wasting
Osteoporosis
Buffalo hump
Hypertension
Facial rounding
Striae
Hirsutism
Type 2 diabetes mellitus
Menstrual irregularity
Impotency
Dilated blood vessels
Thinning subcutaneous tissue on face
Depression to psychosis
Opportunistic infections

porosis gives the appearance of a "buffalo hump." Serial photographs show a rounding of the face. Blood pressure increases mildly. Striae are reliable clinical signs of Cushing's syndrome. Hirsutism consists of excessive fine hair on face, upper back, and arms. Virilization, including clitoromegaly, deep voice, and balding, suggest carcinoma. Glucose intolerance and hyperglycemia are common, and patients develop type 2 diabetes mellitus. Weakness secondary to muscle atrophy occurs, especially in ectopic ACTH syndrome. Menstrual irregularity or amenorrhea is common in women, whereas men have impotency. In children, the most common presenting signs are obesity and short stature. Dilatation of blood vessels and thinning of the subcutaneous tissue give the face a ruddy appearance. Mental changes vary from mild depression to severe psychosis. Hypokalemia exacerbates the weakness and implies carcinoma or ectopic ACTH syndrome. Immunosuppression associated with hypercortisolemia results in opportunistic infections, including cryptococcosis, aspergillosis, nocardiosis, *Pneumocystis carinii*, and necrotizing fasciitis.

The first diagnostic goal is to unequivocally establish the presence of hypercortisolism (Table 56.2). The next step is to exclude the pituitary as a cause, and the final step is to determine the exact etiology. Urinary excretion of free cortisol is directly proportional to the amount of cortisol in the plasma. Determination of 24-hour urinary free cortisol excretion is the single best test to diagnose hypercortisolism. However, some (5%) patients with mild Cushing's syndrome have been

TABLE 56.2. Workup of Cushing's syndrome.

Step	*Goal*	*Method*
1	Diagnose hypercorticolism	24-h urine free cortisol Low-dose dexamethasone
2	Rule out pituitary cause	High-dose dexamethasone MRI of sella Petrosal sinus sampling
3	Find tumor	CT or MRI adrenals Chest CT (ectopic ACTH)

ACTH, adrenocorticotropic hormone.

found to have normal levels of urinary free cortisol. The overnight single-dose (low-dose) dexamethasone test works because patients with hypercortisolism fail to suppress cortisol secretion with low-dose dexamethasone. Normal subjects given 1 mg dexamethasone orally at 11:00 P.M. have plasma cortisol levels less than 5 μg/dL at 8:00 A.M. the next day. Patients with endogenous hypercortisolism do not suppress and have cortisol levels greater than 5 μg/dL. A normal low-dose dexamethasone test and urinary free cortisol (less than 100 μg/day) exclude the diagnosis of hypercortisolism. The standard high-dose dexamethasone suppression test is the most useful test in excluding the pituitary as the cause of hypercortisolism. The expected results are that high-dose dexamethasone (8 mg/day) suppresses urinary levels of free cortisol to less than 50% of baseline levels in patients with pituitary-dependent hypercortisolism (Cushing's disease), but not patients with primary adrenal tumors or ectopic ACTH syndrome. This test diagnoses Cushing's syndrome and determines the cause with an accuracy rate of approximately 95%.

Adrenal computed tomography (CT) can detect normal adrenal glands in most patients. CT can reliably distinguish cortical hyperplasia from tumor. CT has great sensitivity (more than 95%); however, it lacks specificity. CT can be used to image the primary tumor plus local and distant metastases in cancer. Magnetic resonance imaging (MRI) is able to distinguish among adenoma, carcinoma, and pheochromocytoma. Signal loss on chemical shift MRI occurs in adrenal cortical cancer.[9] In a recent study of 204 patients with adrenal masses, the sensitivity of MRI for distinguishing benign from malignant masses was 89%, specificity was 99%, and accuracy was 94%.[10] Fluorodeoxyglucose-positron emission tomography (FDG-PET) has been studied in 10 patients with adrenal cortical cancer. The sensitivity was 100% and the specificity was 95%. In 3 patients, previously unidentified lesions were seen that modified the treatment plan.[11]

Conn's Syndrome

An aldosteronoma is a benign adrenal cortical tumor that secretes excessive amounts of aldosterone. Primary aldosteronism is caused by an aldosterone-producing adenoma, idiopathic hyperplasia, or carcinoma. Secondary aldosteronism, which occurs with renal artery stenosis, is diagnosed by an increase in plasma renin activity, whereas primary has low plasma renin levels. Hypertension, hypokalemia, hyperaldosteronism, and decreased plasma renin levels are essential for the diagnosis of primary aldosteronism. Primary hyperaldosteronism is also associated with weakness, muscle cramps, polyuria, and polydipsia. These clinical signs are caused by hypokalemia (K less than 3.5 mEq/L). Hypertension is usually not severe and is mostly diastolic (diastolic pressure more than 90 mm Hg) (Table 56.3).

Once the diagnosis of primary aldosteronism is established, the next important consideration is the etiology: hyperplasia versus adenoma. CT can image approximately 90% of aldosteronomas but may miss small tumors (Figure 56.1). The contralateral adrenal cortex is thin. Iodocholesterol scans with ^{131}I-β-iodomethyl-19-norcholesterol can distinguish between adenoma and hyperplasia. Hyperplasia has symmetrical uptake in both adrenal glands and adenoma has uptake only in the tumor.[12] If the results are inconclusive, sampling of the adrenal veins for aldosterone is indicated.

TABLE 56.3. Diagnosis and localization of hyperaldosternoism.

Step	Goal	Method
1	Diagnose primary hyperaldosternoism	Measure serum K Blood pressure Serum aldosterone and renin
2	Adenoma vs. hyperplasia (IAH)	CT Iodocholosterol scan Adrenal venous sampling
3	Management Adenoma IAH	 Laparoscopic adrenalectomy Spironolactone

IAH, idiopathic adrenal hyperplasia.

Adrenal venous sampling may be more sensitive than CT and iodocholesterol scans. However, the latter studies usually make the diagnosis.

The management of primary aldosteronism depends on the etiology. Hyperplasia is best managed medically with spironolactone, amiloride or nifedipine. Aldosteronomas are best removed by laparoscopic adrenalectomy, which is associated with less pain and more rapid recovery than open procedures. Aldosterone-producing carcinomas are rare (less than 2% of adrenal cancers) and should be removed by open adrenalectomy.

Incidentaloma

An incidentaloma is an incidental adrenal mass detected by CT. It occurs in 0.6% of abdominal CT scans. The majority are benign adrenal cortical adenomas. Cancer occurs in 7%. Two diagnostic questions arise with incidentalomas. Is it cancer? Does it secrete excessive hormones? If either answer is yes, surgery is indicated (Figure 56.2).

The initial workup of incidentalomas requires a careful history and physical examination, including blood pressure. Weight gain, weakness, signs of hypercortisolism, hypertension, virilization, feminization, change in menstruation, and evidence of occult malignancy (stool guaiac, Pap smear, anemia) should all be noted. Laboratory evaluation consists of a serum potassium level, 24-hour urine collection for free cortisol, vanyl-mandelic acid (VMA), metanephrines, and catecholamines. A low-dose dexamethasone suppression test is indicated, in addition to urinary free cortisol, to rule out hypercortisolism.[13] Some patients have normal urinary levels of free cortisol and fail to suppress with low-dose dexamethasone. Similarly, plasma free metanephrines and normetanephrine levels are indicated in addition to urinary catecholamines to exclude a pheochromocytoma.[13] Hormonal screening for an excess of androgens or estrogens is limited to patients with clinical signs.

Size of an adrenal mass is the single most important criteria for malignancy. Adrenal cancers are generally greater than 6cm in diameter. Nevertheless, a smaller lesion should not be totally ignored. Most recently, because of decreased morbidity with laparoscopic adrenalectomy, experts have advocated resection for 4-cm incidentalomas, especially in younger patients.[13]

Fine-needle aspiration for cytology of an adrenal mass has limited ability to differentiate benign from malignant primary adrenal lesions. Fine-needle aspiration (FNA) may be catastrophic in a patient with an unsuspected pheochromocytoma, so plasma metanephrine and normetanephrine results are required before needle biopsy. FNA may be complicated by hemorrhage and rupture of tumor. In patients with suspected metastatic disease to the adrenal or lymphoma, FNA is diagnostic.[14]

Biochemical assessment should be performed to exclude hormonal function of the tumor. Excessive hormonal secretion (catecholamines, aldosterone, cortisol, sex steroids) is an indication for resection. The size of the tumor is assessed. Size greater than 4cm is an indication for surgical resection. The incidence of cancer in solid adrenal masses equal to 6cm is estimated to be between 35% and 98%. Laparoscopic excision of tumors smaller than 6cm in size is recommended because of less pain and morbidity. Laparoscopic excision of large adrenal tumors (greater than 6cm) is not recommended because a high proportion of these tumors are malignant. If the mass is smaller than 4cm and nonfunctional, a repeat follow-up CT examination in 3 to 6 months is indicated to again determine size. If size increases, surgical excision is necessary.

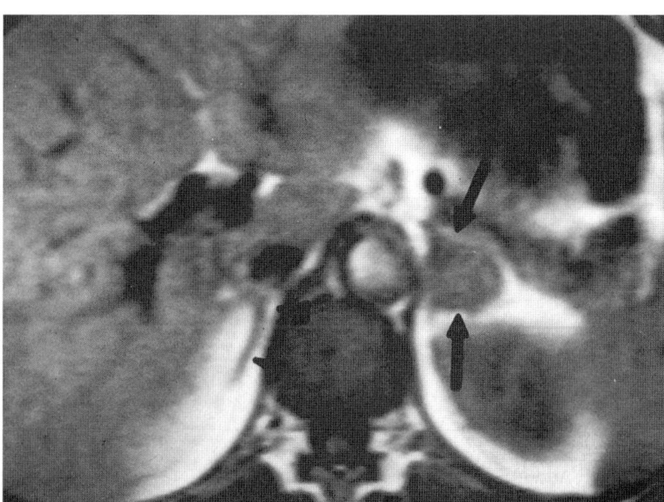

FIGURE 56.1. Computed tomography (CT) of left adrenal aldosteronoma shows a normal right adrenal gland and a small (2-cm) tumor in the left adrenal that was an aldosteronoma.

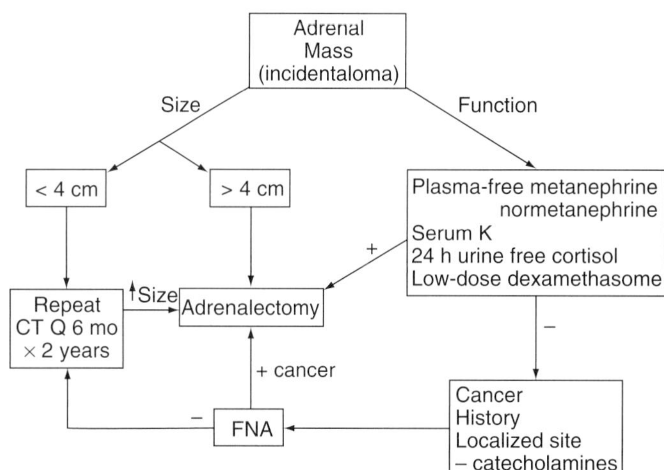

FIGURE 56.2. Flow chart for the management of incidentally discovered adrenal tumors.

TABLE 56.4. Staging of adrenal cancer.

Stage	Tumor size (cm)	Lymph nodes	Local invasion	Distant metastases	Five-year survival (%)
1	Less than 5	–	–	–	More than 80
2	More than 5	–	–	–	50–75
3	Any	+	+	–	50
4	Any	+	+	+	10

Virilization/Feminization

Virilization or feminization may be combined with hypercortisolism, or the tumor may produce only estrogen or testosterone. Sex hormone secretion is often associated with adrenal cancer. In children, the clinical signs of increased androgen production include excessive growth, premature pubic and facial hair, acne, genital enlargement, increased muscle mass, and deep voice. In women, the clinical signs of excess androgen production include hirsutism, acne, amenorrhea, infertility, increased muscle mass, deep voice, and temporal balding. In adult men, hyperestrogenism presents with gynecomastia, decreased sexual drive, impotence, and infertility. In premenopausal women, hyperestrogenism presents with irregular menses. In postmenopausal women, it causes dysfunctional uterine bleeding. The workup includes 24-hour urinary 17-ketosteroids, 17-hydroxysteroids, urinary free cortisol, and, depending on virilization or feminization, serum determination of testosterone or estrogen.

Adrenal Carcinoma

Seventy-five percent of adrenal carcinomas present with excessive glucocorticoid or mineralocorticoid hormone secretion; however, some may be nonfunctional.[15] The mainstay of treatment of adrenal cortical carcinoma is complete surgical resection. If the carcinoma cannot be effectively removed without removing the ipsilateral kidney, concomitant nephrectomy is necessary. CT or MR can image the extent of disease and should include the chest to rule out pulmonary metastases. If the inferior vena cava is involved, imaging studies such as cavography are useful to assess extent of tumor. Tumor size, hemorrhage, and mitotic count each correlate with survival rates for patients undergoing curative resection. Tumors less than 12 cm, mitotic rate less than 6 per high-power field, and absence of hemorrhage are associated with improved survival.[16] Radical, complete resection of all cancer is critical for prolonged survival and potential cure. There is no clearly effective adjuvant therapy.[17] Recurrent or metastatic tumor should also be resected. Recent reports suggest that radiofrequency ablation may be able to control recurrent tumor both inside and outside the liver.[18]

Adrenal carcinoma may occur in children. It occurs in children younger than 6 years, with a higher incidence in girls than boys. The median age in children is 4 years. Virilization is the most common presenting feature (93%), followed by hypercortisolism.[19] The overall 5-year survival rate for children with adrenal cancer is 49%, and following complete resection 70%. Adrenal cancer occurs in adults. The second peak age is between 40 and 50 years, and most present with hormonal syndromes. The staging of patients with adrenal carcinoma is as follows: 20% of patients have stage I, II, and III disease at diagnosis, whereas 80% have metastases[20] (Table 56.4). Many patients (70%) present with stage III or IV disease. The definitive treatment for localized disease including stage III is en bloc resection. Even tumor thrombus within the inferior vena cava is not a contraindication to resection.[21] Surgical resection of localized disease can be curative. The overall 5-year survival rate is between 20% and 35%. In a recent series, the 6-year survival following complete resection of all tumor is 60%.[22] Complete resection of recurrent tumor is also useful and, if achieved, it is associated with a 6-year survival of 40%.[23,24] Patients should undergo monitoring of steroid hormone levels postoperatively to assess for recurrence. CT and MRI are also able to detect local recurrences and pulmonary metastases. If a localized recurrence is detected, it should be removed surgically. Prolonged remissions have been reported after resection of hepatic, pulmonary, and cerebral metastases. Patients with recurrent adrenal cortical carcinoma who can be surgically resected have 5-year survival rates of 50% versus 8% for nonoperated cases. Control of recurrent tumor can be achieved by radiofrequency ablation.[18] Palliation of bony metastases may be achieved by radiation therapy.

Op-DDD (mitotane) is the most commonly used chemotherapy drug for adrenal cancer (Table 56.5). It is administered at a dose of 2 to 6 g daily, and the dose is increased until toxicity occurs. Toxicity includes gastrointestinal, neuromuscular, and skin symptoms. Mitotane prolongs bleeding time and inhibits platelet aggregation. A decrease in urinary steroid excretion is seen in most patients. Partial responses occur in one-third of patients and a few complete responses have been reported. Because mitotane inhibits the multidrug-resistant gene, chemotherapy has been given with mitotane. Patients with metastatic adrenal cortical carcinoma have been given etoposide, cisplatin, and mitotane. The response rate was 33% with some complete responses. Further, when combined with etoposide, doxorubicin, and cisplatin, it had an overall response rate of 22% to 54%.[24,25] Docetaxel and gemcitabine failed to demonstrate a response in 2 patients treated.[26] Irinotecan (CPT-11) at 250 mg/m^2 has been ineffective in 12 patients with metastatic adrenal cortical carcinoma who failed other therapies.[27]

TABLE 56.5. Chemotherapy for adrenal cancer.

Drug	Response rate (%)
Mitotane	30–60
Suramin	15–30
Doxorubicin	19
5-Fluorouracil (5-FU) + doxorubicin + cisplatin	20
Etoposide + doxorubicin + cisplatin	100 (3/3)
Oncovin + cisplatin + epipodophyllotoxin	100 (1/1)
Mitotane + etoposide + doxorubicin + cisplatin	50

Pheochromocytoma

Pheochromocytomas are rare tumors that secrete excessive catecholamines. They arise from chromaffin cells in the adrenal medulla and elsewhere. They occur in about 1 per 100,000 per year.[28] In autopsy series, only 0.005% to 0.1% of persons have unsuspected pheochromocytomas. When urinary catecholamines are measured in hypertensive patients, pheochromocytoma is present in only 0.1% of patients.

Pheochromocytomas may be intraadrenal, extraadrenal, benign, or malignant. Early diagnosis and therapy improve the prognosis. Incidence of malignancy is as low as 5% and as high as 46% in different series. Extraadrenal tumors are more likely to be cancerous. Pheochromocytomas may be associated with endocrine and nonendocrine inherited disorders. Bilateral adrenal medullary pheochromocytomas are components of MEN 2a and MEN 2b. Some families have bilateral adrenal pheochromocytomas and no other manifestation of MEN. In other families, only extraadrenal pheochromocytomas have been reported. Pheochromocytomas occur in approximately 25% of patients with von Hippel–Lindau (VHL) disease and in 1% of patients with neurofibromatosis and von Recklinghausen's disease. Further, recent studies indicate that many patients with apparently sporadic pheochromocytomas really have either MEN-2 (RET gene) or VHL. Among 271 patients, 66 (24%) were found to have mutations of VHL and RET. This finding suggests that patients who present with apparently sporadic nonfamilial pheochromocytoma should be screened for RET and VHL mutations as 25% will have them.[29] Germ-line mutations in three of the succinate dehydrogenase subunits (SDHD, SDHB, and SDHC) cause susceptibility to head and neck paragangliomas (extra-adrenal pheochromocytomas).[30,31]

Pheochromocytomas cause intermittent, episodic, or sustained hypertension. Pheochromocytomas also cause insulin resistance and diabetes.[32] Following resection of the tumor, insulin sensitivity improves.[33] Further, pheochromocytomas may produce other hormones, including ectopic ACTH and Cushing's syndrome. Pheochromocytomas arise from chromaffin cells. Chromaffin cells are widespread and associated with sympathetic ganglia during fetal life. After birth, most chromaffin cells degenerate, and the majority remain in the adrenal medulla; this may explain why approximately 90% of pheochromocytomas are in the adrenal medulla. Extraadrenal pheochromocytomas may arise anywhere, including the carotid body, intracardia, along the aorta (both thoracic and abdominal), and within the urinary bladder. The most common extraadrenal location is the organ of Zuckerkandl that is near the origin of the inferior mesenteric artery to the left of the aortic bifurcation. Data from series of patients with sporadic pheochromocytomas indicate that the right adrenal gland more often harbors a tumor than the left gland. Pheochromocytomas usually measure between 3 and 5 cm in diameter and weigh 100 g. Tumors are tan to gray in color and have a soft consistency. Larger tumors are cystic and have necrosis or calcification. Microscopically, pheochromocytomas are usually arranged in cords or alveolar patterns. Tumors are generally clearly separated from the adrenal cortex by a thin band of fibrous tissue. Extension into the cortex or vascular invasion may occur.

TABLE 56.6. Management of patients with pheochromocytoma.

Step	*Goal*	*Method*
1	Diagnosis	24-h urine for vanyl-mandelic acid (VMA), metanephrines, and catecholamines: plasma free metanephrine, normetanephrine
2	Localization	CT MRI Metaiodobenzylguanidine (MIBG) scan
3	Preparation	Phenoxybenzamine ± propranalol
4	Resection	Laparoscopic adrenalectomy (open for extraadrenal and/or large tumor)
5	Recurrence	Plasma-free metanephrine, normetanephrine

The pathologic distinction between benign and malignant pheochromocytomas is not clear. The only absolute criterion for malignancy is the presence of secondary tumors in sites where chromaffin cells are not usually present and visceral metastases. Malignant tumors tend to be larger and weigh more. Staining for the nuclear proliferation marker MIB-1 is positive in 50% of malignant pheochromocytomas and negative in benign tumors. Benign pheochromocytomas may demonstrate marked nuclear pleomorphism, whereas, paradoxically, malignant ones demonstrate less. Malignant pheochromocytomas usually have many more mitoses, but capsular and vascular invasion occurs with equal frequency in both. Nuclear DNA ploidy may be a predictive indicator of malignant potential. Flow cytometry has been used to identify tetraploidy, polyploidy, and aneuploidy, which are associated with malignancy. Neuropeptide Y gene expression is more common in benign tumors.

Patients with pheochromocytomas can present with a range of symptoms, from mild labile hypertension to sudden death secondary to severe hypertension, myocardial infarction, or cerebral vascular accident. The classic patient describes "spells" of paroxysmal headaches, pallor, palpitations, hypertension, and diaphoresis. In 50% of patients, the hypertension is intermittent, but it may be sustained. In children, hypertension is sustained. Patients may have lactic acidosis. Patients may have weight loss and hyperglycemia.

The diagnosis of pheochromocytoma is based on measuring catecholamines and metabolites in the urine (Table 56.6), which previously required a 24-hour urine for metanephrines and catecholamines.[34] However, plasma free metanephrines and normetanephrines have been used recently to reliably diagnose pheochromocytoma.[35] Certainly the blood measurement greatly facilitates the workup, and it is accurate. Measurements of urinary total metanephrines or VMA are not as reliable as plasma free levels of metanephrines and normetanephrine.[36] If a pheochromocytoma is suspected, the best study is plasma free levels of metanephrine and normetanephrine.[37] Older studies suggest that urinary measurement of catecholamines, VMA, and metanephrine levels are best. It is now clear that plasma free samples have replaced urinary studies as indicated in patients with suspected pheochromocytoma.

CT and MRI are the two nonnuclear medicine procedures of choice to localize pheochromocytomas. Both are noninvasive and sensitive, being able to reliably detect tumors 1 cm in diameter. MRI may be more specific because of findings with different sequences. CT detects more than 95% of pheochromocytomas, including 9 of 10 bilateral tumors. CT also detects most extraadrenal retroperitoneal tumors. However, MRI is similar and may be better. MRI also imaged all pheochromocytomas demonstrated on CT, plus metastases to the chest, retroperitoneum, and liver that were not seen. Because it has no radiation exposure, MRI can be used to image during pregnancy. In one analysis, CT imaged 16 of 19 pheochromocytomas (84%) whereas MRI imaged 12 of 15 (75%) for comparable sensitivity.[38] In addition, MRI successfully imaged an intrapericardial pheochromocytoma and distinguished it from the cardiac chambers and surrounding great vessels, which could not be determined by CT.

The single best technique for localization of pheochromocytomas is nuclear scanning after the administration of labeled metaiodobenzylguanidine (MIBG). The compound is similar to norepinephrine and is taken up by vesicular monoamine transporters.[39] The sensitivity of MIBG scanning with ^{131}I for pheochromocytoma is 100% and the specificity is 95%.[40] It appears that MIBG scanning is safe, noninvasive, and efficacious for the localization of pheochromocytomas, including those that arise in nonadrenal sites, and malignant disease. Bone metastases are best imaged by bone scan. Because MIBG scan is a total body study, it can image tumors wherever they are including unusual locations.[40] Although CT and MRI reflect changes in morphology, scintigraphic imaging relies on tissue function. False-positive results with MIBG are rare, which accounts for the high specificity (98% to 100%). False-negative results do occur, which lowers sensitivity. For patients with suspected pheochromocytoma and negative MIBG, ^{18}F-FDG PET may be useful. Metastases from a predominantly dopamine-secreting pheochromocytoma that did not take up MIBG were imaged with FDG-PET.[41] Further, ^{18}F-DOPA PET has imaged 17 pheochromocytomas in 17 patients. It is highly sensitive and specific and may be very useful if other studies are negative.[41] It has imaged a malignant bladder pheochromocytoma.[42] It may be superior to MIBG for localization of metastatic pheochromocytoma.[43] It is not commonly available, but it can be useful.[44]

Once the diagnosis is established and the tumor localized, preoperative preparation includes α-adrenergic blockade. Patients are started on phenoxybenzamine, 10 mg orally two or three times daily. If tachycardia develops, α-adrenergic blocking agents (propranolol) are added. Propranolol should never be started before α-blockade because unopposed vasoconstriction may worsen hypertension. Phenoxybenzamine increases the total blood and plasma volume and reduces lactic acidosis. Appropriately used calcium channel antagonists and selective alpha$_1$-receptor blockers are also effective and safe.[45]

Small (less than 6 cm) intraadrenal pheochromocytomas are removed using laparoscopic techniques.[46] However, others report that laparoscopic adrenalectomy should still be performed for large tumors (greater than 6 cm). They point out that the operative time, blood loss, and length of stay are the same for either small or large adrenal tumors.[47,48] Laparoscopic procedures appear to decrease pain and shorten the time to recovery.[49] Most pheochromocytomas are well localized, which facilitates laparoscopic removal. Laparoscopic adrenalectomy for familial pheochromocytomas is especially useful because these tumors are small and within the adrenal gland.[50] Adrenal cortical-sparing surgery may be indicated for patients with familial pheochromocytomas who require bilateral adrenalectomy.[51] However, iatrogenic pheochromocytomatosis has been described as a possible complication of laparoscopic removal. Numerous tumor cells are deposited throughout the retroperitoneum near the site of the primary tumor, which may have been caused by laparoscopic excision of a malignant tumor or by spilling benign tumor cells at the time of laparoscopic excision. Despite the exact etiology, this is a rare complication that must be considered if it continues to occur.[52]

Malignant pheochromocytomas are present in approximately 10% of patients with pheochromocytoma. Malignant tumors have high mitotic rate, aneuploidy and high S-phase fraction.[53] EM66 is a novel secretogranin II-derived peptide that is present in the chromaffin cells of the human adrenal gland. EM66 has a higher concentrations in benign pheochromocytomas than malignant tumors.[54] Expression of hTERT, HSP90, and telomerase activity may also be used to detect more-aggressive tumors.[55] SDHB gene is a tumor suppressor gene. Detection of a germ-line SDHB mutation in patients with apparently sporadic pheochromocytomas appears to be associated with a tumor that is high risk for malignancy and recurrence.[56]

The basic principles in the treatment of malignant pheochromocytoma have been to surgically resect recurrences or metastases whenever possible and to treat hypertensive symptoms by catecholamine blockade. Surgical resection of metastatic and recurrent pheochromocytoma has been shown to prolong survival. Soft tissue masses or bony masses may be treated with radiation therapy if doses of 40 Gy or more can be administered.[57] Serum levels of chromogranin A can be used to measure response to therapy.[58] Survival data of patients with malignant pheochromocytoma are difficult to obtain because of the rarity and indolence of the tumor. The 5-year survival rate is between 36% and 60%.

Because of the high sensitivity (85%) and specificity (100%) of ^{131}I-MIBG to image pheochromocytomas, it has been used at higher doses to treat recurrent or metastatic pheochromocytomas. A beneficial response to treatment is observed in 42% to 60% of patients. Paedial remissions as measured by decrease in catecholamine secretion and tumor size have been observed in approximately one-third of patients treated. However, complete responses with ^{131}I-MIBG have been rare.[59] Recently, very high dose (800 mCi) ^{131}I-MIBG resulted in complete antitumor responses in 2 of 12 patients with skeletal and soft tissue metastases from pheochromocytoma and partial responses in most.[60]

Combinations of cyclophosphamide, vincristine, and dacarbazine have been used in patients with metastatic pheochromocytoma. However, the regimen has been abandoned because of toxicity and variability in response rate with few complete responses. Single cases have been reported to have complete responses with cyclophosphamide, vincristine, and dacarbazine (CVD). Long-acting octreotide (sandostatin-LAR) has been used to treat malignant pheochromoctyoma without success. Even tumors that were positive on octreoscan did not respond to LAR.[61] Combination chemotherapy with cyclophosphamide, vincristine, dacarbazine, doxorubicin, and epirubicin resulted in a complete response in a single patient with metastatic pheochromocytoma.[62]

Pancreatic Islet Cell Tumors

Endocrine tumors of the pancreas are classified primarily according to the associated clinical syndrome.[63] Signs and symptoms are caused by uncontrolled excessive secretion of hormone. For example, patients with insulinoma have altered mental status, confusion, seizures, and other neuroglycopenic symptoms related to hypoglycemia caused by excessive uncontrolled insulin secretion.[64] Pancreatic endocrine tumors share a number of common features including similar microscopic appearance, hormonal symptoms, special issues in patients with multiple endocrine neoplasia type 1,[65] and malignant growth affecting survival. Pancreatic endocrine tumors are usually slow growing, and even patients with extensive tumor may still live for long periods. However, if liver metastases occur, survival will be affected by the malignant nature of the tumor. Effective treatment must address the symptoms associated with the clinical syndrome and the malignant potential of the tumor.

Epidemiology

Endocrine tumors of the pancreas are rare, having an incidence of less than 10 per million people per year.[63] Insulinomas are the most common islet cell tumor with a prevalence of approximately 1 per million per year, and gastrinomas are a close second. The remaining islet cell tumors are less common.

Pathology

Pancreatic neuroendocrine tumors arise from cells that have been termed APUDomas (APUD means amine precursor uptake and decarboxylation). Pancreatic neuroendocrine tumors are composed of monotonous sheets of small round cells with uniform nuclei and cytoplasm. Mitotic figures are unusual. Tumors have dense secretory granules. When stained by immunohistochemistry, most pancreatic neuroendocrine tumors are positive for more than one hormone. However, in most instances only one peptide is secreted into the circulation. Pancreatic neuroendocrine tumors are hypervascular, solid, and reddish-brown in color. They occur not only within the pancreas as they have been described in ectopic pancreas tissue.[66] They are usually solid, but cystic and papillary insulinomas have been described.[67] Neuroendocrine tumors may have a "rhabdoid" appearance, which means sheets of monotonous tumor cells with uniform round nuclei.[68] Tumors may be caused by mutations of the tumor suppressor gene DPC4 located on chromosome 18q21 that have been found in 5 of 9 (55%) nonfunctional pancreatic neuroendocrine tumors.[69] X-chromosome loss of heterozygosity is common in gastrinomas from women, and its presence indicates more-aggressive growth and behavior.[70] Aberrant methylation of the APC promoter is strongly involved in the molecular pathogenesis of pancreatic neuroendocrine tumors.[71] Raf-1 activation causes morphologic changes and decrease in secretory granules.[72] One study showed that methylation of the p16^{INK4a} gene is the most common gene alteration in gastrinomas, and it appears to occur early in the time sequence of these tumors and may be a central process in the molecular pathogenesis.[73]

In general, microscopic pathologic analysis of pancreatic endocrine tumors has failed to predict the growth pattern of the tumor and is not able to determine whether a tumor is benign or malignant. In addition, there is no correlation between histologic pattern and clinical syndrome. At present, the only clear determination of malignancy is detection of metastases, either in lymph nodes or liver. However, lymph node metastases do not negatively affect survival, whereas liver metastases clearly do.[74] Microscopic invasion of blood vessels and surrounding pancreas is another indicator of malignancy, but it is not as precise as the detection of distant metastatic disease. Because of this, it is unclear exactly which pancreatic neuroendocrine tumors are malignant. The true nature of an individual tumor can only be determined by careful long-term follow-up studies. In general, few (less than 10%) insulinomas are cancerous,[75] 60% of gastrinomas are malignant (lymph node or liver metastases),[76] and the majority (50% to 90%) of all other islet cell tumors are malignant. Neuroendocrine tumors of the gut are similar and have a similar prognosis. Five-year survival rates for localized neuroendocrine tumors are approximately 80% or greater, whereas for metastatic tumors the rates decrease to 50%.[77] Survival of patients with pancreatic neuroendocrine tumors has been shown to decrease when liver metastases occur. However, surgical excision of liver tumors has salvaged some patients and improved prognosis.[78]

Functional (hormone-producing) pancreatic neuroendocrine tumors are usually malignant (except for insulinomas), but patients have an excellent survival. Most patients who undergo surgery to remove tumor have a 5-year survival of more than 75%.[79] Nonfunctional pancreatic neuroendocrine tumors commonly present as a pancreatic mass lesion. These tumors may be detected incidentally on CT scan ordered for another reason (Figure 56.3). They may cause intestinal bleeding if they invade into the bowel or stomach or they obstruct the splenic vein and cause gastric varices. They may cause gastrointestinal obstruction if they obliterate the lumen of the small bowel or colon. Nonfunctional tumors are distributed evenly throughout the head, body, and tail of the pancreas. The 2-year survival for surgically removed node-negative nonfunctional pancreatic neuroendocrine tumor (NET) is 78%, for node-positive tumors is 72%,

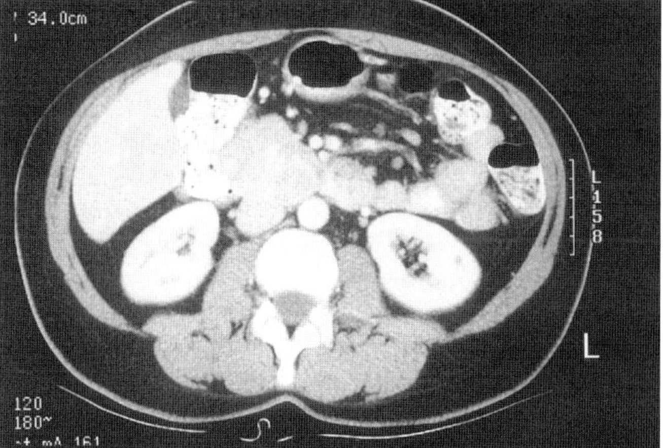

FIGURE 56.3. CT of a large nonfunctional pancreatic neuroendocrine tumor within the head.

and for liver metastases is 36%.[80] Pancreatic neuroendocrine tumors do not usually obstruct the pancreatic duct, but they can be a cause of focal, recurrent pancreatitis.[81,82] The size of an individual islet cell tumor does not appear to correlate with the severity of the hormonally mediated symptoms. There is, however, a clear correlation between the size of the tumor and the occurrence of malignancy; the larger the tumor, the greater the probability of metastases, especially liver metastases. Insulinomas, similar to duodenal gastrinomas, are generally small tumors, less than 2cm. However, duodenal gastrinomas still have a 60% chance of nodal metastases, whereas small insulinomas seldom spread. Glucagonomas, somatostatinomas, pancreatic polypeptidomas, and other islet cell tumors are frequently large at the time of detection, more than 5cm, and are usually malignant. Most pancreatic endocrine tumors are solitary, encapsulated, and within the pancreas. However, islet cell tumors may also occur in the duodenum and other extrapancreatic locations. Primary gastrinomas have been described within the duodenum (Figure 56.4), pancreas, heart, liver, stomach, and ovary. When metastases occur, they are usually found in peripancreatic lymph nodes (60%) or liver (30%). Late in the course of disease, tumor spreads to lung, bone, and even heart.

Pancreatic endocrine tumors occur in either a nonfamilial (sporadic) form or in a familial form associated with multiple endocrine neoplasia type 1 (see section on MEN-1). The exact proportion of patients with pancreatic islet cell tumors who manifest MEN-1 varies in different series from less than 5% to 25%. The recognition of MEN-1 syndrome is important because these patients always have multiple pancreatic neuroendocrine tumors. Furthermore, screening of other family members is indicated. Finally, the presence of one hormonal abnormality in MEN-1 patients may affect another. Primary hyperparathyroidism worsens the manifestations of Zollinger–Ellison syndrome and should be corrected first. Functional islet cell tumors are the second most frequent abnormality in MEN-1 and are present in approximately 80% of individuals. Gastrinomas, insulinomas, glucagonomas, and vasoactive intestinal peptide tumors (VIPomas) occur in decreasing prevalence in MEN-1 patients with gastrinomas in 54% and insulinomas in 20%. In addition to MEN-1, studies suggest that pancreatic islet cell tumors are found more commonly in patients with von Recklinghausen's disease, von Hippel–Lindau syndrome, and tuberous sclerosis. In patients with von Recklinghausen's disease, duodenal somatostatinomas and gastrinomas have been reported. In patients with von Hippel–Lindau syndrome, 17% of patients have pancreatic endocrine tumors, including both adenomas and carcinomas. However, it is unusual for these tumors to be functional and few have a clinical hormonal syndrome. Patients with tuberous sclerosis have insulinomas and nonfunctional pancreatic islet cell tumors.

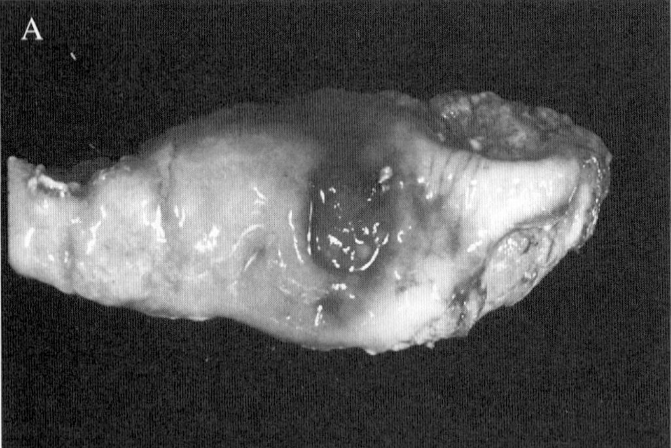

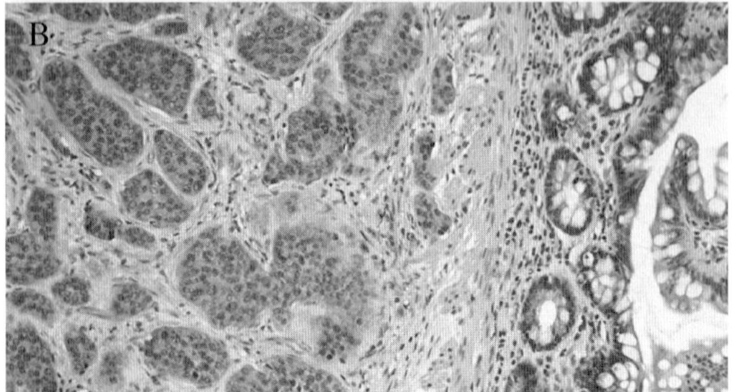

FIGURE 56.4. Gross (A) and microscopic (B) photographs of a duodenal gastrinoma.

Specific Islet Cell Tumors

Insulinomas occur in the pancreas and are evenly distributed among the head, body, and tail.[75] Insulinomas are most often benign, but they can metastasize and be malignant.[83] Glucagonomas also occur within the pancreas (Table 56.7). In contrast, primary gastrinomas usually occur within the duodenum (50%), and the second most common site is the pancreas (20%–40%). Further, approximately 80% to 85% of primary gastrinomas are found within the gastrinoma triangle, an area that includes the head of the pancreas and the duodenum.[84] Vasoactive intestinal peptide-secreting tumors (VIPomas) are usually in the pancreas, but they may also occur within the duodenum. Somatostatinomas are commonly in the pancreas, but may be extrapancreatic. In a recent review of 48 primary somatostatinomas, 56% were in the pancreas and 44% were in the duodenum or jejunum. Similar to glucagonomas, somatostatinomas usually are large, greater than 5cm, and metastases are present at the time of diagnosis.[85]

Patients with insulinoma or gastrinoma have symptoms of hypoglycemia and ulcer diathesis with or without diarrhea, respectively. The diagnosis is established biochemically based on the results of standardized tests. Insulinoma is diagnosed by a 72-hour fast with the development of neuroglycopenic symptoms. Insulinoma is proven by hypoglycemia (glucose less than 45mg/dL) and hyperinsulinism (insulin more than 5μU/mL). Close supervision is necessary to exclude factitious hypoglycemia, use of medications to falsely decrease blood glucose levels. Zollinger–Ellison syndrome (ZES) is diagnosed by measurement of elevated fasting serum levels of gastrin (more than 100pg/mL) and elevated levels of basal acid output (BAO greater than 15mEq/h). All antiacid medications should be discontinued during testing as these drugs may falsely elevate serum gastrin levels. The secretin stimulation test is also used to diagnose ZES; 2U/kg of secretin is given intravenously and serum levels of gastrin are measured before and

TABLE 56.7. Pancreatic neuroendocrine tumor, incidence of multiple endocrine neoplasia (MEN)-1, diagnosis, location, and malignant potential.

Tumor	*MEN-1 (%)*	*Diagnosis*	*Location*	*Malignant (%)*
Insulinoma	10	Fasting glucose Insulin C-peptide Pro-insulin	Pancreas	5–0
Gastrinoma	20	Fasting gastrin Basal acid output (BAO) Secretin test	Duodenum Pancreas Extrapancreatic Extraintestinal	60
Glucagonoma	Rare	Glucagon	Pancreas	100
Somatostatinoma	Rare	Somatostatin	Pancreas Duodenum Jejunum	100
Vasoactive intestinal polypeptide-secreting tumors (VIPoma)	Rare	VIP	Pancreas Duodenum	60
Ppoma (nonfunctional tumor)	Common	Pancreatic polypeptide	Pancreas	60

after. An increase of 200 pg/mL over basal levels of gastrin is consistent with ZES.

After the diagnosis of insulinoma is made based on the results of the fast, localization studies are used to try to image and identify the insulinoma. CT correctly images approximately 50% of these tumors. In a recent study with multiphasic helical CT, 19 of 30 insulinomas were correctly identified; there were no false positives.[86] Most experts agree that multiphasic CT is the imaging study of choice for pancreatic neuroendocrine tumors. It can image all large tumors (more than 2 cm) and it images approximately 50% of tumors as small as 1 cm. Tumors appear as a blush on CT because of increased vascularity.[87] MRI localized 7 of 8 neuroendocrine tumors in one study.[88] Somatostatin receptor scintigraphy (SRS) is the imaging study of choice for all pancreatic neuroendocrine tumors except insulinomas (Figure 56.5). Recent studies suggest that FDG-PET may also be useful, but it is not as good as SRS.[89] SRS is generally believed to be inaccurate for the localization of insulinomas compared to all other pancreatic neuroendocrine tumors. However, in one recent study it was able to identify most insulinomas, and when combined with endoscopic ultrasound (EUS) it correctly demonstrated 15 of 16 insulinomas.[90] EUS is able to identify most insulinomas, more preoperatively than all other studies. However, occasionally it may have false-positive results that lead to misguidance of the surgery. Pancreatic nodules and accessory spleens have been confused with insulinoma. EUS is not a substitute for careful preoperative evaluation and biochemical testing that should be done in every patient.[91] EUS specificity can be improved by needle biopsy, which can be done for primary pancreatic tumors or lymph nodes[92] (Figure 56.6). The best results are seen when one combines thin-section helical CT with EUS. In one study of 18 consecutive patients, this combination identified an insulinoma in each patient.[93]

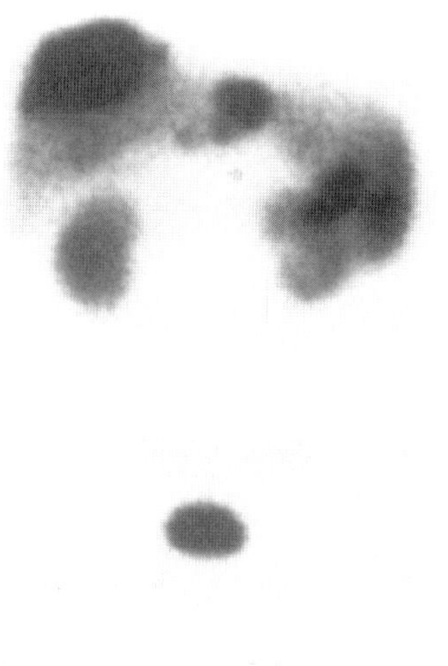

FIGURE 56.5. Somatostatin receptor scintigraphy (octreoscan) of a pancreatic tail neuroendocrine tumor with bilobar liver metastases.

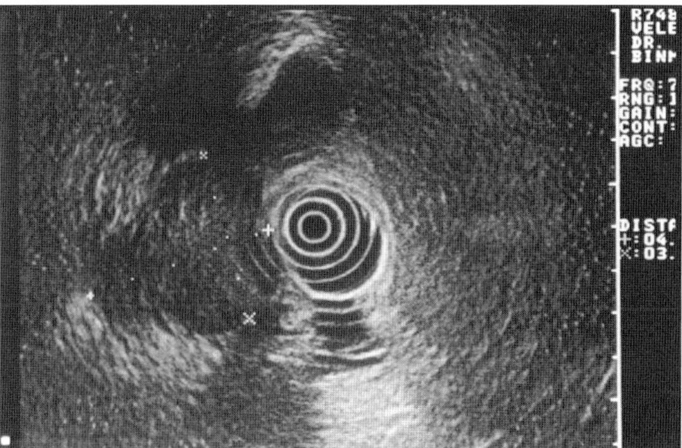

FIGURE 56.6. Endoscopic ultrasound (EUS) of a large nonfunctional neuroendocrine tumor within the head of the pancreas. During EUS, the tumor was aspirated for cells, making the diagnosis of pancreatic neuroendocrine tumor. This tumor is the same tumor seen on CT scan in Figure 56.3.

Because insulinomas are generally benign and located within the pancreas, the goal of surgery is to precisely identify the tumor and remove it preserving as much pancreas as possible. Intraoperative ultrasound has been useful for precise operative localization. It can identify the tumor and its relationship to vital structures such as the common bile duct and the pancreatic duct. It allows the surgeon to decide the best way to remove the tumor and avoid complications. A preoperative calcium angiogram has been shown to localize most (more than 90%) of insulinomas to the head, body, or tail of the pancreas.[94] Similar studies have been done with secretin injection for gastrinomas. However, recently calcium angiogram has been shown to effectively localize most gastrinomas as well.[95] Further, modern methods have allowed laparoscopic enucleation of insulinomas based on laparoscopic ultrasound done during the surgery. If it can be done, this procedure results in less pain and more rapid recovery.[96] However, similar complications such as pancreatic fistula and abscess may occur with laparoscopic pancreatic operations and must be considered. Because of this fact, the length of stay with laparoscopic surgery for NET has not been dramatically different than open operations.[97,98]

The glucagonoma syndrome is a specific hormonally mediated clinical syndrome that includes a characteristic pruritic migratory red excoriating rash called necrolytic migratory erythema (NME), diabetes mellitus, weight loss, anemia, stomatitis, thromboembolic complications, hypoaminoacidemia, and gastrointestinal and neuropsychiatric disturbances.[99] Some patients also have evidence of tachycardia, heart failure, and a dilated cardiomyopathy.[100] These signs and symptoms are relieved by resection of the tumor. Infusions of zinc, amino acids, and total parenteral nutrition have each relieved the NME skin rash in certain cases.[101] It is most likely caused by a nutritional deficiency related to chronic excess levels of glucagon. CT scan and octreoscan image most glucagonomas. PET scan images some tumors as well.[102] Patients commonly have clinical manifestations of the hypercoagulable state, including pulmonary embolus and deep venous thrombosis.[103,104]

Vasoactive intestinal polypeptide-secreting tumors (VIPoma) are rare pancreatic neuroendocrine tumors with remarkable symptoms of severe diarrhea.[105] Most tumors that produce VIP are found within the pancreas, but they can also be extrapancreatic. These tumors are usually malignant. Patients may have liver metastases at the time of diagnosis. MRI is the best imaging study to visualize liver neuroendocrine tumor.[106,107] Octreoscan can also image tumor. VIPoma leads to a syndrome of watery diarrhea, hypokalemia, hypercalcemia, and achlorhydria. It is also called the Verner–Morrison syndrome or the pancreatic cholera syndrome. Dehydration, renal failure, and electrolyte and acid–base abnormalities are so severe that death may ensue if these are not corrected. Octreotide can reverse the diarrhea and correct the fluid–base disturbances and may be lifesaving in some patients. It has few side effects and can be used in the elderly without complications.[108] Interferon-alpha and 5-fluorouracil have been used to treat metastatic VIPoma and have resulted in a dramatic response in one patient.[109]

Nonfunctioning pancreatic islet cell tumors are usually large (more than 5 cm), and symptoms are related to tumor mass. Patients may present with incidentally imaged pancreatic neuroendocrine tumor seen on a CT done for another reason. They may have intestinal bleeding or obstruction or pain. Other less-common functioning islet cell tumors such as those associated with acromegaly (GRFoma), hypercalcemia, or ectopic ACTH production are usually quite large, with liver metastases at diagnosis. Recently, a ghrelin-producing pancreatic neuroendocrine tumor was described. It was not associated with clinical features of acromegaly.[110]

Radiologic Imaging

Despite the fact that there are numerous studies to image pancreatic neuroendocrine tumors, some patients will still have no imageable tumor. CT has been an excellent study for identifying large tumors within the pancreas and liver. It can reliably visualize tumors that are greater than 2 to 3 cm in diameter; however, smaller tumors may be missed. CT is indicated in all patients with suspected islet cell tumors, especially to exclude liver metastases. Multidetector CT has been able to image many neuroendocrine tumors including those within lymph nodes. When coupled with somatostatin receptor scintigraphy, it can reliably detect the majority of neuroendocrine tumors.[111] The results with MRI are similar to CT. MRI has the advantage that no radiation is used; however, it is much more expensive and is not routinely recommended unless small liver metastases are a concern. MRI correctly imaged 29 of 31 neuroendocrine tumors in 19 patients.[112] Somatostatin receptor scintigraphy (SRS) or octreoscan images neuroendocrine tumors based on the density of type 2 somatostatin receptors. The high density of sst2 on pancreatic neuroendocrine tumors and carcinoid tumors makes radiolabeled somatostatin analogues excellent for tumor imaging. If the tumor is imaged by these analogues, the peptide inhibits tumor growth and hormone secretion, making it useful for treatment. Studies are under way to label octreotide with other isotopes to use it for tumor cell destruction.[113] It is an excellent study at identifying both primary and metastatic tumors. It has a sensitivity and specificity of approximately 85% to 90%. It is the imaging study of choice for nearly all neuroendocrine tumors except insulinomas. However, it must be realized that it may fail to identify small tumors within the duodenum. It has been combined with echo-enhanced power Doppler sonography to better image pancreatic neuroendocrine tumors.[114]

Endoscopic ultrasound is best for imaging small pancreatic islet cell tumors within the pancreas such as insulinoma. It has a sensitivity and specificity of 85% for pancreatic islet cell tumors. However, it is observer dependent and not all institutions have had excellent results. Occult insulinomas and gastrinomas can be regionally localized by calcium and/or secretin angiogram. Arteries that perfuse the pancreas are injected with an agent that causes the tumor to secrete hormone that can be measured in the hepatic vein. Calcium is used for both insulinoma and gastrinoma, whereas secretin is only for gastrinoma. These studies provide correct regional localization in approximately 90% of patients. These studies provide less information in gastrinoma, because occult tumors are generally within the gastrinoma triangle, and more information in insulinoma that are uniformly distributed throughout the entire pancreas.

Treatment

Treatment should be designed to control the signs and symptoms of excessive hormone secretion and the malignant growth and spread of the tumor. The only curative treatment is complete surgical resection of all tumor. Gastrinomas are most commonly within the duodenum. Duodenotomy (opening the duodenum) identifies more tumors and results in a greater cure rate, indicating that it should be done routinely in all operations for gastrinoma. These tumors are frequently small, most commonly found in the proximal duodenum, and associated with lymph node metastases in 60% of patients.[115–117]

Resection of primary gastrinoma has been shown to decrease the probability of liver metastases. Even localized liver metastases can be removed for apparent amelioration of symptoms and prolongation of survival.[118] Serum levels of chromogranin A and secretory hormones can be used to assess curative resection, but minor changes in levels are not sensitive enough to assess tumor regression or progression.[119] Repetitive imaging with CT and SRS can be used to follow tumor response to therapy. Aggressive surgery including Whipple pancreaticoduodenectomy has been performed for neuroendocrine tumors (NET) of the pancreas. However, because the prognosis is good with pancreatic neuroendocrine tumors, the operative death rate and morbidity of surgery should be acceptable. A recent report shows that the Whipple for NET had an operative mortality of 10% and a complication rate of 30%. However, the long-term survival was also excellent in that 81% and 70% were alive at 5 and 10 years, respectively.[120]

Chemotherapy treatment is based on tumor differentiation. Differentiation can be assessed by octreoscan and biopsy. Well-differentiated NET are usually positive on SRS, suggesting that somatostatin analogues will be useful in treatment to inhibit both tumor growth and hormone secretion. If the SRS is negative and the tumor is poorly differentiated, chemotherapy treatment is indicated. Drugs such as cisplatin and etoposide are especially useful and have 50% response rates with some dramatic responses.[121] Medical management of the gastric acid hypersecretion in patients with gastrinoma can usually be achieved with 20 to 40 mg of omeprazole twice a day. The hypoglycemic symptoms of insulinoma are treated by more-frequent feedings. Drugs such as diazoxide, octreotide, and verapamil may occasionally be helpful. However, in general, the hypoglycemia of insulinoma is unable to be controlled with drugs. The symptoms of glucagonoma (rash) and VIPoma (diarrhea) can be controlled with octreotide, the long-acting somatostatin analogue. Dopamine agonists have been used to treat the hormonal secretion by some pancreatic NET. Elevated serum levels of pancreatic polypeptide and prolactin have been significantly reduced by either cabergoline or bromocyptine.[122] The malignant tumoral process of islet cell tumors can seldom be controlled with chemotherapy.[123] Approximately 30% to 40% of tumors respond to doxorubicin, 5-FU, and streptozotocin as single drugs or in combination. Interferon-alpha has also produced some partial responses. Chemoembolization of liver metastases using interventional radiology techniques and doxorubicin has had a significant partial response rate. However, there have been no complete responses, and it does not appear to prolong survival. Patients with untreated liver metastases have a 20% 5-year survival. On the other hand, octreotide therapy using long-acting depot slow-release-form sandostatin LAR 20 mg IM every 3 weeks or sandostatin LAR 30 mg IM every 4 weeks does inhibit tumor growth and progression of NET that have high-density somatostatin receptors. This hormonal treatment plus surgical resection and/or radiofrequency ablation of liver neuroendocrine tumors increases the 5-year survival to 80% to 90%.[124,125] Liver transplantation has also been used for patients with metastatic liver NET who do not have tumor outside the liver. In general, the results have been good. Patients are seldom cured by liver transplantation as tumor generally recurs. However, the 5-year survival is between 36% and 83%.[126–128] Bone metastases are usually treated with external-beam radiation therapy. They have also been successfully treated with indium-labeled pentetreotide.[129] Patients may live for many years with distant metastases from neuroendocrine tumors because tumor progression may be slow.

Carcinoid Tumors

Carcinoid tumors are neuroendocrine tumors derived from the diffuse neuroendocrine system. They are composed of monotonous sheets of small round cells with uniform nuclei and cytoplasm. Pathologists cannot differentiate benign from malignant tumors based on histology. Malignancy can only be determined based on the detection of metastases to either lymph nodes or distant sites. Carcinoid tumors synthesize numerous bioactive amines and peptides including neuron-specific enolase (NSE), 5-hydroxytryptamine (serotonin), 5-hydroxytryptophan, synaptophysin, chromogranin A and C, substance P, tachykinins. and hormones such as ACTH, calcitonin, and growth hormone-releasing hormone. Carcinoid tumors are fairly common in autopsy series and are present in approximately 21 per million autopsies. Similarly, 1 in 300 appendectomies will have a carcinoid tumor. Carcinoid tumors occur with greater frequency in patients with the MEN-1 syndrome.

Carcinoid tumors generally originate in four sites: bronchus, appendix, rectum, and small intestine (Table 56.8). Carcinoid tumors most commonly occur in the appendix (40%), small intestine (27%), rectum (13%), and bronchus (12%). Carcinoid tumors may also be divided into foregut, midgut, and hindgut. Foregut tumors include the bronchus, stomach, and thymus, which most commonly produce peptide hormones such as ACTH and calcitonin. These tumors also cause the atypical carcinoid syndrome because they secrete 5-hydroxytryptophan and lack the enzyme to convert it to 5-hydroxytryptamine or serotonin. Midgut carcinoid tumors include the appendix and small intestine (Figure 56.7). These tumors most commonly secrete serotonin that causes the typical carcinoid syndrome. However, because the liver metabolizes serotonin, signs and symptoms of the carcinoid syndrome are not present without liver metastases and the release of serotonin into the systemic circulation. Hindgut carcinoid tumors occur in the rectum and generally secrete no hormones.

Foregut carcinoid tumors most commonly occur in the bronchus and are a common cause of ectopic ACTH syndrome (Cushing's syndrome). The tumors occur in the major bronchi. They appear cherry-red on bronchoscopy because of

TABLE 56.8. **Carcinoid tumors: location, metastases, and carcinoid syndrome.**

Location	*Site*	*Incidence (%)*	*Metastases (%)*	*Carcinoid syndrome*
Foregut	Stomach	2	22	10
	Duodenum	3	20	3
	Bronchus	12	50	13
	Thymus	2	25	0
Midgut	Jejunum	1	35	9
	Ileum	23	35	9
	Appendix	38	2	Less than 1
	Ovary	Less than 1	6	50
Hindgut	Rectum	13	3	0

increased vascularity. Biopsy is contraindicated because of the risk of uncontrolled hemorrhage. MRI of the chest is the best method to diagnose bronchial carcinoid tumors because it can distinguish a tumor from hilar vessels. Lobectomy is the surgical procedure of choice as 50% have lymph node metastases. Thymic carcinoid tumors are another potential cause of ectopic ACTH syndrome. These tumors are commonly malignant. CT and MRI are excellent studies to image the extent of disease and make the diagnosis. The tumor appears as a mass within the anterior superior mediastinum and the thymus. Radical thymectomy is the procedure of choice. Care should be taken to avoid injury to one or both phrenic nerves.

Stomach carcinoid tumors equal only 3 of every 1,000 gastric neoplasms (Figure 56.8). Recent studies suggest that not all gastric carcinoid tumors are similar. Some are associated with chronic hypergastrinemic states such as achlorhydria and Zollinger–Ellison syndrome. These tumors arise from the enterochromaffin cells (ECL) cells, are small, multiple and seldom malignant (9% overall). These are contrasted to sporadic carcinoid tumors of the stomach, which are large, single, and atypical on histology and are associated with the carcinoid syndrome in 15% to 50% of cases. These tumors cause the syndrome without liver metastases as the bioactive substances can enter the systemic circulation; 55% to 66% of these large gastric carcinoid tumors are malignant based on the detection of nodal or liver metastases.

Midgut carcinoid tumors most commonly occur within the appendix. Most carcinoid tumors occur at the tip of the appendix and are totally removed by an appendectomy.

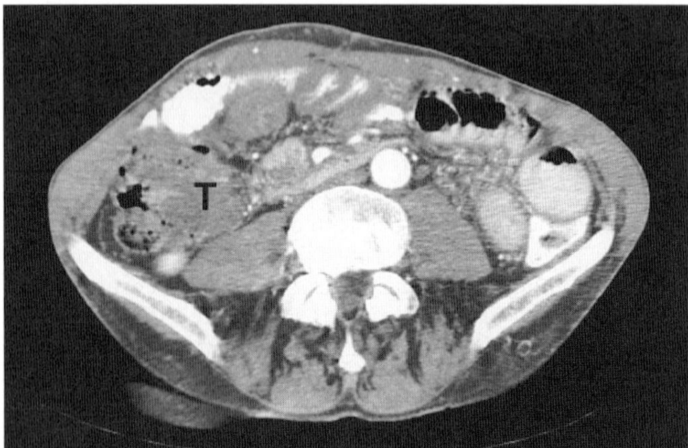

FIGURE 56.7. CT of an ileal carcinoid tumor (T). (From Norton et al.,[76] with permission.)

Appendiceal carcinoid tumors are usually smaller than 1 cm in diameter, and simple appendectomy is adequate. Tumors between 1 and 2 cm are more worrisome, especially when present at the base of the appendix. These tumors have a 50% chance of lymph node metastases and are best treated by right hemicolectomy. Tumors greater than 2 cm in size have a high probability of nodal spread and are also treated by right hemicolectomy. However, most appendiceal carcinoids are smaller than 1 cm, at the tip of the appendix, and only require simple appendectomy. Primary small intestinal carcinoid tumors may be multiple and most occur within the ileum. In fact, 40% are within 2 feet of the ileocecal valve. Unlike appendiceal carcinoid tumors, which are usually benign, these tumors are generally malignant. They spread to local lymph nodes and cause a dense fibrotic reaction that distorts the gut and may cause symptoms of small bowel obstruction. This fibrosis may obliterate venous outflow and result in venous mesenteric infarction. The incidence of nodal metastases from ileal carcinoid tumors is dependent on the size of the tumor. If the tumor is less than 1 cm, nodal metastases are present approximately 15% of the time. If the tumor is between 1 and 2 cm, nodal metastases occur 60% to 80% of the time. If the tumor is larger than 2 cm, metastases nearly always occur. Liver metastases also occur and, if present,

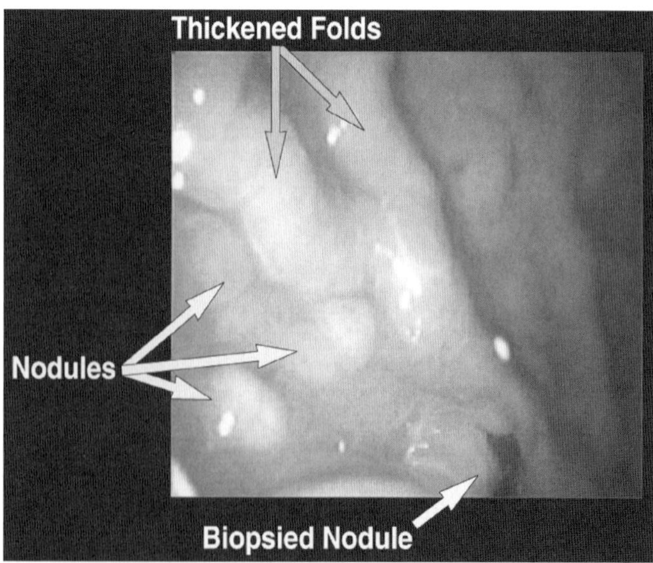

FIGURE 56.8. Multiple stomach carcinoid tumors (nodules) seen on endoscopy. This patient also has thickened gastric folds secondary to Zollinger–Ellison syndrome.

patients have symptoms of the malignant carcinoid syndrome. Duodenal carcinoid tumors may also occur, but most are asymptomatic and are found on endoscopy as an incidental finding. A duodenal carcinoid tumor less than 1 cm is clinically insignificant, whereas approximately one-third of larger tumors spread to lymph nodes. Thus, duodenal carcinoid tumors are rarely clinically significant, but they must be differentiated from gastrinomas and somatostatinomas that can appear like a small duodenal carcinoid. Immunoperoxidase staining for various hormones helps to differentiate the various tumors.

In approximately 1 in every 2,500 sigmoidoscopies, a hindgut carcinoid tumor is identified. Rectal carcinoids occur submucosally on the anterior or lateral walls of the rectum between 4 and 13 cm from the dentate line. Approximately 80% of these tumors are less than 1 cm in size and never metastasize. Tumors greater than 2 cm almost always metastasize. These larger tumors are locally invasive and have a large number of mitoses. Either simple resection with negative margins or low anterior resection is the procedure of choice for rectal carcinoid tumors. Abdominoperineal resection is not recommended as small tumors are seldom malignant and large tumors are usually not cured by surgery. Rectal carcinoid tumors seldom cause the carcinoid syndrome.

Carcinoid Syndrome

The carcinoid syndrome is associated with severe flushing attacks. Flushing attacks are characterized by the sudden onset of a deep red color over the upper part of the body, primarily the neck and face, and an unpleasant feeling of warmth, lacrimation, itching, palpitations, and diarrhea. Flushing spells may be precipitated by stress, certain foods such as cheese or wine, exercise, and drugs. Attacks are generally brief, lasting 2 to 5 minutes, and episodic. Typical flushing attacks are most commonly seen with carcinoid tumors that originate in the midgut and have liver metastases. Diarrhea is also associated with carcinoid syndrome. Ovarian carcinoid tumors also commonly cause the carcinoid syndrome (see Table 56.8). Diarrhea usually occurs with the flushing but it may also occur alone. Typically the stools are watery with the number of movements ranging from 3 to 30 per day. Patients commonly develop wheezing and airway constriction during an attack. Cardiac manifestations are also part of the carcinoid syndrome. The cardiac disease is typically caused by fibrosis that involves primarily the right side of the heart. Fibrous deposits tend to cause constriction of the tricuspid and pulmonic valve that results in regurgitation. In the atypical carcinoid syndrome, the flushing may be prolonged, lasting several days. It is more diffuse over the entire body, and may be a constant red or cyanotic color. The atypical rash is frequently provoked by food and may be associated with intense pruritis.

In general, the signs and symptoms of the carcinoid syndrome are caused by serotonin (5-HT) secretion by the tumor. Most patients (more than 85%) with the carcinoid syndrome have elevated urinary levels of 5-hydroxyindolacetic acid (5-HIAA), the major metabolite of serotonin. The carcinoid syndrome is diagnosed by measurement of elevated urinary levels of 5-HIAA. It is also important to remember that foregut carcinoid tumors may produce the atypical carcinoid syndrome. These tumors lack the appropriate decarboxylase enzyme to convert 5-hydroxytryptophan to serotonin (5-hydroxytryptamine). Therefore, in patients with the atypical carcinoid syndrome, urinary levels of 5-HIAA may be normal but urinary metabolites of tryptophan are elevated. Further, platelet levels of serotonin will be elevated because platelets have the enzyme to convert 5-hydroxytryptophan to serotonin. However, most patients with carcinoid syndrome have midgut carcinoid tumors with liver metastases, and these patients have elevated urinary levels of 5-HIAA.

Localization Studies

Patients with the carcinoid syndrome typically have a mass in the small bowel on CT with cicatrization and narrowing of the bowel with partial obstruction. These patients usually have liver metastases. Tumor is best imaged by somatostatin receptor scintigraphy that has approximately a 90% sensitivity and specificity for the tumor. SRS is especially useful because it will also image bone and other distant metastases. SRS has been shown to be superior to imaging with MIBG.[130]

Prognosis and Treatment

For all patients with the carcinoid syndrome, the 5-year survival is approximately 25% (Table 56.9). The prognosis varies with the site of origin and extent of disease. Patients with the carcinoid syndrome usually have distant metastases. The most immediate life-threatening complication is the carcinoid crisis that may occur during chemotherapy, surgery, or anesthesia. The crisis only happens in patients with 24-hour urinary 5-HIAA levels greater than 200 mg per 24 hours. The crisis initially presents with upper body flush, hypertension, and tachycardia, and subsequently severe hypotension and death may develop. Treatment with intravenous octreotide (long-acting somatostatin analogue) ameliorates the symptoms and signs and can be lifesaving.

The manifestations of the carcinoid syndrome should be managed medically. The flush is initially controlled by avoiding precipitating agents, diarrhea by antidiarrheal drugs, wheezing by bronchial dilators, and valvular heart disease by

TABLE 56.9. Five-year survival (%) with carcinoid tumors by site and stage.

Location	*Site*	*Primary with no metastasis*	*Nodal metastases*	*Distant metastases*
Foregut	Bronchus	96	71	11
	Stomach	93	23	0
Midgut	Appendix	99	99	27
	Ileum	75	60	20
Hindgut	Rectum	92	44	7

inotropic drugs and diuretics. However, the syndrome may not be completely controlled by these measures and eventually patients become more symptomatic. At this point, patients are treated by the somatostatin analogue octreotide 100–150µg SC TID, which markedly improves all symptoms. After 1 to 2 weeks of octreotide, the patient can be given sandostatin LAR 20–30mg IM every 3 to 4 weeks to control the syndrome long term. Patients who are treated chronically with this drug may become refractory to it and require larger and larger doses. Interferon-alpha has also been used to treat the carcinoid syndrome and may be helpful in some patients.

Carcinoid tumors are best managed surgically. However, in patients with liver or locally advanced tumor, surgery is seldom curative. Patients with distant metastases may have symptoms related to a partial small bowel obstruction that warrant surgery. Further, in some reports aggressive surgery to debulk the primary and metastatic tumor is associated with amelioration of symptoms and prolongation of survival. Hepatic metastases may also be treated with chemoembolization, cryotherapy, radiofrequency ablation, and liver transplantation. Each of these procedures may improve symptoms, but none has been shown to clearly prolong survival. Control of liver metastases by surgery is associated with a 5-year survival of 80%.[131] Chemotherapy with adriamycin, 5-fluorouracil, and streptozotocin has a 30% partial response rate. However, there have been no complete responses and no improvement in survival. Immunotherapy with interferon-alpha has also decreased tumor size and may improve symptoms. In general, patients with carcinoid tumors live for long periods (see Table 56.9), and treatments are used to provide specific goals such as relief of symptoms and prolongation of survival. Recent data continue to document that chemotherapy has not been effective in gastroenteropancreatic neuroendocrine tumors. Somatostatin analogues such as sandostatin LAR in doses of 20–30mg IM every 3 to 4 weeks have been able to control the signs and symptoms of carcinoid syndrome and appear to have decreased tumor growth, causing stabilization of disease.[132] A prospective trial of interferon-alpha, lantreotide, or both in 80 patients with metastatic carcinoid tumors demonstrated that each of the drugs and the combination had antitumor activity that decreased symptoms and appeared to prolong survival. However, no treatment group was significantly better than the other groups.[133] Other investigators have criticized this study based on inadequate numbers of patients and the use of lantreotide instead of other somatostain analogues.[134] A new approach that shows promise is based on inhibition of the epidermal growth factor receptor by gefitinib, which induced apoptosis and cell-cycle arrest in in vitro studies of malignant neuroendocrine tumors.[135]

Multiple Endocrine Neoplasia

Multiple endocrine neoplasia type 1 (MEN-1) is an inherited endocrine disorder that includes hyperplasia of the parathyroid glands, tumors of the pancreatic islets and anterior pituitary, and occasionally carcinoid tumors and lipomas. It is inherited as an autosomal dominant disorder with variable penetrance, meaning that 50% of the offspring will develop the disease, but each may not express all the components (Table 56.10).

TABLE 56.10. Multiple endocrine neoplasias: genetics and clinical syndromes.

	MEN-1	*MEN-2A*	*MEN-2B*	*FMTC*
Chromosome	11	10	10	10
Gene	Menin	RET	RET	RET
Autosomal dominant	+	+	+	+
Phenotype	—	—	+	—
MTC	—	+	+	+
Virulence of MTC	—	++	++++	+
Pheochromocytoma	—	+	+	—
Pancreatic NET	+	—	—	—
1° HPT	+	+	—	—
Pituitary tumor	+	–	—	—

MEN, multiple endocrine neoplasia; MTC, medullary thyroid carcinoma; FMTC familial medullary thyroid carcinoma; NET, neuroendocrine tumor; 1° HPT, primary hyperparathyroidism.

Genetic Abnormalities in MEN-1

The causative gene in MEN-1 has been mapped to the long arm of chromosome 11 (see Table 56.10). The exact gene has been identified and named menin. Menin is a tumor suppressor gene, but its exact function is unknown.[136] Screening for the presence of disease should begin during the second or third decade of life. Individuals at risk should be questioned and examined for kidney stones, lipomas, hypercortisolism, hypoglycemia, peptic ulcer disease, headaches, acromegaly, and visual field defects. Blood levels of calcium, glucose, prolactin, gastrin, and pancreatic polypeptide are measured.

Parathyroid Hyperplasia in MEN-1

Primary hyperparathyroidism (HPT) is the most common endocrine disorder in patients with MEN-1.[137,138] The manifestations are similar to those seen in non-MEN-1 patients with HPT and include asymptomatic hypercalcemia, weakness, fatigue, kidney stones, and bone pain from decreased bone density. The prevalence of HPT in MEN-1 increases with age and is nearly 100% after age 50. The age of onset is 25 years, which is younger than sporadic HPT. Primary hyperparathyroidism is diagnosed by measurement of elevated serum levels of total calcium, ionized calcium, and parathyroid hormone (PTH). The intact PTH assay has seldom given false-positive results and is very specific for HPT. These patients always have parathyroid hyperplasia, but at surgery there can be some asymmetry in size.[139] The operation of choice is currently three and one-half gland parathyroidectomy. Half the most normal-appearing parathyroid gland is left intact and marked with a clip. The cervical thymus should also be removed, as supernumerary glands may occur and are usually within the thymus.

Pancreatic Islet Cell Tumors in MEN-1

MEN-1 patients also develop pancreatic or duodenal neuroendocrine tumors. Tissue microdissection techniques show that pancreatic neuroendocrine tumors in MEN-1 originate from the ductal acinar system and not the islets.[140] Endoscopic ultrasound has been used in MEN-1 patients to detect pancreatic neuroendocrine tumors at an early stage before the development of metastases. EUS was able to diagnose the presence of pancreatic neuroendocrine tumors in 14 of 15 MEN-1 patients before they had signs or symptoms of islet cell tumors.[141] These tumors may be malignant, and there is a correlation between the size of the tumor and the chance of metastases.[142] Pancreatic islet cell tumors may be nonfunctional or produce excessive hormones that cause a characteristic clinical syndrome. The most common functional islet cell tumor in MEN-1 is gastrinoma. Moreover, any islet cell tumor can occur in patients with MEN-1, including gastrinoma, insulinoma, glucagonoma, VIPoma, GRFoma, somatostatinoma, and nonfunctional tumor or PPoma.

Surgery is indicated to remove a potentially malignant islet cell tumor and ameliorate hormonal effects. At surgery these patients commonly have multiple pancreatic islet cell tumors and also multiple duodenal neuroendocrine tumors.[143] Recent studies indicate that tumors that produce insulin, glucagon, and VIP are more commonly within the pancreas, whereas tumors that secrete gastrin are usually within the duodenum.[144] The goal of surgery is to remove tumor without excessive morbidity and mortality. Surgical resection seldom cures patients of Zollinger–Ellison syndrome,[145] but it reduces the probability of liver metastases. The concept of early diagnosis of pancreatic neuroendocrine tumors in MEN-1 patients is not supported by the low cure rate and the fact that MEN-1 patients with resected metastatic tumors have the same survival as patients with resected localized tumors.[146]

Pituitary Tumors in MEN-1

The most common pituitary tumor in MEN-1 is a prolactinoma. Elevated serum levels of prolactin are diagnostic and are used as a screening study. Prolactinomas cause galactorrhea and impotence. Pituitary tumors in MEN-1 may also secrete other hormones including corticotropin (ACTH), growth hormone, and thyroid stimulating hormone (TSH). These tumors are associated with Cushing's disease, acromegaly, and hyperthyroidism, respectively. Biochemical diagnosis of each is based on recognition of the clinical signs and symptoms. MRI or CT of the sella and visual field examination are ordered for patients suspected to have pituitary tumors. Bitemporal hemianopsia may occur when large tumors compress the optic chiasm.

Pituitary adenomas that produce prolactin are usually treated with bromocryptine. Pituitary tumors can also be removed surgically or less commonly are treated with irradiation.

Less-Common Tumors in MEN-1

Less-common tumors that may be occur with MEN-1 include bronchial or thymic carcinoids, intestinal carcinoids, gastric carcinoids, lipomas, benign adenomas of the thyroid gland, benign adrenocortical adenomas, and rarely adrenocortical carcinomas. Carcinoid tumors should be removed surgically when identified. Cortical adenomas of the thyroid gland and benign cortical adenomas of the adrenal cortex usually require no treatment, unless there is evidence of excessive hormonal function. Lipomas are usually large and should be excised when symptomatic. Adrenal cortical carcinomas commonly present with signs and symptoms of hypercortisolism and are identified as a large adrenal tumor on CT (6 cm). Surgical resection is the treatment of choice.

Multiple Endocrine Neoplasia Type 2A, 2B, and Familial Medullary Thyroid Carcinoma

Multiple endocrine neoplasia type 2A (MEN-2A) is an autosomal dominant inherited endocrine syndrome that is characterized by medullary thyroid carcinoma (MTC), adrenal pheochromocytoma(s), and parathyroid hyperplasia (see Table 56.10). Multiple endocrine neoplasia type 2B (MEN-2B) is an autosomal dominant inherited endocrine syndrome that is characterized by MTC, adrenal pheochromocytoma(s), and a characteristic phenotype that includes mucosal neuromas, puffy lips, bony abnormalities, marfanoid habitus, intestinal ganglioneuromas, and corneal nerve hypertrophy.[147] Unlike MEN-2A, parathyroid disease is not associated with MEN-2B. Familial medullary thyroid carcinoma (FMTC) is characterized by an autosomal dominant inheritance of only medullary thyroid carcinoma without any other endocrine abnormalities.[148]

Gene Defect in MEN-2

The gene for MEN-2A, MEN-2B, and FMTC has been localized to the pericentromeric region of chromosome 10 (see Table 56.10). The responsible gene is a transmembrane protein kinase receptor called RET.[149,150] RET is an oncogene in that mutations enhance cellular growth. The exact mechanism by which RET enhances cellular growth is unknown. Recent studies have detected missense mutations in RET in all individuals with MEN-2A, MEN-2B, and FMTC.[149,150] MEN-2A and FMTC mutations have been identified within the extracellular portion of the molecule, whereas MEN-2B mutations have been identified within the intracellular domain.

Medullary Thyroid Carcinoma

In patients with MEN-2A, MTC generally appears between the ages of 5 and 25 years before the development of pheochromocytoma or primary hyperparathyroidism.[150] Recently, detection of RET mutations in the peripheral white blood cells of patients from kindreds with MEN-2A has been used as a screening procedure to diagnose an affected individual.[150,151] Because 100% of individuals with MEN-2A will develop MTC, total thyroidectomy has been performed when RET mutations are detected. Before thyroid surgery, it is important to rule out the presence of a pheochromocytoma by measuring 24-hour urine levels of VMA, metanephrines, and total catecholamines. When total thyroidectomy has been performed based solely on genetic testing, either premalignant C-cell hyperplasia or in situ MTC has been identified.

Individuals with MEN-2B have a characteristic phenotype.[147] These patients have prognathism, puffy lips, poor dentition, mucosal neuromas, corneal nerve hypertrophy, and multiple bony abnormalities. The presence of MEN-2B can be ascertained by the observation of corneal nerve hypertrophy on slit-light examination. Patients with MEN-2B usually have locally advanced MTC at presentation.[147] These patients are seldom cured by thyroidectomy and usually die of the MTC.

Individuals with FMTC have the best prognosis.[148] In these patients, MTC occurs at an older age and patients seldom die of MTC. Thus, in the three different familial settings, although the same oncogene is affected, the virulence of the MTC is different. The most virulent form is MEN-2B, the intermediate form is MEN-2A, and the least virulent is FMTC. Total thyroidectomy is indicated for the familial types of MTC as each involves both lobes of the gland.

Pheochromocytoma in MEN-2A and 2B

Individuals with either MEN-2A or MEN-2B may develop bilateral benign intraadrenal pheochromocytomas.[150] The diagnosis of pheochromocytoma is made by detection of elevated 24 hour urinary levels of VMA, metanephrines, or total catecholamines. Urinary metanephrines are the single best diagnostic study. Imaging studies can identify which adrenal gland is involved. CT, MRI, and MIBG scan each have utility. Both MRI and CT can image pheochromocytomas as small as 1 cm. There is controversy as to the extent of adrenalectomy in patients with MEN-2. Some recommend bilateral adrenalectomy for all individuals with biochemical evidence of pheochromocytoma, because studies have shown that 70% are bilateral and sudden death can be caused by an untreated pheochromocytoma. Others remove only the adrenal gland in which a tumor is seen. If a unilateral adrenalectomy is performed, careful follow-up is warranted as some patients may develop another tumor in the contralateral gland. Recent studies have demonstrated that laparoscopic adrenalectomy is the method of choice to remove these tumors. Resection should be performed after the patient has been prepared preoperatively with alpha-adrenergic-blocking drugs such as phenoxybenzamine. Adrenal surgery should be performed before thyroidectomy.

Parathyroid Disease in MEN-2A

Patients with MEN-2A may also develop symptomatic primary hyperparathyroidism (HPT).[152] The diagnosis is ascertained by measurement of elevated serum levels of calcium and parathyroid hormone. HPT is caused by multiple gland disease or parathyroid hyperplasia (see Table 56.10). The proper surgical treatment is three and one-half gland parathyroidectomy.

Gastrointestinal Manifestations of MEN-2A or MEN-2B

Some individuals with MEN-2A may also have Hirschsprung's disease. Recent evidence suggests that Hirschsprung's disease is also associated with RET mutations; however, these mutations are inactivating for RET. Individuals with MEN-2B commonly complain of severe constipation, and megacolon or diverticulosis has been described. MEN-2B patients are known to have abnormal gut motility secondary to intestinal ganglioneuromatosis. Constipation should be treated as symptoms arise. As the MTC becomes metastatic, patients may develop severe secretory diarrhea. MTC can secrete a wide variety of peptide hormones that cause diarrhea. Octreotide has been used to inhibit the diarrhea in this setting.

References

1. Ries LAG, Eisner MP, Kosary CL, et al. (eds). SEER Cancer Statistics Review, 1975–2001. Bethesda, MD: National Cancer Institute, 2004. http://seer.cancer.gov/csr/1975_2001/.
2. Zhao J, Speel E, Muletta-Feurer S, et al. Analysis of genomic alterations in sporadic adrenocortical lesions. Am J Pathol 1999;155:1039–1045.
3. Logie A, Boulle N, Gaston V, et al. Autocrine role of IGF-II in proliferation of human adrenocortical carcinoma NCI H296R cell line. J Mol Endosc 1999;23:23–32.
4. Stojadinovic A, Ghossein R, Hoos A, et al. Adrenocortical carcinoma: clinical, morphologic, and molecular characterization. J Clin Oncol 2002;20:941–950.
5. Hainuat P. Tumor-specific mutations in p53: the acid test. Nat Med 2002;8:21–23.
6. Barzon L, Chilosi M, Fallo F, et al. Molecular analysis of CDKN1C and TP53 in sporadic adrenal tumors. Eur J Endosc 2001;145:207–212.
7. Yamamichi-Nishina M, Ito T, Mizutani T, Yamamichi N, Watanabe H, Iba H. SW13 cells can transition between two distinct subtypes by switching expression of BRG1 and Brm genes at the post-transcriptional level. J Biol Chem 2003;278:7422–7430.
8. Lindholm J, Juul S, Jorgensen JOL, et al. Incidence and late prognosis of Cushing's syndrome: a population-based study. J Clin Endocrinol Metab 2001;86:117–123.
9. Yamada T, Saito H, Moriya T, et al. Adrenal carcinoma with a signal loss on chemical shift magnetic resonance imaging. J Comput Assist Tomogr 2003;27:606–608.
10. Honigschnabl S, Gallo S, Niederle B, et al. How accurate is MR imaging in characterization of adrenal masses: update of a long-term study. Eur J Radiol 2002;41:113–122.
11. Becjerer A, Voerjapper J, Potzi C, et al. FDG PET in adrenocortical carcinoma. Can Biother Radiopharm 2001;16:289–295.
12. Maurea S, Klain M, Caraco C, et al. Diagnostic accuracy of radionuclide imaging using ^{131}I nor-cholesterol or meta-iodobenzylguanidine in patients with hypersecreting or non-hypersecreting adrenal tumours. Nucl Med 2002;23:951–960.
13. Grumbach M, Biller M, Baunstein G, et al. Management of the clinically inapparent adrenal mass. Ann Intern Med 2003;138: 424–429.
14. Lockhard M, Smith J, Kenney P. Imaging of adrenal masses. Eur J Radiol 2002;41:95–112.
15. Fimmano A, Pettinato G, Bonuso C, et al. Giant, nonfunctioning carcinoma of the adrenal cortex. N Engl J Med 2001;345:700.
16. Harrison L, Gaudin P, Brennan M. Pathologic features of prognostic significance for adrenocortical carcinoma after curative resection. Arch Surg 1999;134:181–185.
17. Langer P, Bartsch D, Moebius E, et al. Adrenocortical carcinoma-our experience with 11 cases. Langenbecks Arch Surg 2000;385: 393–397.
18. Wood B, Abraham J, Hvizda J, et al. Radiofrequency ablation of adrenal tumors and adrenocortical carcinoma metastases. Cancer (Phila) 2003;97:554–560.
19. Wajchenberg B, Pereira M, Medonca B, et al. Adrenocortical carcinoma. Cancer (Phila) 2000;88:711–736.
20. Harrison LE, Gaudin PB, Brennan MF. Pathologic features of prognostic significance for adrenocrtical carcinoma after curative resection. Arch Surg 1999;134:181–185.
21. Schulick R, Brennan M. Long-term survival after complete resection and repeat resection in patients with adrenocortical carcinoma. Ann Surg Oncol 1999;6:719–726.
22. Ng L, Libertino J. Adrenocortical carcinoma: diagnosis, evaluation and treatment. J Urol 2003;169:5–11.
23. Abraham J, Bakke S, Rutt A, et al. A phase II trial of combination chemotherapy and surgical resection for the treatment of metastatic adrenocortical carcinoma. Cancer (Phila) 2002;94: 2333–2343.
24. Berruti A, Terzolo M, Angeli A, et al. Mitotane associated with etoposide, doxorubicin, and cisplatin in the treatment of advanced adrenocortical carcinoma. Cancer (Phila) 1998;83: 2194–2200.

25. Williamson S, Lew D, Miller G, et al. Phase II evaluation of cisplatin and etoposide followed by mitotane at disease progression in patients with locally advanced or metastatic adrenocortical carcinoma. Cancer (Phila) 2000;88:1159–1165.
26. Mekhail T, Hutson T, Elson P, et al. Phase I trial of weekly docetaxel and gemcitabine in patients with refractory malignancies. Cancer (Phila) 2003;97:170–178.
27. Baudin E, Docao C, Gicquel C, et al. Use of a topoisomerase I inhibitor (irinotecan, CPT-11) in metastatic adrenocortical carcinoma. Ann Oncol 2002;13:1806–1809.
28. Bravo E, Tagle R. Pheochromocytoma: state-of-the-art and future prospects. Endocr Rev 2003;24:539–553.
29. Neumann H, Bausch B, McWhinney S, et al: Germ-line mutations in nonsyndromic pheochromocytoma. N Engl J Med 2002;346:1459–1466.
30. Maher E, Eng C. The pressure rises: update on the genetics of phaeochromocytoma. Hum Mol Genet 2002;11:2347–2354.
31. Bryant J, Farmer J, Kessler L, et al. Pheochromocytoma: the expanding genetic differential diagnosis. J Natl Cancer Inst 2003;95:1196–1204.
32. La Batide-Alanore A, Chatellier G, Plouin P. Diabetes as a marker of pheochromocytoma in hypertensive patients. J Hypertens 2003;21:1703–1707.
33. Wiesner T, Bluher M, Windgassen M, Paschke R. Improvement of insulin sensitivity after adrenalectomy in patients with pheochromocytoma. J Clin Endocrinol Metab 2003;88:3632–3636.
34. Kudva Y, Sawka A, Young W. The laboratory diagnosis of adrenal pheochromocytoma: the Mayo experience. J Clin Endocrinol Metab 2003;88:4533–4539.
35. Weise M, Merke D, Pacak K, et al. Utility of plasma free metaneprines for detecting childhood pheochromocytoma. J Clin Endocrinol Metab 2002;87:1955–1960.
36. Lenders J, Pacak K, Eisenhofer G. New advances in the biochemical diagnosis of pheochromocytoma. Ann NY Acad Sci 2002;970:29–40.
37. Sawka A, Jaeschke R, Singh R, Young W. A comparison of biochemical tests for pheochromocytoma: measurement of fractionated plasma metanephrines compared with the combination of 24-hour urinary metanephrines and cathecholamines. J Clin Endocrinol Metab 2003;88:553–558.
38. Blake M, Krishnamoorthy S, Boland G, et al. Low-density pheochromocytoma on CT: a mimicker of adrenal adenoma. Am J Radiol 2003;181:1663–1668.
39. Kolby L, Bernhardt P, Levin-Jakobsen A-M, et al. Uptake of meta-iodobenzylguanidine in neuroendocrine tumours is mediated by vesicular monoamine transporters. Br J Cancer 2003;89:1383–1388.
40. Jacob T, Escout J, Bussy E. Malignant diaphragmatic pheochromocytoma. Clin Nucl Med 2002;27:807–809.
41. Taniguchi K, Ishizu K, Torizuka T, et al. Metastases of predominantly dopamine-secreting phaeochromocytoma that did not accumulate meta-iodobenzylguanidine: imaging with whole body positron emission tomography using ^{18}F-labelled deoxyglucose. Eur J Surg 2001;167:866–870.
42. Hoegerle S, Nitzsche E, Altehoefer C, et al. Pheochromocytomas: detection with ^{18}F DOPA whole-body PET: initial results. Radiology 2002;222:507–512.
43. Hwang J, Uchio E, Pate V, et al. Diagnostic localization of malignant bladder pheochromocytoma using 6-[^{18}F]fluorodopamine positron emission tomography. J Urol 2003;169:274–275.
44. Ilias I, Yu J, Carrasquillo J, et al. Superiority of 6-[^{18}F] fluorodopamine positron emission tomography versus [^{131}I]-metaiodobenzylguanidine scintigraphy in the localization of metastatic pheochromocytoma. J Clin Endocrinol Metab 2003;88:4083–4087.
45. Bravo E. Pheochromocytoma an approach to antihypertensive management. Ann NY Acad Sci 2002;970:1–10.
46. Bentrem D, Pappas S, Ahuja Y, et al. Contemporary surgical management of pheochromocytoma. Am J Surg 2002;184:621–625.
47. MacGillivray D, Whalen G, Malchoff C, et al. Laparoscopic resection of large adrenal tumors. Ann Surg Oncol 2002;9:480–485.
48. Porpiglia F, Destefanis P, Fiori C, et al. Does adrenal mass size really affect safety and effectiveness of laparoscopic adrenalectomy? Urology 2002;60:801–805.
49. Zeh H, Udelsman R. One hundred laparoscopic adrenalectomies: a single surgeon's experience. Ann Surg Oncol 2003;10:1012–1017.
50. Brunt L, Lairmore T, Doherty G, et al. Adrenalectomy for familial pheochromocytoma in the laparoscopic era. Ann Surg 2002;235:713–721.
51. Walther M. New therapeutic and surgical approaches for sporadic and hereditary pheochrmocytoma. Ann NY Acad Sci 2002;970:41–53.
52. Li M, Fitzgerald P, Price D, Norton J. Iatrogenic pheochromocytomatosis: a previously unreported result of laparoscopic adrenalectomy. Surgery (St. Louis) 2001;130:1072–1077.
53. Shah M, Karelia N, Patel S, et al. Flow cytometric DNA analysis for determination of malignant potential in adrenal pheochromocytoma or paraganglioma: an Indian experience. Ann Surg Oncol 2003;10:426–431.
54. Yon L, Guillemot J, Montero-Hadjadje M, et al. Identification of the secretogranin II-derived peptide EM66 in pheochromocytomas as a potential marker for discriminating benign versus malignant tumors. J Clin Endocrinol Metab 2003;88:2579–2585.
55. Boltze C, Mundschenk J, Unger N, et al. Expression profile of the telomeric complex discriminates between benign and malignant pheochromocytoma. J Clin Endocrinol Metab 2003;88:4280–4286.
56. Gimenez-Roqueplo A, Favier J, Rustin P, et al. Mutations in the SDHB gene are associated with extra-adrenal and/or malignant phaechromocytomas. Cancer Res 2003;63:5615–5621.
57. Naguib M, Caceres M, Thomas C, et al. Radiation Treatment of recurrent pheochromocytoma of the bladder. Am J Clin Oncol 2002;25:42–44.
58. Rao F, Keiser H, O'Connor D. Malignant and benign pheochromocytoma chromaffin granule transmitters and the response to medical and surgical treatment. Ann NY Acad Sci 2002;971:530–532.
59. Sisson J. Radiopharmaceutical treatment of pheochromocytomas. Ann NY Acad Sci 2002;970:54–60.
60. Rose B, Matthay K, Price D, et al. High-dose ^{131}I-metaiodobenzylguanidine therapy for 12 patients with malignant pheochromocytoma. Cancer (Phila) 2003;98:239–248.
61. Lamarre-Cliché M, Gimenez-Roqueplo A, Billaud E, et al. Effects of slow-release octreotide on urinary metanephrine excretion and plasma chromogranin A and catecholamine levels in patients with malignant or recurrent phaechromocytoma. Clin Endocrinol 2002;57:629–634.
62. Nakane M, Takahashi S, Sekine I, et al. Successful treatment of malignant pheochromocytoma with combination chemotherapy containing anthracycline. Ann Oncol 2003;14:1449–1451.
63. Norton JA. Neuroendocrine tumors of the pancreas and duodenum. Curr Prob Surg 1994;31:77–164.
64. Doherty GM, Doppman JL, Shawker TH, et al. Results of a prospective strategy to diagnose, localize and resect insulinomas. Surgery (St. Louis) 1991;110:989–997.
65. Nakamura Y, Larsson C, Julier C, et al. Localization of the genetic defect in multiple endocrine neoplasia type 1 within a small region of chromosome 11. Am J Hum Genet 1989;44:751–755.
66. Chetty R, Weinreb I. Gastric neuroendocrine carcinoma arising fron heterotopic pancreatic tissue. J Clin Pathol 2004;57:314–317.

67. Pareja-Megia MJ, Rios-Martin JJ, Garcia-Escudero A, Gonzalez-Campora R. Papillary and cystic insulinoma of the pancreas. Histopathology (Oxf) 2002;40:483–494.
68. Perez-Montiel MD, Frankel WL, Suster S. Neuroendocrine carcinomas of the pancreas with "rhabdoid" features. Am J Surg Pathol 2003;27:642–649.
69. Bartsch D, Hahn SA, Danichevski KD, et al. Mutations of the DPC5/Smad4 gene in neuroendocrine pancreatic tumors. Oncogene 1999;18:2367–2371.
70. Chen YJ, Vortmeyer A, Zhuang Z, Gibril F, Jensen RT. X-chromosome loss of heterozygosity frequently occurs in gastrinomas and is correlated with aggressive tumor growth. Cancer (Phila) 2004;100:1379–1387.
71. Arnold C, Sosnowski A, Blum HE. Analysis of molecular pathways in neuroendocrine cancers of the gastroenteropancreatic system. Ann NY Acad Sci 2004;1014:218–219.
72. Sippel RS, Carpenter JE, Kunnimalaiyaan M, Lagerholm S, Chen H. Raf-1 activation suppresses neuroendocrine masker and hormone levels in human gastrointestinal carcinoid cells. Am J Physiol Gastrointestinal 2003;285:G245–G254.
73. Serrano J, Peghini SU, Paolo L, Lubensky IA, Gibril F, Jensen RT. Alterations in the $p16^{INK4a}$ tumor suppressor gene in gastrinomas. J Clin Endocrinol Metab 2000;85:4146–4156.
74. Kisler O, Bastian D, Bartsch D, Nies C, Rothmund M. Localization, malignant potential, and surgical management of gastrinomas. World J Surg 1998;22:651–659.
75. Service FJ, McMahon MM, O'Brien PC, Ballard DJ. Functioning insulinoma: incidence, recurrence, and long-term survival of patients: a 60-year study. Mayo Clin Proc 1991;66:711–719.
76. Norton JA, Doppman JL, Jensen RT. Curative resection in Zollinger-Ellison syndrome: results of a 10 year prospective study. Ann Surg 1992;215:8–18.
77. Pape U, Bohmig M, Berndt U, Tiling N, Wiedenmann B, Plockinger U. Survival and clinical outcome of patients with neuroendocrine tumors of the gastroenteropancreatic tract in a German referral center. Ann NY Acad Sci 2004;1014:222–233.
78. Chu QD, Hill HC, Douglass HO, et al. Predictive factors associated with long-term survival in patients with neuroendocrine tumors of the pancreas. Ann Surg Oncol 2002;9:855–862.
79. Matthews BD, Smith TI, Kercher KW, Holder W Jr, Heniford BT. Surgical experience with functioning pancreatic neuroendocrine tumors. Am Surg 2002;68:660–666.
80. Matthews BD, Heniford BT, Reardon PR, Brunicardi FC, Greene FL. Surgical experience with nonfunctional neuroendocrine tumors of the pancreas. Am Surg 2000;66:1116–1123.
81. Ramsay D, Gibson P, Edmunds S, Mendelson R. Pancreatic islet cell tumours presenting as recurrent acute pancreatitis: imaging features in three cases. Australas Radiol 2001;45:520–523.
82. Grino P, Martinez J, Grino E, et al. Acute pancreatitis secondary to pancreatic neuroendocrine tumors. J Pancreas 2003;4:104–110.
83. Tran TH, Pathak RD, Basa ALP. Metastatic insulinoma: case report and review of the literature. South Med J 2004;97:199–201.
84. Lamberts SW, Bakker WH, Reubi JC, Krenning EP. Somatostatin receptor imaging in the localization of endocrine tumors. N Engl J Med 1990;323:1246–1249.
85. Fraker DL, Norton JA, Alexander HR, Venzon DJ, Jensen RT. Surgery in Zollinger-Ellison syndrome alters the natural history of gastrinoma. Ann Surg 1994;220:320–330.
86. Fidler JL, Fletcher JG, Reading CC, et al. Preoperative detection of pancreatic insulinomas on multiphasic helical CT. AJR 2003;181:775–780.
87. Pereira PL, Wiskirchen J. Morphological and functional investigations of neuroendocrine tumors of the pancreas. Eur Radiol 2003;13:2133–2136.
88. Van Nieuwenhove Y, Vandaele S, Op de Beeck B, Delvaux G. Neuroendocrine tumors of the pancreas. Surg Endosc 2003;17:1658–1662.
89. Sundin A, Eriksson B, Bergstrom M, et al. PET in the diagnosis of neuroendocrine tumors. Ann NY Acad Sci 2004;1014:246–257.
90. Mirallie E, Maunoury V, Huglo D, Proye C. Non-invasive imaging of insulinomas and gastrinomas with endoscopic ultrasonography and somatostatin receptor scintigraphy. Br J Surg 2001;88:1272–1278.
91. Kann PH, Wirkus B, Keth A, Golton K. Pitfalls in endosonographic imaging of suspected insulinomas: pancreatic nodules of unknown dignity. Eur J Endosc 2003;148:531–534.
92. Rathod VD, Binmoeller KF, Thul R, et al. The role of EUS-guided fine needle aspiration-biopsy (FNAB) in the diagnosis of neuroendocrine tumors P280. Gut 1997;25E–26E.
93. Gouya H, Vignaux O, Augui J, et al. CT, endoscopic sonography and a combined protocol for preoperative evaluation of pancreatic insulinomas. AJR 2003;181:987–992.
94. Hiramoto JS, Feldstein VA, LaBerge JM, Norton JA. Intraoperative ultrasound and preoperative localization detects all occult insulinomas. Arch Surg 2001;136:1020–1026.
95. Turner JJO, Wren AM, Jackson JE, Thakker RV, Meeran K. Localization of gastrinomas by selective intra-arterial calcium injection. Clin Endosc 2002;57:821–825.
96. Jaroszewski DE, Schlinkert RT, Thompson GB, Schlinkert DK. Laparoscopic localization and resection of insulinomas. Arch Surg 2004;139:270–274.
97. Fernandez-Cruz L, Saenz A, Astudillo E, et al. Outcome of laparoscopic pancreatic surgery: endocrine and nonendocrine tumors. World J Surg 2002;26:1057–1065.
98. Tagaya N, Kasama K, Suzuki N, et al. Laparoscopic resection of the pancreas and review of the literature. Surg Endosc 2003;17:201–206.
99. Chastain MA. The glucagoma syndrome: a review of its features and discussion of new perspectives. Am J Med Sci 2001;321:306–320.
100. Chang-Chretien K, Chew JT, Judge DP. Reversible dilated cardiomyopathy associated with glucagonoma. Heart 2004;90:1–3.
101. Alexander EK, Robinson M, Staniec M, Dluhy RG. Peripheral amino acid and fatty acid infusion for the treatment of necrolytic migratory erythema in the glucagonoma syndrome. Clin Endocrinol 2002;57:827–831.
102. Fernandez-Represa JA, Rodriguez DF, Contin MJP, et al. Pancreatic glucagonoma: detection by positron emission tomography. Eur J Surg 2000;166:175–176.
103. Johnson DS, Coel MN, Bornemann M. Current imaging and possible therapeutic management of glucagonoma tumors. Clin Nucl Med 2000;25:120–124.
104. Wermers RA, Fatourechi V, Wynne AG, Kvols LK, Lloyd RV. The glucagonoma syndrome: clinical and pathological features in 21 patients. Medicine (Baltimore) 1996;75:53–63.
105. Peng SY, Li JT, Liu YB, et al. Diagnosis and treatment of VIPoma in China. Pancreas 2004;28:93–97.
106. Sofka CM, Semelka RC, Marcos HB, Woosley JT. MR imaging of metastatic pancreatic VIPoma. Magn Reson Imaging 1997;15:1205–1208.
107. Mortele KJ, Oei A, Bauters W, et al. Dynamic gadolinium-enhanced MR imaging of pancreatic VIPoma in a patient with Vermer-Morrison syndrome. Eur Radiol 2001;11:1952–1955.
108. Schoevaerdts D, Favet L, Zekry D, Sieber CC, Michel JP. Vipoma: effective treatment with octreotide in the oldest old. J Am Geriatr Soc 2001;49:496–497.
109. Cellier C, Yaghi C, Cuillerier E, et al. Metastatic jejunal VIPoma: beneficial effect of combination therapy with interferon-alpha and 5-fluorouracil. Am J Gastroenterol 2000;95:289–293.
110. Corbetta S, Peracchi M, Cappiello V, et al. Circulating ghrelin levels in patients with pancreatic and gastrointestinal neuroen-

docrine tumors: identification of one pancreatic ghrelinoma. J Clin Endocrinol Metab 2003;88:3117–3120.

111. Nguyen BD. Scintigraphic and computed tomographic imaging of isolated peripancreatic nodal gastinomas. Clin Nucl Med 2003;28:47–48.
112. Owen NJ, Sohaib SAA, Peppercorn PD, et al. MRI of pancreatic neuroendocrine tumours. Br J Radiol 2001;74:968–973.
113. deHerder WW, Hofland LJ, van der Lely AJ, Lamberts SWJ. Somatostatin receptors in gastroenteropancreatic neuroendocrine tumours. Endocr Relat Cancer 2003;10:451–458.
114. Rickes S, Unkrodt K, Ocran K, Neye H, Wermke W. Differentiation of neuroendocrine tumors from other pancreatic lesions by echo-enhanced power Doppler sonography and somatostatin receptor scintigraphy. Pancreas 2003;1:76–81.
115. McIntyre TP, Stahfels KR, Sell HW Jr. Gastrinoma. Am J Surg 2002;183:666–667.
116. Norton JA, Alexander HR, Fraker D, Venzon D, Gibril F, Jensen RT. Does the use of routine duodenotomy (DUODX) affect rate of cure, development of liver metastases or survival in patients with Zollinger-Ellison Syndrome (ZES)? Ann Surg 2004;239(5):617–625; discussion 626.
117. Zogakis TG, Gibril F, Libutti SK, et al. Management and outcome of patients with sporadic gastrinoma arising in the duodenum. Ann Surg 2003;238:42–48.
118. Norton JA, Sugarbaker PH, Doppman JL, et al. Aggressive resection of metastatic disease in selected patients with malignant gastrinoma. Ann Surg 1986;203:352–359.
119. Abou-Saif A, Gibril F, Ojeaburu JV, et al. Prospective study of the ability of serial measurements of serum chromogranin A and gastrin to detect changes in tumor burden in patients with gastrinomas. Cancer (Phila) 2003;98:249–261.
120. Sarmiento JM, Farnell MB, Que FG, Nagorney DM. Pancreaticoduodenectomy for islet cell tumors of the head of the pancreas: long-term survival analysis. World J Surg 2002;26: 1267–1271.
121. Fjallskog ML, Granberg DPK, Welin SLV, et al. Treatment with cisplatin and etoposide in patients with neuroendocrine tumors. Cancer (Phila) 2001;92:1101–1107.
122. Pathak RD, Tran TH, Burshell AL. A case of dopamine agonists inhibiting pancreatic polypeptide secretion from an islet cell tumor. J Clin Endocrinol Metab 2004;89:581–584.
123. Modlin IM, Lewis JJ, Ahlman H, Bilchik AJ, Kumar RR. Management of unresectable malignant endocrine tumors of the pancreas. Surg Gynecol Obstet 1993;176:507–518.
124. Saito F, Naito H, Funayama Y, et al. Octreotide in control of multiple liver metastases from gastrinoma. J Gastroenterol 2003;38:905–908.
125. Norton JA, Kivlen M, Li M, Schneider D, Chuter T, Jensen R. Morbidity and mortality of aggressive resection in patients with advanced neuroendocrine tumors. Arch Surg 2003;138: 859–866.
126. Ringe B, Lorf T, Dopkens K, Canelo R. Treatment of hepatic metastases from gastroenteropancreatic neuroendocrine tumors: role of liver trasplantation. World J Surg 2001;25:697–699.
127. Ahlman H, Friman S, Cahlin C, et al. Liver transplantation for treatment of metastatic neuroendocrine tumors. Ann NY Acad Sci 2004;1014:265–269.
128. Olausson M, Friman S, Cahlin C, et al. Indication and results of liver transplantation in patients with neuroendocrine tumors. World J Surg 2002;26:998–1004.
129. van der Hiel B, Stokkel MPM, Chiti A, et al. Effective treatment of bone metastases from a tumour of the pancreas with high activities of indium-111-pentetreotide. Eur J Endosc 2003;149: 479–483.
130. Kaltsas G, Korbonits M, Heintz E, et al. Comparison of somatostain analog and metaiodobenzylguanidine radionuclides in the diagnosis and localization of advanced neuroendocrine tumors. J Clin Endocrinol Metab 2001;86:895–902.
131. Norton JA, Warren RS, Kelly MG, Zuraek MB, Jensen RT. Aggressive surgery for metastatic liver neuroendocrine tumors. Surgery (St. Louis) 2003;134:1057–1065.
132. Pelley RJ, Bukowski RM. Recent advances in systemic therapy for gastrointestinal neuroendocrine tumors. Curr Opinion Oncol 1999;11:32–38.
133. Faiss S, Pape UL, Bohmig M, et al. Prospective randomized multicenter trial on the antiproliferative effect of lantreotide, interferon-alpha, and their combination for therapy of metastatic neuroendocrine gastroenteropancreatic tumors: the international lanreotide and interferon alfa study group. J Clin Oncol 2003;21:2689–2696.
134. Volter V, Peschel C. Is lantreotide and/or interferon alfa an adequate therapy for neuroendocrine tumors? J Clin Oncol 2004;22:573–574.
135. Hopfner M, Sutter AP, Gerst B, Zeitz M, Scherubi H. A novel approach in the treatment of neuroendocrine gastrointestinal tumours. Targeting the epidermal growth factor receptor by gefitinib (ZD 1839). Br J Cancer 2003;89:1766–1775.
136. Chandrasekharappa SC, Guru SC, Manickam P, et al. Positional cloning of the gene for multiple endocrine neoplasia type 1. Science 1997;276:404–407.
137. Friedman E, Larsson C, Amorosi A, et al. Multiple endocrine neoplasia type 1 pathology, pathophysiology, molecular genetics and differential diagnosis. In: Bilezikian JP, Levine MA, Marcus R (eds). The Parathyroids. New York: Raven Press, 1994: 647–680.
138. Metz DC, Jensen RT, Bale AE, et al. Multiple endocrine neoplasia type 1 clinical features and management. In: Bilezikian JP, Levine MA, Marcus R (eds). The Parathyroids. New York: Raven Press, 1994:591–646.
139. Marx SJ, Menczel J, Campbell G, Aurbach GD, Spiegel AM, Norton JA. Heterogeneous size of the parathyroid glands in familial multiple endocrine neoplasia type 1. Clin Endocrinol 1991;35:521–526.
140. Vortmeyer AO, Huang S, Lubensky I, Zhuang Z. Non-islet origin of pancreatic islet cell tumors. J Clin Endocrinol Metab 2004;89: 1934–1938.
141. Gauger PG, Scheiman JM, Wamsteker EJ, et al. Role of endoscopic ultrasonography in screening and treatment of pancreatic endocrine tumours in asymptomatic patients with multiple endocrine neoplasia type 1. Br J Surg 2003;90:748–754.
142. Weber HC, Venzon DJ, Jaw-Town L, et al. Determinant of metastatic rate and survival in patients with Zollinger-Ellison syndrome: a prospective long-term study. Gastroenterology 1995;108:1637–1649.
143. Veldhuid JD, Norton JA, Wells SA Jr, Vinik AI, Perry RR. Surgical vs. medical management of multiple endocrine neoplasia type 1. J Clin Endocrinol Metab 1997;82: 357–364.
144. Pipeleers-Marichal M, Somers G, Willems G, et al. Gastrinomas in the duodenums of patients with multiple endocrine neoplasia type 1 and the Zollinger-Ellison syndrome. N Engl J Med 1990;322:723–727.
145. MacFarland MP, Fraker DL, Alexander HR, Norton JA, Lubensky I, Jensen RT. Prospective study of surgical resection of duodenal and pancreatic gastrinomas in multiple endocrine neoplasia type 1. Surgery (St. Louis) 1995;118:973–980.
146. Norton JA, Alexander HR, Fraker DL, et al. Comparison of surgical results in patients with advanced and limited disease with multiple endocrine neoplasia type 1 and Zollinger-Ellison syndrome. Ann Surg 2001;234:495–506.
147. Norton JA, Fromme LC, Farrell RE, Wells SA Jr. Multiple endocrine neoplasia type 2B: the most aggressive form of medullary thyroid carcinoma. Surg Clin N Am 1979;59: 109–119.
148. Farndon JR, Leight GS, Dilley WG, et al. Familial medullary thyroid carcinoma without associated endocrinopathies: a distinct clinical entity. Br J Surg 1986;73:278–282.

149. Mulligan LM, Eng C, Healey CS, et al. Specific mutations of the RET proto-oncogene are related to the disease phenotype in MEN2A and FMTC. Nat Genet 1994;6:70–74.
150. Santoro M, Carlomagno F, Romano A, et al. Activation of RET as a dominant transforming gene by germline mutations of MEN2A and MEN2B. Science 1995;267: 381–383.
151. Lips CJM, Landsvater RM, Hoppener JWM, et al. Clinical screening as compared with DNA analysis in families with multiple endocrine neoplasia type 2A. N Engl J Med 1994;331:828–835.
152. Howe JR, Norton JA, Wells SA Jr. Prevalence of pheochromocytoma and hyperparathyroidism in multiple endocrine neoplasia type 2A: results of long-term follow-up. Surgery (St. Louis) 1993;114:1070–1077.

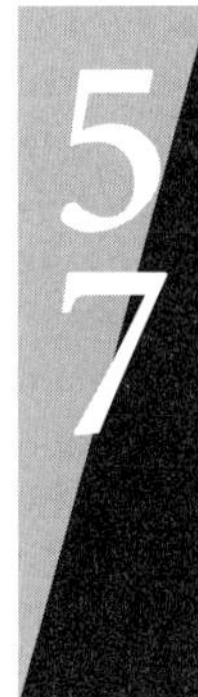

Sarcomas of Bone

Randy N. Rosier and Susan V. Bukata

Sarcomas of bone have a number of distinguishing features that set them apart from primary cancers of many other organ systems. First, they are extremely rare in comparison with other types of cancer, a fact that has impeded the ability of treatment in this field to evolve rapidly in an evidence-based manner because of the small numbers of patients available for studies. Progress in this field has been possible only with multicenter and oncology group trials that can provide sufficient numbers of patients for study. Even so, clinical trials are generally limited to prospective case series at best, and much of the literature is based on retrospective case series. True controlled randomized prospective trials are extremely rare. Nevertheless, a number of clinically useful observations defining the behavior of these tumors and their responses to treatments have derived from the analyses of the numerous case series that have been published, and these results and the associated levels of evidence are reviewed here.

Bone sarcomas are generally characterized by a solitary primary focus with initial local growth being followed by hematogenous patterns of metastasis, with the lungs as the most common initial metastatic site. Metastases to other bones also can occasionally occur, although lymphatic, central nervous system, and other solid organ metastases are distinctly rare. The annual incidence of primary bone malignancies is less than 3,000 cases/year in the United States, excluding marrow cell malignancies such as lymphoma and myeloma.[1] The majority of bone sarcomas fall into three histogenic types: osteosarcoma, Ewing's sarcoma, and chondrosarcoma. Osteosarcoma and Ewing's sarcoma preferentially affect children and young adults, whereas chondrosarcoma is seen more commonly in later adulthood. Far less common sarcomas of bones include fibrosarcoma, malignant fibrous histiocytoma, and extremely rare lesions such as adamantinoma. Because of the extreme rarity and lack of clinical trials with these uncommon lesions, the following material focuses on the three most common tumor types.

Bone sarcomas typically evolve in a single focus, with local centrifugal growth and invasion of the bone and surrounding soft tissues. Although metastases are typically pulmonary in location, metastases within a single bone (so-called skip metastases[2]) or to other bones can occur occasionally.[3] Before the advent of chemotherapy, treatment was generally by surgical amputation proximal to the lesion, and the prognosis for these sarcomas was extremely poor. Use of chemotherapy, in particular for osteosarcoma and Ewing's sarcoma, has markedly improved survival in comparison with historical results. While osteosarcoma and chondrosarcoma are relatively resistant to radiation, Ewing's sarcoma is radiosensitive, and radiation has been used as both a primary or adjuvant treatment for this disease in the past.[4] However, because of late recurrences in bone at the primary site and other complications such as pathologic fracture, the treatment paradigm for this disease has evolved over the past two decades to surgical resection and adjuvant chemotherapy, similar to the approach for osteosarcoma.[5] For chondrosarcoma, because of resistance to both chemotherapy and radiation, surgery remains the only method of treatment.[6]

In addition to the use of adjuvant chemotherapy and radiation, the treatment of bone sarcomas has evolved surgically during the past two to three decades as well. There has been a progressive and well-supported change from amputations to limb-sparing types of surgical procedures for the majority of bone sarcomas.[5,7] A number of factors have contributed to this change, many related to technologic advances. Examples include accurate imaging techniques such as magnetic resonance imaging (MRI), which enable far better assessment of the anatomic location of the tumor than was available previously; free tissue microvascular transfers, enabling coverage of problematic soft tissue defects; and availability of osteochondral allografts and complex prosthetic bone and joint replacement devices for limb reconstruction. These advances have dramatically enhanced the ability to perform limb salvage procedures with preservation of limb function while not compromising treatment of the malignancy. Instruments for limb functional outcomes assessment have been developed[8] and are widely used to evaluate local treatment outcomes, in addition to the traditional measures of disease presence or absence, quantification of disease extent, and performance status.

There are currently two slightly different staging systems used by orthopedic oncologists for bone sarcomas.[9] The surgical staging system of Enneking[10,11] is based on the grade, anatomic extent, and presence of metastases, and has been widely used by musculoskeletal oncologists for many years. It has been adopted by the Musculoskeletal Tumor Society and is also known as the MSTS staging system.[9] The staging correlates well with survival and facilitates surgical planning for the primary lesion. Tumors are graded as either low or high grade (stage I or II, respectively), and as either confined to a single anatomic compartment (A) or involving more than one anatomic compartment (B). Stage III refers to any tumor with metastases. More recently, the American Joint Committee on Cancer has developed a bone tumor staging system

TABLE 57.1. Musculoskeletal Tumor Society staging system.

Stage	*Grade*	*Local extent*	*Metastases*
I-A	Low	Intracompartmental	None
I-B	Low	Extracompartmental	None
II-A	High	Intracompartmental	None
II-B	High	Extracompartmental	None
III	Any	Any	Present, any site

Data from Enneking et al.[10]

that is also in use, the major differences being that tumor size is considered as well as location of metastases.[9] Tables 57.1 and 57.2 outline the bone sarcoma staging systems. Several considerations borne out by both staging systems are that higher-grade tumors, tumors with metastases, and large or anatomically more extensive tumors have worse prognoses. In a recent comparison of the two staging systems, no significant difference in prognosis prediction was found, indicating that at present either system remains acceptable.[9]

Clinical presentation of bone sarcomas usually involves pain, often at rest or at night, and presence of swelling or a mass at the primary site. Systemic symptoms are rare. Occasionally pathologic fracture can occur, although this is fortunately relatively uncommon, presumably because bone sarcomas are generally quite painful and may cause the patient to seek medical attention before bone destruction is sufficient to cause fracture. The most useful study in developing differential diagnosis of the lesion remains the radiograph of the primary site. Osteosarcomas usually exhibit destructive patterns with disorganized bone formation, periosteal reaction, and often extension into the adjacent soft tissues. Ewing's sarcomas tend to have a permeative lytic pattern on radiographs, with periosteal reaction and also with soft tissue extension. Chondrosarcomas may be identified or suspected because of the combination of a destructive radiographic appearance with presence of calcifications. Three-dimensional imaging, generally with MRI, enables evaluation of the anatomic extent, the soft tissue involvement, and proximity to critical neurovascular structures, and helps to determine feasibility of limb-sparing surgical treatment of the tumor. Diagnosis is most commonly achieved by needle biopsy, although occasionally an open biopsy may be necessary to obtain adequate tissue for definitive diagnosis. Biopsy is best performed by an experienced orthopedic oncologist who will ultimately provide the surgical treatment of the primary tumor, because placement of the biopsy site has important anatomic considerations relevant to the definitive resection, and outcomes have been shown to be better in

TABLE 57.2. The American Joint Committee on Cancer (AJCC) staging system for bone tumors.

Stage	*Grade*	*Local extent*	*Metastases*
IA	Low	≤8 cm	None
IB	Low	≥8 cm	None
IIA	High	≤8 cm	None
IIB	High	≥8 cm	None
III	Any	Any	Skip metastases
IVA	Any	Any	Pulmonary metastasis
IVB	Any	Any	Other metastases

Data from *AJCC Cancer Staging Manual*, sixth edition (2002), published by Springer-Verlag New York, www.springer-ny.com.

this circumstance.[12] Additional staging studies besides the imaging of the primary lesion should include computed tomographic (CT) scan of the lungs to detect pulmonary metastases and a whole-body bone scan to help identify bony metastases or skip metastases. Following confirmation of diagnosis and staging, either surgical treatment (for chondrosarcoma) or preoperative adjuvant chemotherapy (for osteosarcoma or Ewing's sarcoma) is initiated. For those tumors treated with adjuvant chemotherapy, surgical resection and reconstruction (if feasible) is carried out after several cycles of preoperative "neoadjuvant" treatment. Following surgical treatment, chemotherapy is resumed for a predetermined number of cycles, depending on the protocol in use. Metastatic pulmonary lesions persisting after chemotherapy or appearing later during posttreatment follow-up may be resected by thoracotomy with salvage of some patients.[13]

After successful completion of therapy, patients are monitored periodically with radiographs and other local imaging modalities at the primary site, as well as with chest CT scans and bone scans. The role of positron emission tomography (PET) scans in evaluation and follow-up of bone sarcomas is still in evolution, and this modality is not yet a component of most standardized protocols. PET scan activity has been shown in chondrosarcoma to correlate with grade and outcome,[14] although CT scans have been shown to be superior to PET scans in detection of pulmonary metastasis of osteosarcoma.[15] PET scan activity has also been shown to correlate with response to chemotherapy for bone sarcomas.[16] However, the role of PET scans in diagnosis and follow-up of bone sarcomas remains to be determined.

Osteosarcoma

Osteosarcoma is by definition a sarcoma composed of bone-forming cells and is the most common of the primary bone sarcomas. Osteosarcoma is characterized by the production by the tumor cells of the matrix of bone, osteoid, which may mineralize to a variable extent. Osteosarcomas may also contain other tissues of mesenchymal origin, such as cartilage and fibrous tissue. Osteosarcoma most commonly affects individuals in the second and third decades and preferentially involves the major long bones, that is, the femur, tibia, and humerus, although essentially any bone can be involved. There are a number of histologic variants of osteosarcoma, including typical central high-grade osteosarcoma, telangiectatic osteosarcoma, parosteal osteosarcoma, periosteal or juxtacortical osteosarcoma, fibroblastic osteosarcoma, chondroblastic osteosarcoma, intramedullary low-grade osteosarcoma, and secondary osteosarcoma (most commonly arising in irradiated bone or in Paget's disease).[17] Parosteal osteosarcomas are low-grade lesions with low metastatic potential arising adjacent to the periosteum, usually of the posterior distal femur, proximal tibia, or of the proximal humerus. These tumors differ from most other osteosarcoma subtypes in that the treatment is generally surgical resection alone.[18] Studies of prognosis versus histogenic subtypes of osteosarcomas have shown that telangiectatic and fibroblastic osteosarcomas have a relatively better prognosis and chondroblastic variants a worse prognosis.[19–22]

The approach to treatment of osteosarcoma for the past two decades has consisted of induction multiagent chemotherapy, surgical resection (whether amputation or limb salvage surgery with reconstruction), and then postoperative chemotherapy. The approach arose from the Rosen T10 protocol, which produced markedly enhanced survival compared with the prior dismal historical results of amputation alone.[23] Although a number of different protocols have been used, the most commonly included drugs in the multiagent regimens have been doxorubicin, methotrexate, cisplatin, cyclophosphamide, and ifosfamide (Table 57.3.[13,24–38] Although other agents have been employed, there has not been a dramatic difference among protocols in outcomes. The recent evidence in the literature is summarized in Table 57.3. Many series consist of small numbers of patients, and most are retrospective or prospective case series, with true randomized clinical trials being extremely rare except for a few Phase III comparative studies. Overall, however, the survival rates with this tumor have not changed dramatically beyond original chemotherapeutic protocols. Comparative studies have determined that local recurrence and survival rates do not differ whether the patient has had limb salvage or amputation.[5] Some of the major advances in the past decade relate to improved ability to salvage functional extremities, with custom and modular prosthetics, enhanced soft tissue reconstructions, and allografting technologies. Recent developments in lengthening prosthetics have enabled salvage of extremities in younger children, despite a relatively high complication rate.[39,40] However, prevention and treatment of metastatic disease remain the major challenges.

Evidence from the literature summarized in Table 57.3 and site-specific evidence presented in Table 57.4[41–45] lead to consensus on a number of issues, which are summarized by the following:

1. Prognosis is worse with metastasis or with local recurrence.
2. Good response to neoadjuvant chemotherapy (greater than 90% necrosis) is associated with a better prognosis.
3. Pelvic and spinal primary sites are associated with a worse prognosis.
4. Older patients have a worse prognosis with osteosarcoma.
5. Pathologic fracture is not associated with a worse prognosis and is no longer believed to be an absolute indication for amputation.
6. Outcome varies among osteosarcoma subtypes.
7. Aggressive treatment with multiagent chemotherapy and surgical resection carries a better prognosis than less-aggressive approaches.

TABLE 57.3. Clinical studies of osteosarcoma.

Study	*Reference*	*Year*	*N*	*Type*	*Study specifics*	*F/U; other*	*EFS*	*OS*	*Conclusions*
Lin	24	2003	50	RCS	Multiagent + surg	47.1 mo	7 years 51%	7 years 68%	
Bacci	25	2003	185	RCS	Cisplatin, dox, ifos, mtx Mets vs. nonmet	w/mets nonmet	2 years 21% 2 years 75%	2 years 55% 2 years 90%	Prog worse w/mets
Wilkins	26	2003	47	PCS	Dox, intraarterial cisplatin preop	92 mo	10 years 84%	10 years 92%	Better prog. w/intraart Rx
Smeland	27	2003	113	PCS	Mtx, cisplatin, dox	83 mo	5 years 63%	5 years 74%	
Kager	28	2003	202	RCS	Multiagent, varied regimens; w/mets	1.9 years	5 years 18% 10 years 16%	5 years 29% 10 years 24%	Supports surg for lung mets
Goorin	29	2003	100	PRCT	Neoadjuvant vs postop chemo	Neoadj Postop	5 years 61% 5 years 65%	5 years 78% (combined)	Neoadj Rx same as postop Rx
Grimer	30	2003	481	RCS	Pt age >40 years; surg + multiagent		NR	5 years 46%	Worse prog. older pts
Tsuchiya	31	2002	280	RCS	Stratified by time of met presentation	Early Late	All metastatic	5 years 18% 5 years 31%	Late mets better prog
Bacci	32	2002	72	PCS	Ifos added to dox, mtx, cisplatin	5 years	5 years 73%	5 years 87%	Increased toxicity; incr. survival
Thompson	13	2002	85	RCS	Multiagent + surg	4 years	4 years 51%	4 years 67%	# mets, early mets worse
Carsi	33	2002	47	RCS	Pt age >40 years		5 years 32%	5 years 42%	Worse prog
Goorin	34	2002	43	phase II/III	Etopo/ifos; pts presenting w/mets	10%CR 49%PR	Lung met Bone met	2 years 39% 2 years 58%	Effective but high toxicity
Berend	35	2001	54	RCS	Neoadj, surg ± postop chemotherapy	Chemo None	NR	5 years 54%	No difference
Bacci	36	2001	162	PCS	Mtx, dox, cisplatin, ifos	6.5 years	5 years 56%	5 years 71%	Ifos no difference
Ferrari	37	2001	300	RCS	Mtx, dox, cisplatin, ifos	9.2 years	8 years 59%	NR	Tumor vol, hi alk phos, poor prognosis
Petrilli	38	1999	33	PCS	Intraarterial carboplatin + multiagent, + mets	No mets + mets	3 years 65% 3 years 14%	3 years 71% 3 years 17%	73%–81% good response to carboplatin

RCS, retrospective case series; PCS, prospective case series; PRCT, prospective randomized clinical trial; EFS, event-free survival; OS, overall survival; NR, not reported; F/U, follow-up; pts, patients; dox, doxorubicin; mtx, methotrexate; etopo, etoposide; ifos, ifosfamide; surg, surgery; mets, metastasis; prog, prognosis; vol, volume; incr, increased; alk phos, alkaline phosphatase.

TABLE 57.4. Site-specific clinical studies of osteosarcoma.

Study	*Reference*	*Year*	*Site*	*N*	*Type*	*Intervention*	*F/U; other*	*EFS*	*OS*	*Conclusions*
Ozaki	41	2003	Pelvis	67	RCS	Multiagent chemo, surg		5 years 19%	5 years 27%	Poor prog; worse w/mets or poor surgical margins
Wittig	42	2002	Humerus	23	RCS	Chemo, surg	Med 10 years	10 years 65%	10 years 65%	Good function w/limb salvage; similar survival to other sites
Ozaki	43	2002	Spine	22	RCS	Chemo, surg, ± XRT	6 years	6 years 14%	6 years 27%	Prog better w/surg or XRT than chemo only
Ham	44	2000	Pelvis	40	RCS	Variable		NR	2 years 35% 5 years 26%	Worse prog. than other sites; best w/chemo + surg
Grimer	45	1999	Pelvis	36	RCS	Variable	Chemo + surg Surgery only	NR	5 years 41% 5 years 18%	Worse prog than other sites; best w/chemo + surg

RCS, retrospective case series; EFS, event-free survival; OS, overall survival; NR, not reported; F/U, follow-up; XRT, radiotherapy; surg, surgery; mets, metastasis; prog, prognosis; alk phos, alkaline phosphatase.

Overall survival with osteosarcoma treated with multiagent chemotherapy and surgery has remained in the 60% to 70% range over the past two decades. Limb salvage has become more prevalent and has not shown an adverse effect on survival, even in the context of pathologic fracture.[5,39,40,46–49] Survival in relapsed or metastatic osteosarcoma is distinctly worse (see Table 57.3) and ranges from 18% to 55%. The prognosis is worse in axial skeletal locations, such as the spine and pelvis (see Table 57.4),[41,43–45] which may relate in part to the technical difficulty of obtaining wide surgical margins in these locations. Prognosis for skip metastases has also been extremely poor.[2]

There has been considerable interest in identifying prognostic markers in osteosarcoma. The RB and p53 genes have long been associated with the pathogenesis and growth dysregulation in osteosarcoma but have not found utility prognostically.[50] Multidrug resistance genes, such as MDR1 (P-glycoprotein), a cellular detoxifying plasma membrane efflux pump that can confer chemotherapeutic resistance on tumor cells, have been fairly widely investigated in osteosarcoma. However, the issue of prognostic relevance remains unresolved, with some studies showing correlation with prognosis[51,52] whereas others have not.[53,54] Bone morphogenetic proteins (BMPs) have been studied, with findings of BMP4 and 7 expression in all osteosarcomas and BMP6 in chondroblastic subtypes.[55,56] Other markers that have been investigated include Her2/neu,[57,58] tenascin,[59] ezrin,[60] LRP5,[61] and telomerase.[62] Although one study suggested overexpression of Her2/neu correlated with poor prognosis,[57] a more-recent study has contradicted that finding.[58] Tenascin, ezrin, LRP5, and telomerase have each been found to correlate with metastasis and worse prognosis in recent single studies.[59–62]

A number of newer agents have been tested for activity against osteosarcoma, including carboplatin, ecteinascidin, liposomal doxorubicin, etoposide, gemcitabine, interleukin 12, topotecan, paclitaxel, and the combination of retinoic acid and interferon alpha, generally in the setting of metastatic and/or recurrent tumor refractory to standard regimens.[38,63–72] Although the studies have been small, ecteinascidin, topotecan, and paclitaxel have exhibited minimum activity.[64,67,71] Ifosfamide, etoposide, and carboplatin have been evaluated in several studies and antitumor efficacy demonstrated, although results are similar to previous multiagent regimens.[34,63,65,69,73] Gemcitabine and interleukin 12 have shown activity against metastatic disease in animal models,[70,74] but interleukin 12 has not been evaluated in clinical trials, and response to gemcitabine in one Phase II trial with refractory disease was modest.[66] Preoperative intraarterial cisplatin has demonstrated improved survival of 92% in a single clinical study,[26] whereas in another study with intraarterial carboplatin the 3-year survival was similar to other multidrug protocols at 71%.[38] Unfortunately, overall the results with newer agents have not shown promise of significantly altering the treatment outcomes with this disease, and further studies are needed.

Ewing's Sarcoma

Ewing's sarcoma is an aggressive, non-matrix-producing primary bone sarcoma that affects individuals mainly in the second and third decades. Many of these tumors are characterized by presence of a specific chromosomal translocation (11:22), resulting in an abnormal transcription factor, EWS-FLI-1, which may contribute to their pathogenesis. Ewing's sarcoma can occur in the soft tissues as well, and both bone and soft tissue lesions often exhibit features of neuroectodermal differentiation, previously termed peripheral neuroectodermal tumors (PNET).[4] The presence of neural differentiation features has not been shown to affect outcome.[75,76] Currently, the term Ewing's sarcoma family of tumors (ESFT, or EFT) is used to encompass the variations of this sarcoma. Ewing's sarcoma is characterized by a permeative pattern of bone destruction, often associated with a periosteal reaction and soft tissue mass. As with other bone sarcomas, the presenting complaint is usually pain at the site of the primary lesion. Involvement of the major long bones is most common, although pelvic, spinal, and rib primary sites also occur.[77] Metastases are hematogenous and usually pulmonary, with bone as a much less common metastatic site. Diagnosis is generally accomplished by needle biopsy, although occasionally an open surgical biopsy may be necessary. The use of immunohistochemistry to identify markers of neural differentiation, cell-surface markers such as CD99, and the specific fusion protein, EWS-FLI-1, which results from the characteristic chromosomal translocation found in most cases of the disease, has made diagnosis more accurate with small tissue specimens.[78–81] The staging studies are similar to those of other bone sarcomas, with magnetic resonance imaging (MRI) of the primary site for surgical planning, CT scan of the chest to assess pulmonary metastasis, and whole-body bone scanning to rule out bone metastases.[77]

Treatment consists of multiagent chemotherapy regimens similar to those used for osteosarcoma, followed by surgical resection and reconstruction if feasible, with or without local radiotherapy, depending on the response of the tumor to neoadjuvant therapy and achievement of wide surgical margins. This regimen represents a shift in approach over the past two decades as previously chemotherapy with local radiation was the most common treatment paradigm. However, late recurrences in irradiated bone in the past led to increasing use of surgical treatment of primary lesions, with improved results.[82–85] In unresectable lesions in difficult locations, such as the spine, chemotherapy with adjuvant radiation treatment remains an acceptable alternative to surgical treatment. Postoperative chemotherapy is then utilized, as for osteosarcoma, with subsequent follow-up using MRI, CT, and bone scan assessments periodically to monitor for recurrent disease.

The published clinical studies of Ewing's family tumors are summarized in Table 57.5[75,82–84,86–101] and Table 57.6,[102–107] and the issues of consensus based on evidence presented in these studies are as follows:

1. Surgical treatment of the primary lesion is associated with a better prognosis than radiotherapy alone.
2. The prognosis of patients presenting with metastatic disease is much worse than those without.
3. Late complications such as relapse and second malignancies occur and must be monitored through long-term follow-up.
4. Addition of etoposide and ifosfamide improves outcome in patients without metastasis but not in those with metastasis at presentation.
5. Pathologic fracture is not associated with worse prognosis and does not necessarily mandate amputation.
6. Chemotherapeutic response of tumor to neoadjuvant chemotherapy is highly correlated with outcome.
7. Prognosis in spinal and pelvic locations is worse than with extremity tumors.
8. Tumor volume is inversely correlated with outcome.
9. Improved survival with stem cell transplantation has not been as yet demonstrated.

The problems associated with interpretation of the data on Ewing's tumors relates in large part to the rarity of the disease. Thus, most of the reported evidence is at the case series level, with few randomized trials. In addition, much of the literature is based on relatively small numbers of cases, with patient and treatment heterogeneity. Furthermore, many reported series have been collected over significant periods of time, introducing the confounding variables of changing treatment paradigms and diagnostic and staging technologies. As can be seen from Table 57.5, reported overall survival rates at 5 years generally are in the range of 50% to 70% for nonmetastatic disease presentation and 20% to 30% for metastatic disease, thus reinforcing the strong prognostic significance of early metastasis. Longer time to relapse has also correlated with improved survival.[92] Surgical treatment of the primary has yielded better outcomes than radiotherapy alone in several studies,[64,83,100,102,108,109] leading to the current shift in paradigm favoring surgical resection whenever possible. Incorporation of surgical treatment for relapsed disease has also been shown to improve survival.[92,110,111] Pathologic fractures occur in Ewing's tumor, particularly in the femur, but have had similar outcomes to disease without fracture whether or not amputation was undertaken.[112,113]

Additional factors that have been found in some studies to correlate with a worse prognosis include tumor volume greater than 100 mL,[94,113,114] nonextremity sites such as the spine and pelvis,[102,103,106,115] elevated serum lactase dehydrogenase (LDH) levels,[76,82,116] and systemic symptoms such as fever and anemia.[116] Apart from the presence of metastatic disease, however, the strongest predictor of prognosis is response to neoadjuvant chemotherapy.[85,94,97,107,113,116,117]

A number of issues remain controversial, such as the prognostic significance of age at diagnosis, concerning which conflicting data have been reported.[97,118] The treatment of metastatic disease does not appear to have improved much over time despite numerous changes in chemotherapeutic protocols, although the value of surgical treatment of the primary lesion has been well supported.[64,83,100,119] Several studies have reported on improved outcomes in nonmetastatic patients with more-recent protocols incorporating ifosfamide and etoposide over previous protocols that did not incorporate these agents.[87,101,120] Some experimental drug regimens evaluated in recent small Phase II studies for relapsed disease include cyclophosphamide + topotecan and irinotecan.[64,121] Although the cyclophosphamide/topotecan study yielded a 35% response rate, further study of larger numbers of patients will likely be needed to determine the possible role of this regimen. Responses in the irinotecan study were minimal,[121] and a Phase II study of pyrazoloacridine yielded no responses.[122]

Although allogeneic and autologous stem cell transplantation for relapsed or advanced disease have not shown improved outcomes over chemotherapy alone,[93,95] a high rate of tumor cell contaminants in autologous stem cells has been reported[93,123] and may be a contributing factor to failures.

One of the serious late complications of Ewing's sarcoma is the occurrence of second malignancies, which ranges from 1 to 6.5% in several series.[82,124–126] The outcomes of secondary osteosarcomas have been reported, with overall survival of the secondary sarcoma 41% at 8 years follow-up.[127] The late surgical complication rates for pelvic Ewing's and limb reconstruction with expanding prostheses in young children have also been high and constitute a longer-term problem requiring ongoing follow-up.[39,104,128,129] Functional studies have supported rotation plasty lower extremity procedures for younger children over prosthetic reconstructions,[130] although multiple reconstructive options have decreased indications for amputation even in younger children.[129,131] One additional

TABLE 57.5. Clinical studies of Ewing's sarcoma family tumors.

Study	*Reference*	*Year*	*N*	*Type*	*Study specifics*	*F/U; other*	*EFS*	*OS*	*Conclusions*
Zogopoulos	86	2004	72	RCS	Multiagent chemo + surg or XRT		7 years 66%	7 years 72%	Nonmetastatic, extremity best outcomes
Bacci	82	2004	402	RCS	Multiagent chemo	18 years	18 years 44%	5 years 57% 10 years 49% 15 years 45% 20 years 38%	Late relapses and 2° malignancies; long-term F/U needed
Miser	87	2004	120	PRCT	Dox, vincr, cyclo, dactin vs. etopo, ifos in pts w/mets	STD Etopo/ifos	8 years 20% 8 years 20%	8 years 32% 8 years 29%	No difference
Bacci	83	2004	268	RCS	XRT vs. surgery	All pts Surgery XRT	5 years 62% 5 years 80% 5 years 48%	5 years 69%	Outcomes better with surgery
Grier	88	2003	518	PRCT	Dox, vincr, cyclo, dactin vs. etopo, ifos; ± met groups	STD Etopo/ifos	5 years 54% 5 years 69%	5 years 61% 5 years 73%	No diff w/mets; etopo/ifos better nonmet
Kolb	89	2003	68	PCS	Dox, cyclo, vincr, etopo, ifos	w/mets no mets	4 years 12% 4 years 82%	4 years 18% 4 years 89%	Metastasis is major prog determinant
Schuck	90	2002	153	RCS	Postop XRT timing	<60 days >60 days	5 years 64% 5 years 64%		LR 2% LR 8%
Marcus	91	2002	144	RCS	Various multidrug regimens	Various Rx groups	NR	5 years 50–63%	No large diff. with regimens; mets poor prog
Rodriguez-Galindo	92	2002	71	RCS	Time to relapse ± surgery for mets	<2 years >2 years Surgery No surg		5 years 18% 5 years 35% 5 years 30% 5 years 9%	Better outcome with late relapse & surgical Rx
Sluga	84	2001	86	RCS	Surgical margins	Wide Nonwide		5 years 60% 5 years 40%	Wider margin better
Meyers	93	2001	32	PCS	TBI, autol. Stem cells in metastatic Ewings		2 years 24%	2 years 0%	No benefit over chemo
Paulussen	94	2001	301	RCS	Ifos vs. cyclo in high- vs. low-risk pts (by tumor volume)		5 years 52%	5 years 57%	No difference; vol >200 mL, poor response worse prognosis
Burdach	95	2000	36	RCS	Stem cell transplant for advanced disease		5 years 24%	5 years 24%	Survival not improved
Cotterill	75	2000	975	RCS	Standard multiagent; ± mets	No mets + mets	5 years 55% 5 years 22%	NR	+mets, earlier relapse worse
Elomaa	96	2000	88	RCS	Vincr/dox/ifos + cisplatin/dox/ifos	Nonmet Met	5 years 58% 5 years 27%	5 years 70% 5 years 28%	Best prog with nonmetastatic, extremity sites
Bacci	97	2000	23	RCS	Age >39 years	8.8 years	5 years 53%	5 years 59%	No difference from age <40
Frolich	98	1999	131	RCS	High-dose melphalan, etopo in relapsed pts	3.7 years	5 years 19%	5 years 27%	No benefit of HDT
Rosito	99	1999	160	RCS	Vincr, dact, dox, cyclo + etopo, ifos	37 months	3 years 78%	3 years 84%	
Givens	100	1999	85	RCS	Multiagent chemo, XRT, ± surgery	10–20 years	NR	5 years 46% 10 years 37%	Results better with surgery
Craft	101	1998	243	RCS	Dox, vincr, dact, ifos	58 months	5 years 56%	5 years 62%	Ifos better compared with historical protocol

RCS, retrospective case series; PCS, prospective case series; PRCT, prospective randomized clinical trial; EFS, event-free survival; LR, local recurrence; OS, overall survival; NR, not reported; F/U, follow-up; dox, doxorubicin; cyclo, cyclophosphamide; vincr, vincristine; dactin, dactinomycin; etopo, etoposide; ifos, ifosfamide; XRT, radiotherapy; surg, surgery; STD, standard multiagent protocol; mets, metastasis; prog, prognosis; vol, volume; incr, increased.

TABLE 57.6. Site-specific clinical studies of Ewing's sarcoma family tumors.

Study	*Reference*	*Year*	*N*	*Site*	*Type*	*Study specifics*	*F/U; other*	*EFS*	*OS*	*Conclusions*
Bacci	102	2003	91	Pelvis	RCS	Multiagent chemo + surgery vs. XRT	XRT Surgery	NR NR	10 years 44% 10 years 64%	Better results w/surgery
Talac	103	2002	7	Spine	RCS	5/7 with positive margins	1/7 recurrence	NR	NR	Poor results with recurrence
Ozaki	104	2002	12	Pelvis	RCS	Chemo + hemipelvic prosthesis; mixed tumors	*n* = 1 Ewings; DOD	5 years 66%	5 years 70%	Poor function; 42% Prosthetic retention
Shamberger	105	2000	53	rRb	RCS	Chemo + resection		5 years 57%	NR	Comparable to sites extremity
Sucato	106	2000	50	Pelvis	RCS	Chemo + surgery or XRT	All Surgery XRT	NR	5 years 44% 5 years 75% 5 years 40%	Better results with surgery; overall pelvis worse prog
Hoffmann	107	1999	241	Pelvis	RCS	Chemo + surgery	Median F/U 26 months	12 years 32%	NR	mets, response = risk factors

RCS, retrospective case series; EFS, event-free survival; OS, overall survival; NR, not reported; F/U, follow-up; XRT, radiotherapy; surg, surgery; mets, metastasis; prog, prognosis; vol, volume; incr, increased.

late complication of treatment that has been reported is diminished bone mineral density, and this may relate to the reported occurrence of late fractures.[124,132,133]

The abnormal fusion protein transcription factor resulting from the 11:22 chromosomal translocation characteristic of many Ewing's family tumors, EWS-FLI1, has been shown to be capable of transforming neuroblastoma tumor cells to a Ewing's sarcoma phenotype, and also drives telomerase expression and cellular proliferation.[134,135] Conversely, inhibition of this factor using small interfering RNA approaches inhibit proliferation and promotes apoptosis of the tumor cells[136]; this has suggested EWS-FLI1 as a possible specific therapeutic target. Expression of cKIT has also been demonstrated in Ewing's tumors, along with associated sensitivity to tyrosine kinase inhibitors such as imatinib (STI571).[137] This has been proposed as a novel clinical treatment, although no clinical trial results have been reported as yet. FLI1 overexpression can aid in the diagnosis of Ewing's immunohistochemically, although it is not entirely specific for this disease.[138]

Chondrosarcoma

Chondrosarcomas are characterized by secretion of a cartilaginous matrix of proteoglycans and chondrocyte-specific collagens such as type II, type IX, and type XI collagens. Unlike osteosarcoma and Ewing's family tumors, chondrosarcoma affects older individuals, most commonly in the fifth to seventh decades, and it is relatively unresponsive to either chemotherapy or radiotherapy.[6] Chondrosarcoma can arise as a primary malignancy or as a secondary malignancy in a preexisting benign cartilage tumor, such as an osteochondroma or enchondroma. Chondrosarcomas vary in histologic grade and are usually graded I–III.[139,140] Dedifferentiated chondrosarcomas also exist, in which other elements such as fibrosarcomatous or osteosarcomatous components may be present.[141] Several clinical and histological subtypes of chondrosarcoma are recognized, including mesenchymal chondrosarcoma,[142] extraskeletal myxoid chondrosarcoma,[143] and clear cell chondrosarcoma.[144] Low-grade chondrosarcomas are slow-growing lesions that can be histologically indistinguishable from benign lesions. In such cases the clinical presentation (pain, enlarging mass) and radiographic or imaging characteristics (bone destruction, soft tissue invasion) are extremely important in diagnosis.[6,145] Chondrosarcoma can also exhibit variable histologic appearance in different areas of the tumor, causing sampling error to be potentially misleading with small biopsy specimens or needle biopsies.[141,145]

Patients generally present with pain or a mass at the primary site, although occasionally the lesion can be identified as an incidental finding detected radiographically. Systemic systems are usually absent. Metastasis of chondrosarcoma is most commonly to the lungs, as with the other bone sarcomas, and is rare in low-grade tumors, although quite common in grade III and dedifferentiated chondrosarcomas. Treatment is surgical excision of the lesion with wide margins, because traditional oncologic adjuvant treatments are not very effective with this tumor. Local adjuvants such as cryotherapy, phenol, and methylmethacrylate implantation have been used with intralesional or marginal excisions, especially with low-grade or borderline malignant lesions, with excellent success in prevention of local recurrence.[145,146] Higher-grade lesions are not amenable to these approaches and carry a substantial local recurrence risk without wide surgical margins.[147]

Radiographically, chondrosarcomas commonly contain calcifications within the cartilaginous matrix, which aids considerably in the differential diagnosis.[148] Staging of the tumor includes a CT scan, or more commonly an MRI scan, to delineate the local extent, a chest CT scan to evaluate for pulmonary metastasis, and a whole-body bone scan to rule out skip metastases or other bony metastases. Although

TABLE 57.7. Clinical studies of chondrosarcoma.

Study	*Reference*	*Year*	*N*	*Site*	*Type*	*Study specifics*	*Other*	*EFS/LR*	*OS*	*Conclusions*
Schniederbauer	149	2004	47	Scapula	RCS	Surgical Rx		LR 40%	5 years 79% 15 years 53%	Wide margins, low grade better outcomes
Mittermayer	150	2004	13	Hand	RCS	Surgical Rx; all grade I	Mean F/U 8 years	LR 13%	8 years 100%	
Patil	151	2003	23	Hand	RCS	Surgical treatment	F/U 8.5 years	LR 22%	100%	No mets despite most lesions gr II–III
Reith	139	2003	109		RCS	Survival vs. grade: surgical Rx	Grade I Grade II Grade III	NR	10 years 92% 10 years 81% 10 years 25%	Significant correlation grade vs outcome
Soderstrom	152	2003	194		RCS	Surgical Rx	9-year min F/U	LR 25%	5 years 70% 10 years 57%	Predictors: histo grade, age >50 years
Ahmed	153	2003	107		RCS	2° CS in osteochondroma		LR 17%	5 years 98% 10 years 95%	90% grI; 10% grII
Kawaguchi	143	2003	42		RCS	Extraskeletal myxoid CS	Mean F/U 7.4 years	5 years 45% 10 years 36%	5 years 100% 10 years 88%	Indolent course, late mets
Fiorenza	154	2002	153		RCS	Surgical Rx	Min F/U 5 years	LR 26%	10 years 70% 15 years 63%	High grade, LR correlated with worse prog
Pring	155	2001	64	Pelvis	RCS	Surgical Rx	Mean F/U 12 years	LR 19%	12 years 71%	High grade poor prog
Bruns	156	2001	42		RCS	Surgical Rx		18% LR	10 years 64%	Worst results in dediff CS
Mitchell	141	2000	22		RCS	Dediff. CS; surgery + chemotherapy	All Surg (n = 11) Surg + chemo (n = 11)	NR	5 years 18% 5 years 0% 5 years 36%	Poor prognosis, better w/chemo
York	157	1999	21	Spine	RCS	Surgery, XRT in 36%		LR 64%	10 years 40%	XRT no benefit
Lee	158	1999	227		RCS	Surgery; XRT in 25%; chemo in 24%		LR 24%	12 years 87%	High grade poor prog; no benefit chemo, XRT
Bjornsson	159	1998	233		RCS	Surgical Rx	Min F/U 5 years	LR 20%	5 years 77%	LR higher in shoulder, pelvis

RCS, retrospective case series; EFS, event-free survival; LR, local recurrence; OS, overall survival; NR, not reported; F/U, follow-up; XRT, radiotherapy; surg, surgery; mets, metastasis; prog, prognosis; vol, volume; incr, increased.

needle biopsy can be used to confirm the histogenesis of the tumor, the results with a small sample can be misleading in terms of the grade of the tumor. Open biopsy may be more helpful in ascertaining absence of higher-grade areas, which may influence the extent of the surgical procedure.[139,145]

Published clinical studies of chondrosarcoma are unfortunately limited to retrospective case series, many with relatively small numbers of patients. There have been no randomized clinical trials involving radiotherapy or chemotherapy, although limited evidence from the few published case series is not encouraging with regard to use of adjuvant modalities. The issues on which there would appear to be consensus in the literature are summarized as follows (see also Table 57.7)[139,141,143,149–159]:

1. Surgical excision of the primary is the accepted method of treatment.
2. Tumor grade is the most significant prognostic variable.

3. Local recurrence is higher than with other bone sarcomas.
4. Progression of disease is often slow, and long-term follow-up is necessary.
5. Prognosis is excellent for the primary lesions in the hand.
6. Wide surgical margins are associated with lower local recurrence rates.
7. Prognosis in surgically difficult areas, such as the spine, scapula, and pelvis, may be worse.

The most striking findings from the published literature, as demonstrated in Table 57.7, are the high local recurrence rates of chondrosarcoma following surgical treatment and the correlation of higher-grade tumors with worse prognoses. The higher local recurrence rate than with osteosarcoma or Ewing's sarcoma may be related to the lack of effective adjuvant therapies such as radiotherapy or chemotherapy. The MDR1 gene and its product P-glycoprotein have been shown to be constitutively expressed in cartilage neoplasms and may account for the lack of sensitivity to chemotherapeutic agents.[160–162] As with other bone sarcomas, current technologic improvements in prosthetic implants for bone and joint reconstruction, availability of allografts, and microvascular techniques enabling free tissue transfer to handle soft tissue coverage problems have led to a shift over the past two decades from amputations to limb salvage procedures for extremity and pelvic chondrosarcomas. Although some studies have found a worse prognosis with pelvic chondrosarcoma,[158] others have not corroborated this,[154,155] so this issue remains unclear. However, there is consensus in the literature that wider margins are associated with lower local recurrence rates and better prognosis, and therefore the difficulty of achieving wide margins in surgically difficult locations such as the pelvis, scapula, and spine may affect outcomes with primaries at these sites.[159] The published case series examining scapular and spinal primaries specifically would support this conclusion.[149,157] In contrast, two series that studied primary chondrosarcomas of the hand both showed an excellent prognosis in all patients in terms of lack of metastasis and long-term survival, regardless of tumor grade.[150,151]

Secondary chondrosarcomas arising in osteochondromas or hereditary multiple exostoses appear to have overall an excellent prognosis, likely because of the preponderance of low-grade lesions.[153] Specific mutations in the EXT1 and EXT2 genes have been identified in more than 80% of individuals with multiple exostoses and in the chondrosarcomas that arise in this condition[163] and may contribute to the pathogenesis of the neoplasm. It is fairly well accepted that the rate of malignant degeneration is substantially higher in patients with multiple exostoses or multiple enchondromas (enchondromatosis, Ollier's disease) than in patients with solitary intraosseous or surface cartilage lesions, although a recent study of a large number of families failed to find an association with disease severity and development of chondrosarcoma.[163]

Possibly because of the diagnostic difficulty in distinguishing between benign and low-grade malignant tumors, considerable investigation of possible markers of malignancy in chondrosarcoma has been undertaken. A number of markers have been associated with increased grade of malignancy, including urokinase-like plasminogen activator,[164,165] cathepsinB,[165] MMP1,[166,167] PTHrP and its receptor,[168,169] INK4A/p16,[170] tenascin-C splice variants,[171] and telomerase reverse transcriptase.[172] Although all these markers are more highly expressed in higher grades of malignancy, none definitively differentiates between benign and malignant low-grade lesions. Her2/neu has been studied and shown no correlation with chondrosarcoma grade.[173] A recent study has found that cyclooxygenase 2 (COX-2) is expressed in all high- and low-grade malignant cartilage tumors whereas it is absent in benign tumors.[174] Although this study involved a small number of specimens ($n = 29$), the absence of expression in benign lesions is in contrast to the continuum of expression from benign to higher-grade tumors observed in all the other published marker studies. This finding could have potential therapeutic as well as diagnostic significance, because prostaglandins stimulate chondrocyte proliferation and COX-2 inhibitors are widely available, but this area requires further study. Because PTHrP also drives chondrocyte proliferation and has been shown in several studies to be more highly expressed in higher-grade lesions,[168,169] potential therapeutic use of antibodies to PTHrP or its receptor has been proposed, and efficacy of this approach in induction of chondrosarcoma cell apoptosis has been demonstrated in vitro.[175] At present, however, use of diagnostic markers has not assumed a place in clinical practice, and new therapeutic options remain theoretical.

References

1. Jemal A, Tiwari RC, Murray T, et al. Cancer statistics, 2004. CA Cancer J Clin 2004;54:8–29.
2. Sajadi K, Heck R, Neel M, et al. The incidence and prognosis of osteosarcoma skip metastases. Clin Orthop 2004;426:92–96.
3. Bacci G, Ferrari S, Longhi A, et al. Pattern of relapse in patients with osteosarcoma of the extremities treated with neoadjuvant chemotherapy. Eur J Cancer 2001;37:32–38.
4. Dunst J, Schuck A. Role of radiotherapy in Ewing tumors. Pediatr Blood Cancer 2004;42:465–470.
5. Bacci G, Ferrari S, Lari S, et al. Osteosarcoma of the limb. Amputation or limb salvage in patients treated by neoadjuvant chemotherapy. J Bone Joint Surg 2002;84B:88–99.
6. Weiner S. Enchondroma and chondrosarcoma of bone: clinical, radiologic and histologic differentiation. Instruct Course Lectures 2004;53:645–649.
7. Givens S, Woo SY, Huang LY, et al. Non-metastatic Ewing's sarcoma: twenty years of experience suggests that surgery is a prime factor for successful multimodality therapy. Int J Oncol 1999;14:1039–1043.
8. Enneking WF, Dunham W, Gebhardt MC, et al. A system for the functional evaluation of reconstructive procedures after surgical treatment of tumors of the musculoskeletal system. Clin Orthop 1993;286:241–246.
9. Heck R, Stacy GS, Flaherty M, et al. A comparison study of staging systems for bone sarcomas. Clin Orthop 2003;415:64–71.
10. Enneking WF, Spanier SS, Goodman MA. A system for the surgical staging of musculoskeletal sarcoma. Clin Orthop 1980;153:106–120.
11. Enneking WF. A system of staging musculoskeletal neoplasms. Clin Orthop 1986;204:9–24.
12. Mankin HJ, Mankin CJ, Simon MA. The hazards of the biopsy, revisited. Members of the Musculoskeletal Tumor Society. J Bone Joint Surg 1996;78A:656–663.
13. Thompson RC Jr, Chent EY, Clohisy DR, et al. Results of treatment for metastatic osteosarcoma with neoadjuvant chemotherapy and surgery. Clin Orthop 2002;397:240–247.
14. Brenner W, Conrad EU, Eary JF. FDG PET imaging for grading and prediction of outcome in chondrosarcoma patients. Eur J Nuclear Med Mol Imaging 2004;31:189–195.

15. Franzius C, Daldrup-Link HE, Sciuk J, et al. FDG-PET for detection of pulmonary metastases from malignant primary bone tumors: comparison with spiral CT. Ann Oncol 2001;12: 479–486.
16. Hawkins DS, Rajendran JG, Conrad EU, et al. Evaluation of chemotherapy response in pediatric bone sarcomas by [F-18]-fluorodeoxy-D-glucose positron emission tomography. Cancer (Phila) 2003;94:3277–3284.
17. McCarthy E, Frassica F. Primary bone tumors. In: Pathology of Bone and Joint Disorders. Philadelphia: Saunders , 1998:205–220.
18. Enneking WF, Springfield D, Gross M. The surgical treatment of parosteal osteosarcoma in long bones. J Bone Joint Surg 1985;67: 125–135.
19. Bacci G, Bertoni F, Longhi A, et al. Neoadjuvant chemotherapy for high-grade central osteosarcoma of the extremity. Histologic response to preoperative chemotherapy correlates with histologic subtype of the tumor. Cancer (Phila) 2003;97:3068–3075.
20. Hauben EI, Weeden S, Pringle J, et al. Does the histological subtype of high-grade central osteosarcoma influence the response to treatment with chemotherapy and does it affect overall survival? A study on 570 patients of two consecutive trials of the European Osteosarcoma Intergroup. Eur J Cancer 2002;38:1218–1225.
21. Bacci G, Ferrari S, Ruggieri P, et al. Telangiectatic osteosarcoma of the extremity: neoadjuvant chemotherapy in 24 cases. Acta Orthop Scand 2001;72:167–172.
22. Bacci G, Ferrari S, Bertoni F, et al. Histologic response of high-grade nonmetastatic osteosarcoma of the extremity to chemotherapy. Clin Orthop 2001;386:186–196.
23. Rosen G, Nirenberg A. Neoadjuvant chemotherapy for osteogenic sarcoma: a five year follow-up (T-10) and preliminary report of new studies (T-12). Prog Clin Biol Res 1985;201:39–51.
24. Lin MT, Lin KH, Lin DT, et al. Unstratified chemotherapy for non-metastatic osteosarcoma of the extremities in children. J. Formos Med Assoc 2003;102:387–393.
25. Bacci G, Briccoli A, Rocca M, et al. Neoadjuvant chemotherapy for osteosarcoma of the extremities with metastases at presentation: recent experience at the Rizzoli Institute in 57 patients treated with cisplatin, doxorubicin, and a high dose of methotrexate and ifosfamide. Ann Oncol 2003;14:1126–1134.
26. Wilkins RM, Cullen JW, Odom L, et al. Superior survival in treatment of primary nonmetastatic pediatric osteosarcoma of the extremity. Ann Surg Oncol 2003;10:498–507.
27. Smeland S, Muller C, Alvegard TA, et al. Scandanavian Sarcoma Group Osteosarcoma Study SSG VIII: prognostic factors for outcome and the role of replacement salvage chemotherapy for poor histological responders. Eur J Cancer 2003;39:488–494.
28. Kager L, Zoubek A, Potschger U, et al. Primary metastatic osteosarcoma: presentation and outcome of patients treated on neoadjuvant Cooperative Osteosarcoma Study Group protocols. J Clin Oncol 2003;21:2011–2018.
29. Goorin AM, Schwartzentruber DJ, Devidas M, et al. Presurgical chemotherapy compared with immediate surgery and adjuvant chemotherapy for nonmetastatic osteosarcoma: Pediatric Oncology Group Study POG-8651. J Clin Oncol 2003;21: 1574–1580.
30. Grimer RJ, Cannon SR, Taminiau AM, et al. Osteosarcoma over the age of forty. Eur J Cancer 2003;39:157–163.
31. Tsuchiya H, Kanazawa Y, Abdel-Wanis ME, et al. Effect of timing of pulmonary metastases identification on prognosis of patients with osteosarcoma: the Japanese Musculoskeletal Oncology Group study. J Clin Oncol 2002;20:3470–3477.
32. Bacci G, Ferrari S, Longhi A, et al. High dose ifosfamide in combination with high dose methotrexate, adriamycin, and cisplatin in the neoadjuvant treatment of extremity osteosarcoma: preliminary results of an Italian Sarcoma Group/Scandinavian Sarcoma Group pilot study. J Chemotherapy 2002;14:198–206.
33. Carsi B, Rock MG. Primary osteosarcoma in adults older than 40 years. Clin Orthop 2002;397:53–61.
34. Goorin AM, Harris MB, Bernstein M, et al. Phase II/III trial of etoposide and high-dose ifosfamide in newly diagnosed metastatic osteosarcoma: a pediatric oncology group trial. J Clin Oncol 2002;20:426–433.
35. Berend KR, Pietrobon A, Moore JO, et al. Adjuvant chemotherapy for osteosarcoma may not increase survival after neoadjuvant chemotherapy and surgical resection. J Surg Oncol 2001;78: 162–170.
36. Bacci G, Briccoli A, Ferrari S, et al. Neoadjuvant chemotherapy for osteosarcoma of the extremity: long-term results of the Rizzoli's 4th protocol. Eur J Cancer 2001;37:2030–2039.
37. Ferrari S, Bertoni F, Mercuri M, et al. Predictive factors of disease-free survival for non-metastatic osteosarcoma of the extremity: an analysis of 300 patients treated at the Rizzoli Institute. Ann Oncol 2001;12:1145–1150.
38. Petrilli AS, Kechichian R, Broniscer A, et al. Activity of intraarterial carboplatin as a single agent in the treatment of newly diagnosed extremity osteosarcoma. Med Pediatr Oncol 1999; 33:71–75.
39. Wilkins RM, Soubeiran A. The Phenix expandable prosthesis: early American experience. Clin Orthop 2001;382:51–58.
40. Eckardt JJ, Kabo JM, Kelley CM, et al. Expandable endoprosthesis reconstruction in skeletally immature patients with tumors. Clin Orthop 2000;373:51–61.
41. Ozaki T, Flege S, Kevric M, et al. Osteosarcoma of the pelvis: experience of the Cooperative Osteosarcoma Study Group. J Clin Oncol 2003;21:334–341.
42. Wittig JC, Bickels J, Kellar-Graney KL, et al. Osteosarcoma of the proximal humerus: long-term results with limb-sparing surgery. Clin Orthop 2002;397:156–176.
43. Ozaki T, Flege S, Liljenqvist U, et al. Osteosarcoma of the spine: experience of the Cooperative Osteosarcoma Study Group. Cancer (Phila) 2002;94:1069–1077.
44. Ham SJ, Kroon HM, Koops HS. Osteosarcoma of the pelvis: oncological results of 40 patients registered by the Netherlands Committee on Bone Tumors. Eur J Surg Oncol 2000;26:53–60.
45. Grimer RJ, Carter SR, Tillman RM, et al. Osteosarcoma of the pelvis. J Bone Joint Surg 1999;81B:796–802.
46. Bacci G, Ferrari S, Longhi A, et al. Nonmetastatic osteosarcoma of the extremity with pathologic fracture at presentation: local and systemic control by amputation of limb salvage after preoperative chemotherapy. Acta Orthop Scand 2003;74:449–454.
47. Brown A, Parsons JA, Martino C, et al. Work status after distal femoral Kotz reconstruction for malignant tumors of bone. Arch Phys Med Rehabil 2003;84:62–68.
48. Scully SP, Ghert MA, Zurakowski D, et al. Pathologic fracture in osteosarcoma: prognostic importance and treatment implications. J Bone Joint Surg 2003;84A:49–57.
49. Davis AM, Devlin M, Griffin AM, et al. Functional outcome in amputation versus limb sparing of patients with lower extremity sarcoma: a matched case-control study. Arch Phys Med Rehabil 1999;80:615–618.
50. Gokgoz N, Wunder JS, Mousses S, et al. Comparison of p53 mutations in patients with localized osteosarcoma and metastatic osteosarcoma. Cancer (Phila) 2001;92:2181–2189.
51. Hornicek FJ, Gebhardt MC, Wolfe MW, et al. P-glycoprotein levels predict poor outcome in patients with osteosarcoma. Clin Orthop 2000;373:11–17.
52. Kumta SM, Zhu QS, Lee KM, et al. Clinical significance of P-glyprotein immunohistochemistry and doxorubicin binding assay in patients with osteosarcoma. Int Orthop 2001;25: 279–282.
53. Gorlick R, Liao AC, Antonescu C, et al. Lack of correlation of functional scintigraphy with (99m)technetium-methoxyisobutylisonitrile with histological necrosis following induction

chemotherapy or measures of P-glyprotein expression in high-grade osteosarcoma. Clin Cancer Res 2001;7:3065–3070.
54. Wunder JS, Bull SB, Aneliunas V, et al. MDR1 gene expression and outcome in osteosarcoma: a prospective, multicenter study. J Clin Oncol 2000;18:2685–2694.
55. Sulzbacher I, Birner P, Trieb K, et al. The expression of bone morphogenetic proteins in osteosarcoma and its relevance as a prognostic parameter. J Clin Pathol 2002;55:381–385.
56. Yoshikawa H, Nakase T, Myoui A, et al. Bone morphogenetic proteins in bone tumors. J Orthop Sci 2004;9:334–340.
57. Zhou H, Randall RL, Brothman AR, et al. Her-2/neu expression in osteosarcoma increases risk of lung metastasis and can be associated with gene amplification. J Pediatr Hematol Oncol 2003;25:27–32.
58. Anninga JK, van de Vijver MJ, Cleton-Jansen AM, et al. Overexpression of the HER-2 oncogene does not play a role in high-grade osteosarcomas. Eur J Cancer 2004;40:963–970.
59. Tanaka M, Yamazaki T, Araki N, et al. Clinical significance of tenascin-C expression in osteosarcoma: tenascin-C promotes distant metastases of osteosarcoma. Int J Mol Med 2000;5: 505–510.
60. Khanna C, Wan X, Bose S, et al. The membrane-cytoskeleton linker ezrin is necessary for osteosarcoma metastasis. Nat Med 2004;10:182–186.
61. Hoang BH, Kubo T, Healey JH, et al. Expression of LDL receptor-related protein 5 (LRP5) as a novel marker for disease progression in high-grade osteosarcoma. Int J Cancer 2004;109: 106–111.
62. Sanders RP, Drissi R, Billups CA, et al. Telomerase expression predicts unfavorable outcome in osteosarcoma. J Clin Oncol 2004;22:3790–3797.
63. Ferguson WS, Harris MB, Goorin AM, et al. Presurgical window of carboplatin and surgery and multidrug chemotherapy for the treatment of newly diagnosed metastatic or unresectable osteosarcoma: Pediatric Oncology Group Trial. J Pediatr Hematol Oncol 2001;23:340–348.
64. Saylors RL III, Stine KC, Sullivan J, et al. Cyclophosphamide plus topotecan in children with recurrent or refractory solid tumors: a Pediatric Oncology Group phase II study. J Clin Oncol 2001;19:3463–3469.
65. Meyer WH, Pratt CB, Poquette CA, et al. Carboplatin/ifosfamide window therapy for osteosarcoma: results of the St Jude Children's Research Hospital OS-91 trial. J Clin Oncol 2001;19: 171–182.
66. Merimsky O, Meller I, Flusser G, et al. Gemcitabine in soft tissue or bone sarcoma resistant to standard chemotherapy: a phase II study. Cancer Chemother Pharm 2000;45:177–181.
67. Laverdiere C, Kolb EA, Supko JG, et al. Phase II study of ecteinascidin 743 in heavily pretreated patients with recurrent osteosarcoma. Cancer (Phila) 2003;98:832–840.
68. Skutitz KM. Phase II trial of pegylated-liposomal doxorubicin (Doxil) in sarcoma. Cancer Invest 2003;21:167–176.
69. Fagioli F, Aglietta M, Tienghi A, et al. High-dose chemotherapy in the treatment of relapsed osteosarcoma: an Italian sarcoma group study. J Clin Oncol 2002;20:2150–2156.
70. Jia SF, Worth LL, Densmore CL, et al. Eradication of osteosarcoma lung metastases following intranasal interleukin-12 gene therapy using a nonviral polyethylenimine vector. Cancer Gene Ther 2002;9:260–266.
71. Patel SR, Papadopoulos NE, Plager C, et al. Phase II study of paclitaxel in patients with previously treated osteosarcoma and its variants. Cancer (Phila) 1996;78:741–744.
72. Todesco A, Carli M, Iacona I, et al. All-*trans* retinoic acid and interferon-alpha in the treatment of a patient with resistant metastatic osteosarcoma. Cancer (Phila) 2000;89:2661–2666.
73. Rodriguez-Galindo C, Daw NC, Kaste SC, et al. Treatment of refractory osteosarcoma with fractionated cyclophosphamide and etoposide. J Pediatr Hematol Oncol 2002;24:250–255.
74. Jia SF, Worth LL, Turan M, et al. Eradication of osteosarcoma lung metastasis using intranasal gemcitabine. Anti-Cancer Drugs 2002;13:155–161.
75. Coterill SJ, Ahrens S, Paulussen M, et al. Prognostic factors in Ewing's tumor of bone: analysis of 975 patients from the European Intergroup Cooperative Ewing's Sarcoma Study Group. J Clin Oncol 2000;18:3108–3114.
76. Luksch R, Sampietro G, Collini P, et al. Prognostic value of clinicopathologic characteristics including neuroectodermal differentiation in osseous Ewing's sarcoma family of tumors. Tumori 1999;85:101–107.
77. McCarthy E, Frassica F. Primary bone tumors. In: Pathology of Bone and Joint Disorders. Philadelphia: Saunders, 1998:258–261.
78. Lee CS, Southey MC, Waters K, et al. EWS/FLI-1 fusion transcript detection and MIC2 immunohistochemical staining in the diagnosis of Ewing's sarcoma. Pediatr Pathol Lab Med 1996;16: 379–392.
79. Machen SK, Fisher C, Gautam RS, et al. Utility of cytokeratin subsets for distinguishing poorly differentiated synovial sarcoma from peripheral primitive neuroectodermal tumour. Histopathology (Oxf) 1998;33:501–507.
80. Halliday BE, Slagel DD, Elsheikh TE, et al. Diagnostic utility of MIC-2 immunocytochemical staining in the differential diagnosis of small blue cell tumors. Diagn Cytopathol 1998;19: 410–416.
81. Collins BT, Cramer HM, Frain BE, et al. Fine-needle aspiration biopsy of metastatic Ewing's sarcoma with MIC2 (CD99) immunocytochemistry. Diagn Cytopathol 1998;19:382–384.
82. Bacci G, Forni C, Longhi A, et al. Long-term outcome for patients with non-metastatic Ewing's sarcoma treated with adjuvant and neoadjuvant chemotherapies: 402 patients treated at Rizzoli between 1972 and 1992. Eur J Cancer 2004;40:73–83.
83. Bacci G, Ferrari S, Longhi A, et al. Role of surgery in local treatment of Ewing's sarcoma of the extremities in patients undergoing adjuvant and neoadjuvant chemotherapy. Oncol Rep 2004; 11:111–120.
84. Sluga M, Windhager R, Lang S, et al. The role of surgery and resection margins in the treatment of Ewing's sarcoma. Clin Orthop 2001;392:394–399.
85. Sluga M, Windhager R, Lang S, et al. A long-term review of the treatment of patients with Ewing's sarcoma in one institution. Eur J Surg Oncol 2001;27:569–573.
86. Zogopoulos G, Teskey L, Sung L, et al. Ewing sarcoma: farourable results with combined modality therapy and conservative use of radiotherapy. Pediatr Blood Cancer 2004;43:35–39.
87. Miser JS, Krailo MD, Tarbell MJ, et al. Treatment of metastatic Ewing's sarcoma or primitive neuroectodermal tumor of bone: evaluation of combination ifosfamide and etoposide—a Children's Cancer Group and Pediatric Oncology Group study. J Clin Oncol 2004;22:2873–2876.
88. Grier HE, Krailo MD, Tarbell NJ, et al. Addition of ifosfamide and etoposide to standard chemotherapy for Ewing's sarcoma and primitive neuroectodermal tumor of bone. N Engl J Med 2003;348:694–701.
89. Kolb EA, Kushner BH, Gorlick R, et al. Long-term event-free survival after intensive chemotherapy for Ewing's family of tumors in children and young adults. J Clin Oncol 2003;21:3423–3430.
90. Schuck A, Rube C, Konemann S, et al. Postoperative radiotherapy in the treatment of Ewing tumors: influence of the interval between surgery and radiotherapy. Strahlenther Onkol 2002;178: 25–31.
91. Marcus RB, Berrey BH, Graham-Pole J, et al. The treatment of Ewing's sarcoma of bone at the University of Florida: 1969–1998. Clin Orthop 2002;397:290–297.
92. Rodriguez-Galindo C, Billups CA, Kun LE, et al. Survival after recurrence of Ewing tumors: the St Jude Children's Research Hospital experience, 1979–1999. Cancer (Phila) 2002;94: 561–569.

93. Meyers PA, Krailo MD, Ladanyi M, et al. High-dose melphalan, etoposide, total-body irradiation, and autologous stem-cell reconstitution as consolidation therapy for high-risk Ewing's sarcoma does not improve prognosis. J Clin Oncol 2001;19:2812–2820.
94. Paulussen M, Ahrens S, Dunst J, et al. Localized Ewing tumor of bone: final results of the cooperative Ewing's Sarcoma Study CESS 86. J Clin Oncol 2001;19:1818–1829.
95. Burdach S, van Kaick B, Laws HJ, et al. Allogeneic and autologous stem-cell transplantation in advanced Ewing tumors. An update after long-term follow-up from two centers of the European Intergroup study EICESS. Stem-cell transplant programs at Dusseldorf University Medical center, Germany, and St. Anna Kinderspital, Vienna, Austria. Ann Oncol 2000;11:1451–1462.
96. Elomaa I, Blomqvist CP, Saeter G, et al. Five-year results in Ewing's sarcoma. The Scandinavian Sarcoma Group experience with the SSG IX protocol. Eur J Cancer 2000;36:875–880.
97. Bacci G, Ferrari S, Comandone A, et al. Neoadjuvant chemotherapy for Ewing's sarcoma of bone in patients older than thirty-nine years. Acta Oncol 2000;39:111–116.
98. Frolich B, Ahrens S, Burdach S, et al. High-dosage chemotherapy in primary metastasized and relapsed Ewing's sarcoma (EI)CESS. Klin Paediatr 1999;211:284–290.
99. Rosito P, Mancini AF, Rondelli R, et al. Italian Cooperative Study for the treatment of children and young adults with localized Ewing sarcoma of bone: a preliminary report of 6 years of experience. Cancer (Phila) 1999;86:421–428.
100. Givens SS, Woo SY, Huang LY, et al. Non-metastatic Ewing's sarcoma: twenty years of experience suggests that surgery is a prime factor for successful multimodality therapy. Int J Oncol 1999;14:1039–1043.
101. Craft A, Cotterill S, Malcolm A, et al. Ifosfamide-containing chemotherapy in Ewing's sarcoma: The Second United Kingdom Children's Cancer Study Group and the Medical Research Council Ewing's Tumor Study. J Clin Oncol 1998;16:3628–3633.
102. Bacci G, Ferrari S, Longhi A, et al. Local and systemic control in Ewing's sarcoma of the femur treated with chemotherapy, and locally by radiotherapy and/or surgery. J Bone Joint Surg 2003; 85B:107–114.
103. Talac R, Yaszemski MJ, Currier BL, et al. Relationship between surgical margins and local recurrence in sarcomas of the spine. Clin Orthop 2002;397:127–132.
104. Ozaki T, Hoffmann C, Hillmann A, et al. Implantation of hemipelvic prosthesis after resection of sarcoma. Clin Orthop 2002;396:197–205.
105. Shamberger RC, Laquaglia MP, Krailo MD, et al. Ewing sarcoma of the rib: results of an intergroup study with analysis of outcome by timing of resection. J Thorac Cardiovasc Surg 2000; 119:1154–1161.
106. Sucato DJ, Rougraff B, McGrath BE, et al. Ewing's sarcoma of the pelvis. Long-term survival and functional outcome. Clin Orthop 2000;373:193–201.
107. Hoffmann C, Ahrens S, Dunst J, et al. Pelvic Ewing sarcoma: a retrospective analysis of 241 cases. Cancer (Phila) 1999;85: 869–877.
108. Paulussen M, Ahrens S, Burdach S, et al. Primary metastatic (stage IV) Ewing tumor: survival analysis of 171 patients from the EICESS studies. European Intergroup Cooperative Ewing Sarcoma Studies. Ann Oncol 1998;9:275–281.
109. San-Julian M, Dolz R, Garcia-Barrecheguren E, et al. Limb salvage in bone sarcomas in patients younger than age 10: a 20-year experience. J Pediatr Orthop 2003;23:753–762.
110. Bacci G, Ferrari S, Longhi A, et al. Therapy and survival after recurrence of Ewing's tumors: the Rizzoli experience in 195 patients treated with adjuvant and neoadjuvant chemotherapy from 1979 to 1997.
111. Briccoli A, Rocca M, Ferrari S, et al. Surgery for lung metastases in Ewing's sarcoma of bone. Eur J Surg Oncol 2004;30:63–67.
112. Fuchs B, Valenzuela RG, Sim FH. Pathologic fracture as a complication in the treatment of Ewing's sarcoma. Clin Orthop 2003;415:25–30.
113. Wunder JS, Paulian G, Huvos AG, et al. The histological response to chemotherapy as a predictor of the oncological outcome of operative treatment of Ewing sarcoma. J Bone Joint Surg 1998;80A:1020–1033.
114. Hense HW, Ahrens S, Paulussen M, et al. Factors associated with tumor volume and primary metastases in Ewing tumors: results from the (EI)CESS studies. Ann Oncol 1999;10:1073–1077.
115. Ahrens S, Hoffmann C, Jabar S, et al. Evaluation of the prognostic factors in a tumor volume-adapted treatment strategy for localized Ewing sarcoma of bone: the CESS 86 experience. Cooperative Ewing Sarcoma Study. Med Pediatr Oncol 1999;32:186–195.
116. Bacci G, Ferrari S, Bertoni F, et al. Prognostic factors in nonmetastatic Ewing's sarcoma of bone treated with adjuvant chemotherapy: analysis of 359 patients at the Istituto Ortopedico Rizzoli. J Clin Oncol 2000;18:4–11.
117. Abudu A, Davies AM, Punsent PB, et al. Tumour volume as a predictor of necrosis after chemotherapy in Ewing's sarcoma. J Bone Joint Surg 1999;81B:317–322.
118. Baldini EH, Demetri GD, Fletcher CD, et al. Adults with Ewing's sarcoma/primitive neuroectodermal tumor: adverse effect of older age and primary extraosseous disease on outcome. Ann Surg 1999;230:79–86.
119. Paulussen M, Ahrens S, Craft AW, et al. Ewing's tumors with primary lung metastases: survival analysis of 114 (European Intergroup) Cooperative Ewing's Sarcoma Studies patients. J Clin Oncol 1998;16:3044–3052.
120. Krasin MJ, Rodriguez-Galindo C, Davidoff AM, et al. Efficacy of combined surgery and irradiation for localized Ewings sarcoma family of tumors. Pediatr Blood Cancer 2004;43:229–236.
121. Cosetti M, Wexler LH, Calleja E, et al. Irinotecan for pediatric solid tumors: the Memorial Sloan-Kettering experience. J Pediatr Hematol Oncol 2002;24:101–105.
122. Berg SL, Blaney SM, Sullivan J, et al. Phase II trial of pyrazoloacridine in children with solid tumors: a Pediatric Oncology Group phase II study. J Pediatr Hematol Oncol 2000;22:506–509.
123. Leung W, Chen AR, Klann RC, et al. Frequent detection of tumor cells in hematopoietic grafts in neuroblastoma and Ewing's sarcoma. Bone Marrow Transplant 1998;22:971–979.
124. Fuchs B, Valenzuela RG, Inwards C, et al. Complications in long-term survivors of Ewing sarcoma. Cancer (Phila) 2003;98:2687–2692.
125. Fuchs B, Valenzuela RG, Petersen IA, et al. Ewing's sarcoma and the development of secondary malignancies. Clin Orthop 2003; 415:82–89.
126. Paulussen M, Ahrens S, Lehnert M, et al. Second malignancies after Ewing tumor treatment in 690 patients from a cooperative German/Austrian/Dutch study. Ann Oncol 2001;12:1619–1630.
127. Tabone MD, Terrier P, Pacquement H, et al. Outcome of radiation-related osteosarcoma after treatment of childhood and adolescent cancer: a study of 23 cases. J Clin Oncol 1999;17: 2789–2795.
128. Grimer RJ, Belthur M, Carter SR, et al. Extendable replacements of the proximal tibia for bone tumours. J Bone Joint Surg 2000; 82B:255–260.
129. Neel MD, Wilkins RM, Rao BN, et al. Early multicenter experience with a noninvasive expandable prosthesis. Clin Orthop 2003;415:72–81.
130. Hillmann A, Hoffmann C, Gosheger G, et al. Malignant tumor of the distal part of the femur or the proximal part of the tibia: endoprosthetic replacement or rotationplasty. Functional outcome and quality-of-life measurements. J Bone Joint Surg 1999; 81A:462–468.

131. Kumta SM, Cheng JC, Li CK, et al. Scope and limitations of limb-sparing surgery in childhood sarcomas. J Pediatr Orthop 2002;22:244–248.
132. Azcona C, Burghard E, Ruza E, et al. Reduced bone mineralization in adolescent survivors of malignant bone tumors: comparison of quantitative ultrasound and dual-energy X-ray absorptiometry. J Pediatr Hematol Oncol 2003;25:297–302.
133. Wagner LM, Neel MD, Pappo AS, et al. Fractures in pediatric Ewing sarcoma. J Pediatr Hematol Oncol 2001;23:568–571.
134. Rorie CJ, Thomas VD, Chen P, et al. The Ews/Fli-1 fusion gene switches the differentiation program of neuroblastomas to Ewing sarcoma/peripheral primitive neuroectodermal tumors. Cancer Res 2004;64:1266–1277.
135. Takahashi A, Higashino F, Aoyagi M, et al. EWS/ETS fusions activate telomerase in Ewing's tumors. Cancer Res 2003;63: 8338–8344.
136. Chansky HA, Barahmand-Pour F, Mei Q, et al. Targeting of EWS/FLI-1 by RNA interference attenuates the tumor phenotype of Ewing's sarcoma cells in vitro. J Orthop Res 2004;22:910–917.
137. Merchant MS, Woo CW, Mackall CL, et al. Potential use of imatinib in Ewing's sarcoma: evidence for in vitro and in vivo activity. J Natl Cancer Inst 2002;94:1673–1679.
138. Rossi S, Orvieto E, Furlanetto A, et al. Utility of immunohistochemical detection of FLI-1 expression in round cell and vascular neoplasms using a monoclonal antibody. Mod Pathol 2004; 17:547–552.
139. Reith JD, Horodyski MB, Scarborough MT. Grade 2 chondrosarcoma: stage I or stage II tumor? Clin Orthop 2003;415:45–51.
140. Welkerling H, Kratz S, Ewerbeck V, et al. A reproducible and simple grading system for classical chondrosarcomas. Analysis of 35 chondrosarcomas and 16 enchondromas with emphasis on recurrence rate and radiological and clinical data. Virchows Arch 2003;443:725–733.
141. Mitchell AD, Ayoub K, Mangham DC, et al. Experience in the treatment of dedifferentiated chondrosarcoma. J Bone Joint Surg 2000;82B:55–61.
142. Brown RE, Boyle JL. Mesenchymal chondrosarcoma: molecular characterization by a proteomic approach, with morphogenic and therapeutic implications. Ann Clin Lab Sci 2003;33: 131–141.
143. Kawaguchi S, Wada T, Nagoya S, et al. Extraskeletal myxoid chondrosarcoma: a multi-institutional study of 42 cases in Japan. Cancer (Phila) 2003;97:1285–1292.
144. Collins MS, Koyama T, Swee RG, et al. Clear cell chondrosarcoma: radiographic, computed tomographic, and magnetic resonance findings in 34 patients with pathologic correlation. Skeletal Radiol 2003;32:687–694.
145. Marco RA, Gitelis S, Brebach GT, et al. Cartilage tumors: evaluation and treatment. J Am Acad Orthop Surg 2000;8:292–304.
146. Schreuder HW, Pruszczynski M, Veth RP, et al. Treatment of benign and low-grade malignant intramedullary chondroid tumors with curettage and cryosurgery. Eur J Surg Oncol 1998; 24:120–126.
147. Ozaki T, Lindner N, Hillmann A, et al. Influence of intralesional surgery on treatment outcome of chondrosarcoma. Cancer (Phila) 1996;77:1292–1297.
148. Murphey MD, Walker EA, Wilson AJ, et al. From the archives of the AFIP: imaging of primary chondrosarcoma: radiologic-pathologic correlation. Radiographics 2003;23:1245–1278.
149. Schneiderbauer MM, Blanchard C, Gullerud R, et al. Scapular chondrosarcomas have high rates of local recurrence and metastasis. Clin Orthop 2004;426:232–238.
150. Mittermayer F, Dominkus M, Krepler P, et al. Chondrosarcoma of the hand: is a wide surgical resection necessary? Clin Orthop 2004;424:211–215.
151. Patil S, deSilva MV, Crossan J, et al. Chondrosarcoma of the small bones of the hand. J Hand Surg 2003;28:602–608.
152. Soderstrom M, Ekfors TO, Bohling TO, et al. No improvement in the overall survival of 194 patients with chondrosarcoma in Finland in 1971–1990. Acta Orthop Scand 2003;74:344–350.
153. Ahmed AR, Tan TS, Unni KK, et al. Secondary chondrosarcoma in osteochondroma: report of 107 patients. Clin Orthop 2003; 411:193–206.
154. Fiorenza F, Abudu A, Grimer RJ, et al. Risk factors for survival and local control in chondrosarcoma of bone. J Bone Joint Surg 2002;84B:93–99.
155. Pring ME, Weber KL, Unni KK, et al. Chondrosarcoma of the pelvis. A review of sixty-four cases. J Bone Joint Surg 2001;83A: 1630–1642.
156. Bruns J, Elbracht M, Niggemeyer O. Chondrosarcoma of bone: an oncological and functional follow-up study. Ann Oncol 2001;12:859–864.
157. York JE, Berk RH, Fuller GN, et al. Chondrosarcoma of the spine: 1954 to 1997. J Neurosurg 1999;90(suppl 1):73–78.
158. Lee FY, Mankin HJ, Fondren G, et al. Chondrosarcoma of bone: an assessment of outcome. J Bone Joint Surg 1999;81A:326–338.
159. Bjornsson J, McLeod RA, Unni KK, et al. Primary chondrosarcoma of long bones and limb girdles. Cancer (Phila) 1998;83: 2105–2119.
160. Rosier RN, O'Keefe RJ, Teot LA, et al. P-glyprotein expression in cartilaginous tumors. J Surg Oncol 1997;65:95–105.
161. Wyman JJ, Hornstein AM, Meitner PA, et al. Multidrug resistance-1 and p-glycoprotein in human chondrosarcoma cell lines: expression correlates with decreased intracellular doxorubicin and in vitro chemoresistance. J Orthop Res 1999;17: 935–940.
162. Terek RM, Schwartz GK, Devaney K, et al. Chemotherapy and P-glycoprotein expression in chondrosarcoma. J Orthop Res 1998;16:585–590.
163. Porter DE, Lonie L, Fraser M, et al. Severity of disease and risk of malignant change in hereditary multiple exostoses. A genotype-phenotype study. J Bone Joint Surg 2004;86:1041–1046.
164. Kobayashi H, Suzuki M, Kanayama N, et al. CD44 stimulation by fragmented hyaluronic acid induces upregulation of urokinase-type plasminogen activator and its receptor and subsequently facilitates invasion of human chondrosarcoma cells. Int J Cancer 2002;102:379–389.
165. Hackel CG, Krueger S, Grote HJ, et al. Overexpression of cathepsin B and urokinase plasminogen activator is associated with increased risk of recurrence and metastasis in patients with chondrosarcoma. Cancer (Phila) 2000;89:995–1003.
166. Berend KR, Toth AP, Harrelson JM, et al. Association between ratio of matrix metalloproteinase-1 to tissue inhibitor of metalloproteinase-1 and local recurrence, metastasis, and survival in human chondrosarcoma. J Bone Joint Surg 1998;90A:11–17.
167. Jiang X, Dutton CM, Qi W, et al. Inhibition of MMP-1 expression by antisense RNA decreases invasiveness of human chondrosarcoma. J Orthop Res 2003;21:1063–1070.
168. Kunisada T, Moseley JM, Slavin JL, et al. Co-expression of parathyroid hormone-related protein (PTHrP) and PTH/PTHrP receptor in cartilaginous tumours: a marker for malignancy? Pathology 2002;34:133–137.
169. Pateder DB, Gish MW, O'Keefe RJ, et al. Parathyroid hormone-related peptide expression in cartilaginous tumors. Clin Orthop 2002;403:198–204.
170. van Beerendonk HM, Rozeman LB, Taminiau AH, et al. Molecular analysis of the INK4A/INK4A-ARF gene locus in conventional (central) chondrosarcomas and enchondromas: indication of an important for tumour progression. J Pathol 2004;202:359–366.
171. Ghert MA, Jung ST, Qi W, et al. The clinical significance of tenascin-C splice variant expression in chondrosarcoma. Oncology 2001;51:306–314.

172. Martin JA, DeYoung BR, Gitelis S, et al. Telomerase reverse transcriptase subunit expression is associated with chondrosarcoma malignancy. Clin Orthop 2004;426:117–124.
173. Park HR, Kim YW, Jung WW, et al. Evaluation of HER-2/neu status by real-time quantitative PCR in malignant cartilaginous tumors. Int J Oncol 2004;24:575–580.
174. Sutton KM, Wright M, Fondren G, et al. Cyclooxygenase-2 expression in chondrosarcoma. Oncology 2004;66:275–280.
175. Miyaji T, Nakase T, Onuma E, et al. Monoclonal antibody to parathyroid hormone-related protein induces differentiation and apoptosis of chondrosarcoma cells. Cancer Lett 2003;199: 147–155.

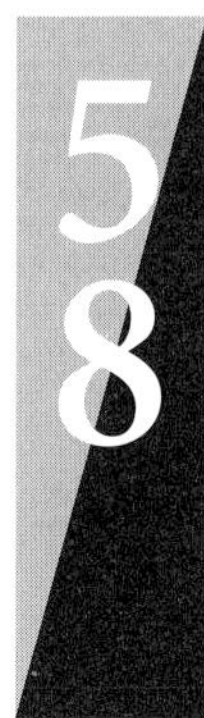

Soft Tissue Sarcoma

T. Christopher Windham and Vernon K. Sondak

Sarcomas are malignant tumors arising from mesenchymal cells. These tumors are usually—but not always—located in muscle, fat, and connective tissues. Sarcomas have varying clinical courses based on their histologic subtype, grade, location and size. These tumors are rare, with approximately 9,400 soft tissue sarcomas diagnosed annually in the United States, representing less than 1% of all newly diagnosed malignancies. In pediatric patients, sarcomas account for a greater percentage of malignancies, 15% of cancer cases. Deaths from soft tissue sarcomas exceed 3,400 and are 1,200 for bone sarcomas.[1] Sarcomas affect both genders equally.

Approximately two-thirds of soft tissue sarcomas are high-grade tumors, and histologic subtypes encountered vary by anatomic location.[2] The rarity of sarcomas, plus the vast array of histologic subtypes, have complicated our understanding of these tumors and impeded the development of effective therapies, as well as hindered efforts to establish "evidence-based" principles of diagnosis, treatment, and follow-up. For example, only 400 to 500 liposarcomas of the thigh (one relatively common histologic type in its most common anatomic site) are diagnosed per year in the United States, and literally only a handful of these patients ever enter onto prospective clinical trials, virtually none of which are randomized trials. Therefore, nearly all recommendations about sarcoma management are based on limited and often anecdotal evidence. Unfortunately, 50% of patients diagnosed with sarcomas ultimately succumb to their disease, and treatment is often associated with significant acute and long-term morbidity and limited if any benefit. Despite these limitations, significant progress has been made in our understanding and treatment of sarcomas. Information about molecular events involved in the development and progress of sarcomas has advanced dramatically during the past 15 years. Improvements in surgical techniques have resulted in significant decreases in morbidity of resection, allowing more-aggressive operations, and active chemotherapeutics have been identified, including the development of biologically targeted therapies. In this chapter, we attempt to take an evidence-based view of all aspects of sarcoma management. It will be readily apparent, however, that much of our clinical practice is based on very scanty, often conflicting data.

Risk Factors for the Development of Sarcomas

Hereditary Syndromes

Several hereditary genetic syndromes have been associated with the development of sarcomas (Table 58.1). Neurofibromatosis type I (c) is the most commonly encountered hereditary genetic syndrome associated with soft tissue sarcoma development. Affected patients usually present early in life with cutaneous findings of café-au-lait spots and freckling in skin folds, particularly in the axilla. These patients go on to develop benign tumors of the soft tissues (dermal neurofibromas) and tumors derived from perineural cells. In a long-term follow-up study of 212 patients with neurofibromatosis type I. Sorenson et al. found that malignant neoplasms or benign central nervous system tumors occurred in 45% of these patients.[3] Neurofibromatosis type I is associated with mutations in the tumor suppressor gene NF1 on chromosome 17, which acts through the negative regulation of *ras*.[4] The protein product of the NF1 gene is neurofibromin. Neurofibromin contains a functional GAP domain, which acts on GTP-*ras*.[5] Homozygous deletion of NF1 in mice is lethal during embryologic development. Heterozygous NF1 knockout mice are viable; however, these mice develop leukemias and pheochromocytomas. Other functions of neurofibromin have yet to be elucidated. The clinically related syndrome of neurofibromatosis type II (NF2) is less common than NF1. This syndrome is associated with mutations of the NF2 gene on chromosome 22. Tumors most commonly encountered in NF2 are schwannomas, ependymomas, and gliomas. The protein product of the NF2 gene is the cytoskeletal protein merlin (also called schwannomin) that acts to link cell-surface glycoproteins to the cytoskeleton.[6,7]

Li and Fraumeni identified an autosomal dominant inheritable syndrome associated with the development of soft tissue and bone sarcomas, breast cancer, brain tumors, acute leukemia, germ cell tumors, and adrenocortical cancer.[8] Subsequent work identified a mutation of the tumor suppressor gene p53 associated with the Li–Fraumeni syndrome.[9] Patients with germ-line inherited mutations of the p53 gene develop cancers at younger ages and at a significantly higher frequency than seen in the general population. The spectrum

TABLE 58.1. Major genetic syndromes associated with sarcoma development.

Syndrome	*Tumors observed*	*Genetic abnormality*	*Studies*
Neurofibromatosis type 1 (von Recklinghausen's disease)	Neurofibromas Gliomas Malignant peripheral nerve sheath tumors Nonlymphocytic leukemia Pheochromocytoma	Mutation of NF1 gene Protein product-neurofibromin	—Cohort/epidemiologic —Molecular studies of small groups of tumor samples and cell lines —Knockout mouse studies
Neurofibromatosis type 2	Schwannoma Ependymoma Meningioma Glioma	Mutation of NF2 gene Protein product–Merlin (schwannomin)	—Cohort/epidemiologic —Molecular studies of small groups of tumor samples and cell lines —Knockout mouse studies
Li–Fraumeni and other p53 mutations	Bone and soft tissue sarcomas Breast cancer (often phyllodes) Adrenocortical cancer Melanoma Gastric cancer Lung cancer Pancreatic cancer	Mutation of p53 gene Protein product p53	—Cohort/epidemiologic —Molecular studies of small groups of tumor samples and cell lines —Knockout mouse studies
Retinoblastoma	Retinoblastoma	Mutation of Rb1 gene Protein product p105 Rb	—Cohort/epidemiologic —Molecular studies of small groups of tumor samples and cell lines —Knockout mouse studies
Gardner syndrome	Colon cancer Desmoid tumors	Mutation of adenomatous polyposis coli gene	—Cohort/epidemiologic —Molecular studies of small groups of tumor samples and cell lines —Knockout mouse studies

Source: Data from references 3–5, 7–14, 13, 15.

of cancer formation varies by the location of mutation within the p53 gene.[10]

Another tumor suppressor gene has been associated with the development of retinoblastoma, a rare neoplasm arising in the epithelium of the retina. Retinoblastoma represents the prototype for inheritable genetic disease involving tumor suppressor genes. As observed by Knudson, patients who inherit a single mutation of the Rb1 gene are at higher risk for developing retinoblastoma in the event of a sporadic mutation of the Rb1 gene occurring in a somatic cell.[11] The Rb1 gene product, p105 protein, plays multiple important regulatory roles in the regulation of cell cycle, survival, proliferation, DNA repair, and DNA replication. The p105 protein has direct interactions with the p53 regulatory pathway.[12] In an analysis of risk of second malignancy in long-term retinoblastoma survivors, Fletcher et al. observed a 69% incidence of second malignancies commonly associated with ionizing radiation or agents causing DNA damage.[11]

Alterations in the adenomatous polyposis coli (APC) gene are found in patients with familial adenomatous polyposis (FAP). These patients have multiple polyps (usually more than 100) of the colon and rectum, as well as variable numbers of polyps in the stomach and small bowel.[13] A subset of patients with FAP has a constellation of findings that has been termed Gardner's syndrome. In addition to the intestinal polyps characteristic of FAP patients, these individuals also have mandibular osteomas and intraabdominal desmoid tumors. Available evidence indicates that Gardner's syndrome is not a distinct entity. Instead, patients with germline APC mutations show a phenotypic spectrum of some or all of the manifestations of classic Gardner's syndrome, and this spectrum correlates with the specific site of the mutation within the APC gene.[14] The APC gene acts to down regulate β-catenin, a regulator of cell proliferation.[13,15]

Current studies of hereditary syndromes rely on cohort reports, epidemiologic studies, and molecular biologic investigations. The validity of these syndromes has been bolstered by the genetic alterations identified through molecular genetic studies identifying specific associations with clinical presentations. Future advances will allow us to better understand genetic alterations involved in sarcomagenesis and assist patients in genetic counseling and also shed light on the biology of sporadic sarcoma cases.

Radiation

The development of sarcomas following radiation exposure was first suggested in the early 1900s. One of the earliest reports was that of Martland, who in 1929 documented the development of bone sarcomas in young girls who painted radioactive luminescent paints onto watch dials.[16] During the past century, other reports relating radiation exposure to sarcoma development began to emerge. Cahan et al. catalogued studies demonstrating the ability to create sarcomas in numerous animal models following treatment with radiation.[17] They further summarized studies documenting development of sarcomas in humans following treatment with radiation therapy and added 11 additional patients from their experience. This was one of the first efforts to describe clinical characteristics of radiation-associated sarcomas. They noted a latent period from 5 to more than 20 years between radiation exposure and the development of sarcoma. Unlike radiation-associated carcinomas, development of sarcomas was primarily seen after higher doses were administered.[18] In this work, Cahan and colleagues set forth criteria still used today for the diagnosis of a "radiation-induced" sarcoma:

1. There must have been microscopic or radiographic evidence of the nonsarcomatous nature of the initial condition.
2. The sarcoma must have arisen in the area included within the radiation field.
3. A relatively long latent period must have elapsed after irradiation before the clinical appearance of the sarcoma, in most cases longer than 5 years.
4. All sarcomas must have been proved histologically.[18–24,25–33]

Sarcomas have been seen after radiation therapy for the treatment of breast cancer, gynecologic malignancies, head and neck diseases, and lymphoma. The incidence of sarcoma following irradiation has been estimated to range from 0.03% to 0.8%.[21,34–36] These sarcomas are frequently high grade, clinically aggressive, and difficult to treat.[19] Histologic sarcoma subtypes most frequently observed following radiation exposure include osteosarcomas, malignant fibrous histiocytomas, and angiosarcomas.[19]

From the 1920s through the early 1950s, the alpha particle-emitting radioactive contrast agent thorium dioxide (Thorotrast) was commonly used in radiologic studies. This compound is selectively taken up by the reticuloendothelial cells of the liver and spleen, where it deposits a very high dose of radiation over many years as a consequence of its very long half-life. Several case-control studies of patients exposed to Thorotrast have found a much higher than expected incidence of liver disease, leukemias, and liver cancers.[37–39] In an updated report summarizing a Japanese Thorotrast follow-up study, Mori et al. reported increased mortality primarily as a result of liver cancers, of which 15% were hemangiosarcomas.[38] In their study, dos Santos Silva and colleagues also found an increased incidence of liver cancers; however, specific histology was not reported.[37] Platz and associates observed increased chromosomal aberrations in the peripheral blood of a group of eight patients exposed to Thorotrast when compared with five patients exposed to nonradioactive contrast during the same time period.[40] The studies to date strongly suggest an association between Thorotrast exposure and the development of sarcomas of the liver.

Although most studies have demonstrated a consistent association between irradiation and sarcoma formation, other factors besides radiation may account for the actual tumor development. Frequently, patients are treated with chemotherapy agents as part of their therapies. A number of studies have documented an increased risk of second malignancy formation following treatment with chemotherapy. Neglia et al., in a large retrospective cohort study, reported 60 bone and soft tissue sarcomas developing as a second malignancy (of 298 second malignancies) in children treated with chemotherapy.[41] Of note, these results were not adjusted to account for patients also treated with radiation therapy. Tucker et al. evaluated bone sarcoma development in children previously treated with chemotherapy or radiation therapy compared with untreated matched controls. They reported an excess number of bone sarcomas in patients who received alkylating agents with or without radiation therapy.[22] In a nonhuman primate study evaluating the effects of procarbazine, Sieber and associates identified 4 sarcomas in 55 monkeys following treatment.[42] Moreover, it is likely that a significant percentage of patients who develop sarcomas after treatment with chemotherapy and/or radiation have underlying genetic susceptibility, as was first observed in sarcomas developing after irradiation for retinoblastoma.

Lymphedema

Sarcoma development has also been associated with chronic lymphedema. A clinical scenario was recognized by Stewart and Treves in which lymphangiosarcoma develops following mastectomy, axillary nodal dissection, and radiation therapy in a chronically lymphedematous limb.[43] Because lymphedema may be associated with radiation therapy, the ultimate association of causation can be difficult or impossible. However, lymphangiosarcomas have been noted to arise in congenitally lymphedematous extremities as well as other settings where no radiation was given, demonstrating that lymphedema alone is sufficient to result in sarcoma formation in some cases.

Foreign Body

Sarcoma formation secondary to the presence of a foreign body has been the subject of numerous case reports. Foreign bodies associated with sarcomas have ranged from shrapnel to medical implants such as vascular conduits and orthopedic hardware.[44–53] Experimental studies have demonstrated foreign body carcinogenesis, identifying a mesenchymal pleuripotent cell lineage in sarcomas arising in association with foreign bodies.[54] Other studies have demonstrated that foreign body tumorigenesis requires a solid material of at least 5 mm and the prolongation of a dense fibrous capsule.[55] Activation of surrounding macrophages, as seen in chronic inflammatory reactions, results in a failure in fibrous capsular formation and subsequent tumor formation.[55] Laboratory studies have demonstrated that surface shape characteristics are important in determining carcinogenic potential; this appears to be a result of variable induction of a dense fibrous capsule by differing surfaces of foreign bodies.[56] The strength of clinical evidence implicating foreign bodies in the development of sarcomas is limited to case reports and small series. Despite these limitations, experimental evidence supports a causative role for foreign body reactions in the induction of rare cases of soft tissue sarcoma.

Viruses

The first viral oncogene, Src, was described by Rous in 1911 and has been confirmed to be tumorigenic.[57] Its significance in humans, however, remains uncertain. The elevated risk for the development of Kaposi's sarcoma in patients diagnosed with acquired immunodeficiency syndrome (AIDS) prompted investigators to determine if viruses could play a causative role in the development of these cancers. Recent studies have implicated the development of Kaposi's sarcoma in AIDS patients who have the herpes simplex virus type 8 (HSV-8). This etiology appears to be secondary to unregulated vascular endothelial cell proliferation in immunosuppressed patients. Dictor et al. found 88% of classical forms of Kaposi's sarcoma and 100% of AIDS–Kaposi's sarcomas with HSV-8.[58]

Epstein–Barr virus (EBV) has been linked to sarcoma development in immunosuppressed patients. McClain and colleagues found evidence of EBV infection in five leiomyosarcomas and two leiomyomas from six human immunodeficiency virus (HIV)-infected patients. They did not find evidence of EBV infection in smooth muscle tumors tested from HIV-negative patients.[59] In a large retrospective study of patients who received a polio vaccine contaminated with simian virus 40 (SV-40), Engels and associates failed to identify an increase in cancer formation.[60] The evidence from case reports, epidemiologic studies, and molecular biology studies supports an association of HSV-8 infection and Kaposi's sarcoma development in HIV-infected patients and probably in sporadic cases as well, and a minor role of EBV infection in other sarcoma formation in HIV-infected patients. Outside the clinical setting of HIV infection and/or immunosuppression, there is a lack of compelling data to support a viral etiology of sarcomas.

Chemical Exposure

A number of studies have evaluated a possible association of chemical exposure and the development of sarcomas. Chemicals implicated by case-control and epidemiologic studies include phenoxy herbicides, chlorinated aromatic compounds (e.g., dioxins), and vinyl chloride. There exist certain limitations inherent in many of these studies. Reporting of visceral sarcomas is often placed under the International Classification of Diseases (ICD) codes assigned to that particular organ rather than as a soft tissue sarcoma.[61] Several large epidemiologic studies of exposed workers have identified an association with chemical exposure, although others have not.[61–71] Public concern surrounding exposure of Vietnam veterans to phenoxy herbicides ("Agent Orange") and subsequent health risks has been addressed through a number of studies. These herbicides contain dioxin, widely reputed to be highly carcinogenic. However, a study by Greenwald and colleagues found no increased risk of sarcomas in veterans exposed to Agent Orange.[72] Subsequent studies, reviewed by Frumkin, have not demonstrated an increase in the development of soft tissue sarcomas in veterans exposed to these herbicides.[73] Further, Cole and colleagues summarized work evaluating dioxin and cancer, concluding that this agent is not a human carcinogen.[74]

Another chemical reported to be associated with the development of sarcomas is vinyl chloride. Case-control, retrospective cohort, and epidemiology studies have linked vinyl chloride exposure with a variety of cancers.[75–79] However, subsequent review by McLaughlin indicated that the increased cancer risk after vinyl chloride exposure was limited to angiosarcomas of the liver.[80] Subsequent review of epidemiologic literature by Bosetti and associates concluded that the only increased cancer risk was that of liver cancers, which they speculate may in fact represent angiosarcomas.[81] At present, studies evaluating exposure to vinyl chloride support an association with the development of angiosarcomas of the liver.

Pathology

There is a wide variety of histologic subtypes of sarcomas, and clinical behavior can be subtly or significantly different depending on histologic type. Pathologists use histogenetic classification schemes, which broadly distinguish soft tissue tumor subtypes based on the tissues they contain or are forming. Light microscopic evaluation is used to seek evidence of specific differentiation as the first step in classification. High-grade sarcomas are poorly differentiated, complicating classification. With advances in immunohistochemistry, cytogenetics, and electron microscopy, non-tissue-specific diagnoses, such as the once-common diagnosis of malignant fibrous histiocytoma, are increasingly being replaced by tissue-specific diagnoses based on direct or indirect evidence of characteristic tissue formation. However, many pleomorphic sarcomas are sufficiently undifferentiated that the tumors cannot be further classified or can only be classified after an extensive (and variably performed clinically) set of tests.

Molecular Pathology

The ultimate evidence of differentiation is provided at the molecular level, and molecular techniques have the potential to profoundly influence our notions regarding the classification and characterization of sarcomas. Our conceptual model of sarcomagenesis has evolved over recent years. Sarcomas are believed to arise de novo in nearly all instances. They rarely arise from preexisting benign neoplasms (one important exception being sarcomas arising within plexiform neurofibromas in patients with neurofibromatosis type I). Sarcomas are thought to develop from mesenchymal stem cells residing in muscle, fat, and connective tissues. The origin of these stem cells remains unclear, and sometimes even their mesenchymal derivation is in question (as for nerve or nerve sheath sarcomas, gastrointestinal stromal tumors, and primitive neuroectodermal tumors (Ewing's sarcomas). Two prevailing theories suggest that mesenchymal stem cells are found in local tissue pools or arise from the bone marrow.[82]

Advances in molecular pathology have enabled us to distinguish two general groups of sarcomas. One group consists of those tumors with simple karyotypes and specific reciprocal chromosomal rearrangements. Specific chromosomal translocations have been identified in a number of pathologic subtypes and may provide a specific diagnosis in the absence of other identifiable evidence of differentiation. Tumors in this group typically occur in younger patients, rarely have p53 mutations, and are not usually associated with genetic syndromes such as Li–Fraumeni syndrome. The second group consists of those tumors with complex karyotypes and random nonreciprocal chromosomal rearrangements; these are typically seen in older patients, frequently have p53 mutations, and are generally the ones seen associated with genetic syndromes.

Molecular signatures, such as provided by cDNA microarray analysis, are increasingly being used to investigate the genetic basis of the histogenetic classification scheme employed for sarcomas. Perhaps not surprising, those sarcomas characterized by specific translocations or mutations have well-defined signatures that correlate strongly with the histopathologic diagnosis. Conversely, the molecular signatures of other sarcomas, notably liposarcomas, leiomyosarcomas, and malignant fibrous histiocytomas, overlap to a significant degree.[83] This finding calls into question the validity of many of the pathologic distinctions that have been

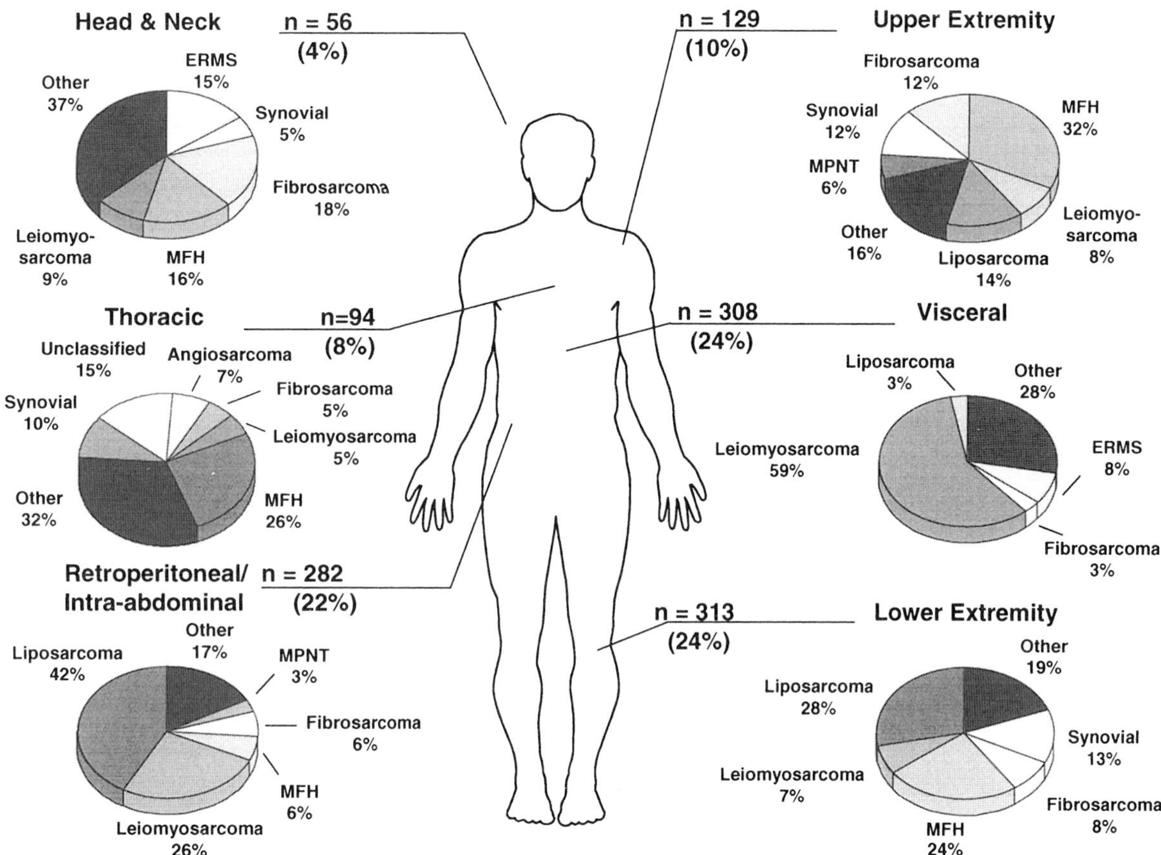

FIGURE 58.1. Certain histologic types of soft tissue sarcoma have a strong predilection for specific anatomic sites. (Pisters, P-Soft Tissue Sarcoma in Surgery Basic Science and Clinical Evidence, New York, Springer 2001. Norton JA, Bollinger R, Chang A, et al. eds.)

made over the years and further suggests that there may be hitherto unrecognized sarcoma categories of clinical relevance.

Patterns of Growth and Anatomic Distribution

Soft tissue sarcomas grow by direct local extension, infiltrating adjacent tissues and structures, occasionally with skip areas. They generally extend along tissue planes and uncommonly transverse or invade major fascial planes or bone. However, on gross inspection, many sarcomas demonstrate a characteristic pattern defined by a *pseudocapsule*, an apparently circumscribed tumor seemingly surrounded by a rim of compressed normal tissue. In fact, this pseudocapsule does not indicate the anatomic extent of the tumor, and removing the main mass from within the pseudocapsule invariably leaves tumor tissue behind. A minority of sarcomas, particularly dermatofibrosarcoma protuberans and cutaneous angiosarcoma, rarely if ever show a pseudocapsule and are instead characterized by very insidious infiltration of surrounding normal tissues that can greatly complicate attempts at complete resection.

Soft tissue sarcomas occur at all anatomic sites of the body, but the majority arise in the extremities.[2] At any given anatomic location, the most commonly encountered histologic subtypes vary. Certain histologic types of soft tissue sarcoma have a strong predilection for specific anatomic sites (Figure 58.1). For example, 40% to 50% of epithelioid sarcomas arise on the forearm or hand, compared to only 14% of soft tissue sarcomas overall presenting anywhere in the upper extremity.[84]

There exist a number of staging systems for soft tissue sarcomas. The most widely used system is the American Joint Commission on Cancer (AJCC) (Table 58.2). This system incorporates the traditional tumor size (T), lymph node status (N), and metastasis (M) categories as well as histologic grade (G). The incorporation of histologic grade reflects the observation that grade is a significant prognostic factor, with survival decreasing with increasing tumor grade.[85] A recent refinement in the staging of soft tissue sarcomas is the distinction of superficial and deep lesions, based on the location of the tumor relative to the investing muscular fascia. Sarcomas arising entirely above the investing fascia (i.e., cutaneous or subcutaneous) are "superficial" and designated in the AJCC system with the T modifier "a." Sarcomas involving the fascia or arising entirely below it are "deep" and given the T modifier "b." The majority (67%) of soft tissue sarcomas are high grade, deep, and more than 5cm in greatest dimension. The evidence base for the AJCC staging system is reviewed subsequently.

TABLE 58.2. American Joint Committee on Cancer (AJCC) GTNM classification and stage grouping of soft tissue sarcomas.

Tumor grade	
GX	Grade cannot be assessed
G1	Well differentiated
G2	Moderately differentiated
G3	Poorly differentiated
G4	Poorly differentiated or undifferentiated (four-tiered systems only)
Primary tumor	
TX	Primary tumor cannot be assessed
T0	No evidence of primary tumor
T1	Tumor 5 cm or less in greatest dimension
T1a	Superficial location
T1b	Deep tumor
T2	Tumor more than 5 cm in greatest dimension
T2a	Superficial location
T2b	Deep tumor
Regional lymph node involvement	
NX	Regional lymph nodes cannot be assessed
N0	No known metastases to lymph nodes
N1[a]	Regional lymph node metastasis
Distant metastasis	
MX	Distant metastasis cannot be assessed
M0	No distant metastasis
M1	Distant metastasis
Stage grouping	
Stage IA	Low grade, small (G1–2, T1a or b, N0, M0)
Stage IB	Low grade, large, superficial (G1–2, T2a, N0, M0)
Stage IIA	Low grade, large, deep (G1–2, T2b, N0, M0)
Stage IIB	High grade, small (G3–4, T1b, N0, M0)
Stage IIC	High grade, large, superficial (G3–4, T2a, N0, M0)
Stage III	High grade, large, deep (G3–4, T2b, N0, M0)
Stage IV	Nodal or distant metastases (any G, any T)

[a]Note: Presence of positive nodes (N1) is considered Stage IV.

Source: Used with the permission of the American Joint Committee on Cancer (AJCC), Chicago, Illinois. The original source for this material is the *AJCC Cancer Staging Manual*, sixth edition (2002), published by Springer-Verlag New York, www.springer-ny.com.

Prognostic Features

Characterization of the heterogeneous group of tumors called sarcomas has been hampered by the relative rarity of each specific subtype. Our understanding of the clinical features and natural history of sarcomas is largely limited to case reports, single-institutional experiences, and a few large-scale surveys of national cancer registries using different methodologies in data collection and reporting. To obtain sufficient numbers of patients with sarcomas, these reports generally combine the data from patients treated over several decades. This practice often results in the inclusion of patients who underwent markedly different treatment regimens, inclusion of bone sarcomas with soft tissue sarcomas, and inclusion of histologic subtypes that are known to have dramatically different clinical behavior. Despite these limitations, we are able to identify a number of salient features associated with sarcomas that are generally supported by studies involving large, often prospectively collected databases. These reports provide the foundation for current grading systems.

The strongest recognized prognostic factors are tumor grade, size, and depth; these key components of widely used clinical staging systems are discussed next (Table 58.3). Other prognostic factors have variably been identified as statistically significantly associated with either local recurrence or metastasis and survival. Local extension of tumor to involve blood vessels and bone has been shown to be associated with decreased survival, as has microscopic vascular invasion.[86,87] Some studies have related worse survival and increased local recurrence rates with increasing age.[88–92] A number of studies have identified that tumor location is of clinical importance.[86,93–95] LeVay and associates noted that local recurrence was higher in patients with sarcomas of the head and neck, likely reflecting difficulties in obtaining negative surgical margins. They also noted higher rates of metastasis in patients with trunk and head and neck sarcomas when compared with extremity sarcomas. In virtually all major studies, patients with extremity tumors fare better than those with sarcomas arising on the trunk, head, neck, or retroperitoneum. Other prognostic factors associated with adverse outcomes identified by researchers in separate studies include skin involvement, lymph node metastasis, pain at presentation, and postoperative fever following resection.[90,95–98]

Another area of controversy is the impact of isolated local recurrence on ultimate prognosis. Presentation with local recurrence has been shown to decrease overall survival in a number of studies.[86,89,92,99] Other studies have indicated a similar outcome for locally recurrent lesions compared to primary sarcomas of the same grade, size, and depth. The available evidence does not clearly support a contention that local recurrence is, in and of itself, an independent negative prognostic factor. Rather, the weight of evidence supports managing most cases of isolated local recurrence of sarcoma in a fashion analogous to the same case presenting for primary treatment.

Histologic grade, widely regarded as the predominant prognostic factor for localized sarcomas, is a subjective determination based on a number of individual microscopic features: these include tumor cellularity, pleomorphism, mitotic rate, degree of differentiation, and the presence or absence of spontaneous necrosis. Some authors have separately evaluated these features and shown them to be independent prognostic factors.[87,88,93,98,100,101] Newly identified molecular markers will likely play an important role in the future. Several molecular markers, such as c-Kit in gastrointestinal stromal tumors, have demonstrated their clinical utility in the diagnosis and treatment of specific sarcomas. Some molecular markers that have been associated with adverse prognosis are ras, c-myc, Ki-67, murine double minute 2 (MDM2), Rb1, and p53.[102–113] Further studies involving larger numbers of patients are required before any of these markers can be regarded to have documented independent prognostic significance.

TABLE 58.3. Major studies evaluating prognostic features of soft tissue sarcomas.

Author	*Study design*	*N*	*Sites*	*Statistically significant factors*			
				Size	*Grade*	*Depth*	*Histology*
Coindre et al., 1996[96]	Retrospective review of prospectively collected data	546	All	(+)* †	(+)* ** †	(+)†	(+)** †
Pisters et al., 1996[89]	Retrospective review of prospectively collected data	1,041	Extremity	(+)**	(+)**	(+)**	(+)*
Zagars et al., 2003[322]	Retrospective case series	1,225	All	(+)* **	(+)* **	NR	(+)* **
LeVay et al., 1993[86]	Retrospective case series	389	All except retroperitoneal and visceral	(+)* ** †	(+)* ** †	NS	NR
Abbas et al., 1981[323]	Retrospective case series	251	All	(+)†	(+)†	NR	(+)†
Tsujimoto et al., 1988[93]	Retrospective case series	236	All	NS	(+)†	(+)†	NR
Trojani et al., 1984[88]	Retrospective case series	155	All	NS	(+)** †	(+)†	NR
Ravaud et al., 1992[94]	Retrospective case series	144	All except visceral	(+)** †	(+)** †	(+)** †	NR
El-Jabbour et al., 1990[100]	Retrospective case series	125	All	(+)†	(+)†	(+)†	(+)†
Mandard et al., 1989[87]	Retrospective case series	109	All except retroperitoneal and visceral	(+)** †	(+)** †	(+)** †	NR
Ruka et. al., 1989[95]	Retrospective case series	267	All except retroperitoneal	(+)** †	NR, all high grade	NR	NR
Lack et al., 1989[101]	Retrospective review of prospectively collected data	300	Extremity	(+)†	(+)** †	NR	NS
Collin et al., 1987[90]	Retrospective case series	423	Extremity	(+)** †	(+)** †	NS	(+)** †
Weitz et al., 2003[91]	Retrospective review of prospectively collected data	1,706	Extremity	(+)**	(+)**	(+)**	(+)**
Singer et al., 1994[92]	Retrospective review of prospectively collected cata	182	Extremity	(+)†	(+)†	NR	(+)†
Ueda et al., 1988[97]	Retrospective case series	163	Extremity and Trunk	(+)†	(+)†	(+)†	NR
Rööser et al., 1987[98]	Retrospective case series	144	Extremity	(+)**	(+)** All intermediate and high grade	NR	NR
Shiu et al., 1975[324]	Retrospective case series	297	Extremity	(+)†	(+)†	NR	NR
Markhede et al., 1982[99]	Retrospective case series	97	Extremity	NS	(+)*	NS	(+)**

(+), statistically significant by univariate or multivariate analysis; NR, not reported; NS, not statistically significant.

*Local recurrence-free survival.

**Disease-free survival.

†Overall survival.

Staging

The importance of staging systems is severalfold. These systems serve as a means to evaluate prognosis, base clinical treatment decisions, and allow comparisons of studies. A staging system needs to be able to discriminate patient outcome in a meaningful and reproducible way. Staging of soft tissue sarcomas remains a work in evolution. Attempts to develop staging systems for soft tissue sarcomas began in earnest in the 1970s. Enneking and colleagues established a staging system for extremity soft tissue sarcomas based on tumor localization within muscular anatomic compartments, histologic grade and metastasis.[114] Subsequent investigators have created new or refined staging systems, each with its strengths and weaknesses.[85,115] Currently, the most widely use staging system is that of the American Joint Committee on Cancer (AJCC), which modifies the familiar TNM system by the addition of grade (G) as a separate component (see Table 58.2).[85] Important caveats related to the AJCC staging system are that it does not apply to Kaposi's sarcoma, dermatofibrosarcoma, infantile fibrosarcoma, and angiosarcomas, as these tumors are known to have unique but often poorly characterized prognostic features. The framers of this staging system also point out that it does not adequately stage sarcomas arising in all anatomic locations. Specifically, sites with unique prognostic features are those sarcomas arising in the dura, brain, parenchymatous organs, gastrointestinal tract, and retroperitoneum. A great deal of evidence forms the basis for the AJCC staging system, but there is also evidence pointing to weaknesses or inadequacies of the current system.

From the studies to date, it is clear that prognosis is inversely proportional to tumor size. The AJCC staging system characterizes size as a dichotomous variable with a breakpoint at 5cm maximum dimension. Available evidence indicates, however, that size should be a considered as a continuous variable. For example, survival with a 6-cm tumor is significantly better than that of a 15-cm sarcoma despite both tumors being staged T2 in the AJCC system. At the very least, it would be appropriate to recognize additional breakpoints (e.g., 10cm, 15cm, 20cm) as defining progressively poorer prognosis categories. Recently, depth was incorporated into the AJCC staging system as a factor secondary in importance to size. Available evidence is inconclusive as to whether depth is truly an independent factor: the apparent prognostic significance of depth may be a reflection of the fact that deeper lesions more often reach larger size (frequently well in excess of the 5-cm cutoff) before diagnosis.

The use of histologic grade as an integral part of the AJCC system is one of the most accepted and time-tested aspects of sarcoma staging, but even this has not been without controversy. Evidence clearly supports that three-part systems (defining low, medium, and high grade) provide additional prognostic information compared to two-part systems.[116] The evidence is much less clear that there is additional information conveyed by four-part systems. The AJCC system uses a four-part grading system but collapses this into a two-part system for assignment of the G classification (that is, grade 1 or 2 sarcomas are G1 while grade 3 or 4 sarcomas are G2). Clinically, it is a widely accepted principle that intermediate- and high-grade sarcomas (in three-part systems) are treated similarly. The rationale for collapsing grade 1 and 2 sarcomas into the same category, especially given how most pathologists discriminate grade 1 and 2 lesions, requires further prospective evaluation and perhaps even revision in future iterations of the system.

The relative significance assigned to grade in stage assignment has also been brought into question. Ramanathan and associates observed that AJCC stage III patients in their study in fact had a higher overall survival than stage II patients.[117] Other investigators similarly found survival rate discrepancies between stages.[118–120]

Lymph node metastasis has been identified as a significant negative prognostic finding,[121,122] as reflected in stage IV assignment in the face of N1 disease, indicating that prognosis for node-positive sarcoma patients is considered similar to those who present with metastatic disease. The frequency of lymph node metastasis has been reported to range from 2% to 13%, with the true incidence likely closer to 5%.[122–126] Although lymph node metastasis is a rare event in soft tissue sarcomas, higher incidence of lymph node metastasis is observed in synovial cell sarcoma, rhabdomyosarcoma, clear cell sarcoma, and alveolar soft parts sarcoma.[126] It remains unclear, based on available data, whether nodal metastasis conveys similarly poor prognosis for all these tumor types and whether the prognosis after nodal metastasis in contemporary series is truly equivalent to metastatic disease beyond the regional nodes.

Validation of the AJCC staging system has been performed through a number of studies. As already discussed, problems with stage discrimination have been identified in several studies. From these reports, it is clear that further modifications will be needed in future iterations. Treatment decisions should incorporate anatomic site, tumor histology, actual tumor size, and, where appropriate, molecular markers rather than restricting decisions to only AJCC stage assignment.

Clinical Evaluation

Extremity Sarcomas

The clinical presentation of patients with soft tissue sarcomas varies by anatomic site. The most common locations for these tumors are shown in Figure 58.1. Patients with soft tissue sarcomas arising in the extremities usually present with a painless mass that is larger than 5cm (Table 58.4). El-Jabbour et al. reported a median duration of symptoms of 6 months before presentation.[100] In a survey of more than 5,800 sarcoma patients, Lawrence and colleagues reported that about half waited at least 4 months before seeing a physician and 20% experienced delays of 6 months or more *after* seeking treatment before a correct diagnosis was made.[127] Often sarcoma patients are diagnosed clinically as having a "chronic hematoma" or "pulled muscle" and undergo prolonged observation or treatment for these conditions. In fact, nonathletic adults rarely develop persistent soft tissue masses from either of these causes in the absence of a history of unusually strenuous activity or significant trauma, unless they are on chronic anticoagulant therapy. When a soft tissue mass arises in a patient with no history of trauma or persists more than 6 weeks after local trauma, further evaluation is indicated.

Virtually all soft tissue masses arising in the extremity that are more than 5cm in diameter and any new, enlarging, or symptomatic lesions should be biopsied. Only small subcutaneous lesions that have persisted unchanged for many years should be considered for observation rather than biopsy.

TABLE 58.4. Major studies reporting clinical presentation of extremity soft tissue sarcomas.

Study	*Age*	*Gender (% male)*	*Pain (%)*	*Less than 5cm (%)*
Donohue et al., 1988[325]	58[a]	46	22	44
Ueda et al., 1988[97]	46[a]	56	30	38
Weitz et al., 2003[91]	55[a]	53	NR	52
Pisters et al., 1996[89]	51[a]	53	19	41
El-Jabbour et al., 1990[100]	58[c]	53	20	33

NR, not recorded.

[a]Median age with metastasis, 48 years without metastasis.

[b]Median.

[c]Mean.

TABLE 58.5. Major studies reporting clinical presentation of retroperitoneal sarcomas.

Study	*N*	*Age*	*Gender (% male)*	*Size greater than 5 cm (%)*	*High grade (%)*
Lewis et al., 1998[129]	500	58[b]	57	94	60
Stöckle et al., 2001[251]	165	54[b]	50	94	43
Ferrario et al., 2003[256]	130	57[b]	53	95	44
Alvarenga et al., 1991[249]	50[b]	50	90	43	
Dalton et al., 1989[247]	116	57[a]	47	98	54
Jaques et al., 1990[239]	114	57[b]	59	100	57
Hassan et al., 2004[254]	97	59[a]	56	97	69
Karakousis et al., 1995[246]	90	58[b]	50	97	40
Zornig et al., 1992[250]	51	44[a]	45	100	42
Wang et al., 1996[255]	40	55[a]	67	100	NR
Makela et al., 2000[252]	32	58[a]	50	91	NR
Pirayesh et al., 2001[253]	22	53[a]	59	100	46
Solla et al., 1986[248]	20	53[a]	40	100	NR

NR, not recorded.

[a]Mean.

[b]Median.

The best way to avoid undue diagnostic delay during evaluation of a soft tissue mass is for the physician always to remain cognizant of the possibility of malignancy. During the physical examination attention should be given to tumor location, size, mobility, tenderness, vascular exam, skin changes, and inspection of all lymphatic basins. It is also relevant to identify often subtle neurologic changes that can result from the mass. If a deep-seated extremity mass is to be biopsied, we prefer that appropriate imaging studies be performed before biopsy; this ensures no tissue distortion that could complicate the interpretation of the study and may assist in the planning of the biopsy to ensure the highest yield samples.

Retroperitoneal and Visceral Sarcomas

Sarcomas arising in the retroperitoneum and from abdominal viscera most commonly present as an abdominal mass often without other symptoms (Table 58.5). Although the median age is around 50, retroperitoneal sarcomas can occur at any age. These tumors usually do not come to the attention of the patient until they are large. Retroperitoneal sarcomas smaller than 5 cm are rarely seen.[128,129] When present, symptoms relate to mass effect of the tumor or local invasion. Early satiety, gastrointestinal obstruction or bleeding, lower extremity swelling, or pain can be the first symptoms leading to the discovery of a retroperitoneal sarcoma. The most useful tool in the evaluation of retroperitoneal tumors is a computed tomographic (CT) scan; this allows assessment of tumor location and relationship to adjacent organs, and can identify metastatic lesions in the liver or peritoneal cavity. Once the initial evaluation identifies a retroperitoneal tumor, the clinician must consider a number of clinical entities, including functioning and nonfunctioning adrenal tumors, renal tumors, pancreatic tumors, advanced gastrointestinal carcinomas, germ cell tumors, and soft tissue sarcomas. Detailed history and physical examination can help distinguish many of these entities and prompt further studies. Serum beta-human chorionic gonadotropin (β-hCG), alpha (α-)fetoprotein, and testicular examination and ultrasonography are indicated in cases of suspected testicular cancer with retroperitoneal metastasis. In patients with lymphadenopathy, either core needle or excisional biopsy of enlarged lymph nodes may be diagnostic for lymphoma. When tumors appear to be arising from the stomach, pancreas, or duodenum, upper gastrointestinal endoscopy with biopsy may be diagnostic. Similarly, colonoscopy with biopsy can be useful in tumors arising from the colon. If these diagnoses are ruled out or low in the differential and sarcoma is the most likely diagnosis, the role of biopsy is controversial.

Pisters and colleagues suggest that surgical exploration is the most appropriate next step for a retroperitoneal mass suspected of being a sarcoma.[130] We advocate a more-cautious approach, as new treatment options may be considered based on the results of a percutaneous biopsy. Examples include the use of imatinib mesylate (Gleevec) in the treatment of gastrointestinal stromal tumors or primary chemotherapy in germ cell tumors or lymphomas. Often the distinction between these diagnoses can be difficult with nonspecific physical findings and imaging studies. Our approach is to have patients undergo CT-guided biopsy of retroperitoneal tumors before treatment planning if the diagnosis is unable to be established through less-invasive means. It is important to note that nondiagnostic biopsies are not uncommon; in such cases, we proceed to surgery.

Head and Neck Sarcomas

The majority of head and neck cancers are epithelial tumors, followed by lymphomas with sarcomas comprising only 1% to 11% of these malignancies.[131] Sarcomas of the head and neck can occur at any age; however, median ages from series are usually in the fourth and fifth decades (Table 58.6). From several series, we observe that the majority of these tumors are less than 5 cm, and they are less often high grade than sarcomas arising in other sites. Bentz et al. reported a series of 111 head and neck sarcomas, noting that half these patients

TABLE 58.6. Major studies reporting clinical features of sarcomas arising in the head and neck.

Study	*N*	*Age*	*Size less than 5 cm (%)*	*High grade (%)*	*Distant metastastes (%)*
Webber et al., 1986[133]	188	50[b]	59	NR	40
Farhood et al., 1990[134]	176	48[a]	52	59	23
Eeles et al., 1993[140]	130	36	78	48	1
Bentz et al., 2004[132]	111	47[a]	72	46	33
Le Vay et al., 1994[135]	73	50[a]	42	NR	16
Dudhat et al., 2000[178]	72	37[b]	29	38	7
Kraus et al., 1994[139]	60	49[b]	72	58	NR

NR, not recorded.
[a] Mean.
[b] Median.

presented with a painless enlarging mass; the remainder reported pain or neurologic dysfunction on presentation.[132] The neck, face, and scalp represent the most frequent subsites for sarcoma formation; however, tumors can arise in the oral cavity, sinuses, orbit, pharynx, and nasopharynx.[131–143]

Imaging

Great advances have occurred during the past two decades through the widespread use of CT and magnetic resonance (MR) scanning. The two modalities have continued to evolve, further refining the quality of these studies. As discussed previously, we strongly encourage imaging of deep soft tissue tumors before any biopsy procedure; this is important in characterizing the lesion before distortion that may accompany the biopsy. Planning the most appropriate biopsy technique, target area, and approach is also facilitated by prebiopsy imaging.

Magnetic resonance images are excellent at delineating tissue planes, neurovascular structures, and characterization of soft tissue tumors without the use of radiation (Figure 58.2). A number of studies have demonstrated the ability of magnetic resonance imaging (MRI) to characterize benign and malignant soft tissue tumors accurately in a high percentage of cases.[144–147] Totty et al. compared MRI with CT scanning for evaluating soft tissue tumors of the extremities.[144] They noted that T_1-weighted MR images better delineated extension of tumors into surrounding fatty tissue. They found that T_2-weighted and spin-density MR images were superior in detecting tumor extension into muscle. Overall, they found MR to yield superior resolution images to CT scanning in 33% of comparisons and equal results in 67%. In their study, MRI never yielded inferior results compared to CT. The only deficiency they identified was the limited ability of MRI to demonstrate soft tissue calcification and gas. In a study comparing MRI with CT in the evaluation of 27 extremity soft tissue tumors, Weeks and associates found that MRI was able to adequately assess neurovascular involvement in 80% of cases compared with 62% of CT scans.[148] Verstraete and colleagues utilized contrast-enhanced techniques in MRI, demonstrating an improved ability to depict tissue vascularization and perfusion.[147] This advantage is relevant in biopsy planning, where the highest yield specimens are more likely to be obtained from viable, well-perfused areas. When bony involvement or destruction is of concern, CT scanning is better suited than MRI (Figure 58.3).

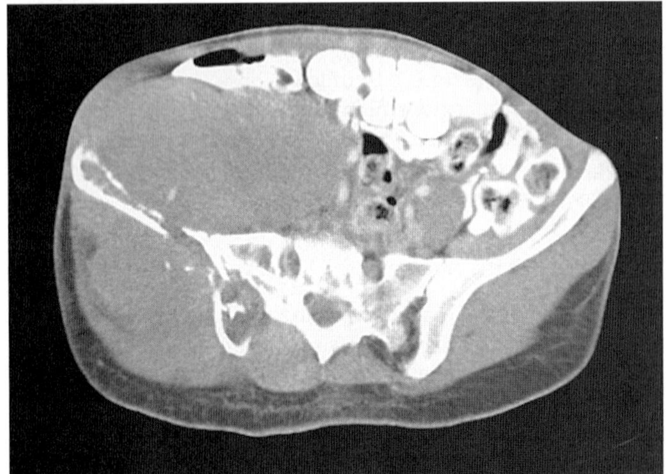

FIGURE 58.2. Magnetic resonance imaging (MRI) of lower extremity high-grade undifferentiated pleomorphic sarcoma with encasement of the sciatic nerve.

Imaging of the head and neck can be accomplished through either CT or MRI. We have usually relied on CT as our initial imaging modality and added MRI when further characterization is required. In imaging the chest, trunk and abdomen, CT scanning is the most commonly employed technique (Figure 58.4). Obtaining high-quality MR scans of the chest and abdomen can be difficult, whereas CT is less sensitive to motion artifact.[149] Characterization of fatty tumors, tumor proximity to adjacent organs, and detection of intraabdominal metastasis are all possible with CT scanning of the abdomen. In the pelvis, all these features of CT are relevant, as well as excellent characterization of bony invasion. Granstrom and Unger reviewed the techniques and interpretation of MR in the evaluation of retroperitoneum.[150] They emphasized the importance of axial images in addition to sagittal and coronal views. Although MR has been investigated in the evaluation of specific organs such as pancreas and adrenal glands, large studies comparing MRI of retroperitoneal sarcomas with CT scanning are lacking. At present, we rely primarily on CT scanning in the evaluation of soft tissue tumors arising in the abdomen and pelvis.

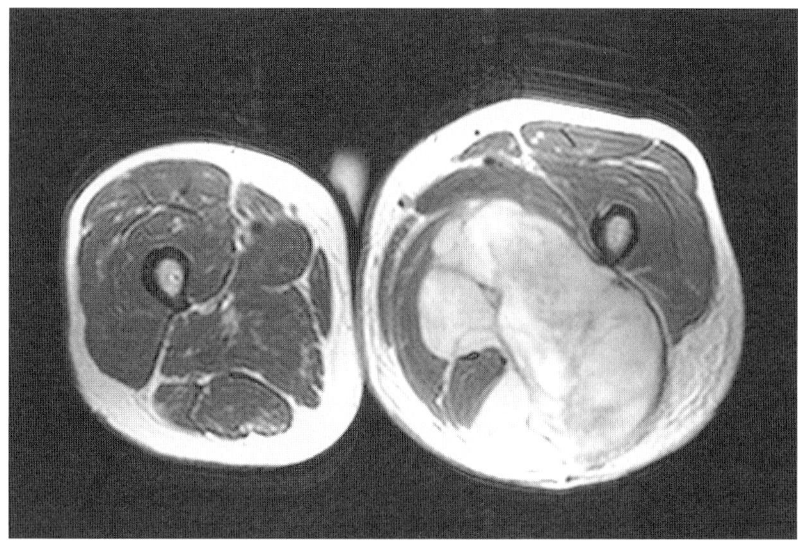

FIGURE 58.3. Computed tomography of a pelvic Ewing's sarcoma showing destruction of the right iliac bone.

Biopsy

The technical details of biopsy in the evaluation and treatment of soft tissue tumors remain the subject of debate, fueled by a surprising lack of high-quality evidence. Concerns surround the technique employed, pathologic interpretation, and treatment implications. Following the initial history and physical examination and appropriate radiologic investigations, the decision regarding biopsy must be carefully considered. Although the technical aspects of the actual performance of the biopsy are not necessarily complex, the decision making can be challenging for even the most experienced surgeon. As Mankin and colleagues pointed out in two similar studies conducted 14 years apart, missteps at this stage can have grave consequences.[151,152] Their initial report identified a 17% complication rate resulting from the biopsy. More concerning was the finding that, in 18% of patients, the treatment or outcome was altered because of some difficulty related to the biopsy. Factors implicated included poorly oriented incisions, made without due regard to the subsequent surgical approach required for definitive resection, and wound complications such as infection or hematoma formation. Perhaps the most distressing finding was that nearly 5% of patients went on to have amputations who might otherwise have been candidates for limb-sparing procedures. The authors concluded that the planning of a biopsy, technique employed, incision orientation, and pathologic interpretation could have significant treatment implications. They also found that patients biopsied at outside referring institutions experienced complications with skin, soft tissue, or bone in 31% whereas only 7% of biopsies performed at specialty centers had similar complications. There was an alteration in treatment as a result of the biopsy in 32% of referring institutions who performed these biopsies and 8% in those performed at the specialty centers. When the authors repeated this study, they found very little had changed in these results despite prior warnings. These issues serve to alert us to the significance a biopsy plays in patients presenting with soft tissue tumors.

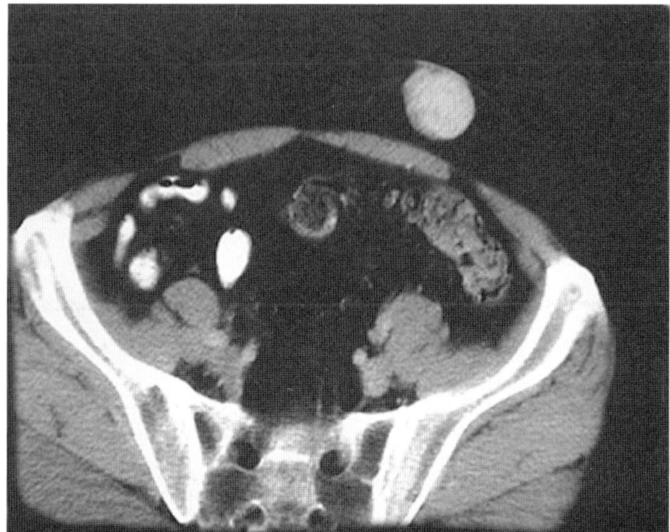

FIGURE 58.4. Computed tomography of abdominal wall solitary fibrous tumor.

In lesions of the extremity, a number of methods can be employed to obtain diagnostic tissue, including fine-needle aspiration (FNA) cytology, core needle biopsy, incisional biopsy, and excisional biopsy. Each technique has its advantages and disadvantages and requires expertise in its performance and, equally importantly, in the pathologic interpretation. FNA is the least invasive, associated with a low complication rate, and can be performed in an outpatient setting. Tumors in both superficial and deep locations can be biopsied using this technique. A number of studies have been able to establish the diagnosis of malignancy in more than 90% of cases; in some series, the majority could be assigned to a specific histologic subtype.[153–157] In a prospective series of 365 consecutive FNA biopsies of soft tissue lesions, Akerman et al. reported correct diagnosis of malignancy in 89% and correct diagnosis of a benign lesion in 96% of lesions.[155] A major concern with the use of FNA remains the occurrence of false-positive diagnoses of malignancy in small numbers of patients in virtually every large series. In Akerman's series, two patients had their care altered as a result of a false diagnosis. The application of ancillary techniques (cytogenetics, immunohistochemistry, flow cytometry, electron microscopy) can achieve a diagnostic accuracy approaching 95% in identifying malignancy.[156] Reported rates of false positives and false negatives range from 1% to 4% with adequate sampling.[153,156,158,159,160–161] Needle tract seeding following FNA biopsy has been reported; however, it appears to be exceptionally rare.[155,157,161–163]

It must also be noted that the majority of studies reporting excellent results with FNA are performed in centers with large volumes of soft tissue tumors, expert cytologists, and individuals with expertise and interest in the cytologic evaluation of soft tissue tumors. Whether these results can be reproduced in institutions without dedicated specialized cytopathologists is doubtful. We currently employ FNA in the evaluation of lesions suspicious for recurrence or metastatic disease, where the prior histology is available and can aid in confirmation, but not for primary extremity lesions.

Core needle biopsy has emerged as the most commonly employed biopsy technique in recent years. Several advantages have been identified when using this approach. This procedure can generally be performed in the outpatient setting with local anesthesia. The complication rate is similar to that of FNA, approximately 1% to 2% in several series.[164–166] Core needle biopsy provides a 1 mm × 10 mm tissue sample, preserving tumor architecture to facilitate pathologic diagnosis and the assignment of histologic grade.[166] Ball and associates evaluated 52 consecutive core needle biopsies of soft tissue tumors, reporting accurate diagnosis in 98% of malignant tumors.[165] They reported correct histologic subtype diagnosis in 85% and correct histologic grade assignment in 88% of sarcomas. In a report comparing 570 core needle and open biopsies, Hoeber and colleagues reported sensitivities of 99.4% and 97.4%, respectively.[166] They found a specificity of 98.7% for core needle biopsy and 100% for incisional biopsy. They were able to assign the histologic subtype and grade in 80% of core needle biopsies. Heslin and associates evaluated 164 primary extremity soft tissue tumors comparing first biopsy attempts of core needle biopsy, incisional biopsy, frozen section, and excisional biopsy,[167] finding that 93% of core needle biopsy samples were adequate to establish the diagnosis. Core needle biopsy was able to identify malignancy in 95%, histologic grade in 88%, and subtype in 75% of biopsies. Taken together, these studies support the accuracy, safety, and utility of core needle biopsy in the evaluation of soft tissue tumors. We utilize core needle biopsy for the initial diagnostic study in most patients presenting with soft tissue tumors larger than 5 cm in both superficial and deep locations.

Incisional biopsies play an important role in evaluation of soft tissue tumors, but decisions regarding when and where to employ this technique require significant experience in the treatment of musculoskeletal tumors. As tumor seeding is a concern, excision of the biopsy scar and tract is required if a sarcoma is diagnosed. Poorly planned incisions may result in added morbidity for sarcoma patients when they undergo definitive resection (Figure 58.5).[168–170] Incisions oriented along the long axis of the extremity do not necessarily yield the best cosmetic result, but they minimize future problems in the event a sarcoma is diagnosed. The incision should be placed directly over the most superficial part of the tumor whenever possible, allowing a surgical approach that avoids crossing through uninvolved compartments to minimize contamination of normal tissues (Figure 58.6).[154] The accuracy in distinguishing benign from malignant tumors is greater than with core needle biopsy; however, risks of hematoma and wound complications are also higher.[151,152,166] Meticulous hemostasis to avoid hematoma and possible contamination of adjacent muscle compartments is imperative. Because the zone of compressed, reactive tissue around a sarcoma can

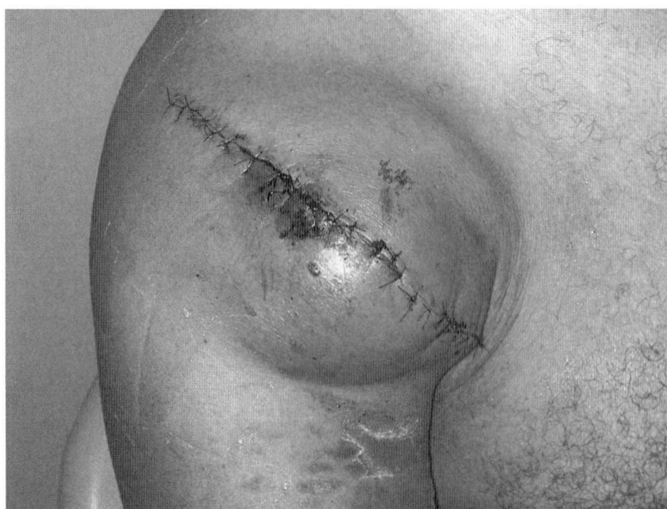

FIGURE 58.5. Poorly oriented biopsy of anterior shoulder with interrupted sutures, hematoma, and infection.

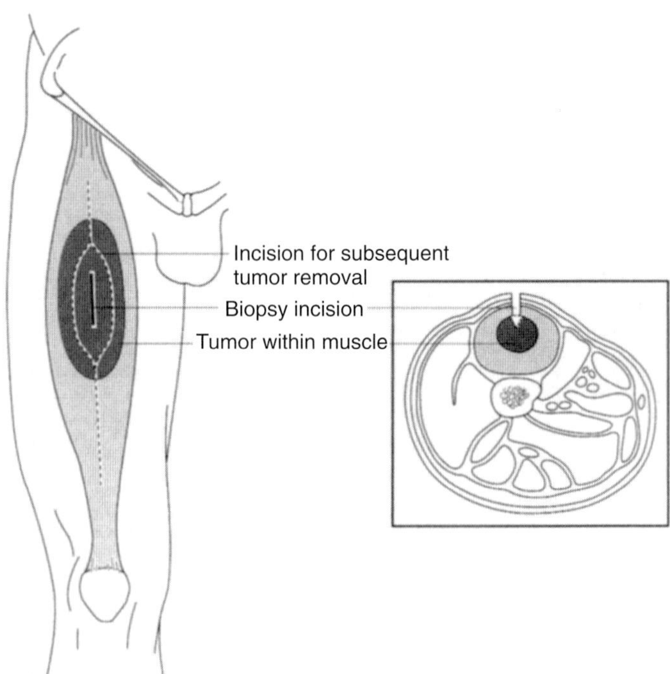

FIGURE 58.6. When making an incision, the incision should be placed directly over the most superficial part of the tumor whenever possible, allowing a surgical approach that avoids crossing through uninvolved compartments to minimize contamination of normal tissues.

look like malignant tumor tissue, we utilize frozen section to ensure adequate tissue for diagnosis has been obtained. The limitations of frozen section histopathology are significant, however, and radical procedures are generally not carried out based on a frozen section diagnosis obtained during incisional biopsy.

Excisional biopsy is reserved for small, superficial lesions. Although most such lesions are benign, the same careful planning is required as described in performing incisional biopsies. The biopsy incision should be oriented in such a way as to allow for uncompromised wide reexcision in the unlikely event of a malignant diagnosis.

When considering biopsy of a large or deep soft tissue tumor, the input of a surgical specialist experienced in the treatment of sarcomas can avoid many of the potential pitfalls reported by Mankin et al.[151,152] Sarcoma treatment centers continue to see patients who have undergone excisional biopsy for large or deep sarcomas. Unplanned excisional biopsy (the so-called oops phenomenon) carries with it a very high risk of leaving gross or microscopic tumor behind, even when the biopsy surgeon believes a complete excision of all tumor has been carried out. Randall and associates reviewed 104 unplanned resections of soft tissue sarcomas referred to a specialty center and found that 82% of excisional biopsies had positive histologic margins.[171] In a retrospective review of 65 patients referred to a specialty care center after unplanned excision of soft tissue sarcomas, Noria and associates documented that 39% of these patients had residual disease when subsequent reresection was performed.[172] None of the patients in this series had identifiable disease on physical examination or by imaging. Noria et al. were unable to identify predictive factors to identify those patients who were most likely to have residual disease. When Davis et al. evaluated their experience performing reexcision in 239 patients after soft tissue sarcoma excisional biopsies, they identified residual disease in 35% to 40% of reresected specimens.[173] Other investigators have similarly found a high incidence of residual disease on reresection.[174,175] Increased local recurrence rates have also been associated with excisional biopsy of soft tissue sarcomas in some but by no means all series.[172,173]

Treatment

Available evidence regarding prognostic and treatment-related factors suggests that treatment decisions for patients with clinically localized soft tissue sarcomas be based on the site and histologic grade of the primary tumor. Traditionally, the mainstay of treatment for soft tissue sarcomas has been surgery.[176–178] Increasingly, it is now recognized that a multidisciplinary, multimodality approach including radiation and at times systemic chemotherapy is associated with improved outcomes for most patients with soft tissue sarcomas. Multimodality therapy in properly selected patients can improve local control rates, decrease the morbidity and quality of life impairment associated with surgery (particularly by decreasing the need for amputation to control extremity sarcomas), and increase the duration of relapse-free survival. Available evidence is insufficient to conclude that multimodality therapy results in increased overall survival durations, but at least some data suggest that it may.

Surgery

The most effective single-modality treatment for localized soft tissue sarcoma in any site is complete resection with histologically negative margins. Because many soft tissue sarcomas manifest a pseudocapsule, "shell out" procedures where tumors are removed from within this apparent capsule are associated with local recurrence rates that approach 100%. Historically, this led to the adoption of extensive radical procedures, frequently in the form of amputations, to ensure adequate local control.

Sarcoma resections are categorized as intracapsular, marginal, wide, or radical.[179] Intracapsular resections are usually a result of "shell out" of an apparently encapsulated tumor when a malignant diagnosis was not anticipated. In a marginal resection, the plane of dissection is outside the pseudocapsule but before or within the surrounding reactive zone. Wide resection consists of resection of surrounding normal tissue outside the reactive zone. In a radical resection, there must exist a natural barrier interposed between the tumor and the margin in all directions. This approach is best illustrated in compartmental resections, where an entire muscle group is resected at its origin and insertion with the fascia intact throughout (Figure 58.7).[179] In this categorization, radical resections are associated with lower local recurrence rates than other procedures when surgery is the sole modality of therapy. In multimodality approaches, however, evidence of the superiority of true radical resections is lacking, and indeed they may be associated with increased complication rates and poorer functional outcomes. For most sarcomas treated with a multimodality approach, wide excisions are the procedure of choice.

The emergence of radiation and systemic chemotherapy as potentially active agents for unresectable sarcomas led to the development of combined modality approaches that could preserve the limb with reasonable function and acceptable local control rates. Rosenberg and associates reported a prospective 2:1 randomized trial of 43 patients comparing limb-sparing surgery (wide excision) and postoperative radiation to amputation; all patients received postoperative systemic chemotherapy.[180] They found that the local recurrence rate was marginally higher in the group undergoing limb-sparing surgery ($P = 0.06$), but a large majority of patients in the limb-sparing surgery group had successful local control of their tumors. There was no statistical difference in overall survival between the two arms, but the study was far too small to reliably detect such a difference. Based on these limited data, multimodality limb-sparing approaches have become the accepted norm for the management of nearly all extremity soft tissue sarcomas. Subsequent studies evaluating limb-sparing surgery in the treatment of soft tissue sarcomas are shown in Table 58.7.

Surprisingly, evidence demonstrating that limb-sparing approaches are associated with measurably improved functional outcomes and/or quality of life compared to amputation is largely nonexistent. Functional outcome comparing patients who had amputation with those who underwent limb-sparing procedures was addressed in a study by Davis et al.,[181] who noted a trend toward increased disability in those patients undergoing amputation versus those who had limb-sparing procedures. Conversely, a study by Sugarbaker and associates found that quality of life assessments failed to

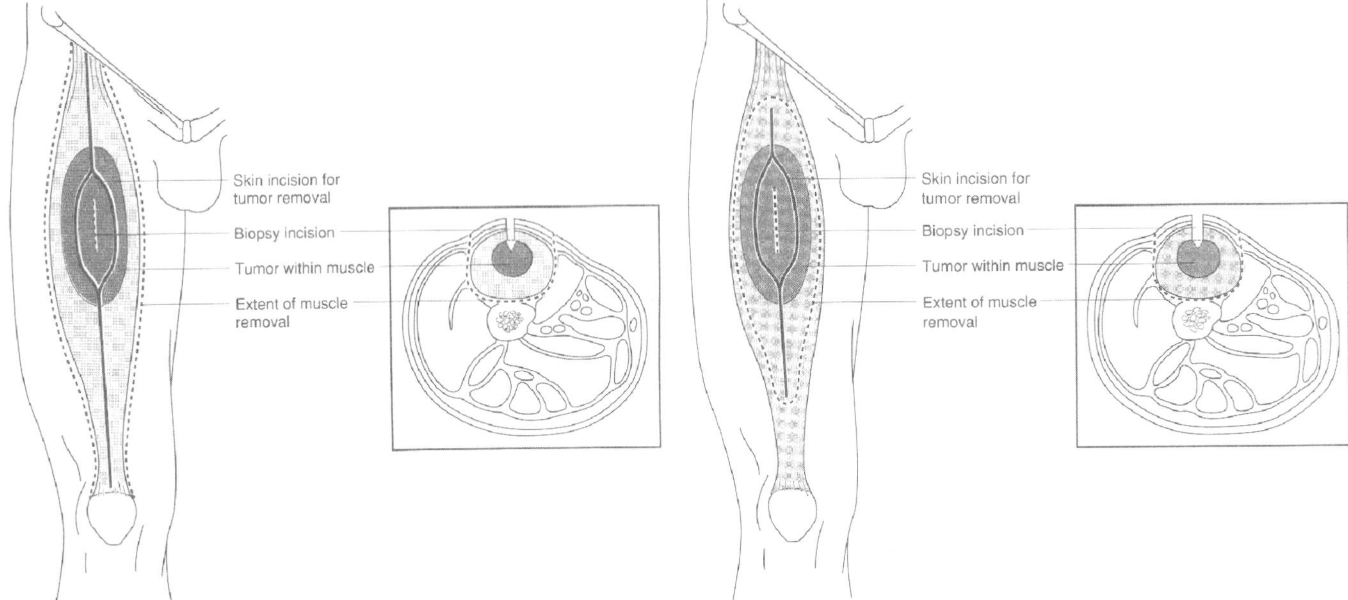

FIGURE 58.7. A compartmental resections is where an entire muscle group is resected at its origin and insertion with the fascia intact throughout.

support a benefit to limb-sparing procedures over amputations.[182] Following radical limb-sparing procedures, many patients have significant functional disability, although most are able to ambulate remarkably well.[183–185] Stinson and colleagues evaluated acute and long-term effects of limb function following limb sparing therapy,[183] reporting that 84% of patient were able to ambulate without assist devices with mild or no pain.

Encasement of nerves or blood vessels by soft tissue sarcomas is uncommon but is not in and of itself an indication for amputation. Complete resection of the sciatic nerve results in loss of knee flexion and dorsiflexion of the foot. With aggressive physical therapy and the use of an ankle-foot orthosis, however, these patients can ambulate. Brooks et al. evaluated functional status of patients following resection of the sciatic, peroneal, or tibial nerves.[186] They reported a post-

TABLE 58.7. Major studies evaluating limb-sparing surgery for soft tissue sarcomas.

Study	*N*	*LR (%)*	*OS (%)*	*Chemo**	*XRT***	*Study design*
Pisters et al., 1996[89]	164					
Brachytherapy		18	84	Yes	Yes	Prospective
No brachytherapy		31	81	Yes	No	Randomized
Brennan et al., 1987[193]	117					
Brachytherapy	52	4	88	Yes	Yes	Prospective
No brachytherapy	65	14	91	Yes	No	Randomized
Yang et al., 1998[196]	91					
Radiation	47	0	75	Yes	Yes	Prospective
No radiation	44	10	74	Yes	No	Randomized
Rosenberg et al., 1982[180]	47					
Amputation	27	0	88	Yes	Yes	Prospective
Limb salvage	16	15	83	Yes	No	Randomized
Williard et al., 1991[326]	649					
Amputation	92	6	NR	Yes	Yes	Retrospective
Limb salvage	557	15				Database Review
Henshaw et al., 2001[191]	33	6	88	Yes	Yes	Retrospective Review
Rydholm et al., 1991[192]	67	12	82	Yes	No	Retrospective Review
Pao et al., 1990[195]	50	8	68	Yes	Yes	Retrospective Review

NR, not recorded; LR, local recurrence; OS, overall survival; chemo, chemotherapy; XRT, radiation therapy.

*Variations in timing, doses, and regimens in different studies.

**Variations in dose, timing, and use in different studies.

operative leg function score of 8 of 10 and added that all patients surveyed preferred their status to amputation. A number of reports have documented the feasibility of en bloc resection of arteries and veins with autologous or prosthetic graft reconstructions.[187,188]

Current multimodality approaches can result in limb preservation with useful function and very high rates of local tumor control. Even though evidence of clear-cut superiority in functional outcome or equivalence in local control and survival when compared to amputation is lacking, sarcoma patients will almost never accept a major amputation if a nonamputative surgery is feasible. This general acceptance of the concept of limb preservation is reflected in the fact that only 5% of patients currently presenting to major centers with primary soft tissue sarcoma of the extremity are treated with amputation.[127] The weight of current evidence supports the use of limb-sparing surgery as part of the multimodality management of soft tissue sarcoma of the extremities. The optimal techniques for limb-sparing treatment have not been defined, and it is undoubtedly true that multiple effective options exist. Matching the proper combination and sequence of therapies to the needs of the individual patient remains one of the major challenges in the treatment of soft tissue sarcomas and often requires the skills of a dedicated multidisciplinary team of physicians and allied health personnel.

Radiation Therapy

Limb-sparing resection alone, particularly marginal or wide excision, has been associated with local recurrence rates up to 50% to 70%,[189,190] which sparked an interest in decreasing local recurrence with the application of radiation. Controversy continues regarding the necessity, type, and timing of radiation therapy; as in so many other situations, prospective comparative clinical trials are few, limited in statistical power, and often contradictory.[118,191,192]

Although most patients with extremity sarcomas do receive some form of radiation along with surgery, available evidence suggests that for some patients, particularly those with small, superficial, or low-grade tumors, wide excision alone is adequate treatment. In a review of 56 patients with extremity sarcoma, Rydholm and associates reported their experience using limb-sparing surgery without radiation.[192] They reported a local recurrence rate of 7%. From their experience, they questioned the necessity of radiation therapy in all extremity sarcoma patients. In contrast, other investigators have demonstrated improved local control rates with the addition of radiation therapy.[119,193–196] Confounding the impact of radiation therapy is the variability in the timing of radiation, surgical margin status, and use of adjuvant chemotherapy. From the studies to date there appears to be a decrease in local recurrence by adding radiation to resection. Studies have generally supported the omission of radiation for low-grade soft tissue sarcomas when surgical margins are widely free of tumor.[118,192,196]

It may be the case that aggressive systemic and/or regional chemotherapy can replace the need for radiation in some cases. In a study by Henshaw and associates, 33 patients were treated with preoperative intraarterial cisplatin and systemic doxorubicin.[191] Ifosfamide was added in the later part of the study. Included in this study were 18 patients with high-grade soft tissue sarcomas of the extremities and pelvis that were deemed unresectable, with the remainder of patients having large but potentially resectable high-grade soft tissue sarcomas in the extremities and pelvis. Variability in the definition of unresectability for extremity sarcomas is a major limitation when comparing studies or trying to generalize results to other institutions. In any event, only 2 of the 18 patients who initially were deemed unresectable actually underwent amputation after receiving chemotherapy. All the remaining patients were able to have limb-sparing resections. Twelve of the patients received radiation therapy, which was reserved for those with close surgical margins or limited degrees of chemotherapy-induced necrosis on histologic evaluation of the resected specimen. Two patients had local recurrences; interestingly, these occurred in the higher-risk patients treated with radiation. Disease-free survival in this study was 88% and 80% at 5 and 10 years, respectively. The authors of this study questioned the need for routine use of adjuvant radiation therapy when using aggressive intra-arterial and systemic preoperative chemotherapy.

The timing of radiation relative to surgery has also been investigated in terms of local disease control, effects on wound complications, and long-term morbidity. The use of preoperative external-beam radiation takes advantage of the presence of an intact tumor mass to delineate and limit the field of treatment. A theoretical advantage of preoperative radiation is the treatment (and presumptive sterilization) of tumor cells outside the pseudocapsule, which might otherwise seed the operative site and result in local recurrence.

Potential disadvantages are that it requires delay of the definitive surgery, which can create a psychologic stress for some patients, and that it may result in higher wound complication rates. Postoperative radiation therapy has the advantages of providing the entire tumor specimen to the pathologist for evaluation before deciding on the need for adjuvant therapy, potentially fewer wound complications, and no delay in surgery.

Taken as a whole, studies have failed to demonstrate that preoperative radiation therapy is superior to postoperative radiation. What has been identified is that preoperative radiation therapy is associated with higher wound complications whereas postoperative radiation has been found in some studies to result in increased fibrosis.[83,197–201] In a prospective randomized trial of 94 patients comparing pre- and postoperative radiation in extremity soft tissue sarcomas, O'Sullivan and colleagues[197] identified wound complications in 35% of the preoperative radiated patients versus 17% of the postoperatively treated patients, a statistically significant difference and strong evidence that wound complication rates are indeed increased after preoperative radiotherapy. No statistically significant difference in local recurrence rates was identified between the two treatment groups. Overall disability was similar between the two groups when assessed one year following therapy. The overwhelming majority of wound complications seen in the preoperatively treated patients occurred in the treatment of lower extremity tumors; wound complication rates were low after preoperative radiation for upper extremity sarcomas. The highest incidence of wound complications (45%) was seen in upper leg tumors treated with preoperative radiation therapy. A confounding element in analyzing wound complications in patients receiving radiation therapy can be the effect of chemotherapy that many patients receive during their treatment. Meric and associates performed a retrospective review of 309 patients and failed to identify an association between chemotherapy use and wound complications.[202]

The optimal method of radiation delivery has not yet been defined. The most commonly used methods are brachytherapy (implanted radiation) and external-beam radiation. Each approach has its advantages and disadvantages. To date there has not been a prospective randomized trial comparing brachytherapy to external-beam radiation. In randomized trials compared to surgery alone, the application of radiation using each technique has been associated with reduction in local recurrences. As such, the primary issues in choosing the best technique is balancing the advantages and disadvantages of each approach for individual patients. Proponents of brachytherapy cite delivery of a high dose of radiation directly to the surgical bed, limited treatment time, limited radiation to surrounding uninvolved tissues, and decreased overall costs.[203,204] Another advantage lies in its potential for use in treatment of recurrent disease in previously radiated tissues. Limitations of brachytherapy lie in its requirement for dedicated surgical and radiation oncologists with experience with this technique and limitations in the ability to treat extremely large resection beds.[119] Because brachytherapy delivers its radiation over a few days instead of many weeks, there is evidence to support the concern that low-grade tumors, with their relatively lower rates of DNA synthesis and cell division, are not well treated by brachytherapy.

With these considerations in mind, the current evidence to date would support preoperative and postoperative external-beam and postoperative brachytherapy radiation as effective methods for local tumor control in large, high-grade soft tissue sarcomas. Our current approach is to tailor therapy to the tumor location, patient ability to complete prescribed therapy, and, most importantly, patient preference.

Adjuvant Systemic Chemotherapy

As with most major issues in the treatment of localized soft tissue sarcomas, the role of chemotherapy remains controversial and the quality of available evidence is variable. Patients with localized soft tissue sarcomas are generally able to achieve local control through surgery and radiation. Unfortunately, roughly 50% will go on to develop distant metastasis, and most of those will die as a direct consequence.[190] Patients with large (more than 5 cm) and high-grade sarcomas are clearly more likely to develop metastatic disease and die than those with smaller or low-grade tumors. Some investigators have observed that local recurrence also places patients at higher risk of distant metastasis, even when all visible disease can be removed by reresection or amputations.[205, 206] This finding suggests but does not prove that lowering local recurrence rates can ultimately enhance relapse-free and overall survival rates. Importantly, adjuvant systemic therapy for osteosarcoma has been shown repeatedly to significantly and markedly improve local control and relapse-free and overall survival rates.

Experience in the treatment of measurable metastatic sarcoma has identified doxorubicin and ifosfamide to have the highest response rates, and the response rates for osteosarcoma and soft tissue sarcoma are relatively similar.[190,207,208] Extrapolating from experience in osteosarcoma, first-generation clinical trials of adjuvant therapy for soft tissue sarcomas were usually doxorubicin based (often with single-agent doxorubicin) and used relatively low doses. Factors that often varied between studies were drug doses, tumor histologic subtypes, anatomic sites, methods of delivery, and timing of therapy. These studies gave inconsistent results; however, there appeared to be some evidence of improvement in relapse-free survival. A meta-analysis was performed evaluating 14 trials composed of 1,568 patients with localized resectable soft tissue sarcomas, including both extremity and nonextremity primary sites.[209] The analysis revealed a 27% relative reduction in local recurrence in patients treated with chemotherapy, translating to an absolute benefit of 6% fewer local recurrences at 10 years. The relative reduction in distant metastasis-free survival was 30%, with an absolute benefit of 10% at 10 years. Adjuvant chemotherapy resulted in a 25% relative reduction in relapse-free survival, with a resultant 10% absolute benefit at 10 years; this corresponded to an overall improvement in recurrence-free survival from 45% without adjuvant chemotherapy to 55% with its use. Overall survival, however, was not improved significantly by the use of chemotherapy. There was a trend toward improved survival with a potential absolute benefit of 4%, which translated to an overall survival improvement from 50% to 54%.

Several criticisms of this meta-analysis have been raised.[190,207,210] The first relates to the time frame of these studies compared to contemporary treatment practices: the most recent study included in the meta-analysis completed accrual in 1990. Since that time, higher doses of chemotherapy and more-effective agents such as ifosfamide have become standard for adjuvant therapy. By grouping patients with extremity and nonextremity sarcomas together, the meta-analysis may have been biased against detecting an impact of adjuvant therapy in extremity sarcoma patients, where surgery and radiation eradicate all local tumor in a higher percentage of patients. Nonetheless, as the primary goals of adjuvant chemotherapy are to improve relapse-free and overall survival, the modest absolute relapse-free survival increase of 10% at 10 years and questionable benefit in overall survival are concerning. These findings suggest that 90% of patients treated with chemotherapy would not gain any advantage from adjuvant treatment compared to providing the same or similar chemotherapy upon relapse; this is an important consideration, in that chemotherapy can result in significant toxicities, diminished overall quality of life, and even in rare cases treatment-related deaths.

In the face of the limitations of the meta-analysis, a subsequent trial from Italy has been widely touted as more contemporary support for the use of chemotherapy in the treatment of soft tissue sarcomas. In this prospective randomized trial of 104 patients with large high-grade soft tissue sarcomas of the extremities, Frustaci and associates evaluated the adjuvant use of epirubicin (an anthracycline cytotoxic drug similar in efficacy and toxicity to doxorubicin) and ifosfamide.[211] The study was closed early secondary to an interim analysis revealing a statistically significant improvement in relapse-free survival in the patients in the chemotherapy arm. The median follow-up was 59 months at the time of this interim analysis, which demonstrated a 41% relative reduction in the risk of disease relapse, translating to an absolute benefit of 27% from chemotherapy at 2 years and 13% at 4 years. Local disease-free survival was not found to be statistically significant between the treatment groups, with the treatment arm having 9 local recurrences and 11 in the control arm ($P = 0.07$). Overall survival favored the treatment arm, with an absolute improvement at 4 years of 19%.

Early termination of a randomized trial due to a highly significant treatment effect requires exceeding a stringent threshold and is the strongest possible evidence of superior efficacy for an investigational therapy. In essence, it means it would be unethical to continue to treat patients on the study with the control regimen (in this case surgery and radiation without systemic adjuvant chemotherapy), and by strong and direct implication, similar patients in the nonprotocol setting as well. Once early termination of a trial takes place, subsequent follow-up of the trial data may be compromised by the smaller than anticipated number of study patients and/or by cross-over of control arm patients to the now recognized superior treatment arm. Indeed, longer-term follow-up of the patients on this study reported at a median of 89 months of follow-up, indicated that the statistically significant survival advantage observed at the interim analysis was no longer present.[212] Time to disease progression, median survival, and survival at 4 years still favored the treatment arm in the extended analysis, which for the reasons described above cannot be considered to invalidate the interim analysis finding.

What are we to take from this body of literature when considering adjuvant chemotherapy for patients with localized disease? The current evidence supports the contention that doxorubicin and ifosfamide are the most active agents currently available and appear to be most effective at relatively high doses, although there is likely a plateau beyond which further dose escalation is not helpful and may be harmful.[190,211–218] These high-dose chemotherapy regimens are toxic and frequently require dose reduction and/or hematopoietic growth factor support to complete therapy. From data compiled through meta-analysis and more-contemporary reports, the benefit from the use of adjuvant chemotherapy may be real. However, this benefit will be confined to a minority of treated patients; others will be cured by local therapy alone or relapse despite the addition of chemotherapy. These factors must be considered when weighing the risks and benefits in adjuvant chemotherapy for an individual patient.

At present, the use of adjuvant chemotherapy in the treatment of intermediate- and high-grade soft tissue sarcomas likely confers a small advantage in local control, time to disease progression, and overall survival when high-dose doxorubicin- and ifosfamide-based regimens are used. Our preference is to provide adjuvant chemotherapy treatment of soft tissue sarcomas under strict protocol-based regimens or in the context of prospective clinical trials. Preoperative or neoadjuvant chemotherapy may have practical advantages over postoperative chemotherapy, not the least of which is the ability to monitor response or lack thereof and alter or terminate therapy in patients who do not appear to be deriving any benefit. Preoperative and postoperative chemotherapy have never been directly compared in randomized trials, however.

Regional Chemotherapy

The fact that so many sarcomas arise in the extremities has prompted investigation of cytotoxic chemotherapeutic agents administered intraarterially. This method has the theoretical advantage of maximizing the dose of drug to the tumor and minimizing the dose delivered systemically to the patient. The relative pharmacologic advantage of intraarterial therapy compared to intravenous administration depends on the degree of "first-pass" extraction of the drug in the perfused tissues. Doxorubicin has a high degree of first-pass extraction in peripheral tissues, conveying a moderate advantage in tumor to systemic drug levels compared to intravenous administration of the same dose. Cisplatin, another drug commonly used for intraarterial therapy of sarcomas, has a much lower degree of first-pass extraction and hence there is relatively little pharmacologic advantage to its intraarterial administration.[219] Intraarterial administration has significant complexity and risks, requires inpatient hospitalization, and results in limiting the systemic antitumor effects of the drug to the same extent that it augments the regional intratumoral effects. Evidence directly supporting the use of intraarterial chemotherapy in extremity soft tissue sarcomas is minimal, essentially anecdotal. One small, randomized trial (90 patients total) compared intravenous to intraarterial doxorubicin when identical doses were administered as part of a preoperative chemoradiation strategy. This trial was only published in abstract form, but insufficient advantage for intraarterial administration was noted and the authors (hitherto the primary advocates for intraarterial doxorubicin administration) abandoned the technique.[220]

Several investigators have attempted to increase the therapeutic advantage of intraarterial drug administration by the use of isolated limb perfusion, a technique commonly applied in the treatment of extremity-confined melanomas. In this technique, surgical isolation of the extremity vasculature and directed circulation of most or all the blood of the extremity through an extracorporeal membrane oxygenator and pump ("heart bypass" machine) minimizes the systemic administration of drug and allows for very high, even otherwise potentially lethal, doses of drug to be circulated intraarterial for a period of time and then extracted in the venous effluent and discarded. Many soft tissue sarcomas present in advanced stages, adjacent to neurovascular structures or with local recurrences where resection may be difficult. From experimental evidence and experiences in the treatment of melanoma patients, most investigators have employed melphalan, tumor necrosis factor-alpha (TNF-α) or occasionally doxorubicin in the treatment of extremity soft tissue sarcomas.[221–231] A multi-institutional experience of 186 patients treated with isolated limb perfusion with TNF-α and melphalan (plus gamma interferon in some cases) for primary or recurrent extremity soft tissue sarcomas was reported by Eggermont and colleagues.[231] Eighty-two patients had an objective tumor response. At a median follow-up of 2 years, the limb salvage rate was 82%. TNF-α is not available in the United States, and results with melphalan or other drugs in the isolation perfusion of sarcomas have been much less encouraging. Studies evaluating the use of isolated limb perfusion are summarized in Table 58.8.

At present evidence supports a possible role for isolated limb perfusion with TNF-α in carefully selected patients with locally advanced or multifocal soft tissue sarcomas when amputation is the only surgical alternative. Whether limb perfusion is worthwhile for sarcoma patients if only melphalan is available is less clear, but it is still advocated by some.[232]

TABLE 58.8. Major studies evaluating isolated limb perfusion for soft tissue sarcomas.

Study	*N*	*Agents*	*Hyperthermia (°C)*	*Limb salvage (%)*	*Design*
Eggermont et al., 1996[231]	186	TNF, melphalan	39–40	82	Review of multiinstitutional experience
McBride et al., 1974[222]	79	Melphalan, dactinomycin	NR	83	Review of institutional experience
Lev-Chelouche et al.,[228]	53	TNF, melphalan	39–40	85	Review of institutional experience
Lejeune et al., 2000[230]	22	TNF, melphalan	38–40	86	Review of institutional experience
Rossi et al., 1999[225]	27	TNF, doxorubicin	40.5–41.5	85	PhaseI/II prospective trial

NR, not recorded; TNF, tumor necrosis factor.

Treatment of Localized Retroperitoneal Soft Tissue Sarcoma

Surgery

Retroperitoneal soft tissue sarcomas have unique clinical characteristics and pose distinct clinical challenges, which distinguish them from the more-common extremity sarcomas. Patients typically present with very large tumors, often with minimal symptoms. Although the most common site of first recurrence for patients with extremity sarcomas is in the form of distant metastatic disease, patients with retroperitoneal sarcomas are more prone to recur within the abdominal cavity. The overall survival for patients with extremity sarcomas is superior to that of patients with retroperitoneal sarcomas. Local failure is evident in nearly 90% of patients who die of retroperitoneal sarcomas,[233] a fact that reflects the large tumor size on presentation, inability to achieve wide surgical margins, and limitations of adjuvant radiation and chemotherapy. Local failure continues to occur beyond 5 and 10 years following resection, leading to some to estimate the overall recurrence rate for resectable retroperitoneal sarcomas exceeds 70%.[234,235]

As for extremity primaries, surgery is the mainstay of treatment for retroperitoneal sarcomas. Because of the limitations of adjuvant therapy, including the inability to deliver high doses of radiation secondary to limited tolerance of bowel, kidneys, liver, and the spinal cord, surgery is somewhat more likely to be used as the only modality for treatment of these tumors. Reports describing experience in the surgical management of primary retroperitoneal soft tissue sarcomas are summarized in Table 58.9. The data in this table

TABLE 58.9. Major studies of the treatment of primary retroperitoneal soft tissue sarcomas.

Study	*N**	*Complete** resection (%)*	*LR*** (%)*	*OS† 5-year (%)*	*OS‡ 10-year (%)*	*Study design*
Lewis et al., 1998[129]	500	80	59	70	NR	Retrospective review of prospectively collected data
Jaques et al., 1990[239]	114	65	49	NR	NR	Retrospective review of prospectively collected data
Stoeckle et al., 2001[251]	165	65	48	46	NR	Registry review
Cody et al., 1981[243]	158	66	33	40	NR	Retrospective case series
Alvarenga et al., 1989[249]	120	30	46	29	NR	Retrospective case series
Dalton et al., 1990[247]	116	54	68	40	22	Retrospective case series
Catton et al., 1994[244]	104	43	50	55	22	Retrospective case series
Hassan et al., 2004[254]	97	78	44	51	NR	Retrospective review
Karakousis et al., 1995[246]	90	100	25	66	57	Retrospective case series
Bevilacqua et al., 1991[245]	80	65	29	57	NR	Retrospective case series
Kilkenny et al., 1996[237]	63	78	40	56	NR	Retrospective case series
Zornig et al., 1991[250]	51	59	24	35	15	Retrospective case series
McGrath et al., 1984[241]	47	38	61	70	58	Retrospective case series
Salvadori et al., 1986[242]	43	42	39	NR	NR	Retrospective case series
Wang et al., 1996[255]	40	70	68	42	NR	Retrospective review
Pirayesh et al., 2001[253]	22	41	45	22	NR	Retrospective review
Solla et al., 1986[248]	20	35	43	43	NR	Retrospective case series

NR, not reported.

*Total patients in study including some presenting with recurrent disease.

**Percent resected with primary retroperitoneal sarcomas.

***Percent local recurrences in those who had complete surgical resection for primary retroperitoneal sarcoma.

†Five-year overall survival of those who had complete surgical resection for primary retroperitoneal sarcoma.

‡Five-year overall survival of those who had complete surgical resection for primary retroperitoneal sarcoma.

focus on primary retroperitoneal sarcomas that have no evidence of metastatic disease. These reports have consistently documented the significance of complete resection of all gross disease in improving local control and disease-specific survival. In most reports, complete excision is achieved less than 70% of the time, with local recurrence occurring in approximately half of patients undergoing complete resection. The impact of local recurrence is reflected in diminished overall survival despite attempts at further resections.[129,236] Results for resection of recurrent retroperitoneal sarcomas are notably worse, in both the percentage of patients who can be resected free of all disease and those who remain recurrence free long term.

With the possible exception of low-grade retroperitoneal liposarcomas, no survival benefit has been observed when incomplete resection is undertaken.[129,237–240] Major complication rates are identical, however, for partial and complete resections. Thus, patients undergoing incomplete resection procedures are exposed to all the morbidity with none of the potential survival benefit of their counterparts who undergo complete excision. This result emphasizes the need for careful preoperative planning as well as determination of unresectability early in the operative procedure so that incomplete resections are not mandated because the surgeon has passed "the point of no return."

Retroperitoneal liposarcomas represent a distinct situation where a more-aggressive surgical approach, including multiple resections for repeated recurrences and even occasionally incomplete resections, may be justified. Liposarcomas in this location have been observed to have a lower incidence of distant metastases (7%) when compared to 15% to 34% for other histologic subtypes.[236,239,241] Shibata and associates observed prolongation in survival in patients with partial resection in patients with liposarcomas when compared with those who only had biopsy.[236] Further, they reported effective palliation of symptoms in 75% of symptomatic patients who underwent debulking procedures.

Identification of prognostic factors other than the adequacy of resection has been inconsistent across studies. Tumor size has not been identified as a predictor of survival, with the recognition that virtually all retroperitoneal sarcomas are larger than 5 cm at presentation. Tumor grade has been found to be significant in some studies but not in others, with the weight of evidence supporting shorter recurrence-free and overall survival for patients with high-grade tumors.[129,233,235,237,239,241–256]

The clinical presentation and imaging evaluation of retroperitoneal sarcomas were discussed previously. Important in the next step is determining resectability from these studies. It is often difficult to determine preoperatively if adjacent vascular structures or organs are involved with tumor. Vascular involvement was noted in 34% of patients undergoing resection in a review by Kilkenny and colleagues.[237] In cases where tumor is near major vessels but routine CT scanning cannot resolve whether the vessels are in fact involved, we have turned to MR angiography or CT angiography. Multivisceral resections are required in the majority of cases (63%–86%), most frequently involving the kidney, colon, small bowel, pancreas, and bladder.[129,237,239,243,248,254] Our experience and that of others have shown that it can difficult to determine whether adjacent organs will be attached or freely separable based on preoperative imaging. In planning resection one must be prepared for the high likelihood of extensive en bloc resections to achieve this goal. No surgeon should operate on a retroperitoneal mass unless he or she is prepared for the magnitude of the resection that may be required.

Radiation

Several investigators have explored methods to decrease the incidence of local failure following resection. Extrapolating from evidence supporting improved local disease control with the use of radiation therapy in the trunk and extremities, radiation therapy is widely used as an adjunct to surgery in retroperitoneal sarcomas. There are important differences, however, that make radiation therapy more problematic and call into question its value for patients with retroperitoneal tumors. To date, no randomized trial has documented the value of adjuvant radiation for retroperitoneal sarcomas, so evaluations of its benefit are confined to retrospective analyses.

Proponents of preoperative radiation therapy cite the theoretical advantages of using the tumors bulk to displace uninvolved intrabdominal viscera, thereby decreasing local toxicity and increasing the ability to administer therapeutic doses.[234,235,257] This approach also allows the target volume to be easily delineated for treatment planning, and treating the tumor before manipulation at the time of surgery could theoretically decrease the likelihood of tumor implantation. Resection is usually performed between 4 to 6 weeks after the completion of radiation. Postoperative external-beam radiation at doses that are most likely to be effective[258,259] can be associated with significant acute and delayed bowel toxicity.[233,260] After removal of the large tumor mass that had been displacing adjacent viscera, the bowel tends to fall into the resection bed and often becomes fixed there by postoperative adhesions. However, as in the extremities, postoperative radiation has advantages, including the ability to examine the entire tumor and the excision margins pathologically before deciding on the need for radiation as well as allowing for the completion of healing and recovery from surgery and complications thereof before instituting radiation. The areas of greatest concern for residual tumor and/or the closest surgical margins can be delineated and given focally higher doses of radiation in many cases. Contrary to some reports, we have successfully used postoperative radiation for retroperitoneal sarcomas over nearly two decades with acceptable acute toxicity and very little in the way of severe chronic toxicity. Radiation should not be automatically withheld from patients who have undergone complete resection, especially with close or involved margins, merely because they are postoperative.

That notwithstanding, the limitations of deliverable dose and the large volumes of the abdomen and pelvis that need to be radiated, whether preoperatively or postoperatively, have led many investigators to explore techniques to augment the effectiveness and/or minimize the toxicity of delivered radiation. Cytotoxic chemotherapy may be combined with radiation, but this combination is often poorly tolerated in patients with a large intraabdominal tumor or convalescing from its recent removal. As reviewed by Storm, studies have generally relied on doxorubicin-based regimens and have not demonstrated convincing improvements in disease-free or overall survival.[261] Nonetheless, a growing body of evidence suggests the combination can be administered to carefully selected patients.[262] The current evidence for the use of adju-

TABLE 58.10. Major studies of the treatment of retroperitoneal soft tissue sarcomas with intraoperative radiation therapy.

*Study**	*N*	*Local recurrence (%)*	*Preoperative XRT*	*Postoperative XRT*
Sindelar et al., 1993**	35			
IORT	15	40	No	Yes
No IORT	20	80	No	Yes
Gieschen et al., 2001***	37			
IORT	20	17	Yes	No
No IORT	17	51	Yes	No
Alektiar et al., 2000***	32	38	No	Yes
Bobin et al., 2003***	22	50	Yes	Yes
Gunderson et al., 1993***	19	15	No	Yes
Willet et al., 1991***	10	10	Yes	No

IORT, intraoperative radiation therapy.

*Studies frequently included primary and recurrent retroperitoneal soft tissue sarcomas. Some patients also treated with chemotherapy regimens.

**Prospective randomized trial.

***Prospective nonrandomized trial.

Sources: References 265, 327–331.

vant chemotherapy in the treatment of sarcomas is reviewed in the section on treatment of extremity sarcomas.

Other approaches have also been evaluated. In a Phase I/II trial using preoperative radiation therapy and the radiosensitizer idoxuridine (also known as IUdR or iododeoxyuridine), which does not have direct antitumor effects, in the treatment of retroperitoneal soft tissue sarcomas, Sondak and associates treated 16 patients with alternating weeks of continuous intravenous infusional iododeoxyuridine and twice-daily radiation therapy before surgery. Patients received a total of five cycles of therapy, either entirely preoperatively or split with three cycles before and two afterward.[263] This effort resulted in an overall local control rate of 45% at 24 months; local control was achieved in 5 of the 8 patients who had complete resection with acceptable toxicity. An alternative approach to intensifying the radiation dose to the tumor bed was conducted in a trial by Jones and associates in which 55 patients with resectable primary or recurrent retroperitoneal sarcomas were treated with preoperative external-beam and postoperative brachytherapy.[264] Forty-six patients had complete resections, with 41 completing preoperative radiation therapy and 23 having brachytherapy. Preoperative radiation therapy was well tolerated, but those treated with brachytherapy experienced significant toxicity, including 1 death. Sondak et al. reported overall 2-year relapse-free and overall survival of 80 and 88%, respectively.

Another approach that has been investigated is the use of intraoperative radiation. Once an enormously complicated undertaking wherein anesthetized surgical patients needed to be transported to treatment machines in the Radiation Oncology Department with their abdomens open, intraoperative radiation is now practically achieved at a number of centers with specially designed and shielded operating rooms equipped with built-in radiation devices. With this technique, the resection bed can be directly targeted to a high dose while nearby radiosensitive tissues are mechanically retracted out of the treatment field. A summary of studies investigating the use of intraoperative radiation therapy is shown in Table 58.10. Unfortunately, the weight of evidence, including one small randomized trial,[265] suggests that intraoperative radiation increases in-field tumor control but not recurrence-free or overall survival, as patients recur just outside the treatment field, and that it adds significant late toxicity.

Local Recurrence

In the absence of metastatic disease, repeat resection when able to remove all gross disease is the treatment of choice for locally recurrent retroperitoneal sarcomas. Many studies have shown that a significant number of patients experience prolonged disease-free survival when all gross disease can be resected. The addition of chemotherapy or radiation in the treatment of locally recurrent disease remains the subject of debate. Given the extremely high risk of further local and distant recurrence, all patients who have not previously received adjuvant therapy should be considered for it after resection of recurrent disease. Subsequent recurrences have progressively diminishing chances for resection. Evidence for the benefit of third and subsequent resections of retroperitoneal sarcomas is scant and largely limited to studies of patients with low-grade liposarcomas. Such aggressive attempts at disease control should almost always be relegated to centers with significant expertise in the management of retroperitoneal tumors.

Treatment of Gastrointestinal Stromal Tumors

Gastrointestinal stromal tumors (GIST) are uncommon tumors believed to originate from the interstitial cells of Cajal in the alimentary tract. These cells form a smooth muscle cellular network to function as a pacemaker of gut motility.[266,267] Gastrointestinal stromal tumors are most commonly found in the stomach (39% to 70%), small intestine (20% to 32%), colon and rectum (5% to 15%), and esophagus (less than 5%) (Figure 58.8).[266–269] The true incidence of these tumors is unclear, because population studies frequently fail to distinguish GIST from gastrointestinal carcinomas.

Traditionally, GIST have been considered to be benign, malignant, or "borderline." The evidentiary basis for this distinction is suspect, but it is clearly difficult to determine if a GIST will metastasize by its light microscopic appearance alone. Studies investigating features most associated with malignant behavior have found tumor size (more than 5 cm), mitotic count (more than 1–5 per 10 high-power fields), tumor necrosis, and most recently immunohistochemical identification of c-Kit (CD117) mutation to be important.[266–270] In most studies that have attempted to use this type of classification, approximately one-third of GIST are classified as "malignant."[271] In nearly all studies, however, tumors classified as "benign" or "borderline" manifest unequivocally malignant behavior (i.e., metastasis) in a small percent of cases. Hence, available evidence would suggest that all GIST should be considered to be malignant neoplasms at low, intermediate, or high risk for developing metastatic disease. Whether there is a subset of GIST that are unequivocally benign, with no propensity whatsoever to metastasize, remains to be proven.

Treatment of GIST has traditionally relied on complete resection. Complete resection of GIST has been reported in the range of 48% to 89% of cases; long-term disease-free survival has been reported to be 18% to 35% and overall survival from 28% to 43%.[271,272] Metastatic GIST are virtually resistant to standard chemotherapeutic agents. Therefore, it is not surprising that the use of adjuvant chemotherapy with cytotoxic agents has been disappointing. In a retrospective review of a multicenter experience in the treatment of GIST with chemotherapy, De Pas and associates found no evident survival benefit from the addition of chemotherapy.[273] The addition of radiation therapy has similarly been limited in its effectiveness in the treatment of GIST.[268]

Identification of c-Kit mutations in GIST has been the focus of extensive recent attention. The Kit protein is a transmembrane protein receptor that is structurally similar to the macrophage colony-stimulating factor receptor. A gain-of-function mutation of exon 11 of the c-Kit gene in GIST tumors was described by Hirota and colleagues, corresponding to the intracellular juxtamembrane region of the c-Kit protein.[274] Additional sites of mutation have been identified within the c-Kit gene in GIST tumors, with the observation that mutated Kit protein products are constitutively activated in the absence of its stem cell factor ligand.[267,275] Alternatively, the platelet-derived growth factor receptor (PDGFR)-α has been found to be mutated and activating in a significant percentage of GIST that lack activating mutations in c-Kit.[276]

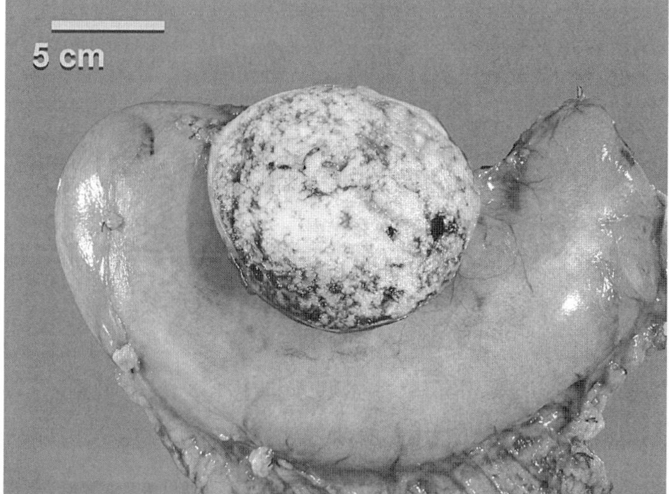

FIGURE 58.8. Bisected gastrointestinal stromal tumor arising from the lesser curvature of the stomach.

Experimental results demonstrated that the use of the tyrosine kinase inhibitor imatinib mesylate (Gleevec) targets the BCR-ABL fusion protein found in chronic myeloid leukemia and is available in an oral formulation.[277] Additional studies of imatinib demonstrated activity against other protein tyrosine receptors including PDGFR-α and Kit. With this background, Joensuu and associates treated a patient with rapidly progressive, chemotherapy-resistant metastatic GIST with imatinib.[278] This protocol resulted in a dramatic response that was sustained for more than 11 months with minimal toxicity. This observation prompted clinical trials using imantinib in the treatment of GIST.[279,280] Results of these studies demonstrated an effective initial dose range of 400 to 800 mg per day, which has since been approved by the U.S. Food and Drug Administration for the treatment of metastatic and/or unresectable GIST.[281] It remains to be determined whether it is better to initiate treatment at the lower end of the effective dose range and increase the dose if necessary because of inadequate efficacy, or to start at the high end of the dose range and decrease the dose in case of toxicity. It is clear, however, that some patients who progress on lower doses of imatinib respond to higher doses, whereas other patients who have prohibitive toxicity at higher doses still derive clinical benefit from doses lower than the usual starting range.

Several investigators have noted that reliance on traditional clinical parameters for measurement of response to imatinib therapy may not be ideal in the treatment of GIST. Benjamin et al. found that time to progression following treatment did not correlate with RECIST criteria of change in size.[208] Instead, these investigators were able to correlate time to progression with changes in glucose uptake detected by positron emission tomography (PET) scanning. They found PET achieved a sensitivity of 94% and specificity of 100% in identifying response to treatment, and was more predictive of time to progression, than CT assessment of tumor size. Other investigators have also highlighted the usefulness of PET in evaluating response to imantinib therapy.[282] Tumors may manifest little if any change in size on CT scans yet show dramatic decreases in activity on PET scans (Figure 58.9). Unfortunately, even tumors that have shown dramatic responses to imatinib eventually progress in most cases, sometimes after several years. Second-line tyrosine kinase inhibitors are in active clinical investigation; if these prove useful, it would be logical to investigate combination therapy with imatinib in future clinical trials.

Although GIST is a rare tumor, it represents an important model for the use of biologically targeted therapy, where an identified molecular alteration is targeted by a specific therapy with clinically relevant results. Another approach currently under investigation is the use of imatinib in the adjuvant and neoadjuvant setting. Whether adjuvant approaches can decrease recurrence, improve survival, and turn unresectable tumors into those that can be completely resected requires prospective testing in clinical trials.

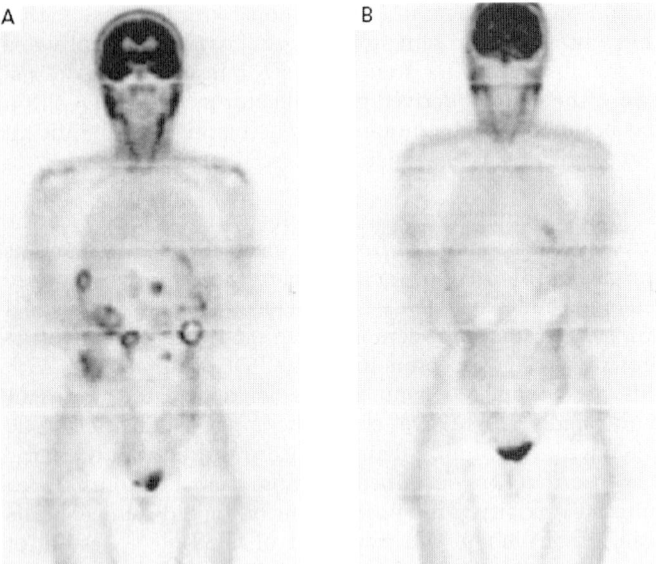

FIGURE 58.9. Positron emission tomography (PET) studies with [18F]fluorodeoxyglucose as the tracer. (A) Before STI571 therapy, multiple metastases are seen in the liver and upper abdomen, with marked retention of [18F]fluorodeoxyglucose in the right renal pelvis and ureter, a finding suggestive of hydronephrosis. (B) After 4 weeks of treatment, no abnormal uptake of tracer is seen in the liver or right kidney.[278]

Treatment of Localized Soft Tissue Sarcomas of Selected Other Sites

Trunk, Heart, and Great Vessels

Sarcomas arising in the soft tissues of the trunk/body wall have been found to follow a clinical course similar to that observed in the extremities. Sarcomas arising in this location account for approximately 10% to 20% of newly diagnosed sarcomas; they are usually over 5cm in size and can involve underlying viscera (Figure 58.10). Treatment principles are derived from the experience with extremity sarcomas, with aggressive attempts at wide excision to achieve clear margins and consideration of chemotherapy and radiation for large high-grade tumors. Soft tissue sarcomas arising from chest wall musculature and diaphragm are quite rare. Treatment of these tumors is based on the general principle of wide resection with clear margins. Radiation therapy can be considered for large lesions, particularly when high grade; however, underlying lung tissue may limit the dose that can be delivered.

Sarcomas are the most common primary malignant neoplasm arising in the heart and are usually angiosarcomas.[189] They may arise from the heart or the pericardium and may be asymptomatic. These tumors are usually advanced when identified, and curative resection is difficult. Surgical removal has been the mainstay of therapy.[283] The rarity of these tumors has not allowed the role of adjuvant therapies to be extensively evaluated. Often surgery is aimed at alleviating symptoms rather than cure. Cardiac allotransplantation, alone or with lung transplantation as well, has been performed in anecdotal cases, but seems to be associated with poor results for high-grade tumors.[284]

The aorta and vena cava are occasionally involved by direct extension of retroperitoneal sarcomas; however, sarcomas arising de novo from the great vessels are rare. Leiomyosarcomas are the predominant histologic type encountered arising from the vena cava and other named veins. Treatment is again based on complete resection with clear surgical margins.[285,286] Mingoli and colleagues reported the results of resection of 218 patients compiled from an international registry of inferior vena cava leiomyosarcomas.[287] Of 120 patients who underwent radical resection with complete removal of all gross disease and clear microscopic margins, caval wall resection with autologous vein or prosthetic patch repair was performed in 44%, and segmental caval resection was performed in 56%. Of the 67 patients who underwent caval resection, 27 had infrarenal caval ligation and 23 had supracaval ligation. The authors reported 3 postoperative deaths, 21 deep venous thromboses, and 7 major complications. There was a local recurrence rate of 57% (mean follow-up of 32 months). These results support a role for resection to clear margins. We have utilized patch repair following caval wall resection or segmental resection with prosthetic graft placement and avoid ligation of the cava if possible (Figure 58.11). The role of adjuvant therapies in the treatment of tumors in this location remains undefined.

Breast

Primary breast sarcomas comprise less than 5% of all soft tissue sarcomas and can be subdivided into two categories. So-called monophasic or stromal sarcomas are identical to their counterparts arising elsewhere in the body. The most commonly encountered histologic types of these primary breast sarcomas are malignant fibrous histiocytoma, angiosarcoma, and liposarcomas.[189,288–290] The second category are sarcomas specific to the breast, entitled cystosarcoma phyllodes or, more generically, phyllodes tumors. Because the pathologic and clinical characteristics of phyllodes tumors are quite distinct from other histologic types they are addressed separately.

From retrospective series, primary breast sarcomas have a peak incidence during the fourth and fifth decades and most commonly present as a painless breast mass. These tumors

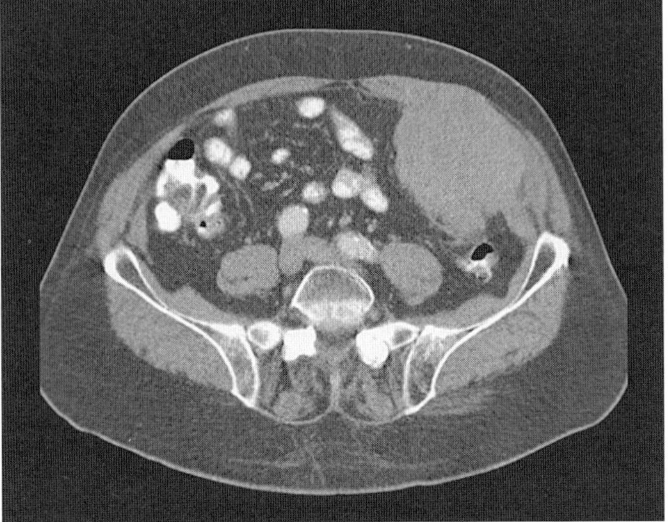

FIGURE 58.10. Computed tomography of high-grade undifferentiated pleomorphic sarcoma arising from the left abdominal wall musculature.

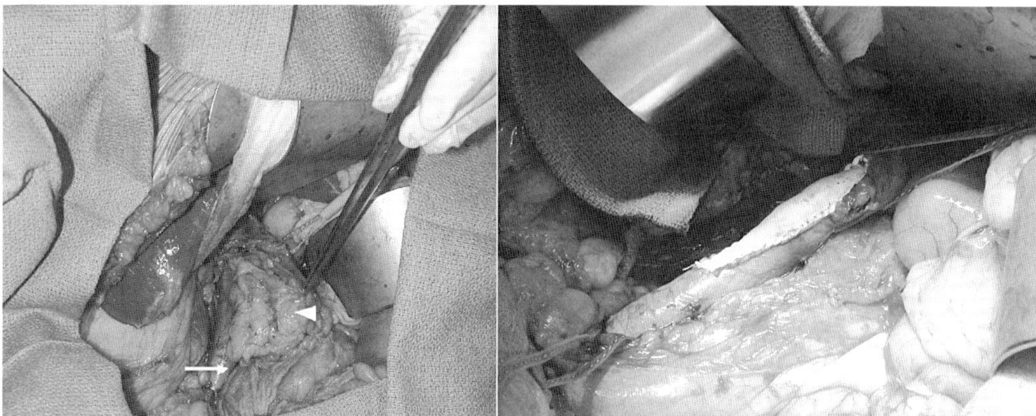

FIGURE 58.11. Left: Leiomyosarcoma (*arrowhead*) arising from the anterior wall of the inferior vena cava (*arrow*). Right: Patch repair of inferior vena cava following resection.

are often mistaken for a fibroadenoma as lymphadenopathy, skin changes, nipple discharge, and other signs typical of breast malignancy are almost always absent. Treatment of primary breast sarcomas is based on experience with extremity and trunk soft tissue sarcomas. Surgical treatment is tailored to breast conservation if the volume of normal breast would be adequate to allow a wide resection of the sarcoma with a 1- to 2-cm circumferential margin. In cases in which breast conservation would not result in a cosmetically acceptable appearance, simple mastectomy is appropriate. Postoperative radiation is often added to decrease local recurrence, particularly if the margin of excision was less than 2 cm (regardless of whether the breast was conserved). Local recurrence, disease-free survival, and overall survival rates following resection are similar to those observed in soft tissue sarcomas arising in other locations. Also, such considerations regarding the addition of adjuvant chemotherapy are the same as discussed in the treatment of extremity sarcomas. As lymph node metastases are exceeding rare in primary breast sarcomas, axillary dissection is not warranted unless clinically palpable nodes are present.[189,288,289]

Phyllodes tumors are fibroepithelial or "biphasic" tumors that arise exclusively in breast tissue. They also have a peak incidence during the fourth and fifth decades of life, typically presenting as a painless breast mass. Some patients report a long-standing mass that begins to grow rapidly. Analogous to gastrointestinal stromal tumors, the propensity to metastasize is often difficult to determine histologically. It has been estimated that 25% of cases are "malignant," but cases deemed to be benign have been associated with the development of distant metastasis. Thus, the evidence would suggest that phyllodes tumors span a spectrum from very low to very high risk of metastasis. Whether any phyllodes tumors can be unequivocally considered to be benign, with no possibility whatsoever of distant metastasis, remains a matter of debate.

Local recurrence of phyllodes tumors is common (16%–22%), so that wide excision with a 1- to 2-cm margin, by mastectomy if necessary, is appropriate therapy.[189,291,292] Radiation and chemotherapy can be considered for cases deemed at high risk of recurrence or metastasis, but the role of each modality is as yet poorly defined in the treatment of phyllodes tumors.

Treatment of Metastatic Disease

Half of all patients with soft tissue sarcomas ultimately develop metastatic disease. Metastases are present in about 10% of patients at time of initial presentation.[127,293] The predominant site of first recurrence is in the lung, seen in 52% of patients who developed local or distant disease (70% of patients with extremity primaries). Patients with retroperitoneal sarcomas have a greater tendency for local recurrence and disseminated disease throughout the abdomen. As reported by Potter and colleagues, 80% of recurrences occur within 5 years.[294]

Approximately 80% of patients with extremity and trunk soft tissue sarcomas who have distant disease have isolated pulmonary metastases.[2,130] The detection of pulmonary metastatic disease is accomplished by either plain film radiographs or CT scanning of the thorax. CT scans have a greater sensitivity in detecting small (3–10) mm pulmonary nodules than plain film radiographs, which has led many clinicians to use CT rather than plain films when evaluating for pulmonary metastases.[189] On the other hand, this greater sensitivity to small nodules means that many subcentimeter benign nodules are identified on CT scans, especially in older patients. Proving these nodules to be benign can be difficult, and their detection often leads to concern for metastasis for patient and physician alike. PET scans were evaluated by Lucas et al. in comparison with CT scans,[295] who reported a sensitivity in detecting pulmonary disease of 87% with a specificity of 100%. Conversely, CT scans had a sensitivity of 100% and a specificity of 96%. PET scanning does poorly at detecting subcentimeter pulmonary nodules and cannot always distinguish malignancy from inflammation or postoperative changes. The available evidence does not support a role for PET in the routine screening for or evaluation of pulmonary metastases, particularly given its limited availability and high cost.

Once detected, pulmonary metastases have associated with median survival rates of 6 to 12 months.[2,296] Because of the strong predilection for sarcoma to metastasize to the lungs and only to the lungs, resection of even multiple pulmonary metastases (metastasectomies) has been shown in multiple reports to be associated with prolonged relapse-free survival in a small but significant percentage of patients (probably at least 25%).[189,293,297–299] Several prognostic features associated with long-term survival in patients undergoing pulmonary metastasectomy have been identified. In an evaluation of soft tissue sarcoma pulmonary metastases, Billingsley and associates observed a more favorable prognosis for those who had complete resection of all metastases, a disease-free interval of more that 12 months or a low-grade primary tumor.[298] Adverse findings included histologies of liposarcomas and malignant peripheral nerve sheath tumors as well as age greater than 50. A relationship between outcome and time interval from initial diagnosis to the development of pulmonary metastases has been observed in multiple studies, although this may be largely or entirely a surrogate for histologic grade of the primary tumor.[189,296–300] Greater numbers of metastatic nodules and rapid tumor doubling times have been associated with diminished survival following resection of soft tissue sarcoma pulmonary metastases.[189] Reported survival rates following complete resection of pulmonary metastases (sometimes with repeated thoracotomies) range from 25% to 39% at 5 years.[189,293,297,299] From published reports to date, an aggressive approach to resection of pulmonary metastases is warranted.

Resection of soft tissue sarcoma hepatic metastases has also been evaluated. Survival rates following hepatic resection have generally been less than observed in pulmonary resections for metastatic disease. One series of soft tissue sarcoma patients undergoing hepatic resections of metastases reported a 100% recurrence rate.[301] Despite this, a median survival time of 30 months for resected patients compared with 11 months for unresected patients was found. The inclusion of many patients with what are now recognized to be gastrointestinal stromal tumors in most series describing sarcoma metastatic to the liver makes interpretation of these series more complex.

The role of chemotherapy in the treatment of unresectable metastatic disease has been extensively reviewed.[190,302] Doxorubicin, ifosfamide, and dacarbazine have all been shown to have significant single-agent activity in the treatment of metastatic soft tissue sarcomas. Although published reports of various combinations of available drugs have suggested them to be superior to single-agent therapy,[303] to date there is little evidence from prospective randomized trials to support that contention. One randomized trial is representative: the addition of ifosfamide to doxorubicin increased response rates at the expense of significantly greater toxicity but did not result in any detectable difference in time to progression or overall survival.[304]

The influence of drug dose intensity has been studied in numerous retrospective and prospective evaluations. There is considerable evidence to support the contention that the two most active drugs, doxorubicin and ifosfamide, yield better results in terms of response rates and time to progression if given at high doses. The range over which increased dose leads to increased benefit is fairly narrow, however, and not entirely defined. One recent report is sobering: patients randomized to receive doxorubicin plus $6\,g/m^2$ ifosfamide actually had slightly superior survival compared to patients randomized to the same dose of doxorubicin plus $12\,g/m^2$ ifosfamide.[218] Reports of even higher doses of chemotherapy along with stem cell rescue have demonstrated the feasibility of this approach; however, its role in the treatment of metastatic soft tissue sarcomas has yet to be determined.[305–307]

There is no consensus whatsoever regarding the ideal second-line chemotherapy regimen for patients with metastatic disease refractory to combination therapy with doxorubicin and ifosfamide. Higher doses of ifosfamide (in the range of $12–14\,g/m^2$) have been associated with objective responses in patients who failed or progressed after chemotherapy with lower doses of ifosfamide, with synovial sarcomas appearing to be particularly responsive to this approach.[308,309] The toxicity of ifosfamide in this range of doses mandates careful patient selection and excludes many older patients and those with impaired renal function. Recently, the combination of gemcitabine and docetaxel in specific sequence has been associated with high objective response rates, even in patients with prior doxorubicin and ifosfamide chemotherapy. This regimen appears to be particularly effective for patients with leiomyosarcomas,[310] but responses in other histologies have been seen as well.[311] Low doses of chemotherapy administered more chronically have received some evaluation in sarcoma subtypes. Low-dose paclitaxel has been used for angiosarcomas[312] and low-dose methotrexate and vinblastine for desmoid tumors.[313,314] Although substantial data attest to differential sensitivities of various sarcoma subtypes to particular chemotherapy regimens, prospective evaluations of specific regimens for individual subtypes have been limited, and it is likely that hitherto unrecognized patterns of susceptibility and resistance exist. Clinical trials remain a highly appropriate option for patients with metastatic soft tissue sarcomas of all histologic subtypes. Novel approaches to clinical trials design are also worthy of exploration, given the multiple potential interactions of drug type, dose, and schedule with histologic subtype and prior treatment status.[315]

Specialty Centers

Several investigators have highlighted the importance of early referral to centers with specialists with experience in treating soft tissue sarcomas.[151,152,316,317] Soft tissue masses are common, with benign soft tissue masses exceeding malignant tumors 100 to 200 fold.[316] As such, physicians frequently treat benign tumor without significant consequence. Unfortunately, malignant soft tissue tumors are more often than not approached with the same lack of concern and are not taken as seriously as masses arising in other locations. In a regional audit of the management of soft tissue sarcomas in England, Clasby and associates found only 21% of patients were investigated adequately and only 60% were treated with wide excision or surgery with radiation.[318] They reported that in 331 patients who had undergone resections, only 104 had a preoperative biopsy and 26% of patients had not had any form of radiologic investigation. They found junior surgeons initially treated two-thirds of soft tissue sarcoma patients, whereas senior surgeons in 80% of cases performed second operations. In an similar audit conducted in France, Ray-Coquard et al. found only 42% of patients had a preoperative biopsy.[319] They identified deficiencies in the initial evaluation in 48% of patients where MRI, chest radiographs, and clinical record of tumor size were frequently omitted. No more than 7% of patients in this study had biopsies planned and performed after formal multidisciplinary review. These studies illustrate a number of difficulties associated with the evaluation and referral of soft tissue tumors. As Clasby and colleagues observed, only 17% of patients were treated with an initial wide margin, with 67% left with an unacceptable margin.[318] Similarly, Ray-Coquard et al. found 74% with inadequate initial resections. As discussed previously, initial failure to achieve clear surgical margins will result in higher local recurrence rates, with the associated poor prognostic implications associated with local recurrences.[319]

Referral to a specialty center with experience in soft tissue sarcomas should be initiated for subfascial masses of any size, tumors greater than 3 to 5 cm, masses that are noted to be changing in size, or any physical findings worrisome for malignancy. These findings may include proximity to neurovascular structures, painful masses, and tumors that are firm or fixed to underlying structures. When evaluating any soft tissue mass one should always consider these factors to maintain an index of suspicion for such lesions. With better education and early referral, we can expect improved oncologic outcomes with less morbidity associated with surgical treatment.

Surveillance Guidelines

When deciding the appropriate surveillance plan for an individual following treatment for soft tissue sarcoma, several considerations arise. The impact of early detection on therapy and patient outcome varies by anatomic location of the recurrent disease. In cases of local recurrence of extremity soft tissue sarcomas, reresection can result in prolonged survival, improved quality of life, and cure in a significant number of patients. The majority (90%) of extremity local recurrences occur during the first 5 years after treatment, of which up to two-thirds are detected during the first 2 years.[300] In a retrospective review of surveillance for follow-up of patients with high-grade extremity sarcomas, Whooley and associates evaluated the efficacy and cost-effectiveness of chest radiographs, CT scans of chest, imaging of the affected extremity, and blood tests.[320] Follow-up evaluations were performed every 3 months during the first 2 years, every 4 to 6 months during the third posttreatment year, every 6 months for years 4 to 5, and annually thereafter. Their review found that physical examination was the most common method of detection of local recurrence (97%), with only one recurrence detected solely by surveillance MR (3%). Pulmonary metastasis was identified in 40% of patients, but only 37% of these patients with pulmonary had symptoms as a basis for detection. Asymptomatic patients had their pulmonary metastasis initially detected with chest radiographs in 83% of cases. In the remainder of patients, pulmonary metastases were detected solely with CT scanning. Metastasectomy was performed on 24 of 36 asymptomatic patients with pulmonary recurrence. Blood tests did not contribute to the detection of any local or distant recurrence.

From their analysis of cost to effectiveness, Whooley et al. concluded that chest radiographs and physical examination were the most useful and cost-effective methods for the detection of local or distant metastasis.[320] They recommended a surveillance program intensified during the early portion of the posttreatment period. They also recommended cross-sectional imaging (CT or MR) every 6 months in cases of deep lesions or in radiated regions where physical examination is difficult.

Similar studies delineating the most useful and cost-effective methods for the detection of local recurrence and distant metastases for other disease sites have not been performed. For soft tissue sarcomas in sites such as head, neck, and trunk, where patterns of failure are similar to those for extremity primaries, it would appear reasonable to follow a similar approach. For intraabdominal and retroperitoneal sarcomas, failure is primarily within the abdomen as in the liver; an additional 20% to 30% of recurrences will occur in the lungs. With this in mind, it would seem appropriate to have the patient undergo physical examination, CT scanning of the abdomen, and chest radiographs as a surveillance strategy. Early detection of local recurrence, metastases to the liver, and pulmonary metastases occasionally results in surgical intervention; it is assumed but not proven that such interventions may prolong survival and improve quality of life.[129,298,299,301] Time to recurrence for intraabdominal and retroperitoneal sarcomas is also highest in the early posttreatment period, and a similar schedule of evaluation used in extremity sarcomas would seem reasonable. These sarcoma surveillance strategies remain to be proven in prospective trials, but are widely used and almost universally recommended, with some controversy remaining as to the incremental value of chest CT scans over radiographs alone. The current National Comprehensive Cancer Network (NCCN) guidelines for the surveillance of soft tissue sarcomas arising in the extremity and retroperitoneum are summarized in Table 58.11.

TABLE 58.11. Surveillance guidelines for extremity soft tissue sarcomas.

Stage I	*Stage II, III*
-H&P every 3–6 mo for 2–3 y, then annually	-H&P every 3–4 mo for 3 y, then every 6 mo for next 2 y, then annually
-Consider imaging surgical site with scan annually based on estimated risk of locoregional recurrence	-Imaging of primary site (MRI, CT, consider US)
-Consider baseline imaging after primary therapy	-Chest imaging (plain radiograph or chest CT) every 3–6 mo for 5 y, then annually
-Consider chest X-ray every 6–12 mo	
Surveillance Guidelines for Retroperitoneal Soft Tissue Sarcomas	
Low grade	*High grade*
Physical exam with imaging (chest/abdomen/pelvis CT) every 3–6 mo for 2–3 y, then annually	Physical exam with imaging (chest/abdomen/pelvis CT) every 3–4 mo for 3 y, then every 6 mo for next 2 y, then annually

MRI, magnetic resonance imaging; CT, computed tomograpy; mo, months; y, years.

Source: Reference 332.

The use of PET scanning in the evaluation and surveillance of GIST is currently under investigation. At present, guidelines do not incorporate PET scans for the routine surveillance of GIST; however, this may change due to the advent of effective therapy (imatinib). To date, there are no compelling data to suggest that PET scanning has a routine role in the initial management or posttreatment surveillance of soft tissue sarcomas other than GIST.

Conclusion

The evaluation and treatment of soft tissue sarcomas remains challenging. Advances in pathology and molecular biology have greatly improved our understanding of this complex and heterogeneous group of tumors. Since the 1980s, aggressive treatment approaches by experienced multidisciplinary teams have improved the outlook for these patients. The widespread acceptance of limb-sparing procedures, the identification of active chemotherapy regimens, and improvements in local disease control from the use of radiation therapy are all examples of the strides that have been made in the treatment of patients with soft tissue sarcoma. Despite these advances, areas of concern remain. Most distressing is the fact that approximately half of patients diagnosed with soft tissue sarcomas will succumb to their disease. Local recurrence remains a difficult problem, with increased associated morbidity and psychologic stress for affected patients. Through improved education, we hope that early biopsy and referral of soft tissue sarcomas will become the norm, and that patients will derive the benefits of multidisciplinary evaluation and treatment of their disease.

References

1. Jemal A, Murray T, Ward E, et al. Cancer statistics, 2005. CA Cancer J Clin 2005;55(1):10–30.
2. Brennan MF, Lewis JJ. Diagnosis and Management of Soft Tissue Sarcoma. London: Dunitz, 2002.
3. Sorensen SA, Mulvihill JJ, Nielsen A. Long-term follow-up of von Recklinghausen neurofibromatosis. Survival and malignant neoplasms. N Engl J Med 1986;314(16):1010–1015.
4. Gutmann DH, Wood DL, Collins FS. Identification of the neurofibromatosis type I gene product. Proc Natl Acad Sci USA 1991;88(21):9658–9662.
5. Korf BR. Malignancy in neurofibromatosis type I. Oncologist 2000;5:477–485.
6. Surace EI, Haipek CA, Gutmann DH. Effect of merlin phosphorylation on neurofibromatosis 2 (NF2) gene function. Oncogene 2004;23(2):580–587.
7. Gutmann DH. The neurofibromatoses: when less is more. Hum Mol Genet 2001;10(7):747–755.
8. Li LP, Fraumeni JF. Soft tissue sarcomas, breast cancer and other neoplasms: a familial syndrome? Ann Intern Med 1969;71:747–752.
9. Malkin D, Li F, Strong LC, et al. Germline p53 mutations in a familial syndrome of sarcomas, breast cancer and other neoplasms. Science 1990;250:1233–1238.
10. Varley JM. Germline TP53 mutations and Li-Fraumeni syndrome. Hum Mutat 2003;21:313–320.
11. Fletcher O, Easton D, Anderson K, Gilham C, Jay M, Peto J. Lifetime risks of common cancers among retinoblastoma survivors. J Natl Cancer Inst 2004;96(5):357–363.
12. Zacksenhaus E. Alternative reading frame suggests an alternative model for retinoblastoma. Cell Cycle 2003;2:27–30.
13. Calvert PM, Frucht H. The genetics of colorectal cancer. Ann Intern Med 2002;137:603–612.
14. Yahanda AM SV, Sass FM, Fearon RM. Etiology of an attenuated colonic polyposis phenotype in familial desmoid disease. Proc Soc Surg Oncol 1988:11.
15. Su L-K, Vogelstein B, Kinzler KW. Association of the APC tumor suppressor protein with catenins. Science 1993;262(5140):1734–1737.
16. Martland HS. Occupational poisoning in manufacture of luminous watch dials. JAMA 1929;92(6):466–473.
17. Cahan WG, Woodard HQ, Higinbotham NL, Stewart FW, Coley BL. Sarcoma arising in irradiated bone: report of eleven cases. Cancer (Phila) 1948;1:3–29.
18. Kim JH, Chu FC, Woodard HQ, Melamed MR, Huvos A, Cantin J. Radiation-induced soft-tissue and bone sarcoma. Radiology 1978;129:501–508.
19. Brady MS, Gaynor JJ, Brennan MF. Radiation-associated sarcoma of bone and soft tissue. Arch Surg 1992;127:1379–1385.
20. Hawkins MM. Second primary tumors following radiotherapy for childhood cancer. Int J Radiat Oncol Biol Phys 1990;19:1297–1301.
21. Taghian A, De Vathaire F, Terrier P, et al. Long-term risk of sarcoma following radiation treatment for breast cancer. Int J Radiat Oncol Biol Phys 1991;21:361–367.
22. Tucker MA, D'Angio GJ, Boice JD Jr, et al. Bone sarcomas linked to radiotherapy and chemotherapy in children. N Engl J Med 1987;317:588–593.
23. Weatherby RP, Dahlin DC, Ivins JC. Postradiation sarcoma of bone. Mayo Clin Proc 1981;56:294–306.
24. Lagrange J-L, Ramaioli A, Chateau M-C, et al. Sarcoma after radiation therapy: retrospective multiinstitutional study of 80 histologically confirmed cases. Radiology 2000;216:197–205.
25. Menu-Branthomme A, Rubino C, Shamsaldin A, et al. Radiation dose, chemotherapy and risk of soft tissue sarcoma after solid tumours during childhood. Int J Cancer 2004;110:87–93.
26. Scanlon EF, Berk RS, Khandekar JD. Postirradiation neoplasia: a symposium. Curr Prob Cancer 1978;111(6):4–35.
27. Amendola BE, Amendola MA, McClatchey KD, Miller CH Jr. Radiation-associated sarcoma: a review of 23 patients with postradiation sarcoma over a 50-year period. Am J Clin Oncol 1989;12(5):411–415.
28. Huvos AG, Woodard HQ, Cahan WG, et al. Postradiation osteogenic sarcoma of bone and soft tissues. Cancer (Phila) 1985;55:1244–1255.
29. Mermershtain W, Cohen AD, Koretz M, Cohen Y. Cutaneous angiosarcoma of breast after lumpectomy, axillary lymph node dissection, and radiotherapy for primary breast carcinoma. Am J Clin Oncol 2002;25(6):597–598.
30. Mark RJ, Poen J, Tran LM, Fu YS, Selch MT, Parker RG. Postirradiation sarcomas. Cancer (Phila) 1994;73(10):2653–2662.
31. Tountas AA, Fornasier VL, Harwood AR, Leung PMK. Postirradiation sarcoma of bone: a perspective. Cancer (Phila) 1979;43:182–187.
32. Laskin WB, Silverman TA, Enzinger FM. Postradiation soft tissue sarcomas. Cancer (Phila) 1988;62:2330–2340.
33. Wiklung TA, Blomqvist CP, Raty J, Elomaa I, Rissanen P, Miettinen M. Postirradiation sarcoma. Cancer (Phila) 1991;68:524–531.
34. Hatfield PM, Schulz MD. Post irradiation sarcoma including 5 cases after x-ray therapy of breast carcinoma. Radiology 1970;96:593–602.
35. Phillips TL, Sheline GE. Bone sarcoma following radiotherapy. Radiology 1963;81:992–996.

36. Doherty MA, Rodger A, Langlands AO. Sarcoma of bone following therapeutic irradiation for breast carcinoma. Int J Radiat Oncol Biol Phys 1986;12:103–106.
37. dos Santos Silva I, Jones M, Malveiro F, Swerdlow A. Mortality in the Portuguese Thorotrast Study. Radiat Res 1999;152:S88–S92.
38. Mori T, Kido C, Fukutomi K, et al. Summary of entire Japanese Thorotrast Follow-up Study: updated 1998. Radiat Res 1999;152:S84–S87.
39. Ron E. Cancer risks from medical radiation. Health Phys 2003;85(1):47–59.
40. Platz EA, Wiencke JK, Kelsey KT, et al. Chromosomal aberrations and hprt mutant frequencies in long-term American thorotrast survivors. Int J Radiat Biol 2000;76(7):955–961.
41. Neglia JP, Friedman DL, Yasui Y, et al. Second malignant neoplasms in five-year survivors of childhood cancer: Childhood Cancer Survivor Study. J Natl Cancer Inst 2001;93(8):618–629.
42. Sieber SM, Correa P, Dalgard DW, Adamson RH. Carcinogenic and other adverse effects of procarbazine in nonhuman primates. Cancer Res 1978;38:2125–2134.
43. Stewart FW, Treves N. Lymphangiosarcoma in postmastectomy lymphedema: a report of six cases in elephantiasis chirurgica. Cancer (Phila) 1948;1:64–81.
44. Lindeman G, McKay MJ, Taubman KL, Bilous AM. Malignant fibrous histiocytoma developing in bone 44 years after shrapnel trauma. Cancer (Phila) 1990;66(10):2229–2232.
45. Ben-Izhak O, Vlodavsky E, Ofer A, Engel A, Nitecky S, Hoffman A. Epithelioid angiosarcoma associated with a dacron vascular graft. Am J Surg Pathol 1999;23(11):1418–1425.
46. Fehrenbacher JW, Bowers W, Strate R, Pittman J. Angiosarcoma of the aorta associated with a dacron graft. Ann Thorac Surg 1980;32(3):297–301.
47. O'Connell TX, Fee HJ, Golding A. Sarcoma associated with dacron prosthetic material. J Thorac Vasc Surg 1976;72(1):94–96.
48. Fyfe BS, Quintana CS, Kaneko M, Griepp RB. Aortic sarcoma four years after dacron graft insertion. Ann Thorac Surg 1994;58:1752–1574.
49. Burns WA, Kanhouwa S, Tillman L, Saini N, Herrmann JB. Fibrosarcoma occurring at the site of a plastic vascular graft. Cancer (Phila)1971;29(1):66–72.
50. Weinberg DS, Maini BS. Primary sarcoma of the aorta associated with a vascular prosthesis: a case report. Cancer (Phila) 1979;46(2):398-402.
51. Hayman J, Huygens H. Angiosarcoma developing around a foreign body. J Clin Pathol 1983;36:515–518.
52. Ben-Izhak O, Kerner H, Brenner B, Lichtig C. Angiosarcoma of the colon developing in a capsule of a foreign body. Am J Clin Pathol 1991;97(3):416–420.
53. Dube VE, Fisher DE. Hemangioendothelioma of the leg following metallic fixation of the tibia. Cancer (Phila) 1972;30(5):1260–1266.
54. Brand KG. Diversity and complexity of carcinogenic processes: conceptual inferences from foreign-body tumorigenesis. J Natl Cancer Inst 1976;57(5):973–976.
55. Ferguseon DJ. Cellular attachment to implanted foreign bodies in relation to tumorigenesis. Cancer Res 1977;37:4367–4371.
56. Moizhess TG, Vasiliev JM. Early and late stages of foreign-body carcinogenesis can be induced by implants of different shapes. Int J Cancer 1989;44:449–453.
57. Rous P. Transmission of a malignant growth by means of a cell free filtrate. JAMA 1911;56:198.
58. Dictor M, Rambech E, Way D, Witte M, Bendsoe N. Human herpesvirus 8 (Kaposi's sarcoma-associated herpesvirus) DNA in Kaposi's sarcoma lesions, AIDS Kaposi's sarcoma cell lines, endothelial Kaposi's sarcoma simulators, and the skin of immunosuppressed patients. Am J Pathol 1996;148(6):2009–2016.
59. McClain KL, Leach CT, Jenson HB, et al. Association of Epstein-Barr virus with leiomyosarcomas in young people with AIDS. N Engl J Med 1995;332(1):12–18.
60. Engels EA, Katki HA, Nielsen NM, et al. Cancer incidence in Denmark following exposure to poliovirus vaccine contaminated with simian virus 40. J Natl Cancer Inst 2003;95(7):532–539.
61. Suruda AJ, Ward EM, Fingerhut MA. Identification of soft tissue sarcoma deaths in cohorts exposed to dioxin and to chlorinated naphthalenes. Epidemiology 1993;4(1):14–19.
62. Wingren G, Fredrikson M, Brage HN, Nordenskjold B, Axelson O. Soft tissue sarcoma and occupational exposures. Cancer (Phila) 1990;66(4):806–811.
63. Eriksson M, Hardell L, Adami H-O. Exposure to dioxins as a risk factor for soft tissue sarcoma: a population-based case-control study. J Natl Cancer Inst 1990;82(6):486–490.
64. Hardell L, Eriksson M. The association between soft tissue sarcomas and exposure to phenoxyacetic acids. Cancer (Phila) 1988;62(3):652–656.
65. Hardell L, Sandstrom A. Case-control study: soft-tissue sarcomas and exposure to phenoxyacetic acids or chlorophenols. Br J Cancer 1979;39:711–717.
66. Coggin D, Acheson ED. Do phenoxy herbicides cause cancer in man? Lancet 1982;1:1057–1059.
67. Smith AH, Pearce NE, Fisher DO, Giles HJ, Teague CA, Howard JK. Soft tissue sarcoma and exposure to phenoxy herbicides and chlorophenols in New Zealand. J Natl Cancer Inst 1984;73(5):1111–1117.
68. Axelson O, Sundell L. Herbicide exposure, mortality and tumor incidence. An epidemiological investigation on Swedish railroad workers. Work Environ Health 1974;11:21–28.
69. Fingerhut MA, Halperin WE, Marlow DA, et al. Cancer mortality in workers exposed to 2,3,7,8-tetrachlorodibenzo-*p*-dioxin. N Engl J Med 1991;324(4):212–218.
70. Bertazzi PA, Consonni D, Bachetti S, et al. Health effects of dioxin exposure: a 20-year mortality study. Am J Epidemiol 2001;153(11):1031–1044.
71. Tuomisto JT, Pekkanen J, Kiviranta H, Tukiainen E, Vartiainen T, Tuomisto J. Soft tissue sarcoma and dioxin: a case-control study. Int J Cancer 2003;108:893–900.
72. Greenwald P, Kovasznay B, Collins DN, Therriault G. Sarcomas of soft tissues after Vietnam Service. J Natl Cancer Inst 1984;73(5):1107–1109.
73. Frumkin H. Agent Orange and cancer: an overview for clinicians. CA Cancer J Clin 2003;53(4):245–255.
74. Cole P, Trichopoulos D, Pastides H, et al. Dioxin and cancer: a critical review. Regul Toxicol Pharmacol 2003;38(3):378–388.
75. Belli S, Bertazzi P, Comba P, et al. A cohort study on vinyl chloride manufacturers in Italy: study design and preliminary results. Cancer Lett 1987;35: 253–261.
76. Buffler PA, Wood S, Eifler C, et al. Mortality experience of workers in a vinyl chloride monomer production plant. J Occup Med 1979;21:195–203.
77. Byren D, Engholm G, Englund A, et al. Mortality and cancer morbidity in a group of Swedish VCM and PVC production workers. Environ Health Perspect 1976;17:167–170.
78. Cooper WC. Epidemiologic study of vinyl chloride workers: mortality through December 31, 1972. Environ Health Perspect 1981;41:101–106.
79. Elliott P, Kleinschmidt I. Angiosarcoma of the liver in Great Britain in proximity to vinyl chloride sites. Occup Environ Med 1997;54:14–18.
80. McLaughlin JK, Lipworth L. A critical review of the epidemiologic literature on health effects of occupational exposure to vinyl chloride. J Epidemiol Biostat 1999;4:253–275.

81. Bosetti C, La Vecchia C, Lipworth L, McLaughlin J. Occupational exposure to vinyl chloride and cancer risk: a review of the epidemiologic literature. Eur J Cancer Prev 2003;12(5):427–430.
82. Helman LJ, Meltzer P. Mechanisms of sarcoma development. Nat Rev 2003;3:685–694.
83. Nielsen OS, Cummings B, O'Sullivan B, Catton C, Bell RS, Fornasier VL. Preoperative and postoperative irradiation of soft tissue sarcomas: effect on radiation field size. Int J Radiat Oncol Biol Phys 1991;21:1595–1599.
84. Enzinger and Weiss's Soft Tissue Tumors, 4th ed. St. Louis: Mosby, 2001.
85. Soft tissue sarcoma. AJCC Cancer Staging Manual, 6th ed. New York: Springer, 2002.
86. LeVay J, O'Sullivan B, Catton C, et al. Outcome and prognostic factors in soft tissue sarcoma in the adult. Int J Radiat Oncol Biol Phys 1993;27(5):1091–1099.
87. Mandard AM, Petiot JF, Marnay J, et al. Prognostic factors in soft tissue sarcomas. Cancer (Phila) 1989;63:1437–1451.
88. Trojani M, Contesso G, Coindre JM, et al. Soft-tissue sarcomas of adults: study of pathological prognostic variables and definition of a histopathological grading system. Int J Cancer 1984;33: 37–42.
89. Pisters PWT, Leung DHY, Woodruff J, Shi W, Brennan MF. Analysis of prognostic factors in 1,041 patients with localized soft tissue sarcomas of the extremities. J Clin Oncol 1996;14(5): 1679–1689.
90. Collin C, Godbold J, Hajdu SI, Brennan MF. Localized extremity soft tissue sarcoma: an analysis of factors affecting survival. J Clin Oncol 1987;5(4):601–612.
91. Weitz J, Antonescu CR, Brennan MF. Localized extremity soft tissue sarcoma: improved knowledge with unchanged survival over time. J Clin Oncol 2003;21(14):2719–2725.
92. Singer S, Corson JM, Gonin R, Labow B, Eberlein TJ. Prognostic factors predictive of survival and local recurrence for extremity soft tissue sarcoma. Ann Surg 1994;219(2):165–173.
93. Tsujimoto M, Aozasa K, Ueda T, Morimura Y, Komatsubara Y, Doi T. Multivariate analysis for histologic prognostic factors in soft tissue sarcomas. Cancer (Phila) 1988;62:994–998.
94. Ravaud A, Bui NB, Coindre JM, et al. Prognostic variables for the selection of patients with operable soft tissue sarcomas to be considered in adjuvant chemotherapy trials. Br J Cancer 1992; 66:961–969.
95. Ruka W, Emrich LJ, Driscoll D, Karakousis CP. Clinical factors and treatment parameters affecting prognosis in adult high-grade soft sarcomas: a retrospective review of 267 cases. Eur J Surg Oncol 1989;15:411–423.
96. Coindre J-M, Terrier P, Bui NB, et al. Prognostic factors in adult patients with locally controlled soft tissue sarcoma: a study of 546 patients from the French Federation of Cancer Centers Sarcoma Group. J Clin Oncol 1996;14(3):869–877.
97. Ueda T, Aozasa K, Tsujimoto M, et al. Multivariate analysis for clinical prognostic factors in 163 patients with soft tissue sarcoma. Cancer (Phila) 1988;62:1444–1450.
98. Rooser B, Attewell R, Rydholm A. Survival in soft tissue sarcoma. Acta Orthop Scand 1987;58:516–522.
99. Markhede G, Angervall L, Stener B. A multivariate analysis of the prognosis after surgical treatment of malignant soft-tissue tumors. Cancer (Phila) 1982;49:1721–1733.
100. El-Jabbour JN, Akhtar SS, Kerr GR, et al. Prognostic factors for survival in soft tissue sarcoma. Br J Cancer 1990;34(6):857–861.
101. Lack EE, Steinberg SM, White DE, et al. Extremity soft tissue sarcomas: analysis of prognostic variables in 300 cases and evaluation of tumor necrosis as a factor in stratifying higher-grade sarcomas. J Surg Oncol 1989;41:263–273.
102. Hill MA, Gong C, Casey TJ, et al. Detection of K-ras mutations in resected primary leiomyosarcoma. Cancer Epidemiol Biomarkers Prev 1997;6(12):1095–1100.
103. Heslin MJ, Cordon-Cardo C, Lewis JJ, Woodruff JM, Brennan MF. Ki-67 detected by MIB-1 predicts distant metastasis and tumor mortality in primary, high grade extremity soft tissue sarcoma. Cancer (Phila) 1998;83:490–497.
104. Duda RB, Cundiff C, August CZ, Wagman LD, Bauer KD. Growth factor receptor and related oncogene determination in mesenchymal tumors. Cancer (Phila) 1993;71:3526–3530.
105. Ozaki T, Ikeda S, Kawai A, et al. Alterations of retinoblastoma susceptible gene accompanied by c-myc amplification in human bone and soft tissue tumors. Mol Cell Biol 1993;39:235–242.
106. Dias P, Kumar P, Marsden HB, et al. n-Myc gene is amplified in alveolar rhabdomyosarcomas (RMS) but not in embryonal RMS. Int J Cancer 1990;45:593–596.
107. Barrios C, Castresana JS, Kreicbergs A. Clinicopathologic correlations and short-term prognosis in musculoskeletal sarcoma with c-myc oncogene amplification. Am J Clin Oncol 1994;17: 273–276.
108. Oliner JD, Kinzler KW, Meltzer PS, George DL, Vogelstein B. Amplification of a gene encoding a p53-associated protein in human sarcomas. Nature (Lond) 1992;358(6381):80–83.
109. Cordon-Cardo C, Latres E, Drobnjak M, et al. Molecular abnormalities of mdm2 and p53 genes in adult soft tissue sarcomas. Cancer Res 1994;54(3):794–799.
110. Nakayama T, Toguchida J, Wadayama B, Kanoe H, Kotoura Y, Sasaki MS. MDM2 gene amplification in bone and soft-tissue tumors: association with tumor progression in differentiated adipose-tissue tumors. Int J Cancer 1995;64:342–346.
111. Leach FS, Tokino T, Meltzer P, et al. p53 Mutation and MDM2 amplification in human soft tissue sarcomas. Cancer Res 1993;53(10):2231–2234.
112. Wadayama B, Toguchida J, Yamaguchi T, Sasaki MS, Kotoura Y, Yamamuro T. p53 expression and its relationship to DNA alterations in bone and soft tissue sarcomas. Br J Cancer 1993;68: 1134–1139.
113. Hieken TJ, Das Gupta TK. Mutant p53 expression: a marker of diminished survival in well-differentiated soft tissue sarcoma. Clin Cancer Res 1996;2(8):1391–1395.
114. Wolf RE, Enneking WF. The staging and surgery of musculoskeletal neoplasms. Orthop Clin N Am 1996;27(3):473–481.
115. Enneking WF, Spanier SS, Goodman MA. A system for the surgical staging of musculoskeletal sarcoma. Clin Orthop 1980;153: 106–120.
116. Myhre J, O., Kaae S, Madsen EH, Sneppen O. Histopathological grading in soft-tissue tumors: relation to survival in 261 surgically treated patients. Acta Pathol Microbiol Immunol Scand 1983;91A:145.
117. Ramanathan RC, A'Hern RA, Fisher C, Thomas JM. Modified staging system for extremity soft tissue sarcomas. Ann Surg Oncol 1999;6(1):57–69.
118. Geer RJ, Woodruff J, Casper ES, Brennan MF. Management of small soft-tissue sarcoma of the extremity in adults. Arch Surg 1992;127:1285–1289.
119. Suit HD, Mankin HJ, Wood WC, Proppe KH. Preoperative, intraoperative, and postoperative radiation in the treatment of primary soft tissue sarcoma. Cancer (Phila) 1985;55:2659–2667.
120. Heise HW, Myers MH, Russell WO, et al. Recurrence-free survival time for surgically treated soft tissue sarcoma patients. Cancer (Phila) 1986;57:172–177.
121. Brennan MF. Staging of soft tissue sarcomas. Ann Surg Oncol 1998;61(1):8–9.
122. Ruka W, Emrich LJ, Driscoll D, Karakousis CP. Prognostic significance of lymph node metastasis and bone, major vessel, or

nerve involvement in adults with high-grade soft tissue sarcomas. Cancer (Phila) 1988;62:999–1006.
123. Weingrad DN, Rosenberg SA. Early lymphatic spread of osteogenic and soft-tissue sarcomas. Surgery (St. Louis) 1978; 84(2):231–240.
124. Fong Y, Coit DG, Woodruff JM. Lymph node metastasis from soft tissue sarcoma in adults. Ann Surg 1993;217:72–77.
125. Lee YT, Moore TM, Schwinn CP. Metastasis of sarcomatous lesion in regional lymph node. J Surg Oncol 1982;20:53–58.
126. Mazeron J-J, Suit HD. Lymph nodes as sites of metastases from sarcomas of soft tissue. Cancer (Phila) 1987;60:1800–1808.
127. Lawrence W, Donegan WL, Natarajan N, Mettlin C, Beart R, Winchester D. Adult soft tissue sarcomas. A pattern of care survey of the American College of Surgeons. Ann Surg 1987;205: 349–359.
128. Senagore AJ, Madbouly KM, Fazio VW, Duepree HJ, Brady KM, Delaney CP. Advantages of laparoscopic colectomy in older patients. Arch Surg 2003;138(3):252–256.
129. Lewis JJ, Leung D, Woodruff JM, Brennan MF. Retroperitoneal soft-tissue sarcoma: analysis of 500 patients treated and followed at a single institution. Ann Surg 1998;228(3):355–365.
130. Pisters PWT. Soft tissue sarcoma. In: Norton JA, Bollinger RR, Chang AE, et al (eds) Surgery: Basic Science and Clinical Evidence. New York: Springer, 2001.
131. Patel SG, Shaha AR, Shah JP. Soft tissue sarcomas of the head and neck: an update. Am J Otolaryngol 2001;22:2–18.
132. Bentz BG, Singh B, Woodruff J, Brennan M, Shah JP, Kraus D. Head and neck soft tissue sarcomas: a multivariate analysis of outcomes. Ann Surg Oncol 2004;11(6):619–628.
133. Weber RS, Benjamin RS, Peters LJ, Ro JY, Achon O, Goepfert H. Soft tissue sarcomas of the head and neck in adolescents and adults. Am J Surg 1986;152:386–392.
134. Farhood AI, Hajdu SI, Shiu MG, Strong EW. Soft tissue sarcomas of the head and neck in adults. Am J Surg 1990;160: 365–369.
135. LeVay J, O'Sullivan B, Catton C, et al. An assessment of prognostic factors in soft-tissue sarcoma of the head and neck. Arch Otolaryngol Head Neck Surg 1994;120(9):981–986.
136. Greager JA, Patel MK, Briele HA, Walker MJ, Das Gupta TK. Soft tissue sarcomas of the adult head and neck. Cancer (Phila) 1985;56:820–824.
137. Tran LM, Mar R, Meier R, Calcaterra TC, Parker RG. Sarcomas of the head and neck: prognostic factors and treatment strategies. Cancer (Phila) 1992;70(1):169–177.
138. Dudhat SB, Mistry RC, Varughese T, Fakih AR, Chinoy RF. Prognostic factors in head and neck soft tissue sarcomas. Cancer (Phila) 2000;89(4):868–872.
139. Krous DH, et al. Prognostic factors for recurrence and survival in head and neck soft tissue sarcomas. Cancer (Phila) 1994;74: 697–702.
140. Eeles RA, Fisher C, A'Hern RA, et al. Head and neck sarcomas: prognostic factors and implications for treatment. Br J Cancer 1993;68:201–207.
141. Willers H, Hug EB, Spiro IJ, Efird JT, Rosenberg AE, Wang CC. Adult soft tissue sarcomas of the head and neck treated by radiation and surgery or radiation alone: patterns of failure and prognostic factors. Int J Radiat Oncol Biol Phys 1995;33(3):585–593.
142. Wanebo HJ, Koness RJ, MacFarlane JK, et al. Head and neck sarcoma: report of the Head and Neck Sarcoma Registry. Society of Head and Neck Surgeons Committee on Research. Head Neck 1992;14:1–7.
143. Kowalski LP, San CI. Prognostic factors in head and neck soft tissue sarcomas: analysis of 128 cases. J Surg Oncol 1994;56:83–88.
144. Totty WG, Murphy WA, Lee JKT. Soft-tissue tumors: MR imaging. Radiology 1986;160(1):135–141.
145. Vanel D, Verstraete KL, Shapeero LG. Primary tumors of the musculoskeletal system. Radiol Clin N Am 1997;35(1):213–237.
146. Gelineck J, Keller J, Jensen OM, Nielsen OS, Christensen T. Evaluation of lipomatous soft tissue tumors by MR Imaging. Acta Radiol 1994;35:367–370.
147. Verstraete KL, Vanzieleghem B, DeDeene Y, et al. Static, dynamic and first-pass MR imaging of musculoskeletal lesions using gadodiamide injection. Acta Radiol 1995;36:27–36.
148. Weeks RG, Berquist TH, McLeod RA, Zimmer WD. Magnetic resonance imaging of soft-tissue tumors: comparison with computed tomography. Magn Reson Imaging 1985;3:345–352.
149. Sanders TG, Parsons TWI. Radiographic imaging of musculoskeletal neoplasia. Cancer Control 2001;8(3):221–231.
150. Granstrom P, Unger E. MR Imaging of the retroperitoneum. MRI Clin N Am 1995;3(1):121–142.
151. Mankin HJ, Lange TA, Spanier SS. The hazards of biopsy in patients with malignant primary bone and soft-tissue tumors. J Bone Joint Surg 1982;64A(8):1121–1127.
152. Mankin HJ, Mankin CJ, Simon MA. The hazards of the biopsy, revisited. J Bone Joint Surg 1996;78A(5):656–663.
153. Costa MJ, Campman SC, Davis RL. Fine-needle aspiration cytology of sarcoma: retrospective review of diagnostic utility and specificity. Diagn Cytopathol 1996;15(1):23–32.
154. Bickels J, Jelinek JS, Shmookler BM, Neff RS, Malawer MM. Biopsy of musculoskeletal tumors. Clin Orthop Relat Res 1999; 368:212–219.
155. Akerman M, Rydholm A, Persson BM. Aspiration cytology of soft-tissue tumors. Acta Orthop Scand 1985;56:407–412.
156. Singh HK, Kilpatrick SE, Silverman JF. Fine needle aspiration biopsy of soft tissue sarcomas. Adv Anat Pathol 2004;11(1): 24–37.
157. Ward WG, Savage P, Boles CA, Kilpatrick SE. Fine-needle aspiration biopsy of sarcomas and related tumors. Cancer Control 2001;8(3):232–238.
158. Abdul-Karim FW, Rader AE. Fine needle aspiration of soft-tissue lesions. Clin Lab Med 1998;18:507–540.
159. Kilpatrick SE, Geisinger KR. Soft tissue sarcomas: the usefulness and limitations of fine needle aspiration biopsy. Am J Clin Pathol 1998;110:50–68.
160. Wakely PEJ, Kneisl JS. Soft tissue aspiration. Cytopathology 2000;90:292–298.
161. Bommer KK, Ramzy I, Mody D. Fine-needle aspiration biopsy in the diagnosis and management of bone lesions. Cancer (Phila) 1997;81:148–156.
162. Ferrucci JT Jr. Malignant seeding of needle tract after thin needle aspiration biopsy: a previously unrecorded complication. Radiology 1979;130:345–346.
163. Davies NM, Livesly PJ, Cannon SR. Recurrence of an osteosarcoma in a needle biopsy tract. J Bone Joint Surg 1993;75B: 977–978.
164. Skrzynski MC, Biermann S, Montag A, Simon MA. Diagnostic accuracy and charge-savings of outpatient core needle biopsy compared with open biopsy of musculoskeletal tumors. J Bone Joint Surg 1996;78A(5):644–649.
165. Ball ABS, Fisher C, Pittam M, Watkins RM, Westbury G. Diagnosis of soft tissue tumours by Tru-Cut biopsy. Br J Surg 1990;77: 756–758.
166. Hoeber I, Spillane AJ, Fisher C, Thomas JM. Accuracy of biopsy techniques for limb and limb girdle soft tissue tumors. Ann Surg Oncol 2001;8(1):80–87.
167. Heslin MJ, Lewis JJ, Woodruff JM, Brennan MF. Core needle biopsy for diagnosis of extremity soft tissue sarcoma. Ann Surg Oncol 1997;4(5):425–431.

168. Huvos AG. The importance of the open surgical biopsy in the diagnosis and treatment of bone and soft-tissue tumors. Hematol Oncol Clin N Am 1995;9(3):541–544.
169. McGrath FP, Gibney RG, Rowley VA, Sedamore CH. Cutaneous seeding following fine needle biopsy of colonic liver metastases. Clin Radiol 1991;43:130–131.
170. Engzell V, Esposti PL, Rubio C, Sigurdson A, Zajicek K. Investigation of tumor spread in connection with aspiration biopsy. Acta Radiol Oncol Radiat Phys Biol 1971;10:385–398.
171. Randall RL, Bruckner JD, Papenhausen MD, Thurman T, Conrad EUI. Errors in diagnosis and margin determination of soft-tissue sarcomas initially treated at non-tertiary centers. Orthopedics 2004;27(2):209–212.
172. Noria S, Davis A, Kandel R, et al. Residual disease following unplanned excision of a soft-tissue sarcoma of an extremity. J Bone Joint Surg 1996;78A(5):650–655.
173. Davis AM, Kandel RA, Wunder JS, et al. The impact of residual disease on local recurrence in patients treated by initial unplanned resection for soft tissue sarcoma of the extremity. J Surg Oncol 1997;66:81–87.
174. Giuliano AE, Eilber FR. The rationale for planned reoperation after unplanned total excision of soft-tissue sarcomas. J Clin Oncol 1985;3:1344–1348.
175. Karakousis CP, Proimakis C, Walsh DL. Primary soft tissue sarcoma of the extremities in adults. Br J Cancer 1995;82:1208–1212.
176. Bowden L, Booher RJ. The principles and technique of resection of soft parts for sarcoma. Surgery (St. Louis) 1958;44(6):963–977.
177. Cantin J, McNeer GP, Chu FC, Booher RJ. The problem of local recurrence after treatment of soft tissue sarcoma. Ann Surg 1968;168(1):47–53.
178. Tanabe KK, Pollock RE, Ellis LM, Murphy A, Sherman N, Romsdahl MM. Influence of surgical margins on outcome in patients with preoperatively irradiated extremity soft tissue sarcomas. Cancer (Phila) 1994;73(6):1652–1659.
179. Sondak V. Sarcomas of bone and soft tissue. In: Greenfield LJ, Mulholland MW, Oldham KT, Zelenock GB, Lillemoe KD (eds) Surgery: Scientific Principles and Practice, 2nd ed. Philadelphia: Lippincott-Raven. 1997:2246–2269.
180. Rosenberg SA, Tepper J, Glatstein E, et al. The treatment of soft-tissue sarcomas of the extremities. Ann Surg 1982;196(3):305–315.
181. Davis AM, Devlin M, Griffin AM, Wunder JS, Bell RS. Functional outcome in amputation versus limb sparing of patients with lower extremity sarcoma: a matched case-control study. Arch Phys Med Rehabil 1999;80:615–618.
182. Sugarbaker PH, Barofsky I, Rosenberg SA, Gianola FJ. Quality of life assessment of patients in extremity sarcoma clinical trials. Surgery (St. Louis) 1982;91:17–23.
183. Stinson SF, DeLaney TF, Greenberg J, et al. Acute and long-term effects on limb function of combined modality limb sparing therapy for extremity soft tissue sarcoma. Int J Radiat Oncol Biol Phys 1991;21:1493–1499.
184. Serletti JM, Carras AJ, O'Keefe RJ, Rosier RN. Functional outcome after soft-tissue reconstruction for limb salvage after sarcoma surgery. Plast Reconstr Surg 1998;102(5):1576–1583.
185. Davis AM. Functional outcome in extremity soft tissue sarcoma. Semin Radiat Oncol 1999;9(4):360–368.
186. Brooks AD, Gold JS, Graham D, et al. Resection of the sciatic, peroneal, or tibial nerves: assessment of functional status. Ann Surg Oncol 2002;9(1):41–47.
187. Hohenberger P, Allenberg JR, Schlag PM, Reichardt P. Results of surgery and multimodal therapy for patients with soft tissue sarcoma invading to vascular structures. Cancer (Phila) 1999;85(2):396–408.
188. Flugstad DL, Wilke CP, McNutt MA, Welk RA, Hart MJ, McQuinn WO. Importance of surgical resection in the successful management of soft tissue sarcoma. Arch Surg 1999;134(8):856–861.
189. Pollock RE. Soft Tissue Sarcomas. London: Decker, 2002.
190. Spira AI, Ettinger DS. The use of chemotherapy in soft-tissue sarcomas. Oncologist 2002;7:348–359.
191. Henshaw RM, Priebat DA, Perry DJ, Shmookler BM, Malawer MM. Survival after induction chemotherapy and surgical resection for high-grade soft tissue sarcoma. Is radiation necessary? Ann Surg Oncol 2001;8(6):484–495.
192. Rydholm A, Gustafson P, Rooser B, et al. Limb-sparing surgery without radiotherapy based on anatomic location of soft tissue sarcoma. J Clin Oncol 1991;9(10):1757–1765.
193. Brennan MF, Hilaris B, Shiu MH, et al. Local recurrence in adult soft-tissue sarcoma. Arch Surg 1987;122:1289–1293.
194. Pisters PW, Harrison LB, Leung DH, Woodruff JM, Casper ES, Brennan MF. Long-term results of a prospective randomized trial of adjuvant brachytherapy in soft tissue sarcoma. J Clin Oncol 1996;14:859–868.
195. Pao WJ, Pilepich MV. Postoperative radiotherapy in the treatment of extremity soft tissue sarcomas. Int J Radiat Oncol Biol Phys 1990;19:907–911.
196. Yang JC, Chang AE, Baker AR, et al. Randomized prospective study of the benefit of adjuvant radiation therapy in the treatment of soft tissue sarcomas of the extremity. J Clin Oncol 1998;16(1):197–203.
197. O'Sullivan B, Davis AM, Turcotte R, et al. Preoperative versus postoperative radiotherapy in soft-tissue sarcoma of the limbs: a randomised trial. Lancet 2002;359:2235–2241.
198. Davis AM, Bell RS, Turcotte R, et al. Function and health status outcomes in a randomized trial comparing preoperative and postoperative radiotherapy in extremity soft tissue sarcoma. J Clin Oncol 2002;20(22):4472–4477.
199. Peat BG, Bell RS, Davis A, et al. Wound-healing complications after soft-tissue sarcoma surgery. Plast Reconstr Surg 1994;93(5):980–987.
200. Ormsby MV, Hilaris BS, Nori D, Brennan MF. Wound complications of adjuvant radiation therapy in patients with soft-tissue sarcomas. Ann Surg 1988;210(1):93–99.
201. Bujko K, Suit HD, Springfield DS, Convery K. Wound healing after preoperative radiation for sarcoma of soft tissues. Surg Gynecol Obstet 1993;176:124–134.
202. Meric F, Milas M, Hunt KK, et al. Impact of neoadjuvant chemotherapy on postoperative morbidity in soft tissue sarcomas. J Clin Oncol 2000;18(19):3378–3383.
203. Hilaris BS, Bodner WR, Mastoras CA. Role of brachytherapy in adult soft tissue sarcomas. Semin Surg Oncol 1997;13:196–203.
204. Janjan NA, Yasko AW, Reece GP, et al. Comparison of charges related to radiotherapy for soft-tissue sarcomas treated by preoperative external-beam irradiation versus interstitial implantation. Ann Surg Oncol 1994;1(5):415–422.
205. Ramanathan RC, A'Hern RA, Fisher C, Thomas JM. Prognostic index for extremity soft tissue sarcomas with isolated local recurrence. Ann Surg Oncol 2001;8(4):278–289.
206. Espat NJ, Lewis JJ. The biological significance of failure at the primary site on ultimate survival in soft tissue sarcoma. Semin Radiat Oncol 1999;9(4):369–377.
207. Cormier JN, Pollock RE. Soft tissue sarcomas. CA Cancer J Clin 2004;54:94–109.
208. Benjamin RS, Choi H, Charnsangavej C, et al. We Should Desist Using Recist, At Least in GIST. Connective Tissue Oncology Society 9th Annual Scientific Meeting, Barcelona, Spain, 2003.
209. Adjuvant chemotherapy for localised resectable soft-tissue sarcoma of adults: meta-analysis of individual data. Sarcoma Meta-analysis Collaboration. Lancet 1997;350(9092):1647–1654.

210. Verweij J. The reason for confining the use of adjuvant chemotherapy in soft tissue sarcoma to the investigational setting. Semin Radiat Oncol 1999;9:352–359.
211. Frustaci S, Gherlinzoni F, De Paoli A, et al. Adjuvant chemotherapy for adult soft tissue sarcomas of the extremities and girdles: results of the Italian Randomized Cooperative Trial. J Clin Oncol 2001;19(5):1238–1247.
212. Frustaci S, De Paoli A, Bidoli E, et al. Ifosfamide in the adjuvant therapy of soft tissue sarcomas. Oncology 2003;65(suppl 2): 80–84.
213. Benjamin RS. Evidence for using adjuvant chemotherapy as standard treatment of soft tissue sarcoma. Semin Radiat Oncol 1999;9:349–351.
214. Maurel J, Fra J, Lopez-Pousa A, et al. Sequential dose-dense doxorubicin and ifosfamide for advanced soft tissue sarcomas. A Phase II trial by the Spanish Group for Research on Sarcomas (GEIS). Cancer (Phila) 2004;100(7):1498–1506.
215. Le Cesne A, Judson I, Crowther D, et al. Randomized phase III study comparing conventional-dose doxorubicin plus ifosfamide versus high-dose doxorubicin plus ifosfamide plus recombinant human granulocyte-macrophage colony-stimulating factor in advanced soft tissue sarcomas: a trial of the European Organization for Research and Treatment of Cancer/Soft Tissue and Bone Sarcoma Group. J Clin Oncol 2000;18:2676–2684.
216. Lopez M, Vici P, Di Lauro L, Carpano S. Increasing single epirubicin doses in advanced soft tissue sarcomas. J Clin Oncol 2002;20:1329–1334.
217. Patel SR, Vanadhan-Raj S, Burgess MA, et al. Results of two consecutive trials of dose-intensive chemotherapy with doxorubicin and ifosfamide in patients with sarcomas. Am J Clin Oncol 1998;21:317–321.
218. Worden FP, Taylor JMG, Bierman JS, et al. A randomized Phase II evaluation of standard dose ifosfamide (IFOS) plus doxorubicin (DOX) versus high dose ifosfamide plus DOX in patients with high-grade soft tissue sarcomas. Proc Am Soc Clin Oncol 2003; 22:817.
219. Bacci G, Ferrari S, Tienghi A, et al. A comparison of methods of loco-regional chemotherapy combined with systemic chemotherapy as neo-adjuvant treatment of osteosarcoma of the extremity. Eur J Surg Oncol 2001;27(1):98–104.
220. Eilber FR, Guiliano AE, Huth JF, Weisenburger TH, Eckardt J. Intravenous (IV) vs. intra-arterial (IA) adriamycin, 2800-rad radiation and surgical excision for extremity soft tissue sarcomas: a randomized prospective trial. Proc Am Soc Clin Oncol 1990;9:A1194.
221. van der Veen AH, de Wilt JHW, Eggermont AMM, van Tiel ST, Seynhaeve ALB, ten Hagen TLM. TNF-α augments intratumoural concentrations of doxorubicin in TNF-α-based isolated limb perfusion in rat sarcoma models and enhances anti-tumour effects. Br J Cancer 2000;82:973–980.
222. McBride CM. Sarcomas of the limbs. Results of adjuvant chemotherapy using isolation perfusion. Arch Surg 1974;109: 304–308.
223. Lienard D, Ewalenko P, Delmotte JJ, Renard N, Lejeune FJ. High-dose recombinant tumor necrosis factor alpha in combination with interferon gamma and melphalan in isolation perfusion of the limbs for melanoma and sarcoma. J Clin Oncol 1992;10(1): 52–60.
224. de Wilt JHW, ten Hagen TLM, de Boeck G, van Tiel ST, de Bruijn EA, Eggermont AMM. Tumour necrosis factor-alpha increases melphalan concentration in tumour tissue after isolated limb perfusion. Br J Cancer 2000;82:1000–1003.
225. Rossi CR, Foletto M, Di Filippo F, et al. Soft tissue limb sarcomas: Italian clinical trials with hyperthermic antiblastic perfusion. Cancer (Phila) 1999;86:1742–1749.
226. Issakov J, Merimsky O, Gutman M, et al. Hyperthermic isolated limb perfusion with tumor necrosis factor-α and melphalan in advanced soft-tissue sarcomas: histopathological considerations. Ann Surg Oncol 2000;7(1):155–159.
227. Gutman M, Inbar M, Lev-Shlush D, et al. High dose tumor necrosis factor-alpha and melphalan administered via isolated limb perfusion for advanced limb soft tissue sarcoma results in a >90% response rate and limb preservation. Cancer (Phila) 1997;79(6):1129–1137.
228. Lev-Chelouche D, Abu-Abid S, Kollender Y, et al. Multifocal soft tissue sarcoma: limb salvage following hyperthermic isolated limb perfusion with high-dose tumor necrosis factor and melphalan. J Surg Oncol 1999;70:185–189.
229. van Etten B, van Geel AN, de Wilt JHW, Eggermont AMM. Fifty tumor necrosis nactor-based isolated limb perfusions for limb salvage in patients older than 75 years with limb-threatening soft tissue sarcomas and other extremity tumors. Ann Surg Oncol 2003;10(1):32–37.
230. Lejueune FJ, Pujol N, Lienard D, et al. Limb salvage by neoadjuvant isolated perfusion with TNF-alpha and melphalan for non-resectable soft tissue sarcoma of the extremities. Eur J Surg Oncol 2000;26:669–678.
231. Eggermont AMM, Koops HS, Schraffordt H, et al. Isolated limb perfusion with tumor necrosis factor and melphalan for limb salvage in 186 patients with locally advanced soft tissue extremity sarcomas: The cumulative multicenter European experience. Ann Surg 1996;224(6):756–765.
232. Kim CJ, Puleo C, Letson GD, Reintgen D. Hyperthermic isolated limb perfusion for extremity sarcomas. Cancer Control 2001;8(3):269–273.
233. Cheifetz R, Catton C, Kandel RA, O'Sullivan B, Couture J, Swallow C. Recent progress in the management of retroperitoneal sarcoma. Sarcoma 2001;5:17–26.
234. Windham TC, Pearson AS, Skibber JM, et al. Significance and management of local recurrences and limited metastatic disease in the abdomen. Surg Clin N Am 2000;80(2):761–774.
235. Heslin MJ, Lewis JJ, Nadler E, et al. Prognostic factors associated with long-term survival for retroperitoneal sarcoma: implications for management. J Clin Oncol 1997;15(8):2832–2839.
236. Shibata D, Lewis JJ, Leung DH, Brennan MF. Is there a role for incomplete resection in the management of retroperitoneal liposarcomas? J Am Coll Surg 2001;193:373–379.
237. Kilkenny JWI, Bland KI, Copeland EMI. Retroperitoneal sarcoma: the University of Florida experience. J Am Coll Surg 1996;182:329–339.
238. Storm FK, Eilber FR, Mirra J, Morton DL. Retroperitoneal sarcomas: a reappraisal of treatment. J Surg Oncol 1981;17: 1–7.
239. Jaques DP, Coit DG, Hajdu SI, Brennan MF. Management of primary and recurrent soft-tissue sarcoma of the retroperitoneum. Ann Surg 1990;212(1):51–59.
240. Malerba M, Doglietto GB, Pacelli F, et al. Primary retroperitoneal soft tissue sarcomas: results of aggressive surgical treatment. World J Surg 1999;23(7):670–675.
241. McGrath PC, Neifeld JP, Lawrence W Jr, et al. Improved survival following complete excision of retroperitoneal sarcomas. Ann Surg 1984;200(2):200–204.
242. Salvadori B, Cusumano F, Delle donne V, De Lellis R, Conti R. Surgical treatment of 43 retroperitoneal sarcomas. Eur J Surg Oncol 1986;12:29–33.
243. Cody HSI, Turnbull AD, Fortner JG, Hajdu SI. The continuing challenge of retroperitoneal sarcomas. Cancer (Phila) 1981;47: 2147–2152.
244. Catton CN, O'Sullivan B, Kotwall C, Cummings B, Hao Y, Fornasier VL. Outcome and prognosis in retroperitoneal soft tissue sarcoma. Int J Radiat Oncol Biol Phys 1994;29(5):1005–1010.
245. Bevilacqua RG, Rogatko A, Hajdu SI, Brennan MF. Prognostic factors in primary retroperitoneal soft-tissue sarcomas. Arch Surg 1991;126:328–334.

246. Karakousis CP, Gerstenbluth R, Kontzoglou K, Driscoll D. Retroperitoneal sarcomas and their management. Arch Surg 1995;130:1104–1109.
247. Dalton RR, Donohue JH, Mucha PJ, van Heerden JA, Reiman HM, Chen S. Management of retroperitoneal sarcomas. Surgery (St. Louis) 1989;106:725–733.
248. Solla JA, Reed K. Primary retroperitoneal sarcomas. Am J Surg 1986;152:496–498.
249. Alvarenga JC, Ball ABS, Fisher C, Fryatt I, Jones L, Thomas JM. Limitations of surgery in the treatment of retroperitoneal sarcoma. Br J Cancer 1991;78:912–916.
250. Zornig C, Weh H-J, Krull A, et al. Retroperitoneal sarcoma in a series of 51 adults. Eur J Surg Oncol 1992;18:475–480.
251. Stoeckle E, Coindre J-M, Bonvalot S, et al. Prognostic factors in retroperitoneal sarcoma: a multivariate analysis of a series of 165 patients of the French Cancer Center Federation Sarcoma Group. Cancer (Phila) 2001;92(2):359–368.
252. Makela J, Kiviniemi H, Laitinen S. Prognostic factors predicting survival in the treatment of retroperitoneal sarcoma. Eur J Surg Oncol 2000;26:552–555.
253. Pirayesh A, Chee Y, Helliwell TR, et al. The management of retroperitoneal soft tissue sarcoma: a single institution experience with a review of the literature. Eur J Surg Oncol 2001;27: 491–497.
254. Hassan I, Park SZ, Donohue JH, et al. Operative management of primary retroperitoneal sarcomas: a reappraisal of an institutional experience. Ann Surg 2004;239(2):244–250.
255. Wang T-Y, Lo S-S, Su C-H, Wu C-W, Lui W-Y. Surgical management of primary retroperitoneal sarcoma. Chin Med J (Taipei) 1996;58:177–182.
256. Ferrario T, Karakousis CP. Retroperitoneal sarcomas: grade and survival. Arch Surg 2003;138:248–251.
257. Pisters PWT, O'Sullivan B. Retroperitoneal sarcomas: combined modality treatment approaches. Curr Opin Oncol 2002;14:400–405.
258. Fein DA, Corn BW, Lanciano RM, Herbert SH, Hoffman JP, Coia LR. Management of retroperitoneal sarcomas: does dose escalation impact on locoregional control? Int J Radiat Oncol Biol Phys 1995;31(1):129–134.
259. Tepper JE, Suit HD, Wood WC, Proppe KH, Harmon D, McNulty P. Radiation therapy of retroperitoneal soft tissue sarcomas. Int J Radiat Oncol Biol Phys 1984;10:825–830.
260. Gleen J, Sindelar WF, Kinsella T, et al. Results of multimodality therapy of resectable soft-tissue sarcomas of the retroperitoneum. Surgery (St. Louis) 1985;97:316–324.
261. Storm FK, Mahvi DM. Diagnosis and management of retroperitoneal soft-tissue sarcoma. Ann Surg 1990;214(1): 2–10.
262. Pisters PW, Shreyaskumar PR, Prieto VG, et al. Phase I trial of preoperative doxorubicin-based concurrent chemoradiation and surgical resection for localized extremity and body wall soft tissue sarcomas. J Clin Oncol 2004;22:3375–3380.
263. Sondak VK, Robertson JM, Sussman JJ, Saran PA, Chang AE, Lawrence TL. Preoperative idoxuridine and radiation for large soft tissue sarcomas: clinical results with five-year follow-up. Ann Surg Oncol 1998;5:106–112.
264. Jones JL, Catton CN, O'Sullivan B, et al. Initial results of a trial of preoperative external-beam radiation therapy and postoperative brachytherapy for retroperitoneal sarcoma. Ann Surg Oncol 2002;9(4):346–354.
265. Sindelar WF, Kinsella TJ, Chen PW, et al. Intraoperative radiotherapy in retroperitoneal sarcomas. Arch Surg 1993;128:402–410.
266. Miettinen M. Diagnostic soft tissue pathology. Philadelphia: Churchill Livingstone, 2003.
267. Strickland L, Letson GD, Muro-Cacho CA. Gastrointestinal stromal tumors. Cancer Control 2001;8(3):252–261.
268. DeMatteo RP, Lewis JJ, Leung D, Mudan SS, Woodruff JM, Brennan MF. Two hundred gastrointestinal stromal tumors: recurrence patterns and prognostic factors for survival. Ann Surg 1999;231(1):51–58.
269. Pidhorecky I, Cheney RT, Kraybill WG, Gibbs JF. Gastrointestinal stromal tumors: current diagnosis, biologic behavior, and management. Ann Surg Oncol 2000;7(9):705–712.
270. Singer S, Rubin BP, Lux ML, et al. Prognostic value of KIT mutation type, mitotic activity, and histologic subtype in gastrointestinal stromal tumors. J Clin Oncol 2002;20(18):3898–3905.
271. Rossi CR, Mocellin S, Mencarelli R, et al. Gastrointestinal stromal tumors: from a surgical to a molecular approach. Int J Cancer 2003;107:171–176.
272. Eisenberg BL, Judson I. Surgery and imatinib in the management of GIST: emerging approaches to adjuvant and neoadjuvant therapy. Ann Surg Oncol 2004;11(5):465–475.
273. De Pas T, Casali PG, Toma S, et al. Gastrointestinal stromal tumors: should they be treated with the same systemic chemotherapy as other soft tissue sarcomas? Oncology 2003; 64(2):186–188.
274. Hirota S, Isozaki K, Moriyama Y, et al. Gain-of-function mutations of c-kit in human gastrointestinal stromal tumors. Science 1998;279:577–580.
275. Judson I. Gastrointestinal stromal tumours (GIST): biology and treatment. Ann Oncol 2002;13(suppl 4):287–289.
276. Heinrich MC, Corless CL, Duensing A, et al. PDGFRA activating mutations in gastrointestinal stromal tumors. Science 2003; 299:708–710.
277. Goldman JM, Melo JV. Targeting the BCR-ABL tyrosine kinase in chronic myeloid leukemia. N Eng J Med 2004;344(14):1084–1086.
278. Joensuu H, Roberts PJ, Sarlomo-Rikala M, et al. Effect of the tyrosine kinase inhibitor STI571 in a patient with a metastatic gastrointestinal tumor. N Engl J Med 2001;344(14):1052–1056.
279. Verweij J, van Oosterom AT, Blay Y, et al. Imatinib mesylate (STI-571 Glivec®, Gleevac™) is an active agent for gastrointestinal stromal tumours, but does not yield responses in other soft-tissue sarcomas that are unselected for a molecular target: results from an EORTC Soft Tissue and Bone Sarcoma Group phase II study. Eur J Cancer 2003;39:2006–2011.
280. Demetri GD, von Mehren M, Blanke CD, et al. Efficacy and safety of imatinib mesylate in advanced gastrointestinal stromal tumors. N Engl J Med 2002;347(7):472–480.
281. Dagher R, Cohen M, Williams G, et al. Approval summary: imatinib mesylate in the treatment of metastatic and/or unresectable malignant gastrointestinal stromal tumors. Clin Cancer Res 2002;8:3034–3088.
282. Van den Abbeele AD, Badawi RD. Use of positron emission tomography in oncology and its potential role to assess response to imatinib mesylate therapy in gastrointestinal stromal tumors (GISTs). Eur J Cancer 2002;38(suppl 5):S60–S65.
283. Harting MT, Messner GN, Igor D, Frazier OH. Sarcoma metastatic to the right ventricle: surgical intervention followed by prolonged survival. Tex Heart Inst J 2004;31(1):93–95.
284. Talbot SM, Taub RN, Keohan ML, Edwards N, Galantowicz ME, Schulman LL. Combined heart and lung transplantation for unresectable primary cardiac sarcoma. J Thorac Cardiovasc Surg 2002;124(6):1145–1148.
285. Sarkar R, Eilber FR, Gelabert HA, Quinones-Baldrich WJ. Prosthetic replacement of the inferior vena cava for malignancy. J Vasc Surg 1998;28(1):75–83.
286. Hollenbeck ST, Grobmyer SR, Kent KC, Brennan MF. Surgical treatment and outcomes of patients with primary inferior vena cava leiomyosarcoma. J Am Coll Surg 2003;197(4):575–579.

287. Mingoli A, Sapienza P, Cavallaro A, et al. The effect of extent of caval resection in the treatment of inferior vena cava leiomyosarcoma. Anticancer Res 1997;17:3877–3882.
288. Zelek L, Llombart-Cussac A, Terrier P, et al. Prognostic factors in primary breast sarcomas: a series of patients with long-term follow-up. J Clin Oncol 2003;21(13):2583–2588.
289. Serralva M, Ramalho A, Oliveira M, Santos G, Veloso V, Silva C. Sarcoma of the breast: a retrospective review of 20 cases. Br J Surg 1997;84(2):21.
290. Teo T, Wee SB. Clinically 'benign' breast lumps: sarcoma in hiding? case reports and literature review. Ann Acad Med Singap 2004;33:270–274.
291. Eroglu E, Irkkan C, Eroglu F. Phyllodes tumor of the breast: case series of 40 patients. Eur J Gynaecol Oncol 2004;25(1):123–125.
292. Soumarova R, Seneklova Z, Horova H, et al. Retrospective analysis of 25 women with malignant cystosarcoma phyllodes: treatment results. Arch Gynecol Obstet 2004;269(4):278–281.
293. Sawyer M, Bramwell V. The treatment of distant metastases in soft tissue sarcoma. Semin Radiat Oncol 1999;9(4):389–400.
294. Potter DA, Glenn J, Kinsella T, et al. Patterns of recurrence in patients with high-grade soft-tissue sarcomas. J Clin Oncol 1985;3:353–366.
295. Lucas JD, O'Doherty MJ, Maguire BM, McKee PH, Smith MA. Evaluation of fluorodeoxyglucose positron tomography in the management of soft tissue sarcomas. Br J Bone Joint Surg 1998; 80:441–447.
296. Billingsley KG, Lewis JJ, Leung D, Casper ES, Woodruff JM, Brennan MF. Multifactorial analysis of the survival of patients with distant metastasis arising from primary extremity sarcoma. Cancer (Phila) 1999;85(2):389–395.
297. van Geel AN, Pastorino U, Jauch KW, et al. Surgical treatment of lung metastases: The European Organization for Research and Treatment of Cancer-Soft Tissue and Bone Sarcoma Group study of 255 patients. Cancer (Phila) 1996;77(4):675–682.
298. Billingsley KG, Burt ME, Jara E, et al. Pulmonary metastases from soft tissue sarcoma. Ann Surg 1999;229(5):602–612.
299. Saltzman DA, Snyder CL, Ferrell KL, Thompson RC, Leonard AS. Aggressive metastasectomy for pulmonic sarcomatous metastases: a follow-up study. Am J Surg 1993;166(5):543–547.
300. Stojadinovic A, Leung DHY, Allen P, Lewis JJ, Jaques DP, Brennan MF. Primary adult soft tissue sarcoma: time-dependent influence of prognostic variables. J Clin Oncol 2002;20(21):4344–4352.
301. Jaques DP, Coit DG, Casper ES, Brennan MF. Hepatic metastases from soft-tissue sarcoma. Ann Surg 1995;221(4):392–397.
302. Brennan MF, Alektiar KM, Maki RG. Sarcomas of Soft Tissue and Bone, 6th ed. Philadelphia: Lippincott, 2001.
303. Elias A, Ryan L, Sulkes A, Collins J, Aisner J, Antman KH. Response to mesna, doxorubicin, ifosfamide, and dacarbazine in 108 patients with metastatic or unresectable sarcoma and no prior chemotherapy. J Clin Oncol 1989;7(9):1208–1216.
304. Antman KH, Crowley J, Balcerzak SP, et al. An intergroup phase III randomized study of doxorubicin and dacarbazine with or without ifosfamide and mesna in advanced soft tissue and bone sarcomas. J Clin Oncol 1993;11(7):1276–1285.
305. Boulad F, Kernan NA, LaQuaglia MP, et al. High-dose induction chemoradiotherapy followed by autologous bone marrow transplantation as consolidation therapy in rhabdomyosarcoma, extraosseous Ewing's sarcoma, and undifferentiated sarcoma. J Clin Oncol 1998;16(5):1697–1706.
306. Carli M, Colombatti R, Oberlin O, et al. High-Dose melphalan with autologous stem-cell rescue in metastatic rhabdomyosarcoma. J Clin Oncol 1999;17(9):2796–2803.
307. Blay J-Y, Bouhour D, Ray-Coquard I, Dumontet C, Philip T, Biron P. High-dose chemotherapy with autologous hematopoietic stem-cell transplantation for advanced soft tissue sarcoma in adults. J Clin Oncol 2000;18(21):3643–3650.
308. Antman KH, Ryan L, Elias A, Sherman D, Grier HE. Response to ifosfamide and mesna: 124 previously treated patients with metastatic or unresectable sarcoma. J Clin Oncol 1989;7(1):126–131.
309. van Oosterom AT, Mouridsen HT, Nielsen OS, et al. Results of randomized studies of the EORTC Soft Tissue and Bone Sarcoma Group (STBSG) with two different ifosfamide regimens in first and second line chemotherapy in advanced soft tissue sarcoma patients. Eur J Cancer 2002;38(18):2397–2406.
310. Hensley ML, Maki R, Venkatraman E, et al. Gemcitabine and docetaxel in patients with unresectable leiomyosarcoma: results of a phase II trial. J Clin Oncol 2002;20(12):2824–2831.
311. Leu KM, Ostruszka LJ, Shewach D, et al. Laboratory and clinical evidence of synergistic cytotoxicity of sequential treatment with gemcitabine followed by docetaxel in the treatment of sarcoma. J Clin Oncol 2004;22:1706–1712.
312. Fata F, O'Reilly E, Ilson D, et al. Paclitaxel in the treatment of patients with angiosarcoma of the scalp or face. Cancer (Phila) 1999;86(10):2034–2037.
313. Weiss AJ, Lackman RD. Low-dose chemotherapy of desmoid tumors. Cancer (Phila) 1989;64(6):1192–1194.
314. Azzarelli A, Gronchi A, Bertulli R, et al. Low-dose chemotherapy with methotrexate and vinblastine for patients with advanced aggressive fibromatosis. Cancer (Phila) 2001;92:1259–1264.
315. Thall PF, Wathen JK, Bekele BN, et al. Hierarchical Bayesian approaches to phase II trials in diseases with multiple subtypes. Stat Med 2003;22:763–780.
316. Rydholm A. Improving the management of soft tissue sarcoma: diagnosis and treatment should be given in specialist centres. Br Med J 1998;317(7151):93–94.
317. Gustafson P, Dreinhofer KE, Rydholm A. Soft tissue sarcoma should be treated at a tumor center. A comparison of quality of surgery in 375 patients. Acta Orthop Scand 1994;65(1):47–50.
318. Clasby R, Tilling K, Smith MA, Fletcher CDM. Variable management of soft tissue sarcoma: regional audit with implications for specialist care. Br J Surg 1997;84(12):1692–1696.
319. Ray-Coquard I, Thiesse P, Ranchere-Vince D, et al. Conformity to clinical practice guidelines, multidisciplinary management and outcome of treatment for soft tissue sarcomas. Ann Oncol 2004;15:307–315.
320. Whooley BP, Mooney MM, Gibbs JF, Kraybill WG. Effective follow-up strategies in soft tissue sarcoma. Semin Surg Oncol 1999;17:83–87.
321. Bennicelli JL, Barr FG. Chromosomal translocations and sarcomas. Curr Opin Oncol 2002;14:412–419.
322. Zagars GK, Ballo MT, Pisters PW, et al. Prognostic factors for patients with localized soft-tissue sarcoma treated with conservation surgery and radiation therapy. Cancer (Phila) 2003;97(10):2530–2543.
323. Abbas JS, Holyoke ED, Moore R, Karakousis CP. The surgical treatment and outcome of soft-tissue sarcoma. Arch Surg 1981; 116:765–769.
324. Shiu MH, Castro EB, Hajdu SI, Fortner JG. Surgical treatment of 297 soft tissue sarcomas of the lower extremity. Ann Surg 1975; 182(5):597–602.
325. Donohue JH, Collin C, Friedrich C, Godbold J, Hajdu SI, Brennan MF. Low-grade soft tissue sarcomas of the extremities. Cancer (Phila) 1988;62:184–193.
326. Williard WC, Hajdu SI, Casper ES, Brennan MF. Comparison of amputation with limb-sparing operations for adult soft tissue sarcoma of the extremity. Ann Surg 1991;215(3):269–275.
327. Gieschen HL, Spiro IJ, Suit HD, et al. Long-term results of intraoperative electron beam radiotherapy for primary and recurrent

retroperitoneal soft tissue sarcoma. Int J Radiat Biol Oncol Phys 2001;50(1):127–131.

328. Alektiar KM, Hu K, Anderson L, Brennan MF, Harrison LB. High-dose-rate intraoperative radiation therapy (HDR-IORT) for retroperitoneal sarcomas. Int J Radiat Biol Oncol Phys 2000; 47(1):157–163.

329. Bobin JY, Al-Lawati T, Granero LE, et al. Surgical management of retroperitoneal sarcomas associated with external and intraoperative electron beam radiotherapy. Eur J Surg Oncol 2003;29:676–681.

330. Gunderson LL, Nagorney DM, McIlrath DC, Fieck JM, Wieand HS, Martinez A. External beam and intraoperative electron irradiation for locally advanced soft tissue sarcomas. Int J Radiat Biol Oncol Phys 1993;25:647–656.

331. Willet GC, Suit HD, Tepper J. Intraoperative electron beam radiation therapy for retroperitomed soft tissue sarcoma. Cancer (Phila) 1991;68:278–283.

332. NCCN Clinical Practice Guidelines in Oncology: CD Rom. 2004.

Cutaneous Melanoma

Mark R. Albertini, B. Jack Longley, Paul M. Harari, and Douglas Reintgen

Epidemiology

The incidence of melanoma has increased dramatically during the past several decades among Caucasian populations.[1] Mortality rates continue to rise overall, but in some populations, such as females, the mortality rate has plateaued or even fallen. The reasons for these trends are not altogether obvious, but may involve changes in attitudes and behaviors with regard to sun exposure or an increased public awareness to the early signs of melanoma diagnosis.

Incidence rates vary from a low of 0.2 (females and males) in China to 34.9 per 100,000 among females in New Zealand and 40.5 per 100,000 among males in Australia.[1] There were 23.1 new cases per 100,000 population in the United States (incidence rate adjusted to the 2000 United States population). Approximately 59,580 new cases of malignant melanoma and 7,770 deaths due to melanoma are predicted for the United States in 2005.[2] Over the past 30 years, the incidence rate has tripled, particularly in the Caucasian male population. Recent data would suggest that the largest proportion contributing to the increased incidence are "thin" melanomas. People born before 1950 show an increased risk of developing melanoma whereas those whose birthdays are after 1950 show stable or declining rates.[1]

Melanoma is a tumor that occurs in the relatively young, with the mean age of diagnosis being 50 years of age, 10 to 15 years before the mean age of diagnosis of some of the more-common cancers such as breast, lung, and colon. In the United States, there has been an increase in the diagnosis of thin melanomas in the young and an increase in the diagnosis of thick lesions in men over the age of 65.[1]

Dermatopathology of Melanoma

The classification of cutaneous melanomas depends on an interaction between the clinical and pathologic features. The commonly recognized melanomas include (1) lentigo maligna melanoma, (2) superficial spreading melanoma, (3) nodular melanoma, and (4) acral lentiginous melanoma. We begin with a discussion of precursors of melanoma followed by a description of the histopathologic features of the various types of melanoma.

Precursors of Malignant Melanoma

It is widely accepted that many if not most melanomas of the superficial spreading type arise in preexisting junctional or compound melanocytic nevi, and benign melanoctic nevi are therefore a risk factor for malignant melanoma.[3] Determining the exact percentage of melanomas arising in nevi is problematic because many melanomas are probably not detected until they have overrun small precursor nevi and because the terminology for early melanoma (in situ) arising in nevi is not standardized (please see following discussion of "dysplastic" nevi). However, most studies that are based on histologic features alone report finding remnants of a preexisting nevus in about 22% of melanomas of the superficial spreading type.[4,5] Studies that include clinical as well as histopathologic criteria report precursors in as many as 39.5% of melanomas.[6]

Several subgroups of precursor nevi have been identified including preexisting congenital nevi, sporadic acquired nevi, and nevi associated with the familial melanoma syndrome. It is commonly accepted that melanomas may arise in large congenital nevi, but a separate study that specifically addressed the size of congenital precursor lesions established that a significant percentage of melanomas may also arise in small congenital nevi less than 1.5 cm in diameter.[4] A representative histologic study found that 59% of the precursor nevi showed features of acquired nevi, 39% showed features of congenital nevi, and the remaining few nevi were not further categorized.[5] Of all these nevi, 54% also showed histologic features of so-called dysplastic nevi, a designation that is controversial.

"Dysplastic nevi" were originally described as a cutaneous marker of familial melanoma.[7] The term "dysplastic nevus" has since been used to describe syndromes of multiple atypical nevi occurring in association with either familial melanomas or sporadic melanomas, and the term has also been used to describe individual atypical nevi occurring in patients without a personal or familial history of melanoma. Several studies have shown a lack of inter-observer reproducibility in the histologic diagnosis of dysplastic nevi, and it is now widely accepted that there is a continuum from ordinary benign (banal) nevi through nevi with moderate and severe dysplasia, to nevi with developing melanoma in situ.[8] Furthermore, the NIH consensus conference recommended excising nevi with histologic features of a dysplastic nevus and moderate to severe cytologic atypia with the 0.5 cm margins, the same margins that they recommended for treatment of melanoma in situ, because developing melanoma in situ may show overlapping histologic characteristics with these nevi.

Types of Malignant Melanoma

Lentigo Maligna and Lentigo Maligna Melanoma

Lentigo maligna is by definition the in situ phase of lentigo maligna melanoma (LMM). Lentigo maligna occurs in chronically sun-exposed skin, usually of the head and neck but occasionally in other sun-exposed areas. Lentigo maligna typically evolves over many years as an unevenly pigmented macular lesion that expands peripherally and that eventually may measure several centimeters in diameter. The histopathologic features in lentigo maligna may be subtle, and partial biopsies may not be diagnostic. Early lentigo maligna may show only epidermal hyperpigmentation and a subtle increase in the number of melanocytes, features that are not easily distinguishable from changes seen in chronically sun-damaged skin. Helpful histologic features include extension of atypical melanocytes down follicular epithelium and spread of melanocytes above the dermal epidermal junction, so-called pagetoid spread of melanocytes.[9–11]

When the dermis is invaded, the lesion is called lentigo maligna melanoma. Dermal invasion is a focal process and may be difficult to recognize. Invasive cells of lentigo maligna melanoma usually have abundant cytoplasm and are epitheliod or spindle shaped in character but may rarely appear as small round cells. Occasionally, lentigo maligna melanoma invades as cells that have spindle-shaped nuclei and relatively little cytoplasm, and induces a fibrotic or "desmoplastic" response in the underlying stroma. This variant, called *desmoplastic malignant melanoma*, may also show neurotropism and may be very difficult to recognize, requiring a high degree of suspicion and the use of immunoperoxidase studies to establish the diagnosis.[12] This morphologic variant of lentigo malignant melanoma is important because it may be difficult to recognize, but it is not associated with a difference in prognosis, compared to other primary melanomas, when adjusted for tumor thickness.[13]

Superficial Spreading Melanoma

Superficial spreading melanomas (SSM) often arise in melanocytic nevi and must be distinguished histologically from normal or atypical nevi. Architecturally, normal nevi are usually symmetric and show relatively uniform nests of cytologically typical melanocytes occurring at the tips and sides of rete ridges. Criteria for a diagnosis for superficial spreading melanoma include both architectural and cytologic features. Architectural features favoring a diagnosis of melanoma include asymmetric growth, a lack of circumscription, and large size. A major criterion for the diagnosis of melanoma is the spread of melanocytes throughout the epidermis as individual cells or nests of cells. Poorly circumscribed lesions also show individual cells at their edges, which are irregularly distributed at and above the dermal epidermal junction.[10,11]

With early invasion, atypical melanocytes extend from the epidermis into the most superficial (papillary) dermis as individual cells, where they start to form nests. Melanoma cells are typically round or polygonal in shape. The dermal component of benign melanocytic nevi is typically composed of melanocytes arranged in nests that are larger in the upper dermis and that gradually decrease in size in the deeper portions of the dermis. Melanocytes of benign nevi may also be arranged in single file, splayed between dermal collagen bundles, and arranged around neurovascular or adnexal structures. In contrast, invasive melanoma cells usually do not decrease in size in the deeper portions of the dermis, a characteristic that distinguishes them from the cells of benign melanocytic nevi. Invasive melanoma more typically grows as irregularly sized and shaped nests of cytologically atypical cells, as irregularly distributed single cells, or as sheets of atypical cells.

Acral Lentiginous Melanoma

The term *acral lentiginous melanoma* (ALM) refers mainly to melanomas occurring in the hairless skin of the palms and soles but also includes those arising in the nail unit and the surrounding periungual areas.[10,11] They are called lentiginous because their early pattern of growth consists of a proliferation of individual cells along the dermal–epidermal junction, a pattern that resembles melanocytic growth in benign lentigines. Features that distinguish ALM from lentigines include the presence of cytologically atypical cells that tend to confluence and the formation of irregularly distributed junctional nests without a benign dermal component. Cytologically, cells in early ALM may be relatively bland and it may be very difficult to establish the diagnosis, particularly if the specimen is a partial biopsy from the edge of a lesion that may show only an increase in pigment and a subtle increase in the number of melanocytes. Invasive ALM usually grows as epitheliod or spindle-shaped cells, or as smaller melanoma cells with less cytoplasm. As with LMM, ALM may show a desmoplastic growth pattern and may preferentially invade and grow along nerves.

Nodular Melanoma

The histologic features of a nodular melanoma (NM) are those of expansile dermal growth with relatively little involvement of the epidermis.[10,11] The epidermal component is often described as spreading no more than three rete ridges beyond the dermal component of the tumor, so whereas the overall architecture of SSM is horizontally oriented as the tumor cells spread within the epidermis and invade the papillary dermis, the orientation of nodular melanoma is vertical and NM typically appear deeper than they do wide. The dermal nests and masses of nodular melanoma cells should be larger than any of the nests present within the epidermis. NM often grow in sheets and may show marked focal differences in pigmentation and cell morphology in different parts of the tumor. Cytologically, the cells of NM are often epithelioid or spindle shaped, but may also be small with a high nuclear to cytoplasmic ratio.

Histologic Features of Prognosis in Cutaneous Melanomas

The only histologic features of primary melanomas that have been consistently shown to be correlated with prognosis in multivariate (Cox regression and Tree structured survival) analyses have been tumor thickness, micrometasases, ulceration, mitotic activity, and incomplete removal of the original lesion with the presence of melanoma on the margins of the primary resection specimen.[13–17] These histologic features are of prognostic significance independent of the age of the patient, the type of the melanoma, or the anatomic location, and it is therefore recommended that these features be specifically mentioned in pathology reports.[18]

Tumor Thickness and Level

The concept that the depth of invasion of a melanoma into the dermis and subcutaneous fat could be related to prognosis was first suggested by Allen and Spitz,[19] and was modified by Clark et al.,[20] who proposed descriptive levels including an in situ level, and levels of invasion involving the papillary dermis, the reticular dermis, and the subcutaneous fat. These studies clearly established the concept that the depth of the tumor was more significant prognostically than its diameter, but these methods resulted in a stepwise classification and were not highly reproducible. In 1970, Alexander Breslow proposed determining the thickness of primary cutaneous melanomas by measuring from the top of the granular layer of the epidermis to the greatest depth of the invasion into the dermis, using an eyepiece micrometer.[15] The resultant continuous variable, usually reported to the hundredth of a millimeter, is variously referred to as the Breslow depth or Breslow thickness, and has been found to be a reproducible and statistically significant prognostic variable in the evaluation of primary cutaneous melanoma.[15]

Vascular Invasion and Micrometastases

The presence of invasion of tumor cells within blood or lymphatic vessels has been shown to be associated with a poor prognosis[21,22] and is generally accepted as a poor prognostic feature. Similarly, micrometastases, defined as discrete masses of tumor cells measuring greater than 0.05 mm in diameter and located in the reticular dermis or subcutaneous fat, separated from the main tumor mass by normal tissue, has been identified as a histologic prognostic feature, and is also generally accepted as an indicator of a poor prognosis.

Ulceration and Other Tissue Reaction Patterns

Spontaneous ulceration of the epidermis has been identified as an independent indicator of poor prognosis in a number of studies.[14,16,17] A second tissue reaction pattern that has been described is the presence or absence of tumor-infiltrating lymphocytes (TILs), which are lymphocytes that infiltrate between the individual melanocytes making up nests and clusters of melanoma cells invading the dermis.[23] Histologic identification of TILs requires interpretation, and the usefulness of this feature has not been as widely validated as have tumor thickness, ulceration, mitoses and margins. A third commonly studied variable is the presence of regression. The histologic feature of partial regression of a primary melanoma are usually observed in the papillary dermis, where there is fibrosis characterized by delicate collagen bundles in the papillary dermis, usually associated with melanophages and lymphocytes, and with melanoma present in the overlying epidermis and/or adjacent papillary dermis. There is also frequently flattening of the overlying epidermis. However, the histologic diagnosis of regression in thin melanomas requires interpretation, and various proposals have been made for the prognostic significance of certain patterns of regression or for stratifying regression based on the percentage of the melanoma that appears to be affected. However, regression of a primary melanoma does not appear to be a robust indicator of clinical outcome.[24]

Mitoses and Proliferative Indices

The presence of mitosis in the invasive component of a melanoma, usually reported as the mitotic rate per millimeter squared (mm^2) or the number of mitoses per 10 high-power fields, has consistently shown to be an independent variable for predicting prognosis.[16] Mitoses are obviously an expression of the proliferative rate of the tumor, and the proliferative capacity has also been estimated by immunohistochemical staining for Ki-67, also known as proliferating nuclear antigen (PNAC).[25,26] Conversely, the level of cyclin A, a cell-cycle regulator, has been reported to be positively associated with disease-free survival.[25]

Melanoma Genetics

Familial Melanoma Syndromes

Two general types of genetic abnormalities are observed in families whose members are at increased risk for melanoma. In one type of abnormality, seen in the multiple primary melanoma syndrome, family members carry an abnormal CDKN2A tumor suppressor gene. This gene, which is located on 9p21, encodes the cell-cycle progression regulator p16, which is part of the cyclin D1/CDK 4/p16/pRb signaling pathway. This cyclin signaling pathway controls proliferation in many cell types,[27–30] and loss of function of genes in this pathway affects individual cells, placing them at increased risk for transformation. In contrast, the mechanism of the second type of familial melanoma susceptibility functions on the level of the whole organism by affecting the ability of pigmented keratinocytes to protect epidermal melanocytes from transformation by ultraviolet irradiation. In this second type of susceptibility, variation in the melanocortin I receptor (MCI R) has been identified as the probable basis for high-risk phenotypes such as pale (type 1) skin, the lack of ability to tan in response to ultraviolet (UV) exposure, and red hair.[31] Thus, these mutations work at the level of the entire organism by decreasing the natural protection afforded by normal epidermal melanin and increasing the risk of damage to melanocytes when the individual is exposed to ultraviolet light.

Genetic Abnormalities in Sporadic Melanoma

In general, sporadic human melanomas show genetic instability, characterized by multiple chromosomal gains and losses, when examined by comparative genomic hybridization,[32–35] but no specific individual gene changes have been associated with the development of sporadic melanomas, other than those directly affecting the cyclin pathway. In sporadic melanomas, loss of the tumor suppressor genes INK 4a/ARF, which are also components of the cyclin pathway, is frequently found.[36] Overexpression of HDM2 is found in 56% of invasive primary and in metastatic melanomas, 27% of melanomas in situ, and in only 6% of "dysplastic nevi," a finding that suggests that this gene may play a role in progression of individual melanomas.[37] Although in vivo animal models of melanoma have been developed by overexpressing HRAS, mutations and increases in copy number of this gene have been found in humans only in Spitz nevi and not in melanomas.

Risk Factors and Prevention

Risk Factors

The identification of risk factors and high-risk populations for melanoma provides opportunities for both primary prevention and early diagnosis. A greatly elevated melanoma risk is present for a changing nevus as well as for dysplastic nevi in the setting of familial melanoma.[38,39] Individuals with a familial melanoma syndrome, as discussed in the previous section on melanoma genetics, are high-risk individuals. An individual with a personal history of melanoma has a lifetime risk of at least 3% of having another primary melanoma.[39,40] Individuals with precursor lesions such as atypical or dysplastic nevi, giant congenital nevi, or numerous common nevi have an increased melanoma risk.[38,39] An elevated risk is also present for patients receiving immunosuppression.[41]

There are numerous studies that suggest the importance of ultraviolet radiation (UVR) on the development of melanoma.[39,42] Geographic location near the equator, especially for individuals with a fair complexion, is associated with an increased risk of melanoma. The phenotype of the typical melanoma patient (fair complexion, tendency to sunburn rather than tan, blond or red hair color, blue or green eyes) is well described.[39] Blistering sunburns, especially in childhood and adolescence, is an identified risk factor. Outdoor recreational habits that include intermittent high ultraviolet radiation (UVR) exposure are associated with an increased melanoma risk. Individuals with the genetic disorder xeroderma pigmentosum, a condition with defective cellular DNA repair mechanisms following UVR, have a significantly increased risk for melanoma compared with age-matched controls.[43]

Prevention

Strategies to prevent melanoma have primarily emphasized primary prevention strategies that target high-risk individuals.[44,45] Because UVR is considered an important modifiable risk factor, efforts have focused on avoidance of excessive sun exposure. The wearing of protective clothing, avoiding blistering sunburns, minimizing peak hours of sun exposure, avoiding tanning parlors, and use of sunscreen with a sun protection factor (SPF) of 15 or higher, are all examples of this sun protective behavior. The topic of sunscreens and melanoma risk remains controversial.[46,47] Several factors confound interpretation of studies evaluating use of sunscreens and melanoma risk. Individuals with a fair complexion and at increased risk for problems with UVR may be more likely to use sunscreens. Sunscreen use may be higher in individuals with a prior history of sunburns. In addition, individuals using sunscreens may allow themselves to have increased UVR. A meta-analysis of 18 case-controlled studies recently addressed this topic, and no association was seen between melanoma and sunscreen use.[48] Direct proof that sunscreens reduce the risk for melanoma is lacking. However, significant indirect evidence supports the recommendations by the American Academy of Dermatology that includes regular use of a broad-spectrum high-SPF sunscreen along with protective clothing and avoiding midday sun as measures to reduce melanoma risk. A prospective randomized study to determine the efficacy of sunscreens would be informative, but this study is unlikely to be performed.

Strategies aimed at chemoprevention of melanoma in individuals with high-risk lesions are also being developed.[49] The possible molecular mechanisms for UV melanogenesis, as well as preliminary data from clinical and preclinical studies, were recently reviewed.[49] Molecular and histologic markers are being identified as surrogate endpoints for melanoma chemoprevention studies. Agents currently receiving clinical testing include retinoids, lovastatin, nonsteroidal antiinflammatory agents, and vitamin E. Many other agents including green tea, perilyl alcohol, COX-2 inhibitors, selinium, and others are receiving preclinical testing. The results of these studies are eagerly awaited, and additional clinical testing is anticipated for melanoma chemoprevention of high-risk precancerous lesions.

Melanoma and Pregnancy or Exogenous Hormone Administration

Melanoma and Pregnancy

A number of clinical observations suggest that pregnancy might have an effect on melanocytes.[50–52] Increased pigmentation is often associated with pregnancy. An increase in levels of melanocytic-stimulating hormone has also been measured in some pregnant women, and receptors that bind the female hormone estrogen can be found on some melanomas. These observations have raised the possibility that the hormonal and other physiologic changes associated with pregnancy may influence the development and course of melanoma. Thus, several investigators utilized available prognostic factors to study women diagnosed with melanoma during their pregnancy as well as evaluate the effect pregnancy might have on women who have previously been diagnosed with melanoma. When patients who are pregnant are compared with patients who are not pregnant and the known prognostic factors are comparable, the outcome of the patients are very similar.[50–52] In addition, the majority of available evidence indicates that women who became pregnant after being previously treated for melanoma do not have a worse outcome or an earlier reactivation of previously diagnosed melanoma.[52]

Melanoma and Exogenous Hormone Administration

The estrogen receptor has been identified in approximately one of five melanomas, which has led some to speculate that the presence of estrogens might influence the course of the disease.[51] However, current studies have not demonstrated any convincing association, either favorable or unfavorable, between the use of oral contraceptives before the diagnosis of melanoma and survival.[51] There are no large, well-conducted studies that have addressed the issue of birth control pills or hormone replacement therapy following the diagnosis of melanoma. Therefore, recommendations are usually made on the basis of clinical need and with the understanding that no evidence currently requires that oral contraceptives or hormone replacement therapy be withheld from these patients.

Classification and Staging: The 2002 AJCC Staging System

The American Joint Committee on Cancer (AJCC) melanoma task force first published the most recent revisions to the melanoma staging system and companion validation prognostic factor analyses in 2001.[53,54] This updated melanoma staging system represents a significant change from the previous system (Table 59.1). These changes are based on a better understanding of the melanoma-associated prognostic factors, derived from an extensive body of literature as well as from the largest melanoma prognostic factor analysis ever conducted, involving complete raw data from 17,600 patients.[54]

The most important criteria for T classification are tumor thickness followed by tumor ulceration (Table 59.2). Analyses of large prospective databases confirmed the importance of tumor thickness as a prognostic factor and found that Clark level of invasion was significant only for melanoma lesions 1 mm thick or less.[54]

In the revised melanoma staging system, four criteria were established as significant prognostic factors for survival in patients with regional metastases: (1) the number of lymph nodes harboring metastatic disease, (2) microscopic versus macroscopic tumor burden in the lymph nodes, (3) the presence of satellite or in-transit metastases, and (4) the presence of ulceration in the primary lesion. These criteria require pathologic confirmation of nodal or regional metastatic disease (see Table 59.2).

Within the M classification there is only one group, M1, because no breakpoints in this classification stratify patients into groups with survival differences sufficient to warrant further subgroupings. Within the M1 group, however, there are three subcategories, "a," "b," and "c," reflecting survival differences that have been reported in other studies or were apparent in 1-year analyses, although not on longer-term analyses, in the AJCC prognostic factors study (see Table 59.2). M1a includes distant skin, subcutaneous, or lymph node metastases; these manifestations of distant disease have been associated with a better prognosis than distant metastases in other anatomic locations.[54] Lung metastases are included in a separate category, M1b, because of the survival advantage at 1 year in the AJCC analysis for patients with lung metastases compared to patients with other visceral metastases (57% versus 41%, P less than 0.0001). Finally, M1c includes all other visceral metastases and cases with any distant metastases and an elevated serum lactate dehydrogenase level. Serum lactate dehydrogenase level is included in the M1c category because it has been identified as one of the

TABLE 59.1. Differences between the previous (1997) version and the present (2002) version of the melanoma staging system.

Factor	*Old system*	*New system*	*Comments*
Thickness	Secondary prognosis factor; thresholds of 0.75, 1.50, 4.0mm	Primary determinant of T staging; thresholds of 1.0, 2.0, 4.0mm	Correlation of metastatic risk is a continuous variable
Level of invasion	Primary determinant of T staging	Used only for defining T1 melanomas	Correlation only significant for thin lesions; variability in interpretation
Ulceration	Not included	Included as a second determinant of T and N staging	Signifies a locally advanced lesion; dominant prognostic factor for grouping stages I, II, and III
Satellite metastases	In T category	In N category	Merged with in-transit lesions
Thick melanomas (>4.0mm)	Stage III	Stage IIC	Stage III defined as regional metastases
Dimensions of nodal metastases	Dominant determinant of N staging	Not used	No evidence of significant prognostic correlation
Number of nodal metastases	Not included	Primary determinant of N staging	Thresholds of 1 vs. 2–3 vs. ≥4 nodes
Metastatic tumor burden	Not included	Included as a second determinant of N staging	Clinically occult ("microscopic") vs. clinically apparent ("macroscopic") nodal volume
Lung metastases	Merged with all other visceral metastases	Separate category as M1b	Has a somewhat better prognosis than other visceral metastases
Elevated serum lactate dehydrogenase (LDH)	Not included	Included as a second determinant of M staging	
Clinical vs. pathologic staging	Did not account for sentinel node technology	Sentinel node results incorporated into definition of pathologic staging	Large variability in outcome between clinical and pathologic staging; pathologic staging encouraged before entry into clinical trials

Source: Adapted from Balch et al.[53] Used with permission of the American Joint Committee on Cancer (AJCC), Chicago, Illinois. The original source for this information is the *AJCC Cancer Staging Manual*, sixth edition (2002), published by Springer-Verlag New York, www.springer-ny.com.

most important predictors of poor prognosis in patients with metastatic disease.[54]

The clinical and pathologic stage groupings for the current staging system are shown in Table 59.3. Stage I includes thin primary lesions with low associated melanoma-specific mortality. The 10-year survival rates for patients with stage IA and IB disease are 88% and 81%, respectively.[53] Stage II includes lesions associated with an intermediate and somewhat higher risk of metastatic disease and melanoma-specific mortality. The 10-year survival rates for patients with stage IIA, IIB, and IIC disease are 64%, 52%, and 32%, respectively.[53] Because of the significant heterogeneity of prognoses in patients with stage III disease, three substages were defined: IIIA, IIIB, and IIIC. The 5-year survival rates for patients with stage IIIA, IIIB, and IIIC disease are 67%, 53%, and 26%, respectively.[53] For patients with stage IV disease, the 1-year survival rates in the M1a, M1b, and M1c groups are 59%, 57%, and 41%, respectively.[53]

TABLE 59.2. Definition of TNM in the 2002 American Joint Committee on Cancer staging system for cutaneous melanoma.

Primary tumor (T)	
TX	Primary tumor cannot be assessed (e.g., shave biopsy or regressed melanoma)
T0	No evidence of primary tumor
Tis	Melanoma in situ
T1	Melanoma ≤1.0mm in thickness with or without ulceration
T1a	Melanoma ≤1.0mm in thickness and level II or III, no ulceration
T1b	Melanoma ≤1.0mm in thickness and level IV or V or with ulceration
T2	Melanoma 1.01–2mm in thickness with or without ulceration
T2a	Melanoma 1.01–2.0mm in thickness, no ulceration
T2b	Melanoma 1.01–2.0mm in thickness, with ulceration
T3	Melanoma 2.01–4mm in thickness with or without ulceration
T3a	Melanoma 2.01–4.0mm in thickness, no ulceration
T3b	Melanoma 2.01–4.0mm in thickness, with ulceration
T4	Melanoma >4.0mm in thickness with or without ulceration
T4a	Melanoma >4.0mm in thickness, no ulceration
T4b	Melanoma >4.0mm in thickness, with ulceration
Regional lymph nodes (N)	
NX	Regional lymph nodes cannot be assessed
N0	No regional lymph node metastasis
N1	Metastasis in one lymph node
N1a	Clinically occult (microscopic) metastasis
N1b	Clinically apparent (macroscopic) metastasis
N2	Metastasis in two to three regional nodes or intralymphatic regional metastasis without nodal metastases
N2a	Clinically occult (microscopic) metastasis
N2b	Clinically apparent (macroscopic) metastasis
N2c	Satellite or in-transit metastasis *without* nodal metastasis
N3	Metastasis in four or more regional nodes, or matted metastatic nodes, or in-transit metastasis or satellite(s) *with* metastasis in regional node(s)
Distant metastasis (M)	
MX	Distant metastasis cannot be assessed
M0	No distant metastasis
M1	Distant metastasis
M1a	Metastasis to skin, subcutaneous tissues, or distant lymph nodes
M1b	Metastasis to lung
M1c	Metastasis to all other visceral sites or distant metastasis at any site associated with an elevated serum lactic dehydrogenase (LDH)

Source: Used with permission of the American Joint Committee on Cancer (AJCC), Chicago, Illinois. The original source for this information is the *AJCC Cancer Staging Manual*, sixth edition (2002), published by Springer-Verlag New York, www.springer-ny.com.

TABLE 59.3. Clinical and pathologic stage grouping in the 2002 American Joint Committee on Cancer staging system for cutaneous melanoma.

	Clinical stage grouping[a]			*Pathologic stage grouping*[b]		
	T	*N*	*M*	*T*	*N*	*M*
Stage 0	Tis	N0	M0	Tis	N0	M0
Stage IA	T1a	N0	M0	T1a	N0	M0
Stage IB	T1b	N0	M0	T1b	N0	M0
	T2a	N0	M0	T2a	N0	M0
Stage IIA	T2b	N0	M0	T2b	N0	M0
	T3a	N0	M0	T3a	N0	M0
Stage IIB	T3b	N0	M0	T3b	N0	M0
	T4a	N0	M0	T4a	N0	M0
Stage IIC	T4b	N0	M0	T4b	N0	M0
Stage III	Any T	N1	M0			
		N2				
		N3				
Stage IIIA				T1–4a	N1a	M0
				T1–4a	N2a	M0
Stage IIIB				T1–4b	N1a	M0
				T1–4b	N2a	M0
				T1–4a	N1b	M0
				T1–4a	N2b	M0
				T1–4a/b	N2c	M0
Stage IIIC				T1–4b	N1b	M0
				T1–4b	N2b	M0
				Any T	N3	M0
Stage IV	Any T	Any N	Any M1	Any T	Any N	Any M1

[a] Clinical staging includes microstaging of the primary melanoma and clinical/radiological evaluation for metastases. By convention, it should be used after complete excision of the primary melanoma with clinical assessment for regional and distant metastases.

[b] Pathologic staging includes microstaging of the primary melanoma and pathologic information about the regional lymph nodes after partial or complete lymphadenectomy. Pathologic stage 0 or stage IA patients are the exception; they do not require pathologic evaluation of their lymph nodes.

Source: Used with permission of the American Joint Committee on Cancer (AJCC), Chicago, Illinois. The original source for this information is the *AJCC Cancer Staging Manual*, sixth edition (2002), published by Springer-Verlag New York.

Surgical Considerations

All lesions with characteristics that are concerning for melanoma should be biopsied. An "ABCD" rule is available to help identify pigmented lesions at risk for melanoma: Asymmetry, Border irregularity, Color inhomogeneity, and diameter greater than 6mm (the size of a pencil eraser).[55] Any pigmented lesion that demonstrates a change in size, color, or shape should be considered clinically suspicious. Although the majority of lesions needing biopsy can be identified by careful visual inspection, additional tools are available to assist in the evaluation of pigmented skin lesions. Serial photography can be used to help follow individuals with a large number of atypical appearing nevi. The use of digital photography especially allows for careful sequential assessment of individual pigmented lesions.[56,57] Lesions that change over time can be identified for diagnostic biopsy. Epiluminescence, or surface microscopy, can be used to examine individual pigmented lesions for features suggestive of malignancy.[56,58,59] Any pigmented lesion with changes or features suggestive of melanoma should be biospied expeditiously.

Biopsy Techniques

The most powerful predictor of survival for primary melanoma is tumor thickness. There is almost a linear relationship between increasing tumor thickness and decreasing survival. The corollary to this is that it is important to biopsy the suspicious pigmented lesion with the proper technique. Shave biopsies should not be performed when a melanoma is suspected because of the risk of cutting through the depth of the lesion and having a positive deep margin. If this occurs, a true tumor thickness cannot be ascertained and prognosis and treatment decisions are hampered; this is particularly pertinent when a shave biopsy straddles the tumor thickness of 0.76–1.0mm. Patients with melanomas less than 0.76mm in thickness have "thin" melanomas and have a high likelihood of cure with simple surgical techniques [1.0-cm-wide local excision (WLE)]. Patients with melanomas thicker than this have a defined rate of nodal and systemic metastases and are candidates for a wide local excision and nodal staging with the new lymphatic mapping techniques. Patients are done a disservice if a true tumor thickness cannot be ascertained. The proper biopsy technique for suspicious pigmented lesions is an excisional biopsy with a 1.0-mm margin. For larger lesions that cannot be completely excised, a 6.0-mm punch or incisional biopsy of the most nodular-appearing area that reaches into the subcutaneous fat beneath the lesion is indicated to make the diagnosis.

Surgical Treatment of the Primary Melanoma

Local management of primary melanoma necessitates wide excision of the lesion with a margin of normal-appearing skin.

TABLE 59.4. Completed prospective randomized trials evaluating surgical excision margins.

Trial	*No. of patients*	*Tumor thickness (mm)*	*Excision margins*	*Overall local recurrence*	*Overall survival*	*Comments*
French Cooperative Group[64]	362	≤2	2 cm vs. 5 cm	NSD[a]	NSD	Margins of 2 cm are safe for melanomas ≤2 mm
World Health Organization, Melanoma Program, trial 10[65–67]	612	≤2	1 cm vs. 3 cm	NSD[b]	NSD	Margins of 1 cm are safe for melanomas ≤1 mm; Follow-up for local failures is ongoing for 1- to 2-mm melanomas
Swedish Melanoma Group[68,69]	989	≤2	2 cm vs. 5 cm	NSD	NSD	Margins of 2 cm are safe for melanomas ≤2 mm
Intergroup Melanoma Surgical Trial[70,71]	486	1–4	2 cm vs. 4 cm	NSD	NSD	Margins of 2 cm are safe for melanomas 1–4 mm
U.K. Melanoma Study Group[72,73]	900	>2	1 cm vs. 3 cm	NSD[c]	NSD	A percentage of nodal or other local/regional events may be reduced by margins >1 cm for melanomas >2 mm

[a] No significant difference.

[b] Trend toward an increase in the absolute number of local recurrences in the narrow excision group for patients in the 1–2 mm subset.

[c] The patients who received a 3-cm excision had an improved relapse-free survival when all local and regional events were grouped together.

Previously, the surgical standard of care was a 3- to 5-cm-wide local excision (WLE) and a split-thickness skin graft. Increasingly, it has become evident that the risk of local recurrence coincides more with the thickness of the lesion and whether it is ulcerated rather than the extent of the surgical margins.[60–62] It may seem more rational, then, to use surgical margins that vary with the ulceration and thickness of the lesion, as these factors seem to correlate best with the risk for local recurrence.

The least advanced form of the disease is melanoma in situ. Although the natural history of this noninvasive melanoma is not completely understood, failure to reexcise the biopsy site may result in a local recurrence as either an invasive melanoma or an in situ lesion.[63] Therefore, it is recommended that the biopsy site of an in situ melanoma be reexcised with at least a 0.5- to 1-cm margin of skin. For "thin" melanomas (less than 1.00 mm in thickness), only a minimum local recurrence rate has been reported in observed patient series,[60–62] despite varying surgical margins. In other words, survival is not influenced by the size of the resection margins. At the present time, a wide excision consisting of no less than 1 cm minimum margin of skin is recommended by many melanoma surgeons.[61] This procedure may be performed as a generous elliptical excision and a primary skin closure. Results from five completed prospective randomized studies, summarized in Table 59.4, have established guidelines for excisional margins for invasive melanomas less than 4.0 mm in thickness.[64–73] Current recommendations are for 1-cm margins for melanomas up to 1 mm, 1- or 2-cm margins for melanomas between 1 and 2 cm, and 2-cm margins for melanomas between 2 and 4 mm.[61] The risk of local recurrence may exceed 10% to 20% for those melanomas more than 4 mm in thickness.[60–62,73] Thus, at least 2-cm margins are recommended for these deep primary melanomas.

Intraoperative Lymphatic Mapping and Sentinel Node Biopsy

A new procedure has been developed to assess the status of the regional lymph nodes more accurately and decrease the morbidity and expense of a complete elective lymph node dissection (ELND). The technique, termed intraoperative lymphatic mapping and selective lymphadenectomy, relies on the concept that regions of the skin have specific patterns of lymphatic drainage, not only to the regional lymphatic basin but also to a specific lymph node (sentinel lymph node, SLN) in the basin.[74] Morton et al. initially proposed the technique[75,76] using a vital blue dye method and showed, in animals and initial human trials, that the SLN is the first node in the lymphatic basin into which the primary site drains. They showed that the SLN histology reflected the histology of the remainder of the nodal basin, so that complete nodal staging could be obtained with a SLN biopsy.[74]

These data have been confirmed by many other institutions, including the Lakeland Regional Cancer Center (LRCC) and Moffitt Cancer Center (MCC),[77] M.D. Anderson Cancer Center,[78] and the Sidney Melanoma Unit.[79] These studies have demonstrated an orderly progression of melanoma nodal metastases. Preoperative lymphoscintigraphy is performed to provide a roadmap for the surgeon as to what basins are at risk for metastatic disease. This nuclear medicine study involves the injection of technetium sulfur colloid into the skin around the melanoma and imaging the patient to ascertain the direction of cutaneous lymphatic flow (Figure 59.1). Two mapping agents are then routinely used intraoperatively, a vital blue dye and a radiocolloid that has the right particle size to be taken up by the cutaneous lymphatics to migrate to the SLN. Upon exposing the lymph nodes in the basin, the SLN will be stained blue and will become "hot" compared to

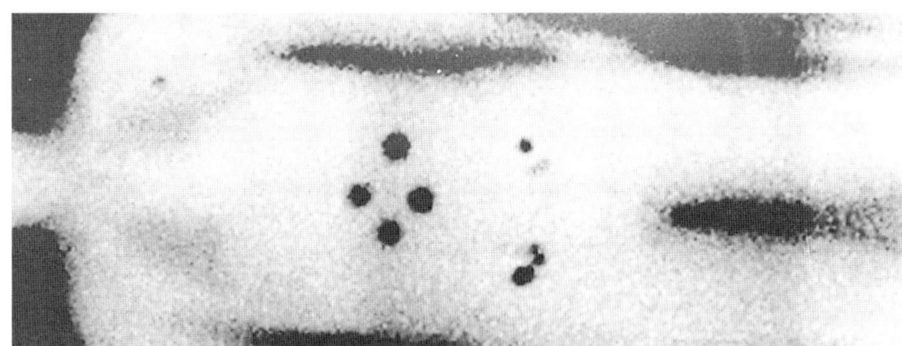

FIGURE 59.1. Preoperative lymphoscinitigraphy in a patient with an intermediate-thickness melanoma around the umbilicus. This region of the skin is a watershed area of the body that can show multidirectional lymphatic flow with more than one basin at risk for metastases. This particular primary melanoma drains to both superficial groins as well as the left axilla.

surrounding neighboring non-SLNs and other tissue in the basin. These hot spots can then be used to direct the dissection with a hand-held gamma probe to the SLN.

This SLN concept was demonstrated in a study involving patients with a primary melanoma tumor thickness greater than 0.76mm and who were considered candidates for an elective lymph node dissection.[76] The SLN was harvested and submitted separately to pathology, followed by a complete node dissection. In this study, 42 patients met the criteria for SLN biopsy based on prognostic factors of their primary melanoma.[76] Thirty-four patients had histologically negative SLNs, with the rest of the nodes in the basin also being negative. Thus, there were no "skip" metastases documented. Eight patients had positive SLNs, with 7 of the 8 having the SLN as the only site of disease. Nodal involvement was compared between the SLN and non-SLN groups based on the binomial distribution. Under the null hypothesis of equality in distribution of nodal metastases, the probability that all seven unpaired observations would demonstrate involvement of the SLN was 0.008. The data presented demonstrates that nodal metastases from cutaneous melanoma are not random events. The SLNs in the lymphatic basins can be mapped and individually identified, and they have been shown to contain the first evidence of melanoma metastases. These findings demonstrate effective pathologic staging, no decrease in standards of care, and a reduction of morbidity with a less-aggressive, rational surgical approach and lower costs for the healthcare system.[74]

Several prospective national trials are in progress to assess whether this surgical strategy provides a survival benefit for patients. In addition, the Florida Melanoma Trial, with the central office and laboratory located at the Lakeland Regional Cancer Center, is a regional industry-sponsored trial that will examine whether all patients with a positive SLN need to undergo a complete lymph node dissection of the affected basin. The results of these ongoing trials will help determine the final role of radioguided surgery in patients with malignant melanoma.

Surgical Management of Regional Metastases

Elective Lymph Node Dissection

Results from four completed prospective randomized studies are available to assess potential survival benefit for patients with clinically negative lymph nodes who receive elective lymph node dissection (ELND) as part of their primary tumor management (Table 59.5).[80–86] These studies clearly demonstrate no overall survival benefit for all patients receiving ELND.[87] However, findings from prospectively stratified subgroups of patients suggest that patients with intermediate-thickness melanomas (1–4mm) that are not ulcerated appear to have a survival advantage with ELND.[84–87] Although surgical management of these patients has been largely replaced with SLN evaluation, these results suggest the potential cura-

TABLE 59.5. Completed prospective randomized trials evaluating elective lymph node dissection (ELND).

Trial	*No. of patients*	*Sites*	*Tumor thickness (mm)*	*Overall group survival benefit*	*Subset survival benefit*	*Comments*
World Health Organization Melanoma Program Trial 1[80,81]	553	Extremities	All thicknesses	NSD[a]	No[b]	All melanoma patients do not benefit from ELND
Mayo Clinic Surgical Trial[82,83]	171	Extremities	All thicknesses	NSD	No[b]	All melanoma patients do not benefit from ELND
Intergroup Melanoma Surgical Trial[84,85]	737	All	1–4	NSD	Yes[c]	Defined subsets may benefit from ELND[c]
World Health Organization Melanoma Program Trial 14[86]	227	Trunk	≥1.5	NSD	Yes[d]	Defined subsets may benefit from ELND[d]

[a] No significant difference.

[b] Prospective stratified subgroup analysis was not performed.

[c] Among the prospectively stratified subgroups of patients, 10-year survival rates were improved in patients who received ELND and had the following characteristics: nonulcerated melanomas, tumor thickness of 1–2mm, extremity melanomas.

[d] Among the prospectively stratified subgroups of patients, overall survival was improved in patients with a tumor thickness of 1.5–4.0mm.

tive potential of surgery for defined subsets of patients with regionally metastatic disease.[87]

Therapeutic Lymph Node Dissection

In patients with gross nodal metastases, the standard of care is to perform a complete lymph node dissection. The 5-year survival of patients with a nonulcerated melanoma and one, microscopically involved lymph node in the regional basin is approximately 75%. For patients with resected gross nodal disease in the regional basin, the 5-year survival rate drops to 25%. Thus, even in the face of gross nodal disease, surgery in and of itself in the nodal basin can cure approximately 25% of the patients.[53,54]

Isolated Limb Perfusion

Isolated limb perfusion (ILP) refers to the regional intravascular delivery of chemotherapeutic agents to an extremity that has had involvement with melanoma.[88] The concept behind ILP is that administration of high drug concentrations is possible with ILP, and the goal with this approach is to improve treatment outcome while limiting systemic toxicities. Major toxicities with ILP have included systemic toxicities related to the infused agent as well as regional toxicities including skin toxicity, limb edema, myopathy, peripheral neuropathy, and vascular toxicity, including arterial embolic events and deep venous thrombosis.[88]

The application of ILP for extremity melanoma has included both adjuvant ILP as well as ILP for established metastatic disease. Unfortunately, most of the literature describing ILP involves nonrandomized single-institution studies that often use a variety of treatment regimens as well as include heterogeneous patient populations.[88] A randomized trial involving 852 patients was performed by an intergroup including the European Organization for Research and Treatment of Cancer (EORTC), World Health Organization (WHO), and the North American Perfusion Group (NAPG) to evaluate the benefit of prophylactic ILP with melphalan for patients with high-risk extremity melanoma.[89] Study results published with a median follow-up of more than 6 years demonstrate an improvement related to disease-free survival, with a decrease in both in-transit metastases (6.6% to 3.3%) as well as a decrease or delay in regional lymph node metastases in the ILP-treated patients.[89] Unfortunately, no benefit in decreasing distant metastases or improving survival was identified. Thus, routine use of adjuvant ILP cannot be recommended for patients with resected high-risk extremity melanoma.

ILP with melphalan has also been administered at normothermic or hyperthermic (HILP) temperatures to melanoma patients who have disease consisting of established in-transit metastases, either with or without additional regional lymph node disease.[88] Results from a number of uncontrolled studies report complete responses ranging from 7% to 82% and overall response rates that range from 48% to 100%.[88] To improve these results, tumor necrosis factor (TNF) alone or with interferon-gamma has been added to melphalan.[88,90,91] Initial results have demonstrated high response rates, and a multiinstitutional Phase III study by the American College of Surgeons Oncology Group (ACSOG) is now in progress to compare ILP using melphalan plus TNF with ILP using melphalan alone.[88] The use of ILP is a treatment of choice for some highly selected patients with in-transit metastases involving an extremity. The optimal treatment agent, treatment time, and limb temperature have not been clearly identified. Palliation can be a goal of this therapy for patients with bulky, symptomatic melanoma of the extremity.

Surgery for Stage IV Melanoma Patients

Patients with systemic metastases (AJCC stage IV) have poor prognoses.[53] Selection of surgery as a treatment option should take into account the general medical condition of the patient, the potential for prevention or relief of symptoms, and improvement in the quality of life. Surgery may be an effective palliative treatment for isolated metastases, especially because melanoma often metastasizes sequentially and effective chemotherapy is not presently available. Surgical excision of metastatic melanoma may give the patient the best, quickest, and longest lasting palliation. On some occasions, the palliative effect can last for 5 to 10 years.[92,93] The obvious limitation of surgery is that it is a local form of treatment, and the patient will very likely die of metastatic disease in another location. Careful patient selection is therefore important.

Mucosal Melanoma

Primary melanomas arising from the mucosal epithelia lining the respiratory, alimentary, and genitourinary tracts are rare, accounting for 3% to 4% of all melanomas diagnosed annually. The lack of large numbers of cases is responsible for the lack of insight into the pathogenesis, natural history, and treatment of mucosal melanomas. Mucosal melanomas are considered to be more aggressive with a worse prognosis than melanomas of the skin, and there are no microstaging data applicable for prognosis for patients with mucosal melanomas. The anatomic sites at which these melanomas originate are the head and neck, followed by vulvar and vaginal mucosa, followed by the anorectum.[94,95] Similar to the primary melanomas that originate in the skin, mucosal melanomas are more common in the Caucasian population and are diagnosed in an older age group. The presence of melanocytes in the mucous membranes is well established, and thus the mucosal melanomas are considered true primary lesions and not metastases. The characteristic growth pattern of cutaneous melanoma is probably not applicable to mucosal melanoma, which is characterized by a rapid vertical growth phase and metastases. Mucosal melanomas act more like the thick, ulcerated cutaneous melanomas. For this reason, the treatment of the primary melanoma should be as conservative as possible, with total excision obtaining clear margins, but avoiding radical resections. For instance, patients with rectal melanoma should be treated with local excisions obtaining clear margins if possible instead of the more radical abdominoperineal resection.[94] A focus in these patients should be on systemic therapy, because many will have systemic metastases at the time of diagnosis. Five-year survival for patients with mucosal melanoma is uncommon regardless of primary site.[95]

Radiation Therapy Considerations

There are several clinical settings in which radiation can provide important benefits for patients with melanoma, the most common involving the palliation of symptomatic regional and distant metastases. Palliative settings frequently include patients with painful bony or soft tissue metastases, as well as patients with metastases to the brain and spinal axis. Furthermore, there are several adjuvant therapy settings for which the role of radiation remains of potential value in an effort to diminish locoregional disease recurrence.

Radiotherapy for Symptomatic Treatment

Focal radiation generally provides excellent pain palliation for patients with metastatic melanoma.[96,97] High rates of palliative pain response for bone metastases have been routinely identified as exemplified by a randomized trial comparing fractionation regimens of 9 Gy × 3 fractions versus 5 Gy × 8 fractions delivered in a twice-weekly schedule. An overall response rate greater than 90% was identified without significant difference between the two arms.[98] Similarly, patients with metastatic melanoma will often have painful soft tissue or in-transit metastases that contribute directly to a reduced quality of life. Symptomatic lesions often can be successfully palliated with small-field electron beam or shallow photon tangent beams for pain relief. In addition, there is a rich literature regarding the use of hyperthermia as an adjuvant to radiation therapy in the treatment of malignant melanoma.[99,100] These reports include studies employing focal hyperthermia with microwave, ultrasound, and interstitial heating devices. Both retrospective and prospective studies suggest an advantage in clinical response for some patients treated with combined hyperthermia and radiation compared with patients treated with radiation alone.[100]

Patients with central nervous system metastases involving the brain or spinal cord present special circumstances for which the emergent use of radiation therapy is often warranted. The heterogeneity of melanoma responsiveness to radiation means that selected patients will have prompt regression of brain metastases following palliative radiotherapy, whereas others will not demonstrate clear response. The combination of high-dose corticosteroids with whole-brain radiation therapy provides effective symptom palliation in one-half to two-thirds of patients as measured by transient improvement in performance status and small extensions in median survival.[101] Despite several studies, no clear benefit of altered fractionation regimens has been clarified, and a convention of 3 Gy × 10 fractions or 4 Gy × 5 fractions is common throughout much of North America. There are emerging reports regarding the potential additional value of stereotactic radiosurgery for patients with one to three melanoma brain metastases, particularly those with lesions of less than 3 cm and no active disease progression in other systemic sites.[102]

Role of Adjuvant Radiotherapy

There are selected circumstances in which locoregional radiotherapy in the adjuvant setting appears particularly promising.[96,103,104] The best described data set examining the use of adjuvant radiotherapy for localized melanoma involves patients with intermediate to thick tumors of the head and neck, with or without regional nodal spread.[96,103] Prospective nonrandomized trials suggest a marked reduction in locoregional disease recurrence in comparison with historic controls treated at the same institution.[103,105] A similar approach has been advocated for melanoma patients with axillary nodal disease, specifically including those patients with extracapsular disease, multiple metastatic nodes, or recurrent disease in a previously dissected axilla. Reports from the M.D. Anderson Cancer Center with more than 5-year median follow-up suggest that the addition of axillary radiation in these high-risk settings can substantially reduce the likelihood of subsequent axillary failure over historical outcome at the same institution.[106]

Adjuvant Interferon Therapy

The only U.S. Food and Drug Administration (FDA)-approved adjuvant therapy following resection of high-risk melanoma remains interferon alpha-2b (IFN-α-2b).[107] Vaccines remain experimental for melanoma patients, and vaccine considerations are presented in a later section of this chapter. Interleukin-2 has been evaluated alone and with other biologic response modifiers and/or chemotherapy in numerous advanced-disease studies (see following sections). Unfortunately, there remains no established adjuvant therapy benefit for high-risk melanoma patients following interleukin-2-based therapy. Although historically controlled studies have suggested benefit for adjuvant therapy with granulocyte-macrophage colony-stimulating factor (GM-CSF),[108] this benefit remains unproven and is now receiving prospective randomized clinical trial testing. Numerous other adjuvant therapies including bacillus Calmette–Guérin (BCG), *Corynebacterium parvum*, dacarbazine, levamisole, megestrol acetate, and interferon-gamma have been evaluated and shown to have limited or no benefit in both randomized and nonrandomized adjuvant therapy trials for melanoma patients.[109–111]

Although high-dose therapy with IFN-α-2b is the only FDA-approved adjuvant treatment for patients with resected high-risk melanoma, significant debate and controversy continue regarding interpretation of the completed interferon adjuvant studies.[112–115] The results of studies evaluating high-dose IFN-α-2b are summarized in Table 59.6. In E1684, the 5-year overall survival rate of patients randomized to observation was 37% and the 5-year overall survival rate of patients randomized to receive IFN-α-2b was 46%.[107] This difference was statistically significant and resulted in FDA approval of high-dose adjuvant IFN-α-2b for melanoma patients following resection of high-risk (stage IIB and III) melanoma. The intergroup trial E1690 was performed to confirm results from E1684, as well as to concurrently compare high-dose IFN-α-2b and low dose IFN-α-2b with observation following resection of high-risk melanoma.[116] Regional lymph node evaluation was not required for patients with T4N0 disease. The 5-year relapse-free survival rate for high-dose IFN-α-2b was 44%, the relapse-free survival rate for low-dose IFN-α-2b was 40%, and the relapse-free survival rate for observation was 35%. However, no significant improvement in overall survival was achieved by either high-dose or low-dose IFN-α-2b in comparison with observation.[116]

The E1694 study compared high-dose IFN-α-2b with a GM2 vaccine based on earlier data suggesting benefit in stage III melanoma patients having GM2 antibodies following vaccination with a GM2 ganglioside vaccine.[117] An independent data monitoring committee evaluated results from the E1694

TABLE 59.6. Completed randomized trials evaluating high-dose interferon alpha-2b (IFN-α-2b) as adjuvant therapy of melanoma.

Trial	*No. of patients*	*Eligibility*	*Treatment regimens*	*HDI[a] overall survival benefit*	*HDI relapse-free survival benefit*	*Comments*
E1684[107]	287	T4 N1-3	HDI vs. observation	Yes	Yes	IFN-α-2b prolonged median survival from 2.8 to 3.8 years compared to observation
E1690[116]	642	T4 N1-3	HDI vs. LDI[b] vs. observation	No	Yes	There was no difference in the estimated 5-year overall survival rates of 52%, 53%, and 55% for HDI, LDI, and observation, respectively
E1694[118]	851	T4 N1-3	HDI vs. GMK vaccine[c]	Yes	Yes	IFN-α-2b is superior to GMK vaccine

[a] High-dose interferon-α-2b (HDI) given at 20 MU/m^2/day IV 5 days per week for 4 weeks, then 3 times weekly at 10 MU/m^2/day subcutaneously for 48 weeks.

[b] Low dose interferon-α-2b (LDI) given 3 times weekly at 3 MU subcutaneously for 2 years.

[c] GMK vaccine (modified GM_2 ganglioside vaccine (Progenics, Inc., Tarrytown, NY) given subcutaneously on a weekly basis for 4 weeks, then every 12 weeks for the next 84 weeks.

study following 16 months of median follow-up. Results from that analysis demonstrated that treatment results had crossed the stopping boundaries specified by the study. The estimated 1- and 2-year relapse-free survival rates for the IFN-α-2b-treated patients were 71% and 62%, and the GM2-KLH/QS21-treated group had 1- and 2-year relapse-free survival rates of 62% and 49%.[118] These results resulted in the recommendation for discontinuation of GM2-KLH/QS21 for patients still receiving it, as it was determined to be inferior to interferon.[118]

The clinical toxicity and economic cost of adjuvant therapy with this high-dose IFN-α-2b regimen are significant. Although the clinical toxicity of high-dose IFN-α-2b is substantial, overall clinical benefit from this treatment has been reported following quality of life adjusted survival analysis.[119] In addition, several investigators are attempting to identify strategies to decrease some of the interferon-associated toxicities.[120] Consensus is not present regarding the "standard" use of this treatment for patients with resected high-risk melanoma.[112,121]

Systemic Chemotherapy

The success of various chemotherapy strategies for patients with metastatic melanoma has been very limited.[110,122–125] Although some patients have certainly benefited from current treatments, additional improvements are critically needed.

Single Agents

The use of single-agent dacarbazine (dimethyl-triazano-imidazol carboxamide, DTIC) has been a "standard" treatment and remains the only FDA-approved cytotoxic drug for metastatic melanoma patients. However, the modest response rate of 15% to 20%, with most of the responses being of brief duration, certainly leaves ample room for improvement.[63,126] The median response duration is only 4 to 6 months, and the likelihood of a complete response is less than 5%. Many other drugs have been evaluated for single-agent activity against melanoma. Overall response rates complete response (CR) + partial response (PR) between 13% and 24% have been reported in single-agent chemotherapy studies utilizing a variety of doses and schedules for temozolomide,[127,128] cisplatin,[129] carboplatin,[130] paclitaxel,[131] docetaxel,[132] carmustine (BCNU),[133] lomustine (CCNU),[134] fotemustine (FTMU),[135] vindesine,[136] vinblastine,[136] and the dihydrofolate-reductase inhibitor piritrexim.[137] Most of these responses are partial, and median response duration is usually measured in units of a few months. Although results from several single-agent Phase II chemotherapy studies appear better than single-agent DTIC, none have been confirmed as superior in a prospective randomized Phase III study.[122,123,128] Thus, combination treatments and novel agents with new mechanisms of action are being actively investigated.

Combination Chemotherapy or Chemohormonal Therapy

Combination chemotherapy regimens have attempted to either combine agents with distinct single-agent activity and/or add tamoxifen as a means to enhance activity of the treatment regimen. A randomized Italian study evaluated treatment with DTIC, either alone or in combination with tamoxifen, for patients with metastatic melanoma.[138] This study reported an improved response rate (28% versus 12%; $P = 0.03$) and an improved median survival (48 weeks versus 29 weeks; $P = 0.02$) in patients receiving DTIC combined with tamoxifen compared with patients receiving DTIC alone (Table 59.7). However, a more-recent study from the Eastern Cooperative Oncology Group (ECOG) randomized 258 eligible patients with metastatic melanoma to receive treatment with dacarbazine either alone or combined with tamoxifen, IFN-α-2b or both tamoxifen and IFN-α-2b. There was no difference between time to treatment failure (median, 2.6 months) or overall survival (median, 8.9 months) between any of the four treatment groups.[139] Thus, neither tamoxifen, IFN-α-2b, nor the combination of tamoxifen and IFN-α-2b was able to improve response rate, time to treatment failure, or survival of melanoma patients when these treatments were added to single-agent therapy with dacarbazine (see Table 59.7). Several studies have reported promising results of tamoxifen in combination with cytotoxic agents including cisplatin,[140] navelbine,[141] and others.[125] Subsequent Phase III testing to determine impact of tamoxifen on the combination treatment either has been negative or has not been performed.[125] Although tamoxifen is still being administered as part of published Phase II protocols, existing data do not demonstrate improved therapeutic outcome with addition of tamoxifen to cytotoxic regimens for melanoma patients.

The three-drug combinations of cisplatin, vinblastine, and DTIC or cisplatin, vindesine, and DTIC achieved response

TABLE 59.7. Randomized Phase III trials comparing chemohormonal or combination chemotherapy with DTIC for patients with advanced melanoma.

Author	No. of patients	Treatment regimens	CR + PR (%)	Median survival (months)	Comments
Cocconi et al.[138]	60	DTIC/TAM DTIC	17 (28)	11	Major benefit of DTIC/TAM appeared to be in
	52		6 (12)	7	women
Falkson et al.[139]	124	DTIC ± IFN-α + TAM	25 (20)	9	This 2 × 2 factorial design showed no advantage
	126	DTIC ± IFN-α	24 (19)	9	for the addition of IFN-α or TAM to DTIC
Buzaid et al.[142]	46	Cisplatin/vinblastine/DTIC	11 (24)	6	No convincing evidence to support combination
	45	DTIC	5 (11)	5	chemotherapy
Chapman et al.[146]	108	Cisplatin/DTIC/BCNU/TAM	20 (18)	7	No convincing evidence to support combination
	118	DTIC	12 (10)	7	chemotherapy

DTIC, dacarbazine; TAM, tamoxifen; IFN-α, interferon-alpha; BCNU, carmustine; CR + PR, complete response + partial response.

rates between 35% and 40% in Phase II testing. Unfortunately, no benefit in response duration or overall survival was seen in subsequent randomized comparison with DTIC (see Table 59.7).[142] The treatment combination of cisplatin, dacarbazine, carmustine, and tamoxifen (CDBT; also known as the Dartmouth regimen) has been suggested for many years to have significant activity for patients with metastatic melanoma. Many of these studies reported response rates up to 30% to 50%, and some of these responses seemed to be durable.[143–145] However, a more recently completed prospective randomized trial compared CDBT with single-agent therapy with DTIC and found no difference in overall survival with either of these treatments (Table 59.7).[146] Although several phase II studies have suggested potential benefit for combination chemotherapy over single agent chemotherapy, results from subsequent phase III testing have been disappointing.

Additional agents are also receiving investigation in combination with standard cytotoxic agents. Thalidomide is an orally bioavailable agent that has both antiangiogenic as well as some immunomodulatory properties. Use of thalidomide as single-agent therapy in melanoma has had limited activity.[147] The combination of thalidomide and temozolomide was tested for patients with metastatic melanoma, as melanoma is a highly vascular tumor that could benefit from this combined approach.[148,149] Current results demonstrate this treatment to be well tolerated and to have some antitumor activity. Overall response rates in small Phase II studies have ranged from 15% to 32%, and durable responses have been reported.[148,149] Further study is needed to determine if this combination regimen offers improved outcome over either single agent alone. Other approaches being tested clinically include the combinaton of chemotherapy with the antisense BCL2 oligonucleotide to inhibit antiapoptotic pathways as well as the combination of chemotherapy with novel agents such as Raf kinase inhibitors. It is anticipated that increased understanding of the many pathways involved in melanoma tumorigenesis will provide new opportunities for melanoma treatment strategies.[150]

Cytokines and Other Immune Activators

Many cytokines and other immune activators are being actively evaluated as therapy for patients with metastatic melanoma.[151] Treatment with high-dose bolus IL-2 is approved by the FDA for the treatment of metastatic melanoma, and many studies are in progress to improve efficacy and/or decrease toxicity of cytokine-based regimens for advanced melanoma patients.

Interferons

As outlined earlier, treatment with IFN-α-2b has received extensive testing as adjuvant therapy for patients with resected stage III melanoma. In addition, measurable responses have been seen with IFN therapy for melanoma patients with advanced metastatic disease.[151] Although the dose and schedule of IFN utilized in the metastatic setting have been quite varied, about 15% of patients have had tumor regression and 5% have been CRs. Although most of these responses last for only a few months, some can be more durable.

Interleukin 2

When peripheral blood mononuclear cells are cultured together with high concentrations of IL-2, a striking proliferation of natural killer (NK) cells and some T cells is observed, with induction of dramatically augmented cytolytic function.[152] This IL-2-induced cytolytic function allows destruction of most cultured tumor cell lines and most populations of fresh tumor cell suspensions. For at least some patients with melanoma, measurable shrinkage of grossly evident tumor metastases can be induced by IL-2 treatment.[153,154] Approximately 6% of these patients achieved complete remission and 10% of patients achieved partial remission in numerous Phase II studies using high-dose bolus IL-2.[151,154,155] These clinical data supported the approval by the FDA of high-dose bolus IL-2 as a treatment for patients with metastatic melanoma.

IL-2 treatment induces NK cell activation, the release of cytokines, and a cytokine syndrome that is associated with capillary leak. This IL-2 therapy has a dose-dependent toxicity profile and has significant toxicity when administered in the approved high-dose bolus regimen.[156] The approved regimen is for administration of IL-2 at 600,000 to 720,000 IU/kg every 8 hours, up to a maximum of 15 doses, on days 1 through 5 and 15 through 19 of a treatment course. Data supporting approval and use of high-dose bolus IL-2 are based on nonrandomized Phase II data.[155] In addition, protocols using lower-dose outpatient regimens of IL-2 have generally had lower response rates as well as few long-term survivors.[151,154] However, the limitations of decision making based on Phase II data for advanced melanoma patients were emphasized with the recently reported results of the randomized Phase III study of combination chemotherapy and biochemotherapy.[157] Thus, use of high-dose bolus IL-2 as a single agent has been primarily at specialized centers with experience in administration of this treatment. Studies involving administration of lymphokine-activated killer (LAK) cells as well as tumor-infiltrating lymphocytes (TILs) together with IL-2 did not demonstrate sufficient additional activity to support noninvestigational use of these approaches.[151] More-recent studies are investigating use of nonmyeloablative chemotherapy before adoptive transfer of cloned T cells and high-dose IL-2 therapy.[158] These studies, as well as integration of vaccine-based approaches given together with IL-2, will receive intense investigation in upcoming years.

Biochemotherapy

Several nonrandomized, single-institution Phase II studies have evaluated combination chemotherapy given together with IL-2 and IFN-α as biochemotherapy for patients with metastatic melanoma. Both inpatient and outpatient regimens have been evaluated, and response rates of 40% to 60% have been reported.[159–162] In addition to the high response rates reported, up to 10% of these patients have achieved a durable complete response. The frequent finding of high response rates in separate Phase II studies, as well as the consistent reporting of durable complete responses in a minority of responders, led to high expectations as well as great enthusiasm for this approach. The potential benefit of IL-2/cisplatin-based biochemotherapy has been investigated in at least six randomized trials (Table 59.8).[157,163–167] The recent intergroup Phase III randomized study was conducted to determine in a definitive fashion whether biotherapy (IL-2, IFN-α-2b, and G-CSF) added to the results of chemotherapy consisting of dacarbazine, cisplatin, and vinblastine when administered in a concurrent fashion. A total of 416 patients without prior treatment for metastatic melanoma were enrolled into the study, and results demonstrated increased toxicity without additional clinical benefit following treatment with the concurrent biochemotherapy regimen (see Table 59.8).[157] It remains unknown whether clinical benefit over chemotherapy alone can be achieved with other biochemotherapy regimens, such as use of some of the sequential biochemotherapy regimens. However, the disappointing result of this carefully performed intergroup study emphasizes the need for Phase III testing of promising approaches before accepting them as standard therapy.

Vaccine Therapy

Numerous advances in molecular biology and immunology provide opportunities for the design and analysis of vaccine-based therapies for melanoma patients.[168–171] Although melanomas contain antigens that can stimulate T-cell responses, the antigen(s) that can stimulate effective in vivo T-cell activation and an antitumor response are not known. Potential sources for antigens to use in melanoma vaccines, listed in Table 59.9, include whole melanoma cells as well as defined melanoma antigens or genes for defined melanoma antigens.

The use of melanoma cellular vaccines has included both autologous as well as allogeneic melanoma cells.[172–175] Dr. Berd and colleagues have been investigating strategies to enhance the immunogenicity of autologous melanoma cell vaccines.[176] A recent update of this nonrandomized experience described 214 clinical stage III (N2 and N3) patients treated adjuvantly with an autologous tumor cell vaccine

TABLE 59.8. Randomized Phase III trials evaluating IL-2/cisplatin-based biochemotherapy for metastatic melanoma patients.

Author	*No. of patients*	*Treatment regimens*	*CR + PR (%)*	*Median survival (months)*	*Comments*
Keilholz et al.[163]	66 60	IL-2/IFN-α CDDP + IL-2/IFN-α	18 33	9 9	Addition of CDDP to cytokine treatment with IFN-α and IL-2 improves response rate without improving survival
Rosenberg et al.[164]	52 50	CDDP/DTIC/TAM CDDP/DTIC/TAM + IL-2/IFN-α	27 44	15.8 10.7	Addition of immunotherapy to combination chemotherapy increased toxicity without improving survival with these treatment regimens
Dorval et al.[165]	49 52	CDDP/IL-2 CDDP/IL-2 + IFN-α	16 24	10.4 10.9	Addition of IFN-α to this CDDP/IL-2 regimen increased toxicity without improving survival
Eton et al.[166]	92 91	CVD Sequential CVD + IL-2/IFN-α	25 48	9.2 11.9	Cytokines improved antitumor activity at the expense of considerable toxicity
Keilholz et al.[167]	363 randomized	CDDP/DTIC/IFN-α CDDP/DTIC/IFN-α + IL-2	23 21	9.0 9.0	Addition of IL-2 to this CDDP/DTIC/IFN-α regimen increased toxicity without improving survival
Atkins et al.[157]	201 204	CVD Concurrent CVD + IL-2/IFN-α	11 17	8.7 8.3	Addition of immunotherapy to combination chemotherapy increased toxicity without improving survival with these treatment regimens

IL-2, interleukin-2; IFN-α, interferon alpha; CDDP, cisplatin; DTIC, dacarbazine; TAM, tamoxifen; CVD, cisplatin/vinblastine/dacarbazine.

TABLE 59.9. Sources of antigen for melanoma vaccines.

Autologous melanoma cells
Allogeneic melanoma cells
Autologous heat shock protein–peptide complexes
Ganglioside antigens
Antiidiotypic monoclonal antibody
Peptides for melanoma-associated antigens
DNA encoding protein containing melanoma-associated antigens

modified with the hapten dinitrophenol (DNP).[177] The 5-year overall survival rate of 44% was better than expected from historical controls, and the 47% of patients with an induced delayed-type hypersensitivity (DTH) to unmodified autologous melanoma had an overall survival that was twice that of the DTH-negative patients (59.3% versus 29.3%; *P* less than 0.001). Additional approaches designed to augment the immunogenicity of autologous melanoma cells include the use of oncolysates of melanoma cells with vaccinia virus and the use of irradiated gene modified melanoma cells as a melanoma vaccine.[173,178–180]

Other investigators are utilizing vaccines based on allogeneic cell lines, as this strategy offers many practical advantages over the use of autologous cells as a cancer vaccine.[173–175] An allogeneic melanoma cell lysate vaccine (Melacine) was compared with combination chemotherapy with the Dartmouth regimen in a randomized clinical trial for patients with metastatic melanoma.[181] Although both treatments had low but similar median survivals (7.2 months for the Dartmouth regimen compared with 6.8 months for Melacine), the improved toxicity profile for Melacine resulted in its approval in Canada. In addition, Melacine was investigated as adjuvant therapy for patients with intermediate-thickness, node-negative melanoma.[182] Although no overall survival benefit for this vaccine was seen in all treated patients, the patient subset with a specific histocompatibility leukocyte antigen (HLA) expression (HLA-A2 and/or HLA-C3) had improved relapse-free and overall survival compared to control patients.[183] Another allogeneic cellular vaccine with promising results in adjuvant studies as well as some antitumor activity in metastatic disease is CancerVax.[184] This vaccine is currently receiving expanded testing in a Phase III adjuvant study comparing CancerVax (with BCG) versus BCG alone for patients with resected stage III melanoma.

Several gangliosides on melanoma cells have been characterized, and these gangliosides provide a target for an antibody response to melanoma.[117] Unfortunately, the GM2-KLH/QS-21 vaccine was inferior to interferon when evaluated in a prospective randomized trial as adjuvant therapy for patients with resected high-risk melanoma.[118] Another approach to stimulate an antibody response to melanoma uses an antiidiotypic antibody as an immunogen. Clinical trials are in progress, and some patients have been shown to develop an antiantiidiotypic antibody following vaccination with an antiidiotypic antibody.[185]

Several clinical studies are now in progress either utilizing immunodominant peptides for melanoma-associated antigens or using DNA-encoding proteins containing melanoma-associated antigens.[186–189] Additional studies are combining these defined vaccines with cytokines or other immune activators. Rosenberg and colleagues reported antitumor activity in HLA-A2-positive melanoma patients receiving GP-100 peptide in combination with IL-2,[190] and Nestle and colleagues reported antitumor activity and antigen-specific T-cell immunity in melanoma patients treated with peptide or tumor lysate pulsed dendritic cells.[191] Thus, ongoing clinical studies will determine the immunogenicity and antitumor activity of defined antigen vaccines given alone or with other immunotherapies. Initial Phase I and Phase II studies will determine promising approaches, but prospective, randomized Phase III studies will be needed to determine clinical benefit.

Imaging and Follow-Up of Melanoma Patients

The use of intensive follow-up of melanoma patients receiving definitive surgical management of primary melanoma is without demonstrated benefit.[192–194] The majority of recurrences for patients with resected melanoma occur in the skin, soft tissues, or lymph nodes. Thus, careful physical examination remains of primary importance in the follow-up of these patients. In addition, the majority of recurrences amenable to surgical resection will be in these regions. Because most recurrences occur in the first 2 years following surgery, the frequency of follow-up is typically greater during the first 2 years following definitive surgery. Typical intervals are every 6 months for patients with melanomas less than 1 mm in thickness and every 3 to 4 months for patients with deeper primary melanomas and/or regional lymph node involvement. Addition of chest X-rays and laboratory studies typically does not take place for patients with melanomas less than 1 mm, but often are obtained at intervals from 3 to 6 months for patients with deeper primary melanomas and/or regional lymph node involvement. Follow-up intervals then become gradually longer between years 3 and 5, and yearly follow-up typically takes places after year 5. Because recurrences can take place more than 10 years from initial resection, some ongoing follow-up is appropriate for these patients.

The use of molecular tumor markers in the blood as early predictors of melanoma recurrence or disease outcome for melanoma patients is also receiving intense investigation.[195,196] The strategy receiving the most intensive investigation involves use of a multiple-marker reverse transcription polymerase chain reaction (RT-PCR) to predict disease outcome. The markers being evaluated include the presence of melanoma-associated mRNA for tyrosinase, melanoma antigen recognized by T cells (MART-1), and the melanoma antigen MAGE. Although preliminary studies suggest potential benefit for this technology, additional evaluation and validation of assay characteristics are needed before incorporation into routine clinical monitoring.

Acknowledgements. Dr. Mark Albertini thanks the Steve Leuthold Family Foundation (Jay Van Sloan Memorial) and Kathy Eagle (Tim Eagle Memorial) for gifts to the University of Wisconsin Comprehensive Cancer Center supporting our research on melanoma immunotherapy. The authors thank Kathy Neish for assistance with manuscript preparation.

References

1. Berwick M, Weinstock MA. Epidemiology: current trends. In: Balch CM, Houghton A, Sober A, Soong S-J (eds). Cutaneous Melanoma. St. Louis: Quality Medical, 2003.
2. Jemal A, Murray T, Ward E, et al. Cancer statistics, 2005. CA Cancer J Clin 2005;55:10–30.
3. Swerdlow AJ, English J, MacKie RM, et al. Benign melanocytic naevi as a risk factor for malignant melanoma. Br Med J (Clin Res Ed) 1986;292:1555–1559.
4. Betti R, Inselvini E, Vergani R, Crosti C. Small congenital nevi associated with melanoma: case reports and considerations. J Dermatol 2000;27:583–590.
5. Kaddu S, Smolle J, Zenahlik P, Hofmann-Wellenhof R, Kerl H. Melanoma with benign melanocytic naevus components: reappraisal of clinicopathological features and prognosis. Melanoma Res 2002;12:271–278.
6. Crucioli V, Stilwell J. The histogenesis of malignant melanoma in relation to pre-existing pigmented lesions. J Cutan Pathol 1982;9:396–404.
7. Clark WH Jr, Reimer RR, Greene M, Ainsworth AM, Mastrangelo MJ. Origin of familial malignant melanomas from heritable melanocytic lesions. "The B-K mole syndrome". Arch Dermatol 1978;114:732–738.
8. Ackerman AB. What naevus is dysplastic, a syndrome and the commonest precursor of malignant melanoma? A riddle and an answer. Histopathology (Oxf) 1988;13:241–256.
9. Barnhill RL, Mihm MC Jr. The histopathology of cutaneous malignant melanoma. Semin Diagn Pathol 1993;10:47–75.
10. Elder D, Elenitsa S. Benign pigmented lesions and malignant melanoma. In: Lever (ed). Histopathology of the Skin. Philadelphia: Lippincott-Raven, 1997.
11. Koh K, Barnhill RL, Rogers G. Melanoma. Cutaneous Medicine and Surgery. Philadelphia: Saunders, 1996.
12. Kibbi AG, Mihm MC Jr. Malignant melanoma with desmoplasia and neurotropism. J Dermatol Surg Oncol 1987;13:1204–1208.
13. Koh HK, Michalik E, Sober AJ, et al. Lentigo maligna melanoma has no better prognosis than other types of melanoma. J Clin Oncol 1984;2:994–1001.
14. Averbook BJ, Fu P, Rao JS, Mansour EG. A long-term analysis of 1018 patients with melanoma by classic Cox regression and tree-structured survival analysis at a major referral center: implications on the future of cancer staging. Surgery (St. Louis) 2002;132:589–602; discussion 602–604.
15. Breslow A. Thickness, cross-sectional areas and depth of invasion in the prognosis of cutaneous melanoma. Ann Surg 1970;172:902–908.
16. Mansson-Brahme E, Carstensen J, Erhardt K, Lagerlof B, Ringborg U, Rutqvist LE. Prognostic factors in thin cutaneous malignant melanoma. Cancer (Phila) 1994;73:2324–2332.
17. Retsas S, Henry K, Mohammed MQ, MacRae K. Prognostic factors of cutaneous melanoma and a new staging system proposed by the American Joint Committee on Cancer (AJCC): validation in a cohort of 1284 patients. Eur J Cancer 2002;38:511–516.
18. Folberg R, Salomao D, Grossniklaus HE, Proia AD, Rao NA, Cameron JD. Recommendations for the reporting of tissues removed as part of the surgical treatment of common malignancies of the eye and its adnexa. Mod Pathol 2003;16:725–730.
19. Allen AC, Spitz S. Malignant melanoma: a clinicopathological analysis of the criteria for diagnosis and prognosis. Cancer (Phila) 1953;6:1–45.
20. Clark WH Jr, Elder DE, Guerry D IV, Epstein MN, Greene MH, Van Horn M. A study of tumor progression: the precursor lesions of superficial spreading and nodular melanoma. Hum Pathol 1984;15:1147–1165.
21. Kashani-Sabet M, Sagebiel RW, Ferreira CM, Nosrati M, Miller JR III. Vascular involvement in the prognosis of primary cutaneous melanoma. Arch Dermatol 2001;137:1169–1173.
22. Kashani-Sabet M, Sagebiel RW, Ferreira CM, Nosrati M, Miller JR III. Tumor vascularity in the prognostic assessment of primary cutaneous melanoma. J Clin Oncol 2002;20:1826–1831.
23. Elder DE, Guerry DT, VanHorn M, et al. The role of lymph node dissection for clinical stage I malignant melanoma of intermediate thickness (1.51–3.99mm). Cancer (Phila) 1985;56:413–418.
24. Cooper PH, Wanebo HJ, Hagar RW. Regression in thin malignant melanoma. Microscopic diagnosis and prognostic importance. Arch Dermatol 1985;121:1127–1131.
25. Florenes VA, Maelandsmo GM, Faye R, Nesland JM, Holm R. Cyclin A expression in superficial spreading malignant melanomas correlates with clinical outcome. J Pathol 2001;195:530–536.
26. Ostmeier H, Fuchs B, Otto F, et al. Prognostic immunohistochemical markers of primary human melanomas. Br J Dermatol 2001;145:203–209.
27. Majore S, Catricala C, Bottoni U, et al. PP-20 molecular characterization of two cases with multiple primary melanomas (MPM). Pigment Cell Res 2003;16:599.
28. Marsh D, Zori R. Genetic insights into familial cancers: update and recent discoveries. Cancer Lett 2002;181:125–164.
29. Masback A, Olsson H, Westerdahl J, et al. Clinical and histopathological features of malignant melanoma in germline CDKN2A mutation families. Melanoma Res 2002;12:549–557.
30. Rulyak SJ, Brentnall TA, Lynch HT, Austin MA. Characterization of the neoplastic phenotype in the familial atypical multiple-mole melanoma-pancreatic carcinoma syndrome. Cancer (Phila) 2003;98:798–804.
31. Gibbs P, Brady BM, Robinson WA. The genes and genetics of malignant melanoma. J Cutan Med Surg 2002;6:229–235.
32. Bastian BC, LeBoit PE, Hamm H, Brocker EB, Pinkel D. Chromosomal gains and losses in primary cutaneous melanomas detected by comparative genomic hybridization. Cancer Res 1998;58:2170–2175.
33. Bastian BC, Kashani-Sabet M, Hamm H, et al. Gene amplifications characterize acral melanoma and permit the detection of occult tumor cells in the surrounding skin. Cancer Res 2000;60:1968–1973.
34. Bastian BC. Molecular cytogenetics as a diagnostic tool for typing melanocytic tumors. Recent Results Cancer Res 2002;160:92–99.
35. Bastian BC. Understanding the progression of melanocytic neoplasia using genomic analysis: from fields to cancer. Oncogene 2003;22:3081–3086.
36. Reed JA, Loganzo F Jr, Shea CR, et al. Loss of expression of the p16/cyclin-dependent kinase inhibitor 2 tumor suppressor gene in melanocytic lesions correlates with invasive stage of tumor progression. Cancer Res 1995;55:2713–2718.
37. Polsky D, Bastian BC, Hazan C, et al. HDM2 protein overexpression, but not gene amplification, is related to tumorigenesis of cutaneous melanoma. Cancer Res 2001;61:7642–7646.
38. Swetter SM. Dermatological perspectives of malignant melanoma. Surg Clin N0 Am 2003;83:77–95.
39. Langley RGB, Fitzpatrick TB, Sober AJ. Clinical characteristics. In: Balch CM, Houghton AN, Sober AJ, Soong SJ (eds). Cutaneous Melanoma, 3rd ed. St. Louis: Quality Medical, 1998:81–101.
40. Nashan D, Kocer B, Schiller M, Luger T, Grabbe S. Significant risk of a second melanoma in patients with a history of melanoma but no further predisposing factors. Dermatology 2003;206:76–77.
41. Euvrard S, Kanitakis J, Claudy A. Skin cancers after organ transplantation. N Engl J Med 2003;348:1681–1691.
42. Veierod MB, Weiderpass E, Thorn M, et al. A prospective study of pigmentation, sun exposure, and risk of cutaneous malignant melanoma in women. J Natl Cancer Inst 2003;95:1530–1538.
43. Wei Q, Lee JE, Gershenwald JE, et al. Repair of UV light-induced DNA damage and risk of cutaneous malignant melanoma. J Natl Cancer Inst 2003;95:308–315.

44. Goggins WB, Tsao H. A population-based analysis of risk factors for a second primary cutaneous melanoma among melanoma survivors. Cancer (Phila) 2003;97:639–643.
45. Geller AC. Screening for melanoma. Dermatol Clin 2002;20: 629–640, viii.
46. Rigel DS. The effect of sunscreen on melanoma risk. Dermatol Clin 2002;20:601–606.
47. Huncharek M, Kupelnick B. Use of topical sunscreens and the risk of malignant melanoma: a meta-analysis of 9067 patients from 11 case-control studies. Am J Public Health 2002;92:1173–1177.
48. Dennis LK, Beane Freeman LE, VanBeek MJ. Sunscreen use and the risk for melanoma: a quantitative review. Ann Intern Med 2003;139:966–978.
49. Demierre MF, Nathanson L. Chemoprevention of melanoma: an unexplored strategy. J Clin Oncol 2003;21:158–165.
50. MacKie RM, Bufalino R, Morabito A, Sutherland C, Cascinelli N. Lack of effect of pregnancy on outcome of melanoma. For The World Health Organisation Melanoma Programme. Lancet 1991;337:653–655.
51. MacKie RM. Pregnancy and hormones. In: Balch CM, Houghton AN, Sober AJ, Soong S-J (eds). Cutaneous Melanoma. St. Louis: Quality Medical, 2003:319–326.
52. Slingluff CL Jr, Reintgen DS, Vollmer RT, Seigler HF. Malignant melanoma arising during pregnancy. A study of 100 patients. Ann Surg 1990;211:552–557; discussion 558–559.
53. Balch CM, Buzaid AC, Soong SJ, et al. Final version of the American Joint Committee on Cancer staging system for cutaneous melanoma. J Clin Oncol 2001;19:3635–3648.
54. Balch CM, Soong SJ, Gershenwald JE, et al. Prognostic factors analysis of 17,600 melanoma patients: validation of the American Joint Committee on Cancer melanoma staging system. J Clin Oncol 2001;19:3622–3634.
55. Friedman RJ, Rigel DS, Silverman MK, Kopf AW, Vossaert KA. Malignant melanoma in the 1990s: the continued importance of early detection and the role of physician examination and self-examination of the skin. CA Cancer J Clin 1991;41: 201–226.
56. Naeyaert JM, Brochez L. Clinical practice. Dysplastic nevi. N Engl J Med 2003;349:2233–2240.
57. Rhodes AR. Intervention strategy to prevent lethal cutaneous melanoma: use of dermatologic photography to aid surveillance of high-risk persons. J Am Acad Dermatol 1998;39:262–267.
58. Pehamberger H, Binder M, Steiner A, Wolff K. In vivo epiluminescence microscopy: improvement of early diagnosis of melanoma. J Invest Dermatol 1993;100:356S–362S.
59. Argenziano G, Fabbrocini G, Carli P, De Giorgi V, Sammarco E, Delfino M. Epiluminescence microscopy for the diagnosis of doubtful melanocytic skin lesions. Comparison of the ABCD rule of dermatoscopy and a new 7-point checklist based on pattern analysis. Arch Dermatol 1998;134:1563–1570.
60. Haddad FF, Costello D, Reintgen DS. Radioguided surgery for melanoma. Surg Oncol Clin N Am 1999;8:413–426.
61. Ross MI, Balch CM, Cascinelli N, Edwards MJ. Excision of primary melanoma. In: Balch CM, Houghton AN, Sober AJ, Soong S-J (eds). Cutaneous Melanoma. St. Louis: Quality Medical, 2003:209–230.
62. Day CL Jr, Mihm MC Jr, Sober AJ, Fitzpatrick TB, Malt RA. Narrower margins for clinical stage I malignant melanoma. N Engl J Med 1982;306:479–482.
63. Balch CM, Reintgen DS, Kirkwood J, Houghton A, Peters L, Ang KK. Cutaneous melanoma. In: Devita VT, Hellman S, Rosenberg SA (eds). Cancer: Principles and Practice of Oncology, 5th ed. Philadelphia: Lippincott-Raven, 1997:1947–1997.
64. Banzet P, Thomas A, Vuillemin E. Wide versus narrow surgical excision in thin (<2 mm) stage I primary cutaneous malignant melanoma: long term results of a French multicentric perspective randomized trial on 319 patients, Proc Am Assoc Clin Oncol 1993, (abstract 387).
65. Veronesi U, Cascinelli N, Adamus J, et al. Thin stage I primary cutaneous malignant melanoma. Comparison of excision with margins of 1 or 3 cm. N Engl J Med 1988;318:1159–1162.
66. Veronesi U, Cascinelli N. Narrow excision (1-cm margin). A safe procedure for thin cutaneous melanoma. Arch Surg 1991;126: 438–441.
67. Cascinelli N. Margin of resection in the management of primary melanoma. Semin Surg Oncol 1998;14:272–275.
68. Ringborg U, Andersson R, Eldh J, et al. Resection margins of 2 versus 5 cm for cutaneous malignant melanoma with a tumor thickness of 0.8 to 2.0 mm: randomized study by the Swedish Melanoma Study Group. Cancer (Phila) 1996;77: 1809–1814.
69. Cohn-Cedermark G, Rutqvist LE, Andersson R, et al. Long term results of a randomized study by the Swedish Melanoma Study Group on 2-cm versus 5-cm resection margins for patients with cutaneous melanoma with a tumor thickness of 0.8–2.0 mm. Cancer (Phila) 2000;89:1495–1501.
70. Balch CM, Urist MM, Karakousis CP, et al. Efficacy of 2-cm surgical margins for intermediate-thickness melanomas (1 to 4 mm). Results of a multi-institutional randomized surgical trial. Ann Surg 1993;218:262–267; discussion 267–269.
71. Karakousis CP, Balch CM, Urist MM, Ross MM, Smith TJ, Bartolucci AA. Local recurrence in malignant melanoma: long-term results of the multiinstitutional randomized surgical trial. Ann Surg Oncol 1996;3:446–452.
72. Thomas JM, Newton-Bishop JA, Timmons M, et al. Surgical margin excision width in high risk (minimum depth 2 mm) cutaneous malignant melanoma: a randomized trial of 1 cm versus 3 cm excision margins in 900 patients. Proc Am Soc Clin Oncol 2002, (abstract 340a).
73. Thomas JM, Newton-Bishop J, A'Hern R, et al. Excision margins in high-risk malignant melanoma. N Engl J Med 2004;350:757–766.
74. Reintgen DS, Thompson JF, Gershenwald JE. Intraoperative mapping and sentinel node technology. In: Balch CM, Houghton AN, Sober AJ, Soong S-J (eds). Cutaneous Melanoma. St. Louis: Quality Medical, 2003:353–377.
75. Morton DL, Wen DR, Wong JH, et al. Technical details of intraoperative lymphatic mapping for early stage melanoma. Arch Surg 1992;127:392–399.
76. Morton DL, Wen DR, Cochran AJ. Management of early-stage melanoma by intraoperative lymphatic mapping and selective lymphadenectomy, an alternative to routine elective lymphadenectomy, or "watch and wait". Surg Oncol Clin N Am 1992;1:247.
77. Reintgen D, Cruse CW, Wells K, et al. The orderly progression of melanoma nodal metastases. Ann Surg 1994;220:759–767.
78. Ross MI, Reintgen D, Balch CM. Selective lymphadenectomy: emerging role for lymphatic mapping and sentinel node biopsy in the management of early stage melanoma. Semin Surg Oncol 1993;9:219–223.
79. Thompson J, McCarthy W, Robinson E. Sentinel lymph node biopsy in 102 patients with clinical stage I melanoma undergoing elective lymph node dissection. In: 47th Cancer Symposium, Society of Surgical Oncology, Houston, TX, 1994 (abstract).
80. Veronesi U, Adamus J, Bandiera DC, et al. Delayed regional lymph node dissection in stage I melanoma of the skin of the lower extremities. Cancer (Phila) 1982;49:2420–2430.
81. Veronesi U, Adamus J, Bandiera DC, et al. Inefficacy of immediate node dissection in stage 1 melanoma of the limbs. N Engl J Med 1977;297:627–630.
82. Sim FH, Taylor WF, Ivins JC, Pritchard DJ, Soule EH. A prospective randomized study of the efficacy of routine elective lymphadenectomy in management of malignant melanoma. Preliminary results. Cancer (Phila) 1978;41:948–956.
83. Sim FH, Taylor WF, Pritchard DJ, Soule EH. Lymphadenectomy in the management of stage I malignant melanoma: a prospective randomized study. Mayo Clin Proc 1986;61:697–705.

84. Balch CM, Soong S, Ross MI, et al. Long-term results of a multi-institutional randomized trial comparing prognostic factors and surgical results for intermediate thickness melanomas (1.0 to 4.0mm). Intergroup Melanoma Surgical Trial. Ann Surg Oncol 2000;7:87–97.
85. Balch CM, Soong SJ, Bartolucci AA, et al. Efficacy of an elective regional lymph node dissection of 1 to 4mm thick melanomas for patients 60 years of age and younger. Ann Surg 1996;224: 255–263; discussion 263–266.
86. Cascinelli N, Morabito A, Santinami M, MacKie RM, Belli F. Immediate or delayed dissection of regional nodes in patients with melanoma of the trunk: a randomised trial. WHO Melanoma Programme. Lancet 1998;351:793–796.
87. Balch CM, Cascinelli N, Sim FH. Elective lymph node dissection: results of prospective randomized surgical trials. In: Balch CM, Houghton AN, Sober AJ, Soong S-J (eds). Cutaneous Melanoma. St. Louis: Quality Medical, 2003:379–395.
88. Fraker DL, Eggermont AMM. Hyperthermic regional perfusion for melanoma of the limbs. In: Balch CM, Houghton AN, Sober AJ, Soong S-J (eds). Cutaneous Melanoma. St. Louis: Quality Medical, 2003:473–493.
89. Koops HS, Vaglini M, Suciu S, et al. Prophylactic isolated limb perfusion for localized, high-risk limb melanoma: results of a multicenter randomized phase III trial. European Organization for Research and Treatment of Cancer Malignant Melanoma Cooperative Group Protocol 18832, the World Health Organization Melanoma Program Trial 15, and the North American Perfusion Group Southwest Oncology Group-8593. J Clin Oncol 1998;16:2906–2912.
90. Lienard D, Ewalenko P, Delmotte JJ, Renard N, Lejeune FJ. High-dose recombinant tumor necrosis factor alpha in combination with interferon gamma and melphalan in isolation perfusion of the limbs for melanoma and sarcoma. J Clin Oncol 1992;10: 52–60.
91. Fraker DL, Alexander HR, Andrich M, Rosenberg SA. Treatment of patients with melanoma of the extremity using hyperthermic isolated limb perfusion with melphalan, tumor necrosis factor, and interferon gamma: results of a tumor necrosis factor dose-escalation study. J Clin Oncol 1996;14:479–489.
92. Feun LG, Gutterman J, Burgess MA, et al. The natural history of resectable metastatic melanoma (stage IVA melanoma). Cancer (Phila) 1982;50:1656–1663.
93. Hena MA, Emrich LJ, Nambisan RN, Karakousis CP. Effect of surgical treatment on stage IV melanoma. Am J Surg 1987;153: 270–275.
94. Ross M, Pezzi C, Pezzi T, Meurer D, Hickey R, Balch C. Patterns of failure in anorectal melanoma. A guide to surgical therapy. Arch Surg 1990;125:313–316.
95. Ross MI, Stern SJ. Mucosal melanomas. In: Balch CM, Houghton A, Sober A, Soong S-J (eds). Current Trends in Cutaneous Melanoma. St. Louis: Quality Medical, 2003:297–308.
96. Geara FB, Ang KK. Radiation therapy for malignant melanoma. Surg Clin N Am 1996;76:1383–1398.
97. Sause WT, Cooper JS, Rush S, et al. Fraction size in external beam radiation therapy in the treatment of melanoma. Int J Radiat Oncol Biol Phys 1991;20:429–432.
98. Overgaard J, von der Maase H, Overgaard M. A randomized study comparing two high-dose per fraction radiation schedules in recurrent or metastatic malignant melanoma. Int J Radiat Oncol Biol Phys 1985;11:1837–1839.
99. Harari PM, Hynynen KH, Roemer RB, et al. Development of scanned focussed ultrasound hyperthermia: clinical response evaluation. Int J Radiat Oncol Biol Phys 1991;21:831–840.
100. Overgaard J, Gonzalez Gonzalez D, Hulshof MC, et al. Randomised trial of hyperthermia as adjuvant to radiotherapy for recurrent or metastatic malignant melanoma. European Society for Hyperthermic Oncology. Lancet 1995;345:540–543.
101. Ziegler JC, Cooper JS. Brain metastases from malignant melanoma: conventional vs. high-dose-per-fraction radiotherapy. Int J Radiat Oncol Biol Phys 1986;12:1839–1842.
102. Somaza S, Kondziolka D, Lunsford LD, Kirkwood JM, Flickinger JC. Stereotactic radiosurgery for cerebral metastatic melanoma. J Neurosurg 1993;79:661–666.
103. Ang KK, Peters LJ, Weber RS, et al. Postoperative radiotherapy for cutaneous melanoma of the head and neck region. Int J Radiat Oncol Biol Phys 1994;30:795–798.
104. Lejeune FJ, Lienard D, Leyvraz S, Mirimanoff RO. Regional therapy of melanoma. Eur J Cancer 1993;29A:606–612.
105. Ballo MT, Ang KK. Radiation therapy for malignant melanoma. Surg Clin N Am 2003;83:323–342.
106. Ballo MT, Strom EA, Zagars GK, et al. Adjuvant irradiation for axillary metastases from malignant melanoma. Int J Radiat Oncol Biol Phys 2002;52:964–972.
107. Kirkwood JM, Strawderman MH, Ernstoff MS, Smith TJ, Borden EC, Blum RH. Interferon alfa-2b adjuvant therapy of high-risk resected cutaneous melanoma: the Eastern Cooperative Oncology Group Trial EST 1684. J Clin Oncol 1996;14:7–17.
108. Spitler LE, Grossbard ML, Ernstoff MS, et al. Adjuvant therapy of stage III and IV malignant melanoma using granulocyte-macrophage colony-stimulating factor. J Clin Oncol 2000;18: 1614–1621.
109. Kirkwood JM, Agarwala SS. Adjuvant systemic therapy. In: Balch CM, Houghton AN, Sober AJ, Soong S-J (eds). Cutaneous Melanoma, 3rd ed. St. Louis: Quality Medical, 1998:451–459.
110. Brown CK, Kirkwood JM. Medical management of melanoma. Surg Clin N Am 2003;83:283–322, viii.
111. Meyskens FL Jr, Kopecky KJ, Taylor CW, et al. Randomized trial of adjuvant human interferon gamma versus observation in high-risk cutaneous melanoma: a Southwest Oncology Group study. J Natl Cancer Inst 1995;87:1710–1713.
112. Schuchter LM. Adjuvant interferon therapy for melanoma: high-dose, low-dose, no dose, which dose? J Clin Oncol 2004;22:7–10.
113. Moschos SJ, Kirkwood JM, Konstantinopoulos PA. Present status and future prospects for adjuvant therapy of melanoma: time to build upon the foundation of high-dose interferon alfa-2b. J Clin Oncol 2004;22:11–14.
114. Wheatley K, Ives N, Hancock B, Gore M, Eggermont A, Suciu S. Does adjuvant interferon-alpha for high-risk melanoma provide a worthwhile benefit? A meta-analysis of the randomised trials. Cancer Treat Rev 2003;29:241–252.
115. Wheatley K, Ives N, Hancock B, Gore M. Need for a quantitative meta-analysis of trials of adjuvant interferon in melanoma. J Clin Oncol 2002;20:4120–4121; author reply 4121–4122.
116. Kirkwood JM, Ibrahim JG, Sondak VK, et al. High- and low-dose interferon alfa-2b in high-risk melanoma: first analysis of intergroup trial E1690/S9111/C9190. J Clin Oncol 2000;18: 2444–2458.
117. Livingston PO, Wong GY, Adluri S, et al. Improved survival in stage III melanoma patients with GM2 antibodies: a randomized trial of adjuvant vaccination with GM2 ganglioside. J Clin Oncol 1994;12:1036–1044.
118. Kirkwood JM, Ibrahim JG, Sosman JA, et al. High-dose interferon alfa-2b significantly prolongs relapse-free and overall survival compared with the GM2-KLH/QS-21 vaccine in patients with resected stage IIB-III melanoma: results of intergroup trial E1694/S9512/C509801. J Clin Oncol 2001;19:2370–2380.
119. Cole BF, Gelber RD, Kirkwood JM, Goldhirsch A, Barylak E, Borden E. Quality-of-life-adjusted survival analysis of interferon alfa-2b adjuvant treatment of high-risk resected cutaneous melanoma: an Eastern Cooperative Oncology Group study. J Clin Oncol 1996;14:2666–2673.
120. Musselman DL, Lawson DH, Gumnick JF, et al. Paroxetine for the prevention of depression induced by high-dose interferon alfa. N Engl J Med 2001;344:961–966.

121. Lens MB, Dawes M. Interferon alfa therapy for malignant melanoma: a systematic review of randomized controlled trials. J Clin Oncol 2002;20:1818–1825.
122. Bajetta E, Del Vecchio M, Bernard-Marty C, et al. Metastatic melanoma: chemotherapy. Semin Oncol 2002;29:427–445.
123. O'Day SJ, Kim CJ, Reintgen DS. Metastatic melanoma: chemotherapy to biochemotherapy. Cancer Control 2002;9: 31–38.
124. Lotze MT, Dallal RM, Kirkwood JM, Flickinger JC. Cutaneous melanoma. In: De Vita VT, Hellman S, Rosenberg SA (eds). Cancer: Principles and Practice of Oncology, 6th ed. Philadelphia: Lippincott, Williams & Wilkins, 2001:2012–2069.
125. Buzaid AC, Bedikian A, Houghton AN. Systemic chemotherapy and biochemotherapy. In: Balch CM, Houghton AN, Sober AJ, Soong S-J (eds). Cutaneous Melanoma, 3rd ed. St. Louis: Quality Medical, 1998:405–418.
126. Hill GJ II, Krementz ET, Hill HZ. Dimethyl triazeno imidazole carboxamide and combination therapy for melanoma. IV. Late results after complete response to chemotherapy (Central Oncology Group protocols 7130, 7131, and 7131A). Cancer (Phila) 1984;53:1299–1305.
127. Bleehen NM, Newlands ES, Lee SM, et al. Cancer Research Campaign phase II trial of temozolomide in metastatic melanoma. J Clin Oncol 1995;13:910–913.
128. Middleton MR, Grob JJ, Aaronson N, et al. Randomized phase III study of temozolomide versus dacarbazine in the treatment of patients with advanced metastatic malignant melanoma. J Clin Oncol 2000;18:158–166.
129. Glover D, Glick JH, Weiler C, Fox K, Guerry D. WR-2721 and high-dose cisplatin: an active combination in the treatment of metastatic melanoma. J Clin Oncol 1987;5:574–578.
130. Chang A, Hunt M, Parkinson DR, Hochster H, Smith TJ. Phase II trial of carboplatin in patients with metastatic malignant melanoma. A report from the Eastern Cooperative Oncology Group. Am J Clin Oncol 1993;16:152–155.
131. Legha SS, Ring S, Papadopoulos N, Raber M, Benjamin RS. A phase II trial of taxol in metastatic melanoma. Cancer (Phila) 1990;65:2478–2481.
132. Bedikian AY, Weiss GR, Legha SS, et al. Phase II trial of docetaxel in patients with advanced cutaneous malignant melanoma previously untreated with chemotherapy. J Clin Oncol 1995;13:2895–2899.
133. Ahmann DL, Hahn RG, Bisel HF. Evaluation of 1-(2-chloroethyl-3-4-methylcyclohexyl)-1-nitrosourea (methyl-CCNU, NSC 95441) versus combined imidazole carboxamide (NSC 45338) and vincristine (NSC 67574) in palliation of disseminated malignant melanoma. Cancer (Phila) 1974;33:615–618.
134. Anderson CM, Buzaid AC, Legha SS. Systemic treatments for advanced cutaneous melanoma. Oncology (Huntingt) 1995;9: 1149–1158; discussion 1163–1164, 1167–1168.
135. Jacquillat C, Khayat D, Banzet P, et al. Final report of the French multicenter phase II study of the nitrosourea fotemustine in 153 evaluable patients with disseminated malignant melanoma including patients with cerebral metastases. Cancer (Phila) 1990;66:1873–1878.
136. Atkins MB. The role of cytotoxic chemotherapeutic agents either alone or in combination with biological response modifiers. In: Kirkwood JK (ed). Molecular Diagnosis, Prevention & Therapy of Melanoma. New York: Dekker, 1997:219.
137. Feun LG, Gonzalez R, Savaraj N, et al. Phase II trial of piritrexim in metastatic melanoma using intermittent, low-dose administration. J Clin Oncol 1991;9:464–467.
138. Cocconi G, Passalacqua R, Foladore S, et al. Treatment of metastatic malignant melanoma with dacarbazine plus tamoxifen, or vindesine plus tamoxifen: a prospective randomized study. Melanoma Res 2003;13:73–79.
139. Falkson CI, Ibrahim J, Kirkwood JM, Coates AS, Atkins MB, Blum RH. Phase III trial of dacarbazine versus dacarbazine with interferon alpha-2b versus dacarbazine with tamoxifen versus dacarbazine with interferon alpha-2b and tamoxifen in patients with metastatic malignant melanoma: an Eastern Cooperative Oncology Group study. J Clin Oncol 1998;16:1743–1751.
140. McClay EF, McClay MT, Monroe L, Jones JA, Winski PJ. A phase II study of high dose tamoxifen and weekly cisplatin in patients with metastatic melanoma. Melanoma Res 2001;11: 309–313.
141. Feun LG, Savaraj N, Hurley J, Marini A, Lai S. A clinical trial of intravenous vinorelbine tartrate plus tamoxifen in the treatment of patients with advanced malignant melanoma. Cancer (Phila) 2000;88:584–588.
142. Buzaid A, Legha S, Winn R, et al. Cisplatin (C), vinblastine (V), and dacarbazine (D) versus dacarbazine alone in metastatic melanoma: preliminary results of a phase III Cancer Community Oncology Program (CCOP) trial. Proc Am Soc Clin Oncol 1993;12.
143. Del Prete SA, Maurer LH, O'Donnell J, Forcier RJ, LeMarbre P. Combination chemotherapy with cisplatin, carmustine, dacarbazine, and tamoxifen in metastatic melanoma. Cancer Treat Rep 1984;68:1403–1405.
144. McClay EF, McClay ME. Tamoxifen: is it useful in the treatment of patients with metastatic melanoma? J Clin Oncol 1994;12: 617–626.
145. Berd D, Mastrangelo MJ. Combination chemotherapy of metastatic melanoma. J Clin Oncol 1995;13:796–797.
146. Chapman PB, Einhorn LH, Meyers ML, et al. Phase III multicenter randomized trial of the Dartmouth regimen versus dacarbazine in patients with metastatic melanoma. J Clin Oncol 1999;17:2745–2751.
147. Eisen T, Boshoff C, Mak I, et al. Continuous low dose thalidomide: a phase II study in advanced melanoma, renal cell, ovarian and breast cancer. Br J Cancer 2000;82:812–817.
148. Danson S, Lorigan P, Arance A, et al. Randomized phase II study of temozolomide given every 8 hours or daily with either interferon alfa-2b or thalidomide in metastatic malignant melanoma. J Clin Oncol 2003;21:2551–2557.
149. Hwu WJ, Krown SE, Menell JH, et al. Phase II study of temozolomide plus thalidomide for the treatment of metastatic melanoma. J Clin Oncol 2003;21:3351–3356.
150. Bogenrieder T, Elder DE, Herlyn M. Molecular and cellular biology. Cutaneous Melanoma. St. Louis: Quality Medical, 2003: 713–751.
151. Chapman PB, Parkinson DR, Kirkwood JM. Biologic therapy. In: Balch CM, Houghton AN, Sober AJ, Soong SJ (eds). Cutaneous Melanoma. St. Louis: Quality Medical, 1998:419–436.
152. Smith KA. Interleukin-2. Curr Opin Immunol 1992;4:271–276.
153. Rosenberg SA. Keynote address: perspectives on the use of interleukin-2 in cancer treatment. Cancer J Sci Am 1997;3(suppl 1): S2–S6.
154. Atkins MB. Interleukin-2: clinical applications. Semin Oncol 2002;29:12–17.
155. Atkins MB, Lotze MT, Dutcher JP, et al. High-dose recombinant interleukin 2 therapy for patients with metastatic melanoma: analysis of 270 patients treated between 1985 and 1993. J Clin Oncol 1999;17:2105–2116.
156. Schwartzentruber DJ. Guidelines for the safe administration of high-dose interleukin-2. J Immunother 2001;24:287–293.
157. Atkins MB, Lee S, Flaherty LE, Sosman JA, Sondak VK, Kirkwood JM. A prospective randomized phase III trial of concurrent biochemotherapy (BCT) with cisplatin, vinblastine, dacarbazine (CVD), IL-2 and interferon alpha-2b (IFN) versus CVD alone in patients with metastatic melanoma (E3695): an ECOG-coordinated intergroup trial. Proc Am Soc Clin Oncol 2003;22.
158. Dudley ME, Wunderlich JR, Robbins PF, et al. Cancer regression and autoimmunity in patients after clonal repopulation with antitumor lymphocytes. Science 2002;298:850–854.

159. Atkins MB, O'Boyle KR, Sosman JA, et al. Multiinstitutional phase II trial of intensive combination chemoimmunotherapy for metastatic melanoma. J Clin Oncol 1994;12:1553–1560.
160. Legha SS. Durable complete responses in metastatic melanoma treated with interleukin-2 in combination with interferon alpha and chemotherapy. Semin Oncol 1997;24:S39–S43.
161. Thompson JA, Gold PJ, Fefer A. Outpatient chemoimmunotherapy for the treatment of metastatic melanoma. Semin Oncol 1997;24:S44–S48.
162. Flaherty LE, Atkins M, Sosman J, et al. Outpatient biochemotherapy with interleukin-2 and interferon alfa-2b in patients with metastatic malignant melanoma: results of two phase II cytokine working group trials. J Clin Oncol 2001;19: 3194–3202.
163. Keilholz U, Goey SH, Punt CJ, et al. Interferon alfa-2a and interleukin-2 with or without cisplatin in metastatic melanoma: a randomized trial of the European Organization for Research and Treatment of Cancer Melanoma Cooperative Group. J Clin Oncol 1997;15:2579–2588.
164. Rosenberg SA, Yang JC, Schwartzentruber DJ, et al. Prospective randomized trial of the treatment of patients with metastatic melanoma using chemotherapy with cisplatin, dacarbazine, and tamoxifen alone or in combination with interleukin-2 and interferon alfa-2b. J Clin Oncol 1999;17:968–975.
165. Dorval T, Negrier S, Chevreau C, et al. Randomized trial of treatment with cisplatin and interleukin-2 either alone or in combination with interferon-alpha-2a in patients with metastatic melanoma: a Federation Nationale des Centres de Lutte Contre le Cancer Multicenter, parallel study. Cancer (Phila) 1999;85:1060–1066.
166. Eton O, Legha SS, Bedikian AY, et al. Sequential biochemotherapy versus chemotherapy for metastatic melanoma: results from a phase III randomized trial. J Clin Oncol 2002;20:2045–2052.
167. Keilholz U, Punt CJ, Gore M, et al. Dacarbazine, cisplatin and IFN-alpha2b with or without IL-2 in advanced melanoma: final analysis of EORTC randomized phase III trial 18951. Proc Am Soc Clin Oncol 2003;22.
168. van der Bruggen P, Traversari C, Chomez P, et al. A gene encoding an antigen recognized by cytolytic T lymphocytes on a human melanoma. Science 1991;254:1643–1647.
169. Rosenberg SA. The development of new cancer therapies based on the molecular identification of cancer regression antigens. Cancer J Sci Am 1995;1:90.
170. Pardoll DM. Cancer vaccines. Nat Med 1998;4:525–531.
171. Pardoll DM. Spinning molecular immunology into successful immunotherapy. Nat Rev Immunol 2002;2:227–238.
172. Livingston P, Sznol M. Vaccine therapy. In: Balch CM, Houghton AN, Sober AJ, Soong S-J (eds). Cutaneous Melanoma. St. Louis: Quality Medical, 1998:437–450.
173. Mitchell MS. Cancer vaccines, a critical review: Part I. Curr Opin Invest Drugs 2002;3:140–149.
174. Mitchell MS. Cancer vaccines, a critical review: Part II. Curr Opin Invest Drugs 2002;3:150–158.
175. Perales MA, Wolchok JD. Melanoma vaccines. Cancer Invest 2002;20:1012–1026.
176. Berd D, Murphy G, Maguire HC Jr, Mastrangelo MJ. Immunization with haptenized, autologous tumor cells induces inflammation of human melanoma metastases. Cancer Res 1991;51:2731–2734.
177. Berd D, Sato T, Maguire HC Jr, Kairys J, Mastrangelo MJ. Immunopharmacologic analysis of an autologous, hapten-modified human melanoma vaccine. J Clin Oncol 2004;22:403–415.
178. Armstrong TD, Jaffee EM. Cytokine modified tumor vaccines. Surg Oncol Clin N Am 2002;11:681–696.
179. Sotomayor MG, Yu H, Antonia S, Sotomayor EM, Pardoll DM. Advances in gene therapy for malignant melanoma. Cancer Control 2002;9:39–48.
180. Mahvi DM, Shi FS, Yang NS, et al. Immunization by particle-mediated transfer of the granulocyte-macrophage colony-stimulating factor gene into autologous tumor cells in melanoma or sarcoma patients: report of a phase I/IB study. Hum Gene Ther 2002;13:1711–1721.
181. Mitchell MS. Perspective on allogeneic melanoma lysates in active specific immunotherapy. Semin Oncol 1998;25:623–635.
182. Sondak VK, Liu PY, Tuthill RJ, et al. Adjuvant immunotherapy of resected, intermediate-thickness, node-negative melanoma with an allogeneic tumor vaccine: overall results of a randomized trial of the Southwest Oncology Group. J Clin Oncol 2002; 20:2058–2066.
183. Sosman JA, Unger JM, Liu PY, et al. Adjuvant immunotherapy of resected, intermediate-thickness, node-negative melanoma with an allogeneic tumor vaccine: impact of HLA class I antigen expression on outcome. J Clin Oncol 2002;20:2067–2075.
184. Hsueh EC, Gupta RK, Qi K, Morton DL. Correlation of specific immune responses with survival in melanoma patients with distant metastases receiving polyvalent melanoma cell vaccine. J Clin Oncol 1998;16:2913–2920.
185. Lutzky J, Gonzalez-Angulo AM, Orzano JA. Antibody-based vaccines for the treatment of melanoma. Semin Oncol 2002;29: 462–470.
186. Sznol M, Holmlund J. Antigen-specific agents in development. Semin Oncol 1997;24:173–186.
187. Albertini MR, King DM, Rakhmilevich AL. The use of particle-mediated gene transfer for immunotherapy of cancer. In: Gerson SL, Lattime ED (eds). Gene Therapy of Cancer: Translational Approaches from Preclinical Studies to Clinical Implementation, vol 2. New York: Academic Press, 2002:225–238.
188. Kim CJ, Dessureault S, Gabrilovich D, Reintgen DS, Slingluff CL Jr. Immunotherapy for melanoma. Cancer Control 2002;9: 22–30.
189. Parmiani G, Castelli C, Dalerba P, et al. Cancer immunotherapy with peptide-based vaccines: what have we achieved? Where are we going? J Natl Cancer Inst 2002;94:805–818.
190. Rosenberg SA, Yang JC, Schwartzentruber DJ, et al. Immunologic and therapeutic evaluation of a synthetic peptide vaccine for the treatment of patients with metastatic melanoma. Nat Med 1998;4:321–327.
191. Nestle FO, Alijagic S, Gilliet M, et al. Vaccination of melanoma patients with peptide- or tumor lysate-pulsed dendritic cells. Nat Med 1998;4:328–332.
192. Virgo KS, Chan D, Handler BS, Johnson DY, Goshima K, Johnson FE. Current practice of patient follow-up after potentially curative resection of cutaneous melanoma. Plast Reconstr Surg 2000; 106:590–597.
193. Hofmann U, Szedlak M, Rittgen W, Jung EG, Schadendorf D. Primary staging and follow-up in melanoma patients: monocenter evaluation of methods, costs and patient survival. Br J Cancer 2002;87:151–157.
194. Coit DG. Patient surveillance and follow-up. In: Balch CM, Houghton AN, Sober AJ, Soong S-J (eds). Cutaneous Melanoma, 3rd ed. St. Louis: Quality Medical, 1998:313–323.
195. Hwu W-J, Balch CM, Houghton AN. Diagnosis of stage IV disease. In: Balch CM, Houghton AN, Sober AJ, Soong S-J (eds). Cutaneous Melanoma. St. Louis: Quality Medical, 2003: 523–546.
196. Wascher RA, Morton DL, Kuo C, et al. Molecular tumor markers in the blood: early prediction of disease outcome in melanoma patients treated with a melanoma vaccine. J Clin Oncol 2003; 21:2558–2563.

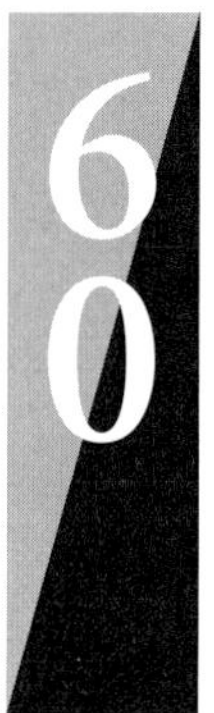

Nonmelanoma Cutaneous Malignancies

Montgomery Gillard, Timothy S. Wang, and Timothy M. Johnson

Facts and Figures

The nonmelanoma skin cancers (NMSC) are the most common human cancer type. More than half of all cancers diagnosed in the United States are NMSC. In the year 2003, more than 1.3 million new cases of NMSC will be diagnosed.[1] One in 5 Americans born in 2003 will be diagnosed with skin cancer in their lifetime. Recent publications and articles in the lay press have labeled nonmelanoma NMSC as "today's epidemic."[2] The incidence of NMSC has been rising since the 1960s at 4% to 8% per year.[3] Basal cell carcinoma (BCC) and squamous cell carcinoma (SCC) account for 96% of new cases of NMSC. The remaining 4% consists of many other types of NMSC, but given their low incidence, discussion of these lesions is beyond the scope of this chapter.

Approximately 80% of skin cancers are BCC and 16% are SCC. Melanoma accounts for 4% of skin cancer diagnoses, but accounts for 75% of skin cancer deaths.[1] NMSC has an excellent prognosis: 90% to 99% of patients are curable following therapy and less than 1% of cases result in death. The number of deaths due to NMSC has been estimated at 2,000 to 2,500 year with three-fourths of these deaths attributed to SCC.[4] However, these tumors are associated with significant morbidity in terms of significant local destruction and disfigurement and medical costs. The annual cost of treating NMSC has been estimated to be more than $500 million.[4] A recent publication described skin cancer among the most costly of all cancers to treat for the Medicare population.[5] Despite the tremendous impact of NMSC on the U.S. population, a limited quality of evidence-based research exists.

Demographics

Increased risk for NMSC is associated with a number of host and environmental risk factors (Table 60.1). Exposure to sunlight is the principal cause of both BCC and SCC. The risk of NMSC varies according to race and ethnic group, with whites of Celtic ancestry having the highest incidence rates.[6] The increased risk phenotype includes fair skin that tans poorly and sunburns easily, extensive freckling, blue or light-colored eyes, and red, blond, or light brown hair. NMSC is uncommon in African Americans, Asians, and Hispanics.[7] As with most malignancies, incidence increases with increasing age. Residence in areas with high levels of ambient ultraviolet B (UVB) radiation (i.e., lower latitudes) is associated with a higher incidence of NMSC.[8] Most NMSC occur on sun-exposed sites, and 80% of lesions arise on the face, head, or neck.[7] Although NMSC usually occurs on sun-exposed sites, these tumors can rarely occur in sun-protected sites such as the anogenital area, mucous membranes, palms, and soles.[9,10]

Genodermatoses and Other Medical Conditions

A number of genetic syndromes are associated with an increased risk of NMSC.[11] Albinism is primarily an autosomal recessive disorder characterized by partial or complete failure to produce ocular and cutaneous protective melanin. Nevoid BCC nevus syndrome (Gorlin's syndrome) is an autosomal dominant or mosaic disorder associated with multiple BCC, jaw cysts, palmoplantar pits, abnormal ribs and vertebrae, and hypertelorism. Xeroderma pigmentosum is an autosomal recessive disorder characterized by hypersensitivity to UV light and high incidence of skin cancer, including melanoma, due to defects in DNA repair. Other less-common genetic syndromes associated with NMSC include epidermodysplasia verruciformis, epidermolysis bullosa, and dyskeratosis congenita. Other conditions associated with an NMSC include burn and vaccination scars, chronic inflammatory processes and ulcers, radiation, photodamaged skin, immunosuppression, and a history of previous NMSC.[12,13]

Environmental Factors

Ultraviolet radiation, particularly UVB (290–320 nm), induces skin cancer as demonstrated in epidemiologic and experimental data.[7,14] Depletion of the earth's ozone layer increases the levels of UVB radiation and the incidence of NMSC by 2% to 4% for each 1% reduction of the ozone layer.[15,16] Ultraviolet B radiation induces NMSC by a variety of mechanism including direct DNA damage, damage to DNA repair systems, and alteration of the local cutaneous immune system.[17] Other environmental/exposure factors associated with NMSC, primarily SCC, include a variety of chemicals: these include hydrocarbons found in coal tars, soot, asphalt, and cutting oils. Chronic exposure to arsenic has been associated with NMSC on both sun-exposed and covered sites.[18] Psoralens used in combination with UVA (PUVA) used for the treatment of psoriasis and other inflammatory dermatoses produce dose-dependent increase in SCC.[19] Cigarette smoking

TABLE 60.1. Risk factors associated with developing nonmelanoma cutaneous malignancy (NMSC).

- Phenotype
  - Skin that tans poorly and sunburns easily
  - Celtic ancestry
  - Freckling
  - Red, blonde, or light brown hair
  - Blue or light-colored eyes
- Demographics
  - Older age
  - Males
  - Outdoor occupation
  - Residence in lower latitudes
  - Immunosuppression
- Genodermatoses
  - Albinism
  - Nevoid basal cell carcinoma (BCC) nevus syndrome
  - Xeroderma pigmentosum
  - Epidermodysplasia verruciformis
- Environmental
  - Ultraviolet light
  - Ionizing radiation
  - Chemicals or drugs
- Cigarette smoking

has been linked to causing SCC of the lip and mouth.[20] Human papillomavirus has been associated with cutaneous SCC.[21] The carcinogenic effect of ionizing radiation inducing NMSC is documented in human and animal models.[22]

Basic Science

Basal Cell Carcinoma

BCC can develop in both a hereditary and sporadic fashion. Mutations in the PTCH gene have been identified as the cause of nevoid BCC syndrome and in sporadic BCC.[23–26] PTCH is a cell membrane receptor for a family of proteins called Hedgehog (Hh).[27] The PTCH protein binds and inhibits a transmembrane protein smoothened (SMO). Mutations in either PTCH or SMO lead to increased smoothened signaling and growth promotion with subsequent cancer formation. The activation of the smoothened pathway leads to induction of a number of proteins via the Gli1 transcription factor, including transforming growth factor-beta (TGF-β), platelet-derived growth factor receptor-α, PTCH, and Gli1, and are relevant to cancer development.[28]

Mutations that inactivate the tumor suppressor gene p53, also known as the guardian of the genome, are one of the most frequently found defects in all tumors.[29] The function of p53 is to sense DNA damage and arrest cell division to allow for DNA repairs or induce an apoptotic response to eliminate defective and potentially malignant cells. Fifty percent to 100% of BCC contain p53 mutations.[30,31] Despite the frequency of p53 mutations in BCC, a causal role for these mutations in BCC development or progression has not been demonstrated. Patients with Li–Fraumeni syndrome, characterized by an inherited mutation in the p53 gene, are susceptible to an increased incidence of a number of malignancies, but an increase in NMSC has not been reported.[28]

Squamous Cell Carcinoma

Squamous cell carcinoma can develop in a hereditary and sporadic fashion. There are several rare syndromes that can predispose individuals to SCC, but there are no monogenic disorders that feature SCC exclusively.[32] Ultraviolet radiation generates specific mutations, thymidine dimers, in p53. The most frequent alteration is the CC→TT mutation, which is a UV signature mutation. Keratinocytes with one mutation in p53 after UV exposure undergo apoptosis. In contrast, keratinocytes with dysfunctional p53 and an additional p53 mutation as a result of UV irradiation cannot undergo apoptosis and instead undergo clonal expansion, which is manifested clinically as the development of an actinic keratosis, a known precursor lesion to SCC. Uncontrolled proliferation of these abnormal keratinocytes eventually leads to SCC in situ and invasive SCC.[33] Brash et al. found that 58% of invasive SCCs of the skin contain mutations in p53.[34] Mutations in other tumor suppressor genes such as RAS and p16/CDKN2A have also been reported.[35,36]

Clinical Presentation

Basal Cell Carcinoma

BCC originate de novo presumably in the bulge area and have no precursor lesion. The presentations of BCC are as varied as the tumor is common. Approximately 80% of BCCs are found on the head and neck.[7] Basal cell carcinoma can be classified into subtypes by their clinical morphology and histopathology. Clinical subtypes vary in appearance and clinical course and include the following more common variants: nodular, superficial, aggressive (infiltrating and morpheaform), and pigmented.[37–39]

The nodular or nodular ulcerative variant is the "classic" BCC. Clinically, this appears as a translucent, flesh-colored or pink, pearly papule with prominent telangiectasias (Figure 60.1). Nodular BCC may ulcerate, forming what was once

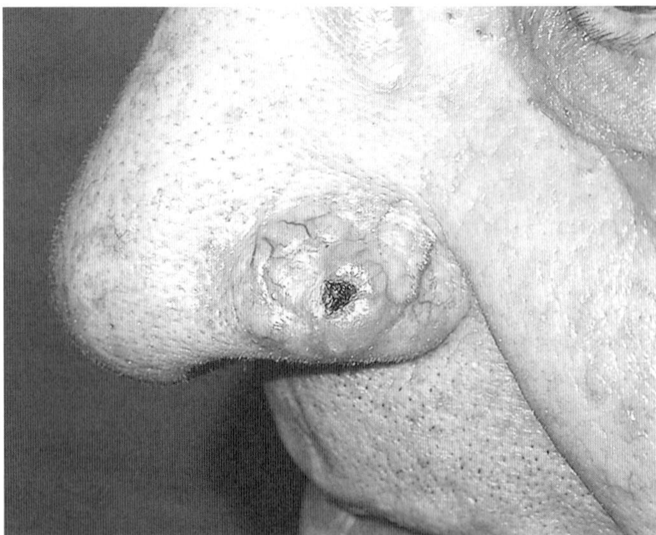

FIGURE 60.1. Nodular pattern basal cell carcinoma of the left nasal ala.

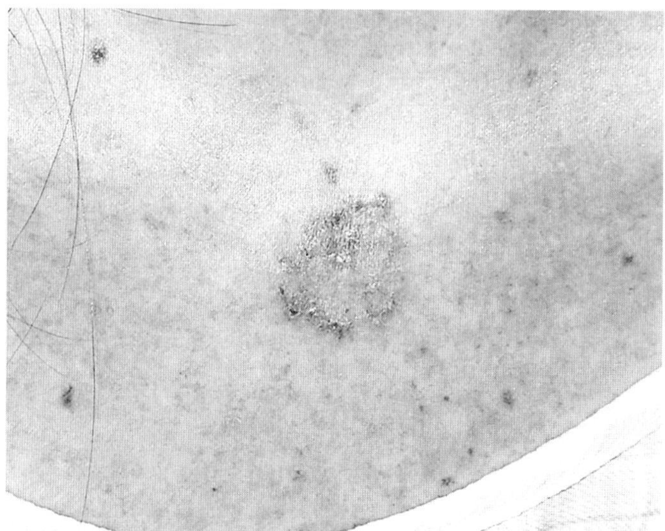

FIGURE 60.2. Superficial pattern basal cell carcinoma on the chest, clinically resembles nummular eczema.

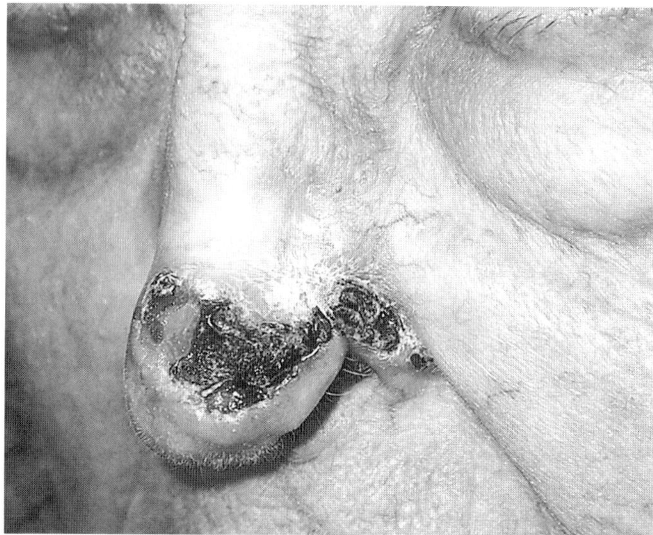

FIGURE 60.3. Locally destructive, recurrent, aggressive growth pattern basal cell carcinoma previously treated with surgical excision and radiation therapy, 9 and 6 years, respectively.

termed a rodent ulcer because of its resemblance to a rat bite. Most lesions are small (less than 1 cm) papules; however, patients do present with very large, disfiguring lesions that have been neglected for many years. Superficial BCC usually presents as a red, scaly macule with a thready translucent border, often with areas of hypopigmentation, atrophy, or scarring. They commonly occur on the trunk and extremities, are sometimes confused with inflammatory skin conditions such as psoriasis and eczema, and may closely resemble Bowen's disease and actinic keratoses (Figure 60.2). The aggressive subtype of BCC usually presents as a flat, indurated, pale, white-to-yellow papule or plaque with indistinct clinical borders and a "scarlike" appearance. As these lesions grow, they often become firm. They are also known as infiltrating, morpheaform, sclerosing, sclerotic, and fibrotic BCC. These lesions often extend well beyond (more than 1 cm) their clinically apparent margins and may ulcerate later in the clinical course (Figure 60.3). Pigmentation within BCC can be variable and can be seen in a variety of subtypes. Some lesions are heavily pigmented, and are categorized as a pigmented BCC and can bear striking resemblance to malignant melanoma or pigmented seborrheic keratoses. Neglected BCC or those with high risk factors described later may result in extensive local tissue destruction and very high morbidity (Figure 60.4).

Squamous Cell Carcinoma

Several precursor lesions to invasive SCC exist, including actinic keratoses, arsenical keratoses, thermal keratoses, radiation keratoses, chronic cicatrix keratoses, Bowen's disease (SCC in situ), and erythroplasia of Queyrat.[40] Actinic keratoses (AK) are both precursors of cutaneous SCC and markers of increased risk for NMSC. Clinically they arise as rough, scaly patches, on average 4 to 10 mm in diameter, on sun-exposed areas. They can be skin colored, erythematous, pink, or brown, and often they are more easily felt than seen. Actinic keratoses occur most commonly on the head and neck and extensor arms and hands. The annual rate of progression of AKs to SCC is unknown and controversial, with estimates of conversion ranging from 0.025% to 20%; the

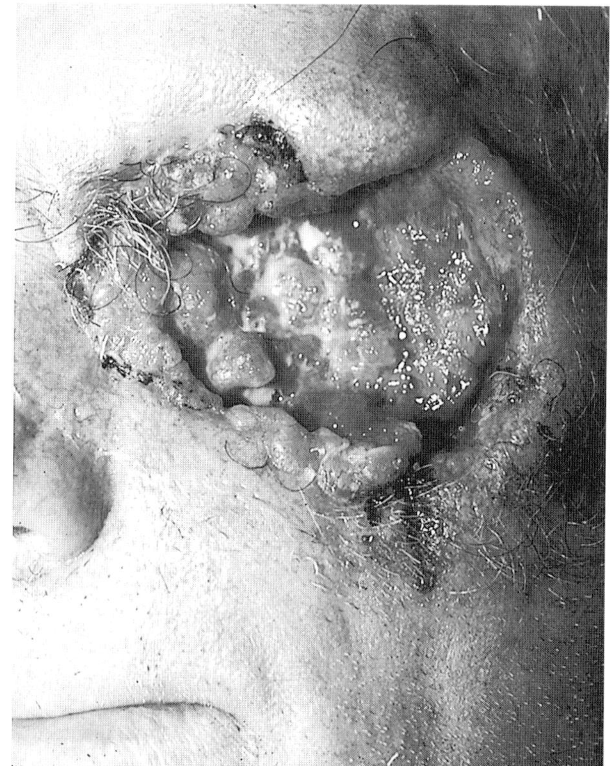

FIGURE 60.4. Multiply recurrent, neglected, basal cell carcinoma involving the eye. Although rarely lethal; tumors with high-risk factors may be associated with local tissue destruction and high morbidity, and even metastasis and death.

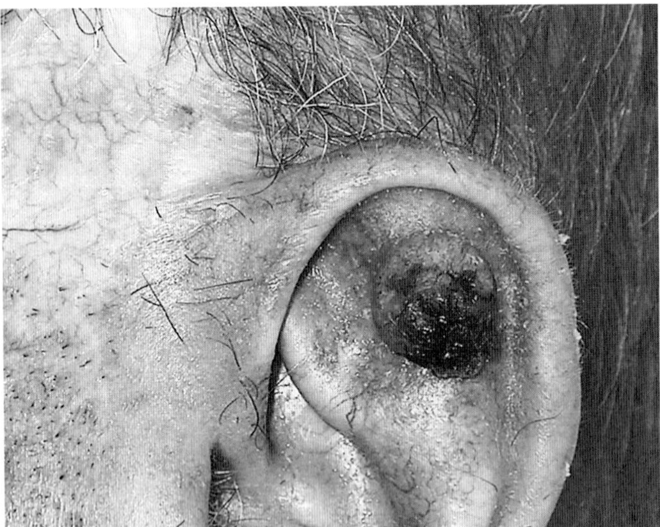

FIGURE 60.5. Squamous cell carcinoma of the left ear, a known high-risk location.

cumulative risk depends on the number or lesions and the length of time they persist.[41–43] Among patients with multiple AKs, the cumulative lifetime risk of having at least one invasive SCC is believed to be 6% to 10%.[44] Clinically, there are two main types of SCC in situ, which include Bowen's disease and erythroplasia of Queyrat. Bowen's disease often presents as a slow-growing, poorly defined, scaly pink patch on sun-exposed sites.[45] Erythroplasia of Queyrat occurs as SCC in situ on the glans penis, often as a smooth, erythematous, plaque. SCC in situ lesions progress to invasive SCC.[21]

Invasive SCC most commonly occurs on the sun-exposed areas of the body. Approximately 80% develop on chronically sun-exposed areas on the head and neck and extremities, followed by the trunk.[21] They vary in their presentation and often appear as 0.5 to 1.5 cm, firm, hyperkeratotic pink papules, nodules, or plaques, sometimes with pain (Figure 60.5). Ulceration is a common finding, and the lesions tend to bleed easily following minor trauma. In darker-skinned patients, SCC may present in nonsun-exposed areas, are often hyperpigmented, and are most commonly associated with chronic inflammatory or scarring processes. Keratoacanthoma (KA) is a well-differentiated subtype of SCC that tends to grow rapidly to form a crateriform nodule.[46] Keratoacanthoma metastasis has been reported.[47]

Histopathology

Basal Cell Carcinoma

The histologic patterns of BCC are as diverse as its clinical appearance. Classic histologic features include presence of multiple basaloid tumor cells islands, cords, or nests with peripheral palisading of nuclei and focal areas of separation or retraction artifact between tumor nodules and mucinous stroma. Many histologic subtypes and classification schemes exist. Nevertheless, there are four major architectural patterns that are useful to identify because of their clinical and prognostic implications. These patterns include superficial, nodular, micronodular, and aggressive-growth (infiltrative and morpheaform) (Table 60.2). Multiple patterns may be found in up to 35% to 50% of lesions, with the most aggressive pattern correlating with biologic behavior.

Numerous, multifocal small buds of basaloid tumor cells that arise in the epidermis and extend into the superficial dermis and down hair follicles characterize superficial BCC. Nodular BCC, also known as solid or well circumscribed, is the most common histologic pattern.[48] It is composed of variable-sized tumor lobules in the dermis that are well circumscribed. Larger lesions that ulcerate are termed nodulocystic BCC and are characterized by centrilobular necrosis or cystic degeneration within the center of the tumor lobules. Smaller tumor islands, approximately the same size as hair bulbs, characterize micronodular BCC.

The aggressive-growth BCC classification merges the histologic pattern with the biologic and clinical behavior. The

TABLE 60.2. Histopathologic features of basal cell carcinoma (BCC) and squamous cell carcinoma (SCC).

Basal cell carcinoma	
Superficial pattern	Numerous, multifocal small buds of basaloid tumor cells that arise in the epidermis and extend into superficial dermis or down hair follicles
Nodular pattern	Well-circumscribed tumor lobules of varying size in dermis
Micronodular pattern	Smaller tumor islands, approximately the size of hair bulbs
Aggressive growth pattern	Narrow linear strands and cords of basaloid tumor cells embedded in a sclerotic stroma
Squamous cell carcinoma	
Conventional type	Malignant proliferation of keratinocytes that extend into dermis with varying degrees of keratinization and anaplasia
Adenoid/acantholytic type	Endophytic invasive lesion with acantholysis of tumor cells leading to a pseudoglandular appearance
Boweniod type	Full-thickness architectural disorder with loss of polarity and absence of orderly keratinocyte maturation with invasion into the dermis
Spindle cell/pleomorphic type	Broad fusiform sheets of atypical spindle cells with rare foci of squamous differentiation
Small cell type	Small round neuroendocrine-like malignant cells, usually associated with overlying SCC in situ lesion
Verrucous type	Well differentiated with little atypia and with pseudoepitheliomatous hyperplasia that "bulldozes" into dermis
Keratoacanthoma type	Well-circumscribed, keratin-filled invaginations, composed of well-differentiated squamous cells with "glassy" eosinophilic cytoplasm
Squamous cell carcinoma in situ type (Bowen's disease)	Full-thickness epidermal dysplasia without invasion into dermis, disordered maturation with "windblown" appearance

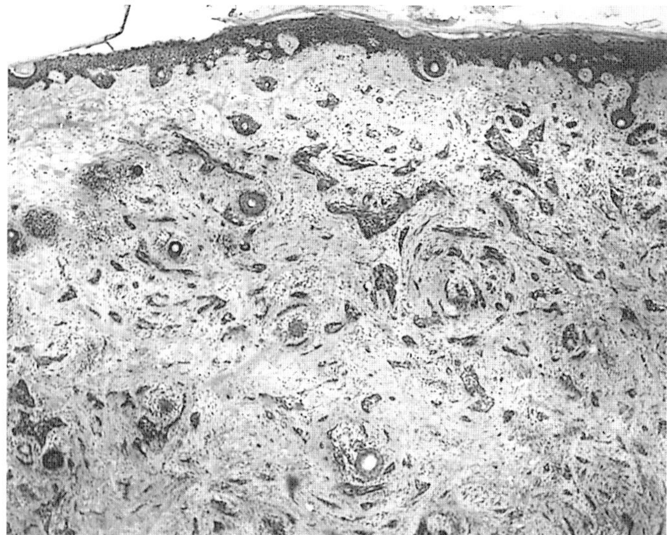

FIGURE 60.6. Mohs' surgery: frozen-section histologic slide of an aggressive growth pattern basal cell carcinoma with numerous tumor cells, often only one cell layer thick, arranged in elongated strands embedded in a dense fibrous stroma. The strands of tumor cells often extend a considerable distance from the clinical lesion and deeply invade the deep dermis and subcutis.

histologic features include small islands and narrow linear strands and cords of basaloid tumor cells embedded in a dense, fibrous to sclerotic stroma. The narrow strands resemble "finger-like" or "spiky" projections; peripheral palisading and stromal retraction are often inconspicuous or absent.[49] It is important for the pathologist to convey to the clinician the growth pattern of all BCC, but it is paramount for aggressive-growth BCC. The aggressive-growth BCC is an infiltrating lesion with extensive subclinical invasion into deep dermis, subcutis, and muscle (Figure 60.6). Aggressive-growth BCC often shelve and skate along muscle and fascial planes, cartilage, and bone. Perineural invasion is also more common.[50] Micronodular BCC similarly often has significant subclinical extension through the dermis or subcutis.[51]

Squamous Cell Carcinoma

There are several histologic subtypes of SCC with the conventional subtype, otherwise known as generic or simplex, being the most common. Other subtypes include adenoid/acantholytic, bowenoid, spindle/pleomorphic, small cell, verrucous, keratoacanthoma, SCC in situ, and microinvasive SCC. The conventional subtype is characterized by lobules and cords of atypical keratinocytes originating from the epidermis and invading the dermis. Cellular features include enlarged, hyperchromatic, variably pleomorphic nuclei with often prominent mitotic activity. Many lesions produce larger amounts of keratin, resulting in keratin-pearl formation, and intercellular bridges are usually easily seen.[52] Perineural invasion occurs in 2.4% to 14% of SCC and is even more frequent in recurrences.[53] The conventional type of SCC may be further subclassified by the degree of differentiation. The Broders system of histologic grading of SCC is based on the degree of cellular differentiation in the neoplasm.[54] Grade I is well differentiated with more than 75% keratinization and grade IV with less than 25% keratinization. More commonly, lesions are referred to as "well differentiated versus poorly differentiated." The underlying trend is that as tumors become less differentiated they behave in a more clinically aggressive mode.

Bowenoid SCC is characterized by architectural disorder of the full thickness of epidermis, with loss of polarity and absence of orderly keratinocyte maturation. The atypical keratinocytes may extend downward along the follicular epithelium to the level of the sebaceous glands. Evidence of invasion into the dermis differentiates bowenoid SCC from Bowen's disease (SCC in situ). Adenoid or acantholytic tumors exhibit a conventional SCC pattern with acantholysis leading to a pseudoglandular appearance. The spindle-cell/pleomorphic variant is composed of intertwining fascicles, and bundles of atypical keratinocytes are surrounded by a myxoid or storiform stroma.[55] Immunohistochemistry is often required to differentiate these neoplasms from spindle cell melanoma and atypical fibroxanthoma. Spindle cell SCC demonstrates positive staining with cytokeratins.[56] The small cell variant of SCC resembles a Merkel cell carcinoma or metastatic small cell neuroendocrine carcinoma.

Prognostic Factors and Risk Status

The majority of NMSC are, fortunately, low-risk lesions that can be treated with relatively high cure rates. "Higher-risk" NMSC lesions are associated with higher incidence of recurrence and/or metastasis. Numerous clinical high-risk factors exist in regard to NMSC. These risk factors include the following: size, location, primary versus recurrent, ill-defined clinical borders, occurrence in immunosuppressed individuals, histologic pattern subtype and depth, perineural invasion, and tumors developing in areas of previous irradiation.

Basal Cell Carcinoma

Most primary BCC are cured by appropriate initial treatment. Recurrent tumors are often locally destructive and more difficult to treat.[57] Several prognostic factors of primary BCC are known to influence whether the tumor will recur after treatment; these include size, anatomic location, histologic subtype, clinically poorly defined tumor borders, perineural invasion, immunosuppression, tumors developing in sites of prior radiotherapy, and recurrent lesions (Table 60.3). BCC located on the head and neck is more likely to recur than

TABLE 60.3. Basal cell carcinoma (BCC) risk factors.

- Anatomic location
  - High risk: mask areas of face, genitalia, hands and feet
  - Medium risk: cheeks, forehead, scalp, and neck
  - Low risk: trunk, extremities
- Size
  - Lesions ≥6 mm on high-risk area: mask areas of face, genitalia, hands and feet
  - Lesions ≥10 mm on medium-risk area: cheeks, forehead, scalp, and neck
  - Lesions ≥20 mm on low-risk area: trunk and extremities
- Histologic subtype patterns
  - Aggressive growth
  - Micronodular
- Poorly defined clinical borders
- Perineural invasion
- Development in sites of prior radiation
- Immunosuppression
- Recurrent tumors

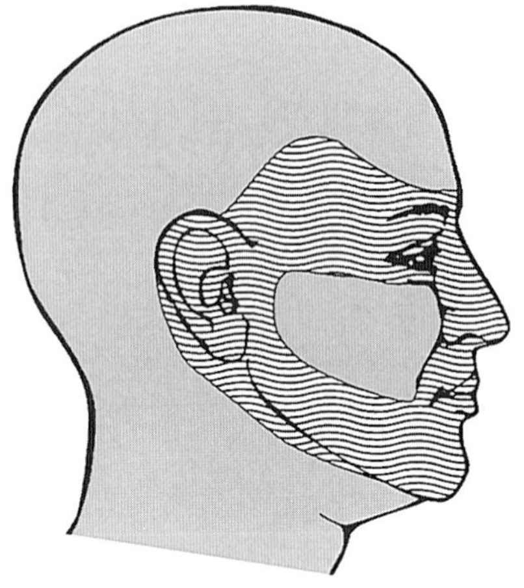
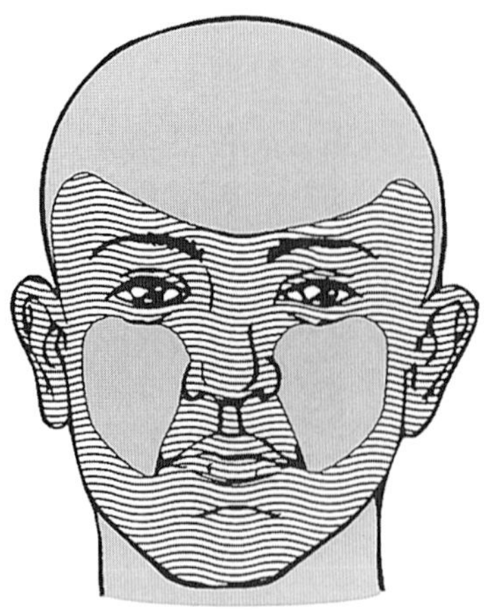

FIGURE 60.7. Lesions located in the high-risk "mask area" of the face (*horizontal lines*) are at increased risk for tumor recurrence. The genitalia, hands, and feet are also high-risk locations. Medium-risk areas of the head and neck shown by *gray shading*.

lesions developing on the trunk and extremities. The high-risk "mask areas" of the face (central face, eyelids, eyebrows, periorbital, nose, lips, chin, mandible, preauricular and postauricular areas, temple and ears) and the genitalia, hands, and feet are at increased risk for tumor recurrence (Figure 60.7). Medium-risk locations include the cheeks, forehead, scalp, and neck, and low-risk sites include the trunk and extremities. The data for size and location are based upon a large 27-year retrospective review from the skin cancer unit at New York University (NYU) published in 1991 and 1992 by Silverman et al.[58–61] The combination of size and location affects recurrence rates. Recurrences in the NYU study were significantly more common when tumors in high-risk locations were 6mm or more in size, in medium-risk areas 10mm or more in diameter, and in low-risk areas, 20mm or more.

An increased risk of tumor recurrence is associated with two histologic subtypes, the aggressive growth (sclerosing, morpheaform, fibrosing, desmoplastic, scirrhous, infiltrative), and micronodular patterns.[62] Poorly defined clinical borders result in higher recurrent rates.[57] Perineural invasion poses a significantly increased risk of recurrence and subclinical invasion, and occurs in up to 3% of all BCC.[63] The incidence of BCC is reportedly increased by a factor of 10 in immunosuppressed transplant recipients.[64] BCC in immunosuppressed patients should be viewed as potentially high-risk tumors. BCC developing in skin previously treated with radiation are at higher risk for significant subclinical invasion and are considered high-risk lesions.[65] Recurrent BCC have rerecurrence rates reported as high as 33% to 50%, regardless of anatomic location or treatment modality used.[66]

Metastatic BCC is a rare event (0.03%).[67] Metastatic spread is most often to the regional lymph nodes, followed by the lungs, bones, and skin.[68] The 5-year survival rate for patients with metastatic disease is poor, and patients with distant disease have a median survival of only between 10 and 14 months.

Squamous Cell Carcinoma

Invasive SCC is the more serious form of NMSC because of its greater potential to metastasize. The majority of SCC are low-risk lesions that are treated with relatively high cure rates. Several variables have been identified as determining risk of local recurrence, metastasis, and survival rates. In 1992, Rowe et al. reviewed the literature since 1940 to identify the most important prognostic factors.[69] Nine variables of cutaneous SCC have been identified as "high-risk" factors for increased likelihood of recurrence, metastasis, and death: size, depth of invasion, histologic differentiation, rapid growth, etiology (scar, radiation, chronic ulcer or inflammatory process, and sinus tract), anatomic site, immunosuppression, perineural invasion, and recurrent lesions (Table 60.4).

SCC is the most common skin cancer in immunosuppressed transplant recipients, occurring 65 to 250 times as frequently as in the general population.[70] Immunosuppression-associated SCC are biologically aggressive and associated with higher risk of rapid growth, local recurrence, regional and distant spread, and mortality.[12,69]

The most common sites of spread are the regional lymph nodes, which occurs in 85% of metastatic cases. Approximately 15% of metastases involve distant sites such as the lungs, liver, brain, bone, and skin.[21,71] Prognosis for patients with metastatic SCC is poor; 10-year survival rates are less than 20% for patients with regional lymph node involvement and less than 10% for patients with distant metastases.

TABLE 60.4. Squamous cell carcinoma (SCC) risk factors.

- Anatomic location
  - High risk: mask areas of face, genitalia, hands and feet, especially ear and lip
  - Medium risk: cheeks, forehead, scalp, and neck
  - Low risk: trunk, extremities
- Size
  - Lesions ≥6mm on high-risk area: mask areas of face, genitalia, hands and feet
  - Lesions ≥10mm on medium-risk area: cheeks, forehead, scalp, and neck
  - Lesions ≥20mm on low-risk area: trunk and extremities
- Histology
  - Poorly differentiated
- Depth of invasion
  - Clark's level IV (lesion that involves the reticular dermis), V (lesion that invades into subcutaneous fat), or ≥4mm
- Perineural invasion
- Rapid growth
- Etiology
  - Scar, chronic ulcer or inflammatory process, sinus tract, sites of prior radiation therapy
- Immunosuppression
- Recurrent tumor

Treatment: Evidence-Based Medicine

Numerous treatment modalities are used for NMSC, both surgical and nonsurgical. Despite the enormous amount of literature involved in the treatment of NMSC, there has been relatively little good-quality research on the efficacy of the treatment modalities used. Rare systematic reviews of treatment modalities and meta-analyses have been reported. This type of analysis may generate misleading results by ignoring the meaningful heterogeneity among studies, fortifying the biases in individual studies, and introducing further biases through the process of finding studies and selecting the results that are pooled.[72] Most of the reported literature is retrospective and not randomized and suffers from selection bias; that is, treatment modality used was influenced by whether the lesion was low or high risk. The selection of therapy is based upon the clinical and histologic risk factors described previously. Randomization is the only way to avoid tumor selection bias, and to date there have been fewer than 30 randomized controlled trials examining treatment modalities in NMSC. Similarly, recurrence rates for different therapies are difficult to compare because of lack of uniformity in methods of reporting. Most of the (short-term) studies report a recurrence rate based on the total number of patients with recurrent NMSC divided by the total number of patients with initial tumors (raw recurrence rate = all recurrences / all tumors treated). This method artificially lowers the recurrence rate because it ignores patients unavailable for follow-up, which is not uncommon for elderly populations who may die of other causes and be unavailable for follow-up.[73] In contrast, most long-term studies report a recurrence rate based on the total number of patients with recurrent NMSC divided by the total number of patients who were observed for at least 5 years (strict 5-year recurrence rate = all recurrences / all nonrecurring tumors followed up for 5 years + all tumors recurring within 5 years). This method excludes nonrecurring patients who were observed for less than 5 years and thereby artificially raises the recurrence rate.[73] From a statistical point of view, recurrence rates are the result of calculating several types of survival curves, such as the Kaplan–Meier survival curve and the life table survival curve according to Cutler and Ederer. The modified life table recurrence rate would be intermediate between the raw and strict recurrence rate in most instances because it uses all available data and gives weighted credit for tumor-free follow-up of less than 5 years.

In this section, the treatment modalities for NMSC are described and the best clinical evidence that currently exists outlines the effectiveness of the therapy described. The Cochrane Collaboration performed a comprehensive evidence-based review of interventions utilized for the treatment of primary BCC in 2003.[74] To be included in their analysis, studies had to meet their strict criteria: adult patients with histologically proven primary BCC, and excluded recurrent lesions or patients with genodermatoses. Primary outcome was recurrence at 3 to 5 years measured clinically (to simulate what happens in clinical practice). Secondary outcomes looked at early treatment failure within 6 months, measured histologically, and esthetic considerations and discomfort to patients. *Clinical Evidence*, an annually updated evidence-based medicine periodical, recently outlined an evidence-based review of squamous cell carcinoma of the skin.[75]

Electrodesiccation and Curettage

Electrodesiccation and curettage (ED&C) is a common treatment modality used primarily by dermatologists and is highly operator dependent. ED&C is a procedure causing local tissue destruction performed under local anesthesia. NMSC have a soft feel that can be differentiated from uninvolved normal surrounding tissue, which feels smooth and firm. First, a larger curette is used to debulk the majority of the soft tumor; this is followed by electrodesiccation of the periphery and base of the wound to destroy residual tumor cells. This process is repeated with both large and small curettes and electrodesiccation for a total of 2 to 4 cycles depending upon the size and feel of the lesion. The experienced operator may provide similar high cure rates with curettage alone, omitting electrodesiccation. The resulting wound heals by secondary intention as a hypopigmented, atrophic scar. If the curette extends into the subcutis or a sclerotic "feel" is noted, excision of the site should be performed. A disadvantage of ED&C is the lack of a surgical specimen in which to examine margins for completeness of tumor removal or to obtain data on histologic depth of invasion.

Clinical Evidence

To date there have been no randomized controlled trials (RCT) comparing ED&C of NMSC with other modalities. Rowe et al. performed a meta-analysis on all the literature from 1947 to the present and reported cure rates for the treatment of primary BCC. They found that the short-term (less than 5 years) recurrence rates for primary BCC in all locations treated with ED&C was 4.7% and the long-term (more than 5 years) recurrence rate was 7.7%.[57] Their findings underscore the fact that short-term follow up (less than 5 years) artificially lowers the recurrence rate and emphasizes the need for standardization of follow up for studying recurrence rates in NMSC. In fact, 18% of recurrences occur after 5 years.[57] Kopf et al. reported on recurrence rates of primary BCC treated with ED&C and noted cumulative 5-year recurrence rates for all lesions ranging from 5.7% to 18.8%.[76] An interesting distinction was that residents in training had higher recurrence rates (18.8%) compared with attending physicians (5.7%); this raises yet another variable in determining tumor recurrence, the degree of experience of the treating physician.

The study by Silverman et al. examined recurrence rate for 2,314 primary BCC treated with ED&C and further examined the role of size and location in recurrence.[59] They found that tumors located in low-risk areas (neck, trunk, extremities) of all sizes responded well to ED&C with a 5-year recurrence rate of 3.5%, whereas tumors located at high-risk locations had a recurrence rate of 4.5% if they were less than 6 mm in size and a 17.6% recurrence rate if they were larger.[59] ED&C has been documented as an effective primary treatment modality for the treatment of low-risk primary BCC. For recurrent BCC, rerecurrence rates with ED&C were 33.3% at 5 years and 40% at more than 5 years.[57]

The treatment of SCC with ED&C is less well documented. In the meta-analysis by Rowe, recurrence rates for primary SCC treated with ED&C was 3.7%.[69] However, these data suffer from the small sample size (82 patients) and treatment bias in selecting for smaller lesions. ED&C of primary SCC is limited to small, low-risk, minimally invasive or in situ lesions in low-risk or nonhair-bearing locations.

In summary, ED&C is an effective primary treatment for primary low-risk BCC and small in situ or minimally invasive SCC in low-risk locations. The technique is operator dependent and the degree of experience with the procedure affects the results. The procedure is easily performed in an office setting with little morbidity.

Cryosurgery

Cryosurgery uses liquid nitrogen delivered by a spray apparatus or cryoprobe that allows for deep-freezing to −50 to −60°C to achieve local destruction and necrosis of tissues. Typically, two freeze-thaw cycles are used. The resulting wound heals by secondary intention. The most common side effects are transient edema, pain, and erythema. Chondritis and cartilage necrosis may occur. Cosmetic results are similar to ED&C. The procedure is performed in an office but requires experience and additional equipment. It is an effective treatment for low-risk BCC as well as for some SCC.[77,78]

Clinical Evidence

A total of four randomized controlled trials (RCTs) have been performed in regard to the use of cryosurgery to treat primary BCC (Table 60.5). One study is omitted from this review because it did not histologically confirm the diagnosis of BCC.[79] One of the studies examined cryosurgery compared to radiotherapy (RT) for 93 patients with primary BCC, excluding lesions on the nose or pinna. Recurrence rates were recorded at only 1 year and not 3 to 5 years.[80] This limitation should be a red flag, and conclusions should be approached with caution because nearly two-thirds of all lesions recur within the first 3 years but may occur at 5 to 10 years. Cryosurgery showed a high recurrence rate (39%) compared with radiotherapy (4%). Cosmetic and discomfort levels were equivalent. Another study of 96 patients compared cryosurgery with surgical excision for superficial and nodular primary BCC of the head and neck.[81] The recurrence rate was 3 in 48 for the cryosurgery group and 0 in 48 for the excision group. The primary outcome was final cosmetic result, and the outcome was better in the excision group. Ninety percent of the cryosurgery group complained of moderate to severe swelling and exudative drainage.

A final study of 88 primary BCC compared cryosurgery with photodynamic therapy (PDT).[82] Lesions were located on the head, neck, and extremities, and the follow-up was 1 year. The recurrence rate at 1-year follow-up was 15% for the cryosurgery group and 25% for the PDT group. This was the only trial to confirm recurrence histologically.

Thissen et al. in 1999 performed a systematic review of noncontrolled prospective studies of primary BCC treated with cryosurgery followed for at least 5 years.[73] They found a cumulative 5-year recurrence rate ranging from 3.5% to 16.5%. A large retrospective study of 3,869 primary BCC, less than 2 cm on all anatomic locations and treated with cryosurgery, were noted to have a 3% to 4% recurrence rate during a follow up period of 1 to 10 years.[83]

No RCT have been performed regarding cryosurgery for the treatment of SCC. Kuflik and Gage reported a series of 3,540 primary skin cancers in 2,220 patients treated over 18 years, of which 188 were SCC.[84] The overall cure rate was 98.4%. Graham and Clarke reported a cure rate of 97.3% for 563 primary SCC; however, the majority of lesions were low risk, ranging in size from 0.5 to 1.2 cm.[85]

In sum, cryosurgery is an effective method to treat small low-risk BCC. However, there is no good direct evidence to show that it is better than other modalities. The cure rates for cryosurgery are less than for surgical excision or radiation therapy. There is even less evidence to recommend cryosurgery as a first-line treatment for SCC. The National Cancer Comprehensive Network (NCCN) does not include cryosurgery as a primary treatment modality in their guidelines for treating NMSC.[86]

Surgical Excision

Surgical excision is an effective treatment modality for all types of NMSC. Recommended margins for excision of NMSC published in the literature range from 2 to 10 mm. A prospective study of 117 patients determined that a surgical excision margin of 4 mm of normal-appearing skin was adequate 95% of the time to clear primary BCC that were less than 2 cm.[87] Similarly, Brodland and Zitelli reported that to achieve clear surgical margins for low-risk SCC (less than 2 cm, Broders histologic grade I, and low-risk location) the minimum surgical margin was 4 mm.[88] Furthermore, a 6-mm margin was needed for higher-risk SCC (Broders histologic grade more than I, more than 2 cm in diameter in a low-risk site and more than 1 cm in a high-risk anatomic site) to obtain a 96% clearance rate. Surgical excision is advantageous because it provides a specimen for histologic margin evaluation, heals rapidly, and is often cosmetically acceptable. The disadvantage of surgical excision is difficulty in estimating the surgical margin need, and the possibility of positive surgical margins following excision. Higher-risk lesions are often associated with significant, asymmetric subclinical extension. Some authors advocate monitoring incompletely

TABLE 60.5. Clinical trials of cryosurgery for primary BCC.

Study	*Year*	*Location*	*No. of patients*	*Follow-up (years)*	*Recurrence rate (%)*	*Aesthetic result*
Wang et al.[82]	2001	Any	41 Cryo 47 PDT	1	15% Cryo 25% PDT	Good
Thissen et al.[81]	2000	Head/neck	48 Cryo 48 Excision	1	6% Cryo 0% Excision	Good for Cryo, better for excision
Hall et al.[80]	1986	Exclude nose/ear	44 Cryo 49 RT	1	39% Cryo 2% RT	Good

Cryo, cryosurgery; RT, radiation therapy; PDT, topical ALA-photodynamic therapy.

TABLE 60.6. Clinical trial of surgical excision for treatment of primary BCC.

Study	*Year*	*No. of patients*	*Randomized*	*Recurrence/persistent tumors*	*Odds ratio*	*Cosmetic result (% good result)*
Avril et al.[92]	1997	347	173 RT 174 Surgery	11/173 (6%) RT 1/174 (<1%) Surgery	0.09 (95% CI, 0.01–0.67)	69% 87%

RT, radiation therapy; CI, confidence interval.

excised NMSC rather then reexcising them or performing Mohs' surgery.[89] We and the NCCN believe that this is not appropriate therapy. Recent reviews have further supported the need to treat incompletely excised NMSC.[90,91]

Clinical Evidence

One RCT by Avril et al. of 347 patients compared surgical excision with frozen section margin control versus radiotherapy in primary BCC.[92] Lesions were less than 40mm in diameter, located on the face, and the growth pattern histology was nodular, ulcerated, superficial, and aggressive. The main outcome measure was histologically confirmed persistent tumor or recurrent tumor at 4 years. A second outcome measure was final cosmetic result. The results demonstrate that there were significantly more persistent or recurrent tumors (11 in 173) at 4 years in the radiotherapy group as compared to the surgery group (1 in 174). This finding equates to an odds ratio of 0.09 [95% confidence interval (CI), 0.01–0.67] in favor of surgery. Cosmetic outcome at 4 years was better in the surgery group. Patients assessed their cosmetic results as good in 87% of the cases following surgery and in 69% after radiotherapy (Table 60.6).

A retrospective review of 588 primary BCC treated with surgical excision demonstrated that BCC less than 6mm in diameter on the head had recurrence rates of 3.2%, whereas larger tumors had recurrence rates of 5% to 9%.[60] Tumors of any size excised from the ear, nasolabial groove, scalp, or forehead had much greater recurrence rates, 42.9%, 20.2%, 14.7%, and 8.4%, respectively.[60] Surgical excision of recurrent BCC is less effective than excision of primary BCC. In the systematic review by Rowe et al., the average 5-year recurrence rate for excision of recurrent tumors was 17.4%.[57]

There has been no RCT assessing the role of surgical excision of cutaneous SCC. The prospective study by Brodland and Zitelli found a 95% clearance rate for SCC less than 2cm in diameter with a margin of 4mm of normal skin and a 96% clearance rate of tumors more than 2cm with a margin of 6mm.[88] The systematic review by Rowe et al. demonstrated that the recurrence rate after excision of low-risk lesions ranges from 5% to 8%.[69] High-risk lesions larger than 2cm had a recurrence rate of 15.7% after excision, and the recurrence rate for tumors less than 2cm in size was 5.8%. Poorly differentiated lesions recurred at a rate of 25% after excision, compared with well-differentiated lesions that recur at a rate of 11.8%.[69]

Mohs' Micrographic Surgery

Histopathologic processing via bread loafing of standard surgical excision specimens examines less than 1% of the true surgical margin; this is problematic in higher-risk NMSC given its high incidence of subclinical extension, which may also be highly asymmetric. Mohs' micrographic surgery (MMS) is an effective procedure in the treatment of NMSC. The tumor is excised with narrow margins and processed using horizontal frozen sectioning, with total (theoretical 100%) margin control. The procedure is named after its inventor, Dr. Frederic E. Mohs. Originally, a zinc chloride chemical paste was applied to the skin to "fix" the tissue in situ. Dr. Mohs and Dr. Theodore Tromovitch modified the technique in the 1970s to its current "fresh tissue" technique. The term chemosurgery is no longer used because of the advent of the fresh tissue technique. The American College of Mohs Micrographic Surgery and Cutaneous Oncology is the "gold standard" body of the field, and certification requires completion of an approved 1- to 2-year fellowship following residency. By definition, the Mohs surgeon functions as both the operative surgeon and pathologist, and through fellowship training the Mohs surgeon becomes adept at microscopic interpretation of horizontally cut frozen sections as well as local flap and graft soft tissue reconstruction techniques.

Mohs' surgery is performed under local anesthesia in an outpatient setting. Briefly, the clinically evident tumor is outlined and anesthetized, and then all gross tumor is removed. Next, a disk of tissue in the shape of a saucer is excised with 1- to 3-mm-deep and peripheral margins. The skin edges are beveled at 45° to assist in tissue processing of the peripheral edges. The specimen is then divided, color-coded, and a schematic map is made for precise anatomic orientation. The specimen is then flipped over and flattened so that the beveled skin edge is placed in the same horizontal plane as the deep margin. The Mohs histotechnician cuts horizontal frozen sections that incorporate the entire undersurface and epidermal skin margin for histologic interpretation. The slides are processed, stained, and reviewed by the Mohs surgeon, who acts as both the surgeon and the pathologist. If residual tumor is noted, the patient returns to the operative suite and the exact area of positivity is again excised, mapped, color-coded, and sent to the Mohs histotechnician for horizontal frozen sectioning. This process is repeated until all margins are free of tumor. In this manner, maximal normal tissue is conserved, and 100% of the margin is examined. Reconstruction can be performed immediately after margins are free (Figure 60.8).

Mohs' surgery is a labor-intensive technique and requires an experienced team. Good-quality Mohs' frozen sections are essential and require additional histotechnician training and experience. Mohs' surgery often requires a multidisciplinary approach for difficult tumors. Collaboration with surgeons from other specialties such as plastic, oculoplastic, and head and neck is important for complex tumors and reconstructions.

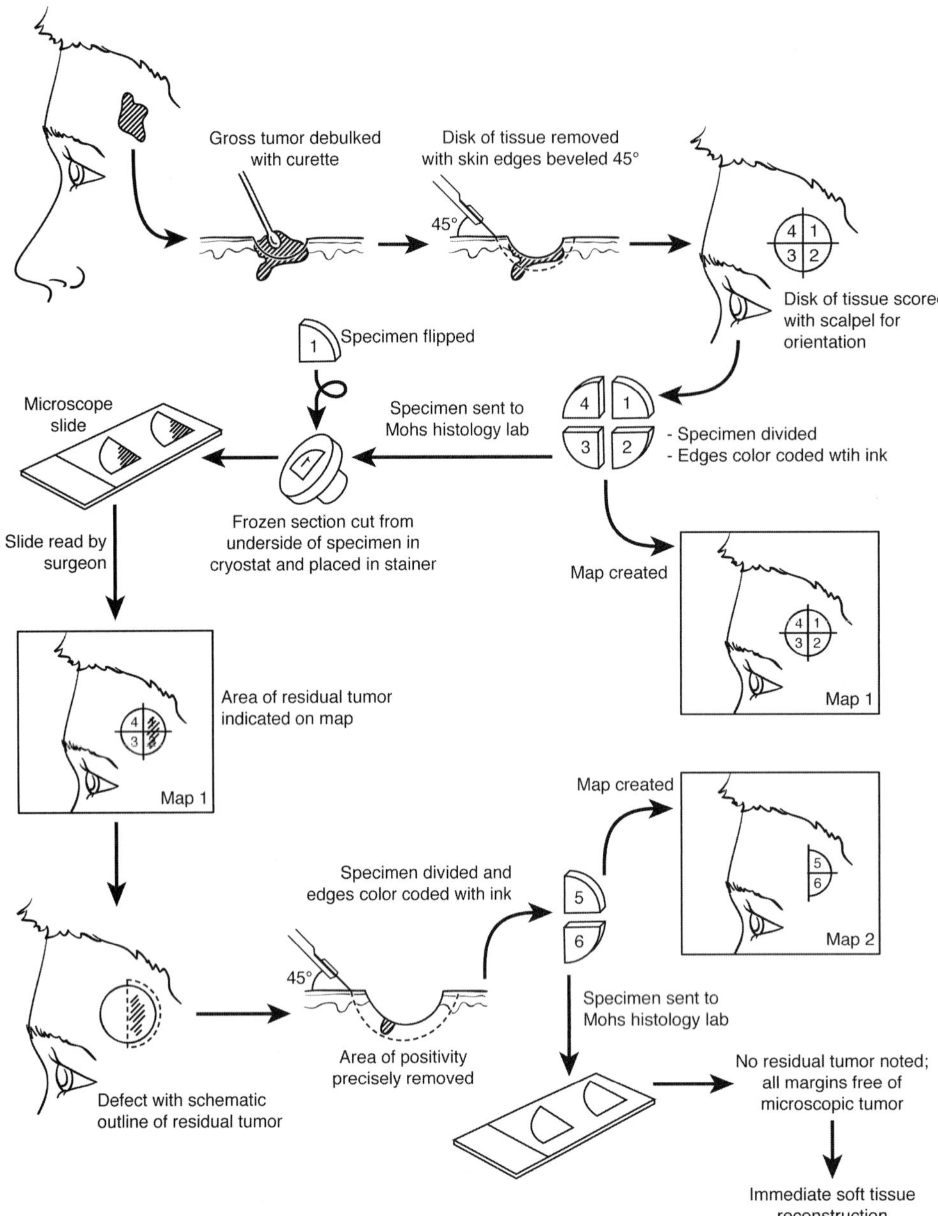

FIGURE 60.8. Schematic diagram of Mohs' surgery technique for the treatment of nonmelanoma cutaneous malignancy (NMSC). Residual tumor is noted in stage I; the area of positivity is delineated and excised in stage II. Once margins are tumor free, reconstruction may occur.

Clinical Evidence

There have been no RCT comparing MMS with other treatment modalities for treatment of NMSC. A systematic review by Rowe et al. analyzed all studies since 1950 that reported recurrence rates for primary BCC.[57] The 5-year cure rate for primary BCC treated with MMS was 99% (based on 7,670 tumors). For recurrent BCC, the 5-year cure rate for MMS was 94%. A study of 145 patients with primary BCC treated with MMS and followed for 5 years demonstrated a raw recurrence rate of 0.7% (1 in 145) and a strict recurrence rate of 0.8% (1 in 117).[93] Mohs et al. reported on the efficacy on MMS for the treatment of primary BCC located on high-risk sites such as the ear and eyelid. A study of 1,032 patients with primary BCC located on the ear, a known high-risk site for recurrence, treated with MMS demonstrated a raw recurrence rate of 1.3% (13 in 1,032) and a strict recurrence rate of 1.7% (13 in 748).[94] A similar study of 1,483 patients with primary BCC of the eyelid, another high-risk site, showed a raw recurrence rate of 0.5% (7 in 1,483) and a strict recurrence rate of 0.6% (7 in 1,124).[95]

An extensive review of all studies since 1940 reported the local recurrence rate for MMS, and standard surgical excision documented a local recurrence rate of 3% for MMS compared with 8% for primary surgical excision of cutaneous SCC.[69] For primary SCC located on the lip, the recurrence rate was

3.1% compared with 10.9% for non-MMS. For SCC located on the ear, the recurrence rate was 5.3% for MMS compared with 18.7% for non-MMS modalities.

In sum, MMS is a highly effective treatment modality for treatment of NMSC. Although there have been no RCT, MMS offers exceptionally high cure rates with maximal preservation of normal tissue. Despite the lack of RCT, the profound benefit of the procedure has been proven and documented in the literature. The NCCN Non-Melanoma skin cancer panel has recognized the benefit of MMS, and it is a primary treatment modality for high-risk and recurrent lesions.

Radiation Therapy

Fractionated radiation therapy (RT) is an effective therapy for NMSC and with proper tumor and patient selection can obtain a cure rate greater than 90% with excellent cosmetic results. Favorable lesion characteristics include low- to medium-risk tumors. Patient characteristics that would favor RT include patients who are poor surgical candidates. Radiation therapy is a primary treatment modality endorsed by the NCCN guidelines. Experience and a clinical understanding of NMSC are vitally important. Contraindications for RT include genodermatoses predisposing to skin cancer (nevoid BCC syndrome and xeroderma pigmentosum) and connective tissue disease (lupus and scleroderma).

Clinical Evidence

Two RCTs have been conducted comparing RT with cryosurgery and surgical excision and have already been described (see Tables 60.5, 60.6).[80,92] Both trials demonstrated low recurrence rates, ranging from 2% to 6%, and excellent cosmetic results for the treatment of primary BCC. RT was superior to cryosurgery but not surgical excision.

A large review of 2,314 patients with primary BCC treated with RT showed a cumulative recurrence rate of 13.2%.[61] Fischbach et al. reviewed 231 patients with BCC and 67 patients with SCC and found 2-year recurrence rates of 7.8% and 14.9%, respectively.[96] Petrovich et al. examined 447 primary BCC treated with RT and noted a 10-year recurrence rate of 2%.[97] In that same study, 115 patients with SCC were treated with RT and had a 10-year recurrence rate of 12%. This study showed a definite relationship in both BCC and SCC between local control at 5 years and tumor size. Local control at 5 years was 99% for lesions less than 2 cm, 92% for tumors 2 to 5 cm, and 60% for tumors more than 5 cm.

Lasers and Photodynamic Therapy

Laser therapy and photodynamic therapy (PDT) have been reported for treating NMSC. Both are new technologies and are considered experimental by the NCCN consensus committee. Zeitouni et al. performed a recent review of the literature, which consists primarily of case reports and small series.[98] Most of these cases involve low-risk, superficial lesions that are easily treated by a variety of modalities. The primary laser used to treat NMSC is the carbon dioxide (CO_2) laser. The CO_2 is essentially a destructive modality similar to ED&C. Photodynamic therapy involves the administration of a photosensitizing drug (either systemic or topical) and its subsequent activation by light (laser or nonlaser light) to produce activated oxygen species that selectively destroy target cells. Light sources include the diode laser and nonlaser light such as filtered halogen or xenon arc lamps, blue light fluorescent tubes, and light-emitting diode (LED) arrays.

Clinical Evidence

There has been no RCT comparing treatment of NMSC by CO_2 laser to other modalities. Early reports concerning the effectiveness of CO_2 laser therapy for primary BCC documented a 50% recurrence rate.[99] However, a more-recent study of 370 superficial BCC demonstrated no recurrences with 20 months of follow up.[100] In this study, however, curettage was also used along with the CO_2 laser. The use of CO_2 laser for the treatment of SCC in situ has been reported.[101] The high recurrence rate is most likely due to follicular extension of the SCC in situ lesions, which is deeper than the depth treated with the CO_2 laser. In certain locations, such as the penis and distal digit, CO_2 laser has been reported to be successful and preserve function and good cosmesis.[102,103] The best indication for CO_2 laser is in the treatment of the precancerous condition actinic cheilitis. CO_2 laser treatment of actinic cheilitis by means of superficial vermilionectomy has been extensively studied and is the treatment of choice.[10]

A RCT comparing PDT with cryosurgery for the treatment of primary BCC was described previously (Table 60.7). The study involved 88 primary BCC and compared cryosurgery with topical photodynamic therapy (PDT) for lesions located on the head, neck, and extremities; the follow up was 1 year.[82] The recurrence rate at 1-year follow-up confirmed histologically was 15% for the cryosurgery group and 25% for the PDT group. The photosensitizer was topically applied 5-aminolevulinic acid (ALA). A systematic review of

TABLE 60.7. Clinical trials for topical photodynamic therapy (ALA-PDT) for treatment of primary NMSC.

Study	*Year*	*Tumor type*	*Randomization*	*No. of patients (number of lesions)*	*Follow-up*	*Recurrence rate (%)*	*Clearance rate (%)*
Wang et al.[82]	2001	BCC	PDT vs. Cryo	47 PDT 41 Cryo	1 year	25% PDT 15% Cryo	
Morton et al.[106]	1996	Bowen's	PDT vs. Cryo	20 PDT 20 Cryo	1 year		75% PDT (1 Tx) 50% Cryo (1 Tx)
Salim et al.[107]	2000	Bowen's	PDT vs. 5-FU	20 PDT (33 lesions) 20 5-FU (33 lesions)	1 year		82% PDT (27/33) 48% 5-FU (16/33)
Morton et al.[108]	2000	Bowen's	Red light vs. green light	32 red 29 green	1 year		94% red (30/32) 72% green (21/29)

Cryo, cryosurgery; PDT, topical ALA-photodynamic therapy; 5-FU, topical 5% 5-fluorouracil; Tx, treatment; BCC, basal cell carcinoma; Bowen's, squamous cell carcinoma in situ.

12 studies by Peng et al. demonstrated a weighted average complete clearance rate of 87% for 826 superficial BCC treated with PDT and a rate of 53% for 208 nodular BCC for a short follow up period of 3 to 36 months.[104] Nodular and aggressive-growth pattern BCC respond poorly.

PDT has been documented to treat Bowen's disease; 13 cases and 3 RCTs have been reported. A single ALA-PDT treatment cleared 86% (6 studies, 71 of 83 patients); this number rose to 93% when one or two treatments were performed (9 studies, 239 of 257 patients).[105] The recurrence rate ranged from 0% to 40% (average, 12%) during a follow-up period of 3 to 36 months, and most lesions were small. A RCT comparing PDT with cryotherapy for the treatment of 40 small Bowen's disease lesions demonstrated the PDT was at least as effective as cryotherapy. PDT displayed a higher rate of clearance, 75% after a single treatment compared with 50% for the cryotherapy group.[106] A RCT comparing ALA-PDT with topical 5-fluorouracil (5-FU) showed a complete clinical response of 82% (27 of 33 lesions) for the ALA-PDT group compared to 48% clearing (16 of 33 lesions) for the 5-FU group at 12 months follow-up.[107] Although these were RCTs, the evidence they provide is suspect because of the short follow-up period and response rates much lower than with standard treatment modalities such as surgery, ED&C, or RT. A RCT comparing different wavelengths of light used as the light source for ALA-PDT demonstrated that the more-penetrating red light (630 ± 15nm) had a significantly higher clearance rate than green light (540 ± 15nm).[108]

The use of ALA-PDT for primary treatment of invasive SCC is controversial. ALA-PDT has also been reported in the treatment of SCC but is noted to have high recurrence rates (up to 69%) and, in light of the metastatic potential, even strong advocates of ALA-PDT do not recommend it for SCC.[105]

In sum, the current evidence does not support the use of laser therapy as a primary treatment modality for NMSC. Similarly, current efficacy data do not support the introduction of PDT for the treatment of BCC, SCC in situ, and invasive SCC without further studies. Currently, there are no 5-year follow-up data, and therefore no direct comparison of ALA-PDT can be made with conventional therapies. However, considerably higher failure rates were associated with PDT when compared to failure rates for surgery, radiotherapy, and cryosurgery described in other studies.

Medical Treatments

Alternatives to surgical treatment of NMSC exist and may be used in certain circumstances, such as debilitated patients or extensive or multifocal lesions. Medical therapy of NMSC includes the biologic response modifiers such as intralesional interferon and topical 5% imiquimod cream, as well as topical chemotherapeutic agents such as topical 5-fluorouracil.

Clinical Evidence

Intralesional Interferon

Three randomized controlled trials have been performed in regard to intralesional interferon (IFN) and BCC (Table 60.8). The first trial, of 165 patients with either nodular or superficial BCC on the head, neck, face, trunk, and extremities, compared interferon-alpha-2b (IFN-α-2a) at 1.5 million units three times weekly for 3 weeks with placebo vehicle in a 3:1 ratio of interferon-treated to placebo-treated patients.[109] Early treatment failure at 20 weeks confirmed by punch biopsy was 14% (17 of 120) in the interferon (IFN) group and 71% (30 of 42) in the placebo group. A second trial of 45 patients with BCC was randomized to receive IFN-α-2a, IFN-β-2a, or a combination.[110] IFN-α-2a is a related cytokine with similar mechanism of action that differs from IFN-α-2b by only one amino acid. Increased effectiveness was not shown with combination therapy. In the third RCT of 65 patients, a single dose of 10 million IU of a sustained-release IFN-β-2a was compared with the same dose weekly for 3 weeks.[111] The early treatment failure measured histologically at 16 weeks was 48% (16 of 33) in the single-injection group and 20% (6 of 30) for the three-times-weekly injection.

The use of intralesional interferon as primary treatment for SCC has been reported; however, no RCT exist. A trial of 28 invasive SCC and 8 SCC in situ were treated with intralesional IFN-α-2b. Lesions ranged in size from 0.5 to 2.0cm.[111] Each patient was injected with 1.5 million IU intralesionally, three times per week. At 18 weeks, treatment sites were excised and examined histologically for tumor persistence. Thirty-three (97.1%) of 34 lesions revealed an absence of SCC histologically after therapy, although three biopsy specimens

TABLE 60.8. Medical therapy: clinical trials of intralesional interferon for treatment of primary BCC.

Study	*Year*	*No. of patients*	*Randomization (number of patients)*	*Early treatment failure (%)*	*Odds ratio*
Cornell et al.[109]	1990	165	123 IFN-α-2a 42 placebo	14% IFN-α-2a 71% placebo	0.07 (95% CI, 0.03–0.15)
Alpsoy et al.[110]	1996	45	15 IFN-α-2a 15 IFN-α-2b 15 IFN-α-2a + IFN-α-2b	33% IFN-α-2a 33% IFN-α-2b 27% IFN-α-2a + IFN-α-2b	No significant differences with monotherapy or combination therapy or between IFN-α-2a and IFN-α-2b
Edwards et al.[111]	1990	65	33 single dose 32 three-times-weekly dose	48% single dose 20% three-times-weekly dose	4.08 (95% CI, 1.33–12.5)

IFN, interferon.

TABLE 60.9. Medical therapy: clinical trials of topical imiquimod 5% cream for treatment of primary NMSC.

Study	*Year*	*No. of patients*	*Tumor type*	*Randomization (number of patients)*	*Duration (weeks)*	*Early treatment failure (%)*	*Odds ratio*
Beutner et al.[112]	1999	35	sBCC nBCC	24 imiquimod (5 dosing regimens) 11 vehicle	16		0.02 (95% CI, 0.00–0.20) imiquimod compared to vehicle
Geisse et al.[113]	2001	128	sBCC	10 b.i.d. 31 q.d. 26 five × week 29 three × week 32 vehicle	12	0% b.i.d. 13% q.d. 11% 5 × week 48% 3 × week 81% vehicle	0.07 (95% CI, 0.03–0.2) imiquimod compared to vehicle
Robinson et al.[114]	2001	92	nBCC	4 b.i.d. 21 q.d. 23 five × week 20 three × week 24 vehicle	12	25% b.i.d. 24% q.d. 30% 5 × week 40% 3 × week 87% vehicle	0.06 (95% CI, 0.02–0.24) imiquimod compared to vehicle
Marks et al.[115]	2001	99	sBCC	3 b.i.d. 33 q.d. 30 six × week 33 three × week	6	0% b.i.d. 12% q.d. 27% six × week 30% three × week	0.31 (95% CI, 0.10–1.01) higher doses compared to lower doses
Shumack et al.[116]	2002	99	nBCC	1 b.i.d. 35 q.d. 31 six × week 32 three × week	6	0% b.i.d. 29% q.d. 58% six × week 41% three × week	0.43 (95% CI, 0.18–1.01) higher doses compared to lower dose
Shumack et al.[116]	2002	92	nBCC	4 b.i.d. 21 q.d. 23 five × week 20 three × week 24 vehicle	12	0% b.i.d. 24% q.d. 30% five × week 40% three × week 87% vehicle	
Sterry et al.[117]	2001a	93	sBCC	Occlusion vs. no occlusion	6		0.66 (95% CI, 0.29–1.52); no significant difference in early treatment failure when occlusion was used
Sterry et al.[117]	2001b	90	nBCC	23 three × week with occlusion 24 three × week without occlusion 22 twice/week with occlusion 21 twice/week without occlusion	6	35% three × week with occlusion 50% three × week without occlusion 50% twice/week with occlusion 43% twice/week without occlusion	1.20 (95% CI, 0.29–1.52); no significant difference in early treatment failure when occlusion used
Mackenzie-Wood et al.[118]	2001	16	SCC in situ	16 b.i.d.	16	7% b.i.d.	

sBCC, superficial BCC; nBCC, nodular BCC; CI, confidence interval; b.i.d., twice a day; q.d., once a day; three × week, three times a week; five × week, five times a week; six × week, six times a week.

(8.8%) obtained after treatment showed actinic keratoses, for an overall complete response rate of 88.2%. The lesion not eliminated after treatment was an invasive squamous cell carcinoma.

In sum, the evidence does not support the use of intralesional IFN as a primary treatment modality for BCC or SCC. Intralesional IFN has a high percentage of early failure rates and does not compare with current standards of surgical or radiotherapy cures.

Imiquimod

A total of 8 RCT were found regarding the use of topical imiquimod 5% cream for primary BCC (Table 60.9). Beutner et al. examined the efficacy and safety of imiquimod in the treatment of superficial and nodular BCC located on the trunk, ranging in size from 0.5 to 2 cm^2.[112] A total of 35 patients were selected, with 24 receiving imiquimod and 11 receiving vehicle in one of five dosing regimens for up to 16 weeks. Treatment failures from the different dosing regimens were combined and compared with the vehicle; there was a significant reduction in early treatment failures with imiquimod as compared to the vehicle [odds ratio (OR) 0.02; 95% confidence interval (CI), 0.00–0.02]. Geisse et al. compared regimens of twice-daily, once-daily, 5 days per week, or 3 days per week versus vehicle for superficial BCC.[113] Lesions ranged in size from 0.5 to 2 cm^2. Early treatment failures were 0% (0 of 10), 13% (4 of 31), 11% (5 of 26), and 48% (14 of 29), respectively; vehicle failure rate was 26 of 32 (81%).

Robinson et al. evaluated imiquimod for nodular BCC using the same four regimens as Geisse for a period of 12 weeks.[114] Early treatment failures were 25% (1 of 4), 24% (5 of 21), 30% (7 of 23), and 40 % (8 of 20), respectively; vehicle early treatment failure rate was 78% (21 of 24). Marks et al. examined imiquimod applied for 6 weeks in 99 patients with superficial BCC.[115] Lesions ranged in size from 0.5 to 2.0 cm^2. Posttreatment biopsy clearance rates were reported as 100% (3 of 3), 88% (29 of 33), 73% (22 of 30), and 70% (23 of 33) for twice-daily, once-daily, 5 days per week, and 3 days per week regimens, respectively. There was a trend toward higher doses of imiquimod having fewer treatment failures as compared to lower doses. Another trial of 99 patients evaluated treatment of nodular BCC with imiquimod using various dosing schemes.[115] Results demonstrate a trend toward fewer treatment failures using higher doses of imiquimod compared with lower doses (OR, 95% CI, 0.18–1.01). Another study of

92 patients with nodular BCC treated with once-daily, 5 days per week, or 3 days per week imiquimod was compared with vehicle.[116] Early treatment failure rates were 24%, 30%, 40%, and 87%, respectively.

Two studies examined the role of occlusion and found no significant difference in early treatment failure rates.[117] Sterry et al. reported 90 patients with nodular BCC with regimens of 3 days per week with and without occlusion and 2 days per week with and without occlusion, respectively.[117] Early treatment failure rates were 35% (8 of 23), 50% (12 of 24), 50% (11 of 22), and 43% (9 of 21), respectively, and there was no significant difference in early treatment failure when occlusion was used (OR 1.20; 95% CI, 0.29–1.52).

Imiquimod has been reported to treat SCC in situ. A Phase II open labeled study examined the use of imiquimod once daily for 16 weeks in 16 patients.[118] Almost all lesions were located on the legs (15 of 16), and lesions ranged in size from 0.7 to 21.6 cm^2. Posttreatment biopsies at 6 weeks revealed no residual tumor in 14 of 15 patients, corresponding to an early treatment failure of 7% (1 of 15). One patient died of an unrelated illness before a biopsy could be obtained. Several case reports have documented the efficacy of imiquimod in treating SCC in situ on the penis.[119,120] Recently, 2 cases of SCC were reported treated with imiquimod.[121]

Side effects and potential drawbacks for topical imiquimod 5% cream include a high rate of significant local skin reaction, such as erythema, pain, edema, vesicles, erosion, and ulceration. In all studies local reactions were common, and some patients were unable to finish studies secondary to moderate to severe local reactions.

No long-term study (3–5 years) of the efficacy of imiquimod in the treatment of NMSC has been performed. As stated previously, 1-year or shorter-duration follow-up periods are inadequate and can falsely improve treatment success rates. No RCT has compared imiquimod with standard treatment modalities such as ED&C, surgery, or radiation.

5-Fluorouracil

Two RCTs were identified in the use of topical 5-fluorouracil (5-FU) for the treatment of BCC (Table 60.10). The first trial compared 5% 5-FU cream in phosphatidyl choline (PC) vehicle with 5% 5-FU in petrolatum for nonsuperficial BCC at least 0.7 cm in greatest diameter, not located on the face.[122] Early treatment failure measured histologically at 16 weeks was 10% for the phosphatidyl choline cream compared with 43% for the petrolatum preparation. The second trial of 122 patients tested the efficacy of six treatment regimens using 5-FU/epinephrine gel.[123] Overall, the six regimens had an average early treatment failure of 9% documented histologically at 3 months after treatment. Side effects included local irritation, erythema, and ulceration.

One RCT comparing 5-FU with PDT has been described previously.[107] The complete clearance rate of the 5-FU group was 48% compared with 82% for the PDT group. Numerous case reports and small series have reported successful treatment of SCC in situ and invasive SCC following treatment with 5-FU. Most of these studies had small numbers of patients with short follow-up periods. Current evidence does not support the use of topical 5-FU as a primary treatment for BCC, SCC in situ, or invasive SCC.

Prevention and Follow-Up

Sun protective measures such as avoiding the sun during the middle of the day, sun protective clothing and shade seeking, and sunscreens are effective for NMSC prevention. A RCT found significantly fewer new actinic keratoses with daily sunscreen use versus placebo.[124] Another RCT found a 40% relative reduction in the incidence of SCC with daily application of sunscreen to the head, neck, arms, and hands compared with discretionary application.[125]

Patients who have been diagnosed with NMSC need continued follow up to facilitate early detection of new tumors or tumor recurrence. Marcil and Stern performed a meta-analysis of the risk of developing a subsequent NMSC in patients with a history of NMSC in 2000.[126] They found an overall 3-year cumulative risk of a subsequent BCC after an index BCC was 44%, which was at least a 10-fold increase in incidence over baseline. Similarly, for SCC, the overall 3-year cumulative risk was 18%, which was also a 10-fold increase in incidence. All patients should be instructed on how to perform self-skin examinations, and these should be performed monthly. Additionally, patients with high-risk SCC should be instructed to palpate the regional lymph nodes monthly to detect for regional metastasis.

TABLE 60.10. Medical therapy: clinical trials of topical 5-fluorouracil for treatment of primary NMSC.

Study	*Year*	*Tumor type*	*No. of patients (number of lesions)*	*Randomization*	*Early treatment failure (%)*	*Conclusions*
Romagosa et al.[122]	2000	BCC	13 (17 lesions)	10 5-FU/PC 7 5-FU/PL	10% 5-FU/PC 43% 5-FU/PL	Increased short-term clearance with 5-FU/PC over 5-FU/PL
Miller et al.[123]	1997	BCC	122	6 different treatment regimens using 5-FU/epi gel	Overall 9%	No statistically significant differences between regimens
Salim et al.[107]	2000	SCC in situ	40 (66 lesions)	20 5-FU (33 lesions) 20 PDT (33 lesions)	52% 18%	5-FU less effective for short-term eradication compared to PDT

5-FU, 5% 5-fluorouracil; 5-FU/PC, = 5% 5- fluorouracil cream in phosphatidyl choline vehicle; 5-FU/PL, 5% 5-fluorouracil in petrolatum; 5-FU/epi gel, 5% 5-fluorouracil/epinephrine gel; PDT, topical ALA-photodynamic therapy.

References

1. Cancer Facts and Figures available at www.cancer.org. Chicago: American Cancer Society, 2002.
2. Limmer BL. Non melanoma skin cancer: today's epidemic. Tex Med 2001;97(2):56–58.
3. Miller D, Weinstock M. Nonmelanoma skin cancer in the United States: incidence. J Am Acad Dermatol 1994;30(5 pt 1): 774–778.
4. Preston D, Stern R. Nonmelanoma cancers of the skin. N Engl J Med 1994;327(23):1649–1662.
5. Housman T, Feldman S, Willford P, et al. Skin cancer is among the most costly of all cancers to treat for the Medicare population. J Am Acad Dermatol 2003;48(3):425–429.
6. Strom S. Epidemiology of basal and squamous cell carcinomas of the skin. In: Weber RSMM, Goepfert H (eds). Basal and Squamous Cell Skin Cancers of the Head and Neck. Philadelphia: Williams & Wilkins, 1996:1–7.
7. Scotto J, Fears TR, Fraumeni JF. Incidence of nonmelanoma skin cancer in the United States, U.S. Department of Health and Human Services, Washington; 1983.
8. Giles G, Marks R, Foley P. Incidence of non-melanocytic skin cancer treated in Australia. Br Med J (Clin Res Ed) 1988; 296(6614):13–17.
9. Robins P, Rabinovitz H, Rigel D. Basal-cell carcinomas on covered or unusual sites of the body. J Dermatol Surg Oncol 1981;7(10):803–806.
10. Johnson TM, Sebastien TS, Lowe L, Nelson BR. Carbon dioxide laser treatment of actinic cheilitis. Clinicohistopathologic correlation to determine the optimal depth of destruction. J Am Acad Dermatol 1992;27:737–740.
11. Kramer K. Heritable diseases with increased sensitivity to cellular injury. In: Fitzpatrick TBEA, Wolff K, Freeberg IM, Austen KF (eds). Dermatology in General Medicine, 5th ed. New York: McGraw-Hill, 1999:1848–1862.
12. Euvrard SKJ, Claudy A. Skin cancers after organ transplantation. N Engl J Med 2003;348:1681–1691.
13. Kaplan R. Cancer complicating ulcerative and scarifying mucocutaneous disorders. Adv Dermatol 1987;2:19.
14. Fitzpatrick T, Sober A. Sunlight and skin cancer. N Engl J Med 1985;313(13):818–820.
15. Kelfkens G, de Gruijl F, van der Leun J. Ozone depletion and increase in annual carcinogenic ultraviolet dose. Photochem Photo Biol 1990;85(4):819–823.
16. Henrickson T, Dahlback A, Larsen S, Moan J. Ultra-violet radiation and skin cancer. Effect of an ozone layer depletion. Photochem Photo Biol 1990;51(5):579–582.
17. Fitzpatrick P, Harwood A. Acute epithelioma—an aggressive squamous cell of the skin. J Am Acad Dermatol 1985;6(8):468–471.
18. Bates M, Smith A, Hopenhayn-Rich C. Arsenic ingestion and internal cancers: a review. Am J Epidemiol 1992;135(5):462–476.
19. Stern R. Non-melanoma skin cancer occurring in patients treated with PUVA five to ten years after first treatment. J Invest Dermatol 1988;91:120–124.
20. Kune G, Bannerman S, Field B, et al. Diet, alcohol, smoking, serum beta carotene, and vitamin A in male nonmelanocytic skin cancer and controls. Nutr Cancer 1992;18(3):237–244.
21. Johnson T, Rowe DM, Nelson BR, et al. Squamous cell carcinoma (excluding lip and oral mucosa). J Am Acad Dermatol 1992;26:467–484.
22. Shore R. Overview of radiation-induced skin cancer in humans. Int Radiat Biol 1990;57(4):809–827.
23. Hahn H, Wicking C, Zaphiropoulous P, et al. Mutations of the human homolog of Drosophila patched in the nevoid basal cell carcinoma syndrome. Cell 1996;85(6):841–851.
24. Johnson R, Rothman A, Xie J, et al. Human homolog of patched, a candidate gene for the basal cell nevus syndrome. Science 1996;27(5268):1668–1671.
25. Gailani M, Stahle-Backdahl M, Leffell D, et al. The role of the human homologue of Drosophila patched sporadic basal cell carcionomas. Nat Genet 1996;14(1):78–81.
26. Unden A, Holmberg E, Lundh-Rozell B, et al. Mutations in the human homologue of Drosophila patched (PTCH) in basal cell carcinomas and the Gorlin syndrome: different in vivo mechanisms of PTCH inactivation. Cancer Res 1996;56(20): 4562–4565.
27. Stone D, Hynes M, Armanini M, et al. The tumor-suppressor gene patched encodes a candidate receptor for Sonic hedgehog. Nature (Lond) 1996;384(6604):129–134.
28. Dicker T, Siller G, Saunders N. Molecular and cellular biology of basal cell carcinoma. Australas J Dermatol 2002;43(4):241–246.
29. Levine A. p53, the cellular gatekeeper for growth and division. Cell 1997;88(3):323–331.
30. Shea C, McNutt N, Volkenandt M, et al. Over expression of p53 protein in basal cell carcinomas of human skin. Am J Epidemiol 1992;141(1):25–29.
31. Ponten F, Berg C, Ahmadian A, et al. Molecular pathology in basal cell cancer with p53 as a genetic marker. Oncogene 1997; 15(9):1059–1067.
32. Tsao H. Genetics of nonmelanoma skin cancer. Arch Dermatol 2001;137(11):1486–1492.
33. Alam M, Ratner D. Cutaneous squamous-cell carcinoma. N Engl J Med 2001;344(13):975–983.
34. Brash D, Rudolph JA, Simon JA et al. A role for sunlight in skin cancer. UV-induced p53 mutations in squamous cell carcinoma. Proc Natl Acad Sci U S A 1991;88:10124–10128.
35. Spencer J, Kahn S, Jiang W, De Leo V, Weinstein I. Activated ras genes occur in human actinic keratoses, premalignant precursors to squamous cell carcinomas. Arch Dermatol 1995; 131(7):796–800.
36. Soufir N, Moles J, Vilmer C, et al. P16 UV mutations in human skin epitelial tumors. Oncogene 1999;18(39):5477–5481.
37. Roenigk R, Ratz J, Bailin P, et al. Trends in the presentation and treatment of basal cell carcinomas. J Am Acad Dermatol 1986; 12(8):860–865.
38. Pearl D, Scott E. The anatomical distribution of skin cancers. Int J Epidemol 1986;15(4):502–506.
39. Emmet A. Surgical analysis and biological behaviour of 2277 basal cell carcinomas. Aust N Z J Surg 1990;60(11):855–863.
40. Schwartz RA, Stoll H. Squamous cell carcinoma. In: Fitzpatrick TBEA, Wolff K, Freeberg IM, Austen KF (eds). Dermatology in General Medicine. New York: McGraw-Hill, 1999:840–857.
41. Glogau R. The risk of progression to invasive disease. J Am Acad Dermatol 2000;42(1 pt 2):23–24.
42. Marks R, Rennie G, Selwood T. Malignant transformation of solar keratoses to squamous cell carcinoma. Lancet 1988; 1(8589):795–797.
43. Callen J, Bickers D, Moy R. Actinic keratoses. J Am Acad Dermatol 1997;36(4):650–653.
44. Salasche S. Epidemiology of actinic keratoses and squamous cell carcinoma. J Am Acad Dermatol 2000;42(1 pt 2):4–7.
45. Lee M, Wick M. Bowen's disease. CA Cancer J Clin 1990; 4(40):237–242.
46. Criber B AP, Grosshans E. Differentiating squamous cell carcinoma from keratoacanthoma using histopathologic criteria: is it possible? Dermatology 1999;199:208–212.
47. Goldenharsh M, Olsen T. Invasive squamous cell carcinoma intitially diagnosed as a giant keratoacanthoma. J Am Acad Dermatol 1984;10(2 pt 2):372–378.
48. Miller S. Biology of basal cell carcinoma (part I). J Am Acad Dermatol 1991;24(1):1–13.
49. Richman T, Penneys N. Analysis of morpheaform basal cell carcinoma. J Cutan Pathol 1988;15(6):359–362.

50. Salasche S, Amonette R. Morpheaform basal-cell epitheliomas. A study of subclinical extensions in a series of 51 cases. J Dermatol Surg Oncol 1981;7(5):987–994.
51. Lang PJ, Maize J. Histologic evolution of recurrent basal cell carcinoma and treatment implications. J Am Acad Dermatol 1986; 14(2 pt 1):186–196.
52. Lohmann C, Solomon A. Clinicopathologic variants of cutaneous cell carcinoma. Adv Anat Pathol 2001;8(1):27–36.
53. Cottel W. Perineural invasion by squamous cell carcinoma. J Dermatol Surg Oncol 1982;8:589–600.
54. Broders A. Squamous cell epithelioma of the skin. Ann Surg 1921;73:141–160.
55. Bernstein S, Lim K, Brodland D, et al. The many faces of squamous cell carcinoma. Dermatol Surg 1996;22(3):243–254.
56. Smith K, Skelton HR, Morgan A, et al. Spindle cell neoplasms coexpressing cytokeratin and vimentin (metaplastic squamous cell carcinoma). J Cutan Pathol 1992;19(4):286–293.
57. Rowe D, Carroll R, Day CJ. Long-term recurrence rates in previously untreated (primary) basal cell carcinoma: implications for patient follow-up. J Dermatol Surg Oncol 1989;15(3): 315–328.
58. Silverman M, Kopf A, Grin C, et al. Recurrence rates of treated basal cell carcinomas. Part 1: Overview. J Dermatol Surg Oncol 1991;17(9):713–718.
59. Silverman M, Kopf A, Grin C, et al. Recurrence rates of treated basal cell carcinomas. Part 2: Curettage-electrodesiccation. J Dermatol Surg Oncol 1991;17(9):720–726.
60. Silverman M, Kopf A, Grin C, et al. Recurrence rates of treated basal cell carcinomas. Part 3: Surgical excision. J Dermatol Surg Oncol 1992;18(6):471–476.
61. Silverman M, Kopf A, Gladstein A, et al. Recurrence rates of treated basal cell carcinomas. Part 4: X-ray therapy. J Dermatol Surg Oncol 1992;18(7):549–554.
62. Lowe L. Histology (basal cell carcinoma). In: Miller S, Maloney ME (eds). Cutaneous Oncology: Pathophysiology, Diagnosis, and Management. London: Blackwell-Science, 1998:609–613.
63. Ratner D, Lowe L, Johnson T, et al. Perineural spread of basal cell carcinomas treated with Mohs micrographic surgery. Cancer (Phila) 2000;88(7):1605–1613.
64. Hartevelt M, Bavinck J, Kootte A, et al. Incidence of skin cancer after renal transplantation in the Netherlands. Transplantation 1990;49(3):506–509.
65. Martin H, Stron E, Spiro R. Radiation-induced skin cancer of the head and neck. Cancer (Phila) 1970;25(1):61–71.
66. Menn H, Robins P, Kopf A, et al. The recurrent basal cell epithelioma. A study of 100 cases of recurrent, re-treated basal cell epitheliomas. Arch Dermatol 1971;103(6):628–631.
67. Lo J, Snow S, Reizner G, et al. Metastatic basal cell carcinoma: Report of twelve cases with a review of the literature. J Am Acad Dermatol 1991;24(5 pt 1):715–719.
68. Snow S. Metastatic basal cell carcinoma: report of five cases. Cancer (Phila) 1994;73:328–335.
69. Rowe D, Carroll RJ, Day CL. Prognostic factors for local recurrence, metastasis, and survival rates in squamous cell carcinoma of the skin, ear, and lip. Implications for treatment modality selection. J Am Acad Dermatol 1992;26(6):976–990.
70. Jensen P, Hansen S, Moller B, et al. Skin cancer in kidney and heart transplant recipients and different long-term immunosuppressive therapy regimens. J Am Acad Dermatol 1999;40(2 pt 1): 177–186.
71. Dinehart S, Pollack S. Metastases from squamous cell carcinoma of the skin and lip. An analysis of twenty-seven cases. J Am Acad Dermatol 1989;21(2 pt 1):241–248.
72. Egger M, Smith G. Bias in location and selection of studies. Br Med J 1998;316(7124):61–66.
73. Thissen M, Neumann M, Schouten L. A systematic review of treatment modalities for primary basal cell carcinomas. Arch Dermatol 1999;135(10):1177–1183.
74. Bath F, Bong J, Perkins W, et al. Interventions for basal cell carcinoma (Cochrane Review). Cochrane Database Syst Rev 2003;(2).
75. Green A, Marks R. Squamous cell carcinoma of the skin: non-metastatic. Clin Evid 2002;1549–1554.
76. Kopf A, Bart R, Schrager D, et al. Curettage-electrodesiccation treatment of basal cell carcionomas. Arch Dermatol 1977;113(4): 439–443.
77. Zacarian S. Cryosurgery of skin cancer: fundamentals of technique and application. Cutis 1975;16:449–460.
78. McIntosh G, Osborne D, Li A, et al. Basal cell carcinoma: a review of treatment results with special reference to cryotherapy. Postgrad Med J 1983;59(697):698–701.
79. Mallon E, Dawber R. Cryosurgery in the treatment of basal cell carcinoma. Assessment of one and two freeze-thaw cycle schedules. Dermatol Surg 1996;22(10):854–858.
80. Hall V, Leppard B, McGill J, et al. Treatment of basal-cell carcinoma: comparison of radiotherapy and cryotherapy. Clin Radiol 1986;37(1):33–34.
81. Thissen M, Nieman F, Ideler A, et al. Cosmetic results of cryosurgery versus surgical excision for primary uncomplicated basal cell carcinomas of the head and neck. Dermatol Surg 2000;26(8):759–764.
82. Wang I, Bendose N, Klinteberg C, et al. Photodynamic therapy vs. cryosurgery of basal cell carcinomas: results of a phase III clinical trial. Br J Dermatol 2001;144(4):832–840.
83. Zacarian S. Cryosurgery of cutaneous carcinomas. An 18-year study of 3,022 patients with 4,228 carcinomas. J Am Acad Dermatol 1983;9(6):947–956.
84. Kuflik E, Gage A. The five-year cure rate achieved by cryosurgery for skin cancer. J Am Acad Dermatol 1991;24(6 pt 1): 1002–1004.
85. Graham G, Clarke LC. Statstical analysis in cryosurgery of skin cancer. In: Breitbart E, Dachow-Siwiec E (eds). Clinics in Dermatology: Advances in Dermatology. New York: Elsevier, 1990:101–107.
86. NCCN Guidelines: Basal and Squamous Cell Skin Cancers. Clinical Practice Guidelines in Oncology. Version 1, 2005. http://www.nccn.org/professionals/physician_gls/PDF/nmsc.pdf
87. Wolf D, Zitelli JA. Surgical margins for basal cell carcinoma. Arch Dermatol 1987;123:340–344.
88. Brodland D, Zitelli JA. Surgical margins for excision of primary cutaneous squamous cell carcinoma. J Am Acad Dermatol 1992;27(2 pt 1):241–248.
89. Gooding C, White G, Yatsuhashi M. Significance of marginal extension in excised basal cell carcinoma. N Engl J Med 1965; 46:549–553.
90. Robinson J, Fisher S. Recurrent basal cell carcinoma after incomplete resection. Arch Dermatol 2000;136(11):1318–1324.
91. Berlin J, Katz K, Helm K, et al. The significance of tumor persistence after incomplete excision of basal cell carcinoma. J Am Acad Dermatol 2002;46(4):549–553.
92. Avril M, Auperin A, Margulis A, et al. Basal cell carcinoma of the face: surgery or radiotherapy? Results of a randomized study. Br J Cancer 1997;76(1):100–106.
93. Julian C, Bowers PW. A prospective study of Mohs' micrographic surgery in two English centres. Br J Dermatol 1997;136(4):515–518.
94. Mohs F, Larson P, Iriondo M. Micrographic surgery for the microscopically controlled excision of carcinoma of the external ear. J Am Acad Dermatol 1988;19:729–737.
95. Mohs F. Micrographic surgery for the microscopically controlled excision of eyelid cancers. Arch Ophthalmol 1986;104(6):901–909.
96. Fischbach AJ, Sauces WT, Plenk HP. Radiation therapy for skin cancer. West J Med 1980;133(5):379–382.

97. Petrovich Z, Parker R, Luxton G, et al. Carcinoma of the lip and selected sites of head and neck and skin. A clinical study of 896 patients. Radiother Oncol 1987;8:11–17.
98. Zeitouni N, Shieh S, Oseroff A. Laser and photodynamic therapy in the management of cutaneous malignancies. Clin Dermatol 2001;19:328–339.
99. Adams E, Price N. Treatment of basal cell carcinomas with carbon dioxide laser. J Dermatol Surg Oncol 1979;5:803–806.
100. Wheeland R, Bailin P, Ratz R, et al. Carbon dioxide laser vaporization and curettage in the treatment of large or multiple superficial basal cell carcinomas. J Dermatol Surg Oncol 1987;13: 119–125.
101. Humphreys T, Malhotra R, Scharf M, et al. Treatment of superficial basal cell carcinoma and squamous cell carcinoma in situ with a high-energy pulsed carbon dioxide laser. Arch Dermatol 1998;134(10):1247–1252.
102. Malek R. Laser Treatment of premalignant and malignant squamous cell lesions of the penis. Lasers Surg Med 1992;12:246–253.
103. Gordon K, Garden J, Robinson J. Bowen's disease of the distal digit. Dermatol Surg 1996;22:723–728.
104. Peng Q, Warloe T, Berg K, et al. 5-ALA based photodynamic therapy. Cancer (Phila) 1997;79:2282–2308.
105. Morton C, Brown S, Collins S, et al. Guidelines for topical photodynamic therapy: report of a workshop of the British Photodermatology Group. Br J Dermatol 2002;146:552–567.
106. Morton CA, Whitehurst C, Moseley H, et al. Comparison of photodynamic therapy with cryotherapy in the treatment of Bowen's disease. Br J Dermatol 1996;135(5):766–771.
107. Salim A, Morton C. Comparison of photodynamic therapy with topical 5-fluorouacil Bowen's disease. Br J Dermatol 2000; 114(suppl 57):114 (abstract).
108. Morton C, Whitehurst C, Moore J, et al. Comparison of red and green light in the treatment of Bowen's disease by photodynamic therapy. Br J Dermatol 2000;143:767–772.
109. Cornell R, Greenway H, Tucker SB, et al. Intestinal interferon therapy for basal cell carcinoma. J Am Acad Dermatol 1990;23: 694–700.
110. Alpsoy E, Yikmaz E, Bassaram E, et al. Comparison of the effects of intralesional interferon alpha-1a, 2b and the combination of 2a and 2b in the treatment of basal cell carcinoma. J Dermatol 1996;23:394–396.
111. Edwards L, Berman B, Rapini R, et al. The effects of intralesional sustained-release formulation of interferon alpha-2b on basal cell carcinoma. Arch Dermatol 1992;126:1029–1032.
112. Beutner K, Geisse J, Helman D, et al. Therapeutic response of basal cell carcinoma to the immune response modifier imiquimod 5% cream for. J Am Acad Dermatol 1999;41: 1002–1007.
113. Geisse J, Marks R, Owens M, et al. Imiquimod 5% cream for 12 weeks treating superficial BCC. The 8th World Congress on Cancer of the Skin, 2001.
114. Robinson J, Marks R, Owens M, et al. Imiquimod 5% cream for 12 weeks treating nodular BCC. The 8th World Congress on Cancer of the Skin, 2001.
115. Marks R, Gebauer K, Shumack S, et al. Imiquimod 5% cream in the treatment of superficial basal cell carcinoma: results of a multicenter 6-week dose-response trial. J Am Acad Dermatol 2001;44:807–813.
116. Shumack S, Robinson J, Kossard S, et al. Efficacy of topical 5% imiquimod cream for the treatment of nodular basal cell carcinoma. Arch Dermatol 2002;138:1165–1171.
117. Sterry W, Ruzicka T, Herrera E, et al. Imiquimod 5% cream for the treatment of superficial and nodular basal cell carcinoma: randomized studies comparing low-frequency dosing with and without occlusion. Br J Dermatol 2002;147(6):1227–1236.
118. Mackenzie-Wood A, Kossard S, de Launey J, et al. Imiquimod 5% cream in the treatment of Bowen's disease. J Am Acad Dermatol 2001;46:462–470.
119. Orengo I, Rosen T, Guill C. Treatment of squamous cell carcinoma in situ of the penis with 5% imiquimod cream: a case report. J Am Acad Dermatol 2002;47:S225–S228.
120. Schroeder T, Sengelmann R. Squamous cell carcinoma in situ of the penis successfully treated with imiquimod 5% cream. J Am Acad Dermatol 2002;46:545–548.
121. Oster-Schmidt C. Two cases of squamous cell carcinoma treated with topical imiquimod 5% cream. J Eur Acad Dermatol Venereol 2004;18(1):93–95.
122. Romagosa R, Saap L, Givens M, et al. A pilot study to evaluate the treatment of basal cell carcinoma with 5-fluorouracil using phosphatidyl choline as a transepidermal carrier. Dermatol Surg 2000;26(4):338–340.
123. Miller B, Shavin J, Shumack S, et al. Nonsurgical treatment of basal cell carcinomas with intralesional 5-fluorouracil/ epinephrine injectable gel. J Am Acad Dermatol 1997;36:72–77.
124. Thompson S, Jolley D, Marks R. Reduction of solar keratoses by regular sunscreen use. N Engl Med 1993;329:1147–1151.
125. Green A, Williams G, Neale R. Daily sunscreen application and betacarotene supplementation in prevention of basal cell and squamous cell carcinomas of the skin: a randomized controlled trial. Lancet 1999;354:723–729.
126. Marcil I, Stern R. Risk of developing a subsequent nonmelanoma skin cancer in patients with a history of nonmelanoma skin cancer: a critical review of the literature and meta-analysis. Arch Dermatol 2000;136:1524–1530.

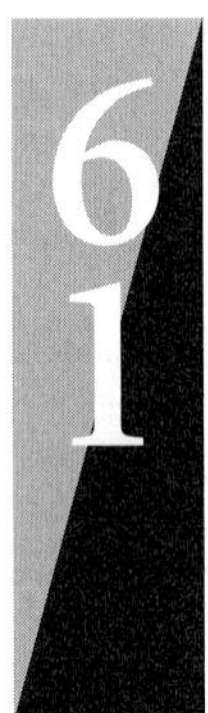

Cancer of Unknown Primary Site

F. Anthony Greco and John D. Hainsworth

In the United States, unknown primary cancers represented about 2% of all cancer diagnoses reported between 1973 and 1987.[1] Registries from seven other countries have listed incidences from 2.3% to 7.8%.[2] These patients are heterogeneous with several clinical presentations and histologic tumor types. Most have metastatic carcinoma of unknown primary site, while others have equivocal pathologic diagnoses with tumors difficult to classify by light microscopic examination. Specialized pathologic studies are essential in diagnosing the type of neoplasm present in many of these patients.

The nature or biology of the primary tumor in patients with unknown primary cancers is enigmatic. The clinical and biologic information suggest that some of these patients represent a distinct entity. Some of these patients have occult primaries found occasionally during the course of their disease, and more commonly at autopsy. Several other possible explanations for the apparent absence of a primary cancer can be contemplated. First, some patients have an unrecognized primary neoplasm (not an unknown primary cancer) inadvertently believed to represent a metastatic lesion. Extragonadal germ cell tumor, lymphoma, melanoma, or sarcoma are examples that arise from these lineages anywhere in the body. Second, primary cancers may inexplicably involute or regress entirely after metastasis has occurred. This notion is supported by the scarring seen occasionally in the testicle of patients with metastatic germ cell neoplasms. Third, tumors may have arisen from embryonic "rest cells" failing to complete their appropriate migration in utero to their appropriate tissue/organ. Extragonadal germ cell tumors with primaries in the mediastinum or undescended testicular cancer are examples of this phenomenon. Fourth, the pathogenesis of these carcinomas may result from a specific genetic lesion present in all cells, and these tumors arise from a second mutation or carcinogenetic event. This mechanism is suggested by the unusual occurrence of metastatic adenocarcinoma of unknown primary site in monozygotic twin brothers with primary immunodeficiency disorder (X-linked hyper IgM syndrome).[3] Finally, some of these cancers may arise from adult stem cells exhibiting plasticity.[4,5] Hematopoietic stem cells are able to transform into several cell types including liver, muscle, gastrointestinal, skin, and brain.[4] Some unknown primary tumors might continue to reflect such a transformation of adult stem cells and may in fact be "tumors of adult stem cells." Seemingly metastatic adenocarcinoma in lymph node, liver, bone, or elsewhere may, in fact, have arisen from an adult stem cell with the capacity to transform into any cell and subsequently develop as a "primary" neoplasm in any of these tissues.[5] Unknown primary tumors all possess a metastatic phenotype. When a primary is clinically undetectable, the natural history may in some patients vary from known primary cancers.

Karyotypic analysis of metastatic carcinoma of unknown primary site usually demonstrates diverse multiple complex random abnormalities not yet helpful in most instances for diagnosis or classification but is more representative of advanced neoplasms of many types.[6] No direct evidence exists to support a common/nonrandom genetic profile for even a portion of unknown primary tumors. Recently, however, gene expression profiles of known primary tumors suggest that the metastatic potential of tumors is encoded in most of the primary tumor, rather than rare cells within the primary tumor.[7] About 10% of poorly differentiated carcinomas of unknown primary strongly express Her-2-neu,[8] and these patients may be reasonable candidates for a trial of anti-Her-2-neu antibody therapy (trastuzumab). The vascular endothelial growth factor (VEGF)[9,10] and the epidermal growth factor receptor (EGFR) are also commonly expressed in several epithelial neoplasms, including unknown primary carcinoma, and therapy with EGFR and VEGF inhibitors is being explored. A much better understanding of unknown primary cancer is likely to arise from the development and study of gene expression profiling of these and other neoplasms.

Several important issues have changed over the past 20 years in oncology. Combination chemotherapy, often used with surgery or radiation therapy, has proved to be potentially curative for some patients with several metastatic tumors. Palliation and prolongation of survival has been possible for some patients with many other tumor types following systemic therapy. Therapy is evolving. Several new and useful biologic targeted agents such as rituximab, trastuzumab, imatinib, and gefitinib are now available. Improving therapies for several known solid tumors is relevant for patients with unknown primary cancer because several of these patients are also likely to respond to these therapies.

Electron microscopy and immunohistochemistry and more recently molecular genetics are responsible for more accurate and precise diagnosis of neoplasms. Several clinical syndromes and features are also being recognized and are helping physicians to better manage these patients.

Patient management requires an understanding of clinicopathologic features that help to identify several subsets of patients with more-responsive tumors. A patient with cancer of unknown primary site usually develops symptoms or signs at a metastatic site, and the diagnosis is made by biopsy of a metastatic lesion. History, physical examination, and other evaluation of the patient fail to identify the primary site. Routine light microscopic histology establishes the neoplastic process and provides a useful classification system on which to further evaluate and manage these patients. There are four major light microscopic diagnoses: (1) poorly differentiated neoplasm, (2) poorly differentiated carcinoma (with or without features of adenocarcinoma), (3) well-differentiated and moderately well differentiated adenocarcinoma, and (4) squamous cell carcinoma.

Poorly Differentiated Neoplasms of Unknown Primary Site

In these patients, the pathologic diagnosis of a neoplasm is clear, but the lineage (e.g., carcinoma, lymphoma, melanoma, sarcoma) is not established. A precise diagnosis is essential for these patients because many have responsive tumors. About 5% of all patients with cancers of unknown primary site present with this diagnosis by initial light microscopic appearance, but most are diagnosed by specialized pathologic study. Thirty-five percent to 65% of poorly differentiated neoplasms have large cell lymphomas after further pathologic study.[11–14] Most of the remaining tumors are carcinomas, with melanoma and sarcoma accounting for less than 15%.

Immunoperoxidase tumor staining, electron microscopy, and genetic analysis are helpful in the diagnosis. An adequate biopsy is essential, and frequently a more-definitive diagnosis can be made by obtaining a larger biopsy. Special tissue processing may be necessary for some pathologic studies. Rarely tumors remain unclassifiable after additional specialized pathologic study.

Specialized Pathology

Immunoperoxidase staining is the most common and widely available specialized pathologic technique for the classification of cancers. Examples of some immunoperoxidase staining patterns that are useful in the differential diagnosis of various neoplasms are listed in Table 61.1.

Many important issues can usually be answered by immunoperoxidase staining. The common leukocyte antigen (CLA) stain is used to make the important distinction between lymphoma and carcinoma.[15,16] Staining for chromogranin and synaptophysin suggests a neuroendocrine carcinoma. Prostate-specific antigen (PSA) staining highly suggests prostate carcinoma.[17,18] Some stains in appropriate clinical situations suggest breast carcinoma (e.g., estrogen or progesterone receptors, gross cystic fluid protein),[15] sarcoma (e.g., positive staining for desmin, vimentin, factor VIII antigen, c-kit-CD117 stain),[19–24] amelanotic melanoma (e.g., positive staining for S-100 protein, vimentin, HMB-45) or germ cell tumor [positive for the human chorionic gonadotropin (HCG)].[25,26]

Poorly differentiated neoplasms identified as lymphoma by positive CLA staining respond well to the combination chemotherapy used for non-Hodgkin's lymphoma.[11] Their survival was similar to a group of concurrently treated patients who had typical non-Hodgkin's lymphomas.

TABLE 61.1. Useful immunoperoxidase tumor staining patterns in the differential diagnosis of neoplasms.

Immunoperoxidase staining	*Tumor type*
Epithelial stains (e.g., CK 7, 20 variable)	Carcinoma
EMA (+) CLA, S-100, vimentin (–)	Lung carcinoma
TTF-1 (+)	Adenocarcinoma
CK 7 (+), CK 20 (–)	Other non-small cell carcinoma
TTF-1 (–)	
TTF-1 (+), chromogranin (+)	Small cell carcinoma
NSE (+)	
CK 7 (–); CK 20 (+)	Colorectal carcinoma
ER, PR (+)	Breast carcinoma
Her-2-neu (+)	
CK 7 (+), CK 20 (–)	
Gross cystic fluid protein 15 (+)	
Epithelial stains (+)	
NSE, chromogranin, synaptophysin (+)	Neuroendocrine carcinoma
Epithelial stains (+)	
HCG, AFP (+)	Germ cell tumor
Placental alkaline phosphatase (+)	
Epithelial stains (+)	
PSA (+), rare false (–) and (+)	Prostate carcinoma
Epithelial stains (+)	
CK 7 (–), CK 20 (–)	Thyroid carcinoma
Thyroglobulin (+), TTF-1 (+)	Follicular/papillary
Calcitonin (+)	Medullary Sarcoma
Vimentin (+)	Mesenchymal
Epithelial stains usually (–)	
Desmin (+)	Rhabdomyosarcoma
Factor VIII antigen (+)	Angiosarcoma
CD117 (C-kit) (+)	Gastrointestinal stromal tumor
S-100, vimentin, HMB-45 (+)	Melanoma
NSE often (+)	
Synaptophysin (–)	
Epithelial stains (–)	
CLA (+), rare false (–)	Lymphoma
EMA occasionally (+)	
All other stains (–)	

+, positive result; –, negative result; AFP, alpha-fetoprotein; CK, cytokeratin; CLA, common leukocyte antigen; EMA, epithelial membrane antigen; ER, estrogen receptor; HCG, human chorionic gonadotropin; NSE, neuron-specific enolase; PR, progesterone receptor; PSA, prostate-specific antigen; TTF-1, thyroid transcription factor-1.

Electron microscopy can be useful in some poorly differentiated neoplasms, although it is not widely available, requires special tissue fixation, and is relatively expensive. If the lineage of a tumor is unclear after routine light microscopy and immunoperoxidase staining, electron microscopy should be done. Electron microscopy is also reliable in differentiating lymphoma from carcinoma. It may be superior to immunoperoxidase staining for diagnosis of poorly differentiated sarcoma. Subcellular structures such as neurosecretory granules (neuroendocrine tumors) or premelanosomes (melanoma) can suggest the tumor.

Genetic analysis (identification of chromosomal abnormalities and specific genetic changes) is becoming important. Tumor-specific chromosomal abnormalities in diagnosis is still limited but will likely become more important in the future.

The majority of B-cell non-Hodgkin's lymphomas are associated with tumor-specific immunoglobulin gene rearrangements, and specific chromosomal changes have been identified in some B-cell and T-cell lymphomas and in Hodgkin's disease.[27,28] If the diagnosis of lymphoma cannot be definitively established with either immunoperoxidase staining or electron microscopy, detection of chromosomal translocations t(14:18); t(8:14); t(11:14) and others or the presence of an immunoglobulin gene rearrangement can be diagnostic.

Other nonrandom chromosomal rearrangements associated with nonlymphoid tumors have been identified but are unusual. Translocation of 11:22 (t11:22) has been found in peripheral neuroepitheliomas, desmoplastic small round cell tumors and in Ewing's tumor.[29–31] An isochromosome of the short arm of chromosome 12 (i12p) and other chromosome 12 abnormalities are frequently found in germ cell tumors.[32–34] Other nonrandom cytogenetic abnormalities found in tumors include t(2:13) in alveolar rhabdomyosarcoma; 3p deletion in small cell lung cancer; 1p deletion in neuroblastoma; t(X:18) in synovial sarcoma; and 11p deletion in Wilm's tumor. Epstein–Barr viral genome found in tumor cells of patients with cervical lymph node metastases of unknown primary site suggests nasopharyngeal primaries.[35,36]

DNA microarrays are being evaluated in several neoplasms[37] and hold promise as a method to classify neoplasms based upon gene expression profiling, perhaps identifying specific genetic patterns independent of previous histologic and biologic knowledge. This technique and others may eventually identify more specific tumor lineages or primary tumor types. Molecular classification of unknown primary carcinoma by gene expression is ongoing and is likely to provide more useful diagnostic and therapeutic information in unknown primary cancers.

Poorly Differentiated Carcinoma, with or Without Features of Adenocarcinoma, of Unknown Primary Site

Various subsets of patients with poorly differentiated carcinoma have been identified in the past 15 years. Specialized pathology has continued to improve and when used with clinical features has resulted in the recognition of several favorable subsets of patients with specific therapeutic implications. Poorly differentiated carcinoma account for about 30% of carcinoma of unknown primary sites, and about 33% have some features of adenocarcinomatous differentiation (poorly differentiated adenocarcinoma). Some patients have extremely responsive neoplasms, and therefore careful clinical and pathologic evaluation is necessary in patients with poorly differentiated carcinoma.

Clinical Characteristics

The clinical characteristics of these patients appear to differ with considerable overlap from the characteristics of patients with well-differentiated adenocarcinoma. When considering the whole group as compared to well-differentiated adenocarcinoma (see subsequent section), the median age is younger and the symptom interval is shorter. Metastasis predominantly involve peripheral lymph nodes, mediastinum, and retroperitoneum.

Pathologic Evaluation

Chemotherapy-responsive tumors cannot be identified by light microscopic features. Immunoperoxidase staining is essential, and for selected tumors electron microscopy and genetic analysis is indicated. Rarely, lymphoma is diagnosed, even though the light microscopic features are more typical of carcinoma. Immunoperoxidase staining is helpful in the routine evaluation of metastatic poorly differentiated carcinoma. Occasionally, it may suggest the lineage of the tumor and have specific therapeutic implications.[38–40]

Electron microscopy can also be useful for a minority of these carcinomas. Electron microscopy should be done for those tumors not diagnosed by immunoperoxidase stains. Lymphoma can be diagnosed reliably, and sarcoma, melanoma, mesothelioma, and neuroendocrine tumors occasionally are defined by subcellular features.

Chromosomal or genetic analysis is continuing to evolve as an important diagnostic method. Several neoplasms have specific abnormalities. Motzer and associates performed genetic analysis on tumors in 40 poorly differentiated carcinoma patients with the extragonadal germ cell syndrome or "midline carcinomas of uncertain histogenesis."[41] In 12 of the 40 patients, abnormalities of chromosome 12 (e.g., i[12p]; del [12p]; multiple copies of 12p) were diagnostic of germ cell tumor. Other abnormalities diagnostic of melanoma (2 patients), lymphoma (1 patient), peripheral neuroepithelioma (1 patient), and desmoplastic small cell tumor (1 patient) were also seen. Of the germinal neoplasms diagnosed on the basis of genetic analysis, 5 achieved a complete response to cisplatin-based chemotherapy. These data confirmed our previously formulated hypothesis that some of these patients have histologically atypical germ cell tumors.[42,43] Additional specific genetic abnormalities or gene expression profiling in solid tumors almost certainly will improve our ability to establish tumor lineage or biology and perhaps also identify specific targets to improve therapy.

In the limited necropsy data available that we have accumulated, it appears that primary sites are found in only a minority of these patients (about 40%). These observations are contrary to those for well-differentiated adenocarcinoma of unknown primary site, in which an occult primary site is found in most patients (about 75%) at autopsy.[44,45]

Diagnostic Evaluation

A history, physical examination, and routine laboratory testing, including a chest radiograph, should be done in each patient. Any abnormalities are followed with appropriate diagnostic testing. Computed tomography (CT) scans of the chest and abdomen should be performed because of the frequency of mediastinal and retroperitoneal involvement. Serum levels of HCG and alpha fetoprotein (AFP) should be measured. Elevations of these markers suggest the diagnosis of germ cell tumor. Serum tumor markers, such as carcinoembryonic antigen (CEA), CA 125, CA 19-9, and CA 15-3 can help in monitoring response to chemotherapy but are not specific enough to be useful in diagnosis. Positron emission tomography (PET) scanning appears to have a role in suggesting the primary cancer in about 20% to 30% of patients.[46–54]

Treatment

Appropriate therapy can be given when additional pathologic studies identify a specific neoplasm (e.g., lymphoma, sarcoma). Patients with clinical features highly suggestive of extragonadal germ cell tumor (e.g., mediastinal or retroperitoneal mass and elevated serum levels of HCG or AFP) should be treated with chemotherapy effective for germ cell tumors. Despite specialized pathologic study, most patients have multiple metastases and are left with the nonspecific diagnoses of poorly differentiated carcinoma or poorly differentiated adenocarcinoma. A small subset of these patients have highly responsive tumors.[43,55–57] These patients were usually young men with mediastinal tumors; serum levels of HCG or AFP were frequently elevated. These patients were thought to have histologically atypical extragonadal germ cell tumors. Other tumor types have also subsequently been identified in some of these patients (i.e., thymoma, neuroendocrine tumors, sarcomas, lymphomas), but many others have not been precisely classified. Further evidence for the responsiveness of many other tumors in patients with poorly differentiated carcinoma of unknown primary site has accumulated since 1978.[38,29,42,58–60]

An update of our initial prospective study in 220 of patients treated with cisplatin-based chemotherapy shows the following: 12% of the entire group have remained alive and free of tumor at a minimum follow-up of 6 years with a range of 6–17 years; the median survival for all patients was 20 months (3 years for complete responders); of the 58 complete responders, 22 patients remain relapse free (38%), representing 10% of the entire group. These results supported the notion that some of this poorly differentiated histology represents more sensitive tumors than well-differentiated adenocarcinoma, and prolongation of life was possible for some of these patients with the expectation of cure for a small minority. In those relatively rare patients with features of an extragonadal germ cell tumor, a standard regimen for the treatment of testicular or extragonadal germ cell tumors should be administered.

We now know that a large number of the 220 patients in the initial study had favorable subsets, each with a relatively good prognosis: these included (a) patients with poorly differentiated neoplasms otherwise not specified; (b) patients with the extragonadal germ cell syndrome; (c) patients with anaplastic lymphoma diagnosed as carcinoma; (d) patients with primary peritoneal carcinoma; (e) patients with poorly differentiated neuroendocrine carcinoma; and (f) patients with predominant sites of tumor involving the retroperitoneum, mediastinum, and peripheral lymph nodes. The nature of many of the other carcinomas remains obscure. Others have also reported the responsiveness of selected poorly differentiated carcinomas.[61–66] Complete responses were seen in 10% to 20% of these patients, and 5% to 10% were long-term disease-free survivors. These results were usually seen with platinum-based chemotherapy.

Our more-recent experience has excluded or stratified these more-favorable subsets of patients in our clinical trials, with the remaining patients having more unfavorable features and poor prognoses. These patients with unfavorable features have a similar prognosis to the large majority of the well-differentiated adenocarcinoma group (discussed later), and thus we now include all these patients in new clinical trials.

The Minnie Pearl Cancer Research Network has treated 396 patients since 1995 on five sequential prospective Phase II clinical trials incorporating several newer drugs (paclitaxel, docetaxel, gemcitabine, irinotecan). Patients with favorable prognostic features were excluded from these trials. As discussed later, the long-term survival seen in these patients suggests a major improvement in survival with these newer therapies.

Neuroendocrine Carcinoma of Unknown Primary Site

These neoplasms have been more readily recognized in recent years with the development of improved pathologic techniques. Well-differentiated or low-grade neuroendocrine tumors such as typical carcinoid or islet cell tumors occasionally present with metastases, without a clinically detectable primary site. These tumors usually have an indolent natural history. Carcinoid tumors of unknown primary have been appreciated for years.[1] There are also two groups of neuroendocrine tumors that are poorly differentiated by light microscopy. The first group of tumors have neuroendocrine light microscopic features (typical small cell, atypical carcinoid, or poorly differentiated neuroendocrine carcinoma) and act aggressively. The second group of neuroendocrine tumors, recently recognized, has high-grade biology and usually no neuroendocrine features by light microscopy. In this group, the diagnosis by light microscopy is poorly differentiated carcinoma, and neuroendocrine features are only recognized when immunoperoxidase staining or electron microscopy is performed.

Low-Grade Neuroendocrine Carcinoma

In these tumors, the metastatic sites usually involves the liver and/or bone, and these are sometimes associated with clinical syndromes produced by the secretion of bioactive substances (e.g., carcinoid syndrome, insulin production, glucogonoma syndrome, vipomas [vasointestinal peptide producing tumors], Zollinger–Ellison syndrome). Primary sites should be sought in the small intestine (particularly the ileum), rectum, pancreas, or bronchus.

These tumors usually exhibit an indolent biology, and slow progression over years is typical. These patients should be managed the same as those with metastatic carcinoid or islet cell tumors from known primary sites. Intensive systemic chemotherapy with cisplatin-based chemotherapy is not useful for most patients as the response rates are low.[67] Appropriate management may include local therapy (resection of isolated metastasis, hepatic artery ligation/embolization, cryotherapy, radiofrequency ablation), treatment with somatostatin analogues, streptozocin, doxorubicin, 5-fluorouracil-based systemic therapy, or symptomatic management.

Small Cell Carcinoma

A lung primary should be suspected, but when no primary is identified, patients with small cell carcinoma should be treated with combination chemotherapy as recommended for small cell lung cancer. Paclitaxel, carboplatin, and oral etoposide is a very active therapy for these patients, and we have continued to evaluate this regimen. Most of these tumors are initially very sensitive to chemotherapy, and major palliative benefit can be derived from treatment. Some patients will enjoy long-term benefit. Rarely these tumors present as a single metastatic site, and the addition of radiation therapy and/or resection to combination chemotherapy should be considered.

Poorly Differentiated Neuroendocrine Carcinoma

In a small minority of poorly differentiated carcinomas, electron microscopy reveals neurosecretory granules, a finding diagnostic of neuroendocrine carcinoma. In the past, these tumors have been called: poorly differentiated neuroendocrine tumors, atypical carcinoids, or primitive neuroectodermal tumors. Electron microscopy is the most definitive diagnostic technique, but most of the tumors also have typical immunoperoxidase staining patterns with positive staining for neuron-specific enolase, chromogranin, or synaptophysin.

We reported 29 patients with poorly differentiated neuroendocrine tumors of unknown primary site[58] and later updated our experience to include a total 51 of patients.[68] These patients had clinical evidence of high-grade tumor, and the majority had metastases in multiple sites; 77% of these patients responded to chemotherapy with a cisplatin-based combination regimen, 13 patients (26%) had complete responses, and 8 patients have remained continuously disease free.

Currently, we are evaluating the combination of paclitaxel, carboplatin, and oral etoposide in patients with poorly differentiated neuroendocrine tumors of unknown primary site.[69] Since 2000, 32 patients have been treated. The majority of these patients had several sites of metastasis, with predominant tumor in the liver (18 patients), nodes (6 patients), and mediastinum (2 patients). These patients also responded well, with 4 complete responders and 12 partial responders. Ten patients remain alive from 12 to 35 months later, and 4 remain progression free.

The origin(s) of these poorly differentiated neuroendocrine tumors remain obscure. Genetic studies may be helpful if an 11:22 translocation (peripheral neuroepithelioma, soft tissue Ewing's sarcoma, or desmoplastic small round cell tumor) or i(12p) abnormality (germ cell tumor) is identified. All these patients without a specific diagnosis should be treated with a trial of combination chemotherapy. Patients with a single site of tumor involvement may be curable with local treatment modalities alone; however, adjuvant chemotherapy should also be administered in these patients if clinically feasible.

Adenocarcinoma of Unknown Primary Site

Clinical Characteristics

Well-differentiated and moderately well differentiated adenocarcinoma represent the most frequent light microscopic diagnoses (60% of patients). Many physicians associate these patients with the entity of unknown primary cancer. The majority are elderly and have metastatic tumors at multiple sites. The sites of tumor often determine the clinical presentation. Common metastatic sites include liver, lung, bone, and lymph nodes.

The primary tumor surfaces in only 15% to 20% of patients during life.[70] However, at autopsy an occult primary site is detected in about 70% to 80% of patients. The most common primaries identified at necropsy are the pancreas and lung (about 40%).[44] Adenocarcinomas from a wide variety of other primary sites are also encountered, but infrequently. An unexpected metastatic pattern is also observed for several of these tumors. Occult pancreatic primaries more frequently involve bone rather than liver, and occult lung and prostate cancer less often involve bone. The clinical course and response to various therapies of occult primary cancers may also differ from that of known primaries.

Patients with metastatic adenocarcinoma of unknown primary site have had a very poor prognosis, with a median survival of only 3 to 4 months. Several patients have widespread metastases and poor performance status at the time of diagnosis. However, within this large group are subsets of patients with more-favorable prognoses, as discussed later. Furthermore, chemotherapy has improved in the past few years, and many patients now are candidates for chemotherapy with an expectation of clinical benefit and improved survival.

Pathology

The light microscopic diagnosis of well-differentiated or moderately well differentiated adenocarcinoma is based on the recognition of glandular structures formed by neoplastic cells. The site of the primary tumor cannot be determined by histologic examination. Certain histologic features typically are associated with some carcinomas, such as signet-ring cells with gastric cancer and papillary features with ovarian cancer, but are not specific enough to be diagnostic. Immunoperoxidase stains and electron microscopy are not helpful in providing additional information in most well-differentiated or moderately well differentiated adenocarcinomas. Prostate-specific antigen stain (PSA) is an exception as it is relatively specific for prostate cancer. Positive immunostaining for estrogen or progesterone receptors, gross cystic fluid protein 15, or Her-2-neu suggests metastatic breast cancer. Neuroendocrine stains [e.g., neuron-specific enolase (NSE), chromogranin, synaptophysin] can occasionally identify an unsuspected neuroendocrine neoplasm. Several other stains or batteries of stains have been evaluated[71–76] and may suggest the primary (see Table 61.1), but none are specific enough to reliably diagnose the primary site. The diagnosis of poorly differentiated adenocarcinoma should be viewed the same as poorly differentiated carcinoma (see previous section).

Diagnostic Evaluation

These patients should be evaluated similarly to that described for patients with poorly differentiated carcinoma. An exhaustive search for the primary site should not be done. Suspicious clinical symptoms or signs and the extent of metastatic disease should be evaluated. A thorough history and physical examination, standard laboratory screening tests (i.e., complete blood count, liver function tests, serum creatinine, urinalysis), and chest radiography are indicated. All women should undergo mammography and all men should have a serum PSA determination. CT scans of the abdomen can identify a primary site in about 20% of patients and frequently are useful in identifying additional sites of metastatic disease.[77,78] Other symptoms, signs, or abnormal physical and laboratory findings should be investigated with appropriate diagnostic studies. An exhaustive evaluation looking for the primary site is rarely useful, is expensive, and often results in false-positive results. A consideration of gastrointestinal endoscopy is appropriate because several of these primary tumor types are now more treatable than before.

PET scanning is an important addition for the evaluation of potential primary sites. Various tumor markers (CEA, CA 15-3, CA 19-9, CA 125, B-HCG, AFP) have not proven to be useful (except in rare instances) for diagnosis or prognosis but can be used to follow the response to therapy.[79,80]

Treatment

This group of patients contains several clinically defined subsets for which useful specific therapy is indicated. Most tumors within these clinically defined subgroups are well- or moderately differentiated adenocarcinomas, but a minority are poorly differentiated carcinomas. Chemotherapy can now be considered, with expectations for good palliation and improved survival for the other patients (discussed later) who do not fit into any of the subsets listed below.

Peritoneal Carcinomatosis in Women

Diffuse peritoneal carcinomatosis is typical of ovarian carcinoma, although carcinomas from the gastrointestinal tract, lung, or breast can occasionally produce this clinical picture. It is now accepted that many of these women have a primary peritoneal carcinoma. Anecdotal case reports from the 1980s documented excellent responses to cisplatin-based chemotherapy in women with this syndrome.[81–84] Similar to ovarian carcinoma, the incidence of primary peritoneal carcinoma is increased in women with BRCA1 mutations.[85]

The clinical features are similar to ovarian carcinoma. Most patients have elevated serum levels of CA-125 antigen. An occasional patient presents with pleural effusion only, but metastases outside the peritoneal cavity are not common. The histologic features are usually similar to ovarian carcinoma. Most of these patients should undergo laparotomy with surgical cytoreduction followed by combination chemotherapy. These patients are now treated as in ovarian cancer and are considered clinically and biologically similar. The overall results from therapy are similar to ovarian cancer. Carboplatin plus paclitaxel or similar regimens considered optimal for the treatment of advanced ovarian cancer would seem a reasonable choice for initial chemotherapy.

Papillary peritoneal carcinomatosis or primary peritoneal carcinoma has also been seen in men.[86] It is difficult to confirm the precise biology, and some of these tumors may be metastatic from an occult primary from elsewhere. The study of gene expression patterns in these patients may solve this dilemma in the future. A trial of chemotherapy should be administered in good performance status patients regardless of gender.

Women with Axillary Lymph Node Metastases

Axillary adenocarcinoma should be considered as arising from an occult primary breast cancer in women. The histology is occasionally poorly differentiated carcinoma. Men with occult breast cancer are very rare. The presence of estrogen and/or progesterone receptors highly suggests the diagnosis of breast cancer.[87] These patients may have stage II breast cancer with an occult primary, which is potentially curable with appropriate therapy. Magnetic resonance imaging (MRI) and PET are superior to mammography in identifying a breast primary.[88–90] In the past, modified radical mastectomy was recommended. A clinically occult breast primary has been identified after mastectomy in about 60% of patients.[91–93] Prognosis is similar to that of other patients with stage II breast cancer.[91–95] Primary radiotherapy to the breast after axillary lymph node dissection is a reasonable alternative therapy. Either neoadjuvant or adjuvant chemotherapy should be administered in this setting, similar to standard therapy for stage II breast cancer.

Women who present with multiple metastatic sites including the axillary lymph nodes may have metastatic breast cancer. They should be considered for therapy for metastatic breast cancer, particularly if serum levels of CA 15-3 or CA 27-29 are elevated and/or estrogen and progesterone receptor and/or Her-2-neu is positive in their tumor.

Prostate Carcinoma

Prostate-specific antigen levels should be measured in men with adenocarcinoma of unknown primary site. In some patients the clinical features (i.e., metastatic pattern) do not suggest prostate cancer, but a positive prostate-specific antigen (serum or tumor stain) is reason for a trial of hormonal therapy.[96,97]

Squamous Carcinoma of Unkown Primary Site

Squamous Carcinoma Involving Cervical and Supraclavicular Lymph Nodes

Cervical lymph nodes are involved more often. These patients are often elderly, and frequently they have abused alcohol or tobacco. When the middle or upper cervical lymph nodes are involved, a primary tumor in the head and neck region should be suspected. These patients should have an examination of the oropharynx, hypopharynx, nasopharynx, larynx, and upper esophagus by direct endoscopy, with biopsy of any suspicious areas. CT of the neck and PET are indicated as these may also identify primary sites.[50–54,98] Epstein–Barr virus genome detected in the tumor tissue suggests a nasopharyngeal primary site.[35,36] When the lower supraclavicular or cervical lymph nodes are involved, lung cancer should be suspected. Fiberoptic bronchoscopy should be performed, because a lung primary is frequently found.[99]

Local treatment should be given to the involved neck when no primary is found. Results in more than 1,400 patients using a variety of treatment modalities have been reviewed.[100–122] About 30% to 40% of patients achieved long-term disease-free survival after local treatment modalities. The results obtained using high-dose radiation therapy, radical neck dissection, or a combination of these therapies have been similar. When resection alone is used in these patients, a primary tumor in the head and neck eventually becomes apparent in 20% to 40%. Radiation therapy techniques should be similar to those used in patients with primary head and neck cancer,[111] and the nasopharynx, oropharynx, and hypopharynx may be included in the irradiated field. Patients with involvement of supraclavicular nodes and low cervical nodes do not do as well (10%–15% long-term survival rates), probably because lung cancer is a frequent occult primary site. Chemotherapy should also be considered, but its role remains controversial, even though it is now clear that combined chemotherapy and radiotherapy are superior to radiotherapy alone in most locally advanced head and neck squamous cancer.

Squamous Carcinoma Involving Inguinal Lymph Nodes

Primary sites in the genital or anorectal areas should be sought. Identification of a primary site is important because curative therapy is available for carcinomas of the vulva, vagina, cervix, and anus, even after spread to regional lymph nodes. About one-half of these patients with inguinal presentations have poorly differentiated carcinoma. In those without identified primary tumors, surgical resection with or without radiation therapy to the inguinal area sometimes results in long-term survival. Neoadjuvant or adjuvant chemotherapy should also be considered.

Squamous Carcinoma Metastatic to Other Sites

Metastatic squamous carcinoma in other areas usually represents metastasis from an occult primary lung cancer, and an appropriate evaluation is indicated. In good performance status patients, chemotherapy with regimens employed in the treatment of non-small cell lung cancer may be considered. Other rare presentations include primaries from the head and neck, esophagus, anus, and skin.

Poorly differentiated squamous carcinoma should be evaluated carefully. Occasionally, breast carcinoma undergo squamous differentiation at metastatic sites. As is the case with poorly differentiated adenocarcinoma, the diagnosis of poorly differentiated squamous cell carcinoma is sometimes based on minimal histologic findings. Specialized pathologic evaluation with immunoperoxidase stains, electron microscopy, and molecular studies should be considered. If the diagnosis remains unclear, these patients should be considered for a trial of therapy for poorly differentiated carcinoma (see previous section).

Chemotherapy for Metastatic Carcinoma of Unknown Primary Site

Most patients with well-differentiated or moderately differentiated adenocarcinoma and poorly differentiated carcinoma do not fit in one of the several favorable prognostic clinical subgroups. Chemotherapy of various types, in the past, has produced low response rates, very few complete responses, and very few long-term survivals.[2,68,122,123] The results of chemotherapy in several reported prospective clinical trial series in 1,515 patients from 1964–2002 have been reviewed.[2,68] The overall response rates from these prospective clinical studies varied from 8% to 39% (mean, 20%); complete responders were less than 1%, median survival 4–15 months (mean, 6 months), survival beyond 2 years was rarely reported, and disease-free survival beyond 3 years was not reported.

We have also reviewed several retrospective reports of survival for 31,419 patients with unknown primary cancer[1,124–131] (Table 61.2) to better define the natural history of this syndrome. Treatment was variable, and some patients received no systemic therapy. These series contained patients now known to fit into specific treatable or favorable subsets. The median survival was 5 months with a 1-year survival of 22% and 5-year survival of 5%. Survival at 1 year and beyond is likely represented by subsets of patients with a more-favorable prognosis who received local therapy (squamous cell carcinoma) or those with very indolent tumors (such as carcinoids). Data in Table 61.3 support this assertion. Squamous (epidermoid) carcinoma and well-differentiated neuroendocrine carcinoma (carcinoid, islet cell type histology) reported in 2,971 patients from some of these series had median, 1-year, and 5-year survival rates of 20 months and 66% and 30%, respectively. All the other patients in these series (total of 26,029 patients) had median, 1-year, and 5-year survival rates of 6 months and 20%, and 5%, respectively.

These historical control data need to be viewed with several factors in mind. Some of the prospective series

TABLE 61.2. Unknown primary cancer survival.[a]

Study	*No. of patients*	*Median survival (months)*	*One-year survival (%)*	*Five-year survival (%)*
Charity Hospital[127]	453	4	13.9	3.3
John's Hopkins[128]	245	3	18	2
Mayo Clinic[129]	150	4	12	0.7
Yale University[124]	1,268	5	23	6
M.D. Anderson[125]	1,000	11	43	11
University of Kansas[126]	686	6	21.5	5.1
SEER[1]	26,050	NR	NR	5
Switzerland[131]	543	4	15	NR
Southeast Netherlands[130]	1,024	2.75	15	NR
Total	31,419	5	22	5

SEER, Surveillance, Epidemiology and End Results registries; NR, not reported.

[a]Includes treated and untreated patient groups, all histologies and clinical presentations.

TABLE 61.3. Survival of patients with well-differentiated neuroendocrine carcinoma and squamous cell carcinoma.[a]

Study	*No. (N)*	*Median survival (months)*	*One-year survival (%)*	*Five-year survival (%)*
Well differentiated neuroendocrine carcinoma:				
M.D. Anderson	43	26	75	34
Squamous cell carcinoma: M.D. Anderson[167]	62	38	85	43
All other patients: M.D. Anderson	895	9	35	8
Squamous cell carcinoma: Yale[166]	148	9	39	15
All other patients: Yale	1,120	5	21	5
Epidermoid carcinoma: SEER[1]	2,670	NR	NR	30
All other patients: SEER	23,380	NR	NR	5
Squamous cell carcinoma: Switzerland[173]	48	10.1	NR	NR
All other patients: Switzerland	495	4	15%	NR
Total Squamous/neuroendocrine	2,971	20[b]	66[b,c]	30[c]
All other patients	25,890	6[b]	20[b]	5[c]

SEER, Surveillance, Epidemiology, and End Results registries; NR, not reported.

[a] = Includes treated and untreated patients.

[b] SEER data not included in calculation (not reported).

[c] Switzerland data not included in calculation (not reported).

are small, and large randomized comparisons are lacking. In addition, patients with all histologic types were included in these series. The patients were not standardly evaluated or compared in reference to sites of metastasis (nodal versus visceral), performance status, sex, age, or other known prognostic factors.

The chemotherapy for patients with adenocarcinoma and poorly differentiated carcinoma who do not fit or conform to a specific "treatable" or favorable subset has recently improved. Several new drugs have been introduced into clinical practice (taxanes, gemcitabine, vinorelbine, and topotecan) with a rather broad spectrum of activity and are changing the standard treatment for patients with several common epithelial cancers.

The Minnie Pearl Cancer Research Network has completed five sequential prospective Phase II trials since 1995 in 396 patients incorporating paclitaxel,[132,133] docetaxel,[133,134] gemcitabine,[135] and irinotecan[136] into first-line therapy. Except for a few exceptions (8 patients in the first two trials), all these patients were considered to have poor prognostic features (i.e., patients with known favorable prognostic features were excluded). The chemotherapy regimens, patient characteristics, response rates, and survivals are summarized in Tables 61.4 and 61.5. The total response rate in the five clin-

TABLE 61.4. Chemotherapy regimens and patient characteristics of five consecutive prospective Phase II studies in 396 patients from 1995 to 2002.

	Study 1 Paclitaxel Carboplatin Etoposide	*Study 2 Docetaxel Cisplatin*	*Study 3 Docetaxel Carboplatin*	*Study 4 Paclitaxel Carboplatin Gemcitabine*	*Study 5 Paclitaxel Carboplatin Etoposide followed by Gemcitabine Irinotecan*	*Total*
Characteristics:						
Number of patients	71	26	47	120	132	396
Male/female	35/36	13/13	25/22	64/56	67/65	203/193
Age, years						
Median	72	60	56	58	59	62
Range	31–82	34–74	23–76	21–85	29–83	21–85
ECOG performance status -0	9 (13%)	10 (38%)	9 (19%)	27 (27%)	24 (18%)	79 (20%)
1	50 (70%)	10 (38%)	26 (55%)	77 (64%)	97 (73%)	260 (66%)
2	12 (17%)	6 (24%)	12 (26%)	16 (14%)	11 (9%)	57 (14%)
Histology						
Adenocarcinoma (well differentiated)	34 (48%)	13 (50%)	18 (38%)	63 (53%)	59 (44%)	187 (47%)
PDC or PDA	30 (42%)	11 (43%)	28 (60%)	56 (46%)	72 (55%)	197 (50%)
Neuroendocrine carcinoma (poorly differentiated)	6 (9%)	2 (7%)	0 (0%)	0 (0%)	0 (0%)	8 (2%)
Squamous carcinoma	1 (1%)	0 (0%)	1 (2%)	1 (1%)	1 (1%)	4 (1%)
Number of organ sites involved-1	28 (39%)	7 (27%)	15 (32%)	42 (35%)	41 (31%)	133 (34%)
≥2	43 (61%)	19 (73%)	32 (68%)	78 (65%)	91 (69%)	263 (66%)

PDC, poorly differentiated carcinoma; PDA, poorly differentiated adenocarcinoma; ECOG, Eastern Cooperative Oncology Group.

TABLE 61.5. Responses and survival.

	Study 1	*Study 2*	*Study 3*	*Study 4*	*Study 5*	*Total*
No. of patients	71	26	47	120	132	396
Partial response/ complete response	48%/15%	22%/4%	22%/0%	21%/4%	23%/6%	30%/6%
1-year survival	48%	40%	33%	42%	35%	38%
2-year survival	20%	28%	28%	23%	16%	19%
3-year survival	14%	16%	15%	14%	Too early	12%
5-year survival	12%	13%	10%	Too early	Too early	10%
8-year survival	8%	Too early	Too early	Too early	Too early	8%
Range of follow-up (years)	6.7–8	6–6.7	4.8–5.8	3–4.6	1–2	1–8
Minimum follow-up (years)	6.7	6	4.8	3	1	1

ical trials was 30% (107 of 353 evaluable patients), with 85 (94%) partial responders and 22 (6%) complete responders. The median survival is 9.1 months, and the 1-, 2-, 3-, 5-, and 8-year survivals are 38%, 19%, 12%, 8%, and 6%, respectively (minimum follow-up, 1 year, maximum 8 years). The median progression-free survival is 5 months, and the 1-, 2-, 3-, 5-, and 8-year progression-free survivals are 17%, 7%, 5%, 4%, and 3%, respectively. There have been no significant differences in survival when comparing the survival curves of all five Phase II studies. There was moderate toxicity, primarily myelosuppression, and 8 (2%) treatment-related deaths.

Trials recently reported by others[2,62,137–140] have confirmed the activity of the newer cytotoxic agents, but long-term follow-up has not yet been reported. The standard therapy for good performance status patients with carcinoma of unknown primary site is with one of the newer cytotoxic combinations as reported in the 396 patients in this chapter, or as reported by others.[137–140]

The more-common patients with unknown primary adenocarcinoma or poorly differentiated carcinoma who do not fit or conform to any previously defined "treatable" or favorable subsets now have the opportunity to attain clinical benefit from the new cytotoxic drug combinations. Randomized trials of treatment versus no treatment have not been done, but the median survival as well as 1-, 2-, 3-, and 5-year survival results are superior to the survivals recorded from the past. The survival for patients with unknown primary carcinoma is now similar to the survival of several other groups of advanced carcinoma patients receiving various types of chemotherapy, such as advanced-stage non-small cell lung cancer.

The Changing Role of Prognostic Factors

The prognoses of the various subsets of patients with poorly differentiated neoplasm (otherwise not classified), poorly differentiated carcinoma, well-differentiated adenocarcinoma, squamous cell carcinoma, neuroendocrine carcinoma, and those with a single small site of metastasis are relatively good. Some other patients with poorly differentiated carcinoma have chemotherapy-responsive tumors, and complete responses and long-term survival have been documented for a minority of these patients. Subsets of patients with a more-favorable prognosis or other "favorable" prognostic factors have been recognized. Many of these patients are managed with specific therapies and have a better prognosis than the group as a whole. Others have features associated with a better prognosis when treated with chemotherapy. Both pathologic and clinical factors can now define several patients with a better prognosis (Table 61.6). For the most part, the larger group of patients with well differentiated adenocarcinoma have had relatively resistant tumors, with virtually no complete responses to chemotherapy, and no long-term survivals in the past. This situation is now changing, as discussed previously.

Most patients who do not fit into a favorable subset have a poor prognosis, regardless of their initial light microscopic diagnosis (well-differentiated adenocarcinoma or poorly differentiated carcinoma). Recently, these patients have been treated with several of the newer cytotoxic combinations (taxanes, gemcitabine, and irinotecan), and modest improvements in the response rate (with some complete responses) and survival have been documented. In addition, the newer cytotoxic combinations appear more effective with less toxicity than cisplatin-based chemotherapy, even for those patients within favorable prognostic subsets who otherwise require chemotherapy. For those rare patients with the extragonadal germ cell syndrome, cisplatin-based therapy remains

TABLE 61.6. Favorable prognostic factors in cancer of unknown primary site.

1. Poorly differentiated malignant neoplasm (otherwise not classified) (60% = lymphomas)
2. Extragonadal germ cell syndrome (PDA or PDC)
3. Retroperitoneal, mediastinal, and/or peripheral lymph node involvement (PDA, PDC, WDA)
4. Squamous cell carcinomas (head/neck or inguinal area)
5. Isolated axillary adenopathy: women, rare in men (WDA, PDC, PDA)
6. Peritoneal carcinoma: women, rare in men (WDA, PDC, PDA)
7. Blastic bone metastases or increased PSA in serum or tumor: men (WDA, PDA, PDC)
8. Neuroendocrine carcinoma: high-grade or poorly differentiated (small cell and others)
9. Neuroendocrine carcinoma: low-grade or well-differentiated (carcinoid/islet cell type)
10. Single site of metastasis (WDA, PDC, PDA)
11. Performance status 0, 1 (with otherwise favorable features)
12. Normal serum LDH (with otherwise favorable features)

PDC, poorly differentiated carcinoma; PDA, poorly differentiated adenocarcinoma; WDA, well-differentiated adenocarcinoma; LDH, lactic dehydrogenase.

TABLE 61.7. Carcinoma of unknown primary site: evaluation and therapy of selected responsive subsets.

	Clinical evaluation[a]	*Special pathologic studies*	*Subsets*	*Therapy*	*Prognosis*
Poorly differentiated carcinoma, poorly differentiated adenocarcinoma	Chest, abdominal CT scans, serum HCG, AFP; PET scan additional studies to evaluate symptoms, signs	Immunoperoxidase staining Electron microscopy Genetic analysis	1. Atypical germ cell tumors (identified by chromosome 12 abnormalities)	Treatment for germ cell tumor	40%–50% cure rate
			2. Extragonadal germ cell syndrome (2 features)	Cisplatin/etoposide	Survival improved; (10%–20% cured)
			3. Lymph node predominant tumors (mediastinum, retroperitoneum, peripheral nodes)	Newer chemotherapy	Survival improved
			4. Gastrointestinal stromal tumors (identified by CD 117 stain)	Imatinib	Survival improved
			5. Other groups (see text)	Newer chemotherapy	Survival improved
Adenocarcinoma (well-differentiated or moderately differentiated)	Chest, abdominal CT scan Men: Serum PSA Women: Mammogram Serum CA 15-3 Serum CA 125 PET scan Additional studies to evaluate symptoms, signs	Men: PSA stain Women: ER, PR	1. Women, axillary node involvement[b]	Treat as primary breast cancer	Survival improved with specific therapy
			2. Women, peritoneal carcinomatosis[b]	Surgical cytoreduction + chemotherapy as in ovarian cancer	
			3. Men, blastic bone metastases, high serum PSA, or PSA tumor staining	Hormonal therapy for prostate cancer	
			4. Single metastatic site[b]	Lymph node dissection radiotherapy	
			5. Other groups (see text)	Newer chemotherapy	Survival improved
Squamous carcinoma	Cervical node presentation[b] Panendoscopy PET scan	Genetic analysis	Cervical adenopathy Nasopharyngeal cancer (identified by PCR for Epstein–Barr viral genes)	Radiation therapy neck dissection chemotherapy	25%–30% 5-year survival
	Supraclavicular presentation[b] Bronchoscopy PET scan		Supraclavicular	Radiation therapy chemotherapy	5%–15% 5-year survival
	Inguinal presentation[b] Pelvic, rectal exams, anoscopy PET scan		Inguinal adenopathy	Inguinal node dissection radiation therapy chemotherapy	15%–20% 5-year survival
Neuroendocrine carcinoma	CT abdomen, chest	Immunoperoxidase Staining Electron microscopy	1. Low-grade 2. Small cell carcinoma 3. Poorly differentiated etoposide	Treat as advanced carcinoid Paclitaxel/carboplatin/ etoposide or platinum/ rarely cured	Indolent biology/long survival High response rate survival improved;

AFP, alpha-fetoprotein; ER, estrogen receptor; HCG, human chorionic gonadotropin; PR, progesterone receptor; PSA, prostate-specific antigen.

[a] In addition to history, physical examination, routine laboratory tests, and chest X-ray films.

[b] May also present with poorly differentiated carcinoma and management and outcome is similar.

the treatment of choice. Additional study of the patients with poor prognoses is important to build on the progress seen with newer cytotoxic agent-based combination chemotherapies.

Conclusion

The recognition of subsets of patients with more treatable cancers within the large heterogeneous population of cancers of unknown primary site represents an improvement in the management of these patients. These patients with more-responsive tumors can often be identified by clinical and pathologic evaluation (Table 61.7). The outcome for patients with cancers of unknown primary site is likely to improve as the therapy for various other cancers improves. Several combination chemotherapy regimens using newer agents have recently found to be useful in previously "unresponsive" patients (i.e., non-small cell lung cancer, colorectal cancer). Recent data, as reported here, also support the benefit of chemotherapy for many unknown primary cancer patients. Improved therapy will likely be developed after a more thorough understanding of the basic biology of these and other cancers is appreciated. Until then, empiric approaches to better manage and treat these patients should continue.

References

1. Muir C. Cancer of unknown primary site. Cancer (Phila) 1995;75:353–356.
2. Pavlidis N, Briasoulis E, Hainsworth J, Greco FA. Diagnostic and therapeutic management of cancer of an unknown primary. Eur J Cancer 2003;39:1990–2005.
3. Wood LA, Venner PM, Pabst HF. Monozygotic twin brothers with primary immunodeficiency presenting with metastatic adenocarcinoma of unknown primary. Acta Oncol 1998;37: 771–772.
4. Korbling M, Katz RL, Khanna A, et al. Hepatocytes and epithelial cells of donor origin in recipients of peripheral blood stem cells. N Engl J Med 2002 346:738–746.
5. McCulloch EA. Stem cells and diversity. Leukemia 2003;17: 1042–1048.
6. Abbruzzese JL, Lenzi R, Raber MN, et al. The biology of unknown primary tumors. Semin Oncol 1993;20:238–243.
7. Ramaswamy S, Ross KN, Lander ES, Golab TR. A molecular signature of metastasis in primary solid tumors. Nat Genet 2003;33:49–54.
8. Hainsworth JD, Lennington WJ, Greco FA. Overexpression of Her-2 in patients with poorly differentiated carcinoma or poorly differentiated adenocarcinoma of unknown primary site. J Clin Oncol 2000;18:632–635.
9. Karavasilis V, Tsanou E, Malamon-Mitsi V, et al. Microvessel density and vascular endothelial growth factor in cancer of unknown primary. An immunohistochemical study. Proc ESMO 2002;51.
10. Hillen HF, Hak LE, Joosten-Achjanie SR, et al. Microvessel density in unknown primary tumors. Int J Cancer 1997;74: 81–85.
11. Horning SJ, Carrier EK, Rouse RV, et al. Lymphomas presenting as histologically unclassified neoplasms: characteristics and response to treament. J Clin Oncol 1989;7:1281–1287.
12. Hales SA, Gatter KC, Heryet A, Mason DY. The value of immunocytochemistry in differentiating high-grade lymphoma from other anaplastic tumours: a study of anaplastic tumours from 1940 to 1960. Leuk Lymphoma 1989;1:59–63.
13. Gatter KC, Alcock C, Heryet A, Mason DY. Clinical importance of analysing malignant tumours of uncertain origin with immunohistochemical techniques. Lancet 1985;1:1302–1305.
14. Azar HA, Espinoza CG, Richman AV, et al. Undifferentiated large cell malignancies: an ultrastructural and immunocytochemical study. Hum Pathol 1982;13:323–333.
15. Warnke RA, Gatter KC, Falini B, et al. Diagnosis of human lymphoma with monoclonal antileukocyte antibodies. N Engl J Med 1983;109:1275–1281.
16. Battifora H, Trowbridge IS. A monoclonal antibody useful for the differential diagnosis between malignant lymphoma and nonhematopoietic neoplasms. Cancer (Phila) 1983;51:816–821.
17. Mackey B, Ordonez NG. Pathological evaluation of neoplasms with unknown primary tumor site. Semin Oncol 1993;20: 206–228.
18. Allhof EP, Proppe KH, Chapman CM. Evaluation of prostate-specific acid phosphatase and prostate-specific antigen. J Urol 1983;57:1084–1086.
19. Denk H, Knepler R, Artlieb U, et al. Proteins of intermediate filaments: an immunohistochemical and biochemical approach to the classification of soft tissue tumors. Am J Pathol 1983; 110:193–208.
20. Osborn M, Weber K. Biology of disease: tumor diagnosis by intermediate filament type—a novel tool for surgical pathology. Lab Invest 1983;48:372–394.
21. Kahn HJ, Marks A, Thom H, et al. Role of antibody to S-100 protein in diagnostic pathology. Am J Clin Pathol 1983;79: 341–347.
22. Gown AM, Vogel AM, Hoak D, et al. Monoclonal antibodies specific for melanocytic tumors distinguish subpopulations of melanocytes. Am J Pathol 1986;123:195–203.
23. Kaufmann O, Deidesteimer T, Muehlenberg M, et al. Immunohistochemical differentiation of metastatic breast carcinomas from metastatic adenocarcinomas of other primary sites. Histopathology (Oxf) 1996;29:233–240.
24. Miettinen M, Lasota J. Gastrointestinal stromal tumors: definition, clinical, histological, immunohistochemical, and molecular genetic features and differential diagnosis. Virchows Arch 2001;438:1–12.
25. Bosman FT, Giard RWM, Nieuwenhuijen-Kruseman AC, et al. Human chorionic gonadotrophin and alpha fetoprotein in testicular germ cell tumors: a retrospective immunohistochemical study. Histopathology (Oxf) 1980;4:673–684.
26. Kurman KJ, Scardino PT, McIntire KR, et al. Cellular localization of alpha fetoprotein and human chorionic gonadotropin in germ cell tumors of the testis using an indirect immunoperoxidase technique: a new approach to classification utilizing tumor markers. Cancer (Phila) 1977;40:2136–2151.
27. Arnold A, Cossman J, Bakhshi A, et al. Immunoglobulin-gene rearrangements as unique clonal markers in human lymphoid neoplasms. N Engl J Med 1983;309:1593–1599.
28. Rowley JD. Recurring chromosome abnormalities in leukemia and lymphoma. Semin Hematol 1990;27:122–130.
29. Turc-Carel C, Philip I, Berger MP, et al. Chromosomal translocation in Ewing's carcoma. N Engl J Med 1983;309:497–498.
30. Whang-Peng J, Triche TJ, Knutsen T, et al. Chromosome translocation in peripheral neuroepithelioma. N Engl J Med 1984; 311:584–585.
31. Gerald WL, Ladanyi M, de Alava E, et al. Clinical, pathologic and molecular spectrum of tumors associated with t(11;22) (p13;q12): desmoplastic small round-cell tumors and its variants. J Clin Oncol 1998;16:3028–3036.
32. Atkin NB, Baker MC. Specific chromosome change, i(12p), in testicular tumors. Lancet 1982;2:1349–1356.
33. Ilson DH, Motzer RJ, Rodriguez E, et al. Genetic analysis in the diagnosis of neoplasms of unknown primary tumor site. Semin Oncol 1993;20:229–237.

34. Summersgill B, Goker H, Osin P, et al. Establishing germ cell origin of undifferentiated tumors by identifying gain of 12p material using comparative genomic hybridization analysis of paraffin-embedded samples. Diagn Mol Pathol 1998;7:260–265.
35. Yuge NK, Mochiki M, Nibu K, et al. Detection of Epstein–Barr virus in metastatic lymph nodes of patients with nasopharyngeal carcinoma and a primary unknown cancer. Arch Otolaryngol Head Neck Surg 2003;129:338–340.
36. Feinmesser R, Miyazaki I, Chenng R, et al. Diagnosis of nasopharyngeal carcinoma by DNA amplification of tissue obtained by fine-needle aspiration. N Engl J Med 1992;326:17–21.
37. Ramaswamy S, Golub TR. DNA microarrays in clinical oncology. J Clin Oncol 2002;20:1932–1941.
38. Hainsworth JD, Wrigth EP, Gray GF Jr, Greco FA. Poorly differentiated carcinoma of unknown primary site: correlation of light microscopic findings with response to cisplatin-based combination chemotherapy. J Clin Oncol 1987;5:1272–1280.
39. Hainsworth JD, Wright EP, Johnson DH, Davis BW, Greco FA. Poorly differentiated carcinoma of unknown primary site; clinical usefulness of immunoperoxidase staining. J Clin Oncol 1991;9:1931–1938.
40. Van der Gaast A, Verweij J, Planting AS, et al. The value of immunohistochemistry in patients with poorly differentiated adenocarcinoma and undifferentiated carcinoma of unknown primary site. J Cancer Res Clin Oncol 1996;122:181–185.
41. Motzer RJ, Rodriguez E, Reuter VE, et al. Molecular and cytogenic studies in the diagnosis of patients with midline carcinomas of unknown primary site. J Clin Oncol 1995;13: 274–283.
42. Greco FA, Vaughn WK, Hainsworth JD. Advanced poorly differentiated carcinoma of unknown primary site: recognition of a treatable syndrome. Ann Intern Med 1986;104:547–556.
43. Richardson RL, Schoumacher RA, Fer MF, et al. The unrecognized extragonadal germ cell cancer syndrome. Ann Intern Med 1981;94:181–186.
44. Nystrom JS, Weiner JM, Hoffelfinger-Juttner J, et al. Metastatic and histologic presentations in unknown primary cancer. Semin Oncol 1977;4:53–58.
45. Mayordomo JI, Guerra JM, Guijarro C, et al. Neoplasms of unknown primary site: a clinicopathological study of autopsied patients. Tumori 1993;79:321–324
46. Kole AC, Nieweg OE, Prium J, et al. Detection of unknown occult primary tumors using positron emission tomography. Cancer (Phila) 1998;82:1160–1166.
47. Lassen U, Daugaard G, Eigtved A, Damgaard K, Friberg L. ^{18}F-FDG whole body positron emission tomography (PET) in patients with unknown primary tumors (UPT). Eur J Cancer 1999;35:1076–1082.
48. Bohuslavizki KH, Klutmann S, Kroger S, Sonnemann U, et al. FDG PET detection of unknown primary tumors. J Nucl Med 2000;41:816–822.
49. Rades D, Kuhnel G, Wildfang I, et al. Localized disease in cancer of unknown primary (CUP): the value of positron emission tomography (PET) for individual therapeutic management. Ann Oncol 2001;12:1605–1609.
50. Stokkel MP, Terhaard CH, Hordijk GJ, van Rijk PP. The detection of unknown primary tumors in patients with cervical metastases by dual-head positron emission tomography. Oral Oncol 1999;35:390–394.
51. Aassar OS, Fischbein NJ, Caputo GR, et al. Metastatic head and neck cancer: role and usefulness of FDG PET in locating occult primary tumors. Radiology 1999;210:177–181.
52. Jungehulsing M, Scheidhauer K, Damm M, Pietrzyk U, Eckel H, Schicha H, Stennert E. 2(F)-fluoro-2-deoxy-D-glucose positron emission tomography is a sensitive tool for detection of occult primary cancer (carcinoma of unknown primary syndrome) with head and neck lymph node manifestation. Otolaryngol Head Neck Surg 2000;123:294–301.
53. Dede F, Ajoedi ND, Ansari SM, et al. Metastatic thyroid cancer occurring as an unknown primary lesion: the role of F-18 FDG positron emission tomography. Clin Nucl Med 2001;26: 396–399.
54. Nieder C, Gregoire V, Ang KK. Cervical lymph node metastases from occult squamous cell carcinoma: cut down a tree to get an apple? Int J Radiat Oncol Biol Phys 2000;50:727–733.
55. Richardson RL, Greco FA, Wolff S, et al. Extragonadal germ cell malignancy: value of tumor markers in metastatic carcinoma of young males. Proc Am Assoc Cancer Res 1979;20:204 (abstract).
56. Hainsworth JD, Greco FA. Poorly differentiated carcinoma of unknown primary site. In: Fer MF, Greco FA, Oldham R (eds). Poorly Differentiated Neoplasms and Tumors of Unknown Origin. Orlando: Grune & Stratton, 1986:189–202.
57. Fox RM, Woods RL, Tattersall MHN. Undifferentiated carcinoma in young men: the atypical teratoma syndrome. Lancet 1979;1:1316–1318.
58. Hainsworth JD, Johnson DH, Greco FA. Poorly differentiated neuroendocrine carcinoma of unknown primary site: a newly recognized clinicopathologic entity. Ann Intern Med 1988;109: 364–371.
59. Hainsworth JD, Greco FA. Treatment of patients with cancer of an unknown primary site. N Engl J Med 1995;329:257–263.
60. Hainsworth JD, Johnson DH, Greco FA. Cisplatin-based combination chemotherapy in the treatment of poorly differentiated carcinoma and poorly differentiated adenocarcinoma of unknown primary site: results of a 12 year experience at a single institution. J Clin Oncol 1992;10:912–922.
61. Falkson CI, Cohen GL. Mitomycin C, epirubicin and cisplatin versus mitomycin C alone as therapy for carcinoma of unknown primary origin. Oncology 1998;55:116–121.
62. Pavlidis N, Kalofonos H, Bafaloukos D, et al. Cisplatin/Taxol combination chemotherapy in 72 patients with metastatic cancer of unknown primary site: a phase II trial of the Hellenic Cooperative Oncology Group. Proc Am Soc Clin Oncol 1999; 18:195a (abstract).
63. Raber MN, Faintuch J, Abbruzzese J, et al. Continuous infusion 5-fluorouracil, etoposide and *cis*-diaminedichloroplatinum in patients with metastatic carcinoma of unknown primary site. Ann Oncol 1991;2:519–520.
64. Pavlidis N, Kosmidis P, Skaros D, et al. Subsets of tumors responsive to cisplatin or combinations in patients with carcinoma of unknown primary site. Ann Oncol 1992:236–241.
65. van der Gaast A, Verweij J, Henzen-Logmans SC, Rodenburg CJ, Stoter G. Carcinoma of unknown primary; identification of a treatable subset. Ann Oncol 1990;1:119–121.
66. Briasoulis E, Txavaris N, Fountzilas G, et al. Combination regimen with carboplatin, epirubicin and etoposide in metastatic carcinomas of unknown primary site: a Hellenic Cooperative Oncology Group phase II trial. Oncology 1998;55:426–430.
67. Moertel CG, Kovals LK, O'Connell MJ, et al. Treatment of neuroendocrine carcinomas with combined etoposide and cisplatin: evidence of major therapeutic activity in the anaplastic variants of these neoplasms. Cancer (Phila) 1991;68:227–233.
68. Greco FA, Hainsworth JD. Cancer of unknown primary site. In: Devita VT, Hellman S, Rosenberg SA (eds). Cancer Principles and Practice of Oncology, 6th ed. Philadelphia: Lippincott, Williams & Wilkins, 2001:2537–2560.
69. McKay CE, Hainsworth JD, Burris AA, et al. Treatment of metastatic poorly differentiated neuroendocrine carcinoma with paclitaxel/carboplatin/etoposide: a Minnie Pearl Cancer Research Network phase II trial. Proc Am Soc Clin Oncol 2002;21:158a.
70. Schildt RA, Kennedy PS, Chen TT, et al. Management of patients with metastatic adenocarcinoma of unknown origin: a Southwest Oncology Group study. Cancer Treat Rep 1983;67: 77–79.

71. Wong NP, Zee S, Zarbo RJ, et al. Coordinate expression of cytokeratins 7 and 20 defines unique subsets of carcinoma. Appl Immunohistochem 1995;3:99–107.
72. Tot T. Cytokeratins 20 and 7 as biomarkers: usefulness in discriminating primary from metastatic adenocarcinoma. Eur J Cancer 2002;38:758–763.
73. Brown RW, Campagna LB, Dunn JK, Cagle PT. Immunohistochemical identification of tumor markers in metastatic adenocarcinoma. A diagnostic adjunct in the determination of primary site. Am J Clin Pathol 1997;107:12–15.
74. Kaufman O, Deidesheimer T, Muehlenberg M, Deicke P, Dietel M. Immunohistochemical differentiation of metastatic breast carcinomas from metastatic adenocarcinomas of other common primary sites. Histopathology (Oxf) 1996;29:233–237.
75. Lagendijk JH, Mullink H, VanDiest PJ, Meijer GA, Meijer CJ. Tracing the origin of adenocarcinomas with unknown primary using immunohistochemistry: differential diagnosis between colonic and ovarian carcinomas as primary sites. Hum Pathol 1998;29:491–495.
76. Tot T. Adenocarcinomas metastatic to the liver: the value of cytokeratins 20 and 7 in the search for unknown primary tumors. Cancer (Phila) 1999;85:171–174.
77. McMillan JH, Levine E, Stephens RH. Computed tomography in the evaluation of metastatic adenocarcinoma from an unknown primary site. Radiology 1982;143:143–146.
78. Karsell PR, Sheedy PF, O'Connell MJ. Computerized tomography in search of cancer of unknown origin. JAMA 1982;248: 340–343.
79. Currow DC, Findlay M, Cox K, Harnett PR. Elevated germ cell markers in carcinoma of unknown primary site do not predict response to platinum-based chemotherapy. Eur J Cancer 1996; 32A:2357–2359.
80. Pavlidis N, Kalef-Ezra J, Briasoulis E, et al. Evaluation of six tumor markers in patients with carcinoma of unknown primary. Med Pediatr Oncol 1994;22:162–165.
81. Hochstere H, Wernz JC, Muggia FM. Intra-abdominal carcinomatosis with histologically normal ovaries [letter]. Cancer Treat Rep 1984;68:931–932.
82. Gooneratne S, Sassone M, Blaustein A, Talerman A. Serous surface papillary carcinoma of the ovary: a clinicopathologic study of 26 cases. Int J Gynecol Pathol 1982;1:258–269.
83. Chen KT, Flam MS. Peritoneal papillary serous carcinoma with long-term survival. Cancer (Phila) 1986;58:1371–1373.
84. August CZ, Murad TM, Newton M. Multiple focal extraovarian serous carcinoma. Int J Gynecol Pathol 1985;4:11–23.
85. Schorge JO, Muto MG, Welch WR, et al. Molecular evidence for multifocal papillary serous carcinoma of the peritoneum in patients with germ-line BRCA1 mutations. J Natl Cancer Inst 1998;90:841.
86. Shah IA, Jayram L, Gani OJ, et al. Papillary serous carcinoma of the peritoneum in a man. Cancer (Phila) 1998;82:860–866.
87. Bhatia SK, Saclarides TJ, Witt TR, et al. Hormone receptor studies in axillary metastases from occult breast cancer. Cancer (Phila) 1987;59:1170–1172.
88. Block EF, Meyer MA. Positron emission tomography in diagnosis of occult adenocarcinoma of the breast. Am Surg 1998;64: 906.
89. Schorn C, Fischer U, Luftner-Nagel S, Westerhof JP, Grabbe E. MRI of the breast in patients with metastatic disease of unknown primary. Eur Radiol 1999;9:470.
90. Henry-Tillman RS, Fischer U, Luftner-Nagel S, et al. MRI of the breast in patients with metastatic disease of unknown primary. Eur Radiol 1999;9:470–474.
91. Ashikari R, Rosen PP, Urban JA, Senoo T. Breast cancer presenting as an axillary mass. Ann Surg 1976;183:415–417.
92. Patel J, Nemoto T, Rosner D, et al. Axillary lymph node metastases from an occult breast cancer. Cancer (Phila) 1981;47: 2923–2927.
93. Merson M, Andreola S, Galimberti V, Bufalina R, Marchini S, Veronesi U. Breast carcinoma presenting as axillary metastases without evidence of a primary tumor. Cancer (Phila) 1992; 70:504.
94. Rosen PP. Axillary lymph node metastases in patients with occult noninvasive breast carcinoma. Cancer (Phila) 1980;46: 1298–1306.
95. Ellerbroek N, Holmes F, Singletary E, Evans H, Oswald M, McNeese M. Treatment of patients with isolated axillary nodal metastases from an occult primary carcinoma consistent with breast origin. Cancer (Phila) 1990;66:1461.
96. Tell DT, Khoury JM, Taylor HG, et al. Atypical metastasis from prostate cancer: clinical utility of the immunoperoxidase technique for prostate-specific antigen. JAMA 1985;253:3574–3575.
97. Gentile PS, Carloss HW, Huang T-Y, et al. Disseminated prostate carcinoma simulating primary lung cancer. Cancer (Phila) 1988;62:711–715.
98. Braams JW, Pruim J, Kole AC, et al. Detection of unknown primary head and neck tumor by positron emission tomography. Int J Oral Maxillofac Surg 1997;26:112–116.
99. Jones AS, Cook JA, Phillips DE, et al. Squamous carcinoma presenting as an enlarged cervical lymph node. Cancer (Phila) 1993;72:1756–1763.
100. Barrie JR, Knapper WH, Strong EW. Cervical nodal metatases of unknown origin. Am J Surg 1970;120:466–470.
101. Jesse RH, Perez CA, Fletcher GH. Cervical lymph node metastasis: unknown primary cancer. Cancer (Phila) 1973;31:854–859.
102. Coker DD, Casterline PF. Chambers RG, Jacques DA. Metastases to lymph nodes of the head and neck from an unknown primary site. Am J Surg 1977;134:517–522.
103. Jose B, Bosch A, Caldwell WL, Frias Z. Metastasis to neck from unknown primary tumor. Acta Radiol Oncol 1979;18:161–170.
104. Nordstrom DG, Tewfik HH, Latourette HB. Cervical lymph node metastases from an unknown primary. Int J Radiat Oncol Biol Phys 1979;5:73–76.
105. Fermont AC. Malignant cervical lymphadenopathy due to an unknown primary. Clin Radiol 1980;31:355–358.
106. Leipzig B, Winter ML, Hokanson JA. Cervical nodal metastases of unknown origin. Laryngoscope 1981;91:593–598.
107. Pacini P, Olmi P, Cellai E, Chiavacci A. Cervical lymph node metastases from an unknown primary tumour. Acta Radiol Oncol 1981;20:311–314.
108. Spiro RH, DeRose G, Strong EW. Cervical node metastasis of occult origin. Am J Surg 1983;146:441–446.
109. Mobit-Tabatabasi MA, Dasmaphapatra KS, Rush BF Jr., Ohanian M. Management of squamous cell carcinoma of unknown origin in cervical lymph nodes. Am Surg 1986;52:152–154.
110. Yang ZY, Hu YH, Yan JH, et al. Lymph node metastases in the neck from an unknown primary: Report on 113 patients. Acta Radiol Oncol 1983;22:17–22.
111. Carlson LS, Fletcher GH, Oswald MJ. Guidelines for the radiotherapeutic techniques for cervical metastases from an unknown primary. Int J Radiat Oncol Biol Phys 1986;12:2101–2110.
112. McCunniff AJ, Raber M. Metastatic carcinoma of the neck from an unknown primary. Int J Radiat Oncol Biol Phys 1986;12: 1849–1852.
113. Bataini JP, Rodriguez J, Jaulerry C, et al. Treatment of metastatic neck nodes secondary to an occult epidermoid carcinoma of the head and neck. Laryngoscope 1987;97:1080–1084.
114. De Braud F, Heilbrun LK, Ahmed K, et al. Metastatic squamous cell carcinoma of an unknown primary localized to the neck: advantages of an aggressive treatment. Cancer (Phila) 1989;64: 510–515.
115. Marcial-Vega VA, Cardenes H, Perez CA, et al. Cervical metastasis from unknown primaries: Radiotherapeutic management

and appearance of subsequent primaries. Int J Radiat Oncol Biol Phys 1990;19:919–928.

116. LeFevre JL, Coche-Dequeant D, Ton Van J, et al. Cervical lymph nodes from unknown primary tumor in 190 patients. Am J Surg 1990;160:443–446.
117. Weir L, Keane T, Cummings B, et al. Radiation treatment of cervical lymph node metastasis from an unknown primary: an analysis of outcome by treatment volume and other prognostic factors. Radiother Oncol 1995;35:206–211.
118. Brizel DM, Albers ME, Fisher SR, et al. Hyperfractionated irradiation with or without concurrent chemotherapy for locally advanced head and neck cancer. N Engl J Med 1998;338:1798–1804.
119. Wendt TG, Grabenbauer GG, Rodel CM, et al. Simultaneous radiochemotherapy versus radiotherapy alone in advanced head and neck cancer: a randomized multicenter study. J Clin Oncol 1998;16:1318–1324.
120. Coletier PJ, Garden AS, Morrison WH, Goepfert H, Geara F, Ang KK. Postoperative radiation for squamous cell carcinoma metastatic to cervical lymph nodes from an unknown primary site: outcomes and patterns of failure. Head Neck 1998;20: 674–679.
121. Fernandez JA, Suarez C, Martinez JA, Llorente JL, Rodrigo JP, Alvarez JC. Metastatic squamous cell carcinoma in cervical lymph nodes from an unknown primary tumor: prognostic factors. Clin Otolaryngol 1998;23:158–163.
122. Medini E, Medini AM, Lee CK, Gapany M, Levitt SR. The management of metastatic squamous cell carcinoma in cervical lymph nodes from an unknown primary. Am J Clin Oncol 1998; 21:121–126.
123. Sporn JR, Greenberg BR. Empirical chemotherapy for adenocarcinoma of unknown primary tumor site. Semin Oncol 1993;20: 261–267.
124. Altman E, Cadman E. An analysis of 1,539 patients with cancer of unknown primary site. Cancer (Phila) 1986;57:120–124.
125. Hess KR, Abbruzzese MC, Lenzi R, et al. Classification and regression free analysis of 1000 consecutive patients with unknown primary carcinoma. Clin Cancer Res 1999;5: 3403–3410.
126. Holmes FT, Fouts TL. Metastatic cancer of unknown primary site. Cancer (Phila) 1970;26:816–820.
127. Krementz ET, Cerise EJ, Foster DC, et al. Metastases of undetermined source. Curr Probl Cancer 1979;4:1–37.
128. Markman M. Metastatic adenocarcinoma of unknown primary site: analysis of 245 patients seen at the Johns Hopkins Hospital from 1965–1979. Med Pediatr Oncol 1982;10:569–574.
129. Moertel CG, Reitmeier RJ, Schutt AJ, et al. Treatment of the patient with adenocarcinoma of unknown primary site. Cancer (Phila) 1972;30:1469–1472.
130. Van de Wouw AJ, Janssen-Heijnen MLC, Coebergh JWW, et al. Epidemiology of unknown primary tumors; incidence and population-based survival of 1285 patients in Southeast Netherlands 1984–1992. Eur J Cancer 2002;38:409–413.
131. Levi F, Te VC, Erler G, et al. Epidemiology of unknown primary tumors. Eur J Cancer 2002;38:1810–1812.
132. Hainsworth JD, Erland JB, Kalman CA, et al. Carcinoma of unknown primary site: treatment with one-hour paclitaxel, carboplatin and extended schedule etoposide. J Clin Oncol 1997;15:2385–2393.
133. Greco FA, Gray J, Burris HA, et al. Taxane-based chemotherapy with carcinoma of unknown primary site. Cancer J 2001;7: 203–212.
134. Greco FA, Erland JB, Morrissey LH, et al. Phase II trials with docetaxel plus cisplatin or carboplatin. Ann Oncol 2000;11: 211–215.
135. Greco FA, Burris HA, Litchy S, et al. Gemcitabine, carboplatin, and paclitaxel for patients with unknown primary site: a Minnie Pearl Cancer Research Network study. J Clin Oncol 2002;20: 1651–1656.
136. Greco FA, Hainsworth JD, Yardley DA, et al. Sequential paclitaxel/carboplatin/etoposide followed by irinotecan/gemcitabine for patients with carcinoma of unknown primary site: a Minnie Pearl Cancer Research Network phase II trial. Proc Am Soc Clin Oncol 2002;21:161a.
137. Briasoulis E, Kalofonos H, Bafaloukos D, et al. Carboplatin plus paclitaxel in unknown primary carcinoma: a phase II Hellenic Cooperative Oncology Group study. J Clin Oncol 2000;18: 3101–3107.
138. Lastra E, Munoz A, Rubio I, et al. Paclitaxel, carboplatin, and oral etoposide in the treatment of patients with carcinoma of unknown primary site. Proc Am Soc Clin Oncol 2000;19: 579a.
139. Mukai H, Watanabe T, Ando M, et al. A safety and efficacy trial of docetaxel and cisplatin in patients with cancer of unknown primary. Proc Am Soc Clin Oncol 2003;22:646.
140. Culine S, Lortholary A, Voigt JJ, et al. Cisplatin in combination with either gemcitabine or irinotecan in carcinomas of unknown primary site: results of a randomized phase II study trial for the French Study Group on Carcinomas of Unknown Primary. J Clin Oncol 2003;21:3479–3482.

62

Solid Tumors of Childhood

Crawford J. Strunk and Sarah W. Alexander

Cancer in children, as compared with adults, is rare. From 1993 to 2000, the incidence of cancer in children and adolescents aged 0 to 19 years was approximately 160 cases per 1 million.[1] Despite the relative rarity of the disease and the progress made in therapy, cancer remains the leading cause of disease-related death in children ages 1 to 19 years[2] (Figure 62.1).

The most common forms of cancer are the acute leukemias and central nervous system tumors. As a group, solid tumors make up approximately one-third of all cancer diagnoses in children. The incidence and types of solid tumors vary by age[1] (Figure 62.2). In general, African-Americans and Asian/Pacific Islanders are less likely to develop cancer than children who are Caucasian.[1] Boys have a higher incidence of cancer than do girls and also have slightly lower overall cure rates.[1]

Screening and Family History

The childhood cancer that has undergone significant study regarding utility of screening is neuroblastoma. Despite extensive efforts, these screening programs have not been shown to decrease disease-related mortality.[3–6] There are, however, children who are at increased risk of developing cancer for whom screening is indicated.[7] For example, patients with Beckwith–Wiedemann syndrome benefit from routine surveillance for Wilm's tumor.[8]

For most children with cancer the disease is a sporadic event; however, for a small fraction the disease is related to a familial cancer syndrome. Certain clinical features should make the clinician consider a familial cancer syndrome, including cancer occurring at an unusually young age (compared with the usual age of presentation for the type of cancer), multifocal development of cancer in a single organ or bilateral development of cancer in paired organs, development of more than one primary tumor of any type in a single individual, family history of cancer of the same type in a close relative, high rate of cancer within a family, and occurrence of cancer in an individual or a family exhibiting congenital anomalies or birth defects.[7]

Environmental Factors

Environmental factors contribute to an increased risk of cancer in children. Exposure to ionizing radiation increases the risk of leukemia, thyroid cancer, and osteosarcoma.[9–12] The risk of ionizing radiation associated with radiographic procedures such as repeated X-rays and computed tomography (CT) has led to considerations of more judicious use of imaging studies in children.[13] There is no measurable increased risk associated with exposure to electromagnetic pulses associated with underground transformers or high-energy electrical stations.[14]

There are an increasing number of childhood cancer survivors who are at risk for secondary malignancies related to the therapy of their primary cancer, such as chemotherapy-related malignancies, most notably topoisomerase and alkylator-related leukemia, and radiation-related secondary neoplasms, including sarcomas, skin cancers, and brain tumors.[15,16]

Clinical Presentation

Persistent low-grade fevers, weight loss, and night sweats are frequent presenting symptoms. Bony tumors often are diagnosed weeks to months after treatment of relatively minor trauma whose symptoms fail to resolve.[17] Most often, however, a lump or mass, with or without pain, first noted by either the parent or the child is usually the first presenting symptom in the child with a solid tumor.[17]

Principles of Therapy

Treatment of solid tumors in pediatrics involves the combination of chemotherapy, surgery, and radiation. In general, children tolerate more intensive therapy than their adult counterparts. Special considerations in children include appropriate dosing of drugs (often based on limited pharmaceutical data); ability to comply with prescribed therapy (for example, the need for anesthesia for radiation), and special concerns for long-term toxicities of therapy.

Late Effects of Therapy

One in 900 adults are survivors of childhood cancer.[18] These individuals are at risk for significant long-term sequelae, including growth impairment, infertility, endocrinopathies, cardiac and pulmonary disease, hearing and visual deficiencies, and orthopedic problems as well as secondary malig-

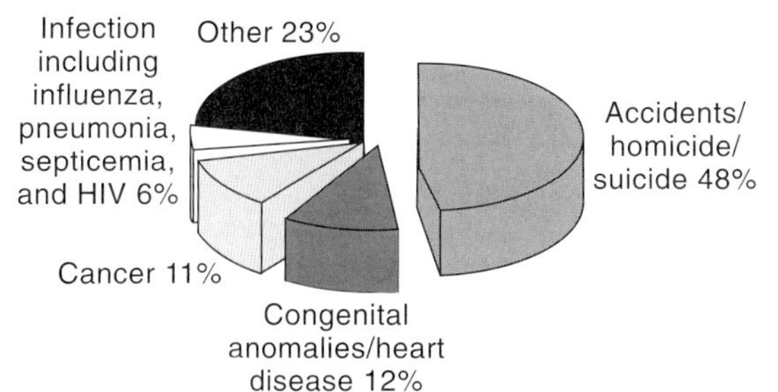

FIGURE 62.1. Leading causes of death in children ages 1 to 14 years.

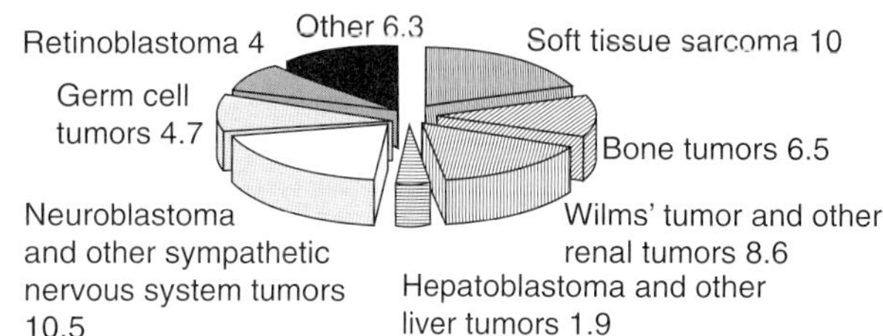

FIGURE 62.2. Incidence rates of solid tumors in children less than 15 years of age.

nancies.[19] In addition, issues of school function and the psychosocial impact of therapy often remain significant years after the completion of therapy. Awareness and surveillance of late effects has improved, and long-term follow-up guidelines for the care of patients who are survivors of childhood cancer have been developed.[20]

Neuroblastoma

Epidemiology

Neuroblastoma (NB) is the most common extracranial solid tumor in children, with a reported incidence of 8 per 1 million children ages 0 to 19 years, which equates to approximately 600 new cases of NB diagnosed in the United States every year.[1] The peak age of incidence is in the 1- to 3-year-old age group. Most cases of NB are considered sporadic; however, approximately 1% to 2% of all cases are familial.[21]

Biology and Histology

Neuroblastoma cells are derived from primitive sympathetic chain cells, and a portion of these tumors have amplification of the n-*myc* oncogene, which resides on the distal end of the short arm of chromosome 2.[22] Some tumors have double minute chromatid bodies in which the region containing the n-*myc* oncogene has become amplified as an extrachromosomal component.[23] Transgenic mice that have targeted expression of n-*myc* develop neuroblastoma-like tumors.[24] Other genetic abnormalities associated with neuroblastoma cells include the chromosome 1p deletions, gain of 17q, and abnormal expression of *Trk-A*, a member of the neurotrophin receptor family important in the regulation of cell survival and growth.[25–27] Histologically, neuroblastomas are small uniformly sized cells with associated neuropil. The presence of Homer Wright pseudorosettes is a common diagnostic feature.

Clinical Presentation

Children with localized neuroblastoma may present only with a painless mass that may be found incidentally by imaging done for unrelated reasons.[17] An advanced disease may present with persistent fevers, bone pain, signs of spinal cord compression, or "raccoon eyes" with disease metastatic to the orbits.[28] Children can present with catecholamine-mediated signs or symptoms, such as hypertension or, rarely, vasoactive intestinal polypeptide(VIP)-induced diarrhea,[28] and rarely paraneoplastic symptoms, including opsoclonus myoclonus.

Diagnosis and Staging

Any patient suspected of having neuroblastoma requires complete staging evaluation including CT of the chest, abdomen, and pelvis, bilateral bone marrow aspirates and biopsies, bone scan and metaiodobenzylguanidine (MIBG) scan, and urine specimens for catecholamines and homovanillic acid (HVA) and vanillylmandelic acid (VMA).[29] Fluorodeoxyglucose-positron emission tomography (FDG-PET) scanning of patients with neuroblastoma is evolving for staging and treatment response.[30–32] Diagnosis is usually by light microscopic evaluation of a biopsy, although some patients with widely disseminated disease are diagnosed by bone marrow evidence of disease and elevated urine catecholamines.

Anatomic staging of neuroblastoma is based on the International Neuroblastoma Staging System (Table 62.1).[29] Special consideration must be made with regard to stage 4S, or "special" disease. Patients with 4S disease are those under 1 year of age who present with tumor that may be metastatic but is limited only to liver, skin, and bone marrow (with less than 10% involvement).[33]

Prognostic Factors

Age (with younger children having a better outcomes) and stage of disease remain critical prognostic determinants. Biologic factors that have been validated to be associated with a

TABLE 62.1. International neuroblastoma staging system.

Stage	*Definition*
1	Localized tumor with gross total resection
2a	Localized tumor with incomplete resection
2b	Localized tumor with or without incomplete resection with ipsilateral positive nodes
3	Tumor that has spread across midline by either direct extension or by lymph node metastasis
4	Disseminated disease with distant metastasis
4s	See text for full description of this stage

Source: Adapted from Brodeur et al.,[29] by permission of *Journal of Clinical Oncology.*

TABLE 62.2. Risk group schema for neuroblastoma.

INSS stage	*Age*	*MYCN status*	*Shimada histology*	*DNA ploidy*	*Risk group*
1	0–21 years	Any	Any	Any	Low
2A/2B	<365 days	Any	Any	Any	Low
	≥365 days–21 years	Nonamplified	Any	—	Low
	≥365 days–21 years	Amplified	Favorable	—	Low
	≥365 days–21 years	Amplified	Unfavorable	—	High
3	<365 days	Nonamplified	Any	Any	Intermediate
	<365 days	Amplified	Any	Any	High
	≥365 days–21 years	Nonamplified	Favorable	—	Intermediate
	≥365 days–21 years	Nonamplified	Unfavorable	—	High
	≥365 days–21 years	Amplified	Any	—	High
4	<365 days	Nonamplified	Any	Any	Intermediate
	<365 days	Amplified	Any	Any	High
	≥365 days–21 years	Any	Any	—	High
4s	<365 days	Nonamplified	Favorable	>1	Low
	<365 days	Nonamplified	Any	= 1	Intermediate
	<365 days	Nonamplified	Unfavorable	Any	Intermediate
	<365 days	Amplified	Any	Any	High

Source: By permission of the Children's Oncology Groups INSS, individual neuroblastoma staging system; MYCN, status of the N-MYC oncogene.

less-favorable prognosis include amplification of the n-*myc* oncogene, hypodiploid cells, and 1p LOH (loss of heterozygosity).[34–38] The staging system developed by Shimada, which includes data regarding patient age, stage, and histopathologic information, has been shown to be a valid prognostic tool.[39]

Current Principles of Therapy

Surgery, radiation, and chemotherapy are all important tools in the therapy of children with neuroblastoma. The Children's Oncology Group (COG) neuroblastoma trial used a risk-based treatment plan (Table 62.2). Age of the patient, stage of the disease, n-*myc* status, Shimada histology of the tumor, and DNA index determine these risk groups. Patients with low-risk disease have an excellent event-free survival and overall survival rate with tumor resection alone, including those who do not have a gross total resection (Table 62.3). In addition, those patients who do relapse are highly likely to be cured with salvage surgery and chemotherapy.[40,41]

Patients with intermediate-risk neuroblastoma also have a very good prognosis, although they require significantly more intensive therapy (see Table 62.3). They are treated with multiagent chemotherapy, most often including cyclophosphamide, doxorubicin, cisplatinum, or carboplatinum and etoposide. Surgery is often done after initial induction

TABLE 62.3. Selected clinical trials for therapy of low- or intermediate-risk neuroblastoma.

Group/date of study closure	*Stage*	*Intervention/chemotherapeutic regimen*	*N*	*EFS/OS/ median F/U*	*Reference*
CCG 3881 1995	1	Surgery alone	374	93%/99% at 4 years for stage 1 81%/98% at 4 years for stage 2	Perez 2000[41]
POG 9047 1998	1	Surgery alone	329	91%/96% at 5 years	Alvarado 2000[40]
POG 8742/9244 1994	2B/3	Complete resection vs. incomplete resection with both groups treated with either VCR/CDDP/VP16/CPM (8742) or VCR/CARBO/VP16/CPM (9244) with second look surgery ± XRT	49	85% EFS with complete resection at 2 years 70% EFS with incomplete resection at 2 years	Strother 1997[274]
CCG 3891 1995	3	Stage 3 patients stratified by age and biologic features Lower-risk patients treated with less-intensive therapy per (CDDP, CPM, DOXO, ETOP) Higher-risk patients treated with dose-intensive therapy and randomized to ABMT vs. chemotherapy	143 lower risk 85 higher risk	Biologically favorable any age 100%/100% at 4 years Biologically unfavorable age <1 90%/93% Biologically unfavorable age >1 54%/65%	Matthay 1998[275]

ABMT, autologous bone marrow transplant; CARBO, carboplatin; CDDP, cisplatin; CPM, cyclophosphamide; DOXO, doxorubicin; CCG, Children's Cancer Group; EFS, event-free survival; OS, overall survival; F/U, follow-up; POG, Pediatric Oncology Group; VCR, vincristine; VP16/ETOP, etoposide; XRT, radiotherapy.

TABLE 62.4. Selected clinical trials of the treatment of high-risk neuroblastoma.

Group/date study closed	*Stage*	*Intervention/chemotherapeutic regimen*	*N*	*Outcomes/comments*	*Reference*
Study Group of Japan 1999	4	Comparison of 3 induction regimens: CDDP, CPM, VCR, DOXO vs. CPPD, CPM, ETOP, DOXO vs. dose intensive CDDP, CPM, ETOP, DOXO with SCT	301	EFS 23%–36%, OS 32%–42% at 5 years, worse outcomes in those with amplified n-*myc*, improved outcomes for those with intensified chemotherapy, of note not all patients underwent SCT	Kaneko 2002[276]
EBMT STR 1992	4	Nonrandomized megatherapy with SCT after induction chemotherapy and surgery	110	26% EFS at 5 years, those patients with evidence of disease in bone or bone marrow at time of SCT fared worse	Ladenstein 1998[43]
CCG 1996	3/4	Induction chemotherapy followed by SCT vs. continued chemotherapy, followed by CRA vs. no CRA	539	Outcomes for those undergoing SCT superior to those treated with chemo alone (EFS at 3 years 34% vs. 22%, respectively) Outcomes for those treated with CRA superior to those with no further therapy (EFS at 3 years 46% vs. 29%	Matthay 1999[42]
DFCI/CHOP/ Emory/Utah 1998	3/4	Single arm induction therapy followed by tandem SCT	39	58% EFS at 3 years (estimated)	Grupp 2000[44]
Chicago Pilot II Study 2000	4	Single arm induction therapy + triple SCT	26	57% EFS at 3 years	Kletzel 2002[46]

SCT, stem cell transplant; CDDP, cisplatin; CPM, cyclophosphamide; CRA, *cis*-retinoic acid; DOXO, doxorubicin; CCG, Children's Cancer Group; VCR, vincristine; ETOP, etoposide; DFCI, Dana-Farber Cancer Institute; CHOP, Children's Hospital of Philadelphia; EBMT STR, European Bone Marrow Transplantation Group Solid Tumor Registry.

chemotherapy. Radiation therapy is used to treat postsurgical residual disease.

Improvement of therapy for patients with high-risk neuroblastomas has been modest, with an overall survival of 30% or less.[42] Treatment usually involves multiagent induction chemotherapy, surgical resection of the primary site of disease, and radiation of residual disease followed by autologous stem cell transplantation (Table 62.4). Autologous stem cell transplant has been shown to have a measurable impact on overall survival.[42–47] In addition, in this high-risk group the use of isotretinoin posttransplantation, which is thought to induce differentiation of neuroblastoma cells, has been shown to be of benefit.[42]

Unique to neuroblastoma is the therapy of stage 4s disease. Despite widely disseminated disease, so long as the biology of the tumor is favorable, infants treated with surgery of the primary tumor site and little if any subsequent chemotherapy have an excellent prognosis (Table 62.5).[48,49]

Late Effects of Therapy

Late effects of treatment for neuroblastoma are dependent on the therapy required. Patients with high-risk disease are at greatest risk of significant long-term morbidity, including cardiac and renal dysfunction, short stature, hearing loss, and secondary malignancies.[50,51]

TABLE 62.5. Selected clinical trials of the treatment of infants with neuroblastoma.

Group/date study closed	*Stage*	*Intervention/regimen*	*N*	*EFS/OS/median F/U/comments*	*Reference*
POG— infant 1987	4/4s	Stage 4 treated with CPM/DOXO. second-look surgery Stage 4s treated with stage 4 regimen vs. observation	Stage 4: 62 Stage 4s: 51	Stage 4: 40%/60% at 5 years (est) Stage 4s: therapy group: 75%/88%, vs. observation group: 50%/92%	Strother 1995[277]
POG 1996	4s	Determine prognostic relevance of age and tumor biology in addition to impact of therapy	110	85% EFS at 3 years No significant difference in those who received therapy vs. observation alone; those with unfavorable biology had a significantly worse outcome	Katzenstein 1998[49]
CCG 1995	4s	Supportive care or low-dose therapy in symptomatic patients	80	86%/92% for all patients at 5 years	Nickerson 2000[48]

CPM, cyclophosphamide; DOXO, doxorubicin; CCG, Children's Cancer Group; POG, Pediatric Oncology Group.

Wilms' Tumor and Other Renal Tumors

Epidemiology

Wilms' tumor is the most common renal cancer in children, with an incidence of 7.6 per million children less than 15 years of age per year.[1] The mean age of presentation is 3 years for unilateral disease and 2 years for bilateral disease.[52]

Wilms' tumor is associated with several congenital syndromes, including WAGR (Wilms' tumor, aniridia, genitourinary malformations, and mental retardation), Beckwith–Wiedeman, sporadic hemihypertrophy, and Denys–Drash syndromes.[53,54] These patients often present at younger ages and have a higher incidence of bilateral disease but have excellent prognosis with modern treatment regimens.[55,56]

Biology and Histology

Wilms' tumor is associated with the loss of function of certain tumor suppressor genes, including Wilms' tumor suppressor genes 1 and 2 (WT1 and WT2), as well as the familial loci FWTI and FWT2.[57] In addition, the loss of heterozygosity of 16q as well as 1p is found in Wilms' tumor patients and may be associated with poor outcome.[58] The histology of Wilms' tumor classically includes three distinct cell types: the blastema, stromal, and epithelial. Anaplasia in Wilms' tumor is described as the presence of cells within the tumor sample with very enlarged polypoid nuclei.[59]

Clinical Presentation

Wilms' tumors most commonly present with parent-detected abdominal distension or an abdominal mass or abdominal pain, gross hematuria, or hypertension.[60]

Diagnosis and Staging

The initial evaluation of a child suspected of having Wilms' tumor should include CT of the chest, abdomen, and pelvis and a renal ultrasound (with evaluation for intravascular tumor spread). Rare perioperative sudden death has been reported from pulmonary emboli from intravascular tumors.[61] Primary nephrectomy is the initial therapy for most children treated in North America, and therefore initial biopsy for diagnosis is usually not undertaken. Patients with clear cell sarcoma and rhabdoid tumors of the kidney should also have radionucleotide bone imaging in addition to magnetic resonance imaging (MRI) evaluation of the brain. The National Wilms Tumor Study Group (NWTSG) has long-standing staging criteria that are used for all pediatric renal tumors, irrespective of histology (Table 62.6).[62]

Prognostic Factors

Tumor stage is an important factor in prognosis, along with tumor histology, with those with anaplastic disease having worse outcomes than others.[59,63] Biologic factors that are associated with worse outcomes include loss of heterozygosity at arms 16q and 1p.[58]

TABLE 62.6. Staging system for renal tumors according to the National Wilms Tumor Study Group.

Stage	*Description*
I	Tumor confined to the kidney and completely resected.
II	Tumor extends beyond the kidney but is completely resected. Includes at least one of the following: penetration of the renal capsule, invasion of the renal sinus vessels, biopsy of the tumor prior to removal, local tumor spill.
III	Gross or residual microscopic tumor postoperatively, including inoperable tumor, positive surgical margins, tumor spillage involving peritoneal surfaces, regional lymph node metastases, or transected tumor thrombus.
IV	Hematogenous or lymphatic metastasis outside the abdomen (e.g., lung, liver, bone, brain)
V	Bilateral renal tumors at onset

Source: From Beckwith,[62] by permission of *Pediatric and Developmental Pathology.*

Current Principles of Therapy

Patients with stage 1 favorable histology (FH) (no anaplasia) WT have an excellent prognosis with primary nephrectomy and short-duration chemotherapy with vincristine and actinomycin and possibly with vincristine alone.[64–67] Small tumors (less than 550g) and age less than 24 months at diagnosis have been shown to be favorable prognostic factors,[68] prompting the evaluation of nephrectomy alone in this population. This strategy was evaluated in the NWTS-V study. The study was closed when the strict stopping rules were met with excess relapse rate in the group who did not receive adjuvant therapy; however, the overall survival (OS) at 2 years in both groups remains 100%.[69]

Patients with stage II or III favorable histology Wilms' tumor have an OS between 80% and 90%.[70] The recent group studies have focused on minimizing long-term risks of therapy, primarily the risks of cardiomyopathy from adriamycin and the risks of second malignant neoplasms and effects on growth and fertility from radiation therapy. For patients with stage II FH WT, neither the addition of adriamycin to actinomycin and vincristine nor the addition of abdominal radiation improved OS.[66,67] For patients with stage III disease, the addition of adriamycin and abdominal radiation both lead to statistically significant although modest improvements in OS, with some protocols using neoadjuvant chemotherapy.[67,71,72]

Patients with stage IV Wilms' tumor (WT) metastatic to lung also have a very good OS of approximately 80%. In NWTS-3, patients received vincristine, actinomycin, and adriamycin in addition to whole-lung irradiation, with abdominal radiation only for those with stage III abdominal disease.[67,70] In an attempt to avoid the acute and chronic toxicities of pulmonary radiation, the International Society of Paediatric Oncology (SIOP) investigated the use of prenephrectomy chemotherapy. Those who obtained a complete response (CR) in terms of their pulmonary disease after 6 weeks of therapy did not receive pulmonary radiation therapy, with a relapse-free survival (RFS) and OS of 83%.[73]

Patients with stage V disease (bilateral disease) provide unique challenges in terms of providing effective cancer therapy while at the same time allowing for the preservation of adequate renal function. For those patients with favorable histology, the use of "nephron-sparing" surgery, with resection of tumor masses, as opposed to nephrectomy in addition to neoadjuvant chemotherapy, has led to overall survival rates approaching 70%, with 80% of survivors having normal renal function in long-term follow-up.[74,75]

The Use of Neoadjuvant Therapy

The use of prenephrectomy chemotherapy has been a source of much controversy, with North American institutions traditionally not pursuing neoadjuvant therapy whereas it is the standard of care in many European centers.[76] A series of studies done by SIOP has investigated various durations of preoperative chemotherapy with the goal of decreasing the need for abdominal irradiation by making more tumors amenable to complete surgical removal and decreasing the rate of intraoperative tumor rupture or spill.[77,78] This strategy has not been followed by the NWTSG because of concerns of misdiagnosis by reliance on initial biopsy alone, difficulty in interpreting histologic information in pretreated tumors, and loss of upfront staging information.[70]

Therapy for Relapsed Disease

Patients with recurrent Wilms' tumor who have not previously received doxorubicin, who have an abdominal recurrence only and did not receive prior abdominal radiation therapy, and those who relapse more than 12 months after completions of primary therapy have a relatively favorable prognosis.[79] Chemotherapeutic agents used in this group include carboplatinum, etoposide, ifosfamide, and cyclophosphamide. The use of stem cell transplant for patients with less-favorable characteristics has been explored, but there are no data to date that reveal superiority of this modality.[80,81]

Late Effects of Therapy

Renal failure posttherapy for Wilms' tumor is relatively rare (less than 1%) and is most often caused by either bilateral nephrectomy done as therapy of bilateral disease, secondary to underlying renal disease (Denys–Drash syndrome), or by radiation nephritis.[82] Other significant late effects include risk of cardiac dysfunction (primarily related to adriamycin), pulmonary disease and infertility (primarily related to radiation), and second malignant neoplasms.[83–85]

Other Renal Tumors

Clear Cell Sarcoma of the Kidney

Clear cell sarcoma of the kidney is the second most common renal neoplasm in children. Mean age of diagnosis is 36 months with a 2:1 male to female preponderance.[86] These tumors metastasize to bone in addition to lung, brain, and other soft tissues.[87] The outcome of patients with clear cell sarcoma is inferior to that for those with a favorable histology Wilms' tumor. Use of doxorubicin in the therapy for patients with clear cell sarcoma appears to be important.[86]

Rhabdoid Tumor

Rhabdoid tumor of the kidney is an extremely aggressive renal neoplasm that usually presents in infancy. The tumor is extremely rare in those over the age of 5 years, with 85% of patients presenting before the age of 2 years.[88] The clinical presentation of children with rhabdoid tumor differs somewhat from those with Wilms' tumor in that they are more likely to have gross or microscopic hematuria, fever, and hypercalcemia.[89]

Rhabdoid tumors, whose cellular origin is unknown, were initially described as a distinct entity in 1978[90] and contain a unique deletion of 22 q11-12, localized to the *h*SNF5/INII gene, which occasionally is a germ-line mutation.[91]

Patients with rhabdoid tumors (majority in stage III or IV) have a dismal prognosis, with 80% of children dead of progressive disease within 1 year of diagnosis[88,92] despite aggressive chemotherapy, surgery, and radiation therapy.[93] A unique association with rhabdoid tumor is the finding of associated brain tumors that may be either from metastatic disease or from synchronous tumors in a susceptible host. Staging at the time of diagnosis must include an MRI of the brain.

Renal Cell Carcinoma

Renal cell carcinoma is extremely rare in children. When it does occur, evaluation and therapy are based on data from adult studies. There are two unique forms of renal cell carcinoma that rarely occur in children. The first is associated with a translocation of Xp11.2.[94,95] The second is renal medullary carcinoma, primarily associated with individuals with sickle cell trait.[96]

Osteosarcoma

Epidemiology

Osteosarcoma is the most common primary bone tumor of children, with an incidence of 5 per 1 million children, with an increased incidence in late adolescence.[1] Osteosarcomas have been reported in patients as old as the sixth decade, but the peak age of incidence is in the second and third decades of life.[97] Boys and African-Americans have a higher predilection for development of osteosarcoma. Ionizing radiation has been associated with an increased risk of developing osteosarcoma.[98] In addition, germ-line defects in the RB1 gene and those patients with Li–Fraumeni syndrome have an increased incidence of osteosarcoma.[7]

Biology and Histology

Osteosarcomas arise from primitive mesenchymal stem cells. Histologically, osteosarcoma, unlike chondrosarcomas and fibrosarcomas, appears as a malignant sarcomatous stroma with evidence of production of osteoid.

The underlying biology of osteosarcoma is not well understood. There is an association with hereditary retinoblastoma syndrome and Li–Fraumeni syndrome. Cytogenetic analysis has shown not only loss of heterozygosity (LOH) at the 13q region (RB gene) and 17p region (p53), but also at the 3q and 18q regions, areas that may harbor additional tumor suppressor genes.[99,100] In approximately 20% of osteosarcomas, the 12q13-14 region, the area that codes for MDM2, is amplified,[101] suggesting increased activity of MDM2 in osteosarcoma. MDM2 is an intracellular protein that interacts with, and renders inactive, the p53 tumor suppressor gene.[97]

Clinical Presentation

Osteosarcoma generally presents as pain or swelling of a bone or joint with or without a soft tissue mass. The usual time from onset of symptoms to time of diagnosis often is prolonged, ranging from 3 to 6 months or longer.[17] Often a sports-related injury is recalled with the initial onset of symptoms. Relatively rarely, osteosarcoma can present secondary to a pathologic fracture. Signs of systemic disease such as weight loss and fevers are rarely noted. The most common site of presentation is in the metaphyses of long bones. The most frequent sites are the distal femur, proximal tibia, and proximal humerus.[102]

Diagnosis and Staging

Plain film examination of the affected area provides clues to the diagnosis. Some osteosarcomas are most often lytic lesions, with a *starburst pattern*, that may have characteristic findings including Codman's triangle. MRI and CT are used to further define the anatomy of the primary site of disease.

Approximately 15% to 20% of patients with osteosarcoma are noted to have metastases at diagnosis.[102] About 80% of those with metastases have pulmonary metastases.[102,103] The majority of the remaining 20% of metastases are bone lesions.[102,103] Because metastatic disease at diagnosis affects not only therapy but also prognosis, all patients should undergo staging evaluation before beginning therapy, including CT of the chest and radionuclide bone scan. Diagnosis of osteosarcoma is made based on histopathologic review of biopsy of the primary lesion.

Prognostic Factors

The single most significant prognostic factor in patients with osteosarcoma remains extent of disease at presentation, with those with metastatic disease at diagnosis continuing to have a poor overall survival.[104] Tumors of the axial skeleton are more difficult to eradicate than those of the extremities, partly related to feasibility of complete surgical resection.[105] Large tumors and those occurring in children less than 10 years old are also associated with poorer outcomes. Biologic factors that may predispose to worse outcomes include LOH of the RB gene locus, overexpression of HER-2, and hyperdiploidy.[106–108] Last, response to neoadjuvant chemotherapy is a powerful prognostic factor with those individuals with less than 10% of residual tumor visible in the resection specimen faring better than those with a larger percentage of viable disease.[109,110]

Current Principles of Therapy

Before 1970, patients with osteosarcoma had a very poor prognosis, with a 5-year event-free survival (EFS) of only 20%.[111] Historically, most patients died of relapsed disease after amputation of the primary tumor. Current principles of therapy include neoadjuvant chemotherapy, surgery for local control, and postsurgical adjuvant chemotherapy; approximately 70% of all patients with nonmetastatic disease at diagnosis can be cured.[102] Radiotherapy remains part of local control measures when tumors are located in sites not amenable to surgery.[112]

Three drugs, methotrexate, cisplatinum, and doxorubicin, are the backbone to chemotherapeutic treatment of osteosarcoma (Table 62.7).[113] Somewhat more recently the addition of ifosfamide and etoposide as a combination regimen has been shown to have therapeutic utility.[114,115] Local control surgery is most commonly performed after 2 to 3 months of neoadjuvant chemotherapy. A recent Pediatric Oncology group study reported no difference in EFS for patients given presurgical chemotherapy for 12 weeks compared to those who underwent primary resection at the time of diagnosis followed by chemotherapy.[116] Advantages to neoadjuvant chemotherapy include tumor shrinkage, facilitating possible limb salvage procedures, and prognostic information based on the histologic response of the excised tumor. Risks of neoadjuvant chemotherapy include progression of disease before surgery.

Patients with metastatic lesions at diagnosis fare poorly, with an overall survival of 21% to 30%.[117,118] Within the group of patients with metastatic disease, favorable characteristics include the site of metastatic disease (with lung only being more favorable than metastatic disease to bone) and completeness of surgical resection of all tumor sites.[104] To date efforts to improve outcomes with intensified chemotherapy have not shown substantial benefit (Table 62.8).[119]

TABLE 62.7. Selected recent clinical trials for primary nonmetastatic osteosarcoma.

Group/date study closed	*Intervention/chemotherapeutic regimen*	*N*	*EFS/OS/median F/U/comments*	*Source*
POG 1993	Presurgical chemotherapy vs. immediate surgery	106	Presurgical chemo 61%/76% at 5 years (est) Immediate surgery 69%/79% No statistical advantage to presurgical chemotherapy	Goorin 2003[116]
Rizzoli Institute 1999	MTX/DOXO/CDDP/IFO vs. dose-intensive IFO/MTX/CDDP/DOXO for pre- and postsurgical chemotherapy	363	Standard vs. dose-intensified: 60%/74% vs. 65%/80% at 5 years (est) No benefit shown with increased dose intensity	Bacci 2003[278]
SSG 1997	MTX/CDDP/DOXO postsurgery in good responders vs. IFO/ETOP in poor responders	113	Good responders 68% EFS at 5 years (est) Poor responders 53% EFS	Smeland 2003[279]

CDDP, cisplatin; DOXO, doxorubicin; ETOP, etoposide; IFO, ifosfamide; MTX, methotrexate; POG, Pediatric Oncology Group; SSG, Scandinavian Sarcoma Study Group.

TABLE 62.8. **Selected clinical trials for treatment of primary metastatic osteosarcoma.**

Group/date study closed	*Intervention/chemotherapeutic regimen*	*N*	*EFS/OS/median F/U*	*Reference*
MSKCC 1984	MTX/DOXO/BCD	62	11% survival; median survival 20 months	Meyers 1993[103]
London Bone and Soft Tissue Tumour Service 1999	CDDP/DOXO/IFO + CDDP + ETOP followed by IFO and SCR	30	17% OS at 3 years	Janinis 2002[118]
Rizzoli Institute 2000	MTX/CDDP/DOXO/IFO	57	21%/55% at 2 years	Bacci 2003[117]
POG Study closed	Dose-intensified ETOP/IFO followed by surgery and MTX/DOXO/CDDP/IFO/ETOP	43	Projected 2-year progression-free survival for those with lung metastases only 39%	Goorin 2002[119]

BCD, bleomycin/cyclophosphamide/dactinomycin; CDDP, cisplatin; DOXO, doxorubicin; ETOP, etoposide; IFO, ifosfamide; MTX, methotrexate, MSKCC, Memorial Sloan-Kettering Cancer Center; POG, Pediatric Oncology Group.

Surgical Management

Historically, amputation was the preferred surgical approach[111]; however, during the 1980s limb-sparing surgical techniques were developed in conjunction with improved diagnostic imaging.[120] By the late 1990s, studies suggested patients with limb salvage surgery had no more local recurrences than those who underwent amputation if surgical margins were adequate, including those initially presenting with pathologic fracture.[121–124]

Therapy of Recurrent Disease

Patients who have recurrent disease generally have a grave prognosis.[125,126] Lungs are the most common site of recurrence, although recurrence can occur locally and at distant bony sites.[127] Prognostic factors that may influence long-term survival in these patients include the relapse-free interval, sites of recurrent disease, number of pulmonary nodules, and feasibility of complete surgical resection.[126,128]

Late Effects of Therapy

Despite surgical advances, orthopedic issues related to amputation or limb salvage procedures can give rise to lifelong impairments. In addition, cardiomyopathy related to anthracycline therapy and hearing deficits related to cisplatinum are common among survivors.[129]

Ewing's Sarcoma Family of Tumors

Epidemiology

Ewing's sarcoma is the second most common primary malignancy of bone in childhood. It is primarily a tumor of bony origin but can also arise from soft tissues. Included in the Ewing's sarcoma family of tumors (ESFT) is the peripheral primitive neuroectodemal tumor (PPNET).

The majority of individuals diagnosed with Ewing's sarcoma are between the ages of 10 and 20 years.[130] Ewing's sarcoma is not associated with any known familial cancer syndromes, nor are there known environmental causes.[131] The disease is significantly more common in Caucasians than in African-Americans and shows a slight male preponderance.[132]

Biology and Histology

The cellular origin of Ewing's sarcoma cells has been controversial over the years, but more recently evidence has revealed that it is most likely derived from primitive neural crest cells. The Ewing's sarcoma family of tumors shares a unique pattern on cytogenetic and molecular characteristics. Ninety percent to 95% of tumors have the EWS-FLI1 (t(11;22)(q24;q12)) translocation.[133] This translocation can be identified as type 1 (65%), type 2 (20%), and others (15%). The second most common translocation, occurring in the remaining 5% to 10% of ESFT, is EWS-ERG, which has several known specific fusion types. Histologically the Ewing's family of tumors represents a spectrum from undifferentiated Ewing's sarcoma to the more-differentiated PPNET.

Clinical Presentation

Typical presenting symptoms in patients with Ewing's sarcoma include pain, palpable mass, fevers, and occasionally pathologic fracture. Many individuals ascribe their pain to a "strain" or recent traumatic event.[134] Some patients present with symptoms related to metastatic sites of disease, including cough from pulmonary disease or multifocal bone pain from extensive bone or bone marrow involvement. The mean time from initial symptoms to diagnosis of Ewing's sarcoma is frequently months, with those individuals with a palpable mass having the shortest interval.[134]

The primary site of disease is axial in approximately 50% of patients and involves the extremities in the other 50%.[135] At the time of diagnosis, approximately 25% of children have metastatic disease, most commonly to lung followed by other bony sites and bone marrow.[136]

Diagnosis and Staging

Early involvement of an orthopedic surgeon skilled in the care of pediatric bone tumors is imperative. Initial biopsy techniques are not only important in providing needed diagnostic material but may have an impact on subsequent local control measures including the possibility of limb salvage surgery.

The complete evaluation of a new patient with Ewing's sarcoma includes a detailed radiographic evaluation of the primary site of disease, assessment for metastatic disease, and a baseline assessment of organ function in anticipation of intensive therapy. The evaluation of the primary site often begins with plain radiographs, followed by MRI and CT, depending on site of disease. The metastatic evaluation needs to include CT scan of the chest, bilateral bone marrow aspirates and biopsies, and radionucleotide bone scan.

Prognostic Factors

The most significant prognostic variable for patients with Ewing's sarcoma is whether the disease is localized or metastatic at the time of diagnosis.[137] Those with localized disease have a 70% chance of disease-free survival (DFS) whereas those with metastatic disease have a DFS of 20% to 30%. Individuals with pulmonary disease as their only site of metastatic disease do more favorably than those with bony or bone marrow involvement.[138] Approximately 20% to 30% of patients with localized disease with morphologically normal bone marrow examination will have detectable disease in the bone marrow when assayed by polymerase chain reaction (PCR), which is associated with a worse prognosis.[139]

Traditionally, both site of primary disease (axial and pelvic tumors being worse than extremity tumors) and size of the primary tumor (tumors greater than 8 cm in longest dimension or greater than 200 cm^3) have been important prognostic factors.[140–142] However, in several more recent cooperative group studies these factors were no longer found to be significant, potentially related to both more-aggressive adjuvant chemotherapy and improved local control measures.[143,144] More recently, histologic response to neoadjuvant chemotherapy has been shown to be an important prognostic tool, with those with less viable disease after neoadjuvant chemotherapy having better outcomes.[145–147]

Last, type of ESFT translocation has been shown to have some prognostic implications. Individuals with EWS-FLI1 type 1 have been shown to have a decreased risk of developing metastatic disease compared to those with other EWS-FLI1 type translocations.[133]

Current Principles of Therapy

The therapy of Ewing's sarcoma has been developed through the investigations performed by several large cooperative groups, beginning in the 1970s (Table 62.9). In most current protocols, multiagent neoadjuvant chemotherapy (most often including adriamycin, vincristine, cyclophosphamide, etoposide, and ifosfamide) is given for 10 to 12 weeks, followed by local control with either surgery, radiation, or a combination of the two modalities followed by further chemotherapy. Early on the addition of doxorubicin was found to be important,[148] whereas more recently the addition of etoposide and ifosfamide to the backbone of vincristine, doxorubicin, and cyclophosphamide was shown to improve outcome.[143]

Dose intensification, either by higher-dose chemotherapy per cycle or by "interval compression," with more frequent chemotherapy cycles, has been investigated. Both methods utilized granulocyte colony-stimulating factor (G-CSF) support. Both methods have been shown to be feasible but without improvement in outcome for those treated with the more-intensive regimens.[149,150]

Historically, surgery was considered superior to radiation therapy for local control therapy in Ewing's sarcoma.[151,152] With advances both in systemic therapy and in radiation planning and surgical techniques, the rates of local recurrence have declined and the difference between surgical and radiation therapy outcomes has become nonsignificant.[153,154] Some studies continue to show somewhat more favorable results with surgery, but this may be biased by risks associated with worse outcomes for those with very large tumors that are not approachable surgically.[155]

Recent attempts to improve outcome in individuals with metastatic disease have largely focused on dose-intensifying chemotherapy, including the evaluation of "megatherapy" with stem cell support.[156] There have been multiple single-institution and cooperative group studies with various conditioning regimens, including the use of total body irradiation (TBI) and tandem transplantation (Table 62.10). One component of stem cell transplant for metastatic Ewing's that may contribute to failure of this modality is evidence of the presence of tumor cells in the stem cell harvests.[157] There continues to be some interest in the use of intensified therapy for subgroups of high-risk patients in whom intensified therapy may prove to have some moderate benefit.

Therapy for Relapsed Disease

Patients with recurrent disease after aggressive primary therapy have a poor prognosis, with EFS at 5 years of 15% to 20%.[158] Those with localized recurrence and those whose

TABLE 62.9. Selected clinical studies for the therapy of nonmetastatic Ewing's sarcoma.

Group/date of study completion	*N*	*Therapy*	*Outcome/comments*	*Source*
Intergroup (IESS) 1978	342	VAC VAC + lung RT VACD	5-year DFS 60% in VACD, 44% in VAC + lung RT, 24% in VAC	Nesbit 1990[148]
Intergroup (IESS) 1982	214	Dose-intensive VACD vs. "standard" VACD	5-year DFS 73% for dose intensive, 56% for "standard" dose	Burgert 1990[148a]
Cooperative (CESS) 1991	301	Standard-risk: VACD High-risk: VAID	10-year DFS survival; no difference with intensified therapy for high-risk patients (52% vs. 51%)	Paulussen 2001[145]
POG-CCG 1993		VACD vs. VACD-IE	Addition of IE afforded superior 5-year DFS (68% vs. 53%)	Grier 2003[143]
UKCCSG/MRC 1993	201	VAID	DFS at 5 years 62%	Craft 1998[144]
POG-CCG 1998	492	VCD-IE with interval compression vs. "standard" VCD-IE	5-year DFS survival no different between two groups (75% vs. 76%)	Granowetter 2001[280]

V, vincristine; A, actinomycin; C, cyclophosplamide; D, doxorubicin; RT, radiation therapy; I, ifosphosplamide; E, etoposide; POG-CCG, Pediatric Oncology Group-Children's Cancer Group.

TABLE 62.10. Selected studies of intensified chemotherapy for metastatic or poor-risk Ewing's sarcoma.

Source	*N*	*Patient characteristics*	*Therapy*	*Outcome/comments*	*Reference*
POG-CCG	123	All patients with metastatic disease	VACD vs. VACD + IE	DFS 20% at 5 years, no benefit of addition of IE	Miser 2004[115]
Meta-EICESS	54	Bone/BM metastases or early relapse	Induction chemotherapy, local control, and single or tandem SCT	EFS of 22% and 29% for single and tandem SCT, respectively, at 5 years	Burdach 2003[281]
Single institution	32 (23 received SCT)	Bone/BM metastases	Induction chemotherapy, local control, followed by SCT	20% for all eligible patients 24% for those who underwent SCT at 2 years	Meyers 2001[282]

POG-CCG, Pediatric Oncology Group-Children's Cancer Group; V, vincristine; A, actinomycin; C, cyclophosphamide; D, doxorubicin; I, ifosphosphamide; E, etoposide; BM, bone marrow; SCT, stem cell transplantation.

recurrence occurs more than 2 years after initial diagnosis have a somewhat better outlook.[158,159] The combination of cyclophosphamide and topotecan has been shown to have significant activity in patients with relapsed Ewing's sarcoma[160] and is often used as part of a reinduction regimen. The use of high-dose therapy and stem cell transplant for this group of patients has not yet shown significant improvement in overall survival.

Late Effects of Therapy

The therapy for Ewing's sarcoma involves intensive use of both alkylators and topoisomerase II inhibitors (etoposide). The intensive use of these agents has been associated with a significant risk of therapy-related acute myelogenous leukemia and myelodysplastic syndromes (t-AML/MDS),[150,161] which may limit any potential additive efficacy of dose-intensified regimens.

Other long-term sequelae for patients treated for Ewing's sarcoma include secondary malignancies related to radiation therapy, orthopedic problems related to local control surgeries, and infertility or early menopause, renal dysfunction, or cardiac dysfunction as sequelae of chemotherapy.[162]

Rhabdomyosarcoma and Undifferentiated Sarcomas

Epidemiology

Rhabdomyosarcoma (RMS) is the third most common extracranial solid tumor in children (Surveillance, Epidemiology, and End Results; SEERS). The median age of diagnosis is 5 years, with the majority presenting by age 10. This tumor arises in virtually all parts of the body; however, certain groupings by age, location, and histology are common. For example, botriod rhabdomyosarcoma tumors of the vagina occur almost exclusively in infants, whereas head and neck tumors with embryonal histology are more common in those under 8 years of age and extremity tumors with alveolar histology are more common in adolescents. Most cases of RMS are sporadic; however, there is an association with neurofibromatosis and with the Li–Fraumeni syndrome.[163–165]

Biology and Histology

Rhabdomyosarcoma is thought to arise from primitive muscle cells. Undifferentiated sarcomas are those of mesenchymal origin that cannot be ascribed to any specific lineage. The two most common histologic types of RMS are alveolar (ARMS) and embryonal (ERMS), which have unique genetic patterns. ARMS has a characteristic translocation of t(2:13)(q35;q14), which juxtaposes PAX 3, a transcription regulator gene, to FKHR, a member of the forkhead family of transcription factors.[166] ERMS is associated with LOH at 11p15.[167] Botriod rhabdomyosarcoma is considered a histologic subtype of ERMS.

Clinical Presentation

The presentation of patients with RMS is variable given that the tumor can involve almost any part of the body. Most often RMS is diagnosed because of the patient presenting with a mass (with or without a history of trauma) or with organ dysfunction related to anatomic disruption from an undetected mass. In the Intergroup Rhabdomyosarcoma Studies (IRS) I, II and III, 35% of the patients had disease involving the head and neck (including parameningeal and orbital), 22% had genitourinary sites of primary disease, 18% had extremity tumors, and the remaining 25% had tumors originating at numerous other sites.[168–170]

Diagnosis and Staging

The evaluation of a child with RMS, not unlike that of other solid tumors, includes radiographic evaluation of the primary site of disease, assessment of possible sites of metastatic disease, and testing for organ function in anticipation of further therapy. The site of local disease is imaged with CT and/or MRI. Evaluation of sites of metastatic disease should include a chest CT, bilateral bone marrow aspirates and biopsies, and technetium-99 bone scan.

Staging of patients with RMS often involves the use of a combination of two systems: the TNM staging systems and the clinical grouping (Tables 62.11, 62.12). Careful and com-

TABLE 62.11. Clinical group staging of rhabdomyosarcoma as defined by Intergroup Rhabdomyosarcoma Studies (IRS) V.

Clinical group	*Extent of disease*
I	A. Completely resected localized disease confined to the muscle or organ of origin
	B. Completely resected localized disease with infiltration outside the muscle or organ of origin
II	A. Gross total resection with microscopic residual
	B. Regional disease with involved nodes, with gross total resection and no microscopic residual
	C. Regional disease with involved nodes, with gross total resection with microscopic residual
III	A. Incomplete resection after biopsy only
	B. Incomplete resection after major resection
IV	Distant metastatic disease

TABLE 62.12. TNM staging for rhabdomyosarcoma as used for IRS IV.

Stage	*Site*	*Invasiveness of tumor (T)*	*Size of tumor (T)*	*Nodes (N)*	*Metastasis (M)*
1	Orbit Head and neck Genitourinary	T1 or T2	A or B	N0 or N1 or Nx	M0
2	Bladder/prostate Extremity Parameningeal Other	T1 or T2	A	N0 or Nx	M0
3	Bladder/prostate Extremity Parameningeal Other	T1 or T2 T1 or T2	A B	N1 N0 or N1 or Nx	M0
4	All	T1 or T2	A or B	N0 or N1 or Nx	M1

T (tumor): T1, confined to anatomic site of origin; T2, extension; A, less than 5cm in diameter; B, more than 5cm in diameter; N (regional nodes): N0, not clinically involved; N1, clinically involved; Nx, unknown; M (metastases): M0, no distant metastases; M1, distant metastases present.

Source: From Lawrence W Jr, Anderson AR, Gehan EA, et al. *Cancer* (Phila) 1997;80:1165, with permission.

plete staging evaluations are critical in that they determine appropriate risk-adapted therapeutic plans.

Prognostic Factors

Several important factors have been identified as useful tools in predicting outcome in patients with RMS: site of primary disease (with the orbit being the most favorable site), surgical resectability (clinical group), extent of disease spread (clinical stage), histology (with embryonal histology associated with a better prognosis that alveolar), and patient age.[170–172] In the IRS-V study, these factors are used to allocate patients into risk categories with risk-adapted therapy.

Current Principles of Therapy

Surgery

Primary surgical resection with regional nodal sampling, when appropriate, is a critical component of the therapy of RMS. Complete initial surgical resection has been shown in multiple studies to be associated with improved outcome.[168–170] For certain disease sites, such as the bladder, the orbit, or biliary tract, aggressive surgical therapy is not reasonable, and biopsy done only to confirm diagnosis is the appropriate surgical approach. Several clinical trials have evaluated the utility of "second-look surgery" following adjuvant chemotherapy for patients with incomplete resections after initial surgery.[168–170,173] The data supporting this approach are mixed, and the question is again being evaluated in IRS-V. In addition, the use of biopsy only at disease outset followed by chemotherapy with no further local control for those with a radiographic complete response was evaluated in an International Society of Pediatric Oncology protocol and was shown to be associated with a higher rate of local disease relapse.[174]

Radiation Therapy

Radiation therapy is an important tool in the therapy of children with RMS. Doses of 50.4 to 54.0Gy for gross disease and 41.4 to 45.0Gy for microscopic residual disease are usually employed. There is clear evidence that the use of radiation in patients with alveolar histology, even with complete resection, provides improvement in local control. The timing of radiation therapy in the multimodality therapy of patients with RMS has varied over time but most often occurs 9 to 12 weeks after the initiation of adjuvant chemotherapy, except for those with invasive parameningeal tumors, for whom therapy usually begins immediately. For young children, the long-term sequelae of radiation therapy, particularly the potential for morbid growth deformities, can make treatment decision difficult.

Chemotherapy

Pioneering studies by Wilbur et al. were the first to show benefit of multiagent chemotherapy in patients with RMS.[175] Many agents have been shown to have activity in treating RMS, including vincristine, actinomycin, cyclophosphamide, doxorubicin, ifosfamide, etoposide, and cisplatinum. More recently, the camptothecin analogues topotecan and irinotecan have shown activity in this disease.[176,177]

Formed in 1972, the Intergroup Rhabdomyosarcoma Studies Group (IRSG) has allowed for well-designed studies of this rare pediatric cancer. The results of IRS studies I–V are summarized in Table 62.13. Despite the improvement in outcomes in each sequential IRS study, progress in treating those with metastatic disease has been marginal, with survival of approximately 30%.[170,178] Patients with embryonal histology who are less than 10 years of age and have pulmonary metastatic disease only are a unique group with a more-favorable prognosis.[170,178] The use of autologous transplant in attempts to intensify therapy and improve outcome in those with clinical group IV disease has not been shown to provide clinical benefit to date.[179–181]

Therapy for Relapsed Disease

The therapy for patients with relapsed RMS is problematic and the outcome poor; 95% of all relapses of RMS occur within 3 years of diagnosis.[182] The median survival time from first relapse is 0.8 years, with 20% of the patients alive at 5 years. Adverse prognostic factors include rapidity of relapse and extent of disease at the time of relapse. Patients with

TABLE 62.13. Sequential IRS studies of the therapy of rhabdomyosarcoma.

IRS study, dates	*Primary study questions*	*N*	*Outcomes/comments*	*Reference*
I 1972–1978	(1) Group I: VAC vs. VAC + XRT (2) Group II: VA + XRT vs. VAC + XRT (3) Groups III and IV: VAC + XRT ± adria	686	(1) For groups I + II: no difference between regimens, OS at 5 years 86% and 72%, respectively (2) No measurable benefit of addition of adria, OS group III 52%, OS group IV 20% (3) Combined OS all patients 63%	Maurer 1988[168]
II 1978–1984	(1) Group I (except EA) had VAC vs. VA (2) Group II (except EA) XRT + intensive VA vs. XRT + VAC (3) Group III and IV: VAC vs. Vadr C/VAC	999	(1) No benefit of VAC vs. VA for group I disease (OS 85% vs. 84%, $P = 0.73$) (2) No difference between regimens for group II disease (OS 88% vs. 79%, $P = 0.17$) (3) No difference in regimens, OS 66% for group III, 26% for group IV (4) Combined OS all patients 71%	Maurer 1993[169]
III 1984–1991	Risk-stratified therapy based on group, histology, and site of disease	1,062	(1) No benefit of VAC over VA for group I disease (2) Improved outcomes for group III patients with more intensive regimen (3) No improvement in outcomes for patients with group IV disease with more complex therapy	Crist 1995[170]
IV 1991–1997	(1) VAC vs. VIE vs. VAI (2) Evaluation of hyperfractionated XRT for group 3 patients (3) "Window" of VAC/IE vs. VM/VAC for patients with metastatic disease	1,056	(1) No significant difference in FFS among three chemotherapy regimens, with FFS at 3 years 75%, 77%, and 77% (2) No difference in OS or FFS for HFRT vs. CFRT (3) 3-year OS and FFS for metastatic disease, 39% and 25%	Crist 2001[283] Donaldson 2001[284] Breneman 2003[178]
V 1997–ongoing	(1) VA vs. VAC + RT in low-risk ERMS (2) VAC vs. VAC/VTC in intermediate-risk RMS (3) Irinotecan/V window in patients with group 4 disease	NA	Data not yet available	NA

VAI, vincristine, actinomycin, ifosfamide; VIE, vincristine, ifosfamide, etoposide; VAC, vincristine, actinomycin, cyclophosphamide; HFRT, hyperfractionated radiation therapy; CRFT, conventionally fractionated radiation therapy; EA, extremity alveolar.

ERMS with localized recurrence have a more-favorable prognosis, with a 5-year OS of 50% with aggressive multimodality therapy.[182]

Late Effects of Therapy

Chemotherapy-related long-term sequelae include infertility or early menopause, renal tubular dysfunction, and secondary leukemias. The increasing role of risk-adapted therapy in RMS is an important strategy in attempting to minimize late effects of therapy.

Hepatoblastoma and Other Liver Tumors

Epidemiology

Primary malignant tumors of the liver in pediatrics are uncommon. According to the SEER program of the National Cancer Institute, liver cancers account for approximately 1% of all pediatric cancers, with hepatoblastoma accounting for 79% of that total, resulting in about 100 new cases of hepatoblastoma per year.[1] The incidence is highest in infants, with most cases occurring before age 5 and males being more commonly affected than females. The incidence of hepatoblastoma has increased during the past 30 years, with incidence in the United States increasing from 0.6 per million (1973–1977) to 1.2 per million (1993–1997).[183]

The incidence of hepatoblastoma is higher in individuals with Beckwith–Wiedemann syndrome (BWS), hemihypertrophy (HH), and familial adenomatous polyposis (FAP). Three percent of patients with BWS or HH develop hepatoblastoma.[184,185] In this group of patients, screening with serial abdominal ultrasounds and alpha fetoprotein (AFP) measurements has been shown to be of benefit.[186]

Recent analysis of the cancer registry in Japan indicates that the incidence of hepatoblastoma is increasing in patients with very low birth weight.[187] Recent analysis of data from both SEER and state registries as well as the unexpectedly high percentage of very low birth weight infants diagnosed with hepatoblastoma on a Children's Cancer Group (CCG) trial appear to confirm those results.[188,189] Of note, the increase in survival of very low birth weight infants has occurred over the same length of time, leading some investigators to conclude that the overall increased incidence of hepatoblastoma is not simply by chance.[190,191]

Biology and Histology

Cytogenetic studies of hepatoblastoma have revealed extra copies of chromosomes 1q, 2q, 7q, 8, 17q, and 20.[192] In addition, loss of heterozygosity (LOH) at the 11p15 site has been observed in one-third of patients with hepatoblastoma.[193] Genes thought to be potentially significant genes on 11p15 include insulin-like growth factor (IGF)-2 and the tumor suppressor genes p57 (KIP2) and H19.[194] The histology of hepatoblastoma ranges from undifferentiated small cells to cells resembling those during embryonal and fetal development. Most tumors have a mixed histologic pattern.

Clinical Presentation

Most patients present with an enlarging abdominal mass, often brought to medical attention by the child's parents' concern over a protuberant or firm abdomen. Systemic symptoms such as weight loss or anorexia are rarely seen. Some boys can present with precocious puberty.[195]

Diagnosis and Staging

On detection of any intraabdominal mass, abdominal ultrasound should be performed to characterize the location and approximate size of the lesion. Doppler flow during ultrasonography can aid in determining the proximity of the tumor to the portal vein. CT scan of the abdomen and pelvis or MRI scan should be undertaken to delineate more accurately the size of the tumor, location, and proximity to the portal vein and inferior vena cava (IVC). The right lobe of the liver is more often involved than the left lobe.[188] The lungs are the most common site of metastatic disease, present in approximately 10% of patients at diagnosis[188]; therefore, CT scan of the chest should also be preformed. Serum AFP levels should be obtained as well as these are elevated in 90% of cases.[196] There is a correlation between AFP level and extent of disease in all stages.[197]

Prognostic Factors

The single most significant prognostic factor for children with hepatoblastoma is feasibility of complete surgical resection. Biologic features that have prognostic implications include histologic subtype (with fetal histology having better outcome than embryonal) and degree of mitotic activity.[198] Patients whose tumors become resectable after neoadjuvant chemotherapy and those whose AFP levels fall quickly have also been shown to have more-favorable outcomes.[199]

Current Principles of Therapy

Historically, surgery was the only curative therapy for hepatoblastoma; however, only about 30% of tumors arc considered resectable at diagnosis.[200,201] The staging system commonly employed is based on the surgical removal of the tumor, such that stage I is complete resection, stage II is microscopic disease after surgery, stage III is unresectable disease or macroscopic disease after surgery, and stage IV is metastatic disease.[188] However, there is no universally accepted staging system for hepatoblastoma.[202]

The utility of chemotherapy in the treatment of hepatoblastoma was first realized in the 1970s.[188] Results of recent group studies are summarized in Table 62.14. Chemotherapy has been shown to increase the overall survival of patients with hepatoblastoma as well as to increase the number of patients with resectable tumors.[203] Early studies documented the benefit of adjuvant therapy with cisplatinum and doxorubicin.[204,205] More recently it has been shown that the use of cisplatinum, 5-fluorouracil, and vincristine was equally effective but less toxic than cisplatinum and doxorubicin.[206] Other chemotherapeutic agents that have been shown to be of utility include carboplatinum, ifosfamide, and etoposide.[207–209]

Therapy of Patients with Unresectable Disease

Orthotopic liver transplantation for patients with unresectable hepatoblastoma has been shown to be an effective therapeutic modality in multiple case series (Table 62.15).[210–212] In these studies, presurgical chemotherapy was

TABLE 62.14. Selected clinical trials of primary hepatoblastoma.

Group/date study closed	*Intervention/chemotherapeutic regimen*	*N*	*DFS/OS/median F/U/comments*	*Reference*
CCSG 1989	CDDP + CI-DOXO	33	67% OS at 2 years (est)	Ortega 1991[197]
POG 1989	CDDP + VCR + 5-FU	46	I-II 80%–90% DFS at 3 years (est) III 67% DFS IV 12.5% DFS Outcome largely dependent on stage	Douglass 1993[285]
CCG/POG 1992	Stage I-FH four cycles of DOXO monotherapy Stage I-UH-IV A (CDDP, 5-FU, VCR × 4) vs. B (CDDP, CI-DOXO × 4)	182	I-FH 100%/100% at 5 years I-UH 91%/98% II 100%/100% III 64%/69% IV 25%/37% No difference between regimen A vs. B	Ortega 2000[206]
POG 1995	CARBO then CARBO/5-FU/VCR × 3 followed by surgery; resectable tumors were removed followed by CARBO/VCR/5-FU; if not resectable or progressed received HDDP/ETOP	III 22 IV 11	All patients 48%/57% at 5 years Stage III 59%/73% Stage IV 27%/27%	Katzenstein 2002[213]
SIOPEL 1 1994	Preoperative chemo with CDDP/ CI-DOXO followed by surgery; some patients were treated with primary surgery	154	All patients 66%/75% at 5 years	Schnater 2002[203] Pritchard 2000[286]
SIOPEL 2 1998	Standard risk: CDDP monotherapy High risk: CDDP/CARBO/DOXO	75 SR 58 HR	SR 89%/91% at 3 years HR 48%/53%	Perilongo 2004[287]

5-FU, 5-fluorouracil; CARBO, carboplatin; CDDP, cisplatin; HDDP, high-dose cisplatin; CI-DOXO, continuous infusion doxorubicin; VCR, vincristine; ETOP, etoposide; CCG, Children's Cancer Group; CCSG, Children's Cancer Study Group; POG, Pediatric Oncology Group; SIOPEL, International Pediatric Oncology Society Liver Tumor Study Group.

TABLE 62.15. Clinical trials for unresectable hepatoblastoma.

Group	*Intervention/chemotherapeutic regimen*	*N*	*Comments*	*Reference*
Children's Medical Center at Dallas	Transplantation for unresectable hepatoblastoma	9	6/9 alive; 1/6 with recurrence of disease	Molmenti 2002[212]
Kings College Hospital, London	Transplantation for unresectable hepatoblastoma	13	11/13 alive with NED	Srinivasan 2002[210]
Birmingham Children's Hospital, Birmingham England	Transplantation vs. surgical resection for extensive hepatoblastoma	34	29/34 (85%) alive with NED 95% OS with hepatectomy 79% OS with transplantation	Pimpalwar 2002[211]

NED, no evidence of disease.

given to reduce the size of the primary tumor. Postoperative chemotherapy or radiotherapy was also performed to consolidate local control. Patients with disease documented to be more responsive to neoadjuvant chemotherapy have a superior overall survival.

Therapy of Patients with Metastatic or Recurrent Disease

The therapy for children with metastatic disease or recurrent disease remains challenging. Intensification of the chemotherapeutic regimen with high-dose cisplatinum and etoposide has shown to be of potential benefit,[207,213] as has surgical removal of isolated pulmonary metastases.[214,215] Several case reports and small case series have reported successful use of high-dose therapy and autologous stem cell rescue for poor-risk patients.[213,216]

Hepatocellular Carcinoma

Although rare, primary liver tumors in children over 3 years of age are more likely to be hepatocellular carcinoma (HCC) than hepatoblastoma.[183] Risk factors for HCC in children include Byler's disease, Wilson's disease, and hepatorenal tyrosinemia.[183] Because of the rarity of this disease in children, studies evaluating the therapy of HCC in pediatric patients have been limited, and most children are treated according to adult therapeutic guidelines. As for adult patients, the primary therapy is surgery, with chemotherapy having limited efficacy.[217,218]

Retinoblastoma

Epidemiology

Retinoblastoma, the most common intraocular tumor in children, is a tumor of developing retinal cells. This tumor has an annual incidence of 11 new cases per million population less than 5 years of age.[1] It occurs as a sporadic and familial tumor, with the former the more common presentation. The majority of children with retinoblastoma present by the age of 2 years, and 95% of cases occur by age 5.[219] Approximately one-quarter of retinoblastomas are bilateral[1]: these are all almost all hereditary, associated with germ-line mutations in the RB1 gene. Another 15% of retinoblastomas are unilateral but hereditary. The remaining 60% are unilateral and nonfamilial.[220] A small number of children present with bilateral retinoblastomas in addition to a pineal blastoma, a combination known as trilateral retinoblastoma.[221]

Biology and Histology

Forty percent of retinoblastomas are hereditary and associated with a germ-line mutation. The epidemiology of the disease prompted the development of the "two hit hypothesis."[222] The specific gene involved is now known as RB1, a tumor suppressor gene located on chromosome 13q14.[223] The defective RB protein leads to a lack of control over cell-cycle regulation.

Histologically, retinoblastoma appears as basophilic cells with scant cytoplasm and having a high mitotic index.[224] Flexner–Winstersteiner rosettes are characteristic, representing a specific orientation of photoreceptor cells.[225]

Clinical Presentation

Children with retinoblastoma most often present with leukokoria. The second most common presentation is strabismus.[226,227] Less-common presentations include decreased vision, ocular inflammation, and family history of the disease.[226]

Diagnosis and Staging

Diagnosis of retinoblastoma is based on direct ophthalmoscopic evaluation. The characteristic finding of the tumor is a chalky, whitish-gray retinal mass with soft, friable consistency.[228] CT scan of the head and orbits may demonstrate a solid intraocular tumor with intratumoral calcifications.[229] Differential diagnosis includes persistent hyperplastic primary vitreous, Coats' disease, and ocular toxoplasmosis.[230]

Staging of retinoblastoma is based most commonly on the Reese–Ellsworth (RE) classification system developed in the 1960s. With more-modern treatment techniques, this system is not clearly prognostic for the ability to save either vision or life; however, it remains the most common staging system in use worldwide. Other staging systems have been developed.[231,232] Metastatic retinoblastoma at the time of initial tumor diagnosis is relatively rare. When metastasis does occur, the disease can spread by direct extension (through the optic nerve or by choroidal invasion), by contamination of the subarachnoid space and dissemination through the cerebrospinal fluid, by hematogenous spread (most commonly to lung, bone, bone marrow, and brain), or by lymphatic spread to the conjunctivae and lids.[228] When metastases are suspected, formal staging evaluation, including bone marrow aspirate and biopsy, lumbar puncture, and radionuclide bone scan should be done.

Prognostic Factors

Prognosis for children with retinoblastoma has improved dramatically over the past decades, with approximately 90% of all children diagnosed being cured of their disease. Patients with overt metastatic disease at the time of diagnosis continue to have a very poor prognosis. Risk factors for development of metastatic disease include extension of the tumor in the optic nerve beyond the lamina cribosa and extrascleral extension into the orbit.[233,234]

Current Principles of Therapy

Traditionally, retinoblastoma was treated with enucleation or with external-beam radiation (EBRT). Recent treatment regimens have tried both to avoid enucleation in attempts to save vision as well as to avoid using external-beam radiation because of the risk of secondary cancers, endocrinopathies, and facial hypoplasia.[235] Low-stage tumors can often be managed with local therapy alone. Local treatment modalities that avoid the need for enucleation include cryotherapy, laser photocoagulation, plaque radiotherapy, and thermotherapy.

Retinoblastoma is a chemotherapy-sensitive tumor, with the active agents currently employed including vincristine, carboplatinum, etoposide, adriamycin, and cyclophosphamide.[236–243] The use of systemic chemotherapy in conjunction with local therapy, without enucleation or EBRT, in the treatment of patients with lower-stage disease has been successful.[237,239,244]

For patients who have RE stage V disease at diagnosis, enucleation remains the standard of care.[237–239,243,245,246] The role of adjuvant chemotherapy for those with poor prognostic features to prevent metastatic disease is generally recommended, although this idea has not undergone rigorous randomized controlled study.[246] There currently are no specific criteria for which patients with intraocular retinoblastoma with extraretinal extension should receive chemotherapy.

Patients with metastatic disease have a grim prognosis, with an average survival of 6 months.[247] For individuals with disseminated disease, the use of myeloablative therapy and autologous stem cell rescue may have some role.[247–250] Patients with trilateral retinoblastoma also fare extremely poorly despite aggressive therapy. Interestingly, those patients with bilateral retinoblastoma who have received neoadjuvant chemotherapy may be protected from developing pineal blastoma.[251]

Late Effects of Therapy

The long-term sequelae of therapy for retinoblastoma include blindness or impaired vision related to extent of initial disease and local control therapies employed. Radiation therapy of the orbit in young children is associated with significant morbidity, including orbital growth abnormalities, endocrinopathies, and risks of secondary tumors. With the increasing use of adjuvant chemotherapy in high-risk patients with retinoblastoma, long-term sequelae of these medications will also become problematic.

Patients with germ-line mutations in the RB1 gene are at increased risk of developing second primary tumors.[223,252,253] Over the course of 50 years after their initial diagnosis, the risk of second primary tumors in those patients with heritable forms of retinoblastoma is 50%.[254] Most commonly, the second tumor is osteogenic sarcoma, followed by other soft tissue sarcomas and malignant melanoma.[223,252,253]

Germ Cell Tumors

Epidemiology

Germ cell tumors (GCT) represent approximately 3% of pediatric malignancies, equaling about 250 new cases per year in the United States.[1] GCT can occur in both gonadal and extragonadal sites. Extragonadal tumors occur more frequently in patients younger than 3 years of age; gonadal tumors occur more often during and after puberty.[255]

Phenotypically, female patients with part or all of the Y chromosome (such as those with gonadal dygenesis, androgen resistance syndromes, or some patients with Turner's syndrome) are at increased risk of developing gonadoblastoma, a benign germ cell tumor found in dysgenetic gonads.[256,257] In addition, males with undescended testes have an increased risk of developing GCTs, with the risk lessened but still elevated in those who undergo orchiopexy.[258–260]

Biology and Histology

Germ cell tumors include a diverse group of neoplasms with a presumed common cell of origin, the primordial germ cell. Extragonadal tumors are thought to arise from aberrancy from the complex migration pattern of germ cells during embryogenesis.

Cytogenetic findings in children with GCTs vary by site, age, and sex of the patient. Abnormalities in I(12p) are very common in adolescent boys with testicular tumors, less common in girls with malignant ovarian GCTs, and rare in younger children with extragonadal GCTs.[261]

The histology of GCTs is diverse and complex and includes teratomas and gonadoblastomas, which most often are benign and malignant GCTs, including yolk sac tumors, germinomas, embryonal carcinomas, and choriocarcinomas.[262]

Clinical Presentation

The clinical presentation of children with germ cell tumors varies by age, sex, and site of the tumor. Boys with testicular tumors most often present with a palpable or visible mass. Girls with ovarian tumors often present with abdominal pain, sometimes mimicking an acute abdomen. The clinical signs associated with extragonadal tumors vary with site of disease, with the most common sites involved including the sacrococcygeal area, the mediastinum, the central nervous system, or the retroperitoneum. Infants with sacrococcygeal tumors are often diagnosed prenatally by routine ultrasonography.

Diagnosis and Staging

Staging evaluation for malignant GCT should include abdominal, pelvic, and chest CT, bone scan, and measurements of beta-human chorionic gonadotropin (β-HCG) and AFP.[263] In the evaluation of infants with GCTs, normative values for AFP must be taken into consideration, with baseline levels falling to adult levels by 8 months of age.[264]

Prognostic Factors

Overall outcomes for children with GCTs are very favorable. In two sequential Intergroup studies that included 515 patients, including 79 with immature teratomas and 436 with malignant CGTs, the OS at 8 years was 92%.[265–267] Adverse prognostic factors include AFP greater than 10,000 kU/L, higher-stage disease, and extragonadal sites.

Current Principles of Therapy

Surgery is the therapy for choice for benign GCTs. For malignant GCTs, surgical resection remains important; however, given the effectiveness of chemotherapy, aggressive primary surgeries are not necessarily warranted. Chemotherapeutic agents known to be active in the therapy of GCTs include actinomycin, bleomycin, doxorubicin, cisplatinum, carboplatinum, and etoposide. The use of combination regimens has been shown to increase the chance of cure. The most common regimen currently employed, developed initially in adults and studied subsequently in children, includes bleomycin, etoposide, and cisplatinum.[268,269]

Recent Children's Cancer Group–Pediatric Oncology Group (CCG-POG) studies have used a risk-based approach to therapeutic decisions. In these studies, patients with stage I testicular malignant tumors and those with immature teratomas are considered low-risk and are treated initially with surgery alone. With this strategy, those with stage I testicular disease had an EFS of 79% and an OS of 100%[270]; those with immature teratomas had an EFS of 95% and OS of 98.7%.[265,266]

Intermediate-risk patients have been defined as those with stage II testicular or stage I or II ovarian malignant GCTs. These patients were treated with surgery and four or six cycles of a modified Einhorn regimen. Patients with stage I ovarian tumors had an EFS and OS of 95% and those with stage II ovarian tumors had EFS and OS of 87% and 93%, respectively; those with stage II testicular tumors had an EFS and OS of 100%.[265,266] Given the data regarding favorable outcome of patients with stage I ovarian tumors treated with surgery, only these patients will be considered low risk in future studies.[271–273]

High-risk patients have been those with stage III or IV gonadal tumors and all stages of extragonadal extracranial malignant GCTs.[255] These patients have been treated with surgery followed by four or six cycles of cisplatinum, etoposide, and bleomycin. The use of higher-dose cisplatinum improves EFS but does not improve OS and is associated with significant toxicity.[267] In addition, the data suggested that those patients with stage III–IV testicular, stage III ovarian, and stage I–II extragonadal GCTs had excellent responses, with EFS 83% to 100% for the various subgroups.[267] In future Intergroup studies, only those with stage IV ovarian and stages III and IV extragonadal GCTs will be considered high risk.

Late Effects of Therapy

The chemotherapy for GCTs is associated with long-term risks of pulmonary toxicity, secondary leukemias, and hearing loss. Risk stratification done in an attempt to minimize exposure to individuals with lower-risk disease with these agents, while preserving excellent cure rates, remains an important focus of the management of children with GCTs.

References

1. Ries L, Eisner M, Kosary C, et al. SEER Cancer Statistics Review, 1975–2000. Bethesda, MD: National Cancer Institute, 2003.
2. Munson M, Sutton P. Births, marriages, divorces, and deaths: pro-visional data for 2003. National Vital Statistics Reports 2004; 52(22).
3. Sawada T, Hirayama M, Nakata T, et al. Mass screening for neuroblastoma in infants in Japan. Interim report of a mass screening study group. Lancet 1984;2(8397):271–273.
4. Schilling FH, Spix C, Berthold F, et al. Neuroblastoma screening at one year of age. N Engl J Med 2002;346(14):1047–1053.
5. Woods WG, Gao RN, Shuster JJ, et al. Screening of infants and mortality due to neuroblastoma. N Engl J Med 2002;346(14): 1041–1046.
6. Kerbl R, Urban CE, Ambros IM, et al. Neuroblastoma mass screening in late infancy: insights into the biology of neuroblastic tumors. J Clin Oncol 2003;21(22):4228–4234.
7. Lindor NM, Greene MH. The concise handbook of family cancer syndromes. Mayo Familial Cancer Program. J Natl Cancer Inst 1998;90(14):1039–1071.
8. Choyke PL, Siegel MJ, Craft AW, Green DM, DeBaun MR. Screening for Wilms tumor in children with Beckwith–W iedemann syndrome or idiopathic hemihypertrophy. Med Pediatr Oncol 1999;32(3):196–200.
9. Preston DL, Kusumi S, Tomonaga M, et al. Cancer incidence in atomic bomb survivors. Part III. Leukemia, lymphoma and multiple myeloma, 1950–1987. Radiat Res 1994;137(suppl 2): S68– S97.
10. Ron E. Ionizing radiation and cancer risk: evidence from epidemiology. Pediatr Radiol 2002;32(4):232–237; discussion 42–44.
11. Hempelmann LH. Epidemiological studies of leukemia in persons exposed to ionizing radiation. Cancer Res 1960;20:18–27.
12. Dahlin DC, Unni KK. Osteosarcoma of bone and its important recognizable varieties. Am J Surg Pathol 1977;1(1):61–72.
13. Berrington de Gonzalez A, Darby S. Risk of cancer from diagnostic X-rays: estimates for the UK and 14 other countries. Lancet 2004;363(9406):345–351.
14. Skinner J, Mee TJ, Blackwell RP, et al. Exposure to power frequency electric fields and the risk of childhood cancer in the UK. Br J Cancer 2002;87(11):1257–1266.
15. Whitlock JA, Greer JP, Lukens JN. Epipodophyllotoxin-related leukemia. Identification of a new subset of secondary leukemia. Cancer (Phila) 1991;68(3):600–604.
16. Loning L, Zimmermann M, Reiter A, et al. Secondary neoplasms subsequent to Berlin-Frankfurt-Munster therapy of acute lymphoblastic leukemia in childhood: significantly lower risk without cranial radiotherapy. Blood 2000;95(9): 2770–2775.

17. Pollock BH, Krischer JP, Vietti TJ. Interval between symptom onset and diagnosis of pediatric solid tumors. J Pediatr 1991; 119(5):725–732.
18. Bottomley SJ, Kassner E. Late effects of childhood cancer therapy. J Pediatr Nurs 2003;18(2):126–133.
19. Lackner H, Benesch M, Schagerl S, Kerbl R, Schwinger W, Urban C. Prospective evaluation of late effects after childhood cancer therapy with a follow-up over 9 years. Eur J Pediatr 2000;159(10): 750–758.
20. Hudson MM, Mertens AC, Yasui Y, et al. Health status of adult long-term survivors of childhood cancer: a report from the Childhood Cancer Survivor Study. JAMA 2003;290(12):1583–1592.
21. Kushner BH, Gilbert F, Helson L. Familial neuroblastoma. Case reports, literature review, and etiologic considerations. Cancer (Phila) 1986;57(9):1887–1893.
22. Schwab M, Ellison J, Busch M, Rosenau W, Varmus HE, Bishop JM. Enhanced expression of the human gene N-myc consequent to amplification of DNA may contribute to malignant progression of neuroblastoma. Proc Natl Acad Sci U S A 1984;81(15): 4940–4944.
23. Brodeur GM, Seeger RC. Gene amplification in human neuroblastomas: basic mechanisms and clinical implications. Cancer Genet Cytogenet 1986;19(1–2):101–111.
24. Weiss WA, Aldape K, Mohapatra G, Feuerstein BG, Bishop JM. Targeted expression of MYCN causes neuroblastoma in transgenic mice. EMBO J 1997;16(11):2985–2995.
25. Brodeur GM, Nakagawara A, Yamashiro DJ, et al. Expression of TrkA, TrkB and TrkC in human neuroblastomas. J Neuro-Oncol 1997;31(1–2):49–55.
26. Caron H, van Sluis P, de Kraker J, et al. Allelic loss of chromosome 1p as a predictor of unfavorable outcome in patients with neuroblastoma. N Engl J Med 1996;334(4):225–230.
27. Bown N, Cotterill S, Lastowska M, et al. Gain of chromosome arm 17q and adverse outcome in patients with neuroblastoma. N Engl J Med 1999;340(25):1954–1961.
28. Weinstein JL, Katzenstein HM, Cohn SL. Advances in the diagnosis and treatment of neuroblastoma. Oncologist 2003;8(3): 278–292.
29. Brodeur GM, Pritchard J, Berthold F, et al. Revisions of the international criteria for neuroblastoma diagnosis, staging, and response to treatment. J Clin Oncol 1993;11(8):1466–1477.
30. Kushner BH, Yeung HW, Larson SM, Kramer K, Cheung NK. Extending positron emission tomography scan utility to high-risk neuroblastoma: fluorine-18 fluorodeoxyglucose positron emission tomography as sole imaging modality in follow-up of patients. J Clin Oncol 2001;19(14):3397–3405.
31. Shulkin BL, Hutchinson RJ, Castle VP, Yanik GA, Shapiro B, Sisson JC. Neuroblastoma: positron emission tomography with 2-[fluorine-18]-fluoro-2-deoxy-D-glucose compared with metaiodobenzylguanidine scintigraphy. Radiology 1996;199(3): 743–750.
32. Scanga DR, Martin WH, Delbeke D. Value of FDG PET imaging in the management of patients with thyroid, neuroendocrine, and neural crest tumors. Clin Nucl Med 2004; 29(2):86–90.
33. Evans AE, D'Angio GJ, Randolph J. A proposed staging for children with neuroblastoma. Children's cancer study group A. Cancer (Phila) 1971;27(2):374–378.
34. Brodeur GM, Seeger RC, Schwab M, Varmus HE, Bishop JM. Amplification of N-myc in untreated human neuroblastomas correlates with advanced disease stage. Science 1984; 224(4653):1121–1124.
35. Cohn SL, Rademaker AW, Salwen HR, et al. Analysis of DNA ploidy and proliferative activity in relation to histology and N-myc amplification in neuroblastoma. Am J Pathol 1990;136(5): 1043–1052.
36. Look AT, Hayes FA, Nitschke R, McWilliams NB, Green AA. Cellular DNA content as a predictor of response to chemotherapy in infants with unresectable neuroblastoma. N Engl J Med 1984;311(4):231–235.
37. Maris JM, Weiss MJ, Guo C, et al. Loss of heterozygosity at 1p36 independently predicts for disease progression but not decreased overall survival probability in neuroblastoma patients: a Children's Cancer Group study. J Clin Oncol 2000;18(9):1888–1899.
38. Seeger RC, Brodeur GM, Sather H, et al. Association of multiple copies of the N-myc oncogene with rapid progression of neuroblastomas. N Engl J Med 1985;313(18):1111–1116.
39. Shimada H, Chatten J, Newton WA Jr, et al. Histopathologic prognostic factors in neuroblastic tumors: definition of subtypes of ganglioneuroblastoma and an age-linked classification of neuroblastomas. J Natl Cancer Inst 1984;73(2):405–416.
40. Alvarado CS, London WB, Look AT, et al. Natural history and biology of stage A neuroblastoma: a Pediatric Oncology Group Study. J Pediatr Hematol Oncol 2000;22(3):197–205.
41. Perez CA, Matthay KK, Atkinson JB, et al. Biologic variables in the outcome of stages I and II neuroblastoma treated with surgery as primary therapy: a children's cancer group study. J Clin Oncol 2000;18(1):18–26.
42. Matthay KK, Villablanca JG, Seeger RC, et al. Treatment of high-risk neuroblastoma with intensive chemotherapy, radiotherapy, autologous bone marrow transplantation, and 13-cis-retinoic acid. Children's Cancer Group. N Engl J Med 1999;341(16):1165– 1173.
43. Ladenstein R, Philip T, Lasset C, et al. Multivariate analysis of risk factors in stage 4 neuroblastoma patients over the age of one year treated with megatherapy and stem-cell transplantation: a report from the European Bone Marrow Transplantation Solid Tumor Registry. J Clin Oncol 1998;16(3):953–965.
44. Grupp SA, Stern JW, Bunin N, et al. Tandem high-dose therapy in rapid sequence for children with high-risk neuroblastoma. J Clin Oncol 2000;18(13):2567–2575.
45. Grupp SA, Stern JW, Bunin N, et al. Rapid-sequence tandem transplant for children with high-risk neuroblastoma. Med Pediatr Oncol 2000;35(6):696–700.
46. Kletzel M, Katzenstein HM, Haut PR, et al. Treatment of high-risk neuroblastoma with triple-tandem high-dose therapy and stem-cell rescue: results of the Chicago Pilot II Study. J Clin Oncol 2002;20(9):2284–2292.
47. Marcus KJ, Shamberger R, Litman H, et al. Primary tumor control in patients with stage 3/4 unfavorable neuroblastoma treated with tandem double autologous stem cell transplants. J Pediatr Hematol Oncol 2003;25(12):934–940.
48. Nickerson HJ, Matthay KK, Seeger RC, et al. Favorable biology and outcome of stage IV-S neuroblastoma with supportive care or minimal therapy: a Children's Cancer Group study. J Clin Oncol 2000;18(3):477–486.
49. Katzenstein HM, Bowman LC, Brodeur GM, et al. Prognostic significance of age, MYCN oncogene amplification, tumor cell ploidy, and histology in 110 infants with stage D(S) neuroblastoma: the pediatric oncology group experience: a pediatric oncology group study. J Clin Oncol 1998;16(6):2007–2017.
50. Parsons SK, Neault MW, Lehmann LE, et al. Severe ototoxicity following carboplatin-containing conditioning regimen for autologous marrow transplantation for neuroblastoma. Bone Marrow Transplant 1998;22(7):669–674.
51. Meadows AT, Tsunematsu Y. Late effects for treatment for neuroblastoma. In: Brodeur GM, Sawada T, Tsuchida Y, Voute PA (eds). Neuroblastoma. Amsterdam: Elsevier, 2000: 561–570.
52. Breslow N, Olshan A, Beckwith JB, Green DM. Epidemiology of Wilms tumor. Med Pediatr Oncol 1993;21(3):172–181.
53. Miller RW, Fraumeni JF Jr, Manning MD. Association of Wilms tumor with aniridia, hemihypertrophy and other congenital anomalies. N Engl J Med 1964;270:922–927.

54. Drash A, Sherman F, Hartmann WH, Blizzard RM. A syndrome of pseudohermaphroditism, Wilms' tumor, hypertension, and degenerative renal disease. J Pediatr 1970;76(4):585–593.
55. Breslow NE, Norris R, Norkool PA, et al. Characteristics and outcomes of children with the Wilms tumor-Aniridia syndrome: a report from the National Wilms Tumor Study Group. J Clin Oncol 2003;21(24):4579–4585.
56. Porteus MH, Narkool P, Neuberg D, et al. Characteristics and outcome of children with Beckwith-Wiedemann syndrome and Wilms' tumor: a report from the National Wilms Tumor Study Group. J Clin Oncol 2000;18(10):2026–2031.
57. Coppes MJ, Williams BR. The molecular genetics of Wilms tumor. Cancer Invest 1994;12(1):57–65.
58. Grundy PE, Telzerow PE, Breslow N, Moksness J, Huff V, Paterson MC. Loss of heterozygosity for chromosomes 16q and 1p in Wilms' tumors predicts an adverse outcome. Cancer Res 1994;54(9):2331–2333.
59. Bonadio JF, Storer B, Norkool P, Farewell VT, Beckwith JB, D'Angio GJ. Anaplastic Wilms' tumor: clinical and pathologic studies. J Clin Oncol 1985;3(4):513–520.
60. Grundy P, Green DM, Coppes MJ, et al. Renal tumors. In: Pizzo PA, Poplack DG (eds). Principles and Practice of Pediatric Oncology, 4th ed. Philadelphia: Lippincott, Williams & Wilkins, 2002: 865–938.
61. Shurin SB, Gauderer MW, Dahms BB, Conrad WG. Fatal intraoperative pulmonary embolization of Wilms tumor. J Pediatr 1982;101(4):559–562.
62. Beckwith JB. National Wilms Tumor Study: an update for pathologists. Pediatr Dev Pathol 1998;1(1):79–84.
63. Coppes MJ, Wolff JE, Ritchey ML. Wilms tumour: diagnosis and treatment. Paediatr Drugs 1999;1(4):251–262.
64. Pritchard J, Imeson J, Barnes J, et al. Results of the United Kingdom Children's Cancer Study Group first Wilms' Tumor Study. J Clin Oncol 1995;13(1):124–133.
65. D'Angio GJ, Evans AE, Breslow N, et al. The treatment of Wilms' tumor: results of the national Wilms' tumor study. Cancer (Phila) 1976;38(2):633–646.
66. D'Angio GJ, Evans A, Breslow N, et al. The treatment of Wilms' tumor: results of the Second National Wilms' Tumor Study. Cancer (Phila) 1981;47(9):2302–2311.
67. D'Angio GJ, Breslow N, Beckwith JB, et al. Treatment of Wilms' tumor. Results of the Third National Wilms' Tumor Study. Cancer (Phila) 1989;64(2):349–360.
68. Green DM, Breslow NE, D'Angio GJ. The treatment of children with unilateral Wilms' tumor. J Clin Oncol 1993;11(6):1009–1010.
69. Green DM, Breslow NE, Beckwith JB, et al. Treatment with nephrectomy only for small, stage I/favorable histology Wilms' tumor: a report from the National Wilms' Tumor Study Group. J Clin Oncol 2001;19(17):3719–3724.
70. Green DM. The treatment of stages I–IV favorable histology Wilms' tumor. J Clin Oncol 2004;22(8):1366–1372.
71. Grundy RG, Hutton C, Middleton H, et al. Outcome of patients with stage III or inoperable WT treated on the second United Kingdom WT protocol (UKWT2); a United Kingdom Children's Cancer Study Group (UKCCSG) study. Pediatr Blood Cancer 2004;42(4):311–319.
72. Tournade MF, Com-Nougue C, Voute PA, et al. Results of the Sixth International Society of Pediatric Oncology Wilms' Tumor Trial and Study: a risk-adapted therapeutic approach in Wilms' tumor. J Clin Oncol 1993;11(6):1014–1023.
73. Green DM. Wilms' tumour. Eur J Cancer 1997;33(3):409–418; discussion 419–420.
74. Cooper CS, Jaffe WI, Huff DS, et al. The role of renal salvage procedures for bilateral Wilms tumor: a 15-year review. J Urol 2000;163(1):265–268.
75. Kumar R, Fitzgerald R, Breatnach F. Conservative surgical management of bilateral Wilms tumor: results of the United Kingdom Children's Cancer Study Group. J Urol 1998;160(4):1450–1453.
76. D'Angio GJ. Pre- or post-operative treatment for Wilms tumor? Who, what, when, where, how, why—and which. Med Pediatr Oncol 2003;41(6):545–549.
77. Lemerle J, Voute PA, Tournade MF, et al. Effectiveness of preoperative chemotherapy in Wilms' tumor: results of an International Society of Paediatric Oncology (SIOP) clinical trial. J Clin Oncol 1983;1(10):604–609.
78. Tournade MF, Com-Nougue C, de Kraker J, et al. Optimal duration of preoperative therapy in unilateral and nonmetastatic Wilms' tumor in children older than 6 months: results of the Ninth International Society of Pediatric Oncology Wilms' Tumor Trial and Study. J Clin Oncol 2001;19(2):488–500.
79. Grundy P, Breslow N, Green DM, Sharples K, Evans A, D'Angio GJ. Prognostic factors for children with recurrent Wilms' tumor: results from the Second and Third National Wilms' Tumor Study. J Clin Oncol 1989;7(5):638–647.
80. Garaventa A, Hartmann O, Bernard JL, et al. Autologous bone marrow transplantation for pediatric Wilms' tumor: the experience of the European Bone Marrow Transplantation Solid Tumor Registry. Med Pediatr Oncol 1994;22(1):11–14.
81. Pein F, Michon J, Valteau-Couanet D, et al. High-dose melphalan, etoposide, and carboplatin followed by autologous stem-cell rescue in pediatric high-risk recurrent Wilms' tumor: a French Society of Pediatric Oncology study. J Clin Oncol 1998;16(10): 3295–3301.
82. Ritchey ML, Green DM, Thomas PR, et al. Renal failure in Wilms' tumor patients: a report from the National Wilms' Tumor Study Group. Med Pediatr Oncol 1996;26(2):75–80.
83. Sorensen K, Levitt G, Sebag-Montefiore D, Bull C, Sullivan I. Cardiac function in Wilms' tumor survivors. J Clin Oncol 1995; 13(7):1546–1556.
84. Green DM, Donckerwolcke R, Evans AE, D'Angio GJ. Late effects of treatment for Wilms tumor. Hematol Oncol Clin N Am 1995;9(6):1317–1327.
85. Breslow NE, Takashima JR, Whitton JA, Moksness J, D'Angio GJ, Green DM. Second malignant neoplasms following treatment for Wilm's tumor: a report from the National Wilms' Tumor Study Group. J Clin Oncol 1995;13(8):1851–1859.
86. Argani P, Perlman EJ, Breslow NE, et al. Clear cell sarcoma of the kidney: a review of 351 cases from the National Wilms Tumor Study Group Pathology Center. Am J Surg Pathol 2000; 24(1):4–18.
87. Green DM, Breslow NE, Beckwith JB, Moksness J, Finklestein JZ, D'Angio GJ. Treatment of children with clear-cell sarcoma of the kidney: a report from the National Wilms' Tumor Study Group. J Clin Oncol 1994;12(10):2132–2137.
88. Palmer NF, Sutow W. Clinical aspects of the rhabdoid tumor of the kidney: a report of the National Wilms' Tumor Study Group. Med Pediatr Oncol 1983;11(4):242–245.
89. Amar AM, Tomlinson G, Green DM, Breslow NE, de Alarcon PA. Clinical presentation of rhabdoid tumors of the kidney. J Pediatr Hematol Oncol 2001;23(2):105–108.
90. Beckwith JB, Palmer NF. Histopathology and prognosis of Wilms tumors: results from the First National Wilms' Tumor Study. Cancer (Phila) 1978;41(5):1937–1948.
91. Versteege I, Sevenet N, Lange J, et al. Truncating mutations of hSNF5/INI1 in aggressive paediatric cancer. Nature (Lond) 1998;394(6689):203–206.
92. Vujanic GM, Sandstedt B, Harms D, Boccon-Gibod L, Delemarre JF. Rhabdoid tumour of the kidney: a clinicopathological study of 22 patients from the International Society of Paediatric Oncology (SIOP) nephroblastoma file. Histopathology (Oxf) 1996;28(4):333–340.
93. Wagner L, Hill DA, Fuller C, et al. Treatment of metastatic rhabdoid tumor of the kidney. J Pediatr Hematol Oncol 2002;24(5):385–388.

94. Tomlinson GE, Nisen PD, Timmons CF, Schneider NR. Cytogenetics of a renal cell carcinoma in a 17-month-old child. Evidence for Xp11.2 as a recurring breakpoint. Cancer Genet Cytogenet 1991;57(1):11–17.
95. Tonk V, Wilson KS, Timmons CF, Schneider NR, Tomlinson GE. Renal cell carcinoma with translocation (X;1). Further evidence for a cytogenetically defined subtype. Cancer Genet Cytogenet 1995;81(1):72–75.
96. Davis CJ Jr, Mostofi FK, Sesterhenn IA. Renal medullary carcinoma. The seventh sickle cell nephropathy. Am J Surg Pathol 1995;19(1):1–11.
97. Sandberg AA, Bridge JA. Updates on the cytogenetics and molecular genetics of bone and soft tissue tumors: osteosarcoma and related tumors. Cancer Genet Cytogenet 2003;145(1):1–30.
98. Fuchs B, Pritchard DJ. Etiology of osteosarcoma. Clin Orthop 2002;397:40–52.
99. Patino-Garcia A, Pineiro ES, Diez MZ, Iturriagagoitia LG, Klussmann FA, Ariznabarreta LS. Genetic and epigenetic alterations of the cell cycle regulators and tumor suppressor genes in pediatric osteosarcomas. J Pediatr Hematol Oncol 2003;25(5): 362–367.
100. Yamaguchi T, Toguchida J, Yamamuro T, et al. Allelotype analysis in osteosarcomas: frequent allele loss on 3q, 13q, 17p, and 18q. Cancer Res 1992;52(9):2419–2423.
101. Tarkkanen M, Karhu R, Kallioniemi A, et al. Gains and losses of DNA sequences in osteosarcomas by comparative genomic hybridization. Cancer Res 1995;55(6):1334–1338.
102. Arndt CA, Crist WM. Common musculoskeletal tumors of childhood and adolescence. N Engl J Med 1999;341(5): 342–352.
103. Meyers PA, Heller G, Healey JH, et al. Osteogenic sarcoma with clinically detectable metastasis at initial presentation. J Clin Oncol 1993;11(3):449–453.
104. Kager L, Zoubek A, Potschger U, et al. Primary metastatic osteosarcoma: presentation and outcome of patients treated on neoadjuvant Cooperative Osteosarcoma Study Group protocols. J Clin Oncol 2003;21(10):2011–2018.
105. Simon R. Clinical prognostic factors in osteosarcoma. Cancer Treat Rep 1978;62(2):193–197.
106. Look AT, Douglass EC, Meyer WH. Clinical importance of near-diploid tumor stem lines in patients with osteosarcoma of an extremity. N Engl J Med 1988;318(24):1567–1572.
107. Feugeas O, Guriec N, Babin-Boilletot A, et al. Loss of heterozygosity of the RB gene is a poor prognostic factor in patients with osteosarcoma. J Clin Oncol 1996;14(2):467–472.
108. Gorlick R, Huvos AG, Heller G, et al. Expression of HER2/erbB-2 correlates with survival in osteosarcoma. J Clin Oncol 1999;17(9):2781–2788.
109. Meyers PA, Gorlick R, Heller G, et al. Intensification of preoperative chemotherapy for osteogenic sarcoma: results of the Memorial Sloan-Kettering (T12) protocol. J Clin Oncol 1998; 16(7):2452–2458.
110. Glasser DB, Lane JM, Huvos AG, Marcove RC, Rosen G. Survival, prognosis, and therapeutic response in osteogenic sarcoma. The Memorial Hospital experience. Cancer (Phila) 1992;69(3):698–708.
111. Friedman MA, Carter SK. The therapy of osteogenic sarcoma: current status and thoughts for the future. J Surg Oncol 1972; 4(5):482–510.
112. Prindull G, Willert HG, Notter G. Local therapy of rhabdomyosarcoma, osteosarcoma and Ewing's sarcoma of children and adolescents. Eur J Pediatr 1985;144(2):120–124.
113. Goorin AM, Abelson HT, Frei E III. Osteosarcoma: fifteen years later. N Engl J Med 1985;313(26):1637–1643.
114. Harris MB, Cantor AB, Goorin AM, et al. Treatment of osteosarcoma with ifosfamide: comparison of response in pediatric patients with recurrent disease versus patients previously untreated: a Pediatric Oncology Group study. Med Pediatr Oncol 1995;24(2):87–92.
115. Miser JS, Krailo MD, Tarbell NJ, et al. Treatment of metastic Ewing's sarcoma of primitive neuroectodermal tumor of bone: evaluation of combination ifosfamide and etoposide—a Children's Cancer Group and Pediatric Oncology Group Study. J Clin Oncol 2004;22(14):2873–2876.
116. Goorin AM, Schwartzentruber DJ, Devidas M, et al. Presurgical chemotherapy compared with immediate surgery and adjuvant chemotherapy for nonmetastatic osteosarcoma: Pediatric Oncology Group Study POG-8651. J Clin Oncol 2003;21(8): 1574–1580.
117. Bacci G, Briccoli A, Rocca M, et al. Neoadjuvant chemotherapy for osteosarcoma of the extremities with metastases at presentation: recent experience at the Rizzoli Institute in 57 patients treated with cisplatin, doxorubicin, and a high dose of methotrexate and ifosfamide. Ann Oncol 2003;14(7):1126–1134.
118. Janinis J, McTiernan A, Driver D, et al. A pilot study of short-course intensive multiagent chemotherapy in metastatic and axial skeletal osteosarcoma. Ann Oncol 2002;13(12):1935–1944.
119. Goorin AM, Harris MB, Bernstein M, et al. Phase II/III trial of etoposide and high-dose ifosfamide in newly diagnosed metastatic osteosarcoma: a pediatric oncology group trial. J Clin Oncol 2002;20(2):426–433.
120. Weis LD. The success of limb-salvage surgery in the adolescent patient with osteogenic sarcoma. Adolesc Med 1999;10(3):451–458, xii.
121. Bacci G, Ruggieri P, Bertoni F, et al. Local and systemic control for osteosarcoma of the extremity treated with neoadjuvant chemotherapy and limb salvage surgery: the Rizzoli experience. Oncol Rep 2000;7(5):1129–1133.
122. Bacci G, Ferrari S, Longhi A, et al. Nonmetastatic osteosarcoma of the extremity with pathologic fracture at presentation: local and systemic control by amputation or limb salvage after preoperative chemotherapy. Acta Orthop Scand 2003;74(4): 449–454.
123. Lindner NJ, Ramm O, Hillmann A, et al. Limb salvage and outcome of osteosarcoma. The University of Muenster experience. Clin Orthop 1999(358):83–89.
124. Rougraff BT, Simon MA, Kneisl JS, Greenberg DB, Mankin HJ. Limb salvage compared with amputation for osteosarcoma of the distal end of the femur. A long-term oncological, functional, and quality-of-life study. J Bone Joint Surg Am 1994; 76(5):649–656.
125. Hawkins DS, Arndt CA. Pattern of disease recurrence and prognostic factors in patients with osteosarcoma treated with contemporary chemotherapy. Cancer (Phila) 2003;98(11):2447–2456.
126. Duffaud F, Digue L, Mercier C, et al. Recurrences following primary osteosarcoma in adolescents and adults previously treated with chemotherapy. Eur J Cancer 2003;39(14):2050–2057.
127. Huth JF, Eilber FR. Patterns of recurrence after resection of osteosarcoma of the extremity. Strategies for treatment of metastases. Arch Surg 1989;124(1):122–126.
128. Ferrari S, Briccoli A, Mercuri M, et al. Postrelapse survival in osteosarcoma of the extremities: prognostic factors for long-term survival. J Clin Oncol 2003;21(4):710–715.
129. Lipshultz SE, Lipsitz SR, Mone SM, et al. Female sex and drug dose as risk factors for late cardiotoxic effects of doxorubicin therapy for childhood cancer. N Engl J Med 1995;332(26):1738–1743.
130. Maygarden SJ, Askin FB, Siegal GP, et al. Ewing sarcoma of bone in infants and toddlers. A clinicopathologic report from the Intergroup Ewing's Study. Cancer (Phila) 1993;71(6):2109–2118.

131. Hartley AL, Birch JM, Blair V, Teare MD, Marsden HB, Harris M. Cancer incidence in the families of children with Ewing's tumor. J Natl Cancer Inst 1991;83(13):955–956.
132. Parkin DM, Stiller CA, Nectoux J. International variations in the incidence of childhood bone tumours. Int J Cancer 1993; 53(3):371–376.
133. de Alava E, Kawai A, Healey JH, et al. EWS-FLI1 fusion transcript structure is an independent determinant of prognosis in Ewing's sarcoma. J Clin Oncol 1998;16(4):1248–1255.
134. Widhe B, Widhe T. Initial symptoms and clinical features in osteosarcoma and Ewing sarcoma. J Bone Joint Surg Am 2000; 82(5):667–674.
135. Grier HE. The Ewing family of tumors. Ewing's sarcoma and primitive neuroectodermal tumors. Pediatr Clin N Am 1997; 44(4):991–1004.
136. Cangir A, Vietti TJ, Gehan EA, et al. Ewing's sarcoma metastatic at diagnosis. Results and comparisons of two intergroup Ewing's sarcoma studies. Cancer (Phila) 1990;66(5):887–893.
137. Cotterill SJ, Ahrens S, Paulussen M, et al. Prognostic factors in Ewing's tumor of bone: analysis of 975 patients from the European Intergroup Cooperative Ewing's Sarcoma Study Group. J Clin Oncol 2000;18(17):3108–3114.
138. Paulussen M, Ahrens S, Burdach S, et al. Primary metastatic (stage IV) Ewing tumor: survival analysis of 171 patients from the EICESS studies. European Intergroup Cooperative Ewing Sarcoma Studies. Ann Oncol 1998;9(3):275–281.
139. Schleiermacher G, Peter M, Oberlin O, et al. Increased risk of systemic relapses associated with bone marrow micrometastasis and circulating tumor cells in localized ewing tumor. J Clin Oncol 2003;21(1):85–91.
140. Jurgens H, Exner U, Gadner H, et al. Multidisciplinary treatment of primary Ewing's sarcoma of bone. A 6-year experience of a European Cooperative Trial. Cancer (Phila) 1988;61(1):23–32.
141. Hayes FA, Thompson EI, Meyer WH, et al. Therapy for localized Ewing's sarcoma of bone. J Clin Oncol 1989;7(2):208–213.
142. Craft AW, Cotterill SJ, Bullimore JA, Pearson D. Long-term results from the first UKCCSG Ewing's Tumour Study (ET-1). United Kingdom Children's Cancer Study Group (UKCCSG) and the Medical Research Council Bone Sarcoma Working Party. Eur J Cancer 1997;33(7):1061–1069.
143. Grier HE, Krailo MD, Tarbell NJ, et al. Addition of ifosfamide and etoposide to standard chemotherapy for Ewing's sarcoma and primitive neuroectodermal tumor of bone. N Engl J Med 2003;348(8):694–701.
144. Craft A, Cotterill S, Malcolm A, et al. Ifosfamide-containing chemotherapy in Ewing's sarcoma: The Second United Kingdom Children's Cancer Study Group and the Medical Research Council Ewing's Tumor Study. J Clin Oncol 1998;16(11):3628– 3633.
145. Paulussen M, Ahrens S, Dunst J, et al. Localized Ewing tumor of bone: final results of the cooperative Ewing's Sarcoma Study CESS 86. J Clin Oncol 2001;19(6):1818–1829.
146. Picci P, Bohling T, Bacci G, et al. Chemotherapy-induced tumor necrosis as a prognostic factor in localized Ewing's sarcoma of the extremities. J Clin Oncol 1997;15(4):1553–1559.
147. Bacci G, Ferrari S, Bertoni F, et al. Prognostic factors in nonmetastatic Ewing's sarcoma of bone treated with adjuvant chemotherapy: analysis of 359 patients at the Istituto Ortopedico Rizzoli. J Clin Oncol 2000;18(1):4–11.
148. Nesbit ME Jr, Gehan EA, Burgert EO Jr, et al. Multimodal therapy for the management of primary, nonmetastatic Ewing's sarcoma of bone: a long-term follow-up of the First Intergroup study. J Clin Oncol 1990;8(10):1664–1674.
148a. Burgert EO Jr, Nesbit ME, Garnsey LA, et al. Multimodal therapy for the management of nonpelvic, localized Ewing's sarcoma of bone: intergroup study IESS-II. J Clin Oncol 1990;8(9):1514–1524.
149. Kushner BH, Meyers PA, Gerald WL, et al. Very-high-dose short-term chemotherapy for poor-risk peripheral primitive neuroectodermal tumors, including Ewing's sarcoma, in children and young adults. J Clin Oncol 1995;13(11):2796–2804.
150. Marina NM, Pappo AS, Parham DM, et al. Chemotherapy dose-intensification for pediatric patients with Ewing's family of tumors and desmoplastic small round-cell tumors: a feasibility study at St. Jude Children's Research Hospital. J Clin Oncol 1999;17(1):180–190.
151. Bacci G, Toni A, Avella M, et al. Long-term results in 144 localized Ewing's sarcoma patients treated with combined therapy. Cancer (Phila) 1989;63(8):1477–1486.
152. Barbieri E, Emiliani E, Zini G, et al. Combined therapy of localized Ewing's sarcoma of bone: analysis of results in 100 patients. Int J Radiat Oncol Biol Phys 1990;19(5):1165–1170.
153. Rosito P, Mancini AF, Rondelli R, et al. Italian Cooperative Study for the treatment of children and young adults with localized Ewing sarcoma of bone: a preliminary report of 6 years of experience. Cancer (Phila) 1999;86(3):421–428.
154. Shankar AG, Pinkerton CR, Atra A, et al. Local therapy and other factors influencing site of relapse in patients with localised Ewing's sarcoma. United Kingdom Children's Cancer Study Group (UKCCSG). Eur J Cancer 1999;35(12):1698–1704.
155. Hoffmann C, Ahrens S, Dunst J, et al. Pelvic Ewing sarcoma: a retrospective analysis of 241 cases. Cancer (Phila) 1999;85(4): 869–877.
156. Kushner BH, Meyers PA. How effective is dose-intensive/myeloablative therapy against Ewing's sarcoma/primitive neuroectodermal tumor metastatic to bone or bone marrow? The Memorial Sloan-Kettering experience and a literature review. J Clin Oncol 2001;19(3):870–880.
157. Yaniv I, Cohen IJ, Stein J, et al. Tumor cells are present in stem cell harvests of Ewings sarcoma patients and their persistence following transplantation is associated with relapse. Pediatr Blood Cancer 2004;42(5):404–409.
158. Rodriguez-Galindo C, Billups CA, Kun LE, et al. Survival after recurrence of Ewing tumors: the St Jude Children's Research Hospital experience, 1979–1999. Cancer (Phila) 2002;94(2): 561–569.
159. Shankar AG, Ashley S, Craft AW, Pinkerton CR. Outcome after relapse in an unselected cohort of children and adolescents with Ewing sarcoma. Med Pediatr Oncol 2003;40(3):141–147.
160. Saylors RL III, Stine KC, Sullivan J, et al. Cyclophosphamide plus topotecan in children with recurrent or refractory solid tumors: a Pediatric Oncology Group phase II study. J Clin Oncol 2001;19(15):3463–3469.
161. Kushner BH, Heller G, Cheung NK, et al. High risk of leukemia after short-term dose-intensive chemotherapy in young patients with solid tumors. J Clin Oncol 1998;16(9):3016–3020.
162. Novakovic B, Fears TR, Horowitz ME, Tucker MA, Wexler LH. Late effects of therapy in survivors of Ewing's sarcoma family tumors. J Pediatr Hematol Oncol 1997;19(3):220–225.
163. Li FP, Fraumeni JF Jr. Rhabdomyosarcoma in children: epidemiologic study and identification of a familial cancer syndrome. J Natl Cancer Inst 1969;43(6):1365–1373.
164. Diller L, Sexsmith E, Gottlieb A, Li FP, Malkin D. Germline p53 mutations are frequently detected in young children with rhabdomyosarcoma. J Clin Invest 1995;95(4):1606–1611.
165. Sung L, Anderson JR, Arndt C, Raney RB, Meyer WH, Pappo AS. Neurofibromatosis in children with rhabdomyosarcoma: a report from the Intergroup Rhabdomyosarcoma study IV. J Pediatr 2004;144(5):666–668.
166. Sublett JE, Jeon IS, Shapiro DN. The alveolar rhabdomyosarcoma PAX3/FKHR fusion protein is a transcriptional activator. Oncogene 1995;11(3):545–552.
167. Scrable H, Witte D, Shimada H, et al. Molecular differential pathology of rhabdomyosarcoma. Genes Chromosomes Cancer 1989;1(1):23–35.

168. Maurer HM, Beltangady M, Gehan EA, et al. The Intergroup Rhabdomyosarcoma Study-I. A final report. Cancer (Phila) 1988; 61(2):209–220.
169. Maurer HM, Gehan EA, Beltangady M, et al. The Intergroup Rhabdomyosarcoma Study-II. Cancer (Phila) 1993;71(5):1904–1922.
170. Crist W, Gehan EA, Ragab AH, et al. The Third Intergroup Rhabdomyosarcoma Study. J Clin Oncol 1995;13(3):610–630.
171. Crist WM, Garnsey L, Beltangady MS, et al. Prognosis in children with rhabdomyosarcoma: a report of the intergroup rhabdomyosarcoma studies I and II. Intergroup Rhabdomyosarcoma Committee. J Clin Oncol 1990;8(3):443–452.
172. Joshi D, Anderson JR, Paidas C, Breneman J, Parham DM, Crist W. Age is an independent prognostic factor in rhabdomyosarcoma: a report from the Soft Tissue Sarcoma Committee of the Children's Oncology Group. Pediatr Blood Cancer 2004;42(1): 64–73.
173. Hays DM, Raney RB, Crist WM, et al. Secondary surgical procedures to evaluate primary tumor status in patients with chemotherapy-responsive stage III and IV sarcomas: a report from the Intergroup Rhabdomyosarcoma Study. J Pediatr Surg 1990;25(10):1100–1105.
174. Godzinski J, Flamant F, Rey A, Praquin MT, Martelli H. Value of postchemotherapy bioptical verification of complete clinical remission in previously incompletely resected (stage I and II pT3) malignant mesenchymal tumors in children: International Society of Pediatric Oncology 1984 Malignant Mesenchymal Tumors Study. Med Pediatr Oncol 1994;22(1):22–26.
175. Wilbur JR. Combination chemotherapy for embryonal rhabdomyosarcoma. Cancer Chemother Rep 1974;58(2):281–284.
176. Kushner BH, Kramer K, Meyers PA, Wollner N, Cheung NK. Pilot study of topotecan and high-dose cyclophosphamide for resistant pediatric solid tumors. Med Pediatr Oncol 2000;35(5): 468–474.
177. Furman WL, Stewart CF, Poquette CA, et al. Direct translation of a protracted irinotecan schedule from a xenograft model to a phase I trial in children. J Clin Oncol 1999;17(6):1815–1824.
178. Breneman JC, Lyden E, Pappo AS, et al. Prognostic factors and clinical outcomes in children and adolescents with metastatic rhabdomyosarcoma: a report from the Intergroup Rhabdomyosarcoma Study IV. J Clin Oncol 2003;21(1):78–84.
179. Carli M, Colombatti R, Oberlin O, et al. High-dose melphalan with autologous stem-cell rescue in metastatic rhabdomyosarcoma. J Clin Oncol 1999;17(9):2796–2803.
180. Boulad F, Kernan NA, LaQuaglia MP, et al. High-dose induction chemoradiotherapy followed by autologous bone marrow transplantation as consolidation therapy in rhabdomyosarcoma, extra-osseous Ewing's sarcoma, and undifferentiated sarcoma. J Clin Oncol 1998;16(5):1697–1706.
181. Walterhouse DO, Hoover ML, Marymont MA, Kletzel M. High-dose chemotherapy followed by peripheral blood stem cell rescue for metastatic rhabdomyosarcoma: the experience at Chicago Children's Memorial Hospital. Med Pediatr Oncol 1999;32(2):88–92.
182. Pappo AS, Anderson JR, Crist WM, et al. Survival after relapse in children and adolescents with rhabdomyosarcoma: a report from the Intergroup Rhabdomyosarcoma Study Group. J Clin Oncol 1999;17(11):3487–3493.
183. Darbari A, Sabin KM, Shapiro CN, Schwarz KB. Epidemiology of primary hepatic malignancies in U.S. children. Hepatology 2003;38(3):560–566.
184. DeBaun MR, Tucker MA. Risk of cancer during the first four years of life in children from The Beckwith-Wiedemann Syndrome Registry. J Pediatr 1998;132(3 pt 1):398–400.
185. Hoyme HE, Seaver LH, Jones KL, Procopio F, Crooks W, Feingold M. Isolated hemihyperplasia (hemihypertrophy): report of a prospective multicenter study of the incidence of neoplasia and review. Am J Med Genet 1998;79(4):274–278.
186. Clericuzio CL, Chen E, McNeil DE, et al. Serum alpha-fetoprotein screening for hepatoblastoma in children with Beckwith-Wiedemann syndrome or isolated hemihyperplasia. J Pediatr 2003;143(2):270–272.
187. Ikeda H, Matsuyama S, Tanimura M. Association between hepatoblastoma and very low birth weight: a trend or a chance? J Pediatr 1997;130(4):557–560.
188. Herzog CE, Andrassy RJ, Eftekhari F. Childhood cancers: hepatoblastoma. Oncologist 2000;5(6):445–453.
189. Reynolds P, Urayama KY, Von Behren J, Feusner J. Birth characteristics and hepatoblastoma risk in young children. Cancer (Phila) 2004;100(5):1070–1076.
190. Ribons LA, Slovis TL. Hepatoblastoma and birth weight. J Pediatr 1998;132(4):750.
191. Feusner J, Buckley J, Robison L, Ross J, Van Tornout J. Prematurity and hepatoblastoma: more than just an association? J Pediatr 1998;133(4):585–586.
192. Schnater JM, Kohler SE, Lamers WH, von Schweinitz D, Aronson DC. Where do we stand with hepatoblastoma? A review. Cancer (Phila) 2003;98(4):668–678.
193. Albrecht S, von Schweinitz D, Waha A, Kraus JA, von Deimling A, Pietsch T. Loss of maternal alleles on chromosome arm 11p in hepatoblastoma. Cancer Res 1994;54(19):5041–5044.
194. Zatkova A, Rouillard JM, Hartmann W, et al. Amplification and overexpression of the IGF2 regulator PLAG1 in hepatoblastoma. Genes Chromosomes Cancer (Phila) 2004;39(2): 126–137.
195. Saxena R, Leake JL, Shafford EA, et al. Chemotherapy effects on hepatoblastoma. A histological study. Am J Surg Pathol 1993;17(12):1266–1271.
196. Lack EE, Neave C, Vawter GF. Hepatoblastoma. A clinical and pathologic study of 54 cases. Am J Surg Pathol 1982;6(8):693–705.
197. Ortega JA, Krailo MD, Haas JE, et al. Effective treatment of unresectable or metastatic hepatoblastoma with cisplatin and continuous infusion doxorubicin chemotherapy: a report from the Childrens Cancer Study Group. J Clin Oncol 1991;9(12): 2167–2176.
198. Haas JE, Feusner JH, Finegold MJ. Small cell undifferentiated histology in hepatoblastoma may be unfavorable. Cancer (Phila) 2001;92(12):3130–3134.
199. Van Tornout JM, Buckley JD, Quinn JJ, et al. Timing and magnitude of decline in alpha-fetoprotein levels in treated children with unresectable or metastatic hepatoblastoma are predictors of outcome: a report from the Children's Cancer Group. J Clin Oncol 1997;15(3):1190–1197.
200. Stringer MD, Hennayake S, Howard ER, et al. Improved outcome for children with hepatoblastoma. Br J Surg 1995; 82(3): 386–391.
201. Seo T, Ando H, Watanabe Y, et al. Treatment of hepatoblastoma: less extensive hepatectomy after effective preoperative chemotherapy with cisplatin and adriamycin. Surgery (St. Louis) 1998; 123(4):407–414.
202. Brown J, Perilongo G, Shafford E, et al. Pretreatment prognostic factors for children with hepatoblastoma: results from the International Society of Paediatric Oncology (SIOP) study SIOPEL 1. Eur J Cancer 2000;36(11):1418–1425.
203. Schnater JM, Aronson DC, Plaschkes J, et al. Surgical view of the treatment of patients with hepatoblastoma: results from the first prospective trial of the International Society of Pediatric Oncology Liver Tumor Study Group. Cancer (Phila) 2002;94(4): 1111–1120.
204. Perilongo G, Shafford E, Plaschkes J. SIOPEL trials using preoperative chemotherapy in hepatoblastoma. Lancet Oncol 2000;1: 94–100.
205. Carceller A, Blanchard H, Champagne J, St-Vil D, Bensoussan AL. Surgical resection and chemotherapy improve survival rate

for patients with hepatoblastoma. J Pediatr Surg 2001;36(5): 755–759.
206. Ortega JA, Douglass EC, Feusner JH, et al. Randomized comparison of cisplatin/vincristine/fluorouracil and cisplatin/continuous infusion doxorubicin for treatment of pediatric hepatoblastoma: a report from the Children's Cancer Group and the Pediatric Oncology Group. J Clin Oncol 2000; 18(14):2665– 2675.
207. Fuchs J, Rydzynski J, Hecker H, et al. The influence of preoperative chemotherapy and surgical technique in the treatment of hepatoblastoma: a report from the German Cooperative Liver Tumour Studies HB 89 and HB 94. Eur J Pediatr Surg 2002;12(4): 255–261.
208. Fuchs J, Rydzynski J, Von Schweinitz D, et al. Pretreatment prognostic factors and treatment results in children with hepatoblastoma: a report from the German Cooperative Pediatric Liver Tumor Study HB 94. Cancer (Phila) 2002; 95(1):172–182.
209. Sasaki F, Matsunaga T, Iwafuchi M, et al. Outcome of hepatoblastoma treated with the JPLT-1 (Japanese Study Group for Pediatric Liver Tumor) Protocol-1: a report from the Japanese Study Group for Pediatric Liver Tumor. J Pediatr Surg 2002;37(6):851– 856.
210. Srinivasan P, McCall J, Pritchard J, et al. Orthotopic liver transplantation for unresectable hepatoblastoma. Transplantation 2002;74(5):652–655.
211. Pimpalwar AP, Sharif K, Ramani P, et al. Strategy for hepatoblastoma management: transplant versus nontransplant surgery. J Pediatr Surg 2002;37(2):240–245.
212. Molmenti EP, Wilkinson K, Molmenti H, et al. Treatment of unresectable hepatoblastoma with liver transplantation in the pediatric population. Am J Transplant 2002;2(6):535–538.
213. Katzenstein HM, London WB, Douglass EC, et al. Treatment of unresectable and metastatic hepatoblastoma: a pediatric oncology group phase II study. J Clin Oncol 2002;20(16):3438–3444.
214. Feusner JH, Krailo MD, Haas JE, Campbell JR, Lloyd DA, Ablin AR. Treatment of pulmonary metastases of initial stage I hepatoblastoma in childhood. Report from the Childrens Cancer Group. Cancer (Phila) 1993;71(3):859–864.
215. Matsunaga T, Sasaki F, Ohira M, et al. Analysis of treatment outcome for children with recurrent or metastatic hepatoblastoma. Pediatr Surg Int 2003;19(3):142–146.
216. Nishimura S, Sato T, Fujita N, et al. High-dose chemotherapy in children with metastatic hepatoblastoma. Pediatr Int 2002;44(3):300–305.
217. Czauderna P, Mackinlay G, Perilongo G, et al. Hepatocellular carcinoma in children: results of the first prospective study of the International Society of Pediatric Oncology group. J Clin Oncol 2002;20(12):2798–2804.
218. Katzenstein HM, Krailo MD, Malogolowkin MH, et al. Hepatocellular carcinoma in children and adolescents: results from the Pediatric Oncology Group and the Children's Cancer Group intergroup study. J Clin Oncol 2002;20(12): 2789–2797.
219. Tamboli A, Podgor MJ, Horm JW. The incidence of retinoblastoma in the United States: 1974 through 1985. Arch Ophthalmol 1990;108(1):128–132.
220. Rubenfeld M, Abramson DH, Ellsworth RM, Kitchin FD. Unilateral vs. bilateral retinoblastoma. Correlations between age at diagnosis and stage of ocular disease. Ophthalmology 1986; 93(8):1016–1019.
221. Paulino AC. Trilateral retinoblastoma: is the location of the intracranial tumor important? Cancer (Phila) 1999;86(1):135–141.
222. Knudson AG Jr. Mutation and cancer: statistical study of retinoblastoma. Proc Natl Acad Sci U S A 1971;68(4):820–823.
223. Friend SH, Bernards R, Rogelj S, et al. A human DNA segment with properties of the gene that predisposes to retinoblastoma and osteosarcoma. Nature (Lond) 1986;323(6089):643–646.
224. Shields J. Retinoblastoma: clinical, and pathological features. In: Intraocular Tumors: A Text and Atlas. Philadelphia: Saunders, 1992:305–332.
225. Tajima Y, Nakajima T, Sugano I, Nagao K, Minoda K, Kondo Y. Cytodiagnostic clues to primary retinoblastoma based on cytologic and histologic correlates of 39 enucleated eyes. Acta Cytol 1994;38(2):151–157.
226. Abramson DH, Beaverson K, Sangani P, et al. Screening for retinoblastoma: presenting signs as prognosticators of patient and ocular survival. Pediatrics 2003;112(6 pt 1):1248–1255.
227. Balmer A, Gailloud C, Munier F, Uffer S, Guex-Crosier Y. Retinoblastoma. Unusual warning and clinical signs. Ophthalmic Paediatr Genet 1993;14(1):33–38.
228. McLean IW, Burnier M, Zimmerman L, Jakobiec F. Tumors of the retina. In: McLean IW, Burnier M, Zimmerman L (eds). Atlas of Tumor Pathology: Tumors of the Eye and Ocular Adnexa. Washington, DC: Armed Forces Institute of Pathology, 1994: 100–135.
229. Char DH, Hedges TR III, Norman D. Retinoblastoma. CT diagnosis. Ophthalmology 1984;91(11):1347–1350.
230. Howard GM, Ellsworth RM. Differential diagnosis of retinoblastoma. A statistical survey of 500 children. I. Relative frequency of the lesions which simulate retinoblastoma. Am J Ophthalmol 1965;60(4):610–618.
231. Pratt CB, Fontanesi J, Lu X, Parham DM, Elfervig J, Meyer D. Proposal for a new staging scheme for intraocular and extraocular retinoblastoma based on an analysis of 103 globes. Oncologist 1997;2(1):1–5.
232. De Sutter E, Hoepping W, Zeller G. Comparison between different retinoblastoma classifications. Bull Soc Belg Ophtalmol 1993;248:19–22.
233. Khelfaoui F, Validire P, Auperin A, et al. Histopathologic risk factors in retinoblastoma: a retrospective study of 172 patients treated in a single institution. Cancer (Phila) 1996;77(6):1206–1213.
234. Kopelman JE, McLean IW, Rosenberg SH. Multivariate analysis of risk factors for metastasis in retinoblastoma treated by enucleation. Ophthalmology 1987;94(4):371–377.
235. Merchant TE, Gould CJ, Hilton NE, et al. Ocular preservation after 36 Gy external beam radiation therapy for retinoblastoma. J Pediatr Hematol Oncol 2002;24(4):246–249.
236. Gallie BL, Budning A, DeBoer G, et al. Chemotherapy with focal therapy can cure intraocular retinoblastoma without radiotherapy. Arch Ophthalmol 1996;114(11):1321–1328.
237. Beck MN, Balmer A, Dessing C, Pica A, Munier F. First-line chemotherapy with local treatment can prevent external-beam irradiation and enucleation in low-stage intraocular retinoblastoma. J Clin Oncol 2000;18(15):2881–2887.
238. Brichard B, De Bruycker JJ, De Potter P, Neven B, Vermylen C, Cornu G. Combined chemotherapy and local treatment in the management of intraocular retinoblastoma. Med Pediatr Oncol 2002;38(6):411–415.
239. Friedman DL, Himelstein B, Shields CL, et al. Chemoreduction and local ophthalmic therapy for intraocular retinoblastoma. J Clin Oncol 2000;18(1):12–17.
240. Lumbroso L, Doz F, Urbieta M, et al. Chemothermotherapy in the management of retinoblastoma. Ophthalmology 2002; 109(6):1130–1136.
241. Shields CL, Shields JA, Needle M, et al. Combined chemoreduction and adjuvant treatment for intraocular retinoblastoma. Ophthalmology 1997;104(12):2101–2111.
242. Shields CL, Honavar SG, Meadows AT, Shields JA, Demirci H, Naduvilath TJ. Chemoreduction for unilateral retinoblastoma. Arch Ophthalmol 2002;120(12):1653–1658.

243. Wilson MW, Rodriguez-Galindo C, Haik BG, Moshfeghi DM, Merchant TE, Pratt CB. Multiagent chemotherapy as neoadjuvant treatment for multifocal intraocular retinoblastoma. Ophthalmology 2001;108(11):2106–2114; discussion 2114–2115.
244. Sussman DA, Escalona-Benz E, Benz MS, et al. Comparison of retinoblastoma reduction for chemotherapy vs. external beam radiotherapy. Arch Ophthalmol 2003;121(7):979–984.
245. Shields CL, Honavar SG, Meadows AT, et al. Chemoreduction plus focal therapy for retinoblastoma: factors predictive of need for treatment with external beam radiotherapy or enucleation. Am J Ophthalmol 2002;133(5):657–664.
246. Honavar SG, Singh AD, Shields CL, et al. Postenucleation adjuvant therapy in high-risk retinoblastoma. Arch Ophthalmol 2002;120(7):923–931.
247. Rodriguez-Galindo C, Wilson MW, Haik BG, et al. Treatment of metastatic retinoblastoma. Ophthalmology 2003;110(6): 1237–1240.
248. Namouni F, Doz F, Tanguy ML, et al. High-dose chemotherapy with carboplatin, etoposide and cyclophosphamide followed by a haematopoietic stem cell rescue in patients with high-risk retinoblastoma: a SFOP and SFGM study. Eur J Cancer 1997; 33(14):2368–2375.
249. Jubran RF, Erdreich-Epstein A, Butturini A, Murphree AL, Villablanca JG. Approaches to treatment for extraocular retinoblastoma: Children's Hospital Los Angeles experience. J Pediatr Hematol Oncol 2004;26(1):31–34.
250. Dunkel IJ, Aledo A, Kernan NA, et al. Successful treatment of metastatic retinoblastoma. Cancer (Phila) 2000;89(10):2117–2121.
251. Shields CL, Meadows AT, Shields JA, Carvalho C, Smith AF. Chemoreduction for retinoblastoma may prevent intracranial neuroblastic malignancy (trilateral retinoblastoma). Arch Ophthalmol 2001;119(9):1269–1272.
252. Draper GJ, Sanders BM, Kingston JE. Second primary neoplasms in patients with retinoblastoma. Br J Cancer 1986;53(5):661–671.
253. Eng C, Li FP, Abramson DH, et al. Mortality from second tumors among long-term survivors of retinoblastoma. J Natl Cancer Inst 1993;85(14):1121–1128.
254. Wong FL, Boice JD Jr, Abramson DH, et al. Cancer incidence after retinoblastoma. Radiation dose and sarcoma risk. JAMA 1997;278(15):1262–1267.
255. Rescorla FJ, Breitfeld PP. Pediatric germ cell tumors. Curr Probl Cancer 1999;23(6):257–303.
256. Lau YF. Gonadoblastoma, testicular and prostate cancers, and the TSPY gene. Am J Hum Genet 1999;64(4):921–927.
257. Lau YF, Lau HW, Komuves LG. Expression pattern of a gonadoblastoma candidate gene suggests a role of the Y chromosome in prostate cancer. Cytogenet Genome Res 2003; 101(3–4):250–260.
258. Fonkalsrud EW. The undescended testis. Curr Probl Surg 1978;15(3):1–56.
259. Fonkalsrud EW. Current management of the undescended testis. Semin Pediatr Surg 1996;5(1):2–7.
260. Jones BJ, Thornhill JA, O'Donnell B, et al. Influence of prior orchiopexy on stage and prognosis of testicular cancer. Eur Urol 1991;19(3):201–203.
261. Bussey KJ, Lawce HJ, Olson SB, et al. Chromosome abnormalities of eighty-one pediatric germ cell tumors: sex-, age-, site-, and histopathology-related differences: a Children's Cancer Group study. Genes Chromosomes Cancer 1999;25(2):134–146.
262. Cushing B, Perlman E, Marina N, Castleberry R. Germ Cell Tumors. In: Pizzo PA, Poplack DG (eds). Principles and Practice of Pediatric Oncology, 4th ed. Lippincott Williams & Wilkins, 2002:1091–1113.
263. Mazumdar M, Bajorin DF, Bacik J, Higgins G, Motzer RJ, Bosl GJ. Predicting outcome to chemotherapy in patients with germ cell tumors: the value of the rate of decline of human chorionic gonadotropin and alpha-fetoprotein during therapy. J Clin Oncol 2001;19(9):2534–2541.
264. Wu JT, Book L, Sudar K. Serum alpha fetoprotein (AFP) levels in normal infants. Pediatr Res 1981;15(1):50–52.
265. Marina NM, Cushing B, Giller R, et al. Complete surgical excision is effective treatment for children with immature teratomas with or without malignant elements: A Pediatric Oncology Group/Children's Cancer Group Intergroup Study. J Clin Oncol 1999;17(7):2137–2143.
266. Cushing B, Giller R, Ablin A, et al. Surgical resection alone is effective treatment for ovarian immature teratoma in children and adolescents: a report of the pediatric oncology group and the children's cancer group. Am J Obstet Gynecol 1999;181(2): 258–353.
267. Cushing B, Giller R, Cullen JW, et al. Randomized comparison of combination chemotherapy with etoposide, bleomycin, and either high-dose or standard-dose cisplatin in children and adolescents with high-risk malignant germ cell tumors: a pediatric intergroup study—Pediatric Oncology Group 9049 and Children's Cancer Group 8882. J Clin Oncol 2004;22(13):2691–2700.
268. Williams S, Blessing J, Slayton R. Ovarian germ cell tumors: adjuvant trials of the gynecologic oncology group. In: Salma S (ed). Proceedings of the Sixth International Conference on the Adjuvant Therapy of Cancer 1990:501–503.
269. Einhorn LH. Chemotherapy of disseminated germ cell tumors. Cancer (Phila) 1987;60(suppl 3l):570–573.
270. Schlatter M, Rescorla F, Giller R, et al. Excellent outcome in patients with stage I germ cell tumors of the testes: a study of the Children's Cancer Group/Pediatric Oncology Group. J Pediatr Surg 2003;38(3):319–324; discussion 324.
271. Gobel U, Schneider DT, Calaminus G, Haas RJ, Schmidt P, Harms D. Germ-cell tumors in childhood and adolescence. GPOH MAKEI and the MAHO study groups. Ann Oncol 2000;11(3):263–271.
272. Baranzelli MC, Bouffet E, Quintana E, Portas M, Thyss A, Patte C. Non-seminomatous ovarian germ cell tumours in children. Eur J Cancer 2000;36(3):376–383.
273. Baranzelli MC, Flamant F, De Lumley L, Le Gall E, Lejars O. Treatment of non-metastatic, non-seminomatous malignant germ-cell tumours in childhood: experience of the "Societe Francaise d'Oncologie Pediatrique" MGCT 1985–1989 study. Med Pediatr Oncol 1993;21(6):395–401.
274. Strother D, van Hoff J, Rao PV, et al. Event-free survival of children with biologically favourable neuroblastoma based on the degree of initial tumour resection: results from the Pediatric Oncology Group. Eur J Cancer 1997;33(12):2121–2125.
275. Matthay KK, Perez C, Seeger RC, et al. Successful treatment of stage III neuroblastoma based on prospective biologic staging: a Children's Cancer Group study. J Clin Oncol 1998;16(4): 1256–1264.
276. Kaneko M, Tsuchida Y, Mugishima H, et al. Intensified chemotherapy increases the survival rates in patients with stage 4 neuroblastoma with MYCN amplification. J Pediatr Hematol Oncol 2002;24(8):613–621.
277. Strother D, Shuster JJ, McWilliams N, et al. Results of pediatric oncology group protocol 8104 for infants with stages D and DS neuroblastoma. J Pediatr Hematol Oncol 1995;17(3): 254–259.
278. Bacci G, Forni C, Ferrari S, et al. Neoadjuvant chemotherapy for osteosarcoma of the extremity: intensification of preoperative treatment does not increase the rate of good histologic response to the primary tumor or improve the final outcome. J Pediatr Hematol Oncol 2003;25(11):845–853.

279. Smeland S, Muller C, Alvegard TA, et al. Scandinavian Sarcoma Group Osteosarcoma Study SSG VIII: prognostic factors for outcome and the role of replacement salvage chemotherapy for poor histological responders. Eur J Cancer 2003;39(4):488–494.

280. Granowetter L, Womer R, Devidas M. Comparison of dose intensified and standard dose chemotherapy for the treatment of non-metastatic Ewing's sarcoma (ES) and primitive neuroectodermal tumor (PNET) of bone and soft tissue: a Pediatric Oncology Group-Children's Cancer Group phase III trial. Med Pediatr Oncol 2001;37:172.

281. Burdach S, Meyer-Bahlburg A, Laws HJ, et al. High-dose therapy for patients with primary multifocal and early relapsed Ewing's tumors: results of two consecutive regimens assessing the role of total-body irradiation. J Clin Oncol 2003;21(16): 3072–3078.

282. Meyers PA, Krailo MD, Ladanyi M, et al. High-dose melphalan, etoposide, total-body irradiation, and autologous stem-cell reconstitution as consolidation therapy for high-risk Ewing's sarcoma does not improve prognosis. J Clin Oncol 2001;19(11): 2812–2820.

283. Crist WM, Anderson JR, Meza JL, et al. Intergroup rhabdomyosarcoma study-IV: results for patients with nonmetastatic disease. J Clin Oncol 2001;19(12):3091–3102.

284. Donaldson SS, Meza J, Breneman JC, et al. Results from the IRS-IV randomized trial of hyperfractionated radiotherapy in children with rhabdomyosarcoma: a report from the IRSG. Int J Radiat Oncol Biol Phys 2001;51(3):718–728.

285. Douglass EC, Reynolds M, Finegold M, Cantor AB, Glicksman A. Cisplatin, vincristine, and fluorouracil therapy for hepatoblastoma: a Pediatric Oncology Group study. J Clin Oncol 1993; 11(1):96–99.

286. Pritchard J, Brown J, Shafford E, et al. Cisplatin, doxorubicin, and delayed surgery for childhood hepatoblastoma: a successful approach. Results of the first prospective study of the International Society of Pediatric Oncology. J Clin Oncol 2000;18(22): 3819–3828.

287. Perilongo G, Shafford E, Maibach R, et al. Risk-adapted treatment for childhood hepatoblastoma. Final report of the second study of the International Society of Paediatric Oncology—SIOPEL 2. Eur J Cancer 2004;40(3):411–421.

SECTION SIX

Hematologic Malignancies

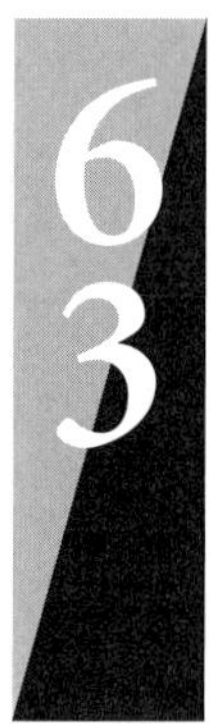

Acute Myeloid Leukemia and the Myelodysplastic Syndromes

Jonathan E. Kolitz

Epidemiology and Etiology of Acute Myeloid Leukemia

The incidence of acute myeloid leukemia (AML) in the United States is about 2.5 per 100,000, with a strong association with increasing age.[1] Males are predominantly affected. There is a predilection for Caucasians in North America and Australasia.[2] The incidence of acute promyelocytic leukemia (APL) is increased in Hispanics and may be associated with a breakpoint in the PML-RARα gene pathognmonic of that disease.[3]

The etiology of most cases of AML is unknown. The Hiroshima and Nagasaki atomic bombings[4] and the Chernobyl nuclear plant disaster[5] have been directly linked with causing AML. Therapeutic radiation alone has been shown to cause a fivefold-increased risk of AML in patients treated for ankylosing spondylitis[6] and has been implicated in causing AML with favorable karyotypes.[7]

Cigarette smoking contributes to inducing AML, especially acute erythroleukemia.[8] Pharmacogenomic studies have associated mutations in enzymes involved in the detoxification of tobacco-derived carcinogens with leukemia risk.[9,10]

Leukemia in identical twins may have a shared clonal derivation, with leukemic progenitors migrating hematogenously within a monochorionic placenta from one twin to the other.[11] Genetic predispositions to developing AML have been documented in hereditary and sporadic diseases associated with numerical abnormalities in chromosome number, instabilities in DNA and chromatin structure, and defects in DNA repair mechanisms.[12–14] Down syndrome has been linked to the development of acute megakaryoblastic leukemia.[12] AML can arise as an end stage in multiple myeloma[15] and myeloproliferative disorders.

Treatment with alkylating agents and topoisomerase II inhibitors can cause AML.[16–19] Among the antimetabolites, hydoxurea induces AML, often harboring 17p mutations, in 3.5% of patients with essential thrombocythemia,[20] whereas methotrexate is probably not leukemogenic in patients treated for rheumatoid arthritis.[21]

Combining radiotherapy and chemotherapy markedly increases the risk of leukemia. The MOPP regimen (mechlorethamine, vincristine, procarbazine, and prednisone) plus radiotherapy for treating Hodgkin's disease is associated with a 2.3% to 13% risk of secondary leukemia at 15 years depending on the extent of the radiation.[22]

Myeloablative treatments have been linked to development of myelodysplastic syndrome (MDS) and AML. A 5% to 10% incidence of secondary MDS/AML has been observed following autologous transplantation for non-Hodgkin's lymphoma.[23,24]

Major differences exist between therapy-related AML due to alkylating agents and those induced by inhibitors of topoisomerase II (anthracyclines, epidophyllotoxins). Alkylating agent-induced AML often has a myelodysplastic phase, a latency period of 3 to 9 years, a strong association with chromosomal deletions, particularly involving chromosomes 5 and/or 7, and a tendency to be chemotherapy resistant. Topoisomerase II-related AML, which was initially observed as a therapy-related complication of childhood ALL,[25] usually presents without a myelodysplastic phase, tends not to display dysplastic changes in the diagnostic marrow, has a short latency period (usually less than 3 years), is often associated with balanced chromosomal translocations involving 11q23, and displays variable chemosensitivity.[26]

Poor-risk secondary AML caused by alkylating agents is associated with deletions of chromosomes 5 and 7.[27,28] Chromosome 5 abnormalities related to alkylating agent exposure are often associated with loss of heterozygosity for the tumor suppressor gene p53.[29] The balanced translocations that occur following exposure to topoisomerase II inhibitors frequently involve the MLL gene in chromosome 11q23[30] and multiple partner chromosomes.[31]

Balanced translocations can create fusion proteins that lead to impaired gene transcription and cellular differentiation; these have been categorized as class II mutations, distinct from class I mutations, which lead to the synthesis of proteins able to stimulate proliferation and/or impede cell death.[32] Figure 63.1 illustrates these two major mutation categories. Class II mutations occur in favorable risk cases of

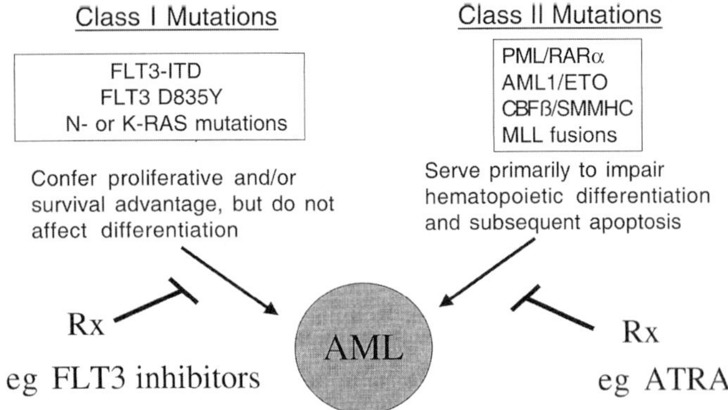

FIGURE 63.1. Class I and II mutations and the origin of acute myeloid leukemia (AML). Class I mutations induce proliferation and enhance survival of leukemic cells whereas class II mutations impede differentiation. Both may be needed to induce acute leukemia. (From Gilliland DG, Griffin JD. *Blood* 2002;100:1532–1542.)

AML, including APL and the core-binding factor (CBF) leukemias marked by t(8;21), inv(16), or t(16;16).

An internal tandem duplication and activation loop mutations in FLT3 (fms-like tyrosine kinase 3) are class I mutations that occur in up to 30% of patients with AML and are often associated with normal cytogenetics and inferior outcomes.[32] Absence of the wild-type FLT3 allele particularly correlates with poor response to therapy.[33] Activating class I mutations also occur in the Ras family of oncoproteins, which transmit downstream signals stimulating cell proliferation after undergoing farnesylation.[34] Ras mutations have a high prevalence (20%–40%) in AML and may strongly contribute to the expansion and myeloid differentiation of early progenitor cells.[35] The Ras pathway has been shown to be stimulated by mutations in SHP-2, a cytoplasmic tyrosine phosphatase.[36] An important common pathway leading to cell proliferation, differentiation, and survival involves signal transducer and activator of transcription (STAT) factors.[37] Mutated FLT3 and other tyrosine kinases can directly phosphorylate and activate STAT molecules.

Survival signals that inhibit programmed cell death, or apoptosis, also contribute to the growth advantage of myeloid leukemia cells.[38] Activation of caspases, enzymes that are final common mediators of cell death following stimulation by proapoptotic signals, is commonly impaired in myeloid leukemic cells, with the degree of dysregulation also correlating with clinical outcomes.[39] NF-kappa B is an antiapoptotic and proliferative stimulus present in leukemic progenitors but not in quiescent, normal pluripotent stem cells.[40] Among proapoptotic mediators, mutations in p53 occur in a minority of patients with AML, most often in the setting of 17p deletions,[41] whereas mutations in the retinoblastoma 1 gene occur in 19% to 55% of cases of AML.[42] p53 mutations have an adverse prognostic impact[43] whereas the clinical impact of Rb-1 mutations is unclear.[42]

Diagnosis and Classification

The use of molecular techniques has helped reclassify the myeloid leukemias using prognostically important clinical and cytogenetic findings. Unlike the French-American-British classification of AML,[44] which depends on morphology and histochemistry, the World Health Organization (WHO) classification (Table 63.1)[45] establishes categories of AML with distinct cytogenetics and more uniform clinical behavior.

The presence of 20% or more marrow blasts is required to diagnose AML because the FAB category of refractory anemia with excess blasts in transformation, which includes 20% to 29% blasts, behaves in a fashion identical to frank AML.[46] Frequently, therapy-related AML presents with dysplastic features reminiscent of RAEB-t, whereas AML with MLD will arise as a de novo disease with similar morphologic features. Of note, AML with MLD and therapy-related AML frequently share similar cytogenetic abnormalities, particularly, deletions of chromosomes 5 and 7 associated with alkylating agent exposure. Such dysplastic features affect prognosis.[47] The analysis of blast populations in bone marrow and peripheral blood smears and marrow biopsies continues to rely on immunohistochemical and flow cytometric techniques.[48] Specific antigen staining patterns characterize erythroleukemia[49] and megakaryoblastic leukemia.[50] Immunophenotyping, rather than morphologic and histochemical findings, is needed to diagnose AML with minimal differentiation (M0).[51] Fluorescence in situ hybridization (FISH)[52] and reverse transcriptase polymerase chain reaction (RT-PCR)[53] are occasionally helpful in identifying distinct subtypes of AML missed by cytogenetics. Spectral karyotyping permits simultaneous visualization of all chromosomes and can also complement classic cytogenetics.[54]

Response criteria for the treatment of AML have been updated to recognize the methodologies available to identify

TABLE 63.1. The World Health Organization (WHO) classification of acute myeloid leukemia.

I. Acute myeloid leukemia with recurrent genetic abnormalities
   i. Acute myeloid leukemia with t(8;21)(q22;q22), (*AML1/ETO*)
   ii. Acute myeloid leukemia with abnormal bone marrow eosinophils and inv(16)(p13q22) or t(16;16)(p13;q22), (*CBFβ/MYH11*)
   iii. Acute promyelocytic leukemia with t(15;17)(q22;q12), (*PML/RARα*) and variants
   iv. Acute myeloid leukemia with 11q23 (*MLL*) abnormalities

II. Acute myeloid leukemia and myelodysplastic syndromes, therapy related
   i. Following myelodysplastic syndrome or MDS/MPD
   ii. Without antecedent myelodysplastic syndrome or MDS/MPD, but with dysplasia in at least 50% of cells in two or more myeloid lineages
   iii. Alkylating agent/radiation-related type
   iv. Topoisomerase II inhibitor-related type (some may be lymphoid)
   v. Others

III. Acute myeloid leukemia, not otherwise categorized
   i. Acute myeloid leukemia, minimally differentiated
   ii. Acute myeloid leukemia without maturation
   iii. Acute myeloid leukemia with maturation
   iv. Acute myelomonocytic leukemia
   v. Acute monoblastic/acute monocytic leukemia
   vi. Acute erythroid leukemia (erythroid/myeloid and pure erythroleukemia)
   vii. Acute megakaryoblastic leukemia
   viii. Acute basophilic leukemia
   ix. Acute panmyelosis with myelofibrosis
   x. Myeloid sarcoma

MRD.[55] In addition to morphologic CR, cytogenetic and molecular CRs are also recognized. Detection of blast populations with the same immunophenotype as the presenting myeloid leukemia puts a patient's remission status in doubt. Persistence of pretreatment cytogenetic abnormalities in an otherwise remission marrow portends very poorly for disease-free survival (DFS).[56] Note is also made of the category of CRi, that is, CR with incomplete peripheral blood count recovery.

Prognostic Factors in AML

Advanced age correlates negatively with outcomes in AML because of the decreased ability of the elderly to withstand intensive chemotherapy and because of an increased prevalence of poor-risk cytogenetics. Furthermore, AML in the elderly has increased expression of multidrug resistance proteins, such as p-glycoprotein (Pgp).[57]

The major factor predictive of CR, disease-free survival, and overall survival in AML, is the cytogenetics at time of diagnosis.[58–60] Analysis of 1,213 patients treated on Cancer and Leukemia Group B (CALGB) trials segregates patients into favorable (CBF leukemias), adverse (including complex karyotypes with three or more abnormalities), and intermediate [normal, t(9;11), among others] risk groups.[60] The cumulative incidence of relapse observed in that analysis is shown in Figure 63.2.

The poor outcomes associated with therapy-related AML are due largely to adverse cytogenetics, with 76% of patients in one large series having abnormalities of chromosomes 5 and/or 7.[18] Secondary AML displaying favorable karyotypes, such as inv(16) and t(15;17) have outcomes similar to de novo AML.[7]

Different series have found that isolated trisomies of chromosomes 8 and 21 have poor[61] and intermediate[58] outcomes in de novo AML. Abnormalities of 3q have inferior responses to induction therapy and poor survival.[58,60] Additional cytogenetic abnormalities, even those that are regarded as prognostically negative, do not alter the favorable risk associated

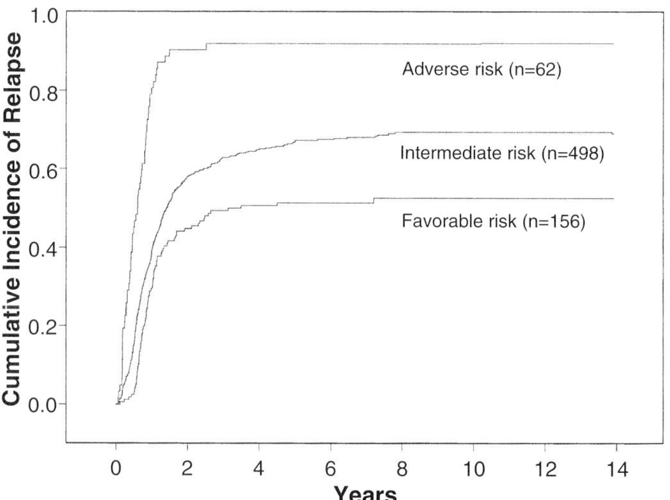

FIGURE 63.2. Cumulative incidence of relapse in 1,213 patients with de novo AML according to cytogenetic risk. (From Byrd et al.,[60] by permission of *Blood*.)

with CBF and APL karyotypes.[58,60] Cytogenetic abnormalities involving 11q23 have been associated with monocytic leukemias and very poor outcomes.[31] An exception may be t(9;11) when treated with intensive postremission therapy.[62]

Partial tandem duplication (PTD) of the MLL gene occurs in up to 11% of patients with AML and normal cytogenetics and is associated with inferior DFS.[63,64] MLL PTD is generally not present in patients with CBF leukemias.[64]

FLT3 is the most frequently constitutively activated kinase in human leukemia.[65] Most such mutations occur in patients with normal karyotypes: they occur in 30% or more of patients with APL without prognostic impact[66–68] and in less than 10% of patients with CBF leukemias.[67,69]

Higher levels of Wilms' tumor 1 (WT1) protein gene expression correlate with inferior outcomes among patients with normal or good-risk cytogenetics.[70] Expression of mRNA for c-mpl, the thrombopoietin receptor, predicts for poor outcomes despite intensive chemotherapy.[71] An example of a loss-of-function mutation associated with improved outcomes occurs in the myeloid transcription factor CCAAT/enhancer binding protein alpha-(C/EBPα).[72]

The in vitro growth of leukemic cells in the absence of exogenous growth factors has prognostic import. Three-year survival was 39% in patients with blasts with a low proliferative capacity, as contrasted with a 3% survival in patients with blasts with the highest proliferative rate.[73]

The presence of dysplastic changes in the presenting bone marrow has no additional negative implications beyond those related to the diagnostic karyotype.[74] Also significantly affecting overall survival (OS) is the presence of residual blasts in bone marrow early after induction chemotherapy,[75] the time taken to attain CR,[76] and persistent cytogenetic abnormalities following treatment.[56]

Once remission is achieved, detection and quantitation of MRD has prognostic significance. Detection by RT-PCR of the PML-RARα transcript associated with the t(15;17) of APL generally presages clinical relapse.[77] On the other hand, prolonged clinical DFS has been seen in patients with AML and t(8;21) despite the presence of the associated AML1-ETO transcript.[78] Studies using real-time RT-PCR for CBFα/MYH11 suggest that there are thresholds above and below which relapse and continued DFS occur in patients with AML and inv(16). Similarly, increased copies of mRNA for WT1 correlates with increasing risk of relapse.[70]

Ultimately, unique gene expression profiles as measured using microarrays may provide more powerful prognostic findings. Early data show that patients with favorable cytogenetics have unique gene expression profiles.[79]

Therapy of AML

The treatment of AML is usually initiated with an induction phase, aimed at eradicating the leukemic population with cytotoxic agents, with or without the use of myeloid growth factors. Once remission is achieved, treatment is directed at eradicating MRD, using moderate- to high-intensity consolidation chemotherapy. Increasing use of myeloablative regimens is occurring in suitable younger patients, while the role of postremission chemotherapy in older patients is unclear.

TABLE 63.2. Results of phase III randomized studies of anthracyclines in induction therapy of AML.

Reference	*N*	*Year*	*Age (years)*	*Drug*	*CR (%)*	*CR duration or DFS*	*Survival duration or OS*	*Comment*
251	200	1990	60	M	63	240 days	328 days	
				D	53	198 days	247 days	
252	180	1991	≤65	A	66*	37%	29%	Similar hematologic toxicities
				D	50	33%	20%	
253	120	1991	16–60	I	80**		19.5 months*	No difference in myelosuppression. I overcomes adverse effect of initial WBC.
				D	58		13.5 months	
254	214	1992	>15	I	70		12.9 months*	CR for I (88%) > D (70%) in patients 18–50 years ($P = 0.035$). ↑ myelosuppression with I. I overcomes adverse effect of initial WBC.
				D	59		8.7 months	
255	220	1996	15–75	I	68			CR for I (83%) > D (58%)** 0.007 in patients 55–65 years old. Trend favoring I for EFS.
				D	61			
143	489	1998	>60	M	47	8%	6%	↓ chemoresistance with M (32% vs. 47%)**
				D	38	8%	9%	

A, aclacinamycin; D, daunorubicin; I, idarubicin; M, mitoxantrone; DFS, disease-free survival; EFS, event-free survival; OS, overall survival.
*$P < 0.05$; **$P < 0.01$.

The Role of Anthracyclines in Induction Therapy of AML

The establishment of the importance of anthracycline-based induction chemotherapy for AML dates back more than 20 years.[80] Doxorubicin caused excess gastrointestinal toxicity as compared with daunorubicin, leading to its abandonment as part of most remission induction therapies.[81]

Multiple agents with similar structural and pharmacodynamic (intracellular topoisomerase II inhibition) properties, but distinct pharmacokinetic and toxicity profiles, are available and have been tested in Phase III trials. As outlined in Table 63.2, several large Phase III trials have pitted newer anthracyclines against daunorubicin in induction regimens for patients with untreated AML. All tested regimens incorporate a course of ara-c given by c.i.v. (continuous IV) for 7 days. Although trends favoring idarubicin have been noted with respect to CR incidence, only one trial has shown a survival advantage.[82] None of these studies took into account a possible dose–response effect attributable to each anthracycline, nor were attempts made to establish comparable dose-limiting toxicities.

High-Dose Cytarabine Therapy

Attempts to overcome drug resistance in blast populations by giving higher than conventional doses of ara-c (high-dose cytarabine, HiDAC) have been evaluated in induction and postremission regimens. With respect to conventional ara-c dosing regimens, a Phase III comparison of two c.i.v. doses showed little difference in outcomes, except in patients less than 60 years of age, where a survival advantage was suggested for patients receiving the higher ara-c dose.[83] A Phase II trial in which 3 days of HiDAC were added to a 7 and 3 induction led to a high (89%) CR incidence and an OS of 55% at 5 years.[84] Patients were consolidated with an autologous or allogeneic transplant. Phase III trials of HiDAC have not shown major improvements in CR rates in patients with de novo AML. A Southwest Oncology Group (SWOG) randomized trial of daunorubicin plus HiDAC, or standard cytarabine and more conventional postremission therapy, showed no difference in CR rates or in OS, although a trend favoring HiDAC with respect to prolongation of DFS was noted.[85] Adding HiDAC to etoposide and daunorubicin led to a modest increase in OS and a far more striking increase in DFS in patients 15 to 60 years of age as compared with conventional doses of cytarabine.[86]

HiDAC given during induction can be toxic and impede the timely delivery of postremission therapy, as seen in the SWOG trial in which more than twice as many patients were unable to receive postremission therapy after a HiDAC induction as compared with a standard dose ara-c induction.[85] HiDAC can cause significant neurotoxicity, especially irreversible cerebellar ataxia, the risk of which is considerably increased by patient age, and adverse renal and hepatic function,[87] as well as cumulative ara-c dose.[88]

Hematopoietic Growth Factors During Induction Therapy

Table 63.3 summarizes results of the major Phase III trials that have evaluated the effect of myeloid growth factors following completion of induction chemotherapy. Modest benefits have been observed, mostly with respect to time in hospital and duration of neutropenia. Although trends favoring growth factor use have been variably noted, only one large Phase III trial showed a strongly significant impact on CR incidence in patients receiving granulocyte colony-stimulating factor (G-CSF).[89] One trial that evaluated marrow response status before starting growth factor also demonstrated an improvement in therapy-related mortality.[90] That trial also described a favorable impact on medical costs using granulocyte-macrophage colony stimulating factor (GM-CSF),[91] while another study showed no such benefit.[92] It can be concluded that use of myeloid growth factors following induction chemotherapy may cause modest reductions in febrile complications and length of hospitalization without stimulating regrowth of leukemic cells.

Two large European studies have shown that reduced probabilities of relapse and increased OS occurs when myeloid growth factors are used concurrently with induction

TABLE 63.3. Phase III trials of myeloid growth factors after induction chemotherapy.

Reference	*N*	*Year*	*Age (years)*	*Induction therapy*[a]	*Growth factor*	*CR*[b]	*Comment*
256	388	1995	≥60	7 + 3	GM-CSF Placebo	51% 54%	↓ days of neutropenia (15 vs. 17) with GM-CSF ($P = 0.02$); no effect on TRM. Nonglycosylated GM-CSF used. No marrow done before starting GM-CSF.
90	124	1995	55–70	7 + 3	GM-CSF Placebo	60% 44%	Doubling of median survival with GM-CSF ($P = 0.048$), with significant ↓ TRM. Glycosylated GM-CSF used. Marrow examined before GM-CSF started.
89	233	1995	≥65	7 + 4	G-CSF Placebo	70% 47%	Glycoslyated G-CSF (lenograstim) used. No effect on OS or TRM. ↓ duration of neutropenia with G-CSF ($P < 0.001$).
257	521	1997	≥16	5 + 3 + etoposide	G-CSF Placebo	69% 68%	No difference in DFS or OS. ↓ days of neutropenia, hospitalization, antibiotics (all $P \leq 0.0001$) and number of patients needing antifungal therapy ($P = 0.04$) with G-CSF.
258	234	1998	≥55	7 + 3	G-CSF Placebo	50% 41%	Incidence of infection, time in hospital, overall survival same. 15% ↓ in time to neutrophil recovery ($P = 0.014$) and duration of infection with G-CSF.

[a] Induction regimens consisted of 5–7 days of cytarabine 100–200 mg/m^2 c.i.v. + daunorubicin 45 mg/m^2 i.v. × 3 or 4 days, as indicated. Etoposide 100 mg/m^2 i.v. × 5 was given concurrently in Ref. 257.

[b] CR differences did not reach $P \leq 0.05$ except in Ref. 89 ($P = 0.002$). A trend favoring GM-CSF was noted in Ref. 90 ($P = 0.08$).

chemotherapy.[93,94] Such "priming" studies aim at increasing the susceptibility of blast cells to cytotoxic agents by increasing the percentage of blast cells in S phase. A U.S. Phase III trial showed no benefit for priming.[95]

Postremission Therapy

An important refinement in the use of postremission therapy has been the recognition that outcomes may differ greatly as a function of the cytogenetics detected in the diagnostic bone marrow. An important example is the susceptibility of the CBF leukemias to HiDAC-based regimens.

There appears to be less therapy-related toxicity when HiDAC is used during postremission as compared with induction therapy, partly because patients enter such therapy with intact cellular barriers against infection and bleeding, and partly because post-CR HiDAC therapy has often been given alone, without an anthracycline. In a three-arm Phase III trial comparing standard (100 mg/m^2), intermediate (400 mg/m^2) ara-c and HiDAC as postremission therapy for patients with de novo AML, patients treated with HiDAC had a 4-year DFS of 44%, versus 29% and 24% for patients treated with intermediate and standard ara-c doses, respectively ($P = 0.002$).[96] Analysis according to cytogenetic risk indicated that patients with the CBF leukemias especially benefited from HiDAC therapy, with a cure fraction well in excess of 50%.[97] Furthermore, the number of courses of HiDAC given during remission correlates with DFS among patients with t(8;21).[98] The large French experience with 271 patients with CBF leukemia suggests that outcomes using diverse postremission therapies, including HiDAC, IDAC, or myeloablative approaches, may be significantly affected by age in patients with inv(16) and t(16;16)[99] and the WBC count among patients with t(8;21).[100]

Among patients not stratified by cytogenetic risk, a randomized comparison of four versus eight courses of intensive consolidation therapy showed no benefit for the more prolonged treatment arm.[101] On the other hand, a large randomized trial concluded that intensive induction and consolidation chemotherapy incorporating daunorubicin, mitoxantrone, conventional dose, and HiDAC, followed by either dose-reduced monthly maintenance or an additional course of intensive consolidation, led to a DFS advantage in patients with poor-risk prognostic features and an overall trend toward improved survival.[102]

Whether the use of sequential, putatively noncross-resistant, significantly myelosuppressive chemotherapy regimens improves outcomes following attainment of CR was evaluated in an early Phase II trial in which HiDAC/asparaginase and amsacrine/etoposide were intercalated between three courses of conventional daunorubicin/cytarabine.[103] Although DFS may have exceeded that seen in historical controls at that time, an 18% incidence of therapy-related mortality in patients in CR proved prohibitive. The EORTC and CALGB have also evaluated noncross-resistant chemotherapy regimens following CR without demonstrating improvements in outcome.[104,105]

The Role of Transplantation in Acute Myeloid Leukemia

Whether transplants using autologous or allogeneic marrow or peripheral blood stem cells (PSC) improve outcomes in AML in first CR continues to be debated even after the completion of several large Phase III trials. A meta-analysis of published trials evaluating autologous transplantation for AML in first CR concluded that DFS is significantly prolonged ($P = 0.006$) but not OS.[106] Such analyses do not weigh variables such as cytogenetic risk, time to transplant, use of marrow rather than PSC, and the chemotherapy used before stem cell harvesting. Studies using an intent-to-treat analysis evaluating transplantation versus chemotherapy have not fully addressed the different risks of relapse among distinct cytogenetic risk groups after initial CR is achieved. Allogeneic transplantation is not easily amenable to randomized analysis: our understanding of the relative benefits of allogeneic transplantation relies on retrospective analyses of outcomes among patients undergoing "genetic randomization" who are assigned allografts if they had a matched sibling donor.

TABLE 63.4. Phase III trials of autotransplantation versus chemotherapy in AML in first CR.

Reference	Year	N	Induction CR, %	Received post-CR therapy	Received autotransplantation[a]	DFS		OS	
						Auto	Chemo	Auto	Chemo
108	1995	990	66%	92%	42%[b]	48%[c]	30%	56%	46%
259	1997	535	73%	62%	51%[d]	44	40	50	55
109	1998	1966	77%	89%	11%[e]	53[f]	40	57	45
107	1998	808	70%	67%	54%	35	35	43	52[g]

[a] Of all CR patients, excluding those assigned to allografts.

[b] Estimate based on 623 patients in CR, 168 assigned to allograft, leaving 455 patients in CR who could have been randomized to autologous transplant vs. chemotherapy: 95 underwent autotransplants.

[c] $P = 0.05$.

[d] Estimate based on 367 CRs minus 73 allografts = 294 patients potentially eligible to be randomized to autograft of whom 75 were autografted patients.

[e] An additional 7% elected to undergo autotransplant and were not randomized.

[f] $P = 0.04$; 381 patients randomized among 1,131 eligible.

[g] $P = 0.05$.

Outcomes from the four large Phase III trials that have compared autologous and allogeneic transplantation and nonmyeloablative chemotherapy are summarized in Tables 63.4 and 63.5. Important differences between the studies include the number and intensity of post-CR consolidation regimens before randomization between chemotherapy and transplant, the length of time between achieving CR and randomization, the transplant conditioning regimens, and therapy-related mortality. Only one study utilized ex vivo purged autologous marrow.[107] Two trials showed a DFS advantage favoring autologous transplant, which did not translate into improved OS because of effective salvage therapies.[108,109] When analyzed according to cytogenetic risk, a DFS and OS benefit was noted in patients with intermediate-risk cytogenetics.[110] The DFS associated with chemotherapy alone was unusually low in one of the trials.[108] On the other hand, therapy-related mortality significantly affected transplant outcome in another trial in which patients who were randomized to receive chemotherapy had significantly improved OS.[107]

In the absence of readily available and reliable methodologies to purge leukemic cells ex vivo, increasing emphasis has been placed on the concept of in vivo purging, for example, utilizing either repeated courses or higher doses of chemotherapy to effect a reduction in the leukemia cell burden below a critical threshold that may result in fewer relapses.

Multiple, sequential courses of moderately intensive therapy were used in the MRC AML 10 trial, leading to a significant improvement in DFS in the relatively small number of patients who completed three courses of postremission therapy before transplant.[109] A single, highly myelosuppressive regimen of HiDAC and high-dose infusional etoposide has been used in patients in first CR for in vivo purging and stem cell mobilization and collection in a Phase II trial.[111] Following an etoposide and busulfan autotransplant, 55% of 128 patients reached 5 years disease free. Whether such brief duration, high-intensity approaches will improve outcomes in a larger cohort of patients uniformly categorized according to cytogenetic risk is undergoing evaluation by the CALGB.

A direct comparison between allogeneic and autologous transplantation in patients 45 years of age or younger in first CR showed that patients with donors had improved DFS and reduced RR, with the benefit confined to patients with adverse risk cytogenetics.[112] These findings are in keeping with disappointing results of high-dose in vivo purging in patients with poor-risk cytogenetics.[111] Data from an intergroup trial show that favorable risk cytogenetics patients benefit from autologous and allogeneic transplantation more so than chemotherapy, whereas poor-risk karyotypes respond best to allografting.[113] Whether outcomes for autotransplant can be improved upon if the approach is limited to patients with minimal tumor burdens remains unclear. DFS has been shown to be inversely related to levels of MRD before autotransplant.[114]

Not surprisingly, tumor burden before allogeneic transplantation is less critical, largely in part of the graft-versus-

TABLE 63.5. Phase III trials of "genetic randomization" comparing allogeneic transplant versus chemotherapy in previously untreated AML.

Reference	Year	DFS		OS		Comment
		Allo	Chemo	Allo	Chemo	
108	1995	46	33	48	40	Age ≤45. Cy-TBI[1] or Bu-Cy[2].
259	1997	44	38	53	53	Age ≤50. Cy-TBI or other-TBI or Bu-Cy.
107	1998	43	36	46	52[3]	Age ≤55. Bu-Cy.
110	2002	47	40	53	45	Age <55. Cy-TBI. ↑ DFS in intermediate cytogenetic risk (50% vs. 39%, $P = 0.02$).

[a] Cyclophosphamide and total body irradiation (TBI) conditioning regimen.

[b] Busulfan and cyclophosphamide conditioning regimen.

[c] $P = 0.04$.

leukemia effect exerted by the allograft.[115] Outcomes following allogeneic transplant performed in patients in early relapse are comparable to those seen in patients in first CR.[116] Furthermore, results following allografts in patients in CR are not improved by administering one course of HiDAC before transplant.[117]

Nonmyeloablative or reduced-intensity (RI) allografts exploit the graft-versus-leukemia effect mediated by donor lymphocytes that occurs after the achievement of partial or full engraftment.[118] Cytotoxic agents are used mainly to inhibit host immune responses before infusion of donor stem cells rather than to exert an antileukemic effect. Immunosuppressive regimens are critically important to modulate what can be severe graft-versus-host disease (GVHD). The degree to which chimerism develops correlates both with antileukemic effects and morbidity and mortality, which may be substantial, from GVHD.[119] Becuase the antileukemic effect mediated by the graft may be aborted by rapidly progressive disease, outcomes are likely to be improved if patients are transplanted in remission.[120] Older patients who may not be candidates for a full allograft could be considered for RI transplantation.

Induction Regimens for Relapsed and Refractory Acute Myeloid Leukemia

HiDAC-Based Regimens

As is the case in untreated AML, cytogenetic abnormalities are predictive of outcome following salvage therapy of patients in relapse or with refractory disease.[121,122] An additional important prognostic factor is the duration of first CR: multivariate analyses point to a 6-month cutoff as being significant,[122,123] whereas a univariate analysis suggests that cytogenetics are particularly important when the CR duration is less than 1 year.[121] Patients who have initial remissions lasting beyond 2 years may have an outlook comparable to that of previously untreated patients.[121] Other prognostic markers include the WBC, blast percentage in blood and/or marrow, serum lactate dehydrogenase (LDH), and bilirubin levels.

HiDAC-containing regimens were first evaluated in relapsed and refractory AML, where CR incidences between 40% and 60% have been reported when given alone or in combination with an anthracycline or etoposide. Representative studies are outlined in Table 63.6.

Multiple salvage regimens for relapsed and refractory AML have been published using intermediate (IDAC) to high doses of cytarabine. Examples include the FLAG and FLAG-Ida regimens,[124–126] and the MEC regimen, which consists of mitoxantrone, etoposide, and IDAC.[127] High-dose mitoxantrone and HiDAC attempts to exploit the potential for a dose response associated with single high doses of mitoxantrone (80 mg/m^2).[128] Topotecan has been combined with IDAC and studied with[129] and without[130,131] cyclophosphamide. A liposomal preparation of daunorubicin (DaunoXome) has gone through a dose-escalation evaluation in combination with IDAC.[132] Although remissions can be achieved with any of these regimens, durable responses occur only for patients undergoing stem cell transplantation. The FLAG and topotecan/cytarabine regimens can occasionally be helpful in older patients who either cannot receive an investigational agent or are precluded from receiving an anthracycline-based reinduction because of comorbidities.

A critical consideration is the lack of tabulation of many earlier trials treating relapsed/refractory AML according to cytogenetic risk. Extrapolating from outcomes seen in previously untreated patients with RAEB, and what is now described as AML with MLD, and poor-risk cytogenetics treated with FLAG or FLAG-Ida,[46] brief remissions and adverse karyotypes are the strongest predictors of poor outcome to conventional salvage regimens. Ideally, therefore, patients with such adverse findings at relapse should be considered for investigational therapies.

Non-HiDAC-Containing Salvage Therapies

Multiple Phase I and II trials have explored the use of alternative induction regimens that do not include HiDAC or, in some instance, dispense with ara-c entirely. Examples of such regimens are outlined in Table 63.7. Regimens using single agents have generally been associated with poor outcomes. Demonstration of antileukemic effects, including achievement of transient marrow aplasia, using these agents may justify further evaluation in combination regimens and in less heavily pretreated patients. Liposomal daunorubicin appears to have single-agent activity and has been combined with IDAC with moderate efficacy in a Phase I–II dose-escalation study.[132] A larger Phase II or III evaluation using the recommended dose of DaunoXome (135 mg/m^2 q d × 3 days) has yet to be performed.

TABLE 63.6. Trials of high-dose cytarabine (HIDAC)-containing regimens in relapsed/refractory AML.

Reference	*Year*	*Phase*	*N*	*Total Ara-C dose*	*Additional agents*	*CR*	*DFS*	*OS*	*Comment*
260	1985	II	76	36	DNR or DOX[a]	53%	5 months		↑ response in refractory patients and ↑ DFS with DNR/DOX
261	1998	III	186	36/12 12/4	Mitox[b]	52%/45% 48%/45%	5.3/3.3[c] 4.5		↑ refractoriness to lower-dose regimens partially offset by ↑ early deaths in higher-dose regimens
262	1999	III	162	36	Mitox[b]	44% 32%	11 days[d] 8	6 8	↑ CR with mitox/HiDAC significant by multivariate analysis
263	2000	II	47	6	Mitox[b]	4 months	4 months		CR in 19/25 patients >60 years

TABLE 63.7. Salvage regimens for relapsed/refractory AML.

Reference	*Year*	*Phase*	*Regimen*	*N*	*CR*	*DFS*	*Comment*
264	1988	II	Mitoxantrone and etoposide[1]	61	42.6%	4.7 months	Severe myelosuppression: median time to CR = 49 days
265	1990	I–II	High-dose cyclophosphamide (CTX) + etoposide (E)	40	42%		MTD 50 mg/kg CTX days 1–4, E 4.2 g/m^2 civ over 29–69 hr. CR in 6/20 HiDAC-resistant patients.
266	1994	I–II	Cladribine	36	8%	2	3 CRs at ≥15 mg/m^2/d civ days 1–5. Delayed sensorimotor peripheral neuropathy in 6/9 patients at ≥19 mg/m^2/day. MTD = 17 mg/m^2/day.
267	1998	II	Carboplatin, etoposide, cyclophosphamide, and cytarabine	25	12%		Tolerable; 3 CRs were in very poor risk patients.
268	2000	II	Cladribine	15	0		Marrow aplasia in 8. No >grade 1 GI toxicity and no neurotoxicity.
269	2002	I	Temozolomide	16	19%	11	MTD = 200 mg/m^2 po qd × 7 days; DLT = prolonged aplasia.
270	2002	I/II	Liposomal daunorubicin	28	46%	6	MTD = 150 mg/m^2 days 1–3; 2 deaths from cardiotoxicity.
271	2002	II	Gemcitabine + mitoxantrone	26	19%	2.5	Recommended dose of G = 10 mg/m^2/hr × 12 hr.
272	2002	I	Gemcitabine	18	0		10 mg/10 mg/m^2/hr × 12 hr × 18 hr well tolerated.
273	2003	I	Gemcitabine (G) + fludarabine (F)	18	16.7%		MTD for G = 9,000 mg/m^2 by civ/15 hr; severe esophagitis, stomatitis, febrile neutropenia

Treatment of Acute Myeloid Leukemia in the Elderly

Because the median age of AML in the United States is 63 years, a major proportion of clinical decision making involves a patient population with frequently significant comorbidities. Furthermore, older patients are more likely than younger patients to present with adverse prognostic features, especially unfavorable cytogenetics, antecedent myelodysplastic syndrome, AML with multilineage dysplasia,[133] and Pgp expression.[57]

Multiple trials have compared the option of best supportive care with that of induction chemotherapy for older patients with AML. A retrospective multivariate analysis of conventional chemotherapy versus best supportive care indicated that chemotherapy administration and LDH less than 400 were significantly associated with prolonged survival.[134] Prospective studies, all nonrandomized, show trends toward better OS with therapy as compared with best supportive care.[135] The very elderly (age 80 or more), on the other hand, may not benefit from chemotherapy as compared with patients who are just 10 years younger.[136]

Once a decision is made to treat an elderly patient with AML, scant evidence exists pointing to the superiority of one regimen over another. Among randomized studies, SWOG has shown that using mitoxantrone and etoposide instead of standard daunorubicin and cytarabine in untreated elderly patients offers no meaningful advantages and may be inferior with respect to OS.[137] The MRC randomized 1,314 older patients between three anthracycline- and cytarabine-containing regimens and showed a significantly higher CR rate for daunorubicin + 6-thioguanine (DAT) but no effect on OS.[138] A small Phase III trial comparing high-dose versus standard-dose mitoxantrone, each in combination with cytarabine, showed no differences with respect to CR incidence, DFS, and OS.[139] Among nonanthracycline-containing regimens, FLAG has been used extensively by hematologists in older patients with untreated and relapsed AML. A Phase III trial that compared Ara-C and G-CSF with and without fludarabine showed that although Ara-CTP incorporation into the DNA of leukemic blast cells is enhanced by fludarabine, no significant differences in CR incidence, DFS, and OS were noted.[140]

Attempts at reversing multidrug resistance using drugs that inhibit Pgp are reviewed above. Gemtuzumab ozogamicin has been used with and without interleukin (IL)-11 in this patient population, with retrospective data indicating that outcomes cannot justify using the regimen in place of conventional idarubicin and cytarabine.[141] The CALGB is planning to study the effect of the bcl-2 antisense inhibitor G3139[142] when combined with daunorubicin and cytarabine in a Phase III trial in untreated elderly patients.

Whether elderly patients in CR should receive postremission therapy is unsettled. Unmaintained remissions of 6 to 9 months have been noted following standard- or high-dose mitoxantrone plus cytarabine induction regimens, results comparable to those seen when postremission therapy is given.[139] The EORTC and ECOG demonstrated a trend toward improved DFS but not OS using courses of low-dose SC ara-c as compared with observation in older patients in CR.[143,144] More intensive consolidations using mitoxantrone and an IDAC variant[145] or HiDAC[96,146] have not improved outcomes in this patient population.

Acute Promyelocytic Leukemia

Acute promyelocytic leukemia (APL) is the most curable of AML subtypes. It is characterized by a pathognmonic translocation, t(15;17), and an associated fusion protein (PML-RARα) that underlies the disease's pathogenesis. PML-RARα promotes histone deacetylation, thereby inhibiting gene transcription, an effect that is reversed by all-*trans* retinoic acid (ATRA).[147]

The efficacy of oral administration of ATRA in inducing CR in APL when used as a single agent is well established.[148] Among large Phase III trials comparing ATRA monotherapy and combination chemotherapy inductions, the North American Intergroup study showed that ATRA improved DFS but not CR incidence whether given before or after chemotherapy.[149] That study also suggested a dose response on the part of APL to anthracycline therapy, a finding consistent with the fact that APL has low expression of p-glycoprotein.[150] Phase II data exist supporting the efficacy of an ATRA and idarubicin induction regimen for APL that omits cytarabine,[151] as well as an ATRA plus arsenic trioxide (ATO) regimen, which dispenses with chemotherapy altogether.[152]

Current practice generally involves concurrent administration of ATRA with anthracycline-based induction therapy on the basis of Phase III trials that have found a superior DFS when ATRA and chemotherapy are given concurrently. A significant improvement in CR incidence (87% versus 70%) for concurrent versus sequential ATRA plus chemotherapy has been seen,[153] whereas a second trial in which a formal ATRA monotherapy induction was followed by chemotherapy and compared with concurrent ATRA/chemotherapy noted no difference in CR rates but found that EFS survival was significantly improved at 2 years (86% versus 75%).[154] The incidence of the ATRA syndrome, a major, potentially lethal complication of ATRA therapy,[155] has been markedly reduced when chemotherapy and ATRA are given together.[156]

In relapsed APL, ATO induced CR in 84% of 41 patients,[157] and the humanized anti-CD33 monoclonal antibody Hum195 effected molecular CR in 11 of 22 relapsed patients reinduced into clinical CR with ATRA.[158] More than 80% of patients attained undetectable levels of the PMR-RARα transcript by RT-PCR following ATO induction and consolidation therapy.[157] The current North American Intergroup study is assessing the effect of ATO consolidation therapy in APL patients in first CR when given before consolidation chemotherapy.

Another question being addressed in the North American Phase III trial is the relative benefit of two forms of maintenance chemotherapy: ATRA given intermittently for 1 year with or without concurrent daily low-dose oral chemotherapy with daily purinethol and weekly methotrexate. The possible benefit of ATRA maintenance has been previously described when given alone[159] and in combination with low-dose chemotherapy.[154]

The studies cited previously indicate that long-term DFS in 80% or so of patients with untreated APL is being realized. In event of relapse, encouraging data demonstrate that autologous transplantation in patients with APL in second remission, who have achieved molecular eradication of the PML-RARα transcript, an outcome often achievable with ATO-based salvage treatment, enjoy prolonged second remissions.[160]

New Agents for the Treatment of Acute Myelogenous Leukemia

Immunotherapy of AML

Monoclonal antibodies can be used to potentiate the effects of combination chemotherapy in the treatment of bulk leukemia, or can serve as a means of eradicating MRD. Although, in principle, unlabeled antibodies can be combined with chemotherapy with little additive toxicity, only one large Phase III has been conducted: patients with relapsed AML over age 60 were randomized to receive salvage chemotherapy with or without Hum195, a humanized anti-CD33 antibody.[161] No definite advantage was seen in the antibody-containing arm.

M195, whether labeled or unlabeled, can cause at least transient antileukemic effects with acceptable toxicity. The replacement of β-emitting radiolabels, such as yttrium and iodine-131 with the pure α-emitter bismuth-214, allows for the retention of significant antileukemic effects with a reduced incidence of myelosuppression.[162]

Gemtuzumab ozogamicin (GO) is a murine anti-CD33 antibody construct that is linked to calicheamycin. Modest single-agent activity for this antibody has been documented in Phase II trials, with the largest overview of its efficacy being a report of 157 older patients in first relapse.[163] Relapsed patients whose first CR lasted more than 1 year had a 35% CR rate, with the probability of CR falling to 9% in patients with first CR durations less than 6 months. In general, the incidence of febrile complications following GO therapy is comparable to that seen with cytotoxic therapy, whereas the incidence of mucositis appears lower and that of hepatotoxicity, including a low but troublesome incidence of venoocclusive disease (VOD), is higher. The likelihood of developing VOD is increased substantially in patients who receive allogeneic transplants within 4 months of treatment with GO.[164]

A Phase II study of GO with or without the thrombopoietic agent interleukin 11 led to CR incidences and remission durations in poor-risk AML and MDS patients that were inferior to those achieved at the same institution using conventional chemotherapy with idarubicin and cytarabine.[141]

GO has been combined with several chemotherapy regimens for treating relapsed and refractory[165,166] as well as previously untreated AML.[167,168] To date, these early data have only demonstrated the feasibility of such combination therapies.

Other monoclonal radiolabeled antibodies which have been used for treating AML, either as salvage therapy or as part of a myeloablative transplantation regimen, include ^{131}I[169] and ^{214}Bi[162] conjugates of M195, ^{131}I-anti CD45,[170] and ^{188}Re-anti CD66.[171]

Interleukin 2 (IL-2), which can induce immune responses on the part of cytotoxic T cells and NK (natural killer) cells against autologous blasts in vitro, and that has exerted antileukemic effects in poor-risk patients, has shown an acceptable safety profile when used as a postremission therapy.[172,173] Evaluations of the effectiveness of IL-2 as a postremission adjuvant therapy for AML are ongoing. A construct of GM-CSF linked to diphtheria toxin has shown modest activity in heavily pretreated, chemotherapy-refractory patients.[174] A noteworthy development has been the observation of significant anti-AML effects following vaccination of AML patients with an HLA-A2-restricted peptide.[175]

Multidrug Resistance (MDR) Modulation

Chemotherapy resistance is partly mediated by P-glycoprotein (Pgp), a cell membrane drug efflux pump encoded by the *MDR1* gene. Significant expression of Pgp is age related, with Pgp positivity noted in close to three-quarters of patients over

TABLE 63.8. New agents for the treatment of AML.

Reference	*Agent*	*Target*	*Toxicity*	*Results*	*Comment*
243, 274, 275	R11577 (Tipifarnib, Zarnestra)	Farnesyl transferase	DLT = neurotoxicity in phase I; minimal toxicity in phase II	About 20% CR in untreated patients; very low CR in previously treated patients	Response associated with inhibition of farnesylation in vivo
276	CEP-701	FLT3	DLT not identified	Transient blast clearance documented in PB and BM	Response correlates with inhibition of FLT3 autophosphorylation
277	SU11248	FLT3	50mg po qd well tolerated; grade 4 cardiac, fatigue, hypertension at 75mg po qd	4/4 brief PR in mutated FLT3; 2/10 in wild type	In vivo inhibition of phosphorylation of tyrosine kinases (c-kit, FLT3, VEGF)
278	PKC412	FLT3	75mg po tid well tolerated; 2 fatal pulmonary events of unclear etiology	7/20 > 2log reduction in blasts, median 13 weeks	FLT3 autophosphorylation inhibited in vivo
234	SU5416	VEGF-R 1, 2	Grade 3/4 in 7%–14%: headaches, infusion-related reactions, dyspnea, thrombotic episodes	3/33 refractory/relapsed AML PR	Marked apoptosis and necrosis in marrows of some patients with AML between days 7 and 14 after beginning therapy
279	Bortezomib (PS-341, Velcade)	Proteasome	DLT ≥3 syncope, orthostatic hypotension, edema, noncardiac chest pain	Transient decreases in blasts noted	44%–63% nonsustained proteasome inhibition documented
142	Oblimersen (G3139, Genasense)	BCL-2	Combined with FLAG; no clear DLT	5/17 CR	75% had BCL-2 mRNA downregulated in vivo

age 55.[57] Multivariate analyses have shown that only Pgp expression and cytogenetics are independent predictors of complete remission (CR) and overall survival (OS) in de novo AML.[176–178]

Favorable effects on CR incidence occurred in patients receiving quinine, a Pgp inhibitor, with idarabucin and ara-c induction therapy who also demonstrated in vitro efflux of the Pgp substrate rhodamine-123.[179] No overall survival advantage was seen, however. Attempts to pharmacologically reverse Pgp activity have centered on the use of cyclosporin A (CsA) and its nonimmunosuppressive analogue, PSC-833 (Valspodar; Novartis). Both drugs competitively inhibit Pgp function and diminish drug efflux in vitro.[180–183] Promising results favoring the use of CsA as a Pgp modulator with infusional daunorubicin and HiDAC in a Phase III trial in poor-risk AML conducted by the Southwest Oncology Group[184] have yet to be duplicated using PSC-833. Three Phase III studies evaluating PSC-833 have been terminated, however. Toxicity concerns halted a trial in older patients with de novo AML,[185] whereas a Phase II trial in relapsed/refractory patients ended because of lack of benefit in the experimental arm.[186] A recent Phase III trial in untreated AML in patients more than 60 years of age conducted by the Medical Research Council (MRC) demonstrated early excess mortality from PSC-833-containing daunorubicin, cytarabine, and 6-thioguanine induction therapy, which became inapparent with further follow-up.[187] On the other hand, nonrandomized Phase I/II data in patients less than 60 years of age with untreated AML suggest a favorable effect on DFS and OS, particularly in patients less than 45 years of age.[188]

New Cytotoxics and Signal Transduction Inhibitors

Among new nucleoside analogues, Clofarabine exerts significant antileukemic effects when used as a single agent in relapsed AML, with toxicity consisting of moderate liver function abnormalities.[189] The l-nucleoside analogue troxacitabine has in vitro antileukemic activity that is complementary to that mediated by ara-c.[190] Disappointingly, troxacitabine when combined with ara-c or with idarubicin, was found highly likely to be inferior to idarubicin and ara-c in the treatment of older patients with AML and poor-risk karyotypes.[191] These studies have shown that the major nonhematologic toxicities of troxacitabine are mucositis and hand–foot syndrome.

A host of interesting new agents that target protein kinases, mediators of angiogenesis, farnesyl transferase, DNA methylation, histone acetylation, and the proteasome are undergoing clinical investigation for the treatment of AML. A representative listing of these agents is found in Table 63.8, along with their targets and early clinical findings. Of great interest will be the determination of optimal means of using these agents and how best to sequence or combine them with chemotherapy.[192]

The Myelodysplastic Syndromes

The myelodysplastic syndromes (MDS) encompass diseases marked by variable abnormalities in hematopoiesis, involving one or more lineages, usually accompanied by dysplastic marrow morphology involving two or three lineages. Marrow cellularity can vary markedly in these diseases, with an important overlap noted between some forms of hypocellular MDS, aplastic anemia, and paroxysmal nocturnal hemoglobinuria.[193] Increasing evidence supports the likelihood that many cases of MDS arise from a mutated hematopoietic stem cell.[194]

MDS is predominantly a disease of the elderly, with 80% of patients diagnosed over age 60 years. Although the etiology of MDS is unknown in most cases, prior chemotherapy is a well-recognized cause. Factors involved in the pathobiology of MDS include abnormalities in apoptotic and growth signals, interactions with bone marrow stromal and vascular

TABLE 63.9. The World Health Organization classification of the myelodysplastic syndromes.

Disease	*Blood findings*	*Bone marrow findings*
Refractory anemia (RA)	Anemia No or rare blasts	Erythroid dysplasia only <5% blasts <15% blasts
Refractory anemia with ringed sideroblasts (RARS)	Anemia No blasts	>15% ringed sideroblasts Erythroid dysplasia only <5% blasts
Refractory cytopenia with multilineage dysplasia (RCMD)	Bi- or pancytopenias No or rare blasts No Auer rods <1 × 10^9/L monocytes	Dysplasia in ≥10% of cells of >2 lineages <5% blasts No Auer rods <15% ringed sideroblasts
Refractory cytopenia with multilineage dysplasia and ringed sideroblasts (RCMD-RS)	Bi- or pancytopenias No or rare blasts No Auer rods <1 × 10^9/L monocytes	Dysplasia in ≥10% of cells of ≥2 lineages <5% blasts No Auer rods ≥15% ringed sideroblasts
Refractory anemia with excess blasts 1 (RAEB-1)	Cytopenias <5% blasts No Auer rods <1 × 10^9/L monocytes	≥1 lineage dysplasia 5%–9% blasts No Auer rods
Refractory anemia with excess blasts 2 (RAEB-2)	Cytopenias 5%–19% blasts Auer rods ± <1 × 10^9/L monocytes	≥1 lineage dysplasia 10%–19% blasts Auer rods ±
Myelodysplastic syndrome—unclassified (MDS-U)	Cytopenias No or rare blasts No Auer rods	Unilineage dysplasia <5% blasts No Auer rods
MDS associated with isolated del(5q)	Anemia Usually normal or increased platelet counts <5% blasts	Normal to increased megakaryocytes with hypolobulated nuclei <5% blasts Isolated del(5q) No Auer rods

Source: Adapted from Vardiman et al.,[45] by permission of *Blood*.

endothelial cells, and, in some cases, T- and NK cell-mediated autoimmune mechanisms. Strategies aimed at interruption of such mechanisms are reviewed next.

Table 63.9 depicts the WHO classification of MDS. Chronic myelomonocytic leukemia (CMML), which shares characteristics of MDS and myeloproliferative diseases and has a variable clinical course,[195] has been placed in a separate category of myelodysplastic/myeloproliferative disorders. To improve the analysis of outcomes following treatment in each of these diseases, the International Prognostic Scoring System (IPSS) has gained acceptance because of its reliance on readily available clinical parameters and reasonable correspondence with prognosis.[196] The IPSS segregates patients into low, intermediate-1 and -2 (INT-1 and INT-2), and high-risk groups (Table 63.10). Figure 63.3 depicts the relationship between the IPSS categories, survival and probability of development of AML observed in 816 patients with MDS.

Standardized response criteria to be used to assess clinical trials in MDS patients have been agreed upon.[197] These criteria emphasize the importance of stratifying patients according to the IPSS and looking at endpoints such as progression-free and disease-free survival.

Role of Hematopoietic Growth Factors in MDS

Erythropoietin (epo) has been shown to benefit a significant minority of patients with MDS. Patients with low marrow blast percentages and serum erythropoietin levels, and without red cell transfusion dependence, are more likely to respond to treatment with epo.[198] Prolonged administration of epo may be needed to effect a response.[199] Of interest is the observation that erythroid progenitors that have normal karyotypes by FISH analysis preferentially undergo expansion in response to epo.[200]

Several studies have utilized G- or GM-CSF in combination with epo, attempting to exploit a possible synergy between these agents with respect to stimulating erythropoiesis while also aiming to expand neutrophil numbers in neutropenic patients. Although not conclusive, the data suggest that the combination of G-CSF and epo may be more

TABLE 63.10. International prognostic scoring system for myelodysplastic syndromes.

	Score value				
Prognostic variable	*0*	*0.5*	*1.0*	*1.5*	*2.0*
BM blasts (%)	<5	5–10	—	11–0	21–3
Karyotype[a]	Good	Intermediate	Poor	—	—
Cytopenias	0–1	2–3	—	—	—

Scores for risk groups: low, 0; INT-1, 0.5–1.0; INT-2, 1.5–2.0; high, ≥2.5.

[a] Good: normal, -Y, del(5q), del(20q); poor: complex (≥3 abnormalities) or chromosome 7 anomalies; intermediate: other abnormalities.

Source: Adapted from Greenberg et al.,[196] by permission of *Blood*.

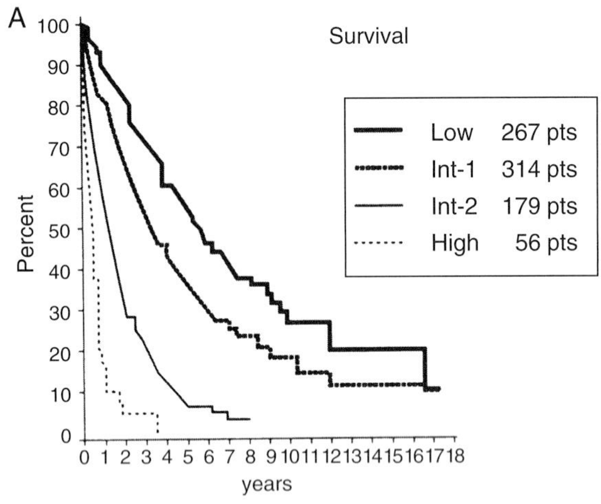

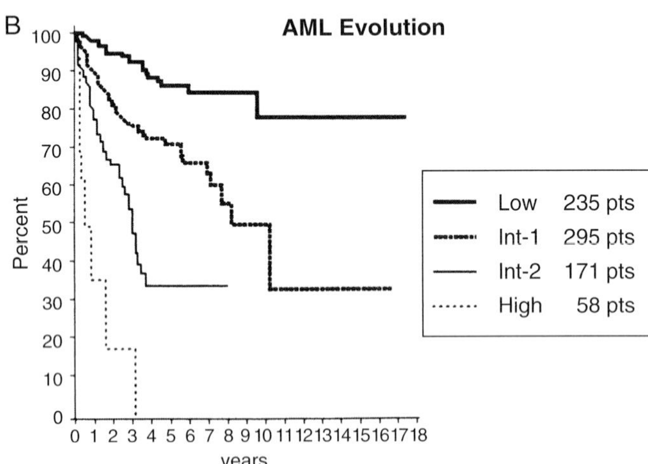

FIGURE 63.3. Probability of survival and evolution into AML according to International Prognostic Scoring System (IPSS) categories. (From Greenberg et al.,[196] by permission of *Blood*.)

effective than epo alone in stimulating erythropoiesis, particularly in patients in more favorable risk groups.[201,202] Transfusion-dependent patients unresponsive to epo do not benefit from the addition of myeloid growth factors.[203] With respect to neutrophil stimulation, one trial has shown that GM-CSF, with or without epo, can increase neutrophil counts by a median of fourfold without inducing an excess risk of conversion to acute leukemia.[204]

Attempts to stimulate thrombopoiesis in MDS and AML have included the use of IL-11, which appears to have modest platelet-stimulating properties,[205] and thrombopoietin, which has not been shown to enhance platelet recovery following induction chemotherapy of AML and about which concerns have been raised regarding potential adverse effects on the biology of myeloid malignancies.[206]

Chemotherapy for High-Risk MDS

Selected patients with MDS with adverse cytogenetics and/or increased blasts who are younger, or who are at unacceptably high risk of infection because of neutropenia or who have an impaired quality of life because of platelet and/or red blood cell transfusion requirements, irrespective of age, may benefit from induction chemotherapy as used for treatment of AML. In general, the benefit is limited, and the toxicity of induction therapy can be prohibitive in older patients.

Topotecan has been used to treat symptomatic patients with MDS either as a single agent[207] or in combination with HiDAC.[208] Although higher CR rates (56% versus 37%) were noted in Phase II trials using the combination as compared to single-agent topotecan, a subsequent large retrospective analysis comparing topotecan and HiDAC and FLAG regimens with standard idarubicin and cytarabine, showed that the newer regimens are likely inferior with respect to CR incidence, DFS, and OS.[209] When adjusted for age, induction therapy of high-risk MDS yields an incidence of CR, and even cytogenetic CR, not very different from that seen in de novo AML. Remission durations, however, tend to be brief.[210]

Pgp-reversal agents have been evaluated in high-risk MDS. Phase III trials comparing anthracycline and ara-c combinations with and without cyclosporine A[211] or quinine,[212] suggested response and DFS benefits in the experimental arms.

An analysis of outcomes following intensive therapies in selected patients with MDS, in some instances incorporating transplantation, and categorized according to the IPSS, indicates patients with intermediate-1, intermediate-2, and high-risk disease had survivals of 2.6, 3.4, and 0.9 years, respectively.[213] A pilot evaluation of myeloablative therapies in patients with MDS demonstrated a 12-month median DFS, with 29% of patients disease free at 4 years[214]; 110 patients who underwent allografts from HLA-matched related or unrelated donors showed a 5-year survival ranging between 8% and 30%, with poor outcomes associated with TBI-containing preparative regimens and the use of cyclophosphamide and targeted blood levels of busulfan without TBI leading to better results.[215] Reduced-intensity allogeneic transplant regimens are being investigated to reduced the toxicity and expand the applicability of transplantation for patients with poor-risk MDS. An innovative and preliminarily effective example of this approach used photopheresis, pentostatin, and TBI as the preparative regimen in patients with MDS (median age, 54), who then received either matched related or unrelated allografts.[216]

Immunosuppressive Therapy for MDS

CsA and antithymocyte globulin (ATG) have been studied in patients with MDS using as a rationale the possible contribution of cytotoxic T-cell-mediated marrow suppression to cytopenias. Oligoclonal expansions of T cells have been linked to the pathogenesis of MDS,[217] with clinical responses to immunosuppressive therapies accompanying suppression of such clonal populations.[218] Combined treatment with ATG and CsA has induced major responses in patients with aplastic anemia who clinically overlap with cases of hypoplastic MDS on the basis of having typical MDS clonal cytogenetic abnormalities.[219] Using either horse or rabbit ATG, significant responses were seen in 10 of 35 patients with MDS, with all responses occurring in patients with refractory anemia (RA), particularly in those with brief disease duration.[220] Ten of 20 patients with MDS and less than 10% marrow blasts (8 of 13 responders had RA) developed transfusion independence following treatment with equine ATG.[221] Durable CRs following ATG therapy were seen in 4 of 18 patients with RA and RARS. Limited efficacy and significant toxicity were observed in another trial of ATG in unselected patients with MDS.[222]

Five of nine patients with hypoplastic RA developed red cell and/or platelet responses to treatment with CsA.[223] A multicenter study of CsA in MDS showed significant erythroid responses irrespective of marrow cellularity that was confined to patients with RA, particularly those positive for HLA-DR15 and without adverse cytogenetics.[224] A higher probability of response to ATG or CsA can be predicted among younger patients who are HLA DR15 positive and have had short periods of red cell transfusion dependence.[225]

Antioangiogenic, Cytokine, and Signal Transduction Modulatory Therapies

As observed in trials of patients with MDS using immunosuppressive therapies, responses to treatments aimed at inhibiting angiogenic mediators are most likely to occur in patients with low-risk MDS and to consist mainly of increments in the hemoglobin. Thalidomide induced such responses in 19% of 83 registered patients, only 51 of whom completed 12 weeks of therapy and were considered evaluable.[226]

CC5013 (Revlimid) is a derivative of thalidomide that has more potent antiangiogenic effects while inducing less neurotoxicity and more myelosuppression. Early data using this orally available agent suggest that tolerable doses can induce major clinical and cytogenetic responses in patients with low and Int-1 MDS.[227] Larger Phase II trials in MDS and in MDS with isolated del(5q) are in progress.

Both thalidomide and Revlimid inhibit angiogenesis while also suppressing the activity of tumor necrosis factor (TNF)-α, death signals such as Fas ligand (CD95) and its receptor,[228,229] and other proapoptotic mediators such as tumor necrosis factor (TNF)-related apoptosis-inducing ligand (TRAIL).[230] Attempts to downregulate such pathways have included small trials of the TNF receptor antagonists Remicade, given as a single agent,[231] and Etanercept, given with low-dose thalidomide.[232] Modest, mostly erythroid responses occurred in a minority of low-risk patients.

Direct inhibition of vascular endothelial growth factor (VEGF) receptors and related tyrosine kinases has been studied using PTK787, an orally available agent. In a trial that included 12 patients with high-risk MDS, a suggestion of slowing of disease progression was noted.[233] Another VEGF receptor family inhibitor that also targets mutant FLT3 and is available only parenterally is SU5416, which induced a PR in 1 of 22 patients with poor-risk MDS.[234]

Amifostine has been used to promote hematopoiesis in MDS, acting through a mechanism that may entail inhibition of p53-mediated apoptosis.[235] Fifteen of 18 patients treated with a twice-weekly IV schedule of this agent developed responses in at least one lineage. Doses above 200 mg/m^2 were associated with fatigue, nausea, and vomiting. All 10 patients treated with amifostine and epo, some of whom also were treated with G-CSF, developed brief responses.[236]

Another therapy that putatively inhibits proapoptotic cytokines is the combination of pentoxyphylline, ciprofloxacin, and dexamethasone, which has induced modest bilineage responses in 9 of 18 patients[237] and transfusion independence in 4 of 17.[238]

Arsenic trioxide (ATO) is an agent that may promote apoptosis of leukemic progenitors while inhibiting production of VEGF-A and the growth of vascular endothelium while promoting nonterminal differentiation of hematopoietic precursors.[239] Six of 25 patients in a Phase II trial responded to APO, some with trilineage responses despite high-risk disease.[240] Eleven had stable disease lasting 2 to 6 months. Moderately severe toxicity was seen, with more than 40% of patients developing febrile neutropenia, thrombocytopenia, and gastrointestinal side effects. Early findings from another Phase II trial of ATO, combined with low-dose thalidomide, showed trilineage responses in a minority of patients, 2 of whom had inv(3)(q21q26.2).[241]

Signaling pathways induced by members of the Ras family of oncogenic proteins have been implicated in the pathogenesis of MDS and CMML and have been targeted using agents that inhibit farnesyl transferase (FT), an enzyme which is crucial to the activation of Ras proteins.[242] R11577 (tipifarnib) is an orally available FT inhibitor that was studied in 21 patients with MDS, with 6 responses (3 hematologic improvement, 2 PR, 1 CR). Although the agent proved myelosuppressive, the DLT consisted of fatigue and confusion. Significant activity (33% major response) was seen in another Phase II trial of tipifarnib in poor-risk AML and MDS.[243] Lonafarnib is another orally available FT inhibitor. In a Phase II trial of 32 patients with advanced MDS and 35 with CMML, half of whom had Int-2 or high-risk disease, there were 2 CR (1 MDS, 1 CMML) and 10 hematologic improvements (3 MDS, 7 CMML). Therapy was discontinued by 26% of patients because of fatigue, nausea, vomiting, and anorexia.[244] Continuous treatment with lonafarnib at a dose of 200 mg po bid was well tolerated; hematologic improvement occurred in 3 of 15 patients with MDS and normalization of monocyte counts in 6 of 12 patients with CMML.[245]

Epigenetic Modulatory Therapies

Transcription of genes important for differentiation and proliferation is affected by the extent of methylation in promoters as well as by the level of acetylation of histones that, in the unacetylated state, entwine DNA into transcriptionally silent euchromatin. These pathways are illustrated in Figure 63.4. Agents that target enzymes involved in these epi-

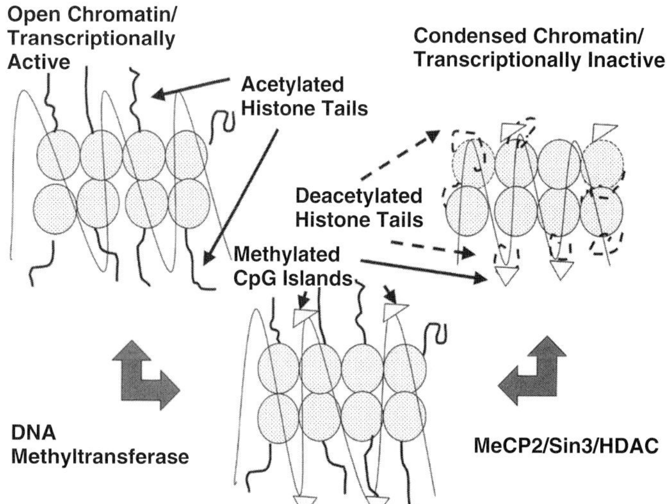

FIGURE 63.4. Epigenetic mechanisms affecting gene transcription: methylation of CpG sequences in promoter regions can prevent gene transcription as can the tightening of DNA into heterochromatic by the coiling of deacetylated histone proteins. (From Mufti et al.,[211] by permission of *Hematology*.)

TABLE 63.11. Epigenetic modulatory therapies of myelodysplastic syndrome (MDS).

Reference	*Year*	*Therapy*	*Target*	*N*	*CR/PR/HI*[b]	*Toxicity*	*Comment*
246	2002	5-Azacytidine[a]	DNA methyl transferase	191	7/16/37[c]	Grade 3,4 cytopenias, 43%–58%	Median time to leukemic transformation 21 months vs. 13 months for observation ($P = 0.007$)
280	2000	Decitabine	DNA methyl transferase	66	13/3/16	Myelosuppression; 7% mortality	20 patients had ≥2 lineage response; median survival = 15 months 3×/week tid schedule[d]
281	2004	Decitabine	DNA methyl transferase	44[e]	11/18 responses at optimal dose	Myelosuppression	Dose escalation studies using low-dose 5×/week schedule[f]
282	2001	Phenylbutyrate	Histone deacetylase	27[g]	0/0/4	None	MTD = 375 mg/kg c.i.v. days 1–7 q 28 days
248	2003	Depsipeptide[g]	Histone deacetylase	9	0/0/0	Grade 3,4 fever, hyponatremia, GI No arrhythmias	Optimal histone acetylation not achieved (100% ↑ acetylation of H3, H4 in all patients)

[a] 75 mg/m² s.c. days 1–7 q 28 days.

[b] HI, hematologic improvement.

[c] Randomized trial vs. observation (5% HI, $P < 0.001$); crossover allowed.

[d] 15 mg/m² i.v./4 hr q 8 hr days 1–3 q 6 weeks.

[e] AML and MDS patients treated.

[f] 5–20 mg/m² i.v./1 hr days 1–5 × 2 weeks; included 16 patients with AML. Prolonged infusions also studied with similar outcomes in AML/MDS, days 1–7 q 2 weeks or days 1–21 q 28 days with 1/23 patients developing neurotoxicity.[283]

[g] Only AML patients treated.

genetic modifications of DNA structure and function have entered clinical trials.

Table 63.11 outlines findings of studies in MDS using agents that target either DNA methylation or histone acetylation. 5-Azacitidine has gained U.S. Food and Drug Administration (FDA) approval for treatment of MDS, largely on the basis of a randomized Phase II trial that demonstrated meaningful benefits with respect to overall survival, time to leukemic transformation,[246] and quality of life.[247] Other agents undergoing investigation include depsipeptide,[248] suberoylanilide hydroxamic acid (SAHA),[249] and valproic acid.[250]

Many interesting compounds are in the process of being studied alone and in combination with chemotherapy in therapies for MDS and AML. The further development of these agents requires well-designed and -conducted clinical trials. Advances in treatment outcomes, it is hoped, will follow.

References

1. Ries I, Kosary C, Hankey B, et al (eds). SEER Cancer Statistics Review 1973–1994. NIH Publication 97–2,789. Bethesda, MD: National Cancer Institute, 1997.
2. Parkin D, Muir, CS, Whelan, SL, et al. Cancer Incidence in Five Continents, vol VII. Lyon, France: IARC Scientific Publications, 1997.
3. Douer D, Santillana S, Ramezani L, et al. Acute promyelocytic leukaemia in patients originating in Latin America is associated with an increased frequency of the bcr1 subtype of the PML/RARalpha fusion gene. Br J Haematol 2003;122:563–570.
4. Preston D. Cancer risks and biomarker studies in the atomic bomb survivors. Stem Cells 1995;13(suppl 1):40–48.
5. Noshchenko AG, Zamostyan PV, Bondar OY, Drozdova VD. Radiation-induced leukemia risk among those aged 0–20 at the time of the Chernobyl accident: a case-control study in the Ukraine. Int J Cancer 2002;99:609–s618.
6. Darby SC, Doll R, Gill SK, Smith PG. Long-term mortality after a single treatment course with X-rays in patients treated for ankylosing spondylitis. Br J Cancer 1987;55:179–190.
7. Andersen MK, Larson RA, Mauritzson N, Schnittger S, Jhanwar SC, Pedersen-Bjergaard J. Balanced chromosome abnormalities inv(16) and t(15;17) in therapy-related myelodysplastic syndromes and acute leukemia: report from an international workshop. Genes Chromosomes Cancer 2002;33:395–400.
8. Bjork J, Albin M, Mauritzson N, Stromberg U, Johansson B, Hagmar L. Smoking and acute myeloid leukemia: associations with morphology and karyotypic patterns and evaluation of dose-response relations. Leuk Res 2001;25:865–872.
9. Lebailly P, Willett EV, Moorman AV, et al. Genetic polymorphisms in microsomal epoxide hydrolase and susceptibility to adult acute myeloid leukaemia with defined cytogenetic abnormalities. Br J Haematol 2002;116:587–594.
10. Bowen DT, Frew ME, Rollinson S, et al. CYP1A1*2B (Val) allele is overrepresented in a subgroup of acute myeloid leukemia patients with poor-risk karyotype associated with NRAS mutation, but not associated with FLT3 internal tandem duplication. Blood 2003;101:2770–2774.
11. Greaves MF, Maia AT, Wiemels JL, Ford AM. Leukemia in twins: lessons in natural history. Blood 2003;102:2321–2333.
12. Hasle H, Clemmensen IH, Mikkelsen M. Risks of leukaemia and solid tumours in individuals with Down's syndrome. Lancet 2000;355:165–169.
13. Poppe B, Van Limbergen H, Van Roy N, et al. Chromosomal aberrations in Bloom syndrome patients with myeloid malignancies. Cancer Genet Cytogenet 2001;128:39–42.
14. Rosenberg PS, Greene MH, Alter BP. Cancer incidence in persons with Fanconi anemia. Blood 2003;101:822–826.
15. Kyle RA. Long-term survival in multiple myeloma. N Engl J Med 1983;308:314–316.
16. Bernard-Marty C, Mano M, Paesmans M, et al. Second malignancies following adjuvant chemotherapy: 6-year results from a Belgian randomized study comparing cyclophosphamide, methotrexate and 5-fluorouracil (CMF) with an anthracycline-based regimen in adjuvant treatment of node-positive breast cancer patients. Ann Oncol 2003;14:693–698.

17. Smith RE, Bryant J, DeCillis A, Anderson S. Acute myeloid leukemia and myelodysplastic syndrome after doxorubicin-cyclophosphamide adjuvant therapy for operable breast cancer: The National Surgical Adjuvant Breast and Bowel Project Experience. J Clin Oncol 2003;21:1195–1204.
18. Smith SM, Le Beau MM, Huo D, et al. Clinical-cytogenetic associations in 306 patients with therapy-related myelodysplasia and myeloid leukemia: the University of Chicago series. Blood 2003; 102:43–52.
19. Crump M, Tu D, Shepherd L, Levine M, Bramwell V, Pritchard K. Risk of acute leukemia following epirubicin-based adjuvant chemotherapy: a report from the National Cancer Institute of Canada Clinical Trials Group. J Clin Oncol 2003;21:3066–3071.
20. Sterkers Y, Preudhomme C, Lai J-L, et al. Acute myeloid leukemia and myelodysplastic syndromes following essential thrombocythemia treated with hydroxyurea: high proportion of cases with 17p deletion. Blood 1998;91:616–622.
21. Kolte B, Baer AN, Sait SN, et al. Acute myeloid leukemia in the setting of low dose weekly methotrexate therapy for rheumatoid arthritis. Leuk Lymphoma 2001;42:371–378.
22. Delwail V, Jais JP, Colonna P, Andrieu JM. Fifteen-year secondary leukaemia risk observed in 761 patients with Hodgkin's disease prospectively treated by MOPP or ABVD chemotherapy plus high-dose irradiation. Br J Haematol 2002;118:189–194.
23. Hosing C, Munsell M, Yazji S, et al. Risk of therapy-related myelodysplastic syndrome/acute leukemia following high-dose therapy and autologous bone marrow transplantation for non-Hodgkin's lymphoma. Ann Oncol 2002;13:450–459.
24. Armitage JO, Carbone PP, Connors JM, Levine A, Bennett JM, Kroll S. Treatment-related myelodysplasia and acute leukemia in non-Hodgkin's lymphoma patients. J Clin Oncol 2003;21: 897–906.
25. Pui CH, Ribeiro RC, Hancock ML, et al. Acute myeloid leukemia in children treated with epipodophyllotoxins for acute lymphoblastic leukemia. N Engl J Med 1991;325:1682–1687.
26. Pedersen-Bjergaard J, Andersen MK, Christiansen DH, Nerlov C. Genetic pathways in therapy-related myelodysplasia and acute myeloid leukemia. Blood 2002;99:1909–1912.
27. Le Beau MM, Espinosa R III, Davis EM, Eisenbart JD, Larson RA, Green ED. Cytogenetic and molecular delineation of a region of chromosome 7 commonly deleted in malignant myeloid diseases. Blood 1996;88:1930–1935.
28. Castro PD, Liang JC, Nagarajan L. Deletions of chromosome 5q13.3 and 17p loci cooperate in myeloid neoplasms. Blood 2000;95:2138–2143.
29. Christiansen DH, Andersen MK, Pedersen-Bjergaard J. Mutations with loss of heterozygosity of p53 are common in therapy-related myelodysplasia and acute myeloid leukemia after exposure to alkylating agents and significantly associated with deletion or loss of 5q, a complex karyotype, and a poor prognosis. J Clin Oncol 2001;19:1405–1413.
30. Strissel PL, Strick R, Rowley JD, Zeleznik-Le NJ. An in vivo topoisomerase II cleavage site and a DNase I hypersensitive site colocalize near exon 9 in the MLL breakpoint cluster region. Blood 1998;92:3793–3803.
31. Schoch C, Schnittger S, Klaus M, Kern W, Hiddemann W, Haferlach T. AML with 11q23/MLL abnormalities as defined by the WHO classification: incidence, partner chromosomes, FAB subtype, age distribution, and prognostic impact in an unselected series of 1897 cytogenetically analyzed AML cases. Blood 2003;102:2395–2402.
32. Gilliland DG. Molecular genetics of human leukemias: new insights into therapy. Semin Hematol 2002;39:6–11.
33. Whitman SP, Archer KJ, Feng L, et al. Absence of the wild-type allele predicts poor prognosis in adult de novo acute myeloid leukemia with normal cytogenetics and the internal tandem duplication of FLT3: a Cancer and Leukemia Group B Study. Cancer Res 2001;61:7233–7239.
34. Lancet JE, Karp JE. Farnesyltransferase inhibitors in hematologic malignancies: new horizons in therapy. Blood 2003;102:3880–3889.
35. Shen SW, Dolnikov A, Passioura T, et al. Mutant N-ras preferentially drives human CD34(+) hematopoietic progenitor cells into myeloid differentiation and proliferation both in vitro and in the NOD/SCID mouse. Exp Hematol 2004;32:852–860.
36. Feng G-S. Mutated SHP and AML in leukemias. Blood 2004;103: 1982–1983.
37. Sternberg DW, Gilliland DG. The role of signal transducer and activator of transcription factors in leukemogenesis. J Clin Oncol 2004;22:361–371.
38. Del Poeta G, Venditti A, Del Principe MI, et al. Amount of spontaneous apoptosis detected by Bax/Bcl-2 ratio predicts outcome in acute myeloid leukemia (AML). Blood 2003;101: 2125–2131.
39. Schimmer AD, Pedersen IM, Kitada S, et al. Functional blocks in caspase activation pathways are common in leukemia and predict patient response to induction chemotherapy. Cancer Res 2003;63:1242–1248.
40. Guzman ML, Neering SJ, Upchurch D, et al. Nuclear factor-κB is constitutively activated in primitive human acute myelogenous leukemia cells. Blood 2001;98:2301–2307.
41. Fenaux P, Jonveaux P, Quiquandon I, et al. p53 gene mutations in acute myeloid leukemia with 17p monosomy. Blood 1991;78: 1652–1657.
42. Sauerbrey A, Stammler G, Zintl F, Volm M. Expression of the retinoblastoma tumor suppressor gene (RB-1) in acute leukemia. Leuk Lymphoma 1998;28:275–283.
43. Stirewalt DL, Kopecky KJ, Meshinchi S, et al. FLT3, RAS, and TP53 mutations in elderly patients with acute myeloid leukemia. Blood 2001;97:3589–3595.
44. Bennett JM, Catovsky D, Daniel MT, et al. Proposals for the classification of the acute leukaemias. French-American-British (FAB) co-operative group. Br J Haematol 1976;33:451–458.
45. Vardiman JW, Harris NL, Brunning RD. The World Health Organization (WHO) classification of the myeloid neoplasms. Blood 2002;100:2292–2302.
46. Estey E, Thall P, Beran M, Kantarjian H, Pierce S, Keating M. Effect of diagnosis (refractory anemia with excess blasts, refractory anemia with excess blasts in transformation, or acute myeloid leukemia [AML]) on outcome of AML-type chemotherapy. Blood 1997;90:2969–2977.
47. Gahn B, Haase D, Unterhalt M, et al. De novo AML with dysplastic hematopoiesis: cytogenetic and prognostic significance. Leukemia 1996;10:946–951.
48. Braylan RC, Orfao A, Borowitz MJ, Davis BH. Optimal number of reagents required to evaluate hematolymphoid neoplasias: results of an international consensus meeting. Cytometry 2001; 46:23–27.
49. Kowal-Vern A, Mazzella FM, Cotelingam JD, Shrit MA, Rector JT, Schumacher HR. Diagnosis and characterization of acute erythroleukemia subsets by determining the percentages of myeloblasts and proerythroblasts in 69 cases. Am J Hematol 2000;65:5–13.
50. Dastugue N, Lafage-Pochitaloff M, Pages M-P, et al. Cytogenetic profile of childhood and adult megakaryoblastic leukemia (M7): a study of the Groupe Francais de Cytogenetique Hematologique (GFCH). Blood 2002;100:618–626.
51. Roumier C, Eclache V, Imbert M, et al. M0 AML, clinical and biologic features of the disease, including AML1 gene mutations: a report of 59 cases by the Groupe Francais d'Hematologie Cellulaire (GFHC) and the Groupe Francais de Cytogenetique Hematologique (GFCH). Blood 2003;101:1277–1283.
52. Frohling S, Skelin S, Liebisch C, et al. Comparison of cytogenetic and molecular cytogenetic detection of chromosome abnormalities in 240 consecutive adult patients with acute myeloid leukemia. J Clin Oncol 2002;20:2480–2485.

53. Mrozek K, Prior TW, Edwards C, et al. Comparison of cytogenetic and molecular genetic detection of t(8;21) and inv(16) in a prospective series of adults with de novo acute myeloid leukemia: a Cancer and Leukemia Group B Study. J Clin Oncol 2001;19:2482–2492.
54. Zhang FF, Murata-Collins JL, Gaytan P, et al. Twenty-four-color spectral karyotyping reveals chromosome aberrations in cytogenetically normal acute myeloid leukemia. Genes Chromosomes Cancer 2000;28:318–328.
55. Cheson BD, Bennett JM, Kopecky KJ, et al. Revised recommendations of the International Working Group for Diagnosis, Standardization of Response Criteria, Treatment Outcomes, and Reporting Standards for Therapeutic Trials in Acute Myeloid Leukemia. J Clin Oncol 2003;21:4642–4649.
56. Marcucci G, Mrozek K, Ruppert AS, et al. Abnormal cytogenetics at date of morphologic complete remission predicts short overall and disease-free survival, and higher relapse rate in adult acute myeloid leukemia: results from cancer and leukemia group B study 8461. J Clin Oncol 2004;22:2410–2418.
57. Leith CP, Kopecky KJ, Godwin J, et al. Acute myeloid leukemia in the elderly: assessment of multidrug resistance (MDR1) and cytogenetics distinguishes biologic subgroups with remarkably distinct responses to standard chemotherapy. A Southwest Oncology Group study. Blood 1997;89:3323–3329.
58. Grimwade D, Walker H, Oliver F, et al. The importance of diagnostic cytogenetics on outcome in AML: analysis of 1,612 patients entered into the MRC AML 10 trial. The Medical Research Council Adult and Children's Leukaemia Working Parties. Blood 1998;92:2322–2333.
59. Schoch C, Haferlach T, Haase D, et al. Patients with de novo acute myeloid leukaemia and complex karyotype aberrations show a poor prognosis despite intensive treatment: a study of 90 patients. Br J Haematol 2001;112:118–126.
60. Byrd JC, Mrozek K, Dodge RK, et al. Pretreatment cytogenetic abnormalities are predictive of induction success, cumulative incidence of relapse, and overall survival in adult patients with de novo acute myeloid leukemia: results from Cancer and Leukemia Group B (CALGB 8461). Blood 2002;100:4325–4336.
61. Farag SS, Archer KJ, Mrozek K, et al. Isolated trisomy of chromosomes 8, 11, 13 and 21 is an adverse prognostic factor in adults with de novo acute myeloid leukemia: results from Cancer and Leukemia Group B 8461. Int J Oncol 2002;21:1041–1051.
62. Mrozek K, Heinonen K, Lawrence D, et al. Adult patients with de novo acute myeloid leukemia and t(9; 11)(p22; q23) have a superior outcome to patients with other translocations involving band 11q23: a cancer and leukemia group B study. Blood 1997;90:4532–4538.
63. Caligiuri MA, Strout MP, Lawrence D, et al. Rearrangement of ALL1 (MLL) in acute myeloid leukemia with normal cytogenetics. Cancer Res 1998;58:55–59.
64. Dohner K, Tobis K, Ulrich R, et al. Prognostic significance of partial tandem duplications of the MLL gene in adult patients 16 to 60 years old with acute myeloid leukemia and normal cytogenetics: a study of the Acute Myeloid Leukemia Study Group Ulm. J Clin Oncol 2002;20:3254–3261.
65. Yamamoto Y, Kiyoi H, Nakano Y, et al. Activating mutation of D835 within the activation loop of FLT3 in human hematologic malignancies. Blood 2001;97:2434–2439.
66. Kainz B, Heintel D, Marculescu R, et al. Variable prognostic value of FLT3 internal tandem duplications in patients with de novo AML and a normal karyotype, t(15;17), t(8;21) or inv(16). Hematol J 2002;3:283–289.
67. Schnittger S, Schoch C, Dugas M, et al. Analysis of FLT3 length mutations in 1,003 patients with acute myeloid leukemia: correlation to cytogenetics, FAB subtype, and prognosis in the AMLCG study and usefulness as a marker for the detection of minimal residual disease. Blood 2002;100:59–66.
68. Thiede C, Steudel C, Mohr B, et al. Analysis of FLT3-activating mutations in 979 patients with acute myelogenous leukemia: association with FAB subtypes and identification of subgroups with poor prognosis. Blood 2002;99:4326–4335.
69. Care RS, Valk PJ, Goodeve AC, et al. Incidence and prognosis of c-KIT and FLT3 mutations in core binding factor (CBF) acute myeloid leukaemias. Br J Haematol 2003;121:775–777.
70. Garg M, Moore H, Tobal K, Liu Yin JA. Prognostic significance of quantitative analysis of WT1 gene transcripts by competitive reverse transcription polymerase chain reaction in acute leukaemia. Br J Haematol 2003;123:49–59.
71. Wetzler M, Baer MR, Bernstein SH, et al. Expression of c-mpl mRNA, the receptor for thrombopoietin, in acute myeloid leukemia blasts identifies a group of patients with poor response to intensive chemotherapy. J Clin Oncol 1997;15:2262–2268.
72. Frohling S, Schlenk, RF, Stolze, I, et al. Mutations in younger adults with acute myeloid leukemia and normal cytogenetics: prognostic relevance and analysis of cooperating mutations. J Clin Oncol 2004;in press.
73. Lowenberg B, van Putten W, Touw IP, Delwel R, Santini V. Autonomous proliferation of leukemic cells in vitro as a determinant of prognosis in adult acute myeloid leukemia. N Engl J Med 1993;328:614–619.
74. Haferlach T, Schoch C, Loffler H, et al. Morphologic dysplasia in de novo acute myeloid leukemia (AML) is related to unfavorable cytogenetics but has no independent prognostic relevance under the conditions of intensive induction therapy: results of a multiparameter analysis from the German AML Cooperative Group Studies. J Clin Oncol 2003;21:256–265.
75. Kern W, Haferlach T, Schoch C, et al. Early blast clearance by remission induction therapy is a major independent prognostic factor for both achievement of complete remission and long-term outcome in acute myeloid leukemia: data from the German AML Cooperative Group (AMLCG) 1992 Trial. Blood 2003;101:64–70.
76. Estey EH, Shen Y, Thall PF. Effect of time to complete remission on subsequent survival and disease-free survival time in AML, RAEB-t, and RAEB. Blood 2000;95:72–77.
77. Grimwade D, Lo Coco F. Acute promyelocytic leukemia: a model for the role of molecular diagnosis and residual disease monitoring in directing treatment approach in acute myeloid leukemia. Leukemia 2002;16:1959–1973.
78. Nucifora G, Larson RA, Rowley JD. Persistence of the 8;21 translocation in patients with acute myeloid leukemia type M2 in long-term remission. Blood 1993;82:712–715.
79. Schoch C, Kohlmann A, Schnittger S, et al. Acute myeloid leukemias with reciprocal rearrangements can be distinguished by specific gene expression profiles. Proc Natl Acad Sci USA 2002;99:10008–10013.
80. Rai KR, Holland JF, Glidewell OJ, et al. Treatment of acute myelocytic leukemia: a study by cancer and leukemia group B. Blood 1981;58:1203–1212.
81. Yates J, Glidewell O, Wiernik P, et al. Cytosine arabinoside with daunorubicin or adriamycin for therapy of acute myelocytic leukemia: a CALGB study. Blood 1982;60:454–462.
82. Berman E, Wiernik P, Vogler R, Velez-Garcia E, Bartolucci A, Whaley FS. Long-term follow-up of three randomized trials comparing idarubicin and daunorubicin as induction therapies for patients with untreated acute myeloid leukemia. Cancer (Phila) 1997;80:2181–2185.
83. Dillman RO, Davis RB, Green MR, et al. A comparative study of two different doses of cytarabine for acute myeloid leukemia: a phase III trial of Cancer and Leukemia Group B. Blood 1991; 78:2520–2526.
84. Mitus A, Miller K, Schenkein D, et al. Improved survival for patients with acute myelogenous leukemia. J Clin Oncol 1995; 13:560–569.

85. Weick JK, Kopecky KJ, Appelbaum FR, et al. A randomized investigation of high-dose versus standard-dose cytosine arabinoside with daunorubicin in patients with previously untreated acute myeloid leukemia: a Southwest Oncology Group study. Blood 1996;88:2841–2851.
86. Bishop JF, Matthews JP, Young GA, et al. A randomized study of high-dose cytarabine in induction in acute myeloid leukemia. Blood 1996;87:1710–1717.
87. Rubin EH, Andersen JW, Berg DT, Schiffer CA, Mayer RJ, Stone RM. Risk factors for high-dose cytarabine neurotoxicity: an analysis of a cancer and leukemia group B trial in patients with acute myeloid leukemia. J Clin Oncol 1992;10:948–953.
88. Jolson HM, Bosco L, Bufton MG, et al. Clustering of adverse drug events: analysis of risk factors for cerebellar toxicity with high-dose cytarabine. J Natl Cancer Inst 1992;84:500–505.
89. Dombret H, Chastang C, Fenaux P, et al. A controlled study of recombinant human granulocyte colony-stimulating factor in elderly patients after treatment for acute myelogenous leukemia. AML Cooperative Study Group. N Engl J Med 1995; 332:1678–1683.
90. Rowe JM, Andersen JW, Mazza JJ, et al. A randomized placebo-controlled phase III study of granulocyte-macrophage colony-stimulating factor in adult patients (>55 to 70 years of age) with acute myelogenous leukemia: a study of the Eastern Cooperative Oncology Group (E1490). Blood 1995;86:457–462.
91. Bennett CL, Stinson TJ, Tallman MS, et al. Economic analysis of a randomized placebo-controlled phase III study of granulocyte macrophage colony stimulating factor in adult patients (>55 to 70 years of age) with acute myelogenous leukemia. Eastern Cooperative Oncology Group (E1490). Ann Oncol 1999;10:177–182.
92. Uyl-de Groot CA, Lowenberg B, Vellenga E, Suciu S, Willemze R, Rutten FF. Cost-effectiveness and quality-of-life assessment of GM-CSF as an adjunct to intensive remission induction chemotherapy in elderly patients with acute myeloid leukemia. Br J Haematol 1998;100:629–636.
93. Witz F, Sadoun A, Perrin MC, et al. A placebo-controlled study of recombinant human granulocyte-macrophage colony-stimulating factor administered during and after induction treatment for de novo acute myelogenous leukemia in elderly patients. Groupe Ouest Est Leucemies Aigues Myeloblastiques (GOELAM). Blood 1998;91:2722–2730.
94. Lowenberg B, van Putten W, Theobald M, et al. Effect of priming with granulocyte colony-stimulating factor on the outcome of chemotherapy for acute myeloid leukemia. N Engl J Med 2003; 349:743–752.
95. Rowe JM, Neuberg D, Friedenberg W, et al. A phase 3 study of three induction regimens and of priming with GM-CSF in older adults with acute myeloid leukemia: a trial by the Eastern Cooperative Oncology Group. Blood 2004;103:479–485.
96. Mayer RJ, Davis RB, Schiffer CA, et al. Intensive postremission chemotherapy in adults with acute myeloid leukemia. Cancer and Leukemia Group B. N Engl J Med 1994;331:896–903.
97. Bloomfield CD, Lawrence D, Byrd JC, et al. Frequency of prolonged remission duration after high-dose cytarabine intensification in acute myeloid leukemia varies by cytogenetic subtype. Cancer Res 1998;58:4173–4179.
98. Byrd JC, Dodge RK, Carroll A, et al. Patients with t(8;21)(q22;q22) and acute myeloid leukemia have superior failure-free and overall survival when repetitive cycles of high-dose cytarabine are administered. J Clin Oncol 1999;17:3767–3775.
99. Delaunay J, Vey N, Leblanc T, et al. Prognosis of inv(16)/t(16;16) acute myeloid leukemia (AML): a survey of 110 cases from the French AML Intergroup. Blood 2003;102:462–469.
100. Nguyen S, Leblanc T, Fenaux P, et al. A white blood cell index as the main prognostic factor in t(8;21) acute myeloid leukemia (AML): a survey of 161 cases from the French AML Intergroup. Blood 2002;99:3517–3523.
101. Elonen E, Almqvist A, Hanninen A, et al. Comparison between four and eight cycles of intensive chemotherapy in adult acute myeloid leukemia: a randomized trial of the Finnish Leukemia Group. Leukemia 1998;12:1041–1048.
102. Buchner T, Hiddemann W, Berdel WE, et al. 6-Thioguanine, cytarabine, and daunorubicin (TAD) and high-dose cytarabine and mitoxantrone (HAM) for induction, TAD for consolidation, and either prolonged maintenance by reduced monthly TAD or TAD-HAM-TAD and one course of intensive consolidation by sequential HAM in adult patients at all ages with de novo acute myeloid leukemia (AML): a randomized trial of the German AML Cooperative Group. J Clin Oncol 2003;21:4496–4504.
103. Tallman MS, Appelbaum FR, Amos D, et al. Evaluation of intensive postremission chemotherapy for adults with acute non-lymphocytic leukemia using high-dose cytosine arabinoside with L-asparaginase and amsacrine with etoposide. J Clin Oncol 1987;5:918–926.
104. Zittoun R, Jehn U, Fiere D, et al. Alternating vs. repeated postremission treatment in adult acute myelogenous leukemia: a randomized phase III study (AML6) of the EORTC Leukemia Cooperative Group. Blood 1989;73:896–906.
105. Moore JO, Powell B, Velez-Garcia E, et al. A comparison of sequential non-cross-resistant therapy or Ara-C consolidation following complete remission in adult patients <60 years with acute myeloid leukemia: CALGB 9222. Proc Am Soc Clin Oncol 1997;16:48.
106. Nathan PC, Sung L, Crump M, Beyene J. Consolidation therapy with autologous bone marrow transplantation in adults with acute myeloid leukemia: a meta-analysis. J Natl Cancer Inst 2004;96:38–45.
107. Cassileth PA, Harrington DP, Appelbaum FR, et al. Chemotherapy compared with autologous or allogeneic bone marrow transplantation in the management of acute myeloid leukemia in first remission. N Engl J Med 1998;339:1649–1656.
108. Zittoun RA, Mandelli F, Willemze R, et al. Autologous or allogeneic bone marrow transplantation compared with intensive chemotherapy in acute myelogenous leukemia. N Engl J Med 1995;332:217–223.
109. Burnett AK, Goldstone AH, Stevens RM, et al. Randomised comparison of addition of autologous bone-marrow transplantation to intensive chemotherapy for acute myeloid leukaemia in first remission: results of MRC AML 10 trial. UK Medical Research Council Adult and Children's Leukaemia Working Parties. Lancet 1998;351:700–708.
110. Burnett AK, Wheatley K, Goldstone AH, et al. The value of allogeneic bone marrow transplant in patients with acute myeloid leukaemia at differing risk of relapse: results of the UK MRC AML 10 trial. Br J Haematol 2002;118:385–400.
111. Linker CA, Ries CA, Damon LE, et al. Autologous stem cell transplantation for acute myeloid leukemia in first remission. Biol Blood Marrow Transplant 2000;6:50–57.
112. Suciu S, Mandelli F, de Witte T, et al. Allogeneic compared with autologous stem cell transplantation in the treatment of patients younger than 46 years with acute myeloid leukemia (AML) in first complete remission (CR1): an intention-to-treat analysis of the EORTC/GIMEMAAML-10 trial. Blood 2003;102:1232–1240.
113. Slovak ML, Kopecky KJ, Cassileth PA, et al. Karyotypic analysis predicts outcome of preremission and postremission therapy in adult acute myeloid leukemia: a Southwest Oncology Group/Eastern Cooperative Oncology Group study. Blood 2000; 96: 4075–4083.
114. Venditti A, Maurillo L, Buccisano F, et al. Pretransplant minimal residual disease level predicts clinical outcome in patients with acute myeloid leukemia receiving high-dose chemotherapy and autologous stem cell transplantation. Leukemia 2003;17:2178–2182.

115. Bleakley M, Riddell SR. Molecules and mechanisms of the graft-versus-leukaemia effect. Nat Rev Cancer 2004;4:371–380.
116. Buckner CD, Sanders J, Appelbaum FR. Allogeneic marrow transplantation for acute non-lymphoblastic leukemia: first remission versus after first relapse. Bone Marrow Transplant 1989;4(suppl 1):244–246.
117. Tallman MS, Rowlings PA, Milone G, et al. Effect of postremission chemotherapy before human leukocyte antigen-identical sibling transplantation for acute myelogenous leukemia in first complete remission. Blood 2000;96:1254–1258.
118. Slavin S, Morecki S, Weiss L, Or R. Immunotherapy of hematologic malignancies and metastatic solid tumors in experimental animals and man. Crit Rev Oncol Hematol 2003;46:139–163.
119. Mattsson J, Uzunel M, Brune M, et al. Mixed chimaerism is common at the time of acute graft-versus-host disease and disease response in patients receiving non-myeloablative conditioning and allogeneic stem cell transplantation. Br J Haematol 2001;115:935–944.
120. Fernandez-Aviles F, Urbano-Ispizua A, Aymerich M, et al. Low-dose total-body irradiation and fludarabine followed by hematopoietic cell transplantation from HLA-identical sibling donors do not induce complete T-cell donor engraftment in most patients with progressive hematologic diseases. Exp Hematol 2003;31:934–940.
121. Estey E. Treatment of refractory AML. Leukemia 1996;10:932–936.
122. Kern W, Schoch C, Haferlach T, et al. Multivariate analysis of prognostic factors in patients with refractory and relapsed acute myeloid leukemia undergoing sequential high-dose cytosine arabinoside and mitoxantrone (S-HAM) salvage therapy: relevance of cytogenetic abnormalities. Leukemia 2000;14:226–231.
123. Archimbaud E, Leblond V, Fenaux P, et al. Timed sequential chemotherapy for advanced acute myeloid leukemia. Hematol Cell Ther 1996;38:161–167.
124. Montillo M, Mirto S, Petti MC, et al. Fludarabine, cytarabine, and G-CSF (FLAG) for the treatment of poor risk acute myeloid leukemia. Am J Hematol 1998;58:105–109.
125. Steinmetz HT, Schulz A, Staib P, et al. Phase-II trial of idarubicin, fludarabine, cytosine arabinoside, and filgrastim (Ida-FLAG) for treatment of refractory, relapsed, and secondary AML. Ann Hematol 1999;78:418–425.
126. Pastore D, Specchia G, Carluccio P, et al. FLAG-IDA in the treatment of refractory/relapsed acute myeloid leukemia: single-center experience. Ann Hematol 2003;82:231–235.
127. Spadea A, Petti MC, Fazi P, et al. Mitoxantrone, etoposide and intermediate-dose Ara-C (MEC): an effective regimen for poor risk acute myeloid leukemia. Leukemia 1993;7:549–552.
128. Feldman EJ, Alberts DS, Arlin Z, et al. Phase I clinical and pharmacokinetic evaluation of high-dose mitoxantrone in combination with cytarabine in patients with acute leukemia. J Clin Oncol 1993;11:2002–2009.
129. Cortes J, Estey E, Beran M, et al. Cyclophosphamide, ara-C and topotecan (CAT) for patients with refractory or relapsed acute leukemia. Leuk Lymphoma 2000;36:479–484.
130. Seiter K, Feldman EJ, Halicka HD, et al. Phase I clinical and laboratory evaluation of topotecan and cytarabine in patients with acute leukemia. J Clin Oncol 1997;15:44–51.
131. Vey N, Kantarjian H, Beran M, et al. Combination of topotecan with cytarabine or etoposide in patients with refractory or relapsed acute myeloid leukemia: results of a randomized phase I/II study. Invest New Drugs 1999;17:89–95.
132. Cortes J, Estey E, O'Brien S, et al. High-dose liposomal daunorubicin and high-dose cytarabine combination in patients with refractory or relapsed acute myelogenous leukemia. Cancer (Phila) 2001;92:7–14.
133. Taylor PR, Reid MM, Stark AN, Bown N, Hamilton PJ, Proctor SJ. De novo acute myeloid leukaemia in patients over 55-years-old: a population-based study of incidence, treatment and outcome. Northern Region Haematology Group. Leukemia 1995;9:231–237.
134. Behringer B, Pitako JA, Kunzmann R, et al. Prognosis of older patients with acute myeloid leukemia receiving either induction or noncurative treatment: a single-center retrospective study. Ann Hematol 2003;82:381–389.
135. Hiddemann W, Kern W, Schoch C, et al. Management of acute myeloid leukemia in elderly patients. J Clin Oncol 1999;17:3569–3576.
136. DeLima M, Ghaddar H, Pierce S, Estey E. Treatment of newly-diagnosed acute myelogenous leukaemia in patients aged 80 years and above. Br J Haematol 1996;93:89–95.
137. Anderson JE, Kopecky KJ, Willman CL, et al. Outcome after induction chemotherapy for older patients with acute myeloid leukemia is not improved with mitoxantrone and etoposide compared to cytarabine and daunorubicin: a Southwest Oncology Group study. Blood 2002;100:3869–3876.
138. Goldstone AH, Burnett AK, Wheatley K, Smith AG, Hutchinson RM, Clark RE. Attempts to improve treatment outcomes in acute myeloid leukemia (AML) in older patients: the results of the United Kingdom Medical Research Council AML11 trial. Blood 2001;98:1302–1311.
139. Feldman EJ, Seiter K, Damon L, et al. A randomized trial of high- vs standard-dose mitoxantrone with cytarabine in elderly patients with acute myeloid leukemia. Leukemia 1997;11:485–489.
140. Ossenkoppele G, Graveland, WJ, Sonneveld, P, et al. The value of Fludarabine in addition to ARA-C and G-CSF in the treatment of patients with high risk myelodysplastic syndromes and elderly AML. Blood 2004;in press.
141. Estey EH, Thall PF, Giles FJ, et al. Gemtuzumab ozogamicin with or without interleukin 11 in patients 65 years of age or older with untreated acute myeloid leukemia and high-risk myelodysplastic syndrome: comparison with idarubicin plus continuous-infusion, high-dose cytosine arabinoside. Blood 2002;99:4343–4349.
142. Marcucci G, Byrd JC, Dai G, et al. Phase 1 and pharmacodynamic studies of G3139, a Bcl-2 antisense oligonucleotide, in combination with chemotherapy in refractory or relapsed acute leukemia. Blood 2003;101:425–432.
143. Lowenberg B, Suciu S, Archimbaud E, et al. Mitoxantrone versus daunorubicin in induction-consolidation chemotherapy: the value of low-dose cytarabine for maintenance of remission, and an assessment of prognostic factors in acute myeloid leukemia in the elderly: final report. European Organization for the Research and Treatment of Cancer and the Dutch-Belgian Hemato-Oncology Cooperative Hovon Group. J Clin Oncol 1998;16:872–881.
144. Robles C, Kim KM, Oken MM, et al. Low-dose cytarabine maintenance therapy vs. observation after remission induction in advanced acute myeloid leukemia: an Eastern Cooperative Oncology Group Trial (E5483). Leukemia 2000;14:1349–1353.
145. Stone RM, Berg DT, George SL, et al. Postremission therapy in older patients with de novo acute myeloid leukemia: a randomized trial comparing mitoxantrone and intermediate-dose cytarabine with standard-dose cytarabine. Blood 2001;98:548–553.
146. Schiller G, Lee M. Long-term outcome of high-dose cytarabine-based consolidation chemotherapy for older patients with acute myelogenous leukemia. Leuk Lymphoma 1997;25:111–119.
147. Grignani F, De Matteis S, Nervi C, et al. Fusion proteins of the retinoic acid receptor-alpha recruit histone deacetylase in promyelocytic leukaemia. Nature (Lond) 1998;391:815–818.
148. Frankel SR, Eardley A, Heller G, et al. All-trans retinoic acid for acute promyelocytic leukemia. Results of the New York Study. Ann Intern Med 1994;120:278–286.

149. Tallman MS, Andersen JW, Schiffer CA, et al. All-*trans* retinoic acid in acute promyelocytic leukemia. N Engl J Med 1997;337: 1021–1028.
150. Paietta E, Andersen J, Gallagher R, et al. The immunophenotype of acute promyelocytic leukemia (APL): an ECOG study. Leukemia 1994;8:1108–1112.
151. Estey E, Thall PF, Pierce S, Kantarjian H, Keating M. Treatment of newly diagnosed acute promyelocytic leukemia without cytarabine. J Clin Oncol 1997;15:483–490.
152. Estey E, Faderl S, Giles F, et al. All-*trans* retinoic acid (ATRA) + arsenic trioxide (ATO) to minimize or eliminate chemotherapy in untreated APL. Blood 2003;
153. Burnett AK, Grimwade D, Solomon E, Wheatley K, Goldstone AH. Presenting white blood cell count and kinetics of molecular remission predict prognosis in acute promyelocytic leukemia treated with all-*trans* retinoic acid: result of the Randomized MRC Trial. Blood 1999;93:4131–4143.
154. Fenaux P, Chastang C, Chevret S, et al. A randomized comparison of all-*trans* retinoic acid (ATRA) followed by chemotherapy and ATRA plus chemotherapy and the role of maintenance therapy in newly diagnosed acute promyelocytic leukemia. Blood 1999;94:1192–1200.
155. Frankel SR, Eardley A, Lauwers G, Weiss M, Warrell RP Jr. The "retinoic acid syndrome" in acute promyelocytic leukemia. Ann Intern Med 1992;117:292–296.
156. de Botton S, Chevret S, Coiteux V, et al. Early onset of chemotherapy can reduce the incidence of ATRA syndrome in newly diagnosed acute promyelocytic leukemia (APL) with low white blood cell counts: results from APL 93 trial. Leukemia 2003;17:339–342.
157. Soignet SL, Frankel SR, Douer D, et al. United States Multicenter Study of Arsenic Trioxide in Relapsed Acute Promyelocytic Leukemia. J Clin Oncol 2001;19:3852–3860.
158. Jurcic JG, DeBlasio T, Dumont L, Yao TJ, Scheinberg DA. Molecular remission induction with retinoic acid and anti-CD33 monoclonal antibody HuM195 in acute promyelocytic leukemia. Clin Cancer Res 2000;6:372–380.
159. Tallman MS, Andersen JW, Schiffer CA, et al. All-*trans* retinoic acid in acute promyelocytic leukemia: long-term outcome and prognostic factor analysis from the North American Intergroup protocol. Blood 2002;100:4298–4302.
160. Meloni G, Diverio D, Vignetti M, et al. Autologous bone marrow transplantation for acute promyelocytic leukemia in second remission: prognostic relevance of pretransplant minimal residual disease assessment by reverse-transcription polymerase chain reaction of the PML/RAR alpha fusion gene. Blood 1997; 90:1321–1325.
161. Feldman E, Stone, RM, Brandwein, J et al. Phase III randomized trial of an anti-CD33 monoclonal antibody (HuM195) in combination with chemotherapy compared to chemotherapy alone in adults with refractory or first-relapse acute myeloid leukemia (AML). Proc Am Soc Clin Oncol 2002;21:261a.
162. Jurcic JG, Larson SM, Sgouros G, et al. Targeted alpha particle immunotherapy for myeloid leukemia. Blood 2002;100:1233–1239.
163. Baldus CD, Tanner SM, Ruppert AS, et al. BAALC expression predicts clinical outcome of de novo acute myeloid leukemia patients with normal cytogenetics: a Cancer and Leukemia Group B Study. Blood 2003;102:1613–1618.
164. Wadleigh M, Richardson PG, Zahrieh D, et al. Prior gemtuzumab ozogamicin exposure significantly increases the risk of veno-occlusive disease in patients who undergo myeloablative allogeneic stem cell transplantation. Blood 2003;102:1578–1582.
165. Cortes J, Tsimberidou AM, Alvarez R, et al. Mylotarg combined with topotecan and cytarabine in patients with refractory acute myelogenous leukemia. Cancer Chemother Pharmacol 2002;50: 497–500.
166. Tsimberidou A, Cortes J, Thomas D, et al. Gemtuzumab ozogamicin, fludarabine, cytarabine and cyclosporine combination regimen in patients with CD33+ primary resistant or relapsed acute myeloid leukemia. Leuk Res 2003;27:893–897.
167. DeAngelo D, Stone, RM, Durrant, S, et al. Gemtuzumab ozogamicin (mylotarg) in combination with induction chemotherapy for the treatment of patients with de novo acute myeloid leukemia: two age-specific phase 2 trials. Blood 2003; 102:65a.
168. Kell WJ, Burnett AK, Chopra R, et al. A feasibility study of simultaneous administration of gemtuzumab ozogamicin with intensive chemotherapy in induction and consolidation in younger patients with acute myeloid leukemia. Blood 2003;102: 4277–4283.
169. Burke JM, Caron PC, Papadopoulos EB, et al. Cytoreduction with iodine-131-anti-CD33 antibodies before bone marrow transplantation for advanced myeloid leukemias. Bone Marrow Transplant 2003;32:549–556.
170. Matthews DC, Appelbaum FR, Eary JF, et al. Phase I study of ^{131}I-anti-CD45 antibody plus cyclophosphamide and total body irradiation for advanced acute leukemia and myelodysplastic syndrome. Blood 1999;94:1237–1247.
171. Bunjes D. ^{188}Re-labeled anti-CD66 monoclonal antibody in stem cell transplantation for patients with high-risk acute myeloid leukemia. Leuk Lymphoma 2002;43:2125–2131.
172. Foa R. Interleukin 2 in the management of acute leukaemia. Br J Haematol 1996;92:1–8.
173. Farag SS, George SL, Lee EJ, et al. Postremission therapy with low-dose interleukin 2 with or without intermediate pulse dose interleukin 2 therapy is well tolerated in elderly patients with acute myeloid leukemia: Cancer and Leukemia Group B Study 9420. Clin Cancer Res 2002;8:2812–2819.
174. Frankel AE, Powell BL, Hall PD, Case LD, Kreitman RJ. Phase I trial of a novel diphtheria toxin/granulocyte macrophage colony-stimulating factor fusion protein (DT388GMCSF) for refractory or relapsed acute myeloid leukemia. Clin Cancer Res 2002;8: 1004–1013.
175. Molldrem J, Kant S, Lu S, et al. Peptide vaccination with PR1 elicits active T cell immunity that induces cytogenetic remission in acute myelogenous leukemia. Blood 2002.
176. van den Heuvel-Eibrink MM, van der Holt B, te Boekhorst PA, et al. MDR 1 expression is an independent prognostic factor for response and survival in de novo acute myeloid leukaemia. Br J Haematol 1997;99:76–83.
177. Samdani A, Vijapurkar U, Grimm MA, et al. Cytogenetics and P-glycoprotein (PGP) are independent predictors of treatment outcome in acute myeloid leukemia (AML). Leuk Res 1996;20:175–180.
178. Wuchter C, Leonid K, Ruppert V, et al. Clinical significance of P-glycoprotein expression and function for response to induction chemotherapy, relapse rate and overall survival in acute leukemia. Haematologica 2000;85:711–721.
179. Solary E, Drenou B, Campos L, et al. Quinine as a multidrug resistance inhibitor: a phase 3 multicentric randomized study in adult de novo acute myelogenous leukemia. Blood 2003;102: 1202–1210.
180. Coley HM, Twentyman PR, Workman P. Improved cellular accumulation is characteristic of anthracyclines which retain high activity in multidrug resistant cell lines, alone or in combination with verapamil or cyclosporin A. Biochem Pharmacol 1989;38:4467–4475.
181. Fukushima T, Yamashita T, Yoshio N, et al. Effect of PSC 833 on the cytotoxicity of idarubicin and idarubicinol in multidrug-resistant K562 cells. Leuk Res 1999;23:37–42.
182. Jiang XR, Kelsey SM, Wu YL, Newland AC. Circumvention of P-glycoprotein-mediated drug resistance in human leukaemic cells by non-immunosuppressive cyclosporin D analogue, SDZ PSC 833. Br J Haematol 1995;90:375–383.

183. Ross DD, Wooten PJ, Sridhara R, Ordonez JV, Lee EJ, Schiffer CA. Enhancement of daunorubicin accumulation, retention, and cytotoxicity by verapamil or cyclosporin A in blast cells from patients with previously untreated acute myeloid leukemia. Blood 1993;82:1288–1299.
184. List AF, Kopecky KJ, Willman CL, et al. Benefit of cyclosporine modulation of drug resistance in patients with poor-risk acute myeloid leukemia: a Southwest Oncology Group study. Blood 2001;98:3212–3220.
185. Baer MR, George SL, Dodge RK, et al. Phase 3 study of the multidrug resistance modulator PSC-833 in previously untreated patients 60 years of age and older with acute myeloid leukemia: Cancer and Leukemia Group B Study 9720. Blood 2002;100: 1224–1232.
186. Greenberg PL, Lee SJ, Advani R, et al. Mitoxantrone, etoposide, and cytarabine with or without valspodar in patients with relapsed or refractory acute myeloid leukemia and high-risk myelodysplastic syndrome: a phase III trial (E2995). J Clin Oncol 2004;22:1078–1086.
187. Ewing JC, Robertson JD, Kell WJ, et al. Autologous peripheral blood stem cell transplantation in first remission adult acute myeloid leukaemia: an intention to treat analysis and comparison of outcome using a predictive model based on the MRC AML10 cohort. Hematology 2003;8:83–90.
188. Kolitz JE, George SL, Dodge RK, et al. Dose escalation studies of ara-C, daunorubicin and etoposide with and without multidrug resistance modulation with PSC-833 in untreated adults with acute myeloid leukemia <60 years: final induction results of CALGB 9621. Blood 2001;98:461a.
189. Kantarjian H, Gandhi V, Cortes J, et al. Phase 2 clinical and pharmacologic study of clofarabine in patients with refractory or relapsed acute leukemia. Blood 2003;102:2379–2386.
190. Bouffard DY, Jolivet J, Leblond L, et al. Complementary antineoplastic activity of the cytosine nucleoside analogues troxacitabine (Troxatyl) and cytarabine in human leukemia cells. Cancer Chemother Pharmacol 2003;52:497–506.
191. Giles FJ, Kantarjian HM, Cortes JE, et al. Adaptive randomized study of idarubicin and cytarabine versus troxacitabine and cytarabine versus troxacitabine and idarubicin in untreated patients 50 years or older with adverse karyotype acute myeloid leukemia. J Clin Oncol 2003;21:1722–1727.
192. Levis M, Pham R, Smith BD, Small D. In vitro studies of a FLT3 inhibitor combined with chemotherapy: sequence of administration is important to achieve synergistic cytotoxic effects. Blood 2004;104:1145–1150.
193. Maciejewski JP, Rivera C, Kook H, Dunn D, Young NS. Relationship between bone marrow failure syndromes and the presence of glycophosphatidyl inositol-anchored protein-deficient clones. Br J Haematol 2001;115:1015–1022.
194. Boultwood J, Wainscoat JS. Clonality in the myelodysplastic syndromes. Int J Hematol 2001;73:411–415.
195. Onida F, Kantarjian HM, Smith TL, et al. Prognostic factors and scoring systems in chronic myelomonocytic leukemia: a retrospective analysis of 213 patients. Blood 2002;99:840–849.
196. Greenberg P, Cox C, LeBeau MM, et al. International scoring system for evaluating prognosis in myelodysplastic syndromes. Blood 1997;89:2079–2088.
197. Cheson BD, Bennett JM, Kantarjian H, et al. Report of an international working group to standardize response criteria for myelodysplastic syndromes. Blood 2000;96:3671–3674.
198. Wallvik J, Stenke L, Bernell P, Nordahl G, Hippe E, Hast R. Serum erythropoietin (EPO) levels correlate with survival and independently predict response to EPO treatment in patients with myelodysplastic syndromes. Eur J Haematol 2002;68:180–185.
199. Terpos E, Mougiou A, Kouraklis A, et al. Prolonged administration of erythropoietin increases erythroid response rate in myelodysplastic syndromes: a phase II trial in 281 patients. Br J Haematol 2002;118:174–180.
200. Rigolin GM, Porta MD, Bigoni R, et al. rHuEpo administration in patients with low-risk myelodysplastic syndromes: evaluation of erythroid precursors' response by fluorescence in situ hybridization on May-Grunwald-Giemsa-stained bone marrow samples. Br J Haematol 2002;119:652–659.
201. Negrin RS, Stein R, Doherty K, et al. Maintenance treatment of the anemia of myelodysplastic syndromes with recombinant human granulocyte colony-stimulating factor and erythropoietin: evidence for in vivo synergy. Blood 1996;87:4076–4081.
202. Kasper C, Zahner J, Sayer HG. Recombinant human erythropoietin in combined treatment with granulocyte- or granulocyte-macrophage colony-stimulating factor in patients with myelodysplastic syndromes. J Cancer Res Clin Oncol 2002;128: 497–502.
203. Musto P, Sanpaolo G, D'Arena G, et al. Adding growth factors or interleukin-3 to erythropoietin has limited effects on anemia of transfusion-dependent patients with myelodysplastic syndromes unresponsive to erythropoietin alone. Haematologica 2001;86:44–51.
204. Thompson JA, Gilliland DG, Prchal JT, et al. Effect of recombinant human erythropoietin combined with granulocyte/ macrophage colony-stimulating factor in the treatment of patients with myelodysplastic syndrome. Blood 2000;95:1175–1179.
205. Kurzrock R, Cortes J, Thomas DA, Jeha S, Pilat S, Talpaz M. Pilot study of low-dose interleukin-11 in patients with bone marrow failure. J Clin Oncol 2001;19:4165–4172.
206. Kaushansky K. Use of thrombopoietic growth factors in acute leukemia. Leukemia 2000;14:505–508.
207. Beran M, Estey E, O'Brien SM, et al. Results of topotecan single-agent therapy in patients with myelodysplastic syndromes and chronic myelomonocytic leukemia. Leuk Lymphoma 1998;31: 521–531.
208. Beran M, Estey E, O'Brien S, et al. Topotecan and cytarabine is an active combination regimen in myelodysplastic syndromes and chronic myelomonocytic leukemia. J Clin Oncol 1999;17: 2819–2830.
209. Estey EH, Thall PF, Cortes JE, et al. Comparison of idarubicin + ara-C-, fludarabine + ara-C-, and topotecan + ara-C-based regimens in treatment of newly diagnosed acute myeloid leukemia, refractory anemia with excess blasts in transformation, or refractory anemia with excess blasts. Blood 2001;98:3575–3583.
210. Estey EH, Kantarjian HM, O'Brien S, et al. High remission rate, short remission duration in patients with refractory anemia with excess blasts (RAEB) in transformation (RAEB-t) given acute myelogenous leukemia (AML)-type chemotherapy in combination with granulocyte-CSF (G-CSF). Cytokines Mol Ther 1995;1:21–28.
211. Mufti G, List AF, Gore SD, Ho AYL. Myelodysplastic syndrome. Hematology 2003;2003:176–199.
212. Wattel E, Solary E, Hecquet B, et al. Quinine improves the results of intensive chemotherapy in myelodysplastic syndromes expressing P glycoprotein: results of a randomized study. Br J Haematol 1998;102:1015–1024.
213. Oosterveld M, Wittebol SH, Lemmens WA, et al. The impact of intensive antileukaemic treatment strategies on prognosis of myelodysplastic syndrome patients aged less than 61 years according to International Prognostic Scoring System risk groups. Br J Haematol 2003;123:81–89.
214. de Witte T, Suciu S, Verhoef G, et al. Intensive chemotherapy followed by allogeneic or autologous stem cell transplantation for patients with myelodysplastic syndromes (MDSs) and acute myeloid leukemia following MDS. Blood 2001;98:2326–2331.
215. Witherspoon RP, Deeg HJ, Storer B, Anasetti C, Storb R, Appelbaum FR. Hematopoietic stem-cell transplantation for treatment-related leukemia or myelodysplasia. J Clin Oncol 2001;19:2134–2141.
216. Chan GW, Foss FM, Klein AK, Sprague K, Miller KB. Reduced-intensity transplantation for patients with myelodysplastic syn-

drome achieves durable remission with less graft-versus-host disease. Biol Blood Marrow Transplant 2003;9:753–759.

217. Epperson DE, Nakamura R, Saunthararajah Y, Melenhorst J, Barrett AJ. Oligoclonal T cell expansion in myelodysplastic syndrome: evidence for an autoimmune process. Leuk Res 2001;25: 1075–1083.
218. Kochenderfer JN, Kobayashi S, Wieder ED, Su C, Molldrem JJ. Loss of T-lymphocyte clonal dominance in patients with myelodysplastic syndrome responsive to immunosuppression. Blood 2002;100:3639–3645.
219. Geary CG, Harrison CJ, Philpott NJ, Hows JM, Gordon-Smith EC, Marsh JC. Abnormal cytogenetic clones in patients with aplastic anaemia: response to immunosuppressive therapy. Br J Haematol 1999;104:271–274.
220. Stadler M, Germing, U, Kliche, KO, et al. A prospective, randomised, phase II study of horse antithymocyte globulin vs rabbit antithymocyte globulin as immune-modulating therapy in patients with low-risk myelodysplastic syndromes. Leukemia 2004; in press.
221. Killick SB, Mufti G, Cavenagh JD, et al. A pilot study of antithymocyte globulin (ATG) in the treatment of patients with 'low-risk' myelodysplasia. Br J Haematol 2003;120:679–684.
222. Steensma DP, Dispenzieri A, Moore SB, Schroeder G, Tefferi A. Antithymocyte globulin has limited efficacy and substantial toxicity in unselected anemic patients with myelodysplastic syndrome. Blood 2003;101:2156–2158.
223. Catalano L, Selleri C, Califano C, et al. Prolonged response to cyclosporin-A in hypoplastic refractory anemia and correlation with in vitro studies. Haematologica 2000;85:133–138.
224. Shimamoto T, Tohyama K, Okamoto T, et al. Cyclosporin A therapy for patients with myelodysplastic syndrome: multicenter pilot studies in Japan. Leuk Res 2003;27:783–788.
225. Saunthararajah Y, Nakamura R, Wesley R, Wang QJ, Barrett AJ. A simple method to predict response to immunosuppressive therapy in patients with myelodysplastic syndrome. Blood 2003; 102:3025–3027.
226. Raza A, Meyer P, Dutt D, et al. Thalidomide produces transfusion independence in long-standing refractory anemias of patients with myelodysplastic syndromes. Blood 2001;98:958–965.
227. List A, Kurtin, SE, Glinsmann-Gibson BJ. High erythropoietic remitting activity of the immunomodulatory thalidomide Analog, CC5013, in patients with myelodysplastic syndrome (MDS). Blood 2002;100:96a.
228. Sawanobori M, Yamaguchi S, Hasegawa M, et al. Expression of TNF receptors and related signaling molecules in the bone marrow from patients with myelodysplastic syndromes. Leuk Res 2003;27:583–591.
229. Gersuk GM, Beckham C, Loken MR, et al. A role for tumour necrosis factor-alpha, Fas and Fas-ligand in marrow failure associated with myelodysplastic syndrome. Br J Haematol 1998;103:176–188.
230. Zang DY, Goodwin RG, Loken MR, Bryant E, Deeg HJ. Expression of tumor necrosis factor-related apoptosis-inducing ligand, Apo2L, and its receptors in myelodysplastic syndrome: effects on in vitro hemopoiesis. Blood 2001;98:3058–3065.
231. Raza A, Lisak, LA, Tahir, S, et al. Hematologic improvement in response to anti-tumor necrosis factor (TNF) therapy with remicade® in patients with myelodysplastic syndromes (MDS). Blood 2002;100:795a.
232. Raza A, Lisak, LA, Tahir, S, et al. Combination of thalidomide and etanercept (tumor necrosis factor receptor or TNFR) effective in improving the cytopenias of some patients with myelodysplastic syndromes (MDS). Blood 2002;100: 340b.
233. Roboz G, List, AF, Giles, F, et al. Phase I Trial of PTK787/ZK 222584, an inhibitor of vascular endothelial growth factor receptor tyrosine kinases, in acute myeloid leukemia and myelodysplastic syndrome. Blood 2002;100:337a.
234. Giles FJ, Stopeck AT, Silverman LR, et al. SU5416, a small molecule tyrosine kinase receptor inhibitor, has biologic activity in patients with refractory acute myeloid leukemia or myelodysplastic syndromes. Blood 2003;102:795–801.
235. Acosta JC, Richard C, Delgado MD, et al. Amifostine impairs p53-mediated apoptosis of human myeloid leukemia cells. Mol Cancer Ther 2003;2:893–900.
236. Neumeister P, Jaeger G, Eibl M, Sormann S, Zinke W, Linkesch W. Amifostine in combination with erythropoietin and G-CSF promotes multilineage hematopoiesis in patients with myelodysplastic syndrome. Leuk Lymphoma 2001;40:345–349.
237. Raza A, Qawi H, Andric T, et al. Pentoxifylline, ciprofloxacin and dexamethasone improve the ineffective hematopoiesis in myelodysplastic syndrome patients; malignancy. Hematology 2000;5:275–284.
238. Novitzky N, Mohamed R, Finlayson J, du Toit C. Increased apoptosis of bone marrow cells and preserved proliferative capacity of selected progenitors predict for clinical response to anti-inflammatory therapy in myelodysplastic syndromes. Exp Hematol 2000;28:941–949.
239. List A, Beran M, DiPersio J, et al. Opportunities for Trisenox (arsenic trioxide) in the treatment of myelodysplastic syndromes. Leukemia 2003;17:1499–1507.
240. List A, Schiller, GJ, Mason, J, et al. Trisenox® (arsenic trioxide, ATO) in patients (pts) with myelodysplastic syndromes (MDS): preliminary findings in a phase II clinical study. Blood 2002; 100:790a.
241. Raza A, Lisak LA, Tahir S, et al. Trilineage responses to arsenic trioxide (Trisenox®) and thalidomide in patients with myelodysplastic syndromes (MDS), particularly those with inv(3)(q21q26.2. Blood 2002;100:795a.
242. Haluska P, Dy GK, Adjei AA. Farnesyl transferase inhibitors as anticancer agents. Eur J Cancer 2002;38:1685–1700.
243. Lancet J, Gojo, I, Gotlib, J, et al. Tipifarnib (ZARNESTRA) in previously untreated poor-risk AML and MDS: interim results of a phase 2 trial. Blood 2003;176a.
244. Feldman E, Cortes, J, Holyoake, TL, et al. Continuous oral lonafarnib (sarasar) for the treatment of patients with myelodysplastic syndrome. Blood 2003;102.
245. Cortes J, Holyoake TL, Silver RT, et al. Continuous oral lonafarnib (Sarasar™) for the treatment of patients with advanced hematologic malignancies: a phase II study. Blood 2002;100.
246. Silverman LR, Demakos EP, Peterson BL, et al. Randomized controlled trial of azacitidine in patients with the myelodysplastic syndrome: a study of the cancer and leukemia group B. J Clin Oncol 2002;20:2429–2440.
247. Kornblith AB, Herndon JE II, Silverman LR, et al. Impact of azacytidine on the quality of life of patients with myelodysplastic syndrome treated in a randomized phase III trial: a Cancer and Leukemia Group B study. J Clin Oncol 2002;20:2441–2452.
248. Marcucci G, Bruner RJ, Binkley PF, et al. Phase I trial of the histone deacetylase inhibitor depsipeptide (FR901228) in acute myeloid leukemia (AML). Blood 2002;100: (abstract).
249. Kelly WK, Richon VM, O'Connor O, et al. Phase I clinical trial of histone deacetylase inhibitor: suberoylanilide hydroxamic acid administered intravenously. Clin Cancer Res 2003;9:3578–3588.
250. Gottlicher M, Minucci S, Zhu P, et al. Valproic acid defines a novel class of HDAC inhibitors inducing differentiation of transformed cells. EMBO J 2001;20:6969–6978.
251. Arlin Z, Case DC Jr, Moore J, et al. Randomized multicenter trial of cytosine arabinoside with mitoxantrone or daunorubicin in previously untreated adult patients with acute nonlymphocytic leukemia (ANLL). Lederle Cooperative Group. Leukemia 1990;4:177–183.
252. Hansen OP, Pedersen-Bjergaard J, Ellegaard J, et al. Aclarubicin plus cytosine arabinoside versus daunorubicin plus cytosine arabinoside in previously untreated patients with acute myeloid leukemia: a Danish national phase III trial. The Danish Society

of Hematology Study Group on AML, Denmark. Leukemia 1991;5:510–516.
253. Berman E, Heller G, Santorsa J, et al. Results of a randomized trial comparing idarubicin and cytosine arabinoside with daunorubicin and cytosine arabinoside in adult patients with newly diagnosed acute myelogenous leukemia. Blood 1991;77: 1666–1674.
254. Wiernik PH, Banks PL, Case DC Jr, et al. Cytarabine plus idarubicin or daunorubicin as induction and consolidation therapy for previously untreated adult patients with acute myeloid leukemia. Blood 1992;79:313–319.
255. Reiffers J, Huguet F, Stoppa AM, et al. A prospective randomized trial of idarubicin vs daunorubicin in combination chemotherapy for acute myelogenous leukemia of the age group 55 to 75. Leukemia 1996;10:389–395.
256. Stone RM, Berg DT, George SL, et al. Granulocyte-macrophage colony-stimulating factor after initial chemotherapy for elderly patients with primary acute myelogenous leukemia. Cancer and Leukemia Group B. N Engl J Med 1995;332:1671–1677.
257. Heil G, Hoelzer D, Sanz MA, et al. A randomized, double-blind, placebo-controlled, phase III study of filgrastim in remission induction and consolidation therapy for adults with de novo acute myeloid leukemia. The International Acute Myeloid Leukemia Study Group. Blood 1997;90:4710–4718.
258. Godwin JE, Kopecky KJ, Head DR, et al. A double-blind placebo-controlled trial of granulocyte colony-stimulating factor in elderly patients with previously untreated acute myeloid leukemia: a Southwest Oncology Group study (9031). Blood 1998;91:3607–3615.
259. Harousseau JL, Cahn JY, Pignon B, et al. Comparison of autologous bone marrow transplantation and intensive chemotherapy as postremission therapy in adult acute myeloid leukemia. The Groupe Ouest Est Leucemies Aigues Myeloblastiques (GOELAM). Blood 1997;90:2978–2986.
260. Herzig RH, Lazarus HM, Wolff SN, Phillips GL, Herzig GP. High-dose cytosine arabinoside therapy with and without anthracycline antibiotics for remission reinduction of acute nonlymphoblastic leukemia. J Clin Oncol 1985;3:992–997.
261. Kern W, Aul C, Maschmeyer G, et al. Superiority of high-dose over intermediate-dose cytosine arabinoside in the treatment of patients with high-risk acute myeloid leukemia: results of an age-adjusted prospective randomized comparison. Leukemia 1998;12:1049–1055.
262. Karanes C, Kopecky KJ, Head DR, et al. A phase III comparison of high dose ARA-C (HIDAC) versus HIDAC plus mitoxantrone in the treatment of first relapsed or refractory acute myeloid leukemia Southwest Oncology Group Study. Leuk Res 1999;23: 787–794.
263. Sternberg DW, Aird W, Neuberg D, et al. Treatment of patients with recurrent and primary refractory acute myelogenous leukemia using mitoxantrone and intermediate-dose cytarabine: a pharmacologically based regimen. Cancer (Phila) 2000;88: 2037–2041.
264. Ho AD, Lipp T, Ehninger G, et al. Combination of mitoxantrone and etoposide in refractory acute myelogenous leukemia: an active and well-tolerated regimen. J Clin Oncol 1988;6:213–217.
265. Brown RA, Herzig RH, Wolff SN, et al. High-dose etoposide and cyclophosphamide without bone marrow transplantation for resistant hematologic malignancy. Blood 1990;76:473–479.
266. Vahdat L, Wong ET, Wile MJ, Rosenblum M, Foley KM, Warrell RP Jr. Therapeutic and neurotoxic effects of 2-chlorodeoxyadenosine in adults with acute myeloid leukemia. Blood 1994;84:3429–3434.
267. Kornblau SM, Kantarjian H, O'Brien S, et al. CECA-cyclophosphamide, etoposide, carboplatin and cytosine arabinoside: a new salvage regimen for relapsed or refractory acute myelogenous leukemia. Leuk Lymphoma 1998;28:371–375.
268. Gordon MS, Young ML, Tallman MS, et al. Phase II trial of 2-chlorodeoxyadenosine in patients with relapsed/refractory acute myeloid leukemia: a study of the Eastern Cooperative Oncology Group (ECOG), E5995. Leuk Res 2000;24:871–875.
269. Seiter K, Liu D, Loughran T, Siddiqui A, Baskind P, Ahmed T. Phase I study of temozolomide in relapsed/refractory acute leukemia. J Clin Oncol 2002;20:3249–3253.
270. Fassas A, Buffels R, Anagnostopoulos A, et al. Safety and early efficacy assessment of liposomal daunorubicin (DaunoXome) in adults with refractory or relapsed acute myeloblastic leukaemia: a phase I-II study. Br J Haematol 2002;116:308–315.
271. Rizzieri DA, Bass AJ, Rosner GL, et al. Phase I evaluation of prolonged-infusion gemcitabine with mitoxantrone for relapsed or refractory acute leukemia. J Clin Oncol 2002;20: 674–679.
272. Gandhi V, Plunkett W, Du M, Ayres M, Estey EH. Prolonged infusion of gemcitabine: clinical and pharmacodynamic studies during a phase I trial in relapsed acute myelogenous leukemia. J Clin Oncol 2002;20:665–673.
273. Rizzieri DA, Ibom VK, Moore JO, et al. Phase I evaluation of prolonged-infusion gemcitabine with fludarabine for relapsed or refractory acute myelogenous leukemia. Clin Cancer Res 2003;9:663–668.
274. Karp JE, Lancet JE, Kaufmann SH, et al. Clinical and biologic activity of the farnesyltransferase inhibitor R115777 in adults with refractory and relapsed acute leukemias: a phase 1 clinical-laboratory correlative trial. Blood 2001;97:3361–3369.
275. Harousseau J, Reiffers, J, Lowenberg B, et al. Zarnestra (R115777) in patients with relapsed and refractory acute myelogenous leukemia (AML): results of a multicenter phase 2 study. Blood 2003;102:176a.
276. Smith B, Levis M, Beran M, et al. Single agent CEP-701, a novel FLT3 inhibitor, shows biologic and clinical activity in patients with relapsed or refractory acute myeloid leukemia. Blood 2004 103(10):3669–3676.
277. Fiedler W, Serve H, Dohner H, et al. A phase I study of SU11248 in the treatment of patients with refractory or resistant acute myeloid leukemia (AML) or not amenable to conventional therapy for the disease. Blood 2004;2004–2005:1846.
278. Stone RM, DeAngelo DJ, Klimek V, et al. Acute myeloid leukemia patients with an activating mutation in FLT3 respond to a small molecule FLT3 tyrosine kinase inhibitor, PKC412. Blood 2004;2003:891.
279. Cortes J, Estey E, Giles F, et al. Phase I study of bortezomib (PS-341, VELCADETM), a proteasome inhibitor, in patients with refractory or relapsed acute leukemias and myelodysplastic syndromes. Blood 2002;100:560a.
280. Wijermans P, Lubbert M, Verhoef G, et al. Low-dose 5-aza-2′-deoxycytidine, a DNA hypomethylating agent, for the treatment of high-risk myelodysplastic syndrome: a multicenter phase II study in elderly patients. J Clin Oncol 2000;18:956–962.
281. Issa J, Garcia-Manero G, Giles FJ, et al. Phase I study of low-dose prolonged exposure schedules of the hypomethylating agent 5-aza-2′-deoxycytidine (Decitabine) in hematopoietic malignancies. Blood 2004; in press.
282. Gore SD, Weng L-J, Zhai S, et al. Impact of the putative differentiating agent sodium phenylbutyrate on myelodysplastic syndromes and acute myeloid leukemia. Clin Cancer Res 2001;7:2330–2339.
283. Gore SD, Weng LJ, Figg WD, et al. Impact of prolonged infusions of the putative differentiating agent sodium phenylbutyrate on myelodysplastic syndromes and acute myeloid leukemia. Clin Cancer Res 2002;8:963–970.

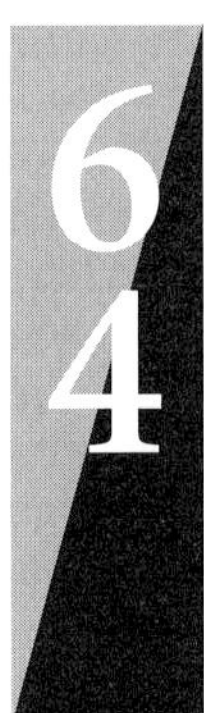

Acute Lymphoblastic Leukemia

Olatoyosi M. Odenike, Laura C. Michaelis, and Wendy Stock

Acute lymphoblastic leukemia (ALL) is a malignant hematologic disease characterized by the accumulation of immature cells within the marrow space that are arrested at the lymphoblast stage of development, with consequent suppression of normal hematopoiesis. ALL is not a biologically uniform disease; rather, it is a collection of heterogeneous entities characterized by distinct phenotypic, cytogenetic, and molecular–genetic profiles. The characterization and study of these subtypes has led to a risk-adapted approach to therapy, an approach pioneered by clinicians involved with the study of ALL in children, which has now been extended to the diagnosis and treatment of adult ALL. Much progress has been made over the years, particularly in pediatric ALL where cure rates are now in the 80% range. In contrast, for adults with ALL, only approximately one-third of patients achieve long-term disease-free survival. Utilization of newer molecular techniques, such as gene expression profiling, will lead to an improved understanding of the biology of the disease, as well as identification of new drug targets and unique drug susceptibility and resistance profiles. Ultimately, these insights will lead to a more refined and targeted approach to therapy with subsequent significant improvement in the cure rates for adults afflicted with this disease.

Etiology and Epidemiology

Incidence

The estimated number of new cases of ALL in the year 2003 in the United States was 3,600. There is a slight male preponderance, with 2,100 of these cases occurring in males.[1] ALL is the most common malignancy diagnosed in children and constitutes 25% of childhood malignancies and more than 70% of all childhood leukemia diagnoses.[2]

ALL is a relatively rare disease in adults; 30% of ALL cases occur in adults, and it represents about 20% of adult acute leukemias. There is a bimodal distribution to the incidence of the disease, with an initial peak in early childhood, which then declines during the adolescence and young adulthood years, and a second smaller peak that occurs in patients older than 50.[2] The age-adjusted incidence is 1.6 in 100,000 in adults (i.e., 16 cases per 1 million people).[3]

Etiology

ALL is largely an acquired disease and, similar to most other malignancies, is a progressive clonal disorder driven by genetic mutations. The inciting event or etiologic agent remains obscure in almost every instance.[4] Various factors have been implicated including hereditary factors, viruses, and environmental factors, such as ionizing radiation. It is likely that a complex interplay of genetic and environmental factors may underlie the development of most cases of ALL.

Congenital Disorders and Heredity

Several inherited genetic syndromes have been associated with an increased predisposition to acute leukemia. Overall, these account for about 5% of acute leukemias (both lymphoid and myeloid) and often involve genes encoding proteins whose functions relate to DNA repair and genomic stability.

One of the best known examples of an inherited predisposing genetic syndrome is Down's syndrome (DS). The incidence of acute leukemia is 10- to 20-fold higher in children with DS when compared with children without DS. Gene dosage, altered folate metabolism, mutations of genes, or disomy of a leukemia predisposition gene on chromosome 21 are among the presumed mechanisms of leukemogenesis in DS patients.[5,6] There are no distinct acquired genetic mutations to date that have been associated with the pathogenesis of ALL occurring in Down's syndrome patients. Klinefelter's syndrome and inherited syndromes associated with excessive chromosomal fragility, such as Fanconi's anemia, Bloom's syndrome, and ataxia-telangiectasia have also been associated with an excess risk of ALL.[7–9]

Apart from congenital inherited predisposition syndromes, other genetic factors, including prenatal factors, may contribute to the development of acute leukemia. Important insight into the prenatal origin of acute leukemia has been gathered from observations regarding the concordance rates of acute leukemia occurring in monozygotic twin pairs. In general, the concordance rate in monozygotic twin pairs aged from birth to 15 years has been reported in a number of surveys to be between 5% and 25%. However, when infant leukemias (less than 1 year of age) are separated from other cases occurring later in childhood, the concordance rate for infant leukemias approaches 100%, in contrast to the concordance rate for childhood ALL, which remains around 10%. Analysis of archived neonatal blood spots (Guthrie cards) demonstrates identical clonal origin of the leukemia in the majority of cases of acute leukemia occurring in monozygotic twin pairs in infants and children and provides crucial evidence supporting the in utero initiation of leukemogenesis.[10] Concordant leukemia has been reported only rarely in adults.[11]

In infant leukemias, the majority of which are characterized by chromosomal rearrangements involving the *MLL* gene, it is probable that by the time the infants are born, the process of leukemogenesis is almost complete. This hypothesis is supported by the very short latency period and almost synchronous diagnosis of leukemia in identical twin infants. Maternal exposure to natural or medicinal topoisomerase II substances, including dietary bioflavinoids, has been implicated as possible etiologic agents in these infant leukemias, particularly, because therapy-related leukemias following prior chemotherapeutic exposure to topoisomerase II inhibitors have also been associated with *MLL* rearrangements.[10,12]

Childhood ALL (more than 1 year of age) occurring in twin pairs may be characterized by chromosomal rearrangements involving the *TEL-AML1* fusion gene and a longer period of postnatal latency, suggesting that additional postnatal genetic mutations or events are necessary for leukemogenesis.[10] The finding on analysis of Guthrie cards that nontwinned children with ALL had detectable clonotypic *TEL-AML1* or rearranged *IGH* sequences at birth supports the concept of prenatal initiation of leukemia in most cases of pediatric ALL.[13,14] In addition, a recent survey of normal cord blood samples revealed the incidence of the *TEL-AML1* fusion transcript to be about 1% (a frequency that is 100 times the incidence of overt ALL involving this fusion transcript), lending further credence to the hypothesis that additional "hits" are required postnatally for the generation of overt acute leukemia in childhood ALL.[15]

Viruses

Epstein–Barr virus (EBV), a human herpesvirus that is the etiologic agent for infectious mononucleosis, is also associated with Burkitt's lymphoma and mature B-cell ALL, as well as lymphomas arising in immunosuppressed patients [such as acquired immunodeficiency syndrome (AIDS)-related and posttransplant lymphoproliferative disorders].[16] EBV efficiently transforms B lymphocytes in vitro, and its role in the pathogenesis of lymphoproliferative disorders in immunosuppressed individuals may occur via aberrant signal transduction mediated by EBV-associated membrane proteins.[17] This virus is not a known etiologic agent for typical (precursor B/precursor T) ALL.

Environmental Factors

Various environmental factors have been postulated as contributing to the development of ALL, but in most cases there is a paucity of direct evidence linking these factors to leukemogenesis. For example, in children of higher socioeconomic status, an increased incidence of ALL has been observed and has been associated with a delayed exposure to common childhood infections as a result of improvements in hygiene, altered patterns of social contacts, and minimal or lack of exposure to breastfeeding. These observations have led to the hypothesis that a rare abnormal response following exposure to common infectious agents may be an important etiologic factor, especially in those cases of childhood ALL occurring in the 2- to 4-year-old age group.[18]

There is a definite relationship between exposure to ionizing radiation and the development of ALL. High acute doses of ionizing radiation, such as occurred in survivors of the atomic bomb explosions in Hiroshima and Nagasaki are more causally linked to leukemogenesis than chronic low-level exposure.[19,20]

Previously, exposure to nonionizing radiation in the form of low-energy electromagnetic fields as occurs with residential high-voltage power lines has been implicated; recently, however, this form of exposure has been largely excluded as an etiologic factor.[21]

Cigarette smoking in adults has been investigated in a case-control study conducted by the Cancer and Leukemia Group B (CALGB). An increased risk of developing ALL was observed in smokers over the age of 60 years (odds ratio, 3.40; 95% confidence interval, 0.97–11.9).[22]

Secondary ALL

Secondary acute leukemias can occur following chemotherapy or radiation therapy for other malignancies. Most of these leukemias are myeloid and occur after prior treatment with alkylating agents or topoisomerase II inhibitors. An increasing number of ALL cases are being reported following exposure to chemotherapy with topoisomerase II inhibitors. These therapy-related ALL cases have been associated with the chromosomal rearrangements involving the *MLL* gene and typically occur within 2 years of initial exposure to the chemotherapeutic agent(s).[23]

Pathology and Pathogenesis

The integrated application of cytochemical stains, immunophenotyping, and cytogenetic and molecular genetic studies, in conjunction with the morphologic evaluation of ALL blasts, has led to a more definitive characterization of the various biologic subtypes of ALL. This comprehensive approach to the classification of ALL has impact on significantly risk group assignment, prognosis, and approach to therapy.

Morphology

FAB Classification

Acute lymphoblastic leukemia cells have historically been subclassified on the basis of the differences in their appearance under the light microscope. The French–American–British (FAB) group described three categories of lymphoblasts

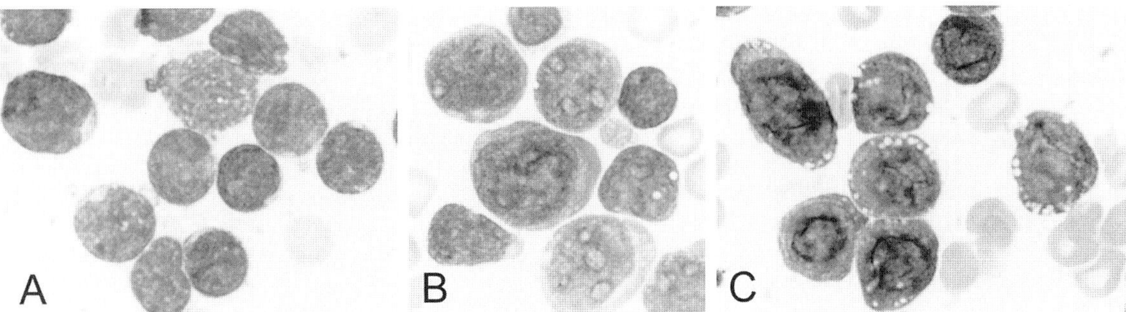

FIGURE 64.1. Cytomorphology of lymphoblasts (Wright-stained bone marrow aspirate smears). (A) Small uniform blasts, previously called "L1" according to French–American–British (FAB) morphologic classification. (B) Lymphoblasts are varied in size with several large blasts with prominent nucleoli, referred to as "L2" according to FAB morphologic classification. (C) Burkitt leukemia cells, previously characterized as "L3" blasts according to FAB morphologic criteria. Blasts are large, with deeply basophilic cytoplasm and prominent vacuoles.

based on cell size, nuclear cytoplasmic ratio, prominence of nucleoli, degree of cytoplasmic basophilia, and vacuolation.[24,25]

L1 lymphoblasts are small and homogeneous with high nuclear to cytoplasmic ratio, inconspicuous nucleoli, and scant pale blue cytoplasm (Figure 64.1). When compared with normal lymphocytes in the peripheral blood or bone marrow aspirate smears, the L1 lymphoblasts are larger, approximately double in size, and the nuclear chromatin is more homogeneous and less condensed. L2 lymphoblasts are larger and pleomorphic with more abundant cytoplasm and prominent nucleoli. There is frequently a combination of these more variable "L2" lymphoblasts in addition to the typical "L1" lymphoblasts. Approximately two-thirds of adults are classified as having L2 ALL.

The distinction between L1 and L2 lymphoblasts does not define specific disease entities because L1 and L2 ALL show no consistent correlation with specific phenotypic or cytogenetic features. These terms (L1 and L2) are now largely descriptive and have not been adopted in the current World Health Organization (WHO) classification of ALL, which is based on immunophenotype and genotype.[26] In contrast, L3 lymphoblasts are quite distinctive. The blasts are large and more homogeneous with deeply basophilic cytoplasm that typically contains well-defined vacuoles. The nuclei are large, with prominent nucleoli and a finely stippled chromatin. These lymphoblasts are characteristic of Burkitt leukemia/lymphoma and have unique immunophenotypic and genotypic features.

WHO Classification[26]

In an attempt to arrive at a classification system that would be more relevant and informative to clinicians, the WHO developed new diagnostic guidelines for malignant diseases of hematopoietic and solid tumors. The WHO has proposed that a 20% or greater number of lymphoblasts is sufficient for a diagnosis of ALL. In addition, the WHO classification scheme has abandoned the distinction between L1 and L2 morphologies (Table 64.1) because of the lack of correlation of these subtypes with specific immunophenotypic, genetic, or clinical characteristics.

Cytochemistry and Immunohistochemistry

Cytochemical stains are a useful adjunct to the phenotypic evaluation of the blast population and facilitate the evaluation of various cytoplasmic constituents.

Myeloperoxidase (MPO) activity is specific for myeloid differentiation and helps to distinguish AML from ALL.

The periodic acid–Schiff (PAS) reaction may be positive in lymphoblasts; usually this staining is localized and the nuclei

TABLE 64.1. Immunophenotype in acute lymphoblastic leukemia (ALL).

World Health Organization (WHO) category	*Lineage*	*Phenotype*
Precursor B-cell lymphoblastic leukemia	B-lineage	
	Pro-B ALL	TdT+, HLA-DR+, CD19/22/79A+, CD10–, cμ–, sIg–
	cALL	TdT+, HLA-DR+, CD19/22/79A+, CD10+, cμ–, sIg–
	Pre-B ALL	TdT+, HLA-DR+, CD19/22/79A+, CD10+, cμ+, sIg–
Burkitt's leukemia	Burkitt	TdT–, HLA-DR+, CD19/22/79A+, CD10+, sIg+
Precursor T-cell acute lymphoblastic leukemia	T-lineage ALL	
	Pro-T ALL	TdT+, HLA-DR±, cCD3+
	Pro-T ALL	TdT+, HLA-DR±, cCD3+, CD2/CD5±, CD7+
	Cortical T ALL	TdT+, HLA-DR–, cCD3+, CD2/5/7+, CD4+/CD8+, CD1a+
	Mature T ALL	TdT±, CD3+, CD2/5/7+, CD4+ or CD8+, CD1a–

TdT, terminal deoxynucleotidyl transferase.

may be partially encircled by a rim of PAS reactivity. In contrast, myeloblasts are usually PAS negative, although block PAS staining may be seen in some cases of AML.[27]

Terminal deoxynucleotidyl transferase (TdT), a nuclear DNA polymerase that inserts nucleotide sequences at splice sites required for recombination of immunoglobulin and T-cell receptor genes, is positive in 95% of L1/L2 lymphoblasts but may also be positive in some cases of AML.[28] Therefore, although no single cytochemical stain is by itself specific, the use of cytochemistry is an important component and integral to the workup that helps to distinguish ALL from AML.

Immunophenotype

Immunophenotypic analysis involves the use of specific monoclonal antibodies to recognize distinct epitopes of surface and intracellular antigens that define stages of maturation of lymphoid and myeloid cells. This technique has significantly improved the classification of acute leukemias.[29] Immunophenotyping may be performed by flow cytometry or by immunohistochemistry and has a central role in confirming a morphologic diagnosis of ALL and in the separation of B- and T-cell ALL.

Immunophenotyping provides information about lineage (myeloid versus lymphoid, B-lineage versus T-lineage), defines the degree of cell maturation, and has contributed to a prognostically relevant view of the leukemic blasts in ALL.[30] Specific immunophenotypic profiles identified at diagnosis may also be useful for the subsequent evaluation of minimal residual disease.[31,32]

B-Lineage Disease

A significant majority of cases of ALL (approximately 70% to 80%) are of B-lineage.[33,34] B-lineage ALL can be further subclassified into subtypes that correspond to different levels of maturation in B-cell development. The WHO classification scheme (see Table 64.1) recognizes the broad categories "precursor B" and "precursor T ALL," because of the lack of conformity and questionable significance of further subclassifying these two groups.[26]

Precursor B ALL includes pre-pre-B ALL (pro-B ALL), common ALL (c-ALL, common precursor-B ALL), and pre-B ALL. Immunophenotypic characteristics are summarized in Table 64.1. The most common subtype of B-lineage ALL is c-ALL, occurring in about 50%, and is positive for CD10 (common ALL antigen, CALLA), B-cell markers (CD19, CD22), TdT, and cytoplasmic CD79A, but lacks cytoplasmic IgM (μ) and surface immunoglobulin (sIg) expression. Pro-B ALL is less common, lacks CALLA expression, is at an earlier level of maturation, and has been associated with a worse prognosis. Pre-B ALL is more mature and is characterized by expression of cytoplasmic μ and lack of expression of sIg.

Burkitt's leukemia (mature B-cell ALL) is characterized by a "mature B" phenotype with surface immunoglobulin (sIg) expression and FAB L3 morphology. This subtype of ALL is also associated with specific cytogenetic changes that are described in more detail next.[35]

T-Lineage Disease

T-lineage ALL accounts for 15% to 25% of adult ALL and can also be further subdivided based on the stage of thymocyte maturation (see Table 64.1).[36] Again, because of the variability in marker expression and lack of conformity of these subdivisions, the WHO recognizes only the "precursor T-group" without further immunophenotypic categorization (Table 64.1).[26]

The most common subtype of T-lineage ALL is cortical T-ALL, which corresponds to an intermediate or cortical thymic stage of development. Cortical T-ALL is characterized by expression of pan-T-cell markers: CD2, cytoplasmic CD3 (cCD3), CD7, CD5, coexpression of CD4 and CD8, and expression of CD1a. More-primitive subtypes of T-ALL include pro-T ALL and pre-T ALL. A subtype that is more mature than cortical T-ALL is the mature T-ALL (see Table 64.1).[37,38] T-ALL typically occurs in young male patients with a high white blood cell (WBC) count and a mediastinal mass.[39]

ALL with Myeloid Antigen Expression

Coexpression of myeloid markers is relatively common in ALL, occurring in about 15% to 50% of adults with the disease, and does not necessarily indicate bilineage involvement. The myeloid markers CD13 and CD33 are the most frequently expressed, but these cases are characteristically myeloperoxidase negative.[26,40] Recently, more uniform grading systems have been instituted with stricter criteria to help define the biphenotypic entity.[41]

Cytogenetics and Molecular Genetics

Recurring nonrandom chromosomal rearrangements occur in the majority (60% to 85%) of ALL cases and confer important prognostic information.[42] In addition, these chromosomal aberrations provide us with a unique insight into the pathobiology of the disease, unraveling critical molecular events, such as the role of oncogenic fusion genes that arise from chromosomal translocations, or tumor suppressor genes that are lost in chromosomal deletions. Cytogenetic analysis is therefore a critical component of the evaluation of any patient with ALL and will often facilitate diagnosis and subtype classification while simultaneously providing prognostic information for treatment planning.

The nonrandom chromosomal aberrations in ALL include both numerical and structural abnormalities. The incidence of common structural abnormalities and the associated molecular correlates are depicted in Table 64.2.

Numerical Abnormalities

Hyperdiploidy is the gain of additional chromosomes so that the total number of chromosomes per cell exceeds the normal complement of 46. In general, hyperdiploidy is more common in pediatric ALL, occurring in about 28% of cases, in contrast to adult ALL, where the incidence is in the 5% range.[43] The good prognosis seen in association with hyperdiploidy (especially in cases with more than 50 chromosomes) in childhood ALL is less obvious in adult ALL with hyperdiploidy. The less favorable prognosis in adult ALL may be explained in part by the presence of associated poor-prognosis structural rearrangements, such as the Philadelphia chromosome.[44]

Hypodiploidy, which occurs when chromosomes are lost, is associated with a poor prognosis. Hypodiploidy is seen in

TABLE 64.2. Molecular and immunophenotypic correlates of common chromosomal translocations in adult ALL.

Phenotype	*Karyotype*	*Genes involved*	*Frequency (%)*
Pro-B	t(4;11)(q21;q23)	*MLL-AF4*	3–6
Pro-B	t(11;19)(q23;p13)	*MLL-ENL*	<1
Pre-B	t(1;19)(q23;p13)	*E2A-PBX1*	3
B-lineage	t(17;19)(q22;p13)	*E2A-HLF*	0.5–1
B-lineage	t(9;22)(q34;q11)	*BCR-ABL*	25–30
B-lineage	t(12;21)(p13;q22)	*TEL-AML1*	1–3
Mature B (sIg+)	t(8;14)(q24;q32)	*IGH-MYC*	5
Mature B (sIg+)	t(2;8)(p12;q24)	*IGK-MYC*	1
Mature B (sIg+)	t(8;22)(q24;q11)	*IGL-MYC*	<1
T-lineage	t(10;14)(q24;q11)	*TCRA-HOX11*	8
T-lineage	t(7;10)(q35;q34)	*TCRB-HOX11*	<1
T-lineage	t(1;14)(p32;q11)	*TCRD-TAL1*	1
T-lineage	t(11;14)(p15;q11)	*TCRA-LMO1*	1
T-lineage	t(11;14)(p13;q11)	*TCRA-LMO2*	1

2% to 8% of ALL, and has been demonstrated to have prognostic significance independent of other presenting variables, such as age and presenting WBC count.[42,44]

Structural Abnormalities

In adult ALL, the most common structural abnormalities are chromosomal translocations that involve the exchange of material between two or more chromosomes. Many of the genes located at translocation breakpoints are known or putative transcription factors or protein kinases. The molecular consequence of several of these translocations is the creation of a chimeric fusion gene that may lead to a block in cellular differentiation and/or aberrant cellular proliferation by disrupting the normal function of the affected transcription factors or by causing aberrant growth factor signaling through constitutively activated protein kinases.[45] Chromosome translocations in ALL may also result in the regulatory element of a gene, such as the immunoglobulin gene (in B-lineage ALL) or the T-cell receptor gene (in T-lineage ALL) being fused to a structurally intact proto-oncogene (such as the *MYC* proto-oncogene in the t(8;14) in mature B cell ALL), resulting in deregulated expression of the latter gene.[46] In the following section, some of the more common structural abnormalities are reviewed.

Chimeric Fusion Genes

t(9;22)(q34;q11) and BCR/ABL

The t(9;22) or the Philadelphia (Ph) chromosome is the most common recurring chromosomal aberration in adult ALL, occurring in 25% to 30% of cases.[42,47] It is rare in childhood ALL, occurring in only about 5% of cases. This translocation, which was initially identified in chronic myelogenous leukemia (CML),[48] results in the fusion of the 3′-region of the *ABL* gene on chromosome 9 to the 5′-region of the BCR gene on chromosome 22. In CML and approximately 20% of Philadelphia chromosome positive (Ph+) ALL cases, the breakpoint in the *BCR* gene is within a 5.8-kb major breakpoint cluster region (M-bcr) and results in a 210-kDa fusion protein (p210). In contrast, in the majority of patients with Ph+ ALL, the breakpoint in the *BCR* gene is upstream of the M-bcr region and a smaller 190-kDa protein (p190) is produced; this fusion rarely occurs in CML.[49] A less common fusion transcript involving a significantly larger portion of the *BCR* gene and encoding for a 230-kDa (p230) protein has also been described.[50]

The incidence of the Ph chromosome may be underestimated by conventional cytogenetic analysis, and the *BCR/ABL* fusion has been detected in up to 40% of newly diagnosed adult ALL patients in some studies utilizing more sensitive PCR techniques.[51] The presence of the Philadelphia chromosome or *BCR/ABL* fusion in ALL portends a poor prognosis and is associated with a higher WBC count, older age, FAB-L2 morphology, and B-lineage phenotype. Expression of CD19, CD10, and CD34 and coexpression of myeloid markers, such as CD13 or CD33 is common.[39]

The fusion protein results in the constitutive activation of the ABL tyrosine kinase with subsequent deregulatory effects on downstream signaling pathways, such as the RAS pathway, and the PI-3 kinase/Akt pathway leading to abnormal cellular proliferation and inhibition of apoptosis.[52] Persuasive evidence that the p210 and p190 proteins are the cause of the phenotypic abnormalities seen in CML and ALL has been obtained from experiments in transgenic mice or mice transduced with the fusion protein by retroviral transfer, which develop myeloproliferative disease and ALL.[53,54] A highly potent and relatively specific inhibitor of the ABL tyrosine kinase, imatinib mesylate (STI-571), has been developed that has emerged as a standard therapy for CML[55] and is now being integrated into clinical trials and treatment regimens in patients with Philadelphia chromosome positive (Ph+) ALL, as discussed next.

11q23 Translocations and MLL

The human chromosome band 11q23 is associated with an astonishing number of recurrent chromosomal abnormalities including translocations, insertions, and deletions. It is involved in more than 20% of acute leukemias. In ALL, the most common translocation involving chromosome band 11q23 is the t(4;11)(q21;q23), which is present in approximately 60% of infant ALL and 10% of adult cases.[56] The cloning of the 11q23 breakpoint region revealed the *MLL* (myeloid-lymphoid leukemia or mixed-lineage leukemia) gene, named for its involvement in both myeloid and lymphoid leukemias.[57] *MLL* is also involved in the myelodysplastic syndrome, biphenotypic leukemias, and in therapy-induced AML and ALL (particularly following treatment with topoisomerase II inhibitors).[58] In general, leukemias involving the *MLL* gene have a poor prognosis.

This gene (also known as *ALL1*, *HRX*, and *HtrX-1*) spans 100 kb and encodes a large and complex protein with several regions of homology to the Drosophila trithorax (trx) protein.[59] Developmental studies using animal models demonstrate that *MLL* positively regulates *HOX* gene expression. *HOX* genes, in general, are important determinants of the mammalian body plan, and are also differentially expressed in subsets of hematopoietic cells. More recent studies suggest that *MLL* is required for normal generation of hematopoietic stem cells in the embryo.[60]

MLL is involved in translocations of at least 50 different partner genes, several of which have now been cloned. In spite of the large size of the gene, the translocation breakpoints in *MLL* cluster around an 8.3-kb region in the 5′-region of the gene. The clustering of the breaks makes it possible to detect virtually all *MLL* rearrangements with a 0.74-kb cDNA probe on Southern blot analysis.[61] The fusion genes that result consist of 5′ *MLL* and 3′ partner gene. Several of the proteins encoded for by these partner genes have transcriptional-effector domains, suggesting that transcriptional dysregulation by these chimeric fusion proteins may be a common pathway facilitating MLL-mediated leukemogenesis.[62]

t(12;21)(p13;q22) and TEL/AML1

The t(12;21)(p13;q22), which results in the *TEL/AML1* fusion transcript, is the most common gene rearrangement in childhood ALL, occurring in about 27% of cases.[63,64] This cryptic translocation between TEL, a member of the ets family of transcription factors, and AML1, a member of the core-binding factor (CBF) transcription complex, is detected only rarely by standard cytogenetics because the translocation does not substantially affect the banding pattern of the chromosomes involved. It is easily detectable by molecular techniques, such as fluorescence in situ hybridization (FISH) and reverse transcriptase-polymerase chain reaction (RT-PCR). Leukemic cells exhibit a precursor B-cell phenotype, and the presence of this fusion transcript is associated with a good prognosis in childhood ALL.[64–66] In adult ALL, the *TEL/AML1* transcript is much less prevalent and was found in only 3% of cases, and little is known about its prognostic significance.[42,67]

19p13 Translocations and E2A

Chromosome band 19p13 is involved in two known translocations in ALL: these include the t(1;19)(q23;p13), which results in the fusion of the *E2A* gene, located on chromosome 19 to the *PBX1* gene located on chromosome 1, and a less common variant, the *t(17;19)(q21;p13)*, which results in the E2A-HLF chimeric fusion gene. The t(1;19)(q23;p13) has been identified in 5% of childhood ALL overall, but is relatively uncommon in adults, with an incidence of about 3%.[45] There is a strong association with the pre-B ALL phenotype (cytoplasmic Ig positive), with the incidence being 25% to 30% in this subgroup of patients with childhood ALL.[68] This fusion gene *(E2A-PBX1)* encodes a potent transcription factor containing the transactivator domains of *E2A* and the DNA-binding homeodomain of *PBX1*, and induces lymphoid malignancies in transgenic mouse models.[69]

The 17;19 translocation that involves E2A and HLF (hepatic leukemia factor), a basic leucine zipper transcription factor on chromosome 17, is relatively rare, occurring in about 0.5% of ALL patients, but has distinct clinical and immunophenotypic correlates. Patients have a pro-B immunophenotype and often present with hypercalcemia and disseminated intravascular coagulation (DIC). Prognosis is poor.

Dysregulated Expression of Structurally Intact Genes

8q24 Translocations and MYC

The translocation t(8;14)(q24;q32) and its less common variants, t(2;8)(p12;q24) and t(8;22)(q24;q11), result in juxtaposition of the *MYC* locus on chromosome band 8q24 to the immunoglobulin gene (*Ig*) regulatory sequences on chromosome bands 14q32 (*IgH*), 2p12 (*IgL*), and 22q11 (*IgK*), respectively.[70,71] *MYC* translocations are associated with virtually all cases of Burkitt's leukemia and lymphoma, and have an overall incidence of less than 5% in both pediatric and adult ALL. The disease has a mature B-cell phenotype and FAB L 3 morphology, and patients frequently present with central nervous system (CNS) involvement and extramedullary disease.[42,72] These translocations bring the translocated *MYC* gene under the control of the transcription regulatory sequences in the proximity of the *Ig* loci, resulting in the dysregulation and constitutive activation of the intact *MYC* proto-oncogene. The normal allele of *MYC* remains silent. *MYC* is frequently associated with human cancers and plays a critical role in regulating cell proliferation, growth, apoptosis, and differentiation. Overexpression or inappropriate expression of the *MYC* protein, a basic loop-helix-loop (bHLH) protein that acts in the nucleus, results in maturation block and abnormal cellular proliferation. Transgenic mice carrying the *MYC* oncogene fused to the *Ig* gene enhancer, develop B-lineage lymphoid malignancies, thus underscoring the central role of *MYC* overexpression in the pathogenesis of these malignancies.[73] The critical genes that are responsible for *MYC*-mediated malignant transformation are poorly defined and remain the subject of ongoing studies.[74]

Translocations Involving the T-Cell Receptor Loci

In T-lineage ALL, several recurring chromosomal rearrangements have been described that involve the T-cell receptor alpha (*TCR*-α) and delta (*TCR*-δ) locus on chromosome 14q11, the T-cell receptor beta (TCR-β) locus on 7q32–36, and rarely, the T-cell receptor gamma (*TCR*-γ) locus on 7p15. These translocations result in the juxtaposition of the enhancer elements of these T-cell receptor genes to one of a variety of transcription factors, resulting in dysregulation or aberrant expression of the latter genes. The genes involved in these reciprocal rearrangements include *MYC (8q24), TAL1/SCL (1p32), TAL2 (9q32), LYL1 (19p13), LMO1/RBTN1(11p15), LMO2/RBTN2 (11p13)*, and *HOX11 (10q24)*.

The t(10;14)(q24;q11) involving the *HOX 11* gene on 10q24 and the *TCR*-α locus on chromosome 14q11 occurs in 4% to 7% of childhood cases and up to 14% of adults, and has been associated with a favorable prognosis.[75,76] The variant translocation t(7;10)(q35;q34) juxtaposes the *HOX 11* gene to the TCR-β.[42]

TAL1, TAL2, LYL1, and *MYC* all encode for transcription factors with a characteristic bHLH motif that allows for protein–protein interaction. These genes are expressed at very low levels in normal thymocytes but at high levels in leukemic cells that have undergone translocations involving these genes. Therefore, it is postulated that inappropriate expression of these genes in a thymocyte triggers leukemic transformation.[77,78] These submicroscopic rearrangements are not detectable by routine cytogenetics but are readily detected using Southern blot or PCR techniques. The *TAL1* gene rearrangements occur in 25% to 30% of pediatric ALL but are very uncommon in adult ALL.[42,79]

Another class of transcription factors involved in chromosomal rearrangements in T-ALL includes *LMO1/RBTN1* and *LMO2/RBTN2*, which belong to the rhombotin gene family. The proteins encoded by these genes contain cysteine-rich regions called LIM domains that are able to bind to nucleic acids or other proteins. LMO2 and TAL1 dimerize and interact in erythroid cells and T-cell leukemias and may act synergistically to induce T-cell leukemias.[80,81] Both genes play a critical role in normal hematopoiesis, and severe defects in erythropoiesis occur in mice that are deficient in either gene.[82]

More recently, dysregulation of the Notch signaling pathway has emerged as an important mechanism of leukemogenesis in patients with T-ALL. *Notch* genes encode transmembrane receptors that are activated by ligand-mediated proteolysis, leading to a cascade of downstream signaling events which regulate differentiation, proliferation, and apoptosis in several tissues.[83] The exact mechanism by which activation of the Notch signaling pathway leads to neoplastic transformation is unknown. Overexpression of the *Notch 3* gene has been demonstrated in all T-ALL patients examined, and is significantly reduced or absent in remission and in other types of ALL.[83,84] *Notch-3* expression in T-ALL is associated with the expression of its target gene *HES1* and of *pT*α (the invariant chain of the pre-T-cell-receptor, TCR), suggesting that a signaling defect at the pre-TCR checkpoint may be responsible for T-cell leukemogenesis.[83]

Tumor Suppressor Genes and Abnormalities of Chromosome 9p

The protein products encoded for by tumor suppression genes normally suppress tumor formation in differentiating cells; therefore, inactivation of such genes would lead to malignant transformation. Loss of the expression of tumor suppressor genes through chromosomal deletions (allelic loss), mutations, or epigenetic changes, such as DNA hypermethylation of promoter regions of such genes is an important pathogenetic mechanism in ALL. Abnormalities of chromosome band 9p, including deletions, unbalanced translocations, mutations, or loss of the entire chromosome, have been reported in 7% to 13% of ALL cases.[42,85] Two candidate tumor suppressor genes, $p16^{INK4A}$ and $p15^{INK4B}$, have been localized to 9p21. These genes encode for proteins that inhibit cyclin-dependent kinases (CDK) 4 or 6 and play a critical role in regulating the cell cycle.

Inactivation of the $p16^{INK4A}$ and $p15^{INK4B}$ genes by deletions or by epigenetic silencing occurs in almost all cases of childhood T-lineage ALL and in a small number of cases of B-lineage ALL.[45,86] Other cell-cycle regulators, such as the CDK inhibitor *p57KIP2*, have also been implicated in ALL pathogenesis. Inactivation of *p57KIP2* via DNA hypermethylation has been reported in approximately half of newly diagnosed and relapsed adult ALL cases, and in combination with other critical cell-cycle regulators such as *p73* and $p15^{INK4B}$ is correlated with a worse overall survival.[87]

RB and TP53 Tumor Suppressor Genes

The *RB* gene, located on chromosome 13q14, controls entry into the cell cycle. Hypophosphorylated RB inhibits the ability of the E2F family of transcription factors to transcribe genes necessary for entry into the S phase. In contrast, hyperphosphorylation of RB, which occurs via the action of CDKs, drives the cell cycle forward, leading to cellular proliferation. Mutations of the RB gene that have been described in 50% to 60% of adult ALL cases cause inactivation of the RB pathway and facilitate malignant transformation.[88,89] In addition, inactivation of the RB pathway can also occur via the loss of expression of $p16^{INK4A}$ and $p15^{INK4B}$ (CDK inhibitors described above), providing an additional mechanism for leukemogenesis.[45]

The *TP53* gene, a prototypic tumor suppressor gene located on chromosome 17p13, encodes the p53 transcription factor. p53 becomes activated in response to DNA damage, hypoxia, or aberrant cellular proliferation, and triggers cell-cycle arrest or apoptosis. Aberrant expression of p53, indicative of mutations in the gene, has been described in approximately one-quarter of patients with adult ALL.[88,89] In addition, components of the p53 pathway such as *HDM2* and $p14^{ARF}$ are frequently mutated.[45]

Cooperative Mutations

ALL probably arises as a result of complex and progressive genetic alterations. The genetic abnormalities arising from chromosomal abnormalities, including translocations have already been described. These genetic aberrations, which impair differentiation, may cooperate with other genetic alterations that confer a proliferative or survival advantage to facilitate leukemogenesis. These cooperating genetic events may include abnormalities in tumor suppressor genes, which have also been discussed, or mutations in receptor tyrosine kinases, such as the FLT-3 mutations, which are described briefly next.[45]

FLT-3 Mutations

FLT-3 is a receptor tyrosine kinase that plays an important role in hematopoietic stem cell development. Constitutive activation of this receptor (via activating mutations or autocrine secretion of the FLT3 ligand) contributes to aberrant signaling and uncontrolled cellular proliferation.[90] FLT-3 overexpression has been described in ALL occurring in infants with MLL rearrangements or hyperdiploidy (more than 50 chromosomes), suggesting that overexpression of the receptor may facilitate the development of leukemia in patients with those chromosomal rearrangements.[91,92]

Gene Expression Profiling

Gene expression profiling utilizing DNA microarrays is a relatively new technique that allows for the simultaneous analysis of thousands of genes within a given specimen and has emerged as a powerful tool for the biologic subclassification of ALL. DNA microarrays can accurately identify known genetic profiles and also provide unique insights into the biology of specific ALL subtypes. For example, using microarray analysis, it was possible to accurately distinguish AML and ALL and also B-lineage versus T-lineage ALL. Distinct gene expression profiles or signatures were associated with specific subsets of ALL and correlated with the presence of specific molecular–genetic aberrations, such as *TEL-AML1*, *BCR-ABL*, *E2A-PBX1*, and *MLL*.[92] Indeed, gene expression profiling demonstrated that leukemias involving the *MLL* gene are characterized by a unique profile of coexpression of early lymphoid- and myeloid-specific genes, suggesting immortalization of an early multipotent progenitor cell.[91] In childhood T-ALL, microchip analysis could identify previously unrecognized molecular subtypes, and the association of activation of particular oncogenes to defined stages of thymocyte development could be made.[93]

Clinical Evaluation

Presenting Features and Diagnostic Evaluation

The accumulation of large numbers of abnormal, immature lymphoid cells in the bone marrow and the subsequent suppression of the normal hematopoietic progenitor cells account for many of the nonspecific symptoms and signs in the adult presenting with acute lymphocytic leukemia (ALL). Most patients present after less than 3 months of symptoms. Symptoms may include, but are not limited to, pallor, dyspnea, fatigue or malaise, bone pains, myalgias, and anorexia. Hepatomegaly and splenomegaly due to leukemic infiltration are present in 40% to 60% of patients with ALL and may lead to complaints of abdominal fullness or early satiety.[94] Lymphadenopathy is more common in ALL than acute myeloid leukemia (AML) but does not typically precede bone marrow or peripheral blood involvement. Fatigue and malaise have multiple overlapping causes, with cytokine release, hypermetabolic demand, and anemia all playing variable roles. Bone pain and myalgias may be due to the increased cell mass in the marrow space.

Objective signs of disease may include petechiae, easy bruising, or mucosal bleeding, all manifestations of thrombocytopenia. Pallor and dyspnea are also commonly seen. Both anemia and thrombocytopenia may be the consequence of redistribution of space and resources in the bone marrow favoring the malignant cell line or because of peripheral blood events, including hemolysis, disseminated intravascular coagulation (DIC), or sequestration in enlarged splenic venuoles. Fever, which occurs in 40% to 50% of adult patients with ALL,[94] may be caused by cytokine release in the setting of accelerated cell turnover, or, more ominously, by infection in the setting of neutropenia. Elevated white blood cell (WBC) counts may be present, but the risk of leukostasis and secondary cerebral and pulmonary complications is somewhat less than it is in AML because of the smaller size and cell-surface characteristics of the lymphoblasts, which render them less "sticky" than myeloblasts.

The heterogeneity of the disease subtypes can also, occasionally, be manifest in the initial clinical presentation. For example, the clinical presentation of mature B-ALL is characterized by a high degree of CNS (12%) and organ (32%) involvement.[95] Adults with B-cell ALL are more often older and the majority are male. In T-cell ALL, the typical patient is a male in his twenties or thirties with an anterior mediastinal mass and leukocytosis. Philadelphia chromosome positive, precursor B-ALL in adults also favors older males, whereas the cytogenetic abnormality of t(4:11) is seen in a younger population. ALL can present at any age in either gender, so a full diagnostic evaluation is imperative whenever leukemia is considered in the differential diagnosis.

The complete evaluation of ALL in the adult requires a full history and physical, focusing, in particular, on physical evidence of occult infection, bleeding disorders, and neurologic dysfunction. Cranial nerves III through VII are the most commonly involved in meningeal leukemia.[94] Full laboratory studies should be performed, including a peripheral blood smear, electrolytes, and a panel of tumor lysis parameters (lactate dehydrogenase, uric acid, phosphorus, and calcium), as well as a search for evidence of possible DIC. All patients should have a chest radiograph and a bone marrow biopsy and aspirate. In the case of patients in the high-risk categories, HLA haplotyping of all siblings should be initiated as soon as feasible. Because ALL treatment is tailored to risk groups, it is vital that accurate cytogenetic, immunohistochemical, immunophenotypic, and molecular studies are performed on the bone marrow aspirate, and bone marrow morphology should be evaluated by an experienced hematopathologist.

Among the initial diagnostic challenges is to exclude non-neoplastic lymphoid proliferative syndromes. On occasion, infectious mononucleosis caused by either Epstein–Barr (EBV) or cytomegalovirus (CMV) can be similar in presentation to ALL. The reactive T cells in EBV can resemble blast cells and, therefore, require adequate stains to exclude the possibility of ALL.

Prognostic Factors and Risk Stratification

ALL is a heterogeneous disease defined by distinct biologic and clinical features that affect the prognosis. The ability to identify groups of ALL patients with differing prognoses based on these features has improved the outcome in childhood ALL[96] and is beginning to translate into risk-adapted therapy in adult ALL. Table 64.3 summarizes both low- and high-risk features that have been identified from a variety of clinical studies in adult ALL. It is important to note that prognostic features may vary according to treatment; for example, mature B-cell ALL (Burkitt's type), once considered a very poor risk subset, is now a curable disease in a significant percentage of patients with the introduction of new therapies that were successfully piloted in children with this disease subset.[95,97,98]

Consistently recognized prognostic factors in adult ALL are discussed briefly next. These prognostic factors can be used to provide a general risk assessment for prognosis and for treatment planning. As many as 75% of adults with ALL can be considered relatively "high risk" with an expected disease-free survival of only 25% to 35%. Only approximately 25% of patients can be considered "standard risk" with anticipated survival rates of more than 50%.

Age at Diagnosis

Most clinical trials[34,99–101] have noted a marked difference in both complete remission (CR) rate and disease-free survival (DFS) in ALL patients, depending on patient age. This is well

TABLE 64.3. Prognostic factors in adult ALL identify risk groups for treatment: stratification.

Prognostic factor	*Good risk*	*Standard risk*	*Poor risk*
Clinical Age Presenting WBC Time to complete remission (CR)	<30 years <30,000/μL CR < 2–4 wks	30–60 years old <30,000/μL CR, 2–4 wks	60 years >30,000/μL (Precursor B) CR > 2–4 weeks
Immunophenotype	Mature B-Burkitt type Precursor T	Precursor B	Pro B Early T (only 1–3 T-cell markers)
Molecular/cytogenetics	High hyperdiploid t(8;14), t(2;8) or t(8;22)	Normal Karyotype	t(9;22)/BCR-ABL t(4;11)/MLL-AF4 +(8) del(7)
Minimal residual disease[a]	$<10^{-4}$ after induction $<10^{-4}$ or negative during first years	—	$>10^{-3}$ after induction $>10^{-4}$ or increasing during first year of therapy

[a] Remains to be validated in a large, prospective series.

illustrated by a combined analysis of the pediatric and adult Medical Research Council (MRC) trials,[102] which demonstrated a progressive decline in CR rate and remission-free survival with increasing age. Older adolescents and young adults fare less well than children ages 2 to 10 years, and with increasing age, survival decreases continuously. Both comorbid medical conditions resulting in increased toxicity of induction and postremission therapy and the presence of higher-risk biologic features contribute to the adverse prognosis of older adults with ALL, for whom disease-free survival is consistently less than 20% in patients over age 60. A higher level of multidrug resistance has been reported in older adults with ALL, which may contribute to lower CR rates. Shorter remission duration in older adults is also a consequence of the higher frequency of adverse cytogenetic features, including the t(9;22)(q34;q11), or Philadelphia chromosome, which may occur in as many as 40% of adults over the age of 50.[103,104] In addition, precursor-T-cell ALL, currently associated with a more favorable prognosis in adult ALL, is less common in older patients.[105]

Leukocyte Count at Presentation

The majority of clinical studies have identified a high presenting WBC count as an adverse prognostic factor that influences both CR rate and duration.[34,106–108] From these studies, the absolute stratification number varies, ranging from more than 15,000 to 30,000/μL, and retains its significance in multivariate analyses in patients with precursor-B ALL. Despite intensification of recent regimens, lower remission durations in this subset of patients persist, particularly in those with WBC counts higher than 100,000/μL.[109] The same degree of hyperleukocytosis has not been as clearly associated with an adverse prognosis in precursor-T ALL, where patients routinely present with higher WBC counts. A cutoff point of more than 100,000/μL has been associated with higher relapse rates in earlier, but not in all, recent adult series.[34,110]

Failure to Attain a Complete Remission in Less Than 4 to 5 Weeks

Several clinical studies have identified the importance of time required to attain first remission as a significant prognostic factor in adult ALL.[101,111] Early clearance of blasts is an important predictor of survival in pediatric ALL; response to chemotherapy is now evaluated as early as 7 days after initiation of treatment as an important prognosticator,[112] and early treatment response to prednisone has been shown to be of importance in adult ALL as well.[113]

Immunophenotype

As treatments have evolved, the prognostic value of specific immunophenotypes has changed. Immunophenotypic classification is an essential component of the diagnostic workup in ALL. As previously noted, the outcome for mature B-cell ALL (surface immunoglobulin+) has improved substantially with specific short-course high-intensity therapies that are described in detail in the risk-adapted treatment section following. Similarly, the addition of cytarabine and cyclophosphamide to adult treatment regimens has produced better outcome for patients with precursor T-ALL.[101,114,115] From childhood ALL studies, it has been suggested that high-dose methotrexate and asparaginase may also be beneficial for postremission therapy in precursor T-ALL.[116,117] However, even this relatively favorable prognostic group can be further subdivided. In a Cancer and Leukemia Group B (CALGB) study, it was demonstrated that the number of T-cell antigens coexpressed by the lymphoblasts correlated with DFS. Patients with coexpression of six or more T-cell markers (indicating a higher degree of lymphoid maturation) on their leukemia cells enjoyed 86% DFS and overall survival (OS) at 3 years in comparison to DFS and OS of only 17% and 30%, respectively, for T-ALLs with expression of only one to three markers (immature or early T-ALL).[39] Similarly, the German study group, German Multicenter Study Group for the Treatment of ALL (GMALL), found that the most relevant prognostic marker in T-ALL was immunologic subtype, with inferior survival noted for patients with early T-ALL characterized by absence of CD2, CD1a, and surface CD3 on the lymphoblasts.[118] In precursor B-lineage ALL, immunophenotypic subset analysis has revealed an inferior DFS for patients with pro-B ALL (TdT+, CD19/22/79a+, CD10–) compared to patients with common precursor B ALL (TdT+, CD19/22/79a+, CD10+).[119–121] Finally, with the advent of multiagent chemotherapy programs, coexpression of myeloid antigens, which occurs in as many as 35% of adult ALL cases and was previously associated with a poor prognosis, is no longer considered an adverse prognostic feature.[34,39,122]

Cytogenetics/Molecular Genetics

Cytogenetic abnormalities occur in about 60% to 70% of adults with ALL and are among the most important prognostic factors in adult ALL.[76,108] The CALGB stratified patients into three prognostic groups based on cytogenetics: poor (including t(9;22), t(4;11), −7 and +8), normal diploid, and miscellaneous (all other structural aberrations) with DFS of 11%, 38%, and 52%, respectively.[47] In this series, a higher frequency (35%) of patients with precursor T-ALL had a normal karyotype. In particular, all larger series have identified that the presence of the Philadelphia chromosome, t(9;22)(q34;q11), and translocations involving the *MLL* gene on chromosome 11q23, the most common of which is the t(4;11)(q21;q23), are independently associated with short CR duration and survival.[42,44,76] The Philadelphia chromosome is the most commonly recurring abnormality (overall, 25% to 30%) in adult ALL and increases in frequency with age. Allogeneic stem cell transplantation in first remission is advocated for these high-risk patients and is discussed next. In contrast, patients with precursor T-ALL and the t(10;14) appear to have durable remissions.[34] Other abnormalities that have been associated with favorable outcomes in pediatric ALL, the *TEL-AML1* fusion gene (1% to 3%), resulting from a cryptic translocation, t(12;21)(p13;q22), and a hyperdiploid karyotype (2% to 5%), occur rarely in adult ALL.[123,124] Furthermore, from the limited data available, it is not clear that adults with a hyperdiploid karyotype have the same excellent prognosis as children.[47] In earlier pediatric and adult studies, an adverse prognosis was associated with translocations involving the *E2A* gene on chromosome 19, the t(1;19)(q23;p13), and a rarer variant, the t(17;19)(q21;p13); however, with more intensive chemotherapy combinations, these patients appear to be faring considerably better and are no longer considered in the poor-risk category.[42,125]

During the past several years, insights into the molecular pathogenesis of ALL are beginning to translate into prognostic information that may be useful for treatment stratification in the future. For example, abnormalities of cell-cycle regulatory genes, including the tumor suppressor genes *p16*, *p53*, and *Rb*, occur frequently in adult ALL and have been associated with a poor prognosis (median survival, 8 months) when at least two of these genes are mutated or deleted in leukemic stem cells. In contrast, patients with zero or one of these genes affected had a median survival time of 25 months.[89] More recently, gene expression array studies have identified a small set of novel genes that confer good or poor outcome in studies of pediatric ALL.[92,93] These studies require further confirmation and must be extended to adult patients, but hold great promise to identify patients at high risk for relapse in whom novel therapies or more intensive consolidation, such as allogeneic stem cell transplant in first remission, may be appropriate.

Minimal Residual Disease Studies

Polymerase chain reaction (PCR) and flow cytometric techniques have recently been used to monitor the persistence of the leukemic clone during treatment in an attempt to identify patients who are in morphologic and cytogenetic remission, but in whom there is persistence of subclinical disease, or minimal residual disease (MRD), and who may be at increased risk for relapse. These sensitive techniques rely on the ability to identify a unique marker of the leukemia cells; for PCR techniques, monitoring of a recurring fusion gene (e.g., *BCR-ABL*) or a clone-specific rearrangement of the immunoglobulin heavy chain or T-cell receptor genes, have been used.[32] For flow cytometric MRD monitoring, an aberrant immunophenotype of the leukemic blasts (e.g., presence of myeloid antigens on a lymphoid progenitor cell) can be identified at diagnosis and used for MRD monitoring. These molecular techniques have far greater sensitivity than standard cytogenetic techniques and may detect from 1 in 10,000 to 1 leukemia cell in a background of 1 million normal cells. Using both semiquantitative and more precise quantitative techniques, a number of studies in both pediatric and adult ALL have now provided preliminary evidence that MRD detection at specific time points following achievement of remission is an independent prognostic factor that may predict early relapse.[126–130]

Although the prognostic value of MRD detection is still under evaluation, improvements in standardization of MRD techniques[131] will provide a better means of comparing MRD data. The goal of MRD monitoring is to design treatment trials where prospective MRD quantification at specific treatment time points can be used to stratify postremission therapy. To date, there is quite convincing evidence in both pediatric and adult ALL studies of MRD that a high level of MRD at the end of induction therapy is associated with a higher relapse rate.[126,127,130] Furthermore, the continuous detection of high levels of MRD during consolidation and maintenance therapy, or the reemergence or increase in MRD, appears to herald relapse. In contrast, declining or negative MRD results are associated with a favorable prognosis.[129] Importantly, MRD levels have been confirmed as an independent prognostic variable in a number of recently published pediatric and adult analyses.[129–132] Therefore, it seems reasonable that quantitative MRD analysis may be incorporated as a prognostic variable considered during risk assessment of postremission treatment options.[133]

Two general strategies for clinical intervention based on MRD monitoring have been proposed and are being piloted in several pediatric and adult ALL trials: intensification of postremission treatment (e.g., allogeneic stem cell transplant in first remission) for patients with high levels of MRD,[134] or decreased duration or intensity of treatment for patients with low or undetectable levels of MRD.[135] For example, the GMALL group has begun a prospective study with MRD-based treatment decisions after 1 year of chemotherapy in patients considered standard risk according to conventional risk factors described previously (Table 64.4). For MRD low-risk patients, defined as MRD levels less than 10^{-4} at all postremission time points, treatment will be stopped after 1 year and maintenance therapy will be omitted, whereas MRD high-risk patients, defined as patients with MRD greater than 10^{-4} at any postremission time point, will have treatment intensification, focusing on allogeneic stem cell transplantation.[135]

TABLE 64.4. Results of recent chemotherapy studies in adult ALL.

Trial	*Reference*	*Year*	*No. of patients*	*Randomized*	*Intervention/design*	*CR rate*	*Progression-free survival (PFS), %*	*Comments*
CALGB 9111	114	1998	198	Yes	Benefit of G-CSF and consolidation	82%	23 months[a]	G-CSF improved CR rates, decreased induction deaths, but did not improve disease-free survival (DFS) or overall survival (OS)
PETHEMA ALL-89	253	1998	108	Yes	Benefit of delayed intensification	86%	41% (5 years)	No benefit to intensification
MDACC	147	2000	203	No	"HYPER-CVAD" alternating cycles of intensive therapy	91%	39% (5 years)	No l-asparaginase/no cranial radiotherapy (RT) administered in this regimen
MRC UKALL XA	161	1991	618	Yes	Benefit of early or late intensification	88%	28% (5 years)	No clear benefit to intensification, but decreased relapses in patients with early intensification
University of California (San Francisco) 8707	142	2002	84	No	Intensified/cyclical but shortened postremission therapy	93%	52% (5 years)	Approach may be effective for standard risk ALL
GMALL 05/93	153	2001	1200	Yes	a) Intensification by risk group b) Intensification of maintenance therapy	86%	47% (5 years)	Long-term follow-up ongoing
GIMEMA ALL 0288	151	2002	794	Yes	a) Addition of cyclophosphamide to induction b) Benefit of early intensification	82%	2 years[a]	Neither induction nor postremission intensification improved CR or DFS

[a] Median survival.

Treatment Strategies in Adult Acute Lymphoblastic Anemia

Treatment programs in adult ALL incorporate multiple active agents into complex regimen-specific sequences that have evolved from the successful strategies employed in pediatric ALL. The goal of these dose-intensive regimens is rapid cytoreduction with restoration of normal hematopoiesis, prevention of the emergence of drug-resistant subclones, prophylaxis of sanctuary sites such as the CNS, and eradication of persistent MRD with prolonged maintenance chemotherapy. Therapy is generally divided into several phases: induction, postremission consolidation or intensification, CNS prophylaxis, and maintenance therapy.

Chemotherapy

Induction Therapy

The combination of prednisone, vincristine, and L-asparaginase, taken directly from pediatric regimens, formed the backbone of early trials in adult ALL. The three-drug combination resulted in CR rates of 40% to 65%, but remission duration was only 3 to 7 months. The addition of an anthracycline, daunorubicin or doxorubicin, increased the CR rate to between 72% and 92% and the median remission duration to approximately 18 months.[99,136–139] In a subsequent study performed by the CALGB, two different anthracyclines, daunorubicin and mitoxantrone, were compared during induction therapy.[140] CR rates in both arms were similar, suggesting that anthracycline choice did not result in a significant therapeutic advantage. More recent Phase II studies have suggested that intensification of the daunorubicin dose during induction may improve CR rates and DFS[141,142] and is the focus of an ongoing trial in the CALGB.[143]

The choice of glucocorticoid may also be important. Several studies from the pediatric groups suggest substitution of dexamethasone for prednisone may provide better antileukemic activity, in part through the achievement of higher drug levels in the cerebrospinal fluid.[144–146] The M.D. Anderson adult ALL trials have utilized dexamethasone during induction and postremission therapy as part of their "HYPER-CVAD" regimen,[147] and the CALGB is exploring the substitution of dexamethasone for prednisone during induction and postremission therapy in their ongoing study for previously untreated adult ALL, CALGB 10102.

The contribution of casparaginase to adult ALL regimens is somewhat controversial, particularly, because significant toxicities, including hepatotoxicity, pancreatitis, and coagulopathy occur with increasing frequency in older adults with ALL. A randomized Japanese study, albeit using a somewhat unconventional dose of L-asparaginase, failed to demonstrate an improvement in CR rate or survival for patients receiving L-asparaginase, vincristine, doxorubicin, and prednisone in comparison to those receiving the latter three drugs without L-asparaginase.[148] A retrospective analysis performed by the CALGB demonstrated a marginal benefit in DFS for adults who received all prescribed doses of L-asparaginase in comparison to those who failed to receive all recommended doses.[149] Recently, optimization of L-asparaginase pharmacokinetics with prolonged asparagine depletion has been studied by the CALGB, utilizing the polyethylene glycol (PEG) conjugate of this agent; however, final analysis of toxicity and efficacy has not yet been reported.

Given the high CR rates of up to 75% to 95% (see Table 64.4) that are now routinely achieved using a four-drug regimen (usually an anthracycline, a glucocorticoid, vincristine, and L-asparaginase), it has been difficult to demonstrate further improvement with additional drugs during induction in the large, heterogeneous groups of adult ALL patients who are enrolled in clinical trials. During the past decade, the German Multicenter ALL cooperative group (GMALL) has also utilized a 5- to 7-day "pro-phase" with prednisone and cyclophosphamide that is given before initiation of standard induction therapy as an effective, gentle method of cytoreduction that decreases the risk of tumor lysis syndrome following initiation of standard induction chemotherapy in this often rapidly proliferating disease.[110] Randomized studies examining the addition of other active agents, such as cyclophosphamide or cytarabine during induction and/or early consolidation, have not documented improved overall response rates.[150,151] Nevertheless, the addition of these agents to specific subsets of ALL may have a positive impact on outcome. For example, the inclusion of cyclophosphamide to the four-drug induction employed by the CALGB, induced a CR rate of 96% in patients with T-ALL and improved DFS as compared to historical studies.[114] A similar result was noted by the German multicenter ALL group (GMALL) with improved outcome of T-ALL with early utilization of cyclophosphamide and cytarabine.[107,152,153]

An effective alternative approach to induction therapy of adult ALL that has been studied at the Memorial Sloan-Kettering Cancer Center avoiding exposure to the toxicities of L-asparaginase, steroids, and vincristine employs high-dose cytarabine and mitoxantrone with 84% of patients achieving CR.[154] Fractionated doses of cyclophosphamide and high doses of methotrexate (without exposure to L-asparaginase) have also been employed successfully with high CR rates of more than 90% by investigators at M.D. Anderson.[147]

Consolidation/Intensification

Despite excellent CR rates of more than 90% in many series of adult ALL, the long-term DFS over the past decade remains relatively low compared to children with ALL, ranging from 25% to 50%. Postremission therapy in adult ALL has employed numerous drugs and schedules, including modification of the standard induction regimens, rotational multiagent consolidation cycles, and intensification of treatment with autologous or allogeneic stem cell transplantation. In addition to the drugs employed for induction, postremission regimens have incorporated numerous active agents, including cytarabine, etoposide, VM26, methotrexate, 6-mercaptopurine (6-MP), and 6-thioguanine (6-TG). Because of the complexity of schedules and heterogeneity of drugs employed, it is difficult to assess the value of any individual treatment component, and further elucidation will undoubtedly require the incorporation of a more biologically defined risk-oriented approach to postremission therapy. Given the relative infrequency and heterogeneity of adult ALL, these advances may only be made in large cooperative group clinical trials.

This discussion focuses on the outcome of postremission consolidation therapy in selective, large prospective studies (summarized in Table 64.4), and the role of stem cell transplantation in first remission is considered below in a separate section.[110,114,141,147,151,155–158] Several recent adult ALL trials have addressed a postremission dose-intensity question. As with induction therapy schema, these chemotherapy regimens have evolved from pediatric ALL studies that have demonstrated improved DFS for high-risk patients[159] when intensive, myelosuppressive treatment modules are incorporated into postremission therapy. In a large Phase II study from the CALGB, patients received both early and late intensification courses of treatment with eight drugs followed by maintenance chemotherapy for 2 years after diagnosis.[114] Compared to previous CALGB trials where less intensive postremission therapy was administered, the median remission duration and survival improved to 29 and 36 months, respectively. Investigators at M.D. Anderson have also explored dose intensification in their "HYPER-CVAD" regimen where eight courses of chemotherapy are given, with alternating cycles composed of fractionated cyclophosphamide, doxorubicin, vincristine, and dexamethasone in cycles 1, 3, 5, and 7 with high-dose methotrexate and high-dose cytarabine in cycles 2, 4, 6, and 8. Using this approach, the median survival for 204 patients treated between 1992 and 1998 was 35 months with a 5-year survival of 39%.[160]

The Italian multicenter group, GIMEMA, addressed the potential benefit of intensive postremission therapy by randomizing 388 patients to receive either postremission intensification followed by maintenance chemotherapy (187 patients) or early progression to maintenance chemotherapy (201 patients).[151] With follow-up of 8 years, there was no difference between the two groups, with 36% DFS in patients receiving consolidation therapy followed by maintenance and 37% DFS in patients randomized to maintenance therapy alone. This outcome may have been influenced by the fact that only 35% of patients randomized to the consolidation/maintenance arm completed therapy according to the recommended schedule because of lack of compliance and treatment-related toxicity. In the Medical Research Council (MRC) UKALL XA, a postremission dose-intensity question was also evaluated. Patients were randomized to receive early combination chemotherapy intensification with cytarabine, etoposide, daunorubicin, and 6-TG at 5 weeks, at 20 weeks, at both time-points, or to no intensification chemotherapy.[155,161] The early block of intensive treatment appeared to prevent disease recurrence; however, the overall improvement in 5-year DFS for patients who received intensification therapy was estimated at only 2%.

Successive German multicenter trials have been evaluating the effect of subset-specific dose intensification during postremission therapy. Recently, patients with standard-risk B-lineage ALL received high-dose methotrexate, T-ALL patients received postremission cyclophosphamide and cytarabine, and high-risk B-lineage patients received both high-dose methotrexate and high-dose cytarabine.[153] The median remission duration was 57 months for standard-risk patients with a 5-year survival of 55%. However, this approach did not appear to improve the outcome of high-risk patients, except for those with pro-B ALL who achieved a continuous CR rate of 41% in contrast to only 19% for other high-risk patients. The outcome for high-risk patients with stem cell transplantation in first complete remission (CR1) has been explored by other groups and is discussed next.

CNS Prophylaxis

Only 2% to 10% of adults with ALL present with CNS involvement at the time of diagnosis[114,162]; however, CNS relapse may be expected in 50% to 75% of patients at 1 year in the absence of CNS-directed therapy.[163,164] The diagnosis of CNS leukemia requires the presence of more than five leukocytes per microliter in the cerebrospinal fluid (CSF) and the identification of lymphoblasts in the CSF differential.[165] Patients with CSF involvement may be asymptomatic or present with headache, meningismus, malaise, fever, or cranial nerve palsies. False-negative CSF results may occur in patients with predominantly cranial nerve involvement. Risk factors for CNS leukemia in children include an age of 1 year or younger, extreme leukocytosis (more than 100,000/μL), T-lineage and mature B-cell immunophenotypes, lymphadenopathy, and organomegaly.[166,167] Mature B-cell ALL, high serum lactate dehydrogenase levels, and high proliferative index (more than 14% of lymphoblasts in the G_2M/S phase of the cell cycle at diagnosis) have been associated with a higher risk of CNS disease in adult ALL.[162]

CNS prophylaxis using intrathecal (IT) methotrexate and 2400 cGy cranial irradiation, widely employed in early pediatric ALL studies, clearly reduced the incidence of CNS disease and was subsequently introduced into early adult ALL treatment studies with demonstration of a decrease in CNS relapses.[168] More recent studies have reduced the radiation dose to 1,800 cGy.[106,169] Combinations of these approaches can reduce CNS relapse rates to less than 5% to 10% and also may decrease the rate of bone marrow relapse.[159] However, long-term follow-up of survivors of pediatric ALL has demonstrated that combined irradiation and IT therapy results in neuropsychiatric sequelae, including seizures, premature dementia, cognitive dysfunction, and growth retardation; however, its long-term effects on adults remain uncertain.[170]

In adult ALL, the concomitant use of cranial irradiation and IT therapy is often quite toxic and may result in delays in delivery of postremission intensification therapy. These toxicities have prompted both the pediatric and adult cooperative groups to evaluate alternative strategies for CNS prophylaxis. Alternative strategies have included triple IT therapy with methotrexate, cytarabine, and a corticosteroid without cranial irradiation,[171] or IT therapy combined with high-dose systemic therapy with CSF-penetrating drugs, including methotrexate, cytarabine, and L-asparaginase and corticosteroids. Systemic administration of dexamethasone achieves higher CSF levels than prednisone and has a longer half-life in the CSF than prednisone[172]; as discussed previously, in a randomized pediatric trial, dexamethasone resulted in a lower incidence of CNS disease compared to prednisone.[144]

Recent studies suggest that effective CNS prophylaxis with CNS relapse rates less than 5% can be achieved in adults with ALL using combination IT and high-dose systemic chemotherapy without cranial irradiation, even in patients at high risk for developing CNS disease.[147,162,173] Other investigators have reported that the use of high-dose cytarabine without any other CNS therapy resulted in only a 4% incidence of CNS relapse in adult ALL.[174] In contrast, in the GMALL studies, attempts to omit or postpone CNS irradiation led to higher CNS relapse rates.[175] Therefore, although several effective strategies for CNS prophylaxis have been described, no single "best" approach for CNS prophylaxis in adult ALL currently exists. Future trials may explore a risk-oriented approach to CNS prophylaxis with the goals of minimizing toxicity and optimizing efficacy. Table 64.5 summarizes CNS prophylaxis regimens and outcome in recent adult ALL clinical trials.

Maintenance Chemotherapy

The use of maintenance therapy in adult ALL, as with all components of therapy discussed thus far, is based upon its efficacy in children with this disease. The theoretical basis for employing maintenance therapy is that prolonged exposure to antimetabolites may kill slowly dividing and potentially drug-resistant subclones that remain after induction and consolidation therapy. In addition, these agents might have a favorable therapeutic index on the leukemic as compared to normal stem cells, thus allowing selective growth of normal marrow with eventual senescence of remaining leukemia cells. Unlike other components of therapy already described, there have been no randomized studies justifying the use of maintenance therapy in adult ALL.

The backbone of maintenance therapy consists of daily 6-MP and weekly methotrexate for 18 to 36 months, often with the addition of periodic "pulses" of vincristine and prednisone or dexamethasone. Only one study has randomized patients between conventional and a dose-intensive maintenance therapy schedule[109]; this study failed to demonstrate any improvement in outcome. However, attempts at omitting maintenance therapy in several different adult ALL studies have yielded unchanged or inferior results.[140,174,176] These studies suggest that maintenance therapy should be included in the treatment plan of patients with ALL. However, the role of maintenance therapy in particular subsets such as T-ALL is uncertain, and there appears to be no benefit to prolonged maintenance therapy for patients with mature B-cell ALL who respond well to short-term dose-intensive regimens (described in a separate section following) and rarely relapse beyond the first year of treatment.

Stem Cell Transplantation

Allogeneic Stem Cell Transplantation in First Remission

As described earlier, the best postremission therapy for adults with ALL is still unclear. For younger patients under the age of 60, allogeneic stem cell transplantation (allo-SCT) has been the treatment of choice for high-risk patients with adverse cytogenetics, including those with a t(9;22) and t(4;11), as discussed next. However, for other adults with ALL, the optimal treatment strategy and indications for allo-SCT in CR1 are being explored in a number of studies.

Survival for adult ALL patients following matched sibling allo-SCT in first remission is approximately 50% (range, 20%–80%).[177] Several studies have tried to compare the outcome of allo-SCT versus chemotherapy in first remission (Table 64.6); however, this comparison has been problematic because of selection bias and lack of available matched sibling donors for as many as 70% of patients. The International Bone Marrow Transplant Registry (IBMTR) compared 251 patients who received intensive postremission chemotherapy with 484 patients who received matched sibling allo-SCT.[178] Adjustments were made for differences in disease characteristics and time to treatment. The 9-year DFS rates were similar, 32% for chemotherapy and 34% for allo-SCT. However, the causes of treatment failure differed with a higher recurrence rate of 66% for chemotherapy patients versus 30% for those receiving allo-SCT. Treatment-related mortality was the main cause of failure in patients who received allo-SCT.

A large French multicenter trial (LALA 87) compared allo-SCT with chemotherapy or autologous stem cell transplantation (auto-SCT) in first remission.[179] After exclusions, 572 patients were analyzed, and 10-year follow-up results were recently published.[158] At 10 years, based on an intent-to-treat analysis, survival was 46% for those receiving allo-SCT compared to 31% for those receiving consolidation chemotherapy alone ($P = 0.04$). In the allo-SCT arm, 92 of 116 patients

TABLE 64.5. Central nervous system (CNS) prophylaxis in large trials.

				CNS prophylaxis				*No. (%) CNS relapse*	
Trial	*Reference*	*Year*	*No. of patients*	*Initiation of CNS Rx (timing)*	*Intrathecal therapy*	*High-dose systemic therapy*	*Radiotherapy (Gy)*	*Isolated*	*With marrow relapse*
SWOG	136	1989	168	Induction[a]	Mtx	—	—	2 (3)	3 (5)
GIMEMA	109	1996	358	Induction	Mtx	Mtx	—	25 (8)	?
MDACC	147	2000	204	Induction	Mtx, ara-C	Mtx, ara-C, Dex	—	1 (1)	4 (2)
UKALLIX	169	1993	266	Postinduction	Mtx	—	18	12 (5)	8 (3)
CALGB 8811	34	1995	197	Postinduction	Mtx	—	24	18 (11)	7 (4)
GMALL	101	1988	368	Postinduction	Mtx	—	24	17 (6)	4 (1)
Mature B-Cell ALL									
MDACC	167	1999	21	Induction	Mtx, ara-C	Mtx, ara-C, Dex	—	0 (0)	?
GMALL	97	1996	24	Induction	Mtx	—	24	3 (20)	1 (7)
CALGB	194	2004	35	Induction	TIT*	Mtx, Dex	24	0 (0)	1 (4)

Therapy initiated during induction and continues throughout maintenance.

Mtx, methotrexate; Dex, dexamethasone; ara-C, cytarabine.

[a] TIT, triple intrathecal therapy (methotrexate, Dex, ara-C).

TABLE 64.6. Studies comparing allogeneic-stem cell transplantation (allo-SCT) SCT with chemotherapy/autologous stem cell transplantation (auto-SCT) in CR1.

Trial/Year	*Reference*	*No. of patients*	*Age (years)*	*Treatment-related mortality (TRM) (%)*	*Relapse rate (%)*	*Five-year DFS (%)*	*P*	*Comments*
IBMTR: 1991								
Allo-SCT	178	234	15–14	39	26	44	—	High-risk features of non-T lineage, WBC predicted poor outcome in both groups
Chemo		404		4	59	36		
BGMT: 1995								
Allo-SCT	182	43	15–55	12	12	68 (3 years)	<0.0001	No benefit of IL-2 maintenance therapy
Auto-CT		77		2	62	26 (3 years)		
LALA 87: 2000								
Allo-SCT	158	116	15–40	16	34	46 (10 years)	0.04	Allo-SCT significantly better than chemo or auto-SCT only for high-risk patients in CRI
High risk		41				44	0.009	
Standard risk		75				49	NS	
Chemo or auto-SCT		141		3	60			
High risk		55	15–50			31 (10 years)		
Standard risk		86				11		
						43		
Japan Adult Leukemia Study Group/IBMTR: 1998								
Allo	254	127	<30	32	22	53	—	Lower relapse rates in allo-SCT patients but high TRM in patients >30
		87	>30	57	37	30		
Chemo		38	<30	3	69	30		
		38	>30	13	70	26		
MRC UKALL 12/ECOG 2993: 2001								
Allo-CT	157	190	15–50	NA	24	52	$P = 0.05$	Preliminary analysis: survival benefit for allo-SCT in CRI in both standard + high-risk groups
Auto-CT + Chem		253	15–50	NA	60	36		

actually received transplantation with a median time of 63 days between achievement of CR and transplantation. The value of allo-SCT appeared clearly after patients were classified into standard-risk and high-risk groups. High risk was defined as having one or more of the following factors: presence of the Ph chromosome, null ALL, age more than 35 years, WBC count more than 30×10^9, time to complete remission more than 4 weeks. In the high-risk group, the overall survival at 10 years was 44% versus only 11% for the control arm ($P = 0.009$). In the standard-risk group, there did not appear to be a distinct survival advantage for allo-SCT over chemotherapy; here, survival rates were 49% and 39%, respectively ($P = 0.6$). These results support the value of allo-SCT in first CR for high-risk patients.

The MRC UKALL12/ECOG 2993 study is the largest prospective randomized trial designed to evaluate the role of allo-SCT as postremission therapy in adult ALL, and accrual is ongoing.[180] All patients received two phases of induction therapy and were assigned in first remission to receive allo-SCT if they had a histocompatible sibling donor, whereas those without a related donor are randomized to auto-SCT versus consolidation and maintenance chemotherapy. To date, more than 1,300 patients have been recruited, and the results reported so far have focused on the Ph+ patients (n = 875). An intention-to-treat analysis showed a significantly reduced relapse rate of 24% in Ph– patients assigned to allograft (I = 190) in comparison to 60% for those randomized to auto-SCT or chemotherapy ($P = 0.0001$). There was a tendency for improved 5-year event-free survival (EFS) in patients assigned to allo-SCT, 52%, versus 36% for the randomized group ($P = 0.05$) that was most noticeable for patients classified as standard risk (5-year EFS of 64% for allo-SCT versus 46%; $P = 0.05$). These data are very preliminary and require further follow-up; however, in contrast to the LALA study, there appears to be a trend toward a beneficial effect for allo-SCT for younger adult ALL patients (age less than 50) in first remission, regardless of risk group.

Autologous Stem Cell Transplantation

Autologous SCT (auto-SCT) has been explored in adult ALL; however, the prospective, randomized studies described above demonstrate that relapse-free survival has been inferior when compared to allo-SCT. Moreover, no advantage in survival has been demonstrated with auto-SCT compared with continued postremission chemotherapy alone.[99,181] Disease-free survival at 3 years following auto-SCT in first remission in two of the largest trials reported was only 28% and 39%, respectively,[158,182,183] which is not better than survival rates reported in recent chemotherapy trials of adult ALL.

Because relapse remains the main cause of failure following auto-SCT, several approaches to eradicate MRD have been

TABLE 64.7. Outcome of allo-SCT in CR2 or beyond.

Study	Reference	No. of patients	Median/age	Donor source	Conditioning regimen	DFS (years)	Transplant-related mortality (%)	Risk of Relapse (%)
CR2 or later CR								
International Bone Marrow Transplant Registry (IBMTR)	255							
High risk		208	NR	Matched, related	Multiple	22 (5)	NR	56
Standard risk		97	NR	Matched, related	Multiple	36 (4)	NR	49
Barret	256	391[a]	19	Matched, related	TBI + Cy ± other drugs	26 (5)	25	52
Mortimer	257	921	NR	Matched, related	Multiple	42 (NR)	NR	NR
Weisdorf	189	106	NR	Matched, related	TBI + Cy ± other drugs	42 (5)	48	17
Doney	258	48	23	Matched, related	TBI + Cy ± other drugs	15 (5)	36	64
Active disease								
IBMTR		281	NR	Matched sib.	Multiple	13 (4)	NR	71
Weisdorf	189	83	NR	Matched, unrelated	TBI + Cy ± other drugs	16 (5)	63	60
Grigg	259	67	28	Matched, unrelated + Matched related	TBI + Cy ± other drugs	<10 (5)	NR	NR

CR2, second complete remission.

[a] Remains to be validated in large, prospective series

explored. One approach to MRD modulation following auto-SCT has been the addition of conventional postremission chemotherapy to auto-SCT programs. Seventy-seven patients in first remission received auto-SCT followed by a maintenance chemotherapy program consisting of pulsed methotrexate, 6-mercaptopurine, vincristine, and prednisone.[184] The 10-year DFS and OS were 50% and 53%, respectively. These results were associated with a better outcome than with historical control patients receiving an auto-SCT, but these data have not been confirmed by other groups.[185] An alternative approach to MRD modulation that has been explored is ex vivo "purging" of the collected autologous stem cells using chemotherapy and/or immunotherapy with monoclonal antibodies directed against the lymphoblast. Although detection of less than 5% leukemia in the autograft has been associated with significantly improved outcome after auto-SCT for ALL,[186] the clinical benefit of ex vivo treatment of the autologous stem cells has not been clearly established and should only be investigated in the context of prospective clinical trials.[187]

Transplantation Beyond First Remission

There are no convincing data suggesting that durable remissions can be achieved with standard chemotherapy for adults with ALL in or beyond CR2 (Table 64.7). It appears that allo-SCT for adults in or beyond CR2 is superior to chemotherapy, with long-term DFS rates of 14% to 43% reported in a number of report studies.[188,189] The outcome of auto-SCT has been compared to matched unrelated donor allo-SCT for ALL for patients in second or later remission.[189] The DFS rate was superior for matched unrelated donor SCT (42% ± 11% versus 20% ± 9%) owing to a significantly higher relapse rate with auto-SCT, suggesting that the graft-versus-leukemia effect of allo-SCT may reduce the incidence of relapse. The outcome of matched unrelated donor allo-SCT for patients with active ALL at the time of transplant was not significantly different from that of patients with unrelated allo-SCT in third or later remission and was 16% ± 8%. In contrast, there were no long-term survivors in patients receiving an auto-SCT in third or later remission. Therefore, at the time of relapse, allo-SCT should be recommended as the treatment of choice for appropriate patients.

Risk-Adapted Therapy

Mature B-Cell ALL

The evolution of treatment for mature B-cell ALL (FAB L3), characterized by the presence of surface immunoglobulin and overexpression of the *MYC* oncogene resulting from chromosomal translocation, illustrates a fundamental paradigm for acute leukemia in general; that is, that the proper assessment of risk, based on immunophenotype and cytogenetics, early response to therapy, and comorbidities, should dictate the choice of treatment regimen. This risk-adapted treatment strategy evolved from the experience in treatment of pediatric leukemias. The adaptation of successful pediatric regimens for mature B-cell ALL to the adult population has dramatically improved the outcome for adults with this aggressive form of ALL.

Mature B-cell ALL is rare in both children and adults. It comprises only 2% to 4% of all cases of adult ALL and 1% to 2% of childhood cases and had been associated with a dismal outcome with very few long-term survivors.[167] But, as was noted as early as 1975, the clinical entity resembles Burkitt's lymphoma, a disease of much higher prevalence in children where several important observations about disease biology prompted the development of a novel treatment approach that capitalized on the rapid growth rate of these cells.[167,190,191] Investigators at St. Jude Children's Hospital postulated that (1) the 48- to 72-hour cell cycle that characterizes Burkitt's growth pattern might be better targeted by a fractionated dosing schedule and (2) the use of a synergistic alternating regimen might prevent emergence of a resistant subclone.[192] The approach employed fractionated high-dose cyclophosphamide, followed by doxorubicin, vincristine, and intensive CNS-directed therapy using combined IT methotrexate, high-dose systemic methotrexate with leucovorin rescue, and cytarabine with alternating cycles given for 24 weeks. Notably, patients did not receive maintenance therapy. Results showed that 93% (27 of 29) achieved a complete remission. Although 81% of patients with stage III Burkitt's lymphoma were disease free for 2 years, only 2 of 10 patients with initial involvement of CNS and/or marrow who achieved a remission were apparently cured of their disease.[192] The addition of high-dose methotrexate and cyclophosphamide or ifosfamide to subsequent regimens improved the CR rate in the pediatric population to approximately 90%, and the leukemia-free survival improved to between 50% and 87%.[97]

This approach was subsequently applied to the adult population, and a series of studies followed that are summarized in Table 64.8. The French SFOP (Societe Francaise d'Oncologie Pediatrique)[95] and German multicenter studies[97] employed a similar strategy to the pediatric approach with the addition of an initial cytoreductive "pre-phase" of treatment, usually consisting of a steroid and cyclophosphamide to minimize the risk of the metabolic complications of tumor lysis syndrome. The schedules did not include the more traditional ALL reinduction or maintenance therapy. Compared to the historical controls treated with more traditional ALL regimens, the adult patients had higher complete remission rates, 63% and 74% versus 44%, and a higher overall survival rate, 49% and 51% versus 0%.

In 1999, researchers at the M.D. Anderson published their experience of using the Hyper-CVAD regimen in adults with mature B-ALL.[167] The median age was 58, much older than previously published trials in adults. The therapeutic protocol consisted of eight courses of alternating intensive chemotherapy using Hyper-CVAD as described previously (in the postremission treatment section): courses 1, 3, 5, and 7 entailed hyperfractionated cyclophosphamide, and dexamethasone with vincristine and doxorubicin in the latter half of the treatment cycle. Even-numbered courses included methotrexate and cytarabine with leucovorin rescue. Prophylactic granulocyte colony-stimulating factor (G-CSF) was administered with the goal of completion of all eight courses within 5 to 6 months of diagnosis. Intrathecal therapy included methotrexate and cytarabine. The Hyper-CVAD protocol produced CR in 21 in 26 patients, or 81%. Female sex, a decreased performance status, albumin less than 3 g/dL, and hepatosplenomegaly were all associated with a lower likelihood of achieving CR. This treatment regimen resulted in a 3-year OS rate of 49%. Survival was much better among patients younger than 60 years: 77% versus 17%. The authors concluded that the addition of hyperfractionated cyclophosphamide and high-dose methotrexate had a superior 3-year survival for patients in comparison to their usual ALL treatment protocol (49% versus 21%; $P = 0.07$). The M.D. Anderson trial was the first to include a high percentage of older patients, and the authors speculated that the poor survival rate in this subset resulted from poor tolerance of the dose

TABLE 64.8. Studies of mature B-cell ALL and small noncleaved cell lymphoma (SNCL).

Cooperative group/institution	*Patients*	*Design*	*Early mortality*	*CR*	*Relapse*	*DFS*	*OS*	*Conclusion*
Societe Francaise d'Oncologie Pediatrique (SFOP)[95]	Untreated adults with SNCL ($n = 41$) or mature B-cell ALL ($n = 24$)	Retrospective Treated with one of three SFOP pediatric regimens	4%	89%	12%	71% 3 years	74% 3 years	Pediatric protocols can be used in adults with efficacy and tolerable toxicities
German Multicenter Study Group for the Treatment of ALL (GMALL)[97]	Untreated adults with mature B-cell ALL ($n = 68$)	Two prospective studies High-dose, short-duration regimens vs. historical treatment	8%–9%	63%–74%	23%–47%	50%–71% 4–8 years	49%–51% 4–8 years	Compared to historical regimens, new protocols adopted from pediatric literature improve CR, DFS, and OS
M.D. Anderson (MDACC)[167]	Untreated adults mature B-cell ALL ($n = 26$)	Prospective, nonrandomized Hyper-CVAD	19%	81%	43%	61% 3 years	49% 3 years	Highly significant association between older age and poor prognosis
Cancer and Leukemia Group B (CALGB)[193,194]	Untreated adults with SNCL ($n = 30$) or mature B-cell ALL ($n = 24$)	Prospective, nonrandomized High-intensity, short duration Alternating courses of chemo With and without prophylactic CNS RT	7%	75%–83%	28%–38%	52% 5 years	46%–57% 5 years	Long-term, disease-free survival possible in about 50% of patients; prophylactic CNS radiation is unacceptably toxic and does not provide added benefit

intensity, requiring subsequent delays and decreases in dose intensity, or a biologically different disease.

A prospective trial of patients with both small noncleaved non-Hodgkin's lymphoma and mature B-cell ALL conducted by the CALGB, has recently been updated.[193,194] A total of 75 patients were enrolled, with a median age of 44 years (range, 18–71 years). The treatment regimen included a "pre-phase," similar to the French and German studies. Subjects then received two alternating treatment regimens at 3-week intervals for a total of seven courses. IT chemotherapy with methotrexate, cytarabine, and hydrocortisone was administered, initially during each treatment cycle. The protocol also initially employed CNS irradiation for all patients, although this was eliminated (and reserved only for patients with active CNS disease at presentation) after interim analysis showed severe neurotoxicity, including transverse myelitis. The CR rate was 80%, and 45% of the mature B-cell ALL patients were long-term survivors. Few relapses occurred more than 1 year after completion of treatment. The CALGB[194] concluded that the individuals who had received CNS irradiation as well as aggressive IT chemotherapy experienced higher degrees of neurotoxicity without a significant DFS advantage and suggested that omission of the cranial radiation was reasonable for patients without overt CNS disease.

The conclusions of the cumulative experience to date argues for the following treatment principles. (1) Mature B-cell ALL should be identified at diagnosis to allow entry into treatment studies that capitalize on this disease's rapid cell cycling and subsequent sensitivity to fractionated cyclophosphamide and high-dose methotrexate. (2) Intensive high-dose methotrexate and aggressive intrathecal chemotherapy can eliminate the need for prophylactic cranial irradiation. (3) Prolonged maintenance therapy does not appear to be necessary. (4) Older age is a consistently poor prognostic indicator.

The addition of hematopoietic growth factor support (e.g., G-CSF) to current trials may decrease toxicity and allow more patients to complete the aggressive treatment that is recommended. Because mature B-cell ALL is strongly CD20+, the use of rituximab (anti-CD20) is a rational addition to treatment that is being explored in ongoing trials in an attempt to improve DFS. The role of autologous or allogeneic SCT as initial consolidation or salvage therapy for high-risk patients (many of them elderly) has not been well defined and requires further study. Those patients with relapse often have rapidly progressive disease that is not amenable to successful tumor reduction necessary for consolidation with auto- or allo-SCT.

Philadelphia Chromosome Positive (Ph+) ALL

Patients with Ph+ ALL pose a great therapeutic challenge to clinicians because the t(9; 22) occurs in 20% to 30% of adult ALL and is not considered curable with standard chemotherapy. The remission rate for these patients is approximately 60% to 80% with intensive induction therapy regimens, but the long-term survival with standard postremission therapy is less than 10%.[47,195] Therefore, attempts to improve outcome in Ph+ ALL have focused on dose intensification with allo-SCT.

Allo-SCT is recommended for patients with Ph+ ALL in first remission. In a preliminary report from the MRC UKALL X11/ECOG E2993 study, the event-free survival (EFS) at 3 years for 35 patients with Ph+ ALL in CR1 was 38%; in comparison, 3-year EFS was only 5% for those patients who received postremission chemotherapy or auto-SCT in CR1.[157] Other studies report survival rates between 30% and 60%.[196–199] It is difficult to draw conclusions from these small series, which vary considerably with respect to median age of the patients, stage of disease (CR1 or beyond), type of transplant preparative regimen, choice of graft-versus-host disease (GVHD) prophylaxis, and supportive care. However, from all these series, it appears that patients fare best when transplanted in first remission. The efficacy of HLA-matched unrelated donor (MUD) transplants has also been explored to allow more patients to undergo this potentially curative treatment. In one small series of 18 young patients (median age, only 25 years) with Ph+ ALL who underwent a MUD allo-SCT, the DFS at 2 years was 49% in this selected group, which is similar to rates reported for HLA-matched sibling transplants.[200] With improvements in GVHD prophylaxis, MUD transplants are also being explored in older patients with Ph+ ALL in CR1.

The most exciting recent development in the treatment of Ph+ ALL has been the intriguing early results observed with imatinib mesylate (STI571, Gleevec; Novartis, East Hanover, NJ). Imatinib is a potent and selective inhibitor of BCR-ABL tyrosine kinase.[201] In a study of 56 patients with recurrent and refractory Ph+ ALL, imatinib at 400 or 600 mg was given once daily.[202] The CR rate was 29%; however, responses were not durable, with only 6% of patients sustaining a response of at least 4 weeks. Nevertheless, the rapidity of response in these refractory patients and the relatively high CR rate has prompted the exploration of the efficacy of this agent in frontline therapy of Ph+ ALL. Imatinib is being combined with standard chemotherapy,[203] where initial reports suggest that CR rates may be higher than with chemotherapy alone, and is also being tested for its ability to reduce disease burden before and after auto- or allo-SCT. Potentially, the most important application of imatinib mesylate will be for older Ph+ patients for whom allo-SCT may not be feasible. The GMALL have initiated a randomized multicenter Phase II study to determine the safety and efficacy of imatinib in Ph+ ALL patients more than 55 years of age as first-line single-agent induction therapy and with concurrent administration of postremission consolidative chemotherapy for a duration of up to 1 year.[204]

ALL with 11q23 (*MLL*) Abnormalities

The t(4;11)(q21;q23) is the most common recurring abnormality involving the *MLL* gene on chromosome 11q23 and occurs in 5% to 10% of adult ALL cases.[61,205,206] These cases are characterized by an early (pro-B) immunophenotype, with expression of CD19, CD22, CD24, and cytoplasmic CD79a and coexpression of myeloid antigens, whereas CD10 is negative. Patients often present with high leukocyte counts, hepatosplenomegaly, and CNS involvement. With standard induction and consolidation chemotherapy, survival for these patients is poor, with less than 15% probability of DFS at 5 years.[47] The GMALL has reported that these patients fare considerably better when an allo-SCT is performed in CR1, with reports of more than 50% of patients achieving long-term DFS.[120] In the GMALL series, the t(4;11) patients had superior outcomes to other high-risk patients receiving allo-SCT in CR1, perhaps as a result of the additional benefit that these patients may have obtained from receiving high-dose cytarabine and mitoxantrone before undergoing allo-SCT. Based on these data, the current recommendation is to identify a donor for allo-SCT early in CR1 for patients with MLL gene rearrangements. In addition, they may benefit from intensive cytoreduction with a high-dose cytarabine-based regimen that may be given as early consolidative therapy while a suitable donor is being identified.

Supportive Care

Improvements in outcome of patients with ALL are, in part, attributable to advances in supportive care of these high-risk patients. Among these advances are new agents for the prevention and treatment of neutropenic infection and its attendant complications, the use of hematopoietic growth factors, and careful prophylaxis against tumor lysis syndrome.

Infectious disease complications secondary to neutropenia are the primary cause of treatment-related morbidity and mortality in acute leukemia, and the risks seem to be especially high in patients over age 60.[114] As such, preventing prolonged neutropenia with prophylactic use of granulocyte-stimulating growth factors has been the target of multiple investigations and clinical practice guidelines.[207–210] Several of these studies have focused on adults with ALL.[114,210] Two sequential studies of G-CSF use during induction therapy performed by the German ALL cooperative group, the GMALL, demonstrated a reduction in the duration of neutropenia, a reduction in the number of nonviral infections, and less frequent interruptions in chemotherapy schedules. These benefits, however, did not translate into improved disease-free or overall survival.[211]

In 1998, the CALGB published results of its large, prospective, randomized trial of G-CSF given during induction and consolidation chemotherapy.[114] Subjects who received G-CSF required fewer days to neutrophil recovery following induction chemotherapy for ALL. Subjects in the G-CSF group also had a shorter hospitalization time, and both a higher CR rate (87% versus 77%) and fewer induction deaths (5% versus 11%) However, G-CSF did not allow for a compressed course of chemotherapy or shorten the overall time required to undergo induction and consolidation. The overall toxicity was not lessened, infectious complications were no different, and there was no significant difference in OS or DFS between individuals who had received the G-CSF and those who had received placebo. Notably, in patients older than age 60, the CR rate for patients receiving G-CSF was 81% compared with 55% in the placebo arm. Induction deaths were also decreased, thus allowing more patients to progress to postremission therapy. In conclusion, the use of G-CSF during intensive treatment of ALL appears reasonable; however, none of the studies has demonstrated improvement in DFS or OS when hematopoietic growth factors are employed during treatment of ALL.[212]

Treatment of Relapse

Currently, more than half of adult patients with ALL will relapse despite the use of intensive combination chemotherapy programs. Most relapse within the first 2 years.[213] More than 80% of relapses occur first in the bone marrow, while the remainder occur in extramedullary sites, primarily the CNS. Relapses in other sites such as lymph nodes, skin, or testes occur much less frequently. Patients with an isolated extramedullary relapse have a very high risk for subsequent bone marrow relapse and should receive systemic chemotherapy following local treatment.

Treatment of Central Nervous System Leukemia

Patients with CNS leukemia at the time of diagnosis usually receive more intensive IT therapy, with or without cranial irradiation and continue planned induction therapy. Frequently, these patients are treated with twice-weekly IT therapy until the CSF is cleared of lymphoblasts, followed by four weekly treatments while continuing with the standard protocol prophylaxis therapy. Thereafter, these patients receive once-monthly injections of intrathecal therapy for 1 year.[147,214] CNS irradiation may be deferred until completion of induction therapy unless patients have evidence of cranial nerve root involvement. With appropriate CNS-directed therapy, patients presenting with CNS involvement can expect a similar outcome compared to patients lacking this complication.[113]

Patients who have an isolated CNS relapse require a different approach. From the pediatric literature, children with a CNS relapse have a dismal prognosis, with fewer than 20% achieving long-term survival.[215] It appears that the poor outcome of these patients is primarily the result of hematologic relapse rather than resistant CNS disease.[216] Therefore, the current approach to CNS relapse in children is to treat with systemic reinduction chemotherapy together with IT chemotherapy, followed by cranial irradiation. Using this approach, the Pediatric Oncology Group treated 83 children with isolated CNS relapses with 6 months of reinduction chemotherapy and consolidation therapy, followed by craniospinal irradiation and maintenance chemotherapy for 2 years from the time of relapse.[217] The EFS at 4 years was 71% for all patients, which approaches the results observed overall for children with newly diagnosed ALL. Insufficient data exist concerning the management of isolated CNS leukemia in adults, but a similar approach may be reasonable. An alternative approach for patients who do not respond to conventional CNS therapy may be the use of depo-cytarabine, a slow-release formulation of cytarabine that may be given every 3 weeks.[218,219]

Although stem cell transplantation is a reasonable approach for adults with CNS relapse, it may not always be an effective means of management of CNS leukemia. In one study, the probability of CNS relapse was 52% for patients with a history of or active CNS disease at the time of transplant.[220] The probability of CNS relapse in this study was less, 17%, for patients who received IT methotrexate after BMT, although the risk of leukoencephalopathy in these patients was significantly higher.

General Strategy for Systemic Relapse of ALL

A variety of treatment protocols have been employed in relapsed or refractory patients. However, in almost every instance, the median remission duration has been less than 6 months, and only a small fraction of these patients become long-term survivors. The best results for such patients have been obtained with allo-SCT in second remission, reviewed earlier in the section on stem cell transplantation, where studies report DFS rates of 14% to 59%. Therefore, when feasible, the goal of salvage therapy is to obtain a second (or subsequent) remission and proceed to allo-SCT.

Chemotherapy Options

The choice of optimal chemotherapy to obtain a second remission is influenced by the initial induction/consolidation regimen, the duration of first remission, features of the disease at relapse, and the availability of a suitable allogeneic donor. Single agents that have been utilized include nucleoside analogues (usually cytarabine), anthracyclines, nonanthracycline intercalators (mitoxantrone), epipodophyllotoxins, alkylating agents (ifosphamide), and antifolates (usually high-dose methotrexate).[221–225] The divergent CR rates range from 0% to 73% and are influenced by the heterogeneity of the patients, as noted earlier. In general, however, combination chemotherapy has been more effective at inducing subsequent remissions and is most successful in patients with prolonged first remissions of more than 1 year. In these cases, reinduction using a regimen identical, or similar, to the initial successful treatment plan can be considered. High-dose cytarabine-containing regimens may be the most successful for achievement of CR, with rates of 38% to 80%. The drug has been combined with mitoxantrone,[188,226,227] with an anthracycline,[228] and with L-asparaginase,[229] or an epipodophyllotoxin.[230,231]

New Drugs in Clinical Trials

Relapse, particularly in older adults (age more than 60 years) with ALL and for those with short CR1 (less than 1 year), is associated with a very poor outcome with median survival of 2 to 4 months[160]; therefore, these poor-risk patients should be encouraged to participate in Phase I/II trials of investigation agents and novel therapeutic approaches.

A unique nucleoside analogue, clofarabine, has been demonstrated to have efficacy in relapsed pediatric and adult ALL, with response rates in the 17% to 32% range as a single agent.[232–234] Its mechanisms of action include the inhibition of ribonucleotide reductase and of DNA polymerase. Combination studies of clofarabine with cytarabine have also demonstrated efficacy in heavily pretreated patients.[235] Based on its efficacy in relapsed pediatric ALL, an application to the Federal Drug Administration is pending, and this may be the first new drug approved for use in relapsed ALL in many years.

Recently, therapy targeted to specific biologic risk groups has been exploited with some success and may be the focus of future novel therapeutics in ALL. Nelarabine (GW506U78) is an analogue of deoxyguanosine. Previous studies have demonstrated that immature T lymphocytes are extremely sensitive to the cytotoxic effects of deoxyguanosine. The toxicity of deoxyguanosine to T cells is related to the accumulation of deoxyguanosine triphosphate (dGTP), with subsequent inhibition of ribonucleotide reductase, inhibition of DNA synthesis, and resultant cell death. Prior Phase I studies determined a maximum tolerated dose of 40 mg/kg/day for 5 days in adult patients.[236,237] The dose-limiting toxicity was neurologic, consisting of seizures, obtundation, and ascending paralysis. As predicted by preclinical studies, the highest response rates were observed in patients with relapsed T-cell ALL and lymphoblastic lymphoma (LBL). To decrease the risk of neurologic toxicities, a dosing regimen of $1.5\,g/m^2$ given IV once per day on an alternate-day schedule (days 1, 3, 5) was recently tested in an intergroup study carried out by the CALGB and the Southwest Oncology Group (SWOG) in adults with relapsed/refractory T-cell ALL or LBL.[238] The overall response rate (CR + PR) for the 38 evaluable patients was 32% (95% CI, 18%–49%). The 1-year OS was 32% (95% CI, 16%–47%) and the 1-year DFS was 40% (95% CI, 10%–70%). These results suggest that nelarabine is well tolerated and has significant antitumor activity in patients with relapsed or refractory T-cell lymphoblastic leukemia/lymphoma, prompting consideration to incorporate nelarabine into frontline therapy for patients with T-lineage ALL.

A similar subset-specific approach is being explored using imatinib mesylate, the BCR-ABL tyrosine kinase inhibitor, in adults with Ph+ ALL in CR1, as described earlier (see section on Ph+ ALL). Although its greatest potential for improving DFS is likely to be in CR1 patients, imatinib as a single agent may induce transient responses in patients with relapsed or refractory disease, allowing such patients to proceed with an allo-SCT in second or subsequent remission. In vitro studies have demonstrated either additive (daunorubicin, interferon-alpha) or synergistic effects (cytarabine)[239]; therefore, combination therapy with imatinib should be tested for patients with relapsed Ph+ ALL. Another tyrosine kinase inhibitor that is directed against CD-19, B-43-Genistein, was shown to demonstrate activity in a Phase I trial of 15 heavily pretreated ALL patients. The CD19 receptor is expressed at high levels on leukemic cells of most ALL patients, is absent on hematopoietic stem cells, and is physically associated with the Src family of protein tyrosine kinases to form a transmembrane tyrosine kinase receptor with important signal transducing properties.[240]

Monoclonal antibodies targeted to epitopes present on the lymphoblasts are also being evaluated. Campath-1H is a monoclonal humanized form of a rat antibody active against CD52, an antigen present on nearly all normal B and T lymphocytes that may be present on the surface of most cases of ALL.[241,242] Although the experience with this antibody in relapsed, refractory ALL has been limited, Campath has been shown to clear blasts from the peripheral blood after failure of traditional chemotherapy.[242,243] The CALGB has recently begun testing the feasibility of incorporating Campath-1H into the initial treatment of adult ALL in an attempt to eradicate MRD in early CR1 (CALGB 10102). Rituximab, a chimeric humanized mouse antibody directed against CD20, which is expressed in approximately 20% of ALL cases, is also being explored as an adjunct to standard chemotherapy in frontline and salvage therapy. Initial reports from the M.D. Anderson suggest that its addition may improve response rates[244]; longer follow-up is needed to determine its potential to improve DFS. Based on decreases in tumor size that were demonstrated using an immunotoxin, anti-B4 blocked ricin (anti-B4-bR); this immunotoxin, which is directed against the surface epitope, CD19, has also been tested in relapsed and frontline ALL.[245,246] Although this approach was feasible as intensification therapy in CR1, there did not appear to be a DFS benefit compared to previous studies. A new generation of conjugated antibodies is being developed, and one of these agents (toxin-conjugated anti-CD22; Wyeth) may soon enter clinical trials in advanced ALL.

The Future: Targeted Agents

Rationale for the use of other novel agents that may target specific pathogenetic pathways in ALL exists. Potential candidates for future study include drugs that target P-glycoprotein, encoded by the multidrug resistance (MDR1) gene, which may be overexpressed in drug-resistant ALL.[247,248] A number of these agents are currently in development and have entered clinical trials in AML but remain to be tested in ALL. Oblimersen (formerly G3139), an antisense oligonucleotide directed against bcl-2, which is frequently overexpressed in ALL,[248] may be combined with standard agents in an attempt to overcome drug resistance and facilitate chemotherapy-induced apoptotic cell death.[249] There is also good rationale for testing the efficacy of hypomethylating agents, such as 5-azacytidine or 2-deoxy 5-azacytidine, because hypermethylation has been associated with drug resistance and is reported in 10% to 50% of de novo and nearly all cases of relapsed or refractory ALL.[160] Overexpression of FLT-3, a receptor tyrosine kinase, occurs in cases of infant ALL with either *MLL* gene rearrangements or hyperdiploidy.[91] Continuous signaling by the receptor contributes to the abnormal growth of leukemia cells, which can be blocked by a small molecule tyrosine kinase inhibitor of FLT-3 in vitro in primary leukemia cells containing MLL gene rearrangements.[91] Thus, the rationale exists for clinical trials of FLT-3 receptor tyrosine kinase inhibitors[250] in these subsets of ALL. In preclinical studies, induction of apoptosis in ALL cell lines has recently been demonstrated after treatment with a histone deacetylase inhibitor.[251,252]

Conclusions

The majority of adults receiving treatment for ALL will achieve remission; however, despite improvements in selected patient subsets, fewer than half of adult ALL patients are long-term survivors. Future advances for this relatively rare group of diseases will require the insights gained from participation in well-designed cooperative group clinical trials. Rapidly emerging insights into the molecular pathogenesis and monitoring of these heterogeneous disorders will improve prognostic ability, aid in risk stratification and treatment choice, and guide new molecularly targeted drug development. Using a risk-adapted approach based on patient characteristics and molecular–cytogenetic features of the disease, as outlined here, will facilitate the development of more individualized and successful treatments to improve outcome for adults with ALL.

References

1. Jemal A, Murray T, Samuels A, Ghafoor A, Ward E, Thun MJ. Cancer statistics, 2003. CA Cancer J Clin 2003;53:5–26.
2. Ries L, Smith MA, Gurney JG. Cancer incidence and survival among children and adolescents: United States SEER Program 1975–1995. Bethesda: National Cancer Institute, 1999.
3. U.S. Cancer Statistics Working Group. United States Cancer Statistics: 2000, Incidence. Atlanta, GA: Department of Health and Human Services, Centers for Disease Control and Prevention and National Cancer Institute, 2003.
4. Sandler DP. Epidemiology and etiology of leukemia. Curr Opin Oncol 1990;2:3–9.
5. Zipursky A, Poon A, Doyle J. Leukemia in Down syndrome: a review. Pediatr Hematol Oncol 1992;9:139–149.
6. Gurbuxani S, Vyas P, Crispino JD. Recent insights into the mechanisms of myeloid leukemogenesis in Down syndrome. Blood 2004;103:399–406.
7. Shaw MP, Eden OB, Grace E, Ellis PM. Acute lymphoblastic leukemia and Klinefelter's syndrome. Pediatr Hematol Oncol 1992;9:81–85.
8. German J, Bloom D, Passarge E, et al. Bloom's syndrome. VI. The disorder in Israel and an estimation of the gene frequency in the Ashkenazim. Am J Hum Genet 1977;29:553–562.
9. Toledano SR, Lange BJ. Ataxia-telangiectasia and acute lymphoblastic leukemia. Cancer (Phila) 1980;45:1675–1678.
10. Greaves MF, Maia AT, Wiemels JL, Ford AM. Leukemia in twins: lessons in natural history. Blood 2003;102:2321–2333.
11. Hecht T, Henke M, Schempp W, Bross KJ, Lohr GW. Acute lymphoblastic leukemia in adult identical twins. Blut 1988;56:261–264.
12. Strick R, Strissel PL, Borgers S, Smith SL, Rowley JD. Dietary bioflavonoids induce cleavage in the MLL gene and may contribute to infant leukemia. Proc Natl Acad Sci U S A 2000;97:4790–4795.
13. Wiemels JL, Cazzaniga G, Daniotti M, et al. Prenatal origin of acute lymphoblastic leukaemia in children. Lancet 1999;354:1499–1503.
14. Fasching K, Panzer S, Haas OA, Marschalek R, Gadner H, Panzer-Grumayer ER. Presence of clone-specific antigen receptor gene rearrangements at birth indicates an in utero origin of diverse types of early childhood acute lymphoblastic leukemia. Blood 2000;95:2722–2724.
15. Mori H, Colman SM, Xiao Z, et al. Chromosome translocations and covert leukemic clones are generated during normal fetal development. Proc Natl Acad Sci U S A 2002;99:8242–8247.
16. Magrath I, Jain V, Bhatia K. Epstein–Barr virus and Burkitt's lymphoma. Semin Cancer Biol 1992;3:285–295.
17. Liebowitz D. Epstein–Barr virus and a cellular signaling pathway in lymphomas from immunosuppressed patients. N Engl J Med 1998;338:1413–1421.
18. Greaves MF, Alexander FE. An infectious etiology for common acute lymphoblastic leukemia in childhood? Leukemia 1993;7:349–360.
19. Preston DL, Kusumi S, Tomonaga M, et al. Cancer incidence in atomic bomb survivors. Part III. Leukemia, lymphoma and multiple myeloma, 1950–1987. Radiat Res 1994;137:S68–S97.
20. Ichimura M, Ishimura T, Belsky JL. Incidence of leukemia in atomic bomb survivors belonging to a fixed cohort in Hiroshima and Nagasaki, 1950–1971: radiation dose, years after exposure, age at exposure, and type of leukemia. J Radiat Res (Tokyo) 1978;19:262–282.
21. UK Childhood Cancer Study Investigators. Br J Cancer 2000;83:1573.
22. Sandler DP, Shore DL, Anderson JR, et al. Cigarette smoking and risk of acute leukemia: associations with morphology and cytogenetic abnormalities in bone marrow. J Natl Cancer Inst 1993;85:1994–2003.
23. Andersen MK, Christiansen DH, Jensen BA, Ernst P, Hauge G, Pedersen-Bjergaard J. Therapy-related acute lymphoblastic leukaemia with MLL rearrangements following DNA topoisomerase II inhibitors, an increasing problem: report on two new cases and review of the literature since 1992. Br J Haematol 2001;114:539–543.
24. Bennett JM, Catovsky D, Daniel MT, et al. Proposals for the classification of the acute leukaemias. French-American-British (FAB) co-operative group. Br J Haematol 1976;33:451–458.
25. Bennett JM, Catovsky D, Daniel MT, et al. The morphological classification of acute lymphoblastic leukaemia: concordance among observers and clinical correlations. Br J Haematol 1981;47:553–561.

26. World Health Organization Classification of Tumours. Pathology and Genetics of Haematopoietic and Lymphoid Tissues. Lyon: IARC Press, 2001.
27. Humphrey GB, Nesbit ME, Brunning RD. Prognostic value of the periodic acid-Schiff (PAS) reaction in acute lymphoblastic leukemia. Am J Clin Pathol 1974;61:393–397.
28. Drexler HG, Sperling C, Ludwig WD. Terminal deoxynucleotidyl transferase (TdT) expression in acute myeloid leukemia. Leukemia 1993;7:1142–1150.
29. Bain BJ, Barnett D, Linch D, Matutes E, Reilly JT. Revised guideline on immunophenotyping in acute leukaemias and chronic lymphoproliferative disorders. Clin Lab Haematol 2002;24:1–13.
30. Bene MC, Castoldi G, Knapp W, et al. Proposals for the immunological classification of acute leukemias. European Group for the Immunological Characterization of Leukemias (EGIL). Leukemia 1995;9:1783–1786.
31. Baer MR. Assessment of minimal residual disease in patients with acute leukemia. Curr Opin Oncol 1998;10:17–22.
32. Stock W, Estrov Z. Studies of minimal residual disease in acute lymphocytic leukemia. Hematol Oncol Clin N Am 2000;14: 1289–305, viii–ix.
33. Boucheix C, David B, Sebban C, et al. Immunophenotype of adult acute lymphoblastic leukemia, clinical parameters, and outcome: an analysis of a prospective trial including 562 tested patients (LALA87). French Group on Therapy for Adult Acute Lymphoblastic Leukemia. Blood 1994;84:1603–1612.
34. Larson RA, Dodge RK, Burns CP, et al. A five-drug remission induction regimen with intensive consolidation for adults with acute lymphoblastic leukemia: cancer and leukemia group B study 8811. Blood 1995;85:2025–2037.
35. Gill PS, Meyer PR, Pavlova Z, Levine AM. B cell acute lymphocytic leukemia in adults. Clinical, morphologic, and immunologic findings. J Clin Oncol 1986;4:737–743.
36. Gassmann W, Loffler H, Thiel E, et al. Morphological and cytochemical findings in 150 cases of T-lineage acute lymphoblastic leukaemia in adults. German Multicentre ALL Study Group (GMALL). Br J Haematol 1997;97:372–382.
37. Kita K, Miwa H, Nakase K, et al. Clinical importance of CD7 expression in acute myelocytic leukemia. The Japan Cooperative Group of Leukemia/Lymphoma. Blood 1993;81:2399–2405.
38. Thalhammer-Scherrer R, Mitterbauer G, Simonitsch I, et al. The immunophenotype of 325 adult acute leukemias: relationship to morphologic and molecular classification and proposal for a minimal screening program highly predictive for lineage discrimination. Am J Clin Pathol 2002;117:380–389.
39. Czuczman MS, Dodge RK, Stewart CC, et al. Value of immunophenotype in intensively treated adult acute lymphoblastic leukemia: cancer and leukemia Group B study 8364. Blood 1999;93:3931–3939.
40. Guyotat D, Campos L, Shi ZH, et al. Myeloid surface antigen expression in adult acute lymphoblastic leukemia. Leukemia 1990;4:664–666.
41. Matutes E, Morilla R, Farahat N, et al. Definition of acute biphenotypic leukemia. Haematologica 1997;82:64–66.
42. Faderl S, Kantarjian HM, Talpaz M, Estrov Z. Clinical significance of cytogenetic abnormalities in adult acute lymphoblastic leukemia. Blood 1998;91:3995–4019.
43. Faderl S, Jeha S, Kantarjian HM. The biology and therapy of adult acute lymphoblastic leukemia. Cancer (Phila) 2003;98:1337–1354.
44. Secker-Walker LM, Prentice HG, Durrant J, Richards S, Hall E, Harrison G. Cytogenetics adds independent prognostic information in adults with acute lymphoblastic leukaemia on MRC trial UKALL XA. MRC Adult Leukaemia Working Party. Br J Haematol 1997;96:601–610.
45. Pui CH, Relling MV, Downing JR. Acute lymphoblastic leukemia. N Engl J Med 2004;350:1535–1548.
46. Klein G. Immunoglobulin gene associated chromosomal translocations in B-cell derived tumors. Curr Top Microbiol Immunol 1999;246:161–167.
47. Wetzler M, Dodge RK, Mrozek K, et al. Prospective karyotype analysis in adult acute lymphoblastic leukemia: the cancer and leukemia Group B experience. Blood 1999;93:3983–3893.
48. Rowley JD. Letter: A new consistent chromosomal abnormality in chronic myelogenous leukaemia identified by quinacrine fluorescence and Giemsa staining. Nature (Lond) 1973;243:290–293.
49. Melo JV. The diversity of BCR-ABL fusion proteins and their relationship to leukemia phenotype. Blood 1996;88:2375–2384.
50. Saglio G, Guerrasio A, Rosso C, et al. New type of Bcr/Abl junction in Philadelphia chromosome-positive chronic myelogenous leukemia. Blood 1990;76:1819–1824.
51. Maurer J, Janssen JW, Thiel E, et al. Detection of chimeric BCR-ABL genes in acute lymphoblastic leukaemia by the polymerase chain reaction. Lancet 1991;337:1055–1058.
52. Skorski T, Kanakaraj P, Nieborowska-Skorska M, et al. Phosphatidylinositol-3 kinase activity is regulated by BCR/ABL and is required for the growth of Philadelphia chromosome-positive cells. Blood 1995;86:726–736.
53. Daley GQ, Van Etten RA, Baltimore D. Induction of chronic myelogenous leukemia in mice by the P210bcr/abl gene of the Philadelphia chromosome. Science 1990;247:824–830.
54. Heisterkamp N, Jenster G, ten Hoeve J, Zovich D, Pattengale PK, Groffen J. Acute leukaemia in bcr/abl transgenic mice. Nature (Lond) 1990;344:251–253.
55. O'Brien SG, Guilhot F, Larson RA, et al. Imatinib compared with interferon and low-dose cytarabine for newly diagnosed chronic-phase chronic myeloid leukemia. N Engl J Med 2003;348:994–1004.
56. Ferrando AA, Look AT. Clinical implications of recurring chromosomal and associated molecular abnormalities in acute lymphoblastic leukemia. Semin Hematol 2000;37:381–395.
57. Ziemin-van der Poel S, McCabe NR, Gill HJ, et al. Identification of a gene, MLL, that spans the breakpoint in 11q23 translocations associated with human leukemias. Proc Natl Acad Sci USA 1991;88:10735–10739.
58. Pedersen-Bjergaard J, Rowley JD. The balanced and the unbalanced chromosome aberrations of acute myeloid leukemia may develop in different ways and may contribute differently to malignant transformation. Blood 1994;83:2780–2786.
59. Djabali M, Selleri L, Parry P, Bower M, Young BD, Evans GA. A trithorax-like gene is interrupted by chromosome 11q23 translocations in acute leukaemias. Nat Genet 1992;2:113–118.
60. Ernst P, Fisher JK, Avery W, Wade S, Foy D, Korsmeyer SJ. Definitive hematopoiesis requires the mixed-lineage leukemia gene. Dev Cell 2004;6:437–443.
61. Thirman MJ, Gill HJ, Burnett RC, et al. Rearrangement of the MLL gene in acute lymphoblastic and acute myeloid leukemias with 11q23 chromosomal translocations. N Engl J Med 1993; 329:909–914.
62. Ayton PM, Cleary ML. Molecular mechanisms of leukemogenesis mediated by MLL fusion proteins. Oncogene 2001;20:5695–5707.
63. Golub TR, Barker GF, Bohlander SK, et al. Fusion of the TEL gene on 12p13 to the AML1 gene on 21q22 in acute lymphoblastic leukemia. Proc Natl Acad Sci USA 1995;92: 4917–4921.
64. Shurtleff SA, Buijs A, Behm FG, et al. TEL/AML1 fusion resulting from a cryptic t(12;21) is the most common genetic lesion in pediatric ALL and defines a subgroup of patients with an excellent prognosis. Leukemia 1995;9:1985–1989.
65. McLean TW, Ringold S, Neuberg D, et al. TEL/AML-1 dimerizes and is associated with a favorable outcome in childhood acute lymphoblastic leukemia. Blood 1996;88:4252–4258.

66. Lanza C, Volpe G, Basso G, et al. Outcome and lineage involvement in t(12;21) childhood acute lymphoblastic leukaemia. Br J Haematol 1997;97:460–462.
67. Aguiar RC, Sohal J, van Rhee F, et al. TEL-AML1 fusion in acute lymphoblastic leukaemia of adults. M.R.C. Adult Leukaemia Working Party. Br J Haematol 1996;95:673–677.
68. Carroll AJ, Crist WM, Parmley RT, Roper M, Cooper MD, Finley WH. Pre-B cell leukemia associated with chromosome translocation 1;19. Blood 1984;63:721–724.
69. Dedera DA, Waller EK, LeBrun DP, et al. Chimeric homeobox gene E2A-PBX1 induces proliferation, apoptosis, and malignant lymphomas in transgenic mice. Cell 1993;74:833–843.
70. Dalla-Favera R, Bregni M, Erikson J, Patterson D, Gallo RC, Croce CM. Human c-myc onc gene is located on the region of chromosome 8 that is translocated in Burkitt lymphoma cells. Proc Natl Acad Sci U S A 1982;79:7824–7827.
71. Taub R, Kirsch I, Morton C, et al. Translocation of the c-myc gene into the immunoglobulin heavy chain locus in human Burkitt lymphoma and murine plasmacytoma cells. Proc Natl Acad Sci U S A 1982;79:7837–7841.
72. Boxer LM, Dang CV. Translocations involving c-myc and c-myc function. Oncogene 2001;20:5595–5610.
73. Adams JM, Harris AW, Pinkert CA, et al. The c-myc oncogene driven by immunoglobulin enhancers induces lymphoid malignancy in transgenic mice. Nature (Lond) 1985;318:533–538.
74. Li Z, Van Calcar S, Qu C, Cavenee WK, Zhang MQ, Ren B. A global transcriptional regulatory role for c-Myc in Burkitt's lymphoma cells. Proc Natl Acad Sci USA 2003;100:8164–8169.
75. Kebriaei P, Anastasi J, Larson RA. Acute lymphoblastic leukaemia: diagnosis and classification. Best Pract Res Clin Haematol 2002;15:597–621.
76. Groupe Francais de. Cytogenetic abnormalities in adult acute lymphoblastic leukemia: correlations with hematologic findings outcome. A Collaborative Study of the Group Francais de Cytogenetique Hematologique. Blood 1996;87:3135–3142.
77. Mellentin JD, Smith SD, Cleary ML. lyl-1, a novel gene altered by chromosomal translocation in T cell leukemia, codes for a protein with a helix-loop-helix DNA binding motif. Cell 1989;58:77–83.
78. Xia Y, Brown L, Yang CY, et al. TAL2, a helix-loop-helix gene activated by the (7;9)(q34;q32) translocation in human T-cell leukemia. Proc Natl Acad Sci USA 1991;88:11416–11420.
79. Stock W, Westbrook CA, Sher DA, et al. Low incidence of TAL1 gene rearrangements in adult acute lymphoblastic leukemia: a cancer and leukemia group B study (8762). Clin Cancer Res 1995;1:459–463.
80. Wadman I, Li J, Bash RO, et al. Specific in vivo association between the bHLH and LIM proteins implicated in human T cell leukemia. EMBO J 1994;13:4831–4839.
81. Valge-Archer VE, Osada H, Warren AJ, et al. The LIM protein RBTN2 and the basic helix-loop-helix protein TAL1 are present in a complex in erythroid cells. Proc Natl Acad Sci USA 1994;91:8617–8621.
82. Shivdasani RA, Mayer EL, Orkin SH. Absence of blood formation in mice lacking the T-cell leukaemia oncoprotein tal-1/SCL. Nature (Lond) 1995;373:432–434.
83. Screpanti I, Bellavia D, Campese AF, Frati L, Gulino A. Notch, a unifying target in T-cell acute lymphoblastic leukemia? Trends Mol Med 2003;9:30–935.
84. Bellavia D, Campese AF, Checquolo S, et al. Combined expression of pTalpha and Notch3 in T cell leukemia identifies the requirement of preTCR for leukemogenesis. Proc Natl Acad Sci USA 2002;99:3788–3793.
85. Chilcote RR, Brown E, Rowley JD. Lymphoblastic leukemia with lymphomatous features associated with abnormalities of the short arm of chromosome 9. N Engl J Med 1985;313:286–291.
86. Omura-Minamisawa M, Diccianni MB, Batova A, et al. Universal inactivation of both p16 and p15 but not downstream components is an essential event in the pathogenesis of T-cell acute lymphoblastic leukemia. Clin Cancer Res 2000;6:1219–1228.
87. Shen L, Toyota M, Kondo Y, et al. Aberrant DNA methylation of p57KIP2 identifies a cell-cycle regulatory pathway with prognostic impact in adult acute lymphocytic leukemia. Blood 2003;101:4131–4136.
88. Tsai T, Davalath S, Rankin C, et al. Tumor suppressor gene alteration in adult acute lymphoblastic leukemia (ALL). Analysis of retinoblastoma (Rb) and p53 gene expression in lymphoblasts of patients with de novo, relapsed, or refractory ALL treated in Southwest Oncology Group studies. Leukemia 1996;10:1901–1910.
89. Stock W, Tsai T, Golden C, et al. Cell cycle regulatory gene abnormalities are important determinants of leukemogenesis and disease biology in adult acute lymphoblastic leukemia. Blood 2000;95:2364–2371.
90. Gilliland DG, Griffin JD. The roles of FLT3 in hematopoiesis and leukemia. Blood 2002;100:1532–1542.
91. Armstrong SA, Staunton JE, Silverman LB, et al. MLL translocations specify a distinct gene expression profile that distinguishes a unique leukemia. Nat Genet 2002;30:41–47.
92. Yeoh EJ, Ross ME, Shurtleff SA, et al. Classification, subtype discovery, and prediction of outcome in pediatric acute lymphoblastic leukemia by gene expression profiling. Cancer Cell 2002;1:133–143.
93. Ferrando AA, Neuberg DS, Staunton J, et al. Gene expression signatures define novel oncogenic pathways in T cell acute lymphoblastic leukemia. Cancer Cell 2002;1:75–87.
94. Stock W, Byrd J, Frankel SR, Bloomfield CD. Adult acute lymphoblastic leukemia. In: Armitage JO, Abeloff M (eds). Clinical Oncology. New York: Churchill-Livingstone, 1999:2451–2489.
95. Soussain C, Patte C, Ostronoff M, et al. Small noncleaved cell lymphoma and leukemia in adults. A retrospective study of 65 adults treated with the LMB pediatric protocols. Blood 1995;85:664–674.
96. Rivera GK, Pinkel D, Simone JV, Hancock ML, Crist WM. Treatment of acute lymphoblastic leukemia. 30 years' experience at St. Jude Children's Research Hospital. N Engl J Med 1993;329:1289–1295.
97. Hoelzer D, Ludwig WD, Thiel E, et al. Improved outcome in adult B-cell acute lymphoblastic leukemia. Blood 1996;87:495–508.
98. Zinzani PL, Bendandi M, Visani G, et al. Adult lymphoblastic lymphoma: clinical features and prognostic factors in 53 patients. Leuk Lymphoma 1996;23:577–582.
99. Kantarjian HM, Walters RS, Keating MJ, et al. Results of the vincristine, doxorubicin, and dexamethasone regimen in adults with standard- and high-risk acute lymphocytic leukemia. J Clin Oncol 1990;8:994–1004.
100. Lazzarino M, Morra E, Alessandrino EP, et al. Adult acute lymphoblastic leukemia. Response to therapy according to presenting features in 62 patients. Eur J Cancer Clin Oncol 1982;18:813–819.
101. Hoelzer D, Thiel E, Loffler H, et al. Prognostic factors in a multicenter study for treatment of acute lymphoblastic leukemia in adults. Blood 1988;71:123–131.
102. Chessells JM, Hall E, Prentice HG, Durrant J, Bailey CC, Richards SM. The impact of age on outcome in lymphoblastic leukaemia; MRC UKALL X and XA compared: a report from the MRC Paediatric and Adult Working Parties. Leukemia 1998;12:463–473.
103. Secker-Walker LM, Craig JM, Hawkins JM, Hoffbrand AV. Philadelphia positive acute lymphoblastic leukemia in adults: age distribution, BCR breakpoint and prognostic significance. Leukemia 1991;5:196–199.

104. Secker-Walker LM. Distribution of Philadelphia positive acute lymphoblastic leukemia: geographical heterogeneity or age related incidence? Genes Chromosomes Cancer 1991;3:320–321.
105. Delannoy A, Ferrant A, Bosly A, et al. Acute lymphoblastic leukemia in the elderly. Eur J Haematol 1990;45:90–93.
106. Linker CA, Levitt LJ, O'Donnell M, Forman SJ, Ries CA. Treatment of adult acute lymphoblastic leukemia with intensive cyclical chemotherapy: a follow-up report. Blood 1991;78:2814–2822.
107. Hoelzer D, Thiel E, Ludwig WD, et al. The German multicentre trials for treatment of acute lymphoblastic leukemia in adults. The German Adult ALL Study Group. Leukemia 1992; 6(suppl 2):175–177.
108. Faderl S, Albitar M. Insights into the biologic and molecular abnormalities in adult acute lymphocytic leukemia. Hematol Oncol Clin N Am 2000;14:1267–1288.
109. Mandelli F, Annino L, Rotoli B. The GIMEMA ALL 0183 trial: analysis of 10-year follow-up. GIMEMA Cooperative Group, Italy. Br J Haematol 1996;92:665–672.
110. Gokbuget N, Hoelzer D, Arnold R, et al. Treatment of adult ALL according to protocols of the German Multicenter Study Group for Adult ALL (GMALL). Hematol Oncol Clin N Am 2000;14: 1307–1325, ix.
111. Gaynor J, Chapman D, Little C, et al. A cause-specific hazard rate analysis of prognostic factors among 199 adults with acute lymphoblastic leukemia: the Memorial Hospital experience since 1969. J Clin Oncol 1988;6:1014–1030.
112. Miller DR, Coccia PF, Bleyer WA, et al. Early response to induction therapy as a predictor of disease-free survival and late recurrence of childhood acute lymphoblastic leukemia: a report from the Childrens Cancer Study Group. J Clin Oncol 1989;7:1807–1815.
113. Cooperative Group. GIMEMA ALL 0183: a multicentric study on adult acute lymphoblastic leukaemia in Italy. GIMEMA Cooperative Group. Br J Haematol 1989;71:377–386.
114. Larson RA, Dodge RK, Linker CA, et al. A randomized controlled trial of filgrastim during remission induction and consolidation chemotherapy for adults with acute lymphoblastic leukemia: CALGB study 9111. Blood 1998;92:1556–1564.
115. Lauer SJ, Pinkel D, Buchanan GR, et al. Cytosine arabinoside/cyclophosphamide pulses during continuation therapy for childhood acute lymphoblastic leukemia. Potential selective effect in T-cell leukemia. Cancer (Phila) 1987;60:2366–2371.
116. Schrappe M, Reiter A, Ludwig WD, et al. Improved outcome in childhood acute lymphoblastic leukemia despite reduced use of anthracyclines and cranial radiotherapy: results of trial ALL-BFM 90. German-Austrian-Swiss ALL-BFM Study Group. Blood 2000;95:3310–3322.
117. Pui CH, Sallan S, Relling MV, Masera G, Evans WE. International Childhood Acute Lymphoblastic Leukemia Workshop, Sausalito, CA, 30 November–1 December 2000. Leukemia 2001; 15:707–715.
118. Hoelzer D, Arnold R, Buechner T, et al. Characteristics, outcome and risk factors in adult T-lineage acute lymphoblastic leukemia. Blood 1999;94:659a.
119. Janssen JW, Ludwig WD, Borkhardt A, et al. Pre-pre-B acute lymphoblastic leukemia: high frequency of alternatively spliced ALL1-AF4 transcripts and absence of minimal residual disease during complete remission. Blood 1994;84:3835–3842.
120. Ludwig WD, Rieder H, Bartram CR, et al. Immunophenotypic and genotypic features, clinical characteristics, and treatment outcome of adult pro-B acute lymphoblastic leukemia: results of the German multicenter trials GMALL 03/87 and 04/89. Blood 1998;92:1898–1909.
121. Pieters R, den Boer ML, Durian M, et al. Relation between age, immunophenotype and in vitro drug resistance in 395 children with acute lymphoblastic leukemia—implications for treatment of infants. Leukemia 1998;12:1344–1348.
122. Pui CH, Behm FG, Singh B, et al. Myeloid-associated antigen expression lacks prognostic value in childhood acute lymphoblastic leukemia treated with intensive multiagent chemotherapy. Blood 1990;75:198–202.
123. Romana SP, Poirel H, Leconiat M, et al. High frequency of t(12;21) in childhood B-lineage acute lymphoblastic leukemia. Blood 1995;86:4263–4269.
124. Raynaud S, Mauvieux L, Cayuela JM, et al. TEL/AML1 fusion gene is a rare event in adult acute lymphoblastic leukemia. Leukemia 1996;10:1529–1530.
125. Hunger SP. Chromosomal translocations involving the E2A gene in acute lymphoblastic leukemia: clinical features and molecular pathogenesis. Blood 1996;87:1211–1224.
126. Cave H, van der Werff ten Bosch J, Suciu S, et al. Clinical significance of minimal residual disease in childhood acute lymphoblastic leukemia. European Organization for Research and Treatment of Cancer—Childhood Leukemia Cooperative Group. N Engl J Med 1998;339:591–598.
127. van Dongen JJ, Seriu T, Panzer-Grumayer ER, et al. Prognostic value of minimal residual disease in acute lymphoblastic leukaemia in childhood. Lancet 1998;352:1731–1738.
128. Foroni L, Coyle LA, Papaioannou M, et al. Molecular detection of minimal residual disease in adult and childhood acute lymphoblastic leukaemia reveals differences in treatment response. Leukemia 1997;11:1732–1741.
129. Mortuza FY, Papaioannou M, Moreira IM, et al. Minimal residual disease tests provide an independent predictor of clinical outcome in adult acute lymphoblastic leukemia. J Clin Oncol 2002;20:1094–1104.
130. Sher D, Dodge R, Bloomfield CD, et al. Clone-specific quantitative real-time PCR of IgH or TCR gene rearrangements in adult ALL following induction chemotherapy identifies patients with a poor prognosis: pilot study from the Cancer and Leukemia Group B (CALGB 20101). Blood 2002;100: 153a.
131. van Dongen JJ, Langerak AW, Bruggemann M, et al. Design and standardization of PCR primers and protocols for detection of clonal immunoglobulin and T-cell receptor gene recombinations in suspect lymphoproliferations: report of the BIOMED-2 Concerted Action BMH4-CT98-3936. Leukemia 2003;17:2257–2317.
132. Brueggemann M, Droese J, Scheuring UJ. Minimal residual disease in adult patients with acute lymphoblastic leukemia during the first year of therapy predicts clinical outcome. Hematol J 2001;1:700a.
133. Biondi A, Valsecchi MG, Seriu T, et al. Molecular detection of minimal residual disease is a strong predictive factor of relapse in childhood B-lineage acute lymphoblastic leukemia with medium risk features. A case control study of the International BFM study group. Leukemia 2000;14:1939–1943.
134. Schrappe M, Flohr T, Beier R, Bartram CR. Risk stratification in childhood acute lymphoblastic leukemias based on clone-specific detection of minimal residual disease (MRD) with molecular genetics: Performance in German Trial ALL-BFM 2000. Hematol J 2001;1:695a.
135. Hoelzer D, Gokbuget N, Bruggemann M. Clinical impact of minimal residual disease in trial design for adult ALL. Blood 2001;98:584.
136. Hussein KK, Dahlberg S, Head D, et al. Treatment of acute lymphoblastic leukemia in adults with intensive induction, consolidation, and maintenance chemotherapy. Blood 1989;73:57–63.
137. Schauer P, Arlin ZA, Mertelsmann R, et al. Treatment of acute lymphoblastic leukemia in adults: results of the L-10 and L-10M protocols. J Clin Oncol 1983;1:462–470.
138. Gottlieb AJ, Weinberg V, Ellison RR, et al. Efficacy of daunorubicin in the therapy of adult acute lymphocytic leukemia: a prospective randomized trial by cancer and leukemia group B. Blood 1984;64:267–274.

139. Radford JE Jr., Burns CP, Jones MP, et al. Adult acute lymphoblastic leukemia: results of the Iowa HOP-L protocol. J Clin Oncol 1989;7:58–66.
140. Cuttner J, Mick R, Budman DR, et al. Phase III trial of brief intensive treatment of adult acute lymphocytic leukemia comparing daunorubicin and mitoxantrone: a CALGB Study. Leukemia 1991;5:425–431.
141. Todeschini G, Tecchio C, Meneghini V, et al. Estimated 6-year event-free survival of 55% in 60 consecutive adult acute lymphoblastic leukemia patients treated with an intensive phase II protocol based on high induction dose of daunorubicin. Leukemia 1998;12:144–149.
142. Linker C, Damon L, Ries C, Navarro W. Intensified and shortened cyclical chemotherapy for adult acute lymphoblastic leukemia. J Clin Oncol 2002;20:2464–2471.
143. Stock W, Yu D, Johnson J, et al. Intensified daunorubicin during induction and post-remission therapy of adult acute lymphoblastic leukemia (ALL): results of CALGB 19802. Blood 2003;102:379a.
144. Jones B, Freeman AI, Shuster JJ, et al. Lower incidence of meningeal leukemia when prednisone is replaced by dexamethasone in the treatment of acute lymphocytic leukemia. Med Pediatr Oncol 1991;19:269–275.
145. Hurwitz CA, Silverman LB, Schorin MA, et al. Substituting dexamethasone for prednisone complicates remission induction in children with acute lymphoblastic leukemia. Cancer (Phila) 2000;88:1964–1669.
146. Bostrom BC, Sensel MR, Sather HN, et al. Dexamethasone versus prednisone and daily oral versus weekly intravenous mercaptopurine for patients with standard-risk acute lymphoblastic leukemia: a report from the Children's Cancer Group. Blood 2003;101:3809–3817.
147. Kantarjian HM, O'Brien S, Smith TL, et al. Results of treatment with hyper-CVAD, a dose-intensive regimen, in adult acute lymphocytic leukemia. J Clin Oncol 2000;18:547–561.
148. Nagura E, Kimura K, Yamada K, et al. Nation-wide randomized comparative study of doxorubicin, vincristine and prednisolone combination therapy with and without L-asparaginase for adult acute lymphoblastic leukemia. Cancer Chemother Pharmacol 1994;33:359–365.
149. Larson RA, Fretzin MH, Dodge RK, Schiffer CA. Hypersensitivity reactions to L-asparaginase do not impact on the remission duration of adults with acute lymphoblastic leukemia. Leukemia 1998;12:660–665.
150. Rohatiner AZ, Bassan R, Battista R, et al. High dose cytosine arabinoside in the initial treatment of adults with acute lymphoblastic leukaemia. Br J Cancer 1990;62:454–458.
151. Annino L, Vegna ML, Camera A, et al. Treatment of adult acute lymphoblastic leukemia (ALL): long-term follow-up of the GIMEMA ALL 0288 randomized study. Blood 2002;99:863–871.
152. Hoelzer D, Thiel E, Ludwig WD, et al. Follow-up of the first two successive German multicentre trials for adult ALL (01/81 and 02/84). German Adult ALL Study Group. Leukemia 1993;7(suppl 2):S130–S134.
153. Goekbuget N, Arnold R, Buechner T, Ganser A. Intensification of induction and consolidation improves only subgroups of adult ALL: analysis of 1200 patients in GMALL Study 05/93. Blood 2001;98:802a.
154. Weiss M, Maslak P, Feldman E, et al. Cytarabine with high-dose mitoxantrone induces rapid complete remissions in adult acute lymphoblastic leukemia without the use of vincristine or prednisone. J Clin Oncol 1996;14:2480–2485.
155. Durrant IJ, Richards SM, Prentice HG, Goldstone AH. The Medical Research Council trials in adult acute lymphocytic leukemia. Hematol Oncol Clin N Am 2000;14:1327–1352.
156. Bassan R, Pogliani E, Casula P, et al. Risk-oriented postremission strategies in adult acute lymphoblastic leukemia: prospective confirmation of anthracycline activity in standard-risk class and role of hematopoietic stem cell transplants in high-risk groups. Hematol J 2001;2:117–126.
157. Rowe JM, Richards SM, Burnett AK, Wiernik P, Harrison G. Favorable results of allogeneic bone marrow transplantation (BMT) for adults with Philadelphia (Ph)-chromosome-negative acute lymphoblastic leukemia (ALL) in first complete remission (CR): results from the International ALL Trial (MRC UKALL XII/ECOG E2993). Blood 2001;98:481a.
158. Thiebaut A, Vernant JP, Degos L, et al. Adult acute lymphocytic leukemia study testing chemotherapy and autologous and allogeneic transplantation. A follow-up report of the French protocol LALA 87. Hematol Oncol Clin N Am 2000;14:1353–1366, x.
159. Nachman JB, Sather HN, Sensel MG, et al. Augmented post-induction therapy for children with high-risk acute lymphoblastic leukemia and a slow response to initial therapy. N Engl J Med 1998;338:1663–1671.
160. Garcia-Manero G, Thomas DA. Salvage therapy for refractory or relapsed acute lymphocytic leukemia. Hematol Oncol Clin N Am 2001;15:163–205.
161. Durrant IJ, Prentice HG, Richards SM. Intensification of treatment for adults with acute lymphoblastic leukaemia: results of U.K. Medical Research Council randomized trial UKALL XA. Medical Research Council Working Party on Leukaemia in Adults. Br J Haematol 1997;99:84–92.
162. Kantarjian HM, Walters RS, Smith TL, et al. Identification of risk groups for development of central nervous system leukemia in adults with acute lymphocytic leukemia. Blood 1988;72:1784–1789.
163. Law IP, Blom J. Adult acute leukemia: frequency of central system involvement in long-term survivors. Cancer (Phila) 1977;40:1304–1306.
164. Cortes J, O'Brien SM, Pierce S, Keating MJ, Freireich EJ, Kantarjian HM. The value of high-dose systemic chemotherapy and intrathecal therapy for central nervous system prophylaxis in different risk groups of adult acute lymphoblastic leukemia. Blood 1995;86:2091–2097.
165. Mastrangelo R. The problem of "staging" in childhood acute lymphoblastic leukemia: a review. Med Pediatr Oncol 1986;14:121–123.
166. Pavlovsky S, Eppinger-Helft M, Sackmann Muriel F. Factors that influence the appearance of central nervous system leukemia. Blood 1973;42:935–938.
167. Thomas DA, Cortes J, O'Brien S, et al. Hyper-CVAD program in Burkitt's-type adult acute lymphoblastic leukemia. J Clin Oncol 1999;17:2461–2470.
168. Omura GA, Moffitt S, Vogler WR, Salter MM. Combination chemotherapy of adult acute lymphoblastic leukemia with randomized central nervous system prophylaxis. Blood 1980;55:199–204.
169. Durrant IJ, Richards SM. Results of Medical Research Council trial UKALL IX in acute lymphoblastic leukaemia in adults: report from the Medical Research Council Working Party on Adult Leukaemia. Br J Haematol 1993;85:84–92.
170. Tucker J, Prior PF, Green CR, et al. Minimal neuropsychological sequelae following prophylactic treatment of the central nervous system in adult leukaemia and lymphoma. Br J Cancer 1989;60:775–780.
171. Pullen J, Boyett J, Shuster J, et al. Extended triple intrathecal chemotherapy trial for prevention of CNS relapse in good-risk and poor-risk patients with B-progenitor acute lymphoblastic leukemia: a Pediatric Oncology Group study. J Clin Oncol 1993;11:839–849.
172. Balis FM, Lester CM, Chrousos GP, Heideman RL, Poplack DG. Differences in cerebrospinal fluid penetration of corticosteroids: possible relationship to the prevention of meningeal leukemia. J Clin Oncol 1987;5:202–207.

173. Mandelli F, Annino L, Vegna ML, et al. GIMEMA ALL 0288: a multicentric study on adult acute lymphoblastic leukemia. Preliminary results. Leukemia 1992;6(suppl 2):182–185.
174. Cassileth PA, Andersen JW, Bennett JM, et al. Adult acute lymphocytic leukemia: the Eastern Cooperative Oncology Group experience. Leukemia 1992;6(suppl 2):178–181.
175. Goekbuget N, Auion-Freire E, Diedrich H, et al. Characteristics and outcome of CNS relapse in patients with adult acute lymphoblastic leukemia. Blood 1999;94:288a.
176. Dekker AW, van't Veer MB, Sizoo W, et al. Intensive postremission chemotherapy without maintenance therapy in adults with acute lymphoblastic leukemia. Dutch Hemato-Oncology Research Group. J Clin Oncol 1997;15:476–482.
177. De Witte T, Awwad B, Boezeman J, et al. Role of allogeneic bone marrow transplantation in adolescent or adult patients with acute lymphoblastic leukaemia or lymphoblastic lymphoma in first remission. Bone Marrow Transplant 1994;14:767–774.
178. Horowitz MM, Messerer D, Hoelzer D, et al. Chemotherapy compared with bone marrow transplantation for adults with acute lymphoblastic leukemia in first remission. Ann Intern Med 1991;115:13–18.
179. Sebban C, Lepage E, Vernant JP, et al. Allogeneic bone marrow transplantation in adult acute lymphoblastic leukemia in first complete remission: a comparative study. French Group of Therapy of Adult Acute Lymphoblastic Leukemia. J Clin Oncol 1994;12:2580–2587.
180. Avivi I, Rowe JM, Goldstone AH. Stem cell transplantation in adult ALL patients. Best Pract Res Clin Haematol 2002;15:653–674.
181. Vey N, Blaise D, Stoppa AM, et al. Bone marrow transplantation in 63 adult patients with acute lymphoblastic leukemia in first complete remission. Bone Marrow Transplant 1994;14:383–388.
182. Attal M, Blaise D, Marit G, et al. Consolidation treatment of adult acute lymphoblastic leukemia: a prospective, randomized trial comparing allogeneic versus autologous bone marrow transplantation and testing the impact of recombinant interleukin-2 after autologous bone marrow transplantation. BGMT Group. Blood 1995;86:1619–1628.
183. Fiere D, Lepage E, Sebban C, et al. Adult acute lymphoblastic leukemia: a multicentric randomized trial testing bone marrow transplantation as postremission therapy. The French Group on Therapy for Adult Acute Lymphoblastic Leukemia. J Clin Oncol 1993;11:1990–2001.
184. Powles R, Sirohi B, Treleaven J, et al. The role of posttransplantation maintenance chemotherapy in improving the outcome of autotransplantation in adult acute lymphoblastic leukemia. Blood 2002;100:1641–1647.
185. Powles R, Mehta J, Singhal S, et al. Autologous bone marrow or peripheral blood stem cell transplantation followed by maintenance chemotherapy for adult acute lymphoblastic leukemia in first remission: 50 cases from a single center. Bone Marrow Transplant 1995;16:241–247.
186. Mizuta S, Ito Y, Kohno A, et al. Accurate quantitation of residual tumor burden at bone marrow harvest predicts timing of subsequent relapse in patients with common ALL treated by autologous bone marrow transplantation. Nagoya BMT Group. Bone Marrow Transplant 1999;24:777–784.
187. Batista AG, Col CF. Autologous stem cell transplantation and purging in adult acute lymphoblastic leukaemia. Best Pract Res Clin Haematol 2003;15:675.
188. Martino R, Brunet S, Sureda A, Mateu R, Altes A, Domingo-Albos A. Treatment of refractory and relapsed adult acute leukemia using a uniform chemotherapy protocol. Leuk Lymphoma 1993;11:393–398.
189. Weisdorf DJ, Billett AL, Hannan P, et al. Autologous versus unrelated donor allogeneic marrow transplantation for acute lymphoblastic leukemia. Blood 1997;90:2962–2968.
190. Berman E. Recent advances in the treatment of acute leukemia: 1999. Curr Opin Hematol 2000;7:205–211.
191. Flandrin G, Brouet JC, Daniel MT, Preud'homme JL. Acute leukemia with Burkitt's tumor cells: a study of six cases with special reference to lymphocyte surface markers. Blood 1975;45:183–188.
192. Murphy SB, Bowman WP, Abromowitch M, et al. Results of treatment of advanced-stage Burkitt's lymphoma and B cell (SIg+) acute lymphoblastic leukemia with high-dose fractionated cyclophosphamide and coordinated high-dose methotrexate and cytarabine. J Clin Oncol 1986;4:1732–1739.
193. Lee EJ, Petroni GR, Schiffer CA, et al. Brief-duration high-intensity chemotherapy for patients with small noncleaved-cell lymphoma or FAB L3 acute lymphocytic leukemia: results of cancer and leukemia group B study 9251. J Clin Oncol 2001;19:4014–4022.
194. Rizzieri DA, Johnson JL, Niedzwiecki D, et al. Intensive chemotherapy with and without cranial radiation for Burkitt leukemia and lymphoma: final results of Cancer and Leukemia Group B Study 9251. Cancer (Phila) 2004;100:1438–1448.
195. Faderl S, Garcia-Manero G, Thomas DA, Kantarjian HM. Philadelphia chromosome-positive acute lymphoblastic leukemia: current concepts and future perspectives. Rev Clin Exp Hematol 2002;6:142–160; discussion 200–202.
196. Dunlop LC, Powles R, Singhal S, et al. Bone marrow transplantation for Philadelphia chromosome-positive acute lymphoblastic leukemia. Bone Marrow Transplant 1996;17:365–369.
197. Stockschlader M, Hegewisch-Becker S, Kruger W, et al. Bone marrow transplantation for Philadelphia-chromosome-positive acute lymphoblastic leukemia. Bone Marrow Transplant 1995;16:663–667.
198. Deane M, Koh M, Foroni L, et al. FLAG-idarubicin and allogeneic stem cell transplantation for Ph-positive ALL beyond first remission. Bone Marrow Transplant 1998;22:1137–1143.
199. Snyder DS, Nademanee AP, O'Donnell MR, et al. Long-term follow-up of 23 patients with Philadelphia chromosome-positive acute lymphoblastic leukemia treated with allogeneic bone marrow transplant in first complete remission. Leukemia 1999;13:2053–2058.
200. Sierra J, Radich J, Hansen JA, et al. Marrow transplants from unrelated donors for treatment of Philadelphia chromosome-positive acute lymphoblastic leukemia. Blood 1997;90:1410–1414.
201. Druker BJ, Tamura S, Buchdunger E, et al. Effects of a selective inhibitor of the Abl tyrosine kinase on the growth of Bcr-Abl positive cells. Nat Med 1996;2:561–566.
202. Ottmann OG, Druker BJ, Sawyers CL, et al. A phase 2 study of imatinib in patients with relapsed or refractory Philadelphia chromosome-positive acute lymphoid leukemias. Blood 2002;100:1965–1971.
203. Thomas DA, Faderl S, Cortes J, et al. Treatment of Philadelphia chromosome-positive acute lymphocytic leukemia with hyper-CVAD and imatinib mesylate. Blood 2004;103:4396–4407.
204. Wassmann B, Gokbuget N, Scheuring UJ, et al. A randomized multicenter open label phase II study to determine the safety and efficacy of induction therapy with imatinib (Glivec, formerly STI571) in comparison with standard induction chemotherapy in elderly (>55 years) patients with Philadelphia chromosome-positive (Ph+/BCR-ABL+) acute lymphoblastic leukemia (ALL) (CSTI571ADE 10). Ann Hematol 2003;82:716–720.
205. Pui CH, Frankel LS, Carroll AJ, et al. Clinical characteristics and treatment outcome of childhood acute lymphoblastic leukemia with the t(4;11)(q21;q23): a collaborative study of 40 cases. Blood 1991;77:440–447.
206. Reiter A, Schrappe M, Ludwig WD, et al. Chemotherapy in 998 unselected childhood acute lymphoblastic leukemia patients.

Results and conclusions of the multicenter trial ALL-BFM 86. Blood 1994;84:3122–3133.

207. Ottmann OG, Hoelzer D. Growth factors in the treatment of acute lymphoblastic leukemia. Leuk Res 1998;22:1171–1178.
208. Papamichael D, Andrews T, Owen D, et al. Intensive chemotherapy for adult acute lymphoblastic leukaemia given with or without granulocyte-macrophage colony stimulating factor. Ann Hematol 1996;73:259–263.
209. Holdsworth MT, Mathew P. Efficacy of colony-stimulating factors in acute leukemia. Ann Pharmacother 2001;35:92–108.
210. Ottmann OG, Hoelzer D, Gracien E, et al. Concomitant granulocyte colony-stimulating factor and induction chemoradiotherapy in adult acute lymphoblastic leukemia: a randomized phase III trial. Blood 1995;86:444–450.
211. Geissler K, Koller E, Hubmann E, et al. Granulocyte colony-stimulating factor as an adjunct to induction chemotherapy for adult acute lymphoblastic leukemia: a randomized phase III study. Blood 1997;90:590–596.
212. Ozer H, Armitage JO, Bennett CL, et al. 2000 update of recommendations for the use of hematopoietic colony-stimulating factors: evidence-based, clinical practice guidelines. American Society of Clinical Oncology Growth Factors Expert Panel. J Clin Oncol 2000;18:3558–3585.
213. Verma A, Stock W. Management of adult acute lymphoblastic leukemia: moving toward a risk-adapted approach. Curr Opin Oncol 2001;13:14–20.
214. Ellison RR, Mick R, Cuttner J, et al. The effects of postinduction intensification treatment with cytarabine and daunorubicin in adult acute lymphocytic leukemia: a prospective randomized clinical trial by Cancer and Leukemia Group B. J Clin Oncol 1991;9:2002–2015.
215. Behrendt H, van Leeuwen EF, Schuwirth C, et al. The significance of an isolated central nervous system relapse, occurring as first relapse in children with acute lymphoblastic leukemia. Cancer (Phila) 1989;63:2066–2072.
216. Ribeiro RC, Rivera GK, Hudson M, et al. An intensive retreatment protocol for children with an isolated CNS relapse of acute lymphoblastic leukemia. J Clin Oncol 1995;13:333–338.
217. Ritchey AK, Pollock BH, Lauer SJ, Andejeski Y, Barredo J, Buchanan GR. Improved survival of children with isolated CNS relapse of acute lymphoblastic leukemia: a Pediatric Oncology Group study. J Clin Oncol 1999;17:3745–3752.
218. Chamberlain MC, Khatibi S, Kim JC, Howell SB, Chatelut E, Kim S. Treatment of leptomeningeal metastasis with intraventricular administration of depot cytarabine (DTC 101). A phase I study. Arch Neurol 1993;50:261–264.
219. Glantz MJ, LaFollette S, Jaeckle KA, et al. Randomized trial of a slow-release versus a standard formulation of cytarabine for the intrathecal treatment of lymphomatous meningitis. J Clin Oncol 1999;17:3110–3116.
220. Thompson CB, Sanders JE, Flournoy N, Buckner CD, Thomas ED. The risks of central nervous system relapse and leukoencephalopathy in patients receiving marrow transplants for acute leukemia. Blood 1986;67:195–199.
221. Barnett MJ, Rohatiner AZ, Ganesan TS, Richards MA, Miller A, Lister TA. A phase II study of high-dose cytosine arabinoside in the treatment of acute leukaemia in adults. Cancer Chemother Pharmacol 1987;19:169–171.
222. Bassan R, Cornelli PE, Battista R, et al. Intensive retreatment of adults and children with acute lymphoblastic leukemia. Hematol Oncol 1992;10:105–110.
223. Bassan R, Lerede T, Barbui T. Strategies for the treatment of recurrent acute lymphoblastic leukemia in adults. Haematologica 1996;81:20–36.
224. Ryan DH, Kopecky KJ, Head D, et al. Phase II evaluation of teniposide and ifosfamide in refractory adult acute lymphocytic leukemia: a Southwest Oncology Group Study. Cancer Treat Rep 1987;71:713–716.
225. Paciucci PA, Keaveney C, Cuttner J, Holland JF. Mitoxantrone, vincristine, and prednisone in adults with relapsed or primarily refractory acute lymphocytic leukemia and terminal deoxynucleotidyl transferase positive blastic phase chronic myelocytic leukemia. Cancer Res 1987;47:5234–5237.
226. Hiddemann W, Buchner T, Heil G, et al. Treatment of refractory acute lymphoblastic leukemia in adults with high dose cytosine arabinoside and mitoxantrone (HAM). Leukemia 1990;4:637–640.
227. Kantarjian HM, Walters RL, Keating MJ, et al. Mitoxantrone and high-dose cytosine arabinoside for the treatment of refractory acute lymphocytic leukemia. Cancer (Phila) 1990;65:5–8.
228. Petti MC, Mandelli F. Idarubicin in acute leukemias: experience of the Italian Cooperative Group GIMEMA. Semin Oncol 1989; 16:10–15.
229. Capizzi RL, Keiser LW, Sartorelli AC. Combination chemotherapy—theory and practice. Semin Oncol 1977;4:227–253.
230. Gore M, Powles R, Lakhani A, et al. Treatment of relapsed and refractory acute leukaemia with high-dose cytosine arabinoside and etoposide. Cancer Chemother Pharmacol 1989;23:373–376.
231. Sanz GF, Sanz MA, Rafecas FJ, Martinez JA, Martin-Aragones G, Marty ML. Teniposide and cytarabine combination chemotherapy in the treatment of relapsed adolescent and adult acute lymphoblastic leukemia. Cancer Treat Rep 1986;70:1321–1323.
232. Jeha S, Gandhi V, Chan KW, et al. Clofarabine, a novel nucleoside analog, is active in pediatric patients with advanced leukemia. Blood 2004;103:784–789.
233. Kantarjian H, Gandhi V, Cortes J, et al. Phase 2 clinical and pharmacologic study of clofarabine in patients with refractory or relapsed acute leukemia. Blood 2003;102:2379–2386.
234. Kantarjian HM, Gandhi V, Kozuch P, et al. Phase I clinical and pharmacology study of clofarabine in patients with solid and hematologic cancers. J Clin Oncol 2003;21:1167–1173.
235. Faderl S, Gandhi V, Garcia-Manero G. Clofarabine is active in combination with cytarabine in adult patients in first relapsed and primary refractory acute leukemia and high-risk myelodysplastic syndrome. Blood 2003;102:615a.
236. Gandhi V, Plunkett W, Rodriguez CO Jr, et al. Compound GW506U78 in refractory hematologic malignancies: relationship between cellular pharmacokinetics and clinical response. J Clin Oncol 1998;16:3607–615.
237. Kisor DF, Plunkett W, Kurtzberg J, et al. Pharmacokinetics of nelarabine and 9-beta-D-arabinofuranosyl guanine in pediatric and adult patients during a phase I study of nelarabine for the treatment of refractory hematologic malignancies. J Clin Oncol 2000;18:995–1003.
238. De Angelo DJ, Yu D, Richards SM. A phase II study of 2-amino-9-alpha-D-arabinosyl-6-methoxy-*9H*-purine (506U78) in patients with relapsed or refractory T-lineage acute lymphoblastic leukemia (ALL) or lymphoblastic lymphoma (LBL): CALGB Study 19801. Blood 2002;100:198a.
239. Thiesing JT, Ohno-Jones S, Kolibaba KS. Efficacy of an ABL tyrosine kinase inhibitor in conjunction with other anti-neoplastic agents against BCR-ABL positive cells. Blood 1999;94.
240. Uckun FM, Messinger Y, Chen CL, et al. Treatment of therapy-refractory B-lineage acute lymphoblastic leukemia with an apoptosis-inducing CD19-directed tyrosine kinase inhibitor. Clin Cancer Res 1999;5:3906–3913.
241. Hale G, Swirsky D, Waldmann H, Chan LC. Reactivity of rat monoclonal antibody CAMPATH-1 with human leukaemia cells and its possible application for autologous bone marrow transplantation. Br J Haematol 1985;60:41–48.
242. Dyer MJ, Hale G, Hayhoe FG, Waldmann H. Effects of CAMPATH-1 antibodies in vivo in patients with lymphoid malignancies: influence of antibody isotype. Blood 1989;73: 1431–1439.
243. Kolitz JE, O'Mara V, Willemze R. Treatment of acute lymphoblastic leukemia with campath. Blood 1994;84:301a.

244. Thomas D, Cortes J, Giles F. The modified hyper-CVAD regimen in newly diagnosed adult acute lymphoblastic leukemia. Blood 2001;98:590a.
245. Grossbard ML, Lambert JM, Goldmacher VS, et al. Anti-B4-blocked ricin: a phase I trial of 7-day continuous infusion in patients with B-cell neoplasms. J Clin Oncol 1993;11:726–737.
246. Szatrowski TP, Dodge RK, Reynolds C, et al. Lineage specific treatment of adult patients with acute lymphoblastic leukemia in first remission with anti-B4-blocked ricin or high-dose cytarabine: Cancer and Leukemia Group B Study 9311. Cancer (Phila) 2003;97:1471–1480.
247. Campos L, Sabido O, Sebban C, et al. Expression of BCL-2 proto-oncogene in adult acute lymphoblastic leukemia. Leukemia 1996;10:434–438.
248. Del Principe MI, Del Poeta G, Maurillo L, et al. P-glycoprotein and BCL-2 levels predict outcome in adult acute lymphoblastic leukaemia. Br J Haematol 2003;121:730–738.
249. Marcucci G, Byrd JC, Dai G, et al. Phase 1 and pharmacodynamic studies of G3139, a Bcl-2 antisense oligonucleotide, in combination with chemotherapy in refractory or relapsed acute leukemia. Blood 2003;101:425–432.
250. Stone RM. Treatment of acute myeloid leukemia: state-of-the-art and future directions. Semin Hematol 2002;39:4–10.
251. Johnstone RW, Licht JD. Histone deacetylase inhibitors in cancer therapy: is transcription the primary target? Cancer Cell 2003;4:13–18.
252. Romanski A, Bacic B, Bug G, et al. Use of a novel histone deacetylase inhibitor to induce apoptosis in cell lines of acute lymphoblastic leukemia. Haematologica 2004;89:419–426.
253. Ribera JM, Ortega JJ, Oriol A, et al. Late intensification chemotherapy has not improved the results of intensive chemotherapy in adult acute lymphoblastic leukemia. Results of a prospective multicenter randomized trial (PETHEMA ALL-89). Spanish Society of Hematology. Haematologica 1998;83: 222–230.
254. Oh H, Gale RP, Zhang MJ, et al. Chemotherapy vs. HLA-identical sibling bone marrow transplants for adults with acute lymphoblastic leukemia in first remission. Bone Marrow Transplant 1998;22:253–257.
255. Report from the International Bone Marrow Transplant Registry. Advisory Committee of the International Bone Marrow Transplant Registry. Bone Marrow Transplant 1989;4:221–228.
256. Barrett AJ, Horowitz MM, Gale RP, et al. Marrow transplantation for acute lymphoblastic leukemia: factors affecting relapse and survival. Blood 1989;74:862–871.
257. Mortimer J, Blinder MA, Schulman S, et al. Relapse of acute leukemia after marrow transplantation: natural history and results of subsequent therapy. J Clin Oncol 1989;7:50–57.
258. Doney K, Fisher LD, Appelbaum FR, et al. Treatment of adult acute lymphoblastic leukemia with allogeneic bone marrow transplantation. Multivariate analysis of factors affecting acute graft-versus-host disease, relapse, and relapse-free survival. Bone Marrow Transplant 1991;7:453–459.
259. Grigg AP, Szer J, Beresford J, et al. Factors affecting the outcome of allogeneic bone marrow transplantation for adult patients with refractory or relapsed acute leukaemia. Br J Haematol 1999;107:409–418.

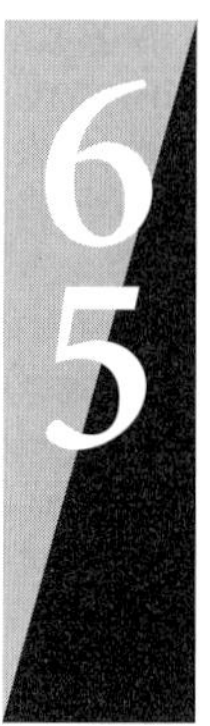

Chronic Lymphocytic Leukemia and Related Chronic Leukemias

Thomas S. Lin and John C. Byrd

The treatment of chronic lymphocytic leukemia (CLL) and related chronic leukemias remains palliative, although long-term survival has been achieved for the subset of patients with hairy cell leukemia. Despite this, the past decade has seen tremendous advancements in the understanding and treatment of these diseases, with the advent of purine analogues, such as fludarabine and monoclonal antibodies, such as rituximab and alemtuzumab. This chapter focuses on recent developments in identifying prognostic factors in CLL, as well as advances in the treatment of these diseases. Particular emphasis is given to the expanding role of monoclonal antibody therapies in these diseases.[1–3]

Chronic Lymphocytic Leukemia

The Disease

Chronic lymphocytic leukemia (CLL) is the most common adult leukemia in the Western world, accounting for a third of newly diagnosed adult leukemia patients; approximately 7,000 patients are diagnosed annually in the United States.[4] The vast majority (95%) of patients present with B-CLL, but a small percentage have T-CLL that, by the current World Health Organization (WHO) classification, would be accorded the title T-cell prolymphocytic leukemia. The optimal treatment for newly diagnosed CLL remains undefined. Although most patients with CLL respond to initial therapy, treatment is not curative, and several large randomized studies failed to show a survival advantage for early treatment of asymptomatic, early-stage patients.[5–7] Despite the advent of new therapeutic agents, such as fludarabine, which have resulted in improved complete response (CR) rates and progression-free survival (PFS), overall survival (OS) has not improved to date.[8–10] The inherent resistance of CLL to cytotoxic therapy is largely the result of defective apoptosis. In contrast to acute leukemias, which are characterized by uncontrolled proliferation, CLL arises from cellular defects in programmed cell death.

CLL is a disease of the elderly with a median age at diagnosis of approximately 65 years; most patients are 50 or older.[4] The male-to-female ratio is approximately 1.7, and men have a poorer prognosis than women. An increasing number of younger patients are being diagnosed at an earlier stage of the disease; however, it is unclear whether this reflects a change in the natural history of the disease or merely a change in surveillance practices. Despite its indolent nature, the impact of CLL on survival in both young and elderly patients is substantial. Median expected life expectancy in patients diagnosed before age 50 is 12.3 years, compared to 31.2 years in the age-matched control group.[11] Although CLL reduces the life expectancy of younger patients, the poorest survival following diagnosis is observed in elderly patients.

Establishing the initial diagnosis of CLL, as defined by the NCI (National Cancer Institute) Working Group, requires an absolute lymphocytosis of more than 5,000/μL.[4] Morphologically, the lymphocytes must appear mature with less than 55% prolymphocytes. The bone marrow aspirate smear must show more than 30% of all nucleated cells to be lymphoid, or the bone marrow core biopsy must show lymphoid infiltrates compatible with marrow involvement by CLL. The overall cellularity must be normocellular or hypercellular. Immunophenotyping must reveal a predominant B-cell monoclonal population sharing a B-cell marker (CD19, CD20, CD22, CD79b) with the CD5 antigen, in the absence of other pan-T-cell markers. Surface immunoglobulin (Ig) density is generally low; CLL cells can rarely have bright-surface Ig expression but almost always express CD23 without overexpression of cyclin D1. The WHO classification includes small lymphocytic lymphoma (SLL) with CLL, as SLL and CLL represent similar immunophenotypic and genetic diseases.

Staging Systems

Patients with CLL are staged utilizing either the Rai or Binet system.[4] Both systems stage patients by the sites of disease and/or degree of cytopenias induced by marrow replacement. Patients can be categorized into three groups. In the modified Rai system, patients in the low-risk group (stage 0) exhibit lymphocytosis alone, intermediate-risk patients also have lymphadenopathy (stage I) and/or splenomegaly (stage II), and high-risk patients have anemia (hemoglobin less than 11.0 g/dL, stage III) and/or thrombocytopenia (platelets fewer than 100×10^9/L, stage IV). The Binet system stages patients by the number of sites involved for low- and intermediate-risk (stage A less than three lymphatic regions, stage B three or more lymphatic regions); advanced-stage C patients have anemia (hemoglobin less than 10.0 g/dL) or thrombocytopenia (platelets fewer than 100×10^9/L). A prospective comparison of these two staging systems by the French Cooperative Group on CLL demonstrated the Binet system to be more effective at discriminating outcome among early-stage patients. Subsequent studies identified a group of patients with smoldering CLL, whose risk of progression to symptomatic CLL was 14% to 17% at 5 years, and whose clinical outcome matched age-matched control population. However, both clinical staging systems fail to discriminate adequately the expected clinical outcome for a large subset of early-stage CLL patients. Improved prognostic discriminating tests are needed to improve our ability to predict clinical outcome and allow adoption of risk-adaptive strategies in this diverse disease.

New Genetic Markers That Identify High-Risk Prognostic Features in CLL

A rapidly evolving area of CLL research is the identification of negative prognostic factors that predict for early progression, poor response to therapy, and inferior survival. CLL is a heterogeneous disease, with a widely varied natural history. New molecular techniques have identified several factors that predict how quickly patients will require therapy or will relapse after treatment. Interphase cytogenetic analysis, using fluorescence in situ hybridization (FISH) probes, is one such useful tool and allows detection of chromosomal abnormalities that may not be seen by traditional metaphase analysis. Interphase FISH analysis of 325 CLL patients detected chromosomal abnormalities in 82% of patients.[12] The most common findings were deletion of 13q14 (55% of patients), trisomy 12 (16%), translocation or deletion of 17p13 (7%), and deletion of 11q22–23 (18%). Deletion of 13q14 leads to loss of a presumed tumor suppressor gene at the D13S25 locus. Deletion of the 13q14 locus predicts a favorable prognosis, with a median survival of 133 months (compared to 111 months for normal karyotype) and a median treatment-free interval of 92 months. Trisomy 12 is often seen in patients with advanced disease and is associated with a higher percentage of prolymphocytes and atypical immunophenotype; however, median survival (114 months) was identical to that of patients with normal karyotype. Deletion of 17p13 results in loss of the p53 tumor suppressor gene at 17p13.1 and predicts for the worst outcome among CLL patients, with poor response to standard alkylator and fludarabine therapy. Median survival was only 32 months, with a treatment-free interval of 9 months. Deletion of 11q22–23 is associated with extensive lymphadenopathy and poor prognosis; median survival was 79 months and treatment-free interval 13 months.[12] As in other hematologic malignancies, complex karyotype, with two or more cytogenetic abnormalities, is associated with a poor prognosis.

V_H Gene Mutations

Studies to date have not shown a uniform correlation between cytogenetic abnormalities and the presence or absence of mutated variable Ig heavy chains (IgV_H) in CLL. However, several publications have demonstrated that unmutated IgV_H correlates with an increased likelihood of requiring early treatment, poorer response to therapy, and inferior survival.[13–20] IgV_H genes of 84 CLL patients were sequenced; 38 patients (45%) had unmutated IgV_H, whereas 46 patients (55%) had mutated IgV_H. Median survival of Binet stage A patients with unmutated IgV_H was 95 months, compared to 293 months for patients with mutated IgV_H; survival was similarly poorer for Binet stage B and C patients with unmutated IgV_H.[13] Correlation between the absence of mutated IgV_H chains and CD38 expression of CD38 has been noted in some studies, but CD38 expression itself is an independent predictor of response to therapy.[14,15,21] Both the intensity of and percentage of CLL cells with CD38 expression (20%–30% or more of total CLL cells) are predictors of survival.[14–17,22,23] CD38 expression has been used as a surrogate marker for unmutated IgV_H, but 28% of CLL patients have discordant CD38 expression and IgV_H mutational status.[16] Median survival was significantly worse in patients with unmutated IgV_H and CD38 expression (8 years) than in patients with mutated IgV_H and absent or low CD38 expression (26 years). The same investigators reported a median survival of 310 months for patients with mutated IgV_H, compared with 119 months for unmutated IgV_H. However, the correlation with CD38 expression and V_H mutation status has not been observed by other groups. By comparison, loss or mutation of p53 in the same group of 205 CLL patients was associated with a median survival of only 47 months.[24]

ZAP-70

Recently, expression of zeta-associated protein 70 (ZAP-70), which is normally expressed in T lymphocytes, has been identified as a surrogate marker of IgV_H mutation status. This expression was initially identified in genomic profile studies, and differential expression was subsequently verified at the mRNA and protein levels.[25] CLL cells with unmutated IgV_H expressed detectable levels of ZAP-70, whereas ZAP-70 could not be detected in CLL cells with mutated IgV_H. Ligation of the B-cell receptor complex resulted in tyrosine phosphorylation of ZAP-70, association of ZAP-70 with the surface Ig, and increased tyrosine phosphorylation of cytosolic proteins, including p72syk.[26] Analysis of 56 CLL patients showed that all 32 patients expressing ZAP-70 on 20% or more of CLL cells had unmutated IgV_H, whereas 21 of 24 patients expressing ZAP-70 on less than 20% of leukemic cells, had mutated IgV_H. ZAP-70 expression did not change over, time and was correlated with rapid progression and inferior survival in Binet stage A patients.[27] A similar analysis of 107 CLL patients demonstrated a 93% correlation between ZAP-70 expression and IgV_H mutation status. CLL cells with unmutated IgV_H had 5.5-fold-higher expression of ZAP-70 than did patients with mutated IgV_H.[25] Thus, ZAP-70 appears to be the gene whose expression best predicts IgV_H mutation status.

p53 and ATM

p53 gene inactivation is a highly predictive marker for drug resistance and inferior survival in patients with CLL.[28–30] Mutations of the p53 tumor suppressor gene are seen in 10% to 20% of patients with untreated CLL, become more frequent with disease progression, and predict for poor response to alkylator or purine analogue therapy.[29–32] Deletion of 17p13.1 results in loss of the p53 gene and predicts for the worst outcome among CLL patients. Median survival with alkylator or fludarabine therapy was only 32 months, with a treatment-free interval of 9 months.[12] A similar study showed that loss or mutation of p53 was associated with a median survival of 47 months.[24]

p53 can be inactivated by mutations of the ATM (ataxia telangiectasia mutated) gene, another potential common high-risk molecular feature of CLL that has been less well characterized. ATM phosphorylates p53, allowing p53 to initiate DNA repair,[33–35] and ATM-deficient cells have increased sensitivity to both X-ray- and free-oxygen-radical-induced DNA damage.[36,37] Diminished or absent ATM protein expression, usually associated with loss or mutation of the ATM gene, negatively affects survival in CLL.[38–41] In one series of 43 CLL patients, tumor cells from all 13 patients with p53 ($n = 6$) or ATM ($n = 7$) mutations failed to undergo apoptosis following ex vivo irradiation.[42] Tumor cells from patients with ATM mutations showed diminished DNA repair and did not undergo apoptosis in response to in vitro radiation, compared to CLL cells with intact ATM and normal stimulated B lymphocytes. Thus, CLL cells with primary or secondary p53 dysfunction are predisposed to increased chromosomal damage with therapy, which leads to additional genetic instability and tumor cell resistance. Identifying therapies that circumvent dysfunctional p53 function is, therefore, a high priority.

Treatment of CLL

When to Treat

In the absence of symptoms, observation is the current practice employed for newly diagnosed patients, based upon several studies demonstrating no improvement in overall survival for asymptomatic CLL patients receiving early therapeutic intervention with chlorambucil therapy.[7] A meta-analysis that included data involving 2,048 patients in six trials demonstrated a slightly higher death rate (42.6%) among those treated early versus those randomized to deferred therapy (41.6%), although this difference was not significant.[7] It must be noted that each of these studies included a large proportion of patients with smoldering or early-stage disease. For this population of patients, therapeutic benefit would require an improvement in overall survival in excess of that observed in the age-matched control population without CLL. Furthermore, each of these studies employed chlorambucil, an agent that yields a low CR rate. With more effective therapies and use of risk stratification with new molecular techniques, reconsideration of this approach in well-designed trials seems quite prudent; this is further substantiated by the now-recognized genetic clonal evolution of CLL that occurs over time from initial diagnosis. This clonal evolution coincides with increasing resistance to apoptosis. Efforts within the German CLL Study Group and several U.S. groups are under way to examine this question with newer CLL therapies.

Determining what constitutes sufficient symptomatology to initiate treatment in CLL is subjective and confounds comparison of clinical trials. To assure uniform study entrance criteria, an NCI-sponsored Working Group on CLL established guidelines for initiation of treatment.[43] These indications include the presence of nonautoimmune cytopenias (Rai stage III and IV), symptomatic lymphadenopathy or hepatosplenomegaly, disease-related B symptoms or fatigue, extreme lymphocytosis (greater than 150–300 × 10^9/L), and autoimmune hemolytic anemia or thrombocytopenia not controlled with steroids. It is imperative to determine if a patient's symptoms are caused by CLL or a comorbid medical condition. The decision of when to start therapy remains one of the most challenging issues physicians caring for patients with CLL must make.

Alkylator Therapy

Chlorambucil and other alkylating agents served as first-line therapy for CLL for many decades.[4] Chlorambucil is generally administered as pulse therapy (40 mg/m^2 orally every 28 days). Although a high-dose (15 mg/day) continuous dosing schedule has been used in several large European studies and has obtained results superior to those of pulse therapy, high-dose therapy is associated with greater myelosuppression and frequently requires dose reduction. Although high-dose therapy may be more effective if maximal cytoreduction is desired, the less intensive pulse dosing schedule should generally be used outside the setting of a clinical study.

Fludarabine Therapy

Fludarabine-based regimens have shown significant clinical efficacy in relapsed and previously untreated CLL.[44–51] The introduction of purine analogues has led to more effective therapies for CLL, as evidenced by improved CR rates and PFS; however, no advantage in OS has been observed to date. Although fludarabine was initially approved for alkylator-refractory CLL, the drug has since become standard therapy for previously untreated CLL, based on several large randomized studies showing improved CR and PFS rates compared to alkylator-based regimens.[8–10] These studies are summarized in Table 65.1. A multicenter European study of 196 evaluable patients randomized to fludarabine or CAP showed a higher overall response rate (ORR) in favor of fludarabine (60% versus 44%). This advantage was true in both previously treated ($n = 96$, 48% versus 27%) and untreated ($n = 100$, 71% versus 60%) patients, although the difference was not statistically significant in the untreated group. Fludarabine achieved a longer median duration of response than did CAP, with a tendency toward longer OS in previously untreated patients.[8] A randomized, multicenter American study confirmed these findings in 509 previously untreated CLL patients, who were randomly assigned to receive fludarabine 25 mg/m^2 IV daily for 5 days every 28 days, chlorambucil 40 mg/m^2 PO every 28 days, or fludarabine 20 mg/m^2 daily for 5 days and chlorambucil 20 mg/m^2 PO every 28 days, for up to 12 cycles. The combination arm was closed for reasons of excessive toxicity. Fludarabine achieved superior CR, ORR, median duration of remission, and median PFS (20%, 63%, 25 months, 20 months, respectively) than did chlorambucil (4%, 37%, 14 months, 14 months, respectively). However, there was no statistically significant difference in OS (66 versus 56 months), although the study employed a cross-over design.[9] Finally, a multicenter French study randomized 938 patients with previously untreated Binet stage B and C CLL to fludarabine, CHOP, or CAP. Although CHOP and fludarabine achieved better response rates than CAP, overall survival (67–70 months) was identical in all three treatment groups.[10]

TABLE 65.1. Selected clinical trial results with fludarabine in previously untreated chronic lymphocytic leukemia (CLL) patients.

Referemce	*Regimen*	*Phase*	*No. of patients*	*CR*	*ORR*	*Mean PFS (months)*	*Mean OS (months)*
8	Flu	III	52	23	71	NR	NR
	CAP		48	17	60	7	54
9	Flu	III	170	20	63	20	66
	CLB		181	4	37	14	56
	Flu + CLB		123	20	61	Not Rep	55
10	Flu	III	341	40	71	32	69
	CHOP		357	30	72	30	67
	CAP		237	15	58	28	70
50	Flu + Cy	II	17	51	92	Not Rep	Not Rep
51	Flu + Cy	II	34	35	88	NR	NR
191	Flu + Cy	II	36	42	64	Not Rep	Not Rep
192	Flu + Cy	II	59	47	78	Not Rep	Not Rep
52	Flu	III	105	9	86	23	NR
	Flu + Cy		104	20	94	28	NR
93	Flu + Ritux	Ran II	51	47	90	NR	NR
	Flu then Ritux		53	28	77	NR	NR
97	Flu + Cy + Ritux	II	202	68	90	NR	NR

Flu, fludarabine; CAP, cyclophosphamide, adriamycin, prednisone; CLB, chlorambucil; CHOP, cyclophosphamide, adriamycin, vincristine, prednisone; Cy, cyclophosphamide; Ritux, rituximab; CR, complete response rate; ORR, overall response rate; PFS, progression-free survival; OS, overall survival; NR, not reached; Not Rep, not reported.

Thus, although large randomized studies demonstrated superior response rates and durations with fludarabine, compared to alkylator-based regimens, no survival advantage was seen with single-agent fludarabine (see Table 65.1).

Fludarabine Combination Regimens

To improve response rates over those seen with single-agent fludarabine, the purine analogue has been combined with cyclophosphamide (Flu/Cy). A large single-institution study administered fludarabine 30 mg/m^2 IV and cyclophosphamide 300–500 mg/m^2 IV daily for 3 days for up to six cycles to 128 patients with CLL (see Table 65.1). Because of myelosuppression, the dose of cyclophosphamide was decreased from 500 mg/m^2 ($n = 11$) to 300 mg/m^2 ($n = 91$). The ORR was 80% in patients naïve or sensitive to fludarabine but only 38% in fludarabine-refractory patients. This regimen achieved a 35% CR rate in previously untreated patients, similar to that expected with single-agent fludarabine. However, only 8% of patients achieving CR had minimal residual disease detectable by flow cytometry, and the median time to progression was not reached despite a median follow-up of 41 months.[51] Retrospective comparison of this result to a previous study of fludarabine and prednisone at this same institution demonstrated Flu/cy to be significantly better. Based in part upon this observation, a large study by the German CLL Study Group randomized 375 previously untreated patients to standard fludarabine versus Flu/Cy (fludarabine 30 mg/m^2 IV and cyclophosphamide 250 mg/m^2 IV daily for 3 days) every 28 days for six cycles. The ORR (94% versus 86%), CR (20% versus 9%), and median PFS (28.2 versus 22.8 months) were better in the Flu/Cy arm,[52] although toxicity was significantly worse in the combination arm. However, it must be noted that the fludarabine arm did poorly in this study, and that the CR rate obtained in the combination arm was less than the 35% rate reported by the M.D. Anderson group.[51] A slightly different regimen (fludarabine 20 mg/m^2 IV days 1–5 and cyclophosphamide 600 mg/m^2 IV day 1 every 28 days for six cycles) was administered to 37 patients with non-Hodgkin's lymphoma (NHL) and 17 patients with CLL. Patients were given granulocyte colony-stimulating factor (G-CSF) support beginning on day 8 of each cycle. The ORR and CR rates were 92% and 51%, respectively; the ORR and CR rates in the 17 CLL patients were 100% and 47%, respectively.[50] This second regimen is currently being tested as part of a large randomized Phase III U.S. Intergroup effort. The choice of fludarabine or Flu/Cy as the backbone upon which to add the monoclonal anti-CD20 antibody rituximab or other monoclonal antibody therapies, depends upon whether one believes that the current data support the contention that Flu/Cy is superior to fludarabine. At the present time, these authors prefer the use of fludarabine alone for such combination approaches.

Monoclonal Antibodies

Monoclonal antibodies offer the potential of targeted therapy with minimal toxicity to normal cells, and clinical studies over the past decade have demonstrated the feasibility, safety, and clinical efficacy of these agents in many solid and hematologic cancers. Monoclonal antibodies are now used to treat diseases as diverse as acute myeloid leukemia (AML), diffuse large B-cell NHL, mycosis fungoides, and CLL.[53–59] Recombinant DNA technology has allowed the generation of chimeric and "humanized" murine monoclonal IgG antibodies. Murine sequences are replaced with the human Fc fragment, resulting in humanized IgG molecules whose Fab portions contain only the murine sequences required to recognize the target antigen. These humanized antibodies are significantly less immunogenic and produce less infusion toxicity.[60–62] The human Fc fragment also allows chimeric antibodies to induce antibody-dependent cellular cytotoxicity (ADCC) and complement-dependent cytotoxicity (CDC). Thus, humanized monoclonal antibodies are better tolerated and more effective.

TABLE 65.2. Summary of monoclonal antibodies available in CLL.

Antibody	*Antigen*	*Description*	*Clinical status*
IDEC-C2B8 (Rituximab)	CD20	Chimeric	FDA approved
Campath-1H (Alemtuzumab)	CD52	Humanized	FDA approved
Hu1D10 (Apolizumab, Remitogen)	1D10 (HLA-DR β)	Humanized	Clinical trials
IDEC-152 (Lumiliximab)	CD23	Primatized	Clinical trials

Role of Monoclonal Antibodies in CLL

The failure of traditional cytotoxic agents to cure CLL may result from the disease's indolent nature, as well as intrinsic resistance mechanisms to chemotherapy. Only a small fraction of CLL cells undergo growth and division at a time. Cytotoxic agents often act only against dividing cells undergoing transcription and DNA replication and thus are ineffective against resting cells. Fludarabine, which acts against both dividing and nondividing cells, is an exception to this rule. The inherent resistance of CLL to chemotherapy is the result of defective apoptosis. Antiapoptotic proteins, such as Bcl-2, Mcl-1, and XIAP are overexpressed, and high levels of Mcl-1 are associated with failure to achieve CR to fludarabine.[63] ADCC and CDC are observed after antibody therapy,[64,65] but monoclonal antibodies may exert their effects in CLL primarily by inducing apoptosis.[66,67] Thus, monoclonal antibodies act directly against the cellular defects in apoptosis that give rise to CLL. Table 65.2 summarizes the major monoclonal antibodies in current clinical use or clinical studies in CLL.

Rituximab

Preclinical Studies Rituximab (Rituxan, IDEC-C2B8), a chimeric murine monoclonal antibody that recognizes the CD20 antigen on the surface of normal and malignant B cells, is the best studied and most widely used monoclonal antibody in lymphoid malignancies. CD20, a calcium channel that interacts with the B-cell receptor complex, is an excellent target; it is expressed in 90% to 100% of CLL and B-cell NHL and is not internalized or shed. However, significant levels of soluble CD20 have been detected in the sera of patients with CLL by one group, and increased circulating CD20 levels correlated with beta-2-microglobulin levels and advanced-stage disease.[68] Circulating CD20 levels correlated with poor survival, and the prognostic value was independent of Rai stage.[69]

Rituximab induces ADCC and CDC, activates caspase 3, and induces apoptosis.[64–67] Rituximab induces apoptosis in vitro within 4 hours; this induction is independent of complement but requires cross-linking with anti-Fcγ antibody. The ratio of the antiapoptotic protein Mcl-1 to the proapoptotic protein Bax was significantly elevated in CLL patients who did not respond to rituximab, compared with responders.[70] Complement activation may be important, as increased expression of complement inhibitors CD55 and CD59 resulted in resistance to rituximab in NHL cell lines and CLL cells.[65,71] Blocking CD55 and CD59 resulted in a fivefold increase in rituximab-induced cell lysis of poorly responding CLL samples, although CD55 and CD59 levels did not predict complement susceptibility.[71] However, baseline expression of CD55 and CD59 was not associated with clinical response to rituximab in 21 treated patients.[70] Thus, although rituximab may act through more than one mechanism, induction of apoptosis appears to be a major contributor to the elimination of CLL cells.

Clinical Studies: Single-Agent Weekly Rituximab Phase I clinical studies in indolent B-cell NHL established a dose of 375 mg/m^2 IV weekly for four doses, although the length of treatment was empirically established. In the pivotal Phase II trial in 166 patients with relapsed or refractory indolent B-cell NHL or CLL, an ORR of 48% was seen (CR 6%) with a median response duration of 12 months.[58] Patients with indolent follicle center B-cell NHL had an ORR of 60%, whereas only 4 of 30 patients with small lymphocytic lymphoma (SLL)/CLL (13%) responded. A British study of 48 patients using the same schedule achieved only 1 partial response (PR) in 10 patients with relapsed or refractory SLL/CLL (10%), although the ORR was only 27% in patients with follicular NHL.[72] A similar study observed only 1 PR in 9 evaluable patients with fludarabine-refractory CLL (11%), although 7 patients had stable disease.[73] A study of 7 patients with refractory or relapsed CLL observed a striking, but transient, reduction (median, 93%) in peripheral lymphocyte count, but nodal disease was not affected.[74] The German CLL Study Group administered weekly rituximab to 28 patients with previously treated CLL; 7 patients (25%) achieved PR with a median duration of 20 weeks. Forty-five percent of patients experienced at least 50% reduction of peripheral lymphocyte count lasting 4 weeks or longer.[57] Finally, a Nordic multicenter study observed an ORR of 35% in 24 heavily pretreated CLL patients, with a median duration of response of only 12.5 weeks. Interestingly, 17 of 20 patients (85%) with adenopathy experienced greater than 50% reduction in nodal disease, whereas only 2 of 18 patients (11%) had reduction of marrow disease.[75]

Thus, weekly rituximab has limited activity in CLL (Table 65.3). Rituximab effectively reduces peripheral blood lymphocytosis but is less effective at reducing bone marrow or nodal disease. The preferential response of peripheral

TABLE 65.3. Selected Phase II trials of weekly rituximab in CLL and small lymphocytic lymphoma (SLL).

Reference	*Doses*	*Prior therapy*	*Evaluable patients*	*Response rate (ORR)*
McLaughlin et al., 1998[58]	4	Yes	30	13%
Nguyen et al., 1999[72]	4	Yes	10	10%
Winkler et al., 1999[73]	4	Yes	9	11%
Ladetto et al., 2000[74]	4	Yes	7	0%
Huhn et al., 2001[57]	4	Yes	28	25%
Hainsworth et al., 2003[77]	4	No	44	58%
Thomas et al., 2001[78]	8	No	21	90%

lymphocyte count may be caused by increased CD20 expression on circulating CLL cells compared to bone marrow cells. In quantitative flow cytometric studies, circulating CLL cells bound an average of 9,050 anti-CD20 molecules compared with only 4,070 molecules for bone marrow CLL cells and 3,950 molecules for lymph node CLL cells.[76] In addition, stromal cells in bone marrow and lymph nodes may provide a survival advantage to CLL cells in these environments over circulating CLL cells.

Initial CLL Therapy with Rituximab Weekly rituximab may be more effective in previously untreated SLL/CLL (see Table 65.3). Forty-four previously untreated patients with SLL/CLL received four weekly doses of rituximab 375 mg/m^2; the ORR after the first course of rituximab was 51% (CR 4%). Twenty-eight patients with stable or responsive disease received additional maintenance therapy with 4-week courses of rituximab every 6 months for up to four cycles, with an increase in the ORR to 58% (CR 9%). However, the median PFS of 19 months was shorter than the 36- to 40-month median PFS obtained by the same group using an identical regimen in previously untreated patients with follicle center NHL.[77] Nonetheless, this response duration was similar to that noted in the intergroup study with fludarabine, suggesting rituximab does have significant efficacy in the treatment of CLL. A second study of eight weekly doses of rituximab 375 mg/m^2 in 31 untreated, early-stage, asymptomatic CLL patients (21 evaluable) not meeting criteria for treatment by the NCI 96 criteria, with a beta-2-microglobulin level of 2.0 mg/dL or more, showed an ORR of 90% (CR, 19%; nodular PR, 19%).[78] The majority of patients achieved only PR, with few patients attaining CR. Toxicity in both studies was minimal except for initial infusion toxicity. Thus, although quite effective and nontoxic as a palliative regimen, rituximab as a single agent is unlikely to significantly alter long-term survival in CLL.

Limitations of Weekly Rituximab in CLL Several theories may explain the inferior efficacy of weekly rituximab in CLL, compared to its activity in indolent follicle center NHL. First, CLL/SLL cells express lower CD20 density than follicle center NHL cells, decreasing the number of target antigen sites and the amount of antibody delivered to individual tumor cells. In an analysis of 70 patients with chronic B-cell leukemias and 17 normal donors, normal B lymphocytes expressed 94,000 CD20 molecules per cell. Although other chronic B-cell leukemias, such as mantle cell lymphoma and hairy cell leukemia expressed between 123,000 and 312,000 CD20 molecules per cell, CLL cells expressed only 65,000 CD20 molecules per cell.[79] However, an analysis of 10 patients with CLL did not identify a correlation between CD20 expression and clinical response to rituximab.[80] A more plausible explanation is that the large intravascular burden of circulating CLL cells may alter the pharmacokinetics of rituximab and result in accelerated clearance of antibody from plasma. Lower trough concentrations of rituximab were observed in CLL patients who did not respond to therapy; the importance of serum rituximab levels was documented in follicle center NHL.[81,82] Serum concentrations of rituximab decrease more rapidly after treatment in CLL than in follicle center NHL. In addition, the presence of soluble CD20 in the sera of CLL patients suggests that free CD20, derived from cell membrane fragments or shed antigen, may contribute to rapid clearance of rituximab. However, a relationship between soluble CD20 levels and response to rituximab has not been demonstrated.[68] Finally, intrinsic mechanisms of resistance, such as overexpression of antiapoptotic proteins or p53 mutations may contribute to the common resistance of CLL to rituximab and cytotoxic therapy.

Rituximab Dose Escalation: Improved Clinical Response Investigators have taken two different strategies to overcome these pharmacokinetic and pharmacodynamic obstacles. Fifty patients with previously treated CLL (n = 40) or other B-cell leukemias (n = 10) received weekly rituximab dose-escalated to 2,250 mg/m^2.[83,84] Although no CLL patient achieved CR, the ORR was 40%, and a statistically significant dose-response relationship was observed; 22% of patients treated with 500 to 850 mg/m^2 responded, compared to 75% of patients treated with 2,250 mg/m^2. The ORR was 36% for CLL and 60% for other B-cell leukemias; median response duration was 8 months. Eight of 12 patients (67%) at 2,250 mg/m^2 developed grade 2 toxicity, primarily fatigue, but no grade 3 or 4 toxicity was observed.

Alternatively, 33 patients with relapsed or refractory SLL/CLL received thrice-weekly rituximab for 4 weeks.[56] Patients received 100 mg over 4 hours on the first day of therapy and 250 mg/m^2 (n = 3) or 375 mg/m^2 (n = 30) thereafter. This "stepped-up" dosing schedule was designed to minimize infusion-related toxicity. The ORR was 45% (CR, 3%), and median response duration was 10 months. Thirteen patients developed transient infusion-related toxicity that appeared to be related to cytokine release [tumor necrosis factor-alpha (TNF-α), interferon-gamma (IFN-γ), interleukin 8 (IL-8), and IL-6] but resolved by the third infusion. Thus, both dose escalation and thrice-weekly dosing improved the response rate in SLL/CLL and established a role for rituximab in the treatment of relapsed CLL. Both approaches produced few complete responses, but no therapeutic agent achieves a significant CR rate in relapsed or refractory CLL.

Toxicity Infusion-related side effects constitute the most common toxicity of rituximab but are manageable, particularly with use of a "stepped-up" dosing schedule. Patients can develop transient hypoxemia, dyspnea, and hypotension, which are partly caused by inflammatory cytokine release. Although initial studies suggested that patients with high lymphocyte counts may be at greater risk of this cytokine release syndrome, subsequent larger studies failed to support this finding. Tumor necrosis factor-alpha (TNF-α) and interleukin-6 (IL-6) peak 90 minutes after start of infusion, and their rise is accompanied by fever, chills, hypotension, and nausea.[73] These side effects are most severe with the first infusion and resolve by the third infusion in the thrice-weekly dosing schedule.[56] An uncommon but potentially severe toxicity is tumor lysis syndrome, which is generally observed in patients with high numbers of circulating CLL cells.[85,86] Patients at risk should receive prophylactic allopurinol, hydration, and careful observation, and it may be necessary to administer the first dose in an in-patient setting. However, patients who develop tumor lysis syndrome to the first dose of rituximab can safely receive subsequent doses, especially after the number of circulating CLL cells is reduced.[85] Other toxicities are minimal and should not affect administration of the antibody.

Combination Therapy There is great interest in combining monoclonal antibody therapy with cytotoxic chemotherapy in the treatment of lymphoid malignancies, and several studies have specifically examined rituximab. The low CR rates to single-agent rituximab indicate that combination with traditional cytotoxic drugs or other monoclonal antibodies may be necessary for rituximab to significantly affect long-term survival in CLL. Several clinical trials examined the use of rituximab in combination regimens against B-cell lymphoid malignancies, including CLL.[54,87–90] Rituximab was successfully combined with fludarabine in both NHL and CLL.[91,92] Concurrent administration of these two agents to 104 previously untreated CLL patients in a randomized phase II CALGB trial yielded a higher CR rate (47%) than did sequential administration (28%).[92] Patients received standard fludarabine 25 mg/m^2 days 1 to 5 every 4 weeks for six cycles (see Table 65.1). Patients were randomized to receive concurrent rituximab 375 mg/m^2 on day 1 of each cycle, with an additional day 4 dose during cycle 1, or sequential rituximab 375 mg/m^2 weekly for four doses beginning 2 months after completion of fludarabine. The median duration of response was not reached at 23 months. The 104 patients in this study experienced improved ORR (84% versus 63%), CR (38% versus 20%), 2-year PFS (67% versus 45%), and 2-year OS (93% versus 81%), compared to 179 previously untreated patients who received single-agent fludarabine in a prior CALGB trial.[93]

A multicenter European Phase II study of concurrent fludarabine and rituximab in 31 evaluable patients with CLL achieved an ORR of 87% (CR 32%), with a median duration of response of 75 weeks. Patients received fludarabine 25 mg/m^2 days 1 to 5 every 4 weeks for four cycles, and rituximab 375 mg/m^2 every 4 weeks for four doses, beginning on day 1 of cycle 3 of fludarabine. ORR and CR were similar in previously treated (ORR 91%, CR 45%) and untreated patients (ORR 85%, CR 25%). Sixteen patients developed a total of 32 infections, and 1 patient died of cerebral hemorrhage caused by prolonged thrombocytopenia.[94] The highest CR rate was achieved by a single-institution study using a combination regimen of fludarabine, cyclophosphamide, and rituximab (FCR). One hundred two evaluable patients received fludarabine 25 mg/m^2 and cyclophosphamide 250 mg/m^2 on days 2 to 4 of cycle 1 and on days 1 to 3 of cycles 2 to 6, in addition to rituximab 375 mg/m^2 on day 1 of cycle 1 and 500 mg/m^2 on day 1 of cycles 2 to 6. The ORR was 73% (CR 23%), and 5 of 13 patients in CR achieved molecular remission.[95] The same authors administered FCR to 202 previously untreated CLL patients with symptomatic disease requiring initiation of therapy by NCI criteria (see Table 65.1), achieving a CR rate of 68%.[96] Molecular remissions were observed in 49 of 100 tested patients who achieved CR (49%) and 9 of 27 patients who achieved nPR or PR (33%); 14 of 33 polymerase chain reaction (PCR)-negative patients developed molecular evidence of relapse, usually within 24 months of completing treatment.[97] The major toxicities of this regimen were grade 4 neutropenia and infection, which occurred in 20% and 17%, respectively, of treatment cycles.[98]

Finally, an aggressive upfront regimen incorporating fludarabine and rituximab has been given to 13 previously untreated patients with CLL, as cytoreductive therapy before autologous stem cell transplantation. Patients received fludarabine 25 mg/m^2 days 1 to 3, cyclophosphamide 200 mg/m^2 days 1 to 3, and mitoxantrone 10 mg/m^2 day 1 every 4 weeks for four to six cycles, followed by rituximab 375 mg/m^2 weekly for four doses. All patients responded (ORR, 100%; CR, 77%), and 4 patients (31%) achieved a molecular remission.[99] The ability of this regimen to induce complete hematologic and molecular remissions is promising, although patients have not been followed long enough to determine if these initial remissions will be durable.

Radioisotope Conjugates of Anti-CD20 Anti-CD20 monoclonal antibody has been conjugated to the radioisotopes yttrium-90 (^{90}Y-ibritumomab; Zevalin) and iodine-131 (^{131}I-tositumomab; Bexxar). Several published clinical trials have demonstrated the efficacy of Zevalin and Bexxar in indolent B-cell NHL, particularly indolent follicle center NHL; the results of these trials have been extensively reviewed elsewhere. There has been reluctance to use Zevalin and Bexxar in patients with SLL/CLL because of concern about myelotoxicity resulting from bystander radiation to normal hematopoietic cells in patients with significant marrow disease. Nonetheless, results of a Phase I dose study indicated that Bexxar is effective in previously treated patients with advanced CLL. Eleven patients with heavily pretreated CLL received a total body dose of 35 to 55 cGy; 3 patients (27%) achieved PR and 6 patients (55%) had stable disease.[100] As expected, myelosuppression was the dose-limiting toxicity and was related to the total radiation dose. A similar study of Zevalin for minimal residual disease was conducted in 13 evaluable CLL patients who had achieved a PR (n = 12) or nodular PR (n = 1) to prior therapy. Significant responses were seen in 2 patients, and prolonged neutropenia (ANC less than 1,000 for median of 42 days) and thrombocytopenia (less than 100,000 for median of 42 days) were observed.[101] Thus, myelosuppression will likely limit the clinical use of Zevalin and Bexxar in patients with significant marrow disease. However, radioisotope conjugates may be more effective than rituximab in SLL/CLL patients with bulky nodal disease, due to delivery of radiation to surrounding tumor cells. Future studies of Zevalin and Bexxar in SLL/CLL should focus on patients with primarily bulky lymphadenopathy and limited marrow involvement. In addition, sequential combination regimens with agents, such as Campath-1H, which effectively reduces blood and marrow disease but has limited activity against nodal disease, should be investigated.

Summary Rituximab is active in CLL, although dose intensification is needed to obtain maximal clinical benefit. Single-agent rituximab produces few CRs and will not, by itself, substantially improve long-term survival in CLL. The combination of rituximab with fludarabine has improved CR rates, and further studies are needed to determine if a higher CR results in improved long-term survival. Although most studies have combined rituximab with traditional cytotoxic agents, several trials are now examining the use of rituximab with other monoclonal antibodies, such as Campath-1H.

Campath-1H

Preclinical Studies Campath-1H (Alemtuzumab) is a humanized anti-CD52 monoclonal antibody that effectively fixes complement and depletes normal lymphocytes and lymphoma cells.[102–104] CD52, a 21- to 28-kDa glycopeptide expressed on the surface of nearly all human lymphocytes, monocytes, and macrophages; a small subset of granulocytes; but not erythrocytes, platelets, or bone marrow stem cells. CD52 is expressed on all CLL cells and indolent B-cell NHL cells.[105,106] Its physiologic function remains unknown, but cross-linking of CD52 on B-cell and T-cell lymphoma cell lines resulted in growth inhibition.[107] Antibody binding of CD52 results in profound complement activation and ADCC. CD52 is not shed, internalized, or modulated. Thus, CD52 is an ideal antigen for targeted immunotherapy. However, the ubiquitous expression of CD52 on normal lymphocytes and monocytes has resulted in increased hematologic and immune toxicity with Campath-1H, manifested by neutropenia, prolonged lymphopenia, and infectious complications.

Campath-1H acts in vivo by inducing programmed cell death. In vivo blood samples showed 19% to 92% reduction in expression of the antiapoptotic protein Bcl-2 in six of eight patients undergoing Campath-1H therapy.[82] In addition, expression of the antiapoptotic proteins Mcl-1 and XIAP was downregulated by treatment with Campath-1H. Campath-1H induced activation of caspase 3 and cleavage of the DNA repair enzyme poly(ADP-ribose) polymerase (PARP), indicating that apoptosis is an important mechanism of action of this antibody.[82]

Clinical Trials Phase I studies established a dose of 30 mg IV three times per week for 4 to 12 weeks. Campath-1H induced significantly more infusion toxicity than rituximab, and a stepped-up dosing schedule was necessary to diminish initial infusion toxicity and make the antibody tolerable. An initial dose of 3mg was given on day 1, 10mg on day 2, and 30mg on day 3; once the full dose of 30mg was achieved, patients were given 30mg thrice weekly. Several clinical studies established the efficacy of Campath-1H in CLL, as summarized in Table 65.4.[59,108–111] A multicenter, European Phase II study administered Campath-1H 30mg thrice weekly for up to 12 weeks to 29 recurrent and refractory CLL patients. The ORR was 42%, but only 1 patient (4%) achieved CR.[59] The antibody cleared CLL cells from the peripheral blood in 97% of patients but was less effective at eliminating marrow (36%) or nodal disease (7%).

The pivotal CAM211 trial administered the same Campath-1H regimen to 93 heavily pretreated, fludarabine-refractory CLL patients; an intent-to-treat ORR of 33% was observed, although only 2% of patients achieved CR.[110] Median time to progression for responders was 9.5 months, with a median overall survival of 16 months for all patients and 32 months for responders. The median peripheral blood CLL count decreased by more than 99.9%, but the antibody was less effective against nodal disease. Although 74% of all patients with nodal disease responded, with 27% experiencing resolution of their adenopathy, patients with bulky lymph nodes did significantly poorer. Although 90% of patients with lymph nodes measuring less than or equal to 2cm responded, with 64% achieving resolution of their adenopathy, only 12% of patients with lymph nodes greater than 5cm responded, with no patients enjoying resolution of their adenopathy. All patients were placed on prophylactic antibacterial and antiviral agents, and toxicity was manageable. Patients with poor performance status did markedly worse than patients with no or minimal symptoms from their disease.

The activity of Campath-1H in CLL was confirmed by a multiinstitutional study in 136 patients with fludarabine-refractory B-CLL who received Campath-1H 30mg thrice weekly for up to 12 weeks on a compassionate basis.[112] The ORR was 40% (CR 7%), and median PFS and OS of responders were 7.3 and 13.4 months, respectively. Similarly, 41 patients with relapsed B-CLL and 1 patient with T-CLL were treated with Campath-1H 30mg IVB thrice weekly for 4 weeks in a single-institution study.[113] Two patients with B-CLL achieved CR (5%), and 9 patients achieved PR (21%), for an ORR of 26%. Interestingly, 7 of 12 patients with B- or T-PLL responded (3 CR, 4 PR, ORR 58%). Although Campath-1H was more effective at eliminating disease in peripheral blood (CR, 36%; PR, 36%) and bone marrow (CR, 41%; PR, 28%) than in lymph nodes (CR, 23%; PR, 13%), a greater response in nodal disease was seen in this study than in previous trials using Campath-1H. A recent update of this study showed an ORR of 35% (CR, 12%) in 78 patients with indolent lymphoproliferative disorders (42 CLL), with a median duration of response of 18 months.[114] Although Campath-1H is effective therapy in previously treated patients with CLL, the antibody is less effective against bulky lymphadenopathy than it is against peripheral blood or bone marrow disease. In addition, patients with an ECOG performance status of 2 or greater had a 0% response rate in the pivotal study, likely the result of inability to tolerate the initial infusion toxicity and worsening of cytopenias often observed with Campath-1H therapy.

Upfront Therapy in Previously Untreated Patients A Phase II clinical trial administered subcutaneous (SC) Campath-1H to 41 previously untreated patients with CLL. Patients received a prolonged course of Campath-1H 30mg SC three times per week for up to 18 weeks. Except for transient grade I–II fever, first-dose reactions were minimal. The

TABLE 65.4. Summary of Campath-1H studies in CLL.

Reference	*No. of patients*	*Weeks of Rx*	*Prior Rx*	*% CR*	*% PR*	*Overall response*
111	9	6–18	No	33	55	89
59	29	6	Yes	4	38	43
108	6	6–12	Yes	0	50	50
193	24	4–16	Yes	0	33	33
194	6*	4–6	Yes	83	N/A	83
195	9*	6	Yes	55	N/A	55
196	29	NR	Yes	34	25	59
197	92	4–12	Yes	2	31	33

ORR was 87% in the 38 patients who received at least 2 weeks of treatment, and the intent-to-treat ORR was 81%.[115] Campath-1H was most effective at clearing disease from peripheral blood (CR 95%), but bone marrow (CR + nodular PR, 66%) and nodal disease (ORR, 87%; CR, 29%) also responded to therapy. Some patients who achieved CR in the marrow required the full 18 weeks of therapy to do so, suggesting that prolonged administration of Campath-1H may be necessary to clear marrow disease. Median time to treatment failure had not been reached at time of study report (18+ months). Thus, SC administration of Campath-1H is feasible, and longer courses of Campath-1H may produce ORR and CR rates similar to those observed with fludarabine. It must be emphasized, however, that SC administration of Campath-1H does not diminish the infectious risk of this agent.

Immunosuppression and Infectious Complications Infections constitute the major complication of Campath-1H therapy.[102,116,117] All 50 previously treated NHL patients in a multicenter European study developed profound lymphopenia. Opportunistic infections and bacterial septicemia occurred in 14% and 18% of patients, respectively, and 6% of patients died of infection.[118] Infections occurred in 55% of patients (27% grade 3–4), and 13% developed septicemia in the CAM211 study.[110] Although Campath-1H also inhibits B cells, CD8+ T cells, natural killer (NK) cells, and monocytes, the most profound effects of the antibody are on CD4+ T lymphocytes.[119–121] Treatment with 5 to 10 daily IV infusions of Campath-1H almost completely depleted lymphocytes, and lymphocyte subsets recovered with varying kinetics. NK cells and monocytes recovered to normal within 1 to 2 months, whereas B-cell numbers returned to normal within 5 months. CD8+ T cells returned to 50% of pretreatment levels by 2 months but did not increase further, and CD4+ T cells never reached 20% of pretreatment levels despite 18 months follow-up.[119] In 41 CLL patients given SC Campath-1H for up to 18 weeks, NK and NK-T cells remained severely suppressed more than 12 months afterward; however, no late infectious complications were observed.[122]

Paroxysmal nocturnal hemoglobinuria (PNH)-like T cells emerge during or immediately after Campath-1H treatment in many patients. These PNH-like cells cannot synthesize glycosylphosphatidylinositol (GPI) anchor glycans, lack GPI-linked surface proteins, such as CD52, and are resistant to CD52-mediated killing. Preliminary studies demonstrated that, despite lacking GPI-linked proteins, these PNH-like T cells are functional immune effector cells.[123] This finding may explain why the great majority of severe opportunistic infections that occur with Campath-1H are observed during active Campath-1H therapy rather than after treatment.

Lymphocyte recovery may depend on the dosing schedule, as the absolute CD4+ T-cell count reached a nadir of 2/μL by week 4 but increased to 84/μL by week 12 in the CAM211 trial.[110] In 42 refractory CLL patients (median CD3+ T-cell count, 1,900/μl) treated with Campath-1H, extreme lymphopenia of less than 30/μL was seen in all patients after a median of 2 weeks of therapy. At a median follow-up of 14 months, the median CD3+ T-cell count recovered to 930/μL and the median CD4+ T-cell count to 320/μL.[123] Campath-1H depleted CD52+ myeloid peripheral blood dendritic cells, resulting in inhibition of the stimulatory activity of peripheral blood mononuclear cells (PBMCs) in allogeneic mixed-lymphocyte reactions. Depletion of CD52+ dendritic cells also inhibited the ability of PBMCs to present antigen to purified CD4+ T lymphocytes.[124] This effect may explain the low rate of graft-versus-host disease (GVHD) in allogeneic stem cell transplants using Campath-1H.[125,126]

This prolonged inhibition of T-lymphocyte and dendritic cell function may limit the clinical use of Campath-1H, particularly in combination regimens with other immunosuppressive agents, such as fludarabine. Patients receiving Campath-1H must be placed on appropriate prophylaxis for *Pneumocystis pneumoniae* (PCP) and varicella zoster virus (VZV). They should be monitored for cytomegalovirus (CMV) reactivation during and for at least 2 to 3 months after therapy. With these prophylactic measures, Campath-1H can be administered safely and with acceptable toxicity.

Infusion Toxicity Infusion-related toxicity occurred in 93% of patients in the CAM211 study, although the majority of reactions were grade 1 or 2. Rigors (90% overall, 14% grade 3), fever (85% overall, 17% grade 3, 3% grade 4) and nausea (53%) were the most common infusion-related toxicities.[110] Similar rates of rigors (71%), fevers (65%), and nausea (45%) were reported in the multicenter study of 136 B-CLL patients, and almost all infusion toxicities were grade 1 or 2.[112] Most toxicity was observed with the first infusion.[110] This first-dose cytokine release syndrome involves TNF-α, IFN-γ, and IL-6.[127] TNF-α levels increase by greater than 1,000-fold after Campath-1H infusion, and TNF-α is a most important cytokine in this syndrome.[128,129] Ligation of the low-affinity Fc receptor for IgG, FcγRIIIa, on NK cells results in release of TNF-α, and may play a central role in inducing infusion toxicity to Campath-1H.[127] These infusion side effects are generally responsive to corticosteroid administration, when severe.

Hematologic Toxicity Campath-1H has significant hematologic toxicity, given the presence of CD52 on many hematopoietic cells. The multicenter study of 136 CLL patients noted 26% neutropenia (22% grade 3 or 4), 35% thrombocytopenia (23% grade 3 or 4), and 21% anemia (11% grade 3).[112] Many patients who develop cytopenias develop grade 3 or 4 toxicity, resulting in severe infectious complications. Although fever, rigors, and nausea may be bothersome and uncomfortable to patients, cytopenias and infectious complications constitute the medically serious toxicities of Campath-1H. However, these toxicities are clinically manageable with proper monitoring of peripheral blood counts and appropriate antibiotic prophylaxis. Granulocyte-macrophage colony-stimulating factor (GM-CSF) should be avoided, as GM-CSF exacerbates infusion-related toxicity, by inducing TNF-α, without significantly improving granulocyte recovery.[128]

Combination Therapy Laboratory evidence from our institution indicates that Campath-1H may synergize with fludarabine in vivo.[82] A small study of 6 CLL patients, refractory to fludarabine alone and Campath-1H alone, suggests that such synergy exists. Fludarabine was given at a dose of 25 mg/m^2 IV for 3 to 5 days, and Campath-1H was given at 30 mg IV three times weekly for 8 to 16 weeks. One patient achieved a CR (17%), and 5 patients achieved a PR, for an ORR of 83%; flow cytometric analysis could not detect residual CLL cells in the 2 patients. Patients received prophylactic co-trimoxazole and acyclovir, and no serious adverse events were noted.[130] A larger study using fludarabine 30mg/m^2 UV and Campath-1H 30mg IV for 3 days every 28 days for 4 cycles achieved 9 CR and 3 PR in 14 evaluable patients with relapsed CLL (ORR 86%). Of note, 1 heavily pretreated patient died of fever of unknown origin. The use of a lower total dose of Campath-1H in this study may diminish long-term toxicity, particularly infections.

The combination of Campath-1H and rituximab can be given safely and may have clinical activity in patients with relapsed CLL. Nine patients received rituximab 375mg/m^2 weeks 1 and 3 to 5, in combination with Campath-1H 3, 10, or 30mg thrice weekly, weeks 2 to 5, in a Phase I dose-escalation study.[131] Toxicity was acceptable, with no opportunistic infections or treatment-related deaths. Eight patients (89%) experienced significant reduction (median, 95% decrease) in peripheral lymphocyte count, but no objective responses by NCI criteria were seen. A second study administered rituximab, 375mg/m^2 weekly for four doses, with Campath-1H 30mg on days 3 and 5 of each week, to 48 patients with relapsed or refractory lymphoproliferative disorders, including 32 patients with CLL and 9 patients with CLL/PLL.[132] The ORR was 52% (CR, 8%), with a median time to progression of 6 months. Nearly all CLL and CLL/PLL patients had resolution of peripheral blood lymphocytosis, but only 11 of 33 patients had clearing of marrow disease (33%), and 24 of 41 patients had more than 50% reduction of nodal disease (59%). Fifty-two percent of patients developed infections, and CMV reactivation was seen in 27% of patients.

Summary As a result of the ubiquitous expression of CD52 on lymphocytes and monocytes, Campath-1H causes significantly more hematologic and immune toxicity than does rituximab. However, infectious complications are manageable with adequate antibiotic prophylaxis. The majority of patients receiving Campath-1H experience infusion toxicity, but toxicity is manageable with a "stepped-up" dosing schedule. In addition, infusion toxicity usually diminishes as therapy progresses. Campath-1H demonstrates greatest activity against CLL cells in peripheral blood, although prolonged therapy may be able to achieve CR in bone marrow. The antibody is less effective against nodal disease; responses are almost exclusively PR. Despite its limitations, Campath-1H is the only approved therapy for CLL that shows activity in relapsed patients with loss or mutation of p53. Thus, further study of Campath-1H is needed. Given its infusion toxicity, future trials will likely center on use of subcutaneous, rather than intravenous, Campath-1H. Despite initial promising results, further studies are needed to determine that subcutaneous administration is as effective as IV dosing in relapsed CLL.

Investigation Agents

Hu1D10

Hu1D10 (Apolizumab, Remitogen) is a humanized murine IgG monoclonal antibody whose antigenic epitope is a polymorphic determinant on the major histocompatibility (MHC) class II HLA-DR beta chain.[133] The 1D10 epitope is present on normal and malignant B lymphocytes, dendritic cells, macrophages, and some activated T lymphocytes. 1D10 is expressed in 50% of acute lymphocytic leukemia, 50% of diffuse large cell NHL, 50% to 70% of follicle center NHL, and 80% to 90% of CLL.[134] Expression is uniformly strong in tumors that are ID10 positive. Hu1D10 induces ADCC and CDC, as well as apoptosis, by a caspase-independent pathway.[133,134]

An initial phase I study in 20 patients with NHL demonstrated that Hu1D10 can be given safely at doses that show potential clinical efficacy.[135] Patients received weekly doses, ranging from 0.15 to 5mg/kg, and a regimen giving the drug on 5 consecutive days was also examined. Infusion-related toxicity was common, but manageable, and included fever, chills, nausea, vomiting, rash, flushing, and hypotension. Four of 8 patients with follicle center NHL responded (1 CR, 3 PR), with a median time to response of 106 days. A Phase II multicenter study in 21 patients with relapsed indolent B-cell lymphoproliferative disorders, including 5 with SLL, treated with Hu1D10 at 0.5 or 1.5mg/kg weekly for four doses, showed good tolerance.[136] Studies in CLL are ongoing.[137]

Anti-CD23

CD23 is another potential target of monoclonal antibody therapy; similar to CD20 and CD5, CD23 is expressed on the overwhelming majority of CLL cells. A chimeric macaque-derived anti-CD23 antibody, p6G5G1, has been developed.[138] Although these antibodies have been developed as possible therapies for asthma and other allergic disorders, the ubiquitous expression of CD23 on CLL cells indicates that preclinical studies of these compounds in CLL should be pursued. Recently, in vitro studies of a humanized anti-CD23 monoclonal antibody, IDEC-152 (Lumiliximab), demonstrated that cross-linked IDEC-152 induced apoptosis in fresh CLL cells from 5 patients. In addition, IDEC-152-induced apoptosis was enhanced in the presence of fludarabine or rituximab.[139] In a Phase I study, 25 evaluable patients with relapsed CLL received IDEC-152 at 125 to 500mg/m^2 IV weekly for four doses. Dose-limiting toxicity was seen in 2 of 10 patients treated at the highest dose, but toxicity was acceptable. Twenty-four patients (96%) achieved a decrease in peripheral lymphocytosis, and 8 of 19 patients (42%) treated at the 375 to 500mg/m^2 doses experienced more than a 50% reduction in their disease.[140]

Flavopiridol

Flavopiridol is an *N*-methylpiperidinyl, chlorophenyl flavone that induces apoptosis in CLL cells by activating caspase 3.[141] Caspase 3 acts distal to p53; thus, induction of apoptosis by flavopiridol is p53 independent.[142] Flavopiridol also induces profound decreases in the levels of Mcl-1 and XIAP in CLL cells in vitro.[143]

Phase I clinical studies determined a safe, tolerable dose of 50mg/m^2/day given as a continuous intravenous infusion (CIVI) over 72 hours.[142] Unfortunately, Phase II studies using this schedule demonstrated no response, including a trial in 10 patients with recurrent or refractory mantle cell lymphoma.[144] Despite plasma flavopiridol concentrations of 200 to 400nM, no apoptosis was seen in peripheral blood mononuclear cells (PBMCs) of patients who received this CIVI schedule.[145,146] This discrepancy is caused by increased binding of flavopiridol to human serum proteins. In vitro assays of apoptosis have used fetal calf serum (FCS) in culture media. However, the free flavopiridol concentration decreased from 63% to 100% to 5% to 8% if human plasma was substituted for FCS, resulting in an increase in 1-hour and 24-hour LC_{50} values from 670 and 120nM to 3,510 and 470nM, respectively.[146,147] Thus, CIVI dosing does not achieve pharmacologically effective drug concentrations, resulting in lack of clinical responses.[145–147] Bolus dosing achieves the necessary LC_{50}, and a Phase II study giving flavopiridol 50mg/m^2 by 1 hour IVB on days 1 to 3 in 36 previously treated, mostly fludarabine-refractory patients, demonstrated activity (14%), with a median response duration of 8 months. Pharmacokinetic modeling indicates an optimal dosing schedule of 30-minute IVB followed by 4-hour CIVI, and initial results of an ongoing Phase I study show activity with clinical response in p53-deficient patients and tumor lysis.[148]

Stem Cell Transplantation

Autologous Stem Cell Transplantation

Studies of autologous stem cell transplantation (SCT) in CLL have produced mixed results because of patient selection and the variable use of stem cell purging. Disease-free survival (DFS) has ranged from 25% to 69%, with similar discrepancies in overall survival (OS).[149–153] A British Medical Research Council (MRC) study recently achieved 5-year DFS and OS of 78% and 52%, respectively, in 65 patients.[149] Sixteen of 20 evaluable patients achieved molecular remission by PCR examination of IgVH gene rearrangement. A retrospective German study of 58 CLL patients (20 mutated, 38 unmutated) showed that unmutated IgVH remained an adverse prognostic factor despite autologous SCT.[154] Median time to clinical relapse was 37 months in the unmutated group, whereas only 1 mutated patient relapsed 4 years post-SCT; 2-year probability of relapse was 19% and 0%, respectively, for unmutated and mutated patients. Nonetheless, unmutated patients still enjoyed a 2-year OS of 89%. A similar German study matched 44 patients who underwent autologous SCT with 44 similar patients who received chemotherapy without SCT.[155] Unmutated IgVH was seen in 66% of both cohorts. Median survival from diagnosis for unmutated patients was 139 months for SCT, versus 73 months for chemotherapy, with a hazard ratio (HR) of 0.31 ($P = 0.02$). Although patients with genetic risk factors such as unmutated IgVH still do poorly compared to good- or intermediate-risk patients who undergo autologous SCT, autologous SCT still confers benefit to high-risk CLL patients.

Despite these promising results, autologous SCT in CLL is limited by several factors. First, patients have significant marrow and blood involvement that may result in contamination of the stem cell product despite cytoreductive therapy.[156] Second, prior fludarabine therapy may cause myelosuppression and hamper collection of an adequate number of autologous stem cells; peripheral stem cell mobilization was unsuccessful in 33% of patients in the MRC study.[149] Third, the high-dose conditioning regimens used in autologous SCT are associated with a significant risk of secondary MDS or AML; 8% of patients in the MRC study developed MDS/AML [149]. Finally, extensive studies in follicle center lymphoma[157] and multiple myeloma[158] have not demonstrated that autologous SCT is curative in hematologic malignancies that are incurable with standard chemotherapy. In particular, this last factor has damped enthusiasm for further studies of autologous SCT for CLL, particularly for patients who have an HLA-identical sibling donor. Given the limitations of autologous SCT, the major focus of clinical research in SCT for CLL has shifted to allogeneic SCT.

Myeloablative Allogeneic SCT

Allogeneic SCT offers theoretical advantages over autologous SCT in CLL. Contamination of the stem cell source and inadequate stem cell collection are not obstacles, and the use of an allogeneic donor allows for an immunologic graft-versus-leukemia (GVL) effect. Limited data suggest that TBI-containing conditioning regimens are superior to BuCy in CLL. A small study of 25 patients by the Seattle group revealed a 100-day treatment-related mortality (TRM) of 57% for BuCy ($n = 7$), compared to 17% for TBI regimens ($n = 18$). Five-year actuarial survival was 56% for 14 patients transplanted with TBI regimens during 1992–1999.[159] An M.D. Anderson study of Cy/TBI in 28 CLL patients observed a 100-day TRM of 11%. Five-year PFS and OS were 78% and 78%, respectively, for chemosensitive patients, compared to 26% and 31% for refractory patients.[160]

A retrospective EBMT study of 135 patients showed 54% 3-year OS and 40% 100-day TRM.[161] Similar findings were reported by the IBMTR, with 45% 3-year OS and 30% 100-day TRM in 242 patients.[162] The high TRM may be explained in part by the late stage of the disease in many of these patients. Median time from diagnosis to SCT was 41 and 46 months, and 37% of patients in the EBMT study were chemorefractory entering transplant.[161,162] Although there are no randomized studies, a retrospective comparison by the M.D. Anderson showed 3-year DFS of 57% for allogeneic SCT, versus 24% for purged autologous SCT.[163]

Thus, myeloablative allogeneic SCT may offer superior DFS in CLL, compared to autologous SCT. Although 3-year DFS after allogeneic SCT is approximately 50%,[159–163] longer follow-up is needed to determine if disease remissions are durable. However, the advantage in markedly decreased relapse rates with allogeneic SCT is offset by a higher TRM,[161,162] decreasing enthusiasm for this treatment modality in CLL. Limited data indicate that Bu/Cy may be particularly toxic in this population; in contrast, TBI regimens have acceptable TRM.[159] To preserve the immunologic GVL effect while reducing TRM, the focus of clinical SCT research in CLL has turned to nonmyeloablative allogeneic SCT.

Nonmyeloablative Allogeneic SCT

Ideally, the GVL effect of allogeneic SCT can be harnessed, while reducing TRM from acute GVHD, acute infection, and organ toxicity associated with myeloablative SCT. Several studies have specifically examined CLL.[2,164–167] Fludarabine, busulfan, and antithymocyte globulin (ATG) were administered to 30 German CLL patients; the stem cell source was a matched related ($n = 15$) or unrelated ($n = 15$) donor.[164,165] Grade 2 to 4 acute GVHD was observed in 56% of patients, whereas 75% developed chronic GVHD.[165] Responses were seen in 93% of patients, with 40% achieving CR. Of note, it took up to 2 years for patients to achieve CR, suggesting a GVL effect. All patients achieved a molecular CR by PCR, but only 6 patients were in continued molecular CR after a median follow-up of 2 years. Two-year TRM, PFS, and OS were 15%, 67%, and 72%, respectively.[165]

The EBMT retrospectively examined 77 CLL patients who received a variety of nonmyeloablative conditioning regimens, following by allogeneic SCT.[2] One-year TRM was 18%, and the 2-year probability of relapse was 31%. Two-year DFS and OS were 56% and 72%, respectively. Nineteen patients received donor lymphocyte infusion (DLI) for relapse or incomplete donor chimerism, but only 7 responded to DLI (37%). Unfortunately, this study was complicated by the heterogeneity of conditioning regimens and the use of ATG or Campath-1H for T-cell depletion in 40% of patients.

A recent German study indicated that nonmyeloablative allogeneic SCT may be superior to autologous SCT in obtaining clinical and molecular remissions in high-risk CLL patients with unmutated IgVH, due to a GVL effect. Seven of 9 patients (78%) became negative by PCR for allele-specific IgVH after day + 100 post-SCT; attainment of molecular CR occurred after DLI or development of chronic GVHD. In contrast, only 6 of 26 control CLL patients (23%) achieved a PCR-negative state after autologous SCT.[166] Thus, an immunologic GVL effect appears to be important in CLL and may confer a long-term survival advantage for allogeneic over autologous SCT, given sufficient time.

Summary CLL remains incurable by standard therapies; thus, SCT should be considered, especially for younger patients and patients with high-risk genetic features who likely will do poorly with chemotherapy. Nonmyeloablative allogeneic SCT is the most promising transplant modality in CLL and is the focus of most SCT studies in CLL. Short-term DFS of 50% to 75% has been obtained with acceptable TRM,[2,165,166] and molecular responses have been obtained with the onset of GVHD or the therapeutic use of DLI.[165] However, long-term follow-up is lacking, and it is unclear whether the DFS observed at 2 years will prove durable over time. Myeloablative allogeneic SCT should be considered for patients with bulky or refractory disease,[160] and a TBI-containing regimen should be utilized to reduce TRM.[159] Finally, autologous SCT should be considered for high-risk CLL patients who do not have an allogeneic option. Although autologous SCT has not proven curative in CLL, autologous SCT still confers a survival advantage to patients with unmutated IgVH.[154,155] However, it is necessary to limit the number of prior therapies, particularly fludarabine-based regimens, given that insufficient stem cells are collected from a third or more of CLL patients being considered for autologous SCT. Several other excellent textbooks and reviews cover this topic in greater detail.[1–3]

The Future: Risk-Stratified Therapy

For decades, treatment of CLL has been based upon clinical staging systems, such as the Rai and Binet systems. However, these staging systems cannot predict the likelihood or duration of clinical response to therapy. The growing wealth of information about the prognostic implications of cytogenetic abnormalities, IgVH mutations, CD38 expression, and ZAP-70 expression in CLL is revolutionizing the clinical management of CLL. A risk-stratified approach is at hand by which therapy can be selected for an individual patient based upon his or her likelihood of achieving a CR and the likely duration of that response. Patients with deletion of 13q14 or mutated IgV_H, who are likely to have an indolent course or enjoy a long duration of response to fludarabine, can be managed conservatively with initial observation and fludarabine-based therapy when treatment is indicated. Patients with deletion of 17p13 or unmutated IgV_H, who are likely to relapse rapidly after therapy, should be treated aggressively. Nonmyeloablative allogeneic SCT should be considered in first remission for patients with deletion of 17p13. Thus, a risk-stratified approach offers the promise of therapy that is best tailored to the medical needs of the individual patient.

Prolymphocytic Leukemia (PLL)

B-PLL

B-cell prolymphocytic leukemia (B-PLL) is a rare disease. B-PLL can be diagnosed de novo or arise by transformation from preexisting B-CLL. A retrospective French study of 41 B-PLL patients revealed a median age of 67 years, median OS of 5 years, and median EFS of 37 months.[168] Age and anemia were the only two factors associated with poor outcome. De novo patients and patients who had transformed from B-CLL had similar outcomes.[168] A similar retrospective Israeli study of 35 B-PLL patients found anemia and lymphocytosis, but not age, to be significant prognostic factors.[169] A 47% PR rate and median response duration of 32 months were observed in 17 patients treated with chlorambucil/prednisone or COP. Two PR and 1 CR, with median response duration of 30 months, were observed in 6 patients treated with CHOP.[169] Impressive results were achieved with 2-chlorodeoxyadenosine (2-CDA, cladribine) in 8 B-PLL patients (4 previously untreated). Patients received 2-CDA 0.1 mg/kg/day by CIVI for 7 days, every 28 to 35 days, for two to five cycles. Responses were observed in all 8 patients (5 CR, 3 PR); however, median response duration was only 14 months for patients achieving CR and 3 months for patients achieving PR.[170]

T-Cell PLL

T-PLL cells are characterized by relatively open chromatin and prominent nucleoli and typically express CD2, CD3, CD5, and CD7. Patients with T-PLL do extremely poorly; analysis of 78 adult T-PLL patients revealed a median survival of only 7.5 months. Fifteen of 31 patients treated with pentostatin responded (48%), with a CR rate of 10% and median survival of 16 months in responders.[171] Fifty-five T-PLL patients received pentostatin 4 mg/m^2/week for 4 weeks, then every 2 weeks until maximal response. The ORR was 45%, with 5 patients (9%) achieving CR.[172]

Campath-1H

Novel therapies are desperately needed in T-PLL. Several studies have demonstrated significant clinical activity of the anti-CD52 monoclonal antibody Campath-1H in T-PLL. Campath-1H was given to 15 T-PLL patients, most of whom had failed pentostatin.[173] The ORR was 73%, and 9 patients achieved CR (60%); in addition, retreatment with Campath-1H induced second CR in 3 patients who relapsed after initial Campath-1H therapy. In comparison, only 3 of 25 similar T-PLL patients (12%) at the same institution achieved CR to pentostatin. Two patients developed severe bone marrow aplasia, and 1 patient died of this complication. A subsequent study by the same authors administered Campath-1H 30 mg IB thrice weekly until maximal response to 39 T-PLL, including 30 who had failed pentostatin.[174] The ORR was 76% (CR, 60%), with a median disease-free interval of 7 months (range, 4–45 months). Finally, a retrospective report of 76 T-PLL patients, who were given Campath-1H thrice weekly for 4 to 12 weeks, demonstrated an ORR of 51% (CR, 40%) with a median duration of CR of 9 months.[175] Median overall survival was 7.5 months, although patients who achieved CR had a median survival of 15 months. Ten patients (13%) developed a total of 15 infections, and severe cytopenias occurred in 6 patients (8%). Two patients (3%) died of treatment-related mortality. Thus, Campath-1H is the most active single agent in T-PLL and, in contrast to its results in CLL, is able to produce CR in up to 60% of patients with relapsed T-PLL.

Correlation of CD52 Expression with Clinical Response

The greater activity of Campath-1H in T-PLL may be due to increased expression of CD52 on T-PLL cells. Quantitative flow cytometry was used to measure CD52 expression in 24 B-CLL patients, 21 T-PLL patients, and 12 normal volunteers.[176] Interestingly, CD52 expression was significantly higher on normal T lymphocytes than on normal B lymphocytes, and T-PLL cells expressed higher levels of CD52 than did B-CLL cells. In addition, CD52 expression was slightly higher in patients who responded to Campath-1H. These results suggest that the likelihood of clinical response to Campath-1H may be related to the level of CD52 expression.

Summary

Although B-PLL is considered to have a poor prognosis, retrospective multicenter studies have shown a median survival of 5 years,[168] with median response duration of 30 to 32 months, to alkylator based chemotherapy.[169] Although very high CR and OR rates were attained with 2-CDA, response duration was surprisingly short.[170] Thus, chlorambucil and COP should be considered first-line therapy for B-PLL, and 2-CDA should be considered for relapsed disease. In contrast to B-PLL, T-PLL exhibits a very poor prognosis, with a median survival of only 7.5 months.[171] Campath-1H and pentostatin are the only two therapies that have shown significant activity in large trials in T-PLL.[174,175] Given the short duration of response to therapy, patients with T-PLL should be referred for allogeneic SCT, preferably on clinical study, in first remission. Although there have been no adequately sized studies of SCT in T-PLL, allogeneic SCT should be considered in light of this disease's grim prognosis. Patients with relapsed T-PLL who are not candidates for SCT should be considered for clinical trials.

Hairy Cell Leukemia

The Disease and Chemotherapy

Hairy cell leukemia (HCL) is another disease within the family of indolent B-cell lymphoproliferative disorders. In contrast to CLL or follicle center NHL, in which standard chemotherapy is strictly palliative, many patients with HCL are cured with conventional chemotherapeutic agents, such as deoxycoformycin (pentostatin) and 2-CDA. Long-term follow-up of 241 HCL patients treated with pentostatin as initial therapy (n = 154) or salvage therapy after failure of interferon-α (n = 87), showed estimated 5- and 10-year survival rates of 90% and 81%, respectively. Five- and 10-year RFS rates were 85% and 67%, respectively, in 173 patients who achieved CR to pentostatin.[177] Analysis of 230 French patients with HCL, two-thirds of whom had failed prior therapy, treated with deoxycoformycin 4 mg/m^2/day every 2 weeks for a median of 9 cycles, demonstrated an ORR of 96% (CR, 79%). Estimated DFS and OS were 88% and 89% at 5 years and 69% and 89% at 10 years, respectively.[178] Similar long-term follow-up of 207 assessable HCL patients treated with 2-CDA 0.1 mg/kg/day by CIVI for 7 days, revealed an ORR of 100% (CR, 95%), with a median duration of first response of 98 months; 37% of patients relapsed at a median of 42 months after therapy. OS was 97% at 108 months.[179] A recent study demonstrated that 2-CDA can be given by SC bolus at a dose of 0.14 mg/kg/day for 5 consecutive days. ORR and CR rates of 97% and 76% were seen in 62 HCL patients (33 previously untreated), with a median time to treatment failure of 38 months.[180] Both cladribine and pentostatin, therefore, remain acceptable therapies for patients with hairy cell leukemia. These authors prefer the use of pentostatin because of the longer remissions observed in multicenter trials as compared to those results derived with cladribine. In addition, pentostatin studies were inclusive of hairy cell leukemia patients with active infection, whereas many of the phase II cladribine studies excluded such patients. However, the period of cladribine administration is shorter and is therefore preferred by many practicing oncologists.

Rituximab

Hairy cell leukemia that is resistant to therapy with purine analogues has a poor prognosis, and treatment options are limited for patients whose disease becomes refractory to pentostatin and/or 2-CDA. Thus, despite the generally favorable prognosis of this disease, monoclonal antibody therapy is a treatment modality of significant interest in HCL. The monoclonal antibody that has been best studied in HCL is the anti-CD20 antibody rituximab. Several case reports and a few series have demonstrated the efficacy of rituximab in this disease. Ten patients with relapsed or progressive HCL who had previously received treatment with 2-CDA or pentostatin/interferon-α received four weekly doses of rituximab at 375 mg/m^2. The ORR was 50%, with 1 patient achieving CR and 4 patients attaining PR. Grade 1–2 infusion toxicity occurred during the first dose of rituximab but extinguished with subsequent doses. Fifty percent of patients experienced greater than 50% reduction of bone marrow involvement, 1, 3, and 6 months after completion of rituximab therapy.[181] A second study administered a similar schedule of rituximab to 8 patients with relapsed HCL and 3 patients with previously untreated HCL. The ORR was 64%, with 6 patients achieving CR and 1 patient PR. The median duration of response was 14 months (range, 0–34 months), and infusion-related toxicity was minimal.[182] A third study gave a similar schedule to 24 HCL patients who had failed prior 2-CDA. ORR and CR rates were 25% and 13%, respectively, and median time to relapse had not been reached at 15 months.[183] To examine whether increase in dosage results in improved clinical response, 8 weekly doses of rituximab 375 mg/m^2 were given to 15 patients with relapsed or primary refractory HCL. Patients who achieved PR, but not CR, received an additional four weekly doses of rituximab. The ORR was 80%; 8 patients (53%) attained CR, 2 patients (13%) achieved hematologic CR but had residual (1%–5%) marrow involvement by HCL, and 2 patients (13%) experienced PR. Median duration of response was not reached after a median follow-up of 32 months; 5 patients relapsed after 8, 12, 18, 23, and 39 months, respectively, and 7 remained in remission. Toxicity was minimal, and no infections were noted.[184]

Thus, in contrast to CLL, weekly dosing of rituximab achieves a significant response rate in HCL, although preliminary data suggest that a longer course of therapy may result in an improved CR rate. Rituximab therapy does not appear to induce greater infusion-related toxicity in HCL than in NHL. The efficacy of weekly rituximab therapy and decreased infusion toxicity in HCL, compared to CLL, may be caused by the lower circulating tumor burden in HCL and the absence of soluble CD20 in HCL patients.

BL-22

The murine IgG 2 monoclonal antibody LL2 recognizes CD22 and has been conjugated to biologic effectors in an attempt to target these toxins to HCL cells.[185] RFB4(dsFv)-PE38 (BL22) is a recombinant immunotoxin generated by fusion of the variable Fv portion of the anti-CD22 monoclonal antibody RFB4 to a truncated form of *Pseudomonas* exotoxin A. Sixteen patients with cladribine-resistant HCL received BL22 every other day for three doses in a Phase I dose-escalation study.[186] Eleven patients achieved CR (69%) and 2 patients attained PR (13%). The 3 patients who failed to respond received low doses of BL22 or had preexisting antibodies that neutralized the toxin. Median follow-up was 16 months, and 3 of the 11 complete responders relapsed but then attained second CR after retreatment with BL22. Common toxicities were transient hypoalbuminemia and transaminitis, but the most serious toxicity was reversible hemolytic uremic syndrome in 2 patients.

LMB-2

LMB-2 (anti-Tac(Fv)-PE38) is a recombinant immunotoxin derived by fusion of the variable Fv portion of the anti-CD25 monoclonal antibody anti-Tac to a truncated form of *Pseudomonas* exotoxin A.[187] CD25 (Tac) is the beta chain of the high-affinity IL-2 receptor and is expressed on the cell surface of T-cell malignancies, as well as HCL.[188,189] In an initial phase I study, LMB-2 induced major responses, including 1 CR, in 4 of 4 patients with refractory HCL who had failed standard therapy.[187] Minimal residual disease was detectable by flow cytometry of the bone marrow aspirate of the patient who achieved hematologic CR. This initial study was expanded to a larger Phase I dose-escalation trial, and 31 additional patients with refractory CD25+ lymphomas and leukemias received LMB-2 at dose levels ranging from 2 to 63 μg/kg IVB every other day for three doses.[190] In contrast to the 100% ORR (25% CR) in HCL, only 4 of the other 31 patients responded, and no other patient achieved CR. Thus, refractory HCL is particularly amenable to therapy with LMB-2.

Summary

Deoxycoformycin and 2-CDA remain the therapies of choice for newly diagnosed HCL. Although 2-CDA is more commonly used because the schedule is more convenient, both drugs achieve similarly excellent results and can be used to treat HCL patients. Patients who relapse after, or are refractory to deoxycoformycin and 2-CDA, should receive rituximab. SCT is rarely used in HCL, given the disease's indolent course and its excellent response to conventional therapies.

Conclusions

The understanding and treatment of CLL and related chronic leukemias constitute a rapidly growing area of clinical research. Great strides are being made toward identifying prognostic genetic factors in CLL, with the goal of developing risk-adapted therapeutic strategies in this disease. The advent of fludarabine and other purine analogues reinvigorated clinical research in CLL and other chronic leukemias, and ongoing trials are examining the optimal treatment regimens in CLL. Monoclonal antibody therapy is perhaps the most exciting area of translational and clinical investigation. Although antibodies such as rituximab and Campath-1H have shown great promise in CLL, studies have clearly demonstrated that monoclonal antibodies as single agents will not produce long-term survival. Thus, ongoing trials are studying the optimal use of rituximab and Campath-1H in combination regimens in CLL. Results of initial studies combining monoclonal antibodies with fludarabine and other cytotoxic agents have been promising, and several trials are currently studying monoclonal antibody combinations. Although studies to date have been conducted primarily in CLL, monoclonal antibodies have also shown significant efficacy and promise in T-PLL and HCL. Each disease must be considered a separate entity; agents and dosing schedules that are effective in lymphoma or a particular chronic leukemia are not necessarily active in other chronic leukemias. Each chronic lymphoid malignancy is different, and diseases should not be "lumped" together.

Acknowledgment. This work was supported by the National Cancer Institute (P01 CA95426-01A1, T.L. and J.C.B.), the Sidney Kimmel Cancer Research Foundation (J.C.B.), The Leukemia and Lymphoma Society of America (J.C.B.), and The D. Warren Brown Foundation (J.C.B.).

References

1. Maloney DG, et al. Non-myeloablative transplantation. Hematology (Am Soc Hematol Educ Program) 2002;392–421.
2. Dreger P, et al. Treatment-related mortality and graft-versus-leukemia activity after allogeneic stem cell transplantation for chronic lymphocytic leukemia using intensity-reduced conditioning. Leukemia 2003;17:841–848.
3. Thomas ED, Blume KG, Forman SJ. Hematopoietic Cell Transplantation, 2nd ed. Malden, MA: Blackwell, 1999.
4. Kay NE, et al. Chronic lymphocytic leukemia. Hematology (Am Soc Hematol Educ Program) 2002;193–213.
5. Brugiatelli M, et al. Treatment of chronic lymphocytic leukemia in early and stable phase of the disease: long-term results of a randomized trial. Eur J Haematol 1995;55:158–163.

6. Dighiero G, et al. Chlorambucil in indolent chronic lymphocytic leukemia: French Cooperative Group on Chronic Lymphocytic Leukemia. N Engl J Med 1998;338:1506–1514.
7. Group CTC. Chemotherapeutic options in chronic lymphocytic leukemia: a meta-analysis of the randomized trials. J Natl Cancer Inst 1999;91:861–868.
8. Johnson S, et al. Multicentre prospective randomised trial of fludarabine versus cyclophosphamide, doxorubicin, and prednisone (CAP) for treatment of advanced-stage chronic lymphocytic leukaemia. The French Cooperative Group on CLL. Lancet 1996;347:1432–1438.
9. Rai KR, et al. Fludarabine compared with chlorambucil as primary therapy for chronic lymphocytic leukemia. N Engl J Med 2000;343:1750–1757.
10. Leporrier M, et al. Randomized comparison of fludarabine, CAP, and CHOP in 938 previously untreated stage B and C chronic lymphocytic leukemia patients. Blood 2001;98:2319–2325.
11. Montserrat E, et al. Presenting features and prognosis of chronic lymphocytic leukemia in younger adults. Blood 1991;78:1545–1551.
12. Dohner H, et al. Genomic aberrations and survival in chronic lymphocytic leukemia. N Engl J Med 2000;343:1910–1916.
13. Hamblin TJ, et al. Unmutated Ig VH genes are associated with a more aggressive form of chronic lymphocytic leukemia. Blood 1999;94:1848–1854.
14. Damie RN, et al. Ig V gene mutation status and CD38 expression as novel prognostic indicators in chronic lymphocytic leukemia. Blood 1999;1840–1847.
15. Jelinek DF, et al. Analysis of clonal B-cell CD38 and immunoglobulin variable region sequence status in relation to clinical outcome for B-chronic lymphocytic leukaemia. Br J Haematol 2001;115:854–861.
16. Hamblin TJ, et al. CD38 expression and immunoglobulin variable region mutations are independent prognostic variables in chronic lymphocytic leukemia, but CD38 expression may vary during the course of the disease. Blood 2002;99:1023–1029.
17. Matrai Z, et al. CD38 expression and Ig VH gene mutation in B-cell chronic lymphocytic leukemia. Blood 2001;97:1902–1903.
18. Thunberg U, et al. CD38 expression is a poor predictor for VH gene mutational status and prognosis in chronic lymphocytic leukemia. Blood 2001;97:1892–1894.
19. Maloum K, et al. Expression of unmutated VH genes is a detrimental prognostic factor in chronic lymphocytic leukemia. Blood 2000;96:377–379.
20. Hamblin TJ, et al. Immunoglobulin V genes and CD38 expression in CLL. Blood 2000;95:2455–2457.
21. Oscier DG, et al. Karyotypic evolution in B-cell chronic lymphocytic leukaemia. Genes Chromosomes Cancer 1991;3:16–20.
22. Del Poeta G, et al. Clinical significance of CD38 expression in chronic lymphocytic leukemia. Blood 2001;98:2633–2639.
23. Ibrahim S, et al. CD38 expression as an important prognostic factor in B-cell chronic lymphocytic leukemia. Blood 2001;98:181–186.
24. Oscier DG, et al. Multivariate analysis of prognostic factors in CLL: clinical stage, IgVH gene mutational status, and loss or mutation of the p53 gene are independent prognostic factors. Blood 2002;100:1177–1184.
25. Wiestner A, et al. ZAP-70 expression identifies a chronic lymphocytic leukemia subtype with unmutated immunoglobulin genes, inferior clinical outcome, and distinct gene expression profile. Blood 2003;101:4944–4951.
26. Chen L, et al. Expression of ZAP-70 is associated with increased B-cell receptor signaling in chronic lymphocytic leukemia. Blood 2002;100:4609–4614.
27. Crespo M, et al. ZAP-70 expression as a surrogate for immunoglobulin variable region mutations in chronic lymphocytic leukemia. N Engl J Med 2003;348:1764–1775.
28. El Rouby S, et al. p53 gene mutation in B-cell chronic lymphocytic leukemia is associated with drug resistance and is independent of MDR1/MDR3 gene expression. Blood 1993;82:3452–3459.
29. Wattel E, et al. p53 mutations are associated with resistance to chemotherapy and short survival in hematologic malignancies. Blood 1994;84:3148–3157.
30. Cordone I, et al. p53 expression in B-cell chronic lymphocytic leukemia: a marker for disease progression and poor prognosis. Blood 1998;91:4342–4349.
31. Stilgenbauer S. Genomic aberrations, p53 abnormalities, and IgV mutation: relationship to disease evolution, resistance to therapy, and clinical course of CLL. Leuk Lymphoma 2000;42(suppl):1–2.
32. Stilgenbauer S, et al. Campath-1H in refractory CLL: complete remission despite p53 gene mutation. Blood 2001;98:771a.
33. Delia D, et al. ATM protein and p53-serine 15 phosphorylation in ataxia-telangiectasia (AT) patients and AT heterozygotes. Br J Cancer 2000;82:1938–1945.
34. Pandita TK, et al. Ionizing radiation activates the ATM kinase throughout the cell cycle. Oncogene 2000;19:1386–1391.
35. Canman CE, et al. Activation of the ATM kinase by ionizing radiation and phosphorylation of p53. Science 1998;281:1677–1679.
36. Takao N, Li Y, Yamamoto K. Protective roles for ATM in cellular response to oxidative stress. FEBS Lett 2000;472:133–136.
37. Morrison C, et al. The controlling role of ATM in homologous recombinational repair of DNA damage. EMBO J 2000;19:463–471.
38. Stankovic T, et al. Inactivation of ataxia telangiectasia mutated gene in B-cell chronic lymphocytic leukaemia. Lancet 1999;353:26–29.
39. Bullrich F, et al. ATM mutations in B-cell chronic lymphocytic leukemia. Cancer Res 1999;59:24–27.
40. Starostik P, et al. Deficiency of the ATM protein expression defines an aggressive subgroup of B-cell chronic lymphocytic leukemia. Cancer Res 1998;58:4552–4557.
41. Schaffner C, et al. Somatic ATM mutations indicate a pathogenic role of ATM in B-cell chronic lymphocytic leukemia. Blood 1999;94:748–753.
42. Pettitt AR, et al. p53 dysfunction in B-cell chronic lymphocytic leukemia: inactivation of ATM as an alternative to TP53 mutation. Blood 2001;98:14–22.
43. Cheson BD, et al. National Cancer Institute-sponsored Working Group guidelines for chronic lymphocytic leukemia: revised guidelines for diagnosis and treatment. Blood 1996;87:4990–4997.
44. Grever MR, et al. A comprehensive phase I and II clinical investigation of fludarabine phosphate. Semin Oncol 1990;17(5 suppl 8):39–48.
45. Keating MJ, et al. Fludarabine: a new agent with major activity against chronic lymphocytic leukemia. Blood 1989;74:19–25.
46. Keating MJ, et al. Fludarabine: a new agent with marked cytoreductive activity in untreated chronic lymphocytic leukemia. J Clin Oncol 1991;9:44–49.
47. Keating MJ, et al. Long-term follow-up of patients with chronic lymphocytic leukemia treated with fludarabine as a single agent. Blood 1993;81:2878–2884.
48. Keating MJ, et al. Long-term follow-up of patients with chronic lymphocytic leukemia (CLL) receiving fludarabine regimens as initial therapy. Blood 1998;92:1165–1171.
49. Boogaerts MA, et al. Activity of oral fludarabine phosphate in previously treated chronic lymphocytic leukemia. J Clin Oncol 2001;19:4252–4258.
50. Flinn IW, et al. Fludarabine and cyclophosphamide with filgrastim support in patients with previously untreated indolent lymphoid malignancies. Blood 2000;96:71–75.

51. O'Brien SM, et al. Results of the fludarabine and cyclophosphamide combination regimen in chronic lymphocytic leukemia. J Clin Oncol 2001;19:1414–1420.
52. Eichhorst BF, et al. Fludarabine plus cyclophosphamide (FC) induces higher remission rates and longer progression free survival (PFS) than fludarabine (F) alone in first line therapy of advanced chronic lymphocytic leukemia (CLL): results of a phase III study (CLL4 protocol) of the German CLL Study Group (GCLLSG). Blood 2003;102:72a.
53. Sievers EL, et al. Efficacy and safety of gemtuzumab ozogamicin in patients with CD33-positive acute myeloid leukemia in first relapse. J Clin Oncol 2001;19:3244–3254.
54. Coiffier B, et al. CHOP chemotherapy plus rituximab compared with CHOP alone in elderly patients with diffuse large B-cell lymphoma. N Engl J Med 2002;346:235–242.
55. Olsen E, et al. Pivotal phase III trial of two dose levels of denileukin diftitox for the treatment of cutaneous T-cell lymphoma. J Clin Oncol 2001;19:376–388.
56. Byrd JC, et al. Rituximab using a thrice weekly dosing schedule in B-cell chronic lymphocytic leukemia and small lymphocytic lymphoma demonstrates clinical activity and acceptable toxicity. J Clin Oncol 2001;19:2153–2164.
57. Huhn D, et al. Rituximab therapy of patients with B-cell chronic lymphocytic leukemia. Blood 2001;98:1326–1331.
58. McLaughlin P, et al. Rituximab chimeric anti-CD20 monoclonal antibody therapy for relapsed indolent lymphoma: half of patients respond to a four-dose treatment program. J Clin Oncol 1998;16:2825–2833.
59. Osterborg A, et al. Phase II multicenter study of human CD52 antibody in previously treated chronic lymphocytic leukemia: European Study Group of CAMPATH-1H Treatment in Chronic Lymphocytic Leukemia. J Clin Oncol 1997;15:1567–1574.
60. Maloney DG, et al. IDEC-C2B8 (Rituximab) anti-CD20 monoclonal antibody therapy in patients with relapsed low-grade non-Hodgkin's lymphoma. Blood 1997;90:2188–2195.
61. Pegram MD, et al. Phase II study of receptor-enhanced chemosensitivity using recombinant humanized anti-p185HER2/neu monoclonal antibody plus cisplatin in patients with HER2/neu-overexpressing metastatic breast cancer refractory to chemotherapy treatment. J Clin Oncol 1998;16:2659–2671.
62. Baselga JM, et al. Phase II study of weekly intravenous trastuzumab (Herceptin) in patients with HER2/neu-overexpressing metastatic breast cancer. Semin Oncol 1999; 26(4 suppl 12):78–83.
63. Kitada S, et al. Expression of apoptosis-regulating proteins in chronic lymphocytic leukemia: correlations with in vitro and in vivo chemoresponses. Blood 1998;91:3379–3389.
64. Golay J, et al. Biologic response of B lymphoma cells to anti-CD20 monoclonal antibody rituximab in vitro: CD55 and CD59 regulate complement-mediated cell lysis. Blood 2000;95:3900–3908.
65. Treon SP, et al. Tumor cell expression of CD59 is associated with resistance to CD20 serotherapy in patients with B-cell malignancies. J Immunother 2001;24:263–271.
66. Byrd JC, et al. The mechanism of tumor cell clearance by rituximab in vivo in patients with B-cell chronic lymphocytic leukemia: evidence of caspase activation and apoptosis induction. Blood 2002;99:1038–1043.
67. Pedersen IM, et al. The chimeric anti-CD20 antibody rituximab induces apoptosis in B-cell chronic lymphocytic leukemia cells through a p38 mitogen activated protein-kinase-dependent mechanism. Blood 2002;99:1314–1319.
68. Keating MJ, O'Brien S, Albitar M. Emerging information on the use of rituximab in chronic lymphocytic leukemia. Semin Oncol 2002;29(1 suppl 2):70–74.
69. Manshouri T, et al. Circulating CD20 is detectable in the plasma of patients with chronic lymphocytic leukemia and is of prognostic significance. Blood 2003;101:2507–2513.
70. Bannerji R, et al. Apoptotic-regulatory and complement-protecting protein expression in chronic lymphocytic leukemia: relationship to in vivo rituximab resistance. J Clin Oncol 2003; 21:1466–1471.
71. Golay J, et al. CD20 levels determine the in vitro susceptibility to rituximab and complement of B-cell chronic lymphocytic leukemia: further regulation by CD55 and CD59. Blood 2001;98: 3383–3389.
72. Nguyen DT, et al. IDEC-C2B8 anti-CD20 (rituximab) immunotherapy in patients with low-grade non-Hodgkin's lymphoma and lymphoproliferative disorders: evaluation of response on 48 patients. Eur J Haematol 1999;62:76–82.
73. Winkler U, et al. Cytokine-release syndrome in patients with B-cell chronic lymphocytic leukemia and high lymphocyte counts after treatment with an anti-CD20 monoclonal antibody (rituximab, IDEC-C2B8). Blood 1999;94:2217–2224.
74. Ladetto M, et al. Rituximab anti-CD20 monoclonal antibody induces marked but transient reductions of peripheral blood lymphocytes in chronic lymphocytic leukaemia patients. Med Oncol 2000;17:203–210.
75. Itala M, et al. Standard-dose anti-CD20 antibody rituximab has efficacy in chronic lymphocytic leukaemia: results from a Nordic multicentre study. Eur J Haematol 2002;69:129–134.
76. Huh YO, et al. Higher levels of surface CD20 expression on circulating lymphocytes compared with bone marrow and lymph nodes in B-cell chronic lymphocytic leukemia. Am J Clin Pathol 2001;116:437–443.
77. Hainsworth JD, et al. Single-agent rituximab as first-line and maintenance treatment for patients with chronic lymphocytic leukemia or small lymphocytic lymphoma: a phase II trial of the Minnie Pearl Cancer Research Network. J Clin Oncol 2003;21: 1746–1751.
78. Thomas DA, et al. Single agent rituxan in early stage chronic lymphocytic leukemia (CLL). Blood 2001;98:364a.
79. Ginaldi L, et al. Levels of expression of CD19 and CD20 in chronic B cell leukaemias. J Clin Pathol 1998;51:364–369.
80. Perz J, et al. Level of CD20 expression and efficacy of rituximab treatment in patients with resistant or relapsing B-cell prolymphocytic leukemia and B-cell chronic lymphocytic leukemia. Leuk Lymphoma 2002;43:149–151.
81. Berinstein NL, et al. Association of serum Rituximab (IDEC-C2B8) concentration and anti-tumor response in the treatment of recurrent low-grade or follicular non-Hodgkin's lymphoma. Ann Oncol 1998;9:995–1001.
82. Byrd JC. Personal communication, 2001.
83. Keating MJ, O'Brien S. High-dose rituximab therapy in chronic lymphocytic leukemia. Semin Oncol 2000;27(6 suppl 12):86–90.
84. O'Brien SM, et al. Rituximab dose-escalation trial in chronic lymphocytic leukemia. J Clin Oncol 2001;19:2165–2170.
85. Byrd JC, et al. Rituximab therapy in hematologic malignancy patients with circulating blood tumor cells: association with increased infusion-related side effects and rapid blood tumor clearance. J Clin Oncol 1999;17:791–795.
86. Jensen, M, et al, Rapid tumor lysis in a patient with B-cell chronic lymphocytic leukemia and lymphocytosis treated with an anti-CD20 monoclonal antibody (IDEC-C2B8, rituximab). Ann Hematol 1998;77:89–91.
87. Czuczman MS, et al. Treatment of patients with low-grade B-cell lymphoma with the combination of chimeric anti-CD20 monoclonal antibody and CHOP chemotherapy. J Clin Oncol 1999;17:268–276.
88. Keating MJ, et al. Combination chemo-antibody therapy with fludarabine (F), cyclophosphamide (C) and rituximab (R) achieves a high CR rate in previously untreated chronic lymphocytic leukemia (CLL). Blood 2000;96:514a.
89. McLaughlin P, et al. Safety of fludarabine, mitoxantrone, and dexamethasone combined with rituximab in the treatment of stage IV indolent lymphoma. Semin Oncol 2000;27:37–41.

90. Vose JM, et al. Phase II study of rituximab in combination with CHOP chemotherapy in patients with previously untreated, aggressive non-Hodgkin's lymphoma. J Clin Oncol 2001;19:389–397.
91. Czuczman MS, et al. Phase II study of Rituximab in combination with Fludarabine in patients (Pts) with low-grade or follicular B-cell lymphoma. Blood 2000;96:729a.
92. Byrd JC, et al. Randomized phase 2 study of fludarabine with concurrent versus sequential treatment with rituximab in symptomatic, untreated patients with B-cell chronic lymphocytic leukemia: results from Cancer and Leukemia Group B 9712 (CALGB 9712). Blood 2003;101:6–14.
93. Byrd JC, et al. The addition of rituximab to fludarabine significantly improves progression-free and overall survival in previously untreated chronic lymphocytic leukemia (CLL) patients. Blood 2003;102:73a.
94. Schulz H, et al. Phase 2 study of a combined immunochemotherapy using rituximab and fludarabine in patients with chronic lymphocytic leukemia. Blood 2002,100:3115–3120.
95. Garcia-Manero G, et al. Update of results of the combination of fludarabine, cyclophosphamide and rituximab for previously treated patients with chronic lymphocytic leukemia (CLL). Blood 2001;98:633a.
96. Keating MJ, et al. A high proportion of molecular remission can be obtained with a fludarabine, cyclophosphamide, rituximab combination (FCR) in chronic lymphocytic leukemia (CLL). Blood 2002;100:205a.
97. Keating MJ, et al. A high proportion of true complete remission can be obtained with a fludarabine, cyclophosphamide, rituximab combination (FCR) in chronic lymphocytic leukemia. Proc Am Soc Clin Oncol, 2003;22:569.
98. Wierda W, et al. Combined fludarabine, cyclophosphamide, and rituximab achieves a high complete remission rate as initial treatment for chronic lymphocytic leukemia. Blood 2001;98:771a.
99. Polliack A, et al. Fludarabine (FLU)-containing regimen and rituximab (RI) as primary therapy with curative intent for younger patients with progressive and advanced B-CLL: high rate of initial response including molecular remissions. Blood 2001;98:364a.
100. Gupta NK, et al. Pilot study of Bexxar in advanced previously heavily treated refractory chronic lymphocytic leukemia (CLL). Blood 2001;98:290b.
101. Liu NS, et al. Yttrium-90 ibritumomab tiuxetan for minimal residual disease in CLL. Blood 2003;102:674a–675a.
102. Flynn JM, Byrd JC. Campath-1H monoclonal antibody therapy. Curr Opin Oncol 2000;12:574–581.
103. Hale G, et al. Removal of T cells from bone marrow for transplantation: a monoclonal antilymphocyte antibody that fixes human complement. Blood 1983;62:873–882.
104. Hale G, et al. Remission induction in non-Hodgkin lymphoma with reshaped human monoclonal antibody CAMPATH-1H. Lancet 1988;2(8625):1394–1399.
105. Hale G, et al. Reactivity of rat monoclonal antibody CAMPATH-1 with human leukaemia cells and its possible application for autologous bone marrow transplantation. Br J Haematol 1985; 60:41–48.
106. Salisbury JR, et al. Immunohistochemical analysis of CDw52 antigen expression in non-Hodgkin's lymphomas. J Clin Pathol 1994;47:313–317.
107. Rowan W, et al. Cross-linking of the CAMPATH-1 antigen (CD52) mediates growth inhibition in human B- and T-lymphoma cell lines, and subsequent emergence of CD52-deficient cells. Immunology 1998;95:427–436.
108. Bowen AL, et al. Subcutaneous CAMPATH-1H in fludarabine-resistant/relapsed chronic lymphocytic and B-prolymphocytic leukaemia. Br J Haematol 1997;96:617–619.
109. Keating MJ, et al. Multicenter study of Campath-1H in patients with chronic lymphocytic leukemia (B-CLL) refractory to fludarabine. Blood 2000;96:722a.
110. Keating MJ, et al. Therapeutic role of alemtuzumab (Campath-1H) in patients who have failed fludarabine: results of a large international study. Blood 2002;99:3554–3561.
111. Osterborg A, et al. Humanized CD52 monoclonal antibody Campath-1H as first-line treatment in chronic lymphocytic leukaemia. Br J Haematol 1996;93:151–153.
112. Rai KR, et al. Efficacy and safety of alemtuzumab (Campath-1H) in refractory B-CLL patients treated on a compassionate basis. Blood 2001;98:365a.
113. Ferrajoli A, et al. Campath-1H in refractory hematological malignancies expressing CD-52: a phase II clinical trial of 68 patients. Blood 2001;98:366a.
114. Ferrajoli A, et al. Phase II study of alemtuzumab in chronic lymphoproliferative disorders. Cancer (Phila) 2003;98:773–778.
115. Lundin J, et al. Phase II trial of subcutaneous anti-CD52 monoclonal antibody alemtuzumab (Campath-1H) as first-line treatment for patients with B-cell chronic lymphocytic leukemia (B-CLL). Blood 2002;100:768–773.
116. Khorana A, et al. A phase II multicenter study of Campath-1H antibody in previously treated patients with nonbulky non-Hodgkin's lymphoma. Leuk Lymphoma 2001;41:77–87.
117. Tang SC, et al. Immunosuppressive toxicity of CAMPATH1H monoclonal antibody in the treatment of patients with recurrent low grade lymphoma. Leuk Lymphoma 1996;24:93–101.
118. Lundin J, et al. CAMPATH-1H monoclonal antibody in therapy for previously treated low-grade non-Hodgkin's lymphoma: a phase II multicenter study. European Study Group of CAMPATH-1H Treatment in Low-Grade Non-Hodgkin's Lymphoma. J Clin Oncol 1998;16:3257–3263.
119. Brett S, et al. Repopulation of blood lymphocyte sub-populations in rheumatoid arthritis patients treated with the depleting humanized monoclonal antibody, CAMPATH-1H. Immunology 1996;88:13–19.
120. Condiotti R, Nagler A. Campath-1G impairs human natural killer (NK) cell-mediated cytotoxicity. Bone Marrow Transplant 1996;18:713–720.
121. Fabian I, et al. Effects of CAMPATH-1 antibodies on the functional activity of monocytes and polymorphonuclear neutrophils. Exp Hematol 1993;21:1522–1527.
122. Rezvany MR, et al. Long-term follow-up of lymphocyte subsets after subcutaneous alemtuzumab (MabCampath) treatment as primary therapy for B-cell chronic lymphocytic leukemia (B-CLL). Blood 2002;100:207a.
123. Kennedy B, et al. Campath-1H in CLL: immune reconstitution and viral infections during and after therapy. Blood 2000;96: 164a.
124. Buggins AGS, et al. Peripheral blood dendritic cells express CD52 and are depleted in vivo by treatment with Campath-1H. Blood 2001;98:366a.
125. Hale G, et al. Improving the outcome of bone marrow transplantation by using CD52 monoclonal antibodies to prevent graft-versus-host disease and graft rejection. Blood 1998;92: 4581–4590.
126. Hale G, et al. CD52 antibodies for prevention of graft-versus-host disease and graft rejection following transplantation of allogeneic peripheral blood stem cells. Bone Marrow Transplant 2000;26:69–76.
127. Wing MG, et al. Mechanism of first-dose cytokine-release syndrome by CAMPATH 1-H: involvement of CD16 (FcgammaRIII) and CD11a/CD18 (LFA-1) on NK cells. J Clin Invest 1996;98: 2819–2826.
128. Flinn IW, et al. Randomized trial of early versus delayed GM-CSF with Campath-1H: preliminary feasibility and correlative biologic studies results. Blood 2000;96:838a.
129. Pruzanski W, et al. Induction of TNF-alpha and proinflammatory secretory phospholipase A2 by intravenous administration of CAMPATH-1H in patients with rheumatoid arthritis. J Rheumatol 1995;22:1816–1819.

130. Kennedy B, et al. Campath-1H and fludarabine in combination are highly active in refractory chronic lymphocytic leukemia. Blood 2002;99:2245–2247.
131. Nabhan C, et al. Phase I study of rituximab and Campath-1H in patients with relapsed or refractory chronic lymphocytic leukemia. Blood 2001;98:365a.
132. Faderl S, et al. Experience with alemtuzumab plus rituximab in patients with relapsed and refractory lymphoid malignancies. Blood 2003;101:3413–3415.
133. Kostelny SA, et al. Humanization and characterization of the anti-HLA-DR antibody 1D10. Int J Cancer 2001;93:556–565.
134. Byrd JC. Personal communication, 2002.
135. Link BK, et al. Phase I study of Hu1D10 monoclonal antibody in patients with B-cell lymphoma. Proc Am Soc Clin Oncol 2001;20:284a.
136. Link BK, et al. A phase II study of Remitogen (Hu1D10), a humanized monoclonal antibody in patients with relapsed or refractory follicular, small lymphocytic, or marginal zone / MALT B-cell lymphoma. Blood 2001;98:606a.
137. Abhyankar VV, et al. Phase I study of escalated thrice weekly dosing of Hu1D10 in chronic lymphocytic leukemia / small lymphocytic lymphoma (CLL/SLL): minimal toxicity and early observation of in vivo tumor cell apoptosis. Proc Am Soc Clin Oncol 2002;21:268a.
138. Yabuuchi S, et al. Anti-CD23 monoclonal antibody inhibits germline Cepsilon transcription in B cells. Int Immunopharmacol 2002;2:453–461.
139. Pathan N, et al. Induction of apoptosis by IDEC-152 (anti-CD23) in chronic lymphocytic leukemia. Leuk Lymphoma 2001; 42(suppl 1):133N.
140. Byrd JC, et al. Interim results from a phase I study of lumiliximab (IDEC-152, anti-CD23 antibody) therapy for relapsed or refractory CLL. Blood 2003;102:74a.
141. Byrd JC, et al. Flavopiridol induces apoptosis in chronic lymphocytic leukemia cells via activation of caspase-3 without evidence of bcl-2 modulation or dependence on functional p53. Blood 1998;92:3804–3816.
142. Parker BW, et al. Early induction of apoptosis in hematopoietic cell lines after exposure to flavopiridol. Blood 1998;91(2):458–465.
143. Kitada S, et al. Protein kinase inhibitors flavopiridol and 7-hydroxy-staurosporine down-regulate antiapoptosis proteins in B-cell chronic lymphocytic leukemia. Blood 2000;96:393–397.
144. Lin TS, et al. Seventy-two hour continuous infusion flavopiridol in relapsed and refractory mantle cell lymphoma. Leuk Lymphoma 2002;43:793–797.
145. Schwartz GK, et al. Phase II study of the cyclin-dependent kinase inhibitor flavopiridol administered to patients with advanced gastric carcinoma. J Clin Oncol 2001;19(7):1985–1992.
146. Innocenti F, et al. Flavopiridol metabolism in cancer patients is associated with the occurrence of diarrhea. Clin Cancer Res 2000;6:3400–3405.
147. Shapiro GI, et al. A phase II trial of the cyclin-dependent kinase inhibitor flavopiridol in patients with previously untreated stage IV non-small cell lung cancer. Clin Cancer Res 2001;7(6): 1590–1599.
148. Lin TS, et al. Flavopiridol given as a 30-min intravenous (IV) bolus followed by 4-hr continuous IV infusion (CIVI) results in clinical activity and tumor lysis in refractory chronic lymphocytic leukemia (CLL). Proc Am Soc Clin Oncol 2004;23: 571.
149. Milligan DW, et al. Autografting for younger patients with chronic lymphocytic leukemia is safe and achieves a high percentage of molecular responses: results of the MRC Pilot Study. Blood (in press).
150. Rabinowe SN, et al. Autologous and allogeneic bone marrow transplantation for poor prognosis patients with B-cell chronic lymphocytic leukemia. Blood 1993;82:1366–1376.
151. Dreger P, et al. Efficacy and prognostic implications of early autologous stem cell transplanation for poor-risk chronic lymphocytic leukemia (CLL). Blood 2000;96:483a.
152. Dreger P, et al. Prognostic factors for survival after autologous stem cell transplantation for chronic lymphocytic leukemia (CLL): the EBMT experience. 2000.
153. Montserrat E, et al. Autologous stem cell transplantation (ASCT) for chronic lymphocytic leukemia (CLL): results in 107 patients. Blood 1999;94:396a.
154. Ritgen M, et al. Unmutated immunoglobulin variable heavy-chain gene status remains an adverse prognostic factor after autologous stem cell transplantation for chronic lymphocytic leukemia. Blood 2003;101:2049–2053.
155. Dreger P, et al. The prognostic impact of autologous stem cell transplantation in patients with chronic lymphocytic leukemia: a risk-matched analysis based on the VH gene mutational status. Blood 2004;103:2850–2858.
156. Jabbour E, et al. Stem cell transplantation for chronic lymphocytic leukemia: should not more patients get a transplant? Bone Marrow Transplant 2004;34:289–297.
157. Lin TS, Copelan EA. Autologous stem cell transplantation for non-Hodgkin's lymphoma. Curr Hematol Rep 2003;2:310–315.
158. Caldera H, Giralt S. Stem cell transplantation for multiple myeloma: current status and future directions. Curr Hematol Rep 2004;3:249–256.
159. Doney KC, et al. Allogeneic related donor hematopoietic stem cell transplantation for treatment of chronic lymphocytic leukemia. Bone Marrow Transplant 2002;29:817–823.
160. Khouri IF, et al. Long-term follow-up of patients with CLL treated with allogeneic hematopoietic transplantation. Cytotherapy 2002;4:217–221.
161. Michallet M, et al. Allogeneic hematopoietic stem cell transplantation (HSCT) for chronic lymphocytic leukemia (CLL): results and prognostic factors for survival after transplantation: analysis from EBMT registry. Blood 2000;96:205a.
162. Horowitz MM, et al. Hematopoietic stem cell transplantation (SCT) for chronic lymphocytic leukemia (CLL). Blood 2000;96: 522a.
163. Khouri IF, Keating MJ, Champlin RE. Hematopoietic stem cell transplantation for chronic lymphocytic leukemia. Curr Opin Hematol 1998;5:454–459.
164. Schetelig J, et al. Reduced non-relapse mortality after reduced intensity conditioning in advanced chronic lymphocytic leukemia. Ann Hematol 2002;81(suppl 2):S47–S48.
165. Schetelig J, et al. Evidence of a graft-versus-leukemia effect in chronic lymphocytic leukemia after reduced-intensity conditioning and allogeneic stem-cell transplantation: the Cooperative German Transplant Study Group. J Clin Oncol 2003;21: 2747–2753.
166. Ritgen M, et al. Graft-versus-leukemia activity may overcome therapeutic resistance of chronic lymphocytic leukemia with unmutated immunoglobulin variable heavy chain gene status: implications of minimal residual disease measurement with quantitative PCR. Blood (in press).
167. Khouri IF, et al. Nonablative allogeneic stem cell transplantation for chronic lymphocytic leukemia: impact of rituximab on immunomodulation and survival. Exp Hematol 2004;32:28–35.
168. Hercher C, et al. A multicentric study of 41 cases of B-prolymphocytic leukemia: two evolutive forms. Leuk Lymphoma 2001;42:981–987.
169. Shvidel L, et al. B-cell prolymphocytic leukemia: a survey of 35 patients emphasizing heterogeneity, prognostic factors and evidence for a group with an indolent course. Leuk Lymphoma 1999;33:169–179.
170. Saven A, et al. Major activity of cladribine in patients with de novo B-cell prolymphocytic leukemia. J Clin Oncol 1997;15: 37–43.

171. Matutes E. et al. Clinical and laboratory features of 78 cases of T-prolymphocytic leukemia. Blood 1991;78:3269–3274.
172. Mercieca J, et al. The role of pentostatin in the treatment of T-cell malignancies: analysis of response rate in 145 patients according to disease subtype. J Clin Oncol 1994;12:2588–2593.
173. Pawson R, et al. Treatment of T-cell prolymphocytic leukemia with human CD52 antibody. J Clin Oncol 1997;15:2667–2672.
174. Dearden CE, et al. High remission rate in T-cell prolymphocytic leukemia with Campath-1H. Blood 2001;98:1721–1726.
175. Keating MJ, et al. Campath-1H treatment of T-cell prolymphocytic leukemia in patients for whom at least one prior chemotherapy regimen has failed. J Clin Oncol 2002;20:205–213.
176. Ginaldi L, et al. Levels of expression of CD52 in normal and leukemic B and T cells: correlation with in vivo therapeutic responses to Campath-1H. Leuk Res 1998;22:185–191.
177. Flinn IW, et al. Long-term follow-up of remission duration, mortality, and second malignancies in hairy cell leukemia patients treated with pentostatin. Blood 2000;96:2981–2986.
178. Maloisel F, et al. Long-term outcome with pentostatin treatment in hairy cell leukemia patients: a French retrospective study of 238 patients. Leukemia 2003;17:45–51.
179. Goodman GR, et al. Extended follow-up of patients with hairy cell leukemia after treatment with cladribine. J Clin Oncol 2003;21:891–896.
180. von Rohr A, et al. Treatment of hairy cell leukemia with cladribine (2-chlorodeoxyadenosine) by subcutaneous bolus injection: a phase II study. Ann Oncol 2002;13:1641–1649.
181. Lauria F, et al. Efficacy of anti-CD20 monoclonal antibodies (Mabthera) in patients with progressed hairy cell leukemia. Haematologica 2001;86:1046–1050.
182. Hagberg H, Lundholm L. Rituximab, a chimaeric anti-CD20 monoclonal antibody, in the treatment of hairy cell leukaemia. Br J Haematol 2001;115:609–611.
183. Nieva J, Bethel K, Saven A. Phase 2 study of rituximab in the treatment of cladribine-failed patients with hairy cell leukemia. Blood 2003;102:810–813.
184. Thomas DA, et al. Rituximab in relapsed or refractory hairy cell leukemia. Blood 2003;in press.
185. Stein R, et al. Epitope specificity of the anti-(B cell lymphoma) monoclonal antibody, LL2. Cancer Immunol Immunother 1993;37:293–298.
186. Kreitman RJ, et al. Efficacy of the anti-CD22 recombinant immunotoxin BL22 in chemotherapy-resistant hairy-cell leukemia. N Engl J Med 2001;345:241–247.
187. Kreitman RJ, et al. Responses in refractory hairy cell leukemia to a recombinant immunotoxin. Blood 1999;94:3340–3348.
188. Uchiyama T, Broder S, Waldmann TA. A monoclonal antibody (anti-Tac) reactive with activated and functionally mature human T cells I: production of anti-Tac monoclonal antibody and distribution of Tac (+) cells. J Immunol 1981;126:1393–1397.
189. Uchiyama T, et al. A monoclonal antibody (anti-Tac) reactive with activated and functionally mature human T cells II: expression of Tac antigen on activated cytotoxic killer T cells, suppressor cells, and on one of two types of helper T cells. J Immunol 1981;126:1398–1403.
190. Kreitman RJ, et al. Phase I trial of recombinant immunotoxin anti-Tac(Fv)-PE38 (LMB-2) in patients with hematologic malignancies. J Clin Oncol 2000;18:1622–1636.
191. Flinn IW, et al. Fludarabine and cyclophosphamide achieves high complete response rate in patients with previously untreated chronic lymphocytic leukemia: ECOG 1997. Blood 2001;98:633a.
192. Cazin B, et al. Oral fludarabine and cyclophosphamide in previously untreated CLL: preliminary data on 59 pts. Blood 2001;98:772a.
193. Rai KR, et al. Alemtuzumab in previously treated chronic lymphocytic leukemia patients who also had received fludarabine. J Clin Oncol 2002;20:3891–3897.
194. Dyer MJ, et al. In vivo 'purging' of residual disease in CLL with Campath-1H. Br J Haematol 1997;97:669–672.
195. Montillo M, et al. Safety and efficacy of subcutaneous Campath-1H for treating residual disease in patients with chronic lymphocytic leukemia responding to fludarabine. Haematologica 2002;87:695–700.
196. Kennedy B, et al. Campath-1H therapy in 29 patients with refractory CLL: "true" complete remission is an attainable goal. Blood 1999;94:603a.
197. Keating MJ, et al. Results of first salvage therapy for patients refractory to a fludarabine regimen in chronic lymphocytic leukemia. Leuk Lymphoma 2002;43:1755–1762.

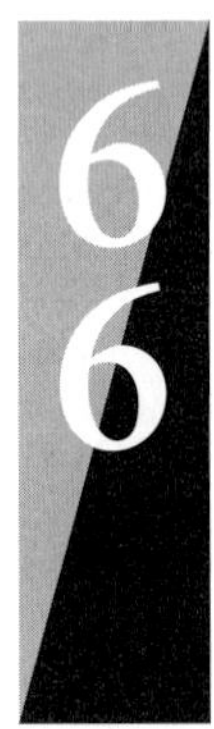

Chronic Myeloid Leukemia

Meir Wetzler

M.T. is a 26-year-old woman with chronic myeloid leukemia (CML) diagnosed during her annual physical examination. Her disease is in the chronic phase, without any high-risk features.[1,2] She has no significant prior medical history. Her sister is a 6/6 HLA antigen match and is in excellent health. Neither sister has been pregnant. M.T. presents for consultation about whether to be treated with imatinib or to undergo allogeneic stem cell transplantation (SCT). She is well informed and has downloaded several articles from the Internet.

In attempting to apply evidence-based medicine in the treatment of chronic myeloid leukemia (CML), it must be acknowledged that a randomized study comparing imatinib mesylate therapy and allogeneic stem cell transplantation (SCT) has not been conducted. The question that will remain at the end of this chapter is whether such a study is feasible, or even ethical. The treatment of CML could represent a paradigm in oncology as well as a unique set of challenges.

Definitions and Molecular Pathogenesis

CML is a clonal expansion of a hematopoietic stem cell resulting from a reciprocal translocation between chromosomes 9 and 22. This translocation results in the head-to-tail fusion of the breakpoint cluster region *(BCR)* gene on chromosome 22q11 with the *ABL* (named after the abelson murine leukemia virus) gene located on chromosome 9q34. Untreated, the disease is characterized by the inevitable transition from a clinically benign chronic phase, often with an interposed accelerated phase, to blast crisis.

The cytogenetic hallmark of CML, found in 90% to 95% of patients, is the t(9;22)(q34;q11.2). The reciprocal 9;22 translocation was originally recognized by the presence of the resultant shortened chromosome 22 (22q–), designated as the *Philadelphia chromosome*. Some patients may have complex translocations (designated as *variant translocations*) involving three, four, or five chromosomes (usually including chromosomes 9 and 22). However, the molecular consequences of these changes appear similar to those resulting from the typical t(9;22). Patients should have evidence of the translocation by either cytogenetics, fluorescence in situ hybridization (FISH), or molecular techniques to make a diagnosis of CML.

The product of the fusion gene resulting from the t(9;22) plays a central role in both the genesis and the treatment of CML. The chimeric gene is transcribed into a hybrid *BCR/ABL* messenger RNA species in which exon 1 of *ABL* is replaced by variable numbers of 5′ *BCR* exons. The Bcr/Abl fusion proteins that then result, $p210^{BCR/ABL}$, contain NH_2-terminal domains of Bcr and COOH-terminal domains of Abl. A rare breakpoint, occurring within the 3′-region of the *BCR* gene, yields a fusion protein of 230 kDa, $p230^{BCR/ABL}$. The role of the Bcr/Abl fusion proteins in leukemogenesis has been substantiated in several laboratory models.

The mechanism(s) by which $p210^{BCR/ABL}$ promotes the transition from the benign state to the fully malignant state is still unclear. Messenger RNA for *BCR/ABL* can occasionally be detected in normal individuals. However, fusion of the *BCR* sequences to *ABL* results in three critical functional changes: (1) the Abl protein becomes constitutively active as a tyrosine kinase enzyme and activates downstream kinases that prevent apoptosis, (2) the DNA protein-binding activity of Abl is attenuated, and (3) the binding of Abl to cytoskeletal actin microfilaments is enhanced.

The molecular events associated with transition to the acute phase, or blast crisis, are poorly understood. Some depend on increased activity of the oncogenic kinase [e.g., an additional t(9;22),[3] deletions adjacent to the translocation breakpoint on the derivative 9 chromosome[4]], and some most probably result from *BCR/ABL*-independent mechanisms [e.g., trisomy 8, or 17p– (p53 loss),[3] lack of production of the retinoblastoma protein, alterations in *RAS*, or presence of an altered *MYC*]. Finally, progressive de novo DNA methylation at the *BCR/ABL* locus has also been shown to herald the onset of blast crisis.[5–7]

Physical Findings

In most patients, the abnormal finding on physical examination at diagnosis is minimal to moderate splenomegaly; mild hepatomegaly is found occasionally. Persistent splenomegaly despite continued therapy is a sign of disease acceleration. Lymphadenopathy and myeloid sarcomas are unusual except late in the course of the disease; when they are present, the prognosis is poor.

Hematologic Findings

Elevated white blood cell counts, with various degrees of immaturity of the granulocytic series, are present at diagnosis. Usually less than 5% circulating blasts and less than 10%

blasts and promyelocytes are noted. Cycling of the counts may be observed in patients followed without treatment. Platelet counts are almost always elevated at diagnosis, and a mild degree of normochromic normocytic anemia is present. Leukocyte alkaline phosphatase is characteristically low in CML cells. Serum levels of vitamin B_{12} and vitamin B_{12}-binding proteins are generally elevated. Phagocytic functions are usually normal at diagnosis and remain normal during the chronic phase. Histamine production secondary to basophilia is increased in later stages, causing pruritus, diarrhea, and flushing.

At diagnosis, bone marrow cellularity, primarily of the myeloid and megakaryocytic lineages, with a greatly altered myeloid to erythroid ratio, is increased in almost all patients with CML. The marrow blast percentage is generally normal or slightly elevated. Marrow or blood basophilia, eosinophilia, and monocytosis may be present. Although collagen fibrosis in the marrow is unusual at presentation, significant degrees of reticulin stain-measured fibrosis are noted in about half the patients.

Disease acceleration is defined by the development of increasing degrees of anemia unaccounted for by bleeding or chemotherapy, cytogenetic clonal evolution, or blood or marrow blasts between 10% and 20%, blood or marrow basophils 20% or greater, or platelet count less than 100,000/μL. *Blast crisis* is defined as acute leukemia, with blood or marrow blasts 20% or more. Hyposegmented neutrophils may appear (Pelger–Huet anomaly). Blast cells can be classified as myeloid, lymphoid, erythroid, or undifferentiated, based on morphologic, cytochemical, and immunologic features. About half the cases are myeloid, one-third lymphoid, 10% erythroid, and the rest are undifferentiated.

Prognostic Factors

Several prognostic models have been developed that identify different risk groups in CML. The most commonly used staging systems were derived from multivariate analyses of prognostic factors. The Sokal index[1] was based on chemotherapy-treated patients and the Hasford system[2] on interferon-treated patients. Table 66.1 compares the two prognostic systems. When applied to a data set of 272 patients treated with interferon-alpha (IFN-α), the Hasford system predicted survival time more accurately than the Sokal score; it identified more low-risk patients but left only a small number of cases in the high-risk group.[8] Preliminary results suggest that the Hasford system is applicable to imatinib-treated patients, but it has not yet been validated in patients undergoing transplantation.

TABLE 66.2. Response criteria in chronic myeloid leukemia (CML).

Hematologic	
Complete response[a]	White blood cell count <10,000/μLl, normal morphology, normal hemoglobin and platelet counts
Incomplete response	White blood cell count ≥10,000/μL
Cytogenetic	Percentage of bone marrow metaphases with t(9;22)
Complete response	0
Partial response	≤35
Minor response	36–85[b]
No response	85–100
Molecular	Presence of *BCR/ABL* transcript by RT-PCR
Complete response	None
Incomplete response	Any
Major response	≥3 log reduction
Minor response	<3 log reduction

[a]Complete hematologic response requires the disappearance of splenomegaly.

[b]Up to 15 normal metaphases are occasionally seen at diagnosis (when 30 metaphases are analyzed).

Treatment

This chapter evaluates the treatment options for CML in chronic phase by a computerized literature search of the MEDLINE database for English-language manuscripts. Observational, retrospective, randomized studies and meta-analyses were reviewed. Case reports were excluded. Survival was the primary objective for defining treatment efficacy, but other measures, such as hematologic, cytogenetic, and molecular responses, were included. At present, the definition of cure in CML is durable, nonneoplastic, nonclonal hematopoiesis, which entails the eradication of cells containing the *BCR/ABL* transcript (Table 66.2). Only recommendations for which there was direct evidence of improved outcome are presented.

Treatment Options

The treatment paradigm for CML is undergoing rapid evolution because of the availability of a curative treatment (allogeneic SCT) that has significant toxicity on the one hand, and on the other, a new, seemingly effective treatment (imatinib) without significant toxicity, but also without long-term follow-up data.

Allogeneic SCT

Allogeneic SCT is currently the only curative therapy for CML and, when feasible, may be the treatment of choice.

TABLE 66.1. Comparison of the Sokal and Hasford prognostic systems.

	Sokal[1] (chemotherapy-based)	*Hasford[2] (interferon-based)*
Age (years)	0.116 (age–43.4)	0.666 when age ≥50
Percentage of blasts	0.0887 (blasts–2.1)	0.0584 × blasts
Spleen size	0.0345 (spleen–7.51)	0.042 × spleen
Platelet count	0.188 [(platelet/700)^2–0.563]	1.0956 when ≥1.5 × 10^9/L
Percentage of eosinophils		0.0413 × eosinophils
Percentage of basophils		0.20399 × basophils ≥3%

TABLE 66.3. Comparison of peripheral blood and bone marrow in recipients of matched sibling allogeneic transplantation for CML.

Study	*Design*	*No. of patients*	*Results*
Couban[18]	Multicenter randomized trial	109[a]	Benefit in overall survival favoring PBSC[b]
Champlin[19]	Retrospective database cohort	346[c]	Similar 1-year cumulative incidence of relapse, probability of leukemia-free survival, and risk of treatment failure
Elmaagacli[20]	Retrospective analysis	41[c]	Similar 3-year survival with a trend toward increased acute GVHD in patients undergoing PBSC transplantation

GVHD, graft-versus-host disease; PBSC, peripheral blood stem cell.

[a]First chronic-phase and more-advanced stages were presented together.

[b]At 30 months.

[c]Patients in first chronic phase only.

However, it is complicated by a high mortality rate. Outcome of SCT depends on multiple factors associated with (1) the patient (age, comorbidities, and phase of disease); (2) the type of donor [syngeneic (monozygotic twins) or HLA-compatible allogeneic, related or unrelated]; (3) the preparative regimen; (4) presence and severity of graft-versus-host disease (GVHD), and (5) the ability to prevent or treat relapse after transplantation.

The Patient

As experience has been gained and safety and efficacy of transplantation have been established, it has become clear that patients should have acceptable end-organ function, be younger than 65 to 75 years, and have a healthy and histocompatible donor. Furthermore, observational studies have demonstrated that survival after SCT in the accelerated and blastic phases of the disease is significantly inferior because of a very high rate of relapse.[9,10] The pre-imatinib Seattle data demonstrated that bone marrow transplantation (BMT) has a better outcome in early chronic phase (1 to 2 years from diagnosis) compared to later in the course of the disease.[11] Another issue in young patients, and particularly, young female patients, is the very high likelihood of infertility following transplantation.

The Donor

Transplantation from a related donor who is either fully matched or mismatched at only one HLA locus should be considered the optimal curative treatment for CML. With HLA-identical sibling BMT in the chronic phase, observational studies have reported 5-year disease-free survival in 40% to 70% of patients, with a 25% relapse rate.[9,10,12,13] Retrospective analysis revealed that male recipients with female donors have an increased risk of developing chronic GVHD, leading to a lower relapse rate but increased mortality.[14] Moreover, for patients in chronic phase less than 1 year from diagnosis and younger than 30 years, BMT from an HLA-matched unrelated donor resulted in similar 5-year disease-free survival as matched sibling donor transplantation in comparative analyses.[15–17] For all other groups, patients receiving transplants from unrelated individuals have higher rates of graft failure (odds ratio, 5.39) and acute (relative risk, 1.31) and chronic (relative risk, 1.48) GVHD, compared to those who receive allogeneic transplants from related individuals.[17]

Peripheral blood is now being studied as a source of hematopoietic progenitor cells; it may offer less risk for the donor as well as more rapid engraftment. One randomized study[18] and two retrospective studies[19,20] compared bone marrow and peripheral blood in recipients of matched sibling allogeneic transplants (Table 66.3). These studies demonstrated an overall survival benefit for recipients receiving peripheral blood stem cells (PBSC) in the randomized study,[18] but similar survival in the two retrospective studies.[19,20] In unrelated donors, a retrospective study[21] demonstrated no difference in incidence and severity of GVHD and improved disease-free survival for peripheral blood compared to bone marrow stem cell transplants (Table 66.4). No randomized studies have been reported so far. At the present time, some centers collect bone marrow and some collect peripheral blood from donors for newly diagnosed CML patients. Umbilical cord blood may permit mismatched SCT with notably less GVHD; graft-versus-leukemia (GVL) effects do not appear to be impaired.[22,23] A problem with cord blood as a source is obtaining an appropriate number of progenitor cells to reconstitute hematopoiesis in an adult.

Preparative Regimens

Four randomized studies compared cyclophosphamide and total-body irradiation with busulphan and cyclophosphamide.[24–27] Long-term follow-up in these studies[28] demonstrated (Table 66.5) no significant differences in the incidence

TABLE 66.4. Comparison of peripheral blood and bone marrow in recipients of unrelated allogeneic transplantation in CML.

	BMT	*PBSC*	*P*
Number	54	37	
Acute GVHD grade III–IV	13 (24)	3 (8)	<0.05
DFS at 1,000 days (%)	64	91	<0.05
Overall survival at 1,000 days (%)	66	94	<0.02

BMT, bone marrow transplant; DFS, disease-free survival; GVHD, graft-versus-host disease; PBSC, peripheral blood stem cells.

Source: Data from Elmaagacli et al.[21]

TABLE 66.5. Long-term follow-up of four randomized studies comparing busulphan and cylophosphamide with total body irradiation and cyclophosphamide.

	Busulphan Cyclophosphamide[a]	*Total body irradiation Cyclophosphamide*[a]
Projected 10-year survival	65*	63
(95% CI)	57–74	54–73
DFS	52	46
(95% CI)	43–61	36–56
5-year cumulative incidence of clinical extensive GVHD	37	39
7-year cumulative incidence of cataracts*	16	47
7-year cumulative incidence of pulmonary disease	15	15
7-year cumulative incidence of avascular osteonecrosis**	3	10

CI, confidence interval; GVHD, graft-versus-host disease.

[a]Numbers represent percentages.

*$P = 0.0003$; remained statistically significant even after adjustment for age and acute and chronic GVHD.

**$P = 0.03$.

Source: Data from Socie et al.[28]

of venoocclusive disease of the liver, speed of engraftment, or the 3-year probabilities of relapse, event-free survival, or overall survival. Significantly, more patients in the total-body irradiation arm experienced cataracts and avascular necrosis. However, chronic GVHD was associated with increased risk of irreversible alopecia in patients treated with busulphan. There was no significant association between busulphan levels and regimen-related toxicity,[29,30] but low levels were associated with an increased risk of relapse in one study.[29] Intravenous busulphan allows better control of plasma levels.[31,32] Nonmyeloblative transplants in which the preparative regimen is aimed at eliminating host lymphocytes rather than eradicated bone marrow and maximizing GVL effect are being tested.[33,44] Reduced toxicity with preserved antitumor efficacy is the goal. Table 66.6 summarizes the published observational studies. Interestingly, for studies that included only patients in chronic phase,[38,40,44] overall survival was 75%, 85%, and 87%, and disease-free survival was 63%, 85%, and 80%. However, the follow-up is relatively short and no randomized studies have been published so far.

Chances of pregnancy after conditioning with busulfan and cyclophosphamide are slim.[45,46] Reduced-intensity transplantation may prevent alopecia, but little is known about its effects on fertility, nor are there long-term data on overall and disease-free survival following this conditioning method.

Development and Type of GVHD

Development of grade I GVHD (mild maculopapular rash involving less than 25% of body surface area, or less than 1000mL diarrhea/day, or bilirubin less than 3mg/dL[47]), as compared to no GVHD, decreases the risk of relapse.[48] A lower relapse rate is observed also in patients with grade II GVHD, but these patients have a substantially higher transplant-related mortality rate.[48] The decreased relapse rate may be caused by a GVL effect. Depletion of T lymphocytes from donor marrow can prevent GVHD but results in an increased risk of relapse, exceeding the relapse rate after syngeneic SCT. Thus, T lymphocytes from the donor marrow mediate a significant antileukemic, or GVL, effect, and even syngeneic marrow[49,50] may exhibit limited GVL activity in CML.

Treatment and Prevention of Posttransplant Relapse

Further support for the existence of an immunologically mediated GVL effect came from the observation that donor

TABLE 66.6. Reduced-intensity conditioning for allografting in CML.

	No. of patients	*Stage of disease*	*Related/ unrelated*	*Acute GVHD (>grade II; %)*	*DFS*[a] *(%)*	*OS*[a] *(%)*
Childs[33]	2	2 CP	2/0	0	—[b]	—[b]
Raiola[34]	15	9 CP/4 AP/2 BP	15/0	N/A	60	80
Giralt[35]	27	6 CP/21 TP	N/A	N/A	34[c]	32[c]
Bornhäuser[36]	44	26 CP/11 AP/7 BP	21/23	14	41	52
Khoury[37]	30	28 CP/2 BP	30/0	17	N/A	83
Okamoto[38]	8	8 CP	8/0	13	63	75
Kreuzer[39]	14	11 CP/2 AP/1 BP	4[d]/0	14	71	N/A
Or[40]	24	24 CP	19/5	21	85	85
Das[41]	17	16 CP/1 AP	17/0	18	29	35
Wong[42]	9	1 CP/2 3rd CP/[d] 4 AP/2 BP	0/9	20	44[c]	56[c]
Sloand[43]	12	7 CP/5 2nd CP	12/0	25	33[e]	67[f]
Uzunel[44]	15	15 CP	10/5	7	80[e]	87

AP, accelerated phase; BP, blastic phase, CP, chronic phase; DFS, disease-free survival; GVHD, graft-versus-host disease; N/A, not available; OS, overall survival; TP, transformed (accelerated and blastic) phase.

[a]Available time points specified in the table.

[b]At 7 and 14 months, both patients are alive in molecular remission.

[c]At 1 year.

[d]Two were nonidentical family members.

[e]By reverse transcriptase-polymerase chain reaction (RT-PCR) at 12 months.

[f]For at least 24 months.

TABLE 66.7. **Factors predicting molecular response after donor-lymphocyte infusions.**

	Probability of molecular response (%)		
Variable	*52*	*53*	*54*
Type of relapse			
Molecular	100[a]	100	
Cytogenetic	84	88	
Hematologic (CP)	55	N/A	63
Interval SCT to relapse			
<9 months	56	N/A	N/A
≥9 months	76		
Dose of T lymphocytes			
CD3 <1 × 108/kg	N/A	N/A	90[a]
CD3 >1 × 108/kg			47

CP, chronic phase; GVHD, graft-versus-host disease; N/A, not available; SCT, stem cell transplant.

[a]Statistically significant.

TABLE 66.9. **Imatinib compared with interferon-alpha (IFN-α) + cytarabine in newly diagnosed CML.**

	Imatinib (n = 553)	*IFN-α + cytarabine (n = 553)*
Age (median)	50	51
Sokal risk groups (%)		
Low	52.5	48.2
Intermediate	29.0	29.7
High	18.5	22.1
Hasford risk groups (%)		
Low	45.6	44.6
Intermediate	44.3	45.4
High	10.1	10.1
Complete hematologic response at 18 months (95% CI)	95.3* 93.2–96.9	55.5 51.3–59.7
Complete cytogenetic response at 18 months (95% CI)	73.8* 69.9–77.4	8.5 6.3–11.1
Reduction of ≥3 log in *BCR/ABL* transcripts from baseline after 12 months of treatment (%)	39*	2
Improvement in quality of life from baseline to 12 months (%)	41*	16

*$P < 0.001$.

Source: Data from References 64–66.

leukocyte infusions (without any preparative chemotherapy or GVHD prophylaxis) can induce hematologic and cytogenetic remissions in patients with CML who have relapsed after allogeneic SCT (Table 66.7).[51–54]

The effect of imatinib in the chronic phase of the disease prompted its study in patients who relapse after allogeneic SCT.[55–57] Retrospective studies (Table 66.8) with small numbers of patients have shown that imatinib can control CML that has recurred after allogeneic SCT but is associated with myelosuppression and recurrence of GVHD. Studies of imatinib treatment after allogeneic SCT to prevent relapse in patients with advanced disease at the time of transplantation (patients at high risk for relapse) or patients undergoing non-myeloblative transplants are under way. No randomized trials have compared donor lymphocyte infusions to imatinib for patients who relapse after allogeneic SCT.

Imatinib Mesylate

Imatinib mesylate (Gleevec, STI571) functions through competitive inhibition at the adenosine triphosphate (ATP)-binding site of the Abl kinase, which leads to inhibition of tyrosine phosphorylation of proteins involved in Bcr/Abl signal transduction.[58] It shows a high degree of specificity for Bcr/Abl, the platelet-derived growth factor receptors and c-*kit* tyrosine kinases. Imatinib induces apoptosis in cells expressing Bcr/Abl. Based on its antileukemic activity in vitro, it was tested in clinical trials.

Most patients with CML in chronic phase have a rapid hematologic response to imatinib therapy. In the initial studies[59] with imatinib in patients with chronic-phase CML who have been intolerant to IFN-α, 95% of patients achieved complete hematologic remissions, 60% achieved major cytogenetic remissions, and 41% achieved complete cytogenetic remissions. Those who did not achieve at least a major cytogenetic remission following 3 months of imatinib therapy had a higher risk of progression of the disease to the accelerated/blastic phases. The accelerated[60]/blastic[61–63] phases of the disease are less responsive to imatinib and the outcome of treatment is less favorable (overall survival at 12 months: accelerated phase, 74%[60]; blastic phase, 22%[61]/32%[62]/28%[63]). These studies led to U.S. Food and Drug Administration approval of imatinib for patients who were intolerant or unresponsive to IFN-α or for patients in the accelerated/blast crisis phases of the disease.

In newly diagnosed CML, a recent randomized phase III study of imatinib (400 mg/day) versus IFN-α and cytarabine,[64,65] demonstrated complete hematologic remission rates of 95.3% with imatinib, compared to 55.5% with IFN-α and cytarabine, after 18 months of treatment (Table 66.9). Similarly, the complete cytogenetic remission rate was 73.8% in patients treated with imatinib, compared to 8.5% in patients treated with IFN-α and cytarabine. Progression to accelerated/blastic phases of the disease was noted in 3% of patients treated with imatinib compared to 8.5% of patients treated

TABLE 66.8. **Imatinib for relapse following allogeneic transplantation.**

	No. of patients	*Stage of disease*	*CHR*	*CCGR*
Kantarjian[55]	28	5 CP/15 AP/8 BP	17	10
Au[56]	8	5 CP/3 BP	7	6
Ollavarria[57]	123	50 CP/29 AP/44 BP	87	44
Total	159	60 (38%) CP/44 (28%) AP/61 55 (35%[a]) BP	111 (70%)	60 (38%)

AP, accelerated phase; BP, blastic phase; CCGR, complete cytogenetic response; CHR, complete hematologic response; CP, chronic phase.

[a]Numbers exceed 100% due to rounding.

with IFN-α and cytarabine.[64] In addition, levels of *BCR/ABL* transcripts were studied in patients who had a complete cytogenetic remission following 12 months of treatment.[65] The levels decreased by at least 3 log in 57% of those on the imatinib arm, compared to 24% of those on the IFN-α and cytarabine arm. No survival data will be available from this study as it had a cross-over option and most patients on the IFN-α and cytarabine arm have crossed over to imatinib. Finally, imatinib offered a clear quality of life advantage as compared to IFN-α and cytarabine in newly diagnosed CML.[66] These results led to rapid U.S. Food and Drug Administration approval of imatinib for newly diagnosed CML patients.

Imatinib is administered orally and has an acceptable toxicity profile. The main side effects are fluid retention, nausea, muscle cramps, diarrhea, and skin rashes. The management of these side effects is usually supportive. Myelosuppression is the most common hematologic toxicity and patients with longer time from diagnosis, those previously treated with busulphan, and those who had cytopenias induced by IFN-α, are at higher risk.[67] Myelosuppression may result from eradication of the malignant clone and delayed recovery of the normal nonclonal progenitor cells. Blood and platelet support should be provided, and the imatinib dose should rarely be reduced in the absence of infection. Use of erythropoietin to treat anemia during imatinib therapy has become standard practice despite the absence of clinical studies, but there is concern that erythropoietin will promote resistance against imatinib.[68] Similarly, the use of granulocyte colony-stimulating factor (G-CSF) has gained acceptance with only small observational studies to support it.[69,70] Imatinib doses below 300 mg per day seem ineffective and may lead to development of resistance.[71]

Resistance to imatinib occurs by mechanisms that are either *BCR/ABL* dependent (gene amplification, mutations at the kinase site, enhanced expression of multidrug exporter proteins) or *BCR/ABL* independent (alternative signaling pathways functionally compensating for the imatinib-sensitive mechanisms). Imatinib resistance has been shown to have an unfavorable prognosis in the accelerated and blast crisis phases of the disease. Specifically, patients who do not achieve major cytogenetic remission within 3 months of initiation of imatinib have shorter survival than patients who achieve that level of remission.[60–63] Both *BCR/ABL*-dependent and *BCR/ABL*-independent mechanisms of imatinib resistance are being targeted in clinical trials. Although no randomized studies have been published, a phase II clinical trial of high-dose imatinib in newly diagnosed patients with chronic-phase CML was recently published.[72] In comparison to a historical control group receiving standard-dose imatinib, patients treated with high-dose imatinib had significantly higher rates of complete cytogenetic response and molecular response.[72]

Interferons

When allogeneic SCT was not feasible, IFN-α therapy was previously the treatment of choice before the availability of imatinib. Only longer follow-up of patients treated with imatinib will demonstrate whether IFN-α will still have a role in the treatment of CML. The interferons are a complex group of naturally occurring proteins produced by eukaryotic cells in response to viruses, antigens, and mitogens. Three distinct groups of IFN species have been identified: IFN-α, IFN-β, and IFN-γ. Although various interferons have become available for clinical investigation, most data have been generated with IFN-α preparations.

Interferons have potent, pleiotropic biologic effects, with a spectrum of antiviral, microbicidal, immunomodulatory, and antiproliferative properties. Although interferons downregulate the expression of several oncogenes and cytokines, they also upregulate the expression of IFN regulatory factor 1 (a transcriptional activator with antioncogenic activity), adhesion molecules, and the histocompatibility genes. Interferons also inhibit angiogenesis and induce a cellular immune response. However, their mode(s) of action in CML is still unknown.

Meta-analysis of seven randomized studies revealed that patients treated with high-dose (5×10^6 units/m^2/day) IFN-α survived longer than patients treated with hydroxyurea or busulphan,[73] with 5-year survival rates of 51% and 42%, respectively. Interestingly, pegylated recombinant IFN-α and recombinant IFN-α had similar efficacy and toxicity profiles in a randomized study.[74] In addition, the combination of high-dose IFN-α with cytarabine produced better results in one randomized study[75] but not in another (Table 66.10).[76] At least two randomized trials[77,78] did not detect any significant difference between high- and low-dose (2.5×10^6 units/m^2/day or 3×10^6 units/5 days/week) IFN-α with regard to complete cytogenetic response, survival, and transformation rates. Furthermore, low-dose IFN-α with cytarabine failed to show any benefit over low-dose IFN-α with or without the addition of hydroyurea in two randomized studies.[79,80] In summary, low-dose, as opposed to high-dose, IFN-α may be used in combination with imatinib in future clinical trials aimed at increased response to imatinib or preventing imatinib resistance.

Patients develop both acute and chronic side effects from IFN-α therapy. Acute side effects (flu-like symptoms) appear early in the course of the treatment. Most flu-like symptoms respond to acetaminophen, and tachyphylaxis develops within 1 to 2 weeks. Chronic reactions, such as fatigue and lethargy, depression, weight loss, myalgias, and arthralgias, occur in about half of patients and often require dose reduction. Patients also report cough, postnasal drip, and dry skin. Infrequently, immune-mediated thrombocytopenia and anemia develop. In addition, long-term therapy has been associated with late autoimmune side effects, such

TABLE 66.10. Comparison of two randomized trials of IFN-α versus IFN-α and low-dose cytarabine for newly diagnosed chronic-phase CML patients.

	IFN-α	*IFN-α + cytarabine*
	Major cytogenetic response (%)	
Guilhot[75a]	41	24[b]
Baccarani[76c]	28	18[b]
	Overall survival (%)	
Guilhot[75d]	85.7	79.1
Baccarani[76c]	68	65

[a]Results at 12 months.
[b]Results are statistically significant.
[c]Results at 24 months.
[d]Results at 36 months.

as hypothyroidism and occasional generalized autoimmune phenomena.

The most important persistent side effects in patients with CML who are treated with IFN-α are neuropsychiatric. All patients treated with IFN-α are subject to some neurologic toxicity, the most common symptom being lethargy. Up to 20% of patients have neurologic side effects that are associated with compromised quality of life and reduced ability to carry out their regular activity, such as full-time work. From at least one observational study,[81] it seems that patients with a pretreatment neurologic or psychiatric diagnosis are at significantly increased risk of developing severe neuropsychiatric toxicity.

Chemotherapy

Innovative approaches are still important in CML because the exact role of imatinib in the armamentarium of CML is still not clear. Initial management of patients with chemotherapy is currently reserved for rapid lowering of white blood cell counts, reduction of symptoms, and reversal of symptomatic splenomegaly. Hydroxyurea, a ribonucleotide reductase inhibitor, induces rapid disease control. The initial dose is 1 to 4 g/day, and the dosage should be reduced by half with each 50% reduction of the leukocyte count. Unfortunately, cytogenetic remissions with hydroxyurea are uncommon. Busulphan, an alkylating agent that acts on early progenitor cells, has a more prolonged effect. However, it is rarely used because of its serious side effects, which include unexpected, and occasionally fatal, myelosuppression in 5% to 10% of patients, as well as pulmonary, endocardial, and marrow fibrosis and an Addison-like wasting syndrome.

Intensive combination chemotherapy has also been used in chronic-phase CML, with 30% to 50% of patients achieving complete cytogenetic responses. However, these cytogenetic remissions have been short-lived. Consequently, intensive combination chemotherapy regimens are being used today only to mobilize normal progenitors in the blood to collect circulating stem cells for autologous transplantation.

Autologous SCT

Autologous SCT could potentially cure CML if a means to select the residual normal progenitors, which coexist with their malignant counterparts, could be developed. As a source of autologous hematopoietic stem cells for transplantation, blood offers certain advantages over marrow (e.g., faster engraftment and no necessity for general anesthesia). Normal hematopoietic stem cells appear with increased frequency in the blood of patients with CML during the recovery phase after chemotherapy, with G-CSF priming. A role for imatinib prestem cell collection to achieve minimal residual disease and to maintain this status following transplantation is being currently investigated.[82–84] However, only a few patients have been reported to successfully engraft following imatinib therapy. Therefore, such approaches should be implemented only in clinical trials.

Leukapheresis and Splenectomy

Intensive leukapheresis may control the blood counts in chronic-phase CML; but this procedure is expensive and cumbersome. It is useful in emergency situations in which leukostasis-related complications, such as pulmonary failure or cerebrovascular accidents are likely. It may also have a role in the treatment of pregnant women in whom it is important to avoid potentially teratogenic drugs.

Splenectomy was used in CML in the past because of the suggestion that evolution to the acute phase might occur in the spleen. However, this does not appear to be the case, and splenectomy is now reserved for relief of pain associated with splenomegaly unresponsive to chemotherapy or with recurrent splenic infarcts, or improvement of significant anemia or thrombocytopenia associated with hypersplenism. Splenic radiation is used rarely to reduce the size of the spleen.

Minimal Residual Disease

After allogeneic SCT, residual disease may be detected by reverse transcriptase-polymerase chain reaction (RT-PCR) analysis during the first 6 months in patients who subsequently achieve a long-lasting remission, according to a multivariate analysis of 346 patients.[85] However, RT-PCR results, by 6 months, classified as negative, positive at a low level (less than 100 *BCR/ABL* transcripts/μg RNA and/or *BCR/ABL-ABL* ratio of less than 0.02%), or positive at a high level (transcripts levels exceeding the above) did predict outcome in one observational study,[86] with probabilities of relapse of 16.7%, 42.9%, and 86.4%, respectively. Late persistence of RT-PCR positivity appears to indicate a reduced probability of cure.[85,87] Therefore, after allogeneic SCT, patients are often divided according to RT-PCR results into one of three groups: (1) persistently positive, (2) intermittently negative, and (3) persistently negative. These three groups have low, intermediate, and high probability of disease-free survival, respectively. Although these data suggest that patients who are persistently RT-PCR positive more than 6 months after allogeneic SCT need additional therapeutic interventions, this conclusion has not been rigorously established. The studies have used an assortment of techniques for measuring minimal residual disease, the level of sensitivity has been variable, and the durations of patient follow-up have been short. For example, quantitative real-time RT-PCR may provide a less sensitive tool (sensitivity in the range of $1:10^4$ to $1:10^5$) to predict relapse in CML as compared to competitive nested PCR (sensitivity in the range of $1:10^5$ to $1:10^6$).[88] In patients who do not have any evidence of GVHD and are intermittently or persistently RT-PCR positive, GVL may be induced by administering donor lymphocytes to eradicate the residual leukemia cells.[51–54] Another approach is the use of imatinib to eradicate minimal residual disease.[55–57]

In contrast to the results achieved with allogeneic SCT, only a minority (5% to 10%) of patients develop molecular remission following imatinib therapy.[65,89–92] Extrapolating from the SCT data, patients without molecular remission are likely to be at high risk of relapse. However, patients with AML with t(8;21) who are in long-term remission have persistent multipotent progenitor cells expressing *AML1/ETO* transcripts.[93] Therefore, it is unclear whether achieving durable molecular remission with imatinib should indeed be the goal of treatment in CML. This question will be answered only with long-term follow-up of imatinib-treated patients.

Recommendations

The encouraging results with imatinib have steered many clinicians to offer it as a first-line therapy for newly diagnosed CML patients, including those who otherwise would have benefited from transplant (e.g., young patients with sibling-matched donors). This approach may be unwise because the clinical studies so far have very short follow-up, thus limiting knowledge regarding the cure rate associated with imatinib. There is a risk that, by delaying transplantation, either new clonal cytogenetic abnormalites will develop in Philadelphia chromosome-negative cells[94–106] or transplantation after the development of resistance may be associated with worse outcome.[107,108]

If transplantation is selected, evidence-based data are available to recommend BMT with a preparatory regimen that includes busulphan and cyclophosphamide. Only one randomized trial[18] with 30 months follow-up demonstrated better survival with PBSC versus bone marrow as a source of stem cells. Further, the data from reduced-intensity preparative regimens are intriguing, but no randomized studies or long-term follow-up data are available at this point. Therefore, physician experience and patient preference must be factored into the treatment selection process.

Discussion of both treatment options with a patient is indicated. The decision should focus on the outcomes, risks, and toxicities of the two approaches. Some centers would employ allogeneic SCT in patients younger than 30 years of age, as the risk of transplant-related toxicity is minimal in that population. A proposed treatment plan for the newly diagnosed patient with CML is presented in Figure 66.1.

There is no clear answer for M.T. However, if she elects to start treatment with imatinib, it is imperative that her response be followed carefully. Consensus based on clinical experience suggests monitoring cytogenetics or peripheral blood FISH every 3 to 6 months. Patients who achieve a complete cytogenetic remission should have bone marrow cytogenetics every 6 months, alternating with peripheral blood quantitative RT-PCR. SCT will be revisited at any sign of disease progression, for example, increasing BCR/ABL transcript levels.

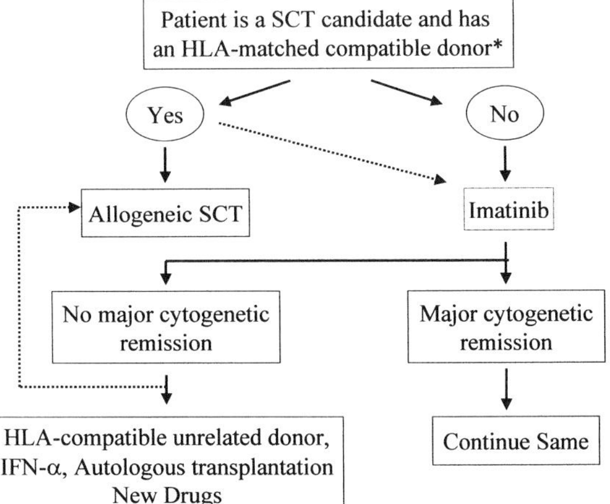

FIGURE 66.1. Flow chart for the therapy of newly diagnosed chronic myeloid leukemia (CML). Patients with an HLA-compatible donor have the possibility to undergo allogeneic stem cell transplantation (SCT) as initial therapy or treatment with Imatinib. The *asterisk* denotes centers that employ allogeneic SCT only if Imatinib fails to induce a response. *Dotted lines* denote lack of long-term survival data.

References

1. Sokal JE. Prognosis in chronic myeloid leukaemia: biology of the disease vs. treatment. Baillieres Clin Haematol 1981;907–929.
2. Hasford J, Pfirrmann M, Hehlmann R, et al. A new prognostic score for survival of patients with chronic myeloid leukemia treated with interferon alfa. Writing Committee for the Collaborative CML Prognostic Factors Project Group. J Natl Cancer Inst 1998;90:850–858.
3. Swolin B, Weinfeld A, Westin J, et al. Karyotypic evolution in Ph-positive chronic myeloid leukemia in relation to management and disease progression. Cancer Genet Cytogenet 1985; 18:65–79.
4. Sinclair PB, Nacheva EP, Leversha M, et al. Large deletions at the t(9;22) breakpoint are common and may identify a poor-prognosis subgroup of patients with chronic myeloid leukemia. Blood 2000;95:738–743.
5. Zion M, Ben-Yehuda D, Avraham A, et al. Progressive de novo DNA methylation at the bcr-abl locus in the course of chronic myelogenous leukemia. Proc Natl Acad Sci USA 1994;91: 10722–10726.
6. Asimakopoulos FA, Shteper PJ, Krichevsky S, et al. ABL1 methylation is a distinct molecular event associated with clonal evolution of chronic myeloid leukemia. Blood 1999;94:2452–2460.
7. Issa JP, Kantarjian H, Mohan A, et al. Methylation of the ABL1 promoter in chronic myelogenous leukemia: lack of prognostic significance. Blood 1999;93:2075–2080.
8. Bonifazi F, De Vivo A, Rosti G, et al. Testing Sokal's and the new prognostic score for chronic myeloid leukaemia treated with alpha-interferon. Italian Cooperative Study Group on Chronic Myeloid Leukaemia. Br J Haematol 2000;111:587–595.
9. Clift RA, Storb R. Marrow transplantation for CML: the Seattle experience. Bone Marrow Transplant 1996;3:S1–S3.
10. Horowitz MM, Rowlings PA, Passweg JR. Allogeneic bone marrow transplantation for CML: a report from the International Bone Marrow Transplant Registry. Bone Marrow Transplant 1996;3:S5–S6.
11. Thomas ED, Clift RA, Fefer A, et al. Marrow transplantation for the treatment of chronic myelogenous leukemia. Ann Intern Med 1986;104:155–163.
12. van Rhee F, Szydlo RM, Hermans J, et al. Long-term results after allogeneic bone marrow transplantation for chronic myelogenous leukemia in chronic phase: a report from the Chronic Leukemia Working Party of the European Group for Blood and Marrow Transplantation. Bone Marrow Transplant 1997;20: 553–560.
13. Koh LP, Hwang WY, Tan CH, et al. Long term follow-up of Asian patients with chronic myeloid leukemia (CML) receiving allogeneic hematopoietic stem cell transplantation (HSCT) from HLA-identical sibling: evaluation of risks and benefits. Ann Hematol 2004;83:286–294.
14. Gratwohl A, Brand R, Apperley J, et al. Chronic Leukemia Working Party of the European Group for Blood and Marrow Transplantation (CLWP-EBMT). Graft-versus-host disease and outcome in HLA-identical sibling transplantations for chronic myeloid leukemia. Blood 2002;100:3877–3886.
15. Hansen JA, Gooley TA, Martin PJ, et al. Bone marrow transplants from unrelated donors for patients with chronic myeloid leukemia. N Engl J Med 1998;338:962–968.
16. Davies SM, DeFor TE, McGlave PB, et al. Equivalent outcomes in patients with chronic myelogenous leukemia after early transplantation of phenotypically matched bone marrow from related or unrelated donors. Am J Med 2001;110:339–346.

17. Weisdorf DJ, Anasetti C, Antin JH, et al. Allogeneic bone marrow transplantation for chronic myelogenous leukemia: comparative analysis of unrelated versus matched sibling donor transplantation. Blood 2002;99:1971–1977.
18. Couban S, Simpson DR, Barnett MJ, et al. Canadian Bone Marrow Transplant Group. A randomized multicenter comparison of bone marrow and peripheral blood in recipients of matched sibling allogeneic transplants for myeloid malignancies. Blood 2002;100:1525–1531.
19. Champlin RE, Schmitz N, Horowitz MM, et al. Blood stem cells compared with bone marrow as a source of hematopoietic cells for allogeneic transplantation. IBMTR Histocompatibility and Stem Cell Sources Working Committee and the European Group for Blood and Marrow Transplantation (EBMT). Blood 2000;95: 3702–3709.
20. Elmaagacli AH, Peceny R, Steckel N, et al. Outcome of transplantation of highly purified peripheral blood $CD34^+$ cells with T-cell add-back compared with unmanipulated bone marrow or peripheral blood stem cells from HLA-identical sibling donors in patients with first chronic phase chronic myeloid leukemia. Blood 2003;101:446–453.
21. Elmaagacli AH, Basoglu S, Peceny R, et al. Improved disease-free-survival after transplantation of peripheral blood stem cells as compared with bone marrow from HLA-identical unrelated donors in patients with first chronic phase chronic myeloid leukemia. Blood 2002;99:1130–1135.
22. Sanz GF, Saavedra S, Jimenez C, et al. Unrelated donor cord blood transplantation in adults with chronic myelogenous leukemia: results in nine patients from a single institution. Bone Marrow Transplant 2001;27:693–701.
23. Laughlin MJ, Barker J, Bambach B, et al. Hematopoietic engraftment and survival in adult recipients of umbilical-cord blood from unrelated donors. N Engl J Med 2001;344:1815–1822.
24. Blaise D, Maraninchi D, Archimbaud E, et al. Allogeneic bone marrow transplantation for acute myeloid leukemia in first remission: a randomized trial of a busulfan-Cytoxan versus Cytoxan-total body irradiation as preparative regimen: a report from the Group d'Etudes de la Greffe de Moelle Osseuse. Blood 1992;79:2578–2582.
25. Ringden O, Ruutu T, Remberger M, et al. A randomized trial comparing busulfan with total body irradiation as conditioning in allogeneic marrow transplant recipients with leukemia: a report from the Nordic Bone Marrow Transplantation Group. Blood 1994;83:2723–2730.
26. Clift RA, Buckner CD, Thomas ED, et al. Marrow transplantation for chronic myeloid leukemia: a randomized study comparing cyclophosphamide and total body irradiation with busulfan and cyclophosphamide. Blood 1994;84:2036–2043.
27. Devergie A, Blaise D, Attal M, et al. Allogeneic bone marrow transplantation for chronic myeloid leukemia in first chronic phase: a randomized trial of busulfan-cytoxan versus cytoxan-total body irradiation as preparative regimen: a report from the French Society of Bone Marrow Graft (SFGM). Blood 1995; 85:2263–2268.
28. Socie G, Clift RA, Blaise D, et al. Busulfan plus cyclophosphamide compared with total-body irradiation plus cyclophosphamide before marrow transplantation for myeloid leukemia: long-term follow-up of 4 randomized studies. Blood 2001;98: 3569–3574.
29. Slattery JT, Clift RA, Buckner CD, et al. Marrow transplantation for chronic myeloid leukemia: the influence of plasma busulfan levels on the outcome of transplantation. Blood 1997;89: 3055–3060.
30. Radich JP, Gooley T, Bensinger W, et al. HLA-matched related hematopoietic cell transplantation for chronic-phase CML using a targeted busulfan and cyclophosphamide preparative regimen. Blood 2003;102:31–35.
31. Olavarria E, Hassan M, Eades A, et al. A phase I/II study of multiple-dose intravenous busulfan as myeloablation prior to stem cell transplantation. Leukemia 2000;14:1954–1959.
32. Schuler US, Renner UD, Kroschinsky F, et al. Intravenous busulphan for conditioning before autologous or allogeneic human blood stem cell transplantation. Br J Haematol 2001;114: 944–950.
33. Childs R, Epperson D, Bahceci E, et al. Molecular remission of chronic myeloid leukaemia following a nonmyeloablative allogeneic peripheral blood stem cell transplant: in vivo and in vitro evidence for a graft-versus-leukaemia effect. Br J Haematol 1999;107:396–400.
34. Raiola AM, Van Lint MT, Lamparelli T, et al. Reduced intensity thiotepa-cyclophosphamide conditioning for allogeneic haemopoietic stem cell transplants (HSCT) in patients up to 60 years of age. Br J Haematol 2000;109:716–721.
35. Giralt S, Thall PF, Khouri I, et al. Melphalan and purine analog-containing preparative regimens: reduced-intensity conditioning for patients with hematologic malignancies undergoing allogeneic progenitor cell transplantation. Blood 2001;97:631–637.
36. Bornhauser M, Kiehl M, Siegert W, et al. Cooperative German Transplant Study Group. Dose-reduced conditioning for allografting in 44 patients with chronic myeloid leukaemia: a retrospective analysis. Br J Haematol 2001;115:119–124.
37. Khoury H, Adkins D, Brown R, et al. Low incidence of transplantation-related acute complications in patients with chronic myeloid leukemia undergoing allogeneic stem cell transplantation with a low-dose (550 cGy) total body irradiation conditioning regimen. Biol Blood Marrow Transplant 2001;7:352–358.
38. Okamoto S, Watanabe R, Takahashi S, et al. Long-term follow-up of allogeneic bone marrow transplantation after reduced-intensity conditioning in patients with chronic myelogenous leukemia in the chronic phase. Int J Hematol 2002;75:493–498.
39. Kreuzer KA, Schmidt CA, Schetelig J, et al. Kinetics of stem cell engraftment and clearance of leukaemia cells after allogeneic stem cell transplantation with reduced intensity conditioning in chronic myeloid leukaemia. Eur J Haematol 2002;69:7–10.
40. Or R, Shapira MY, Resnick I, Amar A, et al. Nonmyeloablative allogeneic stem cell transplantation for the treatment of chronic myeloid leukemia in first chronic phase. Blood 2003;101: 441–445.
41. Das M, Saikia TK, Advani SH et al. Use of a reduced-intensity conditioning regimen for allogeneic transplantation in patients with chronic myeloid leukemia. Bone Marrow Transplant 2003; 32:125–129.
42. Wong R, Giralt SA, Martin T, et al. Reduced-intensity conditioning for unrelated donor hematopoietic stem cell transplantation as treatment for myeloid malignancies in patients older than 55 years. Blood 2003;102:3052–3059.
43. Sloand E, Childs RW, Solomon S, et al. The graft-versus-leukemia effect of nonmyeloablative stem cell allografts may not be sufficient to cure chronic myelogenous leukemia. Bone Marrow Transplant 2003;32:897–901.
44. Uzunel M, Mattsson J, Brune M, et al. Kinetics of minimal residual disease and chimerism in patients with chronic myeloid leukemia after nonmyeloablative conditioning and allogeneic stem cell transplantation. Blood 2003;101:469–472.
45. Sanders JE, Hawley J, Levy W, et al. Pregnancies following high-dose cyclophosphamide with or without high-dose busulfan or total-body irradiation and bone marrow transplantation. Blood 1996;87:3045–3052.
46. Salooja N, Szydlo RM, Socie G, et al. Late Effects Working Party of the European Group for Blood and Marrow Transplantation. Pregnancy outcomes after peripheral blood or bone marrow transplantation: a retrospective survey. Lancet 2001;358: 271–276.
47. Glucksberg H, Storb R, Fefer A, et al. Clinical manifestations of graft-versus-host disease in human recipients of marrow from

HL-A-matched sibling donors. Transplantation 1974;18: 295–304.
48. McGlave P. Bone marrow transplants in chronic myelogenous leukemia: an overview of determinants of survival. Semin Hematol 1990;27(3 suppl 4):23–30.
49. Wolin MJ, Rigor RL. Acute graft-versus-host disease in a recipient of a twin blood cell transplant. Bone Marrow Transplant 1996;17:125–126.
50. Reiter E, Greinix HT, Mitterbauer G, et al. Graft-versus-host disease following second syngeneic stem cell transplantation for relapsed chronic myeloid leukemia. Ann Hematol 1998;77: 283–286.
51. Roman J, Alvarez MA, Torres A. Molecular basis for therapeutic decisions in chronic myeloid leukemia patients after allogeneic bone marrow transplantation. Haematologica 2000;85: 1072–1082.
52. Dazzi F, Szydlo RM, Cross NC, et al. Durability of responses following donor lymphocyte infusions for patients who relapse after allogeneic stem cell transplantation for chronic myeloid leukemia. Blood 2000;96:2712–2716.
53. Raiola AM, Van Lint MT, Valbonesi M, et al. Factors predicting response and graft-versus-host disease after donor lymphocyte infusions: a study on 593 infusions. Bone Marrow Transplant 2003;8:687–893.
54. Vela-Ojeda J, Garcia-Ruiz Esparza MA, Reyes-Maldonado E, et al. Donor lymphocyte infusions for relapse of chronic myeloid leukemia after allogeneic stem cell transplantation: prognostic significance of the dose of CD3(+) and CD4(+) lymphocytes. Ann Hematol 2004;83:295–301.
55. Kantarjian HM, O'Brien S, Cortes JE, et al. Imatinib mesylate therapy for relapse after allogeneic stem cell transplantation for chronic myelogenous leukemia. Blood 2002;100:1590–1595.
56. Au WY, Lie AK, Ma SK, et al. Tyrosine kinase inhibitor STI571 in the treatment of Philadelphia chromosome-positive leukaemia failing myeloablative stem cell transplantation. Bone Marrow Transplant 2002;7:453–457.
57. Olavarria E, Ottmann OG, Deininger M, et al. Leukaemia Working Party of the European Group of Bone and Marrow Transplantation (EBMT). Response to imatinib in patients who relapse after allogeneic stem cell transplantation for chronic myeloid leukemia. Leukemia 2003;17:1707–1712.
58. Goldman JM, Melo JV. Chronic myeloid leukemia advances in biology and new approaches to treatment. N Engl J Med 2003; 349:1451–1464.
59. Kantarjian H, Sawyers C, Hochhaus A, et al. International STI571 CML Study Group. Hematologic and cytogenetic responses to imatinib mesylate in chronic myelogenous leukemia. N Engl J Med 2002;346:645–652.
60. Talpaz M, Silver RT, Druker BJ, et al. Imatinib induces durable hematologic and cytogenetic responses in patients with accelerated phase chronic myeloid leukemia: results of a phase 2 study. Blood 2002;99:1928–1937.
61. Kantarjian HM, Cortes J, O'Brien S, et al. Imatinib mesylate (STI571) therapy for Philadelphia chromosome-positive chronic myelogenous leukemia in blast phase. Blood 2002;99: 3547–3553.
62. Sawyers CL, Hochhaus A, Feldman E, et al. Imatinib induces hematologic and cytogenetic responses in patients with chronic myelogenous leukemia in myeloid blast crisis: results of a phase II study. Blood 2002;99:3530–3539.
63. Sureda A, Carrasco M, de Miguel M, et al. Imatinib mesylate as treatment for blastic transformation of Philadelphia chromosome positive chronic myelogenous leukemia. Haematologica 2003;11:1213–1220.
64. O'Brien SG, Guilhot F, Larson RA, et al. Imatinib compared with interferon and low-dose cytarabine for newly diagnosed chronic-phase chronic myeloid leukemia. N Engl J Med 2003;348: 994–1004.
65. Hughes TP, Kaeda J, Branford S, et al. International Randomised Study of Interferon versus STI571 (IRIS) Study Group. Frequency of major molecular responses to imatinib or interferon alfa plus cytarabine in newly diagnosed chronic myeloid leukemia. N Engl J Med 2003;349:1423–1432.
66. Hahn EA, Glendenning GA, Sorensen MV, et al. Quality of life in patients with newly diagnosed chronic phase chronic myeloid leukemia on imatinib versus interferon alfa plus low-dose cytarabine: results from the IRIS Study. J Clin Oncol 2003; 21:2138–2146.
67. Deininger MW, O'Brien SG, Ford JM, et al. Practical management of patients with chronic myeloid leukemia receiving imatinib. J Clin Oncol 2003;21:1637–1647.
68. Kirschner KM, Baltensperger K. Erythropoietin promotes resistance against the Abl tyrosine kinase inhibitor imatinib (STI571) in K562 human leukemia cells. Mol Cancer Res 2003;1:970–980.
69. Marin D, Marktel S, Foot N, et al. Granulocyte colony-stimulating factor reverses cytopenia and may permit cytogenetic responses in patients with chronic myeloid leukemia treated with imatinib mesylate. Haematologica 2003;88:227–229.
70. Heim D, Ebnother M, Meyer-Monard S, et al. G-CSF for imatinib-induced neutropenia. Leukemia 2003;17:805–807.
71. Peng B, Hayes M, Resta D, et al. Pharmacokinetics and pharmacodynamics of imatinib in a phase I trial with chronic myeloid leukemia patients. J Clin Oncol 2004;22:935–942.
72. Kantarjian H, Talpaz M, O'Brien S, et al. High-dose imatinib mesylate therapy in newly diagnosed Philadelphia chromosome-positive chronic phase chronic myeloid leukemia. Blood 2003; Dec 24 [Epub ahead of print.]
73. Anonymous. Interferon alfa versus chemotherapy for chronic myeloid leukemia: a meta-analysis of seven randomized trials: Chronic Myeloid Leukemia Trialists' Collaborative Group. J Natl Cancer Inst 1997;89:1616–1620.
74. Michallet M, Maloisel F, Delain M, et al. PEG-Intron CML Study Group. Pegylated recombinant interferon alpha-2b vs. recombinant interferon alpha-2b for the initial treatment of chronic-phase chronic myelogenous leukemia: a phase III study. Leukemia 2004;18:309–315.
75. Guilhot F, Chastang C, Michallet M, et al. Interferon alfa-2b combined with cytarabine versus interferon alone in chronic myelogenous leukemia. French Chronic Myeloid Leukemia Study Group. N Engl J Med 1997;3374:223–229.
76. Baccarani M, Rosti G, de Vivo A, et al. Italian Cooperative Study Group on Myeloid Leukemia. A randomized study of interferon-alpha versus interferon-alpha and low-dose arabinosyl cytosine in chronic myeloid leukemia. Blood 2002;99:1527–1535.
77. Kluin-Nelemans HC, Buck G, Le Cessie S, et al. Randomized comparison of low dose versus high dose interferon-alfa in chronic myeloid leukemia: prospective collaboration of three joint trials by the MRC and HOVON groups. Blood 2004; Mar 9 [Epub ahead of print.]
78. Penarrubia MJ, Odriozola J, Gonzalez C, et al. A randomized study of intermediate as compared with high doses of interferon-alpha for chronic myeloid leukemia: no differences in cytogenetic responses. Ann Hematol 2003;82:750–758.
79. Giles FJ, Shan J, Chen S, et al. A prospective randomized study of alpha-2b interferon plus hydroxyurea or cytarabine for patients with early chronic phase chronic myelogenous leukemia: the International Oncology Study Group CML1 study. Leuk Lymphoma 2000;37:367–377.
80. Kuhr T, Burgstaller S, Apfelbeck U, et al. Austrian CML Study Group. A randomized study comparing interferon (IFN alpha) plus low-dose cytarabine and interferon plus hydroxyurea (HU) in early chronic-phase chronic myeloid leukemia (CML). Leuk Res 2003;27:405–411.
81. Hensley ML, Peterson B, Silver RT, et al. Risk factors for severe neuropsychiatric toxicity in patients receiving interferon alfa-2b and low-dose cytarabine for chronic myelogenous leukemia:

analysis of Cancer and Leukemia Group B 9013. J Clin Oncol 2000;18:1301–1308.

82. Drummond MW, Marin D, Clark RE, et al. United Kingdom Chronic Myeloid Leukaemia (UK CML) Working Party. Mobilization of Ph chromosome-negative peripheral blood stem cells in chronic myeloid leukaemia patients with imatinib mesylate-induced complete cytogenetic remission. Br J Haematol 2003; 123:479–483.
83. Hui CH, Goh KY, White D, et al. Successful peripheral blood stem cell mobilisation with filgrastim in patients with chronic myeloid leukaemia achieving complete cytogenetic response with imatinib, without increasing disease burden as measured by quantitative real-time PCR. Leukemia 2003;17: 821–828.
84. Kreuzer KA, Kluhs C, Baskaynak G, et al. Filgrastim-induced stem cell mobilization in chronic myeloid leukaemia patients during imatinib therapy: safety, feasibility and evidence for an efficient in vivo purging. Br J Haematol 2004;124:195–199.
85. Radich JP, Gehly G, Gooley T, et al. Polymerase chain reaction detection of the BCR-ABL fusion transcript after allogeneic marrow transplantation for chronic myeloid leukemia: results and implications in 346 patients. Blood 1995;85:2632–2638.
86. Olavarria E, Kanfer E, Szydlo R, et al. Early detection of BCR-ABL transcripts by quantitative reverse transcriptase-polymerase chain reaction predicts outcome after allogeneic stem cell transplantation for chronic myeloid leukemia Blood 2001; 97:1560–1565.
87. Faderl S, Talpaz M, Kantarjian HM, et al. Should polymerase chain reaction analysis to detect minimal residual disease in patients with chronic myelogenous leukemia be used in clinical decision making? Blood 1999;93:2755–2759.
88. Guo JQ, Lin H, Kantarjian H, et al. Comparison of competitive-nested PCR and real-time PCR in detecting BCR-ABL fusion transcripts in chronic myeloid leukemia patients. Leukemia 2002;16:2447–2453.
89. Merx K, Muller MC, Kreil S, et al. Early reduction of BCR-ABL mRNA transcript levels predicts cytogenetic response in chronic phase CML patients treated with imatinib after failure of interferon alpha. Leukemia 2002;16:1579–1583.
90. Kantarjian HM, Talpaz M, Cortes J, et al. Quantitative polymerase chain reaction monitoring of BCR-ABL during therapy with imatinib mesylate (STI571; gleevec) in chronic-phase chronic myelogenous leukemia. Clin Cancer Res 2003;9: 160–166.
91. Wu CJ, Neuberg D, Chillemi A, McLaughlin S, et al. Quantitative monitoring of BCR/ABL transcript during STI-571 therapy. Leuk Lymphoma 2002;43:2281–2289.
92. Paschka P, Muller MC, Merx K, et al. Molecular monitoring of response to imatinib (Glivec) in CML patients pretreated with interferon alpha. Low levels of residual disease are associated with continuous remission. Leukemia 2003;17:1687–1694.
93. Miyamoto T, Weissman IL, Akashi K. AML1/ETO-expressing nonleukemic stem cells in acute myelogenous leukemia with 8;21 chromosomal translocation. Proc Natl Acad Sci USA 2000; 97:7521–7526.
94. Andersen MK, Pedersen-Bjergaard J, Kjeldsen L, et al. Clonal Ph-negative hematopoiesis in CML after therapy with imatinib mesylate is frequently characterized by trisomy 8. Leukemia 2002;16:1390–1393.
95. Bumm T, Muller C, Al-Ali HK, et al. Emergence of clonal cytogenetic abnormalities in Ph cells in some CML patients in cytogenetic remission to imatinib but restoration of polyclonal hematopoiesis in the majority. Blood 2003;101:1941–1949.
96. Besalduch J, Guti Rrez A, Parody R, et al. Chromosomal abnormalities in Philadelphia (Ph)-negative cells of patients with chronic myeloid leukemia treated with Imatinib (ST1571). Haematologica 2003;88:ELT03.
97. O'Dwyer ME, Gatter KM, Loriaux M, et al. Demonstration of Philadelphia chromosome negative abnormal clones in patients with chronic myelogenous leukemia during major cytogenetic responses induced by imatinib mesylate. Leukemia 2003; 17:481–487.
98. Chee YL, Vickers MA, Stevenson D, et al. Fatal myelodysplastic syndrome developing during therapy with imatinib mesylate and characterised by the emergence of complex Philadelphia negative clones. Leukemia 2003;17:634–635.
99. Gozzetti A, Tozzuoli D, Crupi R, et al. Emergence of Ph negative clones in chronic myeloid leukemia (CML) patients in complete cytogenetic remission after therapy with imatinib mesylate (STI). Eur J Haematol 2003;71:313–314.
100. Mozziconacci MJ, Cailleres S, Maurice C, et al. Myelodysplastic features developing in Philadephia-negative cells during imatinib mesylate therapy for CML: report of a new case. Leukemia 2003;7:1901–1902.
101. Cherrier-De Wilde S, Rack K, Vannuffel P, et al. Philadelphia-negative acute lymphoblastic leukemia developing in a CML patient in imatinib mesylate-induced complete cytogenetic remission. Leukemia 2003;17:2046–2048.
102. Herens C, Baron F, Croisiau C, et al. Clonal chromosome aberrations in Philadelphia-negative cells from chronic myelocytic leukemia patients treated with imatinib mesylate: report of two cases. Cancer Genet Cytogenet 2003;147:78–80.
103. Medina J, Kantarjian H, Talpaz M, et al. Chromosomal abnormalities in Philadelphia chromosome-negative metaphases appearing during imatinib mesylate therapy in patients with Philadelphia chromosome-positive chronic myelogenous leukemia in chronic phase. Cancer (Phila) 2003;98:1905–1911.
104. Jin Huh H, Won Huh J, Myong Seong C, et al. Acute lymphoblastic leukemia without the Philadelphia chromosome occurring in chronic myelogenous leukemia with the Philadelphia chromosome. Am J Hematol 2003;74:218–220.
105. Alimena G, Breccia M, Mancini M, et al. Clonal evolution in Philadelphia chromosome negative cells following successful treatment with Imatinib of a CML patient: clinical and biological features of a myelodysplastic syndrome. Leukemia 2004; 18:361–362.
106. Gozzetti A, Tozzuoli D, Crupi R, et al. A novel t(6;7)(p24;q21) in a chronic myelocytic leukemia in complete cytogenetic remission after therapy with imatinib mesylate. Cancer Genet Cytogenet 2004;148:152–154.
107. Bornhauser M, Jenke A, Freiberg-Richter J, et al. CNS blast crisis of chronic myelogenous leukemia in a patient with a major cytogenetic response in bone marrow associated with low levels of imatinib mesylate and its N-desmethylated metabolite in cerebral spinal fluid. Ann Hematol 2003; Dec 12 [Epub ahead of print.]
108. Avery S, Nadal E, Marin D, et al. Lymphoid transformation in a CML patient in complete cytogenetic remission following treatment with imatinib. Leuk Res 2004;28:75–77.

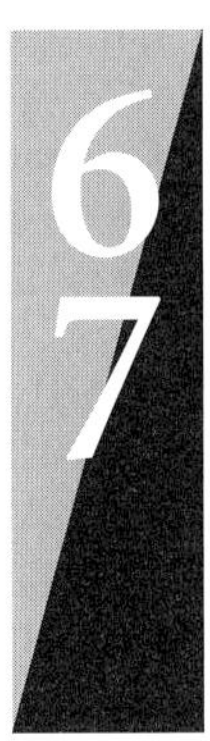

An Evidence-Based Approach to the Management of Hodgkin's Lymphoma

Craig H. Moskowitz

Thomas Hodgkin reported the initial cases of this distinct malignant lymphoma in 1832. The term *Hodgkin's disease* (HD) was used because of the uncertainty as to whether this entity was a tumor or an infection. Based on the evidence proving that the Hodgkin Reed–Sternberg cell is a B cell, the term *Hodgkin's lymphoma* (HL) is the correct term, although physicians are reluctant to change to this terminology.

Approximately 7,500 new cases of HL are diagnosed each year in the United States; slightly more men than women develop this disease. Successive refinements in therapy have led to a continuous improvement in survival, which now exceeds 80% at 5 years (see Chapter 103, Medical and Psychosocial Issues in Hodgkin's Disease Survivors). There is a fine balance, however, on achieving these excellent results without excessive toxicity. Appropriately, the focus on therapy has shifted toward tailoring management based on pretreatment prognostic factors. Treatment strategies must try to reduce toxicity in patients expected to do well while at the same time to not compromise or even intensify therapy in those with poor risk features.

The following chapter critically evaluates the evidence regarding the optimal management for patients with HL. This is not an exhaustive review of HL; the goal of this chapter is to make appropriate treatment recommendations based on the available evidence, and attempt to identify areas for needed clinical research. Treatment recommendations concerning the management of untreated HL are made by reviewing important multicenter randomized studies, as well as other supporting evidence that investigates specific subgroups. For relapsed and refractory patients, there are only two random assignment clinical trials evaluating autotransplantation. Therefore, to fully understand the role of autologous and allogeneic transplantation, large single-institution or registry-based studies are also reviewed. Areas of special interest, including the origin of the Hodgkin Reed–Sternberg cell, the role of Epstein–Barr virus in the pathogenesis of HL, and the use of positron emission tomography (PET) imaging in the staging evaluation of HL are evaluated. For the important topic of secondary breast cancer, large registry-based series are summarized and recommendations to decrease the incidence of this unfortunate complication are discussed.

What Is the Evidence That the Hodgkin's–Reed–Sternberg Cell Is a B Cell?

In the HL lymph node biopsy specimen, a small number of the neoplastic Hodgkin and Reed–Sternberg (HRS) cells, usually less than 2%, are admixed with a major population of B cells, T cells, plasma cells, eosinophils, neutrophils, histiocytes, and stromal cells.[1] Modern pathologic classification includes two major subtypes: 95% of patients have classic HL (nodular sclerosis, mixed cellularity, lymphocyte-rich, and lymphocyte-depleted) and 5% have lymphocyte-predominant HL.[2] In classic HL (cHL), the HRS cells express the activation markers CD30 and CD15 and generally lack B-lineage antigens. In lymphocyte-predominant HL (LPHL), the situation is opposite: B-cell markers are expressed and CD30 and CD15 are absent.[3]

During the past 5 to 10 years, elegant papers describing the clonality of the HRS cell were reported.[4–8] A given V (D) J gene rearrangement is specific for a B cell and its descendants; sequence analysis of V gene rearrangements determines clonality. Standard molecular biologic techniques, such as Southern blotting or the polymerase chain reaction (PCR), using total DNA from an involved lymph node have been successful in determining clonality in non-Hodgkin's lymphoma (NHL). However, because there are so few HRS cells within the lymph node specimen in HL, these standard techniques have failed in HL. The clonal nature of the HRS cell was made possible by the combination of micromanipulation of HRS cells from frozen samples and PCR amplification of genes from these single cells.[9,10]

Two groups, one from Cologne and the other from Berlin, have published the majority of the evidence concerning the clonal nature of the HRS cell. Analysis of the Ig and T-cell receptor loci of single HRS cells revealed that these cells are a monoclonal population of tumor cells and that nearly all are derived from B cells. These clonal B cells are different in cHL and LPHL.

Upon antigen-dependent activation in lymphoid tissues, B cells enter the primary follicle and form a germinal center (GC). B-cell proliferation and selection are driven by the process of somatic hypermutation. Only cells producing Ig with high affinity to the antigen survive in the GC; the rest are eliminated by apoptosis. Specific stages of B-cell development can be identified by sequence analysis of the rearranged V genes. Immature B cells carry unmutated V genes; GC B cells accumulate somatic mutations and have ongoing somatic mutations, whereas GC-derived memory B cells no longer acquire somatic mutations.[11,12]

The HRS cells of both types of HL have somatic mutations in their V region genes.[13,14] In cHL there is usually no evidence of ongoing somatic mutation, but in 25% of cases analyzed by Rajewsky et al., mutations were found that rendered the original functional Ig rearrangement nonfunctional.[15] These are called crippling mutations and include mutations resulting in the generation of stop codons or reading frame shifts. These HRS cells should be removed by apoptosis but are not[16] (see discussion in section on Epstein–Barr virus). Recently, a study using gene expression profiling reported that a series of B-cell-specific genes are downregulated in cHL. The authors speculate that the HRS cell in cHL downregulates surface immunoglobulin (BCR) and its downstream signals.[17] In most cases of LPHL, the rearranged Ig genes carry no crippling mutation, and in fact there is evidence of ongoing somatic mutations.[18,19] Also, in contrast to cHL, the LPHL tumor clone shows evidence of selection for expression of a functional antigen receptor; this is supported by the detection of mRNA for kappa or lambda light chains in the HRS cells in LPHL but not cHL. Based on the foregoing evidence, it is clear the HRS cells of both cHL and LPHL are clonally derived GC B cells.[20] Further research is needed to determine why the HRS is not removed by apoptosis.

What Is the Evidence That Epstein–Barr Virus Has a Role in the Pathogenesis of Hodgkin's Lymphoma?

The age–incidence curve in cHL is described as bimodal. In developing countries, the first peak is seen in childhood and the second in the older age group, whereas in developed countries the first peak is seen in young adulthood.[21] This finding suggests an infectious etiology as the cause of the disease.[22,23] A severalfold increase in the risk of HL occurs after infectious mononucleosis (IM), which is the typical clinical manifestation to primary Epstein–Barr virus (EBV) infection in adolescent children.[24,25]

EBV-positive and -negative cases of HL have different age distributions, with EBV-negative cases having a unimodal age distribution in young adulthood. Recently, Hjalgrim et al. compared incidence rates of HL in two population-based Danish cohorts of patients who were tested for IM: 17,045 patients with serologic evidence of EBV infection and 24,614 with no evidence.[26] Biopsy specimens of HL occurring during this time were also tested for EBV. The data suggest that only serologically confirmed IM was associated with an increased incidence of HL. Sixteen of 29 tumors obtained from patients with a history of IM had evidence of EBV. There was no evidence of an increased risk of EBV-negative HL after IM. The relative risk for EBV-positive HL after IM was 4, and the median incubation time from IM to HL was only 4.1 years.

The literature suggests that there is an altered antibody pattern to EBV in patients before clinically presenting with HL, with elevated titers against viral capsid antigen and EBV nuclear antigens compared with controls. This finding may suggest a more severe primary EBV infection. In situ hybridization methods to detect EBV DNA provided the first demonstration of its existence in HRS cells. Subsequently, the demonstration of EBV early RNA (EBER1 and EBER 2) sequences in the HRS cells provided a sensitive method for detecting latent infection. This technique is the accepted test to determine latent EBV infection in lymph node samples.[27] The linear genome of EBV has a variable number of 500-base-pair tandem repeat sequences at both ends. Because the number of repeats varies between patients but is constant within an individual patient, it can be used as a clonal marker in EBV-infected cells.

Three different patterns of expression of EBV latent genes and cellular antigens have been described in vitro and are referred to latency types I, II, and III. HRS cells exhibit the type II form of latency gene expression being limited to the EBERs, Epstein–Barr nuclear antigen I (EBNA1), and latent membrane proteins 1 and 2 (LMP1 and -2). What is the evidence that EBV is important in the pathogenesis of HL? There is a high level of LMP1 expression in HRS that can induce B-cell activation markers as well as IL-10 production. IL-10 production is more frequent in EBV-positive HRS cells when compared with EBV-negative counterparts, and some groups speculate that this accounts for the failure of cytotoxic T lymphocytes (CTL) to recognize the HRS cell. LMP1 also protects B cells from cell death by upregulating several anti-apoptosis genes, including bcl-2. LMP1 appears to function as a constitutively activated tumor necrosis factor receptor and, as a result, can activate a variety of signaling pathways, including NF-kB.[28–32] Members of the NF-kB family of transcription factors play a role in cellular activation, immune responses, and oncogenesis.[33–35] In most cells they are kept inactive by complexing with members of the IkB family, whose degradation activates NF-kB. Constitutive NF-kB activation has been consistently detected in HRS cells, and nuclear NF-kB expression can be stained for by immunohistochemistry.[36]

Although NF-kB activation is a common feature in HRS cells, the molecular route is different in EBV-positive and -negative HL. In single HRS cells, Jungnickel et al. detected clonal mutations in two of three cases of EBV-negative cases of IkBα gene but none in EBV-positive cases.[37] This finding suggests that the constitutive activation of NF-kB by LMP1 in EBV-positive cases may be substituted by IkBα gene mutations in HRS cells not infected by EBV. Despite improvements in our understanding of the pathogenesis of HL, the precise contribution of EBV remains unknown. Many questions concerning EBV and HL need to be resolved but two appear critical: (1) Why is there no effective immune response to LMP1 and -2 expressing HRS cells, and (2) What is the reason we are unable to detect EBV in all cases of HL?

What Is the Evidence That There Is a Standard Management for Early-Stage Disease?

Multiple treatment options exist for early-stage (ES) HL, and the standard approach is controversial.[38–40] The reason for the controversy stems from the premise that despite diverse initial therapeutic options with different disease control rates, outcome is excellent in patients who relapse; therefore, overall survival tends to be the same. There are supporters of radiation therapy (RT) for initial therapy who argue that many ESHL patients avoid chemotherapy, which can be reserved for patients who fail RT. Supporters of combined modality therapy (CMT), in which the number of cycles of chemotherapy, as well as the RT fields, continue to be reduced, argue that disease control is best with this approach despite the fact that patients who fail need to receive an autologous stem cell transplant. Finally, there is a recent trend to use full-course chemotherapy alone. The rationale for this approach is to decrease the incidence of secondary solid tumors, specifically, breast cancer. In deciding the optimal treatment strategy, one must understand that ESHL encompasses distinct subgroups of patients with different prognostic factors. These prognostic factors can help tailor therapy with the goal to ensure an excellent progression-free survival (PFS) with minimal long-term side effects.

Prognostic Factors Help Guide Treatment Decisions in ESHL

Historically, patients with stage I–II HL with favorable prognostic features were candidates for short primary RT, whereas patients with unfavorable prognostic factors tended to receive full-course CMT.[41–45] This section evaluates if this approach is correct on the basis of the evidence of prospective randomized trials.

Many factors that originally predicted for a high risk of occult abdominal disease in pathologically staged patients are no longer relevant in the era of clinical staging with subsequent CMT. These factors are still important in the design of prospective clinical trials in which the goal is to reduce therapy but maintain a high PFS rate. The factors that are commonly reported include male sex, age greater than 40 years, B symptoms or an ESR greater than 50, mixed-cellularity HL (MCHL) or lymphocyte-depleted HL (LDHL) histology, large mediastinal mass (LMA), extranodal extension, infradiaphragmatic disease, and three or four sites of lymph node involvement above the diaphragm. Using these prognostic factors, three groups of early-stage patients are usually defined: very favorable, favorable, and unfavorable ESHL. Very favorable ESHL accounts for only 5% of cases, with no specific randomized studies addressing this cohort of patients, and it is not discussed further (Table 67.1).

A number of multicenter randomized clinical trials are reported in favorable/unfavorable ESHL. The concepts of these trials include the following: decrease the number of chemotherapy cycles, avoidance of leukemogenic chemotherapeutic agents, reduce the dose of RT, decrease the size of the RT field or eliminate RT altogether.

Extended-Field Radiotherapy as Primary Therapy for ESHL Is Replaced by Combined Modality Therapy

In general, before the 1990s, extended-field primary RT was the treatment of choice for ESHL. Complete response rates were greater than 90%, but 30% of patients relapsed. Although the majority of these relapsing patients can be cured with standard-dose chemotherapy, there is a higher risk of secondary cancers and cardiac complications in these patients.

The HD7 trial of the German Hodgkin's Disease Study Group (GHSG) consisted of ABVD for two cycles and subtotal nodal irradiation (STLI) versus STLI alone. At a planned interim analysis, the complete response rates were the same, but freedom from treatment failure (FFTF) was 96% in the CMT arm versus 87% in the STLI arm.[46]

The Southwest Oncology Group (SWOG) recently published the results of a randomized trial of doxorubicin and vinblastine × 3 and STLI versus STLI alone in ESHL. The study was closed at the second planned interim analysis because of superior failure-free survival (FFS) in the CMT arm (94% versus 81%).[47]

The EORTC/GELA H7F and H8F trials significantly reduced the irradiated volume in the combined modality arm to include only the site of the originally involved nodes (involved field) as opposed to STLI on the radiation-alone arm. Still, the combined modality arm yielded significantly better relapse-free survival rate than radiation alone.[48,49] Based on the results of the GHSG, EORTC, and SWOG studies, STLI for the treatment ESHL is no longer recommended (Table 67.2).

TABLE 67.1. Risk factors and treatment groups in early-stage Hodgkin's lymphoma (ESHL).

Risk factors (RF)	*EORTC*	*GHSG*	*NCCN*
	A. Large MM B. Age ≥50 years C. B symptoms[a] or ESR ≥50 D. ≥4 involved sites	A. Large MM B. Extranodal disease C. B symptoms[a] or ESR ≥50 D. ≥3 involved sites	A. Large MM / any >10cm B. B symptoms or ESR ≥50 C. ≥4 involved sites
Treatment groups			
Early stage favorable		CS I-II with no RF	CS I–II with no RF
Early stage unfavorable		CS I-II with any RF	CS I, CSIIA with any RF; CS IIB with C/D but without A/B
Advanced stage		CS III-IV	CS IIB with A/B; CS III–IV

CS, clinical stage; EORTC, European Organization for Research and Treatment of Cancer; GHSG, German Hodgkin Lymphoma Study Group; MM, mediastinal mass; NCCN, National Comprehensive Cancer Network.

[a]If B symptoms, ESR should be ≥30.

TABLE 67.2. Studies comparing radiotherapy (RT) alone with combined modality therapy in favorable patients.

Study	Treatment regimens	FFTF or RFS	OS (years)
GHSG HD7[17] (617 pts)	EF	75%	94% (5)
	ABVD (2) + EF	91%	94%
	$P < 0.001$		NS
SWOG 9133[18] (326 pts)	STLI	81%	96% (3)
	AV (3) + STLI	94%	98%
	$P < 0.001$		NS
EORTC/GELA H7F[19] (333 pts)	STLI	81%	95% (5)
	EBVP (6) + IFRT	90%	98%
	$P = 0.0001$		NS
EORTC/GELA H8F[20] (543 pts)	STLI	80%	(4)
	MOPP/ABV (3) + IFRT	99%	
	$P < 0.0001$	$P < 0.02$	

EFRT, extended-field radiotherapy; IFRT, involved-field radiotherapy; STLI; subtotal lymphoid irradiation; pts, patients.

MOPP Is Replaced by ABVD as the Standard Chemotherapy Regimen in ESHL

The EORTC H6 twin randomized studies were reported 10 years ago. The study was divided into favorable and unfavorable groups.[50] Focusing on the unfavorable group (H6U), patients were clinically staged and randomized to receive ABVD × 3/mantle RT/ABVD × 3 versus MOPP × 3/mantle RT/MOPP × 3. ABVD achieved better results with less hematologic and gonadal toxicity.

Our group at Memorial Sloan-Kettering Cancer Center (MSKCC) conducted a randomized trial of MOPP × 4 and involved-field RT versus four cycles of thiotepa, bleomycin, and vinblastine (TBV) and involved-field RT. For MOPP and RT, the CR percentage was 98% (60 of 61), and at 5 years, the percentage of patients remaining in CR was 90%, with freedom from progression of 89% and overall survival of 91%. For TBV and RT, the CR percentage was 93% (55 of 59), with a 5-year duration of CR of 83%, freedom from progression of 81%, and overall survival of 91% (P greater than 0.15). The median follow-up at the time of the publication was 65 months (range, 7 to 96 months). Short-term toxicity, except for transient leukopenia, was far less for TBV and RT than for MOPP and RT.[51] Based on these results, standard MOPP chemotherapy is no longer used in the management of ESHL.

Can the Dose of RT be Reduced in CMT in ESHL?

Although the treatment results obtained with chemotherapy and RT are superior to STLI in favorable early-stage HD, the next objective was to see if the radiation field could be reduced safely in an effort to reduce toxicity. Several randomized studies were conducted in this setting; however, the majority of patients have a large mediastinal mass (LMA) and are at unfavorable risk. The Istituto Nazionale Tumorie Milan Trial has provided the clearest data regarding the adequacy of radiation volume reduction. From 1990 to 1996, 140 patients with ESHL (IA bulky IB; IIA bulky; and IIEA) were randomly assigned to four cycles of ABVD, followed by STLI with the same regimen followed by involved-field radiotherapy (IFRT). The dose of RT ranged from 30 to 36 Gy to uninvolved and involved sites, respectively. After a median follow-up of 87 months, CR rates were 100% after ABVD + STLI versus 97% after ABVD + IFRT; freedom from treatment failure (FFTF) was 97% versus 94% and overall survival (OS) 93% versus 94%, respectively.[52]

The EORTC H8U trial randomly assigned unfavorable patients to four cycles of MOPP/ABVD plus IFRT (36–40 Gy) with the same chemotherapy followed by STLI (36–40 GY). FFTF was the same in both groups, 92% in each arm.[53]

The GHSG HD8 study randomly assigned unfavorable early-stage patients to receive four cycles of cyclophosphamide, vincristine, procarbazine, and prednisone (COPP)/ABVD followed by either extended or involved field. At a median follow-up of 56 months, FFTF was 86% (in each arm), and no difference in relapse rate or survival was observed. Acute side effects were more frequent in patients who received the extended-field RT.[54] Based on these clinical trials, CMT using extended-field RT is no longer recommended (Table 67.3).

Can the Number of Chemotherapy Cycles and Dose of RT Be Reduced in ESHL?

An important study that just finished accruing patients is the HD10 trial of the GHSG. In this trial, reduction of the number of ABVD chemotherapy cycles, as well as reduction of RT dose in the IFRT, was tested in favorable ESHL patients. Thus, patients were randomly assigned between four cycles of ABVD followed by IFRT (30 Gy, arm A), four cycles ABVD + 20 Gy IFRT (arm B), two cycles ABVD + 30 Gy IFRT (arm C), and two cycles ABVD + 20 Gy IFRT (arm D). Between May 1998 and June 2000, 486 HL patients with ESHL [i.e., CS I, II without risk factors (favorable)] received one of these four treatments, and 390 patients (80%) are currently evaluable. At the first interim analysis in 2001 when the median observation time was 18 months, the CR rate was 98% and only 1% of patients had either progressive disease or no change. Overall survival (SV) rate was 98% and FFTF was 96%. The trial reached the target recruitment and was closed in January 2003. This critical study hopes to determine if less chemotherapy and RT can maintain the high FFTF rates with less toxicity in patients with favorable ESHL.[55]

TABLE 67.3. Studies comparing involved field radiation with extended radiation in combined modality programs for favorable and unfavorable early-stage Hodgkin's lymphoma (ESHL).

Study	Treatment regimens	FFTF or RFS	OS (years)
Milan[21] (140 pts)	ABVD (4) + STLI	97%	93% (5)
	ABVD (4) + IFRT	94%	94%
		NS	NS
GHSG HD8[22] (1,064 pts)	COPP/ABVD (4) + EFRT	86%	91% (5)
	COPP/ABVD (4) + IFRT	84%	92%
		NS	NS
EORTC/GELA H8U[23] (995 pts)	MOPP/ABV (6) + IFRT	94%	90% (4)
	MOPP/ABV (4) + IFRT	95%	95%
	MOPP/ABV (4) + STLI	96%	93%
		NS	NS

EFRT, extended-field radiotherapy; IFRT, involved-field radiotherapy; STLI, subtotal lymphoid irradiation; FFTF, freedom from treatment failure; RFS, relapse-free survival; OS, overall survival.

Can Chemotherapy Alone Be Used in the Management of ESHL?

Three important randomized studies evaluated the use of chemotherapy alone in ESHL. These patients have favorable and unfavorable features, but no patients have large mediastinal masses. At Memorial Sloan-Kettering Cancer Center (MSKCC), we tested the hypothesis that CMT was superior to ABVD alone in ESHL. We randomly assigned 152 patients to six cycles of ABVD alone or ABVD for six cycles and extended-field RT (EFRT). In intent-to-treat analysis, the CR rates were 94% in both cohorts. At 5 years, 91% of patients receiving CMT and 87% receiving ABVD alone continue in CR (P = 0.61). FFTF at 5 years is 86% for CMT and 81% for ABVD alone (P = 0.6). Interestingly, the overall survival (OS) trends are in favor of CMT (97% for CMT versus 91% for ABVD alone; P = 0.08).[56] Nachman et al., for the Children's Cancer Group (CCG), randomly assigned 501 patients who achieved an initial CR to risk-adapted combination chemotherapy to low-dose IFRT (21 Gy) or no further treatment. Patients receiving CMT had an OS of 92% versus 87% for patients treated with chemotherapy alone (P = 0.057). However, if one analyzes the data by therapy received there is a survival benefit for CMT (P = 0.0024).[57] An intergroup study [NCI of Canada and Eastern Cooperative Oncology Group (ECOG)] compared standard therapy STLI (favorable patients) or ABVD × 2 and STLI (unfavorable patients) to ABVD × 4 alone for both favorable and unfavorable patients. The median duration of follow-up is 4.2 years. The experimental arm, ABVD × 4, had an inferior PFS to that of standard therapy (P = 0.006).[58] There is a large ongoing trial in favorable early-stage patients with classic HL. All patients receive six cycles of EBVP (epirubicin, bleomycin, vinblastine, and prednisone). Only patients who achieve a CR are randomized to either IFRT of 36 Gy, IFRT of 20 Gy, or no radiation. Last year, the EORTC/GELA groups closed the no RT arm due to an excessive number of relapses in this group. The study remains open for randomization on the two combined modality arms.[55]

The evidence from these three studies suggests that, for patients with ESHL without a large mediastinal mass, four to six cycles of chemotherapy alone is inferior to the same chemotherapy and consolidative RT.

Summary

The following recommendations can be made concerning ESHL: all the previously mentioned randomized studies indicate that CMT should be standard therapy. Although short-course chemotherapy and extended-field RT are superior to chemotherapy alone, this strategy is unlikely to reduce long-term treatment-related morbidity and mortality. Although it has been shown that the radiation field can be safely reduced in unfavorable patients receiving CMT, we await follow-up of the HD10 trial if this can be achieved in favorable ESHL patients. There is no evidence that four to six cycles of chemotherapy is equivalent to the same chemotherapy and IFRT. At the present time, four cycles of chemotherapy, preferably ABVD, followed by IFRT (30–36 Gy), should be considered standard therapy for favorable and unfavorable patients with ESHL. These recommendations must be made with caution, however, in the light of the increased incidence of secondary breast cancer in young women treated with CMT (discussed in a later section).

What Is the Evidence That There Is a Standard Management for Advanced-Stage Disease?

ABVD Replaces MOPP as Standard Therapy for Advanced-Stage HL

Advanced-stage HL (ASHL) comprises all stage III and IV disease as well as selected patients with stage IIB disease, including those with a LMA, extranodal disease, or massive splenic involvement. The landmark report by DeVita et al., 36 years ago, determined that more than 80% of patients with ASHL achieved a CR to the MOPP chemotherapy program; 50% of patients have had long-term PFS.[40,59,60] The ABVD regimen has replaced MOPP as the standard chemotherapy program of HL, primarily because of a more favorable toxicity profile.[61] The modern era of ASHL begins with the results of a three-arm randomized CALGB study reported by Canellos et al. In this multicenter trial, three regimens were compared: ABVD for 6 to 8 cycles, MOPP for 6 to 8 cycles, and MOPP alternating with ABVD for 12 cycles. RT was not administered. Patients who relapsed after either MOPP or ABVD alone were switched to the opposite regimen. The CR rate to MOPP was inferior to the other arms (67%, 82%, and 83%, respectively; P = 0.006). FFTF was also inferior with MOPP (50%, 61%, and 65%, respectively); however, OS was the same in each arm.[62] Although this prospective trial shows an improved FFTF with the ABVD regimens even at a median follow-up of 10 years, OS is the same, reflecting the ability of high-dose therapy and autologous stem cell transplantation to salvage these patients. Based on the equivalent efficacy of ABVD and MOPP alternating with ABVD, the better short- and long-term toxicity profile seen with ABVD alone makes ABVD the benchmark against which newer regimens need to be compared. Three important questions need to be addressed: (1) Can prognostic factors help tailor therapy for patients with ASHL? (2) Are there randomized data showing that newer regimens are superior to ABVD or an ABVD equivalent? (3) Should adjuvant RT be used for patients with ASHL?

Can Prognostic Factors Guide Therapy in ASHL?

Therapy with ABVD or an ABVD-equivalent chemotherapy program fails to cure patients with ASHL one-third of the time, but just as important is the fact that some patients are overtreated unnecessarily. A number of pretreatment clinical prognostic factors have been identified to have independent prognostic value.[63] An international database on HL was developed to help define a prognostic model for ASHL. The factors defined are based on more than 5,000 patients treated with ABVD or an ABVD-equivalent chemotherapy program, and include age greater than 45 years, male sex, stage IV versus III disease, serum albumin less than 4 g/dL, hemoglobin less than 10.5 mg/dL, white blood cell count more than 15,000/mm^3, and absolute lymphocyte count less than 600/mm^3. These seven factors comprise the international prognostic index (IPI) for ASHL developed by Hasenclever et al.[64] (Table 67.4). Clinically, patients can be divided into three risk groups. Patients with an IPI score of 0–2 (low risk), accounting for 57% of ASHL, have a freedom from progression rate (FFP) of 74%. Patients with an IPI score of 3 (intermediate risk), accounting for 23% of ASHL, have an FFP of 60%. Patients with an IPI score of 4 or more (high risk), only

TABLE 67.4. Risk factors and survival for advanced-stage Hodgkin's lymphoma (ASHL).

	IPI model	MSKCC model
Risk factors (RF)	Age >45, male sex, albumin <4, hemoglobin <10.5 WBC >15 K, ALC < 600 Stage IV disease	Age >45, elevated LDH, large mediastinal mass, >1 extranodal site, low hematocrit, inguinal nodal involvement
Good risk	0–2 RF, FFTF (74%)	<2 RF, FFTF (>90%)
Intermediate risk	3 RF, FFTF (60%)	
Poor risk	>4 RF, FFTF (47%)	≥2 RF, FFTF (<50%)

IPI, international prognostic index, MSKCC, Memorial Sloan-Kettering Cancer Center; WBC, white blood count; ALC, absolute lymphocyte count; LDH, lactate dehydrogenase; FFTF, freedom from treatment failure.

19% of ASHL, have an FFP of 47%. When reviewing studies in ASHL, it is important to evaluate these risk factors. Patients with high-risk disease may benefit from a more aggressive chemotherapy program and, conversely, low-risk patients do not need to be overtreated with more toxic regimens.

MOPP/ABV Hybrid Is No Better Than ABVD in ASHL

In 1985, Klimo and Connors reported the results of the MOPP/ABV hybrid regimen. MOPP is administered on day 1 and 7 and ABV on day 8; dacarbazine was omitted in this regimen, and the dose of doxorubicin was increased from 25 mg/m^2 to 35 mg/m^2. IFRT was administered to some patients postchemotherapy. At 4 years, the OS rate was 90%.[65,66] This Phase II study led to two randomized studies comparing the hybrid to alternating MOPP/ABVD. The National Cancer Institute of Canada (NCIC) randomly assigned 301 patients who failed extended-field RT to the hybrid versus the alternating regimen. The OS rates at 5 years were not statistically different, but the hybrid regimen had more hematologic toxicity.[66] An intergroup trial of 737 patients compared the hybrid to six cycles of MOPP followed by three cycles of ABVD. At 8 years, FFS was superior with the hybrid regimen (64% versus 54%%; $P = 0.01$).[67] Although prognostic factors were not evaluated in this study, many physicians at the time considered the hybrid the standard of care for ASHL.

Recently, Duggan et al. reported the results of a randomized intergroup study of the ABVD versus MOPP/ABV hybrid. The major endpoints of the study were FFS and OS. Patients were eligible if they had untreated ASHL or if they relapsed after RT alone. All patients received 8 to 10 cycles of chemotherapy. Eight hundred fifty-six patients were randomly assigned to one of the two regimens, and the median follow-up at the time of the publication was 6 years. The CR rate, FFS, and OS were the same with the two regimens. When evaluating these endpoints based on the IPI score, there were no differences between the two cohorts. Although the efficacy endpoints between the two regimens are the same, the toxicity endpoints were quite different. There was a statistically significant increase in acute pulmonary and hematologic toxicity seen with the hybrid regimen ($P = 0.06$ and 0.001, respectively). More important, there was an increased incidence of myelodysplasia or secondary acute leukemia with the hybrid regimen as compared to ABVD. There was a total of 13 cases of MDS or AML; 11 of these patients were treated with the hybrid.[68] The results of this study are clear: the two regimens have equal efficacy, but the hybrid regimen is more toxic and its use can no longer be recommended. ABVD continues to be the standard regimen for ASHL.

HD9 Trial of the GHSG: Escalated BEACOPP Improves Survival in Poor-Risk Patients with ASHL

To improve on the results with ABVD in ASHL, subsequent studies involved two different treatment strategies. The first is dose intensification with the active agents in HL and the second is a change in the scheduling similar to some of the weekly chemotherapy programs for aggressive NHL, such as MACOP-B.[69]

Intensification of therapy can be via two distinct pathways: the first is to give higher doses of chemotherapy using a standard schedule and the second is to consolidate with upfront high-dose chemotherapy and autologous stem cell transplantation. From 1993 to 1998, the GHSG randomly assigned 1,201 patients with ASHL to eight cycles of COPP/ABVD (ABVD equivalent) to that of either standard doses of BEACOPP (bleomycin, etoposide, doxorubicin, cyclophosphamide, vincristine, prednisone, and procarbazine) or escalated BEACOPP (Figure 67.1). Patients in any of the three cohorts were eligible to receive IFRT postchemotherapy if a residual nodal mass was at least 2 cm postchemotherapy or if there was bulky disease at presentation. At the first interim analysis, the COPP/ABVD arm was stopped due to inferior results. The final analysis included 260 patients

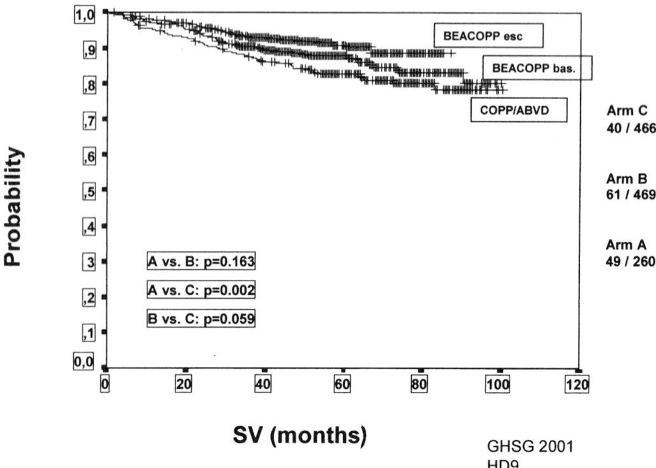

FIGURE 67.1. Survival by treatment arm.

receiving COPP/ABVD, 469 receiving standard-dose BEACOPP, and 466 patients receiving escalated BEACOPP. At 5 years, FFTF and OS rates for COPP/ABVD, standard-dose BEACOPP, and escalated BEACOPP were 69% and 83%, 76% and 88%, and 87% and 91%, respectively. FFTF and OS were statistically significantly superior for escalated BEACOPP when compared to COPP/ABVD (P = 0.04 and 0.002, respectively). There was, however, a higher incidence of grade three/four hematologic toxicity for the escalated BEACOPP regimen despite universal use of granulocyte colony-stimulating factor (G-CSF). The IPI score was available for only a minority of patients. Interestingly, 5-year OS for patients with IPI scores of 0–3 are similar for COPP/ABVD, BEACOPP, and escalated BEACOPP: 84% to 92%, 86% to 93%, and 90% to 95%, respectively. The critical result, however, is the 5-year FFTF for patients with at least four risk factors. The results are as follows: 59% for COPP/ABVD, 74% for standard BEACOPP, and 82% for escalated BEACOPP.[70] This randomized clinical trial has two obvious conclusions: a randomized study is required for patients with 0 to 3 risk factors comparing ABVD and escalated BEACOPP with all patients receiving RT for bulky or residual disease, and the available evidence suggests that escalated BEACOPP is a standard treatment option for patients with four or more IPI risk factors.

Consolidative Upfront ASCT Is No Better Than ABVD for Patients with ASHL

As described in a later section (see What Is the Evidence That There Is a Standard Management for Relapsed/Refractory Disease?), high-dose therapy and autologous stem transplantation is the treatment of choice for relapsed and primary refractory HL. If dose escalation of standard-dose chemotherapy can improve FFTF, then it is possible that high-dose therapy (HDT) and autologous stem transplantation (ASCT) may have a role as consolidation treatment for patients with unfavorable ASHL. The underlying question is identifying which patients were most likely to fail standard treatment. Before the publication of the IPI, another similar prognostic model was in use. The lymphoma service at MSKCC found that the following six risk factors were predictive for CR duration and relapse-free survival in ASHL: age greater than 45, elevated LDH, an LMA, at least two extranodal sites of disease, inguinal node involvement, and a low hematocrit.[71,72] Patients with at least two factors were considered poor risk. Based on this model, an intergroup study randomly assigned patients to eight cycles of ABVD-equivalent chemotherapy or four cycles of the same chemotherapy followed by HDT and ASCT. All patients were eligible to receive postchemotherapy RT if they had initial bulky disease or residual nodal masses.[73] There was no difference in the CR rate, FFS, or OS between the two arms. Based on these results, one can conclude that unfavorable patients defined by the MSKCC index do not benefit from a consolidative upfront ASCT.

Weekly Chemotherapy and Consolidative RT for ASHL

A scheduling change of the active chemotherapeutic agents in HL to weekly schedule is the principle of the Stanford V regimen.[74] The concept is threefold: decrease the cumulative doses of doxorubicin, nitrogen mustard, and bleomycin, add etoposide, and consolidate with more intensive radiotherapy. By definition, all lymph nodes greater than 5 cm pretreatment receive full-dose RT (36 Gy) at the conclusion of the 12 weeks of chemotherapy. An update of the Stanford experience was recently published in which 142 patients with ASHL were treated. The 5-year FFP and OS rates were 89% and 96%, respectively. Patients with an IPI score of 0–2 had a significantly superior FFP to those with scores of 3 or greater (94% versus 75%; P = 0.0001). There were no cases of secondary leukemia.[75] We analyzed our 7-year experience at MSKCC in 126 patients treated with the Stanford V combined modality regimen. Sixty-seven patients (53%) had extensive local disease, 26 patients (21%) had stage III, and 33 patients (26%) had stage IV. Seventy-five patients (58%) had B symptoms and 20 patients (16%) had at least four adverse factors included in the IPI score. At a median follow-up of 36 months (range, 12 to 92 months), the 3-year FFTF was 80% and OS was 91%. Patients with none to three IPI factors had FFTF and OS of 86% and 95%, respectively; patients with four or more factors had FFTF and OS of 50% and 75%, respectively. Cox regression analysis indicated that IPI of 4 or more is a significant predictor for both FFTF and OS (P less than 0.0001). There were 25 (20%) failures of treatment (9 patients had primary refractory HL, 1 died of hepatic failure, and 15 patients relapsed). Of the 25 failures, 14 patients were successfully salvaged with high-dose chemoradiotherapy and ASCT. The 3-year freedom-from-second-relapse for all patients who failed Stanford V was 55%. No secondary leukemia was observed, and 7 successful pregnancies were reported by our 65 female patients. Our study confirms the excellent results reported with Stanford V and radiotherapy by the Stanford group, indicates the relevance of the IPI model in determining outcome of this program, and demonstrates that failures of Stanford V remain highly salvageable with high-dose chemoradiotherapy.[76]

Randomized Data of Weekly Combined Modality Therapy Versus Standard Schedule Combined Modality Therapy in ASHL

Unfortunately, weekly therapy has not been successful in two prospective randomized studies. Radford et al. reported the results of weekly chemotherapy with the VAPEC-B (bleomycin, etoposide, doxorubicin, cyclophosphamide, vincristine, and prednisolone) versus ChlVPP/EVA (chlorambucil, vinblastine, procarbazine, prednisolone, etoposide, vincristine, and doxorubicin) hybrid. There were 282 patients randomized; RT was administered to sites of bulky disease or residual nodal involvement postchemotherapy. At 5 years, FFP and OS was significantly better for the hybrid arm (82% and 89% versus 62% and 82%; P less than 0.001). When analyzing the IPI score, all risk groups had improved survival with the hybrid.[77] The Italian Lymphoma Study group reported the results of 355 patients randomly assigned to ABVD, Stanford V, or a novel 10-drug regimen. Patients received RT only if they had bulky disease; hence, a variation of the standard RT practices for Stanford V as described previously. Only CR and relapse rates are available but they are inferior for Stanford V (CR rates: 89% for ABVD, 83% for the 10-drug regimen, and 74% for Stanford V; relapse rates: 6% for ABVD, 4% for the 10-drug regimen, and 16% for Stanford

V).[78] Despite these issues, there is an ongoing United States Intergroup trial comparing ABVD and Stanford V in ASHL. Until these results are available, weekly therapy cannot be recommended as standard of care for any patient with ASHL.

Does Adjuvant or Consolidative RT Improve Outcome in Patients with ASHL?

As described previously, many treatment programs included RT after full-course chemotherapy in ASHL. The evidence for this approach is controversial. The contribution of RT tends to be used as part of a planned CMT approach, as with Stanford V, or to convert an uncertain CR to a CR, as with escalated BEACOPP. The premise is that patients with ASHL relapse at bulky or residual sites and, if radiated, FFTF can be improved. The results of the early large randomized studies are conflicting.

Pavlovsky et al. randomly assigned 151 patients to six cycles of MOPP-equivalent chemotherapy (CVPP, CCNU, vinblastine, procarbazine, and prednisone) or the same therapy with RT interspersed between cycles 3 and 4. The CR and FFS rates were significantly better for CMT approach ($P = 0.01$ and 0.001).[79] The results for chemotherapy alone in this study were extremely poor and difficult to explain.

The SWOG treated 278 patients with six cycles of an alternating regimen and then randomly assigned patients to low-dose RT to all lymph node sites or observation. There was no difference in remission duration, relapse-free survival, or OS between the two groups. In a planned subset analysis, patients with either nodular sclerosis pathology or bulky disease had significantly better remission duration with the addition of RT.[80]

Diehl et al. treated 288 patients with an alternating regimen, and patients achieving a CR were randomly assigned to 20 Gy RT to initially involved fields or to an additional cycle of COPP/ABVD chemotherapy. There were no statistically significant differences in the two treatment programs.[81]

The CALGB treated 258 patients with one of four treatment programs: CVPP alone for 6 cycles, CVPP for 12 cycles, CVPP for 6 cycles followed by 25 Gy RT, or CVPP for 3 cycles followed by 25 Gy RT and then 3 more cycles of CVPP. Relapse in irradiated sites occurred in only 6% of responding patients, but there was no impact on OS. In fact, doubling the number of cycles of CVPP also had no impact on OS.[82]

Because the data were confusing after these publications, a meta-analysis of the randomized studies performed from 1972 to 1988 was reported by Loeffler et al. Data were available on 1,740 patients treated on 14 different trials. There were two distinct study designs. RT was randomly assigned after chemotherapy or patients were randomly assigned to RT or additional chemotherapy. Nearly all the chemotherapy regimens used in these studies were MOPP or MOPP-equivalent regimens. In the additional RT design, there was 11% improvement in CR duration in the RT groups (P less than 0.001); OS was the same. In contrast, when CMT was compared with the cohorts that received additional chemotherapy, CR duration was the same but OS was superior with patients who did not receive RT ($P = 0.045$). The conclusion of this meta-analysis should be approached with caution because MOPP or MOPP-equivalents are no longer used.[83]

Three recent random assignment studies have been published, adding to the confusion. The GELA (Groupe d'etudes des Lymphomes) reported the results of a randomized study comparing two different chemotherapy regimens [MOPP/ABV to ABVPP (doxorubicin, bleomycin, vinblastine, procarbazine, and prednisone)] followed by a second randomization for patients achieving a complete or partial response to two more cycles of the same chemotherapy or subtotal nodal irradiation. The study included 559 patients. After induction chemotherapy, 418 patients were evaluated for the consolidation phase. OS at 5 years in the MOPP/ABV groups were the same between additional chemotherapy and RT (85% versus 88%). After ABVPP, OS was superior for the chemotherapy arm (94% versus 78%; $P = 0.002$).[84]

The Children's Cancer Group (CCG) randomly assigned 501 patients achieving a CR to low-dose IFRT or observation. The 3-year FFTF was 87% for all patients, 92% for those randomized to receive RT and 87% randomized to observation ($P = 0.06$). An alternative analysis based on therapy actually received was undertaken that excluded the patients randomized to receive RT who refused the intervention. In this "as-treated" analysis, there was a significant improvement in FFTF for those patients who received RT (93% versus 85%; $P = 0.002$).[57]

Most recently, the EORTC randomly assigned 421 patients in CR after MOPP/ABV chemotherapy to RT or observation. The dose of RT was 24 Gy administered to all initially involved nodal sites and 16–24 Gy to all initially involved extranodal sites. Patients in partial remission were all treated with 30 Gy to nodal areas and 18–24 Gy to extranodal sites. The median follow-up is 6.5 years. The 5-year OS rates for the RT and observation groups were 85% and 91%, respectively ($P = 0.07$). Those patients who had a partial response to MOPP/ABV had event-free and OS rates after RT of 79% and 87%. Based on these three studies using ABVD-equivalent chemotherapy, RT clearly did not improve the outcome for patients in CR after full-course chemotherapy[85] (Table 67.5).

Summary

The IPI score can help guide standard management in ASHL; this is the concept of risk-adapted therapy. The goal is to use optimal management such that the IPI score is no longer rel-

TABLE 67.5. Randomized cooperative group studies of adjuvant RT in ASHL.

Study	*Patients randomized*	*Chemo*	*RT*	*FFTF—RT—no RT*	*OS RT—no RT*
SWOG	278	MOP-BAP × 6	IF	79%–68%	79%–86%
GHSG	100	COPP/ABVD × 4	IF	76%–79%	92%–96%
CCG	501	Doxorubicin based	IF	92%–87%	
EORTC	421	MOPP/ABV	EFRT		85%–91%

SWOG, Southwest Oncology Group; GHSG, German HD study group; CCG, Children's Cancer Group; FFTF, freedom from treatment failure; IFRT, involved-field RT; EF, extended-field RT; OS, overall survival.

evant. It is clear that 80% of patients with an IPI score of 0–3 do well with ABVD and if not, are highly salvageable with high-dose therapy and ASCT (see following discussion). There is no evidence that any of the new treatment programs are superior to ABVD in this subset of patients. In patients who require CMT with zero to three risk factors because of bulky disease, the Stanford V regimen is a reasonable alternative to ABVD, although randomized data are lacking. In the subset of patients with four to seven risk factors, escalated BEACOPP offers a survival advantage. It is important to remember that this is a combined modality treatment program and these excellent results include the use of adjuvant RT. In patients receiving ABVD or ABVD-equivalent treatment programs, such as alternating or hybrid regimens, there is no evidence to use adjuvant RT in patients who achieve a complete remission to full-course chemotherapy.

What Is the Evidence That Positron-Emission Tomography Imaging Should Be Used to Determine If Additional Therapy Is Needed After the Completion of the Standard Chemotherapy Program?

Careful staging in HL is critical to determine the prognosis of the patient and to design an optimal treatment strategy. Standard staging evaluation includes history, physical examination, routine laboratory studies, including a CBC, liver function tests, ESR, bone marrow biopsy, chest X-ray, and computed tomography (CT) scanning of the chest, abdomen, and pelvis with contrast. CT scanning has limited utility in discerning active disease in normal-size lymph nodes or in some extranodal sites, particularly bone. In addition, CT scans cannot differentiate between posttreatment fibrosis from active HD. Functional imaging improves the accuracy of HL staging. For many years, gallium scanning has complemented CT for staging and response evaluation. Fluorine-18 fluorodeoxyglucose positron emission tomography (PET) has virtually replaced gallium scanning in the United States as the functional imaging test of choice for a variety of reasons that include improved resolution, reduced nonspecific abdominal uptake, and ease of administration. There are at least three small single-center reports prospectively comparing gallium and PET scanning in lymphoma patients; both NHL and HL patients were included. In each study, PET scanning had a significantly higher sensitivity for depicting active disease. The major problem with PET is the high rate of false-positive results.[86–88]

The critical questions facing physicians regarding PET imaging include the following: What is the positive predictive value (PPV) and negative predictive value (NPV) of PET imaging in evaluation of a residual mass after initial therapy, and does a positive PET scan posttreatment preclude the need for biopsy confirmation of active disease? Most patients with HL have a residual mass on CT scan following the completion of initial therapy. These masses contain one of the following: fibrosis, necrotic tissue, residual HL, or an unsuspected concurrent diffuse large B-cell lymphoma. There are a number of publications specifically addressing the role of PET imaging in this situation. Many of these series contain patients with both HL and NHL.

First, NPV is defined as a negative PET result in a patient who is progression free and PPV is defined as a positive PET result in a patient who has a subsequent relapse. There are six studies with more than 25 patients reported. The NPV ranges between 90% and 96%. Summarizing, 178 patients had a negative PET scan at the end of treatment of which 15 relapsed corresponding to a NPV or 91.6%. The PPV ranges from 46% to 100%. Summarizing, 65 patients had a positive PET scan at the end of treatment of which 50 relapsed, corresponding to a PPV of only 77%.[89–97] Because therapy for relapsed or primary refractory HL generally includes stem cell transplantation, the following recommendation is reasonable: all patients should have a pretreatment and posttreatment CT and PET scan. If the PET scan is positive, a biopsy is mandatory. In patients with a normal PET scan, monitoring of any size residual mass, by CT, is warranted.

What Is the Evidence That There Is a Standard Management for Relapsed/Refractory Disease?

The majority of patients with HL are cured with radiation therapy and/or combination chemotherapy. However, patients who relapse after attaining a complete remission with chemotherapy and those with primary refractory disease have a poor outcome with conventional salvage regimens. Treatment results with standard-dose second-line regimens produce low complete remission rates and minimal survival benefit. Longo et al. reported a median survival of only 16 months in 51 patients treated with MOPP chemotherapy who never achieved a complete remission; similar results were seen in patients who failed MOPP/ABV hybrid or alternating regimens with a long-term event-free survival of 8%.[98,99] Over the past 15 years, many clinical trials using high-dose chemotherapy or chemoradiotherapy (HDT) with autologous stem cell transplantation (ASCT) in this setting have been reported, and approximately 40% of patients appear to be cured using this approach.[100]

Most early transplant studies included heavily pretreated patients, which influenced the morbidity and mortality of HDT. The introduction of G-CSF, peripheral blood progenitor cells as opposed to bone marrow as the stem cell graft, better transfusion practices, and more effective antibiotics have decreased transplant-related mortality from 15% to less than 3% in most series. Despite this improvement in supportive care, long-term FFTF has improved by at most 10% in recent studies. Therefore, there are a number of prognostic factors that predict for outcome.

Chemosensitive Disease Is Required to Achieve Benefit from HDT/ASCT

Two randomized studies comparing standard-dose second-line chemotherapy (SDSC) with high-dose therapy (HDT) and ASCT have been reported. The British National Lymphoma Investigation (BNLI) randomly assigned relapsed and primary refractory patients to either BEAM (carmustine, etoposide, cytarabine, and melphalan) HDT followed by ABMT or up to three cycles of mini-BEAM with standard support.[101] The German Lymphoma study group randomly assigned patients with relapsed HL to either two cycles of dexa-BEAM and BEAM and ASCT or four cycles of dexa-BEAM.[102] Each study demonstrated a statistically significant improvement in both EFS and PFS for the patients treated on the HDT arms, but neither was powered to show an OS advantage.

The importance of pretransplant cytoreduction with SDSC has been demonstrated in numerous previous reports. In 1993, we published our results using high-dose combined modality therapy in patients with biopsy-proven relapsed and primary refractory HD in our first-generation programs (MSKCC protocols 85-97 and 86-86).[103,104] The program used accelerated fractionation radiotherapy either as total lymphoid irradiation (TLI) or as an IFRT followed by HDT and bone marrow infusion. The strategy of incorporating radiation into the high-dose treatment regimen is based on the premise that the pattern of relapse post-HDT is similar to relapse following front-line chemotherapy; it most commonly occurs at sites of initial nodal involvement and is therefore amenable to treatment with radiotherapy. One hundred fifty-six patients with relapsed or primary refractory disease were treated; chemosensitive disease to SDSC was not a requirement for subsequent HDT. At a median follow-up of 11 years, the EFS is 45% with no relapses occurring later than 36 months posttransplant. After the introduction of G-CSF, overall mortality of the program decreased from 18% to 6%. These results demonstrated the feasibility of incorporating dose-intensive radiotherapy into HDT for HL and most importantly determined that patients with chemosensitive disease to SDSC had a marked improvement in EFS compared with patients with refractory disease at the time of HDT.

As with aggressive non-Hodgkin's lymphoma, chemosensitive disease to SDSC is now required for transplant eligibility in the United States. There is limited information regarding the optimal SDSC regimen. The following requirements for a SDSC regimen are adequate cytoreduction in at least 75% of patients without extramedullary toxicity or severe bone marrow suppression with subsequent inability to collect an adequate stem cell harvest.[105] Specifically, in the Phase III randomized German study described previously, of the 161 patients enrolled, 13 could not be randomized secondary to dexa-BEAM related mortality (8 patients) or severe infection.

We recently reported the results of a comprehensive program for the treatment of 82 patients with relapsed and primary refractory HL (MSKCC protocol 94-68).[106] All patients received uniform cytoreductive chemotherapy with ifosfamide, carboplatin, and etoposide (ICE), and only responders were subsequently offered HDT and ASCT. All patients in this trial had biopsy-proven relapsed or refractory disease, and our data were analyzed by intent to treat. ICE chemotherapy was a highly effective SDSC regimen in HD. The response rate to ICE was 90% with no ICE-related extramedullary toxicity. The median number of CD34+ cells/kg collected was 7 × 106/kg. The Kaplan–Meier estimate of the proportion of patients who are alive, event free, and analyzed by intent to treat at a median follow-up for surviving patients of 6 years is 55%. In the subset of patients who received HDT/ASCT (75 of 82 patients), the EFS is 61%.

Do Patients with Primary Refractory Disease Have a Suboptimal Outcome with ASCT?

Although response to SDSC is the major selection criteria to proceed to ASCT, other prognostic factors may also predict for long-term EFS in patients with relapsed and refractory HD. Some groups have suggested that patients with primary refractory disease do less well than those patients who achieved an initial remission to frontline therapy. Conflicting data have been reported by the North American Autologous Blood and Bone Marrow Transplant Registry (ABMTR), German Hodgkin's Lymphoma Study Group (GHSG), and the Groupe d'Etudes des Lymphoma de l'Adulte (GELA).[107–110]

The ABMTR series of 122 primary refractory patients had 3-year PFS and OS rates of 38% and 50%, respectively, using a variety of HDT regimens. Although chemosensitivity status was unknown in one-third of patients, it was concluded that only B symptoms at diagnosis and a poor performance status at ASCT predicted a poor outcome.

In the GELA data, primary refractory patients were defined as progression of disease on therapy, less than 50% response, or persistent bone marrow involvement after four cycles of induction chemotherapy. These patients had poor outcomes with HDT and ASCT, with 5-year freedom from second failure of 23%, even though most patients (62%) had chemosensitive disease to SDSC.

The GHSG evaluated 206 primary refractory patients defined as progression of disease or biopsy confirmation of active disease within 90 days postinduction therapy. Although only 70 of these 206 patients actually received HDT and ASCT, the authors concluded that HDT was no better than standard chemoradiotherapy when the data were analyzed by intent to treat.

We recently reported our data for 75 patients with primary refractory HL, which has longer median follow-up than any other reported series. With a median follow-up of 10 years, our results indicate that HDT/ASCT should be considered as standard treatment for patients with primary refractory HD if chemosensitive disease to SDSC is established. We found no difference in EFS for patients with chemosensitive primary refractory versus chemosensitive relapsed disease[111] (Table 67.6).

TABLE 67.6. Outcome in primary refractory Hodgkin's lymphoma (HL).

Series	*Patients (n)*	*Median follow-up (months)*	*Biopsy proven*	*PFS*	*OS*	*TD*	*Chemosensitivity*
Vancouver	30	42	55%	42%	30%	18%	N/A
ABMTR	122	28	N/A	38%	50%	12%	NS
GELA	157	50	36%	23%–66%	30%–76%	12%	$P = 0.05$
GHSG	70	52	57%	31%	43%	9%	$P = 0.0001$
SFGM	86	29	None	25%	35%	8%	$P = 0.0001$
MSKCC	75	120	100%	49%	48%	9%	$P < 0.0001$

TABLE 67.7. Adverse prognostic factors for treatment outcome after ASCT for HL.

Vancouver	B symptoms at relapse, extranodal disease at relapse, duration of 1st CR <12 months
Stanford	B symptoms at relapse, pulmonary/bone marrow involvement, more than minimal disease at ASCT
City of Hope	>2 prior regimens, extranodal disease at relapse, PSC as sole stem cell source
M.D. Anderson	>2 prior regimens, extranodal involvement, abnormal performance status, chemorefractory
Boston	>1 extranodal site, ECOG classification >0, progressive disease at ASCT
SFGM	Extranodal relapse, duration of 1st CR <12 months
ABMTR	Chemorefractory, abnormal LDH, KPS <90%
Nebraska	Second-line IPI

CR, complete remission.

Multiple Factors Predict Survival in Relapsed and Primary Refractory HL

Many groups have suggested that a variety of prognostic factors other than refractory disease predicts survival, as summarized in Table 67.7.[112–116] In our study of ICE SDSC followed by HDT and ASCT discussed previously, Cox regression analysis determined that the three factors associated with a poor outcome pre-ICE were extranodal sites of disease (ENS), P less than 0.001, initial response duration less than 1 year ($P = 0.001$), and B symptoms (P less than 0.001). Using this three-factor model, we identified three groups of patients with widely disparate outcomes with this treatment approach (Figure 67.2). A favorable risk group having zero or one of these risk factors (65% of the patients) had an EFS of 80% measured from initiation of ICE therapy. Patients with two and three risk factors fared less well, with an EFS of 34% and 12%, respectively.

This three-factor model was the basis of our third-generation risk-adapted comprehensive study (MSKCC protocol 98-71). In this study, patients with zero or one risk factor (ENS, initial response duration less than 1 year or B symptoms at time of study enrollment), group A, were treated exactly the same as in the second-generation program; in that study EFS was 80%. Patients with two risk factors, group B, received one dose of standard-dose ICE followed by a dose of augmented ICE second-line therapy, as well as a more dose-intense transplant conditioning regimen. Finally, patients with all three risk factors, group C, received a completely different regimen. Cytoreduction was done with transplant doses of ICE followed by stem cell support, which was followed by a second autotransplant. This three-arm study, however, uses one universal theme: patients must have disease chemosensitive to their "ICE" therapy; that is, group A to standard doses of ICE, group B to augmented ICE, and group C to transplant doses of ICE. The median follow-up of the patients is now 30 months, and patients with multiple risk factors have improved EFS as compared to our previous report.

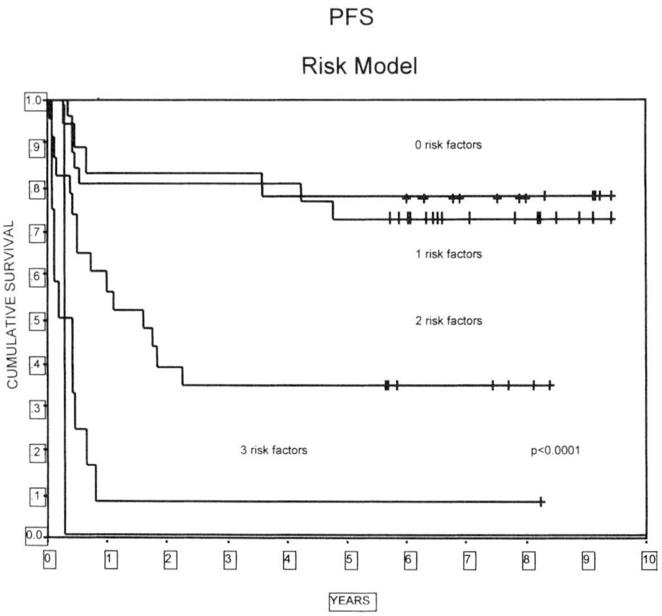

FIGURE 67.2. Progression-free survival (PFS) risk model.

Summary

In conclusion, HDT and ASCT are standard therapy for patients with relapsed and primary refractory HD, provided chemosensitivity is established. Future studies need to evaluate functional imaging in the transplant setting. In addition, the role of radiotherapy as part of transplant conditioning regimens is not defined in HL, and prospective trials are needed to assess if involved-field radiotherapy can decrease the relapse rate post-ASCT.[117–119]

What Is the Evidence That Allogeneic Transplantation Has a Place in the Management of HL?

As described previously, the use of HDT and ASCT is standard therapy for chemosensitive relapsed and primary refractory HL. The indications for and the use of allogeneic stem cell transplantation (allo-SCT) in these patients are poorly defined. The low morbidity with concomitant 40% to 50% long-term PFS rates seen with ASCT has precluded widespread use of allo-SCT. The two main reasons to consider allo-SCT are (1) infusion of a lymphoma-free stem cell product (not a concern in HL), and (2) the graft-versus-lymphoma effect. The major problem with allo-SCT is the high treatment-related mortality compared with ASCT. The EBMT registry recently reported the results of a matched study of allo-SCT for lymphoma for patients treated between 1982 and 1998[120] that analyzed 1,185 lymphoma transplants. All patients received ablative allo-SCT. All lymphomas were included in the analysis of which 167 patients had HL. Unfortunately, transplant-related mortality in the group of HL patients was extremely high at 51.7%. In addition, HL was the only lymphoma that showed an inferior relapse-free survival as compared with ASCT. From these data, the conservative use of allo-SCT in patients with HL is correct. Importantly, however, allo-SCT has changed dramatically in the past 5 years with the use of nonmyeloablative approaches.

Reduced-Intensity and Nonmyeloablative Conditioning Regimens

The transplant conditioning regimen in allo-SCT was originally intended to cytoreduce lymphoma while providing immunosuppression to prevent graft rejection. It has become clear in the past decade that the benefit for allo-SCT is largely related to immune-mediated graft-versus-tumor or -lymphoma effect. This premise has led to the use of reduced-intensity (RI) or nonmyeloablative (NMT) conditioning regimens to achieve engraftment and allow for the development of a graft-versus-lymphoma effect as the main form of therapy for the tumor.[121] A few general approaches are currently being used. The nonmyeloablative approaches include using immunosuppressive chemotherapy agents, generally fludarabine, in combination with an alkylating agent. Another technique is based on using low-dose total-body irradiation with or without fludarabine.[122,123] Last, Mackinnon et al. have led the effort using a T-cell-depleted approach by incorporating the humanized monoclonal antibody alemtuzumab for T-cell depletion, followed by fludarabine and melphalan. Donor lymphocyte infusions are added in patients with residual disease or those not evolving to 100% donor chimerism.[124] The reduced-intensity conditioning regimen approaches have used standard ASCT conditioning regimens, most commonly BEAM (carmustine, etoposide, cytarabine, and melphalan).[125] ASCT conditioning regimens can cytoreduce lymphoma, with very low transplant toxicity, and support allogeneic engraftment.

Most reports using either NMT or RI regimens in lymphoma are single-institution studies with fewer than 50 patients, of whom 5 to 15 have HL. It is fairly clear from these reports that NMT offers a reduced risk of early transplant-related mortality compared with conventional transplantation. Despite the lower toxicity, graft-versus-host disease (GVHD) still remains the major limitation of NMT. HL patients with chemorefractory disease achieve minimal benefit. Patients who receive alemtuzumab have a higher incidence of cytomegalovirus reactivation but a lower incidence of GVHD, both acute and chronic. Alemtuzumab-based regimens often require donor lymphocyte infusions to achieve similar tumor control to that of standard regimens.

Reduced-intensity (RI) regimens offer the possibility of early complete donor chimerism as opposed to mixed chimerism often seen with NMT. The largest report is by Faulkner et al., evaluating a BEAM-alemtuzumab RI regimen in patients with lymphoproliferative disorders in which only 5 patients had HL. Sustained, full donor chimerism was seen in 35 of 36 patients.[126] Treatment-related mortality was 8% in patients who had not failed ASCT but was 50% in those who had failed ASCT. Cooney et al. evaluated BEAM alone in 10 patients with HL who failed ASCT. One year postallograft, 9 of 10 patients are alive, with 7 progression free.[125]

Only general recommendations can be made using allo-SCT. (1) A conventional allo-SCT should not be administered in patients who have failed ASCT. (2) NMT is reasonable therapy for patients who have failed ASCT provided that the disease responds to some form of salvage chemotherapy. (3) In patients with an HLA-identical sibling donor who have poor-risk disease as defined as initial remission duration of less than 1 year with concomitant B symptoms and stage IV disease, RI allo-SCT with regimens, such as BEAM, should be considered instead of ASCT. The use of ASCT for cytoreduction followed by NMT in these poor-risk patients is a reasonable study alternative to RI allo-SCT.

What Is the Evidence That Mantle Radiotherapy Causes Secondary Breast Cancer?

As survival in HL increases, because of the success of initial and second-line therapy, the long-term side effects of this therapy have had a major impact on morbidity and mortality of patients. Recently, Aleman et al. analyzed a group of 1,261 patients with a median follow-up of 18 years post-HL therapy and determined cause-specific mortality. The main cause of death was HL, but after 10 years the main causes of death are similar to the general population; that is, cancer and cardiovascular disease. Unfortunately, the relative and absolute risk of solid tumors and AML, compared to age-matched controls, are markedly increased in HL patients.[127]

The Late Effects Study Group evaluated 1,380 children with HL and determined the incidence of secondary cancers (SC) and the risk factors associated with them. There was 88 SC, either secondary leukemia or solid tumors.[128] The incidence of secondary leukemia has markedly decreased in the past decade because of the minimal leukemogenic potential of the ABVD regimen as compared to alkylator-based therapy. The focus of this section is to critically review large registry-based databases on secondary breast cancer and recommend strategies to minimize its occurrence without compromising PFS.

In the Late Effects Study Group publication in the *New England Journal of Medicine* in 1996, cumulative incidence of SC was 7.0%, 15 years posttherapy. Solid tumors generally began 12 years postdiagnosis of HL and developed in 56 patients. Breast cancer was the most common solid tumor, occurring in 17 patients. All patients received radiotherapy as part of their HL management. In this young cohort, the risk of breast cancer was 75 times greater than that in age-matched controls and occurred at even a higher rate in those girls radiated between ages 10 and 16. The dose of radiotherapy to the mantle region ranged from 2,000 to 4,750 cGy. The high incidence of breast cancer in this population is most likely related to the effect of radiotherapy on proliferating breast tissue.

The risk of SC was evaluated in a large British cohort of 5,519 patients treated from 1963 to 1993. There was 322 SC in this cohort, but the incidence of breast cancer was very low and was only increased in patients who received radiotherapy alone for the management of their HL. The incidence of breast cancer was also only increased in those women treated with radiotherapy before the age of 25.[129]

Van Leeuwen et al. evaluated 1,253 survivors of HL treated during adolescence or young adulthood in the Netherlands. The median follow-up of these patients at the time of the publication was 14 years. The risk of SC was 7.0; patients treated before the age of 20 had a 14-fold increase in relative risk of developing a solid tumor, which decreased to 6.5 and 4.2 for patients treated at ages 21 to 30 years and 31 to 39 years, respectively. Once again, for breast cancer, the absolute excess risk increased with decreasing age of initial treatment. Breast cancer risk was increased in all treatment categories except for those patients treated with chemotherapy alone.[130] Unfortunately, the relative risk of breast cancer in this study was 40, confirming the data of the Late Effects Study Group.

What is likely the definitive study evaluating the risk of breast cancer following radiotherapy and chemotherapy among young women, was recently published by Travis et al.[131] The risk of breast cancer was evaluated in 3,817 women diagnosed before the age of 30, and the goal was to determine estimates of relative and absolute excess risk of breast cancer. Nearly all patients received radiotherapy, with a mean dose of radiation delivered to the breast of 25.1 Gy (range, 12.0–61.3 Gy). The median age at diagnosis of HL was 22, and breast cancer developed in 105 patients at a mean of 18 years posttherapy. Treatment with radiotherapy alone was associated with a 3.2-fold-increased risk of breast cancer, which decreased to 1.4-fold if patients received combined modality therapy consisting of radiotherapy and alkylator-based chemotherapy. The few patients who received chemotherapy alone in this series experienced a reduced risk of breast cancer (relative risk, 0.6). The increased risk of breast cancer occurred at all radiation dose categories but was greatest for patients receiving more than 41 Gy. Interestingly, a decreased risk of breast cancer was associated with the percentage of women who became menopausal from either chemotherapy or radiation to the pelvis. The authors suggest that, if lower doses of radiation to the chest are administered, the relative risk of secondary breast cancer can be attenuated.

In summary, for women who have a history of HL and were successfully treated at a young age, the most significant long-term side effect of therapy is secondary breast cancer. The data are clear: The risk is related to mantle radiotherapy. This risk is increased by the dose of the radiotherapy administered, develops late, usually 15 years or more after initial treatment, and is age related. The highest risk is associated when radiotherapy is administered to young women aged 10 to 20 years; unfortunately, the risk remains markedly increased until the age of 30. Fortunately, primary therapy for HL has changed. All patients now receive chemotherapy as primary treatment of HL, so the role of radiation therapy in management of ESHL is that of consolidation. Hence, the radiation fields are much smaller than in the previously reported registry databases. In fact, the dose of radiotherapy used in modern combined modality series is closer to 25–30 Gy, not 40 Gy as described previously. One hopes that this change in treatment strategy will decrease the risk of secondary breast cancer without compromising PFS.

References

1. Drexler HG. Recent results on the biology of Hodgkin and Reed–Sternberg cells. II. Continuous cell lines. Leuk Lymphoma 1993;9:1–25.
2. Harris NL. Hodgkin's lymphomas: classification, diagnosis, and grading. Semin Hematol 1999;36:220–232.
3. Mason DY, Banks PM, Chan J, et al. Nodular lymphocyte predominance in Hodgkin's disease. A distinct clinicopathological entity. Am J Surg Pathol 1994;18:526–530.
4. Kuppers R, Hansmann ML, Diehl V, Rajewsky K. Molecular single-cell analysis of Hodgkin and Reed–Sternberg cells. Mol Med Today 1995;1:26–30.
5. Kuppers R, Hansmann ML, Rajewsky K. Clonality and germinal centre B-cell derivation of Hodgkin/Reed–Sternberg cells in Hodgkin's disease. Ann Oncol 1998;9(suppl 5):S17–S20.
6. Kuppers R, Rajewsky K. The origin of Hodgkin and Reed/Sternberg cells in Hodgkin's disease. Annu Rev Immunol 1998;16: 471–493.
7. Stein H, Hummel M. Cellular origin and clonality of classic Hodgkin's lymphoma: immunophenotypic and molecular studies. Semin Hematol 1999;36:233–241.
8. Brauninger A, Hansmann ML, Strickler JG, et al. Identification of common germinal-center B-cell precursors in two patients with both Hodgkin's disease and non-Hodgkin's lymphoma. N Engl J Med 1999;340:1239–1247.
9. Marafioti T, Hummel M, Anagnostopoulos I, et al. Origin of nodular lymphocyte-predominant Hodgkin's disease from a clonal expansion of highly mutated germinal-center B cells. N Engl J Med 1997;337:453–458.
10. Ohno T, Stribley JA, Wu G, Hinrichs SH, Weisenburger DD, Chan WC. Clonality in nodular lymphocyte-predominant Hodgkin's disease. N Engl J Med 1997;337:459–465.
11. Martinez-Valdez H, Guret C, de Bouteiller O, et al. Human germinal center B cells express the apoptosis genes Fas, c-myc, P53, and Bax but not the survival gene bcl-2. J Exp Med 1996;183:991–997.
12. Rajewsky K. Clonal selection and learning in the antibody system. Nature (Lond) 1996;381:751–758.
13. Kanzler H, Kuppers R, Hansmann ML, Rajewsky K. Hodgkin and Reed–Sternberg cells in Hodgkin's disease represent the outgrowth of a dominant tumor clone derived from (crippled) germinal center B cells. J Exp Med 1996;184:1495–1505.
14. Kuppers R, Rajewsky K, Zhao M, et al. Hodgkin's disease: clonal Ig gene rearrangements in Hodgkin and Reed–Sternberg cells picked from histological sections. Ann N Y Acad Sci 1995;764: 523–524.
15. Kuppers R. Molecular biology of Hodgkin's lymphoma. Adv Cancer Res 2002;84:277–312.
16. Marafioti T, Hummel M, Foss HD, et al. Hodgkin and Reed–Sternberg cells represent an expansion of a single clone originating from a germinal center B-cell with functional immunoglobulin gene rearrangements but defective immunoglobulin transcription. Blood 2000;95:1443–1450.
17. Schwering I, Brauninger A, Distler V, et al. Profiling of Hodgkin's lymphoma cell line L1236 and germinal center B cells: identification of Hodgkin's lymphoma-specific genes. Mol Med 2003;9: 85–95.
18. Rajewsky K, Kanzler H, Hansmann ML, Kuppers R. Normal and malignant B-cell development with special reference to Hodgkin's disease. Ann Oncol 1997;8(suppl 2):79–81.
19. Chan WC. Cellular origin of nodular lymphocyte-predominant Hodgkin's lymphoma: immunophenotypic and molecular studies. Semin Hematol 1999;36:242–252.
20. Kuppers R, Schwering I, Brauninger A, Rajewsky K, Hansmann ML. Biology of Hodgkin's lymphoma. Ann Oncol 2002;13(suppl 1):11–18.
21. Gutensohn NM. Social class and age at diagnosis of Hodgkin's disease: new epidemiologic evidence for the "two-disease hypothesis." Cancer Treat Rep 1982;66:689–695.
22. Alexander FE, McKinney PA, Williams J, Ricketts TJ, Cartwright RA. Epidemiological evidence for the 'two-disease hypothesis' in Hodgkin's disease. Int J Epidemiol 1991;20:354–361.
23. Alexander FE. Clustering and Hodgkin's disease. Br J Cancer 1990;62:708–711.
24. Mueller N. Epidemiologic studies assessing the role of the Epstein–Barr virus in Hodgkin's disease. Yale J Biol Med 1987;60: 321–332.

25. Hjalgrim H, Askling J, Sorensen P, et al. Risk of Hodgkin's disease and other cancers after infectious mononucleosis. J Natl Cancer Inst 2000;92:1522–1528.
26. Hjalgrim H, Askling J, Rostgaard M, et al. Characteristics of Hodgkin's Lymphoma after infectious mononucleosis. N Engl J Med 2003;349:1324–1332.
27. Jarrett RF, MacKenzie J. Epstein–Barr virus and other candidate viruses in the pathogenesis of Hodgkin's disease. Semin Hematol 1999;36:260–269.
28. Poppema S, Visser L. Absence of HLA class I expression by Reed–Sternberg cells. Am J Pathol 1994;145:37–41.
29. Oudejans JJ, Jiwa NM, Kummer JA, et al. Analysis of major histocompatibility complex class I expression on Reed–Sternberg cells in relation to the cytotoxic T-cell response in Epstein–Barr virus-positive and -negative Hodgkin's disease. Blood 1996;87:3844–3851.
30. Murray PG, Constandinou CM, Crocker J, Young LS, Ambinder RF. Analysis of major histocompatibility complex class I, TAP expression, and LMP2 epitope sequence in Epstein–Barr virus-positive Hodgkin's disease. Blood 1998;92:2477–2483.
31. Sing AP, Ambinder RF, Hong DJ, et al. Isolation of Epstein–Barr virus (EBV)-specific cytotoxic T lymphocytes that lyse Reed–Sternberg cells: implications for immune-mediated therapy of EBV+ Hodgkin's disease. Blood 1997;89:1978–1986.
32. Herbst H, Foss HD, Samol J, et al. Frequent expression of interleukin-10 by Epstein–Barr virus-harboring tumor cells of Hodgkin's disease. Blood 1996;87:2918–2929.
33. Herbst H, Dallenbach F, Hummel M, et al. Epstein–Barr virus DNA and latent gene products in Ki-1 (CD30)-positive anaplastic large cell lymphomas. Blood 1991;78:2666–2673.
34. Niedobitek G, Kremmer E, Herbst H, et al. Immunohistochemical detection of the Epstein–Barr virus-encoded latent membrane protein 2A in Hodgkin's disease and infectious mononucleosis. Blood 1997;90:1664–1672.
35. Staratschek-Jox A, Kotkowski S, Belge G, et al. Detection of Epstein–Barr virus in Hodgkin–Reed–Sternberg cells: no evidence for the persistence of integrated viral fragments in latent membrane protein-1 (LMP-1)-negative classical Hodgkin's disease. Am J Pathol 2000;156:209–216.
36. Flavell KJ, Murray PG. Hodgkin's disease and the Epstein–Barr virus. Mol Pathol 2000;53:262–269.
37. Jungnickel B, Staratschek-Jox A, Brauninger A, et al. Clonal deleterious mutations in the Ikappa-Balpha gene in the malignant cells in Hodgkin's lymphoma. J Exp Med 2000;191:395–402.
38. Diehl V. Chemotherapy or combined modality treatment: the optimal treatment for Hodgkin's disease. J Clin Oncol 2004;22:15–18.
39. Longo DL. Radiation therapy in the treatment of Hodgkin's disease: do you see what I see? J Natl Cancer Inst 2003;95:928–929.
40. DeVita VT Jr. Hodgkin's disease: clinical trials and travails. N Engl J Med 2003;348:2375–2376.
41. Mendenhall NP, Cantor AB, Barre DM, Lynch JW Jr., Million RR. The role of prognostic factors in treatment selection for early-stage Hodgkin's disease. Am J Clin Oncol 1994;17:189–195.
42. Tubiana M, Henry-Amar M, Hayat M, et al. Prognostic significance of the number of involved areas in the early stages of Hodgkin's disease. Cancer (Phila) 1984;54:885–894.
43. Tubiana M, Henry-Amar M, Burgers MV, van der Werf-Messing B, Hayat M. Prognostic significance of erythrocyte sedimentation rate in clinical stages I–II of Hodgkin's disease. J Clin Oncol 1984;2:194–200.
44. Lee CK, Aeppli DM, Bloomfield CD, Levitt SH. Hodgkin's disease: a reassessment of prognostic factors following modification of radiotherapy. Int J Radiat Oncol Biol Phys 1987;13:983–991.
45. Mauch P, Tarbell N, Weinstein H, et al. Stage IA and IIA supradiaphragmatic Hodgkin's disease: prognostic factors in surgically staged patients treated with mantle and paraaortic irradiation. J Clin Oncol 1988;6:1576–1583.
46. Sieber M, Franklin J, Tesch H, et al. Two cycles of ABVD plus extended field radiotherapy is superior to radiotherapy alone in early stage Hodgkin's disease: Blood 2002;a341.
47. Press OW, LeBlanc M, Lichter AS, et al. Phase III randomized intergroup trial of subtotal lymphoid irradiation versus doxorubicin, vinblastine, and subtotal lymphoid irradiation for stage IA to IIA Hodgkin's disease. J Clin Oncol 2001;19:4238–4244.
48. Hagenbeek A, Eghbali H, Ferme C, et al. Three cycles of MOPP/ABV hybrid and involved-field irradiation is more effective than subtotal nodal irradiation in favorable supradiaphragmatic clinical stages I–II Hodgkin's disease: preliminary results of the EORTC-GELA H9-F randomized trial in 543 patients. Blood 2000;96(11):A575.
49. Carde P, Noordijk E, Hagenbeek A, et al. Superiority of EBVP chemotherapy in combination with involved field irradiation over subtotal nodal irradiation in favorable clinical stage I–II Hodgkin's disease: the EORTC-GPMC H7F randomized trial. Proc ASCO 1997;16:13.
50. Carde P, Hagenbeek A, Hayat M, et al. Clinical staging versus laparotomy and combined modality with MOPP versus ABVD in early-stage Hodgkin's disease: the H6 twin randomized trials from the European Organization for Research and Treatment of Cancer Lymphoma Cooperative Group. J Clin Oncol 1993;11:2258–2272.
51. Straus DJ, Yahalom J, Gaynor J, et al. Four cycles of chemotherapy and regional radiation therapy for clinical early-stage and intermediate-stage Hodgkin's disease. Cancer (Phila) 1992;69:1052–1060.
52. Bonfante V, Viviani S, Devizz I, et al. 10 year experience with ABVD and radiotherapy in early stage HD. Proc ASCO 2001.
53. Ferme C, Eghbali H, Hagenbeek A, et al. MOPP/ABV hybrid and RT in unfavorable supradiaphragmatic clinical stage I/II HD. Comparison of 3 treatment modalities. Blood 2000;A576.
54. Engert A, Schiller P, Josting A, et al. Involved-field radiotherapy is equally effective and less toxic compared with extended-field radiotherapy after four cycles of chemotherapy in patients with early-stage unfavorable Hodgkin's lymphoma: results of the HD8 Trial of the German Hodgkin's Lymphoma Study Group. J Clin Oncol 2003;21(19):3601–3608.
55. Diehl V, Stein H, Hummel M. Hodgkin S. Lymphoma: biology and treatment strategies for primary, refractory, and relapsed disease. Am Soc Hematol Educ Program 2003:225–247.
56. Straus D, Portlock CS, Qin J, et al. Results of a prospective randomized clinical trial of doxorubicin, bleomycin, vinblastine, and dacarbazine (ABVD) followed by radiation therapy (RT) versus ABVD alone for stages I, II, and IIIA nonbulky Hodgkin disease. Blood 2004;104(12):3483–3489.
57. Nachman JB, Sposto R, Herzog P, et al. Randomized comparison of low-dose involved-field radiotherapy and no radiotherapy for children with Hodgkin's disease who achieve a complete response to chemotherapy. J Clin Oncol 2002;20:3765–3771.
58. Meyer R, Gospodarwicz M, Connors J, et al. Randomized phase III comparison of single modality ABVD with a strategy that includes RT in patients with early stage Hodgkin's disease. Blood 2003;A81.
59. DeVita VT Jr. Hodgkin's disease: conference summary and future directions. Cancer Treat Rep 1982;66:1045–1055.
60. Longo DL, Young RC, Wesley M, et al. Twenty years of MOPP therapy for Hodgkin's disease. J Clin Oncol 1986;4:1295–1306.
61. Bonadonna G, Santoro A. ABVD chemotherapy in the treatment of Hodgkin's disease. Cancer Treat Rev 1982;9:21–35.
62. Canellos GP, Anderson JR, Propert KJ, et al. Chemotherapy of advanced Hodgkin's disease with MOPP, ABVD, or MOPP alternating with ABVD. N Engl J Med 1992;327:1478–1484.
63. Straus DJ, Gaynor JJ, Myers J, et al. Prognostic factors among 185 adults with newly diagnosed advanced Hodgkin's disease treated with alternating potentially noncross-resistant

chemotherapy and intermediate-dose radiation therapy. J Clin Oncol 1990;8:1173–1186.
64. Hasenclever D, Diehl V. A prognostic score for advanced Hodgkin's disease. International Prognostic Factors Project on Advanced Hodgkin's Disease. N Engl J Med 1998;339:1506–1514.
65. Klimo P, Connors JM. MOPP/ABV hybrid program: combination chemotherapy based on early introduction of seven effective drugs for advanced Hodgkin's disease. J Clin Oncol 1985;3:1174–1182.
66. Connors JM, Klimo P, Adams G, et al. Treatment of advanced Hodgkin's disease with chemotherapy: comparison of MOPP/ABV hybrid regimen with alternating courses of MOPP and ABVD. A report from the National Cancer Institute of Canada clinical trials group. J Clin Oncol 1997;15:1638–1645.
67. Glick JH, Young ML, Harrington D, et al. MOPP/ABV hybrid chemotherapy for advanced Hodgkin's disease significantly improves failure-free and overall survival: the 8-year results of the intergroup trial. J Clin Oncol 1998;16:19–26.
68. Duggan DB, Petroni GR, Johnson JL, et al. Randomized comparison of ABVD and MOPP/ABV hybrid for the treatment of advanced Hodgkin's disease: report of an intergroup trial. J Clin Oncol 2003;21:607–614.
69. Klimo P, Connors JM. Updated clinical experience with MACOP-B. Semin Hematol 1987;24:26–34.
70. Diehl V, Franklin J, Pfreundschuh M, et al. Standard and increased-dose BEACOPP chemotherapy compared with COPP-ABVD for advanced Hodgkin's disease. N Engl J Med 2003;348:2386–2395.
71. Straus DJ, Gaynor J, Myers J, et al. Results and prognostic factors following optimal treatment of advanced Hodgkin's disease. Recent Results Cancer Res 1989;117:191–196.
72. Straus DJ. High-risk Hodgkin's disease prognostic factors. Leuk Lymphoma 1995;15(suppl 1):41–42.
73. Federico M, Bellei M, Brice P, et al. High-dose therapy and autologous stem-cell transplantation versus conventional therapy for patients with advanced Hodgkin's lymphoma responding to front-line therapy. J Clin Oncol 2003;21:2320–2325.
74. Bartlett NL, Rosenberg SA, Hoppe RT, Hancock SL, Horning SJ. Brief chemotherapy, Stanford V, and adjuvant radiotherapy for bulky or advanced-stage Hodgkin's disease: a preliminary report. J Clin Oncol 1995;13:1080–1088.
75. Horning SJ, Hoppe RT, Breslin S, Bartlett NL, Brown BW, Rosenberg SA. Stanford V and radiotherapy for locally extensive and advanced Hodgkin's disease: mature results of a prospective clinical trial. J Clin Oncol 2002;20:630–637.
76. Yahalom J, Moskowitz C, Horwitz S, et al. Stanford V and radiotherapy for advanced and locally extensive Hodgkins disease (HD): the Memorial Sloan-Kettering Cancer Center (MSKCC) experience. In: BLOOD ed. ASH; 2003.
77. Radford JA, Rohatiner AZ, Ryder WD, et al. ChlVPP/EVA hybrid versus the weekly VAPEC-B regimen for previously untreated Hodgkin's disease. J Clin Oncol 2002;20:2988–2994.
78. Chisesi T, Federico M, Levis A, et al. ABVD versus Stanford V versus MEC in unfavourable Hodgkin's lymphoma: results of a randomised trial. Ann Oncol 2002;13(suppl 1):102–106.
79. Pavlovsky S, Santarelli MT, Muriel FS, et al. Randomized trial of chemotherapy versus chemotherapy plus radiotherapy for stage III-IV A & B Hodgkin's disease. Ann Oncol 1992;3:533–537.
80. Fabian C, Mansfield C, Dahlberg S, et al. Low dose involved field radiation after chemotherapy in advanced stage HD. Ann Intern Med 1994;120:903–912.
81. Diehl V, Loeffler M, Pfreundschuh M, et al. Further chemotherapy versus low-dose involved-field radiotherapy as consolidation of complete remission after six cycles of alternating chemotherapy in patients with advanced Hodgkin's disease. German Hodgkins' Study Group (GHSG). Ann Oncol 1995;6:901–910.
82. Coleman M, Rafla S, Propert KJ, et al. Augmented therapy of extensive Hodgkin's disease: radiation to known disease or prolongation of induction chemotherapy did not improve survival: results of a Cancer and Leukemia Group B study. Int J Radiat Oncol Biol Phys 1998;41:639–645.
83. Loeffler M, Brosteanu O, Hasenclever D, et al. Meta-analysis of chemotherapy versus combined modality treatment trials in Hodgkin's disease. International Database on Hodgkin's Disease Overview Study Group. J Clin Oncol 1998;16:818–829.
84. Ferme C, Sebban C, Hennequin C, et al. Comparison of chemotherapy to radiotherapy as consolidation of complete or good partial response after six cycles of chemotherapy for patients with advanced Hodgkin's disease: results of the Groupe d'Etudes des Lymphomes de l'Adulte H89 trial. Blood 2000;95:2246–2252.
85. Aleman BM, Raemaekers JM, Tirelli U, et al. Involved-field radiotherapy for advanced Hodgkin's lymphoma. N Engl J Med 2003;348:2396–2406.
86. Kostakoglu L, Leonard J, Kuji I, et al. Comparison of PET and Ga-67 in evaluation of lymphoma. Cancer (Phila) 2002;94:879–888.
87. Bossche B, Lambert B, De Winter F, et al. PET versus Ga scintigraphy for restaging and treatment follow-up of lymphoma patients. Nucl Med Commun 2002;23:1079–1083.
88. Wirth A, Seymour JF, Hicks RJ, et al. Fluorine-18 fluorodeoxyglucose positron emission tomography, gallium-67 scintigraphy, and conventional staging for Hodgkin's disease and non-Hodgkin's lymphoma. Am J Med 2002;112:262–268.
89. Jerusalem G, Warland V, Najjar F, et al. Whole-body 18F-FDG PET for the evaluation of patients with Hodgkin's disease and non-Hodgkin's lymphoma. Nucl Med Commun 1999;20:13–20.
90. Jerusalem G, Beguin Y, Fassotte MF, et al. Whole-body positron emission tomography using 18F-fluorodeoxyglucose for post-treatment evaluation in Hodgkin's disease and non-Hodgkin's lymphoma has higher diagnostic and prognostic value than classical computed tomography scan imaging. Blood 1999;94:429–433.
91. Jerusalem G, Beguin Y, Najjar F, et al. Positron emission tomography (PET) with 18F-fluorodeoxyglucose (18F-FDG) for the staging of low-grade non-Hodgkin's lymphoma (NHL). Ann Oncol 2001;12:825–830.
92. Weihrauch M, Re D, Scheidhauer K, et al. Thoracic PET for evaluation of residual mediastinal HD. Blood 2001;98:2930–2934.
93. Zinzani P, Magagnoli M, Chieichetti F, et al. The role of PET in the management of lymphoma patients. Ann Oncol 1999;10:1181–1184.
94. Spaepen K, Mortelmans L. Evaluation of treatment response in patients with lymphoma using [18F]FDG-PET: differences between non-Hodgkin's lymphoma and Hodgkin's disease. Q J Nucl Med 2001;45:269–273.
95. Spaepen K, Stroobants S, Dupont P, et al. Can positron emission tomography with [(18)F]-fluorodeoxyglucose after first-line treatment distinguish Hodgkin's disease patients who need additional therapy from others in whom additional therapy would mean avoidable toxicity? Br J Haematol 2001;115:272–278.
96. de Wit M, Bohuslavizki KH, Buchert R, Bumann D, Clausen M, Hossfeld DK. ^{18}FDG-PET following treatment as valid predictor for disease-free survival in Hodgkin's lymphoma. Ann Oncol 2001;12:29–37.
97. Mikhaeel NG, Timothy AR, Hain SF, O'Doherty MJ. 18-FDG-PET for the assessment of residual masses on CT following treatment of lymphomas. Ann Oncol 2000;11(suppl 1):147–150.
98. Longo DL, Duffey PL, Young RC, et al. Conventional-dose salvage combination chemotherapy in patients relapsing with Hodgkin's disease after combination chemotherapy: the low probability for cure. J Clin Oncol 1992;10:210–218.

99. Bonfante V, Santoro A, Viviani S, et al. Outcome of patients with Hodgkin's disease failing after primary MOPP-ABVD. J Clin Oncol 1997;15:528–534.
100. Linch DC, Goldstone AH. High-dose therapy for Hodgkin's disease. Br J Haematol 1999;107:685–690.
101. Linch DC, Winfield D, Goldstone AH, et al. Dose intensification with autologous bone-marrow transplantation in relapsed and resistant Hodgkin's disease: results of a BNLI randomised trial. Lancet 1993;341:1051–1054.
102. Schmitz N, Pfistner B, Sextro M, et al. Aggressive conventional chemotherapy compared with high-dose chemotherapy with autologous haemopoietic stem-cell transplantation for relapsed chemosensitive Hodgkin's disease: a randomised trial. Lancet 2002;359:2065–2071.
103. Yahalom J, Gulati SC, Toia M, et al. Accelerated hyperfractionated total-lymphoid irradiation, high-dose chemotherapy, and autologous bone marrow transplantation for refractory and relapsing patients with Hodgkin's disease. J Clin Oncol 1993;11: 1062–1070.
104. Yahalom J. Integrating radiotherapy into bone marrow transplantation programs for Hodgkin's disease. Int J Radiat Oncol Biol Phys 1995;33:525–528.
105. Zelenetz AD, Hamlin P, Kewalramani T, Yahalom J, Nimer S, Moskowitz CH. Ifosfamide, carboplatin, etoposide (ICE)-based second-line chemotherapy for the management of relapsed and refractory aggressive non-Hodgkin's lymphoma. Ann Oncol 2003;14(suppl 1):i5–i10.
106. Moskowitz CH, Nimer SD, Zelenetz AD, et al. A 2-step comprehensive high-dose chemoradiotherapy second-line program for relapsed and refractory Hodgkin disease: analysis by intent to treat and development of a prognostic model. Blood 2001;97: 616–623.
107. Sweetenham JW, Carella AM, Taghipour G, et al. High-dose therapy and autologous stem-cell transplantation for adult patients with Hodgkin's disease who do not enter remission after induction chemotherapy: results in 175 patients reported to the European Group for Blood and Marrow Transplantation. Lymphoma Working Party. J Clin Oncol 1999;17:3101–3109.
108. Josting A, Reiser M, Rueffer U, Salzberger B, Diehl V, Engert A. Treatment of primary progressive Hodgkin's and aggressive non-Hodgkin's lymphoma: is there a chance for cure? J Clin Oncol 2000;18:332–339.
109. Ferme C, Mounier N, Divine M, et al. Intensive salvage therapy with high-dose chemotherapy for patients with advanced Hodgkin's disease in relapse or failure after initial chemotherapy: results of the Groupe d'Etudes des Lymphomes de l'Adulte H89 Trial. J Clin Oncol 2002;20:467–475.
110. Lazarus HM, Rowlings PA, Zhang MJ, et al. Autotransplants for Hodgkin's disease in patients never achieving remission: a report from the Autologous Blood and Marrow Transplant Registry. J Clin Oncol 1999;17:534–545.
111. Moskowitz C, Nimer S, Zelenetz A, Jing Q, Yahalom J. Effectiveness of high dose therapy and ASCT for patients with biopsy proven relapsed and primary refractory Hodgkin's disease. Br J Hematol 2004;in press.
112. Wheeler C, Eickhoff C, Elias A, et al. High-dose cyclophosphamide, carmustine, and etoposide with autologous transplantation in Hodgkin's disease: a prognostic model for treatment outcomes. Biol Blood Marrow Transplant 1997;3:98–106.
113. Bierman PJ, Lynch JC, Bociek RG, et al. The International Prognostic Factors Project score for advanced Hodgkin's disease is useful for predicting outcome of autologous hematopoietic stem cell transplantation. Ann Oncol 2002;13:1370–1377.
114. Horning SJ, Chao NJ, Negrin RS, et al. High-dose therapy and autologous hematopoietic progenitor cell transplantation for recurrent or refractory Hodgkin's disease: analysis of the Stanford University results and prognostic indices. Blood 1997;89: 801–813.
115. Reece DE, Barnett MJ, Shepherd JD, et al. High-dose cyclophosphamide, carmustine (BCNU), and etoposide (VP16-213) with or without cisplatin (CBV +/– P) and autologous transplantation for patients with Hodgkin's disease who fail to enter a complete remission after combination chemotherapy. Blood 1995;86:451–456.
116. Josting A, Franklin J, May M, et al. New prognostic score based on treatment outcome of patients with relapsed Hodgkin's lymphoma registered in the database of the German Hodgkin's lymphoma study group. J Clin Oncol 2002;20:221–230.
117. Wadhwa P, Shina DC, Schenkein D, Lazarus HM. Should involved-field radiation therapy be used as an adjunct to lymphoma autotransplantation? Bone Marrow Transplant 2002;29: 183–189.
118. Mundt AJ, Sibley G, Williams S, Hallahan D, Nautiyal J, Weichselbaum RR. Patterns of failure following high-dose chemotherapy and autologous bone marrow transplantation with involved field radiotherapy for relapsed/refractory Hodgkin's disease. Int J Radiat Oncol Biol Phys 1995;33:261–270.
119. Yahalom J. Changing role and decreasing size: current trends in radiotherapy for Hodgkin's disease. Curr Oncol Rep 2002;4:415–423.
120. Peniket AJ, Ruiz de Elvira MC, Taghipour G, et al. An EBMT registry matched study of allogeneic stem cell transplants for lymphoma: allogeneic transplantation is associated with a lower relapse rate but a higher procedure-related mortality rate than autologous transplantation. Bone Marrow Transplant 2003;31: 667–678.
121. Mollee P, Lazarus HM, Lipton J. Why aren't we performing more allografts for aggressive non-Hodgkin's lymphoma? Bone Marrow Transplant 2003;31:953–960.
122. Giralt S, Aleman A, Anagnostopoulos A, et al. Fludarabine/melphalan conditioning for allogeneic transplantation in patients with multiple myeloma. Bone Marrow Transplant 2002;30: 367–373.
123. Tanimoto TE, Kusumi E, Hamaki T, et al. High complete response rate after allogeneic hematopoietic stem cell transplantation with reduced-intensity conditioning regimens in advanced malignant lymphoma. Bone Marrow Transplant 2003; 32:131–137.
124. Perez J, Kottaridis P, Martino R, et al. Nonmyeloablative transplantation with or without alemtuzumab: comparison between 2 prospective studies in patients with lymphoproliferative disorders. Blood 2002;100:3121–3127.
125. Cooney J, Stiff P, Toor A, et al. BEAM allogeneic transplantation for patients with HD who relapse after ASCT is safe and effective. Biol Blood Marrow Transplant 2003;9:177–182.
126. Faulkner R, Craddock C, Byrne J, et al. BEAM-alemtuzumab reduced-intensity allogeneic stem cell transplantation for lymphoproliferative diseases: GVHD, toxicity, and survival in 65 patients. Blood 2004;103:428–434.
127. Aleman BM, Van Den Belt-Dusebout AW, Klokman WJ, Van't Veer MB, Bartelink H, Van Leeuwen FE. Long-term cause-specific mortality of patients treated for Hodgkin's disease. J Clin Oncol 2003;21(18):3431–3439.
128. Bhatia S, Robison LL, Oberlin O, et al. Breast cancer and other second neoplasms after childhood Hodgkin's disease. N Engl J Med 1996;334:745–751.
129. Swerdlow AJ, Higgins CD, Adlard P, Preece MA. Risk of cancer in patients treated with human pituitary growth hormone in the UK, 1959–85: a cohort study. Lancet 2002;360:273–277.
130. van Leeuwen FE, Klokman WJ, Veer MB, et al. Long-term risk of second malignancy in survivors of Hodgkin's disease treated during adolescence or young adulthood. J Clin Oncol 2000;18: 487–497.
131. Travis L, Hill D, Dores G, et al. Breast cancer following radiotherapy and chemotherapy among young women with Hodgkin's disease. JAMA 2003;290:465–475.

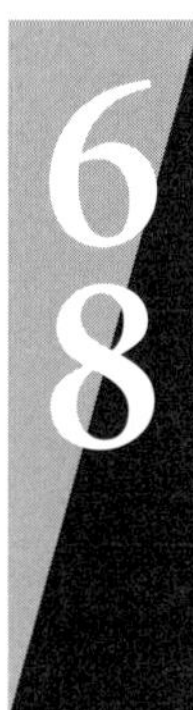

The Non-Hodgkin's Lymphomas

Andrew D. Zelenetz and Steven Horwitz

The non-Hodgkin's lymphomas (NHLs) represent a group of diseases arising from clonal proliferation of lymphocytes. NHL is the most common hematologic malignancy, with an estimated new patient incidence of 54,000 with 14,000 deaths from disease,[1] accounting for 4% of the new cancer diagnosed in 2004. The NHLs represent a diverse group of diseases with distinctive natural histories and clinical presentations.[2] This diversity arises from the fact that each of the lymphomas is derived from distinct stages of the complex process of lymphocyte ontogeny. Morphology was the mainstay of diagnosis and classification of NHL for many years. In 1994, the authors of the Revised European and American Lymphoma (REAL)[3] sought to create a classification system that defined distinct clinical entities. To accomplish this, the morphologic appearance was supplemented by the incorporation of additional information derived from immunophenotyping, genetics, and clinical features. This classification was the basis for the World Health Organization (WHO) classification of the neoplastic diseases of the hematopoietic and lymphoid tissues.[4,5] There are 27 entities included in the WHO classification of the non-Hodgkin's lymphoid neoplasms; this number excludes subtypes and subcategories recognized in the WHO classification. The major categories of the WHO classification are shown in Table 68.1.

An exhaustive overview of the management of NHL is beyond the scope of this chapter. Rather, the material herein focuses on the diagnosis, staging, prognostication, and management of the most common diseases and presentations. Very rare entities such as the T/NK (natural killer) lymphoma, adult T-cell lymphoma/leukemia (HTLV)-1-associated adult T-cell lymphoma/leukemia, and Burkitt's lymphoma, among others, are so uncommon that practicing oncologists are likely to encounter them only a few times, if ever, during their career. For these very rare tumors, consultation with a dedicated lymphoma specialist is warranted. Lymphoblastic lymphoma is managed similar to acute lymphoblastic leukemia, as discussed in Chapter 67. The diagnosis and evaluation of small lymphocytic lymphoma (SLL) is similar to that of other indolent lymphoma (see following), although the clinical management is similar to chronic lymphocytic leukemia, as will be reviewed here.

Pathology

In the WHO classification, the initial major discriminator is the cell of origin: B cell versus T/NK cell. The B- and T-cell neoplasms are further classified as being either precursor cell (lymphoblastic) versus mature or peripheral cell. Further discussion of the precursor cell neoplasms is in Chapter 67. The mature or peripheral cell neoplasms of B and T/NK origin make up the vast majority of the cases of NHL. Currently, there is no comprehensive description of the natural history and clinical features of all the NHL diagnoses recognized in the current WHO classification. The characteristics and natural history of the 13 most common entities, comprising about 90% of all the diagnoses of NHL in the United States, have been detailed by the International Lymphoma Classification Project[2] (Table 68.2).

The distribution of histologic types among 1,403 lymphoma cases has been investigated in the International Lymphoma Classification Project.[2] Two lymphomas represent more than half of all the cases of NHL in the United States: diffuse large B-cell (DLBCL), 31%; and follicular lymphoma (FL), 22%. Several other types are common (>5%): these include mucosa-associated lymphoid tissue lymphoma (MALTL), 5%; small lymphocytic lymphoma (chronic lymphocytic lymphoma type), 6%; peripheral T-cell lymphoma, 6%; mantle cell lymphoma, 6%. All other subtypes are rare or very rare with none seen in more than 2% of cases. The 12 most common subtypes (combining Burkitt's and Burkitt's-like, as is done in the WHO Classification) account for 88% of the diagnoses of NHL in the United States.

Diagnosis

Proper management of NHL begins with an accurate diagnosis, which has traditionally meant an incisional or excisional biopsy to provide adequate material. As already discussed, the WHO classification is not solely dependent on morphology and incorporates immunophenotyping and, in some cases, genetics and clinical information to establish a diagnosis. This change has raised the possibility that the traditional lymph node biopsy could be replaced by fine-needle aspiration (FNA) in conjunction with flow cytometry, which would

TABLE 68.1. World Health Organization (WHO) classification of the non-Hodgkin's lymphomas.

B-Cell Neoplasms
- Precursor B-cell neoplasm
  - Precursor B-lymphoblastic leukemia/lymphoma (precursor B-cell acute lymphoblastic leukemia)
- Mature (peripheral) B-cell neoplasms[a]
  - B-cell chronic lymphocytic leukemia/small lymphocytic lymphoma
  - B-cell prolymphocytic leukemia
  - Lymphoplasmacytic lymphoma
  - Splenic marginal zone B-cell lymphoma (± villous lymphocytes)
  - Hairy cell leukemia
  - Plasma cell myeloma/plasmacytoma
  - Extranodal marginal zone B-cell lymphoma of MALT type
  - Nodal marginal zone B-cell lymphoma (± monocytoid B cells)
  - Follicular lymphoma
  - Mantle cell lymphoma
  - Diffuse large B-cell lymphoma
    - Mediastinal large B-cell lymphoma
    - Primary effusion lymphoma
- Burkitt's lymphoma/Burkitt cell leukemia

T-Cell and NK-Cell Neoplasms
- Precursor T-cell neoplasm
  - Precursor T-lymphoblastic lymphoma/leukemia (precursor T-cell acute lymphoblastic leukemia)
- Mature (peripheral) T-cell neoplasms
  - T-cell prolymphocytic leukemia
  - T-cell granular lymphocytic leukemia
  - Aggressive NK-cell leukemia
  - Adult T-cell lymphoma/leukemia (HTLV-1+)
  - Extranodal NK/T-cell lymphoma, nasal type
  - Enteropathy-type T-cell lymphoma
  - Hepatosplenic gamma-delta T-cell lymphoma
  - Subcutaneous panniculitis-like T-cell lymphoma
  - Mycosis fungoides/Sézary syndrome
  - Anaplastic large-cell lymphoma, T/null cell, primary cutaneous type
  - Peripheral T-cell lymphoma, not otherwise characterized
  - Angioimmunoblastic T-cell lymphoma
  - Anaplastic large-cell lymphoma, T/null cell, primary systemic type

HTLV1+, human T-cell leukemia virus; MALT, mucosa-associated lymphoid tissue; NK, natural killer.

[a] B-cell and T-cell/NK-cell neoplasms are grouped according to major clinical presentations (predominantly disseminated/leukemic, primary extranodal, predominantly nodal).

Source: Data from Jaffe et al.[4]

TABLE 68.2. Characteristics of most common lymphomas.

Subtype	*Immunophenotype*	*Molecular lesions*	*Frequency (%)*
DLBCL	CD20+	BCL2, BCL6, CMYC	31
FL	CD20+, CD10+, CD5–	BCL2	22
SLL/CLL	CD20 weak, CD5+, CD23+	+12, 11q–, p53, V gene	6
PTCL	CD20–, CD3+	Variable	6
MCL	CD20+, CD5+, CD23–	CYCLIN D1	6
MZL (MALT)	CD20+, CD5–, CD23–	BCL10, MALT1	5
Mediastinal LCL	CD20+	Variable	2
ALCL	CD20–, CD3+, CD30+, CD15–, EMA+	ALK	2
LL (T/B)	T cell CD3+, B cell CD19+	Variable, TCL1-3	2
MZL (nodal)	CD20+, CD10–, CD23–, CD5–	+3, +18	1
SLL, PL	CD20+, cIg+, CD5–, CD23–	PAX-5	1
BL	CD20+, CD10+, CD5–	CMYC	3[a]

SLL, small lymphocytic lymphoma.

[a] This category includes both Burkitt's and Burkitt's-like, which are combined in the WHO.

have the potential benefit of reduced costs and morbidity. The cytologic diagnosis of lymphoma by FNA has been examined in a large number of series, which have been reviewed.[6] Overall, a precise NHL diagnosis could be established in 70% of cases representing both initial diagnosis and relapse. There was clearly greater accuracy in diagnosis among the cases suspicious for relapse compared to the initial diagnosis. It is clear that some diagnoses were readily established by the combination of flow cytometry and cytopathology: acute lymphoblastic leukemia/lymphoma as well as SLL/CLL (chronic lymphocytic leukemia). A problem with most of the published series is that they are based on classifying tumors in the International Working Formulation[7] rather than the REAL or WHO classification in current use. In a series reported by Mourad et al.,[8] the accuracy of FNA for initial diagnosis was evaluated in a series of 74 cases with classification according to the WHO. This study further evaluated accuracy in diagnosis based on the background and training of the pathologists, comparing dedicated cytopathologists and/or hematopathologists to surgical pathologists lacking this specialized training. The diagnosis of lymphoma was rendered in all cases; however, in only 63% of the cases could the lymphoma be accurately categorized according to the WHO. Flow cytometry significantly enhanced the diagnostic accuracy (84% versus 33%), as did specialized expertise (80% versus 56%). Based on these data, the use of FNA for the initial diagnosis of lymphoma should be discouraged because of the potential for inaccuracy is making a specific diagnosis; however, it can expedite the diagnosis of recurrent disease.[8–10]

In institutions where cytopathologists and/or hematopathologists have appropriate specialized training, FNA may have a greater role, but the surgical biopsy remains the gold standard for diagnosis. The exception to this recommendation is in cases of acute lymphoblastic lymphoma (ALL) and SLL/CLL where a combination of cytopathology and flow cytometry can routinely provide accurate diagnoses. Furthermore, FNA has a role when the differential diagnosis includes lymphoma but an epithelial tumor is considered more likely.[11] Given the high potential for a false-negative result in cases that ultimately prove to be lymphoma, it is important that a nondiagnostic FNA be followed by an excisional biopsy.[11]

Staging and Prognosis

The clinical staging of NHL is taken from the Ann Arbor (AA) staging system developed for Hodgkin's disease as modified at the Cotswold meeting in 1989[12] (Table 68.3). The modification retained the well-known four-stage Ann Arbor system. adding a modifier for bulk (X), and recommending that computed tomography (CT) be included as the method of evaluation of intrathoracic and infradiaphragmatic adenopathy. The staging system is based on the extent of involvement of nodal groups: stage I is a single lymph node group; stage II is multiple lymph node groups on a single side of the diaphragm; stage III disease involves nodal groups on both sides of the diaphragm; and stage IV includes noncontiguous extranodal involvement (e.g., lung nodules, bone marrow). The E modifier denotes direct extension to an extranodal site or isolated involvement of a single extranodal site. A stage is denoted clinical (CS) if it is based on physical examination, imaging, and a bone marrow biopsy and denoted pathologic (PS) if confirmed by one more additional biopsy (as in a staging laparotomy). However, in contrast to Hodgkin's disease, NHL does not tend to move through adjacent lymph node groups, thus reducing the general utility of clinical staging. In some of the indolent lymphomas, such as SLL/CLL and FL, bone marrow involvement is so common that most patients have stage IV disease. Furthermore, bone marrow involvement in the indolent lymphomas is not clearly associated with outcome, thereby rendering the clinical staging system of limited value. Frequently, patients are categorized as having early-stage (AA CS I/II) versus advanced-stage disease (AA CS III/IV) as this has been more clinically valuable.

TABLE 68.3. Cotswold modification of Ann Arbor Staging System.

Stage	*Area of involvement*
I	Single lymph node group
II	Multiple lymph node groups on same side of diaphragm
III	Multiple lymph node groups on both sides of diaphragm
IV	Multiple extranodal sites or lymph nodes and extranodal disease
Modifier	***Description***
X	Bulk >10 cm
E	Extranodal extension or single isolated site of extranodal disease
A/B	B symptoms: weight loss >10%, fever, drenching night sweats

Source: Data from Lister et al.[12]

Given the limited value of clinical staging, significant efforts have been undertaken to establish prognostic models that can help guide clinical management and clinical trial design and interpretation. Throughout the decade of the 1980s, a vast number of clinical prognostic models were published that were often developed on limited data sets without validation. Given institutional differences in treatment and patient variables, validation across centers was often difficult. However, these models did identify a number of clinical variables that were important in the prognosis of aggressive lymphoma. To circumvent the limitation of small patient numbers and institutional variation, an international effort was undertaken to identify prognostic factors in patients with aggressive lymphoma treated with anthracycline-based regimens.[13] From a group of 2,031 patients, five clinical factors [age, performance status, serum lactate dehydrogenase (LDH), extranodal disease, stage] were identified that predicted for both disease-free survival (DFS) and overall survival (OS) (Table 68.4). The 95% confidence intervals of the relative risks of these five variables overlapped, allowing a simple model to be derived based on the number of adverse risk factors: 0–1, low risk; 2, low-intermediate risk; 3, high-intermediate risk; 4–5, high risk. The model divides patients into four similar-sized risk groups with 5-year OS ranging from 26% in high-risk patients to 73% in low-risk patients. A second, age-adjusted prognostic model was derived for patients no more than 60 years of age with only three clinical factors (performance status, LDH, stage) (see Table 68.4). Similar to the full index, the number of risk factors corresponded to the risk group: 0, low risk; 1, low-intermediate; 2,

TABLE 68.4. International Prognostic Index for aggressive lymphoma.

A. Full index

Factor	Adverse
Age	>60 years
PS	≥2
LDH	>Normal
Extranodal sites	≥2
Stage (AA)	III–IV

Risk group	No. of factors present	Five-year DFS (%)	Five-year OS (%)
Low	0–1	70	73
Low/intermediate	2	50	51
High/intermediate	3	49	43
High	4–5	40	26

B. Age-adjusted index

Factor	Adverse
PS	≥2
LDH	>Normal
Stage (AA)	III–IV

Risk group	No. of factors present	Five-year OS, age >60 years (%)	Five-year OS, age ≤60 years (%)
Low	0	56	83
Low/intermediate	1	44	69
High/intermediate	2	37	46
High	3	21	32

LDH, lactate dehydrogenase; DFS, disease-free survival; OS, overall survival.

Source: From The International Non-Hodgkin's Lymphoma Prognostic Factors Project,[13] by permission of *New England Journal of Medicine*.

high-intermediate; 3, high risk. The validation and total samples again divided into four groups, ranging in outcome from 32% in high-risk to 83% in low-risk patients. Although based on retrospective data, both models were derived on a subset of the patients and validated on the remaining patients with similar results. The models have been validated in both aggressive lymphoma as well as other histologies, including follicular lymphoma and mantle cell lymphoma,[14–16] as well as in relapsed DLBCL.[17–19] This prognostic model has been very valuable in interpreting trial results as well as in the prospective design of clinical trials for patients with uniform risk.

In patients with follicular lymphoma, the International Prognostic Index (IPI) has more limited clinical utility.[20] Although IPI stratifies patients with follicular lymphoma into four risk groups with significantly different outcomes in both progression-free and overall survival, only 11% and 2% of patients fall into the high-intermediate (three factors) and high (four to five factors) risk groups. Others have obtained very similar results when applying the IPI to patients with FL.[15,21,22] The lack of balance between risk groups limits the utility of the IPI for use in the design of clinical trials. Recently, a prognostic index specific for patients with follicular lymphoma was published that addresses this limitation.[23] Similar to the IPI, this was an international collaborative effort and included complete data on 4,167 patients. A multivariate analysis identified eight factors that were independent predictors of outcome. To create an easier-to-use index, a subindex containing five variables was evaluated and found to have a very similar predictive value as the eight-factor model. The five factors that comprise the Follicular Lymphoma International Prognostic Index (FLIPI), include number of nodal sites (adverse, five or more); LDH (adverse, greater than normal); age (adverse, age greater than 60 years); stage (adverse, AA III–IV); hemoglobin (less than 12g/dL) (Table 68.5). Of note, the number of nodal sites is based on a mannequin distinct from that used in the Ann Arbor staging (Figure 68.1). Patients with low-risk disease (zero or one factor, 10-year OS, 70.7%), intermediate risk (two factors, 10-year OS, 50.9%), and high-risk disease (three to five factors, 10-year OS, 35.5%) are divided into similar-sized groups. The IPI and FLIPI share three factors but each is unique in two factors (Figure 68.2); however, these changes enable the FLIPI to be a more clinically useful prognostic model for patients with FL. Thus, the FLIPI could be used to stratify or select patients for risk-adapted therapy trials. The utility of the FLIPI has been validated at relapse in another dataset.[24] In a study from Memorial Sloan-Kettering Cancer Center (MSKCC), involving an analysis of 260 patients with FL, the utility of the FLIPI as a reliable means of stratifying prognostic groups was confirmed and, furthermore, histologic grade (1, 2, 3a, 3b) added no additional prognostic information.[25]

As useful as the IPI has been in serving as a "Rosetta Stone" in the interpretation of clinical trials with differing patient populations and for the design of clinical trials, it does not identify the molecular basis for the prognostic differences. It is through the identification of molecular determinants of prognosis that novel therapeutic targets may be identified. Nonetheless, clinical markers of prognosis represent a very powerful tool in clinical care of the patient.

TABLE 68.5. Follicular Lymphoma International Prognostic Index: risk factors and outcome.

Risk Factors

Factor	Adverse
Age	>60 years
Hgb	<12g/dL
LDH	>Normal
Number of nodal sites	≥5
Stage (AA)	III–IV

Risk group	No. of factors	Fraction of patients (%)	Five-year OS (%)	Ten-year OS (%)
Low	0, 1	36	90.6	70.7
Intermediate	2	37	77.6	50.9
High	3–5	27	52.5	35.5

Source: From Solal-Celigny et al.,[23] by permission of *Blood*.

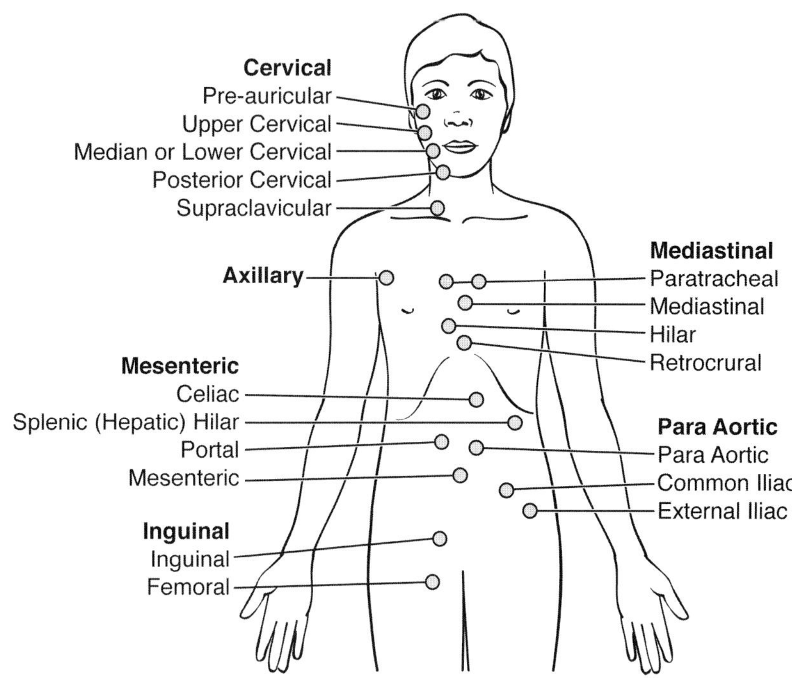

FIGURE 68.1. Nodal mannequin for the Follicular Lymphoma International Prognostic Index. (From Solal-Celigny et al.,[23] by permission of *Blood*.)

Prognostic Models Based on Gene Expression Profiles

Gene expression profiling has emerged as an important tool in the identification of prognostic subtypes in hematologic malignancies. A detailed description of the methodology is beyond the scope of this chapter, and the reader is referred to a number of excellent review articles.[26–29] Briefly, this technology interrogates a tissue or tumor for the expression of thousands of genes simultaneously. The resulting gene expression profile can be analyzed in a number of ways. The two most common analyses are hierarchical clustering and supervised analysis. In hierarchical clustering analysis, specimens are grouped by the relatedness of their overall expression pattern and distinct patterns identified by the construction of dendrograms. The ability of this method to identify distinct subgroups is dependent on the number of subgroups, the sample size, and the distinctiveness of the gene expression profile. This method does not necessarily identify groups with distinct clinical outcome. In supervised analysis, the samples are divided on the basis of known feature of the data set, for example, cured versus refractory. Patterns of gene expression that distinguish between the subgroups are identified. Given the enormous number of genes being examined at one time, an adequate sample size is necessary to identify a robust prognostic model. Furthermore, an

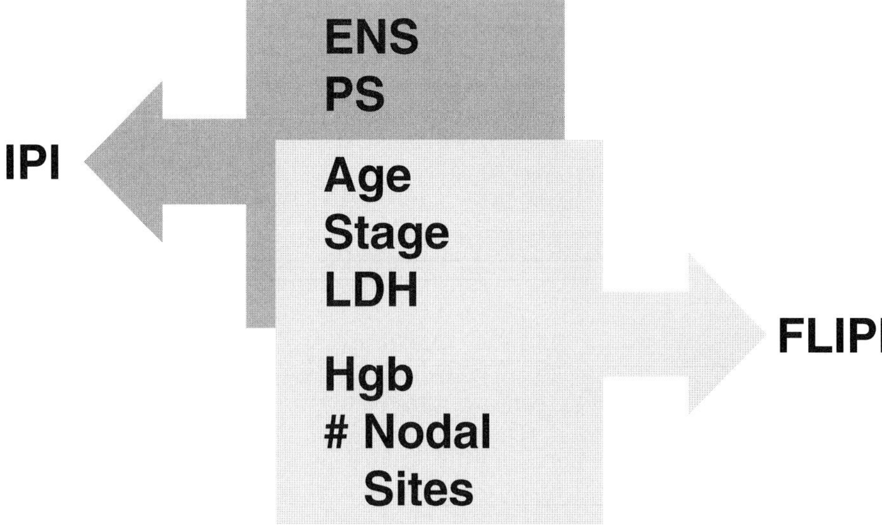

FIGURE 68.2. Similarities and differences between the International Prognostic Index (IPI) and Follicular Lymphoma International Prognostic Index (FLIPI).

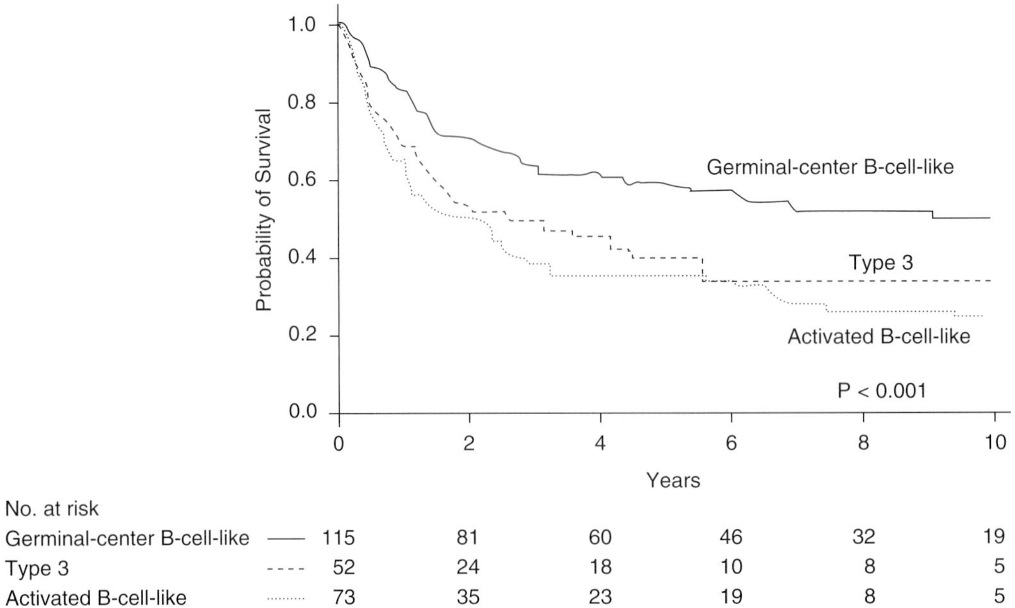

FIGURE 68.3. Outcome of patients with diffuse large B-cell lymphoma (DLBCL) according to the gene expression profile. (From Rosenwald et al.,[32] by permission of *New England Journal of Medicine*.)

independent validation sample is ideally needed to confirm the significance of the genes selected in the prognostic model. Both of these approaches have been used to construct prognostic models for NHL.

The initial application of gene expression profiling in lymphoma was conducted by the Leukemia and Lymphoma Molecular Profiling Project (LLMPP). Using the LymphoChip,[30] the LLMPP initially identified two molecular subtypes of DLBLC by hierarchical clustering that were named on the basis of the similarity of gene expression with normal B-cell counterparts: germinal center B-cell and active B-cell lymphomas.[31] This approach was later refined with additional samples into three subgroups with the addition of type III lymphoma.[32] Hierarchical clustering per se does not dictate that identified subgroups should have distinct prognoses. Nonetheless, patients with the germinal center B-cell phenotype were demonstrated to have a superior outcome compared to patients with either the activated B-cell or type III, which were very similar (Figure 68.3).[32] Currently, gene expression profiling is an investigational tool. Until a simplified technology can be validated in a multicenter setting, the clinical utility of gene expression profiling is limited. This realization led investigators in the LLMPP to determine if routine immunohistochemical markers could differentiate the tumors into germinal center (GC) versus nongerminal center (non-GC) origins. It has been shown that the results from three antibodies directed at CD10, BCL6, and MUM1 can adequately identify GC versus non-GC.[33]

It is very interesting that the molecular prognostic models developed for DLBCL, either based on cell of origin[31–33] or by supervised analysis to identify genes associated with a poor outcome,[34] can subdivide IPI risk groups. This finding suggests that the molecular signatures identified are independent of the IPI and that additional molecular markers remain to be identified that correlate with the clinic prognostic model.

Aggressive NHL: Initial Management of Advanced Stage

The International Working Formulation (IWF) classified NHL by its natural history into three broad groups: low-, intermediate-, and high-grade.[7] This was an important step in providing some uniformity to clinical trials for NHL. However, IWF intermediate-grade lymphoma, which is referred to here as aggressive NHL, represents a heterogeneous group of disorders, including both B- and T-cell lymphomas. When classified by WHO criteria, aggressive NHL is dominated by DLBCL, with about 10% having peripheral T-cell lymphoma and about 5% other lymphomas. Thus, the results of large-scale trials reviewed here are largely applicable to patients with DLBCL. Patients with DLBCL (including anaplastic B-cell lymphoma) have often been exclusively included in trials developed since the widespread acceptance of the REAL/WHO classification and the development of targeted therapy. Thus, one must be aware that the conclusions drawn from the evidence reviewed here largely apply to DLBCL. A brief discussion of the T-cell lymphoma is included below to help clarify that these entities have unique natural histories and outcomes with therapy.

Evidence for CHOP as the Standard for Aggressive Lymphoma

The publication of the cyclophosphamide, doxorubicin, vincristine, prednisone (CHOP) regimen in 1976[35] and the COMLA (cyclophosphamide, vincristine, methotrexate with leucovorin rescue, and cytarabine) regimen in 1980[36] ushered in the era of curative therapy for aggressive large-cell lymphoma with approximately 30% of patient achieving long-term remission. In subsequent years, a number of second- and third-generation regimens were introduced for the management of aggressive NHL that reported curative outcomes in 55% to 65% of patients. The m-BACOD (methotrexate, bleomycin, doxorubicin, cyclophosphasmide, vincristine, and dexamethasone) regimen was typical of a second-generation regimen.[37] MACOP-B (methotrexate, doxorubicin, cyclophosphamide, vincristine, prednisone, and bleomycin)[38] and ProMACE-CytaBOM (prednisone, methotrexate, cyclophosphamide, etoposide, cytarabine, bleomycin, vincristine, and methotrexate)[39] were representative third-generation regimens. However, many of these studies were performed in single centers with relatively small patient numbers. In 1993, the national high priority intergroup Phase III trial compared CHOP, MACOP-B, ProMACE-Cytabom, and m-BACOD, demonstrating that the outcomes of the four regimens were equivalent and that CHOP was associated with the most modest toxicity. Thus, following this trial, CHOP chemotherapy emerged as the standard regimen for treatment in the United States.

Improvement of Outcome with Increased Dose Intensity and Dose Density

In Europe, the Groupe d'Etude des Lymphomes de l'Adulte (GELA) developed the ACVBP regimen (doxorubicin, cyclophosphamide, vindesine, bleomycin, and prednisone), consisting of an induction phase of intensified chemotherapy and central nervous system (CNS) prophylaxis followed by a sequential consolidation phase.[40] The GELA conducted a randomized trial to compare the ACVBP regimen to CHOP in previously untreated patients (aged 61 to 69 years) with poor-risk aggressive lymphoma (at least one adverse factor in the age-adjusted IPI). Although there was no difference in complete response rate, the 5-year event-free survival (EFS; 39% versus 29%) and overall survival (OS; 46% versus 38%) significantly favored the ACVBP arm.[41] Building on the CHOP regimen, the German High-Grade Non-Hodgkin's Lymphoma Study Group tested both, the addition of etoposide (CHOEP) to the regimen, as well as increased dose density, comparing standard 21-day cycles to accelerated 14-day cycles (DSHNHL) in both younger and older patients.[42,43] The toxicity of the CHOEP (when given at both 14- and 21-day intervals) limited the effectiveness of these regimens for patients more than 60 years of age (61 to 75). However, CHOP-14 was superior to CHOP-21 for both EFS (44% versus 33%) and OS (53% versus 41%). For patients younger than 60 years of age, the results were less clear. The 2-week interval did not improve EFS, although there was a marginally significant improvement in OS (85% versus 79%). In the CHOP versus CHOEP comparison, there was a significant improvement in the 5-year estimated EFS (58% versus 69%) but not in the OS. Thus, these data suggest intensification of chemotherapy as with ACVBP, CHOP-14 (in patients 61 to 75), or CHOEP can improve outcomes compared to conventional CHOP given at 21-day intervals. Nonetheless, the failure of multiple second- and third-generation regimens to improve upon the outcomes obtained with CHOP chemotherapy point to the limitation of additional chemotherapy for improving outcome.

Another approach to improving outcome has been the use of infusional chemotherapy. The EPOCH (infusional etoposide, doxorubicin, vincristine with bolus prednisone and cyclophosphamide) was initially tested in 74% of patients with relapsed and refractory disease; 92% of the patients had had at least four of the drugs previously. The overall response rate was 87%, with complete responses in 27%. A modified regimen, dose-adjusted (DA) EPOCH, was tested in patients with untreated aggressive lymphoma. The dose adjustment was to account for interpatient variability in drug metabolism.[44] The target was a nadir absolute neutrophil count below 0.5×10^9/L. Using this approach in 50 patients with newly diagnosed DLBCL, the complete remission rate was 92%. At the median follow-up of 62 months, the progression-free survival (PFS) and OS were 70% and 73%, respectively. Provocatively, the IPI was not associated with outcome. Rituximab has been added to this regimen with improved outcome in selected patients (see following).[45]

High-Dose Therapy as a Component of Initial Therapy

A number of trials have tried to evaluate the role of high-dose therapy with autologous stem cell transplant (HDT/ASCT) in first consolidation for patients with aggressive NHL. The report of the jury of the international consensus conference on high-dose therapy concluded that there were conflicting data regarding the role of HDT/ASCT as consolidation following induction chemotherapy for high-risk patients.[46] In a subset analysis of the LNH-87 study, patients with high-intermediate and high-risk disease by the age-adjusted IPI had an improved outcome with consolidative HDT/ASCT compared to the conventional therapy in 5-year DFS (57% versus 36%; $P = 0.01$), but the OS benefit was marginally significant (65% versus 52%; $P = 0.06$).[47,48] In a subset analysis of the Italian Non-Hodgkin's Lymphoma Study Group trial, a similar result was seen in patients with age-adjusted IPI high-intermediate and high-risk disease.[49] However, in two other studies using an abbreviated course of induction chemotherapy, followed by HDT/ASCT on the investigation arm, compared to conventional chemotherapy on the control arm, demonstrated no superiority for HDT/ASCT consolidation.[50,51] At the time of the presentation of the LNH-93 trial, the conventional chemotherapy arm had superior EFS (54% versus 41%; $P = 0.01$) and OS (63% versus 47%; $P = 0.003$) compared to the induction chemotherapy followed by HDT/ASCT.[50] In the German High-Grade Lymphoma Study Group trial, CHOEP × 5 with involved field radiation therapy (IFRT) was compared to CHOEP × 3 followed by HDT/ASCT. In this study, survival after relapse was significantly inferior in the HDT/ASCT arm.[51] Another approach to poor-risk aggressive lymphoma has been to intensify the initial therapy. A study from Milan compared MACOP-B to a high-dose sequential (HDS) therapy consisting of high-dose single agents: cyclophosphamide, methotrexate, and etoposide followed by melphalan/total body irradiation with ASCT.[52] The 7-year EFS (76% versus 49%; $P = 0.004$) favored HDS therapy over MACOP-B. However, there was significant survival advantage for HDS (81% versus 55%; $P = 0.09$), in part, because of the cross-over design of the study. This result raises an important question as to the timing of HDT/ASCT. Is there an advantage to integration of HDT/ASCT as part of initial therapy or is it better to use this approach for patients with recurrent disease after conventional chemotherapy? This question is the subject of ongoing clinical trials; thus, the role of HDT/ASCT as a component of initial therapy for

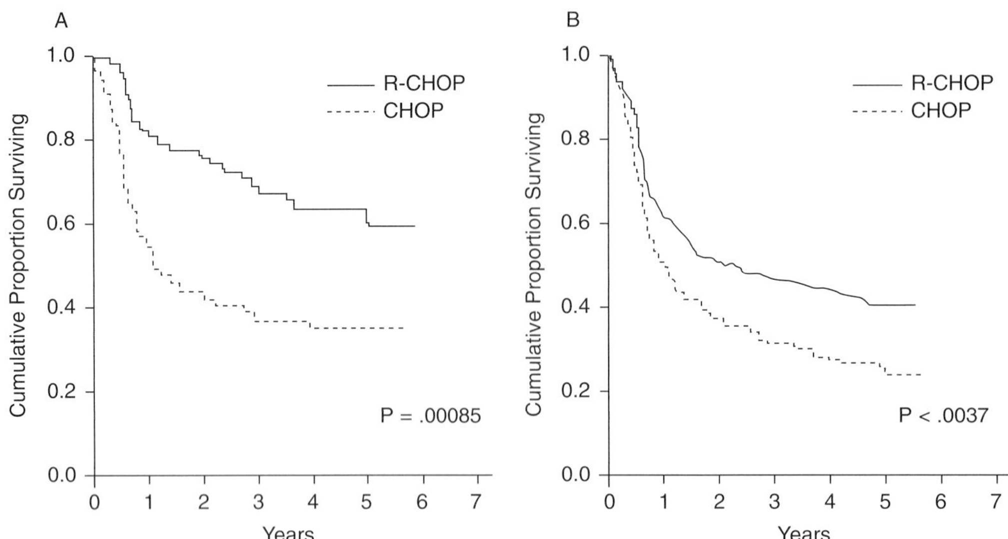

FIGURE 68.4. R-CHOP versus cyclophosphamide, doxorubicin, vincristine, prednisone (CHOP) in patients aged 60–80 with DLBLC: event-free survival (EFS) by age-adjusted IPI. (A) Low-risk patients with IPI scores of 0 or 1; (B) high-risk patients with IPI scores of 2 or 3. (From Coiffier et al.,[59] by permission of *Blood*.)

poor-risk patients remains investigational as the evidence just discussed does not provide a clear answer.

Addition of Rituximab to Induction Therapy

Rituximab is a recombinant chimeric monoclonal antibody with specificity for the human pan-B-cell antigen CD20; it has the original murine variable domain of the parent antibody 2B8 with human IgG-1 heavy-chain and human kappa light-chain constant regions.[53] The GELA demonstrated that rituximab had modest single-agent activity with 37% overall response rate in patients with relapsed and refractory DLBCL.[54] The principal toxicity seen is associated primarily with the initial infusions and, importantly, there is no significant myelotoxicity. The combination of single-agent activity without overlapping toxicity provided a rationale for the combination of rituximab with conventional chemotherapy. A multicenter Phase II study of rituximab (day 1 of each cycle) and CHOP (day 3 of each cycle) for patients with untreated DLBCL was conducted to evaluate safety and efficacy.[55] Thirty-three patients were treated with six cycles of R-CHOP at 21-day intervals, and the principal toxicities were infusional reactions during the first dose of rituximab and the expected toxicities of CHOP. The addition of the rituximab did not appear to augment the toxicity of the chemotherapy. The overall response rate was 94% with 61% complete responders. At the time of the publication, the follow-up was short (26 months) and the median time to progression had not been reached. Among 13 patients who had a t(14;18) translocation identified by polymerase chain reaction (PCR) at baseline, 11 had molecular remission at the end of therapy. The efficacy was believed to be at least as good as that expected for patients treated with CHOP. Based on these favorable Phase II results, several randomized studies were conducted to see if rituximab enhanced the efficacy of CHOP chemotherapy.[56–58]

In LNH 98.5, the GELA compared eight cycles of conventional CHOP chemotherapy to eight cycles of the combination of rituximab (day 1 of each cycle) with CHOP (day 1 of each cycle) for patients aged 60 to 80 years.[56] Addition of rituximab to the CHOP chemotherapy resulted in significant improvement in complete response (76% versus 53%; P = 0.005), as well as 5-year EFS (47% versus 29%; P less than 0.00001) and OS (58% versus 45%; P = 0.0073).[59] The benefit has been durable, with increased separation of the Kaplan–Meier survival curves with increasing length of follow-up. The relative benefit of the chemoimmunotherapy is greater in the patients with low- and low- to intermediate-risk disease determined by the age-adjusted IPI; nonetheless, even among the poor-risk patients there is a significant improvement in the outcome (Figure 68.4).

ECOG 4494 examined a very similar patient population (aged 60 and over), although the dosing of the rituximab was different (Figure 68.5).[57] Two doses of rituximab were administered before cycle 1 and one dose of rituximab was administered before cycles 3, 5, and 7 (if necessary). Treatment was given for six to eight cycles; those in a complete response after four cycles received six cycles and all other patients received eight. In addition to posing the question regarding the role of adding rituximab to CHOP, the trial evaluated the effect of maintenance rituximab (MR) administered for four doses

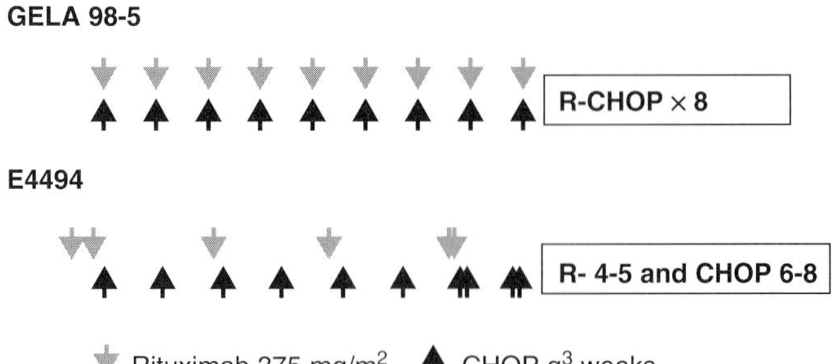

FIGURE 68.5. Comparison of the schedule of the chemoimmunotherapy arms therapy in the GELA 98-5 and ECOG 4494 trials comparing R-CHOP to CHOP for patients. (GELA, Groupe d'Etude des Lymphomes de l'Adulte; R, rituximab; CHOP, cyclophosphamide, doxorubicin, vincristine, prednisone.)

every 6 months for 2 years. Interpretation of the trial results was complicated by the 2 × 2 trial design, because it was based on the erroneous assumption that there was no interaction between the randomizations. The overall response rate was unaffected by the second randomization. In contrast to the GELA LNH 98.5 trial, there was no difference in the response rate between the R-CHOP and CHOP (79% versus 76%). Interestingly, the response of the control arm in this trial is similar to the chemoimmunotherapy arm of LNH 98.5. In the pairwise analysis of induction, R-CHOP demonstrated a small benefit at 3 years in EFS (53% versus 46%; $P = 0.04$) but not overall survival. However, this analysis was complicated by the interaction between the induction and maintenance therapies. Because the induction therapy influenced the results of the maintenance, a weighted analysis was performed to elucidate the effect of induction therapy without influence from the maintenance. In this analysis, R-CHOP improved 3-year EFS (52% versus 39%; $P = 0.003$) and OS (67% versus 58%; $P = 0.05$). In the pairwise analysis evaluating maintenance, patients receiving MR had a significant increase in time to treatment failure but not in overall survival. Importantly, the benefit of MR was restricted to patients treated with CHOP induction. The event-free survivals at 2 years for the four treatment groups were R-CHOP, 77%; R-CHOP + MR, 79%; CHOP, 47%; and CHOP+MR, 74%. Thus, E4494 confirmed the benefit of R-CHOP for patients over the age of 60 and demonstrated that in DLBCL MR has no added benefit to induction therapy with chemoimmunotherapy.

Both the GELA LNH 98.5 and ECOG 4494 studies focus on patients 60 years of age and older. Two additional studies have examined the benefit of chemoimmunotherapy for DLBCL in younger patients.[58,60] The Mint trial was an international intergroup study for patients with untreated DLBCL aged 18 to 60 with low-risk disease (IPI 0 or 1, stages II–IV, and stage I with bulk). Patients were randomized to receive six cycles of a CHOP-like regimen or the same chemotherapy plus rituximab 375 mg/m^2 given on days 1, 22, 43, 64, 85, and 106. Radiotherapy was planned to sites of initial bulk and/or extranodal involvement.[58] CHOP-like chemotherapy included CHOEP (44%), CHOP (48%), MACOP-B (4%), and PMitCEBO (prednisolone, mitoxantrone, cyclophosphamide, etoposide, bleomycin, vincristine)[61] (4%); the use of these regimens was balanced in the chemotherapy-alone (CHEMO) and rituximab plus chemotherapy (R-CHEMO) arms. As in the GELA study, the R-CHEMO arm had a higher complete response (CR) (86% versus 68%; P less than 0.0001). This response was associated with an improvement in the estimated 2-year EFS (76% versus 60%; P less than 0.0001) and OS (94% versus 87%; P less than 0.001). This study supports the use of rituximab plus anthracycline-based chemotherapy in the initial management of young patients with very favorable DLBCL; however, it does not directly address patients with poor-risk disease.

Based on the early results of the GELA LNH 98.5 study, the British Columbia Cancer Agency (BCCA) implemented a policy on March 1, 2001, recommending the use of R-CHOP for newly diagnosed patients with advanced-stage DLBCL. To analyze the impact of that policy recommendation, the investigators at the BCCA performed a retrospective analysis comparing the outcomes of patients with newly diagnosed DLBCL for a 3-year period spanning the 18 months before (Pre-R) and 18 months after (Post-R) the policy change.[60] In the Pre-R group, 9% of the patients received rituximab and in the Post-R group, 85% of the patients received rituximab. Significantly more patients received radiation therapy in the Pre-R group compared to the Post-R (25% versus 15%; $P = 0.04$). For the entire population, the Post-R group had a superior estimated 2-year PFS (71% versus 52%; $P = 0.00009$) and OS (77% versus 53%; $P = 0.0001$) compared to the Pre-R group. However, in the patients younger than 60, the 2-year estimated EFS was not statistically significant (70% post-R versus 60% pre-R; $P = 0.18$). In this subset, the OS was superior (87% post-R versus 69% pre-R; $P = 0.018$), but this finding may reflect differences in second-line therapy in patients treated in different time spans. Although these results confirm the efficacy of R-CHOP in a community setting, they raise a question about the management of younger patients. Clearly, a more careful prospective evaluation of the role of adding rituximab to chemotherapy for young patients with poor-risk DLBCL is necessary.

Rituximab has also been added to the DA-EPOCH regimen.[45] The complete response rate (CR/CRu) of the 61 evaluable patients was 92%. At the median follow-up of 22 months, the estimated PFS and OS where 79% and 84%, respectively, quite similar to the historical control.[44] However, in a subset analysis based on the expression of BCL2 as judged by immunohistochemistry, there was an improved outcome in patients whose tumors expressed the BCL2 gene product if they were treated with DA-EPOCH-R compared to DA-EPOCH. Addition of rituximab did not improve the outcome in patients whose tumors did not express BCL2 protein. A similar observation has been made in a retrospective analysis of the GELA LNH 98.5 study.[62] An analysis of E4494 did not find this relationship between BCL2 protein expression and benefit with rituximab. In E4494, the lack of BCL6 expression was associated with a poorer outcome for patients receiving CHOP (without maintenance) that was not seen in patients receiving rituximab.[63] It is possible that in these studies, BCL2 expression or lack of BCL6 expression, is a surrogate for another distinguishing feature, such as nongerminal center lymphomas.[33] Based on these data, it is premature to use the expression of BCL2 protein or the lack of expression of BCL6 protein to select patients for treatment with chemotherapy alone versus chemoimmunotherapy.

Aggressive NHL: Initial Management of Limited-Stage Disease

Radiotherapy Alone for Limited-Stage Aggressive NHL

Before the 1980s, early-stage aggressive lymphoma was initially managed with radiation therapy alone and results depended on the stage at presentation. Patients with clinical stage I disease treated with regional or extended fields could achieve cure rates of approximately 50%. The overall survival of patients with clinical stage II disease treated in a parallel manner was approximately 20%, despite sterilization of the primary site of disease. Selection of patients with pathologic staging and use of total lymphoid irradiation increased the cure rate, but failure was still common.[64] The failure of radiation therapy to cure early-stage aggressive lymphoma is evidence that systemic disease undetected by clinical staging is commonly present.

Combined Modality Therapy Versus Chemotherapy Alone

Development of effective chemotherapy for advanced-stage aggressive lymphoma led to clinical trials testing the hypothesis that adding chemotherapy to the radiation therapy could improve the control of the systemic, undetected disease through a strategy of combined modality therapy (CMT). A randomized trial of radiation therapy followed by adjuvant CHOP chemotherapy or observation for clinical stage I patients, resulted in significant improvement in 7-year relapse-free survival (RFS) (86% versus 20%) and OS (92% versus 47%).[65] In this trial, the sequence of CMT was radiation followed by chemotherapy. Although effective, this approach has several practical drawbacks, including the potential of radiation recall with doxorubicin-based chemotherapy, the use of larger fields, and higher doses of radiation to control the primary site of disease. The alternative sequence, chemotherapy followed by radiation, allows for simultaneous cytoreduction of the primary site of disease and treatment of microscopic systemic disease with the potential benefit of permitting smaller radiation fields and lower doses. This approach to CMT is most commonly used in current practice. Chemotherapy followed by involved-field radiation therapy was evaluated in several Phase II studies with favorable results.[66–69] This approach was investigated in a Southwest Oncology Group (SWOG) Phase III randomized trial comparing a course of eight cycles of CHOP chemotherapy versus three cycles of CHOP followed by involved-field radiation therapy. When the study was initially published with a median of 5 years of follow-up, there was a significant advantage for PFS (77% versus 64%) and OS (82% versus 72%).[70] However, subsequent analysis with a median follow-up of 8 years, demonstrated that the advantage of combined modality therapy disappeared as a consequence of late events in the combined modality arm.[71] A stage-modified IPI has been proposed for patients with early-stage disease: CS I versus II; normal versus abnormal LDH; age 60 years or less versus over 60 years; ECOG PS 1 or less versus 2 or more. Patients with zero adverse factors define a very limited-stage group with a 5-year median OS of approximately 90%. Patients with nonbulky disease but having one or more risk factors define a limited-stage group with a 5-year median OS of approximately 70%.[72] Patients with bulky disease [bulk with mass greater than 10cm or mediastinal mass larger than one-third of the maximal thoracic diameter on posteroanterior (PA) chest radiography] have outcomes similar to those with advanced-stage disease.[73] The Eastern Cooperative Oncology Group (ECOG) conducted a randomized study evaluating the role of adjuvant radiation therapy following a full course of eight cycles of CHOP chemotherapy. Patients with a radiographic CR were randomly assigned to involved-field radiation therapy or observation; the study failed to demonstrate a survival advantage for adjuvant low-dose radiation (30Gy) despite a significant improvement in DFS (73% versus 56%) and local control in the CMT arm at 6 years.[74] The GELA conducted a randomized Phase III trial of ACVBP chemotherapy versus CHOP × 3 and IFRT for patients with CS I or II aggressive lymphoma and no risk factors by the age-adjusted IPI (all patients were 60 years of age or less). At a median follow-up of 7.7 years, the 5-year EFS (82% versus 74%) and OS (90% versus 81%) favored the ACVBP arm. Bulky disease was a poor prognostic factor for both event-free and overall survival. However, in a subset analysis of the patients without bulky disease, EFS and OS still favored the ACVBP arm although the magnitude of the benefit was reduced. The results of these studies are summarized in Table 68.6.

TABLE 68.6. Management of early-stage aggressive lymphoma.

Study	*N*	*Comparison*	*Five years*	*Five-year OS*
SWOG	401	R CHOP [3] → IFRT vs. CHOP [8]	PFS 64 vs. 77	72 vs. 82
ECOG	399	CHOP[8] → R CRs IFRT vs. observation	DFS 56 vs. 73[a]	NS
GELA	647	R CHOP [3] → IFRT vs. ACVBP	EFS 82 vs. 74*	90 vs. 81

SWOG, Southwest Oncology Group; ECOG, Eastern Cooperative Oncology Group; GELA, Groupe d'Etude des Lymphomes de l'Adulte; R, rituximab; CHOP, cyclophosphamide, doxorubicin, vincristine, prednisone; IFRT, involved field radiation therapy; CR, complete response; ACVBP, doxorubicin, cyclophosphamide, vindesine, bleomycin, prednisone; PFS, progression-free survival; DFS, disease-free survival; EFS, event-free survival.

[a] Six years.

*No significant difference.

Rituximab as a Component of Early-Stage Disease

The SWOG have presented results of a pilot study investigating the role of chemoimmunotherapy with R-CHOP for three cycles followed by IFRT.[75] Patients with one or more risk factors in the stage-modified IPI were eligible. Early results suggest an improvement in PFS but not OS compared to historical controls at 2 years. Outside the setting of a clinical trial, the evidence would support the use of R-CHOP × 3 and IFRT for patients with limited-stage disease with risk factors. For patients with very limited stage disease (CS I, no risk factors), CHOP × 3 and IFRT has excellent results. In practice, the very limited-stage patients are not likely to be distinguished from the limited-stage patients and therefore, the addition of rituximab to CHOP would be appropriate, understanding that there is no trial evidence to support this approach. However, definitive evidence of superiority of this approach requires a randomized comparison of chemoimmunotherapy versus chemoimmunotherapy and IFRT. For patients with bulky disease, treatment with regimens appropriate for aggressive lymphoma should be used. Because vindesine is not available in the United States, the ACVBP regimen cannot be used.

Primary Mediastinal Lymphoma

Primary mediastinal large B-cell lymphoma (PMLBL) is a distinct subtype of diffuse large B-cell lymphoma (DLBCL) that accounts for 6% of all non-Hodgkin's lymphoma (NHL).[76] PMLBL possesses distinctive clinical features, justifying its inclusion as a specific NHL entity in the WHO/REAL classification.[2,3,5] In contrast to other types of DLBCL, in PMLBL there is a slight female predominance, younger median age, bulky disease, and uncommon extrathoracic spread at presentation.[77] Direct extension to the lung, pericardium, chest wall, or pleura is common at presentation and may adversely affect outcomes.[77,78] Prognostic factor analyses have been inconsistent, and a lack of consensus exists concerning the prognostic utility of the IPI in this disease entity.[77–80]

Recently, the genetic relationship between PMLBL and DLBCL has been examined using comparative genomic hybridization (CGH). Not surprisingly, similar patterns of BCL-6 gene mutations in the two groups were demonstrated, suggesting a germinal center origin for PMLBL.[81] Expression microarray analysis of PMLBL demonstrates striking similarity to that observed in Hodgkin's disease, which may explain some of the clinical similarities between the two entities.[82,83]

In general, this entity has been managed similar to DLBCL. There are no trials that have prospectively treated patients with this diagnosis. Therefore, our knowledge about this entity is based on retrospective series, occasionally with conflicting conclusions. The areas of controversy include use of anthracycline-based chemotherapy, upfront HDT/ASCT, dose-dense strategies, and the role of radiation therapy. In the 43 patients identified at the University of Nebraska, the outcome of the patients with PMLBL was similar to those of a large control group of DLBCL.[84] The GELA identified 141 patients and also concluded that outcome was similar to DLBCL and the management should also be similar.[77] In a retrospective analysis of 138 patients managed at multiple centers in Italy, treatment with the dose-dense regimens MACOP-B and VACOP-B were associated with superior outcomes compared to CHOP: EFS was 76% versus 40% at *P* less than 0.001; the OS is not given.[80] Independent of treatment, there was also a benefit for IFRT versus no radiation ($P = 0.04$), although this was not significant in the multivariate analysis (only attaining a CR and type of chemotherapy were significant). In 141 patients seen at MSKCC, a dose-dense regimen NHL-15[85] was superior to CHOP and CHOP-like regimens for both EFS (60% versus 34%; *P* less than 0.001 and OS (84% versus 51%; *P* less than 0.001).[86] The effect of RT in this analysis could not be assessed.

The role of rituximab in the management of PMLBL is unknown. The data support the use of dose-dense regimens, such as MACOP-B, VACOP-B, or NHL-15. However, clinical trials specifically for PMLBL or large studies with planned analysis of these patients are necessary to confirm these retrospective conclusions. Furthermore, the role of radiation therapy would require evaluation in Phase III trials.

Aggressive T-Cell Lymphoma

T-cell lymphomas form a heterogeneous group of NHLs. They are relatively uncommon, comprising 10% to 15% of all newly diagnosed NHL in the United States. The proportions are reversed in Asia where 70% to 80% of NHL may be of T-cell phenotype. Under the World Health Organization (WHO) classification schema, T-cell lymphomas are divided into disorders that have precursor T cells or are predominantly extranodal or predominantly nodal lymphomas (Table 68.7).

Peripheral T-cell lymphoma (PTCL) represents the largest group of the T-cell lymphomas. PTCL comprised 6% of all NHL in the REAL classification.[2] In general, T-cell lymphomas are aggressive and have a poor prognosis, with the exception of a few more indolent or favorable subtypes, such as mycosis fungoides, ALK-1-positive anaplastic large-cell lymphoma, and primary cutaneous anaplastic large-cell lymphoma. Most patients with T-cell NHL have a poorer prognosis than their B-cell counterparts. Larger clinical series of T-cell lymphomas report median survivals of less than 2 years and 5-year survival rates between 20% and 30%.[2,87–89] Failure-free survival for intermediate- and high-risk patients is between 0% and 10% in the larger series with no plateau on the curves for these populations. This poor prognosis is related to both poor sensitivity to chemotherapy, as well as a propensity for T-cell lymphomas to present with poor risk factors.

There are no prospective randomized trials for patients with aggressive forms of T-cell lymphoma. As a result, available outcome data for patients with aggressive T-cell lymphomas are based upon retrospective or subset analyses. In the prerituximab era, patients with aggressive T-cell lymphoma were generally included in trials for aggressive NHL and received the same treatment as patients with DLBCL. In a series from Spain, only 43% (62/144) of patients with non-anaplastic large cell lymphoma (ALCL) T-cell NHL achieved a complete response, whereas a nearly equivalent number, 41% (59/144), were nonresponders to therapy.[87] In data from the GELA and Mayo Clinic, poor-risk patients had similarly poor response rates in other studies, with CR rates of 42% and 39% when the more favorable patients are excluded.[89,90]

TABLE 68.7. Classification of the T-cell lymphomas.

Precursor T-cell lymphoma/leukemia	*Predominantly nodal*	*Predominantly extranodal*
T-lymphoblastic lymphoma	PTCL, unspecified	Mycosis fungoides
Blastic NK	Angioimmunoblastic-type	Sezary syndrome
LGL	Anaplastic large cell, Alk-1–	ALCL-cutaneous
NK/T-cell leukemia/lymphoma	Anaplastic large cell, Alk-1+	Lymphomatoid papulosis
T-cell CLL/PLL		Subcutaneous panniculitis-like
Adult T-cell		Nasal T/NK Enteropathy-type T-cell

PTCL, peripheral T-cell lymphoma; ALCL, anaplastic T-cell lymphoma; CLL, chronic lymphocytic leukemia; PLL, prolymphocytic leukemia; LGL, Large granular lymphocytic lymphoma.

Source: Adapted from Zelenetz et al.,[107] by permission of *Annals of Oncology*.

Separating and evaluating less favorable patients can be achieved by eliminating favorable histologic subtypes from the analysis and by utilizing the international prognostic index (IPI). As with diffuse large B-cell lymphoma, the IPI can help cull a group of patients with the poorest prognosis.[13] The simple clinical factors of age (greater than 60 or less than 60 years of age), Stage (I–II versus III–IV), performance status (0–1 versus 2–4), extranodal disease (0–1 site versus 2+ sites), and LDH (normal versus elevated) can separate patients into low, low-intermediate, high-intermediate, and high-risk subgroups. Moreover, the higher-risk patients are overrepresented among the T-cell patients, with 63% to 83% having high-intermediate or high-risk disease at presentation.[2,89,90] Not surprisingly, the poorest prognosis comes from the higher-risk subgroups. In the GELA series, only 35% of patients with two adverse risk factors and 23% of those with three adverse factors were alive at 5 years.[89] Similarly poor survival was seen in the Mayo clinic series with 9% of patients with high-risk disease, 28% of patients with high-intermediate risk disease, and only 32% of patients with low-intermediate risk being alive at 5 years.[90] In the NHL Classification Project, only 10% of high-intermediate or high-risk patients were free from progression at 2 years.[88]

There are few studies on initial therapy specifically for patients with T-cell lymphomas, as most have been treated alongside aggressive B-cell lymphomas with the T-cell patients retrospectively analyzed, as in the series described here. There are no published prospective trials for untreated T-cell lymphoma patients. In a large randomized trial of intermediate-grade lymphoma, CHOP was found to be similar to other combination regimens.[91] Immunophenotype was not assessed, but patients with PTCL were included in this study and CHOP became, and remains, a standard treatment for them. The most homogeneously treated group of T-cell lymphoma patients comes from the GELA series, in which 288 patients with T-cell histology were included in several prospective trials where patients were randomized according to age, to comparative arms of mBACOD, or ACVB followed by autologous BMT for those in CR, or for older patients, ACVB followed by maintenance therapy or CV(T)P.[89] It is not possible to conclude a preferred treatment approach from these retrospective series of T-cell patients. However, several principles do emerge. As above, the prognosis for T-cell lymphomas was worse than for B-cell patients, and this difference was primarily seen among the poorer-prognosis patients. Favorable IPI T-cell patients may do as well as their B-cell counterparts. High-dose therapy and autologous stem cell transplantation provided similar results in T- and B-cell patients achieving a CR to initial therapy (see following). Although the outcomes of the transplanted patients are encouraging, only 35% (16/46) patients in this arm achieved a CR, and thus, the majority never became eligible for high-dose therapy.[89] Hence, the difficulty in treating T-cell lymphomas can be simplified to two problems: poor response to initial therapy, as demonstrated by poor CR rates, and frequent relapses with poor long-term survival for those who do respond.

Aggressive NHL: Treatment at Progression

About half of all patients with aggressive lymphoma either have persistence of tumor following initial therapy (primary refractory disease) or have a relapse after a complete remission. For these patients, high-dose therapy and autologous stem cell transplantation (HDT/ASCT) has been demonstrated to have the greatest potential for a curative outcome (Figure 68.6).[92] However, this treatment approach has typically been restricted to patients with disease sensitive to second-line chemotherapy.[93] For patients in whom HDT/ASCT is not an option because of comorbidities or lack of stem cells, conventional dose chemotherapy has been used with palliative benefit.[94,95]

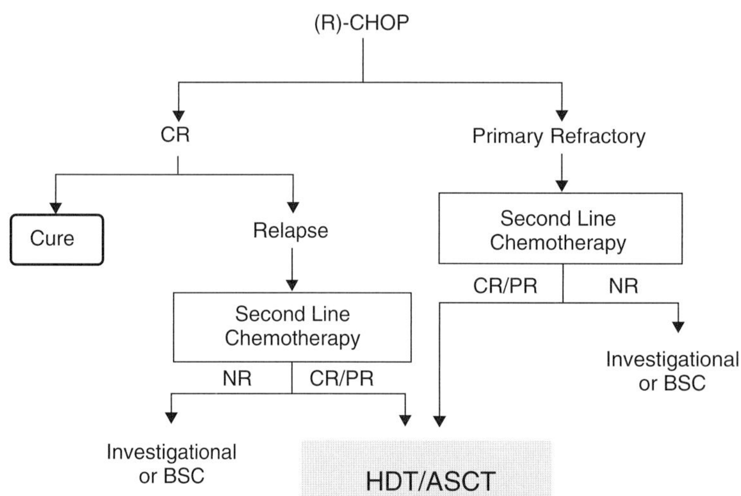

FIGURE 68.6. Approach to the management of relapsed refractory aggressive lymphoma. (From Zelenetz et al.,[107] by permission of *Annals of Oncology*.)

TABLE 68.8. Second-line therapy for non-Hodgkin's lymphoma (NHL).

Regimen	*Disease*	N	*ORR*	*CR*	*PR*	*Aphereses, median (range)*	*Median CD34+ × 10^6/kg*	*Percent failed mobilization (<2 × 10^6/kg)*	*MARR*	*Reference*
ICE	NHL	163	66.3	24	42	3 (1–5)	8.4	14	52	101
RICE	NHL	31	81	55	26		6.3	17	64	105
Ifos/Vino	NHL, HD	10	40	0	40		10.9	<11[a]	29–40	102
MINE	NHL, HD	27	67	38	29	3	13.3	8	59	103
VIM	NHL, HD	46	56	39	17	3	10.6	8	48	103
ESHAP	HD, NHL	84	64[a]	37[a]	27[a]	(1–4)	4.9	15	~49	104
CY 1.5 g/m^2	HD, NHL	78	64[a]	37[a]	27[a]	(1–4)	3.3	29	~35	104
DHAP	NHL	38	63.9	25	38.9	2 (1–3)	5.9	14.7	49.2	106
CPM	NHL	34	63.9	25	38.9	2 (1–3)	7.1	10.5	53.4	106

[a] ESHAP response rate is based on their historic data.

HD, Hodgkin's Disease; ICE, ifosfamide, carboplatin, etoposide; RICE, rituximab with ICE; Ifos/Vino, ifosfamide, vinorebine; MINE, mitoguazone, ifosfamide, vinorelbine and etoposide; VIM, etoposide, ifosfamide, methotrexate; ESHAP, etoposide, solumedrol, cytarabine, cis-platin; CY, cyclophosphamide; DHAP, dexamethasone, cytarabine, cis-platin); CPM, cyclophosphamide; ORR, overall response rate; CR, complete response; PR, partial response.

MARR, mobilization adjusted response rate ([CR] + [PR] − mobilization failure).[107]

Second-Line Chemotherapy

The curative potential of HDT/ASCT is restricted to patients with chemosensitive relapsed disease.[96] Thus, the effectiveness of the second-line regimen is of paramount importance. To be suitable as pretransplant therapy, a second-line regimen should have the following features: effective cytoreduction, a low incidence of nonhematologic toxicity, a brief duration of therapy, and ability to mobilize peripheral blood progenitor cells.[97–100] Numerous second-line regimens have been evaluated for the treatment of relapsed and refractory NHL.[101–107] Some of the most commonly used regimens, ESHAP, DHAP, and mini-BEAM, have some potential limitations that may preclude stem cell transplantation (SCT), including poor stem cell mobilization and nonhematologic toxicities, such as nephrotoxicity (DHAP and ESHAP) and pulmonary toxicity (mini-BEAM). However, these regimens have been used effectively as cytoreduction before HDT/ASCT. The ICE (ifosfamide, carboplatin, etoposide) regimen was developed to minimize the nonhematologic toxicity associated with second-line therapy.[101] Overall response rates for various second-line regimens range from 40% to 84% (Table 68.8). There have been limited data on the role of rituximab in second-line therapy. Addition of rituximab to the ICE regimen[105] improved the CR rate compared to a historical control and provided a trend to improve long-term outcome. However, this was in a group of rituximab-naïve patients; the effectiveness in patients already failing chemoimmunotherapy is unknown. There have been no completed randomized comparative trials to determine the standard for second-line therapy.

The second-line regimens have varied in overall response rate and the ability to mobilize peripheral blood progenitor cells, a critical step for successful completion of HDT/ASCT. These are the two most significant parameters in evaluating the effectiveness of a pretransplant cytoreductive regimen. These parameters can be incorporated into a single value, the Mobilization-Adjusted Response Rate [MARR = ORR (%) − Mobilization Failures (%)]; (ORR, overall response rate)] to evaluate the effectiveness of a cytoreductive regimen.[107] The MARR can be used to evaluate the effectiveness of a second-line therapy as cytoreduction before HDT/ASCT; it is a primary endpoint in the ongoing CORAL study evaluating R-DHAP versus R-ICE.[108]

High-Dose Chemotherapy and Stem Cell Transplant

Patients with relapsed NHL were shown to have favorable outcomes when treated with HDT/ASCT compared to historical controls.[93,96] Successful cytoreduction by second-line therapy (CR or partial response, PR) was essential to a favorable outcome following HDT/ASCT.[96] The PARMA study group conducted a randomized Phase III trial of HDT/ASCT versus chemotherapy in patients having had a CR or PR to two courses of second-line chemotherapy. Two hundred fifteen patients were registered to the study and 109 responding patients were randomized: chemotherapy with IFRT (n = 54) versus HDT/ASCT (n = 55). At 5 years, the EFS (46% versus 12%, $P = 0.001$) and OS (53% versus 32%; $P = 0.038$) favored the patients receiving the HDT/ASCT.[92] This pivotal study established the curative potential for HDT/ASCT in recurrent disease.

The PARMA study established the role of HDT/ASCT in patients with chemosensitive, relapsed aggressive lymphoma. However, the effectiveness of this approach in patients with chemorefractory disease was not established. Investigators at MSKCC undertook a retrospective analysis of patients treated with ICE followed by HDT/ASCT for refractory aggressive lymphoma.[109] Patients were classified as induction partial responders (IPR; $n = 40$) if they attained a partial response to doxorubicin-based front-line therapy or as induction failures (IF; $n = 45$) if they had less than partial response. Patients in the IPR group had confirmation of active disease by repeat biopsy. The overall response to ICE was 51% with no difference between IF and IPR subsets. In the intent-to-treat analysis (from start of ICE), the estimated 3-year EFS and OS were 22% and 25%, respectively. Among the 42 patients who underwent HDT/ASCT, the estimated 3-year EFS and OS were 44% and 52%, respectively. Thus, the outcome of patients with primary refractory aggressive lymphoma is very similar to those patients with relapsed disease when determined from the time of HDT/ASCT; however, the response to second-line therapy is lower.

Allogeneic stem cell transplantation offers a tumor-free graft but there is a risk of graft-versus-host disease (GVHD) and graft rejection. A potential benefit is the development of a graft-versus-lymphoma (GVL) effect. Most of the experience is derived from data submitted to transplant registries or retrospective analyses from single centers. No multicenter randomized studies have been conducted comparing autologous and allogeneic sources of stem cells. A review of cases in the European Bone Marrow Transplant registry (EBMT) provided support for a GVL effect with a reduced relapse rate compared to autologous grafts. However, the benefit was outweighed by increased transplant-related mortality with the allogeneic transplants.[110] Results from the Ontario transplant registry demonstrated similar survival in patients receiving allogeneic and autologous sources of stem cells despite a lower relapse rate in patients receiving allogeneic stem cells.[111] In a report from the International Bone Marrow Transplant Registry (IBMTR), 114 patients with recurrent NHL following autologous transplant were analyzed, demonstrating that the transplant was technically feasible, but the 5-year PFS was only 5%, suggesting at best a palliative benefit.[112] There has been limited experience with nonmyeloablative allogeneic stem cell transplants for aggressive lymphoma because of the risk of rapid regrowth. A study from the University of Göttingen explored a regimen with intermediate intensity.[113] In this study, the investigators initially T-cell depleted the grafts, followed by unmanipulated grafts with immunosuppression. Although T-cell depletion was associated with a lack of GVHD, the relapse rate was very high; when the T cells were not depleted, the relapse rate was very low but GVHD was problematic. These results support the existence of GVL but point to the difficulty in balancing the GVHD and GVL.[113] Further prospective studies are necessary to determine the role of allogeneic stem cell transplant in the management of recurrent aggressive lymphoma.

Investigators at Stanford University have evaluated the role of rituximab administered as an adjuvant (two 4-weekly courses at day 42 and day 180) following HDT/ASCT in NHL.[114] This study included various histologies including DLBCL (71%, n = 25), mantle cell lymphoma (MCL) (9%, n = 3), and other B-cell lymphomas (20%, n = 7). In a subset analysis restricted to the patients with relapsed (n = 13) or refractory (n = 8) DLBCL, the 2-year estimated EFS and OS were 81% and 85%, respectively. These are very intriguing results, but interpretation is limited because the patients were rituximab naïve; thus, the impact of prior rituximab is unknown. Similar results have been reported for adjuvant rituximab after both autologous and allogeneic stem cell transplant.[115] This approach is being tested in an ongoing ECOG trial comparing adjuvant rituximab to observation.

A variety of prognostic models have been developed that have predicted for a favorable outcome post-HDT/ASCT.[17,19,116,117] In the series from MSKCC, the IPI determined at the start of second-line therapy (sIPI) predicted for estimated 2.5-year failure-free survival (FFS): 45% in patients with low (L) and low-intermediate (LI) risk disease versus 9% in patients with high-intermediate (HI) and high (H) risk disease (P less than 0.001). This analysis was undertaken on a larger group of patients with relapsed and refractory DLBCL and the best discriminator for outcome was saaIPI L/LI versus HI/H risk disease.[19] The predictive significance of the IPI was confirmed in an analysis confined to those patients who underwent HDT/ASCT.[18,19] Another important factor was the quality of response to second-line therapy, with superior outcome for patients in CR at time of transplant versus those in PR.[19,117] Thus, it is possible to identify patients with poor outcome with sequential second-line therapy followed by HDT/ASCT. The patients with low- and low-intermediate risk disease do very well with conventional treatment. However, patients with high-intermediate and high-risk disease are poorly served with the conventional approach and should be enrolled in clinical trials.

Indolent Lymphoma: General Considerations

Indolent NHL can be of either B-cell or T-cell phenotype, although the B-cell tumors are far more common. With conventional chemotherapy, patients with indolent B-cell lymphoma have a chronic remitting and relapsing course with a median survival of 10 years and a steady drop in the survival curve without a plateau. Furthermore, the outcome did not change substantially from the 1960s to the early 1990s.[118] The introduction of targeted therapy with rituximab and subsequently, with yittrium-90 ibritumomab tiuxetan and iodine-131-tositumomab has provided important new therapeutic modalities but evidence of curative outcomes remains elusive. Therefore, management of indolent lymphoma requires clinicians, like chess players, to think a few moves ahead to try to optimize the sequence of therapy over the course of a chronic illness. Considerations, such as age, comorbidities, prior therapy, symptoms, extent of disease, and impact on end-organ function all affect therapeutic decisions (Table 68.9). The data discussed in the section emphasize approaches to treatment rather than the sequence of therapy, because the treatment sequence is often highly individualized in the absence of curative outcome.

The reader should note that it is impossible to be exhaustive in this review of the management of indolent lymphoma because of space constraints. The reader is referred to excellent reviews on the role of interferon alpha in the management of indolent lymphoma.[119–124] Interferon-alpha is a therapy that has not gained wide acceptance in the United States. No information regarding vaccine is presented because the critical randomized trials are ongoing and without them, understanding the effectiveness of vaccine is impossible.

The indolent lymphomas are characterized by a risk of transformation to an aggressive lymphoma, generally recognized as a poor prognosis with short survival.[125] However, in the retrospective review of 74 patients with transformation

TABLE 68.9. Factors influencing therapy choice in indolent lymphoma.

Patient characteristics	*Disease characteristics*
Age	Stage
Symptoms	FL IPI risk group
Comorbid conditions	Sites of involvement
Preservation of future options	Prior therapy Time from prior therapy Transformation

FL, follicular lymphoma; IPI, international prognostic index.

at Stanford, a subgroup of patients with a favorable outcome after transformation could be identified.[126] The median time to transformation was 66 months. Factors associated with a good prognosis following transformation, included limited prior therapy (none versus any), limited stage (I/II versus III/IV), and response to prior therapy (CR versus PR or none). Thirty of the patients had a CR after treatment for transformation, and the response duration (RD) was 81 months.

Indolent Lymphoma: Initial Management

Early Stage

MALT lymphoma is the prototype of a localized indolent lymphoma. In contrast, limited-stage early-stage follicular lymphoma is uncommon. Gastric MALT lymphoma, the most common subtype, is associated with *Helicobacter pylori* infection. Numerous studies have demonstrated that clinical remissions can be induced in most cases; however, molecular testing reveals persistence of disease in at least 50% of cases.[127] Late relapses occur, which are sometimes self-limited, and careful clinical monitoring is essential. A subset of patients fail to respond to or recur following antibiotic therapy; this can be seen particularly in patients with a t(11;18) translocation activating API2-MLT1.[128,129] These patients can be effectively managed with IFRT with excellent long-term disease control.[130] MALT lymphoma at other sites can also be effectively controlled by IFRT.[131]

About 15% of patients with follicular lymphoma (FL) presented with localized disease, and retrospective studies have demonstrated excellent disease control with IFRT.[132,133] In the Stanford series, 177 patients with FL, grades 1 and 2, were treated (CS I, $n = 73$; CS II, $n = 104$) with IFRT, and the median OS was 13.8 years; relapse after 10 years was uncommon. In a provocative retrospective analysis, the Stanford group identified 43 patients (CS I, $n = 11$; CS II, $n = 32$) who were observed for early-stage FL, grades 1 and 2.[134] Radiation was deferred for a variety of reasons. At the median follow-up of 86 months, 63% had not been treated and survival was similar to patients who had undergone IFRT.

The European Organization for Research and Treatment of Cancer (EORTC) conducted a study of radiation in early-stage NHL. Patients with stage I disease were randomized to IFRT or IFRT followed by CVP.[135] Although FFS favored the combined modality (CMT) arm, it did not affect on overall survival. The MDACC did a study of CHOP-B (CHOP with bleomycin) with IRFT for localized low-grade lymphoma and have reported long-term results; the 10-year time to treatment failure (TTTF) and OS were 76% and 82%, respectively.[136] A randomized trial is required to determine if CMT has a survival advantage over IFRT alone.

Management of Advanced Stage

Observation

Long-term follow-up has confirmed the incurability of this disease with conventional therapy.[118] Because indolent lymphoma is a chronic illness, it is reasonable to postpone initial therapy in asymptomatic patients. The natural history of patients without bulky lymphadenopathy or symptoms was examined. The overall survival at 10 years was 73%, and the median time to first treatment was 3 years; spontaneous remissions were seen in 23% of patients.[137,138] The deferral of initial therapy has been examined in prospective randomized trials.[139,140] The National Cancer Institute (NCI) conducted a study of observation ($n = 44$) (which permitted limited radiation therapy) versus an aggressive regimen of ProMACE-MOPP (prednisone, methotrexate, doxorubicin, cyclophosphamide, etoposide alternating with mechlorethamine, vincristine, procarbazine, prednisone) followed by total nodal irradiation (TNI; $n = 45$) in patients with indolent lymphoma.[139] At 34 months, 56% of the patients on the observation arm had not required therapy. There was no survival disadvantage to the patients on the observation arm compared to the chemoradiotherapy arm. The Groupe d'Etude des Lymphomes Folliculaires (GELF) compared observation to prednimustine or interferon-alpha for patients with low tumor burden lymphomas.[140] One hundred ninety-three patients were randomized to the three arms with well-balanced clinical characteristics. The median time to treatment was 24 months in the deferred treatment arm. The overall response to treatment, when started in the deferred treatment arm was 70%, which was not different from the overall response in the two treatment arms (78% for prednimustine, 70% for interferon-alpha). Estimated 5-year OS was not affected by deferred therapy (78% observation, 70% prednimustine, 84% interferon-alpha). Selection of patients is important, and the GELF has proposed criteria predicting poor outcomes that have been modified by the National Comprehensive Cancer Network (Table 68.10).[140,141] The limitation of these data is that all predate the era of immunotherapy in the management of indolent lymphoma. However, since the use of immunotherapy has not affected OS (see following), observation is an appropriate option for selected patients. Deferral of therapy preserves future treatment options without compromising survival.

TABLE 68.10. Indication for therapy in indolent lymphoma.

Cytopenias associated with bone marrow infiltration
Compromised end-organ function
Three or more nodal masses >3 cm
One nodal mass >7 cm
Massive splenomegaly
Symptoms attributable to disease
Concurrent histologic transformation to aggressive lymphoma
Steady progression over a period of more than 6 months
Malignant pleural effusions[a]

[a] This entity is in the original description of the Groupe d'Etude des Lymphomes de l'Adulte (GELF) criteria, but it is clinically very rare and is not in the National Comprehensive Cancer Network (NCCN) criteria.

Source: Data from references 140 and 141.

Chemotherapy

Indolent lymphomas are sensitive to a wide range of chemotherapy, either alone or in combination. It is beyond the scope of this chapter to review the extensive literature regarding the activity of lymphoma in indolent lymphoma. Rather, the focus is on higher-level evidence from randomized trials that help us understand the comparative benefits of different chemotherapy. In the indolent lymphoma, it is very important to have long-term follow-up because high remission rates are not always associated with superior survival.

The Cancer and Leukemia Group B compared two approaches for the initial management of follicular lymphoma, grades 1 to 2: single-agent therapy versus combination therapy with known curative potential in aggressive disease.[142] The study randomized 228 patients between cyclophosphamide (arm 1) and CHOP-B (CHOP with bleomycin) (arm 2), and the complete response rates were the same in the two arms (66% versus 60%; $P = 0.36$). The 10-year FFS (25% versus 33%; $P = 0.107$) and OS (44% versus 46%; $P = 0.79$) were also not affected by the treatment arm. In a subset analysis of 46 patients with FL, grade 2, the combination therapy was associated with better FFS (9% versus 48%; $P = 0.005$) and OS (25% versus 61%; $P = 0.24$). These results were from an unplanned subset analysis, and the benefit should be confirmed in a larger study. However, it is interesting that a similar observation was reported by the NCI using ProMACE-MOPP.[143]

The role of doxorubicin as a component of initial therapy in indolent lymphoma has been an area of controversy. Retrospective studies have suggested that the addition of doxorubicin did not add to the median overall survival in patient with indolent lymphoma.[144] A trial from the Hospital Saint-Louis in France compared C-MOPP (cyclophosphamide, vincristine, prednisone, procarbazine) to the same regimen with doxorubin added.[145] The trial identified no difference in EFS or OS with the addition of rituximab to initial therapy; interestingly, the study also found no difference in the risk of transformation to aggressive lymphoma.

Multiple Phase II studies demonstrated activity of fludarabine in patients with untreated as well as relapsed indolent lymphoma. An Italian multicenter trial group evaluated the role of fludarabine in the management of indolent lymphoma in two randomized trials.[146,147] The first trial compared the single agent fludarabine (F) to the combination of fludarabine and idarubicin (FI) in patients with newly diagnosed indolent and mantle cell lymphoma.[146] The addition of idarubicin did not change overall survival for the entire population, again suggesting that initial therapy with an anthracycline dose did not improve survival in indolent lymphoma. In the follicular lymphoma subset (the only group large enough to be analyzed by itself), there were more CRs (60% versus 40%; $P = 0.007$) with F versus FI, although PFS was greater in the FI arm. This result is difficult to explain. Nonetheless, it establishes fludarabine as an active drug for indolent lymphoma. The second trial compared fludarabine and mitroxantrone (FM, $n = 72$) (with or without rituximab) to CHOP ($n = 68$) (with or without rituximab) in patients with follicular lymphoma.[147] In this trial, molecular remissions were determined by PCR amplification of the t(14;18) translocation. If patients achieved a molecular remission (CR–), they received no further therapy. However, if the molecular test was positive (CR+), patients received adjuvant rituximab. FM had a higher rate of both CR (68% versus 42%; $P = 0.003$) and CR– (39% versus 19%; $P = 0.001$) than the CHOP arm. Rituximab increased the CR– rate in both arms, but the final CR– rate favored the FM ± R arm (71% versus 51%; $P = 001$). However, in a short follow-up of only 19 months, there is no difference in PFS or OS.

Rituximab Immunotherapy

The development of the chimeric monoclonal antibody rituximab (C2B8) has been altering the therapy of indolent lymphoma.[53] In the early Phase I single-dose, dose-escalation trials, tumor regressions were seen (2 PR and 4 minor responses in 15 patients).[148] A subsequent four weekly dose-finding study identified a biologically effective dose of $375\,mg/m^2$, again with clinical responses that were particularly frequent in patients with indolent lymphoma.[149] The subsequent "pivotal" study was a Phase II design that included 166 patients with relapsed and refractory indolent lymphoma treated with four weekly doses of rituximab.[150] The overall response rate was 48%, and the median time to progression was 13 months. The overall response rate was higher in patients with follicular lymphoma (60%) than in the patients with SLL (IWF A) (12%). Based on these data, the U.S. Food and Drug Administration (FDA) approved the clinical use of rituximab for patients with relapsed and recurrent follicular lymphoma. A subsequent Phase II study at the same dose and schedule demonstrated that patients initially responding to rituximab could be retreated at time of progression but the response rate was only 40%.[151] These data ushered in the era of immunotherapy that has fundamentally altered the treatment of B-cell NHL. Although these data demonstrate that rituximab has substantial activity, they do not inform us as to the optimal use of this agent.

Rituximab has been used to treat newly diagnosed indolent lymphoma with response rates ranging from 52% to 73% with a PFS of about 12 months.[152–154] Building upon the single-agent activity in indolent lymphoma, investigators from the Sarah Cannon Cancer Center, evaluated planned retreatment with four weekly courses of rituximab at 6-month intervals.[155] This study demonstrated a 34-month PFS and an increasing CR rate with time. However, the Phase II study design made it difficult to ascertain if either of these observations was superior to a single four week course. The Swiss Group for Clinical Cancer Research (SAKK)[156] examined the role of extended dosing in a randomized trial. Patients were treated with a standard 4-week course of rituximab, followed by a randomization to observation or prolonged therapy given as one dose of rituximab every 8 weeks for four doses; patients with progression after the initial rituximab were excluded from the randomization. Of 185 patients enrolled, the ORR to the rituximab was 67% in chemotherapy naïve patients and 46% in previously treated patients; 151 patients were eligible for randomization. At a median follow-up of 35 months, the median EFS favored the prolonged therapy group (23 months versus 12 months; $P = 0.02$) with a larger benefit in the chemo-naïve subset (36 months versus 19 months; $P = 0.004$). Interestingly, the CR rate was identical in both treatment groups, suggesting that achievement of CR did not require additional rituximab. IgM plasma levels decreased for a significantly longer time after prolonged treatment, but this was not associated with an increased infectious risk. These data support the idea that EFS can be extended with maintenance or prolonged rituximab.

A randomized Phase II study was conducted to determine if maintenance rituximab (four weekly doses every 6 months) was superior to retreatment with four weekly doses of rituximab at disease progression.[157] Patients ($n = 114$) were treated with rituximab and randomized ($n = 90$) if they had stable or responding disease. The endpoint of the study was the duration of rituximab benefit, which was the same between the two arms: maintenance, 31 months versus retreatment groups, 27 months. However, this randomized Phase II trial does not have sufficient power to draw definitive conclusions, and the ECOG is conducting a large Phase III study (RESORT) to address the question of maintenance versus retreatment at progression.

Chemoimmunotherapy

Phase II studies have suggested that rituximab can add to the clinical benefit of combination chemotherapy in patients with indolent lymphoma. For example, compared to historical controls, rituximab improved the EFS with single-agent fludarabine as well as CHOP.[158,159] However, small trial sizes and potential selection biases make definitive conclusions impossible to draw. A series of randomized studies have been undertaken to address this question in untreated and relapsed indolent lymphoma.

The German Low Grade Lymphoma Study Group (GLSG) examined the impact of adding rituximab to the FCM (fludarabine, cyclophosphamide, mitroxantrone) regimen in patients with relapsed or refractory FL and MCL.[160] Of 147 patients randomized, 128 were evaluable. In the FL patients, the ORR (94% versus 70%) favored the R-FCM arms. In the FL patient subgroup, there was a benefit in median PFS for the R-FCM, patients (not reached at 3 years) versus FCM (21 months), at $P = 0.0139$. At 2 years, the estimated OS is 90% in R-FCM, as compared with 70% on the FCM arm ($P = 0.0943$). Thus, in rituximab-naïve patients with recurrent disease, rituximab adds a palliative benefit to chemotherapy (no impact on OS) in patients with FL.

A multicenter study in England examined the addition of rituximab to CVP chemotherapy.[161] The chemotherapy was a modified CVP with a low dose of cyclophosphamide (750 mg/m^2) and prednisone (40 mg/m^2). Patients treated with R-CVP had significantly improved OR and CR rates, as well as TTF. However, the study had an unusual definition of time to treatment failure (TTF), considering patients with less than a PR after four cycles as a treatment failure, and this had an disproportionate impact on the chemotherapy arm. Therefore, the TTP is a more reliable comparison in this trial. TTP for R-CVP and CVP was 32 months and 15 months (P less than 0.0001. Alhough the results in the control arm seem to be suboptimal, this was a study with about 50% of patients with FLIPI high-risk disease. Thus, cross-trials comparisons must be made carefully and take into account the differences in study populations.

The rationale for the combination of rituximab with chemotherapy has been in vitro demonstration with various chemotherapeutic agents.[162–164] One of the demonstrated synergies was with doxorubicin,[162] which provided the rationale for the R-CHOP regimen.[159] The GLSG conducted a randomized trial of CHOP versus R-CHOP in FL.[165] The study has a second randomization evaluating two doses of interferon-alpha in patients over 60 years of age and evaluating HDT/ASCT versus interferon-alpha in patients 60 years of age or younger. Preliminary results have demonstrated that R-CHOP has superior OR and CR rates. In this study, 606 patients were randomized. However, at the time of presentation, only 394 patients were evaluable. R-CHOP provided only a modest increase in OR and CR rates. However, R-CHOP significantly increased the median TTF (P less than 0.0007). In the R-CHOP arm at a median follow-up of 3 years, the median TTF had not been reached, compared to 2.6 years for CHOP. However, the analysis is complicated by the second randomization, and further follow-up is necessary to determine if there is a survival benefit.

These randomized trials indicate that rituximab added to chemotherapy can improve OR, CR, and EFS or PFS, but the impact on OS is not yet clear, which is in contrast to the data presented earlier for DLBCL. The long natural history of FL confounds the survival endpoints in these studies. If the data ultimately demonstrate a survival advantage, there will be no controversy regarding the inclusion of rituximab in upfront treatment. However, if the benefit is only on PFS or EFS and not OS, then the timing of the use of rituximab may become crucial. Because patients develop resistance to rituximab, its use early in the course may compromise the later effectiveness of the drug. Thus, further follow up of the chemoimmunotherapy trials is essential.

External-Beam Radiation Therapy and Radioimmunotherapy

Radiation Alone

The role of radiation therapy in the management of indolent lymphoma has been studied for many years. The limitation has been the systemic nature of the disease and the limitation of external-beam radiation therapy (EBRT). Nonetheless, several randomized studies have evaluated the role of EBTR in indolent lymphoma. Radioimmunotherapy (RIT) can be delivered to multiple sites and is effective. However, there are limited randomized data that examine the relative potential of RIT in different patient populations.

Advanced-stage indolent lymphoma is a systemic disease, and when EBRT is used alone total-body irradiation (TBI) is necessary. This approach has been studied in a number of Phase II studies demonstrating feasibility and efficacy.[166–168] A randomized comparison of chlorambucil and prednisone (CP) versus TBI was conducted in 108 patients with indolent lymphoma.[169] The various histologic subtypes were stratified to the two treatment arms. The CR rate and OS for all histologies were not different between the two arms: 59% for CP versus 52% for TBI, and 53 months for CP versus 57 months for TBI. In the subset of patients with FL, there were no significant differences in CR rate or OS. The EORTC conducted a similar trial comparing low-dose TBI to CHVmP (cyclophosphamide, doxorubicin, teniposide, prednisone) in patients with FL.[170] There were 93 patients (84 evaluable): 44 received TBI and 40 CHVmP. The ORR rates, EFS, and OS were not different between the arms. These data support that TBI can be effective for the treatment of indolent lymphoma but that the technical limitations are significant. However, the results provide a sound rationale for the development of the use of RIT.

Two anti-CD20 radioimmunotherapy agents have been approved by the FDA: ^{90}Y-ibritumomab tiuxetan and ^{131}I-tositumomab. In Phase II studies, both agents have demonstrated activity in patients with relapsed and refractory indolent lymphoma, in rituximab-refractory patients, and in transformed lymphoma with ORR (40%–84%) and TTP of 8 to 16 months.[171–177] The remissions following RIT can be very durable in a subset of patients.[178] Toxicity of the treatment is largely hematologic. The risk of secondary leukemia is similar to other patients with multiply recurrent indolent lymphoma.[179]

Two randomized studies have been conducted to demonstrate superiority over unlabeled antibody. A comparison of the murine antibody tositumomab was compared to ^{131}I-tositumomab to determine if the radioisotope contributed to the efficacy of the drug.[180] Seventy-eight patients were randomized. ORR significantly favored the radiolabeled antibody compared to the unlabeled antibody: 55% versus 19%, P = 0.002. Median response duration (not reached versus 28.1 months) and TTP (6.3 months versus 5.3 months; P = 0.031) favored the radiolabeled antibody. Patients with disease progression after tositumomab could cross over to the ^{131}I-tositumomab arm. Following cross-over to RIT, the ORR (68% versus 16%; P = 0.002), median response duration (12.6 versus 7.6 months; P = 0.001), and median TTP (12.4 versus 5.5 months; P = 0.01) were superior to results with prior unlabeled antibody response. This trial clearly demonstrates that the radioisotope adds efficacy to the treatment.

The second randomized trial rituximab was compared to ^{90}Y-ibrituomab tiuxetan to determine if the radioantibody was superior to the chimeric unlabeled antibody.[181] The primary endpoint was ORR, and it was underpowered to identify differences in PFS. One hundred forty-three patients were randomized to R alone (70) or RIT (73). The OR and CR rates favored the RIT arm: 80% versus 56%, P = 0.002; 30% versus 16%, P = 0.04. TTP was not different between arms, but durable responses of 6 months or greater were seen more often following RIT than R (64% versus 47%; P = 0.03). These data support the conclusion that RIT provides superior responses, but larger randomized trials are needed to demonstrate if there are benefits in EFS and OS.

Chemotherapy Followed by Radiation

Investigators from Mexico evaluated the role of adjuvant radiation in patients with follicular lymphoma (FL) achieving a CR after initial therapy.[182] Four hundred sixty-nine patients were randomized to observation (control) or to adjuvant radiation therapy to initial sites of bulky disease. At 20 years, there was an advantage for both EFS (41% versus 68%; P less than 0.01) and OS (71% versus 89%; P = 0.01). Treatment-related mortality and the secondary myelodysplastic syndrome/acute myelogenous leukemia (MDS/AML) were identical in the two arms.

RIT could provide radiation to all sites of disease without the toxicity and technical difficulty of TBI. SWOG conducted a pilot study (S9911) to evaluate the safety and efficacy of adjuvant ^{131}I-tositumomab following a course of six cycles of CHOP chemotherapy.[183] Toxicity was primarily hematologic and was more severe during the chemotherapy than during the RIT. The ORR was 90%. The final response after RIT improved in 57% of the patients who had had less than a CR to CHOP. The estimated 2-year EFS and OS were 81% and 97%, respectively. This trial established the feasibility of sequential chemotherapy and RIT. It is currently being evaluated in a Phase III comparison to rituximab and CHOP chemotherapy (SWOG S0016).

RIT Summary

The optimal use of RIT has not been determined. A recent provocative study of ^{131}I-tositumomab as initial therapy for FL from the University of Michigan demonstrated high response (OR 95%, CR 75%).[184] Using PCR for the t(14;18) translocation, 80% of the informative patients had molecular remissions. The median PFS was 6.1 years. Toxicity was principally hematologic. These results suggest that in selected patients a single course of RIT can have substantial long-term benefit. Taken together with the CHOP followed by the RIT study already cited, results suggest that RIT may have an important role in the management of indolent lymphoma. However, to determine the appropriate placement in the treatment algorithm for FL, additional randomized trials are necessary.

Transplant

The role of stem cell transplant has been somewhat limited in indolent lymphoma for several reasons. First, these lymphomas are generally seen in older patients for whom stem cell transplant may not be appropriate. Second, the natural history is long, and determining when in the course of treatment to use these therapies is not always clear. Retrospective data from the University of Nebraska suggest the HDT/ASCT should be done in second or third remission; the use of this approach later is no different from in other salvage chemotherapy.[185] Several randomized studies have tried to address the role of stem cell transplant in indolent lymphoma.

The European CUP trial posed the question whether conventional chemotherapy (C) versus HDT/ASCT with unpurged (U) or purged (P) stem cell products was superior for relapsed FL.[186,187] Of 140 patients registered, 89 patients were randomized. Patients were initially treated with three cycles of CHOP. Responding patients were eligible to proceed to the randomized arm. At the median follow-up of 69 months, HDT/ASCT (both U and P) by the log rank test were significantly superior in PFS (P = 0.0037) and OS (P = 0.079). The estimated 2-year PFS for C, U, and P were 26%, 58%, and 55%, respectively. Estimated 4-year OS for C, U, and P are 46%, 71%, and 77%, respectively. Thus, in young patients with chemosensitive recurrent FL, HDT/ASCT appears to provide a survival advantage. Purging did not appear to have an effect on outcome.

The GLSG conducted a trial of HDT/ASCT or interferon (INF) in first remission of patients with FL younger than 60 years of age.[188] Three hundred seven patients underwent induction chemotherapy with two cycles of CHOP or MCP (mitroxantrone, chlorambucil, prednisone) and were then randomized to the HDT/ASCT or INF groups. Induction chemotherapy continued until patients had achieved a CR or PR. Two hundred forty patients with FL were evaluable for the comparison of INF versus HDT/ASCT. Of note, patients progressing after INF could cross over to HDT/ASCT, complicating the OS analysis. The PFS favored the HDT/ASCT arm (65% versus 33%; P less than 0.0001). The overall survival curves are identical between the arms, but longer follow-up is necessary. Late transplant complications have not been seen.

A very similar study has been conducted by the Group Ouest Est Leucemies Aigues Myeloblastiques (GOELAM) study group of a randomized trial comparing CHVmP-INF and induction chemotherapy followed by HDT with purged ASCT in newly diagnosed advanced-stage FL patients.[189] One hundred seventy-two patients were randomized. The HDT arm has a superior OR rate (81% versus 69%; $P = 0.045$) and a longer median EFS (not reached versus 45 months). However, there was no OS advantage because of an excess of secondary malignancies after transplantation. Thus, in neither randomized study of upfront HDT/ASCT has a survival advantage been seen; therefore, this approach should still be considered investigational in the treatment of advanced-stage indolent lymphoma.

Allogeneic stem cell transplant has been used to treat recurrent and refractory indolent lymphoma. However, most reports are small case series. No randomized trials have been conducted. The best quality evidence we have available is from the transplant registry. A joint report from the IBMTR and ABMTR identified 904 patients transplanted with FL, and sought to compare outcome following autologous and allogeneic stem cell transplant.[190] A total of 176 (19%) received allogeneic, 131 (14%) received purged autologous, and 597 (67%) received unpurged autologous transplants. Treatment-related mortality at 5 years was allogeneic SCT, 30%; purged ASCT, 14%; and unpurged ASCT, 8%. Recurrence at 5 years was allogeneic SCT, 21%; purged ASCT, 43%; and unpurged ASCT, 58%. Estimated 5-year survival was allogeneic, 51%; purged ASCT, 62%; and unpurged ASCT, 55%. TBI was associated with higher treatment-related mortality (TRM) but lower recurrence. In this retrospective registry analysis, there was a suggestion of a benefit for purged stem cells not seen in the CUP trial (see above). The toxicity of allogeneic SCT appears to offset the benefit; thus, unless TRM can be significantly reduced, HDT/ASCT appears to be the preferred choice if autologous stem cells can be mobilized.

Mycosis Fungoides

Mycosis fungoides (MF) is an often indolent cutaneous lymphoma composed of CD4+ T cells. It accounts for about 2% of new cases of NHL in the United States, but because of the long survival of many patients, the prevalence is considerably higher.[191] Staging for mycosis fungoides utilizes a unique TNM system. Prognosis for mycosis fungoides is stage dependent with stage IA patients having an overall survival similar to unaffected age-matched controls.[192] Moreover, less than 10% of patients with stage IA disease will progress to a higher stage. Patients with stage IIB–IV disease have a much poorer survival and, in contrast to their early-stage counterparts, most of these patients will die of their disease.

Mycosis fungoides generally behaves as a chronic, relapsing illness. Although not curative, many effective treatment strategies have been studied in this disease. These Phase II experiences demonstrate the efficacy of topical therapies, phototherapy, radiation, retinoids, extracorporeal photopheresis, interferon-alpha, fusion proteins, and single-agent and combination chemotherapy. A randomized study compared electron-beam radiation therapy and a combination chemotherapy to sequential topical therapies, showing improved response but no survival benefit for the aggressive approach.[193]

Mantle Cell Lymphoma

Mantle cell lymphoma (MCL) was originally described based on its morphologic appearance variously as centrocytic lymphoma, lymphocytic lymphoma of intermediate differentiation, intermediate lymphocytic lymphoma, or mantle zone lymphoma; unfortunately, the morphology overlapped significantly with other entities, making this diagnosis very difficult to make. It was recognized to be a CD5+ B-cell tumor but was difficult to distinguish from other CD5+ lymphocytic lymphomas on morphologic grounds.[194,195] The tumors were characterized by a chromosomal translocation t(11;14), and the breakpoint was cloned in the early 1990s and found to juxtapose the immunoglobulin heavy chain (IgH) gene on chromosome 14 to the BCL1/PRAD1/CYCLIN D1 locus on chromosome 11.[196–199] It became possible to reliably and reproducibly diagnose MCL following the development of immunohistochemical reagents able to identify cyclin D1 in paraffin-embedded tissue sections.[200] By flow cytometry, these tumors express the pan-B-cell antigens CD19 and CD20 in addition to CD5. They typically do not express CD23 and FMC7 in contrast focus. The SWOG retrospective study analyzed the outcome of patients previously diagnosed as IWF groups A–E to determine the incidence and natural history of MCL.[201] MCL represents about 6% of the cases of NHL in the United States[2] and was typically categorized as diffuse small cleaved cell lymphoma (IWF E). However, some cases were confused with small lymphocytic lymphoma (IWF A) and follicular small cleaved cell lymphoma (IWF B). This study demonstrated that MCL has a tumor with significantly shorter progression-free and overall survival when compared to other small lymphocytic lymphomas.

The role of cyclin D1 expression in the definitive diagnosis of MCL is controversial. There are some cases of lymphoma that have the typical phenotype by flow cytometry (CD20+, CD5+, CD23–) that fail to express cyclin D1. A series from Japan suggests that these tumors have a natural history identical to other small lymphocytic lymphoma,[202,203] whereas others suggest the outcome is no different.[204] However, in many trials, expression of cyclin D1 has been considered necessary for inclusion on trials for MCL.

Much of our knowledge of the natural history of MCL lymphoma has been derived from retrospective studies. The disease has a striking male predominance, for unknown reasons. Although most patients have an aggressive clinical course, a small portion of patients can have an indolent course,[205] but these patients have been difficult to identify prospectively. Presentation as early-stage disease (CS I or II) is very uncommon, and information regarding management is either retrospective or anecdotal. Data on 26 patients with limited-stage MCL treated in Vancouver, have been reported,[206] with a variety of treatments with 5-year PFS and OS of 45% and 70%, respectively. Age (less than 60 years) and initial use of radiation were found to have a positive effect. Bone marrow, peripheral blood, and gastrointestinal tract involvement is common. In general, the retrospective studies suggest that MCL is responsive to chemotherapy, but remission durations are brief, and median overall survival is about 3 years with no plateau on survival curves.[207–212] In CHOP-treated patients, the 10-year EFS and OS were 6% and 8%, respectively.[201] More recently, prospective trials have tried to determine if the natural history can be altered by intensification of therapy and addition of immunotherapy.

Chemotherapy for MCL

There are few randomized trials of chemotherapy that include patients with MCL. In general, when patients with MCL have been included, it has been as a minor population in larger trials, and it is not possible to draw definitive comparative conclusions regarding the treatment arms.[146,213] However, in both the comparison of prednimustine and mitroxantrone versus cyclophosphamide[213] and that of fludarabine versus fludarabine idarubicin,[146] the patients with MCL had similar overall response rates as the patients with FL, but the complete response rate was lower.

Investigators at the M.D. Anderson Cancer Center (MDACC) have used alternating regimens of hyperCVAD regimen (fractionated cyclophosphamide, vincristine, doxorubicin, dexamethasone) with MA (methotrexate, cytarabine) as treatment for MCL. They initially treated a group of 45 patients (25 patients as initial therapy), alternating chemotherapy with hyperCVAD and MA followed by high-dose therapy and autologous stem cell transplant (HDT/ASCT). Among the 25 previously untreated patients, the 3-year EFS and OS were 72% and 92%, respectively.[214] These results have been updated and include an analysis restricted to 33 patients who underwent transplant; it did not include patients treated with hyperCVAD/MA who did not proceed to HDT/ASCT. Among the transplanted patients, the DFS and OS were 43% and 77%, respectively.[215]

Rituximab for MCL

Single Agent

A European intergroup conducted a study of single-agent rituximab in patients with newly diagnosed and recurrent MCL.[216] In a total of 74 patients (34 untreated, 40 relapsed), the overall response rate was 38%, which was unaffected by prior treatment. The median duration of response was 1.2 years. These results were similar to a small pilot trial using 8 consecutive weeks of treatment, and some patients were treated at a higher dose.[54] Thus, neither the longer treatment duration nor the higher dose appeared to be important for the single-agent activity in MCL.

The Swiss Group for Clinical Cancer Research (SAKK) conducted a study to determine if prolonged dosing of rituximab could improve the outcome of patients with untreated and relapsed MCL treated with single-agent rituximab.[217] All patients received four weekly doses of rituximab at the standard dose of 375 mg/m^2. Patients with stable or responding disease were randomized to observation versus rituximab given at a dose of 375 mg/m^2 every 8 weeks for an additional four doses. One hundred four patients were treated in this trial with a response rate of 27%. After the induction therapy, PCR amplification of the t(11;14) translocation breakpoint became negative in the peripheral blood of 4 of 20 informative patients and only 1 of 14 informative bone marrows. Sixty-one patients were randomized (stable or responding disease), and there was no difference in outcome (EFS, RD, OS) between the prolonged therapy group and the observation group. These data demonstrate modest single-agent activity for rituximab in MCL.

Chemoimmunotherapy

The MDACC group built on their experience with the alternating hyperCVAD and MA with the addition of rituximab. Rituximab was added to both the alternating regimens that were administered for a total of six to eight cycles (hyper-CVAD and MA are counted as separate cycles).[218] Ninety-seven patients were treated, and the CR/CRu rate after six cycles was 87%. The estimated 3-year EFS and OS were 67% and 81%, respectively. Despite these encouraging results, the survival curve has no plateau, and there is a steady relapse rate over time, suggesting that the R-hyperCVAD/R-MA regimen alone was not curative. The toxicity of the regimen was significant, with 5 deaths in the study (5%), and 4 patients subsequently developing myelodysplasia syndrome (MDS), with 3 deaths.

Investigators at the Dana Farber Cancer Institute (DFCI) investigated the addition of rituximab to CHOP chemotherapy.[219] Forty patients were treated in this trial with an overall response rate of 96% (CR, 48%). The median PFS was 16.6 months, no different from historical controls. Twenty-five of the patients had a t(11;14) translocation breakpoint that was amplifiable by the PCR. Nine of 25 patients who had informative PCR, achieved a molecular remission. The median PFS was the same in patients who achieved a molecular remission as those who did not.

The German Low Grade Lymphoma Study Group (GLSG) undertook a large randomized Phase III study of CHOP, with or without rituximab, for patients with untreated MCL.[220] There was a secondary randomization that was stratified by age: patients over 60 were randomized to two doses of adjuvant interferon-alpha and the younger patients were randomized to adjuvant HDT/ASCT or interferon-alpha. One hundred twenty-two patients were randomized: CHOP, n = 60; R-CHOP, n = 62. Analyzed according to initial randomization, R-CHOP was significantly superior to CHOP in overall response rate (94% versus 75%; $P = 0.0054$) and complete remission rate (34% versus 7%; $P = 0.00024$). There was also a significant benefit in the median TTF (21 versus 14 months; $P = 0.0131$). Despite the improvement in TTF, there was no advantage to the chemoimmunotherapy arm in progression-free or overall survival.

GLSG also evaluated the addition of rituximab to FCM (fludarabine, cyclophosphamide, mitroxantrone) for patients with relapsed and refractory FL and MCL (24 patients in each of the arms).[160] Addition of rituximab did not significantly improve the overall response rate (FCM-R, 58%, versus FCM, 46%; $P = 0.282$), but there was 29% complete remissions with rituximab versus none without. Although there was no difference in the median PFS (FCM-R, 8 months, versus FCM, 4 months; $P = 0.3887$), there was a difference in median OS (FCM-R, not reached, versus FCM, 11 months; $P = 0.0042$). It is unclear why the treatment could result in a significant improvement of OS without an improvement in PFS. Given the small sample size, it is possible the survival benefit reflects an unintentional selection bias.

The National Cancer Institute (NCI) investigators evaluated DA-EPOCH-R with idiotype vaccination in patients with untreated MCL.[221] Twenty-six patients were treated with DA-EPOCH-R with an overall response rate of 100% (complete response, 92%). Interestingly, the proliferation signature that had been identified to be important in the outcome of patients with MCL treated with CHOP-based regimens[204,222] was not predictive of outcome with DA-EPOCH-R. The mechanism by which this regimen would overcome the proliferation signature is unknown. The impact of the idiotype vaccination on outcome is unknown. The DA-EPOCH-R regimen profoundly affected on humoral responses although T-cell responses to the Id-KLH/GM-CSF vaccine were seen.

Stem Cell Transplantation

The role of HDT/ASCT in the management of MCL has been controversial. Investigators at the DFCI undertook a retrospective analysis of the outcome of those who underwent high-dose chemoradiotherapy and anti-B-cell monoclonal antibody-purged autologous bone marrow transplantation (ABMT) for MCL in first or subsequent remission.[223] The results were very discouraging, with no evidence of a plateau on the survival curve, and an estimated DFS and OS at 4 years of only 31% and 62%, respectively. In another small study of 24 patients, the EFS was 55% at 5 years, but again there was no evidence of a plateau on the survival curve.[224] The data between 1988 and 1998 for 195 patients with MCL provided to the European Blood and Marrow Transplant Registry (EBMT), or the Autologous Blood and Marrow Transplant Registry (ABMTR) were reviewed.[225] At the median follow-up of 3.9 years, the estimated 5-year PFS and OS were 33% and 55%, respectively. There was a significantly worse outcome for patients not in first complete remission (CR1) compared to those in CR1 (relative risk, 2.99; $P = 0.001$).

The European MCL network undertook a randomized Phase III study to evaluate the role of consolidation of the first remission with HDT/ASCT.[226] Patients were initially treated with four to six cycles of CHOP-like chemotherapy. Patients achieving a PR or CR were randomized to either two additional cycles of the same chemotherapy, followed by interferon-alpha, or to stem cell mobilization with dexa-BEAM (dexamethasone, carmustine, etoposide, cytarabine, melphalan), followed by total-body irradiation (TBI) and cyclophosphamide. Patients who progressed after the interferon arm were eligible to cross over to the high-dose therapy arm. One hundred twenty-two patients were randomized: 60 to HDT/ASCT and 62 to interferon-alpha. Induction therapy included CHOP in 61%, R-CHOP in 26%, and other CHOP-like regimens in 13%, and these were relatively well balanced between arms. Patients receiving consolidation with HDT/ASCT versus interferon-alpha had a superior median PFS (36 months versus 17 months; $P = 0.0108$). Despite a trend in improvement in OS, this was not statistically significant; however, the survival analysis was complicated by the cross-over design. Despite the improvement in PFS with HDT/ASCT in first remission, there is no plateau on the survival curve to suggest a group of patients being cured with this therapy.

Allogeneic stem cell transplantation has also been investigated for patients with relapsed/refractory MCL. Anecdotal experience with conventional myeloablative allogeneic transplantation, suggests that some patients can have long-term disease-free benefit.[227,228] Investigators at Johns Hopkins identified 58 patients with MCL in their transplant registry who received either autologous or allogeneic stem cells.[229] Nineteen patients received an allograft. In this analysis, there was no clear evidence of a graft-versus-tumor effect, because the actuarial risk of relapse was similar between those who received either autologous or allogeneic stem cells. There was no difference in 3-year EFS (70%) between allogeneic and autologous transplant performed in CR1.

A trial of nonmyeloablative allogeneic stem cell transplantions was conducted at the MDACC.[230] Eighteen patients were treated in two trials that differed in the chemotherapy regimen: fludarabine, cyclophosphamide, high-dose rituximab ($n = 13$), and cisplatin, fludarabine, cytarabine ($n = 5$). The median number of prior treatments was three, and 5 patients had prior HDT/ASCT. Complete remissions were seen in 94%, and 3 patients progressed. One of the 3 was reinduced into CR with donor lymphocyte infusions. The estimated 3-year current EFS was 82% (this includes the patient reinduced into CR). Investigators at the Fred Hutchinson Cancer Research Center (FHCRC), evaluated a nonmyeloablative approach using fludarabine and 2 Gy TBI for patients with relapsed and refractory MCL.[231] Thirty-three patients were treated (HLA-matched related, $n = 16$; unrelated, $n = 17$), including 14 patients who had had a prior HDT/ASCT. Stable engraftment occurred in 31 of the patients. Of the 30 patients undergoing the procedure in CR ($n = 13$), or with responding disease ($n = 17$), only 1 patient had relapse. The relapse mortality was 9%, but regimen-related mortality was 24% at 2 years. The estimated 2-year DFS and OS were 60% and 65%, respectively.

New Approaches

Radioimmunotherapy

Mantle cell lymphoma is sensitive to radiation; however, the role of external-beam radiation is limited in the management of the disease because of the systemic nature of the disease. Radioimmunotherapy is a means of providing systemic radiation therapy to multiple sites of disease. Preliminary results of two trials have been presented. Untreated patients with MCL were treated with sequential radioimmunotherapy (RIT) with ^{131}I-tositumomab (65–75 cGy, whole body) followed by conventional CHOP chemotherapy.[232] There was an overall response rate to the RIT of 83% (CR, 50%) and the chemotherapy improved the CR to 90%. Investigators at MDACC treated a group of 15 patients with relapsed and refractory MCL with ^{90}Y-ibritumomab tiuxetan (0.3–0.4 mCi ^{90}Y/kg).[233] There was an overall response rate of 33% (all CR/CRu). These trials are very preliminary and response durations are not available, although they suggest conventional-dose RIT has activity in both untreated and relapsed/refractory disease.

At the FHCRC, the role of high-dose RIT with stem cell support for MCL was investigated.[234] The systemic distribution of disease, with extensive bone marrow and peripheral blood involvement, raised the concern that the dosimetry of RIT in MCL would be different from that in other tumors. In 25 patients with MCL treated with high-dose RIT, the biodistribution and dosimetry were similar to other histologies.[235] Sixteen patients were treated with ^{131}I-tositumomab at a dose calibrated to deliver 20 to 25 Gy to normal organs, followed

10 days later by high-dose etoposide (30–60 mg/kg) and cyclophosphamide (60–100 mg/kg). Patients then had autologous stem cells reinfused. At 3 years, the PFS and OS are 61% and 91%, respectively, in a population that had a median of three prior treatment and 7 patients with chemorefractory disease. Substitution of high-dose RIT is a promising approach, but larger controlled studies are necessary to validate these findings.

Novel Agents

Bortezomib is a reversible inhibitor of the protease approved for the treatment of relapsed and refractory multiple myeloma.[236] This drug has been evaluated in the treatment of MCL at both MSKCC and MDACC. Both centers used a dose of bortezomib (1.5 mg/m^2 on days 1, 4, 8, and 11 every 21 days) that was associated with significant asthenia, neuropathy, and thrombocytopenia.[237,238] However, in a limited number of patients, the response rate was reported to be approximately 50%. Additional data have been presented by the NCIC and St. Bartholomew's.[239,240] In these trials, the schedule was the same but the dose was 1.3 mg/m^2, and this appeared to be mildly less toxic; asthenia, thrombocytopenia, and neuropathy remained significant toxicities. The activity was maintained at the lower dose, with overall response rates of 36% (St. Bartholomew's, $n = 11$) and 33% (NCIC, $n = 24$). A multicenter confirmatory Phase II trial is ongoing in the United States. However, additional schedules and integration with other therapy are necessary.

There have been anecdotal reports of thalidomide inducing remissions in patients with refractory MCL.[241,242] Based on the rationale that thalidomide might target the microenvironment and rituximab the tumor, investigators from Austria examined the combination in patients with MCL.[243] Sixteen patients were treated with rituximab 375 mg/m^2 weekly × 4 with thalidomide 200 mg po/day for 2 weeks, then increased to 400 mg po/day until progression or relapse. Thirteen (81%) of the patients responded, with CR in 31%. Median PFS was 20.4 months, with an estimated 3-year OS of 75%. Toxicity was primarily related to the thalidomide, with thromboembolic events in 2 patients and grade IV neutropenia in 1.

Summary

The clinical management of MCL remains a major challenge. Early-stage disease is uncommon, and other than small retrospective cases series, there is no high-level evidence to guide the management of these patients. These patients should be extensively evaluated for occult sites of extranodal disease with inclusion of gastrointestinal tract evaluation with blind biopsies (if not gross disease). It appears that involved-field radiation should be a component of the therapy. In advanced-stage disease, outside of a clinical trial, effective cytoreductive therapy (R-HyperCVAD/R-MA; R-CHOP) should be followed by HDT/ASCT in appropriate candidates. However, it should be cautioned that this is an effective palliative, and not a curative approach. For this reason, when possible patients with MCL should be referred for clinical trial. The effectiveness of HDT/ASCT at relapse is controversial, but most data suggest that it is not as effective for relapsed/refractory disease as it is for consolidation in first remission. Off study, the fludarabine-based FCM (±R) is justified on the basis of the evidence presented, but the benefit is relatively brief. The data with investigational approaches, such as bortezomib, rituximab plus thalidomide, high-dose radioimmunotherapy, and allogeneic stem cell transplantation are all promising, but further trials are necessary to determine how these treatments fit into the management of MCL. Other agents, such as the MTOR inhibitor CCI779 and flavopiridol, also may have activity in MCL. Thus, patients with relapsed disease have no standard therapy and when possible should be referred for clinical trials.

Conclusions

The non-Hodgkin's lymphomas represent a clinically diverse array of diseases with some entities being incurable chronic illnesses and others progressing rapidly but having the potential for cure. Owing to the relative rarity of some of these entities, such as T-cell lymphoma, high-level evidence does not exist, and therapeutic decisions are based on small retrospective studies and the clinical impression of experts. In contrast, there is high-level evidence to guide the therapy of DLBCL in most clinical situations. Poor-risk young patients remain an area of controversy. Even in aggressive lymphoma relapse, randomized data support the use of HDT/ASCT. Among the indolent lymphomas, FL remains the greatest challenge in day-to-day practice because of the chronic nature of the disease and lack of clear guidance as to an optimal order of therapy. In these cases, it is important to extract the lessons learned from the high-level evidence and apply these to the particulars of the patient's clinical situation. FL is a disease, barring a major breakthrough resulting in curative outcomes, in which individual considerations will shape treatment choices. In MCL, much of the high-level evidence informs the clinician of what not to do. Despite intensive study over the past decade, consistent curative outcome has not been achieved. It remains very important that these patients be referred for clinical trials. Many lymphoma entities were not covered in this chapter because they are very uncommon. Regrettably, in many of these entities, high-level evidence may never exist to guide the management of these patients. In those circumstances, we must rely on the experience of highly specialized consultants who may be able to provide insight on a case-by-case basis.

References

1. Jemal A, Tiwari RC, Murray T, et al. Cancer statistics, 2004. CA Cancer J Clin 2004;54(1):8–29.
2. Armitage JO, Weisenburger DD. New approach to classifying non-Hodgkin's lymphomas: clinical features of the major histologic subtypes. Non-Hodgkin's Lymphoma Classification Project. J Clin Oncol 1998;16(8):2780–2795.
3. Harris NL, Jaffe ES, Stein H, et al. A revised European-American classification of lymphoid neoplasms: a proposal from the International Lymphoma Study Group. Blood 1994;84(5): 1361–1392.
4. Jaffe ES, Harris NL, Diebold J, et al. World Health Organization Classification of lymphomas: a work in progress. Ann Oncol 1998;9(suppl 5):S25–S30.
5. Harris NL, Jaffe ES, Diebold J, et al. The World Health Organization classification of neoplastic diseases of the hematopoietic and lymphoid tissues. Report of the Clinical Advisory Com-

mittee Meeting, Airlie House, Virginia, November, 1997. Ann Oncol 1999;10(12):1419–1432.
6. Wakely PE, Jr. Fine-needle aspiration cytopathology in diagnosis and classification of malignant lymphoma: accurate and reliable? Diagn Cytopathol 2000;22(2):120–125.
7. Classification of non-Hodgkin's lymphomas. Reproducibility of major classification systems. NCI non-Hodgkin's Classification Project Writing Committee. Cancer, 1985;55(1):91–95.
8. Mourad WA, Tulbah A, Shoukri M, et al. Primary diagnosis and REAL/WHO classification of non-Hodgkin's lymphoma by fine-needle aspiration: cytomorphologic and immunophenotypic approach. Diagn Cytopathol 2003;28(4):191–195.
9. Mann GB, Conlon KC, LaQuaglia M, et al. Emerging role of laparoscopy in the diagnosis of lymphoma. J Clin Oncol 1998;16(5):1909–1915.
10. Dong HY, Harris NL, Preffer FI, et al. Fine-needle aspiration biopsy in the diagnosis and classification of primary and recurrent lymphoma: a retrospective analysis of the utility of cytomorphology and flow cytometry. Mod Pathol 2001;14(5): 472–481.
11. Lioe TF, Elliott H, Allen DC, et al. The role of fine needle aspiration cytology (FNAC) in the investigation of superficial lymphadenopathy; uses and limitations of the technique. Cytopathology 1999;10(5):291–297.
12. Lister TA, Crowther D, Sutcliffe SB, et al. Report of a committee convened to discuss the evaluation and staging of patients with Hodgkin's disease: Cotswolds meeting. J Clin Oncol 1989;7(11):1630–1636.
13. A predictive model for aggressive non-Hodgkin's lymphoma. The International Non-Hodgkin's Lymphoma Prognostic Factors Project. N Engl J Med 1993;329(14):987–994.
14. Hermans J, Krol AD, van Groningen K, et al. International Prognostic Index for aggressive non-Hodgkin's lymphoma is valid for all malignancy grades. Blood 1995;86(4):1460–1463.
15. Foussard C, Desablens B, Sensebe L, et al. Is the International Prognostic Index for aggressive lymphomas useful for low-grade lymphoma patients? Applicability to stage III-IV patients. The GOELAMS Group, France. Ann Oncol 1997;8(suppl 1): 49–52.
16. Wilder RB, Rodriguez MA, Medeiros LJ, et al. International prognostic index-based outcomes for diffuse large B-cell lymphomas. Cancer (Phila) 2002;94(12):3083–3088.
17. Moskowitz CH, Nimer SD, Glassman JR, et al. The International Prognostic Index predicts for outcome following autologous stem cell transplantation in patients with relapsed and primary refractory intermediate-grade lymphoma. Bone Marrow Transplant 1999; 23(6):561–567.
18. Blay J, Gomez F, Sebban C, et al. The International Prognostic Index correlates to survival in patients with aggressive lymphoma in relapse: analysis of the PARMA trial. Parma Group. Blood 1998;92(10): 3562–3568.
19. Hamlin PA, Zelenetz AD, Kewalramani T, et al. Age-adjusted International Prognostic Index predicts autologous stem cell transplantation outcome for patients with relapsed or primary refractory diffuse large B-cell lymphoma. Blood 2003;102(6): 1989–1996.
20. Decaudin D, Lepage E, Brousse N, et al. Low-grade stage III-IV follicular lymphoma: multivariate analysis of prognostic factors in 484 patients: a study of the groupe d'Etude des lymphomes de l'Adulte. J Clin Oncol 1999;17(8):2499–2505.
21. Stelitano C, Baldini L, Pieresca C, et al. Validation of the international prognostic index in working formulation group A low-grade non-Hodgkin's lymphoma: retrospective analysis of 137 patients from the Gruppo Italiano per lo Studio dei Linfomi registry. Haematologica 2000;85(2):154–159.
22. Kondo E, Ogura M, Kagami Y, et al. Assessment of prognostic factors in follicular lymphoma patients. Int J Hematol 2001;73(3):363–368.
23. Solal-Celigny P, Roy P, Colombat P, et al. Follicular lymphoma international prognostic index. Blood 2004;104(5):1258–1265.
24. Montoto S, Lopez-Guillermo A, Altes A, et al. Predictive value of Follicular Lymphoma International Prognostic Index (FLIPI) in patients with follicular lymphoma at first progression. Ann Oncol 2004;15(10):1484–1489.
25. Halaas JL, Teruya-Feldstein J, Filippa DA, et al. The Follicular Lymphoma International Prognostic Index (FLIPI) is superior to WHO/REAL histological grade for identifying high-risk patients: a retrospective review of the MSKCC experience in 260 patients with follicular lymphoma. Blood 2004;104(11):3268.
26. Golub TR. Genomic approaches to the pathogenesis of hematologic malignancy. Curr Opin Hematol 2001;8(4):252–261.
27. Shaughnessy J, Jr. Primer on medical genomics. Part IX: Scientific and clinical applications of DNA microarrays: multiple myeloma as a disease model. Mayo Clin Proc 2003; 78(9):1098–1109.
28. Staudt LM. Molecular diagnosis of the hematologic cancers. N Engl J Med 2003;348(18):1777–1785.
29. Rosenwald A. DNA microarrays in lymphoid malignancies. Oncology (Huntingt) 2003;17(12):1743–1748; discussion 1750, 1755, 1758–1759 passim.
30. Alizadeh A, Eisen M, Davis RE, et al. The lymphochip: a specialized cDNA microarray for the genomic-scale analysis of gene expression in normal and malignant lymphocytes. Cold Spring Harb Symp Quant Biol 1999;4:71–78.
31. Alizadeh AA, Eisen MB, Davis RE, et al. Distinct types of diffuse large B-cell lymphoma identified by gene expression profiling. Nature (Lond) 2000;403(6769):503–511.
32. Rosenwald A, Wright G, Chan WC, et al. The use of molecular profiling to predict survival after chemotherapy for diffuse large-B-cell lymphoma. N Engl J Med 2002;346(25):1937–1947.
33. Hans CP, Weisenburger DD, Greiner TC, et al. Confirmation of the molecular classification of diffuse large B-cell lymphoma by immunohistochemistry using a tissue microarray. Blood 2004;103(1):275–282.
34. Shipp MA, Ross KN, Tamayo P, et al. Diffuse large B-cell lymphoma outcome prediction by gene-expression profiling and supervised machine learning. Nat Med 2002;8(1):68–74.
35. McKelvey EM, Gottlieb JA, Wilson HE, et al. Hydroxyldaunomycin (Adriamycin) combination chemotherapy in malignant lymphoma. Cancer (Phila) 1976;38(4):1484–1493.
36. Sweet DL, Golomb HM, Ultmann JE, et al. Cyclophosphamide, vincristine, methotrexate with leucovorin rescue, and cytarabine (COMLA) combination sequential chemotherapy for advanced diffuse histiocytic lymphoma. Ann Intern Med 1980;92(6):785–790.
37. Shipp MA, Harrington DP, Klatt MM, et al. Identification of major prognostic subgroups of patients with large-cell lymphoma treated with m-BACOD or M-BACOD. Ann Intern Med 1986;104(6):757–765.
38. Klimo P, Connors JM. MACOP-B chemotherapy for the treatment of diffuse large-cell lymphoma. Ann Intern Med 1985; 102(5):596–602.
39. Fisher RI, Longo DL, DeVita, VJ Jr., et al. Long-term follow-up of ProMACE-CytaBOM in non-Hodgkin's lymphomas. Ann Oncol 1991;2(suppl 1):33–35.
40. Coiffier B, Gisselbrecht C, Herbrecht R, et al. LNH-84 regimen: a multicenter study of intensive chemotherapy in 737 patients with aggressive malignant lymphoma. J Clin Oncol 1989;7(8): 1018–1026.
41. Tilly H, Lepage E, Coiffier B, et al. Intensive conventional chemotherapy (ACVBP regimen) compared with standard CHOP for poor-prognosis aggressive non-Hodgkin lymphoma. Blood 2003;102(13):4284–4289.
42. Pfreundschuh M, Trumper L, Kloess M, et al. Two-weekly or 3-weekly CHOP chemotherapy with or without etoposide for the treatment of elderly patients with aggressive lymphomas:

results of the NHL-B2 trial of the DSHNHL. Blood 2004;104(3): 634–641.
43. Pfreundschuh M, Trumper L, Kloess M, et al. Two-weekly or 3-weekly CHOP chemotherapy with or without etoposide for the treatment of young patients with good-prognosis (normal LDH) aggressive lymphomas: results of the NHL-B1 trial of the DSHNHL. Blood 2004;104(3):626–633.
44. Wilson WH, Grossbard ML, Pittaluga S, et al. Dose-adjusted EPOCH chemotherapy for untreated large B-cell lymphomas: a pharmacodynamic approach with high efficacy. Blood 2002; 99(8):2685–2693.
45. Wilson WH, Pittaluga S, Gutierrez M, et al. Dose-adjusted EPOCH-rituximab in untreated diffuse large B-cell lymphoma: benefit of rituximab appears restricted to tumors harboring anti-apoptotic mechanisms. Blood 2003;102(11):abstract 356.
46. Shipp MA, Abeloff MD, Antman KH, et al. International Consensus Conference on High-Dose Therapy with Hematopoietic Stem Cell Transplantation in Aggressive Non-Hodgkin's Lymphomas: report of the jury. J Clin Oncol 1999;17(1):423–429.
47. Haioun C, Lepage E, Gisselbrecht C, et al. Benefit of autologous bone marrow transplantation over sequential chemotherapy in poor-risk aggressive non-Hodgkin's lymphoma: updated results of the prospective study LNH87-2. Groupe d'Etude des Lymphomes de l'Adulte. J Clin Oncol 1997;15(3):1131–1137.
48. Haioun C, Lepage E, Gisselbrecht C, et al. Survival benefit of high-dose therapy in poor-risk aggressive non-Hodgkin's lymphoma: final analysis of the prospective LNH87-2 protocol. A Groupe d'Etude des Lymphomes de l'Adulte study. J Clin Oncol 2000;18(16):3025– 3030.
49. Santini G, Salvagno L, Leoni P, et al. VACOP-B versus VACOP-B plus autologous bone marrow transplantation for advanced diffuse non-Hodgkin's lymphoma: results of a prospective randomized trial by the non-Hodgkin's Lymphoma Cooperative Study Group. J Clin Oncol 1998;16(8):2796–2802.
50. Reyes F, Lepage E, Morel P, et al. Failure of first-line inductive high-dose chemotherapy (HDC) in poor-risk patients (PTS) with aggressive lymphoma: updated results of the randomized LNH93-3 study. Blood 1997;90(11 suppl 1):594a.
51. Kaiser U, Uebelacker I, Abel U, et al. Randomized study to evaluate the use of high-dose therapy as part of primary treatment for "aggressive" lymphoma. J Clin Oncol 2002;20(22):4413–4419.
52. Gianni AM, Bregni M, Siena S, et al. High-dose chemotherapy and autologous bone marrow transplantation compared with MACOP-B in aggressive B-cell lymphoma. N Engl J Med, 1997;336(18):1290–1297.
53. Reff ME, Carner K, Chambers KS, et al. Depletion of B cells in vivo by a chimeric mouse human monoclonal antibody to CD20. Blood 1994;83(2):435–445.
54. Coiffier B, Haioun C, Ketterer N, et al. Rituximab (anti-CD20 monoclonal antibody) for the treatment of patients with relapsing or refractory aggressive lymphoma: a multicenter phase II study. Blood 1998;92(6):1927–1932.
55. Vose JM, Link BK, Grossbard ML, et al. Phase II study of rituximab in combination with CHOP chemotherapy in patients with previously untreated, aggressive non-Hodgkin's lymphoma. J Clin Oncol 2001;19(2):389–397.
56. Coiffier B, Lepage E, Briere J, et al. CHOP chemotherapy plus rituximab compared with CHOP alone in elderly patients with diffuse large-B-cell lymphoma. N Engl J Med 2002;346(4): 235–242.
57. Habermann TM, Weller E, Morrison VA, et al. Rituximab-CHOP versus CHOP with or without maintenance rtituximab in patients 60 years of age or older with diffuse large B-cell lymphoma (DLBCL): an update. Blood 2004;104(11):abstract 127.
58. Pfreundschuh M, Truemper L, Gill D, et al. First analysis of the completed Mabthera International (MInT) trial in young patients with low-risk diffuse large B-cell lymphoma (DLBCL): addition of rituximab to a CHOP-like regimen significantly improves outcome of all patients with the identification of a very favorable subgroup with IPI = 0 and no bulky disease. Blood 2004;104(11):abstract 157.
59. Coiffier B, Feugier P, Sebban C, et al. Long-term results of the GELA study: R-CHOP vs. CHOP in elderly patients with diffuse large B-cell lymphoma. Blood 2004;104(11):abstract 1383.
60. Sehn LH, Donaldson J, Chhanabhai M, et al. Introduction of combined CHOP-rituximab therapy dramatically improved outcome of diffuse large B-cell lymphoma (DLBC) in British Columbia (BC). Blood 2003;102(11):abstract 88.
61. Hoskin PJ. Weekly chemotherapy using PMitCEBO in the palliation of recurrent non-Hodgkin's lymphoma. Acta Oncol 1997;36(6):573–576.
62. Mounier N, Briere J, Gisselbrecht C, et al. Rituximab plus CHOP (R-CHOP) overcomes bcl-2-associated resistance to chemotherapy in elderly patients with diffuse large B-cell lymphoma (DLBCL). Blood 2003;101(11):4279–4284.
63. Winter JN, Weller E, Horning SJ, et al. Rituximab (R) alters the prognostic indicator profile in diffuse aggressive non-Hodgkin lymphomas. Blood 2003;102(11):abstract 345.
64. Yahalom J. Radiation therapy in the treatment of lymphoma. Curr Opin Oncol 1999;11(5):370–374.
65. Yahalom J, Varsos G, Fuks Z, et al. Adjuvant cyclophosphamide, doxorubicin, vincristine, and prednisone chemotherapy after radiation therapy in stage I low-grade and intermediate-grade non-Hodgkin lymphoma. Results of a prospective randomized study. Cancer (Phila) 1993;71(7):2342–2350.
66. Kaminski MS, Coleman CN, Colby TV, et al. Factors predicting survival in adults with stage I and II large-cell lymphoma treated with primary radiation therapy. Ann Intern Med 1986;104(6): 747–756.
67. Jones SE, Miller TP, Connors JM. Long-term follow-up and analysis for prognostic factors for patients with limited-stage diffuse large-cell lymphoma treated with initial chemotherapy with or without adjuvant radiotherapy. J Clin Oncol 1989;7(9): 1186–1191.
68. Connors JM, Klimo P, Fairey RN, et al. Brief chemotherapy and involved field radiation therapy for limited-stage, histologically aggressive lymphoma. Ann Intern Med 1987;107(1):25–30.
69. Longo DL, Glatstein E, Duffey PL, et al. Treatment of localized aggressive lymphomas with combination chemotherapy followed by involved-field radiation therapy. J Clin Oncol 1989;7(9):1295–1302.
70. Miller TP, Dahlberg S, Cassady JR, et al. Chemotherapy alone compared with chemotherapy plus radiotherapy for localized intermediate- and high-grade non-Hodgkin's lymphoma. N Engl J Med 1998;339(1):21–26.
71. Miller TP, LeBlanc M, Spier CM, et al. CHOP alone compared to CHOP plus radiotherapy for early stage aggressive non-Hodgkin's lymphomas: an update of the Southwest Oncology Group (SWOG) randomized trial. Blood 2001;98(11):742a (abstract).
72. Miller TP. The limits of limited stage lymphoma. J Clin Oncol 2004;22(15):2982–2984.
73. Fisher RI, DeVita VT Jr., Johnson BL, et al. Prognostic factors for advanced diffuse histiocytic lymphoma following treatment with combination chemotherapy. Am J Med 1977;63(2):177–182.
74. Horning SJ, Weller E, Kim K, et al. Chemotherapy with or without radiotherapy in limited-stage diffuse aggressive non-Hodgkin's lymphoma: Eastern Cooperative Oncology Group study 1484. J Clin Oncol 2004;22(15):3032–3038.
75. Miller TP, Unger JM, Spier C, et al. Effect of adding rituximab to three cycles of CHOP plus involved-field radiotherapy for limited-stage aggressive diffuse B-cell lymphoma (SWOG-0014). Blood 2004;104(11):abstract 158.
76. Lichtenstein AK, Levine A, Taylor CR, et al. Primary mediastinal lymphoma in adults. Am J Med 1980;68(4):509–514.
77. Cazals-Hatem D, Lepage E, Brice P, et al. Primary mediastinal large B-cell lymphoma. A clinicopathologic study of 141 cases

compared with 916 nonmediastinal large B-cell lymphomas, a GELA ("Groupe d'Etude des Lymphomes de l'Adulte") study. Am J Surg Pathol 1996;20(7):877–888.
78. Lazzarino M, Orlandi E, Paulli M, et al. Treatment outcome and prognostic factors for primary mediastinal (thymic) B-cell lymphoma: a multicenter study of 106 patients. J Clin Oncol 1997;15(4):1646–1653.
79. Zinzani PL, Stefoni V, Tani M, et al. MACOP-B regimen followed by involved-field radiation therapy in early-stage aggressive non-Hodgkin's lymphoma patients: 14-year update results. Leuk Lymphoma 2001;42(5):989–995.
80. Todeschini G, Secchi S, Morra E, et al. Primary mediastinal large B-cell lymphoma (PMLBCL): long-term results from a retrospective multicentre Italian experience in 138 patients treated with CHOP or MACOP-B/VACOP-B. Br J Cancer 2004;90(2): 372–376.
81. Palanisamy N, Abou-Elella AA, Chaganti SR, et al. Similar patterns of genomic alterations characterize primary mediastinal large-B-cell lymphoma and diffuse large-B-cell lymphoma. Genes Chromosomes Cancer 2002;33(2):114–122.
82. Rosenwald A, Wright G, Leroy K, et al. Molecular diagnosis of primary mediastinal B cell lymphoma identifies a clinically favorable subgroup of diffuse large B cell lymphoma related to Hodgkin lymphoma. J Exp Med 2003;198(6):851–862.
83. Savage KJ, Monti S, Kutok JL, et al. The molecular signature of mediastinal large B-cell lymphoma differs from that of other diffuse large B-cell lymphomas and shares features with classical Hodgkin lymphoma. Blood 2003;102(12):3871–3879.
84. Abou-Elella AA, Weisenburger DD, Vose JM, et al. Primary mediastinal large B-cell lymphoma: a clinicopathologic study of 43 patients from the Nebraska Lymphoma Study Group. J Clin Oncol 1999;17(3):784–790.
85. Portlock CS, Qin J, Schaindlin P, et al. The NHL-15 protocol for aggressive non-Hodgkin's lymphomas: a sequential dose-dense, dose-intense regimen of doxorubicin, vincristine and high-dose cyclophosphamide. Ann Oncol 2004;15(10):1495–1503.
86. Hamlin PA, Portlock CS, Straus DJ, et al. Primary mediastinal large B cell lymphoma: elucidating optimal therapy and prognostic factors; an analysis in 141 consecutive patients treated at Memorial Sloan Kettering from 1980–1999. Blood 2004; 104(11):abstract 614.
87. Lopez-Guillermo A, Cid J, Salar A, et al. Peripheral T-cell lymphomas: initial features, natural history, and prognostic factors in a series of 174 patients diagnosed according to the R.E.A.L. Classification. Ann Oncol 1998;9(8):849–855.
88. Rudiger T, Weisenburger DD, Anderson JR, et al. Peripheral T-cell lymphoma (excluding anaplastic large-cell lymphoma): results from the Non-Hodgkin's Lymphoma Classification Project. Ann Oncol 2002;13(1):140–149.
89. Gisselbrecht C, Gaulard P, Lepage E, et al. Prognostic significance of T-cell phenotype in aggressive non-Hodgkin's lymphomas. Groupe d'Etude des Lymphomes de l'Adulte (GELA). Blood 1998;92(1):76–82.
90. Ansell SM, Habermann TM, Kurtin PJ, et al. Predictive capacity of the International Prognostic Factor Index in patients with peripheral T-cell lymphoma. J Clin Oncol 1997;15(6):2296–2301.
91. Fisher RI, Gaynor ER, Dahlberg S, et al. Comparison of a standard regimen (CHOP) with three intensive chemotherapy regimens for advanced non-Hodgkin's lymphoma. N Engl J Med 1993;328(14):1002–1006.
92. Philip T, Guglielmi C, Hagenbeek A, et al. Autologous bone marrow transplantation as compared with salvage chemotherapy in relapses of chemo-therapy-sensitive non-Hodgkin's lymphoma. N Engl J Med 1995;333(23):1540–1545.
93. Philip T, Chauvin F, Armitage J, et al. Parma international protocol: pilot study of DHAP followed by involved-field radiotherapy and BEAC with autologous bone marrow transplantation. Blood 1991; 77(7):1587–1592.
94. Chao NJ, Rosenberg SA, Horning SJ. CEPP(B): an effective and well-tolerated regimen in poor-risk, aggressive non-Hodgkin's lymphoma. Blood 1990;76(7):1293–1298.
95. Wilson WH, Bryant G, Bates S, et al. EPOCH chemotherapy: toxicity and efficacy in relapsed and refractory non-Hodgkin's lymphoma. J Clin Oncol 1993;11(8):1573–1582.
96. Philip T, Armitage JO, Spitzer G, et al. High-dose therapy and autologous bone marrow transplantation after failure of conventional chemotherapy in adults with intermediate-grade or high-grade non-Hodgkin's lymphoma. N Engl J Med 1987; 316(24):1493–1498.
97. Velasquez WS, Cabanillas F, Salvador P, et al. Effective salvage therapy for lymphoma with cisplatin in combination with high-dose Ara-C and dexamethasone (DHAP). Blood 1988;71(1): 117–122.
98. Velasquez WS, McLaughlin P, Tucker S, et al. ESHAP—an effective chemotherapy regimen in refractory and relapsing lymphoma: a 4-year follow-up study. J Clin Oncol 1994;12(6): 1169–1176.
99. Colwill R, Crump M, Couture F, et al. Mini-BEAM as salvage therapy for relapsed or refractory Hodgkin's disease before intensive therapy and autologous bone marrow transplantation. J Clin Oncol 1995;13(2):396–402.
100. Girouard C, Dufresne J, Imrie K, et al. Salvage chemotherapy with mini-BEAM for relapsed or refractory non-Hodgkin's lymphoma prior to autologous bone marrow transplantation. Ann Oncol 1997;8(7):675–680.
101. Moskowitz CH, Bertino JR, Glassman JR, et al. Ifosfamide, carboplatin, and etoposide: a highly effective cytoreduction and peripheral-blood progenitor-cell mobilization regimen for transplant-eligible patients with non-Hodgkin's lymphoma. J Clin Oncol 1999;17(12):3776–3785.
102. Magagnoli M, Sarina B, Balzarotti M, et al. Mobilizing potential of ifosfamide/vinorelbine-based chemotherapy in prereated malignant lymphoma. Bone Marrow Transplant 2001;28(10): 923–927.
103. Mayer J, Vasova I, Koristek Z, et al. Ifosfamide- and etoposide-based chemotherapy as salvage and mobilizing regimens for poor prognosis lymphoma. Eur J Haematol Suppl 2001;64:21–27.
104. Watts MJ, Ings SJ, Leverett D, et al. ESHAP and G-CSF is a superior blood stem cell mobilizing regimen compared to cyclophosphamide 1.5 $g m^2$ and G-CSF for pre-treated lymphoma patients: a matched pairs analysis of 78 patients. Br J Cancer 2000;82(2):278–282.
105. Kewalramani T, Zelenetz AD, Nimer SD, et al. Rituximab and ICE as second-line therapy before autologous stem cell transplantation for relapsed or primary refractory diffuse large B-cell lymphoma. Blood 2004;103(10):3684–3688.
106. Pavone V, Gaudio F, Guarini A, et al. Mobilization of peripheral blood stem cells with high-dose cyclophosphamide or the DHAP regimen plus G-CSF in non-Hodgkin's lymphoma. Bone Marrow Transplant 2002;29(4):285–290.
107. Zelenetz AD, Hamlin P, Kewalramani T, et al. Ifosfamide, carboplatin, etoposide (ICE)-based second-line chemotherapy for the management of relapsed and refractory aggressive non-Hodgkin's lymphoma. Ann Oncol 2003;14(suppl 1):i5–i10.
108. Gisselbrecht C, Mounier N. Improving second-line therapy in aggressive non-Hodgkin's lymphoma. Semin Oncol 2004;31(1 suppl 2):12–16.
109. Kewalramani T, Zelenetz AD, Hedrick EE, et al. High-dose chemoradiotherapy and autologous stem cell transplantation for patients with primary refractory aggressive non-Hodgkin lymphoma: an intention-to-treat analysis. Blood 2000;96(7): 2399–2404.
110. Peniket AJ, Ruiz de Elvira MC, Taghipour G, et al. An EBMT registry matched study of allogeneic stem cell transplants for lymphoma: allogeneic transplantation is associated with a lower relapse rate but a higher procedure-related mortality rate than

autologous transplantation. Bone Marrow Transplant 2003;31(8): 667–678.
111. Schimmer AD, Jamal S, Messner H, et al. Allogeneic or autologous bone marrow transplantation (BMT) for non-Hodgkin's lymphoma (NHL): results of a provincial strategy. Ontario BMT Network, Canada. Bone Marrow Transplant 2000;26(8): 859–864.
112. Freytes CO, Loberiza FR, Rizzo JD, et al. Myeloablative allogeneic hematopoietic stem cell transplantation in patients who experience relapse after autologous stem cell transplantation for lymphoma: a report of the International Bone Marrow Transplant Registry. Blood 2004;104(12):3797–3803.
113. Glass B, Nickelsen M, Dreger P, et al. Reduced-intensity conditioning prior to allogeneic transplantation of hematopoietic stem cells: the need for T cells early after transplantation to induce a graft-versus-lymphoma effect. Bone Marrow Transplant 2004;34(5):391–397.
114. Horwitz SM, Negrin RS, Blume KG, et al. Rituximab as adjuvant to high-dose therapy and autologous hematopoietic cell transplantation for aggressive non-Hodgkin lymphoma. Blood 2004;103(3):777–783.
115. Shimoni A, Hardan I, Avigdor A, et al. Rituximab reduces relapse risk after allogeneic and autologous stem cell transplantation in patients with high-risk aggressive non-Hodgkin's lymphoma. Br J Haematol 2003;122(3):457–464.
116. Vose JM, Anderson JR, Kessinger A, et al. High-dose chemotherapy and autologous hematopoietic stem-cell transplantation for aggressive non-Hodgkin's lymphoma. J Clin Oncol 1993;11(10): 1846–1851.
117. Prince HM, Imrie K, Crump M, et al. The role of intensive therapy and autologous blood and marrow transplantation for chemotherapy-sensitive relapsed and primary refractory non-Hodgkin's lymphoma: identification of major prognostic groups. Br J Haematol 1996;92(4):880–889.
118. Horning SJ. Natural history of and therapy for the indolent non-Hodgkin's lymphomas. Semin Oncol 1993;20(5 suppl 5):75–88.
119. McLaughlin P. The role of interferon in the therapy of malignant lymphoma. Biomed Pharmacother 1996;50(3–4):140–148.
120. Hiddemann W, Griesinger F, Unterhalt M. Interferon alfa for the treatment of follicular lymphomas. Cancer J Sci Am 1998;4(suppl 2):S13–S18.
121. Allen IE, Ross SD, Borden SP, et al. Meta-analysis to assess the efficacy of interferon-alpha in patients with follicular non-Hodgkin's lymphoma. J Immunother 2001;24(1):58–65.
122. Coiffier B, Neidhardt-Berard EM, Tilly H, et al. Fludarabine alone compared to CHVP plus interferon in elderly patients with follicular lymphoma and adverse prognostic parameters: a GELA study. Groupe d'Etudes des Lymphomes de l'Adulte. Ann Oncol 1999;10(10):1191–1197.
123. Rohatiner A, Radford J, Deakin D, et al. A randomized controlled trial to evaluate the role of interferon as initial and maintenance therapy in patients with follicular lymphoma. Br J Cancer 2001;85(1):29–35.
124. Aviles A, Neri N, Huerta-Guzman J, et al. Interferon alpha 2b as maintenance therapy improves outcome in follicular lymphoma. Leuk Lymphoma 2004;45(11):2247–2251.
125. Acker B, Hoppe RT, Colby TV, et al. Histologic conversion in the non-Hodgkin's lymphomas. J Clin Oncol 1983;1(1): 11–16.
126. Yuen AR, Kamel OW, Halpern J, et al. Long-term survival after histologic transformation of low-grade follicular lymphoma. J Clin Oncol 1995;13(7):1726–1733.
127. Zucca E, Cavalli F. Are antibiotics the treatment of choice for gastric lymphoma? Curr Hematol Rep 2004;3(1):11–16.
128. Liu H, Ruskon-Fourmestraux A, Lavergne-Slove A, et al. Resistance of t(11;18) positive gastric mucosa-associated lymphoid tissue lymphoma to *Helicobacter pylori* eradication therapy. Lancet 2001;357(9249):39–40.
129. Ye H, Liu H, Raderer M, et al. High incidence of t(11;18)(q21;q21) in *Helicobacter pylori*-negative gastric MALT lymphoma. Blood 2003;101(7):2547–2550.
130. Schechter NR, Portlock CS, Yahalom J. Treatment of mucosa-associated lymphoid tissue lymphoma of the stomach with radiation alone. J Clin Oncol 1998;16(5):1916–1921.
131. Tsang RW, Gospodarowicz MK, Pintilie M, et al. Localized mucosa-associated lymphoid tissue lymphoma treated with radiation therapy has excellent clinical outcome. J Clin Oncol 2003;21(22):4157–4164.
132. MacManus MP, Hoppe RT. Is radiotherapy curative for stage I and II low-grade follicular lymphoma? Results of a long-term follow-up study of patients treated at Stanford University. J Clin Oncol 1996;14(4):1282–1290.
133. Tsang RW, Gospodarowicz MK, O'Sullivan B. Staging and management of localized non-Hodgkin's lymphomas: variations among experts in radiation oncology. Int J Radiat Oncol Biol Phys 2002;52(3):643–651.
134. Advani R, Rosenberg SA, Horning SJ. Stage I and II follicular non-Hodgkin's lymphoma: long-term follow-up of no initial therapy. J Clin Oncol 2004;22(8):1454–1459.
135. Carde P, Burgers JM, van Glabbeke M, et al. Combined radiotherapy-chemotherapy for early stages non-Hodgkin's lymphoma: the 1975–1980 EORTC controlled lymphoma trial. Radiother Oncol 1984;2(4):301–312.
136. Seymour JF, Pro B, Fuller LM, et al. Long-term follow-up of a prospective study of combined modality therapy for stage I–II indolent non-Hodgkin's lymphoma. J Clin Oncol 2003;21(11): 2115–2122.
137. Portlock CS. Deferral of initial therapy for advanced indolent lymphomas. Cancer Treat Rep 1982;66(3):417–419.
138. Horning SJ, Rosenberg SA. The natural history of initially untreated low-grade non-Hodgkin's lymphomas. N Engl J Med 1984;311(23):1471–1475.
139. Young RC, Longo DL, Glatstein E, et al. The treatment of indolent lymphomas: watchful waiting vs. aggressive combined modality treatment. Semin Hematol 1988;25(2 suppl 2): 11–16.
140. Brice P, Bastion Y, Lepage E, et al. Comparison in low-tumor-burden follicular lymphomas between an initial no-treatment policy, prednimustine, or interferon alfa: a randomized study from the Groupe d'Etude des Lymphomes Folliculaires. Groupe d'Etude des Lymphomes de l'Adulte. J Clin Oncol 1997;15(3): 1110–1107.
141. Zelenetz AD, Hoppe RT. NCCN: non-Hodgkin's lymphoma. Cancer Control 2001;8(6 suppl 2):102–113.
142. Peterson BA, Petroni GR, Frizzera G, et al. Prolonged single-agent versus combination chemotherapy in indolent follicular lymphomas: a study of the cancer and leukemia group B. J Clin Oncol 2003;21(1):5–15.
143. Longo DL, Young RC, Hubbard SM, et al. Prolonged initial remission in patients with nodular mixed lymphoma. Ann Intern Med 1984;100(5):651–656.
144. Dana BW, Dahlberg S, Nathwani BN, et al. Long-term follow-up of patients with low-grade malignant lymphomas treated with doxorubicin-based chemotherapy or chemoimmunotherapy. J Clin Oncol 1993; 11(4):644–651.
145. Lepage E, Sebban C, Gisselbrecht C, et al. Treatment of low-grade non-Hodgkin's lymphomas: assessment of doxorubicin in a controlled trial. Hematol Oncol 1990;8(1):31–39.
146. Zinzani PL, Magagnoli M, Moretti L, et al. Randomized trial of fludarabine versus fludarabine and idarubicin as frontline treatment in patients with indolent or mantle-cell lymphoma. J Clin Oncol 2000;18(4):773–779.
147. Zinzani PL, Pulsoni A, Perrotti A, et al. Fludarabine plus mitoxantrone with and without rituximab versus CHOP with and without rituximab as front-line treatment for patients with follicular lymphoma. J Clin Oncol 2004;22(13):2654–2661.

148. Maloney DG, Liles TM, Czerwinski DK, et al. Phase I clinical trial using escalating single-dose infusion of chimeric anti-CD20 monoclonal antibody (IDEC-C2B8) in patients with recurrent B-cell lymphoma. Blood 1994;84(8):2457–2466.
149. Maloney DG, Grillo-Lopez AJ, Bodkin DJ, et al. IDEC-C2B8: results of a phase I multiple-dose trial in patients with relapsed non-Hodgkin's lymphoma. J Clin Oncol 1997;15(10):3266–274.
150. McLaughlin P, Grillo-Lopez AK, Link BK, et al. Rituximab chimeric anti-CD20 monoclonal antibody therapy for relapsed indolent lymphoma: half of patients respond to a four-dose treatment program. J Clin Oncol 1998;16(8):2825–2833.
151. Davis TA, Grillo-Lopez AJ, White CA, et al. Rituximab anti-CD20 monoclonal antibody therapy in non-Hodgkin's lymphoma: safety and efficacy of re-treatment. J Clin Oncol 2000;18(17):3135–3143.
152. Hainsworth JD, Burris, HA 3rd, Morrissey LH, et al. Rituximab monoclonal antibody as initial systemic therapy for patients with low-grade non-Hodgkin lymphoma. Blood 2000;95(10): 3052–30526.
153. Colombat P, Salles G, Brousse M, et al. Rituximab (anti-CD20 monoclonal antibody) as single first-line therapy for patients with follicular lymphoma with a low tumor burden: clinical and molecular evaluation. Blood 2001;97(1):101–106.
154. Witzig TE, Vukov AM, Habermann TM, et al. Rituximab therapy for patients with newly diagnosed, advanced-stage, follicular grade I non-Hodgkin's lymphoma: a phase II trial in the North Central Cancer Treatment Group. J Clin Oncol 2005;23(6):1103–1108.
155. Hainsworth JD, Litchy S, Burris HA 3rd, et al. Rituximab as first-line and maintenance therapy for patients with indolent non-Hodgkin's lymphoma. J Clin Oncol 2002;20(20):4261–4267.
156. Ghielmini M, Schmitz SF, Cogliatti SB, et al. Prolonged treatment with rituximab in patients with follicular lymphoma significantly increases event-free survival and response duration compared with the standard weekly x 4 schedule. Blood 2004;103(12):4416–4423.
157. Hainsworth JD, Litchy S, Shaffer DW, et al. Maximizing therapeutic benefit of rituximab: maintenance therapy versus re-treatment at progression in patients with indolent non-Hodgkin's lymphoma: a randomized phase II trial of the Minnie Pearl Cancer Research Network. J Clin Oncol 2005; 23(6):1088–1095.
158. Czuczman MS, Grillo-Lopez AJ, White CA, et al. Treatment of patients with low-grade B-cell lymphoma with the combination of chimeric anti-CD20 monoclonal antibody and CHOP chemotherapy. J Clin Oncol 1999;17(1):268–276.
159. Czuczman MS, Weaver R, Alkuzweny B, et al. Prolonged clinical and molecular remission in patients with low-grade or follicular non-Hodgkin's lymphoma treated with rituximab plus CHOP chemotherapy: 9-year follow-up. J Clin Oncol 2004;22(23):4711–4716.
160. Forstpointner R, Dreyling M, Repp R, et al. The addition of rituximab to a combination of fludarabine, cyclophosphamide, mitoxantrone (FCM) significantly increases the response rate and prolongs survival as compared with FCM alone in patients with relapsed and refractory follicular and mantle cell lymphomas: results of a prospective randomized study of the German Low-Grade Lymphoma Study Group. Blood 2004; 104(10):3064–3071.
161. Marcus R, Imrie K, Belch A, et al. CVP chemotherapy plus rituximab compared with CVP as first-line treatment for advanced follicular lymphoma. Blood 2005;105(4):1417–1423.
162. Demidem A, Lam T, Alas S, et al. Chimeric anti-CD20 (IDEC-C2B8) monoclonal antibody sensitizes a B cell lymphoma cell line to cell killing by cytotoxic drugs. Cancer Biother Radiopharm 1997;12(3):177–186.
163. Emmanouilides C, Jazirehi AR, Bonavida B. Rituximab-mediated sensitization of B-non-Hodgkin's lymphoma (NHL) to cytotoxicity induced by paclitaxel, gemcitabine, and vinorelbine. Cancer Biother Radiopharm 2002;17(6):621–630.
164. Chinn P, Braslawsky G, White C, et al. Antibody therapy of non-Hodgkin's B-cell lymphoma. Cancer Immunol Immunother 2003;52(5):257–280.
165. Hiddemann W, Dreyling MH, Forstpointner R, et al. Combined immuno-chemotherapy (R-CHOP) significantly improves time to treatment failure in first line therapy of follicular lymphoma. Results of a prospective randomized trial of the German Low Grade Lymphoma Study Group (GLSG). Blood 2003;102(11): abstract 352.
166. Richaud P, Hoerni-Simon G, Denepoux R, et al. Total body irradiation (T.B.I.). Preliminary results of a new technique in 30 patients with hematologic malignancy. Strahlentherapie 1979;155(11):736–739.
167. Rees GJ, Bullimore JA, Lever JV, et al. Total body irradiation as a secondary therapy in non-Hodgkin's lymphoma. Clin Radiol 1980;31(4):437–439.
168. Lybeert ML, Meerwaldt JH, Deneve W. Long-term results of low dose total body irradiation for advanced non-Hodgkin lymphoma. Int J Radiat Oncol Biol Phys 1987;13(8):1167–1172.
169. Jacobs P, King HS. A randomized prospective comparison of chemotherapy to total body irradiation as initial treatment for the indolent lymphoproliferative diseases. Blood 1987;69(6): 1642–1646.
170. Meerwaldt JH, Carde P, Burgers JM, et al. Low-dose total body irradiation versus combination chemotherapy for lymphomas with follicular growth pattern. Int J Radiat Oncol Biol Phys 1991;21(5):1167–1172.
171. Zelenetz AD. Radioimmunotherapy for lymphoma. Curr Opin Oncol 1999;11(5):375–380.
172. Witzig TE, White CA, Wiseman GA, et al. Phase I/II trial of IDEC-Y2B8 radioimmunotherapy for treatment of relapsed or refractory CD20(+) B-cell non-Hodgkin's lymphoma. J Clin Oncol 1999;17(12):3793–3803.
173. Vose JM, Wahl RL, Saleh M, et al. Multicenter phase II study of iodine-131 tositumomab for chemotherapy-relapsed/refractory low-grade and transformed low-grade B-cell non-Hodgkin's lymphomas. J Clin Oncol 2000;18(6):1316–1323.
174. Kaminski MS, Zelenetz AD, Press OW, et al. Pivotal study of iodine I-131 tositumomab for chemotherapy-refractory low-grade or transformed low-grade B-cell non-Hodgkin's lymphomas. J Clin Oncol 2001;19(19):3918–3928.
175. Witzig TE, Flinn IW, Gordon LI, et al. Treatment with ibritumomab tiuxetan radioimmunotherapy in patients with rituximab-refractory follicular non-Hodgkin's lymphoma. J Clin Oncol 2002;20(15):3262–3269.
176. Zelenetz AD. A clinical and scientific overview of tositumomab and iodine I-131 tositumomab. Semin Oncol 2003;30(2 suppl 4): 22–30.
177. Horning SJ, Younes A, Jain V, et al. Efficacy and safety of tositumomab and iodine-131 tositumomab (Bexxar) in B-cell lymphoma, progressive after rituximab. J Clin Oncol 2005;23(4): 712–719.
178. Gordon LI, Witzig T, Molina A, et al. Yttrium 90-labeled ibritumomab tiuxetan radioimmunotherapy produces high response rates and durable remissions in patients with previously treated B-cell lymphoma. Clin Lymphoma 2004;5(2):98–101.
179. Bennett JM, Kaminski MS, Leonard JP, et al. Assessment of treatment-related myelodysplastic syndromes and acute myeloid leukemia in patients with non-Hodgkin's lymphoma treated with Tositumomab and Iodine I-131 Tositumomab (BEXXAR(R)). Blood 2005;105(12):4576–4582.
180. Davis TA, Kaminski MS, Leonard JP, et al. The radioisotope contributes significantly to the activity of radioimmunotherapy. Clin Cancer Res 2004;10(23):7792–7798.
181. Witzig TE, Gordon LI, Cabanillas F, et al. Randomized controlled trial of yttrium-90-labeled ibritumomab tiuxetan radioim-

munotherapy versus rituximab immunotherapy for patients with relapsed or refractory low-grade, follicular, or transformed B-cell non-Hodgkin's lymphoma. J Clin Oncol 2002;20(10): 2453–2463.

182. Aviles A, Delgado S, Fernandez R, et al. Combined therapy in advanced stages (III and IV) of follicular lymphoma increases the possibility of cure: results of a large controlled clinical trial. Eur J Haematol 2002; 68(3):144–149.
183. Press OW, Unger JM, Braziel RM, et al. A phase 2 trial of CHOP chemotherapy followed by tositumomab/iodine I-131 tositumomab for previously untreated follicular non-Hodgkin lymphoma: Southwest Oncology Group Protocol S9911. Blood 2003;102(5):1606–1612.
184. Kaminski MS, Tuck M, Estes J, et al. ^{131}I-tositumomab therapy as initial treatment for follicular lymphoma. N Engl J Med 2005;352(5): 441–449.
185. Bierman PJ, Vose JM, Anderson JR, et al. High-dose therapy with autologous hematopoietic rescue for follicular low-grade non-Hodgkin's lymphoma. J Clin Oncol 1997;15(2):445–450.
186. Schouten HC, Kvaloy S, Sydes M, et al. The CUP trial: a randomized study analyzing the efficacy of high dose therapy and purging in low-grade non-Hodgkin's lymphoma (NHL). Ann Oncol 2000;11(suppl 1):91–94.
187. Schouten HC, Qian W, Kvaloy S, et al. High-dose therapy improves progression-free survival and survival in relapsed follicular non-Hodgkin's lymphoma: results from the randomized European CUP trial. J Clin Oncol 2003;21(21): 3918–3927.
188. Lenz G, Dreyling M, Schiegnitz E, et al. Myeloablative radiochemotherapy followed by autologous stem cell transplantation in first remission prolongs progression-free survival in follicular lymphoma: results of a prospective, randomized trial of the German Low-Grade Lymphoma Study Group. Blood 2004;104(9):2667–2674.
189. Deconinck E, Foussard C, Milpied N, et al. High dose therapy followed by autologous purged stem cell transplantation and doxorubicin based chemotherapy in patients with advanced follicular lymphoma: a randomized multicenter study by the GOELAMS. Blood 2005;105(10):3817–3823.
190. van Besien K, Loberiza FR Jr, Bajorunaite R, et al. Comparison of autologous and allogeneic hematopoietic stem cell transplantation for follicular lymphoma. Blood 2003;102(10):3521–3529.
191. Weinstock MA, Horm JW. Mycosis fungoides in the United States. Increasing incidence and descriptive epidemiology. JAMA 1988;260(1):42–46.
192. Kim, YH, Jensen RA, Watanabe GL, et al. Clinical stage IA (limited patch and plaque) mycosis fungoides. A long-term outcome analysis. Arch Dermatol 1996;132(11):1309–1313.
193. Kaye FJ, Bunn PA Jr, Steinberg SM, et al. A randomized trial comparing combination electron-beam radiation and chemotherapy with topical therapy in the initial treatment of mycosis fungoides. N Engl J Med 1989; 321(26):1784–1790.
194. Plank L, Hansmann ML, Lennert K. Centrocytic lymphoma. Am J Surg Pathol 1993;17(6):638–639; author reply 641.
195. Banks PM, Chan J, Cleary ML, et al. Mantle cell lymphoma. A proposal for unification of morphologic, immunologic, and molecular data. Am J Surg Pathol 1992;16(7):637–640.
196. Tsujimoto Y, Yunis J, Onorato-Showe L, et al. Molecular cloning of the chromosomal breakpoint of B-cell lymphomas and leukemias with the t(11;14) chromosome translocation. Science 1984;224(4656):1403–1406.
197. Motokura T, Bloom T, Kim HG, et al. A novel cyclin encoded by a bcl1-linked candidate oncogene. Nature (Lond) 1991; 350(6318):512–515.
198. Williams ME, Meeker TC, Swerdlow SH. Rearrangement of the chromosome 11 bcl-1 locus in centrocytic lymphoma: analysis with multiple breakpoint probes. Blood 1991;78(2):493–498.
199. Coignet LJ, Schuuring E, Kibbelaar RE, et al. Detection of 11q13 rearrangements in hematologic neoplasias by double-color fluorescence in situ hybridization. Blood 1996;87(4):1512–1519.
200. Yang WI, Zukerberg LR, Motokura T, et al. Cyclin D1 (Bcl-1, PRAD1) protein expression in low-grade B-cell lymphomas and reactive hyperplasia. Am J Pathol 1994;145(1):86–96.
201. Fisher RI, Dahlberg S, Nathwani BN, et al. A clinical analysis of two indolent lymphoma entities: mantle cell lymphoma and marginal zone lymphoma (including the mucosa-associated lymphoid tissue and monocytoid B-cell subcategories): a Southwest Oncology Group study. Blood 1995;85(4):1075–1082.
202. Yatabe Y, Nakamura S, Seto M, et al. Clinicopathologic study of PRAD1/cyclin D1 overexpressing lymphoma with special reference to mantle cell lymphoma. A distinct molecular pathologic entity. Am J Surg Pathol 1996;20(9):1110–1122.
203. Yatabe Y, Suzuki R, Tobinai K, et al. Significance of cyclin D1 overexpression for the diagnosis of mantle cell lymphoma: a clinicopathologic comparison of cyclin D1-positive MCL and cyclin D1-negative MCL-like B-cell lymphoma. Blood 2000; 95(7):2253–2261.
204. Rosenwald A, Wright G, Wiestner A, et al. The proliferation gene expression signature is a quantitative integrator of oncogenic events that predicts survival in mantle cell lymphoma. Cancer Cell 2003;3(2):185–197.
205. Bookman MA, Lardelli P, Jaffe ES, et al. Lymphocytic lymphoma of intermediate differentiation: morphologic, immunophenotypic, and prognostic factors. J Natl Cancer Inst 1990;82(9): 742–748.
206. Leitch HA, Gascoyne RD, Chhanabhai M, et al. Limited-stage mantle-cell lymphoma. Ann Oncol 2003;14(10):1555–1561.
207. Teodorovic I, Pittaluga S, Kluin-Nelemans JC, et al. Efficacy of four different regimens in 64 mantle-cell lymphoma cases: clinicopathologic comparison with 498 other non-Hodgkin's lymphoma subtypes. European Organization for the Research and Treatment of Cancer Lymphoma Cooperative Group. J Clin Oncol 1995;13(11):2819–2826.
208. Pittaluga S, Bijnens L, Teodorovic I, et al. Clinical analysis of 670 cases in two trials of the European Organization for the Research and Treatment of Cancer Lymphoma Cooperative Group subtyped according to the Revised European-American Classification of Lymphoid Neoplasms: a comparison with the Working Formulation. Blood 1996;87(10):4358–4367.
209. Argatoff LH, Connors JM, Klasa RJ, et al. Mantle cell lymphoma: a clinicopathologic study of 80 cases. Blood 1997;89(6): 2067–2078.
210. Bosch F, Lopez-Guillermo A, Campo E, et al. Mantle cell lymphoma: presenting features, response to therapy, and prognostic factors. Cancer (Phila) 1998;82(3):567–575.
211. Oinonen R, Franssila K, Teerenhovi L, et al. Mantle cell lymphoma: clinical features, treatment and prognosis of 94 patients. Eur J Cancer 1998;34(3):329–336.
212. Hiddemann W, Unterhalt M, Herrmann R, et al. Mantle-cell lymphomas have more widespread disease and a slower response to chemotherapy compared with follicle-center lymphomas: results of a prospective comparative analysis of the German Low-Grade Lymphoma Study Group. J Clin Oncol 1998;16(5): 1922–1930.
213. Unterhalt M, Herrmann R, Tiemann M, et al. Prednimustine, mitoxantrone (PmM) vs. cyclophosphamide, vincristine, prednisone (COP) for the treatment of advanced low-grade non-Hodgkin's lymphoma. German Low-Grade Lymphoma Study Group. Leukemia 1996; 10(5):836–843.
214. Khouri IF, Romaguera J, Kantarjian H, et al. Hyper-CVAD and high-dose methotrexate/ cytarabine followed by stem-cell transplantation: an active regimen for aggressive mantle-cell lymphoma. J Clin Oncol 1998;16(12):3803–3809.

215. Khouri IF, Saliba RM, Okoroji GJ, et al. Long-term follow-up of autologous stem cell transplantation in patients with diffuse mantle cell lymphoma in first disease remission: the prognostic value of beta2-microglobulin and the tumor score. Cancer (Phila) 2003; 98(12):2630–2635.
216. Foran JM, Rohatiner AZ, Cunningham D, et al. European phase II study of rituximab (chimeric anti-CD20 monoclonal antibody) for patients with newly diagnosed mantle-cell lymphoma and previously treated mantle-cell lymphoma, immunocytoma, and small B-cell lymphocytic lymphoma. J Clin Oncol 2000; 18(2):317–324.
217. Ghielmini M, Schmitz SF, Cogliatti S, et al. Effect of single-agent rituximab given at the standard schedule or as prolonged treatment in patients with mantle cell lymphoma: a study of the Swiss Group for Clinical Cancer Research (SAKK). J Clin Oncol 2005;23(4):705–711.
218. Romaguera JE, Fayad L, Rodriguez MA, et al. Rituximab plus hyperCVAd (R-HCVAD) alternating with rituximab plus high-dose methotrexate-cytarabine (R-M/A) in untreated mantle cell lymphoma (MCL): prolonged follow-up confirms high rates of failure-free survival (FFS) and overall survival (OS). Blood 2004;104(11):abstract 128.
219. Howard OM, Gribben JG, Neuberg DS, et al. Rituximab and CHOP induction therapy for newly diagnosed mantle-cell lymphoma: molecular complete responses are not predictive of progression-free survival. J Clin Oncol 2002;20(5):1288–1294.
220. Lenz G, Dreyling M, Hoster E, et al. Immunochemotherapy with rituximab and cyclophosphamide, doxorubicin, vincristine, and prednisone significantly improves response and time to treatment failure, but not long-term outcome in patients with previously untreated mantle cell lymphoma: results of a prospective randomized trial of the German Low Grade Lymphoma Study Group (GLSG). J Clin Oncol 2005;23(9):1984–1992.
221. Wilson WH, Neelapu S, Rosenwald A, et al. Idiotype vaccine and dose-adjusted EPOCH-rituximab treatment in untreated mantle cell lymphoma: preliminary report on clinical outcome and analysis of immune response. Blood 2003;102(11):abstract 358.
222. Martinez N, Camacho FI, Algara P, et al. The molecular signature of mantle cell lymphoma reveals multiple signals favoring cell survival. Cancer Res 2003;63(23):8226–8232.
223. Freedman AS, Neuberg D, Gribben JG, et al. High-dose chemoradiotherapy and anti-B-cell monoclonal antibody-purged autologous bone marrow transplantation in mantle-cell lymphoma: no evidence for long-term remission. J Clin Oncol 1998;16(1):13–18.
224. Decaudin D, Brousse N, Brice P, et al. Efficacy of autologous stem cell transplantation in mantle cell lymphoma: a 3-year follow-up study. Bone Marrow Transplant 2000;25(3):251–256.
225. Vandenberghe E, Ruiz de Elvira C, Loberiza FR, et al. Outcome of autologous transplantation for mantle cell lymphoma: a study by the European Blood and Bone Marrow Transplant and Autologous Blood and Marrow Transplant Registries. Br J Haematol 2003;120(5):793–800.
226. Dreyling M, Lenz G, Hoster E, et al. Early consolidation by myeloablative radiochemotherapy followed by autologous stem cell transplantation in first remission significantly prolongs progression-free survival in mantle-cell lymphoma: results of a prospective randomized trial of the European MCL Network. Blood 2005;105(7):2677–2684.
227. Kroger N, Hoffknecht M, Kruger W, et al. marrow transplantation for refractory mantle c Ann Hematol 2000;79(10):578–580.
228. Milpied N, Gaillard F, Moreau P, et al.High-dose t stem cell transplantation for mantle cell lymphoma: prognostic factors, a single center experience. Bone Transplant 1998;22(7):645–650.
229. Kasamon YL, Jones RJ, Diehl LF, et al. Outcomes of autol and allogeneic blood or marrow transplantation for mantle lymphoma. Biol Blood Marrow Transplant 2005;11(1):39–46.
230. Khouri IF, Lee MS, Saliba RM, et al. Nonablative allogene stem-cell transplantation for advanced/recurrent mantle-cell lymphoma. J Clin Oncol 2003;21(23):4407–4412.
231. Maris MB, Sandmaier BM, Storer BE, et al. Allogeneic hematopoietic cell transplantation after fludarabine and 2 Gy total body irradiation for relapsed and refractory mantle cell lymphoma. Blood 2004;104(12):3535– 3542.
232. Zelenetz AD, Donnelly G, Halaas J, et al. Initial treatment of mantle cell lymphoma with sequential radioimmunotherapy with tositumomab/iodine I-131 I-tositumomab followed by CHOP chemotherapy results in a high complete remission rate. Blood 2003;102(11):abstract 1477.
233. Oki Y, Pro B, Delpassand E, et al. A phase II study of yttrium 90 (^{90}Y) ibritumomab tiuxetan (Zevalin®) for treatment of patients with relapsed and refractory mantle cell lymphoma (MCL). Blood 2004;104(11):abstract 2632.
234. Gopal AK, Rajendran JG, Petersdorf SH, et al. High-dose chemo-radioimmunotherapy with autologous stem cell support for relapsed mantle cell lymphoma. Blood 2002;99(9):3158–3162.
235. Rajendran J, Gopal A, Durack L, et al. Comparison of radiation dose estimation for myeloablative radioimmunotherapy for relapsed or recurrent mantle cell lymphoma using (131)I tositumomab to that of other types of non-Hodgkin's lymphoma. Cancer Biother Radiopharm 2004;19(6):738–745.
236. Schenkein D. Proteasome inhibitors in the treatment of B-cell malignancies. Clin Lymphoma 2002;3(1):49–55.
237. O'Connor OA, Wright J, Moskowitz C, et al. Phase II clinical experience with the novel proteasome inhibitor bortezomib in patients with indolent non-Hodgkin's lymphoma and mantle cell lymphoma. J Clin Oncol 2005;23(4):676–684.
238. Goy A, Younes A, McLaughlin P, et al. Phase II study of proteasome inhibitor bortezomib in relapsed or refractory B-cell non-Hodgkin's lymphoma. J Clin Oncol 2005;23(4):667–675.
239. Belch A, Kouroukis CT, Crump M, et al. Phase II trial of bortezomib in mantle cell lymphoma. Blood 2004;104(abstract 608).
240. Strauss SJ, Maharaj L, Stec J, et al. Phase II clinical study of bortezomib (VELCADE®) in patients (pts) with relapsed/refractory non-Hodgkin's lymphoma (NHL) and Hodgkin's Disease (HD). Blood 2004;104(11):abstract 1386.
241. Wilson EA, Jobanputra S, Jackson R, et al. Response to thalidomide in chemotherapy-resistant mantle cell lymphoma: a case report. Br J Haematol 2002;119(1):128–130.
242. Damaj G, Lefrere F, Delarue R, et al. Thalidomide therapy induces response in relapsed mantle cell lymphoma. Leukemia 2003;17(9):1914–1915.
243. Kaufmann H, Raderer M, Wohrer S, et al. Antitumor activity of rituximab plus thalidomide in patients with relapsed/refractory mantle cell lymphoma. Blood 2004;104(8):2269–2271.

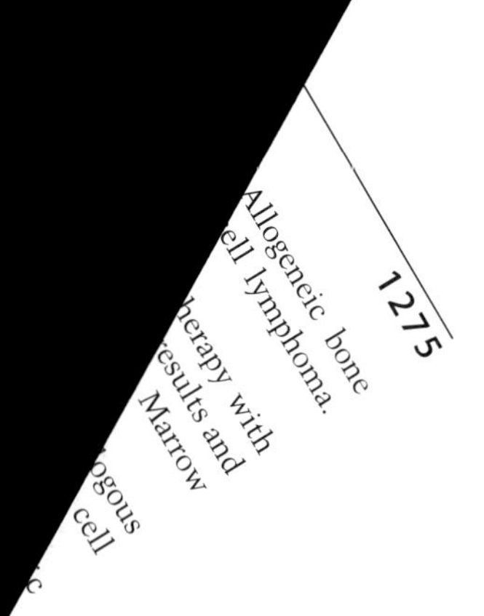

ltiple Myeloma

Robert L. Schlossman

Multiple myeloma (MM) is an incurable plasma cell neoplasm characterized by the accumulation of malignant plasma cells in the bone marrow. In the vast majority of cases, this neoplastic proliferation of plasma cells produces a monoclonal protein or immunoglobulin fragment that can be detected in the blood, urine, or both. Signs and symptoms of MM can be related to the location of these cells as well as the excessive production of irrelevant monoclonal immunoglobulin. As the malignant plasma cells expand in the marrow, normal surrounding bone can dissolve as a result of stimulation of osteoclasts by a variety of cytokines. Damage to the bone can lead to pain, pathologic fractures, and hypercalcemia. Furthermore, normal bone marrow can be suppressed, in particular, erythropoiesis. Impairment of the immune system leads to decreased humoral immunity with increased risk of infection, particularly encapsulated organisms. The paraprotein itself can lead to problems, including hyperviscosity, amyloid, and renal damage. This disease typically occurs in individuals in the sixth or seventh decades, but can also be seen in younger people. Systemic therapy is palliative. For decades, chemotherapy was based on single agents or combinations of alkylating agents and steroids. Despite great enthusiasm, dose intensification is not curative in the majority of cases, but can prolong overall survival (OS) and event-free survival (EFS). Newer drugs, based on antiangiogenesis approaches and targeting cytokine pathways, have generated a great deal of interest.

Epidemiology and Etiology

The estimated number of new cases of MM in the United States for 2004 was 15,270, for an incidence rate of 4 per 100,000 per year. The estimated number of deaths from the disease in 2004 was 11,070.[1] The prevalence is approximately 50,000. Although not considered a common disease, MM does account for 20% of deaths caused by hematologic malignancies in the United States. Although MM represents 1% of all malignancies, it is the second most common hematologic malignancy after non-Hodgkin's lymphomas. The disease does appear to be increasing slowly in incidence. This increase may be in part due to increased screening by routine blood work and more sensitive tests. One hypothesis is that the increased incidence may be real and the results of increasing environmental toxins known and unknown.[2,3]

Increased risk of developing MM may be related to the interaction of genetic and environmental factors, neither of which alone is enough to lead to disease. Environmental risk factors associated with an increased incidence of MM, include excessive exposure to petroleum products, organic solvents, pesticides, herbicides, Agent Orange, and radiation. Groups particularly at increased risk of exposure to these compounds include farmers, woodworkers, and paper producers.[4,5] An increased risk of MM was also noted in atomic bomb survivors exposed to more than 50 Gy radiation.[6] Although the genetic predisposition to the disease is not so strong as seen in other related lymphoproliferative disorders, MM has been described in first-degree relatives. Whether these associations represent a true genetic predisposition or a common environmental exposure remains unclear.

The Biology of MM

A process of immunoglobulin gene rearrangement characterizes normal B-cell development. As the B cell matures from a naïve pre-B to memory B cell and plasma cell, a number of genetic events occur. This process involves immunoglobulin VDJ rearrangement, somatic mutation, and immunoglobulin class switching.[7] The hypermutated sequences of joining regions of the VDJ can provide molecular markers for identifying the presence of clonotypic myeloma cells even in low numbers. Using CDR3 polymerase chain reaction technology, the malignant clone can be identified with greater sensitivity.[8]

MM is characterized by sheets of mature-looking plasma cells. The malignant cell is a B lymphocyte with a plasma cell morphology. These malignant plasma cells are cIg+, CD38+, CD56+, and BB-4+ (CD138+). MM cells can aberrantly express CD10, HLA-DR, and CD20.[7,9] The final oncogenic event leading to the development of MM appears to occur late in B-cell development based on immunoglobulin gene sequence analysis. The MM cell is postfollicular with the mutated homogeneous clonal sequences indicating no continuing exposure to somatic hypermutation.[9]

Chromosomal abnormalities occur in the range of 30% to 80%, but the true incidence is difficult to ascertain because of the low proliferative potential of MM cells and the methodology used to perform the analysis. Conventional cytogenetic analysis demonstrates abnormal karyotypes in 30% to 40% of patients,[10] whereas fluorescence in situ hybridization (FISH) analysis increases this figure to 80%.[11] Spectral karyotyping (SKY) purportedly detects chromosomal abnormalities in almost 100% of MM cells.[12]

The most common chromosomal abnormalities involve 14q32, which is the heavy-chain locus. In many cases, the translocation involves genes on the partner chromosome that encode growth or transcription factors. These nonimmunoglobulin chromosomes include 11q13, 4p16, 8q24, 16q23, and 6p25.[7] Deletions of the short arm of chromosome 13 correlate with a poorer outcome, although the associated genes remain to be identified.

The Bone Marrow Microenvironment

In addition to intrinsic genetic abnormalities, the role of the bone marrow environment in the pathogenesis of MM has come to be appreciated. Both normal and neoplastic plasma cells are attracted to the bone marrow via adhesion molecules and ligands. Once these cells enter the bone marrow microenviromment, they are exposed to a variety of cytokines that promote growth, migration, and survival. Specifically, bone marrow stromal cells (BMSC) secrete a variety of cytokines, including interleukin 6 (IL-6), vascular endothelial growth factor (VEGF), stromal cell-derived growth factor (SDF-1), and insulin growth factor (IGF-1).[13–15] In addition to attracting MM cells to the bone marrow, adhesion of MM cells to BMSCs results in paracrine secretion of IL-6 as well as VEGF. IL-6 is secreted via a NF-kB dependent pathway. IL-6 is a major growth factor for MM cells and results in increased survival and resistance to dexamethasone-induced apoptosis via a number of signaling pathways.

Another cytokine that plays an important role in MM is tumor necrosis factor-alpha (TNF-α). Although TNF-α does not act directly on MM cells, it does increase expression of cell-surface adhesion molecules via an NF-kB-dependent pathway. The adhesion molecules ICAM-1 and VCAM-1 are found on both BMSC and MM cells. Increased expression of these adhesion molecules results in binding of the MM cells to the bone marrow and secretion of IL-6.[16]

Clinical Presentation

The majority of symptomatic patients present with a combination of bone pain, fatigue, and recurrent infections. Cortical bone destruction leads to pain in the back and chest. The pain worsens with weight bearing and typically does not involve the joints. Compression fractures of the vertebral bodies can lead to neurologic complications, including weakness, neuropathies, muscle spasm, and the signs and symptoms of cord compression. Loss of height can occur if multiple vertebrae are compressed. Often, back pain is present for weeks to months before a patient seeks medical evaluation. Extensive bone involvement can result in hypercalcemia, which in turn can result in weakness, constipation, confusion, and arrhythmias and potentiate renal dysfunction. Other complications include anemia caused by marrow suppression, immune dysfunction, and end-organ toxicity secondary to paraprotein deposition. The paraprotein can be directly nephrotoxic as well as neurotoxic and can be deposited in a variety of tissues as amyloid. Fevers and night sweats are rare but occasionally seen. Organomegally is also rarely seen as a presented symptom. A subset of patients are diagnosed while asymptomatic when laboratory abnormalities are noted incidentally on annual physicals or during the course of a workup to evaluate other issues.

Bone Disease

One of the dreaded complications of MM is cortical bone destruction, which leads to bone pain and pathologic fractures. Bone damage appears to be mediated by osteoclast activation by a host of cytokines released by MM cells and bone marrow stromal cells (BMSC). These cytokines include lymphotoxin (LT), TNF-α, hepatocyte growth factor (HGF), IL-6, metalloproteinases, and insulin-like growth factor-binding protein 4.[17–21] Excessive production of these cytokines upsets the normal balance of bone modeling and favors bone reabsorption.

Approximately 70% to 80% of patients will experience bone pain during the course of their disease. The bone survey remains the standard imaging study. The classic abnormality is a punched-out lytic lesion typically seen in the axial skeleton, including the vertebrae, calvarium, ribs, and proximal long bones. Additional studies include computed tomography (CT) scans (although the risk of renal dysfunction due to contrast dye makes this imaging modality problematic), magnetic resonance imaging (MRI), and positron emission tomography (PET) scans. Extensive lytic bone disease is associated with hypercalcemia, which in turn can lead to constipation, weakness, and confusion. Bone scans are of limited use because of the pure lytic nature of these lesions. Osteosclerosis is uncommon and represents callus formation in healing of the POEMS variant of MM.

Another feared complication of MM is renal failure. Up to 25% of MM patients may experience some degree of renal dysfunction. The etiology of renal damage can be multifactorial and includes myeloma kidney, light-chain deposition disease, uric acid nephropathy, infection, hypercalcemia, dehydration, medication toxicity, and amyloid. In myeloma kidney, monoclonal light chains and intact immunoglobulin precipitate in the distal and collecting renal tubules, resulting in waxy casts. In light-chain deposition disease, monoclonal light chains deposit on the glomerular membrane. Another pattern of renal damage is due to the deposition of amyloid. These mechanisms of damage can be potentiated by dehydration. Also contributing to the damage caused by these mechanisms is hyperuricemia and medications. Nonsteroidal antinflammatory agents can potentiate renal damage by modulating afferent blood flow into the glomerulus.

Anemia is common and can result in profound fatigue. Factors that contribute to anemia, include bone marrow infiltration by MM, suppressed erythropoietin production in part caused by renal dysfunction, and chemotherapy. In some cases, anemia may be a consequence of iron deficiency, which may in turn be caused by chronic gastrointestinal blood loss from nonsteroidal antiinflammatory drugs (NSAIDs) or steroid-induced gastritis. Also contributing may be the anemia of chronic disease.

Sensorimotor neuropathies are common in MM. Neurotoxic agents used in the therapy of myeloma exacerbate these neuropathies. Neurotoxic agents commonly used in the therapy of MM, include vinca alkaloids, steroids, thalidomide, and bortezomib. Sensory neuropathy is a common presenting symptom in POEMS. The mechanism of nerve damage includes amyloid deposition, paraprotein directed against myelin,[22] and nerve root damage secondary to compression fractures. Other causes of neurologic involvement include carpal tunnel syndrome due to amyloid.

Recurrent infections with encapsulated organisms are common and result from compromised humoral-mediated immunity. In advanced disease, further immunosuppression can be caused by steroid use and neutropenia. Aggressive antibiotic therapy for bacterial, viral, and fungal infections is essential in reducing the risk of life-threatening sepsis. All patients should receive pneumococcal vaccine at diagnosis and influenza vaccines annually. Prophylaxis for *Pneumocystis carinii* pneumonia should be considered for all patients on steroid-based regimens. In addition, antiviral therapy is advised for patients at increased risk of reactivation of varicella zoster virus. This prophylaxis is particularly important following high-dose therapy. For individuals with recurrent life-threatening or debilitating infections, intravenous immunoglobulin infusions may be indicated for passive immunization and to help clear existing infections.

Less common complications include hepatomegaly, malignant pleural effusions, subcutaneous plasmacytomas, and blood clots. Hyperviscosity symptoms can occur in patients with IgM paraproteins, or rarely, in those with hyperviscosity are seen extremely high IgG levels (IgG subclass 3).

Laboratory Findings: Diagnostic Tests

- Complete blood count
- Measurement of electrolytes, BUN, creatinine, calcium, LDH
- Serum protein electrophoresis
- Serum protein immunoelectrophoresis
- Metastatic series
- Bone marrow aspirate and biopsy
- 24-hour urine collection for urine immunoelectrophoresis
- Free serum light chains
- B2 microglobulin, C-reactive protein, plasma cell labeling index

The evaluation proceeds in a stepwise fashion and includes routine blood work and radiographic studies. A normocytic normochromic anemia is seen in 62% of cases.[23] Usually the remainder of the complete blood count (CBC) is normal. On peripheral blood smear, rouleaux formation is common and can account for a falsely elevated mean corpuscular volume (MCV) on automated CBC determinations. Approximately 55% of patients have some degree of renal insufficiency, and 76% have a monoclonal spike of serum electrophoresis.[23] If the preliminary workup is suspicious, then a more detailed workup is undertaken to establish the diagnosis and estimate tumor burden. Additional tests can be utilized to evaluate the biologic aggressiveness of the disease. Patients with more aggressive appearing disease at initial diagnosis can then be counseled about the need for sooner intervention and the possible benefit of more aggressive therapy.

Establishing the diagnosis is the first step in evaluating a patient suspected of having MM. Combinations of major or minor criteria are then evaluated.[24] This evaluation includes defining a monoclonal protein in the serum, urine or both, presence of depressed normal immunoglobulins, presence of monotypic plasma cells, and lytic bone lesions. These diagnostic tests include a serum protein electrophoresis and urine immunoelectrophoresis to evaluate for a monoclonal protein in the blood, urine, or both. Quantitative immunoglobulins with immunofixation can further identify and quantitate the paraprotein. A monoclonal spike in the blood, urine, or both is found in 99% of patients with only 0.3% being nonsecretory.[23] While it remains unclear whether different types of monoclonal spikes are associated with different survival, they are associated with different complications. IgM and IgA myeloma have a higher association with hyperviscosity syndromes, whereas light chains have a higher association with renal dysfunction and amyloid.

Essential to the diagnosis is the demonstration of increased numbers of clonogenic plasma cell cells in the bone marrow. MM cells usually make up at least 10% to 30% of the bone marrow cellularity. Further identification of the plasma cell can be made with immunoperoxidase studies demonstrating light-chain restriction. In early-stage disease and some cases, involvement of the marrow can be patchy. Sampling error can lead to falsely elevated or reduced estimates of involvement when looking only at the percentage involvement in the marrow.

Once the diagnosis is established, other tests are performed to evaluate the extent of disease. Other tests used in staging, include a complete blood count (CBC) and chemistry panel, including blood urea nitrogen (BUN), creatinine, and calcium. For evaluating bone damage in MM, a skeletal survey remains the standard of care. Although the classic finding is a punched-out lytic lesion, other patterns can include diffuse osteopenia or a normal appearance to the bones. Typically, MM lesions involve the axial skeleton but can also be seen in the long bones. Other imaging studies useful in the evaluation of MM, include MRI. MRIs are particularly useful in evaluating bone damage that is not readily apparent on plain films. In addition, MRI is particularly sensitive for evaluating disease in the spine and defining the anatomy of the spinal cord and nerve roots. Myeloma lesions are commonly dark on T_1-weighted images and bright on T_2 images. Positron emission tomography (PET) is less well defined in MM. It may play a role in whole-body imaging of patients with nonsecretory disease and to evaluate extramedullary disease.

Differential Diagnosis

Although the diagnosis of MM is often clear once the tests are performed, monoclonal proteins can be associated with other disorders. The differential diagnosis for a monoclonal gammopathy includes monoclonal gammopathy of unknown significance (MGUS), smoldering myeloma, non-Hodgkin's lymphoma, chronic lymphocytic leukemia, primary amyloidosis, light-chain deposition disease, and Waldenstrom's macroglobulinemia. All but the MGUS, smoldering myeloma, and primary amyloid are fairly easy to distinguish when additional workup is pursued, including CT scans and flow cytometry.

The distinction between MGUS and smoldering MM is based on the amount of paraprotein and extent of bone marrow involvement. These disorders represent steps leading to the development of symptomatic MM, whereas primary amyloid represents a complication related to the biochemical properties of the paraprotein itself. Amyloid can develop in the context of both MGUS and MM. A MGUS is characterized by a M-spike of less than 3 g/dL and minimal involvement of the bone marrow by plasma cells. This disorder affects approximately 2% to 3% of individuals over 50 years old and increases in incidence with age. Commonly, the bone marrow looks normal but can have up to 10% involvement by plasma cells. Given the low number of plasma cells, a metastatic series should be normal, as well as the blood work, with the exception of the M-component. The diagnosis of a MGUS is associated with an increased risk of evolving into a malignant lymphoproliferative disorder. This risk is 24% overall and 1% per year in a large series from the Mayo Clinic.[25] Increasing paraprotein, elevated erythrocyte sedimentation rate (ESR), and presence of light chains are associated with an increased risk of transformation.[5] Thus, MGUS represents a premalignant B-cell disorder.

Smoldering MM may represent the next step in the evolution of a MGUS into MM. In smoldering MM, the M-component is more than 3 g/dL, and there is a greater degree of involvement on the bone marrow with more than 10% activity.[26] The development of smoldering MM from MGUS, may reflect changes occurring in the bone marrow that result in increased stimulation of plasma cells by cytokines and paracrine signaling.

Additional laboratory evaluation can be used to define how aggressive a particular patient's myeloma cells may behave. These factors include the B_2-microglobulin (β2M), level chromosome 13 abnormalities, C-reactive protein (CRP), IL-6 levels, plasma cell labeling index (PCLI), lactate dehydrogenase (LDH), plasmablastic morphology, and presence of circulating plasma cells in the peripheral blood. Of these tests, the β2M is the single most important prognostic factor. The β2M represents the light chain of the major histocompatibility complex of the cell membrane on lymphocytes. Increased plasma cell turnover, associated with a rapid growth fraction, results in increased β2M being shed into the serum. An elevated β2M in a patient with normal renal function is associated with poorer survival and a rising level is associated with disease progression.[27] Because β2M is renal excreted, renal insufficiency can falsely elevate the value.

Recently, chromosome 13 abnormalities have been shown to be an adverse prognostic factor. Deletions of the short arm of chromosome 13 (13q−) have been shown by FISH in approximately 40% of patients, and are associated with survivals of 27 months, compared to 65 months in patients without the deletion (P less than 0.001).[12,28,29] An elevated CRP correlates with shorter survival and elevated IL-6 levels.[30] As in NHL, an elevated LDH is also a predictor of poorer outcome.[31] The PCLI is a measure of plasma cell turnover in the bone marrow. Normally, plasma cells have a low mitotic fraction of less than 1%. A PCLI of 1% or greater is associated with more aggressive disease.[31] Plasmablastic morphology also correlates with more aggressive disease and shorter survival.[32]

For 30 years, MM has been classified based on the Durie–Salmon staging system.[33] This system was based on tumor burden and complications based on the evaluation. While this staging system was predictive of survival, it was not based on biologic features. The International Staging System for MM attempts to correct the deficiencies of the Durie–Salmon Staging system by utilizing only the beta-2 microglobulin and albumin.[34]

Initial Management

Once the diagnosis of MM is made, the next step is to initiate supportive care and decide whether systemic chemotherapy is warranted. Additional interventions include patient education, establishing a follow-up routine, and determining suitability for clinical trials. Supportive care includes reviewing the patient's history and updating immunizations, particularly for encapsulated organisms. These patients should be immunized against pneumococcal pneumonia and *Hemophilus influenzae* as well as influenza.

Newly diagnosed patients should be offered bisphosphonate therapy with either pamidronate or zolendronic acid as prophylaxis against bone disease. Bisphosphonates are analogues of normal pyrophosphonates involved in bone formation. These side-group substitutions allow pamidronate and zolendronic acid to be incorporated into bone but to prevent hydrolysis by osteoclasts. Pamidronate reduces the risk of skeletal-related events in patients undergoing chemotherapy from 42% to 24%, based on results from a randomized trial.[35] In this study, skeletal-related events were defined as pathologic fractures, bone pain, and bone damage requiring intervention. Based on this study and others, pamidronate has been approved for use in patients who meet diagnostic criteria for MM, demonstrate bone disease, and who are being started on systemic therapy. Bisphosphonate therapy in patients not requiring systemic therapy is controversial. Preclinical studies have demonstrated an antimyeloma effect for bisphosphonates in cell culture. This activity has been hard to demonstrate in the clinical setting. The newer bisphosphonate, zolendronic acid, has gained widespread use. While zolendronic acid is a more potent bisphosphonate in the laboratory, it has not been demonstrated to be superior to pamidronate in the clinical setting. Zolendronic acid is typically given over 20 minutes rather than the 2 hours recommended for pamidronate.

Although well tolerated, bisphosphonates have a number of potential side effects. The main concern is the risk of renal dysfunction. In patients with multiple risk factors for renal dysfunction, the relative contributions are not always apparent. This risk is low and may be related to rate of infusion. Initially, the incidence of renal dysfunction was believed to be higher with zolendronic acid than pamidronate, although some concerns did not materialize into a real problem. With more experience, this increased risk does not appear to be borne out. Possible explanations for the increased incidence of renal dysfunction associated with zolendronic acid, include rapid infusion rates and higher doses. When zolendronic acid was first evaluated, it was given in higher doses and over shorter periods. The current dosing recommendations of 4 mg over 20 minutes appear to be safe. In renal dysfunction due to pamidronate, patients sometimes develop an asymptomatic proteinuria. With zolendronic acid, this warning sign is not typically seen.

Other side effects seen with bisphosphonate therapy, include low-grade temperatures and bone pain. These complaints can begin within 24 to 48 hours of the infusion and are often self-limited. When these symptoms occur, prophylactic Tylenol can be useful. Another risk associated with pamidronate, in particular, is thrombophlebitis. This complication typically occurs at the site of a peripheral intravenous catheter and can be avoided with central lines. Hypocalcemia is another potential risk of bisphosphonate use. Given that many of these patients are normocalcemic at initiation of the therapy, it is common for calcium levels to run in the 8.0–8.4 range. In patients with renal insufficiency who are not receiving adequate calcium repletion, clinically significant hypocalcemia may occur. For patients with stable to responding disease, cautious calcium repletion is reasonable.

Duration of Therapy

Initially, there was much enthusiasm for bisphosphonates and the consensus recommendation is to continue therapy so long as the patient benefits.[36] This initial enthusiasm has been tempered by the recognition of long-term complications. Osteonecrosis of the jaw (ONJ) presents as pain in the maxilla or mandible. This pain can be associated with a draining sinus. Initial workup should include MRI or detailed radiographic studies. These lesions are frequently biopsied to distinguish between abscess, plasmacytoma, and osteomyelitis. Pathology is consistent with bone necrosis and superinfection. Intervention typically focuses on antibiotic therapy but can include debridement and reconstruction in more advanced cases. In patients with suspected ONJ, the bisphosphonate should be stopped immediately and the patient referred to a dentist or oral surgeon familiar with the complication.

Other Interventions

Newly diagnosed patients or those already receiving care may benefit from further interventions. Lytic bone disease is a particularly dreaded complication. In addition to systemic therapy, patients may benefit from more-localized interventions. These approaches can include surgical stabilization, kyphoplasty/vertebroplasty, and radiation therapy (XRT). XRT can be used to reduce the risk of a pathologic fracture, as well as palliatively to treat pain. In addition, it can be used with curative intent in the setting of an isolated osseous or extraosseous plasmacytoma. MM is sensitive to even low doses of XRT. Indications for XRT include palliation of an impending pathologic fracture of a weight-bearing bone or intractable pain in a non-weight-bearing bone. For patients with a solitary osseous plasmacytoma, definitive XRT can result in long-term disease-free survival in up to 50% of patients.[37] In these patients, the XRT is given with curative intent at higher doses. The typical palliative dose is 2,500 to 3,000 cGy, whereas in curative intent the goal is 4,250 cGy.

Indications for invasive stabilization of bones include pathologic fractures, impending pathologic fracture of a weight-bearing bone, or intractable pain in a non-weight-bearing bone. Interventions are most successful before a fracture occurs. Surgical stabilization of a long bone can often be accomplished via rodding and relatively small incisions. Once a long bone is fractured, then the surgery becomes more extensive. Vertebroplasty and kyphoplasty are less invasive interventions directed at stabilizing vertebral compression fractures. Indications include significant pain at a neurologic level and a compression fracture documented by MRI. Furthermore, the endplates of the vertebra must be intact with adequate space to insert the needles. Finally, the lesion must be relatively recent to avoid excessive calcification. If these requirements are met, then large-bore needles are inserted into the space between the endplates, avoiding the spinal cord. Balloon catheters are then inserted and inflated. The catheters are then removed and methyl methacrylate injected. A vertebroplasty differs only in omitting the balloon catheter step.

For patients not amenable to noninvasive intervention, then surgical stabilization is an option. Concerns about extensive surgery, include bleeding, inadequate anchoring of the devices, delayed wound healing, and increased risk of infection.

Other interventions considered supportive care, include hemodialysis (HD), plasmapheresis, and leukapheresis. The latter technique is reserved for patients with plasma cell leukemia (PCL) and the therapy of leukostasis. For patients with life-threatening complications of renal failure, HD is essential. Duration and etiology of renal failure can be predictive of which patients may recover function. The longer the duration of renal failure, the less likely patients are to recover. If patients are treated aggressively and promptly, the renal dysfunction may to some extent reverse over time. Plasmapheresis is controversial but does play a role in the treatment of hyperviscosity. It is most effective in IgA and IgM MM, because the majority of paraprotein is intravascular. Effective plasmapharesis can remove up to approximately 90% of circulating paraprotein and relieve the symptoms of hyperviscosity. The diagnosis is made clinically in a patient with more than 3 g paraprotein and appropriate symptoms, such as fatigue disproportionate to the degree of anemia, epistaxis, bruising, renal dysfunction, blurred vision, headaches, and pain. IgG paraproteins are less successfully managed with this strategy owing to a much larger volume of distribution. The role of plasmapheresis in the management of renal dysfunction and neuropathies caused by IgG or light-chain MM is much more controversial. Studies show both benefit and no advantage to plasmapheresis in this setting. Given that IgG and light-chain paraproteins have a much larger volume of distribution with a significant extravascular component, plasmapheresis should be accompanied by aggressive systemic therapy. Timing of chemotherapy with plasmapheresis is always difficult.

Conventional Therapy

Initial Treatment for Nontransplant Candidates

An important distinction to be made when initiating chemotherapy is whether the patient is a transplant candidate or not. For patients more than 70 years old or with significant comorbid illness, an alkylating agent is a reasonable choice. The combination of oral melphalan and predinisone (MP) has been used for three decades. MP is associated with a response rate of 50% to 60%,[38,39] is well tolerated, and is convenient. Typically, therapy is continued for 6 to 12 months until the monoclonal proteins stabilize in a plateau.

Once the patient enters a plateau, the therapy is discontinued and the patient monitored. Typical oral doses are 6 to 12 mg/m^2 by mouth each day for 4 days, repeated every 4 to 6 weeks. Other dosing schema include 0.15 mg/kg daily for 7 days. The prednisone is dosed at a fixed dose of 40 mg per day for 4 to 7 days to 40 to 60 mg/m^2. Because absorption of melphalan is unpredictable, the dose is often adjusted based on the degree of neutropenia at 3 weeks. Even in the absence of objective paraprotein response, patients may benefit in terms of symptoms and progression-free survival.

Although patients clearly benefited from MP, it was clear that other forms of therapy were needed. For patients with stable to responsive disease, median survival was of the order of 4 years. In patients with progressive disease, survival dropped to approximately 1 year. In an attempt to salvage MP failures and improve response rates, a number of combination chemotherapy regimens (CCT) were developed for MM. In single-institution trials, response rates in excess of 80% were reported. Popular regimens included vincristine, adriamcycin, and dexamethasone (VAD),[40] as well as vincristine, BCNU, melphalan, cytoxan, and prednisone (VBMCP or M2).[41] Multiple other regimens were developed, including alternating regimens. When these combination regimens were compared to MP, no difference was seen in efficacy. Gregory and colleagues conducted a meta-analysis of 18 randomized controlled trials comparing CCT with MP that showed no difference in response rates.[42] Further analysis suggested that patients with high-risk disease did benefit in terms of survival with CCT but that patients with standard-risk disease did not benefit.

Initial Treatment for Transplant Candidates

For patients being considered for transplant, induction therapy ideally should be effective and have minimal stem cell toxicity. Although many patients have received induction chemotherapy containing alkylating agents, there is evidence that this approach has quantitative and qualitative implications concerning the ability to collect stem cells. For individuals failing initial therapy based on thalidomide or dexamethasone, up to several cycles of cyclophosphamide-based therapy is a reasonable strategy. Before the widespread adoption of front-line thalidomide-based therapy, induction therapy was often accomplished using VAD. Typically, the VAD was administered for 4 months or up to 6 to 8 months until the patient entered a plateau. Risks associated with VAD include neutropenia, alopecia, hyperpigmentation, myocardial injury, neuropathies, and constipation. In addition to the side effects associated with chemotherapy, are those of clotting and infections due to an indwelling catheter. Another approach is single-agent dexamethasone. While the response rate may be lower with single-agent dexamethasone (Webber), this strategy is convenient and avoids the toxicity of vincristine and adriamycin, as well as the need for placement of an indwelling catheter.

Over the past several years, the antiangiogenic drug thalidomide has gained widespread use. Single-agent thalidomide was first shown to have activity in heavily pretreated patients.[43] Recently, studies evaluating the combination of thalidomide and dexamethasone in newly diagnosed patients have revealed it to be highly active with response rates of 80%.[44] Importantly, the combination does not appear to compromise the ability to collect adequate numbers of stem cells to perform single or tandem transplants. The common risks include sedation, constipation, neuropathies, and hypercoagulability. There are several dosing schedules using thalidomide in doses of 100 to 200 mg orally each night and dexamethasone 40 mg orally once a week to days 1 to 4, 9 to 12, and 17 to 20.

The toxicity of thalidomide and dexamethasone appears to be dose related. Lower doses in general are associated with fewer side effects. Sedation is addressed by using reduced doses and instructing the patient take the drug at night. Sedation occurs within 1 to 2 hours of taking the drug and can last for 8 to 10 hours. To reduce the incidence of constipation, patients are advised to take a combination of stool softeners and laxatives; more aggressive interventions may be necessary. Neuropathies are inevitable with thalidomide. The risk appears to be related to dose and duration of exposure. The neuropathy typically occurs as a sensorimotor neuropathy that occurs in a stocking-and-glove distribution. This complication can take weeks to months to develop and often begins as intermittent parathesias. The sensations can progress to become constant, severe in intensity, and progress proximally. Anecdotal evidence suggests that B vitamin supplementation may ameliorate the symptoms in some patients. In addition, nutritional supplements and electrolyte repletion may benefit selected patients. Other side effects include tachyarrhythmias, bradyarrhythmias, drug rashes including toxic epidermal necrolysis, and Stevens–Johnsons syndrome, visceral neuropathies, and fatigue.

Should patients not plateau in a minimal disease state following thalidomide-based therapy, options include single-agent cyclophosphomide, burtgonis, infusional doxorubutrin-based therapy, or investigational studies. Once a patient achieves adequate disease control, then there are three options. These options include observation, maintenance therapy, and consolidation with dose intensification and stem cell support. The argument for observation is based on the sense that the disease is incurable and that the response seen with initial therapy can last for 6 to 12 months without further intervention. Continuing initial therapy longer can be associated with increased treatment-related toxicity, stem cell damage, and the selection of a greater number of resistant MM cells. Any of these options requires ongoing observation and supportive care, including bisphosphonates and monitoring by blood work, urine studies, radiographic studies, and bone marrows when warranted. Should there be consistent evidence of disease progression, therapy can be reinstituted. If the relapse occurs more than 6 to 12 months after discontinuing therapy, then there can be benefit to another trial of the same therapy. If the progression occurs within 6 to 12 months, then another therapeutic option is a reasonable next step.

Numerous studies have evaluated the role of a variety of medications for maintenance. The rationale behind maintenance is to continue therapy in a reduced dose or schedule to prolong the response seen with the initial combination. The majority of studies evaluating the role of acintanse therapy, continue the chemotherapy in full dose or reduced dose, or consider other agents, such as interferon-alpha-2 (IFN-α). Although the main benefit appears to be in terms of prolonging the progression-free survival, none of these studies has shown a consistent benefit in terms of prolonging overall survival. When this modest benefit is weighed against the toxicity of some of these agents, the utility is questionable. Although IFN-α has been shown to prolong survival, the benefit was tempered by the decrement of quality of life in Quality Adjusted Time Without Symptoms of Toxicity (Q-TWIST) analysis.[45,46] In an update of the tandem transplant experience, maintenance therapy with thalidomide and bisphosphonate therapy was associated with a prolongation in overall survival.

Maintenance therapy with low-dose thalidomide is appealing because it is well tolerated, oral, and does not damage stem cells. For patients who wish to be proactive but are ambivalent about transplant, thalidomide maintenance is a reasonable compromise. Newer forms of thalidomide will be even more appealing in this role given the reduced toxicity. Unfortunately, one of several outcomes is inevitable on thalidomide maintenance. Typically, thalidomide is discontinued because of disease progression or neurotoxicity. Maintenance therapy with steroids has also been evaluated. In a Southwest Oncology Group (SWOG) study, alternating-day prednisone was associated with improved overall and event-free survival.[47]

Dose Intensification Followed by Stem Cell Rescue

High-dose therapy followed by infusion of autologous marrow or stem cells has become the standard of care in young and relatively healthy patients with MM. Despite high response rates and favorable side-effect profiles, MM remains an incurable illness. In addition, resistance can be overcome by dose intensification. As a consequence, the administration of alkylating agents in high doses with or without total-body irradiation, followed by infusion of allogeneic or autologous stem cells, is an appealing approach.

Autologous Stem Cell Transplantation

The rationale behind autologous transplantation is dose intensification to overcome resistance. Early studies performed at the Royal Marsden Hospital demonstrated that resistance to oral melphalan could be overcome by higher doses administered intravenously.[48] Unfortunately, this approach was associated with a high incidence of neutropenic complications. The addition of stem cell support was associated with shorter durations of neutropenia and a low risk of fatal infectious complications. Dose intensification is also associated with higher response rates when compared to conventional dose therapy. Although not curative, randomized studies demonstrate that patients treated with transplant have a prolonged overall and event-free survival compared to patients receiving conventional chemotherapy.

The first randomized study to demonstrate the benefits of autologous transplantation was the Intergroupe Francophone du Myelome 90 study, which enrolled 200 patients.[49] These patients received four to six cycles of vincristine, melphalan, cyclophosphamide, and prednisone (VMCP) alternating with carmustine, vincristin, doxorubicin, and prednisone (BVAP) for cytoreduction. They were then randomized to eight more cycles of VMCP/BVAP or autologous bone marrow transplant using melphalan and total-body irradiation (TBI). The results demonstrated a statistically significant prolongation in event-free and overall survival in those receiving transplant. Estimated overall survival at 5 years was 52% for the transplant arm versus 12% on the chemotherapy arm ($P = 0.03$). Another randomized study demonstrating the benefits of autologous transplantation is the Medical Research Council Myeloma VII study.[50] This study also demonstrated a superior outcome in terms of overall and event-free survival. The median survival was 54 months with transplantation versus 42 months with chemotherapy ($P = 0.04$). Additional Phase II and Phase III studies of single transplants have at best shown no benefit in survival or only an advantage in terms of response rates or progression-free survival.[51–53] Interpreting these studies is difficult. Although few if any patients are cured, at a minimum, transplant appears to improve response rates, prolong progression-free survival, and in some patients, prolong overall survival. The benefit appears to be on the order of 1 to 2 years at best. Importantly, this benefit must be weighed against the substantial toxicity of the process itself. It also appears that patients who may derive the most benefit are those who are less heavily pretreated and who have sensitive disease.

Strategies to Improve Outcome

Timing

Although there are an increasing number of therapeutic options for treating MM utilizing newer drugs and combinations, the emphasis remains to perform the transplant earlier in the disease course rather than later. The strategy to transplant in first or second remission is based on subset analysis of transplant trials, which suggested that the sooner patients were transplanted, the better the outcome. Ease and speed in bringing a patient to transplant selects for those who have sensitive disease and who are in a minimal disease state. Heavily treated patients are more likely not to achieve a minimal disease state and to have more resistant disease. The recommendation for earlier transplant is also a consequence of therapeutic options before the availability of thalidomide and velcade. Before these agents, first-line therapy consisted of dexamethasone-based therapy whereas cyclophosphamide-based therapy was utilized in second-line regimens. Obtaining a third remission and preserving stem cell function was not always possible. Only one large randomized study addresses the issue of timing. The Myelome Autogreffe study compared transplant in first remission versus second remission.[54] In this study, no difference was seen in survival. The overall survival was 64 months in both groups. The main benefit to early transplant in this study was in terms of quality of life analysis. Quality Adjusted Time Without Symptoms and Toxicity (Q-TWIST) analysis as reported by the early-transplant group was superior compared to the late-transplant arm. One explanation for this finding is that, although the patients in the second remission arm received milder upfront therapy, because of the relapse they required combination chemotherapy and transplant.

Conditioning

A variety of regimens are used in conditioning patients for high-dose therapy. These regimens typically rely on alkylating agents with or without TBI. TBI was included because of the radiosensitive nature of myeloma and different mechanism of action. Moreau et al., in an Intergroupe Francophone du Myelome (IFM) study, evaluated the role of TBI and determined that, although response rates were comparable, there was increased toxicity associated with melphalan plus TBI versus melphalan alone.[55]

Purging of Bone Marrow or Stem Cells

One explanation for relapses following autologous transplantation, is reintroduction of tumor cells at the time of stem cell reinfusion. Several strategies have been employed to reduce contamination of the bone marrow or stem cell product by tumor cells. First, patients are not even evaluated for transplant until they have demonstrated a clinically significant response to conventional therapy. An indirect benefit of using peripheral blood stem cells as compared to bone marrow is that there may be less contamination by tumor cells. Using polymerase chain reaction (PCR) analysis of the hypervariable joining regions of the immunoglobulin heavy-chain gene (CDR3 PCR), sensitive probes can be created to measure minimal disease.[8] CDR3 PCR analysis has demonstrated significantly less tumor cell contamination in the peripheral blood versus the bone marrow. Another approach taken to reduce contamination of the stem cell product by tumor cells is further manipulation to remove tumor cells or to select the normal stem cells. One approach was to use a cocktail of monoclonal antibodies directed at B-cell antigens combined with rabbit complement[56–58] to kill contaminating tumor cells. Another approach was to select for normal hematopoietic stem cells using an anti-CD34 monoclonal antibody combined with a biotin and avidin system.[59] Unfortunately, these approaches do not address residual systemic disease and did not translate into improved response rates or survival.

Multiple Transplants

In an attempt to improve outcome following single transplants, a number of strategies have evolved to do multiple transplants. These approaches range from performing second or even third transplants as salvage for relapsed disease to planning second transplants in a sequential fashion. A further refinement to this approach is an autologous transplant followed by allogeneic transplant. A number of studies have demonstrated that multiple transplants can result in higher response rates when compared to single transplants and conventional dose chemotherapy.[60–62] A number of groups have published studies suggesting improved outcome with tandem transplants.[63–65] While the Myeloma Autogreffe 95[65] fails to show a benefit and the Bologna 96 trial[64] only shows an event-free survival benefit of 44 versus 27 months ($P = 0.005$), the Intergroupe Francophone du Myeloma 94[66] does show both an event-free and overall survival benefit for the tandem transplant arm versus the single arm. The authors concluded that the survival benefit required at least 5 years of follow-up to reach statistical significance. At 7 years, the tandem arm demonstrated an overall survival of 42% versus 21% of the single-transplant arm ($P = 0.01$). This benefit becomes more impressive in patients who have a poorer response to the first transplant. In patients with less than a very good partial response within 3 months of the first transplant, the probability of surviving 7 years was 11% in the single-transplant group and 43% in the double-transplant group (P less than 0.001). This study illustrates several points. The most important message is that it may take longer follow-up to see a benefit from tandem transplants. Although it is early, a substantial number of patients still relapse. Although the transplant-related mortality is comparable between the two groups, the tandem arms may experience increased morbidity. Finally, the single arm in the study received less dose intensity than many single transplants use.

Allogeneic Stem Cell Transplantation

Allogeneic transplant has a number of theoretical advantages over autologous transplantation. Using stem cells from a normal donor avoids the risk of contamination by tumor cells and concerns of stem cell function resulting from exposure to chemotherapy. Importantly, donor stem cell products contain immunocompetent lymphocytes that can initiate a graft-versus-myeloma effect. These benefits come at a cost in terms of increased morbidity and mortality. The 1-year transplant-related mortality of an autologous peripheral blood stem cell transplant is approximately 0.5% to 2% in large centers. The transplant-related mortality of an allogeneic transplant depends on the source of the stem cells and the degree of match but ranges from 8% to an excess of 50%. This increased risk is due to a greater degree of immunosuppression and complications associated with graft-versus-host disease (GVHD) and its therapy. There is no larger randomized, prospective trial comparing autologous to allogeneic transplantation. Allowing for the initial increase in transplant-related mortality, survival curves appear similar.[67]

The single largest allogeneic transplant experience comes from the European Bone Marrow Transplant Group (EBMT).[68] For the 44% of patients who achieved a complete remission to allogeneic transplant, the overall survival was 32% at 4 years and 28% at 7 years. Overall progression-free survival was 36% at 6 years with only a handful of patients in continuing CR more than 4 years after transplant. The transplant-related mortality was 41%. In this study, favorable prognostic factors included being in a CR before transplant, fewer lines of conventional therapy, earlier stage at diagnosis, female, low β2m, and IgA isotype. In another large allogeneic experience from Seattle,[69] the transplant-related mortality was 44%. For the 36% of patients achieving a CR, the overall survival and event-free survival at 54 months were 20% and 24%, respectively. A smaller experience using T-cell depletion as the GVHD is from the Dana Farber Cancer Institute.[70] In this study, the early treatment-related mortality was 5%, with a CR rate of 28%; overall survival at 36 months was 40% and event-free survival at 38 months was 20%.

Donor Lymphocyte Infusion

The existence of a significant graft-versus-myeloma (GVM) effect was inferred from the increased incidence of CRs in allogeneic transplant, as well as delayed responses in some cases.[71–73] Donor lymphocyte infusion (DLI) has been used to treat relapsed disease as well as being used prophylactically posttransplant before a documented relapse. The use of DLI was particularly appealing in the setting of T-cell depletion for GVHD prophylaxis because of the reduced GVM effect resulting from T-cell depletion.[74] In this study, CD8-depleted DLI was utilized to further reduce the risk of GVHD. The DLI was performed at 6 months following a T-cell-depleted matched related donor transplant. In this setting, DLI accounted for addition responses but could only be performed in 58% of patients because of treatment-related mortality (TRM) and active GVHD.

Nonmyeloablative Transplants

The rationale behind a nonmyeloablative transplant is to reduce the toxicity of the transplant while maintaining a GVM effect. The reduced-dose conditioning therapy essentially represents immunosuppression to reduce the risk of graft rejection although melphalan-containing regimens have antimyeloma activity. The goal of this approach is to establish a chimera and to rely on the GVM for long-term disease control. In this setting, the use of DLI is even more appealing. Because of the reduced cytoreduction, nonmyeloablative transplants may be more appropriate for patients with indolent low-volume disease. Patients with aggressive high-volume disease may progress long before a GVM effect can be established. Preliminary results have demonstrated that nonmyeloablative transplants are associated with reduced immediate transplant-related morbidity and mortality.[75–77] These studies also demonstrate substantial acute and chronic GVHD.

Related Disorders

Osteosclerotic MM

Osteosclerotic MM is characterized by a polyneuropathy, organomegaly, endocrinopathy, M-spike, and skin changes (POEMS syndrome).[78] It is rare to see all these features present at once. These patients usually seek medical attention because of a progressive motor neuropathy. Renal dysfunction is rare, as is a significant anemia. Gynecomastia and testicular atrophy can be seen. The M-spike is often relatively low given the degree of symptoms. These patients respond to therapy although rarely does the neuropathy resolve.

Nonsecretory MM

Approximately 2% to 5% of patients with MM have no measurable M-spike. Prognosis does not appear to be different compared to patients with a M-spike.[79] Monitoring of the disease can be challenging but is not impossible. Disease response and progression can be measured following the anemia, change in reciprocal depressions of the serum immunoglobulins, and B2M. In addition, serial bone marrow examinations can add useful information. Free serum light-chain tests may be sensitive enough to detect free light chains not seen on 24-hour urine immunoelectrophoresis.

Plasma Cell Leukemia

Plasma cell leukemia (PCL) can occur during the course of therapy or be the presenting diagnosis. PCL is defined as a peripheral plasmacytosis of more than 20% or an absolute plasma cell count greater than 2×10^9/L. PCL is associated with a poor prognosis, although the median survival of patients with primary PCL may be better than those with secondary PCL. Median survivals are of the order of a year; although rare, patients can survive longer.

Solitary Plasmacytomas

Solitary plasmacytomas consist of isolated collections of plasma cells in bone or extramedullary tissues. Extramedullary plasmacytomas are associated with a median survival of 100.8 months versus 86.4 months for solitary osseous plasmacytomas.[80] Involved-field XRT is indicated and can be curative in selected patients.[37,81] Disappearance of the M-spike following XRT predicts for long-term disease-free survival.

Primary Amyloidosis

Primary amyloidosis is characterized by the accumulation of a homogeneous amorphous material consisting of the variable portion of light chains. Free lambda light chains predominate, and the formation of amyloid is associated with the degradation of light chains, which then form beta pleated sheets. The clinical manifestation of the disease correlates to the extent of end-organ damage.[82,83] Amyloid is relatively rare and can be divided into five categories. Primary amyloid is associated with lymphoproliferative disorders. Secondary amyloid is seen with chronic inflammation or infection. The other types are associated with inherited disorders, aging, and other malignancies. The clinical manifestations of amyloid include cardiac involvement with congestive heart failure and conduction disturbances, renal failure, and gastrointestinal involvement with malabsorption. The prognosis is dismal, and therapy is limited by organ toxicity. Therapy is palliative, and melphalan and prednisone remain the standard of care.[84] In selected patients, transplant is feasible and may improve symptoms.[85,86]

New Therapies

The treatment of MM has been revolutionized by the development of new drugs and combinations. At the root of this activity has been a growing understanding of the biology of MM cells and their complex interactions with the bone marrow microenvironment. This knowledge has led to new paradigms of drug development. Despite these developments, no drug appears to be curative. Rather than replacing the older agents, newer approaches allow additional lines of therapy and prolongation of survival. Although an old drug, thalidomide has been resurrected with MM. Based on an appreciation of the increased density of blood vessels in the bone marrow in myeloma and novel approach of attacking angiogenesis, thalidomide was evaluated in MM.[43,87] The mechanism of action does not appear to be suppression of neovascularization but rather, induction of apoptosis, inhibition of cytokine production and angiogenesis, and immunomodulation.[14,88,89] Response rates in relapsed patients were 25% to 30%.[43,87] In newly diagnosed patients in combination with dexamethasone, RR are in excess of 63% to 72%.[44,90]

Bortezomib is a proteosome inhibitor approved for second-line therapy in MM. Proteosomes play an important role in the regulation of intracellular proteins vital to cell function. In addition to dysregulation of cell-cycling proteins, bortezomib has been shown to have several other effects on both myeloma cells and stromal cells in the bone marrow. By inhibiting degradation of regulatory proteins that have been targeted for destruction by ubiquination, the cell can no longer remain viable. Molecular effects include stabilization of the inhibitory protein of the nuclear factor kappaB (NF-kB).[91] This effect blocks downstream activities of proliferation, survival, and angiogenesis. Bortezomib as a single agent in relapsed refractory patients has a response rate of 27%.[92] Studies combining bortezomib with other agents show even higher response rates.

Based on a growing understanding of the interactions between MM cells and the bone marrow microenvironment, new molecular targets are being identified. Novel agents are being evaluated that target the MM cell by interrupting MM cell growth, survival, drug resistance, and migration. These approaches include combining available drugs as well as novel drugs and analogues of thalidomide.

References

1. Jemal A, et al. Cancer statistics, 2004. CA Cancer J Clin 2004; 54(1):8–29.
2. Bourguet CC, et al. Multiple myeloma and family history of cancer. Cancer (Phila) 1985;56:2133–2139.
3. Kyle RA, et al. Incidence of multiple myeloma in Olmsted County, Minnesota: 1978 through 1990, with a review of the trend since 1945. J Clin Oncol 1994;12:1577–1583.
4. Bergsagel DE, et al. Benzene and multiple myeloma: appraisal of the scientific evidence. Blood 1999;94:1174–1182.
5. Cesana C, et al. Prognostic factors for malignant transformation in monoclonal gammopathy of undetermined significance and smoldering multiple myeloma. J Clin Oncol 2002;20:1625–1634.
6. Kyle RA, et al. A long-term study of prognosis in monoclonal gammopathy of undetermined significance. N Engl J Med 2002; 346:564–569.
7. Kuehl WM, Bergsagel PL. Multiple myeloma: evolving genetic events and host interactions. Nat Rev Cancer 2002;2(3):175–187.
8. Billadeau D, et al. Detection and quantitation of malignant cells in the peripheral blood of multiple myeloma patients. Blood 1992;80(7):1818–1824.
9. Vescio RA, et al. Myeloma Ig heavy chain V region sequences reveal prior antigenic selection and marked somatic mutation but no intraclonal diversity. J Immunol 1995;155:2487–2497.
10. San Miguel JF, et al. Immunological phenotype of neoplasms involving the B cell in the last step of differentiation. Br J Haematol 1986;62:75–83.
11. Harada H, et al. Phenotypic difference of normal plasma cells from mature myeloma cells. Blood 1993;81(1):2658–2663.
12. Facon T, et al. Chromosome 13 abnormalities identified by FISH analysis and serum beta2-microglobulin produce a powerful myeloma staging system for patients receiving high-dose therapy. Blood 2001;97:1566–1571.
13. Hallek M, Bergsagel PL, Anderson KC. Multiple myeloma: increasing evidence for a multistep transformation process. Blood 1998;91:3–21.
14. Mitsiades N, et al. Apoptotic signaling induced by immunomodulatory thalidomide analogs in human multiple myeloma cells: therapeutic implications. Blood 2002;99(12):4525–4530.
15. Hideshima T, et al. NF-kappa B as a therapeutic target in multiple myeloma. J Biol Chem 2002;277(19):16639–16647.
16. Hideshima T, et al. Biologic sequelae of interleukin-6 induced PI3-K/Akt signaling in multiple myeloma. Oncogene 2001;20(42):5991–6000.
17. Cozzolino F, et al. Production of interleukin-1 by bone marrow myeloma cells. Blood 1989;74:380–387.
18. Garrett IR, et al. Production of lymphotoxin, a bone-resorbing cytokine, by cultured human myeloma cells. N Engl J Med 1987;317:526–532.
19. Barille S, et al. Production of metalloproteinase-7 (matrilysin) by human myeloma cells and its potential involvement in metalloproteinase-2 activation. J Immunol 1999;163(10):5723–5728.
20. Hjertner O, et al. Hepatocyte growth factor (HGF) induces interleukin-11 secretion from osteoblasts: a possible role for HGF in myeloma-associated osteolytic bone disease. Blood 1999;94:3883–3888.
21. Lacey DL, et al. Osteoprotegerin ligand is a cytokine that regulates osteoclast differentiation and activation. Cell 1998;93: 165–176.
22. Latov N, et al. Plasma-cell dyscrasia and peripheral neuropathy with a monoclonal antibody to peripheral-nerve myelin. N Engl J Med 1980;303:618–621.
23. Kyle RA. Multiple myeloma: review of 869 cases. Mayo Clin Proc 1975;50:29–40.
24. Durie BGM. Staging and kinetics of multiple myeloma. Semin Oncol 1986;13:300–309.
25. Kyle RA. Monoclonal gammopathy of undetermined significance and solitary plasmacytoma. Implications for progression to overt multiple myeloma. Hematol Oncol Clin N Am 1997; 11(1):71–87.
26. Kyle RA, Greipp PR. Smoldering multiple myeloma. N Engl J Med 1980;302:1347–1349.
27. Durie BG, et al. Prognostic value of pretreatment serum beta 2 microglobulin in myeloma: a Southwest Oncology Group Study. Blood 1990;75:823–830.
28. Tricot G., et al. Unique role of cytogenetics in the prognosis of patients with myeloma receiving high-dose therapy and autotransplants. J Clin Oncol 1997;15:2659–2666.
29. Fonseca R, et al. Myeloma and the t(11;14)(q13;q32); evidence for a biologically defined unique subset of patients. Blood 2002; 99(10):3735–3741.
30. Bataille R, et al. C-reactive protein and b-2 microglobulin produce a simple and powerful myeloma staging system. Blood 1992;80:733–737.
31. Greipp P, et al. Plasma cell labeling index and b2-microglobulin predict survival independent of thymidine kinase and C-reactive protein in multiple myeloma. Blood 1993;81:3382–3387.
32. Greipp PR, et al. Plasmablastic morphology: an independent prognostic factor with clinical and laboratory correlates. Eastern Cooperative Oncology Group (ECOG) myeloma trial E9486 report by the ECOG Myeloma Laboratory Group. Blood 1998;91: 2501–2507.
33. Durie BGM, Salmon SE. A clinical staging system for multiple myeloma. Correlation of measured cell mass with presenting clinical features, response to treatment and survival. Cancer (Phila) 1975;36:842–854.
34. Greipp P, et al. International staging system for multiple myeloma. J Clin Oncol 2005;23(15):1–9.
35. Berenson J, et al. Pamidronate disodium reduces the occurrence of skeletal events in patients with advanced multiple myeloma. N Engl J Med 1996;334:488–493.
36. Berenson J, et al. American Society of Clinical Oncology Clinical Practice Guidelines: the role of bisphosphonates in multiple myeloma. J Clin Oncol 2002;20(17):3719–3736.
37. Moulopoulos LA, et al. Magnetic resonance imaging in the staging of solitary plasmacytoma of bone. J Clin Oncol 1993; 11(7):1311–1315.

38. Alexanian R, Dimopoulos M. The treatment of multiple myeloma. N Engl J Med 1994;330:484–489.
39. Kyle RA. Long-term survival in multiple myeloma. N Engl J Med 1983;308:314–316.
40. Barlogie B, Smith L, Alexanian R. Effective treatment of advanced multiple myeloma refractory to alkylating agents. N Engl J Med 1984;310:1353–1356.
41. Case DCJ, Lee DJI, Clarkson BD. Improved survival times in multiple myeloma treated with melphalan, prednisone, cyclophosphamide, vincristine and BCNU: M-2 protocol. Am J Med 1977;63:897–903.
42. Gregory WM, Richards MA, Malpas JS. Combination chemotherapy versus melphalan and prednisolone in the treatment of multiple myeloma: an overview of published trials. J Clin Oncol 1992;10:334–342.
43. Singhal S, et al. Antitumor activity of thalidomide in refractory multiple myeloma [published erratum appears in N Engl J Med 2000;342(5):364]. N Engl J Med 1999;341(21):1565–1571.
44. Rajkumar SV, et al. Combination therapy with thalidomide plus dexamethasone for newly diagnosed myeloma. J Clin Oncol 2002;20:4319–4323.
45. Ludwig H, et al. Patient preferences for interferon-α in multiple myeloma. J Clin Oncol 1997;15:1672–1679.
46. Zee B, et al. Quality-adjusted time without symptoms or toxicity analysis of interferon maintenance in multiple myeloma. J Clin Oncol 1998;16:2834–2839.
47. Berenson JR, et al. Maintenance therapy with alternate-day prednisone improves survival in multiple myeloma patients. Blood 2002;99(9):3163–3168.
48. McElwain TJ, Powles RL. High-dose intravenous melphalan for plasma-cell leukemia and myeloma. Lancet 1983;II(8354):822–824.
49. Attal M, et al. Autologous bone marrow transplantation versus conventional chemotherapy in multiple myeloma: a prospective, randomized trial. N Engl J Med 1996;335:91–97.
50. Child JA, et al. High-dose chemotherapy with hematopoietic stem-cell rescue for multiple myeloma. N Engl J Med 2003;348:1875–1883.
51. Fermand J-P, et al. High-dose chemoradiotherapy and autologous blood stem cell transplantation in multiple myeloma: results of a phase II trial involving 63 patients. Blood 1993;82(7):2005–2009.
52. Barlogie B, et al. High-dose melphalan with autologous bone marrow transplantation for multiple myeloma. Blood 1986;67(5):1298–1301.
53. Blade J, et al. High-dose therapy autotransplantation/intensification vs. continued conventional chemotherapy in multiple myeloma in patients responding to initial treatment chemotherapy. Results of a prospective randomized trial from the Spanish Cooperative Group PETHEMA. Blood 2001;98:815a.
54. Fermand J-P, et al. High-dose therapy and autologous peripheral blood stem cell transplantation in multiple myeloma: up-front or rescue treatment? Results of a multicenter sequential randomized clinical trial. Blood 1998;92(9):3131–3136.
55. Moreau P, et al. Comparison of 200 mg/m^2 melphalan and 8 Gy total body irradiation plus 140 mg/m^2 melphalan as conditioning regimens for peripheral blood stem cell transplantation in patients with newly diagnosed multiple myeloma: final analysis of the Intergroupe Francophone du Myelome 9502 randomized trial. Blood 2002;99:731–735.
56. Anderson KC, et al. Monoclonal antibody purged autologous bone marrow transplantation therapy for multiple myeloma. Blood 1991;77:712–720.
57. Anderson KC, et al. Monoclonal antibody-purged bone marrow transplantation therapy for multiple myeloma. Blood 1993;82(8):2568–2576.
58. Seiden M, et al. Monoclonal antibody-purged bone marrow transplantation therapy for multiple myeloma. Leuk Lymphoma 1995;17:87–93.
59. Schiller G, et al. Transplantation of CD34 positive peripheral blood progenitor cells following high dose chemotherapy for patients with advanced multiple myeloma. Blood 1995;86:390–397.
60. Barlogie B, et al. Total therapy with tandem transplants for newly diagnosed multiple myeloma. Blood 1999;93:55–65.
61. Vesole DH, et al. Autotransplants in multiple myeloma: what have we learned? Blood 1996;88:838–847.
62. Desikan R, et al. Results of high-dose therapy for 1000 patients with multiple myeloma: durable complete remissions and superior survival in the absence of chromosome 13 abnormalities. Blood 2000;95:4008–4010.
63. Attal M, et al. Single versus double transplant in myeloma: a randomized trial of the Intergroupe Francais du Myelome (IMF). Blood 2002;100:418a.
64. Cavo M, et al. The "Bologna 96" clinical trial of single vs. double autotransplants for previously untreated multiple myeloma patients. Blood 2002;100(11):179a (abstract).
65. Fermand JP, et al. In single versus tandem high dose therapy (HDT) supported with autologous blood stem cell (ABSC) transplantation using unselected or CD34 enriched ABSC: preliminary results of a two by two designed randomized trial in 230 young patients with multiple myeloma. Blood 2002;100:815a.
66. Attal M, et al. Single versus double autologous stem-cell transplantation for multiple myeloma. N Engl J Med 2003;349(26):2495–2502.
67. Alyea E, et al. Outcome after autologous and allogeneic stem cell transplantation for patients with multiple myeloma: impact of graft versus myeloma effect. 2002.
68. Gahrton G, et al. Progress in allogeneic bone marrow and peripheral blood stem cell transplantation for multiple myeloma: a comparison between transplants performed 1983–1993 and 1994–1998 at European Group for Blood and Marrow Centers. Br J Haematol 2001;113:209–216.
69. Bensinger WI, Maloney D, Storb R. Allogeneic hematopoietic cell transplantation for multiple myeloma. Semin Hematol 2001;38(3):243–249.
70. Alyea E, et al. T-cell-depleted allogeneic bone marrow transplantation followed by donor lymphocyte infusion in patients with multiple myeloma: induction of graft-versus-myeloma effect. Blood 2001;98:934–939.
71. Corradini P, et al. Molecular and clinical remissions in multiple myeloma: role of autologous and allogeneic transplantation of hematopoietic cells. J Clin Oncol 1999;17(1):208–215.
72. Martinelli G, et al. Molecular remission after allogeneic or autologous transplantation of hematopoietic stem cells for multiple myeloma. J Clin Oncol 2000;18(11):2273–2281.
73. Cavo M, et al. Allogeneic BMT for multiple myeloma (MM). The Italian experience. Bone Marrow Transplant 1991;7(suppl 2):31.
74. Alyea EP, et al. CD-8 depleted donor lymphocyte infusions mediate graft-versus multiple myeloma (MM) effect. Blood 2002;88(suppl).
75. Maloney D, et al. Combining an allogeneic graft versus myeloma effect with high dose autologous stem cell rescue in the treatment of multiple myeloma. Blood 2001;98:434a.
76. Kroger N, et al. Autologous stem cell transplantation followed by a dose-reduced allograft induces high complete remission rate in multiple myeloma. Blood 2002;100:755–760.
77. Badros A, et al. High response rate in refractory and poor-risk multiple myeloma after allotransplantation using a nonmyeloablative conditioning regimen and donor lymphocyte infusions. Blood 2001;97:2574–2579.
78. Bardwick PA, et al. Plasma cell dyscrasia with polyneuropathy, organomegaly, endocrinopathy, M protein, and skin changes: the

POEMS syndrome. Report on two cases and a review of the literature. Medicine (Baltim) 1980;59:311–322.

79. Cavo M, et al. Nonsecretory multiple myeloma. Presenting findings, clinical course and prognosis. Acta Haematol 1985;74: 27–30.
80. Knowling MA, Harwood AR, Bergsagel DE. Comparison of extramedullary plasmactyomas with solitary and multiple plasma cell tumors of bone. J Clin Oncol 1983;1(4):255–262.
81. Dimopoulos MA, et al. Curability of solitary bone plasmacytoma. J Clin Oncol 1992;10:587–590.
82. Kyle RA.,Amyloidosis. Introduction and overview. J Intern Med 1992;232:507–508.
83. Gillmore JD, Hawkins PN, Pepys MB. Amyloidosis: a review of recent diagnostic and therapeutic developments. Br J Haematol 1997;99:245–256.
84. Kyle RA, et al. Long-term survival (10 years or more) in 30 patients with primary amyloidosis. Blood 1999;93(3):1062–1066.
85. Comenzo RL, et al. Dose-intensive melphalan with blood stem cell support for the treatment of AL amyloidosis: one-year follow-up in five patients. Blood 1996;88:2801–2806.
86. Comenzo RL, et al. Stem cell contamination predicts post-transplant survival in AL amyloidosis. Blood 1999;94(suppl 1): 575a.
87. Weber DM, et al. Thalidomide alone or with dexamethasone for multiple myeloma. Blood (Suppl) 1999;94:604a.
88. Hideshima T, et al. Thalidomide and its analogues overcome drug resistance of human multiple myeloma cells to conventional therapy. Blood 2000;96:2943–2950.
89. Davies FE, et al. Thalidomide and immunomodulatory derivatives augment natural killer cell cytotoxicity in multiple myeloma. Blood 2001;98(1):210–216.
90. Weber D, et al. Thalidomide alone or with dexamethasone for previously untreated multiple myeloma. J Clin Oncol 2003;21: 16–19.
91. Mitsiades N, et al. Molecular sequelae of proteasome inhibition in human multiple myeloma cells. Proc Natl Acad Sci USA 2002;99:14374–14379.
92. Richardson P, et al. A phase 2 study of bortezomib in relapsed, refractory myeloma. New Engl J Med 2003;348(26):2609–2617.

SECTION SEVEN

Practice of Oncology

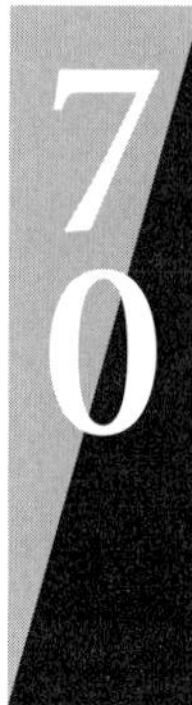

Superior Vena Cava Syndrome

Michael S. Kent and Jeffrey L. Port

Obstruction of the superior vena cava (SVC) is a common complication of thoracic malignancy and of bronchogenic cancer in particular. Although the condition was first described in 1757,[1] little progress had been made in the treatment of these patients until the first report of surgical reconstruction in 1951.[2] However, over the past decade there has been a remarkable evolution in the successful management of this disease, in large measure as a result of the refinement of endovascular techniques, such as stent placement and thrombolysis.

Superior vena cava obstruction is a disease with a wide range of clinical presentation and treatment. Caval obstruction may be an incidental finding on computed tomography (CT), with the development of collateral venous channels, or may be the fulminant, initial presentation of a malignancy. Furthermore, SVC obstruction may also arise as a consequence of benign conditions, such as mediastinal fibrosis or thrombosis related to indwelling central catheters. The successful management of this disease requires a familiarity with the wide variety of treatment options available and an appreciation of the significant disparity in prognosis between those with benign and malignant causes of SVC obstruction.

This chapter reviews the relevant anatomy and pathophysiology of SVC obstruction and discusses the current treatment options, including surgical reconstruction, radiation and/or chemotherapy, and endovascular therapies. Unfortunately, the majority of reports are single-institution case series. When available, data from clinical trials in which treatment modalities are directly compared are emphasized.

Clinical Presentation

The first reported case of SVC obstruction, by William Hunter in 1757, described a patient with an aneurysm of the ascending aorta. Although such benign causes of SVC obstruction were common in the 19th century, the increasing incidence of bronchogenic cancer has led to the overwhelming association of this condition with malignancy. For example, nearly 40% of cases reported in the first half of the 20th century were associated with infectious conditions, such as mycotic aortic aneurysms, tuberculosis, or syphilis.[3] In contrast, malignant causes of SVC obstruction now account for more than 90% of cases.[4] Bronchogenic carcinomas, both small cell (SCLC) and non-small cell (NSCLC) histologies, are responsible for 65% to 80% of these cases. Mediastinal tumors, particularly thymoma and thyroid cancer, account for 20% of malignant cases, and metastatic solid tumors are responsible for the remainder.[5] Although far less common, benign etiologies of SVC obstruction must also be considered. Thrombosis of the SVC from central venous catheters or pacemaker leads has been well described.[6,7] Rare causes of SVC occlusion include mediastinal fibrosis and late effects of external-beam radiation therapy (Table 70.1).[8]

Superior vena cava obstruction is not an uncommon condition when all causes are considered. The disease is estimated to affect as many as 15,000 patients in the United States annually.[9] Although only 3% of all patients with lung cancer develop SVC obstruction, the condition may develop in up to 10% of those with right-sided malignancies.[10] SVC obstruction is especially common in small cell lung cancer, with a reported prevalence as high as 11%.[11]

The pathogenesis of SVC occlusion is typically one of extraluminal compression. Direct extension of a malignancy, classically a non-small cell lung cancer arising from the right upper lobe, may lead to circumferential involvement of the cava and obstruction of venous return to the heart. The compressibility of the SVC and its central location within the mediastinum render it particularly susceptible to this process. SVC occlusion may also develop from mediastinal lymphadenopathy, particularly metastases from a NSCLC to the right paratracheal lymph node stations. Similarly, the central lymphadenopathy associated with small cell lung cancer leads to the high prevalence of SVC obstruction with this disease. A final mechanism of SVC occlusion is that of intraluminal thrombosis. The presence of indwelling central catheters has been shown to induce endothelial damage and turbulent blood flow, leading to catheter encapsulation and venous thrombosis.[12] In cases of malignant disease, a tumor that invades into the lumen of the cava may serve as the nidus for thrombus formation.

The development of SVC occlusion leads to a characteristic syndrome of facial and upper extremity edema, along with the development of tortuous collateral veins on the anterior chest wall. Headache, dizziness, and nausea are not infrequent. Rare signs of SVC occlusion include obtundation from cerebral edema and airway compromise from edema of the epiglottis (Table 70.2). Patients rarely present with acute symptoms; more commonly, they describe the gradual onset of symptoms over several weeks.[13] The symptoms of SVC occlusion may be quite distressing for the patient and affect quality of life significantly. Fortunately, life-threatening symptoms are extremely rare. Severe neurologic symptoms and airway compromise have been reported to occur in less

TABLE 70.1. **Common causes of superior vena cava (SVC) obstruction.**

Malignant
Non-small cell lung cancer
Small cell lung cancer
Thymoma
Lymphoma
Thyroid cancer
Mediastinal germ cell tumors
Metastatic cancer (breast, colon)
Benign
Fibrosing mediastinitis
SVC thrombosis from indwelling catheters or hypercoagulability
Sarcoidosis
Histoplasmosis

TABLE 70.2. **Symptoms of SVC obstruction.**

Symptoms	*Frequency*
Facial swelling	72%
Dyspnea	60%
Cough	38%
Arm swelling	28%
Dysphagia	11%
Headache	6%
Stridor	4%

Source: From Wudel and Nesbitt.[9]

than 5% of patients.[14] Furthermore, central nervous system (CNS) symptoms may be secondary to cerebral metastases rather than SVC occlusion, and should be ruled out by CT or magnetic resonance imaging (MRI).

The belief that SVC syndrome represents an oncologic emergency has not been supported by modern series. Early reports suggested a high mortality associated with SVC occlusion; however, the majority of patients from these series had end-stage disease and the cause of death was not clear.[15] Recent series have documented an early mortality of 2% or less.[11,13,16] Furthermore, diagnostic studies may be safely performed in patients with SVC obstruction, and thus, adequate information may be obtained before embarking upon therapy.[17,18]

Although patients rarely die as a direct consequence of SVC occlusion, the overall prognosis for these patients is quite poor, especially for those with lung cancer. In a review of 337 patients with malignant causes of SVC obstruction, patients with lung cancer had an overall 5-year survival of only 2%, compared with a 10% survival for those with breast cancer and a 40% survival for patients with lymphoma.[14] Median survival is typically only 6 to 9 months following treatment.[19] In contrast, the majority of patients with SVC syndrome from nonmalignant causes can anticipate a normal life expectancy.

Evaluation

The appropriate treatment of SVC obstruction depends greatly on the underlying cause of the syndrome. Often, patients with malignant causes of SVC obstruction have a known cancer diagnosis. However, SVC obstruction may be the presenting sign of a malignancy in up to 10% of patients with SCLC and 2% of those with NSCLC.[19] In these situations, a tissue biopsy is necessary to clarify the diagnosis. In older series, fear of uncontrollable hemorrhage led to empiric treatment of patients without a tissue diagnosis. However, noninvasive techniques, such as sputum cytology, can yield a diagnosis in two-thirds of patients.[20] Furthermore, invasive procedures have been shown to be safe in patients with SVC obstruction. For instance, in a series of 88 patients who underwent a variety of sampling techniques, including CT-guided biopsy and mediastinoscopy, no mortalities and only 1 treatment-related morbidity were reported.[18] Although mediastinoscopy has been shown to be safe in this patient population, the incidence of complications is indeed higher than in those without SVC obstruction. Clinical series have documented the need for salvage sternotomy because of bleeding to be between 1% and 3%,[18,21,22] compared with the 0.3% sternotomy rate reported for patients without SVC obstruction.[23]

Physical examination is sufficient to establish the diagnosis of SVC obstruction. Radiologic assessment, such as CT and venography, is not necessary to confirm the diagnosis but is valuable in treatment planning. CT defines the anatomic extent of the mass, determines whether the obstruction is from a primary tumor or malignant lymphadenopathy, and allows for a CT-guided biopsy (Figure 70.1). Rarely, patients with malignant tumors and SVC invasion may be resected for cure.[24,25] CT in this setting would be essential for operative planning.

In addition, both CT and venography provide anatomic detail of the venous system that can define the severity of the SVC obstruction. In the presence of SVC obstruction, the major pathway for collateral flow to the heart is the azygos vein. The azygos vein runs parallel to the superior and infe-

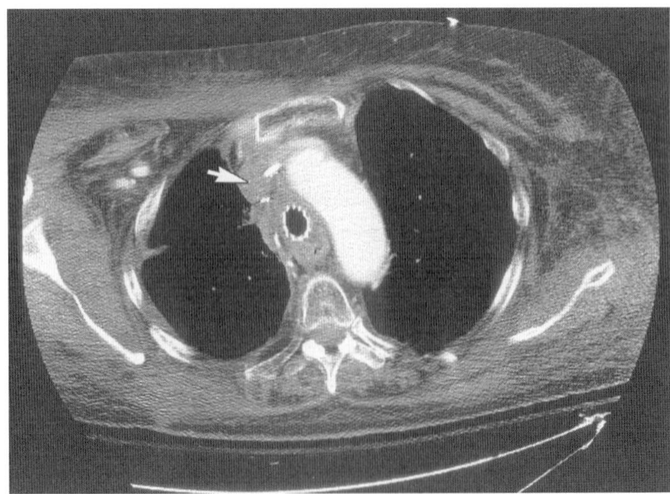

FIGURE 70.1. Computed tomography (CT) scan of a patient with recurrent non-small cell (NSCLC) and superior vena cava (SVC) obstruction. The tip of a subclavian catheter is seen within the thrombosed SVC (*arrow*). A tracheal stent and adjacent paratracheal lymphadenopathy are also appreciated.

TABLE 70.3. Classification of SVC obstruction by computed tomography (CT) and venography.

	Finding
CT classification	
Type IA	Moderate SVC narrowing without collateral flow
Type IB	Severe SVC narrowing with retrograde flow in azygos vein
Type II	SVC obstruction above azygos with retrograde flow into thoracic, vertebral, or other collateral channels
Type III	SVC obstruction below azygos with retrograde flow through azygos into the inferior vena cava (IVC)
Type IV	SVC obstruction at azygos vein with multiple small peripheral collaterals
Venogram classification	
Type I	Partial obstruction of the SVC with patency of the azygos vein
Type 2	Near-complete to complete obstruction of the SVC with antegrade flow in the azygos vein
Type 3	Near-complete to complete obstruction of the SVC with retrograde flow in the azygos vein to the IVC
Type 4	Complete obstruction of the SVC and azygos vein

rior vena cavae and drains into both the right common iliac vein and SVC just above the pericardial reflection. Obstruction of the SVC below the insertion of the azygos vein leads to retrograde flow through the azygos vein, into the inferior vena cava, and ultimately into the right atrium. When the obstruction is above the azygos vein, collateral venous beds, such as the cervical and paravertebral plexuses dilate. These collateral vessels then drain into the azygos vein. The most severe cases of SVC syndrome occur when the obstruction is at the level of the azygos vein. In these cases, small vessels overlying the thoracic wall dilate and serve to return venous blood to the inferior vena cava. Dilation of these vessels only occurs over a period of several weeks. Consequently, obstruction at the azygo–caval junction that occurs acutely may lead to severe symptoms.

Evaluation of the azygos vein is therefore critical in documenting the severity of SVC obstruction. Higher grades of SVC obstruction in current classification systems are those in which the azygos vein is not visualized. The schemes developed by Stanford and Doty for venography[26] and Raptopoulos for CT[27] are those most commonly referenced (Table 70.3).

Unfortunately, a similar classification of clinical symptoms has not been universally accepted. Such a scheme would allow for the means to objectively compare the degree of symptomatic relief between different methods of treatment. An illustrative scoring system is presented in Table 70.4; however, this scale has not been validated in a prospective fashion.[28]

TABLE 70.4. Clinical scoring system for SVC obstruction.

Symptom	*Points*
Arm/head/extremity swelling	1
Neck or chest vein distension	1
Cough	1
Blurred vision	1
Tinnitus	1
Headache	1
Dizziness	1
Dyspnea	1
Plethora	1
Vocal cord paralysis	1
Total	Up to 10 points

Treatment

Historically, the treatment of SVC occlusion has included head elevation and the administration of steroids and diuretics. These measures are largely ineffective,[4] and the standard treatment for patients with malignant causes of SVC obstruction has been radiation therapy and/or chemotherapy. Surgical bypass is an option for those who fail medical therapy, although the morbidity of such a procedure in patients with a limited life expectancy was often thought to be prohibitive. Endovascular stenting of SVC was first reported in 1992[29] and has gained increasing popularity since then. Many now consider stenting to be the mainstay of treatment for patients with malignant SVC obstruction. For benign causes of SVC occlusion, the most appropriate role for stenting or surgical bypass has not been well defined. As no standard treatment exists for all patients with SVC occlusion, a review of all the methods of available therapy is appropriate.

Chemotherapy and Radiotherapy

Chemotherapy and radiation therapy (CRT) have been the first-line therapy for patients with SVC occlusion of malignant etiology. The majority of reports of CRT are retrospective and include patients who undergo therapy for a variety of tumor subtypes, making a direct comparison of different protocols extremely difficult. Analysis is further complicated by the fact that patients are often treated with both radiotherapy and chemotherapy, so the two modalities cannot be directly compared.

Recently, a review of current therapy for SVC obstruction caused by bronchogenic cancer was published.[19] In this review, 22 studies of CRT that included 746 patients were analyzed, and the results were stratified by small cell or non-small cell histology. For SCLC, 77% of patients experienced symptomatic relief of SVC obstruction after chemotherapy or radiation therapy. For NSCLC, the rates of symptomatic relief were lower: 59% for chemotherapy alone and 63% for radiotherapy alone. The rapidity of symptom relief after CRT was not well documented. Overall, a clinical response generally occurred within 2 to 3 weeks after the initiation of therapy. However, one study found that 25% of clinical responses occurred 3 weeks after starting treatment.[11] Data regarding relapse were provided in a smaller subset of series. Overall, clinical relapse occurred in 17% of patients with SCLC and 19% of those with NSCLC.

Endovascular Therapy

The entire spectrum of endovascular technology, including thrombolysis, angioplasty, and stenting, has found an application in the management of patients with SVC obstruction. The era of endovascular therapy for this condition began in 1986. In that year, the first successful angioplasty of SVC stenosis caused by a transvenous pacemaker was reported.[30] In that same year, the first patient with malignant SVC obstruction was treated by placement of an SVC stent.[31] Since these early reports, endovascular therapy has essentially replaced surgery as the treatment for patients with malignant SVC obstruction who fail CRT. The role of endovascular technology as first-line therapy remains controversial, although many centers have recently adopted this approach.

Thrombolysis is rarely the sole method of treatment of SVC obstruction, because the majority of patients have external compression of the cava, for which thrombolysis alone is ineffective.[32] On occasion, patients may have thrombosis of the SVC from benign causes, most often indwelling central lines, for which thrombolytic therapy may be effective. In this case, infusion of agents, such as tissue plasminogen activator (tPA), has been shown to be 88% successful if used within 5 days of the occlusion, but only 25% successful if used thereafter.[33] Thus, for subacute or long-standing thrombosis, pharmacologic therapy alone is insufficient. Similarly, angioplasty alone has a high rate of restenosis and failure because of the elastic nature of the cava.[34] Therefore, stenting in combination with angioplasty or thrombolysis is the more common treatment paradigm.

A wide variety of stents designed for peripheral vascular disease may be deployed within the SVC. Stents may be categorized as self-expanding or balloon-expanding. Most authors prefer to use self-expanding stents in the venous system. Self-expanding stents typically are more flexible and have greater radial force than balloon-expanding stents. In addition, the diameter of the cava often increases after successful stenting. Balloon-mounted stents that lack self-expansion are more likely to migrate in this circumstance.[36] Some of the more commonly used self-expanding stents include the Gianturco Z-stent, the Wallstent, and the Smartstent. The Z-stent was the first device used to stent the SVC; however, it has a relatively large profile compared to more recent devices. In addition, the Z-stent has a propensity to migrate or fracture.[36] The Wallstent is less likely to migrate; however, it has a tendency to shorten after deployment, which makes precise placement of the stent difficult. Foreshortening of the stent may be significant to the point of uncovering the point of obstruction, leading to restenosis.[37] The Smartstent is a further evolution of stent technology based on nitinol (Figure 70.2). Nitinol is a nickel-titanium alloy that assumes a predetermined shape at a certain temperature. It has been found to have a high radial strength, a very low risk of fracture, and is not prone to foreshortening.

Access for stent deployment is usually obtained from the basilic vein. If larger sheaths are required or access via the brachial route is not possible, then the femoral vein may be cannulated. A guidewire is then passed beyond the obstruction under fluoroscopic guidance. A venogram is then obtained to document the areas of stenosis and thombus formation within the cava (Figure 70.3). Thrombus formation is associated with SVC obstruction in up to 37% of cases[38]; however, the majority of patients have a nonocclusive clot that does not require thrombolysis. Given the risk of bleeding complications, thrombolytic therapy is usually reserved for patients with extensive thrombus within the caval system. Angioplasty is occasionally performed if the stenosis is significant enough to prevent stent deployment. In general, however, angioplasty is avoided and immediate stenting is performed (Figure 70.4). This practice results from the concern that angioplasty may dislodge a thrombus along the caval wall and lead to distant embolism.[35] Patients who require thrombolysis are routinely placed on intravenous heparin and then warfarin for a period of 3 to 6 months. Many authors recommend coumadin or antiplatelet therapy for all

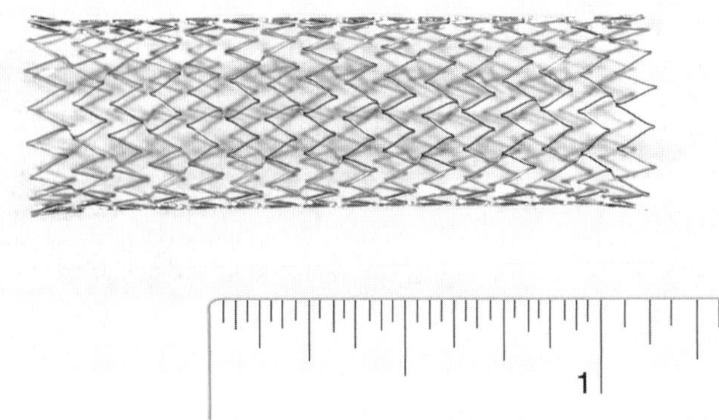

FIGURE 70.2. Self-expanding nitinol stent used for SVC obstruction.

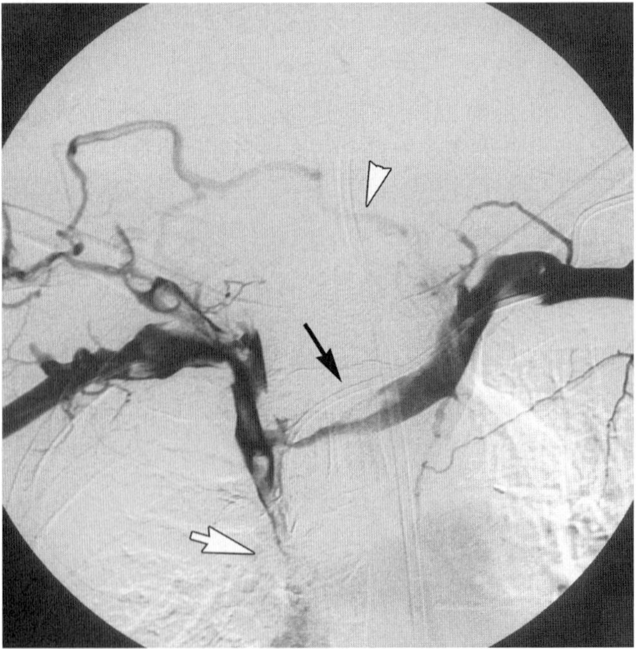

FIGURE 70.3. Pretreatment angiogram of a patient with SVC obstruction (*white arrow*) from NSCLC. A catheter with surrounding thrombus is visible within the left brachiocephalic vein (*black arrow*). Also present are small collateral channels (*white arrowhead*) that cross the midline.

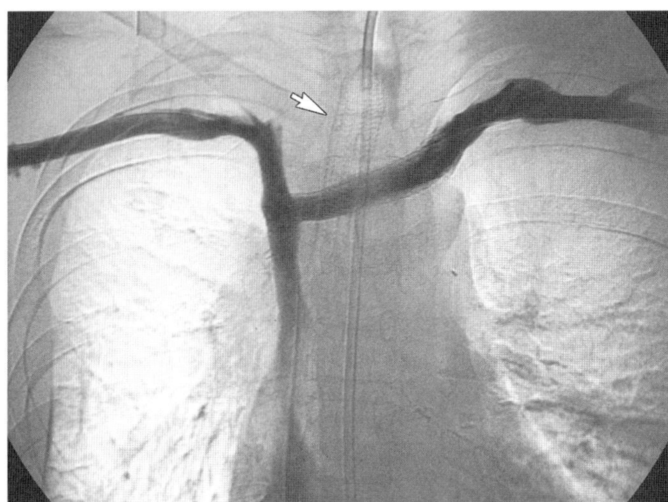

FIGURE 70.4. Completion angiography in the same patient after thrombolysis and placement of an SVC stent. A tracheal stent (*arrow*) is also seen.

patients after SVC stenting,[39,40] although there is no clear justification for this practice.

Stent deployment is technically successful in 95% of cases[19] (Table 70.5). The majority of patients report immediate relief of headache.[41] Other symptoms, such as arm and facial edema, usually resolve within 72 hours. Dyspnea is the most resistant symptom to improvement after stent placement and may persist in up to 40% of patients.[39] The rate of relapse following stent placement is also quite low. In a review of 23 series of SVC stenting in patients with lung cancer, the relapse rate was 11%.[19] The majority of patients with recurrent symptoms may be treated with additional stent placement or thrombolysis. Given the success of subsequent interventions, the secondary patency rate after stenting in this review was 93%. The median survival for these patients, however, was less than 1 year, and thus the long-term patency of SVC stenting could not be determined.

Although uncommon, several complications have been associated with SVC stenting. Transient chest pain is often seen with stent deployment. Bleeding complications, such as puncture site hematoma, melena, and epistaxis, have also been reported in those who require thrombolysis. Other complications, such as stent fracture or migration, were reported in earlier studies. Dislodged stents have even been documented to migrate to the pulmonary artery,[42] although this is extremely rare. SVC rupture with pericardial tamponade has also been reported.[42] Thankfully, these mechanical complications are uncommon in more recent series. No deaths have been recently reported with SVC stent deployment.[19]

TABLE 70.5. Results of endovascular stenting for SVC obstruction.

Author	*N*	*Restoration of patency*	*Recurrence*
Garcia Monaco (2003)[50]	44	100%	14%
Courtheoux (2003)[40]	20	95%	15%
Chatziioannou (2003)[49]	18	100%	NS
Wilson (2002)[51]	18	100%	6%
Lanciego (2001)[39]	52	100%	6%
Smayra (2001)[35]	30	100%	43%
Miller (2000)[52]	23	82%	17%
Tanigawa (1998)[53]	23	78%	21%
Gross (1997)[54]	13	100%	NS
Nicholson (1997)[28]	76	100%	9%

Surgery

Surgery is rarely indicated for patients with SVC occlusion. Infrequently, patients may require contiguous resection of the SVC in the context of a malignancy that is otherwise resectable. However, the majority of patients with symptomatic SVC occlusion have locally advanced or distant disease and are not resectable for cure. Thus, surgery is often performed as a purely palliative procedure.

Venocavography is essential before undertaking surgical reconstruction; this allows for a precise determination of the proximal degree of obstruction and the presence of intraluminal thrombus. Usually the bypass is constructed between a single vein, such as the right or left brachiocephalic vein, and the right atrium (Figure 70.5). Bilateral bypasses are rarely required because collateral channels that cross the midline are sufficient to drain the contralateral side.

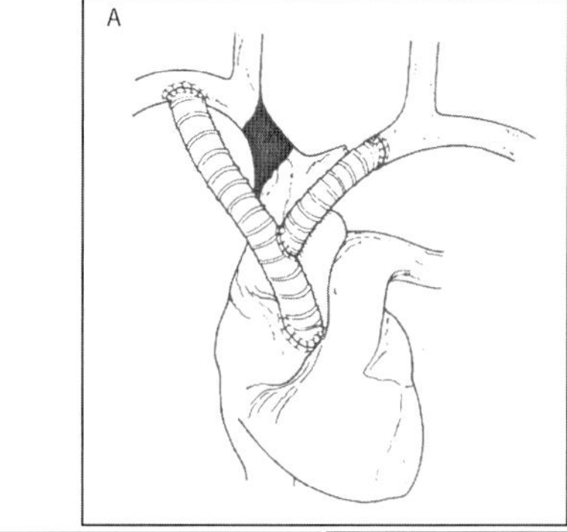

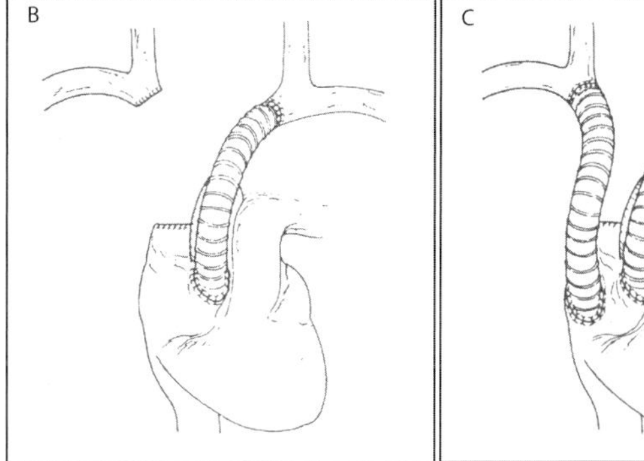

FIGURE 70.5. Polytetrafluoroethylene (PTFE) bypass grafts for SVC obstruction. (A) Y-shaped graft from the right and left innominate veins to the right atrial appendage. (B) Graft from the left innominate vein to the right atrial appendage. (C) Dual grafts from the right innominate vein to the right atrium and from the left innominate vein to the right atrial appendage. (Reprinted with permission from Magnan P, Thomas P, Giudicelli R, et al. Surgical reconstruction of the superior vena cava. Cardiovasc Surg 1994;2:598–604.[45])

Several conduits are available to bypass the SVC. Conduits may be autologous vein, such as the saphenous or common femoral vein, or synthetic material, such as polytetrafluoroethylene (PTFE). The femoral vein was the first conduit used to relieve SVC obstruction[34]; however, its use has declined significantly since the description of the technique in 1951. The size discrepancy between the femoral vein and SVC is significant, and removal of the femoral vein may lead to venous insufficiency of the leg. However, composite grafts of the smaller saphenous vein have found widespread applicability. In the initial report, the saphenous vein was incised along its length and "panels" of vein were sewn together to create a conduit of larger diameter.[43] A subsequent modification of the technique was the creation of a "spiral graft" in which the vein was sewn to itself in a spiral fashion around a chest tube or other stent.[44] The disadvantage of autologous vein, however, is its easy compressibility; this may lead to early occlusion, especially if the cause is a thoracic malignancy that may continue to progress. For this reason, some authors have preferred to use ringed PTFE, which has an intrinsic skeleton that renders it relatively resistant to external compression. Ringed PTFE has a 5-year patency of 86%,[25] which is comparable to that of spiral saphenous vein.[44] The equivalent long-term patency and the simplicity of the technique have led to a preference for synthetic grafts among many authors.[25,45]

Surgical bypass for SVC obstruction is performed through a median sternotomy. Although bypass procedures using the azygos vein have been reported through a right thoracotomy,[22] a sternotomy provides superior exposure to structures within the anterior mediastinum. The innominate vein is mobilized to the origin of the interior jugular vein and is encircled with tourniquets. After the patient has been systemically heparinized, a small venotomy is made. If present, thrombus within the vein is removed using a Fogarty catheter. Next, the conduit is sutured to the vein in an end-to-side fashion. The graft is flushed with heparinized saline, and an anastomosis is constructed to either the right atrial appendage or the right atrium.

It should be noted that patients who undergo caval resection and replacement (Figure 70.6), as opposed to surgical bypass, require a more-complex procedure. In this setting, the SVC is rarely occluded and clamping of the vein may lead to significant hemodynamic instability.[46] Techniques, such as intraluminal shunting or cardiopulmonary bypass, may be required; these are outside the scope of this chapter.

Although patients with SVC obstruction are often moribund, the operative mortality has been low (Table 70.6). In the largest report of 43 patients who underwent bypass for malignant SVC obstruction, the operative mortality was only 4%.[47] Furthermore, relief of symptoms is nearly immediate and early thrombosis of the graft is uncommon. For patients with SVC obstruction from benign causes, the long-term patency of the bypass is critical. The largest series of SVC bypass for nonmalignant disease documented an overall 5-year patency of 80%.[48] Among the 29 patients, 5 required reoperation for early graft failure. Eight patients required additional interventions for late graft failure. The majority of these interventions were endovascular, although 3 patients required surgical revision. In this series, spiral saphenous vein had a superior patency and was preferred over PTFE conduits.

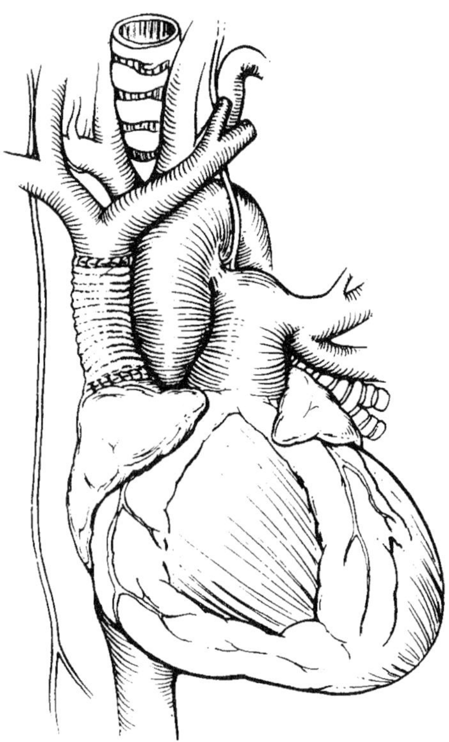

FIGURE 70.6. Resection of the SVC and replacement with an interposition PTFE graft. (Reprinted with permission from Nesbitt J. Surgical management of superior vena cava syndrome. In: Lung Cancer: Principles and Practice. Philadelphia: Lippincott-Raven, 1996.[14])

Management Controversies

There are no randomized studies that compare treatment options for patients with SVC obstruction. Nonetheless, the

TABLE 70.6. Results of open surgical bypass for SVC obstruction.

Author	*N*	*Etiology*	*Conduit*	*Operative mortality*	*Early graft failures*	*Five-year patency*
Kalra (2003)[48]	29	Benign	Both	0%	17%	80%
Doty (1999)[44]	16	Benign	SSVG	0%	19%	88%
Magnan (1994)[45]	10	Both	PTFE	0%	0%	NS
Moore (1991)[55]	10	Benign	Both	0%	10%	NS
Dartevelle (1991)[25]	22	Malignancy	PTFE	4.5%	5%	NS

NS, not stated.

high success rate of stenting reported in case series, has led to a reduction in open surgical bypass, at least for patients with malignant SVC occlusion. However, two areas of controversy still exist in the management of this syndrome. The first is whether stenting should be first-line therapy for patients with malignant SVC obstruction, or reserved for those who fail radiation or chemotherapy. The second relates to the proper role of stenting versus open surgery for patients with benign causes of SVC obstruction.

Despite the lack of prospective data, there is evidence to support the use of stenting as primary therapy for patients with malignant SVC obstruction. Stenting has clearly demonstrated superiority over CRT in terms of the initial response to therapy. Stenting relieved symptoms in 95% of patients with bronchogenic cancer compared with 59% (for NSCLC) and 77% (for SCLC) of those treated with radiation or chemotherapy. Furthermore, relief of symptoms with stenting was nearly immediate, compared to days to weeks with chemotherapy. This difference is particularly significant in a patient population whose median survival is less than 1 year. Perhaps most important, fewer patients developed a recurrence of symptoms when treated with stenting. Thus, the relapse-free rate, defined as the response rate minus the recurrence rate, was estimated at 84% for stenting, compared with 41% (NSCLC) to 60% (SCLC) among those treated with radiation or chemotherapy.[19] Certainly, for patients with NSCLC, these data would support the use of stenting as primary therapy. Although the response to CRT is somewhat higher for those with SCLC, stenting would still be justifiable as primary therapy in this patient population.

Additional data support stenting as primary therapy for malignant SVC syndrome. First, stenting in no way precludes further administration of CRT.[49] In fact, stenting may allow for the easier administration of intravenous fluids required for chemotherapy. Second, stenting has been estimated to incur only a marginal increase in the cost of treating these patients due to the expense of end-of-life care.[37,41] Finally, most patients who develop a recurrence after stenting may be retreated, either with thrombolytics or additional stenting, leading to a secondary patency rate of nearly 100%.[39,40]

The long-term results of stenting are not as well documented, and for this reason, the best treatment for patients with benign SVC occlusion remains controversial. In comparison with stenting, surgical bypass has been shown to yield excellent long-term results. For example, Doty reported on a series of 16 patients who underwent spiral saphenous vein bypass for benign SVC obstruction, most commonly caused by fibrosing mediastinitis. With a mean follow-up of nearly 11 years, 14 of the 16 grafts were patent. Only 3 patients had early graft occlusion, and reoperation restored flow in all but 1.[44] The only other large series of patients treated for benign SVC obstruction was from the Mayo Clinic. This report described similar results, with a 5-year patency of 80%.[48]

The durability of stenting the SVC for benign disease does not seem to be as impressive. For example, in the Mayo Clinic series 3, additional patients were described who underwent stenting as primary therapy. All 3 patients required repeat interventions for restenosis, and 1 patient ultimately required open surgical bypass. Similarly, a recent report from Toulouse, described 14 patients who underwent stenting for benign disease, the majority related to venous access for hemodialysis.[35] Stenting *failed* to restore patency in 11 of these patients. After repeat interventions, only 9 patients had restoration of flow. Furthermore, the follow-up of these patients was only 14 months, and so the rate of late restenosis is not known.

For several reasons, stenting will remain an option for patients with benign disease. First, it is certain that refinements in stent technology will improve on these relatively poor early results. Second, patients may prefer a minimally invasive therapy, even though the rate of early failure and the need for repeat intervention will be high. Perhaps most important, few centers have a large enough experience with open bypass to achieve long-term success. As experience with SVC stenting for malignancy increases, it may become the first option for benign disease as well, simply because of ease of insertion and familiarity with the technique.

References

1. Hunter W. History of aneurysm of the aorta with some remarks on aneurysms in general. Medical Observations and Inquires (London) 1757;1:323.
2. Klassen K, Andrews N, Curtis G. Diagnosis and treatment of superior vena cava obstruction. Arch Surg 1951;63:311–325.
3. Markman W. Diagnosis and management of superior vena cava syndrome. Cleve Clin J Med 1999;66:59.
4. Ostler P, Clarke D, Watkinson A, Gaze M. Superior vena cava obstruction: a modern management strategy. Clin Oncol 1997; 9:83–89.
5. Chen J, Bongard F, Klein S. A contemporary perspective on superior vena cava syndrome. Am J Surg 1990;160:207–211.
6. Otten T, Stein P, Patel K, et al. Thromboembolic disease involving the superior vena cava and brachiocephalic veins. Chest 2003;123:809–812.
7. Spitell P, Hayes D. Venous complications after insertion of transvenous pacemaker. Mayo Clin Proc 1992;37:258–265.
8. Van Putten J, Schlosser N, Vujaskovic Z et al. Superior vena cava obstruction caused by radiation-induced venous fibrosis. Thorax 2000;55:245–246.
9. Wudel L, Nesbitt J. Superior vena cava syndrome. Curr Treat Options Oncol 2001;2:77–91.
10. Escalante C. Causes and management of superior vena cava syndrome. Oncology 1993;7:61–68.
11. Chan R, Dar A, Yu E, et al. Superior vena cava obstruction in small-cell lung cancer. Int J Radiat Oncol Biol Phys 1997;38: 513–520.
12. Stokes K, Chem B, Anderson J, et al. The encapsulation of polyurethane-insulated transvenous cardiac pacemaker leads. Cardiovasc Pathol 1995;4:163–171.
13. Yellin A, Rosen A, Reichert N, et al. Superior vena cava syndrome: the myth, the facts. Am Rev Respir Dis 1990;141:1114.
14. Nesbitt J. Surgical management of superior vena cava syndrome. In: Lung Cancer: Principles and Practice. Philadephia: Lippincott-Raven, 1996.
15. Maddox A, Valdivieso M, Lukeman J, et al. Superior vena cava syndrome in small-cell bronchogenic carcinoma: clinical parameters and survival. Cancer (Phila) 1983;52:2165–2172.
16. Schraufnagel D, Hill R, Leech J, et al. Superior vena cava obstruction: is it a medical emergency? Am J Med 1981;70:1169–1174.
17. Ahmann F. A reassessment of the clinical implications of the superior vena cava syndrome. J Clin Oncol 1984;2:961–969.
18. Porte H, Metois D, Finzi L, et al. Superior vena cava syndrome of malignant origin. Which surgical procedure for which diagnosis? Eur J Cardiothorac Surg 2000;17:384–388.
19. Rowell N, Gleeson F. Steroids, radiotherapy, chemotherapy and stents for superior vena caval obstruction in carcinoma of the bronchus: a systematic review. Clin Oncol 2002;14:338–351.

20. Armstrong B, Perez C, Simpson J et al. Role of irradiation in the management of superior vena cava syndrome. Int J Radiat Oncol Biol Phys 1987;3:531.
21. Mineo T, Ambrogi V, Nofroni I, et al. Mediastinoscopy in superior vena cava obstruction: analysis of 80 consecutive patients. Ann Thorac Surg 1999;68:223–226.
22. Jahangiri M, Goldstraw P. The role of mediastinoscopy in superior vena cava obstruction. Ann Thorac Surg 1995;59:453–455.
23. Ginsberg R. Evaluation of the mediastinum by invasive techniques. Surg Clin N Am 1987;67:1025–1035.
24. Spaggiari L, Thomas P, Magdeleinat P. Superior vena cava resection with prosthetic replacement for non-small cell lung cancer: long-term results of a multicentric study. Eur J Cardiothorac Surg 2002;2:1080–1086.
25. Dartevelle P, Chapelier A, Pastorini U, et al. Long-term follow-up after prosthetic replacement of the superior vena cava combined with resection of mediastinal-pulmonary malignant tumors. J Thorac Cardiovasc Surg 1991;102:259–265.
26. Stanford W, Doty D. The role of venography and surgery in the management of patients with superior vena cava obstruction. Ann Thorac Surg 1986;41:158.
27. Raptopoulos V. Computed tomography of the superior vena cava. CRC Crit Rev Diagn Imaging 1986;25;373.
28. Nicholson A, Ettles D, Arnold A, et al. Treatment of malignant superior vena cava obstruction: metal stents or radiation therapy? J Vasc Intervent Radiol 1997;8:781–788.
29. Rocchini A, Meliones J, Beekman R et al. Use of balloon-expandable stents to treat peripheral pulmonary artery and superior vena cava stenoses: preliminary experience. Pediatr Cardiol 1992;13:92–96.
30. Sherry C. Successful treatment of SVC syndrome by venous angioplasty. Am J Roentgenol 1986;147:834–835.
31. Charnsangavej C, Carrasco C, Wallace S, et al. Stenosis of the vena cava: preliminary assessment of treatment with expandable metallic stents. Radiology 1986;161:295–298.
32. Schindler N, Vogelzang R. Superior vena cava syndrome: experience with endovascular stents and surgical therapy. Surg Clin N Am 1999;79:983–994.
33. Gray B, Olin J, Graor R, et al. Safety and efficacy of thrombolytic therapy for superior vena cava syndrome. Chest 1991;99:54–59.
34. Klassen K, Andrews N, Curtis G. Diagnosis and treatment of superior vena cava obstruction. Arch Surg 1951;63:311–325.
35. Smayra T, Otal P, Chabbert V, et al. Long-term results of endovascular stent placement in the superior caval venous system. Cardiovasc Intervent Radiol 2001;24:388–394.
36. Rosch J, Uchida B, Hall L, et al. Gianturco-Rosch expandable Z-stent in the treatment of superior vena cava syndrome. Cardiovasc Intervent Radiol 1992;15:319–327.
37. Dyet J, Nicholson A, Cook A. The use of the Wallstent endovascular prosthesis in the treatment of malignant obstruction of the superior vena cava. Clin Radiol 1993;48:381–385.
38. Thony F, Moro D, Witmeyer P, Angiolini S, et al. Endovascular treatment of superior vena cava obstruction in patients with malignancies. Eur Radiol 1999;9:965–971.
39. Lanciego C, Chacon J, Julian A, et al. Stenting as first option for endovascular treatment of malignant superior vena cava syndrome. AJR 2001;177:585–593.
40. Courtheoux P, Alkofer B, Al Refai M, et al. Stent placement in superior vena cava syndrome. Ann Thorac Surg 2003;75; 158–161.
41. Irving J, Dondelinger R, Reidy J, et al. Gianturco self-expanding stents: clinical experience in the vena cava and large veins. Cardiovasc Intervent Radiol 1992;15:328–333.
42. Kee S, Kinoshita L, Razavi M, et al. Superior vena cava syndrome: treatment with catheter-directed thrombolysis and endovascular stent placement. Radiology 1998;206:187–193.
43. Benvenunto R, Rodman F, Gilmour J, et al. Composite venous graft for replacement of the superior vena cava. Arch Surg 1962;84:100–103.
44. Doty J, Flores J, Doty D. Superior vena cava obstruction: bypass using spiral vein graft. Ann Thorac Surg 1999;67:1111–1116.
45. Magnan P, Thomas P, Giudicelli R et al. Surgical reconstruction of the superior vena cava. Cardiovasc Surg 1994;2:598–604.
46. Gonzalez-Fajardo J, Garcia-Yuste M, Florez S, et al. Hemodynamic and cerebral repercussions arising from surgical interruption of the superior vena cava: an experimental model. J Thorac Cardiovasc Surg 1994;107:1044–1049.
47. Moghissi K, Dhumale R, Sench M. Innominate to right atrium bypass graft for malignant superior vena caval obstruction. Paper presented to the Society of Thoracic and Cardiovascular Surgeons of Great Britain and Ireland, London, 1983.
48. Kalra M, Gloviczki P, Andrews J, et al. Open and endovascular treatment of superior vena cava syndrome caused by nonmalignant disease. J Vasc Surg 2003;38:215–223.
49. Chatziioannou A, Alexopoulos T, Mourikis D, et al. Stent therapy for malignant superior vena cava syndrome: should be first-line therapy or simple adjunct to radiotherapy? Eur J Radiol 2003;47:247–250.
50. Garcia Monaco R, Bertoni H, Pallota G. Use of self-expanding vascular endoprostheses in superior vena cava syndrome. Eur J Cardiothorac Surg 2003;24:208–211.
51. Wilson E, Lyn E, Lynn A, Khan S. Radiological stenting provides effective palliation in malignant central venous obstruction. Clin Oncol 2002;14:228–232.
52. Miller J, McBride K, Little F, et al. Malignant superior vena cava obstruction: stent placement via the subclavian route. Cardiovasc Intervent Radiol 2000;23:155–158.
53. Tanigawa N, Sawada S, Mishima K, et al. Clinical outcome of stenting in superior vena cava syndrome associated with malignant tumors, comparison with conventional treatment. Acta Radiol 1998;39:669–674.
54. Gross C, Kramer J, Waigand J, et al. Stent implantation in patients with superior vena cava syndrome. Am J Roentgenol 1997;169:429–432.
55. Moore W, Hollier L, Pickett T. Superior vena cava and central venous reconstruction. Surgery (St. Louis) 1991;110:35–41.

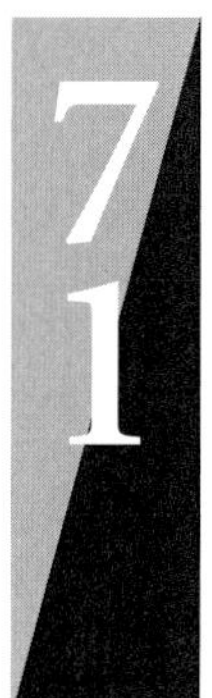

Central Nervous System Emergencies

Kevin P. McMullen, Edward G. Shaw, and Volker W. Stieber

Emergency management of central nervous system malignancies is an unfortunate reality facing the oncologist. Although expeditious treatment is certainly the cornerstone of management, the astute clinician should carefully weigh a combination of multidisciplinary therapeutic options to ensure optimal outcome for the patient, with an eye toward both treatment sequelae and anticipation of future need for further treatment.

Malignant Spinal Cord Compression

Epidemiology and Pathology

Malignant spinal cord compression (MSCC) is a medical emergency, with incidence second only to brain metastases for cancer emergencies in the central nervous system. Spinal cord compression from epidural metastases occurs in 5% to 10% of cancer patients, and in up to 40% of patients with preexisting nonspinal bone metastases.[1–4] Of those with bony spinal disease, 10% to 20% develop symptomatic spinal cord compression, resulting in more than 25,000 cases per year.[5,6] Symptoms depend on location of the compression and can involve the spinal cord at any level. If not rapidly diagnosed and treated, paralysis, incontinence, and severe chronic pain may be the inevitable result.

The spine is the most common site of bony metastases overall, with a reported incidence in cancer patients of 40%.[4] It has been estimated that the incidence of MSCC in the United States is approximately 25,000 cases annually.[5,6] Approximately 5% to 10% of patients who die of their malignancy experience an MSCC.[6,7] A recent population-based cohort study of cancer patients in Ontario, Canada, from 1990 to 1995, is the most comprehensive study available in the peer-reviewed literature on epidemiology for MSCC.[8] In this study, overall incidence of MSCC within 5 years of death from cancer was 2.5% overall. Based on the American Cancer Society estimate of 563,700 cancer deaths expected in 2004,[9] and assuming this population cohort is similar to the U.S. population, then an overall incidence for MSCC of 2.5% or 5% would estimate the number of cases of MSCC in 2004 to be between 14,100 and 28,200.

MSCC is slightly more common in male patients than in female patients (60:40 ratio).[10] This difference may reflect the relative incidence of primary breast cancer compared with primary prostate cancer. All ages of patients may be affected, but the period of highest prevalence coincides with the relatively high cancer risk period that occurs between 40 and 65 years of age.[9]

The histology of MSCC follows the incidence patterns of malignant disease, with the most common histologic diagnoses (breast, lung, and prostate) accounting for approximately half of all cases.[4,9] Approximately 25% of all patients with MSCC have breast cancer, 15% have lung cancer, and 10% have prostate carcinomas. In the Ontario study, the overall incidence of MSCC ranged from 0.2% to 7.9%, depending on primary disease site.[8] Overall, 5.5% of breast cancer patients, 2.6% of lung cancer patients, 7.2% of prostate cancer patients, and 0.8% of colorectal cancer patients experienced a MSCC. Other commonly reported histologic diagnoses in adults include, by order of cumulative incidence, multiple myeloma, nasopharynx, renal cell, melanoma, small cell lung, lymphoma, and cervix.[4,8,11]

Seventy percent of cases occur at the thoracic level, 20% at the lumbar region, and 10% at the cervical region, approximately corresponding to the vertebral body bone volume in each region of the spine.[12,13] Metastatic lesions present initially at multiple, noncontiguous levels in 10% to 38% of cases.[12,14,15] In a recent prospective trial of surgical decompression and radiation therapy, the incidence of MSCC by vertebral level was 10% to 16% cervical, 35% to 40% in T1–T6, and 44% to 55% in T7–T12.[16] By vertebral location, 56% to 64% were in the anterior vertebral body, 18% to 22% in the lateral elements, and 14% to 26% in the posterior elements, with a spine instability rate of 35% to 40% at the time of presentation.

Pathophysiology

A complicated cascade of events occurs with compression of the spinal cord and nerve roots. Epidural venous plexus compression can lead to cord edema and the secondary increase in inflammatory mediators, such as prostaglandin E_2 and interleukins 1 and 6. This cascade of events, if left unchecked, will eventually lead to ischemia, neuronal death, and permanent neurologic injury.[4,17]

Anterior tumors can cause compression by growing posteriorly from the vertebral body into the epidural space, or by vertebral body collapse, causing tumor/bone retropulsion into the spinal canal. Lateral and posterior elements are less commonly, sites of origin for tumor that causes MSCC. Paravertebral tumors can cause compression by entering the spinal canal through the intervertebral foramina, and in rare instances, metastases can be intramedullary or in the epidural space without bony involvement.[4,18] If not addressed rapidly upon the appearance of suspicious symptoms, it has been reported that roughly only 10% to 25% of patients who are not ambulatory before treatment will regain the ability to walk, as pretreatment ambulatory function is the main determinant for posttreatment gait function.[19–21] In addition, patients who have a slow loss of function are significantly more likely to ambulate again after treatment than those with rapid decline when treated with radiation therapy.[22]

Clinical Presentation and Diagnosis

The clinical presentation of tumors metastatic to the spinal axis is a function of the local anatomy.[23] Within the spinal canal there exists a well-defined extradural space containing epidural fat and blood vessels. Metastatic lesions are most commonly found in the extradural space. The extradural space communicates with adjacent extraspinal compartments via the intervertebral foramina. A spinal cord tumor produces local and distal symptoms and signs; the latter reflect involvement of motor and sensory long tracts within the spinal cord. These signs allow localization of the level of the lesion based on clinical findings.[23] However, the clinical presentation of a spinal tumor rarely indicates if it is extradural or intradural. Loss of sphincter control and ambulation before initiation of treatment are poor prognostic factors for recovery of function, so expeditious imaging and subsequent treatment must be initiated without delay when MSCC is suspected. Ninety percent or more of patients present with local and/or radicular pain.[4,20,24,25] Weakness (76%) and sensory findings (51%) are common at diagnosis but are rarely, if ever, a presenting symptom.[12]

Lesions at the conus medullaris can produce several symptoms, including saddle anesthesia, acute urinary retention, incontinence of bowel and bladder, and impotence. If the lesion remains confined to the conus, it will not cause paralysis of the lower limbs and the ankle reflexes are preserved. However, rarely is a conus tumor diagnosed when it is this small, but rather, when some extension upward has occurred and there are additional cord signs.

Flaccid weakness, atrophy, fasciculations, and reduced deep tendon reflexes are seen in corresponding myotomes, with involvement of the anterior horn cells and the ventral roots (lower motor neuron lesions). A tumor involving the lateral corticospinal tracts can cause weakness, spasticity, hyperreflexia, and an extensor plantar response (Babinski's sign). Motor weakness and spasticity are seen with tumors above the conus medullaris. Weakness and flaccidity are seen with tumors below the conus. A tumor restricted to the conus should not cause weakness, although one also involving the cauda equina will.

Sensory impairment often helps to localize the level of the tumor based on loss of dermatome function, although the upper level of impaired long tract function may be several segments below the actual tumor. A lesion involving the lateral spinothalamic tract will cause numbness, paresthesias, and decreased temperature sensation over the contralateral limb or trunk below the lesion; this produces the classic finding of a sensory level, which is best demonstrated with a pin observation for absence of perspiration or of temperature (cold) sensation. A lesion in the posterior column can cause gait ataxia. Standing posture is affected with the eyes closed (Romberg's sign). Paresthesias can occur below the level of the lesion.

Because pain and temperature pathways cross over in the spinal cord and proprioceptive and motor pathways do not, a unilateral spinal cord lesion can result in ipsilateral paralysis and proprioceptive loss, as well as contralateral pain–temperature loss below the level of the lesion. Because light touch travels in two pathways, one that crosses in the spinal cord (spinothalamic tract) and one that does not (posterior columns), it is usually spared in unilateral lesions. This combination of findings is known as the Brown–Sequard syndrome.

Both bladder and bowel symptoms can result from a spinal cord tumor. Bladder symptoms include hesitancy, dribbling, incontinence, urgency with incontinence, or acute retention. Most of the time, if the bowel is affected, constipation rather than incontinence occurs. Loss of bladder control is seen early in the presentation of tumors in or below the conus and later in tumors above the conus. Cord lesions above L1 can lead to impotence or reflex priapism. Lesions involving S2–S4 may produce loss of erection and ejaculation ability. Decreased genital sensation can occur from lesions affecting the S2 nerve roots.

Pain from spinal canal tumors can be either radicular, midline, or central. Radicular pain is secondary to involvement of the posterior roots and is typically described as shooting pain in a dermatomal distribution. The nerve can be compressed inside or outside the dura. Midline spinal pain causes discomfort localized to the area of the tumor and is thought to arise from pain-sensitive structures in the dura and extradural tissues. Characteristically, pain is more severe in extradural lesions. Sometimes, with spinal cord compression, a dull or burning pain, more widespread than segmental spinal or radicular pain, occurs. This type of pain, although relatively rare, has numerous designations, including central pain, causalgia, and deafferentation pain; it involves a limb or trunk below the lesion.

Cauda equina lesions can cause radicular pain in the thigh, weakness, and atrophy of muscles, including the glutei, hamstrings, gastrocnemius, and the anterior tibialis. Saddle anesthesia, absent ankle reflexes, impotence, urinary urgency, or acute retention and constipation are also commonly seen. Depending upon the location of the lesion, other reflexes may be affected.

Intramedullary metastases are exceedingly rare. In this location, they can cause a characteristic neurologic syndrome. Early on, decreased temperature and pain sensation occurs in the dermatomes of the spinal segments occupied by the tumor and two to three segments caudal to the lesion. No other sensory modality is affected while the tumor is confined to the central cord. This "dissociated" sensory loss is rarely seen with extramedullary tumors. Additionally, weakness and atrophy are early findings in the myotomes of the corresponding cord segments involved by tumor. As the tumor grows transversely, reflexes produced at the level of the tumor disappear, and spastic paralysis with hyperreflexia develops below the lesion. Eventually, all sensory modalities are affected. Cervical tumors can produce Horner's syndrome by interrupting unilateral autonomic pathways.

Magnetic Resonance Imaging of The Spine: Evidence Level III, Recommendation Grade A

The most important modality in the workup of suspected MSCC is magnetic resonance imaging (MRI) of the entire spinal axis with gadolinium enhancement. With the exception of a primary paraspinal or neuraxis tumor, MSCC occurs most often in the setting of disseminated disease from a distant primary site. A potential pitfall in the initial evaluation of a patient with suspected spinal cord compression, is imaging only the symptomatic area of the spine. Frequently, patients with lower body or extremity symptoms, and/or radicular pain in the lumbar distribution, present for evaluation and management with only partial spine imaging. Helweg-Larson et al. reported on a series of patients with MSCC diagnosed by myelography.[26] Their data showed that 35% of patients with MSCC had multiple metastases at presentation, and 7.5% developed a second episode of MSCC in an untreated portion of the spine during follow-up. Today, myelography has been replaced by magnetic resonance imaging. Husband et al. published a prospective study evaluating the value of MRI of the entire spine in the workup of suspected MSCC.[27] In this study of 201 patients, 25% of patients evaluated had spinal cord compression verified at multiple levels, and approximately two-thirds of these had involvement of different regions of the spine. The authors determined that when a sensory level was present on patient evaluation, it was two or more segments different from the actual lesion on MRI in 28% of patients, and four or more levels distant from the lesion in 21%. These data confirm that the entire spine must be imaged with MRI with gadolinium enhancement to make early diagnosis of occult lesions in other segments of the spinal axis.

Treatment

Medical Management

Use of Steroids: Evidence Level II, Recommendation Grade A

Dexamethasone is the most commonly used agent. Maranzano et al. reported on a consecutive series of 209 patients who received different steroid regimens based on pretreatment clinical assessment of extent of motor deficit.[28] All patients received 30 Gy radiation therapy, but paraparetic and paraplegic patients received 1 g/day methylprednisolone, whereas patients with better motor function received 16 mg/day dexamethasone, with results comparing favorably across the literature. No direct comparison has ever been attempted with methylprednisolone and dexamethasone.

Dexamethasone is typically given at an initial dosage of 16 mg divided into four daily doses, with a subsequent taper lasting a few weeks to several months (usually a dose reduction of 2 mg every 3–7 days), as guided by the patient's symptoms.[29,30] The lowest possible dose should be used. Patients not on corticosteroids at the beginning of radiation may be observed and dexamethasone added if they become symptomatic. Side effects of intermediate- to long-term steroid use include hyperglycemia, insomnia, emotional lability, thrush, gastric irritation and intestinal ulceration, proximal muscle wasting, weight gain and adiposity (moon facies, buffalo hump, centripetal obesity), osteoporotic compression fractures, and aseptic necrosis of the hip joints.[31]

The efficacy of steroids has been well demonstrated. In a single blind, randomized trial of 57 patients by Sorenson et al., patients with MSCC from solid tumors, were assigned to radiation therapy with or without high-dose dexamethasone (96 mg bolus; 96 mg per day given orally in qid dosing for 3 days, followed by a 10-day taper).[19] The primary endpoint was maintaining pretreatment gait function and/or the recovery of lost function. Radiation therapy to both groups was 28 Gy in 7 consecutive days of 4 Gy per day. Results showed improved rates of surviving with intact gait function at 3 months (81% versus 63%), 6 months (59% versus 33%), and 1 year (30% versus 20%).[32]

The optimal dose of steroids has not been completely defined. The concern with the use of high-dose steroids is the associated toxicity, and some data exist that moderate-dose steroids in the treatment of MSCC may be just as effective as a high dose. A small randomized trial by Vecht et al., comparing high (100 mg) and modest (10 mg) initial bolus dose dexamethasone in patients with MSCC, reported no difference between the two regimens in terms of continence, ambulation, or pain.[33] However, the number of patients was small and there was no stratification by pretreatment motor function.[18] In the trial by Sorenson et al., 11% of patients suffered significant toxicity in the high-dose steroid treatment arm.[19] Heimdal et al. reported overall steroid-related toxicity of 28.6%, 14.3% of which was rated as serious.[19,34] When these authors abandoned higher-dose steroids for moderate dose (16 mg/day tapered over 2 weeks), there were no serious steroid-related side effects reported. On the other hand, Greenberg et al. reported only 1 of 89 patients on a high-dose regimen of dexamethasone with RT who suffered a serious steroid-related complication.[25]

Select patients may not require steroids during treatment. Maranzano et al. reported a Phase II trial of 20 consecutive patients with good baseline motor function and without major invasion of the spinal cord.[35] Of the 20 patients, 80% were ambulatory without need for support, and 20% needed support for ambulation as a result of radiculopathy or pain. Patients received 3,000 cGy in 10 fractions initiated within 24 hours of diagnosis, and no steroids were given. All 16 ambulatory patients retained gait function, and the other 4 patients regained the ability to walk. This study suggests that some patients with good performance status who have rapid local treatment may be considered candidates to manage without steroids, although the majority of published data with radiation therapy are in combination with steroids. This management strategy may be considered reasonable if a patient is at high risk of complication from steroids because of underlying medical comorbidities, such as peptic ulcer disease, uncontrolled diabetes, or other medical problems that may cause severe or life-threatening problems if steroids are initiated.

Surgery

Surgical Decompression: Evidence Level II, Recommendation Grade A

Laminectomy has historically been the standard surgery for MSCC, with most series in the literature showing no benefit to laminectomy-treated patients over patients managed with radiation therapy.[4,12,36,37] Laminectomy traditionally had not only failed to showed a benefit but also was reported to have high rates of spinal instability and postoperative morbidity.[4,8] Because most spinal cord compression is from sources anterior to the spinal canal, it stands to reason that simply enlarging the spinal canal with laminectomy would usually fail. Vertebral body resection offers the possibility of truly decompressing the spine and resecting tumor and bone fragments. No studies have ever compared these two modalities, but the morbidity is greater in vertebral body resection series (10%–54%) than in laminectomy series (0%–10%).[8] Figure 71.1 shows an example of an anterior vertebral body resection of MSCC with surgical stabilization.

Despite the risk of morbidity, emergency surgery is not without support as initial management for MSCC. Harris et al. reported retrospectively on 84 patients with MSCC and compared outcomes based on whether the patient received emergent decompressive surgery or routine surgery (within 24 hours).[38] There were no reported postoperative deaths, and most of the surgical procedures were laminectomy or laminectomy with fusion (98%). Functional improvement, as defined by continence and/or mobility, was more commonly seen in patients who underwent emergency decompression (62% versus 25%). In this series, almost half (49%) of 35 incontinent and immobile patients regained function, with most of those regaining function (77%) being in the emergency surgery group. Furthermore, Sundaresan et al. retrospectively reviewed 110 surgical patients, 78% of whom underwent higher-risk surgery of anterior or anterior/posterior resection with instrumentation. The overall success rate, measured as maintaining or regaining ambulatory function, was 82% with decompressive surgery.[39] Strikingly, 67% of nonambulatory patients recovered gait, and in a subgroup of patients rated as having severe paresis, 55% regained gait function.

Radiation Therapy

Radiation Therapy Alone: Evidence Level II, Recommendation Grade A

In reality, many patients with spinal cord compression are not surgical candidates and are best treated with steroids and radiation therapy as their primary modality. Even patients with very poor initial performance or mobility/continence status can be helped by receiving emergent radiation therapy. Although no randomized trials exist comparing radiotherapy to best supportive care or medical therapy alone, every published radiotherapy series for MSCC has shown efficacy of radiation therapy in helping patients to retain or regain lost function and to relieve pain. Steroids are always initiated at the time of diagnosis, and as already discussed, the strongest evidence suggests that high-dose dexamethasone is the preferred regimen.

Selection of Radiation Therapy Dose: Evidence Level III, Recommendation Grade B

Treatment outcomes reported in the literature vary only a small amount from series to series, regardless of fractionation schedule. Multiple fractionation schedules, ranging from $8\,Gy \times 1$ to $2\,Gy \times 20$, have been proposed and evaluated both prospectively and retrospectively[21,25,28,40–42] (Table 71.1). Morbidity is generally low and is well tolerated even by patients with a poor performance status. Approximately 89% of patients who are ambulatory before radiation therapy can expect to retain gait function, while an average of 39% of paretic patients and 10% of paraplegic patients can expect to see an improvement after treatment.[8] Although 30 Gy in 10 fractions and 37.50 Gy in 15 fractions are commonly used regimens, no compelling data are available to point to poorer outcomes with hypofractionated regimens.[40] Most recently,

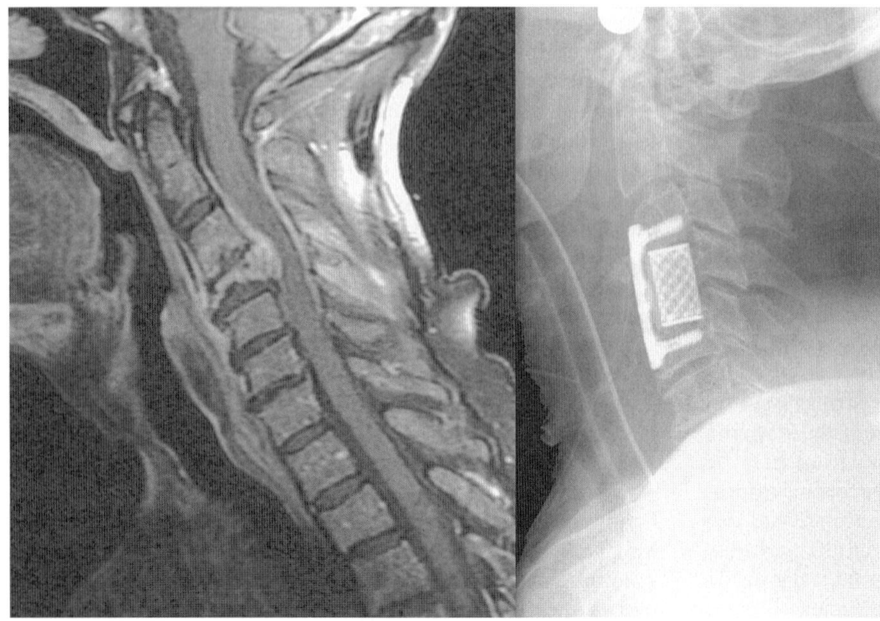

FIGURE 71.1. This patient presented with upper extremity weakness and numbness, and magnetic resonance imaging (MRI) revealed tumor with vertebral body collapse and a spinal cord compression at the C4 level. Surgery was recommended, and the patient's vertebral column was stabilized with resection of the gross tumor.

TABLE 71.1. Typical fractionation schedules for treatment of spinal cord compression and subsequent functional outcomes.

Author	*Total dose*	*Fraction size*	*Overall percentage of patients ambulatory after irradiation*
Greenberg[25] Maranzano[97]	15 Gy, followed by 15 Gy for responders	5 Gy, followed by 3 Gy for responders	57%–75%
Helweg-Larson[21] Sorensen[19]	28 Gy	4 Gy	61%–72%
Hoskin[42]	8 Gy 20 Gy	8 Gy 4 Gy	71%
Maranzano[98]	16 Gy (1 week split)	8 Gy	63%
Maranzano[28]	15 Gy, then 15 Gy 30 Gy	5 Gy, then 3 Gy 3 Gy	76%
Rades[99]	30 Gy 40 Gy	3 Gy 2 Gy	56%–60%

Gy, gray.

Maranzano et al. have reported preliminary data of a randomized trial comparing 16 Gy in 2 fractions to a 30-Gy split-course regimen (15 Gy in 3 fractions followed by 15 Gy in 5 fractions for responders), showing no difference in efficacy or toxicity.[43]

Reirradiation of a spinal metastasis may be necessary in some long-term survivors with recurrent disease. Schiff et al. reviewed 54 reirradiated patients with at least two courses of radiation therapy to the same segment of the spine for the risk of radiation-induced myelopathy.[44] The median initial dose was 3,000 cGy in 10 fractions and the median reirradiation dose was 2,200 cGy in 11 fractions, with a median time of 9.1 months elapsing between treatment courses. Ninety percent of ambulatory patients retained gait function by the end of treatment, 43% regained ambulatory status, and 88% of ambulatory patients at the end of reirradiation were still ambulatory at the last documented follow-up.

Treatment Techniques

Common treatment approaches include a single posterior field (PA), opposed lateral fields, a PA field with opposed laterals, opposed anteroposterior/posteroanterior (AP/PA) fields, and oblique wedge-pair fields.[45,46] Normal tissue constraints and potential toxicity must be considered when defining field arrangements. For tumors in the cervical region, an opposed lateral-beam approach can be employed to minimize dose to the anterior neck. For tumors in the cervicolumbar region, a split-beam technique can be employed with the central axis placed above the upper limit of the shoulders. Opposed lateral beams are used to treat the upper spine, whereas a PA field is used for the area of the spine below the central axis. Tumors in the thoracic region can be treated with opposed lateral beams: a three-field approach using a PA field and opposed lateral beams, a two-field approach using anteroposterior beams, or a posterior beam prescribed to an appropriate depth. The tolerance of dose-limiting organs, most commonly, the spinal cord and esophagus, may need to be taken into account by the radiation oncologist, depending upon the clinical scenario. In the lumbar region, care should be taken to minimize dose to the kidneys; AP/PA or PA fields are often used here, but a four-field approach using AP/PA and opposed lateral beams with the AP/PA beams preferentially weighted may be useful.

Tolerance of the Spinal Cord and Lumbosacral Nerve Roots: Evidence Level II, Recommendation Grade A

Radiation myelopathy may present as a transient early delayed or as a late delayed reaction. Transient radiation myelopathy is clinically manifested by momentary, electrical shocklike paresthesias or numbness radiating from the neck to the extremities, precipitated by neck flexion (Lhermitte's sign).[47] The syndrome typically develops 3 to 4 months after treatment and spontaneously resolves over the following 3 to 6 months without therapy. It is attributed to transient demyelination caused by radiation-induced inhibition of myelin-producing oligodendroglial cells in the irradiated spinal cord segment.[47–49]

Irreversible radiation myelopathy typically is not seen earlier than 6 to 12 months after completion of treatment. It is thought to be multifactorial, involving demyelination and white matter necrosis ultimately caused by oligodendroglial cell depletion and microvascular injury. The signs and symptoms are typically progressive over several months, but acute onset of plegia over several hours or a few days is possible. The diagnosis of radiation myelopathy is one of exclusion that first requires a history of radiation therapy in doses sufficient to result in injury. The region of the irradiated cord must lie slightly above the dermatome level of expression of the lesion; the latent period from the completion of treatment to the onset of injury must be consistent with that observed in radiation myelopathy, and local tumor progression must be ruled out. There are no pathognomonic laboratory tests or imaging studies that conclusively diagnose radiation myelopathy. MRI findings include swelling of the spinal cord with hyperintensity on the T_2-weighted images with or without areas of contrast enhancement.[49,50] There is no known consistently effective treatment for radiation myelitis.[51,52] The probability of dying of radiation myelopathy is approximately 70% in cervical lesions and 30% with thoracic spinal cord injury.[53] Figure 71.2 shows the characteristic MRI findings of radiation-induced myelitis.

There is no convincing evidence that the cervical and thoracic cord differ in their radiosensitivity, and there appears to be little change in tolerance with variations in the length of cord irradiated.[54] Typically, half the patients who develop radiation-induced myelopathy in the cervical or thoracic cord region will do so within 20 months of treatment and 75% of

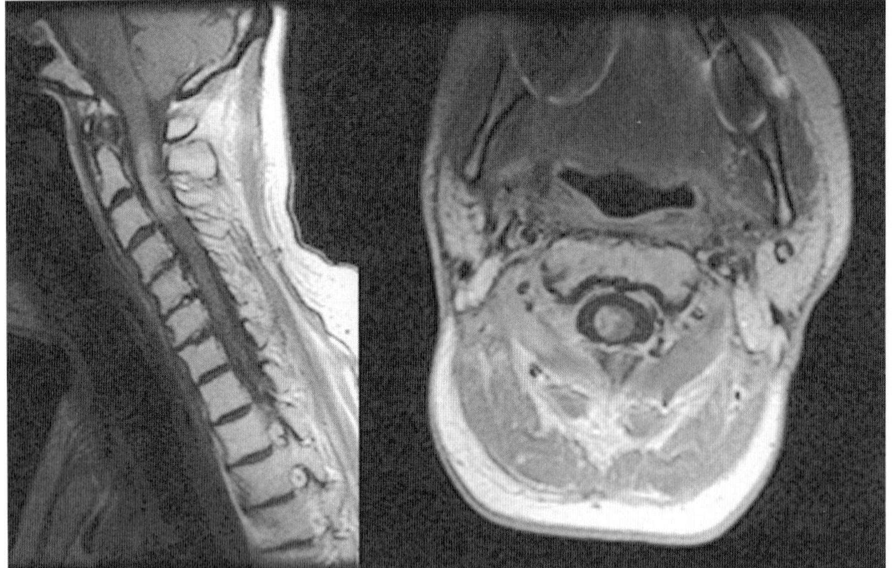

FIGURE 71.2. This patient received 50 Gy (at 200 cGy per fraction) of radiation therapy to the cervical spine. His expected risk of myelitis was less than 5%. At 2.5 years after treatment, he developed pain, extremity weakness, and numbness, and eventually urinary retention. The patient's imaging revealed increased T2 signal with an expansile region showing poorly defined gadolinium enhancement. These findings, along with the clinical history and symptoms, were consistent with radiation myelitis.

the cases will occur within 30 months.[55] Table 71.2 shows a range of iso-morbid fractionation schemes, all of which carry a 5% risk of radiation myelopathy.[56–65] The tolerance of the lumbosacral nerve roots appears to be somewhat higher than that of the spinal cord.[66–68] Given that the overall survival of patients presenting with MSCC is 6 months or less, selecting the shortest feasible fractionation schedule may be reasonable for the majority of patients.

Multimodality Therapy

Surgical Decompression Followed by Adjuvant Radiation Therapy: Evidence Level I, Recommendation Grade A

Randomized and retrospective data historically have shown the benefit of surgery before radiation therapy to be of questionable benefit.[12,36] Because the most common surgical procedure in the past for decompression of MSCC has been laminectomy, it stands to reason that most of the time the tumor is not adequately debulked. This is purely an anatomic issue, because a laminectomy will merely remove the posterior elements of the spinal column, and in most cases, the tumor is growing posteriorly toward the spinal cord from a tumor burden within the vertebral body. Thus, a posterior approach would not ordinarily lend itself to removal of tumor in these cases and would only allow the cord to be displaced posteriorly without compression by the posterior rim of the bony spinal canal.

Patchell et al. recently reported the results of a randomized trial evaluating the benefit of adding surgical decompression to the radiotherapeutic management of metastatic spinal cord compression.[16] Patients with symptomatic malignant spinal cord compression documented by clinical examination and MRI, were randomized to decompressive surgery with high-dose dexamethasone and adjuvant radiation therapy or the same radiation therapy and steroids without surgery. Dexamethasone dose was 100 mg on day 1 followed by 24 mg per day thereafter. Surgery was a decompressive procedure of the surgeon's discretion, and radiation therapy was given as 30 Gy in 10 fractions over 2 weeks. Patients treated with radiation alone were allowed to undergo surgery if they had a significant decrease in neurologic function; this did not apply to patients who were completely paraplegic at the start of treatment. The primary endpoint of the trial was the length of time patients maintained their ambulatory status after treatment. Secondary endpoints were the length of time patients were able to maintain continence, overall survival, and narcotic and steroid dose requirements. The trial initially was planned to accrue approximately 200 patients, but a planned interim analysis forced an early stoppage of the trial after accruing the first 100 patients when an improvement in gait maintenance was demonstrated in the surgery arm (P = 0.0045). Patients who underwent decompressive surgery had a median time of gait retention of 126 days versus 35 days for those receiving only radiation therapy. More strikingly, 56% of surgical patients who were not ambulatory at the start of treatment regained gait function, but only 19% in the radiation-alone arm regained gait function, and 30% of those who underwent surgical salvage walked again. Continence was

TABLE 71.2. Fractionation schemes with a 5% iso-effective risk of radiation-induced spinal cord myelopathy.

Dose per fraction (Gy)	*No. of fractions*	*Total dose (Gy)*
2.00	29	58.00
3.00	13	39.00
3.30	11	33.00
4.00	7	28.00
5.00	5	25.00
10.00	1	10.00

Gy, gray.

Source: Adapted from Stieber et al.,[100] by permission of McGraw-Hill, 2005.

TABLE 71.3. Randomized and nonrandomized data showing the benefit of the addition of surgical decompression to radiation therapy in the management of malignant spinal cord compression (MSCC).

Author	*Randomized*	*N*	*Endpoint*	*RT*	*RT + Sx*	*Significant difference in outcome?*
Patchell et al.[16]	Yes	101	Days of ambulation retention	35	126	Yes
			Percent regaining ambulation	19%	56%	Yes
Young et al.[36]	Yes	29	Ambulatory posttreatment			
			Immediately	54%	45%	
			Alive and ambulatory at 4 months	83%	66%	No
Gilbert et al.[12]	No	235	Ambulatory posttreatment	49%	46%	
			Percent alive and ambulatory (at 6 months/12 months)			
			At 6 months	78%	75%	
			At 12 months	46%	54%	(n/a)

RT, radiation therapy; Sx, surgery.

maintained for 142 versus 12 days, favoring the surgery arm. Overall survival was not significantly different at 129 (surgery) versus 100 days ($P = 0.08$). The median steroid dose given to patients who received only radiation therapy was one-third of that given to those who underwent surgery (0.0093), and narcotic dosages were 12-fold less in surgical patients (0.002). The surgical complication rate was 12% among those patients who underwent planned surgery but 40% for those who received surgery because of treatment failure after radiation therapy alone. Overall, this trial suggests that all patients presenting with MSCC of short duration should undergo decompressive surgery, if feasible. Table 71.3 compares these outcomes to older historical data.

Emergent Management of Brain Tumors and Their Sequelae

Epidemiology and Pathology

Patients with primary brain tumors or brain metastases may occasionally present with potentially life-threatening symptoms requiring emergent management. Although either primary or metastatic tumors can cause symptoms requiring emergent management, this scenario is most commonly associated with metastatic lesions because of the 10:1 ratio of incidence each year of metastatic tumors compared to primary brain tumors.[69] Besides brain metastases, similar problems can also be encountered with posterior fossa tumors, such as medulloblastoma or ependymoma, tumors with a tendency to sudden hemorrhage with subsequent rapid enlargement, such as metastatic melanoma or choriocarcinoma, leukemic involvement of the central nervous system, and highly infiltrative tumors that commonly exhibit significant surrounding brain edema, such as glioblastoma multiforme. Primary brain tumors can frequently be distinguished from brain metastases based on imaging characteristics, location, number of lesions, and a previous diagnosis of extracranial malignancy. Primary brain tumors, once resected and the patient stabilized, are managed according to accepted treatment pathways and/or clinical trials that are not specifically the subject of the following review.

Pathophysiology

A tumor can obstruct cerebrospinal fluid (CSF) flow directly by sheer size and location or indirectly, as a result of secondary edema in the normal brain tissue that then leads to mass effect and subsequent CSF obstruction. Obstruction of normal CSF flow and cerebral edema can lead rapidly to increased intracranial pressure, which in turn results in headaches, nausea, vomiting, and, ultimately, lethargy, coma, and death.

Clinical Presentation and Diagnosis

Presenting signs and symptoms of an intracranial mass include headache (70%), miscellaneous focal neurologic deficits, seizures (30%–60%), cognitive impairment (30%), papilledema (8%), and intracranial hemorrhage, among others.[11,18] Patients may develop obstructive hydrocephalus, particularly those with lesions in proximity to crucial areas of narrow CSF flow, such as the third or fourth ventricle or the foramen of Munro.

Diagnostic Workup

Patients with signs and symptoms of an intracranial emergency need rapid evaluation to assess the cause (Figure 71.3). Among the possible causes of central nervous system (CNS) intracranial emergency in cancer patients, are metastases or primary brain tumor, hemorrhage, infarction, as well as infectious, inflammatory, drug-related, or metabolic etiologies.[18] Computed tomography (CT) gives inferior imaging of brain parenchyma but can give good baseline information initially and can be done quickly in a tenuously stable patient or a patient in whom a hemorrhage is suspected. Once the patient's condition has stabilized, the brain imaging modality of choice is MRI of the brain with and without gadolinium enhancement. Lumbar puncture should be avoided if at all possible until intracranial pressure has normalized because of the risk of herniation and death.

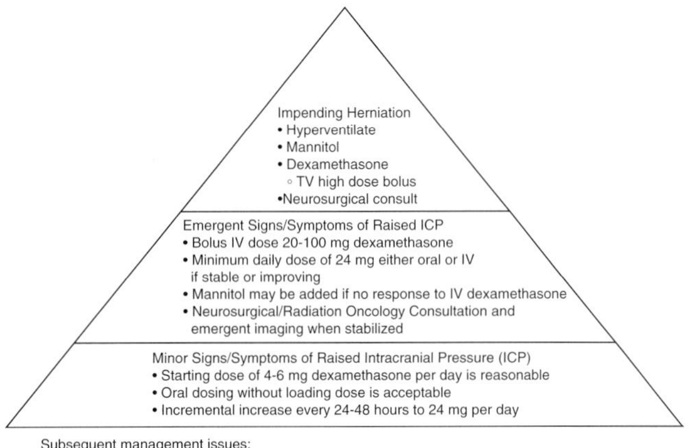

Subsequent management issues:

- GI prophylaxis with H2 blocker/proton pump inhibitor until off steroids
- Monitor for hyperglycemia, thrush, anticonvulsant levels, electrolyte disorders
- Taper dexamethasone after surgical resection or initiation of radiation therapy
    - Taper over 2-4 weeks based on symptom control, starting dose and toxicity of steroid therapy
    - If neurological symptoms recur, increase dexamethasone to last dose at which patient was neurologically stable and taper more slowly
- Monitor for infections in immunocompromised patients; PCP prophylaxis justified in some patients

FIGURE 71.3. Recommended management of raised intracranial pressure (ICP) from emergent (*top*) to minor (*bottom*).

Treatment

Medical Management

The initial emergent management consists of hyperventilation, which, through a series of changes induced by decreased partial pressure of CO_2, leads to vasoconstriction and a subsequent transient drop in intracranial pressure (ICP).[11,18] Because of the potentially deleterious effects of prolonged hyperventilation, namely, acidosis and potential ischemic brain injury due to vasoconstriction, other medical measures to decrease ICP must be rapidly employed.

Steroids/Osmotic Agents: Evidence Level I, Recommendation Grade A

Medical decompressive therapy (MDT) generally consists of steroids with or without mannitol.[70] Mannitol functions by decreasing peritumoral brain edema, whereas dexamethasone does not, indicating different pathways in their mechanism of action in reducing the effects of cerebral edema.[71] Mannitol has been shown to be of value for decreasing cerebral edema from sources other than brain tumors (head injury, hepatic failure).[72,73] The only randomized data evaluating the combined usage of mannitol and dexamethasone for cerebral edema are from Canalese et al. for patients with cerebral edema from fulminant hepatic failure.[73] In this study, 44 patients were randomized to mannitol, dexamethasone, both drugs, or no treatment when they developed or presented with encephalopathy. Patients given mannitol had significantly better response in the presence of cerebral edema than those who did not. A common regimen of mannitol is 20% to 25% solution given intravenously over approximately 30 minutes dosed at 0.5 to 2.0 g/kg.[18]

The general value of dexamethasone has been discussed in the section on spinal cord compression. For obvious ethical reasons, no randomized data exist comparing steroids with placebo in patients with emergent symptoms from intracranial malignancy. The first large experience demonstrating the effectiveness of dexamethasone in decreasing cerebral edema in the setting of intracranial malignancies, came from the University of Minnesota.[74,75] Here, 249 patients with intracranial neoplasms were treated with steroids, with 212 having clinical signs of ICP and 31 being comatose. A response to therapy was noted within 12 to 18 hours of administration and more than 80% of patients showed dramatic improvement by 3 to 4 days after initiation of therapy.

Prospective data do exist evaluating the relative risks and benefits of varying dosing regimens of dexamethasone in the emergent management of cranial emergencies.[76,77] Wolfson et al. published a small trial of 12 patients receiving 30 Gy cranial radiation and dexamethasone.[77] All patients received high-dose dexamethasone (24 mg IV every 6 hours) for 48 hours and were then randomized to further steroids (4 mg po every 6 hours) or no further steroids. The study could not confirm a clear benefit to either arm in terms of performance status or neurologic functional status, although the study had a surprisingly low rate of only 33% of patients having any clear response to the high-dose therapy.

Vecht et al. performed two separate randomized trials investigating different dose regimens of dexamethasone in patients with brain metastases who had an impaired performance status.[76] In addition to radiation therapy, all patients received oral dosing of dexamethasone with patients in the first trial randomized to 8 versus 16 mg/day. A tapering schedule with dexamethasone dose reductions every 4 days was initiated at day 7 of steroid therapy. Although the patients did not show a difference in Karnofsky Performance Status (KPS) after 1 week, after 28 days, the low-dose group had a lower rate of KPS improvement (53% versus 81%). The authors hypothesized that the tapering schedule may have been started too early to allow the low-dose patients to maintain their KPS as the tapering schedule was initiated before radiation therapy. They therefore initiated a second study substituting 4 mg per day as the low-dose arm, but continued the steroid dosing unchanged in both arms for the full 28 days before tapering. The results of this trial showed no improvement in KPS for the high-dose arm so long as the steroids were given over a longer period before tapering. A higher percentage of patients (41%) in the 4-mg arm had to have their tapering schedules extended due to recurrence of neurologic symptoms during or after tapering. The authors also found that the incidence of side effects was higher in the high-dose arm, significantly, the development of cushingoid features, peripheral edema, and steroid myopathy. The authors concluded that 4 mg dosing per day of steroids was adequate for treatment of symptomatic edema from brain metastases provided that the patients were tapered over a 28-day period. The outcomes for all treatment groups in these two trials are summarized in Table 71.4. Other studies have raised concerns also over the incidence of steroid-induced toxicity with steroid dosing longer than 21 days in duration.[78] Higher doses and longer tapering schedules should be based on physician assessment of response.

The frequency of dexamethasone dosing is controversial. The plasma half-life in both humans and animal models is relatively short, on the order of 3 to 6 hours, but the biologic half-life may be twice that, and drug-related effects last much longer.[79,80] The most common dosing regimen of dexamethasone is every 6 hours, but a pilot study of twice-daily dexamethasone with radiation therapy, showed good responses with acceptable toxicity.[78] No randomized study comparing the common qid dosing to less-frequent daily dose regimens has been published. An excellent evidence-based review of

TABLE 71.4. The results of two randomized trials investigating different dose regimens of dexamethasone in patients with brain metastases who had an impaired performance status.

	Trial 1		*Trial 2*	
Dexamethasone dose	*8 mg*	*16 mg*	*4 mg*	*16 mg*
Number of patients	20	22	24	23
KPS improvement at 7 days (%)	60	54	67	70
Number of patients	15	16	21	18
KPS improvement at 28 days (%)	53	81	62	50
Elevated glucose (%)	25		18	21[a]
Infections (%)	6		9	9[a]
GI toxicity (%)	6		18	24[a]
Peripheral edema (%)	13		14	26[a]
Cushingoid features (%)	69		32	65[a]
Steroid myopathy (%)	38		14	38[a]

KPS, Karnofsky Performance Status.
[a]Percentage includes patients in high-dose arm on both trials.
Source: Data from references 33, 76.

medical decompressive therapy and dosing literature, including the aforementioned Dutch trial, was published by Sarin and Murthy.[70] This review provides recommendations for starting doses, dose escalation, and tapering schedules based on symptoms and response. Based on this publication and our own review of the peer-reviewed literature, we propose a management scheme as depicted in Figure 71.4.

Anticonvulsants: Evidence Level I, Recommendation Grade A

The routine use of prophylactic anticonvulsants for patients diagnosed with a brain mass is not recommended based on Level 1 evidence. Glantz et al. reported on a randomized, double-blind placebo-controlled study of 74 patients with newly diagnosed brain mass and no history of seizures.[81] Patients received either divalproex sodium or placebo, with an equivalent risk of a first seizure. In addition, Forsyth et al. reported on a prospective, randomized, nonblinded study of 100 patients newly diagnosed with a brain tumor and having no history of prior seizures.[82] Patients were randomized to prophylactic anticonvulsants or placebo and followed for incidence of seizures, seizure-free interval, and survival. Although the study was truncated early for statistical reasons, there was no significant difference between the groups for any of these endpoints.

Stabilization of the patient in status epilepticus to perform imaging and make management decisions is critical.[83] After securing the airway and stabilizing the patient, seizure activity must be terminated as rapidly as possible. Phenytoin and rapid-onset/short-acting benzodiazepines are commonly used to quickly control seizure activity. Recommended initial regimens include 0.1 mg/kg at 2 mg/min lorazepam or diazepam at 0.2 mg/kg at 5 mg/min. Phenytoin infusion of 15 to 20 mg/kg at 50 mg/min or less in adults is indicated for seizure activity refractory to benzodiazepines or after truncation of seizures with diazepam.[83] Failure to control seizures can potentially lead to physical injuries, airway compromise, and secondary brain hypoxia/injury, or coma.[18] From a practical standpoint, no randomized data exist comparing emergent medical treatment of seizure activity to observation because failure to treat is unacceptable.

There is Level 1 evidence for optimization of phenytoin dosing from a recent randomized study investigating the most rapid method of achieving therapeutic phenytoin levels in the emergency setting.[84] This study compared rapid intravenous infusion of fosphenytoin versus traditional phenytoin infusion. Fosphenytoin, a prodrug of phenytoin without the polyethylene glycol (PEG) vehicle, could be infused at a faster rate and was shown to more rapidly achieve therapeutic phenytoin serum levels.

Surgery

Decompressive Surgery: Evidence Level I, Recommendation Grade A

Surgical resection and/or placement of a shunt is often required for emergent management of brain masses causing life-threatening hydrocephalus, mass effect, or profound neurologic impairment. In all instances, attempts at patient stabilization before surgery with the use of high-dose glucocorticoids with or without mannitol should be made. Patients often exhibit rapid recovery of neurologic and/or cognitive function, which may allow time for more effective diagnostic studies. Medical decompression, in many cases, may also relieve symptoms enough that other modalities such as whole-brain radiation therapy or radiosurgery may be considered as alternate management strategies. Good imaging also can better define the lesion(s) in question to allow stereotactic planning for more accurate surgery. Symptoms are usually related to mass effect, so resection or debulking are often the only logical choices if medical therapy fails to provide improvement in neurologic symptoms. Rapid surgical decompression is the treatment of choice for such prob-

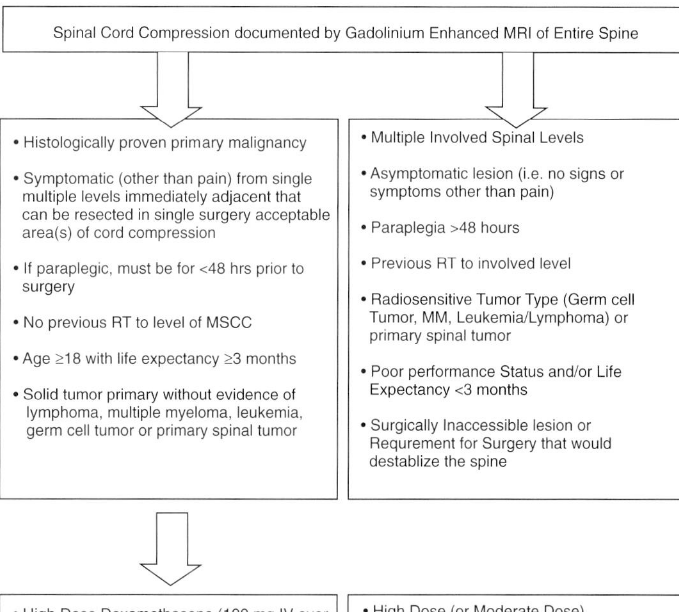

FIGURE 71.4. Evidence-based decision tree graph for malignant spinal cord compression.

lems when surgery can be performed safely based on patient performance status or tumor location. If no neurosurgical team is available, transfer of the patient should be initiated while medical measures are undertaken to stabilize the patient.

Radiation Therapy

Palliative Radiation Therapy: Evidence Level I, Recommendation Grade A

Multimodality therapy for emergent brain tumors routinely takes the form of medical decompression followed by radiation therapy or surgery if there is no response to medical therapy or for most single, bulky resectable lesions. Patients who are medically inoperable, refuse surgery, or have multiple and/or unresectable lesions typically receive whole-brain radiation therapy for palliation of their symptoms. The fact that 60% to 70% of patients who present with brain metastases have multiple lesions makes radiotherapy the primary modality for palliation in the majority of cases.[69,85] Many patients will respond dramatically to medical therapy and radiation in the emergent setting with an improvement in their performance status, particularly if their symptoms are largely caused by edema or rapidly correctable problems, such as electrolyte abnormalities. With this in mind, radiation therapy dosing schedules for the treatment of emergent patients can be tailored to patient parameters, such as initial response to steroids, extent of extracranial disease, primary site, and purported response of primary to systemic therapy.

The Radiation Therapy Oncology Group (RTOG) has reported on several large trials with differing fractionation schedules of whole-brain radiotherapy (Table 71.5). In the specific setting of emergent management, however, there are no randomized trials to specifically address the issues of dose; 50 Gy in conventional fractionation has been used for postoperative treatment,[69] but in the emergent setting, larger daily fraction sizes are typically used to achieve a more rapid response. Doses of 30 to 37.5 Gy using fraction sizes in the range of 2.5 to 3 Gy per day are commonly used but may be adjusted based on patient response. One should keep in mind that larger fraction sizes do seem to predict for a higher incidence of radiation-induced dementia if the patient survives for an extended period of time.[18,69]

Multimodality Therapy

Adjuvant Treatment After Surgery: Level 1 Evidence, Recommendation Grade A

In the context of truly emergent management, there are no randomized data for emergent surgery. If surgery is recommended, this routinely addresses the emergent situation; postoperative radiation therapy as already described is then added on a routine basis once the patient has recovered.[86,87] However, because the treatment of brain metastases is for all practical purposes palliative in its nature, the preservation of functional independence is a valid and strong argument for patients with a solitary metastasis to undergo surgery, if such a benefit can be clearly demonstrated. In this regard, the issue of surgery for patients with solitary brain metastases who have been medically stabilized with MDT remains somewhat controversial. Hazuka et al. retrospectively reviewed patients with one or more metastases who underwent surgery and radiation therapy.[85] Patients with one lesion had excellent median, 1-, and 2-year survivals. Level 1 evidence from two randomized trials comparing radiotherapy with or without surgical resection in the management of solitary brain metastases has documented a survival advantage with the addition of surgery over radiation alone.[86,88] However, another randomized trial failed to show any survival advantage for surgery in addition to radiotherapy alone, the reason for which remains unclear.[89] Table 71.6 summarizes the pertinent data from these three randomized trials. There is no Level 1 evidence demonstrating any survival benefit from operating on patients with multiple metastases. Retrospective data from M.D. Anderson suggest that patients with two or three metastases benefit from having them all resected, even when requiring multiple craniotomies.[90] However, conflicting retrospective data have not been able to confirm this conclusion.[85] Patients with multiple lesions and severe neurologic symptoms from a dominant metastasis that is unresponsive to medical decompressive therapy may benefit from a craniotomy for the reasons just described. An improvement in the patient's performance status may then allow further aggressive therapy with external-beam radiation therapy and/or radiosurgery.

TABLE 71.5. Overview of Radiation Therapy Oncology Group (RTOG) trials evaluating various fractionation regimens for the palliation of brain metastases.

Trial	*Total dose*	*Fraction size*
RTOG 79-16[101]	30 Gy	3 Gy
	30 Gy	5 Gy
RTOG 85-28[102]	48 → 54.4 → 64 → 70.4 Gy	1.6 Gy bid
RTOG 89-05[103]	37.5 Gy	2.5 Gy
RTOG 91-04[104]	54.4	1.6 Gy bid
	30 Gy	3 Gy

Treatment was given once daily unless otherwise noted.
Gy, gray; bid, twice daily.

TABLE 71.6. Randomized and nonrandomized data showing the benefit of the addition of surgical resection to radiation therapy in the management of the solitary brain metastasis.

	Author	*No. of patients*	*Median survival (months)*	*Months of functional independence*	*Rate of death from CNS progression*	*No. of patients with initial KPS less than 70*	*Percentage of patients with extracranial disease*
Sx + RT	Patchell	25	10	9.5	29%	0	36%
	Vecht	32	10	8.25	35%	8	31%
	Mintz	41	5.62	1.8	46%	8	42%
RT alone	Patchell	23	3.75	2	50%	0	39%
	Vecht	31	6	3.75	33%	9	32%
	Mintz	43	6.28	2.1	63%	10	49%

Source: Adapted from Patchell,[69] by permission of *Cancer Treatment Reviews*.

Chemotherapy: No Evidence

There is currently no role for chemotherapy in the emergent management of brain tumors. A Japanese trial evaluated the use of whole-brain radiotherapy with or without chemotherapy after surgical resection, but demonstrated no compelling benefit from the additional therapy.[91]

Nonmetastatic Intracranial Disease

Patients with malignant glioma who require emergent treatment are typically treated with regimens similar to those used for brain metastases. Surgical debulking is the mainstay of emergent treatment, as is the initiation of steroid therapy. Patients who are unable to undergo surgical debulking may be treated with a short course of whole-brain radiation similar to that used for brain metastases. Varying fractionation schedules ranging from 30 Gy in 6 fractions to 50 Gy in 20 fractions have been described in the palliative setting.[92–95] Typically, the prognosis for these patients is quite poor; if they survive long enough to complete their initial course of treatment, their survival time typically ranges from 3 to 9 months under the most favorable circumstances.

Leukemic brain infiltration causing acute mental status changes and/or impending herniation is a rare entity. There are virtually no data in the literature defining the optimal radiation therapy dosing for treatment of this uncommon problem. Most data describing the treatment of CNS leukemia with radiation therapy are from the pediatric experience and typically describe nonemergent craniospinal axis irradiation. One series from M.D. Anderson described the management of recurrent CNS leukemia in adults.[96] The median dose to the cranium was 24 Gy in 1.8-Gy fractions, with a median dose of 18 Gy given to the spine. Most patients also received chemotherapy in some form. The median times to progression and to death from CNS relapse were 7 and 9 months, respectively. Based on this experience, patients presenting with leukemic brain involvement requiring emergent palliative therapy could be treated with total doses ranging from 24 to 30 Gy in 1.8- to 3.0-Gy fractions.

Conclusion

Fortunately, reasonable data exist to guide the oncologist in the therapeutic management of most CNS emergencies. For both malignant spinal cord compression and brain metastases, emergent therapy typically consists of initiation of steroid therapy, evaluation for emergent decompressive surgery, and a relatively short course of palliative radiation therapy. In addition, the astute clinician will learn to recognize the nuances of each case that will require therapeutic decisions based not on randomized trials, but on hindsight and foresight, that is, past clinical experience and anticipation of future problems.

References

1. Wong DA, Fornasier VL, MacNab I. Spinal metastases: the obvious, the occult, and the impostors. Spine 1990;15(1):1–4.
2. Healey JH, Brown HK. Complications of bone metastases: surgical management. Cancer (Phila) 2000;88(suppl 12):2940–2951.
3. Bilsky MH, Lis E, Raizer J, Lee H, Boland P. The diagnosis and treatment of metastatic spinal tumor. Oncologist 1999;4(6):459–469.
4. Byrne TN. Spinal cord compression from epidural metastases. N Engl J Med 1992;327(9):614–619.
5. Gerszten PC, Welch WC. Current surgical management of metastatic spinal disease. Oncology (Huntingt) 2000;14(7):1013–1024.
6. Schaberg J, Gainor BJ. A profile of metastatic carcinoma of the spine. Spine 1985;10(1):19–20.
7. Sucher E, Margulies JY, Floman Y, Robin GC. Prognostic factors in anterior decompression for metastatic cord compression. An analysis of results. Eur Spine J 1994;3(2):70–75.
8. Loblaw DA, Laperriere NJ, Mackillop WJ. A population-based study of malignant spinal cord compression in Ontario. Clin Oncol (R Coll Radiol) 2003;15(4):211–217.
9. American Cancer Society I. Cancer Facts and Figures 2004. Chicago: American Cancer Society, 2004.
10. Constans JP, de Divitiis E, Donzelli R, Spaziante R, Meder JF, Haye C. Spinal metastases with neurological manifestations. Review of 600 cases. J Neurosurg 1983;59(1):111–118.
11. Schiff D, Batchelor T, Wen PY. Neurologic emergencies in cancer patients. Neurol Clin 1998;16(2):449–483.
12. Gilbert RW, Kim JH, Posner JB. Epidural spinal cord compression from metastatic tumor: diagnosis and treatment. Ann Neurol 1978;3(1):40–51.
13. Pigott KH, Baddeley H, Maher EJ. Pattern of disease in spinal cord compression on MRI scan and implications for treatment. Clin Oncol (R Coll Radiol) 1994;6(1):7–10.
14. Ruff RL, Lanska DJ. Epidural metastases in prospectively evaluated veterans with cancer and back pain. Cancer (Phila) 1989;63(11):2234–2241.
15. O'Rourke T, George CB, Redmond J III, et al. Spinal computed tomography and computed tomographic metrizamide myelography in the early diagnosis of metastatic disease. J Clin Oncol 1986;4(4):576–583.
16. Patchell R, Tibbs PA, Regine WF, et al. A randomized trial of direct decompressive surgical resection in the treatment of spinal cord compression caused by metastasis. J Clin Oncol 2003;21(90230):237s-a.
17. Siegal T. Spinal cord compression: from laboratory to clinic. Eur J Cancer 1995;31A(11):1748–1753.
18. Quinn JA, DeAngelis LM. Neurologic emergencies in the cancer patient. Semin Oncol 2000;27(3):311–321.
19. Sorensen S, Helweg-Larsen S, Mouridsen H, Hansen HH. Effect of high-dose dexamethasone in carcinomatous metastatic spinal cord compression treated with radiotherapy: a randomised trial. Eur J Cancer 1994;30A(1):22–27.
20. Black P. Spinal metastasis: current status and recommended guidelines for management. Neurosurgery 1979;5(6):726–746.
21. Helweg-Larsen S, Sorensen PS, Kreiner S. Prognostic factors in metastatic spinal cord compression: a prospective study using multivariate analysis of variables influencing survival and gait function in 153 patients. Int J Radiat Oncol Biol Phys 2000;46(5):1163–1169.
22. Rades D, Heidenreich F, Karstens JH. Final results of a prospective study of the prognostic value of the time to develop motor deficits before irradiation in metastatic spinal cord compression. Int J Radiat Oncol Biol Phys 2002;53(4):975–979.
23. Mumenthaler M. Diseases affecting mainly the spinal cord. In: Mumenthaler M (ed). Neurology. New York: Thieme, 1990:181–232.
24. Rodichok LD, Harper GR, Ruckdeschel JC, et al. Early diagnosis of spinal epidural metastases. Am J Med 1981;70(6):1181–1188.
25. Greenberg HS, Kim JH, Posner JB. Epidural spinal cord compression from metastatic tumor: results with a new treatment protocol. Ann Neurol 1980;8(4):361–366.

26. Helweg-Larsen S, Hansen SW, Sorensen PS. Second occurrence of symptomatic metastatic spinal cord compression and findings of multiple spinal epidural metastases. Int J Radiat Oncol Biol Phys 1995;33(3):595–598.
27. Husband DJ, Grant KA, Romaniuk CS. MRI in the diagnosis and treatment of suspected malignant spinal cord compression. Br J Radiol 2001;74(877):15–23.
28. Maranzano E, Latini P. Effectiveness of radiation therapy without surgery in metastatic spinal cord compression: final results from a prospective trial. Int J Radiat Oncol Biol Phys 1995;32(4):959–967.
29. Thapar K, Taylor MD, Laws ER. Brain edema, increased intracranial pressure, and vascular effects of human brain tumors. In: Kaye AH, Laws ER (eds). Brain Tumors: An Encyclopedic Approach. London: Churchill Livingstone (Elsevier Science), 2001:189–215.
30. Tatter SB. Neurosurgical management of low- and intermediate-grade gliomas. Semin Radiat Oncol 2001;11(2):113–123.
31. Bilsky M, Posner JB. Intensive and postoperative care of intracranial tumors. In: Ropper AH (ed). Neurological and Neurosurgical Intensive Care. New York: Raven Press, 1993:309–329.
32. Kalkanis SN, Eskandar EN, Carter BS, Barker FG. Microvascular decompression surgery in the United States, 1996 to 2000: mortality rates, morbidity rates, and the effects of hospital and surgeon volumes. Neurosurgery 2003;52(6):1251–1261.
33. Vecht CJ, Haaxma-Reiche H, van Putten WL, de Visser M, Vries EP, Twijnstra A. Initial bolus of conventional versus high-dose dexamethasone in metastatic spinal cord compression. Neurology 1989;39(9):1255–1257.
34. Heimdal K, Hirschberg H, Slettebo H, Watne K, Nome O. High incidence of serious side effects of high-dose dexamethasone treatment in patients with epidural spinal cord compression. J Neuro-oncol 1992;12(2):141–144.
35. Maranzano E, Latini P, Beneventi S, et al. Radiotherapy without steroids in selected metastatic spinal cord compression patients. A phase II trial. Am J Clin Oncol 1996;19(2):179–183.
36. Young RF, Post EM, King GA. Treatment of spinal epidural metastases. Randomized prospective comparison of laminectomy and radiotherapy. J Neurosurg 1980;53(6):741–748.
37. Loblaw DA, Laperriere NJ. Emergency treatment of malignant extradural spinal cord compression: an evidence-based guideline. J Clin Oncol 1998;16(4):1613–1624.
38. Harris JK, Sutcliffe JC, Robinson NE. The role of emergency surgery in malignant spinal extradural compression: assessment of functional outcome. Br J Neurosurg 1996;10(1):27–33.
39. Sundaresan N, Sachdev VP, Holland JF, et al. Surgical treatment of spinal cord compression from epidural metastasis. J Clin Oncol 1995;13(9):2330–2335.
40. Rades D, Karstens JH, Alberti W. Role of radiotherapy in the treatment of motor dysfunction due to metastatic spinal cord compression: comparison of three different fractionation schedules. Int J Radiat Oncol Biol Phys 2002;54(4):1160–1164.
41. Rades D, Karstens JH. A comparison of two different radiation schedules for metastatic spinal cord compression considering a new prognostic factor. Strahlenther Onkol 2002;178(10): 556–561.
42. Hoskin PJ, Grover A, Bhana R. Metastatic spinal cord compression: radiotherapy outcome and dose fractionation. Radiother Oncol 2003;68(2):175–180.
43. Maranzano E, Frattegiani A, Rossi R, et al. Randomized trial of two different hypofractionated radiotherapy (RT) schedules (8 Gy × 2 vs. 5 Gy × 3; 3 Gy × 5) in metastatic spinal cord compression (MSCC). Radiother Oncol 2002;64(suppl 1):82–83.
44. Schiff D, Shaw EG, Cascino TL. Outcome after spinal reirradiation for malignant epidural spinal cord compression. Ann Neurol 1995;37(5):583–589.
45. Michalski JM. Spinal canal. In: Leibel SA, Phillips TL (eds). Textbook of Radiation Oncology. Philadelphia: Saunders, 1998: 860–875.
46. Minehan KJ, Shaw EG, Scheithauer BW, Davis DL, Onofrio BM. Spinal cord astrocytoma: pathological and treatment considerations. J Neurosurg 1995;83(4):590–595.
47. Esik O, Csere T, Stefanits K, et al. A review on radiogenic Lhermitte's sign. Pathol Oncol Res 2003;9(2):115–120.
48. Okada S, Okeda R. Pathology of radiation myelopathy. Neuropathology 2001;21(4):247–265.
49. Nieder C, Ataman F, Price RE, Ang KK. Radiation myelopathy: new perspective on an old problem. Radiat Oncol Invest 1999;7(4):193–203.
50. Wang PY, Shen WC, Jan JS. MR imaging in radiation myelopathy. AJNR Am J Neuroradiol 1992;13(4):1049–1055.
51. Feldmeier JJ, Lange JD, Cox SD, Chou LJ, Ciaravino V. Hyperbaric oxygen as prophylaxis or treatment for radiation myelitis. Undersea Hyperb Med 1993;20(3):249–255.
52. Liu CY, Yim BT, Wozniak AJ. Anticoagulation therapy for radiation-induced myelopathy. Ann Pharmacother 2001;35(2): 188–191.
53. Schultheiss TE, Stephens LC, Peters LJ. Survival in radiation myelopathy. Int J Radiat Oncol Biol Phys 1986;12(10): 1765–1769.
54. Schultheiss TE, Kun LE, Ang KK, Stephens LC. Radiation response of the central nervous system. Int J Radiat Oncol Biol Phys 1995;31(5):1093–1112.
55. Schultheiss TE, Higgins EM, El Mahdi AM. The latent period in clinical radiation myelopathy. Int J Radiat Oncol Biol Phys 1984;10(7):1109–1115.
56. Ang KK, Jiang GL, Feng Y, Stephens LC, Tucker SL, Price RE. Extent and kinetics of recovery of occult spinal cord injury. Int J Radiat Oncol Biol Phys 2001;50(4):1013–1020.
57. Cohen L, Creditor M. An iso-effect table for radiation tolerance of the human spinal cord. Int J Radiat Oncol Biol Phys 1981;7(7):961–966.
58. Jeremic B, Djuric L, Mijatovic L. Incidence of radiation myelitis of the cervical spinal cord at doses of 5,500 cGy or greater. Cancer (Phila) 1991;68(10):2138–2141.
59. Macbeth FR, Wheldon TE, Girling DJ, et al. Radiation myelopathy: estimates of risk in 1,048 patients in three randomized trials of palliative radiotherapy for non-small cell lung cancer. The Medical Research Council Lung Cancer Working Party. Clin Oncol (R Coll Radiol) 1996;8(3):176–181.
60. Marcus RB Jr, Million RR. The incidence of myelitis after irradiation of the cervical spinal cord. Int J Radiat Oncol Biol Phys 1990;19(1):3–8.
61. McCunniff AJ, Liang MJ. Radiation tolerance of the cervical spinal cord. Int J Radiat Oncol Biol Phys 1989;16(3):675–678.
62. Nieder C, Milas L, Ang KK. Tissue tolerance to reirradiation. Semin Radiat Oncol 2000;10(3):200–209.
63. Niewald M, Feldmann U, Feiden W, et al. Multivariate logistic analysis of dose-effect relationship and latency of radiomyelopathy after hyperfractionated and conventionally fractionated radiotherapy in animal experiments. Int J Radiat Oncol Biol Phys 1998;41(3):681–688.
64. Schultheiss TE. The radiation dose response of the human cervical spinal cord. Int J Radiat Oncol Biol Phys 1999;45(3 suppl 1).
65. Wara WM, Phillips TL, Sheline GE, Schwade JG. Radiation tolerance of the spinal cord. Cancer (Phila) 1975;35(6):1558–1562.
66. Pieters RS, O'Farrell D, Fullerton B. Cauda equina tolerance to radiation therapy. Int J Radiat Oncol Biol Phys 1996; 38(suppl).
67. Fuller DB, Bloom JG. Radiotherapy for chordoma. Int J Radiat Oncol Biol Phys 1988;15(2):331–339.
68. Schoenthaler R, Castro JR, Petti PL, Baken-Brown K, Phillips TL. Charged particle irradiation of sacral chordomas. Int J Radiat Oncol Biol Phys 1993;26(2):291–298.
69. Patchell RA. The management of brain metastases. Cancer Treat Rev 2003;29(6):533–540.

70. Sarin R, Murthy V. Medical decompressive therapy for primary and metastatic intracranial tumours. Lancet Neurol 2003;2(6): 357–365.
71. Bell BA, Smith MA, Kean DM, et al. Brain water measured by magnetic resonance imaging. Correlation with direct estimation and changes after mannitol and dexamethasone. Lancet 1987; 1(8524):66–69.
72. Cruz J, Minoja G, Okuchi K. Improving clinical outcomes from acute subdural hematomas with the emergency preoperative administration of high doses of mannitol: a randomized trial. Neurosurgery 2001;49(4):864–871.
73. Canalese J, Gimson AE, Davis C, Mellon PJ, Davis M, Williams R. Controlled trial of dexamethasone and mannitol for the cerebral oedema of fulminant hepatic failure. Gut 1982;23(7): 625–629.
74. French L. The use of steroids in the treatment of cerebral edema. Bull N Y Acad Med 1966;42(4):301–311.
75. Long DM, Hartmann JF, French LA. The response of experimental cerebral edema to glucosteroid administration. J Neurosurg 1966;24(5):843–854.
76. Vecht CJ, Hovestadt A, Verbiest HB, van Vliet JJ, van Putten WL. Dose-effect relationship of dexamethasone on Karnofsky performance in metastatic brain tumors: a randomized study of doses of 4, 8, and 16 mg per day. Neurology 1994;44(4):675–680.
77. Wolfson AH, Snodgrass SM, Schwade JG, et al. The role of steroids in the management of metastatic carcinoma to the brain. A pilot prospective trial. Am J Clin Oncol 1994;17(3): 234–238.
78. Weissman DE, Janjan NA, Erickson B, et al. Twice-daily tapering dexamethasone treatment during cranial radiation for newly diagnosed brain metastases. J Neuro-Oncol 1991;11(3): 235–239.
79. Cassidy F, Ritchie JC, Verghese K, Carroll BJ. Dexamethasone metabolism in dexamethasone suppression test suppressors and nonsuppressors. Biol Psychiatry 2000;47(7):677–680.
80. Al Katheeri NA, Wasfi IA, Lambert M, Saeed A. Pharmacokinetics and pharmacodynamics of dexamethasone after intravenous administration in camels: effect of dose. Vet Res Commun 2004;28(6):525–542.
81. Glantz MJ, Cole BF, Friedberg MH, et al. A randomized, blinded, placebo-controlled trial of divalproex sodium prophylaxis in adults with newly diagnosed brain tumors. Neurology 1996; 46(4):985–991.
82. Forsyth PA, Weaver S, Fulton D, et al. Prophylactic anticonvulsants in patients with brain tumour. Can J Neurol Sci 2003;30(2):106–112.
83. Working Group on Status Epilepticus, Epilepsy Foundation of America. Treatment of convulsive status epilepticus. Recommendations of the Epilepsy Foundation of America's Working Group on Status Epilepticus. JAMA 1993;270(7):854–859.
84. Swadron SP, Rudis MI, Azimian K, Beringer P, Fort D, Orlinsky M. A comparison of phenytoin-loading techniques in the emergency department. Acad Emerg Med 2004;11(3):244–252.
85. Hazuka MB, Burleson WD, Stroud DN, Leonard CE, Lillehei KO, Kinzie JJ. Multiple brain metastases are associated with poor survival in patients treated with surgery and radiotherapy. J Clin Oncol 1993;11(2):369–373.
86. Patchell RA, Tibbs PA, Walsh JW, et al. A randomized trial of surgery in the treatment of single metastases to the brain. N Engl J Med 1990;322(8):494–500.
87. Patchell RA, Tibbs PA, Regine WF, et al. Postoperative radiotherapy in the treatment of single metastases to the brain: a randomized trial. JAMA 1998;280(17):1485–1489.
88. Vecht CJ, Haaxma-Reiche H, Noordijk EM, et al. Treatment of single brain metastasis: radiotherapy alone or combined with neurosurgery? Ann Neurol 1993;33(6):583–590.
89. Mintz AH, Kestle J, Rathbone MP, et al. A randomized trial to assess the efficacy of surgery in addition to radiotherapy in patients with a single cerebral metastasis. Cancer (Phila) 1996;78(7):1470–1476.
90. Bindal RK, Sawaya R, Leavens ME, Lee JJ. Surgical treatment of multiple brain metastases. J Neurosurg 1993;79(2):210–216.
91. Ushio Y, Arita N, Hayakawa T, et al. Chemotherapy of brain metastases from lung carcinoma: a controlled randomized study. Neurosurgery 1991;28(2):201–205.
92. Phillips C, Guiney M, Smith J, Hughes P, Narayan K, Quong G. A randomized trial comparing 35 Gy in ten fractions with 60 Gy in 30 fractions of cerebral irradiation for glioblastoma multiforme and older patients with anaplastic astrocytoma. Radiother Oncol 2003;68(1):23–26.
93. Chang EL, Yi W, Allen PK, Levin VA, Sawaya RE, Maor MH. Hypofractionated radiotherapy for elderly or younger low-performance status glioblastoma patients: outcome and prognostic factors. Int J Radiat Oncol Biol Phys 2003;56(2):519–528.
94. Roa W, Brasher PM, Bauman G, et al. Abbreviated course of radiation therapy in older patients with glioblastoma multiforme: a prospective randomized clinical trial. J Clin Oncol 2004;22(9): 1583–1588.
95. McAleese JJ, Stenning SP, Ashley S, et al. Hypofractionated radiotherapy for poor prognosis malignant glioma: matched pair survival analysis with MRC controls. Radiother Oncol 2003; 67(2):177–182.
96. Sanders KE, Ha CS, Cortes-Franco JE, Koller CA, Kantarjian HM, Cox JD. The role of craniospinal irradiation in adults with a central nervous system recurrence of leukemia. Cancer (Phila) 2004;100(10):2176–2180.
97. Maranzano E, Latini P, Checcaglini F, et al. Radiation therapy of spinal cord compression caused by breast cancer: report of a prospective trial. Int J Radiat Oncol Biol Phys 1992;24(2): 301–306.
98. Maranzano E, Latini P, Perrucci E, Beneventi S, Lupattelli M, Corgna E. Short-course radiotherapy (8 Gy × 2) in metastatic spinal cord compression: an effective and feasible treatment. Int J Radiat Oncol Biol Phys 1997;38(5):1037–1044.
99. Rades D, Fehlauer F, Hartmann A, Wildfang I, Karstens JH, Alberti W. Reducing the overall treatment time for radiotherapy of metastatic spinal cord compression (MSCC): 3-year results of a prospective observational multi-center study. J Neuro-oncol 2004;70(1):77–82.
100. Stieber V, Tatter S, Shaw EG. Primary spinal tumors. In: Schiff D (ed). Cancer of the Nervous System: Principles and Practice of Neuro-Oncology. Columbus: McGraw-Hill, 2005.
101. Komarnicky LT, Phillips TL, Martz K, Asbell S, Isaacson S, Urtasun R. A randomized phase III protocol for the evaluation of misonidazole combined with radiation in the treatment of patients with brain metastases (RTOG-7916). Int J Radiat Oncol Biol Phys 1991;20(1):53–58.
102. Sause WT, Scott C, Krisch R, Rotman M, et al. Phase I/II trial of accelerated fractionation in brain metastases RTOG 85-28. Int J Radiat Oncol Biol Phys 1993;26(4):653–657.
103. Phillips TL, Scott CB, Leibel SA, Rotman M, Weigensberg IJ. Results of a randomized comparison of radiotherapy and bromodeoxyuridine with radiotherapy alone for brain metastases: report of RTOG trial 89-05. Int J Radiat Oncol Biol Phys 1995;33(2):339–348.
104. Murray KJ, Scott C, Greenberg HM, et al. A randomized phase III study of accelerated hyperfractionation versus standard in patients with unresected brain metastases: a report of the Radiation Therapy Oncology Group (RTOG) 9104. Int J Radiat Oncol Biol Phys 1997;39(3):571–574.

72

Metabolic Emergencies in Oncology

Daniel J. De Angelo

Tumor Lysis Syndrome

Tumor lysis syndrome (TLS) refers to the constellation of electrolyte abnormalities that occur as a result of the rapid and immediate release of intracellular contents into the bloodstream. The syndrome is characterized by hyperuricemia, hyperkalemia, hyperphosphatemia, and hypocalcemia (Table 72.1).[1–4] Metabolic acidosis and acute renal failure may also occur. The release of intracellular potassium and organic, as well as inorganic, phosphate into the bloodstream from cells undergoing apoptosis, results in the development of hyperkalemia and hyperphosphatemia, respectively.[5,6] Prolonged and severe hyperphosphatemia may result in a marked decrease of the serum calcium concentration, but symptomatic hypocalcemia rarely develops. It is the rapid breakdown of nucleic acids that leads to hyperuricemia.[7] TLS may develop before the administration of chemotherapy in patients with rapidly proliferating hematologic neoplasms; however, TLS usually occurs after the administration of high doses of chemotherapy, which results in the rapid destruction of tumor cells.[8–11]

Patients with large tumor burdens are at an increased risk for TLS (Table 72.2), especially if the malignancy is sensitive to chemotherapy. These disorders include acute myelogenous and lymphoblastic leukemias, especially those with high circulating blast counts.[4,12,13] In addition, TLS is commonly seen in patients with acute lymphoblastic and Burkitt's lymphomas or other high-grade lymphoproliferative disorders (Table 72.3).[14] Large bulky solid tumors that undergo rapid cellular destruction also place patients at a significant risk for the development of TLS.[15–20] TLS is more common in patients with elevated lactate dehydrogenase (LDH) levels. Elevated LDH levels are usually caused by ongoing cell lysis and are most commonly seen in patients with aggressive hematologic malignancies. TLS has also been described after the use of nonchemotherapy agents, such as α-interferon or with hormonal therapy for breast cancer.[21,22] The risk of developing TLS is greater in older patients or patients with poor renal function at baseline. These patients have a lower glomerular filtration rate and are more susceptible to electrolyte disturbances as compared to patients with normal renal function.

Hyperuricemia

Purine nucleotides and deoxynucleotides are broken down within the liver. Xanthine oxidase catalyzes the breakdown of hypoxanthine and xanthine to uric acid[23] (Figure 72.1). With the exception of primates, all other mammals convert uric acid to allantoin, which is 10 times more soluble than uric acid. The pK_a of uric acid is approximately 5.75 at 37°C. Therefore, in the serum where the pH is higher, uric acid is usually present in the acid-soluble form. Within the acidic environment of the renal tubules, uric acid is present in the nonionized and therefore less soluble form.[24] Hyperuricemia can be present as an isolated abnormality without the other characteristic metabolic findings associated with TLS (Table 72.4)[6,9,25] Renal insufficiency develops when the urine becomes supersaturated with urate, which is caused by the development of uric acid crystals in the renal tubules and the distal renal collecting system.[26,27] The development of uric acid stones is uncommon and usually develops only in patients with chronic hyperuricemia. Before the development of renal failure, patients with hyperuricemia may develop nausea, vomiting, diarrhea, and anorexia. As renal function declines, patients may develop edema and lethargy. In addition to renal failure, gouty arthritis is the other most important consequence of both acute and chronic hyperuricemia. It is important to recognize that certain medications, namely, diuretics, such as thiazides, as well as antituberculous drugs and certain cytotoxic agents, can aggravate hyperuricemia.

The single most important factor in the treatment of hyperuricemia is first to recognize the patients who are most at risk for its development and then initiate appropriate prophylactic measures (Figure 72.2). Drugs that elevate serum uric acid levels should be discontinued if at all possible. Intravenous hydration should be initiated, preferably before the start of chemotherapy.[28] It is important to correct any preexisting intravascular volume deficits. By increasing urinary outflow, the concentration of uric acid is substantially decreased, thereby decreasing the problems typically associated with its poor solubility. The main focus in the treatment of hyperuricemia is to attempt to maintain adequate urinary volume. Alkalinization of the urine will further decrease uric acid solubility, which can usually be achieved with the addition of sodium bicarbonate (50–100 mmol/L) to the intravenous fluids. The admixture can be adjusted so that the urine pH is maintained above 7.0 without overalkalinizing the serum.[29–31] This latter complication may further complicate hypocalcemia when present.[25] Acetazolamide is a carbonic anhydrase inhibitor that may be added to increase the effects of alkalinization. Nevertheless, the most important factor in decreasing uric acid levels is the maintenance of adequate urine output, and alkalinization remains a secondary factor. Although furosemide increases the renal tubular reab-

TABLE 72.1. Tumor lysis syndrome.

Metabolic complications
Hyperuricemia
Hyperkalemia
Hyperphosphatemia
Hypocalcemia
Metabolic acidosis
Acute renal failure may also result

sorption of uric acid, this is offset by the preservation of increased urinary flow rates. Therefore, furosemide can be used safely to maintain a proper total body fluid balance.

Allopurinol (Zyloprim, Aloprim) is the standard medical treatment for both the prevention and treatment of hyperuricemia.[32] Allopurinol is an inhibitor of xanthine oxidase and is extremely well tolerated. The most common adverse reaction is an erythematous skin rash due to a hypersensitivity reaction. Fortunately, this reaction is usually delayed by several days, and allopurinol can be given safely during the most critical period for patients who are at a high risk for the development of TLS. There have been rare reports of interstitial nephritis developing after the administration of allopurinol. Allopurinol will increase the serum levels of both hypoxanthine and xanthine; however, this has rarely been associated with the development of acute renal failure.[33–35] Allopurinol (Zyloprim) is usually administered orally at a dose of 200 to 300 mg/m^2/day. For patients who receive a dose greater than 300 mg/day, allopurinol should be administered in divided doses. Typical doses of allopurinol range from 300 to 600 mg/day with a maximum oral dose of 800 mg/day. Allopurinol is cleared renally, and the dose should be adjusted in older patients or patients with chronic renal failure. In addition, allopurinol is now available intravenously (Aloprim).[36] The typical dose of intravenous allopurinol is 200 to 400 mg/m^2/day as either a single infusion or in divided doses with a maximum adult dose of 600 mg/day. The starting dose of intravenous allopurinol in pediatric patients is slightly lower at 200 mg/m^2/day. Both azathioprine (Imuran) and 6-mercaptopurine (Purinthol) are metabolized by xanthine oxidase; therefore, the dose of these agents must be reduced by one-third to one-fourth during treatment with allopurinol.[23]

Rasburicase (Elitek), a recombinant urate oxidase enzyme, catalyzes the enzymatic oxidation of uric acid into the inactive, water-soluble metabolite, allantoin (see Figure 72.2).[37–40] Rasburicase is well tolerated and has a rapid onset of action as a uricolytic agent. The typical dose of rasburicase is 0.15 to 0.2 mg/kg IV over 30 minutes daily for 1 to 5 days. The safety and efficacy of rasburicase dosing beyond 5 days or for more than one course has not been well established and this should not be recommended. Rasburicase is contraindicated in patients with glucose-6-phosphatase dehydrogenase (G6PD) deficiency.

Rasburicase is effective in both the prophylaxis and treatment of hyperuricemia associated with malignancy.[41,42] With regard to prophylaxis, chemotherapy should begin 4 to 24 hours after the first dose of rasburicase. In patients at high risk of TLS, that is, when uric acid is greater than 8 mg/dL or other criteria consistent with TLS, rasburicase may be substituted for allopurinol. Rasburicase is usually administered at a dose of 0.2 mg/kg IV every 24 hours and is typically required for approximately 1 to 3 doses over a 72-hour period. Allopurinol should not be administered concomitantly with rasburicase. Intravenous hydration should be administered at 3,000 mL/m^2/day during the initial few days of therapy. Alkalinization is not necessary with recombinant urate oxidase therapy.

It is important to evaluate patients who develop oliguria or acute renal failure with ultrasonography or computed tomography (CT) scans to rule out ureteral obstruction caused by uric acid stones. Intravenous contrast agents should be avoided because of the risk of developing acute tubular necrosis.[43] Hemodialysis and continuous venous–venous hemofiltration (CVVH) are both effective in reversing severe uric acid nephropathy and states of fluid overload.[44] Rapid and early

TABLE 72.2. Risk factors for tumor lysis syndrome.

Large tumor burden
Acute leukemias
High-grade lymphomas
Large, bulky solid tumors
High tumor growth fraction
Tumors highly sensitive to chemotherapy
Markedly elevated lactate dehydrogenase (LDH)
Baseline renal insufficiency

TABLE 72.3. Risk for tumor lysis syndrome by tumor type.

Frequent cases
Acute myelogenous leukemia
Acute lymphoblastic leukemia or lymphoma
Burkitt's and other high-grade lymphomas
Less frequent occurrences
Diffuse large B-cell lymphoma
Chronic myelogenous leukemia
Low-grade lymphoma
Small-cell lung cancer
Breast cancer
Germ cell tumor
Non-seminoma, seminoma, mediastinal, ovarian
Rare case reports
Merkel's cell carcinoma
Adenocarcinoma
Medulloblastoma

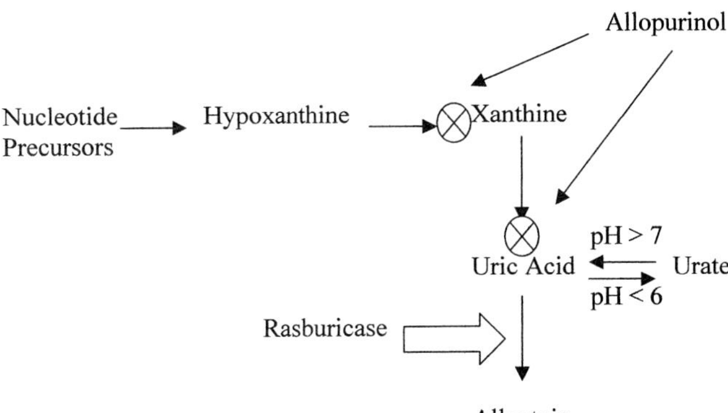

FIGURE 72.1. The oxidation of nucleotide precursors.

TABLE 72.4. Signs and symptoms of tumor lysis syndrome.

Laboratory abnormality	*Clinical symptoms*
Hyperuricemia	Nausea, vomiting, diarrhea, joint pain, oliguria, anuria, azotemia, flank pain, hematuria, crystalluria
Hyperkalemia	Muscle cramps, nausea, weakness, paresthesias, paralysis, EKG changes, bradyarrhythmias, tachyarrhythmias, cardiac arrest
Hyperphosphatemia	Oliguria, anuria, azotemia, renal failure
Hypocalcemia	Muscle twitching, tetany, laryngospasm, paresthesias, hypotension, ventricular arrhythmias, heart block

consultation of the nephrology team should be initiated once the renal function starts to deteriorate or in the case of severe hypervolemia that is not responsive to loop diuretics.

Hyperkalemia

Hyperkalemia is the principal life-threatening electrolyte abnormality that develops during tumor lysis syndrome.[45–47] Hyperkalemia, defined as plasma concentration greater than 5.0mmol/L, results from the release of large intracellular stores due to cell lysis. Iatrogenic causes, which result from administration of potassium, especially in patients with renal insufficiency, must be excluded. Pseudohyperkalemia may result from poor phlebotomy technique, hemolysis, or marked leukocytosis or thrombocytosis. The latter two are caused by the release of intracellular potassium into the serum following clot formation. Measuring the plasma potassium using a heparinized tube may be required in the setting of a markedly elevated platelet count.

The intracellular and extracellular potassium ion concentrations maintain the resting membrane potential.[48] Hyperkalemia will cause a partial depolarization of the resting membrane potential, and prolonged depolarization will eventually lead to impaired excitability, resulting in muscular weakness, which may progress to flaccid paralysis.

The most serious and life-threatening manifestation of hyperkalemia is ventricular arrhythmia (see Table 72.4). Unfortunately, cardiac toxicity does not necessarily correlate with the degree of hyperkalemia. The initial electrocardiographic abnormalities include increased amplitude of the T-waves, which are often referred to as "peaked" T-waves. Subsequent EKG changes include prolongation of the PR and QRS intervals, A-V conduction blocks, and flattening of the P-waves. Eventually the QRS complex will merge with the T-wave, resulting in a sine wave pattern, which will often terminate in ventricular fibrillation or asystole. Fatal

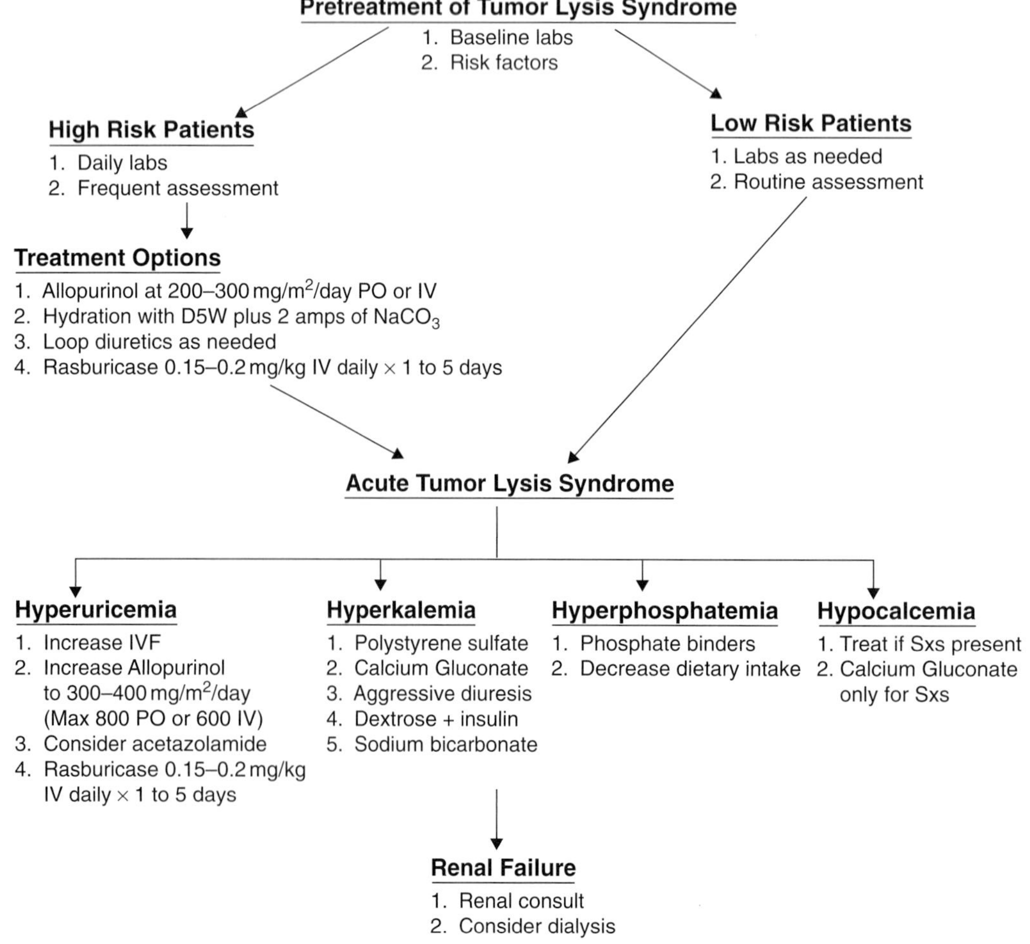

FIGURE 72.2. The treatment of tumor lysis syndrome.

hyperkalemia rarely occurs at a plasma potassium concentration less than 7.5 mmol/L.

The treatment of hyperkalemia largely depends upon the potassium serum concentration (see Figure 72.2). All patients with hyperkalemia, regardless of the degree of elevation, require an electrocardiogram. Furthermore, medications that interfere with potassium metabolism, such as nonsteroidal antiinflammatory drugs (NSAIDS) and angiotensin-converting enzyme inhibitors (ACEI), should be discontinued. Oral cation-exchange resins promote the exchange of potassium and sodium ions within the lumen of the gastrointestinal (GI) tract; this is an easy and effective initial strategy for patients with mild asymptomatic hyperkalemia. A dose of 15 to 30 g sodium polystyrene sulfonate (Kayexalate) will generally lower the serum potassium concentration by 0.5 to 1.0 mmol/L within 1 to 2 hours and last for about 4 hours.

Severe hyperkalemia requires more emergent treatment. Calcium gluconate should be given to decrease cellular membrane excitability. The usual dose is 10 mL 10% solution administered over 1 to 3 minutes. The effect, which can be seen in minutes, is unfortunately short-lived. The administration of insulin with glucose will cause potassium to shift into cells. The usual combination is 10 to 20 units of regular insulin with 25 to 50 g glucose. Glucose should be avoided if the patient is already severely hyperglycemic. This method typically results in the lowering of the serum potassium concentration by 0.5 to 1.5 mmol/L and will last for several hours. Alkalinization of the serum with bicarbonate will also lead to a shift of potassium into cells. Hemodialysis and continuous venous–venous hemofiltration (CVVH) are the most effective methods for effectively lowering the serum potassium levels, especially in patients with either preexisting or acute renal failure. Peritoneal dialysis is not as effective as hemodialysis in lowering the serum potassium level, and its initiation should be avoided in patients receiving chemotherapy.

Hyperphosphatemia

Similar to hyperkalemia, hyperphosphatemia results from the release of intracellular phosphate stores into the serum as a result of cell lysis.[30] Hyperphosphatemia is defined as a serum phosphate level above 1.67 mmol/L (5.0 mg/dL). Spurious hyperphosphatemia may occur in patients with a marked thrombocytosis, and the phosphorus levels should be confirmed in a heparinized tube. In addition, positively charged paraproteins, as in plasma cell dyscrasias, may cause marked elevations in the serum phosphate levels.

Hyperphosphatemia is a potentially dangerous condition because of extraosseous calcification. Although it should only serve as a guideline, a calcium–phosphorus product [serum Ca (mg/dL) × serum P (mg/dL)] greater than 70, suggests a potential risk of metastatic calcification.[49] Prolonged hyperphosphatemia may result in lowering the serum calcium levels. Except in those patients with renal failure, the initial treatment of hyperphosphatemia includes volume expansion (see Figure 72.2), which effectively results in the increase of the fractional clearance of phosphorus by the kidney. Aluminum-based antacids bind to phosphorus in the gut and prevents further absorption. Although the chronic use of these agents may lead to aluminum toxicity, they are safe and effective for short-term use. Other phosphate binders, such as calcium acetate (PhosLo) or sevalamer (Renagel) may also be used. Calcium acetate is dispensed as two tablets or gelcaps (667 mg) with each meal, and the dose can be increased so long as hypercalcemia does not develop. Sevalamer, a cross-linked polyallylamine hydrochloride, is a cationic polymer that binds intestinal phosphate. The recommended starting dose of sevelamer is 800 to 1,000 mg three times daily. The treatment of hyperphosphatemia in the setting of renal failure often requires hemodialysis.

Hypocalcemia

Unlike the other metabolic alterations resulting from TLS, hypocalcemia is a direct manifestation of hyperphosphatemia.[1–3,6] Many oncology patients have hypocalcemia, defined as a serum calcium level less than 2.1 mmol/L (8.5 mg/dL); however, only 10% of these patients will have a reduction in ionized calcium.[50] Hypoalbuminemia is the principal cause of a reduced total serum calcium level in severely ill patients. Overalkalinization of the serum will increase the binding of calcium to proteins and result in a further reduction of the serum calcium level. In these cases, an ionized calcium level should be measured. Transient hypocalcemia also may arise from repeated transfusions of blood products due to the use of citrate as an anticoagulant. Although parathyroid hormone (PTH) is responsible for the regulation of serum calcium levels, it is overwhelmed in patients with TLS by the excessive loss of calcium from the extracellular fluid. Transient hypocalcemia is seldom clinically significant, but if long-standing, it can lead to several serious clinical manifestations (see Table 72.4); these include muscle spasms, carpopedal spasms, and in severe cases, tetany, laryngeal spasms, or convulsions. The QT interval on the EKG can become prolonged, which may lead to serious ventricular arrhythmias. Rarely, patients may become irritable, depressed, or psychotic as a consequence of severe prolonged hypocalcemia.

The principal focus on correcting the hypocalcemia of TLS revolves around the treatment of the hyperphosphatemia (see Figure 72.2). Calcium supplementation with oral calcium or calcium gluconate in severe symptomatic cases must be taken with caution, especially if the calcium–phosphate product is greater than 70 (see above). In general, calcium should not be given in asymptomatic patients, as this may precipitate calcium phosphate deposition. The correction of serum phosphate levels will usually improve the serum calcium levels. For patients who have persistent hypocalcemia, calcitrol may be used until the serum calcium level normalizes.[51]

Hypercalcemia

The single most common metabolic disorder in patients with cancer is hypercalcemia.[52] Hypercalcemia caused by an underlying malignancy must be differentiated from hypercalcemia as a result of primary hyperparathyroidism. Patients who present with cancer-related hypercalcemia often have signs and symptoms of the underlying malignant tumor that include the recent onset of weight loss and is associated with a shortened median survival.[53] Patients with primary hyperparathyroidism are often asymptomatic or present with recurrent nephrolithiasis.[54] The association of elevated serum

TABLE 72.5. **Signs and symptoms of hypercalcemia.**

Category	*Clinical symptoms*
Constitutional	Weight loss, anorexia, polydipsia
Neurologic	Fatigue, lethargy, muscle weakness, confusion, seizure, coma
Gastrointestinal	Nausea, vomiting, constipation, ileus, abdominal pain, obstipation
Renal	Polyuria, azotemia, renal failure
Cardiac	Bradycardia, prolonged PR interval, shortened QT interval, wide T wave, arrhythmias

calcium with a low or normal parathyroid hormone (PTH) level excludes the diagnosis of primary hyperparathyroidism.

Serum calcium is highly bound to albumin; therefore, the total serum concentration will vary depending on serum protein concentrations.[55] Measurement of the ionized calcium level can often assist in sorting out difficult cases.[56,57] An adjustment for the total serum calcium concentration based on the serum albumin concentration can be made as follows:

$$\text{Corrected calcium (mg/dL)} = \text{measured calcium (mg/dL)} - \text{albumin(g/dL)} + 4.0$$

Clinical symptoms that arise from hypercalcemia are a direct result of both the rate of rise and the absolute serum calcium level (Table 72.5).[58] The most common constitutional symptoms include weight loss, anorexia, polydipsia, which may progress into nausea, vomiting, polyuria, azotemia, renal failure, constipation, ileus, abdominal pain, and even obstipation. With continued rise, patients may begin to experience neurologic symptoms, such as fatigue, lethargy, muscle weakness, confusion, seizure, and even coma. Cardiac symptoms are rare, but when they occur, can lead to fatal arrhythmias. The initial electrocardiographic changes include bradycardia, prolonged PR interval, shortened QT interval, and widening of the T-wave.

Most patients remain asymptomatic even with a serum calcium level as high as 14 mg/dL. However, if the serum calcium levels remain at a level of 13 mg/dL for an extended period of time, dehydration, renal insufficiency, and calcifications may begin to occur, especially if the serum phosphate levels are also elevated. When the serum calcium level exceeds 16 mg/dL, severe neurologic and cardiac changes begin to occur that may prove life threatening, and should be treated as a medical emergency, with prompt hospitalization and immediate initiation of appropriate therapy to correct the electrolyte abnormalities.

The cause of cancer-related hypercalcemia depends marginally upon the underlying malignancy. In patients with widespread bone metastasis, hypercalcemia is believed to be associated with direct bone destruction by the cancer cells[59]; this is referred to as local osteolytic hypercalcemia. More commonly however, are the various humorally mediated causes for hypercalcemia.[60–62] Even in patients with extensive bone metastasis, humorally mediated factors often are most important. In many cases of cancer-related hypercalcemia, PTH stimulation induces significant biochemical changes. These changes include increased renal tubular reabsorption of calcium and the development of hypophosphatemia, as well as an increase in urinary output of phosphate.[63,64] The predominant cause of the cancer-related hypercalcemia in these cases is ectopic PTH production with a PTH-related protein (PTH-RP). The genes encoding PTH-RP have been mapped to the short arm of chromosome 12.[65,66] Authentic human PTH has been mapped to the short arm of chromosome 11. Both the authentic PTH, as well as the PTH-RP, have much in common. The most important similarity is within the amino terminal portion where 8 of the first 13 of the amino acids are homologous. This portion of PTH corresponds to the receptor-binding domain. PTH-RP is the most common cause of cancer-related hypercalcemia and is found in many patients with solid tumors, particularly those with squamous cell carcinomas.[67,68] In addition, high levels of PTH-RP have been reported in the human T-cell leukemia/lymphoma virus (HTLV)-1-associated adult T-cell leukemia/lymphoma syndrome (ATLL).[69] In this case, it is thought that the viral *TAX* activates the PTH-RP gene promoter. PTH-RP has also been associated with patients with cancer-related hypercalcemia and patients with bone metastasis from breast carcinoma[70] and prostate cancer.[71] Patients with high levels of PTH-RP in the primary tumor seem more likely to develop bone metastasis. PTH-RP does not seem to be involved in most hematologic cancers, such as multiple myeloma or lymphoma.[67]

Elevated serum levels of 1,25-$(OH)_2$-vitamin D_3 have been reported in patients with Hodgkin's disease, non-Hodgkin's lymphoma, and multiple myeloma.[72,73] The increase of the vitamin D_3 level results from an increase in 1-α-vitamin D-hydroxylase, thereby increasing enzymatic conversion to vitamin D_3.

Osteoclast-activating factors are important molecules that induce bone reabsorption. For example, interleukin 6 (IL-6) is an autocytokine growth factor in patients with multiple myeloma and has been shown to increase bone reabsorption in vitro.[74,75] IL-6 administration can induce remarkably high levels of serum calcium, which can be blocked by specific neutralizing antibodies. Other cytokines can also serve as osteoclast-activating factors, such as interleukin-1, tumor-derived hematopoietic colony-stimulating factor (CSF), tumor necrosis factor, and transforming growth factors (TGFs).[76–78]

It is important to know that the treatment of cancer-related hypercalcemia should be directed at the underlying malignancy. Hypercalcemia most commonly affects older patients, as well as patients with an underlying renal insufficiency, and those patients with advanced disease. It is important to take note of several supportive issues that can exacerbate hypercalcemia, such as immobilization, as well as to review the patient's medication list to avoid drugs that inhibit the usual calcium excretion, such as thiazide diuretics, nonsteroidal antiinflammatory agents, and histamine receptor antagonists.[52]

Most patients with hypercalcemia present with marked dehydration resulting from anorexia, nausea, and vomiting, as well as polyurea caused by calciuresis. Therefore, aggressive fluid repletion with normal saline is the first line of therapy. Appropriate volume expansion not only increases renal blood flow but will also improve calcium excretion. The rate of fluid administration will depend upon the clinical situation, keeping in mind many patients may have renal and cardiac dysfunction at baseline. Once euvolemia has been established, forced diuresis with furosemide can be initiated. One must be extremely careful because furosemide can reestablish a volume-depleted state. The effect of calcium reduction with forced diuresis is only minimal and therefore, the use of furosemide should be limited to balancing fluid intake and urine output, as patients are volume depleted.

Bisphosphonates form the basis of most therapeutic endeavors in the treatment of cancer-related hypercalcemia.[79] Older agents, such as etidronate,[80] and clodronate[81] have been largely replaced with pamidronate (Aredia)[82,83] and zoledronic acid (Zometa).[84–87] The typical onset of action is within 24 to 48 hours. Bisphosphonates work by absorbing to the surface of hydroxyapatite, thereby inhibiting calcium released from bone. Bisphosphonates also interfere with the metabolic activity of osteoclasts. Interestingly, bisphosphonates may not be as effective in the management of cancer-related hypercalcemia in patients and those mediated by PTH-RP.

Both pamidronate and zoledronic acid should be administered intravenously. Pamidronate is typically infused at a dose of 60 to 90mg over 2 to 4 hours, and zoledronic acid is administered at a dose of 4mg in patients with normal renal function. Peak levels of both pamidronate and zoledronic acid have been associated with renal tubular dysfunction.[84,88,89] Although zoledronic acid was initially infused at a rate of less than 15 minutes, infusion rates between 30 and 45 minutes are now being recommended, and zoledronic acid should be dose reduced in patients with renal insufficiency.

Gallium nitrate is a potent inhibitor of bone absorption.[90] Gallium is incorporated into the bone, thereby rendering hydroxyapatite resistant to cell-mediated reabsorption. Calcitonin (Miacalcin) is particularly advantageous, given its rapid onset of action, 2 to 4 hours.[91,92] Calcitonin reduces serum calcium by increasing renal calcium excretion and also by inhibiting bone reabsorption. Unfortunately, the hypocalcemic effect of calcitonin is relatively weak, and the acute response peaks at approximately 48 hours even with continued treatment. Randomized clinical trials have demonstrated the superiority of gallium nitrate over calcitonin for the treatment of resistant hypercalcemia.[93]

The use of corticosteroids is most useful in patients with malignancies that respond to cortical steroid therapy[91,94]; these include multiple myeloma, lymphoma, and acute lymphoblastic leukemia. Unfortunately, corticosteroids do not seem to have a consistent effect on serum calcium levels in other malignancies.

Hyponatremia

Hyponatremia is a potentially life-threatening abnormality that has many causes. One must first differentiate between true hyponatremia and pseudohyponatremia, which is a lowering of the measured serum sodium level that is not physiologic.[95] Because sodium ions are dissolved in plasma, any increase in the nonaqueous phase will artificially lower the serum sodium concentration. This point is important, as the plasma osmolality typically remains normal. The most common cause of pseudohyponatremia is hyperproteinemia or hyperlipidemia. Other causes of pseudohyponatremia as a result of increased plasma osmolality, include hyperglycemia and mannitol administration.

The differential diagnosis of hyponatremia cannot be made until the patient's volume status is accurately determined.[96,97] Hypotonic hyponatremia is typically caused either by a primary water gain or as a result of primary or secondary sodium loss. In the absence of water intake, it is important to realize that hyponatremia is not a disease, but a manifestation of a variety of underlying clinical disorders. To ascertain the cause of hyponatremia, it is important also to measure the plasma osmolality, the urine osmolality, and the urine sodium concentration, as well as the urine potassium concentration.

In patients with hyponatremia, who are volume overloaded, the expanded extracellular fluid (ECF) status is typically caused by a decrease in the effective circulating volume, as in patients with congestive heart failure, hepatic cirrhosis, or nephrotic syndrome. Patients with hyponatremia that occurs as a result of a reduced ECF volume or dehydration, include those with significant sodium losses from sweating, large body area burns, or gastrointestinal losses due to vomiting, fistula or visceral tube drainage, or diarrhea. Diuretic-induced hyponatremia is usually as a result of thiazide-type diuretics, as the loop diuretics impair maximal urinary concentrating capacity.

The syndrome of inappropriate antidiuretic hormone secretion (SIADH) is the most common cause of hyponatremia that occurs in the euvolemic state.[97–99] SIADH is a result of the nonphysiologic release of arginine vasopressin (AVP) either secreted from the posterior pituitary or an ectopic source. SIADH is usually caused by the production of an ADH-like substance through ectopic production, although nonmalignant causes must be excluded (Table 72.6). Although only approximately 10% to 15% of patients with small cell lung cancer present with SIADH, the majority of patients with small cell lung tumors stain positively for AVP. SIADH can be caused by a variety of other tumors, including non-small cell lung cancer, head and neck tumors, brain tumors, and rarely, hematologic malignancies, such as leukemia and lymphoma (Table 72.7).

In addition to malignant cause for SIADH, there are several nonmalignant causes that must be excluded; these include central nervous system infections or vasculitis. Rarely, head injury or benign tumors can also cause SIADH, and numerous pulmonary infections and a variety of drugs have been implicated in causing SIADH. It is important to remember that tumor-associated SIADH remains a diagnosis of exclusion; however, the treatment of both tumor-related SIADH and SIADH from other causes is similar.

The clinical manifestations of hyponatremia are a direct relationship to the rate of change in the serum plasma sodium concentration.[100] Plasma sodium concentrations that fall

TABLE 72.6. Common causes of syndrome of inappropriate antidiuretic hormones secretion (SIADH).

	Drugs
Central nervous system (CNS)	
Infection	Vincristine
Vasculitis	Cytotoxan
Stroke	Cisplatin
Head trauma	Morphine
Tumors	Carbomazepines
	Thiazides
Pulmonary	
Infection	
Tumors	

TABLE 72.7. Causes of SIADH by tumor type.

Lung cancer (small and non-small cell)
Head and neck cancer
Primary CNS tumors
Rare tumors
Mesothelioma
Lymphoma
Leukemia
Gastrointestinal tumors
Gynecologic tumors
Prostate
Bladder

slowly over long periods of time are often well tolerated and patients usually remain asymptomatic. As the plasma sodium concentration falls to below 120mmol/L, patients may develop neurologic symptoms. These symptoms include headache, lethargy, and confusion, and if left uncorrected, may develop into seizures and coma.

The goal of therapy is to increase the serum sodium concentration. In patients with mild to moderate hyponatremia, this can be efficiently corrected by restricting the patient's free water intake.[97,98,101] In the event that free water restriction is ineffective in raising the sodium level, demeclocycline can be used. Demeclocycline (Declomycin) has a modest effect on inhibiting the effect of arginine vasopressin (AVP) on the kidneys. The typical dose of demeclocycline is 600 mg/day. However, one must be cognizant that the overall goal of therapy, specifically in a patient with SIADH, is to effectively treat the underlying malignancy. In patients who have hypovolemia, restoration of normal volume status typically initiates AVP release, allowing free water excretion. In patients with severe hyponatremia that results in the development of neurologic symptoms, it may be necessary to administer hypertonic saline. One must be extremely careful with the administration of hypertonic saline to avoid central pontine myelinolysis.[102] This devastating neurologic syndrome can be avoided by ensuring that the plasma sodium concentration is raised by no more than 1 to 2mmol/L per hour.

Adrenal Failure

Adrenal failure as a result of destruction of adrenal cortical tissue by metastatic tumor is extremely uncommon.[103–105] Bilateral adrenal hemorrhage may also result in severe adrenal insufficiency, and patients with the antiphospholipid antibody syndrome are at high risk of adrenal hemorrhage and infarction.[106,107] In autopsy series, metastases to the pituitary or hypothalamus are found in up to 5% of patients with cancer, but associated adrenal insufficiency is rarely reported. Other causes of adrenal failure include the long-term use of chronic corticosteroid therapy. Patients on long-term corticosteroids may develop suppression of adrenal cortical function and require a taper of their corticosteroids to maintain baseline adrenal function. Patients at the highest risk for adrenal failure caused by chronic corticosteroid therapy are those patients with central nervous system tumors or spinal column tumors or patients undergoing treatment for acute lymphoblastic leukemia, non-Hodgkin's lymphoma, or Hodgkin's disease. Chemotherapeutics that may result in adrenal failure include mitotane (Lysodren), ketoconazole (Nizoral), and aminoglutethemide (Cytadren); the latter inhibits adrenal steroid synthesis.[108]

Symptoms of adrenal insufficiency are rather insidious. Classic signs include weakness, weight loss, and anorexia. In patients with long-standing adrenal insufficiency, hyperpigmentation as well as postural hypertension may also develop. Shock as a result of circulatory collapse is extremely uncommon and may develop in the setting of clinical infection. Laboratory abnormalities include nonanion gap metabolic acidosis, mild hyponatremia, and hypokalemia.

To make the diagnosis of adrenal insufficiency, patients should receive an injection of cosyntropin (Cortrosyn) at a dose of 0.25mg intravenously with measurement of serum cortisone levels at baseline and at 30 minutes and 1 hour after injection. An increase of the serum cortisone level of 5 to 7mg/dL over baseline is considered normal. In patients who are suspected to have adrenal insufficiency based on clinical symptoms, stress-dose steroid replacement should be initiated immediately; this is typically administered as hydrocortisone 100mg intravenously every 8 hours and tapered as tolerated. Physiologic cortisol replacement is administered as prednisone at a dose of 25mg in the morning and 12.5mg in the evening. During periods of stress, such as infection and or an operation, the doses may need to be increased substantially. Occasionally, the addition of a mineralocorticoid, such as fludrocortisone at a dose of 0.1mg/day is required.

Disorders of Blood Glucose

Hypoglycemia as a result of an underlying malignancy is extremely rare. The most frequent cause is as a result of an insulin-producing islet cell tumor. However, several cases of hypoglycemia as a result of non-islet cell tumors have also been reported.[109] Non-islet cell tumors that are associated with hypoglycemia tend to be extremely large and are often mesenchymal in origin, such as fibrosarcomas, leiomyomas, rhabdomyosarcomas, liposarcomas, and even mesotheliomas.[109] There have also been reports of hepatomas causing tumor-related hypoglycemia.

Patients with hypoglycemia usually present with symptoms of tachycardia, diaphoresis, nausea, weakness, and dizziness; these are extremely nonspecific findings, and only if the clinician is extremely compulsive will a diagnosis of hypoglycemia be entertained. For most patients, symptoms are usually worse early in the morning after an overnight fast and improve only after a meal. In patients with severe hypoglycemia, mental status changes may develop that can result in focal neurologic deficits, which may lead to the development of a seizure or coma. Islet cell tumors induce hypoglycemia as a result of abundant ectopic insulin secretion. In most patients with non-islet cell tumor-induced hypoglycemia, the secretion of substances with nonsuppressible insulin-like activity has been detected; these are usually a result of a secretion of insulin-like growth factors, such as IGF-1, IGF-2, somatomedian A, and somatomedian C.[109,110] The IGF proteins are similar to pro-insulin but have only 1% of its biologic activity. Similar to pro-insulin, IGFs are bound by circulating proteins and induce specific biologic activities only after binding to cell-surface receptors.[110–117]

Increased glucose utilization by large tumors may also account for several episodes of cancer-related hypoglycemia. Tumor sizes greater than 1 kg may utilize 50 to 200 g glucose per day.[118] In a healthy patient, the liver can produce approximately 700 g of glucose per day; however, patients with cancer-related hypoglycemia have tumors that weigh several kilograms and may also have extensive hepatic metastasis, which impairs hepatic glucose production. In addition, patients with cancer-related hypoglycemia may have dysfunctional counterregulatory mechanisms that induce hypoglycemia.[118] For example, impaired hepatic function can lead to a decrease in both glycogenolysis and gluconeogenesis.

The treatment of severe hypoglycemia is the immediate infusion of 50 mL 50% dextrose (D50). In patients who have a serum glucose level less than 40 mg/dL, the administration of continuous glucose after an infusion of D50 may prove beneficial. Patients with mild hypoglycemia can usually be managed by increasing the frequency of their meals. In addition, the coadministration of corticosteroids may provide some symptomatic relief, and the use of a continuous infusion of glucagon via a portable pump has met with some success.[119]

The most common glycemic abnormality in patients with cancer is hyperglycemia. Hyperglycemia may result from long-term corticosteroid administration, especially in patients with underlying glucose intolerance or diabetes mellitus.[120] Patients at highest risk are those patients who receive high-dose corticosteroids as part of their chemotherapy or antiemetic regimen, such as those patients with non-Hodgkin's lymphoma, Hodgkin's disease, acute lymphoblastic leukemia, or lymphoma, as well as those patients with metastatic tumors to the central nervous system and spinal column. Long-term corticosteroid administration may result in dysregulated glucose utilization, leading to states of hyperglycemia. For most patients, hyperglycemia is mild and the only metabolic abnormality, but in other patients long-term hyperglycemia may result in hyperosmolar states requiring insulin administration. Rarely will hyperglycemia lead to ketoacidosis unless the patient already has an underlying type 1 diabetes mellitus that is either poorly controlled or inappropriately monitored.[121]

References

1. Arrambide K, Toto R. Tumor lysis syndrome. Semin Nephrol 1993;13:273–280.
2. Abramson E, Gajardo H, Kukreja S. Hypocalcemia in cancer. Bone Miner 1990;10(3):161–169.
3. Flomenbaum C. Metabolic emergencies in the cancer patient. Semin Oncol 2000;27:322–334.
4. Fleming D, Doukas M. Acute tumor lysis syndrome in hematologic malignancies. Leuk Lymph 1992;8:315–318.
5. Hogan D, Rosenthal L. Oncologic emergencies in the patient with lymphoma. Semin Oncol Nurs 1998;14:312–320.
6. Jones D, Mahmoud H, Chesney R. Tumor lysis syndrome: pathogenesis and management. Pediatr Nephrol 1995;9:206–212.
7. O'Connor NT, Prentice HG, Hoffbrand AV. Prevention of urate nephropathy in the tumour lysis syndrome. Clin Lab Haematol 1989;11:97–100.
8. Bunin NJ, Pui CH. Differing complications of hyperleukocytosis in children with acute lymphoblastic or acute nonlymphoblastic leukemia. J Clin Oncol 1985;3:1590–1595.
9. Cohen LF, Balow JE, Magrath IT, Poplack DG, Ziegler JL. Acute tumor lysis syndrome. A review of 37 patients with Burkitt's lymphoma. Am J Med 1980;68:486–491.
10. Frei E III, Bentzel CJ, Rieselbach R, Block JB. Renal complications of neoplastic disease. J Chronic Dis 1963;16:757–776.
11. Rieselbach RE, Bentzel CJ, Cotlove E, Frei E III, Freireich EJ. Uric acid excretion and renal function in the acute hyperuricemia of leukemia. Pathogenesis and therapy of uric acid nephropathy. Am J Med 1964;37:872–883.
12. Razis E, Arlin Z, Ahmed T, et al. Incidence and treatment of tumor lysis syndrome in patients with acute leukemia. Acta Haematol 1994;91:171–174.
13. Tsokos G, Balow J, Spiegel R, Magrath I. Renal and metabolic complications of undifferentiated and lymphoblastic lymphomas. Medicine (Baltim) 1981;60:218–229.
14. Boccia R, Longo D, Lieher M, Jaffe E, Fisher R. Multiple recurrences of acute tumor lysis syndrome in an indolent non-Hodgkin's lymphoma. Cancer (Phila) 1985;56:2295–2297.
15. Drakos P, Bar-Ziv J, Catane R. Tumor lysis syndrome in nonhematologic malignancies. Am J Clin Oncol 1994;17:502–505.
16. Barton J. Tumor lysis syndrome in nonhematopoietic neoplasms. Cancer (Phila) 1989;64:738–740.
17. Dirix LY, Prove A, Becquart D, Wouters E, Vermeulen P, Van Oosterom A. Tumor lysis syndrome in a patient with metastatic Merkel cell carcinoma. Cancer (Phila)1991;67:2207–2210.
18. Crittenden DR, Ackerman GL. Hyperuricemic acute renal failure in disseminated carcinoma. Arch Intern Med 197;137:97–99.
19. Hussein AM, Feun LG. Tumor lysis syndrome after induction chemotherapy in small-cell lung carcinoma. Am J Clin Oncol 1990;13:10–13.
20. Ultmann JE. Hyperuricemia in disseminated neoplastic disease other than lymphomas and leukemias. Cancer (Phila) 1962;15: 122–129.
21. Fer M, Bottino G, Sherwin S, et al. Atypical tumor lysis syndrome in a patient's T-cell lymphoma treated with recombinant leukocyte interferon. Am J Med 1984;77:953–956.
22. Cech P, Block JB, Cone LA, Stone R. Tumor lysis syndrome after tamoxifen flare. N Engl J Med 1986;315:263–264.
23. Conger JD. Acute uric acid nephropathy. Med Clin N Am 1990; 74:859–871.
24. Klinenberg JR, Kippen I, Bluestone R. Hyperuricemic nephropathy: pathologic features and factors influencing urate deposition. Nephron 1975;14:88–98.
25. Lorigan P, Woodings P, Morgenstern G, Scarffe J. Tumor lysis syndrome, case report and review of the literature. Ann Oncol 1996;7:631–636.
26. Wolf G, Hegewisch-Becker S, Hossfeld DK, Stahl RA. Hyperuricemia and renal insufficiency associated with malignant disease: urate oxidase as an efficient therapy? Am J Kidney Dis 1999;34:E20.
27. Mahmoud HH, Leverger G, Patte C, Harvey E, Lascombes F. Advances in the management of malignancy-associated hyperuricaemia. Br J Cancer, 1998;77(suppl 4):18–20.
28. Conger JD, Falk SA. Intrarenal dynamics in the pathogenesis and prevention of acute urate nephropathy. J Clin Invest 1977; 59:786–793.
29. Holland P, Holland NH. Prevention and management of acute hyperuricemia in childhood leukemia. J Pediatr 1968;72: 358–366.
30. Kjellstrand CM, Cambell DC II, von Hartitzsch B, Buselmeier TJ. Hyperuricemic acute renal failure. Arch Intern Med 1974;133:349–359.
31. Garnick MB, Mayer RJ. Acute renal failure associated with neoplastic disease and its treatment. Semin Oncol 1978;5:155–165.
32. Krakoff IH, Meyer RL. Prevention of hyperuricemia in leukemia and lymphoma: use of alopurinol, a xanthine oxidase inhibitor. JAMA 1965;193:1–6.

33. Hande KR, Hixson CV, Chabner BA. Postchemotherapy purine excretion in lymphoma patients receiving allopurinol. Cancer Res 1981;41:2273–2279.
34. Band PR, Silverberg DS, Henderson JF, et al. Xanthine nephropathy in a patient with lymphosarcoma treated with allopurinol. N Engl J Med 1970;283:354–357.
35. Landgrebe AR, Nyhan WL, Coleman M. Urinary-tract stones resulting from the excretion of oxypurinol. N Engl J Med 1975;292:626–627.
36. Smalley RV, Guaspari A, Haase-Statz S, Anderson SA, Cederberg D, Hohneker JA. Allopurinol: intravenous use for prevention and treatment of hyperuricemia. J Clin Oncol 2000;18:1758–1763.
37. Goldman SC, Holcenberg JS, Finklestein JZ, et al. A randomized comparison between rasburicase and allopurinol in children with lymphoma or leukemia at high risk for tumor lysis. Blood 2001;97:2998–3003.
38. Pui CH, Jeha S, Irwin D, Camitta B. Recombinant urate oxidase (rasburicase) in the prevention and treatment of malignancy-associated hyperuricemia in pediatric and adult patients: results of a compassionate-use trial. Leukemia 2001;15:1505–1509.
39. Pui CH, Mahmoud HH, Wiley JM, et al. Recombinant urate oxidase for the prophylaxis or treatment of hyperuricemia in patients with leukemia or lymphoma. J Clin Oncol 2001;19:697–704.
40. Bosly A, Sonet A, Pinkerton CR, et al. Rasburicase (recombinant urate oxidase) for the management of hyperuricemia in patients with cancer: report of an international compassionate use study. Cancer (Phila) 2003;98:1048–1054.
41. Pui CH. Urate oxidase in the prophylaxis or treatment of hyperuricemia: the United States experience. Semin Hematol 2001; 38:13–21.
42. Lee AC, Li CH, So KT, Chan R. Treatment of impending tumor lysis with single-dose rasburicase. Ann Pharmacother 2003;37: 1614–1617.
43. Mandell GA, Swacus JR, Rosenstock J, Buck BE. Danger of urography in hyperuricemic children with Burkitt's lymphoma. J Can Assoc Radiol 1983;34:273–277.
44. Steinberg SM, Galen MA, Lazarus JM, Lowrie EG, Hampers CL, Jaffe N. Hemodialysis for acute anuric uric acid nephropathy. Am J Dis Child 1975;129:956–958.
45. Lobe TE, Karkera MS, Custer MD, Shenefelt RE, Douglass EC. Fatal refractory hyperkalemia due to tumor lysis during primary resection for hepatoblastoma. J Pediatr Surg 1990;25: 249–250.
46. Arseneau JC, Bagley CM, Anderson T, Canellos GP. Hyperkalaemia, a sequel to chemotherapy of Burkitt's lymphoma. Lancet 1973;1:10–14.
47. Wilson D, Stewart A, Szwed J, Einhorn LH. Cardiac arrest due to hyperkalemia following therapy for acute lymphoblastic leukemia. Cancer (Phila) 1977;39:2290–2293.
48. DeFronzo R, Smith J. Clinical Disorders of Hyperkalemia, 5th ed. New York: McGraw-Hill, 1994:697–754.
49. Holick M, Krane S. Introduction to Bone and Mineral Metabolism, 15th ed. New York: McGraw-Hill, 2001:2192–2204.
50. Potts J. Diseases of the Parathyroid Gland and Other Hyper- and Hypocalcemic Disorders, 15th ed. New York: McGraw-Hill, 2001:2205–2225.
51. Dunlay RW, Camp MA, Allon M, Fanti P, Malluche HH, Llach F. Calcitriol in prolonged hypocalcemia due to the tumor lysis syndrome. Ann Intern Med 1989;110:162–164.
52. Stewart AF. Clinical practice. Hypercalcemia associated with cancer. N Engl J Med 2005;352:373–379.
53. Ralston SH, Gallacher SJ, Patel U, Campbell J, Boyle IT. Cancer-associated hypercalcemia: morbidity and mortality. Clinical experience in 126 treated patients. Ann Intern Med 1990;112: 499–504.
54. Bilezikian JP, Silverberg SJ. Clinical practice. Asymptomatic primary hyperparathyroidism. N Engl J Med 2004;350:1746–1751.
55. John R, Oleesky D, Issa B, et al. Pseudohypercalcaemia in two patients with IgM paraproteinaemia. Ann Clin Biochem 1997;34(pt 6):694–696.
56. Ladenson JH, Lewis JW, Boyd JC. Failure of total calcium corrected for protein, albumin, and pH to correctly assess free calcium status. J Clin Endocrinol Metab 1978;46:986–993.
57. Ladenson JH, Lewis JW, McDonald JM, Slatopolsky E, Boyd JC. Relationship of free and total calcium in hypercalcemic conditions. J Clin Endocrinol Metab 1979;48:393–397.
58. LeBoff MS, Mikulec KH. Hypercalcemia: Clinical Manifestations, Pathogenesis, Diagnosis, and Management, 5th ed. Washington, DC: American Society for Bone and Mineral Research, 2003:225–230.
59. Roodman GD. Mechanisms of bone metastasis. N Engl J Med 2004;350:1655–1664.
60. Nakayama K, Fukumoto S, Takeda S, et al. Differences in bone and vitamin D metabolism between primary hyperparathyroidism and malignancy-associated hypercalcemia. J Clin Endocrinol Metab 1996;81:607–611.
61. Godsall JW, Burtis WJ, Insogna KL, Broadus AE, Stewart AF. Nephrogenous cyclic AMP, adenylate cyclase-stimulating activity, and the humoral hypercalcemia of malignancy. Recent Prog Horm Res 1986;42:705–750.
62. Stewart AF, Vignery A, Silverglate A, Ravin ND, LiVolsi V, Broadus AE, Baron R. Quantitative bone histomorphometry in humoral hypercalcemia of malignancy: uncoupling of bone cell activity. J Clin Endocrinol Metab 1982;55:219–227.
63. Horwitz MJ, Tedesco MB, Sereika SM, Hollis BW, Garcia-Ocana A, Stewart AF. Direct comparison of sustained infusion of human parathyroid hormone-related protein-(1-36) [hPTHrP-(1-36)] versus hPTH-(1-34) on serum calcium, plasma 1,25-dihydroxyvitamin D concentrations, and fractional calcium excretion in healthy human volunteers. J Clin Endocrinol Metab 2003;88:1603–1609.
64. Bonjour JP, Philippe J, Guelpa G, et al. Bone and renal components in hypercalcemia of malignancy and responses to a single infusion of clodronate. Bone (NY) 1988;9:123–130.
65. Moseley JM, Kubota M, Diefenbach-Jagger H, et al. Parathyroid hormone-related protein purified from a human lung cancer cell line. Proc Natl Acad Sci U S A 1987;84:5048–5052.
66. Suva LJ, Winslow GA, Wettenhall RE, et al. A parathyroid hormone-related protein implicated in malignant hypercalcemia: cloning and expression. Science 1987;237:893–896.
67. Burtis WJ, Brady TG, Orloff JJ, et al. Immunochemical characterization of circulating parathyroid hormone-related protein in patients with humoral hypercalcemia of cancer. N Engl J Med 1990;322:1106–1112.
68. Wysolmerski JJ, Broadus AE. Hypercalcemia of malignancy: the central role of parathyroid hormone-related protein. Annu Rev Med 1994;45:189–200.
69. Motokura T, Fukumoto S, Matsumoto T, et al. Parathyroid hormone-related protein in adult T-cell leukemia-lymphoma. Ann Intern Med 1989;111:484–488.
70. Powell GJ, Southby J, Danks JA, et al. Localization of parathyroid hormone-related protein in breast cancer metastases: increased incidence in bone compared with other sites. Cancer Res 1991;51:3059–3061.
71. Iwamura M, di Sant'Agnese PA, Wu G, et al. Immunohistochemical localization of parathyroid hormone-related protein in human prostate cancer. Cancer Res 1993;53:1724–1726.
72. Seymour JF, Gagel RF. Calcitriol: the major humoral mediator of hypercalcemia in Hodgkin's disease and non-Hodgkin's lymphomas. Blood 1993;82:1383–1394.

73. Seymour JF, Gagel RF, Hagemeister FB, Dimopoulos MA, Cabanillas F. Calcitriol production in hypercalcemic and normocalcemic patients with non-Hodgkin lymphoma. Ann Intern Med 1994;121:633–640.
74. Bataille R, Jourdan M, Zhang XG, Klein B. Serum levels of interleukin 6, a potent myeloma cell growth factor, as a reflection of disease severity in plasma cell dyscrasias. J Clin Invest 1989; 84:2008–2011.
75. Ishimi Y, Matsumoto K. Model system for DNA replication of a plasmid DNA containing the autonomously replicating sequence from *Saccharomyces cerevisiae*. Proc Natl Acad Sci USA 1993;90:5399–5403.
76. Sato K, Mimura H, Han DC, et al. Production of bone-resorbing activity and colony-stimulating activity in vivo and in vitro by a human squamous cell carcinoma associated with hypercalcemia and leukocytosis. J Clin Invest 1986;78:145–154.
77. Stashenko P, Dewhirst FE, Peros WJ, Kent RL, Ago JM. Synergistic interactions between interleukin 1, tumor necrosis factor, and lymphotoxin in bone resorption. J Immunol 1987; 138:1464–1468.
78. Garrett IR, Durie BG, Nedwin GE, et al. Production of lymphotoxin, a bone-resorbing cytokine, by cultured human myeloma cells. N Engl J Med 1987;317:526–532.
79. Fleisch H. Bisphosphonates: mechanisms of action. Endocr Rev 1998;19:80–100.
80. Gucalp R, Ritch P, Wiernik PH, et al. Comparative study of pamidronate disodium and etidronate disodium in the treatment of cancer-related hypercalcemia. J Clin Oncol 1992;10: 134–142.
81. Shah S, Hardy J, Rees E, et al. Is there a dose response relationship for clodronate in the treatment of tumour induced hypercalcaemia? Br J Cancer 2002;86:1235–1237.
82. Nussbaum SR, Younger J, Vandepol CJ, et al. Single-dose intravenous therapy with pamidronate for the treatment of hypercalcemia of malignancy: comparison of 30-, 60-, and 90-mg dosages. Am J Med 1993;95:297–304.
83. Berenson JR, Rosen L, Vescio R, et al. Pharmacokinetics of pamidronate disodium in patients with cancer with normal or impaired renal function. J Clin Pharmacol 197;37:285–290.
84. Cheer SM, Noble S. Zoledronic acid. Drugs 2001;61:799–805; discussion 806.
85. Body JJ, Lortholary A, Romieu G, Vigneron AM, Ford J. A dose-finding study of zoledronate in hypercalcemic cancer patients. J Bone Miner Res 1999;14:1557–1561.
86. Major PP, Coleman RE. Zoledronic acid in the treatment of hypercalcemia of malignancy: results of the international clinical development program. Semin Oncol 2001;28:17–24.
87. Major P, Lortholary A, Hon J, et al. Zoledronic acid is superior to pamidronate in the treatment of hypercalcemia of malignancy: a pooled analysis of two randomized, controlled clinical trials. J Clin Oncol 2001;19:558–567.
88. Machado CE, Flombaum CD. Safety of pamidronate in patients with renal failure and hypercalcemia. Clin Nephrol 1996;45: 175–179.
89. Markowitz GS, Fine PL, Stack JI, et al. Toxic acute tubular necrosis following treatment with zoledronate (Zometa). Kidney Int 2003;64:281–289.
90. Leyland-Jones B. Treatment of cancer-related hypercalcemia: the role of gallium nitrate. Semin Oncol 2003;30:13–19.
91. Binstock ML, Mundy GR. Effect of calcitonin and glutocorticoids in combination on the hypercalcemia of malignancy. Ann Intern Med 1980;93:269–272.
92. Wisneski LA, Croom WP, Silva OL, Becker KL. Salmon calcitonin in hypercalcemia. Clin Pharmacol Ther 1978;24:219–222.
93. Warrell RP Jr, Israel R, Frisone M, Snyder T, Gaynor JJ, Bockman RS. Gallium nitrate for acute treatment of cancer-related hypercalcemia. A randomized, double blind comparison to calcitonin. Ann Intern Med 1988;108:669–674.
94. Watson L, Moxham J, Fraser P. Hydrocortisone suppression test and discriminant analysis in differential diagnosis of hypercalcaemia. Lancet 1980;1:1320–1325.
95. Kumar S, Berl T. Sodium. Lancet 1988;352:220–228.
96. Gines P, Abraham WT, Schrier RW. Vasopressin in pathophysiological states. Semin Nephrol 1994;14:384–397.
97. Verbalis JG. Hyponatremia: epidemiology, pathophysiology, and therapy. Curr Opin Nephrol Hypertens 1993;2:636–652.
98. Kovacs L, Robertson GL. Syndrome of inappropriate antidiuresis. Endocrinol Metab Clin N Am 1992;21:859–875.
99. Kovacs L, Robertson GL. Disorders of water balance: hyponatraemia and hypernatraemia. Baillieres Clin Endocrinol Metab 1992;6:107–127.
100. Verbalis JG. Adaptation to acute and chronic hyponatremia: implications for symptomatology, diagnosis, and therapy. Semin Nephrol 1998;18:3–19.
101. Goldszmidt MA, Iliescu EA. DDAVP to prevent rapid correction in hyponatremia. Clin Nephrol 2000;53:226–229.
102. Sterns RH, Cappuccio JD, Silver SM, Cohen EP. Neurologic sequelae after treatment of severe hyponatremia: a multicenter perspective. J Am Soc Nephrol 1994;4:1522–1530.
103. Seidenwurm DJ, Elmer EB, Kaplan LM, Williams EK, Morris DG, Hoffman AR. Metastases to the adrenal glands and the development of Addison's disease. Cancer (Phila) 1984;54:552–557.
104. Redman BG, Pazdur R, Zingas AP, Loredo R. Prospective evaluation of adrenal insufficiency in patients with adrenal metastasis. Cancer (Phila) 1987;60:103–107.
105. Gamelin E, Beldent V, Rousselet MC, et al. Non-Hodgkin's lymphoma presenting with primary adrenal insufficiency. A disease with an underestimated frequency? Cancer (Phila) 1992;69: 2333–2336.
106. Dahlberg PJ, Goellner MH, Pehling GB. Adrenal insufficiency secondary to adrenal hemorrhage. Two case reports and a review of cases confirmed by computed tomography. Arch Intern Med 1990;150:905–909.
107. Siu SC, Kitzman DW, Sheedy PF II, Northcutt RC. Adrenal insufficiency from bilateral adrenal hemorrhage. Mayo Clin Proc 1990;65:664–670.
108. Hoffken K, Kempf H, Miller AA, et al. Aminoglutethimide without hydrocortisone in the treatment of postmenopausal patients with advanced breast cancer. Cancer Treat Rep 1986;70:1153–1157.
109. Daughaday WH. Hypoglycemia in patients with non-islet cell tumors. Endocrinol Metab Clin N Am 1989;18:91–101.
110. LeRoith D, Clemmons D, Nissley P, Rechler M M. NIH conference. Insulin-like growth factors in health and disease. Ann Intern Med 1992;116:854–862.
111. Macaulay VM. Insulin-like growth factors and cancer. Br J Cancer 1992;65:311–320.
112. Daughaday WH, Emanuele MA, Brooks MH., Barbato AL, Kapadia M, Rotwein P. Synthesis and secretion of insulin-like growth factor II by a leiomyosarcoma with associated hypoglycemia. N Engl J Med 1988;319:1434–1440.
113. Daughaday WH, Kapadia M. Significance of abnormal serum binding of insulin-like growth factor II in the development of hypoglycemia in patients with non-islet-cell tumors. Proc Natl Acad Sci USA 1989;86:6778–6782.
114. Shapiro ET, Bell GI, Polonsky KS, Rubenstein AH, Kew MC, Tager HS. Tumor hypoglycemia: relationship to high molecular weight insulin-like growth factor-II. J Clin Invest 1990;85: 1672–1679.
115. Zapf J, Schmid C, Guler HP, et al. Regulation of binding proteins for insulin-like growth factors (IGF) in humans. Increased expression of IGF binding protein 2 during IGF I treatment of

healthy adults and in patients with extrapancreatic tumor hypoglycemia. J Clin Invest 1990;86:952–961.

116. Zapf J, Futo E, Peter M, Froesch ER. Can "big" insulin-like growth factor II in serum of tumor patients account for the development of extrapancreatic tumor hypoglycemia? J Clin Invest 1992;90:2574–2584.
117. Zapf J. Role of insulin-like growth factor (IGF) II and IGF binding proteins in extrapancreatic tumour hypoglycaemia. J Intern Med 1993;234:543–552.
118. Tisdale MJ, Brennan RA. Metabolic substrate utilization by a tumour cell line which induces cachexia in vivo. Br J Cancer 1986;54:601–606.
119. Samaan NA, Pham FK, Sellin RV, Fernandez JF, Benjamin RS. Successful treatment of hypoglycemia using glucagon in a patient with an extrapancreatic tumor. Ann Intern Med 1990;113:404–406.
120. Harris MI, Flegal KM, Cowie CC, et al. Prevalence of diabetes, impaired fasting glucose, and impaired glucose tolerance in U.S. adults. The Third National Health and Nutrition Examination Survey, 1988–1994. Diabetes Care 1998;21:518–524.
121. Umpierrez GE, Khajavi M, Kitabchi AE. Review: diabetic ketoacidosis and hyperglycemic hyperosmolar nonketotic syndrome. Am J Med Sci 1996;311:225–233.

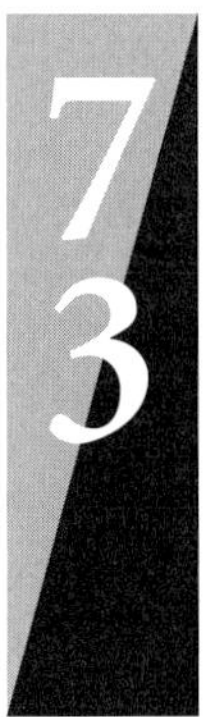

Surgical Emergencies

David A. August, Thomas Kearney, and Roderich E. Schwarz

Most surgical problems in cancer patients are not urgent. Tumors rarely grow or metastasize rapidly. Surgical evaluation can usually proceed at a measured pace over a number of weeks to accurately assess the patient's underlying cancer, to define associated comorbidities that may modify treatment decisions, to consult various disciplines to devise multimodal therapies, and to work with patients and families to create care plans that account for patient preferences and family needs. In light of this panoply of issues that affect surgical decision making in cancer patients, the presence of a surgical emergency requiring prompt evaluation and intervention is especially problematic. Thorough evaluation of cardiac, pulmonary, and other comorbidities may not be feasible. Discussions with medical and radiation oncologists and other consultants may be constrained by time and availability. Attempts to inform and understand patient and family wishes may be confounded by changes in emotional state and cognitive ability caused by pain, anxiety, fear, and the need to intervene promptly.

This chapter discusses the evaluation and treatment of general surgery oncologic emergencies. Attention is focused upon those problems likely to be treated by a general surgeon or general surgical oncologist, including the acute abdomen; surgical complications of radiation therapy and chemotherapy; gastrointestinal obstruction, bleeding, and perforation; abdominal and anorectal emergencies in the setting of neutropenia; and problems peculiar to bone marrow transplant patients.

For the purposes of this chapter, a surgical emergency is defined as an acute medical problem necessitating surgical evaluation for urgent intervention; by this definition, many "surgical emergencies" do not require surgery. The term acute abdomen implies the presence of a life-threatening situation causing abdominal signs and/or symptoms that needs to be evaluated for potential surgical intervention.[1] In many instances, patients with an acute abdomen do not require immediate surgery (e.g., abdominal pain resulting from an evolving inferior wall myocardial infarction or lower lobe pneumonia, or free air introduced by transmigration during an otherwise uncomplicated colonoscopy). All cancer patients may be considered immunocompromised. Especially problematic are those patients with absolute neutropenia (absolute neutrophil count less than 1,000 cells/mm^3) secondary to bone marrow suppression from chemotherapy, radiation therapy, and/or the underlying malignancy. They may fail to exhibit the classic signs of an emergent surgical problem, such as pain, tenderness, fever, and leukocytosis. Often, more subtle manifestations such as intolerance of oral intake, abdominal distension, diarrhea, changes in mental status, or isolated hyperbilirubinemia may be the only indications of an evolving, life-threatening situation.

General Considerations

An initial diagnosis of cancer is made in less than 1% of cases seen in a typical emergency department.[2] Such a presentation, however, is ominous. The prognosis of patients newly diagnosed with cancer during an emergency room evaluation is poor. In comparison with other newly diagnosed cancer patients, they are more likely to have metastatic disease and they are more likely to die during their initial hospital admission. Median survival for these patients is less than 1 year.[3–5] This poorer prognosis likely relates to poor access to medical care in these patients (resulting in inadequate screening and fewer opportunities to recognize signs and symptoms early), increased morbidity and mortality frequently observed in patients presenting with any type of emergency problem, and advanced stage of disease at presentation.[6] Overall, approximately 5% of cancer cases are initially diagnosed in an emergency room setting.[4] This number may be significantly higher for certain sites, such as the gastrointestinal tract.[5]

In patients being treated for cancer, surgical emergencies may arise as a consequence of their antitumor therapy. In a review of 213 cancer patients requiring exploration for an acute abdomen, approximately one-third had problems relating directly to chemotherapy or the cancer itself (Table 73.1).[7,8] It has been observed that emergent abdominal complications are more likely to arise in patients with acute leukemia during or immediately following treatment with chemotherapy.[9] Corticosteroids administered as part of a chemotherapy regimen are also a common offender.[10] Radiation therapy may contribute to the development of surgical emergencies. Injury to irradiated tissues may lead to necrosis or vascular catastrophes (thrombosis or rupture) requiring acute intervention. Radiotherapy is implicated in approximately one-third of enterocutaneous fistulae.[11] As many as 15% of patients receiving abdominal irradiation may experience related complications, although most will not require an operation.[12] Most radiation-induced surgical emergencies arise well after the therapy is completed. With increased fractionation and a greater number of ports used, the less likely it is that normal tissue injury will occur.[13]

TABLE 73.1. The spectrum of diagnoses in 213 cancer patients requiring emergency laparotomy.

Diagnosis	*Location*	*% (n)*
Obstruction	Not specified	39% (83)
Hemorrhage	Intraabdominal tumor	4% (8)
	Gastrointestinal (stomach, 6; duodenum, 5; small bowel, 3; colon, 9)	11% (23)
Perforation	Stomach, 7; duodenum, 9; small bowel, 11; colon, 20	22% (47)
Infection	Cholecystitis, 7; appendicitis, 5; bile peritonitis, 4; cholangitis, 3; ascites, 1; neutropenic enterocolitis, 1; other, 1	10% (22)
Incarcerated hernia	Not specified	3% (6)
Vascular occlusion	Mesenteric	3% (6)
Other	Not specified	1% (3)
Negative laparotomy	Not specified	7% (15)

Source: From Turnbull.[7]

Abdominal pain is a common presenting complaint for a variety of illnesses. Distension of hollow organs, bowel or organ ischemia, and irritation of the peritoneum by infection or gastrointestinal contents can cause abdominal pain. For all patients presenting to an emergency room with abdominal pain, the most common diagnosis is nonspecific pain (35%). Appendicitis (17%), bowel obstruction (15%), renal calculi (6%), and gallstones (5%) are the most common specific diagnoses.[14]

Evaluation of patients with an initial or known diagnosis of cancer who present with a potential surgical emergency may be difficult. Neutropenia, corticosteroids, narcotic analgesics, and malnutrition may all blunt the signs and symptoms of a surgical emergency. Pain may be obscured, the patient's ability to mount an inflammatory response may be muted, and preexisting poor performance status may hide functional consequences of an evolving catastrophe. Conversely, cytokine support [granulocyte colony-stimulating factor (G-CSF) and granulocyte macrophage colony-stimulating factor (GM-CSF)] may confound the interpretation of standard laboratory tests, such as a complete blood count.

These factors notwithstanding, pain is usually the most important symptom heralding a surgical emergency. Particularly in the setting of a preexisting malignancy, pain and other complaints, such as vomiting, abdominal distension, fever, anorexia, constipation, melena/hematochezia, perianal symptoms, and even subtle stigmata of soft tissue infections, must be evaluated promptly and thoroughly. Although the need for emergent operations in cancer patients is relatively uncommon, failure to intervene in a timely fashion can increase morbidity and mortality in these compromised hosts.[15]

Physical examination remains the mainstay of diagnosis. Constitutional signs, such as fever, tachypnea, and tachycardia, on occasion, are the only objective findings present. Their presence is significant, because they represent a systemic reaction, connoting a more generalized process. Although immunocompromised hosts may not demonstrate localized tenderness, more diffuse abdominal or soft tissue tenderness is usually present. Paradoxically, it may be easier to palpate organomegaly or an abdominal mass in these patients because of the blunting of involuntary guarding. Care must be taken when examining open wounds or considering digital rectal or vaginal examination in neutropenic patients, as these examinations may result in transient bacteremia. Given the prevalence of anorectal and soft tissue infections in these patients, however, a careful visual inspection of the perineum, vaginal introitus, anoderm, and anal canal, and of soft tissue wounds, is mandatory.

Laboratory and imaging studies are also helpful. A complete blood count with differential is necessary to determine whether absolute neutropenia or leukocytosis is present. It will also demonstrate the presence of thrombocytopenia, which is important in bleeding patients and in those in whom an operation is considered. Liver function tests and serum amylase and lipase often help to direct evaluation of the acute abdomen. Standard laboratory studies are also necessary to direct preoperative resuscitation and operative risk assessment. Because of the immunocompromised status of these patients, plain X-rays (chest X-ray and abdominal films to look for pneumonia, pleural effusion, intestinal obstruction, pneumoperitoneum, and soft tissue air) and cross-sectional imaging with ultrasound, computed tomography (CT), and/or magnetic resonance imaging (MRI) are usually indicated, even though immune compromise may blunt some of the subtle inflammatory findings that can be helpful with these imaging modalities. Localization of a bleeding source in patients with gastrointestinal or other hemorrhage using endoscopy or arteriography is important and may even be therapeutic. The roles of these studies are discussed here in relationship to specific clinical situations. Critical care issues in cancer patients undergoing emergency operations are important but are beyond the scope of this chapter.[16]

When Is Operative Therapy Not Appropriate?

Acute surgical interventions in cancer patients should improve patients' well-being. In patients being treated for cancer with curative intent, decisions to operate should be guided by the medical circumstances. Although an operation may be high risk, successful acute intervention can result in long-term survival.

More problematic are surgical emergencies in a patient in whom cancer cure is not possible (Table 73.2).[17] It is important that the patient's definition and assessment of well-being be understood by the treating clinicians and incorporated into medical decision making. If an operation is unlikely to improve the patient's well-being according to his or her definition, even though it may be technically indicated (e.g., plication of a perforated duodenal ulcer in a patient with metastatic melanoma), it may be inappropriate.[17] In this circumstance, likelihood of survival to discharge (although often difficult to predict) can be an important parameter. Futile procedures that are unlikely to have a beneficial outcome are contraindicated, although few data exist to assist with these decisions.[17] There are some data concerning the efficacy of

TABLE 73.2. Factors that identify situations in which surgical treatment may not be appropriate.

Factor	*Comment*
Surgical indication vs. palliation	Operations undertaken in patients with potentially curable acute complications and potentially curable cancers are more likely to be beneficial. Operations undertaken to palliate symptoms should be carefully considered in light of potential nonoperative alternatives and in accordance with patients' preferences and values.
Likely outcome	Procedures should not be undertaken when the likelihood of survival to discharge is low (e.g., cardiopulmonary resuscitation in patients with metastatic disease, emergency laparotomy in patients with widespread metastatic disease).
Futility	When therapy is as unlikely to lead to a desirable outcome as supportive care, the latter is preferred. It is not the physician's duty to attempt to do "everything possible."

cardiopulmonary resuscitation in patients with metastatic cancer. In one review, fewer than 3% of patients with metastatic cancer survived to actually be discharged from the hospital.[18] Emergency abdominal operations in patients with metastatic cancer may be equally futile. In a series of 21 such patients receiving chemotherapy, 17 died in the immediate postoperative period. Only 3 survived to discharge, and only 1 lived beyond 5 months.[19] Generally, invasive treatments are not appropriate when the patient's definition of well-being is unlikely to be achieved, or when the intervention is doomed to failure because of its inherent medical futility. In this light, decisions to treat or not treat must be made using the medical knowledge and experience of the treating clinicians (surgeons, medical oncologists, primary care physicians, nurses, and other involved clinicians and support staff) in combination with the values and wishes of the patient and family.

Gastrointestinal Obstruction

Gastrointestinal obstruction is the most common problem that requires urgent surgical evaluation in cancer patients, and this is especially true in patients with solid tumors of intraabdominal and pelvic origin. At one institution, 39% of cancer patients requiring emergency abdominal operation suffered from intestinal obstruction.[8,20] In most patients, cancer is the cause of the obstruction. However, obstruction is secondary to a benign process in approximately 30% of cases; most often, this occurs as a result of adhesions that develop after a previous operation. Cancer-related obstruction is seen most often in patients with a history of gastrointestinal cancer, followed by gynecologic malignancy. Obstruction from metastases is less common. Acute intestinal obstruction may be the initial presentation of gastrointestinal cancer, comprising up to 30% of cases of malignant bowel obstruction.[16] In patients with primary small bowel neoplasms, as many as 64% require emergency treatment; obstruction is the most common presenting finding (22%), followed by bleeding in 17%, and perforation in 6%.[21]

Clinical Presentation, Evaluation, and Stabilization

Crampy abdominal pain, nausea, and vomiting are characteristic symptoms of intestinal obstruction. Dysphagia or early postprandial vomiting suggest esophagogastric obstruction. Bilious vomiting is encountered when small bowel or proximal colon are involved. More distal large bowel obstruction usually presents with distension, pain, and constipation before vomiting occurs. So-called paralytic ileus and intestinal pseudoobstruction (Ogilvie's syndrome) are the main differential diagnoses; they are usually characterized by the absence of bowel sounds, which is only a late finding in patients with true gastrointestinal obstruction. Peritonitis in the setting of obstruction is ominous and is associated with bacterial translocation, perforation, or bowel necrosis.

Laboratory tests are often nonspecific. Leukocytosis can reflect the degree of inflammation or infection associated with obstruction but may not be present in immunocompromised hosts. Sometimes, a subtle left shift alone may be the only laboratory finding. Metabolic acidosis, especially if not correctable, should raise concern over tissue ischemia or necrosis. Plain abdominal radiographs can confirm a clinical diagnosis of obstruction and help define the anatomic site. Upper gastrointestinal (GI) contrast studies should be avoided except when esophageal or gastric obstruction is suspected. If these studies are performed, aspiration precautions must be implemented. A water-soluble contrast diagnostic enema study can be very helpful to rule out colon obstruction and to facilitate intraoperative decision making. For example, a water-soluble contrast enema can assess left-sided colorectal patency and may avoid the need for a colostomy in a patient explored for small bowel obstruction with peritoneal carcinomatosis. In addition, it may differentiate a true obstruction from a pseudoobstructive process.[22] CT is almost always helpful to assess the extent of the underlying malignancy. This information can inform decisions of whether to operate and whether the goal of an operation should be palliation or cure.

Initial management of the cancer patient with intestinal obstruction should include cessation of oral intake, intravenous hydration, nasogastric decompression, pain management, and nutrition status assessment. If signs of peritonitis or sepsis (fever, tachycardia, leukocytosis, acidosis, peritoneal signs on abdominal examination) are absent, most patients can be stabilized and undergo deliberate evaluation. Emergency operations, necessitated by the presence of infection or compromised bowel, are accompanied by greater morbidity and mortality.[23,24] Avoidance of emergency operations, when possible, also allows assessment of potentially curative resection options and of palliative nonoperative approaches for incurable tumors.

Treatment

Endoscopic ablation techniques can provide temporary control of localized obstruction caused by large tumor masses, especially in cases of esophageal or distal colorectal obstruction.[25–27] Endoscopic or interventional intestinal stent placement offer additional nonoperative options. With judicious use of these techniques, operations for partial esophagogastric, duodenal, and colorectal obstruction can frequently be avoided in patients with advanced disease. Unfortunately, most patients with small bowel obstruction who fail to respond to hydration and nasogastric decompression, or those with complete intestinal obstruction at any level, require operative therapy (Figure 73.1). Nasogastric decompression and supportive care alone may succeed in 25% to 35% of cancer patients with intestinal obstruction; unfortunately, as many as 50% of these patients will develop subsequent recurrent bowel obstruction. An exception is those situations in which intestinal obstruction is caused by a malignancy that is likely to respond well to either chemotherapy and/or radiation therapy, such as lymphoma and testicular cancer; operations are best avoided in this setting, in favor of cytotoxic treatment.

Operative techniques include resection of the obstructed intestinal segment, intestinal bypass, and external diversion (ileostomy, colostomy, esophageal spit fistula). The decision whether to stage decompression, resection, and/or reconstruction, or combine these steps within a one-stage procedure, must be individualized. Patient physiologic status (hemodynamic stability, organ function, presence of ascites, nutrition status, performance status, and presence of comorbidities) and operative factors (tissue viability, contamination, extent of cancer) must be considered.[28]

There is ongoing controversy over whether a colon resection with primary anastomosis should be performed in cases of left-sided large bowel obstruction. When the primary presentation of colon cancer is obstruction, and resection for cure is possible, it may be considered, but available trial-based evidence is sparse.[29] Intraoperative bowel cleansing can be performed and may reduce the risk of anastomotic leak.[30] Alternatively, subtotal colectomy with ileorectal anastomosis apparently can be performed with acceptable morbidity and functional outcome.[31,32] Alternatively, an endoscopic colon stent may achieve decompression, after which a definitive resection can be performed electively.[33–35]

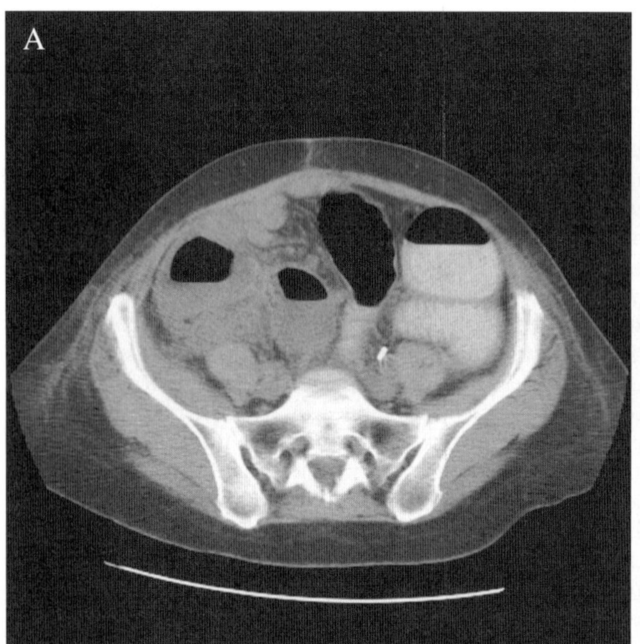

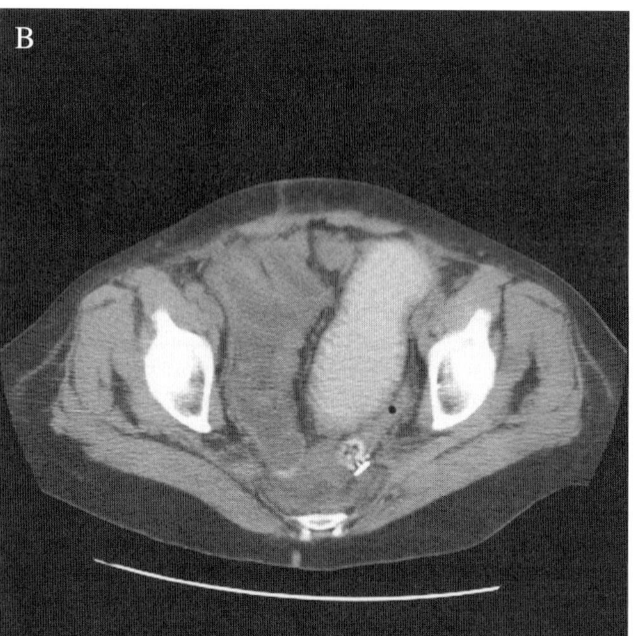

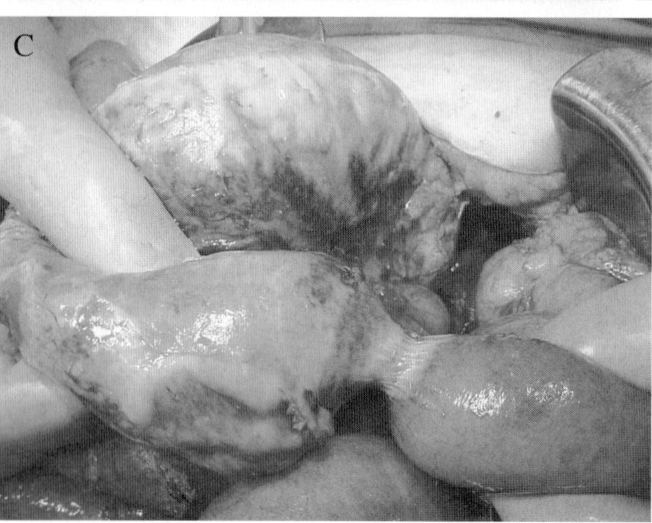

FIGURE 73.1. A 59-year-old woman presented with small bowel obstruction 2 years after low anterior resection for a T1N0M0 rectal cancer. Computed tomography demonstrated distended small bowel loops (A, B). Laparotomy revealed distal small bowel strangulation, with a gangrenous segment (C). After segmental resection and reanastomosis, the patient recovered uneventfully.

TABLE 73.3. Outcomes of operative treatment for palliation of malignant bowel obstruction in the setting of peritoneal carcinomatosis.

Reference	*Interval*	*Patients with carcinomatosis (n)*	*Morbidity (%)*	*Mortality (%)*	*Hospital stay (days)*	*Successful palliation (%)*	*Recurrent obstruction (%)*	*Median survival*
Sadeghi[38]	1995–1997	370	37	21				3.1 months
Chu[39]	1984–1987	100		29				Colorectal: 6 months; other nonsarcoma: 1 month
Turnbull[40]	1977–1986	89	44	13	25 (median)	74	38	98 days
Tang[41]	1985–1993	43	45	12		50		5 months
Woolfson[42]	1987–1995	32		22	21 (mean)	53	48	1 month
Blair[16]	1995–2000	63	44	21	12 (median)	45	24	90 days

Source: From Blair et al.[16]

Tube gastrostomy may be helpful in patients with extensive peritoneal carcinomatosis, or those at risk for recurrence of obstruction. In patients with inoperable malignant bowel obstruction, operative or percutaneous endoscopic gastrostomy can avoid the need for prolonged or even lifelong nasogastric tube decompression. A feeding jejunostomy tube can assist the management of patients with proximal gastrointestinal dysfunction or if sufficient oral food tolerance remains unlikely. Feeding tubes, however, should be reserved for those patients with active treatment options (chemotherapy or radiation therapy).

Outcomes after operations for malignant bowel obstruction vary considerably, based on the patient's physiologic and functional status and extent of underlying disease. In general, however, mortality rates are high (10% to 25%). Postoperative complications may occur in as many as 50% of patients. Success rates for palliative operations are rarely reported. The median survival for these patients ranges between 3 and 7 months. A systematic review of available clinical trials concludes that surgical therapy for malignant bowel obstruction remains problematic: symptom control is achieved in only 40% to 80% of patients; reobstruction occurs frequently (10% to 50% of the time); and perioperative morbidity and mortality are formidable. Especially disappointing is the lack of validated outcome.[36,37] A recent review reported outcomes of palliative operations in 63 patients with malignant bowel obstruction. The complication rate was 44%, with a 15% mortality rate, and a median length of hospital stay of 12 days. Patients with colorectal primaries had somewhat better survival. Absence of ascites, obstruction site outside of the small bowel, and a serum albumin greater than 3 mg/dL correlated with the ability to tolerate solid food postoperatively. Prolonged successful palliation was observed in only one-third of patients.[16] Comparable outcomes in patients with peritoneal carcinomatosis and malignant bowel obstruction have been reported in other operative series (Table 73.3). Emergency gastrectomy for gastric obstruction as compared to acute bleeding is rare.[43,44]

Nonoperative therapy of bowel obstruction beyond that of general supportive care may be indicated, especially in patients with advanced-stage disease, or without specific anticancer therapy options, or whose physiologic status will not permit a safe operation. Corticosteroid treatment has been advocated to improve intestinal obstruction and alleviate associated symptoms. Outcome data are limited.[37] In several prospective trials, octreotide has been effective, controlling vomiting or reducing the volume of nasogastric drainage.[45–48] Symptomatic improvement has also been described in a series of 20 patients with inoperable intestinal obstruction with the combined use of morphine sulfate, scopolamine, and haloperidol.[49]

Colonoscopic placement of self-expanding metallic stents for large bowel obstruction is safe and effective (perforation rate less than 5%; 17% need for subsequent intestinal stoma) (Table 73.4).[50] Stent reobstruction (29%) and migration (9%) have been reported, but may be managed with further endo-

TABLE 73.4. Outcomes of stent placement for cancer-related colorectal obstruction.

Reference	*Year*	*Patients (n)*	*Successful placement (n)*	*Migration (n)*	*Reobstruction (n)*	*Perforation (n)*
Saida[51]	1996	15	12	1	0	2
Baron[52]	1998	27	23	5	2	4
Choo[53]	1998	20	18	4	0	0
de Gregorio[54]	1998	24	23	2	1	0
Mainar[55]	1999	71	66	0	0	1
Repici[56]	2000	16	15	2	0	1
Law[50]	2000	24	23	3	3	1
Aviv[57]	2002	13	11	2	3	0
Wong[35]	2002	16	14	0	0	3
Dauphin[58]	2002	26	22	1	4	0
Clark[59]	2003	16	13	0	0	0
Law[60]	2004	52	50	8	2	1
Total		320	290 (91%)	28 (9%)	15 (5%)	13 (4%)

TABLE 73.5. Outcomes of stent placement for cancer-related gastroduodenal obstruction.

Reference	*Year*	*Patients (n)*	*Successful placement (n)*	*Migration (n)*	*Reobstruction (n)*	*Perforation (n)*
Jung[61]	2000	19	18	5	2	0
Kim[62]	2001	29	26	2	2	0
Pinto[63]	2001	31	27	1	2	0
Park[64]	2001	24	18	5	2	0
Yim[65]	2001	29	25	0	2	0
Aviv[66]	2002	15	14	1	2	0
Schiefke[67]	2003	20	20	2	4	0
Kaw[68]	2003	33	32	1	3	0
Tang[69]	2003	21	18	0	0	0
Nassif[70]	2003	63	60	4	13	2
Total		284	258/284 (91%)	21/284 (7%)	32/284 (11%)	2/284 (0.7%)

scopic manipulation.[58] The majority of patients stented with palliative intent achieve long-term relief of obstruction.[35] Experience with stents for gastric outlet obstruction is more limited (Table 73.5).[66–70] Even with simultaneous biliary stenting in many patients, immediate success rates are reported as high as 95%, with 70% of patients remaining free of gastrointestinal symptoms during their remaining lifetime.[70] Among positive effects are: ability to tolerate solid food (77%), weight gain (71%), and improvement of reflux esophagitis (92%).[67] Late complications include tumor ingrowth and stent occlusion in about 20% of patients, but restenting is possible and often successful.[66,68] In all series, median survival is limited to around 4 months.[71] A small retrospective series suggests patients who undergo endoscopic stenting may achieve oral intake and hospital discharge sooner than those who undergo open or laparoscopic gastrojejunostomy for gastroduodenal obstruction.[72]

Biliary Tract Obstruction

Biliary obstruction in patients with cancer is rarely an emergency and is not discussed here in detail. Obstructive jaundice itself does not require urgent treatment. Secondary cholangitis is an emergency, but rarely, if ever, occurs absent prior manipulation of the biliary tree either surgically or by endoscopic or transhepatic maneuvers.[73–75] In most cases of painless obstructive jaundice, primary or recurrent neoplasms of the pancreatic head, extrahepatic biliary tree, or other periampullary tissues are identified; secondary lesions in retroperitoneal lymph nodes causing biliary obstruction most often metastasize, in decreasing order of frequency, from gastric, colonic, breast, or lung cancer primaries.[73] Endoscopic retrograde cholangiopancreatography (ERCP) or transhepatic imaging or stent placement upon initial presentation in a patient without signs of infection is rarely indicated, especially because preoperative biliary manipulation may increase operative mortality.[74] Biliary sepsis in the setting of biliary obstruction does necessitate emergent biliary decompression. Under these circumstances, endoscopic stenting via ERCP, when feasible, appears preferable to percutaneous transhepatic stent placement. For patients with metastatic disease, endoscopic stents should always be considered first.[76]

Gastrointestinal Hemorrhage

Acute gastrointestinal hemorrhage is the third most frequent problem requiring emergency abdominal operation in cancer patients.[7,8] Both benign causes and tumor-related etiologies occur in patients with cancer.

Clinical Presentation, Evaluation, and Stabilization

In a review of five case series encompassing 121 cancer patients, the most common causes for upper gastrointestinal hemorrhage were gastritis (36%), ulcer disease (26%), and tumor-related bleeding (23%).[77] Other reports support these findings, and they are true even today despite a dramatic decrease in the need for emergency operations for benign peptic disease in noncancer patients with the advent of H2 blockers and proton pump inhibitors.[78–80] It is unusual for upper GI bleeding to require operative intervention (11%), and in only one-fourth of cases is the need for operation a true emergency.[81]

Lower gastrointestinal hemorrhage resulting from noncancerous conditions has an 80% likelihood of stopping spontaneously, but the rebleeding rate is 50%. Colonoscopy or scintigraphic bleeding scan alone fail to localize a bleeding site in up to 50% of cases, but they complement each other.[82] Angiographic localization succeeds in more than 80% of patients.[83,84] The prevalence of lower GI bleeding and of both benign and malignant lesions that may cause lower GI hemorrhage increase with greater age. Arteriovenous malformation, diverticulosis, hemorrhoids, and cancer are therefore the most common causes of lower gastrointestinal bleeding.[85]

In a study of 377 patients with advanced malignancy receiving palliative care at home, 18 developed gastrointestinal bleeding, resulting in 3 deaths. Metastatic liver disease was common in these patients.[86] Many factors present in cancer patients may increase the risk of a bleeding diathesis. Direct tumor growth and/or invasion can cause mucosal ulceration and vascular invasion. Intestinal ulceration and bleeding can also be caused by chemotherapy or corticosteroids. Chemotherapy-induced thrombocytopenia, coagulation disturbances from tumor- or treatment-induced hepatopathy, and use of aspirin, other nonnarcotic analgesics, and therapeutic anticoagulants in patients with cancer-related thromboembolic complications can all predispose to and exacerbate GI hemorrhage. Gastrointestinal hemorrhage can result from *Candida*, cytomegalovirus, or *Clostridium difficile* infections in the GI tract, or from systemic sepsis resulting from immunosuppressive side effects of cancer and systemic cancer therapy. Direct chemical or physical injury to the GI tract by chemotherapy and radiation therapy can cause bleeding. Radiation-related bleeding risk is directly related to the dose administered.[87] Other factors increasing the bleeding risk in cancer patients relate to underlying conditions, such as variceal bleeds in cirrhotic patients with hepatocellular cancer.[88]

Postoperative gastrointestinal hemorrhage can occur after visceral resection, as well as GI bypass procedures.[89] Acute hemorrhage by far outweighs obstruction among the indications for urgent reoperations after previous gastrectomy.[44] Massive GI hemorrhage, occurring in 3.2% of patients with previous abdominal cancer operations, can result from arterial erosions related to anastomotic leaks or from anastomotic mucosal suture line bleeding, at roughly equal frequency.[90] The mortality for anastomotic leak-associated hemorrhage may approach 50%, but is much lower for suture line bleeds. Hemorrhage can also be encountered postoperatively in the presence of uncontrolled infection or sepsis, although these are rare events even after major visceral resections for cancer.[91–93]

Treatment

Immediate therapeutic efforts must focus on hemodynamic resuscitation and correction of coagulopathy. Venous access, fluid resuscitation, and transfusion of blood products (including packed red blood cells, platelets, and plasma to optimize coagulation) must be accomplished rapidly. As always, disease extent, patient physiologic and performance status, and advanced directives must be considered before complex treatment decisions are made. When the patient is stabilized, diagnostic studies should be initiated without delay, for reactivation of bleeding is common. These studies may include upper or lower gastrointestinal endoscopy, or contrast arteriography, based on the suspected site, bleeding rate, and underlying mechanism. Both endoscopy and angiography may also be therapeutic. Endoscopic variceal ligation is more effective for acute upper gastrointestinal bleeding in patients with hepatocellular cancer than conservative therapy.[94] For other sites, less-rapid bleeding from the intestinal mucosal surface suggests initial attempt at control by endoscopy. Techniques include argon beam plasma coagulation or laser application.[25,26] Bleeding from radiation proctitis has been effectively controlled with topical formalin application.[95] More rapid bleeds in the presence of a larger tumor mass, or other local tissue compromise, such as infection, are more likely to respond to angiographic embolization.[96] If less-rapid bleeding originates from tumor tissue, especially large, unresectable lesions with gastrointestinal erosion, external-beam radiation therapy may be effective. For example, a single fraction of 10 Gy to patients with advanced uterine cancer controls pelvic bleeding in 90% of cases.[97] Similarly, rectal bleeding can be controlled in 85% of patients with ovarian cancer and tumor erosion with the use of radiation therapy.[98,99]

Operative treatment for cancer-related hemorrhage should be considered only when tumor bleeding can be treated by complete resection, when less-invasive therapeutic modalities have failed, or when endoscopy, angiography, and radiation are unlikely to be effective. It is imperative that the source of bleeding be unambiguously identified and localized before laparotomy. In cases of tumor bleeding, preoperative understanding of organ resectability is of great help as well, but obtaining the desirable imaging study may not always be feasible.

In a review of 427 patients with gastric cancer, 36 presented with upper gastrointestinal bleeding; among these, hemorrhage was self-limited in 44%, but an emergency operation was required in 56%; the resulting mortality after gastrectomy was 28%.[100] Bleeding gastric cancers tend to be larger in size, but resection is indicated whenever technically and physiologically feasible.[101] Most emergency gastrectomies in cancer patients are performed for massive, intractable bleeding. The majority of these patients do not have adenocarcinoma; lymphomas, gastrointestinal stromal tumors, and other soft tissue neoplasms are the more frequent cause of massive neoplastic gastric hemorrhage. The mortality rate for emergency gastrectomy under these circumstances is 50% compared to 4% for nonemergent procedures.[23] Mortality among elderly cancer patients requiring emergency gastrectomy is reported to be as high as 67%.[43]

Bleeding is not as common an indication as obstruction for small bowel resection in cancer patients, as both primary neoplasms and metastases to the small intestine cause hemorrhage in fewer than 20% of cases.[102–104] An exception seems to be melanoma metastatic to the small intestine; equal numbers of patients require emergency resection for hemorrhage and for obstruction.[105–107] Emergency abdominal colectomy for bleeding is associated with a high mortality rate. In one series, 5 of 11 patients undergoing emergency colectomy died, primarily of infectious complications.[108] In a larger series of emergency colectomies, only 6% (10 of 170) were indicated because of bleeding. Overall mortality after a one-stage procedure was 11%.[109] Massive gastrointestinal bleeding as first presentation of other visceral tumors is rare, but has been reported for pancreatic cancers and others.[110]

In rare cases of bleeding arteriodigestive fistulae, usually related to previous operations and/or radiation therapy, selective angiography, if feasible, can be both diagnostic and therapeutic.[111] When bleeding is massive, immediate operation with intrathoracic aortic inflow control, temporizing suture hemostasis, and subsequent vascularized tissue flap coverage may lead to a rare treatment success.[112] Similarly, visceral parenchymal hemorrhage from tumor is infrequent. Perhaps the most common occurrence of this rare event is from the liver secondary to intraparenchymal or intraperitoneal rupture of a hepatocellular carcinoma. Mortality is high. Angiographic embolization seems to offer the best chance for initial control and stabilization, followed by subsequent resection.[113,114] Rarely, emergency surgery with resection is successful, but cancer recurrence is likely.[115]

Gastrointestinal Perforation

Perforations of the gastrointestinal tract constitute the second most common indication for urgent abdominal surgical intervention in cancer patients. In a series of 47 patients, the sites of perforation were located in the colon ($n = 20$), small intestine ($n = 11$), duodenum ($n = 9$), and stomach ($n = 7$) patients.[7,8] Primary small bowel tumors often present with an emergent problem, In a series of 32 patients with emergent presentations, 8 were perforated, 7 were bleeding, and 17 were obstructed.[107] Gastrointestinal perforation in cancer patients occurs by various mechanisms. Tumor may erode through the wall of the GI tract. Treatment-related perforations may occur after endoscopic or operative procedures. They may also result from rapid tumor regression following administration of chemotherapy or radiation therapy; these types of perforations, although rare, are seen most often during treatment of bulky, chemotherapy-sensitive tumors (i.e., lymphoma, testicular cancer, germ cell tumors) involving the gastrointestinal tract. Perforations may also occur secondary to treatment-related toxicity, such as nonsteroidal antiinflammatory drug (NSAID)- or corticosteroid-induced ulcer diatheses, immunosuppression-induced cytomegalovirus or other infections, inadvertent embolization of arteries that supply the bowel during chemoembolization angiographic procedures, and inadvertent perfusion of gastrointestinal mucosa with cytotoxic drugs during hepatic artery infusion therapy. Finally, other causes altogether unrelated to the underlying malignancy, such as peptic ulcer disease or diverticular perforation, can occur as well. Iatrogenic perforations relating to endoscopic procedures are probably underreported; they may occur during colonic or duodenal stent placement (1%–4%) and esophageal photodynamic therapy procedures (2%).[27,50,70]

Clinical Presentation, Evaluation, and Stabilization

Cancer patients with gastrointestinal perforation may present with as little sign as subtle abdominal discomfort or with overwhelming signs of peritonitis, including sepsis and shock. Acute pain from a perforation may be masked by medications.[116] Findings on physical examination may include abdominal wall crepitus, distension, firmness, and rebound tenderness. Clinical findings and laboratory studies reflect the severity of infection, systemic inflammatory response, and compromise of organ function only in patients who are not immunocompromised. Chest and abdominal X-rays can detect free air, the most accurate sign of visceral perforation (Figure 73.2). CT is a more sensitive test to detect extraluminal air; it can define the extent of the underlying cancer and assess local resectability of the diseased bowel at the same time. Tissue pneumatosis or intravenous air can be the result of an intestinal perforation due to cancer.[117] As noted for obstruction and hemorrhage, initial therapy should include establishment of adequate venous access and hemodynamic monitoring, vigorous hydration, initiation of antibiotics, and assessment of the patient's overall physiologic and oncologic status.

Treatment

Intestinal perforation almost always requires operative therapy to remediate, in contradistinction to obstruction or bleeding. Whether a patient is a candidate for an operation is determined by the presence of comorbidities, the overall cancer burden, and the patient's values and goals (cure, palliation, comfort). These issues must be addressed early in the presentation. The prognosis for a meaningful postoperative recovery is influenced by the patient's underlying immune function, nutrition status, and performance status, as well as his/her physiologic and oncologic status. Even in patients without cancer, operations for "benign" ulcer perforations are attended by significant morbidity and mortality.[78] In a report of 170 urgent surgical procedures for colorectal conditions, not specifically limited to cancer patients, 71% were performed for obstruction, 23% for perforation, and 6% for massive bleeding, with an overall mortality rate of 18%.[109] In cancer patients, the choice of surgical procedure to treat a perforation largely depends on the patient's acute physiologic status, the technical resectability of the diseased bowel, and the extent of the cancer. In general, resection of the site of perforation is preferable to suture repair or simple drainage. Intestinal resection may be followed by anastomotic reconstruction, if the severity of the associated peritonitis and physiologic and nutrition status permit.[28] Otherwise, intestinal diversion with a stoma or enterostomy is necessary.

The mortality of spontaneous gastrointestinal perforation in cancer patients is high. In one series of 36 patients, 84% died. Factors responsible for this high mortality include delayed diagnosis, perforation through tumor, advanced stage of disease, and multiple organ failure. Even in patients able to undergo surgery, only 32% survived.[118] In a subsequent review of 30 cancer patients with gastrointestinal perforation treated operatively, steroid therapy was implicated in 77% and chemotherapy in 23%. Sites of perforation were almost evenly divided between the small and large bowel. In half the patients, cancer was identified at the perforation site. Operative mortality was 53%.[119] Tumor involvement at the perforation site appears to be especially ominous.

Spontaneous gastroduodenal perforations in patients with various cancers, but mostly without tumor at the perforation site, are amenable to nonresectional surgical treatment, such as simple closure, omental patch, vagotomy, and pyloroplasty. In this setting, mortality may be as low as 10% to 20%.[120] Surgical treatment of gynecologic cancers presenting with intestinal pneumatosis or perforation has been reported to be associated with 67% mortality. Again, tumor involvement appears crucial. In this series, cancer was not present in any of the survivors.[121] Not surprisingly, patients with spontaneous perforations of gastric cancer are likely to present with advanced disease. Good outcomes can be achieved if the perforation and associated cancer are amenable to complete resection.[23,101] Tumors metastatic to the intestines rarely cause perforation. One of 32 patients with melanoma metastases to the small bowel presented with a perforation.[106] Among 24 patients with melanoma metastatic to the large intestine, perforation and obstruction predicted poor median survival (less than 10 months).[122] Gastrointestinal lymphomas have been linked to perforation as a result of treatment-induced tumor necrosis. However, the perception that this is a common problem is probably not true. Upon initial presentation of gastrointestinal lymphomas, perforation is seen in 2% (gastric non-Hodgkin's lymphoma, NHL) to 9% of cases (intestinal NHL), compared to bleeding rates of 19% and 6%, respectively.[123] Among intestinal NHLs, T-cell lymphomas appear to present more frequently with perforation (37% versus 5%) or bleeding (17% versus 10%) than B-cell lymphomas.[124] In the same series, the rate of emergency operations upon presentation of the intestinal NHL was 46% for T-cell lymphomas, compared to 14% for B-cell lymphomas. However, actual treatment-induced perforation is seen in only 4% of patients (Table 73.6).

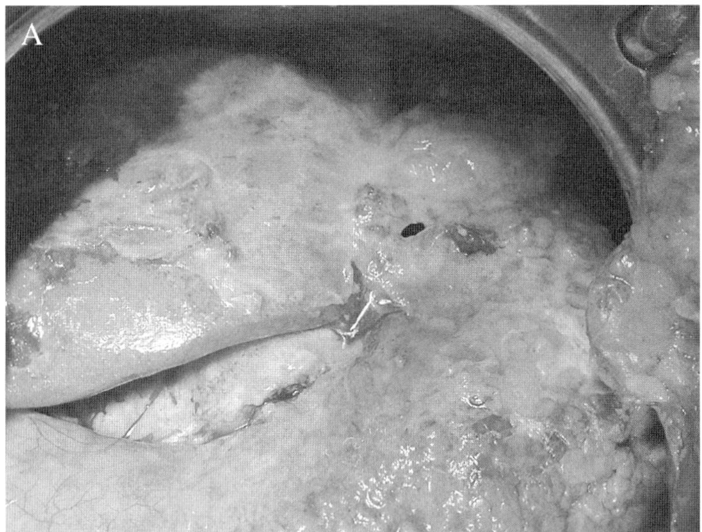

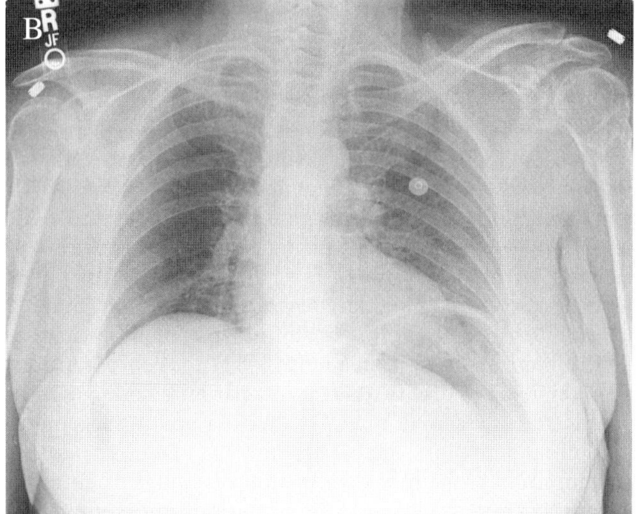

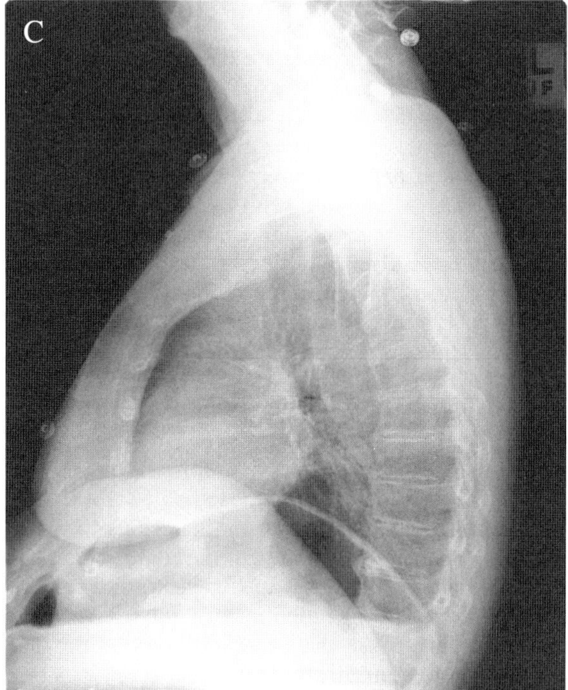

FIGURE 73.2. Operative findings in a woman with metastatic gastric cancer who presented with acute abdominal pain. A gastric perforation was identified (A). A palliative gastrectomy with esophagojejunostomy was performed. The patient was discharged tolerating solid food. One month later after discharge, she presented again with abdominal discomfort. Chest radiographs showed pneumoperitoneum on both posteroanterior (B) and lateral views (C), which was secondary to an anastomotic leak. The patient received supportive care only and died after 4 weeks.

TABLE 73.6. Complications of gastrointestinal lymphomas: frequency of perforation and hemorrhage when surgical resection is not performed before initiation of cytotoxic therapy.

				Complication (n)	
Reference	*Year*	*Patients (n)*	*Type of lymphoma*	*Perforation*	*Bleeding*
Kemeny[167]	1982	41	Burkitt's	0	5
Meyers[168]	1985	92	Non-Hodgkin's	4	NR
Talamonti[104]	1990	24	Non-Hodgkin's	2	4
Maor[169]	1990	34	Gastric non-Hodgkin's	0	0
Salles[170]	1991	77	Non-Hodgkin's	1	1
Rackner[171]	1991	15	Non-Hodgkin's	2	0
Haim[172]	1995	26	Gastric non-Hodgkin's		
Gale[173]	2000	24	T cell	4	1
Total		333		13 (4%)	14 (4%)

NR, not reported.

Neutropenic Patients

Abdominal Pain

In the oncology setting, surgeons are frequently asked to evaluate patients with abdominal pain who are neutropenic. The neutropenia is often a side effect of the patient's therapy. Most commonly, this occurs in patients with leukemia or other hematologic malignancies, although it also may be seen in patients with solid tumors.[125] The neutropenia in patients with hematologic malignancies can be quite profound and prolonged, especially following autologous or allogeneic stem cell or bone marrow transplant (BMT).[126] The potential for graft-versus-host disease (GVHD) in patients undergoing allogeneic transplant may make evaluation and management of abdominal pain particularly difficult. It must be remembered that common problems occur commonly and the neutropenic patient may be suffering from a common problem, such as cholecystitis or appendicitis.

After a detailed history is obtained and the patient is examined, imaging studies are useful. Because patients with neutropenia often fail to exhibit the classic signs and symptoms of an acute abdomen, CT is almost always indicated. Plain abdominal films may also be helpful.

The abdominal pain may be caused by obstruction or ileus; vascular problems, such as infarct or ischemia; infectious or inflammatory conditions; or other miscellaneous causes. Ileus is occasionally seen secondary to chemotherapeutic agents. Vincristine is classically linked with ileus; more than 40% of patients receiving the drug describe abdominal pain and constipation. Fortunately, this complication is almost always self-limited. Hydration, bowel rest, and decompression usually suffice. Arterial insufficiency causing bowel ischemia or infarct can occur in neutropenic patients but is not common. Venous thrombosis is associated with cancer as a result of the hypercoagulable state that is present, often coupled with dehydration. Infectious or inflammatory problems causing abdominal pain in neutropenic patients are the major focus of the rest of this section. These conditions can be divided into problems unique to the neutropenic cancer patient, those that affect the general population, and posttransplant complications.

Causes of Abdominal Pain Unique to Neutropenic Cancer Patients

Neutropenic enterocolitis (NE) is the most common cause of abdominal pain in neutropenic cancer patients.[127,128] This syndrome has many synonyms, including typhlitis, necrotizing or neutropenic enteropathy. and ileocecal syndrome. The syndrome was initially described in 1970 as a complication of leukemia treatment in children.[129] NE is characterized by fever, abdominal pain (usually right-sided), nausea, and vomiting, occurring in the setting of a low or falling neutrophil count. Adult patients are usually neutropenic secondary to myeloablative chemotherapy for leukemia or other hematologic malignancy.[130,131] Occasionally, NE can be seen in adult patients being treated for solid tumors, particularly when high-dose chemotherapy is used with BMT.[126,132] Although NE is probably the most common cause of abdominal pain requiring surgical intervention in neutropenic patients, few neutropenic patients develop NE and even fewer require operation (Table 73.7).[128,133] In case series of several hundred adult leukemias, the incidence of NE ranged between 2% and 6%.[127,128,134–136] In childhood leukemia, the incidence appears to be lower.[137–139]

The site of inflammation is usually the right colon, cecum, and terminal ileum. The cecum is usually the area most severely affected. The pathologic basis for this anatomic location is unclear. Proposed reasons include relative ischemia, greater distensibility, and stasis of GI contents. Infection with bacterial pathogens plays some role as evidenced by frequent recovery of enteric bacteria from blood cultures in NE patients. Commonly cultured organisms include *Pseudomonas aeruginosa*, *Klebsiella pneumoniae*, *Escherichia coli*, and *Candida* species as well as *Clostridia* species.[138,140] The most likely inciting factor is mucosal injury with ulceration and subsequent invasion of the bowel wall with enteric bacteria and/or opportunistic pathogens[126]; this sets the stage for breakdown of gut mucosal barrier function, further invasion, and (rarely) perforation.

The clinical picture of abdominal pain, fever, and neutropenia usually suggests NE, although other conditions can be present. The symptoms usually appear a few days to weeks after the onset of neutropenia. Laboratory evaluation reveals

TABLE 73.7. Incidence of neutropenic enterocolitis and mortality of surgery in patients with neutropenia and abdominal pain.

Reference	*Patients (n)*	*Incidence*	*Surgery*	*Mortality*[a]
Gorschluter 2001[127]	16	16/553 (2.9%)	5 (31%)	8 (50%)
Cartoni 2001[136]	88	88/1,450 (6.1%)	1 (1.1%)	13 (14.7%)
Neto 2000[137]	12	NA	8 (67%)	1 (8.3%)
Song 1998[131]	14	NA	2 (14%)	1 (7.1%)
Gomez 1998[125]	29	NA	1 (3%)	5 (17.2%)
Buyukasik 1997[144]	20	NA	3 (15%)	12 (60%)
Sloas 1993[138]	24	24/6,911 (0.35%)[b]	3 (12%)	2 (8.3%)
Villar 1987[128]	19	19/438 (4.3%)	4 (21%)	15 (78%)
Mower 1986[135]	13	13/499 (2.6%)	8 (61%)	12 (92%)

[a] Pediatric center.

[b] Denominator includes all patients seen at hospital; incidence for acute myclogenous leukemia patients was 2.1%.

AML, acute myelogenous leukemia.

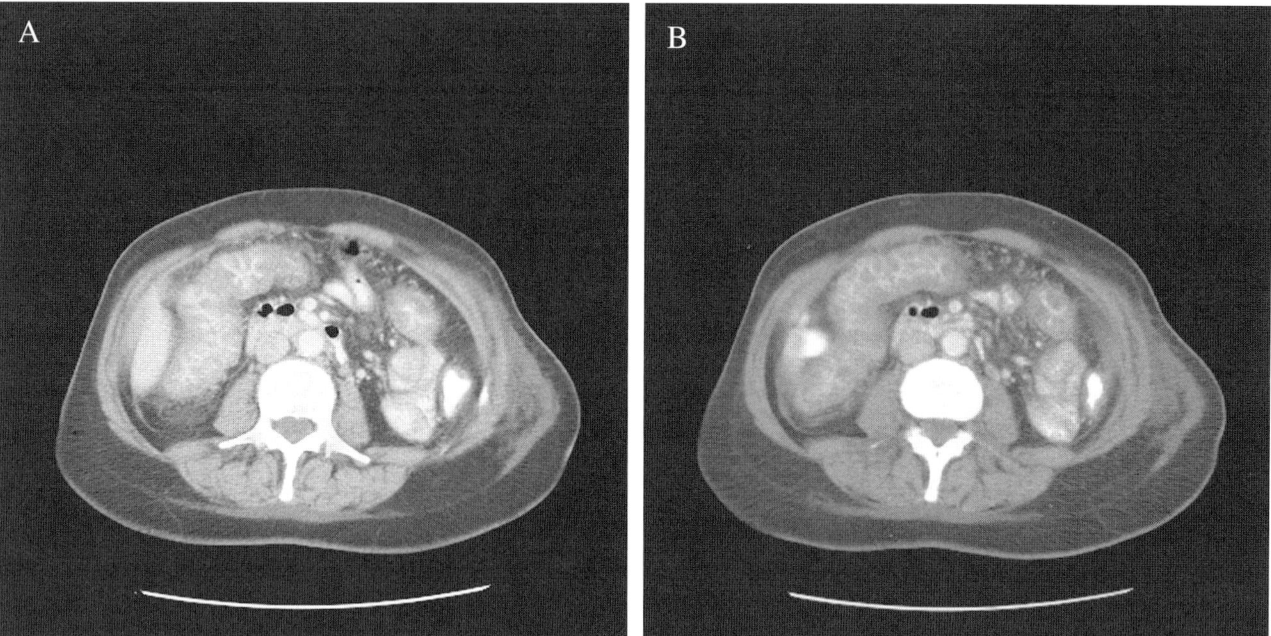

FIGURE 73.3. Computed tomography (CT) scan panels (A, B) show marked bowel wall edema in the terminal ileum in a patient with neutropenic colitis.

absolute neutropenia as well as anemia and thrombocytopenia.[138] The total bilirubin can be elevated and probably reflects ongoing sepsis and hepatic dysfunction. Positive blood cultures are associated with higher mortality.[135] Stool cultures can be positive for *Clostridium difficile*, *E. coli*, *Pseudomonas*, and adenovirus.[125,138] In the past, plain radiographs were usually obtained and signs of bowel wall thickening, such as thumb printing, were associated with the diagnosis of NE. However, only 50% of patients have this radiologic sign.[135] Pneumatosis can be seen as well as distension and cecal fluid. Free air is a sign of perforation and an indication for surgery.[141] CT scan with intravenous and oral contrast is the study of choice to evaluate patients with suspected NE. In a review of 289 neutropenic patients undergoing abdominal CT scan, 76 had abnormal scans. NE was present in 53 patients. *C. difficile* colitis was seen in 14 and 7 had GVHD.[142] Bowel wall thickening was seen in all NE patients, and also in all *C. difficile* colitis patients and 86% of the GVHD patients (Figure 73.3). Pneumatosis intestinalis was seen only in NE and occurred in 21% of the patients. Abnormalities in the cecum alone were only seen in NE although entire right colon involvement was seen with the other conditions. *C. difficile* colitis was characterized by the most wall thickening, more pancolitis, and wall nodularity. Ultrasound has been used to evaluate NE. In a review of 88 leukemic patients with clinical signs of NE, 50% had bowel wall thickening on ultrasound; this was associated with higher mortality (29% versus 0%) and longer duration of symptoms (7.9 days versus 3.8 days).[136] In another study, ultrasonic bowel wall thickening was observed in 6 of 36 patients (16%). Three patients had acute cholecystitis diagnosed by ultrasound.[143]

The treatment of NE is controversial. There are no prospective randomized trials. Varying criteria for diagnosis make comparisons between reports difficult. Some series include both adult and pediatric patients. Some reports focus solely on NE.[125,131,135–138,144] Other reports discuss all abdominal problems in neutropenic patients.[127,128,142,143] These caveats notwithstanding, recommendations have changed over the past decade. Initial reports emphasized prohibitive surgical mortality and recommended medical management.[145,146] Nonoperative therapy usually includes broad-spectrum antibiotics, hydration, bowel rest with or without nasogastric decompression, and frequent clinical reevaluation. Subsequent investigators recommended operative management.[125,128,135] More recent reports once again emphasize nonoperative treatment. Gomez et al. reported on 29 cases from two institutions between 1992 and 1996,[125] of which 18 had definite NE while 11 had possible NE, and 28 patients received nonoperative management. One patient underwent exploratory laparotomy for suspected intussusception; NE was found, no resection was performed, and the patient was treated medically. Overall mortality was 17%. Cartoni et al. reported on 88 patients. All were managed medically except one who underwent right colectomy after neutropenia resolved. Mortality was 14%.[136]

Current recommendations for patients with suspected NE include initial evaluation by physical examination, routine laboratory tests, stool cultures, and CT imaging. Patients with clearly defined surgical problems other then NE, such as cholecystitis or appendicitis, should have surgery. Patients with clearly defined medical problems other then NE, such as *C. difficile* or fungal colitis should receive specific appropriate medical management. Patients with presumed NE without clear surgical indications should be managed medically. Indications for surgery include evidence of free perforation, pneumoperitoneum, pneumatosis, associated hemorrhage, or clinical progression despite maximum medical therapy. When surgery is performed and NE is discovered, most authors recommend resection of grossly involved colon and small bowel because of the degree of necrosis typically seen. Anastomosis is risky and should be avoided through use of a stoma.

Causes of Abdominal Pain in Bone Marrow Transplant Patients

Autologous bone marrow or stem cell transplantation (BMT) following high-dose chemotherapy is a treatment modality for many hematologic malignancies. The role of BMT in the treatment of solid tumors remains controversial. Patients undergoing autologous transplant are profoundly neutropenic at the initiation of their therapy and are subject to all the complications seen in the typical neutropenic patient. Marrow recovery secondary to reinfusion of stem cells eventually resolves the neutropenia. Allogeneic bone marrow transplant has been used to treat a variety of hematologic malignancies, aplastic anemia, immunodeficiencies, and other congenital disorders. Allogeneic transplant patients are subject to profound neutropenia but have additional problems related to the infusion of donor marrow or stem cells. Pharmacologic immunosuppression is required after transplant to control rejection. Approximately 50% of BMT patients experience abdominal pain during their treatment. It is helpful to consider three phases of BMT in relation to the etiology of abdominal pain in these patients.[147]

The marrow ablative chemotherapy and radiation therapy that are used during the induction phase of BMT is toxic to gastrointestinal mucosa and often causes diarrhea and colicky pain. Nausea, vomiting, and dysphagia are also common. These symptoms are usually present starting 3 to 7 days following induction therapy and may last as long as 2 weeks.[148] Overt GI bleeding occurs in about 8% of patients, with gastritis and esophagitis being the most common endoscopic findings.[149] When neutropenia evolves 7 to 10 days following induction therapy, patients are subject to all the causes of abdominal pain previously discussed, including neutropenic enterocolitis, fungal or viral enteritis, and more run-of-the-mill entities, such as pancreatitis or cholecystitis; this represents the second phase of BMT-related abdominal pain. As in non-BMT patients with NE, management is usually conservative, but surgery may be required for perforation or hemorrhage.[126]

After 2 to 10 weeks, bone marrow engraftment with resolution of neutropenia occurs. The patient enters the third phase of BMT-related abdominal pain. This phase is characterized by the possibility of the presence of graft-versus-host disease (GVHD) in patients undergoing allogeneic transplant (although GVHD may be seen as soon as 7 days posttransplant).[2,148] In acute GVHD, donor T cells attack the host. The presence and course of the disease is determined by the degree of histocompatibility mismatch between the donor and the recipient and the extent of immunosuppression in the recipient. Patients with acute GVHD may experience diarrhea, abdominal pain, and GI bleeding along with skin rash and hepatopathy characterized by hyperbilirubinemia.[149] It is occasionally difficult to differentiate GVHD from infectious complications. Biopsy of the gastric or rectal mucosa or the skin can be helpful. GVHD is thought to occur in 30% to 80% of BMT patients.[148,150] Despite the frequency with which GVHD appears, most patients do not require surgical intervention. Severe bleeding, obstruction, or perforation are the most common indications for operation.[149–151] Pneumatosis intestinalis has been reported in up to 20% of BMT patients with acute GVHD.[152] In this setting, associated pneumoperitoneum may be managed nonoperatively, as a frank bowel perforation or necrosis may not be present; persistent evidence of peritonitis, hemodynamic instability, sepsis, or acidosis necessitate surgery.[153,154] Chronic GVHD appears several months to a year after transplant and is usually preceded by acute GVHD; it is seen in 20% to 40% of BMT patients. Most patients with chronic GVHD have liver function abnormalities, as well as chronic abdominal pain, diarrhea, and malnutrition.

Veno-occlusive disease (VOD) is another condition specific to BMT patients. It is seen in 20% to 50% of BMT patients and usually occurs several weeks posttransplant secondary to the intense chemoradiation preparative regimen.[155] In 15% of patients the VOD is severe, with mortality approaching 100%. The pathogenesis is thought to be secondary to hepatic endothelial damage from chemotherapy and radiation therapy with resulting postsinusoidal obstruction. Patients with preexisting liver disease have a higher incidence. Patients may experience fluid retention, weight gain, hepatomegaly, ascites, jaundice, and encephalopathy. The diagnosis can be confirmed with liver biopsy that reveals centrolobular necrosis with obliteration of the sinusoids and terminal venules. VOD resolves in most patients but can lead to multisystem organ failure. Treatment is primarily supportive with attention to maintaining fluid volume and renal function. There are case reports of successful liver transplantation to salvage patients dying of severe VOD.[156] Anticoagulant and thrombolytic agents have also been used to treat VOD. Tissue plasminogen activator was used to treat 42 patients with VOD and was successful in 29%. However, therapy had to be started before multiorgan failure appeared and was associated with a significant risk of hemorrhage.[157] In a small study with historical controls, antithrombin III concentrate was associated with clinical improvement and increased survival in patients with severe VOD.[158] VOD is not treated surgically but may be confused with surgical diagnoses. It can mimic myriad other entities, including cholecystitis, hepatitis, cholangitis, sepsis, and GVHD. The ultrasound findings in patients with VOD may suggest the presence of cholecystitis.[159] As noted previously, in cases of suspected VOD, liver biopsy is confirmatory. It is worth noting that jaundice is observed in as many as one-fourth of all patients undergoing BMT and is rarely the result of a problem requiring surgery.[160]

Perianal Problems in Neutropenic Patients

Perianal problems occur with some frequency in neutropenic patients. The incidence of perianal problems among patients with leukemia ranges from 5% to 8%.[161–163] The diagnosis and management of these disorders in neutropenic patients must be modified because of their immunocompromised status. Patients present with perirectal pain, pain with defecation, and fever in 70% of cases.[161] The most common physical findings are tenderness, erythema, and induration; they are present in almost all patients.[163] Most common is perirectal infection (what would otherwise be an abscess in an immunocompetent host), seen in 30% of neutropenic patients with perianal problems, followed by fissures and hemorrhoids.[161]

TABLE 73.8. Incidence of perianal disorders and mortality of surgery in patients with neutropenia.

Reference	*Patients (n)*	*Incidence*	*Surgery*	*Mortality*[a]
Lehrnbecher 2002[165]	64 (82)	NA	30 (47%)	0
Buyukasik 1997[144]	20	20/367 (5.4%)	10 (50%)	4 (20%)
North 1996[161b]	83 (92)	83/1214 (6.8%)	13 (16%)	NA
Glenn 1984[164]	44 (57)	NA	26 (59%)	17 (37%)
Barnes 1984[162]	16	16/202 (7.9%)	10 (63%)	2 (13%)

[a] Death from leukemia versus death from perianal sepsis may not be specified in the article.
[b] Includes noninfectious perianal problems.

Fistula in ano is much less common. In advanced cases of perianal infection, tissue necrosis and fasciitis (Fournier's gangrene) can develop. Most perianal infections are polymicrobial, based on the results of needle aspiration for culture or surgical incision and drainage. Common organisms include *Pseudomonas aeruginosa*, *Escherichia coli*, *Streptococcus*, and *Klebsiella*. Anaerobic organisms and *Candida* may also be involved.[161,162,164]

The etiology of these perianal problems is not definitively known but probably involves the translocation of normal microbial flora through physiologically and immunologically compromised mucosal and dermal barriers on the perineum. The diarrhea often seen in neutropenic patients can lead to breakdown of perianal skin and transitional epithelium in the anal canal, forming a nidus that is particularly problematic in the setting of compromised immune function. Once established, an infection can spread through the perirectal tissue planes. Although historically observed in patients with hematologic malignancies, solid tumor patients are increasingly prone to these problems, perhaps reflecting the use of more aggressive chemotherapeutic regimens.[165]

Upon initial evaluation, examination of the perianal area is often limited by tenderness. Historically, digital rectal examination and instrumentation with anoscopes has been avoided because of concern over traumatic microbial seeding. More recent studies suggest this may not be the case.[163,166] There is little information concerning the use of CT scans or other imaging modalities in the evaluation of perianal infections. Radiographic as well as physical examination findings are often limited by the absence of the usual stigmata of inflammation and infection.[163,166] The host is simply incapable of mounting an effective immune response. Aspiration of an indurated area may be performed with culture results used to guide antibiotic coverage. One report suggested this practice leads to modification of the antibiotic regimen in up to 50% of cases.[165] Antibiotic treatment alone is usually adequate, as return of immunocompetence with resolution of the neutropenia almost always clears the process. Specific antibiotics targeted to anaerobic infection are beneficial, increasing resolution from 55% to 88% in cases that do not require surgery.[164] Symptomatic treatment with sitzbaths, stool softeners, and analgesia is usually also recommended.

Despite adequate antibiotic coverage, in some patients infection will progress. Surgical intervention may be required, although the need is less common in more recent series (Table 73.8). Absolute indications for surgery include fluctuance, worsening sepsis, extension of erythema, soft tissue necrosis, and crepitus. Fluctuance indicates the presence of pus in the perianal tissues. Incision and drainage is the most common procedure performed in all studies reviewed. In severe cases, debridement of tissue and diverting colostomy may be necessary. Overall mortality appears to be lower currently in comparison to older studies,[164,165] which may be the result of earlier recognition of perianal sepsis, improved antibiotic therapy, and more prompt surgical intervention when indicated. It is important to undertake a more thorough examination when the neutropenia resolves. At that time, patients can be evaluated for hemorrhoids or fissures that may require therapy, particularly if further chemotherapy is planned.

References

1. Chang AE, August DA. Acute abdomen, bowel obstruction, and fistula. In: Abeloff MD, Armitage JO, Lichter AS, Niederhuber JE (eds). Clinical Oncology. New York: Churchill Livingstone, 1995:583–597.
2. Yahanda AM. Surgical emergencies in the cancer patient. In: Norton JA, Bollinger RR, Chang AE, et al (eds). Surgery: Basic Science and Clinical Evidence. New York: Springer-Verlag, 2001: 1823–1839.
3. Swenson K, Rose M, Ritz L, Murray C, Adlis S. Recognition and evaluation of oncology-related symptoms in the emergency department. Ann Emerg Med 1995;26:12–17.
4. Hargarten S, Roberts M, Anderson A. Cancer presentation in the emergency department: a failure of primary care. Am J Emerg Med 1992;10:290–293.
5. Porta M, Fernandez E, Belloc J, Malats N, Gallen N, Alonso J. Emergency admission for cancer: a matter of survival? Br J Cancer 1998;77:477–484.
6. Smothers L, Hynan L, Fleming J, Turnage R, Simmang C, Anthony T. Emergency surgery for colon carcinoma. Dis Colon Rectum 2003;46:24–30.
7. Turnbull ADM. Abdominal and upper gastrointestinal emergencies. In: Turnbull ADM (ed). Surgical Emergencies in the Cancer Patient. Chicago: Yearbook Medical, 1987:152.
8. Starnes HF, Turnbull ADM, Daly JM. Colon and rectal emergencies. In: Turnbull ADM (ed). Surgical Emergencies in the Cancer Patient. Chicago: Yearbook Medical, 1987:195–204.
9. Hawkins JA, Mower WR, Nelson EW. Acute abdominal conditions in patients with leukemia. Am J Surg 1985;150:739–742.
10. Torosian MH, Turnbull ADM. Emergency laparotomy of spontaneous intestinal and colonic perforations in cancer patients receiving corticosteroids and chemotherapy. J Clin Oncol 1988; 6:291–296.
11. Reber H, Roberts C, Way LW, Dunphy JE. Management of external gastrointestinal fistulas. Ann Surg 1978;188:460–467.
12. Jahnson S, Westerborn O, Gerdin B. Prognosis of surgically treated radiation damage to the intestine. Eur J Surg Oncol 1992;18:487–493.
13. Novak J, Collins J, Donowitz M, et al. Effects of radiation on the human gastrointestinal tract. J Clin Gastroenterol 1979;3:9–39.

14. Irvin TT. Abdominal pain: a surgical audit of 1190 emergency admissions. Br J Surg 1989;76:1121.
15. Swenson A, Glenn J, Funkhouser WK, Schneider P. Acute illnesses necessitating urgent abdominal surgery in neutropenic cancer patients: description of 14 cases and review of the literature. Surgery (St. Louis) 1989;105:778–789.
16. Blair SL, Chu DZ, Schwarz RE. Outcome of palliative operations for malignant bowel obstruction in patients with peritoneal carcinomatosis from nongynecological cancer. Ann Surg Oncol 2001;8:632–637.
17. Easson AM, Asch M, Swallow CJ. Palliative general surgical procedures. Surg Oncol Clin N Am 2001;10:161–184.
18. Faber-Langendoen K. Resuscitation of patients with metastatic cancer: is transient benefit still futile? Arch Intern Med 1991; 151:235–239.
19. Ferrara J, Martin E, Carey L. Morbidity of emergency operations in patients with metastatic cancer receiving chemotherapy. Surgery (St. Louis) 1982;92:605–609.
20. Turnbull AD, Guerra J, Starnes HF. Results of surgery for obstructing carcinomatosis of gastrointestinal, pancreatic, or biliary origin. J Clin Oncol 1989;7:381–386.
21. Brophy C, Cahow CE. Primary small bowel malignant tumors. Unrecognized until emergent laparotomy. Am Surg 1989:55: 408–412.
22. Farmer K, Phillips R. True and false large bowel obstruction. Baillieres Clin Gastroenterol 1991;5:563–585.
23. Schwarz RE, Zagala-Nevarez K. Gastrectomy circumstances that influence early postoperative outcome. Hepatogastroenterology 2002;49:1742–1746.
24. Smothers L, Hynan L, Fleming J, Turnage R, Simmang C, Anthony T. Emergency surgery for colon carcinoma. Dis Colon Rectum 2003:46:24–30.
25. Akhtar K, Byrne J, Bancewicz J. Argon beam plasma coagulation in the management of cancers of the esophagus and stomach. Surg Endosc 2000;14:1127–1130.
26. Jakobs R, Miola J, Altwood SR. Endoscopic laser palliation for rectal cancer: therapeutic outcome and complications in eighty-three consecutive patients. Gastroenterology 2002;40:551–556.
27. Litle VR, Luketich JD, Christie NA, et al. Photodynamic therapy as palliation for esophageal cancer: experience in 215 patients. Ann Thorac Surg 2003;76:1687–1692.
28. Myrvold H. Surgical procedures in colorectal cancer emergencies. Scand J Gastroenterol 1988;149:120S–124S.
29. De SG, Gava C, et al. Curative surgery for obstruction from primary left colorectal carcinoma: primary or staged resection? Cochrane Database Syst Rev 2002.
30. Lee YM, Law WL, Chu KW, Poon RT. Emergency surgery for obstructing colorectal cancers: a comparison between right-sided and left-sided lesions. J Am Coll Surg 2001;192:719–725.
31. Arnaud J, Bergamaschi R. Emergency subtotal/total colectomy with anastomosis for acutely obstructed carcinoma of the left colon. Dis Colon Rectum 1994;37:685–688.
32. Halevy A, Levi J, Orda R. Emergency subtotal colectomy. A new trend for treatment of obstructing carcinoma of the left colon. Ann Surg 1989;210:220–223.
33. Dauphine CE, Tan P, Beart RW, Jr., Vukasin P, Cohen H, Corman ML. Placement of self-expanding metal stents for acute malignant large-bowel obstruction: a collective review. Ann Surg Oncol 2002;9:574–579.
34. Morino M, Bertello A, Garbarini A, Rozzio G, Repici A. Malignant colonic obstruction managed by endoscopic stent decompression followed by laparoscopic resections. Surg Endosc 2002;16:1483–1487.
35. Wong K, Cheong D, Wong D. Treatment of acute malignant colorectal obstruction with self-expandable metallic stents. A N Z J Surg 2002;72:385–388.
36. Feuer DJ, Broadley KE, Shepherd JH, Barton DP. Systematic review of surgery in malignant bowel obstruction in advanced gynecological and gastrointestinal cancer. The Systematic Review Steering Committee. Gynecol Oncol 1999;75:313–322.
37. Feuer DJ, Broadley KE, Shepherd JH, Barton DP. Surgery for the resolution of symptoms in malignant bowel obstruction in advanced gynaecological and gastrointestinal cancer. Cochrane Database Syst Rev 2000;4:CD002764.
38. Sadeghi B, Arvieux C, Glehen O, et al. Peritoneal carcinomatosis from non-gynecologic malignancies: results of the EVOCAPE 1 multicentric prospective study. Cancer (Phila) 2000;88:358–363.
39. Chu DZ, Lang NP, Thompson C, Osteen PK, Westbrook KC. Peritoneal carcinomatosis in nongynecologic malignancy. A prospective study of prognostic factors. Cancer (Phila) 1989;63: 364–367.
40. Turnbull AD, Guerra J, Starnes HF. Results of surgery for obstructing carcinomatosis of gastrointestinal, pancreatic, or biliary origin. J Clin Oncol 1989;7:381–386.
41. Tang T, Allison M, Dunkley I, Roberts P, Dickinson R. Enteral stenting in 21 patients with malignant gastroduodenal obstruction. J R Soc Med 2003;96: 494–496.
42. Woolfson RG, Jennings K, Whalen GR. Management of bowel obstruction in patients with abdominal cancer. Arch Surg 1997;132: 1093–1097.
43. Alexander HR, Turnbull AD, Salamone J, Keefe D, Melendez J. Upper abdominal cancer surgery in the very elderly. J Surg Oncol 1991;47:82–86.
44. Familiari G, Paternollo R, Agabiti E, Earatti BC, Costeri S, Libezio D. Gastric re-resection in emergency. Hepatogastroenterology 1998;45:1172–1176.
45. Mercadante S, Spoldi E, Caraceni A, Maddaloni S, Simonetti MT. Octreotide in relieving gastrointestinal symptoms due to bowel obstruction. Palliat Med 1993;7:295–299.
46. Khoo D, Hall E, Motson R, Riley J, Denman K, Waxman J. Palliation of malignant intestinal obstruction using octreotide. Eur J Cancer 1994;30A:28–30.
47. Ripamonti C, Mercadante S, Groff L, Zecca E, De Conno F, Casuccio A. Role of octreotide, scopolamine butylbromide, and hydration in symptom control of patients with inoperable bowel obstruction and nasogastric tubes: a prospective randomized trial. J Pain Symptom Manag 2000;19:23–34.
48. Mystakidou K, Tsilika E, Kalaidopoulou O, Chondros K, Georgaki S, Papadimitriou L. Comparison of octreotide administration vs. conservative treatment in the management of inoperable bowel obstruction in patients with far advanced cancer: a randomized, double-blind, controlled clinical trial. Anticancer Res 2002;22:1187–1192.
49. Ventafridda V, Ripamonti C, Caraceni A, Spoldi E, Messina L, De Conno F. The management of inoperable gastrointestinal obstruction in terminal cancer patients. Tumori 1990;76:389–393.
50. Law WL, Chu KW, Ho JW, Tung HM, Law SY, Chu KM. Self-expanding metallic stent in the treatment of colonic obstruction caused by advanced malignancies. Dis Colon Rectum 2000;43: 1522–1527.
51. Saida Y, Sumiyama Y, Nagao J, Takase M. Stent endoprosthesis for obstructing colorectal cancers. Dis Colon Rectum 1996;39: 552–555.
52. Baron TH, Dean PA, Yates MR, 3rd, Canon C, Koehler RE. Expandable metal stents for the treatment of colonic obstruction: techniques and outcomes. Gastrointest Endosc 1998;47: 277–286.
53. Choo IW, Do YS, Sch W, et al. Malignant colorectal obstruction: treatment with a flexible covered stent. Radiology 1998;206: 415–421.
54. de Gregorio MA, Mainar A, Tejero E, et al. Acute colorectal obstruction: stent placement for palliative treatment—results of a multicenter study. Radiology 1998;209:117–120.

55. Mainar A, de Gregorio MA, Tejero E, et al. Acute colorectal obstruction: treatment with self-expandable metallic stents before scheduled surgery—results of a multicenter study. Radiology 1999;210:65–69.
56. Repici A, Reggio D, De Angelis C, et al. Self-expanding covered esophageal ultraflex stent for palliation of malignant colorectal anastomotic obstruction complicated by multiple fistulas. Gastrointest Endosc 2000;51:346–348.
57. Aviv RI, Shyamalan G, Watkinson A, Tibballs J, Ogunbaye G. Radiological palliation of malignant colonic obstruction. Clin Radiol 2002;57:347–351.
58. Dauphine CE, Tan P, Beart RW, Jr., Vukasin P, Cohen H, Corman ML. Placement of self-expanding metal stents for acute malignant large-bowel obstruction: a collective review. Ann Surg Oncol 2002;9:574–579.
59. Clark JS, Buchanan GN, Khawaja AR, et al. Use of the Bard Memotherm self-expanding metal stent in the palliation of colonic obstruction. Abdom Imaging 2003;28:518–524.
60. Law WL, Choi HK, Lee YM, Chu KW. Palliation for advanced malignant colorectal obstruction by self-expanding metallic stents: prospective evaluation of outcomes. Dis Colon Rectum 2004;47:39–43.
61. Jung GS, Song HY, Seo TS, et al. Malignant gastroduodenal obstructions: treatment by means of a covered expandable metallic stent-initial experience. Radiology 2000;216(3):758–763.
62. Kim JH, Yoo BM, Lee KJ. Self-expanding coil stent with a long delivery system for palliation of unresectable malignant gastric outlet obstruction: a prospective study. Endoscopy 2001;33:838–842.
63. Pinto Pabon IT, Diaz LP, et al. Gastric and duodenal stents: follow-up and complications. Cardiovasc Intervent Radiol 2001;24:147–153.
64. Park KB, Do YS, Kang WK, et al. Malignant obstruction of gastric outlet and duodenum: palliation with flexible covered metallic stents. Radiology 2001;219:679–683.
65. Yim HB, Jacobson BC, Saltzman JR, et al. Clinical outcome of the use of enteral stents for palliation of patients with malignant upper GI obstruction. Gastrointest Endosc 2001;53:329–332.
66. Aviv R, Shyamalan G, Khan FM, et al. Use of stents in the palliative treatment of malignant gastric outlet and duodenal obstruction. Clin Radiol 2002;57:587–592.
67. Schiefke I, Zabel-Langhennig A, Wiedmann M, et al. Self-expandable metallic stents for malignant duodenal obstruction caused by biliary tract cancer. Gastrointest Endosc 2003;58:213–219.
68. Kaw M, Singh S, Gagneja H, Azad P. Role of self-expandable metal stents in the palliation of malignant duodenal obstruction. Surg Endosc 2003;17:646–650.
69. Tang T, Allison M, Dunkley I, Roberts P, Dickinson R. Enteral stenting in 21 patients with malignant gastroduodenal obstruction. J R Soc Med 2003;96:494–496.
70. Nassif T, Prat F, Meduri B. Endoscopic palliation of malignant gastric outlet obstruction using self-expandable metallic stents: results of a multicenter study. Endoscopy 2003;35:483–489.
71. Born P, Neuhaus H, Rosch T, Lorenz R, Classen M. A minimally invasive palliative approach to advanced pancreatic and papillary cancer causing both biliary and duodenal obstruction. Z Gastroenterol 1996;34:416–420.
72. Mittal A, Windsor J, Woodfield J, Casey P, Lane M. Matched study of three methods for palliation of malignant pyloroduodenal obstruction. Br J Surg 2004;91:205–209.
73. Lokich JJ, Kane RA, Harrison DA, McDermott WV. Biliary tract obstruction secondary to cancer: management guidelines and selected literature review. J Clin Oncol 1987;5:969–581.
74. Povoski SP, Karpeh MS, Jr., Conlon KC, Blumgart LH, Brennan MF. Preoperative biliary drainage: impact on intraoperative bile cultures and infectious morbidity and mortality after pancreaticoduodenectomy. J Gastrointest Surg 1999;3:496–505.
75. Schwarz RE. Technical considerations to maintain a low frequency of postoperative biliary stent-associated infections. J Hepatobiliary Pancreat Surg 2002;9:93–97.
76. Fainsinger RL. Integrating medical and surgical treatments in gastrointestinal, genitourinary, and biliary obstruction in patients with cancer. Hematol Oncol Clin N Am 1996;10:173–188.
77. Kemeny MM, Brennan MF. The surgical complications of chemotherapy in the cancer patient. Curr Probl Surg 1987;24:609–675.
78. Welch CE, Rodkey GV, von Ryll Gryska P. A thousand operations for ulcer disease. Ann Surg 1986;204:454–467.
79. Rockall T. Management and outcome of patients undergoing surgery after acute upper gastrointestinal haemorrhage. Steering Group for the National Audit of Acute Upper Gastrointestinal Haemorrhage. J R Soc Med 1998;91:518–523.
80. Padmanabhan A, Douglass H, Nava HR. Role of endoscopy in upper gastrointestinal bleeding in patients with malignancy. Endoscopy 1980;12:101–104.
81. Sugawa C, Steffes C, Nakamura R. Upper GI bleeding in an urban hospital. Etiology, recurrence, and prognosis. Ann Surg 1990;212:521–526.
82. Kouraklis G, Misiakos E, Karatzas G, Gogas J, Skalkeas G. Diagnostic approach and management of active lower gastrointestinal hemorrhage. Int Surg 1995;80:138–140.
83. Nath RL, Sequeira JC, Weitzman AF, Birkett DH, Williams LF Jr. Lower gastrointestinal bleeding. Diagnostic approach and management conclusions. Am J Surg 1981;141:478–481.
84. Rosch J, Kozak BE, Keller FS, Dotter CT. Interventional angiography in the diagnosis of acute lower gastrointestinal bleeding. Eur J Radiol 1986;6:136–141.
85. Miller LS, Barbarevech C, Friedman LS. Less frequent causes of lower gastrointestinal bleeding. Gastroenterol Clin North Am 1994;23:21–52.
86. Mercadante S, Fusco F, Valle A, et al. Factors involved in gastrointestinal bleeding in advanced cancer patients followed at home. Support Care Cancer 2004;12:95–98.
87. Fiorino C, Cozzarini C, Vavassori V, et al. Relationships between DVHs and late rectal bleeding after radiotherapy for prostate cancer: analysis of a large group of patients pooled from three institutions. Radiother Oncol 2002;64:1–12.
88. Desautels SG, Slivka A, Schoen RE, Carr B, Rabinovitz M, Silverman W. Gastrointestinal bleeding in cirrhotic patients with hepatocellular carcinoma undergoing intrahepatic artery chemotherapy. Gastrointest Endosc 1997;46:430–434.
89. Meinke WB, Twomey PL, Guernsey JM, et al. Gastrointestinal bleeding after operation for pancreatic cancer. Am J Surg 1983;146:57–60.
90. van Berge Henegouwen MI, Allema JH, et al. Delayed massive haemorrhage after pancreatic and biliary surgery. Br J Surg 1995;82:1527–1531.
91. Jarnagin W, Gonen M, Fong Y, et al. Improvement in perioperative outcome after hepatic resection: analysis of 1,803 consecutive cases over the past decade. Ann Surg 2002;236:397–406.
92. Jimenez RE, Shoup M, Cohen AM, Paty PB, Guillem J, Wong WD. Contemporary outcomes of total pelvic exenteration in the treatment of colorectal cancer. Dis Colon Rectum 2003;46:1619–1625.
93. Rizk N, Bach P, Schrog D, et al. The impact of complications on outcomes after resection for esophageal and gastroesophageal junction carcinoma. J Am Coll Surg 2004;198:42–50.
94. Chen C, Chang T, et al. Endoscopic variceal ligation versus conservative treatment for patients with hepatocellular carcinoma and bleeding esophageal varices. Gastrointest Endosc 1995;42:535–539.
95. Yegappan M, Ho YH, Nyam D, Leong A, Eu KW, Seow C. The surgical management of colorectal complications from irradia-

tion for carcinoma of the cervix. Ann Acad Med Singap 1998;27: 627–630.
96. Spinosa DJ, Angle JF, McGraw JK, Maurer EJ, Hagspiel KD, Matsumoto AH. Transcatheter treatment of life-threatening lower gastrointestinal bleeding due to advanced pelvic malignancy. Cardiovasc Intervent Radiol 1998;21:503–505.
97. Onsrud M, Hagen B, Strickert T. 10-Gy single-fraction pelvic irradiation for palliation and life prolongation in patients with cancer of the cervix and corpus uteri. Gynecol Oncol 2001;82: 167–171.
98. Tinger A, Waldron T, Peluso N. Effective palliative radiation therapy in advanced and recurrent ovarian carcinoma. Int J Radiat Oncol Biol Phys 2001;51:1256–1263.
99. Corn BW, Lanciano RM, Boente M, Hunter WM, Ladazack J, Ozols RF. Recurrent ovarian cancer. Effective radiotherapeutic palliation after chemotherapy failure. Cancer (Phila) 1994;74: 2979–2983.
100. Moreno-Otero R, Rodriguez S, Carbo J, Mearin F, Pajares JM. Acute upper gastrointestinal bleeding as primary symptom of gastric carcinoma. J Surg Oncol 1987;36:130–133.
101. Kasakura Y, Ajani JA, Mochizuki F, Morishita Y, Fujii M, Takayama T. Outcomes after emergency surgery for gastric perforation or severe bleeding in patients with gastric cancer. J Surg Oncol 2002;80:181–185.
102. Johnson A, Harman P, Hanks JB. Primary small bowel malignancies. Am Surg 1985;51:31–36.
103. Berger A, Cellier C, Daniel C, et al. Small bowel metastases from primary carcinoma of the lung: clinical findings and outcome. Am J Gastroenterol 1999;94:1884–1887.
104. Talamonti MS, Dawes LG, Joehl RJ, Nahrwold DL. Gastrointestinal lymphoma. A case for primary surgical resection. Arch Surg 1990;125:972–976.
105. Branum G, Seigler H. Role of surgical intervention in the management of intestinal metastases from malignant melanoma. Am J Surg 1991;162:428–431.
106. Ihde J, Coit D. Melanoma metastatic to stomach, small bowel, or colon. Am J Surg 1991;162:208–211.
107. Serour F, Dona G, Birkenfeld S, Balassiano M, Krispin M. Primary neoplasms of the small bowel. J Surg Oncol 1992;49:29–34.
108. Terry B, Beart R. Emergency abdominal colectomy with primary anastomosis. Dis Colon Rectum 1981;24:1–4.
109. Repse S, Calic M, Zakelj B, Stor Z, Juvan R, Jelenc F. Emergency colorectal surgery: our results and complications. Ann Ital Chir 1996;67:205–209.
110. Lee P, Sutherland D. Massive gastrointestinal bleeding as the initial manifestation of pancreatic carcinoma. Int J Pancreatol 1994;15:223–237.
111. de Villa VH, Calvo FA, Bilbao JI, et al. Arteriodigestive fistula: a complication associated with intraoperative and external beam radiotherapy following surgery for gastric cancer. J Surg Oncol 1992;49:52–57.
112. Schwarz RE, Marx HF, Andersen JS. Successful management and outcome of a postoperative aortogastric fistula in a patient with recurrent gastric cancer: report of a case. Surg Today 2002; 32:816–820.
113. Liu C-L, Fan S-T, Lo C-M, et al. Management of spontaneous rupture of hepatocellular carcinoma: single-center experience. J Clin Oncol 2001;19:3725–3732.
114. Castells L, Moreiras M, Quiroga S, et al. Hemoperitoneum as a first manifestation of hepatocellular carcinoma in western patients with cirrhosis: effectiveness of emergency treatment with transcatheter arterial embolization. Dig Dis Sci 2001;46:555–562.
115. Yeh C-N, Lee W-C, Jeng L-B, et al. Spontaneous tumour rupture and prognosis in patients with hepatocellular carcinoma. Br J Surg 2002;89:1125–1129.
116. Morita T, Tsunoda J, Inoue S, Chihara S. Intestinal perforation in terminally ill cancer patients: clinical characteristics. Am J Gastroenterol 1999;94:541–542.
117. Schwarz RE, Strair RK. Complications of malignancy: case 2. Infectious tissue pneumatosis as a result of colon cancer perforation in a survivor of Hodgkin's disease. J Clin Oncol 2004;22: 373–374.
118. Lundy J, Sherlock P, Kurtz R, Fortner JG, Turnbull AD. Spontaneous perforation of the gastrointestinal tract in patients with cancer. Am J Gastroenterol 1975;63:447–450.
119. Torosian MH, Turnbull AD. Emergency laparotomy for spontaneous intestinal and colonic perforations in cancer patients receiving corticosteroids and chemotherapy. J Clin Oncol 1988; 6:291–296.
120. Chao T, Wang C, Chen MF. Gastroduodenal perforation in cancer patients. Hepatogastroenterology 1999;46:2878–2881.
121. Horowitz N, Cohn D, Mezog TJ, et al. The significance of pneumatosis intestinalis or bowel perforation in patients with gynecologic malignancies. Gynecol Oncol 2002;86:79–84.
122. Tessier DJ, McConnell EJ, Young-Fadok T, Wolff BG. Melanoma metastatic to the colon: case series and review of the literature with outcome analysis. Dis Colon Rectum 2003;46:441–447.
123. Koch P, del Valle F, Berdel WE, et al. Primary gastrointestinal non-Hodgkin's lymphoma: I. Anatomic and histologic distribution, clinical features, and survival data of 371 patients registered in the German Multicenter Study GIT NHL 01/92. J Clin Oncol 2001;19:3861–3873.
124. Daum S, Ullrich R, Heise W, et al. Intestinal non-Hodgkin's lymphoma: a multicenter prospective clinical study from the German Study Group on Intestinal non-Hodgkin's Lymphoma. J Clin Oncol 2003;21:2740–2746.
125. Gomez L, Martino R, Rolston KV. Neutropenic enterocolitis: spectrum of the disease and comparison of definite and possible causes. Clin Infect Dis 1998;27:695–699.
126. Avignan D, Richardson P, Elias A, et al. Neutropenic enterocolitis as a complication of high dose chemotherapy with stem cell rescue in patients with solid tumors: a case series with a review of the literature. Cancer (Phila) 1998;83:409–414.
127. Gorschluter M, Glasmacher A, Hahn C, et al. Severe abdominal infections in neutropenic patients. Cancer Invest 2001;19: 669–677.
128. Villar HV, Warnecke JA, Peck MD, et al. Role of surgical treatment in the management of complications of the gastrointestinal tract in patients with leukemia. Surg Gynecol Obstet 1987; 165:217–222.
129. Wagner ML, Rosenberg HS, Ferbach DJ, et al. Typhlitis: a complication of leukemia in childhood. Am J Roentgenol 1970;109:341.
130. Wade DS, Nava HR, Douglass HO. Neutropenic enterocolitis: clinical diagnosis and treatment. Cancer (Phila) 1992;69:17–23.
131. Song HK, Kreisel D, Canter R, et al. Changing presentation and management of neutropenic enterocolitis. Arch Surg 1998;133: 979–982.
132. Abbasoglu O, Cakmakci K. Neutropenic enterocolitis in patients without leukemia. Surg 1993;113:113–116.
133. Glenn J, Funkhouser WK, Schneider PS. Acute illnesses necessitating urgent abdominal surgery in neutropenic cancer patients: description of 14 cases and review of the literature. Surgery (St. Louis) 1989;105:778–789.
134. Moir CR, Scudamore CH, Benny WB. Typhlitis: selective surgical management. Am J Surg 11986;51:563–566.
135. Mower WJ, Hawkins JA, Nelson EW. Neutropenic enterocolitis in adults with acute leukemia. Arch Surg 1986;121:571–574.
136. Cartoni C, Dragoni F, Micozzi A, et al. Neutropenic enterocolitis in patients with acute leukemia: prognostic significance of bowel wall thickening detected by ultrasonography. J Clin Oncol 2001;19:756–761.
137. Neto LS, Oliviera-Filho AG, Epelman A, et al. Selective surgical indications in the management of neutropenic children presenting with acute abdomen. Pediatr Hematol Oncol 2000;17: 483–487.

138. Sloas MM, Flynn PM, Kaste SC, et al. Typhlitis in children with cancer: a 30 year experience. Clin Infect Dis 1993;17:484–490.
139. Skibber J, Matter G, Pizzo P. Right lower quadrant pain in young patients with leukemia. Ann Surg 1987;206:711.
140. Sayfan J, Shoavi O, Koltun L, et al. Acute abdomen caused by neutropenic enterocolitis: surgeon's dilemma. Eur J Surg 1999; 165:502–504.
141. Quigley MM, Bethel K, Nowacki M, et al. Neutropenic enterocolitis: a rare presenting complication of acute leukemia. Am J Hematol 2001;66:213–219.
142. Kirkpatrick ID, Greenberg HM. Gastrointestinal complications in neutropenic patients: characterization and differentiation with abdominal CT. Radiology 2003;226:668–674.
143. Gorschluter M, Marklein G, Hofling K, et al. Abdominal infections in patients with acute leukemia: a prospective study applying ultrasonography and microbiology. Br J Haematol 2002;117: 351–358.
144. Buyukasik Y, Ozcebe O, Haznedaroglu I, et al. Neutropenic enterocolitis in adult leukemias. Int J Hematol 1997;66: 47–55.
145. Gandy W, Greenberg BR. Successful medical management of neutropenic enterocolitis. Cancer (Phila) 1983;51:1551–1555.
146. Shaked A, Shinar E, Freund H. Neutropenic enterocolitis: a plea for conservatism. Dis Colon Rectum 1983;26:351–352.
147. Wolford JL, McDonald GB. A problem oriented approach to intestinal and liver disease after marrow transplantation for leukemia. J Clin Gastroenterol 1988;10:419–433.
148. Bortin MM, Ringden O, Horowitz MM, et al. Temporal relationships between the major complications of bone marrow transplantation for leukemia. Bone Marrow Transplant 1989;4: 339–344.
149. Evans J, Percy J, Eckstein R, et al. Surgery for intestinal graft-versus-host disease: report of two cases. Dis Colon Rectum 1998;41:1573–1576.
150. McGregor GI, Shepherd JD, Phillips GL. Acute graft-versus-host disease of the intestine: a surgical perspective. Am J Surg 1988;155:680–682.
151. Kaur S, Cooper G, Fakult S, et al. Incidence and outcome of overt gastrointestinal bleeding in patients undergoing bone marrow transplantation. Dig Dis Sci 1996;41:598–603.
152. Maile CW, Frick MP, Crass JR, et al. The plain abdominal radiograph in acute gastrointestinal graft-vs.-host disease. AJR Am J Roentgenol 1985;145:289–292.
153. Day DL, Ramsay NKC, Letourneau JG. Pneumotosis intestinalis after bone marrow transplantation. AJR Am J Roentgenol 1988; 151:85–87.
154. Lipton J, Patterson B, Mustard R, et al. Pneumotosis intestinalis with free air mimicking intestinal perforation in a bone marrow transplant patient. Bone Marrow Transplant 1994;14:323–326.
155. McDonald GB, Hinds MS, Fisher LD, et al. Veno-occlusive disease of the liver and multiorgan failure after bone marrow transplantation: a cohort study of 355 patients. Ann Intern Med 1993;118:255–267.
156. Rosen HR, Martin P, Schiller GJ, et al. Orthotopic liver transplantation for bone-marrow transplant-associated veno-occlusive disease and graft-versus-host disease of the liver. Liver Transplant Surg 1996;2:225–232.
157. Bearman SI, Lee JL, Baron AE, et al. Treatment of hepatic venoocclusive disease with recombinant human tissue plasminogen activator and heparin in 42 marrow transplant patients. Blood 1997;89:1501–1506.
158. Morris JD, Harris RE, Hashmi R, et al. Anti-thrombin III for the treatment of chemotherapy-induced organ dysfunction following bone marrow transplantation. Bone Marrow Transplant 1997;20:871–878.
159. Herbetko J, Grigg AP, Buckley AR, Phillips GL. Venoocclusive liver disease after bone marrow transplantation: Findings at duplex sonography. AJR Am J Roentgenol 1992;158:1001–1005.
160. Wasserheit C, Acaba L, Gulati S. Abnormal liver function in patients undergoing autologous bone marrow transplantation for hematologic malignancies. Cancer Invest 1995;13:347–354.
161. North JH, Weber TK, Rodriguez-Bigas MA, et al. The management of infectious and noninfectious anorectal complications in patients with leukemia. J Am Coll Surg 1996;183:322–328.
162. Barnes GG, Sattler FR, Ballard JO. Perirectal infections in acute leukemia. Ann Intern Med 1984;100:515–518.
163. Buyukasik Y, Ozcebe OI, Sayinalp N, et al. Perianal infections in patients with leukemia: importance of the course of neutrophil counts. Dis Colon Rectum 1998;41:81–85.
164. Glenn J, Cotton D, Wesley R, et al. Anorectal infections in patients with malignant disease. Rev Infect Dis 1984;10:42–52.
165. Lehrnbecher T, Marshall D, Gao C, et al. A second look at anorectal infections in cancer patients in a large cancer institute: the success of early intervention with antibiotics and surgery. Infection 2002;30:272–276.
166. Cohen JS, Paz BI, O'Donnell MR, et al. Treatment of perianal infection following bone marrow transplantation. Dis Colon Rectum 1996;39:981–985.
167. Kemeny MM, Magrath IT, Brennan MF. The role of surgery in the management of American Burkitt's lymphoma and its treatment. Ann Surg 1982;196:82–86.
168. Meyers PA, Potter VP, Wollner N, Exelby P. Bowel perforation during initial treatment for childhood non-Hodgkin's lymphoma. Cancer (Phila) 1985;56:259–261.
169. Maor MH, Velasquez WS, Fuller LM, Silvermintz KB. Stomach conservation in stages IE and IIE gastric non-Hodgkin's lymphoma. J Clin Oncol 1990;8:266–271.
170. Salles G, Herbrecht R, Tilly M. et al. Aggressive primary gastrointestinal lymphomas: review of 91 patients treated with the LNH-84 regimen. A study of the Groupe d'Etude des Lymphomes Agressifs. Am J Med 1991;90:77–84.
171. Rackner VL, Thirlby RC, Ryan JA. Role of surgery in multimodality therapy for gastrointestinal lymphoma. Am J Surg 1991;161:570–575.
172. Haim N, Leviov M, Ben-Arieh Y, et al. Intermediate and high-grade gastric non-Hodgkin's lymphoma: a prospective study of non-surgical treatment with primary chemotherapy, with or without radiotherapy. Leuk Lymphoma 1995;17:321–326.
173. Gale J, Simmonds PD, Mead GM, Sweetenham JW, Wright DH. Enteropathy-type intestinal T-cell lymphoma: clinical features and treatment of 31 patients in a single center. J Clin Oncol 2000;18:795–803.

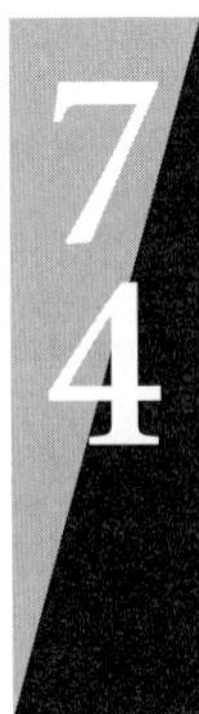

Oral Complications of Cancer Therapy

Mark S. Chambers and Adam S. Garden

Many patients receive cytotoxic therapies that result in complications to the oral mucosa. Other patients receive either radiation or surgery as treatment of malignancies involving the head and neck region, with resultant consequences to the normal structures of the oral cavity and pharynx.

Strategies for managing these sequelae of therapy include a combination of preventive measures, treatment directed at reversal of the insults to the oral tissues, and supportive care interventions. Few objective scales on oral morbidity have been reliably evaluated in clinical measure studies.

General Considerations

Overview

Evaluation, treatment, and prevention of any oral and dental preexisting pathology is an important aspect of the overall treatment outcome for cancer patients.[1,2] Patients undergoing aggressive anticancer treatment encounter preventable, if not treatable, oral mucosal and dental sequelae that could produce morbid events.[3] Complications vary with each patient, depending on the individual's oral and dental status, the type of malignancy, and the therapeutic approach (i.e., surgery, radiation therapy, chemotherapy, or a combination of these treatments).[4]

Oral complications associated with cancer therapy can be classified into seven general types: stomatitis, infection, bleeding, mucositis, pain, loss of function, and xerostomia.[5] Such complications arise primarily in three anatomic sites: the mucosa, periodontium, and teeth.[4] Management algorithms for these complications are reviewed in the following sections dedicated to the causative modalities.

Pretherapy Evaluation and Management

An oral and dental consultation before chemotherapy, radiation therapy, or head and neck surgery is extremely important in the oral management of cancer patients.[2,6–11] Addressing the dental needs at the outset allows for more careful planning of the timing of the overall treatment; as with regard to nonsurgical therapies, timing can influence outcome. Necessary dental work can be managed at the same time as the surgery, and in the immediate postsurgical period, the oral cavity should be prepared for appropriate prosthetic rehabilitation to correct postsurgical deficits. The following sections describe methods of integrating dental and oral treatment into specific oncologic therapies.

Radiation Therapy

Radiation-Induced Oral Complications

The complications from radiation therapy are categorized as either acute (e.g., mucositis, infectious stomatitis, alteration of taste or smell acuity, dermatitis, pain, inflammation, and difficulty swallowing) or late (e.g., xerostomia, caries, abnormal development, fibrosis, trismus, osteoradionecrosis, and pain).[2,12,13] The term *late* refers to effects that either affect slowly responding tissues, such as muscles and bone, or effects that persist and are generally irreversible, such as xerostomia.

The severity of treatment-induced morbidity depends on multiple factors, such as the radiation dose, energy source, volume of tissue treated, pretreatment performance status, and pretreatment periodontal condition.[14] In addition, treatment intensification by altered fractionation or the use of concurrent chemotherapy can increase the morbidity to the oral mucosa. The volume of tissue irradiated is susceptible to dermatitis and mucositis, which are often accompanied by salivary gland hypofunction, dysgeusia, dysphagia, odynophagia, hypovascularity of soft and hard tissues, fibrosis, or trismus.[2,14–16] Widespread oral melanotic hyperpigmentation and hypopigmentation have been reported.[17] Developmental abnormalities of the dentition and jaws may occur in children undergoing head and neck radiation therapy.[17–25] In patients of all ages, altered tissues within the volume of tissue radiated are highly susceptible to infectious processes, especially with fungal organisms (*Candida* species)[26,27]; bacterial infections, especially with streptococci and staphylococci; and viral infections, especially with herpes simplex virus (HSV).[28,29]

Mucositis

Oral mucositis generally occurs 5 to 7 days after initiation of external-beam radiation therapy by accelerating the rate of destruction of the basal cell layer compared with the proliferation of new cells. Subepithelial edema can provoke an epithelial breakdown, beginning with erythema of the involved mucosa in the second week of therapy. As treatment continues, the epithelial surface cells shed, but their replacement by cells from the basal level does not occur. The mucosa becomes thin and superficially ulcerated, appearing as white patches, commonly mistaken for a yeast infection. As radiation progresses, the patches coalesce, forming large fields of superficial ulceration, referred to as *confluent mucositis*. Infrequently, radiation-induced mucositis can form deep ulceration with necrosis and hemorrhage. By the end of treatment, diffuse erythema, ulceration, spontaneous bleeding, and white or yellow pseudomembrane formation may be present.[30–32] Following a course of fractionated radiation, the mucositis heals, generally in 6 weeks after therapy, but ulceration can last for 2 or 3 months and occasionally longer.[33,34]

The definitions of the degree and intensity of mucositis are quite varied. Numerous scoring systems, none universally accepted, have been proposed and are used in clinical trials.[35] The most common are the World Health Organization (WHO) system that incorporates subjective symptoms (dysphagia) into the scores, and the NCI CTC system, a simple 0–4 system based on the observed degree of mucositis. This lack of uniformity, as well as the question of the validity of these systems despite their common usage, further compounds the difficulty in assessing trials exploring mucositis.

Management of mucositis is twofold. Agents are used or are being developed to either prevent or delay both the onset and severity of mucositis. The primary mode of mucositis management, however, is on symptom management. These agents are being used or tested for mucositis, but they fall into one of three categories: drugs designed to protect damage to the proliferating cells, drugs that are antiinflammatory, or drugs that are antiinfective.

Mucosal Protectors

Amifostine (WR-2721), a radioprotector, is a phosphorylated aminothiol pro-drug.[36] In tissue, membrane-bound alkaline phosphatase dephosphorylates the drug to its active metabolite, the free thiol WR-1065. The postulated mechanism of action of WR-1065 is scavenging of free radicals created by the action of radiation. The drug is currently approved for the prevention of radiation-induced xerostomia, but investigators have also been interested in using the drug to prevent or reduce the severity of mucositis.

To date, the impact of amifostine on mucositis is controversial. In more than 300 patients randomized in a trial whose primary endpoint was xerostomia, amifostine did not reduce the incidence of mucositis.[37] Mucositis grade 3 occurred in 35% of the amifostine group and in 39% of the radiotherapy-alone patients. The median duration of mucositis was also similar in the two groups of patients (41 days versus 38 days, respectively).

Several smaller randomized trials have also investigated the role of amifostine for patients with head and neck cancer, with mucositis as a primary endpoint. Bourhis and colleagues randomized 26 patients treated with an extremely accelerated course of radiation.[38] Patients randomized to amifostine had a lower incidence of grade 4 mucositis and required their feeding tubes for a shorter duration. Buntzel et al. investigated the role of amifostine with concurrent chemotherapy and radiation. Randomizing 28 patients, they report a significant reduction in mucositis, as none of the patients receiving amifostine had grade 3 or 4 mucositis, compared with 86% of patients treated with radiation alone.[39] Despite the conflicting reports, the question is likely moot; as amifostine has been demonstrated to reduce xerostomia, it will be administered to many patients undergoing radiation for head and neck cancers.

Growth factors and/or cytokines can either stimulate or suppress proliferation, including interleukin 11 and transforming growth factor-beta.[40–43] Some, through a variety of mechanisms, may reduce mucositis either by interfering with epithelial proliferation or through other effects. Clinical use of these agents for radiation-induced mucositis remains highly investigational.

Keratinocyte growth factor (KGF) is another growth factor speculated to have a role in prevention of mucositis. KGF has stem cell stimulatory properties. Recombinant human keratinocyte growth factor (rHuKGF)[44] has been demonstrated to cause a marked increase in oral mucosal radiation tolerance in mice. However, preliminary reports of a Phase 2 testing rHuKGF in patients receiving head and neck irradiation are mixed, and Phase 3 trials still are to be conducted.[45]

Preclinical data have demonstrated granulocyte macrophage colony-stimulating factor (GM-CSF) can influence the proliferation of keratinocytes.[46] Clinical observations that patients receiving GM-CSF, with myeloablative chemotherapy for hematologic malignancies, appeared to have a lower incidence of grade 3 and 4 mucositis, compared with placebo controls[47] have also garnered interest. However, small trials using this agent via a subcutaneous route that have been conducted[48,49] have not demonstrated a benefit with regard to mucositis reduction. Topical administration of GM-CSF is also under investigation. Despite encouraging results in single-arm trials testing topical GM-CSF,[50] a trial randomizing patients receiving concurrent chemoradiation to topical administration of GM-CSF or a control solution, was discontinued when preliminary results did not demonstrate any benefit.[51]

Sucralfate, an agent that has little systemic absorption and adheres to ulcer bases, has been postulated to be of use in the prevention or amelioration of mucositis. It is believed that the coating action provides some protection from injury and also promotes healing. The majority of studies (Table 74.1), including double-blinded, placebo-controlled randomized trials, show little if any benefit of sucralfate in reducing radiation-induced oral side effects.[52–59]

Antiinflammatory Agents

Despite the recognition that a severe inflammatory response ensues following radiation injury, few investigations and few data support the use of classic (steroids and nonsteroidal) antiinflammatory agents. Topical prostaglandins are believed to have antiinflammatory properties that may benefit patients who develop radiation-induced mucositis. However, both prostaglandin E_1 (misoprostol), and prostaglandin E_2 (prostin) have been evaluated in small trials, and neither has been demonstrated to either prevent or reduce the severity of radiation-induced mucositis.[60,61]

Benzydamine hydrochloride (HCl) is a topical agent that has been studied for preventing or alleviating radiation-induced mucositis. The primary mode of action is believed to be antiinflammatory, and it has been demonstrated[62] that benzydamine HCl inhibits the production and effects of inflammatory cytokines.

TABLE 74.1. Randomized trials evaluating sucralfate versus placebo for the prevention or alleviation of mucositis secondary to radiation therapy to the head and neck.

Authors	*No. of patients*	*Endpoint(s)*[a]	*Results*	*P value*
Scherlacher et al.[52]	45	1: Absence (minimal) mucosal inflammation 2: Absence (minimal) pain	1: 88% (S) vs. 43% (Pl) 2: 79% (S) vs. 28% (Pl)	ND
Epstein et al.[53]	33	1: Mucositis score 2: Severity of pain	No differences	NS
Makkonen et al.[59]	40	Mucosal changes	No differences	0.79
Franzen et al.[57]	48	1: Mucosal reactions weeks 1–3 2: Pain	1: Less mucositis (S) 2: No differences	<0.05 >0.1
Lievens et al.[58]	102	1: Mean peak reactions 2: Subjective intolerance	No differences	NS
Carter et al.[55]	102	1: Grade 3 mucositis 2: Pain	No differences	0.31 0.88
Cengiz et al.[56]	18	Degree of mucositis	Less mucositis (S)	<0.05
Etiz et al.[54]	44	1: Oral mucositis score 2: Pain score	Lower scores (S)	<0.0002 <0.09

S, sucralfate; Pl, placebos; ND, not described; NS, not significant [value(s) not provided].

[a] Several studies evaluated more than two endpoints; in those cases, only two are provided for the table.

[b] In general, scoring systems and descriptions of mucositis were study specific.

In a randomized trial of nearly 150 patients,[63] for conventionally fractionated radiation up to cumulative doses of 50 Gy, benzydamine significantly ($P = 0.006$) reduced erythema and ulceration by approximately 30% compared with the placebo, and more than 33% of benzydamine subjects remained ulcer free compared with 18% of placebo subjects ($P = 0.037$). However, benzydamine was not effective in subjects receiving accelerated radiation doses. Further studies are under way.

Targeting Infection

It has been theorized that the formation of ulcerative mucositis, combined with changes in the pH of the oral cavity caused by effects of radiation on salivary glands, creates a favorable environment for microbials and local infections. These infections create additional stress on the tissues and thereby intensify the severity of mucositis. Based on this theory, topical antimicrobials have been studied as a strategy to minimize mucositis.

Chlorhexidine, a broad-spectrum rinse effective against both gram-positive and gram-negative bacilli and yeast, has been tested in several randomized trials for preventing or alleviating oral mucositis. No trial has demonstrated it to be efficacious,[64,65] and it may even be detrimental for some patients undergoing radiation for head and neck cancer.[66]

Several centers have studied rinses or pastilles using a combination of agents. Typically, the combinations have included an antifungal (amphotericin B or clotrimazole) and antibacterials, particularly those to combat gram-negative organisms. PTA, a combination of polymyxin B, tobramycin, and amphotericin B,[67] has been tested in several centers as an antimicrobial strategy for mucositis prevention, with both randomized placebo-controlled trials having mixed results, using either a lozenge or pastille.[68,69] Differences in several measured secondary endpoints including a lower incidence of worse reported grade of mucositis, dysphagia, and weight loss in patients treated with the drug have been reported. Wijers et al. also tested a PTA paste in a randomized placebo-controlled double-blind study and did not find that PTA reduced the incidence of mucositis.[70] El-Sayed et al. randomized patients to either a lozenge of bacitracin, clotrimazole, and gentamicin, or placebo, and found no differences in the severity of mucositis in patients receiving conventionally fractionated radiation between the two groups.[71]

A trial investigating iseganan HCl, a broad-spectrum antimicrobial rinse, randomized patients in a Phase III multiinstitutional trial to active drug, placebo rinse, or best standard of care. There was no benefit to the active drug compared with placebo.[72] A summary of randomized trials testing antibiotic therapy is shown in Table 74.2.

Mucositis Symptom Management

The management of radiation-induced mucositis primarily involves managing pain. Mucositis that is not severe can be managed with topical agents, although their efficacy has not been proven. Baking soda rinses, with or without salt, are advocated, although they too have not been proven to alleviate mucositis. However, they are important in maintaining good oral hygiene.

Lidocaine gel (2%) is occasionally useful particularly for anterior oral sores. Diluting lidocaine in *magic mouthwashes* is a common practice. These mouthwashes combine aluminum hydroxide antacid, benadryl, and lidocaine. Although prophylactic antifungal agents are not needed, some practices include nystatin in the mouthwash. Again, it should be emphasized that no significant evidence-based studies exist to support the use of these mouthwashes.[73]

Other topical agents with soothing properties, including aloe vera and the bioadherent Gelclair, have not demonstrated benefit in randomized trials. Neither aloe vera nor Gelclair has been shown in randomized Phase III trials to benefit patients with radiation-induced mucositis.

Ultimately, mucositis is managed with analgesics including acetaminophen or nonsteroidal antiinflammatory agents and, eventually, narcotics. Our pain regimens begin with codeine-based products, then progress to morphine-based products, primarily hydromorphone or morphine sulfate or methadone. Recently, we have found fentanyl transdermal patches are effective for many patients, as they are long-acting and avoid contact with oral mucous membranes.

Osteoradionecrosis

Radiation can permanently destroy cellular elements of bone and thus limit the potential for wound maintenance and the ability to heal after infection or trauma (e.g., dental extraction, alveoloplasty).[74,75] Further, the risk of complications following trauma or oral surgical procedures in an irradiated field can be highly significant, depending on a predetermined threshold of irradiation, and result in osteoradionecrosis (ORN).[14,16,75,76] For these reasons, elective oral surgical procedures, such as extractions or soft tissue surgery, are contraindicated within an irradiated field owing to hypovascularity, hypocellularity, and hypoxia.[2] However, nonsurgical dental procedures that can safely be performed include routine restorative procedures, oral prophylaxis, radiography, endodontic, and prosthodontic procedures.[2,12,13]

If oral or periodontal surgical intervention is required after radiation therapy, the clinician should discuss the volume of tissue radiated and specific treatment parameters with the treating radiation therapist and should request a copy of the simulation or port films and treatment summary. Preoperative hyperbaric oxygen (HBO) therapy may increase the potential of wound healing while minimizing the risk of ORN by promoting angiogenesis and osteogenesis.[77–79] HBO therapy must be used as an adjunct to debridement (sequestrectomy), wound care, parenteral antibiotics (as dictated by bone culture results), and composite bone and muscle grafts by free tissue transfer (subject to the availability of the requisite microvascular skills).[78,79]

Optimal oral health must be maintained during and after radiation therapy. However, to avoid soft tissue injury during the postradiation healing period, patients must curtail all but the most basic oral hygiene procedures (i.e., brushing, flossing, and fluoride therapy). Conventional oral physiotherapy (oral opening exercises) can be performed during and after radiation treatment, especially if the pterygoid regions are involved in the radiation treatment fields, resulting in increased fibrosis of masticatory musculature and trismus.[80–82] Trismus is a challenging problem and may prove to be irreversible. Therefore, patients should be encouraged to perform mouth-stretching exercises before, during, and after radiation therapy.[2,6,80,83,84] Sophisticated means of oral opening exercises may need to be employed with opening devices. In addition to exercising, other supportive care adjuncts should include nutritional counseling and smoking cessation therapy, as indicated.

Following initial recovery from radiation effects, nonsurgical periodontal therapy, usually with prophylactic antibiotic coverage, is appropriate for treatment of the periodontium within the radiation field. It is important to detect and treat dental caries or traumatic dental injury that could lead to pathosis. However, ORN can occur spontaneously if wound healing is compromised.[85–89] If postradiation extractions are necessary, HBO therapy, along with a specific oral care regimen, is indicated to augment wound healing. In such cases, tissues should be managed gently, and antibiotic coverage is required. Local anesthetics containing epinephrine should be avoided, when possible, to prevent further vascular constriction.[11] Workers have reported successful placement of endosseous implants in irradiated fields, with a pretreatment regimen of hyperbaric oxygen.[90,91] In contrast, ORN has been initiated by such elective surgical intervention.[86,88,91]

TABLE 74.2. Randomized trials evaluating topical antibiotic therapy versus placebo for the prevention or alleviation of mucositis secondary to radiation therapy to the head and neck.

Authors	*No. of patients*	*Regimen*	*Endpoint(s)*[a]	*Differences detected between regimen and placebo*	*P value*
Spijkervet et al.[65]	30	Chlorhexidine	Mucositis scores[b]	No	ND
Ferretti et al.[64]	30	Chlorhexidine	Mucositis incidence and severity	No	ND
Foote et al.[66]	52	Chlorhexidine	Objective stomatitis	No	0.82
			Subjective stomatitis	No	0.06
Okuno et al.[68]	108	PTA	Objective mucositis	No	NS
			Subjective mucositis	Yes	0.02
Symonds et al.[69]	275	PTA	Mucositis distribution	Yes	0.002
			Severity of dysphagia	Yes	0.007
Wijers et al.[70]	77	PTA	Mucositis scores week 4	No	0.33
			Pain duration week 4	No	0.36
Stokman et al.[81]	55	PTA	Mean mucositis score	No	>0.2
El-Sayed et al.[71]	137	BcoG	Time to develop mucositis	No	0.61
Trotti et al.[72]	545	Iseganan HCl	Proportion of patients without ulcerative mucositis	No (9% vs. 9%)	0.998

PTA, polymyxin E, tobramycin, and amphotericin B; BcoG, bacitracin, clotrimazole, and gentamicin.

[a] Several studies evaluated more than two endpoints; In those cases only two are provided for this table.

[b] In general, scoring systems and descriptions of mucositis were study specific.

Xerostomia

When the major salivary glands are involved in the volume of tissue irradiated, the quality and quantity of salivary secretions decrease.[2,92,93] Serous cells, found predominantly in the parotid glands, are extremely radiosensitive, and undergo apoptosis when exposed to low doses of radiation.[94] Salivary gland dysfunction to the direct effects of radiation on the vascular and connective tissues of the glands[92,93] may account for the effects on the submandibular glands, which have a high proportion of mucinous cells and are essential for resting saliva.

Radiation damage to the major glands results in either a transient or permanent decreased salivary flow.[92] Saliva is a complex bodily fluid that consists of multiple small organic molecules, electrolytes, and immunoglobulins that defend the oral cavity from contamination and promote healing. Salivary hypofunction can increase the risk for dental caries and compromise mucosal integrity.[2] Dryness of the mucosal tissues may increase the susceptibility to oral infections and lead to difficulty in chewing, swallowing, and speech.[76,93] Therefore, when the salivary glands are within the radiation field, irreversible damage due to the cytotoxic effects of the radiation is imminent, as are the clinical manifestations of xerostomia.

Dental caries is a common postradiation morbid sequela that is often exacerbated by xerostomia.[95] Irradiation of major salivary glands leads to qualitative and quantitative changes in salivary secretions, thus increasing plaque and mucoid debris accumulation, reducing the salivary pH, and reducing the buffering capacity of saliva.[96] This sequence creates a cariogenic oral environment, particularly in patients ingesting a diet high in carbohydrates or sucrose. Susceptibility to caries is not limited to the dentition within the volume of tissue irradiated. Because of the harmful effect of postradiation caries, patients who have undergone radiation should be treated with a specific prophylactic regimen consisting of flossing, brushing, and fluoride therapy. An effective combination of oral hygiene, frequent dental follow-up examinations, and appropriate prophylactic treatment procedures are essential to caries prevention, as is fluoride treatment consisting of a daily application of 0.4% stannous fluoride or 1.1% sodium fluoride to the dentition using a brush-on technique or gel-filled trays (i.e., fluoride carriers).[2,14,96,97] In adults with xerostomia, fluoride leaches out of the enamel within 24 hours; thus, the fluoride regimen must be performed daily for optimal protection. The most efficient method of fluoride application is to use a custom-made polypropylene fluoride carrier that completely covers, and extends slightly beyond, the tooth surface.[14] Patients who receive low doses of radiation and are expected to have a slight degree of xerostomia can use a toothbrush to apply the fluoride gel.[98] Sensitivity and pain are common side effects of fluoride and may necessitate a change in the fluoride concentration or the method of application. A daily fluoride program can decrease postradiation dentinal hypersensitivity, remineralize cavitated enamel matrices, and, more importantly, inhibit caries-forming organisms.[2,14]

Managing Xerostomia

Radiation-induced reductions in salivary flow are worrisome because saliva protects the oral mucosa from dehydration and assists in the mechanical lavage of food and microbial debris from the oral cavity.[93] To avoid oral infections and to reduce the mucositis that may arise during radiation therapy, patients must frequently rinse the oral cavity to reduce oral microorganisms and to maintain mucosal hydration. Such oral lavage can be performed by rinsing with a solution of 1 tsp sodium bicarbonate dissolved in 1 quart water several times each day to alkalinize the oral cavity and keep the oral and oropharyngeal tissues moist.[2,12]

The traditional treatment for radiation-induced xerostomia and mucositis is inadequate, as no effective salivary substitute for patients with these conditions can replicate natural salivary mucin and protective salivary components.[14,99] Mouth rinses, saliva substitutes, and gustatory stimulants have not been tested in Phase III trials to clearly demonstrate their efficacy. Oral Balance or Biotene were found to have palliative effects superior to the effects of a placebo.[100]

Sialogogue therapy, such as with cholinergic agonists (e.g., pilocarpine hydrochloride and cevimeline), has been shown to provide clinically significant relief of symptoms of postradiation xerostomia in randomized trials.[101–103]

Preventing Xerostomia

Cholinergic agonists, primarily pilocarpine, have been tested in the postradiation setting, and the evidence is fairly convincing that they have a palliative benefit in a subset of patients who experience radiation-induced xerostomia. Pilocarpine has also been tested during radiation to determine if stimulation of salivary glands can result in either improvement in quality of life during radiation or long-term benefits.

Two randomized trials conducted in North America tested pilocarpine compared with placebo administered during radiotherapy. Warde et al. found no improvement in quality of life measures or differences in subjective measures of xerostomia or mucositis.[104] The Radiation Therapy Oncology Group (RTOG) did find objective measures of increased salivary flow when pilocarpine was administered during radiation, but this finding did not translate into improved subjective scores.[105] The authors concluded that during and immediately following radiation, mucositis plays such a dominant role in patient quality of life that xerostomia was not a critical issue. Rode et al. not only studied the effects of salivary stimulation during radiation but also salivary inhibition with biperiden.[106] In a small randomized trial, the authors concluded that patients benefited the most from salivary inhibition with biperiden during radiation followed by stimulation with pilocarpine following radiation treatment. In conclusion, the evidence for prevention of xerostomia by salivary stimulation is weak. Table 74.3 summarizes randomized trials evaluating agents tested for prevention or alleviation of xerostomia.

The main efforts for prevention of xerostomia are either with drugs that are true radioprotectors or by using methods to limit the dose to some of the major glands. When administered intravenously, during radiation therapy, amifostine, a free radical scavenger, has been shown to diminish toxic effects of irradiation on salivary glands.[37] Amifostine, described in the mucositis section, has been tested in several randomized trials. Brizel et al. demonstrated an absolute reduction of grade 2 xerostomia in approximately 20% of patients treated with amifostine daily before delivery of fractionated radiation. Quality of life measures were also

TABLE 74.3. Randomized trials evaluating agents for prevention or alleviation of xerostomia.

Authors	*No. of patients*	*Drug and timing*	*Endpoint(s)*	*Differences detected between regimen and placebo*[a]	*P value*
Brizel et al.[37]	303	Amifostine during radiation	Acute and late grade 2 xerostomia	51% vs. 78% 34% vs. 57%	<0.0001 0.002
Antonadou et al.[139]	50	Amifostine during radiochemotherapy	Grade 2 xerostomia (2 years)	5% vs. 30%	0.047
Warde et al.[104]	130	Pilocarpine during radiation	Subjective measure in severity of xerostomia	No difference	
Fisher et al.[105]	214	Pilocarpine during radiation	Quality of life assessment of amount of saliva	No difference	
Johnson et al.[101]	207	Pilocarpine after radiation	Subjective improvement in oral dryness	44% vs. 25%	0.027
Leveque et al.[102]	162	Pilocarpine after radiation	Improvement in overall global assessment		0.035

[a]Amifostine trials with no treatment rather than placebo arm.

improved in the amifostine-treated patients.[107] The study, however, was neither blinded nor placebo controlled.

When administered intravenously, amifostine has a modest toxicity profile, with a small incidence of hypotension that can potentially be severe and a high incidence of drug-induced nausea. To decrease the toxicity, the drug can be administered subcutaneously,[108] and smaller trials have suggested it is efficacious when delivered via this route with a lower incidence of both nausea and severe hypotension.[109,110] Preliminary results of a randomized trial comparing the two routes of administration suggest that the subcutaneous route is safer with a lower incidence of hypotension, and to date, it is as efficacious with respect to xerostomia.[111]

An intriguing method to prevent xerostomia is to transfer surgically one gland away from the proposed radiation field. Jha et al. have conducted a Phase II trial.[112] During patients' oncologic surgery, one submandibular gland was transferred into the submental space, an area that routinely is not irradiated. The gland was not transferred in 20% of patients and was not shielded in an additional 16% of patients. In those patients in whom the gland was transferred and shielded from radiation, only 20% experienced severe late xerostomia. Further evaluation of this technique is planned in a multiinstitutional setting.

Conformal radiation, and, in particular, intensity-modulated radiation, are radiation techniques that potentially can minimize the dose to salivary glands and thereby decrease the incidence of xerostomia. Unfortunately, the threshold dose for salivary gland sparing is unclear. It is recognized that high doses (50 Gy and above) result in a high incidence of xerostomia, but the effects of intermediate doses (between 15 and 35 Gy) are less clear. Eisbruch et al., using conformal techniques, stated that keeping the mean parotid dose below 26 Gy minimized the incidence of xerostomia,[113] whereas Chao and colleagues, using complex mathematical modeling, have stated the threshold dose is 32 Gy, and each gray results in a 4% reduction in salivary flow.[114]

Eisbruch et al. have used conformal techniques with parotid gland sparing in their treatment of patients with head and neck cancer and report a reduction in the incidence of xerostomia.[115] Similarly, Chao et al. have reported similar results with the use of intensity-modulated radiation.[116] Lee et al. analyzed the results of intensity-modulated radiation in the treatment of patients with nasopharynx cancer.[117] Although the goal of the technique was improved tumor coverage, a by-product has been lower doses to the parotid glands, and the group described a low incidence of grade 2 or greater xerostomia. The RTOG is now testing intensity-modulated radiation in the multiinstitutional setting.

Chemotherapy and Bone Marrow Transplantation

Most cytotoxic drugs are effective in destroying cancer cells because they interfere, through various mechanisms, with the synthesis or function of DNA.[118] Thus, it is not surprising that these drugs are in general more toxic to proliferating cells than to those incapable of replication and are most effective against tumors with high growth fractions.[12] Chemotherapeutic agents have gained a certain notoriety for damaging normal tissue, resulting in such effects as hematologic suppression, mucositis, and hair loss. In many patients, these drugs also cause nausea and vomiting with marked oral effects.

Malignancy coupled with aggressive chemotherapeutic regimens profoundly compromises the immune system, leading to multiple serious infections with varying potential to involve the oral cavity. Empirical use of prophylactic antimicrobial agents may substantially alter the risk of infection of the oral cavity and the presenting signs and symptoms of infection during chemotherapy.[12,119,120] Oncologic physicians and treatment centers vary in their treatment philosophies on the use of such antiinfectious agents.

The dentoalveolar complex should be thoroughly evaluated for microbial reservoirs or sanctuaries (e.g., plaque, calculus, or periodontal pockets), and these infectious foci should be eliminated before the start of chemotherapy.[12,119–121] A compromised periodontal status presents a risk of infection.[122,123] Clinically, however, the risk of infection depends on multiple interacting factors, such as oral hygiene, immunomyelosuppressive status, chemotherapeutic agents used, prophylactic or therapeutic antimicrobial agents used, and the degree of periodontal pathology.

To minimize the risks of periodontal infection, it is important to develop simple and practical guidelines for maintaining periodontal health and for diagnosing, preventing, and treating periodontal infections during therapy.[2,12] Cancer patients should make regular dental visits for overall dental and periodontal assessment. Patients receiving chemotherapy can undergo a dental cleaning, provided that they meet the following hematologic conditions: first, an absolute neutrophil count of approximately 1,000/mm^3 (white blood cell count times % neutrophils equals the absolute neutrophil count), a level at which the risk of developing an infection is minimal, and second, a platelet count greater than 50,000/mm^3 with a normal coagulation profile.[124] The administration of prophylactic antibiotics is essential, owing to the induced bacteremia, immunocompromised status, and potential for hypofunctioning white blood cells introduced by chemotherapy.

Patients with an uninfected dentition and good periodontal health do not pose a diagnostic treatment challenge, nor do patients with advanced periodontal disease that mandates immediate surgical intervention. However, patients with increased loss of attachment, with bone loss at the junction of the roots of molar dentition and frank bone exposure without gingival coverage (furcation) or periodontal pocket formation with furcation involvement, pose a treatment dilemma.[12] Patients in whom the soft tissue parallels the bone loss and in whom pocket depth is normal can be treated with regular periodontal care and maintenance. Extraction should be considered only for patients with pathologic mobility of dentition or with a fulminant periapical abscess.[2,12] Patients with moderate to advanced periodontal disease, present a greater challenge and would, under usual circumstances, receive instructions for infection prophylaxis and dental hygiene, as well as surgical correction. However, the feasibility of such comprehensive therapy during chemotherapy can be limited by several factors, including performance status, type of malignant disease, cycling of chemotherapy, and hematologic competence. The clinician should strive to provide a thorough scaling and to encourage maintenance through exceptional plaque control (i.e., brushing, flossing, and use of chlorhexidine gluconate).[12,125–130] To reduce the risk of a septic foci, extractions should be considered for patients with any exacerbated acute periodontal infection. This oral surgical correction should be performed at the appropriate time in the treatment cycle (beginning of cycle or during recovery phase with hematological/chemistry stability) or when the patient's cancer is in complete remission. If chemotherapy is on hold, oral surgical intervention could be considered provided that the hematologic status is appropriate. The oral surgeon must discuss with the treating medical oncologist the patient's oral status, treatment plan, and contraindications to surgical intervention, as well as the appropriate timing of oral treatment intervention.[12,118,131]

Toothbrushing and flossing should be the standard of dental care for patients who routinely brush and floss. However, as in the general population, many patients with cancer either do not floss or floss only infrequently. Thus, clinicians either may instruct patients to floss or may stress brushing techniques only. In most cases, patient factors and limited time parameters do not permit the patient to become proficient in flossing techniques. However, if the clinician identifies an area where food continually lodges, the patient should be encouraged to floss the area to reduce the risk of gingival inflammation.[13,132–136] Patients who floss on a regular basis are instructed to modify the flossing technique in certain clinical situations. First, patients are instructed to floss gently when the lining of the oral cavity starts to become sensitive to thermal changes or food substances, indicating mucosal thinning caused by suppressive effects of chemotherapy on the normally proliferative epithelium.[134,136] Second, patients are instructed to floss only to the gingiva when the platelet count falls below 50,000/mm^3. This technique removes most of the debris from this area.[12]

Toothbrushing is imperative for plaque control. The patient should be instructed to always brush after each meal. In certain clinical situations, such as increased mucosal sensitivity to food or thermal changes, increased sensitivity to toothbrush bristles, irritation of the gingival tissues by the toothbrush, or profound thrombocytopenia (less than 20,000/mm^3), patients should change from a soft to an ultrasoft-bristled or sensitive-bristled toothbrush.[2,12,13,29] In controlling plaque accumulation, it is important to minimize the risk of gingival inflammation, the oral bacterial load, and the potential for infection.[137] Along with routine brushing and flossing, rinsing with chlorhexidine gluconate should be initiated when patients begin chemotherapy. Such rinsing is an adjunct to ideal oral periodontal care and can also be used when indications arise, such as oral mucosal changes secondary to chemotherapy and subsequent increased soft tissue sensitivity.[12,125–130,138] Patients undergoing chemotherapy should be encouraged to rinse with a dilute saline and sodium bicarbonate solution (5%) to reduce adherent mucoid debris on oral soft tissues, lubricate oral mucosal and oropharyngeal tissues, and elevate the pH of oral fluids.[13,139] Patients encountering nausea and anorexia should be encouraged to rinse with the sodium bicarbonate and salt water solution several times throughout the day to reduce oral acidity and minimize the mucosal insult.[140,141]

Another challenge cancer patients face is the risk of local infection or septicemia associated with dental implants. If an implant with its restorative component poses a risk of infection for patients under normal circumstances, this risk will be intensified during chemotherapy. Interventional antibiotics and aggressive hygiene have limited ability to control infection caused by a poorly integrated endosseous implant, whereas a well-integrated implant should not pose problems if its integrity is maintained with effective dental hygiene practices.[142–144]

Aggressive anticancer therapy severely undermines the integrity of the mucosal epithelium of the oral cavity. In addition, the oral cavity is a focused area for trauma from teeth, denture prostheses, and hot or cold dietary substances.[4] Many patients are at risk for infection from resident microflora or opportunistic pathogens sequestered in sanctuary areas. Furthermore, cancer patients share with the general population common problems of the oral cavity, such as poor hygiene, poorly maintained dentition, periodontal disease, and prostheses in poor repair, with the associated mucosal pathology.[12] With all these interactive injurious influences in such close proximity, even small alterations in the area could cause a problem. Each course of chemotherapy introduces this threat of oral complication, and the risk of developing complications with subsequent courses increases as local or systematic resistance is challenged. Appropriate evaluation of the oral cavity and correction of existing oral and dental pathology can minimize, and in some cases eliminate, treatment-limiting toxicities, such as mucositis, oral infections, and bleeding, that necessitate chemotherapy dose reduction or termination.[12,118,145]

Mucositis

The oral mucosal response to cancer therapy is varied and unpredictable. Mucositis, the most common acute complication of chemotherapy, has a specific, defined mechanism of progression: mucosal erythema progresses to oral sensitivity and then to mucosal denudation[3,136,146] Several grading scales for oral mucositis have been developed to assess the severity of the mucosal reaction during each course of chemotherapy. These grading scales allow the clinicians to prescribe appropriate preventive or therapeutic measures to treat mucosal situations after chemotherapy or during subsequent treatment courses. Grading scales range from the simple to the complex.[35,147,148]

Mucosal HSV infections occurring early in the chemotherapy cycle can mimic mucositis. Failure to collect diagnostic cultures with each mucosal reaction can lead to a misdiagnosis of mucositis, in which case the infection goes untreated.[149–153] Culturing at this early stage of therapy is essential for differentiating mucositis from infectious stomatitis that can be caused by a bacterial, fungal, or viral agent and that is usually associated with low hematologic values (i.e., the nadir).[2,12] Oral mucosal infectious agents must be correctly identified and treated, because the loss of mucosal integrity creates a portal of entry for systemic infection in immunocompromised patients.[154–156]

Unlike the approach to oral stomatitis, effective therapy for oral mucositis has not been standardized. All the interventional agents are aimed at either the prevention and reduction or the palliation of chemotherapy toxicity. The many agents used vary widely in their mechanisms of action.[146,157] When mucositis can be controlled as a dose-limiting toxicity, chemotherapy agents, alone or in combination regimens, are escalated to higher doses to achieve the ultimate goal of cure. Chemotherapy-induced pancytopenia, combined with mucositis, can develop oral infection and bleeding events. Severe thrombocytopenia (less than 20,000/mm^3) and neutropenia (less than 500/mm^3) may exist with normal-appearing oral mucosa. Serious complications, such as hemorrhagic diathesis or sepsis, can occur if hematologic parameters are not considered in the treatment of the oral cavity. Thus, clinicians should conduct a benefit-versus-risk analysis of the intended therapy and should thoroughly assess the hematologic values before each treatment intervention. Treatment guidelines based on such assessments have been established.[2,3,12,121,145]

Drug-related mucositis can be severe, with onset occurring within 7 days after initiation of chemotherapy and with duration varying from several days to weeks. Compared with single-agent therapy, combination drug therapy or chemoradiation therapy is more likely to induce intensified mucosal morbidity. Maximal myelosuppression can induce thrombocytopenia, thereby causing gingivitis and gingival bleeding. Drugs most frequently associated with mucositis and myelosuppression include cytoxan, etoposide, cyclophosphamide, doxorubicin, dactinomycin, daunorubicin, 5-fluorouracil, bleomycin, melphalan, and methotrexate.[3,6,19,118,131,158–163]

Gingival hemorrhage can usually be controlled by such local measures as the application of pressure, cool water, periodontal dressings, topical thrombin, gelatin sponges, oxidized cellulose, prefabricated stents lined with a hemostatic agent, or tranexamic acid.[2] Persistent hemorrhage may require platelet support.[6,11,12,139]

As previously mentioned, any emergent oral treatment given while patients undergo myelosuppressive chemotherapy requires prophylactic antibiotic coverage, and all patients with in-dwelling central venous catheters require prophylactic antibiotic coverage for procedures likely to induce bacteremia.[13,164] The dental specialist should consult with the patient's treating oncologist to select the most appropriate antibiotic.

Although grossly overlooked, diet profoundly influences the stability of the oral tissues and can cause mucosal problems when a patient is undergoing cancer therapy.[2,131] During the myelosuppressive phase of therapy or when the mucosa is thinned owing to chemotherapy, the diet should consist of nontraumatizing, soft foods that cannot puncture, abrade, or otherwise damage the compromised mucosal epithelium. Hard or abrasive food items can lead to increased pain, infection, or bleeding episodes as they interact with the oral mucosa.

Although all patients with cancer and on chemotherapy are at risk for oral complications, some patients are at a greater risk than others, depending primarily on the type of malignancy and the aggressiveness of the cancer treatment. Patents with hematologic malignancies (e.g., leukemia and lymphoma) have a greater risk than do patients with solid tumors (e.g., breast cancer, lung cancer, and sarcomas), because the protective elements that maintain bodily homeostasis are part of the malignant process of hematologic malignancies.[14,131]

Viral reactivity may lead to severe oral or disseminated infections during periods of myeloimmunosuppression. In particular, HSV infections are often associated with severe, painful, and prolonged ulcerations atypical of those found in immunocompetent hosts.[149–151,153,165,166] Suspected HSV lesions should be treated with antiviral agents, such as acylovir administered orally or intravenously and managed as described previously for irradiated patients. The diagnosis should be established using viral cultures, direct immunofluorescence, or other rapid diagnostic tests, and the lesions.[149–153,163,165]

Bacterial infections following chemotherapy can cause localized mucosal lesions, sialoadenitis, periodontal abscesses, pericoronitis, or acute necrotizing ulcerative gingivitis.[12,158] Because systemic infection is a serious complication in neutropenic patients, constant vigilance must be maintained to prevent or manage oral infections of any type.[2,12,13,163,167] Because antileukemic therapy is designed to achieve myelosuppression, this risk may be higher among patients with leukemia than among those with solid tumors.[163,168] Oral infections should be treated with selected antibiotic combinations (broad-spectrum antibiotics), including an agent effective against anaerobic gram-negative bacilli such as *Pseudomonas*, *Klebsiella*, or enterobacteria, which are often found in the oral cavity of immunocompromised individuals.[12,13,132,135,158,161] Oral microbial culture testing should be used to ensure antibiotic sensitivity and resistance selection and to assist in identification of the causative organisms.[139,169]

Bone Marrow Transplant

The risk of oral complications from an autologous transplant is similar, possibly slightly higher, to that of conventional chemotherapy because patients receive their own cells after undergoing an intensified chemotherapy regimen. Thus, the risk is highest during immunomyelosuppression and engraftment of the stem cells.[170–173] In contrast, patients who undergo an allogeneic transplant face ponderous complications during the conditioning chemotherapy, infusion of the donor's stem cells, and engraftment. Allogeneic transplant patients, with all the interactive dynamic clinical signs and symptoms, patient factors, and topical and systemic medicines used to treat their conditions, challenge the diagnostic acumen of oral healthcare practitioners.

Patients with bone marrow transplantation (BMT) are at high risk for the development of candidiasis, viral infections (most commonly HSV, varicella zoster, and cytomegalovirus),[29,138,174–179] and bacterial infections, including those associated with microorganisms of periodontal origin.[123,180,181] Workers have reported hairy leukoplakia caused by Epstein–Barr viral infection in human immunodeficiency virus-negative BMT patients.[182] Atypical, potentially life-threatening pathogenic organisms have been isolated in cultures from sites of preexisting periodontitis in patients with myelosuppression, a finding that emphasizes the importance of establishing periodontal health status before cancer therapy.[12,13,183]

Graft-versus-host disease (GVHD)[184–188] is associated with a spectrum of intraoral presentations, ranging from atrophy/erythema to lichenoid hyperkeratosis resembling lichen planus to ulceration-pseudomembrane reaction.[147] The associated symptoms vary widely depending on the mucosal changes, thus making oral care and dietary support difficult. Additional chemotherapeutic agents, such as methotrexate and cyclosporin, may be required to prevent severe GVHD following BMT.[175]

For patients undergoing chemotherapy or BMT, proper oral care is imperative to preventing complications. Because of the varying clinical presentations, oral infections are exceedingly difficult to diagnose. Clinicians must constantly be vigilant and suspect any mucosal change or symptom as infection.[176,189–191] Oral and dental care depend on the degree of mucosal sensitivity and the patient's tolerance to treatment. Exceptional plaque control with topical fluoride is imperative in the treatment of rampant caries. The use of typical steroid-containing rinses provides additional oral comfort when mucosal changes develop in BMT patients.[126–128]

Conclusion

The oral cavity should be thoroughly evaluated in all patients diagnosed with cancer, as well as in patients undergoing any immunomyelosuppressive therapy. Preventing and treating the oral complications of cancer are important responsibilities of the treating physicians, and anticipating primary and secondary mucosal insults and recognizing oral complications promptly in this setting, can decrease the incidence of such complications or ameliorate their morbid side effects. By fostering communication and compliance among the multidisciplinary team, the cancer patient can receive optimal oral care while undergoing oncologic treatment.

References

1. King G, Toth B, Fleming T. Oral dental care of the cancer patient. Texas Dent J 1988;105:10–11.
2. Chambers M, Toth BB, Martin JW, Fleming TJ, Lemon JC. Oral and dental management of the cancer patient: prevention and treatment of complications. Support Care Cancer 1995;3:168–175.
3. National Institutes of Health Consensus Development Conference Statement. Oral complications of cancer therapies: diagnosis, prevention, and treatment. J Am Dent Assoc 1989;119:179–183.
4. Toth B, Martin JW, Fleming TJ. Oral and dental care associated with cancer therapy. Cancer Bull 1991;43:397–402.
5. Toth B, Fleming TJ. Oral care for the patient with cancer. Highlights Antineoplastic Drugs 1990;8:27–35.
6. Hurst P. Dental considerations in management of head and neck cancer. Otolaryngol Clin N Am 1985;18:573–603.
7. Lockhart P, Clark J. Pretherapy dental status of patients with malignant conditions of the head and neck. Oral Surg Oral Med Oral Pathol 1994;77:236–241.
8. Marciani R, Ownby HE. Treating patients before and after irradiation. J Am Dent Assoc 1992;123:108–112.
9. Niehaus C, Meiller TF, Peterson DE, Overholser CD. Oral complications in children during cancer therapy. Cancer Nurs 1987;10:15–20.
10. Peters E, Monopoli M, Woo SB, Sonis S. Assessment of the need for treatment of postendodontic asymptomatic periapical radiolucencies in bone marrow transplant recipients. Oral Surg Oral Med Oral Pathol 1993;76:45–48.
11. Wescott W. Dental management of patients being treated for oral cancer. Can Dent Asssoc J 1987;13:42–47.
12. Toth B, Chambers M, Fleming T, et al. Minimizing oral complications of cancer treatment. Oncology 1995;9:851–858.
13. Toth B, Chambers MS, Fleming TJ. Prevention and management of oral complications associated with cancer therapies: radiotherapy/chemotherapy. Texas Dent J 1996;113:23–29.
14. Fleming T. Oral tissue changes of radiation-oncology and their management. Dent Clin N Am 1990;34:223–237.
15. Shrout M. Managing patients undergoing radiation. J Am Dent Assoc 1991;122:69–70, 72.
16. Marciani RH. Osteoradionecrosis of the jaws. J Oral Maxillofac Surg 1986;4:218–223.
17. Barrett A, Porter SR, Scully C, Eveson JW, Griffiths MJ. Oral melanotic macules that develop after radiation therapy. Oral Surg Oral Med Oral Pathol 194;77:431–434.
18. Rothwell B. Prevention and treatment of the orofacial complications of radiotherapy. J Am Dent Assoc 1987;114:316–322.
19. Fleming P. Dental management of the pediatric oncology patient. Curr Opin Dent 1991;1:577–582.
20. Brown A, Sims RE, Raybould TP, Lillich TT, Henslee PJ, Feretti GA. Oral gram-negative bacilli in bone marrow transplant patients given chlorhexidine rinses. J Dent Res 19889;68:1199–1204.
21. Dahllöf G, Krekmanova L, Kopp S, Borgström B, Forsberg CM, Ringden O. Craniomandibular dysfunction in children treated with total-body irradiation and bone marrow transplantation. Acta Odontol Scand 1994;52:99–105.
22. Dahllöf G, Rozell B, Forsberg CM, Borgström B. Histologic changes in dental morphology induced by high dose chemotherapy and total body irradiation. Oral Surg Oral Med Oral Pathol 1994;77:56–60.
23. Dury D, Roberts NW, Miser JS, Folio J. Dental root agenesis secondary to irradiation therapy in a case of rhabdomyosarcoma

of the middle ear. Oral Surg Oral Med Oral Pathol 1984;57: 595–599.

24. Dahllöf G, Barr M, Bolme P, et al. Disturbances in dental development after total body irradiation in bone marrow transplant recipients. Oral Surg Oral Med Oral Pathol 1988;65:41–44.
25. Dahllöf G, Forsberg CM, Ringden O, et al. Facial growth and morphology in long-term survivors after bone marrow transplantation. Eur J Orthod 1989;11:332–340.
26. Grotz K, Genitsariotis S, Vehling D, Al-Nawas B. Long-term oral *Candida* colonization, mucositis and salivary function after head and neck radiotherapy. Support Care Cancer 2003;11(11): 717–721.
27. Dahiya M, Redding SW, Dahiya RS, et al. Oropharyngeal candidiasis caused by non-*albicans* yeast in patients receiving external beam radiotherapy for head-and-neck cancer. Int J Radiat Oncol Biol Phys 2003;57:79–83.
28. Bergman O. Oral infections and septicemia in immunocompromised patients with hematologic malignancies. J Clin Microbiol 1988;26:2105–2109.
29. Toth B, Martin JW, Chambers MS, Robinson KA, Andersson BS. Oral candidiasis: a morbid sequelae of anticancer therapy. Texas Dent J 1998;115:24–29.
30. Denham J, Hauer-Jensen M. The radiotherapeutic injury—a complex 'wound'. Radiother Oncol 2002;63:129–145.
31. Garden A. Mucositis: current management and investigations. Semin Radiat Oncol 2003;13:267–273.
32. Sonis S, Clark J. Prevention and management of oral mucositis induced by antineoplastic therapy. Oncology 1991;5:11–18.
33. Poulsen M, Denham JW, Peters LJ, et al. A randomised trial of accelerated and conventional radiotherapy for stage III and IV squamous carcinoma of the head and neck: a Trans-Tasman Radiation Oncology Group Study. Radiother Oncol 2001;60:113–122.
34. Bentzen S, Saunders MI, Dische S, Bond SJ. Radiotherapy-related early morbidity in head and neck cancer: quantitative clinical radiobiology as deduced from the CHART trial. Radiother Oncol 2001;60:123–125.
35. Parulekar W, Mackenzie R, Bjarnason G, Jordan RCK. Scoring oral mucositis. Oral Oncol 1998;34:63–71.
36. Capizzi R. Amifostine: the preclinical basis for broad-spectrum selective cytoprotection of normal tissues from cytotoxic therapies. Semin Oncol 1996;23:2–16.
37. Brizel D, Wasserman TH, Henke M, et al. Phase III randomized trial of amifostine as a radioprotector in head and neck cancer. J Clin Oncol 2000;18:3339–3345.
38. Bourhis J, De Crevoisier R, Abdulkarim B, et al. A randomized study of very accelerated radiotherapy with and without amifostine in head and neck squamous cell carcinoma. Int J Radiat Oncol Biol Phys 2000;46:1105–1108.
39. Buntzel J, Schuth J, Kuttner K, et al. Radiochemotherapy with amifostine cytoprotection for head and neck cancer. Support Care Cancer 1998;6:155–160.
40. Sonis S, Peterson RL, Edwards LJ, et al. Defining mechanisms of action of interleukin-11 on the progression of radiation-induced oral mucositis in hamsters. Oral Oncol 2000;36:373–381.
41. Potten C. Protection of the small intestinal clonogenic stem cells from radiation-induced damage by pretreatment with interleukin 11 also increases murine survivial time. Stem Cells 1996;14:452–459.
42. Booth D, Haley J, Bruskin A, et al. Transforming growth factor b3 protects murine small intestinal crypt stem cells and animal survival after irradiation, possibly by reducing stem cell cycling. Int J Cancer 2000;86:53–59.
43. Sonis S. Transforming growth factor-beta 3 mediated modulation of cell cycling and attenuation of 5-fluorouracil induced mucositis. Oral Oncol 1997;33:47–54.
44. Dorr W, Hamilton CS, Boyd T, Reed B, Denham JW. Radiation-induced changes in cellularity and proliferation in human oral mucosa. Int J Radiat Oncol Biol Phys 2002;52:911–917.
45. Spielberger R, Still P, Emmanouilides C, et al. Efficacy of recombinant human keratinocyte growth factor (rHuKGF) in reducing mucositis in patients with hematologic malignancies undergoing peripheral progenitor cell transplantation (auto-PBPCT) after radiation-based conditioning: results of a phase 2 trial. Proc ASCO 2001;20:7a.
46. Kaplan G, Walsh G, Guido L, et al. Novel responses of human skin to intradermal recombinant granulocyte/macrophage-colony-stimulating factor: Langerhans cell recruitment, keratinocyte growth, and enhanced wound healing. J Exp Med 1992;175:1717–1728.
47. Nemunaitis J, Rosenfeld C, Ash R, et al. Phase III randomized, double-blind placebo-controlled trial of rhGM-CSF following allogeneic bone marrow transplantation. Bone Marrow Transplant 1995;15:949–954.
48. Makkonen T. Granulocyte macrophage-colony stimulating factor (GM-CSF) and sucralfate in prevention of radiation-induced mucositis: a prospective randomized study. Int J Radiat Oncol Biol Phys 2000;46:525–534.
49. Rosso M. Effect of granulocyte-macrophage colony-stimulating factor on prevention of mucositis in head and neck cancer patients treated with chemo-radiotherapy. J Chemother 1997;9:382–385.
50. Mantovani G, Massa E, Astara G, et al. Phase II clinical trial of local use of GM-CSF for prevention and treatment of chemotherapy- and concomitant chemoradiotherapy-induced severe oral mucositis in advanced head and neck cancer patients: an evaluation of effectiveness, safety and costs. Oncol Rep 2003;10:197–206.
51. Sprinzl G, Galvan O, De Vries A, et al. Local application of granulocyte-macrophage stimulating factor (GM-CSF) for the treatment of oral mucositis. Eur J Cancer 2001;37:2003–2009.
52. Scherlacher A, Beaufort-Spontin F. Radiotherapy of head-neck neoplasms: prevention of inflammation of the mucosa by sucralfate treatment. HNO 1990;38:24–28.
53. Epstein J, Wong F. The efficacy of sucralfate suspension in the prevention of oral mucositis due to radiation therapy. Int J Radiat Oncol Biol Phys 1994;28:693–698.
54. Etiz D, Erkal H, Serin M, et al. Clinical and histopathological evaluation of sucralfate in prevention of oral mucositis induced by radiation therapy in patients with head and neck malignancies. Oral Oncol 2000;36:116–120.
55. Carter D, Hebert M, Smink K, et al. Double blind randomized trial of sucralfate vs. placebo during radiotherapy for head and neck cancers. Head Neck 1999;21:760–766.
56. Cengiz M, Ozyar E, Akol F, et al. Sucralfate in the prevention of radiation-induced oral mucositis. J Clin Gastroenterol 1999;28:40–43.
57. Franzen L, Henriksson R, Littbrand B, et al. Effects of sucralfate on mucositis during and following radiotherapy of malignancies in the head and neck region. Acta Oncol 1995;34:219–223.
58. Lievens Y, Haustermans K, Van der Weyngaert D, et al. Does sucralfate reduce the acute side-effects in head and neck cancer treated with radiotherapy? A double-blind randomized trial. Radiother Oncol 1998;47:149–153.
59. Makkonen T, Bostrom P, Vilja P, et al. Sucralfate mouth washing in the prevention of radiation-induced mucositis: a placebo-controlled double-blind randomized study. Int J Radiat Oncol Biol Phys 1994;30:177–182.
60. Matejka M, Nell A, Kment G, et al. Local benefit of prostaglandin E2 in radiochemotherapy-induced oral mucositis. Br J Oral Maxillofac Surg 1990;28:89–91.
61. Porteder H, Rausch E, Kment G, et al. Local prostaglandin E2 in patients with oral malignancies undergoing chemo- and radiotherapy. J Craniomaxillofac Surg 1988;16:371–374.
62. Sironi M, Pozzi P, Polentarutti N, et al. Inhibition of inflammatory cytokine production and protection against endotoxin toxicity by benzydamine. Cytokine 1996;8:710–716.

63. Epstein JB, Silverman S Jr, Paggiarino DA, et al. Benzydamine HCl for prophylaxis of radiation-induced oral mucositis: results from a multicenter, randomized, double-blind, placebo-controlled clinical trial. Cancer (Phila) 2001;92:875–885.
64. Ferretti G, Raybould TP, Brown AT, et al. Chlorhexidine prophylaxis for chemotherapy- and radiotherapy-induced stomatitis: a randomized double-blind trial. Oral Surg Oral Med Oral Pathol 1990;69:331–338.
65. Spijkervet F, van Saene HK, Panders AK, et al. Effect of chlorhexidine rinsing on the oropharyngeal ecology in patients with head and neck cancer who have irradiation mucositis. Oral Surg Oral Med Oral Pathol 1989;67:154–161.
66. Foote R, Loprinzi C, Frank A, et al. Randomized trial of a chlorhexidine mouthwash for alleviation of radiation-induced mucositis. J Clin Oncol 1994;12:2630–2633.
67. Spijkervet F, van Saene HK, van Saene JJ, et al. Effect of selective elimination of the oral flora on mucositis in irradiated head and neck cancer patients. J Surg Oncol 1991;46:167–173.
68. Okuno S, Foote RL, Loprinzi CL, et al. A randomized trial of a nonabsorbable antibiotic lozenge given to alleviate radiation-induced mucositis. Cancer (Phila) 1997;79:2193–2199.
69. Symonds R, McIlroy P, Khorrami J, et al. The reduction of radiation mucositis by selective decontamination antibiotic pastilles: a placebo-controlled double-blind trial. Br J Cancer 1996;74:312–317.
70. Wijers O, Levendag P, Harms E, et al. Mucositis reduction by selective elimination of oral flora in irradiated cancers of the head and neck: a placebo-controlled double-blind randomized study. Int J Radiat Oncol Biol Phys 2001;50:343 352.
71. El-Sayed S, Nabid A, Shelley W, et al. Prophylaxis of radiation-associated mucositis in conventionally treated patients with head and neck cancer: a double-blind, phase III, randomized, controlled trial evaluating the clinical efficacy of an antimicrobial lozenge using a validated mucositis scoring system. J Clin Oncol 2002;20:3956–3963.
72. Trotti A, Garden A, Warde P, et al. A multinational, randomized phase III trial of iseganan HCl oral solution for reducing the severity of oral mucositis in patients receiving radiotherapy for head and neck malignancy. Int J Radiat Oncol Biol Phys 2004;58:674–681.
73. Dodd M, Dibble S, Miaskowski C, et al. Randomized clinical trial of the effectiveness of 3 commonly used mouthwashes to treat chemotherapy-induced mucositis. Oral Surg Oral Med Oral Pathol Oral Radiol Endod 2000;90:39–47.
74. Beumer J, Silverman S Jr, Benak SB Jr. Hard and soft tissue necrosis following radiation therapy for oral cancer. J Prosthet Dent 1972;27:640–644.
75. Epstein J, Rea, G, Wong, FL, Spinelli J, Stevenson-Moore P. Osteoradionecrosis: study of the relationship of dental extractions in patients receiving radiotherapy. Head Neck Surg 1987;10:48–54.
76. Schweiger J. Oral complications following radiation therapy: A five-year retrospective report. J Prosthet Dent 1987;58: 78–82.
77. Marx R, Johnson RP. Studies in the radiobiology of osteoradionecrosis and their clinical significance. Oral Surg Oral Med Oral Pathol Oral Radiol Endod 1987;64:379–390.
78. Mansfield M, Sanders DW, Heimbach RD. Hyperbaric oxygen as an adjunct in the treatment of osteoradionecrosis of the mandible. J Oral Surg 1981;39:585–589.
79. Farmer J, Shelton PL, Angelillo JF. Treatment of radiation induced tissue injury by hyperbaric oxygen. Ann Otolaryngol 1978;87:707–715.
80. Barrett V, Martin JW, Jacob RF. Physical therapy techniques in the treatment of the head and neck patient. J Prosthet Dent 1988;59:343–346.
81. Rocabardo M, Johnston BE, Blakney MG. Physical therapy and dentistry: an overview. J Craniomand Pract 1983;1:46–49.
82. Morton M, Simpson W. The management of osteoradionecrosis of the jaws. Br J Oral Maxillofac Surg 1986;24:332–341.
83. Ritchie J, Brown JR, Guerra LR, Mason G. Dental care for the irradiated dental patient. Quintessence Int 1985;12:837–842.
84. Mealey B, Semba SE, Hallmon WW. The head and neck radiotherapy patient. Part 2. Management of oral complications. Compendium Cont Educ Dent 1994;15:442–458.
85. Fattore L, Strauss R, Bruno J. The management of periodontal disease in patients who have received radiation therapy for head and neck cancer. Spec Care Dentist 1987;120–123.
86. Epstein J, Wong FL, Stevenson-Moore P. Osteoradionecrosis: clinical experience and a proposal for classification. J Oral Maxillofac Surg 1987;45:104–110.
87. Fujita M, Tanimoto K, Wada T. Early radiographic changes in radiation bone injury. Oral Surg Oral Med Oral Pathol 1986;61:641–644.
88. McClure D, Barker G, Barker B, Feil P. Oral management of the cancer patient. Part II. Oral complications of radiation therapy. Compendium Cont Educ Dent 1987;8:88–92.
89. Pappas G. Oral roentgenology. Bone changes in osteoradionecrosis: a review. Oral Surg Oral Med Oral Pathol 1969;27: 622–630.
90. Bundgaard T, Tandrup O, Elbrond O. A functional evaluation of patients treated for oral cancer. A prospective study. Int J Oral Maxillofac Surg 1993;22:28–34.
91. Granstrom G, Jacobsson M, Tjellstrom A. Titanium implants in irradiated tissues: benefits from hyperbaric oxygen. Int J Oral Maxillofac Impl 1992;7:15–25.
92. Liu R, Fleming TJ, Toth BB. Salivary flow rates in patients with head and neck cancer 0.5 to 25 years after radiotherapy. Oral Surg Oral Med Oral Pathol Oral Radiol Endod 1990;70:724–729.
93. Mandel I. The role of saliva in maintaining oral homeostasis. J Am Dent Assoc 1989;119:298–303.
94. Stephens L, Schultheiss TE, Price RE, Ang KK, Peters LJ. Radiation apoptosis of serous acinar cells of salivary and lacrimal glands. Cancer (Phila) 1991;67:1539–1543.
95. Schubert M, Izutsu KT. Iatrogenic causes of salivary gland dysfunction. J Dent Res 1987;66(S):680–688.
96. Keene H, Fleming TJ. Prevalence of caries-associated microflora after radiotherapy in patients with cancer of the head and neck. Oral Surg Oral Med Oral Pathol Oral Radiol Endod 1987;64:421–426.
97. Toljanic J, Saunders VW Jr. Radiation therapy and management of the irradiated patient. J Prosthet Dent 1984;52:852–858.
98. Keene H, Fleming TJ, Toth BB. Cariogenic microflora in patients with Hodgkin's disease before and after mantle field radiotherapy. Oral Surg Oral Med Oral Pathol Oral Radiol Endod 1994;78:577–581.
99. Engelmeier R. A dental protocol for patients receiving radiation therapy for cancer of the head and neck. Spec Care Dentist 1987;7:54–58.
100. Warde P, Kroll B, O'Sullivan B, et al. A phase II study of Biotene in the treatment of postradiation xerostomia in patients with head and neck cancer. Support Care Cancer 2000;8:203–208.
101. Johnson J, Feretti GA, Nethery WJ, et al. Oral pilocarpine for post-irradiation xerostomia in patients with head and neck cancer. N Engl J Med 1993;329:390–395.
102. LeVeque F, Montgomery M, Potter D, et al. A multicenter, randomized, double-blind, placebo-controlled, dose-titration study of oral pilocarpine for treatment of radiation-induced xerostomia in head and neck cancer patients. J Clin Oncol 1993;11: 1124–1131.
103. Fife R, Chase WF, Dore RK, et al. Cevimeline for the treatment of xerostomia in patients with Sjogren syndrome: a randomized trial. Arch Intern Med 2002;162:1293–1300.
104. Warde P, O'Sullivan B, Aslanidis J, et al. A Phase III placebo-controlled trial of oral pilocarpine in patients undergoing radio-

therapy for head-and-neck cancer. Int J Radiat Oncol Biol Phys 2002;54:9–13.
105. Fisher J, Scott C, Scarantino CW, et al. Phase III quality-of-life study results: impact on patients' quality of life to reducing xerostomia after radiotherapy for head-and-neck cancer: RTOG 97-09. Int J Radiat Oncol Biol Phys 2003;56:832–836.
106. Rode M, Smid L, Budihna M, Soba E, Rode M, Gaspersic D. The effect of pilocarpine and biperiden on salivary secretion during and after radiotherapy in head and neck cancer patients. Int J Radiat Oncol Biol Phys 1999;45:373–378.
107. Wasserman T, Mackowiak JI, Brizel DM, et al. Effect of amifostine on patient assessed clinical benefit in irradiated head and neck cancer. Int J Radiat Oncol Biol Phys 2000;48:1035–1039.
108. Cassatt D, Fazenbaker C, Kifle G, et al. Subcutaneous administration of amifostine (ethyol) is equivalent to intravenous administration in a rat mucositis model. Int J Radiat Oncol Biol Phys 2003;57:794–802.
109. Anne P. Phase II trial of subcutaneous amifostine in patients undergoing radiation therapy for head and neck cancer. Semin Oncol 2002;29:80–83.
110. Koukourakis M, Kyrias G, Kakolyris S, et al. Subcutaneous administration of amifostine during fractionated radiotherapy: a randomized phase II study. J Clin Oncol 2002;18:2226–2233.
111. Bardet E, Martin L, Calais G, et al. Preliminary data of the GORTEC 2000-02 phase III trial comparing intravenous and subcutaneous administration of amifostine for head and neck tumors treated by external radiotherapy. Semin Oncol 2002;29: 57–60.
112. Jha N, Seikaly H, Harris J, et al. Prevention of radiation induced xerostomia by surgical transfer of submandibular salivary gland into the submental space. Radiother Oncol 2003;66:283–289.
113. Eisbruch A, Ten Haken RK, Kim HM, et al. Dose, volume, and function relationships in parotid salivary glands following conformal and intensity-modulated irradiation of head and neck cancer. Int J Radiat Oncol Biol Phys 1999;45:577–587.
114. Chao KSC, Deasy JO, Markman J, et al. A prospective study of salivary function sparing in patients with head-and-neck cancers receiving intensity-modulated or three-dimensional radiation therapy: initial results. Int J Radiat Oncol Biol Phys 2001;49: 907–916.
115. Eisbruch A, Kim H, Terrell J, et al. Xerostomia and its predictors following parotid-sparing irradiation of head-and-neck cancer. Int J Radiat Oncol Biol Phys 2001;50:695–704.
116. Chao K, Majhail N, Huang CJ, et al. Intensity-modulated radiation therapy reduces late salivary toxicity without compromising tumor control in patients with oropharyngeal carcinoma: a comparison with conventional techniques. Radiother Oncol 2001;61:275–280.
117. Lee N, Xia P, Quivey J, et al. Intensity-modulated radiotherapy in the treatment of nasopharyngeal carcinoma: an update of the UCSF experience. Int J Radiat Oncol Biol Phys 2002;53: 12–22.
118. Fleming I, Brady LW, Mieszkalski GB, Cooper MR. Basis for major current therapies for cancer. In: Murphy GPLW, Lenhard RE (eds). American Cancer Society Textbook of Clinical Oncology, 2nd ed. Atlanta: The American Cancer Society, 1995: 96–134.
119. Heimdahl A, Mattsson T, Dahllöf G, Lonnquist B, Ringdén O. The oral cavity as a port of entry for early infections in patients treated with bone marrow transplantation. Oral Surg Oral Med Oral Pathol 1989;68:711–716.
120. Cutler L. Evaluation and management of the dental patient with cancer. I. Complications associated with chemotherapy or bone marrow transplantation. J Conn State Dent Assoc 1987;61: 236–238.
121. Toth B, Martin JW, Fleming TJ. Oral complications associated with cancer therapy: an M.D. Anderson Cancer Center experience. J Clin Periodontol 1990;17:508–515.
122. Overholser C, Peterson DE, Williams LT, Schimpff SC. Periodontal infection of patients with acute nonlymphocyte leukemia: prevalence of acute exacerbations. Arch Intern Med 1982;142:551–554.
123. Peterson D, Minah GE, Overholser CD, et al. Microbiology of acute periodontal infection in myelosuppressed cancer patients. J Clin Oncol 1987;5:1461–1468.
124. Bodey G. Quantitative relationship between circulating leukocytes and infection in patients with acute leukemia. Ann Intern Med 1966;64:328–340.
125. Epstein J, Vickars L, Spinelli J, Reece D. Efficacy of chlorhexidine and nystatin rinses in prevention of oral complications in leukemia and bone marrow transplantation. Oral Surg Oral Med Oral Pathol 1992;73:682–689.
126. Ferretti G, Hansen IA, Whittenburg K, Brown AT, Lillich TT, Ash RC. Therapeutic use of chlorhexidine in bone marrow transplant patients: case studies. Oral Surg Oral Med Oral Pathol Oral Radiol Endod 1987;63:683–687.
127. Ferretti G, Ash RC, Brown AT, Largent BM, Kaplan A, Lillich TT. Chlorhexidine for prophylaxis against oral infections and associated complications in patients receiving bone marrow transplants. J Am Dent Assoc 1987;114:461–467.
128. Raether D, Walker PO, Bostrum B, Weisdorf D. Effectiveness of oral chlorhexidine for reducing stomatitis in a pediatric bone marrow transplant population. Pediatr Dent 1989;11:37–42.
129. Rutkauskas J, Davis JW. Effects of chlorhexidine during immunosuppressive chemotherapy. A preliminary report. Oral Surg Oral Med Oral Pathol 1993;76:441–448.
130. Thurmond J, Brown AT, Sims RE, et al. Oral *Candida albicans* in bone marrow transplant patients given chlorhexidine rinses: occurrence and susceptibilities to the agent. Oral Surg Oral Med Oral Pathol 1991;72:291–295.
131. Lenhard R, Lawrence W, McKenna RJ. General approach to the patient. In: Murphy GPLW, Lenhard RE (eds). American Cancer Society Textbook of Clinical Oncology, 2nd ed. Atlanta: The American Cancer Society, 1995:64–74.
132. Cheatham B, Henry RJ. A dental complication involving *Pseudomonas* during chemotherapy for acute lymphoblastic leukemia. J Clin Pediatr Dent 1994;18:215–217.
133. Kaminski S, Gillette WB, O'Leary TJ. Sodium absorption associated with oral hygiene procedures. J Am Dent Assoc 1987;114: 644–646.
134. Maeda H, Kameyama Y, Nakane S, Takehana S, Sato E. Epithelial dysplasia produced by carcinogen pretreatment and subsequent wounding. Oral Surg Oral Med Oral Pathol 1989;68:50–56.
135. O'Sullivan E, Duggal MS, Bailey CC, Curzon MEJ, Hart P. Changes in the oral microflora during cytotoxic chemotherapy in children being treated for acute leukemia. Oral Surg Oral Med Oral Pathol 1993;76:161–168.
136. Borowski B, Benhamou E, Pico JL, Laplanche A, Margainaud JP, Hayat M. Prevention of oral mucositis in patients treated with high-dose chemotherapy and bone marrow transplantation: a randomized controlled trial comparing two protocols of dental care. Eur J Cancer B Oral Oncol 1994;30B:93–97.
137. Lefkoff M, Beck FM, Horton JE. The effectiveness of a disposable tooth cleansing device on plaque. J Periodontol 1995;66: 218–221.
138. Brown A, Shupe JA, Sims RE, et al. In vitro effect of chlorhexidine and amikacin on oral gram-negative bacilli from bone marrow transplant recipients. Oral Surg Oral Med Oral Pathol 1990;70:715–719.
139. Semba S, Mealey BL, Hallmon WW. Dentistry and the cancer patient. Part 2. Oral health management of the chemotherapy patient. Compendium Cont Educ Dent 1994;15:1378–1388.
140. Drugs of choice for cancer chemotherapy. Med Lett 1995;37: 25–32.
141. Pizzo P. Management of fever in patients with cancer and treatment-induced neutropenia. N Engl J Med 1993;328:1323–1332.

142. Sager R, Theis RM. Dental implants placed in a patient with multiple myeloma: report of a case. J Am Dent Assoc 1990;121:699–701.
143. Vassos D. Dental implant treatment in a severely compromised (irradiated) patient. J Oral Implantol 1992;18:142–147.
144. Karr R, Kramer DC. You can treat the chemotherapy patient. Texas Dent J 1992;109:15–20.
145. Toth B, Frame RT. Dental oncology: the management of disease and treatment-related oral/dental complications associated with chemotherapy. Curr Probl Cancer 1983;7:7–35.
146. Sonis S. Mucositis as a biological process: a new hypothesis for the development of chemotherapy-induced stomatotoxicity. Oral Oncol 1998;34:39–43.
147. Schubert M, Williams BE, Lloid ME, Donaldson G, Chapko MK. Clinical assessment scale for the rating of oral mucosal changes associated with bone marrow transplantation: development of an oral mucositis index. Cancer (Phila) 1991;69:2469–2477.
148. Sonis S, Eilers JP, Epstein JB, et al. Validation of a new scoring system for the assessment of clinical trial research of oral mucositis induced by radiation or chemotherapy. Mucositis Study Group. Cancer (Phila) 1999;85:2103–2113.
149. Montgomery M, Redding SW, LeMaistre CF. The incidence of oral herpes simplex virus infection in patients undergoing cancer chemotherapy. Oral Surg Oral Med Oral Pathol 1986;61: 238–242.
150. MacPhail L, Hilton JF, Heinic GS, Greenspan D. Direct immunofluorescence vs. culture for detecting HSV in oral ulcers: a comparison. J Am Dent Assoc 1995;126:74–78.
151. Tang I, Shepp DH. Herpes simplex virus infection in cancer patients: prevention and treatment. Oncology 1992;6:101–109.
152. Flaitz C, Hammond HL. The immunoperoxidase method for the rapid diagnosis of intraoral herpes simplex virus infection in patients receiving bone marrow transplants. Spec Care Dentist 1988;8:82–85.
153. Greenberg M. Oral herpes simplex infections in patients with leukemia. J Am Dent Assoc 1987;114:483–486.
154. Wade J, Schmiff SC, Newman KA. *Staphylococcus epidermidis*: an increasing cause of infection in patients with granulocytopenia. Ann Intern Med 1982;97:503–508.
155. Meurman J, Pyrhönen S, Teerenhovi L, Lindqvist C. Oral sources of septicaemia in patients with malignancies. Oral Oncol 1997;33:389–397.
156. Eting L, Bodey GP, Keefe BH. Septicema and shock syndrome due to viridans streptococci: a case-control study of predisposing factors. Clin Infect Dis 1992;14:1201–1207.
157. Bez C, Demarosi F, Sardella A, et al. GM-CSF mouthrinses in the treatment of severe oral mucositis: a pilot study. Oral Surg Oral Med Oral Pathol Oral Radiol Endod 1999;88:311–315.
158. Rosenberg S. Oral care of chemotherapy patients. Dent Clin N Am 1990;34:239–250.
159. Allard W, el-Akkad S, Chatmas JC. Obtaining pre-radiation therapy dental clearance. J Am Dent Assoc 1993;124:88–91.
160. Barrett A, Buckley DJ. Oral complications of high-dose melphalan in multiple myeloma. Oral Surg Oral Med Oral Pathol 1987;64:264–267.
161. Carl W. Managing the oral manifestations of cancer therapy. Part II. Chemotherapy. Compendium Cont Educ Dent 1988; 9:376–386.
162. McCarthy G, Skillings JR. Orofacial complications of chemotherapy for breast cancer. Oral Surg Oral Med Oral Pathol 1992;74:172–178.
163. Mealey B, Semba SE, Hallmon WW. Dentistry and the cancer patient. Part I. Oral manifestations and complications of chemotherapy. Compendium Cont Educ Dent 1994;xv: 1252–1256.
164. Ramos L. Oral aspects of chemotherapy: patient information. Texas Dent J 1994;111(6):42–45.
165. Poland J. Prevention and treatment of oral complications in the cancer patient. Oncology 191;5:45–62.
166. Epstein J, Sherlock CH, Page JL, Spinelli J, Phillips G. Clinical study of herpes simplex virus infection in leukemia. Oral Surg Oral Med Oral Pathol 1990;70:38–43.
167. Toth B, Martin JW, Chambers MS, Lippman SM. Oral cancer, leukoplakia, and chemoprevention. Oral Disease Update 1997;3:8–9.
168. Cooper B. New concepts in management of acute leukemia. BUMC Proc 1990;3:31–33.
169. Mattsson T, Arvidson K, Heimdahl A, Ljungman P, Dahllöf G, Ringdén O. Alterations in test acuity associated with allogeneic bone marrow transplantation. J Oral Pathol Med 1992;21:33–37.
170. Barasch A, Safford MM. Management of oral pain in patients with malignant diseases. Compendium Cont Educ Dent 1993;14:1376–1383.
171. Collins R, Miller GW, Fay JW. Autologous bone marrow transplantation: a review. BUMC Proc 1991;4:3–12.
172. Dahllöf G, Heimdahl A, Modéer T, Twetman S, Bolme P, Ringdén O. Oral mucous membrane lesions in children treated with bone marrow transplantation. Scand J Dent Res 1989;97:268–277.
173. Maxymiw W, Wood RE. The role of dentistry in patients undergoing bone marrow transplantation. Br Dent J 1989;167:229–234.
174. Birck C, Patterson B, Maximi WC, Minden MD. EBV and HSV infections in a patient who had undergone bone marrow transplantation: oral manifestations and diagnosis by in situ nucleic acid hybridization. Oral Surg Oral Med Oral Pathol 1989;68:612–617.
175. LeVeque F, Ratanatharathorn V, Danielsson KH, Orville B, Coleman DN, Turner S. Oral cytomegalovirus infection in an unrelated bone marrow transplantation with possible mediation by graft-versus-host disease and the use of cyclosporin? Oral Surg Oral Med Oral Pathol 1994;77:248–253.
176. Schubert M, Peterson DE, Flournoy N, Meyers J, Truelove EL. Oral and pharyngeal herpes simplex virus infection following bone marrow transplantation: analysis of factors associated with infection. Oral Surg Oral Med Oral Pathol 1990;70:286–293.
177. Schuchter L, Wingard JR, Piantadosi S, Burns WH, Santos GW, Saral R. Herpes zoster infection after autologous bone marrow transplantation. Blood 1989;74:1424–1427.
178. Vose J, Kennedy BC, Bierman PJ, Kessinger A, Armitage JO. Long-term sequelae of autologous bone marrow or peripheral stem cell transplantation for lymphoid malignancies. Cancer (Phila) 1992;69:784–789.
179. Schubert M, Epstein JB, Lloyd ME, Cooney E. Oral infections due to cytomegalovirus in immunocompromised patients. J Oral Pathol Med 1993;22:268–273.
180. Barrett A, Schifter M. Antibiotic strategy in orofacial/head and neck infections in severe neutropenia. Oral Surg Oral Med Oral Pathol 1994;77:350–355.
181. Mattsson T, Heimdahl A, Dahllöf G, Ma DQ, Ringden O. Oral and nutritional status in allogeneic marrow recipients treated with T-cell depletion or cyclosporine combined with methotrexate to prevent graft-versus-host disease. Oral Surg Oral Med Oral Pathol 1992;74:34–40.
182. Epstein J, Sherlock CH, Wolber RA. Hairy leukoplakia after bone marrow transplantation. Oral Surg Oral Med Oral Pathol 1993;75:690–695.
183. Peterson D. Pretreatment strategies for infection prevention in chemotherapy patients. NCI Monogr 1990;9:61–71.
184. Ferrara J, Deeg HJ. Graft-versus-host disease. N Engl J Med 1991;324:667–674.

185. Curtis JJ, Caughman GB. An apparent unusual relationship between rampant caries and graft-versus-host disease. Oral Surg Oral Med Oral Pathol Oral Radiol Endod 1991;78:267–272.
186. Hiroki A, Nakamura S, Shinohara M, Oka M. Significance of oral examination in chronic graft-versus-host disease. J Oral Pathol Med 194;23:209–215.
187. Heimdahl A, Johnson G, Danielsson KH, Lönnquist B, Sundelin P, Ringdén O. Oral condition of patients with leukemia and severe aplastic anemia. Follow-up one year after bone marrow transplantation. Oral Surg Oral Med Oral Pathol 1985;60:498–504.
188. LeVeque F. An unusual presentation of chronic graft-versus-host disease in an unrelated bone marrow transplantation. Oral Surg Oral Med Oral Pathol 1990;69:581–584.
189. Barrett A. Graft-versus-host disease. A clinicopathologic review. Ann Dent 1987;46:7–11.
190. Allen C, Kapoor N. Verruciform xanthoma in a bone marrow transplant recipient. Oral Surg Oral Med Oral Pathol 1993;75: 591–594.
191. Wingard J, Niehaus CS, Peterson DE, et al. Oral mucositis after bone marrow transplantation. A marker of treatment toxicity and predictor of hepatic veno-occlusive disease. Oral Surg Oral Med Oral Pathol 1991;72:419–424.

75

Alopecia and Cutaneous Complications of Chemotherapy

Faith M. Durden and Paradi Mirmirani

Alopecia and Chemotherapy

The hair growth cycle is composed of three well-recognized phases: anagen (growth), catagen (deconstruction), and telogen (resting) phases. At any time, approximately 90% of the 100,000 to 150,000 scalp hairs are in the anagen phase An in-depth discussion of hair cycling is beyond the scope of this chapter, but please refer to the referenced article for an excellent review on the current thinking on the subject.[1]

Only the hair follicle has the unique ability to destruct via apoptosis, remodel, and reconstruct a hair shaft on a continuous, cyclic, and relatively rapid basis, occurring, in most cases, throughout the life of the individual. Remarkably, however, it does so with such precision that malignancies of the hair shaft are rare. This fact, coupled with the fact that the hair growth rate rivals many malignancies, makes the hair follicle an important organ to understand. In addition, despite perturbations, such as insult via chemotherapeutic agents, the hair frequently deconstructs, biding its time until the insult has ceased, before resuming its growth cycle once again.

Alopecia is the most common side effect of cancer chemotherapy. Known as anagen effluvium, or anagen arrest, this typically begins in the first 1 to 4 weeks after instituting cancer chemotherapy, becoming most noticeable 1 to 2 months after therapy begins. As the name implies, hairs in the anagen phase are predominantly affected. Long-term or repeated treatment often results in complete, but usually reversible, hair loss. It is because of the hair follicle epithelium's high replication rate that it is exquisitely susceptible to insult from chemotherapeutic agents. Although loss of scalp hair is more readily noted by the patient, loss of body hair, such as the axillae, pubic region, beard, and lashes and brows may occur as well. The hair loss occurs as a result of dystrophic hair shaft development, resulting in hair fragility and easy breakage proximal to the scalp.[2]

Transduction signals results in accelerated apoptotic activity in chemotherapy patients. This induced programmed cell death (cell suicide) results in a dystrophic hair. Apoptosis appears to occur either as a result of direct action of the drug on the cell or as a result of cell-cycle events resulting in delayed activation. The apoptosis regulatory gene, bcl-2, exhibits increased expression in mice treated with cyclophosphamide, promoting catagen and subsequent alopecia. Bcl-2 is most strongly expressed during the anagen phase.[3]

p53 also plays a major role in chemotherapy-induced hair follicle apoptosis. The mechanism of p53 in inducing hair follicle apoptosis is unknown but may be secondary to upregulation of IGF–BP3, coupled with upregulation of Fas/Apo-1 and alteration of the bcl-2/Bax ratio, resulting in the presence of endonucleases and upregulation of interleukin 1-beta-converting enzyme.[4–7]

Microscopic evaluation of the affected hair shaft reveals a decrease in hair shaft diameter, with separation of the protective outer layer (cuticle) from the inner core (cortex). Depigmentation occurs frequently. Splaying of the hair shaft, swelling of the inner and outer root sheath, and cuticular fragmentation also occur.[8]

Although these findings are usually temporary, 58% of women found possible hair loss the most concerning side effect of chemotherapy, and in some cases, were at risk for not accepting therapy as a result of this potential complication. In addition, those who experience hair loss reported feelings of alienation, isolation, and embarrassment because of personal feelings and reactions from others. Others felt shame, loss of privacy while trying to cope with cancer therapy, and loss of self-esteem. Social interactions may become impaired or avoided altogether. Alopecia caused a significant number of women to exhibit evidence of poor body image and sexual dysfunction.[9–16]

Studies are being conducted to determine the validity of using computer-generated images to allow patients to view how they will look without hair as a modality to have patients adjust to the possibility of alopecia. The patient may also generate multiple images using wigs, scarves, and other coverings. This technique allows the patient to not only view herself as bald before this actually occurs but to have a plan of adaptive strategies before chemotherapy has begun.[17]

If treatment regimens have no differing efficacy, considerations of side effects, including potential for a regimen to induce alopecia, should be considered. However, one must keep in mind that the majority of patients adjust well to the hair loss, with appropriate counseling. Additionally, hair may even regrow during the course of long-term chemotherapy. Recovery typically occurs in 6 to 12 months after chemotherapy has ended. Occasionally, the hair may have an altered texture and/or color. The degree of hair loss is dependent on the type of drug used, its half-life, and the dose of the drug, as well as the duration of use, duration of infusion, and use

TABLE 75.1. Frequency of alopecia from various chemotherapeutic agents.

Frequency of alopecia	*Drug*
Common	Cyclophosphamide Daunorubicin Docetaxel Doxorubicin Idarubicin Ifosfamide Paclitaxel
Often	Bleomycin Etoposide Mechlorethamine Methotrexate Mitoxantrone
Infrequent	5-Fluorouracil Hydroxyurea Thiotepa Vinblastine Vincristine Vinorelbine
Rare	Procarbazine

Source: From Alley et al.,[18] by permission of *Current Opinion in Oncology*.

of combination regimens. Chemotherapeutic agents typically producing alopecia are listed in Table 75.1.[18]

One study reviewed the incidence of irreversible alopecia in patients receiving high-dose chemotherapy using carboplatin, thiotepa, and cyclophosphamide. Although these patients had received previous chemotherapy and cyclophosphamide was also part of the regimen, it was thought that carboplatin and thiotepa may have played the principal role in the hair loss. Thus, it may be advisable to warn patients of the possibility of permanent alopecia if chemotherapy employing carboplatin and thiotepa is offered.[19]

By contrast, a study of 17 patients with Hodgkin's disease with ABVD or MOPP/ABV suggested that those who fail to experience alopecia may have a poorer response than those who do.[20]

Unfortunately, there are currently no preventative treatments available in the United States to prevent the alopecia common to chemotherapy patients. Scalp hypothermia for prevention of alopecia, being investigated in other countries, is thought to work by limiting the follicular uptake of chemotherapy due to vasoconstriction. Factors influencing efficacy of hypothermic devices include rapidity, dose, type of chemotherapy, route of administration, and duration and degree of cooling of the scalp. Three recently studied devices used outside the United States are reviewed in Table 75.2. Previously used in the United States, scalp cooling has been banned by the U.S. Food and Drug Administration (FDA) secondary to reports of scalp metastases occurring in patients. However, benefits versus risks remain controversial. There may be an eventual role in using such a modality in patients receiving palliative therapy who are concerned about hair loss. However, should an indication receive approval, well-controlled studies will be required to determine optimal temperature, type of device to use, optimal cooling agent, duration of treatment, and objective measurement of the degree of alopecia.[21–25]

Other modalities to prevent loss and/or induce growth have been studied as well. Preliminary studies suggest topical 2% minoxidil may decrease the duration of alopecia. It is well tolerated. Topical 1,25-dihydroxyvitamin D_3 was not effective in preventing hair loss in humans in one small series. However, murine models suggest that use of 1,25-dihydroxyvitamin D_3 may help accelerate the hair regrowth process. Further studies are necessary to evaluate these very safe options.[26] Antioxidants not only fail to prevent alopecia, they may actually impede response to chemotherapy.[27]

On the horizon: The primary approach in preventing chemotherapy-induced alopecia has been to alter or manipulate the hair cycle either before or after a chemotherapeutic insult. Typically, candidate agents are those compounds known to affect the follicular cycle. The data presented here have been derived from animal models but may hold promise for future developments for viable treatment options (murine models predominating).

TABLE 75.2. Treatment modalities for prevention/treatment of chemotherapy-induced alopecia.

Treatment	*Reference*	*Year*	*No. of patients*	*Randomized*	*Placebo*	*Intervention/design*	*Median follow-up*	*Conclusions*
Hypothermia	21	2003	74	No	No	Digitized, scalp cooling system	15 months	100% prevention of hair loss in anthracycline-treated patients
Hypothermia	22	2002	83	No	No	MSC Cold Cap	Unknown	69%–88% effective in preventing alopecia from anthracycline, etoposide, or taxane
Hypothermia	23	2000	70	No	No	Cold cap system	Unknown	92% effective in prevention of alopecia from anthracycline and taxane
Minoxidil topical solution	26	1996	22	Yes	Yes	2% Minoxidil topical solution	N/A	Decreased duration of alopecia caused by chemotherapy
Topical calcitriol	27	1999	14	Yes	Yes	Topical topitriol (calcitriol, 1,25-dihydroxyvitamin D_3) at various dosages 7 days before and 5 days after chemotherapy	30 days after chemotherapy	All patients developed grade 2 alopecia 20–30 days post-chemotherapy demonstrating lack of efficacy of calcitriol in this schedule of administration.

Murine studies suggest a role for a topical sonic hedgehog expression therapy, which appears to induce hair regrowth after treatment with cyclophosphamide. Similarly, the immunophilins cyclosporine A and tacrolimus were found to transiently induce anagen and to decrease cyclophosphamide-induced alopecia in mice. Although cyclosporine response was dose dependent, response to tacrolimus was not. In addition, tacrolimus was more effective in decreasing cyclophosphamide-induced hair loss. Importantly, however, hair loss occurred eventually. Further studies in humans are warranted.[28,29]

Pretreatment with calcitriol decreased, but failed to completely inhibit, follicular apoptosis postcyclophosphamide therapy in mice. Although the exact mechanism of action of inhibition unknown, it may be secondary to calcium-dependent effects.[30–32]

The parathormone/parathormone receptor protein (PTH/PTHrP) antagonist aided in hair retention in cyclophosphamide-treated mice. In addition, the PTH/PTHrPR agonist resulted in hair growth promotion after chemotherapy. Similar findings of hair loss reduction have been reported in mice treated with topical p53 inhibitors, CDK2 antagonists, fas/fasl inhibitors, and caspase-3. These latter agents are known to impede apoptosis.[33,34]

N-Acetylcysteine may provide a protective effect against alopecia in mice and rats receiving chemotherapy, as hair was retained.[35]

Cutaneous Complications of Chemotherapy

The following section of this chapter is devoted to the common cutaneous side effects of chemotherapy.

Hypersensitivity Reactions

Fortunately, allergic reactions are relatively rare, but can be severe enough to change or alter the dose of the offending drug. Although type I hypersensitivity reactions (HSR) are most common, type II, III, and IV reactions may occur as well. Manifestations include urticaria, angioedema, anaphylaxis, eczematous dermatitis, vasculitis, and variants of erythema multiforme. Table 75.3 summarizes common chemotherapeutic agents causing hypersensitivity reactions.[18]

L-Asparaginase is the most common cause of type I hypersensitivity, followed by cisplatin, carboplatin (intravenous), docetaxel, and paclitaxel. The former has been reported mainly in children. Although rare, rasburicase, used to prevent tumor lysis syndrome, may cause hypersensitivity reactions, in some cases, severe. In addition, this medication is contraindicated in persons who are G6PD deficient.[36–38]

Using a test dose for taxanes has proven beneficial in decreasing the severity of hypersensitivity reactions, medication waste, and costs associated with managing patients suffering from such reactions. *Escherichia coli* asparaginase is generally well tolerated, but *Erwinia* asparaginase may be substituted in individuals sensitive to the *E. coli* derivative without sacrificing efficacy.[39]

Of note, mechlorethamine ranks as one of the major causes of type IV hypersensitivity reaction. These eruptions are eczematous in presentation, resembling the eruption one might see with a nickel- or poison ivy-type rash.

TABLE 75.3. Common chemotherapeutic agents causing hypersensitivity reactions.

Drug	*Type of reaction*[a]
Alemtuzumab	Type I
L-Asparaginase	Type I
Bleomycin	Type I
Carboplatin	Type I
Cisplatin	Type I, II
Chlorambucil	Type I, II
Cyclophosphamide	Type I
Cytarabine	Type I
Docetaxel	Type I
Daunorubicin	Type I
Doxorubicin	Type I
Dacarbazine	Type I
Etoposide	Type I, III
5-Fluorouracil	Type I
Ifosfamide	Type I
Mechlorethamine (topical)	Type IV
Melphalan	Type I
Methotrexate	Type I, III
Mitomycin	Type I, III, IV
Mitoxantrone	Type I
Paclitaxel	Type I
Procarbazine	Type I, III
Pentostatin	Type I
Rituximab	Type I, III
Teniposide	Type I
Trastuzumab	Type I

[a] Type I, immediate hypersensitivity reaction (mediated by IgE antibody to specific antigens); type II, cytotoxic antibody reaction (mediated by IgG and IgM to specific antigens); type III, immune complex reaction (antigen–antibody complexes deposit in tissue); type IV, delayed-type hypersensitivity (mediated by T lymphocytes to specific antigens).

Source: From Alley et al.,[18] by permission of *Current Opinion in Oncology*.

In summary, hypersensitivity reactions are idiosyncratic. However, if feasible, test doses may be given to try to identify patients who may be at risk for HSR type I. In those patients with a positive reaction, desensitization, prophylaxis, or use of an efficacious alternative may be employed. Indeed, prophylaxis is highly recommended before treatment with the aforementioned agents associated with HSR type 1, using H_1 with H_2 blockers and systemic corticosteroids. Treatment of reactions include use of epinephrine, systemic corticosteroids, antihistamines, and stable maintenance of the patient's hemodynamic status. In some instances, cisplatin may be successfully substituted for carboplatin-hypersensitive individuals; again, skin testing should be performed first.[40]

Extravasation Reactions

Extravasation reactions occur in approximately 0.1% to 6% of adults, and the rate is higher in children. The two types of reactions include irritant and vesicant reactions.[41] Clinically, irritant reactions present with erythema, tenderness, and swelling at the infusion site, with associated phlebitis. Necrosis does not occur. Later, sclerosis and hyperpigmentation may occur. Treatment includes discontinuation of the drug and aspiration to remove as much residua as possible. The extremity should be elevated. Use of hot or cold compresses may prove beneficial; cold compresses help alleviate associated discomfort.

Extravasation with vesicating agents are typically similar to irritant extravasation reactions. They may occur days to weeks after exposure to an offending drug. In addition to erythema, pain, hyperpigmentation, and superficial desquamation, bullae may form. Extensive extravasation may result in ulcer formation. If small, these ulcers typically heal with routine wound management. By contrast, larger ulcers may remain indolent or enlarge. Thus, prompt management may help reduce the risk of involvement of tendons, nerves, and blood vessels, which, in turn, could further complicate wound healing and result in disabling outcomes, including joint contractures. Fortunately, secondary local and systemic infection is rare, even in persons with extensive ulceration.[42–44]

Common vesicants include the vinca alkaloids, the anthracyclines, nitrogen mustard, paclitaxel, and cisplatin. Reactions are treated with extremity elevation and cold compresses. The exception to this is in the case of the vinca alkaloid. As cold compresses have been associated with increased necrosis in animal models, hot compresses are preferred. Surgery is indicated only for failure to respond to conservative therapy or if ulceration and/or necrosis occur. Corticosteroids, lidocaine, hyaluronidase, and phentolamine are ineffective in preventing necrosis associated with extravasation of vesicating agents.[45–47]

Hyperpigmentation

Hyperpigmentation is common, occurring locally secondary to mechanical stress (i.e., electrodes, monitors, bandages), or diffusely. Increased pigmentation may be identified not only in the skin but in hair, mucous membranes, and nails as well.[48] The exact mechanism of diffuse hyperpigmentation is unknown. Serpiginous and linear streaks of hyperpigmentation have been associated with bleomycin therapy. Pigmentation will usually resolve spontaneously in 6 to 12 months after discontinuation of therapy. However, a single case report of permanent hyperpigmentation occurred in a patient treated with bleomycin and cisplatin. Serpentine supravenous hyperpigmentation has been reported as well. Diffuse pigmentation may be seen with persons receiving busulfan, hence the term "busulfan tan."[48–52]

Acral Erythema

Also known as Burgdorf's syndrome, toxic erythema of the palms and soles, palmar-plantar erythema, palmoplantar erythrodysesthesia, and hand–foot syndrome, this condition occurs most commonly with cytarabine, doxorubicin, and fluorouracil, but may occur with many other chemotherapeutic agents, including tegafur, a derivative of fluorouracil. The frequency varies from 6% to 42% of patients, and it occurs almost exclusively in adults but may occur in children receiving high-dose methotrexate therapy. Lesions typically develop 1 to 90 days after chemotherapy.[53]

Capecitabine, an oral derivative of fluorouracil, has a long tissue half-life. It is associated with acral erythema in up to 10% of treated patients, with 57% of patients having some symptomatology of acral erythema.

The patient typically complains of a burning sensation of the palms and soles, followed by exquisite tenderness and/or pruritus and swelling. Subsequently, discrete, intensely red plaques develop on the thenar and hypothenar eminence, and/or the lateral fingers, with occasional extension to the dorsum of the hands. Periungual erythema and erythematous bands over the joint surfaces may occur. The hands are affected more than the feet. A morbilliform eruption may occur on the head, neck, chest, and extremities; periorbital swelling may also occur. Symptoms resolve with discontinuation of the offending agent, but subsequent desquamation is not uncommon. Complete recovery occurs in approximately 1 month.[54–56]

The bullous variant, reported in persons receiving cytarabine and methotrexate, is associated with necrosis, sloughing, and subsequent reepithelialization. The exact cause is unknown but may be dose related. The condition is typically more severe with short-term bolus infusions compared with low-dose infusions.

Acral erythema resembles early graft-versus-host disease of the hands and feet and may be quite difficult to distinguish in patients who have undergone bone marrow transplant. Similarly, the two diseases may occur simultaneously. Serial biopsies, performed 3 to 5 days apart, will eventually elucidate the cause, allowing for appropriate management. There are no evidence-based protocols for treatment of acral erythema, but pyridoxine and corticosteroids have been reported beneficial anecdotally.

Pain management, elevation of the extremities, and cold compresses help relieve symptoms. Cold immersion of the hands and feet may also decrease the incidence and severity of the reaction, presumably secondary to vasoconstriction resulting in lower drug levels being delivered to the extremities. Acral erythema might also be prevented by using lower drug dosages, when feasible, coupled with use of pyridoxine. Some patients may resume their chemotherapy with subsequent decreased severity of the condition.

Inflammation of Keratosis

Precancerous actinic keratoses and, occasionally, benign seborrheic keratoses become inflamed when patients receive systemic fluorouracil (most common) and other types of chemotherapy. The reaction is thought to be secondary to the lesions' relative rapidly dividing nature, compared to uninvolved skin. The lesions are characterized by focal, scaly papules or plaques in sun-exposed areas that become inflamed and/or eroded. No intervention is necessary, unless the lesions become bothersome for the patient, as removal of actinic keratosis will prevent subsequent development of cutaneous squamous cell carcinoma, which might otherwise occur in these lesions. The patient may use low-potency topical corticosteroids if the lesions become symptomatic.

Graft-Versus-Host Disease

Although mild graft-versus-host disease (GVHD) may have a therapeutic effect against malignant cells, severe reactions may result in significant morbidity and mortality. GVHD is divided into acute and chronic GVHD, occurring within and after 100 days posttransplant, respectively.

Acute GVHD estimates are 6% to 90%. Factors increasing risk include patient's age, prevention protocols, and HLA type. In HLA-matched adults, the incidence is approximately 35%. The selective epithelial inflammation typically affects the skin, digestive tract, and liver, with cutaneous involvement being the most common. Patients frequently complain of itching, but pain and tenderness may also occur. Patients develop a morbilliform eruption, often with folliculocentric prominence. Involvement of the palms, soles, and ears is common. In rare cases, a toxic epidermal necrolysis-type presentation may occur, presenting either with erythema with superficial desquamation, or in a vesicular pattern.[57,58]

Lymphocytic infiltration and cytopathic changes of keratinocytes are the major features of acute GVHD. However, histopathologic diagnosis is difficult because of other factors that can cause a similar histopathologic picture in these patients, and thus the biopsy results must be interpreted in the context of the clinical findings in the patient, as well as other sites of presumed involvement, such as the liver and gut. Histologic signs are classified into four grades, as summarized in Table 75.4.

One school of thought suggests GVHD develops when the donor T lymphocytes are recognized as foreign, resulting in activation of recipient T cells and recipient IL-2 secretion. The recipient IL-2/donor IL-2 receptor binding results in expansion and proliferation of the T lymphocytes, and in release of tumor necrosis factor-alpha (TNF-α), which, in turn, recruits effector cells, including natural killer cells, macrophages, and mast cells, in concert with fas/fasl (the latter found only in TH-1 lymphocytes), perforingranzyme, and tumor necrosis factor. Interleukin (IL)-1, -2, and -6, as well as interferon-gamma, may also play a role. Cellular apoptosis and tissue damage ensues, resulting in continued activation; thus, the cycle perpetuates itself. Acute GVHD is thought to be predominantly TH-1 mediated.

Conditioning regimens themselves cause release of cytokines, promoting GVHD; these are amplified in the "second phase" when the marrow or PBSCs are infused. Subsequently, the aforementioned mediators are released, potentiating the entire cascade. Patients with high IL-10 production have partial protection from GVHD.[59–61]

Current treatment options include psoralens/UVA photochemotherapy (PUVA; improves cutaneous GVHD only). Other drugs used include oral and topical corticosteroids,

TABLE 75.4. Histologic grading of cutaneous graft-versus-host disease (GVHD).

Grade	*Histologic description*
Grade I	Basal cell vacuolization
Grade II	Basal cell vacuolization and single necrotic keratinocytes
Grade III	Superepidermal clefts and numerous necrotic keratinocytes
Grade IV	Necrosis of the entire epidermis and complete separation from the dermis

Source: From Aractingi et al.,[57] by permission of *Archives of Dermatology*.

calcineurin inhibitors, and cyclosporine A. The role of extracorporeal photochemotherapy remains unclear.

On the horizon: One murine study demonstrated blockade if only the fas was associated with effective inhibition of GVHD without inducing graft versus leukemia. In addition, blockade of fasl in mouse models was associated with improvement of GVHD. Thus, further study into blockade of fas/fasl is warranted.[62–64]

Antithymocyte antibody improves the cutaneous stigmata of acute GVHD but not advanced internal GVHD. Thus, there was no difference in survival outcomes in those treated with antithymocyte globulin and those who were not.[65]

"Mega-dose" CD34+ cells, coupled with a conditioning regimen of thiotepa, antithymocyte globulin, cyclophosphamide, and total-body irradiation, was well tolerated and appeared to allow for inhibition of GVHD without inhibiting a graft-versus-leukemia effect. Similar findings have been found in vitro.[66]

Chronic graft-versus-host disease (c-GVHD) occurs in 60% to 80% of allogeneic hematopoietic stem cell transplant recipients, and is also associated with a high morbidity and mortality rate. It is unclear if it is TH-2 mediated. Chronic GVHD occurs more frequently in those with previous acute GVHD (a-GVHD) (11-fold increase, compared with those without a history of a-GVHD, older donor or recipients, males receiving alloimmune female donor marrow, and those receiving non-T-cell-depleted bone marrow). Because c-GVHD involving skin only is associated with only mild morbidity, some question the utility of treating under this scenario. Mortality is as high as 40% in those with visceral involvement, usually secondary to liver failure, infection, and/or wasting. Chronic GVHD may occur in a continuum of acute GVHD, de novo, or as an intermittent finding.[67–72]

The two types of c-GVHD are lichenoid and sclerodermatous. In early c-GVHD, the lichenoid form predominates, typically with involvement of the palms, soles, ears, and periorbital region, and occasionally the penis, foreskin, and vaginal mucosa. Again, the eruption may be folliculocentric. The sclerodermatous form occurs later and is characterized by erythematous plaques and papules occurring on the extremities, with progressive involvement of the trunk. Conjunctivitis, mucositis, esophageal, and genital strictures are associated findings also. Nail changes, including onycholysis, vertical ridging, and periungual telangiectasias, may occur as well. Secondary onychomycosis may develop. The sclerodermatous pattern is characterized by firm, indurated, pearl-white papules and plaques, often with a surrounding border of erythema. These lesions may remain localized but can become generalized and debilitating. As a result of the constriction associated with the sclerodermatous skin changes, patients are at risk for chronic leg ulcers, peripheral neuropathy, joint constriction and retraction, and lung constriction.[73,74]

Treatment options include oral and topical tacrolimus (the latter for skin involvement only), cyclosporine A, corticosteroids, thalidomide, hydroxychloroquine, UVB and PUVA, and mycophenylate mofetil. Although thalidomide for c-GVHD may decrease the need for long-term corticosteroid therapy, it increases the risk of c-GVHD if used prophylactically. The dose ranges from 1,200 to 1,600 mg/day. Complete or partial response occurs in up to 20% of conventional therapy nonresponders. However, the side effects, including somnolence and neuropathy, are great.[75–82] The prognosis is poor in those with generalized sclerodermatous changes, due in great part to lung constriction.

On the horizon: TNF antagonists show promise, even in systemic disease. Depletion of cd20-positive B lymphocytes via monoclonal antibodies may prove beneficial as well.[83–85]

Radiation Recall

Radiation recall occurs in a previously irradiated site after receiving chemotherapy. It occurs most often after use of doxorubicin and dactinomycin but may occur in association with other chemotherapeutic agents as well.[86–88]

The condition usually occurs after the first 1 to 2 weeks after ionizing radiation therapy and hours to days after receiving the corresponding chemotherapeutic agent. Recall reactions occur after first exposure to the drug. Although erythema is present, symptoms vary from none to extreme pain. Pruritus and swelling may also occur. The erythema is well demarcated, corresponding to the radiation field. Rarely, ulcer formation and necrosis may occur.[89,90]

There should be a reasonable interval between radiation therapy and chemotherapy. Elicitation of a reaction seems predicated on the time interval between radiation and administration of chemotherapy. Two case reports in the literature suggest that the magnitude of radiation therapy dictates the severity of the radiation recall reaction. The mechanism of action is unknown, but it may be secondary to defects associated with DNA repair mechanisms.[91,92]

Recall reactions seem to occur more rapidly with infused medications, compared with oral agents. By contrast, recovery time is longer for oral medications, compared with infused agents. Resolution occurs with discontinuation of the drug and, in some cases, will resolve despite continuation of the offending agent. Additionally, recurrence on rechallenge is often associated with an attenuated reaction. Although dosages are often altered and/or systemic corticosteroids are used, this practice has not undergone scrutiny.

Standardization of reporting would help better delineate the pathophysiology of this phenomenon. Those radiation reactions occurring within 7 days after radiation therapy may represent radiation enhancement reactions; therefore, these would represent an insult to tissue undergoing repair and thus, should not be included with true radiation recall reactions.

Radiation Enhancement

In contrast to radiation recall, radiation enhancement represents the phenomenon associated with increased toxicity of radiation in a patient receiving chemotherapy than would be expected if radiation had been used alone. The effect may be additive or synergistic.

The radiation therapy and the chemotherapy occur within 7 days of one another; the reaction may occur in nearly any organ tissue. It is dose dependent, related to the time between chemotherapy and radiation therapy, the treated tissue, and the mechanism of action of the drug. The most common agents associated with this phenomenon are listed next.

Although radiation enhancement may have a beneficial effect on solid tumors, and may be part of the therapeutic regimen, significant cutaneous side effects may occur. Erythema, swelling, blister formation, and erosions may develop; ulceration and necrosis may occur in severe cases. Although typically involving only the area irradiated, local extension may occur. Mucositis may occur if a mucous membrane is within the radiation port. Eventually, the eruption clears, with subsequent pigmentary changes, atrophy, scarring, and telangiectasias. Treatment is supportive, with avoidance of further injury to the involved area.

Ultraviolet/Photosensitivity

Photosensitivity reactions occur in patients receiving chemotherapy, followed by intentional or unintentional ultraviolet (UV) exposure. Most of these reactions resemble an exaggerated sunburn, with erythema, swelling, pruritus and/or pain, superficial desquamation, and occasionally, blister formation. Subsequent hyperpigmentation is not uncommon. Diagnosis is aided when the eruption occurs in areas typically receiving the greatest sun exposure, such as the face, posterior neck, the "V" of the chest (upper medial region), dorsum of the arms, and anterior legs.

Treatment consists of discontinuation of the offending agent and complete avoidance of UV light for 2 weeks. Physical sunblocks providing at least SPF 30 afford the greatest protection; these include those containing zinc oxide and titanium dioxide. Treatment is supportive, and includes systemic antihistamines, cold compresses, and topical immunomodulators, such as corticosteroids or calcineurin inhibitors (tacrolimus, pimecrolimus).[93]

Porphyrins, used for photodynamic therapy in the treatment of solid tumors, are known cutaneous photosensitizers. Thus, patients treated with these compounds are at great risk for photoxicity, even after taking the appropriate precautions to avoid UV exposure, including bright lights. The photosensitivity is of longer duration, lasting up to 6 weeks after discontinuing the porphyrins.

Nails can be affected in a process called photo-onycholysis in which the distal third of the nail plate separates from the nail bed. This effect has been reported in patients receiving mercaptopurine.

UV recall may occur with use of methotrexate, after a previous episode of recent phototoxicity, such as a sunburn (within 5 days). Similar reactions have been reported with use of suramin. In contrast to recall associated with methotrexate, however, often there is no history of previous sun exposure.[94]

Cutaneous Eruption of Lymphocyte Recovery

This condition develops in some individuals receiving ablative chemotherapy for subsequent bone marrow transplant, typically 6 to 21 days after receiving chemotherapy. Peripheral lymphocytes in the skin recover, becoming immunocompetent once again and subsequently causing cutaneous toxicity, characterized by erythematous macules, papules, and possible erythroderma. Fever is common. The rash usually clears within 1 week, with desquamation and hyperpigmentation.

Histologic findings are nonspecific and may resemble GVHD.

The Role of Skin Biopsies in Therapeutic Outcomes

In a retrospective study performed by Chren et al., the outcomes of 123 adult hospital inpatients with 190 episodes of skin rashes were reviewed. The study revealed that although the utility of biopsy for diagnostic purposes might alter the clinical impression of the rash, it does little in altering management strategies. Interestingly, none of the patients receiving biopsy to evaluate for an infectious etiology for the rash required change in their management. In addition, even in cases when the prebiopsy and postbiopsy diagnosis differed, therapeutic changes occurred in only 22% of patients: Change of systemic management occurred in 14%. Comparatively, changes in systemic therapy occurred in 12% of individuals where the pre- and postbiopsy diagnoses were the same. Additionally, follow-up of patients not receiving biopsy revealed no incidence that later deemed a biopsy should have been performed. Nevertheless, the article points out that biopsy can prove beneficial for reasons other than planning therapeutic strategies.[95]

References

1. Paus R. Principles of hair cycle control. J Dermatol 1998;25:793–802.
2. Susser WS, et al. Mucocutaneous reactions to chemotherapy. J Am Acad Dermatol 1999;40:367–398.
3. Botchkarev VA. Molecular mechanisms of chemotherapy-induced hair loss. J Invest Dermatol 2003;8:72–75.
4. Barry MA, et al. Activation of programmed cell death (apoptosis) by cisplatin, other anticancer drugs, toxins and hyperthermia. Biochem Pharmacol 1990;40:2353–2362.
5. Botchkarev VA, et al. p53 is essential for chemotherapy-induced hair loss. Cancer Res 2000;60:5002–5006.
6. Rudman SM, et al. The role of IGF-1 in human skin and its appendages: morphogen as well as mitogen? J Invest Dermatol 1997;109:770–777.
7. Lindner G, et al. Analysis of apoptosis during hair follicle regression (catagen). Am J Pathol 1997;151:1121–1127.
8. Linder G, et al. Analysis of apoptosis during hair follicle regression (catagen). Am J Pathol 1997;151:1601–1617.
9. Pai GS, et al. Occurrence and severity of alopecia in patients on combination chemotherapy. Indian J Cancer 2000;37:94–104.
10. McGarvey EL, et al. Psychological sequelae and alopecia among women with cancer. Cancer Pract 2001;9:283–289.
11. Munstedt K, et al. Changes in self-concept and body image during alopecia induced cancer chemotherapy. Support Care Cancer 1997;5:139–143.
12. Tierney AJ, et al. Knowledge, expectations and experiences of patients receiving chemotherapy for breast cancer. Scand J Caring Sci 1992;6:75–80.
13. Williams J, et al. A narrative study of chemotherapy-induced alopecia. Oncol Nurs Forum 1999;26:1463–1468.
14. Pickard-Holley S. The symptom experience of alopecia. Semin Oncol Nurs 1995;11:235–238.
15. Baxley KO, et al. Alopecia: effect on cancer patients' body image. Cancer Nurs 1984;7:499–503.
16. Batchelor D. Hair and cancer chemotherapy: consequences and nursing care—a literature study. Eur J Can 2001;10:147–163.
17. Edelstyn GA, et al. Improvement of life quality in cancer patients undergoing chemotherapy. Clin Oncol 1979;5:43–49.
18. Alley E, et al. Cutaneous toxicities of cancer chemotherapy. Curr Opin Oncol 2002;14:212–216.
19. de Jonge ME, et al. Relationship between irreversible alopecia and exposure to cyclophosphamide, thiotepa, and carboplatin (CTC) in high-dose chemotherapy. Bone Marrow Transplant 2002;30:593–597.
20. Lishner M, et al. Association between alopecia and response to aggressive chemotherapy in patients with Hodgkin's disease. Med Hypotheses 1999;53:447–449.
21. Ridderheim M, et al. Scalp hypothermia to prevent chemotherapy-induced alopecia is effective and safe: a pilot study of a new digitized scalp-cooling system used in 74 patients. Support Care Cancer 2003;11:371–377.
22. Christodoulou C, et al. Effectiveness of the MSC cold cap system in the prevention of chemotherapy-induced alopecia. Oncology 2002;62:97–102.
23. Katsimbri P, et al. Prevention of chemotherapy-induced alopecia using an effective scalp cooling system. Eur J Cancer 2000;36:766–771.
24. Ron IG, et al. Scalp cooling in the prevention of alopecia in patients receiving depilating chemotherapy. Support Care Cancer 1997;5:136–138.
25. Tierney AJ. Preventing chemotherapy-induced alopecia in cancer patient: is scalp cooling worthwhile? J Adv Nurs 1987;12:303–310.
26. Duvic M, et al. A randomized trial of minoxidil in chemotherapy-induced alopecia. J Am Acad Dermatol 1996;35:74–78.
27. Conklin KA. Dietary antioxidants during cancer chemotherapy: impact on chemotherapeutic effectiveness and development of side effects. Nutr Cancer 2000;37(1):1–18.
28. Sato, Noboru, et al. Effect of adenovirus-mediated expression of sonic hedgehog gene on hair regrowth in mice with chemotherapy-induced alopecia. J Nat Cancer Inst 2001;93:1858–1864.
29. Maurer M, et al. Hair growth modulation by topical immunophilin ligands: induction of anagen, inhibition of massive catagen development, and relative protection from chemotherapy-induced alopecia. Am J Pathol 1997;150:1433–1441.
30. Paus R, et al. Topical calitriol enhances normal hair regrowth but does not prevent chemotherapy-induced alopecia in mice. Cancer Res 1996;56:4438–4443.
31. Jimenez JJ, et al. Protection from chemotherapy-induced alopecia by 1,25-dihydroxyvitamin D3. Cancer Res 1992;52:5123–5125.
32. Schilli MB, et al. Reduction of intrafollicular apoptosis in chemotherapy-induced alopecia by topical calcitriol analogs. J Invest Dermatol 1998;111:598–604.
33. Peters EMJ, et al. A new strategy for modulating chemotherapy-induced alopecia, using PTH/PTHrP receptor agonist and antagonist. J Invest Dermatol 2001;117:173–178.
34. Davis ST, et al. Prevention of chemotherapy-induced alopecia in rats by cdk inhibitors. Science 2001;291:134–137.
35. D'Agostini F, et al. Induction of alopecia in mice exposed to cigarette smoke. Toxicol Lett 2000;114:117–123.
36. Polyzos A, et al. Hypersensitivity reactions to carboplatin administration are common but not always severe: a 10-year experience. Oncology 2001;61:129–133.
37. Larson RA, et al. Hypersensitivity reactions to L-asparaginase do not impact on the remission duration of adults with acute lymphoblastic leukemia. Leukemia 1998;12:660–665.
38. Brant JM. Rasburicase: an innovative new treatment for hyperuricemia associated with tumor lysis syndrome. Clin J Oncol Nurs 2002;6:12–16.
39. Krieger JA, et al. Implementation and results of a test dose program with taxanes. Cancer J 2002;8:337–341.
40. Porzio G, et al. Hypersensitivity reaction to carboplatin: successful resolution by replacement with cisplatin. Eur J Gynaecol Oncol 2002;4:335–336.
41. Heckler F. Current thoughts on extravasation injuries. Clin Plast Surg 1989;16:557–563.
42. Boyle D, et al. Vesicant extravasation: myths and realities. Oncol Nurs Forum 1995;22:57–67.

43. Richardson DS, et al. Anthracyclines in haematology: preclinical studies, toxicity, and delivery systems. Blood Rev 1997;11: 201–223.
44. Hood AF. Cutaneous side effects of cancer chemotherapy. Med Clin N Am 1986;70:187–208.
45. Bertelli G. Prevention and management of extravasation of cytotoxic drugs. Drug Saf 1995;12:245–255.
46. Scuderi N, et al. Antitumor agents: extravasation, management, and surgical treatment. Ann Plast Surg 1994;32:39–44.
47. Tsavaris N, et al. Prevention of tissue necrosis due to accidental extravasation of cytostatic drugs by a conservative approach. Cancer Chemother Pharmacol 1992;30:330–333.
48. Lang K, et al. Supravenous hyperpigmentation, transverse leukonychia and transverse melanonychia after chemotherapy for Hodgkins's disease. J Eur Acad Dermatol-Venereol 2002;16: 162–163.
49. Harrold BP, Syndrome resembling Addison's disease following prolonged treatment with busulfan. Br Med J 1966;1:463–464
50. Mutafoglu-Uysal, et al. Bleomycin-induced hyperpigmentation and hypersensitivity reactions to etoposide and vinblastine in a child with endodermal sinus tumor. Turkish J Pedatr 2001;43:172–174.
51. Marcoux D, et al. Persistent serpentine supravenous hyperpigmented eruption as an adverse reaction to chemotherapy combining actinomycin and vincristine. J Am Acad Dermatol 2000;43:540–546.
52. Al Lamki Z, et al. Localized cisplatin hyperpigmentation induced by pressure. Cancer (Phila) 1996;77:1578–1581.
53. Bastida J, et al. Chemotherapy-induced acral erythema due to tegafur. Acta Dermato-Venereol 1997;77:72–94.
54. Vargas-Diez E, et al. Chemotherapy-induced acral erytherma. Acta Dermato-Venereol 79:173–175.
55. Millot F, et al. Acral erythema in children receiving high-dose methotrexate. Pediatr Dermatol 1999;16:398–400.
56. Demircay Z, et al. Chemotherapy-induced acral erythema in leukemic patients: a report of 15 cases. Int J Dermatol 1997;35: 593–598.
57. Aractingi S, et al. Cutaneous graft versus host disease. Arch Dermatol 1998;134:602–612.
58. Hiscott A, et al. Graft versus host disease in allogeneic bone marrow transplantation: the role of monoclonal antibodies in prevention and treatment. Br J Biomed Sci 2000;57:163–169.
59. Foss FM, et al. Extracorporeal photopheresis in chronic graft versus host disease. Bone Marrow Transplant 2000;29:719–725.
60. Dickinson AM, et al. Predicting outcome in hematological stem cell transplantation. Arch Immunol Ther Exp 2002;50:371–378.
61. Wehrli P, et al. Death receptors in cutaneous biology and disease. J Invest Dermatol 2000;115:141–148.
62. Tsukada N, et al. Graft-versus-leukemia effect and graft-versus-host disease can be differentiated by cytotoxic mechanisms in a murine model of allogeneic bone marrow transplantation. Blood 1999;93:2738–2747.
63. Hattori K, et al. Differential effects of anti-Fas ligand and anti-tumor necrosis factor alpha antibodies on acute graft-versus-host disease pathologies. Blood 1998;91:4051–4055.
64. Miwa K, et al. Therapeutic effect of an anti-fas ligand mAb on lethal graft-versus-host disease. Int Immunol 1999;11:925–931.
65. Remberger M, et al. Treatment of severe acute graft versus host disease with anti-thymocyte globulin. Clin Transplantation, 2001;15:147–153.
66. Reisner Y, et al. Transplantation tolerance induced by "mega dose" cd34+ cell transplants. Exp Hematol 2000;28:119–127.
67. Ratanatharathorn V, et al. Chronic graft-versus-host disease: clinical manifestation and therapy. Bone Marrow Transplant 2001;28:121–129.
68. Ratanatharathorn V, et al. Phase III study comparing methotrexate and tacrolimus (prograf, fk506) with methotrexate and cyclosporine for graft versus-host disease prophylaxis after HLA-identical sibling bone marrow transplantation. Blood 1998;92: 2303–2314.
69. Nash RA, et al. Phase 3 study comparing methotrexate and tacrolimus with methotrexate and cyclosporine for prophylaxis of acute graft-versus-host disease after marrow transplantation from unrelated donors. Blood 2000;96:2062–2068.
70. Woo SB, et al. Graft-vs.-host disease. Crit Rev Oral Biol Med 1997;8:201–216.
71. DeLord C, et al. Vaginal stenosis following allogeneic bone marrow transplantation for acute myeloid leukaemia. Bone Marrow Transplant 1999;23:52–55.
72. Kami M, et al. Phimosis as a manifestation of chronic graft-versus-host disease after allogeneic bone marrow transplantation. Bone Marrow Transplant 1998;21:721–723.
73. Singhal S, et al. Oral pilocarpine hydrochloride for the treatment of refractory xerostomia associated with chronic graft-versus-host disease. Blood 1995;85:1147–1148.
74. Parker PM, et al. Thalidomide as salvage therapy for chronic graft-versus-host disease. Blood 1995;86:3604–3609.
75. Rovelli A, et al. The role of thalidomide in the treatment of refractory chronic graft-versus-host disease following bone marrow transplantation in children. Bone Marrow Transplant 1998;21:577–581.
76. Vogelsang GB, et al. Thalidomide for the treatment of chronic graft-versus-host disease. N Engl J Med 1992;326:1055–1058.
77. Gilman AL, et al. Hydroxychloroquine for the treatment of chronic graft versus host disease. Biol Blood Marrow Transplant 2000;6:327–334.
78. Enk CD, et al. Chronic graft-versus-host disease treated with UVB phototherapy. Bone Marrow Transplant 1998;22: 1179–1183.
79. Eriksson T, et al. Clinical pharmacology of thalidomide. Eur J Clin Pharmacol 2001;57:365–376.
80. Okafor MC. Thalidomide for erythema nodosum leprosum and other applications. Pharmacotherapy 2003;23:481–493.
81. Vogelsgang GB, et al. Treatment of chronic graft-versus-host disease with ultraviolet irradiation and psoralen (puva). Bone Marrow Transplant 1996;17:1061–1067.
82. Couriel DR, et al. Infliximab for the treatment of graft-versus-host disease in allogeneic transplant recipients: an update. Blood 2001;96:400a.
83. Chiang KY, et al. Recombinant human soluble tumor necrosis factor receptor fusion protein (enbrel) as a treatment for chronic graft-versus host disease (CGvHD) following allogeneic bone marrow transplantation. Blood 2001;96:401a.
84. Ratanatharanthorn V, et al. Anti-CD20 chimeric monoclonal antibody treatment of refractory immune-mediated thrombocytopenia in a patient with chronic graft-versus-host disease. Ann Intern Med 2000;133:275–279.
85. Wallenborn P, et al. Radiation recall supraglottitis: a hazard in head and neck chemotherapy. Arch Otolaryngol 1984;110: 614–617.
86. DeSpain JD. Dermatologic toxicity of chemotherapy. Semin Oncol 1992;19:501–507.
87. Kellie S, et al. Radiation recall and radiosensitization with alkylating agents. Lancet 1987;1:1149–1150.
88. Schweitzer V, et al. Radiation recall dermatitis and pneumonitis in a patient treated with paclitaxel. Cancer (Phila) 1995;76:1069–1072.
89. Perez E, et al. Radiation recall dermatitis induced by edatrexate in a patient with breast cancer. Cancer Invest 1995;13: 604–607.
90. Camidge, Ross, et al. Characterizing the phenomenon of radiation recall dermatitis. Radiother Oncol 2001;59:237–245.
91. Bostrom A, et al. Radiation recall: another call with tamoxifen. Acta Oncol 1999;38:955–959.

92. Extermann M, et al. Radiation recall in a patient with breast cancer treated for tuberculosis. Eur J Clin Pharmacol 1993;48: 77–78.
93. Yeo W, Johnson PJ. Radiation-recall skin disorders associated with the use of antineoplastic drugs: pathogenesis, prevalence and management. Am J Clin Dermatol 2000;2:113–116.
94. Potter T, et al. Cutaneous photosensitivity to medications. Comp Ther 1994;20:414–417.
95. Chren MM, et al. Rashes in immunocompromised cancer patients: the diagnostic yield of skin biopsy and its effects on therapy. Arch Dermatol 1993;129:175–181.

Infectious Complications of Cancer Therapy

Nasia Safdar, Christopher J. Crnich, and Dennis G. Maki

Advances in the management of cancer, particularly the development of new chemotherapeutic agents, have greatly improved the survival and outcome of patients with hematologic malignancies and solid tumors; overall 5-year survival rates in cancer patients have improved from 39% in the 1960s to 60% in the 1990s.[1] However, infection, caused by both the underlying malignancy and cancer chemotherapy, particularly myelosuppressive chemotherapy, remains a persistent challenge.[2]

Impairment of Immunity with Cancer and Treatment of Cancer

Infection occurs commonly during treatment of cancer; 80% of patients with acute leukemia, 40% to 60% of those with lung cancer, and 50% of those with lymphoma, develop an infection at some point in the course of the illness.[3] A number of factors account for the increased risk of infection in the cancer patient: poor nutritional status, mechanical obstruction by the tumor, breach of anatomic barriers by surgery, intravascular devices (IVDs), or mucositis caused by cytotoxic chemotherapy, and defects of humoral and cell-mediated immunity that are either disease associated or follow myelosuppressive chemotherapy (Table 76.1).

Granulocytes are the most critical component of the host innate defense against infection. Granulocytopenia is defined as a neutrophil count less than 500 cells/mm^3 or less than 1,000 cells/mm^3 with expected decrease to less than 500 cells/mm^3 within 48 hours, and it is the main immune defect of cancer patients following chemotherapy.[4]

The inverse relationship between the magnitude of granulocytopenia and subsequent infection was first delineated in the 1960s by Bodey et al., in patients with acute leukemia[5]: the incidence of infection was 14% if the absolute granulocyte count fell below 500 to 1,000/mm^3 and 24% to 60% if it fell below 100/mm^3 (Figure 76.1).[5] Prolonged granulocytopenia, especially a rapid decline in circulating granulocytes, also increases the risk of deep fungal infection.[5] Absolute granulocyte counts less than 500 cells/mm^3 for more than 10 days is now viewed as the threshold for a greatly increased risk of severe infection.[6] Common pathogens causing infection in granulocytopenia include a wide array of gram-negative and gram-positive bacteria, *Candida* species, and filamentous fungi, such as *Aspergillus* and *Fusarium*.[1]

In general, with the exception of lymphoproliferative malignancies, defects of humoral immunity are not seen in most patients with cancer. However, globulin dysfunction or depletion is common in chronic lymphocytic leukemia (CLL) and nearly universal in multiple myeloma, predisposing to invasive infection with encapsulated organisms, particularly *Streptococcus pneumoniae*.[7]

Impairment of cell-mediated immunity (CMI) occurs with selected chemotherapeutic agents, such as the purine analogues,[8] and has also been described with novel therapies for cancer, such as monoclonal antibodies. Pathogens typically associated with impaired CMI include *Pneumocystis jiroveci* (formerly *carinii*), the herpesviruses, especially cytomegalovirus (CMV) and varicella-zoster virus (VZV), and atypical mycobacteria, *Candida*, and *Nocardia*.

Infections Associated with Chemotherapeutic Agents

Purine Analogues

Purine analogues, particularly fludarabine, and to a lesser extent, cladribine (2-chlorodeoxyadenosine, 2-CdA) and pentostatin (2′-deoxycoformycin, 2′-DCF), are potent chemotherapeutic agents for the treatment of lymphoproliferative malignancies, such as CLL, Waldenstrom's macroglobulinemia, non-Hodgkin's lymphoma, T-cell leukemia, Sezary syndrome, and hairy cell leukemia (HCL). This class of drugs produces profound lymphocytopenia and a marked decrease in CD4 cells that can persist for several years following the discontinuation of treatment, which, in the case of fludarabine, has been associated with a high incidence of severe opportunistic infections, as high as 50% in some series, most occurring during the first 6 weeks of therapy.[8]

Early reports on the spectrum of infections associated with purine analogues emphasized, in addition to the usual bacterial pathogens causing infection in granulocytopenic patients, an increased incidence of infections caused by pathogens associated with impaired cell-mediated immunity (CMI), particularly *Listeria monocytogenes* and *Pneumocystis jiroveci (carinii)*, occurring most often in patients who were heavily pretreated with alkylating agents and may also have received concomitant corticosteroids. Invasive infections with opportunistic pathogens, such as *Nocardia*,

TABLE 76.1. Defects in host defense mechanisms and common infections associated with malignant diseases.

Disease	*Proportion (%) of patients developing infection*	*Predominant defect*	*Common infections*
Acute leukemia, aplastic anemia	80	Granulocytopenia	Gram-positive cocci, gram-negative bacilli, *Candida, Aspergillus, Fusarium, Trichosporon*
Hairy cell leukemia	60	Granulocytopenia, impaired lymphocyte function, monocytopenia	Gram-negative bacilli, gram-positive cocci, mycobacteria (including nontuberculous)
Chronic lymphatic leukemia, multiple myeloma	50	Hypogammaglobulinemia	*Streptococcus pneumoniae; Haemophilus influenzae; Neisseria meningitidis*
Hodgkin's disease	75	Impaired T-lymphocyte response	*Pneumocystis, Cryptococcus,* mycobacteria, *Toxoplasma, Listeria, Cryptosporidum, Candida,* cytomegalovirus
Bone marrow transplant recipient	90	Granulocytopenia, increased activity of suppressor T lymphocytes	Gram-positive cocci, gram-negative bacilli, cytomegalovirus, *Candida, Aspergillus,* other herpes viruses
Breast cancer	35	Tissue necrosis	Staphylococci and gram-negative bacilli
Lung cancer	46–62	Local obstruction, tissue necrosis	Gram-positive cocci, gram-negative bacilli, anaerobic bacteria
Gynecologic malignancy	25	Local obstruction, tissue necrosis	Mixed aerobic and anaerobic enteric bacteria

Source: Adapted from Rolston and Bodey,[1] by permission of *Cancer Medicine.*

Mycobacterium tuberculosis, and atypical mycobacteria and fungi have also been reported.[9] The most frequent late infection has been herpes zoster, both localized and disseminated, with a median time to onset following treatment of 7 to 8 months.[9]

Factors that further increase the risk of infection with purine analogue therapy include organ damage, such as severe mucositis, renal or hepatic failure, prior therapy with antineoplastic agents, advanced stage of underlying cancer, advanced age and poor performance status, pretreatment pancytopenia, high doses of purine analogue therapy, and failure of the cancer to respond to purine analogue therapy.[9]

Strategies suggested to prevent opportunistic infection in patients receiving purine analogue therapy include prophylaxis against *P. jiroveci (carinii).* No placebo-controlled trials have been conducted to address the issue; however, some authorities recommend trimethoprim-sulfamethoxazole (160/800mg by mouth) thrice weekly for 2 months following fludarabine therapy.[8]

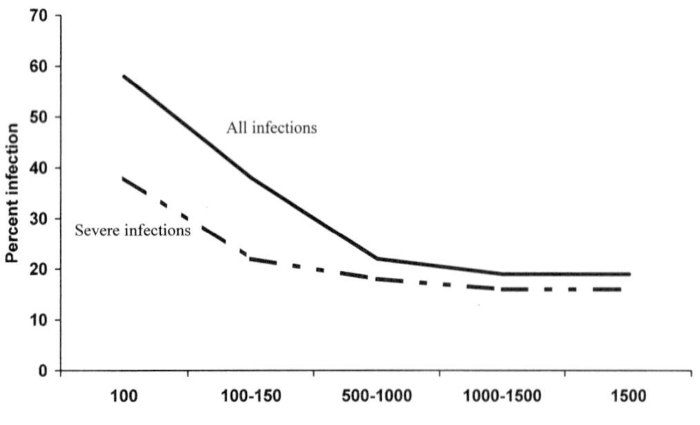

FIGURE 76.1. Relationship between granulocyte count and infection in patients with acute leukemia. The incidence of infection is inversely related to the level of circulating granulocytes. (Adapted from Bodey et al.,[5] by permission of *Annals of Internal Medicine.*)

Immunotherapy

Monoclonal antibodies are a new class of biologic anticancer agents targeted at specific receptors on tumor cells. Five monoclonal antibodies—rituximab, trastuzumab, gemtuzumab, ozagamicin, alemtuzumab, and ibritumonab tiuxetan—are in clinical trials with a variety of hematologic malignancies, especially lymphomas and solid tumors.[10] Infusion-related fever, chills, and hypotension may occur with any of the monoclonal antibodies. However, the incidence and microbiology of infections vary according to the cell line affected by the monoclonal antibody. The only commercially available monoclonal antibodies at the present time are rituximab (Rituxan), for the treatment of lymphoma and relapsed HCL, and alemtuzumab (Campath), for the treatment of CLL.

Rituximab, a chimeric monoclonal antibody, targets the B-cell antigen CD20, resulting in the depletion of peripheral B-lymphocyte counts by approximately 90% within 3 days; B-cell recovery occurs slowly, over 9 to 12 months. Mild transient reductions in granulocyte count may also be seen. Infections have been reported with the use of rituximab; however, the incidence of infections with rituximab appears to be no higher than that seen with conventional cytotoxic chemotherapy.[11]

Alemtuzumab is a chimeric monoclonal antibody that binds to the CD52 antigen. Because this antigen is present on the surface of all lymphocytes, alemtuzumab significantly depletes both B and T cells and is associated with infections caused by organisms similar to those seen with purine analogue therapy, including *P. jiroveci (carinii)* pneumonia and invasive infection caused by *Candida, Aspergillus,* VZV, and

TABLE 76.2. Bacterial infections in 4,452 febrile episodes in granulocytopenic cancer patients.

	1975–1977		*1986–1989*		*1994–1995*		*1999–2000*	
Infection type	*No.*	*(%)*	*No.*	*(%)*	*No.*	*(%)*	*No.*	*(%)*
Microbiologically documented	318	(31)	344	(27)	189	(28)	207	(30)
Gram-positive	65	(21)	170	(51)	86	(46)	99	(48)
Gram-negative	201	(63)	110	(33)	54	(28)	51	(25)
Polymicrobial	42	(13)	54	(16)	49	(26)	51	(25)
Anaerobic	10	—	—	—	—	—	—	—
Unexplained fever	481	(47)	644	(53)	373	(56)	390	(57)

Source: Adapted from Rolston and Bodey,[1] by permission of *Cancer Medicine.*

CMV. All patients receiving alemtuzumab should receive trimethoprim-sulfamethoxazole (TMP-SMZ) prophylaxis against *Pneumocystis carinii* pneumonia (PCP) and acyclovir for prevention of herpes simplex virus (HSV).

Myeloablative Chemotherapy and Bone Marrow Transplantation

An increasing number of cancers are now being treated with myeloablative chemotherapy, followed by autologous or allogeneic bone marrow transplantation.[12,13] The intense immunosuppression incurred by this approach, which involves high-dose cytotoxic chemotherapy and total-body irradiation, places the cancer patient at extremely high risk of infection. Typically, profound marrow suppression lasts 2 to 3 weeks until the newly infused marrow engrafts. Severe granulocytopenia and mucositis during this period, often necessitating parenteral nutrition, are major risk factors for infection. Gram-negative bacilli, fungi including *Candida* spp. and *Aspergillus*, herpesviruses, and CMV are the major pathogens causing invasive infection following bone marrow transplantation. In allogeneic bone marrow transplantation, well-conducted studies have shown that acyclovir, given prophylactically for 3 months, almost completely prevents an otherwise very high incidence of severe HSV mucosal infection.[14]

Infection in the Granulocytopenic Patient

General Considerations

Infection remains the most frequent life-threatening complication in patients with hematologic malignancies or solid tumors. Infection is the cause of death of 50% of patients with solid tumors and lymphomas and 75% of patients with leukemia.[15,16]

Microbiology

The epidemiology and microbiology of infections in patients with granulocytopenia and malignancy has undergone a shift from predominantly gram-negative bacilli in the 1960s and 1970s, to a preponderance of gram-positive organisms in more recent years[17] (Table 76.2). Between 30% and 50% of febrile episodes in granulocytopenic patients can be confirmed microbiologically, and of these, most represent bacteremia.[6] Causes of fever in the granulocytopenic patient are shown in Figure 76.2.[18]

The emergence of gram-positive bacteria as pathogens in patients with granulocytopenia is most striking for bloodstream infections (BSIs) (see Table 76.2).[19] This dramatic shift in the ecology of invasive infection reflects greatly increased use of IVDs for long-term access, the wide use of antibiotic prophylaxis against gram-negative infections, most often with TMP-sulfa or fluoroquinolones, intense antineoplastic therapy, which produces severe mucositis, and initiation of broad-spectrum empiric antiinfective therapy at the first sign of fever in the cancer patient.

Nevertheless, gram-negative bacilli continue to be associated with major morbidity and mortality in granulocytopenic patients, and the emergence of strains highly resistant to multiple antibiotics, such as *Acinetobacter* spp., *Stenotrophomonas maltophilia*, and *Alcaligenes xylosoxidans*, is of great concern. Resistance in all nosocomial gram-negative bacilli is increasing: data from the U.S. Centers for Disease Control and Prevention, show that nosocomial infections in intensive care unit (ICU) patients caused by gram-

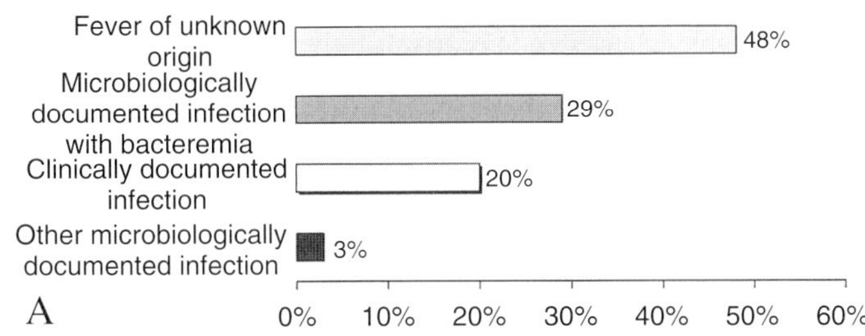

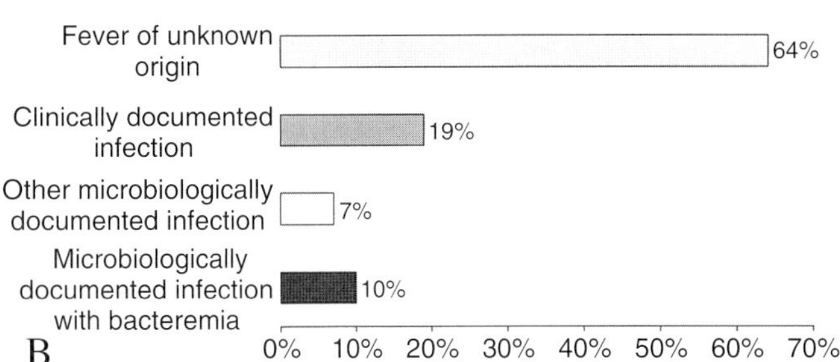

FIGURE 76.2. (A, B) Causes of fever in granulocytopenic patients with hematologic malignancies or solid tumors. Data derived from four consecutive European Organization for Research and Treatment of Cancer studies between 1991 and 2000, and from a North American Study conducted between 1992 and 1997.[212,293,294,303,304] [By permission of Marchetti O, Calandra T. Infections in the neutropenic cancer patient. In: Cohen J, Powderly WG (eds) Infectious Diseases, 2nd ed. St. Louis: Mosby, 2004:1083.]

negative bacilli resistant to third-generation cephalosporins, have risen to 32.2% of all *Enterobacter* infections and 14% of all *Klebsiella pneumoniae* infections.[20]

Moreover, new and emerging pathogens, such as *Chryseobacterium meningosepticum*, *Aeromonas* spp., *Fusobacterium nucleatum*, *Burkholderia cepacia*, *Roseomonas*, *Agrobacterium radiobacter*, and *Sphingomonas paucimobilis*, many of which are associated with significant attributable mortality, are being increasingly encountered in granulocytopenic patients.[21] The major pathogens that cause infection in granulocytopenic cancer patients are shown in Table 76.3.

Major Bacterial Pathogens in Patients with Granulocytopenia

Enterobacteriaceae

Enterobacteriaceae are the leading gram-negative pathogens implicated in bacteremia in granulocytopenic patients. Although in recent years the overall frequency of gram-negative infections has declined, the proportion of gram-negative infections caused by *Enterobacteriaceae* has remained remarkably unchanged. Data from several surveillance studies show that *Enterobacteriaceae* cause 65% to 80% of documented gram-negative infections in cancer patients, with *Escherichia coli* and *Klebsiella pneumoniae* most commonly isolated. The bloodstream is the most frequent site of infection, followed by the urinary tract and the lung.

TABLE 76.3. The most common pathogens in granulocytopenic cancer patients.

Gram-positive aerobic bacteria
- Coagulase-negative staphylococci[a]
- Viridans streptococci[a]
- *Staphylococcus aureus*[a]
- Other streptococci (*Streptococcus pneumoniae, Streptococcus pyogenes*)[a]
- *Enterococcus* spp.[a]
- *Corynebacterium jeikeium*[a]
- *Bacillus* spp.
- *Listeria monocytogenes*

Gram-negative aerobic bacteria
- *Enterobacteriaceae*
  - *Escherichia coli*[a]
  - *Klebsiella* spp.[a]
  - *Enterobacter*
  - Other (*Proteus, Serratia, Citrobacter* spp.)
- *Pseudomonas aeruginosa*[a]
- *Legionella* spp.

Anaerobic bacteria
- *Bacteroides* spp.
- *Clostridium* spp.
- *Fusobacterium* spp.
- *Propionibacterium* spp.

Fungi
- *Candida* spp.
- *Aspergillus* spp.
- Other molds (*Fusarium, Pseudoallescheria boydii, Scedosporium*, Mucorales)

Viruses
- Herpes simplex
- Varicella-zoster
- Respiratory viruses (influenza, respiratory syncytial virus)

Parasites
- *Strongyloides stercoralis*

[a]Common causes of bacteremia.

The recent widespread emergence of resistance to beta-lactams, mediated by inducible and extended-spectrum beta-lactamases, poses a major problem.[22] Risk factors for infection caused by an extended-spectrum beta-lactamase-producing organism, include exposure to broad-spectrum cephalosporins, prolonged hospitalization, invasive devices, and immunocompromised state.[23] Although the majority of infections caused by *Enterobacteriaceae* can yet be treated with standard therapy, most often, a third-generation cephalosporin or a fluoroquinolone, a carbapenem should be used if infection with an extended-spectrum beta-lactamase-producing organism is suspected or confirmed.[24]

Pseudomonas Aeruginosa

Historically, *Pseudomonas aeruginosa* has been the leading cause of life-threatening invasive infection and bacteremia in the granulocytopenic cancer patient.[25] In recent years, however, the incidence of bacteremia caused by *P. aeruginosa* has declined. A recent large retrospective cohort study of *P. aeruginosa* bacteremia in a cancer hospital, found that the incidence of BSI fell from 4.7 to 2.1 per 1,000 admissions in 1991 to 1995; however, no decline was noted in patients with acute leukemia, and *P. aeruginosa* accounted for 15% to 20% of gram-negative infections in leukemic patients.[26]

Pseudomonas aeruginosa rarely causes serious infection in the normal host but is capable of causing devastating, invasive disease if host defenses are breached by mucositis or myelosuppression from chemotherapy or the underlying malignancy, IVDs, or other invasive devices. However, the most important risk factor for life-threatening *P. aeruginosa* infection in patients with cancer is granulocytopenia.[26,27]

Pseudomonas aeruginosa causes a wide spectrum of infections in the granulocytopenic patient. Pneumonia and bacteremia are most common, but involvement of the urinary tract and skin also occurs. Skin lesions are present in approximately 20% of cancer patients with bacteremia. Ecthyma grangrenosum, the classic skin lesion historically associated with *P. aeruginosa* in patients with granulocytopenia, occurs most commonly in the axilla, groin, and perianal region[28] (Figure 76.3). Histologically, these lesions show a septic vasculitis with dense bacillary infiltration of the blood vessel walls. *P. aeruginosa* septicemia may also be associated with subcutaneous nodules, deep abscesses, cellulitis, vesicular or pustular lesions, bullae, or necrotizing fasciitis.[29]

In general, treatment of *P. aeruginosa* sepsis represents a formidable challenge, because of the intrinsic resistance of the organism to most antimicrobials, and the capacity to rapidly develop resistance during therapy. Factors associated with an unfavorable outcome include persistent neutropenia, especially an absolute granulocyte count of less than 100 cells/mm^3, septic shock, lung, skin, or soft tissue involvement, or unidentified source, renal failure, metastatic foci, rapidly or ultimately fatal underlying disease, and inappropriate antibiotic therapy.[26,27,30] Most studies have found a higher mortality rate among patients with *P. aeruginosa* bacteremia compared with other bacteremias.[26,27] It is not clear to what extent a higher mortality rate reflects the more severe underlying illnesses affecting patients susceptible to

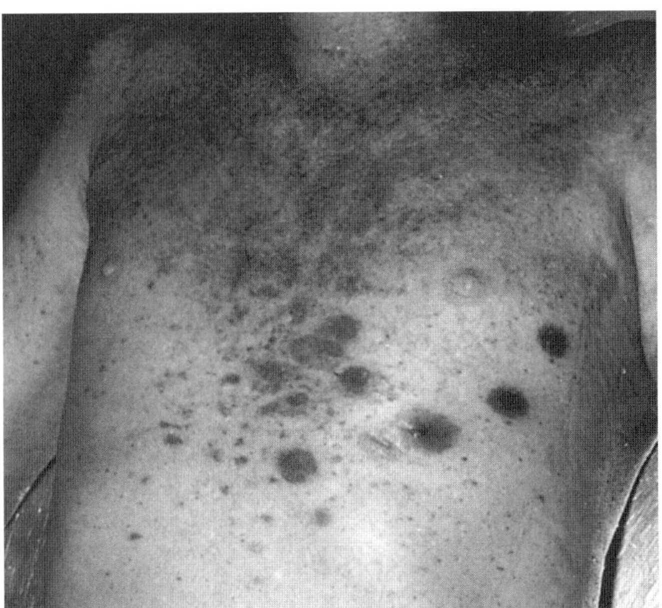

FIGURE 76.3. Classic ecthyma gangrenosum secondary to *Pseudomonas aeruginosa* infection. [By permission of Fekety R. External manifestations of systemic infections. In: Mandell GL (ed). Essential Atlas of Infectious Diseases for Primary Care. Current Medicine, vol. 1. Philadelphia: Churchill-Livingstone, 1997:45.]

Pseudomonas bacteremia as contrasted with the greater inherent virulence of the organism.

It is absolutely essential that empiric antimicrobial therapy for granulocytopenic patients with fever always include a drug or drugs active against *P. aeruginosa*. The number and choice of antibiotics in this setting are controversial, however. In a recent meta-analysis of five studies of *P. aeruginosa* bacteremia, mortality was reduced with combination therapy [relative risk (RR), 0.65; *P* less than 0.05].[31] The conventional approach to presumptive therapy in the face of granulocytopenia, or other settings in which *Pseudomonas* is a potential pathogen, is to combine treatment with an aminoglycoside or fluoroquinolone plus an extended-spectrum antipseudomonal penicillin (e.g., piperacillin-tazobactam or ticarcillin-clavulanate) or antipseudomonal cephalosporin (ceftazidime or cefepime) or a carbapenem (imipenem or meropenem). The specific choice of agents should be guided by institutional antibiotic susceptibility patterns and guidelines. Although the subject of intense debate, cohort studies and a recent meta-analysis suggest that, in patients with *P. aeruginosa* sepsis, there is a survival advantage with combination therapy as contrasted with treatment with one antimicrobial to which the infecting strain is susceptible.[31]

Staphylococcal Infections

Coagulase-negative staphylococci have emerged as major pathogens in granulocytopenic patients; two large multicenter studies in patients with hematologic malignancy or solid tumor, identified coagulase-negative staphylococci to be the most common cause of bacteremia in granulocytopenic cancer patients.[19] This increase in incidence clearly reflects an ever increasing use of long-term IVDs in this population.

Although widely regarded as organisms of low virulence, recent studies have shown that infections caused by coagulase-negative staphylococci are associated with considerable morbidity and mortality in immunocompromised patients.[32] Primary bacteremia is the major site of infection; complications, such as abscesses and septic phlebitis, have been well described.

Virtually all *Staphylococcus epidermidis* infections are health care associated and most are multiresistant, reflecting the selection pressure of widespread antibiotic use in that setting. Vancomycin remains the mainstay of therapy for coagulase-negative bacteremia.

Staphylococcus aureus is still a major pathogen causing intravascular device-related (IVDR) BSI in granulocytopenic patients and is associated with severe morbidity and mortality. Metastatic infection to distant sites, particularly endocarditis, always poses a threat. In the healthcare setting, approximately 50% of *S. aureus* isolates are resistant to methicillin (MRSA).[33] Until recently, vancomycin was the only available treatment for MRSA; however, recently, two new antimicrobials, linezolid and daptomycin, have been approved for treatment of MRSA infections. In two large randomized trials, linezolid has been shown to reduce mortality from MRSA pneumonia in ICU patients.[34] The optimal duration of therapy for *S. aureus* uncomplicated or complicated bacteremia has not been studied thus far; in most instances, a prolonged course (4–6 weeks) of parenteral antimicrobial therapy is desirable for complicated *S. aureus* bacteremia. An echocardiogram to rule out endocarditis in *S. aureus* bacteremia is highly recommended to determine whether prolonged therapy is necessary, as discussed next.

Alpha-Hemolytic (Viridans) Streptococci

Viridans streptococci have become increasingly important pathogens in cancer patients, particularly, patients with acute leukemia undergoing intensive chemotherapy and allogeneic bone marrow transplant recipients; *Streptococcus mitis*, *Streptococcus sanguis*, and *Streptococcus salivarius* are the predominant infecting species.[35–37] Viridans streptococci are now a leading cause of bacteremia in febrile, neutropenic patients. At the M.D. Anderson Cancer Center in Houston, the incidence of streptococcal bacteremia increased from 1 case per 10,000 admissions in 1972 to 47 per 10,000 in 1989.

A number of studies have examined risk factors for viridans streptococcal bacteremia in patients with cancer.[36–38] Bacteremia usually occurs in association with aggressive cytoreductive therapy for acute leukemia or allogeneic bone marrow transplantation, especially after treatment with high-dose cytosine arabinoside.[39] In a case-controlled study, the risk of viridans streptococcal bacteremia was reported to increase with profound neutropenia, prophylactic administration of trimethoprim-sulfamethoxazole or a fluoroquinolone, and use of antacids or histamine type 2 (H_2) receptor antagonists (e.g., cimetidine).[36] Another risk factor strongly implicated is the presence of mucositis[38,40,41]; in one noncomparative study of 32 patients, 78% had oral inflammation or ulceration at the onset of infection.[40] Bostrom and Weisdorf reported an association of viridans streptococcal bacteremia with an increased radiation dose to the oral cavity,[42] whereas Ringden and colleagues described an association with herpes simplex infection[43]; prophylactic acyclovir reduced the frequency of all bacteremias following allogeneic bone marrow transplantation.

Although the most common clinical presentation of viridans streptococcal infection in patients with cancer is primary bacteremia, in many patients, the infection is fulminant, producing septic shock and acute respiratory distress syndrome (ARDS) akin to toxic shock syndrome, resulting in a 25% to 35% mortality, despite prompt and appropriate antimicrobial therapy.[44,45]

Also of great concern is the fact that 20% to 60% of alpha-hemolytic streptococci now exhibit high-level penicillin resistance in some centers.[46,47] All these strains remain susceptible to vancomycin, although tolerance to glycopeptides has been described, and the use of antibiotic combinations, such as vancomycin plus rifampin, with or without gentamicin, may be needed to control infections caused by resistant strains.[35]

Enterococci

Enterococcal infections, distinctly uncommon in cancer patients until the mid-1970s, are now the second most common gram-positive species, after coagulase-negative staphylococci, isolated from granulocytopenic patients. Their increased frequency almost certainly derives from the very heavy use of cephalosporins over the past 25 years, drugs to which all enterococci are intrinsically resistant. The most common infections caused by enterococci are bacteremias, urinary tract infections, and postoperative surgical site infections; endocarditis is seen only rarely in patients being treated for cancer.[48] *Enterococcus faecalis* is the predominant species, accounting for 75% to 80% of enterococcal infections; however, infections caused by *Enterococcus faecium* are rapidly rising. This finding is of great concern, because 25% of all enterococcal isolates in U.S. hospitals are now resistant to vancomycin, and most of the vancomycin-resistant strains are *E. faecium*.[49] In the setting of granulocytopenia, bacteremia with vancomycin-resistant enterococci (VRE) has been associated with mortality greater than 70%.[50]

Major Infectious Syndromes in the Granulocytopenic Patient

Numerous studies have shown that infection can be clinically or microbiologically documented in only 50% of patients with granulocytopenia and fever.[51] A large multicenter study from 1985 to 1990 found, in 1,573 patients with granulocytopenic fever, that pulmonary infections were most frequent (17%), followed by BSI and fungemia; in only 5% of cases was an infection clinically and microbiologically diagnosed. The response to treatment was significantly poorer in documented infections than in unexplained fever, with the worse outcomes for pulmonary infections (crude mortality, 21%).

Perianal Infection

Perianal infections occur in 10% to 25% of patients with leukemia undergoing chemotherapy and are associated with a 15% to 35% mortality.[52] Most patients with perirectal infection have underlying hematologic malignancy, although the incidence of these infections appears to be increasing in patients with solid tumors, probably because of more intensive myelosuppressive chemotherapy. Although fever is near universal, the predominant local presenting symptom is rectal pain; fewer than half of the patients, however, have frank fluctuance or drainage. Because hypotension or septic shock occurs in 10% of patients, a high index of suspicion for this condition is essential.

The majority of anorectal infections are caused by gram-negative bacilli, particularly, *P. aeruginosa* and *E. coli*; the role of anaerobes is much less clear (Table 76.4). Computed tomography (CT) imaging should be performed to ascertain

TABLE 76.4. Major infectious disease syndromes in patients with granulocytopenia.

Syndrome	*Microbial etiology*	*Differential diagnosis*	*Diagnostic tests*
Skin and soft tissue infection			
Perirectal infection	*Pseudomonas aeruginosa* *Aeromonas* spp.		Clinical; computed tomography to determine extent of infection
Complicated cellulitis	Staphylococci, streptococci, gram-negative bacilli		Percutaneous aspirate, biopsy; computed tomography
Pulmonary infections	*P. aeruginosa, Klebsiella, Escherichia coli, Enterobacteriaceae, Streptococcus pneumoniae, Staphylococcus aureus, Aspergillus, Fusarium, Mucor*	Aspiration Pulmonary edema Pulmonary embolus Atelectasis Alveolar hemorrhage Acute respiratory distress syndrome Pulmonary toxicity from chemotherapy	Chest radiograph, high-resolution computed tomography, sputum stains and cultures, bronchoalveolar lavage, biopsy if platelet count permits
Granulocytopenic typhlitis	Gram-negative bacilli	*C. difficile* infection	Plain films and computed tomography of abdomen
Intravascular device-related BSI	Coagulase-negative staphylococci, *S. aureus*, enterococci	Sepsis from another source	Paired quantitative or qualitative blood cultures
Antibiotic-associated colitis	*Clostridium difficile*	Typhlitis Peritonitis	Stool toxin A and B; cytotoxin B; flexible sigmoidoscopy
Oropharyngeal-esophageal mucositis	Herpes simplex *Candida* spp.	Aphthous ulceration	Biopsy, culture for herpes simplex virus (HSV) and *Candida*

BSI, bloodstream infection.

the extent of necrotic tissue and inflammation. Combination regimens with antipseudomonal drugs should be administered, including an agent with activity against anaerobic bacteria. Surgical intervention should be considered only if the disease progresses despite adequate antimicrobial therapy. With simple cellulitis, without fluctuance or abscess, most patients will do well without surgical debridement, if granulocyte function is returning or can be anticipated to return in the immediate future. The occurrence of severe gram-negative soft tissue infection in patients with refractory profound granulocytopenia may be an indication for allogeneic granulocyte transfusion therapy to keep the infection under control until granulocyte function returns. The main predictor of improvement is recovery of granulocyte function.

Patients with fissures or hemorrhoids should undergo fissurectomy or hemorrhoidectomy when their malignancy is in remission; failure to do so will result in an increased risk of perianal infection with myelosuppression.[52]

Other Skin and Soft Tissue Infections

Skin infections in patients with cancer may also occur secondary to necrotic tumor masses, postoperative wound infection, extravasation of vesicant drugs, infected IVDs, folliculitis, infected pressure ulcers, or as a manifestation of systemic bacteremic infection. Bacterial cellulitis in granulocytopenic patients is most often caused by staphylococci or streptococci, the leading causes of cellulitis in immunocompetent patients. However, gram-negative bacilli, such as *P. aeruginosa*, which rarely cause de novo skin and soft tissue infection in normal hosts, commonly cause severe soft tissue infections in the granulocytopenic patient.

Antineoplastic therapy makes cancer patients more vulnerable to necrotizing soft tissue infections, "necrotizing fascitis," which may involve underlying muscle. These infections are usually polymicrobial, caused by gram-positive bacteria, gram-negative bacilli, and anaerobic organisms. Bacteremia occurs in up to 40% of cases.[53] In contrast to uncomplicated monomicrobial gram-negative cellulitis in the granulocytopenic patient, which can usually be managed nonsurgically, with necrotizing polymicrobial soft tissue infections, early surgical debridement is imperative to avert otherwise very high mortality.[54]

Any soft tissue inflammation occurring in patients at risk for complex cellulitis must be vigorously evaluated diagnostically, at the minimum with Gram stain and culture of percutaneous aspirates or biopsies[55]; in most cases, the Gram stain will show the infecting organisms. If a grayish hue or frank necrosis is seen or gas is present in the deep tissues on radiographic examination, surgical debridement is imperative at the outset.

Intraabdominal Infections

Focal enterocolitis (typhlitis) is a life-threatening condition occurring primarily in granulocytopenic patients.[56] Although the pathogenesis is poorly understood, mucosal injury by cytotoxic drugs in the setting of profound granulocytopenia is thought to foster microbial invasion of the bowel wall, leading to necrosis. The cecum is almost always affected but the infection may involve the entire colon. This infection is assumed to be polymicrobial; however, the presence of *Clostridium septicum*, in association with typhlitis, has been described.[57]

Typhlitis must be considered in the differential diagnosis of any profoundly granulocytopenic patient (absolute granulocyte count less than 500/μL) who presents with fever and abdominal pain, usually in the right lower quadrant. More than 60% of patients have bloody diarrhea; two-thirds develop gram-negative bacteremia. Peritoneal signs and shock suggest full-thickness necrosis with perforation of the bowel wall. Stomatitis and pharyngitis, suggesting widespread mucositis, may be present. Symptoms typically appear 10 to 14 days after cytotoxic chemotherapy, at a time when granulocytopenia is most profound and the patient is febrile.

Computed tomography is the preferred diagnostic modality; findings include presence of a fluid-filled dilated and distended cecum, diffuse cecal wall thickening, or the presence of intramural edema, air, or hemorrhage; localized perforation with free air or a soft tissue mass, suggesting abscess formation, may also be seen.[58] Other diagnoses to be excluded, include appendicitis, cholecystitis, intraabdominal abscess, pseudomembranous colitis, and Ogilvie's syndrome (colonic pseudoobstruction). In patients with uncomplicated typhlitis, that is, without peritonitis, perforation, or bleeding, nonsurgical management, with combination antimicrobial therapy, bowel rest, nasogastric suction, and IV fluids, is usually effective if there is a return of granulocyte function; in one study, 70% of affected patients survived with medical therapy alone.[59]

Surgical intervention is reserved for patients with generalized peritonitis, free perforation, persistent gastrointestinal bleeding despite correction of coagulopathy, or clinical deterioration despite medical treatment. If surgery is necessary, a two-stage right hemicolectomy is preferred, and further chemotherapy should be delayed until recovery. Resection of all necrotic tissue is essential; incomplete removal of necrotic tissue is almost always fatal.[56]

Pulmonary Infections

Pulmonary infiltrates occur in 15% to 25% of all patients with profound granulocytopenia following intensive chemotherapy.[60] In approximately two-thirds of cases, they become apparent within the first 5 days after the onset of fever. Pulmonary infections in granulocytopenic patients are associated with the highest mortality and remain a formidable challenge, diagnostically and therapeutically.[60] Noninfectious causes of pulmonary infiltrates that mimic infectious pneumonitis include aspiration, alveolitis, fluid overload, alveolar hemorrhage, malignant infiltration, and pneumonitis caused by chemotherapy or radiotherapy. Although pneumonia has become less frequent in patients with granulocytopenia because of earlier initiation of empiric antibiotic therapy with the onset of fever, gram-negative pneumonia is still common, although there has been an increased incidence of gram-positive pneumonia caused by *Streptococcus pneumoniae*, viridans streptococci, and *Staphylococcus aureus*.[61] Pneumonia caused by viridans streptococci has been encountered most commonly in patients with severe oropharyngeal mucositis following chemotherapy with high-dose ARA-C.[35] Hematogenous pneumonia occurs in 3% to 31% of patients with bacteremia, whereas a fatal ARDS syndrome is noted with about the same incidence.

Accurate microbiologic diagnosis of pneumonia poses the greatest challenge to optimal management. In 20% to 30% of patients with gram-positive and gram-negative bacteremia, there is radiographic evidence of pneumonia, and it is usually assumed to be caused by the same organisms causing bacteremia; this is not necessarily the case, particularly with bacteremia caused by bacteria, such as enterococci, coagulase-negative staphylococci, *Bacillus* species, or *Corynebacterium jeikium*, which rarely cause pneumonia. Conventional chest radiographs show pulmonary infiltrates in less than 10% of patients who remain febrile despite antibacterial therapy, whereas CT, particularly the use of high-resolution scans, shows lung infiltrates in 50% of these patients.[62] Microbiologic diagnosis is based on blood cultures and cultures of specimens obtained by bronchoscopy or bronchoalveolar lavage. However, the role of invasive diagnostic procedures in granulocytopenic patients remains controversial; moreover, many bronchoscopists are reluctant to perform bronchoscopy, especially transbronchial biopsy, in patients with severe thrombocytopenia. During the past decade, molecular diagnostic methods have become available for the diagnosis of pneumonia caused by *S. pneumoniae*, *Aspergillus*, and *Legionella*.[63] However, the predictive value of these tests in patients with granulocytopenia and pneumonia has not been adequately characterized at this time.

The initial step in the management of a patient with a focal infiltrate early in the granulocytopenic period begins with early intensive empiric antimicrobial therapy, providing coverage for gram-positive and gram-negative pathogens. In institutions where MRSA is a common pathogen in granulocytopenic patients, the initial regimen should include vancomycin or linezolid.[34] In our institution, a fourth-generation cephalosporin (cefepime), combined with a fluoroquinolone, is most often used, but a carbapenem is also acceptable. Patients who are clinically stable and have a small infiltrate may be observed for 48 hours. If the chest radiograph is suggestive of fluid overload, a trial of diuretics may be given, but continued observation of diffuse infiltrates is not recommended, as rapid clinical deterioration tends to occur when the problem is diffuse pneumonitis.[64]

If rapid clinical improvement does not ensue, and the infiltrate has not changed, the patient may continue to be observed on therapy, and follow-up pulmonary imaging should be considered. If the infiltrate progresses on antimicrobial therapy, more aggressive diagnostic procedures are strongly recommended, preferably fiberoptic bronchoscopy with bronchoalveolar lavage (BAL).[64]

In many centers, if no improvement is noted after 5 to 7 days of antibiotics, empiric therapy with amphotericin B is started. In general, fungal infections are rarely documented before the patient has received at least 5 days of therapy.

Finally, if an infiltrate appears during antimicrobial or antifungal therapy, the approach needs to be modified in favor of an early bronchoscopy because of the high likelihood of infection caused by a fungus or a bacteria resistant to the empiric therapy, or another process altogether, such as viral pneumonitis or a noninfectious process.

In a large prospective study conducted by the Paul Ehrlich Society, supplementation of antibiotics with amphotericin B in all persistently febrile granulocytopenic patients with pulmonary lung infiltrates resulted in a favorable response rate of 78%.[65] This finding has led to the recommendation that empiric treatment with amphotericin B should be given early for all febrile granulocytopenic patients with pulmonary infiltrates, especially if there is not an early clinical response to empiric antimicrobial therapy.

Clostridium Difficile-Associated Diarrhea

Clostridium difficile is the major infectious cause of nosocomial diarrhea[66] and is associated with prolonged hospitalization and increased hospital costs.[67] The incidence of infection with this organism is increasing in hospitals worldwide as a result of the widespread use of broad-spectrum antibiotics, with reported rates ranging from 1 to 10 cases per 1,000 discharges and 17 to 60 cases per 100,000 bed-days.[68]

Patients with hematologic malignancies are at particularly high risk of developing *C. difficile*-associated diarrhea, and outbreaks have been reported.[69–71] The majority of these patients receive antimicrobial therapy; mucositis and surgical procedures also increase risk.[23] Studies have also implicated chemotherapeutic agents as independent risk factors for *C. difficile*-associated diarrhea, even in the absence of antibiotic therapy, presumably because of alteration of the normal bowel flora and extensive mucosal inflammation caused by chemotherapy, facilitating colonization by *C. difficile*.[71] A recent case-control study in hematology and oncology patients showed that antineoplastic therapy was associated with a fivefold-greater risk of developing *C. difficile* colitis [adjusted odds ratio (OR) 5.1; $P = 0.01$].[72]

Clostridium difficile infection encompasses a spectrum of conditions ranging from asymptomatic colonization to fulminant disease with toxic megacolon.[73] The usual presentation is acute watery diarrhea with lower abdominal pain and fever occurring during or shortly after beginning antimicrobial therapy. The antibiotics that most predispose to *C. difficile* infection are third- or fourth-generation cephalosporins, clindamycin, and penicillins[74]; however, virtually any antimicrobial may trigger *C. difficile* infection.

Diagnosis of *C. difficile*-associated diarrhea can be reliably made by detection of *C. difficile* toxins A and/or B by enzyme-linked immunosorbent assay (ELISA) in a stool sample.[75] If this test is negative and *C. difficile* infection is strongly suspected, then cytotoxin testing, widely regarded as the reference standard, should be performed. This test, although 94% to 100% sensitive and 99% specific, takes at least 48 to 72 hours before results are available. In severely ill patients, flexible sigmoidoscopy provides a rapid means of diagnosis, because 90% of cases of pseudomembranous colitis involve the left side of the colon; the visualization of colonic pseudomembranes is essentially pathognomonic for *C. difficile* infection (Figure 76.4). CT of the abdomen, although useful for identifying bowel wall thickness, does not differentiate between *C. difficile* and other causes of bowel wall thickening, such as ischemic colitis.[76]

The most important step in the treatment of *C. difficile* is discontinuation of the culpable antimicrobial, if possible; in approximately 25% of cases of antibiotic-associated diarrhea, this will prove sufficient to resolve the infection. However, discontinuation may not always be possible in a profoundly granulocytopenic patient who is infected or febrile. Modification of the regimen to exclude drugs with

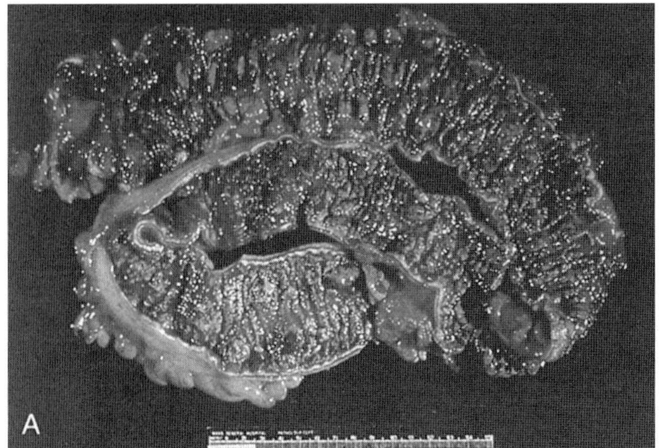

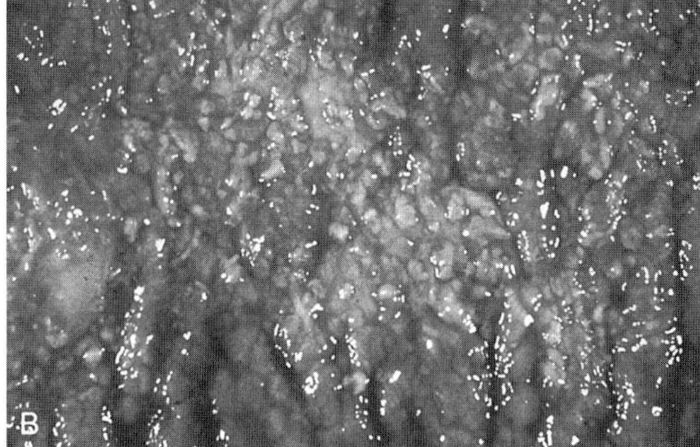

FIGURE 76.4. (A, B) Diffuse hemorrhagic colitis is seen in the resected colon. (B) Closeup reveals the diffuse mucosal irregularity and pseudomembrane formation seen with *Clostridium difficile* infection. [By permission of Stone DR, Gorbach SL (eds) Atlas of Infectious Diseases. Philadelphia: Saunders, 2000.]

unnecessary antianaerobic activity is strongly recommended if antimicrobials cannot be discontinued.

Oral metronidazole in a dose of 500mg three times daily for 7 to 10 days is the treatment of choice for symptomatic *C. difficile* infection; vancomycin given orally should be restricted to patients who fail to respond to metronidazole or who have had relapses.[77] In critically ill patients unable to take oral medications, intravenous metronidazole should be given in conjunction with vancomycin given either by intracolonic instillation or by enema.[78] *C. difficile* colitis cannot be treated with an agent that fails to achieve high intraluminal concentrations; vancomycin given intravenously is ineffective. In most clinical situations, it is not necessary to repeat stool toxin assays in patients who are responding satisfactorily to therapy.

Clostridium difficile has now become a major nosocomial pathogen widely prevalent in healthcare institutions, and control of nosocomial transmission is also essential. A growing body of literature suggests that the inanimate environment may contribute to nosocomial transmission of *C. difficile*. Commonly used hospital disinfectants are not germicidal against *C. difficile* spores, which may persist for very prolonged periods on surfaces. A recent before–after study using sodium hypochlorite solution to disinfect a bone marrow transplant ward found that rates of *C. difficile* infection decreased from 8.3 per 1,000 patient-days to 3.4 per 1,000 patient-days; when hypochlorite disinfection was discontinued, rates rose to the baseline level.[79]

The Society for Healthcare Epidemiology of America has published a guideline for prevention and treatment of *C. difficile* infections (Table 76.5).[80] Patients with *C. difficile* should be placed in private rooms and gowns and gloves should be worn for all contacts with the patient. Hand hygiene with an antiseptic agent is essential. It is important to note that alcohol-based handrubs do *not* have activity against the spore form of *C. difficile*. Equipment, such as stethoscopes and sphygmomanometers, should be dedicated to the patient, and the environment should be terminally disinfected with an agent active against spores, such as sodium hypochlorite.

Intravascular Device-Related Bloodstream Infection

The use of IVDs has become an essential component of care to patients with cancer. Unfortunately, vascular access is associated with substantial and generally underappreciated potential for producing iatrogenic disease, particularly BSI originating from infection of the percutaneous device used for vascular access. Nearly 40% of all nosocomial bacteremias derive from vascular access in some form[81] and are associated with excess mortality,[82] increased length of hospitalization, and excess healthcare costs.[83] Different types of IVDs pose widely ranging risks of infection (Table 76.6).[84]

Figure 76.5 summarizes the microbial profile of IVD-related BSIs from 159 published prospective studies.[85] As might be expected from knowledge of the pathogenesis of these infections, skin microorganisms account for the largest proportion of IVDR BSIs.

Recent evidence-based guidelines provide the best current information on the evaluation of the ICU patient with fever or other signs of sepsis (Table 76.7).[86] Before any decision regarding initiation of antimicrobial therapy or removal of an IVD, the patient must be thoroughly examined to identify *all* plausible sites of nosocomial infection, including pneumonia, urinary tract infection, surgical site infection, or antibiotic-associated colitis, as well as line sepsis.

Despite the challenge of identifying the source of a patient's signs of sepsis,[86] several clinical, epidemiologic, and microbiologic findings point strongly toward an IVD as the source of a fever: patients with abrupt onset of signs and symptoms of sepsis without any other identifiable source should prompt suspicion of infection of an IVD; the presence of inflammation or purulence at the catheter insertion site is now uncommon in patients with IVDR BSI[87]; however, if purulence is seen, it is highly likely the patient has IVDR BSI, and this finding should prompt removal of the IVD. Finally, recovery of certain microorganisms in multiple blood cultures, such as staphylococci, *Corynebacterium* or *Bacillus* species, or *Candida* or *Malassezia* species, strongly suggests infection of the IVD.[81]

TABLE 76.5. Recommendations for prevention and treatment of *Clostridium difficile*-associated diarrhea (CDAD) in the healthcare institution.

Recommendation	*Strength of recommendation*[a]
Surveillance and diagnosis	
Surveillance for CDAD should be performed in every institution	B-III
Appropriate and prompt diagnostic testing should be performed in patients with antibiotic-associated diarrhea	A-II
Diagnostic tests for *Clostridium difficile* should be performed only on diarrheal (soft or unformed) stool specimens, unless ileus is suspected	B-III
Testing of stool specimens from asymptomatic patients for *C. difficile* (including "test of cure" after treatment)	B-II
Treatment	
If possible, discontinuation of the offending antimicrobial agent is recommended	A-I
Oral metronidazole should be considered the treatment of choice for CDAD; oral vancomycin should be administered only if there has been failure to respond to metronidazole, or if the patient cannot tolerate or is allergic to metronidazole	A-I
Treatment of asymptomatic patients with *C. difficile* colonization is not recommended	A-I
First recurrences of CDAD following treatment of initial episode should be retreated as for the initial episode	B-III
Prevention and control	
Implement policies to ensure prudent antimicrobial use	A-II
Surveillance of antimicrobial utilization in the facility should be conducted	B-III
Healthcare providers in the facility should be educated about the epidemiology of CDAD	B-III
Patients with CDAD and fecal incontinence should be in a private room; if possible, all patients with CDAD should be in private rooms	B-III
Meticulous hand hygiene with soap or an antiseptic agent is recommended after contact with patients, their body substances, or their potentially contaminated environment	B-III
Healthcare providers should wear gloves for contact with patients with CDAD	A-I
Use of disposable, single-use thermometers (rather than shared electronic thermometers) is recommended	A-II
Patient care items, such as stethoscopes and sphygmomanometers should be dedicated; if they must be shared, they should be disinfected between patients	B-III
Disinfection of the environment of a patient with CDAD should be done using sporocidal agents, such as a diluted sodium hypochlorite solution	B-II
Patients with CDAD may be removed from contact isolation when their diarrhea has resolved	B-III

[a]Data in part from the 2002 Society for Healthcare Epidemiology of America guidelines for the prevention of *Clostridium difficile*-associated diarrhea; Simor et al.,[80] *Infection Control and Hospital Epidemiology* 2002;23:696–703; from the Infectious Diseases Society of America Guidelines for weighting recommendations based on the quality of scientific evidence.[283] Category: A, good evidence to support a recommendation for use; B, moderate evidence to support a recommendation for use; C, poor evidence to support a recommendation for use. Quality of evidence: I, evidence from one or more properly randomized controlled trial; II, evidence from one or more well-designed observational study, multiple time-series, or dramatic results of uncontrolled experiments; III, expert opinion, descriptive studies.

It is indefensible to start antiinfective drugs for suspected or presumed infection in the critically ill patient without first obtaining blood cultures from two separate sites, at least one of which is drawn from a peripheral vein by percutaneous venipuncture. In adults, if at least 30mL blood is cultured, 99% of detectable BSIs should be identified.[88] Similar operating characteristics are achieved in the pediatric population using a weight-based graduated volume approach to blood cultures.[89] Standard blood cultures drawn through central venous catheters (CVCs) provide excellent sensitivity for diagnosis of

TABLE 76.6. Rates of bloodstream infection (BSI) caused by various types of devices used for vascular access.

	Rates of device-related BSI			
	Per 100 catheters		*Per 1,000 catheter-days*	
Device (number of prospective studies)	*Pooled mean*	*95% CI*	*Pooled mean*	*95% CI*
Peripheral venous catheters (13)	0.16	0.08–0.23	0.60	0.31–0.88
Arterial catheters (17)	0.75	0.49–1.02	1.78	1.17–2.40
Short-term, nonmedicated central venous catheters (CVCs) (88)	4.48	4.19–4.78	2.51	2.34–2.68
Pulmonary-artery catheters (15)	1.45	1.06–1.85	5.50	4.00–7.01
Hemodialysis catheters Noncuffed (17)	7.41	6.43–8.39	2.62	2.26–2.98
Cuffed (19)	18.48	17.13–19.82	1.81	1.67–1.96
Peripherally inserted central catheters (14)	2.49	1.76–3.21	0.75	0.53–0.97
Long-term tunneled and cuffed CVCs (48)	21.25	20.13–22.38	1.53	1.44–1.62
Subcutaneous central venous ports (18)	3.91	3.22–4.59	0.13	0.11–0.15

CI, confidence interval.

Source: Data in part from Kluger and Maki,[84] based on 245 published prospective studies where every device was evaluated for infection.

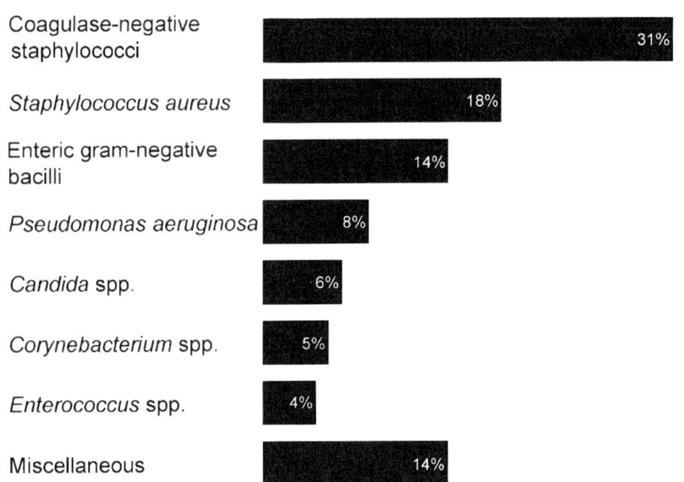

FIGURE 76.5. Microbial profile of intravascular device-related bloodstream infection based on an analysis of 159 published prospective studies. (From Maki DG, Crnich CJ,[85] by permission of *Seminars in Respiratory and Critical Care Medicine*.)

BSI but are less specific than cultures obtained from a peripheral vein.[90]

Short-term IVDs should be removed from the outset in unstable patients with suspected IVDR BSI or if IVDR BSI is documented (see Table 76.7); however, it is difficult or, more often, unnecessary to arbitrarily remove surgically implanted IVDs, such as Hickman and Broviac catheters or central venous ports. Only 15% to 45% of long-term IVDs that are removed for suspected infection are truly colonized or infected at the time of removal.[91,92] To avoid unnecessary removal of IVDs, novel methods have been developed to identify IVDR BSI without removing the device: (1) paired quantitative blood cultures drawn from the IVD and percutaneously from a peripheral vein[93]; (2) differential time-to-positivity (DTP) of paired standard blood cultures, one drawn from the IVD, the second from a peripheral vein[94]; and (3) Gram stain[95] or acridine orange staining[96] of blood samples drawn through the IVD.

Quantitative blood cultures are labor intensive and cost almost twice as much as standard blood cultures. The differential-time-to-positivity (DTP) of paired blood cultures, one drawn through the IVD and the second concomitantly from a peripheral vein, has been shown to reliably identify IVDR BSI of long-term IVDs if the blood culture drawn from the IVD turns positive 2 or more hours before the culture drawn peripherally. In studies of patients with long-term IVDs, the sensitivity and specificity of DTP are 92% and 75%, respectively.[94]

If a short-term vascular catheter is suspected of being infected because the patient has no obvious other source of infection to explain fever, there is inflammation at the insertion site, or cryptogenic staphylococcal bacteremia or candidemia has been documented, blood cultures should be obtained and the catheter should be removed and cultured (see Table 76.7). Failure to remove an infected IVD puts the patient at risk of developing septic thrombophlebitis with peripheral

TABLE 76.7. Algorithm for diagnosis and management of intravascular device (IVD)-related bloodstream infection.

- Examine the patient thoroughly to identify unrelated sources of infection.
- Carefully examine all catheter insertion sites; Gram stain and culture any expressible purulence from sites.
  - Obtain *two* 10- to 15-mL cultures:

  If standard (nonquantitative) blood cultures, draw one by *percutaneous peripheral* venipuncture and one through the suspect IVD.

  If quantitative blood culture techniques are available (e.g., the Isolator system), catheter-drawn cultures can enhance the diagnostic specificity of blood culturing in diagnosis of line sepsis. However, a peripheral percutaneous quantitative blood culture *must* be drawn *concomitantly.*
- Option regarding a peripheral IV or arterial catheter: *remove and culture catheter.*
  - Options regarding a short-term central venous catheter:

  Purulence at insertion site or no purulence, but patient *floridly septic, without obvious source*:
    - *Remove and culture catheter.*
    - Gram stain purulence.
    - Reestablish access at new site.

  No purulence, patient not floridly septic:
    - *Leave catheter in place,* pending results of blood cultures.
    - or

  Remove and culture catheter, reestablish needed access at new site.
  - Options regarding surgically implanted, cuffed Hickman-type catheters.

  Remove at outset if:
    - Infecting organism known to be *S. aureus, Bacillus* spp., JK *Diptheroid, Mycobacterium* species, or filamentous fungus.
    - Refractory or progressive exit-site infection, despite antimicrobial therapy, especially with *Pseudomonas aeruginosa.*
    - Tunnel infected.
    - Evidence of septic thrombosis of cannulated central vein or septic pulmonary emboli.
    - Evidence of endocarditis.

  Remove later on if:
    - Any of the above become manifest.
    - BSI persists 3 days or more, despite IV antimicrobial therapy through catheter.
  - Options regarding surgically implanted subcutaneous central ports (e.g., Portacath):

  Cellulitis without documented bacteremia: begin antimicrobial therapy, *withhold removing port.*

  Aspirate from port shows organisms on Gram stain or heavy growth in quantitative culture, or documented port-related bacteremia: *remove port.*
- Decision on whether to begin antimicrobial therapy, before culture results available, based on clinical assessment and/or Gram stain of exit site or the blood drawn from a long-term IVD.
- With no microbiologic data to guide antimicrobial selection in a septic patient with suspected line sepsis, consider: *IV vancomycin and ciprofloxacin, cefepime, or imipenem/meropenem.*

Source: Adapted from Maki,[213] by permission of Lippincott Williams & Wilkins.

IV catheters, septic thrombosis of a great central vein with CVCs,[97] or even endocarditis. Continued access, if necessary, can be established with a new catheter inserted in a new site. Although small studies have found some utility in catheter exchange over a guidewire in the management of CVCs suspected of being infected,[98] we believe that, in the absence of randomized studies demonstrating its safety, guidewire exchange generally should not be performed if there is strong suspicion of IVDR BSI, especially if there are signs of local infection, such as purulence or erythema at the insertion site or signs of systemic sepsis without a source (see Table 76.7). In these cases, the old catheter should be removed and cultured, and a new catheter should be inserted in a new site.

Bloodstream infection that might have originated from a long-term IVD, such as a Hickman catheter or subcutaneous port, does not automatically mandate removal of the device, unless (see Table 76.7) there has been persistent exit site infection; the tunnel is obviously infected; there is evidence of complicating endocarditis, septic thrombosis, or septic pulmonary emboli; the infecting pathogen is *S. aureus*, *Corynebacterium* JK, a *Bacillus* species, *Stenotrophomonas* spp., *Burkholderia cepacia* and all pseudomonal species, a filamentous fungus or *Malassezia* species, or a mycobacterial species; or bacteremia or candidemia persists for more than 3 days despite adequate therapy.[99] Intravascular device-related BSI caused by *S. aureus* must always prompt removal of the IVD, even if signs of bacteremia have resolved following antimicrobial therapy, because of the significant risk of infectious endocarditis (IE) or other metastatic infection if bacteremia recurs.[100,101] Similarly, we believe that patients with documented for presumed IVDR candidemia should have their catheter removed in most situations.[102–104]

In small, uncontrolled clinical trials of "antibiotic lock therapy" (ALT), usually in conjunction with systemic antibiotic therapy, cure rates of infected IVDs in excess of 90% have been reported.[105–107] Most of the IVDs reported in these studies were infected with coagulase-negative staphylococci and fermenting gram-negative bacilli; therefore, at this time ALT cannot be recommended for the management of long-term IVDs infected by *S. aureus*, *Bacillus* sp., *Corynebacterium* JK, *Stenotrophomonas* spp., *B. cepacia*, all *Pseudomonas* species, fungi, or mycobacterial species. Obviously, if IVDR BSI recurs after an attempt to salvage an IVD with ALT, the device should be removed.

Infected surgically implanted subcutaneous central ports have rarely proven to be curable with medical therapy alone, especially if it is clear that the device is infected (e.g., an aspirate from the port shows heavy growth).[108] A recent study of patients with acquired immunodeficiency syndrome (AIDS), with surgically implanted ports who developed IVDR BSI, found that ALT, combined with systemic antibiotic therapy, resulted in 70% of the ports being salvaged; however, long-term follow-up data on surveillance cultures of the ports were not reported.[109] The only other clinical study of the utilization of ALT in subcutaneous central port infections achieved salvage rates less than 50%.[110] Based on the marginal efficacy of ALT in these two studies and the historically poor cure rate achieved with systemic antibiotics alone, we believe that definitive therapy of infected subcutaneous central ports mandates removal of the infected device.

If IVDR BSI is suspected, after cultures have been obtained, the combination of IV vancomycin (for staphylococci resistant to methicillin, i.e., MRSA) with a fluoroquinolone, cefepime, or imipenem/meropenem (for multiresistant nosocomial gram-negative bacilli) (see Table 76.7), should prove effective against the bacterial pathogens most likely to be encountered (see Figure 76.5). Initial therapy can then be modified based on the ultimate microbiologic identification and susceptibilities of the infecting organisms.

How long to treat IVDR BSI will be influenced by the infecting microorganism, and by whether the patient has underlying valvular heart disease, already has evidence of endocarditis or septic thrombosis, or shows evidence of metastatic infection. If endocarditis is suspected, transesophageal echocardiography offers superior sensitivity and discrimination for detecting vegetations, as compared with transthoracic echocardiography.[101] In patients with high-grade bacteremia or fungemia, but without clinical or echocardiographic evidence of endocarditis, septic thrombosis should be suspected.[97] Central venous thrombosis can now be diagnosed by venography, ultrasonography, magnetic resonance imaging, or CT.[111]

Although there are no prospective studies to guide the optimal duration of antimicrobial therapy for IVDR BSIs, most coagulase-negative staphylococcal infections can be cured with 5 to 7 days of therapy,[112,113] whereas most infections caused by other microorganisms are adequately treated with 10 to 14 days of antimicrobial therapy.[113] These recommendations hold only as long as there are no complications related to the infection and the BSI clears within 72 hours of initiating therapy. Nosocomial enterococcal bacteremia deriving from an IVD is rarely associated with persistent endovascular infection, and unless there is clinical or echocardiographic evidence of endocarditis, treatment with IV ampicillin or vancomycin alone for 7 to 14 days should suffice.[48]

The management of *S. aureus* device-related infection deserves special mention, as there have been no prospective studies to evaluate the optimal duration of therapy for IVDR BSIs caused by this ubiquitous human pathogen. Historically, high rates of associated IE and late complications led to a universal policy of 4 to 6 weeks of antimicrobial therapy for *all* patients with *S. aureus* bacteremia. Earlier diagnosis and initiation of bactericidal therapy of nosocomial *S. aureus* BSIs in recent years have been associated with lower rates of IE and metastatic complications, prompting suggestions that short-course therapy (i.e., 14 days) is effective and safe for most patients with *S. aureus* IVDR BSI, so long as the patient defervesces within 72 hours and there is no evidence of metastatic infection.[114] In a study of transesophageal echocardiography (TEE) in 103 hospitalized patients with *S. aureus* bacteremia, 69 related to an IVD, Fowler et al. found a surprisingly high incidence of endocarditis, 23% with IVDR *S. aureus* BSI.[101] In a more recent report, these authors have reported that the routine use of TEE with IVDR *S. aureus* BSI, as a means to stratify patients into short-course or long-course therapy, is cost-effective.[115] However, at this time, there are no prospective studies to affirm this approach. Until more data are available, short-course therapy for IVDR *S. aureus* bacteremia therapy should be approached with caution, and used only when the TEE is unequivocally negative and the patient has defervesced within 72 hours of removing the IVD and starting antiinfective therapy.

All patients with an IVDR BSI must be monitored closely, for at least 6 weeks after completing therapy, especially if they have had high-grade bacteremia or candidemia, to detect late-appearing endocarditis or other metastatic infection, such as vertebral osteomyelitis.

An updated guideline for the prevention of intravascular device-related bloodstream infections (IVDR BSIs) was published in 2002 by the CDC's Healthcare Infection Control Practices Advisory Committee.[116] The use of antimicrobial lock solutions for prevention of BSIs caused by long-term IVDs has been of particular interest in cancer patients. Seven randomized, prospective trials have examined a vancomycin-containing antibiotic lock solution for the prevention of IVDR BSI,[117] the largest of which found that use of a vancomycin or vancomycin/ciprofloxacin lock solution reduced the risk of IVDR BSI nearly 80% (P equal to or less than 0.005).[118] Concern about the emergence of resistance with prophylactic antibiotic-containing lock solutions has limited their acceptance to date. Three of the seven studies performed serial surveillance cultures for vancomycin-resistant enterococcus; VRE was not found in any of these studies. However, the use of prophylactic antibiotic lock solution is considered acceptable in the HICPAC Guideline if a patient with an essential long-term IVD has continued to experience recurrent IVDR BSIs despite consistent application of recommended infection control practices.[116]

Viral Infections

Patients who have inherited or acquired impairment of cell-mediated immunity are at risk of opportunistic viral infections. Not surprisingly, patients who are treated with agents with potent activity against this arm of the immune system, such as glucocorticoids, calcineurin inhibitors (i.e., cyclosporine A and tacrolimus),[119] alkylating agents (i.e., cyclophosphamide),[120] selected antimetabolites (i.e., azathioprine, methotrexate, and fludarabine),[121] and monoclonal antibodies [i.e., alemtuzumab (anti-CD52) and basiliximab and daclizumab (anti-CD25)][122] are at greatest risk. In general, reactivation of latent herpesviruses account for the majority of viral infections in this population, although community- and nosocomial-acquired infections caused by other common viral pathogens occur at an increased frequency, compared to the general population, and may be associated with increased patient morbidity and mortality.

Herpesviruses

Currently, there are eight herpesviruses that can infect humans and cause disease (Table 76.8). All members of this family demonstrate a tropism for human cells and share the

TABLE 76.8. The human herpesviruses.

Alphaherpesviruses
Herpes simplex virus type 1 (HSV-1)
Herpes simplex virus type 2 (HSV-2)
Varicella-zoster virus (VZV)
Betaherpesviruses
Cytomegalovirus (CMV)
Human herpesvirus type 6 (HHV-6)
Human herpesvirus type 7 (HHV-7)
Gammaherpesviruses
Epstein–Barr virus (EBV)
Human herpesvirus type 8 (HHV-8)

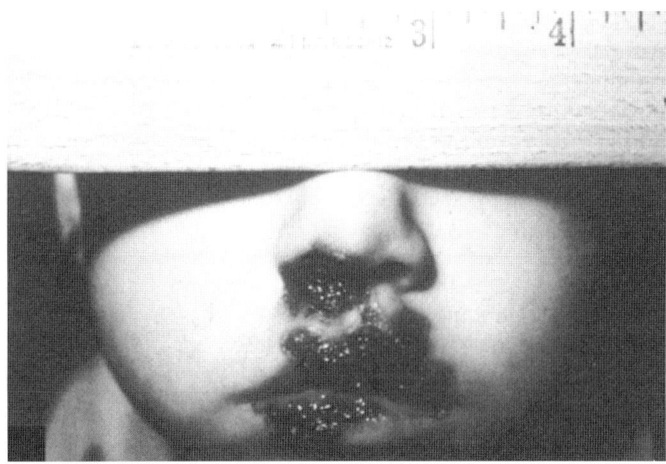

FIGURE 76.6. Herpes simplex mucositis in an immunocompromised patient. [By permission of Yogev R. Pediatric HIV infection. In: Mandell GL (ed). Essential Atlas of Infectious Diseases for Primary Care. Current Medicine, vol. 1. Philadelphia: Churchill-Livingstone, 1997:45.]

ability to establish themselves in a state of latency following acute infection. Reactivation of latent infection, characterized by viral replication and shedding, tends to occur most often during periods of immunosuppression, although there is variability in the clinical manifestations of reactivated infection, depending on the virus.

Herpes Simplex Virus Type 1 and 2

Herpes simplex virus type 1 and 2 (HSV-1 and HSV-2) are widely distributed in the population, seroprevalence in adults approaching 95% for HSV-1 and 25% for HSV-2. Upward of 70% to 80% of seropositive stem cell transplant (SCT) patients begin to shed HSV following transplantation,[123] a finding that has led to recommendations for routine acyclovir prophylaxis in bone marrow transplantation (BMT) and patients with hematologic malignancies who are receiving chemotherapy.[124]

Herpes simplex virus infection typically manifests as localized mucocutaneous disease, most commonly involving the oral cavity, which can be necrotizing in the immunocompromised patient (Figure 76.6), less commonly the genital area. Extensive mucocutaneous disease involving the esophagus may occur in up to 10% of cancer patients with upper gastrointestinal symptoms.[123] Life-threatening disease is rare, even in this population; however, HSV pneumonia, hepatitis, encephalitis, and disseminated disease are seen, and are associated with a high mortality, despite appropriate antiviral therapy.

The diagnosis of HSV infection is usually made on clinical grounds in immunocompetent individuals; however, identification of HSV infection is complicated in cancer patients because extensive mucocutaneous disease can be caused by chemotherapeutic drugs, as well as a number of other opportunistic infections. It is thus important that the clinician strive to determine the etiology of the patient's mucocutaneous signs and symptoms.

In the case of acute mucocutaneous disease, viral culture of a swab of an unroofed vesicle or open ulcer offers the best method of confirming HSV infection, with results available in most cases within 48 to 96 hours. Direct Giesma staining (Tzanck preparation) of fluid from an unroofed vesicle, seeking giant cells or intranuclear inclusions, cannot reliably differentiate between varicella-zoster virus (VZV) infection and HSV infection, is insensitive, and should *not* be used to rule out HSV infection. When feasible, every attempt should be made to obtain specimens for pathologic examination and viral culture or polymerase chain reaction (PCR) in patients with suspected HSV esophagitis or pneumonitis, although empiric treatment based on clinical symptoms may be necessary in patients in whom the risks of invasive tests are too high. In patients with suspected HSV encephalitis, PCR testing of cerebrospinal fluid (CSF) has shown sensitivity and specificity approaching 100%,[125] although the yield has been shown to be laboratory dependent.[126]

The treatment of HSV infections is dependent on the location and severity of infection (Table 76.9).[123] Valaciclovir and famciclovir have an oral bioavailability three to five times that of oral acyclovir, making oral therapy of serious disease a technical feasibility. Nevertheless, the use of oral therapy from the outset should be restricted to immunocompromised patients who have limited mucocutaneous disease. In the presence of extensive mucocutaneous disease, esophagitis, pneumonitis, or disseminated disease, initial therapy should begin with intravenous acyclovir, 5 to 10mg/kg every 8 hours, to ensure adequate tissue levels, particularly in patients in whom intestinal absorption is in question. Once the patient has shown a favorable response to therapy, therapy may be completed with a highly bioavailable oral agent such as valaciclovir or famciclovir.

Varicella-Zoster Virus

Primary varicella-zoster virus (VZV) infection, in the form of chicken pox, is a ubiquitous childhood infection, most commonly associated with a diffuse vesicular rash, and is associated with secondary reactivation later in life, in the form of a painful, localized eruption, herpes zoster. Primary infection usually occurs in children under the age of 13; however, morbidity and mortality related to primary infection occurs disproportionately in susceptible adults over the age of 23.

Immunocompromised persons are at high risk of primary and reactivation disease,[127] and these patients are more likely to experience visceral dissemination, with involvement of the lungs, liver, or brain.[127] Primary VZV infection usually occurs in children with hematologic malignancy where infection is associated with pneumonia in up to 32% of untreated cases.[128] In contrast, herpes zoster is a delayed reactivated infection that occurs most commonly in adults undergoing chemotherapy and is associated with visceral involvement in up to 13% of cases.[129]

The diagnosis of varicella and herpes zoster infection is usually made on clinical grounds, with a generalized vesicular centripetal rash in lesions in varying stages of development seen in chicken pox and a unilateral dermatomal eruption with herpes zoster (Figure 76.7). Cutaneous dissemination can follow a dermatomal eruption in up to 35% of cancer patients, in contrast to only 4% in persons without cancer. Involvement of adjacent dermatomes is not unusual in immunocompetent patients and does not usually represent disseminated disease. Viral culture of lesions fails to detect the virus in 40% to 70% of cases.[130] Fluorescent antibody staining appears to be easier and far more sensitive diagnostically. Amplification of VZV DNA is of limited value in the diagnosis of cutaneous disease, but PCR of bronchoalveolar lavage and cerebrospinal fluid can be a useful adjunct in the diagnosis of VZV pneumonia or meningoencephalitis.[131,132]

Treatment of immunodeficient patients with varicella or herpes zoster is described in Table 76.9. Intravenous acyclovir, 10mg/kg every 8 hours, is recommended for most patients; however, oral therapy with valaciclovir or famciclovir may be used in patients with mild to moderate immunosuppression who do not have evidence of disseminated or visceral disease. Resistance to acyclovir, mediated by mutation of the viral thymidine kinase, has been seen almost exclusively in patients with AIDS, but should be suspected in any patient not responding to therapy, in which case the use of foscarnet or cidofovir is recommended (see Table 76.9).[123]

The median time to onset of herpes zoster in BMT patients is 5 months[123]; as a result, preventive therapy with acyclovir or its congeners is not recommended. The use of varicella zoster-immunoglobulin (VZIG) can reduce the risk of primary infection and its attendant complications, but must be given to susceptible immunodeficient individuals within 96 hours of exposure at a dose of 125U/10kg (maximum dose, 625U).[133] The use of live, attenuated varicella virus vaccine is contraindicated in immunocompromised adults at the present time, although a clinical trial of the vaccine is under way in susceptible children.[133] Household contacts of immunodeficient patients at risk should be vaccinated if they are known to be susceptible to varicella infection (i.e., children and adults with no known history of varicella).[134]

Cytomegalovirus

Cytomegalovirus (CMV) is a herpesvirus that may infect up to 50% to 70% of the population in developed countries.[123] Cytomegalovirus infection is seen mainly in patients undergoing BMT or solid organ transplantation,[135,136] although there have been increasing reports of CMV infection among

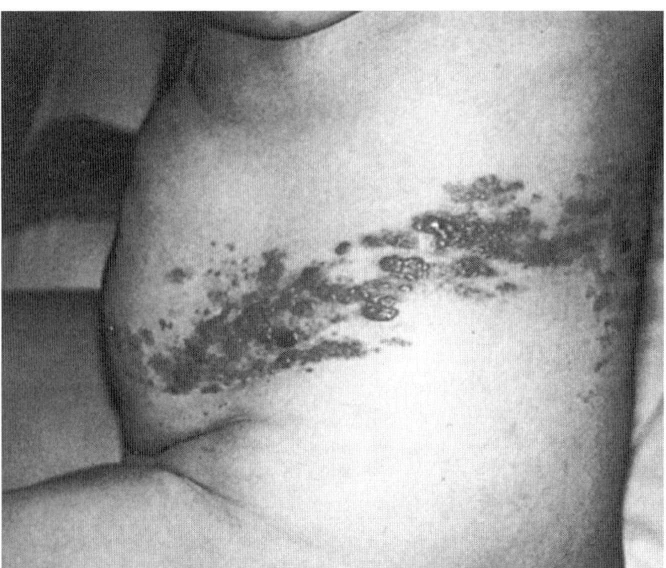

FIGURE 76.7. Herpes zoster infection in immunosuppressed adult. Note the dermatomal distribution of the eruption. [By permission of Stone DR, Gorbach SL (eds). Atlas of Infectious Diseases. Philadelphia: Saunders, 2000.]

TABLE 76.9. Treatment and prophylaxis of infections caused by viral pathogens.

Indication	*Drug*	*Route*	*Dosage*	*Duration*
HSV 1 and 2				
Prophylaxis	Acyclovir	IV	5 mg/kg q12	For the period of the most severe immunosuppression (usually 2–3 months)
		PO	200–400 mg q8 to 800 mg q12	Same
	Valacyclovir	PO	500–1,000 q12	Same
	Famciclovir	PO	500 mg q12	Same
Treatment				
Mucocutaneous disease	Acyclovir	IV	5 mg/kg q8	7–10 days
		PO	200–400 mg 5×/day	7–10 days
	Valacyclovir	PO	500–1,000 mg q12	7 days
	Famciclovir	PO	500 mg q12 or 250 mg q8	7 days
Esophageal disease	Acyclovir	IV	5 mg/kg q8	10 days
Encephalitis or pneumonia	Acyclovir	IV	10–15 mg/kg q8	14–21 days
Resistant infection	Foscarnet	IV	60 mg/kg q12 or 40 mg/kg q8	As above
	Cidofovir	IV	5 mg/kg once weekly for 2 weeks	Continue every 2 weeks until healing
VZV				
First prophylaxis (patient VZV seronegative)	VZIG immunoglobulin	IV	125 U/10 kg once	Must be given within 96 hours of exposure
Second prophylaxis (patient VZV seropositive)	Not recommended			
Treatment				
Disseminated or invasive disease	Acyclovir	IV	10 mg/kg q8	7–10 days
Localized mucocutaneous disease	Acyclovir	PO	800 mg 5×/day	7–10 days
	Valacyclovir	PO	1,000 mg q8	7–10 days
	Famciclovir	PO	500 mg q8	7–10 days
Resistant infection	Foscarnet	IV	60 mg/kg q8–q12	7–14 days or until complete healing
CMV				
Prophylaxis	Ganciclovir	IV	5 mg/kg q12 then 5 mg/kg daily	5 days From engraftment until day 100 after bone marrow transplantation (BMT)
Preemptive therapy	Ganciclovir	IV	5 mg/kg q12 then 6 mg/kg daily 5 days per week	14 days Until CMV surveillance test negative
	Foscarnet	IV	60 mg/kg q12 then 90 mg/kg daily 5 days per week	14 days Until CMV surveillance test negative
Treatment	Ganciclovir	IV	5 mg/kg q12 then 5–6 mg/kg daily	14 days 30 days or until complete recovery
Resistant infection	Foscarnet	IV	90 mg/kg q12 or 60 mg/kg q8 for 2 weeks, then 90–120 mg/kg once daily	Until complete recovery
Influenza A				
Prophylaxis	Amantidine	PO	200 mg daily	For duration of peak influenza activity in community
	Rimantidine	PO	100 mg bid	For duration of peak influenza activity in community
Treatment	Amantidine	PO	200 mg daily	4–5 days or until 24–48 hours after symptomatic improvement
	Rimantidine	PO	100 mg bid	4–5 days or until 24–48 hours after symptomatic improvement
Influenza A & B				
Prophylaxis	Oseltamivir	PO	75 qd	For duration of peak influenza activity in community
Treatment	Oseltamivir	PO	75 mg bid	5 days
	Zanamavir	inhaled	2 inhalations bid	5 days
RSV	Ribavirin	Inhaled	55 mg/h for 12 hours	7–14 days
	RSV IVIG	IV	1.5 g/kg	Once

VZV, varicella-zoster virus; CMV, cytomegalovirus; RSV, respiratory syncytial virus.

Source: Adapted in part from Reusser,[123] by permission of Mosby.

patients with leukemia, as a result of exposure to powerful immunosuppressive drugs, such as fludarabine and cytoxan.[137] Seropositive patients undergoing BMT or those who receive marrow from a seropositive donor without preventive therapy, develop infection in 60% to 70% of cases.[123] The likelihood of CMV infection is greatly increased in patients who develop graft-versus-host disease, those who receive an HLA-mismatched transplant, or those who receive antithymocyte immunoglobulin.[138,139]

Clinically, CMV infection in immunosuppressed patients can range from asymptomatic excretion to fulminant disseminated disease. Cytomegalovirus viremia often presents as unexplained fever without specific end-organ involvement but usually manifests as pneumonia or gastroenteritis. Without therapy, CMV pneumonia is fatal in up to 85% of cases.[139] Less common manifestations include esophagitis, myocarditis, hepatitis, encephalitis, and retinitis.

The diagnosis of CMV infection requires documentation of CMV in blood, tissue, or bronchoalveolar fluid specimens. Serologic, histopathologic, and direct culture methods have proven to be insensitive for diagnostic purposes, as highlighted in BMT patients where CMV cultures of blood may be negative in up to 30% of cases of proven invasive disease.[140] Newer molecular techniques, including pp65 CMV antigen detection, PCR, branched-chain DNA, and hybrid capture CMV DNA assay, have revolutionized the diagnosis of invasive CMV disease.[141] Studies of quantitative CMV antigen assays and real-time PCR have found that these tests have negative predictive values that range from 90% to 95%, with positive predictive values ranging from 50% to 84%.[141,142]

Ganciclovir should be used for the initial treatment of all suspected or established CMV disease in immunocompromised patients (see Table 76.9). Many transplant centers also use CMV immunoglobulin for the treatment of patients with CMV pneumonia; however, this recommendation is based on older studies utilizing historical controls,[143] and at least one contemporary study has failed to find additional benefit over ganciclovir therapy alone.[144] As a result, we do not recommend the adjunctive use of CMV immunoglobulin in the treatment of invasive CMV disease.

The prophylactic use of antivirals in patients at risk for developing invasive CMV disease is also another area of controversy. Many transplant centers routinely give prophylactic ganciclovir to patients who are CMV seropositive or who have received a transplant from a CMV-positive donor. Although this approach does lead to a reduction in documented episodes of invasive CMV, no study has shown a survival advantage.[123] An alternative approach, which relies on preemptive ganciclovir therapy in patients with documented CMV viremia, as determined by use of one or more of the molecular techniques already described, has been found to be associated with a survival advantage in several prospective trials.[145,146] However, studies have found that up to 86% of patients with evidence of CMV shedding, based on molecular surveillance studies, ultimately do not require therapy.[147] As a result, whether to use a prophylactic or preemptive strategy remains controversial, and the approach used will be influenced by institutional rates of CMV infection. The prevention of primary CMV infection in susceptible (antibody-negative) patients is best approached by using CMV-negative marrow and blood products.

Epstein–Barr Virus

Epstein–Barr virus (EBV) occurs in more than 90% of the population. In developed countries, primary infection occurs principally in adolescents and teenagers, and as a result primary infection is a rare phenomenon in adults with cancer. However, EBV-induced posttransplant lymphoproliferative disease (PTLD) is a threat to patients who have undergone solid organ or allogeneic BMT. The incidence of this disorder in patients with solid organ transplants varies by the degree of immunosuppression; renal transplant patients have an incidence of PTLD of 1%, whereas the incidence in small bowel transplant patients is as high as 14%.[123] In contrast, the incidence of PTLD in BMT patients appears to be lower, around 1.3%.[148] The mortality from PTLD ranges from 30% to 80%, although mortality in BMT patients approaches 90%.[149] Treatment of patients with PTLD is difficult and generally requires a reduction or, better, total cessation of immunosuppressive therapy.[150] Use of antiviral agents is generally of little benefit, although anecdotal success has been reported with infusions of donor-derived leukocytes and the use of anti-B-cell antibodies.[149]

Human Herpesvirus 6

Human herpesvirus 6 (HHV-6) causes exanthem subitum in children, and shedding of the virus may be seen in up to 60% of patients undergoing BMT.[123] Human herpesvirus 6 has been implicated as a cause of rejection, marrow suppression, encephalitis, and interstitial pneumonia in this population; however, clear evidence of a causal role has only been established clearly for encephalitis.[151] There have been no prospective trials reported to evaluate the effectiveness of antiviral therapy in infections thought to be caused by HHV-6, although both foscarnet and ganciclovir exhibit in vitro activity, and successful treatment of patients with HHV-6 encephalitis with ganciclovir and foscarnet has been reported anecdotally.[152]

Community-Acquired Viral Respiratory Pathogens

Community-acquired viral respiratory pathogens (Table 76.10) are increasingly recognized causes of infection in immunocompromised patients. In one study at the M.D. Anderson Cancer Center, a respiratory virus was isolated from 33% of adult patients presenting with a respiratory illness, 31% caused by respiratory syncytial virus (RSV), 28% by rhinoviruses or picornaviruses, 18% by influenza A or B, and 23% by parainfluenza or adenoviruses.[153] Parainfluenza, rhinoviruses, and andenovirus infections occur year round, whereas infections caused by influenza A and B and RSV peak during the winter months. Although many respiratory viral infections are community acquired, several studies have clearly demonstrated the potential for nosocomial acquisi-

TABLE 76.10. Community-acquired respiratory pathogens.

Influenza A and B
Respiratory syncytial virus A & B
Parainfluenza viruses 1, 2, & 3
Rhinoviruses
Adenoviruses
Coronaviruses

tion, most likely as a result of transmission from visitors or healthcare workers.[154,155]

Mortality associated with these infections is difficult to establish, because many patients infected by these viruses die with, rather than of, their viral infection. Nevertheless, studies examining mortality in immunocompromised patients from whom a viral respiratory pathogen has been isolated have found case-fatality rates ranging from 22% to 44%.[153] Mortality appears to be higher for patients infected with RSV; Whimby et al. found that 60% of leukemic patients who developed RSV died of complications related to their infection.[156]

Diagnostic tests for most of the major respiratory viral pathogens, such as influenza A and B, parainfluenza 1, 2, and 3, RSV, and adenovirus, are commercially available. A description of individual tests is beyond the scope of this text; however, a new rapid reverse transcriptase PCR test (Hexaplex; Prodesse, Waukesha, WI), which simultaneously tests for the presence of both influenza subtypes, the three parainfluenza subtypes, and the two RSV subtypes, has shown high diagnostic accuracy.[157]

The treatment of most respiratory viral infections is supportive; however, there are viable treatment options for influenza and RSV.[158] The neuraminidase inhibitor, oseltamivir, is active against both influenza A and B, whereas amantidine and rimantidine possess activity only against influenza A; therapeutic impact appears to be negligible if the antiviral agent cannot be started within 48 to 72 hours of onset of clinical symptoms.[158] Aerosolized ribavirin has traditionally been used in patients with RSV; however, its benefit appears to be marginal in patients with established infection. The concomitant use of RSV immunoglobulin with aerosolized ribavirin has been shown to reduce mortality in leukemic adults by 30% compared to historical controls (70% to 50%).[155] The results from an ongoing randomized trial of aerosolized ribavirin versus ribavirin plus RSV immunoglobulin are still unavailable. The use of intravenous ribavirin does not appear to be of clinical benefit and can be associated with hemolysis, limiting its utility in this population.[159]

The prevention of nosocomial transmission of community-acquired respiratory viral infections, such as influenza and RSV deserves mention, given the number of reports of institutional outbreaks.[160,161] Minimum infection control practices to prevent nosocomial respiratory viral infections include (1) timely immunization of patients and staff against influenza[162]; (2) prevention of patient contact with persons (friends, family, and healthcare staff) who have active respiratory symptoms; (3) use of rapid diagnostic tests to quickly identify symptomatic patients with potentially transmissible viral pathogens; (4) grouping patients with confirmed infection when single rooms are not available; and (5) placement of patients with suspected community-acquired respiratory viral infections in droplet isolation precautions. The use of more aggressive isolation procedures, such as contact and airborne isolation precautions, with or without the use of prophylactic antiviral agents, may require consideration with outbreaks among very high risk patients.

Fungal Pathogens

The growing problem of devastating fungal infections in cancer patients necessitates a major focus on the leading fungal pathogens in patients with malignant disease. Most fungal infections occur in patients with hematologic malignancies as a result of the intrinsic nature of the disease and the chemotherapeutic regimens that result in severe and prolonged granulocytopenia, which correlate very strongly with an increased risk of infections caused by the filamentous fungi, such as *Aspergillus* and *Fusarium*. Filamentous fungal infections are far less common in patients with lymphoma and rare in patients with solid tumors. Regardless of the type of malignancy, all patients with cancer are at increased risk of infection caused by *Candida* spp., primarily as a result of the widespread use of IVDs and the intensive chemotherapeutic regimens used in this patient population.

Candida

The risk of developing a *Candida* infection is closely associated with the type of cancer; candidiasis occurs in 9% to 25% of patients undergoing BMT, 1% to 13% of patients with granulocytopenia as a result of chemotherapy and hematologic malignancies, 1% to 2% in patients being treated for lymphoma, and 0.5% in patients undergoing treatment for solid tumors.[163] *Candida albicans* is most commonly isolated; however, many centers are experiencing a sharp rise in infections cause by non-*albicans* species, including *Candida glabrata*, *Candida tropicalis*, *Candida krusei*, and *Candida parapsilosis*.[164] The clinical relevance of this finding is that most non-*albicans* species are relatively resistant to azoles, including fluconazole and itraconazole, necessitating the use of alternative therapeutic agents, such as amphotericin and caspofungin.

There is a wide spectrum of diseases caused by *Candida* spp., including oropharyngeal mucosal infection, esophagitis, BSI, and hepatosplenic candidiasis. Pulmonary and neurologic involvement are rarely seen as isolated disease and most often occur in conjunction with disseminated infection.

Oropharyngeal candidiasis is characterized by the presence of typical adherent white plaques on the tongue, palate, or buccal mucosa. Staining or cultures of the adherent material usually is not necessary unless infection caused by non-*albicans* species is suspected. Treatment with clotrimazole troches is usually sufficient with limited oropharyngeal disease, although systemic therapy with fluconazole or itraconazole is mandatory in patients with severe disease or when concomitant esophagitis is suspected (Table 76.11).[165] Intravenous amphotericin or caspofungin may be necessary in patients with severe oropharyngeal disease caused by azole-resistant non-*albicans* species.

Candida esophagitis often presents with dysphagia, but retrosternal pain, nausea, vomiting, and gastrointestinal bleeding are other common complaints. Contrast radiographic studies are nonspecific and may be negative in up to 25% of cases; therefore, the diagnosis of candida esophagitis rests on detection of characteristic pseudomembranes and ulcerations by endoscopy. Examination of biopsy specimens, if obtained, confirms the diagnosis. Topical therapy with nonabsorbable antifungals is ineffective in patients with esophagitis, and systemic therapy with fluconazole, caspofungin, or IV amphotericin B is mandatory. The latter two agents are preferred in institutions with high rates of infections caused by non-*albicans* species or in patients with candida esophagitis who have received azoles in the past.

TABLE 76.11. Treatment of selected infections caused by *Candida* species.

Infection	*Drug*	*Route*	*Dosage*	*Duration*
Oropharyngeal	Clotrimazole	PO	10 mg troche 5¥/day	7–14 days
	Fluconazole	PO	100 mg daily	7–14 days
	Itraconazole	PO	200 mg daily	7–14 days
	Amphotericin B	IV	0.3 mg/kg daily	7–14 days
	Caspofungin	IV	70 mg loading dose 50 mg daily thereafter	7–14 days
Esophagitis	Fluconazole	IV/PO	200–400 mg loading dose 100–200 mg daily	14–21 days
	Amphotericin B	IV	0.3–0.7 mg/kg daily	14–21 days
	Caspofungin	IV	70 mg loading dose 50 mg daily thereafter	14–21 days
Candidemia	Amphotericin	IV	0.3–0.5 mg/kg daily	14 days after last positive culture
	Fluconazole	IV	400 mg daily	14 days after last positive culture
	Caspofungin	IV	70 mg loading dose 50 mg daily thereafter	14 days after last positive culture
Visceral candidiasis	Amphotericin	IV	0.5–0.7 mg/kg daily	Until lesions have resolved or calcified
	Fluconazole	IV	400 mg daily	Until lesions have resolved or calcified
	Caspofungin	IV	70 mg loading dose 50 mg daily thereafter	Until lesions have resolved or calcified

Source: Adapted in part from Pappas et al.,[173] by permission of *Clinical Infectious Diseases.*

Candida spp. are also an increasingly common cause of nosocomial BSI,[166] associated with case-fatality rates ranging from 30% to 60%.[167,168] Disseminated infection usually occurs as a complication of candidemia and may be associated with cutaneous lesions, retinitis or endophthalmitis, osteomyelitis, and even endocarditis. Most episodes of candidemia in nongranulocytopenic patients originate from IVDs.[169] However, controversy exists over the relative role of IVDs versus intestinal translocation in patients with granulocytopenia or who have received intensive cytotoxic chemotherapy.[170]

Studies performed two decades ago found that blood cultures are negative in more than 50% of patients with disseminated *Candida* infections confirmed at autopsy.[171] In contrast, recent studies have found that automated blood culturing systems detect up to 93% of cases of active candidemia.[172]

Recovery of *Candida* spp. from a blood culture should never be regarded as a contaminant in decisions regarding treatment. Controversies about the source of candidemia aside, a considerable body of literature suggests that retention of an IVD is associated with prolonged candidemia and excess mortality.[102–104] As a result, we believe that IVDs should be removed from most patients with proven candidemia. Candidemia that responds rapidly to removal of the device and institution of IV amphotericin B can be reliably treated with a daily dose of 0.3 to 0.5 mg/kg and a total dose of 3 to 5 mg/kg.[173] If a lipid-associated formulation of amphotericin B is being used, a daily dose of 1 to 2 mg/kg and a total dose of 10 to 20 mg/kg should be sufficient in most cases.[104] If the patient has septic thrombosis of the central vein, associated with high-grade candidemia and florid sepsis, or infection caused by non-*albicans* species, a higher dose of IV amphotericin B is recommended, 0.7 mg/kg/day and 20 mg/kg or more total conventional amphotericin, 2 to 3 mg/kg/day and 20 to 30 mg/kg total, for a lipid-associated formulation.[173]

Fluconazole (400 mg/day) has been shown to be as effective as IV amphotericin B in randomized trials in nongranulocytopenic patients,[174,175] and has further been shown to be comparable to amphotericin B in observational studies of granulocytopenic patients with *Candida* IVDR BSIs,[104] but should not be used in IVDR BSIs associated with septic thrombosis and high-grade candidemia or in BSIs caused by azole-resistant species.

Infections caused by fluconazole-resistant organisms, such as *Candida krusei* and *Candida glabrata*, have become all too common, with many centers reporting that more than 50% of their *Candida* isolates are non-*albicans* species that are usually resistant to azoles.[164] Caspofungin was recently shown to be at least as effective as IV amphotericin B in a prospective randomized double-blind trial in patients with deep *Candida* infections, most of whom had candidemia[176]; most notably, caspofungin was associated with a greatly reduced rate of study drug withdrawal because of adverse events (2.6% versus 23.2%; $P = 0.003$). Intravenous caspofungin, which has a low incidence of side effects and can be given once daily, can now be considered a first-line drug for initial treatment of deep invasive candidal infection in centers with high rates of infection caused by non-*albicans* species, pending identification and susceptibility of the bloodstream isolate.

Hepatosplenic candidiasis is a more indolent form of visceral candidiasis that typically presents as persistent fever in a cancer patient who is recovering from granulocytopenia.[177] Blood cultures are usually negative; however, imaging with CT demonstrates multiple small nodules in the liver and spleen (Figure 76.8), and occasionally in the lungs, kidneys, or bone as well. Cultures of material obtained by percutaneous aspiration or biopsy can confirm the diagnosis but because of the small size of the infected nodules may be negative. Therefore, most clinicians initiate therapy (see Table 76.11) on the basis of radiographic findings and only proceed to invasive diagnostic procedures when patients remain refractory to treatment.

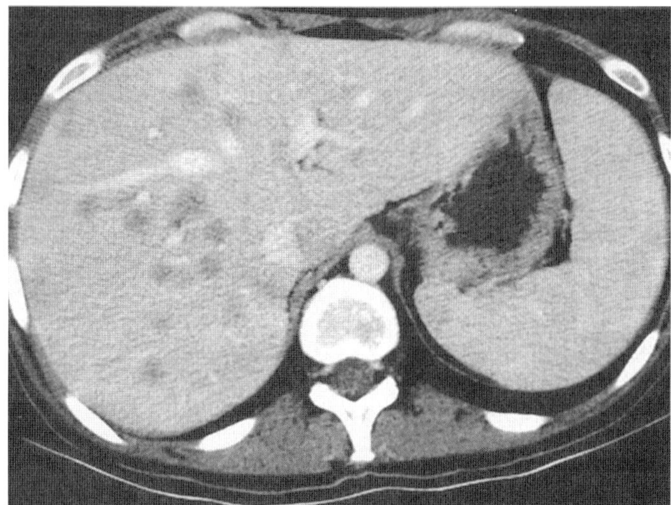

FIGURE 76.8. Hepatosplenic candidiasis in a patient with acute myelogenous leukemia seen on computed tomography (CT) scan. Multiple nodules can be seen in the liver and spleen. [By permission of Marchetti O, Calandra T. Infections in the neutropenic cancer patient. In: Cohen J, Powderly WG (eds) Infectious Diseases, 2nd ed. St. Louis: Mosby, 2004:1083.]

Aspergillus

Aspergillus spp. are ubiquitous environmental organisms, encountered most often in rural areas but also found throughout most hospitals. Invasive infections caused by *Aspergillus* spp. are an increasing problem in many hematology and solid organ transplant centers, with incidence rates of 5% to 24% among patients with acute leukemia.[178] Invasive aspergillosis is most often a complication of severe and prolonged granulocytopenia, and the duration of granulocytopenia is the most powerful predictor of risk of invasive aspergillosis. The median time to onset of disease in patients with severe granulocytopenia is 17 days and, historically, the majority of cases occur within 90 days in patients undergoing BMT,[163] although recent studies have found an increasing number of patients with invasive aspergillus that developed in 90 days or more.[179,180] Other risk factors associated with invasive aspergillosis include receipt of OKT3 antibodies, active CMV disease, and renal failure.[163] The most commonly isolated species have been *Aspergillus fumigatus* (more than 90% of all proven infections), *Aspergillus flavus*, *Aspergillus niger*, and *Aspergillus terreus*.

Aspergillus can infect any organ, but sinopulmonary disease is the most common manifestation. Infections often present insidiously in patients with granulocytopenia and fever may be the only manifestation. Dull chest pain that may become pleuritic in nature, cough, and sinus congestion are also common. Hemoptysis, although suspicious for invasive pulmonary aspergillosis, is relatively uncommon. Up to half of patients with lung involvement have disseminated disease that can involve the central nervous system, gastrointestinal tract, kidney, liver, or skin.[163] Less common presentations include isolated skin lesions, often at sites of vascular catheter insertions[181] or isolated gastrointestinal involvement,[163] possibly the result of ingestion of water containing these organisms.[182] Despite advances in diagnosis and treatment, mortality in patients with invasive aspergillosis remains high, 90% in BMT patients and nearly 80% in patients with leukemia.[183]

The diagnosis of invasive *Aspergillus* infection remains a formidable challenge. Chest radiographs are completely normal in 10% of patients with documented infection.[184] Chest CT is read as normal in only 3% of cases, and up to 85% of infected patients have characteristic radiographic findings, such as a "halo"[185] or "crescent"[186] sign. *Aspergillus* species are rarely isolated from expectorated sputum, and cultures of bronchoalveolar lavage (BAL) fluid are positive in only 20% of cases in most series; however, a positive culture for *Aspergillus fumigatus* has a very high positive predictive value for invasive disease in high-risk patients, in excess of 75%.[187] Transbronchial biopsy increases the diagnostic yield to 75%.[184] Molecular diagnostic tests that detect the presence of circulating galactomannan, a fungal cell wall constituent, and PCR techniques to detect ribosomal genetic material conserved across *Aspergillus* species, may eventually abrogate the need for invasive tests.[163] The sequential use of an ELISA to detect galactomannan was found to have an 87.5% positive predictive value and a 98.4% negative predictive value in a recent prospective trial in neutropenic BMT patients.[188]

The treatment of invasive aspergillosis has also undergone evolution. Traditional therapy has relied upon IV amphotericin B deoxycholate in doses of 1 to 1.5 mg/kg/day (Table 76.12); however, at these doses, nephrotoxicity is ubiquitous.

TABLE 76.12. Treatment options for patients with invasive infections caused by *Aspergillus* species.

Drug	*Route*	*Dose*	*Duration*
Amphotericin B deoxycholate	IV	1.0–1.5 mg/kg daily	Until evidence of infection has resolved
Liposomal amphotericin B (Ambisome)	IV	5.0–7.5 mg/kg daily; doses as high as 15 mg/kg daily have been used safely	Same
Amphotericin B lipid complex (ABLC)	IV	5.0 mg/kg daily	Same
Amphotericin B colloidal dispersion (ABCD)	IV	3–4 mg/kg daily	Same
Caspofungin	IV	70 mg loading dose 50 mg daily	Same
Itraconazole (suspension)	IV	6–12 mg/kg daily 200 mg bid	Same
	PO		Same
Voriconazole	IV	6 mg/kg q12 for 2 doses 4 mg/kg bid thereafter	Same
	PO	IV load as above 200 mg bid thereafter	Same
Combination therapy	Investigational		

Despite the use of lipid-based agents, such as liposomal amphotericin B and amphotericin B lipid complex, in daily doses of 5 to 10 mg/kg, treatment-related side effects have remained high, prompting a search for less toxic alternatives. Caspofungin, a member of a new class of drugs that inhibit the synthesis of 1,3-β-glucan, an integral component of the fungal cell wall, was approved for the treatment of invasive aspergillosis refractory to treatment with other agents in 2001.[189] Itraconazole also possesses activity against *Aspergillus* spp. and appeared to be equivalent to amphotericin B deoxycholate in a retrospective analysis[190]; however, bias toward treatment of less severely ill patients limits the generalizability of this report, and we do not believe that clinicians should rely upon itraconazole alone for the treatment of invasive aspergillus infections at this time.[190] On the other hand, the newly released triazole, voriconazole, was recently shown to be superior, in terms of fewer side effects and improved clinical response (53% versus 32%) and patient survival (71% versus 58%), compared to amphotericin B deoxycholate in a large multicenter randomized trial.[191] As a result, voriconazole is now widely considered the standard of therapy for patients with documented *Aspergillus* infections. The use of antifungal drug combinations for treatment of invasive aspergillosis is currently under investigation, with caspofungin combined with lipid-based amphotericin B or voriconazole showing the most promise.[192,193]

Zygomycetes

Zycomycosis, known more commonly as mucormycosis, is a devastating infection caused by a variety of filamentous fungi in the order Mucorales. Risk factors for mucormycosis include diabetic ketoacidosis, iron overload, and, increasingly, prolonged granulocytopenia.[194] Rhinocerebral disease is the most common presentation in patients with diabetic ketoacidosis; however, pulmonary involvement, very similar to that seen with invasive aspergillosis, appears to be the most common manifestation of Mucorales infection in patients with cancer.[194] A black eschar may be seen on the nasal mucosa or soft palate in rhinocerebral disease, or on the skin in disseminated disease (Figure 76.9), or at sites of intravascular catheter insertion.[195] Involvement of the central nervous system can occur either as a result of direct extension from the sinuses, with rhinocerebral disease, or hematogenously, in disseminated disease.

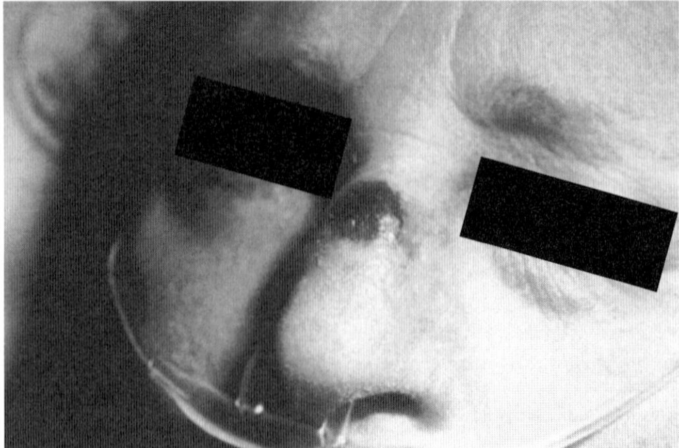

FIGURE 76.9. Necrotizing rhinocerebral infection with *Rhizopus*. Note the black eschar on the nose. [By permission of Stone DR, Gorbach SL (eds) Atlas of Infectious Diseases. Philadelphia: Saunders, 2000.]

Diagnosis of Mucorales infection rests on histopathologic examination or culture of a biopsy specimen, as blood and respiratory tract specimens are almost always culture negative, and the radiographic presentation may not be distinguishable from that seen with invasive pulmonary aspergillosis. It is important to recognize that the newer antifungals, voriconazole and caspofungin, have no activity against zygomycetes. Treatment begins with aggressive debridement whenever possible, combined with the use of conventional (1.0 to 1.5 mg/kg/day) or lipid-based amphotericin B (5 to 7.5 mg/kg/day). Despite treatment, mortality is greater than 75% in cancer patients.[163]

Fusarium

Fusarium species are soil saprophytes that have been increasingly implicated as a cause of fatal infection in patients with cancer, primarily patients with acute leukemia or those undergoing BMT.[196] Colonization originating from contaminated hospital water systems has been described,[197] although the significance of this finding has been challenged.[198] Fusariosis may be acquired either as a result of inhalation, with the development of pulmonary disease indistinguishable from invasive pulmonary aspergillosis, or from direct inoculation through the skin or an IVD access site. In all settings, hematogenous dissemination with widespread cutaneous involvement is common, and blood cultures are positive in up to 50% of patients with documented systemic fusariosis.[163] Recovery from granulocytopenia is critical to patient survival: a recent study found that all patients who had refractory granulocytopenia died of fusarium infection.[199]

Fluconazole and itraconazole are inactive against *Fusarium* species, and amphotericin B (1.0 to 1.5 mg/kg/day) is still considered the first line of therapy. Voriconazole possesses activity against *Fusarium* species in vitro, and its clinical use was associated with a complete or partial response in 43% of patients in a recent small trial.[194] Granulocyte infusions may have an important adjunctive role in infected patients with refractory granulocytopenia.[199]

Other Fungal Infections

A variety of unusual fungal organisms has been increasingly reported in infected patients with cancer.[163] Infections caused by these rare organisms have recently been reviewed by Walsh and Groll.[200] Table 76.13 lists some of the more prevalent emerging fungal pathogens and possible therapeutic options, although it is important to note that the outcome with most of these infections has been poor, and reported successes with treatment modalities have been anecdotal.

Evaluation of the Granulocytopenic Patient with Fever[6]

Infection in the granulocytopenic patient can progress very rapidly; hence, a thorough evaluation of the granulocytopenic patient with fever must be undertaken without delay. Characteristic signs and symptoms of inflammation may be minimal or absent,[201] and careful examination is necessary to detect subtle findings, especially in the periodontium; the

TABLE 76.13. Emerging fungal pathogens in patients with cancer.

Organism	*Treatment*
Dematiaceous (dark-walled) fungi	
Alternaria	Amphotericin B + flucytosine, itraconazole
Bipolaris	Itraconazole, voriconazole
Cladosporium	Amphotericin B, itraconazole
Curvularia	Amphotericin B, itraconazole, terbinafine
Scedosporium apiospermum (Pseudallescheria boydii)	Voriconazole, amphotericin B + itraconazole
Wangiella (Exophilia) dermatidis	Amphotericin + itraconazole, itraconazole
Hyaline fungi	
Acremonium	Amphotericin B, voriconazole
Geotrichum	Amphotericin B ± 5-flucytosine, itraconazole
Paecilomyces lilacinus	Amphotericin B, terbinafine
Paecilomyces variotii	Itraconazole or fluconazole
Penicillium	Amphotericin B, fluconazole, itraconazole
Trichophyton	Itraconazole or fluconazole
Yeasts	
Blastoschizomyces capitatus	Fluconazole
Trichosporon beigelii	Amphotericin B

pharynx; the lower esophagus; the lung; the perineum, including the anus; the eye (fundus); and the skin, including bone marrow aspiration sites, vascular catheter access sites, and tissue around the nails.

Bacterial cultures of blood should be obtained, including one drawn through the IVD; if a catheter insertion site has exudate, the material should be also be sent for Gram stain and culture. If the exudate is chronic, the material should also be analyzed for fungi and mycobacteria. A sample for urine microscopy and culture should also be obtained.

The evaluation of infectious diarrhea is based on whether it is community acquired, nosocomial, or chronic. For community-acquired diarrhea, stool specimens should be cultured for *Salmonella*, *Shigella*, *Campylobacter*, and *Escherichia coli* O157:H7. The major cause of nosocomial diarrhea is *Clostridium difficile*, which has been addressed in an earlier section; for diarrhea after 3 or more days of hospitalization, stool cultures for common community-acquired enteric pathogens have very low yield and are rarely necessary.[202] Persistent infectious cryptogenic diarrhea may warrant evaluation for giardia and cryptosporidium infection.

New, abnormal skin lesions in granulocytopenic patients often represent invasive bacterial or fungal infection and should be aspirated, or better, biopsied, and a Gram stain, bacterial and fungal culture, and histopathologic examination should be performed.

Chest radiographs should be obtained whenever signs or symptoms point toward a respiratory tract process. Some experts recommend chest radiography for all persons who are to be treated as outpatients, even without clinical evidence of pulmonary infection. A baseline radiograph may be helpful for granulocytopenic patients who subsequently develop respiratory symptoms or evidence of an infiltrate but may not be cost-effective on a routine basis. Of note, high-resolution CT will reveal evidence of pneumonia in more than one-half of febrile granulocytopenic patients who have normal findings on chest radiograph.

Examination of CSF is not recommended as a routine procedure unless the patient has severe headache, meningismus, or altered mental status. However, in general, a CT scan with and without intravenous contrast should be obtained before performing a lumbar puncture because of the risk of intracranial hemorrhage in patients with drug-induced thrombocytopenia and to rule out central fungal infection.

Complete blood cell counts and determination of the levels of serum creatinine and urea nitrogen are needed to plan supportive care and to monitor antiinfective drug toxicity. These tests should be done at least every 3 days during the course of intensive antiinfective therapy; more frequent monitoring may be required if amphotericin B is also being given.

Initial Empiric Antimicrobial Therapy

Empiric antimicrobial therapy should be instituted without delay in all granulocytopenic patients with fever, ideally, within 2 hours of the clinical evaluation. Afebrile patients who are granulocytopenic, but who have signs or symptoms suggestive of infection, should also receive empirical antimicrobial therapy, begun in the same manner as for febrile patients. The choice of initial antimicrobial regimens should be based on knowledge of the most common infecting pathogens in that center or patient population and the antibiotic susceptibilities at that institution. The major pathogens causing infection in granulocytopenic patients are shown in Table 76.3. *Because of the ever-present risk of life-threatening infection by* Pseudomonas aeruginosa, *all initial antimicrobial regimens must include at least one drug with antipseudomonal activity.*

Despite a plethora of randomized trials, no single empiric regimen can be recommended for the treatment of all patients with granulocytopenic fever. Comparing numerous studies is difficult because of differing definitions of disease and criteria used to assess the response to treatment.

The 2002 IDSA Guideline offers three options for initial intravenous antimicrobial therapy that are considered to be of comparable efficacy,[6] with the caveat that one may be more appropriate for certain patients or in certain institutions than the others: single-drug therapy (monotherapy), two-drug therapy without a glycopeptide (vancomycin), and therapy with glycopeptide (vancomycin) plus one or two other antiinfective drugs.

MONOTHERAPY

Multiple studies have shown no outcome differences between monotherapy and multidrug combinations for empiric treatment of uncomplicated fever in granulocytopenic patients, that is, those without clinical evidence of local infection or sepsis at the outset. Two recent meta-analyses encompassing more than 4,000 patients, found that patients with uncomplicated granulocytopenic fever treated with a beta-lactam alone, as contrasted with a beta-lactam plus an aminoglycoside found no significant difference in all-cause mortality (RR, 0.85–0.87; $P = 0.057$).[203,204] Although rates of superinfection in both groups were similar, the frequency of adverse events was higher in patients receiving combination therapy. Another meta-analysis, using clinical failure of antimicrobial therapy as the outcome measure, also found beta-lactam monotherapy to be comparable to aminoglycoside-containing combinations in uncomplicated granulocytopenic fever.[205]

The antimicrobial agents that have been best studied for monotherapy include a third-generation (ceftazidime) or fourth-generation cephalosporin (cefepime) or a carbapenem (imipenem-cilastatin or meropenem). The emergence of extended-spectrum β-lactamases (ESBL) in *Enterobacteriaceae* has reduced the utility of ceftazidime for monotherapy.[206] Imipenem-cilastatin, meropenem, and cefepime, unlike ceftazidime, are active against ESBL-producing *Enterobacteriaceae* and also have excellent activity against viridans streptococci and pneumococci. A prospective double-blind study of 411 patients with cancer showed that the rate of clinical response was higher in febrile granulocytopenic patients treated with meropenem than it was in those treated with ceftazidime.[207]

It is important to recognize that the spectrum of any of these drugs does not usually encompass coagulase-negative staphylococci, methicillin-resistant *Staphylococcus aureus*, vancomycin-resistant enterococci, and some strains of multiresistant *Streptococcus pneumoniae* or viridans streptococci. Therefore, close monitoring of the clinical response to treatment is important, and antiinfective therapy may need to be adapted to institutional susceptibilities, and modified, based on the susceptibilities of the organisms recovered in culture.

Current evidence to support the use of fluoroquinolones as monotherapy is limited and the results of the few studies have been conflicting.[208] The widespread use of fluoroquinolones for prophylaxis in granulocytopenic patients also limits their utility for initial empiric therapy, and this class of drugs cannot be recommended for initial monotherapy in patients with granulocytopenia and fever. Treatment with aminoglycosides alone is also suboptimal and not recommended.

TWO-DRUG COMBINATION THERAPY

Two-drug combination therapy most often comprises an aminoglycoside (gentamicin, tobramycin, or amikacin) plus an antipseudomonal penicillin (ticarcillin-clavulanate or piperacillin-tazobactam) or an antipseudomonal cephalosporin (cefepime or ceftazidime), or an an aminoglycoside plus a carbapenem (imipenem-cilastatin or meropenem). These regimens have been shown to have comparable efficacy in numerous trials.[204] Because of intrinsic and growing acquired resistance in many species of gram-negative bacteria causing serious infections,[209] and the high mortality associated with these infections, combination antimicrobial therapy, most commonly with two drugs, is intuitively appealing. However, as noted, the studies to date have not shown combination therapy to be superior to monotherapy *if there is no clinical obvious source of infection at the time therapy is begun.*[31,204] Moreover, there are disadvantages to using combination antiinfective therapy, including increased toxicity and cost and, possibly, an increased likelihood of a superinfection with even more resistant bacteria or fungi.

Although the combination of ciprofloxacin with piperacillin-tazobactam was found to have efficacy comparable to tobramycin and piperacillin-tazobactam in a large multicenter randomized trial,[210] in our opinion, fluoroquinolones in initial empiric regimens should not be used *if* the patient has had heavy exposure to this class of drugs in the past, such as for prophylaxis or treatment of a recent infection.

VANCOMYCIN-CONTAINING REGIMENS

There has been much controversy regarding the inclusion of vancomycin in the initial empiric regimen for the febrile granulocytopenic patient to provide a drug active against methicillin-resistant staphylococci, enterococci, and *Corynebacterium* species. Comparative trials have found that inclusion of vancomycin in the initial regimen does reduce the frequency of secondary nosocomial BSIs with these organisms during therapy[211]; however, these studies have not shown reduced morbidity and mortality. A recent prospective trial randomized 165 granulocytopenic patients with persistent fever despite piperacillin/tazobactam to the addition of vancomycin or placebo; no statistically significant differences were noted regarding time to defervescence or additional episodes of gram-positive bacteremia.[212]

In general, heavy use of vancomycin in the absence of a clear clinical indication is undesirable because of the risk of promoting vancomycin resistance in enterococci or *S. aureus*. Thus, routine use of vancomycin in the initial antimicrobial regimen for the febrile granulocytopenic patient is not recommended unless (1) the hospital has a high rate of nosocomial infection with MRSA or the patient is known to have previously been colonized or infected by MRSA, (2) there are reasons to suspect overwhelming alpha-hemolytic viridans streptococcal bacteremia, that is, shock with respiratory distress, (3) the patient shows evidence of infection at the exit site or tunnel of a CVC, or (4) the patient is at risk for endocarditis, that is, has a prosthetic heart valve.[213]

For microbiologically confirmed infections with coagulase-negative staphylococci or other resistant gram-positive organisms, vancomycin should be added to the initial regimen. Linezolid, the first U.S. Food and Drug Administration (FDA)-approved oxazolidinone, offers promise for treatment of resistant gram-positive bacterial infections, including those caused by VRE, although reversible drug-related myelosuppression can be seen, mainly with prolonged courses. Quinupristin-dalfopristin, another drug that has recently been approved by the FDA, is also effective against vancomycin-resistant *E. faecium* (but not *E. fecalis*) and other gram-positive bacteria.[214] However, further studies are needed before recommendations can be made for the use of these drugs in initial empiric regimens in patients with cancer.

Oral Antimicrobial Therapy

Until recently, the accepted standard of care for the cancer patient with granulocytopenic fever, has been immediate hospitalization for parenteral administration of antibiotics, with close monitoring for complications and response to therapy.[215] As a result, there has been a dramatic decrease in mortality among febrile granulocytopenic patients. Recent investigations have shown that granulocytopenic patients with fever are a heterogeneous population, with varying risks relative to the response to therapy, the occurrence of serious medical complications, and mortality.[216,217]

Over the past decade, subsets of febrile granulocytopenic patients at low risk for complications have been identified, which have impelled studies of using oral antimicrobials, entirely in the outpatient setting or in the hospital, usually following a brief course of parenteral broad-spectrum antiinfective therapy. Table 76.14 summarizes the randomized controlled trials that have been undertaken to examine the efficacy and safety of oral antimicrobial therapy for low-risk patients with granulocytopenic fever.

These trials should be interpreted within the context of their limitations. Assessment of risk of infection, antimicrobial regimens used, and location of antimicrobial therapy (inpatient or outpatient) varied widely. Moreover, the outcome "success of therapy" was not uniformly defined. Nonetheless, the results of these important studies show

TABLE 76.14. Randomized controlled trials assessing the efficacy of oral antibiotic therapy in granulocytopenic patients with fever.

Author	*Patient population*	*Location of group treated orally*	*Antimicrobial regimen Oral treatment*	*Resolution of infection Inpatient parenteral*	*Oral treatment parenteral*	*RR Inpatient*	*Relative risk*
Minotti 1999[284]	Adults	Outpatient	Ciprofloxacin	Ceftriaxone	82%	75%	1.09
Paganini 2000[285]	Children	Outpatient	Ceftriaxone then cefixime	Ceftriaxone + amikacin	98%	98%	1.00
Paganini 2001[286]	Children	Outpatient	Initial ceftriaxone then ciprofloxacin	Ceftriaxone + amikacin followed by cefixime	100%	98%	1.02
Paganini 2003[287]	Children	Outpatient	Ciprofloxacin	Ceftriaxone[a]	85%	82%	1.03
Shenep 2001[288]	Children	Inpatient	Cefixime	Ticarcillin + tobramcyin + vancomycin	72%	73%	0.98
Mullen 1999[289]	Children	Outpatient	Ciprofloxacin	Ceftazidime[a]	80%	94%	0.85
Hidalgo 1999[290]	Adults	Outpatient	Ofloxacin	Ceftazidime + amikacin	89%	91%	0.97
Innes 2003[291]	Adults	Outpatient	Ciprofloxacin + amoxicillin-clavulanate	Gentamicin + piperacillin-tazobactam	84%	90%	0.93
Petrilli 2000[292]	Children	Outpatient	Ciprofloxacin	Ceftriaxone[a]	83%	75%	1.16
Freifeld 1999[293]	Adults	Inpatient	Ciprofloxacin + amoxicillin-clavulanate	Ceftazidime	71%	67%	1.05
Kern 1999[294]	Adults	Inpatient	Ciprofloxacin + amoxicillin-clavulanate	Ceftriaxone + amikacin	86%	84%	1.02
Engervall 1996[295]	Adults	Outpatient	Trimethoprim-sulfamethoxazole + amikacin	Ceftazidime	30%	36%	0.83
Velasco 1995[296]	Adults	Inpatient	Ciprofloxacin and penicillin	Amikacin + carbenicillin	94%	93%	1.01
Giamarellou 2000[208]	Adults	Inpatient	Ciprofloxacin	Ceftazidime + amikacin	50%	50%	1.00
Malik 1992[297]	Adults	Inpatient	Ofloxacin as outpatient	Ofloxacin as inpatient	81%	83%	0.97
Rubenstein 1993[298]	Adults	Inpatient	Ciprofloxacin + clindamycin	Clindamycin + aztreonam[a]	88%	95%	0.92
Johnson 1992[299]	Adults	Outpatient	Ciprofloxacin	Azlocillin + netilmicin	38%	42%	0.90
Flaherty 1989[300]	Adults	Outpatient	Ciprofloxacin + azlocillin	Ceftazidime + amikacin	35%	56%	0.62
Chan 1989[301]	Adults	Outpatient	Ciprofloxacin + netilmicin	Piperacillin + netilmicin	59%	62%	0.95
Rolston 1995[302]	Adults	Outpatient	Ciprofloxacin + amoxicillin-clavulanate	Clindamycin + aztreonam	90%	87%	1.03

[a] Parenteral regimen was provided on an outpatient basis.

that, in general, the outcomes for low-risk patients treated with oral antimicrobial therapy are generally equivalent to those for similar-risk patients treated with intravenously administered therapy. Oral therapy has the advantages of reduced cost, the potential for outpatient management, and avoidance of intravenous access, thereby obviating the risk of IVDR BSI. The oral regimens that have been most thoroughly evaluated are ofloxacin alone, ciprofloxacin alone, and ciprofloxacin plus amoxicillin-clavulanate.

Pivotal to the success of this approach in clinical practice is to accurately identify patients at low risk. Clinical prediction rules have been developed for this purpose. The hypothesis of Talcott et al. that granulocytopenic patients with controlled cancer and no serious comorbidity who developed fever in an outpatient setting are at low risk and can safely be treated as outpatients, was validated in a prospective study.[217] Klastersky et al. developed a Multinational Association for Supportive Care in Cancer risk index; a score of more than 21 identified low-risk patients with a positive predictive value of 91%, specificity of 68%, and sensitivity of 71%.[218] The variables comprising this index are summarized in Table 76.15.

Summary Recommendations for Initial Empiric Therapy

Figure 76.10 summarizes the IDSA 2002 Guideline Recommendations for Initial Empiric Antimicrobial Therapy in Granulocytopenic Patients with Fever.[6] The first step is to determine whether the patient is at low or high risk for serious life-threatening infection, on the basis of the criteria observed at the time of presentation (see Table 76.15). If the risk is high, IV antimicrobials must be used; if risk is low, the patient may be treated with either intravenous or oral drugs. Second, decide whether the patient qualifies for vancomycin therapy. If the patient qualifies, begin treatment with a two- or three-drug combination, with vancomycin plus cefepime, ceftazidime, or a carbapenem, with or without an aminoglycoside. If vancomycin is not indicated, begin monotherapy with a cephalosporin (cefepime or ceftazidime) or a carbapenem (meropenem or imipenem-cilastatin), administered

TABLE 76.15. Scoring index for identification of low-risk febrile granulocytopenic patients at time of presentation with fever.[a]

Characteristic	*Score*
Extent of illness[b]	
No symptoms	5
Mild symptoms	5
Moderate symptoms	3
No hypotension	5
No chronic obstructive pulmonary disease	4
Solid tumor or no fungal infection	4
No dehydration	3
Outpatient at onset of fever	3
Age less than 60 years	2

[a] Does not apply to patients 16 years of age or less. Initial monocyte count of 100 cells/mm^3 or more, no comorbidity, and normal chest radiograph findings indicate children at low risk for significant bacterial infections.

[b] Choose one item only. Highest theoretical score is 26. A risk index score of 21 or more indicates that the patient is likely to be at low risk for complications and morbidity.

Source: Adapted from Hughes et al.,[6] by permission of *Clinical Infectious Diseases.*

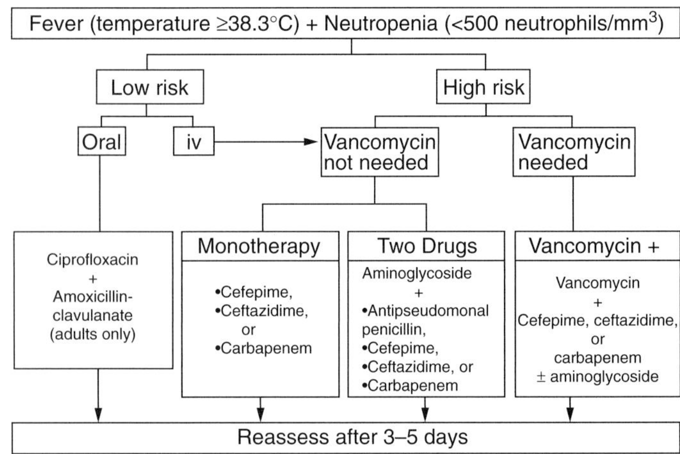

FIGURE 76.10. Algorithm for initial management of febrile granulocytopenic patients. (From Hughes et al.,[6] by permission of *Clinical Infectious Diseases.*)

intravenously for uncomplicated cases. Two-drug combinations are recommended for management of complicated cases or if antimicrobial resistance is strongly suspected.

Adults selected for oral therapy may receive ciprofloxacin plus amoxicillin-clavulanate. Selection of patients for outpatient therapy must be done carefully from the low-risk group, depending on the capabilities of the medical center and the feasibility of close follow-up. Initial therapy with oral antimicrobials alone in the outpatient setting is not recommended for children because of a lack of sufficient evidence.

Modification of Empiric Therapy

The majority of patients with febrile granulocytopenia will not have a microbiologically documented infection. Therefore, duration of therapy usually cannot be guided by monitoring clinical resolution of a local infection or clearance of bacteremia. Scientific evidence to answer this important question is scant and does not permit definitive conclusions. The evidence-based 2002 IDSA Guideline for the management of granulocytopenic fever stratifies patients by duration of fever and, for patients who become afebrile by day 3, recommends discontinuation of antiinfective therapy if the patient's granulocyte count is 500 cells/mm^3 or higher for 2 consecutive days, there is no definite site of infection, and cultures remain negative. If the patient's granulocyte count is still less than 500 cells/mm^3 by day 7, but the patient was initially at low risk and there are no subsequent complications, therapy may be stopped when the patient is afebrile for 5 to 7 days. However, if the patient was initially considered to be high risk, antiinfective therapy should be continued (Figure 76.11).[6]

Patients with persistent fever for more than 3 days after initial therapy, for whom no infected site of organism has been identified, pose the greatest challenge. Persistent fever suggests that the patient has a nonbacterial, especially fungal, infection, a bacterial infection resistant to or slow to respond to the drug or drugs being given, the emergence of a superinfection, inadequate serum and tissue levels of the antibiotic(s), drug fever, or need for source control (e.g., an abscess or infected IVD). Although some patients with microbiologically defined bacterial infections, even when appropriately

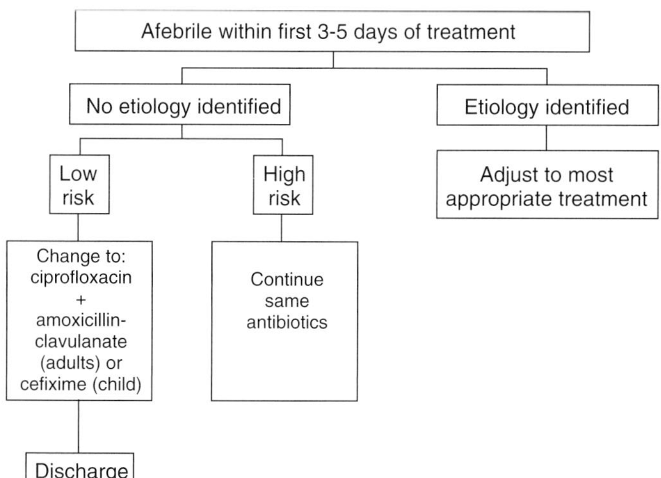

FIGURE 76.11. Guide for management of patients who become afebrile in the first 3 to 5 days of initial antibiotic therapy. See Table 7.15 for rating patients at low risk. (From Hughes et al.,[6] by permission of *Clinical Infectious Diseases*.)

treated, may require 5 days of therapy before defervescence occurs, a comprehensive reassessment should be undertaken if the patient fails to respond to initial therapy within 3 days, to include a review of all culture results, physical examination, chest radiograph, culturing of additional blood samples, and samples from clinically suspected sites of infection, and diagnostic imaging of any deep organ suspected of harboring infection. Ultrasonography or high-resolution CT are especially helpful for patients with suspected pneumonia, sinusitis, or typhlitis.

If fever persists after 5 days of antimicrobial therapy and reassessment does not yield a cause, there are three possible approaches (Figure 76.12): (1) continue treatment with the initial antibiotics, (2) modify the initial regimen, or (3) add an antifungal agent to the regimen, with or without modification of the antibacterial regimen.

If no discernible improvement in the patient's condition has occurred (i.e., the patient remains febrile but stable) during the first 4 to 5 days of initial antimicrobial therapy, and if reevaluation yields no new information to the contrary,

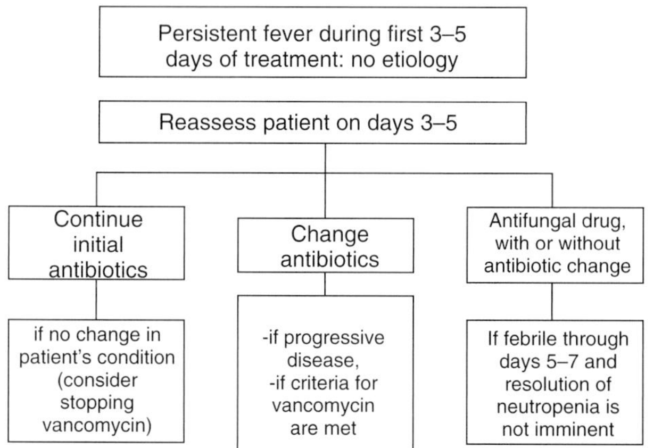

FIGURE 76.12. Guide to treatment of patients who have persistent fever after 3 to 5 days of treatment and for whom the cause of the fever is not found. (From Hughes et al.,[6] by permission of *Clinical Infectious Diseases*.)

the initial regimen can be continued. This decision will be strengthened if the granulocytopenia can be expected to resolve within the ensuing 5 days.

If evidence suggests clinical deterioration or a complication (such as the onset of abdominal pain from enterocolitis or typhlitis, new or worsening mucosal lesions, or drainage from an IVD exit site or pulmonary infiltrates) during the initial antimicrobial course, consideration should be given to adding appropriate antibiotics or changing to a different regimen.

If the initial regimen is monotherapy or two drugs without vancomycin, vancomycin may be considered if any of the criteria for use of vancomycin previously mentioned has been met. If a blood- or site-specific pathogen is isolated, the most appropriate antibiotic should be used while continuing broad-spectrum coverage.

The third decision to consider is the addition of empiric antifungal therapy. Amphotericin B is usually the drug of first choice (see Figure 76.12). Studies in 1982[219]and 1989[220] suggested that up to one-third of febrile granulocytopenic patients who do not respond to a 1-week course of empiric antimicrobial therapy have a systemic fungal infection that, in most cases, is caused by *Candida* or *Aspergillus* species. The empiric use of IV amphotericin B deoxycholate in patients with prolonged febrile granulocytopenia, was shown to reduce the incidence of invasive fungal infection and improve patient survival.[221,222] Although clinicians disagree when amphotericin B therapy should be initiated empirically, most believe that the patient who remains febrile and profoundly granulocytopenic for 5 days, despite administration of antimicrobial therapy in adequate doses, is a candidate for antifungal therapy.[6] However, every effort should be made to determine whether systemic fungal infection exists, by biopsy of suspicious lesions, radiographs of chest and sinuses, nasal endoscopy to investigate sinusitis, and CT of the abdomen and chest, before amphotericin B therapy is started.

Comparative trials show that lipid formulations of amphotericin B can be used as alternatives to amphotericin B deoxycholate for empiric therapy. Although they do not appear to be any more effective therapeutically,[223] lipid formulations of amphotericin are associated with much less infusion-related toxicity and, especially, nephrotoxicity.[224,225]

The use of azoles—fluconazole, itraconazole, or voriconazole—in patients with febrile granulocytopenia has been less well studied. Small trials have demonstrated equivalency between amphotericin B deoxycholate and fluconazole[226] or itraconazole[227]; however, both these studies were performed in populations with low rates of filamentous fungal infection.

The new triazole, voriconazole, has also been compared to liposomal amphotericin B in a large randomized multicenter study.[228] The use of voriconazole was associated with a reduced incidence of documented invasive fungal infections; however, voriconazole was found to be inferior to liposomal amphotericin, based on a five-part composite primary endpoint. As a result, voriconazole has not been licensed by the FDA for the empiric therapy of febrile granulocytopenia.[229]

Duration of Antimicrobial Therapy

The most important guides to successful discontinuation of antibiotics are the granulocyte count and defervescence

TABLE 76.16. Recommendations for duration of empiric antimicrobial therapy for patients with granulocytopenic fever.

Duration	*Recommendation*
Afebrile by day 3–5	
ANC >500 per 2 consecutive days	Stop antibiotics 48 hours after afebrile and ANC >500
ANC <500 by day 7	
Initially considered low-risk patient and clinically well	Stop antibiotics when afebrile for 5–7 days
Initially considered high risk, or profoundly granulocytopenic, or with mucositis or clinically unstable	Continue antibiotics
Persistent fever without identifiable source or pathogen	
ANC >500	Stop antibiotics 4–5 days after ANC >500 and reassess
ANC <500	Continue antibiotics for 2 weeks; reassess and stop if no disease is found

Source: Adapted from Hughes et al.,[6] by permission of *Clinical Infectious Diseases.*

(Table 76.16). As noted earlier, if no infection is identified, if the granulocyte count is 500 cells/mm^3 or more for 2 consecutive days, and the patient is afebrile for 48 hours or more, empiric antimicrobial therapy may be stopped at that time.

If the patient becomes afebrile but remains granulocytopenic, the best course is less well defined and no consensus exists. Some authorities recommend continuation of antibiotics, given intravenously or orally, until granulocytopenia has resolved; others suggest that for granulocytopenic patients who appear healthy clinically, who are in a low-risk category at onset of treatment, and who have no radiographic or laboratory evidence of infection may have systemic antimicrobial therapy stopped after 5 to 7 afebrile days, or sooner with hematologic recovery.[230] If antibiotics are stopped while the patient has granulocytopenia, the patient must be monitored very closely and intravenous antibiotics resumed immediately with the recurrence of fever or other evidence of bacterial infection.[231] *In general, antibiotic therapy should be continued throughout the granulocytopenic period in patients with profound granulocytopenia (less than 100 cells/mm^3), mucous membrane lesions of the mouth or gastrointestinal tract, unstable vital signs, or other identified risk factors.*

In patients with prolonged granulocytopenia in whom hematologic recovery cannot be anticipated, one can consider stopping antibiotic therapy after 2 weeks if no site of infection has been identified and the patient can be observed carefully (see Table 76.16).

The duration of amphotericin B therapy differs. If a systemic fungal infection has been identified, the course of antifungal therapy will be determined by the causative agent, the extent of the disease, and the clinical and microbiologic response. However, if no fungal infection is found, it is less clear how long empiric amphotericin B or other antifungal drugs should be continued. Experience is limited predominantly to amphotericin B. When granulocytopenia has resolved, the patient is clinically well, and CT of the abdomen and chest reveal no suspicious lesions, amphotericin B may be discontinued.[232] For clinically well patients with prolonged granulocytopenia, it is suggested that, after 2 weeks of daily doses of amphotericin B, if no discernible lesions can be found by clinical evaluation, chest radiography (or CT of the chest), and CT of the intraabdominal organs,[233] the drug can be stopped. In the patient who appears ill or is at high risk, one should consider continuation of therapy with antibiotics *and* amphotericin B throughout the period of granulocytopenia, assuming that hematologic recovery can be anticipated.

Predictors of Response to Antimicrobial Therapy

Elting et al. assessed predictors of outcome in 909 episodes of bacteremia selected from 10 randomized clinical trials of antimicrobial therapy for infection in patients with cancer and granulocytopenia.[234] Extensive tissue infection significantly compromised response to initial therapy (74% versus 38%; *P* less than 0.0001), ultimate outcome of infection (94% versus 73%; *P* less than 0.0001), and survival (94% versus 75%; *P* less than 0.0001). Log regression showed that shock (OR, 18.0; *P* less than 0.0001) and bacteremia caused by *P. aeruginosa* species (OR, 7.0; *P* = 0.03), *Clostridium* species (OR, 9.0; *P* = 0.006), or a pathogen resistant to antibiotics used for initial therapy (OR, 3.0; *P* less than 0.0001), were each independently associated with a poor outcome. Recovery of the granulocyte count predicted a favorable outcome (OR, 0.4; *P* less than 0.0001). Although the overall mortality rate was not significantly increased when patients with bacteremia caused by gram-negative organisms initially received monotherapy or when patients with bacteremia due to gram-positive organisms received delayed vancomycin therapy, these strategies increased the duration of therapy by 25%. Patients with bacteremia caused by alpha-hemolytic streptococcus were more likely to die if vancomycin was not included in the initial empirical regimen (*P* = 0.004).

Hematopoietic Growth Factors

Hematopoietic growth factors have been studied as an adjunct to antimicrobial therapy for granulocytopenic fever in several randomized trials. Although the duration of granulocytopenia was consistently shorter in these studies, it did not translate into clinically relevant improved outcomes. In a meta-analysis of 13 randomized, controlled trials comparing antibiotics and granulocyte colony-stimulating factor (G-CSF) with antibiotics alone for granulocytopenic fever, Clark et al. found a decrease in length of hospitalization [RR, 0.63; 95% confidence interval (CI), 0.40–0.82; *P* less than 0.001] and a shorter time to granulocyte recovery (RR, 0.32; 95% CI, 0.23–0.46; *P* less than 0.001); however, no effect on either overall mortality (OR, 0.68; 95% CI, 0.43–1.08; *P* = 0.05) or infection-related mortality (OR, 0.85; 95% CI, 0.33–2.20; *P* = 0.7) was observed.[235] Based on the available evidence, recent guidelines[6,236] that have addressed the use of G-CSF and granulocyte macrophage colony-stimulating factors (GM-CSF) in patients with cancer recommend against the routine use of hematopoietic growth factors. However, under certain conditions, with a worsening of the course and expected delay in marrow recovery, use of these agents may be appropriate with pneumonia, hypotension, or shock, severe cellulitis or sinusitis, systemic fungal infections, or multiorgan dysfunction secondary to sepsis.[6] Therapy with colony-stimulating factors could also be considered for patients who remain severely granulocytopenic and have documented infections that have failed to respond to appropriate antimicrobial therapy, such as gram-negative cellulitis.

Granulocyte Transfusions

Existing evidence does not support the routine use of granulocyte transfusions in patients with granulocytopenic fever. The major indication for granulocyte transfusion support at the present time is the patient with profound granulocytopenia and overwhelming gram-negative bacillary infection, especially major soft tissue infection that is unresponsive to antiinfective therapy.[237]

Supportive Therapy

Treatment of infection, especially associated with sepsis or early multiple organ dysfunction (MODS) syndrome, does not stop with source control and antiinfective therapy but demands the highest skills of the clinician to keep the patient alive until the infection can be controlled.

Circulatory Support

The importance of very early and aggressive circulatory support of the septic patient with large volumes of fluids, with or without cardiovascular pressor drugs, cannot be overemphasized.[238] The most experienced clinician cannot by physical examination alone reliably assess a critically ill patient's cardiac performance vis-à-vis ventricular filling pressures or cardiac output. Thus, if an infected patient exhibits hypoxemia or hypotension refractory to initial fluid resuscitation, a flow-directed, balloon-tipped, pulmonary artery catheter (PAC) can be helpful to guide fluid therapy and decisions on choice of pressors and inotropic drugs, with the physiologic goal of optimizing oxygen delivery and uptake. Recent fear, based on a retrospective study, that PACs increase mortality in critically ill patients[239] has been dispelled by a large, multicenter randomized trial in older adult surgical patients showing that PACs can be used safely without increased mortality.[240]

There are no data to indicate that colloid solutions, such as albumin, plasma protein fraction, or hydroxyethyl starch (hetastarch) are superior to crystalloids, such as 0.9% normal saline or Ringer's lactate, for support of the failing circulation in the patient with septic shock. Crystalloids should be the IV fluid of choice for treatment of sepsis and in the patient with shock and should be given aggressively in the first 4 to 6 hours, guided by the central venous pressure, to minimize mortality.[238]

Novel Adjunctive Therapies

For nearly 40 years, despite advances in antiinfective therapy and in ICU care, the mortality of septic shock has declined only marginally, pointing up the need to modulate the severe systemic inflammatory response syndrome that underlies shock, multiorgan dysfunction, and death.[213]

Patients who have been receiving long-term corticosteroid therapy who develop sepsis need supplemental stress doses of corticosteroids, hydrocortisone 50 to 75 mg IV every 6 hours, to prevent acute adrenal crisis. However, there is growing evidence to suggest that these doses of hydrocortisone will improve survival in patients with severe sepsis. A recent multicenter, double-blind randomized trial in France found, in patients with severe sepsis or septic shock, that adjunctive therapy with hydrocortisone 50 mg IV every 6 hours and fludrocortisone 5 μg per day orally reduced mortality 30%.[241]

It has long been recognized that most patients with septic shock have low levels of the essential physiologic anticoagulant, protein C. A recent international, multicenter trial was undertaken to assess the therapeutic effect of repleting protein C with a recombinant activated form (rhAPC) in patients with severe sepsis, 75% with shock.[242] The choice of protein C was influenced by knowledge of its capacity to modulate inflammation through inhibition of monocyte production of tumor necrosis factor-alpha (TNF-α) and interleukin (IL)-1b, inhibition of neutrophil activation, and downregulation of endothelial expression molecules, intercellular adhesion molecule ICAM-1, E-selectin, and VCAM-1. In the double-blind trial in 1,640 patients, a continuous infusion of rhAPC 24 μg/kg/min, begun within 24 hours of the onset of severe sepsis and continued for 96 hours, was associated with a 19% reduction in 28-day all-cause mortality ($P = 0.005$). There was a slight increase in bleeding complications in recipients of rhAPC (serious bleeding, 3.5% versus 2.0%; $P = 0.06$); however, rhAPC was well tolerated, considering the critical illness of most of the recipients.[242] The major contraindications to adjuvant use of rhAPC in cancer patients are active bleeding, severe thrombocytopenia (less than 30,000), or chronic renal or hepatic failure.

Prevention of Infection in the Patient with Cancer[213]

Protective Isolation

Profound and prolonged granulocytopenia, whether caused by the primary hematologic malignancy or its therapy, puts the patient at great risk for severe infection. Approximately 70% of deaths from acute nonlymphoblastic leukemia (ANLL) are ascribed to infection, the risk of which is inversely related to the absolute granulocyte count. Prevention of infection may allow patients to receive more intensive chemotherapy and thereby increase the rates of remission and overall survival. Concerted efforts have been made to protect the granulocytopenic patient from nosocomial infection during chemotherapy or bone marrow transplantation. Randomized trials have prospectively evaluated various procedures for protection of the granulocytopenic patient, including protective environments, the use of prophylactic nonabsorbable antibiotics, or both.[243]

Most programs have been based on elaborate protocols for protection against both extrinsic and endogenous pathogens, typically isolating the patient in a room or tent with filtered ultraclean air and requiring persons entering the room to wear sterile overgarments, gloves, shoe covers, and masks. Such protocols have been supplemented by regular applications of cutaneous and orificial disinfectants, use of food and water low in microbial content, and continuous administration of prophylactic oral nonabsorbable antibiotics. Because the expense of such complex programs is prohibitive for most hospitals, simple protective isolation (or reverse precautions) requiring that the person entering the room wear a clean gown, gloves, and mask is widely used as an alternative means to protect the granulocytopenic patient from infection. A prospective, randomized unblinded study to assess the efficacy of protective isolation in 37 granulocytopenic patients with 43 episodes of infection found no statistically significant differences in the overall incidence of infection, time to onset of first infection, or days with fever.[244] Neither response to antileukemic therapy nor survival was improved with isolation.

These randomized trials are difficult to compare because of differing isolation protocols, different antileukemic or antibiotic regimens; moreover, criteria of infection have not been consistently defined. In general, however, comparative studies have shown that patients in whom some method or protection was used, either a protective environment or antibiotics alone or in combination, had fewer infections, fewer days of fever, and often reduced mortality from infection. However, more importantly, these measures have failed to find improvement in rates of leukemic remission or overall survival.

Prevention of Nosocomial Transmission of Resistant Organisms

Isolation of infected and colonized patients is widely regarded as the most important measure to prevent spread of resistant pathogens through the healthcare institution.[245,246] The most recent CDC Guideline categorizes isolation precautions: (1) standard precautions and (2) transmission-based precautions.[247] Standard precautions specify the use of gloves for any anticipated contact with blood, any body fluid, secretions or excretions (except sweat), nonintact, skin or mucous membranes. Gowns are recommended if patient care activities are likely to generate splashes of blood, body fluids, and secretions. Hand hygiene is expected after removing gloves and between patients. Standard precautions apply to *all* patients, without regard to clinical diagnosis.

Transmission-based precautions include contact, droplet, and airborne precautions, each based on the mode of transmission of the infectious agent within the healthcare setting. Acknowledging that multiresistant nosocomial pathogens, particularly MRSA and VRE, are spread primarily by direct (and indirect) contact with healthcare workers, the Guideline specifies that patients known to be colonized or infected by resistant bacteria are to be placed in contact isolation, which requires a private room for the patient (or pairing the patient in a semiprivate room with another patient who is also colonized or infected by the same organism). Healthcare workers are expected to wear gloves on entry to the room, and gowns as well if substantial contact with the patient or the environment is anticipated. Gloves and gowns should be removed and hands treated with a medicated hand hygiene product while still in the isolation room. Noncritical patient care items should be dedicated; if reused, they must be disinfected between patients.

Unfortunately, the existent paradigm for preventing spread of resistant organisms in the hospital—waiting until colonization or infection by MRSA, VRE, or some other resistant organism is serendipitously identified by the clinical laboratory, following which the patient is placed in isolation, usually in a single room, requiring gloves, with or without a gown, for all contacts with the patient—is failing dismally, viewing the inexorable growth in antimicrobial resistance.[49,248,249]

A recent Guideline from the Society for Healthcare Epidemiology of America[250] recommends that surveillance cultures to detect silent VRE or MRSA carriage be performed in roommates of VRE- or MRSA-colonized or -infected patients and other high-risk patients, at the discretion of infection control staff; patients found to be colonized must *also* be placed in contact isolation.[250] If these measures fail to contain spread, efforts should be intensified in the highest risk areas, such as the ICU. Grouping of staff and screening of staff for carriage, if epidemiologic data point to a link, is recommended. Verification that environmental disinfection procedures are effective, by environmental surveillance cultures before and after cleaning areas containing VRE- or MRSA-colonized or -infected patients, is also recommended.

Strategies designed to proactively identify the reservoir of asymptomatic colonized patients by routine surveillance cultures of patients at high risk for MRSA or VRE carriage, rather than relying solely on clinical cultures driven by suspicion of infection, followed by isolation only if cultures indicate the presence of a resistant organism,[251,252] have had variable results; most before-and-after studies have shown that this strategy has been useful in containing institutional spread of multiresistant organisms,[251,253,254] but others have found limited benefit.[255–257] It is notable that no randomized trial has yet been undertaken to assess the effectiveness of prospective microbiologic surveillance beyond the outbreak setting.

Eradication of VRE or MRSA from the hospital is most likely to succeed when the rate of colonization or infection is still low or confined to a single unit.[258,259] A comprehensive multifaceted infection control program, consisting of contact isolation (gowns, gloves) for patients found to be colonized in weekly screening of all patients, handwashing, dedicated use of noncritical equipment, and intensive education, was highly successful in reducing the prevalence of VRE colonization from 2.2% to 0.5% in the Siouxland region of Iowa, Nebraska, and South Dakota, where VRE was only recently detected for the first time.[258] Once hyperendemicity has occurred, eradication is very difficult and costly. The continued reintroduction of new multiresistant strains into the institution from interinstitutional transfers of unrecognized colonized patients has fueled the continued spread of multiresistant nosocomial organisms. Infection control policies must find ways to prevent both intra- and interinstitutional spread.

The majority of patients admitted to ICUs have multiple risk factors for colonization or infection by resistant organisms,[23] which mandates screening a very large proportion of the patients or, better, all of them. Weekly surveillance cultures, as performed in the majority of studies that have used this approach, requires substantial microbiologic support and is labor intensive.[260] By the time the results of surveillance cultures showing colonization by a resistant organism become available, and isolation precautions can be implemented, precious time has passed, providing opportunities for further spread of the organism. Moreover, targeted screening for only one nosocomial pathogen, such as VRE, ignores the possibility that the patient might be colonized by nosocomial pathogens other than VRE, such as MRSA, resistant gram-negative bacteria, or *Clostridium difficile*, which obviously facilitates their spread.

We believe that a simpler strategy for preventing spread of all types of multiresistant bacteria, is the preemptive use of barrier isolation precautions (gowns and gloves) and dedicated patient care items, such as stethoscopes and sphygmomanometers, in *all* high-risk patients from the time of admission, to prevent healthcare workers from acquiring hand contamination by multiresistant organisms when having contact with patients with unrecognized colonization or infection, and thus, to block transmission to other, as yet uncolonized, patients. Numerous studies have shown that the preemptive use of barrier precautions, also called "protective isolation," can effectively prevent the spread of multiresistant organisms, such as MRSA or VRE, in an epidemic setting,[261,262] and other studies have shown the effectiveness of protective isolation in high-risk populations, such as patients in an ICU, for prevention of endemic nosocomial infection, including spread by multiresistant organisms.[256,263–267] Three prospective randomized trials have been conducted to assess the efficacy of preemptive barrier precautions[263,264,268]; two showed benefit with a reduction in all nosocomial infections in ICU patients (relative risk reduction, 52% to 81%).[263,264]

Antimicrobial Prophylaxis

Prophylactic antimicrobials during granulocytopenia have been shown to reduce the frequency of febrile episodes; however, enthusiasm for the use of prophylactic antimicrobials has been damped by the adverse consequences of such a strategy, particularly emergence of multiresistant bacteria, superinfection by fungi, and toxicity from the antimicrobials used.

Combinations of nonabsorbable drugs, such as aminoglycosides, polymyxins, and vancomycin, have been used for infection prophylaxis in the past. However, recent prospective, randomized trials have consistently found that trimethoprim-sulfamethoxazole (TMP-SMZ) and fluoroquinolones are more effective and better tolerated.[269,270]

A recent meta-analysis of nine prospective, randomized trials (1,202 patients) to assess the benefit of adding an agent for gram-positive coverage (vancomycin, penicillin, amoxicillin, roxithromycin, or rifampin) to prophylactic fluoroquinolones found that although the frequency of infections caused by gram-positive bacteria (coagulase-negative staphylococci and streptococci) was reduced, overall mortality attributable to infection was similar in both groups.[271] Side effects occurred twice as frequently in the group receiving additional prophylaxis against gram-positive bacteria. As such, the routine use of prophylactic antibiotics for prevention of infection in patients with cancer and granulocytopenia is not recommended.

Invasive fungal infection is associated with considerable morbidity and mortality especially in patients with hematologic malignancy. Because these infections are difficult to diagnose and have high mortality, prophylaxis against fungal infections is an attractive approach for patients expected to have prolonged granulocytopenia. Numerous randomized trials assessing the efficacy of antifungal agents, most often fluconazole, itraconazole, or amphotericin have been undertaken. The results are difficult to compare because of differing patient populations, myelosuppressive regimens, drug dosage and routes of administration, varying durations of prophylaxis, and lack of uniform case definitions. Nonetheless, most trials have found benefit for prevention of invasive fungal infections; however, a survival benefit was not consistently demonstrated.[272,273]

The risk of developing a potentially fatal invasive fungal infection increases in patients with hematologic (rather than solid organ) malignancy, duration of granulocytopenia, prolonged corticosteroid therapy, allogeneic and autologous bone marrow and stem cell transplantation, graft-versus-host disease, and concomitant viral infections.[274,275] Therefore, the best studies of antifungal prophylaxis have focused on these high-risk groups. Fluconazole has been the most widely studied agent for prophylaxis in doses ranging from 50 to 400 mg daily. Goodman et al. found that 400 mg/day of fluconazole was superior to placebo in reducing both the incidence of invasive fungal infection and attributable mortality.[276] In the second trial, performed in pediatric and adult bone marrow transplant recipients, fluconazole, given for 100 days posttransplantation, reduced the incidence of invasive fungal infection when compared with clotrimazole troches.[277]

Based on results from these and other studies that reported similar results, 400 mg/day fluconazole is recommended for patients undergoing allogeneic bone marrow or stem cell transplantation.

Fluconazole has dose-dependent activity against *Candida glabrata* and no activity against *Candida krusei* and *Aspergillus* species. An azole with a broader spectrum, itraconazole, has been studied in several trials. The oral suspension has superior bioavailability than capsules and has been shown to be more efficacious. The results of randomized trials indicate a reduction in the incidence of fungal infection; however, a mortality benefit was not consistently demonstrated. A recent meta-analysis of 13 randomized trials (3,597 patients) found that prophylaxis with itraconazole reduced the incidence of invasive fungal infection (RR, 40%; $P = 0.002$) and mortality from invasive fungal infection; however, no impact on overall mortality was observed.[278] As yet, the benefit of prophylaxis with itraconazole remains controversial, and it cannot be recommended universally.

Amphotericin B deoxycholate and lipid-based amphotericin B have each been studied in a limited number of trials, most of which employed historical controls or a small number of subjects.[279,280] Infusion-related toxicity with amphotericin B and the high cost of lipid-associated amphotericin B have limited the prophylactic use of these agents.

Two new antifungal agents, voriconazole and caspofungin, have recently become available for treatment of fungal infection; however, data on prophylaxis are as yet too limited to draw conclusions.[281] Recent recommendations regarding the use of antifungal prophyalxis have been published by the German Society of Hematology and Oncology[282] and are summarized in Table 76.17.

Acknowledgment. This work was supported by an unrestricted gift for research from the Oscar Rennebohm Foundation of Madison, Wisconsin.

TABLE 76.17. **Summary of recommendations for antifungal prophylaxis in patients with malignancy.**

Patient population	*Drug*	*Dosage*	*Level of evidence*
Conventional chemotherapy	Fluconazole	50–400 mg/day	C-I
	Itraconazole oral suspension	≤5 mg/kg/day	C-I
	Itraconazole capsules parenteral	Any dose	C-I
	amphotericin B deoxycholate parenteral	0.5–1.0 mg/kg every 48 hours	C-II
	amphotericin B deoxycholate	<0.5 mg /kg every 48 hours	C-II
Allogeneic transplant	Fluconazole	400 mg/day	A-I
	Fluconazole	50–200 mg/day	C-I
	Itraconazole	400 mg/day oral solution	C-I
	Liposomal amphotericin B	1.0 mg/kg/day	C-I
Solid tumors	Any antifungal	Any dose	C-I

Source: Adapted from Cornely et al.,[282] by permission of *Annals of Hematology*.

From the Infectious Diseases Society of America Guidelines for weighting recommendations based on the quality of scientific evidence.[283] Category: A, good evidence to support a recommendation for use; B, moderate evidence to support a recommendation for use; C, poor evidence to support a recommendation for use. Quality of evidence: I, evidence from one or more properly randomized controlled trial; II, evidence from one or more well-designed observational study, multiple time-series, or dramatic results of uncontrolled experiments; III, expert opinion, descriptive studies.

References

1. Rolston KVI, Bodey GP. Infections in patients with cancer. In: Frei E (ed) Cancer Medicine. Hamilton, Ontario: Decker, 2003.
2. Crawford J, Dale DC, Lyman GH. Chemotherapy-induced neutropenia: risks, consequences, and new directions for its management. Cancer (Phila) 2004;100:228–237.
3. Casazza AR, Duvall CP, Carbone PP. Infection in lymphoma. Histology, treatment, and duration in relation to incidence and survival. JAMA 1966;197:710–716.
4. Bodey GP. Infection in cancer patients. A continuing association. Am J Med 1986;81:11–26.
5. Bodey GP, Buckley M, Sathe YS, Freireich EJ. Quantitative relationships between circulating leukocytes and infection in patients with acute leukemia. Ann Intern Med. 1966;64:328–340.
6. Hughes WT, Armstrong D, Bodey GP, et al. 2002 guidelines for the use of antimicrobial agents in neutropenic patients with cancer. Clin Infect Dis 2002;34:730–751.
7. Egerer G, Hensel M, Ho AD. Infectious complications in chronic lymphoid malignancy. Curr Treat Options Oncol 2001;2:237–244.
8. Samonis G, Kontoyiannis DP. Infectious complications of purine analog therapy. Curr Opin Infect Dis 2001;14:409–413.
9. Anaissie EJ, Kontoyiannis DP, O'Brien S, et al. Infections in patients with chronic lymphocytic leukemia treated with fludarabine. Ann Intern Med 1998;129:559–566.
10. Harris M. Monoclonal antibodies as therapeutic agents for cancer. Lancet Oncol 2004;5:292–302.
11. Coiffier B, Lepage E, Briere J, et al. CHOP chemotherapy plus rituximab compared with CHOP alone in elderly patients with diffuse large-B-cell lymphoma. N Engl J Med 2002;346:235–242.
12. Maness LJ, McSweeney PA. Treatment options for newly diagnosed patients with chronic myeloid leukemia. Curr Hematol Rep 2004;3:54–61.
13. Lamanna N, Weiss M. Treatment options for newly diagnosed patients with adult acute lymphoblastic leukemia. Curr Hematol Rep 2004;3:40–46.
14. Wade JC, Newton B, Flournoy N, Meyers JD. Oral acyclovir for prevention of herpes simplex virus reactivation after marrow transplantation. Ann Intern Med 1984;100:823–828.
15. Chang HY, Rodriguez V, Narboni G, Bodey GP, Luna MA, Freireich EJ. Causes of death in adults with acute leukemia. Medicine (Baltim) 1976;55:259–268.
16. Feld R, Bodey GP, Rodriguez V, Luna M. Causes of death in patients with malignant lymphoma. Am J Med Sci 1974; 268:97–106.
17. Zinner SH. Changing epidemiology of infections in patients with neutropenia and cancer: emphasis on gram-positive and resistant bacteria. Clin Infect Dis 1999;29:490–494.
18. Rolston KVI, Bodey GP. Infections in patients with cancer. In: Holland JF, Frei E (eds) Cancer Medicine. Hamilton, Ontario: Decker, 2000.
19. Wisplinghoff H, Seifert H, Wenzel RP, Edmond MB. Current trends in the epidemiology of nosocomial bloodstream infections in patients with hematological malignancies and solid neoplasms in hospitals in the United States. Clin Infect Dis 2003;36:1103–1110.
20. Anonymous. National Nosocomial Infections Surveillance (NNIS) System report, data summary from January 1990–May 1999, issued June 1999. Am J Infect Control 1999;27:520–532.
21. Farr BM. Vascular catheter related infections in cancer patients. Surg Oncol Clin N Am 1995;4:493–503.
22. Rupp ME, Fey PD. Extended spectrum beta-lactamase (ESBL)-producing *Enterobacteriaceae*: considerations for diagnosis, prevention and drug treatment. Drugs 2003;63:353–365.
23. Safdar N, Maki DG. The commonality of risk factors for nosocomial colonization and infection with antimicrobial-resistant *Staphylococcus aureus*, enterococcus, gram-negative bacilli, *Clostridium difficile*, and *Candida*. Ann Intern Med 2002;136:834–844.
24. Endimiani A, Luzzaro F, Perilli M, et al. Bacteremia due to *Klebsiella pneumoniae* isolates producing the TEM-52 extended-spectrum beta-lactamase: treatment outcome of patients receiving imipenem or ciprofloxacin. Clin Infect Dis 2004;38:243–251.
25. Schimpff S, Satterlee W, Young VM, Serpick A. Empiric therapy with carbenicillin and gentamicin for febrile patients with cancer and granulocytopenia. N Engl J Med 1971;284:1061–1065.
26. Chatzinikolaou I, Abi-Said D, Bodey GP, Rolston KV, Tarrand JJ, Samonis G. Recent experience with *Pseudomonas aeruginosa* bacteremia in patients with cancer: Retrospective analysis of 245 episodes. Arch Intern Med 2000;160:501–509.
27. Pagano L, Tacconelli E, Tumbarello M, et al. Bacteremia in patients with hematological malignancies. Analysis of risk factors, etiological agents and prognostic indicators. Haematologica 1997;82:415–419.
28. Agger WA, Mardan A. *Pseudomonas aeruginosa* infections of intact skin. Clin Infect Dis 1995;20:302–308.
29. Rolston KV, Bodey GP. *Pseudomonas aeruginosa* infection in cancer patients. Cancer Invest 1992;10:43–59.
30. Carmeli Y, Troillet N, Karchmer AW, Samore MH. Health and economic outcomes of antibiotic resistance in *Pseudomonas aeruginosa*. Arch Intern Med 1999;159:1127–1132.

31. Safdar N, Handelsman J, Maki DG. Does combination therapy reduce mortality in gram-negative bacteremia: a meta-analysis. In: 43rd InterScience Conference on Antimicrobial Agents and Chemotherapy, 2003.
32. Spanik S, Trupl J, Kunova A, et al. Risk factors, aetiology, therapy and outcome in 123 episodes of breakthrough bacteraemia and fungaemia during antimicrobial prophylaxis and therapy in cancer patients. J Med Microbiol 1997;46:517–523.
33. National Nosocomial Infections Surveillance (NNIS) System Report. Data summary from January 1992 to June 2002, issued August 2002. Am J Infect Control 2002;30:458–475.
34. Wunderink RG, Rello J, Cammarata SK, Croos-Dabrera RV, Kollef MH. Linezolid vs. vancomycin: analysis of two double-blind studies of patients with methicillin-resistant *Staphylococcus aureus* nosocomial pneumonia. Chest 2003;124: 1789–1797.
35. Tunkel AR, Sepkowitz KA. Infections caused by viridans streptococci in patients with neutropenia. Clin Infect Dis 2002;34:1524–1529.
36. Elting LS, Bodey GP, Keefe BH. Septicemia and shock syndrome due to viridans streptococci: a case-control study of predisposing factors. Clin Infect Dis 1992;14:1201–1207.
37. Bilgrami S, Feingold JM, Dorsky D, Edwards RL, Clive J, Tutschka PJ. *Streptococcus viridans* bacteremia following autologous peripheral blood stem cell transplantation. Bone Marrow Transplant 1998;21:591–595.
38. Cohen J, Donnelly JP, Worsley AM, Catovsky D, Goldman JM, Galton DA. Septicaemia caused by viridans streptococci in neutropenic patients with leukaemia. Lancet 1983;2:1452–1454.
39. Paganini H, Staffolani V, Zubizarreta P, Casimir L, Lopardo H, Luppino V. Viridans streptococci bacteraemia in children with fever and neutropenia: a case-control study of predisposing factors. Eur J Cancer 2003;39:1284–1289.
40. Ruescher TJ, Sodeifi A, Scrivani SJ, Kaban LB, Sonis ST. The impact of mucositis on alpha-hemolytic streptococcal infection in patients undergoing autologous bone marrow transplantation for hematologic malignancies. Cancer (Phila) 1998;82:2275–2281.
41. Richard P, Amador Del Valle G, Moreau P, et al. Viridans streptococcal bacteraemia in patients with neutropenia. Lancet 1995;345:1607–1609.
42. Bostrom B, Weisdorf D. Mucositis and alpha-streptococcal sepsis in bone marrow transplant recipients. Lancet 1984;1: 1120–1121.
43. Ringden O, Heimdahl A, Lonnqvist B, Malmborg AS, Wilczek H. Decreased incidence of viridans streptococcal septicaemia in allogeneic bone marrow transplant recipients after the introduction of acyclovir. Lancet 1984;1:744.
44. Bochud PY, Eggiman P, Calandra T, Van Melle G, Saghafi L, Francioli P. Bacteremia due to viridans streptococcus in neutropenic patients with cancer: clinical spectrum and risk factors. Clin Infect Dis 1994;18:25–31.
45. Shenep JL. Viridans-group streptococcal infections in immunocompromised hosts. Int J Antimicrob Agents 2000;14:129–135.
46. Marron A, Carratala J, Alcaide F, Fernandez-Sevilla A, Gudiol F. High rates of resistance to cephalosporins among viridans-group streptococci causing bacteremia in neutropenic cancer patients. J Antimicrob Chemother 2001;47:87–91.
47. Lyytikainen O, Rautio M, Carlson P, et al. Nosocomial bloodstream infections due to viridans streptococci in haematological and non-haematological patients: species distribution and antimicrobial resistance. J Antimicrob Chemother 2004;53: 631–634.
48. Maki DG, Agger WA. Enterococcal bacteremia: clinical features, the risk of endocarditis, and management. Medicine (Baltim) 1988;67:248–269.
49. Anonymous. National Nosocomial Infections Surveillance (NNIS) System Report. Data summary from January 1992 through June 2003, issued August 2003. Am J Infect Control 2003;31:481–498.
50. Lautenbach E, Bilker WB, Brennan PJ. Enterococcal bacteremia: risk factors for vancomycin resistance and predictors of mortality. Infect Control Hosp Epidemiol 1999;20:318–323.
51. Chanock SJ, Pizzo PA. Fever in the neutropenic host. Infect Dis Clin N Am 1996;10:777–796.
52. Rolston KV, Bodey GP. Diagnosis and management of perianal and perirectal infection in the granulocytopenic patient. Curr Clin Top Infect Dis 1993;13:164–171.
53. Lopez FA, Sanders CV. Dermatologic infections in the immunocompromised (non-HIV) host. Infect Dis Clin N Am 2001;15: 671–702, xi.
54. File TM. Necrotizing soft tissue infections. Curr Infect Dis Rep 2003;5:407–415.
55. Stamenkovic I, Lew PD. Early recognition of potentially fatal necrotizing fasciitis. The use of frozen-section biopsy. N Engl J Med 1984;310:1689–1693.
56. Bodey GP. Unusual presentations of infection in neutropenic patients. Int J Antimicrob Agents 2000;16:93–95.
57. Johnson S, Driks MR, Tweten RK, et al. Clinical courses of seven survivors of *Clostridium septicum* infection and their immunologic responses to alpha toxin. Clin Infect Dis 1994;19: 761–764.
58. Horton KM, Corl FM, Fishman EK. CT evaluation of the colon: inflammatory disease. Radiographics 2000;20:399–418.
59. Schlatter M, Snyder K, Freyer D. Successful nonoperative management of typhlitis in pediatric oncology patients. J Pediatr Surg 2002;37:1151–1155.
60. Rolston KV. The spectrum of pulmonary infections in cancer patients. Curr Opin Oncol 2001;13:218–223.
61. Okamoto Y, Ribeiro RC, Srivastava DK, Shenep JL, Pui CH, Razzouk BI. Viridans streptococcal sepsis: clinical features and complications in childhood acute myeloid leukemia. J Pediatr Hematol Oncol 2003;25:696–703.
62. Maschmeyer G. Pneumonia in febrile neutropenic patients: radiologic diagnosis. Curr Opin Oncol 2001;13:229–235.
63. Rano A, Agusti C, Jimenez P, et al. Pulmonary infiltrates in non-HIV immunocompromised patients: a diagnostic approach using non-invasive and bronchoscopic procedures. Thorax 2001; 56:379–387.
64. Ninane V. Bronchoscopic invasive diagnostic techniques in the cancer patient. Curr Opin Oncol 2001;13:236–241.
65. Maschmeyer G, Link H, Hiddemann W, Meyer P, Helmerking M, Adam D. Interventional antimicrobial strategy in febrile neutropenic patients. Results of a multicenter study in 1,260 patients with hematological malignancies. The Interventional Antimicrobial Strategy Study Group, Paul Ehrlich Society for Chemotherapy. Onkologie 1990;13:38–42.
66. Kyne L, Farrell RJ, Kelly CP. *Clostridium difficile*. Gastroenterol Clin N Am 2001;30:753–777, ix–x.
67. Kyne L, Hamel MB, Polavaram R, Kelly CP. Health care costs and mortality associated with nosocomial diarrhea due to *Clostridium difficile*. Clin Infect Dis 2002;34:346–353.
68. Archibald LK, Banerjee SN, Jarvis WR. Secular trends in hospital-acquired *Clostridium difficile* disease in the United States, 1987–2001. J Infect Dis 2004;189:1585–1589.
69. Pituch H, van Belkum A, van den Braak N, et al. Clindamycin-resistant, toxin A-negative, toxin B-positive *Clostridium difficile* strains cause antibiotic-associated diarrhea among children hospitalized in a hematology unit. Clin Microbiol Infect 2003;9:903–904.
70. Blot E, Escande MC, Besson D, et al. Outbreak of *Clostridium difficile*-related diarrhoea in an adult oncology unit: risk factors and microbiological characteristics. J Hosp Infect 2003; 53:187–192.
71. Hornbuckle K, Chak A, Lazarus HM, et al. Determination and validation of a predictive model for *Clostridium difficile*

diarrhea in hospitalized oncology patients. Ann Oncol 1998;9: 307–311.

72. Komatsu M, Kato H, Aihara M, et al. High frequency of antibiotic-associated diarrhea due to toxin A-negative, toxin B-positive *Clostridium difficile* in a hospital in Japan and risk factors for infection. Eur J Clin Microbiol Infect Dis 2003;22:525–529.
73. Bartlett JG. *Clostridium difficile* infection: pathophysiology and diagnosis. Semin Gastrointest Dis 1997;8:12–21.
74. Bartlett JG. Antimicrobial agents implicated in *Clostridium difficile* toxin-associated diarrhea of colitis. Johns Hopkins Med J 1981;149:6–9.
75. Delmee M. Laboratory diagnosis of *Clostridium difficile* disease. Clin Microbiol Infect 2001;7:411–416.
76. Kawamoto S, Horton KM, Fishman EK. Pseudomembranous colitis: spectrum of imaging findings with clinical and pathologic correlation. Radiographics 1999;19:887–897.
77. Bartlett JG. Management of *Clostridium difficile* infection and other antibiotic-associated diarrhoeas. Eur J Gastroenterol Hepatol 1996;8:1054–1061.
78. Apisarnthanarak A, Razavi B, Mundy LM. Adjunctive intracolonic vancomycin for severe *Clostridium difficile* colitis: case series and review of the literature. Clin Infect Dis 2002;35: 690–696.
79. Mayfield JL, Leet T, Miller J, Mundy LM. Environmental control to reduce transmission of *Clostridium difficile*. Clin Infect Dis 2000;31:995–1000.
80. Simor AE, Bradley SF, Strausbaugh LJ, Crossley K, Nicolle LE. *Clostridium difficile* in long-term-care facilities for the elderly. Infect Control Hosp Epidemiol 2002;23:696–703.
81. Crnich CJ, Maki DG. The role of intravascular devices in sepsis. Current Infect Dis Rep 2001;3:497–506.
82. Pittet D, Tarara D, Wenzel R. Nosocomial bloodstream infection in critically ill patients. Excess length of stay, extra costs, and attributable mortality. JAMA 1994;271:1598–1601.
83. Rello J, Ochagavia A, Sabanes E, et al. Evaluation of outcome of intravenous catheter-related infections in critically ill patients. Am J Respir Crit Care Med 2000;162:1027–1030.
84. Kluger D, Maki D. The relative risk of intravascular device-related bloodstream infections with different types of intravascular devices in adults. A meta-analysis of 206 published studies [abstract]. Infect Control Hosp Epidemiol 2000;21:95–96.
85. Maki DG, Crnich CJ. Line sepsis in the ICU. Semin Respir Crit Care Med 2002;24:22–36.
86. O'Grady NP, Barie PS, Bartlett JG, et al. Practice guidelines for evaluating new fever in critically ill adult patients. Task Force of the Society of Critical Care Medicine and the Infectious Diseases Society of America. Clin Infect Dis 1998;26:1042–1059.
87. Safdar N, Maki DG. Inflammation at the insertion site is not predictive of catheter-related bloodstream infection with short-term, noncuffed central venous catheters [comment]. Crit Care Med 2002;30:2632–2635.
88. Mermel LA, Maki DG. Detection of bacteremia in adults: consequences of culturing an inadequate volume of blood. Ann Intern Med 1993;119:270–272.
89. Gaur AH, Giannini MA, Flynn PM, et al. Optimizing blood culture practices in pediatric immunocompromised patients: evaluation of media types and blood culture volume. Pediatr Infect Dis J 2003;22:545–552.
90. Beutz M, Sherman G, Mayfield J, Fraser VJ, Kollef MH. Clinical utility of blood cultures drawn from central vein catheters and peripheral venipuncture in critically ill medical patients. Chest 2003;123:854–861.
91. Tacconelli E, Tumbarello M, Pittiruti M, et al. Central venous catheter-related sepsis in a cohort of 366 hospitalised patients. Eur J Clin Microbiol Infect Dis 1997;16:203–209.
92. Gowardman JR, Montgomery C, Thirlwell S, et al. Central venous catheter-related bloodstream infections: an analysis of incidence and risk factors in a cohort of 400 patients. Intens Care Med 1998;24:1034–1039.
93. Bouza E, Burillo A, Munoz P. Catheter-related infections: diagnosis and intravascular treatment. Clin Microbiol Infect 2002;8:265–274.
94. Raad I, Hanna HA, Alakech B, Chatzinikolaou I, Johnson MM, Tarrand J. Differential time to positivity: a useful method for diagnosing catheter-related bloodstream infections. Ann Intern Med 2003;140:18–25.
95. Moonens F, el Alami S, Van Gossum A, Struelens MJ, Serruys E. Usefulness of gram staining of blood collected from total parenteral nutrition catheter for rapid diagnosis of catheter-related sepsis. J Clin Microbiol 1994;32:1578–1579.
96. Kite P, Dobbins BM, Wilcox MH, McMahon MJ. Rapid diagnosis of central-venous-catheter-related bloodstream infection without catheter removal. Lancet 1999;354:1504–1507.
97. Verghese A, Widrich WC, Arbeit RD. Central venous septic thrombophlebitis: the role of medical therapy. Medicine (Baltim) 1985;64:394–400.
98. Martinez E, Mensa J, Rovira M, et al. Central venous catheter exchange by guidewire for treatment of catheter-related bacteraemia in patients undergoing BMT or intensive chemotherapy. Bone Marrow Transplantat 1999;23:41–44.
99. Maki DG. Managment of life-threatening infection in the intensive care unit. In: Prough DS (ed) Critical Care Medicine: Preoperative Management, 2nd ed. Philadelphia: Lippincott Williams & Williams, 2002:616–648.
100. Malanoski GJ, Samore MH, Pefanis A, Karchmer AW. *Staphylococcus aureus* catheter-associated bacteremia. Minimal effective therapy and unusual infectious complications associated with arterial sheath catheters. Arch Intern Med 1995;155:1161–1166.
101. Fowler VG Jr, Li J, Corey GR, et al. Role of echocardiography in evaluation of patients with *Staphylococcus aureus* bacteremia: experience in 103 patients. J Am Coll Cardiol 1997;30: 1072–1078.
102. Nguyen MH, Peacock JE Jr, Tanner DC, et al. Therapeutic approaches in patients with candidemia. Evaluation in a multicenter, prospective, observational study. Arch Intern Med 1995;155:2429–2435.
103. Rex JH, Bennett JE, Sugar AM, et al. Intravascular catheter exchange and duration of candidemia. Clin Infect Dis 1995;21:994–996.
104. Anaissie EJ, Rex JH, Uzun O, Vartivarian S. Predictors of adverse outcome in cancer patients with candidemia. Am J Med 1998;104:238–245.
105. Messing B, Man F, Colimon R, Thuillier F, Beliah M. Antibiotic lock technique is an effective treatment of bacterial catheter-related sepsis during parenteral nutrition. Clin Nutr 1990;9:220–224.
106. Cuntz D, Michaud L, Guimber D, Husson MO, Gottrand F, Turck D. Local antibiotic lock for the treatment of infections related to central catheters in parenteral nutrition in children. JPEN (J Parenter Enteral Nutr) 2002;26:104–108.
107. Guedon C, Nouvellon M, Lalaude O, Lerebours E. Efficacy of antibiotic-lock technique with teicoplanin in *Staphylococcus epidermidis* catheter-related sepsis during long-term parenteral nutrition. J JPEN (J Parenter Enteral Nutr) 2002;26:109–113.
108. Brothers TE, Von Moll LK, Niederhuber JE, Roberts JA, Walker-Andrews S, Ensminger WD. Experience with subcutaneous infusion ports in three hundred patients. Surg Gynecol Obstet 1988;166:295–301.
109. Domingo P, Fontanet A, Sanchez F, Allende L, Vazquez G. Morbidity associated with long-term use of totally implantable ports in patients with AIDS. Clin Infect Dis 1999;29:346–351.
110. Longuet P, Douard MC, Maslo C, Benoit C, Arlet G, Leport C. Limited efficacy of antibiotic lock techniques (ALT) in catheter related bacteremia of totally implanted ports (TIP) in HIV infected oncologic patients [abstract]. Abstracts and Proceedings

from the 35th Interscience Conference of Antimicrobial Agents and Chemotherapy. Washington, DC: ASM Press, 1995:J5.
111. Crnich CJ, Maki DG. Infections of vascular devices. In: Cohen J (ed) Infectious Diseases, 2nd ed. Philadelphia: Mosby, 2003:722–743.
112. Raad I, Davis S, Khan A, Tarrand J, Elting L, Bodey GP. Impact of central venous catheter removal on the recurrence of catheter-related coagulase-negative staphylococcal bacteremia. Infect Control Hosp Epidemiol 1992;13:215–221.
113. Mermel LA, Farr BM, Sherertz RJ, et al. Guidelines for the management of intravascular catheter-related infections. Clin Infect Dis 2001;32:1249–1272.
114. Raad, II, Sabbagh MF. Optimal duration of therapy for catheter-related *Staphylococcus aureus* bacteremia: a study of 55 cases and review. Clin Infect Dis 1992;14:75–82.
115. Rosen AB, Fowler VG, Jr., Corey GR, et al. Cost-effectiveness of transesophageal echocardiography to determine the duration of therapy for intravascular catheter-associated *Staphylococcus aureus* bacteremia. Ann Intern Med 1999;130:810–820.
116. O'Grady NP, Alexander M, Dellinger EP, et al. Guidelines for the prevention of intravascular catheter-related infections. Clin Infect Dis 2002;35:1281–1307.
117. Crnich CJ, Maki DG. The promise of novel technology for the prevention of intravascular device-related bloodstream infection. II. Long-term devices. Clin Infect Dis 2002;34:1362–1368.
118. Henrickson KJ, Axtell RA, Hoover SM, et al. Prevention of central venous catheter-related infections and thrombotic events in immunocompromised children by the use of vancomycin/ciprofloxacin/heparin flush solution: a randomized, multicenter, double-blind trial. J Clin Oncol 2000;18:1269–1278.
119. Kuypers DR, Evenepoel P, Maes BD, Coosemans W, Pirenne J, Vanrenterghem YF. Role of immunosuppressive drugs in the development of tissue-invasive cytomegalovirus infection in renal transplant recipients. Transplant Proc 2002;34:1164–1170.
120. Rasoul-Rockenschaub S, Zielinski CC, Muller C, Tichatschek E, Popow-Kraupp T, Kunz C. Viral reactivation as a cause of unexplained fever in patients with progressive metastatic breast cancer. Cancer Immunol Immunother 1990;31:191–195.
121. Perkins JG, Flynn JM, Howard RS, Byrd JC. Frequency and type of serious infections in fludarabine-refractory B-cell chronic lymphocytic leukemia and small lymphocytic lymphoma: implications for clinical trials in this patient population. Cancer (Phila) 2002;94:2033–2039.
122. Perez-Simon JA, Kottaridis PD, Martino R, et al. Nonmyeloablative transplantation with or without alemtuzumab: comparison between 2 prospective studies in patients with lymphoproliferative disorders. Blood 2002;100:3121–3127.
123. Reusser P. Opportunistic viral infections. In: Powderly WG (ed) Infectious Diseases, vol 1. New York: Mosby, 2003:1169–1181.
124. Dykewicz CA. Summary of the Guidelines for Preventing Opportunistic Infections among Hematopoietic Stem Cell Transplant Recipients. Clin Infect Dis 2001;33:139–144.
125. Mitchell PS, Espy MJ, Smith TF, et al. Laboratory diagnosis of central nervous system infections with herpes simplex virus by PCR performed with cerebrospinal fluid specimens. J Clin Microbiol 1997;35:2873–2877.
126. Schloss L, van Loon AM, Cinque P, et al. An international external quality assessment of nucleic acid amplification of herpes simplex virus. J Clin Virol 2003;28:175–185.
127. Gnann JW. Varicella-zoster virus: atypical presentations and unusual complications. J Infect Dis 2002;186:S91–S98.
128. Feldman S, Lott L. Varicella in children with cancer. Impact of antiviral therapy and prophylaxis. Pediatrics 1987;80:465–472.
129. Wood MJ. Viral infections in neutropenia: current problems and chemotherapeutic control. J Antimicrob Chemother 1998;41:81–93.
130. Cohen JI, Brunell PA, Straus SE, Krause PR. Recent advances in varicella-zoster virus infection. Ann Intern Med 1999;130:922–932.
131. Saito S, Yano T, Koga H, Arikawa K, Koyanagi N, Oizumi K. Case of varicella-zoster pneumonia with bronchioalveolar lavage confirmed by the detection of VZV DNA in the bronchial washing by the polymerase chain reaction. Kansenshogaku Zasshi (J the Japanese Association for Infectious Diseases) 1999;73:346–350.
132. Kleinschmidt-DeMasters BK, Gilden DH. Varicella-Zoster virus infections of the nervous system: clinical and pathologic correlates. Arch Pathol Lab Med 2001;125:770–780.
133. Prevention of varicella: recommendations of the Advisory Committee on Immunization Practices (ACIP). (MMWR Morb Mortal Wkly Rep) 1996;45:1–25.
134. Prevention of varicella. Updated recommendations of the Advisory Committee on Immunizations Practices (ACIP). MMWR (Morb Mortal Wkly Rep) 1999;48:1–5.
135. Patel R, Paya CV. Infections in solid-organ transplant recipients. Clin Microbiol Rev 1997;10:86–124.
136. Konoplev S, Champlin RE, Giralt S, et al. Cytomegalovirus pneumonia in adult autologous blood and marrow transplant recipients. Bone Marrow Transplant 2001;27:877–881.
137. Nguyen Q, Estey E, Raad I, et al. Cytomegalovirus pneumonia in adults with leukemia: an emerging problem. Clin Infect Dis 2001;32:539–545.
138. Meyers JD, Ljungman P, Fisher LD. Cytomegalovirus excretion as a predictor of cytomegalovirus disease after marrow transplantation: importance of cytomegalovirus viremia. J Infect Dis 1990;162:373–380.
139. Enright H, Haake R, Weisdorf D, et al. Cytomegalovirus pneumonia after bone marrow transplantation. Risk factors and response to therapy. Transplantation 1993;55:1339–1346.
140. Goodrich JM, Bowden RA, Fisher L, Keller C, Schoch G, Meyers JD. Ganciclovir prophylaxis to prevent cytomegalovirus disease after allogeneic marrow transplant. Ann Intern Med 193;118:173–178.
141. Boeckh M, Boivin G. Quantitation of cytomegalovirus: methodologic aspects and clinical applications. Clin Microbiol 1998;11:533–554.
142. Cortez KJ, Fischer SH, Fahle GA, et al. Clinical trial of quantitative real-time polymerase chain reaction for detection of cytomegalovirus in peripheral blood of allogeneic hematopoietic stem-cell transplant recipients. J Infect Dis 2003;188:967–972.
143. Reed EC, Bowden RA, Dandliker PS, Lilleby KE, Meyers JD. Treatment of cytomegalovirus pneumonia with ganciclovir and intravenous cytomegalovirus immunoglobulin in patients with bone marrow transplants. Ann Intern Med 1988;109:783–788.
144. Machado CM, Dulley FL, Boas LS, et al. CMV pneumonia in allogeneic BMT recipients undergoing early treatment of pre-emptive ganciclovir therapy. Bone Marrow Transplant 2000;26:413–417.
145. Goodrich JM, Mori M, Gleaves CA, et al. Early treatment with ganciclovir to prevent cytomegalovirus disease after allogeneic bone marrow transplantation. N Engl J Med 1991;325:1601–1607.
146. Schmidt GM, Horak DA, Niland JC, Duncan SR, Forman SJ, Zaia JA. A randomized, controlled trial of prophylactic ganciclovir for cytomegalovirus pulmonary infection in recipients of allogeneic bone marrow transplants. The City of Hope-Stanford-Syntex CMV Study Group [comment]. N Engl J Med 1991;324:1005–1011.
147. Singhal S, Powles R, Treleaven J, et al. Cytomegaloviremia after autografting for leukemia: clinical significance and lack of effect on engraftment. Leukemia 1997;117:835–838.
148. Baker KS, DeFor TE, Burns LJ, Ramsay NK, Neglia JP, Robison LL. New malignancies after blood or marrow stem-cell transplantation in children and adults: incidence and risk factors

[erratum appears in J Clin Oncol 2003;21(16):3181]. J Clin Oncol 2003;21:1352–1358.
149. Loren AW, Porter DL, Stadtmauer EA, Tsai DE. Post-transplant lymphoproliferative disorder: a review. Bone Marrow Transplant 2003;31:145–155.
150. Cohen JI. Epstein-Barr virus infection. N Engl J Med 2000;343:481–492.
151. Singh N, Paterson DL. Encephalitis caused by human herpesvirus-6 in transplant recipients: relevance of a novel neurotropic virus. Transplantation 2000;69:2474–2479.
152. Cole PD, Stiles J, Boulad F, et al. Successful treatment of human herpesvirus 6 encephalitis in a bone marrow transplant recipient. Clin Infect Dis 1998;27:653–654.
153. Couch RB, Englund JA, Whimbey E. Respiratory viral infections in immunocompetent and immunocompromised persons. Am J Med 1997;102:2–9; discussion 25–26.
154. Englund JA, Anderson LJ, Rhame FS. Nosocomial transmission of respiratory syncytial virus in immunocompromised adults. J Clin Microbiol 1991;29:115–119.
155. Whimbey E, Champlin RE, Couch RB, et al. Community respiratory virus infections among hospitalized adult bone marrow transplant recipients. Clin Infect Dis 1996;22:778–782.
156. Whimbey E, Couch RB, Englund JA, et al. Respiratory syncytial virus pneumonia in hospitalized adult patients with leukemia. Clin Infect Dis 1995;21:376–379.
157. Hindiyeh M, Hillyard DR, Carroll KC. Evaluation of the Prodesse Hexaplex multiplex PCR assay for direct detection of seven respiratory viruses in clinical specimens. Am J Clin Pathol 2001;116:218–224.
158. Ison MG, Hayden FG. Viral infections in immunocompromised patients: what's new with respiratory viruses? Curr Opin Infect Dis 2002;15:355–367.
159. Nichols WG, Gooley T, Boeckh M. Community-acquired respiratory syncytial virus and parainfluenza virus infections after hematopoietic stem cell transplantation: the Fred Hutchinson Cancer Research Center experience. Biol Blood Marrow Transplant 2001;7:11S–15S.
160. Salgado CD, Farr BM, Hall KK, Hayden FG. Influenza in the acute hospital setting. Lancet Infect Dis 2002;2:145–155.
161. Hall CB. Nosocomial respiratory syncytial virus infections: the "Cold War" has not ended. Clin Infect Dis 2000;31:590–596.
162. Bridges CB, Harper SA, Fukuda K, et al. Prevention and control of influenza. Recommendations of the Advisory Committee on Immunization Practices (ACIP). Morb Mortal Wkly Rep Recommend Rep 2003;52:1–34; quiz CE31–CE34.
163. Wheat LJ, Goldman M, Sarosi GA. Fungal infections in the immunocompromised host. In: Young LS (ed) Clinical Approach to Infection in the Compromised Host, 4th ed. New York: Kluwer/Plenum, 2002:215–247.
164. Colombo AL, Perfect J, DiNubile M, et al. Global distribution and outcomes for *Candida* species causing invasive candidiasis: results from an international randomized double-blind study of caspofungin versus amphotericin B for the treatment of invasive candidiasis. Eur J Clin Microbiol Infect Dis 2003;22: 470–474.
165. Rex JH, Walsh TJ, Sobel JD, et al. Practice guidelines for the treatment of candidiasis. Infectious Diseases Society of America. Clin Infect Dis 2000;30:662–678.
166. National Nosocomial Infections Surveillance (NNIS) System Report. Data summary from January 1992 to June 2002, issued August 2002. AJIC Am J Infect Control 2002;30:2002:458–475.
167. Pittet D, Li N, Woolson R, Wenzel R. Microbiological factors influencing the outcome of nosocomial bloodstream infections: a 6-year validated, population-based model. Clin Infect Dis 1997;24:1068–1078.
168. Viscoli C, Girmenia C, Marinus A, et al. Candidemia in cancer patients: a prospective, multicenter surveillance study by the Invasive Fungal Infection Group (IFIG) of the European Organization for Research and Treatment of Cancer (EORTC). Clin Infect Dis 1999;28:1071–1079.
169. Wey SB, Mori M, Pfaller MA, Woolson RF, Wenzel RP. Risk factors for hospital-acquired candidemia. A matched case-control study. Arch Intern Med 1989;149:2349–2353.
170. Walsh TJ, Rex JH. All catheter-related candidemia is not the same: assessment of the balance between the risks and benefits of removal of vascular catheters. Clin Infect Dis 2002;34: 600–602.
171. Hockey LJ, Fujita NK, Gibson TR, Rotrosen D, Montgomerie JZ, Edwards JE Jr. Detection of fungemia obscured by concomitant bacteremia: in vitro and in vivo studies. J Clin Microbiol 1982;16:1080–1085.
172. Munoz P, Bernaldo de Quiros JC, Berenguer J, Rodriguez Creixems M, Picazo JJ, Bouza E. Impact of the BACTEC NR system in detecting *Candida* fungemia. J Clin Microbiol 1990; 28:639–641.
173. Pappas PG, Rex JH, Sobel JD, et al. Guidelines for treatment of candidiasis. Clin Infect Dis 2004;38:161–189.
174. Rex JH, Bennett JE, Sugar AM, et al. A randomized trial comparing fluconazole with amphotericin B for the treatment of candidemia in patients without neutropenia. N Engl J Med 1994;331:1325–1330.
175. Phillips P, Shafran S, Garber G, et al. Multicenter randomized trial of fluconazole versus amphotericin B for treatment of candidemia in non-neutropenic patients. Canadian Candidemia Study Group. Eur J Clin Microbiol Infect Dis 1997;16:337–345.
176. Mora-Duarte J, Betts R, Rotstein C, et al. Comparison of caspofungin and amphotericin B for invasive candidiasis. N Engl J Med 2002;347:2020–2029.
177. Thaler M, Pastakia B, Shawker TH, O'Leary T, Pizzo PA. Hepatic candidiasis in cancer patients: the evolving picture of the syndrome. Ann Intern Med 1988;108:88–100.
178. Denning DW. Invasive aspergillosis. Clin Infect Dis 1998;26: 781–805.
179. Baddley JW, Stroud TP, Salzman D, Pappas PG. Invasive mold infections in allogeneic bone marrow transplant recipients. Clin Infect Dis 2001;32:1319–1324.
180. Marr KA, Carter RA, Boeckh M, Martin P, Corey L. Invasive aspergillosis in allogeneic stem cell transplant recipients: changes in epidemiology and risk factors. Blood 202;100: 4358–4366.
181. Allo MD, Miller J, Townsend T, Tan C. Primary cutaneous aspergillosis associated with Hickman intravenous catheters. N Engl J Med 1987;317:1105–1108.
182. Warris A, Gaustad P, Meis JF, Voss A, Verweij PE, Abrahamsen TG. Recovery of filamentous fungi from water in a paediatric bone marrow transplantation unit. J Hosp Infect 2001;47: 143–148.
183. Denning DW. Therapeutic outcomes in invasive aspergillosis. Clin Infect Dis 1996;23:608–615.
184. Denning DW, Marinus A, Cohen J, et al. An EORTC multicentre prospective survey of invasive aspergillosis in haematological patients: diagnosis and therapeutic outcome. EORTC Invasive Fungal Infections Cooperative Group. J Infect 1998;37:173–180.
185. Kuhlman JE, Fishman EK, Siegelman SS. Invasive pulmonary aspergillosis in acute leukemia: characteristic findings on CT, the CT halo sign, and the role of CT in early diagnosis. Radiology 1985;157:611–614.
186. Curtis AM, Smith GJ, Ravin CE. Air crescent sign of invasive aspergillosis. Radiology 1979;133:17–21.
187. Perfect JR, Cox GM, Lee JY, et al. The impact of culture isolation of *Aspergillus* species: a hospital-based survey of aspergillosis. Clin Infect Dis 2001;33:1824–1833.
188. Maertens J, Verhaegen J, Lagrou K, Van Eldere J, Boogaerts M. Screening for circulating galactomannan as a noninvasive diagnostic tool for invasive aspergillosis in prolonged neutropenic

patients and stem cell transplantation recipients: a prospective validation. Blood 2001;97:1604–1610.

189. Denning DW. Echinocandins: a new class of antifungal. J Antimicrob Chemother 2002;49:889–891.
190. Patterson TF, Kirkpatrick WR, White M, et al. Invasive aspergillosis: a disease spectrum, treatment practices, and outcomes. Medicine (Baltim) 2000;79:250–260.
191. Herbrecht R, Denning DW, Patterson TF, et al. Voriconazole versus amphotericin B for primary therapy of invasive aspergillosis. N Engl J Med 2002;347:408–415.
192. Manavathu EK, Alangaden GJ, Chandrasekar PH. Differential activity of triazoles in two-drug combinations with the echinocandin caspofungin against *Aspergillus fumigatus*. J Antimicrob Chemother 2003;51:1423–1425.
193. Dannaoui E, Lortholary O, Dromer F. In vitro evaluation of double and triple combinations of antifungal drugs against *Aspergillus fumigatus* and *Aspergillus terreus*. Antimicrob Agents Chemother 2004;48:970–978.
194. Segal BH, Walsh TJ. Opportunistic fungal infections. In: Powderly WG (ed) Infectious Diseases, vol 1. New York: Mosby, 2003:1155–1167.
195. Leong KW, Crowley B, White B, et al. Cutaneous mucormycosis due to *Absidia corymbifera* occurring after bone marrow transplantation. Bone Marrow Transplant 1997;19:513–515.
196. Fleming RV, Walsh TJ, Anaissie EJ. Emerging and less common fungal pathogens. Infect Dis Clin N Am 2002;16:915–933, vi–vii.
197. Anaissie EJ, Penzak SR, Dignani MC. The hospital water supply as a source of nosocomial infections: a plea for action. Arch Intern Med 2002;162:1483–1492.
198. Raad I, Tarrand J, Hanna H, et al. Epidemiology, molecular mycology, and environmental sources of *Fusarium* infection in patients with cancer. Infect Control Hosp Epidemiol 2002;23:532–537.
199. Boutati EI, Anaissie EJ. *Fusarium*, a significant emerging pathogen in patients with hematologic malignancy: ten years' experience at a cancer center and implications for management. Blood 1997;90:999–1008.
200. Walsh TJ, Groll AH. Emerging fungal pathogens: evolving challenges to immunocompromised patients for the twenty-first century. Transplant Infect Dis 1999;1:247–261.
201. Sickles EA, Greene WH, Wiernik PH. Clinical presentation of infection in granulocytopenic patients. Arch Intern Med 1975;135:715–719.
202. Siegel DL, Edelstein PH, Nachamkin I. Inappropriate testing for diarrheal diseases in the hospital. JAMA 1990;263:979–982.
203. Furno P, Bucaneve G, Del Favero A. Monotherapy or aminoglycoside-containing combinations for empirical antibiotic treatment of febrile neutropenic patients: a meta-analysis. Lancet Infect Dis 2002;2:231–242.
204. Paul M, Soares-Weiser K, Leibovici L. Beta lactam monotherapy versus beta lactam-aminoglycoside combination therapy for fever with neutropenia: systematic review and meta-analysis. BMJ 2003;326:1111.
205. Paul M, Soares-Weiser K, Grozinsky S, Leibovici L. Beta-lactam versus beta-lactam-aminoglycoside combination therapy in cancer patients with neutropaenia. Cochrane Database Syst Rev 2003:CD003038.
206. Smith CE, Tillman BS, Howell AW, Longfield RN, Jorgensen JH. Failure of ceftazidime-amikacin therapy for bacteremia and meningitis due to *Klebsiella pneumoniae* producing an extended-spectrum beta-lactamase. Antimicrob Agents Chemother 1990;34:1290–1293.
207. Fleischhack G, Hartmann C, Simon A, et al. Meropenem versus ceftazidime as empirical monotherapy in febrile neutropenia of paediatric patients with cancer. J Antimicrob Chemother 2001;47:841–853.
208. Giamarellou H, Bassaris HP, Petrikkos G, et al. Monotherapy with intravenous followed by oral high-dose ciprofloxacin versus combination therapy with ceftazidime plus amikacin as initial empiric therapy for granulocytopenic patients with fever. Antimicrob Agents Chemother 2000;44:3264–3271.
209. Livermore DM. Multiple mechanisms of antimicrobial resistance in *Pseudomonas aeruginosa*: our worst nightmare? Clin Infect Dis 2002;34:634–640.
210. Peacock JE, Herrington DA, Wade JC, et al. Ciprofloxacin plus piperacillin compared with tobramycin plus piperacillin as empirical therapy in febrile neutropenic patients. A randomized, double-blind trial. Ann Intern Med 2002;137:77–87.
211. Rubin M, Hathorn JW, Marshall D, Gress J, Steinberg SM, Pizzo PA. Gram-positive infections and the use of vancomycin in 550 episodes of fever and neutropenia. Ann Intern Med 1988;108:30–35.
212. Cometta A, Kern WV, De Bock R, et al. Vancomycin versus placebo for treating persistent fever in patients with neutropenic cancer receiving piperacillin-tazobactam monotherapy. Clin Infect Dis 2003;37:382–389.
213. Maki DG. Management of life-threatening infection in the intensive care unit. In: Murray MJ, Coursin DB (eds) Critical Care Medicine: Preoperative Management. Philadelphia: Lippincott, Williams & Wilkins, 2002.
214. Rybak MJ. Therapeutic options for gram-positive infections. J Hosp Infect 2001;49(suppl A):S25–S32.
215. Hughes WT, Armstrong D, Bodey GP, et al. From the Infectious Diseases Society of America. Guidelines for the use of antimicrobial agents in neutropenic patients with unexplained fever. J Infect Dis 1990;161:381–396.
216. Talcott JA, Finberg R, Mayer RJ, Goldman L. The medical course of cancer patients with fever and neutropenia. Clinical identification of a low-risk subgroup at presentation. Arch Intern Med 1988;148:2561–2568.
217. Talcott JA, Siegel RD, Finberg R, Goldman L. Risk assessment in cancer patients with fever and neutropenia: a prospective, two-center validation of a prediction rule. J Clin Oncol 1992;10:316–322.
218. Klastersky J, Paesmans M, Rubenstein EB, et al. The Multinational Association for Supportive Care in Cancer risk index: a multinational scoring system for identifying low-risk febrile neutropenic cancer patients. J Clin Oncol 2000;18:3038–3051.
219. DeGregorio MW, Lee WM, Linker CA, Jacobs RA, Ries CA. Fungal infections in patients with acute leukemia. Am J Med 1982;73:543–548.
220. Davies SV, Murray JA. Amphotericin and abolition of fever in neutropenic sepsis. Br Med J 1989;299:1339–1340.
221. Pizzo PA, Ribichaud KJ, Gill FA, Witebsky FG. Empiric antibiotic and antifungal therapy for cancer patients with prolonged fever and granulocytopenia. Am J Med 1982;72:101–111.
222. Stein RS, Kayser J, Flexner JM. Clinical value of empirical amphotericin B in patients with acute myelogenous leukemia. Cancer (Phila) 1982;50:2247–2251.
223. Subira M, Martino R, Gomez L, Marti JM, Estany C, Sierra J. Low-dose amphotericin B lipid complex vs. conventional amphotericin B for empirical antifungal therapy of neutropenic fever in patients with hematologic malignancies: a randomized, controlled trial. Eur J Haematol 2004;72:342–347.
224. Walsh TJ, Finberg RW, Arndt C, et al. Liposomal amphotericin B for empirical therapy in patients with persistent fever and neutropenia. N Engl J Med 1999;340:764–771.
225. Wingard JR, White MH, Anaissie E, et al. A randomized, double-blind comparative trial evaluating the safety of liposomal amphotericin B versus amphotericin B lipid complex in the empirical treatment of febrile neutropenia. L Amph/ABLC Collaborative Study Group [comment]. Clin Infect Dis 2000;31:1155–1163.
226. Winston DJ, Hathorn JW, Schuster MG, et al. A multicenter, randomized trial of fluconazole versus amphotericin B for

empiric antifungal therapy of febrile neutropenic patients with cancer. Am J Med 2000;108:282–289.

227. Boogaerts M, Winston DJ, Bow EJ, et al. Intravenous and oral itraconazole versus intravenous amphotericin B deoxycholate as empirical antifungal therapy for persistent fever in neutropenic patients with cancer who are receiving broad-spectrum antibacterial therapy. A randomized, controlled trial. Ann Intern Med 2001;135:412–422.
228. Walsh TJ, Pappas P, Winston DJ, et al. Voriconazole compared with liposomal amphotericin B for empirical antifungal therapy in patients with neutropenia and persistent fever. N Engl J Med 2002;346:225–234.
229. Powers JH, Dixon CA, Goldberger MJ. Voriconazole versus liposomal amphotericin B in patients with neutropenia and persistent fever. N Engl J Med 2002;346:289–290.
230. Aquino VM, Tkaczewski I, Buchanan GR. Early discharge of low-risk febrile neutropenic children and adolescents with cancer. Clin Infect Dis 1997;25:74–78.
231. Joshi JH, Schimpff SC, Tenney JH, Newman KA, de Jongh CA. Can antibacterial therapy be discontinued in persistently febrile granulocytopenic cancer patients? Am J Med 1984;76:450–457.
232. Talbot GH, Provencher M, Cassileth PA. Persistent fever after recovery from granulocytopenia in acute leukemia. Arch Intern Med 1988;148:129–135.
233. Flynn PM, Shenep JL, Crawford R, Hughes WT. Use of abdominal computed tomography for identifying disseminated fungal infection in pediatric cancer patients. Clin Infect Dis 1995;20:964–970.
234. Elting LS, Rubenstein EB, Rolston KV, Bodey GP. Outcomes of bacteremia in patients with cancer and neutropenia: observations from two decades of epidemiological and clinical trials. Clin Infect Dis 1997;25:247–259.
235. Clark OA, Lyman G, Castro AA, Clark LG, Djulbegovic B. Colony stimulating factors for chemotherapy induced febrile neutropenia. Cochrane Database Syst Rev 2003:CD003039.
236. Link H, Bohme A, Cornely OA, et al. Antimicrobial therapy of unexplained fever in neutropenic patients: guidelines of the Infectious Diseases Working Party (AGIHO) of the German Society of Hematology and Oncology (DGHO), Study Group Interventional Therapy of Unexplained Fever, Arbeitsgemeinschaft Supportivmassnahmen in der Onkologie (ASO) of the Deutsche Krebsgesellschaft (DKG-German Cancer Society). Ann Hematol 2003;82(suppl 2):S105–S117.
237. Lucas KG. Another look at granulocyte transfusions in neutropenic patients with cancer. Infect Med 1996;13.
238. Rivers E, Nguyen B, Havstad S, et al. Early goal-directed therapy in the treatment of severe sepsis and septic shock. N Engl J Med 2001;345:1368–1377.
239. Connors AF Jr, Speroff T, Dawson NV, et al. The effectiveness of right heart catheterization in the initial care of critically ill patients. SUPPORT Investigators. JAMA 1996;276:889–897.
240. Sandham JD, Hull RD, Brant RF, et al. A randomized, controlled trial of the use of pulmonary-artery catheters in high-risk surgical patients. N Engl J Med 2003;348:5–14.
241. Annane D, Sebille V, Charpentier C, et al. Effect of treatment with low doses of hydrocortisone and fludrocortisone on mortality in patients with septic shock. JAMA 2002;288:862–871.
242. Bernard GR, Vincent JL, Laterre PF, et al. Efficacy and safety of recombinant human activated protein C for severe sepsis. N Engl J Med 2001;344:699–709.
243. Shelton BK. Evidence-based care for the neutropenic patient with leukemia. Semin Oncol Nurs 2003;19:133–141.
244. Nauseef WM, Maki DG. A study of the value of simple protective isolation in patients with granulocytopenia. N Engl J Med 1981;304:448–453.
245. Boyce JM. Understanding and controlling methicillin-resistant *Staphylococcus aureus* infections. Infect Control Hosp Epidemiol 2001;23(9):485–487.
246. Wenzel RP, Reagan DR, Bertino JS Jr, Baron EJ, Arias K. Methicillin-resistant *Staphylococcus aureus* outbreak: a consensus panel's definition and management guidelines. Am J Infect Control 1998;26:102–110.
247. Garner JS. Guideline for isolation precautions in hospitals. The Hospital Infection Control Practices Advisory Committee. Infect Control Hosp Epidemiol 1996;17:53–80.
248. Fridkin SK. Increasing prevalence of antimicrobial resistance in intensive care units. Crit Care Med 2001;29:N64–N68.
249. Warren DK, Fraser VJ. Infection control measures to limit antimicrobial resistance. Crit Care Med 2001;29:N128–N134.
250. Muto CA, Jernigan JA, Ostrowsky BE, et al. SHEA guideline for preventing nosocomial transmission of multidrug-resistant strains of *Staphylococcus aureus* and enterococcus. Infect Control Hosp Epidemiol 2003;24:362–386.
251. Jernigan JA, Clemence MA, Stott GA, et al. Control of methicillin-resistant *Staphylococcus aureus* at a university hospital: one decade later. Infect Control Hospital Epidemiol 1995;16:686–696.
252. Farr BM. Hospital wards spreading vancomycin-resistant enterococci to intensive care units: returning coals to Newcastle. Crit Care Med 1998;26:1942–1943.
253. Walsh TJ, Vlahov D, Hansen SL, et al. Prospective microbiologic surveillance in control of nosocomial methicillin-resistant *Staphylococcus aureus*. Infect Control 1987;8:7–14.
254. Jernigan JA, Titus MG, Groschel DH, Getchell-White S, Farr BM. Effectiveness of contact isolation during a hospital outbreak of methicillin-resistant *Staphylococcus aureus*. Am J Epidemiol 1996;143:496–504.
255. Murray-Leisure KA, Geib S, Graceley D, et al. Control of epidemic methicillin-resistant *Staphylococcus aureus*. Infect Control Hosp Epidemiol 1990;11:343–350.
256. Morris JG Jr, Shay DK, Hebden JN, et al. Enterococci resistant to multiple antimicrobial agents, including vancomycin. Establishment of endemicity in a university medical center. Ann Intern Med 1995;123:250–259.
257. Goetz AM, Rihs JD, Wagener MM, Muder RR. Infection and colonization with vancomycin-resistant *Enterococcus faecium* in an acute care Veterans Affairs Medical Center: a 2-year survey. Am J Infect Control 1998;26:558–562.
258. Ostrowsky BE, Trick WE, Sohn AH, et al. Control of vancomycin-resistant enterococcus in health care facilities in a region. N Engl J Med 2001;344:1427–1433.
259. Kotilainen P, Routamaa M, Peltonen R, et al. Eradication of methicillin-resistant *Staphylococcus aureus* from a health center ward and associated nursing home. Arch Intern Med 2001;161:859–863.
260. Zuckerman RA, Steele L, Venezia RA, Tobin EH. Undetected vancomycin-resistant *Enterococcus* in surgical intensive care unit patients. Infect Control Hosp Epidemiol 1999;20:685–686.
261. Maki DG, Zilz MA, McComick R. The effectiveness of using preemptive barrier precautions routinely (protective isolation) in all high-risk patients to prevent nosocomial infection with resistant organisms, especially MRSA, VRE and *C. difficile*. In: Thirty-fourth Annual Meeting of the Infectious Disease Society of North America, 1996, New Orleans, Louisiana.
262. van Voorhis J, Destefano L, Sobek S, et al. Impact of barrier precautions and cohorting on a monoclonal outbreak of vancomycin-resistant *Enterococcus faecium* (VRE). In: Society for Healthcare Epidemiology of America, 1997.
263. Klein BS, Perloff WH, Maki DG. Reduction of nosocomial infection during pediatric intensive care by protective isolation. N Engl J Med 1989;320:1714–1721.
264. Slota M, Green M, Farley A, Janosky J, Carcillo J. The role of gown and glove isolation and strict handwashing in the reduction of nosocomial infection in children with solid organ transplantation. Crit Care Med 2001;29:405–412.

265. Safdar N, Marx J, Meyer N, Maki DG. The effectiveness of preemptive enhanced barrier precautions for controlling MRSA in a burn unit. In: 43rd InterScience Conference on Antimicrobial Agents and Chemotherapy, 2003, Chicago, Illinois.
266. Srinivasan A, Song X, Ross T, Merz W, Brower R, Perl TM. A prospective study to determine whether cover gowns in addition to gloves decrease nosocomial transmission of vancomycin-resistant enterococci in an intensive care unit. Infect Control Hosp Epidemiol 2002;23:424–428.
267. Montecalvo MA, Jarvis WR, Uman J, et al. Infection-control measures reduce transmission of vancomycin-resistant enterococci in an endemic setting. Ann Intern Med 1999;131:269–272.
268. Koss WG, Khalili TM, Lemus JF, Chelly MM, Margulies DR, Shabot MM. Nosocomial pneumonia is not prevented by protective contact isolation in the surgical intensive care unit. Am Surg 2001;67.
269. Lew MA, Kehoe K, Ritz J, et al. Ciprofloxacin versus trimethoprim/sulfamethoxazole for prophylaxis of bacterial infections in bone marrow transplant recipients: a randomized, controlled trial. J Clin Oncol 1995;13:239–250.
270. Prentice HG, Hann IM, Nazareth B, Paterson P, Bhamra A, Kibbler CC. Oral ciprofloxacin plus colistin: prophylaxis against bacterial infection in neutropenic patients. A strategy for the prevention of emergence of antimicrobial resistance. Br J Haematol 2001;115:46–52.
271. Cruciani M, Malena M, Bosco O, Nardi S, Serpelloni G, Mengoli C. Reappraisal with meta-analysis of the addition of gram-positive prophylaxis to fluoroquinolone in neutropenic patients. J Clin Oncol 2003;21:4127–4137.
272. Bow EJ, Laverdiere M, Lussier N, Rotstein C, Cheang MS, Ioannou S. Antifungal prophylaxis for severely neutropenic chemotherapy recipients: a meta-analysis of randomized-controlled clinical trials. Cancer (Phila) 2002;94:3230–3246.
273. Kanda Y, Yamamoto R, Chizuka A, et al. Prophylactic action of oral fluconazole against fungal infection in neutropenic patients. A meta-analysis of 16 randomized, controlled trials. Cancer (Phila) 2000;89:1611–1625.
274. Wiederhold NP, Lewis RE, Kontoyiannis DP. Invasive aspergillosis in patients with hematologic malignancies. Pharmacotherapy 2003;23:1592–1610.
275. Fukuda T, Boeckh M, Carter RA, et al. Risks and outcomes of invasive fungal infections in recipients of allogeneic hematopoietic stem cell transplants after nonmyeloablative conditioning. Blood 2003;102:827–833.
276. Goodman JL, Winston DJ, Greenfield RA, et al. A controlled trial of fluconazole to prevent fungal infections in patients undergoing bone marrow transplantation. N Engl J Med 1992;326:845–851.
277. MacMillan ML, Goodman JL, DeFor TE, Weisdorf DJ. Fluconazole to prevent yeast infections in bone marrow transplantation patients: a randomized trial of high versus reduced dose, and determination of the value of maintenance therapy. Am J Med 2002;112:369–379.
278. Glasmacher A, Prentice A, Gorschluter M, et al. Itraconazole prevents invasive fungal infections in neutropenic patients treated for hematologic malignancies: evidence from a meta-analysis of 3,597 patients. J Clin Oncol 2003;21:4615–4626.
279. Mattiuzzi GN, Kantarjian H, Faderl S, et al. Amphotericin B lipid complex as prophylaxis of invasive fungal infections in patients with acute myelogenous leukemia and myelodysplastic syndrome undergoing induction chemotherapy. Cancer (Phila) 2004;100:581–589.
280. Bodey GP, Anaissie EJ, Elting LS, Estey E, O'Brien S, Kantarjian H. Antifungal prophylaxis during remission induction therapy for acute leukemia fluconazole versus intravenous amphotericin B. Cancer (Phila) 1994;73:2099–2106.
281. Walsh TJ, Pappas P, Winston DJ, et al. Voriconazole compared with liposomal amphotericin B for empirical antifungal therapy in patients with neutropenia and persistent fever. N Engl J Med 2002;346:225–234.
282. Cornely OA, Bohme A, Buchheidt D, et al. Prophylaxis of invasive fungal infections in patients with hematological malignancies and solid tumors: guidelines of the Infectious Diseases Working Party (AGIHO) of the German Society of Hematology and Oncology (DGHO). Ann Hematol 2003;82(suppl 2):S186–S200.
283. Kish MA. Guide to development of practice guidelines. Clin Infect Dis 2001;32:851–854.
284. Minotti V, Gentile G, Bucaneve G, et al. Domiciliary treatment of febrile episodes in cancer patients: a prospective randomized trial comparing oral versus parenteral empirical antibiotic treatment. Support Care Cancer 1999;7:134–139.
285. Paganini HR, Sarkis CM, De Martino MG, et al. Oral administration of cefixime to lower risk febrile neutropenic children with cancer. Cancer (Phila) 2000;88:2848–2852.
286. Paganini H, Rodriguez-Brieshcke T, Zubizarreta P, et al. Oral ciprofloxacin in the management of children with cancer with lower risk febrile neutropenia. Cancer (Phila) 2001;91:1563–1567.
287. Paganini H, Gomez S, Ruvinsky S, et al. Outpatient, sequential, parenteral-oral antibiotic therapy for lower risk febrile neutropenia in children with malignant disease: a single-center, randomized, controlled trial in Argentina. Cancer (Phila) 2003;97:1775–1780.
288. Shenep JL, Flynn PM, Baker DK, et al. Oral cefixime is similar to continued intravenous antibiotics in the empirical treatment of febrile neutropenic children with cancer. Clin Infect Dis 2001;32:36–43.
289. Mullen CA, Petropoulos D, Roberts WM, et al. Outpatient treatment of fever and neutropenia for low risk pediatric cancer patients. Cancer (Phila) 1999;86:126–134.
290. Hidalgo M, Hornedo J, Lumbreras C, et al. Outpatient therapy with oral ciprofloxacin for patients with low risk neutropenia and fever: a prospective, randomized clinical trial. Cancer (Phila) 1999;85:213–219.
291. Innes HE, Smith DB, O'Reilly SM, Clark PI, Kelly V, Marshall E. Oral antibiotics with early hospital discharge compared with in-patient intravenous antibiotics for low-risk febrile neutropenia in patients with cancer: a prospective randomised controlled single centre study. Br J Cancer 2003;89:43–49.
292. Petrilli AS, Dantas LS, Campos MC, Tanaka C, Ginani VC, Seber A. Oral ciprofloxacin vs. intravenous ceftriaxone administered in an outpatient setting for fever and neutropenia in low-risk pediatric oncology patients: randomized prospective trial. Med Pediatr Oncol 2000;34:87–91.
293. Freifeld A, Marchigiani D, Walsh T, et al. A double-blind comparison of empirical oral and intravenous antibiotic therapy for low-risk febrile patients with neutropenia during cancer chemotherapy. N Engl J Med 1999;341:305–311.
294. Kern WV, Cometta A, De Bock R, Langenaeken J, Paesmans M, Gaya H. Oral versus intravenous empirical antimicrobial therapy for fever in patients with granulocytopenia who are receiving cancer chemotherapy. International Antimicrobial Therapy Cooperative Group of the European Organization for Research and Treatment of Cancer. N Engl J Med 1999;341:312–318.
295. Engervall P, Gunther G, Ljungman P, et al. Trimethoprim-sulfamethoxazole plus amikacin versus ceftazidime monotherapy as empirical treatment in patients with neutropenia and fever. Scand J Infect Dis 1996;28:297–303.
296. Velasco E, Costa MA, Martins CA, Nucci M. Randomized trial comparing oral ciprofloxacin plus penicillin V with amikacin plus carbenicillin or ceftazidime for empirical treatment of febrile neutropenic cancer patients. Am J Clin Oncol 1995;18:429–435.
297. Malik IA, Abbas Z, Karim M. Randomised comparison of oral ciprofloxacin alone with combination of parenteral antibiotics in neutropenic febrile patients. Lancet 1992;339:1092–1096.

298. Rubenstein EB, Rolston K, Benjamin RS, et al. Outpatient treatment of febrile episodes in low-risk neutropenic patients with cancer. Cancer (Phila) 1993;71:3640–3646.
299. Johnson PR, Liu Yin JA, Tooth JA. A randomized trial of high-dose ciprofloxacin versus azlocillin and netilmicin in the empirical therapy of febrile neutropenic patients. J Antimicrob Chemother 1992;30:203–214.
300. Flaherty JP, Waitley D, Edlin B, et al. Multicenter, randomized trial of ciprofloxacin plus azlocillin versus ceftazidime plus amikacin for empiric treatment of febrile neutropenic patients. Am J Med 1989;87:278S–282S.
301. Chan CC, Oppenheim BA, Anderson H, Swindell R, Scarffe JH. Randomized trial comparing ciprofloxacin plus netilmicin versus piperacillin plus netilmicin for empiric treatment of fever in neutropenic patients. Antimicrob Agents Chemother 1989;33:87–91.
302. Rolston KVI, Rubenstein E, Elting L. Ambulatory management of febrile episodes in low-risk patients. In: 35th InterScience Conference of Antimicrobial Agents and Chemotherapy, 1995, San Francisco, California.
303. Cometta A, Zinner S, de Bock R, et al. Piperacillin-tazobactam plus amikacin versus ceftazidime plus amikacin as empiric therapy for fever in granulocytopenic patients with cancer. The International Antimicrobial Therapy Cooperative Group of the European Organization for Research and Treatment of Cancer. Antimicrob Agents Chemother 1995;39:445–452.
304. Cometta A, Calandra T, Gaya H, et al. Monotherapy with meropenem versus combination therapy with ceftazidime plus amikacin as empiric therapy for fever in granulocytopenic patients with cancer. The International Antimicrobial Therapy Cooperative Group of the European Organization for Research and Treatment of Cancer and the Gruppo Italiano Malattie Ematologiche Maligne dell'Adulto Infection Program. Antimicrob Agents Chemother 1996;40:1108–1115.

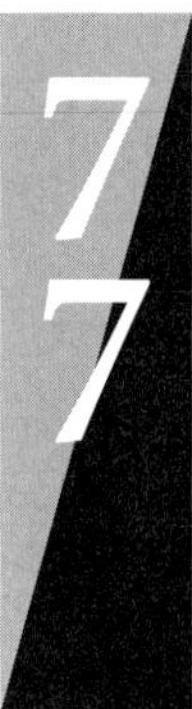

Acute Toxicities of Therapy: Pulmonary Complications

Scott E. Evans and Andrew H. Limper

Surveillance data indicate that adverse drug reactions result in between 3.5% and 32.9% of hospitalizations.[1–3] Of the more than 350 medications known or suspected of causing pulmonary complications, a substantial number are chemotherapeutic agents.

Twenty percent of patients receiving cytotoxic chemotherapeutic agents (10% or less for noncytotoxic drugs) develop symptoms of untoward pulmonary reactions.[4,5] Up to 3% of patients on some cytotoxic regimens will succumb to pulmonary-related mortality.[6,7] An estimated 5% to 30% of pulmonary disorders in cancer patients are directly attributed to chemotherapy.[8] Further, a Mayo Clinic study of lung biopsies from immunocompromised patients with diffuse lung disease, implicated chemotherapeutic agents as causative 21% of the time.[9]

Despite the prevalence of chemotherapy-associated pulmonary toxicity (CAPT), the assessment of these effects remains difficult. The myriad presentations of CAPT are often nonspecific and vary both by drug and by individual patient.[4,10] Further, although unrecognized CAPT may be fatal, so too are the conditions from which it must most often be differentiated: progression or metastasis of the underlying malignancy and pulmonary infections in the immunocompromised cancer patient. Unfortunately, neither blood tests nor even biopsy can alone confirm the diagnosis of CAPT,[9,11] and, accordingly, the diagnosis of CAPT is sometimes a diagnosis of exclusion.[11,12]

Typical Presentations

The first indications of CAPT often arise weeks to years after the initial administration of chemotherapeutic drugs. The most consistently described symptoms in CAPT are dyspnea, nonproductive cough, and, notably, fever. Chills are typically absent. Although the physical examination varies with the underlying process, the most common finding in CAPT is the presence of fine crackles.

With the possible exception of methotrexate pneumonitis-related hilar lymphadenopathy, specific X-ray presentations cannot be reliably used to predict the offending chemotherapeutic agent.[13] The most frequently described chest X-ray findings are diffuse interstitial changes,[13,14] and a diffuse mixed alveolar-interstitial pattern may also be observed in some forms of CAPT (Figure 77.1).

High-resolution computed tomography (HRCT) of the chest may help exclude common CAPT mimics, such as some lower respiratory tract infection, radiation pneumonitis, or progression of malignancy.[15] Although nonspecific, identification of suggestive HRCT findings may aid in the diagnosis of CAPT.[16–18] The most common findings in CAPT are diffuse or multifocal ground-glass opacities, patchy areas of consolidation, interlobular septal thickening, centrilobular nodules, pleural effusion, and pulmonary nodules.[13,14,18]

Gallium (^{67}Ga) uptake is elevated in most chemotherapy-induced pulmonary reactions.[9] One study also prospectively showed that technetium (^{99m}Tc) pentetic acid (DTPA) scintigraphy can discriminate patients with methotrexate pneumonitis from those not receiving methotrexate.[19]

Routine pulmonary function testing is often recommended for patients managed with agents known to have pulmonary toxicities, particularly, bleomycin. Plethysmographic testing of lung volumes in CAPT can reveal evidence of restrictive lung disease, although spirometry does not generally demonstrate airflow obstruction.[9] Probably the most sensitive pulmonary function parameter for identifying preclinical CAPT is the carbon monoxide diffusing capacity (D_{LCO}). Decrements in the D_{LCO} have been prospectively noted days to weeks before symptoms or radiographic changes of CAPT are evident,[20] and may offer an opportunity to minimize disease progression through drug withdrawal. Conflicting data exist, however, and some authors argue that isolated D_{LCO} decreases rarely progress to clinically relevant disease and improve after completion of therapy.[21]

Fiberoptic bronchoscopy with bronchoalveolar lavage and/or transbronchial biopsy is commonly performed in cases of suspected CAPT. The utility of this approach remains unproved in a prospective manner, although valuable information may be gained.[5] In particular, the presence of lower respiratory tract infections may be excluded by either bronchoalveolar lavage or transbronchial biopsy with a reasonably strong negative predictive value. Either test may reveal alternate pulmonary diagnoses, and transbronchial biopsy may identify lymphangitic tumor spread. Although sampling error is always a concern with transbronchial biopsy, it has also been reported that lymphocytic alveolitis identified in a bronchoscopically obtained sample may be suggestive of CAPT.[22]

The determination for open versus thoracoscopic biopsy must be made on a case-by-case basis, determined by features, such as clinical stability, location of infiltrates, and coagulopathies.[23]

Largely as a result of differing mechanisms of injury and interindividual variations, no single histologic pattern has been identified to conclusively prove CAPT. In this respect, the most informative element of pathologic reports is often the exclusion of alternate conditions when CAPT is suspected.[24]

Several classic histologic patterns have been described in CAPT. Most commonly described are "bizarre" changes of type II pneumocytes with marked cellular atypia and hyperplasia, but no changes suggestive of malignancy, and a reduction in the type I pneumocyte population. The simple presence of cytological atypia cannot by itself definitively establish chemotherapy-associated lung injury.

Interstitial inflammation is also frequently reported during CAPT and can be associated with septal thickening caused by fibrin and collagen deposition. Such extracellular matrix deposition can eventually progress to severe fibrosis, such as occurs during long-term bleomycin therapy (Figure 77.2). Other forms of CAPT, including that associated with cytosine arabinoside, demonstrate a pattern of diffuse alveolar damage. In addition, bronchiolitis obliterans-organizing pneumonia has also been described with chemotherapeutic agents. Because of the limited number of toxic responses the lung is capable of generating, many biopsy specimens in CAPT can be characterized no more precisely than interstitial pneumonia.[24]

Also complicating the pathologic assessment of patients with CAPT, is incomplete understanding of the correlation between histologic changes and clinical disease. More precisely, the relevance of atypical epithelial cells recovered from bronchial washings or sputum samples remains unclear. Even when classic type II pneumocyte changes are observed, the rate of progression to symptomatic CAPT is unknown.

An understanding of the typical timing of various CAPT syndromes often facilitates determination of the significance of radiographic and pathologic findings. The majority of patients who develop CAPT present more than 2 months after the completion of therapy. Hypersensitivity pneumonitis and hypersensitivity-like inflammatory interstitial pneumonias, however, are most often reported in the early days to weeks of therapy and are most commonly described with methotrexate, procarbazine, carmustine (BCNU), paclitaxel, and bleomycin.[25] These patients present with features typical of hypersensitivity of other causes, including nonproductive cough, exertional dyspnea, fine crackles on examination, interstitial or mixed interstitial-alveolar infiltrates on radiographs, and often with peripheral and parenchymal eosinophilia. As with many other CAPT presentations, they also tend to have low-grade fevers. Another commonly problematic early-onset presentation of CAPT, is noncardiogenic pulmonary edema, with chemotherapy-induced endothelial inflammation leading to vascular leak. Cytosine arabinoside (ara-C), interleukin-2, all-*trans*-retinoic acid (ATRA), and bleomycin, are the most common culprits in this type of reaction.[25] Other well-characterized early presentations include bronchospasm (vinblastine, methotrexate), pleural effusion

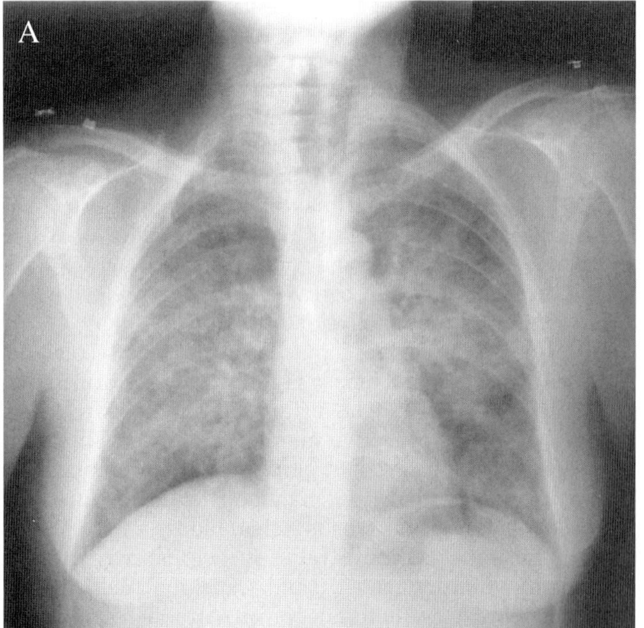

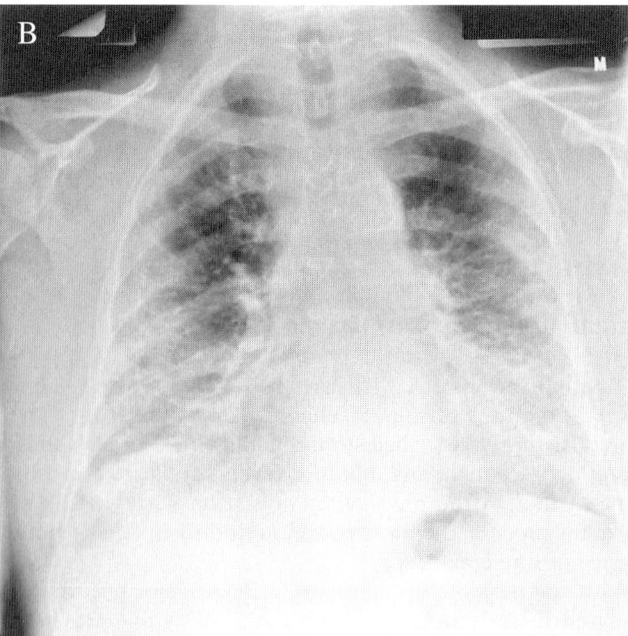

FIGURE 77.1. Radiographic patterns of chemotherapy-associated pulmonary toxicity. (A) Chest radiograph of a patient receiving busulfan therapy. The X-ray demonstrates diffuse mixed alveolar and interstitial infiltrates. (B) Chest radiograph shows chronic interstitial fibrotic infiltrates in patient receiving long-term chlorambucil therapy.

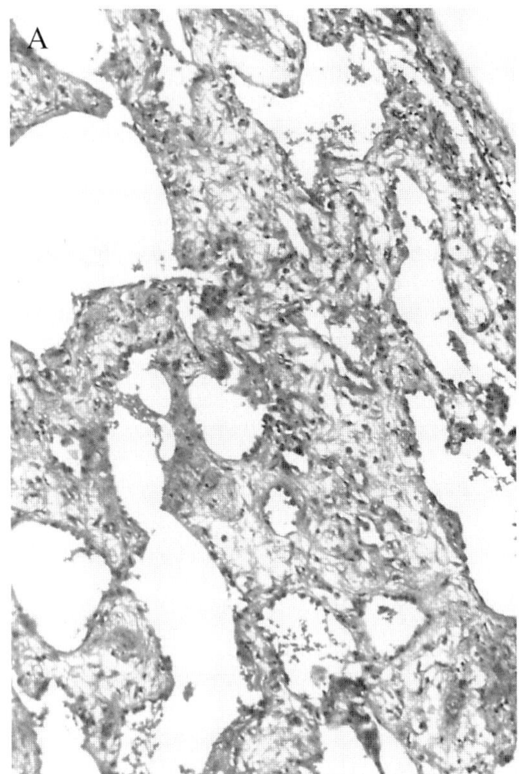

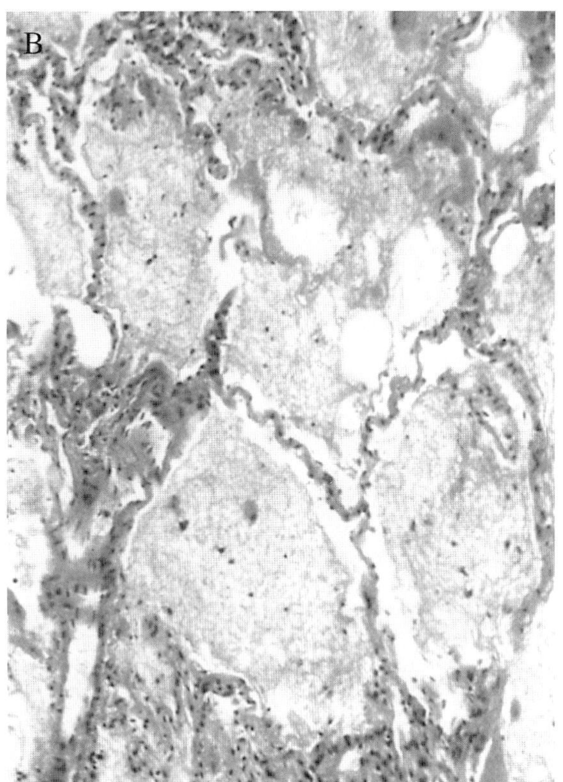

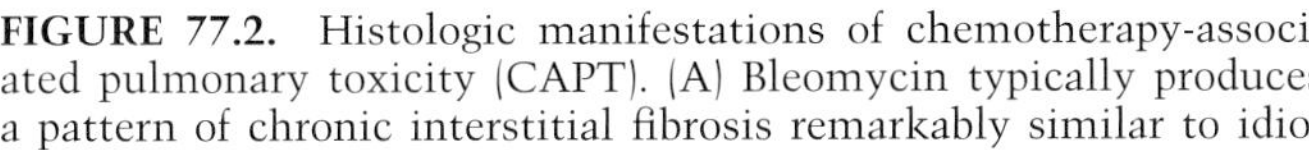

FIGURE 77.2. Histologic manifestations of chemotherapy-associated pulmonary toxicity (CAPT). (A) Bleomycin typically produces a pattern of chronic interstitial fibrosis remarkably similar to idiopathic usual interstitial pneumonia. (B) Certain types of CAPT, such as associated with high-dose cytosine arabinoside (ARA-C), produce a histologic pattern of diffuse alveolar damage.

(methotrexate, ATRA, mitomycin-C), and early-onset pulmonary fibrosis (ATRA, rarely bleomycin).

The norm is CAPT presentation months to years after initiation of therapy.[9,25] Interstitial fibrosis is undoubtedly the most common manifestation of late-stage CAPT, with bleomycin, BCNU, busulfan, and mitomycin-C the biggest offenders.[4,26] Although the radiographic distribution may be somewhat atypical, the histologic features of CAPT-induced fibrosis are generally identical to those in idiopathic pulmonary fibrosis. In addition to interstitial fibrosis, both pleural thickening and pulmonary nodules have been described with late-stage extracellular matrix deposition and bronchiolitis obliterans-organizing pneumonia. Intriguingly, cytotoxic chemotherapeutic agents have also been associated with exacerbations of previously established radiation pneumonitis with fibrosis, so-called radiation recall effects.[6] And, conversely, patients with cytotoxic agent-induced fibrosis have been shown to display accelerated collagen deposition following exposure to high inspired oxygen concentrations for at least 6 months after completion of therapy.[6]

Regardless of the specific agent, the central tenets of CAPT management are cessation of exposure to the drug and supportive care. Oxygen supplementation, mechanical ventilation, diuresis, and even lung transplantation have been used when clinically necessary. Corticosteroid therapy is also widely advocated for many severe reactions, although data are lacking to show proof of effect for most CAPT reactions.[9,10,12,26]

Specific Agents

Antibiotics

Bleomycin

With reports of 20% to 46%[6] of treated patients demonstrating clinically relevant CAPT and 1% to 3% mortality,[7,27] bleomycin is both the most common cause of CAPT and the prototypical example. Although other uncommon presentations abound, pulmonary fibrosis is the characteristic manifestation of bleomycin toxicity (Table 77.1).

Bleomycin toxicity appears to result from direct cellular damage by the drug.[6] The predilection for bleomycin to affect lung and skin, results from relatively low levels of the inactivating enzyme bleomycin hydrolase in these cells,[6] and allows for drug accumulation and DNA fragmentation in pneumocytes. Type I pneumocytes are typically affected first, but because type II cells proliferate to replace injured type I cells, they are affected as well. The cell-cycle-dependent manner of type II cell injury results in increased risk of type II cell injury with repeated dosing. The fibroblast proliferation in bleomycin-induced fibrosis occurs both by direct stimulation of fibroblasts by the drug and as a secondary consequence of pneumocyte depletion. An additional component of free radical-related injury almost certainly exists and likely accounts for subsequent sensitivity to oxygen therapy.

TABLE 77.1. Reported manifestations of bleomycin-induced pulmonary toxicity.

Chronic interstitial pneumonia/chronic fibrosis
Acute interstitial pneumonia/acute fibrosis
Bronchiolitis obliterans-organizing pneumonia
Hypersensitivity pneumonitis
Single or multiple pulmonary nodules
Chest pain
"Radiation recall"/exacerbation of prior radiation fibrosis
Chronic eosinophilic pneumonia
Pneumothorax (rare)

Many studies have been undertaken to identify those most at risk for bleomycin-induced disease, and cumulative dose is among the most convincing risk factors. Although toxicity has been described with as little as 20 units, most bleomycin-induced fibrosis occurs in patients who have received more than 450 units.[27] At doses greater than 550 units, the mortality rates can exceed 10%. Age also appears to affect the likelihood of bleomycin-induced lung disease. Bleomycin-treated patients over 70 years of age demonstrate a significant increase in the incidence of fibrosis.[6] Conversely, children also may be at elevated risk, with up to 70% of patients treated for rhabdomyosarcomas developing some fibrosis.[25] Human studies predict risk factors based on polymorphisms of the tumor necrosis factor-α_2 domain,[28] and animal investigations have implicated numerous foci in bleomycin susceptibility, including p53.[29]

In addition to the direct effects of the drug, bleomycin is uniquely prone to synergistic effects with other pulmonary toxic agents.[9,25,26] As already described, pneumonitis related to prior or concomitant radiotherapy can be exacerbated, or even induced, by bleomycin. Inspiring high oxygen concentrations during or after bleomycin treatment can foster progression of bleomycin injury,[6] often encountered during surgery or during episodes of acute respiratory failure. The durability of this effect is unclear, but this oxygen sensitivity has been clearly noted for months to years after therapy with bleomycin. Further, a host of other chemotherapeutic agents are reported to have enhanced pulmonary toxicities when coadministered with bleomycin. Implicated drugs include cyclophosphamide, vincristine, doxorubicin, methotrexate, and possibly, granulocyte colony-stimulating factor (G-CSF).[25]

Although prospective evidence of benefit is lacking, many clinicians advocate frequent monitoring of the diffusing capacity to predict the development of clinically apparent bleomycin toxicity. Drug withdrawal is generally recommended when there is a progressive fall in D_{LCO}. Studies have failed to conclusively link subtle gas exchange abnormalities with dose-limiting toxicity, with some authors arguing that changes in the vital capacity and pulmonary capillary blood volume are better predictors of impending CAPT.[21] CT scanning appears somewhat helpful in the diagnosis of subclinical bleomycin fibrosis, with one series showing 38% abnormal CT scans but only 15% abnormal chest X-rays.[6] This finding bears unclear relevance, as up to 20% of patients with findings indicative of bleomycin toxicity are asymptomatic.[30]

After discontinuation of the drug, any additional therapy for bleomycin-induced fibrosis is strictly empiric. Expert, mostly anecdotal, opinion suggests dosing prednisone equivalents of approximately 60mg per day for worsening fibrosis. Outcomes data following corticosteroid therapy are widely variable.

In addition to the characteristic fibrosis, bleomycin toxicity manifests in many other, less common presentations. Numerous radiographic patterns are described, including acute interstitial changes and rare pneumothoraces. Among the most troublesome presentations, is the development of single or multiple pulmonary nodules. Because the primary diagnosis from which this must be differentiated is the progression of malignancy, essentially all suspected bleomycin-induced nodules must be biopsied. Most nodules that prove nonmalignant demonstrate histologic features of bronchiolitis obliterans-organizing pneumonia. Hypersensitivity pneumonitis and chronic eosinophilic pneumonia have also been rarely reported during bleomycin therapy, with abrupt onset symptoms, cough, fever, exertional dyspnea, and eosinophilia.[31]

Mitomycin C

Mitomycin C-related CAPT has been estimated to occur in the range of 8% to 39% of treated patients.[25,26] In many ways, mitomycin-induced changes are similar to those of bleomycin, with toxicity commonly evident as an interstitial pneumonitis with fibrosis that occurs 3 to 12 months after completion of therapy. As with bleomycin, mitomycin-treated patients appear more likely to develop significant toxicities when exposed to high inspired oxygen concentrations or radiation therapy. Additionally, prior or concomitant therapy with bleomycin, cisplatin, cyclophosphamide, doxorubicin, or vinca alkaloids is a risk factor for mitomycin-induced fibrosis. As with bleomycin, the D_{LCO} often falls before the development of fibrosis-related symptoms. However, the development of symptoms after a decline in the D_{LCO} is less common than with bleomycin (in one series, 28% of treated patients had a reduction in the D_{LCO}, but only 5% developed symptoms).[32] Suggested therapy for mitomycin-induced fibrosis is identical to that of bleomycin: drug discontinuation, avoidance of high oxygen tensions, and supportive care. Corticosteroids are reported to be somewhat more beneficial in mitomycin toxicity than with bleomycin.

Unique to mitomycin toxicity are accumulating case reports of a microangiopathic hemolytic anemia; this is associated with renal failure and noncardiogenic pulmonary edema, with perhaps half of these patients progressing to acute respiratory distress syndrome. Pathologic review demonstrates arteriolar intimal hyperplasia, capillary cellular atypia, and fibrin thrombi in the kidneys and lungs. Risk factors for this syndrome appear to include fluorouracil therapy and blood transfusions.[33]

Other Antibiotics

Actinomycin D appears particularly prone to radiation recall effects, even when the drug is given long after completion of radiation therapy.[25,26] It otherwise behaves similarly to the other antineoplastic antibiotics. Mitoxantrone occasionally induces interstitial pneumonia.[26] Phase I trials of the mitomycin C analog KW-2149 have also induced dose-limiting CAPT that was not prevented by prophylactic corticosteroid administration.[34]

Alkylating Agents

Busulfan

First identified in 1961, busulfan was the first chemotherapeutic agent linked to pulmonary toxicity. Although the alkylating agents often demonstrate less CAPT when used as monotherapy than many other agents, prediction of patients who will develop busulfan toxicity remains very difficult. No risk factors have been convincingly identified,[11] and no relationship to cumulative dose has been demonstrated. Further, symptom development averages 3.5 years after completion of therapy and is reported as much as a decade later. Even more troubling is the fact that mortality rates from busulfan CAPT are exceedingly high (estimated 80%), and no therapies are known to improve this.[25]

Busulfan toxicity probably occurs in about 4% to 6% of patients (reported range, 2.5% to 43%).[35] In general, the clinical findings are similar to those of bleomycin toxicity, with progressive fibrosis. These patients may have a greater predilection for mixed alveolar-interstitial patterns on radiographs. Accordingly, histologic findings often demonstrate lymphocytic and plasma cell infiltration, in addition to fibrosis and type II pneumocyte hyperplasia with atypia. Alveolar proteinosis is also occasionally described with busulfan toxicity. By report, the proteinosis is more refractory to lavage therapy than primary alveolar lipoproteinosis. No data exist regarding corticosteroid therapy in busulfan-induced alveolar proteinosis.[9]

Cyclophosphamide

Alhough some experts have suggested that the incidence of cyclophosphamide-induced pulmonary toxicity is underestimated, current estimates indicate that less than 1% of patients develop fibrosis with therapy.[25] A review of 20 years experience at the Mayo Clinic identified only six cases in which cyclophosphamide was the only factor contributing to pulmonary toxicity.[36]

Cyclophosphamide toxicity typically presents as one of two temporally distinct variants.[36] Both present with dyspnea, fever, nonproductive cough, and new parenchymal infiltrates. The early-onset variety (6 months or less of initiation of therapy) is often mistaken for an infectious pneumonia because of its rapidity of onset. This variety responds well to drug withdrawal alone and may resolve entirely without additional intervention. The late-onset form (months to years after initiating therapy) displays less encouraging outcomes. The interstitial radiographic changes in late-onset cyclophosphamide toxicity include marked, progressive fibrosis, often with honeycombing, and may be associated with bilateral pleural thickening. On histologic section, the fibrosis in cyclophosphamide toxicity is associated with lymphocytic and plasma cell infiltrates and organizing pneumonia. In this form of toxicity, the pulmonary-related mortality approaches 60% despite drug withdrawal and corticosteroids.[36]

It appears that cumulative dosing of greater than 150 to 250 mg may be associated with CAPT, although this association is not universally accepted. The risk of cyclophosphamide toxicity is likely elevated when used in conjunction with carmustine (BCNU) for conditioning before bone marrow transplantation, but no other drugs have been implicated in inducing cyclophosphamide toxicity. For additionally unclear reasons, some patients with a history of resolved cyclophosphamide toxicity can be rechallenged with the drug and not redevelop the syndrome. For safety reasons, this practice is not recommended. As previously noted, cyclophosphamide may exacerbate bleomycin toxicity.

Ifosfamide

Ifosfamide has rarely been reported to cause pulmonary toxicity. These occasional reports describe fibrosis similar to that seen in cyclophosphamide, as might be expected given the chemical similarities of the two agents.

Vinblastine

Aside from anecdotal reports of noncardiogenic pulmonary edema,[37] vinblastine has not historically been associated with significant pulmonary toxicities, despite many years of use. In recent years, however, combination therapies that include vinblastine have resulted in increased reports of CAPT. Approximately 2% of patients treated with concurrent vinblastine and mitomycin C present with noncardiogenic pulmonary edema, interstitial fibrosis, or bronchospasm.[37]

Chlorambucil

Chlorambucil occasionally induces an interstitial pneumonitis similar to that seen with busulfan and cyclophosphamide. Peak timing for this complication occurs in the range of 6 to 12 months after initiating therapy; this generally occurs with doses between 2 and 7.5 g and is associated with high mortality rates.[25,26]

Melphalan

Rare cases of pulmonary toxicity have been described with high-dose (200 mg/m^2 or more) melphalan use.[38] Some experts have argued that the incidence is underestimated, although given the chronicity of use for many melphalan-treated diseases, this seems unlikely. Similar to chlorambucil, when present, melphalan toxicity is associated with high mortality rates.

Antimetabolites

Methotrexate

Methotrexate pneumonitis has been confirmed in several hundred cases[8] but represents a quite unusual phenomenon.[39,40] Further, methotrexate pneumonitis-related fatalities are reported in less than 10% of affected patients.[26,39]

The CAPT associated with methotrexate is unique in many aspects. The timing of symptoms is earlier than with most chemotherapeutic agents. Most patients who eventually experience cough, dyspnea, and nonproductive cough, do so in the first days to weeks of therapy, and only rarely in subsequent weeks or months. The histologic features on biopsy are usually more consistent with hypersensitivity pneumonitis than with fibrosis. More than half of affected patients have a peripheral eosinophilia, also supporting a hypersensitivity state. The radiographic presentation of methotrexate pneumonitis is usually homogeneous interstitial infiltrates, although methotrexate is also uniquely prone to causing pleural effusions or hilar lymphadenopathy.

Most cases of methotrexate pneumonitis resolve with drug withdrawal alone. In the rare cases of acute fibrotic reactions, corticosteroid therapy is thought to reduce sequelae and to improve mortality.[39] The development of methotrexate pneumonitis does not appear to be dose related, and fatalities have been described following intrathecal as well as oral administration. Fatal noncardiogenic pulmonary edema has also been seen after intrathecal administration.[37] As with a handful of other chemotherapeutic drugs, patients with confirmed cases of methotrexate pneumonitis have been later rechallenged without redevelopment of the toxicity. In general, we do not, however, recommend rechallenge with methotrexate or any other agent causing CAPT.

Cytosine Arabinoside (Ara-C)

Noncardiogenic pulmonary edema is the respiratory complication most frequently reported with ara-C therapy and has a high mortality.[41] Pathologic review typically demonstrates proteinaceous material filling alveolar airspaces but not the pneumocyte atypia or inflammatory infiltrates described with most other chemotherapeutic agents. An estimated 13% to 28% of patients develop respiratory complaints during administration of ara-C, and more than 40% develop symptoms within 1 month. Clinical management relies on oxygen supplementation and mechanical ventilation, if needed. Diuretics may be beneficial, and some have suggested that clearance is enhanced by corticosteroids.[41]

Gemcitabine

Although often regarded as minimally toxic to the lungs, gemcitabine has also been associated with fatal noncardiogenic pulmonary edema.[37,42] This event results from a vascular leak syndrome, comparable to that seen with chemically similar ara-C.[41] Gemcitabine therapy induces severe dyspnea in 3% to 5% of treated patients,[41] and pulmonary edema affects 0.1% to 7%, usually after multiple doses.[43] Pulmonary edema may occur more frequently when gemcitabine is combined with docetaxel.[37] The early introduction of corticosteroids has been advised for gemcitabine-related pulmonary edema.[41] Interstitial pneumonitis has been rarely reported with gemcitabine and also appears to improve with steroid therapy.[44]

Other Antimetabolites

Azathioprine and its metabolite 6-mercaptopurine have both been occasionally reported to cause interstitial pneumonias, although many cases are confounded by the coadministration of other drugs that may have similar toxicities. Most cases of azathioprine-associated pulmonary fibrosis have been reported following solid organ transplants.[26] Similarly, fludarabine has rarely been reported to cause chronic interstitial fibrosis, acute eosinophilic pneumonia, and hypersensitivity pneumonitis, with apparent corticosteroid benefit.[45–47]

Nitrosoureas

Carmustine (BCNU)

BCNU has been associated with several distinct CAPT syndromes, with an overall incidence estimated between 1.5% and 20% of treated patients. Some patients experience an early-onset alveolitis and fibrosis, as can be seen with bleomycin. This phenomenon appears dose related, likely at dosages greater than 1,400 mg/m^2,[48] although this has clearly occurred among patients receiving much lower doses.[49] Some experts note that fever is less prominent with BCNU than in other CAPT syndromes.

BCNU also results in late-phase pulmonary fibrosis, 6 months to 3 years after completion of therapy. All the nitrosoureas have been reported to cause fibrosis, but BCNU has been most often described to produce this effect. It is also uniquely predisposed to cause upper lobe predominant fibrosis. In fact, one small long-term series suggested the incidence of upper lobe fibrosis might surpass 70% if patients are followed long enough. In general, patients with BCNU-related fibrosis experience clinical courses similar to that seen with bleomycin-related fibrosis, although the response to corticosteroids is reportedly more robust.[49]

Another unique feature of BCNU-related CAPT is the occurrence of drug-induced pneumothoraces, which is seldom described with any other chemotherapeutic agent; this may be related to the upper lobe fibrobullous changes induced by this agent.

BCNU synergistically induces pulmonary toxicity with other antineoplastic interventions, including cyclophosphamide and radiation therapy, as mentioned previously. BCNU-containing regimens also exacerbate bone marrow transplant-related pulmonary toxicity, with up to 40% incidence.[26] Underlying lung diseases, especially chronic obstructive pulmonary disease and certain pneumoconioses, also place patients at higher risk of BCNU toxicity.

Other Nitrosoureas

Occasional reports of inflammatory pneumonitis and chronic fibrosis have been associated with lomustine (CCNU), semustine (methyl-CCNU), fotemustine (CENU), and chlorozotocin. Rare reports of pneumothoraces have also surfaced with these agents. Their pulmonary toxicities are expected to be closely aligned with those of BCNU, given their chemical similarities.

Interleukin 2 (IL-2)

Most patients receiving IL-2 develop some manifestation of pulmonary toxicity, primarily because of its induction of severe vascular leakage. Early experience with IL-2 resulted in pulmonary resulted radiologic infiltrates in up to 80% of patients and pleural effusions in more than half. More recent data place the risk of severe vascular effects in the range of 3% to 20% of treated patients. Risk factors for development of the vascular phenomenon include reduction in pretreatment airflows, previous chemotherapy, and bolus infusion of IL-2.

The noncardiogenic pulmonary edema resulting from IL-2-induced vascular leak can lead to acute respiratory distress syndrome. Complicating the management of NCPE/ARDS is the potential for IL-2 to cause cardiac toxicity, thereby inducing cardiogenic pulmonary edema. Fortunately, even in the case of severe toxicity, the process resolves in most patients within days of cessation of therapy.[37] There may be a role for prostaglandins or cyclooxygenase-2 inhibitors in management of this toxicity, although clinicians are increasingly aware that it may often be avoided through careful patient selection.[37]

IL-2 is also responsible for inducing hypersensitivity pneumonitis, as well as bronchospasm in patients without preexisting asthma. Both conditions tend to resolve with discontinuation of therapy.

Gefitinib

Considerable recent attention has been paid to the pulmonary toxicity of gefitinib, the selective epidermal growth factor receptor-tyrosine kinase inhibitor recently approved in the United States for management of salvage therapy of non-small cell lung carcinoma. By mid-2003, nearly 200 deaths had been reported as a result of respiratory failure among more than 10,000 patients in Japan.[50,51] The best characterized series reports 4 patients among 18 gefitinib-treated patients who developed severe acute interstitial pneumonia. All 4 patients had undergone previous thoracic radiation and/or had a low performance score; 2 subsequently improved with corticosteroids, and 2 patients died.[52] Although this agent is restricted in use to patients who have failed platinum-based therapy, post-marketing experience will certainly enhance the understanding of its CAPT.

Miscellaneous Chemotherapeutic Agents with Pulmonary Toxicities

Procarbazine infrequently causes CAPT, usually after the third or fourth dose. The characteristic toxicity seen with procarbazine is hypersensitivity pneumonitis, with marked eosinophilia. In most cases, this syndrome resolves following discontinuation of procarbazine therapy. Reports of procarbazine-induced fibrosis are exceedingly rare.[53]

Zinostatin is described to occasionally result in an interstitial pneumonia, particularly among patients receiving long-term therapy. One histologic feature distinguishing zinostatin-related CAPT from that of other drugs, is its propensity to induce endothelial hypertrophy in the pulmonary vasculature.[9]

Case reports implicate etoposide (VP-16) as having pulmonary toxic effects.[54] However, its frequent use in the management of small cell lung cancer (especially in combination with known pulmonary toxic agents, such as methotrexate and cyclophosphamide) has confounded the comprehensive evaluation of it pulmonary toxicity.

The pulmonary effects of tumor necrosis factor-α in antineoplastic therapy remain unclear. One small study prospectively showed statistically significant reductions in the D_{Lco} in all patients studied but did not identify other physiologic manifestations of CAPT.[55]

Roughly one-quarter of patients receiving all-*trans* retinoic acid (ATRA) for acute promyelocytic leukemia develop a vascular leak syndrome similar to that seen with IL-2; this is believed to result from the sudden differentiation of blasts into mature granulocytes that then adhere to the pulmonary endothelium. Absolute blast count is the only identified risk factor for this syndrome, although a specific number below which ATRA is safe remains unidentified. ATRA can also induce acute pulmonary fibrosis in a smaller percentage of patients. In addition to drug withdrawal, steroids appear beneficial if started early.[37]

The taxanes paclitaxel and docetaxel have both been reported to cause noncardiogenic pulmonary edema,[25,37] and numerous radiographic patterns have been described for treated patients.[14] Hypersensitivity pneumonitis occurs in 3% to 5% of paclitaxel treated patients,[56] although some of the reported patients were likely hypersensitive to the suspension vehicle (Cremophor EL) rather than the antineoplastic agent.[26] The concurrent use of thoracic radiation has been shown to exacerbate the pulmonary toxicity of paclitaxel.[57]

Monotherapy with granulocyte colony-stimulating factor (G-CSF) occasionally induces noncardiogenic pulmonary edema.[37] More frequently, however, it exacerbates preexisting lung injury, whether caused by CAPT or acute lung injury associated with previous critical illness.[58,59] This effect likely occurs by a neutrophil-dependent mechanism, and it responds well to corticosteroids in most cases.[60] Further understanding of G-CSF-induced toxicities is hindered by the rarity with which it is used as monotherapy.[60]

When used in combination with radiation therapy, irinotecan (CPT-11) results in more respiratory symptoms than are seen among patients receiving radiotherapy alone. This finding is notable, given the already high incidence (17.4% to 22%) of cough and dyspnea with CPT-11 therapy.[61] A wide range of radiographic patterns accompany the respiratory symptoms, including very rare pleural effusions.[14] Fatal respiratory insufficiency has been reported with CPT-11 treatment.[61]

Hormone therapy is generally regarded as having little pulmonary toxicity. However, one well-characterized case report describes severe pulmonary fibrosis following therapy with nilutamide and buserelin.[62]

Combination Therapies

Many specific combinations of chemotherapeutic agents are reported to induce pulmonary toxicities at rates greater than expected from their additive effects. Several are described in the foregoing chapter. Additionally, Table 77.2 describes several additional combinations of agents with their reported toxicities.

Radiation Effects

The acute effects of radiation can produce tissue changes that mimic cytotoxic lung responses and may on occasion involve areas of lung outside the port of radiation. The process is generally initiated with fever beginning 3 to 8 weeks after initiation of radiation therapy and may progress rapidly to a respiratory failure despite corticosteroid therapy. The disease may improve spontaneously but usually progresses to chronic radiation effects. Bronchoalveolar lavage predominantly demonstrates lymphocytes, not only in the involved lung but also in the opposite lung.[63] The chronic effects of radiation are well known: they begin 3 to 6 months or later after radiation therapy, and their primary effect is vascular obliteration and fibrosis.[64] Recently, a form of radiation pneumonitis has been observed outside the treatment fields, usually in patients with breast cancer.[65] Tissue examination has revealed bronchiolitis obliterans with organizing pneumonitis in these cases.[65]

TABLE 77.2. Chemotherapeutic combinations reported to induce pulmonary toxicity.

Combination	*Toxicity*
Adriamycin, bleomycin, vincristine, dexamethasone (ABVD)	Interstitial fibrosis
Cyclophosphamide, cisplatin, carmustine (CPB)	Interstitial fibrosis
Mitoxantrone, methotrexate, mitomycin C (3M)	Radiation sensitivity
Carmustine, etoposide, melphalan (BEM)	Acute interstitial pneumonia
Carmustine, etoposide, cyclophosphamide (BVC, CBV)	Acute interstitial pneumonia
Doxorubicin, cyclophosphamide, 5-fluorouracil (CAF)	Interstitial fibrosis
Fludarabine, cytarabine, idarubicin, G-CSF (FLAG-ida)	Interstitial fibrosis
Cyclophosphamide, dexamethasone, etoposide, cisplatin (CDEP)	Acute interstitial pneumonia
Cyclophosphamide, methotrexate, etoposide	Acute interstitial pneumonia
Docetaxel, gemcitabine	Pulmonary edema
Docetaxel, estramustine	Acute interstitial pneumonia
Paclitaxel, carboplatin	Interstitial fibrosis
Doxorubicin, G-CSF	Acute interstitial pneumonia
Doxorubicin, vindesine	Acute interstitial pneumonia
Vinblastine, mitomycin C	Pulmonary edema

Listed are combinations of agents with toxicities reported to occur with greater frequency than would be anticipated from the summative effects of the components, along with their described effects.

Conclusions

Uniformity in reporting untoward pulmonary effects of chemotherapy, thereby enhancing our collective ability to diagnose and manage CAPT, is essential in advancing our understanding of these processes. One system proposed by the authors is outlined in Table 77.3. The goal of this approach is to standardize the commonly used clinical criteria for diagnosis of drug-induced lung disease, including drug exposure, usual clinical symptoms, and time course consistent with the suspected drug, exclusion of competing diagnoses, and beneficial response to withdrawal of the agent. Widespread use of such a system would promote a more uniform approach to reporting CAPT and enhance critical appraisal of the available literature. In addition to better defining CAPT, authors must also be challenged to describe its severity. This practice will help evaluate the success of interventions and provide data by which one can weigh the risks and benefits of a therapeutic regimen. Such a scoring system has been endorsed for studies of radiation-induced lung toxicity[66] but has not been defined for CAPT.

State-of-the-art management for CAPT relies on early recognition of consistent syndromes and prompt drug withdrawal when necessary. Supportive care and empiric antiinflammatory therapies are utilized when removal of the offending agent is insufficient. As CAPT is better defined, the systematic assessment of risk factors will certainly assist clinicians to avoid the induction of CAPT syndromes before they develop.

TABLE 77.3. Clinical criteria for diagnosis of chemotherapy-associated pulmonary toxicity (CAPT).

Symptom complex consistent with suspect drug
The time course (acute, subacute, chronic, delayed) is compatible with that suspect drug
Reasonable competing diagnoses have been excluded
Objective improvement after drug D/C'ed
BAL and tissue compatible
Occurs after rechallenge: the latter is NOT recommended

Definite CAPT requires five criteria are met; probable CAPT requires four criteria are met; suspected CAPT requires three criteria are met.

References

1. Hallas J, Davidsen O, Grodum E, Damsbo N, Gram LF. Drug-related illness as a cause of admission to a department of respiratory medicine. Respiration 1992;59:30–34.
2. Hallas J, Gram LF, Grodum E, et al. Drug related admissions to medical wards: a population based survey. Br J Clin Pharmacol 1992;33:61–68.
3. Nelson KM, Talbert RL. Drug-related hospital admissions. Pharmacotherapy 1996;16:701–707.
4. Rosenow EC III, Limper AH. Drug-induced pulmonary disease. Semin Respir Infect 1995;10:86–95.
5. Snyder LS, Hertz MI. Cytotoxic drug-induced lung injury. Semin Respir Infect 1988;3:217–228.
6. Sleijfer S. Bleomycin-induced pneumonitis. Chest 2001;120: 617–624.
7. Simpson AB, Paul J, Graham J, Kaye SB. Fatal bleomycin pulmonary toxicity in the west of Scotland 1991–1995: a review of patients with germ cell tumours. Br J Cancer 1998;78:1061–1066.
8. Rosenow EC III. Drug-induced pulmonary disease. Disease-A-Month 1994;40:253–310.
9. Limper AH, Rosenow EC III. Drug-induced pulmonary disease. In: Murray JF, Nadel JA (eds) Textbook of Respiratory Medicine, 3rd ed. New York: Saunders, 2000.
10. Camus PH, Foucher P, Bonniaud PH, Ask K. Drug-induced infiltrative lung disease. Eur Respir J (Suppl) 2001;32:93s–100s.
11. Wesselius LJ. Pulmonary complications of cancer therapy. Comprehens Ther 1999;25:272–277.
12. Limper AH, Rosenow EC III. Drug-induced interstitial lung disease. Curr Opin Pulmon Med 1996;2:396–404.
13. Cleverley JR, Screaton NJ, Hiorns MP, Flint JD, Muller NL. Drug-induced lung disease: high-resolution CT and histological findings. Clin Radiol 2002;57:292–299.

14. Akira M, Ishikawa H, Yamamoto S. Drug-induced pneumonitis: thin-section CT findings in 60 patients. Radiology 2002;224: 852–860.
15. Rice KL. Pulmonary infiltrates associated with noncytotoxic drugs. Semin Respir Infecti 988;3:229–239.
16. Erasmus JJ, McAdams HP, Rossi SE. High-resolution CT of drug-induced lung disease. Radiol Clin N Am 2002;40:61–72.
17. Erasmus JJ, McAdams HP, Rossi SE. Drug-induced lung injury. Semin Roentgenol 2002;37:72–81.
18. Ellis SJ, Cleverley JR, Muller NL. Drug-induced lung disease: high-resolution CT findings. AJR (Am J Roentgenol) 2000;175: 1019–1024.
19. Lin WY, Kao CH, Wang SJ, Yeh SH. Lung toxicity of chemotherapeutic agents detected by TC-99m DTPA radioaerosol inhalation lung scintigraphy. Neoplasma 1995;42:133–135.
20. Petersen PM, Hansen SW. The course of long-term toxicity in patients treated with cisplatin-based chemotherapy for non-seminomatous germ-cell cancer. Ann Oncol 1999;10:1475–1483.
21. Sleijfer S, van der Mark TW, Schraffordt Koops H, Mulder NH. Decrease in pulmonary function during bleomycin-containing combination chemotherapy for testicular cancer: not only a bleomycin effect. Br J Cancer 1995;71:120–123.
22. White DA, Rankin JA, Stover DE, Gellene RA, Gupta S. Methotrexate pneumonitis. Bronchoalveolar lavage findings suggest an immunologic disorder. Am Rev Respir Dis 1989;139: 18–21.
23. White DA, Wong PW, Downey R. The utility of open lung biopsy in patients with hematologic malignancies. Am J Respir Crit Care Med 2000;161:723–729.
24. Smith GJ. The histopathology of pulmonary reactions to drugs. Clin Chest Med 1990;11:95–117.
25. Abid SH, Malhotra V, Perry MC. Radiation-induced and chemotherapy-induced pulmonary injury. Curr Opin Oncol 2001;13:242–248.
26. Hinson JM, McKibben AW. Chemotherapy-associated lung injury. In: Perry MC (ed) The Chemotherapy Source Book, 3rd ed. New York: Lippincott Williams & Wilkins, 2001.
27. Ferrozzi F, Schiavi A, Ganzetti A, Bassi P, Campani R. Pulmonary iatrogenic lesions in chemotherapy: computerized tomography findings (in Italian). Radiol Med 1998;96:62–67.
28. Libura J, Bettens F, Radkowski A, Tiercy JM, Piguet PF. Risk of chemotherapy-induced pulmonary fibrosis is associated with polymorphic tumour necrosis factor-a2 gene. Eur Respir J 2002;19:912–918.
29. Mishra A, Doyle NA, Martin WJC. Bleomycin-mediated pulmonary toxicity: evidence for a p53-mediated response. Am J Respir Cell Mol Biol 2000;22:543–549.
30. Hirsch A, Vander Els N, Straus DJ, et al. Effect of ABVD chemotherapy with and without mantle or mediastinal irradiation on pulmonary function and symptoms in early-stage Hodgkin's disease. J Clin Oncol 1996;14:1297–1305.
31. Yousem SA, Lifson JD, Colby TV. Chemotherapy-induced eosinophilic pneumonia. Relation to bleomycin. Chest 1985;88: 103–106.
32. Castro M, Veeder MH, Mailliard JA, Tazelaar HD, Jett JR. A prospective study of pulmonary function in patients receiving mitomycin. Chest 1996;109:939–944.
33. Sheldon R, Slaughter D. A syndrome of microangiopathic hemolytic anemia, renal impairment, and pulmonary edema in chemotherapy-treated patients with adenocarcinoma. Cancer (Phila) 1986;58:1428–1436.
34. Schrijvers D, Catimel G, Highley M, et al. KW-2149-induced pulmonary toxicity is not prevented by corticosteroids: a phase I and pharmacokinetic study. Anti-Cancer Drugs 1999;10: 633–639.
35. Massin F, Fur A, Reybet-Degat O, Camus P, Jeannin L. Busulfan-induced pneumopathy (in French). Rev Malad Respir 1987;4: 3–10.
36. Malik SW, Myers JL, DeRemee RA, Specks U. Lung toxicity associated with cyclophosphamide use. Two distinct patterns. Am J Respir Crit Care Med 1996;154:1851–1856.
37. Briasoulis E, Pavlidis N. Noncardiogenic pulmonary edema: an unusual and serious complication of anticancer therapy. Oncologist 2001;6:153–161.
38. Akasheh MS, Freytes CO, Vesole DH. Melphalan-associated pulmonary toxicity following high-dose therapy with autologous hematopoietic stem cell transplantation. Bone Marrow Transplant 2000;26:1107–1109.
39. Zisman DA, McCune WJ, Tino G, Lynch JP III. Drug-induced pneumonitis: the role of methotrexate. Sarcoidosis Vasculitis Diffuse Lung Dis 2001;18:243–252.
40. Dawson JK, Graham DR, Desmond J, Fewins HE, Lynch MP. Investigation of the chronic pulmonary effects of low-dose oral methotrexate in patients with rheumatoid arthritis: a prospective study incorporating HRCT scanning and pulmonary function tests [comment]. [Erratum appears in Rheumatology (Oxford) 2002;41(5):597]. Rheumatology 2002;41:262–267.
41. Pavlakis N, Bell DR, Millward MJ, Levi JA. Fatal pulmonary toxicity resulting from treatment with gemcitabine [comment]. Cancer (Phila) 1997;80:286–291.
42. Gupta N, Ahmed I, Steinberg H, Patel D, Nissel-Horowitz S, Mehrotra B. Gemcitabine-induced pulmonary toxicity: case report and review of the literature. Am J Clin Oncol 2002;25: 96–100.
43. Sauer-Heilborn A, Kath R, Schneider CP, Hoffken K. Severe non-haematological toxicity after treatment with gemcitabine. J Cancer Res Clin Oncol 1999;125:637–640.
44. Ash-Bernal R, Browner I, Erlich R. Early detection and successful treatment of drug-induced pneumonitis with corticosteroids. Cancer Invest 2002;20:876–879.
45. Garg S, Garg MS, Basmaji N. Multiple pulmonary nodules: an unusual presentation of fludarabine pulmonary toxicity: case report and review of literature. Am J Hematol 2002;70:241–245.
46. Stoica GS, Greenberg HE, Rossoff LJ. Corticosteroid responsive fludarabine pulmonary toxicity. Am J Clin Oncol 2002;25: 340–341.
47. Trojan A, Meier R, Licht A, Taverna C. Eosinophilic pneumonia after administration of fludarabine for the treatment of non-Hodgkin's lymphoma. Ann Hematol 2002;81:535–537.
48. Weinstein AS, Diener-West M, Nelson DF, Pakuris E. Pulmonary toxicity of carmustine in patients treated for malignant glioma. Cancer Treat Rep 1986;70:943–946.
49. Kalaycioglu M, Kavuru M, Tuason L, Bolwell B. Empiric prednisone therapy for pulmonary toxic reaction after high-dose chemotherapy containing carmustine (BCNU). Chest 1995;107:482–487.
50. Schultz J. Apparent adverse drug reactions prompt concern about Iressa. J Natl Cancer Inst 2003;95:577–579.
51. Okamoto I, Fujii K, Matsumoto M, et al. Diffuse alveolar damage after ZD1839 therapy in a patient with non-small cell lung cancer. Lung Cancer 2003;40:339–342.
52. Inoue A, Saijo Y, Maemondo M, et al. Severe acute interstitial pneumonia and gefitinib [comment]. Lancet 2003;361:137–139.
53. Mahmood T, Mudad R. Pulmonary toxicity secondary to procarbazine. Am J Clin Oncol 2002;25:187–188.
54. Gurjal A, An T, Valdivieso M, Kalemkerian GP. Etoposide-induced pulmonary toxicity. Lung Cancer 1999;26:109–112.
55. Kuei JH, Tashkin DP, Figlin RA. Pulmonary toxicity of recombinant human tumor necrosis factor. Chest 1989;96:334–338.
56. Fujimori K, Yokoyama A, Kurita Y, Uno K, Saijo N. Paclitaxel-induced cell-mediated hypersensitivity pneumonitis. Diagnosis using leukocyte migration test, bronchoalveolar lavage and transbronchial lung biopsy. Oncology 1998;55:340–344.
57. Hanna YM, Baglan KL, Stromberg JS, et al. Acute and subacute toxicity associated with concurrent adjuvant radiation therapy

and paclitaxel in primary breast cancer therapy. Breast J 2002;8:149–153.
58. Azoulay E, Attalah H, Yang K, et al. Exacerbation by granulocyte colony-stimulating factor of prior acute lung injury: implication of neutrophils. Crit Care Med 2002;30:2115–2122.
59. Iki S, Yoshinaga K, Ohbayashi Y, Urabe A. Cytotoxic drug-induced pneumonia and possible augmentation by G-CSF: clinical attention. Ann Hematol 1993;66:217–218.
60. Yokose N, Ogata K, Tamura H, et al. Pulmonary toxicity after granulocyte colony-stimulating factor-combined chemotherapy for non-Hodgkin's lymphoma. Br J Cancer 1998;77:2286–2290.
61. Madarnas Y, Webster P, Shorter AM, Bjarnason GA. Irinotecan-associated pulmonary toxicity. Anti-Cancer Drugs 2000;11: 709–713.
62. Seigneur J, Trechot PF, Hubert J, Lamy P. Pulmonary complications of hormone treatment in prostate carcinoma. Chest 1988; 93:1106.
63. Roberts CM, Foulcher E, Zaunders JJ, et al. Radiation pneumonitis: a possible lymphocyte-mediated hypersensitivity reaction. Ann Intern Med 1993;118:696–700.
64. Boyars MC. Clinical management of radiation-induced lung disease. J Respir Dis 1990;11:167–183.
65. Arbetter KR, Prakash UBS, Tazelaar HD, Douglas WW. Radiation-induced pneumonitis in the "nonirradiated" lung. Mayo Clin Proc 1999;74:27–36.
66. McDonald S, Rubin P, Phillips TL, Marks LB. Injury to the lung from cancer therapy: clinical syndromes, measurable endpoints, and potential scoring systems. Int J Radiat Oncol Biol Phys 1995;31:1187–1203.

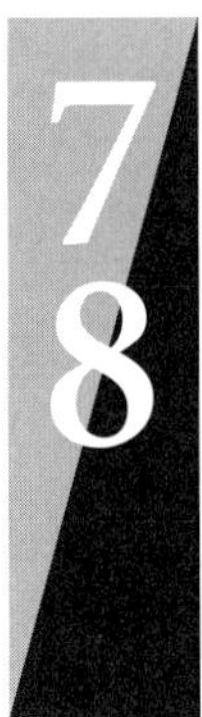

Cardiac Complications

Maged I. Gharib and Alan K. Burnett

Cardiac toxicity is a well-recognized serious side effect of chemotherapy. Since early reports of heart failure in children treated with doxorubicin,[1] anthracyclines remain the best known chemotherapeutic agents clearly linked to cardiotoxicity. There are, however, a number of other chemotherapeutic agents that cause cardiotoxicity which are still not so well recognized in clinical practice.

Cardiac toxicity may occur acutely, during, or up to 1 week following the administration of chemotherapy, usually as mild transient blood pressure and/or electrocardiographic (ECG) changes. More serious acute cardiotoxicity, such as arrhythmias, myocarditis, pericarditis, or myocardial infarction occur less commonly. The most clinically significant, however, is the anthracycline-induced chronic progressive cardiomyopathy, which may end in left ventricular failure (LVF) or congestive heart failure (CHF).

Cytotoxic Antibiotics (Anthracyclines and Mitoxantrone)

Anthracyclines

The cytotoxic antibiotics daunorubicin and doxorubicin were originally extracted from fungi belonging to the species *Streptomyces*. They are very efficacious broad-spectrum antineoplastic agents that demonstrate a clear dose–response relationship in several curative chemotherapeutic regimens.[2,3] Their cardiotoxicity, however, remains the major limiting factor for their use at high doses that could substantially improve the cure rates of various cancers. Two distinct subtypes of cardiotoxicity could follow anthracycline use.

Acute/Subacute Cardiotoxicity

This form of cardiotoxicity occurs within a week of anthracycline administration. Although rare, it may occur after only one dose. It seldom leads to serious clinical consequences. Transient electrophysiologic abnormalities detected as ECG changes may be seen in 20% to 30% of the patients as nonspecific ST- and T-wave changes, T-wave flattening, decreased QRS voltage, and/or prolongation of the QT interval. Arrhythmias, including ventricular, supraventricular, and junctional tachycardias, are seen in 0.5% to 3% of patients with an overall incidence of 0.7%.[4] More serious arrhythmias, such as atrial flutter or atrial fibrillation, are rare. Subacute cardiotoxicity has resulted in acute left ventricular failure, pericarditis, or a fatal pericarditis-myocarditis syndrome in some rare cases.[5] No clear risk factors have been linked to this form of cardiotoxicity, and it does not appear to be related to the chronic progressive form.[6]

Chronic Progressive Cardiotoxicity

Chronic progressive cardiotoxicity is the more recognized and clinically significant subtype of cardiotoxicity. Authors used to subdivide chronic anthracycline-induced cardiomyopathy into early-onset[7] and late-onset subtypes.[6,8] This designation originated from the earliest work published on this subject by Von Hoff and associates,[7] who reported that heart failure as a result of anthracycline-induced cardiomyopathy occurred 0 to 231 days after the completion of therapy. They retrospectively analyzed 4,018 records of patients treated with anthracyclines; their endpoint was "clinically manifest" congestive heart failure as "recorded" by the treating clinician. With accumulation of data over the years, it became apparent that cardiotoxicity remained subclinical but progressed over time only to become "clinically manifest" years after completion of the treatment. Steinherz and coworkers have shown that the both the incidence and severity of systolic ventricular dysfunction increased with the length of follow-up.[9] It therefore seems logical not to use this artificial classification.

Pathogenesis

The exact mechanism through which anthracyclines cause cardiac damage is still debatable and is probably multifactorial. There is a general consensus that doxorubicin undergoes redox cycling to generate free radicals that are responsible for mediating the myocyte damage. The quinone form of doxorubicin is reduced to the free radical semiquinone form by cytochrome P-450 reductase, particularly in myocardial cells with a high level of flavin-centered reductases.[6] The subcellular targets continue to be debated, however. Anthracyclines have been shown to alter transcription of myocellular proteins.[10]

Incidence

Because of the variability of treatment protocols (doses, rates of administration, and combination with other chemotherapeutic agents and/or mediastinal irradiation), parameters used for the assessment of cardiac functions and endpoints in different reports (clinically manifest or subclinical echocardiographic finding), age at exposure, and the time lapsed since exposure, it is not surprising to see a lack of consensus on the reported incidence of this complication.[9–25] An incidence of

65% of increased afterload or decreased contractility has been reported with cumulative doxorubicin doses as low as 228 mg/m^2 in children treated for leukemia 15 years after treatment.[11] In the majority of cases, this effect remains subclinical. The incidence of symptomatic heart failure during or within the first year of completing anthracycline therapy is less than 3%.[7,9,12] It should be emphasized, however, that early-onset cardiotoxicity (occurring during or within 1 year of anthracycline therapy) is the largest predictor of the deterioration over time.[9,11,13,14] At 15 years after treatment, up to 5% of children treated with anthracyclines at cumulative dose higher than 300 mg/m^2 develop heart failure.[25]

Risk Factors

Risk factors for anthracycline-related chronic progressive cardiotoxicity include the following:

- Total cumulative dose[7,9,10,25]; this, by far, is the most important risk factor
- Age at anthracycline administration[7,11,13,20]
- Rate of administration[7,15–20]
- Female gender[13,21]
- Preexisting heart disease and hypertension[7]
- Mediastinal irradiation[22–24]
- Interval since anthracycline chemotherapy should also be considered as a risk factor, particularly in those who received the drug in their childhood[9,11,13,14]

The incidence of CHF secondary to doxorubicin-induced cardiomyopathy is strongly linked to the cumulative dose of the drug.[7,8,9,11–14] In adults, with a cumulative dose of less than 400 mg/m^2, the incidence of *early* CHF was 0.14%, compared with 7% at a dose of more than 550 mg/m^2 and to 18% at a dose of more than 700 mg/m^2.[7] This rapid increase in the clinical cardiotoxicity at doses greater than 550 mg/m^2 has made it a common empirical maximum allowable cumulative dose in clinical practice. There appears to be great individual variability in the tolerable anthracycline dose in both adults and children. Five patients in Von Hoff's series (3,941 patients) received more than 1,000 mg/m^2; none of them sustained early CHF.[7] A cumulative dose of anthracycline guaranteed not to lead to cardiomyopathy has not been established.[14]

Children appear to be at higher risk of developing anthracycline-induced cardiotoxicity.[11,13,20] Age less than 4 years at the time of exposure has been shown to be a significant risk factor for abnormal cardiac function; it was mainly predictive of increased afterload caused by reduced ventricular wall thickness.[11] Anthracyclines have been shown to alter transcription of myocellular proteins.[10] The inappropriate reduction in the left ventricular wall thickness found in children previously treated with anthracyclines[11,14] could be the result of such an effect. In adults, an increasing risk of doxorubicin-induced CHF with increasing patient age has been observed ($P = 0.0027$).[7] Previous cardiac disease and hypertension may also potentially increase the risk of doxorubicin-induced CHF ($P = 0.08$).[7]

Anthracycline-induced cardiotoxicity seems to be related to the peak plasma drug concentration. The antineoplastic activity seems, however, to be dependent on the total systemic exposure or the tissue concentration over time and not the peak plasma concentration.[15] Doxorubicin appears to be less cardiotoxic when administered as a prolonged, continuous intravenous infusion over more than 48 to 96 hours.[15] A 2.81-fold-greater risk of developing cardiomyopathy after a maximum single dose of 50 mg/m^2/dose has been reported as compared with lower dosing schedules,[20] which is probably why anthracycline regimens given as weekly injections instead of a single bolus injection every 3 weeks were found to be less cardiotoxic.[16–19] Also, female patients appear to be more vulnerable to the cardiotoxic effects of anthracyclines.[13,21]

Radiotherapy is frequently used in combination with multidrug chemotherapy protocols in patients with various hematologic and solid neoplasms. Mediastinal irradiation is believed to increase anthracycline-induced cardiotoxicity.[22–24] Severity of histopathologic changes evaluated by endomyocardial biopsy were significantly higher (P less than 0.01) in patients pretreated with mediastinal irradiation before anthracycline compared with those who did not receive radiation therapy.[23]

A relatively recently published study on a cohort of 607 children with long-term follow-up (mean, 6.3 years) has shown the only independent risk factor is a cumulative dose greater than 300 mg/m^2. The other possible risk factors (i.e., female sex, younger age at diagnosis, radiotherapy involving the heart, and ifosfamide or cyclophosphamide treatment) were not associated with increased risk in this cohort.[25]

Management

Monitoring and Prevention In clinical practice, regular monitoring of the cardiac functions to stop further exposure, once evidence of deterioration starts to appear, is still the only management action. Theoretically, the following measures could prevent (or minimize) cardiotoxicity:

- Identifying individuals at risk before commencing anthracycline chemotherapy to modify the dose, formulation (e.g., liposomal encapsulated daunorubicin), and administration rate and schedule.
- Regular patient monitoring during and following completion of anthracycline therapy.
- Anthracycline modification:
  - Use of anthracycline analogues of less cardiotoxicity
  - Use of cardioprotective drugs (dexrazoxane)
  - Liposomal encapsulation (this is likely to supersede the previous two)

Identifying patients at risk of cardiotoxicity is the first and crucial step for prophylaxis. The difficulty starts as early as this because there appears to be a great variation in the individual sensitivity to anthracyclines. Histopathologic changes consistent with anthracycline-induced cardiotoxicity have been noted at doses as low as 183 mg/m^2 (less than one-third of what is considered the allowable maximum cumulative dose),[26] whereas doses greater than 1,000 mg/m^2 have been tolerated by others.[7,27] There is so far no test to detect those at high risk. Monitoring still depends on signs of early (subclinical) reduction of left ventricular systolic function aiming at early discontinuation of anthracyclines.

Noninvasive echocardiographic measurement of left ventricular ejection fraction (LVEF) and fractional shorting (FS) is by far the most commonly used method in most centers. Complete recovery of echocardiographic LVEF and FS may occur if anthracycline therapy is discontinued at an early stage,[28] although this does not necessarily exclude long-term reductions in functional reserve.[29] Radionuclide angiocardiography is also widely used in monitoring for early anthracycline-induced cardiotoxicity. Schwartz et al. proposed guidelines for prophylaxis against anthracycline-induced heart failure based on serial radionuclide measurement of LVEF.[30] Patients with a baseline LVEF of 30% or less should not receive anthracycline therapy. Those with LVEF greater than 30%, but less than 50%, can receive doxorubicin, but measures should be repeated before each dose. For patients with LVEF of 50% or more, evaluations should be repeated after a cumulative dose of 250 to 300 mg/m^2, and thereafter at 450 mg/m^2 if they have no risk factors. Doxorubicin therapy should be stopped if there is a 10% or greater absolute decrease in the EF, with decrease of the LVEF to 50% or less in patients with baseline LVEF of 50% or more, and to 30% or less in those with a baseline LVEF less than 50% but more than 30%. Multivariate analysis demonstrated a fourfold reduction in the incidence of CHF in those patients whose management was concordant with the proposed guideline criteria.[30] Unfortunately, resting LVEF obtained by radionuclide angiocardiography is relatively insensitive in detecting early anthracycline cardiotoxicity. Both LVEF and FS are load-dependent indices that give an estimate of the overall left ventricular systolic performance rather than the absolute contractility. Sensitivity could be increased by using load-independent contractility indices, for example, the stress velocity index. Exercise radionuclide studies may also increase the chance of detecting subclinical anthracycline-induced cardiotoxicity.[22,31] Failure to increase the ejection fraction by 5% over the resting value has been suggested to be a marker of high risk for developing anthracycline-induced ventricular dysfunction.[32] Serial testing is, however, required to improve the low specificity of a single test, and maximal exercise is often difficult for patients receiving chemotherapy, because most of them are debilitated.

Measuring diastolic parameters has been found useful in early detection of anthracycline-induced cardiomyopathy. Results have been inconsistent as to whether this precedes systolic dysfunction.[33–40] This inconsistency probably reflects the fact that in some patients, anthracyclines cause extensive endocardial fibrous thickening, which gives a restrictive cardiomyopathic picture.[41]

Endomyocardial biopsy is a fairly sensitive indicator of chronic anthracycline-induced cardiotoxicity. A semiquantitative histologic scoring system that correlated well with the cumulative anthracycline dose has been available since 1984.[42] Such a monitoring strategy did not find its way to clinical practice for clear reasons, being invasive with concerns about safety of its repetition, particularly in children.[43] Moreover, underestimation of cardiac damage with right ventricular biopsy may occur because of scattered cardiomyopathic changes[44] or the predominance of left ventricular injury.[41] Finally, expertise in obtaining and interpreting biopsy specimens is not widely available.

Prospects for Ideal Monitoring

No ideal screening or monitoring technique has yet been found. One would speculate that this might aim at detection of susceptible genotype(s), probably by using one of the recent molecular techniques or a biochemical marker. The former might explain the great individual tolerability variation, and so define individuals in whom anthracyclines should be avoided. The latter, on the other hand, aims at reliable prediction of early irreversible myocardioctye damage in a way very similar to the elevation of liver enzymes many years before the cirrhosis in chronic active hepatitis. Natriuretic peptides could be useful in this respect, as shown by preliminary studies.[45–48] These studies are, however, of small size and of short-term follow-up. A relatively recent study, on the other hand, suggested that serial natriuretic peptide measurements cannot be used in predicting the impairment of left ventricular function. It was found that the decrease in LVEF started very early and could already be seen after the cumulative doxorubicin dose of 200 mg/m^2, whereas the increase in plasma natriuretic peptides was not evident until the cumulative doxorubicin dose of 400 mg/m^2.[49]

Endothelin 1 could also be a potential predictor. In a single small-scale study so far, progressive elevation of its plasma levels occurred before deterioration of LVEF in patients who subsequently developed CHF.[50,51] Cardiac troponins also warrant further investigation to evaluate their potential use for monitoring patients during and after anthracycline therapy.[52,53]

Anthracycline Semisynthetic Analogues

Epirubicin is an epimer of doxorubicin with comparable antitumor activity and less cardiotoxicity.[54–56] Cardiotoxicity appears to occur at a higher cumulative dose greater than 900 mg/m^2.

Idarubicin is a lipophilic semisynthetic derivative of daunorubicin that can be orally administered.[6] It was shown to be less cardiotoxic than doxorubicin.[57,58]

Cardioprotective Agents

Dexrazoxane is a derivative of ethylenediaminetetraacetic acid (EDTA) that readily penetrates cell membranes and acts as an intracellular chelating agent.[6] Its proposed mechanism of cardioprotection is through the chelation of intracellular iron, which may decrease anthracycline-induced free radical generation. Dexrazoxane (ICRF-187) has been shown to decrease the incidence of clinical CHF in patients treated with anthracyclines.[59,60] Neither the normal antioxidant mechanisms nor the pharmacokinetics of doxorubicin or its metabolites is affected by dexrazoxane.[61] It is given via slow IV push or rapid infusion not more than 30 minutes before doxorubicin administration. The recommended dose is 10 times that of the scheduled doxorubicin dose. It is generally well tolerated, but side effects include enhanced myelosuppression and pain on injection.[60]

Concerns, however, exist concerning possible interference of dexrazoxane with the efficacy of the anthracycline antitumour effect.[60,62] It is therefore *not routinely recommended with anthracycline therapy*, at least at the present time. Recent guidelines by the American Society of Clinical Oncology advised that dexrazoxane *may only be considered* for patients with *metastatic breast cancer* who have received a *cumulative doxorubicin dose 300 mg/m^2 or more in the metastatic setting* and who may benefit from further anthracycline therapy. Patients receiving dexrazoxane should continue to be monitored for anthracycline-induced cardiotoxicity.[63]

Liposomal Anthracyclines

Liposomal encapsulation of daunorubicin improves its pharmacokinetic properties. Encapsulation reduces its volume of distribution, the total body clearance, and interindividual variability.[64,65] Experimentally, it has been shown that liposomal encapsulation reduces the intracellular accumulation speed of daunorubicin, and therefore, diminishes free radical generation, ATP depletion, and necrotic (but not apoptotic) cell death[66]; however, this does not affect its efficacy on tumor cells. Both free and encapsulated forms induce activation of caspases 9 and 3. The sensitivity of leukemic cells correlates with caspase activation and reduction of mitochondrial membrane potential but not depletion of ATP and the generation of free radicals.[66] In fact, experimentally, liposomal encapsulation overcomes resistance to the free drug in certain resistant breast (MCF7ADR), ovarian (SKOV3), and small-cell lung (H69VP) carcinoma cell lines, probably by escaping the membrane pumps, such as P-glycoprotein.[67] Early clinical studies suggest that liposomal daunorubicin is safer with much less early cardiotoxicity. These results are encouraging, but as mentioned earlier, cardiomyopathy can appear years after exposure, and therefore, long-term follow-up for larger number of patients is essential to give a better profile of its cardiac safety.

Mitoxantrone

This non-cell-cycle-specific anthraquinone derivative was developed to provide broad-spectrum antitumor activity, similar to anthracyclines, without cardiotoxicity. Although initial animal studies revealed a lack of cardiotoxicity,[68,69] its cardiotoxicity soon became evident in clinical trials. It has been shown to have an anthracycline-like spectrum of cardiotoxicity. Prior doxorubicin therapy and mitoxantrone cumulative dose are the main risk factors.[70] The incidence of CHF significantly increases (more than 5%) beyond a cumulative dose of 160 mg/m^2, even in the absence of previous doxorubicin exposure.[71]

Prophylaxis should follow the same lines of anthracyclines therapy, and mitoxantrone therapy to a patient previously treated with an anthracycline, should be based on the risk-to-benefit balance for each individual case and the awareness of the heart failure risk prediction curves[60] for anthracyclines and mitoxantrone.

Alkylating Agents

Cyclophosphamide

Cyclophosphamide is a non-cell-cycle-specific alkylating agent that is a mainstay of most pretransplant conditioning regimens. High-dose cyclophosphamide can cause an acute form of cardiotoxicity within 10 days of its administration.[72–74] Cyclophosphamide-induced cardiotoxicity presents as a combination of symptoms and signs of myopericarditis, which could lead to fatal complications (e.g., CHF, arrhythmias, cardiac tamponade).[72,74,75] The total dose of cyclophosphamide per course is so far the only reproducible risk factor.[73] The incidence of symptomatic cyclophosphamide-induced cardiotoxicity in two series,[75,76] when combined, was 22% (16/72), and that of fatal cardiotoxicity was 11%. A total dose greater than 170 to 180 mg/kg per course (over 4 to 7 days) was the risk factor. Goldberg et al. found that doses based on body surface area, rather than body weight, correlate well with incidence of cyclophosphamide-induced cardiotoxicity.[72] The incidence of symptomatic cyclophosphamide-induced cardiotoxicity in a group of patients who never had prior anthracycline therapy was 25% (13/52), with 12% (6/52) mortality when cyclophosphamide dose exceeded 1.55 mg/m^2/day. Those who received less than 1.55 mg/m^2/day had 3% (1/32) symptomatic cardiotoxicity with no mortality.[72] The fact that young children have a relatively higher body surface area probably explains the lower incidence and severity of cyclophosphamide-induced effects in them compared with adolescent and adult cardiotoxicity.[6,72] Cyclophosphamide-induced cardiotoxicity may last from 1 to 6 days and, despite the relatively high mortality, there are no long-term sequelae or late cardiotoxicity in patients who survive the initial acute event.[75] So far, there is no evidence of cumulative cyclophosphamide cardiotoxicity.

Prevention

Ideal prevention would depend on the avoidance of exceeding a certain critical dose, beyond which the incidence and severity of cardiotoxicity becomes unacceptably high. Identification of this critical dose warrants further large-scale studies, but it is likely to be around 1.55 g/m^2/day, as shown by the Goldberg group.[77] We, therefore, recommend that hematopoietic stem cell transplant protocols should be modified to use cyclophosphamide doses calculated per body surface area/day to limit the daily dose to less than 1.55 g/m^2. The current evidence shows that this will significantly reduce this potentially fatal cardiotoxicity without affecting engraftment success.[77]

Secondary prevention of cyclophosphamide-induced cardiotoxicity necessitates awareness by the clinicians of this potential complication. They should keep it in mind when looking after patients who received high-dose cyclophosphamide within the past 2 weeks.

Ifosfamide

Ifosfamide, structurally similar to cyclophosphamide, seems to have a similar cardiotoxicity pattern with a 30% incidence of cardiotoxicity with doses beyond 20 g/m^2.[78] Further studies are needed to confirm the critical dose that should not be exceeded, as this will be the efficient route of prophylaxis.

Mitomycin

There is strong evidence that mitomycin (MMC) enhances doxorubicin-induced cardiomyopathy when administered in combination with or following such agent.[79,80] MMC-related cardiotoxicity is dose dependent, occurring at cumulative dose levels of 30 mg/m^2, mainly in patients treated, previously or simultaneously, with doxorubicin.[81] Careful monitoring of left ventricular function is therefore essential as with anthracycline chemotherapy.

Miscellaneous Agents

The previously mentioned chemotherapeutic agents are the most significant as far as cardiotoxicity in clinical practice is concerned. It is worth mentioning, however, that many other chemotherapeutic agents could sometimes cause transient cardiotoxicity, such as transient ECG change, arrhythmias, or blood pressure changes. Although these are rarely of clinical significance, clinicians should be aware of them.

Fluorouracil (5-FU)

Care should be taken with this synthetic pyrimidine antimetabolite as it can cause myocardial ischemia.[82] Although rare (1.6%), the possibility must be taken into account in practice, particularly in those patients already affected with cardiac diseases, as cases of massive myocardial infarctions have occurred.[82–84] 5-FU cardiotoxicity is more common following high-dose continuous infusion than after IV bolus administration.[85] Prophylaxis starts with identifying those with ischemic heart disease in whom the agent should be avoided. Using IV bolus administration rather than continuous administration is advisable based on the current available evidence. Taking this potential cardiotoxicity into account in practice should be of prophylactic benefit.

Taxanes (Paclitaxel and Docetaxel)

This is a group of antimicrotubule agents originally extracted from the bark of the western yew tree, *Taxus brevifolia*. Paclitaxel has been linked to cardiotoxicity in two ways: early arrhythmias during or soon after administration and possible aggravation of anthracycline-induced cardiomyopathy when given in combination. Both ways warrant closer scientific examination.

As regards arrhythmias, critical evaluation of reports show that in early Phase I studies, paclitaxel was associated with a high incidence of serious hypersensitivity reactions.[7,86] Premedication with antihistamines, and a slower rate of infusion, reduced the frequency and severity of this side effect, but it also led to routine continuous cardiac monitoring during paclitaxel administration in Phase II studies in an attempt to evaluate hypersensitivity reactions more efficiently. This approach had led to unintentional overreporting of cardiac *arrhythmias* in patients receiving paclitaxel, with "asymptomatic sinus bradycardia" being the most frequently reported cardiac event.[87] Paclitaxel-associated cardiac rhythm disturbances described in the literature, included nearly every known arrhythmia, but seldom led to clinically significant sequelae, and the reported incidence of life-threatening ventricular arrhythmias (fibrillation or tachycardia) is only 0.26%.[88] Ventricular arrhythmias could occur at any time during the drug infusion. It can occur during first-dose infusion although it is most often seen during second and subsequent doses.[88] Patients revert to normal sinus rhythm after discontinuation of paclitaxel, but some patients may continue to exhibit infrequent, brief episodes of supraventricular tachycardia or rare ventricular premature beats up to 10 days after discontinuation of paclitaxel. As mentioned previously, paclitaxel-induced arrhythmias seldom led to clinically significant sequelae.

Paclitaxel and doxorubicin is a highly effective combination in advanced breast cancer. The unexpectedly high incidence of CHF reported in two of the early trials caused some concern. It is likely that a pharmacokinetic interaction between doxorubicin and paclitaxel is responsible for the higher than expected incidence of congestive heart failure observed in these studies, as paclitaxel decreases the clearance of doxorubicin by approximately 30% when the two drugs are administered in close succession.[89] A recent review of results from 10 studies (657 patients) was, however, reassuring that the use of combination doxorubicin and paclitaxel is safe up to a cumulative doxorubicin dose of 340 to 380 mg/m^2.[90]

The paclitaxel closely related antimicrotubule, docetaxel, does not seem to induce arrhythmias.[91] No concerns were raised to its use in combination with anthracyclines.

References

1. Tan C, Tasaka H, Kou-Ping Y, et al. Daunomycin, an antitumor antibiotic, in the treatment of neoplastic disease: clinical evaluation with special reference to childhood leukemia. Cancer (Phila) 1967;20:333–353.
2. Hitchcock-Bryan S, Jeal GRC. The impact of induction anthracyclines on long-term failure-free survival in childhood acute lymphoblastic leukemia. Med Pediatr Oncol 1986;14:211–215.
3. Ettinghausen SE, Bonow RO, Palmeri ST, et al. Prospective study of cardiomyopathy induced by adjuvant doxorubicin therapy in patients with soft-tissue sarcomas. Arch Surg 1986;121:1445–1451.
4. Frishman WH, Sung HM, Yee HC, et al. Cardiovascular toxicity with cancer chemotherapy. Curr Probl Cancer 1997;21:301–360.
5. Ferrans VJ. Overview of cardiac pathology in relation to anthracycline cardiotoxicity. Cancer Treat Rep 1978;62:955–961.
6. Pai VB, Nahata MC. Cardiotoxicity of chemotherapeutic agents: incidence, treatment and prevention. Drug Saf 2000;22:263–302.
7. Von Hoff DD, Layard MW, Basa P, et al. Risk factors for doxorubicin-induced congestive heart failure. Ann Intern Med 1979;91:710–717.
8. Shan K, Lincoff AM, Young JB. Anthracycline-induced cardiotoxicity. Ann Intern Med 1996;125:47–58.
9. Steinherz LJ, Steinherz PG, Tan CT, Heller G, Murphy ML. Cardiac toxicity 4 to 20 years after completing anthracycline therapy. JAMA 1991;266:1672–1677.
10. Boucek RJ, Miracle A, Anderson M, Engelman R, Atkinson J, Dodd DA. Persistent effects of doxorubicin on cardiac gene expression. J Mol Cell Cardiol 1999;31:1435–1446.
11. Lipshultz SE, Colan SD, Gelber RD, Perez-Atayde AR, Sallan SE, Sanders SP. Late cardiac effects of doxorubicin therapy for acute lymphoblastic leukemia in childhood. N Engl J Med 1991;324:808–815.
12. Bu'Lock FA, Mott MG, Oakhill A, Martin RP. Left ventricular diastolic filling patterns associated with progressive anthracycline-induced myocardial damage: a prospective study. Pediatr Cardiol 1999;20:252–263.
13. Lipshultz SE, Lipsitz SR, Mone SM, et al. Female sex and drug dose as risk factors for late cardiotoxic effects of doxorubicin therapy for childhood cancer. N Engl J Med 1995;332:1738–1743.
14. Grenier MA, Lipshultz SE. Epidemiology of anthracycline cardiotoxicity in children and adults. Semin Oncol 1998;25:72–85.
15. Legha SS, Benjamin RS, Mackay B, et al. Reduction of doxorubicin cardiotoxicity by prolonged continuous intravenous infusion. Ann Intern Med 1982;96:133–139.
16. Torti FM, Bristow MR, Howes AE, et al. Reduced cardiotoxicity of doxorubicin delivered on a weekly schedule. Assessment by endomyocardial biopsy. Ann Intern Med 1983;99:745–749.
17. Weiss AJ, Metter GE, Fletcher WS, Wilson WL, Grage TB, Ramirez G. Studies on adriamycin using a weekly regimen demonstrating its clinical effectiveness and lack of cardiac toxicity. Cancer Treat Rep 1976;60:813–822.
18. Weiss AJ, Manthel RW. Experience with the use of adriamycin in combination with other anticancer agents using a weekly schedule, with particular reference to lack of cardiac toxicity. Cancer (Phila) 1977;40:2046–2052.

19. Chlebowski RT, Paroly WS, Pugh RP, et al. Adriamycin given as a weekly schedule without a loading course: clinically effective with reduced incidence of cardiotoxicity. Cancer Treat Rep 1980;64:47–51.
20. Krischer JP, Epstein S, Cuthbertson DD, Goorin AM, Epstein ML, Lipshultz SE. Clinical cardiotoxicity following anthracycline treatment for childhood cancer: the Pediatric Oncology Group experience. J Clin Oncol 1997;15:1544–1552.
21. Silber JH, Jakacki RI, Larsen RL, Goldwein JW, Barber G. Increased risk of cardiac dysfunction after anthracyclines in girls. Med Pediatr Oncol 1993;21:477–479.
22. Bristow MR, Mason JW, Billingham ME, Daniels JR. Doxorubicin cardiomyopathy: evaluation by phonocardiography, endomyocardial biopsy, and cardiac catheterization. Ann Intern Med 1978;88:168–175.
23. Praga C, Beretta G, Vigo PL, et al. Adriamycin cardiotoxicity: a survey of 1,273 patients. Cancer Treat Rep 1979;63:827–834.
24. Pihkala J, Saarinen UM, Lundstrom U, et al. Myocardial function in children and adolescents after therapy with anthracyclines and chest irradiation. Eur J Cancer 1996;32A:97–103.
25. Kremer LC, van Dalen EC, Offringa M, Ottenkamp J, Voute PA. Anthracycline-induced clinical heart failure in a cohort of 607 children: long-term follow-up study. J Clin Oncol 2001;19:191–196.
26. Friedman MA, Bozdech MJ, Billingham ME, Rider AK. Doxorubicin cardiotoxicity. Serial endomyocardial biopsies and systolic time intervals. JAMA 1978;240:1603–1606.
27. Bristow MR, Thompson PD, Martin RP, Mason JW, Billingham ME, Harrison DC. Early anthracycline cardiotoxicity. Am J Med 1978;65:823–832.
28. Lewis AB, Crouse VL, Evans W, Takahashi M, Siegel SE. Recovery of left ventricular function following discontinuation of anthracycline chemotherapy in children. Pediatrics 1981;68:67–72.
29. Moreb JS, Oblon DJ. Outcome of clinical congestive heart failure induced by anthracycline chemotherapy. Cancer (Phila) 1992;70:2637–2641.
30. Schwartz RG, McKenzie WB, Alexander J, et al. Congestive heart failure and left ventricular dysfunction complicating doxorubicin therapy. Seven-year experience using serial radionuclide angiocardiography. Am J Med 1987;82:1109–1118.
31. Bristow MR, Mason JW, Billingham ME, Daniels JR. Dose-effect and structure-function relationships in doxorubicin cardiomyopathy. Am Heart J 1981;102:709–718.
32. McKillop JH, Bristow MR, Goris ML, Billingham ME, Bockemuehl K. Sensitivity and specificity of radionuclide ejection fractions in doxorubicin cardiotoxicity. Am Heart J 1983;106:1048–1056.
33. Lee BH, Goodenday LS, Muswick GJ, Yasnoff WA, Leighton RF, Skeel RT. Alterations in left ventricular diastolic function with doxorubicin therapy. J Am Coll Cardiol 1987;9:184–188.
34. Hausdorf G, Morf G, Beron G, et al. Long term doxorubicin cardiotoxicity in childhood: non-invasive evaluation of the contractile state and diastolic filling. Br Heart J 1988;60:309–315.
35. Marchandise B, Schroeder E, Bosly A, et al. Early detection of doxorubicin cardiotoxicity: interest of Doppler echocardiographic analysis of left ventricular filling dynamics. Am Heart J 1989;118:92–98.
36. Stoddard MF, Seeger J, Liddell NE, Hadley TJ, Sullivan DM, Kupersmith J. Prolongation of isovolumetric relaxation time as assessed by Doppler echocardiography predicts doxorubicin-induced systolic dysfunction in humans. J Am Coll Cardiol 1992;20:62–69.
37. Ganz WI, Sridhar KS, Forness TJ. Detection of early anthracycline cardiotoxicity by monitoring the peak filling rate. Am J Clin Oncol 1993;16:109–112.
38. Ewer MS, Ali MK, Gibbs HR, et al. Cardiac diastolic function in pediatric patients receiving doxorubicin. Acta Oncol 1994;33:645–649.
39. Cottin Y, Touzery C, Coudert B, et al. Impairment of diastolic function during short-term anthracycline chemotherapy. Br Heart J 1995;73:61–64.
40. Schmitt K, Tulzer G, Merl M, et al. Early detection of doxorubicin and daunorubicin cardiotoxicity by echocardiography: diastolic versus systolic parameters. Eur J Pediatr 1995;154:201–204.
41. Mortensen SA, Olsen HS, Baandrup U. Chronic anthracycline cardiotoxicity: haemodynamic and histopathological manifestations suggesting a restrictive endomyocardial disease. Br Heart J 1986;55:274–282.
42. Billingham ME, Bristow MR. Evaluation of anthracycline cardiotoxicity: predictive ability and functional correlation of endomyocardial biopsy. Cancer Treat Symp 1984;3:71–76.
43. Pegelow CH, Popper RW, de Wit SA, King OY, Wilbur JR. Endomyocardial biopsy to monitor anthracycline therapy in children. J Clin Oncol 1984;2:443–446.
44. Isner JM, Ferrans VJ, Cohen SR, et al. Clinical and morphologic cardiac findings after anthracycline chemotherapy. Analysis of 64 patients studied at necropsy. Am J Cardiol 1983;51:1167–1174.
45. Neri B, De Scalzi M, De Leonardis V, Gemelli MT, Ghezzi P, Pacini P. Preliminary study on behaviour of atrial natriuretic factor in anthracycline-related cardiac toxicity. Int J Clin Pharmacol Res 1991;11:75–81.
46. Bauch M, Ester A, Kimura B, Victorica BE, Kedar A, Phillips MI. Atrial natriuretic peptide as a marker for doxorubicin-induced cardiotoxic effects. Cancer (Phila) 1992;69:1492–1497.
47. Tikanoja T, Riikonen P, Perkkio M, Helenius T. Serum N-terminal atrial natriuretic peptide (NT-ANP) in the cardiac follow-up in children with cancer. Med Pediatr Oncol 1998;31:73–78.
48. Suzuki T, Hayashi D, Yamazaki T, et al. Elevated B-type natriuretic peptide levels after anthracycline administration. Am Heart J 1998;136:362–363.
49. Nousiainen T, Jantunen E, Vanninen E, Remes J, Vuolteenaho O, Hartikainen J. Natriuretic peptides as markers of cardiotoxicity during doxorubicin treatment for non-Hodgkin's lymphoma. Eur J Haematol 1999;62:135–141.
50. Yamashita J, Ogawa M, Nomura K. Plasma endothelin-1 and doxorubicin cardiotoxicity. N Engl J Med 1994;331:1528–1529.
51. Yamashita J, Ogawa M, Shirakusa T. Plasma endothelin-1 as a marker for doxorubicin cardiotoxicity. Int J Cancer 1995;62:542–547.
52. Lipshultz SE, Rifai N, Sallan SE, et al. Predictive value of cardiac troponin T in pediatric patients at risk for myocardial injury. Circulation 1997;96:2641–2648.
53. Missov E, Calzolari C, Davy JM, Leclercq F, Rossi M, Pau B. Cardiac troponin I in patients with hematologic malignancies. Coron Artery Dis 1997;8:537–541.
54. Ganzina F. 4′-epi-Doxorubicin, a new analogue of doxorubicin: a preliminary overview of preclinical and clinical data. Cancer Treat Rev 1983;10:1–22.
55. Jain KK, Casper ES, Geller NL, et al. A prospective randomized comparison of epirubicin and doxorubicin in patients with advanced breast cancer. J Clin Oncol 1985;3:818–826.
56. Brambilla C, Rossi A, Bonfante V, et al. Phase II study of doxorubicin versus epirubicin in advanced breast cancer. Cancer Treat Rep 1986;70:261–266.
57. Villani F, Galimberti M, Comazzi R, Crippa F. Evaluation of cardiac toxicity of idarubicin (4-demethoxydaunorubicin). Eur J Cancer Clin Oncol 1989;25:13–18.
58. Lopez M, Contegiacomo A, Vici P, et al. A prospective randomized trial of doxorubicin versus idarubicin in the treatment of advanced breast cancer. Cancer (Phila) 1989;64:2431–2436.

59. Speyer JL, Green MD, Kramer E, et al. Protective effect of the bispiperazinedione ICRF-187 against doxorubicin-induced cardiac toxicity in women with advanced breast cancer. N Engl J Med 1988;319:745–752.
60. Speyer JL, Green MD, Zeleniuch-Jacquotte A, et al. ICRF-187 permits longer treatment with doxorubicin in women with breast cancer. J Clin Oncol 1992;10:117–127.
61. Hochster H, Liebes L, Wadler S, et al. Pharmacokinetics of the cardioprotector ADR-529 (ICRF-187) in escalating doses combined with fixed-dose doxorubicin. J Natl Cancer Inst 1992;84:1725–1730.
62. Swain SM, Whaley FS, Gerber MC, et al. Cardioprotection with dexrazoxane for doxorubicin-containing therapy in advanced breast cancer. J Clin Oncol 1997;15:1318–1332.
63. Hensley ML, Schuchter LM, Lindley C, et al. American Society of Clinical Oncology clinical practice guidelines for the use of chemotherapy and radiotherapy protectants. J Clin Oncol 1999;17:3333–3355.
64. Gill PS, Espina BM, Muggia F, et al. Phase I/II clinical and pharmacokinetic evaluation of liposomal daunorubicin. J Clin Oncol 1995;13:996–1003.
65. Hempel G, Reinhardt D, Creutzig U, et al. Population pharmacokinetics of liposomal daunorubicin in children. Br J Clin Pharmacol 2003;56(4):370–377.
66. Liu FT, Kelsey SM, Newland AC, et al. Liposomal encapsulation diminishes daunorubicin-induced generation of reactive oxygen species, depletion of ATP, and necrotic cell death in human leukaemic cells. Br J Haematol 2002;117(2):333–342.
67. Sadava D, Coleman A, Kane SE. Liposomal daunorubicin overcomes drug resistance in human breast, ovarian, and lung carcinoma cells. J Liposome Res 2002;12(4):301–309.
68. Henderson BM, Dougherty WJ, James VC, Tilley LP, Noble JF. Safety assessment of a new anticancer compound, mitoxantrone, in beagle dogs: comparison with doxorubicin. I. Clinical observations. Cancer Treat Rep 1982;66:1139–1143.
69. Sparano BM, Gordon G, Hall C, Iatropoulos MJ, Noble JF. Safety assessment of new anticancer compound, mitoxantrone, in beagle dogs: comparison with doxorubicin. II. Histologic and ultrastructural pathology. Cancer Treat Rep 1982;66:1145–1158.
70. Mather FJ, Simon RM, Clark GM, Von Hoff DD. Cardiotoxicity in patients treated with mitoxantrone: Southwest Oncology Group phase II studies. Cancer Treat Rep 1987;71:609–613.
71. Posner LE, Dukart G, Goldberg J, Bernstein T, Cartwright K. Mitoxantrone: an overview of safety and toxicity. Invest New Drugs 1985;3:123–132.
72. Goldberg MA, Antin JH, Guinan EC, Rappeport JM. Cyclophosphamide cardiotoxicity: an analysis of dosing as a risk factor. Blood 1986;68:1114–1118.
73. Dow E, Schulman H, Agura E. Cyclophosphamide cardiac injury mimicking acute myocardial infarction. Bone Marrow Transplant 1993;12:169–172.
74. Gardner SF, Lazarus HM, Bednarczyk EM, et al. High-dose cyclophosphamide-induced myocardial damage during BMT: assessment by positron emission tomography. Bone Marrow Transplant 1993;12:139–144.
75. Gottdiener JS, Appelbaum FR, Ferrans VJ, Deisseroth A, Ziegler J. Cardiotoxicity associated with high-dose cyclophosphamide therapy. Arch Intern Med 1981;141:758–763.
76. Steinherz LJ, Steinherz PG, Mangiacasale D, et al. Cardiac changes with cyclophosphamide. Med Pediatr Oncol 1981;9:417–422.
77. Goldberg MA, Antin JH, Guinan EC, Rappeport JM. Cyclophosphamide cardiotoxicity: an analysis of dosing as a risk factor. Blood 1986;68:1114–1118.
78. Quezado ZM, Wilson WH, Cunnion RE, et al. High-dose ifosfamide is associated with severe, reversible cardiac dysfunction. Ann Intern Med 1993;118:31–36.
79. Buzdar AU, Legha SS, Tashima CK, et al. Adriamycin and mitomycin C: possible synergistic cardiotoxicity. Cancer Treat Rep 1978;62:1005–1008.
80. Villani F, Comazzi R, Lacaita G, et al. Possible enhancement of the cardiotoxicity of doxorubicin when combined with mitomycin C. Med Oncol Tumor Pharmacother 1985;2:93–97.
81. Verweij J, Funke-Kupper AJ, Teule GJ, Pinedo HM. A prospective study on the dose dependency of cardiotoxicity induced by mitomycin C. Med Oncol Tumor Pharmacother 1988;5:159–163.
82. Labianca R, Beretta G, Clerici M, Fraschini P, Luporini G. Cardiac toxicity of 5-fluorouracil: a study on 1083 patients. Tumori 1982;68:505–510.
83. Patel B, Kloner RA, Ensley J, Al Sarraf M, Kish J, Wynne J. 5-Fluorouracil cardiotoxicity: left ventricular dysfunction and effect of coronary vasodilators. Am J Med Sci 1987;294:238–243.
84. Rezkalla S, Kloner RA, Ensley J, et al. Continuous ambulatory ECG monitoring during fluorouracil therapy: a prospective study. J Clin Oncol 1989;7:509–514.
85. De Forni M, Malet-Martino MC, Jaillais P, et al. Cardiotoxicity of high-dose continuous infusion fluorouracil: a prospective clinical study. J Clin Oncol 1992;10:1795–1801.
86. Weiss RB, Donehower RC, Wiernik PH, et al. Hypersensitivity reactions from taxol. J Clin Oncol 1990;8:1263–1268.
87. Rowinsky EK, McGuire WP, Guarnieri T, et al. Cardiac disturbances during the administration of taxol. J Clin Oncol 1991;9:1704–1712.
88. Arbuck SG, Strauss H, Rowinsky E, et al. A reassessment of cardiac toxicity associated with taxol. J Natl Cancer Inst Monogr 1993;15:117–130.
89. Perez EA. Doxorubicin and paclitaxel in the treatment of advanced breast cancer: efficacy and cardiac considerations. Cancer Invest 2001;19(2):155–164.
90. Gianni L, Dombernowsky P, Sledge G, et al. Cardiac function following combination therapy with paclitaxel and doxorubicin: an analysis of 657 women with advanced breast cancer. Ann Oncol 2001;12(8):1067–1073.
91. Ekholm E, Rantanen V, Syvanen K, Jalonen J, Antila K, Salminen E. Docetaxel does not impair cardiac autonomic function in breast cancer patients previously treated with anthracyclines. Anticancer Drugs 2002;13(4):425–429.

79

Neurologic Complications of Therapy

Kristin Bradley and H. Ian Robins

The etiology of neurotoxicity following treatment with chemotherapy and/or radiation therapy is not always obvious. Neurologic complications can be difficult to identify, diagnose appropriately, and measure. In addition, neurotoxicity may be delayed and patients may experience tumor-related mortality before the diagnosis of treatment-related complications. Furthermore, the signs and symptoms of neurotoxicity may resemble those of disease progression. Finally, underlying diseases, such as diabetes mellitus, infections, hypertension, paraneoplastic syndromes, age-related dementia, seizures, concomitant medications, such as antiepileptic agents, and metabolic disorders can be confounding factors.

Neurotoxicity following treatment spans a spectrum from acute to chronic, and from reversible to irreversible; neurotoxicity may involve the central nervous system (CNS), the peripheral nervous system (PNS), or both. The complications can range in grade from subclinical to severe. In the following sections, we discuss the neurotoxicities of chemotherapy and radiation therapy individually, as well as the neurologic complications of combined chemoradiation. In specific areas, the limited information regarding prophylaxis and/or treatment of therapy-related neurotoxicity is similarly presented.

In the text to follow, an attempt is made to critically summarize an extensive literature. In this regard, many of the available data pertaining to this significant treatment-limiting morbidity are observational. In spite of this, a substantial database has been accrued by investigators. Thus, it is the intention of this review to provide a synopsis to reinforce early clinical recognition of these toxicities. It was further envisioned that this review might serve to stimulate further laboratory and controlled clinical research.

Chemotherapy-Induced Neurotoxicity

Vinca Alkaloids

Vincristine was the first chemotherapeutic agent described as having neurotoxicity,[1] which, it is dose-limiting for this drug. Other *Vinca* alkaloids, for example, vinblastine and vinorelbine, share this same predisposition, but to a lesser extent.[2] Such neurotoxicity can involve the peripheral, autonomic, or central nervous system.[1–7] Toxicity can be dose related and/or cumulative. Peripheral neuropathy is well recognized by clinicians, and it tends to be reversible over the course of years.[7] Severe constipation and bladder atony are not uncommonly observed. Rarely, cranial nerves can be affected, resulting in ophthalmoplegia and facial palsies; laryngeal nerve paralysis and cortical blindness have also been reported.[5,6] Although many physicians treat these complications with vitamin therapy (including the B group), there are no data to support this practice. The use of metoclopramide has been used and reported for gastrointestinal (GI) motility dysfunction.[8]

5-Fluorouracil

Historically, 5-fluorouracil (5-FU) was also an early chemotherapy drug for which neurotoxicity became readily apparent,[9–17] with an incidence up to 5%. Clinically, patients can experience loss of coordination, ataxia of the trunk and extremities, slurred speech, nystagmus, optic neuropathy, and hypotonia. Peripheral neuropathy and acute encephalopathy have also been reported.[12,13] It has been postulated that the use of 5-FU in conjunction with levamisole or leucovorin (both of which can be neurotoxins[18,19]) may add to the neurotoxic potential of 5-FU.[16] The neurotoxicity observed is not necessarily dose or schedule dependent, and it is often reversible on drug cessation. It has also been postulated[20] that 5-FU toxicity may relate to 5-FU-induced thiamine deficiency (observed in a series of 35 patients[21]); this may be particularly relevant to the syndrome of 5-FU-cerebellar ataxia. Pathologically, some toxic events can be correlated with multifocal cerebral demyelination. In extreme cases, patients can become encephalopathic.[12] This life-threatening complication may be associated with dihydropyrimidine dehydrogenase deficiency. This enzyme deficiency, which may exist in up to 3% of the population, affects 5-FU metabolism and places patients at extreme risk for any and all 5-FU complications.[22] Takimoto et al.[23] reported such a case in which a comatose state was reversible with infusional thymidine.

Platinum Agents

With the introduction of cisplatin more than two decades ago, its neurotoxic potential was immediately recognized. The toxicity of this heavy metal is generally dose related and in part, may be related to segmental demyelination of sensory nerves.[24] Neurologic complications in addition to peripheral sensory loss, with paresthesias severe enough to result in loss of fine motor skills, include loss of motor reflexes; foot drop; leg cramping; neuropathic pain (as an extension of the sensory neuropathy); Lhermittes's sign (also induced by radiation); auditory and visual cranial nerve injury; and autonomic neuropathy.[24–32] Although cisplatin-induced hypomagnesmia is correlated with increased risk for neurotoxicity,[29] it is not clear that diligent magnesium repletion prevents progression of peripheral neuropathy. Hearing deficits begin the majority of the time with reversible tinnitus, progress to asymptomatic loss of high-frequency tones, and finally to symptomatic permanent mid-frequency loss. Vision compromise can range from color alteration to retinal inflammation and/or damage, transient blindness, and papilledema. The sensory neuropathy can result in severe gait disturbances. These observations taken collectively, often necessitate the modification or discontinuation of the drug, particularly in patients not being treated with curative intent. Consideration of a less neurotoxic analogue, that is, carboplatin, represents an alternative option. Amifostine, primarily used as a renal protectant, provides limited neuropathy protection relative to cisplatin,[33] but its use is limited by the amifostine-related side effects. Most recently, a new platinum analogue, oxaliplatin, has entered clinical practice. It too has sensory neuropathy and cramping, but also can produce pharyngolaryngeal dysesthesias.[34,35] The appearance of the pharyngolaryngeal dysesthesias is often acute, as is the appearance of cold intolerance. Extending the period of oxaliplatin infusion can minimize the toxicities. The sensory neuropathy is late, cumulative, and dose dependent, but often reverses to some extent at approximately 6 months. Some clinicians believe that calcium and magnesium supplementation is beneficial in palliating and preventing this complication.

Taxanes

At this point in the discussion, it is appropriate to highlight that the combined use of two neurotoxic agents produces enhancement of neurotoxicity. Examples include doublets of platinum agents, *Vinca* alkaloids, and/or taxanes.[2,36–43] Relative to the taxanes as a class, the two approved analogues, paclitaxel and docetaxel, also have treatment-limiting peripheral neuropathy much the same as the platinum-based drugs and the *Vinca* alkaloids.[44–50] Taxane-related neuropathy is cumulative and dose dependent. In general, neurosensory and neuromuscular effects are less severe and less frequent with docetaxel than with paclitaxel. The toxicity relates in part to axonal degeneration and demyelination related to a direct effect on microtubules.[51] Motor myopathy also has been associated with the taxanes. It is difficult, however, to differentiate this sequela of therapy from the effect of corticosteroids usually given with the taxanes to prevent allergic reactions. Rare reports of visual disturbances and encephalopathy also exist.[52,53] There is some controversy as to whether preexisting conditions, such as diabetes mellitus, can predispose patients to increased neuropathy.[44] As in the case of the previously discussed peripheral neuropathies, no intervention to date has been demonstrated to be efficacious in alleviating symptoms, although the empiric use of amitriptyline is popular. Early work has reported that glutamine may be beneficial in reducing neuropathy associated with paclitaxel administration.[54] These early results, however, need to be confirmed by a placebo-controlled trial. Occasionally, symptoms may reverse several months after drug cessation. In contrast to cisplatin, amifostine is not effective for taxane-induced neuropathy.[55]

Cytosine Arabinoside

Cytosine arabinoside (Ara-C), given systemically or intrathecally (IT), can cause an acute dose-dependent cerebellar neuropathy defined by specific pathologic changes.[56–61] Although this toxicity is reversible with drug cessation, permanent truncal and gait ataxia can develop. The neurotoxicity of Ara-C is dose and schedule dependent, and is related to the cumulative dose of the drug. Early clinical signs include nystagmus, dysarthria, tremors, and dysmetria. Mental status changes including encephalopathy and seizures may follow. Additionally, spinal myopathy, basal ganglia necrosis, and pseudobulbar palsy have been reported.[60] If the need for drug cessation is not recognized early in the patient's clinical course, any of these complications can progress to death.

Methotrexate

Methotrexate (MTX), which can also be given intravenously (IV) or IT, also can produce significant neurologic symptoms (both acute and late), ranging from meningeal irritation and/or transient paraparesis to encephalopathy.[62–65] Such complications typically are only seen with IV use at high doses and probably are directly related to levels in the cerebrospinal fluid. The physician treating a CNS manifestation of malignancy with MTX (as is also the case with ara-C) must be careful not to mistake drug toxicity for disease progression, as the symptoms (e.g., seizures, somnolence, nuchal rigidity, nausea and vomiting, headache) may overlap. Aminophylline has been reported to reverse MTX neurotoxicity.[66] In general, the major neurologic complications encountered with MTX relate to its use (high-dose IV or IT) in combination with ionizing irradiation.[67,68] Leukoencephalopathy is a well-recognized complication following combined modality therapy. In this regard, children may be at increased risk for such toxicity.[69]

Alkylating Agents

The alkylating agent ifosfamide can produce an array of neurologic complications, probably as a result of degradation metabolites.[70] Acute clinical manifestations can include hallucinations, confusion, seizures, hemiparesis, lethargy, coma, personality changes, cerebellar and cranial nerve deficits, peripheral neuropathy, and extrapyramidal problems.[71–75] Although cumulative dose neurotoxic effects have not been reported, rechallenge with the drug can again precipitate acute neurotoxicity. Reversal of such CNS toxicity has been achieved with the use of IV methylene blue.[70,71] Altretamine, another alkylating agent, predominantly produces peripheral neuropathy-related toxicity, but central effects similar to ifosfamide, including parkinsonian tremors, have been reported.[76]

Radiation Therapy Toxicities

Central Nervous System Toxicity

The neurotoxicities of radiation therapy, similar to those from chemotherapy, can be broadly classified as acute (within the first 3 months), subacute (from 3 months to 1 year), and chronic (years after irradiation).

A person may suffer from headache, nausea, vomiting, lethargy, fever, and occasionally, exacerbation of their neurologic symptoms within 2 weeks of finishing radiation therapy. This acute phenomenon is broadly attributed to breakdown of the blood–brain barrier with subsequent development of increased intracranial pressure caused by edema. Experimental models in large animals support the hypothesis of radiation-induced breakdown of the blood–brain barrier with accumulation of vasogenic edema; in humans, large fraction radiation, as seen with radiosurgery, supports this observation.[77,78] Rarely, early neurologic toxicity may be more severe in patients with multiple metastases, a large posterior fossa tumor, or with large radiation fraction sizes.[79]

Subacute CNS toxicity generally manifests between 1 to 6 months after radiation therapy and is not limited to a single clinical presentation; both the brain and the spinal cord can be affected. In the spinal cord, Lhermitte's sign, in which neck flexion triggers fleeting, electrical shocklike paresthesias radiating from the neck to the extremities, typifies the onset of radiation myelopathy. Believed to be caused by transient demyelination, the syndrome is self-limiting, gradually improves over 2 to 9 months, and does not predict for the development of later, irreversible myelopathy.[80,81]

Early-delayed brain injury following cranial irradiation is marked by a somnolence syndrome and is most prominent in children. Up to three-quarters of children receiving prophylactic or therapeutic CNS irradiation for acute lymphoblastic leukemia, may develop a somnolence syndrome characterized by hypersomnia, irritability, anorexia, headache, and fever.[82,83] Adults rarely experience the somnolence syndrome.[84] The pathogenesis of the somnolence syndrome is believed to be due to oligodendroglial cell injury and altered capillary permeability resulting in transient demyelination.[80,81,85] The syndrome may go undiagnosed, with the patient improving spontaneously over weeks or months. Rarely, subacute CNS toxicity following irradiation may be severe, or even fatal.[81]

The manifestations of late-delayed radiation-induced CNS toxicity can appear months to years after irradiation.[86] Radiation necrosis is one of the most serious delayed CNS complications. It typically presents 1 to 2 years following external-beam radiation therapy and 6 to 9 months after interstitial brachytherapy or radiosurgery.[87] The reappearance of prior neurologic deficits, as well as the emergence of new focal neurologic problems, can simulate tumor recurrence. The use of positron emission tomography (PET) scanning and/or magnetic resonance imaging (MRI) spectroscopy can be useful in distinguishing recurrent or progressive disease from necrosis. Radiation necrosis tends to be progressive and may be irreversible, with prominent edema and mass effect caused by coagulative necrosis of cerebral white matter.[88] Another delayed neurotoxicity following irradiation is leukoencephalopathic cognitive dysfunction without necrosis.[89,90] Some reports have estimated that there is a 10% to 15% risk of leukoencephalopathy following whole-brain radiotherapy. Children whose brains are still developing are at particularly high risk of developing profound neurocognitive sequelae; the risk is greatest for children irradiated before 3 to 4 years of age, the age when CNS myelination is complete.[91,92] Radiation-induced neurocognitive dysfunction ranges from mild changes in attention span, short-term memory, and problem-solving ability that do not affect overall performance status, to more profound functional deficits. Severe decline and alterations of IQ, memory, response times, problem-solving ability, emotional state, balance, and gait trend toward progressive deterioration, with death 1 to 48 months after the onset of symptoms.[87] The pathophysiology of late cognitive and intellectual decline following cranial irradiation is not fully understood, but clinical, radiographic, and neuropathologic findings incriminate white matter changes.[87,93–95]

Spinal cord radiation myelopathy, another delayed neurotoxicity, has a median latency of 20 months after irradiation, but this varies with radiation dose, region and length of spinal cord irradiated, patient age, and prior treatment.[81,96] Clinically, delayed myelopathy may be gradual or sudden and may result in partial or complete functional deficits, but is generally progressive and irreversible, often resulting in bowel and bladder dysfunction, paraplegia or quadriplegia, paresthesias, partial Brown–Séquard syndrome, and lower motor neuron dysfunction.[81,97] As many as one-half of patients die of secondary complications, including infection, pulmonary embolism, and respiratory compromise.[98]

Other chronic radiation-induced CNS toxicities may include hypothalamic-pituitary axis (HPA) dysfunction with endocrinopathies, cranial nerve injuries, vascular abnormalities, and second malignancies.

Peripheral Nervous System Toxicity

Shortly after receiving radiotherapy, patients may note paresthesias following irradiation of peripheral nerves. More significant, however, are the early- and late-delayed complications of PNS irradiation. Fortunately, reports of peripheral nerve injury have decreased as a result of the use of three-dimensional, computer-based planning and improved quality control.[99] Brachial plexopathy following radiotherapy for locally advanced breast cancer manifests as paresthesias, pain, and weakness in the distribution of the brachial plexus nerve roots. The injury may be transient or may develop into an irreversible, progressive brachial plexopathy, typically a year or more after receiving 60Gy or greater. Lumbosacral plexopathy, presenting as unilateral or bilateral lower extremity sensory or motor deficits following pelvic irradiation, has been reported less frequently than brachial plexus injury. Paresthesias and pain may or may not accompany muscle atrophy and weakness.[99] Identifying the etiology of plexopathies can be a challenge for the treating physician because the findings of treatment-induced injury may resemble those of tumor recurrence.

Toxicities of Combined Chemotherapy and Radiation Therapy

Neurotoxicity, in particular CNS toxicity, following combined treatment with chemotherapy and radiation therapy, is a challenging problem for the oncologist. Although chemotherapy and radiation have their own independent toxicities, overlapping toxicities make it difficult to clearly identify the offending modality. Complications of other illnesses, such as diabetes and hypertension, as well as neurotoxicity resulting from disease recurrence or progression, must be eliminated before ascribing a complication to chemoradiotherapy. The neurotoxicities of two important drug–radiation interactions are discussed in detail next.

Methotrexate and Cranial Irradiation

There are three widely recognized late syndromes following the combined use of methotrexate (MTX) and cranial irradiation: necrotizing leukoencephalopathy, mineralizing microangiopathy, and cognitive impairment.[100] Necrotizing leukoencephalopathy results from white matter necrosis with sparing of grey matter and is generally without an inflammatory response. The risk of its development appears to be greatest if MTX is given concurrently with or after radiation therapy. Usually occurring within 1 year of treatment, it manifests as a change in personality, dementia, seizures, ataxia, hemiparesis or quadriparesis, and pseudobulbar palsy. The clinical course may stabilize, or rarely, improve, but for the majority of patients, it is severe, progressive, and potentially fatal. Leukoencephalopathy following treatment with MTX and cranial radiation has been extensively reported in children receiving CNS treatment or prophylaxis for acute lymphoblastic leukemia (ALL).[101–103] The dose of radiation and intravenous MTX, rather than intrathecal MTX, is correlated with the risk of its development.[103]

In contrast to necrotizing leukoencephalopathy, mineralizing microangiopathy generally has longer latency periods and usually produces milder neurologic dysfunction.[101] Its course may be subclinical, or it may produce headaches, incoordination, and seizures. Similar to most neurologic sequelae of chemoradiation, younger children are at greater risk. Grey matter changes are seen, resulting from the mineral deposition in the walls of the small vessels of grey matter.[104]

A third syndrome seen following the combined use of MTX and cranial irradiation is cognitive impairment.[105–109] In adults, the use of high-dose MTX, along with whole-brain radiotherapy for primary CNS lymphoma, has resulted in a 15% to 32% overall incidence of late neurotoxicity.[108,109] In the recently reported Radiation Therapy Oncology Group (RTOG) study (93-10), a neurotoxicity rate of 15% was seen.[109] In children treated with chemoradiation for ALL, medulloblastoma, or other intracranial tumors, neurocognitive toxicity typically manifests as a decline in IQ with impaired school performance resulting from learning disabilities.[92,105–107] In children 3 to 7 years of age treated for medulloblastoma, a 20- to 30-point decline in IQ score over a 3- to 4-year period has been reported.[92] A debate continues about whether cranial irradiation or intrathecal MTX is the primary causative factor.[110,111]

Cisplatin and Cranial Irradiation

As discussed in a previous section, cisplatin alone can result in neurotoxicity. One of the most recognized neurotoxicities of cisplatin is ototoxicity, a high-frequency hearing loss resulting from hair cell damage. When cranial irradiation is combined with cisplatin, either sequentially or concurrently, the risk of severe ototoxicity increases significantly.[112,113] As the sensorineural hearing loss progresses from high frequencies to frequencies required for speech perception and recognition, a child's ability to understand and learn is impaired. In an attempt to decrease the audiotoxicity of combined cisplatin and irradiation, intensity-modulated radiation therapy (IMRT), which provides for more conformal radiation delivery, has been employed to decrease radiation dose to the auditory apparatus.[114] A retrospective comparison of patients with medulloblastoma who received either conventional radiotherapy or IMRT showed that IMRT delivered 32% less radiation dose to the auditory apparatus while delivering full doses to the target volume. Children treated with IMRT experienced lower ototoxicity: 13% of the IMRT patients had grade 3 or 4 hearing loss compared with 64% of the conventional radiotherapy patients.[114]

Management of Neurotoxicity Following Chemotherapy and Radiation Therapy

The first and most important step in the management of neurotoxicity related to chemotherapy and/or radiation therapy is to recognize its existence and, subsequently, to make attempts at prophylaxis. Prevention begins with the elucidation of factors that predict such toxicity, including age; medical comorbidities; use of concomitant chemoradiotherapy; and the specifics of dose, dose-per-fraction, and volume treated. Whenever possible, an attempt should be made to mitigate these risk factors.

Symptomatic Management

Corticosteroids are commonly used in the symptomatic management of treatment-related, and particularly radiation-induced, neurotoxicity. They are employed to decrease the edema seen after radiation.[115] Although beneficial in decreasing vasogenic edema, dexamethasone is less effective for treatment-related brain necrosis. Animal and human studies have shown, at best, only a minor delay in the development of radiation necrosis with dexamethasone.[116,117] Similarly, following spinal cord irradiation, some studies have demonstrated that corticosteroids can temporarily delay the progression of radiation myelitis but do not prevent or successfully treat it.[85,118] Other pharmacologic agents, including deferrioxamine, anticoagulants, lipid peroxidase inhibitors, and antioxidants, have been investigated with mixed results.[119–121]

Management of Radiation Necrosis

Because corticosteroids have a limited role in the symptomatic management of brain necrosis following chemoradiation, other strategies have been explored as treatment options. Resection of the necrotic tissue may or may not lead to recovery of impaired neurologic functions. Surgical resection is more successful for discrete areas of necrosis than for areas of diffuse necrosis.[122,123] Hyperbaric oxygen (HBO) therapy also has been used to treat complications of radiation therapy. By increasing tissue oxygenation concentration, HBO stimulates angiogenesis and improves capillary function.[124,125] Small reports have detailed improvement of radiation myelitis and cerebral radiation necrosis with HBO therapy.[126–128] Additional study of the application of HBO therapy in adults and children suffering from nervous system necrosis after chemoradiation is required before a conclusion can be reached about its effectiveness. Controlled clinical trials of innovative therapeutic interventions for radiation necrosis are difficult to design and execute. Nevertheless, such studies are now being designed by the RTOG.

Amifostine

In considering the collective neurotoxicities of chemotherapy, it is the peripheral neurotoxicities that represent the major clinical problem, as they are often dose limiting. Many attempts have been made to develop strategies for treatment and prevention. Amifostine (WR 2721) has been explored as a neuroprotective agent. Amifostine is a thiol compound that requires endothelial dephosphorylation to be activated. Because normal endothelium dephosphorylates the drug more efficiently than tumor endothelium, amifostine may exert a preferential protective effect in normal tissue.[129,130] However, the intracranial permeability and localization of amifostine in normal brain are very limited; hence its value as a radioprotector for the CNS is limited. Amifostine provides some protection against cisplatin-related peripheral neurotoxicity, but its utility is limited by vomiting and significant hypotension.[33,38]

Conclusions

Neurotoxicity can occur following chemotherapy, radiation therapy, or the combined use of both therapeutic modalities. Neurologic complications can develop during the course of therapy, weeks to months after finishing therapy, and even years following treatment. Similarly, their severity covers a wide range, with a reported spectrum of mild to function impairing to potentially fatal. The clinical and radiographic signs and symptoms of neurotoxicity often are not unique to the etiology. As a consequence, distinguishing treatment-related toxicities from recurrent tumor or from complications of other medical illnesses can be difficult. Currently, management of the neurotoxicities of chemotherapy and radiation therapy is mostly symptomatic, with initial efforts being undertaken at prevention and prophylaxis. Further elucidation of the mechanisms of these toxicities (via preclinical and controlled clinical studies), coupled to the investigation of patient- and treatment-related factors that predict for or increase the risk of their development, are needed. Only when these mechanisms and predictive factors are better understood will significant success at prevention and prophylaxis be achieved. The elucidation of both mechanistic and predictive factors should provide a foundation for future research encompassing prevention, prophylaxis, and treatment.

References

1. Weiden PL, Wright SE. Vincristine neurotoxicity. N Engl J Med 1972;286:1369–1370.
2. Le Chevalier T, Brisgand D, Douillard JY, et al. Randomized study of vinorelbine and cisplatin versus vindesine and cisplatin versus vinorelbine alone in advanced non-small-cell lung cancer: results of a European multicenter trial including 612 patients. J Clin Oncol 1994;12:360–367.
3. Roca E, Bruera E, Politi PM, et al. Vinca alkaloid-induced cardiovascular autonomic neuropathy. Cancer Treat Rep 1985;69:149–151.
4. Haim N, Epelbaum R, Ben-Shahar M, et al. Full dose vincristine (without 2-mg dose limit) in the treatment of lymphomas. Cancer (Phila) 1994;73:2515–2519.
5. Merimsky O, Loewenstein A, Chaitchik S. Cortical blindness: a catastrophic side effect of vincristine. Anti-Cancer Drugs 1992;3:371–373.
6. Burns BV, Shotton JC. Vocal fold palsy following vinca alkaloid treatment. J Laryngol Otol 1998;112:485–487.
7. Postma TJ, Benard BA, Huijgens PC, et al. Long-term effects of vincristine on the peripheral nervous system. J Neuro-Oncol 1993;15:23–27.
8. Garewal HS, Dalton WS. Metoclopramide in vincristine-induced ileus. Cancer Treat Rep 1985;69:1309–1311.
9. Allegra CJ, Grem JL. Antimetabolites. In: De Vita V Jr, Hellman S, Rosenberg SA (eds) Cancer: Principles and Practice of Oncology. Philadelphia: Lippincott-Raven, 1997:432–452.
10. Moertal CG, Fleming TR, MacDonald JS, et al. Levamisol and fluorouracil for adjuvant therapy of resected colon carcinoma. N Engl J Med 1990;322:352–358.
11. Bygrave HA, Geh JI, Jani Y, et al. Neurological complications of 5-fluorouracil-associated peripheral neuropathy: a report and review of the literature. Clin Oncol (R Coll Radiol) 1998;10:334.
12. Langer CJ, Hageboutros A, Kloth DD, et al. Acute encephalopathy attributed to 5-FU. Pharmacotherapy 1996;16:311–313.
13. Stein ME, Drumea K, Yarnitsky D, et al. A rare event of 5-fluorouracil and levamisole. Am J Clin Oncol 1998;21:248–249.
14. Saletti P, Pagani O, Sessa C, et al. Two cases of neurotoxicity possibly related to 5-fluorouracil and FA administration. Ann Oncol 1996;7:213–214.
15. Kimmel DW, Schutt AJ. Multifocal leukoencephalopathy: occurrence during 5-fluorouracil and levamisole therapy and resolution after discontinuation of chemotherapy. Mayo Clin Proc 1993;68:363–365.
16. Hook CC, Kimmel DW, Kvols LK, et al. Multifocal inflammatory leukoencephalopathy with 5-fluorouracil and levamisole. Ann Neurol 1992;31:262–267.
17. Bixenman WW, Nicholls JV, Warwick OH. Oculomotor disturbances associated with 5-fluorouracil chemotherapy. Am J Ophthalmol 1977;83:789–793.
18. Meropol NJ, Creaven PJ, Petrelli NJ, et al. Seizures associated with leucovorin administration in cancer patients. J Natl Cancer Inst 1995;87:56.
19. Fassas AB, Gattani AM, Morgello S. Cerebral demyelination with 5-fluorouracil and levamisole. Cancer Invest 1994;12:379–383.
20. Koenig H, Patel A. Biochemical basis for fluorouracil neurotoxicity. The role of Krebs cycle inhibition by fluoroacetate. Arch Neurol 1970;23(2):155–160.
21. Askoy M, Basu T, Brint J, et al. Thiamine status of patients treated with drug combinations containing 5-fluorouracil. Eur J Cancer 1980;16:1041–1045.
22. Milano G, Etienne MC, Vierrefite V, et al. Dihydropyrimidine dehydrogenase deficiency and fluorouracil-related toxicity. Br J Cancer 1999;79:627–630.
23. Takimoto CH, Lu ZH, Zhang R, et al. Severe neurotoxicity following 5-fluorouracil-based chemotherapy in a patient with dihydropyrimidine dehydrogenase activity. Clin Cancer Res 1996;2:477–481.
24. Berry JM, Jacobs C, Sikic B, et al. Modification of cisplatin chemotherapy with diethyliathiocarbamate. J Clin Oncol 1990;8:1585–590.
25. Gerritsen van der Hoop R, van der Burg MEL, ten Bokkel Huinink WW, et al. Incidence of neuropathy in 395 patients with

ovarian cancer treated with or without cisplatin. Cancer (Phila) 1990;66:1697–1702.
26. Cersosimo RJ. Cisplatin neurotoxicity. Cancer Treat Rev 1989;16:195–211.
27. Cavaletti G, Marzorati L, Bogliun G, et al. Cisplatin-induced peripheral neurotoxicity is dependent on total dose intensity and single-dose intensity. Cancer (Phila) 1992;69:203–207.
28. Hilkens PHE, van der Burg MEL, Moll JWB, et al. Neurotoxicity is not enhanced by increased dose intensities of cisplatin administration. Eur J Cancer 1995;31A:678–681.
29. Ashraf M, Scotel RN, Krall JM, et al. Cis-platinum-induced hypomagnesemia and peripheral neuropathy. Gynecol Oncol 1983;16:309–318.
30. Forman A. Peripheral neuropathy in cancer patients: incidence, features, and pathophysiology. Oncology 1990;4:57–62.
31. Wilding G, Caruso R, Lawrence T, et al. Retinal toxicity after high-dose cisplatin therapy. J Clin Oncol 1985;3:1683–1689.
32. Holden S, Felde G. Nursing care of patients experiencing cisplatin-related peripheral neuropathies. Oncol Nurs Forum 1987;14:13–19.
33. Kemp G, Rose P, Lurain J, et al. Amifostine pretreatment for protection against cyclophosphamide-induced and cisplatin-induced toxicities: results of a randomized control trial in patients with advanced ovarian cancer. J Clin Oncol 1996;14:2101–2112.
34. Becouarn Y, Ychou M, Ducreux M, et al. Phase II trial of oxaliplatin as first-line chemotherapy in metastatic colorectal cancer patients. J Clin Oncol 1998;16:2739–2744.
35. Gilles-Amar V, Garcia ML, Seille A, et al. Evolution of severe sensory neuropathy with oxaliplatin combined to the bimonthly 48-h leucovorin (LV) and 5-fluorouracil (5FU) regimens (FOLFOX) in metastatic colorectal cancer. Proc ASCO 1999;18:246a.
36. Parimoo D, Jeffers S, Muggia FM. Severe neurotoxicity from vinorelbine-paclitaxel combinations. J Natl Cancer Inst 1996;88: 1079–1080.
37. Fazeny B, Zifki U, Meryn S, et al. Vinorelbine-induced neurotoxicity in patients with advanced breast cancer pretreated with paclitaxel: a phase II study. Cancer Chemother Pharmacol 1996;39:150–156.
38. Selvaggi G, Belani CP. Carboplatin and paclitaxel in non-small cell lung cancer: the role of amifostine. Semin Oncol 1999; 26(suppl 7):51–60.
39. Wasserheit C, Frazein A, Oratz R, et al. Phase II trial of paclitaxel and cisplatin in women with advanced breast cancer: an active regimen with limiting neurotoxicity. J Clin Oncol 1996;14:1993–1999.
40. Berger T, Malayeri R, Doppelbauer A, et al. Neurological monitoring for neurotoxicity induced by paclitaxel/cisplatin chemotherapy. Eur J Cancer 1997;33:1393–1399.
41. Connelly E, Markman M, Kennedy A, et al. Paclitaxel delivered as a 3-hr infusion with cisplatin in patients with gynecologic cancers: unexpected incidence of neurotoxicity. Gynecol Oncol 1966;62:166–168.
42. Cavaletti G, Boglium G, Marzorati L, et al. Peripheral neurotoxicity of taxol in patients previously treated with cisplatin. Cancer (Phila) 1995;75:1141–1150.
43. Faivre S, Kalla S, Cvitkovic E, et al. Oxaliplatin and paclitaxel combination in patients with platinum-pretreated ovarian carcinoma: an investigator-originated compassionate-use experience. Ann Oncol 1999;10:1125–1128.
44. Rowinsky EK, Chaudhry V, Cornblath DR, et al. Neurotoxicity of taxol. Monog Natl Cancer Inst 1993;15:107–115.
45. Postma TJ, Vermoken JB, Liefting AJM, et al. Paclitaxel-induced neuropathy. Ann Oncol 1995;6:489–494.
46. Forsyth PA, Balmaceda C, Peterson K, et al. Prospective study of paclitaxel-induced peripheral neuropathy with quantitative sensory testing. J Neuro-Oncol 1997;35:47–53.
47. Hilkens PHE, Verweij J, Vecht CJ, et al. Clinical characteristics of severe peripheral neuropathy induced by docetaxel (Taxotere). Ann Oncol 1997;8:187–190.
48. New PZ, Jackson CE, Rinaldi D, et al. Peripheral neuropathy secondary to docetaxel (Taxotere). Neurology 1996;46:108–111.
49. Quasthoff S, Hartung HP. Chemotherapy-induced peripheral neuropathy. J Neurol 2002;249:9–17.
50. Freilich RJ, Balmaceda C, Seidman AD, et al. Motor neuropathy due to docetaxel and paclitaxel. Neurology 1996;47:115–118.
51. Noone MH, Fioravanti SG. Taxol: past, present, and future. Oncol Nurs 1994;1:4.
52. Capri G, Munzone E, Trarenzi E, et al. Optic nerve disturbances: a new form of paclitaxel neurotoxicity. J Natl Cancer Inst 1994;86:1099–1101.
53. Perry JR, Warner E. Transient encephalopathy after paclitaxel (Taxol) infusion. Neurology 1996;46:1596–1599.
54. Vahdat L, Papadopoulos K, Lange D, et al. Reduction of paclitaxel-induced peripheral neuropathy with glutamine. Clin Cancer Res 2001;7:1192–1197.
55. Gelmon K, Eisenhauer E, Bryce C, et al. Randomized phase II study of high-dose paclitaxel with or without amifostine in patients with metastatic breast cancer. J Clin Oncol 1999;17:3038–3047.
56. Rubin EH, Anderson JW, Berg DT, et al. Risk factors for high-dose cytarabine neurotoxicity: an analysis of a cancer and leukemia trial of patients with acute myeloid leukemia. J Clin Oncol 1992;10:948–953.
57. Barnett MJ, Richards MA, Ganesan TS, et al. Central nervous system toxicity of high-dose cytosine arabinoside. Semin Oncol 1985;12:571–575.
58. Nand S, Messmore HL, Patel R, et al. Neurotoxicity associated with systemic high-dose cytosine arabinoside. J Clin Oncol 1986;4:571–575.
59. Baker WJ, Royer GL, Weiss RB. Cytarabine and neurologic toxicity. J Clin Oncol 1991;9:679–693.
60. Graves T, Hooks MA. Drug-induced toxicities associated with high-dose cytosine arabinoside infusions. Pharmacotherapy 1989;9:23–28.
61. Chabner VA. Cytatine analogues. In: Chabner BA, Longo DL (eds) Cancer Chemotherapy and Biotherapy. Philadelphia: Lippincott-Raven, 1996:213–233.
62. Nelson RW, Frank JT. Intrathecal methotrexate-induced neurotoxicities. Am J Hosp Pharm 1981;38:65–68.
63. Rubnitz JE, Relling MV, Harrison PL, et al. Transient encephalopathy following high-dose methotrexate treatment in childhood acute lymphoblastic leukemia. Leukemia 1998;12: 1176–1181.
64. Shore T, Barnett MJ, Phillips GL. Sudden neurologic death after intrathecal methotrexate. Med Pediatr Oncol 1990;18:159–161.
65. Lovblad K, Kelkar P, Ozdoba C, et al. Pure methotrexate encephalopathy presenting with seizures: CT and MRI features. Pediatr Radiol 1998;28:86–91.
66. Bernini JC, Fort DW, Griener JC, et al. Aminophylline for methotrexate-induced neurotoxicity. Lancet 1995;345:544–547.
67. Bleyer WA. Neurological sequelae of methotrexate and ionizing radiation: a new classification. Cancer Treat Rep 1981;65(suppl): 89–98.
68. Evans A. Central nervous system workshop. Cancer Clin Trials 1981;4(suppl):31–35.
69. Brown RT, Madan-Swain A, Walco GA, et al. Cognitive and academic late effects among children previously treated for acute lymphocytic leukemia receiving chemotherapy as CNS prophylaxis. J Pediatr Psychol 1998;23:333–340.
70. Kupfer A, Aeschlimann C, Cerny T. Methylene blue and the neurotoxic mechanisms of ifosfamide encephalopathy. Eur J Clin Pharmacol 1996;50:249–252.

71. Kupfer A, Aeschlimann C, Wermuth B, et al. Prophylaxis and reversal of ifosfamide encephalopathy with methylene-blue. Lancet 1994;343:763–764.
72. Merimsky O, Inbar M, Reider-Grosswasser I, et al. Ifosfamide-related acute encephalopathy: clinical and radiological aspects. Eur J Cancer 1991;27:1188–1189.
73. Miller LJ, Eaton VE. Ifosfamide-induced neurotoxicity: a case report and review of the literature. Ann Pharmacother 1992;26:183–187.
74. Cerny T, Kupfer A. The enigma of ifosfamide encephalopathy. Ann Oncol 1992;3:679–681.
75. Patel SR, Forman AD, Benjamin RS. High-dose ifosfamide-induced exacerbation of peripheral neuropathy. J Natl Cancer Inst 1994;86:305–306.
76. Weiss RB. The role of hexamethylmelamine in advanced ovarian carcinoma treatment. Gynecol Oncol 1981;12:141–149.
77. Fike JR, Gobbel GT. Central nervous system radiation injury in large animal models. In: Gutin PH, Leibel SA, Sheline GE (eds) Radiation Injury to the Nervous System. New York: Raven Press, 1991:113–135.
78. Caveness WF, Tanaka A, Hess KH, et al. Delayed brain swelling and functional derangement after X-irradiation of the right visual cortex in the *Macaca mulatta*. Radiat Res 1974;57: 104–120.
79. Young DF, Posner JB, Chu F, et al. Rapid-course radiation therapy of cerebral metastases: results and complications. Cancer (Phila) 1974;34:1069–1076.
80. Jones A. Transient radiation myelopathy (with reference to Lhermitte's sign of electrical paraesthesia). Br J Radiol 1964;37: 727–744.
81. Leibel SA, Sheline GE. Tolerance of the brain and spinal cord to conventional irradiation. In: Gutin PH, Leibel SA, Sheline GE (eds) Radiation Injury to the Nervous System. New York: Raven Press, 1991:239–256.
82. Freeman JE, Johnston PGB, Voke JM. Somnolence after prophylactic cranial irradiation in children with acute lymphoblastic leukaemia. Br Med J 1973;4:523–525.
83. Littman P, Rosenstock J, Gale G, et al. The somnolence syndrome in leukemic children following reduced daily dose fractions of cranial radiation. Int J Radiat Oncol Biol Phys 1979;5:367–371.
84. Boldry E, Sheline GE. Delayed transitory clinical manifestations after radiation treatment of intracranial tumors. Acta Radiol (Ther) 1966;5:5–10.
85. Delattre JY, Rosenblum MK, Thaler HT, et al. A model of radiation myelopathy in the rat. Pathology, regional capillary permeability changes and treatment with dexamethasone. Brain 1988;111:1319–1336.
86. Sheline GE, Wara WM, Smith V. Therapeutic irradiation and brain injury. Int J Radiat Oncol Biol Phys 1980;6:1215–1228.
87. Keime-Guibert F, Napolitano M, Delattre JY. Neurological complications of radiotherapy and chemotherapy. J Neurol 1998;245: 695–708.
88. Burger PC, Boyko OB. The pathology of central nervous system radiation injury. In: Gutin PH, Leibel SA, Sheline GE (eds) Radiation Injury to the Nervous System. New York: Raven Press, 1991:191–208.
89. Crossen JR, Garwood D, Glastein E, Neuwelt EA. Neurobehavioral sequelae of cranial irradiation in adults: a review of radiation-induced encephalopathy. J Clin Oncol 1994;12:627–642.
90. Packer RJ, Mehta M. Neurocognitive sequelae of cancer treatment. Neurology 2002;59:8–10.
91. Silber JH, Radcliffe J, Peckham V, et al. Whole-brain irradiation and decline in intelligence: the influence of dose and age on IQ score. J Clin Oncol 1992;10:1390–1396.
92. Ris MD, Packer R, Goldwein J, et al. Intellectual outcome after reduced-dose radiation therapy plus adjuvant chemotherapy for medulloblastoma. J Clin Oncol 2001;19:3470–3476.
93. Mulhern RK, Ochs J, Kun LE. Changes in intellect associated with cranial radiation therapy. In: Gutin PH, Leibel SA, Sheline GE (eds) Radiation Injury to the Nervous System. New York: Raven Press, 1991:325–340.
94. Caveness WF. Experimental observations: delayed necrosis in normal monkey brain. In: Gilbert HA, Kagen AR (eds) Radiation Damage to the Nervous System. A Delayed Therapeutic Hazard. New York: Raven Press, 1980:1–26.
95. Burger PC, Mahaley MS, Dudka L, et al. The morphologic effects of radiation administered therapeutically for intracranial gliomas: a postmortem study of 25 cases. Cancer (Phila) 1979;44: 1256–1272.
96. Schultheiss TE, Higgins EM, El-Mahdi AM. The latent period in clinical radiation myelopathy. Int J Radiat Oncol Biol Phys 1984;10:1109–1115.
97. St. Clair WH, Arnold SM, Sloan AE, Regine WF. Spinal cord and peripheral nerve injury: current management and investigations. Semin Radiat Oncol 2003;13:322–332.
98. Schultheiss TE, Stephens LC, Peters LJ. Survival in radiation myelopathy. Int J Radiat Oncol Biol Phys 1986;12:1765–1769.
99. Giese WL, Kinsella TJ. Radiation injury to peripheral and cranial nerves. In: Gutin PH, Leibel SA, Sheline GE (eds) Radiation Injury to the Nervous System. New York: Raven Press, 1991:383–403.
100. DeAngelis LM, Shapiro WR. Drug/radiation interactions and central nervous system injury. In: Gutin PH, Leibel SA, Sheline GE (eds) Radiation Injury to the Nervous System. New York: Raven Press, 1991:361–382.
101. Bleyer WA, Griffin TW. White matter necrosis, mineralizing microangiopathy, and intellectual abilities in survivors of childhood leukemia: associations with central nervous system irradiation and methotrexate therapy. In: Gilbert HA, Kagan AR (eds) Radiation Damage to the Nervous System. A Delayed Therapeutic Hazard. New York: Raven Press, 1980:155–174.
102. Rubinstein LJ, Herman MM, Long TF, et al. Disseminated necrotizing leukoencephalopathy: a complication of treated central nervous system leukemia and lymphoma. Cancer (Phila) 1975; 35:291–305.
103. Price RA, Jamieson PA. The central nervous system in childhood leukemia. II. Subacute leukoencephalopathy. Cancer (Phila) 1975;35:306–318.
104. Price RA, Birdwell DA. The central nervous system in childhood leukemia. III. Mineralizing microangiopathy and dystrophic calcification. Cancer (Phila) 1978;42:717–728.
105. Meadows AT, Massari DJ, Fergusson J. Declines in IQ scores and cognitive dysfunctions in children with acute lymphocytic leukaemia treated with cranial irradiation. Lancet 1981;2: 1015–1018.
106. Butler RW, Hill JM, Steinherz PG, et al. Neuropsychologic effects of cranial irradiation, intrathecal methotrexate and systemic methotrexate in childhood cancer. J Clin Oncol 1994;12: 2621–2629.
107. Duffner PK, Cohen ME, Thomas P. Late effects of treatment on the intelligence of children with posterior fossa tumors. Cancer (Phila) 1983;51:233–237.
108. Abrey LE, DeAngelis LM, Yahalom J. Long-term survival in primary CNS lymphoma. J Clin Oncol 1998;16:859–863.
109. DeAngelis LM, Seiferheld W, Schold SC, et al. Combination chemotherapy and radiotherapy for primary central nervous system lymphoma: Radiation Therapy Oncology Group Study 93-10. J Clin Oncol 2002;20:4643–4648.
110. Rodgers J, Marckus R, Kearns P, Windebank K. Attentional ability among survivors of leukaemia treated without cranial irradiation. Arch Dis Child 2003;88:147–150.
111. Riva D, Giorgi C, Nichelli F, et al. Intrathecal methotrexate affects cognitive function in children with medulloblastoma. Neurology 2002;59:48–53.

112. Miettinen S, Laurikainen E, Johansson R, et al. Radiotherapy enhanced ototoxicity of cisplatin in children. Acta Otolaryngol Suppl 1997;529:90–94.
113. Walker DA, Pillow J, Waters KD, et al. Enhanced cis-platinum ototoxicity in children with brain tumors who have received simultaneous or prior cranial irradiation. Med Pediatr Oncol 1989;17:48–52.
114. Huang E, Teh BS, Strother DR, et al. Intensity-modulated radiation therapy for pediatric medulloblastoma: early report on the reduction of ototoxicity. Int J Radiat Oncol Biol Phys 2002;52:599–605.
115. Michalowski AS. On radiation damage to normal tissues and its treatment. II. Anti-inflammatory drugs. Acta Oncol 1994;33: 139–157.
116. Moulder JE. Pharmacological intervention to prevent or ameliorate chronic radiation injuries. Semin Radiat Oncol 2003;13: 73–84.
117. Tada E, Matsumoto K, Kinoshita K, et al. The protective effect of dexamethasone against radiation damage induced by interstitial irradiation in normal monkey brain. Neurosurgery 1997;41: 217–219.
118. Schultheiss TE, Stevens LC. Radiation myelopathy. Am J Neuroradiol 1992;13:1056–1058.
119. Hornsey S, Myers R, Jenkinson T, et al. The reduction of radiation damage to the spinal cord by post-irradiation administration of vasoactive drugs. Int J Radiat Oncol Biol Phys 1990;18: 1437–1442.
120. Glantz MJ, Burger PC, Friedman AH, et al. Treatment of radiation-induced nervous system injury with heparin and warfarin. Neurology 1994;44:2020–2027.
121. Buatti JM, Friedman WA, Theele DP, et al. The lazaroid U74389G protects normal brain from stereotactic radiosurgery-induced radiation injury. Int J Radiat Oncol Biol Phys 1996;34: 591–597.
122. Cross NE, Glantz MJ. Neurologic complications of radiation therapy. Neurol Clin N Am 2003;21:249–277.
123. Di Lorenzo N, Nolletti A, Palma L. Late cerebral radionecrosis. Surg Neurol 1978;10:281–289.
124. Knighton DR, Hunt TK, Schenestuhl H, et al. Oxygen tension regulates the expression of angiogenesis factor by macrophages. Science 1983;221:1283–1289.
125. Marx RE, Ehler WJ, Tayapongsak PT, et al. Relationship of oxygen dose to angiogenesis induction in irradiated tissue. Am J Surg 1990;160:519–524.
126. Calabro F, Jinkins JR. MRI of radiation myelitis: a report of a case treated with hyperbaric oxygen. Eur Radiol 2000;101:1079–1084.
127. Ashamalla HL, Thom SR, Goldwin JW, et al. Hyperbaric oxygen therapy for the treatment of radiation-induced sequelae in children. The University of Pennsylvania experience. Cancer (Phila) 1996;77:2407–2412.
128. Chuba RJ, Aronin P, Bhambhani K, et al. Hyperbaric oxygen therapy for radiation-induced brain injury in children. Cancer (Phila) 1997;80:2005–2012.
129. Bergstrom P, Johnsson A, Begenheim T, et al. Effects of amifostine on cisplatin induced DNA adduct formation and toxicity in malignant glioma and normal tissues in rat. J Neuro-Oncol 1999;42:13–21.
130. Forman A. Peripheral neuropathy. In: Levin VA (ed) Cancer in the Nervous System. New York: Oxford University Press, 2002:397–412.

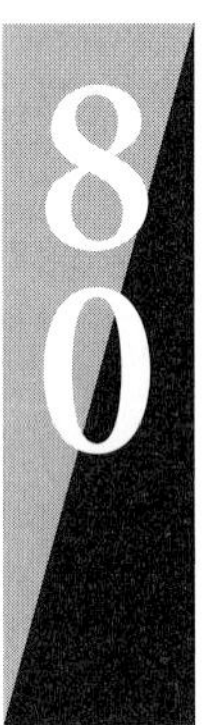

Acute Toxicities of Therapy: Urologic Complications

Sandy Srinivas

Acute urologic complications of therapy could arise from any of the three modalities that are used to treat cancers: surgery, radiation and chemotherapy.

Hemorrhagic Cystitis

Hemorrhagic cystitis is defined as acute, diffuse bladder inflammation and ulceration with hemorrhage. It can be a serious, and sometimes life threatening, complication of a multitude of toxic agents. However, pelvic irradiation for urologic and gynecologic malignancies and treatment with chemotherapeutic agents account for the majority of severe cases of bladder hemorrhage (Table 80.1). The most common class of chemotherapeutic compounds causing hemorrhagic cystitis are the oxazaphosphorine alkylating agents, namely, cyclophosphamide and ifosphamide. Other less common agents are temozolamide, bleomycin, and doxorubicin.[1]

Pathology of Hemorrhagic Cystitis Secondary to Oxazaphosphorine Compounds

The metabolite of oxazaphosphorines responsible for hemorrhagic cystitis (HC) is acrolein, which is excreted by the kidney and becomes highly concentrated in the bladder. It causes edema and hyperemia of the bladder mucosa within 4 hours of administration, with progression to ulceration, exposure, and rupture of the submucosal blood vessels, with bleeding for up to 36 hours after one dose. Despite aggressive therapy, 2% to 4% mortality from severe hemorrhage has been reported.[2]

Healing eventually begins with mucosal hyperplasia, papillary formation, smooth muscle edema and contraction, and fibrosis. With high doses and repeated exposure, bladder damage progresses and becomes irreversible. Patients may develop small, contracted, poorly compliant bladders. Transitional cell carcinoma has also been reported.

The incidence of severe HC is about 6% in patients undergoing bone marrow transplantation and receiving high-dose cyclophosphamide.[3] Ifosphamide has a higher incidence of HC compared to cyclophosphamide, presumably because of the excretion of chloroacetaldehyde.

Incidence and Pathology of Radiation Cystitis

Patients receiving radiation therapy for pelvic malignancies are also at risk for developing HC that may be accompanied by symptoms of dysuria, urgency, and urinary frequency secondary to reduced bladder capacity and compliance. Approximately 20% of patients develop bladder complications.[4] In one study, 9% of patients who received full-dose radiation suffered hemorrhage.[5] Hematuria may develop months to years after treatment and can range from mild and only microscopic to catastrophic. It is often impossible to predict in advance which patients will develop significant complications.

Diagnosis

Patients present with dysuria and urinary frequency. As the hemorrhage increases, patients can develop urinary retention from clot formation and may complain of severe suprapubic and flank pain. Cystoscopy reveals mucosal hyperemia and diffuse bleeding and, in severe cases, ulcerations. In radiation cystitis, the bladder mucosa is pale and studded with telangectatic vessels. Ulcerations may also be present.

Prevention

All attempts must be made to prevent this complication from occurring; this can be accomplished by aggressive hydration and the use of mesna.

Fluids

Hydration with intravenous normal saline at 250 mL/h and furosemide sufficient to maintain urinary output above 150 mL/h was evaluated in a series of 100 consecutive patients undergoing bone marrow transplantation with high-dose cyclophosphamide, and this was found to be very effective in preventing this complication.[6]

Mesna

Mesna is a thiol compound that is rapidly oxidized in plasma to mesna disulfide (dimesna), its major metabolite. Dimesna is hydrophilic and remains in the intravascular compartment and is rapidly eliminated by the kidneys. In the kidney,

TABLE 80.1. Causes of hemorrhagic cystitis.

I. Cytotoxic agents
 Ifosfamide
 Cyclophosphamide
 Temozolomide
 Bleomycin
 Doxorubicin
II. Radiation

dimesna is reduced to the free thiol compound, which reacts chemically with urotoxic ifosfamide metabolites (acrolein and 4-hydroxyifosfamide), resulting in their detoxification.[7]

Mesna has been compared to hydration in preventing HC. In a randomized trial conducted in 100 patients undergoing bone marrow transplantation (BMT), both treatments were equally effective in preventing the incidence of cyclophosphamide-induced hemorrhagic cystitis.[8] The most frequently reported adverse reactions of mesna alone are headache, injection-site reactions, flushing, dizziness, nausea, vomiting, somnolence, diarrhea, anorexia, fever, pharyngitis, hyperesthesia, influenza-like symptoms, and coughing.[9]

Treatment

In addition to aggressive supportive care with hydration, bladder irrigation, saline lavage with clot removal, and transfusion, several intravesical agents have been used in the treatment of HC (Table 80.2).

Intravesicular Treatments

Instillation into the bladder of agents to help control the bleeding locally has been used. The agents most commonly used are formalin and prostaglandins.

Intravesical Formalin

Dewan et al. treated 35 patients who developed HC after radiation with 1% and 4% intravesical formalin.[10] Complete response was achieved in 89% and partial response in 8% after a single instillation. The 1% strength was associated with less morbidity compared to 4% formalin. Vicente et al. reviewed the data on 25 patients treated with intravesical formalin.[11] Hemostasis was obtained in 88% of cases, during a mean of 4 months. Complications included 1 case of vesicorectal fistula, 1 case of ureterohydronephrosis, and 1 case of vesical extravasation of formalin when a concentration of 10% was used. The only complication seen with 4% formalin was 1 case of upper urinary tract dilatation. Donahue and Frank reviewed the literature and reported on 235 patients treated with intravesical formalin.[12] Evaluating the effectiveness, rate of recurrence, and complications of therapy, they concluded that increasing concentrations of formalin improved effectiveness but resulted in higher morbidity.

TABLE 80.2. Treatment of hemorrhagic cystitis.

I. Bladder irrigations
II. Intravesical agents
 Formalin
 Prostaglandins
III. Epsilon-aminocaproic acid
IV. Conjugated estrogens
V. Hyperbaric oxygen

Intravesical Instillation of Prostaglandins

The proposed mechanism of action of prostaglandin E_2 (PGE_2) in controlling HC, is an increase in smooth muscle contractions in mucosal and submucosal blood vessels.[13] Ippoliti et al. reported on 24 patients treated with carboprost, a PGE_2, to determine the optimum intravesical dose and demonstrated a response of 62%, some of which were seen by day 7 at doses greater than 0.8 mg/dL.[14] They concluded that intravesicular carboprost at 1.0 mg/dL every 6 hours for no more than 7 days, was a reasonable choice for the treatment of refractory hemorrhagic cystitis. Levine and colleagues reported on their experience on 18 patients with refractory hemorrhagic cystitis treated with intravesical instillation of 0.4 to 1.0 mg% carboprost for 2 hours four times per day, alternating with continuous saline bladder irrigation for 2 hours.[15] Complete resolution of gross hematuria occurred in 9 patients (50%). Eight patients had a partial response, with decreased transfusion requirements. No changes in renal or bladder function were noted during the mean follow-up of 17 weeks. Side effects were limited to bladder spasm in 14 of the 18 patients (78%), with no systemic complications. Prostaglandin E_1 intravesically has also been used successfully in patients with adenovirus-induced hemorrhagic cystitis, with resolution of the hematuria in 5 of the 6 patients who were treated.[16]

Epsilon-Aminocaproic Acid (EACA)

EACA, an antifibrinolytic agent, has been used in the treatment of hemorrhagic cystitis. A loading dose of 5 g is administered orally or parenterally, followed by 1.0 to 1.25 g hourly to a maximum of 30 g in a 24-hour period. Maximal response was achieved in 8 to 12 hours. Singh et al. treated 37 patients with IV EACA, of whom 34 responded with no major complications.[17] There are other case reports of resolution of hematuria in patients with hemorrhagic cystitis treated with antifibrinolytic therapy.[3,18]

Conjugated Estrogens

Conjugated estrogens at 1 mg/kg, given intravenously, followed by 5 mg/day, has been used in the treatment of HC. Complications, such as thromboembolism and other side effects associated with conjugated estrogen, were not seen.[19] The mechanism of action of conjugated estrogens for the treatment of HC is unclear. It is postulated that estrogens may have an effect on the capillary wall that results in decreased vascular fragility. Miller et al. treated seven patients with conjugated estrogens and reported a response in five patients.[20]

Hyperbaric Oxygen

Hyperbaric oxygen improves angiogenesis and promotes healing in radiation-induced tissues. In general, patients are treated every day in a chamber until hematuria resolves. It appears that the treatment may be more successful when instituted earlier rather than later. Resolution of hematuria occurs in 27% to 92%.[21–23]

Cystoscopies done at resolution of HC demonstrated resolution of the underlying pathology and return to normal

TABLE 80.3. Published data on the treatment of HC.

Author	*Reference*	*Type of intervention*	*No. of patients*	*Type of study*	*Endpoint*	*Results*
Ballen	6	Hyperhydration	100	Phase II	Prevention of HC	7% incidence
Shephard	8	Mesna vs. hyperhydration	100	Randomized	Prevention of hematuria	Incidence of 33% vs. 20% ($P = 0.31$)
Dewan	10	Intravesical formalin	35	Retrospective	Complete resolution of hematuria	89%
Vicente	11	Intravesical formalin	25	Retrospective	Resolution of hematuria	88%
Ippoliti	14	Intravesicular carboprost	24	Prospective	Resolution of hematuria	62%
Levine	15	Intravesicular carboprost	18	Retrospective	Complete resolution of hematuria	50%
Singh	17	Intravenous epsilon-aminocaproic acid	37	Retrospective	Resolution of hematuria	92%
Miller	20	Conjugated estrogens	7	Retrospective	Resolution of hematuria	71%
Del Pizzo	21	Hyperbaric oxygen	11	Retrospective	Complete resolution of symptoms	27%
Lee	22	Hyperbaric oxygen	20	Retrospective	Complete resolution of hematuria	80%
Weiss	23	Hyperbaric oxygen	13	Retrospective	Complete resolution of hematuria	92%

bladder mucosa and function. There were no adverse events referable to the hyperbaric oxygen therapy in these reports. Hyperbaric oxygen therapy appears to be effective, but it is limited to stable patients and those with access to a hyperbaric chamber.

In conclusion, there are several agents available to treat HC (Table 80.3). If these measures fail, some patients are taken to urinary diversion. Because of the rarity of this entity, the therapies that are recommended are based on small series and case reports.

Impotence

Definition

Impotence is defined as the inability to maintain an erection with sufficient rigidity for vaginal penetration half or more of the times attempted.

Patients at Risk

Patients with diabetes mellitus, atherosclerosis, and hypertension are at risk of developing erectile dysfunction. In the field of urologic oncology, impotence is a complication of radical prostatectomy for prostate cancer, cystoprostatectomy for bladder cancer, radiation therapy for prostate cancer, and treatment with hormonal therapy for prostate cancer.

Incidence

In the general population, impotence is related to age. It is estimated that 50% of men over age 50 suffer from some degree of erectile dysfunction, and the incidence increases with age. The incidence with radical prostatectomy and cystoprostatectomy varies from 100% in non-nerve-sparing procedures to 20% with nerve-sparing surgery in young and preoperatively potent men who have organ-confined prostate cancer operated on by experienced surgeons.[24] The onset of impotence with radiation therapy is more gradual than it is with surgery. It is estimated that 60% of men are potent 5 years following external-beam radiation to the prostate. Patients receiving antiandrogen therapy lose libido in addition to erectile dysfunction.

Mechanism of Erection

The mechanism of erection is mediated by both nervous and vascular systems. Sexual stimulation releases nitric oxide (NO) from the nonadrenergic noncholinergic nerve endings and the vascular endothelium of the cavernous tissue in the corpora cavernosa of the penis. NO stimulates guanyl cyclase, which converts guanosine triphosphate (GTP) to cyclic guanosine monophosphate (cGMP). cGMP is a potent smooth muscle relaxant that causes arteriolar dilation and, therefore, penile rigidity. The process of detumescence occurs with the degradation or breakdown of cGMP by the phosphodiesterase 5-enzyme system.

Any condition that interferes with the nerve or vascular supply of the corpora cavernosa will cause impotence. Radical surgery interrupts the nerves to the corpora cavernosa that run very close to the prostate gland, and radiation therapy interferes with both the blood supply and the nerve supply to the penis.

Therapy

Choice of therapy for men rendered impotent by radical surgery depends on the ease of administration of the drug, motivation of the patient and partner, side effects of the

TABLE 80.4. Treatment of impotence.

Oral agents
Sildenafil
Tadalafil
Vardenafil
Yohimbine
Vacuum devices
Intraurethral alprostadil
Intracavernous alprostadil
Other intracavernous injections
Penile prosthesis

agent, and other comorbidities. In general, a step-up approach is used with minimally invasive therapies initially, followed by more-invasive therapies. Oral agents are used as monotherapy first, followed by combination therapy, followed by the use of vacuum devices, intraurethral suppositories, intracorporal injection, then surgical implants as a last resort (Tables 80.4, 80.5).

Oral Agents

Phosphodiesterase 5 inhibitors, sildenafil, tadalafil, and vardenafil, prevent the breakdown of cGMP, which accumulates in the cavernous tissues and causes sustained vasodilation and rigidity. Sildenafil was the first of this class of agents and received the most evaluation. It has been extensively used in postprostatectomy patients with erectile dysfunction. Response appears to be related to the extent to which the neurovascular bundles have been left intact.[25] Men who have had a nerve-sparing prostatectomy respond much better than those whose neurovascular bundles were resected. Zelefsky et al. evaluated the efficacy of sildenafil in 50 patients with erectile dysfunction after radiotherapy.[26] Patients were initially given 50mg sildenafil and instructed to use the medication on at least three occasions and were then contacted to ascertain the efficacy. Significant improvement in the firmness of the erection was reported in 37 patients (74%), and improvement in the durability of the erection was reported in 33 patients (66%). Patients with partial or moderate erectile function before using sildenafil were more likely to benefit from the medication compared with those with absent function.

Weber et al. treated 35 patients after external-beam radiotherapy who had erectile dysfunction, with 100mg sildenafil and reported a 77% success in sexual intercourse.[27] Failure to respond was higher in patients receiving concomitant hormones (50% versus 15%). Rates of success as high as 81% have been reported in the use of sildenafil after brachytherapy-induced erectile dysfunction.[28]

Caution must be exercised in patients with underlying cardiovascular disease and concomitant use of nitrates.[29] Sildenafil is contraindicated in men taking nitrates. In men with preexisting coronary disease, risk of cardiac ischemia during sexual intercourse must be evaluated. The newer agents, tadalafil and vardenafil, may have fewer cardiovascular side effects; however, they have not been as extensively studied as sildenafil.[30,31]

Apomorphine is a selective dopamine receptor agonist that generates an arousal response with penile erection by stimulating the central nervous system (CNS). The U.S. Food and Drug Administration (FDA) has not yet approved it.

Yohimbine is an indolalquinolonic alkaloid that acts centrally by blocking alpha-adrenergic stimulation and enhances cholinergic and dopaminergic stimulation. It is also used as a mydriatic. It increases peripheral blood flow. The usual dose is 6mg three times a day. It may be effective for the treatment of side effects caused by serotonin reuptake blockers.[32] There are several reports on its benefit in men with psychogenic impotence.[33,34] However, results from a randomized placebo-controlled trial showed no significant benefit over placebo.[35] Lebret et al. reported on the combination of yohimbine with L-arginine as being effective in mild to moderate forms of erectile dysfunction.[36]

Vacuum Devices

These devices are the least invasive, most affordable, and safest of the treatment options for erectile dysfunction. Commercially available devices consist of a plastic cylinder that fits over the penis and a vacuum pump that generates negative pressure into the cylinder, drawing blood into the penis and producing an erection. An elastic band slipped around the base of the penis maintains the erection. This method is safe, inexpensive, and reasonably effective; however, it requires partner cooperation and lacks spontaneity.

Intraurethral Alprostadil

The FDA approved intraurethral alprostadil in January 1997. Its success rate is reported to be between 50% and 65%. The dose required to give a good erection is 500 to 1,000μg.[37] The side effects include penile pain and urethral bleeding. The combination of sildenafil and intraurethral alprostadil is more effective than monotherapy.[38,39]

Intracavernous Injection

Prostaglandins are injected into the corpus cavernosum either alone or in combination with papaverine and phentolamine. Prostaglandins are powerful vasodilators, papaverine causes

TABLE 80.5. Drug therapy for impotence.

Author	*Reference*	*Type of intervention*	*No. of patients*	*Type of study*	*Endpoint*	*Results*
Zelefsky	26	Oral sildenafil	50	Prospective	Durability of erection	66%
Weber	27	Oral sildenafil	35	Prospective	Successful intercourse	77%
Brock	31	Oral tadalafil vs. placebo	1,112	Randomized	Improved erections	81% vs. 35% $P = 0.0001$
Kunelius	35	Yohimbine vs. placebo	29	Randomized	Erectile function	44% vs. 34% P = NS

smooth muscle relaxation and vasodilation, and phentolamine causes adrenergic blockade that leads to erection. It is an effective treatment but has less patient desirability because of its invasiveness. Its complications include fibrosis of the cavernous tissues and prolonged erections and priapism.

Penile Implants

These implants are the last resort, offered to patients who have failed less invasive treatments. Penile prostheses are artificial devices implanted within the corpora cavernosa to provide rigidity for penetration and sexual intercourse. An ideal device should be one that is erect only when desired, with few complications or infections, and pain free. There are two types of prostheses: the semirigid and the inflatable. The semirigid type is bendable but remains sufficiently firm in the penis to permit vaginal penetration. The inflatable has a pump placed in the scrotum, which in turn is connected to a reservoir placed in the prevesical space or, alternatively, as part of the pump mechanism in the scrotum. The two cylinders placed in the corpora cavernosa are connected to this mechanism and can be distended ("inflated") with sterile solution from the reservoir by use of the pump. Penile implants are effective but have the disadvantage of requiring a surgical procedure, which, when combined with the price of the prosthesis, is costly. Mechanical failures with the inflatable prosthesis are significant and can occur in 25% of cases.[40] Failures require reoperation, and there is also a 10% incidence of infection.

In conclusion, impotency is very common after treatment of prostate, bladder, and rectal cancer. A variety of treatment options exist. Oral agents are the preferred first choice, and if they fail more invasive options are used.

Chemotherapy-Induced Renal Dysfunction

Nephrotoxicity is an inherent adverse effect of certain anticancer drugs.[41] We discuss here specific syndromes causing renal failure by chemotherapeutic agents and their management (Tables 80.6 and 80.7).

Renal dysfunction in patients with cancer results from the following three causes:

Prerenal causes: hypoperfusion
Renal causes: Hypoperfusion; exposure to nephrotoxins; renotubular precipitation of compounds; renovascular damage; tubulointerstitial damage

TABLE 80.6. Chemotherapy agents causing renal dysfunction.

Drug	*Class*	*Mechanism*
Carmustine	Alkylator	Glomerular sclerosis
Cisplatin	Alkylator	Tubulointerstitial damage
Cyclophosphamide	Alkylator	Distal tubular damage
Ifosfamide	Alkylator	Proximal tubular damage
Interferon-α	Immunomodulator	ATN
IL-2	Immunomodulator	Hypoperfusion
Lomustine	Alkylator	Glomerular sclerosis
Methotrexate	Antimetabolite	Intratubular deposition
Mitomycin C	Antibiotic	Microangiopathic changes
Pentostatin	Antimetabolite	ATN
Streptozocin	Alkylator	Proximal tubular damage

ATN, acute tubular necrosis.

Postrenal causes: Urinary obstruction
Factors potentiating renal dysfunction include age, nutritional status, intravascular volume depletion, preexisting renal dysfunction, and concomitant use of other nephrotoxic drugs.

Cisplatin-Induced Renal Insufficiency

Cisplatin, one of the most effective chemotherapeutic agents, is associated with nephrotoxicity. Its effect is dose related and cumulative and can result in renal dysfunction in about 20% to 25% of patients. The toxicity is manifested by a decrease in the glomerular filtration rate and clinically, by an increase in serum creatine and a fall in the creatinine clearance. It affects the proximal and distal renal tubules and the collecting duct. Tubular damage results in a salt-wasting syndrome that resolves with time.

Prevention

There is evidence that the nephrotoxicity of cisplatin can be diminished by vigorous hydration with infusion of isotonic saline at 250 mL/h. Hydration reduces cisplatin concentration and the contact time with the tubular epithelium.

Amifostine

Amifostine is an aminothiol that improves renal tolerance to cisplatin.[42] Studies in both ovarian and non-small cell lung cancer have shown lack of interference with chemotherapy

TABLE 80.7. Drug therapy for chemotherapy-induced renal dysfunction.

Author	*Reference*	*Type of intervention*	*No. of patients*	*Type of study*	*Endpoint*	*Results*
Kemp	60	Cisplatin, cyclophosphamide ± IV amifostine	242	Phase III randomized	Renal dysfunction	40% reduction in creatine clearance in untreated group $P = 0.001$
Bosly	53	Rasburicase 0.2 mg/kg IV days 1–7	280	Prospective	Decrease in serum uric acid	100% reduction in uric acid
Saito	61	V2 arginine vasopeptide antagonist	11	Case series	Increase in serum sodium	100%

TABLE 80.8. Dose modification for renal dysfunction.

Drugs	*Greater than 60 mL/min*	*301–60 mL/min*	*Less than 30 mL/min*
Bleomycin	100%	75%	75%
Methotrexate	100%	50%	Omit
Cisplatin	100%	50%	Omit
Cyclophosphamide	100%	50%	Omit
Mitomycin C	100%	75%	Omit
Nitrosourea	100%	75%	50%

efficacy. Amifostine, unfortunately, has several side effects, such as hypotension, nausea, and vomiting, limiting its use.

Acute Capillary Leak Syndrome

This syndrome is characterized by episodes of hypotension with hemoconcentration and hypoproteinemia. It is caused by unexplained episodic capillary hyperpermeabilty that results in fluid and protein shift from the intravascular to the interstitial space, resulting in generalized edema, shock, and renal failure. This syndrome has most commonly been described with interleukin 2 (IL-2) therapy.[43]

Hemolytic Uremic Syndrome

Definition

Hemolytic uremic syndrome (HUS) is a multisystem disorder characterized by thrombocytopenia, microangiopathic hemolytic anemia, renal failure, and ischemic manifestations, resulting from platelet agglutination in the arterial microvasculature.

Etiology

Initially described as an association with mucinous adenocarcinomas, HUS is now known to occur as an acute complication of chemotherapy. The drugs most commonly associated with this are mitomycin C and cisplatin with or without bleomycin. The risk of developing HUS with mitomycin C is about 4% to 15%.[44] Newer agents, such as gemcitabine and biologic agents, such as interferon-α have been reported to be causative agents as well.[45,46]

Diagnosis

Patients typically present with microangiopathic hemolytic anemia, thrombocytopenia, and acute renal failure. The onset of HUS can be delayed, usually occurring months after discontinuing chemotherapy.

Management

Before the introduction of plasma exchange, the mortality associated with this disease was greater than 90%. The indication of plasmapheresis is based on case series without a control group, experimental results, case reports, and pathophysiologic reasoning.[47] Plasma exchange with fresh frozen plasma (FFP) appears to be superior to plasma transfusion in the management of HUS, resulting in significant reduction in mortality. The prognosis is dependent on the severity of symptoms, but most patients respond to immunoadsorption and plasma exchange with FFP.[48]

Tumor Lysis Syndrome

Definition

Acute tumor lysis syndrome (ATLS) is a metabolic derangement with hyperuricemia, hyperphosphatemia, hyperkalemia, and hypocalcemia associated with lymphoproliferative malignancies with a high cell turnover. It is characterized by the increased release of intracellular contents (uric acid, potassium, phosphorus) into the extracellular compartment, overwhelming the body's capacity for clearance.

Etiology

Although initially reported with hematologic malignancies, ATLS is now reported with many solid tumors, including small cell, breast cancer, metastatic melanoma, and ovarian cancer.[49–51]

Incidence

In a report by Hande et al., the incidence in non-Hodgkin's lymphoma of laboratory tumor lysis was 42% and clinical tumor lysis was 6%.[52] Clinical tumor lysis occurred more frequently in patients with pretreatment renal insufficiency and high pretreatment serum lactate dehydrogenase (LDH). Additional findings of hyperkalemia, hyperphosphatemia, hypocalcemia, and increased serum LDH were reported in more than 75% of patients.[50]

Diagnosis

The tumor lysis syndrome should be suspected in patients with a large tumor burden who develop acute renal failure in the presence of marked hyperuricemia greater than 15 mg/dL and/or hyperphosphatemia greater than 8 mg/dL.

Management

Management of ATLS includes prophylaxis, prevention, and treatment. Before the start of chemotherapy, patients with bulky tumors should receive aggressive hydration, alkalinization of the urine, diuretics, and the reduction of uric acid levels using allopurinol or urate oxidase. Allopurinol inhibits xanthine oxidase, an enzyme that catalyzes the conversion of hypoxanthine and xanthine to uric acid.

Rasburicase, a recombinant urate oxidase that converts uric acid (UA) into the soluble compound allantoin, has been shown to control hyperuricemia faster and more reliably than allopurinol. At a dose of 0.20 mg/kg, administered intravenously once a day for 1 to 7 days, rasburicase decreased uric acid levels in 100% of patients and was safe in the treatment of hyperuricemia in adults and children.[53]

A randomized trial comparing allopurinol to rasburicase in children with leukemia or lymphoma has been reported.[54] Fifty-two patients were randomized to either rasburicase or allopurinol, and in 4 hours after the first dose, patients randomized to rasburicase compared to allopurinol, achieved an 86% versus 12% reduction of initial plasma uric acid levels.

An entity called spontaneous tumor lysis exists and occurs in patients with cancers before initiation of chemotherapy. It has been described with leukemias and lymphomas and also with breast cancer.[55] An important distinction between spontaneous tumor lysis and that occurring after therapy is the lack of hyperphosphatemia in the spontaneous form.

Syndrome of Inappropriate Antidiuretic Hormone Secretion

Definition

The syndrome of inappropriate antidiuretic hormone secretion (SIADH) represents a constellation of laboratory findings of hyponatremia, hypoosmolality, inappropriately elevated urine osmolality, a urine sodium concentration that is usually above 40 mEq/L, normal acid–base and potassium balance, and a low plasma uric acid concentration, in the absence of hypothyroidism and normal adrenal function.

Etiology

SIADH is most often seen in small cell lung cancer. It can be a complication following chemotherapy. High-dose cyclophosphamide, vinca alkaloids, and cisplatin are the most common agents associated with this syndrome. Vinorelbine, thiotepa, and chlorambucil have also been implicated.[56–58]

Treatment

In the absence of neurologic symptoms, all that is needed is water restriction. Salt administration is done in resistant hyponatremic and symptomatic patients. A loop diuretic may be added to enhance the effect of saline administration. Therapeutic agents, such as democlocycline, lithium, and V_2 receptor antagonist, are sometimes used to treat this entity.

Nonpeptide vasopressin V_2 receptor antagonists represents a promising treatment option to directly antagonize the effects of elevated plasma arginine vasopressin (AVP) concentrations by increasing the water permeability of renal collecting tubules, thereby promoting excretion of retained water and normalizing hypoosmolar hyponatremia. This treatment may be of benefit in patients with congestive heart failure and cirrhosis.[59]

In conclusion, chemotherapeutic agents can result in renal dysfunction and specific syndromes that have been well described. Awareness and best supportive care is essential in managing these patients.

References

1. Islam R, Isaacson BJ, Zickerman PM, Ratanawong C, Tipping SJ. Hemorrhagic cystitis as an unexpected adverse reaction to temozolomide: case report. Am J Clin Oncol 2002;25:513–514.
2. Ilhan O, Koc H, Akan H, et al. Hemorrhagic cystitis as a complication of bone marrow transplantation. J Chemother 1997;9:56–61.
3. Aroney RS, Dalley DN, Levi JA. Haemorrhagic cystitis treated with epsilon-aminocaproic acid. Med J Aust 1980;2:92.
4. Dean RJ, Lytton B. Urologic complications of pelvic irradiation. J Urol 1978;119:64–67.
5. Ram MD. Complications of radiotherapy for carcinoma of the bladder. Proc R Soc Med 1970;63:93–95.
6. Ballen KK, Becker P, Levebvre K, et al. Safety and cost of hyperhydration for the prevention of hemorrhagic cystitis in bone marrow transplant recipients. Oncology 1999;57:287–292.
7. Goren MP, McKenna LM, Goodman TL. Combined intravenous and oral mesna in outpatients treated with ifosfamide. Cancer Chemother Pharmacol 1997;40:371–375.
8. Shepherd JD, Pringle LE, Barnett MJ, Klingemann HG, Reece DE, Phillips GL. Mesna versus hyperhydration for the prevention of cyclophosphamide-induced hemorrhagic cystitis in bone marrow transplantation. J Clin Oncol 1991;9:2016–2020.
9. Cohen MH, Dagher R, Griebel DJ, et al. U.S. Food and Drug Administration drug approval summaries: imatinib mesylate, mesna tablets, and zoledronic acid. Oncologist 2002;7:393–400.
10. Dewan AK, Mohan GM, Ravi R. Intravesical formalin for hemorrhagic cystitis following irradiation of cancer of the cervix. Int J Gynaecol Obstet 1993;42:131–135.
11. Vicente J, Rios G, Caffaratti J. Intravesical formalin for the treatment of massive hemorrhagic cystitis: retrospective review of 25 cases. Eur Urol 1990;18:204–206.
12. Donahue LA, Frank IN. Intravesical formalin for hemorrhagic cystitis: analysis of therapy. J Urol 1989;141:809–812.
13. Levine LA, Kranc DM. Evaluation of carboprost tromethamine in the treatment of cyclophosphamide-induced hemorrhagic cystitis. Cancer (Phila) 1990;66:242–245.
14. Ippoliti C, Przepiorka D, Mehra R, et al. Intravesicular carboprost for the treatment of hemorrhagic cystitis after marrow transplantation. Urology 1995;46:811–815.
15. Levine LA, Jarrard DF. Treatment of cyclophosphamide-induced hemorrhagic cystitis with intravesical carboprost tromethamine. J Urol 1993;149:719–723.
16. Trigg ME, O'Reilly J, Rumelhart S, Morgan D, Holida M, de Alarcon P. Prostaglandin E1 bladder instillations to control severe hemorrhagic cystitis. J Urol 1990;143:92–94.
17. Singh I, Laungani GB. Intravesical epsilon aminocaproic acid in management of intractable bladder hemorrhage. Urology 1992;40:227–229.
18. Lakhani A, Raptis A, Frame D, et al. Intravesicular instillation of E-aminocaproic acid for patients with adenovirus-induced hemorrhagic cystitis. Bone Marrow Transplant 1999;24:1259–1260.
19. Liu YK, Harty JI, Steinbock GS, Holt HA Jr, Goldstein DH, Amin M. Treatment of radiation or cyclophosphamide induced hemorrhagic cystitis using conjugated estrogen. J Urol 1990;144:41–43.
20. Miller J, Burfield GD, Moretti KL. Oral conjugated estrogen therapy for treatment of hemorrhagic cystitis. J Urol 1994;151:1348–1350.
21. Del Pizzo JJ, Chew BH, Jacobs SC, Sklar GN. Treatment of radiation induced hemorrhagic cystitis with hyperbaric oxygen: long-term follow-up. J Urol 1998;160:731–733.
22. Lee HC, Liu CS, Chiao C, Lin SN. Hyperbaric oxygen therapy in hemorrhagic radiation cystitis: a report of 20 cases. Undersea Hyper Med 1994;21:321–327.
23. Weiss JP, Mattei DM, Neville EC, Hanno PM. Primary treatment of radiation-induced hemorrhagic cystitis with hyperbaric oxygen: 10-year experience. J Urol 1994;151:1514–1517.
24. McCullough AR. Prevention and management of erectile dysfunction following radical prostatectomy. Urol Clin N Am 2001;28:613–627.
25. Zippe CD, Jhaveri FM, Klein EA, et al. Role of Viagra after radical prostatectomy. Urology 2000;55:241–245.
26. Zelefsky MJ, McKee AB, Lee H, Leibel SA. Efficacy of oral sildenafil in patients with erectile dysfunction after radiotherapy for carcinoma of the prostate. Urology 1999;53:775–778.
27. Weber DC, Bieri S, Kurtz JM, Miralbell R. Prospective pilot study of sildenafil for treatment of postradiotherapy erectile dysfunction in patients with prostate cancer. J Clin Oncol 1999;17:3444–3449.
28. Merrick GS, Butler WM, Lief JH, Stipetich RL, Abel LJ, Dorsey AT. Efficacy of sildenafil citrate in prostate brachytherapy patients with erectile dysfunction. Urology 1999;53:1112–1116.

29. Cheitlin MD, Hutter AM Jr, Brindis RG, et al. Use of sildenafil (Viagra) in patients with cardiovascular disease. Technology and Practice Executive Committee. Circulation 1999;99:168–177.
30. Thadani U, Smith W, Nash S, et al. The effect of vardenafil, a potent and highly selective phosphodiesterase-5 inhibitor for the treatment of erectile dysfunction, on the cardiovascular response to exercise in patients with coronary artery disease. J Am Coll Cardiol 2002;40:2006–2012.
31. Brock GB, McMahon CG, Chen KK, et al. Efficacy and safety of tadalafil for the treatment of erectile dysfunction: results of integrated analyses. J Urol 2002;168:1332–1336.
32. Hollander E, McCarley A. Yohimbine treatment of sexual side effects induced by serotonin reuptake blockers. J Clin Psychiatry 1992;53:207–209.
33. Montorsi F, Strambi LF, Guazzoni G, et al. Effect of yohimbine-trazodone on psychogenic impotence: a randomized, double-blind, placebo-controlled study. Urology 1994;44:732–736.
34. Susset JG, Tessier CD, Wincze J, Bansal S, Malhotra C, Schwacha MG. Effect of yohimbine hydrochloride on erectile impotence: a double-blind study. J Urol 1989;141:1360–1363.
35. Kunelius P, Hakkinen J, Lukkarinen O. Is high-dose yohimbine hydrochloride effective in the treatment of mixed-type impotence? A prospective, randomized, controlled double-blind crossover study. Urology 1997;49:441–414.
36. Lebret T, Herve JM, Gorny P, Worcel M, Botto H. Efficacy and safety of a novel combination of L-arginine glutamate and yohimbine hydrochloride: a new oral therapy for erectile dysfunction. Eur Urol 2002;41:608–613; discussion 613.
37. Guay AT, Perez JB, Velasquez E, Newton RA, Jacobson JP. Clinical experience with intraurethral alprostadil (MUSE) in the treatment of men with erectile dysfunction. A retrospective study. Medicated urethral system for erection. Eur Urol 2000;38:671–676.
38. Mydlo JH, Volpe MA, MacChia RJ. Results from different patient populations using combined therapy with alprostadil and sildenafil: predictors of satisfaction. BJU Int 2000;86:469–473.
39. Mydlo JH, Volpe MA, Macchia RJ. Initial results utilizing combination therapy for patients with a suboptimal response to either alprostadil or sildenafil monotherapy. Eur Urol 2000;38:30–34.
40. Merrill DC. Clinical experience with Scott inflatable penile prosthesis in 150 patients. Urology 1983;22:371–375.
41. Kintzel PE. Anticancer drug-induced kidney disorders. Drug Saf 2001;24:19–38.
42. Glover D, Glick JH, Weiler C, Fox K, Turrisi A, Kligerman MM. Phase I/II trials of WR-2721 and cis-platinum. Int J Radiat Oncol Biol Phys 1986;12:1509–1512.
43. Castro MP, VanAuken J, Spencer-Cisek P, Legha S, Sponzo RW. Acute tumor lysis syndrome associated with concurrent biochemotherapy of metastatic melanoma: a case report and review of the literature. Cancer (Phila) 1999;85:1055–1059.
44. Lesesne JB, Rothschild N, Erickson B, et al. Cancer-associated hemolytic-uremic syndrome: analysis of 85 cases from a national registry. J Clin Oncol 1989;7:781–789.
45. Walter RB, Joerger M, Pestalozzi BC. Gemcitabine-associated hemolytic-uremic syndrome. Am J Kidney Dis 2002;40:E16.
46. Al-Zahrani H, Gupta V, Minden MD, Messner HA, Lipton JH. Vascular events associated with alpha interferon therapy. Leuk Lymphoma 2003;44:471–475.
47. von Baeyer H. Plasmapheresis in thrombotic microangiopathy-associated syndromes: review of outcome data derived from clinical trials and open studies. Ther Apher 2002;6:320–328.
48. Kaplan AA. Therapeutic apheresis for cancer related hemolytic uremic syndrome. Ther Apher 2000;4:201–206.
49. Bilgrami SF, Fallon BG. Tumor lysis syndrome after combination chemotherapy for ovarian cancer. Med Pediatr Oncol 1993;21:521–524.
50. Kalemkerian GP, Darwish B, Varterasian ML. Tumor lysis syndrome in small cell carcinoma and other solid tumors. Am J Med 1997;103:363–367.
51. Drakos P, Bar-Ziv J, Catane R. Tumor lysis syndrome in nonhematologic malignancies. Report of a case and review of the literature. Am J Clin Oncol 1994;17:502–505.
52. Hande KR, Garrow GC. Acute tumor lysis syndrome in patients with high-grade non-Hodgkin's lymphoma. Am J Med 1993;94:133–139.
53. Bosly A, Sonet A, Pinkerton CR, et al. Rasburicase (recombinant urate oxidase) for the management of hyperuricemia in patients with cancer: report of an international compassionate use study. Cancer (Phila) 2003;98:1048–1054.
54. Goldman SC, Holcenberg JS, Finklestein JZ, et al. A randomized comparison between rasburicase and allopurinol in children with lymphoma or leukemia at high risk for tumor lysis. Blood 2001;97:2998–3003.
55. Sklarin NT, Markham M. Spontaneous recurrent tumor lysis syndrome in breast cancer. Am J Clin Oncol 1995;18:71–73.
56. Garrett CA, Simpson TA Jr. Syndrome of inappropriate antidiuretic hormone associated with vinorelbine therapy. Ann Pharmacother 1998;32:1306–1309.
57. Sica S, Cicconi S, Sora F, et al. Inappropriate antidiuretic hormone secretion after high-dose thiotepa. Bone Marrow Transplant 1999;24:571–572.
58. Wagner AM, Brunet S, Puig J, Ortega E, Subira M, Puig M. Chlorambucil-induced inappropriate antidiuresis in a man with chronic lymphocytic leukemia. Ann Hematol 1999;78:37–38.
59. Palm C, Reimann D, Gross P. The role of V2 vasopressin antagonists in hyponatremia. Cardiovasc Res 2001;51:403–408.
60. Kemp G, Rose P, Lurain J, et al. Amifostine pretreatment for protection against cyclophosphamide-induced and cisplatin-induced toxicities: results of a randomized control trial in patients with advanced ovarian cancer. J Clin Oncol 1996;14:2101–2112.
61. Saito T, Ishikawa S, Abe K, et al. Acute aquaresis by the nonpeptide arginine vasopressin (AVP) antagonist OPC-31260 improves hyponatremia in patients with syndrome of inappropriate secretion of antidiuretic hormone (SIADH). J Clin Endocrinol Metab 1997;82:1054–1057.

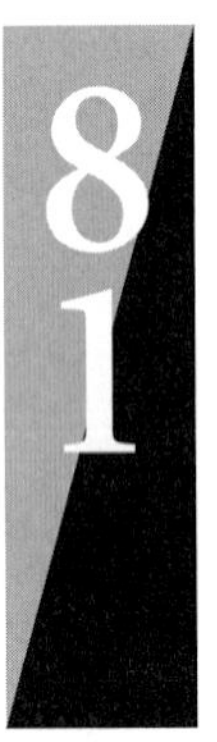

Issues in Vascular Access with Special Emphasis on the Cancer Patient

Paul F. Mansfield and David L. Smith

Vascular Access in the Cancer Patient

The management of the cancer patient is often complex and involves multiple disciplines. The complexity of the care that is required often necessitates venous access for the administration of myriad therapies and the acquisition of blood samples. Reliable venous access is critical for the optimal management of the many aspects of care of a patient with cancer. Although the exact number of catheters inserted annually in the United States for care of cancer patients is unknown, it is likely that it represents a significant percentage of the more than 5 million central venous catheters placed.[1]

Many chemotherapeutic agents require prolonged venous access for continuous infusion, which may last several days, and a full course of treatment may last a year or more. Critically ill patients may require monitoring of central venous pressure or central access for administration of vasoactive agents. In addition, maintaining adequate nutrition in the cancer patient is often a difficult issue. Although the use of total parenteral nutrition (TPN) in the cancer patient may be controversial, we generally believe it is a reasonable option in the patient actively undergoing therapy. Although the alimentary tract is always the preferred route of feeding in patients, in the cancer patient, TPN is often necessary, because the gastrointestinal side effects of chemotherapeutic agents can be severe, and complications of surgery may render the gastrointestinal tract unusable for various periods of time. The selection of patients for the use of TPN is a complex one that requires careful consideration of the patient's treatment, the response of the malignancy to therapy and physical factors, and in some rare circumstances, such as appendiceal cancer, a patient may live for several years on TPN. TPN, vesicant or protracted infusion chemotherapy, or central pressure monitoring and resuscitation, all require consistent and durable access to the central venous system.

Peripheral venous access is not often reliable or available for long in cancer patients. Some patients simply have very poor peripheral veins to start with, whereas others lose their venous access from repeated use and caustic agents. The multiple episodes of venipuncture for blood draws and administration of medications and fluids often result in sclerosis of the vessels. In a randomized trial between peripherally inserted central catheters (PICC) and peripheral IVs for the postoperative management of pediatric patients, Schwengel et al. found, not surprisingly, that there were fewer venipunctures in the PICC group and that both patient and parent satisfaction were higher in the PICC group (P less than 0.05).[2] Major complications were rare in both groups but minor ones were common in the IV group. The authors advocated the use of PICC lines whenever postoperative hospitalization was anticipated to last 4 or more days.

In general, the choice of peripheral venous access versus central venous access is determined by the following factors: the nature of the planned therapy, the length of time of administration, the number of agents and the nature of their compatibilities, the patients' desire for a particular type of access, which may be based on lifestyle, and the status of the patients' peripheral venous system versus their central venous system. Patients with multiple prior central venous catheters may require investigation of the patency of the central vasculature as a part of their assessment. Peripheral access is certainly appropriate in a patient with excellent peripheral veins requiring a short-term course of therapy or a weekly infusion with nonsclerosing agents.

Catheter Types

We initially globally review some of the various issues of access and then examine studies that address the major issues which apply to all access approaches, specifically, those related to the insertion, and then the complications of thrombosis and infection. There are many venous access devices available, which have been designed to fit pediatric and adult patients with various body types and various clinical scenarios. The catheters are also designed to accommodate infusions at different rates, allow for blood draws, accommodate patients' daily activities, and, more recently, to withstand the pressures of bolus infusions for radiographic imaging. The types of central venous catheters can be divided in several different ways:

- External versus implanted
- Tunneled versus nontunneled
- Peripheral versus central
- Single lumen versus multilumen
- Untreated versus antibiotic-coated or antibiotic-impregnated

Each of these choices has specific benefits and downsides, and there are also some unusual situations that can arise in the patient who has lost the use of the major venous branches feeding into the superior vena cava. The common approaches to central access are via the subclavian, jugular, or femoral approaches. In addition, some of the most difficult access cases may require direct inferior vena cava (IVC) puncture through a translumbar or a transhepatic approach, or through the azygous system or directly into the right atrium (RA) via thoracotomy.

Devices that have an external component have a higher risk of infection than totally implanted ones but can be inserted or exchanged more easily. This higher rate of infection comes from two potential sources: first, from the repeated manipulation and accessing of the hub of the catheter, and second, from the area where the catheter transits the skin. Implanted ports require flushing with heparin for thrombosis prevention only once a month, whereas external devices generally are flushed once a day. The implanted port has a silicon diaphragm that can sustain repeated penetrations by an offset (Huber) needle. One should never use a standard needle for accessing these devices. For an active person who likes to participate in water sports, an implanted port may be better. However, if a patient is facing a bone marrow or stem cell transplant, a percutaneous catheter may be a better choice, as one can exchange the catheter over a wire and not lose access if a catheter-related bloodstream infection (CRBSI) is suspected. Implanted ports are usually placed in the operating room, and patients may require a trip back to the operating room for removal, both with obviously added expense. If frequent, repeated, and prolonged instrumentation of the port is anticipated, this may increase the risk of infection. There has never been a prospective randomized trial of implanted ports versus percutaneous catheters, and thus, the decisions are often based on patient and local clinical practice patterns.

External catheters may be tunneled (usually with a cuff) or percutaneous. Cuffed catheters are designed to be tunneled, with the cuff in a subcutaneous position. The cuff encourages significant fibrosis in the surrounding tissue. This fibrotic rim of tissues provides a mechanical barrier to pathogens, which can gain access via the external components of the device. In a small prospective randomized trial of cuffed versus noncuffed catheters, Flowers et al. found a significant reduction in both the rate of colonization (34.5% to 7.7%) and that of CRBSI (13.8% to 0%).[3] One of the major problems with this study is that most of the infections were fungal, as an antibacterial (not fungicidal) ointment was used for dressings. Tunneled catheters may have a lower rate of infection than percutaneous catheters, but in patient populations where intense education and training in catheter care are performed, the rates are similar. One area where this may not be accurate was revealed in a randomized trial of tunneled versus nontunneled femoral catheters by Timsit et al.[4] In a study of 336 evaluable intensive care unit (ICU) patients, they found probable systemic catheter-related sepsis occurred in 15 of 168 nontunneled catheters and 5 of 168 tunneled catheters (*P* less than 0.025). The relative risk of actual CRBSI in the tunneled group was 0.28 [confidence interval (CI), 0.03 to 0.72; *P* = 0.005]. Whether this approach would also benefit sites with lower general risk of infection, such as the subclavian approach, is unknown. Cuffed, tunneled catheters are usually placed in the operating room or interventional radiology, whereas percutaneous ones may be placed at the patient bedside. It should be noted that both implanted catheters and implanted ports should be placed with fluoroscopic guidance. Similar to implanted ports, if a catheter-related infection is suspected, a cuffed or tunneled catheter generally cannot be exchanged over a wire as can a percutaneous catheter, as we do for suspected CRBSI. This approach was endorsed in a small prospective (and partially randomized) trial by Michel et al., in which they found fewer insertion problems in the exchange group, when compared with the new insertion group and no difference in infection rates.[5]

Peripherally inserted catheters generally eliminate the risk of puncture of the lung, or arterial or nerve structures, during insertion, but carry a 15% incidence of thrombophlebitis. In our experience, in 3% of patients this is severe enough to necessitate removal. Centrally inserted catheters also have the risk of puncture (or less frequently, laceration) of the subclavian artery or injury to nerves (brachial plexus, phrenic, and vagus have all been reported) or the thoracic duct. These concerns are discussed in more detail next.

Single-lumen catheters are used for the simplest of therapies, such as antibiotic therapy or single-agent chemotherapy. Multilumen catheters (two or three) are used for more complex therapies, particularly when there are problems of compatibility. When there is a choice about the number of lumens that will be necessary, it is generally considered best to use the fewest lumens (which is generally a reflection of catheter diameter and has been associated with increased risk of thrombosis).[6] Farkas et al. conducted a randomized trial of single- versus triple-lumen catheters.[7] They found it was much more likely that patients with a single-lumen catheter would need additional peripheral access (25/68 versus 1/61, respectively; *P* less than 0.001). However, they found no difference in the incidence of catheter-related sepsis. In contrast, Clark-Christoff et al. randomized 204 patients to either a single- or double-lumen catheter, and found a substantial increase in the incidence of catheter-related sepsis when using the triple-lumen catheter, compared with a single-lumen catheter [2/78 (3%) versus 13/99 (13%); *P* less than 0.01].[8] Ma et al. found no difference among single-, double-, and triple-lumen catheters used to administer TPN.[9] Implanted ports and tunneled catheters also come as single- or double-lumen constructions. In this chapter, we examine the common complications of central venous catheters and ways to prevent or treat them or minimize their risk: these include (1) risks of insertion, (2) infection, and (3) thrombosis.

Site Selection

The first issue with central venous access is to determine the site of placement. We find the subclavian approach to be the best for long-term access; however, other sites may have specific advantages and disadvantages. Ruesch et al. conducted a systematic review of internal jugular (IJ) versus subclavian approaches in 17 prospective randomized trials (comprising more than 4,500 patients).[10] They found there were more arterial punctures in the IJ group (3.0% versus 0.5%) but more malpositioned catheters with the subclavian approach (5.3% versus 9.3%). In our own experience, from a prospective trial of more than 800 subclavian catheters alone, the risk of arterial puncture occurred in approximately 3% of patients and the risk of malposition was about 4%.[11] The authors found the risk of CRBSI was roughly twice as high with the IJ approach compared to the subclavian (8.3% versus 4.0%). Curiously, in this study the risk of hemothorax or pneumothorax was nearly the same, at 1.3% versus 1.5%, whereas the rate of pneumothorax is generally assumed to be lower with the jugular approach. Martin et al. conducted a comparative, nonrandomized trial of IJ compared with subclavian catheters, and found no difference in a series of 141 patient (catheter-related infection, 8.1% for subclavian and 7.6 for IJ, respectively).[12] Merrer et al. conducted a randomized trial of femoral and subclavian approaches for central access in eight ICUs across France.[13] They examined mechanical, infectious, and thrombotic complications in 289 patients. Overall infection rates were 19.8% in the femoral group and 4.5% in the subclavian group (P less than 0.001); however, the risk of sepsis was 4.4% versus 1.5% ($P = 0.07$). The risk of thrombotic complications was 21.5% and 1.9%, respectively. Complete thrombosis of the vessel occurred in 6% of the femoral approach and none of the subclavian group ($P = 0.01$). Although this study underscores the increased thrombotic and infectious risks with the femoral approach, there are still occasions (such as the coagulopathic patient) where this approach is necessary. As in all of medicine, it is a weighing of the relative risks and benefits.

Insertion Technique

Once a decision is made to place a central venous catheter, there are some specific and general considerations. In general, implanted ports and catheters (tunneled) should be placed in the operating room (for maximal sterility) with fluoroscopic assistance. Several authors have examined the role of sterile barriers. Hu et al. conducted a systematic review of the use of maximal sterile barriers and found three primary research studies.[14] Although each study seemed to support the use of the barriers and gowns, the authors seemed lukewarm in their endorsement of the approach. In a prospective randomized trial from our institution, Raad et al. found a significant reduction in catheter-related infections when using the barriers, and following patients for up to 3 months (4/176 test group versus 12/167 in the control group; $P = 0.03$).[15] This was a controlled population of cancer patients; however, anyone who has placed a central venous catheter recognizes the ease with which the wire may easily brush against a forearm or nonsterile sheet if the whole site is not protected. Different institutions handle patient education in different ways, from minimal or none to extensive programs. For external devices, intensive training of patients and their caregivers can dramatically decrease the incidence of infection. In preparation for placement of the venous access device, the patient and a caregiver should be instructed on the placement and long-term care of the device. This procedure allows the patient an opportunity to determine what lifestyle changes may be necessary as well as which device would be best suited to the patient. At University of Texas M.D. Anderson Cancer Center, the patients are shown a detailed video regarding implantation and care of the device. Patients and their caregivers (typically the spouse or other family member) also receive personal detailed instruction in the care of the catheter and must even pass a test, demonstrating competency.

Before arriving for line placement, patients should be assessed for the appropriate form of access to be used. This assessment includes an evaluation of the coagulation profile [prothrombin time (PT) and platelet count] as well as the intended use of the catheter. Table 81.1 is a copy of the guidelines used at M.D. Anderson Cancer Center for the management of various coagulation situations one may encounter. These may seem a bit liberal for some but have proved to be quite safe in a setting where more than 6,000 subclavian insertions are performed annually. If a patient's coagulation profile cannot be corrected, a safer alternative, such as a jugular or femoral approach, where pressure can be applied directly, may be used. After a detailed history, including number of previous catheters or attempts and prior operations, such as axillary or neck dissection, has been obtained, a physical examination is performed and a suitable site is selected. The factors important in this decision include anatomic factors, such as evidence of occlusion (prominent collaterals) or location of tumor or open wounds or irritated skin, whether the patient is left- or right-handed, as well as preferences of the healthcare provider placing the device. In the case of central venous catheter placements, a chest radiograph is also obtained to confirm the absence of any anatomic abnormalities that might alter the side of placement (bony abnormali-

TABLE 81.1. Coagulation profile and platelet count guidelines for insertion of central venous catheters (CVCs) procedure.

Platelet count	*PT less than or equal to 16 s*	*PT greater than 16 s*
More than 50 K	Place line	Give 2 units of FFP (or vitamin K if indicated) If PT remains greater than 16 s, consider femoral or jugular line
More than 20 K but less than 50 K	Place line while 6 units of platelets are infusing	Give 4–6 units of platelets If platelet count and/or PT improve, then reassess If PT remains more than 16 s, consider femoral jugular line Then 4–6 more units of platelets should be infused while line is placed
Less than 20 K	Give 4–6 units of platelets If platelet counts remain less than 20,000, primary medical team should contact surgical team for line placement; then 4–6 units of platelets should be infused while line being placed	Give 4–6 units of platelets and 2 units of FFP If platelet count and PT remain out of range, then femoral or jugular line may be placed with additional 4–6 units of platelets

Large-bore subclavian and jugular catheters have more risk and require platelet transfusion when necessary. Large-bore catheter placement in patients with abnormal coagulation carries increased risk, to be weighed against the need for access.

PT, prothrombin time; FFP, fresh frozen plasma.

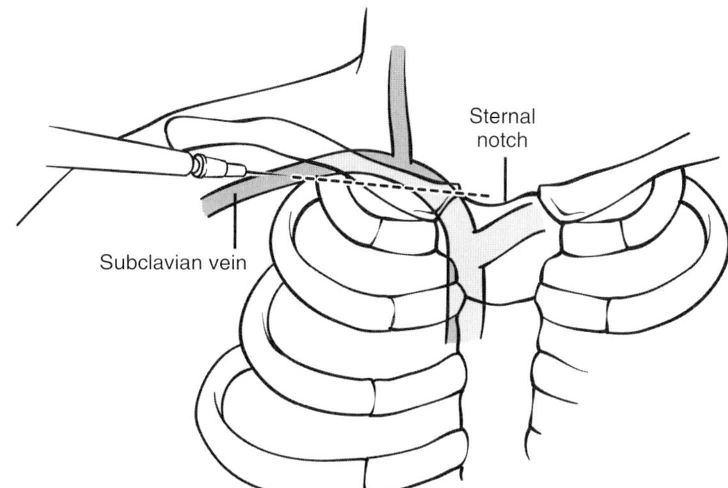

FIGURE 81.1. Approach to subclavian vein, aiming to just above the sternal notch. (By permission of Chen H, Sonneday CJ, Lillemoe KD. *Manual of Common Bedside Surgical Procedures*. Philadelphia: Lippincott Williams & Wilkins, 2003.)

ties or pleural effusions). Patient anxiety level and the ability to tolerate only local anesthesia also may determine the need for sedation during the planned procedure. Over the past few years, we have significantly increased the availability of conscious sedation for patients undergoing this procedure. Patients should also be instructed to be off any antiplatelet therapy for several days before insertion.

Several factors have been found to increase the risk of complications or failure during insertion: these include the experience of the inserter as well as patient factors, including previous catheters, prior radiation, surgery at the site, or a body mass index greater than 30 or less than 20.[1,11]

Technique for Specific Sites

Subclavian Vein

All patients for elective line placement are encouraged to hydrate themselves well the night before the procedure and to not eat or drink for at least 8 hours before if they are to receive sedation. Although most surgeons are trained to place a rolled towel between the shoulder blades, Jesseph et al. performed a magnetic resonance imaging (MRI) and cadaver dissection study, and found that such practice actually distorted the regional anatomy and would make the risk of failure or malposition greater.[16] Boyd et al. conducted a prospective randomized trial by a single house staff officer of placing a shoulder roll (bump); of 105 randomized patients, 93 had a successful outcome (98% in the bump group and 83% in the no-bump group; *P* less than 0.04).[17] The limitations of a single practitioner study cannot be overemphasized, although the results are intriguing. Fortune and Feustel examined five different patient positions with ultrasound in healthy volunteers, and found that the Trendelenburg's position with the shoulders flat and head neutral maximized the diameter of the subclavian vein at the level of the clavicle, whereas arching the back (roll or bump) caused the vein to be closer to the clavicle.[18] We prefer to use a neutral position. The patient's chest is prepped and draped in a sterile fashion with the patient in the supine position. Minimal draping and only sterile gloves for the person inserting the catheter should be discouraged. Parienti et al. conducted a randomized trial of alcoholic 5% povidone-iodine solution with aqueous 10% povidone-iodine solution.[19] This study, which was conducted over a 2-year period, randomized two different ICUs and alternated therapy by unit every 3 months to achieve randomization. Catheter colonization and catheter-related infection were both less in the alcohol group [relative risk (RR), 0.38 (*P* less than 0.001) and 0.34 (*P* less than 0.04)], respectively. Catheter-related bacteremia was similar in both arms of the study, however. For the reasons already mentioned, we generally do not use a shoulder roll and keep the head in the neutral position. The patient's bed is then placed in Trendelenburg's position to facilitate distension of the subclavian vein. Although the vein is technically fixed as it courses between the clavicle and first rib, some distension does occur, as noted in the study by Fortune and Feustel.[18] Using local anesthesia, the area of the chest wall at the site of the bend in the clavicle, as well as the periosteum of the clavicle is anesthetized. If the patient is not too obese, we often try to find the vein with the 1.5-in. local anesthetic needle; this will provide information about the location depth and angle of entry to the vein while minimizing any risk should an arterial puncture or puncture of the lung occur. The introducer needle with syringe attached is then inserted under the clavicle, entering the skin 2 cm from the inferior edge of the clavicle, in the direction of the suprasternal notch (Figure 81.1).

Once under the clavicle with negative pressure applied to the syringe, the subclavian vein is punctured. Upon obtaining good venous blood flow, the syringe is removed and the guidewire is inserted into the subclavian vein. The color and nature (pressure or flow) of the blood return must be carefully noted to make sure that it is not arterial. The needle is then withdrawn over the guidewire and a small incision is made in the skin at the site of entry of the guidewire. Ectopy is generally considered evidence that the wire is in the correct location. A dilator is passed over the guidewire with gentle pressure to avoid penetrating the back wall of the vein while keeping the wire straight to prevent kinking of the wire in the subcutaneous tissues. The dilator is removed and the catheter is inserted over the guidewire to the predetermined length. Several studies have looked at ways to confirm the best location of the tip of the catheter. The system we use was developed by a nurse in our infusion therapy unit and is

TABLE 81.2. Lum's CVC measurement guide.

Height (in)	*Height (cm)*	*R. SC (cm)*	*L. SC (cm)*	*R. JGC (cm)*	*R. PICC (cm)*	*L. PICC (cm)*	*Height (cm)*	*Height (in)*
4 ft 8 in.	142	14.0	18.0	13.0	43.0	47.0	142	4 ft 8 in.
4 ft 10 in.	147	14.5	18.5	13.5	44.0	48.0	147	4 ft 10 in.
5 ft	152	15.0	19.0	14.0	45.5	49.5	152	5 ft
5 ft 2 in.	157	15.5	19.5	14.5	47.0	51.0	157	5 ft 2 in.
5 ft 4 in.	163	16.0	20.0	15.0	48.5	52.5	163	5 ft 4 in.
5 ft 6 in.	168	16.5	20.5	15.5	50.0	54.0	168	5 ft 6 in.
5 ft 8 in.	173	17.0	21.0	16.0	51.5	55.5	173	5 ft 8 in.
5 ft 10 in.	178	17.5	21.5	16.5	53.0	57.0	178	5 ft 10 in.
6 ft	183	18.0	22.0	17.0	54.5	58.5	183	6 ft
6 ft 2 in.	188	18.5	22.5	17.5	56.0	60.0	188	6 ft 2 in.
6 ft 4 in.	193	19.0	23.0	18.0	57.5	61.5	193	6 ft 4 in.

CVC, central venous catheter; R, right; L, left; JGC, jugular catheter; SC, subclavian cathether; PICC, peripheral inserted central catheter; for "JGC," insertion is at the apex of the sternocleidomastoid m. triangle or cricoid level.

Source: From Lum PL. A new formula-based measurement guide for optimal positioning of central venous catheters. *Journal of the Association for Vascular Access* 2004;9:80–85. Reprinted with permission from the Association for Vascular Access.

reproduced as Table 81.2. Using these lengths, based on patient height and site of insertion, in a series of 382 insertions, 373 (97%) were correctly placed.[20] Several studies have shown that the optimal location of the catheter tip is in the distal superior vena cava (SVC) or at the junction of the SVC and RA; tip placement outside this area leads to much higher risk of thrombosis. If an implanted port or tunneled catheter is being placed, this should always be done with fluoroscopic guidance to confirm the position of the tip of the catheter, as it cannot easily be corrected after final placement.

Internal Jugular Vein

The neck is palpated and examined before the insertion. Attention must be addressed to the location of the carotid artery and the heads of the sternocleidomastoid muscle. The patient's head is turned to face the direction away from the site of insertion. The area is prepped and draped in sterile fashion and the patient's bed is placed in Trendelenburg's position.

With the operator standing at the head of the bed, the carotid artery is palpated. The area is anesthetized, and the internal jugular vein is accessed with a small-gauge needle by directing the venipuncture lateral to the location of the carotid artery in a direction toward the ipsilateral nipple. A larger-gauge needle mounted on a syringe is then used to access the internal jugular vein. Once adequate blood flow is obtained, Seldinger's technique is once again used to pass the guidewire and subsequently place the catheter. As with the subclavian vein placement, fluoroscopy can be used to determine catheter location, although this is only truly necessary for tunneled catheters. At this time, the exit area for a tunneled device is determined. The subcutaneous pocket or the exit site for external devices that are tunneled is situated on the midanterior chest wall within 5 to 10 cm of the midclavicle area. This area is anesthetized, as well as the tract of the tunnel between the planned exit site of the device or the subcutaneous pocket for the port. The subcutaneous tunnel is created by passing the tunneling device from the site of insertion of the guidewire to the planned exit site or the subcutaneous pocket. The catheter is attached to the tunneling device, which is then withdrawn, bringing the catheter to the site of insertion of the guidewire. The catheter is then passed over the guidewire and secured as previously described.

Complications

Insertion Related

Several factors are associated with an increased risk of complications. For jugular catheters, a short neck or obese patient makes the insertion more difficult and the risk of complications (principally arterial puncture) greater. For subclavian venipuncture, the most common complications include pneumothorax, arterial puncture, hemothorax, malposition of the catheter, and injury to the regional nerves (including brachial plexus, vagus, and phrenic nerves). Although injury to the nerves is extremely rare (approximately 1:20,000–1:30,000 procedures), injuries can happen and typically are associated with less experienced practitioners or persistence beyond a reasonable chance of success. As mentioned previously, factors that are associated with an increased risk of complications, include a very thin patient, prior surgery or radiotherapy in the area, and an inexperienced practitioner. The incidence of insertion-related pneumothorax, which is continuously monitored on an ongoing basis at M.D. Anderson Cancer Center (MDACC), is between 1% and 1.5%. Most pneumothoraces are asymptomatic and a postprocedure chest X-ray (CXR) is mandatory. Although most of these CXRs are negative, it is important to confirm the location of the tip of the catheter. A malpositioned catheter can oftentimes be corrected by either patient positioning or a power flush.[21] Sometimes a partial withdrawal over a wire or fluoroscopic correction is needed. In a study by Laronga et al. from our institution, 100 pneumothoraces were detected in a consecutive series of 9,637 patients (1.04%), suggesting that the yield of routine CXR to be very low for pneumothorax in the asymptomatic patient.[22] If one were able to confirm catheter tip by another means, this could then lead to a challenge of the practice of obtaining routine CXR following central venous access placement. However, we have not yet reached that state. CXR performed in patients with symptoms appears to be a more pertinent approach, and in fact, both the patient and clinician must be aware of the risk of delayed pneumothorax, which we find comprises about 10% of our pneumothoraces. If the line is inserted as an outpatient procedure, the patient may not develop the symptoms of pneumothorax for 12 to 24 hours. It is imperative that such patients seek medical attention urgently. Laronga et al. also developed a treatment algorithm for the management of postcentral venous catheter (post-CVC) pneumothorax, whereby some patients, based on size of pneumothorax, presence of symptoms, difficulty of insertion, and prior history of a CVC, may safely be observed with follow-up CXR[22] (Figure 81.2).

Hemorrhage is another potential complication of central venous access placement. As with pneumothorax, this occurs infrequently, and although most are self-limited, the outcome of this complication can be fatal. Hemorrhage can be a consequence of either accidental arterial puncture or result from a venous puncture. Major vessel injury can occur during placement of the introducer sheath. As mentioned in the Insertion section, the introducer sheath should be placed with gentle pressure. When this placement occurs too vigorously the sheath can accidentally penetrate the back wall of the vessel. The loss of blood into the chest cavity may also go unrecognized before the patient develops symptoms. In roughly 1 of 10,000 procedures, the artery may be injured in such a fashion as to become an emergency requiring either surgical, or in some cases, interventional radiology, correction.

The proximity of the brachial plexus to both the subclavian and internal jugular veins, places these nerves at risk for laceration by the introducer needle, although fortunately, this risk is quite low. Another mode of injury can occur as a result of compression by a hematoma. This effect is usually associated with neuropraxia as opposed to paralysis. The symptoms associated with nerve injury from compression are usually self-limiting and usually resolve without any sequelae.

An unusual, and more annoying than life-threatening complication of central venous access, is that of a chyle leak. This complication can be encountered while accessing the left subclavian vein or the left internal jugular vein. Perforation of the thoracic duct results in leakage of chyle, which tracks back out around the catheter. Chyle leaks are treated with direct pressure dressing, and if this fails, the catheter may need to be removed and a new stick performed. Only on the rarest of occasions may surgical exploration with ligation of the thoracic duct become necessary.

Numerous efforts have been undertaken in an attempt to minimize the risks of central venous catheter placement. Most often these attempts have involved the use of imaging guidance of the insertion attempt. Although some have found the use of ultrasound beneficial, this advantage may be site dependent. In a randomized trial of more than 800 patients, we found that ultrasound localization (but not real-time guidance) was of no benefit for subclavian catheter placement.[11] Other investigators have found varying results. In a randomized study, in which a single clinician inserted the catheters, Lefrant et al. found only modest benefit from ultrasound guidance.[23] Although the overall risk of complications was decreased by using ultrasound guidance from 16.8% to 5.6% (P less than 0.01), most of this benefit was actually for malpositioned catheters (7.7% to 0.7%; P less than 0.01). In fact, failures, immediate complications, and total number of skin punctures were similar in the two arms, whereas the Doppler ultrasound arm took six times as long for insertion (300 versus 27 seconds). Bold et al. conducted a randomized trial of Doppler-guided placement of subclavian catheters in approximately 500 patients, and found no benefit to the technology.[24] Clinicians inserting the catheters were either highly efficient with and without the technology or they were not. This is one of the problems with applying technology across the board; there is significant operator variation. Conversely, Teichgraber et al., in a randomized trial of 100 patients undergoing IJ venipuncture, found that ultrasound markedly decreased time of insertion, failure rate, and complications.[25]

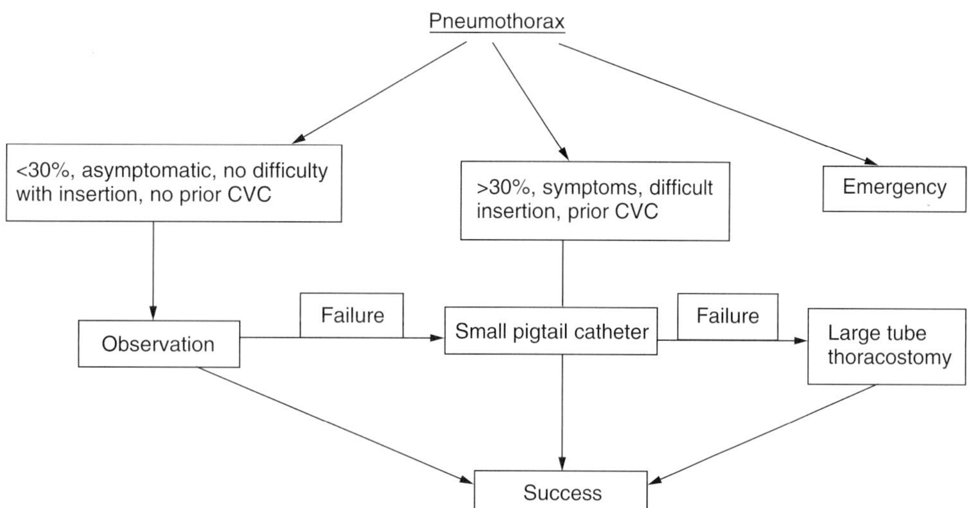

FIGURE 81.2. Algorithm for management of pneumothorax occurring secondary to central venous catheter (CVC) placement. (From Laronga et al.,[22] by permission of *American Journal of Surgery.*)

Randolph et al. performed a meta-analysis of real-time ultrasound guidance for both subclavian and IJ catheter placement and found improvements in failure rate (RR, 0.32; 95% confidence interval, 0.18–0.55) and complications (RR, 0.22; 95% confidence interval, 0.10–0.45).[26]

Catheter Related

The two main considerations here, are CRBSI and venous thrombosis, although there is some overlap between the two. We examine first the issue of thrombosis and then move to infection.

Thrombosis

Venous thrombosis is a serious and relatively common catheter-related complication. Although studies have examined the use of various anticoagulants to prevent thrombosis, perhaps one of the most important interventions to prevent them is to make sure the catheter tip is in the correct position (distal superior vena cava to junction of superior vena cava and right atrium).[27] In patients with central venous access, this may present with upper extremity swelling or difficulty withdrawing blood from the device. One must differentiate between an occluded catheter and an occluded vein or determine if both are present, with the latter causing the former. The evaluation of this would include either a nuclear or contrast venogram, although duplex Doppler can also be helpful. Once the diagnosis is made, the decision on how to treat is heavily influenced by the need of the patient for the device. If it is suspected that a clot or a fibrin sheath obstructs the catheter, tissue plasminogen activator (tPA) may be instilled in the device with a high success rate.[28] Recombinant urokinase has also been shown to be better than placebo at restoring catheter patency.[29] If the thrombosis involves the subclavian vein, anticoagulation with heparin, followed by warfarin therapy, may be necessary as these clots can also lead to pulmonary embolism. If one has an aggressive interventional radiology unit, and the patient is anticipated to have long-term needs for venous access and loss of this vessel would be extremely detrimental to that care, a peripheral catheter can be inserted and tPA used to lyse the clot and the patient is then placed on long-term anticoagulation.

Several efforts have been made to prevent the formation of clots. It is helpful to know how frequent the problem is before trying to prevent it. In a prospective study by Martin et al., it was found that 47% of patients developed a fibrin sheath and that partial vein occlusion occurred in 8% of patients.[30] An additional 3% of patients developed evidence of a radiographic complete occlusion. In addition, the authors examined the duration of catheter presence and found that catheters in place less than 2 weeks were unlikely to develop thrombosis. Abdelkefi et al. examined the use of continuous-infusion low-dose heparin (compared with saline) to prevent catheter-related thrombosis in patients with hematologic malignancies.[31] They found, in 128 randomized patients, that catheter-related thrombosis occurred in 1.5% of the heparin group and 12.6% of the control group ($P = 0.03$). There was no difference in bleeding complications (2 in the heparin group and 3 in the control group). Massicotte et al. conducted a randomized trial of low molecular weight heparin for prevention of CVC-related thrombosis.[32] This study, conducted in children, was closed early for slow accrual; no difference was found in the rate of venous thromboembolism between standard care and reviparin-sodium (12.5% and 14.1%, respectively, in 80 and 78 patients), and there was also no difference in bleeding complications.

Infection

There are several components to the issue of catheter-related infections. Some of these, including skin preparation and draping the patient, we have already discussed. Contrary to the suggestion in the study by Ma et al. mentioned earlier, regarding the risk of infection and TPN, Tokars et al. evaluated risk factors for infection in catheters maintained in an outpatient setting.[33] Of 988 catheters maintained in 827 patients, they found five factors associated with an increased risk of infection, including (1) recent bone marrow transplant (RR, 5.8), (2) TPN (RR, 4.1), (3) receipt of therapy outside the home (such as at a physician's office) (RR, 3.6), (4) use of a multilumen catheter (RR, 2.8), and (5) history of a previous bloodstream infection (RR, 2.5). Patients who had three or more of these risk factors had an approximately 40-fold-increased risk of infection when compared with those with none of these risk factors. In addition, catheter maintenance (including the site and connections), the various uses of the catheter, prophylactic antibiotics, routine catheter exchange, antimicrobial flushes, and use of catheters impregnated or coated with various antimicrobial agents, all may have roles. This section examines these issues.

Prophylactic Antibiotics

Bock et al. conducted a prospective randomized trial of preinsertion intravenous antibiotics compared with placebo or routine catheter exchange in 92 patients undergoing therapy with interleukin 2 (IL-2).[34] They found a significant decrease in catheter-related sepsis in the oxacillin group ($P = 0.05$), as well as a decrease in bacterial colonization (P less than 0.001) when compared with the other two arms.

Catheter Exchange

Bonawitz et al. randomized 85 patients with 159 catheters to have a replacement at 3 or 7 days and whether or not a cuffed catheter was used.[35] They found no benefit to either the earlier exchange or the use of the cuff, although the size of the study may have been limiting. Nevertheless, there was certainly no obvious benefit to routine exchange. Cobb et al. also examined the role of routine catheter exchange in a four-arm randomized trial.[36] Patients were randomized to either having the catheter exchanged or replaced every 3 days or when clinically indicated. They found that there was no decrease in infections with replacement or exchange every 3 days. Exchange over a wire was associated with an increase in infections, and new placement every 3 days was associated with an increased risk of complications of insertion. Eyer et al. conducted a prospective randomized trial among every-7-days over-wire exchange, every-7-days new catheter placement, and change based only on clinical need in 112 patients.[37] Although there was no difference in catheter-related infections, the size of the study does limit conclusions to some degree.

Catheter Dressings, Connections, and Tubing

As noted earlier in the study of catheter cuffs by Flowers et al., in fact the topical antimicrobial may have been responsible for fungal infections.[3] Other investigators have examined various aspects of the local care of catheters. Conly et al. randomized 115 patients between a transparent or gauze dressing, and found that colonization was far less in the gauze group (P = 0.009).[38] Local catheter-related infection and catheter-related bacteremia were both significantly more common in the transparent group (P = 0.002 and P = 0.15, respectively). Maki et al. randomized 442 patients to one of three local dressing approaches: (1) sterile gauze and tape replaced every 2 days, (2) conventional polyurethane dressing replaced every 5 days, or (3) a highly permeable polyurethane dressing replaced every 5 days.[39] Although they found no difference in catheter colonization or CRBSI, bacterial colonization under the dressing was greatest with the standard polyurethane dressing, and least with the gauze dressing (P less than 0.001). Laura et al. compared two different time intervals for CVC dressing changes in a bone marrow transplant population.[40] This multiinstitutional study evaluated 399 patients with either a tunneled or nontunneled catheter. The randomized times were different for the two types of catheters (5 or 10 days for the tunneled and 2 or 5 for the nontunneled). They found no difference in local infection rates based on duration of dressing, but did find more local skin reactions in the every-2-day group. Crawford et al. conducted a cost–benefit analysis based on randomized controlled trial data of chlorhexidine dressings when compared with standard dressings.[41] Considering averted cost of treatment of both local infections and CRBSI at all Philadelphia area hospitals, they calculated that the standard use of a chlorhexidine gluconate dressing would result in potential savings of $275 million to $1.97 billion, with 329 to 3,906 lives saved annually across the United States. Rickard et al. examined the practice of routine changing of the intravenous administration sets on colonization or infection of CVCs.[42] In this study, 251 patients with 404 catheters were randomized to have their IV administration sets changed at 4 days or not. There were 10 colonized CVCs in the change group and 19 in the no-change group, the difference not being statistically different (P less than 0.1). All lines were removed by day 7. One of the major considerations of trying to extrapolate from these data, is that all the patients had chlorhexidine gluconate and silver sulfadiazine-coated catheters. Henrickson et al. conducted a three-arm randomized trial in 126 pediatric patients comparing the impact of flushing the catheter with vancomycin, heparin, and ciprofloxicin (VHC), with vancomycin and heparin (VH), and heparin alone.[43] Both the VHC and VH groups had substantially fewer CRBSIs than the heparin-alone group (heparin, 31; VH, 3; VHC, 6). Interestingly, there were significantly fewer episodes of occlusion in the VHC group when compared with the heparin-alone group (P less than 0.001). Two reports of the use of needle-less connectors found somewhat divergent results. Cookson et al. found a significant increase in the risk of BSIs in patients after the introduction of a needle-less system (9.4 versus 5.0/1,000 CVC days).[44] The authors conjectured that much of the increase was likely the result of nurses' unfamiliarity with the devices and departure from manufacturers' recommendations. Casey et al. conducted a randomized trial of needle-less versus standard cap in 77 cardiac patients.[45] After 72 hours, the caps/connectors were cultured; 55 of 306 (18%) of the standard Luer group were contaminated, whereas 18 of 274 (6.6%) of the needle-less group were contaminated (P less than 0.001). The authors also randomized patients to receive various disinfectants for the external surfaces and found the combination of chlorhexidine and alcohol was far superior to alcohol alone (30.8% versus 69.2%, respectively; P less than 0.001).

At M.D. Anderson, line care is done according to very specific treatment guidelines to minimize site infections and prolong catheter life. However, site problems will occur, and these are managed at our institution according to the algorithm shown in Figure 81.3, based on the severity of the site problem.

Impregnated or Coated Catheters

In what seems to be the pinnacle of attempts to prevent CRBSI, several investigators have either coated or impregnated catheters with various agents to prevent the development of the biofilm that coats catheters and serves as a nidis for infections, as well as to prevent the severe toxicity of CRBSI. A summary of reported trials with at least 100 randomized patients is included in Table 81.3. Maki et al. conducted a randomized trial of a chlorhexidine/silver sulfadiazine-impregnated polyurethane catheter with a standard polyurethane catheter[46] that studied 403 catheters in 158 adult patients. Catheter colonization, bloodstream infection, and CRBSI were all significantly less common in the treated-catheter group. There were in fact no instances of CRBSI in the treatment group, whereas 8 occurred in the control group (P = 0.003). Carrasco et al. performed a randomized trial between a heparin-coated catheter and a chlorhexidine/silver sulfadiazine-coated one in 180 patients requiring a triple-lumen catheter.[47] Of the 132 heparin catheters, 29 were colonized, whereas 13 of the 128 chlorhexidine/silver sulfadiazine catheters were (P = 0.03). The incidence of CRBSI was similar in the two arms, 3.24 per 1,000 catheter-days and 2.6 per 1,000 catheter-days, respectively. Corral et al. evaluated a silver central venous catheter in 206 patients randomized to receive a standard catheter or the silver one.[48] Colonization was less in the silver group, with 30 of 103 compared with 45 of 103, respectively (P = 0.04), whereas the rates of CRBSI were 0.8 and 2.8 per 1,000 catheter-days (P less than 0.001). Darouiche et al. conducted a multiinstitutional randomized trial comparing minocycline/rifampin (MR)-impregnated catheters with those impregnated with chlorhexidine/silver sulfadiazine (CSS),[49] in which 865 catheters were inserted and 85% were evaluable. Colonization occurred in 28 of 356 (7.9%) MR catheters and 87 of 382 (22.8%) in the CSS group (P less than 0.001). Most importantly, CRBSI occurred in only 1 of 356 (0.3%) MR catheters and 13 of 382 (3.4%) of the CSS catheters (P less than 0.002). All these studies utilized polyurethane catheters, which are generally associated with a greater risk of thrombosis and generally have a much shorter functional life than silicone catheters. Hanna et al. randomized 370 patients to receive either a standard silicone catheter or one impregnated with minocycline and rifampin.[50] There were

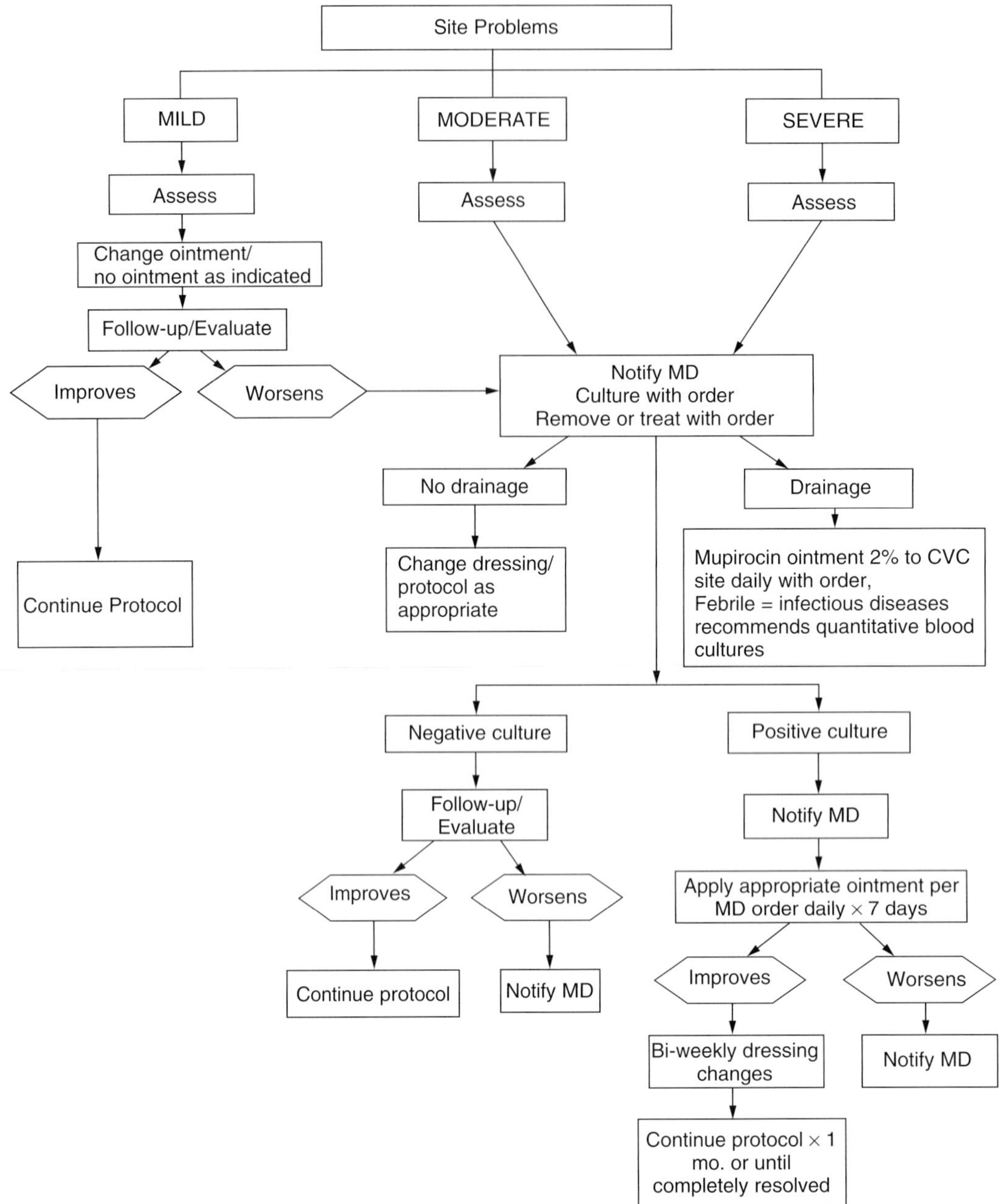

FIGURE 81.3. Algorithm for management of CVC site problems. (By permission of Raad IL. *Guidelines for Managing VAD Site Complications*. Infusion Therapy Team, The University of Texas M.D. Anderson Cancer Center, June 25, 1996.)

356 evaluable catheters in 355 patients. In this study, the mean duration was more than 2 months in both groups, and the risk of CRBSI was substantially less in the impregnated catheters than the standard ones (0.25 and 1.28/1,000 catheter-days; $P = 0.003$). The importance of these results should not be minimized as silicone catheters generally have a much longer duration of use than polyurethane ones. At M.D. Anderson, we generally restrict their use to patients receiving a marrow or stem cell transplant or IL-2-based therapy; those who are having a catheter exchanged for suspected infection; long-term ICU patients; and those patients who are known to have poor access options and have had catheter-related infections in the past.

General Infection Recommendations

Based on some of the data presented here, in 2002, the Centers for Disease Control and Prevention (CDC), issued guidelines for the prevention of catheter-related infections.[51] Their major points were (1) education and training of those placing and maintaining the catheters, (2) use of maximal sterile barrier at time of insertion, (3) use of a 2% chlorhexidine skin preparation, (4) avoidance of routine catheter replacement, and (5) use of antiseptic/antibiotic-impregnated catheters if the rate of infection is high despite the other interventions.

TABLE 81.3. Summary of randomized trials of 100 or more patients using impregnated or coated catheters.

Author	No. of patients randomized	Year	No. of catheters total	Control arm	Treatment arm	No. of lumens	Catheter material	Median catheter duration, Tx/Cont	Coated (C) vs. impregnated (I)	Catheter colonization (%treatment over %control)	CRBSI/1,000 catheter days (or %CRBSI) treatment/control
Brun-Buisson[52]	363	2004	363	Noncoated	Chlorhexidine/silber sulfadiazine (CSS)	1 or 2	Polyurethane	10.5/12.0	C	3.7/13.1 ($P = 0.01$)	2/5.2 ($P = 0.1$)
Carrasco[47]	180	2004	260	Heparin coated	CSS	3	Polyurethane	9.5/9.0	C	10.1/22.0 ($P = 0.03$)	2.6/3.24 ($P = 0.79$)
Jaeger[53]	106	2005	106	Uncoated triple lumen	CSS	3	Polyurethane	14.3/16.6	I	9.8/16.4 ($P + 0.035$)	2.0% vs.14.5% ($P = 0.02$)
Hanna[50]	356	2004	356	Uncoated silicone	Minocycline-rifampin (MR)	1 or 2	Silicone	66.2/63.0	I	Not specified	0.25/1.28 ($P = 0.003$)
Leon[54]	465	2004	465	Nonimpregnated	MR	3	Polyurethane	10.3/10.4	I	10.4/24 (RR, 0.43; CI, 0.26–0.73)	3.1/5.9 (RR, 0.53; CI, 0.2–1.44)
Darouiche[49]	698	1999	738	CSS	MR	3	Polyurethane	6.0/7.0	I	7.9%/22.8% $P < 0.001$	0.3% vs. 3.4% $P < 0.002$
Logghe[55]	538	1997	680	Nonimpregnated	CSS	>1	Polyurethane	19/19	I	Not specified	5% vs. 4.4% P = NS
Maki[46]	158	1997	403	Standard	CSS	3	Polyurethane	6.0/6.0	I	13.5%/24.1% ($P = 0.005$)	1.6/7.6 (RR, 0.21; CI, 0.03–0.95) $P = 0.03$
Heard[56]	251	1998	308	Uncoated	CSS	3	Polyurethane	8.5/9.0	C	40%/52% ($P < 0.05$)	3.3% vs. 3.8% P = NS
Tennenberg[57]	282	1997	282	Uncoated	CSS	>1	Polyurethane	5.2/7.8	C	28% vs. 49% $P < 0.001$	3.8% vs. 6.4% P = NS
Raad[58]	281	1997	298	Uncoated	MR	3	Polyurethane	6.0/6.0	C	8% vs. 26% $P < 0.001$	0% vs. 5% $P < 0.01$
Thornton[59]	110	1996	176	Nonbonded	Vancomycin	3	Not specified	Not specified	C	62% vs. 80% ($P = 0.01$)	

Tx., treatment; Cont, control; RR, relative risk; CI, confidence interval.

Conclusions

With all the progress that has been made, issues that remain of concern for venous access in patients with cancer are the optimal way to minimize the risk of thrombosis, the best way to minimize the risks of insertion, and balancing the competing concerns of minimizing complications and the costs of these interventions, particularly in those populations which may be at lower risk. Although there are many efforts to increase the use of oral agents in the treatment of the cancer patient, it is unlikely that the need for central venous access will diminish during our lifetime.

References

1. McGee DC, Gould MK. Preventing complications of central venous catheterization. N Engl J Med 2003;348:1123–1133.
2. Schwengel DA, McGready J, Berenholtz SM, et al. Peripherally inserted central catheters: a randomized, controlled, prospective trial in pediatric surgical patients. Anesth Analg 2004;99: 1038–1043, table of contents.
3. Flowers RH III, Schwenzer KJ, Kopel RF, et al. Efficacy of an attachable subcutaneous cuff for the prevention of intravascular catheter-related infection. A randomized, controlled trial. JAMA 1989;261:878–883.
4. Timsit JF, Bruneel F, Cheval C, et al. Use of tunneled femoral catheters to prevent catheter-related infection. A randomized, controlled trial. Ann Intern Med 1999;130:729–735.
5. Michel LA, Bradpiece HA, Randour P, et al. Safety of central venous catheter change over guidewire for suspected catheter-related sepsis. A prospective randomized trial. Int Surg 1988;73:180–186.
6. Grove JR, Pevec WC. Venous thrombosis related to peripherally inserted central catheters. J Vasc Intervent Radiol 2000;11: 837–840.
7. Farkas JC, Liu N, Bleriot JP, et al. Single- versus triple-lumen central catheter-related sepsis: a prospective randomized study in a critically ill population. Am J Med 1992;93:277–282.
8. Clark-Christoff N, Watters VA, Sparks W, et al. Use of triple-lumen subclavian catheters for administration of total parenteral nutrition. JPEN J Parenter Enteral Nutr 1992;16:403–407.
9. Ma TY, Yoshinaka R, Banaag A, et al. Total parenteral nutrition via multilumen catheters does not increase the risk of catheter-related sepsis: a randomized, prospective study. Clin Infect Dis 1998;27:500–503.
10. Ruesch S, Walder B, Tramer MR. Complications of central venous catheters: internal jugular versus subclavian access: a systematic review. Crit Care Med 2002;30:454–460.
11. Mansfield PF, Hohn DC, Fornage BD, et al. Complications and failures of subclavian-vein catheterization. N Engl J Med 1994;331:1735–1738.
12. Martin C, Bruder N, Papazian L, et al. Catheter-related infections following axillary vein catheterization. Acta Anaesthesiol Scand 198;42:52–56.
13. Merrer J, De Jonghe B, Golliot F, et al. Complications of femoral and subclavian venous catheterization in critically ill patients: a randomized controlled trial. JAMA 2001;286:700–707.
14. Hu KK, Lipsky BA, Veenstra DL, et al. Using maximal sterile barriers to prevent central venous catheter-related infection: a systematic evidence-based review. Am J Infect Control 2004;32: 142–146.
15. Raad IL, Hohn DC, Gilbreath BJ, et al. Prevention of central venous catheter-related infections by using maximal sterile barrier precautions during insertion. Infect Control Hosp Epidemiol 1993; 415:231–238.
16. Jesseph JM, Conces DJ Jr, Augustyn GT. Patient positioning for subclavian vein catheterization. Arch Surg 1987;122:1207–1209.
17. Boyd R, Saxe A, Phillips E. Effect of patient position upon success in placing central venous catheters. Am J Surg 1996;172:380–382.
18. Fortune JB, Feustel P. Effect of patient position on size and location of the subclavian vein for percutaneous puncture. Arch Surg 2003;138:996–1000; discussion 1001.
19. Parienti JJ, du Cheyron D, Ramakers M, et al. Alcoholic povidone-iodine to prevent central venous catheter colonization: a randomized unit-crossover study. Crit Care Med 2004;32: 708–713.
20. Lum P. A new formula-based measurement guide for optimal positioning of central venous catheters. J Assoc Vasc Access 2004;9:80–85.
21. Lum PS, Soski M. Management of malpositioned central venous catheters. J Intraven Nurs 1989;12:356–365.
22. Laronga C, Meric F, Truong MT, et al. A treatment algorithm for pneumothoraces complicating central venous catheter insertion. Am J Surg 2000;180:523–526; discussion 526–527.
23. Lefrant JY, Cuvillon P, Benezet JF, et al. Pulsed Doppler ultrasonography guidance for catheterization of the subclavian vein: a randomized study. Anesthesiology 1998;88:1195–1201.
24. Bold RJ, Winchester DJ, Madary AR, et al. Prospective, randomized trial of Doppler-assisted subclavian vein catheterization. Arch Surg 1998;133:1089–1093.
25. Teichgraber UK, Benter T, Gebel M, et al. A sonographically guided technique for central venous access. AJR Am J Roentgenol 1997;169:731–733.
26. Randolph AG, Cook DJ, Gonzales CA, et al. Ultrasound guidance for placement of central venous catheters: a meta-analysis of the literature. Crit Care Med 1996;24:2053–2058.
27. Luciani A, Clement O, Halimi P, et al. Catheter-related upper extremity deep venous thrombosis in cancer patients: a prospective study based on Doppler US. Radiology 2001;220:655–660.
28. Middleton G, Ruzevick B. Alteplase (Cathflo Activase). Clin J Oncol Nurs 2004;8:417–418, 420.
29. Haire WD, Deitcher SR, Mullane KM, et al. Recombinant urokinase for restoration of patency in occluded central venous access devices. A double-blind, placebo-controlled trial. Thromb Haemostasis 2004;92:575–582.
30. Martin C, Viviand X, Saux P, et al. Upper-extremity deep vein thrombosis after central venous catheterization via the axillary vein. Crit Care Med 1999;27:2626–629.
31. Abdelkefi A, Ben Othman T, Kammoun L, et al. Prevention of central venous line-related thrombosis by continuous infusion of low-dose unfractionated heparin, in patients with haemato-oncological disease. A randomized controlled trial. Thromb Haemostasis 2004;92:654–661.
32. Massicotte P, Julian JA, Gent M, et al. An open-label randomized controlled trial of low molecular weight heparin compared to heparin and coumadin for the treatment of venous thromboembolic events in children: the REVIVE trial. Thromb Res 2003;109:85–92.
33. Tokars JI, Cookson ST, McArthur MA, et al. Prospective evaluation of risk factors for bloodstream infection in patients receiving home infusion therapy. Ann Intern Med 1999;131: 340–347.
34. Bock SN, Lee RE, Fisher B, et al. A prospective randomized trial evaluating prophylactic antibiotics to prevent triple-lumen catheter-related sepsis in patients treated with immunotherapy. J Clin Oncol 1990;8:161–169.
35. Bonawitz SC, Hammell EJ, Kirkpatrick JR. Prevention of central venous catheter sepsis: a prospective randomized trial. Am Surg 1991;57:618–623.
36. Cobb DK, High KP, Sawyer RG, et al. A controlled trial of scheduled replacement of central venous and pulmonary-artery catheters. N Engl J Med 1992;327:1062–1068.

37. Eyer S, Brummitt C, Crossley K, et al. Catheter-related sepsis: prospective, randomized study of three methods of long-term catheter maintenance. Crit Care Med 1990;18:1073–1079.
38. Conly JM, Grieves K, Peters B. A prospective, randomized study comparing transparent and dry gauze dressings for central venous catheters. J Infect Dis 1989;159:310–319.
39. Maki DG, Stolz SS, Wheeler S, et al. A prospective, randomized trial of gauze and two polyurethane dressings for site care of pulmonary artery catheters: implications for catheter management. Crit Care Med 1994;22:1729–1737.
40. Laura R, Degl'Innocenti M, Mocali M, et al. Comparison of two different time interval protocols for central venous catheter dressing in bone marrow transplant patients: results of a randomized, multicenter study. The Italian Nurse Bone Marrow Transplant Group (GITMO). Haematologica 2000;85:275–279.
41. Crawford AG, Fuhr JP Jr, Rao B. Cost-benefit analysis of chlorhexidine gluconate dressing in the prevention of catheter-related bloodstream infections. Infect Control Hosp Epidemiol 2004;25:668–674.
42. Rickard CM, Lipman J, Courtney M, et al. Routine changing of intravenous administration sets does not reduce colonization or infection in central venous catheters. Infect Control Hosp Epidemiol 2004;25:650–655.
43. Henrickson KJ, Axtell RA, Hoover SM, et al. Prevention of central venous catheter-related infections and thrombotic events in immunocompromised children by the use of vancomycin/ciprofloxacin/heparin flush solution: a randomized, multicenter, double-blind trial. J Clin Oncol 2000;18:1269–1278.
44. Cookson ST, Ihrig M, O'Mara EM, et al. Increased bloodstream infection rates in surgical patients associated with variation from recommended use and care following implementation of a needleless device. Infect Control Hosp Epidemiol 1998;19:23–27.
45. Casey AL, Worthington T, Lambert PA, et al. A randomized, prospective clinical trial to assess the potential infection risk associated with the PosiFlow needleless connector. J Hosp Infect 2003;54:288–293.
46. Maki DG, Stolz SM, Wheeler S, et al. Prevention of central venous catheter-related bloodstream infection by use of an antiseptic-impregnated catheter. A randomized, controlled trial. Ann Intern Med 1997;127:257–266.
47. Carrasco MN, Bueno A, de las Cuevas C, et al. Evaluation of a triple-lumen central venous heparin-coated catheter versus a catheter coated with chlorhexidine and silver sulfadiazine in critically ill patients. Intensive Care Med 2004;30:633–638.
48. Corral L, Nolla-Salas M, Ibanez-Nolla J, et al. A prospective, randomized study in critically ill patients using the Oligon Vantex catheter. J Hosp Infect 2003;55:212–219.
49. Darouiche RO, Raad, II, Heard SO, et al. A comparison of two antimicrobial-impregnated central venous catheters. Catheter Study Group. N Engl J Med 1999;340:1–8.
50. Hanna H, Benjamin R, Chatzinikolaou I, et al. Long-term silicone central venous catheters impregnated with minocycline and rifampin decrease rates of catheter-related bloodstream infection in cancer patients: a prospective randomized clinical trial. J Clin Oncol 2004;22:3163–3171.
51. O'Grady NP, Alexander M, Dellinger EP, et al. Guidelines for the prevention of intravascular catheter-related infections. Centers for Disease Control and Prevention. MMWR Recomm Rep 2002;51:1–29.
52. Bruin-Buisson C, Doyon F, Sollet JP, et al. Prevention of intravascular catheter-related infection with newer chlorhexidine-silver sulfadiazine-coated catheters: a randomized controlled trial. Intensive Care Med 2004;30(5):837–843.
53. Jaeger J, Zenz S, Juttner B, et al. Reduction of catheter-related infections in neutropenic patients: a prospective controlled randomized trial using a chlorhexidine and silver sulfadiazine-impregnated central venous catheter. Ann Hematol 2005;84(4): 258–262.
54. Leon Leon C, Ruiz-Santana S, Rello J. Benefits of minocycline and rifampin-impregnated central venous catheters. A prospective, randomized, double-blind, controlled, multicenter trial. Intensive Care Med 2004;30(10):1891–1899.
55. Logghe C, Van Ossel C, D'Hoove W, et al. Evaluation of chlorhexidine and silver-sulfadiazine impregnated central venous catheters for the prevention of bloodstream infection in leukaemic patients: a randomized controlled trial. J Hosp Infect 1997;37(2):145–156.
56. Heard SO, Wagle M, Vijayakumar E, et al. Influence of triple-lumen central venous catheters coated with chlorhexidine and silver sulfadiazine on the incidence of catheter-related bacteremia. Arch Intern Med 1998;158(1):81–87.
57. Tennenberg S, Lieser M, McCurdy B, et al. A prospective randomized trial of an antibiotic- and antiseptic-coated central venous catheter in the prevention of catheter-related infections. Arch Surg 1997;132(12):1348–1351.
58. Raad IL. Vascular catheters impregnated with antimicrobial agents: present knowledge and future direction. Infect Control Hosp Epidemiol 1997;18(4):227–229.
59. Thornton J, Todd NJ, Webster NC. Central venous line sepsis in the intensive care unit. A study comparing antibiotic coated catheters with plain catheters. Anaesthesia 1996;51(11): 1018–1020.

82

Management of Cancer Pain

Donald P. Lawrence, Leonidas C. Goudas, Andrew J. Lipman, Joseph Lau, Rina M. Bloch, and Daniel B. Carr

Enormous advances have occurred in the past two decades in our understanding of cancer pain and in our capacity to relieve it in most cases. Progress has been made in our understanding of the pathogenesis of nociception, the epidemiology of cancer pain, the validation of effective treatment algorithms, and the evaluation of novel pharmacologic and nonpharmacologic approaches to ameliorate pain. Paralleling these developments in research,[1] pain management has emerged as a priority in healthcare policy and medical education.[2]

Despite these advances, pain remains the aspect of cancer perhaps most feared by patients. Substantial barriers to optimal pain management persist, including the expense of appropriate medications or lack of access to them, healthcare disparities based on age, gender, and race,[3] inadequate awareness or expertise on the part of practitioners, and the stigma still attached to opioid analgesics.[4]

This chapter is an updated synopsis of two recently published comprehensive evidence reports focusing on three broad areas of cancer pain: occurrence (i.e., prevalence and incidence), methods of assessment, and treatment.

Cancer Pain: Definitions

Cancer pain may be a manifestation of the disease itself, or may result from treatments, including surgery, radiotherapy, and chemotherapy. Acute pain, chronic pain, tumor-specific pain, and treatment-related pain may exist simultaneously or sequentially.

The experience of pain is profoundly influenced by cultural[5] and psychologic factors,[6] and therefore a distinction can be made between pain and the distress and suffering that may result from it.[7–9] In cancer, pain may be a reminder of mortality and carries profound personal, social, cultural, and religious implications.[10,11]

Cancer pain shares mechanisms with both acute and chronic noncancer pain. Traditional definitions of chronic pain require duration of 3 to 6 months.[12–15] Yet, current pain research[16] confirms that every physiologic feature considered essential for chronic pain—central sensitization, hyperalgesia, novel gene expression, synaptic remodeling ("plasticity"), "pain memory" formation, and behavioral adjustment—is triggered within days of acute, ongoing tissue injury.[17] Thus, pain of relatively brief duration has the potential to provoke the physiologic responses associated with chronic pain. Furthermore, when a new painful stimulus occurs in a patient with cancer, the intensity of the pain and its response to analgesics may be modulated by a nervous system sensitized by prior nociception.

Tumors cause pain by the local release of inflammatory mediators and by exerting pressure on surrounding tissues, including nerves.[18,19] Inflammatory mediators associated with cancer include prostaglandins, cytokines, such as tumor necrosis factor,[20] growth factors, and other tumor-derived products, such as endothelin,[21] each of which can excite nociceptors.[22] Some cancers induce the production of autoantibodies that are implicated in painful paraneoplastic syndromes.[23,24] Animal models of bone cancer pain have suggested a distinctive neurochemical and histologic "signature" in afferent nerves and their spinal cord connections.[25]

Cancer pain frequently has neuropathic components, in which damage to the nervous system causes pain,[26] as well as nociceptive components, in which injury to nonneural tissue is conveyed through an intact nervous system. Common causes of neuropathic pain in cancer patients include nerve entrapment syndromes, postprocedural pain, and neuropathies due to chemotherapy and radiation therapy.

Current therapeutic options for cancer pain relief overlap substantially with those for noncancer pain. However, there is increasing evidence to support the use of modalities that are specific for cancer pain. The palliative benefit of external-beam radiation for cancer pain is well established. The use of bisphosphonates, radiofrequency tumor ablation, and systemic radionuclides has been shown to improve pain in specific cancer types. Improved pain control also has been demonstrated in clinical trials of chemotherapy and hormonal therapy for certain advanced cancers.

Methodology of Finding, Retrieving, and Evaluating the Evidence on Cancer-Related Pain

A comprehensive, systematic review of cancer pain is beyond the scope of this chapter. The material presented represents a summary and selective update of two recent evidence reports on cancer pain prepared for the Agency for Healthcare Research and Quality (AHRQ) at the request of the American Pain Society[27] and, subsequently, the National Cancer Institute.[28] The purpose of the evidence reports was to provide a comprehensive overview of published studies on the occurrence, assessment, and treatment of cancer pain. In preparing the evidence reports, a sensitive search strategy was applied to the Medline and CancerLit databases and the Cochrane Controlled Trials Registry. This strategy yielded 24,822 reports published in English. Studies selected for inclusion in the evidence reports met all the following criteria: (a) all or part of the population studied suffered from cancer, (b) pain was a measured primary or secondary outcome, and (c) pain was attributed to the cancer itself or to cancer treatment. Studies with the primary purpose of assessing the prevalence or incidence of cancer pain, were used to obtain information about the occurrence of cancer pain. Both retrospective and prospective studies were used to obtain information about the methods of assessment of cancer pain. Randomized controlled trials were used to assess the efficacy of interventions. The characteristics of the retrieved studies were analyzed with respect to population and disease characteristics, patient demographics, treatment comparisons, outcome measures, and methodological features. The methodological quality, the applicability of the reported findings, and the magnitude of treatment effects of randomized controlled trials (RCTs) were assessed. For the purposes of this text, a selective review of the evidence included in these two evidence reports is provided, and more recent studies of particular importance are highlighted.

Occurrence of Cancer-Related Pain

Twenty-nine studies were identified reporting the prevalence and/or incidence of cancer-related pain[29–57] (Table 82.1). More than half the studies were conducted in the United States. The majority of the remaining studies were conducted in Europe; 2 were from Asia and 1 was from South Africa. Two studies focused on pain in pediatric cancer patients.[32,33] In two studies, the prevalence of pain in patients with recently diagnosed cancers was reported.[44,52] Three studies focused on hospice or end-of-life care.[35,43,55] We identified only 2 studies that provided a quantitative estimate of the prevalence of pain in minority groups (African-Americans, Hispanics, Asians, and American Indians)[42,51] and 1 study that reported the prevalence of pain in elderly cancer patients.[51]

The patient populations were heterogeneous in the majority of studies, representing a mixture of demographics, cancer types, stages of disease, and mechanisms of pain. Two studies focused on the occurrence of a specific pain syndrome, pain after surgery for breast cancer.[46,49] Four studies focused on specific malignancies: one on patients with colon or lung cancer,[38] and one each on ovarian cancer,[41] lung cancer,[43] and pancreatic cancer.[44]

The large majority of the studies involved selected cohorts, ranging from 60 to 2,266 subjects, from hospitals, clinics, pain services, and hospices. The largest study by far (and the only one that could be considered population based) was a national survey from Japan of 35,683 hospitalized patients with cancer.[37] In this study, the incidence of pain was defined as the percentage of patients receiving analgesics (32.6%), a definition that excludes untreated pain and therefore, almost certainly represents an underestimate of the true incidence.

By any measure, pain is extremely common among cancer patients, and a large majority experience pain during the course of their illness. None of the studies identified a pain prevalence rate less than 14% of the patients surveyed, and rates of up to 100% were found in selected populations. As might be expected, pain appears to be more common in metastatic than in localized cancer. It is difficult, however, to determine other reliable correlations between the prevalence or incidence of pain and patient factors, disease characteristics, the setting in which care is provided (e.g., primary care or specialized oncology or pain treatment clinics), or specific treatments directed toward the underlying disease. Various methods were used to assess pain, and therefore the reported rates in different studies are not readily comparable.

The total number of patients surveyed in studies on the occurrence of cancer pain is a minuscule fraction of those affected, a much lower fraction than has been studied in other conditions of comparable frequency and impact. Few of the studies were longitudinal and none focused on cancer survivors. Only one study was population based; the others were cohort studies. Studies of selected cohorts may underestimate the true burden of pain because patients with the most intense pain may have been too symptomatic to participate or perhaps less likely to receive their care in the academic referral centers where the majority of the studies were conducted. Although much has been learned about the prevalence of cancer pain, the picture remains far from complete. Little is known about the variations in the prevalence, severity, and course of cancer pain with respect to patient factors (age, gender, race, socioeconomic status, ethnicity), disease characteristics (type, stage, and phenotypic or genotypic classifications), treatment modalities, provider attributes, and the setting in which care is provided.

Assessment of Cancer-Related Pain

Simple patient self-report instruments, such as numeric, verbal, or pictorial scales and brief questionnaires have proven to be a rapid, reliable way to assess cancer pain. The U.S. Joint Commission on Accreditation of Healthcare Organizations includes the assessment of pain using such methods among its standards for accreditation of hospitals. The Brief Pain Inventory (BPI) has been validated in at least 18 languages and is perhaps the most widely used multiple-item pain assessment instrument. Despite the availability of reliable methods of assessment and the mandate for their use as a matter of healthcare policy, it remains uncertain how effectively and consistently cancer pain is assessed in various practice settings. A number of studies have suggested that inadequate assessment is a major contributing factor to the undertreatment of cancer pain, particularly in children, the elderly, and minorities (see following).[42,51,58]

In clinical practice, regular evaluation of pain is the foundation of effective treatment.[12,59,60] Patients with cancer may experience acute or chronic pain related to their primary diagnosis, from treatment, or from unrelated, even preexisting disorders. The initial evaluation of a patient with cancer pain should include assessment of the pain intensity by patient self-report, using a numerical, verbal, or pictorial scale. Assessment of cancer pain intensity serially, using a standard,

TABLE 82.1. Summary of studies reporting the prevalence and/or incidence of cancer pain.

Author	*Setting*	*Population*	*Aim of the study*	*Type of cancer*	*Incidence or prevalence of pain, etiology, characteristics (comments)*
Daut 1982[29]	Country: USA Setting: hospital clinic (inpatients and outpatients) Specialty: oncology, urology, and gynecology	$N = 667$ Age: 19–88 years Symptoms: pain Sx duration: 9 months Source of data: questionnaire, charts	To evaluate the incidence of pain at the time of diagnosis and in progression of disease. Also evaluated were intensity, location, and perceived cause, treatment, and efficacy, interference with life.	Breast (289/667 = 43.3%) Prostate (48/667 = 7.2%) Colon/rectal (127/667 = 19.0%) Cervix (91/667 = 13.6%) Uterine (27/667 = 4.0%) Ovary (85/667 = 12.0%)	Met Non-met Breast 64% 40% Prostate 75% 30% Colon/rectal 47% 40% Cervix ND 35% Uterine 40% 14% Ovary 59% 39% Total (pain due directly to tumor): 33% 6% 6%–7% pain due to other etiologies
Ahles 1984[30]	Country: USA Setting: clinic outpatients Specialty: oncology	$N = 208$ Age: 17–86 years Symptoms: pain Sx duration: 7 months Source of data: questionnaire, charts	To determine prevalence of pain and relation of pain to cancer, treatment of cancer, or other. The study also evaluated the incidence of pain according to the stage (local, regional, metastatic).	Breast (62/208 = 29.8%) Lung (26/208 = 12.5%) Lymphoma (22/208 = 10.6%) Colon (19/208 = 9.1%) Other (79/208 = 38.0%)	33.5% pain due to cancer 6.7% cancer-related procedures 11.0% non-cancer-related pain commonly associated with metastatic disease.
Gilbert 1986[31]	Country: USA Setting: clinic inpatients Specialty: oncology	$N = 162$ Age: >18 years Symptoms: neurologic Sx duration: 3 months Source of data: questionnaire, charts	To determine the incidence and nature of pain and other major neurologic problems (e.g., disorientation) in cancer patients.	Non-Hodgkin's lymphoma (26/162 = 16.0%) Breast (17/162 = 10.5%) Hepatoma (15/162 = 9.2%) Small-cell lung (13/162 = 8.0%) Multiple myeloma (13/162 = 8.0%) Colon (10/162 = 6.1%) (All others <10)	34/162 21% overall
Miser 1987[32]	Country: USA Setting: hospital, clinic (in- and outpatients) Specialty: pediatric oncology	$N = 139$ 161 inpatient days, 195 outpatient clinic visits (in- and outpatients) Age: >7 years Symptoms: pain Sx duration: 6 months Source of data: questionnaires	To investigate the prevalence and nature of pain in children and young adults with malignancy.	Leukemia (44/139 = 31%) Soft tissue sarcoma (33/139 = 23.7%) Ewing's sarcoma (28/139 = 20.1%) Osteosarcoma (20/139 = 14.4%) Lymphoma (12/139 = 8.6%) Other (2/139 = 1.4%)	In 356 patient visits, pain present in 54% of total inpatient population and 26% of outpatient population: 46% pain due to tumor alone, 14% pain due to both tumor and therapy 40% pain due to cancer Tx Only tumor-related pain was due to bone invasion 68%, cord compression 5%, and multiple causes 11%. Pain was associated with lower functional status (Karnofsky score).

TABLE 82.1. (continued)

Author	*Setting*	*Population*	*Aim of the study*	*Type of cancer*	*Incidence or prevalence of pain, etiology, characteristics (comments)*
Miser 1987[33]	Country: USA Setting: hospital, clinic (in- and outpatients) Specialty: pediatric oncology	*N* = 92 Age: children and young adults (age not stated) Symptoms: pain Sx duration: 26 months Source of data: questionnaires	To investigate the incidence of pain in children and young adults presenting with newly diagnosed malignancy.	Soft tissue sarcoma (23/92 = 25%) Ewing's sarcoma (21/92 = 22.8%) Osteosarcoma (14/92 = 15.2%) Leukemia (12/92 = 13%) Lymphoma (10/92 = 10.9%) Neuroblastoma (1/92 = 1.0%) Other (11)	Soft tissue sarcoma 52.2% Ewing's sarcoma 60.0% Osteosarcoma 78.3% Leukemia 100% Lymphoma 100% Neuroblastoma 100% On initial evaluation 72 of 92 patients were experiencing pain that had been present for median 74 days (3–21 days, range); 42 had experienced sleep disturbances due to pain. Pain was associated with lower functional status (Karnofsky score).
Greenwald 1987[34]	Country: USA Setting: hospital (outpatients) Specialty: anesthesiology and pain management	*N* = 536 Age: 20–80 years Symptoms: neurologic Sx duration: 18 months Source of data: Cancer Surveillance System registry, graphic rating scales, McGill Pain Questionnaire	To determine the prevalence and characteristics of pain in four types of primary cancer restricted to recently diagnosed patients (within 3 months of the survey).	Lung (260/536 = 48.5%) Prostate (201/536 = 37.5%) Uterine/cervix (50/536 = 9.3%) Pancreas (25/536 = 4.7%)	Lung 50.7% Prostate 38.3% Uterine/cervix 38.0% Pancreas 60.0% % of patients reporting moderate to very bad pain in past week by cancer site; % by stage also reported.
Coyle 1990[35]	Country: USA Setting: pain service (outpatients) Specialty: neurology	*N* = 90 (40 M, 50 F) Median age: 59 (23–82) years Symptoms: pain Sx duration: 6 years (retrospective) Source of data: retrospective/ patient charts	To retrospectively evaluate the prevalence of pain by intensity, type, analgesic consumption, and suicidal ideation in cancer patients during the 4 weeks preceding death.	Lung (23/90 = 25.6%) Colon (18/90 = 20.0%) Breast (18/90 = 20.0%) Head/neck (9/90 = 10.0%) Gynecologic (6/90 = 6.7%) (All others <5%)	For all sites: 100% had pain 80% mild to moderate 20% moderate to severe 67% more than one type of pain (40% somatic and neuropathic)
Portenoy 1990[36]	Country: USA Setting: pain service Specialty: neurology	*N* = 63, 41 (64%) with breakthrough pain episodes (19 M, 22 F) Median age: 51 (15–81) years Symptoms: breakthrough pain Sx duration: 3 months Source of data: prospective survey	To evaluate prevalence and characteristics of breakthrough pain.	Genitourinary (11/41 = 26.8%) Head/neck (5/41 = 12.2%) GI (4/41 = 9.8%) Lung (3/41 = 7.3%) Sarcoma (3/41 = 7.3%) Other (13)	Patients with breakthrough pain, 1 type (32), 2 distinct types (8), and 3 types (1). Characteristics: (median 4 pains/day; range 1–3,600) 22 (43%) had rapid onset (<3 min) Duration: (median 30 min; range 1–240) 21 (41%) both paroxysmal and brief 15 (29%) began or worsened at end of a fixed opioid dose interval Type of pain: somatic 17 (33%) visceral 10 (20%) neuropathic 14 (27%) mixed 10 (20%)
Hiraga 1991[37]	Country: Japan Setting: nationwide hospitals (inpatients) Specialty: all	*N* = 35,683 (31.6% of all hospitalized patients at the time of survey) Age: not reported Symptoms: pain Sx duration: not reported Source of data: nationwide questionnaire by nurses	To determine the incidence of pain in different stages of illness, analgesic methods, and rate of pain relief in cancer patients in Japan (incidence was defined as the percentage of patients receiving pain medication).	Stomach (5,882/35,683 = 16.4%) Liver/biliary/pancreas (4,578/35,683 = 12.8%) Lung (4,428/35,683 = 12.4%) Colon/rectal (3,332/35,683 = 9.3%) Oral/pharynx/larynx (2,966/35,683 = 8.3%) Ovary/cervix/corpus (2,765/35,683 = 7.7%)	32.6%

(continued)

TABLE 82.1. Summary of studies reporting the prevalence and/or incidence of cancer pain. (continued)

Author	*Setting*	*Population*	*Aim of the study*	*Type of cancer*	*Incidence or prevalence of pain, etiology, characteristics (comments)*
				Genitourinary (2,746/35,683 = 7.7%) Lymphoma/leukemia (2,686/35,683 = 7.5%) Breast (1,925/35,683 = 5.4%) Other (9675)	
Portenoy 1992[38]	Country: USA Setting: three physicians' outpatient practices Specialty: oncology, two specialists in lung cancer and one in colon cancer	N = 398 patients with lung or colon cancer Age: 57 ± 10.4 years (average for 91 patients who reported pain during the 2 previous weeks and consented to an interview) Symptoms: pain, mood (0–100 mm VAS for pain intensity, pain relief, and mood and 8-point categorical scale for pain intensity) Sx duration: 9 months Source of data: prospective survey with face-to-face interviews	To evaluate the prevalence and characteristics of pain in ambulatory patients with colon and lung cancer during active antitumor therapy. A prospective survey using face-to-face and telephone interviews by trained quality assurance analysts.	Lung (185/398 = 46.4%) Colon (213/398 = 55.6%)	"Persistent or frequent pain" during the previous 2 weeks was reported by: 57/145(39.3%) with lung cancer and 52/181(28.7%) with colon cancer. 91 of the above patients (47 lung, 44 colon) were interviewed in detail. There were no significant differences in pain with the exception of pain location between the two tumor types. One-third of patients had more than one discrete pain. Median pain duration was 4 weeks (range, less than 1 week-468 weeks), and average pain intensity was moderate. Approximately 90% of patients experienced pain more than 25% of the time. Regarding pain treatment: 56/91(61.5%) were prescribed no medication; 4/91(4.4%) were prescribed nonopioid medication; 31/91(34.1%) were given opioids. Of patients reporting that pain in general was moderate or greater, 57.8% were prescribed no pain medications and 37.3% received opioids.
Brescia 1992[39]	Country: USA Setting: a 200-bed "specialty hospital for advanced cancer" Specialty: terminal care	N = 1,103 patients admitted during the survey period, and 1,017 patients who died within 6 months of the end of the survey Age: mean, 68; range, 24–94 years; 62% of patients were older than 65. Symptoms: pain intensity (none, mild, or severe) Severe pain was defined as recorded pain of moderate or greater intensity that occurred with regularity throughout the day. Mild pain was noted when the record stated that pain was relieved without the use of analgesics, by nonopioid agents, or by the "weak" opioids such as	To develop a clinical database for advanced cancer patients and to survey data to determine (1) pain severity at admission, (2) opioid use at admission, (3) change in opioid use during the hospital stay, and (4) survival in the hospital. Data were collected prospectively within 72 h after admission and soon after death or discharge.	Primary sites: Lung 19% Breast 13% Colon 10% Colon-rectum 6% Other sites 33%–55% Bone metastases: (pain-producing) in 38% Other sites of metastases: Lung 24% Liver 28% Brain 17%	73% of patients had pain at admission. Severe pain was inversely related to age; patients younger than 55 were twice as likely to have severe pain as older patients. Frequency of severe pain by type of cancer: cervix (68%, prostate 57%, colon-rectum 49%; severe pain was noted by nearly one-half (49%) of the patients with bone metastases. At baseline, 25% of patients were receiving morphine, 18% codeine, 6% hydromorphone, and 3% methadone or levorphanol. Most (71.7%) patients had a stable dosing pattern; only 4.2% required opioid dose increases of 10% or more per day.

TABLE 82.1. (continued)

Author	Setting	Population	Aim of the study	Type of cancer	Incidence or prevalence of pain, etiology, characteristics (comments)
		codeine. No pain was recorded when the record stated explicitly that the patient offered no complaint of pain or was comfortable. Sx duration: 12 months Source of data: prospective chart review at baseline (72h after admission) and again "soon after the patient's death or discharge."			
Vuorinen 1993[40]	Country: Finland Setting: pain clinic (outpatients) Specialty: anesthesiology	*N* = 378 (240 evaluable, 40% M, 60% F) Median age: 64 (27–89) years Symptoms: pain Sx duration: 9 months. Source of data: questionnaire	To investigate the prevalence and causes of pain at the early stages of cancer (0–6 months from diagnosis).	Genitourinary (73/240 = 31%) GI (38/240 = 16%) Breast (63/240 = 26%) Hematologic (26/240 = 11%) Lung (14/240 = 6%) Skin (13/240 = 5%) Other (13/240 = 5%)	66/240 (28%) at time of questionnaire; 42/240 (24%) as first sign of cancer. Cause: 46% direct tumor growth 67% conditions secondary to cancer 18% unrelated to cancer
Portenoy 1994[41]	Country: USA Setting: hospital clinic (inpatients and outpatients) Specialty: neurology, pain	*N* = 151 (111 inpatients, 40 outpatients) Median age: 55 (23–86) years Symptoms: pain Sx duration: 18 months. Source of data: questionnaires	To investigate the prevalence, characteristics, and impact of pain in ovarian cancer patients.	Ovarian cancer	62% had pain before diagnosis 42% had pain during last 2 weeks. Most patients had pain-related interference with function.
Cleeland 1994[42]	Country: USA Setting: outpatients in 54 oncology clinics Specialty: medical research, neurology	*N* = 1,308 (376M, 495F) 871 with pain or taking analgesics during week before to study Median age: 62 (19–90) years Symptoms: pain Sx duration: 12 months Source of data: questionnaire	To assess adequacy of analgesic drug prescribing according to WHO guidelines, factors that influence whether analgesia was adequate, and the effects of inadequate analgesia on patients' perception of pain relief and function status.	Breast (270/871 = 60%) GI (148/871 = 58%) Lung (124/871 = 63%) genitourinary (86/871 = 66%) Lymphoma (55/871 = 71%) Gyn (23/871 = 63%) [% of patients by site (see prior column) with substantial pain; pooled figure = 67%]	Physicians commonly underestimated the severity of pain; 42% of patients with pain were not given adequate analgesic therapy according to WHO guidelines. Independent risk factors for inadequate pain management included pain not attributed to cancer, better performance status, age 70 or older, female sex, and minority status. Underrated pain impaired function.
Mercadante 1994[43]	Country: Italy Setting: palliative care service (outpatients) Specialty: pain management	*N* = 60 (52 evaluable, 44M, 8F) Age: 64.2 ± 2 (42–82) years Symptoms: pain Sx duration: unclear, 51.3 ± 9.4 days observation period Source of data: questionnaires	To obtain the prevalence, characteristics, and localization of pain in lung cancer and also to determine response to treatment by WHO analgesic ladder.	Lung	46 of 52 (88.4%) experienced pain. Pain was localized in: Chest 26/52 Legs/lumbar 1/52 Abdomen/arms 8/52 Head 6/52 The type of pain was: Somatic 85.7% Visceral 42.8% Neuropathic 30.9% Incident 23.8%
Kelsen 1995[44]	Country: USA Setting: oncology and palliative care service, in- and outpatients	*N* = 189 (130 evaluable, 79M, 51F, total screened 277) Patients were divided into two groups, those who	To evaluate the prevalence of pain and depression, their correlation and their effect on quality of life in	Adenocarcinoma of the pancreas	At study entrance: 37% no pain 34% mild or minimal pain; 29% moderate to severe pain. Of patients who reported pain at entry, its duration ranged

(continued)

TABLE 82.1. Summary of studies reporting the prevalence and/or incidence of cancer pain. (continued)

Author	*Setting*	*Population*	*Aim of the study*	*Type of cancer*	*Incidence or prevalence of pain, etiology, characteristics (comments)*
	Specialty: neurology and medicine	underwent surgery (83/130) and those who received chemotherapy (47/130). Median age: 63 years Symptoms: pain Sx duration: unclear Source of data: questionnaires	patients with recently diagnosed adenocarcinoma of the pancreas.		from 1 to >5 months, 67% described a diffuse abdominal pain. Chemotherapy patients had more intense pain than preoperative patients. Patients with moderate or greater pain had more impairment of functional activity than patients with mild or no pain. Significant correlations between increasing pain and depression, and between pain/depressive symptoms and quality of life.
Larue 1995[45]	Country: France Setting: 20 cancer treatment services, in- and outpatients Specialty: not specified	*N* = 605 (601 evaluable, 252 M, 347 F, ?2) Mean age: 57.8 ± 14 SD Symptoms: pain Sx duration: unclear Source of data: questionnaires by patients and physicians	To describe the treatment of cancer pain in France and to evaluate the predictive factors for inadequate management.	Breast (211/605 = 34.8%) GI (108/605 = 17.9% Genitourinary (80/605 = 13.2%) Lung (77/605 = 12.7%) Head/neck (57/605 = 9.4%) Lymphoma (26/605 = 4.2%) Other (46/605 = 7.6%)	57% (340/601) reported pain due to their disease. 69% (224/325) of those with pain rated their worst pain at a level that impaired their ability to function. 30% (84/279) were not receiving pain medication. 51% (137/200) of those receiving pain medication found relief was inadequate. Doctors' pain ratings were consistently less than patients'.
Stevens 1995[46]	Country: USA Setting: 16 ambulatory care services Specialty: nursing	*N* = 95 (435 oncology patients screened) Mean age: 49.16 ± 13 SD and 52.6 ± 12.4 SD (with and without pain, respectively) Symptoms: postmastectomy pain Sx duration: unclear Source of data: medical records, questionnaires	To investigate prevalence, characteristics, and impact of postmastectomy pain.	Breast (postmastectomy)	65% reported no pain 15% reported pain of somatic or visceral type associated with the tumor 20% postmastectomy pain. All with pain reported interference with work or home activities. All with pain reported exacerbation on movement. Patients used weak, nonopioid analgesics (25%) or none (75%). 85% used nonpharmacologic pain control.
Vainio 1996[47]	Country: Switzerland (data from UK, Switzerland, Finland, USA, and Australia) Setting: 7 hospices, in- and outpatients Specialty: multiple	*N* = 1640 Age: ≥18 years Symptoms: pain and other symptoms Sx duration: 3 months to 3 years Source of data: questionnaire by nurse or doctor	To estimate the prevalence of pain and eight other common symptoms in a large population of patients with advanced cancer from different palliative care centers.	Lung (343/1,640 = 21% Breast (174/1,640 = 11%) Colorectal (121/1,640 = 7%) Head/neck (92/1,640 = 6%) Stomach (86/1,640 = 5%) Prostate (76/1,640 = 5%) Gynecologic (83/1,640 = 5%) Lympho-hematologic (60/1,640 = 4%) Esophagus (36/1,640 = 2%) Other, unknown (569/1,640 = 35%)	The prevalence of moderate to severe pain was 51%, ranging from 43% (stomach) to 80% (gynecologic). Wide intercenter differences (e.g., 10%–50% with severe pain).
Grond 1996[48]	Country: Germany Setting: pain service Specialty: anesthesiology; unclear if	*N* = 2266 (53% M, 47% F) Mean age: 59 ± 13 SD Symptoms: pain Sx duration: 9 years (1983–1992)	To evaluate the localization, etiologies, and pathophysiologic mechanisms of cancer-related pain syndromes.	GI (663/2,266 = 29%) Genitourinary (379/2,266 = 17%) Head/neck (377/2,266 = 17%) Breast (227/2,266 = 10%)	30% 1 pain location 39% 2 pain location 31% 3 pain location Etiology: cancer 85% antineoplastic Tx 17% Type of pain: bone 35% soft tissue 45%

TABLE 82.1. (continued)

Author	*Setting*	*Population*	*Aim of the study*	*Type of cancer*	*Incidence or prevalence of pain, etiology, characteristics (comments)*
	inpatient or outpatient	Source of data: questionnaire by nurse or doctor		Lung (218/2,266 = 10%) Lymphatic-hematopoietic (114/2,266 = 5%) Skin, bone, connective (121/2,266 = 5%) Others or multiple (167/2,266 = 7%)	visceral 33% neuropathic 34% Localization: lower back 36%; abdominal 27%; thorax 23%; legs 21% head 17%; pelvis 15%
Tasmuth 1996[49]	Country: Finland Setting: university hospital, surgical outpatient clinic Specialty: anesthesiology	*N* = 93 (105 screened) Median age: 59 (29–85) and 57 (40–86) years [two groups, mastectomy, resection] Symptoms: pain Sx duration: 1 year (1993–1994) Source of data: questionnaire by nurse or doctor	To assess pain, neurologic symptoms, edema of the ipsilateral arm, depression, and anxiety in women treated with mastectomy or limited resection (plus axillary dissection for either), and the impact of these symptoms in daily life.	Breast (postmastectomy)	Incidence of pain before surgery: 36% (mastectomy) 23% (resection) After surgery: 26%, 15%, and 17% (1 month, 6 months, and 1 year postmastectomy) 28%, 33%, and 33% (postresection at same times)
Higginson 1997[50]	Country: UK, Ireland Setting: multi-disciplinary palliative care centers (6 in England, 5 in London), in- and outpatients Specialty: palliative medicine and oncology (nursing with special training)	*N* = 695 (55% M, 45% F [Irl], 54% M, 46% F [UK]) Median age: 67 (5–95) years UK and 67 (32–90) years Irl [two ethnic groups] Symptoms: pain Sx duration: not reported Source of data: questionnaire by nurse	To investigate the prevalence and intensity of pain in advanced cancer patients.	Lung/ENT (110/418 = 16.3% & 73/277 = 26%) GI (144/418 = 34% & 84/277 = 30%) Genitourinary (58/418 = 13.8% & 44/277 = 15.8%) Breast/bone (48/418 = 11.4% & 26/277 = 09.4%) Lymph/hematopoietic (13/418 = 3.1% & 10/277 = 3.6%) Other (45/418 = 10.8% & 40/277 = 14%)	UK Ireland Lung/ENT 69% 74% GI 68% 68% Genitourinary 66% 84% Breast/bone 71% 85% Lymph/hemato 62% 90% Other 62% 63% Overall prevalence of pain at referral in the two settings was 68% and 74% (similar figures for home hospice patients as for hospitalized cancer patients).
Bernabei 1998[51]	Country: USA Setting: 1492 nursing homes Specialty: multiple	*N* = 13,625 Age: >65 (65–74 years, 45% M) 65–84 years (44% M) >85 years (40% M) Symptoms: pain Sx duration: 1992–1995 Source of data: systematic assessment of geriatric drug use via epidemiology database	To evaluate the adequacy of pain management in elderly and minority cancer patients admitted to nursing homes.	Not provided	4,003/13,625 (27.38%) reported daily pain. Age, gender, race, marital status, physical function, depression, and cognitive status were all independently associated with presence of pain. 26% of those in pain received no analgesic agent. Predictors for not receiving any analgesic agent despite daily pain were age >85, minority race, impaired cognition, and receiving multiple medications concurrently.

(*continued*)

TABLE 82.1. Summary of studies reporting the prevalence and/or incidence of cancer pain. (continued)

Author	*Setting*	*Population*	*Aim of the study*	*Type of cancer*	*Incidence or prevalence of pain, etiology, characteristics (comments)*
Ger 1998[52]	Country: Taiwan Setting: three outpatient oncology clinics Specialty: anesthesiology	N = 296 (194 M, 66%, 102 F, 34%) 69% interviewed within 14 days from cancer diagnosis. Age: 56.4 ± 16 SD (10–80) years Symptoms: pain Sx duration: 18 months Source of data: questionnaire	To evaluate the prevalence and severity of cancer pain in newly diagnosed cancer patients.	Lung (63/296 = 21%) Upper GI (58/296 = 20%) Colorectal (36/296 = 12%) Head/neck (29/296 = 10%) Other (76/296 = 36%)	113/296 (38%) had pain Of those, 92% cancer related, 5% treatment related, 3% both cancer and treatment related. Ethnic minority status, lower-grade insurance status, excellent prior pain tolerance, impaired function status (ECOG scale), and distant spread of disease each separately predicted the presence of pain.
Petzke 1999[53]	Part I Country: Germany Setting: 1 Outpatient clinic Specialty: Anesthesiology	N = 243 (39% of 613 consecutive cancer pts with pain; 270 M, 361 F) Age: 59.2 ± 13.8 (16–97) years Symptoms: Transitory exacerbations of pain Duration: Within past week Source of data: Patient interview	To identify and evaluate the incidence of transitory pain in cancer pain patients	GI 26%, GU 17%, Head/neck 16%, Breast 12%, Other 29%	Location of cancer, tumor stage, presence/absence of metastasis, and type of therapy were not significantly different in patients with or without transitory pain. The intensity of baseline pain was higher in pts **without** transitory pain: 68% reported severe-maximal pain vs 54%. However, the intensity in those **with** transitory pain was rated severe to maximal in 92% of pts.
	Part II Country: Germany Setting: Clinic as above Specialty: Anesthesiology	N = 55 (68% of 81 pts, 33 M, 22 F) reported transitory pain on admission. Age: 59 ± 12.1 (30–85) years Symptoms: Pain similar in frequency, duration, and intensity to those in Part I.	To further describe and quantify transitory pain experienced by these patients.	Comparable to those in Part I.	Transitory pain was characterized by rapid onset (within 3 min) in 47% of pts; 58% of these pts reported a duration of less than 15 min. 97% of these pts had either neuropathic (35%) or nociceptive pain (62%). 40% of patients identified no precipitating event, while movements or timing of analgesic regimen were named as known triggers for 2/3 of the others. Additional or regular medication was effective in relieving transitory pain in 75% of patient. Analgesic preparations with novel delivery mechanisms-i.e., oral transmucosal have recently been found effective for breakthough pain.
Chang 2000[54]	Country: USA Setting: VA Medical Center, NJ Specialty: Medical oncology	N = 240 (232 M, 8 F): 100 consecutive outpatients, 140 consecutive inpatients who reported pain symptoms. Age: Median 68 (27–89) years; Symptoms: median of 8	To assess symptom prevalence, symptom intensity and their relationship to QOL in this population.	Solid tumors: 201 (139 metastatic); Hematologic disease: 39	Symptom assessment: MSAS found median number of symptoms/pt to be 8. Fatigue/lack of energy and pain were most prevalent symptoms: 62% and 52%, respectively. Number of symptoms, intensity, and resulting level of distress were correlated with extent of disease. Lower Karnofsky scores indicated a likelihood of intense and/or distressing symptoms. Authors noted that pain was never a solitary symptom, and should be considered a marker for presence of other symptoms.

TABLE 82.1. (continued)

Author	*Setting*	*Population*	*Aim of the study*	*Type of cancer*	*Incidence or prevalence of pain, etiology, characteristics (comments)*
Zepetella 2000[55]	Country: UK Setting: Hospice Specialty: Palliative medicine	*N* = 245 (59%of 414 consecutive cancer admissions; 185 M, 229 F) Age: 71(33–100) years Symptoms: Chronic pain of variable duration	To examine the prevalence and characteristics of breakthrough pain in terminally ill pts admitted to hospice. Satisfaction with treatment was also assessed.	Lung 27%, Breast, Prostate, and Unknown Primary 9% each. Most breakthrough pain was tumor related; 38% rated as severe-excruciating, and related to patient dissatisfaction, underlining the value of ongoing assessment.	Of the 245 participants, 89% had breakthrough pain, most of which was frequent and short-lasting, suggesting that effective treatment would include medications that are fast-acting, readily and quickly absorbed
Meuser 2001[56]	Country: Germany Setting: Academic Medical Center Specialty: Anesthesiology pain service	*N* = 593 (all patients treated by the service between August 1992 and July 1994; 46.8% M, 43.2% F). Age: 59 ± 14 years Symptoms: Pain + at least one other symptom	To survey symptom prevalence, etiology, and severity, taking all possibilities of symptom relief into consideration.	Percentages: GI 24.6, Respiratory 19.8, GU 18.9, Head/neck 16.9 most prevalent. 98.3% of patients referred suffered pain and at least one other symptom.	Nonopioid analgesics were used most frequently—initially by 94.3% of pts, finally by 78.3%. WHO step guidelines were used throughout, plus other palliative treatment in 50% of pts: chemo, hormonal therapy, radiation, and surgery in 15.5%, 21.4%, 26.9%, and 8/9%, respectively. Efficacy was good in 70%, satisfactory in 16% of pts and inadequate in 14%, and all caused a significant reduction in other symptoms, demonstrating that pain relief can be achieved without increasing most symptoms.
Beck 2001[57]	Country: South Africa Setting: Inpatient and outpatient areas of two healthcare facilities in Pretoria: a 120 bed private hospital, a 1000 bed public hospital Specialty: Medical oncology	Phase I: *N* = 263 (98.5% of 267 pts seen during study period; 103 M, 160 F; 75% white) Age: mean 55 (18–87) years Symptoms: Pain Sx Duration: Not stated Source of Data: Survey of Cancer Pain in South Africa (BPI translated into five local languages)	To document the prevalence of pain among cancer patients in inpatient and outpatient settings	All types represented in patients of the two participating facilities	Cancer type and pain prevalence were determined. Of cancer in males (105) top distribution was as follows: lymphoma 14, head/neck and prostate each 11, lung and melanoma each 10, colorectal 9. In females (158) distribution was breast 86, ovary 14, uterus 13, lymphoma 12, head/neck 6, lung 3.
		Phase II: *N* = 479 were eligible; 426 completed the questionnaire (163 M, 251 F), 46% white, 42% black, 12% colored or Asian Age: mean 56.7 (18–90) years Symptoms: Pain	To describe patterns of cancer pain and pain management in South Africa	In male pts, prostate, lung, head/neck, and esophagus accounted for 50.5%, in females, breast and cervix alone accounted for 53.3%; lymphoma, colorectal, and esophageal afflicted most of the rest in both.	57.4% of pts experienced pain 7 d/wk; 23.6% were in pain 24 h/day. Ratings of 'worst pain' were highest in community-based pts (38.1%), lowest in hospices (23.6%). Almost twice as many pts were in moderate or severe 'pain now' in public (39%) vs. private (20%) settings. Of nonwhites (black/colored/Asian), 81% experienced 'worst pain' of moderate-severe intensity vs. 65% of whites ($P < 0.0001$).

Met, metastatic; Non-met, nonmetastatic; GI, gastrointestinal; Sx, symptoms; Tx, therapy; WHO, World Health Organization.

validated measure is essential to judge the efficacy of treatment.[61–63] Recent studies suggest that patients identify a decline in pain intensity of about 30% as the threshold for clinical pain relief.[1,64,65]

The reduction of pain to a single parameter (intensity) is pragmatic, perhaps essential, for purposes of assessment and treatment, but intensity should be simply a starting point in pain assessment. The characteristics of the pain (location, intensity, quality, temporal characteristics, exacerbating and relieving factors, and responses to prior treatments) should be assessed, together with a review of treatment, psychosocial assessment, physical examination, and appropriate diagnostic studies.[66,67] Efforts should be made to determine the etiology of the pain, and in particular, to determine whether it represents an emergency, such as spinal cord compression or an impeding or existing bone fracture. Psychosocial assessment should address the mood of the patient, his or her coping skills, family support structure, signs and symptoms of anxiety or depression, expectations regarding pain management, risk factors for undertreatment of pain, and the meaning of the pain for the patient and family.

The majority of clinical trials evaluating treatments for cancer pain have employed single-variable pain intensity scales. The diverse mechanisms of pain, its quality and time course, and its impact on quality of life were not reported in most treatment trials. Furthermore, the instruments used to capture information about pain are sufficiently heterogeneous to preclude merging of results.[28]

Figure 82.1 depicts the contribution of various patient- and disease-related factors to the occurrence of cancer symptoms. Fundamental to this model is the fact that the methods of assessment affect the observed prevalence rate of any symptom. Evaluating the clinical evidence on cancer pain is complicated by the heterogeneity of instruments or scales used to assess pain. This problem is of more than academic interest. In a cohort study of 313 cancer patients with pain, the proportion of patients whose pain was inadequately treated varied very widely, from 16% to 91%, depending on which of four different assessment measures was used. This variability was entirely due to the choice of measure, rather than the approach to treatment of the pain.[68]

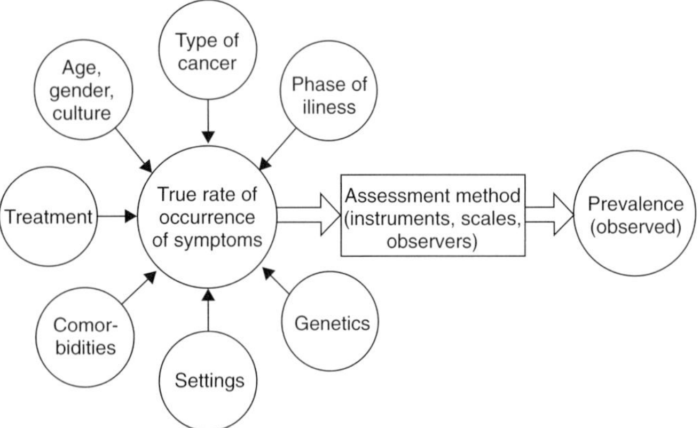

FIGURE 82.1. Relationship among factors that contribute to the occurrence of cancer symptoms, methods of assessment, and prevalence of symptoms.

Treatment of Cancer Pain

Systemic analgesic therapy is the foundation for treating cancer pain because of its relative low risk and cost, dependability, and ease of administration.[66,69] Nonpharmacologic measures, such as patient education and cognitive-behavioral strategies, are also important components of treatment. Because patients differ in their acceptance of, and responses to, specific analgesics and to different behavioral strategies, it is essential that treatment be individualized.[70,71]

The three principal families of drugs used to manage cancer pain are nonsteroidal antiinflammatory drugs (NSAIDs; acetaminophen is usually included in this category although it is not an NSAID), opioid analgesics, and adjuvant medications. Adjuvants treat concurrent symptoms that exacerbate pain (e.g., insomnia), enhance the analgesic efficacy of opioids, or provide analgesia for specific types of pain (e.g., antidepressants and anticonvulsants for neuropathic pain). Medicines to prevent or treat the adverse effects of opioids, such as constipation and nausea, also have a critical role.

Clinical consensus and common sense dictate initial use of the least invasive delivery method and simplest dosing regimen.[72] Oral administration of drugs is effective for most cancer pain, but may be problematic for reasons of dysphagia, odynophagia, nausea from chemotherapy or radiation therapy, malabsorption from gastrointestinal dysfunction, or the need to swallow an unwieldy number of tablets. The rectal, transdermal,[73] sublingual, transmucosal,[74–76] and pulmonary routes are other relatively noninvasive options for the delivery of systemic analgesics. Some of these routes are not influenced by first-pass hepatic metabolism, so, for example, an oral dose of a drug is not expected to be equianalgesic with the same dose administered rectally.

Systemic Opioids

Few studies have evaluated systemic opioids for cancer pain using a randomized, placebo-controlled trial design.[76–78] Placebo-controlled studies involving people in pain are ethically problematic, unless a rescue medication is provided. Furthermore, the effective palliation of pain with opioids has a strong historical record of efficacy of several millennia, thus obviating the need for placebo-controlled assessment.

Numerous opioids with various pharmacologic features are available; however, no one opioid has consistently been demonstrated to provide either a superior toxicity profile or superior efficacy. A heterogeneous group of 10 trials compared the efficacy and adverse effects of different opioids administered by the same route within each study.[77,79–87] The applicability of these studies is generally low, and therefore, there is little evidence to support the use of one opioid over another. Exceptions exist to this generalization. Meperidine is generally considered inferior to other opioids for cancer pain because of the potential for accumulation of toxic metabolites with repeated dosing. In patients with renal failure who are treated with morphine, metabolites of the drug (particularly morphine-6-glucuronide) may accumulate, leading to hyperalgesia and central nervous system (CNS) toxicity, so other opioids, such as hydromorphone may be preferable in that setting.

There do not appear to be any advantages for sustained-release formulations of opioids over immediate-release formulations, except possibly for convenience, patient preference, and, by extension, patient adherence. Eight studies have been performed comparing controlled-release morphine with immediate-release oral morphine.[88–95] No significant differences were observed between the two formulations with respect to analgesic efficacy (reduction of pain intensity or increased pain relief). The studies also found no difference with respect to adverse effects or other outcomes. Three hundred seventeen patients, with a wide range of cancer types as well as pain types, were enrolled in these trials, of which 244 were evaluated (78.7%). The foregoing studies all addressed the same study question; therefore, a meta-analysis could be performed using pain intensity as the outcome of interest. All eight studies provided numerical data on mean pain intensities and standard errors or confidence intervals. Differences in average pain intensity between the two study arms (over 4 to 14 days), measured on a continuous visual analogue scale (VAS) (0–100 mm), were combined using a random effects model. No significant difference in average pain intensity was found between controlled-release morphine and morphine sulfate solution [1.18 mm; 95% confidence interval (CI), −1.62 to 3.98 mm]. More extended sustained-release formulations of oral morphine, administered once daily, provide analgesia that is comparable to twice-daily sustained-release formulations but may be preferred by patients.[96,97]

Transdermal fentanyl was compared with oral controlled-release morphine in two studies, neither of which demonstrated a significant difference in pain intensity.[98,99] In one of the studies, more patients expressed a preference for the fentanyl patch, which was associated with less constipation and daytime drowsiness, but greater sleep disturbance and shorter sleep duration. There were no differences in quality of life measures.

In a given patient, the analgesic effect and adverse effects of the different opioids may vary substantially, even when given at theoretically equianalgesic doses.[100] Although the pharmacologic basis of these observations is not well understood, they have led to the empiric practice of drug rotation to improve analgesia or ameliorate adverse effects. If unacceptable side effects occur before an effective dose of an opioid is reached, another one can often be substituted with good effect.[101] Elucidation of genetic variability in the analgesic response to opioids, and in their pharmacokinetics, could potentially give rise to pain treatment that is targeted to the individual patient, rather than be strictly empiric.

Equianalgesic dosing of different opioids is not necessarily straightforward. In the 1960s and 1970s, the relative analgesic potency of single doses of a variety of opioid analgesics (morphine, profadol, oxymorphone, codeine, methotrimeprazine, and oxycodone) was evaluated in patients with cancer.[102–107] Reproducible estimates were generated for the relative potency of opioids in this context, which provide part of the basis for equianalgesic dosing. Several issues complicate the interpretation of these studies. Baseline pain intensity and information about the pathophysiologic substrate of pain were not reported. Thus, relative potency ratios of opioid analgesics are assumed to apply in the whole range of baseline pain (mild, moderate, and severe) and pathophysiologic mechanisms (nociceptive or neuropathic). The majority of patients in these studies had been exposed to opioid analgesics before enrollment, suggesting potential tolerance to opioid test drugs. However, the existence or precise influence of tolerance on the results cannot be estimated because the duration of previous exposure and type of opioids used were not reported.

Adverse effects that limit opioid dosing include constipation, nausea, sedation, confusion, urinary retention, pruritus, myoclonus, dysphoria, sleep disturbance, and respiratory depression. Persistent respiratory depression is rare in opioid-tolerant individuals. Treatment of these adverse effects was the subject of a recent systematic review.[101] Nine uncontrolled studies of at least 180 subjects reported on adverse events of oral opioids.[108–116] Seven were prospective cohort studies, each examining one to five oral opioids used for treatment of cancer pain. Pain relief and quality of life were the primary outcomes in seven of the studies. Two studies primarily examined adverse events: constipation and laxative use[108] and emesis.[109] A total of seven opioids were evaluated at a wide range of average daily dosages (for example, from approximately 19 to 60 mg/day oxycodone and from approximately 80 to 380 mg/day morphine). Subjects were followed from a minimum of 3 days to a maximum of 4 months. In these studies, reported rates of nausea were 7% to 25%; vomiting, 6% to 40%; constipation, 11% to 73%; and sedation, 2% to 54%. The extreme variability of these rates probably reflects the heterogeneous study designs and methods of assessment.

Seven uncontrolled studies of at least 50 subjects reported on adverse events of parenteral opioids.[117–123] Five were prospective cohort studies. One studied subcutaneous oxycodone[121]; the rest studied morphine and/or hydromorphone given subcutaneously or intravenously at a wide range of doses. All the studies examined pain relief or quality of life as primary outcomes. Few studies provided explicit definitions for the symptoms that were being reported. The studies that included both morphine and hydromorphone, or subcutaneous or intravenous injections, did not report different adverse event rates for the different drugs or routes. Six studies reported on nausea and/or vomiting. Nausea (including vomiting) occurred in 0% to 15% percent of subjects; vomiting, when reported separately from nausea, occurred in 0% to 1% percent of subjects. Constipation occurred in 0% to 70% of subjects in five studies. The large range of rates of constipation is likely due to unreported differences in definitions for constipation and different laxative regimens. Fatigue occurred in 17% of subjects and mild sedation in 51% of subjects; otherwise, uncharacterized sedation occurred in 0% to 12% of subjects, and severe sedation in 4% to 6% of subjects. Adverse effects occurring in less than 10% of subjects included local skin irritation or bleeding, skin infections, myoclonus, confusion, dizziness, and seizures. Depending on the methods of assessment and reporting, hallucinations, mental clouding, dry mouth, and sweating ranged from very rare (0% to 6%) to common (15% to 32%). Respiratory depression occurred in 0% to 2% of the subjects in studies evaluating subcutaneous opioids and in 18% of the subjects receiving intravenous morphine.

Tolerance and physical dependence are common, and to some extent, even predictable during chronic opioid administration.[124] These terms are often confused with psychologic dependence ("addiction"), which causes drug abuse or drug-seeking behavior. However, tolerance simply refers to the requirement for escalating and/or more frequent doses of an agent to sustain therapeutic effectiveness during chronic administration. Physical dependence indicates that, for certain chronically administered drugs (e.g., benzodiazepines or opioids), sudden discontinuation or the administration of an antagonist drug will precipitate an abstinence syndrome. Addiction rarely occurs in patients with cancer or other medical illness in the absence of a history of substance abuse.

Nonsteroidal Antiinflammatory Drugs

Eighteen studies were identified addressing the question of relative efficacy of one NSAID in comparison to another or to placebo.[27,28] A total of 1,302 patients were enrolled in these studies (range, 18 to 145), and 15 different NSAIDs were evaluated. The applicability of these studies to the everyday care of patients with cancer is generally low. One study examined the administration of a single dose of the study drug; the duration of treatment in the remaining studies was 7 to 14 days. NSAIDs were consistently found to be superior to placebo. However, only one study suggested a difference in efficacy between different NSAIDs.[125]

Adverse effects of NSAIDs include gastrointestinal distress, ulceration, and bleeding, renal insufficiency or failure, interference with platelet function, and less commonly, allergic reactions, impaired hepatic function, fluid retention, and central nervous system dysfunction. The incidence of adverse effects caused by NSAIDs was generally found to be low in trials of brief duration, but there are limited data on the toxicity of extended use of NSAIDs. Valentini et al. compared misoprostol to ranitidine for prevention of gastrointestinal toxicity in cancer patients receiving high-dose diclofenac.[126] After 4 weeks, gastric ulcers developed in 7 of 49 evaluable patients; 6 of 7 patients with ulcers were asymptomatic. Ulceration was associated with older age and higher doses of diclofenac. Misoprostol was more effective than ranitidine in preventing gastroduodenal lesions (8.7% versus 38.5%, P less than 0.02). The overall 14% incidence of (mostly asymptomatic) gastric ulcers is of concern and suggests that serious gastrointestinal toxicity from NSAIDs may be more common in this population than the rates reported in short-term studies.

Studies comparing NSAIDs with combinations of NSAIDs plus weak opioids, or with opioids alone, are heterogeneous with respect to design characteristics, agents used, route of administration, and type of pain. A meta-analysis of studies to evaluate the relative efficacy of NSAIDs and combinations of opioids was possible with only 3 of the 29 studies assessed.[127–129] The treatment arms included in these studies were diclofenac, naproxen or dipyrone (NSAID arm), and diclofenac plus codeine, controlled-release morphine, and morphine (NSAIDs plus weak opioid, or strong opioid). The evaluated outcome was pain intensity differences between NSAIDs and NSAIDs plus weak opioids or opioids alone, expressed on a VAS scale (0–100mm). Outcomes were combined using a random effects model. No difference was found between NSAIDs and NSAIDs plus weak opioids or opioids alone, 3.8mm (95% CI, –4.7 to 12.4mm]. These results are in agreement with the findings of other meta-analyses on this topic.[130,131]

What is the evidence for an opioid-sparing effect, improved analgesia, or a reduction in opioid-related adverse effects as a result of the coadministration of an NSAID with an opioid? The combination of an NSAID and an opioid is recommended by the World Health Organization (WHO) guidelines for cancer pain. In the large, prospective cohort studies that validated the efficacy of the WHO strategy (see following), however, the specific contribution of NSAIDs and adjunctive analgesics could not be determined. Few randomized studies have addressed these questions. The most convincing evidence for an opioid-sparing effect from an NSAID is based on a study of 156 patients with cancer pain, who, after 1 week of stabilization with opioids, were randomized to continued opioid escalation based on their clinical needs, with or without oral ketorolac. The ketorolac group was found to have significantly better analgesia after 1 week, with slower opioid escalation, and required lower doses of opioids. Gastric discomfort was more common in the group receiving ketorolac and morphine, whereas constipation was more common in the group receiving morphine only. Dropout was substantial in this study, with only 47 of the original 156 patients assessable for the main endpoints.[132]

The World Health Organization Analgesic Ladder

A simple, widely applied approach to managing cancer pain, developed by the World Health Organization (WHO), is the "three-step analgesic ladder" (Figure 82.2).[133] The first tier, for mild to moderate pain, consists of an NSAID or acetaminophen with or without adjuvant medications. As pain escalates or persists, treatment progresses to the second tier, in which a "weak" opioid, such as codeine or hydrocodone, is added to the NSAID, with or without an adjuvant drug. If pain still persists, treatment progresses to the third tier, substitution of a "strong" opioid (i.e., one more readily titrated to doses with greater analgesic efficacy) for the "weak" opioid; the "strong" opioid category includes morphine, hydromorphone, methadone, fentanyl, and levorphanol. The WHO approach to managing cancer pain emphasizes by-the-clock rather than as-needed dosing and therapy individualized to each patient.

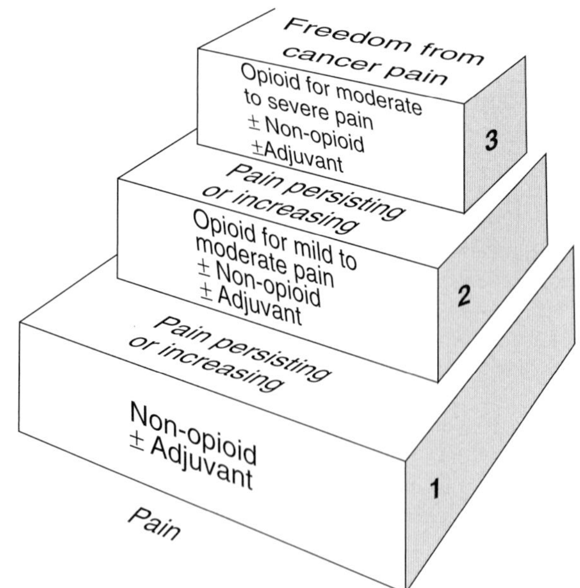

FIGURE 82.2. The World Health Organization analgesic ladder. (From World Health Organization,[133] by permission of the World Health Organization.)

In several large case series, the WHO method yielded satisfactory pain relief in a majority (80% to 90%) of patients with cancer pain. However, validation trials of the specific choice of agents and the sequence of their application within the WHO ladder have been limited.[131,134,135] The common clinical impressions that NSAIDs are particularly beneficial for bone pain, or that opioids are of little benefit for neuropathic pain, are either unconfirmed in systematic literature reviews[131] or are unsupported by direct clinical trials of mechanism-based drug selection.[136]

Mercadante reported results of implementing the WHO guidelines in 3,678 consecutive cancer patients referred to a home palliative care program.[137] Pain intensity improved rapidly, and the improvement was sustained until death for most patients; 89% of patients achieved adequate pain control (a score of less than 4 on a visual analogue scale, VAS) by week 2. In another large cohort study, 2,118 patients referred to a pain service in a university hospital were treated according to the WHO guidelines over 140,478 treatment days.[138] Pain reduction was highly significant within the first week; at the time of enrollment, 78% had severe, very severe, or maximal pain. At the first follow-up evaluation (an average of 6 days later), the proportion with severe, very severe, or maximal pain had declined to 13%. The benefits were sustained with an average follow-up of 66 days, and in a smaller cohort that was followed until death, 84% rated their pain as moderate or less in the final days of life. Over the entire treatment period, pain control was reported to be good in 76% of patients, satisfactory in 12%, and inadequate in 12%.

Nausea and vomiting were reported in 6% to 22% of subjects in these studies, more commonly in subjects in step 3 than in step 2 and in step 2 than in step 1. Constipation occurred among 3% to 36% of subjects and sedation occurred in 14% to 46%.

Summary of the Evidence on Adjuvant Medications

Twenty-two RCTs evaluated the efficacy of various adjuvant medications for cancer pain, including anticonvulsants, antidepressants, local anesthetics, calcium channel blockers, psychostimulants, alpha-adrenergic agonists, and *N*-methyl-D-aspartate (NMDA) antagonists.

Stimulant medications have generated interest as adjuvants to opioids because of their potential to ameliorate sedation, as well as suggestions that they may potentiate analgesia. Three double-blind, cross over studies have been performed comparing adjuvant administration of the stimulant methylphenidate to placebo in patients receiving systemic opioids for cancer pain.[139–141] These studies were small (20 to 43 subjects) and the populations heterogeneous. In one of these studies, pain intensity, activity, drowsiness, and the average number of rescue doses of analgesics all improved with methylphenidate compared with placebo. Interestingly, placebo alone significantly decreased pain intensity. Patients and investigators (all blinded) preferred methylphenidate to placebo.[139] Another study by the same group found that methylphenidate improved cognitive function and decreased drowsiness and confusion but did not alter pain intensity, nausea, or activity. Again, significantly more investigators and patients preferred methylphenidate to placebo.[140] In a third study, however, no statistically significant benefit for methylphenidate was observed in terms of pain intensity, appetite, anxiety/agitation, drowsiness, well-being/mood, sleep, pain medication use, or patient preference for drug or placebo.[141]

The anticonvulsant gabapentin appears to be effective for neuropathic pain in patients with diabetic neuropathy and spinal cord injury based on randomized, controlled trials, but the evidence for its use in cancer pain is limited. Two studies have evaluated gabapentin for acute pain after breast cancer surgery. In one, 70 patients were randomized to a single dose of oral gabapentin (1,200 mg) or placebo 1 hour before radical mastectomy. Patients then received patient-controlled analgesia (PCA) morphine postoperatively. The group receiving gabapentin required significantly less morphine and had lower scores on a visual analogue scale of pain during movement at 2 and 4 hours after surgery. There was no difference in pain at rest or in adverse effects.[142] Gabapentin, 1,200 mg/day for 10 days, was compared to mexilitine, 600 mg/day, or placebo in a randomized study of 75 patients undergoing surgery for breast cancer. Both drugs were associated with a reduction in the consumption of codeine and acetaminophen, and with a reduction in pain on the third postoperative day, compared to placebo. The prevalence and intensity of chronic pain 3 months later was similar in the three groups.[143]

Phenytoin (100 mg orally twice daily) was compared with buprenorphine (0.2 mg sublingually twice daily) and the combination of phenytoin and buprenorphine (50 mg orally plus 0.1 mg sublingually, respectively, twice daily) in a double-blind study of 75 patients with moderate to severe cancer pain. The combination of buprenorphine and phenytoin appeared to provide better pain relief than buprenorphine alone.[144]

The NMDA antagonist ketamine has shown promising analgesic efficacy in small studies. Ketamine (0.25 or 0.50 mg/kg intravenously) was evaluated in 10 cancer patients whose pain was unrelieved by morphine in a randomized, double-blind, crossover, double-dose study. Ketamine, but not saline solution, significantly reduced the pain intensity in almost all the patients at both doses. Ketamine caused mental status changes that were reversible with diazepam.[145] Oral ketamine has been compared to a transdermal nitroglycerin polymer, the NSAID dipyrone, or escalating doses of morphine in 60 patients with cancer pain who had been stabilized on morphine. The VAS pain intensity scores after the test drug was introduced were similar among the groups; however, both oral ketamine and transdermal nitroglycerine appeared to be associated with a morphine-sparing effect.[146,147] Intranasal ketamine has also been found to be efficacious for "malignant breakthrough pain" in a small (n = 20) randomized, double-blind cross over trial of patients with either cancer-related or other types of pain.[148]

Ventafridda et al.[149] compared trazodone (225 mg) with amitriptyline (75 mg) in a randomized, double-blind trial in 45 patients with neuropathic pain from cancer (n = 27) and noncancer causes (n = 18). Ninety-five percent were receiving NSAIDs, alone or with weak or strong opioids. The integrated pain score decreased significantly from baseline in both groups.

Two small, placebo-controlled trials of the calcium channel blocker nimodipine have been performed in patients with cancer pain. In one study, nimodipine limited escalation of morphine dosages in more patients than did placebo (four versus nine). Daily morphine consumption declined significantly more with nimodipine than placebo.[150] The second study reported no benefit in pain intensity or relief with nimodipine compared to placebo.[151]

In small trials, no benefit has been observed for cancer pain with a number of other potential adjuvants, including the somatostatin analogue octreotide,[152] the cholecystokinin antagonist proglumide,[153] intravenous lidocaine,[154] and oral cocaine.[155]

Complementary Approaches for Cancer Pain

Five RCTs examined the effects of hypnosis and cognitive behavioral interventions on various types of cancer pain.[156–160] These studies, although small, provide preliminary indications that these techniques may ameliorate acute procedural pain and pain related to mucositis.

Auricular acupuncture was shown to reduce pain intensity by 36% over a 2-month period and was statistically superior to two placebo treatments in a cohort of 90 patients.[161] Acupuncture may also improve postoperative mobility and pain in breast cancer patients.[162] The effects of Chinese herbs, ear acupuncture, and epidural morphine on postoperative pain were evaluated in 16 men with liver cancer. Any combination that included at least one of the three treatments provided better pain relief than placebo.[163]

Neuraxial Drug Delivery

For the minority of cancer patients whose pain is refractory to systemic opioids and adjuvants, or in whom adverse effects are intolerable, neuraxial (epidural or intrathecal) drug delivery can provide effective pain control.[164–166] Considerations as to whether to employ central routes for drug delivery include the site(s), nature, and character of pain; life expectancy; therapeutic preferences of the patient and family; ability of the infrastructure to manage the device and catheter; and stage of the underlying disease.[167]

Numerous nonrandomized studies support the efficacy of intrathecal or epidural opioids, with or without adjuvants. We reviewed the eight studies with the largest sample sizes (at least 100) that reported on adverse events of spinal opioids.[168–175] Six studies examined pain relief or quality of life as primary outcomes. Two reported primarily on complications of spinal opioid treatment. Only three studies described collection of information about adverse events in a prospective manner. Most studies followed subjects for a mean of 3 to 5 months. The definition of adverse events varied across studies. Catheter-related infections occurred in 0% to 9% of subjects and meningitis in 0% to 4%. In the four studies that reported removal of catheters and discontinuation of spinal opioids due to adverse events, the rates ranged from 0.3% to 10%. Few studies explicitly defined symptoms. Four studies reported on nausea and/or vomiting, which occurred in 9% to 40% of subjects. Three studies reported on constipation, which occurred in 17% to 34% of subjects. Variable rates were reported for pruritus or skin inflammation (1% to 38%), urinary retention (4% to 73%), and headache (3% to 18%). Sedation was reported in only two studies, at rates of 1% and 2%, and respiratory depression was also uncommon.

Smith et al. reported the results of the only RCT to date evaluating intrathecal opioids in patients with unrelieved cancer pain.[176] Patients were eligible if they had pain scores of 5/10 or more on a VAS on two occasions within a week of randomization, despite 200mg/day oral morphine or its equivalent, or if they had refractory adverse effects from systemic opioids. They were randomly assigned to "comprehensive medical management" (CMM), with or without intrathecal analgesia via an implantable drug delivery system (IDDS); 202 patients were enrolled, 200 were analyzed, and 148 were evaluable after 4 weeks. The majority had pain that was characterized as a mixture of neuropathic and nociceptive. CMM was provided according to guidelines published by the Agency for Health Care Policy and Research.[66] The IDDS patients received intrathecal morphine (94%) or hydromorphone (6%); 29% also received intrathecal bupivicaine. The primary endpoint was the proportion of patients with a reduction in their VAS score of 20% or more regardless of increased toxicity or an equal VAS score with a 20% or greater reduction in toxicity; 84.5% in the IDDS and 70.8% in the CMM group achieved this endpoint ($P = 0.05$). The IDDS group had a greater reduction in VAS pain scores (3.90 ± 3.42 versus 3.05 ± 3.16, $P = 0.055$). All common opioid adverse effects, except impotence and pruritis, were reduced to a greater degree in the IDDS group, with statistically significant advantages in fatigue, depressed level of consciousness, and an aggregate score of opioid toxicity compared to CMM alone. Six-month survival was found to favor IDDM (53.9% versus 37.2%, $P = 0.06$). This finding must be interpreted cautiously because survival was not a prospectively defined endpoint of this study.

Several issues complicate the interpretation of this important study. Among 101 patients randomized to IDDS, only 51 actually had a drug delivery device implanted. Five patients assigned to CMM eventually crossed over and received an implanted device. Sixteen serious adverse events associated with the devices were reported in the 56 patients who received them. Key results were reported as a percentage of those for whom data were available at 4 weeks, not on an intent-to-treat basis. Despite the questions raised by these issues, this study may lead to greater acceptance of interventional approaches for cancer pain in the 5% to 15% of patients whose pain responds inadequately to medical management or who are intolerant of opioids.

A number of adjuvants administered by the intrathecal or epidural route have been evaluated in small, randomized studies. When combined with morphine, epidural infusion of the alpha-2-adrenergic agonist clonidine at 10µg/h was found to be superior to placebo in providing successful analgesia, particularly in pain that was characterized as neuropathic.[177] Intrathecal bupivacaine has been reported to provide an opioid-sparing effect.[178] Epidural morphine, combined with low doses of ketamine, neostigmine, or midazolam, was evaluated in a randomized double-blind study of 48 terminal cancer patients.[179] Pain was initially treated with epidural morphine to maintain the VAS score below 4/10. Thereafter, pain escalation was treated by the addition of the epidural study drug (morphine, 2mg; ketamine, 0.2mg/kg, neostigmine 100µg, or midazolam, 500µg) on a daily basis. Only the patients in the ketamine group had lower VAS pain scores compared to the morphine group ($P = 0.018$). Those receiving ketamine required less epidural morphine during the 25-day period of study ($P = 0.003$). Based on findings such as these, clinical practice in patients treated with neuraxial drug infusions for otherwise intractable pain is evolving toward the administration of several agents simultaneously.[180,181]

Neurolytic Approaches

Nondestructive analgesia generally precedes tissue-damaging forms of palliation, such as neurolytic blocks and other anesthetic techniques or neurosurgical division of afferent pathways. Among the consensus exceptions, supported by randomized trials, is celiac block for patients with pancreatic or other retroperitoneal tumors who have moderate to severe pain.[182–187] The decision to employ neurolytic blocks normally follows inadequate pain control with more conservative therapy, lack of other efficacious options, access to medical and social support systems afterward, and a favorable result from a test block using local anesthetic.[165,188] The evidence for other ablative procedures, such as cordotomy, myelotomy, and rhizotomy, is based on uncontrolled cohort studies.

Treatments for Neuropathic Cancer Pain

Few studies have focused specifically on cancer patients suffering from neuropathic pain. We identified three RCTs reporting on analgesic effects of amantadine, amitriptyline, and capsaicin for the treatment of surgical or postmastectomy neuropathic pain.[189–191] All three agents were reported to be significantly superior to placebo; however, the numbers of subjects involved were small and the results must be considered preliminary. Clinical trials[192] and systematic reviews[193,194] have documented the efficacy of antidepressants and anticonvulsants for a spectrum of neuropathic pain, but not specifically in cancer patients. Anticonvulsant medications have been shown to be effective in the management of postherpetic neuralgia. A multicenter, placebo-controlled RCT in 229 patients demonstrated a significant reduction in pain intensity in those receiving gabapentin versus placebo for 8 weeks.[195] There is as yet no evidence from RCTs that cancer patients with painful neuropathies caused by chemotherapy, radiotherapy, surgery, or nerve entrapment benefit from gabapentin.

Oral Mucositis-Related Pain

The incidence of oral mucositis ranges from 40% in patients undergoing chemotherapy treatment to more than 80% in patients receiving radiation treatment to the head and neck.[196] The treatment and prevention of mucositis have been the subject of recent systematic reviews.[197–199]

Treatments that have been evaluated for the prevention of oral mucositis include chlorhexidine,[200–203] ice chips,[204,205] prostaglandins,[206,207] glutamine,[208,209] sucralfate,[210] recombinant human granulocyte macrophage colony-stimulating factor (GM-CSF),[211] chamomile,[212] and allupurinol mouthwash.[213] The conclusion of a Cochrane Review[199] was that there is some evidence that oral ice chips may have a beneficial effect for the prevention of mucositis. However, this conclusion is based on two studies involving 117 subjects who were not blinded to treatment. More recently, recombinant human keratinocyte growth factor (KGF) was evaluated for prevention of mucositis and its symptoms in a randomized Phase I study of 81 patients receiving 5-fluorouracil and leucovorin.[214] The rates of grade two to four mucositis were 43% with KGF and 67% with placebo ($P = 0.06$). However, cutaneous toxicity was dose limiting in 3 patients. This trial, although not designed to be definitive, should stimulate further research on the use of KGF for mucositis.

A systematic review and meta-analysis of prophylaxis for oral mucositis in irradiated head and neck cancer included 15 randomized, controlled trials involving a total of 1,022 patients.[197] Nine studies assessed direct cytoprotectants. Of these, 5 evaluated the barrier sucralfate and 4 evaluated protectants that are thought to stimulate epithelial response (1 trial each of prostaglandin, beta-carotene, hydrogen peroxide, and laser therapy). One assessed indirect cytoprotectants (benzydamine) and 5 trials considered antibacterials. Of those, 3 studied broad-spectrum antibacterials and 2 evaluated narrow-spectrum antibiotic lozenges. In the meta-analysis, the odds ratio (OR) favored antibacterial agents over placebo (OR 0.47; 95% CI, 0.25, 0.92), and within this grouping, the only significant effect was for the narrow-spectrum antibacterials, and only when assessed by the physician (OR 0.45; 95% CI, 0.23, 0.86). Based on patient self-assessments, none of the agents was found to provide effective prophylaxis. Furthermore, a subsequent RCT of 137 patients undergoing radiotherapy for head and neck cancer found no benefit for an antimicrobial lozenge compared with placebo.[215] Amifostine, a thiophosphate cytoprotective agent, has been found to ameliorate acute and chronic xerostomia associated with radiotherapy but does not prevent mucositis.[216]

Treatment of established oral mucositis, and the pain associated with it, has also been the subject of a separate Cochrane Systematic Review[198]; 25 RCTs involving 1,292 patients were reviewed. Allopurinol, immunoglobulin, and human placental extract were found (in a single trial of each) to ameliorate mucositis, but 2 of these studies were judged to be at moderate risk for bias and one at high risk. Mucositis was found to heal significantly more quickly with allopurinol compared to placebo and with GM-CSF compared to povidone iodine. In head and neck cancer patients with severe, painful mucositis resulting from concurrent chemotherapy and radiotherapy, a morphine mouthwash was found to reduce significantly the intensity and duration of oral pain, and the duration of functional impairment, compared to a mouthwash containing lidocaine, diphenhydramine, and magnesium aluminum hydroxide ("magic mouthwash").[217] This trial, although small (26 patients), focused on a highly symptomatic cohort and provides perhaps the best evidence to support a specific treatment for pain due to mucositis.

The Roles of Systemic Chemotherapy and Hormonal Therapy in Treating Cancer Pain

For patients with cancers that can potentially be cured by chemotherapy, the optimal approach to cancer pain may be prompt and aggressive treatment of the underlying disease with the most effective systemic therapy. The number of tumors that fall into this category is, unfortunately, small (e.g., germ cell tumors, choriocarcinoma, non-Hodgkin's lymphoma, Hodgkin's disease). For many common cancers, however, such as non-small cell lung cancer, colorectal cancer, and hormone-refractory prostate cancer (HRPC), the response rates for chemotherapy are generally less than 30%, and complete or durable responses are rare. Despite relatively low objective response rates, a number of recent studies have demonstrated the potential for chemotherapy to ameliorate cancer pain. In a clinical trial of chemotherapy for metastatic breast cancer, 73.7% of those who responded to treatment experienced an improvement in pain (although it should be noted that, even among patients with disease progression on treatment, 22.7% had improvement in pain, suggesting either a placebo effect for chemotherapy or an improvement in patients' analgesic regimens).[218]

Three RCTs have evaluated the impact of the chemotherapeutic agent mitoxantrone on pain in HRPC.[219–221] Tannock et al. randomized 161 patients to prednisone with or without mitoxantrone.[219] The primary response variable was pain and analgesic use. Pain declined in 29% of patients receiving combination therapy and in 12% of those receiving prednisone alone ($P = 0.01$). An additional 7 patients in each group reduced analgesic consumption by at least 50% without an increase in pain. The response to combination therapy lasted 15 weeks, twice as long as that to prednisone alone (P less than 0.001). Possible cardiac toxicity was reported in 5 of 130 patients in the mitoxantrone group. In another study of 242 patients with HRPC, there was an indication that health-related quality of life (HRQOL) was better with mitoxantrone and hydrocortisone versus hydrocortisone alone, particularly with respect to pain control.[220] In a third randomized trial comparing mitoxantrone plus prednisone to prednisone alone in HRPC, patients taking prednisone showed no improvement in HRQOL scores after 6 weeks, whereas those taking mitoxantrone plus prednisone showed significant and durable improvement in global quality of life, four functioning domains, and nine symptoms, including pain. The addition of mitoxantrone to prednisone after failure of prednisone alone was associated with improvement in pain, pain impact, pain relief, and global quality of life.[221] These three studies present consistent evidence for better relief of pain when using mitoxantrone plus a corticosteroid compared to a corticosteroid alone in selected patients with advanced HRPC. More recently, two large randomized studies suggested that docetaxel is superior to mitoxantrone in HRPC in terms of both pain control and survival.[222,223]

Advanced pancreatic cancer is notoriously refractory to treatment, rapidly progressive, and often associated with a multiplicity of symptoms. In this context, the results of a study by Burris et al., comparing two chemotherapy regimens, is very striking and has certainly changed the standard of care for this disease.[224] In this study, 126 patients with advanced, symptomatic pancreatic cancer were randomized to treatment with weekly intravenous fluorouracil (5-FU) or intravenous gemcitabine given weekly for 7 of the first 8 weeks and then weekly for 3 weeks of every 4. The primary endpoint was "clinical benefit," a composite measure of pain, analgesic consumption, Karnofsky performance status, and weight. The criterion for clinical benefit was an improvement in any of these parameters for at least 4 weeks, without worsening in the other parameters; 23.8% of patients in the gemcitabine arm had a clinical benefit, compared to 4.8% in the 5-FU arm ($P = 0.0022$). There was also a survival benefit associated with gemcitabine, with 18% of patients alive at 12 months compared to 2% of those treated with 5-FU.

Despite these promising indications that chemotherapy can ameliorate cancer pain under certain circumstances, the number of trials specifically addressing this question is limited, and other published studies reported negative findings.[224,225] The potential palliative impact of chemotherapy on pain is only one variable that must be weighed in the decision to pursue such treatment. The decision depends on a multitude of other factors including the patient's wishes, his or her underlying medical condition, and the likelihood of an impact on survival and on overall quality of life.

Less controversial is the role of hormonal therapy in breast and prostate cancer. Androgen deprivation has been recognized to be an effective, albeit palliative, treatment for advanced prostate cancer for more than 60 years. Only a handful of studies have compared the relative efficacy of different types of hormonal therapy for pain caused by prostate cancer.[226–229] Based on the available data, there is no clear advantage for luteinizing hormone-releasing hormone (LHRH) analogues compared to surgical orchiectomy in achieving castrate levels of testosterone, and thus, the choice of method can be made on the basis of patient preference, cost, and convenience. The addition of a nonsteroidal antiandrogen can lead to more rapid resolution of bone pain and can prevent pain and other complications resulting from the tumor flare phenomenon that may accompany the initiation of therapy with LHRH analogues. In men who progress symptomatically after medical or surgical androgen ablation, low-dose prednisone appears to provide better pain relief than the antiandrogen flutamide, with similar time to progression and overall survival.[230] In advanced breast cancer, hormonal therapy is usually the treatment of choice for patients whose tumors express the estrogen receptor, with responses to first-line treatment in the 50% to 60% range and generally favorable toxicity profiles. In patients who respond to it, hormonal therapy for metastatic breast cancer may provide excellent palliation of pain and other symptoms.

External-Beam Radiation and Systemic Radionuclides in Treating Cancer Pain

Fourteen trials involving a total of 3,859 patients compared various fractional dosing schedules of palliative radiotherapy, most often given for painful bone metastases.[231–244] High rates of pain relief were reported. Meta-analysis is problematic due to the heterogeneity of the dosing schedules, the variability in the anatomic sites and fields involved, and the outcomes assessed. Short courses of treatment with moderate doses appear to yield results similar to longer courses and seem preferable for convenience. Some studies suggest the possibility that a single dose may be sufficient. In one small study, the addition of a corticosteroid to radiotherapy did not improve pain control.[245]

Few studies have focused specifically on the incidence of pain resulting from radiation therapy. The effect of breast irradiation on HRQOL, including pain and cosmetic outcome, was evaluated in a clinical trial in which 416 patients were randomly allocated to radiation therapy and 421 to no further treatment.[246] A modified version of the Breast Cancer Chemotherapy Questionnaire was administered at baseline, 4 weeks, and 8 weeks after randomization. Irritation of the skin of the breast, breast pain, and appearance of the breast to the patient were also assessed every 3 months for the first 2 years of the study. Breast irradiation therapy had a negative effect on quality of life during treatment. After treatment, irradiated patients reported increased breast symptoms compared with controls. However, no difference was detected between groups after 2 years in the rates of skin irritation, breast pain, and being upset by the appearance of the breast.

Systemic Radionuclide Therapy

Porter et al. evaluated the efficacy of external-beam radiation with or without systemic ^{89}Sr in reducing pain among men with HRPC.[247] Pain was assessed by analgesic use and by the Radiation Therapy Oncology Group analgesic and pain scoring system. At 6 months, the ^{89}Sr group had better pain scores, although the difference between groups was not significant. However, the ^{89}Sr group had significantly fewer new pain sites and did not require further radiotherapy for a mean of 35 weeks compared with 20 weeks for the radiotherapy-alone group. The ^{89}Sr group also had significantly higher rates of hematologic toxicity.

Samarium-153 ethylenediaminetetramethylene phosphonate (^{153}Sm EDTMP) was evaluated in 118 patients, most with breast or prostate cancer, who had painful bone metastases.[248] They were randomized in a blinded fashion to receive a single dose of placebo or 0.5 or 1.0 mCi/kg of the active drug. Those on the placebo arm who did not respond by week 4 were eligible to cross over to treatment at 1.0 mCi/kg. There was a benefit in integrated pain scores and opioid analgesic use at 4 weeks in patients receiving the higher dose of ^{153}Sm EDTMP. Only 30% of patients completed the 16-week follow-up period. In another study of a single dose of ^{153}Sm EDTMP (either 37 or 18.5 MBq/kg) in patients with painful bone metastases, 58 of 70 patients in the high-dose group, and 30 of 35 in the low-dose group, had a reduction in pain, and Karnofsky indices improved at both doses. Of 72 patients who had been receiving analgesics, 63 reduced their consumption.[249]

Bisphosphonates in the Treatment and Prevention of Pain Caused by Bone Metastases

Bisphosphonates, inhibitors of bone resorption by osteoclasts, have been evaluated extensively in patients with (primarily osteolytic) bone metastases. Many of the larger and more recent studies have focused on the impact of these agents on skeletal complications, including pathologic fractures, spinal cord compression, and the need for surgery or radiation therapy. Pain was most often reported as a secondary endpoint, without providing detailed information. The main role of bisphosphonates appears to be the prevention of skeletal morbidity in patients with bone involvement from breast cancer and multiple myeloma. Their role in other cancers is not as well established.

A recent Cochrane Systematic Review identified eight RCTs of bisphosphonates involving 1,962 women with breast cancer metastatic to bone.[250] Bisphosphonates reduced the risk of a skeletal event by 14% (*P* less than 0.00001). Compared to placebo or no bisphosphonate, pain was improved significantly in four studies.

The combined results of two prospective, multicenter, randomized, double-blind, placebo-controlled trials of pamidronate, involving 751 evaluable patients, strongly support a protective effect in women with breast cancer and bone metastases receiving hormonal therapy or chemotherapy.[251] Skeletal complications occurred in 51% of those receiving pamidronate, 90 mg, intravenously every 3 to 4 weeks and 64% of the placebo group (*P* less than 0.001). Pain and analgesic requirements were also significantly worse in the placebo groups at 24 months and at the last study visit compared with the pamidronate groups.

A randomized, placebo-controlled, multicenter study in Sweden and Norway evaluated the efficacy of 60 mg pamidronate in 404 women with advanced breast cancer with skeletal metastases.[252] Pain scores, using a VAS, and analgesic consumption were recorded every third month. There was a significantly increased time to progression of pain (*P* less than 0.01) in favor for the pamidronate group; this group also fared better with respect to performance status (*P* less than 0.05). There was a lower consumption of opioid analgesics in the pamidronate group, but this was not statistically significant ($P = 0.14$).

A Cochrane Review focusing on bisphosphonates in multiple myeloma identified 11 RCTs.[253] In aggregate, there was a highly statistically significant amelioration of pain (as well as skeletal events) associated with bisphosphonates in patients with multiple myeloma. The odds ratio for pain was 0.59 (95% CI, 0.46–0.76); however, the authors of the review stated that the data on pain were heterogeneous and should be interpreted with caution.

The higher-potency bisphosphonate zoledronic acid was shown to be as effective as pamidronate in reducing skeletal complications in a large RCT of patients with breast cancer or multiple myeloma, but its impact on pain is less well documented.[254]

Because of the tropism of prostate cancer for bone, bisphosphonates have been extensively evaluated for their potential to reduce morbidity from osseous metastases in that disease. In contrast to breast cancer and multiple myeloma, however, the data on the efficacy of these agents in prostate cancer are mixed; this may be because the bone metastases produced by prostate cancer are predominantly blastic rather than lytic. Also, the evaluation of pain or analgesic use as an outcome for bisphosphonate therapy may be confounded by many factors, such as the concurrent use of chemotherapy, hormonal therapy, radiotherapy, and conventional analgesics.

Despite some early promising results, several recent large RCTs have failed to support a role for bisphosphonates in prostate cancer, other than perhaps to slow the progression of osteopenia. Oral clodronate was evaluated in 311 patients on hormonal therapy for bone metastases from prostate cancer.[255] There were no significant differences in symptomatic bone progression-free survival (absence of increase in analgesic use, treatment with radiotherapy, change in hormonal therapy, pathologic fracture, or spinal cord compression) associated with clodronate compared to placebo. Similarly, when combined with mitoxantrone and prednisone, intravenous clodronate was no more effective than placebo in reducing pain intensity in an RCT of 209 patients with metastatic hormone-refractory prostate cancer.[256] A pooled analysis was performed of two clinical trials in which 378 patients were randomly assigned to 90 mg pamidronate or placebo every 3 weeks for 27 weeks.[257] All patients had pain due to metastatic prostate cancer that had progressed on first-line hormonal therapy, and reduction in pain was the primary endpoint of the studies. No sustained differences were observed between the pamidronate and placebo groups in scores on the Brief Pain Inventory, analgesic consumption, or adverse skeletal events.

The best evidence (albeit equivocal) for a benefit from a bisphosphonate in prostate cancer comes from an RCT evaluating zoledronic acid in subjects with bone metastases and a rising prostate-specific antigen level while on hormonal therapy.[258] Those requiring "strong narcotic therapy" were excluded. Six hundred forty-three patients were randomly assigned to receive 8 mg zoledronic acid (subsequently reduced to 4 mg due to renal toxicity), 4 mg zoledronic acid, or placebo, given intravenously every 3 weeks for 15 months. The primary outcome variable was the proportion of patients with at least one skeletal event (pathologic bone fracture, spinal cord compression, surgery or radiotherapy to bone, or a change in antineoplastic therapy to treat bone pain). A smaller proportion of patients in both zoledronic acid arms experienced skeletal events, but the difference was only statistically significant in those on the 4-mg arm (33.2% versus 44.2% for placebo; $P = 0.021$). Pain, as assessed by the Brief Pain Inventory every 6 weeks, increased in all three groups. The mean increase from the baseline pain score after 15 months was less in both active treatment groups than the placebo group, but, unlike the primary outcome, the difference was statistically significant only in the group initially assigned to receive the 8-mg dose of zoledronic acid and subsequently reduced to 4 mg. The observation of significantly fewer skeletal events only in the 4-mg arm, but significantly smaller increments in pain only in the arm initially assigned to receive 8 mg, remains unexplained. There were no significant differences in analgesic use or quality of life among the three groups.

Given the inconsistencies in the data, and the fact that bisphosphonates are not without toxicity (adverse effects include myalgias, fevers, nausea, and renal insufficiency), this class of drugs cannot be considered part of standard care in metastatic prostate cancer. Limited evidence supports a possible benefit in reducing skeletal morbidity, rather than an analgesic or opioid-sparing effect. Few studies have evaluated bisphosphonates in cancers other than breast, prostate, and multiple myeloma, and the results are not definitive.[259]

Undertreatment of Cancer Pain

Despite the prospect of achieving control of cancer pain in the great majority of patients, cancer pain remains undertreated even in oncology specialty clinics within wealthy, industrialized nations.[42] A substantial body of research indicates that undertreatment is multifactorial. Inadequacy of clinicians' knowledge of effective pain assessment and management, negative attitudes of patients and clinicians toward the use of drugs (particularly opioids) for pain relief,[260–262] and problems of access, cost, and reimbursement,[263,264] each contribute. Issues of culture and ethnicity[265–267] have considerable importance for cancer pain assessment and management but have until recently received little attention in clinical trials. The elderly, women, children, and members of racial minorities are at increased risk for unsatisfactory pain relief.[51,58,268–272] A finding of considerable concern was that, among nursing home patients with cancer in the United States, 26% of those with daily pain received no analgesics.[51] The predictors for undertreatment or nontreatment of pain included age greater than 85, impaired cognitive status, and minority race. This study and others indicate that disparities exist in pain assessment and treatment based on demographic factors, such as age and race.[3] In addition, pilot studies suggest clinically relevant gender[273–275] and genetic[276,277] differences in the efficacy and adverse effects of opioid analgesics.

The Role of Patient Education

Lack of adherence with prescribed analgesic regimens represents a significant barrier to effective management of cancer pain.[278] The reasons for patients' lack of adherence are complex, including issues of access and cost, the narrow therapeutic index of opioids, and the fear and misperceptions attached to them. In light of these barriers, educating cancer patients about their pain and its treatment is an essential component of effective management.

The impact of pain education programs has been evaluated in a small number of RCTs. In a study of 313 cancer patients with chronic pain, the educational intervention consisted of verbal, written, and audiotaped instruction on pain management and a pain diary. Among the 67% of patients not receiving home nursing care, there was a statistically significant decrease in pain intensity associated with patient education.[279] Miaskowski et al.[280] randomized 174 patients with cancer pain to standard care or to a "PRO-SELF" intervention in which patients received individualized counseling by specially trained nurses and written instructions on the management of pain and the adverse effects of their medicines. The patients kept pain diaries and were taught to use a pill box and to communicate effectively with their caregivers about unrelieved pain. Pain intensity scores (worst, average, and least pain) declined significantly in the PRO-SELF group but not in those receiving standard care. "Standard care" in this study consisted of providing subjects with the patient version of the Cancer Pain Guidelines,[66] instructing them in the maintenance of a daily pain diary, and providing home visits and telephone contacts from a nurse on the same schedule as the PRO-SELF group. As the control group received educational support superior to that provided in most practice settings, the positive results achieved with the PRO-SELF intervention are even more striking.

Conclusion

The studies reviewed here provide unequivocal evidence that cancer pain is highly prevalent yet can be ameliorated in the large majority of people who suffer from it. In the face of this evidence, neglect and therapeutic nihilism are not justifiable. Straightforward algorithms for assessing pain have been validated. Treatment according to the WHO analgesic ladder provides effective pain relief in 80% to 90% of cases. Neuraxial drug delivery and other invasive techniques may be options for the minority of patients who have inadequate relief or intolerable adverse effects with systemic opioid therapy, NSAIDs, and adjuvants. For selected subsets of patients, radiotherapy, chemotherapy, hormonal therapy, and bisphosphonates may provide relief from pain or prevent its escalation.

Further progress in cancer pain depends on dissemination and implementation of methods of assessment and treatment that are known to be effective. The evidence suggests that pain is inadequately assessed and undertreated in many practice settings, and that women, children, the elderly, and minorities are less likely to receive effective pain management. Education of caregivers is needed to address these disparities. Educational support for patients and their families has been shown to play an important role in optimal pain management.

Investigations of the mechanisms of pain have led to an increasingly detailed understanding of its pathogenesis, yet treatment remains largely empiric rather than mechanism based. Various routes of drug administration have been explored, but no new, generally effective agents have been added to the traditional pharmacopeia of opioids, acetaminophen, NSAIDs, and adjuvants. Variations in individual responses to the different agents in these classes are poorly understood, leading to empiric rotation of drugs. There is little evidence to support specific, "targeted" therapies for defined pain syndromes, such as postmastectomy or postthoracotomy pain. The narrow therapeutic index of opioids means that, for many patients, pain relief comes at the cost of opioid-related adverse effects including sedation, constipation, and nausea, which themselves require treatment.

The development of new drugs and other treatment modalities for cancer pain, and the more efficacious use of existing modalities, depend on their evaluation in well-designed, adequately powered clinical trials. The performance of such trials presents several challenges, including the heterogeneity of cancer pain, difficulties in accruing symptomatic patients, the ethical problems associated with placebo controls in patients with pain, high dropout rates, and the choice of appropriate assessment measures and endpoints. Researchers concerned with improving symptoms in cancer patients have already demonstrated the capacity to surmount these and other obstacles. They have provided a strong evidence base for daily clinical care and a foundation for continued progress against cancer pain.

References

1. Cepeda MS, Carr DB. Overview of pain management. In: Berman S (ed) Approaches to Pain Management: An Essential Guide for Clinical Leaders. Oakbrook Terrace, IL: Joint Commission on Accreditation of Healthcare Organizations, 2003:1–20.
2. Lasch KE, Greenhill A, Wilkes G, Carr D, Lee M, Blanchard R. Why study pain? A qualitative analysis of medical and nursing faculty and students' knowledge of and attitudes to cancer pain management. J Palliat Med 2002;5:57–71.
3. Green CR, Anderson KO, Baker TA, et al. The unequal burden of pain: confronting racial and ethnic disparities in pain. Pain Med 2003;4:277–294.
4. Bennett D, Carr D. Opiophobia as a barrier to the treatment of pain. J Pain Palliat Care Pharmacother 2002;16:105–109.
5. Morris DB. The Culture of Pain. Berkeley: University of California Press, 1991.
6. Turk DC, Gatchel RJ (eds) Psychosocial Factors in Pain: Critical Perspectives. New York: Guilford Press, 1999.
7. Bonica JJ. Treatment of cancer pain: current status and future need. In: Fields ML, Dubner R, Cerrero F, Jones LE (eds) Proceedings of the Fourth World Congress on Pain. Advances in Pain Research and Therapy, vol 9. New York: Raven Press, 1985.
8. Chapman CR, Garvin J. Suffering: the contributions of persistent pain. Lancet 1999;353(9171):2233–2237.
9. Loeser JD, Melzack R. Pain: an overview. Lancet 1999; 353(9164):1607–1609.
10. Field MJ, Cassel CK (eds) Approaching Death. Improving Care at the End of Life. Institute of Medicine. Washington, DC: National Academy Press, 1997.
11. Cassel C, Foley KM. Principles for Care of Patients at the End of Life: An Emerging Consensus Among the Specialties of Medicine. New York: Milbank Memorial Fund, 1999.
12. Fields HL. Core Curriculum for Professional Education in Pain. A Report of the Task Force on Professional Education of the International Association for the Study of Pain. Seattle: IASP Press, 1995.
13. Task Force on Pain Management. Practice guidelines for chronic pain management. A report by the American Society of Anesthesiologists Task Force on Pain Management, Chronic Pain Section. Anesthesiology 1997;86(4):995–1004.
14. Aronoff GM. Evaluation and Treatment of Chronic Pain, 3rd ed. Baltimore: Williams & Wilkins, 1999.
15. Ashburn MA, Staats PS. Management of chronic pain. Lancet 1999;353(9167):1865–1869.
16. Hunt SP, Mantyh PW. The molecular dynamics of pain control. Nat Rev Neurosci 2001;2:83–90.
17. Carr DB, Goudas LC. Acute pain. Lancet 1999;353(9169): 2051–2058.
18. Ashburn MA, Rice LJ (eds) The Management of Pain. New York: Churchill Livingstone, 1998.
19. Wall PD, Melzack R (eds) Textbook of Pain. Edinburgh: Churchill Livingstone, 1984.
20. Sorkin LS, Xiao WH, Wagner R, Myers RR. Tumour necrosis factor-alpha induces ectopic activity in nociceptive primary afferent fibres. Neuroscience 1997;81:255–262.
21. Davar G, Hans G, Fareed MU, Sinnott C, Strichartz G. Behavioral signs of acute pain produced by application of endothelin-1 to rat sciatic nerve. Neuroreport 1998;9(10): 2279–2283.
22. Schwei MJ, Honore P, Rogers SD, et al. Neurochemical and cellular reorganization of the spinal cord in a murine model of bone cancer pain. J Neurosci 1999;19(24):1086–1097.
23. Start R, Yu AL, Yaksh TL, Sorkin LS. An animal model of pain produced by systemic administration of an immunotherapeutic anti-ganglioside antibody. Pain 1997;69:119–125.
24. Sorkin LS. Antibody activation and immune reactions: potential linkage to pain and neuropathy. Pain Med 2000;1:296–302.
25. Honore P, Mantyh PW. Bone cancer pain: from mechanism to model to therapy. Pain Med 2000;1:303–309.
26. Woolf CJ, Mannion RJ. Neuropathic pain: aetiology, symptoms, mechanisms, and management. Lancet 1999;353(9168): 1959–1964.
27. Goudas LC, Carr DB, Bloch R, et al. Management of Cancer Pain. Evidence Report/Technology Assessment No. 35 (Contract 290-97-0019 to the New England Medical Center). Rockville, MD: Agency for Health Care Research and Quality, 2001.
28. Carr DB, Goudas LC, Lawrence D, et al. Management of Cancer Symptoms: Pain, Depression and Fatigue. Evidence Report/ Technology Assessment No. 61 (Contract 290-97-0019 to the New England Medical Center). Rockville, MD: Agency for Health Care Research and Quality, 2002.
29. Daut RL, Cleeland CS. The prevalence and severity of pain in cancer. Cancer (Phila) 1982;50(9):1913–1918.
30. Ahles TA, Ruckdeschel JC, Blanchard EB. Cancer-related pain. I. Prevalence in an outpatient setting as a function of stage of disease and type of cancer. J Psychosom Res 1984;28(2):115–119.
31. Gilbert MR, Grossman SA. Incidence and nature of neurologic problems in patients with solid tumors. Am J Med 1986;81(6): 951–954.
32. Miser AW, Dothage JA, Wesley RA, Miser JS. The prevalence of pain in a pediatric and young adult cancer population. Pain 1987;29(1):73–83.

33. Miser AW, McCalla J, Dothage JA, Wesley M, Miser JS. Pain as a presenting symptom in children and young adults with newly diagnosed malignancy. Pain 1987;29(1):85–90.
34. Greenwald HP, Bonica JJ, Bergner M. The prevalence of pain in four cancers. Cancer (Phila) 1987;60(10):2563–2569.
35. Coyle N, Adelhardt J, Foley KM, Portenoy RK. Character of terminal illness in the advanced cancer patient: pain and other symptoms during the last four weeks of life [see comments]. J Pain Symptom Manag 1990;5(2):83–93.
36. Portenoy RK, Hagen NA. Breakthrough pain: definition, prevalence and characteristics [see comments]. Pain 1990;41(3): 273–281.
37. Hiraga K, Mizuguchi T, Takeda F. The incidence of cancer pain and improvement of pain management in Japan. Postgrad Med J 1991;67(suppl 2):S14–S25.
38. Portenoy RK, Miransky J, Thaler HT, et al. Pain in ambulatory patients with lung or colon cancer. Prevalence, characteristics, and effect. Cancer (Phila) 1992;70(6):1616–1624.
39. Brescia FJ, Portenoy RK, Ryan M, Krasnoff L, Gray G. Pain, opioid use, and survival in hospitalized patients with advanced cancer. J Clin Oncol 1992;10(1):149–155.
40. Vuorinen E. Pain as an early symptom in cancer. Clin J Pain 1993;9(4):272–278.
41. Portenoy RK, Kornblith AB, Wong G, et al. Pain in ovarian cancer patients. Prevalence, characteristics, and associated symptoms. Cancer (Phila) 1994;74(3):907–915.
42. Cleeland CS, Gonin R, Hatfield AK, et al. Pain and its treatment in outpatients with metastatic cancer. N Engl J Med 1994; 330(9):592–596.
43. Mercadante S, Armata M, Salvaggio L. Pain characteristics of advanced lung cancer patients referred to a palliative care service. Pain 1994;59(1):141–145.
44. Kelsen DP, Portenoy RK, Thaler HT, et al. Pain and depression in patients with newly diagnosed pancreas cancer. J Clin Oncol 1995;13(3):748–755.
45. Larue F, Colleau SM, Brasseur L, Cleeland CS. Multicentre study of cancer pain and its treatment in France [see comments]. BMJ 1995;310(6986):1034–1037.
46. Stevens PE, Dibble SL, Miaskowski C. Prevalence, characteristics, and impact of postmastectomy pain syndrome: an investigation of women's experiences. Pain 1995;61(1):61–68.
47. Vainio A, Auvinen A. Prevalence of symptoms among patients with advanced cancer: an international collaborative study. Symptom Prevalence Group. J Pain Symptom Manag 1996; 12(1):3–10.
48. Grond S, Zech D, Diefenbach C, Radbruch L, Lehmann KA. Assessment of cancer pain: a prospective evaluation in 2266 cancer patients referred to a pain service. Pain 1996;64(1): 107–14.
49. Tasmuth T, von Smitten K, Kalso E. Pain and other symptoms during the first year after radical and conservative surgery for breast cancer. Br J Cancer 1996;74(12):2024–2031.
50. Higginson IJ, Hearn J. A multicenter evaluation of cancer pain control by palliative care teams. J Pain Symptom Manag 1997; 14(1):29–35.
51. Bernabei R, Gambassi G, Lapane K, et al. Management of pain in elderly patients with cancer. SAGE Study Group. Systematic Assessment of Geriatric Drug Use via Epidemiology [see comments]. JAMA 1998;279(23):1877–1882.
52. Ger LP, Ho ST, Wang JJ, Cherng CH. The prevalence and severity of cancer pain: a study of newly diagnosed cancer patients in Taiwan. J Pain Symptom Manag 1998;15(5):285–293.
53. Petzke F, Radbruch L, Zech D, Loick G, Grond S. Temporal presentation of chronic cancer pain: transitory pains on admission to a multidisciplinary pain clinic. J Pain Symptom Manag 1999; 17(6):391–401.
54. Chang VT, Hwang SS, Feuerman M, Kasimis BS. Symptom and quality of life survey of medical oncology patients at a veterans affairs medical center: a role for symptom assessment. Cancer (Phila) 2000;88(5):1175–1183.
55. Zeppetella G, O'Doherty CA, Collins S. Prevalence and characteristics of breakthrough pain in cancer patients admitted to a hospice. J Pain Symptom Manag 2000;20(2):87–92.
56. Meuser T, Pietruck C, Radbruch L, Stute P, Lehmann KA. Grond S. Symptoms during cancer pain treatment following WHO guidelines: a longitudinal follow-up study of symptom prevalence, severity and etiology. Pain 2001;93(3):247–257.
57. Beck SL, Falkson G. Prevalence and management of cancer pain in South Africa. Pain 2001;94(1):75–84.
58. Wolfe J, Grier HE, Klar N, et al. Symptoms and suffering at the end of life in children with cancer. N Engl J Med 2000; 342(5):326–333.
59. Spross JA, McGuire DB, Schmitt RM. Oncology Nursing Society position paper on cancer pain. Part I: Introduction and Background. Oncol Nurs Forum 1990;17(4):595–614.
60. Spross JA, McGuire DB, Schmitt RM. Oncology Nursing Society position paper on cancer pain. Part II: Education. Oncol Nurs Forum 1990;17(5):751–760.
61. Jadad-Bechara AR. Meta-analysis of randomised clinical trials in pain relief. Doctoral thesis. Oxford: University of Oxford, 1994.
62. Max B. Collecting better data about drug treatment? In: Cohen MJM, Campbell JN (eds) Pain Treatment Centers at the Crossroads: A Practical and Conceptual Reappraisal. Seattle: IASP Press, 1996.
63. McQuay H, Moore A. An Evidence-Based Resource for Pain Relief. Oxford: Oxford University Press, 1998.
64. Farrar JT, Portenoy RK, Berlin JA, Kinman JL, Strom BL. Defining the clinically important difference in pain outcome measures. Pain 2000;88:27–94.
65. Farrar JT, Young JP, LaMoreaux L, Werth JL. Poole RM. Clinical importance of changes in pain intensity measured on an 11-point numerical pain rating scale. Pain 2001;94:149–158.
66. Jacox A, Carr DB, Payne R, et al. Management of Cancer Pain. Clinical Practice Guideline. AHCPR Publication 94-0592. Rockville, MD: Agency for Health Care Policy and Research, U.S. Department of Health and Human Services, 1994.
67. Cancer Pain. NCCN Practice Guidelines in Oncology, Version 1. 2004, 01-21-04 © 2004 National Comprehensive Cancer Network, Inc., http://www.nccn.org/professionals/physician_gls/PDF/pain.pdf.
68. de Wit R, van Dam R, Abu-Saad HH, et al. Empirical comparison of commonly used measures to evaluate pain treatment in cancer patients with chronic pain. J Clin Oncol 1999;17(4):1280.
69. American Pain Society. Principles of Analgesic Use in the Treatment of Acute Pain and Cancer Pain, 4th ed. Glenview IL: American Pain Society, 1999.
70. McQuay H. Opioids in pain management. Lancet 1999; 353(9171):2229–2233.
71. Warfield CA (ed) Principles and Practice of Pain Management. New York: McGraw-Hill, 1993.
72. Cherny NI, Chang V, Frager G, et al. Opioid pharmacotherapy in the management of cancer pain: a survey of strategies used by pain physicians for the selection of analgesic drugs and routes of administration. Cancer (Phila) 1995;76:1288–1293.
73. Breitbart W, Chandler S, Eagel B, et al. An alternative algorithm for dosing transdermal fentanyl for cancer-related pain. Oncology (Huntingt) 2000;14:695–705.
74. Payne R, Coluzzi P, Hart L, et al. Long-term safety of oral transmucosal fentanyl citrate for breakthrough cancer pain. J Pain Symptom Manag 2001;22(1):575–583.
75. Coluzzi PH, Schwartzberg L, Conroy JD, et al. Breakthrough cancer pain: a randomized trial comparing oral transmucosal fentanyl citrate (OTFC) and morphine sulfate immediate release (MSIR). Pain 2001;91(1–2):123–130.
76. Farrar JT, Cleary J, Rauck R, Busch M, Nordbrock E. Oral transmucosal fentanyl citrate: randomized, double-blinded, placebo-

controlled trial for treatment of breakthrough pain in cancer patients. J Natl Cancer Inst 1998;90(8):611–616.
77. Stambaugh JE Jr, McAdams J. Comparison of intramuscular dezocine with butorphanol and placebo in chronic cancer pain: a method to evaluate analgesia after both single and repeated doses. Clin Pharmacol Ther 1987;42(2):210–219.
78. Dhaliwal HS, Sloan P, Arkinstall WW, et al. Randomized evaluation of controlled-release codeine and placebo in chronic cancer pain. J Pain Symptom Manag 1995;10(8):612–623.
79. Heiskanen T, Kalso E. Controlled-release oxycodone and morphine in cancer related pain. Pain 1997;73(1):37–45.
80. Wilder-Smith CH, Schimke J, Osterwalder B, Senn HJ. Oral tramadol, a mu-opioid agonist and monoamine reuptake-blocker, and morphine for strong cancer-related pain. Ann Oncol 1994; 5(2):141–146.
81. Grochow L, Sheidler V, Grossman S, Green L, Enterline J. Does intravenous methadone provide longer lasting analgesia than intravenous morphine? A randomized, double-blind study. Pain 1989;38(2):151–157.
82. Ventafridda V, Ripamonti C, Bianchi M, Sbanotto A, De Conno F. A randomized study on oral administration of morphine and methadone in the treatment of cancer pain. J Pain Symptom Manag 1986;1(4):203–207.
83. Mercadante S, Casuccio A, Agnello A, Serretta R, Calderone L, Barresi L. Morphine versus methadone in the pain treatment of advanced-cancer patients followed up at home. J Clin Oncol 1998;16:3656–3661.
84. Pasqualucci V, Tantucci C, Paoletti F, et al. Buprenorphine vs. morphine via the epidural route: a controlled comparative clinical study of respiratory effects and analgesic activity. Pain 1987;29(3):273–286.
85. Ventafridda V, De Conno F, Guarise G, Tamburini M, Savio G. Chronic analgesic study on buprenorphine action in cancer pain. Comparison with pentazocine. Arzneimittel-Forschung 1983; 33(4):587–590.
86. Mercadante S, Salvaggio L, Dardanoni G, Agnello A, Garofalo S. Dextropropoxyphene versus morphine in opioid-naive cancer patients with pain. J Pain Symptom Manag 1998;15(2):76–81.
87. Twycross RG. The measurement of pain in terminal carcinoma. J Int Med Res 1976;4(suppl 2):58–67.
88. Hanks GW, Twycross RG, Bliss JM. Controlled release morphine tablets: a double-blind trial in patients with advanced cancer. Anaesthesia 1987;42(8):840–844.
89. Goughnour BR, Arkinstall WW, Stewart JH. Analgesic response to single and multiple doses of controlled-release morphine tablets and morphine oral solution in cancer patients. Cancer (Phila) 1989;63(suppl 11):2294–2297.
90. Thirlwell MP, Sloan PA, Maroun JA, et al. Pharmacokinetics and clinical efficacy of oral morphine solution and controlled-release morphine tablets in cancer patients. Cancer (Phila) 1989; 63(suppl 11):2275–2283.
91. Ventafridda V, Saita L, Barletta L, Sbanotto A, De Conno F. Clinical observations on controlled-release morphine in cancer pain. J Pain Symptom Manag 1989;4(3):124–129.
92. Walsh TD, MacDonald N, Bruera E, Shepard KV, Michaud M, Zanes R. A controlled study of sustained-release morphine sulfate tablets in chronic pain from advanced cancer. Am J Clin Oncol 1992;15(3):268–272.
93. Deschamps M, Band PR, Hislop TG, Rusthoven J, Iscoe N, Warr D. The evaluation of analgesic effects in cancer patients as exemplified by a double-blind, crossover study of immediate-release versus controlled-release morphine. J Pain Symptom Manag 1992;7(7):384–392.
94. Panich A, Charnvej L. Comparison of morphine slow release tablet (MST) and morphine sulphate solution (MSS) in the treatment of cancer pain. J Med Assoc Thailand 1993;76(12):672–676.
95. Finn JW, Walsh TD, MacDonald N, Bruera E, Krebs LU, Shepard KV. Placebo-blinded study of morphine sulfate sustained-release tablets and immediate-release morphine sulfate solution in outpatients with chronic pain due to advanced cancer. J Clin Oncol 1993;11(5):967–972.
96. O'Brien T, Mortimer PG, McDonald CJ, Miller AJ. A randomized crossover study comparing the efficacy and tolerability of a novel once-daily morphine preparation (MXL capsules) with MST continuous tablets in cancer patients with severe pain. Palliat Med 1997;11(6):475–482.
97. Broomhead A, Kerr R, Tester W, et al. Comparison of a once-a-day sustained-release morphine formulation with standard oral morphine treatment for cancer pain. J Pain Symptom Manag 1997;14(2):63–73.
98. Wong JO, Chiu GL, Tsao CJ, Chang CL. Comparison of oral controlled-release morphine with transdermal fentanyl in terminal cancer pain [published erratum appears in Acta Anaesthesiol Sin 1997;35(3):191]. Acta Anaesth Sin 1997;35(1):25–32.
99. Ahmedzai S, Brooks D. Transdermal fentanyl versus sustained-release oral morphine in cancer pain: preference, efficacy, and quality of life. J Pain Symptom Manag 1997;13(5):254–261.
100. Lipkowski AW, Carr DB. Rethinking opioid equivalence. Pain Clin Updates 2002:10(4):1–4.
101. McNicol E, Horowicz-Mehler N, Fisk RA, et al. Management of opioid side effects in cancer-related and chronic noncancer pain: a systematic review. J Pain 2003;4:231–256.
102. Beaver WT, Wallenstein SL, Houde RW, Rogers A. A comparison of the analgesic effects of pentazocine and morphine in patients with cancer. Clin Pharmacol Ther 1966;7(6):740–751.
103. Beaver WT, Wallenstein SL, Houde RW, Rogers A. A comparison of the analgesic effects of methotrimeprazine and morphine in patients with cancer. Clin Pharmacol Ther 1966;7(4):436–446.
104. Beaver WT, Wallenstein SL, Houde RW, Rogers A. A comparison of the analgesic effects of profadol and morphine in patients with cancer. Clin Pharmacol Ther 1969;10(3):314–319.
105. Beaver WT, Wallenstein SL, Houde RW, Rogers A. Comparisons of the analgesic effects of oral and intramuscular oxymorphone and of intramuscular oxymorphone and morphine in patients with cancer. J Clin Pharmacol 1977;17(4):186–198.
106. Beaver WT, Wallenstein SL, Rogers A, Houde RW. Analgesic studies of codeine and oxycodone in patients with cancer. I. Comparisons of oral with intramuscular codeine and of oral with intramuscular oxycodone. J Pharmacol Exp Ther 1978; 207(1):92–100.
107. Beaver WT, Wallenstein SL, Rogers A, Houde RW. Analgesic studies of codeine and oxycodone in patients with cancer. II. Comparisons of intramuscular oxycodone with intramuscular morphine and codeine. J Pharmacol Exp Ther 1978;207(1): 101–108.
108. Sykes NP. The relationship between opioid use and laxative use in terminally ill cancer patients. Palliat Med 1998;12(5): 375–382.
109. Campora E, Merlini L, Pace M, et al. The incidence of narcotic-induced emesis. J Pain Symptom Manag 1991;6:428–430.
110. De Conno F, Ripamonti C, Sbanotto A, et al. A clinical study on the use of codeine, oxycodone, dextropropoxyphene, buprenorphine, and pentazocine in cancer pain. J Pain Symptom Manag 1991;6:423–427.
111. De Conno F, Groff L, Brunelli C, Zecca E, Ventafridda V, Ripamonti C. Clinical experience with oral methadone administration in the treatment of pain in 196 advanced cancer patients. J Clin Oncol 1996;14:2836–2842.
112. Schug SA, Zech D, Grond S, Jung H, Meuser T, Stobbe B. A long-term survey of morphine in cancer pain patients. J Pain Symptom Manag 1992;7:259–266.
113. Ventafridda V, Oliveri E, Caraceni A, et al. A retrospective study on the use of oral morphine in cancer pain. J Pain Symptom Manag 1987;2:77–81.
114. Payne R, Mathias SD, Pasta DJ, Wanke LA, Williams R, Mahmoud R. Quality of life and cancer pain: satisfaction and

side effects with transdermal fentanyl versus oral morphine. J Clin Oncol 1998;16:1588–1193.
115. Warfield CA. Guidelines for the use of MS Contin tablets in the management of cancer pain. Postgrad Med J 1991;67:S9–S12.
116. Vijayaram S, Ramamani PV, Chandrashekhar NS, et al. Continuing care for cancer pain relief with oral morphine solution. One-year experience in a regional cancer center. Cancer (Phila) 1990;66:1590–1595.
117. Meuret G, Jocham H. Patient-controlled analgesia (PCA) in the domiciliary care of tumour patients. Cancer Treat Rev 1996; 22(suppl A):137–140.
118. Ferris FD, Kerr IG, De Angelis C, Sone M, Hume S. Inpatient narcotic infusions for patients with cancer pain. J Palliat Care 1990;6(2):51–59.
119. Bruera E, Brenneis C, Michaud M, et al. Use of the subcutaneous route for the administration of narcotics in patients with cancer pain. Cancer (Phila) 1988;62:407–411.
120. Stuart GJ, Davey EB, Wight SE. Continuous intravenous morphine infusions for terminal pain control: a retrospective review. Drug Intell Clin Pharm 1986;20:968–972.
121. Gagnon B, Bielech M, Watanabe S, Walker P, Hanson J, Bruera E. The use of intermittent subcutaneous injections of oxycodone for opioid rotation in patients with cancer pain. Support Care Cancer 1999;7:265–270.
122. Moulin DE, Johnson NG, Murray-Parsons N, Geoghegan MF, Goodwin VA, Chester MA. Subcutaneous narcotic infusions for cancer pain: treatment outcome and guidelines for use. Can Med Assoc J 1992;146:891–897.
123. Bruera E, Brenneis C, Michaud M, Chadwick S, MacDonald RN. Continuous sc infusion of narcotics using a portable disposable device in patients with advanced cancer. Cancer Treat Rep 1987; 71:635–657.
124. Basbaum AI. Insights into the development of opioid tolerance. Pain 1995;61:349–352.
125. Yalcin S, Gullu IH, Tekuzman G, Savas C, Firat D. A comparison of two nonsteroidal antiinflammatory drugs (diflunisal versus dipyrone in the treatment of moderate to severe cancer pain: a randomized crossover study. Am J Clin Oncol 1998; 21(2):185–188.
126. Valentini M, Cannizzaro R, Poletti M, et al. Nonsteroidal antiinflammatory drugs for cancer pain: comparison between misoprostol and ranitidine in prevention of upper gastrointestinal damage. J Clin Oncol 1995;13:2637–2642.
127. Dellemijn PL, Verbiest HB, van Vliet JJ, Roos PJ, Vecht CJ. Medical therapy of malignant nerve pain. A randomised double-blind explanatory trial with naproxen versus slow-release morphine. Eur J Cancer 1994;30A(9):1244–1250.
128. Minotti V, De Angelis V, Righetti E, et al. Double-blind evaluation of short-term analgesic efficacy of orally administered diclofenac, diclofenac plus codeine, and diclofenac plus imipramine in chronic cancer pain. Pain 1998;74(2–3):133–137.
129. Rodriguez M, Barutell C, Rull M, et al. Efficacy and tolerance of oral dipyrone versus oral morphine for cancer pain. Eur J Cancer 1994;30A(5):584–587.
130. McNicol E, Strassels S, Goudas L, Lau J, Carr DB. Nonsteroidal anti-inflammatory drugs, alone or combined with opioids, for cancer pain: a systematic review. J Clin Oncol 2004;22: 1975–1992.
131. Eisenberg E, Berkey CS, Carr DB, Mosteller F, Chalmers T. Efficacy and safety of nonsteroidal antiinflammatory drugs for cancer pain: a meta-analysis. J Clin Oncol 1994;12(12): 2756–2765.
132. Mercadante S, Fulfaro F, Casuccio A. A randomised controlled study on the use of anti-inflammatory drugs in patients with cancer pain on morphine therapy: effects on dose-escalation and a pharmacoeconomic analysis. Eur J Cancer 2002;38(10): 1358–1363.
133. World Health Organization. Cancer Pain Relief and Palliative Care. Report of a WHO expert committee. World Health Organization Technical Report Series 804. Geneva: World Health Organization, 1990:1–75.
134. Jadad AR, Browman GP. The WHO analgesic ladder for cancer pain management. Stepping up the quality of its evaluation. JAMA 1995;274(23):1870–1873.
135. Mercadante S. World Health Organization Guidelines: problem areas in cancer pain management. Cancer Control J Moffitt Cancer Center 1999;6(2):191–197.
136. Ashby MA, Fleming BG, Brooksbank M, et al. Description of a mechanistic approach to pain management in advanced cancer. Preliminary report. Pain 1992;51(2):153–162.
137. Mercadante S. Pain treatment and outcomes for patients with advanced cancer who receive follow-up care at home [see comments]. Cancer (Phila) 1999;85(8):1849–1858.
138. Zech DF, Grond S, Lynch J, Hertel D, Lehmann KA. Validation of World Health Organization Guidelines for cancer pain relief: a 10-year prospective study. Pain 1995;63(1):65–76.
139. Bruera E, Chadwick S, Brenneis C, Hanson J, MacDonald RN. Methylphenidate associated with narcotics for the treatment of cancer pain. Cancer Treat Rep 1987;71(1):67–70.
140. Bruera E, Miller MJ, Macmillan K, Kuehn N. Neuropsychological effects of methylphenidate in patients receiving a continuous infusion of narcotics for cancer pain. Pain 1992;48(2): 163–166.
141. Wilwerding MB, Loprinzi CL, Mailliard JA, et al. A randomized, crossover evaluation of methylphenidate in cancer patients receiving strong narcotics. Support Care Cancer 1995;3(2): 135–138.
142. Dirks J, Fredensborg BB, Christensen D, Fomsgaard JS, Flyger H, Dahl JB. A randomized study of the effects of single-dose gabapentin versus placebo on postoperative pain and morphine consumption after mastectomy. Anesthesiology 2002;97(3): 560–564.
143. Fassoulaki A, Patris K, Sarantopoulos C, Hogan O. The analgesic effect of gabapentin and mexiletine after breast surgery for cancer. Anesth Analg 2002;95(4):985–991.
144. Yajnik S, Singh GP, Singh G, Kumar M. Phenytoin as a coanalgesic in cancer pain. J Pain Symptom Manag 1992;7(4):200–213.
145. Mercadante S, Arcuri E, Tirelli W, Casuccio A. Analgesic effect of intravenous ketamine in cancer patients on morphine therapy: a randomized, controlled, double-blind, crossover, double-dose study. J Pain Symptom Manag 2000;20(4):246–252.
146. Lauretti GR, Lima IC, Reis MP, Prado WA, Pereira NL. Oral ketamine and transdermal nitroglycerin as analgesic adjuvants to oral morphine therapy for cancer pain management. Anesthesiology 1999;90(6):1528–1533.
147. Lauretti GR, Perez MV, Reis MP, Pereira NL. Double-blind evaluation of transdermal nitroglycerine as adjuvant to oral morphine for cancer pain management [see comment]. J Clin Anesth 2002;14(2):83–86.
148. Carr DB, Goudas LC, Denman WT, et al. Safety and efficacy of intranasal ketamine for the treatment of breakthrough pain in patients with chronic pain: a randomized, double blind, placebo-controlled, crossover study. Pain 2004;108:17–27.
149. Ventafridda V, Bonezzi C, Caraceni A, et al. Antidepressants for cancer pain and other painful syndromes with deafferentation component: comparison of amitriptyline and trazodone. Ital J Neurol Sci 1987;8(6):579–587.
150. Santillan R, Hurle MA, Armijo JA, de los Mozos, Florez J. Nimodipine-enhanced opiate analgesia in cancer patients requiring morphine dose escalation: a double-blind, placebo-controlled study. Pain 1998;76(1–2):17–26.
151. Roca G, Aguilar JL, Gomar C, Mazo V, Costa J, Vidal F. Nimodipine fails to enhance the analgesic effect of slow release morphine in the early phases of cancer pain treatment. Pain 1996;68(2–3):239–243.

152. De Conno F, Saita L, Ripamonti C, Ventafridda V. Subcutaneous octreotide in the treatment of pain in advanced cancer patients. J Pain Symptom Manag 1994;9:34–38.
153. Bernstein ZP, Yucht S, Battista E, Lema M, Spaulding MB. Proglumide as a morphine adjunct in cancer pain management. J Pain Symptom Manag 1998;15:314–320.
154. Ellemann K, Sjogren P, Banning AM, Jensen TS, Smith T, Geertsen P. Trial of intravenous lidocaine on painful neuropathy in cancer patients. Clin J Pain 1989;5:291–294.
155. Kaiko RF, Kanner R, Foley KM, et al. Cocaine and morphine interaction in acute and chronic cancer pain. Pain 1987;31:35–45.
156. Zeltzer L, LeBaron S. Hypnosis and nonhypnotic techniques for reduction of pain and anxiety during painful procedures in children and adolescents with cancer. J Pediatr 1982;101(6): 1032–1035.
157. Wall VJ, Womack W. Hypnotic versus active cognitive strategies for alleviation of procedural distress in pediatric oncology patients. Am J Clin Hypnosis 1989;31(3):181–191.
158. Syrjala KL, Cummings C, Donaldson GW. Hypnosis or cognitive behavioral training for the reduction of pain and nausea during cancer treatment: a controlled clinical trial [see comments]. Pain 1992;48(2):137–146.
159. Syrjala KL, Donaldson GW, Davis MW, Kippes ME, Carr JE. Relaxation and imagery and cognitive-behavioral training reduce pain during cancer treatment: a controlled clinical trial. Pain 1995;63(2):189–198.
160. Sloman R, Brown P, Aldana E, Chee E. The use of relaxation for the promotion of comfort and pain relief in persons with advanced cancer. Contemp Nurse 1994;3(1):6–12.
161. Alimi D, Rubino C, Pichard-Leandri E, et al. Analgesic effect of auricular acupuncture for cancer pain: a randomized, blinded, controlled trial. J Clin Oncol 2003;21:4120–4126.
162. He JP, Friedrich M, Ertan AK, Muller K, Schmidt W. Pain-relief and movement improvement by acupuncture after ablation and axillary lymphadenectomy in patients with mammary cancer. Clin Exp Obstet Gynecol 1999;26:81–84.
163. Li QS, Cao SH, Xie GM, et al. Combined traditional Chinese medicine and Western medicine. Relieving effects of Chinese herbs, ear-acupuncture and epidural morphine on postoperative pain in liver cancer. Chin Med J 1994;107(4):289–294.
164. Bennett G, Serafini M, Burchiel K, et al. Evidence-based review of the literature on intrathecal delivery of pain medication [review]. J Pain Symptom Manag 2000;20(2):S12–S36.
165. Brown DL. Regional Anesthesia and Analgesia. Philadelphia: Saunders, 1996.
166. Carr DB, Cousins MJ. Spinal route of analgesia and opioids and future options. In: Cousins MJ, Bridenbaugh PO (eds) Neural Blockade in Clinical Anesthesia and Management of Pain, 3rd ed. Philadelphia: Lippincott-Raven, 1998:915–984.
167. Dougherty PM, Staats PS. Intrathecal drug therapy for chronic pain: from basic science to clinical practice. Anesthesiology 1999;91(6):1891–1918.
168. Madrid JL, Fatela LV, Alcorta J, Guillen F, Lobato RD. Intermittent intrathecal morphine by means of an implantable reservoir: a survey of 100 cases. J Pain Symptom Manag 1988;3(2):67–71.
169. Cheng KI, Tang CS, Chu KS, Yip NS, Yu KL, Tseng CK. Retrospective investigation of intermittent bolus intrathecal morphine for cancer pain patients. Kao-Hsiung i Hsueh Ko Hsueh Tsa Chih (Kaohsiung Journal of Medical Sciences) 1993;9(11): 632–642.
170. Nitescu P, Sjoberg M, Appelgren L, Curelaru I. Complications of intrathecal opioids and bupivacaine in the treatment of "refractory" cancer pain. Clin J Pain 1995;11(1):45–62.
171. Zenz M, Piepenbrock S, Tryba M. Epidural opiates: long-term experiences in cancer pain. Klin Wochenschr 1985;63(5): 225–229.
172. Liew E, Hui YL. A preliminary study of long-term epidural morphine for cancer pain via a subcutaneously implanted reservoir. Ma Tsui Hsueh Tsa Chi (Anaesthesiologica Sinica) 1989; 27(1):5–12.
173. Du Pen SL, Peterson DG, Williams A, Bogosian AJ. Infection during chronic epidural catheterization: diagnosis and treatment. Anesthesiology 1990;73(5):905–909.
174. Plummer JL, Cherry DA, Cousins MJ, Gourlay GK, Onley MM, Evans KH. Long-term spinal administration of morphine in cancer and non-cancer pain: a retrospective study. Pain 1991; 44(3):215–220.
175. Samuelsson H, Malmberg F, Eriksson M, Hedner T. Outcomes of epidural morphine treatment in cancer pain: nine years of clinical experience. J Pain Symptom Manag 1995;10(2):105–112.
176. Smith TJ, Staats PS, Deer T, et al. Implantable Drug Delivery Systems Study Group. Randomized clinical trial of an implantable drug delivery system compared with comprehensive medical management for refractory cancer pain: impact on pain, drug-related toxicity, and survival. J Clin Oncol 2002; 20:4040–4049.
177. Eisenach JC, DuPen S, Dubois M, Miguel R, Allin D. Epidural clonidine analgesia for intractable cancer pain. Pain 1995; 61(3):391–399.
178. van Dongen RT, Crul BJ, van Egmond J. Intrathecal coadministration of bupivacaine diminishes morphine dose progression during long-term intrathecal infusion in cancer patients. Clin J Pain 1999;15(3):166–172.
179. Lauretti GR, Gomes JM, Reis MP, Pereira NL. Low doses of epidural ketamine or neostigmine, but not midazolam, improve morphine analgesia in epidural terminal cancer pain therapy. J Clin Anesth 1999;11(8):663–668.
180. Bennett G, Burchiel K, Buchser E, et al. Clinical guidelines for intraspinal infusion: report of an expert panel: PolyAnalgesic Consensus Conference 2000. J Pain Symptom Manag 2000; 20:S37–S43.
181. Walker SM, Goudas LC, Cousins MJ, Carr DB. Combination spinal analgesic chemotherapy: a systematic review. Anesth Analg 2002;95:674–715.
182. Brown DL, Bulley CK, Quiel EL. Neurolytic celiac plexus block for pancreatic cancer pain. Anesth Analg 1987;66(9):869–873.
183. Brown DL. A retrospective analysis of neurolytic celiac plexus block for nonpancreatic intra-abdominal cancer pain. Reg Anesth 1989;14(2):63–65.
184. Eisenberg E, Carr DB, Chalmers TC. Neurolytic celiac plexus block for treatment of cancer. Anesth Analg 1995;80(290): 295.
185. Kawamata M, Ishitani K, Ishikawa K, et al. Comparison between celiac plexus block and morphine treatment on quality of life in patients with pancreatic cancer pain. Pain 1996;64(3):597–602.
186. Mercadante S. Celiac plexus block versus analgesics in pancreatic cancer pain. Pain 1993;52:187–192.
187. Lillemoe KD, Cameron JL, Kaufman HS, Yeo CJ, Pitt HA, Sauter PK. Chemical splanchnicectomy in patients with unresectable pancreatic cancer. A prospective randomized trial. Ann Surg 1993;217(5):447–457.
188. Cousins M, Bridenbaugh P (eds) Neural Blockade in Clinical Anesthesia and Management of Pain, 3rd ed. Philadelphia: Lippincott-Raven, 1998.
189. Pud D, Eisenberg E, Spitzer A, Adler R, Fried G, Yarnitsky D. The NMDA receptor antagonist amantadine reduces surgical neuropathic pain in cancer patients: a double blind, randomized, placebo controlled trial. Pain 1998;75(2–3):349–354.
190. Kalso E, Tasmuth T, Neuvonen P. Amitriptyline effectively relieves neuropathic pain following treatment of breast cancer. Pain 1996;64(2):293–302.
191. Sloan JA, Wender DB, Rowland KM, et al. Phase III placebo-controlled trial of capsaicin cream in the management of surgical neuropathic pain in cancer patients. J Clin Oncol 1997; 15(8):2974–2980.

192. Max MB. Thirteen consecutive well-designed randomized trials show that antidepressants reduce pain in diabetic neuropathy and postherpetic neuralgia. Pain Forum 1995;4(4):248–253.
193. McQuay HJ, Tramer M, Nye BA, Carroll D, Wiffen PJ, Moore RA. A systematic review of antidepressants in neuropathic pain [see comments]. Pain 1996;68(2–3):217–227.
194. McQuay H, Carroll D, Jadad AR, et al. Anticonvulsant drugs for management of pain: a systematic review [see comments]. Br Med J 1995;311(7012):1047–1052.
195. Rowbotham M, Harden N, Stacey B, et al. Gabapentin for the treatment of postherpetic neuralgia: a randomized controlled trial. JAMA 1998;280(21):1837–1842.
196. Carl W, Havens J. The cancer patient with severe mucositis. Curr Rev Pain 2000;4(3):197–202.
197. Sutherland SE, Browman GP. Prophylaxis of oral mucositis in irradiated head-and-neck cancer patients: a proposed classification scheme of interventions and meta-analysis of randomized controlled trials. Int J Radiat Oncol Biol Phys 2001; 49(4):917–930.
198. Worthington HV, Clarkson JE, Eden OB. Interventions for Treating Oral Mucositis for Patients with Cancer Receiving Treatment (Cochrane Review). The Cochrane Library, issue 2. Chichester, UK: Wiley, 2004.
199. Clarkson JE, Worthington HV, Eden OB. Prevention of oral mucositis or oral candidiasis for patients with cancer receiving chemotherapy (excluding head and neck cancer). Cochrane Database Syst Rev 2000;(2):CD000978.
200. Dodd MJ, Larson PJ, Dibble SL, et al. Randomized clinical trial of chlorhexidine versus placebo for prevention of oral mucositis in patients receiving chemotherapy. Oncol Nurs Forum 1996;23(6):921–927.
201. Ferretti GA, Ash RC, Brown AT, Parr MD, Romond EH, Lillich TT. Control of oral mucositis and candidiasis in marrow transplantation: a prospective, double-blind trial of chlorhexidine digluconate oral rinse. Bone Marrow Transplant 1988; 3(5):483–493.
202. Ferretti GA, Raybould TP, Brown AT, et al. Chlorhexidine prophylaxis for chemotherapy- and radiotherapy-induced stomatitis: a randomized double-blind trial. Oral Surg Oral Med Oral Pathol 1990;69(3):331–338.
203. Wahlin YB. Effects of chlorhexidine mouthrinse on oral health in patients with acute leukemia. Oral Surg Oral Med Oral Pathol 1989;68(3):279–287.
204. Cascinu S, Fedeli A, Fedeli SL, Catalano G. Oral cooling (cryotherapy), an effective treatment for the prevention of 5-fluorouracil-induced stomatitis. Eur J Cancer B Oral Oncol 1994;30B(4):234–236.
205. Mahood DJ, Dose AM, Loprinzi CL, et al. Inhibition of fluorouracil-induced stomatitis by oral cryotherapy. J Clin Oncol 1991;9(3):449–452.
206. Duenas-Gonzalez A, Sobrevilla-Calvo P, Frias-Mendivil M, et al. Misoprostol prophylaxis for high-dose chemotherapy-induced mucositis: a randomized double-blind study. Bone Marrow Transplant 1996;17(5):809–812.
207. Labar B, Mrsic M, Pavletic Z, et al. Prostaglandin E_2 for prophylaxis of oral mucositis following BMT. Bone Marrow Transplant 1993;11(5):379–382.
208. Anderson PM, Schroeder G, Skubitz KM. Oral glutamine reduces the duration and severity of stomatitis after cytotoxic cancer chemotherapy. Cancer (Phila) 1998;83(7):1433–1439.
209. Jebb SA, Osborne RJ, Maughan TS, et al. 5-Fluorouracil and folinic acid-induced mucositis: no effect of oral glutamine supplementation. Br J Cancer 1994;70(4):732–735.
210. Shenep JL, Kalwinsky DK, Hutson PR, et al. Efficacy of oral sucralfate suspension in prevention and treatment of chemotherapy-induced mucositis. J Pediatr 1988;113(4): 758–763.
211. Cartee L, Petros WP, Rosner GL, et al. Evaluation of GM-CSF mouthwash for prevention of chemotherapy-induced mucositis: a randomized, double-blind, dose-ranging study. Cytokine 1995;7(5):471–477.
212. Fidler P, Loprinzi CL, O'Fallon JR, et al. Prospective evaluation of a chamomile mouthwash for prevention of 5-FU-induced oral mucositis. Cancer (Phila) 1996;77(3):522–525.
213. Loprinzi CL, Cianflone SG, Dose AM, et al. A controlled evaluation of an allopurinol mouthwash as prophylaxis against 5-fluorouracil-induced stomatitis. Cancer (Phila) 1990; 65(8):1879–1882.
214. Meropol NJ, Somer RA, Gutheil J, et al. Randomized phase I trial of recombinant human keratinocyte growth factor plus chemotherapy: potential role as mucosal protectant [see comment]. J Clin Oncol 2003;21(8):1452–1458.
215. El-Sayed S, Nabid A, Shelley W, et al. Prophylaxis of radiation-associated mucositis in conventionally treated patients with head and neck cancer: a double-blind, phase III, randomized, controlled trial evaluating the clinical efficacy of an antimicrobial lozenge using a validated mucositis scoring system. J Clin Oncol 2002;20(19):3956–3963.
216. Brizel DM, Wasserman TH, Henke M, et al. Phase III randomized trial of amifostine as a radioprotector in head and neck cancer [see comment] [erratum appears in J Clin Oncol 2000;18(24):4110–4111]. J Clin Oncol 2000;18(19):3339–3345.
217. Cerchietti LC, Navigante AH, Bonomi MR, et al. Effect of topical morphine for mucositis-associated pain following concomitant chemoradiotherapy for head and neck carcinoma [erratum appears in Cancer 2003;97(4):1137]. Cancer (Phila) 2002;95(10):2230–2236.
218. Geels P, Eisenhauer E, Bezjak A, et al. Palliative effect of chemotherapy: objective tumor response is associated with symptom improvement in patients with metastatic breast cancer. J Clin Oncol 2000;18(12):2395–2405.
219. Tannock IF, Osoba D, Stockler MR, et al. Chemotherapy with mitoxantrone plus prednisone or prednisone alone for symptomatic hormone-resistant prostate cancer: a Canadian randomized trial with palliative end points. J Clin Oncol 1996; 14(6):1756–1764.
220. Kantoff PW, Halabi S, Conaway M, et al. Hydrocortisone with or without mitoxantrone in men with hormone-refractory prostate cancer: results of the cancer and leukemia group B 9182 study. J Clin Oncol 1999;17(8):2506–2513.
221. Osoba D, Tannock IF, Ernst DS, et al. Health-related quality of life in men with metastatic prostate cancer treated with prednisone alone or mitoxantrone and prednisone [see comments]. J Clin Oncol 1999;17(6):1654–1663.
222. Petrylak DP, Tangen C, Hussain M, et al. SWOG 99-16: randomized phase III trial of docetaxel (D)/estramustine (E) versus mitoxantrone(M)/prednisone(p) in men with androgen-independent prostate cancer (AIPCA). Proc Am Soc Clin Oncol 2004;23:2 (abstract 3).
223. Eisenberger MA, De Wit R, Berry W, et al. A multicenter phase III comparison of docetaxel (D) + prednisone (P) and mitoxantrone (MTZ) + P in patients with hormone-refractory prostate cancer (HRPC). Proc Am Soc Clin Oncol 2004;23:2 (abstract 4).
224. Burris HA, Moore MJ, Andersen J, et al. Improvements in survival and clinical benefit with gemcitabine as first-line therapy for patients with advanced pancreas cancer: a randomized trial. J Clin Oncol 1997;15:2403–2413.
225. Fossa SD, Aaronson NK, Newling D, et al. Quality of life and treatment of hormone resistant metastatic prostatic cancer. The EORTC Genito-Urinary Group. Eur J Cancer 1990; 26(11–12):1133–1136.
226. Labianca R, Pancera G, Aitini E, et al. Folinic acid + 5-fluorouracil (5-FU) versus equidose 5-FU in advanced colorectal cancer. Phase III study of GISCAD (Italian Group for the Study of Digestive Tract Cancer). Ann Oncol 1991;2(9):673–679.

227. da Silva FC. Quality of life in prostatic carcinoma. Eur Urol 1993;24(suppl 2):113–117.
228. Rizzo M, Mazzei T, Mini E, Bartoletti R, Periti P. Leuprorelin acetate depot in advanced prostatic cancer: a phase II multicentre trial. J Int Med Res 1990;18(suppl 1):114–125.
229. Boccardo F, Decensi A, Guarneri D, et al. Zoladex with or without flutamide in the treatment of locally advanced or metastatic prostate cancer: interim analysis of an ongoing PONCAP study. Italian Prostatic Cancer Project (PONCAP). Eur Urol 1990;18(suppl 3):48–53.
230. Fossa SD, Slee PH, Brausi M, et al. Flutamide versus prednisone in patients with prostate cancer symptomatically progressing after androgen-ablative therapy: a phase III study of the European organization for research and treatment of cancer genitourinary group. J Clin Oncol 2001;19(1):62–71.
231. Anonymous. 8 Gy single fraction radiotherapy for the treatment of metastatic skeletal pain: randomised comparison with a multifraction schedule over 12 months of patient follow-up. Bone Pain Trial Working Party. Radiother Oncol 1999;52(2):111–121.
232. Roos DE, O'Brien PC, Smith JG, et al. A role for radiotherapy in neuropathic bone pain: preliminary response rates from a prospective trial (Trans-Tasman Radiation Oncology Group, TROG 96.05) [published erratum appears in Int J Radiat Oncol Biol Phys 2000;47(2):545]. Int J Radiat Oncol Biol Phys 2000; 46(4):975–981.
233. Steenland E, Leer JW, van Houwelingen H, et al. The effect of a single fraction compared to multiple fractions on painful bone metastases: a global analysis of the Dutch Bone Metastasis Study [see comments] [published erratum appears in Radiother Oncol 1999;53(2):167]. Radiother Oncol 1999;52(2):101–109.
234. Tong D, Gillick L, Hendrickson FR. The palliation of symptomatic osseous metastases: final results of the study by the Radiation Therapy Oncology Group. Cancer (Phila) 1982;50(5): 893–899.
235. Madsen EL. Painful bone metastasis: efficacy of radiotherapy assessed by the patients: a randomized trial comparing 4 Gy × 6 versus 10 Gy × 2. Int J Radiat Oncol Biol Phys 1983;9(12): 1775–1779.
236. Price P, Hoskin PJ, Easton D, Austin D, Palmer SG, Yarnold JR. Prospective randomised trial of single and multifraction radiotherapy schedules in the treatment of painful bony metastases. Radiother Oncol 1986;6(4):247–255.
237. Okawa T, Kita M, Goto M, Nishijima H, Miyaji N. Randomized prospective clinical study of small, large and twice-a-day fraction radiotherapy for painful bone metastases. Radiother Oncol 1988;13(2):99–104.
238. Hoskin PJ, Price P, Easton D, et al. A prospective randomised trial of 4 Gy or 8 Gy single doses in the treatment of metastatic bone pain. Radiother Oncol 1992;23(2):74–78.
239. Niewald M, Tkocz HJ, Abel U, et al. Rapid course radiation therapy vs. more standard treatment: a randomized trial for bone metastases. Int J Radiat Oncol Biol Phys 1996;36(5):1085–1089.
240. Rees GJ, Devrell CE, Barley VL, Newman HF. Palliative radiotherapy for lung cancer: two versus five fractions. Clin Oncol (R Coll Radiol) 1997;9(2):90–95.
241. Nielsen OS, Bentzen SM, Sandberg E, Gadeberg CC, Timothy AR. Randomized trial of single dose versus fractionated palliative radiotherapy of bone metastases. Radiother Oncol 1998; 47(3):233–240.
242. Jeremic B, Shibamoto Y, Acimovic L, et al. A randomized trial of three single-dose radiation therapy regimens in the treatment of metastatic bone pain. Int J Radiat Oncol Biol Phys 1998; 42(1):161–167.
243. Medical Research Council Lung Cancer Working Party. Medical Research Council (MRC) randomised trial of palliative radiotherapy with two fractions or a single fraction in patients with inoperable non-small-cell lung cancer (NSCLC) and poor performance status. Br J Cancer 1992;65(6):934–941.
244. Macbeth FR, Bolger JJ, Hopwood P, et al. Randomized trial of palliative two-fraction versus more intensive 13-fraction radiotherapy for patients with inoperable non-small cell lung cancer and good performance status. Medical Research Council Lung Cancer Working Party [see comments]. Clin Oncol (R Coll Radiol) 1996;8(3):167–175.
245. Teshima T, Inoue T, Ikeda H, et al. Symptomatic relief for patients with osseous metastasis treated with radiation and methylprednisolone: a prospective randomized study. Radiat Med 1996;14(4):185–188.
246. Whelan TJ, Levine M, Julian J, et al. The effects of radiation therapy on quality of life of women with breast carcinoma: results of a randomized trial. Ontario Clinical Oncology Group. Cancer (Phila) 2000;88(10):2260–2266.
247. Porter AT, McEwan AJ, Powe JE, et al. Results of a randomized phase-III trial to evaluate the efficacy of strontium-89 adjuvant to local field external beam irradiation in the management of endocrine resistant metastatic prostate cancer. Int J Radiat Oncol Biol Phys 1993;25(5):805–813.
248. Serafini AN, Houston SJ, Resche I, et al. Palliation of pain associated with metastatic bone cancer using samarium-153 lexidronam: a double-blind placebo-controlled clinical trial. J Clin Oncol 1998;16(4):1574–1581.
249. Tian JH, Zhang JM, Hou QT, et al. Multicentre trial on the efficacy and toxicity of single-dose samarium-153-ethylene diamine tetramethylene phosphonate as a palliative treatment for painful skeletal metastases in China. Eur J Nucl Med 1999;26(1):2–7.
250. Pavlakis N, Stockler M. Bisphosphonates for breast cancer. Cochrane Lib 2004;2.
251. Lipton A, Theriault RL, Hortobagyi GN, et al. Pamidronate prevents skeletal complications and is effective palliative treatment in women with breast carcinoma and osteolytic bone metastases: long-term follow-up of two randomized, placebo-controlled trials. Cancer (Phila) 2000;88(5):1082–1090.
252. Hultborn R, Gundersen S, Ryden S, et al. Efficacy of pamidronate in breast cancer with bone metastases: a randomized, double-blind placebo-controlled multicenter study. Anticancer Res 1999;19(4C):3383–3392.
253. Djulbegovic B, Wheatley K, Ross J, et al. Bisphosphonates in multiple myeloma [update of Cochrane Database Syst Rev 2001;4:CD003188; PMID 11687178]. Cochrane Database System Rev 2002;3:CD003188.
254. Rosen LS, Gordon D, Kaminski M, et al. Long-term efficacy and safety of zoledronic acid compared with pamidronate disodium in the treatment of skeletal complications in patients with advanced multiple myeloma or breast carcinoma: a randomized, double-blind, multicenter, comparative trial. Cancer (Phila) 2003;98(8):1735–1744.
255. Dearnaley DP, Sydes MR, Mason MD, et al. Mrc Pr05 Collaborators. A double-blind, placebo-controlled, randomized trial of oral sodium clodronate for metastatic prostate cancer (MRC PR05 Trial) [see comment]. J Natl Cancer Inst 2003;95(17): 1300–1311.
256. Ernst DS, Tannock IF, Winquist EW, et al. Randomized, double-blind, controlled trial of mitoxantrone/prednisone and clodronate versus mitoxantrone/prednisone and placebo in patients with hormone-refractory prostate cancer and pain. J Clin Oncol 2003;21(17):3335–3342.
257. Small EJ, Smith MR, Seaman JJ, Petrone S, Kowalski MO. Combined analysis of two multicenter, randomized, placebo-controlled studies of pamidronate disodium for the palliation of bone pain in men with metastatic prostate cancer [see comment]. J Clin Oncol 2003;21(23):4277–4284.
258. Saad F, Gleason DM, Murray R, et al. Zoledronic Acid Prostate Cancer Study Group. A randomized, placebo-controlled trial of zoledronic acid in patients with hormone-refractory metastatic prostate carcinoma [see comment]. J Natl Cancer Inst 2002; 94(19):1458–1468.

259. Rosen LS, Gordon D, Tchekmedyian S, et al. Zoledronic acid versus placebo in the treatment of skeletal metastases in patients with lung cancer and other solid tumors: a phase III, double-blind, randomized trial: the Zoledronic Acid Lung Cancer and Other Solid Tumors Study Group. J Clin Oncol 2003;21(16):3150–3157.
260. Hill CS Jr, Fields WS (eds) Drug Treatment of Cancer Pain in a Drug-Oriented Society, vol 11. New York: Raven Press, 1989.
261. Crothers TD. Criminal morphomania. JAMA 100 years ago. JAMA 1999;282(6):590.
262. Joranson DE, Ryan KM, Gilson AM, Dahl JL. Trends in medical use and abuse of opioid analgesics. JAMA 2000;283(13): 1710–1714.
263. Hoffman DE. Pain management and palliative care in the era of managed care: issues for health insurers. J Neurosurg 1998; 26(267):289.
264. Bonica JJ. The Management of Pain, 2nd ed. Philadelphia: Lea & Febiger, 1990.
265. Lasch KE. Culture and pain. Pain Clin Updates 2002;10(5):1–4.
266. Fadiman A. The Spirit Catches You and You Fall Down. A Hmong Child, Her American Doctors, and the Collision of Two Cultures. New York: Farrar, Straus & Giroux, 1997.
267. Morris DB. Ethnicity and pain. Pain Clin Updates 2001;9(4):1–4.
268. Blendon RJ, Aiken LH, Freeman HE, Corey CR. Access to medical care for black and white Americans. A matter of continuing concern. JAMA 1989;261(2):278–281.
269. Cleeland CS, Gonin R, Baez L, Loehrer P, Pandya KJ. Pain and treatment of pain in minority patients with cancer. Ann Intern Med 1997;127(9):813–816.
270. Walsh D. Palliative medicine and supportive care of the cancer patient. Semin Oncol 2000;1–108.
271. Cooper-Smith L, Gallo JJ, Gonzales MD, et al. Race, gender, and partnership in the patient-physician relationship. JAMA 1999;282(6):583–589.
272. Anderson KO, Richman SP, Hurley J, et al. Cancer pain management among underserved minority outpatients: perceived needs and barriers to optimal control. Cancer (Phila) 2002; 94(8):2295–2304.
273. Unruh AM. Gender variations in clinical pain experience. Pain 1996;65:123–167.
274. Giles BE, Walker JS. Gender differences in pain. Curr Opin Anaesthesiol 1999;12:591–595.
275. Miaskowski C, Levine JD. Does opioid analgesia show a gender preference for females? Pain Forum 1999;8:34–44.
276. Gershon E, Vatine JJ, Shir Y, et al. Correlation between phantom limb pain and other phantom sensory phenomena in human amputees. In: III European Federation of IASP Chapters Congress, Nice, France, September 2000.
277. Mogil JS. The genetic mediation of individual differences in sensitivity to pain and its inhibition. Proc Natl Acad Sci USA 1999;96:7744–7751.
278. Miaskowski C, Dodd MJ, West C, Paul SM, Tripathy D, Koo P, Schumacher K. Lack of adherence with the analgesic regimen: a significant barrier to effective cancer pain management [see comment]. J Clin Oncol 2001;19(23):4275–4279.
279. de Wit R, van Dam F, Zandbelt L, et al. A pain education program for chronic cancer pain patients: follow-up results from a randomized controlled trial. Pain 1997;73(1):55–69.
280. Miaskowski C, Dodd M, West C, et al. Randomized clinical trial of the effectiveness of a self-care intervention to improve cancer pain management. J Clin Oncol 2004;22(9):1713–1720.

83

Nausea and Vomiting in the Cancer Patient

Paula Gill, Axel Grothey, and Charles Loprinzi

Nausea and vomiting are two of the most feared cancer treatment-related side effects for cancer patients and their families. In 1983, Coates et al. found that patients receiving chemotherapy ranked nausea and vomiting as the first and second most severe side effects, respectively.[1] Up to 20% of patients receiving highly emetogenic agents in this era postponed, or even refused, potentially curable treatments.[2] Despite the availability of more than 20 different antiemetics, nausea and vomiting in cancer patients remain problematic and continue to pose tremendous challenges to practicing oncologists.

The broad scope of this problem and the vast number of ways to intervene may seem overwhelming to the busy oncologist whose patient is in the examination room waiting for a solution. This is a reason to take an evidence-based approach when tackling this problem. This chapter presents options based on data and experience gathered over the past several decades in different clinical settings and discusses the importance of using cost-effective antiemetic regimens.

Chemotherapy-Induced Nausea and Vomiting Syndromes

Investigations into the control of chemotherapy-related nausea and vomiting have led to the description of three distinct, widely accepted, emetic syndromes: acute, delayed, and anticipatory.[3,4] Despite many theories and hypotheses, the exact pathophysiology behind each syndrome is not known (Figure 83.1).

Acute

Acute nausea and vomiting has been, for no convincing pathophysiologic reason, considered as that which occurs within the first 24 hours of chemotherapy initiation. It has been hypothesized that the chemostimulated release of serotonin binds to 5-hydroxytriptamine 3 (5-HT3) receptors on gut vagal afferent neurons and initiates the emetic reflex arch.[3,4] Within 18 hours postinfusion, the serum serotonin concentration returns to "normal," that is, prechemotherapy levels.[5]

Several factors have been identified for predicting chemotherapy-induced nausea and vomiting (CINV). The most important factor is the emetogenicity of the chemotherapeutic agents being used. In 1997, Hesketh et al. proposed a classification for the acute emetogenicity of cancer chemotherapy, both single agents and combination chemotherapy.[6] They proposed that the emetogenic potential of chemotherapy, without the use of antiemetics, be divided into five levels based on frequency (Table 83.1).[6] An algorithm for the emetogenic potential of combined regimens was also outlined (Table 83.2). Part of the problem with utilizing this emetogenic classification system, particularly with newer chemotherapy agents, is that antiemetics are given to patients as a standard of care; this makes it difficult to know the true emetogenic potential of individual cytotoxic agents. In 1998, the Anti-emetic Subcommittee of the Multinational Association of Supportive Care in Cancer held a consensus conference, whereby the foregoing classification was reviewed.[7] Although the use of the classification was encouraged by the panel, the lack of evidence regarding the emetogenicity of specific agents or chemotherapy combinations rendered them unable to come to a consensus.[8,9]

There are also well-described patient factors, predisposing for more or less emetic trouble with specific chemotherapy regimens, that have been supported in multiple studies. Factors predicting for more emetic troubles include poor emetic control with prior chemotherapy,[10] female gender, low alcohol intake (current or chronic, less than 100g EtOH/day),[11–13] younger age (less than 50 to 65 years),[11–14] and, although less consistent, low social functioning or high fatigue scores.[12] CINV increases almost fourfold in those with any four of six risk factors they described (female, prechemotherapy nausea, highly emetogenic chemotherapy, lack of maintenance antiemetics, low social functioning, history of low alcohol use).

Delayed

Delayed nausea and vomiting is arbitrarily defined as occurring more than 24 hours after chemotherapy. As little as we know about the pathophysiology of acute CINV, we know even less about that of delayed.[15] The neurokinin substance P, however, has recently been implicated in the pathogenesis of acute and delayed CINV. Neurokinins (NK) are a family of peptides found in mammals that share a common carboxy-terminal amino acid sequence (Phe-X-Gly-Leu-Met•NH2). Three neurokinins have been identified to date (substance P, neurokinin A, and neurokinin B), along with three NK recep-

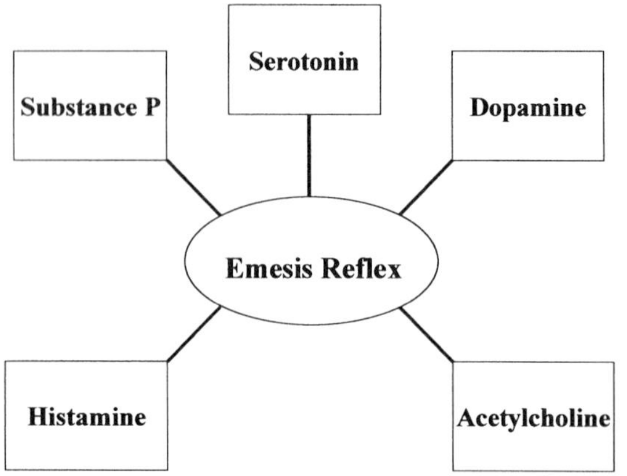

FIGURE 83.1. Proposed endogenous mediators of chemotherapy-induced nausea and vomiting (CINV).

tors (NK1, NK2, NK3). NK1 receptors are found throughout the central nervous system, peripheral nervous system, and gut, with a very high density located in the chemoreceptor trigger zone (CTZ) of the medulla oblongata.[16] NK1-receptor antagonists have been shown to be helpful in the treatment of both acute and delayed CINV (discussed next).

As with acute CINV, the emetogenic potential of chemotherapy regimens and certain patient characteristics can help oncologists predict which patients are at risk for developing delayed CINV. Delayed CINV is well described in patients receiving cisplatin chemotherapy. Only recently has this risk been formally assessed with moderately emetogenic agents, such as cyclophosphamide (750–1,500 mg/m^2).[17]

In some models, one patient characteristic that predicts for an increased risk of delayed CINV is poor control of acute CINV.[3,8,11] Those who experience acute nausea and/or emesis with chemotherapy are much more likely to develop these complications 24 hours or more after treatment. It makes sense, therefore, that patient characteristics that increase the risk of acute CINV (poor emetic control with prior chemotherapy, female gender, low alcohol intake, younger age) will also increase their risk of delayed CINV.

Anticipatory

Anticipatory nausea and/or vomiting is a conditioned response that has a tendency to occur when nausea and vomiting have been poorly controlled with previous cycles of chemotherapy.[7,18,19] Previously neutral stimuli become conditioned stimuli and can thereby elicit anticipatory nausea and/or vomiting. This event can occur before, during, or after chemotherapy and can be brought on by sights (the clinic, the oncologist), smells (smell of the hospital), or environments (the chemotherapy suite).

Several studies have shown acute or delayed CINV with previous cycles, highly emetogenic drugs, and a patient receiving chemotherapy over an extended period of time (i.e., several months) are associated with a higher incidence of anticipatory nausea and/or vomiting.[4] Some studies have shown that younger patients (less than 50 years old), as well as those with a history of anxiety or depression, have more difficulty with anticipatory nausea and/or vomiting.[18] One of the most well supported predictors is a history of motion sick-

TABLE 83.1. Emetogenicity of chemotherapeutic agents.

Level 1 (<10%)
Androgens
Bleomycin
Busulfan (po, <4 mg/kg/day)
Chlorambucil (po)
Cladribine
Corticosteroids
Fludarabine
Hydroxyurea
Interferon
Melphalan (po)
Mercaptopurine
Methotrexate (<50 mg/m^2)
Thioguanine (po)
Tretinoin
Vinblastine
Vincristine
Vinorelbine
Level 2 (10%–30%)
Asparaginase
Cytarabine (<1 g/m^2)
Docetaxel
Doxorubicin hydrochloride (<20 mg/m^2)
Etoposide
Fluorouracil (1,000 mg/m^2)
Gemcitabine
Methotrexate (>50 mg/m^2; <250 mg/m^2)
Mitomycin
Paclitaxel
Teniposide
Thiotepa
Topotecan
Level 3 (30%–60%)
Aldesleukin
Cyclophosphamide (IV <750 mg/m^2)
Dactinomycin (<1.5 mg/m^2)
Doxorubicin hydrochloride (20–60 mg/m^2)
Epirubicin hydrochloride (<90 mg/m^2)
Idarubicin
Ifosfamide
Methenamine (po)
Methotrexate (250–1,000 mg/m^2)
Mitoxantrone (<15 mg/m^2)
Level 4 (60%–90%)
Carboplatin
Carmustine (<250 mg/m^2)
Cisplatin (<50 mg/m^2)
Cyclophosphamide (>750 mg/m^2 to <1,500 mg/m^2)
Cytarabine (>1 g/m^2)
Dactinomycin (>1.5 mg/m^2)
Doxorubicin hydrochloride (>60 mg/m^2)
Irinotecan
Melphalan (IV)
Methotrexate (>1,000 mg/m^2)
Mitoxantrone (>15 mg/m^2)
Procarbazine (po)
Level 5 (>90%)
Carmustine (>250 mg/m^2)
Cisplatin (>50 mg/m^2)
Cyclophosphamide (>1,500 mg/m^2)
Dacarbazine (>500 mg/m^2)
Lomustine (>60 mg/m^2)
Mechlorethamine
Pentostatin
Streptozocin

Source: From Hesketh et al.,[6] by permission of *Journal of Clinical Oncology*.

TABLE 83.2. Algorithm for estimation of emetogenic potential of combination chemotherapy regimens.

1. Use Table 83.1 to assign emetic level to each agent in the regimen.
2. Identify most emetogenic agent.
3. When considering the other components of the regimen, use the following rules:
   a. Level 1 agents do not contribute to emetogenicity.
   b. Adding level 3 or 4 agents increases emetogenicity by one level/agent.
   c. Adding level 2 agents (regardless of number) increases emetogenicity by one level greater than the most emetogenic agent.

Source: From Hesketh et al.,[6] by permission of *Journal of Clinical Oncology*.

ness.[19,20] It is important to realize that anticipatory nausea and/or vomiting is not a sign of underlying psychopathology but is a classically conditioned, Pavlovian-type response that may be avoided if nausea and/or vomiting does not occur with previous cycles of chemotherapy.

Treatment of Chemotherapy-Induced Nausea and Vomiting

Treatment of Acute Nausea and Vomiting (Table 83.3)

Serotonin Receptor Antagonists

Which antiemetic agents are most effective? Is intravenous administration superior to oral application? Which dose is best? The improved efficacy of highly emetogenic antineo-

TABLE 83.3. Level of evidence for treatment recommendations.

Comparison	*Result*	*Evidence level*	*Reference*
A. Highly emetogenic chemotherapy: acute emesis			
5-HT3 antagonist vs. no 5-HT3 antagonist			
Ondansetron vs. metoclopramide	Ondansetron superior	I	90–92
Ondansetron/dexamethasone vs. metoclopramide/dexamethasone	Ondansetron/dexamethasone superior	I	28, 93, 94
Granisetron vs. metoclopramide/dexamethasone	Equivalent	II	95, 96
Granisetron/dexamethasone vs. metoclopramide/dexamethasone	Granisetron/dexamethasone superior	I	95, 97
Dolasetron vs. metoclopramide	Dolasetron superior	II	30
5-HT3 antagonist vs. 5-HT3 antagonist + dexamethasone			
Ondansetron vs. ondansetron/dexamethasone	Ondansetron/dexamethasone superior	I	98, 99
Granisetron vs. granisetron/dexamethasone	Granisetron/dexamethasone superior	I	68, 95
5-HT3 antagonist vs. other 5-HT3 antagonist			
Ondansetron vs. granisetron	Equivalent	I	24, 25, 29
Ondansetron vs. dolasetron	Equivalent	II	26
Ondansetron vs. palonosetron	Equivalent	II	42
B. Moderately emetogenic chemotherapy: acute emesis			
5-HT3 antagonist vs. no 5-HT3 antagonist			
Ondansetron vs. metoclopramide	Ondansetron superior	I	100–102
Ondansetron vs. metoclopramide/dexamethasone	Equivalent	II	103
Granisetron/dexamethasone vs. metoclopramide/dexamethasone	Granisetron/dexamethasone superior	II	104
5-HT3 antagonist vs. other 5-HT3 antagonist			
Ondansetron vs. granisetron	Equivalent	I	13, 105, 106
Dolasetron vs. palonosetron (single doses of each agent)	Palonosetron superior	II	41
Ondansetron vs. palonosetron (single doses of each agent)	Palonosetron superior	II	56
C. Delayed emesis			
Dexamethasone vs. no dexamethasone			
Dexamethasone combination vs. non-dexamethasone combination	Dexamethasone superior	I	43, 50, 107, 108
5-HT3 antagonist vs. no 5-HT3 antagonist			
5-HT3 antagonist/dexamethasone vs. metoclopramide/dexamethasone	Equivalent	I	27, 95, 109, 110
5-HT3 antagonist vs. metoclopramide	Equivalent	II	90
5-HT3 antagonist vs. other 5-HT3 antagonist			
Ondansetron vs. granisetron	Equivalent	I	105
Ondansetron vs. palonosetron (single doses of each agent)	Palonosetron superior	II	41, 56
Aprepitant vs. no aprepitant			
Aprepitant combination vs. 5-HT3-antagonist combination	Aprepitant combination superior	I	45, 46, 57, 58, 111

5-HT3, 5-hydroxytriptamine 3.

plastic agents, such as cisplatin and ifosfamide, led to their increased use worldwide. As stated previously, despite higher cure rates with these effective antineoplastic agents, a drawback was their association with a marked increase in chemotherapy-related nausea and vomiting. Clinicians responded by raising the dose of metoclopramide (2–3 mg/kg IV), a potent antagonist of type 2 dopamine receptors and very weak inhibitor of serotonin receptors.[21] In response to the intolerable extrapyramidal side effects that occurred at high doses of metoclopramide,[22] investigators searched for more selective 5-HT3 receptor antagonists.[23] The successful discovery of selective receptor antagonists led to clinical trials, which then proved their efficacy and safety. As of 2004, five such 5-HT3 receptor-selective antagonists had found their way into clinical practice: granisetron, ondansetron, tropisetron, dolasetron, and, most recently, palonosetron. Granisetron, ondansetron, tropisetron, and dolasetron share similar low side effect profiles, which include headache, transient asymptomatic elevation in transaminases, and constipation.[11] Therefore, toxicity criteria do not help the practicing physician decide which serotonin receptor antagonist to use. Multiple large, randomized, well-controlled studies compared these agents to each other.[24–31] The overall conclusion is that their efficacy is relatively equivalent.

Following initial trials that supported comparable effectiveness of the agents in this class, subsequent studies were conducted to address the issues of route (po or IV), dose, and schedule. Serotonin receptor antagonists have excellent oral bioavailability. In a multicenter, double-blind, randomized parallel study, Perez et al. showed that a single oral dose of granisetron (2 mg) was equivalent to a single IV dose of ondansetron (32 mg) for the prevention of acute CINV with moderately emetogenic chemotherapy (cyclophosphamide 500–1,200 mg/m^2 or carboplatin).[13] Gralla et al. reported similar results when comparing the same antiemetic regimens (granisetron 2 mg po versus ondansetron 32 mg IV) for highly emetogenic cisplatin-based chemotherapy.[24] Multiple studies were also done comparing oral ondansetron (16–24 mg po) to an intravenous dose (32 mg IV) of the same agent.[31–33] Again, equal effectiveness was shown. Given the comparable efficacy of oral and intravenous routes, current recommendations are based upon ease of administration and cost-effectiveness, concluding that the oral use of these 5-HT3 receptor-selective antagonists is preferred above intravenous administration, unless the patient is unable to tolerate oral medications. Part of the rationale for this preference relates to medication cost. At the time that these studies were reported (1998), a single dose of oral granisetron (2 mg) was US $62 whereas a dose of IV ondansetron was US $129.[8,21] Although the specific prices may have changed over time, a similar gap between the oral and intravenous costs remains.

The optimal dose of serotonin receptor antagonists has been investigated as well. Many studies have shown that it is possible to give too little of a particular 5-HT3 antagonist, resulting in poor emetic control.[34–37] On the other hand, given the physiology of serotonin receptor antagonists, most experts concur that there is likely a threshold effect, meaning that once all receptors are saturated, higher doses will not increase antiemetic activity. An illustration of this phenomenon is provided in Figure 83.2. The threshold dose of each serotonin receptor antagonist may vary based on the emetogenicity of a particular chemotherapy treatment regimen; this has led to the current recommendation that the lowest fully effective dose of each agent should be used for CINV.[8,11,27]

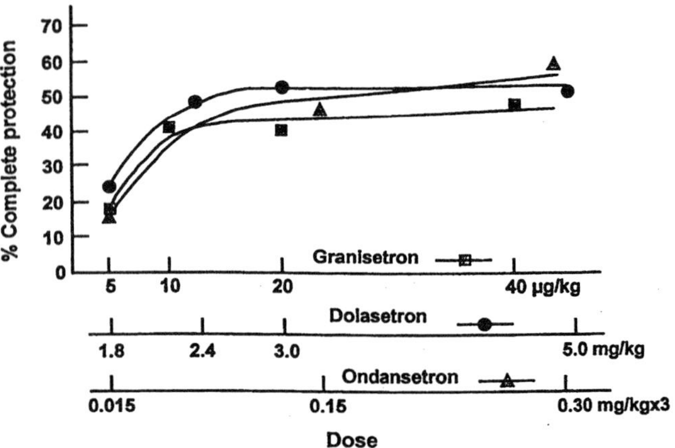

FIGURE 83.2. Protection from cisplatin-induced emesis by various 5HT3 antagonists. (From Grunberg et al.,[37] by permission of *Cancer Chemotherapy and Pharmacology*.)

Several large, randomized trials have been conducted to study whether serotonin receptor antagonists are best given in a single daily dose versus dividing the total daily dose and administering as multiple doses. Beck et al. compared IV ondansetron, given as a single 32 mg dose, to ondansetron dosed at 0.15 mg/m^2 every 4 hours, in a stratified, randomized, double-blind, multicenter study.[35] The single IV dose regimen was as effective as the multiple dose regimen. Once the equivalent efficacy of oral 5-HT3 antagonists was established, similar studies were performed to examine dosing schedules. Ettinger et al. compared a single, 2 mg oral dose of granisetron to two divided doses (1 mg 1 hour before chemotherapy, 1 mg 12 hours after chemotherapy).[38] Both regimens were equally effective in controlling CINV. Harman et al. looked at the same question, single dose versus divided dose, with dolasetron.[39] Once again, both dosing schedules appeared equivalent. Current guidelines for the use of 5-HT3 antagonists for acute CINV, taking the aforementioned factors (lowest effective dose, ease of administration, and cost-effectiveness) into consideration, are outlined in Tables 83.2, 83.3, and 83.4. Although there are many similarities between the recommendations of

TABLE 83.4. Levels of evidence.

Level	*Type of evidence*
I	Evidence is obtained from meta-analysis of multiple, well-designed, controlled studies. Randomized trials have low false-positive and low false-negative errors (high power).
II	Evidence is obtained from at least one well-designed experimental study. Randomized trials have high false-positive and/or false-negative errors (low power).
III	Evidence is obtained from well-designed, quasi-experimental studies, such as nonrandomized, controlled, single-group, prepost, cohort, time, or matched case-control series.
IV	Evidence is from well-designed, nonexperimental studies, such as comparative and correlational descriptive and case studies.
V	Evidence is from case reports and clinical examples.

the American Society for Clinical Oncology, the National Comprehensive Cancer Network (NCCN), and the American Society of Health-System Pharmacists, there are also some notable differences. For example, the NCCN guidelines include aprepitant, an NK-1 antagonist further discussed next, for prevention of acute and delayed CINV.[8,11,40]

Palonosetron is a new antiemetic agent, approved by the U.S. Food and Drug Administration (FDA) in the fall of 2003, that shows high selectivity and strong binding affinity for 5-HT3 receptor sites. Of particular significance, compared to other serotonin receptor antagonists, is its substantially higher binding capacity to the targeted serotonin receptor and its extended plasma half-life of approximately 40 hours, which presumably contributes to its prolonged antiemetic effects. Phase III studies have shown that palonosetron is safe and effective in treating both acute and delayed CINV.[41,42] Palonosetron decreases both acute and delayed nausea and emesis with a single intravenous dose, given before chemotherapy. In one trial, it appeared to be better than dolasetron (100 mg orally) for diminishing both acute and delayed nausea/vomiting, although this trial did not utilize corticosteroids.[41,42] Beneficial effects remained through multiple cycles of chemotherapy. The most common adverse effect was headache, with a frequency similar to other 5-HT3 antagonists. The eventual role of palonosetron in relationship to the other available serotonin receptor antagonists is yet to be determined.

Corticosteroids

Corticosteroids are among the most frequently used antiemetics because of their efficacy, low cost, and wide availability.[7,8] Dexamethasone and methylprednisolone are the most thoroughly studied. Dexamethasone is used most often due to its wide availability and its variety of dosage formulations. The efficacy of oral and IV corticosteroids appears to be equivalent, so oral formulations are recommended based on ease of use and cost.

Recently, a meta-analysis was performed to identify randomized evidence of the efficacy of dexamethasone in protecting against acute and delayed nausea and vomiting in patients who received highly or moderately emetic chemotherapy. Data were collected from a search of the medical literature. All randomized studies that compared dexamethasone to placebo, no treatment, or other antiemetic therapy, qualified for inclusion in this analysis. A search of 1,200 citations revealed 32 studies that included 42 pertinent comparisons involving a total population of 5,613 patients. Results of the meta-analysis revealed that dexamethasone was superior to placebo or to no treatment for complete protection from acute and delayed emesis and nausea.[43]

To determine the optimal dose of dexamethasone for control of nausea and vomiting associated with highly emetogenic chemotherapy, a double-blind dose-finding study was undertaken. A total of 531 patients were randomized to receive either 4, 8, 12, or 20 mg dexamethasone, administered by IV infusion, along with 8 mg ondansetron.[44] The 4 mg and 8-mg doses of dexamethasone provided complete control of acute vomiting in 69% of patients and complete control of acute nausea in 61%. For patients receiving the 12-mg dose, complete control rates were 79% for vomiting and 67% for nausea. The 20-mg dose provided the highest control rates of 83% for vomiting and 71% for nausea. Complete protection from vomiting was substantially significantly better for patients receiving 20 mg dexamethasone compared to those receiving 4 or 8 mg (P less than 0.005) and somewhat better, but not statistically significant, than results for patients receiving 12 mg dexamethasone. There was no difference between groups in the frequency of side effects. Treatment guidelines currently recommend dexamethasone 10 to 20 mg po/IV or methylprednisolone 40 to 125 mg administered once, before chemotherapy, to control acute emesis.[7–9,11,40] When the NK1 receptor antagonist aprepitant (discussed next) is given, the corticosteroid dose should be cut in half, as aprepitant decreases dexamethasone metabolism.[45,46]

Combined Regimens

Given that both corticosteroids and 5-HT3 antagonists are effective in reducing acute CINV, the obvious question arises as to whether combining the two classes of antiemetics would be more efficacious than either alone. Several well-designed randomized studies were performed to address this question. A meta-analysis evaluated 30 randomized studies comparing 5-HT3 antagonists with conventional antiemetics in patients receiving moderately and highly emetogenic chemotherapy. In 11 of these trials, 5-HT3 antagonists used as single agents were compared to combination therapy with 5-HT3 antagonists plus dexamethasone. Combination therapy with dexamethasone was superior to treatment with a 5-HT3 antagonist alone in 10 of 11 trials.[31] Current recommendations, therefore, suggest the use of 5-HT3 antagonists and dexamethasone for emetic prophylaxis when using highly or moderately emetogenic chemotherapy regimens.[7,8,11,40]

Other Agents

Other antiemetic classes, such as benzamides, phenothiazines, butyrophenones, and cannibinoids, have a lower therapeutic index and are only recommended for use with highly emetogenic treatments in patients who are refractory to, or intolerant of, 5-HT3 receptor antagonists or corticosteroids for the treatment of acute CINV. Chemotherapy regimens that have a lower risk of inducing nausea or vomiting do not require as aggressive prophylaxis. The minimal benefit that may exist with using serotonin receptor antagonists in this situation has not been shown to be cost-effective.[9] In fact, for treatments with level 1 and 2 emetogenicity, most guidelines suggest that antiemetics should be used on an as-needed basis.

Benzamides

Metoclopramide is the most commonly used drug in this class. Since the advent of serotonin receptor antagonists, the use of high-dose metoclopramide has become almost obsolete. Metoclopramide blocks type 2 dopamine receptors in the chemoreceptor trigger zone (CTZ), increases lower esophageal sphincter tone, and enhances bowel and gastric motility. At lower doses (20–40 mg po q 4–6 h), metoclopramide may be a useful tool for treating less severe CINV.

Phenothiazines

Phenothiazines, such as prochlorperazine, thiethylperazine, and promethazine, are widely prescribed antiemetic agents.

They act on dopamine receptors centrally and peripherally, and, similar to the benzamides, are useful in treating mild CINV. Side effects include extrapyramidal symptoms (EPS; acute dystonia, akathisias, dyskinesias), anticholinergic effects (dry mouth, drowsiness, urinary retention, tachycardia), and sedation. As with metoclopramide, diphenhydramine or hydroxyzine may be used prophylactically or therapeutically to antagonize extrapyramidal system receptors. Intravenous prochlorperazine can cause marked hypotension if administered too rapidly. Phenothiazines can be given IV, IM, po, or rectally, making them very useful in patients who are having trouble with oral intake or who have difficult IV access.

Butyrophenones

The two drugs in this class, droperidol and haloperidol, are type 2 dopamine receptor antagonists. Their side effect profile is similar to the phenothiazines, including extrapyramidal reactions, sedation, and hypotension. Although they have stronger anitemetic effects than the phenothiazines, the incidence of EPS is higher. Droperidol can be given IM or IV, and haloperidol can be administered orally as well.

Cannabinoids

Despite the controversy that surrounds the use of cannabinoids for CINV, several studies have shown them to be effective antiemetics alone or in combination with other agents.[11,47,48] However, cannabinoids have not been proven effective as prophylaxis against highly emetogenic chemotherapies. Drugs in this class are available as plant extracts (dronabinol) and semisynthetic substances (nabilone, levonantradol). Side effects include dizziness, sedation, hypotension, and dysphoria, which are more pronounced in older patients. As with the other agents having a lower therapeutic index, cannabinoids are only recommended for the treatment of acute CINV as an adjunct to serotonin receptor antagonists and corticosteroids, or in those who are intolerant of more standard antiemetics.

Neurokinin 1 Antagonists

As discussed earlier in this chapter, the neurokinin substance P has been implicated in the pathogenesis of acute and delayed CINV.[16] This discovery has led to the development of a novel NK-1 antagonist, such as aprepitant, which has recently been approved by the FDA for use in preventing acute and delayed CINV related to highly emetogenic chemotherapy. The rationale for the use of NK-1 antagonists is discussed in the next section.

Treatment of Delayed Nausea and Vomiting

Corticosteroids

In 1985, D'Olimpio et al. demonstrated that dexamethasone is better than placebo when used as single agent for preventing delayed CINV.[49] In a randomized, double-blind trial, 64 patients receiving cisplatin-based chemotherapy were given either high-dose intravenous dexamethasone (20mg IV precisplatin and 20mg IV at 3, 6, and 9 hours postcisplatin) or an intravenous placebo. Although there was no clinically significant difference in episodes of emesis between the two arms, those receiving dexamethasone experienced much less nausea, and had it for a shorter duration, than the patients in the placebo group (25% for 30 minutes versus 53% for 3.5 hours, respectively).

Current treatment guidelines recommend the use of oral corticosteroids to reduce or prevent delayed emesis (Tables 83.5, 83.6, and 83.7). Optimal dosing regimens need further study, but typical regimens currently include 8mg administered twice daily for 2 to 3 days, with the continued use of 4mg bid for 1 or 2 more days, as needed. Long-term use of corticosteroids may cause adrenal insufficiency, but the short duration of corticosteroids for antiemetic therapy does not result in this side effect. However, adrenal insufficiency can occur in patients receiving dexamethasone in multiple daily chemotherapy regimens. In addition, corticosteroid use may cause hyperglycemia and insomnia.

Clinical studies have shown that dexamethasone provides improved control of delayed emesis when used alone, but improved efficacy may occur when it is used in combination with another antiemetic agent.[27,43,50,51]

Metoclopramide

Metoclopramide (20mg po q 6h days 2–5) added to dexamethasone (8mg po bid days 2–3, 4mg po bid days 4–5) has been reported to be better than dexamethasone alone.[52,53] Two large, randomized trials showed complete protection from delayed vomiting in 52% and 70% of patients treated with metoclopramide and dexamethasone, after receiving cisplatin chemotherapy, compared to only 35% and 44% of patients treated with dexamethasone alone.[54] Nonetheless, the toxicities of metoclopramide, as already discussed, can be quite problematic in some patients.[9]

Serotonin Receptor Antagonists

Given that delayed CINV was successfully preempted only 50% to 70% of the time with corticosteroids, the role of serotonin receptor antagonists in this setting has also been investigated. Initially, ondansetron and granisetron were compared to placebo. Although they did provide some symptom improvement in patients receiving highly emetogenic chemotherapy, this benefit was only modest. Further studies compared 5-HT3 antagonists plus dexamethasone to dexamethasone alone. Large, randomized, double-blind trials, however, were unable to demonstrate an improvement in control of delayed CINV with the addition of serotonin receptor antagonists.[54] In 1997, the Italian Group for Antiemetic Research compared dexamethasone plus metoclopramide versus dexamethasone plus ondansetron (8mg po bid days 2–4) in a randomized, double-blind study of 322 patients receiving cisplatin.[27] The two treatment regimens offered similar protection from delayed CINV associated with highly emetogenic chemotherapy.

The only study to compare antiemetic regimens, in patients receiving moderately emetogenic treatments, comes, again, from the Italian Group for Antiemetic Research: 705 patients were divided into two groups 24 hours after moderately emetogenic chemotherapy.[55] The low-risk group, defined as those who had no vomiting and only minimal nausea, included 618 patients. The high-risk group, those who had either emesis or moderate to severe nausea, numbered

TABLE 83.5. Summary of American Society of Clinical Oncology (ASCO) antiemetic guidelines.

I. Chemotherapy-Induced Emesis
  A. Acute Emesis (vomiting occurring 0 to 24 hours after chemotherapy)
    1. Antiemetic Agents: Highest Therapeutic Index
      a. Serotonin Receptor Antagonists
        i. Agent equivalence: At equivalent doses, serotonin receptor antagonists have equivalent safety and efficacy and can be used interchangeably based on convenience, availability, and cost.
        ii. Drug dosage: Established, proven doses of all agents are recommended.
        iii. Drug schedule: Single doses of antiemetics are effective and preferred for convenience and cost.
        iv. Route of administration: At biologically equivalent doses, oral agents are equally effective and are as safe as intravenous antiemetics. In most settings, oral agents are less costly and more convenient; for these reasons, they are recommended over intravenous therapy.
      b. Corticosteroids
        i. Agent equivalence and route of administration: At equivalent doses, corticosteroids have equivalent safety and efficacy and can be used interchangeably.
        ii. Drug dose and schedule: Single doses of corticosteroids are recommended.
    2. Antiemetic Agents: Lower Therapeutic Index—Dopamine Antagonists, Butyrophenones, Phenothiazines, and Cannabinoids: For chemotherapy with a high risk of emesis, selective serotonin antagonists (with dexamethasone) are recommended.
    3. Antiemetic Agents: Adjunctive Drugs—Benzodiazepines and Antihistamines: Benzodiazepines and antihistamines are useful adjuncts to antiemetic drugs but are not recommended as single agents.
    4. Antiemetic Agents: Combinations of Antiemetics: It is recommended that serotonin antagonists be given with corticosteroids.
    5. Risk Factors for Acute Emesis
      a. Patient Characteristics
      b. Chemotherapeutic Agents
      c. Guidelines
        i(a). High risk: Cisplatin: The combination of a 5-HT3 antagonist plus a corticosteroid is recommended before chemotherapy.
        i(b). High risk: Noncisplatin: The combination of a 5-HT3 antagonist plus a corticosteroid is recommended before chemotherapy.
        ii. Intermediate risk: A corticosteroid is suggested for patients being treated with agents of intermediate emetic risk.
        iii. Low risk: It is suggested that, for patients being treated with agents of low emetic risk, no antiemetic be routinely administered before chemotherapy.
        iv. Combination chemotherapy: It is suggested that, when combination chemotherapy is given, the patient be given antiemetics appropriate for the chemotherapeutic agent of greatest emetic risk.
        v. Multiple consecutive days of chemotherapy: It is suggested that antiemetics appropriate for the risk class of the chemotherapy, as outlined above, be administered for each day of the chemotherapy.
  B. Delayed Emesis (vomiting occurring >24 hours after chemotherapy)
    1. Antiemetic Agents
      a. Single Agents
        i. Corticosteroids
        ii. Metoclopramide and serotonin receptor antagonists
      c. Guidelines
        i(a). High risk: Cisplatin
        For all patients receiving cisplatin, a corticosteroid plus metoclopramide or plus a 5-HT3 antagonist is recommended for the prevention of delayed emesis.
        i(b). High risk: Noncisplatin
        A prophylactic corticosteroid as a single agent, a prophylactic corticosteroid plus metoclopramide, and a prophylactic corticosteroid plus a 5-HT3 antagonist are regimens suggested for the prevention of delayed emesis.
        ii. Intermediate—low risk

No regular preventive use of antiemetics for patients receiving these chemotherapeutic agents or delayed emesis is suggested for patients.

  C. Anticipatory Emesis
    1. Prevention: Use of the most active antiemetic regimens appropriate for the chemotherapy being given to prevent acute or delayed emesis is suggested. Such regimens must be used with the initial chemotherapy, rather than after assessment of the patient's emetic response to less effective treatment.
    2. Treatment: If anticipatory emesis occurs, behavioral therapy with systematic desensitization is effective and is suggested.

II. Radiation-Induced Emesis
  A. Risk Factors for Radiation-Induced Emesis
    1. Guidelines
      a. High Risk: Total-Body Irradiation
      A serotonin receptor antagonist should be given with or without a corticosteroid before each fraction and for at least 24 hours after.
      b. Intermediate Risk: Hemibody Irradiation, Upper Abdomen, Abdominal-Pelvic, Mantle, Cranial Radiosurgery, and Craniospinal Radiotherapy
      A serotonin receptor antagonist or a dopamine receptor antagonist should be given before each fraction.
      c. Low Risk: Radiation of the Cranium Only, Breast, Head and Neck, Extremities, Pelvis, and Thorax
      Treatment should be given on an as-needed basis only. Dopamine or serotonin receptor antagonists are advised. Antiemetics should be continued prophylactically for each remaining radiation treatment day.

Source: From Gralla et al.,[11] by permission of *J of Clinical Oncology*.

TABLE 83.6. Summary of American Society of Health-System Pharmacists (ASHP) antiemetic recommendations.

1. The emetic potential of the chemotherapeutic agent is the primary factor to consider when deciding whether to administer pharmacologic prophylaxis and which antiemetic(s) to select.
2. Adult and pediatric patients receiving chemotherapeutic agent(s) with emetic potential classified as level 2 through 5 should receive pharmacologic prophylaxis against nausea and vomiting each day on which chemotherapy is given. Antiemetic prophylaxis is not required when the level of emetogenicity is 1.
   (a) Adult and pediatric patients receiving level 2 chemotherapeutic regimens can receive dexamethasone or methylprednisolone alone for prophylaxis of nausea and vomiting. Prochlorperazine is also an option for adults.
   (b) Adult and pediatric patients receiving chemotherapeutic agent(s) with emetic potential of level 3 through 5 should receive a corticosteroid (dexamethasone or methylprednisolone) in combination with a 5-HT3 receptor antagonist.
   (c) Orally and intravenously administered antiemetics are generally equivalent in efficacy and safety for both adult and pediatric patients. The decision as to which formulation to use should be based on patient-specific factors and cost.
   (d) The decision as to which 5-HT3 receptor antagonist to use should be based on the acquisition cost of comparable doses. Dosage recommendations for adult and pediatric patients differ.
3. All patients receiving chemotherapy should have antiemetics available on an as-needed basis for rescue for breakthrough nausea and vomiting. Patients should be educated about the appropriate administration of and expectations for therapy and should be reassured that every effort is being made to prevent symptoms. In adults, lorazepam, methylprednisolone, prochlorperazine, metoclopramide, dexamethasone, haloperidol, and dronabinol are effective. In pediatric patients, chlorpromazine, lorazepam, or methylprednisolone (or dexamethasone) is recommended. The choice of agent should be based on patient-specific factors (e.g., anticipated adverse effects, past success) and cost.
4. For the prevention of delayed emesis after cisplatin therapy in adults, dexamethasone with metoclopramide or a 5-HT3 receptor antagonist is recommended. The choice of agent should be based on patient-specific factors and cost. For delayed emesis after cyclophosphamide, doxorubicin, or carboplatin therapy, a 5-HT3 receptor antagonist with dexamethasone is recommended. Prochlorperazine in combination with dexamethasone has also been used and is available in extended-release and rectal dosage forms, but the evidence to support this combination is limited. In pediatric patients, chlorpromazine, lorazepam, or a 5-HT3 receptor antagonist can be used in combination with a corticosteroid.
5. Patients receiving total or hemibody irradiation (with or without concomitant chemotherapeutic agents) or single-exposure, high-dose radiation therapy to the upper abdomen should receive preventive therapy for nausea and vomiting with each day of therapy. A 5-HT3 receptor antagonist should be used both in adults and in pediatric patients. Oral therapy should be encouraged; however, IV therapy is an acceptable option. There is no evidence to support the use of 5-HT3 receptor antagonists 24 hours beyond the last dose of radiation.
6. If an agent is needed to treat established radiation therapy-induced emesis in adults, prochlorperazine, metoclopramide, or thiethylperazine is recommended. 5-HT3 receptor antagonists are also an option. Chlorpromazine and lorazepam can be used in pediatric patients.
7. When patients do not respond to initial therapy with an antiemetic agent, it is recommended that an agent from another pharmacologic class be added, that the dose of the antiemetic be increased to the maximum within an accepted range, or that a combination of both approaches be used.

Source: From American Society of Health-System Pharmacists,[8] by permission of *American Journal of Health System Pharmacists.*

TABLE 83.7. Summary of National Comprehensive Cancer Network (NCCN) antiemetic guidelines.

1. **Highly emetogenic chemotherapy (level 5)**
   - Aprepitant (NK-1 antagonist) pre- and postchemotherapy **AND**
   - Dexamethasone pre- and postchemotherapy **AND**
   - 5-HT3 inhibitor pre- and postchemotherapy
   - ± Benzodiazepine if needed
2. **Moderately emetogenic chemotherapy (level 3–4)**
   Day 1
   - Dexamethasone **AND**
   - 5-HT3 inhibitor **OR**
   - 5-HT3 inhibitor
   - ± Benzodiazepine if needed
   - ± Aprepitant if needed

   Days 2–4
   - Dexamethasone **OR**
   - 5-HT3 inhibitor pre- and postchemotherapy **OR**
   - Metoclopramide ± diphenhydramine **OR**
   - Aprepitant **AND** dexamethasone
   - ± Benzodiazepine if needed
3. **Low emetogenic potential chemotherapy (level 2)**
   a. Dexamethasone prechemotherapy **OR**
   b. Phenothiazine as needed **OR**
   c. Metoclopramide + diphenhydramine as needed
   d. ± Benzodiazepine as needed
4. **Minimal emetogenic potential chemotherapy (level 1)**
   a. No prechemotherapy emesis prevention
   b. Use phenothiazines/metoclopramide/benzodiazepines as needed

Source: NCNN Antiemesis Practice Guidelines in Oncology. Version 1.2004, 03-30-04. National Comprehensive Cancer Network; 2004. Available at http//www.nccn.org. Accessed April 10, 2004.

87 patients. Patients in the low-risk group were randomly assigned to receive placebo, dexamethasone (4 mg po bid), or ondansetron (8 mg po bid) plus dexamethasone on days 2 to 5 after chemotherapy. The high-risk patients were randomly assigned to receive oral dexamethasone only or dexamethasone plus ondansetron at the same doses given in the low-risk group. In the low-risk group, 92% of those receiving combined treatment (dexamethasone and ondansetron) had complete protection from significant delayed CINV; 87% of those who received dexamethasone only, and 77% of the placebo group, achieved complete protection. For the patients in the high-risk group, 41% of those treated with ondansetron and dexamethasone achieved complete protection, whereas only 23% using dexamethasone alone had complete protection. Nonetheless, the results in the high-risk group were not statistically significant. What this study suggested, above all else, is that the best way to prevent delayed CINV with moderately emetogenic chemotherapy regimens is to control acute CINV.

Palonosetron

As noted previously, palonosetron is the newest approved 5-HT3 receptor antagonist. When compared to dolasetron and ondansetron in prospective clinical trials, a single prechemotherapy dose of palonosetron was more effective at decreasing delayed CINV.[41,56] These trials have been criticized, however, as no corticosteroids were routinely utilized.

However, palonosetron was recently approved by the FDA for the prophylaxis of delayed nausea and vomiting associated with initial and repeated courses of moderately emetogenic chemotherapy.

Neurokinin 1 Antagonists

In March 2003, the FDA approved aprepitant, a neurokinin 1 antagonist, for the prevention of acute and delayed nausea and vomiting associated with highly emetogenic chemotherapy. The implication of neurokinin, substance P, in the pathogenesis of acute and delayed CINV led to the development of aprepitant, a novel neurokinin 1 antagonist that demonstrated antiemetic activity in humans receiving chemotherapy. Early trials conducted in the late 1990s demonstrated the high clinical efficacy of neurokinin receptor blockage for the prophylaxis of acute and delayed emesis associated with highly emetogenic chemotherapy.[57,58] Subsequently, Campos et al. demonstrated, in a multicenter, double-blind, parallel group trial, that once-daily oral administration of aprepitant was effective in reducing delayed nausea and vomiting after high-dose cisplatin[46]; 351 patients receiving high-dose cisplatin chemotherapy were divided into four groups (I–IV). Group I received an oral placebo on day −1 (the evening before cisplatin), granisetron (10µg/kg IV) prechemotherapy, and an oral placebo days 2 to 5 after cisplatin; group II received an oral placebo on day −1, granisetron (10µg/kg) IV and aprepitant (400mg po) prechemotherapy, and aprepitant (300mg po qd) on days 2 to 5. Group III received aprepitant (400mg po) on day −1, an intravenous placebo and aprepitant (400mg po) prechemotherapy, and aprepitant (300mg poqd) on days 2 to 5; and group IV received an oral placebo on day −1, an intravenous placebo and aprepitant (400mg po) prechemotherapy, and aprepitant (300mg poqd) on days 2 to 5. All groups received dexamethasone 20mg po precisplatin. Results showed that, in the delayed-period groups I, II, III, and IV, 27%, 63%, 51%, and 57%, respectively, had no emesis and minimal nausea (P less than 0.01). The overall conclusion was that once-daily oral administration of aprepitant was effective in reducing delayed nausea and vomiting after high-dose cisplatin. This study also showed that the triple combination of a 5-HT3 antagonist, aprepitant, and dexamethasone provided superior control of acute emesis.

Poli-Bigelli et al. reported remarkably similar results in a randomized, double-blind, placebo-controlled trial conducted in Latin America,[45] in which 523 patients receiving high-dose cisplatin were randomized to one of two regimens: standard therapy (ondansetron 32mg IV, dexamethasone 20mg po day 1 and 8mg pobid days 2–4) or standard therapy plus aprepitant (125mg po day 1, 80mg po days 2–3). Complete protection from delayed CINV was achieved in 68% of the aprepitant group, compared to 47% with standard therapy (P less than 0.001). Similar results were seen with acute CINV, with 83% completely protected in the aprepitant group versus 68% with standard therapy (P less than 0.001). Although optimal dosage and schedule have yet to be determined, NK-1 antagonists, such as aprepitant, appear very promising for the prevention of acute and delayed CINV. Aprepitant is the only NK1 antagonist approved for treatment of CINV. However, other NK1 antagonists are being investigated: L-758, 298, a prodrug of aprepitant, CP-122,721, and CJ-11,974 all appear promising in Phase I and Phase II trials.

Although aprepitant is being incorporated into clinical practice in some settings, the cost of hundreds of dollars for a single course has limited a more universal acceptance of this therapeutic addition. The eventual role for this therapy in antiemetic guidelines has yet to be determined.

Treatment of Anticipatory Nausea and Vomiting

Although acute and delayed nausea and vomiting are direct effects of the chemotherapy drugs used, anticipatory nausea/vomiting is not, making standard antiemetics ineffective. Given that a major risk factor for the development of anticipatory nausea/vomiting is poor control of nausea/emesis with prior treatments, prevention is the key. Appropriate antiemetic regimens used to decrease acute and delayed CINV should also decrease the risk of anticipatory nausea/vomiting with subsequent cycles.

Anxiolytics

A double-blind, placebo-controlled study by RAZIVI et al. compared alprazolam versus placebo in 57 breast cancer patients.[59] Despite a much higher occurrence of anticipatory nausea/vomiting (18% versus 0%) in the placebo arm before the third treatment, this difference was not maintained with a subsequent treatment cycle. Thus, although anxiolytics may appear to help individual patients with anticipatory nausea/vomiting, its usefulness should be evaluated on a case-by-case basis.

Aside from prevention, behavioral therapies are the mainstay of treatment for anticipatory nausea/vomiting. Systemic desensitization has been shown to be very effective in managing this problem. This technique is covered in detail in a subsequent section titled Unconventional Therapies for Nausea and Vomiting.

Radiation-Associated Nausea and Vomiting

Incidence, Etiology, and Predictive Factors

Nausea and vomiting in patients receiving radiation therapy is, in general, less problematic than that associated with chemotherapy but also less predictable. As with CINV, the exact mechanism by which patients receiving radiation develop nausea or vomiting is unclear. It has been postulated to be a combination of direct mucosal injury and neurotransmitter release, specifically, serotonin.[60]

Whether antiemetics should be given on a preventive basis at the initiation of radiation therapy, versus as needed if nausea or vomiting becomes a problem, depends on the emetogenic potential of the radiation therapy being given. The major determinants of the emetogenicity of radiation appear to be irradiation site, dose, dose rate, and field size. Of these, the site plays the largest role predicting for the onset, peak, and duration of nausea and/or vomiting. Total-body irradiation carries the highest risk, with 90% developing nausea and 80% vomiting within 40 to 90 minutes.[61] Intermediate-risk sites include hemibody irradiation (40%–83%) and radiation therapy to the upper abdomen (50%). Abdomen-pelvis, mantle, craniospinal, and cranial radiation therapy appear to cause nausea and vomiting in 40% to 50% of recipients. Single-port irradiation of the extremities, cranium, breast, head and neck, pelvis, and thorax carries the lowest risk of nausea and vomiting.[4,11]

Relative to dose functions, radiation delivered as a single high dose has more emetogenic potential than do smaller, fractionated doses. Higher dose rates and larger field size also carry increased risk, as does chemotherapy given immediately before, or concurrent with, radiation.

Treatment of Radiation-Associated Nausea and Vomiting

As with CINV, antidopaminergic agents were the mainstay of treatment, before the advent of 5-HT3 antagonists. The use of metoclopramide or chlorpromazine for radiation-induced nausea and/or vomiting (RINV) produced response rates of only 50%. Cannabinoid derivatives were also tried with similar results.[62]

In 1990, Priestman et al. performed a prospective, double-blind, randomized trial comparing ondansetron to metoclopramide for the prevention of nausea and vomiting in patients receiving high-dose upper abdominal irradiation.[63] Complete control was achieved in 97% of patients receiving ondansetron (8 mg po tid) versus 47% with metoclopramide (10 mg po tid). Several studies have shown 5-HT3 receptor antagonists (ondansetron, granisetron) to be superior to placebo for treating radiation-induced nausea/vomiting related to total-body irradiation or upper abdominal radiation.[64,65] However, there have been few studies comparing different antiemetic regimens or the role of nausea/vomiting prophylaxis in patients receiving intermediate- or low-risk radiotherapy.[66] In 2000, the National Cancer Institute of Canada Clinical Trials Group, performed a Phase III study investigating the efficacy of dexamethasone for radiation-induced emesis (RIE).[67] In this study, 150 patients receiving radiotherapy to the upper abdomen were accrued and randomized to dexamethasone (2 mg po tid) versus placebo; 70% of patients in the dexamethasone arm had complete protection from radiation-induced vomiting versus 49% of those receiving placebo. Recently, Matsuoka et al. performed a small, prospective randomized study comparing granisetron plus dexamethasone versus granisetron alone in the prevention of vomiting caused by stem cell transplant conditioning regimens.[68] For patients receiving total-body irradiation on day 1 of conditioning, complete emetic control was achieved in all patients (100%) in the granisetron plus dexamethasone group, compared with 63% in the granisetron only group ($P = 0.02$).

Current guidelines suggest using serotonin receptor antagonists (ondansetron 8 mg po bid-tid or granisetron 2 mg po qd), with or without corticosteroids, for patients receiving total body irradiation. For those in the intermediate-risk category, dexamethasone, serotonin, or dopamine receptor antagonists are recommended before each fraction. For patients receiving radiation to low-risk areas, antiemetics are suggested for use on an as-needed basis only.[7,8,11,40]

Nausea and Vomiting in Patients with Advanced Cancer: A Common Problem

Independent of cytotoxic therapy and radiation therapy, patients with advanced incurable cancer can have prominent problems with nausea and vomiting. An illustration of this situation became apparent in a clinical trial that evaluated megestrol acetate versus a placebo for patients with cancer anorexia/cachexia.[69] In this clinical trial, patients were asked whether they perceived nausea or vomiting to be problems that they attributed to the study medication that they were receiving. In reply to this question, 38% of the placebo recipients blamed nausea on the placebo they were taking (while they were blinded as to what they were receiving). Additionally, 25% of the respondents blamed vomiting on the placebo they were receiving. Another group of investigators, also evaluating megestrol acetate versus placebo, noted a similarly high instance of nausea and vomiting in these patients.[70] This latter group of investigators asked the patients about nausea and vomiting before starting any study medication and then after they were receiving study medications. They noted a similar high incidence of nausea and vomiting in patients before and after they started taking placebos. The conclusions of these investigators were that nausea and vomiting were common clinical problems in patients independent of anticancer treatments. The effect of megestrol acetate on nausea and vomiting in these two trials is described in a subsequent paragraph.

Etiology

The etiology of nausea and vomiting in patients with advanced incurable cancer is multifactorial. One of the causes relates to gastrointestinal structural changes, including tumor impingement and bowel obstruction. In addition, multiple electrolyte abnormalities, brain metastases, and multiple medications (including narcotics) can be responsible for causing nausea and vomiting. It is possible also that the tumor itself releases yet undefined substances that lead to nausea and vomiting in these patients.

Treatment of Nausea and Vomiting Related to Advanced Cancer

Remarkably little has been done to evaluate potential treatments for nausea and vomiting, independent of chemotherapy- or radiation therapy-induced causes, in patients with advanced incurable cancer. Nonetheless, the most obvious thing to do is to try to treat the underlying cause of the nausea and vomiting. Unfortunately, oftentimes this is not very feasible. If underlying causes have been treated as effectively as possible (for example, treatment of brain metastases, hypercalcemia, and/or bowel obstruction), there are some dietary suggestions that can be provided, including the intake of frequent small feedings, as opposed to less frequent larger meals. In addition, it has been recommended to keep patients away from food odors, as these may induce nausea. These dietary recommendations, however, have not been properly studied, and any clinician can relate that they have limited efficacy overall.

Medications that have been commonly utilized to treat such nausea and vomiting in patients with advanced incurable cancer, include prochlorperazine and haloperidol. Theoretically, dexamethasone may also have a role in this situation. However, this has not been well studied, and the long-term use of this drug causes its own set of problems.

Megestrol Acetate

One medication that is not well appreciated as being an antiemetic in this situation is megestrol acetate. In the two noted trials described previously,[69,70] significantly reduced incidences of nausea and vomiting were seen with megestrol acetate compared to placebos. In one of these trials, the incidence of nausea was 38% in placebo-receiving patients versus 13% in those receiving megestrol acetate ($P = 0.001$).[69] Correspondingly, the incidence of vomiting was 25% in placebo-receiving patients versus 8% in those receiving megestrol acetate ($P = 0.009$). Similar numbers were observed in the other trial.[71] Additionally, another trial also demonstrated that patients randomized to receive megestrol acetate had significantly less trouble with nausea and vomiting than did patients receiving a placebo.[72] Thus, megestrol acetate is a reasonable recommendation for attempting to control nausea and vomiting in this situation. Although these three described trials examined doses of 800 to 1,600 mg/day provided as tablets, it appears reasonable to utilize liquid megestrol acetate doses of 160 to 400 mg/day. The liquid preparation is a more bioavailable preparation and is more economically priced.

Serotonin Receptor Antagonists

Interestingly, there have not been good data to establish the pros and cons of using serotonin receptor antagonists for nausea and vomiting associated with advanced malignancies in this situation. Anecdotal reports have suggested that serotonin receptor antagonists may provide reduction or relief of nausea and vomiting, unrelated to chemotherapy or radiation therapy, in patients with advanced cancer.[73–77] Anecdotal information also suggests that the use of serotonin receptor antagonists may provide benefit in treating chronic nausea and vomiting in patients without advanced cancer.[76–78] Nonetheless, anecdotal reports can be fraught with error, and no placebo-controlled study has been successfully performed to assess the efficacy of serotonin receptor antagonists in patients with advanced cancer who have chronic nausea and vomiting unrelated to chemotherapy. This lack of success is not from lack of effort, as the North Central Cancer Treatment Group (NCCTG), for example, developed a placebo-controlled, double-blind trial to address this question, but it was closed for lack of patient accrual.

Factors speaking against the use of chronic 5-HT3 receptor antagonists in patients with nausea and vomiting from advanced cancer are that these agents do not appear to work very well for delayed nausea and vomiting from chemotherapy, as opposed to their substantial benefit in ameliorating chemotherapy-induced acute nausea and vomiting. In addition, these medications are quite expensive and do have their own set of side effects (mostly headache and constipation), as discussed previously. If such medications are started, some patients will consider them to have some efficacy. However, in clinical practice it is very difficult to determine whether a medication, such as this, is having a placebo effect versus being an effective antidote.

Metoclopramide

Pilot trials have suggested that prokinetic agents, such as metoclopramide might reduce chronic nausea in patients with advanced cancer.[71,79,80] In follow-up to this, one small double-blind crossover, placebo-controlled trial of metoclopramide was conducted for patients with chronic nausea and dyspepsia associated with advanced cancer.[81] This trial entered 26 patients, 20 of whom were evaluable, to study a controlled-release dose of metoclopramide (40 mg bid). Patients were treated for 4 days with metoclopramide versus placebo and then crossed-over to the alternative regimen on the subsequent 4 days. This trial reported that the patients receiving metoclopramide had a very modest reduction in nausea (12 ± 10 on a 100-point visual analogue scale versus 17 ± 12; $P = 0.04$). However, no reduction in vomiting was seen, and there was no reduction in the use of rescue medications for nausea or vomiting. The small size of this clinical trial, the borderline statistical results regarding nausea, and the lack of any effect on vomiting, provide suggestive evidence that metoclopramide, in this dosage, might be helpful in patients with chronic cancer-associated nausea. Further work is necessary to better confirm or refute this contention.

Other Agents

There is no information available concerning the use of NK1 receptor antagonists in this situation. Last, there is some information to suggest that somatostatin analogue therapy may be of some value in patients with nausea and vomiting related to a small bowel obstruction that is not surgically approachable.[82] However, better information regarding its use in this situation is needed.

Cost-Effective Management of Nausea and Vomiting

In the early 1990s, 5-HT3 receptor antagonists were the highest ticket drug item in many oncology practices because they were relatively expensive medications that were used across a wide variety of chemotherapy agents. Chemotherapy drugs themselves were a bit less expensive at that time compared to the prices of some chemotherapy drugs used today.

In addition to being a high-cost item, there was tremendous variation in practice, regarding the use of antiemetics, within and between different oncology groups. The high cost of these drugs, and the variation in their use, led to the development of guidelines by some large group practices.[9] Guidelines were subsequently developed by different associations, such as the American Society of Clinical Oncology (ASCO), American Society of Health-System Pharmacists (ASHP), and National Comprehensive Cancer Network (NCCN) (see Tables 83.5, 83.6, and 83.7).[8,11,40] These guidelines provide an algorithm for the utilization of antiemetics based on the emetogenic potential of different chemotherapeutic agents and regimens. Ideally, such guidelines provide for the relatively automated use of the different antiemetic regimens for chemotherapy treatments of similar emetogenic potential. When developed, these guidelines need to be updated at regular intervals as new information, and new agents, become available.

Unconventional Therapies for Nausea and Vomiting

The use of unconventional therapies for the control of cancer-related symptoms has gained increased acceptance over the past several decades. Rather than remaining on the medical fringe, interventions, such as acupuncture, massage, and hypnosis, are making their way into mainstream health care. Increasing patient and physician interest in unconventional supportive treatments created the need for randomized studies investigating their merit. In 2001, Vickers and Cassileth published a review of unconventional therapies for cancer-related symptoms.[83] In this, they made the important distinction between "alternative medicine" and "complementary medicine." The former was defined as "those commonly promoted for use instead of, rather than as an adjunct to, mainstream therapy," whereas complementary therapies were those "used together with mainstream care for management of symptoms to improve quality of life." The advantages of alternative therapies remain largely unproven and, therefore, are not discussed in this text. However, many complementary therapies have been investigated in well-designed clinical trials and are of proven benefit.

Hypnosis

Hypnosis has been an area of interest for decades. It has been used for smoking cessation, phobia management, and anxiety. Its utility in the treatment of nausea and vomiting in cancer patients has been well described, mainly in children and adolescents.[84] Redd et al. describe it as a self-control technique, in which patients learn to invoke a physiologic state incompatible with nausea and/or vomiting.[85] With this method an altered state of consciousness is induced, followed by total-body relaxation. In this relaxed state patients are asked to visualize events associated with nausea/vomiting. The goal is teaching patients to relax despite the presence of anxiety-provoking stimuli.

Systematic Desensitization

Systematic desensitization, a subcategory of hypnosis, appears to be particularly effective in the management of anticipatory nausea and vomiting.[86,87] The mainstay of this intervention is construction of a hierarchy of events related to the known stimulus, that is, chemotherapy.[84] To conduct this therapy, patients describe triggers for anticipatory nausea/vomiting and rank them from strongest to weakest triggers. A relaxed state is then induced, after which the patients use guided imagery to imagine the nausea-inducing situations. They are asked to start at the bottom of the list, with the least threatening trigger, and remain relaxed while picturing the scene. As the intensity of the triggers increases, the patients concentrate on remaining relaxed. Systematic desensitization can be taught to patients in about 20 minutes. Properly trained nurses and oncologists can be as effective instructors, as are behavioral consultants.[84] The goal of systematic desensitization is to create a sense of relaxation using guided imagery that can be accessed when patients encounter the actual trigger.

Acupuncture

Acupuncture may be the most well-studied complementary therapy for cancer- or chemotherapy-related nausea and vomiting. In 1996, Vickers performed a systematic review of acupuncture for nausea and emesis related to chemotherapy, pregnancy, or anesthetics. In that review, 11 of 12 placebo-controlled, randomized, double-blind studies showed benefit with acupuncture.[88] More recently, Shen et al. showed, in a randomized controlled trial, significant benefit in the use of electroacupuncture for control of myeloablative chemotherapy-induced emesis.[89] In the review by Vickers and Cassileth, they cited 16 clinical trials investigating potential benefits of acupuncture as a complementary therapy for nausea and vomiting. Of these, 11 found "significant differences or trends in favor of acupuncture."[83] Therefore, at institutions where this therapy is available, acupuncture is reasonable to try.

Conclusion

Despite our best efforts, nausea and vomiting in cancer patients continue to challenge us. Those receiving chemotherapy and radiation are most certainly affected, as are patients with advanced malignancies. We are able to control this problem, to some degree, with medications and other therapeutic interventions. However, we are far from solving it. As oncologists, one of our ever-present goals is to relieve our patients' symptoms related to cancer and its treatment. As our ability to do this improves, so too, should the quality of our patients' lives.

References

1. Coates A, Dillenbeck CF, McNeil DR, et al. On the receiving end. II. Linear analogue self-assessment (LASA) in evaluation of aspects of the quality of life of cancer patients receiving therapy. Eur J Cancer Clin Oncol 1983;19:1633–1637.
2. Wilcox PM, Fetting JH, Nettesheim KM, et al. Anticipatory vomiting in women receiving cyclophosphamide, methotrexate, and 5-FU (CMF) adjuvant chemotherapy for breast carcinoma. Cancer Treat Rep 1982;66:1601–1604.
3. Herrstedt J. Nausea and emesis: still an unsolved problem in cancer patients? Support Care Cancer 2002;10:85–87.
4. Berger AEA. Cancer: Principles and Practice of Oncology. 6th ed. Philadelphia: Lippincott Williams & Wilkins, 2001.
5. Roila F, Boschetti E, Tonato M, et al. Predictive factors of delayed emesis in cisplatin-treated patients and antiemetic activity and tolerability of metoclopramide or dexamethasone. A randomized single-blind study. Am J Clin Oncol 1991;14:238–242.
6. Hesketh PJ, Kris MG, Grunberg SM, et al. Proposal for classifying the acute emetogenicity of cancer chemotherapy. J Clin Oncol 1997;15:103–109.
7. Antiemetic Subcommittee of the Multinational Association of Supportive Care in Cancer (MASCC). Prevention of chemotherapy- and radiotherapy-induced emesis: results of Perugia Consensus Conference. Ann Oncol 1998;9:811–819.
8. American Society of Health-System Pharmacists. ASHP Therapeutic Guidelines on the Pharmacologic Management of Nausea and Vomiting in Adult and Pediatric Patients Receiving Chemotherapy or Radiation Therapy or Undergoing Surgery. Am J Health Syst Pharm 1999;56:729–764.
9. Loprinzi CL, Alberts SR, Christensen BJ, et al. History of the development of antiemetic guidelines at Mayo Clinic Rochester. Mayo Clin Proc 2000;75:303–309.

10. de Wit R, Schmitz PI, Verweij J, et al. Analysis of cumulative probabilities shows that the efficacy of 5-HT3 antagonist prophylaxis is not maintained. J Clin Oncol 1996;14:644–651.
11. Gralla RJ, Osoba D, Kris MG, et al. Recommendations for the use of antiemetics: evidence-based, clinical practice guidelines. American Society of Clinical Oncology. J Clin Oncol 1999;17: 2971–2994.
12. Osoba D, Zee B, Pater J, et al. Determinants of postchemotherapy nausea and vomiting in patients with cancer. Quality of Life and Symptom Control Committees of the National Cancer Institute of Canada Clinical Trials Group. J Clin Oncol 1997;15: 116–123.
13. Perez EA, Hesketh P, Sandbach J, et al. Comparison of single-dose oral granisetron versus intravenous ondansetron in the prevention of nausea and vomiting induced by moderately emetogenic chemotherapy: a multicenter, double-blind, randomized parallel study. J Clin Oncol 1998;16:754–760.
14. Dodd MJ, Onishi K, Dibble SL, et al. Differences in nausea, vomiting, and retching between younger and older outpatients receiving cancer chemotherapy. Cancer Nurs 1996;19:155–161.
15. Tavorath R, Hesketh PJ. Drug treatment of chemotherapy-induced delayed emesis. Drugs 1996;52:639–648.
16. Saria A. The tachykinin NK1 receptor in the brain: pharmacology and putative functions. Eur J Pharmacol 375:51–60, 1999.
17. Kaizer L, Warr D, Hoskins P, et al. Effect of schedule and maintenance on the antiemetic efficacy of ondansetron combined with dexamethasone in acute and delayed nausea and emesis in patients receiving moderately emetogenic chemotherapy: a phase III trial by the National Cancer Institute of Canada Clinical Trials Group. J Clin Oncol 1994;12:1050–1057.
18. Andrykowski MA, Jacobsen PB, Marks E, et al. Prevalence, predictors, and course of anticipatory nausea in women receiving adjuvant chemotherapy for breast cancer. Cancer (Phila) 1988;62:2607–2613.
19. Morrow GR, Lindke J, Black PM. Anticipatory nausea development in cancer patients: replication and extension of a learning model. Br J Psychol 1991;82(pt 1):61–72.
20. Morrow GR. Susceptibility to motion sickness and chemotherapy-induced side-effects. Lancet 1984;1:390–391.
21. Perez EA. A risk-benefit assessment of serotonin 5-HT3 receptor antagonists in antineoplastic therapy-induced emesis. Drug Saf 1998;18:43–56.
22. Miner WD, Sanger GJ. Inhibition of cisplatin-induced vomiting by selective 5-hydroxytryptamine M-receptor antagonism. Br J Pharmacol 1986;88:497–499.
23. Miner WD, Sanger GJ, Turner DH. Evidence that 5-hydroxytryptamine 3 receptors mediate cytotoxic drug and radiation-evoked emesis. Br J Cancer 1987;56:159–162.
24. Gralla RJ, Navari RM, Hesketh PJ, et al. Single-dose oral granisetron has equivalent antiemetic efficacy to intravenous ondansetron for highly emetogenic cisplatin-based chemotherapy. J Clin Oncol 1998;16:1568–7315.
25. Navari R, Gandara D, Hesketh P, et al. Comparative clinical trial of granisetron and ondansetron in the prophylaxis of cisplatin-induced emesis. The Granisetron Study Group. J Clin Oncol 1996;13:1242–1248.
26. Hesketh P, Navari R, Grote T, et al. Double-blind, randomized comparison of the antiemetic efficacy of intravenous dolasetron mesylate and intravenous ondansetron in the prevention of acute cisplatin-induced emesis in patients with cancer. Dolasetron Comparative Chemotherapy-induced Emesis Prevention Group. J Clin Oncol 1996;14:2242–2249.
27. Italian Group for Antiemetic Research. Ondansetron versus metoclopramide, both combined with dexamethasone, in the prevention of cisplatin-induced delayed emesis. J Clin Oncol 1997;15:124–130.
28. Italian Group for Antiemetic Research. Ondansetron + dexamethasone vs. metoclopramide + dexamethasone + diphenhydramine in prevention of cisplatin-induced emesis. Lancet 1992;340:96–99.
29. Italian Group of Antiemetic Research. Ondansetron versus granisetron, both combined with dexamethasone, in the prevention of cisplatin-induced emesis. Ann Oncol 1995;6:805–810.
30. Chevallier B, Cappelaere P, Splinter T, et al. A double-blind, multicentre comparison of intravenous dolasetron mesilate and metoclopramide in the prevention of nausea and vomiting in cancer patients receiving high-dose cisplatin chemotherapy. Support Care Cancer 1997;5:22–30.
31. Jantunen IT, Kataja VV, Muhonen TT. An overview of randomised studies comparing 5-HT3 receptor antagonists to conventional anti-emetics in the prophylaxis of acute chemotherapy-induced vomiting. Eur J Cancer 1997;33:66–74.
32. Perez EA. 5-HT3 antiemetic therapy for patients with breast cancer. Breast Cancer Res Treat 1999;57:207–214.
33. Hesketh PJ. Comparative review of 5-HT3 receptor antagonists in the treatment of acute chemotherapy-induced nausea and vomiting. Cancer Invest 2000;18:163–173.
34. Seynaeve C, Schuller J, Buser K, et al. Comparison of the antiemetic efficacy of different doses of ondansetron, given as either a continuous infusion or a single intravenous dose, in acute cisplatin-induced emesis. A multicentre, double-blind, randomised, parallel group study. Ondansetron Study Group. Br J Cancer 1992;66:192–197.
35. Beck TM, Hesketh PJ, Madajewicz S, et al. Stratified, randomized, double-blind comparison of intravenous ondansetron administered as a multiple-dose regimen versus two single-dose regimens in the prevention of cisplatin-induced nausea and vomiting. J Clin Oncol 1992;10:1969–1975.
36. Grunberg SM. Phase I and other dose-ranging studies of ondansetron. Semin Oncol 1992;19:16–22.
37. Grunberg SM, Lane M, Lester EP, et al. Randomized double-blind comparison of three dose levels of intravenous ondansetron in the prevention of cisplatin-induced emesis. Cancer Chemother Pharmacol 1993;32:268–272.
38. Ettinger DS, Eisenberg PD, Fitts D, et al. A double-blind comparison of the efficacy of two dose regimens of oral granisetron in preventing acute emesis in patients receiving moderately emetogenic chemotherapy. Cancer (Phila) 1996;78:144–151.
39. Harman GS, Omura GA, Ryan K, et al. A randomized, double-blind comparison of single-dose and divided multiple-dose dolasetron for cisplatin-induced emesis. Cancer Chemother Pharmacol 1996;38:323–328.
40. National Comprehensive Cancer Network. NCCN Practice Guidelines in Oncology, lst ed, 03-30-04.
41. Eisenberg P, Figueroa-Vadillo J, Zamora R, et al. Improved prevention of moderately emetogenic chemotherapy-induced nausea and vomiting with palonosetron, a pharmacologically novel 5-HT3 receptor antagonist: results of a phase III, single-dose trial versus dolasetron. Cancer (Phila) 2003;98:2473–2482.
42. Aapro M, Bertoli L, Lyer P. Palonosetron is as effective as ondansetron in preventing chemotherapy-induced nausea and vomiting in patients receiving highly emetogenic chemotherapy: results of a phase III trial. Support Care Cancer 2003.
43. Ioannidis JP, Hesketh PJ, Lau J. Contribution of dexamethasone to control of chemotherapy-induced nausea and vomiting: a meta-analysis of randomized evidence. J Clin Oncol 2000;18: 3409–3422.
44. Italian Group for Antiemetic Research. Double-blind, dose-finding study of four intravenous doses of dexamethasone in the prevention of cisplatin-induced acute emesis. J Clin Oncol 1998;16:2937–2942.
45. Poli-Bigelli S, Rodrigues-Pereira J, Carides AD, et al. Addition of the neurokinin 1 receptor antagonist aprepitant to standard antiemetic therapy improves control of chemotherapy-induced nausea and vomiting. Results from a randomized, double-blind,

placebo-controlled trial in Latin America. Cancer (Phila) 2003; 97:3090–3098.
46. Campos D, Pereira JR, Reinhardt RR, et al. Prevention of cisplatin-induced emesis by the oral neurokinin-1 antagonist, MK-869, in combination with granisetron and dexamethasone or with dexamethasone alone. J Clin Oncol 2001;19:1759–1767.
47. Darmani NA, Johnson JC. Central and peripheral mechanisms contribute to the antiemetic actions of delta-9-tetrahydrocannabinol against 5-hydroxytryptophan-induced emesis. Eur J Pharmacol 2004;488:201–212.
48. Walsh D, Nelson KA, Mahmoud FA. Established and potential therapeutic applications of cannabinoids in oncology. Support Care Cancer 2003;11:137–143.
49. D'Olimpio JT, Camacho F, Chandra P, et al. Antiemetic efficacy of high-dose dexamethasone versus placebo in patients receiving cisplatin-based chemotherapy: a randomized double-blind controlled clinical trial. J Clin Oncol 1985;3:1133–1135.
50. Koo WH, Ang PT. Role of maintenance oral dexamethasone in prophylaxis of delayed emesis caused by moderately emetogenic chemotherapy. Ann Oncol 1996;7:71–74.
51. Lofters WS, Pater JL, Zee B, et al. Phase III double-blind comparison of dolasetron mesylate and ondansetron and an evaluation of the additive role of dexamethasone in the prevention of acute and delayed nausea and vomiting due to moderately emetogenic chemotherapy. J Clin Oncol 1997;15:2966–2973.
52. Stephens SH, Silvey VL, Wheeler RH. A randomized, double-blind comparison of the antiemetic effect of metoclopramide and lorazepam with or without dexamethasone in patients receiving high-dose cisplatin. Cancer (Phila) 1990;66:443–446.
53. Strum SB, McDermed JE, Liponi DF. High-dose intravenous metoclopramide versus combination high-dose metoclopramide and intravenous dexamethasone in preventing cisplatin-induced nausea and emesis: a single-blind crossover comparison of antiemetic efficacy. J Clin Oncol 1985;3:245–251.
54. Roila F, Donati D, Tamberi S, et al. Delayed emesis: incidence, pattern, prognostic factors and optimal treatment. Support Care Cancer 2002;10:88–95.
55. Italian Group for Antiemetic Research. Delayed emesis induced by moderately emetogenic chemotherapy: do we need to treat all patients? Ann Oncol 1997;8:561–567.
56. Gralla R, Lichinitser M, Van Der Vegt S, et al. Palonosetron improves prevention of chemotherapy-induced nausea and vomiting following moderately emetogenic chemotherapy: results of a double-blind randomized phase III trial comparing single doses of palonosetron with ondansetron. Ann Oncol 2003;14: 1570–1577.
57. Navari RM, Reinhardt RR, Gralla RJ, et al. Reduction of cisplatin-induced emesis by a selective neurokinin-1-receptor antagonist. L-754,030 Antiemetic Trials Group. N Engl J Med 1999;340:190–195.
58. Roila F, Ballatori E, Del Favero A. Prevention of cisplatin-induced emesis by a neurokinin-1-receptor antagonist. N Engl J Med 1999;340:1926–1928.
59. Razavi D, Delvaux N, Farvacques C, et al. Prevention of adjustment disorders and anticipatory nausea secondary to adjuvant chemotherapy: a double-blind, placebo-controlled study assessing the usefulness of alprazolam. J Clin Oncol 1993;11: 1384–1390.
60. Dubois A, Fiala N, Boward CA, et al. Prevention and treatment of the gastric symptoms of radiation sickness. Radiat Res 1988;115:595–604.
61. Chaillet MP, Cosset JM, Socie G, et al. Prospective study of the clinical symptoms of therapeutic whole body irradiation. Health Phys 1993;64:370–374.
62. Priestman TJ, Priestman SG. An initial evaluation of Nabilone in the control of radiotherapy-induced nausea and vomiting. Clin Radiol 1984;35:265–266.
63. Priestman TJ, Roberts JT, Lucraft H, et al. Results of a randomized, double-blind comparative study of ondansetron and metoclopramide in the prevention of nausea and vomiting following high-dose upper abdominal irradiation. Clin Oncol (R Coll Radiol) 1990;2:71–75.
64. Lanciano R, Sherman DM, Michalski J, et al. The efficacy and safety of once-daily Kytril (granisetron hydrochloride) tablets in the prophylaxis of nausea and emesis following fractionated upper abdominal radiotherapy. Cancer Invest 2001;19:763–772.
65. Spitzer TR, Friedman CJ, Bushnell W, et al. Double-blind, randomized, parallel-group study on the efficacy and safety of oral granisetron and oral ondansetron in the prophylaxis of nausea and vomiting in patients receiving hyperfractionated total body irradiation. Bone Marrow Transplant 2000;26:203–210.
66. Maranzano E. Radiation-induced emesis: a problem with many open questions. Tumori 2001;87:213–218.
67. Kirkbride P, Bezjak A, Pater J, et al. Dexamethasone for the prophylaxis of radiation-induced emesis: a National Cancer Institute of Canada Clinical Trials Group phase III study. J Clin Oncol 2000;18:1960–1966.
68. Matsuoka S, Okamoto S, Watanabe R, et al. Granisetron plus dexamethasone versus granisetron alone in the prevention of vomiting induced by conditioning for stem cell transplantation: a prospective randomized study. Int J Hematol 2003;77:86–90.
69. Loprinzi CL, Kugler JW, Sloan JA, et al. Randomized comparison of megestrol acetate versus dexamethasone versus fluoxymesterone for the treatment of cancer anorexia/cachexia. J Clin Oncol 1999;17:3299–3306.
70. Tchekmedyian NS, Hickman M, Siau J, et al. Megestrol acetate in cancer anorexia and weight loss. Cancer (Phila) 1992;69: 1268–1274.
71. Pereira J, Bruera E. Chronic nausea. In: Bruera EHI (ed) Cachexia-Anorexia in Cancer Patients. Oxford: Oxford University Press, 1996:23–37.
72. Rowland KM Jr, Loprinzi CL, Shaw EG, et al. Randomized double-blind placebo-controlled trial of cisplatin and etoposide plus megestrol acetate/placebo in extensive-stage small-cell lung cancer: a North Central Cancer Treatment Group study. J Clin Oncol 1996;14:135–141.
73. Porcel JM, Salud A, Porta J, et al. Antiemetic efficacy of subcutaneous 5-HT3 receptor antagonists in terminal cancer patients. J Pain Symptom Manag 1998;15:265–266.
74. Philpot CR. Ondansetron by subcutaneous infusion. Med J Aust 1993;159:213.
75. Mulvenna PM, Regnard CF. Subcutaneous ondansetron. Lancet 1992;339:1059.
76. Currow DC, Coughlan M, Fardell B, et al. Use of ondansetron in palliative medicine. J Pain Symptom Manag 1997;13:302–307.
77. Wilde MI, Markham A. Ondansetron. A review of its pharmacology and preliminary clinical findings in novel applications. Drugs 1996;52:773–794.
78. Macario A, Ronquillo RB, Brose WG, et al. Improved outcome with chronic subcutaneous infusion of odansetron for intractable nausea and vomiting. Anesth Analg 1996;83:194–195.
79. Bruera E, Seifert L, Watanabe S, et al. Chronic nausea in advanced cancer patients: a retrospective assessment of a metoclopramide-based antiemetic regimen. J Pain Symptom Manag 1996;11:147–153.
80. Nelson KA, Walsh TD, Sheehan FG, et al. Assessment of upper gastrointestinal motility in the cancer-associated dyspepsia syndrome. J Palliat Care 1993;9:27–31.
81. Bruera E, Belzile M, Neumann C, et al. A double-blind, crossover study of controlled-release metoclopramide and placebo for the chronic nausea and dyspepsia of advanced cancer. J Pain Symptom Manag 2000;19:427–435.

82. Khoo D, Hall E, Motson R, et al. Palliation of malignant intestinal obstruction using octreotide. Eur J Cancer 1994;30A:28–30.
83. Vickers AJ, Cassileth BR. Unconventional therapies for cancer and cancer-related symptoms. Lancet Oncol 2001;2:226–232.
84. Morrow GR, Roscoe JA, Hickok JT, et al. Nausea and emesis: evidence for a biobehavioral perspective. Support Care Cancer 2002;10:96–105.
85. Redd WH, Andresen GV, Minagawa RY. Hypnotic control of anticipatory emesis in patients receiving cancer chemotherapy. J Consult Clin Psychol 1982;50:14–19.
86. Vasterling J, Jenkins RA, Tope DM, et al. Cognitive distraction and relaxation training for the control of side effects due to cancer chemotherapy. J Behav Med 1993;16:65–80.
87. Morrow GR. Clinical characteristics associated with the development of anticipatory nausea and vomiting in cancer patients undergoing chemotherapy treatment. J Clin Oncol 1984;2:1170–1176.
88. Vickers AJ. Can acupuncture have specific effects on health? A systematic review of acupuncture antiemesis trials. J R Soc Med 1996;89:303–311.
89. Shen J, Wenger N, Glaspy J, et al. Electroacupuncture for control of myeloablative chemotherapy-induced emesis: a randomized controlled trial. JAMA 2000;284:2755–2761.
90. De Mulder PH, Seynaeve C, Vermorken JB, et al. Ondansetron compared with high-dose metoclopramide in prophylaxis of acute and delayed cisplatin-induced nausea and vomiting. A multicenter, randomized, double-blind, crossover study. Ann Intern Med 1990;113:834–840.
91. Hainsworth J, Harvey W, Pendergrass K, et al. A single-blind comparison of intravenous ondansetron, a selective serotonin antagonist, with intravenous metoclopramide in the prevention of nausea and vomiting associated with high-dose cisplatin chemotherapy. J Clin Oncol 1991;9:721–728.
92. Sledge GW Jr, Einhorn L, Nagy C, et al. Phase III double-blind comparison of intravenous ondansetron and metoclopramide as antiemetic therapy for patients receiving multiple-day cisplatin-based chemotherapy. Cancer (Phila) 1992;70:2524–2528.
93. Italian Group for Antiemetic Research. Difference in persistence of efficacy of two antiemetic regimens on acute emesis during cisplatin chemotherapy. J Clin Oncol 1993;11:2396–2404.
94. Italian Group for Antiemetic Research. Ondansetron plus dexamethasone versus metoclopramide plus dexamethasone plus diphenhydramine in cisplatin-treated patients with ovarian cancer. Support Care Cancer 1994;2:167–170.
95. Heron JF, Goedhals L, Jordaan JP, et al. Oral granisetron alone and in combination with dexamethasone: a double-blind randomized comparison against high-dose metoclopramide plus dexamethasone in prevention of cisplatin-induced emesis. The Granisetron Study Group. Ann Oncol 1994;5:579–574.
96. Warr D, Wilan A, Venner P, et al. A randomised, double-blind comparison of granisetron with high-dose metoclopramide, dexamethasone and diphenhydramine for cisplatin-induced emesis. An NCI Canada Clinical Trials Group Phase III Trial. Eur J Cancer 1992;29A:33–36.
97. Ohmatsu H, Eguchi K, Shinkai T, et al. A randomized cross-over study of high-dose metoclopramide plus dexamethasone versus granisetron plus dexamethasone in patients receiving chemotherapy with high-dose cisplatin. Jpn J Cancer Res 1994;85:1151–1158.
98. Joss RA, Bacchi M, Buser K, et al. Ondansetron plus dexamethasone is superior to ondansetron alone in the prevention of emesis in chemotherapy-naive and previously treated patients. Swiss Group for Clinical Cancer Research (SAKK). Ann Oncol 1994;5:253–258.
99. Roila F, Tonato M, Cognetti F, et al. Prevention of cisplatin-induced emesis: a double-blind multicenter randomized crossover study comparing ondansetron and ondansetron plus dexamethasone. J Clin Oncol 1991;9:675–678.
100. Kaasa S, Kvaloy S, Dicato MA, et al. A comparison of ondansetron with metoclopramide in the prophylaxis of chemotherapy-induced nausea and vomiting: a randomized, double-blind study. International Emesis Study Group. Eur J Cancer 1990;26:311–314.
101. Bonneterre J, Chevallier B, Metz R, et al. A randomized double-blind comparison of ondansetron and metoclopramide in the prophylaxis of emesis induced by cyclophosphamide, fluorouracil, and doxorubicin or epirubicin chemotherapy. J Clin Oncol 1990;8:1063–1069.
102. Marschner NW, Adler M, Nagel GA, et al. Double-blind randomised trial of the antiemetic efficacy and safety of ondansetron and metoclopramide in advanced breast cancer patients treated with epirubicin and cyclophosphamide. Eur J Cancer 1991;27:1137–1140.
103. Levitt M, Warr D, Yelle L, et al. Ondansetron compared with dexamethasone and metoclopramide as antiemetics in the chemotherapy of breast cancer with cyclophosphamide, methotrexate, and fluorouracil. N Engl J Med 1993;328:1081–1084.
104. Numbenjapon T, Sriswasdi C, Mongkonsritragoon W, et al. Comparative study of low-dose oral granisetron plus dexamethasone and high-dose metoclopramide plus dexamethasone in prevention of nausea and vomiting induced by CHOP-therapy in young patients with non-Hodgkin's lymphoma. J Med Assoc Thai 2002;85:1156–1163.
105. del Giglio A, Soares HP, Caparroz C, et al. Granisetron is equivalent to ondansetron for prophylaxis of chemotherapy-induced nausea and vomiting: results of a meta-analysis of randomized controlled trials. Cancer (Phila) 89:2301–2308.
106. Stewart A, McQuade B, Cronje JD, et al. Ondansetron compared with granisetron in the prophylaxis of cyclophosphamide-induced emesis in out-patients: a multicentre, double-blind, double-dummy, randomised, parallel-group study. Emesis Study Group for Ondansetron and Granisetron in Breast Cancer Patients. Oncology 1995;52:202–210.
107. Chevallier B, Marty M, Paillarse JM. Methylprednisolone enhances the efficacy of ondansetron in acute and delayed cisplatin-induced emesis over at least three cycles. Ondansetron Study Group. Br J Cancer 1994;70:1171–1175.
108. Olver I, Paska W, Depierre A, et al. A multicentre, double-blind study comparing placebo, ondansetron and ondansetron plus dexamethasone for the control of cisplatin-induced delayed emesis. Ondansetron Delayed Emesis Study Group. Ann Oncol 1996;7:945–952.
109. Aapro MS, Thuerlimann B, Sessa C, et al. A randomized double-blind trial to compare the clinical efficacy of granisetron with metoclopramide, both combined with dexamethasone in the prophylaxis of chemotherapy-induced delayed emesis. Ann Oncol 2003;14:291–297.
110. Campora E, Giudici S, Merlini L, et al. Ondansetron and dexamethasone versus standard combination antiemetic therapy. A randomized trial for the prevention of acute and delayed emesis induced by cyclophosphamide-doxorubicin chemotherapy and maintenance of antiemetic effect at subsequent courses. Am J Clin Oncol 1994;17:522–526.
111. Van Belle S, Lichinitser MR, Navari RM, et al. Prevention of cisplatin-induced acute and delayed emesis by the selective neurokinin-1 antagonists, L-758,298 and MK-869. Cancer (Phila) 2002;94:3032–3041.

84

Nutritional Support for the Cancer Patient

Lawrence E. Harrison

Cancer cachexia is a complex syndrome clinically manifest by progressive involuntary weight loss and diminished food intake and characterized by a variety of biochemical alterations. Importantly, cancer cachexia has been associated with increased morbidity and mortality and decreased response to therapy. The impact of cancer cachexia on patient outcome and healthcare resources continues to be significant. It is therefore important to identify those cancer patients who are malnourished in an attempt to reverse or at least abate the progression of malnutrition. The goal of nutritional supplementation is to translate repletion into clinical benefit, thereby decreasing morbidity or mortality and increasing the response rate to treatment. The focus of this chapter is to review the etiology of cancer cachexia, summarize the biologic and clinical effects of nutrition, define specific indications for nutrition in the cancer patient population, and explore new therapies available to reverse cancer cachexia.

Prevalence and Clinical Implications of Malnutrition in the Cancer Patient

Cancer patients are at high risk for malnutrition, and cachexia is often a presenting manifestation of malignancy. As early as 1932, cancer cachexia was noted to be a common syndrome. In an autopsy series of 500 cancer patients, Warren reported that the immediate cause of death was inanition in 22%, and that as many as two-thirds of these cancer patients exhibited some degree of cachexia.[1] The predictive nature of outcome from wasting and malnutrition associated with malignancy has been well documented. In a large series, 3,047 patients that were enrolled in 12 Eastern Cooperative Oncology Group (ECOG) chemotherapy protocols for a variety of tumor types, were assessed for weight loss before initiation of chemotherapy. Survival was significantly shorter in patients who demonstrated weight loss compared with those who had not lost any weight before chemotherapy treatment.[2]

In addition to the presence of cancer, the type and stage of malignancy is an important determinant for weight loss. In the ECOG study, patients with breast cancer, acute nonlymphocytic leukemia, sarcomas, and favorable subtypes of non-Hodgkin's lymphoma, had the lowest frequency of weight loss (31%–40%), whereas those with colon cancer, prostate cancer, lung cancer, and unfavorable non-Hodgkin's lymphoma, presented with an intermediate frequency of weight loss (48%–61%). Patients with pancreatic and gastric cancer had the highest frequency of weight loss (83%–87%), with about one-third having greater than 10% weight loss[3] (Table 84.1). In a prospective study of 280 cancer patients, malnutrition was related mainly to the type and site of the tumor, with stomach and esophageal cancer patients demonstrating significant malnutrition as compared with other groups. As expected, malnutrition became more severe as the disease advanced.[3] In an additional study of gastrointestinal cancer patients, almost one-half of the 365 patients were determined to be malnourished, and the incidence of malnutrition was related to site of disease. Stage also predicted weight loss, with more than 50% of stage III patients manifesting malnutrition.[4]

Assessment of Malnutrition

Malnutrition has been associated with increased morbidity and mortality, and therefore, assessment of treatment risk should include a nutritional evaluation. Clinical assessment is the simplest method of nutritional evaluation. The usefulness of a good history and physical examination in this regard cannot be overstated. Prior medical history provides clues to nutritional deficiencies. For example, previous gastrectomy may lead to dumping syndrome, diarrhea, or folate insufficiency, whereas ileal resection or chronic pancreatitis may be associated with steatorrhea and deficiencies in fat-soluble vitamins. A history of alcoholism is associated with protein-calorie malnutrition as well as deficits in niacin and zinc. A history of perioperative chemotherapy or radiation treatment may indicate a malnourished state. A careful review of systems should focus on recent weight loss, weakness, fatigue, and anorexia. Gastrointestinal symptoms, such as nausea, vomiting, abdominal pains, diarrhea, melena, and dysphagia, may also provide insight in determining the presence and magnitude of malnutrition.

The physical examination should include overall appearance, noting muscle and fat wasting. Although muscle wasting is commonly associated with protein-calorie malnutrition, most patients are not overtly emaciated, and evaluation of muscle atrophy may be more readily appreciated in the hypothenar muscles of the hand and the muscles of facial expression. Other indicators of malnutrition include loss of subcutaneous adipose tissue, peripheral edema, skin lesions, and loss of skin turgor.

Weight loss has been shown to be an important index of the presence, severity, and progression of malignancy. The

TABLE 84.1. Incidence of weight loss and effect on survival.

		Percentage of weight loss in previous 6 months				*Median survival (weeks)*	
Tumor type	*N*	*0*	*0–5*	*5–10*	*>10*	*No. weight loss*	*Weight loss*
Favorable NHL 138*		290	69	14	8	10	—
Breast 45*	289	64	22	8	6	70	
Acute leukemia 4		129	61	27	8	4	8
Sarcoma 25*	189	60	21	11	7	46	
Unfavorable NHL 55*	311	52	20	13	15	107	
Colon 21*	307	46	26	14	14	43	
Prostate 24*		78	44	28	18	10	46
Small cell lung 27*		436	43	23	20	14	34
Non-small cell lung 14*	590	39	25	21	15	20	
Pancreas 12	111	17	29	28	26	14	
Gastric (nonmeasurable) 27*	179	17	21	32	30	41	
Gastric (measurable) 16	138	13	20	29	38	18	
Total:	**3,047**	**46**	**22**	**17**	**15**		

NHL, non-Hodgkin's lymphoma.

*$P < 0.05$, survival of patients with weight loss versus no weight loss.

Source: Adapted with permission from DeWys et al.,[2] *American Journal of Medicine* 1980;69:491–497.

importance of weight loss was noted early in the classic study of Studley, who reported that patients who had lost more than 20% of their body weight before surgery for peptic ulcer disease had a higher operative mortality.[5] Although body weight is the most commonly used anthropometric measurement, its interpretation as a sole indicator of malnutrition should be tempered. Weight is highly dependent on the hydration status of the patient and offers no information about the composition of the individual compartments of the body.

Laboratory measurements may provide additional insight for the diagnosis and extent of malnutrition. Albumin is the most commonly used laboratory parameter to evaluate malnutrition. Multiple studies associate increased morbidity and mortality in patients with decreased serum albumin levels.[6,7] The use of albumin as a nutritional index is limited by the fact that (1) use of albumin levels as an indicator of visceral protein synthesis assumes steady-state synthetic rates, which is not the case during acute illness; (2) the long half-life makes it a poor marker to follow acute nutritional changes; (3) reduced serum levels are seen with multiple conditions besides malnutrition; and (4) serum levels are changed by altering hydration status and redistribution. Nevertheless, albumin levels remain the most frequently used index of visceral protein synthesis because this test is widely available and relatively inexpensive.

The diagnosis of malnutrition is based generally on subjective and objective measurements of nutritional status already described, including history of appetite, weight loss, changes in body weight, and serum albumin levels. Although these indicators are useful, alone they do not have significant predictive value for malnutrition and, more importantly, patient outcome with treatment. Based on the unsatisfactory performance of any single assessment value to determine outcome with malnutrition, attention has been turned to combinations of nutritional assessment values to improve the sensitivity and specificity. Various nutritional indices have been examined with the goal of identifying these malnourished patients. Buzby et al. developed a linear predictive model that related nutritional status with risk of operative morbidity or mortality that was based on a variety of parameters from 161 patients undergoing elective general surgery procedures. Using multivariate analysis, the authors developed a weighted combination of four prognostic factors that predicted the risk of operative mortality and morbidity. The index, termed prognostic nutritional index (PNI), is defined as

$$\text{PNI}(\%) = 158 - 16.6\ (\text{ALB}) - 0.78\ (\text{TSF}) - 0.20\ (\text{TFN}) - 5.8\ (\text{DH})$$

where ALB is serum albumin level (g/100 mL), TSF is triceps skinfold (mm), TFN is serum transferrin level (mg/100 mL), and DH is cutaneous delayed-type hypersensitivity reactivity to any three recall antigens graded as 0 (nonreactive), 1 (less than 5 mm induration), or 2 (5 mm or more induration). Patients determined to be high risk have a PNI of 50% or more, those of intermediate risk, 40% to 49%, and low-risk patients, less than 40%. In the subsequent validation of this model, 62% of the 100 patients undergoing similar procedures were determined to be intermediate- or high-risk patients and 89% of these ultimately developed complications. Of note, 27 of the 44 cancer patients (61%) studied were either intermediate or high risk.[8] Subsequently, Buzby et al. also reported the nutritional risk index (NRI), which is derived from the serum albumin and the ratio of actual to usual weight:

$$\text{NRI} = 1.519\ (\text{serum albumin, g/dL}) + 41.7\ (\text{present weight/usual weight})$$

where an NRI greater than 100 indicates that the patient is not malnourished, 97.5 to 100 means mild nutrition, 83.5 to 97.5 relates to moderate malnutrition, and less than 83.5 means severe malnutrition.[9]

Nutritional status is conventionally assessed by a means of a combination of anthropometric and laboratory measurements. Clinically, these methods, such as skin-fold thickness, are time consuming and not readily available. To address this issue, the Subjective Global Assessment (SGA) was developed, which provided a clinical score based on a standardized questionnaire concerning food intake and complaints, such as weight change, gastrointestinal symptoms, edema, ascites, and performance status. Based on these data, patients are classified as well nourished (SGA-A) or mildly (SGA-B) or severely malnourished (SGA-C). Importantly, this tool does not use any anthropometric measurements or laboratory tests.[10] SGA has been validated in surgical patients, and a modified form has been developed for use in cancer patients.[11,12] In addition to the scores already described, a variety of other indices, including the Gassull classification, Mini Nutritional Assessment, and Instant Nutritional Assessment, have also been reported.[13–15] Currently, there is no consensus on the best method for assessment of nutritional status. However, the use of clinical scores may assist in the detection of malnourished patients, and clinical scores are probably more accurate than any single nutritional parameter.

In summary, all cancer patients being evaluated for treatment should have evaluation of nutritional status. By whatever means, it is important to assess and identify all patients who are at risk for malnutrition. Although there is no single parameter that distinguishes the depleted patient, combinations of parameters, incorporating the previously mentioned techniques, are useful in defining this patient population.

Mechanisms of Cancer Cachexia

Host tissue depletion is dependent on the imbalance between nutrient intake and metabolic demands of the host and tumor. Although diminished food intake is one feature of cancer cachexia, nutrients must also transgress the gastrointestinal tract into the portal system and ultimately be utilized systematically to maintain host body mass. Alterations in food intake, absorption, and nutrient utilization ultimately lead to cachexia (Figure 84.1).

Abnormalities in Host Metabolism

Although anorexia is a component of cancer cachexia, restoration of caloric intake does not reverse these alterations. The tumor-bearing state is often associated with abnormalities in energy, protein, carbohydrate, and fat metabolism, and therefore, additional factors must be involved. Although increased nutrient demand by the tumor mass has been suggested as a contributing mechanism, tumor substrate consumption is rarely significant enough to account solely for host weight loss and metabolic alterations (Table 84.2).

Alterations in Protein Metabolism

It has been hypothesized that tumors act as "nitrogen sinks," depleting the host of protein mass, resulting in characteristic alterations in protein metabolism. This tumor avidity for nitrogen accompanies cancer cachexia and involves alterations in whole-body, liver, and skeletal muscle protein metabolism. In general, although whole-body and hepatic protein synthesis is elevated, muscle protein synthesis is depressed. This pattern is unlike simple starvation, where liver and muscle protein synthetic rates are decreased. Tumors derive protein at the expense of the host, resulting in an increased whole-body protein turnover. With few exceptions, whole-body protein turnover, synthesis, and catabolism have been reported to be elevated in both weight-stable and weight-losing cancer patients. Jeevanandam and colleagues compared whole-body protein kinetics in malnourished cancer patients with malnourished patients with benign disease, and with starved normal controls. They found whole-

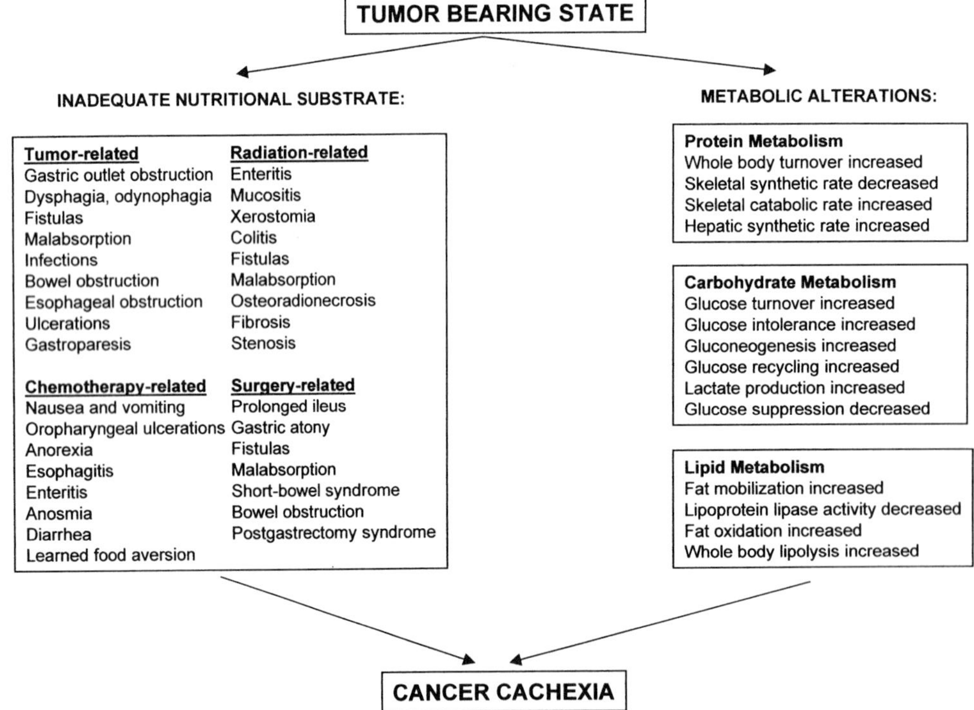

FIGURE 84.1. Inadequate nutritional substrate and metabolic alterations can lead to cachexia.

TABLE 84.2. Metabolic effects of malignancy.

Metabolic component	*Parameter*	*Effect*	*Reference*
Energy expenditure	Resting energy expenditure	±	66, 133–140
Protein metabolism	Whole-body turnover	↑	26, 141–144
	Skeletal synthetic rate	↓	145
	Skeletal catabolic rate	↑	145
	Hepatic synthetic rate	↑	16, 146–148
Carbohydrate metabolism	Glucose turnover	↑	149, 150
	Glucose intolerance	↑	151, 152
	Gluconeogenesis	↑	153
	Glucose recycling	↑	17, 154–157
	Lactate production	↑	21
	Glucose suppression	↓	22, 23, 24, 150
Lipid metabolism	Fat mobilization	↑	20, 158
	Lipoprotein lipase activity	↓	18, 152, 159
	Fat oxidation	↑	19, 140
	Whole-body lipolysis	↑	158

body protein turnover to be 32% and 35% higher in the cancer patients compared to those with benign disease and starvation, respectively. In addition, the rate of protein synthesis was 35% and 54% higher in the cancer group compared to those with benign disease and normal starved controls.[16] Depression of muscle protein synthetic rates and overall muscle wasting is commonly seen in cancer patients. Comparing rectus abdominus muscle biopsied from a heterogeneous group of 43 cancer patients with 55 age- and sex-matched controls, Lundholm demonstrated a decreased rate of protein synthesis and increased rate of protein catabolism.[17]

Carbohydrate Metabolism

The literature is replete with evidence documenting alterations of carbohydrate metabolism in the cancer patient and is the basis for the ability of positron emission tomography (PET) scans to detect malignancy. The changes seen are similar to a type II diabetic state, but also share elements similar to the stress state. Specifically, these abnormalities include the following:

1. Increased hepatic glucose production[18,19]
2. Decreased skeletal muscle glucose utilization[20]
3. Increased tumor glucose utilization with increased lactate production[21]
4. Increased glucose recycling (Cori cycle)[22–25]

Cancer patients, similar to diabetic patients, have a 25% to 40% increase in hepatic glucose production compared to normal controls. However, in contrast to diabetics, cancer patients continue to produce increased hepatic glucose in the face of starvation. The mechanism for this increased glucose production has been implicated as either upregulation of gluconeogenic enzyme activity or increased availability of gluconeogenic precursors, such as alanine, lactate, and glycerol.

The tumor-bearing state is also associated with reduced suppression of endogenous hepatic glucose production by adequate glucose availability. In normal volunteers, a glucose infusion completely suppresses endogenous glucose production. However, in patients with advanced gastrointestinal cancers, gluconeogenesis is suppressed only 70%. Patients with sarcoma and leukemia demonstrate approximately 30% suppression of hepatic glucose production. Most solid tumors produce large amounts of lactate, which is subsequently converted to glucose in the liver through the Cori cycle. Gluconeogenesis from lactate is a very energy inefficient pathway, and this futile cycle may be responsible, in part, for the increased energy expenditure observed in cancer patients.

Lipid Metabolism

Although reduced food intake contributes to the depletion of host fat reserves, alterations in lipid metabolism resulting from tumor burden have also been implicated. Increased fat mobilization has been demonstrated in the cancer patient. The tumor-bearing state is associated with increased lipid mobilization, as well as decreased serum clearance. As a result, hyperlipidemia has been reported to be associated with some tumor types.[26] The hypertriglyceridemia associated with the tumor-bearing state is due, in part, to suppression of lipoprotein lipase (LPL).[27] LPL is synthesized by adipose and muscle parenchymal cells and is responsible for triglyceride clearance from plasma. In the uncomplicated starved state, LPL is decreased as a result of reduction in insulin levels. In cancer patients, a reduction of LPL activity is seen without a change in insulin levels. Vlassara et al. reported a 35% decreased lipoprotein lipase activity in a group of 28 cancer patients with weight loss while maintaining normal or elevated insulin levels. In addition, the degree of reduction correlated with weight loss.[28]

Studies in human and animals models provide evidence for a lipid-mobilizing factor (LMF), which is elevated in the tumor-bearing state. An LMF was recently isolated from a cachexia-inducing tumor and from the urine of patients with advanced cancer.[29,30] This factor acts directly on adipocytes to stimulate lipolysis in a cyclic adenosine monophosphate (AMP)-dependent manner by a mechanism similar to that of lipolytic hormones, and may account, in part, for the lipid metabolic abnormalities observed in cancer patients. Treatment of mice with LMF caused a decrease in body weight that consisted entirely of loss of carcass lipid without any change in food or water intake.[30] Another factor, leptin, is a hormone secreted by adipose tissue that appears to play an important role in triggering the adaptive response to weight loss. In addition, leptin acts as a negative feedback signal critical to the normal control of food intake and body weight. Leptin modifies the gene expression and synthetic pathway of both orexigenic (appetite-stimulating) and anorexigenic (appetite-suppressing) molecules in the hypothalamus, thereby controlling adipocyte energy stores. Further studies are needed to elucidate the role of leptin in cancer cachexia.[31,32]

Routes of Nutritional Support

Nutritional supplementation is an important aspect in the treatment of cancer. Although parenteral nutrition is indicated for patients with nonfunctioning gastrointestinal (GI) tracts, disadvantages of total parenteral nutrition (TPN) include the high cost of parenteral solutions, catheter maintenance, and increased need for absolute sterile technique. In addition, prolonged TPN administration leads to intestinal mucosal atrophy, enterocyte hypoplasia, and decreased intestinal enzyme activity.[33] These changes are associated with a break in the enterocyte barrier, allowing transgression of bacteria and endotoxin into the portal and lymph systems.[34] These observations led to the hypothesis that the intestinal tract is a source of sepsis in the critically ill patient, and there are data to support that TPN is associated with higher rates of infection in certain patient populations.[35,36]

Therefore, enteral feeding, when possible, is the preferred route of nutrition. Enteral feeds, either by oral supplementation or tube feedings, are less costly, easier to maintain, and are more physiologic. Luminal nutrient in the small bowel maintains normal villous architecture and function. Enteral feeding also has been reported to decrease infectious complications and sepsis compared to TPN,[35] which is most likely the result of maintenance of the enterocyte barrier and splanchnic immune function. Studies have demonstrated that enteral nutrition is superior to TPN in maintaining the host immunologic function. Fong et al.[37] demonstrated that endotoxin administered to human volunteers maintained on either TPN or enteral nutrition, resulted in an exaggerated counterregulatory hormone response and hepatic and splanchnic production of TNF in the TPN group. In summary, enteral feeding is at least as efficient as, if not more efficient than, parenteral alimentation in terms of nutritional repletion. Feeding via the gut is cheaper, easier, and offers a method of maintaining intestinal enterocyte integrity. This advantage translates into a decreased incidence of bacterial translocation, affecting on sepsis in a patient population that is already at high risk for infectious complications.

Site-Specific Cancer Therapy and Nutrition

Malnourished cancer patients are at a higher risk for treatment morbidity and mortality compared to well-nourished patients. Although nutrition support has been shown to be important in sustaining patients with "benign" causes of malnutrition, it remains unclear whether feeding of patients with cancer will reduce the morbidity and mortality associated with therapy. A variety of studies have attempted to define the role of nutrition in the cancer patient (Table 84.3).

Head and Neck Cancer

Approximately 40% of patients with advanced head and neck cancers initially present with some form of protein depletion. Although malignancy itself contributes to their malnutrition, they often have an associated history of chronic alcohol abuse, which places them at an even higher nutritional risk. To compound the problem, treatment of head and neck cancer significantly contributes to the severe malnutrition seen in these patients. Head and neck cancer patients are a high-risk group for malnutrition and are perfect candidates for enteral feeding because the majority of the gastrointestinal tract is not involved by tumor or affected by treatment. Therefore, these patients may be fed enterally, either by small-bore nasogastric tubes or percutaneously placed gastrostomies or jejunostomies. If anatomy does not allow entry into the gastrointestinal tract through an endoscopic route, surgical placement of a gastrostomy or jejunostomy tube is a viable option. Sako et al. prospectively randomized 69 patients with head and neck cancer to either preoperative TPN or enteral tube feeding. Nutritional support was given for 14 days. Nitrogen balance was improved in the TPN group, but they were unable to demonstrate any differences in terms of immune parameters, wound healing, complications, or survival.[38] In a report of nutritional supplementation in head and neck cancer patients, Daly et al. compared nasogastric tube feedings versus optimal oral nutrition during radiation therapy. Caloric intake was higher in the tube-fed group, with significant improvement in body weight and normalization of serum albumin at the completion of radiotherapy. However, there was no significant difference in survival between the two groups.[39]

Esophageal Cancer

Malnutrition is a common finding in patients with esophageal cancer. The malnutrition associated with esophageal cancer is, in part, caused by mechanical obstruction and anorexia, but tumor-dependent metabolic alterations also contribute to the cachexia syndrome.[40] Therapy associated with esophageal cancer also contributes to worsening nutritional conditions. Radiation may induce esophagitis and subsequently, fibrosis and stricture. Chemotherapy induces nausea, vomiting, and anorexia, which further worsen the patient's nutritional status. Surgical treatments interfere with the normal anatomy and invariably result in decreased food intake. In addition, esophageal anastomotic leak, regurgitation, early satiety, decreased gastric emptying, and diarrhea are common complications and sequelae after surgery. A few studies have attempted to study the effects of nutrition in the esophageal cancer patient. Lim et al. treated a small group of esophageal cancer patients with preoperative gastric tube feeds and reported weight gain after approximately 1 week and a positive nitrogen balance after 5 days. After 4 weeks of nutrition, albumin levels increased 7.4%. However, the TPN group demonstrated a greater weight gain (although this study did not differentiate whether this reflected protein accrual or just water retention) and early positive nitrogen balance.[41] In another study, Burt et al. randomized patients with localized squamous cell carcinoma of the esophagus to three nutritional regimens: oral feeding, jejunal feeding, or TPN. After 2 weeks of therapy, both jejunal feeding and TPN were efficacious in markedly suppressing gluconeogenesis while increasing glucose turnover, pool size, and clearance rate.[25] Haffejee studied 20 patients with esophageal carcinoma. Patients were evaluated for nutritional status, as well as immune status 1 week before and 3 weeks after enteral supplementation. After supplementation, the average weight gain was almost 4 kg,

TABLE 84.3. Trials of nutrition and treatment.

Author	*Reference*	*Year*	*N*	*Tumor type*	*Nutrition*	*Comments*
VA study[a]	160	1991	395	Heterogeneous	TPN vs. IV fluid	Severely malnourished patients had fewer noninfectious complications
Muller[a]	161	1982	125	Heterogeneous	TPN vs. oral diet	High incidence of complications in control patients Increased weight gain
Holter[a]	162	1977	56	Gastrointestinal	TPN vs. oral diet	Increased weight Increased albumin
Thompson[a]	163	1981	21	Gastrointestinal	TPN vs. IV fluids	Decreased weight loss
Young[a]	164	1980	20	Colon	TPN vs. IV fluids vs. amino acids alone	Mixture of malignant and benign patients Spare lean body mass Decreased length of stay
Brennan[a]	44	1994	117	Pancreatic	TPN vs. IV fluid	No difference in overall survival
Moghissi[a]	165	1977	15	Esophageal	TPN vs. IV fluid	Improved nitrogen balance
Heatley[a]	166	1979	74	Esophageal	TPN vs. oral diet	TPN decreased morbidity but increased wound infections
Lim	41	1981	19	Esophageal	TPN vs. enteral	Control = enteral feeding Improved weight gain
Sako[a]	38	1981	68	Head and neck	TPN vs. enteral	TPN improved weight gain, nitrogen balance
Fan	167	1994	124	Hepatic	TPN	TPN decreased postoperative deterioration of indocyanine green hepatic clearance
Daly[a]	39	1984	40	Head and neck/ radiation	Enteral vs. optimal oral nutrition	Increased caloric intake Increased weight gain Increased serum albumin No difference in survival
Burt[a]	25	1982		Esophageal	Oral feedings vs. TPN vs. enteral	Enteral/TPN: decreased gluconeogenesis Decreased glucose turnover
Lim[a]	41	1981	19	Esophageal	TPN vs. enteral	TPN>Enteral: weight gain Earlier positive nitrogen balance
Haffejee	42	1979	20	Esophageal	Enteral: pre- vs. posttreatment	Increased weight gain Increased serum albumin Increased cellular + humoral immune parameters
Daly[a]	168	1987	28	Bladder cancer	Postoperative enteral vs. IV Low vs. high BCAA	Increased caloric intake Less negative nitrogen balance No difference in hospital stay

TPN, total parenteral nutrition; BCAA, branched-chain amino acids.

[a] Randomized control trial.

nitrogen balance became positive, and serum albumin and total iron-binding capacity were also improved. In addition, both cellular and humoral parameters were improved.[42] Although the cited studies report improved biologic endpoints, they do not demonstrate improved survival or decreased morbidity associated with supplemental nutrition.[43]

Pancreatic Cancer

Pancreatic cancer is associated with a high incidence of malnutrition and weight loss. Numerous etiologies are identified. Mechanical impingement of the tumor can result in gastric outlet obstruction with associated nausea and vomiting, and biliary obstruction can cause fat malabsorption and vitamin K deficiency. With these potential mechanical and endocrine problems, it is not surprising that patients with pancreatic cancer often have malnutrition. Unfortunately, there is no evidence to support perioperative nutritional support for patients with pancreatic cancer. Brennan et al. studied a homogeneous patient population undergoing a pancreatic resection, to test the hypothesis that TPN could reduce postoperative morbidity and decrease length of hospital stay in patients with pancreatic malignancy. Pancreatic resection was chosen based on the assumption that the operative procedure produces a significant catabolic insult with a definable morbidity and mortality that could be ameliorated by TPN. One hundred seventeen patients were randomized to either postoperative TPN ($n = 60$) or IV hydration ($n = 57$). The average preoperative weight loss in this cohort was 6%. Treatment in both groups continued until oral intake exceeded 1,000 kcal/day. Ten patients in the control arm required cross-over to TPN secondary to complications. The authors reported no significant differences in length of hospital stay (16 days for TPN versus 14 days for control), postoperative mortality (7% in TPN versus 2% in control), or overall survival (mean, 24 months). However, the incidence of intraabdominal abscess formation was significantly higher in the TPN group. A trend toward significance in the incidence of peritonitis and intestinal obstruction was also seen in the TPN group.[44] In summary, the data suggest that perioperative parenteral nutrition may be detrimental, and few data exist examining the efficacy of enteral nutrition in this setting.

Chemotherapy

Chemotherapeutic agents contribute to host malnutrition by a variety of mechanisms, including nausea and vomiting,

TABLE 84.4. Trials of nutrition and chemotherapy.

Author	*Reference*	*Year*	*N*	*Tumor type*	*Nutrition*	*Response*	*Survival*	*Comments*
DeVries[a]	169	1982	55	Leukemia	Enteral vs. oral diet	↑ Serum albumin ↓ Weight loss		
Popp[a]	50	1981	41	Lymphoma	TPN vs. oral diet	NS		Weight gain improved No change in lean body mass No change in nutritional indices
Shamberger[a]	170	1983	27	Metastatic sarcoma	TPN vs. oral diet	NS		No difference in infectious complications Time of myelosuppression not changed
Nixon[a]	171, 172	1981	45	Colon cancer	TPN vs. oral diet		↓ with TPN	Weight gain improved
Samuels	173	1981	30	Testicular	TPN	NS	NS	Protein levels unchanged Weight loss improved
Drott[a]	174	1988	23	Testicular	TPN vs. oral diet			Nitrogen balance improved No difference in toxicity Lean body mass unchanged
Evans[a]	55	1987	192	Advanced colorectal and lung cancer	Enteral vs. oral diet	NS	NS	No difference in toxicity
Shike[a]	51, 175	1984	31	SCLC	TPN vs. oral diet			No effect on lean body mass
Clamon[a]	53	1985	119	SCLC	TPN vs. oral diet	NS	NS	Increased febrile episodes
Weiner[a]	54	1985	120	SCLC	TPN vs. oral diet			Weight loss decreased Significant number of TPN-related complications
Jordan[a]	176	1981	65	Lung cancer	TPN vs. oral diet	NS	↓ with TPN	
Weisdorf[a]	59	1987	137	BMT	TPN vs. IV fluids		↑ with TPN	No difference in engraftment, length of stay, graft vs. host disease, or bacteremia
Szeluga[a]	58	1987	61	BMT	TPN vs. enteral		NS	TPN > enteral maintaining body cell mass No difference in hematopoietic recovery No difference in length of stay
Mulder[a]	57	1989	22	BMT	TPN vs. enteral			No difference in nitrogen balance Enteral nutrition as efficacious as TPN

SCSL, small cell lung cancer; BMT, bone marrow transplant; NS, not significant.

[a] Randomized control trial.

mucositis, gastrointestinal dysfunction, and learned food aversions. These effects may compound the already malnourished cancer patient, ultimately influencing the outcome after chemotherapy and leading to increased morbidity and mortality. In addition, increased toxicity from chemotherapy is associated with poor nutritional status of the patient.[45]

Although the impact of malnutrition on survival in cancer patients is well documented, the ability of nutritional intervention to influence clinical outcome in patients undergoing chemotherapy is yet to be defined (Table 84.4). TPN was first suggested by Schwartz et al. to potentially decrease chemotherapy-related toxicity and improve host tolerance.[46] Early retrospective studies suggested that nutritional repletion might allow patients to undergo chemotherapy with improved results and less morbidity.[47–49] These encouraging results prompted prospective, randomized nutrition trials in a variety of malignancies; however, these trials have not demonstrated improved tumor response or longer survival in patients receiving nutritional support.[50–55] Summarized in a position paper by the American College of Physicians, a meta-analysis of 12 randomized TPN trials resulted in an odds ratio for overall survival of 0.81. In other words, patients receiving TPN were only 81% as likely to survive as control patients. For short-term survival (3 months), the odds ratio fell to 0.74. In patients receiving TPN, tumor response rate was 68%. They recommended that "routine use of parenteral nutrition for patients undergoing chemotherapy should be strongly discouraged, and, in deciding to use such therapy in individual patients whose malnutrition is judged to be life threatening, physicians should take into account the possible exposure to increased risk."[56] Enteral nutrition studies have demonstrated improvement in biologic endpoints in patients undergoing chemotherapy but have not demonstrated any significant improvement in response or survival.

Nutritional support has been shown to affect positively clinical outcome in one particular cancer patient population undergoing chemotherapy. Bone marrow transplantation (BMT) requires intensive chemotherapy, resulting in severe adverse nutritional effects. At least 50% of BMT patients suffer enteritis severe enough to result in protein-losing enteropathy, as well as frequent bouts of mucositis and esophagitis. As a result, these patients seem to benefit from nutritional support.[57,58] In a prospective randomized trial, Szeluga et al. randomized 61 patients requiring BMT to either TPN or individualized enteral feed program. Although the enteral feeding program was less effective in maintaining body cell mass, there was no difference in rates of hematopoietic recovery, length of hospital stay, or overall survival between the two groups.[58] In another randomized, prospective trial, 137 patients were randomized to receive either TPN 1 week before BM transplantation or standard hydration. TPN was continued for 4 weeks after BMT. Overall survival, disease-free survival, and time to relapse were significantly improved in those patients receiving TPN. Average protein and calorie intake was also increased in the TPN group. No differences in engraftment, duration of hospitalization, bacteremia, or graft-versus-host disease were noted. Importantly, 40 of 66 control patients were crossed over to TPN when nutritional depletion was documented, and these patients were still analyzed with the control group.[59]

Nutritional support has not been shown to improve accrual of lean body mass, improve nutritional parameters, or ameliorate chemotherapy-related gastrointestinal and hematologic toxicity. Importantly, randomized trials have not demonstrated an improvement in response rate or overall survival in patients receiving nutritional support during courses of chemotherapy, with the exception of patients undergoing BMT. Based on these data, there is relatively little indication that enteral feedings or TPN have any role as an adjunct for chemotherapy.

Radiation Therapy

In addition to chemotherapy, radiation therapy contributes to the cancer patient's malnourished state. The severity and incidence of malnutrition and weight loss are determined by the body region undergoing radiation and by dose, duration, and volume of therapy. Retrospective studies have supported the use of nutrition supplementation in patients undergoing radiation, claiming to improve the nutritional state, as well as offering a protective effect against acute and chronic radiation changes. However, there are no randomized prospective studies demonstrating improvement in local control or survival with nutritional support.

There is experimental evidence to support enteral nutrition as a form of prophylaxis against radiation injury.[60] Bounous reported that elemental nutrition works by suppressing pancreatic and biliary secretions. In addition, he states that it prevents alterations in microvilli, reduction in the enterocyte glycocalyx, and suppression of brush border enzymes.[61] Some of these findings have been reproduced in human trials. McArdle et al. fed 20 patients 3 days before and 4 days during radiotherapy for bladder cancer. All patients underwent cystectomy and ileal conduit. Tube feedings were restarted on the first postoperative day. These patients were compared with treatment-, age-, sex-, and grade-matched historical controls. The authors concluded that the control group had increased amounts of diarrhea, nausea, and vomiting in both the pre- and postoperative period, and that the time for the return of gastrointestinal function was decreased. In addition, histologic examination of biopsy specimens of the terminal ileum in 3 patients who were not fed the elemental diet, demonstrated moderate to severe radiation damage compared to those receiving enteral feedings, who demonstrated normal morphologic findings.[62]

In summary, there is good evidence that nutrition positively affects the cancer patient in terms of metabolic parameters.[63,64] However, at the present time, there is a paucity of data demonstrating a positive clinical impact (Tables 84.3, 84.4, 84.5). Reasons for this are many. Most importantly,

TABLE 84.5. Trials of nutrition and radiation.

Author	*Reference*	*Year*	*N*	*Tumor type*	*Nutrition*	*Response*	*Survival*	*Comments*
Kinsella[a]	177	1981	32	Pelvic malignancy	TPN vs. oral intake			Mixture of curative and palliative treatment Improved transferrin levels No improvement in quality of life or complications Improved weight gain
Ghavimi[a]	178	1982	25	Pediatric pelvis/ abdominal malignancy	TPN vs. oral diet		NS	Some patients received chemotherapy No difference in anthropometrics Increased diarrhea with TPN Depression of WBC increased with TPN
Valerio[a]	179	1978	20	Pelvic malignancy	TPN vs. oral diet			Increase in transferring Improved weight gain
Solassol[a]	180	1980	81	Ovarian malignancy	TPN vs. oral diet		NS	Treatment interruptions decreased with TPN
McArdle	62	1985	20	Bladder cancer	Enteral compared to historical controls			↓ GI symptoms Improved nitrogen balance Terminal ileum histology: improved radiation changes
Douglass[a]	181	1978	30	Locally advanced GI cancers	Enteral vs. oral diet		NS	Improved delayed-type hypersensitivity
Daly[a]	39	1984	40	Head and neck cancers	Enteral vs. oral diet	NS	NS	↑ caloric intake ↑ protein intake ↓ weight loss ↑ recovery of serum albumin

[a] Randomized control trial.

studies demonstrating improvement in survival and morbidity require a large number of patients with significant follow-up time. Unfortunately, there are few studies large enough and with homogeneous populations and sufficient follow-up time to definitively state conclusions about nutrition and its impact on overall survival. Although promising, large prospective, randomized studies are still required before nutrition is instituted globally in cancer patients in an attempt to improve outcome and overall survival.

Pharmacologic Support

Enteral or parenteral nutritional supplementation is one approach to overcome nutritional impairment, but "force feeding" alone cannot always reverse the effects of cancer cachexia. It is possible that the failure of conventional nutritional interventions to improve clinical outcome in cancer patients may be because standard formulations do not affect or reverse the abnormalities of intermediate metabolism seen in cancer cachexia. Therefore, there has been an interest in developing certain pharmacologic agents to improve weight gain and nutritional status in cancer patients by addressing these issues (Figure 84.2; Table 84.6).

Promotility Agents

Patients with advanced cancers experience early satiety based, in part, on delayed upper gastrointestinal motility. In addition, factors, such as postoperative ileus and opiate-associated dysmotility, contribute to delayed emptying.[65] The cancer-associated dyspepsia syndrome, including nausea, vomiting, loss of appetite, and bloating, is related to autonomic dysfunction. Metaclopramide is a benzamide derivative with marked dopamine receptor antagonism and weak antagonism of the 5-hydroxytryptamine-3 receptor. It has direct effects on gastrointestinal motility, as well as having an antiemetic effect. Metaclopramide has been shown to relieve anorexia and early satiety in small trials.[66,67] A controlled release form of metaclopramide studied in a cancer patient population, showed the drug to be moderately effective, with improvement in nausea.[68,69] Although it has been shown to improve gastric emptying and provide symptomatic improvement, demonstration of an effect on clinical nutritional endpoints is necessary before metaclopramide is used in routine clinical practice. Erythromycin and other macrolide antibiotics have also been studied as anticachectic agents.[70] In addition to their promotiliy effects, macrolides also posses antiinflammatory properties. In a small trial, 33 patients with unresectable primary non-small cell lung cancer were treated with clarithromycin for 3 months. As compared to a similar cohort of patients not receiving clarithromycin, patients receiving the macrolide demonstrated reduced serum interleukin (IL)-6 levels, which correlated with improved weight gain.[71]

Orexigenic Agents

Orexigenic agents are drugs that stimulate appetite. The most studied orexigenic agent is megestrol acetate. Megestrol acetate (Megace), a synthetic progestational agent, has been used for hormonal management of breast cancer. Studies with megestrol acetate noted that the drug produced weight gain, increased appetite, and promoted a sense of well-being, unrelated to its antitumor effect.[72] In a randomized, double-blinded study, 133 cancer patients with anorexia and weight

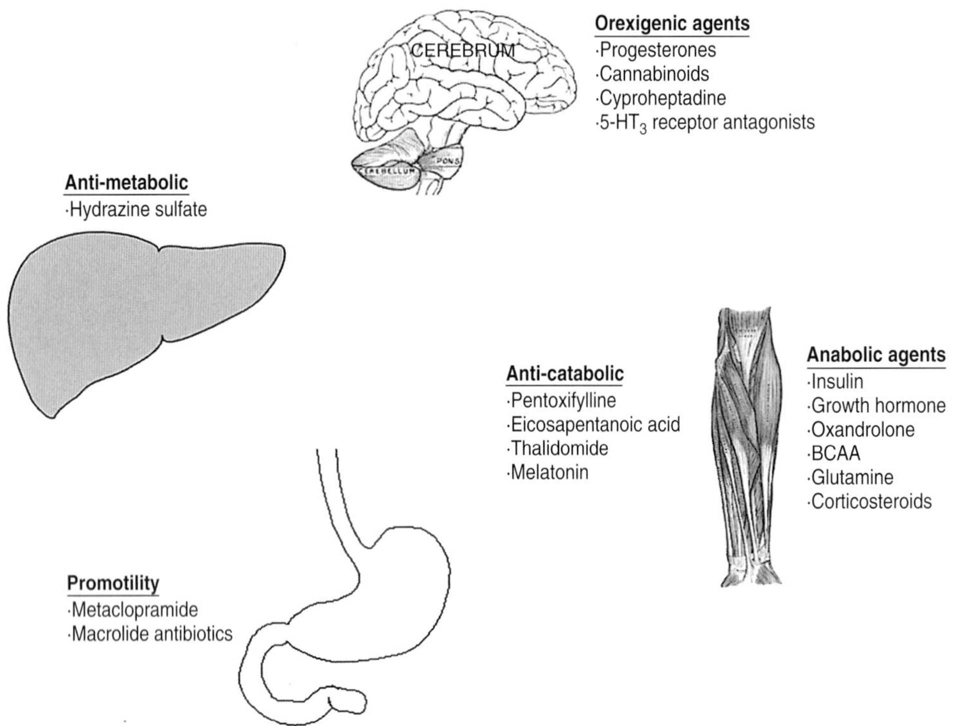

FIGURE 84.2. Pharmacologic agents have been developed to improve weight gain and nutritional status in cancer patients.

TABLE 84.6. Pharmacologic support.

	Agent	*Author*	*Reference*	*Year*	*N*	*Tumor type*	*Trial type*	*Comments*
Promotility:	Metaclopramide	Bruera	68	2000	26	Heterogeneous	Crossover	Nausea improved compared to placebo
		Wilson	69	2002	48	Heterogeneous	Phase II	Appetite and bloating improved
	Macrolide antibiotics	Sakamoto	71	2001	33	NSCLC	Case-control	Weight gain IL-6 serum level decreased
		Mikasa	70	1997	49	NSCLC	RCT	Improved survival
Orexigenic:	Progestational	Loprinzi	73	1990	133	Heterogeneous	RCT	Megase improved food intake and weight gain
		Erkurt	74	2000	100	Heterogeneous	RCT	Megase improved weight gain, performance status, and appetite
		Simons	77	1998	54	Heterogeneous	RCT	MPA increased energy intake and fat mass
	Cannabinoids	Jatoi	80	2002	469	Heterogeneous	RCT	Compared megase and dronabinol and combination Equal effect, no benefit from combination therapy
	Antiserotonin	Kardinal	81	1990	295	Heterogeneous	RCT	Cyproheptadine decreased nausea and vomiting No effect on weight loss
		Edelman	82	1999	20	Heterogeneous	Phase II	Ondansetron Failed to prevent weight loss
Anabolic:	Steroids	Willox	83	1984	300	Heterogeneous	RCT	Improved appetite
		Loprinzi	85	1999	475	Heterogeneous	Phase III	Compared dexamethasone, megase, and fluoxymesterone: Megase = Dex > Fluo
		Moertel	84	1974		Heterogeneous	RCT	Dexamethasone improved appetite No effect on weight gain
	Insulin	Minn	86	1994	6	Lymphoma	Observational	Insulin improved glucose uptake in skeletal muscle but not tumor by PET scan
		Pearlstone	182	1994	11	Postoperative	Crossover	Insulin improved protein kinetics
	Growth hormone	Berman	91	1999	30	Postoperative	Randomized	GH improved protein kinetics
	Amino acids	Tayek	95	1986	10	Advanced abdominal	Crossover	BCAA enriched TPN improved whole-body protein kinetics
		Hunter	96	1989	9	Intraabdominal adenocarcinoma	RCT	BCAA enriched TPN improved protein kinetics
		Ziegler	99	1992	45	Hematologic malignancies	RCT	Glutamine enriched TPN improved nitrogen balance and decreased length of stay
		May	97	2002	32	Solid tumors	RCT	Nonessential amino acids vs. beta-hydroxy-beta methylbutyrate arginine and glutamine Improved fat free mass
Other:	Pentoxifylline	Goldberg	104	1995	70	Heterogeneous	RCT	Failed to improve appetite
	Hydrazine	Loprinzi	107	1994	127	NSCLC	RCT	Failed to demonstrate any benefit
			108	1994	243	Advanced colorectal	RCT	Failed to demonstrate any benefit
	Fatty acids	Wigmore	109	1996	18	Pancreas	Phase II	Stabilization of energy expenditure
		Burns	183	1999	22	Heterogeneous	Phase I	
		Gogos	112	1998	60	Solid tumors	RCT	PUFA had an immunomodulating effect and prolonged survival
	Thalidomide	Khan	115	2003	11	Esophageal	Phase II	Reversed weight loss
		Bruera	113	1999				
	Melatonin	Lissoni	116	2002	1,440	Heterogeneous	Phase II	Decreased weight loss
		Lissoni	118	2003	100	NSCLC	Randomized	Improved survival Chemotherapy better tolerated

RCT, randomized control trial; NSCLC, non-small cell lung cancer; BCAA, branched-chain amino acids; GH, growth hormone.

loss were treated with megestrol acetate (800 mg/day) or placebo. Megestrol acetate resulted in a significantly improved appetite and food intake, while leading to less nausea and vomiting. Although overall weight gain was no different, weight gain greater than 10% was reported in more patients taking megestrol acetate (16%) compared to placebo (2%). The only side effect noted was mild edema.[73] In a multiinstitutional, placebo-controlled trial, megestrol acetate was also found to improve weight gain and appetite.[74] The primary concern with megestrol acetate has been that weight gain results from the deposition of fat and not lean body mass.[75] Related to megestrol acetate, medroxyprogesterone acetate (MPA) is a synthetic progesterone derivative that has also been studied as an appetite stimulant, as well as a modulator of cytokine release.[76] In a randomized, prospective trial, Simons et al. report that MPA stimulated food intake and reversed fat loss in 54 nonhormone-sensitive cancers.[77]

Another orexigenic agent considered for use in cancer patients is dronabinol (marinol), which is the major active ingredient of marijuana (tetrahydrocannabinol). It is currently approved as a treatment of refractory nausea and vomiting. It has also been noted to be an appetite stimulant. In a small study, patients with advanced cancers were treated with dronabinol and, although there was improvement in appetite, weight loss continued unabated.[78] In a similar study, dronabinol improved both appetite and reduced the rate of weight loss.[79] Dronabinol has recently been compared to megestrol acetate in a prospective study of 469 patients with advanced cancer. Patients were randomized to megestrol acetate, dronabinol, or a combination of both agents. Although 75% of patients taking megestrol acetate reported an improved appetite, only 49% of the patients receiving dronabinol had significant improvements. The combination therapy did not confer any additional benefit over megestrol acetate alone.[80] Further prospective trials are needed to ascertain the utility of this agent in clinical practice.

Cyproheptadine is an antiserotonin agent with known appetite stimulatory effects. In a randomized, double-blinded, placebo-controlled study, 295 patients with advanced malignancy were treated with cyproheptadine or placebo. Patients receiving the active drug demonstrated a slight improvement in appetite.[81] However, no increase in weight gain was noted. Other antiseritonergic agents have also been studied. Ondansetron and granisetron are newer 5-HT3 receptor antagonists and powerful antiemetics. In a study of 20 metastatic cancer patients, ondansetron improved the ability of patients to enjoy eating, but this effect did not translate into weight gain or improvement of other biochemical parameters of cachexia.[82] Future trials with antiseritonergic agents are needed to define their role in the treatment of cancer cachexia.

Anabolic Agents

Anabolic agents have the potential to improve body composition by maintaining or enhancing lean body mass. This class of agents includes growth hormone (GH), insulin, steroids, and amino acids.

Corticosteroids have been used in the palliative setting for cancer patients because they have been shown to possess a significant antinausea effect and to improve appetite and pain control. In a double-blinded cross-over study comparing placebo to prednisolone in more than 300 cancer patients with advanced disease, 80% of the patients experienced improved appetite and a sense of well-being, compared with 50% on placebo. However, no increase in caloric intake or body weight resulted.[83] In a randomized, double-blinded placebo-controlled study, dexamethasone was studied in preterminal gastrointestinal cancer patients and found to improve appetite, but it had no effect on weight gain.[84] Advanced cancer patients randomized to megestrol acetate, fluoxymesterone, and dexamethasone, demonstrated equal weight gain and appetite enhancement in the megestrol acetate and dexamethasone groups, but toxicity of dexamethasone was somewhat greater.[85] Although the short-term toxicity of steroids is well tolerated, chronic use of steroids would be necessary to achieve clinical improvement. The long-term side effects and morbidity associated with steroid use outweigh its potential benefit.

Insulin has been extensively investigated as an anabolic agent in cachectic animal models, demonstrating decreased weight loss, preservation of normal host composition, and improved survival after tumor resection. When administered to rats, insulin increased host weight and muscle weight compared to controls. The mechanism of the effects of insulin in these studies included improved food intake, but insulin may also be involved in overcoming tumor-induced metabolic defects, which promote protein catabolism.[86,87] Although both animal and human data have demonstrated that insulin can improve protein and carbohydrate metabolism in the tumor-bearing state, and despite that it is an inexpensive, readily available agent, the clinical correlates have never been demonstrated.

Growth hormone (GH) has been shown to attenuate both the loss of body protein and body cell mass when administered to noncancer, catabolic patients. However, there is a paucity of studies using GH in the cancer population. The relatively few studies using GH as a nutritional adjunct in cancer patients may be because many investigators are reticent to administer GH to cancer patients, because of the potential for stimulating tumor growth. There are limited data to suggest that GH and/or its mediator, insulin-like growth factor (IGF)-I, may support tumor growth, and it is possible that the potentially salutary effects of GH may be offset by a tumor-promoting effect.[88] Concerns regarding potential stimulation of tumor growth by GH have not been substantiated. Numerous in vivo animal studies provide no evidence to suggest that studies of GH in the cancer patient should not be performed.[89,90]

In a prospective, randomized trial, Berman et al. treated cancer patients following surgical resection of upper gastrointestinal malignancies with GH (0.1 mg/kg) daily for 4 postoperative days in conjunction with standard TPN ($n = 10$). Patients receiving standard TPN served as a control ($n = 10$). Patients underwent a whole-body and skeletal muscle protein kinetic study. Patients receiving GH demonstrated improved whole-body protein net balance. While the patients receiving only TPN demonstrated a decrease in serum IGF-1 levels postoperatively, GH was able to normalize IGF-1 levels back to preoperative levels.[91]

Growth hormone has been shown to improve protein metabolism, wound healing, and immunologic status in the surgical patient.[92] Although expensive and inconvenient to administer, GH still has potential to improve the clinical response in malnourished cancer patients. Further studies are needed to define the role of GH in the nutritional supplementation of cancer patients.

Branched-chain amino acids (BCAA) have been proposed as modulators of protein metabolism. Infusion of BCAA has been shown to reduce protein catabolism in healthy as well as cancer-bearing animals and humans.[93,94] Tayek et al. studied 10 malnourished cancer patients using a cross-over design, providing conventional TPN and BCAA-enriched TPN (50% of amino acids as BCAA) for 2 to 5 days. The authors reported an increase in whole-body protein synthesis, with no difference in protein breakdown, in patients receiving the BCAA-enriched TPN.[95] This beneficial effect on protein metabolism has been confirmed in a subsequent study.[96] Although these clinical trials have reported improvements in protein kinetics, studies addressing clinical outcome are required before BCAA-enriched TPN should be routinely administered to cancer patients.

Other amino acids have been studied as supplements. Glutamine is a nonessential amino acid that is often depleted in cancer patients. The mechanism of this depletion is unknown, but likely is caused by alterations in host protein metabolism, avidity of tumors for host glutamine, and the catabolic effects of cancer therapy.[97] The glutamine-depleted state may have a negative impact on the patient's clinical course.[98] In a double-blinded, prospective trial, Ziegler et al. randomized 45 patients undergoing BMT for hematologic malignancies to either conventional TPN or isonitrogenous, isocaloric TPN supplemented with glutamine. Patients were treated for 4 weeks posttransplantation. Those patients who had received the glutamine-enriched TPN had an improved nitrogen balance, significantly fewer infectious complications, and shortened length of hospitalization.[99]

There is an extensive literature suggesting low circulating levels of serum testosterone in patients with malignancy.[100,101] Most data related to testosterone replacement are derived from human immunodeficiency virus (HIV) studies. Oxandrolone is a testosterone derivative approved by the U.S. Food and Drug Administration for weight gain in chronic wasting diseases. Oxandrolone increases lean body mass, strength, weight gain, and perhaps quality of life in men with acquired immunodeficiency syndrome (AIDS)-related cachexia,[102,103] and ongoing studies are evaluating the use of oxandrolone in the cancer cachexia population.

Anticatabolic Agents

Pentoxifylline is a methylxanthine derivative that is approved for intermittent claudication. Based on the observation that pentoxifylline blocks tumor necrosis factor-alpha (TNF-α), which is believed to be a mediator of cancer cachexia, a randomized, double-blinded, placebo-controlled study was performed to evaluate its use in treating cancer cachexia. Seventy patients with documented cancer cachexia were randomized to pentoxifylline or placebo. Although well tolerated, pentoxifylline failed to improve the appetites of study patients.[104] Hydrazine sulfate inhibits the enzyme PEP-CK, and interferes with gluconeogenesis, and has been reported to normalize the carbohydrate metabolism of cancer patients with cachexia.[105] Athough some have claimed it improves appetite and has anititumor effects,[106] multiple clinical studies have not shown any benefit from the drug.[107–109]

The polyunsaturated fatty acids, such as eicosapentanoic acid (EPA), have been shown to inhibit lipolysis and muscle degradation in cancer cachexia animal models. In a study of patients with unresectable pancreatic cancer, dietary fish oil supplements, including EPA, were administered. After 3 months, patients showed decreased fatigue, a median weight gain of 0.3 kg/month, and stabilization of resting energy expenditure.[110,111] The effects of EPA on inflammatory cytokines, prostaglandin E_2, and the proteolytic cachectic factor may explain, at least in part, the reversal of weight loss reported in cachectic pancreatic cancer patients and tumor-bearing mice supplemented with fish oil.[100] In another study by Gogos and colleagues, 60 patients with advanced solid tumors were randomized to supplemental omega-3 polyunsaturated fatty acids or placebo. Patients receiving the fish oil supplementation demonstrated an improved immune response, as well as a longer mean survival.[112] These findings suggest a potential role of EPA as a useful supplement to treat or prevent cancer cachexia.

Forty years since its worldwide withdrawal for its teratogenic effects, thalidomide is currently undergoing a remarkable renaissance as a powerful immunomodulatory agent. Over the past decade, it has been found to be active in a wide variety of inflammatory and malignant disorders. One of the effects of thalidomide is its ability to inhibit TNF-α, and it has recently been studied as a drug to treat HIV-associated wasting and cancer cachexia.[113,114] Khan and colleagues reported on 10 patients with nonobstructing and inoperable esophageal cancer who were established on an isocaloric diet for 2 weeks, followed by 2 weeks on thalidomide, 200 mg daily. Thalidomide treatment appeared to reverse the loss of weight and lean body mass over the 2-week trial period, with a mean gain in lean body mass of 1.75 kg.[115] Thalidomide is very well tolerated, and further randomized clinical trials are warranted. Melatonin is the main hormone released from the pineal gland and has been shown to have antitumor and anticachectic effects.[116] One potential mechanism is through melatonin's ability to decrease circulating levels of TNF in patients with advanced cancers.[117] In a large trial, Lissoni et al. studied 1,440 patients with untreatable advanced solid tumor who received supportive care alone versus supportive care with melatonin. They demonstrated that melatonin decreased the frequency of cachexia in those patients taking supplemental melatonin.[116] In a randomized trial of 100 patients with non-small cell lung cancer undergoing chemotherapy, patients receiving concomitant melatonin demonstrated a higher tumor response and survival.[118] These trials provide early evidence to support further trials evaluating melatonin in the supportive care of patients with cancer-related malnutrition.

Despite being an attractive concept, there is no universally accepted "cocktail" of nutritional supplementation, coupled with pharmacologic support, that improves the nutritional status of patients with cancer cachexia. Further work with these and newer agents is needed before the standard of care changes.

Nutritional Support and Tumor Stimulation

Nutritional status plays an important role in the complex relationship between tumor and host, and nutritional repletion in cancer patients elicits a potential concern of stimulation of tumor growth. Tumors may preferentially extract exogenous nutrients at the expense of the host, resulting in accelerated tumor growth. Numerous laboratory and clinical studies have addressed the effect of nutritional supplementation on tumor development, tumor growth, and metastasis. Animal studies have shown that both intravenous and oral nutritional repletion of malnourished tumor-bearing animals restores host body weight, immunocompetence, and serum protein to normal, but tumor growth has also been shown to be concomitantly stimulated.[119–121] Few human trials address the effects of nutritional repletion on tumor growth. In a study of head and neck cancer patients with a weight loss greater than 10%, Baron et al. reported that tumors aspirated before and after 3 to 17 days of TPN, demonstrated an increase in hyperdiploid cells after TPN, by flow cytometry. In contrast, there was no difference in cell-cycle kinetics in adjacent normal mucosa.[122] Frank et al. also studied head and neck cancer patients before and after 7 days of TPN and reported similar results. They observed an increase in incorporation of bromodeoxyuridine into the tumor cells after completion of TPN.[123] Tumor protein kinetics has been studied in patients undergoing nutritional support. In a prospective randomized study of gastrointestinal malignancies, Mullen et al. reported on 25 patients randomized to either oral diet or TPN for 7 to 10 days before operation. On the day of surgery, patients were infused with ^{15}N-glycine, and tumor biopsies were analyzed for protein fractional synthetic rate. No differences in protein fractional synthetic rates were observed between patients receiving TPN (14.2%/day) versus oral diet (15.1%/day). In addition, the rate of protein synthesis was independent of the extent of disease and was related to the rate of protein synthesis of the adjacent normal tissue.[124]

Overall, most animal studies support the findings that tumor growth is stimulated with nutritional repletion. Definitive conclusions from these animal models, however, are limited by the fact that they use rapidly growing, nonmetastasizing transplantable tumors with tumor burdens reaching nonphysiologic proportions. Therefore, the effects of nutritional repletion on host and neoplastic tissues observed in animal models may be different in humans. There is no objective evidence that nutritional support in humans actually stimulates tumor growth and, utilizing clinical endpoints, there is no evidence that nutritional support increases tumor growth or promotes metastatic potential. Therefore, the selective use of nutritional support in the cancer patient population, where indicated for nutritional repletion, should not be discouraged based on this theoretical concern.

Ethics

There is little debate about providing nutritional support for a reversible acute illness. However, the controversy exists in initiating and sustaining nutritional support for patients with incurable or end-stage cancer with little prospect of reversing the underlying disease and regaining nutritional independence. Patients with cancer may fall anywhere within this spectrum, and careful consideration of patient, family, and physician expectations should be included in the decision-making process.

Through the ages, the act of giving food and drink has been symbolic of caring and compassion. Supplemental nutrition is believed by some to be a logical continuation of this basic tenet, while others feel that "forced feeding" is an invasive medical intervention, requiring definitive indications and consent. The debate has yet to be resolved, and each case needs to be evaluated by its own merits and circumstances. Although nutritional support is considered ethically similar to any other life-sustaining treatment, such as ventilator support, dialysis, and antibiotics, physicians are not obligated to offer nutritional support and hydration unless potential benefit is anticipated. In terms of legal considerations, almost every court has ruled in favor that nutritional support is a medical intervention that can be refused by either a competent patient or a surrogate (when there is clear and convincing evidence that the patient would want therapy withdrawn). Excellent reviews and essays on the legal precedent are available.[125–127]

In addition to a life-prolonging intervention, there is also debate regarding the palliative effects of nutritional support in the terminal cancer patient. The placement of a gastrostomy tube can provide suitable nutrition and hydration and may also be useful for palliative decompression of the gastrointestinal tract.[128] Bozzetti et al. report that home TPN in severely malnourished, almost aphagic terminal cancer patients improved their quality of life, especially in patients surviving more than 3 months.[129] Home TPN or enteral nutrition also may be useful interventions to facilitate hospital discharge so that, if so desired, patients can die at home rather than in the hospital. On the other hand, the salutatory aspects of palliative nutritional support must be tempered.[130] While it is difficult to "watch some one starve to death," investigators have shown that contrary to popular belief, patients with terminal illness can be made quite comfortable despite very limited food and fluid intake.[131] Importantly, the use of nutritional support should not provide unrealistic hope and prevent the involvement of hospice services.

Overall, several principles can be used to direct the decision process, which are based on active patient, family, and physician participation[132]:

1. A patient's expressed wishes, either in the present or through a prior directive, should be the primary guiding force when nutritional support is a medical option.
2. Although nutrition may prevent dehydration and malnutrition, there are no data supporting its efficacy in providing comfort by alleviating the subjective conditions of thirst or hunger.
3. The decision to use nutritional support must be made by assessing the benefits and burdens for each individual case.
4. A therapeutic trial of nutritional support should be discontinued when the burdens clearly outweigh the benefits.
5. The patient should be the final arbiter in assessing benefits and burdens.

In summary, a thoughtful approach is necessary in the initiation and continuation of nutritional support in the cancer patient. Potential benefits must be weighed against burdens, and realistic goals must be evaluated. Although the patient is the final arbiter, the family and physician must participate and communicate in the decision-making process.

References

1. Warren S. The immediate causes of death in cancer. Am J Med Sci 1932;184:610–615.
2. DeWys WD, Begg C, Lavin PT, et al. Prognostic effect of weight loss prior to chemotherapy in cancer patients. Am J Med 1980;69:491–497.
3. Bozzetti F, Migliavacca S, Scotti A, et al. Impact of cancer, type, site, stage and treatment on the nutritional status of patients. Ann Surg 1982;196:170–179.
4. Meguid MM, Meguid V. Preoperative identification of the surgical cancer patient in need of postoperative supportive total parenteral nutrition. Cancer (Phila) 1985;55:258–262.

5. Studley HO. Percentage of weight loss: a basic indicator of surgical risk in patients with chronic peptic ulcer. JAMA 1936;106:458–460.
6. Pettigrew RA, Hill GL. Indicators of surgical risk and clinical judgement. Br J Surg 1986;73:47–51.
7. Reeds PJ, Laditan AAO. Serum albumin and transferrin in protein-energy malnutrition. Br J Nutr 1976;36:255–263.
8. Buzby GP, Mullen JL, Matthews DC, Hobbs CL, Rosato EF. Prognostic nutritional index in gastrointestinal surgery. Am J Surg 1980;139:160–167.
9. Buzby GP, Williford WO, Peterson OL, et al. A randomized clinical trial of total parenteral nutrition in malnourished surgical patients: the rationale and impact of previous clinical trials and pilot study on protocol design. Am J Clin Nutr 1988;47:357–363.
10. Baker JP, Detsky AS, Wesson DE, et al. Nutritional assessment: a comparison of clinical judgement and objective measurements. N Engl J Med 1982;306(16):969–972.
11. Ottery FD. Definition of standardized nutritional assessment and interventional pathways in oncology. Nutrition 1996;12: S15–S19.
12. Bauer J, Capra S, Ferguson M. Use of the scored Patient-Generated Subjective Global Assessment (PG-SGA) as a nutrition assessment tool in patients with cancer. Eur J Clin Nutr 2002;56:779–785.
13. Pablo AM, Izaga MA, Alday LA. Assessment of nutritional status on hospital admission: nutritional scores. Eur J Clin Nutr 2003;57:824–831.
14. Thoresen L, Fjeldstad I, Krogstad K, Kaasa S, Falkmer UG. Nutritional status of patients with advanced cancer: the value of using the subjective global assessment of nutritional status as a screening tool. Palliat Med 2002;16:33–42.
15. Schneider SM, Hebuterne X. Use of nutritional scores to predict clinical outcomes in chronic diseases. Nutr Rev 2000;58: 31–38.
16. Jeevanandam M, Legaspi A, Lowry SF, Horowitz GD, Brennan MF. Effect of total parenteral nutrition on whole body protein kinetics in cachectic patients with benign or malignant disease. J Parenter Enteral Nutr 1988;12(3):229–236.
17. Lundholm K, Edstrom S, Ekman L, Karlberg I, Bylund A, Schersten T. A comparative study of the influence of malignant tumor on host metabolism in mice and man. Evaluation of an experimental model. Cancer 1978;42:453–461.
18. Shaw JHF, Humberstone DM, Wolfe RR. Energy and protein metabolism in sarcoma patients. Ann Surg 1988;207:283–289.
19. Long CL, Spenser JL, Kinney JM, Geiger JW. Carbohydrate metabolism in normal man and effect of glucose infusion. J Appl Physiol 1971;31:102–109.
20. Glicksman AS, Rawson RW. Diabetes and altered carbohydrate metabolism in patients with cancer. Cancer (Phila) 1956;9:1127–1134.
21. Kokal WA, McCulloch A, Wright PD, Johnston IDA. Glucose turnover and recycling in colorectal cancer. Ann Surg 1983;198: 601–604.
22. Eden E, Edstrom S, Bennegard K, Scersten T, Lundholm K. Glucose flux in relation to energy expenditure in malnourished patients with and without cancer during periods of fasting and feeding. Cancer Res 1984;44:1718–1724.
23. Lundholm K, Edstrom S, Karlberg I, Ekman L, Schersten T. Glucose turnover, gluconeogenesis from glycerol, and estimation of net glucose cycling in cancer patients. Cancer (Phila) 1982;50:1142–1150.
24. Heber D, Chlebowski RT, Ishibashi DE, Herrold JN, Block JB. Abnormalities in glucose and protein metabolism in noncachectic lung cancer patients. Cancer Res 1982;42:4815–4819.
25. Burt ME, Gorschboth CM, Brennan MF. A controlled, prospective, randomized trial evaluating the metabolic effects of enteral and parenteral nutrition in the cancer patient. Cancer (Phila) 1982;49(6):1092–1105.
26. Falconer JS, Fearon KCH, Plester CE, Ross JA, Carter DC. Cytokines, the acute-phase response, and resting energy expenditure in cachectic patients with pancreatic cancer. Ann Surg 1994;219(4):325–331.
27. Waterhouse C. Oxidation and metabolic interconversion in malignant cachexia. Cancer Treat Rep 1981;65(suppl 5):61–66.
28. Vlassara H, Spiegel RJ, Doval DS. Reduced plasma lipoprotein lipase activity in patients with malignancy associated weight loss. Horm Metab Res 1986;18:698–703.
29. Hirai K, Hussey HJ, Barber MD, Price SA, Tisdale MJ. Biological evaluation of a lipid-mobilizing factor isolated from the urine of cancer patients. Cancer Res 1998;58:2359–2365.
30. McDevitt TM, Todorov PT, Beck SA, Khan SH, Tisdale MJ. Purification and characterization of a lipid-mobilizing factor associated with cachexia-inducing tumors in mice and humans. Cancer Res 1995;55:1458–1463.
31. Friedman JM, Halaas JL. Leptin and the regulation of body weight in mammals. Nature (Lond) 1998;395:763–770.
32. Iniu A. Cancer anorexia-cachexia syndrome: are neuropeptides the key? Cancer Res 1999;22:62–67.
33. Rombeau JL, Lew JI. Nutritional-metabolic support of the intestine: implications for the critically ill patient. In: Kinney JM, Tucker HN (eds) Organ Metabolism and Nutrition: Ideas for Future Critical Care. New York: Raven Press, 1994:197–229.
34. Deitch EA. Role of the gut lymphatic system in multiple organ failure. Curr Opin Crit Care 2001;7:92–98.
35. Kudsk KA, Croce MA, Fabian TC, et al. Enteral versus parenteral feeding: effects on septic morbidity after blunt and penetrating abdominal trauma. Ann Surg 1992;215:503–511.
36. Sandstrom R, Drott C, Hyltander A, Arfvidsson B. The effect of postoperative intravenous feeding (TPN) on outcome following major surgery evaluated in a randomized study. Ann Surg 1993; 217:185–195.
37. Fong Y, Marano MA, Barber A, et al. Total parenteral nutrition and bowel rest modify the metabolic response to endotoxin in humans. Ann Surg 1989;210(4):449–457.
38. Sako K, Lore JM, Kaufman S, Razack M, Bakamjian V, Reese P. Parenteral hyperalimentation in surgical patients with head and neck cancer: a randomized study. J Surg Oncol 1981;16: 391–402.
39. Daly JM, Hearne B, Dunaj J, et al. Nutritional rehabilitation in patients with advanced head and neck cancer receiving radiation therapy. Am J Surg 1984;148:514–520.
40. Burt ME, Brennan MF. Nutritional support of the patient with esophageal cancer. Semin Oncol 1984;11(2):127–135.
41. Lim STK, Choa RG, Lam KH, Wong J, Ong GB. Total parenteral nutrition versus gastrostomy in the preoperative preparation of patients with carcinoma of the oesophagus. Br J Surg 1981;68: 69–72.
42. Haffejee AA, Angorn IB. Nutritional status and the nonspecific cellular and humoral immune response in esophageal carcinoma. Ann Surg 1979;189(4):475–479.
43. Page RD, Oo AY, Russell GN, Pennefather SH. Intravenous hydration versus naso-jejunal enteral feeding after esophagectomy: a randomised study. Eur J Cardiothorac Surg 2002;22: 666–672.
44. Brennan MF, Pisters PWT, Posner M, Quesada O, Shike M. A prospective randomized trial of total parenteral nutrition after major pancreatic resection for malignancy. Ann Surg 1994;220(4):436–444.
45. Kokal WA. The impact of antitumor therapy on nutrition. Cancer (Phila) 1985;55:273–278.
46. Schwartz GF, Green HL, Bendon ML. Combined parenteral hyperalimentation and chemotherapy in the treatment of disseminated solid tumors. Am J Surg 1971;121:169–173.
47. Souchan EA, Copeland EM, Watson P. Intravenous hyperalimentation as an adjunct to cancer chemotherapy with 5-fluorouracil. J Surg Res 1975;18:451–454.

48. Issell BF, Valdivieso M, Zaren HA, et al. Protection against chemotherapy toxicity by IV hyperalimentation. Cancer Treat Rep 1978;62(8):1139–1143.
49. Serrou B, Cupissol D, Plagne R, Boutin P, Carcassone Y, Michel FB. Parenteral intravenous nutrition (PIVN) as an adjunct to chemotherapy in small cell anaplastic lung carcinoma. Cancer Treat Rep 1981;65(suppl 5):151–155.
50. Popp MB, Fisher RI, Wesley R. A prospective randomized study of adjuvant parenteral nutrition in the treatment of advanced diffuse lymphoma: Influence on survival. Surgery (St. Louis) 1981;90:195–203.
51. Shike M, Russell DM, Detsky AS, et al. Changes in body composition in patients with small-cell lung cancer. Ann Intern Med 1984;101:303–309.
52. Lopez MJ, Robinson P, Madden T, Highbarger T. Nutritional support and prognosis in patients with head and neck cancer. J Surg Oncol 1994;55:33–36.
53. Clamon GH, Feld R, Evans WK, et al. Effect of adjuvant central IV hyperalimentation on the survival and response to treatment of patients with small cell lung cancer: a randomized trial. Cancer Treat Rep 1985;69(2):167–177.
54. Weiner RS, Kramer BS, Clamon GH, et al. Effects of intravenous hyperalimentation during treatment in patients with small-cell lung cancer. J Clin Oncol 1985;3(7):949–957.
55. Evans WK, Nixon DW, Daly JM, et al. A randomized study of oral nutritional support versus ad lib nutritional intake during chemotherapy for advanced colorectal and non-small-cell lung cancer. J Clin Oncol 1987;5(1):113–124.
56. McGeer AJ, Detsky AS, O'Rourke K. Parenteral nutrition in patients receiving cancer chemotherapy. Ann Intern Med 1989;110(9):734–736.
57. Mulder PO, Bouman JG, Gietema JA, et al. Hyperalimentation in autologous bone marrow transplantation for solid tumors. Cancer (Phila) 1989;64:2045–2052.
58. Szeluga DJ, Stuart RK, Brookmeyer R, Utermohlen V, Santos GW. Nutritional support of bone marrow transplant recipients: prospective, randomized clinical trial comparing total parenteral nutrition to an enteral feeding program. Cancer Res 1987;47: 3309–3316.
59. Weisdorf SA, Lysne J, Wind D, et al. Positive effect of prophylactic total parenteral nutrition on long-term outcome of bone marrow transplantation. Transplantation 1987;43(6):833–838.
60. McArdle AH, Wittnich C, Freeman CR. Elemental diet as prophylaxis against radiation injury: histologic and ultrastructural studies. Arch Surg 1985;120:1026–1032.
61. Bounous G. The use of elemental diets during cancer therapy. AntiCancer Res 1983;3:299–304.
62. McArdle AH, Reid EC, Laplante MP, Freeman CR. Prophylaxis against radiation injury. Arch Surg 1986;121:879–885.
63. Hochwald S, Harrison LE, Heslin MJ, Burt ME, Brennan MF. Early postoperative enteral feeding improves whole body protein kinetics in upper gastrointestinal cancer patients. Am J Surg 1997;174:325–330.
64. Harrison LE, Brennan MF. The role of total parenteral nutrition in the patient with cancer. Curr Probl Surg 1995;32:833–917.
65. Grosvenor M, Bulcavage L, Chlebowski RT. Symptoms potentially influencing weight loss in a cancer population. Cancer (Phila) 1989;63:330–334.
66. Shivshanker K, Bennet RW, Haynie TP. Tumor-associated gastroparesis: correction with metaclopramide. Am J Surg 1983;145:221–225.
67. Nelson KA, Walsh TD. Metaclopramide in anorexia caused by cancer-associated dyspepsia syndrome (CADS). J Palliat Care 1993;9:14–18.
68. Bruera E, Belzile M, Neumann C, Harsanyi Z, Babul N, Darke A. A double-blind, crossover study of controlled-release metaclopramide and placebo for the chronic nausea and dyspepsia of advanced cancer. J Pain Symptom Manag 2000;19: 427–435.
69. Wilson J, Plourde JY, Marshall D, et al. Long-term safety and clinical effectiveness of controlled-release metaclopramide in cancer-associated dyspepsia syndrome: a multicentre evaluation. J Palliat Care 2002;18:84–91.
70. Mikasa K, Sawaki M, Kita E, et al. Significant survival benefit to patients with advanced non-small-cell lung cancer from treatment with clarithromycin. Chemotherapy 1997;43: 288–296.
71. Sakamoto M, Mikasa K, Majima T, et al. Anti-cachectic effect of clarithromycin for patients with unresectable non-small cell lung cancer. Chemotherapy 2001;47:444–451.
72. Aisner J, Tchekmedyian NS, Moody M. High-dose megestrol acetate for the treatment of advanced breast cancer: dose and toxicities. Semin Hematol 1987;24(suppl 1):48–55.
73. Loprinzi CL, Ellison NM, Schaid DJ, al. Controlled trial of megestrol acetate in patients with cancer anorexia and cachexia. J Natl Cancer Inst 1990;82:1127–1132.
74. Erkurt E, Erkisi M, Tunali C. Supportive treatment in weight-losing cancer patients due to the additive adverse effects of radiation treatment and/or chemotherapy. J Exp Clin Cancer Res 2000;19:431–439.
75. Loprinzi CL, Schaid DJ, Dose AM, Burnham NL, Jensen MD. Body-composition changes in patients who gain weight while receiving megestrol acetate. J Clin Oncol 1993;11:152–154.
76. Nishimura R, Nagao K, Miyayama H, et al. An analysis of serum interleukin-6 levels to predict benefits of medroxyprogesterone acetate in advanced or recurrent breast cancer. Oncology 2000; 59:166–173.
77. Simons JP, Schols AM, Hoefnagels JM, Westerterp KR, ten Velde GP, Wouters EF. Effects of medroxyprogesterone acetate on food intake, body composition, and resting energy expenditure in patients with advanced, nonhormone-sensitive cancer: a randomized, placebo controlled trial. Cancer (Phila) 1998;82:553–560.
78. Wadleigh R, Spaulding M, Lembersky B. Dronabinol enhancement of appetite in cancer patients. Proc Am Soc Clin Oncol 1990;9:1280.
79. Plasse TF, Gorter RW, Krasnow SH, Lane M, Shepard KV, Wadleigh RG. Recent clinical experience with dronabinol. Pharmacol Biochem Behav 1991;40:695–700.
80. Jatoi A, Windschitl HE, Loprinzi CL, et al. Dronabinol versus megestrol acetate versus combination therapy for cancer-associated anorexia: a North Central Cancer Treatment Group study. J Clin Oncol 2002;20:567–573.
81. Kardinal CG, Loprinzi CL, Schaid DJ. A controlled trial of cyproheptadine in cancer patients with anorexia and/or cachexia. Cancer (Phila) 1990;65:2657–2662.
82. Edelman MJ, Gandara DR, Meyers FJ, al. Serotonergic blockade in the treatment of the cancer anorexia-cachexia syndrome. Cancer (Phila) 1999;86:684–688.
83. Willox JC, Corr J, Shaw J. Prednisilone as an appetite stimulant in patients with cancer. Br Med J 1984;228:17–31.
84. Moertel CG, Schutt AJ, Reitemeier RJ. Corticosteroid therapy of preterminal gastrointestinal cancer. Cancer (Phila) 1974;33: 1607–1609.
85. Loprinzi CL, Kugler JW, Sloan JA, et al. Randomized comparison of megestrol acetate versus dexamethasone versus fluoxymesterone for the treatment of cancer anorexia/cachexia. J Clin Oncol 1999;17:3299–3306.
86. Minn H, Nuutila P, Lindholm P, et al. In vivo effects of insulin on tumor and skeletal muscle glucose metabolism in patients with lymphoma. Cancer (Phila) 1994;73:1490–1498.
87. Moley JF, Morrison SD, Norton JA. Insulin reversal of cancer cachexia in rats. Cancer Res 1985;45:4925–4931.
88. Ohmura E, Okada M, Onoda N, et al. Insulin-like growth factor I and transforming growth factor alpha as autocrine growth

factors in human pancreatic cancer cell growth. Cancer Res 1990;50:103–107.
89. Ng B, Wolf RF, Weksler B, Brennan MF, Burt ME. Growth hormone administration preserves lean body mass in sarcoma-bearing rats treated with doxorubicin. Cancer Res 1993;53:5483–5486.
90. Harrison LE, Blumberg D, Berman RS, et al. Exogenous human growth hormone does not influence growth, protein kinetics, or cell cycle kinetics of human pancreatic carcinoma in vivo. Surg Forum 1994;65:469–471.
91. Berman RS, Harrison LE, Pearlstone DB, Burt ME, Brennan MF. Growth hormone, alone and in combination with insulin, increases whole body and skeletal muscle protein kinetics in cancer patients after surgery. Ann Surg 1999;229:1–10.
92. Harrison LE, Port JL, Hochwald S, Blumberg D, Burt ME. Perioperative growth hormone improves wound healing and immunologic function in rats receiving adriamycin. J Surg Res 1995;58:646–650.
93. Louard RJ, Barrett EJ, Gelfand RA. Effect of infused branched-chain amino acids on muscle and whole-body amino acid metabolism in man. Clin Sci 1990;79:457–466.
94. Crosby LE, Bistrian BR, Ling P, Istfan NW, Blackburn GL, Hoffman SB. Effects of branched chain amino acid-enriched total parenteral nutrition on amino acid utilization in rats bearing Yoshida sarcoma. Cancer Res 1988;48:2698–2702.
95. Tayek JA, Bistrian BR, Hehir DJ, Martin R, Moldawer LL, Blackburn GL. Improved protein kinetics and albumin synthesis by branched chain amino acid-enriched total parenteral nutrition in cancer cachexia. Cancer (Phila) 1986;58:147–157.
96. Hunter DC, Weintraub M, Blackburn GL, Bistrian BR. Branched chain amino acids as the protein component of parenteral nutrition in cancer cachexia. Br J Surg 1989;76:149–153.
97. May PE, Barber A, D'Olimpio JT, Hourihane A, Abumrad NN. Reversal of cancer-related wasting using oral supplementation with a combination of beta-hydroxy-beta-methylbutyrate, arginine, and glutamine. Am J Surg 2002;183:471–479.
98. Souba WW. Glutamine and cancer. Ann Surg 1993;218(6): 715–728.
99. Ziegler TR, Young LS, Benfell K. Glutamine-supplemented parenteral nutrition improves nitrogen retention and reduces hospital mortality versus standard parenteral nutrition following bone marrow transplantation: a randomized, double-blinded trial. Ann Intern Med 1992;116:821–828.
100. MacDonald N, Easson AM, Mazurak VC, Dunn GP, Baracos VE. Understanding and managing cancer cachexia. J Am Coll Surg 2003;197:143–161.
101. Langer CJ, Hoffman JP, Ottery FD. Clinical significance of weight loss in cancer patients: rationale for the use of anabolic agents in the treatment of cancer-related cachexia. Nutrition 2001;17:S1–S21.
102. Bhasin S, Storer TW, Javanbakht M, et al. Testosterone replacement and resistance exercise in HIV-infected men with weight loss and low testosterone levels. JAMA 2000;283:763–770.
103. Kong A, Edmonds P. Testosterone therapy in HIV wasting syndrome: systematic review and meta-analysis. Lancet Infect Dis 2002;2:692–699.
104. Goldberg RM, Loprinzi CL, Mailliard JA, et al. Pentoxifylline for treatment of cancer anorexia and cachexia? A randomized, double-blind, placebo-controlled trial. J Clin Oncol 1995;13: 2856–2859.
105. Chlebowski RT, Heber D, Richardson B, Block JB. Influence of hydrazine sulfate on abnormal carbohydrate metabolism in cancer patients with weight loss. Cancer Res 1984;44:857–861.
106. Gold J. Hydrazine: a current prospective. Nutr Cancer 1987; 9(2,3):59–66.
107. Loprinzi CL, Goldberg RM, Su JQ, et al. Placebo-controlled trial of hydrazine sulfate in patients with newly diagnosed non-small-cell lung cancer. J Clin Oncol 1994;12:1126–1129.
108. Loprinzi CL, Kuross SA, O'Fallon JR, et al. Randomized placebo-controlled evaluation of hydrazine sulfate in patients with advanced colorectal cancer. J Clin Oncol 1994;12:1121–1125.
109. Kost MP, Fleishman SB, Herndon JE, et al. Cisplatin, vinblastine, and hydrazine sulfate in advanced, non-small-cell lung cancer: a randomized placebo-controlled, double-blind phase III study of the Cancer and Leukemia Group B. J Clin Oncol 1994;12:1113–1120.
110. Wigmore SJ, Ross JA, Falconer JS, et al. The effect of polyunsaturated fatty acids on the progress of cachexia in patients with pancreatic cancer. Nutrition 1996;12:S27–S30.
111. Barber MD, Fearon KCH, Tisdale MJ, McMillan DC, Ross JA. Effect of a fish oil-enriched nutritional supplement on metabolic mediators in patients with pancreatic cancer cachexia. Nutr Cancer 2001;40:118–124.
112. Gogos CA, Salsa B, Apostolidou E, Zoumbos NC, Kalfarentzos F. Dietary omega-3 polyunsaturated fatty acids plus vitamin E restore immunodeficiency and prolong survival for severely ill patients with generalized malignancy: a randomized control trial. Cancer (Phila) 1998;82:395–402.
113. Bruera E, Neumann CM, Pituskin E, Calder K, Ball G, Hanson J. Thalidomide in patients with cachexia due to terminal cancer: preliminary report. Ann Onc 1999;10:857–859.
114. Kaplan G, Thomas S, Fierer DS, et al. Thalidomide for the treatment of AIDS-associated wasting. AIDS Res Hum Retroviruses 2000;16:1345–1355.
115. Khan ZH, Simpson EJ, Cole AT, et al. Oesophageal cancer and cachexia: the effect of short-term treatment with thalidomide on weight loss and lean body mass. Aliment Pharmacol Ther 2003;17:677–682.
116. Lissoni P. Is there a role for melatonin in supportive care? Support Care Cancer 2002;10:110–116.
117. Lissoni P, Barni S, Tancini G, et al. Role of the pineal gland in the control of macrophage functions and its possible implication in cancer: a study of interactions between tumor necrosis factor-alpha and the pineal hormone melatonin. J Biol Regul Homeos Agents 1994;8:126–129.
118. Lissoni P, Chilelli M, Villa S, Cerizza L, Tancini G. Five years survival in metastatic non-small cell lung cancer patients treated with chemotherapy alone or chemotherapy and melatonin: a randomized trial. J Pineal Res 2003;35: 12–15.
119. Daly J, Copeland EM, Dudrick SJ, Delaney JM. Nutritional repletion of malnourished tumor-bearing and non-tumor bearing rats: effects on body water weight, liver muscle and tumor. J Surg Res 1980;28:507–518.
120. Daly J, Reynolds HM, Rowlands BJ, Dudrick SJ, Copeland EM. Tumor growth in experimental animals: nutritional manipulation and chemotherapeutic responses in the rat. Ann Surg 1980;191(3):316–322.
121. Torosian MH, Donoway RB. Total parenteral nutrition and tumor metastasis. Surgery (St. Louis) 1991;109:597–601.
122. Baron PL, Lawrence W, Chan WMY. Effect of parenteral nutrition on cell cycle kinetics of head and neck cancer. Arch Surg 1986;121:1231–1236.
123. Frank JL, Lawrence W, Banks WL. Modulation of cell cycle kinetics in human cancer with total parenteral nutrition. Proc Assoc Acad Surg 1991;25:128.
124. Mullen JL, Buzby GP, Gertner MH. Protein synthesis dynamics in human gastrointestinal malignancies. Surgery (St. Louis) 1980;87:331–338.
125. Annas GJ. Do feeding tubes have more rights than patients? Hastings Cent Rep 1986;16:26–28.
126. Paris JL. When burdens of feeding outweigh benefits. Hastings Cent Rep 1986;16:30–32.
127. King DG, Maillet JO. Position of the American Dietetic Association: Issues in feeding the terminally ill adult. J Am Diet Assoc 1987;87:78–85.

128. Angus F, Burakoff R. The percutaneous endoscopic gastrostomy tube: medical and ethical issues in placement. Am J Gastroenterol 2003;98:272–277.
129. Bozzetti F, Cozzaglio L, Biganzoli E, et al. Quality of life and length of survival in advanced cancer patients on home parenteral nutrition. Clin Nutr 2002;21:281–288.
130. Buchman AL. Must every cancer patient die with a central venous catheter? Clin Nutr 2002;21:269–271.
131. McCann RM, Hall WJ, Groth-Juncker A. Comfort care for terminally ill patients. The appropriate use of nutrition and hydration. JAMA 1994;272:1263–1266.
132. Quill TE. Utilization of nasogastric feeding tubes in a group of chronically ill, elderly patients in a community hospital. Arch Intern Med 1989;149:1937–1941.
133. DeWys WD. Abnormalities of taste as a remote effect of a neoplasm. Ann NY Acad Sci 1974;230:427.
134. Theologides A. Pathogenesis of cachexia in cancer. Cancer (Phila) 1972;29(2):484–488.
135. Norton JA, Moley JF, Green MV, Carson RE, Morrison SD. Parabiotic transfer of cancer anorexia/cachexia in male rats. Cancer Res 1985;45:5547–5552.
136. Illig KA, Maronian N, Peacock JL. Cancer cachexia is transmissible in plasma. J Surg Res 1992;52:353–358.
137. Pittinger T, Maronian N, Illig K, Peacock J. Induction of cachexia in rats by plasma from cancer-bearing patients. SSO 47th Cancer Symp 1994;138 (abstract).
138. Langstein HN, Norton JA. Mechanisms of cancer cachexia. Hematol Oncol Clin N Am 1991;5(1):103 123.
139. Brennan MF. Uncomplicated starvation versus cancer cachexia. Cancer Res 1977;37:2359–2364.
140. Burke M, Bryson EI, Kark AE. Dietary intakes, resting metabolic rates, and body composition in benign and malignant gastrointestinal disease. Br Med J 1980;280:211–215.
141. Macfie J, Burkinshaw L, Oxby C, Holmfield JHM, Hill GL. The effect of gastrointestinal malignancy on resting energy expenditure. Br J Surg 1982;69:443–446.
142. Frederix EWHM, Soeters PB, Wouters EFM, Deerenberg IM, von Meyenfeldt MF, Saris WHM. Effect of different tumor types on resting energy expenditure. Cancer Res 1991;6138–6141.
143. Dempsey DT, Feurer ID, Knox LS, Mullen JL. Energy expenditure in malnourished gastrointestinal cancer patients. Cancer (Phila) 1984;53:1265–1273.
144. Hansell DT, Davies JWL, Burns HJG. The effects on resting energy expenditure of different tumor types. Cancer (Phila) 1986;58:1739–1744.
145. Luketich JD, Mullen JL, Feurer ID, Sternlieb J, Fried RC. Ablation of abnormal energy expenditure by curative tumor resection. Arch Surg 1990;125:337–341.
146. Arbeit JM, Lees DE, Corsey R, Brennan MF. Resting energy expenditure in controls and cancer patients with localized and diffuse disease. Ann Surg 1984;199(3):292–298.
147. Eden E, Ekman L, Bennegard K, Lindmark L, Lundholm K. Whole-body tyrosine flux in relation to energy expenditure in weight-losing cancer patients. Metabolism 1984;33(11):1020–1027.
148. Burt ME, Stein TP, Schwade JG, Brennan MF. Whole-body protein metabolism in cancer-bearing patients. Effect of total parenteral nutrition and associated serum insulin response. Cancer (Phila) 1984;53(6):1246–1252.
149. Shaw JHF, Wolfe RR. Whole-body protein kinetics in patients with early and advanced gastrointestinal cancer: the response to glucose infusion and total parenteral nutrition. Surgery (St. Louis) 1988;103(2):148–155.
150. Tayek JA, Bistrian BR, Hehir D, Martin R, Moldawer LL, Blackburn GL. Improved protein kinetics and albumin synthesis by branched chain amino acid-enriched total parenteral nutrition in cancer cachexia. Cancer (Phila) 1986;58:147–157.
151. Stein TP, Oram-Smith JC, Leskiw MJ, Wallace HW, Miller EE. Tumor-caused changes in host protein synthesis under different dietary situations. Cancer Res 1976;36:3936–3940.
152. Pain VM, Randall DP, Garlick PJ. Protein synthesis in liver and skeletal muscle of mice bearing an ascites tumor. Cancer Res 1984;44:1054–1057.
153. Torosian MH, Mullen JL. Nutritional assessment. In: Kaminski I, Mitchell V (eds) Hyperalimentation: A Guide for Clinicians. New York: Dekker, 1985:47–76.
154. Lukaski HC. Methods for the assessment of human body composition: traditional and new. Am J Clin Nutr 1987;46:537–556.
155. Shaw JHF, Humberstone DM, Douglas RG, Koea J. Leucine kinetics in patients with benign disease, non-weight-losing cancer, and cancer cachexia: studies at the whole-body and tissue level and the response to nutritional support. Surgery (St. Louis) 1991;109(1):37–50.
156. Lundholm K, Ekman L, Karlberg I, Jagenburg R, Schersten T. Protein synthesis in liver tissue under the influence of a methylcholanthrene-induced sarcoma in mice. Cancer Res 1979;39:4657–4661.
157. Norton JA, Shamberger R, Stein P, Milne GWA, Brennan MF. The influence of tumor-bearing on protein metabolism in the rat. J Surg Res 1981;30:456–462.
158. Richtsmeier WJ, Dauchy R, Sauer LA. In vivo nutrient uptake by head and neck cancers. Cancer Res 1987;47:5230–5233.
159. Nolop KB, Rhodes CG, Brudin LH, et al. Glucose utilization in vivo by human pulmonary neoplasms. Cancer (Phila) 1987;60:2682–2689.
160. The Veterans Affairs Total Parenteral Nutrition Cooperative Study Group. Perioperative total parenteral nutrition in surgical patients. N Engl J Med 1991;325:525–532.
161. Muller JM, Brenner U, Dienst C, Pichlmaier H. Preoperative parenteral feeding in patients with gastrointestinal carcinoma. Lancet 1982;1:68–71.
162. Holter AR, Fischer JE. The effects of perioperative hyperalimentation on complications in patients with carcinoma and weight loss. J Surg Res 1977;23:31–34.
163. Thompson BR, Julian TB, Stremple JF. Perioperative total parenteral nutrition in patients with gastrointestinal cancer. J Surg Res 1981;30:497–500.
164. Young GA, Hill GL. A controlled study of protein-sparing therapy after excision of the rectum. Ann Surg 1980;192(2):183–191.
165. Moghissi K, Hornshaw J, Teasdale PR, Dawes EA. Parenteral nutrition in carcinoma of the oesophagus treated by surgery: nitrogen balance and clinical studies. Br J Surg 1977;64:125–128.
166. Heatley RV, Williams RHP, Lewis MH. Pre-operative intravenous feeding: a controlled trial. Postgrad Med J 1979;55:541–545.
167. Fan S, Lo C, Lai E, Chu K, Liu C, Wong J. Perioperative nutritional support in patients undergoing hepatectomy for hepatocellular carcinoma. N Engl J Med 1994;331(23):1547–1552.
168. Daly JM, Bonau R, Stofberg P, Bloch A, Jeevanandam M, Morse M. Immediate postoperative jejunostomy feeding: clinical and metabolic results in a prospective trial. Am J Surg 1987;153:198–206.
169. DeVries EGE, Mulder NH, Houwen B, deVries-Hospers HG. Enteral nutrition by nasogastric tube in adult patients treated with intensive chemotherapy for acute leukemia. Am J Clin Nutr 1982;35:1490–1496.
170. Shamberger RC, Pizzo PA, Goodgame JT, et al. The effect of total parenteral nutrition on chemotherapy-induced myelosuppression. Am J Med 1983;74:40–48.
171. Nixon DW, Moffitt S, Lawson DH, et al. Total parenteral nutrition as an adjunct to chemotherapy of metastatic colorectal cancer. Cancer Treat Rep 1981;65(suppl 5):121–128.

172. Nixon DW, Lawson D, Kutner MH, et al. Effect of total parenteral nutrition on survival in advanced colon cancer. Cancer Detect Prev 1981;4:421–427.
173. Samuels ML, Selig DE, Ogden S, Grant C, Brown B. IV hyperalimentation and chemotherapy for stage III testicular cancer: a randomized study. Cancer Treat Rep 1981;65(7–8):615–627.
174. Drott C, Unsgaard B, Schersten T, Lundholm K. Total parenteral nutrition as an adjuvant to patients undergoing chemotherapy for testicular cancer: protection of body composition. A randomized, prospective trial. Surgery (St. Louis) 1988;103(5): 499–506.
175. Shike M, Russel DM, Detsky AS, et al. Changes in body composition in patients with small-cell lung cancer. The effect of total parenteral nutrition as an adjunct to chemotherapy. Ann Intern Med 1984;101:303–309.
176. Jordan WM, Valdivieso M, Frankmann C, et al. Treatment of advanced adenocarcinoma of the lung with ftorafur, doxorubicin, cyclophosphamide, and cisplatin (FACP) and intensive IV hyperalimentation. Cancer Treat Rep 1981;65(3–4):197–205.
177. Kinsella TJ, Malcolm AW, Bothe A, Valerio D, Blackburn GL. Prospective study of nutritional support during pelvic irradiation. Int J Radiat Oncol Biol Phys 1981;7:543–548.
178. Ghavimi F, Shils ME, Scott BF, Brown M, Tamaroff M. Comparison of morbidity in children requiring abdominal radiation and chemotherapy, with and without total parenteral nutrition. J Pediatr 1982;101(4):530–537.
179. Valerio D, Overett L, Malcom A, Blackburn GL. Nutritional support for cancer patients receiving abdominal and pelvic radiotherapy: a randomized prospective clinical experiment of intravenous versus oral feeding. Surg Forum 1978;29:145–148.
180. Solassol C, Joyeux H, Dubois JB. Total parenteral nutrition (TPN) with complete nutritive mixtures: an artificial gut in cancer patients. Nutr Cancer 1980;1:13–18.
181. Douglass HO, Milliron S, Nava H. Elemental diet as an adjuvant for patients with locally advanced gastrointestinal cancer receiving radiation therapy: a prospectively randomized study. J Parenter Enteral Nutr 1978;2:682–686.
182. Pearlstone DB, Wolf RF, Berman RS, Burt ME, Brennan MF. Effect of systemic insulin on protein kinetics in postoperative cancer patients. Ann Surg Oncol 1994;1(4):321–332.
183. Burns CP, Halabi S, Clamon GH, et al. Phase I clinical study of fish oil fatty acid capsules for patients with cancer cachexia: cancer and leukemia group B study 9473. Clin Cancer Res 1999;5:3942–3947.

Paraneoplastic Syndromes

Shirish M. Gadgeel and Antoinette J. Wozniak

Malignancies most often produce symptoms by local tumor growth and invasion, or by metastatic spread. However, there are remote effects of the primary cancer termed paraneoplastic that can result in significant symptomatology and organ dysfunction.[1] It is postulated that these syndromes result from the production of substances, such as hormones or their precursors, steroid metabolites, enzymes, and various cytokines.[2] Neurologic syndromes associated with neoplasms may be the result of antibody production related to immunoaccessible antigens produced by the neoplasm.

In general, it is common for malignancies to produce these substances, but it is less common that actual clinically relevant paraneoplastic syndromes develop. About 7% to 10% of cancer patients present with a paraneoplastic syndrome as the first manifestation of disease.[3] If one considers some of the more common problems associated with malignancy, such as anemia, anorexia, and fever as paraneoplastic, a significant number of patients are affected by these syndromes. This chapter discusses some of the more common paraneoplastic syndromes associated with malignancies.

Endocrinologic Syndromes

The manifestations of the endocrinologic paraneoplastic syndromes are associated with the production of hormones or hormone-like substances. Table 85.1 lists the syndromes that have been reported and some of the malignancies with which they are associated.[4–6]

Hypercalcemia

Hypercalcemia is a fairly common metabolic problem that can occur in the presence of osseous metastases or as a result of a paraneoplastic process. A number of different cancers, including breast, lung, head and neck, kidney, and hematologic malignancies can cause hypercalcemia.[7] Associated humoral and cytokine etiologic factors include parathyroid hormone-related protein (PTH-RP), transforming growth factor-alpha, interleukin 1, tumor necrosis factor, prostaglandins, and lymphotoxin.[8] The clinician should be aware that benign conditions, such as hyperparathyroidism can coexist with malignancy and be the source of the hypercalcemia. The interaction of PTH, calcitonin, and 1,25-dihydroxyvitamin D in the bone, kidney, and gastrointestinal tract physiologically controls body calcium. Intact PTH is generally normal or suppressed in malignancy-related hypercalcemia, indicating that there are other causative factors. PTH-RP is a small peptide homologous with the amino-terminus of PTH, which is also the portion that binds to the PTH receptor.[9] PTH-RP can stimulate bone resorption and renal phosphate wasting resulting in hypercalcemia and hypophosphatemia. PTH-RP production is often found in squamous cell carcinomas and other solid tumors. Hematologic malignancies may cause hypercalcemia by production of several cytokines, including osteoclast-activating factor (OAF), lymphotoxin, and tumor necrosis factor (TNF).[10] Lymphomas can produce 1,25-dihydroxycholecalciferol, promoting gastrointestinal (GI) absorption of calcium, resulting in suppressed PTH, normal to increased phosphorus, and hypercalcemia.[6]

Hypercalcemia is a significant source of morbidity and mortality in the cancer patient. Early manifestations can include anorexia, fatigue, lethargy, nausea, constipation, pruritis, polydypsia, and polyuria. These symptoms may not always be recognized because of attribution to the existing malignancy, other comorbid conditions, and treatment toxicities. If left untreated, symptoms can progress, resulting in severe dehydration, renal insufficiency, constipation, ileus, confusion, obtundation, seizures, and coma.

Patients who have a serum calcium level greater than 13 mg/dL usually exhibit symptoms. The degree of symptomology is variable depending on the level of serum calcium, the rapidity with which the level was achieved, and the patient's overall health (i.e., performance status, age, preexisting organ dysfunction). The initial goal of treatment is restoration of intravascular volume and promotion of calcuresis, which can be accomplished with normal saline hydration (100–400 mL/h). Slower hydration may be more appropriate in patients with cardiovascular or renal impairment. Diuretics, such as furosemide, should be used judiciously to balance fluid intake and output. Dialysis may be necessary in cases of renal failure.

The bisphosphonates are the most common pharmaceutical agents used to treat hypercalcemia. These agents are analogues of pyrophosphate and inhibit osteoclast activity by binding to hydroxyapatite. Pamidronate and the newer generation, zoledronic acid, are the bisphosphonates used in the treatment of hypercalcemia. In randomized trials, zoledronic acid (4 and 8 mg) proved to be superior to pamidronate (90 mg), by yielding a more rapid and sustained decrease in serum calcium.[11] The current recommended dose of zoledronic acid is 4 mg intravenously over 15 minutes. The bisphosphonates

TABLE 85.1. Endocrinologic paraneoplastic syndromes.

Syndrome	*Etiologic factors*	*Common associated tumors*	*Biochemical presentation*	*Clinical presentation*
Hypercalcemia	PTH-RP; lymphotoxin; TGF; IL-1; TNF; PGE; OAF; IL-6; 1,25-OHD	Squamous cell carcinomas, lung, breast, kidney, ovary, myeloma, lymphoma, and others	↑ Serum calcium, variable serum phosphate, calcuria	Fatigue, anorexia, constipation, dehydration, neurologic symptoms, cardiac arrhythmias
Ectopic ACTH	ACTH production via POMC or CRH	SCLC, carcinoid, medullary thyroid, thymus, islet cell, pheochromocytoma, ganglioneuroma, and others	↑ ACTH Hypokalemia Metabolic alkalosis Hyperglycemia	Cushing's syndrome
SIADH	ADH (vasopression)	Lung (especially SCLC), head and neck, brain, GI, prostate, breast, sarcoma, carcinoid, hematologic	Hyponatremia, serum hyposmolality, inappropriately high urine osmolality and urine sodium	Anorexia, headache, lethargy, mental status changes, seizure, coma
Gonadotropin Production	HCG	Germ cell tumors, lung, GI, melanoma, kidney, breast, islet of pancreas	↑ β-HCG	Gynecomastia (adult males), precocious puberty (young females), hyperthyroidism
Hypoglycemia	(1) Insulin (2) Insulin-like substance	(1) Insulinoma, islet (2) Sarcoma mesothelioma hepatoma, GI, adrenal, hematologic	↓ Fasting glucose	Symptoms of hypoglycemia
Hypocalcemia	Calcitonin	Medullary thyroid	Hypocalcemia	Rare clinical symptoms
Prolactin Production	Prolactin	Kidney, lung, breast, cervix, colorectal, others	↑ Prolactin	Asymptomatic loss of libido, galactorrhea
Osteomalacia	Inhibition 1,25-OHD, phosphaturic substance	Mesenchymal tumors, lung, prostate	Hypophosphatemia, phosphaturia, ↓ 1,25-OHD, glycosuria	Myopathy, bone pain

See text for explanation of abbreviations.

Source: Data from references 4, 5, 6.

should be administered with caution in patients with renal insufficiency.

Gallium nitrate is another agent that can inhibit bone resorption via inhibition of osteoclast activity. It is administered at a dose of 100 to 200 mg/m^2/day by continuous infusion for up to 5 days. Gallium nitrate was proven to be superior to pamidronate in a randomized clinical trial,[12] but it has not been compared to zoledronic acid. As with the bisphophonates, there is potential for nephrotoxicity. Calcitonin has a rapid onset of action and can be used in critically ill patients with renal insufficiency. The main disadvantage to this agent is that its hypocalcemic effect diminishes and it is rarely effective long term. Plicamycin (mithramycin) is an antineoplastic agent, toxic to osteoclasts, that was used in the prebisphophonate era. Because of its toxic side effects and the availability of other agents, it is no longer commercially available. Corticosteroids can inhibit calcium resorption and are frequently used in hypercalcemia related to hematologic malignancies, where they are part of the systemic therapy.

The pharmaceutical agents used to treat hypercalcemia are a temporary "fix" for the situation, and ultimately, successful treatment of the malignancy controls hypercalcemia. This aim may not be achievable in patients who have disease that is refractory to treatment, and eventually, inability to treat the malignancy will result in death.

Ectopic ACTH Production

The precursor of adrenocorticotropic hormone (ACTH), proopiomelanocortin (POMC), is made by normal tissue but malignancies can produce this same precursor in much larger quantities. Some neoplasms are capable of converting POMC to biologically active ACTH, resulting in ectopic ACTH syndrome.[6] Excessive ACTH can also occur via tumor production of corticotropin-releasing hormone (CRH).[13] Small cell carcinoma of the lung (SCLC) is the most common tumor associated with ectopic ACTH production, although most patients do not develop clinically apparent Cushing's syndrome. A number of other malignancies that are also capable of producing ACTH are listed in Table 85.1.

The clinical syndrome is characterized by features associated with Cushing's disease, including centripetal obesity, hypertension, easy bruisability, muscle weakness, hyperpigmentation, glucose intolerance, and metabolic alkalosis. In patients with a rapidly growing tumor such as SCLC, the metabolic abnormalities, muscle wasting, and hypertension predominate. When overproduction of ACTH is clinically suspected it is important to distinguish between pituitary or adrenal disorders or ectopic ACTH production. An elevated ACTH plasma level often rules out primary adrenal disease as a causative factor. The high-dose dexamethasone suppression test generally suppresses cortisol production in pituitary-related Cushing's disease but not in ectopic ACTH related to tumors. Unfortunately, there are false positives and false negatives associated with the testing. The metyrapone suppression and CRH stimulation tests add to the accuracy of the dexamethasone suppression test.[14,15] Other techniques, such as petrosal venous sinus sampling, continuous dexamethasone suppression, and serum chromagranin have been used with some success, but the results have not been verified.[5]

In patients who have early-stage tumors, with the exception of SCLC, surgery with removal of the primary tumor is the treatment of choice. In one series, 75% of patients with ACTH production and localized primary tumors were cured of their Cushing's syndrome with surgery.[16] In patients who have disease that is not surgically resectable, symptoms can be palliated by bilateral adrenalectomy or medical therapy. Medical intervention can include cytotoxic chemotherapy with or without other medications, such as aminoglutethimide, metyrapone, mitotane, or ketoconazole, all of which suppress cortisol production. Ketoconazole (400 to 1,200 mg/day), because of its effectiveness and favorable toxicity profile, is probably the medical treatment of choice.[17] Treatment of SCLC involves cytotoxic chemotherapy. Treatment outcomes with SCLC patients who have ectopic ACTH secretion appear to be inferior, possibly secondary to increased complications (i.e., infection) related to high levels of corticosteroid.[18]

Syndrome of Inappropriate Antidiuretic Hormone

The syndrome of inappropriate antidiuretic hormone (SIADH) is caused by excessive release of vasopressin or ADH, which binds to receptors in the renal collecting ducts and the ascending loop of Henle, resulting in increased water reabsorption and increased sodium excretion via decreased proximal reabsorption. SCLC is the most common malignancy associated with SIADH. Most small cell cancers demonstrate positive staining for vasopressin, but only 15% or less actually have the clinical syndrome.[19] Other malignancies that can have excessive ADH secretion are mentioned in Table 85.1. There are a number of nonmalignant conditions associated with SIADH, including intracranial processes (i.e., cerebral vascular accident, trauma, infection), pulmonary disease, and drug treatment (i.e., narcotics, chlorpropramide, chlorflibrate, carbomazepines, vincas, cisplatin, cyclophosphamide).[20] When evaluating patients for hyponatremia, other causes in addition to SIADH should be considered, such as congestive heart failure, renal and liver disease, hypothyroidism, and adrenal insufficiency.

The hallmark features of SIADH include hyponatremia, euvolemia, low serum osmolality, inappropriately elevated urine osmolality and sodium, and normal renal, adrenal, and thyroid function. Most patients are asymptomatic or complain of weakness, lethargy, anorexia, and headache. As the serum sodium level drops, patients may develop mental status changes, seizures, focal neurologic signs, and coma. Mild hyponatremia can be managed with fluid restriction, whereas patients with severe symptoms may require treatment with 3% hypertonic saline; this requires careful monitoring, usually in an intensive care unit. The correction rate should be no more than 1 mEq/L/h to avoid the potential complication of central pontine demyelinosis.[21] Demeclocyline (600 mg/day), which can inhibit the action of vasopressin, may also be used.[22] Patients with SCLC are treated with cytotoxic chemotherapy. The presence of SIADH does not necessarily portend a poor prognosis.[23] Redevelopment of low sodium after treatment completion may herald disease recurrence.

Gonadotropins

The gonadotropins include follicle-stimulating hormone (FSH), luteinizing hormone (LH), and human chorionic gonadotropin (HGG).[24] They have a common subunit and a hormone specific β-subunit that determines biologic specificity. HCG production is found in a number of malignancies (see Table 85.1), and the β-subunit of HCG is measured in the serum. The most common clinical presentation in adults is unexplained gynecomastia, usually as a result of a germ cell tumor or lung cancer. In young women, precocious puberty can develop from ovarian stimulation. When β-HCG is present at high levels, hyperthyroidism can result from stimulation of thyroid-stimulating hormone.

Hypoglycemia

Hypoglycemia is an uncommon paraneoplastic syndrome most often associated with sarcomas and mesothelioma. Other tumors that reportedly can cause hypoglycemia are listed in Table 85.1. A number of etiologies have been proposed, but the suspected cause is the tumor secretion of a nonsuppressible insulin-like substance.[25] Insulin itself can be produced by insulinomas and islet cell malignancies. Fasting hypoglycemia is the most common clinical presentation. Patients are treated by surgical resection of the tumor or antineoplastic therapy. When this is not possible, symptoms of hypoglycemia can be palliated by frequent meals and the use of various agents, including glucagon, corticosteroids, diazoxide (inhibits insulin secretion), and growth hormone.

Other Endocrine Paraneoplastic Syndromes

Calcitonin is secreted by the cells of the thyroid and can be produced by medullary thyroid carcinoma and a number of other tumors. Clinically apparent hypocalcemia is rare. Acromegaly has been attributed to the secretion of a growth hormone-releasing factor.[26] Elevated prolactin levels have been reported in a variety of tumors. Clinical symptoms are uncommon, but galactorrhea has been reported.[27] Tumor-induced osteomalacia is a syndrome characterized by severe hypophosphatemia, phosphaturia, glycosuria, bone pain, myopathy, and inadequate bone mineralization.[28] It is thought to be caused by inhibition of the conversion of 1,25-hydroxyvitamin D and phosphaturic substance.[5] It is most commonly seen in benign mesenchymal tumors and has rarely been reported in other malignancies (see Table 85.1).

Paraneoplastic Syndromes of the Nervous System

Paraneoplastic syndromes can affect any part of the nervous system (Table 85.2). The frequency of clearly defined symptomatic neurologic paraneoplastic syndromes is less than 1% of cancer patients.[29] However, the frequency is underestimated because in many patients the neurologic disorder may precede the diagnosis of the underlying cancer. Interestingly, clinical and electrophysiologic studies in cancer patients often disclose neuromuscular dysfunction in otherwise asymptomatic patients. In some, the signs and symptoms of

TABLE 85.2. Neurologic paraneoplastic syndromes.

Antibody	*Targeted neuron*	*Paraneoplastic syndrome*	*Tumors*
Anti-Hu (ANNA-1)	All neurons	Encephalomyelitis, sensory neuronopathy, cerebellar degeneration	Small cell, neuroblastoma, prostate cancer, sarcoma
Anti-Yo (PCA-1)	Purkinje cell	Cerebellar degeneration	Small cell, breast, ovarian
Anti-Ri (ANNA-2)	Central nervous system neurons	Opsoclonus-myoclonus, cerebellar degeneration	Small cell, breast, ovarian, bladder
Anti-Tr	Purkinje cell	Cerebellar degeneration	Hodgkin's and non-Hodgkin's Lymphoma
Anti-CAR	Photoreceptors	Cancer-associated retinopathy	Small cell, Melanoma
Anti-VGCC	Presynaptic neuromuscular junction	Lambert–Eaton myasthenic syndrome	Small cell, Hodgkins Lymphoma
Anti-Ta	Neurons (nucleus)	Limbic encephalitis	Testis
Anti-MAG	Peripheral nerve	Peripheral neuropathy	Waldenstrom's macroglobulinemia
Antiamphiphysin	Presynaptic nerve terminals, central nervous system neurons	Encephalomyelitis, stiff-man syndrome	Breast cancer, small cell
Anti-AchR	Postsynaptic neuromuscular junction	Myasthenia gravis	Thymoma

Ach, acetylcholine; CAR, cancer-associated retinopathy; MAG, myelin-associated glycoprotein; VGCC, voltage gated calcium channel.

the neurologic disorder appear months or even a few years before the underlying tumor is diagnosed. The probability that a neurologic syndrome is associated with a tumor varies with the specific type of paraneoplastic syndrome.

Pathogenesis

There is increasing evidence that most if not all the paraneoplastic neurologic disorders are immune mediated. The pathogenic mechanism involves the ectopic expression by the tumor of an antigen that is normally expressed in the nervous system. The immune system, for reasons that are not entirely clear, recognizes these antigens as foreign and mounts an immune response, in the form of antibodies and/or cytotoxic T cells. These antibodies and T cells then attack the neural tissues that express the antigens shared with the tumor.

The relative role of humorally mediated immunity and cellular immunity in paraneoplastic neurologic disorders is unresolved. In disorders, such as Lambert–Eaton syndrome, myasthenia gravis, opsoclonus-myoclonus, and cerebellar degeneration surface receptors serve as target antigens and antibodies appear to have a dominant role. The actual role of the antibodies is unproven. There have been several attempts to reproduce these paraneoplastic neurologic syndromes by passive transfer of antibodies, such as anti-Hu and anti-Yo, and by immunization of animals with recombinant antigens.[30,31] These experiments did not result in neurologic dysfunction. However, most patients with antibody-associated paraneoplastic syndromes of the central nervous system have continuous intrathecal synthesis of antibodies.

Many studies have also documented the role of cellular immunity in neurologic paraneoplastic disorders. Tumors of patients with neurologic disorders have an intense inflammatory infiltrate that have been recently shown to contain CD4 and CD8 lymphocytes.[32,33] Receptor studies of T cells in these infiltrates show that they are specifically targeted to the neuronal antigens. Activated T cells have been found in the peripheral blood of patients with acute paraneoplastic cerebellar degeneration that react to cells with the Yo (cdr2) antigen. In many cases, the antibodies and T cells are directed against the same neuronal antigen, suggesting that the neurologic paraneoplastic disorders may result from the combined effect of the two arms of the immune system.

The presence of antibodies in the serum or particularly in the cerebrospinal fluid (CSF), may aid in the diagnosis of paraneoplastic neurologic disorders.[34] This fact may focus attention on certain neoplasms, and it is important to consider that these antibodies may be present in the serum of patients without paraneoplastic syndromes.

The clinical spectrum of paraneoplastic syndromes is varied. Many patients present with rapid development and progression of symptoms. Therefore, by the time a diagnosis is made, many patients may have irreversible pathologic changes. This may be the reason that patients with disorders involving the peripheral nerves or neuromuscular junction may respond to therapy, whereas disorders with neuronal damage may be permanent.

Paraneoplastic Encephalomyelitis

Paraneoplastic encephalomyelitis is characterized by multifocal involvement of the nervous system with signs of inflammation demonstrated by radiologic studies, such as magnetic resonance imaging (MRI), CSF examination, or biopsy. The manifestations of this disorder are varied. Some patients present with focal encephalitis involving the limbic system or brainstem. However, when these cases have been analyzed there is pathologic evidence of multifocal involvement.[35,36] Paraneoplastic encephalomyelitis is most often associated with small cell lung cancer. Young patients with symptoms of limbic and/or brainstem dysfunction may have associated germ cell tumors. They often have Ma antibodies in the peripheral blood.

Encephalomyelitis responds poorly to therapy. Stabilization of the symptoms could be expected if the tumor responds well to anticancer treatment. Limbic encephalitis is an exception because it may improve with therapy.[35] The role of immunosuppressive therapy, such as plasma exchange, cyclophosphamide, and steroids in the treatment of encephalomyelitis is questionable.[37] Patients with encephalomyelitis could die of the consequences of the paraneoplastic disorder. Factors that are likely to increase the possibility of death are older age, multiple sites of involvement, and impaired performance status.

Cerebellar Degeneration

Paraneoplastic cerebellar degeneration is the most common paraneoplastic disorder affecting the central nervous system. A variety of tumors, especially SCLC, breast cancer, and ovarian cancer, are the most frequent sources. Paraneoplastic antibodies are associated with this disorder.[38] The predominant pathologic feature is the loss of Purkinje cells, with a variable involvement of the other neurons. Clinical presentation of this disorder is characterized by symmetric cerebellar ataxia but patients may also have dysarthria, dysphagia, and diplopia. The onset of symptoms is usually sudden, and progression occurs over weeks to months. Patients with paraneoplastic antibodies progress much more rapidly.[39] Radiologic studies in the early stages of the disease are generally unremarkable. Cerebellar atrophy may be observed on MRI and computed tomography (CT) scans in patients who have had the disease for a long period. CSF studies may show evidence of pleocytosis and, in seropositive cases, higher titers of antibodies than appear in serum. The best therapeutic approach to this disorder is prompt treatment of the tumor. Unfortunately, most patients do not respond to antitumor therapy or to immunosuppression.

Opsoclonus-Myoclonus

Opsoclonus consists of involuntary conjugate saccadic eye movements. The paraneoplastic syndrome is often associated with focal myoclonic movements and ataxia. The syndrome is more common among children than adults. In children, almost 50% who present with opsoclonus have an underlying neuroblastoma.[40,41] Opsoclonus can also occur following a viral infection. Paraneoplastic opsoclonus responds to treatment of the tumor and steroids; however, the majority of the patients have residual neurologic deficits including behavioral abnormalities. In adults, only 20% of the opsoclonus cases are associated with tumors. The most common tumor type is lung cancer.[42] Prompt therapy of the tumor results in a better prognosis, but most adult patients have persistent deficits. Some patients may respond to the use of steroids.

Limbic Encephalitis

Limbic encephalitis is a rare paraneoplastic disorder characterized by personality changes, short-term memory loss, and, occasionally, seizures and hallucinations. Pathologic changes predominantly involve the amygdala, hippocampus, and insular cortex. The syndrome can occur with testicular cancers, small cell lung cancer, and other tumors. In testicular cancer, it is associated with antibodies to Ma1 and Ma2 proteins, which are neuronal proteins with unknown function. Patients with seropositive disease may have good responses to antitumor therapy and immunosuppression.[43]

Sensory and Motor Neuronopathies

Paraneoplastic sensory neuronopathy is characterized by progressive sensory loss in limbs, trunk, and face. The sensory loss progresses over weeks and then stabilizes after several months. The vibration and joint position sensations may be more affected than nociceptive sensation. The sensory loss can affect the patient's ability to ambulate. The associated tumor is usually small cell lung cancer and these patients often harbor anti-Hu antibodies.[44] Pathologic findings consist of neuronal loss in the dorsal root ganglia. Response to therapy is limited, and patients often remain disabled.

Motor neuronopathy is associated primarily with lymphomas.[45] Pathologic findings consist of neuronal degeneration in the anterior horn with demyelination of the anterior nerve roots. Patients have a progressive motor weakness, primarily in the lower extremities. In contrast to other paraneoplastic disorders, patients may develop this syndrome after the diagnosis of the underlying neoplasm.

Sensorimotor Neuropathy

Differentiating the various causes of neuropathies in cancer patients could be challenging. Peripheral neuropathy can occur in cancer patients from a variety of sources, including cytotoxic therapy and metabolic and nutritional etiologies. A paraneoplastic chronic sensorimotor neuropathy has been described with lung cancer.[46] Patients usually have mild symptoms in a typical glove-and-stocking distribution.

In patients with osteosclerotic myeloma, a group of symptoms referred to as POEMS may develop. POEMS consists of neuropathy, organomegaly, endocrine dysfunctions, and skin changes. The pathologic basis of this syndrome is unclear. Symptoms including neuropathy may respond to myeloma therapy.

Stiff-Man Syndrome

This syndrome is characterized by chronic muscle rigidity with superimposed muscle spasms. It results from autoimmunity affecting synaptic antigens, and the majority of patients with this disorder do not have an underlying tumor. Paraneoplastic stiff-man syndrome is associated with antibodies to amphiphysin, a protein expressed at high levels in the brain and skeletal muscle.[47] The tumor type most commonly associated with the paraneoplastic stiff-man syndrome is breast cancer. Treatment of the tumor and steroids may improve the symptoms.[47,48]

Myopathies

Various myopathic syndromes may have a paraneoplastic origin. However, in most patients with these syndromes there is no underlying tumor. Lambert–Eaton syndrome (LES) could be nonparaneoplastic in 50% of the cases.[49] It results from an antibody directed against the voltage-dependent calcium channels in the presynaptic nerve terminal.[50] These antibodies block calcium entry into the channels, resulting in reduced acetylcholine release and thus, reduced muscle activity. The tumor type most commonly associated is small cell lung cancer, although other malignancies, such as lymphoma have been reported with this syndrome. The clinical features are characterized by muscle weakness, particularly in the proximal muscles with easy fatigability. This syndrome does respond to immunosuppressive therapy, plasmapheresis, and intravenous immunoglobulin (IVIG). Treatment of the underlying tumor is most important.

Myasthenia gravis is a myopathy characterized by increasing muscle weakness with repeated use of the muscles. The most commonly involved muscles are the bulbar muscles, muscles of the face and neck, and the distal muscles of the extremities. In 90% of the patients with myasthenia gravis, there is no underlying tumor. The most common tumor type associated with paraneoplastic myasthenia is thymoma.

Dermatomyositis and polymyositis are inflammatory myopathies with features of pain, muscle tenderness, and symmetric proximal muscle weakness. The rash in dermatomyositis is on the face, elbows, and knees. The disorders are paraneoplastic in only about 10% of the cases.[51] The probability that an underlying cancer is present is higher in older individuals. The most common associated tumor types are lung and breast cancer. These myopathies may respond to steroids.

Cutaneous Paraneoplastic Disorders

Similar to other paraneoplastic disorders, cutaneous syndromes may precede, occur concurrently, or follow the diagnosis of cancer (Table 85.3). In 1976, Curth set out criteria regarding paraneoplastic dermatoses: (1) both start at approximately the same time; (2) both follow a parallel course; (3) a specific tumor is associated with a specific skin manifestation; (5) the dermatoses are not common in the general population; and a high percentage of association is observed between the cancer and the dermatoses.[52]

Acanthosis Nigrans

Acanthosis nigrans is characterized by velvety hyperpigmentation and papillomatosis of the skin folds. The neck, axillae, antecubital, popliteal, and anogenital region are the areas commonly affected. Acanthosis nigrans may be idiopathic or could be associated with endocrine disorders, such as diabetes, obesity, and polycystic ovary syndrome. Paraneoplastic acanthosis nigrans is most commonly linked with abdominal adenocarcinomas, such as gastric cancer.[53] It has also been observed with other adenocarcinomas, such as lung, breast, ovarian, and endometrial as well as lymphomas. The malignant form of acanthosis nigrans progresses rapidly and diffusely. In one series, it preceded the diagnosis of the associated cancer in 69% of the cases.[53] The condition may improve with the therapy of the underlying tumor.

Tripe palms are hyperkeratotic palms with exaggerated ridges and a velvety texture. They commonly occur with acanthosis nigrans. Tripe palms are associated with malignancy in almost 90% of the cases.[53,54] Lung cancer and gastric cancer are the most common malignancies.

Ichthyosis

Ichthyosis is characterized by dry skin with rhomboidal scales having free edges. There are two forms of ichthyosis, congenital and acquired. Acquired ichthyosis is associated with many disorders, such as cancer, acquired immunodeficiency syndrome (AIDS), sarcoidosis, and leprosy and can be drug induced. The most common malignancy is non-Hodgkin's lymphoma but the syndrome has been seen in breast cancer, lung cancer, leiomyosarcomas, and Kaposi's sarcoma (with or without AIDS).[55] In cancer-related ichthyosis, the areas most commonly affected are extensor surfaces of extremities, with relative sparing of the flexor surfaces and palms and soles. The condition in most patients follows the diagnosis of the cancer and usually is observed in the late stages of the disease.[56] Treatment is

TABLE 85.3. Cutaneous paraneoplastic syndromes.

Cutaneous syndrome	*Features*	*Tumors*
Acanthosis nigrans	Velvety pigmentation and papillomatosis in the neck, axilla, flexor areas, and anogenital area	Adenocarcinomas, mainly gastric, but also seen with lung, ovarian
Ichthyosis	Dry skin with rhomboidal scales having free edges; extensor surfaces of extremities	Non-Hodgkin's lymphoma, lung cancer, breast cancer
Bazex's syndrome	Dry and scaly skin plaques on the acral surfaces of ears, nose, hands, and feet	Squamous cell carcinomas of the aerodigestive tract
Sign of Leser–Trelat	Seborrheic keratoses on the trunk with pruritus	Gastric, colon, breast, lung adenocarcinomas
Paraneoplastic pemphigus	Bullous lesions that may erode, present over the trunk and the extremities; internal organ involvement may also occur	Lymphomas, Waldenstrom's macroglobulinemia
Erythroderma	Exfoliative dermatitis with erythema and scaling of the skin	Leukemias and lymphomas
Necrotizing migratory erythema	Erythematous macules and papules, which may erode, in the inguinal area, thighs, buttocks, perineum, and central face	Glucagonomas
Erythema gyratum repens	Migrating concentric rings of erythema with trailing scale on the trunk and extremities	Lung cancer
Paget's disease	Erythematous keratotic patches at the affected sites, which include breast, vulva, perianal area, male genitalia	Breast, prostate, bladder, vaginal, endometrial, rectal
Sweet's syndrome	Erythematous plaques on the face, neck, and extremities	Acute myeloid leukemia

primarily directed at the underlying cancer. Application of lubricating agents and keratolytic agents, such as 2% salicylic acid may help reduce the symptoms of dry skin and pruritus. Use of antihistamines and nonsteroidal antiinflammatory drugs (NSAIDS) to treat pruritus may also be helpful.

Bazex's Syndrome

Bazex's syndrome, also known as acrokeratosis paraneoplastica, is characterized by dry, scaly skin plaques on the acral surfaces of the ears, nose, hands, and feet. These lesions may exhibit a violaceous erythema. Nail changes, including ridging, discoloration, thickening, and paronychia, may also occur. The syndrome is almost always associated with squamous cell carcinoma of the aerodigestive tract.[57] Males are affected much more frequently than females.

The pathogenic mechanism of the disorder is unknown but is postulated to be a result of cross-reactivity between tumor antigens and epidermal or basement membrane antigens. Tumor secretion of growth factors, such as transforming growth factor or insulin-like growth factor may contribute to the development of the syndrome.[58] The syndrome may precede, occur with, or follow the diagnosis of the cancer. In patients with Bazex's syndrome without a known malignancy, a search for an underlying tumor should be done. The condition generally tends to improve with effective tumor therapy, although the nail changes may persist. Good skin care and antibiotic therapy in the event of a secondary infection are crucial.

Sign of Leser–Trelat

Sign of Leser–Trelat is the sudden appearance of seborrheic keratoses. The keratoses often erupt on the trunk and can be pruritic. The significance of this condition is thought to be controversial but its presence is generally considered to require a cancer workup. This sign is most often found in patients with adenocarcinoma of the stomach and colon but has been reported in other tumors, such as breast, lung, and ovary.[59,60]

Paraneoplastic Pemphigus

In this disorder, there are bullous lesions that may erode and which are present on the skin over the trunk and the extremities. Internal organ involvement may also occur, and respiratory failure causes death in some patients with this disorder. The tumors with which this paraneoplastic syndrome is associated are lymphomas, Waldenstrom's macroglobulinemia, and spindle cell tumors.[61] The course of the disease is independent of the underlying tumor. Corticosteroids, cyclosporine, and mycophenolate mofetil have been recommended as therapy.[61,62]

Erythroderma

Erythroderma is an exfoliative dermatitis characterized by erythema and scaling of the skin. It usually starts as scattered erythematous pruritic patches that become generalized. Inflammatory lymphadenopathy may be present in association with the erythema.[63] Leukemias and lymphomas are most commonly associated with this disorder.[63,64] Solid tumors that have been implicated include liver, lung, and colon.

Necrotizing Migratory Erythema

Necrotizing migratory erythema is the skin manifestation of glucagonomas.[65] Patients develop a dermatitis characterized by erythematous macules and papules in the inguinal area, thighs, buttocks, perineum, and central face. These lesions may progress to erosions secondary to epidermal necrosis. Opportunistic infections including *Candida* may occur. The skin disease has a waxing and a waning course. It tends to occur late in the course of the tumor although it could occur before the diagnosis. The pathogenesis of the skin condition is believed to be from the catabolism induced by glucagons.[66] Treatment for the condition is usually surgical resection of the glucagonoma. Somatostatin or chemotherapy may be used in an attempt to reduce glucagon secretion if surgery is not feasible. The catabolic state induced by glucagon hypersecretion may result in amino acid deficiencies. Therefore, it has been suggested that an amino acid infusion may correct the underlying catabolic state and help the cutaneous condition.

Erythema Gyratum Repens

Erythema gyratum repens consists of migrating concentric rings of erythema with trailing scale on the trunk and extremities.[6] It is often pruritic by nature. The most common underlying malignancy is lung cancer, although other tumors, such as breast, cervix, and stomach cancers have been reported with this skin condition.[67,68] Treatment involves management of the underlying tumor and antipruritic measures.

Paget's Disease

Paget's disease may be mammary or extramammary and consists of erythematous keratotic patches at the affected site.[69] Histologic examination of the skin reveals large round cells with clear cytoplasm in the epidermis of the skin and often in the cutaneous appendages. Mammary Paget's disease is associated with breast cancer and involves the areola and the nipple. The presenting symptom may vary from a "pimple" to scaling with rash and erosion. Crusting and weeping exudates may occur. Extramammary Paget's disease occurs in the vulva, the genitals in men, and perianal area in both sexes. It is associated with tumor in 50% of the cases.[55] Most of the cancers arise from a site close to the Paget's disease. The most common tumor types are rectal, prostate, bladder, vaginal, and endometrial. Surgical resection of the underlying malignancy is the treatment of choice.

Sweet's Syndrome

Sweet first reported this syndrome in 1964[70]; it consists of erythematous plaques on the face, neck and extremities resulting from dermal infiltration of neutrophils. The skin changes occur with fever and neutrophilia. This syndrome may be associated with an underlying malignancy, particularly acute myeloid leukemia (AML).[71] AML patients may develop leukemia cutis, which is characterized by infiltration of the skin with leukemic blasts; however, in Sweet's syndrome there is only infiltration with mature neutrophils. This syndrome may be associated with other hematologic malignancies as well as solid tumors.[52] Treatment with steroids usually resolves the symptoms promptly.

Paraneoplastic Rheumatic Disorders

Rheumatic disorders may occur in cancer patients either as direct invasion by the tumor or as a paraneoplastic phenomenon. Antineoplastic drugs may also induce rheumatic disorders. Patients with certain rheumatic disorders, such as rheumatoid arthritis and Sjogren's syndrome may have a higher risk of developing cancer.[72,73]

Polyarthritis Syndrome (Including Hypertrophic Osteoarthropathy)

Cancer-associated polyarthritis is generally seronegative, asymmetric, and can occur suddenly. Polyarthritis has been associated with solid tumors, such as lung, breast, ovarian, and pancreatic tumors, and lymphoma and leukemias.[74,75] In leukemias and, rarely, in lymphomas patients may have infiltration of the joint with malignant cells.

Hypertrophic osteoarthropathy (HOA) is the best known cancer-associated arthropathy. Patients are required to have both clubbing and periostitis to make the diagnosis. Clubbing results from paronychial soft tissue expansion, which in turn results from an increase in vascular and connective tissues in the nail bed. Periostitis develops from periosteal proliferation in the long bones, particularly the tibia and femurs. Patients may present with only certain components of the syndrome, such as clubbing.

HOA may be primary or secondary. Secondary HOA is seen in pulmonary, cardiac, intestinal, and hepatic disorders. The common link among disorders associated with HOA appears to be right to left shunting either in the heart or in the lung parenchyma, which permits megakaryocytes to access the peripheral circulation instead of being fragmented in the pulmonary circulation. These megak aryocytes in the distal digital circulation possibly release platelet-derived growth factor, which induces the changes observed with clubbing.[76,77] It is unclear if the same mechanism explains the periostitis. The tumors most commonly associated with HOA are pulmonary or mediastinal tumors, such as lung and esophageal cancers and thymoma. The symptoms with HOA may cause significant morbidity. Treatment is primarily focused toward the underlying cancer. NSAIDs may relieve the pain associated with HOA.[78]

Several studies have shown that patients with rheumatoid arthritis (RA) have higher rates of cancer than the general population. Lymphomas and myeloma are most commonly associated with RA.[79] The increased observed rate may be related to the use of immunosuppressive therapy.

Nonarticular Syndromes

Cancer patients may develop various inflammatory muscle conditions or vasculitis. Dermatomyositis, the most common paraneoplastic muscular syndrome, was discussed earlier. Other myositis syndromes observed in cancer patients include body myositis and paraneoplastic necrotizing myopathy.[80,81]

Patients with hematologic malignancies, such as myelodysplasia, lymphoma, or leukemia and sometimes patients with solid tumors may develop vasculitis. Patients can present with lupus-like symptoms including arthralgias/arthritis, neuropathy, and skin rashes. Cancer patients may also have Raynaud's phenomenon, which may be associated with the presence of cryoglobulins, and improves with cancer treatment.

Paraneoplastic Renal Syndromes

Renal complications of cancer can develop through many mechanisms, including tumor infiltration (leukemias, lymphomas), treatment-related complications, tumor lysis, and fluid and electrolyte disturbances. Paraneoplastic renal syndromes consist primarily of glomerular disorders resulting in renal dysfunction and/or nephrotic syndrome. Membranous nephropathy is the most common form of paraneoplastic glomerular disease.[82] Patients present with proteinuria in the nephrotic range, hypertension, and miroscopic hematuria. Immune complexes appear to play a role in the pathogenesis of this nephropathy.[83] Tumors commonly associated with membranous nephropathy are lung, ovarian, and gastric cancers.

Other glomerular diseases include membranoproliferative glomerulonephritis associated with chronic lymphocytic leukemia (CLL), hairy cell leukemia, and lymphomas; an IgA nephropathy with pancreatic and lung cancers; minimal change disease in Hodgkin's lymphoma; and focal and segmental glomerulosclerosis with CLL, T-cell lymphomas, and AML. Patients may also develop hemolytic uremic syndrome with prostate, gastric, and pancreatic cancers. Renal vasculitis with cryoglobulinemia can be seen in patients with hepatomas associated with hepatitis C.[84]

Hematologic and Vascular Syndromes

Erythrocyte Disorders

A number of hematologic abnormalities and vascular complications have been associated with malignancies (Table 85.4), and are presumed to be paraneoplastic in nature. One of the most common problems is anemia. Cancer-related anemia can be multifactorial, resulting from nutritional deficiency, bone marrow involvement by tumor, bleeding, treatment-related marrow depression, and coexisting comorbid conditions. Anemia with no other apparent cause can be termed neoplastic. The anemia is characterized by normochromic or slightly hypochromic red blood cells. Ferritin levels and iron stores are normal to increased, and both reticulocytes and erythropoietin levels are inappropriately low. Normal bone marrow morphology is usually present. A number of cytokines (tumor necrosis factor, interleukin 1, transforming growth factor-β) are thought to blunt erythropoietin response.[85] There are other rarer causes of anemia. Autoimmune hemolytic anemias are usually associated with chronic lymphocytic leukemia and lymphomas and rarely with solid tumors.[86,87] Both warm and cold antibodies can be

TABLE 85.4. Hematologic paraneoplastic syndromes.

Erythrocyte disorders
- Anemia
- Autoimmune hemolytic anemia
- Microangiopathic hemolytic anemia
- Erthrocytosis

Leukocyte disorders
- Leukocytosis
- Eosinophilia
- Monocytosis

Platelet disorders
- Thrombocytosis
- Idiopathic thrombocytopenic purpura
- Platelet function disorders

Coagulation and vascular disorders
- Thrombophlebitis/Trousseau's syndrome
- Disseminated intravascular coagulation
- Amyloidosis
- Acquired von Willebrand's disease
- Nonbacterial thrombotic endocarditis

present. They may arise secondary to immunoregulatory problems rather than production of an abnormal substance by the tumor.[86] Steroids often control hemolysis but are less effective when carcinomas are involved. Even less common is microangiopathic hemolytic anemia, which can occur with mucinous adenocarcinomas.[88] Pure red cell aplasia is rare and has been associated with thymoma and hematologic malignancies.[89,90]

Erythrocytosis can be caused by overproduction of erythropoietin and is most commonly associated with renal cell carcinoma. A number of other tumors, such as hepatomas and hemangioblastomas have also been reported to cause erythrocytosis.[86] This condition is controlled by management of the primary neoplasm, but phlebotomy may also be necessary.

Leukocytosis/Leukopenia

Leukocytosis has been associated with malignancies. At times the leukocyte count can be fairly high, and myeloproliferative disorders and infection should be part of the differential diagnoses. Leukocytosis has been linked to cytokines, such as interleukin 1 and granulocyte-stimulating factor.[91] Leukopenia has rarely been reported as a paraneoplastic syndrome. Monocytosis and/or eosinophilia are more commonly seen with a number of malignancies.

Thrombocytosis/Thrombocytopenia

Thrombocytosis, excluding other etiologies, such as iron deficiency anemia and inflammatory disorders, is a common occurrence in a number of malignancies. It may be related to prevalence of cytokine growth factors, such as thrombopoietin and interleukin[92,93] and it may have a role in the hypercoagulable state associated with malignancies. Thrombocytopenia usually occurs with nonparaneoplastic causes, such as the effects of treatment, drug-induced thrombocytopenia, and marrow involvement by tumor. Idiopathic thrombocytopenic purpura has been found in hematologic malignancies but rarely in solid tumors.

Coagulation/Vascular Disorders

Thrombophlebitis is commonly associated with malignancies. It can be migratory in nature (Trousseau's syndrome) and can present at unusual sites. It is most often seen in pancreatic cancer and other GI malignancies, as well as other adenocarcinomas, including lung, breast, ovarian, and prostate cancers.[94] The etiology of the hypercoagulable state in malignancy is quite complex. Contributing factors can include release of procoagulant materials, such as a sialic acid from mucin, release of cytokines with procoagulant activity, platelet hyperactivity, and the release of tissue factors via abnormal tumor vasculature.[95] Unless the underlying malignancy is controlled, treatment can be difficult in that heparin and particularly, warfarin resistance is often encountered.

Disseminated intravascular coagulation (DIC) with consumption of platelet and clotting factors resulting in hemorrhage and/or thrombosis is associated with malignancy. Overt DIC is uncommon and is most often seen in association with acute promyelocytic leukemia.[96] A lower grade of DIC can be found in a number of solid tumors, particularly adenocarcinomas. Therapy involves treatment of the underlying malignancy as well as other interventions, such as heparin, platelets, and cryoprecipitate, depending on the situation. Other bleeding disorders that have been reported, include hemostatic disruptions related to the paraproteins in plasma cell dyscrasias and acquired von Willebrand's disease in association with hematologic malignancies. Nonbacterial thrombotic endocarditis presents with sterile verrucous fibrin platelet lesions in the left-sided heart valve. Emboli to the brain and other organs can occur, and hemorrhage may also be seen at a number of sites. Adenocarcinoma of the lung is the most common etiology but other malignancies have also been implicated.[97] Anticoagulation is not beneficial in this disorder.

Other Paraneoplastic Syndromes

Fever can be seen in cancer patients as a paraneoplastic process. Before this diagnosis is considered, other etiologies, particularly infections, need to be ruled out. Renal carcinoma is the most common cancer associated with fever.[98] Fever can also occur in a number of hematologic malignancies, particularly Hodgkin's and non-Hodgkin's lymphoma, and is indicative of a worse prognostic category.

A number of other malignancies have also been reported to produce fever.[99] Pyrogenic cytokines produced by the tumor cells or induced via white blood cells are thought to be the source of "tumor fever." Some of these cytokines include interleukin 1, tumor necrosis factor, interleukin 6, and the interferons.[99] The production of the pyrogen cytokines can result in an acute response by the host. The pyrogen cytokines induce prostaglandin 2 (PGE_2) synthesis as an important part of fever production, which is likely the reason nonsteroidal antiinflammatory drugs (NSAIDs) have been effective at managing fever. It has been suggested that the NSAID naproxen can be used to distinguish fever related to tumor versus that of an infectious nature.[100] One randomized trial found three different NSAIDs to be equally effective.[101] Corticosteroids are also useful antipyretics. Similar to the NSAIDs, they reduce prostaglandin synthesis and can block the transcription of the mRNA for the pyrogenic cytokines.[99]

Cancer cachexia is one of the most frequent and difficult to manage problems encountered in the cancer patient. The cancer cachexia syndrome is characterized by anorexia, weight loss, and weakness resulting in impaired immune status, tissue wasting, and a decline in performance status.[102] The most obvious clinical manifestation is weight loss. A study from the Eastern Cooperative Oncology Group showed that weight loss was associated with a significantly shorter survival and was dependent on the tumor type.[103] Anorexia resulting in decreased caloric intake is the main symptom contributing to the weight loss. Patients develop altered taste sensation and food aversions, particularly for protein-rich foods.[104] The anorexia and weight loss can be potentiated by location of the tumor (i.e., involvement of the GI tract, obstruction), pain, effects of cancer treatment, and psychologic factors.

The etiology of cancer cachexia is not totally understood but is believed to be multifactorial. There are a number of metabolic abnormalities that are characteristic of the cancer patient. Glucose metabolism is abnormal. There is increased hepatic production of glucose, increased use of glucose by the tumor, and the development of insulin resistance. There are also problems with protein, amino acid, and lipid metabolism, all favoring the nutritional needs of the tumor over the host.[102] A number of cytokines, tumor factors, and hormones have been implicated in cancer cachexia, including tumor necrosis factors, interleukins, proteoglycan, insulin, corticotropin, epinephrine, human growth factor, and insulin-like growth factor.[105,106] The management of cancer cachexia is particularly challenging. Despite the fact that malnutrition is evident, a number of trials failed to show any significant clinical benefit for nutritional support. In a review of more than 70 prospective randomized controlled trials that evaluated the clinical efficacy of parenteral and enteral nutrition in cancer patients, the data fail to show a therapeutic effect.[107] Parenteral and enteral nutritional support should still be considered in patients who have complications from therapy (e.g., esophagitis) or in those who cannot maintain adequate nutrition secondary to tumor obstruction. A number of pharmacologic agents have been evaluated in the treatment of cancer cachexia. The most commonly utilized drug is megestrol acetate (MA). In a trial by Loprinzi et al., a positive dose–response effect on appetite resulted with increasing doses of MA (no benefit beyond 800 mg/day) and a trend toward nonfluid weight gain was apparent.[108] Steroids are frequently used but they generally do not have any prolonged benefit. Some of the other agents that have been evaluated include cannabinol derivatives, hydrazine sulfate, metaclopramide, cyproheptadine, melatonin, and pentoxifyllene. The studies utilizing those drugs either have been too small or did not show significant clinical benefit. Eicosapentaenoic acid (EPA), an omega-3 fatty acid, appeared to have promising results in early trials. Unfortunately, in a recent randomized study, EPA supplement, either alone or in combination with MA, did not improve weight or appetite better than MA alone.[109] Clearly, a better understanding of the etiology of cancer anorexia/cachexia and improved cancer treatment is needed before advances can be made.

References

1. Hall TC (ed) Paraneoplastic syndromes. Ann NY Acad Sci Ann 1974;230:1–577.
2. Odell WD. Paraneoplastic syndromes. In: Bast RC Jr, Kufe DW, Pollock RE, et al (eds) Cancer Medicine, 5th ed. New York: Dekker, 2000:777–789.
3. Nathanson L, Hall TC. Introduction: paraneoplastic syndromes. Semin Oncol 1997;24:265–268.
4. Odell WD. Endocrine/metabolic syndromes of cancer. Semin Oncol 1997;24:299–317.
5. Arnold SM, Lowy AM, Patchell R, Foon KA. Paraneoplastic syndromes. In: DeVita VT Jr, Hellman S, Rosenberg SA (eds) Cancer: Principles and Practice of Oncology, 6th ed. Philadelphia: Lippincott, 2001:2511–2536.
6. Yeung S-C J, Gagel RF. Endocrine complications and paraneoplastic syndromes. In: Kufe DW, Pollock RE, Weichselbaum RR, et al (eds) Cancer Medicine, 6th ed. New York: Dekker, 2003: 2609–2622.
7. Mundy GR, Martin TJ. The hypercalcemia of malignancy: pathogenesis and management. Metabolism 1982;31:1247–1277.
8. Mundy GR. Hypercalcemic factors other than parathyroid hormone-related protein. Endocrinol Metab Clin N Am 1989;18: 795–806.
9. Rankin W, Grill V, Martin TJ. Parathyroid hormone-related protein and hypercalcemia. Cancer (Phila) 1997;80(suppl 8): 1564–1571.
10. Garrett IR, Durie BG, Nedwin GE, et al. Production of lymphotoxin, a bone-resorbing cytokine, by cultured human myeloma cells. N Engl J Med 1987;317:526–532.
11. Major P, Lortholary A, Hon J, et al. Zoledronic acid is superior to pamidronate in the treatment of hypercalcemia of malignancy: a pooled analysis of two randomized, controlled clinical trials. J Clin Oncol 2001;19:558–567.
12. Bertheault-Cvitkovic F, Armand J-P, Tubiana-Hulin M, et al. Randomized, double-blind comparison of pamidronate vs. gallium nitrate for acute control of cancer-related hypercalcemia. Proc EORTC/NCI Symp New Drugs Cancer Ther 1996;9:140.
13. Newell-Price J, Trainer P, Besser M, Grossman A. The diagnosis and differential diagnosis of Cushing's syndrome and pseudo-Cushing's states. Endocr Rev 1998;19:647–672.
14. Avgerinos PC, Vanovski JA, Oldfield EH, et al. The metyrapone and dexamethasone suppression tests for the differential diagnosis of the adrenocorticotropin-dependent Cushing syndrome: a comparison. Ann Intern Med 1994;121:318–327.
15. Nieman LK, Chrousos GP, Oldfield EH, et al. The ovine corticotropin-releasing hormone stimulation test and the dexamethasone suppression test in the differential diagnosis of Cushing's syndrome. Ann Intern Med 1986;105:862–867.
16. Zeiger MA, Pass HI, Doppman JD, et al. Surgical strategy in the management of non-small cell ectopic adrenocorticotropic hormone syndrome. Surgery (St. Louis) 1992;112:994–1000.
17. Winquist EW, Laskey J, Crump M, et al. Ketoconazole in the management of paraneoplastic Cushing's syndrome secondary to ectopic adrenocorticotropin production. J Clin Oncol 1995;13: 157–164.
18. Shepherd FA, Laskey J, Evans WK, et al. Cushing's syndrome associated with ectopic corticotropin production and small-cell lung cancer. J Clin Oncol 1992;10:21–27.
19. Lokich JJ. The frequency and clinical biology of ectopic hormone syndromes of small cell carcinoma. Cancer (Phila) 1982;50: 2111–2114.
20. Glover DJ, Glick JH. Metabolic oncologic emergencies. CA Cancer J Clin 1987;37:302–320.
21. Ayus JC, Krothapalli RK, Areiff AI. Treatment of symptomatic hyponatremia and its relation to brain damage. A prospective study. N Engl J Med 1987;317:1190–1195.

22. Cherrill DA, Stote RM, Birge JR, et al. Demeclocycline treatment in the syndrome of inappropriate antidiuretic hormone secretion. Ann Intern Med 1975;83:654–656.
23. Bondy PK, Gilby ED. Endocrine function in small cell undifferentiated carcinoma of the lung. Cancer (Phila) 1982;50: 2147–2153.
24. Blackman MR, Weintraub BD, Rosen SW, et al. Human placental and pituitary glycoprotein hormones and their subunits as tumor markers: a quantitative assessment. J Natl Cancer Inst 1980;65:81–93.
25. Gorden P, Hendricks CM, Kahn CR, et al. Hypoglycemia associated with non-islet cell tumor and insulin-like growth factors. N Engl J Med 1981;305:1452–1455.
26. Scheithauer BW, Carpenter PC, Bloch B, et al. Ectopic secretion of a growth hormone-releasing factor. Report of a case of acromegaly with bronchial carcinoid tumor. Am J Med 1984;76: 605–616.
27. Kallenberg GA, Pesce CM, Norman B, et al. Ectopic hyperprolactinemia resulting from an ovarian teratoma. JAMA 1990;263: 2472–2474.
28. Ryan EA, Reiss E. Oncogenous osteomalacia. Review of the world literature of 42 cases and report of two new cases. Am J Med 1984;77:501–512.
29. Darnell R, Posner J. Paraneoplastic syndromes involving the nervous system. N Engl J Med 2003;349:1543–1554.
30. Tanaka K, Tanaka M, Onodera O, et al. Passive transfer and active immunization with the recombinant leucine-zipper (Yo) protein as an attempt to establish an animal model of paraneoplastic cerebellar degeneration. J Neurol Sci 1994;127:153–158.
31. Graus F, Illa I, Agusti M, et al. Effect of intraventricular injection of an anti-Purkinje cell antibody (anti-Yo) in a guinea pig model. J Neurol Sci 1991;106:82–87.
32. Graus F, Ribalta T, Campo E, et al. Immunohistochemical analysis of the immune reaction in the nervous system in paraneoplastic encephalomyelitis. Neurology 1990;40:219–222.
33. Jean W, Dalmau J, Ho A, et al. Analysis of the IgG subclass distribution and inflammatory infiltrates in patients with anti-Hu associated paraneoplastic encephalomyelitis. Neurology 1994; 44:140–147.
34. Vega F, Graus F, Chen QM, et al. Intrathecal synthesis of the anti-Hu antibody in patients with paraneoplastic encephalomyelitis or sensory neuronopathy: clinical-immunologic correlation. Neurology 1994;44:2145–2147.
35. Gultekin S, Rosenfeld M, Voltz R, et al. Paraneoplastic limbic encephalitis: neurological symptoms, immunological findings and tumor association in 50 patients. Brain 2000;123: 1481–1494.
36. Rosenfeld M, Eichen J, Wade D, et al. Molecular and clinical diversity in paraneoplastic immunity to Ma proteins. Ann Neurol 2001;50:339–348.
37. Graus F, Keime-Guibert F, Rene R, et al. Anti-Hu-associated paraneoplastic encephalomyelitis: analysis of 200 patients. Brain 2001;124:1138–1148.
38. Peterson K, Rosenblum M, Kotenides H, et al. Paraneoplastic cerebellar degeneration I: a clinical analysis of 55 anti-Yo antibody positive patients. Neurology 1992;42:1931–1937.
39. Anderson N, Rosenblum M, Posner J. Paraneoplastic cerebellar degeneration: clinical-immunological correlations. Ann Neurol 1988;24:559–567.
40. Russo C, Cohn S, Petruzzi M, et al. Long-term neurologic outcome in children with opsoclonus-myoclonus associated with neuroblastoma: a report from the Pediatric Oncology Group. Med Pediatr Oncol 1997;28:284–288.
41. Hammer MS, Larsen MB, Stack CV. Outcome of children with opsoclonus-myoclonus regardless of etiology. Pediatr Neurol 1995;13:21–24.
42. Digre K. Opsoclonus in adults. Arch Neurol 1986;43:1165–1175.
43. Rosenfeld M, Eichen J, Wade D, et al. Molecular and clinical diversity in paraneoplastic immunity to Ma proteins. Ann Neurol 2001;50:339–348.
44. Molinuevo J, Graus F, Rene R, et al. Utility of anti-Hu antibodies in the diagnosis of paraneoplastic sensory neuropathy. Ann Neurol 1998;44:976–980.
45. Schold S, Cho E, Somasundaram M, et al. Subacute motor neuronopathy: a remote effect of lymphoma. Ann Neurol 1979;5: 271–287.
46. Croft P, Urich H, Wilkinson M. Peripheral neuropathy of sensorimotor type associated with malignant disease. Brain 1967; 90:31–66.
47. Folli F, Solimena M, Cofiell R, et al. Autoantibodies to a 128-kd synaptic protein in three women with stiff-man syndrome. N Engl J Med 1993;328:546–551.
48. Schmierer K, Valdueza J, Bender A, et al. Atypical stiff-person syndrome with spinal MRI findings, amphiphysin autoantibodies, and immunosuppression. Neurology 1998;51:250–252.
49. O'Neill J, Murray N, Newsom-Davis J. The Lambert-Eaton myasthenic syndrome. A review of 50 cases. Brain 1988;111: 577–596.
50. Leys K, Lang B, Johnston I, et al. Calcium channel autoantibodies in the Lambert-Eaton myasthenic syndrome. Ann Neurol 1991;29:307–314.
51. Dalakas M. In: Polymyositis and Dermatomyositis. Boston: Butterworth, 1988.
52. Cohen P, Kurzrock R. Mucocutaneous paraneoplastic syndromes. Semin Oncol 1997;24:334–359.
53. Gross G, Pfister H, Hellenthal B, et al. Acanthosis nigricans maligna: clinical and virological investigations. Dermatologica 1984;168:265–272.
54. Schwartz R. Acanthosis nigricans. J Am Acad Dermatol 1994; 31:1–19.
55. McLean D, Haynes H. Cutaneous manifestations of internal malignant disease. In: Freedberg I, Eisen K, Wolfe K, et al (eds) Dermatology in General Medicine. New York: McGraw-Hill, 1999:2106–2120.
56. Griffin L, Massa M. Acquired ichthyosis and pityriasis rotunda. Clin Dermatol 1993;11:27–32.
57. Bolognia J. Bazex's syndrome: acrokeratosis paraneoplastica. Semin Dermatol 1995;14:84–89.
58. Bolognia J, Brewer Y, Cooper D. Bazex's syndrome (acrokeratosis paraneoplastica): an analytical review. Medicine (Baltim) 1991;70:269–280.
59. Schwartz R. Sign of Leser-Trelat. J Am Acad Dermatol 1996;35: 88–95.
60. Holdiness M. The sign of Leser-Trelat. Int J Dermatol 1986;25: 564–572.
61. Anhalt G. Paraneoplastic pemphigus. Adv Dermatol 1997;12: 77–96.
62. Williams J, Marks J, Billingsley E. Use of mycophenolate mofetil in the treatment of paraneoplastic pemphigus. Br J Dermatol 2000;142:506–508.
63. Karakayli G, Beckham G, Orengo I, et al. Exfoliative dermatitis. Am Fam Physician 1999;59:625–630.
64. Pal S, Haroon T. Erythroderma: a clinicoetiologic study of 90 cases. Int J Dermatol 1998;37:104–107.
65. Shepherd M, Raimer S, Tyring S, et al. Treatment of necrolytic migratory erythema in glucagonoma syndrome. J Am Acad Dermatol 1991;25:925–928.
66. Thorisdottir K, Camisa C, Tomecki K, et al. Necrolytic migratory erythema: a report of three cases. J Am Acad Dermatol 1994;30:324–329.
67. Tyring SK. Reactive erythemas: erythema annulare centrifugum and erythema gyratum repens. Clin Dermatol 1993;11: 1135–1139.
68. Appell M, Ward W, Tyring S. Erythema gyratum repens: a cutaneous marker of malignancy. Cancer (Phila) 1988;62:548–550.

69. McDonald A. Skin ulceration. In: Groenwald S, Frogge M, Goodman M, Yarbro C (eds) Cancer Symptom Management. Boston: Jones and Bartlett, 1996:364–381.
70. Sweet R. An acute febrile neutrophilic dermatosis. Br J Dermatol 1964;76:349–356.
71. Cooper P, Innes D, Greer K. Acute febrile neutrophilic dermatosis (Sweet's syndrome) and myeloproliferative disorders. Cancer (Phila) 1983;51:1518–1526.
72. Rosenthal A, McLaughlin J, Gridley G, et al. Incidence of cancer among patients with systemic sclerosis. Cancer (Phila) 1995;76: 910–914.
73. Porter D, Madhok R, Capell H. Non-Hodgkin's lymphoma in rheumatoid arthritis. Ann Rheum Dis 1991;50:275–276.
74. Bennet R, Ginsberg M, Thomsen S. Carcinomatous polyarthritis. The presenting symptom of an ovarian tumor and association with a platelet activating factor. Arthritis Rheum 1976;19: 953–958.
75. Drenth J, de Kleijn E, de Mulder P. Metastatic breast cancer presenting as rash, fever, and arthritis. Cancer (Phila) 1995;75: 1608–1611.
76. Dickinson C. The aetiology of clubbing and hypertrophic osteoarthropathy. Eur J Clin Invest 1993;23:330–338.
77. Martinez-Lavin M. Pathogenesis of hypertrophic osteoarthropathy. Clin Exp Rheumatol 1992;10(suppl 7):49–50.
78. Martinez-Lavin M, Weisman M, Pineda C. Hypertrophic osteoarthropathy. In: Schumacher H (ed) Primer on Rheumatic Diseases. Atlanta: Arthritis Foundation, 1988:240.
79. Carson S. The association of malignancy with rheumatic and connective tissue diseases. Semin Oncol 1997;24:360–372.
80. Ytterberg S, Roelofs R, Mahowald M. Inclusion body myositis and renal cell carcinoma: report of two cases and review of literature. Arthritis Rheum 1993;36:416–421.
81. Vosskamper M, Korf B, Franke F, et al. Paraneoplastic necrotizing myopathy: a rare disorder to be differentiated from polymyositis. J Neurol 1989;236:489–492.
82. Lee J, Yamauchi H, Hooper J. The association of cancer and nephritic syndrome. Ann Intern Med 1966;64:41–51.
83. Dinh B, Brassard A. Renal lesion associated with the Walker 256 adenocarcinoma in the rat. Br J Exp Pathol 1968;49:145–151.
84. Maesaka J, Mittal S, Fishbane S. Paraneoplastic syndromes of the kidney. Semin Oncol 1997;24:273–281.
85. Spivak JL. Cancer-related anemia: its causes and characteristics. Semin Oncol 1994;21(2 suppl 3):3–8.
86. Staszewski H. Hematologic paraneoplastic syndromes. Semin Oncol 1997;24:329–333.
87. Spira MA, Lynch EC. Autoimmune hemolytic anemia and carcinoma: an unusual association. Am J Med 1979;67:753–758.
88. Lohrmann HP, Adam W, Heymer B, et al. Microangiopathic hemolytic anemia in metastatic carcinoma. Report of eight cases. Ann Intern Med 1973; 79:368–375.
89. Vasavada PJ, Bournigal LJ, Reynolds RW. Thymoma associated with pure red cell aplasia and hypogammaglobulinemia. Postgrad Med 1973;54:93–98.
90. Akard LP, Brandt J, Lu L, et al. Chronic T cell lymphoproliferative disorders and pure red cell aplasia. Am J Med 1987;83: 1069–1074.
91. Shimasaki AK, Hirata T, Kawamura T, et al. The level of granulocyte colony-stimulating factor in cancer patients with leukocytosis. Intern Med 1992;31:861–865.
92. Estrov Z, Talpaz M, Mavligit G, et al. Elevated plasma thrombopoietic activity in patients with cancer related thrombocytosis. Am J Med 1995;98:551–558.
93. Gastl G, Plante, Finstad CL, et al. High IL-6 levels in ascitic fluid correlate with reactive thrombocytosis in patients with epithelial ovarian cancer. Br J Haematol 1993;83:433–441.
94. Sack GH Jr, Levin J, Bell WR. Trousseau's syndrome and other manifestations of chronic disseminated coagulopathy in patients with neoplasms: clinical, pathophysiologic, and therapeutic factors. Medicine (Baltim) 1977;56:1–37.
95. Green KB, Silverstein RL. Hypercoagulability in cancer. Hematol Oncol Clin N Am 1996;10:499–530.
96. Gralnick HR, Abrell E. Studies of the procoagulant and fibrinolytic activity of promyelocytes in acute promyelocytic leukemia. Br J Haematol 1973;24:89–99.
97. Gonzalez Quintela A, Candela MJ, Vidal C, et al. Non-bacterial thrombotic endocarditis in cancer patients. Acta Cardiol 1991; 46:1–9.
98. Laski ME, Vugrin D. Paraneoplastic syndromes in hypernephroma. Semin Nephrol 1987;7:123–130.
99. Dinarello CA, Bunn PA Jr. Fever. Semin Oncol 1997;24:288–298.
100. Chang JC, Gross HM. Utility of naproxen in the differential diagnosis of fever of undetermined origin in patients with cancer. Am J Med 1984;76:597–603.
101. Tsavaris N, Zinelis A, Karabelis A, et al. A randomized trial of the effect of three non-steroidal antinflammatory agents in ameliorating fever in cancer-induced fever. J Intern Med 1990; 228:451–455.
102. Puccio M, Nathanson L. The cancer cachexia syndrome. Semin Oncol 1997;24:277–287.
103. Dewys WD, Begg D, Lavin PT, et al. Prognostic effect of weight loss prior to chemotherapy in cancer patients. Eastern Cooperative Oncology Group. Am J Med 1980;69:491–497.
104. Nelson KA, Walsh D, Sheehan FA. The cancer anorexia-cachexia syndrome. J Clin Oncol 1994;12:213–225.
105. Langstein HN, Norton JA. Mechanisms of cancer cachexia. Hematol Oncol Clin N Am 1991;5:103–123.
106. Todorov P, Cariuk P, McDevitt T, et al. Characterization of cancer cachectic factor. Nature (Lond) 1996;379:739–742.
107. Klein S, Koretz RL. Nutrition support in patients with cancer: what do the data really show? Nutr Clin Pract 1994;9:91–100.
108. Loprinzi CL, Michalak JC, Schaid DJ, et al. Phase III evaluation of four doses of megestrol acetate as therapy for patients with cancer anorexia and/or cachexia. J Clin Oncol 1993;11:762–767.
109. Jatoi A, Rowland K, Loprinzi CL, et al. An eicosapentaenoic acid supplement versus megestrol acetate versus both for patients with cancer-associated wasting: a North Central Cancer Treatment Group and National Cancer Institute of Canada collaborative effort. J Clin Oncol 2004;22:2469–2476.

Malignant Effusions

Shamus R. Carr and Joseph S. Friedberg

Epidemiology

Malignant pleural effusions are a common clinical problem. The estimated annual incidence of malignant pleural effusions in the United States is greater than 150,000 cases per year, with lung cancer accounting for nearly half.[1–3] Breast cancer, lymphoma, and ovarian cancer round out the top four leading causes of malignant pleural effusions.[4–7]

Anatomy and Physiology

The pleura has a dual innervation and blood supply. The visceral pleura lacks somatic innervation, whereas the parietal pleura has extensive somatic innervation, in addition to sympathetic and parasympathetic fibers. Although the visceral pleura is insensate, irritation of the parietal pleura can elicit pain, or "pleurisy."[8] The visceral pleura receives arterial blood from both bronchial and pulmonary arteries, whereas the parietal pleura receives it from systemic arteries.[9]

Significant differences also exist between the lymphatic drainage routes of the visceral and parietal pleurae. Lymph from the visceral pleura drains into the pulmonary lymphatic network and is directed toward the pulmonary hilum. Depending upon the region of the parietal pleura, lymph from the parietal pleura drains into the corresponding internal thoracic, mediastinal, tracheobronchial, axillary, intercostal, or phrenic lymph nodes. Drainage into transverse cervical, celiac, or retrosternal lymph nodes also may occur. The visceral pleura has the majority of its lymphatic drainage concentrated in the lower lobes and is relatively sparse in the upper lobes; this is thought to be compensation for the greater connective tissue separation and higher venous pressure in the lower lobes compared to the upper lobes.[10]

The pleura is also important for maintaining local fluid homeostasis. The exact mechanisms of pleural fluid production and absorption are complex and not fully understood.[11,12] Pleural fluid originates from parietal pleura capillaries and is produced at a rate of 0.01 mL/kg/h under normal conditions[13] and is in equilibrium with reabsorption. The potential reabsorptive capabilities of normal pleura may be well in excess of 0.20 to 0.40 mL/kg/h, making it possible to process more than 700 mL fluid per day.[14,15]

Pleural effusions accumulate when the balance between fluid formation and uptake favors the former. Causes of increased production of pleural fluid include increased hydrostatic or decreased oncotic pressures within the interstitial microvasculature, loss of pulmonary volume, inflammation, increase in microvascular permeability, pleural involvement with metastatic malignancies, and either direct or indirect transfer of peritoneal fluid to the pleural cavity.[15,16] In addition, obstruction of the thoracic duct or direct pleural invasion may result in fluid accumulation and are considered mechanisms leading to the formation of malignant pleural effusions.[6,7]

Clinical Evaluation and Diagnostic Considerations

Patients with malignant pleural effusions are frequently symptomatic, but up to 25% of patients may be asymptomatic with effusions noted incidentally on a chest radiograph.[6,17] Patients with pleural effusions may complain of cough, shortness of breath, dyspnea on exertion, or chest pain. Dyspnea may be caused by diminished chest wall compliance, decreased lung volumes, diaphragmatic depression, and/or contralateral mediastinal shift.[18] Pleuritic chest pain may indicate involvement of the parietal pleura or direct chest wall involvement by underlying malignancy.[8] As many as a third of patients with malignant pleural effusions present with weight loss and cachexia and appear debilitated by chronic illness.[19] The presence of a malignant pleural effusion usually indicates advanced disease that is incurable with surgery alone.

Physical examination of patients with pleural effusions may reveal diminished breath sounds, pleural rub, dullness on percussion, reduced tactile fremitus, or decreased diaphragmatic excursion. Shift of the trachea or heart sounds to the contralateral side may be present with large effusions.

A chest radiograph is an excellent first test for a patient with a suspected pleural effusion. It can establish the diagnosis of pleural effusion, its size, if there is tracheal or mediastinal shift, and, with a lateral decubitus film, if it is free flowing. Blunting of the costophrenic angle is suggestive of a small pleural effusion and can be present with as little as 200 mL free fluid.[20] Complete opacification of the hemithorax may be present with massive effusions. Large pleural effusions are frequently associated with some contralateral mediastinal shift. When mediastinal shift is absent, it may be due to several reasons: volume loss of the ipsilateral lung secondary to bronchial occlusion or fixation of the mediastinal structures by pleural carcinomatosis/mesothelioma or malignant lymph nodes.[19]

Currently, the most useful radiographic study is a chest computed tomography (CT) scan. CT scans help establish the presence of a loculated pleural effusion, allow for evaluation of the pulmonary parenchyma if there is not complete lung compression, and distinguish pleural thickening from effusion. It also provides an excellent way to evaluate the mediastinum for the presence of masses or lymphadenopathy and permits detection of pleural-based nodules.[21] The role of magnetic resonance imaging (MRI) in the evaluation of pleural effusions is limited, but it may be beneficial in better characterizing possible tumor involvement of the chest wall or diaphragm.[22] Positron emission tomography (PET scan) with ^{18}F-fluorodeoxyglucose provides less anatomic information but has the potential advantage of providing diagnostic information about the effusion. In one study of 35 patients with biopsy-proven lung cancer, PET scans had a sensitivity and specificity of 88.8% and 94.1%, respectively, in distinguishing between benign and malignant pleural effusions.[23] It is our feeling that this information may prove useful, but the true value of a PET scan in this setting would be to provide additional information about disease elsewhere, not to give a diagnosis of malignancy. In addition, treatment of a malignant effusion will depend on the type of cancer, and this cannot be determined with a PET scan.

Once a pleural effusion is documented, diagnostic or therapeutic thoracentesis should be performed to establish the nature of the effusion. Effusions are classified as either exudative or transudative based on established criteria:[24]

1. Ratio of pleural fluid protein to serum protein concentration is greater than 0.5
2. Ratio of pleural fluid lactate dehydrogenase (LDH) to its serum concentration is greater than 0.6
3. LDH concentration in pleural effusion is greater than two-thirds of the upper normal value for the serum LDH

The overall accuracy of these criteria is 93% to 95%.[25,26] Patients with congestive heart failure treated with diuretics, may benefit from pleural fluid cholesterol measurements because the accuracy of Light's criteria is decreased in this setting and transudates can be mistakenly classified as exudates. A pleural cholesterol level greater than 60mg/dL is indicative of an exudate and seems to be independent of the serum level.[27] In addition, the appearance of the fluid, its consistency and color, should be noted. Sanguinous effusions are commonly malignant. Measurements of pleural pH, glucose level, and differential cell count are routinely performed as well. In the absence of esophageal rupture, elevation of amylase and its salivary isotype is associated with lung cancer.[28] A prospective study of 841 patients with pleural effusions evaluated the cause and relative frequency of amylase-rich pleural effusions. High amylase levels were associated with three times the likelihood of finding tumor cells, most frequently, with adenocarcinomas of lung origin.[29]

Pleural effusions are malignant when cancer cells are found on cytologic examination.[30] Malignant pleural effusions may be serous, serosanguineous, or bloody, and usually are exudative in nature,[19] but about 5% to 10% of malignant pleural effusions are transudative. This finding is most commonly seen in patients with underlying conditions that may cause transudative effusions, such as renal failure, congestive heart failure, or early stages of lymphatic or bronchial obstruction.[31]

In addition to classifying pleural effusions as transudative or exudative, specific immunohistochemical tests and tumor markers have been evaluated to aid in the diagnosis of malignant pleural effusions. Immunohistochemical markers, such as anti-CEA, anti-B72.3, and anti-Leu M1, tend to be positive with metastatic adenocarcinoma and negative with either reactive or malignant mesothelial cells. More than 95% of adenocarcinomas are positive for at least two of the three listed antigens.[32] Tumor markers, such as alpha fetoprotein (AFP), CA 19-9, CA 15-3, CYFRA 21-1, and CA 125 have been evaluated, but none has proven reliable to establish the diagnosis of malignant pleural effusion.[33,34]

Cytology establishes the diagnosis of a malignancy in approximately half the patients during first cytologic examination.[35] The yield is increased to 65% to 70% with two subsequent thoracenteses, if examined by an experienced cytopathologist[35–38]; this results in a positive diagnosis in 80% of patients.[39] The type of primary malignancy affects the diagnostic yield of cytology. The diagnosis of adenocarcinomas can be established in nearly all patients, whereas patients with pleural effusions secondary to Hodgkin's disease, have a positive cytologic exam in less than 25% of cases.[15,40–43]

Blind percutaneous pleural biopsy is another method to ascertain the diagnosis of pleural malignancy. It carries an 8% risk of pneumothorax, and adds little to the workup of the patient with suspected malignancy, because fluid cytology is much more sensitive in establishing the diagnosis of malignant pleural effusion. In a series of 118 patients with pleural effusions and negative cytology, closed pleural biopsy established the diagnosis of malignant pleural effusion in only 17% of cases.[35] The low diagnostic yield of closed pleural biopsy in patients with malignant pleural effusions can be explained by the fact that costal pleura is not involved by cancer in about 50% of patients, as initial metastatic disease most commonly occurs on the visceral, mediastinal, and diaphragmatic pleurae.[44]

Video-assisted thoracic surgery (VATS) can be used to investigate the nature of pleural effusions. In a study of 620 patients where VATS was utilized to diagnose the underlying cause of effusion, only 8% percent remained without a diagnosis after the procedure.[45] The advantages of VATS include visually directed and selective biopsies of parietal, mediastinal, and visceral pleura, direct visualization and examination of the entire hemithorax, and simultaneous lung or lymph node biopsy if required. The procedure is well tolerated with less than 1% mortality.[46,47] In addition, VATS provides the ability to divide adhesions and perform pleurodesis at the time of the operation with excellent results.[47] Thoracotomy for diagnostic purposes is almost never indicated, because less invasive methods can provide diagnosis in up to 97% of cases.[48–50]

Management

Once the diagnosis of malignant pleural effusion is established, palliative therapy is usually indicated because life expectancy in these patients is typically limited to a few months.[15,19] Treatment should be directed toward symptomatic relief of dyspnea, control of the effusion, prevention of its recurrence, improvement of performance status, reducing duration and the number of hospitalizations, and patient and

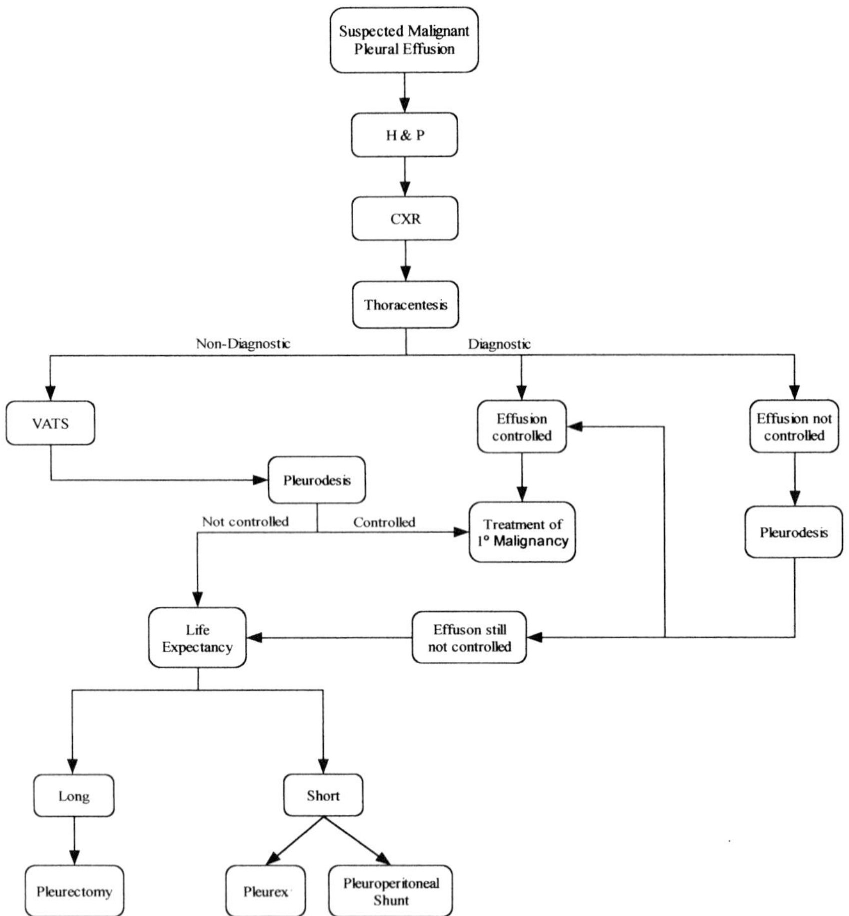

FIGURE 86.1. Algorithm for treatment options for pleural effusion.

family support (Figure 86.1). Prolonged survival has been documented in a few studies, if control of the primary tumor can be achieved.[51] Several options are available to achieve these goals and are summarized in Table 86.1. There is rarely a role for aggressive surgery in these patients outside a protocol setting.

Therapeutic thoracentesis is the first step in the management of patients with symptomatic malignant pleural effu-

TABLE 86.1. Options to prolonged survival if the primary tumor can be controlled.

	Advantages	*Disadvantages*
Thoracentesis	Rapid relief of symptoms, if lung is not trapped Potentially diagnostic Outpatient procedure	High recurrence rate Formation of loculations with repeat procedures
Pleurodesis	60%–93% success rate, based on sclerosant Can be done immediately after drainage, if lung reexpands	Morbidities based on sclerosants (see Table 86.2)
Pleurex catheter	Can be placed as outpatient Can be used with trapped lung Greater than 90% efficacy Up to 46% have spontaneous pleurodesis	10% need to be replaced for either infection or occlusion Risk of nutritional depletion
Pleuroperitoneal shunt	Relatively easy to use Can be used with trapped lung	Up to 15% rate of occlusion or infection Risk of nutritional depletion Pumping transfers only 2 mL fluid per pump; therefore, it is time consuming
VATS with pleurodesis	Directed biopsies provide the highest yield for diagnosis; 93% success rate when combined with pleurodesis	General anesthesia
Pleurectomy	Successful when effusion is refractory to other measures, if lung will reexpand	Painful High morbidity and mortality Very limited indications

VATS, video-assisted thoracic surgery.

sions and can be easily accomplished with a standard central venous line catheter, a commercially available thoracentesis kit, or image-guided drainage. The goal is to determine if drainage of the fluid will improve the patient's breathing. Drainage alone is very unlikely to prevent the recurrence of the effusion.[41,52] Those who demonstrate symptomatic improvement and have reexpansion of the lung should be considered for pleurodesis. For this to be successful, obliteration of the pleural space, creating symphysis between the parietal and visceral pleura, is paramount to prevent the recurrence of the effusion. Although many clinicians believe there must be only minimal drainage to achieve pleurodesis, a randomized trial evaluating the volume of chest tube drainage before pleurodesis, demonstrated that, regardless of the amount of chest tube output, pleurodesis was successful 80% of the time.[53] This approach allows for earlier ambulation, shorter hospitalization, and better cost containment. Pleurodesis is appropriate for all patients with malignant pleural effusions who respond to thoracentesis except, perhaps, those with a life expectancy of less than 1 month.

Since the 1930s, more than 30 sclerosing agents have been evaluated and proved either ineffective, toxic, expensive, or inconvenient and, therefore, are no longer used.[54–56] In 1972, tetracycline was introduced and remained the agent of choice until 1993, when it became unavailable in the United States.[57] Currently, sterile talc, bleomycin, and doxycycline are approved by the U.S. Food and Drug Administration for pleurodesis and are the most commonly used pleurodesing agents in the United States (Table 86.2).[58] There is an ongoing debate about which of these sclerosing agents provides the highest success rate. Multiple studies have shown talc to be effective in up to 93% of the cases, whereas bleomycin has a reported response rate between 60% and 80%. Doxycycline has a similar efficacy when compared to bleomycin.[59–61]

When undergoing pleurodesis, it was previously assumed that patients should remain in bed and be frequently turned from side to side to provide equal dispersion of the sclerosing agent within the pleural space. A randomized trial using radiolabeled talc examined its dispersion and the success rate of pleurodesis in patients who were subjected to a standard turning protocol and those who were not. There was no difference in talc dispersion, and the success rate of pleurodesis for both groups was 85% at 1 month.[62] These data echo animal studies that showed no evidence of improved distribution of pleural injectant with rotation.[63] Based on these studies, it is not recommended that patients be restricted to bed or posturally rotated after pleurodesis. Elimination of these protocols has increased patient comfort and decreased time consumed by medical personnel in turning patients.[64]

Fever and chest pain are the most common side effects of pleurodesis.[60] In addition, talc and bleomycin have been reported to cause acute pneumonitis and acute respiratory distress syndrome.[65–68] A major disadvantage of bleomycin is its cost. Bleomycin costs nearly $1,200 per 60 unit dose, whereas the cost of 500 mg doxycycline is about $75 and that of 4 g talc is less than $5.

Another modality that can be used in the treatment of malignant pleural effusions, with or without pleurodesis, is pleurectomy. Pleurectomy involves removal of the parietal pleura and, if required, decortication of the lung. With pleurectomy, it is possible to control pleural effusions in more than 90% of cases, but with a documented morbidity of 23%, and a mortality of 10%,[20,52,69] there are very limited indications. It has been reported that pleurectomy should be considered in a patient who is undergoing a surgical intervention for undiagnosed pleural effusion and malignant disease is found, or when chemical or mechanical pleurodesis is likely to fail, as in patients with persistent or recurrent pleural effusions and patients with trapped lung.[20] Some authors have stated that pleurectomy should not be undertaken in patients with a poor performance status or an expected survival of less than 6 months.[58] It is our preference that pleurectomy should be employed extremely selectively, either as part of a protocol or in unusual cases where the pleural malignancy has demonstrated a very indolent course but is causing symptoms refractory to other palliative measures.

In some institutions, VATS has become the procedure of choice in the management of patients with malignant pleural effusion, with a reported mortality of less than 1%.[47,70,71] VATS allows for complete evacuation of the pleural fluid, precise biopsies, division of adhesions, implantation of indwelling catheters, mechanical or talc pleurodesis, and parietal pleurectomy. When VATS is combined with a maneuver to obliterate the pleural space, success rates as high as 93% have been reported.[71,72]

An alternative to pleurodesis or pleurectomy is intermittent drainage. In the past, selected patients with malignant pleural effusions were managed by repeated therapeutic thoracentesis for symptomatic relief. The disadvantages of this method include rapid reaccumulation of the pleural effusion, development of intrapleural adhesions, resulting in a trapped lung, risk of infection, and the need for repeating the procedure, sometimes as often as weekly.[41] Analysis of the fluid removed with serial thoracenteses has shown biochemical and cytologic evidence of an increased pleural inflammatory response and could explain the phenomenon of spontaneous pleurodesis and ultimate resolution of the effusion in a small percentage of patients.[73]

TABLE 86.2. Sclerosants.

	Talc	*Doxycycline*	*Bleomycin*
Success rate[60]	93%	60%–80%	50%–60%
Cost	Less than $5 for 4 g	$75 for 500 mg	$1,200 for 60 units
Pain[83–86]	Painful (10%–30%)	Probably most painful (40%–80%)	Least painful (5%–20%)
Fever[84–90]	35%	20%–30%	5%–20%
Morbidities[91]	Empyema, pulmonary edema: less than 5%	None reported in literature	None reported in literature
Mortalities[92,93]	ARDS 1.2%	None reported in literature	Three cases of diffuse alveolar injury

ARDS, acute respiratory distress syndrome.

TABLE 86.3. Phase III randomized trials for treatment of malignant pleural effusion.

Author	*Agents*	*No. of patients*	*Result*
Bayly[94]	TCN vs. quinacrine	20	Equivalence
Fentiman[95]	Nitrogen mustard vs. talc	46	Talc better
Leahy[96]	CP vs. TCN	32	Equivalence
Fentiman[97]	TCN vs. talc	41	Talc better
Kessinger[86]	Bleo vs. TCN	34	Equivalence
Hamed[98]	Bleo vs. talc	29	Talc
Masuno[99]	Doxorubicin vs. doxorubicin and LC 9018	95	Doxorubicin and LC9018 better
Ruckdeschel[100]	Bleo vs. TCN	85	Bleo better
Hartman[59]	Bleo vs. TCN vs. talc	99	Talc better than Bleo better than TCN
Loutsidis[101]	Talc vs. metchlorethamine	40	Talc
Yim[102]	VATS talc vs. talc slurry	57	Equivalence
Emad[103]	Talc vs. Bleo vs. talc and Bleo	60	Talc and Bleo best
Zimmer[104]	Talc slurry vs. Bleo	29	Equivalence
Martinez-Moragon[105]	TCN vs. Bleo	62	Equivalence
Patz[106]	Bleo vs. doxycycline	106	Equivalence
Putnam[79]	Pleurex vs. doxycycline	144	Equivalence
Diacon[89]	VATS talc vs. Bleo	36	VATS talc better
Sartori[107]	Bleo vs. interferon	160	Bleo better

Bleo, bleomycin.

The pleuroperitoneal shunt was introduced in 1982 for the management of pleural effusions.[74] Several series have shown that effective palliation can be achieved in up to 90% of cases.[70,75–77] It is used for patients who have failed pleurodesis or systemic chemotherapy, are not surgical candidates, or have trapped lung. The major disadvantage of the pleuroperitoneal shunt is the length of time required to drain the pleural space. The volume of pumping chamber is only 1.5 to 2mL, which translates into the necessity for frequent and protracted pumping sessions, a major inconvenience for patients. Infection and shunt occlusion are the most common complications, occurring in up to 15% of cases.[78]

Recently, the Pleurex catheter (Denver Biomedical, Golden, CO, USA) was added to the armamentarium for the treatment of symptomatic, recurrent malignant pleural effusions. The catheter is placed into the pleural cavity under either local or general anesthesia, and allows for rapid drainage of pleural fluid by connecting the catheter to a drainage bottle or system as often as necessary to relieve symptoms. Additionally, spontaneous pleurodesis occurs in up to 46% of patients within 1 month of insertion of the catheter.[79] Compared to the pleuroperitoneal shunt, it is possible to drain the effusion quickly, manual pumping is not required, the catheters are well tolerated by the patients, and they are easy to manage by caregivers in outpatient settings. In prospective randomized multiinstitutional trials, the Pleurx catheters have been proved to be safe, practical, and cost-effective.[80,81]

Table 86.3 shows the randomized trials for the management of malignant pleural effusion since 1983. One is struck by the small number of patients in the trials, leading to potentially misleading conclusions based on inadequate power. Nevertheless, it is generally agreed that talc is as good if not better than most agents and has the best cost profile. There does not seem to be an advantage to performing talc poudrage as a VATS procedure. The Pleurex catheter, as already described, however, is becoming increasingly popular for these individuals because of its equivalent performance of effusion management, as well as the minimal toxicity profile and the ability to perform the procedure as an outpatient. There has been some concern in isolated centers about infectious complications with the catheter. Whether a randomized trial of the Pleurex catheter versus talc slurry will be performed is under discussion at a number of institutions.

Summary

Malignant pleural effusions remain a significant cause of morbidity for patients with cancers metastatic to the pleura or primary pleural malignancies. Once the diagnosis of malignant effusion is ascertained, a therapeutic thoracentesis should be performed to provide relief if the patient is symptomatic. If dyspnea resolves, chemical pleurodesis should be considered for permanent control of symptoms. Several methods of pleurodesis are available, and careful patient selection is a prerequisite for successful management. For an effusion that has defied diagnosis, or even as a primary diagnostic procedure, VATS should be considered. This operation can usually be performed through a single "chest tube" incision and can allow unification of the pleural space, complete drainage of the effusion, a diagnostic biopsy, instillation of talc, and accurate chest tube placement. Pleurectomy and/or decortication have a very limited role and should generally be considered in the setting of a protocol. External or internal drainage of effusions are other options, generally considered for patients who have failed pleurodesis. Future investigative efforts should be directed toward improved diagnosis, evaluation of novel immunomodulation methods, gene therapy, and clarification of current management protocols.[82]

References

1. Antony VB, Loddenkemper R, Astoul P, et al. Management of malignant pleural effusions. Eur Respir J 2001;18(2):402–419.
2. Light RW, Erozan YS, Ball WC Jr. Cells in pleural fluid. Their value in differential diagnosis. Arch Intern Med 1973;132(6): 854–860.
3. Marel M, Zrustova M, Stasny B, Light RW. The incidence of pleural effusion in a well-defined region. Epidemiologic study in central Bohemia. Chest 1993;104(5):1486–1489.
4. Belani CP, Pajeau TS, Bennett CL. Treating malignant pleural effusions cost consciously. Chest 1998;113(suppl 1):78S–85S.
5. Fracchia AA, Knapper WH, Carey JT, Farrow JH. Intrapleural chemotherapy for effusion from metastatic breast carcinoma. Cancer (Phila) 1970;26(3):626–629.
6. Chernow B, Sahn SA. Carcinomatous involvement of the pleura: an analysis of 96 patients. Am J Med 1977;63(5):695–702.
7. Meyer PC. Metastatic carcinoma of the pleura. Thorax 1966; 21(5):437–443.
8. Stein PD, Terrin ML, Hales CA, et al. Clinical, laboratory, roentgenographic, and electrocardiographic findings in patients with acute pulmonary embolism and no pre-existing cardiac or pulmonary disease. Chest 1991;100(3):598–603.
9. Albertine KH, Wiener-Kronish JP, Roos PJ, Staub NC. Structure, blood supply, and lymphatic vessels of the sheep's visceral pleura. Am J Anat 1982;165(3):277–294.
10. Lee KF, Olak J. Anatomy and physiology of the pleural space. Chest Surg Clin N Am 1994;4(3):391–403.
11. Staub NC. Lung liquid and protein exchange: the four inhomogeneities. Ann Biomed Eng 1987;15(2):115–126.
12. Miserocchi G. Physiology and pathophysiology of pleural fluid turnover. Eur Respir J 1997;10(1):219–225.
13. Broaddus VC, Wiener-Kronish JP, Staub NC. Clearance of lung edema into the pleural space of volume-loaded anesthetized sheep. J Appl Physiol 1990;68(6):2623–2630.
14. Wang NS. Anatomy and physiology of the pleural space. Clin Chest Med 1985;6(1):3–16.
15. Light RW. Management of pleural effusions. J Formos Med Assoc 2000;99(7):523–531.
16. Moores DW. Management of the malignant pleural effusion. Chest Surg Clin N Am 1994;4(3):481–495.
17. Weick JK, Kiely JM, Harrison EG Jr, Carr DT, Scanlon PW. Pleural effusion in lymphoma. Cancer (Phila) 1973;31(4): 848–853.
18. Estenne M, Yernault JC, De Troyer A. Mechanism of relief of dyspnea after thoracocentesis in patients with large pleural effusions. Am J Med 1983;74(5):813–819.
19. Sahn SA. Malignancy metastatic to the pleura. Clin Chest Med 1998;19(2):351–361.
20. Martini N, Bains M, Beattie E Jr. Indications for pleurectomy in malignant effusion. Cancer (Phila) 1975;35:734–738.
21. Mori K, Hirose T, Machida S, et al. Helical computed tomography diagnosis of pleural dissemination in lung cancer: comparison of thick-section and thin-section helical computed tomography. J Thorac Imaging 1998;13(3):211–218.
22. Marom EM, Erasmus JJ, Pass HI, Patz EF Jr. The role of imaging in malignant pleural mesothelioma. Semin Oncol 2002;29(1): 26–35.
23. Gupta NC, Rogers JS, Graeber GM, et al. Clinical role of F-18 fluorodeoxyglucose positron emission tomography imaging in patients with lung cancer and suspected malignant pleural effusion. Chest 2002;122(6):1918–1924.
24. Light RW, MacGregor MI, Luchsinger PC, Ball WC Jr. Pleural effusions: the diagnostic separation of transudates and exudates. Ann Intern Med 1972;77(4):507–513.
25. Burgess LJ, Maritz FJ, Taljaard JJ. Comparative analysis of the biochemical parameters used to distinguish between pleural transudates and exudates. Chest 1995;107(6):1604–1609.
26. Romero S, Candela A, Martin C, Hernandez L, Trigo C, Gil J. Evaluation of different criteria for the separation of pleural transudates from exudates. Chest 1993;104(2):399–404.
27. Hamm H, Brohan U, Bohmer R, Missmahl HP. Cholesterol in pleural effusions. A diagnostic aid. Chest 1987;92(2):296–302.
28. Light RW. Diagnostic principles in pleural disease. Eur Respir J 1997;10(2):476–481.
29. Villena V, Perez V, Pozo F, et al. Amylase levels in pleural effusions: a consecutive unselected series of 841 patients. Chest 2002;121(2):470–474.
30. Light RW, Rodriguez RM. Management of parapneumonic effusions. Clin Chest Med 1998;19(2):373–382.
31. Ashchi M, Golish J, Eng P, O'Donovan P. Transudative malignant pleural effusions: prevalence and mechanisms. South Med J 1998;91(1):23–26.
32. Brown RW, Clark GM, Tandon AK, Allred DC. Multiple-marker immunohistochemical phenotypes distinguishing malignant pleural mesothelioma from pulmonary adenocarcinoma. Hum Pathol 1993;24(4):347–354.
33. Villena V, Lopez-Encuentra A, Echave-Sustaeta J, Martin-Escribano P, Ortuno-de-Solo B, Estenoz-Alfaro J. Diagnostic value of CA 72-4, carcinoembryonic antigen, CA 15-3, and CA 19-9 assay in pleural fluid. A study of 207 patients. Cancer (Phila) 1996;78(4):736–740.
34. Ferrer J, Villarino MA, Encabo G, et al. Diagnostic utility of CYFRA 21-1, carcinoembryonic antigen, CA 125, neuron specific enolase, and squamous cell antigen level determinations in the serum and pleural fluid of patients with pleural effusions. Cancer (Phila) 1999;86(8):1488–1495.
35. Prakash UB, Reiman HM. Comparison of needle biopsy with cytologic analysis for the evaluation of pleural effusion: analysis of 414 cases. Mayo Clin Proc 1985;60(3):158–164.
36. Jarvi O, Kunnas R, Laitio M, Tyrkko J. The accuracy and significance of cytologic cancer diagnosis of pleural effusions. (A follow-up study of 338 patients.) Acta Cytol 1972;16(2):152–158.
37. Grunze H. Cytologic diagnosis of tumors of the chest. Acta Cytol 1973;17(2):148–159.
38. Dekker A, Bupp P. Cytology of serous effusions. An investigation into the usefulness of cell blocks versus smears. Am J Clin Pathol 1978;70(6):855–860.
39. Hsu C. Cytologic detection of malignancy in pleural effusion: a review of 5,255 samples from 3,811 patients. Diagn Cytopathol 1987;3(1):8–12.
40. Melamed M. The cytological presentation of malignant lymphomas and related disease in effusions. Cancer (Phila) 1963; 16:413–431.
41. Anderson CB, Philpott GW, Ferguson TB. The treatment of malignant pleural effusions. Cancer (Phila) 1974;33(4):916–922.
42. Yousem SA, Weiss LM, Colby TV. Primary pulmonary Hodgkin's disease. A clinicopathologic study of 15 cases. Cancer (Phila) 1986;57(6):1217–1224.
43. Celikoglu F, Teirstein AS, Krellenstein DJ, Strauchen JA. Pleural effusion in non-Hodgkin's lymphoma. Chest 1992;101(5): 1357–1360.
44. Canto A, Rivas J, Saumench J, Morera R, Moya J. Points to consider when choosing a biopsy method in cases of pleurisy of unknown origin. Chest 1983;84(2):176–179.
45. Kendall S, Bryan A, Large S, Wells F. Pleural effusions: is thoracoscopy a reliable investigation? A retrospective review. Respir Med 1992;86(5):437–440.
46. Lewis RJ, Caccavale RJ, Sisler GE, MacKenzie JW. Video-assisted thoracic surgical resection of malignant lung tumors. J Thorac Cardiovasc Surg 1992;104(6):1679–1685; discussion 1685–1687.
47. Cardillo G, Facciolo F, Carbone L, et al. Long-term follow-up of video-assisted talc pleurodesis in malignant recurrent pleural effusions. Eur J Cardiothorac Surg 2002;21(2):302–305; discussion 305–306.

48. Boutin C, Viallat JR, Cargnino P, Farisse P. Thoracoscopy in malignant pleural effusions. Am Rev Respir Dis 1981;124(5): 588–592.
49. Rusch VW, Mountain C. Thoracoscopy under regional anesthesia for the diagnosis and management of pleural disease. Am J Surg 1987;154(3):274–278.
50. Hucker J, Bhatnagar NK, al-Jilaihawi AN, Forrester-Wood CP. Thoracoscopy in the diagnosis and management of recurrent pleural effusions. Ann Thorac Surg 1991;52(5):1145–1147.
51. Osaki T, Sugio K, Hanagiri T, et al. Survival and prognostic factors of surgically resected T4 non-small cell lung cancer. Ann Thorac Surg 2003;75(6):1745–1751; discussion 1751.
52. Grossi F, Pennucci MC, Tixi L, Cafferata MA, Ardizzoni A. Management of malignant pleural effusions. Drugs 1998;55(1): 47–58.
53. Villanueva A, Gray A Jr, Shahian D, Williamson W, Beamis J Jr. Efficacy of short-term versus long-term tube thoracostomy drainage before tetracycline pleurodesis in the treatment of malignant pleural effusions. Thorax 1994;49(1):23–25.
54. Ariel IM, Oropeza R, Pack GT. Intracavitary administration of radioactive isotopes in the control of effusions due to cancer. Results in 267 patients. Cancer (Phila) 1966;19(8):1096–1102.
55. Adler RH, Sayek I. Treatment of malignant pleural effusion: a method using tube thoracostomy and talc. Ann Thorac Surg 1976;22(1):8–15.
56. Austin EH, Flye MW. The treatment of recurrent malignant pleural effusion. Ann Thorac Surg 1979;28(2):190–203.
57. Heffner JE, Unruh LC. Tetracycline pleurodesis. Adios, farewell, adieu. Chest 1992;101(1):5–7.
58. Sahn SA. Management of malignant pleural effusions. Monaldi Arch Chest Dis 2001;56(5):394–399.
59. Hartman D, Gaither J, Kesler K, Mylet D, Brown J, Mathur P. Comparison of insufflated talc under thoracoscopic guidance with standard tetracycline and bleomycin pleurodesis for control of malignant pleural effusions. J Thorac Cardiovasc Surg 1993;105(4):743–747; discussion 747–748.
60. Walker-Renard PB, Vaughan LM, Sahn SA. Chemical pleurodesis for malignant pleural effusions. Ann Intern Med 1994;120(1): 56–64.
61. Aelony Y, King R, Boutin C. Thoracoscopic talc poudrage pleurodesis for chronic recurrent pleural effusions. Ann Intern Med 1991;115(10):778–782.
62. Mager H, Maesen B, Verzijlbergen F, Schramel F. Distribution of talc suspension during treatment of malignant pleural effusion with talc pleurodesis. Lung Cancer 2002;36(1):77–81.
63. Vargas FS, Teixeira LR, Coelho IJ, Braga GA, Terra-Filho M, Light RW. Distribution of pleural injectate. Effect of volume of injectate and animal rotation. Chest 1994;106(4):1246–1249.
64. Lorch DG, Gordon L, Wooten S, Cooper JF, Strange C, Sahn SA. Effect of patient positioning on distribution of tetracycline in the pleural space during pleurodesis. Chest 1988;93(3): 527–529.
65. Kennedy L, Rusch V, Strange C, Ginsberg R, Sahn S. Pleurodesis using talc slurry. Chest 1994;106(2):342–346.
66. Bouchama A, Chastre J, Gaudichet A, Soler P, Gibert C. Acute pneumonitis with bilateral pleural effusion after talc pleurodesis. Chest 1984;86(5):795–797.
67. Rinaldo J, Owens G, Rogers R. Adult respiratory distress syndrome following intrapleural instillation of talc. J Thorac Cardiovasc Surg 1983;85(4):523–526.
68. Audu P, Sing R, Mette S, Fallahnejhad M. Fatal diffuse alveolar injury following use of intrapleural bleomycin. Chest 1993; 103(5):1638.
69. Fry WA, Khandekar JD. Parietal pleurectomy for malignant pleural effusion. Ann Surg Oncol 1995;2(2):160–164.
70. Putnam JB Jr. Malignant pleural effusions. Surg Clin N Am 2002;82(4):867–883.
71. de Campos JR, Vargas FS, de Campos Werebe E, et al. Thoracoscopy talc poudrage: a 15-year experience. Chest 2001;119(3): 801–806.
72. Schulze M, Boehle AS, Kurdow R, Dohrmann P, Henne-Bruns D. Effective treatment of malignant pleural effusion by minimal invasive thoracic surgery: thoracoscopic talc pleurodesis and pleuroperitoneal shunts in 101 patients. Ann Thorac Surg 2001;71(6):1809–1812.
73. Chung CL, Chen YC, Chang SC. Effect of repeated thoracenteses on fluid characteristics, cytokines, and fibrinolytic activity in malignant pleural effusion. Chest 2003;123(4):1188–1195.
74. Weese JL, Schouten JT. Pleural peritoneal shunts for the treatment of malignant pleural effusions. Surg Gynecol Obstet 1982; 154(3):391–392.
75. Petrou M, Kaplan D, Goldstraw P. Management of recurrent malignant pleural effusions. The complementary role of talc pleurodesis and pleuroperitoneal shunting. Cancer (Phila) 1995;75(3):801–805.
76. Cimochowski GE, Joyner LR, Fardin R, Sarama R, Maran A. Pleuroperitoneal shunting for recalcitrant pleural effusions. J Thorac Cardiovasc Surg 1986;92(5):866–870.
77. Lee KA, Harvey JC, Reich H, Beattie EJ. Management of malignant pleural effusions with pleuroperitoneal shunting. J Am Coll Surg 1994;178(6):568–586.
78. Ponn RB, Blancaflor J, D'Agostino RS, Kiernan ME, Toole AL, Stern H. Pleuroperitoneal shunting for intractable pleural effusions. Ann Thorac Surg 1991;51(4):605–609.
79. Putnam JB Jr, Light RW, Rodriguez RM, et al. A randomized comparison of indwelling pleural catheter and doxycycline pleurodesis in the management of malignant pleural effusions. Cancer (Phila) 1999;86(10):1992–1999.
80. Putnam JB Jr, Walsh GL, Swisher SG, et al. Outpatient management of malignant pleural effusion by a chronic indwelling pleural catheter. Ann Thorac Surg 2000;69(2):369–375.
81. Ohm C, Park D, Vogen M, et al. Use of an indwelling pleural catheter compared with thorascopic talc pleurodesis in the management of malignant pleural effusions. Am Surg 2003; 69(3):198–202; discussion 202.
82. American Thoracic Society. Management of malignant pleural effusions. Am J Respir Crit Care Med 2000;162(5):1987–2001.
83. Herrington JD, Gora-Harper ML, Salley RK. Chemical pleurodesis with doxycycline 1 g. Pharmacotherapy 1996;16(2): 280–285.
84. Ostrowski MJ, Halsall GM. Intracavitary bleomycin in the management of malignant effusions: a multicenter study. Cancer Treat Rep 1982;66(11):1903–1907.
85. Brant A, Eaton T. Serious complications with talc slurry pleurodesis. Respirology 2001;6(3):181–185.
86. Kessinger A, Wigton RS. Intracavitary bleomycin and tetracycline in the management of malignant pleural effusions: a randomized study. J Surg Oncol 1987;36(2):81–83.
87. Ong KC, Indumathi V, Raghuram J, Ong YY. A comparative study of pleurodesis using talc slurry and bleomycin in the management of malignant pleural effusions. Respirology 2000;5(2): 99–103.
88. Pulsiripunya C, Youngchaiyud P, Pushpakom R, Maranetra N, Nana A, Charoenratanakul S. The efficacy of doxycycline as a pleural sclerosing agent in malignant pleural effusion: a prospective study. Respirology 1996;1(1):69–72.
89. Diacon AH, Wyser C, Bolliger CT, et al. Prospective randomized comparison of thoracoscopic talc poudrage under local anesthesia versus bleomycin instillation for pleurodesis in malignant pleural effusions. Am J Respir Crit Care Med 2000;162(4 pt 1): 1445–1449.
90. Ostrowski MJ, Priestman TJ, Houston RF, Martin WM. A randomized trial of intracavitary bleomycin and *Corynebacterium parvum* in the control of malignant pleural effusions. Radiother Oncol 1989;14(1):19–26.

91. Viallat JR, Rey F, Astoul P, Boutin C. Thoracoscopic talc poudrage pleurodesis for malignant effusions. A review of 360 cases. Chest 1996;110(6):1387–1393.
92. Campos JR, Werebe EC, Vargas FS, Jatene FB, Light RW. Respiratory failure due to insufflated talc. Lancet 1997; 349(9047):251–252.
93. Schafers SJ, Dresler CM. Update on talc, bleomycin, and the tetracyclines in the treatment of malignant pleural effusions. Pharmacotherapy 1995;15(2):228–235.
94. Bayly TC, Kisner DL, Sybert A, MacDonald JS, Tsou E, Schein PS. Tetracycline and quinacrine in the control of malignant pleural effusions. A randomized trial. Cancer (Phila) 1978;41: 1188–1192.
95. Fentiman IS, Rubens RD, Hayward JL. Control of pleural effusions in patients with breast cancer. A randomized trial. Cancer (Phila) 1983;52:737–739.
96. Leahy BC, Honeybourne D, Brear SG, Carroll KB, Thatcher N, Stretton TB. Treatment of malignant pleural effusions with intrapleural *Corynebacterium parvum* or tetracycline, Eur J Respir Dis 1985;66:50–54.
97. Fentiman IS, Rubens RD, Hayward JL. A comparison of intracavitary talc and tetracycline for the control of pleural effusions secondary to breast cancer. Eur J Cancer Clin Oncol 1986;22: 1079–1081.
98. Hamed H, Fentiman IS, Chaudary MA, Rubens RD. Comparison of intracavitary bleomycin and talc for control of pleural effusions secondary to carcinoma of the breast. Br J Surg 1989;76:1266–1267.
99. Masuno T, Kishimoto S, Ogura T, et al. A comparative trial of LC9018 plus doxorubicin and doxorubicin alone for the treatment of malignant pleural effusion secondary to lung cancer. Cancer (Phila) 1991;68:1495–1500.
100. Ruckdeschel JC, Moores D, Lee JY, et al. Intrapleural therapy for malignant pleural effusions. A randomized comparison of bleomycin and tetracycline. Chest 1991;100:1528–1535.
101. Loutsidis A, Bellenis I, Argiriou M, Exarchos N. Tetracycline compared with mechlorethamine in the treatment of malignant pleural effusions. A randomized trial. Respir Med 1994;88: 523–526.
102. Yim AP, Chan AT, Lee TW, Wan IY, Ho JK. Thoracoscopic talc insufflation versus talc slurry for symptomatic malignant pleural effusion. Ann Thorac Surg 1996;62:1655–1658.
103. Emad A, Rezaian GR. Treatment of malignant pleural effusions with a combination of bleomycin and tetracycline. A comparison of bleomycin or tetracycline alone versus a combination of bleomycin and tetracycline. Cancer (Phila) 1996;78:2498–2501.
104. Zimmer PW, Hill M, Casey K, Harvey E, Low DE. Prospective randomized trial of talc slurry vs. bleomycin in pleurodesis for symptomatic malignant pleural effusions. Chest 1997;112: 430–434.
105. Martinez-Moragon E, Aparicio J, Rogado MC, Sanchis J, Sanchis F, Gil-Suay V. Pleurodesis in malignant pleural effusions: a randomized study of tetracycline versus bleomycin. Eur Respir J 1997;10:2380–2383.
106. Patz EF Jr, McAdams HP, Erasmus JJ, et al. Sclerotherapy for malignant pleural effusions: a prospective randomized trial of bleomycin vs. doxycycline with small-bore catheter drainage. Chest 1998;113:1305–1311.
107. Sartori S, Tassinari D, Ceccotti P, et al. Prospective randomized trial of intrapleural bleomycin versus interferon alfa-2b via ultrasound-guided small-bore chest tube in the palliative treatment of malignant pleural effusions. J Clin Oncol 2004;22:1228–1233.

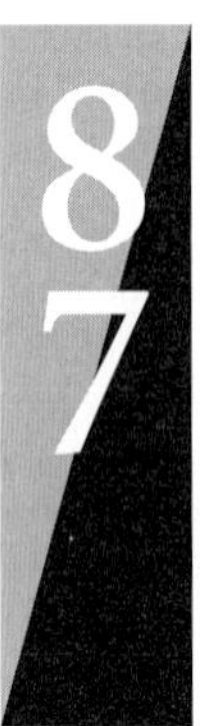

Evidence-Based Use of Hematopoietic Growth Factors for Optimal Supportive Care of Patients with Cancer

George D. Demetri

Hematopoiesis, the production and maintenance of blood elements, is critical to life. Many of the complications of cancer and anticancer therapies can be clinically damaging to patients as a result of adverse effects on normal hematopoietic mechanisms. Since the early 1990s, it has been possible for physicians to intervene with genetically engineered biotherapies, such as hematopoietic growth factors to mitigate the hematopoietic dysfunction of cancer patients.[1–4] In this chapter, the evidence is examined upon which physicians and other caregivers may base rational clinical decision making to provide patients with optimal supportive care to improve the hematopoietic problems associated with cancer.

Mechanisms and Differential Diagnosis of Cancer-Associated Hematopoietic Dysfunction

Cancer and its treatment may alter normal blood cell production, either by direct effects on hematopoietic stem and progenitor cells or by indirect mechanisms, such as inadequate nutritional status. The physical interactions in the marrow microenvironment among hematopoietic cells, microvascular endothelial cells, and connective tissue stromal cells, can be disrupted by hematologic cancers or metastatic solid tumor cells, leading to abnormal function. The anemia of cancer is a remarkably common feature of many diseases, likely representing a form of the complex syndrome known as the anemia of chronic disease. One of the most common causes of hematopoietic dysfunction in patients with cancer is iatrogenic, as a side effect of the cytotoxic therapies commonly used to treat many malignancies. Many variables can determine the hematopoietic impact of anticancer therapy, such as (i) the cytotoxic insult itself (e.g., chemotherapies with various mechanisms or radiation therapy), (ii) the doses and duration of therapy administered, and (iii) host factors reflecting variables, such as nutritional adequacy and marrow functional reserve.

An understanding of the normal physiologic function of the hematopoietic elements can help explain the negative impact of cytotoxic therapies and can also allow physicians to predict how hematopoietic cytokines can mitigate the damage from such factors. Bone marrow "stem cells" generally exist in a relatively inactive, nonproliferative state. Selective expansion of a few clones of stem cells leads to a sizeable marrow-based compartment of proliferating cells at various stages of differentiation. This proliferative compartment of progenitor cells can supply the mature elements of the peripheral blood for up to 8 to 10 days after a cytotoxic insult; this can explain the delayed nadirs seen with most cytotoxic chemotherapy treatments, with repopulation of the cycling progenitor cell compartment ultimately leading to full recovery of normal blood cell levels.

The timing of hematopoietic dysfunction may vary depending on the mechanism of action of the chemotherapy, because cell-cycle-active agents affect the proliferating progenitor pool, whereas "stem cell poisons" (G_0 active agents, such as BCNU and busulfan) typically cause a much more delayed nadir and recovery (e.g., occurring 4 to 6 weeks after drug administration). The adverse impact of radiation on hematopoiesis will also vary based on the amount of radiation (dose and size of the irradiated field) as well as the duration of exposure.

It is essential to keep in mind the numerous derangements in normal physiology that may occur in the setting of cancer and/or cytotoxic treatment and which may contribute to pancytopenia. These factors may include deficiencies or lack or bioavailability of nutritional factors, such as folate, iron, or other vitamins. There may be abnormal regulatory mechanisms in hematopoiesis, such as cell-mediated suppression of hematopoiesis in aplastic anemia,[5] the blunted response to erythropoietin with anemia in cancer patients,[6] or the stimulation of thrombopoiesis associated with iron deficiency anemia. Marrow fibrosis and stromal damage can occur either as part of a disease process or as a reaction to therapy, thereby compromising bone marrow reserve and function. Immunologically mediated destruction of cells, as well as other factors, such as splenomegaly, can result in clinically significant cytopenias. Most importantly, occult bleeding must always be considered in the differential diagnosis of persistent anemia and refractory thrombocytopenia. These clinical examples emphasize the importance of assessing cancer patients carefully for reversible medical etiologies of their hematologic complications before attributing these effects to the underlying neoplasms as a diagnosis of exclusion.

Hematopoietic Dysfunction by Cell Lineage

Leukopenias and the Risk of Fatal Infections or Other Adverse Outcomes

Cancer and the nonspecific cytotoxic approaches to treating cancers commonly result in abnormally low levels of white blood cells, leaving the patient vulnerable to an increased risk of infection. The immunocompromised status of leukopenic cancer patients has been recognized since the mid-1960s, when Hersh et al.[7] and Bodey et al.[8] reported that leukemia patients treated at the National Cancer Institute, had a significant risk of fatal infections, especially marked with lower levels of circulating leukocytes. Both the severity and duration of leukopenia were noted to be key variables which defined the risk of these immunocompromised cancer patients for fatal outcomes from the infections. This work has served as the basis for the subsequent evolution of clinical management of leukopenic cancer patients.

Patients with leukemias generally have more severe leukopenia that extends for a longer period of time than patients with common solid tumors, such as cancers of the prostate, gastrointestinal tract, breast, or lung. Nonetheless, the relationship between leukopenia and risk of fatal outcome has been assumed to be essentially the same in patients with leukemias, as well as those with solid tumors despite the shorter duration of risk in the latter group. This raises the issue of whether all cancer patients really are equally at risk for adverse outcomes from leukopenia. Clinical predictive models have been developed and tested by investigators, such as Talcott et al.[9] and Klastersky et al.,[10] in an effort to identify key clinical criteria that would reliably predict subsequent outcomes at the time a patient presents with fever and neutropenia, but these models have not been widely applied in practice. Cancer patients differ broadly, from young, otherwise healthy individuals with sarcomas and germ cell tumors, to frail elderly patients with multiple coexisting medical problems and multiorgan dysfunction. These individual patient-specific differences can also change the risks of leukopenia markedly. The risk of even a single patient having an adverse or fatal outcome from a potentially treatable infectious event has led to a widespread conservativism in this field, with conventional supportive care generally based on the administration of empiric broad-spectrum antibiotics, often with hospitalization. Research in this field has also been challenging because large numbers of very heterogeneous patients are required to assess rare events: the incidence of fatal complications of leukopenia has, thankfully, been very low in most clinical trials over the past two decades. Reducing iatrogenic morbidity, such as hospitalization and potential toxicities of nephrotoxic antibiotics, is a reasonable goal to justify the use of hematopoietic growth factors; the costs of inpatient hospitalizations and other expensive interventions also may be sufficiently high to serve as an alternative rationale to change practice.

Leukopenia may also affect clinical outcomes for cancer patients in other indirect ways. The safe administration of cytotoxic chemotherapy is dependent upon a functional immune system, most often measured by the level of circulating neutrophils. In the setting of severe neutropenia, chemotherapy administration may be delayed or reduced to subtherapeutic doses. The impact of inadequate chemotherapy dosing may be particularly acute with malignancies in which chemotherapy is highly effective, such as patients with lymphomas[11] or even in the adjuvant therapy of breast cancer.[12] The importance of chemotherapy dose and schedule remains an area of active clinical investigation for many malignancies, and the availability of hematopoietic growth factor support has allowed many clinical trials to answer novel questions about dose and schedule of myelotoxic therapies.

Applications of Hematopoietic Growth Factors to Neutropenia

Table 87.1 lists the bioengineered human hematopoietic growth factors that are currently approved by the U.S. Food and Drug Administration (FDA) for clinical use. These agents have been widely adopted as a standard of practice in many clinical settings. However, the substantial costs of these agents as supportive care for patients receiving myelosuppressive chemotherapy makes it imperative to understand the benefits and limitations of the evidence, as well as to identify the optimal settings in which their use can make a significant difference in patient outcomes.

A more detailed review of recommendations for the use of the hematopoietic growth factors that act to mitigate leukopenia has been prepared by a clinical practice guidelines subcommittee of the American Society of Clinical Oncology (ASCO). These guidelines for the use of "colony-stimulating factors (CSFs)" were initially developed in 1994 and have subsequently been updated biennially.[13–16] The ASCO guidelines were developed to encourage best practice, specifically, to encourage evidence-based use of CSFs in situations where efficacy was well documented, and also to discourage inappropriate use when no meaningful improvements in clinical outcomes were expected. These clinical practice guidelines have been published[13–16] and can be accessed easily at the official Web site of ASCO (www.asco.org).

The first hematopoietic growth factors with the ability to increase the levels of circulating neutrophils to be tested in the clinic were granulocyte colony-stimulating factor (G-CSF) and granulocyte-macrophage colony-stimulating factor (GM-CSF). These agents proved remarkably effective in increasing the circulating levels of leukocytes, particularly neutrophils,[1–4,17–20] even in the earliest stages of clinical testing. Administration of pharmacologic doses of these recombinant molecules was well tolerated overall: dose-limiting toxicities at very high doses of GM-CSF were identified as

TABLE 87.1. Hematopoietic growth factors commercially available for oncology indications in the United States.

Growth factor	*Generic name*	*Trade name*	*Distributor(s)/ manufacturer(s)*	*Indication(s)*
G-CSF	Filgrastim	Neupogen	Amgen	Cancer patients receiving myelosuppressive chemotherapy Patients with nonmyeloid malignancy following progenitor/stem cell transplantation For mobilization of PBPCs Patients with severe cyclic/chronic neutropenia Following induction chemotherapy in AML
Pegylated G-CSF	Pegfilgrastim	Neulasta	Amgen	Cancer patients receiving myelosuppressive chemotherapy
GM-CSFs	Argramostim	Leukine	Berlex	Following autologous or allogeneic progenitor/stem cell transplantation engraftment delay or failure following autologous progenitor/stem cell transplantation Following induction chemotherapy in older patients with AML Allogeneic stem cell transplantation For mobilization of PBPCs
EPO	Epoietin alfa	Procrit	Ortho Biotech	Anemia in patients with nonmyeloid malignancies receiving chemotherapy
NESP	Darbepoietin alfa	Aranesp	Amgen	Anemia in patients with nonmyeloid malignancies receiving chemotherapy
IL-11	Oprelvekin	Neumega	Wyeth	Mitigation of thrombocytopenia following myelosuppressive chemotherapy in patients with nonmyeloid malignancy who are at high risk of severe thrombocytopenia

AML, acute myelogenous leukemia; G-CSF, granulocyte colony-stimulating factor; EPO, erythropoietin; PBPC, peripheral blood progenitor cell.

pleuropericarditis, capillary leak, and venous thromboses, whereas clinical activity was clearly documented at doses far below the high doses associated with these adverse effects.[21] Interestingly, no true dose-limiting toxicities have ever been described for G-CSF, even at massive doses (e.g., greater than 100μg/kg/day) higher than one would ever use in the clinic.[18,22,23]

G-CSF was first approved by the FDA in 1991, which gave it a very broad indication for commercial distribution and clinical application: reducing the incidence of febrile neutropenia in cancer patients with nonmyeloid malignancies receiving any sort of myelosuppressive chemotherapy. GM-CSF received a more narrow FDA approval in 1991, which limited the initial therapeutic indication to accelerating the hematopoietic recover, of patients with nonmyeloid malignancies undergoing autologous bone marrow transplantation (BMT). However, since the initial FDA approval, the clinical indications for GM-CSF have been expanded to include other indications, such as accelerating the recovery from myelosuppression in patients with leukemia who are undergoing induction chemotherapy, as well as indications in other transplantation-related settings.

A new formulation of G-CSF has been developed to modify the pharmacology of the recombinant protein. Pegylated G-CSF (pegfilgrastim) has a longer circulating half-life due to the pegylation of the protein backbone of the molecule, allowing a single injection per chemotherapy cycle to suffice, rather than the multiple daily injections required of unmodified G-CSF or GM-CSF. The convenience of this agent has driven its rapid acceptance by physicians and patients, and the safety and efficacy profile appears to justify the utility of this agent as equally effective as multiple daily doses of G-CSF. However, because a single dose of pegfilgrastim is the pharmacodynamic equivalent of G-CSF given in multiple doses, there may still be clinical indications for G-CSF, such as in the support of less intensive or more frequent chemotherapy where more flexibility of hematopoietic support would be desired. The decision about whether to use filgrastim or pegfilgrastim is a complex one that must therefore, take into account the expected number of days for which hematopoietic support would be needed. In general, if approximately 7 or more days of filgrastim would be required, pegfilgrastim would be a reasonable agent to use for patient convenience. However, if frequent dosing or complex dosing schedules are required, filgrastim may offer the needed flexibility to avoid the concurrent administration of cell-cycle-active cytotoxics with CSF dosing. Concurrent dosing of CSF with chemotherapy may result in excessively severe myelosuppression, as the hematopoietic progenitors are shifted into proliferation at the same time that high levels of cytotoxic drug circulate in the patient.

Defining the Indication for Neutrophil-Stimulating Hematopoietic Growth Factors

Clinicians may be faced with several situations in which hematopoietic stimulation of neutrophil production might be advantageous for the patient. Broadly defined, the two major settings can be classified as either *prophylactic use* or *therapeutic use*. Prophylactic use of hematopoietic growth factors is defined as the use of an agent to prevent or minimize neutropenia that could be therapeutically detrimental (e.g., to prevent fever with neutropenia or other infections, or to allow continued dosing of chemotherapy on a specific dosing schedule). Prophylaxis is further subcategorized into *primary* or *secondary* prophylaxis. Primary prophylaxis is the setting in which patients who have never previously suffered any infectious episode (i.e., no prior fever or infectious episode during neutropenia) receive hematopoietic growth factor dosing in an effort to prevent any future occurrence. Secondary prophylaxis is defined as administering hematopoietic growth factor to a patient who previously experienced some infectious complication (e.g., prior episode of fever with neutropenia), with the goal of preventing recurrent episodes of any infectious complication. The therapeutic use of hematopoietic growth factors may be defined as the administration of these agents to a patient once an infection or infectious complication is actively in progress, especially in the absence of prior prophylactic use of the agent (e.g., attempting to minimize the duration of ongoing fever with neutropenia).

Evidence Supporting the Use of Hematopoietic Growth Factors as Primary Prophylaxis

Extensive data from well-designed prospective randomized studies[24,25] support the use of hematopoietic growth factors to minimize the risks of aggressively dosed cytotoxic chemotherapy to patients with cancer. Both the incidence and the duration of myelotoxicity have consistently been documented to be improved with the support of CSFs. A meta-analysis of eight randomized controlled trials that tested primary prophylaxis with CSFs in a range of malignancies treated with aggressively dosed chemotherapy regimens, supported the finding that primary prophylaxis could be quite effective at minimizing toxicities, with a reduction in the risk of fever with neutropenia [odds ratio (OR) = 0.38), fewer documented infections (OR = 0.51), and less infection-related mortality (OR = 0.60).[26] Similar benefits have been noted with a single injection of the longer-acting pegylated form of G-CSF as with multiple daily injections of G-CSF.[27,28]

The costs of CSF support have driven much debate about the appropriate utilization of these agents. Previous editions of the ASCO CSF Practice Guidelines have emphasized that the expected incidence of fever with neutropenia or other expected complications would have to be 40% or more to justify the costs of CSF administration as primary prophylaxis. However, more recent data have noted that CSF support can be effective also in decreasing the incidence of infectious complications of chemotherapy, such as fever with neutropenia, in clinical settings where the expected risk is approximately 20%.[29] Despite the fact that the expected cost of CSF support is in the range of US $2,800 per cycle, there are economic analyses that suggest that primary prophylaxis can be economically justified and favorable (given the alternative costs of inpatient hospitalization and management of infectious morbidity) for patients in whom the expected risk of fever with neutropenia exceeds 20% per cycle.[30,31] It is noteworthy that, for many chemotherapy regimens in standard practice, the incidence of fever with neutropenia or other infectious complications, remains less than 10%. Therefore, for most chemotherapy regimens, the use of CSF support as primary prophylaxis is generally neither required nor suggested by the ASCO Guidelines. However, it is also important to note that there may, nonetheless, be advantages to the use of primary CSF prophylaxis in certain special populations, including the frail elderly with multiple comorbid diseases, patients with past history of serious infection, patients with bulky or very symptomatic disease with poor performance status or organ dysfunction, and others. Medical judgment should always be used in assessing the relative risks of chemotherapy in any given patient.

Although other clinical strategies also may be used in place of CSF support as primary prophylaxis, none are particularly relevant for broad use. Chemotherapy dose reduction is probably the most widely used technique to minimize chemotherapy toxicity in the first cycle of administration, but this could conceivably compromise therapeutic outcomes. The use of prophylactic oral antibiotics has been tested with varying success, but this strategy induces other toxicities [including gastrointestinal (GI) toxicities and rash from the antibiotics] and may facilitate the development of antibiotic-resistant organisms. Based on these concerns, the Infectious Disease Society of America has recommended against the routine use of antibiotics such as fluoroquinolones as prophylaxis of chemotherapy-associated infections.[32]

The initial registration trial for GM-CSF used that agent to accelerate hematopoietic recovery from high-dose chemoradiotherapy with autologous bone marrow transplantation. To date, this agent has not been formally approved by the FDA for use in the broader context of chemotherapy-induced myelosuppression outside of transplantation or aggressive chemotherapy for acute leukemias.

Special Cases of "Prophylaxis"

Use of CSF Support to Deliver High-Dose or More Frequent ("Dose Dense") Chemotherapy

Traditional schedules of administration for many cytotoxic chemotherapy agents were generally developed in the era before the availability of CSF support. The "cycling" of chemotherapy was designed to induce damage to tumor (along with the hematopoietic and mucosal pools of stem and progenitor cells) with subsequent recovery of normal hematopoietic and mucosal elements, but with less recovery of malignant cells. Although preclinical models have demonstrated a steep dose–response relationship for many chemotherapy agents, these findings have generally failed to translate into meaningful clinical benefits for most common solid tumors. In the adjuvant systemic therapy of breast cancer, for example, improvements can be demonstrated for delivering standard versus substandard doses, although higher delivered doses requiring CSF support do not appear to result in major additional benefits.[33,34] In a large number of clinical trials for solid tumors, administration of higher doses of chemotherapy with CSF support has failed to result in major improvements in clinical outcomes, although toxicities and costs have increased along with the doses. However, modest increases in "dose density" (defined as increasing drug delivery per unit time) have been more tolerable and may be associated with improved outcomes in some studies.[12] A judicious recommendation would be to consider as investigational the use of CSF support to increase chemotherapy doses above "conventional levels" unless well-designed prospective trials have confirmed the benefits in meaningful clinical outcomes of this approach.

Use of CSF Support for Patients Undergoing High-Dose Chemotherapy or Chemoradiotherapy with Stem Cell Transplantation

CSF support is critical to enable the modern approach to hematopoietic cell transplantation, both autologous transplantation of peripheral blood progenitor cells as well as conventional allogeneic marrow transplantation. The use of CSFs in the autologous setting is at least twofold: first, to mobilize the circulation of high numbers of hematopoietic stem and progenitor cells into the bloodstream where they can be collected for subsequent transplantation use, and second, to stimulate the hematopoietic functions (proliferation and differentiation) of the transplanted stem and progenitor cells. The use of a CSF (either G-CSF or GM-CSF) in the setting of hematopoietic stem cell transplantation is generally considered a standard of care for these procedures associated with prolonged myelosuppression.[13–16]

Use of CSF Support for Patients with Acute Leukemia Undergoing Aggressive Induction Chemotherapy

Several studies worldwide have evaluated the use of CSF support to mitigate the enormous and expected myelotoxicity of induction chemotherapy for acute leukemias [both acute lymphocytic leukemia (ALL) and acute myeloid leukemia (AML)]. The results of these studies have shown that there is no major impact on the CSF support with regard to the malignant leukemic clones: no major impact to improve or reduce the incidence or duration of remissions has been observed. This finding is in many ways reassuring: there is no apparent antiapoptotic effect on the leukemic clones that might lead to an adverse impact on survival in these clinical trials. In fact, although there is no overall impact on survival, there does appear to be some modest ability of CSF support to decrease the lengthy inpatient hospitalizations that characterize the induction therapy for acute leukemias. These benefits might be justifiable purely on the basis of cost-saving, and certainly on the basis of allowing these patients more time out of hospital, with expected improvements in their function and quality of life,[35] as would be particularly true for elderly patients or those with poor performance status. Again, patient-specific variables are best applied to this important therapeutic decision.

In the setting of pediatric leukemias, especially ALL, extreme caution is warranted in the use of CSF as supportive care because this is a situation in which high levels of cure are expected. Although CSF support can improve certain acute toxicities, such as duration of neutropenia and hospitalization,[36] there may also be a higher risk of subsequent secondary myeloid leukemias or myelodysplastic marrow failures.[37] Based on this potential risk, the routine use of CSF support for pediatric patients with ALL treated with curative intent, generally has not been recommended.

Evidence Supporting the Use of Hematopoietic Growth Factors as Secondary Prophylaxis

Once a patient experiences an infectious complication of chemotherapy, such as fever with neutropenia, that patient is at increased risk of subsequent recurrences of infectious episodes. Hematopoietic growth factor support may decrease the risk of subsequent infectious complications if given prophylactically after chemotherapy ("secondary prophylaxis"). Analyses of the placebo-controlled trials of G-CSF support for patients receiving chemotherapy provided data that secondary prophylaxis can effectively decrease the risk of subsequent myelotoxicity from chemotherapy.[24,26,29] An alternative approach, of course, might be to reduce the doses of chemotherapy administered, and no trial to date has proven that the "full dose, on time" strategy (with CSF support) leads to significant improvements in meaningful patient outcomes, such as overall survival, progression-free survival, or improved patient-reported quality of life. However, these hypotheses have not been fully tested in appropriately powered trials, and there may be some effect of dose and schedule on survival outcomes, especially for patients with very chemosensitive diseases, such as lymphomas or adjuvant breast cancer in which curative intent is being pursued.[11,33] Therefore, medical judgment and specific clinical details are critical to guide practice regarding the choice between dose reduction, CSF support, or possibly both in highly compromised patients treated for palliation.

Evidence Supporting the Therapeutic Use of Hematopoietic Growth Factors

Although the foregoing studies evaluated the prophylactic use of CSF support, another logical option might be to treat only that subset of patients who suffer an active infectious episode once it has already occurred (so-called therapeutic intent). Multiple studies have been performed in this setting. Overall, the data suggest that, although there may be limited clinical benefit to this approach in certain patient subsets, the total benefit appeared to be less than if the CSF support were to have been used as prophylaxis.[38] Several reviews have summarized the results of many trials testing whether therapeutic application of CSF support during a period of fever with neutropenia would result in improved clinical outcomes.[39,40] Although some marginal decrease in the duration of hospitalization was occasionally reported, overall there have not been major differences in the outcomes of patients who did or did not receive CSF support during hospitalizations for fever with neutropenia. It is again important to note that selected subsets of very high risk patients may nonetheless obtain benefit from the judicious use of CSF given with therapeutic intent in addition to standard antibiotics and supportive care. Predictive features of patients at very high risk for adverse outcomes during an episode of fever with neutropenia include such variables as the severity of neutropenia (e.g., fewer than 1,000 neutrophils/mL), the expected duration of neutropenia (with more than 7 days being an adverse prognostic indicator), poor performance status with sepsis features, and multiorgan dysfunction.[9,10] Physicians must take all this into account when deciding whether therapeutic use of CSF support is indicated for any given patient presenting with an infectious complication of chemotherapy.

One area in which there is definitive evidence against the use of CSF support is in the setting of asymptomatic neutropenia without fever. In this setting, a randomized prospective clinical trial has definitively shown that there is no impact on clinical outcomes from the administration of CSF support to improve neutrophil levels in the absence of clinical problems.[41] There is no reason to give CSF support to patients simply because of asymptomatic low neutrophil counts.

Special Cases of "Therapeutic Intent": Use of CSF Support for Patients with Myelodysplastic Syndromes or Congenital Neutropenias

In patients with myelodysplastic syndromes (MDS) and other rare congenital neutropenias (such as cyclic neutropenias), marrow failure can lead to chronic or intermittent neutropenia, with occasional clinical problems of recurrent or severe infections. In these situations, intermittent dosing of CSF support may help alleviate the problems. In the case of cyclic neutropenia, intermittent dosing with G-CSF can effectively eliminate clinical problems with this disease.[42] For other forms of MDS, intermittent dosing with CSF support may be appropriate, with the caveat that there are still no definitive data about whether CSF stimulation might accelerate further malignant transformation of the abnormal clones in MDS and lead to more rapid onset of secondary leukemias.

Dosing of Myeloid CSFs

The conventional dosing of G-CSF (filgrastim) is on a flat daily dose scale (5µg/kg/day), administered subcutaneously, beginning approximately 24 hours after the last dose of chemotherapy and continuing until hematologic recovery (generally defined as a peripheral neutrophil count of 2,000–3,000 cells/µL). Dosing for pegfilgrastim is also on a flat basis, given as a single dose of 6mg subcutaneously, approximately 24 hours after the last dose of chemotherapy. Dosing of GM-CSF (sargramostim) is recommended to be based on patient size, given as 250µg/m^2/day, subcutaneously, approximately 24 hours after the last dose of chemotherapy. Higher doses of G-CSF (10µg/kg/day) are used generally for mobilization of peripheral blood progenitor/stem cells in patients preparing for transplant procedures.

Toxicities of Myeloid Hematopoietic Growth Factors

All genetically engineered versions of myeloid CSFs (G-CSF, pegylated G-CSF, and GM-CSF) have been remarkably well-tolerated agents overall, based on extensive clinical experience with these agents over the past 15 years. Nonetheless, as for any drug, certain side effects have been noted occasionally.

Bone Pain

The most common side effect observed with the use of G-CSF is mild to moderate bone pain, which typically occurs in the marrow-containing bones (such as the lower back, pelvis, or sternum) in about one-third of treated patients. Bone pain is usually noted at the initiation of G-CSF therapy or at the early phases of neutrophil recovery. Rarely, the pain can be severe and may even require analgesics for control. The pegylated version of G-CSF (pegfilgrastim) appears to have somewhat less prominent bone pain associated with its use. Bone pain has also been reported with GM-CSF, although it seems less pronounced with that agent.

Laboratory Abnormalities

Laboratory abnormalities observed with the rise in white blood cell (WBC) count that occurs during CSF administration, include elevations in serum lactate dehydrogenase (LDH), uric acid, and alkaline phosphatase levels (from leukocyte alkaline phosphatase sources).

Uncommon Side Effects

Uncommon side effects associated with the use of G-CSF include stimulation of preexisting psoriasis, Sweet's syndrome (neutrophilic dermatitis), and cutaneous vasculitis. Chronic administration of G-CSF to patients with congenital or idiopathic neutropenia has been associated with splenomegaly, which could be dangerous in the case of traumatic rupture. Less frequently observed side effects associated with the use of GM-CSF, include diarrhea, anorexia, facial flushing, dyspnea, and edema. Other side effects that have been reported with the older *Escherichia coli*-derived version of GM-CSF, such as the first-dose phenomenon (hypoxemia within minutes of taking the first dose, resulting from leukostasis within pulmonary capillaries) and capillary leak syndrome, but these rarely have been observed with the currently available yeast-derived version of GM-CSF (sargramostim). Constitutional side effects, such as fevers, myalgias, headaches, and chills were reported in some of the earliest trials of GM-CSF, although these appear to be related to higher doses of GM-CSF.

In summary, the extensive clinical research in the development and application of CSFs to clinical oncology have led to many lines of high-quality evidence upon which to base practice.

Although survival outcomes are relatively easy to quantify, another dimension of improving clinical outcomes is the potential to increase the quality of life for patients undergoing myelosuppressive therapy. CSF support of myelosuppressive regimens may allow patients to tolerate these treatments with quantifiable improvements in their quality of life. To date, however, this has not been studied prospectively in a rigorous manner. Although costly in absolute terms, judicious use of CSF support has proven to add value and to be cost-effective (and even cost-saving) for certain clinically important outcomes.[43] Exhaustive analyses of evidence supporting the appropriate clinical utilization of hematopoietic growth factors for cancer patients have been developed and disseminated by the American Society of Clinical Oncology.[13–16] These evidence-based clinical practice guidelines should be used as a practical reference as they are reviewed and updated on a regular basis.

Anemia in Patients with Cancer: Approach to the Problem and Practical Management with Hematopoietic Growth Factors

Anemia in patients with cancer is exceedingly common, ranges from mild to severe, and often is caused by multifactorial etiologies.[44] Both the incidence and severity of anemia in patients with cancer increase as the stage of the disease progresses. Cancer-associated anemia may be designated as an "anemia of chronic disease" only with a normal cellular pattern in the marrow, low to normal serum iron and iron-binding capacity is demonstrated, the iron content of the marrow is normal or increased, and the serum ferritin is elevated.[45] Other causes of anemia, such as active hemolysis, occult bleeding, nutritional deficiencies, or marrow replacement by tumor, must be considered also in the diagnostic evaluation of anemia in cancer patients.

Serum erythropoietin (EPO) levels have been noted to be inappropriately low for a given level of anemia in patients with cancer compared to anemic patients without cancer.[6] The expected increases in serum EPO levels can be further blunted by the administration of chemotherapy regimens with or without nephrotoxic agents, such as cisplatin.

Because the endogenous EPO response to anemia is inadequate in patients with cancer,[44,46] treatment of the anemia of cancer with pharmacologic dosing of recombinant versions of human EPO represents a highly targeted and rational therapeutic approach. The logic is related to the "replacement therapies" that are often used in endocrine deficiency syndromes: in the case of erythropoiesis in cancer patients, the "inadequate hormone" is EPO itself, which can be replaced pharmacologically by provision of recombinant versions of this molecule. This hypothesis has been tested extensively in prospective, randomized, placebo-controlled trials, and the beneficial effects of supplemental EPO dosing are consistent and reliably documented, as discussed next. The ability of EPO to stimulate erythropoiesis in cancer patients and improve clinical outcomes, such as decrease, transfusion requirements, led the FDA to approve this agent in the early 1990s for the supportive care of anemic cancer patients with nonmyeloid malignancies receiving concurrent chemotherapy.

Prospective, randomized, placebo-controlled studies have been performed in heterogeneous populations of anemic cancer patients, either untreated with cytotoxic therapy or undergoing treatment with a wide variety of cytotoxic regimens. These trials generally have shown that EPO dosing induces a gradual increase in hemoglobin levels (occurring after approximately 3 to 4 weeks of EPO supplementation) in patients receiving pharmacologic dosing with EPO.[44]

These initial findings have been confirmed and expanded in large community-based practice studies in approximately 7,000 cancer patients.[44,47–49] In these large trials, one major goal was to quantify the patient-assessed quality of life using indicator scales measuring such dimensions as energy level, activity level, and overall sense of well-being. These studies confirmed preliminary findings from the initial placebo-controlled studies and showed that patients who respond to EPO dosing with an increase in hemoglobin levels, report clinically meaningful benefits in their quality of life parameters.[47–49] Newer molecules based on the native molecular structure of human EPO, such as darbepoetin, have also been developed and tested. Darbepoetin was genetically engineered to increase the number of glycosylation sites exhibited by normal human EPO, and these extra carbohydrate residues increase the circulating half-life of darbepoetin by approximately threefold over the previous recombinant versions of human erythropoietin (either epoetin-alpha or epoetin-beta). In placebo-controlled studies, darbepoetin has also proven to have beneficial effects in stimulating erythropoiesis similar to the effects of EPO.[50–52]

The clinical value of treating cancer patients with EPO is based on the sustained clinical benefits that have now been demonstrated in thousands of cancer patients receiving this supportive care. The costs of alternative strategies, such as transfusional support, as well as the opportunity costs of ignoring symptomatic yet mild anemias, allow the judicious use of EPO or darbepoetin to be cost-effective if appropriate metrics of value and utility are used to judge the benefits. Nonetheless, given the relatively high cost of optimal use of EPO or other recombinant versions of this agent, careful clinical assessments and data-based decision making on behalf of the prescribing physician is still warranted.[53] It is especially important to note the clinical situations in which EPO does not have the desired benefits for a patient, so that other elements in the differential diagnosis of persistent anemia can be evaluated and, if possible, resolved. Adequate iron levels, for example, are absolutely necessary for patients to achieve the full benefits of EPO supplementation. The optimal way to supplement iron, or even to measure functional iron reserves in cancer patients, remains controversial.

Besides patients with cancer, other forms of hematologic dysfunction also commonly exhibit anemia, either as the sole clinical manifestation or as part of a multilineage marrow failure state. Patients with myelodysplastic syndromes (MDS) are most often anemic and frequently have elevated levels of endogenous EPO. Several small pilot trials have attempted to stimulate more effective erythropoiesis in MDS patients by pharmacologic dosing of EPO.[45–57] These clinical trials have consistently demonstrated clinical benefits with EPO supplementation in approximately 25% of patients with MDS. Although the prognostic factors that might predict a response to EPO supplementation remain poorly understood, most trials suggest that patients with exceedingly high endogenous EPO levels (generally defined as greater than 50 to 100 U/mm^3 blood) have a very low probability of responding to EPO. EPO may also synergize with G-CSF supplementation in MDS patients, and attempts have been made to define the predictive factors for benefit.[57]

For MDS patients who suffer from anemia and transfusion dependency, yet who exhibit relatively low, normal, or only slightly elevated levels of endogenous EPO, a trial of pharmacologic dosing with EPO is a very reasonable therapeutic strategy.

Dosing Considerations with EPO

The conventional dose and schedule with EPO was 150 units/kg given subcutaneously three times each week. However, EPO has also been approved by the FDA to be given as once-weekly subcutaneous injection of 40,000 units as a flat dose. Darbepoetin is recommended by the FDA in the package label to be given at the dose of 2.25 μg/kg administered subcutaneously on a once-weekly basis. However, less frequent administration has also been tested, and a flat dose of 200 μg every other week given subcutaneously is being widely promulgated for darbepoetin.

Safety Concerns in the Use of Erythropoietic Growth Factors in Cancer Patients

Certain safety considerations have arisen in recent years in specific clinical areas, particularly around the investigational use of EPO in settings, such as combined chemoradiotherapy.

First, a small number of patients in France treated with a recombinant version of EPO that is not commercially available in the United States, developed pure red cell aplasia,[58] which appeared to be caused by the presence of neutralizing antierythropoietin antibodies that arose during the EPO therapy.

This toxicity has not been reported with either epoietin-alpha or darbepoietin-alpha, the two EPO-related products that are available in the United States. It remains unclear what stimulated the low but real incidence of pure red cell aplasia in the European patients, but it was likely an issue of drug formulation that was unique to the European marketplace.

A more general concern was raised from other clinical trials that were testing EPO with the goal of achieving higher-than-standard levels of hemoglobin in cancer patients. The rationale for these studies was that higher levels of hemoglobin might improve the therapeutic effects of chemotherapy and/or radiotherapy by increasing oxygen delivery to tumor sites. Paradoxically, however, in a heterogeneous population of head and neck cancer patients, statistically worse survival was noted in the patients who achieved the higher hemoglobin levels with EPO supplementation.[59] Although the reasons for these observations remain obscure, it is possible that there may be potentially negative impact from the overly aggressive increases in hemoglobin levels targeted in this trial. It is likely that such excessively high hemoglobin levels might facilitate thrombotic and/or other vascular complications, especially because cancer patients have an excess incidence of clot formation and thrombovascular adverse events even in the absence of EPO. A public advisory board was held with the FDA based on these concerns, but the decision of the advisory board was that EPO and EPO-related molecules are safe when used as directed in the commercially approved labeling. Other clinical variables, such as the use of EPO with combination chemoradiotherapy, or the use of overly high hemoglobin target levels, may decrease the favorable safety profile of EPO, and therefore, these should be used only in well-defined and strictly monitored clinical trials.

Overall, EPO has been proven to have a very favorable safety profile when used in thousands of cancer patients worldwide. The appropriate utilization of agents to stimulate erythropoiesis has demonstrable and quantifiable clinical benefits for cancer patients in many settings.

Thrombocytopenia in Cancer Patients

Thrombocytopenia in cancer patients is usually attributable to iatrogenic issues, such as cytotoxic chemotherapy and radiation therapy, although impaired marrow reserve or marrow replacement by tumor can also lead to clinically relevant thrombocytopenia. Platelet function can be abnormal in cancer patients, even if normal numbers of platelets are observed. Bleeding and/or clotting complications are observed at an excess rate in cancer patients, most likely because of an underlying activation of inflammatory pathways and perhaps the release of tissue factors from proliferating tumor cells.

Data from 1960s trials in leukemia patients at the National Cancer Institute, demonstrated the quantitative relationship between platelet count and hemorrhage.[60,61] These early studies proved that low circulating platelet counts increase the risk of potentially fatal bleeding complications.

Thrombocytopenia can also indirectly affect the outcomes of cancer patients by causing dose delays or dose reductions of planned cytotoxic drug regimens. Additionally, for patients receiving very aggressive chemotherapy, and certainly in the setting of induction therapy for leukemia or stem cell transplantation, thrombocytopenia can present major clinical challenges.

Hematopoietic Growth Factors to Stimulate Platelet Production in Cancer Patients: Challenges in Developing Clinically Useful Thrombopoietic Agents

The only thrombopoietic agent approved by the FDA to date is recombinant human interleukin 11 (IL-11) (Oprevelkin). Oprevelkin is a relatively nonspecific and pleiotropic cytokine that demonstrates some thrombopoietic activity.

IL-11 was approved by the FDA to prevent severe thrombocytopenia and to reduce the need for platelet transfusions following myelosuppressive chemotherapy in patients with nonmyeloid malignancies. This approval was based on the results of a randomized clinical trial of IL-11 in cancer patients who required at least one platelet transfusion after a prior chemotherapy cycle. In this trial, the use of IL-11 as secondary prophylaxis, reduced the need for platelet transfusions in a subsequent cycle of chemotherapy.[62]

It is critical to recognize that severe thrombocytopenia requiring platelet transfusions is a relatively uncommon problem with administration of standard-dose chemotherapy. Nonetheless, thrombocytopenia can represent an increasingly severe problem over time, with cumulative damage to marrow cells developing with time.

Adverse Reactions

Patients treated with IL-11 commonly experience at least mild to moderate fluid retention, as manifested by peripheral edema and/or dyspnea. In some patients, preexisting pleural effusions have increased during IL-11 administration. Therefore, patients with a history of pleural or pericardial effusions or ascites, should be carefully monitored during IL-11 therapy. In addition, fluids and electrolytes should be monitored very carefully in any patients requiring diuretic therapy. Particular caution should be taken with the use of IL-11 in patients with a history of cardiac arrhythmias because palpitations, tachycardia, and atrial arrhythmias (atrial fibrillation or flutter) have been reported in association with this agent.

Future Directions for Stimulation of Thrombopoiesis

Improving the therapeutic index for thrombopoietic growth factors has proven difficult. Many of the adverse effects of IL-11 likely relate to the fact that this is an inflammatory cytokine, to some degree. Other more selective agents have been tested but have encountered problems. In particular, recombinant human thrombopoietin (TPO) has been tested extensively, with some early promising results.[63] However, the recombinant version also induced cross-reacting autoantibodies against native thrombopoietin in certain clinical trial subjects, and this safety concern led to discontinuation of the development plans for this agent.[64] Newer agonists of the TPO receptor are in clinical development, and it is hoped that these might offer some improved activity for this hematopoietic lineage in the future.

Summary

The translation of basic scientific research into effective therapeutics has been a hallmark of the field of hematopoietic growth factors. Basic scientific inquiry has given us the knowledge and the recombinant proteins to manipulate human hematopoiesis for therapeutic use. The use of hematopoietic growth factors, coupled with an improved understanding of stem cell physiology and the signaling pathways that govern proliferation, differentiation, and apoptosis in hematopoietic cells, has already resulted in improved outcomes for patients, and new insights into basic mechanisms of physiology. Careful review of the data in this field will allow physicians to prescribe hematopoietic growth factors in a responsible, judicious manner to improve patient outcomes while being sensitive to economic values and costs of these agents.

References

1. Metcalf D. The granulocyte-macrophage colony-stimulating factors. Science 1985;229:16.
2. Morstyn G, Burgess AW. Hemopoietic growth factors: a review. Cancer Res 1988;48:5624.
3. Lieschke GJ, Burgess AW. Granulocyte colony-stimulating factor and granulocyte-macrophage colony-stimulating factor (parts I and II). N Engl J Med 1992;327:28, 99.
4. Wingard JR, Demetri GD (eds). Clinical Applications of Cytokines and Growth Factors. Dordrecht: Kluwer, 1999.
5. Zoumbos NC, Gascon P, Djue J, et al. Circulating activated suppressor T lymphocytes in aplastic anemia. N Engl J Med 1985;312:257.
6. Miller CB, Jones RJ, Piantadose S, et al. Decreased erythropoietin response in patients with the anemia of cancer. N Engl J Med 1990;322:1689.
7. Hersh EM, Bodey GP, Niles BA, Freireich EJ. Causes of death in acute leukemia. A ten year study of 414 patients from 1954–1963. JAMA 1965;193:99.
8. Bodey GP, Buckley M, Sathe YS, Freireich EJ. Quantitative relationships between circulating leukocytes and infection in patients with acute leukemia. Ann Intern Med 1966;64:328.
9. Talcott JA, Siegel RD, Finberg R, Goldman L. Risk assessment in cancer patients with fever and neutropenia: a prospective, two-center validation of a prediction rule. J Clin Oncol 1992; 10:316.
10. Klastersky J, Paesmans M, Rubenstein EB, et al. The Multinational Association for Supportive Care in Cancer risk index: a multinational scoring system for identifying low-risk febrile neutropenic cancer patients. J Clin Oncol 2000;18:3038–3051.
11. Chrischilles EA, Link BK, Scott SD, et al. Factors associated with early termination of CHOP therapy and the impact on survival among patients with chemosensitive intermediate-grade non-Hodgkin's lymphoma. Cancer Control 2003;10:396–403.
12. Citron ML, Berry DA, Cirrincione C, et al. Randomized trial of dose-dense versus conventionally scheduled and sequential versus concurrent combination chemotherapy as postoperative adjuvant treatment of node-positive primary breast cancer: first report of Intergroup Trial C9741/Cancer and Leukemia Group B Trial 9741. J Clin Oncol 2003;21(8):1431–1439.
13. ASCO Ad Hoc Committee. American Society of Clinical Oncology Recommendations for the Use of Hematopoietic Colony-Stimulating Factors: Evidence-Based, Practice Guidelines. J Clin Oncol 1994;12:2471–2508.
14. ASCO Ad Hoc Committee. Update of recommendations for the use of hematopoietic colony-stimulating factors: evidence-based, clinical practice guidelines. J Clin Oncol 1996;14:1957–1960.
15. ASCO Ad Hoc Committee. 1997 update of recommendations for the use of hematopoietic colony-stimulating factors: evidence-based, clinical practice guidelines. J Clin Oncol 1997;15:3288–3289.
16. Ozer H, Armitage JO, Bennett CL, et al. American Society of Clinical Oncology. 2000 update of recommendations for the use of hematopoietic colony-stimulating factors: evidence-based, clinical practice guidelines. American Society of Clinical Oncology Growth Factors Expert Panel. J Clin Oncol 2000; 18(20):3558–3585.
17. Welte K, Gabrilove J, Bronchud MH, Platzer E, Morstyn G. Filgrastim (r-metHuG-CSF): the first 10 years. Blood 1996;88: 1907–1929.
18. Gabrilove JL, Jakubowski A, Fain K, et al. Phase I study of granulocyte colony-stimulating factor in patients with transitional cell carcinoma of the urothelium. J Clin Invest 1988;82: 1454.
19. Bronchud MH, Scarffe JH, Thatcher N, et al. Phase I/II study of recombinant human granulocyte colony-stimulating factor in patients receiving intensive chemotherapy for small cell lung cancer. Br J Cancer 1987;56:809.
20. Groopman JE, Mitsuyasu RT, DeLeo MJ, et al. Effect of recombinant human granulocyte-macrophage colony-stimulating factor on myelopoiesis in the acquired immunodeficiency syndrome. N Engl J Med 1987;317:593.
21. Antman K, Griffin J, Elias A, et al: Effect of recombinant human granulocyte-macrophage colony-stimulating factor on chemotherapy-induced myelosuppression. N Engl J Med 1988; 319:593.
22. Morstyn G, Campbell L, Souza LM, et al. Effect of granulocyte colony stimulating factor on neutropenia induced by cytotoxic chemotherapy. Lancet 1988;1:667.
23. Gabrilove JL, Jakubowski A, Scher H, et al. Effect of granulocyte colony-stimulating factor on neutropenia and associated morbidity due to chemotherapy for transitional-cell carcinoma of the urothelium. N Engl J Med 1988;318:1414.
24. Crawford J, Ozer H, Stoller R, et al. Reduction by granulocyte colony-stimulating factor of fever and neutropenia induced by chemotherapy in patients with small-cell lung cancer. N Engl J Med 1991;325:164.
25. Trillet-Lenoir V, Green J, Manegold C, et al. Recombinant granulocyte colony stimulating factor reduces the infectious complications of cytotoxic chemotherapy. Eur J Cancer 1993; 29A:319.
26. Lyman GH, Kuderer NM, Djulbegovic B. Prophylactic granulocyte colony-stimulating factor in patients receiving dose-intensive cancer chemotherapy: a meta-analysis. Am J Med 2002;112:406–411.
27. Holmes FA, O'Shaughnessy JA, Vukelja S, et al. Blinded, randomized, multicenter study to evaluate single administration pegfilgrastim once per cycle versus daily filgrastim as an adjunct to chemotherapy in patients with high-risk stage II or stage III/IV breast cancer. J Clin Oncol 2002;20:727–731.
28. Green MD, Koelbl H, Baselga J, et al. A randomized double-blind multicenter phase III study of fixed-dose single-administration pegfilgrastim versus daily filgrastim in patients receiving myelosuppressive chemotherapy. Ann Oncol 2003;14:29–35.
29. Vogel CL, Wojtukiewicz MZ, Carroll RR, et al. First and subsequent cycle use of pegfilgrastim prevents febrile neutropenia in patients with breast cancer: a multicenter, double-blind,

placebo-controlled phase III study. J Clin Oncol 2005;23(6):1178–1184.

30. Esser M, Brunner H. Economic evaluations of granulocyte colony-stimulating factor: in the prevention and treatment of chemotherapy-induced neutropenia. Pharmacoeconomics 2003; 21:1295–1313.
31. Komrokji RS, Lyman GH. Biological response modifiers used to prevent and treat neutropenia and its complications. Expert Opin Biol Ther 2004;4:1897–1910.
32. Hughes WT, Armstrong D, Bodey GP, et al. 2002 guidelines for the use of antimicrobial agents in neutropenic patients with cancer [comment]. Clin Infect Dis 2002;34:730–751.
33. Budman DR, Berry DA, Cirrincione CT, et al. Dose and dose intensity as determinants of outcome in the adjuvant treatment of breast cancer: The Cancer and Leukemia Group B. J Natl Cancer Inst 1998;90:1205–1211.
34. Henderson IC, Berry DA, Demetri GD, et al. Improved outcomes from adding sequential Paclitaxel but not from escalating Doxorubicin dose in an adjuvant chemotherapy regimen for patients with node-positive primary breast cancer. J Clin Oncol 2003;21(6):976–983.
35. Bennett CL, Stinson TJ, Laver JH, et al. Cost analyses of adjunct colony stimulating factors for acute leukemia: can they improve clinical decision making. Leuk Lymphoma 2000;37:65–70.
36. Sung L, et al. Prophylactic granulocyte colony-stimulating factor and granulocyte-macrophage colony-stimulating factor decrease febrile neutropenia after chemotherapy in children with cancer: a meta-analysis of randomized controlled trials. J Clin Oncol 2004;22:3350–3356.
37. Relling MV, Boyett JM, Blanco JG, et al. Granulocyte colony-stimulating factor and the risk of secondary myeloid malignancy after etoposide treatment. Blood 2003;101:3862–3867.
38. Maher DW, Lieschke GJ, Green M, et al. Filgrastim in patients with chemotherapy-induced febrile neutropenia. A double-blind, placebo-controlled trial. Ann Intern Med 1994;121(7):492–501.
39. Clark OA, Lyman G, Castro AA, et al. Colony stimulating factors for chemotherapy induced febrile neutropenia. Cochrane Database Systematic Review: CD003039, 2004.
40. Berghmans T, Paesmans M, Lafitte JJ, et al. Therapeutic use of granulocyte and granulocyte-macrophage colony-stimulating factors in febrile neutropenic cancer patients. A systematic review of the literature with meta-analysis. Support Care Cancer 2002;10:181–188.
41. Hartmann LC, Tschetter LK, Habermann TM, et al. Granulocyte colony-stimulating factor in severe chemotherapy-induced afebrile neutropenia. N Engl J Med 1997;336(25):1776–1780.
42. Dale DC, Bolyard AA, Aprikyan A. Cyclic neutropenia. Semin Hematol 2002;39(2):89–94.
43. Lyman GH, Kuderer NM. The economics of the colony-stimulating factors for the prevention and treatment of febrile neutropenia. Crit Rev Oncol Hematol 2004;50:129–146.
44. Desai J, Demetri GD. Recombinant human erythropoietin in cancer-related anemia: an evidence-based review. Best Pract Res Clin Haematol 2005;18(3):389–406.
45. Lee GR. The anemia of chronic disease. Semin Hematol 1983;20: 61.
46. Cazzola M, Mercuriali F, Brugnara C. Use of recombinant human erythropoietin outside the setting of uremia. Blood 1997;89:4248–4267.
47. Glaspy J, Bukowski R, Steinberg D, et al. Impact of therapy with epoetin alfa on clinical outcomes in patients with nonmyeloid malignancies during cancer chemotherapy in community oncology practice. J Clin Oncol 1997;15:1218–1234.
48. Demetri GD, Kris M, Wade J, Degos L, Cella D. Quality-of-life benefit in chemotherapy patients treated with epoetin alfa is independent of disease response or tumor type: results from a prospective community oncology study. J Clin Oncol 1998;16: 3412–3425.
49. Gabrilove JL, Cleeland CS, Livingston RB, Sarokhan B, Winer E, Einhorn LH. Clinical evaluation of once-weekly dosing of epoetin alfa in chemotherapy patients: improvements in hemoglobin and quality of life are similar to three-times-weekly dosing, J Clin Oncol 2001;19:2875–2882.
50. Vansteenkiste J, Pirker R, Massuti B. Aranesp 980297 Study Group. Double-blind, placebo-controlled, randomized phase III trial of darbepoetin alfa in lung cancer patients receiving chemotherapy. J Natl Cancer Inst 2002;94(16):1211–1220.
51. Pirker R. Darbepoetin alfa for the treatment of cancer-related anemia: an update. Expert Rev Anticancer Ther 2004;4(5): 735–744.
52. Schwartzberg LS, Yee LK, Senecal FM, et al. A randomized comparison of every-2-week darbepoetin alfa and weekly epoetin alfa for the treatment of chemotherapy-induced anemia in patients with breast, lung, or gynecologic cancer. Oncologist 2004;9(6): 696–707.
53. Finkelstein SN, Huber SL, Greenberg PE. Comment: cost comparison of recombinant human erythropoietin and blood transfusion in cancer chemotherapy-induced anemia. Ann Pharmacother 1997;31(9):1094–1095.
54. Kurzrock R, Talpaz M, Estey E, et al. Erythropoietin treatment in patients with myelodysplastic syndrome and anemia. Leukemia 1990;5:985.
55. Stein RS, Abels RI, Krantz SB. Pharmacologic doses of recombinant human erythropoietin in the treatment of myelodysplastic syndromes. Blood 1991;78:1658.
56. Negrin RS, Stein R, Doherty K, et al. Maintenance treatment of the anemia of myelodysplastic syndromes with recombinant human granulocyte colony-stimulating factor and erythropoietin: evidence for in vivo synergy. Blood 1996;87(10):4076–4081.
57. Hellstrom-Lindberg E, Negrin R, Stein R, et al. Erythroid response to treatment with G-CSF plus erythropoietin for the anaemia of patients with myelodysplastic syndromes: proposal for a predictive model. Br J Haematol 1997;99(2):344–351.
58. Bennett CL, Luminari S, Nissenson AR, et al. Pure red-cell aplasia and epoetin therapy. N Engl J Med 2004;351(14): 1403–1408.
59. Henke M, Laszig R, Rube C, et al. Erythropoietin to treat head and neck cancer patients with anaemia undergoing radiotherapy: randomised, double-blind, placebo-controlled trial. Lancet 2003; 362:1255–1260.
60. Hersh EM, Bodey GP, Niles BA, Freireich EJ. Causes of death in acute leukemia. A ten year study of 414 patients from 1954–1963. JAMA 1965;193:99.
61. Gaydos LA, Freireich EJ, Mantel N. The quantitative relation between platelet count and hemorrhage in patients with acute leukemia. N Engl J Med 1962;266:905.
62. Tepler I, Elias L, Smith JW II, et al. A randomized placebo-controlled trial of recombinant human interleukin-11 in cancer patients with severe thrombocytopenia due to chemotherapy. Blood 1996;87(9):3607–3614.
63. Kuter DJ, Begley CG. Recombinant human thrombopoietin: basic biology and evaluation of clinical studies. Blood 2002; 100(10):3457–3469.
64. Li J, Yang C, Xia Y, et al. Thrombocytopenia caused by the development of antibodies to thrombopoietin. Blood 2001;98(12): 3241–3248.

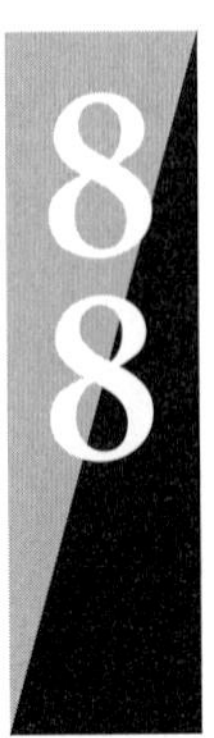

Management of the Bone Marrow Transplant Patient

Daniel J. Weisdorf and Marcie Tomblyn

Progressive experience and success in application of blood and marrow transplantation has heightened attention to clinical management of the complications and long-term outcomes of such procedures. More than 20,000 patients yearly undergo transplant therapy and more than 25,000 patients survive beyond 5 years after transplantation. The recognition, prophylaxis, management, and screening for early complications and for late effects following successful transplant have developed by extrapolation of procedures for intensive therapy of hematologic malignancy (e.g., acute leukemia) and by recognition of specific toxicities, immunodeficiencies and problems encountered uniquely by the transplant recipient.[1] Similar to other hematology/oncology procedures, most management strategies are supported principally by empirically derived and some experience-supported evidence. Overall, less than one-quarter of transplant decision making is supported by Level 1 evidence.[2] We review the approach to transplant complications through the phases of therapy emphasizing the available evidence, the frequently held consensus opinions, and areas for future study.

Early Posttransplant Toxicities

Pretransplant chemotherapy and radiation are used for their immunosuppressive and antineoplastic impact but can be toxic to host tissues and organs, substantially augmenting peritransplant morbidity.[3] Direct conditioning-associated toxicity may include oral mucositis,[4] interstitial pneumonitis,[5] hepatic veno-occlusive disease,[6] gastrointestinal toxicity with nausea, vomiting, or diarrhea,[7] desquamative dermatitis,[8] and hemorrhagic cystitis.[9] Much more infrequently, myocardial injury[10] or central nervous system toxic encephalopathy[11] may occur. These toxicities may each mimic or be complicated by local or regional infection and can be compounded by delayed neutrophil recovery, poor tissue healing, and secondary infection.[12]

Delayed Engraftment/Graft Failure

Slow or incomplete hematopoietic recovery after transplantation yields ongoing neutropenia, transfusion dependence for platelets and red cells, and slow recovery from the initial toxicity of transplantation.[13] Poor graft function can prolong and exacerbate the risks of infection and directly increase peritransplant mortality. Criteria for a satisfactory autologous graft have been described in numerous, prospective single-arm studies (Level 2 evidence).[14,15] Only a few comparative trials have addressed graft source or supportive techniques to improve the speed and completeness of autologous reconstitution.[16–19]

A suitable autograft should include at least 1×10^8 marrow aspirated mononuclear cells/kg. Since the late 1980s, blood-derived stem cell and progenitor cells have been collected by apheresis. Only a few formal comparisons of blood versus marrow autografts have been performed.[17,19] Autologous marrow harvest was, for the most part, abandoned in the early 1990s.

Although direct quantitation of the hematopoietic stem cell content of autografts is still clinically unavailable, the surrogate measure of CD34+ cells/kg is used to judge the adequacy of an apheresis-collected progenitor population. A minimum of 2×10^6 CD34+ cells/kg is accepted as a suitable autologous graft likely to yield prompt neutrophil, platelet, and red cell recovery.[15] Distribution of the cell infusion over several days[20] has been prospectively tested with no benefit. Similarly, formally testing delay in administration of granulocyte colony-stimulating factor (G-CSF) postgraft infusion to day 5,[21] or use of higher daily doses of G-CSF,[22] did not change the timing of multilineage recovery. No consensus about the dose or timing of G-CSF administration posttransplant has been well documented. Level 3 evidence from numerous retrospectively reported series,[15,23,24] suggests that G-CSF may be unneeded if an autograft contains 5×10^6 CD34+ cells/kg, but still may have some supportive benefit if daily G-CSF (5–10 μg/kg/day) is administered for grafts containing 2 to 5×10^6 CD34+/kg. Growth factor-stimulated bone marrow-harvested autografts have been studied,[18,25,26] but have not been pursued, largely because of suggested, although undocumented, concerns about tumor contamination in a marrow harvest or hypocellularity and difficult collections in heavily treated patients.

Engraftment After Allogeneic Transplantation

Allogeneic transplantation poses additional barriers to successful lymphohematopoietic reconstitution beyond the progenitor content of the infused graft. Supporting lymphoid and stromal elements may be essential as well as immunosuppression sufficient to overcome histocompatibility barriers for a successful allograft. The intensity of immunosuppression, degree of histocompatibility between donor and host, and perhaps other poorly studied factors, such as NK-mediated rejection modulated by killer immunoglobulin receptor (KIR) alloreactivity or marrow stromal damage, may further limit the speed or completeness of alloengraftment. Extensive retrospective analysis suggests that alternative donor transplants (closely matched unrelated donor, URD) have limited graft failure risks (less than 5%),[27] although haploidentical-related transplants yield more frequent graft failure, which might be overcome by variant conditioning, megadose progenitor grafts, or favorable NK-mediated alloreactivity.[28,29] No prospective data comparing strategies to limit risks of graft failure after allotransplant are available, although extensive single-arm and retrospective reports support these conclusions.

Peripheral Blood Versus Bone Marrow Allografts

After widespread adoption of peripheral blood stem cells (PBSC) for autologous transplants, G-CSF-mobilized allografts became extensively studied. Numerous prospective randomized trials comparing blood to marrow sibling donor allografts have been reported (Table 88.1). Although neutrophil recovery is generally quicker using PBSC, acute and, more often, chronic graft-versus-host disease (GVHD) occur more frequently after peripheral blood (PB) allografts.[30,31] Few data support any long-term survival advantage for the use of G-CSF-mobilized PBSC for sibling donor transplantation. Nonetheless, early improvements in morbidity and mortality, reported in some series, accelerated worldwide adoption of G-CSF-mobilized PBSC for nearly all sibling donor transplants, at least in adults. Prospective studies are under way addressing these techniques in URD transplantation.

TABLE 88.1. Peripheral blood versus bone marrow allografts.

Trial	*Reference*	*Year*	*N*	*Randomized*	*GVHD*	*DFS/survival*	*Conclusions*
Bensinger	159	2001	172	G-PB vs. BM	II–IV: 64% vs. 57%, NS III–IV: 15% vs. 12%, NS Extensive cGVHD: 46% vs. 35%, NS	2-year DFS: 65% vs. 45%, $P = 0.03$ 2-year OS: 66% vs. 54%, $P = 0.06$	Shorter time to PMN and platelet recovery; equivalent GVHD
Blaise	160	2000	111	G-PB vs. BM	II–IV: 44% vs. 42%, NS cGVHD: 50% vs. 29%, $P < 0.03$	2-year DFS: 67% vs. 66%, NS 2-year OS: 67% vs. 65%, NS	Shorter time to PMN and platelet recovery; increased cGVHD with PB; equal survival
Champlin	161	2000	824	Retrospective PB = 288 BM = 536	II–IV: 40% vs. 35%, NS III–IV: 13% vs. 19%, NS cGVHD: 65% vs. 53%, $P = 0.02$	1-year DFS AL, CR1: 70% vs. 61%, NS AL, ≥CR2: 77% vs. 57%, $P = 0.03$ CML CP: 63% vs. 74%, NS CML AP 68% vs. 23%, $P > 0.01$	Shorter time to PMN and platelet recovery; increased cGVHD with PB; improved DFS with PB in advanced leukemias
Couban	162	2002	227	G-PB vs. BM	II–IV: 44% vs. 44%, NS III–IV: 26% vs. 18%, NS cGVHD: 85% vs. 69%, NS Extensive cGVHD: 40% vs. 30%, NS	30 month OS: 68% vs. 60%, $P = 0.04$	Shorter time to PMN and platelet recovery; equivalent GVHD; improved OS with PB
Morton	33	2001	57	G-PB vs. G-BM	II–IV: 52% vs. 54%, NS III–IV: 22% vs. 43%, $P < 0.09$ Steroid refractory-year aGVHD: 18% vs. 47%, $P < 0.02$ cGVHD: 47% vs. 90%, $P < 0.02$ Extensive cGVHD: 22% vs. 80%, $P < 0.002$	18 month OS: 67% vs. 64%, NS	Equal PMN and platelet recovery; equal survival
Schmitz	163	1998	66	G-PB vs. BM	II–IV: 54% vs. 48% III–IV: 21% vs. 18%	12 month OS: 73% vs. 82%, NS	Shorter time to platelet recovery
Vigorito	164	1998	37	G-PB vs. BM	II–IV: 27% vs. 19%, NS cGVHD: 71% vs. 53%, NS Extensive cGVHD: 100% vs. 50%, $P = 0.02$	1000 day DFS: 58% vs. 52%, NS 1,000-day OS: 47% vs. 51%, NS	Shorter time to platelet recovery; similar AcGVHD similar, but increased extensive cGVHD; no survival differences

G-PB, granulocyte colony-stimulating factor (G-CSF)-mobilized peripheral blood; BM, bone marrow; DFS, disease-free survival; OS, overall survival; PMN, polymorphonuclear neutrophil leukocytes; AL, acute leukemia; CML, chronic myelogenous leukemia; aGVHD, acute graft-versus-host disease; cGVHD, chronic GVHD; NS, not significant.

Children may suffer excessive GVHD after PB-derived allografting.[32]

A newer approach, G-CSF-mobilized bone marrow harvest compared to G-CSF-mobilized PBSC apheresis, has been reported in a limited series[33] with equivalent survival, equally speedy engraftment, and more-frequent GVHD in PBSC recipients (see Table 88.1). Ji et al.[34] compared G-CSF-mobilized bone marrow to unprimed bone marrow harvest for sibling transplantation for chronic myelogenous leukemia (CML). The mobilized grafts had three-fold-higher CD34 content and lower CD4:CD8 ratios. Use of the cytokine-mobilized harvests led to significantly accelerated neutrophil (15 versus 20 days) and platelet (17 versus 24 days) recovery, and significantly less acute (6% versus 27%) and chronic (24% versus 33%) GVHD, although with similar relapse risks and similar survival. Additional experience from these small preliminary reports and others, suggests that G-CSF-mobilized bone marrow may add modestly to donor morbidity but yield possibly promising outcomes for the recipient.

G-CSF administration after allotransplantation is widely used but is not well supported by prospective study. Lee et al.[35] prospectively tested delayed administration of G-CSF post-PBSC allograft and observed equivalent neutrophil and platelet engraftment, although suggestively poorer survival in those receiving G-CSF starting day 0, but no other reports corroborate this negative effect. A single report[36] evaluated G-CSF initiated at either day 0, 5, or 10 after URD transplantation, and showed no differences in hematologic recovery, fever, use of antibiotics, relapse, or survival, although costs were reduced using later-onset G-CSF.

Overall, G-CSF-mobilized PBSC allografts result in prompt hematopoietic recovery and, if more than 5×10^6 CD34+ cells/kg are infused, posttransplant G-CSF may be unneeded. Uncertain risks of acute, and particularly, long-term development of chronic GVHD suggest that continuing follow-up of previous randomized trials and the prospective randomized trial currently under way in URD transplantation, will be necessary to conclude the equivalence or superiority of one graft source or another. Partial matched related donor transplants (haploidentical or better) are usually performed with PBSC, although no formal comparisons are available.

Umbilical Cord Blood Allografts

Unrelated donor umbilical cord blood (UCB) is increasingly frequently used to support allotransplanted patients without available HLA-compatible sibling or volunteer unrelated donors (URD).[37–39] Used primarily for smaller or pediatric patients, increasing experience in adults shows promise, although delayed recovery or graft failure is frequent.[40] Infusion of two closely matched grafts may promote engraftment in adults.[41] Only retrospective data are available, which suggest that both higher cell dose (more than $2–3 \times 10^7$ nucleated cells/kg) and progenitor content (more than $2–3 \times 10^5$ CD34+ cells/kg) are dominant predictors of satisfactory donor-derived neutrophil engraftment after UCB transplantation.[37,39] Some retrospective data reported from Minnesota[42] and France,[43] suggest that closely HLA-matched UCB donors yield more effective engraftment and survival, although only low-resolution HLA typing and matching have been studied. The impact of HLA-C or other locus matching has not been analyzed or reported in depth. Developing experience, although limited, offers no strong evidence except to confirm that high cell dose and close HLA matching (four to five matched loci of six HLA-A, -B, -DRB1) is preferred, to expect prompt hematopoietic recovery after UCB transplantation.

Added host factors (myelofibrosis or splenomegaly) can augment risks of graft failure. Graft manipulation (T-lymphocyte depletion) may deplete stem cells or deplete essential, although uncertain, donor cellular elements necessary for satisfactory immunosuppression of the recipient and prevention of active graft allorejection. Treatment of graft failure most often involves administration of G-CSF or granulocyte macrophage colony-stimulating factor (GM-CSF) in different doses or dose schedules. Randomized trials of growth factors given for delayed engraftment[13] demonstrated acceleration of leukocyte, but not platelet, reconstitution. Limited testing of thrombopoietin or erythropoietin has been inconclusive in supporting their value. Additional stem cell infusions can be effective if graft failure develops.[44] Intensified immunosuppression, most often high-dose corticosteroids or antithymocyte globulin (ATG), has been used to prepare recipients for second allograft infusions. When the original donor (sibling or URD) is unavailable, such as with UCB, alternative donor sources (other UCB, volunteer URD, or partial matched related donors) have been tried, although only anecdotal and retrospective experience is available for review.

Oropharyngeal Mucositis

Direct toxicity to the oropharyngeal epithelium follows chemoradiotherapy conditioning and may be complicated by localized minimally invasive infection (viral, yeast, or bacterial), GVHD prophylaxis agents (e.g., methotrexate), or by GVHD.[4] Prolonged neutropenia compounds the risk of local infections and delays oral healing. Painful swallowing, eating, talking, or airway compromise can follow severe oral mucositis, and its severity can directly augment risks of fever, systemic infection, requirement for parenteral nutrition or narcotics, prolonged hospitalization, peritransplant mortality, and increased costs of care.[45,46]

The intensity of conditioning and use of methotrexate directly promotes greater epithelial trauma, apoptosis, and mucosal ulceration, yielding more frequent and more severe oropharyngeal mucositis. High-dose total-body irradiation (TBI) and etoposide are particularly mucosal toxic, but melphalan, especially if combined with TBI, yields severe mucositis as well. Management using local rinse debridement, topical anesthetics, and coating agents (magic mouthwash containing diphenhydramine), antiacid solutions, or ice chips are largely supportive, and little formal study has documented their value. Formal prospective, and usually blinded, trials of antimicrobials (chlorhexidine, isoganan, calcium phosphate) have been undertaken with inconclusive results.[4,47,48] Systemic cytokines have accelerated neutrophil recovery and concomitantly limited the duration of mucositis. Interleukin (IL)-11 worsened systemic toxicity and had no benefit.[49] Keratinocyte growth factor (KGF, palifermin) has significantly shortened the severity, duration, accompanying pain, and peritransplant morbidities of mucositis after intensively conditioning autografts.[50,51] Similarly, amifostine has reduced the direct mucosal cytotoxicity of high-dose alkylators and has been used to facilitate intensive, augmented chemotherapy conditioning regimens.[52] Only KGF and amifostine are of demonstrable benefit, but these have not been studied in widespread fashion nor yet been adopted for general use.

Hepatic Veno-Occlusive Disease

Jaundice, hepatomegaly, and fluid retention, resulting from stenosis or obliteration of terminal hepatic venules, comprises the syndrome of hepatic veno-occlusive disease (VOD) that follows high-dose chemotherapy and radiation conditioning for transplantation.[53,54] Most often developing within the first month, this syndrome has been reported with extremely variable incidence because of differences in diagnostic stringency and specific criteria. Ten percent to 60% of patients may be affected with VOD, and this looseness in definition complicates interpretation of any and all literature about VOD.[53,55] Generally recognized risk factors include intensive transplant conditioning or pretransplant chemotherapy (particularly including previous therapy with mylotarg), abnormal transaminase values, chronic hepatic viral infection, and other uncertain factors. Case series with more liberal definitions (reporting 30% to 50% incidence) include peritransplant liver toxicity without all the histologic and hemodynamic changes characteristic of florid VOD, whereas those with more stringent definitions (reporting 5% to 10% incidence) most often demonstrate all the clinical diagnostic features, plus hepatic reversal of flow by Doppler ultrasound and perivenular necrosis and fibrous obliteration on liver biopsy.[56] This severe VOD results in high mortality.

Prevention of VOD has been tested in several prospective trials, most frequently evaluating ursodeoxycholic acid, although corticosteroids, supplementation of hepatic glutathione, antithrombin III concentrates, prostaglandin E_1, and tumor necrosis factor-alpha (TNF-α) neutralization have all been studied; heparin[57] and pentoxifylline[58] were studied in modest size, prospective randomized trials.

Ursodeoxycholic acid was shown of benefit in several small trials but not confirmed in a larger Phase III prospective study.[59] Ursodeoxycholic acid is the only suggestively beneficial agent recognized to reduce VOD incidence and might be recommended, at least in high-risk patients displaying some pretransplant risk factors augmenting their hazards of VOD. The combination of ursodeoxycholic acid and heparin was not additive in its protective effect.[60]

Therapy of VOD is uncertain. The thrombotic nature of its findings has led to uncontrolled testing of heparin, recombinant human tissue plasminogen activator,[61,62] and supplementation of the anticoagulants antithrombin III and activated protein C, but no conclusive findings or comparative trials with strong evidence supporting its use are available. Defibrotide (DF) reduces the thrombogenicity of endothelium through numerous effects and has activity in reducing vascular injury and thrombosis in a variety of settings. Limited prospective noncomparative trials suggest its potential value,[63] although no clear evidence of efficacy is available. Other treatments supportive of liver dysfunction from other causes [plasmapheresis, intrahepatic portasystemic shunting (TIPS), and hemodialysis] have been used without specific literature available to document their value in this setting.

Interstitial Pneumonitis

Although most lung complications following transplantation are infectious, two specific syndromes, idiopathic interstitial pneumonitis [sometimes called idiopathic pneumonia syndrome (IPS)] and diffuse alveolar hemorrhage (DAH) occur without infection.

The first, IPS, typically occurs in the first 2 to 6 weeks following transplantation, and is seen more frequently in patients with extensive pretransplant chemotherapy receiving high-dose cyclophosphamide or high-dose total-body irradiation (TBI), but it may be associated with blood transfusions, methotrexate, and GVHD.[64,65] Some reports suggest that IPS occurs as frequently in syngeneic as allogeneic recipients, and postulate that immunodeficiency is a lesser risk factor for IPS than for infectious pneumonitis.[66,67] Drug and radiation toxicities have been reported as major contributors, although no clear conclusions regarding this syndrome can be determined from formal trials comparing TBI or non-TBI conditioning regimens. In some trials, higher-dose TBI has been associated with more frequent IPS, although this is not consistently reported.[68,69] Corticosteroids or anticytokines (etanercept or infliximab), have been proposed as cytokine shields and antiinflammatory protective agents, but their use has not been validated in prospective trials.

Diffuse alveolar hemorrhage (DAH) was initially reported in autograft recipients, but a similar syndrome occurs following allotransplantation that is, at times, included in the syndrome of IPS.[70,71] Its specific diagnosis requires diffuse consolidation on chest X-ray, hypoxemia, and progressively bloody alveolar lavage obtained through bronchoscopy. Because bloody bronchoalveolar lavage (BAL), but not hemoptysis, is required for diagnosis, it is less frequently described in children (for whom bronchoscopy is performed less frequently), but true incidence figures are difficult to discern. Its presentation with dyspnea, hypoxemia, respiratory distress, and nonproductive cough, is usually rapid in onset and has an associated mortality of 70% to 100%. Supportive measures include correction of coagulopathy and aggressive ventilatory support. High-dose corticosteroids are regularly offered, but no controlled data and only limited, anecdotal series are available to support their use.[70,72] Recombinant factor VIIa and other hemostatic agents have been evaluated informally, but no data beyond anecdotal reports have been published.

Posttransplant Host Defense and Infection

The initial chemotherapy and radiation insult blunts mechanical barriers to invasive infection through disruption of cutaneous mucosal and epithelial membranes.[12,73] Neutropenia and hypogammaglobulinemia further limit defense against aerobic organisms. Severe cellular immune dysfunction, including T-cell lymphopenia and ineffective T-cell function persists for 6 to 12 months following transplantation.[74] These defects are more intense and more prolonged in patients developing GVHD. Natural killer cell recovery is early, within 4 weeks of transplant, although its importance

TABLE 88.2. Fungal prophylaxis.

Trial	*Reference*	*Year*	*N*	*Randomized*	*DFS/survival*	*Conclusions*
Goodman	77	1992	356	Placebo vs. Fluc	Superficial fungal 33% vs. 8%, $P < 0.001$ Systemic fungal 16% vs. 3%, $P < 0.001$	Prophylactic Fluc decreases the incidence of both superficial and systemic fungal infections
Marr	79	2000	300	Placebo vs. Fluc for 75 days post-BMT	Invasive candidiasis 20% vs. 3%, $P < 0.001$ 8-year OS: 28% vs. 45%, $P = 0.0001$	Improved survival; decreased GVHD of the gut
Marr	80	2004	304	Itra vs. Fluc	Invasive fungal 13% vs. 16%, NS; invasive mold 5% vs. 12%, $P = 0.03$	Survival NS; increased GI toxicity with Itra; improved prevention of invasive mold infection with Itra
Nucci	81	2000	210	Placebo vs. Itra	Empiric Ampho 61% vs. 22%, $P = 0.001$ Definite fungal 19% vs. 6%, $P = 0.04$; molds 12% vs. 5%, $P = 0.03$	Itra prophylaxis decreased the frequency of systemic fungal infections and decreased the use of empiric Ampho
Slavin	78	1995	300	Placebo vs. Fluc for 75 days post-BMT	Systemic fungal 18% vs. 7%, $P = 0.004$ OS to day +110 65% vs. 80%, $P = 0.004$	Fluconazole decreases the incidence of systemic fungal infections and improves survival to day +110
Winston	165	2003	140	Fluc vs. Itra	Invasive fungal 25% vs. 9%, $P = 0.01$ Overall survival: 42% vs. 45%, NS	Itraconazole decreases the risk of invasive fungal infections

Fluc, fluconazole; Itra, itraconazole; Ampho, amphotericin; BMT, bone marrow transplantation.

in host defense at that stage is undetermined.[75] In some reports, greater risks of infection follow alternative donor transplantation, even in the absence of clinical GVHD.[76]

In the preengraftment 1 to 3 weeks posttransplant, neutropenia and oral/enteric mucosal disruption predominate. Fever is frequent, although only 50% of patients have specific pathogens identified. Tissue injury, transfusions, amphotericin, or other drug fevers may explain some of these culture-negative febrile episodes. Usual supportive care includes protective isolation, in many centers using high-efficiency particulate air (HEPA) filtration to reduce inhalation of airborne fungal pathogenic spores, although its use has never been formally tested. Early experience suggested reduction in febrile days for patients transplanted, using more extensive protective isolation including laminar airflow environments, broad-spectrum decontaminating antibiotics, and sterile food, but no reduction in defined infection or early mortality was observed.[12,73] Recent experience, particularly with reduced-intensity allotransplantation and the brief neutropenia accompanying autografting, has led to abandonment of or at least diminished attention to protective isolation because many patients are cared for as outpatients.

Antibacterial prophylaxis directed toward aerobic bacteria using trimethoprim sulfa has been tested but has not been shown to be efficacious in leukemia or transplant recipients.[73,77] Quinolones, especially those with gram-positive and gram-negative activity, have been more widely used, although definitive trials demonstrating their value in reduction in defined infection or reduced hospital days, 30-day mortality, or other proximate benefits remain uncertain. Some series suggest that their use limits febrile episodes and a need for systemic broad-spectrum antibiotic therapy, but these results have not been confirmed. Empiric broad-spectrum antibiotic therapy for neutropenic fever remains the norm, supported by numerous, although small, studies in the 1970s. Alternative strategies, for the most part, have not been formally tested. Varying antibiotic combinations have been studied extensively, although none has emerged as superior. Attention to local hospital flora and antibiotic resistance patterns, formulary determinations, and associated other medication use (avoidance of nephrotoxic aminoglycosides in patients treated with calcineurin inhibitors) should determine choice of empiric antibiotic therapy.

Fungal infections have emerged during the past 15 years as the dominant and most frequently lethal pathogens affecting the transplant recipient (Table 88.2). Several studies documented the value of fluconazole in reducing yeast infections and overall peritransplant mortality,[77–79] but concerns about inadequate prophylaxis against molds, especially *Aspergillus*, persist. Recent evaluations of itraconazole have shown promise in prophylaxis,[80,81] but variable and uncertain absorption has limited its widespread use.

Controlled testing of voriconazole with its favorable oral absorption, pharmacokinetics, and efficacy have documented its value as empiric treatment for neutropenic fever and treatment of established aspergillosis.[82,83] Large multicenter trials are currently assessing its efficacy compared to fluconazole for prophylaxis in allogeneic transplant recipients. Echinocandins (caspofungin, micafungin) have been recognized effective in some settings, but no formal prophylaxis trials document their utility for antimold prophylaxis in the high-risk allotransplant patient.[84,85]

Therapy of invasive fungal infection remains imperfect despite the array of agents now available to supplement or replace amphotericin, the previous therapeutic gold standard. As above, voriconazole has proven superior in both efficacy and reduced toxicity when compared to amphotericin (conventional or lipid-based) as treatment for neutropenic fever or for established aspergillosis.[82,83] Ongoing investigations with itraconazole, caspofungin, and several as yet unlicensed antimold agents suggest that the toxicities accompanying conventional amphotericin may be undesirable because the other agents have less multiorgan toxicity and similar efficacy. Ongoing controlled study is essential for continued informed choices, recently made more difficult by the array of available antifungal agents.

Superior antimold activity of newer antibiotics may be supplemented with a change in strategy to preemptive treatment rather than broad and intensive therapy for all patients with culture-negative neutropenic fever. Serum galactomannan[86,87] has been licensed for early diagnosis of aspergillosis and, although needing confirmation in additional multicenter trials, may prove valuable to supplement culture-negative fever, focal pulmonary infiltrates, or upper airway and sinus inflammation as early warning of the development of invasive *Aspergillus* or other mold infections.

Posttransplant Viral Infections

Three groups of viruses plague the immunocompromised transplant recipient. The herpes group viruses (herpes simplex, varicella-zoster, cytomegalovirus, Epstein–Barr virus, and possibly human herpesvirus 6) all need specific attention, screening, consideration of prophylaxis, and therapy if they reactivate following blood or marrow transplantation.[12,73] Oral or genital herpes simplex virus (HSV) reactivates in nearly two-thirds of transplant recipients not receiving specific antiviral prophylaxis.[88] The efficacy of acyclovir or valacyclovir has been demonstrated in other settings, and their use is widely applied to the HSV seropositive transplant recipient. Therapy with such antivirals is generally highly effective and is associated with limited toxicity. Disseminated HSV (pneumonitis, esophagitis, encephalitis) is uncommon with effective prophylaxis, prompt monitoring, and treatment.

Cytomegalovirus (CMV) risks are primarily determined by the patient's pretransplant exposure.[89] Highest risks of reactivation infection and disease are observed in CMV seropositive recipients, intermediate risks in seronegative allograft recipients receiving CMV seropositive donor transplants, and lowest risks in those who are CMV seronegative recipient and donor.[90] The seronegative recipient (with seronegative donor) requires protection against transfusion-associated transmission of CMV, and controlled studies have supported the value of CMV seronegative transfusion support,[91–93] leukocyte-depleted transfusion support, or the combination. The risks of CMV infection remain less than 5% in appropriately protected patients and CMV disease is rare, although one recent report highlighted the imperfect protection against transfusion-associated CMV transmission by leukoreduction.[94]

The seropositive recipient or patient receiving a seropositive graft requires specific CMV management: either antiviral prophylaxis or aggressive and prolonged screening to detect early infection and initiation of preemptive therapy. Early randomized studies supported the value of acyclovir, despite its limited anti-CMV activity in vitro, as suggestively effective in preventing and delaying CMV infection after allotransplantation (Table 88.3). In many centers, its use in the

TABLE 88.3. Prevention of cytomegalovirus (CMV) reactivation.

Trial	*Reference*	*Year*	*I*	*Randomized*	*Responses*	*Conclusions*
Boeckh	97	1996	226	Preemptive ganciclovir vs. prophylactic ganciclovir	CMV disease +100 14% vs. 2.7%, $P = 0.002$ CMV disease +180 equal	Survival equal
Burns	95	2002	91	Acyclovir vs. ganciclovir	Antigenemia 41% vs. 31%, $P = 0.22$; CMV disease 17% vs. 13%, $P = 0.59$	Bacterial infection and neutropenia more common with ganciclovir
Ljungman	166	2002	727	Valacyclovir vs. acyclovir	CMV infection/disease 28% vs. 40%, $P = 0.0001$	Survival equal
Meyers	167	1988	151	Acyclovir vs. placebo for CMV seropositive	70% vs. 87% CMV infection, $P = 0.0001$; 22% vs. 38% CMV disease, $P = 0.008$	Superior 100-day survival
Prentice	168	1997	310	Acyclovir vs. placebo	Reduced risk of CMV infection	19% better survival at 1 year
Reusser	98	2002	213	Foscarnet vs. ganciclovir	CMV disease or death and EFS equal	More neutropenia, thrombocytopenia with ganciclovir
Schmidt	169	1991	104	Ganciclovir vs. placebo for asymptomatic CMV + BAL	25% vs. 70% CMV infection or death, $P = .01$	Preemptive ganciclovir prevents pneumonitis
Verdonck	180	1997	41	Risk-adapted ganciclovir	No CMV pneumonitis using ganciclovir for antigenemia or for acute GVHD	Effective strategy
Winston	99	2003	168	Valacyclovir vs. ganciclovir	CMV infection 12% vs. 19%, $P = 0.93$	Equal CMV disease
Zikos	100	1998	128	IV IgG vs. CMV-IgG	Antigenemia 71% vs. 61%, $P = 0.37$	Time to antigenemia 47 vs. 48 days, $P = 0.9$

EFS, event-free survival; BAL, bronchoalveolar lavage.

early posttransplant period continues despite only limited data supporting its value.[95,96] Better tested is the more effective antiviral, ganciclovir, as specific CMV prophylaxis in the early posttransplant months. Its greater myelosuppressive activity confounds its superior antiviral effectiveness, and formal prospective trials[97] have suggested that its use as preemptive treatment following early detection of infection may be as effective as generally applied ganciclovir prophylaxis to the seropositive recipient. Foscarnet and valacyclovir had demonstrable efficacy as prophylaxis,[98,99] but high-titer anti-CMV IgG did not[100] (see Table 88.3).

Therapy of CMV reactivation includes ganciclovir, usually in high dose for a minimum of 2 to 3 weeks induction and an extended 4- to 6-week maintenance period of antiviral suppression. Treatment of antigenemia ($n = 60$) compared to treatment of CMV isolated from alveolar lavage ($n = 58$) reduced CMV disease to 1.7% versus 12% ($P = 0.02$).[101] This preemptive strategy led to CMV treatment in 48% versus only 13.8% of patients ($P = 0.001$), but GVHD and bacterial and fungal infections as well as survival were equivalent. Small comparative studies suggest efficacy of foscarnet for preemptive therapy as well, although its nephrotoxicity and metabolic disturbances (hypocalcemia, hypophosphatemia) complicate its general applicability and limit its efficacy for outpatient parenteral antiviral therapy. A comparison of foscarnet ($n = 110$) versus ganciclovir ($n = 113$) for antigenemia led to equivalent CMV disease and mortality, but neutropenia (4% versus 11%; $P = 0.04$) and stopping therapy for cytopenia (0% versus 6%; $P = 0.03$) was more common with ganciclovir.[98] Another smaller trial ($n = 39$) showed more CMV breakthrough with ganciclovir but similar CMV disease and treatment-related mortality.[102]

Equally important as the efficacy of the antiviral preemptive therapy is regular and prolonged effective screening for CMV reactivation. CMV antigenemia (pp65 testing of circulating leukocytes) is highly sensitive although ineffective during the first few weeks of leukopenia following transplant, even though this period is rarely associated with CMV reactivation and infection. Polymerase chain reaction (PCR) assays (which may be more specific but are not available in all centers) have high specificity and sensitivity and demonstrate the same indications for preemptive antiviral therapy when detectable in posttransplant blood samples.[103] Detection of late CMV infection (beyond day 100 posttransplant) requires continuing surveillance, particularly for patients with ongoing GVHD and immunosuppression, but the strategic specifics of antiviral screening in the late posttransplant period have not been well tested.[104] Generally, CMV blood reactivation in a patient with ongoing chronic GVHD would be treated, although all surveillance series recognize that a small fraction of patients with low-level antigenemia or low PCR burden will fail to progress to CMV disease despite lack of effective antiviral therapy.[105] This anecdotal experience does not define the appropriate duration for aggressive surveillance and initiation of therapy for high-risk GVHD patients with CMV reactivation.

CMV disease, usually pneumonitis or enteritis, demands treatment, most often with high-dose ganciclovir plus IV immunoglobulin (IVIG).[106–108] Studies in the 1980s defined the high mortality of CMV pneumonitis. These risks are reduced by IV IgG, although viral neutralization but higher anti-CMV IgG titers in the infused product have not been associated with the efficacy of IVIG therapy.[107] Immunomodulation and reduction of lung injury through IVIG, along with effective antiviral antibiotics, can reduce the mortality of CMV pneumonitis to less than 50%, particularly if therapy is initiated before ventilator support for respiratory failure is required.

CMV enteritis has been poorly studied, and only limited prospective data support a therapeutic approach similar to that used for CMV pneumonitis. Retrospective data[108] emphasize the variable effectiveness of such treatment, but highlight the limited evidence upon which to choose therapeutic approaches to biopsy-documented CMV enteritis. An anti-CMV monoclonal antibody was tested prospectively,[109] but failed to prevent or modulate the severity of CMV disease.

Epstein–Barr virus is most often associated with posttransplant lymphoproliferative disorders (PTLD),[110,111] which are best treated with antiviral therapy, IgG, and rituximab to lyse the virally infected CD20+ B-lymphoid neoplasm.[112,113] No controlled data support these approaches, nor have these been formally tested in comparison, but promising retrospective series strongly suggest that rituximab, reduction in immunosuppression, and possibly antiviral treatment represent the best therapeutic approach to these otherwise highly lethal disorders. Infusion of donor lymphocytes (from allograft donors) also may be highly effective in treating PTLD.[114,115]

Human herpesvirus (HHV) 6 has been associated with graft failure, encephalitis, enteritis, pneumonitis, and febrile posttransplant syndromes.[116,117] Its detection through the PCR method is not always associated with notable symptomatology. Clear understanding of the HHV 6-associated syndromes and their management and therapy is still lacking. Center-specific approaches rather than evidence-based comprehension of their pathophysiology remains the norm in most transplant centers.

Respiratory viruses, including respiratory syncytial virus (RSV), parainfluenza virus (PIV), and other agents associated with upper or lower respiratory community-acquired infections, are frequent and threatening to the transplant recipient.[118] RSV, because of its rapid diagnostic test (enzyme-linked immunosorbent assay, ELISA) and available therapy with inhaled ribavirin, has been most studied.[119,120] Its seasonal occurrence has caused regular outbreaks in transplant units worldwide. Protection of patients from visitors and staff with upper respiratory infection (URI) symptoms (mask and handwashing) and isolation of URI-infected patients to prevent horizontal transmission is essential. A similar, nonseasonal syndrome caused by PIV has been described, but the lack of rapid testing has prevented definitive assessment of the efficacy of antiviral therapy.[121] For both agents, alternative antivirals—IVIG and hyperimmune globulins—have been suggested, although no clear demonstrations of efficacy have been reported. Yearly influenza vaccine of transplant recipients and, perhaps more importantly, their immediate household contacts, is essential to reduce exposure and infection during seasonal influenza outbreaks.

Late Infections

Infections of 3 to 12 months or longer in the transplant recipient are well recognized,[76] especially in those with ongoing chronic GVHD who have defective opsonization of encapsulated bacteria (*Pneumococcus* and *Haemophilus influenza*). Poor T-cell function leaves patients at risk for *Pneumocystis carinii* or late fungal infection. Reactivation of varicella-zoster virus (VZV) or CMV are well-recognized risks. Vaccine strategies for *Haemophilus* and *Pneumococcus* have been investigated but not widely adopted.[73,77] Donor vaccine and posttransplant recipient booster vaccines, particularly with protein adjuvant, newer-generation vaccines, are promising[122,123] in augmenting antibody titers, although clinical efficacy has not been reported. Antibiotic prophylaxis against *Pneumocystis carinii* pneumonia (PCP) with trimethoprim sulfa, atovaquone, or dapsone is well recognized as effective in other populations. Limited reports in stem cell transplant patients, generally retrospective, support their continued use through 6 to 12 months posttransplant and 3 to 6 months after discontinuation of immunosuppression for chronic GVHD. Antipneumococcal antibiotic prophylaxis is essential for the chronic GVHD patient, but no formal reports of its efficacy are available. Widespread development of pneumococcal resistance to penicillin suggests that alternate agents (extended-spectrum quinolones) might be of value. Neither ciprofloxacin nor trimethoprim sulfa is effective as pneumococcal prophylaxis in the postsplenectomy or chronic GVHD setting. Ongoing antibiotic prophylaxis against VZV or CMV is not standardized although, as stated earlier, continuing CMV surveillance for the chronic GVHD patient under active immunosuppression is advisable, based upon the perceived risk and morbidity associated with viral reactivation.

Graft-Versus-Host Disease

Acute graft-versus-host disease (GVHD) is the most frequent life-threatening complication occurring following allogeneic transplantation.[124] Typically developing 3 weeks to 3 months after grafting, GVHD can produce a desquamative or even blistering erythematous skin rash, cholestatic hepatitis, and/or gastrointestinal (GI) involvement with nausea, vomiting, or large-volume secretory diarrhea. Its pathogenesis involves donor T-cell allorecognition, T-cell activation, and expansion in response to host alloantigens. GVHD is more frequent and more severe following partially matched or unrelated donor transplantation.[125] Some reports suggest its incidence and severity may be less in UCB transplants, despite their greater HLA donor–recipient mismatch.[38,39,41] GVHD can be directly life threatening, can further confound host defense, and thus be complicated by infection. A chronic GVHD syndrome can develop with a sicca syndrome, hepatitis, GI involvement with esophageal dysmotility and weight loss, cutaneous scleroderma changes, contractures and arthralgias, and myopathy or genitourinary involvement.[126,127]

GVHD requires specific prophylaxis, and numerous strategies have been studied in small and large prospective Phase III trials. Nearly three decades of experience extending from the acknowledgment that T lymphocytes are essential for initiating GVHD, led to graft manipulations to limit, eliminate, or inactivate the donor T cells within the graft as GVHD prophylaxis.[124,128] Varying intensities of T-cell depletion using anti-T-cell antibody plus complement, elutriation for mechanical cell fractionation, CD34 selection with resultant T-cell depletion, or anti-T-cell antisera "in the bag," have all shown variable effectiveness in limiting the frequency and severity of GVHD. Despite frequent studies of this approach, no consensus about its value, efficacy, or long-term advantage for use as GVHD prophylaxis remains. T-cell depletion regularly increases risks of graft failure, limits the allogeneic antitumor effect, sometimes resulting in more relapse, and may delay immune recovery, thereby augmenting risks of continuing opportunistic posttransplant infections. Despite ample evidence and extensive clinical testing, the heterogeneity of clinical settings (HLA-matched donor, unrelated donor, partial-matched haploidentical donor) and T-cell depletion strategies yields no clear evidence to conclude that T-cell depletion is either effective or ineffective at improving outcomes after transplantation. Extensive T-cell depletion can limit GVHD, but most reports demonstrate augmented alternative morbidity and similar mortality using T-cell depletion versus posttransplant immunosuppressive therapy for GVHD prophylaxis after any type of allogeneic transplant.

Pharmacologic GVHD prophylaxis is also widely studied (Table 88.4). Prevention of acute GVHD has been tested using single or combination therapies most frequently with corticosteroids, methotrexate, cyclosporine, tacrolimus, and mycophenolate mofetil (MMF). Newer anticytokine therapies (interleukin 1 receptor antagonist, anti-TNF antibodies, TNF receptor antagonists, IL-11) and newer drugs (sirolimus, pentostatin, fludarabine) have also been studied without clear conclusions as to their utility. This specific topic is the most frequent subject for prospective randomized trials in all allogeneic transplantation, yet there is continued variability across transplant centers because the evidence is uncertain.

In the 1980s, methotrexate (short course) plus cyclosporine was definitively demonstrated as superior to either cyclosporine alone, methotrexate alone, or either in combination with corticosteroids.[129–131] Subsequent trials suggested value for addition of low-dose prednisone, although these results are unconfirmed.[132,133] Long-term follow-up shows no continuing advantage for the addition of prednisone. Two large trials in the 1990s (one in sibling donors, one in URD), tested tacrolimus versus cyclosporine in conjunction with short-course methotrexate as GVHD prophylaxis.[134,135] In both studies, GVHD was less frequent using tacrolimus, but alternative morbidities and other complications yielded statistically similar survival and disease-free survival in both cohorts. Because of inhomogeneity in the randomized strata (particularly in the HLA-matched sibling trial), many centers adopted tacrolimus as superior. Frequently, lower therapeutic (5–10 ng/mL) targeted blood levels are used, although follow-up trials have not been reported to confirm its superiority.

Similarly, methotrexate, long a mainstay of GVHD prophylaxis, has had modifications to the originally reported four-dose, short-course regimen (15 mg/m^2 day 1, 10 mg/m^2 days 3, 6, and 11 posttransplant). Shorter courses and smaller doses (often 5 mg/m^2) have been reported with less mucositis

TABLE 88.4. Prevention of acute GVHD.

Trial	*Reference*	*Year*	*N*	*Randomized*	*DFS/survival*	*Conclusions*
Antin	170	2002	186	IL1RA vs. placebo	61% vs. 59% B–D aGVHD	No effect of IL1RA on OS or DFS
Bacigalupo	171	2001	109	ATG vs. control	11% vs. 50% III/IV aGVHD with high dose ATG, $P = 0.001$; 39% vs. 50% cGVHD	OS equal; more infections with ATG
Bolwell	172	2004	40	CSA/Mtx vs. CSA/MMF	65% vs. 21% severe mucositis, $P = 0.008$; 18 vs. 11 days neutrophil engraftment, $P < 0.001$; equal GVHD	Less toxicity with MMF
Chao	133	2000	186	CSA/Mtx/Pred vs. CSA/Mtx	18% vs. 20% II–IV aGVHD, $P = 0.6$; 46% vs. 62% cGVHD, $P = 0.83$	Similar OS, DFS
Deeg	131	1997	122	CSA vs. CSA/prednisone	73% vs. 60% II/IV aGVHD, $P = 0.01$; 21% vs. 44% cGVHD, $P = 0.02$	OS equal
Locatelli	173	2000	59	Low-dose CSA vs. CSA	57% vs. 38% II/IV aGVHD, $P = 0.06$; 30% vs. 26% cGVHD, P = NS	Similar outcomes with low dose
Nash	135	2000	180	FK/Mtx vs. CSA/Mtx	56% vs. 74% II/IV aGVHD, $P = 0.0002$; 76% vs. 50% cGVHD, $P = 0.06$	Relapse 15% vs. 41%, $P = 0.03$; OS equal
Ratanath-arathorn	134	1998	329	FK/Mtx vs. CSA/Mtx	32% vs. 44% II/IV aGVHD, $P = 0.01$; 56% vs. 49% cGVHD, P = NS	More toxicity with FK
Ruutu	132	2000	108	CSA/Mtx/methylprednisolone vs. CSA/Mtx	19% vs. 56% aGVHD, $P = 0.0001$	Trend to less GVHD; equal survival
Storb	129	1989	67	Mtx vs. CSA/Mtx	53% vs. 33% II/IV aGVHD, $P = 0.012$; 80% vs. 42% cGVHD, P = NS	Less acute GVHD
Storb	130	1986	46	Mtx vs. CSA/Mtx	18% vs. 53% II/IV aGVHD, $P = 0.012$; 82% vs. 60% 2-year survival, $P = 0.062$	Less acute GVHD

IL1RA, interleukin 1 receptor antagonist; FK, FK506 (tacrolimus); CSA, cyclosporine; Mtx, methotrexate; MMF, mycophenolate mofetil.

and sometimes quicker neutropenia, but all studies have been too small and thus underpowered to recognize limitations in GVHD prophylaxis using these mini-methotrexate approaches.[136] They remain, however, increasingly frequently used. Individual center habits and local protocols, often thoughtfully but empirically derived from evidence-based literature, remain the norm in defining GVHD prophylaxis strategies across many centers.

Therapy of Acute Graft-Versus-Host Disease

In addition to potent immunosuppressive therapy to blunt the immunologically based tissue injury, critical elements for treatment of acute GVHD, include aggressive infection prophylaxis, nutritional support, mineral balance, and avoidance of polypharmacy and drug-associated toxicities. Specific GVHD therapy relies upon corticosteroids and has done so for more than two-and-a-half decades. Several formal trials have tested added immunosuppressive reagents for initial therapy of acute GVHD, but none has sustained a demonstrable therapeutic advantage (Table 88.5). Antithymocyte globulin, ABX-CBL, daclizumab, and infliximab have been tested in formal prospective randomized trials with neither better GVHD symptom control nor reduced infections, lesser steroid requirements, nor improved short-term survival. Numerous other agents, including anti-TNF antibodies, pentostatin, etanercept, MMF, and denileukin diftitox (Ontax) have all showed promise in unconfirmed, single-arm, and small Phase II trials, but additional therapy evaluation in a more formal setting is required to accept any agent as promising for acute GVHD therapy.[137]

Steroid dosing (1–2 mg/kg/day) of prednisone or methylprednisolone has been the most commonly applied initial therapy, with limited testing of higher doses not confirmed as superior. One formal trial compared shorter (8-week) versus longer (16-week) defined corticosteroid tapering and showed equivalent GVHD control, shorter total therapy, and no added risks of the quicker tapering schedule.[138] Little other evidence is available to strongly support the use of other reagents as primary or salvage therapy for flares of acute GVHD (anti-CD5 immunotoxin, interleukin 1 receptor antagonist, etanercept, infliximab).

TABLE 88.5. Treatment of acute GVHD.

Trial	*Reference*	*Year*	*I*	*Randomized*	*Response*	*Conclusions*
Couriel	174	2004	134	Infliximab vs. control	67% response; 62% CR	Many infections
Cragg	175	2000	100	Prednisone vs. ATG/Pred	76% responses in both groups	Equal survival; no advantage to ATG
Deeg	176	2001	27	ABX-CBL for steroid refractory GVHD	51% response; 26% CR	44% 6-month survival
Doney	177	1981	37	Prednisone vs. ATG/Pred	Equal response and survival	
Hings	138	1993	30	Long- vs. short-course prednisone	Similar control of GVHD with shorter course prednisone	Shorter therapy course preferable
Lee	178	2004	102	Daclizumab vs. prednisone	53% vs. 51% response, $P = 0.85$ 77% vs. 94% 100-day survival, $P = 0.02$ 29% vs. 60% 1-year survival, $P = 0.002$	Unsafe combination GVHD therapy
Martin	179	1996	243	CD5 immunotoxin vs. placebo	40% vs. 25% CR at 4 weeks but equal response at 6 weeks, 49% vs. 45% 1-year survival, $P = 0.68$	No net benefit of immunotoxin

ATG, antithymocyte globulin; CR, complete remission.

Chronic Graft-Versus-Host Disease

The continuing donor-derived immune attack on recipient tissues manifest as chronic GVHD develops in 30% to 40% of allograft recipients, more often in adults and recipients of mismatched transplants.[126,127,139] Resembling scleroderma or lupus to some extent, but also including failure to thrive, intestinal dysfunction, bronchiolitis obliterans, and an ocular and oral sicca syndrome, chronic GVHD is often accompanied by autoantibody formation, hypogammaglobulinemia, and secondary infection. Its therapy requires long-term, low-dose immunosuppressive treatment with aggressive attention to hydration, nutrition, infection prophylaxis, and attempts to minimize the cumulative and chronic effects of long-term immunosuppression, including the consequences of extended steroid therapy. Diabetes, osteopenia, cataracts, and avascular necrosis of bone all complicate such extended therapy. Ongoing studies are required to minimize these toxicities.

In addition to corticosteroids, cyclosporine, azathioprine, MMF, pentostatin, hydroxychloroquine, and thalidomide have all been used as adjunct immunosuppressive therapies, most in limited single-arm Phase II trials. The promise of thalidomide was not confirmed in two prospective randomized trials.[140,141] The first showed no advantage in disease control, infection prophylaxis, limited steroid use, duration of immunosuppressive therapy, or survival for patients treated with thalidomide, cyclosporine, and alternate-day prednisone compared to the latter two agents without thalidomide.[140] The other trial demonstrated intolerance of thalidomide for the majority of patients and incomplete continuation of therapy.[141] Newer approaches to chronic GVHD show some, albeit limited, activity in a variety of small series, but no clear-cut guidelines for initiation or continuation of therapy beyond low-dose alternate-day steroids and calcineurin inhibitors have been recognized. Continuation of therapy for 6 to 9 months beyond active symptoms followed by slow withdrawal of therapy is the general recommended schedule. Several series have shown no advantage to even cyclosporine beyond alternate-day steroids for patients with standard-risk chronic GVHD.[139,142]

Late Complications of Transplantation

Study of late transplant complications has, for the most part, been directed toward identification of the possible toxicities, comprehension of specific risk factors, and recommendation of screening strategies to identify late toxicities. TBI, alkylating agents, and corticosteroids all contribute to cataract formation, but long-term results of TBI-sparing conditioning regimens and the incidence of such complications are not reported.[143] Hypothyroidism (30% to 50% of patients) and hypogonadism (60% to 90% of patients) develop and need periodic assessment through careful history-taking and occasional biochemical screening.[144,145] Menopausal symptomatology and sexual dysfunction may develop requiring appropriate attention, sometimes hormone replacement and attention to prophylaxis against ongoing and progressive osteoporosis.[145–149] No techniques, including gonadotropic inhibitors or pretransplant hormonal replacement for gonadal suppression, have proved effective at preventing or reducing the incidence of posttransplant gonadal failure for women. Nearly all men are azoospermic and thus infertile after transplantation. Transplantation without TBI can be fertility sparing in nearly one-third of patients, particularly in prepubertal transplant recipients, although secondary sexual development may be delayed.[150]

The most dramatic, although not most frequent, posttransplant complication is secondary carcinogenesis as a consequence of prolonged immunosuppression, pre- and peritransplant alkylator and radiation mutagenesis, and viral-associated neoplasia.[110,111] Greater than eightfold-higher risk of cancer for transplant recipients has been reported, most involving non-Hodgkin's lymphomas and secondary myelodysplastic syndromes or acute myelogenous leukemia (AML), but no formal studies have addressed peritransplant techniques to reduce the incidence of posttransplant secondary neoplasia.[151–154] Limited use of irradiation, reduced exposure to alkylators or other DNA-damaging agents, and earlier transplantation before years of alkylator exposure (e.g., for lymphoma or chronic lymphocytic leukemia) have occurred, might be effective in these goals, but definitive evidence to support these contentions is lacking.[154]

Recovery and Quality of Life

Stem cell transplant survivors generally return to full and complete functional status.[148,155–157] Numerous quality of life reports have shown that, within 1 year of transplantation, the vast majority of patients return to work and nearly 90% of autologous transplant recipients show high quality of life in formal testing.[157] Allogeneic transplant recipients recover more slowly, especially those beyond 35 or 40 years of age, those with chronic GVHD, and those in whom physical and ongoing psychologic problems delay their return to full health and good performance status. A recent report[158] emphasized that full recovery after transplant requires 3 to 5 years for the majority of patients. Patients with slower physical recovery had higher medical risks and were more depressed before bone marrow transplantation. Patients with chronic GVHD, those with less pretransplant social support, and women had more posttransplant depression. Encouragingly, even patients who had extended cancer therapy before transplantation had rapid recovery from depression and overall treatment-related distress.

Summary

Overall, the life-saving potential of transplant therapy remains unchallenged by many new advances in cancer therapy. Continued efforts to reduce peritransplant morbidity and mortality require less empiricism, less reliance on experience, and additional focus on formal testing of diagnostic therapeutic and long-term supportive care approaches that can definitively improve the outcome and augment the applicability of transplantation to a larger patient population, although complex medical care in this field, as in many others, relies on expanded experience and specialty expertise. Coalescence of that expertise into defined clinical protocols, followed by testing in prospective therapeutic trials, can help remove the lore and support the physiologically based best practices in managing recipients of transplantation.

References

1. Antin JH. Clinical practice. Long-term care after hematopoietic-cell transplantation in adults. N Engl J Med 2002;347:36–42.
2. Djulbegovic B, Loughran TP Jr, Hornung CA, et al. The quality of medical evidence in hematology-oncology. Am J Med 1999;106:198–205.
3. Bearman SI, Appelbaum FR, Buckner CD, et al. Regimen-related toxicity in patients undergoing bone marrow transplantation. J Clin Oncol 1988;6:1562–1568.
4. Weisdorf DJ, Bostrom B, Raether D, et al. Oropharyngeal mucositis complicating bone marrow transplantation: prognostic factors and the effect of chlorhexidine mouth rinse. Bone Marrow Transplant 1989;4:89–95.
5. Shankar G, Cohen DA. Idiopathic pneumonia syndrome after bone marrow transplantation: the role of pre-transplant radiation conditioning and local cytokine dysregulation in promoting lung inflammation and fibrosis. Int J Exp Pathol 2001;82:101–113.
6. Carreras E, Bertz H, Arcese W, et al. Incidence and outcome of hepatic veno-occlusive disease after blood or marrow transplantation: a prospective cohort study of the European Group for Blood and Marrow Transplantation. European Group for Blood and Marrow Transplantation Chronic Leukemia Working Party. Blood 1998;92:3599–3604.
7. Wolford JL, McDonald GB. A problem-oriented approach to intestinal and liver disease after marrow transplantation. J Clin Gastroenterol 1988;10:419–433.
8. Beyer J, Grabbe J, Lenz K, et al. Cutaneous toxicity of high-dose carboplatin, etoposide and ifosfamide followed by autologous stem cell reinfusion. Bone Marrow Transplant 1992;10:491–494.
9. Sencer SF, Haake RJ, Weisdorf DJ. Hemorrhagic cystitis after bone marrow transplantation. Risk factors and complications. Transplantation 1993;56:875–879.
10. Murdych T, Weisdorf DJ. Serious cardiac complications during bone marrow transplantation at the University of Minnesota, 1977–1997. Bone Marrow Transplant 2001;28:283–287.
11. Krouwer HG, Wijdicks EF. Neurologic complications of bone marrow transplantation. Neurol Clin 2003;21:319–352.
12. van Burik JA, Weisdorf DJ. Infections in recipients of blood and marrow transplantation. Hematol Oncol Clin N Am 1999;13:1065–1089.
13. Weisdorf DJ, Verfaillie CM, Davies SM, et al. Hematopoietic growth factors for graft failure after bone marrow transplantation: a randomized trial of granulocyte-macrophage colony-stimulating factor (GM-CSF) versus sequential GM-CSF plus granulocyte-CSF. Blood 1995;85:3452–3456.
14. Bensinger W, Appelbaum F, Rowley S, et al. Factors that influence collection and engraftment of autologous peripheral-blood stem cells. J Clin Oncol 1995;13:2547–2555.
15. Weaver CH, Hazelton B, Birch R, et al. An analysis of engraftment kinetics as a function of the CD34 content of peripheral blood progenitor cell collections in 692 patients after the administration of myeloablative chemotherapy. Blood 1995;86:3961–3969.
16. Schmitz N, Linch DC, Dreger P, et al. Randomised trial of filgrastim-mobilised peripheral blood progenitor cell transplantation versus autologous bone-marrow transplantation in lymphoma patients. Lancet 1996;347:353–357.
17. Weisdorf DJ, Verfailli CM, Miller WJ, et al. Autologous bone marrow versus non-mobilized peripheral blood stem cell transplantation for lymphoid malignancies: a prospective, comparative trial. Am J Hematol 1997;54:202–208.
18. Weisdorf D, Miller J, Verfaillie C, et al. Cytokine-primed bone marrow stem cells vs. peripheral blood stem cells for autologous transplantation: a randomized comparison of GM-CSF vs. G-CSF. Biol Blood Marrow Transplant 1997;3:217–223.
19. Beyer J, Schwella N, Zingsem J, et al. Hematopoietic rescue after high-dose chemotherapy using autologous peripheral-blood progenitor cells or bone marrow: a randomized comparison. J Clin Oncol 1995;13:1328–1335.
20. Abdel-Razeq H, Pohlman B, Andresen S, et al. A randomized study of multi-day infusion of autologous peripheral blood progenitor cells. Bone Marrow Transplant 1998;21:221–223.
21. Bolwell BJ, Pohlman B, Andresen S, et al. Delayed G-CSF after autologous progenitor cell transplantation: a prospective randomized trial. Bone Marrow Transplant 1998;21:369–373.
22. Bolwell B, Goormastic M, Dannley R, et al. G-CSF post-autologous progenitor cell transplantation: a randomized study of 5, 10, and 16 micrograms/kg/day. Bone Marrow Transplant 1997;19:215–219.

23. Sheridan WP, Begley CG, To LB, et al. Phase II study of autologous filgrastim (G-CSF)-mobilized peripheral blood progenitor cells to restore hemopoiesis after high-dose chemotherapy for lymphoid malignancies. Bone Marrow Transplant 1994;14:105–111.
24. Hogge DE, Lambie K, Sutherland HJ, et al. Quantitation of primitive and lineage-committed progenitors in mobilized peripheral blood for prediction of platelet recovery postautologous transplant. Bone Marrow Transplant 2000;25:589–598.
25. Dicke KA, Hood DL, Arneson M, et al. Effects of short-term in vivo administration of G-CSF on bone marrow prior to harvesting. Exp Hematol 1997;25:34–38.
26. Gyger M, Sahovic E, Aslam M. Randomized trial of autologous filgrastim-primed bone marrow transplantation versus filgrastim-mobilized peripheral blood stem cell transplantation in lymphoma patients. Blood 1998;92:3489–3490.
27. Davies SM, Kollman C, Anasetti C, et al. Engraftment and survival after unrelated-donor bone marrow transplantation: a report from the National Marrow Donor Program. Blood 2000;96:4096–4102.
28. Aversa F, Velardi A, Tabilio A, et al. Haploidentical stem cell transplantation in leukemia. Blood Rev 2001;15:111–119.
29. Yamasaki S, Ohno Y, Taniguchi S, et al. Allogeneic peripheral blood stem cell transplantation from two- or three-loci-mismatched related donors in adult Japanese patients with high-risk hematologic malignancies. Bone Marrow Transplant 2004;33:279–289.
30. Cutler C, Giri S, Jeyapalan S, Paniagua D, Viswanathan A, Antin JH. Acute and chronic graft-versus-host disease after allogeneic peripheral-blood stem-cell and bone marrow transplantation: a meta-analysis. J Clin Oncol 2001;19:3685–3691.
31. Anderson D, DeFor T, Burns L, et al. A comparison of related donor peripheral blood and bone marrow transplants: importance of late-onset chronic graft-versus-host disease and infections. Biol Blood Marrow Transplant 2003;9:52–59.
32. Eapen M, Horowitz MM, Klein JP, et al. Higher mortality after allogeneic peripheral blood transplantation compared to bone marrow in children and adolescents. J Clin Oncol 2004;22(24):4865–4866.
33. Morton J, Hutchins C, Durrant S. Granulocyte-colony-stimulating factor (G-CSF)-primed allogeneic bone marrow: significantly less graft-versus-host disease and comparable engraftment to G-CSF-mobilized peripheral blood stem cells. Blood 2001;98:3186–3191.
34. Ji SQ, Chen HR, Wang HX, Yan HM, Pan SP, Xun CQ. Comparison of outcome of allogeneic bone marrow transplantation with and without granulocyte colony-stimulating factor (lenograstim) donor-marrow priming in patients with chronic myelogenous leukemia. Biol Blood Marrow Transplant 2002;8:261–267.
35. Lee KH, Lee JH, Choi SJ, et al. Randomized comparison of two different schedules of granulocyte colony-stimulating factor administration after allogeneic bone marrow transplantation. Bone Marrow Transplant 1999;24:591–599.
36. Hagglund H, Ringden O, Oman S, Remberger M, Carlens S, Mattsson J. A prospective randomized trial of Filgrastim (r-metHuG-CSF) given at different times after unrelated bone marrow transplantation. Bone Marrow Transplant 1999;24:831–836.
37. Rubenstein P, Carrier C, Scaradavou, et al. Outcomes among 562 recipients of placental-blood transplants from unrelated donors. N Engl J Med 1998;339:1565–1577.
38. Michel G, Rocha V, Chevret S, et al. Unrelated cord blood transplantation for childhood acute myeloid leukemia: a Eurocord Group analysis. Blood 2003;102:4290–4297.
39. Barker JN, Davies SM, DeFor T, Ramsay NK, Weisdorf DJ, Wagner JE. Survival after transplantation of unrelated donor umbilical cord blood is comparable to that of human leukocyte antigen-matched unrelated donor bone marrow: results of a matched-pair analysis. Blood 2001;97:2957–2961.
40. Laughlin MJ, Barker J, Bambach B, et al. Hematopoietic engraftment and survival in adult recipients of umbilical-cord blood from unrelated donors. N Engl J Med 2001;344:1815–1822.
41. Barker JN, Weisdorf DJ, DeFor TE, et al. Transplantation of two partially HLA-matched umbilical cord blood units to enhance engraftment in adults with hematologic malignancy. Blood 2005;105:1343–1347.
42. Wagner JE, Barker JN, DeFor TE, et al. Transplantation of unrelated donor umbilical cord blood in 102 patients with malignant and nonmalignant diseases: influence of CD34 cell dose and HLA disparity on treatment-related mortality and survival. Blood 2002;100:1611–1618.
43. Gluckman E, Rocha V, Arcese W, et al. Factors associated with outcomes of unrelated cord blood transplant: guidelines for donor choice. Exp Hematol 2004;32:397–407.
44. Davies SM, Weisdorf DJ, Haake RJ, et al. Second infusion of bone marrow for treatment of graft failure after allogeneic bone marrow transplantation. Bone Marrow Transplant 1994;14:73–77.
45. Sonis ST, Oster G, Fuchs H, et al. Oral mucositis and the clinical and economic outcomes of hematopoietic stem-cell transplantation. J Clin Oncol 2001;19:2201–2205.
46. Wardley AM, Jayson GC, Swindell R, et al. Prospective evaluation of oral mucositis in patients receiving myeloablative conditioning regimens and haemopoietic progenitor rescue. Br J Haematol 2000;110:292–299.
47. Giles FJ, Rodriguez R, Weisdorf D, et al. A phase III, randomized, double-blind, placebo-controlled, study of isoganan for the reduction of stomatitis in patients receiving stomatotoxic chemotherapy. Leuk Res 2004;28:559–565.
48. Papas AS, Clark RE, Martuscelli G, O'Loughlin KT, Johansen E, Miller KB. A prospective, randomized trial for the prevention of mucositis in patients undergoing hematopoietic stem cell transplantation. Bone Marrow Transplant 2003;31:705–712.
49. Antin JH, Lee SJ, Neuberg D, et al. A phase I/II double-blind, placebo-controlled study of recombinant human interleukin-11 for mucositis and acute GVHD prevention in allogeneic stem cell transplantation. Bone Marrow Transplant 2002;29:373–377.
50. Meropol NJ, Somer RA, Gutheil J, et al. Randomized phase I trial of recombinant human keratinocyte growth factor plus chemotherapy: potential role as mucosal protectant. J Clin Oncol 2003;21:1452–1458.
51. Spielberger R, Stiff P, Bensinger W, et al. Palifermin for oral mucositis after intensive therapy for hematologic cancers. N Engl J Med 2004;351:2590–2598.
52. Phillips GL, Meisenberg B, Reece DE, et al. Amifostine and autologous hematopoietic stem cell support of escalating-dose melphalan: A phase I study. Biol Blood Marrow Transplant 2004;10:473–483.
53. McDonald GB, Hinds MS, Fisher LD, et al. Veno-occlusive disease of the liver and multiorgan failure after bone marrow transplantation: a cohort study of 355 patients. Ann Intern Med 1993;118:255–267.
54. Bearman SI. The syndrome of hepatic veno-occlusive disease after marrow transplantation. Blood 1995;85:3005–3020.
55. Jones RJ, Lee KS, Beschorner WE, et al. Venoocclusive disease of the liver following bone marrow transplantation. Transplantation 1987;44:778–783.
56. Sharafuddin MJ, Foshager MC, Steinbuch M, Weisdorf DJ, Hunter DW. Sonographic findings in bone marrow transplant patients with symptomatic hepatic venoocclusive disease. J Ultrasound Med 1997;16:575–586.
57. Attal M, Huguet F, Rubie H, et al. Prevention of hepatic veno-occlusive disease after bone marrow transplantation by contin-

uous infusion of low-dose heparin: a prospective, randomized trial. Blood 1992;79:2834–2840.
58. Attal M, Huguet F, Rubie H, et al. Prevention of regimen-related toxicities after bone marrow transplantation by pentoxifylline: a prospective, randomized trial. Blood 1993;82:732–736.
59. Essell JH, Schroeder MT, Harman GS, et al. Ursodiol prophylaxis against hepatic complications of allogeneic bone marrow transplantation. A randomized, double-blind, placebo-controlled trial. Ann Intern Med 1998;128:975–981.
60. Park SH, Lee MH, Lee H, et al. A randomized trial of heparin plus ursodiol vs. heparin alone to prevent hepatic veno-occlusive disease after hematopoietic stem cell transplantation. Bone Marrow Transplant 2002;29:137–143.
61. Bearman SI, Lee JL, Baron AE, McDonald GB. Treatment of hepatic venocclusive disease with recombinant human tissue plasminogen activator and heparin in 42 marrow transplant patients. Blood 1997;89:1501–1506.
62. Schriber J, Milk B, Shaw D, et al. Tissue plasminogen activator (tPA) as therapy for hepatotoxicity following bone marrow transplantation. Bone Marrow Transplant 1999;24:1311–1314.
63. Richardson PG, Murakami C, Jin Z, et al. Multi-institutional use of defibrotide in 88 patients after stem cell transplantation with severe veno-occlusive disease and multisystem organ failure: response without significant toxicity in a high-risk population and factors predictive of outcome. Blood 2002;100:4337–4343.
64. Robbins RA, Linder J, Stahl MG, et al. Diffuse alveolar hemorrhage in autologous bone marrow transplant recipients. Am J Med 1989;87:511–518.
65. Ho VT, Weller E, Lee SJ, Alyea EP, Antin JH, Soiffer RJ. Prognostic factors for early severe pulmonary complications after hematopoietic stem cell transplantation. Biol Blood Marrow Transplant 2001;7:223–229.
66. Applebaum FR, Meyers JD, Fefer A, et al. Nonbacterial nonfungal pneumonia following marrow transplantation in 100 identical twins. Transplantation 1982;33:265–268.
67. Chen CS, Boeckh M, Seidel K, et al. Incidence, risk factors, and mortality from pneumonia developing late after hematopoietic stem cell transplantation. Bone Marrow Transplant 2003;32: 515–522.
68. Ringden O, Remberger M, Ruutu T, et al. Increased risk of chronic graft-versus-host disease, obstructive bronchiolitis, and alopecia with busulfan versus total body irradiation: long-term results of a randomized trial in allogeneic marrow recipients with leukemia. Nordic Bone Marrow Transplantation Group. Blood 1999;93:2196–2201.
69. Gopal R, Ha CS, Tucker SL, et al. Comparison of two total body irradiation fractionation regimens with respect to acute and late pulmonary toxicity. Cancer (Phila) 2001;92:1949–1958.
70. Metcalf JP, Rennard SI, Reed EC, et al. Corticosteroids as adjunctive therapy for diffuse alveolar hemorrhage associated with bone marrow transplantation. University of Nebraska Medical Center Bone Marrow Transplant Group. Am J Med 1994;96: 327–334.
71. Lewis ID, DeFor T, Weisdorf DJ. Increasing incidence of diffuse alveolar hemorrhage following allogeneic bone marrow transplantation: cryptic etiology and uncertain therapy. Bone Marrow Transplant 2000;26:539–543.
72. Chao NJ, Duncan SR, Long GD, Horning SJ, Blume KG. Corticosteroid therapy for diffuse alveolar hemorrhage in autologous bone marrow transplant recipients. Ann Intern Med 1991;114: 145–146.
73. Sullivan KM, Dykewicz CA, Longworth DL, et al. Preventing opportunistic infections after hematopoietic stem cell transplantation: the Centers for Disease Control and Prevention, Infectious Diseases Society of America, and American Society for Blood and Marrow Transplantation Practice Guidelines and beyond. Hematology (Am Soc Hematol Educ Program) 2001; 392–421.
74. Storek J, Dawson MA, Storer B, et al. Immune reconstitution after allogeneic marrow transplantation compared with blood stem cell transplantation. Blood 2001;97:3380–3389.
75. Storek J, Gooley T, Witherspoon RP, Sullivan KM, Storb R. Infectious morbidity in long-term survivors of allogeneic marrow transplantation is associated with low CD4 T cell counts. Am J Hematol 1997;54:131–138.
76. Ochs L, Shu XO, Miller J, et al. Late infections after allogeneic bone marrow transplantations: comparison of incidence in related and unrelated donor transplant recipients. Blood 1995;86: 3979–3986.
77. Goodman JL, Winston DJ, Greenfield RA, et al. A controlled trial of fluconazole to prevent fungal infections in patients undergoing bone marrow transplantation. N Engl J Med 1992;326:845–851.
78. Slavin MA, Osborne B, Adams R, et al. Efficacy and safety of fluconazole prophylaxis for fungal infections after marrow transplantation—a prospective, randomized, double-blind study. J Infect Dis 1995;171:1545–1552.
79. Marr KA, Seidel K, Slavin MA, et al. Prolonged fluconazole prophylaxis is associated with persistent protection against candidiasis-related death in allogeneic marrow transplant recipients: long-term follow-up of a randomized, placebo-controlled trial. Blood 2000;96:2055–2061.
80. Marr KA, Crippa F, Leisenring W, et al. Itraconazole versus fluconazole for prevention of fungal infections in patients receiving allogeneic stem cell transplants. Blood 2004;103:1527–1533.
81. Nucci M, Biasoli I, Akiti T, et al. A double-blind, randomized, placebo-controlled trial of itraconazole capsules as antifungal prophylaxis for neutropenic patients. Clin Infect Dis 2000;30: 300–305.
82. Walsh TJ, Pappas P, Winston DJ, et al. Voriconazole compared with liposomal amphotericin B for empirical antifungal therapy in patients with neutropenia and persistent fever. N Engl J Med 2002;346:225–234.
83. Herbrecht R, Denning DW, Patterson TF, et al. Voriconazole versus amphotericin B for primary therapy of invasive aspergillosis. N Engl J Med 2002;347:408–415.
84. Mora-Duarte J, Betts R, Rotstein C, et al. Comparison of caspofungin and amphotericin B for invasive candidiasis. N Engl J Med 2002;347:2020–2029.
85. Denning DW. Echinocandin antifungal drugs. Lancet 2003; 362:1142–1151.
86. Marr KA, Balajee SA, McLaughlin L, et al. Detection of galactomannan antigenemia by enzyme immunoassay for the diagnosis of invasive aspergillosis: variables that affect performance. J Infect Dis 2004;190:641–649.
87. Rovira M, Jimenez M, De La Bellacasa JP, et al. Detection of *Aspergillus galactomannan* by enzyme immunoabsorbent assay in recipients of allogeneic hematopoietic stem cell transplantation: a prospective study. Transplantation 2004;77:1260–1264.
88. Wade JC, Newton B, Flournoy N, Meyers JD. Oral acyclovir for prevention of herpes simplex virus reactivation after marrow transplantation. Ann Intern Med 1984;100:823–828.
89. Zaia JA. Prevention of cytomegalovirus disease in hematopoietic stem cell transplantation. Clin Infect Dis 2002;35:999–1004.
90. Boeckh M, Nichols WG. The impact of cytomegalovirus serostatus of donor and recipient before hematopoietic stem cell transplantation in the era of antiviral prophylaxis and preemptive therapy. Blood 2004;103:2003–2008.
91. Miller WJ, McCullough J, Balfour HH Jr, et al. Prevention of cytomegalovirus infection following bone marrow transplantation: a randomized trial of blood product screening. Bone Marrow Transplant 1991;7:227–234.
92. Bowden RA, Sayers M, Flournoy N, et al. Cytomegalovirus immune globulin and seronegative blood products to prevent primary cytomegalovirus infection after marrow transplantation. N Engl J Med 1986;314:1006–1010.

93. Bowden RA, Slichter SJ, Sayers M, et al. A comparison of filtered leukocyte-reduced and cytomegalovirus (CMV) seronegative blood products for the prevention of transfusion-associated CMV infection after marrow transplant. Blood 1995;86:3598–3603.
94. Nichols WG, Price TH, Gooley T, Corey L, Boeckh M. Transfusion-transmitted cytomegalovirus infection after receipt of leukoreduced blood products. Blood 2003;101:4195–4200.
95. Burns LJ, Miller W, Kandaswamy C, et al. Randomized clinical trial of ganciclovir vs acyclovir for prevention of cytomegalovirus antigenemia after allogeneic transplantation. Bone Marrow Transplant 2002;30:945–951.
96. Ljungman P, Aschan J, Lewensohn-Fuchs I, et al. Results of different strategies for reducing cytomegalovirus-associated mortality in allogeneic stem cell transplant recipients. Transplantation 1998;66:1330–1334.
97. Boeckh M, Gooley TA, Myerson D, Cunningham T, Schoch G, Bowden RA. Cytomegalovirus pp65 antigenemia-guided early treatment with ganciclovir versus ganciclovir at engraftment after allogeneic marrow transplantation: a randomized double-blind study. Blood 1996;88:4063–4071.
98. Reusser P, Einsele H, Lee J, et al. Randomized multicenter trial of foscarnet versus ganciclovir for preemptive therapy of cytomegalovirus infection after allogeneic stem cell transplantation. Blood 2002;99:1159–1164.
99. Winston DJ, Yeager AM, Chandrasekar PH, Snydman DR, Petersen FB, Territo MC. Randomized comparison of oral valacyclovir and intravenous ganciclovir for prevention of cytomegalovirus disease after allogeneic bone marrow transplantation. Clin Infect Dis 2003;36:749–758.
100. Zikos P, Van Lint MT, Frassoni F, et al. Low transplant mortality in allogeneic bone marrow transplantation for acute myeloid leukemia: a randomized study of low-dose cyclosporin versus low-dose cyclosporin and low-dose methotrexate. Blood 1998; 91:3503–3508.
101. Humar A, Lipton J, Welsh S, Moussa G, Messner H, Mazzulli T. A randomized trial comparing cytomegalovirus antigenemia assay vs. screening bronchoscopy for the early detection and prevention of disease in allogeneic bone marrow and peripheral blood stem cell transplant recipients. Bone Marrow Transplant 2001;28:485–490.
102. Moretti S, Zikos P, Van Lint MT, et al. Foscarnet vs. ganciclovir for cytomegalovirus (CMV) antigenemia after allogeneic hematopoietic stem cell transplantation (HSCT): a randomized study. Bone Marrow Transplant 1998;22:175–180.
103. Einsele H, Ehninger G, Hebart H, et al. Polymerase chain reaction monitoring reduces the incidence of cytomegalovirus disease and the duration and side effects of antiviral therapy after bone marrow transplantation. Blood 1995;86:2815–2820.
104. Boeckh M, Leisenring W, Riddell SR, et al. Late cytomegalovirus disease and mortality in recipients of allogeneic hematopoietic stem cell transplants: importance of viral load and T-cell immunity. Blood 2003;101:407–414.
105. Osarogiagbon RU, Defor TE, Weisdorf MA, Erice A, Weisdorf DJ. CMV antigenemia following bone marrow transplantation: risk factors and outcomes. Biol Blood Marrow Transplant 2000;6: 280–288.
106. Emanuel D, Cunningham I, Jules-Elysee K, et al. Cytomegalovirus after bone marrow transplantation successfully treated with the combination of ganciclovir and high-dose intravenous immune globulin. Ann Intern Med 1988;109: 777–782.
107. Enright H, Haake R, Weisdorf D, et al. Cytomegalovirus pneumonia after bone marrow transplantation: risk factors and response to therapy. Transplantation 1993;55:1339–1346.
108. van Burik JA, Lawatsch EJ, DeFor T, et al. Cytomegalovirus enteritis among hematopoietic stem cell transplant recipients. Biol Blood Marrow Transplant 2001;7:674–679.
109. Boeckh M, Bowden RA, Storer B, et al. Randomized, placebo-controlled, double-blind study of a cytomegalovirus-specific monoclonal antibody (MSL-109) for prevention of cytomegalovirus infection after allogeneic hematopoietic stem cell transplantation. Biol Blood Marrow Transplant 2001;7: 343–351.
110. Bhatia S, Ramsay NKC, Steinbuch M, et al. Malignant neoplasms following bone marrow transplantation. Blood 1996;87:3633–3639.
111. Curtis RE, Travis LB, Rowlings PA, et al. Risk of lymphoproliferative disorders after bone marrow transplantation: a multi-institutional study. Blood 1999;94:2208–2216.
112. Preiksaitis JK, Cockfield SM. Epstein-Barr virus and lymphoproliferative disorders after transplantation. In: Bowden RA, Ljungman P, Paya CV (eds) Transplant Infections. Philadelphia: Lippincott-Raven, 1998:245–263.
113. Kuehnle I, Huls MH, Liu Z, et al. CD20 monoclonal antibody (rituximab) for therapy of Epstein-Barr virus lymphoma after hematopoietic stem-cell transplantation. Blood 2000;95: 1502–1505.
114. Papadopoulos EB, Ladanyi M, Emanuel D, et al. Infusions of donor leukocytes to treat Epstein-Barr virus-associated lymphoproliferative disorders after allogeneic bone marrow transplantation. N Engl J Med 1994;330:1185–1191.
115. Loren AW, Porter DL, Stadtmauer EA, et al. Post-transplant lymphoproliferative disorder: a review. Bone Marrow Transplant 2003;31:145–155.
116. Yoshikawa T, Asano Y, Ihira M, et al. Human herpesvirus 6 viremia in bone marrow transplant recipients: clinical features and risk factors. J Infect Dis 2002;185:847–853.
117. Cone RW, Huang ML, Corey L, et al. Human herpesvirus 6 infections after bone marrow transplantation: clinical and virologic manifestations. J Infect Dis 1999;179:311–318.
118. Ljungman P. Prevention and treatment of viral infections in stem cell transplant recipients. Br J Haematol 2002;118:44–57.
119. Whimbey E, Englund JA, Couch RB. Community respiratory virus infections in immunocompromised patients with cancer. Am J Med 1997;102:10–18.
120. Ghosh S, Champlin RE, Englund J, et al. Respiratory syncytial virus upper respiratory tract illnesses in adult blood and marrow transplant recipients: combination therapy with aerosolized ribavirin and intravenous immunoglobulin. Bone Marrow Transplant 2000;25:751–755.
121. Wendt CH, Weisdorf DJ, Jordan CM, et al. Parainfluenza virus respiratory infection after bone marrow transplantation. N Engl J Med 1992;326:921–926.
122. Arvin AM. Varicella-zoster virus: Pathogenesis, immunity, and clinical management in hematopoietic stem cell transplant recipients. Biol Blood Marrow Transplant 2000;6:219–230.
123. Hata A, Asanuma H, Rinki M, et al. Use of an inactivated varicella vaccine in recipients of hematopoietic-cell transplants. N Engl J Med 202;347:26–34.
124. Ferrara JL, Levy R, Chao NJ. Pathophysiologic mechanisms of acute graft-vs.-host disease (review). Biol Blood Marrow Transplant 1999;5:347–356.
125. Remberger M, Beelen DW, Fauser A, et al. Increased risk of extensive chronic graft-versus-host disease after allogeneic peripheral blood stem cell transplantation using unrelated donors. Blood 2005;105:548–551.
126. Arora M, Burns LJ, Davies SM, et al. Chronic graft-versus-host disease: a prospective cohort study. Biol Blood Marrow Transplant 2003;9:38–45.
127. Vogelsang GB. How I treat chronic graft-versus-host disease. Blood 2001;97:1196–1201.
128. Ho VT, Soiffer RJ. The history and future of T-cell depletion as graft-versus-host disease prophylaxis for allogeneic hematopoietic stem cell transplantation (review). Blood 2001;98: 3192–3204.

129. Storb R, Deeg HJ, Pepe M, et al. Methotrexate and cyclosporine versus cyclosporine alone for prophylaxis of graft-versus-host disease in patients given HLA-identical marrow grafts for leukemia: long-term follow-up of a controlled trial. Blood 1989;73:1729–1734.
130. Storb R, Deeg HJ, Farewell V, et al. Marrow transplantation for severe aplastic anemia: methotrexate alone compared with a combination of methotrexate and cyclosporine for prevention of acute graft-versus-host disease. Blood 1986;68:119–125.
131. Deeg HJ, Lin D, Leisenring W, et al. Cyclosporine or cyclosporine plus methylprednisolone for prophylaxis of graft-versus-host disease: a prospective, randomized trial. Blood 1997;89:3880–3887.
132. Ruutu T, Volin L, Parkkali T, et al. Cyclosporine, methotrexate, and methylprednisolone compared with cyclosporine and methotrexate for the prevention of graft-versus-host disease in bone marrow transplantation from HLA-identical sibling donor: a prospective randomized study. Blood 2000;96:2391–2398.
133. Chao NJ, Snyder DS, Jain M, et al. Equivalence of 2 effective graft-versus-host disease prophylaxis regimens: results of a prospective double-blind randomized trial. Biol Blood Marrow Transplant 2000;6:254–261.
134. Ratanatharathorn V, Nash RA, Przepiorka D, et al. Phase III study comparing methotrexate and tacrolimus (prograf, FK506) with methotrexate and cyclosporine for graft-versus-host disease prophylaxis after HLA-identical sibling bone marrow transplantation. Blood 1998;92:2303–2314.
135. Nash RA, Antin JH, Karanes C, et al. Phase 3 study comparing methotrexate and tacrolimus with methotrexate and cyclosporine for prophylaxis of acute graft-versus-host disease after marrow transplantation from unrelated donors. Blood 2000;96:2062–2068.
136. Zikos P, Van Lint MT, Frassoni F, et al. Low transplant mortality in allogeneic bone marrow transplantation for acute myeloid leukemia: a randomized study of low-dose cyclosporin versus low-dose cyclosporin and low-dose methotrexate. Blood 1998; 91:3503–3508.
137. Antin J, Chen AR, Couriel DR, et al. Novel approaches to the therapy of steroid-resistant acute graft-versus-host disease. Biol Blood Marrow Transplant 2004;10(10):655–668.
138. Hings IM, Filipovich AH, Miller WJ, et al. Prednisone therapy for acute graft-versus-host disease: short- versus long-term treatment. A prospective randomized trial. Transplantation 1993;56:577–580.
139. Koc S, Leisenring W, Flowers ME, et al. Therapy for chronic graft-versus-host disease: a randomized trial comparing cyclosporine plus prednisone versus prednisone alone. Blood 2002;100:48–51.
140. Arora M, Wagner JE, Davies SM, et al. Randomized clinical trial of thalidomide, cyclosporine, and prednisone versus cyclosporine and prednisone as initial therapy for chronic graft-versus-host disease. Biol Blood Marrow Transplant 2001; 7:265–273.
141. Koc S, Leisenring W, Flowers ME, et al. Thalidomide for treatment of patients with chronic graft-versus-host disease. Blood 2000;96:3995–3996.
142. Kansu E, Gooley T, Flowers ME, et al. Administration of cyclosporine for 24 months compared with 6 months for prevention of chronic graft-versus-host disease: a prospective randomized clinical trial. Blood 2001;98:3868–3870.
143. Deeg HJ, Flournoy N, Sullivan KM, et al. Cataracts after total body irradiation and marrow transplantation: a sparing effect of dose fractionation. Int J Radiat Oncol Biol Phys 1984;10: 957–964.
144. Katsanis E, Shapiro RS, Robison LL, et al. Thyroid dysfunction following bone marrow transplantation: long-term follow-up of 80 pediatric patients. Bone Marrow Transplant 1990;5:335–340.
145. Tauchmanova L, Selleri C, Rosa GD, et al. High prevalence of endocrine dysfunction in long-term survivors after allogeneic bone marrow transplantation for hematologic diseases. Cancer (Phila) 2002;95:1076–1084.
146. Enright H, Haake R, Weisdorf D. Avascular necrosis of bone: a common serious complication of allogeneic bone marrow transplantation. Am J Med 1990;89:733–738.
147. Socie G, Cahn JY, Carmelo J, et al. Avascular necrosis of bone after allogeneic bone marrow transplantation: analysis of risk factors for 4388 patients by the Societe Francaise de Grefe de Moelle (SFGM). Br J Haematol 1997;97:865–870.
148. Deeg HJ. Delayed complications and long-term effects after bone marrow transplantation. Hematol Oncol Clin N Am 1990;4: 641–657.
149. Stern JM, Sullivan KM, Ott SM, et al. Bone density loss after allogeneic hematopoietic stem cell transplantation: a prospective study. Biol Blood Marrow Transplant 2001;7:257–264.
150. Wingard JR, Plotnik LP, Freemer CS, et al. Growth in children after bone marrow transplantation: busulfan and cyclophosphamide versus cyclophosphamide plus total body irradiation. Blood 1992;79:1068–1073.
151. Curtis RE, Rowlings PA, Deeg HJ, et al. Solid cancers after bone marrow transplantation. N Engl J Med 1997;336:897–904.
152. Socie G, Stone JV, Wingard JR, et al. Long-term survival and late deaths after allogeneic bone marrow transplantation: late effects working committee of the International Bone Marrow Transplant Registry. N Engl J Med 1999;341:14–21.
153. Witherspoon RP, Fisher LD, Schoch G, et al. Secondary cancers after bone marrow transplantation for leukemia or aplastic anemia. N Engl J Med 2003;321:784–789.
154. Metayer C, Curtis RE, Vose J, et al. Myelodysplastic syndrome and acute myeloid leukemia after autotransplantation for lymphoma: a multicenter case-control study. Blood 2003;101: 2015–2023.
155. Hjermstad MJ, Evensen SA, Kvaloy SO, et al. Health-related quality of life 1 year after allogeneic or autologous stem-cell transplantation: a prospective study. J Clin Oncol 1999;17: 706–718.
156. Fife BL, Huster GA, Cornetta KG, et al. Longitudinal study of adaptation to the stress of bone marrow transplantation. J Clin Oncol 2000;18:1539–1549.
157. Lee SJ, Fairclough D, Parsons SJ, et al. Recovery after stem-cell transplantation for hematologic diseases. J Clin Oncol 2001;19: 242–252.
158. Syrjala KL, Langer SL, Abrams JR, et al. Recovery and long-term function after hematopoietic cell transplantation for leukemia or lymphoma. JAMA 2004;291:2335–2343.
159. Bensinger WI, Martin PJ, Storer B, et al. Transplantation of bone marrow as compared with peripheral-blood cells from HLA-identical relatives in patients with hematologic cancers. N Engl J Med 2001;344:175–181.
160. Blaise D, Kuentz M, Fortanier C, et al. Randomized trial of bone marrow versus lenograstim-primed blood cell allogeneic transplantation in patients with early-stage leukemia: a report from the Societe Francaise de Greffe de Moelle. J Clin Oncol 2000; 18:537–546.
161. Champlin RE, Schmitz N, Horowitz MM, et al. Blood stem cells compared with bone marrow as a source of hematopoietic cells for allogeneic transplantation. IBMTR Histocompatibility and Stem Cell Sources Working Committee and the European Group for Blood and Marrow Transplantation (EBMT). Blood 2000; 95:3702–3709.
162. Couban S, Simpson DR, Barnett MJ, et al. A randomized multicenter comparison of bone marrow and peripheral blood in recipients of matched sibling allogeneic transplants for myeloid malignancies. Blood 2002;100:1525–1531.
163. Schmitz N, Bacigalupo A, Hasenclever D, et al. Allogeneic bone marrow transplantation vs. filgrastim-mobilised peripheral

blood progenitor cell transplantation in patients with early leukaemia: first results of a randomised multicentre trial of the European Group for Blood and Marrow Transplantation. Bone Marrow Transplant 1998;21:995–1003.
164. Vigorito AC, Azevedo WM, Marques JF, et al. A randomised, prospective comparison of allogeneic bone marrow and peripheral blood progenitor cell transplantation in the treatment of haematological malignancies. Bone Marrow Transplant 1998;22: 1145–1151.
165. Winston DJ, Maziarz RT, Chandrasekar PH, et al. Intravenous and oral itraconazole versus intravenous and oral fluconazole for long-term antifungal prophylaxis in allogeneic hematopoietic stem-cell transplant recipients. A multicenter, randomized trial. Ann Intern Med 2003;138:705–713.
166. Ljungman P, de La Camara R, Milpied N, et al. Randomized study of valacyclovir as prophylaxis against cytomegalovirus reactivation in recipients of allogeneic bone marrow transplants. Blood 2002;99:3050–3056.
167. Meyers JD, Reed EC, Shepp DH, et al. Acyclovir for prevention of cytomegalovirus infection and disease after allogeneic marrow transplantation. N Engl J Med 1988;318:70–75.
168. Prentice HG, Gluckman E, Powles RL, et al. Long-term survival in allogeneic bone marrow transplant recipients following acyclovir prophylaxis for CMV infection. The European Acyclovir for CMV Prophylaxis Study Group. Bone Marrow Transplant 1997;19:129–133.
169. Schmidt GM, Horak DA, Niland JC, Duncan SR, Forman SJ, Zaia JA. A randomized, controlled trial of prophylactic ganciclovir for cytomegalovirus pulmonary infection in recipients of allogeneic bone marrow transplants; The City of Hope-Stanford-Syntex CMV Study Group. N Engl J Med 1991;324:1005–1011.
170. Antin JH, Weisdorf D, Neuberg D, et al. Interleukin-1 blockade does not prevent acute graft-versus-host disease: results of a randomized, double-blind, placebo-controlled trial of interleukin-1 receptor antagonist in allogeneic bone marrow transplantation. Blood 2002;100:3479–3482.
171. Bacigalupo A, Lamparelli T, Bruzzi P, et al. Antithymocyte globulin for graft-versus-host disease prophylaxis in transplants from unrelated donors: 2 randomized studies from Gruppo Italiano Trapianti Midollo Osseo (GITMO). Blood 2001;98:2942–2947.
172. Bolwell B, Sobecks R, Pohlman B, et al. A prospective randomized trial comparing cyclosporine and short course methotrexate with cyclosporine and mycophenolate mofetil for GVHD prophylaxis in myeloablative allogeneic bone marrow transplantation. Bone Marrow Transplant 2004;34:621–625.
173. Locatelli F, Bruno B, Zecca M, et al. Cyclosporin A and short-term methotrexate versus cyclosporin A as graft versus host disease prophylaxis in patients with severe aplastic anemia given allogeneic bone marrow transplantation from an HLA-identical sibling: results of a GITMO/EBMT randomized trial. Blood 2000;96:1690–1697.
174. Couriel D, Saliba R, Hicks K, et al. Tumor necrosis factor alpha blockade for the treatment of acute GVHD. Blood 2004;104: 649–654.
175. Cragg L, Blazar BR, Defor T, et al. A randomized trial comparing prednisone with antithymocyte globulin/prednisone as an initial systemic therapy for moderately severe acute graft-versus-host disease. Biol Blood Marrow Transplant 2000;6: 441–447.
176. Deeg HJ, Blazar BR, Bolwell BJ, et al. Treatment of steroid-refractory acute graft-versus-host disease and anti-CD147 monoclonal antibody ABX-CBL. Blood 2001;98:2052–2058.
177. Doney KC, Weiden PL, Storb R, Thomas ED. Treatment of graft-versus-host disease in human allogeneic marrow graft recipients: a randomized trial comparing antithymocyte globulin and corticosteroids. Am J Hematol 1981;11:1–8.
178. Lee SJ, Zahrieh D, Agura E, et al. Effect of up-front daclizumab when combined with steroids for the treatment of acute graft-versus-host disease: results of a randomized trial. Blood 2004; 104:1559–1564.
179. Martin PJ, Nelson BJ, Appelbaum FR, et al. Evaluation of a CD5-specific immunotoxin for treatment of acute graft-versus-host disease after allogeneic marrow transplantation. Blood 1996; 88:824–830.
180. Verdonck LF, Dekker AW, Rozenberg-Arska M, van den Hoek MR. A risk-adapted approach with a short course of ganciclovir to prevent cytomegalovirus (CMV) pneumonia in CMV-seropositive recipients of allogeneic bone marrow transplants. Clin Infect Dis 1997;24:901–907.

Management of Anxiety and Depression in Adult Cancer Patients: Toward an Evidence-Based Approach

Paul B. Jacobsen, Kristine A. Donovan, Zoë N. Swaine, and Iryna S. Watson

Anxiety and depression can be viewed as part of a broader construct of psychologic distress. We chose to focus on anxiety and depression rather than on psychologic distress for several reasons. First, the literature on anxiety and depression can be more readily identified than the literature on the broader and less well defined construct of psychologic distress. Second, as described in the following, criteria have been established for the diagnosis of clinical syndromes of anxiety and depression; no similar criteria exist for the diagnosis of clinical syndromes of psychologic distress. Third, as described here, this approach allows us to build upon the findings of several previous systematic reviews and meta-analyses that also have focused on psychosocial and pharmacologic approaches to the management of anxiety and depression in adult cancer patients.

Heightened anxiety or depression in individuals diagnosed with cancer is well documented.[1,2] Possible sources of anxiety or depression in these individuals are varied and include preexisting psychologic problems (i.e., problems predating cancer diagnosis), reactions to the diagnosis of a severe and/or life-threatening illness, and concerns about or reactions to disruptions in life plans, diminished quality of life, and disease recurrence or progression. In addition, anxiety and depression can occur as a reaction to adverse disease symptoms or treatment side effects (e.g., pain, nausea, and fatigue) or as a direct result of the effects of disease or treatments on the central nervous system. Observational studies indicate that heightened anxiety and depression are not limited to the active treatment period but can persist for months or even years following successful treatment.[3]

Estimates of the prevalence of anxiety and depression in cancer patients vary widely. For example, one review reports prevalence rates for depression in cancer patients ranging from 1.5% to 50%.[4] This variability in prevalence is most likely a reflection of differences across studies in the characteristics of the samples recruited, and the methods used to assess anxiety and depression. With regard to sample characteristics, differences across studies in patient factors, such as age and disease severity, are likely to influence prevalence estimates; research consistently indicates greater anxiety and depression in younger patients and patients with more advanced disease. Concerning the methods used, differences in prevalence may reflect whether anxiety and depression were assessed using a single-symptom approach, a symptom cluster approach, or a clinical syndrome approach. The single-symptom approach refers to assessment methods that focus specifically on measuring anxious or depressed mood as a continuous variable (e.g., visual analogue scales measuring severity of anxious or depressed mood) or a categorical variable (e.g., clinical interview items measuring presence/absence of anxious or depressed mood).

The symptom cluster approach refers to assessment methods that focus on measuring constellations of anxiety or depressive symptoms theorized to reflect the construct of interest. Common symptom cluster approaches to measuring anxiety and depression in cancer patients, include self-report scales such as the State-Trait Anxiety Inventory[5] and the Beck Depression Inventory.[6] The content of the State-Trait Anxiety Inventory consists primarily of affective symptoms whose presence is either consistent with the presence of anxiety (e.g., "I feel frightened") or inconsistent with the presence of anxiety (e.g., "I am relaxed"); the latter are reversed coded for scoring purposes such that higher scores on the State-Trait Anxiety Inventory reflect greater anxiety. The content of the Beck Depression Inventory includes cognitive symptoms of depression (e.g., pessimism), affective symptoms of depression (e.g., sadness), and somatic symptoms of depression (e.g., changes in appetite).

The clinical syndrome approach refers to assessment methods used to detect the presence of an anxiety disorder (e.g., generalized anxiety disorder) or a mood disorder (e.g., major depressive disorder). In the United States, this approach usually involves the application of criteria identified in the fourth edition of the American Psychiatric Association's *Diagnostic and Statistical Manual of Mental Disorders* (DSM-IV).[7] For example, a diagnosis of a major depressive episode requires the presence of five or more symptoms of depression, at least one of which is either depressed mood or loss of interest or pleasure in usual activities; additional symptoms may include somatic symptoms (e.g., changes in appetite) or cognitive symptoms (e.g., feeling of worthlessness or excessive or inappropriate guilt). A diagnosis of a generalized anxiety disorder requires the presence of excessive anxiety and worry, difficulty controlling the worry, plus three or more additional symptoms of anxiety (e.g., difficulty concentrating, irritability, or muscle tension). Studies of the prevalence of anxiety and depression in cancer patients have typically relied on a clinical syndrome approach. Prevalence has also occasionally been estimated using cutoff scores for clinically significant symptomatology on symptom cluster measures, such as the Hospital Anxiety and Depression Scale.[8]

Although prevalence estimates vary widely, there is general agreement that anxiety and depression are among the most common symptoms experienced by cancer patients. This assertion is supported by recent surveys of symptom prevalence among cancer patients.[9,10] The importance of these symptoms is also reflected in the relatively large number of studies identified here that have evaluated the effects of psychosocial and pharmacologic interventions for anxiety and depression in cancer patients. Before discussing the methods used to identify these studies and reviewing their findings, we describe previous systematic reviews and meta-analyses that have examined the effects of interventions for anxiety and depression in cancer patients.

Existing Clinical Practice Guidelines for Management of Anxiety and Depression in Cancer Patients

In recent years, several organizations have proposed clinical practice guidelines that include recommendations for the management of anxiety and depression in cancer patients. Two of these guidelines are described next to illustrate different approaches to the development of such guidelines.

National Comprehensive Cancer Network Guidelines

The National Comprehensive Cancer Network (NCCN) Guidelines for Distress Management,[11] which were updated annually, consist primarily of recommendations for evaluation, treatment, and follow-up care organized in terms of clinical pathways. Most of the recommendations represent a uniform consensus among panel members based on lower-level evidence, such as clinical experience, as opposed to higher-level evidence, such as randomized clinical trials.

Recommendations for the management of symptoms of anxiety and depression appear primarily in the sections of the guidelines devoted to adjustment disorder, anxiety disorder, and mood disorder. Underlying each recommendation is the assumption that, before initiating treatment, patients have been referred to a mental health team for psychologic/psychiatric evaluation. Nevertheless, the guidelines recognize that variations exist across clinical sites in the resources and personnel available to implement these recommendations. Accordingly, the guidelines stipulate that multidisciplinary institutional committees be formed to implement local standards for distress management.

The NCCN guidelines recommend an initial determination of suicide risk for patients with symptoms of adjustment disorder and mood disorder. If the patient is at risk for suicide, patient safety should first be assured and hospitalization should be considered.

For patients with a mild adjustment disorder, the initial recommendation is to initiate psychotherapy or counseling before follow-up or reevaluation. For patients with a moderate to severe adjustment disorder, the initial recommendation is to prescribe psychotropic medications and begin psychotherapy before follow-up or reevaluation. For patients with a mood disorder, the initial recommendation is for evaluation, diagnostic studies, and modification of factors potentially contributing to mood disorder symptoms, such as concurrent medications, pain, and withdrawal states. Based on findings, subsequent recommendations include initiation of antidepressant medication and psychotherapy (with or without concurrent initiation of anxiolytic medication) and consideration of referral to social work services or pastoral counseling before follow-up or reevaluation. For patients with signs and symptoms of an anxiety disorder, the initial recommendation is for evaluation, diagnostic studies, and modification of factors potentially contributing to the presenting symptoms, such as concurrent medications, pain, and withdrawal states. Based on findings, subsequent recommendations include psychotherapy (with or without anxiolytic medication and/or antidepressant medication) before follow-up or reevaluation.

National Breast Cancer Centre and National Cancer Control Initiative Guidelines

In 2003, the National Breast Cancer Centre and the National Cancer Control Initiative in Australia, published the first edition of "Clinical Practice Guidelines for the Psychosocial Care of Adults with Cancer."[12] The guidelines are presented in the form of a series of recommendations accompanied by identification of the levels and sources of research support. Numerous recommendations relevant to the present review appear throughout the document, and a complete summary of these recommendations is well beyond the scope of the current review. A table included in the document provides a succinct summary of all recommendations for psychosocial care of cancer patients that are based on systematic review of all relevant randomized controlled trials (Level I evidence) or at least one properly designed randomized controlled trial (Level II evidence). Those recommendations that relate primarily to the management of anxiety and depression are reproduced in adapted form in Table 89.1. It should be noted that the Level I evidence and Level II evidence cited in support of these recommendations, includes several systematic reviews and randomized trials that were conducted on populations other than cancer patients.

TABLE 89.1. National Breast Cancer Centre and National Cancer Control Initiative recommendations relevant to management of anxiety and depression supported by Level I or Level II evidence.

Recommendation	*Evidence level*
Providing question prompt sheets to patients with cancer during an initial consultation promotes patient questions, reduces anxiety, improves recall, and shortens the consultation.	II
Providing patients with information about the procedure they are about to undergo reduces emotional distress and improves psychological and physical recovery.	I
Providing patients with practical details about the procedure (procedural information), a booklet, and/or a videotape decreases anxiety and psychological distress.	II
Providing patients with information about what they are likely to experience before, during, and after a procedure (sensory information) decreases anxiety.	I
Providing patients with psychological support before undergoing surgery reduces psychological distress.	I
Cognitive behavioral, psycho-educational, and crisis interventions, as well as combinations of education and behavioral or nonbehavioral interventions and antianxiety medications, are effective in the treatment of anxiety.	I
Cognitive behavioral, psychoeducational, and supportive interventions, as well as combinations of education and behavioral or nonbehavioral interventions and cognitive behavioral interventions and antidepressants, are effective in the treatment of depression.	I
Supportive psychotherapy, in combination with antidepressants, such as selective serotonin reuptake inhibitors, is effective for the management of posttraumatic stress disorder.	I
Depression can be managed by incorporating a combination of supportive psychotherapy, cognitive and behavioral techniques, and pharmacotherapy.	I
There is no evidence that any particular antidepressant is superior to another in the management of depression in people with cancer.	I

Source: Adapted from National Breast Cancer Centre and National Cancer Control Initiative,[12] by permission of National Breast Cancer Centre.

Previous Systematic Reviews and Meta-Analyses of the Effects of Psychosocial Interventions on Anxiety and Depression

Using search methods described next, two publications[13,14] were identified that reported the results of meta-analyses performed on studies examining the effects of psychosocial interventions on anxiety and depression in cancer patients (Table 89.2). In addition, one publication was identified that reported the results of a systematic review of studies examining the effects of psychosocial interventions on depression in cancer patients,[15] and one publication was identified that reported the results of a systematic review of studies examining the effects of pharmacologic interventions on depression in cancer patients.[16]

Effects on Anxiety

Devine and Westlake[13] identified 68 studies that used randomized, quasi-experimental, or single-group pretest–posttest designs to evaluate the effects of "psychoeducational care" on anxiety in adults with cancer. The authors determined that, in 95% of these studies, a positive (although not statistically significant) treatment effect existed. The average effect size reported (0.56) was characterized as medium in magnitude. There was evidence of considerable heterogeneity among the effect sizes for the individual studies. Analyses based on type of psychoeducational care indicated that studies of progressive muscle relaxation were the major source of heterogeneity. Further analyses with corrected effect size values suggested that the effects of the different types of psychoeducational care on anxiety were not significantly different from each other. Based on these findings, the authors concluded that many types of psychoeducational care have beneficial effects on anxiety in cancer patients.

Sheard and Maguire[14] identified 19 studies that featured a control condition and evaluated the effects of "psychosocial or psychiatric interventions" on anxiety in cancer patients. The average effect size reported for these studies (0.42) was characterized as being of moderate clinical significance.

TABLE 89.2. Results of meta-analyses of effects of psychosocial interventions on anxiety and depression in cancer patients.

Authors	*Reference*	*Designs of studies included*	*Types of publications included*	*Outcome*	*Mean effect size*
Devine and Westlake[13]	68	Randomized, quasi-experimental, and pre–post designs	Journal articles, dissertations	Anxiety	0.56 (heterogeneous)
Devine and Westlake[13]	48	Randomized, quasi-experimental, and pre–post designs	Journal articles, dissertations	Depression	0.54 (homogeneous)
Sheard and Maguire[14]	19	Randomized and nonrandomized designs with control group	Journal articles, dissertations	Anxiety	0.42 (heterogeneous) 0.27 with positive outliers removed
Sheard and Maguire[14]	20	Randomized and nonrandomized designs with control group	Journal articles, dissertations	Depression	0.36 (heterogeneous) 0.19 with positive outliers removed

Restriction of the analysis to 10 studies determined to be of more reliable design resulted in a slightly lower average effect size (0.36). As in the analysis reported by Devine and Westlake,[13] there was evidence of considerable heterogeneity among the effect sizes for the 19 studies. Examination of potential moderator variables suggested that effect sizes were larger for group interventions (particularly group psychoeducational interventions), more time-intensive interventions, and interventions conducted by more experienced therapists. The authors note that few of the studies reviewed included patients experiencing significant distress. Characterizing most of the psychologic interventions reviewed as "preventative," they concluded these interventions may have a moderate clinical effect on anxiety.

Effects on Depression

Devine and Westlake[13] identified 48 studies that used randomized, quasi-experimental, or single-group pretest–posttest designs to evaluate the effects of "psychoeducational care" on depression in adults with cancer. The authors determined that, in 92% of these studies, a positive (although not statistically significant) treatment effect existed. The average effect size reported (0.54) was characterized as medium in magnitude. Analyses did not suggest the presence of considerable heterogeneity among the effect sizes for the individual studies. Based on these findings, the authors reached the same conclusions for depression as they did for anxiety. That is, they concluded that many types of psychoeducational care have beneficial effects on depression in cancer patients.

Sheard and Maguire[14] identified 20 studies that featured a control condition and evaluated the effects of "psychosocial or psychiatric interventions" on depression in cancer patients. The average effect size reported for these studies (0.36) was noted to be not as robust as the value these authors reported for anxiety (0.42). Limitation of the analysis to 8 studies of "more reliable design" resulted in a much lower average effect size (0.21). Analyses indicated the presence of considerable heterogeneity among the effect sizes for the 20 studies. Examination of potential moderator variables suggested that effect sizes were larger for interventions conducted by more experienced therapists and interventions provided to patients with more advanced disease. Based on these findings, particularly the lower mean effect size for studies using more reliable designs, the authors concluded that the effects of psychosocial interventions on depression in cancer patients are "weak to negligible."

Barsevick and colleagues[15] conducted a systematic review of studies that evaluated "psychoeducational interventions" for depression in cancer patients. The review, which included articles published between 1980 and 2000, did not place limitations on study design. Of the 48 studies identified, 36 were randomized clinical trials, 7 were quasi-experimental studies, and 5 were descriptive studies. The authors observed that 30 of these studies (63%) provided evidence in support of the benefit of psychoeducational interventions for depression. Based on these findings, the authors concluded that psychoeducational interventions were effective in reducing depression.

Carr and colleagues[16] conducted a systematic review of controlled studies that evaluated the effects of pharmacologic interventions on depressive symptoms in cancer patients. Eleven studies dating back to 1972 were identified. These studies evaluated a variety of agents, including antipsychotics, anxiolytics, psychostimulants, and corticosteroids, as well as antidepressants. The authors observe that, with the exception of 2 studies, all medications classified as antidepressants showed benefit. In contrast, medications other than antidepressants did not appear to be effective against depressive symptoms in cancer patients.

Methodology Used in the Current Review to Identify Relevant Empirical Literature

A variety of methods were used to identify relevant published research. As an initial strategy, we sought to identify systematic reviews and meta-analyses published since 1980 that covered topics overlapping with the topic of the current study. These publications were identified through electronic searches of MedLine and PsycINFO, using search terms described next, and limits were placed on the searches to identify review papers and meta-analyses. This method identified five systematic reviews (including the one cited previously) and three publications reporting the results of meta-analyses (including the two cited previously). The systematic reviews were of psychologic treatments for cancer patients[17]; behavioral interventions for cancer treatment side effects[18]; psychologic therapies for cancer patients[19]; psychoeducational interventions for depression in patients with cancer[15]; and depression in palliative care.[20] The meta-analyses were of psychosocial interventions for adult cancer patients[21,22]; psychoeducational care provided to adults with cancer[13]; psychologic interventions for anxiety in cancer patients[14]; and psychologic interventions for depression in cancer patients.[14] In addition to these published works, we identified a systematic review of the treatment of depression in cancer patients prepared for the Agency for Health Care Research and Quality.[16] All these sources were examined to identify studies that evaluated the impact of psychosocial and pharmacologic interventions on anxiety or depression in adult cancer patients. Studies identified in this manner were then obtained to determine if they met eligibility criteria (described next) for the current systematic review.

To identify studies published since the publication of the most recent systematic reviews, we also conducted electronic searches using MedLine and PsycINFO. This search was limited to studies published between January 2000 and March 2003 (MedLine) or August 2003 (PsycINFO). For MedLine, the search terms used were neoplasms AND antianxiety agents, depression, antidepressive agents, cognitive therapy, counseling, relaxation, techniques, patient education, psychotherapy, self-help groups, group psychotherapy, OR hypnosis. For PsychINFO, the search terms used were neoplasms AND tricyclic antidepressant drugs, antidepressant drugs, anxiety disorders, anxiety, anxiety management, drug therapy, benzodiazepines, depression, cognitive therapy, behavior therapy, counseling, relaxation therapy, client education, psychotherapy, support groups, self-help techniques, OR group psychotherapy.

Abstracts of studies identified through inspection of systematic reviews and meta-analyses or searches of MedLine and PsychINFO, were then reviewed to determine if they met criteria for inclusion in the current review. In the case of studies involving psychosocial interventions, the inclusion criteria were (1) published in English in journal form since 1980; (2) focused on adults (individuals aged 18 years or older); (3) included an evaluation of a psychosocial or educational intervention; (4) involved randomization to intervention and control condition(s); (5) had a usual care, wait-list, or no treatment control condition or a design in which all forms of care other than the intervention under evaluation were administered to all participants; (6) involved use of individuals as the unit of randomization; (7) used an outcome measure labeled "anxiety" or "depression"; (8) reported results in terms of statistical significance; and (9) included comparisons of an individual intervention condition with a control condition. In the case of studies involving pharmacologic interventions, the inclusion criteria were (1) published in English in journal form since 1980; (2) focused on adults (individuals aged 18 years or older); (3) included an evaluation of a pharmacologic agent; (4) involved randomization to intervention and control condition(s); (5) had a placebo control condition or a design in which all pharmacologic agents other than the agent under evaluation were administered to all participants; (6) involved use of individuals as the unit of randomization; (7) used an outcome measure labeled "anxiety" or "depression"; and (8) reported results in terms of statistical significance. This process resulted in identification of 60 studies that examined the effects of psychosocial interventions (Table 89.3) and 12 studies that examined the effects of pharmacologic interventions (Table 89.4).

Characteristics of the Psychosocial Intervention Studies

Of the 60 psychosocial studies identified, 62% (n = 37) included men and women, 30% (n = 18) included only women, 5% (n = 3) included only men, and 3% (n = 2) did not provide sufficient information to identify the gender of participants. Among studies that included men and women, the average percentage of males was 43%.

With regard to disease site, 57% of the studies (n = 34) included patients with a mix of different cancers. Twenty-seven percent (n = 16) included only breast cancer patients. The remaining studies included samples consisting only of patients with gynecologic malignancies (n = 2), melanoma (n = 2), Hodgkin's lymphoma (n = 2), bladder cancer (n = 1), testicular cancer (n = 1), renal cell cancer (n = 1), or colorectal cancer (n = 1). Although some of the most commonly diagnosed cancers (e.g., lung cancer and prostate cancer) were not the focus of specific studies, these cancers were often represented in samples of patients with mixed cancers.

Stage of disease and illness progression were widely distributed across study samples. Seventy-three percent (n = 44) included patients diagnosed with stage I to stage IV cancer. Fifteen percent (n = 9) of studies limited their samples to certain stages: five included patients with stage I or II disease, one included patients with stage I, II, or III disease, one included patients with stage II, III, or IV disease, one included patients with stage II disease, and one included patients with stage IV disease. Of the remaining 12%, 3% (n = 2) included patients with nonmetastatic disease, 7% (n = 4) included patients with metastatic disease, and 2% (n = 1) included only patients considered to be in the terminal phase of illness.

As shown in Table 89.5, 25% of the studies (n = 15) included patients who were in various stages of treatment. That is, these studies enrolled patients actively undergoing treatment (e.g., chemotherapy, radiotherapy, or hormonal therapy) as well as patients not in active treatment. Seventeen percent (n = 10) of the studies enrolled patients just before or immediately after surgery. Of the remaining studies, 23% (n = 14) enrolled patients during chemotherapy, 12% (n = 7) enrolled patients during radiotherapy, and 10% (n = 6) enrolled newly diagnosed patients who had not yet begun treatment. The remaining 8% (n = 5) enrolled patients who were not currently receiving treatment. Of the 14 studies that enrolled patients during chemotherapy, 5 focused on patients who were experiencing anticipatory symptoms (anxiety, nausea, or vomiting). There were few studies designed specifically to include more select groups of patients. For example, only 1 study each was limited to patients reporting pain, undergoing vaccine therapy, or undergoing bone marrow transplantation.

Four studies enrolled patients based on their degree of anxiety, depression, or distress at randomization. One study included only those patients who were considered to be at high risk for psychologic distress based on their scores on a self-report questionnaire. Three studies included patients who met criteria for psychologic morbidity based on their scores on measures of anxiety and depression and a measure of adjustment to cancer.

Across studies, sample sizes for each condition ranged widely, from as few as 8 patients to as many as 158 patients. The median sample size for both experimental and control conditions was 29 patients. Four studies failed to specify the number of subjects enrolled in the control or intervention conditions.

Usual care was the most frequently employed control condition, with 87% of the studies (n = 52) using this control condition. Other control conditions included attentional control (2%), wait-list control (2%), and usual care accompanied by limited forms of intervention (e.g., informational brochure) (5%). One study (2%) used a pharmacotherapy-only intervention as its control condition, with comparisons made to pharmacotherapy plus psychosocial intervention.

A total of 80 interventions were evaluated in the 60 studies reviewed. The majority of interventions (71%; n = 57) were provided in an individual format. The group format accounted for 25% of the interventions (n = 20), with the remaining 4% (n = 3) provided in either a group or individual format, depending upon the availability of participants. The intervention most commonly evaluated was relaxation training combined with an education component and/or skills training, accounting for 33% of the interventions evaluated (n = 26). Relaxation training alone, typically progressive muscle relaxation, was the second most commonly evaluated intervention (20%; n = 16), followed by education (18%; n = 14), supportive-expressive therapies (13%; n = 10), problem-solving therapies (10%; n = 8), various forms of counseling (6%; n = 5), and provision of audiotaped music (1%; n = 1).

Fifty-five percent of the studies (n = 33) reviewed included one follow-up assessment, 27% (n = 16) involved two follow-up assessments, and the remaining 18% (n = 11) included three or more follow-up assessments. The length of time between intervention and the final follow-up assessment ranged from immediately after intervention to 2 years. Of the 60 studies reviewed, 27% (n = 16) conducted the final follow-up immediately postintervention, 37% (n = 22) conducted it from 1 week to less than 3 months postintervention, 15% (n = 9) conducted it from 3 to 5 months postintervention, 8% (n = 5) conducted it 6 months postintervention, 13% (n = 8) conducted it between 7 and 12 months postintervention, and 2% (n = 1) conducted it more than 12 months postintervention. The median interval between intervention and the final follow-up assessment was 6 weeks.

Findings from the Psychosocial Intervention Studies

Thirteen of the 60 psychosocial studies targeted anxiety, 6 targeted depression, and 41 targeted both anxiety and depression. Outcomes were measured via patient self-report on various psychometric instruments that have been used extensively with cancer patients. Anxiety, for example, was commonly measured using the State-Trait Anxiety Inventory,[5] the Tension-Anxiety subscale of the Profile of Mood States,[23] or the anxiety subscale of the Hospital Anxiety and Depression Scale.[8] Measures of depression used included the Beck Depression Inventory,[24] the Center for Epidemiological Studies Depression Scale,[25] the Depression-Dejection subscale of the Profile of Mood States,[23] and the depression scale of the Hospital Anxiety and Depression Scale.[8]

The total number of anxiety outcomes, when all follow-up assessments were taken into account, was 135. Forty-nine or 36% of the total were statistically significant at P less than 0.05. As presented in Table 89.6, independent of patients' treatment status, 37% (n = 14) of the anxiety outcomes in studies utilizing relaxation combined with education and/or skills training (the most common type of intervention studied) were statistically significant. When compared across treatment status, the percentage of significant results ranged from 0% (0 of 1 outcome) for bone marrow transplantation (BMT) to 66% (2 of 3 outcomes) for patients receiving radiotherapy. When relaxation only was evaluated, 51% (n = 18) of the anxiety outcomes were significant. The percentage of significant results across treatment status ranged from 0% (0 of 1 outcome) for patients not in active treatment to 100% (7 of 7 outcomes) for newly diagnosed patients. Among those studies utilizing education-based interventions, 32% (n = 7) of the anxiety outcomes were significant. The percentage of significant results across treatment status ranged from 0% (0 of 7 outcomes) for patients undergoing radiotherapy to 66% (2 of 3 outcomes) for patients just before or immediately after surgery. Seventy percent (n = 7) of the outcomes for the supportive-expressive intervention were significant and ranged from 0% (0 of 1 outcome) for patients not in active treatment and patients receiving vaccine therapy to 100% (2 of 2 outcomes) for patients receiving chemotherapy and patients receiving radiotherapy. Twenty-five percent (n = 3) of the anxiety outcomes for the various problem-solving interventions were significant. The percentage of significant outcomes ranged from 0% (0 of 3 outcomes) for patients receiving chemotherapy to 40% (2 of 5 outcomes) for mixed/unspecified treatment. The percentage of significant anxiety outcomes for the counseling interventions was zero (0 of 9 outcomes for patients receiving chemotherapy and 0 of 1 outcome for patients before or immediately after surgery). There were also no significant outcomes for anxiety for patients receiving radiotherapy who were provided with audiotaped music (0 of 8 anxiety outcomes).

The total number of depression outcomes, when all follow-up assessments were taken into account, was 102. Forty-two or 41% of the total were statistically significant at P less than 0.05. Independent of treatment status, 38% (n = 17) of the outcomes for the relaxation combined with education and/or skills training interventions were significant. Compared across treatment status, the percentage of significant results ranged from 0% (0 of 1 outcome) for BMT to 64% (7 of 11 outcomes) for mixed/unspecified treatment. Sixty-seven percent (n = 10) of the depression outcomes for the relaxation-only interventions were statistically significant. The percentage of significant outcomes across treatment status ranged from 0% (0 of 1 outcome) for patients not in active treatment to 100% (6 of 6 outcomes) for newly diagnosed patients. Forty-three percent (n = 3) of the outcomes for education-based interventions were significant. Across treatment status, the percentage of significant results ranged from 0% (0 of 1 outcome) to 100% (1 of 1 outcome) for newly diagnosed patients and patients before and immediately after surgery. Forty-four percent (n = 7) of the depression outcomes for the supportive-expressive interventions were significant. Across treatment status, the results ranged from 0% (0 of 1 outcome) for patients receiving vaccine therapy and for newly diagnosed patients (0 of 3 outcomes) to 100% (2 of 2 outcomes) for patients receiving chemotherapy and patients receiving radiotherapy. Twenty-nine percent (n = 2) of the outcomes for the various counseling interventions were significant. The percentage of significant results across treatment status ranged from 0% (0 of 1 outcome) for patients receiving chemotherapy to 100% (1 of 1 outcome) for patients before and immediately after surgery. Eighteen percent (n = 2) of the depression outcomes were significant for problem-solving interventions. Across treatment status, significant results ranged from 0% for mixed treatment/unspecified (0 of 5 outcomes) and for patients before and immediately after surgery (0 of 3 outcomes) to 100% (1 of 1 outcome) for patients receiving radiotherapy. With respect to cognitive therapy, there was only 1 depression outcome (n = 1), and it was statistically significant for patients receiving chemotherapy.

Characteristics of the Pharmacologic Intervention Studies

Of the 12 pharmacologic studies identified, 75% (n = 9) included men and women and 25% (n = 3) included only women. Among studies that included men and women, the average percentage of males was 51%.

With regard to disease site, 67% of the studies (n = 8) included patients with a mix of different cancers. Of the remaining studies, 17% (n = 2) included only breast cancer patients, 8% (n = 1) included melanoma patients, and 8% (n = 1) included lymphoma patients.

Stage of disease and disease status were widely distributed across study samples. Sixty-seven percent of studies (n = 8) included patients diagnosed with stage I to IV cancer. Eight percent of studies (n = 1) limited their samples to patients with stage I or II disease. Seventeen percent of studies (n = 2) included only patients considered to be in the terminal phase

TABLE 89.3. Randomized clinical trials of psychosocial interventions with adult cancer patients.

			Patient characteristics		*Study design*			*Comparisons of intervention and control groups: number of statistically significant measures favoring intervention group (P < 0.05)/number of measures*	
Investigators	*Year*	*Reference*	*Eligibility criteria*	*Percent male*	*Control (C) groups (number of subjects at baseline)*	*Intervention groups (number of subjects at baseline)*	*Timing of follow-ups (F)*	*Anxiety*	*Depression*
Ali and Khalil	1989	35	Patients with bladder cancer undergoing urinary diversion surgery	77%	C1: Usual care (n = 15)	I1: Therapist administered individual intervention (information, visit by ostomy patient, opportunity for emotional expression);1 30- to 60-minute session 1–2 days preoperatively (n = 15)	F1: 3 days postoperative F2: 12 days postoperative	F1: 1/1 F2: 1/1	
Arakawa	1997	36	Patients with mixed cancers scheduled for chemotherapy	60%	C1: Attentional control (n = 30)	I1: Therapist administered individual intervention (progressive muscle relaxation); 45- to 60-minute session 1 week before chemotherapy and guided practice once a day until chemotherapy (n = 30)	F1: 72 hours after first chemotherapy treatment	F1: 1/1	
Arathuzik	1994	37	Patients with metastatic breast cancer experiencing pain	0%	C1: Usual care (n = 8)	I1: Therapist administered individual intervention (progressive muscle relaxation and guided imagery); 75-minute session (n = 8) I2: Therapist administered individual intervention (progressive muscle relaxation, guided imagery, and cognitive coping skills); 2-hour session (n = 8)	F1: postintervention (post-I)	F1: I1 0/1 F1: I2 0/1	F1: I1 0/1 F1: I2 0/1
Berglund et al.	1994	38	Patients with mixed cancers within 2 months of completing chemotherapy or radiotherapy	4%	C1: Usual care with or without a single information session with an oncologist and dietician (n = 101)	I1: Therapist administered group intervention (physical training, progressive muscle relaxation with guided imagery, information, coping skills training); 11 2-hour sessions over 7 weeks (n = 98)	F1: post-I (2–6 weeks and 3 months)	F1: 0/1	F1: 0/1
Bindemann et al.	1991	39	Patients with mixed cancers newly diagnosed	44%	C1: Usual care (n = 40)	I1: Therapist administered individual intervention (progressive muscle relaxation and hypnosis); 12 25-minute sessions at varying intervals over 12 weeks (n = 40)	F1: 6 weeks F2: 12 weeks	F1: 3/3 F2: 3/3	F1: 3/3 (women only) F2: 3/3 (women only)

Brown et al.	2001	40	Patients with mixed cancers attending initial consultation with medical or radiation oncologist	56%	C1: Usual care ($n = 158$)	I1: Patient provided with question prompt sheet that is actively addressed by oncologist ($n = 81$) I2: Patient provided with question prompt sheet that is not actively addressed by oncologist ($n = 79$)	F1: post-I F2: 1 week	F1: I1 0/1 F1: I2 0/1 F2: I1 0/1 F2: I2 0/1	
Burish and Lyles	1981	41	Patients with mixed cancers undergoing chemotherapy experiencing anticipatory anxiety nausea or vomiting	13%	C1: Usual care ($n = 8$)	I1: Therapist administered individual intervention (progressive muscle relaxation and guided imagery training); 5 45-minute sessions coinciding with chemotherapy treatment ($n = 8$)	F1: 4th chemotherapy treatment F2: 5th chemotherapy treatment	F1: 2/2 F2: 2/2	F1: 1/1 F2: 0/1
Burish et al.	1987	42	Patients with mixed cancers undergoing chemotherapy	?	C1: Usual care ($n = 12$)	I1: Therapist administered individual intervention (progressive muscle relaxation and guided imagery training); 6–8 45-minute sessions coinciding with chemotherapy treatment ($n = 12$)	F1: 4th chemotherapy treatment F2: 5th chemotherapy treatment	F1: 1/1 F2: 1/1	F1: 1/1 F2: 1/1
Cain et al.	1986	43	Patients with gynecologic cancer, expected to survive at least 1 year	0%	C1: Usual care ($n = 28$)	I1: Therapist administered group intervention (structured thematic counseling including health education and information, problem solving, coping, and relaxation); 8 weekly sessions ($n = 28$) I2: Therapist administered individual intervention (structured thematic counseling including health education and information, problem solving, coping, and relaxation); 8 weekly sessions ($n = 21$)	F1: 1–2 weeks F2: 6 months	F1: I1 0/1 F1: I2 1/1 F2: I1 1/1 F2: I2 1/1	F1: I1 0/1 F1: I2 0/1 F2: I1 1/1 F2: I2 1/1
Carey and Burish	1987	44	Patients with mixed cancers undergoing chemotherapy experiencing conditioned anxiety and nausea or receiving agents expected to produce nausea and vomiting	44%	C1: Usual care ($n = ?$)	I1: Therapist administered individual intervention (progressive muscle relaxation and guided imagery provided by professional therapist); 3 sessions of varying duration (15–45 minutes) coinciding with chemotherapy administration ($n = ?$) I2: Therapist administered individual intervention (progressive muscle relaxation and guided imagery provided by paraprofessional); 3 sessions of varying duration (15–45 minutes) coinciding with chemotherapy administration ($n = ?$)	F1: (during and following intervention)	F1: I1 1/1 F1: I2 0/1 F1: I3 0/1	

(*continued*)

TABLE 89.3. Randomized clinical trials of psychosocial interventions with adult cancer patients. (continued)

			Patient characteristics		Study design			Comparisons of intervention and control groups: number of statistically significant measures favoring intervention group ($P < 0.05$)/number of measures	
Investigators	*Year*	*Reference*	*Eligibility criteria*	*Percent male*	*Control (C) groups (number of subjects at baseline)*	*Intervention groups (number of subjects at baseline)*	*Timing of follow-ups (F)*	*Anxiety*	*Depression*
						I3: Audiotaped administered intervention (progressive muscle relaxation and guided imagery delivered via audiotape); 3 sessions of varying duration (15–45 minutes) coinciding with chemotherapy (n = ?)			
Cheung et al.	2003	45	Patients with colorectal cancer who have undergone stoma surgery for cancer	68%	C1: Usual care (n = 30)	I1: Therapist administered individual intervention (progressive muscle relaxation and controlled breathing); 2 sessions (n = 29)	F1: post-I (5 and 10 weeks)	F1: 1/1	
Christensen	1983	46	Patients with breast cancer treated with mastectomy	0%	C1: Usual care (n = 10)	I1: Therapist administered couples intervention (counseling focusing on marital relationship and adjustment); 4 weekly sessions (n = 10)	F1: 6 weeks	F1: 0/1	F1: 1/1
de Moor et al.	2002	47	Patients with metastatic renal cell carcinoma expected to survive at least 4 months participating in a Phase II clinical trial of vaccine therapy	86%	C1: Usual care plus neutral writing assignments (n = 21)	I1: Patients asked to write their deepest thoughts and feelings about their cancer; 4 writing sessions during consecutive clinic visits for vaccine treatment (n = 21)	F1: post-I (day of 4th writing session and 4, 6, 8, and 10 weeks later	F1: 0/1	F2: 0/1
Decker et al.	1992	48	Patients with mixed cancers undergoing radiotherapy	37%	C1: Usual care (n = 29)	I1: Therapist administered individual intervention (progressive muscle relaxation, cue-controlled relaxation and psychoeducation); 6 60-minute sessions (n = 34)	F1: post-I	F1: 1/1	F1: 1/1
Dodd	1987	49	Patients with mixed cancers undergoing radiotherapy	57%	C1: Usual care (n = 30)	I1: Therapist administered individual intervention (information on side effect management techniques) (n = 30)	F1: 6 weeks	F1: 0/2	

Edelman et al.	1999	50	Patients with metastatic breast cancer	0%	C1: Usual care ($n = 62$)	I1: Therapist administered group intervention (cognitive skills training, deep relaxation/meditation); 8 weekly sessions, family night, and 3 monthly sessions ($n = 62$)	F1: post-I F2: 3 months F3: 6 months	F1: 0/1 F2: 0/1 F3: 0/1	F1: 1/1 F2: 0/1 F3: 0/1
Edgar et al.	2001	51	Patients with breast or colon cancer about to begin treatment	18%	C1: Usual care ($n = 59$)	I1: Therapist administered individual intervention (problem-solving, goal setting, cognitive reappraisal, relaxation training, use of social support and resources); 5 90-minute sessions over a 6-month period ($n = 57$) I2: Therapist administered group intervention (problem-solving, goal setting, cognitive reappraisal, relaxation training, use of social support and resources); 5 90-minute sessions over a 6-month period ($n = 52$) I3: Therapist administered group intervention (supportive unstructured approach); 5 90-minute sessions over a 6-month period ($n = 57$)	F1: 4 months F2: 8 months F3: 12 months		F1: I1 0/1 F1: I2 0/1 F1: I3 0/1 F2: I1 1/1 (breast only) F2: I2 0/1 F2: I3 0/1 F3: I1 0/1 F3: I2 0/1 F3: I3 0/1
Elsesser et al.	1994	52	Patients with mixed cancers not receiving active cancer treatment	15%	C1: Wait-list control ($n = 10$)	I1: Therapist administered individual intervention (anxiety-management training and stress inoculation training); 8 sessions over a 6-week period (duration of sessions not reported) ($n= 10$)	F1: mid-I and post-I	F1: 2/2	F1: 0/1
Evans and Connis	1995	53	Patients with mixed stage II cancers undergoing radiotherapy	65%	C1: Usual care ($n = 26$)	I1: Therapist administered group intervention (cognitive behavioral therapy); 8 weekly 60-minute sessions ($n = 29$) I2: Therapist administered group intervention (social support); 8 weekly 60-minute sessions ($n = 23$)	F1: post-I F2: 6 months	F1: I1 1/1 F1: I2 1/1 F2: I1 0/1 F2: I2 1/1	F1: I1 1/1 F1: I2 1/1 F2: I1 0/1 F2: I2 1/1
Fawzy	1995	54	Patients with stage I or II melanoma being treated surgically	55%	C1: Usual care ($n = 33$)	I1: Therapist administered individual intervention (progressive muscle relaxation, educational manual, and instruction on its use); 3 hours total duration over 2 sessions ($n = 29$)	F1: 6 weeks F2: 3 months	F1: 0/2 F2: 0/2	F1: 0/2 F2: 0/2
Fawzy et al.	1990	106	Patients with stage I or II melanoma treated surgically and not undergoing immunotherapy, chemotherapy, or radiotherapy	47%	C1: Usual care ($n = 40$)	I1: Therapist administered group intervention (health education, problem-solving skills, relaxation, and social support); 6 weekly 90-minute sessions ($n = 40$)	F1: post-I F2: 6 months	F1: 0/1 F2: 0/1	F1: 0/1 F2: 1/1

(continued)

TABLE 89.3. **Randomized clinical trials of psychosocial interventions with adult cancer patients.** (continued)

			Patient characteristics		*Study design*			*Comparisons of intervention and control groups: number of statistically significant measures favoring intervention group ($P < 0.05$)/number of measures*	
Investigators	*Year*	*Reference*	*Eligibility criteria*	*Percent male*	*Control (C) groups (number of subjects at baseline)*	*Intervention groups (number of subjects at baseline)*	*Timing of follow-ups (F)*	*Anxiety*	*Depression*
Fukui et al.	2000	55	Patients with breast cancer at high risk of recurrence	0%	C1: Wait-list control ($n = 25$)	I1: Therapist administered group intervention (health education, coping skills training, stress management, psychosocial support); 6 weekly 90-minute sessions ($n = 25$)	F1: post-I (6 weeks and 6 months)	F1: 0/2	F1: 0/2
Gaston-Johansson et al.	2000	56	Patients with stage II–IV breast cancer undergoing autologous bone marrow transplantation	0%	C1: Usual care ($n = 58$)	I1: Therapist administered individual intervention (comprehensive coping strategy program including relaxation with guided imagery); intervention delivered at least 2 weeks before admission for transplant ($n = 52$)	F1: post-I (2 days before and 7 days after transplant)	F1: 0/1	F1: 0/1
Goodwin et al.	2001	57	Patients with metastatic breast cancer expected to survive at least 3 months	0%	C1: Usual care ($n = 77$)	I1: Therapist administered group intervention (supportive-expressive therapy); weekly 90-minute sessions for at least 1 year ($n = 158$)	F1: change during the year after randomization	F1: 1/1	F1: 1/1
Greer et al.	1992	58	Patients with mixed cancers expected to survive at least 1 year who met criteria for psychologic morbidity	21%	C1: Usual care ($n = 84$)	I1: Therapist administered individual intervention (problem-focused cognitive-behavioral therapy); 6 sessions of at least 60 minutes over 8 weeks ($n = 72$)	F1: 8 weeks F2: 4 months	F1: 1/1 F2: 1/1	F1: 0/1 F2: 0/1
Häggmark et al.	2001	59	Patients with breast, bladder, or prostate cancer undergoing curative radiotherapy	11%	C1: Usual care ($n = 69$)	I1: Nurse administered group intervention (information and practical advice); 1 60-minute session ($n = 69$) I2: Informational brochure mailed to home ($n = 72$)	F1: 1 hour before start of radiotherapy	F1: 0/1	F1: 0/1
Hagopian and Rubenstein	1990	60	Patients with mixed cancers undergoing radiotherapy	42%	C1: Usual care ($n = 28$)	I1: Telephone calls from a nurse to assess problems and reinforce teaching about management of side effects; weekly until 1 month after treatment completion ($n = 27$)	F1: early in radiotherapy treatment F2: midway through radiotherapy treatment F3: late in radiotherapy treatment	F1: 0/1 F2: 0/1 F3: 0/1	

Heinrich and Schag	1985	61	Patients with mixed cancers	68%	C1: Usual care ($n = 25$)	I1: Therapist administered group intervention (education and information, relaxation, cognitive therapy and problem-solving, and activity management); weekly 2-hour sessions over a 6-week period ($n = 26$)	F1: 2 months post-I	F1: 0/1	F1: 0/1
Jacobs et al.	1983	62	Patients with Hodgkin's disease receiving chemotherapy or within 2 years of completing chemotherapy	66%	C1: Usual care ($n = 26$)	I1: Informational booklet and periodic newsletters ($n = 21$)	F1: 3 months	F1: 1/1	
Jacobs et al.	1983	62	Patients with Hodgkin's disease receiving chemotherapy or within 2 years of completing chemotherapy	41%	C1: Usual care ($n = 18$)	I1: Therapist administered group intervention (discussion of common problems); 8 weekly 90-minute sessions ($n = 16$)	F1: post-I	F1: 0/1	
Jacobsen et al.	2002	63	Patients with mixed cancers receiving chemotherapy but not radiotherapy	24%	C1: Usual care ($n = 132$)	I1: Therapist administered individual intervention (progressive muscle relaxation, abdominal breathing, coping self-statements); 1 60-minute session ($n = 125$) I2: Patient self-administered individual intervention (progressive muscle relaxation, abdominal breathing, coping self-statements) ($n = 125$)	F1: post-I (before cycles 2, 3, 4)	F1: I1 0/1 F1: I2 1/1	F1: I1 0/1 F1: I2 1/1
Larson et al.	2000	64	Patients with breast cancer awaiting surgery or surgery plus radiotherapy or chemotherapy	0%	C1: Usual care ($n = 18$)	I1: Therapist administered individual or small group intervention (education, problem-solving, relaxation, and support); 2 90-minute sessions ($n = 23$)	F1: post-I (1–3 days before surgery)		F1: 0/1
Lerman et al.	1990	65	Patients with mixed cancers undergoing chemotherapy	33%	C1: Usual care ($n = 23$)	I1: Therapist administered individual intervention (progressive muscle relaxation, deep breathing, and education and information about chemotherapy); 1 30-minute session before start of chemotherapy ($n = 25$)	F1: before 3rd chemotherapy treatment	F1: 0/1	F1: 0/1
Linn et al.	1982	66	Men with stage IV cancer expected to survive between 3 and 12 months	100%	C1: Usual care ($n = 58$)	I1: Therapist administered individual intervention (counseling including "life review"); sessions at least once a week until death or for 12 months ($n = 62$)	F1: 1 month F2: 3 months F3: 6 months F4: 9 months F5: 12 months		F1: 0/1 F2: 1/1 F3: 0/1 F4: 0/1 F5: 0/1

(continued)

TABLE 89.3. Randomized clinical trials of psychosocial interventions with adult cancer patients. (continued)

			Patient characteristics		*Study design*			*Comparisons of intervention and control groups: number of statistically significant measures favoring intervention group (P < 0.05)/number of measures*	
Investigators	*Year*	*Reference*	*Eligibility criteria*	*Percent male*	*Control (C) groups (number of subjects at baseline)*	*Intervention groups (number of subjects at baseline)*	*Timing of follow-ups (F)*	*Anxiety*	*Depression*
Liossi and White	2001	67	Patients with mixed cancers in terminal stage of illness expected to survive at least 4 months	54%	C1: Usual care that included 4 weekly 30-minute sessions of supportive counseling (n = ?)	I1: Therapist administered individual intervention (hypnotic suggestions for symptom management and ego-strengthening); 4 weekly 30-minute sessions (n = ?)	F1: post-I	F1: 1/1	F1: 1/1
Lyles et al.	1982	68	Patients with mixed cancers undergoing chemotherapy experiencing anticipatory anxiety, nausea, or vomiting	38%	C1: Usual care (n = ?)	I1: Therapist administered individual relaxation training (progressive muscle relaxation and guided imagery); 3 sessions (n = ?) I2: Therapist led discussion with patient; 3 sessions (n = ?)	F1: 4th chemotherapy treatment after initial intervention	F1: I1 0/1 F1: I2 0/1	F1: I1 0/1 F1: I2 0/1
Mantovani et al.	1996	69	Patients with mixed cancers over age 65 with symptoms of anxiety or depression receiving chemotherapy	58%	C1: Psychopharmacologic treatment (alprazolam 3 mg daily (po) and sulpride 150 mg daily po) (n = 25)	I1: C1 plus social support carried out by volunteers (n = 23) I2: C1 plus therapist administered individual psychotherapy with autogenic training with guided imagery); weekly 60-minute sessions for 6 months (n = 24)	F1: 2.5 months F2: 5 months	F1: I1 2/2 F1: I2 1/2 F2: I2 2/2	F1: I1 1/1 F1: I2 1/1 F2: I1 1/1 F2: I2 1/1
Marchioro et al.	1996	70	Patients with nonmetastatic breast cancer undergoing adjuvant chemotherapy after surgery	0%	C1: Usual care (n = 18)	I1: Therapist administered intervention (individual cognitive psychotherapy and family counseling); weekly 50-minute cognitive therapy sessions and bimonthly family counseling sessions (n = 18)	F1: post-I (1, 3, 6, 9 months)		F1: 1/1
McArdle et al.	1996	71	Patients with breast cancer undergoing surgery	0%	C1: Usual care (n = 67)	I1: Nurse administered individual intervention (information and emotional reassurance); at least 1 20- to 30-minute session (n = 70); I2: Support from a voluntary organization (information, counseling and group meetings based on counselor decision); (n = 66) I3: Combination of I1 and I2; (n = 69)	F1: post-I (postoperative clinic visit and 3, 6, and 12 months after surgery)	F1: I1 0/1 F1: I2 0/1 F1: I3 0/1	F1: I1 1/1 F1: I2 0/1 F1: I3 0/1

McHugh et al.	1995	72	Patients with mixed cancers receiving potentially distressing information about diagnosis or prognosis	41%	C1: Usual care ($n = 54$)	I1: Patients provided audiotapes of interviews with treating clinicians (information about diagnosis, treatment, and prognosis); 2 taped interviews 4 weeks apart ($n = 63$)	F1: before second interview F2: 5 months	F1: 0/1 F2: 0/1	F1: 0/1 F2: 0/1
McQuellon et al.	1998	73	Patients with mixed cancers presenting for initial oncology consultation	49%	C1: Usual care ($n = 78$)	I1: Therapist administered individual intervention (clinic tour, description of clinic procedures, general information, question and answer session); 1 15- to 20-minute session ($n = 72$)	F1: within 1 week	F1: 1/1	F1: 1/1
Molassiotis et al.	2002	74	Patients with breast cancer receiving first cycle of doxorubicin and cyclophosphamide	0%	C1: Usual care ($n = 33$)	I1: Therapist administered individual intervention (progressive muscle relaxation training with guided imagery); 1 session before chemotherapy and 5 daily sessions after chemotherapy ($n = 38$)	F1: post-I (7 and 14 days)	F1: 0/2	F1: 0/1
Moorey et al.	1994	75	Patients with mixed cancers expected to survive at least 1 year who met criteria for psychologic morbidity	?	C1: Usual care ($n = 72$)	I1: Therapist administered individual intervention (problem-focused cognitive-behavioral therapy); 6 60-minute sessions over 8 weeks ($n = 62$)	F1: 1 year	F1: 0/1	F1: 0/1
Morrow	1986	76	Patients with mixed cancers experiencing anticipatory side effects after three chemotherapy cycles	34%	C1: Usual care ($n = 20$)	I1: Therapist administered individual intervention (progressive muscle relaxation and guided imagery within context of systematic desensitization); 2 60-minute sessions between the 4th and 5th chemotherapy cycle ($n = 26$) I2: Therapist administered individual intervention (progressive muscle relaxation training and guided imagery but no attempt at systematic desensitization); 2 sessions 60-minute between 4th and 5th chemotherapy cycle ($n = 26$)	F1: post-I (after 6th cycle) F2: 2–4 weeks (after 7th cycle)	F1: I1 1/2 F1: I2 0/2 F1: I3 0/2 F2: I1 1/2 F2: I2 0/2 F2: I3 0/2	

(continued)

TABLE 89.3. Randomized clinical trials of psychosocial interventions with adult cancer patients. (continued)

			Patient characteristics		*Study design*			*Comparisons of intervention and control groups: number of statistically significant measures favoring intervention group ($P < 0.05$)/number of measures*	
Investigators	*Year*	*Reference*	*Eligibility criteria*	*Percent male*	*Control (C) groups (number of subjects at baseline)*	*Intervention groups (number of subjects at baseline)*	*Timing of follow-ups (F)*	*Anxiety*	*Depression*
						I3: Therapist administered individual intervention (person-centered Rogerian counseling); 2 60-minute sessions between 4th and 5th chemotherapy cycles ($n = 20$)			
Morrow and Morrell	1982	77	Patients with mixed cancers undergoing chemotherapy and experiencing anticipatory nausea or vomiting	30%	C1: Usual care ($n = 20$)	I1: Therapist administered individual intervention (progressive muscle relaxation and guided imagery within context of systematic desensitization); 2 sessions 60-minute between 4th and 5th chemotherapy cycles ($n = 20$) I2: Therapist administered individual intervention (person-centered Rogerian counseling); 2 60-minute between 4th and 5th chemotherapy cycles ($n = 20$)	F1: post-I (after 6th cycle) F2: 2–4 weeks (after 7th cycle)	F1: I1 0/2 F1: I2 0/2 F2: I1 0/2 F2: I2 0/2	
Moynihan et al.	1998	78	Patients with newly diagnosed testicular cancer treated with unilateral orchidectomy	100%	C1: Usual care ($n = 37$)	I1: Therapist administered individual intervention (problem-focused cognitive behavioral therapy); 6 60-minute sessions over 8 weeks ($n = 36$)	F1: 2 months F2: 4 months F3: 1 year	F1: 1/1 F2: 0/1 F3: 0/1	F1: 0/1 F2: 0/1 F3: 0/1
Petersen and Quinlivan	2002	79	Patients with gynecologic cancer undergoing surgery	0%	C1: Usual care ($n = 26$)	I1: Physician administered individual intervention (relaxation and counseling); 1 60-minute session ($n = 27$)	F1: 6 weeks after surgery	F1: 2/2	F1: 1/2

Pruitt et al.	1993	80	Patients with mixed cancers diagnosed within the previous 6 weeks undergoing radiotherapy with curative intent and considered to be at high risk for psychologic distress	71%	C1: Usual care ($n = 16$)	I1: Therapist administered individual intervention (information, discussion of effective coping strategies and common areas of concern); 3 weekly 60-minute sessions ($n = 15$)	F1: post-I (1 and 3 months)	F1: 0/1	F1: 1/1
Rawl et al.	2002	81	Patients with newly diagnosed breast, colorectal, or lung cancer undergoing chemotherapy	23%	C1: Usual care ($n = 54$)	I1: Therapist administered individual computer-based nursing intervention (program used to guide clinical assessment, problem identification, selection of interventions, and outcome measurement); 5 face-to-face 1-hour meetings and 4 20-minute telephone sessions over an 18-week period ($n = 55$)	F1: mid-I F2: (mid-I and 1 month post-I)	F1: 0/1 F2: 0/1	F1: 1/1 F2: 0/1
Richardson et al.	1997	82	Patients with nonmetastatic breast cancer who have completed treatment	0%	C1: Usual care ($n = 15$)	I1: Therapist administered group intervention (unstructured, support oriented); 6 weekly 60-minute sessions ($n = 16$) I2: Therapist administered group intervention (training in relaxation, imagery, and breathing); 6 weekly 60-minute sessions ($n = 16$)	F1: 1 week post-I	F1: I1 0/1 F1: I2 0/1	F1: I1 0/1 F1: I2 0/1
Sandgren and McCaul	2003	83	Patients with stage I–III breast cancer undergoing adjuvant chemotherapy, radiotherapy, or hormonal therapy	0%	C1: Usual care ($n = 55$)	I1: Nurse administered individual intervention (telephone counseling regarding disease and treatment-related information, managing side effects, and maintaining a healthy lifestyle); 5 weekly 30-minute telephone calls and 6th call 3 months later ($n = 78$) I2: Nurse administered individual intervention (telephone counseling regarding encouragement of emotional expression); 5 weekly 30-minute telephone calls and 6th call 3 months later ($n = 89$)	F1: 5 months	F1: I1 0/1 F1: I2 0/1	F1: I1 0/1 F1: I2 0/1

(continued)

TABLE 89.3. **Randomized clinical trials of psychosocial interventions with adult cancer patients.** (continued)

			Patient characteristics		*Study design*			*Comparisons of intervention and control groups: number of statistically significant measures favoring intervention group (P < 0.05)/number of measures*	
Investigators	*Year*	*Reference*	*Eligibility criteria*	*Percent male*	*Control (C) groups (number of subjects at baseline)*	*Intervention groups (number of subjects at baseline)*	*Timing of follow-ups (F)*	*Anxiety*	*Depression*
Sandgren et al.	2000	84	Patients with stage I or II breast cancer diagnosed within prior 3–4 months	0%	C1: Usual care ($n = 29$)	I1: Therapist administered individual intervention (telephone counseling regarding support, managing anxiety and stress, and problem solving); 1 call weekly for 4 weeks followed by 1 call every 2 weeks for 12 weeks ($n = 24$)	F1: 4 months F2: 10 months	F1: 0/1 F2: 0/1	F1: 0/1 F2: 0/1
Simpson et al.	2001	85	Patients with stage 0–II breast cancer who have completed treatment	0%	C1: Usual care ($n = 43$)	I: Therapist administered group intervention (relaxation, stress management, goal setting, planning and achieving change); 6 weekly 90-minute sessions ($n = 46$)	F1: post-I F2: 1 year F3: 2 years		F1: 1/1 F2: 0/1 F3: 1/1
Smith et al.	2001	86	Patients with mixed cancers receiving at least 5 weeks of radiotherapy for pelvic or abdominal malignancies	100%	C1: Usual care ($n = 23$)	I1: Patient access to music of their choice during radiotherapy simulation and treatment ($n = 19$)	F1: postsimulation F2: 1 week F3: 3 weeks F4: 5 weeks	F1: 0/2 F2: 0/2 F3: 0/2 F4: 0/2	
Speca et al.	2000	87	Patients with mixed cancers	17%	C1: Wait-list control ($n = 48$)	I1: Therapist administered group intervention (information, practice of meditation, problem solving); 7 weekly 90-minute sessions ($n = 61$)	F1: 7 weeks	F1: 0/2	F1: 2/2

Spiegel et al.	1981	88	Patients with metastatic breast cancer	0%	C1: Usual care ($n = 36$)	I1: Therapist administered group intervention (supportive-expressive therapy); weekly 90-minute sessions for 1 year ($n = 50$)	F1: post-I (4, 8, and 12 months)	F1: 1/1	F1: 0/1
Telch and Telch	1986	89	Patients with mixed cancers receiving outpatient care	34%	C1: Usual care ($n = 14$)	I1: Therapist administered group intervention (discussion of feelings, concerns, and problems); 6 weekly 60-minute sessions ($n = 14$) I2: Therapist administered group intervention (relaxation and stress management, communication and assertion, problem solving and constructive thinking, feelings management, and pleasant activity planning); 6 weekly 60-minute sessions ($n = 13$)	F1: 6 weeks	F1: I1 1/1 F1: I2 1/1	F1: I1 1/1 F1: I2 1/1
Thomas et al.	2000	90	Patients with mixed cancers receiving chemotherapy or radiotherapy	42%	C1: Usual care ($n = 107$)	I1: Patient viewed film providing preparatory information about chemotherapy and radiotherapy ($n = 113$)	F1: 3 weeks	F1: 1/1	F1: 1/1
Watson et al.	1988	91	Patients with early-stage breast cancer undergoing mastectomy	0%	C1: Usual care ($n = ?$)	I1: Therapist administered individual intervention (emotional support and facilitation of adjustment, information about physical state, and practical advice on breast prostheses); at least 4 sessions ($n = ?$)	F1: 1 week postoperative F2: 3 months postoperative F3: 12 months postoperative		F1: 0/1 F2: 1/1 F3: 0/1
Wells et al.	1995	92	Newly diagnosed patients with mixed cancers making first visit to hematology/oncology clinic	45%	C1: Usual care ($n = 16$)	I1: Brief clinic orientation (clinic tour and information and discussion session) ($n = 17$)	F1: post-I	F1: 2/2	

TABLE 89.4. Randomized clinical trials of pharmacological interventions with cancer patients.

Investigators	*Year*	*Reference*	*Eligibility criteria*	*Percent male*	*Design*	*Control groups (number of subjects at baseline)*	*Intervention groups (number of subjects at baseline)*	*Timing of follow-ups*	*Anxiety*	*Depression*
Bruera et al.	1985	93	Patients with mixed cancers in terminal phase of illness (no treatment within last month)	45%	Randomized double-blind placebo-controlled crossover trial	C1: Placebo ($n = 40$)	I1: Methylprednisolone po 32 mg/day × 5 days ($n = 40$)	F1: 5 and 13 days	F1: 0/1	F2: 1/1
Bruera et al.	1986	94	Patients with mixed cancers in terminal phase of illness (no treatment within last month)	70%	Randomized double-blind placebo-controlled crossover trial	C1: Placebo ($n = 30$)	I1: Mazindol po 3 mg/day × 5 days ($n = 30$)	F1: 6 and 12 days	F1: 0/1	F2: 0/1
Clerico et al.	1993	95	Patients with mixed cancers undergoing cisplatin-based chemotherapy	85%	Randomized double-blind placebo-controlled crossover trial	C1: Placebo ($n = 60$)	I1: Lorazepam po 2.5 mg evening before chemotherapy and just before start of chemotherapy ($n = 60$)	F1: After 1st and 2nd infusion	F1: 1/1	
Costa et al.	1985	96	Patients with mixed cancers diagnosed with major depression and having depression symptoms exceeding cutoff score	0%	Randomized double-blind placebo-controlled trial	C1: Placebo ($n = 37$)	I1: Mianserin po 30 mg/day × 1 week then 60 mg/day × 3 weeks ($n = 36$)	F1: 1 week F2: 2 weeks F3: 3 weeks F4: 4 weeks		F1: 2/2 F2: 0/2 F3: 1/2 F4: 2/2
Fisch et al.	2003	97	Patients with mixed cancers expected to survive 3–24 months and having depressed mood or anhedonia	50%	Randomized double-blind placebo-controlled trial	C1: Placebo ($n = 80$)	I1: Fluoxetine po 20 mg/day ($n = 83$)	F1: post-I (every 3–6 weeks for 12 weeks) F2: post-I (best change)		F1: 1/1 F2: 0/1
González Barón et al.	1991	98	Patients with mixed cancers undergoing chemotherapy	71%	Randomized controlled trial	C1: Standardized antiemetic regimen (high-dose metaclopramide plus methylprednisolone) at each infusion ($n = 85$)	I1: Standardized antiemetic regimen at each infusion plus lorazepam 0.02 mg/kg 30 minutes before and 8 hours after each infusion ($n = 78$)	F1: first day postchemotherapy F2: third day postchemotherapy	F1: 1/1 F2: 0/1	

Musselman et al. Capuron et al.	2001 2002	99 100	Patients with melanoma treated surgically and about to be treated with interferon alfa	50%	Randomized double-blind placebo-controlled trial	C1: Placebo ($n = 20$)	I1: Paroxetine po 10 mg/day × 1 week then 20 mg/day × 1 week then up to 40 mg/day ($n = 20$)	F1: 2 weeks F2: 4 weeks F3: 8 weeks F4: 12 weeks	F1: 0/1 F2: 1/1 F3: 1/2 F4: 2/2	F1: 0/1 F2: 0/1 F3: 2/2 F4: 2/2
Razavi et al.	1996	101	Patients with mixed cancers diagnosed with adjustment disorder (with depressive mood or mixed features) or major depressive disorder	20%	Randomized double-blind placebo-controlled trial with 1-week placebo run-in	C1: Placebo ($n = 46$)	I1: Fluoxetine po 20 mg/day ($n = 45$)	F1: 5 weeks	F1: 1/2	F1: 0/2
Tarrier et al.	1984	102	Patients with breast cancer treated with mastectomy consecutively referred for treatment of depression and poor adaptation	0%	Randomized controlled trial	C1: Behavioral intervention ($n = 5$)	I1: Behavioral intervention plus mianserin po 30–90 mg/day ($n = 5$)	F1: 1 week after completion of behavioral intervention F2: 3 months after completion of behavioral intervention		F1: 0/1 F2: 0/1
Van Heeringen and Zivkov	1996	103	Patients with stage I–II breast cancer and depression symptoms exceeding cutoff score	0%	Randomized double-blind placebo-controlled trial with 1-week placebo run-in	C1: Placebo ($n = 27$)	I1: Mianserin po 30 mg/day × 1 week then 60 mg/day ($n = 28$)	F1: 14 days F2: 28 days F3: 42 days		F1: 0/1 F2: 1/1 F3: 1/1
Wald et al.	1993	104	Patients with mixed cancers diagnosed with generalized anxiety disorder, panic disorder or adjustment disorder (with anxious mood), and having anxiety symptoms exceeding cutoff score	47%	Randomized double-blind placebo-controlled trial	C1: Placebo ($n = 18$)	I1: Alprazolam po at dose between 0.5 mg/day and 3.4 mg/day ($n = 18$)	F1: 1, 2, 3, and 4 weeks	F1: 0/1	F1: 0/1
Wolanskyj et al.	2000	105	Patients newly diagnosed with lymphoma undergoing first bone marrow biopsy and aspiration (BMBA)	68%	Randomized double-blind placebo-controlled trial	C1: Placebo at first and second BMBA ($n = 12$)	I1: Placebo at first BMBA followed by lorazepam po 2 mg and hydromorphone po 2 mg before second BMBA 1 hour later ($n = 13$)	F1: Difference between first and second BMBA	F1: 0/2	

TABLE 89.5. Number of psychosocial studies by cancer site and treatment status.

	Cancer site									
Treatment status	*Breast*	*Gynecologic*	*Testicular*	*Bladder*	*Colorectal*	*Melanoma*	*Hodgkin's*	*Renal cell*	*Mixed*	*Total*
Newly diagnosed									6	6
During chemotherapy	2						2		10	14
During radiotherapy									7	7
Before/immediately after surgery	4	1	1	1	1	2				10
Not in active treatment	3								2	5
Mixed treatment or not specified	6	1							9	16
Vaccine therapy								1		1
Bone marrow transplantation	1									1
Total	16	2	1	1	1	2	2	1	34	60

of cancer. Eight percent of studies (n = 1) included patients with "advanced" cancer.

With regard to treatment status, 33% of the studies (n = 4) included patients who were in various stages of treatment; that is, these studies enrolled patients actively undergoing treatment (e.g., chemotherapy, radiotherapy, or hormonal therapy), as well as patients not in active treatment. Seventeen percent (n = 2) of the studies enrolled patients during chemotherapy and 17% (n = 2) of the studies enrolled patients who had undergone surgery. Seventeen percent (n = 2) enrolled patients who were in the terminal phase of their illness and had not had treatment within the past month. Eight percent (n = 1) enrolled patients who were undergoing bone marrow biopsy and aspiration, and 8% (n = 1) did not provide enough detail to determine patients' treatment status.

Five of the 12 studies (42%) enrolled and randomized only those patients reporting significant symptoms of depression or anxiety. With respect to depression, two studies enrolled patients who met or exceeded a cutoff score on a screening measure of depressive symptomatology. Three studies enrolled patients who met diagnostic criteria for Major Depressive Disorder. With respect to anxiety, one study enrolled patients who met diagnostic criteria for an anxiety disorder and exceeded a cutoff score on a self-report measure of anxiety. The remainder of the studies (n = 7) did not enroll patients based on the presence of significant depressive or anxious symptomatology.

Across studies, sample sizes for each condition ranged widely, from as few as 5 patients to as many as 85 patients. The median sample size was 33.5 patients for the experimental conditions and 33 for the control conditions.

Ten of the 12 studies (83%) were double-blind studies. Placebo-controlled was the most frequently employed control condition, with 83% of the studies (n = 10) using this condition. Two of the 10 placebo-controlled studies included a 1-week placebo run-in. Three of the 10 studies utilized a crossover design. The other control conditions included a standardized antiemetic regimen (8%; n = 1) and a behavioral intervention (8%; n = 1).

Each of the 12 studies evaluated a standardized pharmacologic intervention. Six of the studies evaluated antidepressant agents, 4 evaluated antianxiety agents, 1 evaluated mazindol, a psychostimulant, and 1 evaluated methylprednisolone, a corticosteroid. Specifically, 17% (n = 2) evaluated fluoxetine, 8% (n = 1) evaluated paroxetine, 17% (n = 2) evaluated mianserin only, and 8% (n = 1) evaluated mianserin plus a behavioral intervention compared to the behavioral intervention alone. One study (8%) evaluated alprazolam, 2 (17%) evaluated lorazepam, and 1 (8%) evaluated a standardized antiemetic regimen (metoclopramide plus methylprednisolone) plus lorazepam compared to the standardized antiemetic regimen. Finally, 1 study (n = 8%) evaluated mazindol and 1 (n = 8%) evaluated methylprednisolone.

Fifty percent (n = 6) of the studies reviewed included one follow-up assessment, 25% (n = 3) involved two follow-up assessments, 8% (n = 1) included three follow-up assessments, and 17% (n = 2) included four follow-up assessments.

TABLE 89.6. Outcomes of psychosocial interventions studies by intervention type and treatment status [number of studies].

	Combination		*Relaxation only*		*Psychoeducation*	
	Anxiety	*Depression*	*Anxiety*	*Depression*	*Anxiety*	*Depression*
Newly diagnosed		1/6 [2]	7/7 [2]	6/6 [1]	3/7 [3]	1/1 [1]
During chemotherapy	4/7 [3]	3/5 [3]	9/24 [7]	3/6 [4]	1/1 [1]	
During radiotherapy	2/3 [2]	2/3 [2]			0/7 [3]	0/1 [1]
Before/immediately after surgery	2/10 [4]	2/11 [5]	1/1 [1]		2/3 [2]	1/1 [1]
Not in active treatment	2/5 [3]	2/7 [4]	0/1 [1]	0/1 [1]		
Mixed treatment or not specified	4/11 [6]	7/11 [6]	1/2 [2]	1/2 [2]	1/4 [3]	1/4 [3]
Vaccine therapy						
Bone marrow transplantation	0/1 [1]	0/1 [1]				
Total	14/38	17/45	18/35	10/15	7/22	3/7

Supportive-expressive		*Problem-solving*		*Counseling*		*Cognitive therapy*		*Music*	
Anxiety	*Depression*	*Anxiety*	*Depression*	*Anxiety*	*Depression*	*Anxiety*	*Depression*	*Anxiety*	*Depression*
	0/3 [1]								
2/2 [1]	2/2 [1]	0/3 [2]	1/2 [1]	0/9 [2]	0/1 [1]		1/1 [1]		
2/2 [1]	2/2 [1]	0/1 [1]	1/1 [1]					0/8 [1]	
	1/3 [1]	1/3 [1]	0/3 [1]	0/1 [1]	1/1 [1]				
	0/1 [1]	0/1 [1]							
3/4 [4]	2/4 [4]	2/5 [3]	0/5 [3]		1/5 [1]				
0/1 [1]	0/1 [1]								
7/10	7/16	3/12	2/11	0/10	2/7		1/1 [1]	0/8	

The length of time between intervention and the final follow-up assessment ranged from immediately postintervention to 12 weeks. Of the 12 studies reviewed, 17% ($n = 2$) conducted the final follow-up immediately postintervention, 25% ($n = 3$) conducted it from 3 days to 12 days after the intervention, 33% ($n = 4$) conducted it from 4 to 6 months postintervention, and 25% ($n = 3$) conducted it 12 weeks postintervention. The median interval between commencement of the intervention and the final follow-up assessment was 4 weeks.

Findings from the Pharmacologic Studies

Three of the 12 pharmacologic studies targeted anxiety only, 4 targeted depression only, and 5 targeted both anxiety and depression. Outcomes were measured via observer report and patient self-report on various psychometric instruments that have been used extensively with cancer patients. Anxiety, for example, was most commonly measured using the observer-rated Hamilton Anxiety Scale.[26] Patient's self-report of anxiety was recorded using instruments, such as the State-Trait Anxiety Inventory[5] or the anxiety subscale of the Hospital Anxiety and Depression Scale.[8] Measures of depression used included the observer rated Hamilton Rating Scale for Depression.[27] Patient's self-report was recorded using instruments such as the Beck Depression Inventory,[24] the Zung Self-rating Depression Scale,[28] and the depression scale of the Hospital Anxiety and Depression Scale.[8]

The total number of anxiety outcomes, when all follow-up assessments were taken into account, was 16. Seven or 44% of the total were statistically significant at P less than 0.05. The total number of depression outcomes, when all follow-up assessments were taken into account, was 26. Thirteen or 48% of the total were statistically significant at P less than 0.05.

As presented in Table 89.7, when the six studies examining an antidepressant agent were evaluated, 52% (12 of 23 outcomes) of the depression outcomes were significant and 63% of the anxiety outcomes (5 of 8 outcomes) were significant. With respect to the agents' antidepressant effect, the percentage of significant results ranged from 0% (0 of 2 outcomes) for mianserin and fluoxetine to 67% (4 of 6 outcomes and 2 of 3 outcomes) for paroxetine and mianserin, respectively. With respect to the agents' antianxiety effect, the percentage of significant results ranged from 50% (1 of 2 outcomes) for fluoxetine and 67% (4 of 6 outcomes) for paroxetine. When the four studies examining an antianxiety agent were evaluated, 33% (2 of 6 outcomes) of the anxiety outcomes were significant and 0% of the depression outcomes (0 of 1 outcome) were significant. With respect to the agents' antianxiety effect, the percentage of significant results ranged from 0% (0 of 1 outcome and 0 of 2 outcomes) for alprazolam and lorazepam, respectively, to 100% (1 of 1 outcome) for lorazepam. The percentage of significant results for the agents' antidepressant effect was 0% (0 of 1 outcome) for alprazolam. In the study examining the effects of mazindol, 0% (0 of 1 outcome) of the depression outcomes and 0% (0 of 1 outcome) of the anxiety outcomes were significant. In the study examining methylprednisolone, 0% (0 of 1 outcome) of the anxiety outcomes were significant and 100% (1 of 1 outcome) of the depression outcomes were significant.

Evidence-Based Recommendations for Management of Anxiety and Depression in Cancer Patients

This comprehensive review of published research provides considerable support for the use of psychosocial interventions to effectively manage anxiety and depression in adult patients with cancer. As shown in Table 89.3, the research was conducted across a broad range of cancer types, disease stages, and treatment status. The interventions were as varied as a 1-hour group-based information and orientation session, several months of weekly individual psychotherapy to explore end-of-life concerns, and self-administered relaxation. Despite the diversity of patients and the wide variety of interventions, careful reading of the research results suggests

TABLE 89.7. Outcomes for pharmacologic studies by medication type [number of studies].

	Anxiety	*Depression*
Antidepressants		
Fluoxetine	1/2 [1]	1/4 [2]
Paroxetine	4/6 [1]	4/6 [1]
Mianserin		7/13 [3]
Anxiolytics		
Lorazepam	2/5 [3]	
Alprazolam	0/1 [1]	0/1 [1]
Corticosteroid		
Methylprednisolone	0/1 [1]	1/1 [1]
Amphetamine		
Mazindol	0/1 [1]	0/1 [1]

TABLE 89.8. Evidence-based recommendations on the use of psychosocial interventions.

GENERAL RECOMMENDATIONS

Psychosocial interventions are effective in preventing or relieving anxiety and depression in cancer patients[13,15]

Psychosocial interventions are effective in preventing or relieving anxiety and depression in both male and female cancer patients[35,36,39,41,44–46,48,52,53,58,62,63,67,69,73,76,80,81,87,89,90,92,106]

RECOMMENDATIONS BASED ON DISEASE STATUS

Psychosocial interventions are effective in preventing or relieving anxiety in newly diagnosed patients[39,73,92]

Psychosocial interventions are effective in preventing or relieving depression in newly diagnosed patients[36,39,51,73]

Psychosocial interventions are effective in preventing or relieving anxiety in breast cancer patients with metastatic disease[57,88]

Psychosocial interventions are effective in preventing or relieving depression for breast cancer patients with metastatic disease[50,57]

Psychosocial interventions are effective in preventing or relieving anxiety and depression in patients in the terminal phase of illness[67]

RECOMMENDATIONS BASED ON TREATMENT STATUS

Psychosocial interventions are effective in preventing or relieving anxiety in patients undergoing chemotherapy[41,42,44,62,63,69,76]

Psychosocial interventions are effective in preventing or relieving depression in patients undergoing chemotherapy[41,42,63,69,70,81]

Psychosocial interventions are effective in preventing or relieving anxiety in patients undergoing radiotherapy[48,53]

Psychosocial interventions are effective in preventing or relieving depression in patients undergoing radiotherapy[48,53,80]

Psychosocial interventions are effective in preventing or relieving anxiety in patients before and after surgery[35,45,78,79]

Psychosocial interventions are effective in preventing or relieving depression in patients before and after surgery[46,79,106]

Psychosocial interventions are effective in preventing or relieving anxiety following completion of active treatment[52]

Psychosocial interventions are effective in preventing or relieving depression following completion of active treatment[85]

RECOMMENDATIONS BASED ON TYPE OF INTERVENTION

Relaxation techniques are effective in preventing or relieving anxiety in cancer patients[36,39,41,42,44,45,67,76]

Relaxation techniques are effective in preventing or relieving depression in cancer patients[39,41,42,67]

Relaxation techniques, in combination with education and skills training, are effective in preventing or relieving anxiety in cancer patients[43,48,52,63,69,79,89]

Relaxation techniques, in combination with education and skills training, are effective in preventing or relieving depression in cancer patients[43,48,50,51,63,69,79,85,87,89,106]

Psychoeducation is effective in preventing or relieving anxiety in cancer patients[35,62,73,90,92]

Psychoeducation is effective in preventing or relieving depression in cancer patients[71,73,90]

Supportive and supportive-expressive therapies are effective in preventing or relieving anxiety in cancer patients[53,57,69,88,89]

Supportive and supportive-expressive therapies are effective in preventing or relieving depression in cancer patients[53,57,69,89]

Problem-solving therapies are effective in preventing or relieving anxiety in cancer patients[58,78]

Problem-solving therapies are effective in preventing or relieving depression in cancer patients[80,81]

Counseling is effective in preventing or relieving depression in cancer patients[46,66]

Cognitive therapy is effective in preventing or relieving depression in cancer patients[70]

RECOMMENDATIONS BASED ON INTERVENTION TYPE AND DISEASE OR TREATMENT STATUS

Relaxation techniques, alone or in combination with education and skills training, are effective in preventing or relieving anxiety in newly diagnosed cancer patients[36,39]

Relaxation techniques, alone or in combination with education and skills training, are effective in preventing or relieving depression in newly diagnosed cancer patients[39,51]

Relaxation techniques, alone or in combination with education and skills training, are effective in preventing or relieving anxiety in patients undergoing chemotherapy[41,42,44,63,69,76]

Relaxation techniques, alone or in combination with education and skills training, are effective in preventing or relieving depression in patients undergoing chemotherapy[41,42,63,69]

Relaxation techniques, alone or in combination with education and skills training, are effective in preventing or relieving anxiety in patients undergoing radiotherapy[48,53]

Relaxation techniques, alone or in combination with education and skills training, are effective in preventing or relieving depression in patients undergoing radiotherapy[48,53]

Relaxation techniques, alone or in combination with education and skills training, are effective in preventing or relieving anxiety in patients before and after surgery[45,79]

Relaxation techniques, alone or in combination with education and skills training, are effective in preventing or relieving depression in patients before and after surgery[79,106]

Relaxation techniques, alone or in combination with education and skills training, are effective in preventing or relieving anxiety following completion of active treatment[52]

Relaxation techniques, alone or in combination with education and skills training, are effective in preventing or relieving depression following completion of active treatment[85]

Relaxation techniques, alone or in combination with education and skills training, are effective in preventing or relieving anxiety in patients in the terminal phase of illness[67]

Relaxation techniques, alone or in combination with education and skills training, are effective in preventing or relieving depression in patients in the terminal phase of illness[67]

Psychoeducation is effective in preventing or relieving anxiety in newly diagnosed patients[73]

Psychoeducation is effective in preventing or relieving depression in newly diagnosed patients[73]

Psychoeducation is effective in preventing or relieving anxiety in patients before and after surgery[35]

Psychoeducation is effective in preventing or relieving depression in patients before and after surgery[71]

Psychoeducation is effective in preventing or relieving anxiety in patients undergoing chemotherapy[62]

Supportive and supportive-expressive therapies are effective in preventing or relieving anxiety in patients undergoing chemotherapy[69]

Supportive and supportive-expressive therapies are effective in preventing or relieving depression in patients undergoing chemotherapy[69]

Supportive and supportive-expressive therapies are effective in preventing or relieving anxiety in patients undergoing radiotherapy[53]

Supportive and supportive-expressive therapies are effective in preventing or relieving depression in patients undergoing radiotherapy[53]

Supportive and supportive-expressive therapies are effective in preventing or relieving depression in patients before and after surgery[91]

Problem-solving therapies are effective in preventing or relieving anxiety in patients before and after surgery[78]

Problem-solving therapies are effective in preventing or relieving depression in patients undergoing chemotherapy[81]

Problem-solving therapies are effective in preventing or relieving depression in patients undergoing radiotherapy[80]

Counseling is effective in preventing or relieving depression in cancer patients before and after surgery[46]

Cognitive therapy is effective in preventing or relieving depression in patients undergoing chemotherapy[70]

TABLE 89.9. Evidence-based recommendations on the use of pharmacologic interventions.

Recommendation:
Antidepressants are effective in preventing or relieving depression in cancer patients[96,97,99,100,103]
Antidepressants are effective in preventing or relieving anxiety in cancer patients[99–101]
Anxiolytics are effective in preventing or relieving anxiety in cancer patients[95,98]
Corticosteroids are effective in preventing or relieving depression in cancer patients in the terminal phase of illness[93]

a number of recommendations for preventing or relieving anxiety and depression in cancer patients. The recommendations presented in Table 89.8 are based on statistically significant, clinically relevant evidence provided by both previous systematic reviews and meta-analyses and our systematic review of randomized controlled trials.

The review of published research designed to evaluate pharmacologic interventions for the management of anxiety and depression in cancer patients is considerably narrower in scope. Nevertheless, the best available evidence supports the use of pharmacologic interventions in adult patients with cancer. The recommendations presented in Table 89.9 are based on statistically significant, clinically relevant evidence provided by our systematic review of randomized controlled trials.

Limitations of Existing Research Base for Developing an Evidence-Based Approach to Management of Anxiety and Depression in Cancer Patients

The relatively large number of randomized clinical trials listed in Tables 89.3 and 89.4, provides a strong foundation for developing an evidence-based approach to the management of anxiety and depression in cancer patients. The recommendations listed in Tables 89.8 and 89.9, which follow directly from the results of these many studies, address numerous aspects of the psychologic and psychiatric care of cancer patients. It should be noted, however, that several recommendations listed in Tables 89.8 and 89.9, are based on a very few studies. In addition, important gaps in the existing research literature can be identified that limit the type and scope of recommendations that can be offered.

Limitations in Research on Psychosocial Interventions

Inspection of the evidence and recommendation tables included in this chapter, suggests several areas where evidence regarding the use of psychosocial interventions to manage anxiety and depression in cancer patients is sparse. With respect to patient characteristics, we noted that in only 5% of the studies were the samples limited to male cancer patients. Although these studies and studies of samples including both men and women suggest that psychosocial interventions are effective in male patients, important questions regarding the relative effectiveness and acceptability of psychosocial interventions in male and female cancer patients remain unanswered. Clinicians often report that male cancer patients can be more difficult to engage in psychosocial interventions and, once engaged, are more likely to benefit from educational interventions than interventions focusing on expression of emotions and group support. Clearly, more research is needed to either confirm or disconfirm beliefs that male cancer patients are less likely than female cancer patients to benefit from psychosocial approaches to the management of anxiety and depression.

Limitations in the evidence base also exist regarding the effectiveness of psychosocial interventions in specific forms of cancer. We noted that 57% of psychosocial intervention studies were based on patient samples that included more than one form of cancer. Although breast cancer was the focus of 27% of the remaining studies, no other single form of cancer was the focus of more than two studies. The significance of this issue lies in the possibility that the sources of anxiety and depression and the methods needed to treat it psychologically, may vary considerably across different cancers. For example, the psychologic issues raised by having a disease in a part of the body closely related to sexual functioning (e.g., breast cancer) are likely to differ from those associated with having a disease linked to smoking behavior (e.g., lung cancer) or a disease that may lead to significant changes in facial appearance (e.g., head and neck cancer) or cognitive abilities (e.g., brain cancer). To address this gap, more studies are needed that focus on forms of cancer other than breast cancer, as well as studies that examine whether generic interventions (e.g., relaxation training) are more effective if adapted or tailored for different forms of cancer.

A similar situation exists with regard to disease stage or status. Most of the studies identified (73%) did not focus on patients at a specific stage of disease. Information included in many of these studies suggests that they were composed primarily of patients with early-stage disease. Of those studies in which eligibility was limited by disease stage or status, just 9% focused on patients with stage IV or metastatic disease and only 2% focused on patients in the terminal phase of their disease. Although these studies provide preliminary evidence that psychosocial interventions are effective in patients with more advanced disease, the issue merits closer study in light of evidence suggesting the presence of more severe psychologic symptoms in patients with more advanced disease.[29]

Examination of treatment status also leads to identification of gaps in the research base. In general, studies of psychosocial interventions for anxiety and depression have focused on patients in the period during which they are being actively treated with surgery, chemotherapy, and/or radiotherapy. Just 8% of the studies identified were limited to patients not currently receiving treatment. A growing body of research has documented the presence of anxiety and depression in patients who have successfully completed treatment for cancer.[30,31] Although preliminary evidence suggests that psychosocial interventions are effective in the posttreatment period, a number of important issues have yet to be examined. For example, no randomized clinical trials could be identified that have evaluated interventions designed specifically to address symptoms of posttraumatic stress in patients who had completed treatment for cancer.

Another consideration involves the types of interventions that have been evaluated. Our systematic review found that 53% of the psychosocial studies evaluated the effectiveness of relaxation training, either alone or in combination with education and skills training. Other forms of psychosocial intervention, such as problem-solving therapy, were found to be effective in a limited number of studies and merit further evaluation. In addition, there are several major forms of psychotherapy found to be effective against anxiety and depression in outpatient psychiatric settings that received little or no attention in research with cancer patients. These approaches, which include interpersonal therapy[32] and cognitive therapy,[33] may be particularly well suited to cancer patients experiencing more severe symptoms of anxiety and depression.

The issue of symptom severity is one that has received relatively little attention in prior psychosocial research with cancer patients. Our systematic review found that only 5% of studies restricted eligibility to patients experiencing heightened levels of psychologic distress. As a consequence, the average pretreatment levels of anxiety and depression in these studies are likely to have been relatively low. In contrast, clinical practice guidelines, such as those developed by NCCN,[11] recommend the use of psychosocial interventions for cancer patients experiencing the heightened distress characteristic of adjustment, mood, or anxiety disorders. By evaluating psychosocial interventions with patients experiencing more severe symptoms of anxiety and depression, future research is likely to yield results of greater relevance to the evaluation of current clinical practice.

Limitations in Research on Pharmacologic Interventions

The primary limitation in the evidence base for pharmacologic interventions is the relative paucity of randomized clinical trials. Only 12 such studies could be identified, and these studies encompassed the evaluation of several different classes of pharmacologic agents, including antidepressants, anxiolytics, psychostimulants, and corticosteroids. Five of the studies were of an antidepressant agent and included eligibility criteria based on level or presence of depressive symptomatology. These studies yield evidence that supports the NCCN guideline recommendation that antidepressants be prescribed for cancer patients experiencing severe adjustment reactions or mood disorders.[11] The principal gap in the evidence base is the lack of research on the effectiveness of anxiolytic agents in cancer patients experiencing heightened anxiety. Although 4 studies were identified that evaluated anxiolytic agents, 3 of these studies focused on the use of lorazepam in combination with antiemetic or analgesic medications for relief of treatment-related symptoms. Another important gap in the evidence base is research on the effectiveness of psychostimulants for the treatment of depression in cancer patients. Although nonrandomized studies suggest that psychostimulants, such as methylphenidate, are effective as antidepressants in patients with advanced disease,[34] evidence from randomized clinical trials is lacking.

In addition to the need for more research on pharmacologic interventions for anxiety and depression in cancer patients, there is a need for research about the relative efficacy of pharmacologic and psychologic approaches with cancer patients. One type of research needed is studies that evaluate whether the combined psychosocial and pharmacologic intervention results in better management of anxiety and depression than the use of psychosocial or pharmacologic interventions alone. This type of research would allow for evaluation and possible refinement of recommendations, such as those contained in NCCN guidelines,[11] that patients with mood disorders be treated initially with antidepressant agents plus psychotherapy, as well as recommendations that patients with anxiety disorders be treated initially with psychotherapy with or without psychotropic medication. Another type of research needed is studies that directly compare the effectiveness of pharmacologic and psychosocial approaches in treating anxiety and depression in cancer patients. This type of research would allow for evaluation of recommendations, such as those contained in NCCN guidelines,[11] that patients with mild adjustment disorders be treated initially with psychotherapy alone.

Summary

Anxiety and depression, which are among the most common symptoms experienced by cancer patients, have been the focus of considerable attention and research. In recent years, clinical practice guidelines have appeared that include specific recommendations for the management of anxiety and depression in cancer patients. These efforts have been limited, however, by reliance on a consensus-based approach rather than an evidence-based approach,[11] or by inclusion of evidence from studies conducted on populations other than cancer patients.[12] To address these issues, the present chapter focused on evidence from randomized clinical trials of psychosocial and pharmacologic interventions with cancer patients, in which anxiety or depression was measured as outcomes.

Aided by previous systematic reviews and meta-analyses, we were able to identify 60 randomized clinical trials of psychosocial interventions and 12 randomized clinical trials of pharmacologic interventions. The relatively large number of psychosocial studies yielded numerous evidence-based recommendations regarding the use of psychosocial interventions in the management of anxiety and depression. Indeed, the quantity and quality of the research permitted not only general recommendations, but recommendations based on disease status, treatment status, type of intervention, and the combination of type of intervention and disease or treatment status. Because of the much smaller number of studies, far fewer evidence-based recommendations could be offered regarding the use of pharmacologic interventions for anxiety and depression in cancer patients.

Despite the relatively large number of psychosocial intervention studies that have been conducted, several important gaps in this evidence base could be identified: these include the limited number of studies that have focused on male patients, patients with cancers other than breast cancer, patients with more advanced disease, patients who have completed cancer treatment, and patients with more severe symptoms of anxiety and depression. The primary limitation in the evidence base for pharmacologic interventions is the relative paucity of randomized clinical trials. Notable gaps in the evidence base include the lack of placebo-controlled studies of anxiolytic agents in the treatment of anxiety symptoms and of psychostimulant agents in the treatment of depressive symptoms. In addition to these types of pharmacologic studies, there is a need for studies that evaluate the relative and combined efficacy of psychosocial and pharmacologic interventions with cancer patients. These types of studies will allow for the evaluation of patterns of care for which there appears to be a general clinical consensus, as suggested by NCCN guidelines,[11] but no direct empirical evidence. This approach would also allow us to proceed from individual evidence-based recommendations to a more comprehensive evidence-based approach to treatment selection and delivery of care for the management of anxiety and depression in cancer patients.

References

1. Newport DJ, Nemeroff CB. Assessment and treatment of depression in the cancer patient. J Psychosom Res 1998;45:215–237.
2. Stark DPH, House A. Anxiety in cancer patients. Br J Cancer 2000;83:1261–1267.
3. Cordova MJ, Andrykowski MA, Kenady DE, et al. Frequency and correlates of posttraumatic-stress-disorder-like symptoms after treatment for breast cancer. J Consult Clin Psychol 1995; 63:981–986.
4. Bottomley A. Depression in cancer patients: a literature review. Eur J Cancer Care 1998;7:181–191.
5. Speilberger CD. Manual for the State-Trait Anxiety Inventory (Form Y). Palo Alto, CA: Consulting Psychologists Press, 1983.
6. Beck A, Mendelson M, Mock J, et al. Inventory for measuring depression. Arch Gen Psychiatry 1961;4:561–571.
7. Diagnostic and Statistical Manual of Mental Disorders, 4th ed. Washington, DC: American Psychiatric Association, 1994.
8. Zigmond AS, Snaith RP. The hospital anxiety and depression scale. Acta Psychiatr Scand 1983;67:361–370.
9. Cleeland CS, Mendoza TR, Wang XS, et al. Assessing symptom distress in cancer patients: the M.D. Anderson Symptom Inventory. Cancer (Phila) 2000;89:1634–1646.
10. Chang VT, Hwang SS, Feuerman MS, et al. The Memorial Symptom Assessment Scale Short Form (MSAS-SF). Cancer (Phila) 2000;89:1162–1171.
11. Distress Management Guidelines Panel. Distress management clinical practice guidelines in oncology. J Natl Compr Cancer Netw 2003;1:344–393.
12. National Breast Cancer Centre and National Cancer Control Initiative. Clinical practice guidelines for the psychosocial care of adults with cancer. Camperdown, Australia: National Breast Cancer Centre, 2003.
13. Devine EC, Westlake SK. The effects of psychoeducational care provided to adults with cancer: meta-analysis of 116 studies. Oncol Nurs Forum 1995;22:1369–1381.
14. Sheard T, Maguire P. The effect of psychological interventions on anxiety and depression in cancer patients: results of two meta-analyses. Br J Cancer 1999;80:1770–1780.
15. Barsevick AM, Sweeney C, Haney E, et al. A systematic qualitative analysis of psychoeducational interventions for depression in patients with cancer. Oncol Nurs Forum 2002;29:73–84.
16. Carr D, Goudas L, Lawrence D, et al. Management of Cancer Symptoms: Pain, Depression, and Fatigue. Evidence Report/Technology Assessment No. 61. AHRQ Publication No. 02-E032. Rockville, MD: Agency for Health Care Research and Quality, 2002.
17. Trijsburg RW, van Knippenberg FC, Rijpma SE. Effects of psychological treatment on cancer patients: a critical review. Psychosom Med 1992;54:489–517.
18. Redd WH, Montgomery GH, DuHamel KN. Behavioral intervention for cancer treatment side effects. J Natl Cancer Inst 2001;93:810–823.
19. Newell SA, Sanson-Fisher RW, Savolainen NJ. Systematic review of psychological therapies for cancer patients: overview and recommendations for future research. J Natl Cancer Inst 2002;94:558–584.
20. Ly KL, Chidgey J, Addington-Hall J, et al. Depression in palliative care: a systematic review. Part 2. Treatment. Palliat Med 2002;16:279–284.
21. Meyer TJ, Mark MM. Effects of psychosocial interventions with adult cancer patients: A meta-analysis of randomized experiments. Health Psychol 1995;14:101–108.
22. Rehse B, Pukrop R. Effects of psychosocial interventions on quality of life in adult cancer patients: meta-analysis of 37 published controlled outcome studies. Patient Educ Couns 2003;50:179–186.
23. McNair DM, Lorr M, Droppleman L. Profile of Mood States. San Diego, CA: Educational and Industrial Testing Service, 1992.
24. Beck AT, Ward CH, Mendelson M, et al. An inventory for measuring depression. Arch Gen Psychiatry 1961;4:561–571.
25. Radloff LS. The CES-D Scale: a self-report depression scale for research in the general population. Appl Psychol Meas 1977;1:385–401.
26. Maier W, Buller R, Philipp M, et al. The Hamilton Anxiety Scale: reliability, validity and sensitivity to change in anxiety and depressive disorders. J Affect Disord 1988;14:61–68.
27. Hamilton M. A rating scale for depression. J Neurol Neurosurg Psychiatry 1960;23:56–62.
28. Zung WW. A self-rating depression scale. Arch Gen Psychiatry 1965;12:63–70.
29. Minagawa H, Uchitomi Y, Yamawaki S, et al. Psychiatric morbidity in terminally ill cancer patients. A prospective study. Cancer (Phila) 1996;78:1131–1137.
30. Smith MY, Redd WH, Peyser C, et al. Post-traumatic stress disorder in cancer: a review. Psycho-Oncology 1999;8:521–537.
31. Deimling GT, Kahana B, Bowman KF, et al. Cancer survivorship and psychological distress in later life. Psycho-Oncology 2002; 11:479–494.
32. Weissman MM, Markowitz JC. Interpersonal psychotherapy for depression. In: Gotlib IH, Hammen CL (eds) Handbook of Depression. New York: Guilford Press, 2002:404–421.
33. Beck AT. Cognitive therapy: past, present, and future. In: Mahoney MJ (ed) Cognitive and Constructive Psychotherapies: Theory, Research, and Practice. New York: Springer, 1995:29–40.
34. Rozans M, Dreisbach A, Letora JJ, et al. Palliative uses of methylphenidate in patients with cancer: a review. J Clin Oncol 2002;20:335–339.
35. Ali NS, Khalil HZ. Effect of psychoeducational intervention on anxiety among Egyptian bladder cancer patients. Cancer Nurs 1989;12:236–242.
36. Arakawa S. Relaxation to reduce nausea, vomiting, and anxiety induced by chemotherapy in Japanese patients. Cancer Nurs 1997;20:342–349.
37. Arathuzik D. Effects of cognitive-behavioral strategies on pain in cancer patients. Cancer Nurs 1994;17:207–214.
38. Berglund G, Bolund C, Gustafsson U, et al. A randomized study of a rehabilitation program for cancer patients: the 'starting again' group. Psycho-Oncology 1994;3:109–120.
39. Bindemann S, Soukop M, Kaye SB. Randomised controlled study of relaxation training. Eur J Cancer 1991;27:170–174.
40. Brown RF, Butow PN, Dunn SM, et al. Promoting patient participation and shortening cancer consultations: a randomised trial. Br J Cancer 2001;85:1273–1279.
41. Burish TG, Lyles JN. Effectiveness of relaxation training in reducing adverse reactions to cancer chemotherapy. J Behav Med 1981;4:65–78.

42. Burish TG, Carey MP, Krozely MG, et al. Conditioned side effects induced by cancer chemotherapy: prevention through behavioral treatment. J Consult Clin Psychol 1987;55:42–48.
43. Cain EN, Kohorn EI, Quinlan DM, et al. Psychosocial benefits of a cancer support group. Cancer (Phila) 1986;57:183–189.
44. Carey MP, Burish TG. Providing relaxation training to cancer chemotherapy patients: a comparison of three delivery techniques. J Consult Clin Psychol 1987;55:732–737.
45. Cheung YL, Molassiotis A, Chang AM. The effect of progressive muscle relaxation training on anxiety and quality of life after stoma surgery in colorectal cancer patients. Psycho-Oncology 2003;12:254–266.
46. Christensen DN. Postmastectomy couple counseling: an outcome study of a structured treatment protocol. J Sex Marital Ther 1983;9:266–275.
47. de Moor C, Sterner J, Hall M, et al. A pilot study of the effects of expressive writing on psychological and behavioral adjustment in patients enrolled in a Phase II trial of vaccine therapy for metastatic renal cell carcinoma. Health Psychol 2002;21:615–619.
48. Decker TW, Cline-Elsen J, Gallagher M. Relaxation therapy as an adjunct in radiation oncology. J Clin Psychol 1992;48:388–393.
49. Dodd MJ. Efficacy of proactive information on self-care in radiation therapy patients. Heart Lung 1987;16:538–544.
50. Edelman S, Bell DR, Kidman AD. A group cognitive behaviour therapy programme with metastatic breast cancer patients. Psycho-Oncology 1999;8:295–305.
51. Edgar L, Rosberger Z, Collet JP. Lessons learned: outcomes and methodology of a coping skills intervention trial comparing individual and group formats for patients with cancer. Int J Psychiatry Med 2001;31:289–304.
52. Elsesser K, van Berkel M, Sartory G. The effects of anxiety management training on psychological variables and immune parameters in cancer patients: a pilot study. Behav Cognit Psychother 1994;22:13–23.
53. Evans RL, Connis RT. Comparison of brief group therapies for depressed cancer patients receiving radiation treatment. Public Health Rep 1995;110:306–311.
54. Fawzy NW. A psychoeducational nursing intervention to enhance coping and affective state in newly diagnosed malignant melanoma patients. Cancer Nurs 1995;18:427–438.
55. Fukui S, Kugaya A, Okamura H, et al. A psychosocial group intervention for Japanese women with primary breast carcinoma. Cancer (Phila) 2000;89:1026–1036.
56. Gaston-Johansson F, Fall-Dickson JM, Nanda J, et al. The effectiveness of the comprehensive coping strategy program on clinical outcomes in breast cancer autologous bone marrow transplantation. Cancer Nurs 2000;23:277–285.
57. Goodwin PJ, Leszcz M, Ennis M, et al. The effect of group psychosocial support on survival in metastatic breast cancer. N Engl J Med 2001;345:1719–1726.
58. Greer S, Moorey S, Baruch JD, et al. Adjuvant psychological therapy for patients with cancer: a prospective randomised trial. Br Med J 1992;304:675–680.
59. Haggmark C, Bohman L, Ilmoni-Brandt K, et al. Effects of information supply on satisfaction with information and quality of life in cancer patients receiving curative radiation therapy. Patient Educ Couns 2001;45:173–179.
60. Hagopian GA, Rubenstein JH. Effects of telephone call interventions on patients' well-being in a radiation therapy department. Cancer Nurs 1990;13:339–344.
61. Heinrich RL, Schag CC. Stress and activity management: group treatment for cancer patients and spouses. J Consult Clin Psychol 1985;53:439–446.
62. Jacobs C, Ross RD, Walker IM, et al. Behavior of cancer patients: a randomized study of the effects of education and peer support groups. Am J Clin Oncol 1983;6:347–353.
63. Jacobsen PB, Meade CD, Stein KD, et al. Efficacy and costs of two forms of stress management training for cancer patients undergoing chemotherapy. J Clin Oncol 2002;20:2851–2862.
64. Larson MR, Duberstein PR, Talbot NL, et al. A presurgical psychosocial intervention for breast cancer patients. Psychological distress and the immune response. J Psychosom Res 2000;48:187–194.
65. Lerman C, Rimer B, Blumberg B, et al. Effects of coping style and relaxation on cancer chemotherapy side effects and emotional responses. Cancer Nurs 1990;13:308–315.
66. Linn MW, Linn BS, Harris R. Effects of counseling for late stage cancer patients. Cancer (Phila) 1982;49:1048–1055.
67. Liossi C, White P. Efficacy of clinical hypnosis in the enhancement of quality of life of terminally ill cancer patients. Contemp Hypnosis 2001;18:145–160.
68. Lyles JN, Burish TG, Krozely MG, et al. Efficacy of relaxation training and guided imagery in reducing the aversiveness of cancer chemotherapy. J Consult Clin Psychol 1982;50:509–524.
69. Mantovani G, Astara G, Lampis B, et al. Evaluation by multidimensional instruments of health-related quality of life of elderly cancer patients undergoing three different "psychosocial" treatment approaches. A randomized clinical trial. Support Care Cancer 1996;4:129–140.
70. Marchioro G, Azzarello G, Checchin F, et al. The impact of a psychological intervention on quality of life in non-metastatic breast cancer. Eur J Cancer 1996;32A:1612–1615.
71. McArdle JM, George WD, McArdle CS, et al. Psychological support for patients undergoing breast cancer surgery: a randomised study. Br Med J 1996;312:813–816.
72. McHugh P, Lewis S, Ford S, et al. The efficacy of audiotapes in promoting psychological well-being in cancer patients: a randomised, controlled trial. Br J Cancer 1995;71:388–392.
73. McQuellon RP, Wells M, Hoffman S, et al. Reducing distress in cancer patients with an orientation program. Psycho-Oncology 1998;7:207–217.
74. Molassiotis A, Yung HP, Yam BM, et al. The effectiveness of progressive muscle relaxation training in managing chemotherapy-induced nausea and vomiting in Chinese breast cancer patients: a randomised controlled trial. Support Care Cancer 2002;10:237–246.
75. Moorey S, Greer S, Watson M, et al. Adjuvant psychological therapy for patients with cancer: outcome at one year. Psycho-Oncology 1994;3:39–46.
76. Morrow GR. Effect of the cognitive hierarchy in the systematic desensitization treatment of anticipatory nausea in cancer patients: a component comparison with relaxation only, counseling, and no treatment. Cognit Ther Res 1986;10:421–446.
77. Morrow GR, Morrell C. Behavioral treatment for the anticipatory nausea and vomiting induced by cancer chemotherapy. N Engl J Med 1982;307:1476–1480.
78. Moynihan C, Bliss JM, Davidson J, et al. Evaluation of adjuvant psychological therapy in patients with testicular cancer: randomised controlled trial. Br Med J 1998;316:429–435.
79. Petersen RW, Quinlivan JA. Preventing anxiety and depression in gynaecological cancer: A randomised controlled trial. Br J Obstet Gynaecol 2002;109:386–394.
80. Pruitt BT, Waligora-Serafin B, McMahon T, et al. An educational intervention for newly-diagnosed cancer patients undergoing radiotherapy. Psycho-Oncology 1993;2:55–62.
81. Rawl SM, Given BA, Given CW, et al. Intervention to improve psychological functioning for newly diagnosed patients with cancer. Oncol Nurs Forum 2002;29:967–975.
82. Richardson MA, Post-White J, Grimm EA, et al. Coping, life attitudes, and immune responses to imagery and group support after breast cancer treatment. Altern Ther Health Med 1997;3:62–70.
83. Sandgren AK, McCaul KD. Short-term effects of telephone therapy for breast cancer patients. Health Psychol 2003;22:310–315.

84. Sandgren AK, McCaul KD, King B, et al. Telephone therapy for patients with breast cancer. Oncol Nurs Forum 2000;27:683–638.
85. Simpson JS, Carlson LE, Trew ME. Effect of group therapy for breast cancer on healthcare utilization. Cancer Pract 2001;9:19–26.
86. Smith M, Casey L, Johnson D, et al. Music as a therapeutic intervention for anxiety in patients receiving radiation therapy. Oncol Nurs Forum 2001;28:855–862.
87. Speca M, Carlson LE, Goodey E, et al. A randomized, wait-list controlled clinical trial: the effect of a mindfulness meditation-based stress reduction program on mood and symptoms of stress in cancer outpatients. Psychosom Med 2000;62: 613–622.
88. Spiegel D, Bloom JR, Yalom I. Group support for patients with metastatic cancer. A randomized outcome study. Arch Gen Psychiatry 1981;38:527–533.
89. Telch CF, Telch MJ. Group coping skills instruction and supportive group therapy for cancer patients: a comparison of strategies. J Consult Clin Psychol 1986;54:802–808.
90. Thomas R, Daly M, Perryman B, et al. Forewarned is forearmed: benefits of preparatory information on video cassette for patients receiving chemotherapy or radiotherapy. A randomised controlled trial. Eur J Cancer 2000;36:1536–1543.
91. Watson M, Denton S, Baum M, et al. Counselling breast cancer patients: a specialist nurse service. Counsel Psychol Q 1988;1: 25–34.
92. Wells ME, McQuellon RP, Hinkle JS, et al. Reducing anxiety in newly diagnosed cancer patients: a pilot program. Cancer Pract 1995;3:100–104.
93. Bruera E, Roca E, Cedaro L, et al. Action of oral methylprednisolone in terminal cancer patients: a prospective randomized double-blind study. Cancer Treat Rep 1985;69:751–754.
94. Bruera E, Carraro S, Roca E, et al. Double-blind evaluation of the effects of mazindol on pain, depression, anxiety, appetite, and activity in terminal cancer patients. Cancer Treat Rep 1986;70:295–298.
95. Clerico M, Bertetto O, Morandini MP, et al. Antiemetic activity of oral lorazepam in addition to methylprednisolone and metoclopramide in the prophylactic treatment of vomiting induced by cisplatin. A double-blind, placebo-controlled study with crossover design. Tumori 1993;79:119–122.
96. Costa D, Mogos I, Toma T. Efficacy and safety of mianserin in the treatment of depression of women with cancer. Acta Psychiatr Scand Suppl 1985;320:85–92.
97. Fisch MJ, Loehrer PJ, Kristeller J, et al. Fluoxetine versus placebo in advanced cancer outpatients: a double-blinded trial of the Hoosier Oncology Group. J Clin Oncol 2003;21:1937–1943.
98. González Barón M, Chacon JI, Garcia Giron C, et al. Antiemetic regimens in outpatients receiving cisplatin and non-cisplatin chemotherapy. A randomized trial comparing high-dose metoclopramide plus methylprednisolone with and without lorazepam. Acta Oncol 1991;30:623–627.
99. Musselman DL, Lawson DH, Gumnick JF, et al. Paroxetine for the prevention of depression induced by high-dose interferon alfa. N Engl J Med 2001;344:961–966.
100. Capuron L, Gumnick JF, Musselman DL, et al. Neurobehavioral effects of interferon-alpha in cancer patients: phenomenology and paroxetine responsiveness of symptom dimensions. Neuropsychopharmacology 2002;26:643–652.
101. Razavi D, Allilaire JF, Smith M, et al. The effect of fluoxetine on anxiety and depression symptoms in cancer patients. Acta Psychiatr Scand 1996;94:205–210.
102. Tarrier N, Maguire P. Treatment of psychological distress following mastectomy: an initial report. Behav Res Ther 1984;22:81–84.
103. van Heeringen K, Zivkov M. Pharmacological treatment of depression in cancer patients. A placebo-controlled study of mianserin. Br J Psychiatry 1996;169:440–443.
104. Wald TG, Kathol RG, Noyes R Jr, et al. Rapid relief of anxiety in cancer patients with both alprazolam and placebo. Psychosomatics 1993;34:324–332.
105. Wolanskyj AP, Schroeder G, Wilson PR, et al. A randomized, placebo-controlled study of outpatient premedication for bone marrow biopsy in adults with lymphoma. Clin Lymphoma 2000;1:154–157.
106. Fawzy FI, Cousins N, Fawzy NW, et al. A structured psychiatric intervention for cancer patients. I. Changes over time in methods of coping and affective disturbance. Arch Gen Psychiatry 1990;47:720–725.

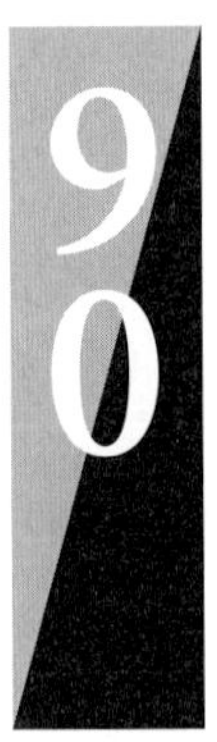

Reproductive Complications and Sexual Dysfunction in the Cancer Patient

Leslie R. Schover

Defining the Population at Risk for Reproductive Complications

This chapter will review risk factors and management for three types of reproductive complications of cancer treatment: infertility, menopausal symptoms, and sexual dysfunction. Each problem area affects unique, albeit overlapping, populations of cancer patients and survivors.

Risk Factors for Cancer-Related Infertility

The demographics of cancer survivorship and delayed childbearing ensure that increasing numbers of patients will have their family-building disrupted by cancer treatment. The success of cancer treatment for malignancies that affect young people, such as pediatric cancers, testicular cancer, and Hodgkin's Disease, has yielded a large population of cancer survivors. According to the National Health Information Survey of 2001,[1] 2.2% of adults aged 18 to 44 in the United States have been diagnosed with cancer. Extrapolating based on statistics for this age group from the United States 2000 Census,[2] approximately 2.5 million adults of childbearing age are cancer survivors. It is more difficult to specify how many have faced infertility, but most probably had treatment with gonadotoxic chemotherapy, and smaller numbers would be at risk for infertility because of surgery or radiation therapy affecting the reproductive system.

Another trend that increases the salience of cancer and fertility is delayed childbearing in American families. Birth rates for women in their thirties have been climbing steadily, reaching a high in 2001 of 95.6 per 1,000 women aged 30–34 and 41.4 per 1,000 women aged 35–39.[3] Births to women aged 40–44 have more than doubled since 1981 to 8.1 per 1,000 women. According to the United States Census report for 2000, the percentage of childless women age 30–34 has jumped from 19.8% in 1980 to 28.1% in 2000, and for women aged 35–39 from 12.1% in 1980 to 20.1% in 2000.[4] When these women are ready to conceive, some will receive the unwelcome news of a malignancy. Data on paternal age are not readily available, but in 1995 in the United States, men at marriage were on the average 2.7 years older than their brides so that men, too, would be more at risk currently to have cancer interfere with their fertility.[5]

Infertility Related Directly to a Malignancy

For a few types of malignancy, for example testicular cancer, the risk of infertility and risk of cancer are related. In a cohort of 3,530 Danish men who were born between 1945 and 1980 and developed testicular cancer from 1960 to 1993, the standardized fertility rate was significantly lower (ratio 0.93) than for all 1,488,957 Danish men born in the same era.[6] Fertility was particularly reduced in the two years leading up to cancer diagnosis, and for men with nonseminomatous tumors (ratio 0.87). Furthermore, men who developed testicular cancer were less likely than men in the general population to conceive male children, possibly indicating a genetic or environmental factor.

Skakkebæk and his colleagues believe that a testicular dysgenesis syndrome (TDS) is increasing in frequency in Western countries because of environmental influences in utero, perhaps combined with a genetic susceptibility factor. The syndrome includes testicular cancer, undescended testes, hypospadias, and decreased semen quality.[7] Although the evidence for TDS, and in particular the influence of endocrine disrupting pollutants, remains controversial, it is clear that men with testis cancer have a high percentage of abnormalities in the contralateral testis suggesting abnormal fetal development of these tissues.[8] The standardized incidence ratios of testis cancer in 32,442 men who had a semen analysis at the laboratory in Copenhagen between the years of 1963 and 1995 were compared with rates in the general population of Danish men.[9] Parameters of poor semen quality, including low count, poor motility, and abnormal morphology, were all associated with increased risk of testis cancer (standardized incidence ratios of 2.3–3.0).

In women, a recent evidence-based review of the link between infertility and cancer risk concluded that borderline ovarian tumors are slightly more common in women diagnosed with infertility.[10] It is less clear whether infertile women are at increased risk for invasive ovarian cancer, but rates may be elevated in those who never achieve a pregnancy or among women with endometriosis. In contrast, infertility does not appear to be a risk factor for breast cancer.[10] Although most cohort and case-control studies have not demonstrated a link between using ovarian stimulating drugs to treat female infertility and subsequent cancer risk for any site,[11] a recent comparison of 4,575 women with breast cancer and 4,682 controls found that women who used human menopausal gonadotropin for at least 6 cycles had a greater relative risk of breast cancer (2.7–3.8).[12]

Infertility Caused by Cancer Treatment

Many cancer patients are put at risk for infertility by the therapies used to eradicate or control their malignancy. Surgical treatment for pelvic cancer may remove a critical part of the reproductive organ system, e.g. bilateral orchiectomy for prostate cancer or for asynchronous testicular tumors, or bilateral oophorectomy as part of treatment for gynecological malignancies or as prevention for breast or ovarian cancer in women with BRCA mutations.[13] Treatment of prostate or bladder cancer may entail removal of the prostate and seminal vesicles and the vagina or uterus may be removed to treat vaginal, cervical, or uterine cancer. Nerves controlling antegrade ejaculation of semen may be damaged in retroperitoneal lymphadenectomy for testicular cancer[14] or in surgery for colorectal cancer.[15]

Radiation therapy to the pelvis damages fertility because developing gametes and ovarian follicles, like cancer cells, are more likely to be in the genetically vulnerable, proliferative state.[16] Patients treated for prostate or cervical cancer, or those who have total body irradiation as preparation for bone marrow transplant, are the most common groups to experience radiation-associated infertility.

Chemotherapy drugs also interfere with gametogenesis because maturing sperm and oocytes are vulnerable to the toxins that damage rapidly-growing cancer cells.[17,18] Alkylating drugs (including the platinum-based chemotherapies) are most likely to damage fertility. The likelihood of permanent ovarian failure in women increases with cumulative dose and age, and is manifested as decreased numbers of follicles, atretic follicles, and fibrotic changes in the ovary.[19] Spermatogenesis is even more vulnerable to disruption by chemotherapy, with a similar pattern of risk factors in terms of dosage and type of drugs.[20] The impact of male age on fertility after cancer is unclear, but in general men over age 45 take longer to establish a pregnancy and have decreased conception rates.[21]

Preventing and Managing Cancer-Related Infertility

Preserving fertility is highly important to men and women diagnosed with cancer before completing their families. Although research on the psychosocial aspects of cancer-related infertility is limited, surveys and qualitative interview studies concur that most survivors feel healthy enough to be good parents, believe that their experience of cancer has increased the value they place on family closeness, are particularly distressed about infertility if childless, and are not getting enough information on options to spare or treat fertility.[22–26]

Utilization of infertility services in the United States is limited even for the population at large. Less than 50% of women with infertility seek medical consultation and only 1.6% use assisted reproductive technology.[27] Although male factors explain roughly half of infertility, no statistics are available on men's use of infertility services.[28] This gives some context for help-seeking among cancer survivors with infertility.

Preventing Cancer-Related Infertility

Obviously it is preferable to prevent cancer-related infertility rather than to try treating it after the fact. Hormonal manipulation during chemotherapy may be used to try to minimize damage to the gonads. In addition, when treatment of a particular malignancy has become highly successful, efforts have been made to spare fertility in younger patients by using less toxic chemotherapy drugs or by limiting cancer surgery. Several options are available to cryopreserve gametes or embryos before cancer treatment for later use in conception, although assisted reproductive technology is typically required. Each of these options will be reviewed, and the level of evidence for its efficacy examined.

Hormonal Prevention

In men, efforts during chemotherapy to protect the spermatogonia A cells that produce mature spermatozoa have included prescribing GnRH analogues with or without accompanying testosterone. Despite promising results in animals, human trials have been uniformly disappointing.[29] Howell and Shalet speculate that continuing hormonal treatment for several months after finishing chemotherapy might have more success, allowing surviving stem cells to recover and renew spermatogenesis. If no spermatogonia survive chemotherapy or radiation therapy, however, continuing hormonal treatment will be fruitless. Even in the prepubertal testis, cancer therapies damage fertility because the Leydig, Sertoli, and germ cells are not truly quiescent, but continue to develop,[30] making them vulnerable to toxic cancer therapies

Efforts at hormonal protection of the ovaries during chemotherapy in women have had more promising results, but double-blind randomized trials are still lacking. The largest case-control cohort has been followed by Blumenfeld in Israel.[31] An injectable GnRH agonist was administered, beginning 1 to 2 weeks before chemotherapy and continuing for up to 6 months, to a group of 60 women aged 15 to 40 being treated for lymphoma. All but 3 of the surviving women resumed menstruation by the end of the first year, compared to only 45% of 60 women treated with chemotherapy alone, without hormonal protection. Inhibin –A and –B levels decreased during GnRH administration, normalizing only in the women who resumed menstruation.[18] Although the GnRH and comparison groups did not differ on age, tumor type, cumulative dose of chemotherapy drugs, or exposure to radiation therapy, the comparison group consisted either of historical controls or women who were not seen in time to start the GnRH-agonist before chemotherapy.[31] Obviously, selection bias is possible.

The use of a GnRH-agonist during adjuvant chemotherapy for breast cancer is attractive because it not only may protect against ovarian failure in young women, but could potentially add to cancer control. In a Phase II pilot study, a group in Rome administered the long-acting GnRH analog goserelin for one year during adjuvant chemotherapy to 64 newly diagnosed women with breast cancer, aged 18 to 50 and without distant metastases.[32] Dosage and drug regimen depended on cancer stage. At a median follow-up time of 55 months, 86% of women had resumed menstruation after chemotherapy, including five who had stem cell transplantation. Although this was a lower rate of ovarian failure than would be expected, no comparison group was provided.

Chemoprotection Strategies

Even if hormonal protection helps preserve a greater number of primordial follicles during chemotherapy, many of those remaining would be damaged.[33] Another type of chemoprotection is suggested by advances in understanding how toxins like chemotherapy influence signaling pathways in the testis and ovary. A small lipid molecule, sphingosine 1-phosphate, may be able to prevent damage to the follicles as well as protecting against genetic damage to the oocyte.[34] Even more tantalizing is the recent discovery of stem cells in the human ovary, suggesting that females are not limited to the number of oocytes that survive fetal development, but have ongoing replenishment of primordial follicles.[35]

Cryopreservation of Reproductive Tissue for Future Conception

The most well established form of reproductive tissue cryopreservation in cancer patients is sperm banking. Measures of the effectiveness of sperm banking include the success of using sperm cryopreserved by cancer patients in conceiving healthy offspring and the utilization of stored samples by cancer survivors.

Conception rates from banked sperm have increased radically since the advent of intracytoplasmic sperm injection (ICSI) in 1992. In this technique, only one live sperm is injected into each oocyte retrieved from in vitro fertilization (IVF). Rates of fertilization with ICSI do not differ when using sperm that was cryopreserved versus from a fresh ejaculate, nor has the use of cryopreserved sperm resulted in increased birth defects.[36]

Although many men diagnosed with cancer have impaired semen quality, samples from patients with suboptimal semen parameters survive freezing and thawing just as well as sperm from men of normal fertility.[37,38] Several prospective case series of men who cryopreserved sperm are presented in Table 90.1. Only about 6% to 18% of cancer patients are azoospermic and unable to bank at the time of attempted semen collection.[39,41,42,44] The most efficient use of stored samples is to attempt to conceive with IVF-ICSI,[41,43] unless the semen quality is unusually good.

It appears that less than 10% of men who store semen actually use their samples to try to conceive, but this rate may be accelerating with the availability of IVF-ICSI.[42–44] The percentage of couples who use their cryopreserved sperm with assisted reproductive technology (ART) and actually have a live birth varies widely from center to center, but is comparable to results for the general population of infertile couples.[41,43] With all cohorts in Table 90.1 combined, 37 healthy babies were born, with only one pregnancy terminated because a major fetal malformation was detected.[42]

Although specific rates of impaired fertility have been reported for a variety of chemotherapy combinations or radiation therapy doses and fields,[29] it is not possible to accurately predict recovery of fertility in any one man treated for cancer.[36] Therefore, sperm banking should be routinely offered when men are about to begin treatments that put fertility at risk. An adequate number of specimens can be banked without delaying cancer treatment in all but the most

TABLE 90.1. Long-term Follow-Ups of Cohorts of Consecutive Cancer Patients Who Cryopreserved Sperm.

Reference	*Year*	*No. of Patients*	*Years follow-up*	*% able to store sperm*	*% using samples*	*Cycles of ART*	*Pregnancies per cycle*	*Live births*	*% couples attempting conception who achieved parenthood*	*Birth defects*
Lass et al.[39]	1998	191	8	83%	3%	IUI: 2 IVF: 9 ICSI: 4	100% 22% 50%	7	83%	0
Audrins et al.[40]	1999	258*	20	—	2%	IUI: 53 IVF: 14	4% 36%	7	33%	0
Kelleher et al.[41]	2001	930	22	90%	10%	IUI: 28 IVF: 28 ICSI: 35	43% 31% 21%	39	45%	2
Blackhall et al.[42]	2002	122*	22	94%	27%	—	—	11	27%	1
Agarwal et al.[43]	2002	318**	20	—	9% (26% in past 4 yrs.)	IUI: 37 IVF: 23 ICSI: 20	8% 26% 35%	12	44%	0
Ragni et al.[44]	2003	776	15	88%	5%***	IUI: 40 IVF: 6 ICSI: 42	8% 0% 26%	14	43%	1

*Hodgkin's disease only

**Only N cryopreserving sperm was reported

***Rates increase with duration of follow-up to 12% at 12 years emergent cases. A study of 95 cancer patients found that acceptable post-thaw semen quality could be obtained when men abstained for only 24 to 48 hours between collecting ejaculates.[45]

Despite low rates of usage of stored sperm, men do not appear to regret the trouble or expense. Hallak and colleagues examined the reasons that 56 (16%) of 342 cancer men who had banked sperm before cancer treatment in their clinic discarded their cryopreserved specimens.[46] Out of the 56 men, 21 had died and the families discarded the samples, 23 had already conceived all the children they wanted without using their stored sperm, 8 had a return of good semen parameters, and 4 had decided not to have children. The cost of banking sperm was not a factor in these decisions.

Unfortunately, recent surveys of oncologists reveal that many fail to give men information about sperm-banking, underestimating its importance to their male patients and overestimating the barriers of cost and availability of sperm banking facilities.[47–49] For those cancer patients interested in having future children, the most common reason cited for failure to bank sperm is lack of timely information. In our recent survey of young male survivors, only half recalled their oncology health care providers discussing the possibility of banking sperm.[23]

The pediatric oncology community has shown an increasing interest in giving teens with cancer the option of banking sperm. Out of 238 boys aged 12 to 19 referred to one center in London, 87% were able to produce an ejaculate for semen storage, with semen quality similar to that in adult cancer survivors.[50] A new experimental technique uses testicular biopsies to obtain spermatogonia from prepubertal boys for cryopreservation before cancer treatment, in the hope that they can be replaced through autografting to restore fertility later. Attempts at replacement in adult men have been disappointing, however, since it is not possible to inject the thawed suspension of cells directly into the fibrous seminiferous tubules.[29] Cryopreserved human spermatogonial stem cells have been transplanted into mouse testes and survived for up to 6 months, suggesting that xenotransplantation could some day be another option for producing mature sperm cells for IVF-ICSI, or at least for providing a research model.[51]

In women, progress is also being made with the use of a rapid freezing technique called *vitrification* to freeze mature, unfertilized oocytes, although pregnancy rates still do not approach those with cryopreserved embryos.[52] Another promising avenue is the use of sugars as cryoprotectants during freezing.[53] To have a true analogue to sperm banking in men, it would be necessary to cryopreserve primordial follicles and then to mature them in the laboratory. Although such techniques remain years away,[54] researchers are having some preliminary success with in vitro maturation of freshly retrieved antral follicles that are approaching full maturity.[55]

A number of centers around the world are removing and cryopreserving ovarian tissue for women about to undergo cancer treatment that could impair fertility.[54] Several cases of auto-transplantation have taken place, with promising results.[56,57] Technical problems include minimizing injury to ovarian tissue during the freezing itself and ischemia causing damage to follicles while the graft grows a new vascular system.[58] For some malignancies, concern about reintroducing cancer cells along with the ovarian tissue may limit this option.[58] An alternative use of the tissue could be in xenotransplantation to immunodeficient mice with subsequent harvest of mature oocytes. Recently an embryo was produced using an oocyte retrieved from transplanted ovarian tissue in a female cancer survivor, but no pregnancy resulted when the embryo was transferred to the woman's uterus.[59] Furthermore, the first primate has been born using this technique—a rhesus monkey.[60] Still, an ethical dilemma is that women facing cancer treatment and desperate to protect their future fertility are paying several thousand dollars in out-of-pocket costs to harvest, freeze, and store ovarian tissue with very low odds that a pregnancy will ever result.

Ovarian Transposition During Pelvic Radiation Therapy

When radiation therapy fields include the pelvis, the ovaries can be moved surgically to a more protected location. Although both medial positioning behind the uterus and lateral movement to the pelvic sidewall have been used, currently the most common procedure is to use laparoscopy to move the ovaries laterally just prior to starting radiotherapy. Although ovarian transposition can be performed during a staging laparotomy, it is less effective because the ovaries tend to migrate back to their original position.[61] The ideal position is above the pelvic brim, with the fallopian tubes remaining attached to the uterus.[62]

A recent literature review of the outcome of laparoscopic lateral ovarian transposition included only 44 cases of women under age 40 with a variety of malignancies. However, 89% had preserved menstrual function.[62] Oophoropexy can be complicated by vascular injury, infarction of the fallopian tube, or ovarian cyst formation. IVF is often required to conceive. Women with adenocarcinoma of the cervix or with more advanced stage disease may be at some risk for metastasis to a transposed ovary or to the site of trocar insertion for the laparoscopy.[63] Successful transposition may still be followed by early menopause because of reduced ovarian reserve after radiation therapy.[64]

Fertility-Sparing Surgery for Early-Stage Gynecological Malignancies

Young women diagnosed with early stage cervical or ovarian cancer may opt for conservative surgical procedures that allow them to retain fertility. For women with squamous cell carcinoma of the cervix that is invasive but still early stage, a trachelectomy can be substituted for a radical hysterectomy.[65–68] After the majority of the cervix is removed, the vaginal cuff is sewn back to the cervical remnants. As long as lymph nodes and surgical margins are clear, recurrence rates are comparable to those after radical hysterectomy. Although many women are able to become pregnant after trachelectomy, rates of miscarriage and prematurity are higher than normal. The cervical mucous plug that prevents infection of the amniotic membranes may be inadequate and there is an increased risk of cervical incompetence.

Women with adenocarcinoma of the cervix that is either in situ or very early stage can be treated with conization alone to preserve fertility, as long as surgical margins are clear.[69,70] Adenocarcinoma of the cervix is often multifocal or located high in the endocervical canal, however, and about 20% of women with negative margins at the time of conization will have local recurrences.

In conservative surgery for young women with borderline or germ cell ovarian tumors, only the affected ovary is removed, preserving the uterus and contralateral ovary.[66] Results have been good, both in terms of fertility and cancer control, but only small case series have been published.[71,72] Recurrence rates after conservative surgery for borderline tumors are higher than after radical surgery, but survival rates remain similar[71] Conservative surgery has also been utilized for Stage I epithelial tumors.[73] The largest cohort study included women treated for germ cell tumors with a median follow-up of 122 months.[74] Of those who tried to conceive (N = 38), 76% have become pregnant.

Other Fertility-Sparing Modifications of Cancer Treatment

Other modifications made to cancer treatment to spare fertility have not been evaluated in randomized clinical trials, but instead have been compared to historical controls. Examples include the less gonadotoxic chemotherapy regimens for Hodgkin's disease[75]; surveillance protocols and nerve-sparing retroperitoneal lymphadenectomy for early stage testicular cancer[76]; and orthotopic bladder reconstruction with fertility preservation for men with bladder cancer.[77]

The Safety of Pregnancy After Cancer Treatment

It would be of little utility to promote fertility in women after cancer if pregnancy were a risk factor for cancer recurrence. However, evidence has accumulated that becoming pregnant after successful cancer treatment does not affect women's survival, even those who have had breast cancer.[78] Women diagnosed with breast cancer during pregnancy often have more advanced disease but do not have a survival disadvantage when matched to nonpregnant controls on medical factors such as cancer stage and histology.[79]

An area much in need of study is the psychosocial impact of experiencing cancer during pregnancy, and the development of supportive interventions for women in this predicament.[80] One recent survey found that reproductive concerns remain salient in women successfully treated for gestational trophoblastic disease and that 75% would have attended support groups if they had been available during treatment.[81] Young survivors often lack accurate information about pregnancy after cancer. In our pilot survey, 20% of breast cancer survivors and 18% of women with other cancer sites worried at least "a fair amount" that pregnancy could trigger a recurrence of cancer. Only 53% of women recalled any discussion by their oncology team of pregnancy after cancer.[22]

Survivors also lack knowledge about potential pregnancy complications related to impaired cardiac, pulmonary, or uterine function after cancer treatment. Few would plan evaluation by a high-risk obstetrician before trying to conceive.[22] In the largest study to date, 4,029 pregnancies of participants in the Childhood Cancer Survivor Study were reviewed.[82] A woman's history of chemotherapy was not associated with adverse outcomes, but women who had pelvic irradiation were more likely to have low birthweight infants. A higher than expected rate of voluntary pregnancy termination was observed, again suggesting that women may be worried about the safety of pregnancy or about the likelihood of having healthy offspring. Some women may also have been told in error that they were infertile, and thus did not use contraception to prevent an unwanted pregnancy. Higher rates of miscarriage and prematurity have also been observed in women with uterine exposure to radiotherapy as young adults, although the damage from childhood exposure is more severe.[83]

The Use of Assisted Reproductive Technology (ART) and Cancer

Although cryopreservation of embryos is far more successful than freezing unfertilized oocytes or ovarian tissue, undergoing IVF before cancer treatment presents some difficulties.[84,85] Women with a very aggressive malignancy such as acute leukemia may not have time to delay chemotherapy for several weeks of ovarian stimulation. Women who do not have a committed male partner have to use an anonymous sperm donor to create embryos. Women recently diagnosed with cancer often do not produce many mature oocytes in response to IVF. Women with untreated breast cancer risk exacerbating their disease by taking hormones for IVF. One alternative is natural cycle IVF, in which the one or two oocytes that mature without exogenous hormones are harvested and fertilized. Recently Oktay and colleagues developed an IVF protocol especially for women newly diagnosed with breast cancer, using tamoxifen for ovarian stimulation. The average number of embryos per cycle was 1.6 compared to 0.6 with a natural cycle, yielding a higher chance of an eventual pregnancy.[86] Ovarian stimulation regimens combining tamoxifen and follicle stimulating hormone (FSH) are yielding even better results.[87]

Women who wait until after chemotherapy to try IVF typically have a suboptimal response to the hormone stimulating drugs.[85] Creating embryos with oocytes from a donor is another option for the woman who has diminished fertility or is in ovarian failure after cancer treatment, but can still carry a pregnancy.[88,89] The cancer survivor herself does not undergo the risks of ovarian stimulation. If she is in ovarian failure, she may need some hormonal support to prepare her uterus for embryo transfer, as well as during the first weeks of a pregnancy, until the placenta begins to produce its own hormones. The hormone levels during these intervals are similar to those in a natural pregnancy. Pregnancy rates per cycle with donated oocytes are high, especially when both egg donor and recipient are under age 35. Women who have had pelvic irradiation still suffer the risk of prematurity and miscarriage, however. Along with survivors who have lost their uterus to cancer but have stored embryos or ovarian tissue, they may work with a gestational carrier to have a child. Only isolated case reports are available in the literature, however.[90]

For men with poor semen quality after cancer, IVF with ICSI is the preferred method of treatment. Some men do not have any mature spermatozoa in their semen, or no longer ejaculate seminal fluid after their cancer treatment. If they did not bank sperm before treatment, some options are still open to them. Men who do not ejaculate after node dissection for testis cancer or surgery for colorectal tumors may respond to medications that temporarily restore antegrade ejaculation. Viable sperm may also be retrieved from urine voided just after orgasm. Perhaps the most reliable means of obtaining sperm from these men is via electrical stimulation of ejaculation with a probe in the anal canal.[91] This procedure must be performed under anesthesia, but yields samples that typically can be used for IVF with ICSI.[92] Some urologists have used electroejaculation to obtain ejaculates from young teens who are unable to collect semen through masturbation due to anxiety or religious constraints.[93]

About half of men with no sperm in their semen after chemotherapy do have islands of spermatogenesis in their testes. A few viable sperm can be retrieved in testicular biopsies and used for successful IVF with ICSI.[94,95] Although increased aneuploidy has been observed in the sperm of men recently treated for cancer,[96] and aneuploidy has been associated with poorer fertilization rates with ICSI,[97] the pregnancy rates using ICSI with testicular sperm from cancer survivors have been comparable to those with other causes of male factor infertility, with a quarter to a third of cycles resulting in a healthy baby.[94,95] In a recent case series of 33 male childhood cancer survivors, only 33% of had normal semen quality but the integrity of DNA in their spermatozoa did not differ from that in a group of control men, suggesting that offspring would not be at increased risk of birth defects or other health problems.[98]

Health of Offspring of Cancer Survivors

Despite concerns that children born to men or women who had been treated for cancer would have unusual rates of genetic abnormalities or fetal malformations,[99] the available data suggest reasonable cause for optimism. Karyotypes of 2,630 live-born children with a parent who had survived childhood cancer were available from the Danish Cytogenetic Registry.[100] The rate of abnormal karyotypes was not significantly greater than those in the children born to the siblings of the childhood cancer patients. No study has thus far documented an excess rate of birth defects in children born after one parent's cancer treatment, with the caveats that 1) a limited number of offspring have been studied; and 2) the nature and duration of follow-up of offspring has been limited.

Genetic damage from cancer treatment may impact rates of early miscarriage or the gender of surviving infants. In addition to the results of pregnancies from the females in the Childhood Cancer Survivor Study,[82] 2,323 pregnancies sired by the male cancer survivors were documented. The live birth rate of 69% was significantly less than that for the survivors' brothers, and a deficit of male offspring born to the survivors was also observed.[101] Partners of men exposed to more than 5,000 mg/m^2 of procarbazine had an increased risk of miscarriage. A large Scandinavian registry study did not document any increased lifetime cancer risk in offspring, except in families with known, autosomal dominant inherited cancer syndromes.[102] Most offspring in these studies have been born to childhood cancer survivors long removed from their active treatment when they conceived. On the other hand, some types of chemotherapy can be administered to pregnant women in the second and third trimesters without causing fetal malformations.[103]

A new issue is the impact on young adults' childbearing decisions of knowing they carry a mutation that increases lifetime cancer risk. For example, women with BRCA mutations increase their risk of breast cancer by having a pregnancy before age 40 and decrease their risk by early oophorectomy without estrogen replacement.[104,105] Technologies such as prenatal diagnosis and preimplantation genetic diagnosis are also available to identify known autosomal dominant mutations responsible for hereditary cancer syndromes,[106] bringing potential ethical dilemmas, especially whether they should be used for those syndromes with a relatively late onset.

Risk Factors for Cancer-Related Menopausal Symptoms

Since the incidence of cancer increases with aging, menopausal symptoms are probably of high concern for more survivors than infertility. Women treated for breast cancer and men receiving hormonal therapy for advanced prostate cancer are particularly at risk for troublesome hot flashes. Vaginal atrophy and dyspareunia are the major sexual consequences of menopause for women[107] and will be discussed in the sections on sexual function. Menopause-related risks for cardiovascular disease and osteoporosis fall outside of the scope of this chapter.

Psychosocial Factors and Hot Flashes

It is unclear whether cancer survivors experience more severe menopause symptoms than women in the community without a cancer history. The prevalence of menopausal symptoms has generally been overestimated. The Massachusetts Women's Health Study followed a large cohort of women through the transition to menopause.[108,109] Most women did not have hot flashes or depression, had neutral or positive attitudes to menopause, and did not seek any medical attention for menopausal symptoms. Women who had hysterectomy were a more distressed group, with indications that women with pre-existing psychological problems are more likely to have this surgery.[110] An analysis of sexual function in 200 of the participants found that estrogen levels were significantly correlated with reports of dyspareunia, but not with any other sexual problem. A woman's perceptions of her overall health and the quality of her dyadic relationship were stronger predictors of her sexual function than was her menopausal status.[111]

Psychosocial factors play an important role in women's menopause complaints. The best predictors of depression, general health, and utilization of medical services after menopause are a woman's physical and psychological health and history of medical consultation before menopause.[109,110,112,113] Hot flashes and the use of hormone replacement therapy (HRT) are both correlated with psychological distress.[114,115] More educated women are consistently less likely to report hot flashes,[114,115] and cultural beliefs and expectations about menopause affect women's symptom reporting.[116]

The Prevalence of Hot Flashes After Breast Cancer

Women with breast cancer are the group most at risk for troublesome hot flashes after cancer treatment because they are advised not to use systemic estrogen replacement. No large case-control study has compared hot flashes in breast cancer survivors and other women. Carpenter and colleagues surveyed breast cancer survivors from a tumor registry, with about a third responding (N = 69), and compared them to a convenience sample of women with no history of breast cancer but similar age. Hot flashes were more frequent, severe, and distressing for the breast cancer sample. This finding may reflect selection bias in women who chose to participate, as well as the fact that women in the breast cancer group were significantly more likely to be menopausal and less likely to be using estrogen replacement.[117] Within the breast cancer group, hot flash severity and indices of emotional distress were related, parallel to findings in the general population of postmenopausal women.[117,118]

Among 860 breast cancer survivors surveyed by Ganz and colleagues at an average of 3 years post-diagnosis, 55% reported problems with hot flashes, a higher rate than expected from similar studies in healthy postmenopausal non-users of HRT.[119] Women who are premenopausal at breast cancer diagnosis and become menopausal because of cancer treatment are at highest risk to have hot flashes.[119–121] Although women taking tamoxifen experience hot flashes, they decrease after therapy ceases if women resume menses.[122,123] When adjuvant chemotherapy causes permanent menopause, however, hot flashes, vaginal dryness, and decreased quality of life persist even at long-term follow-up.[122,124]

Menopause Symptoms After Other Malignancies

Very little information is available on the prevalence and severity of menopausal symptoms in young women treated for other malignancies with chemotherapy or pelvic radiation that causes ovarian failure, although hot flashes and vaginal dryness are classic symptoms in women who become menopausal after treatment for gynecological cancer[125,126] or after intensive chemotherapy for hematological malignancies.[127] Women whose tumors are not hormone-sensitive may be less reluctant than breast cancer survivors to use estrogen replacement,[127] although publicity about the results of the Women's Health Initiative[128] has many women questioning the benefits of estrogen to manage all but the most short-term menopausal symptoms.

Hot Flashes in Male Cancer Survivors

A final group of cancer survivors at risk for menopausal symptoms are men who have androgen ablation to treat prostate cancer or take hormonal therapy for male breast cancer. Whether prostate cancer treatment involves orchiectomy or administration of a gonadotropin-releasing-hormone (GnRH) agonist, half to three-quarters of men report troublesome hot flashes.[129] As in the literature on menopausal women, there is not convincing evidence that androgen ablation increases depression in men, although sexual dysfunction is quite common.[129] Although in the year 2002, 189,000 new cases of prostate cancer were expected compared to only 1,500 men diagnosed with breast cancer,[130] the symptoms of hot flashes and sexual dysfunction are also common when men are treated with tamoxifen for advanced breast malignancies.[131]

Managing Menopausal Symptoms in Cancer Survivors

A variety of treatments are available for menopausal symptoms, ranging from relaxation treatment to antidepressant medication or hormonal replacement therapy. Only a few have been validated in double-blind randomized trials, a crucial design given the large and enduring placebo effect observed when breast cancer survivors are presented with a credible treatment for hot flashes.[132] Most intervention studies have used breast cancer survivors, the principal group at risk because of their concern about using estrogen replacement and their high rates of hot flashes. Men on hormonal therapy for prostate cancer have been another target group.

Estrogen Replacement for Hot Flashes

Estrogen replacement has consistently been shown to reduce hot flashes in 80% to 90% of postmenopausal women.[132] Nevertheless, an estimated 56% of all American women on HRT tried to stop within the first 8 months after publication of the Women's Health Initiative findings.[133] This randomized trial not only failed to confirm health benefits of HRT[128] but showed that HRT increases the risk of breast cancer.

The literature on using estrogen replacement after treatment for breast cancer also showed clear benefits in alleviating menopausal symptoms.[134–136] Case control studies failed to find an impact on survivors' cancer recurrence or decreased survival,[134,135,137–143] including a meta-analysis comparing 717 breast cancer survivors using some form of HRT to 2,545 nonusers. The relative risk of recurrence for women on HRT was 0.72 (95% confidence interval 0.47–1.10).[144] The relative risk of death for women on HRT after breast cancer was 0.18 (95% confidence interval, 0.10–0.31).

The first randomized trial[145] to be conducted confirmed these results, but included only 56 women in the estrogen-treated group. Women who agree to participate in such a trial may be a very select sample, since most survivors of breast cancer are highly anxious about the risks of taking estrogen.[145,146] More recently, the HABITS trial of the safety of hormone replacement therapy after breast cancer was stopped after 345 women had been followed for a median of about 2 years. An excess of new breast cancer events showed up in the hormone-treated group.[147]

One alternative hormonal therapy for hot flashes is to use progestins alone. Depomedroxyprogesterone acetate was effective in reducing hot flashes in a randomized clinical trial of breast and prostate survivors, and 45% continued using the medication for up to three years, despite some side effects.[148]

Nonhormonal Therapies for Hot Flashes

Trials of nonhormonal approaches to treating hot flashes are summarized in Table 90.2, with a focus on trials that include cancer survivors. Newer antidepressants appear to be the most promising nonhormonal therapy for both breast and prostate cancer survivors with hot flashes, producing greater relief and fewer side effects than older treatments such as progestins, clonidine, or bellergal.[132] Some other widely touted remedies such as isoflavones, black cohosh, and magnetic therapy have proved disappointing when tested in placebo-controlled trials.[153–155,158,159]

TABLE 90.2. Trials of Nonhormonal Therapies for Hot Flashes.

Reference	*Year*	*Type of trial*	*No. of patients*	*Type of treatment*	*Type of patients*	*Average length of follow-up*	*Impact on hot flashes*
Pandya et al.[149]	2000	Randomized, double-blind trial	194	Oral clonidine, 0.1 mg./day	Postmenopausal women on tamoxifen for breast cancer	12 weeks	38% reduction on clonidine vs. 24% on placebo
Stearns et al.[150]	2003	Randomized, double-blind trial	165	Paroxetine, 12.5 or 25.0 mg./day	Postmenopausal women without active cancer or cancer treatment	6 weeks	62% reduction on 12.5-mg./day and 65% on 25.0 mg./day
Loprinzi et al.[151]	2000	Randomized, double-blind trial	191	Venlaxafine, 75 mg./day or 150 mg/day	Breast cancer survivors or women scared to use HRT	4 weeks	37% reduction on 75 mg./day, 49% on 150 mg./day and 27% on placebo
Quella et al.[152]	1999	Pilot trial	16	Venlaxafine, 25 mg./day	Prostate cancer patients on androgen ablation with hot flashes	4 weeks	54% reduction in hot flashes
Quella et al.[153]	2000	Randomized, double-blind trial	149	50 mg. soy isoflavone/day	Breast cancer survivors with severe hot flashes	9 weeks	24% of women had 50% reduction on soy, 36% on placebo
Tice et al.[154]	2003	Randomized, double-blind trial	246	57 mg. or 82 mg. of isoflavone/day	Recently postmenopausal with severe hot flashes	12 weeks	No significant group differences
Nikander et al.[155]	2003	Randomized, double-blind trial	62	114 mg.isoflavone/day	Postmenopausal breast cancer survivors with hot flashes	12 weeks	No significant group differences
Muñoz et al.[156]	2003	Random, open-label trial	136	20 mg. *Cimicifuga racemosa*	Premenopausal breast cancer survivors on tamoxifen	52 weeks	Treatment group improved significantly more than usual care group in number and frequency of hot flashes
Wuttke et al.[157]	2003	Randomized, double-blind placebo-controlled	62	40 mg. *Cimicifuga racemosa* vs. 6 mg. conjugated estrogens vs. placebo	Postmenopausal women	13 weeks	Herbal preparation and estrogen gave equal symptom relief and both were better than placebo
Jacobson et al.[158]	2001	Randomized placebo-controlled, stratified on tamoxifen use	69	Black cohosh	Breast cancer survivors who had completed primary treatment	8 weeks	No significant group differences
Carpenter et al.[159]	2002	Randomized, placebo-controlled crossover study	11	Magnetic device	Breast cancer survivors	3 days	Placebo group improved more than magnet group
Porzio et al.[160]	2002	Pilot trial	15	Acupuncture	Breast cancer patients on tamoxifen	26 weeks	Emotional distress and hot flashes decreased significantly

Given the magnitude of the placebo effect, promising results using herbal remedies or acupuncture must be confirmed with randomized, placebo-controlled trials. For example, acupuncture using clinically recommended points could be tested against acupuncture using sites judged inactive according to traditional Chinese medicine. The duration of therapies tested has also been quite short, particularly given the stubborn nature of hot flashes in breast and prostate cancer survivors. Since some studies focused on cancer survivors with severe symptoms while others used unselected samples, the efficacy of various treatments cannot be directly compared. Although not yet tested in cancer survivors, behavioral modalities such as relaxation training[132,161] and engaging in regular aerobic exercise[162] show promise in decreasing hot flashes in postmenopausal women unselected for cancer history.

One small, randomized trial has examined the efficacy of a brief, nursing intervention in reducing menopausal symptoms in 76 postmenopausal breast cancer survivors chosen because they had at least one severe problem of hot flashes, vaginal dryness, or urinary stress incontinence.[163] Women were randomized to receive usual care or to have a special session with a nurse practitioner to assess symptoms and apply treatment algorithms such as prescribing medication or advising on the use of vaginal lubricants and moisturizers. Telephone follow-up calls were included. All three target symptoms improved in the treated group compared to the usual care group. This type of inexpensive, brief intervention should be replicated, and then tested in further studies to evaluate its effectiveness and dissemination into a variety of health care settings.

Risk Factors for Cancer-Related Sexual Dysfunction

To understand the prevalence of sexual dysfunction after cancer, it is important to realize how common these problems are in otherwise healthy adults.

Prevalence of Sexual Dysfunction in the General Population

The National Health and Social Life Survey (NHSLS) conducted in1992 still provides the best estimates of the prevalence of sexual problems in American adults 18 to 59, because the researchers used probability sampling and achieved a high response rate (79%).[107,164] Thirty-one percent of men and 43% of women had experienced a sexual dysfunction in the past year. Factors associated with sexual problems included poor physical and mental health, aging, past sexual trauma, and relationship satisfaction.

More recently, the Pfizer Global Study of Sexual Attitudes and Behaviors has used similar interview techniques to sample over 26,000 men and women aged 40 to 80 in 28 countries around the world. Although response rates were much lower than in the NHSLS, the sheer volume of data is impressive. Again, one-third to one-half of men and women reported having sexual dysfunctions during the past year.[165] In the data subsets from the United States, Canada, Australia and New Zealand, lack of sexual desire was the most frequent female problem (29%) whereas premature ejaculation was the most common male dysfunction (26%)[166] Overall, women were twice as likely as men to experience difficulty with sexual desire, experiencing pleasure, and reaching orgasm. Most large surveys agree that erectile dysfunction (ED) increases dramatically with age and cardiovascular risk factors in men, so that by age 70, about half of men experience it.[167–168] In contrast, sexual problems in sexually active women (other than vaginal dryness) do not increase consistently with age or ill health.[107,166] Elderly women are more likely than men of the same age to be without a sexual partner, however.[169]

Risk Factors for Sexual Dysfunction After Cancer

Within groups of cancer survivors, sexual dysfunction is usually related to the impact of cancer treatment, rather than being a function of the cancer itself, with a few notable exceptions. Prostate cancer that is locally advanced may damage nerves essential for erection.[170] Women with gynecological cancer, especially cancer of the cervix, vagina, or vulva, may experience pain and bleeding with sexual activity as a presenting symptom of their malignancy.[171] Cancer survivors most at risk for treatment-related sexual dysfunction are those with pelvic tumors and/or those whose treatments damage the hormonal systems mediating sexual desire and pleasure.

Psychosocial factors are also crucial. The risk of sexual dysfunction for any individual cancer survivor is heightened by overall emotional distress, relationship conflict, and having a partner who is sexually dysfunctional. It is also important to remember that medications used to treat depression, anxiety, pain, and nausea during and after cancer treatment frequently have sexual side effects.[167–169]

Treatment-Related Sexual Problems in Men

Men treated for prostate cancer are the group at highest risk for sexual dysfunction. In a prospective study of 31,742 nonphysician health professionals aged 53 to 90, rates of ED for the 2,109 men who had been diagnosed with prostate cancer were 10 to 15 times higher than for men of comparable age.[168] Despite attempts to modify surgery or radiation therapy for prostate cancer to spare sexual function, recent large cohort studies suggest that 75% to 85% of men treated for localized disease have long-term problems with ED.[172–175] Rates of ED are similar after radical cystectomy[176] but somewhat lower with treatment for colorectal cancer.[177] Men on hormonal therapy for advanced prostate cancer have even more severe sexual dysfunction because of the impact of androgen ablation on sexual desire and arousability.[129,175]

Men treated for testicular cancer are often assumed to be at increased risk for sexual problems. Two extensive recent reviews of the literature on this topic concur that few studies of high quality are available.[178,179] Nevertheless, both reviews conclude that the only clear sexual morbidity of treatment for testicular cancer is the interference of retroperitoneal node dissection with antegrade ejaculation. When the lymph nodes are fully dissected along the bifurcation of the aorta, nerves are disrupted that control the smooth muscle contractions of the prostate and seminal vesicles during the emission phase of male orgasm. The result is that men experience the pleasure of orgasm, but with no expulsion of semen. Most retroperitoneal lymphadenectomies now spare crucial nerves by limiting the dissection, preserving normal ejaculation of semen in 75% to 90% of patients.[180,181]

Prospective data on sexual function from a very recent Norwegian randomized trial of chemotherapy for 666 men with metastatic germ cell tumors found that sexual problems rose somewhat 3 months after treatment began, but by 2-year follow-up had subsided to normal levels.[182] The quality of the sexual relationship with a partner had also not suffered. In the longer term, however, testicular cancer survivors who had higher doses of external beam radiation therapy may have an increased risk of ED with aging[178] because of the potential for reduced blood flow in an irradiated pelvic vascular bed.

Higher than expected rates of sexual dysfunction have been reported in longer-term survivors of renal cell carcinoma[183] and bone marrow transplantation.[184] Low-normal to frankly low levels of testosterone are common in young men treated with high-dose chemotherapy for lymphoma or Hodgkin's Disease, which could be a factor in loss of sexual interest and arousal.[29]

Treatment-Related Sexual Problems in Women

Breast cancer is often assumed to be the site most associated with female sexual dysfunction. Although sexual problems are present in about half of long-term survivors of breast cancer, rates are comparable to those in age-matched women who have not had cancer.[119] Frequency of sexual activity is also similar to that of community-dwelling women of similar age.[119,123,185] Premenopausal women whose chemotherapy results in ovarian failure cancer do have unusually high rates of sexual dysfunction, however,[119,123,186] including a long-term loss of desire for sex, increased vaginal dryness, and dyspareunia. In a sample of 153 women interviewed 20 years after having chemotherapy for premenopausal breast cancer, 29% attributed current sexual problems to past cancer treatment.[187] In contrast to chemotherapy, tamoxifen is not associated with decreased desire for sex or impaired lubrication with sexual arousal.[119,186–188] Breast loss is not a crucial factor in these problems, contrary to conventional wisdom. Comparisons of women after various breast surgeries have been highly consistent in showing that breast conservation and reconstruction are not superior to mastectomy in preserving women's sexual function or satisfaction.[119,123,188,189]

Indeed, young women treated for leukemia or Hodgkin's disease are as likely as breast cancer survivors to report sexual dysfunction.[187] About a quarter to a third of women have sexual dysfunction after treatment for hematological malignancies. Although both psychosocial trauma and ovarian failure can contribute to their sexual problems,[190,191] in at least one, small randomized trial, a less gonadotoxic chemotherapy was not superior in sparing sexual function.[192]

A gender difference in sexual function seen both in unselected, healthy women[193] and in cancer survivors[119,194] is that women's sexual satisfaction is not tightly linked to physical functioning like men's, but rather to overall well-being and the quality of intimacy and affection with the sexual partner. For example, in women treated for vulvar cancer, the extent of the tissue excised is less important than relationship happiness in predicting sexual satisfaction.[194] Among breast cancer survivors, those who had found new partners after their cancer treatment had the happiest sex lives.[119]

Nevertheless, it is clear that treatment for gynecological malignancies, including cancer of the cervix, vulva, or uterus, does increase the prevalence of sexual dysfunction beyond that seen in healthy, community-dwelling peers, particularly rates of vaginal dryness and pain with sexual activity.[195] In women treated for localized cervical cancer, pelvic radiation therapy has a more negative impact than radical hysterectomy in reducing vaginal lubrication and expansion with sexual arousal, as seen in two small, but carefully monitored, prospective studies.[196,197] The literature on hysterectomy for benign disease also demonstrates no detriment of surgery to sexual function, even when the cervix is removed, as long as the woman's hormonal status remains unchanged.[198,199] The risk of painful sex and loss of erotic pleasure increases when bilateral oophorectomy is included, or if pelvic surgery affects vaginal caliber or depth, as in abdomino-perineal resection,[177] radical cystectomy,[200] or total pelvic exenteration.[201]

Management of Sexual Symptoms in Cancer Survivors

Despite increased attention in the past 20 years to sexual dysfunction as a consequence of cancer treatment, pitifully little progress has been made in developing cost-effective treatment programs to alleviate these symptoms. The entire field of behavior therapy for sexual dysfunction has seen scant innovation in techniques or new outcome research since the 1970s.[202] Although standard sex therapy programs have been modified for cancer patients,[203] prospective studies of efficacy are lacking.

In 1987 we published a retrospective chart review of detailed clinical notes on consultations in a sexual rehabilitation program within a cancer center over a 4-year period.[203] Out of 384 individuals or couples, 73% were seen only once or twice. Of the index patients seen, 308 were men and 76 were women. Male cancer patients were older, and were more likely to include a partner in their visits (56%) than were the women (28%). Seventy-nine percent of the patients had pelvic malignancies, but this probably reflected referral bias, since the program was located within a urology department and also had strong ties to gynecology. According to their retrospective reports, the prevalence of sexual dysfunctions had increased after cancer treatment in the index patients, but not in their partners. Most men sought help for ED whereas women typically had a combination of loss of desire and vaginal dryness/dyspareunia.

About half of patients were seen prior to or during cancer treatment, and half were first evaluated after treatment had been completed. Follow-up data on outcome were available for only 118 cases. The therapist rating of improvement was "somewhat to much better" for 63% of this group. Factors correlated with better outcome included having more counseling sessions, younger age, absence of depression, and absence of marital conflict.

Prospective clinical trials of sex therapy for specific types of sexual dysfunctions after cancer, using standardized outcome measures, should have followed this report. They are strikingly absent from the literature, however. The majority of people with sexual dysfunction after cancer never seek professional help. In the Pfizer Global Study of Sexuality, less than 20% of men or women unselected for health who had sexual problems consulted a physician about them, although roughly half discussed the problem with a partner, friend, or family member.[204]

Physicians are often urged to initiate discussions of sexuality with all patients, but an analysis of data from the same survey on 5,250 men aged 40 to 80 from 7 countries in Europe revealed that less than 7% had a physician who initiated an assessment of sexual function in the past year, although the majority of men believed such dialogues should be routine.[205] Medical schools in North America only devote an average of 3 to 10 hours to sexuality in the entire 4-year curriculum,[206] so that a physician who wants to counsel patients on sexual rehabilitation must be essentially self-taught. Qualitative interviews of nurses and physicians on an ovarian cancer treatment unit in England confirmed that less than a quarter ever discussed sexuality with patients,[207] despite knowing that sexual problems were prevalent.

We will discuss evidence-based management of sexual problems after cancer using the minimal empirical evidence that exists in the literature on treatment of dysfunctions in men and women unselected for health, and in the literature on sexual rehabilitation after cancer.

Modifying Cancer Treatment to Spare Male Sexual Function

One approach to managing cancer-related sexual dysfunction is to modify cancer treatment to prevent damage to hormonal, vascular, or neurologic systems needed for a healthy sexual response.

In men, hormonal therapy for advanced prostate cancer results in a profound loss of desire for sex, as well as erectile dysfunction and difficulty reaching orgasm.[175,208,209] Tactics to avoid this morbidity have included delaying treatment in asymptomatic men, using intermittent hormonal therapy to keep prostate specific antigen (PSA) values close to zero while allowing improved sexual function during intervals off treatment, or prescribing an androgen-blocker such as bicalutamide either alone or in combination with finasteride. Unfortunately, delayed treatment may compromise ultimate survival time,[210] and both androgen production and sexual function appear to be permanently impaired by a period of months on androgen ablation.[175,211] Bicalutamide is more promising, but considerable sexual morbidity still occurs.[212]

Perhaps the best-validated attempt to preserve sexual function after cancer is the nerve-sparing modification of radical prostatectomy, cystectomy, and colorectal cancer surgery.[213] Although avoiding damage to the nerves near the prostate and posterior urethra helps preserve penile hemodynamics and erection in some men, up to 80% do not recover erections firm enough to allow vaginal penetration on most attempts.[172–175,214] Success depends on the skill of the surgeon, the ability to spare nerves bilaterally, and younger patient age. Although nerve-sparing may not restore normal erections, it does increase the percentage of men who can effectively use oral medications such as sildenafil.[175,214] Similarly, using brachytherapy instead of external beam irradiation to treat localized prostate cancers is only slightly more successful in preserving erectile function.[175,215]

Modifying cancer surgery to conserve or reconstruct pelvic organs does appear superior in terms of impact on sexuality. For example, conserving the bladder by using a combination of transurethral resection, chemotherapy, and radiation leaves men with better sexual function compared to radical cystectomy.[216] Procedures to reconstruct a continent, internal urinary pouch combined with nerve-sparing also appear to result in better sex lives for men compared to the traditional, radical cystectomy with ileal conduit.[217,218]

Modifying Cancer Treatment to Spare Female Sexual Function

In women, the main approaches that spare hormonal function are aimed at fertility, i.e. the conservative surgical approaches to gynecologic cancers.[66,71–74] The sexual consequences of such modifications have not been examined. Likewise, researchers have not studied the sexual impact of efforts to spare ovarian function by using ovarian transposition prior to radiation therapy, or GnRH agonists during chemotherapy.

In contrast to results after radical cystectomy, women who have orthotopic bladder reconstruction with preservation of the anterior vaginal wall do not report sexual dysfunction.[176,219] Surgery for colorectal cancer that avoids creation of an ostomy also results in better quality of life and sexual satisfaction.[220] Despite some controversy about the value of vaginal reconstruction after total pelvic exenteration for cervical cancer, the majority of women stay sexually active with their neovagina[201] and the use of myocutaneous flaps helps fill in the surgical defect and promotes healing.

Unfortunately, these reports focus on small series of highly selected patients treated at academic centers. It would be virtually impossible to conduct randomized trials of more vs. less radical surgical procedures, keeping patient age, education, socioeconomic status, and tumor variables equal between groups. Yet, when several randomized trials did compare mastectomy to breast conservation, researchers were surprised to find that neither sexual variables nor quality of life differed according to the extent of breast surgery.[119,188]

Treatment of Desire Disorders

Loss of desire for sex is one of the most common sexual problems seen in both male and female cancer survivors. The efficacy of androgen in alleviating these problems is controversial. Decreased androgen levels are an important factor in men on androgen ablation, some men treated for testicular cancer, or men who have sustained gonadal damage from high-dose chemotherapy.[221] Ovarian failure in women and chronic use of opioid therapy[222] in both genders also can reduce circulating androgens and sexual desire.

Unfortunately, androgen replacement therapy remains more of an art than a science. In young men who are clearly hypogonadal, testosterone replacement restores sexual motivation and pleasure.[223,224] Only two double-blinded, randomized, placebo-controlled trials of the newer testosterone gel or patch formulations have been published, however, with contrasting outcomes.[225,226] Androgens were administered to hypogonadal men unselected for cancer history. The study showing no benefit focused on men over age 65 with testosterone in low-normal range.[225] Men in the more successful trial were more hypogonadal.[226]

In men, loss of desire for sex is often linked to frustration and low self-esteem when erectile function is impaired.[175] One research group has had success in treating ED by combining testosterone with sildenafil for men with low circulating androgen levels.[227] The same strategy was helpful to eight severely hypogonadal men who had testicular failure after bone marrow transplant.[221] Whereas testosterone replacement is a viable option for young , hypogonadal, cancer survivors, men treated for prostate cancer are obviously not candidates. Although elevated luteinizing hormone levels combined with low-normal testosterone levels are common in young men after high-dose chemotherapy, a recent trial of the testosterone patch in 35 such survivors failed to document positive changes in mood or sexual function.[228]

Loss of desire for sex is common after systemic treatment for breast cancer,[119,124,188] As reviewed in the previous section of this chapter, there is reasonable evidence for the safety of short-term estrogen replacement in breast cancer survivors, but no studies have examined the impact of androgen replacement in this population, despite suggestions that such treatment might improve women's sexual function.[229] Yet, high androgen levels are clearly associated with breast cancer risk in postmenopausal women, and have also been observed post-diagnosis.[230]

In fact, the level of androgens needed to maintain normal sexual function in women, particularly after menopause, is unknown.[231] Several methodologically sound studies have not found any correlation between endogenous androgen levels and sexual function in naturally postmenopausal women.[232–234] The only randomized, placebo-controlled trials that have shown a sexual benefit of testosterone replacement in women have studied surgically menopausal women and have raised testosterone above the normal physiological level.[235–237] No published trials of testosterone replacement have focused on female cancer survivors, although studies of safety and efficacy would be appropriate in women in ovarian failure after treatment for tumors that are not hormone sensitive. However, female survivors of Hodgkin's disease exposed to radiation would be poor candidates because of their already elevated risk of breast cancer, which appears to be potentiated by ovarian hormones.[238]

In the future, selective androgen receptor modifiers may provide a safer modality to treat desire problems in women with abnormally low testosterone. A recent randomized, double-blind cross-over trial of tibolone vs. placebo in 44 postmenopausal women who did not have sexual complaints found in a laboratory paradigm that women taking tibolone had increased sexual desire, fantasies, and arousability, as well as improved vaginal lubrication.[239] Unfortunately, tibolone also appears to increase the risk of breast cancer in postmenopausal women.[240]

Loss of sexual desire after cancer treatment is often multifactorial, rather than a purely hormonal problem, particularly in women. Risk factors can include lingering post-treatment fatigue, pain, or nausea; perceiving oneself as less attractive after cancer; loss of sexual pleasure because of changes in skin sensitivity or genital blood flow; dreading sex because of dyspareunia; medication side effects; mild depression; and relationship conflict exacerbated by cancer treatment. Empirical studies suggest that sexual desire and arousability are linked in women, not only with each other, but with chronic mood disorders, low self-esteem, and guilt about sexuality.[241] Andersen developed a questionnaire to measure negative sexual self-image and found women's scores correlated with failure to resume sex comfortably after gynecological cancer.[242] Treating low desire in women may involve cognitive-behavioral psychotherapeutic interventions rather than a simple, pharmaceutical approach. Such treatment programs should also be evaluated in randomized, controlled trials.[243,244]

Treatment of Erectile Dysfunction (ED) After Cancer

Most efforts at sexual rehabilitation for men after cancer have had the goal of mechanically restoring erectile rigidity. Despite the revolution in treating ED in the past 20 years, yielding not only the various types of penile prosthesis, medications to inject into the penis, vacuum devices, urethral suppositories, and more recently several oral prostaglandin E5-inhibiting drugs (PDE5-inibitors), the majority of men who seek help for ED are not satisfied in the long term. In three studies of outcome in impotence clinics where men were not selected for health or the etiology of their ED, only 30% to 40% of men were sexually active and considered their problem resolved by one to five years after their initial evaluation despite trying a mean of two treatment modalities.[245–247]

Men prefer noninvasive, "natural" therapies, such as oral medication, and often will not try more invasive treatments for ED if PDE-5 inhibitors do not restore reliable, firm erections. Men's adherence even to taking a pill is limited. In two case series of men prescribed sildenafil for ED of varied etiology, over half were no longer taking it by 2-year follow-up.[248,249] In a cohort of 197 consecutive patients, the most significant correlate of discontinuing sildenafil was a history of radical prostatectomy, primarily because the drug was less effective for these men.[249] Only 56% of the men who stopped using sildenafil tried a second treatment.

The importance of encouraging men who fail a first-line treatment to try a more invasive method is reinforced by data from 89 men with ED prospectively followed over 12 months.[250] Men tried an average of two treatments for ED, and those who found an effective medical treatment for ED reported better quality of life and less emotional distress about ED. Prostate cancer survivors were more likely to report trying more than one ED treatment.

In our own retrospective cohort study of men in the prostate cancer registry at the Cleveland Clinic Foundation, half of consecutive men surveyed filled out questionnaires.[214] At an average of 4.5 years after cancer treatment, 59% of 1,188 respondents with ED had tried at least one treatment for it. Only 38% of men found a medical treatment that was at least somewhat helpful in improving their sex lives, however, and just 30% of respondents were still using an ED treatment at the time of the survey. Seventy-nine percent of men had stopped using intraurethral prostaglandin suppositories, 66% no longer used penile injections, 61% stopped taking sildenafil, 59% discarded a vacuum erection device, and 19% no longer had sex with their implanted penile prosthesis. The most important factor in men continuing to use a treatment for ED was that it worked effectively. As in the case series above, men who tried a greater number of treatments were more likely to have positive scores on the International Index of Erectile Function.

A man's motivation to progress from taking a pill to trying a more invasive therapy may be a particularly important factor in the ultimate success of sexual rehabilitation. Penile injection therapy is one of the most effective treatments for men after prostate cancer.[214,250] Other correlates of a good sexual outcome in our survey included younger age, having a sexual partner who still enjoyed sex, having a cancer treatment that was more likely to spare some erectile function (e.g. bilateral nerve-sparing prostatectomy or brachytherapy), and no historical or current use of anti-androgen therapy.[175,214]

Surgeons who perform radical prostatectomy frequently encourage men to begin attempts within 6 weeks to get an erection through use of penile injections, a vacuum device, or a PDE5-inhibitor.[251] The theory is that regular increases of blood circulating to the penis will oxygenate the tissues of the cavernous bodies, preventing fibrosis and atrophy and enhancing the chance of nerve regeneration. This popular theory is based on one very small randomized trial using early penile injection therapy after prostatectomy, published in 1997.[252] Despite a number of attempts to replicate the results using oral medication or vacuum devices, no other peer-reviewed randomized trial has been published

Treating Female Sexual Arousal Disorder (FSAD)

Men can observe their erections, but women are often unaware of vaginal expansion and lubrication, and subjective ratings of sexual arousal do not always correlate well with physiological measures.[253] When women complain of poor sexual arousability after cancer, they typically report a loss of desire for sex, along with a lack of subjective excitement and symptoms of vaginal dryness and tightness. Ovarian failure is a frequent medical factor.

In recent years, researchers testing pharmacological treatments for women's sexual problems have created the "diagnosis" of female sexual arousal disorder (FSAD), an isolated sexual complaint characterized by lack of genital vasocongestion. Nine randomized, placebo-controlled trials of therapies for FSAD in postmenopausal women have been published, including those reviewed above on androgen replacement.[254–257] None focus on cancer populations. Two randomized, placebo-controlled clinical trials of sildenafil for FSAD have not produced convincing results on its efficacy,[255,258] and Pfizer no longer intends to seek approval of the drug for women.[259] Another trial examined the efficacy of alprostadil cream applied to the vulva before intercourse. This is the same medication most commonly used in penile injection therapy, but no significant impact on female sexual function was observed.[256] The remaining trial compared a proprietary vulvar herbal lotion to placebo oil.[257] Only 20 women participated. The outcome measure was a sexual diary created for the study, which was conducted by the company marketing the lotion.

Thinking that FSAD might be caused by inadequate blood flow to the clitoris, researchers created a special vacuum device, the Eros, to increase clitoral engorgement.[260] In a sample of 19 women, use of the Eros over 6 weeks significantly increased reports of erotic sensation, lubrication, ability to reach orgasm, and overall sexual satisfaction, regardless of whether a woman had sexual dysfunction at baseline. The device has received FDA approval and has been shown to increase genital engorgement on repeated use.[261]

Women's subjective pleasure as well as objective changes in genital blood flow should be measured in a randomized trial comparing the Eros device to a handheld vibrator, or even to a woman's own manual self-stimulation. Although a placebo-controlled trial may not be possible, these two other conditions would presumably also induce sexual arousal and increased genital blood flow, as well as giving the woman tacit permission to enjoy genital stimulation. It is possible that these are the active components of the Eros intervention, rather than the vacuum-induced clitoral vasocongestion.

Managing Sexual Pain After Cancer Treatment

For women, pain with sexual activity is one of the most frequent problems after cancer treatment. Postmenopausal vaginal atrophy is frequently the cause. As noted in the previous section on managing menopausal symptoms, systemic or local estrogen replacement is highly effective in reversing vaginal atrophy as well as decreasing hot flashes. Although many female cancer survivors have concerns about using systemic estrogen, new forms of topical estrogen may be safer options.

The Estring® is a vaginal ring delivering a low dose of estradiol time-released over three months. It is effective in reversing vaginal atrophy with little impact on plasma estrogen levels.[262–264] In the dosage that would be used in breast cancer survivors, the Estring® may not reduce hot flashes but has been shown in randomized, placebo-controlled trials to reduce urinary incontinence in about 50% of women.[264] A higher dose could be used in women who had not had a history of hormone-sensitive tumors. Women prefer the Estring® to vaginal suppositories[265] or creams. Many can insert the Estring® themselves but others may need a medical visit to replace the ring. Women with significant vaginal prolapse may not be able to tolerate the ring. Another form of vaginal estrogen replacement that is superior to estrogen cream in patient acceptance and does not elevate plasma estradiol is the Vagifem® suppository[266] which contains 17beta-estradiol.

Trials of these localized estrogen therapies should be conducted specifically in cancer survivors. One goal would be to ascertain the safety of long-term use in women prematurely menopausal after breast cancer. Another would be to test efficacy in women whose vaginal atrophy is not just the result of estrogen deficiency, but is complicated by tissue damage from pelvic radiotherapy[267] or post-transplant graft vs. host disease.[268] These women are particularly vulnerable to dyspareunia. Recently a case report has described successful treatment of vaginal agglutination after allogeneic bone marrow transplant, using a combination of surgical dissection of adhesions, estrogen cream, and vaginal dilation.[269]

Although regular vaginal stretching by intercourse or use of a dilator has been assumed to prevent loss of depth and caliber after pelvic radiation therapy, remarkably little evidence exists to demonstrate this effect. A recent Cochrane Library review of interventions for female sexual dysfunction after pelvic radiotherapy[270] found only two references on dilators. Both were retrospective case series, although they presented evidence that dilators could help maintain or restore vaginal patency. The most recent reference was published in 1999. Furthermore, most women are probably not adherent with the classic recommendation to have sexual intercourse or use a dilator three times weekly. In one small study, 32 cervical cancer survivors were randomized to one session of counseling plus a booklet on sex and cancer, or to a 3-hour psychoeducational group designed to increase adherence to vaginal dilation.[271] Group participation increased the percentage of women under age 41 who met the criterion of dilator/intercourse use from 6% to 44%. About half of the older women met the criterion, whether they were in the intervention or control group. For all women, rates of dilation decreased over the year of the study. Since the fibrosis after radiation therapy continues to progress for several years,[267] long-term adherence to vaginal stretching would be necessary to ensure continued ability to enjoy sexual intercourse and to allow adequate pelvic examinations—assuming that vaginal stretching is indeed physiologically effective.

Perhaps the simplest and most conservative intervention for dyspareunia after cancer is instruction on the use of water-based lubricants during sexual activity. Yet, the only study that evaluates the outcome of giving advice on lubricants is Ganz' nursing intervention, which did reduce vaginal pain and dryness.[163] This trial and several others also included the use of Replens®, a polycarbophil-based vaginal moisturizer that adheres to the vaginal mucosa and is designed to be used three times weekly, independent of any sexual activity. One double-blind, crossover, randomized clinical trial compared 4 weeks of Replens® to a "placebo" water-based lubricant[272] in 45 postmenopausal breast cancer survivors. Although both preparations relieved vaginal dryness, Replens® was signifi-

TABLE 90.3. Treatment Algorithms for Common Reproductive Problems after Cancer.

Level of Intervention	*Hot Flashes*	*Loss of Sexual Desire*	*Erectile Dysfunction*	*Vaginal Dryness/Dyspareunia*
Written pamphlet, video, internet, or nurse	Education about diet, dress, sleep, hygiene	Assessment of depression, fatigue, and medications with sexual side effects	Education about impact of cancer treatment and availability of medical treatments	Education on use of water-based lubricants and vaginal moisturizers[280]
Peer counseling or counseling by a mental health professional	Stress management with focus on relaxation training	Promote positive body image, permission to have sexual fantasies, activities that increase desire, and erotic material such as stories or films[280]	Intervention to enhance couple's sexual communication, improve partner's sexual satisfaction[280]	Education on positioning, Kegel exercises to gain voluntary control over circumvaginal muscles[280]
Intervention by a physician	Prescription of antidepressant medication, and consideration of risk/benefit ratio of using estrogen replacement	Change medications that may be interfering with desire; Consideration of androgen replacement, but only if survivor's levels are in the clinically hypogonadal range and the survivor is not at high risk for breast or prostate cancer as a recurrence or second primary tumor	Try medical treatments that are acceptable to both partners, starting with least invasive[281]	Prescription of graduated vaginal dilators with instructions on use to maximize control over vaginal muscles[280]; Prescription of local vaginal estrogen replacement if appropriate; Consideration of vaginal reconstructive surgery in rare cases

cantly more effective in reducing dyspareunia scores. In two open-label studies of women unselected for cancer history, Replens® was just as effective as estrogen cream in treating vaginal atrophy and dyspareunia.[273,274]

In women with chronic pelvic pain and dyspareunia unrelated to a history of cancer treatment, successful comprehensive treatment programs have combined sexual counseling with specific biofeedback and physical therapy modalities designed to increase awareness of and control over muscle tension in the pelvic floor.[275] Trials applying these techniques are needed with women who have dyspareunia related to surgical adhesions or anatomic changes, radiation damage to the vagina, or vaginal complications of graft vs. host disease.

Similar treatments have been helpful in a pilot study of men with chronic pelvic pain.[276] Pelvic pain has been reported to be more common than usual after treatment for testicular cancer[277] or after radical prostatectomy.[175,278] This type of pain is very recalcitrant to treatment and may include aching in the testes or groin, and/or urethral pain exacerbated by urination or ejaculation. Non-steroidal anti-inflammatory or alpha-blocking drugs, low-dose antidepressants, and nerve blocks are occasionally helpful, but more extreme surgical procedures do not produce results that justify routine use.[279] Randomized trials of treatments for male pelvic pain have not been published.

Table 90.3 presents treatment algorithms for the most common reproductive symptoms seen in cancer survivors: hot flashes, loss of sexual desire, erectile dysfunction, and vaginal dryness/dyspareunia. The first level of intervention involves giving patient education materials in written, video, or interactive computerized format. If more help is needed, brief counseling can be provided either by a trained peer counselor or by a member of the oncology team, such as a nurse clinician or social worker. At the third level, a health care provider specialist is consulted. Many brief counseling interventions can be found in a self-help format[280] and algorithms for treating ED are also available.[281]

Conclusions

Reproductive health problems, including sexual dysfunction, menopausal symptoms, and infertility are common, long-term consequences of cancer treatment for both men and women. Until targeted cancer therapies are more common, systemic chemotherapy is likely to entail considerable gonadal toxicity. Efforts to modify pelvic surgery and radiation therapy to spare the reproductive system are ongoing, but remain limited in applicability and efficacy. Because sexuality and childbearing are such sensitive issues, psychosocial counseling and education may increase the efficacy of purely physiological interventions As this review highlights, very little evidence-based knowledge is available to guide oncology clinicians in remediating reproductive health issues. For many problems, pilot studies of efficacy of innovative treatments are needed before randomized trials can be justified. Hopefully our increasing knowledge about the prevalence, causes, and impact on quality of life of reproductive health problems will soon generate more research.

References

1. Lucas JW, Schiller JS, Benson V. Summary health statistics for United States adults: National Health Interview Survey, 2001. National Center for Health Statistics, Vital Health Stat 2004; 10(218).
2. United States Census Bureau. US Summary 2000: Census 2000 Profile. Washington, DC: Government publication C2KPROF00US; 2002.
3. MacDorman MF, Minino AM, Strobino DM, et al. Annual summary of vital statistics—2001. Pediatrics 2002;110: 1037–1052.
4. Bachu A, O'Connell M. Fertility of American women: June 2000. Current Population Reports, P20-543RV. U.S. Census Bureau, Washington, DC, 2001.
5. United Nations Population Division of the Department of Economic and Social Affairs. Wall chart: World Marriage

Patterns 2000. http://www.un.org/esa/population/publications/worldmarriage/worldmarriage.htm, accessed 12/7/04.
6. Jacobsen R, Bostofte E, Engholm G, et al. Fertility and offspring sex ratio of men who develop testicular cancer: a record linkage study. Hum Reprod 2000;15:1958–1961.
7. Skakkebæk NE, Rajpert-De Meyts E, Main KM. Testicular dysgenesis syndrome: an increasingly common developmental disorder with environmental aspects. Hum Reprod 2001;16: 972–978.
8. Hoei-Hansen, CE, Holm M, Rajpert-De Meyts E, Skakkebæk NE. Histological evidence of testicular dysgenesis in contralateral biopsies from 218 patients with testicular germ cell cancer. J Pathol 2003;200:370–374.
9. Jacobsen R, Bostofte E., Engholm G, et al. Risk of testicular cancer in men with abnormal semen characteristics: cohort study. Brit Med J 2000;321:789–792.
10. Venn A, Healy D, McLachlan R. Cancer risks associated with the diagnosis of infertility. Best Practice & Res Clin Obstet Gynecol 2003;17:343–367.
11. Doyle P, Maconochie N, Beral V, et al. Cancer incidence following treatment for infertility at a clinic in the UK. Hum Reprod 2002;17:2209–2213.
12. Burkman RT, Tang MTC, Malone KE, et al. Infertility drugs and the risk of breast cancer: findings from the National Institute of Child Health and Human Development Women's Contraceptive and Reproductive Experiences Study. Fertil Steril 2003;79: 844–851.
13. Kauff ND, Satagopan JM, Robson ME, et al. Risk-reducing salpingo-oophorectomy in women with a BRCA1 or BRCA2 mutation. N Eng J Med 2002;346:1609–1615.
14. Heidenreich A, Albers P, Hartmann M, et al. Complications of primary nerve sparing retroperitoneal lymph node dissection for clinical stage I nonseminomatous germ cell tumors of the testis: experience of the German Testicular Cancer Study Group. J Urol 2003;169:1710–1714.
15. Havenga K, Maas CP, DeRuiter MC, Welvaart K, Trimbos JB. Avoiding long-term disturbance to bladder and sexual function in pelvic surgery, particularly with rectal cancer. Sem Surg Oncol 2000;18:235–243.
16. Meirow D, Nugent D. The effects of radiotherapy and chemotherapy on female reproduction. Hum Reprod 2001;7: 535–543.
17. Tilly JL, Kolesnick RN. Sphingolipids, apoptosis, cancer treatments and the ovary: investigating a crime against female fertility. Biochim Biophys Acta 2002;1585:135–138.
18. Blumenfeld Z. Preservation of fertility and ovarian function and minimalization of chemotherapy associated gonadotoxicity and premature ovarian failure: the role of inhibin–A and –B as markers. Molecular Cellular Endocrinol 2002;187:93–105.
19. Minton SE, Munster PN. Chemotherapy-induced amenorrhea and fertility in women undergoing adjuvant treatment for breast cancer. Cancer Control 2002;9:466–472.
20. Thomson AB, Critchley HOD, Wallace WHB. Paediatric update: fertility and progeny. Eur J Cancer 2002;38:1634–1644.
21. Hassan MA, Killick SR. Effect of male age on fertility: evidence for the decline in male fertility with increasing age. Fertil Steril 2003;79 (Suppl 3):1520–1527.
22. Schover LR, Rybicki LA, Martin BA, et al. Having children after cancer: a pilot survey of survivors' attitudes and experiences. Cancer 1999;86:697–709.
23. Schover, LR Brey K, Lichtin A, et al. Knowledge and experience regarding cancer, infertility, and sperm banking in younger male survivors. J Clin Oncol 2002;20:1880–1889.
24. Green D, Galvin H, Horne B. The psycho-social impact of infertility on young male cancer survivors: a qualitative investigation. Psycho-Oncology 2003;12:141–152.
25. Thewes B, Meiser B, Rickard J, et al. The fertility- and menopause-related information needs of younger women with a diagnosis of breast cancer: a qualitative study. Psycho-Oncology 2003;12:500–511.
26. Dow KH. Having children after breast cancer. Cancer Practice 1994;2:407–413.
27. Stephen EH, Chandra A. Use of infertility services in the United States: 1995. Family Planning Perspect 2000;32:132–137.
28. Schover LR, Thomas AJ. Overcoming Male Infertility. New York: John Wiley & Sons, 2000.
29. Howell SJ, Shalet SM. Fertility preservation and management of gonadal failure associated with lymphoma therapy. Curr Oncol Rep 2002;4:443–452.
30. Kelnar CJ, McKinnell C, Walker M, et al. Testicular changes during infantile 'quiescence' in the marmoset and their gonadotrophin dependence: a model for investigating susceptibility of the prepubertal human testis to cancer therapy. Hum Reprod 2002;17:1367–1378.
31. Blumenfeld Z, Dann E, Avivi R, et al. Fertility after treatment for Hodgkin's disease. Ann Oncol 2002;13 (Suppl 1):138–147.
32. Recchia F, Sica G, De Filippis S, et al. Goserelin as ovarian protection in the adjuvant treatment of premenopausal breast cancer: a phase II pilot study. Anti-Cancer Drugs 2002;13: 417–424.
33. Familiari G, Caggiati, A, Nottola SA, et al. Ultrastructure of human ovarian primordial follicles after combination chemotherapy for Hodgkin's disease. Hum Reprod 1993;8: 2080–2087.
34. Tilly JL. Molecular and genetic basis of normal and toxicant-induced apoptosis in female germ cells. Toxicol Lett 1998; 102–103:497–501.
35. Johnson J, Canning J, Kaneko T, Pru JK, Tilly J. Germline stem cells and follicular renewal in the postnatal mammalian ovary. Nature 2004;428:145–150.
36. Anger JT, Gilbert BR, Goldstein M. Cryopreservation of sperm: Indications, methods and results. J Urol 2003;170:1079–1084.
37. Agarwal A, Tolentine MV, Sidhu RS, et al. Effect of cryopreservation on semen quality of patients with testicular cancer. Urol 1995;46:382–389.
38. Padron OF, Sharma RK, Thomas AJ, et al. Effects of cancer on spermatozoa quality after cryopreservation: a 12–year experience. Fertil Steril 1997;67:326–331.
39. Lass A, Akagbosu F, Abusheikha N, et al. A programme of semen cryopreservation for patients with malignant disease in a tertiary infertility centre: lessons from 8 years' experience. Hum Reprod 1998;13:3256–3261.
40. Audrins P, Holden CA, McLachlan RI, Kovacs GT. Semen storage for special purposes at Monash IVF from 1977 to 1997. Fertil Steril 1999;72:179–181.
41. Kelleher S, Wishart SM, Liu PY, et al. Long-term outcomes of elective human sperm cryostorage. Hum Reprod 2001;16: 2632–2639.
42. Blackhall FH, Atkinson AD, Maaya MB et al. Semen cryopreservation, utilization and reproductive outcome in men treated for Hodgkin's disease. Brit J Cancer 2002;87:381–384.
43. Agarwal A, Ranganathan P, Kattal N, et al. Fertility after cancer: a prospective review of assisted reproductive outcome with banked semen specimens. Fertil Steril 2004;81:342–348.
44. Ragni G, Somigliana E, Restelli L, et al. Sperm banking and rate of assisted reproduction treatment: insights from a 15–year cryopreservation program for male cancer patients. Cancer 2003;97:1624–1629.
45. Agarwal A, Sidhu RK, Shekarriz M, et al. Optimum abstinence time for cryopreservation of semen in cancer patients. J Urol 1995;54:86–88.
46. Hallak J, Sharma RK, Thomas AJ, et al. Why cancer patients request disposal of cryopreserved semen specimens post-therapy: a retrospective study. Fertil Steril 1998;69:889–893.

47. Schover LR, Brey K, Lichtin A, et al. Oncologists' attitudes and practices regarding banking sperm before cancer treatment. J Clin Oncol 2002;20:1890–1897.
48. Wilford H, Hunt J. An overview of sperm cryopreservation services for adolescent cancer patients in the United Kingdom. Eur J Oncol Nurs 2003;7:24–32.
49. Allen C, Keane D, Harrison, RF. A survey of Irish consultants regarding awareness of sperm freezing and assisted reproduction. Ir Med J 2003;96:23–25.
50. Hallak J, Hendin B, Bahadur G, et al. Semen quality and cryopreservation in adolescent cancer patients. Hum Reprod 2002; 17:3157–3161.
51. Nagano M, Patrizio P, Brinster RL. Long-term survival of human spermatogonial stem cells in mouse testes. Fertil Steril 2002; 78:1225–1233.
52. Yoon TK, Kim TJ, Park SE, et al. Live births after vitrification of oocytes in a stimulated in vitro fertilization-embryo transfer program. Fertil Steril 2003;79:1323–1326.
53. Eroglu A, Toner M, Toth TL. Beneficial effect of microinjected trehalose on the cryosurvival of human oocytes. Fertil Steril 2002;77:152–158.
54. Gosden R, Nagano M. Preservation of fertility in nature and ART. Reprod 2002;123:3–11.
55. Liu J, Ju G, Qian Y, et al. Pregnancies and births achieved from in vitro matured oocytes retrieved from poor responders undergoing stimulation in in vitro fertilization cycles. Fertil Steril 2003;80:447–449.
56. Oktay K, Economos K, Khan M, et al. Endocrine function and oocyte retrieval after autologous transplantation of ovarian cortical strips to the forearm. JAMA 2001;286:1490–1493.
57. Radford JA, Leiberman BA, Brison RB, et al. Orthotopic reimplantation of cryopreserved ovarian cortical strips after high-dose chemotherapy for Hodgkin's lymphoma. Lancet 2001;57:1172–1175.
58. Kim SS. Ovarian tissue banking for cancer patients: to do or not to do? Hum Reprod 2003;18:1759–1761.
59. Oktay K, Buyuk E, Veeck L, et al. Embryo development after heterotopic transplantation of cryopreserved ovarian tissue. Lancet 2004;363:837–840.
60. Lee DM, Yeoman RR, Battaglia DE, et al. Brief Communication: live birth after ovarian tissue transplant. Nature 2004;428: 137–138.
61. Williams RS, Littell RD, Mendenhall NP. Laparoscopic oophoropexy and ovarian function in the treatment of Hodgkin disease. Cancer 1999;86:2138–2142.
62. Bisharah M, Tulandi T. Laparoscopic preservation of ovarian function: an underused procedure. Am J Obstet Gynecol 2003; 188:367–370.
63. Picone O, Aucouturier JS, Louboutin A, et al. Abdominal wall metastasis of a cervical adenocarcinoma at the laparoscopic trocar insertion site after ovarian transposition: case report and review of the literature. Gynecol Oncol 2003;90:446–449.
64. Buekers TE, Anderson B, Sorosky JI, et al. Ovarian function after surgical treatment for ovarian cancer. Gynecol Oncol 2001;80:85–88.
65. Burnett AF, Roman LD, O'Meara AT, Morrow CP. Radical vaginal trachelectomy and pelvic lymphadenectomy for preservation of fertility in early cervical carcinoma. Gyn Oncol 2003; 88:419–423.
66. Plante, M. Fertility preservation in the management of gynecologic cancers. Curr Opin Oncol 2000;12:497–507.
67. Schlaerth JB, Spritos NM, Schlaerth AC. Radical trachelectomy and pelvic lymphadenectomy with uterine preservation in the treatment of cervical cancer. Am J Obstet Gynecol 2003; 188:29–34.
68. Shepherd JH, Mould T, Oram DH. Radical trachelectomy in early stage carcinoma of the cervix: outcome as judged by recurrence and fertility rates. BJOG 2001;108:882–885.
69. McHale MT, Le TD, Burger RA, et al. Fertility sparing treatment for in situ and early invasive adenocarcinoma of the cervix. Obstet Gynecol 2001;98:726–731.
70. Soutter WP, Haidopoulos D, Gornall, RJ, et al. Is conservative treatment for adenocarcinoma in situ of the cervix safe? BJOG 2001;108:1184–1189.
71. Morris RT, Gershenson DM, Silva EG, et al. Outcome and reproductive function after conservative surgery for borderline ovarian tumors. Obstet Gynecol 2000;95:541–547.
72. Brewer M, Gershenson DM, Herzog CE, et al. Outcome and reproductive function after chemotherapy for ovarian dysgerminoma. J Clin Oncol 1999;17:2670–2675.
73. Schilder JM, Thompson AM DePriest PD, et al. Outcome of reproductive age women with stage IA or IC invasive epithelial ovarian cancer treated with fertility-sparing therapy. Gynecol Oncol 2002;87:1–7.
74. Tangir J, Zelterman D, Ma W, Schwartz PE. Reproductive function after conservative surgery and chemotherapy for malignant germ cell tumors of the ovary. Obstet Gynecol 2003;101:251–257.
75. Meistrich ML, Wilson G, Mathur K, et al. Rapid recovery of spermatogenesis after mitoxantrone, vincristine, vinblastine, and prednisone chemotherapy for Hodgkin's disease. J Clin Oncol 1997;15:3488–3495.
76. Ohl DA, Sonksen J. What are the chances of infertility and should sperm be banked? Sem Urol Oncol 1996;14:36–44.
77. Colombo R, Bertini R, Salonia A, et al. Nerve and seminal sparing radical cystectomy with orthotopic urinary diversion for select patients with superficial bladder cancer: an innovative surgical approach. J Urol 2001;165:51–55.
78. Weisz B, Schiff E, Lishner M. Cancer in pregnancy: maternal and fetal implications. Hum Reprod Update 2001;7:384–393.
79. Gwyn KM, Theriault RL. Breast cancer during pregnancy. Curr Treat Options Oncol 2000;1:239–243.
80. Schover LR. Psychosocial issues associated with cancer in pregnancy. Sem Oncol 2000;27:699–703.
81. Wenzel L, Berkowitz RS, Newlands E, et al. Quality of life after gestational trophoblastic disease. J Reprod Med 2002;47:387–394.
82. Green DM, Whitton JA, Stovall M, et al. Pregnancy outcome of female survivors of childhood cancer: a report from the Childhood Cancer Survivor Study. Am J Obstet Gynecol 2002;187: 1070–1080.
83. Critchley HO, Bath LE, Wallace WH. Radiation damage to the uterus: Review of the effects of treatment of childhood cancer. Hum Fertil 2002;5:61–66.
84. Surbone A, Petrek JA. Childbearing issues in breast carcinoma survivors. Cancer 1997;79:1271–1278.
85. Ginsburg ES, Yanushpolsky EH, Jackson KV. In vitro fertilization for cancer patients and survivors. Fertil Steril 2001;75: 705–710.
86. Oktay KH, Buyuk E, Yermakova I, Veeck L, Rosenwaks Z. Fertility preservation in breast cancer patients: IVF and embryo cryopreservation after ovarian stimulation with tamoxifen. Hum Reprod 2003;18:90–95.
87. Oktay K. Further evidence on the safety and success of ovarian stimulation with letrozole and tamoxifen in breast cancer patients undergoing in vitro fertilization to cryopreserve their embryos for fertility preservation. J Clin Oncol 2005;23:3858–3859.
88. Anselmo AP, Cavalieri E, Aragona C, et al. Successful pregnancies following an egg donation program in women with previously treated Hodgkin's disease. Haematologia 2001;86:624–628.
89. Larsen EC, Loft A, Holm K, et al. Oocyte donation in women cured of cancer with bone marrow transplantation including total body irradiation in adolescence. Hum Reprod 2000; 15:1505–1508.
90. Giacalone PL, Laffargue F, Benos P, et al. Successful in vitro fertilization-surrogate pregnancy in a patient with ovarian

transposition who had undergone chemotherapy and pelvic irradiation. Fertil Steril 2001;76:388–389.
91. Ohl DA, Denil J, Bennett CJ, et al. Electroejaculation following retroperitoneal lymphadenectomy. J Urol 1991;145:980–983.
92. Ohl DA, Wolf LJ, Menge AC, et al. Electroejaculation and assisted reproductive technologies in the treatment of anejaculatory infertility. Fertil Steril 2001;76:1249–1255.
93. Hovav Y, Dan-Goor M, Yaffe H, et al. Electroejaculation before chemotherapy in adolescents and young men with cancer. Fertil Steril 2001;75:811–813.
94. Damani MN, Master V, Meng MV, et al. Postchemotherapy ejaculatory azoospermia: fatherhood with sperm from testis tissue with intracytoplasmic sperm injection. J Clin Oncol 2002;20:930–936.
95. Chan PT, Palermo GD, Veeck LL, Rosenwaks Z, et al. Testicular sperm extraction combined with intracytoplasmic sperm injection in the treatment of men with persistent azoospermia postchemotherapy. Cancer 2001;92:1632–1637.
96. Robbins WA, Meistrich ML, Moore D, et al. Chemotherapy induces transient sex chromosomal and autosomal aneuploidy in human sperm. Nat Genet 1997;16:74–78.
97. Burrello N, Vicari E, Shin P, et al. Lower sperm aneuploidy frequency is associated with high pregnancy rates in ICSI programmes. Hum Reprod 2003;18:1371–1376.
98. Thomson AB, Campbell AJ, Irvine DC, et al. Semen quality and spermatozoal DNA integrity in survivors of childhood cancer: a case-control Study. Lancet 2002;360(9330):361–367.
99. Arnon J, Meirow D, Lewis-Roness H, et al. Genetic and teratogenic effects of cancer treatments on gametes and embryos. Hum Reprod 2001;7:394–403.
100. Winther JF, Boice JD, Mulvihill JJ, et al. Chromosomal abnormalities among offspring of childhood-cancer survivors in Denmark: a population-based study. Am J Hum Genet 2004;74: 1282–1285.
101. Green DM, Whitton JA, Stovall M, et al. Pregnancy outcome of partners of male survivors of childhood cancer: a report from the Childhood Cancer Survivor Study. J Clin Oncol 2003;21: 716–721.
102. Sankila R, Olson JH, Anderson H, et al. Risk of cancer among offspring of childhood-cancer survivors. Association of the Nordic Cancer Registries and the Nordic Society of Paediatric Haematology and Oncology. N Engl J Med 1998;38:1339–1344.
103. Berry DL, Theriault RL, Holmes FA, et al. Management of breast cancer during pregnancy using a standardized protocol. J Clin Oncol 1999;7:855–861.
104. Narod SA. Hormonal prevention of hereditary breast cancer. Ann NY Acad Sci 2001;952:36–43.
105. Rebbeck TR, Lynch HT, Neuhausen SL, et al. The Prevention and Observation of Surgical End Points Study Group. Prophylactic oophorectomy in carriers of BRCA1 or BRCA2 mutations. N Eng J Med 2002;346:1616–1622.
106. Rechitsky S, Verlinsky O, Chistokhina A, et al. Preimplantation genetic diagnosis for cancer predisposition. Reprod Biomed 2002; 5:148–155.
107. Laumann EO, Paik A, Rosen RC. Sexual dysfunction in the United States: Prevalence and predictors. JAMA 1999;281: 537–544.
108. Avis NE, McKinlay SM. The Massachusetts Women's Health Study: an epidemiologic investigation of the menopause. J Amer Med Women's Association 1995;50:45–49.
109. Avis NE, McKinlay SM. A longitudinal analysis of women's attitudes toward the menopause: results from the Massachusetts Women's Health Study. Maturitas 1991;13:65–79.
110. McKinlay JB, McKinlay SM, Brambilla DJ. Health status and utilization behavior associated with menopause. Amer J Epidemiol 1987;125:111–121.
111. Avis NE, Stellato R, Crawford S, Johannes C, et al. Is there an association between menopause status and sexual functioning? Menopause 2000;7:286–288.
112. McKinlay JB, McKinlay SM, Brambilla D. The relative contributions of endocrine changes and social circumstances to depression in mid-aged women. J Health Soc Behav 1987;28: 345–363.
113. Avis NE, Crawford S, McKinlay SM. Psychosocial, behavioral, and health factors related to menopause symptomatology. Womens Health 1997;3:103–120.
114. Sternfeld B, Quesenberry CP Jr., Husson G. Habitual physical activity and menopausal symptoms: a case-control study. J Women's Health 1999;8:115–123.
115. Keating NL, Cleary PD, Rossi AS, et al. Use of hormone replacement therapy by postmenopausal women in the United States. Annals Internal Med 1999;130:545–553.
116. Staropoli CA, Flaws JA, Bush TL, et al. Predictors of menopausal hot flashes. J Women's Health 1998;7:1149–1155.
117. Carpenter JS, Johnson D, Wagner L, et al. Hot flashes and related outcomes in breast cancer survivors and matched comparison women. Oncol Nurs Forum 2002;29:E16–25.
118. Carpenter JS, Andrykowski MA, Cordova M, et al. Hot flashes in postmenopausal women treated for breast carcinoma: prevalence severity, correlates, management, and relation to quality of life. Cancer 1998;82:1682–1691.
119. Ganz PA, Rowland JH, Desmond K, et al. Life after breast cancer: understanding women's health-related quality of life and sexual functioning. J Clin Oncol 1998;16:501–514.
120. Biglia N, Cozzarella M, Cacciari F, et al. Menopause after breast cancer: a survey on breast cancer survivors. Maturitas 2003;45: 29–38.
121. Stein KD, Jacobsen PB, Hann DM, et al. Impact of hot flashes on quality of life among postmenopausal women being treated for breast cancer. Pain Symptom Manage 2000;19:436–445.
122. Nystedt M, Berglund G, Bolund C, et al. Side effects of adjuvant endocrine treatment in premenopausal breast cancer patients: a prospective randomized study. J Clin Oncol 2003;21:1836–1844.
123. Mourits MJ, Bockermann I, de Vries EG, et al. Tamoxifen effects on subjective and psychosexual well-being, in a randomized breast cancer study comparing high-dose and standard-dose chemotherapy. Br J Cancer 2002;86:1546–1550.
124. Ganz PA, Desmond KA, Leedham B, et al. Quality of life in long-term disease-free survivors of breast cancer: a follow-up study. J Natl Cancer Inst 2002;94:39–49.
125. Jensen PT, Klee MC, Groenvold M. Validation of a questionnaire for self-rating of urological and gynaecological morbidity after treatment of gynaecological cancer. Radiother Oncol 2002;65: 29–38.
126. Denton AS, Maher EJ. Interventions for the physical aspects of sexual dysfunction in women following pelvic radiotherapy (Cochrane Review). In: The Cochrane Library 2003;3:1–26. Oxford: Update Software.
127. Schimmer AD, Quatermain M, Imrie D, et al. Ovarian function after autologous bone marrow transplantation. J Clin Oncol 1998;16:2359–2363.
128. Rossouw JE, Anderson GL, Prentice RL, et al. Risks and benefits of estrogen plus progestin in healthy postmenopausal women: principal results from the Women's Health Initiative randomized controlled trial. JAMA 2002;288:321–333.
129. Thompson CA, Shanafelt TD, Loprinzi CL. Andropause: symptom management for prostate cancer patients treated with hormonal ablation. The Oncologist 2003;8:474–487.
130. American Cancer Society. Cancer facts and figures: 2002. American Cancer Society, Atlanta, GA.
131. Smolin Y, Massie MJ. Male breast cancer: a review of the literature and a case report. Psychomatics 2002;43:326–330.
132. Hoda D, Perez DG, Loprinzi CL. Hot flashes in breast cancer survivors. Breast J 2003;9:431–438.
133. Ettinger B, Grady D, Tosteson ANA, et al. Effect of the Women's Health Initiative on women's decisions to discontinue postmenopausal hormone therapy. Obstet Gynecol 2003;102: 1225–1232.

134. Beckmann MW, Jap D, Djahansouzi S, et al. Hormone replacement therapy after treatment of breast cancer: effects on postmenopausal symptoms, bone mineral density and recurrence rates. Oncol 2001;60:199–206.
135. Durna EM, Wren BG, Heller GZ, et al. Hormone replacement therapy after a diagnosis of breast cancer: cancer recurrence and mortality. Med J Australia 2002;177:347–351.
136. Decker DA, Pettinga JE, VanderVelde N, et al. Estrogen replacement therapy in breast cancer survivors: a matched-controlled series. Menopause 2003;10:277–285.
137. Wile AG, Opfell RW, Margileth DA. Hormone replacement therapy in previously treated breast cancer patients. Am J Surg 1993;165:372–375.
138. DiSaia PJ, Grosen EA, Kurosaki T, et al. Hormone replacement therapy in breast cancer survivors: a cohort study. Am J Obstet Gynecol 1996;174:1494–1498.
139. Dew J, Eden J, Beller E, et al. A cohort study of hormone replacement therapy given to women previously treated for breast cancer. Climacteric 1998;1:137–142.
140. Ursic-Vrscaj M, Bebar S. A case-control study of hormone replacement therapy after primary surgical breast cancer treatment. Eur J Surg Oncol 1999;25:146–151.
141. O'Meara ES, Rossing MA, Daling JR, et al. Hormone replacement therapy after a diagnosis of breast cancer in relation to recurrence and mortality. JNCI 2001;93:754–762.
142. Peters GN, Fodera T, Sabol J, et al. Estrogen replacement therapy after breast cancer: a 12-year follow-up. Ann Surg Oncol 2001; 8:828–832.
143. Natrajan PK, Gambrell RD Jr. Estrogen replacement therapy in patients with early breast cancer. Am J Obstet Gynecol 2002; 187:289–294.
144. Meurer LN, Lena S. Cancer recurrence and mortality in women using hormone replacement therapy after breast cancer: meta-analysis. J Fam Pract 2002;51:1056–1062.
145. Vassilopoulou-Sellin R, Cohen DS, Hortobagyi GN, et al. Estrogen replacement therapy for menopausal women with a history of breast carcinoma: results of a 5-year, prospective study. Cancer 2002;95:1817–1826.
146. Ganz PA, Greendale GA, Kahn B, et al. Are older breast carcinoma survivors willing to take hormone replacement therapy? Cancer 1999;86:814–820.
147. Holmberg L, Anderson H. The HABITS steering and data monitoring committee. Lancet 2004;363:453–455.
148. Quella SK, Loprinzi CL, Sloan JA, et al. Long term use of megestrol acetate by cancer survivors for the treatment of hot flashes. Cancer 1998;82:1784–1788.
149. Pandya KJ, Raubertas RF, Flynn PJ et al. Oral clonidine in postmenopausal patients with breast cancer experiencing tamoxifen-induced hot flashes: a University of Rochester Cancer Center Community Clinical Oncology Program study. Ann Inten Med 2000; 32:788–793.
150. Stearns V, Beebe KL, Iyengar M, et al. Paroxetine controlled release in the treatment of menopausal hot flashes: a randomized controlled trial. JAMA 2003;289:2827–2834.
151. Loprinzi CL, Kugler JW, Sloan JA, et al. Venlafaxine in management of hot flashes in survivors of breast cancer: a randomised controlled trial. Lancet 2000;356:2059–2063.
152. Quella SK, Loprinzi CL, Sloan J, et al. Pilot evaluation of venlafaxine for the treatment of hot flashes in men undergoing androgen ablation therapy for prostate cancer. J Urol 1999;162: 98–102.
153. Quella SK, Loprinzi CL, Barton DL, et al. Evaluation of soy phytoestrogens for the treatment of hot flashes in breast cancer survivors: a North Center Cancer Treatment Group Trial. J Clin Oncol 2000;18:1068–1074.
154. Tice JA, Ettinger B, Ensrud K, et al. Phytoestrogen supplements for the treatment of hot flashes: the Isoflavone Clover Extract (ICE) Study: a randomized controlled trial. JAMA 2003;290: 207–214.
155. Nikander E, Kilkkinen A, Metsa-Heikkila M, et al. A randomized placebo-controlled crossover trial with phytoestrogens in treatment of menopause in breast cancer patients. Obstet Gynecol 2003;101:1213–1220.
156. Muñoz GH, Pluchino S. *Cimicifuga racemosa* for the treatment of hot flushes in women surviving breast cancer. Maturitas 2003;44(Suppl 1):S59–65.
157. Wuttke W, Seidlove-Wuttke D, Gorkow C. The Cimicifuga preparation BNO 1055 vs. conjugated estrogens in a double-blind placebo-controlled study: effects on menopause symptoms and bone markers. Maturitas 2003;44(Suppl 1):S67–77.
158. Jacobson J, Traxel AB, Evans J, et al. Randomized trial of black cohosh for the treatment of hot flashes among women with a history of breast cancer. J Clin Oncol 2001;19:2739–2745.
159. Carpenter JS, Wells N, Lambert B, et al. A pilot study of magnetic therapy for hot flashes after breast cancer. Cancer Nurs 2002;25:104–109.
160. Porzio G, Trapasso T, Martelli S, et al. Acupuncture in the treatment of menopause-related symptoms in women taking tamoxifen. Tumori 2002;88:128–130.
161. Irvin JH, Domar AD, Clark C, et al. The effects of relaxation response training on menopausal symptoms. J Psychosom Obstet Gynaecol 1996;17:202–207.
162. Ivarsson T, Spetz AC, Hammar M. Physical exercise and vasomotor symptoms in postmenopausal women. Maturitas 1998; 29:139–146.
163. Ganz PA, Greendale GA, Petersen L, et al. Managing menopausal symptoms in breast cancer survivors: Results of a randomized controlled trial. J Nat Cancer Inst 2000; 92:1054–1064.
164. Rosen RC, Laumann EO. The prevalence of sexual problems in women: How valid are comparisons across studies? Arch Sex Behav 2003;32:209–211.
165. Laumann EO, Nicolosi A, Glasser DB, et al. GSSAB Investigators' Group. Sexual problems among women and men aged 40–80 years: prevalence and correlates identified in the global study of sexual attitudes and behaviors. Int J Impot Res 2005;17:39–57.
166. Nicolosi A, Laumann EO, Glasser DB, et al. Global Study of Sexual Attitudes and Behaviors Investigators' Group. Sexual behavior and sexual dysfunctions after age 40: the global study of sexual attitudes and behaviors. Urology 2004;64:991–997.
167. Feldman HA, Goldstein I, Hatzichristou DG, et al. Impotence and its medical and psychosocial correlates: results of the Massachusetts Male Aging Study. J Urol 1994;151:54–61.
168. Bacon CG, Mittleman MA, Kawachi I, et al. Sexual function in men older than 50 years of age: results from the Health Professionals Follow-Up Study. Ann Intern Med 2003;139: 161–168.
169. Laumann EO, Gagnon JH, Michael RT, et al. The social organization of sexuality. Chicago: The University of Chicago Press, 1994:184–185.
170. Hollenbeck BK, Dunn RL, Wei JT, et al. Determinants of long-term sexual health outcome after radical prostatectomy measured by a validated instrument. J Urol 2003;169:1453–1457.
171. Andersen BL, Lachenbruch PA, Anderson B, et al. Sexual dysfunction and signs of gynecologic cancer. Cancer 1986;7: 1880–1886.
172. Cooperberg MR, Koppie TM, Lubeck DP et al. How potent is potent? Evaluation of sexual function and bother in men who report potency after treatment for prostate cancer. Data from CaPSURE. Urol 2003;61:190–196.
173. Potosky AL, Davis WW, Hoffman RM, et al. Five-year outcomes after prostatectomy or radiotherapy for prostate cancer: the prostate cancer outcomes study. J Natl Cancer Inst 2004;96:1358–1367.
174. Steineck G, Helgesen F, Adolfsson J, et al. Quality of life after radical prostatectomy or watchful waiting. N Eng J Med 2002; 347:790–796.

175. Schover LR, Fouladi RT, Warneke CL, et al. Defining sexual outcomes after treatment for localized prostate cancer. Cancer 2002;95:1773–1778.
176. Henningsohn L, Steven K, Kallestrup EB, et al. Distressful symptoms and well-being after radical cystectomy and orthotopic bladder substitution compared with a matched control population. J Urol 2002;168:168–175.
177. Havenga K, Maas CP, DeRuiter MC, Welvaart K, Trimbos JB. Avoiding long-term disturbance to bladder and sexual function in pelvic surgery, particularly with rectal cancer. Sem Surg Oncol 2000;18:235–243.
178. Jonker-Pool G, Van de Wile HBM, Hoekstra HJ, et al. Sexual functioning after treatment for testicular cancer: review and meta-analysis of 36 empirical studies between 1975–2000. Arch Sex Behav 2001;30:55–74.
179. Nazareth I, Lewin J, King M. Sexual dysfunction after treatment for testicular cancer: a systemic review. J Psychosom Res 2001; 51:735–743.
180. Coogan CL, Hejase MJ, Wahle FR, et al. Nerve sparing post-chemotherapy retroperitoneal lymph node dissection for advanced testicular cancer. J Urol 1996;156:1656–1658.
181. Jacobsen KD, Ous S, Waehre H, et al. Ejaculation in testicular cancer patients after post-chemotherapy retroperitoneal lymph node dissection. Br J Cancer 1999;80:249–255.
182. Fossa SD, de Wit R, Roberts T, et al. Quality of life in good prognosis patients with metastatic germ cell cancer: a prospective study of the European Organization for Research and Treatment of Cancer Genitourinary Group/Medical Research Council Testicular Cancer study Group (30941/TE20). J Clin Oncol 2003;21:1107–1118.
183. Anatasiadis AG, Davis AR, Sawczuk IS, et al. Quality of life aspects in kidney cancer patients: data from a national registry. Supportive Care in Cancer 2003;11:700–706.
184. Syrjala KL, Roth-Roemer SL, Abrams JR, et al. Prevalence and predictors of sexual dysfunction in long-term survivors of marrow transplantation. J Clin Oncol 1998;16:3148–3157.
185. Dorval M, Maunsell E, Deschenes L, et al. Long-term quality of life after breast cancer: comparison of 8-year survivors with population controls. J Clin Oncol 1998;16:487–494.
186. Berglund G, Nystedt M, Bolund C, et al. Effect of endocrine treatment on sexuality in premenopausal breast cancer patients: a prospective randomized study. J Clin Oncol 2001;19: 2788–2796.
187. Kornblith AB, Herndon JE II, Weiss RB, et al. Long-term adjustment of survivors of early-stage breast carcinoma, 20 years after adjuvant chemotherapy. Cancer 2003;98:679–689.
188. Schover LR, Yetman RJ, Tuason LJ, et al. Partial mastectomy and breast reconstruction: a comparison of their effects on psychosocial adjustment, body image, and sexuality. Cancer 1995;75:54–64.
189. Rowland JH, Desmond KA, Meyerowitz BE, et al. Role of breast reconstructive surgery in physical and emotional outcomes among breast cancer survivors. J Ntl Cancer Inst 2000;92: 1422–1429.
190. Abrahamsen AF, Loge JH, Hannisdal E, et al. Socio-medical situation for long-term survivors of Hodgkin's disease: a survey of 459 patients treated at one institution. Eur J Cancer 1998;34: 1865–1870.
191. van Tulder MW, Aaronson NK, Bruning PF. The quality of life of long-term survivors of Hodgkin's disease. Ann Oncol. 1994; 5(2):153–158.
192. Kornblith AB, Anderson J, Cella DF, et al. Comparison of psychosocial adaptation and sexual function of survivors of advanced Hodgkin disease treated by MOPP, ABVD, or MOPP alternating with ABVD. Cancer 1992;15:2508–2516.
193. Bancroft J, Loftus J, Long JS. Distress about sex: a national survey of women in heterosexual relationships. Arch Sex Beh 2003; 32:193–208.
194. Weijmar Schultz WCM, Van De Wiel HBM, Hahn DEE, et al. Psychosexual functioning after treatment for gynecological cancer: an integrative model, review of determinant factors and clinical guidelines. Int J Gynecol Cancer 1992;2:281–290.
195. Andersen BL, Anderson B, deProsse C. Controlled prospective longitudinal study of women with cancer: I. Sexual functioning outcomes. J Consult Clin Psychol. 1989;57:683–691.
196. Grumann M, Robertson R, Hacker NF, et al. Sexual functioning in patients following radical hysterectomy for stage IB cancer of the cervix. Int J Gynecol Cancer 2001;11:372–380.
197. Schover LR, Fife M, Gershenson DM. Sexual dysfunction and treatment for early stage cervical cancer. Cancer 1989; 63:204–212.
198. Rhodes JC, Kjerulff KH, Langenberg PW, et al. Hysterectomy and sexual functioning. JAMA 1999;282:1934–1941.
199. Thakar R, Ayers S, Clarkson P, et al. Outcomes after total versus subtotal abdominal hysterectomy. N Engl J Med 2002;347: 1318–1325.
200. Schover, LR, von Eschenbach, AC. Sexual function and female radical cystectomy: a case series. J Urol 1985;134:465–468.
201. Ratliff CR, Gershenson DM, Morris M, et al. Sexual adjustment in patients undergoing gracilis myocutaneous flap vaginal reconstruction in conjunction with pelvic exenteration. Cancer 1996; 78:2229–2235.
202. Heiman JR. Sexual dysfunction: overview of prevalence, etiological factors, and treatments. J Sex Res 2002;39:73–78.
203. Schover LR, Evans RB, von Eschenbach AC. Sexual rehabilitation in a cancer center: diagnosis and outcome in 384 consultations. Arch Sex Beh 1987;16:445–461.
204. Moreira ED Jr, Brock G, Glasser DB, et al. GSSAB Investigators' Group. Help-seeking behaviour for sexual problems: the global study of sexual attitudes and behaviors. Int J Clin Pract 2005;59:6–16.
205. Gingell C, Nicolosi A, Buvat J, et al. Preliminary results from the Global Study of Sexual Attitudes and Behaviors: patient-physician communication. Presented at the 18th Congress of the European Association of Urology, February 2002, Birmingham, UK.
206. Solursh DS, Ernst JL, Lewis RW, et al. The human sexuality education of physicians in North American medical schools. Int J Impot Res 2003;15(Suppl 5): S41–45.
207. Stead ML, Brown JM, Fallowfield L, et al. Lack of communication between healthcare professionals and women with ovarian cancer about sexual issues. Br J Cancer 2003;88:666–667.
208. Fossa SD, Woehre H, Kurth KH, et al. Influence of urological morbidity on quality of life in patients with prostate cancer. Eur Urol 1997;31(Suppl 3):S3–8.
209. Helgason AR, Adolfsson J, Dickman P, et al. Factors associated with waning sexual function among elderly men and prostate cancer patients. J Urol 1997;158:155–159.
210. Messing E. The timing of hormone therapy for men with asymptomatic advanced prostate cancer. Urol Oncol 2003;21: 245–254.
211. Shahidi M, Norman AR, Gadd J, et al. Recovery of serum testosterone, LH and FSH levels following neoadjuvant hormone cytoreduction and radical radiotherapy in localized prostate cancer. Clin Oncol 2001;13:291–295.
212. Iversen P. Bicalutamide monotherapy for early stage prostate cancer: an update. J Urol 2003;170:S48–52.
213. Schover LR. Lesson 24: sexuality after pelvic cancer. AUA Updates, 2005.
214. Schover LR, Fouladi RT, Warneke CL, et al. Utilization of medical treatments for erectile dysfunction in prostate cancer survivors. Cancer 2002;95:2397–2407.
215. Merrick GS, Butler WM, Galbreath RW, et al. Erectile function after permanent prostate brachytherapy. Int J Radiation Oncology Biol Phys 2002;52:893–902.

216. Zietman AL, Sacco D, Skowronski U, et al. Organ conservation in invasive bladder cancer by transurethral resection, chemotherapy and radiation: results of a urodynamic and quality of life study on long-term survivors. J Urol 2003;170: 1772–1776.
217. Bjerre BD, Johansen, C, Steven K. Sexological problems after cystectomy: bladder substitution compared with ileal conduit diversion. A questionnaire study of male patients. Scand J Urol Nephrol 1998;32:187–193.
218. Spitz A, Stein JP, Lieskovsky G, et al. Orthotopic urinary diversion with preservation of erectile and ejaculatory function in men requiring radical cystectomy for nonurothelial malignancy: a new technique. J Urol 1999;161:1761–1764.
219. Horenblas S, Meinhardt W, Ijzerman W, et al. Sexuality preserving cystectomy and neobladder: initial results. J Urol 2001;166:837–840.
220. Engel J, Kerr J, Schlesinger-Raab A, et al. Quality of life in rectal cancer patients: A four-year prospective study. Ann Surg 2003; 238:203–213.
221. Chatterjee R, Kottaridis PD, McGarrigle HH, et al. Management of erectile dysfunction by combination therapy with testosterone and sildenafil in recipients of high-dose therapy for haematological malignancies. Bone Marrow Trans 2002;29: 607–610.
222. Rajagopal A, Vassilopoulou-Sellin R, Palmer JL, et al. Hypogonadism and sexual dysfunction in male cancer survivors receiving chronic opioid therapy. J Pain Symptom Manage 2003;26: 1055–1061.
223. Wang C, Swerdloff SR, Iranmanesh A, et al. Transdermal testosterone gel improves sexual function, mood, muscle strength, and body composition parameters in hypogonadal men. J Clin Endocrinol Metab 2000;85:2839–2853.
224. McNicholas TA, Mulder DH, Carnegie C, et al. A novel testosterone gel formulation normalizes androgen levels in hypogonadal men, with improvements in body composition and sexual function. BJU Int 2003;91:69–74.
225. Snyder PJ, Peachey H, Hannoush P, et al. Effect of testosterone treatment on body composition and muscle strength in men over 65 years of age. J Clin Endocrinol Metab 1999;84: 2647–2653.
226. Steidle C, Schwartz S, Jacoby K, et al. for the North American AA2500 T Gel Study Group. AA2500 testosterone gel normalizes androgen levels in aging males with improvements in body composition and sexual function. J Clin Endocrinol Metab 2003;88:2673–2681.
227. Aversa A, Isidori AM, Spera G, et al. Androgens improve cavernous vasodilation and response to sildenafil in patients with erectile dysfunction. Clin Endocrinol (Oxf) 2003;58:632–638.
228. Howell SJ, Radford JA, Adams JE, et al. Randomized placebo-controlled trial of testosterone replacement in men with mild Leydig cell insufficiency following cytotoxic chemotherapy. Clin Endocrinol (Oxf) 2001;55:315–324.
229. Kaplan HS. A neglected issue: the sexual side effects of current treatments for breast cancer. J Sex Marital Ther 1992;18:3–19.
230. Lillie EO, Bernstein L, Ursin G. The role of androgens and polymorphisms in the androgen receptor in the epidemiology of breast cancer. Breast Cancer Res 2003;5:164–173.
231. Padero MC, Bhasin S, Friedman TC. Androgen supplementation in older women: too much hype, not enough data. J Am Geriatr Soc 2002;50:1131–1140.
232. Cawood EHH, Bancroft J. Steroid hormones, the menopause, sexuality and well-being of women. Psychol Med 1996;26: 925–936.
233. Bachmann GA, Leiblum SR, Kemmann E, et al. Sexual expression and its determinants in the post-menopausal woman. Maturitas 1984;6:19–29.
234. Dennerstein L, Dudley EC, Hoppel JL. Sexuality, hormones and the menopausal transition. Maturitas 1977;26:83–93.
235. Sherwin BB. Use of combined estrogen-androgen preparations in the postmenopause: evidence from clinical studies. Int J Fertil 1998;43:98–103.
236. Shifren JL, Braunstein GD, Simon JA, et al. Transdermal testosterone treatment in women with impaired sexual function after oophorectomy. N Eng J Med 2000;343:682–688.
237. Floter A, Nathorst-Boos J, Carlsrom K, et al. Addition of testosterone to estrogen replacement therapy in oophorectomized women: effects on sexuality and well-being. Climacteric 2002;5: 357–365.
238. van Leeuwen FE, Klokman WJ, Stovall M, et al. Roles of radiation dose, chemotherapy, and hormonal factors in breast cancer following Hodgkin's disease. J Natl Cancer Inst 2003;95: 971–980.
239. Laan E, van Lunsen RHW, Everaerd W. The effects of tibolone on vaginal blood flow, sexual desire and arousability in postmenopausal women. Climacteric 2001;4:28–41.
240. Stahlberg C, Tønnes Pedersen A, Lynge E, et al. Increased risk of breast cancer following different regimens of hormone replacement therapy frequently used in Europe. Int J Cancer 2004;109:721–727.
241. Hartmann U, Heiser K, Ruffer-Hesse C, et al. Female sexual desire disorders: subtypes, classification, personality factors and new directions for treatment. World J Urol 2002;20:79–88.
242. Andersen BL. Surviving cancer: the importance of sexual self-concept. Med Pediatr Oncol 1999;33:15–23.
243. Schover LR, LoPiccolo J. Treatment effectiveness for dysfunctions of sexual desire. J Sex Marital Therapy 1982;8:179–197.
244. Hawton K, Catalan J, Fagg J. Low sexual desire: sex therapy results and prognostic factors. Behav Res Ther 1992;29:217–224.
245. Dewire DM, Todd E, Meyers P. Patient satisfaction with current impotence therapy. Wis Med J 1995;94:542–544.
246. Jarow JP, Nana-Sinkam P, Sabbagh M, et al. Outcome analysis of goal directed therapy for impotence. J Urol 1996;155: 1609–1612.
247. Hanash KA. Comparative results of goal oriented therapy for erectile dysfunction. J Urol 1997;157:2135–2138.
248. El-Galley R, Rutland H, Talic R, et al. Long-term efficacy of sildenafil and tachyphylaxis effect. J Urol 2001;166:927–931.
249. Gonzalgo ML, Brotzman M, Trock et al. Clinical efficacy of sildenafil citrate and predictors of long-term response. J Urol 2003;170:503–506.
250. McCullough AR, Kau EL, Kaci L, et al. A 12-month longitudinal study of treatment seeking behavior in 200 men after radical retropubic prostatectomy. American Urological Association Abstracts (#1418), 2003.
251. Gontero P, Fontana F, Bagnasacco A, et al. Is there an optimal time for intracavernous Prostaglandin E1 rehabilitation following nonnerve sparing radical prostatectomy? Results from a hemodynamic prospective study. J Urol 2003;169:2166–2169.
252. Montorsi F, Guazzoni G, Strambi LF, et al. Recovery of spontaneous erectile function after nerve-sparing radical retropubic prostatectomy with and without early intracavernous injections of alprostadil: results of a prospective, randomized trial. J Urol 1997;158:1408–1410.
253. Brody S, Laan E, van Lunsen RH. Concordance between women's physiological and subjective sexual arousal is associated with consistency of orgasm during intercourse but not other sexual behavior. J Sex Marital Ther 2003;29:15–23.
254. Modelska K, Cummings S. Female sexual dysfunction in postmenopausal women: Systematic review of placebo-controlled trials. Am J Obstet Gynecol 2003;188:286–293.
255. Berman JR, Berman LA, Toler SM, et al. Safety and efficacy of sildenafil citrate for the treatment of female sexual arousal disorder: a double-blind placebo-controlled study. J Urol 2003; 170:2333–2338.
256. Padma-Nathan H, Brown C, Fendl J, et al. Efficacy and safety of topical alprostadil cream for the treatment of female sexual

arousal disorder (FSAD): a double-blind, multicenter, randomized, and placebo-controlled clinical trial. J Sex Marital Ther 2003;29:329–344.
257. Ferguson DM, Steidle CP, Singh GS et al. Randomized, placebo-controlled, double blind, crossover design trial of the efficacy and safety of Zestra for Women in women with and without female sexual arousal disorder. J Sex Marital Ther 2003; 29(Supple 1):33–44.
258. Basson R, McInnes R, Smith MD, et al. Efficacy and safety of sildenafil citrate in women with sexual dysfunction associated with female sexual arousal disorder. J Womens Health Gend Base Med 2002;11:367–377.
259. Mayor S. News roundup: Pfizer will not apply for a licence for sildenafil for women. BMJ 2004;328:542.
260. Wilson SK, Delk JR, Billups KL. Treating symptoms of female sexual arousal disorder with the Eros-Clitoral Therapy Device. J Gend Specif Med 2001;4:54–58.
261. Munarriz R, Maitland S, Garcia Sp, et al. A prospective duplex Doppler ultrasonographic study in women with sexual arousal disorder to objectively assess genital engorgement induced by EROS therapy. J Sex Marital Ther 2003;29(Suppl 1):85–94.
262. Bachmann G. Estradiol-releasing vaginal ring delivery system for urogenital atrophy. Experience over the past decade. J Reprod Med 1998;43:991–998.
263. Gabrielsson J, Wallen beck I, Birgerson L. Pharmacokinetic data on estradiol in light of the estring concept. Estradiol and estring pharmacokinetics. Acta Obstet Gynecol Scand Suppl 1996; 163:26–34.
264. Buckler H, Al-Azzawi F for the UK VR Multicentre Trial Group. The effect of a novel vaginal ring delivering oestradiol acetate on climacteric symptoms in postmenopausal women. BJOG 2003;110:753–759.
265. Casper F, Petri E. Local treatment of urogenital atrophy with an estradiol-releasing vaginal ring: a comparative and a placebo-controlled multicenter study. Vaginal Ring Study Group. Int Urogynecol J & Pelvic Floor Dysfunct 1999;10:171–176.
266. Rioux JE, Devlin C, Gelfand MM, et al. 17beta-Estradiol vaginal tablet versus conjugated equine estrogen vaginal cream to relieve menopausal atrophic vaginitis. Menopause 2000;7: 156–161.
267. Bruner DW, Lanciano R, Keegan M, et al. Vaginal stenosis and sexual function following intracavitary radiation for the treatment of cervical and endometrial carcinoma. Int J Radiat Oncol Biol Phys 1993;27:825–830.
268. Balleari E, Garre S,Van Lint MT, et al. Hormone replacement therapy and chronic graft-versus-host disease activity in women treated with bone marrow transplantation for hematologic malignancies. Ann N Y Acad Sci 2002;966:187–192.
269. Hayes EC, Rock JA. Treatment of vaginal agglutination associated with chronic graft-versus-host disease. Fertil Steril 2002; 78:1125–1126.
270. Denton AS, Maher EJ. Interventions for the physical aspects of sexual dysfunction in women following pelvic radiotherapy. Cochrane Library 2003;3:1–26.
271. Robinson JW, Faris PD, Scott CB. Psychoeducational group increases vaginal dilation for younger women and reduced sexual fears for women of all ages with gynecological carcinoma treated with radiotherapy. Int J Radiation Oncology Biol Phys 1999;44:497–506.
272. Loprinzi CL, Abu-Ghazaleh S, Sloan JA, et al. Phase III randomized double-blind study to evaluate the efficacy of a polycarbophil-based vaginal moisturizer in women with breast cancer. J Clin Oncol 1997;15:969–973.
273. Nachtigall LE. Comparative study: replens versus local estrogen in menopausal women. Fertil Steril 1994;61:178–180.
274. Bygdemen M, Swahn ML. Replens versus dienoestrol cream in the symptomatic treatment of vaginal atrophy in postmenopausal women. Maturitas 1996;23:259–263.
275. Beji NK, Yalcin O, Erkan HA. The effect of pelvic floor training on sexual function of treated patients. Int Urogynecol J Pelvic Floor Dysfunct 2003;14:234–238.
276. Clemens JQ, Nadler RB, Schaeffer AJ, et al. Biofeedback, pelvic floor re-education, and bladder training for male chronic pelvic pain syndrome. Urol 2000;56:951–955.
277. Schover LR, von Eschenbach AC. Sexual and marital relationships after treatment for nonseminomatous testicular cancer. Urol 1985;25:251–255.
278. Sall M, Madsen FA, Rhodes PR, et al. Pelvic pain following radical retropubic prostatectomy: A prospective study. Urol 1997;49:575–579.
279. Masarani M, Cox R. The aetiology, pathophysiology and management of chronic orchialgia. BJU International 2003;91: 435–437.
280. Schover LR. Sexuality and fertility after cancer. New York, John Wiley & Sons, 1997:122–130.
281. Padma-Nathan H. Diagnostic and treatment strategies for erectile dysfunction: the 'Process of Care' model. Int J Impot Res 2000;12 (Suppl 4):S119–121.

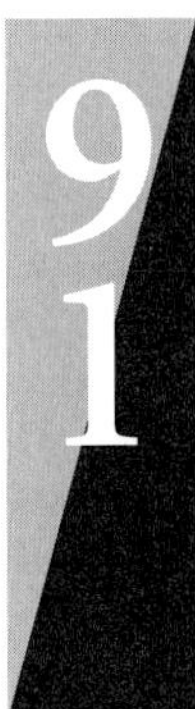

The Care of the Terminal Patient

Andrew Putnam

According to the Institute of Medicine, "at the beginning of the 21st century, half of all patients diagnosed with cancer will die of their disease within a few years."[1] This statistic does not fully explain the reality of the illness and its repercussions for the individuals living with cancer and their families and friends.[2] Many patients live through a final period of life when health professionals, in concert with the patient, must acknowledge that there are no reasonable treatments that remain untried. The patient will most probably die of complications of the cancer. This is a stressful period when health professionals must continue their efforts to treat the patient's suffering and alleviate onerous symptoms.

Palliative care, as part of good medical practice, is delivered in various amounts throughout the disease process, but at different times the goals of care may differ. This chapter discusses palliative care as delivered by oncologists, palliative care teams, and hospice, concentrating on adult cancer patients in the United States. In the interest of brevity, there is very little discussion pertaining to palliative care outside the United States. There also is no discussion of pediatric palliative care. Palliative care in that population faces many of the same challenges as in adults, but also others that pertain specifically to the pediatric population.

Palliative care has been defined as follows: "The active total care of patients whose disease is not responsive to curative treatment. Control of pain, of other symptoms, and of psychological, social and spiritual problems, is paramount. The goal of palliative care is achievement of the best quality of life for patients and their families. Many aspects of palliative care are also applicable earlier in the course of the illness in conjunction with anticancer treatment."[3]

Although all oncologists must have some skills in palliative care, an expert team often has a role. A key aspect of palliative care is that it should be integrated throughout the course of illness and not only at the end of life. Symptom management, family support, skilled communication, and other aspects of palliative care clearly have important roles throughout the care of a patient with cancer. An important tenet of palliative care is taking care of the whole person and the family, not only the disease. Whether an oncologist or a palliative care specialist is taking care of the patient, treating the *entire* patient requires considering how to identify and best care for the patient's medical, physical, psychologic, spiritual, and social concerns. With this wide spectrum of concerns in mind, the aspects of medicine and care that are embraced under the "umbrella" of palliative care cover a very broad area.

This chapter focuses on reviewing research in some key areas of palliative care: the role of the palliative care team, shifting goals in cancer care, aspects of communication, symptom management, systems of care, end-of-life care, and also discussions of some ethical questions. Because palliative care is a broad topic, a full review of all evidence related to the many aspects of palliative care is beyond the scope of this chapter. That stated, key evidence is reviewed for many aspects of care; where the evidence for aspects of care is highly complex or detailed, the reader is referred to specialized reviews of particular topics.

Palliative medicine is the medical specialty whose practitioners specialize in treating symptoms throughout a patient's illness, but certainly their focus is commonly on the later phases of illness. One of the goals of the palliative care team is to improve or maintain the patient's quality of life, making the end of that person's life as comfortable as possible. There is evidence to show that specialized palliative care teams can improve patient care in a number of different domains, including patient and caregiver satisfaction, number of inpatient hospital days, and overall cost to the system.[4]

Because no single healthcare professional can be an expert in all the necessary areas of palliative care, the skills of members of an interdisciplinary team are required to address the array of needs that arise in patients with cancer. These teams usually include physicians, nurses, social workers, chaplains, and sometimes physical therapists, music therapists, and other paramedical practitioners.

Research in Palliative Medicine

Before proceeding with this chapter, it is important for the reader to be aware that much of our understanding of optimal approaches to end-of-life care to date has been based on anecdote or case reports. In fact, some people believe that careful research, which may affect a patient's comfort, defies the spirit of palliative care.[5] Researchers might even be concerned about charges of experimentation on the dying.[5] Recently, however, investigators are turning increasingly to evidence-based studies to research the efficacy of palliative care interventions and improve the understanding of the care of the patient near the end of life.

In attempting research on seriously ill palliative care patients, there are several problems that have to do with the complicated nature of the end of life. Steinhauser wrote that "end-of-life is a complex multidimensional experience in which understanding of the interrelatedness of domains is unclear."[6] Even the most basic question of what defines "the end of life" does not have a satisfactory answer.[7] It is not easy in a given patient to predict the date of death, which makes it difficult to find patients who fit criteria for a study but who are also still able to participate.[8] This restriction adds to the problem of clinicians' lack of comfort in labeling a patient "terminal." Another problem is the interconnectedness of patient and family, which makes research at this time more complicated as the experience of each person affects the other in ways that are unclear.[6] It is not always easy to sort out the feelings of the patient from those of the family.

Research in end-of-life care has often seemed to be a low priority for funding agencies, but often also for those patients who are close to dying, as they have other concerns. In addition, it is often difficult to retain the seriously ill patients who do decide to enroll. The numbers of patients who complete palliative care studies are often low, and those patients who do survive to that point may be the healthier ones as compared to the entire population.[8]

Other problems for palliative care research that have been suggested have to do with study design, such as (1) possible suboptimal care, (2) biased results, and (3) enrollment and retention.[9] There is also the problem that patients often find it difficult to communicate effectively during the last days to weeks of life.[6]

Many palliative care studies use death as a marker. This criterion complicates the results of a study, as any heterogeneity of diagnoses and problems can lead to a wide variety of results, thus reducing its applicability.[9] This difficulty, as well as the other problems already mentioned, has caused research into end-of-life care to lag as a scientific discipline.

Active Treatment to Palliative Care

At diagnosis, or as cancer progresses, a patient may run out of realistic options to prolong life. Life-sustaining goals are often a priority even at the very end of life, but for many, there comes a time when the likely burdens of any remaining treatments may far outweigh the benefits. Some patients may still wish to participate in clinical trials, feeling that any chance of sustaining life is better than no chance at all. Other patients may not desire to participate with such a small likelihood of success.

Certainly, however, in many cases, a physician might reasonably advise an end to active treatment and a change to a purely palliative mode of care. Despite this, many patients and physicians are, however, reluctant to shift, or recommend a shift, to care in which the primary focus is quality of life and comfort. The reasons behind physicians' apparent hesitancy to discuss these topics are complex, and some of these are discussed next.

One of the common barriers to shifting to palliative care is acknowledging when to begin it.[10] Often a patient has undergone multiple different therapies, and the time to make the switch to therapies focused on patient comfort may not be obvious. At other times, the barrier may be that it is difficult for the oncologist to actually suggest this change to a dying patient. This difficulty may be greater in a patient who has progressed through many treatments but wishes to continue with another treatment. There is evidence demonstrating that the longer a physician knows a patient, the more likely it is that the physician will be overly optimistic in predicting the patient's prognosis.[11]

There is some evidence to suggest that patients welcome discussions of end-of-life care[12–14]; however, most of these discussions took place with relatively healthy patients. There is little evidence involving a population of sick cancer patients, but a recent study by Straton et al., provided evidence that individuals with significant functional impairment may be more likely than those without impairment to endorse the use of "high-burden" treatments.[15]

Helping the patients to reframe their hopes once significant life extension seems no longer possible is very important. This is a process that takes time and is not linear. Reframing hope may include focusing on the present and specifics that can be done in the present, rather than vague uncertainties about the future. This refocusing may create the form of encouraging the patient to create a legacy to leave behind, resolving conflicts with friends or relatives, or creating special memories with one's spouse. Patients may hope for improved quality of life and, as death approaches, possibly for release from suffering or for a painless death. Clinicians may find it helpful to discuss the idea of hope with their patients early in treatment because that discussion can become more threatening later if the disease does progress. Physicians and patients alike consider it important that the physician be comfortable discussing death and dying as part of end-of-life care.[16]

Some patients interpret their individual culture or religion[17] as requiring a continued fight for life instead of a peaceful death.[6] It may be necessary to request a chaplain or an authority figure for that culture or religion to discuss the patient's views. These views may serve as another barrier when trying to move from care aimed at cure, to care or sustaining life, to care where the primary focus is quality of life.

The Importance of Communication

One area of importance in terminal care is consistent open communication among the medical team, the patients, and their caregivers (Table 91.1). There is evidence that different patients[18,19] and families want varying amounts and types of information from their physicians. While also receiving active treatment, these individuals often have many psychosocial needs, but the number of these needs often increases once the main focus shifts to palliative care.[20] Patients whose needs are

TABLE 91.1. Six areas of central importance in communicating with dying patients.

1. Talking with patients in an honest and straightforward way
2. Being willing to talk about dying
3. Giving bad news in a sensitive way
4. Listening to patients
5. Encouraging questions from patients
6. Being sensitive to when patients are ready to talk about death

Source: From Wenrich et al.,[27] by permission of *Archives of Internal Medicine*.

TABLE 91.2. Losses in the process of dying.

1. Physical health
2. The belief in remaining healthy indefinitely—of living indefinitely
3. Confidence in the certainty, order, predictability, and security of life
4. Family
5. Roles, identity
6. Job, employment
7. Being productive, feeling competent
8. Independence
9. Control (of bowels, of life—everything)
10. People thought to be friends
11. Things (i.e., possessions)
12. The future
13. Superficial relationship with God
14. Hope
15. Meaning

Source: From Kemp,[22] by permission of Lippincott, Williams & Wilkins.

not met may later report higher levels of distress[21] and possibly dissatisfaction with care received.

Patients are thought to suffer through a number of losses as their illnesses advance (Table 91.2). The first loss is usually that of physical health when an illness that may end life at some time in the future is diagnosed. As illness progresses, many people are faced with having to give up their work, their identities in society, and even their independence once they need others to assist them with even the most basic activities of daily living.[22] Patients may also struggle with thoughts of leaving everything behind, or from finding that despite all the medical advances, they are still going to die.[23] Patients frequently want open and honest discussion about their end-of-life concerns.[24,25] Detmar et al., found, however, that often clinicians missed opportunities to address those concerns.[26] There may be a desire not to upset the patient, but this minimizes the patient's needs and feelings. Patients want physicians who are sensitive to these needs.[16,27]

Family and close friends also need opportunities to communicate their suffering, which is often overlooked because of the necessary focus on the patient.[28] Lederberg has referred to family caregivers as second-order patients. Although they in essence have been part of the healthcare team, they need as much support and care as the patient.[29] While taking into account the importance of patient trust and privacy, clinicians should consider the role of discussing such desires with patients and, with permission, facilitating these discussions. Lilly et al. found that when caregivers spent more time meeting with patients and families, they were more effective at meeting the goals of the patient.[30]

Communication may become more difficult when bad news must be given to the patient and/or family. While there is little evidence about the best way to deliver bad news, there are a variety of ways that seem to be effective.[31,32] How the news is presented may affect how the patient and others interpret the news. However it is presented, it is optimal to find a quiet comfortable place to deliver the news[33]; this will help those present feel that there is enough time for discussion. Prefacing the bad news with "forewarning words" such as "I'm afraid I have some bad news" or "This result is not as good as we had hoped for" is speculated to help listeners prepare mentally for what is to follow.[34] Such words also help the physician gauge whether the patient and/or family members wish to hear more. Lilly et al. found that when caregivers spent more time meeting with patients and families they were more effective at meeting the goals of the patient.[30] The physician's skill at communicating can greatly assist in the care of the patient and family. One crucial skill is being able to explain the situation in everyday language. Patients and families often misunderstand the meaning of any discussion if there is too much medical jargon.[35] A clear and careful explanation by the clinician, in terms that are understood by the patient and family will facilitate a better understanding of what to expect and how to act during such a sad situation.

Symptom Management

Treating symptoms should be a priority throughout the course of cancer. As a patient's condition worsens, the causes of symptoms may become more complex, and there may be limits on clinicians' ability to treat the primary etiologic factors. In certain situations, an approach that directly treats the cause of the symptom and provides relief may still be obvious. Examples include the draining of a pleural effusion to treat dyspnea or the use of whole-brain radiation to shrink brain metastases and eliminate the disability that had resulted from the lesion. Often, however, the cause of a symptom may be multifactorial or unclear and/or the cause may not be amenable to treatment. In these cases, the best course may be to bring the patient relief by treating the symptom itself, whether it is caused by the disease or is a side effect of a necessary medication. It is beyond the scope of this chapter to provide a comprehensive guide to the treatment of all the symptoms that patients experience. Table 91.3 provides a brief list of some of the more frequently encountered symptoms and some common treatments in the terminal patient.[36–62] Evidence for the different treatments varies, but use is often the result of anecdote or clinical experience.

TABLE 91.3. Frequently encountered symptoms and some common treatments in the terminal patient.

Symptom	*Class*	*Examples of agents*	*Comments*
Anorexia	Corticosteroids Cannabinoid derivative	Megestrol[36] Dronabinol[37]	
Anxiety	Benzodiazepines Neuroleptics[38]	Lorazepam Clonazepam diazepam Quetiapine olanzapine Haloperidol	IV formulation
Asthenia/ fatigue	Corticosteroids[39] Psychostimulant	Dexamethasone Methylphenidate Dextroamphetamine	Also used for opioid-induced sedation[39]
Bowel obstruction	Opioids Corticosteroids Somatostatin analogue	Morphine Others Dexamethasone Octreotide[40,41]	For pain Uncertain effectiveness[42] Dries out GI tract
Constipation	Stool softeners Bulking agents Stimulants	Docusate sodium Polyethylene glycol Lactulose Senna Casanthranol	No conclusive evidence to determine if any medications for constipation are more effective than any others[43,44]
Cough	Opioids Tetracaine derivative	Codeine Morphine Benzonatate[45]	
Delirium	Neuroleptics[46] Benzodiazepines	Quetiapine Risperidone Haloperidol *Not recommended*	Risk of paradoxical agitation
Depression	Selective seritonin reuptake inhibitor (SSRI) antidepressants Psychostimulant	Sertraline Citalopram Escitalopram Methylphenidate[47]	Depression is common in terminal patients[48,49] Effective for short periods of time
Dyspnea	Open window or a fan blowing on the face[50,51] Oral or parenteral opioids[53,53] Benzodiazepines[50,54]	Morphine Others Lorazepam	Dyspnea is compatible with normal O_2 saturation[54] Poor evidence for their use in most patients
Hiccups		Metoclopramide, baclofen chlorpromazine nifedipine[55,56]	There is little good evidence for any pharmacologic therapy
Myoclonus		Clonazepam[44]	
Nausea/ vomiting		Metoclopramide hydroxyzine Haloperidol Octreotide[40]	
Pain	Opioids NSAIDS Tricyclic antidepressants Anticonvulsants	Many choices Many choices Amitriptyline Desipramine Gabapentin Carbamazepine	Neuropathic pain Neuropathic pain
Pruritus	Corticosteroids[57,58] Antihistamines[57,58]	Various Various	Symptomatic treatment depends on cause
Restless legs syndrome	Catecholamine precursor Benzodiazepines	Levodopa[59] Clonazepam	Some evidence Nighttime symptoms
Somnolence	Stimulant	Methylphenidate[60]	
Terminal restlessness	Benzodiazepines[61] Antipsychotics[61] Barbiturates[61]	Lorazepam Haloperidol Pentobarbital	Sedation may be necessary
Xerostomia	Sialagogues Saliva replacements Vaseline	Pilocarpine[62] Various	If saliva glands have residual function Symptomatic Keeps lips moist

Hospice and Palliative Care

The term *hospice* has been used in Europe since medieval times. The first known hospice specifically for the dying was begun in Lyons, France, in 1842. The Irish Sisters of Charity opened hospices in Dublin in 1879 and London in 1905.[63] There were other important efforts, but the first modern hospice is generally considered to be St. Christopher's in London, which opened in 1967.[63] The first modern hospice in the United States is frequently considered to have opened in 1974, in Branford, Connecticut.[63] The hospice movement in the United States has expanded so that in 1999 about 25% of all deaths in the United States involved hospice.[64]

When the likely burdens of any remaining life-prolonging options outweigh the likely benefits, the clinician may refer the patient to hospice, depending on that patient's care needs and resources. The term hospice can be confusing for patients because it has been used in several different ways. An inpatient hospice can be a free-standing building or beds in a hospital reserved for end-of-life care. A home hospice program supports terminal patients in the home or in institutions, such as nursing homes.

Although there are few data for the United States, it is generally thought that most people would prefer to die at home.[65] In 2002, 25% of Americans died at home, whereas 50% died in hospitals and another 25% died in other institutions, such as nursing homes.[66] Wherever they die, patients, their families and other caregivers often experience economic, physical, and social burdens imposed by the terminal illness.[67,68] Hospice can assist in many ways to overcome those burdens.

The philosophy of hospice involves interdisciplinary care, as already mentioned. To relieve suffering in all aspects of the patient's life, the hospice team may include doctors, nurses, physical therapists, chaplains, social workers, volunteers, and many others. The goals of care are to preserve the patient's dignity, function, and control for as long as possible. Encouraging realistic personal goals is an important aspect of care. Caregivers can help fit the goal to the current condition of a patient, for example, whether the patient has the stamina for a long-desired trip or for making a videotape for children or grandchildren.

A cancer patient's spiritual beliefs can be a major source of support. Many patients are actively supported by members of their faith group during their disease. It is important to explore patients' beliefs because they can be important indicators of how patients will manage the terminal phase of their lives.[17]

Under the original rules, the Medicare hospice benefit did not allow payment for any antineoplastic treatment for a hospice patient. Over the past decade, many hospices have moved more toward a palliative care model, getting involved earlier in the disease process. This shift means that in some instances, hospices may accept patients who are still undergoing chemotherapy or radiation, especially if the treatment is palliative. Sometimes a patient's insurance may contribute to the payment for such treatments in addition to covering hospice services. The total time in hospice still remains short; however, as in 2002, the median length of stay in hospice was only about 21 days.[69]

A home hospice referral is appropriate when a patient requires symptom management or support and there is a likely possibility of death from the disease within 6 months, as required by the Medicare Hospice Benefit. The advantages of being in a home hospice program include home visits by hospice nurses who specialize in symptom control and other hospice professionals, such as social workers and chaplains. The hospice program also usually covers all medications used to treat symptoms related to the terminal disease.

When a home hospice program cares for a patient, family members remain the primary caregivers, taking care of the patient for more than 90% of each day. In general, although it varies, a hospice program in the United States supplies regular short nursing visits a few days a week and possibly a home health aide who will come to the house for 1 to 2 hours a day to provide patient care.

A hospice program's psychosocial and emotional support can be very helpful to a family's success in caring for a patient at home because many families find it hard to take care of a dying family member. For some, the trauma of the disease or discomfort with performing various intimate aspects of care can be significant barriers to caring for the patient at home.

Living at home and ultimately dying there is usually the hospice patient's goal, but in certain cases, inpatient hospice referral is appropriate. These situations include patients with symptoms that are difficult to treat, such as severe pain or dyspnea. Another instance is when caregivers are exhausted and need a break. Admitting the patient for a few days of inpatient "respite care" allows the caregivers necessary rest.

Whether directed beds in a hospital or a free-standing building, inpatient hospices usually are small and have few beds. These are normally held for patients who are thought to be in the final 2 weeks of life or for whom staying at home can mean great suffering. If a patient is nearing death and has accepted that idea, an inpatient hospice may be a better place than an acute care hospital. In such a case, the goals of the hospice are often in line with those of the dying patients and decrease the possibility of unwanted aggressive workups or treatments. If a patient's symptoms are severe and require around-the-clock professional nursing, remaining at home can put the patient at risk for a very uncomfortable death. At those times, admission to inpatient hospice can be the best option for both patient and caregivers.

The discomfort with conversations about death and the stigma of hospice may prevent referrals early enough for the patient to benefit fully from hospice services.[70] Although receiving an accurate prognosis is important to many patients, medical professionals have a bias toward overly optimistic predictions.[71] This attitude reduces a patient's ability to make informed choices regarding quality of life. Patients may, however, also wish to continue antineoplastic treatments until they are dying, which is another important barrier to hospice referrals. If the goals of care are frequently revisited with patients and concerns and ways of addressing those concerns are defined, patients and caregivers may take more advantage of what hospice programs have to offer. In addition, another change that could affect the timing of referrals would occur if the ability of hospices to accept patients receiving anticancer treatment for the relief of symptoms were more widespread.

The Final Days

When a patient is dying, clear communication with the patient, if possible, and with caregivers is crucial. Time used by clinicians to explain the dying process can make an important difference in end-of-life care, both for the patient and also in how the family is affected by the experience.[72,73] Manfredi et al. showed that discussions about goals of care were helpful in implementing advanced directives and making decisions to forgo specific interventions.[73] The medical community generally focuses on the patient, but the caregivers, many of

TABLE 91.4. Concerns important at the end of life.[a]

1. Be kept clean
2. Name a decision maker
3. Have a nurse with whom one feels comfortable
4. Know what to expect about one's physical condition
5. Have someone who will listen
6. Maintain one's dignity
7. Trust one's physician
8. Have financial affairs in order
9. Be free of pain
10. Maintain sense of humor
11. Say goodbye to important people
12. Be free of shortness of breath
13. Be free of anxiety
14. Have a physician with whom one can discuss fears

[a]These concerns were rated very important by more than 90% of patients and more than 70% of bereaved family members, physicians, and other care providers.

Source: From Steinhauser et al.,[16] by permission of *Journal of the American Medical Association.*

whom may not have seen someone die before, in the midst of their own suffering also need support.

Unspoken fears and anxieties are often close to the surface for both patient and family (Table 91.4). Some patients fear that their lives will be technologically prolonged at the expense of quality of life.[74] Other patients fear being a financial drain on their families,[75] as well as the loss of independence.[44] The Support Study showed that as cancer patients approached the end of life, increasing numbers preferred care that focused on quality of life.[44] Other studies have found that the opposite can be true. In these studies, as the patients' conditions worsened, they became more likely to choose more aggressive treatments.[15,76] These thoughts and others are often what the patient wishes to discuss, but they often need encouragement from family or clinicians to do so.

"Comfort measures only" is often written by physicians to describe care provided near the end of life that focuses on quality of life. This description means that clinicians must weigh the benefits against the burdens of any proposed intervention to determine the effect on patient comfort. As a person nears death, certain interventions are less likely to be beneficial than they might be for a healthier patient. For example, blood draws and other needle sticks are obviously painful. Unless the result might direct a change in treatment, such as demonstrating hypercalcemia as a treatable cause of delirium, blood draws can usually be discontinued as they are more burdensome than beneficial to the patient. The decrease in pain from stopping unnecessary needle sticks is fairly clear, but other changes that may provide increased comfort to dying patients are not always so easily recognized.

It is usually necessary at this time to reevaluate the patient's goals. As death approaches, patients often will not benefit from various interventions in the way they might have earlier in the disease process. These medical interventions, although necessary in sick patients, can increase discomfort in the dying. Although medical nutrition, gastric tube feedings, and even intravenous fluids can be important in some settings, such as in a patient with an obstructed bowel and in some instances of delirium, they do not necessarily increase a dying person's comfort. These medical interventions not only are capable of prolonging the dying process but also have the potential to increase patient suffering. Typical rates of intravenous fluids may cause increased rates of vomiting, urination, and defecation that may require painful moving and cleaning of the patient.[77] The fluid also commonly does not stay intravascular and so it may cause or even worsen peripheral and pulmonary edema. Vullo-Navich et al. found that dehydration near the end of life causes fairly benign symptoms and, by decreasing the risk of all the factors just mentioned, often leaves the patient more comfortable.[78] In one study, almost all discomfort caused by the lack of nutrition or hydration was relieved with either small amounts of food or appropriate mouth care.[79]

Medical nutrition in the dying patient can also be counterproductive. In most cultures, feeding the sick is part of normal care of that person. This concept may lead to the concern that a patient near the end of life might "starve" unless given proper nutrition. One study appeared to show that allowing dying patients to eat and drink as they wish, but not attempting artificial life-prolonging therapies, usually leads to more comfortable and peaceful deaths.[79] Stopping medical feedings may also be beneficial because the body then produces ketones, which can provide an additional sense of well-being as a patient approaches death.[72]

Patients with diminished renal function are often more comfortable with decreased amounts of various medications as well as fluids. Decreasing body mass or dehydration can lead to increasing side effects that may require lowering the doses of medications, including the pain medications that a dying patient receives. However, if the patient is already comfortable, options include changing to as-needed dosing or treating the side effects rather than risking increased pain from a dose reduction.

One common end-of-life intervention in the hospital setting is a "morphine drip." Continuous intravenous morphine may be indicated to treat existing pain or dyspnea, but it is not necessary for all dying patients. The fact that a person is close to death is not a sufficient reason to start intravenous morphine if pain is not already a problem. Patients, who have not experienced pain as a major problem during their disease rarely develop severe pain near the end. Morphine and other opioids, although important for comfort, can also cause side effects. Somnolence, myoclonus, and urinary retention can become problems as the dose of opioid is increased. However, use of an opioid at high doses, if indicated for relief of symptoms, is generally considered to be acceptable. The use of morphine and other opioids at this time are governed by the principle of double effect. This principle holds that it is the clinician's intention of providing comfort that determines the ethics of appropriate opioids use at the end of life and not any possible unintended hastening of the patient's death.[80]

Bereavement

An important but often-overlooked aspect of caring for the family of a terminal patient is following up with them after their loved one dies.[81] After the intensity of the final days of a patient's life, the family will often benefit from and be grateful for communication from the physician. An early phone call or letter of sympathy to family members from the physician or some other known member of the medical team can mean a great deal. Later on, verbal contact can be helpful in distinguishing normal from pathologic grief.[81]

Studies have demonstrated the possibility of significant morbidity during the bereavement period.[82,83] So far, however, there is little evidence that lends support to any specific intervention. Hospices are required to offer bereavement follow-up to anyone who lives in the areas they serve even if the deceased loved one was not involved with hospice.

Ethical and Legal Issues

Decision Making

Difficult ethical issues can arise while taking care of a terminal patient. The range of issues includes requests to withhold information from the patient, requests for futile treatment, withholding or withdrawing life-sustaining treatments, and requests for physician-assisted suicide.

One issue that can arise is a request by the family to withhold distressing information from the patient. In the United States, the patient "of sound mind and adult years" holds the legal right to make medical decisions.[84] The patient does have the option to delegate that responsibility to someone else and request not to be told, but that ought to be an explicit decision.

One approach to a request to withhold information from the patient is to explore with the family their reasons.[85] Often clinicians can allay their fears of the patient losing hope or not wanting to know. Using open-ended statements allows patients to ask questions or to express the desire not to know. Occasionally there may be a valid reason for concern, such as a patient's suicide threat following previous distressing news. Although cultural differences can have a great impact in this area, specific cases are beyond the scope of this chapter.

Medical Futility

Another ethical issue involves the concept of *medically futile treatment*. The medical team may view certain procedures or treatments as futile for an end-stage patient while the family's view may be quite different. The reverse may also occur. There may be a point at which the treating team should decide that they have done everything medically indicated to support a patient's life. Determining that any specific treatment is futile and needs to be stopped requires careful communication and possibly an ethics consult if the family and medical team disagree.

Withholding or withdrawing any life-sustaining treatment can lead to major disagreement, whether the medical team views it as futile or the patient does not want it. In most states, stopping a treatment or never starting it are legally equivalent and also viewed as ethically equal.[86] Once a patient starts receiving intravenous fluids or a feeding tube, however, the experience of stopping the treatment often appears far more difficult emotionally. It is best to try to discuss those possibilities long before they may become reality.

Physician-Assisted Suicide

"Doctor, will you help me end my suffering?" According to one study in 1998, this is not a rare question. Of a national sample of 1,902 physicians, 18.3% had received a request for a prescription to end suffering by ending life, with a median of three requests per physician since entering practice.[87] Of these physicians, 3.3% had written at least one of these prescriptions.

Well-respected leaders have expressed support both for and against physician-assisted suicide (PAS). As of this writing, the state of Oregon is the only American jurisdiction that has legalized PAS. There are formal criteria that must be met before the act may occur (Table 91.5). Valid arguments exist both for and against the legalization of PAS, and it would require more than the space allowed here to do full justice to the topic. Some of the arguments for each side are listed in Table 91.6 and are also briefly described next. For more complete presentations on the subject, there are several good references.[88–90]

Although there is some disagreement as to the exact meaning of the term physician-assisted suicide, here the meaning of PAS is as used in the Oregon law. PAS occurs if a person commits suicide using a method supplied by a physician specifically for that purpose (Table 91.7). In Oregon, the physician supplies a prescription for medication, which the patient fills and later uses to commit suicide either with the doctor present or not. This is not the same as euthanasia, which is when the physician physically performs the action that ends the life of the patient, such as with a lethal injection. Euthanasia is considered murder in all parts of the United States today.

TABLE 91.5. Requirements for physician-assisted suicide.

1. The person must be a capable adult resident of Oregon.
2. The person must have a terminal disease.
3. There must be less than 6 months to live.
4. The person must make two oral requests for assistance in dying.
5. The person must make one written request for assistance in dying.
6. The person must convince two physicians that he or she is capable, acting voluntarily, and making an informed decision.
7. The person is not making the decision because of a depression or other psychiatric or psychologic disorder.
8. The person must be informed of the diagnosis, prognosis, potential risks of medication, probable result of taking the medication, and "the feasible alternatives, including but not limited to, comfort care, hospice care, and pain control."
9. The person must wait 15 days.

Source: From The Oregon Death with Dignity Act of the Oregon Revised Statutes.

TABLE 91.6. Arguments in favor of and against physician-assisted suicide.

Arguments in favor of physician-assisted suicide:
1. Respect for patient autonomy
2. Relief of suffering
3. Legalization allows controls
4. Society allows some killing

Arguments against physician-assisted suicide:
1. Intrinsic value of life
2. Legalization would reduce efforts at palliative care
3. Slippery slope
4. Professional ethics

TABLE 91.7. Some definitions of terms.

Suicide signifies that a person knowingly performs an action that takes his or her own life.

Physician-assisted suicide is suicide as above in that the person commits the act of knowingly ending his or her own life, but has been assisted by a physician in obtaining the means, usually a medication.

Euthanasia is the ending of a person's life by another. In the medical sense, usually the patient has expressed a wish to die and someone else performs the act.

Execution is commonly used in the setting of a government-sanctioned act as a form of capital punishment.

Murder is involuntary euthanasia, which is illegal everywhere in the United States.

Turning off a ventilator or stopping some other form of life-sustaining treatment at the patient's or family's request, with the intention of allowing life to end, is not usually considered PAS. Benjamin Cardozo, a New York judge, in 1914, ruled that "every human being of adult years and sound mind has the right to determine what shall be done with his own body."[84] If a ventilator, or other life-sustaining treatment, is determined by the patient or other legal decision maker to be excessively burdensome, then removing it is not PAS but a legal request in most states that ought to be respected. In these cases, the life-sustaining treatment is considered as holding back death and, when stopped, the patient dies of his disease or medical problem, not from the withdrawal of the treatment. In some states, the law limits the ability of a decision maker, but not the patient, to withdraw certain treatments.

Although not a legal part of end-of-life care in most of the country at this time, PAS is an ongoing question. Below are presented some of the arguments supporting PAS followed by some that oppose it.

The Case in Favor of Physician-Assisted Suicide

Some of the arguments for PAS are based on respect for patient autonomy, which is generally considered to be the preeminent principle in American medical ethics today. Respect for autonomy is the basis for informed consent, which is necessary for any procedure performed on a patient. If a patient wishes to die to escape uncontrollable suffering, or being an extreme burden on the family, some would argue that the patient's physician has a responsibility to try all possible legal means to achieve patient comfort. Various forms of suffering are, however, extremely difficult to control. Even the provision of excellent palliative care may not relieve all types of psychologic, emotional, existential, or even physical pain. Proponents of PAS argue that duty requires that the physician not abandon the patient whose suffering remains intolerable, claiming that there are no other palliative treatments. This argument continues that the logical continuation of a physician's responsibility, after ensuring that the patient neither is depressed nor has otherwise compromised decision making, is to provide the means for a comfortable death.

Many are afraid that dying must be a painful experience. When a clinician is unable to prevent unbearable suffering in a dying patient, proponents would argue that PAS should be an option on the continuum of total care of a patient. They would say that a physician is responsible for treating that suffering by any possible means and that refusing to explore what may be the only way to prevent that suffering could be viewed as abandoning the patient. Proponents could also argue that giving a patient control over the process of dying would reduce some suffering. Most of the requests for PAS in Oregon have been made to try and control the circumstances of dying, not because of physical symptoms, which are more easily treated.[75]

To some extent PAS or even euthanasia is widespread already. A national survey in 1998 reported that 4.7% of physicians stated that they had given at least one patient a lethal injection.[87] These situations already exist in the privacy of the doctor–patient relationship, and some would say that they should be allowed to continue without interference. This argument continues that legalizing PAS would allow society to acknowledge and regulate these actions, thereby providing protections for all involved parties. Currently, in all states except Oregon, any physician involved in PAS is legally at risk, whereas the patient, if interrupted or unsuccessful in the act, is at risk for unwanted aggressive measures and increased physical handicaps.

Intentionally ending the life of a person, while usually proscribed by society, is allowed in a few specific instances. Killing another human being while fighting for one's country is often defended as a responsible act, or even a required one for a member of the military. Capital punishment is legal in 38 states for those whom society has deemed deserving of that ultimate punishment. Some say that PAS should be included in this class of "justifiable killing."

The Case Against Physician-Assisted Suicide

The case against PAS also follows several avenues, a few of which are presented below. Two of the main arguments involve the effect of PAS on society as a whole.

The first argument states that life has intrinsic value and that physicians are viewed as guardians of those lives. They attempt to heal the sick, but when cure is not possible, proponents would say that their role is to comfort the sick until a patient succumbs to his or her inevitable death. Their role is either trying to prolong life or bearing witness to the end of patients' lives they cannot prolong because of the value of those lives. It would follow that they are not charged by society *intentionally* to shorten life. Many argue that the public's views of the profession would change were physicians allowed to intend death while supplying the means. It is certainly possible for a physician to hasten a patient's death while struggling to make a dying patient comfortable with opioids and benzodiazepines, but the intention here is to relieve suffering. The alternative is uncontrolled pain and suffering followed by a difficult death. Proponents would argue that the role of physicians is to protect the lives of patients and not purposely try to end them.

Opponents of PAS might also say that legalizing PAS could allow the medical profession not to work so hard to provide the best palliative care. Instead, if comfort were not achieved easily, there would be an alternative to continued serious efforts. Currently, with the choice of either increasing or decreasing levels of comfort, the only option is to continue trying to reduce any patient's suffering. PAS would serve as an "easy way out" for some physicians if they found end-of-life care too challenging.

Some would argue that legalizing PAS could be the beginning of a slippery slope. It might begin as a way for people with a serious illness to avoid a bad end and could proceed to a time when people with serious disabilities or the very old would be encouraged to end their lives and cease being a burden to their families or to society. PAS could become viewed as the way to rid society of those who were no longer capable of being contributing members. Some might even argue that it could eventually open the door for euthanasia.

PAS could also lead to decisions burdened by conflicts of interest. Patients who may not be ready to die, but who also do not wish to deplete their family's resources, might feel pressure not based on the medical situation. On the other side, physicians in certain situations might eventually find financial incentives involved in the decision. Legalizing PAS could lead to society having serious questions about how the decisions are influenced.

Physicians are not required to provide care that they believe is unethical, and many people feel that killing a human being under any circumstances is evil in itself. Legalizing PAS would cause some physicians to be seen as not helping those who suffer because of their beliefs. This could cause a difficult split within the community of physicians. Of course, there is also the question of whether humans should decide when to end their own lives. At this time, American society has not fully resolved this larger question.

End-of-life care in the United States is changing rapidly as palliative care and hospice both develop and become more well known. Oncologists and other physicians are becoming more aware of the needs of terminal patients and their families, and there is more literature about those situations. Palliative care specialists and teams are becoming more widespread, and hospice now takes care of about 50% of the dying people in the United States. One common idea is that good palliative care will prevent the need for PAS. Although this concept seems as though it might be valid, there is little evidence to prove it. As terminal care continues to improve, it will be interesting to watch what happens to the debate over PAS.

References

1. Foley K, Gelband H (eds). Improving Palliative Care for Cancer. Washington, DC: National Academy Press, 2001.
2. Emanuel LL, von Gunten CF, Ferris FD. Gaps in end-of-life care. Arch Fam Med 2000;9(10):1176–1180.
3. Doyle D, Hanks GW, MacDonald N. Introduction. In: Doyle D, Hanks GW, MacDonald N (eds) Oxford Textbook of Palliative Medicine, 2nd ed. New York: Oxford University Press, 1998: 3–8.
4. Hearn J, Higginson IJ. Do specialist palliative care teams improve outcomes for cancer patients? A systematic literature review. Palliat Med 1998;12(5):317–332.
5. Calman K, Hanks GW. Clinical and health services research. In: Doyle D, Hanks GW, MacDonald N (eds) Oxford Textbook of Palliative Medicine. New York: Oxford University Press, 1998:159–165.
6. Steinhauser KE. Measuring outcomes prospectively. In: Improving End-of-Life Care. Bethesda, MD: National Institutes of Health, 2004:33–34.
7. Finucane T. Preferences and changes in the goals of care. In: Improving End-of-Life Care. Bethesda, MD: National Institutes of Health, 2004:23–27.
8. Teno J. Measuring outcomes retrospectively. In: Improving End-of-Life Care. Bethesda, MD: National Institutes of Health, 2004:35–37.
9. Grande GE, Todd CJ. Why are trials in palliative care so difficult? Palliat Med 2000;14(1):69–74.
10. Zyabroff KR, Mandelblatt JS, Ingham J. The quality of medical care at the end-of-life in the USA: existing barriers and examples of process and outcome measures. Palliat Med 2004;18(3):202–216.
11. Lamont EB, Christakis NA. Prognostic disclosure to patients with cancer near the end of life. Ann Intern Med 2001; 134(12):1096–1105.
12. Lo B, McLeod GA, Saika G. Patient attitudes to discussing life-sustaining treatment. Arch Intern Med 1986;146(8):1613–1615.
13. Emanuel LL, Barry MJ, Stoeckle JD, Ettelson LM, Emanuel EJ. Advance directives for medical care: a case for greater use. N Engl J Med 1991;324(13):889–895.
14. Song MK. Effects of end-of-life discussions on patients' affective outcomes. Nurs Outlook 2004;52(3):118–125.
15. Straton JB, Wang NY, Meoni LA, et al. Physical functioning, depression, and preferences for treatment at the end of life: the Johns Hopkins Precursors Study. J Am Geriatr Soc 2004; 52(4):577–582.
16. Steinhauser KE, Christakis NA, Clipp EC, McNeilly M, McIntyre L, Tulsky JA. Factors considered important at the end of life by patients, family, physicians, and other care providers. JAMA 2000;284(19):2476–2482.
17. Lo B, Ruston D, Kates LW, et al. Discussing religious and spiritual issues at the end of life: a practical guide for physicians. JAMA 2002;287(6):749–754.
18. Kutner JS, Steiner JF, Corbett KK, Jahnigen DW, Barton PL. Information needs in terminal illness. Soc Sci Med 1999;48(10):1341–1352.
19. Leydon GM, Boulton M, Moynihan C, et al. Cancer patients' information needs and information seeking behaviour: in depth interview study. Br Med J 2000;320(7239):909–913.
20. Osse BH, Vernooij-Dassen MJ, Schade E, de Vree B, van den Muijsenbergh ME, Grol RP. Problems to discuss with cancer patients in palliative care: a comprehensive approach. Patient Educ Couns 2002;47(3):195–204.
21. Morasso G, Capelli M, Viterbori P, et al. Psychological and symptom distress in terminal cancer patients with met and unmet needs. J Pain Symptom Manag 1999;17(6):402–409.
22. Kemp C. Terminal Illness: A Guide to Nursing Care. Philadelphia: Lippincott, 1999.
23. Buckman R. Communication in palliative care: a practical guide. In: Doyle D, Hanks GW, MacDonald N (eds) Oxford Textbook of Palliative Medicine, 2nd ed. New York: Oxford University Press, 1998:141–156.
24. Finucane TE, Shumway JM, Powers RL, D'Alessandri RM. Planning with elderly outpatients for contingencies of severe illness: a survey and clinical trial. J Gen Intern Med 1988;3(4): 322–325.
25. Tierney WM, Dexter PR, Gramelspacher GP, Perkins AJ, Zhou XH, Wolinsky FD. The effect of discussions about advance directives on patients' satisfaction with primary care. J Gen Intern Med 2001;16(1):32–40.
26. Detmar SB, Muller MJ, Wever LD, Schornagel JH, Aaronson NK. The patient-physician relationship. Patient-physician communication during outpatient palliative treatment visits: an observational study. JAMA 2001;285(10):1351–1357.
27. Wenrich MD, Curtis JR, Shannon SE, Carline JD, Ambrozy DM, Ramsey PG. Communicating with dying patients within the spectrum of medical care from terminal diagnosis to death. Arch Intern Med 2001;161(6):868–874.
28. Ingham J, Cullen J, Ogdie AR, Mangan PA, Taylor KL. A cohort study of desired services and barriers to service access among informal caregivers of patients with advanced cancer. In:

American Society of Clinical Oncology Annual Meeting Proceedings, 2004, New Orleans, LA. Chicago: American Society of Clinical Oncology, 2004:728.
29. Lederberg M. The family of the cancer patient. In: Holland J (ed) Psycho-oncology. New York: Oxford University Press, 1998: 981–993.
30. Lilly CM, De Meo DL, Sonna LA, et al. An intensive communication intervention for the critically ill. Am J Med 2000; 109(6):469–475.
31. Friedrichsen MJ, Strang PM. Doctors' strategies when breaking bad news to terminally ill patients. J Palliat Med 2003;6(4): 565–574.
32. Girgis A, Sanson-Fisher RW. Breaking bad news: consensus guidelines for medical practitioners. J Clin Oncol 1995;13(9): 2449–2456.
33. Faulkner A. ABC of palliative care. Communication with patients, families, and other professionals. Br Med J 1998; 316(7125):130–132.
34. Friedrichsen MJ, Strang PM, Carlsson ME. Cancer patients' interpretations of verbal expressions when given information about ending cancer treatment. Palliat Med 2002;16(4): 323–330.
35. Ambuel B, Mazzone MF. Breaking bad news and discussing death. Prim Care 2001;28(2):249–267.
36. Loprinzi CL, Kugler JW, Sloan JA, et al. Randomized comparison of megestrol acetate versus dexamethasone versus fluoxymesterone for the treatment of cancer anorexia/cachexia. J Clin Oncol 1999;17(10):3299–3306.
37. Jatoi A, Windschitl HE, Loprinzi CL, et al. Dronabinol versus megestrol acetate versus combination therapy for cancer-associated anorexia: a North Central Cancer Treatment Group study. J Clin Oncol 2002;20(2):567–573.
38. Breitbart W, Chochinov HM, Passik SD. Psychiatric aspects of palliative care. In: Doyle D, Hanks GW, MacDonald N (eds) Oxford Textbook of Palliative Medicine. New York: Oxford University Press, 1998:933–954.
39. Bruera E, Sweeney C. Cachexia and asthenia in cancer patients. Lancet Oncol 2000;1:138–147.
40. Ripamonti C, Mercadante S, Groff L, Zecca E, De Conno F, Casuccio A. Role of octreotide, scopolamine butylbromide, and hydration in symptom control of patients with inoperable bowel obstruction and nasogastric tubes: a prospective randomized trial. J Pain Symptom Manag 2000;19(1):23–34.
41. Muir JC, von Gunten CF. Antisecretory agents in gastrointestinal obstruction. Clin Geriatr Med 2000;16(2):327–334.
42. Ripamonti C, Twycross R, Baines M, et al. Clinical-practice recommendations for the management of bowel obstruction in patients with end-stage cancer. Support Care Cancer 2001; 9(4):223–233.
43. McNicol E, Horowicz-Mehler N, Fisk RA, et al. Management of opioid side effects in cancer-related and chronic noncancer pain: a systematic review. J Pain 2003;4(5):231–256.
44. Heaven CM, Maguire P. The relationship between patients' concerns and psychological distress in a hospice setting. Psycho-oncology 1998;7(6):502–507.
45. Doona M, Walsh D. Benzonatate for opioid-resistant cough in advanced cancer. Palliat Med 1998;12(1):55–58.
46. Breitbart W, Marotta R, Platt MM, et al. A double-blind trial of haloperidol, chlorpromazine, and lorazepam in the treatment of delirium in hospitalized AIDS patients. Am J Psychiatry 1996; 153(2):231–237.
47. Macleod A. Methylphenidate in terminal depression. J Pain Symptom Manag 1998;16:193–198.
48. Hotopf M, Chidgey J, Addington-Hall J, Ly KL. Depression in advanced disease: a systematic review Part 1. Prevalence and case finding. Palliat Med 2002;16(2):81–97.
49. Passik SD, Dugan W, McDonald MV, Rosenfeld B, Theobald DE, Edgerton S. Oncologists' recognition of depression in their patients with cancer. J Clin Oncol 1998;16(4):1594–1600.
50. Thomas JR, von Gunten CF. Clinical management of dyspnoea. Lancet Oncol 2002;3(4):223–228.
51. Bredin M, Corner J, Krishnasamy M, Plant H, Bailey C, A'Hern R. Multicentre randomised controlled trial of nursing intervention for breathlessness in patients with lung cancer. Br Med J 1999;318(7188):901–904.
52. Boyd KJ, Kelly M. Oral morphine as symptomatic treatment of dyspnoea in patients with advanced cancer. Palliat Med 1997; 11(4):277–281.
53. Bruera E, MacEachern T, Ripamonti C, Hanson J. Subcutaneous morphine for dyspnea in cancer patients. Ann Intern Med 1993;119(9):906–907.
54. Ripamonti C. Management of dyspnea in advanced cancer patients. Support Care Cancer 1999;7(4):233–243.
55. Friedman NL. Hiccups: a treatment review. Pharmacotherapy 1996;16(6):986–995.
56. Launois S, Bizec JL, Whitelaw WA, Cabane J, Derenne JP. Hiccup in adults: an overview. Eur Respir J 1993;6(4):563–575.
57. Krajnik M, Zylicz Z. Understanding pruritus in systemic disease. J Pain Symptom Manag 2001;21(2):151–168.
58. Twycross R, Greaves MW, Handwerker H, et al. Itch: scratching more than the surface. Q J Med 2003;96(1):7–26.
59. Hening WA. Restless legs syndrome. Curr Treat Options Neurol 1999;1(4):309–319.
60. Wilwerding MB, Loprinzi CL, Mailliard JA, et al. A randomized, crossover evaluation of methylphenidate in cancer patients receiving strong narcotics. Support Care Cancer 1995;3(2): 135–138.
61. Shuster JL. Delirium, confusion and agitation at the end of life. J Palliat Med 1998;1(2):177–186.
62. Hancock PJ, Epstein JB, Sadler G. Oral and dental management related to radiation therapy for head and neck cancer. J Can Dent Assoc 2003;69(9):585–590.
63. Saunders C. Foreword. In: Doyle D, Hanks GW, MacDonald N (eds) Oxford Textbook of Palliative Medicine. New York: Oxford University Press, 1998:v–ix.
64. Lynn J. Perspectives on care at the close of life. Serving patients who may die soon and their families: the role of hospice and other services. JAMA 2001;285(7):925–932.
65. Doyle D. Domiciliary palliative care. In: Doyle D, Hanks GW, MacDonald N (eds) Oxford Textbook of Palliative Medicine, 2nd ed. New York: Oxford University Press, 1998: 957–973.
66. NHPCO Facts and Figures. Alexandria, VA: National Hospice and Palliative Care Organization, 2004.
67. Emanuel EJ, Fairclough DL, Slutsman J, Emanuel LL. Understanding economic and other burdens of terminal illness: the experience of patients and their caregivers. Ann Intern Med 2000;132(6):451–459.
68. Emanuel EJ, Fairclough DL, Slutsman J, Alpert H, Baldwin D, Emanuel LL. Assistance from family members, friends, paid care givers, and volunteers in the care of terminally ill patients. N Engl J Med 1999;341(13):956–963.
69. NHPCO Facts and Figures. Alexandria, VA: National Hospice and Palliative Care Organization, 2004.
70. Friedman BT, Harwood MK, Shields M. Barriers and enablers to hospice referrals: an expert overview. J Palliat Med 2002; 5(1):73–84.
71. Christakis NA, Lamont EB. Extent and determinants of error in doctors' prognoses in terminally ill patients: prospective cohort study. Br Med J 2000;320(7233):469–472.
72. Ferris FD, von Gunten CF, Emanuel LL. Competency in end-of-life care: last hours of life. J Palliat Med 2003;6(4): 605–613.
73. Manfredi PL, Morrison RS, Morris J, Goldhirsch SL, Carter JM, Meier DE. Palliative care consultations: how do they impact the

care of hospitalized patients? J Pain Symptom Manag 2000; 20(3):166–173.

74. Felt DH, Early JL, Welk TA. Attitudes, values, beliefs, and practices surrounding end-of-life care in selected Kansas communities. Am J Hosp Palliat Care 2000;17(6):401–406.
75. Ganzini L, Harvath TA, Jackson A, Goy ER, Miller LL, Delorit MA. Experiences of Oregon nurses and social workers with hospice patients who requested assistance with suicide. N Engl J Med 2002;347(8):582–588.
76. Slevin ML, Stubbs L, Plant HJ, et al. Attitudes to chemotherapy: comparing views of patients with cancer with those of doctors, nurses, and general public. Br Med J 1990;300(6737):1458–1460.
77. Long MC. Death and dying and recognizing approaching death. Clin Geriatr Med 1996;12(2):359–368.
78. Vullo-Navich K, Smith S, Andrews M, Levine AM, Tischler JF, Veglia JM. Comfort and incidence of abnormal serum sodium, BUN, creatinine and osmolality in dehydration of terminal illness. Am J Hosp Palliat Care 1998;15(2):77–84.
79. McCann RM, Hall WJ, Groth-Juncker A. Comfort care for terminally ill patients. The appropriate use of nutrition and hydration. JAMA 1994;272(16):1263–1266.
80. Sulmasy DP, Pellegrino ED. The rule of double effect: clearing up the double talk. Arch Intern Med 1999;159(6):545–550.
81. Prigerson HG, Jacobs SC. Perspectives on care at the close of life. Caring for bereaved patients: "all the doctors just suddenly go." JAMA 2001;286(11):1369–1376.
82. Raphael B, Minkov C, Dobson M. Psychotherapeutic and pharmacological intervention for bereaved persons. In: Stroebe M, Hansson R, Stroebe W, Schut H (eds) Handbook of Bereavement Research: Consequences, Coping and Care. Washington, DC: American Psychological Association, 2001.
83. Stroebe W, Stroebe M. Determinants of adjustment to bereavement in younger widows and widowers. In: Stroebe M, Stroebe W, Hansson R (eds) Handbook of Bereavement Research. New York: Cambridge University Press, 1993.
84. Mary E. Schloendorff, Appellant v. The Society of the New York Hospital, Respondent. In: Court of Appeals of New York, 211 N.Y. 125; 105 N.E. 92 Decided April 14, 1914.
85. Hallenbeck JL. Intercultural differences and communication at the end of life. Prim Care 2001;28(2):401–413.
86. Beauchamp TL, Childress JF. Principles of Biomedical Ethics, 3rd ed. New York: Oxford University Press, 1989.
87. Meier DE, Emmons CA, Wallenstein S, Quill T, Morrison RS, Cassel CK. A national survey of physician-assisted suicide and euthanasia in the United States. N Engl J Med 1998;338(17): 1193–1201.
88. Foley K, Hendin H (eds). The Case Against Assisted Suicide, 1st ed. Baltimore: The Johns Hopkins University Press, 2002.
89. Beauchamp TL (ed). Intending Death, 1st ed. Upper Saddle River, NJ: Prentice-Hall, 1996.
90. Emanuel L (ed). Regulating How We Die, 1st ed. Cambridge: Harvard University Press, 1998.

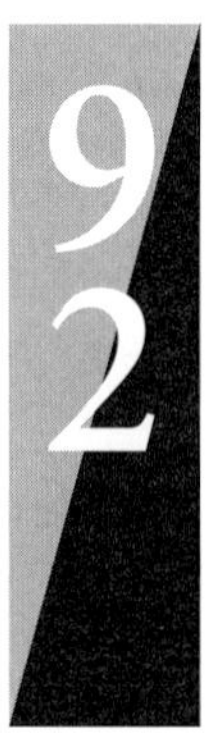

Metastatic Cancer to the Central Nervous System

Douglas B. Einstein

Epidemiology

Brain metastases are the most common intracranial solid tumors identified in adults, with 150,000 to 170,000 newly diagnosed cases of brain metastases per year in the United States.[1] Ten percent to 30% of adult cancer patients develop brain metastases in their lifetime with an incidence of up to 25% to 40% at time of autopsy.[2,3] The mean age of patients diagnosed with brain metastases is 60 years.[4] Brain metastases are much less frequent in children, affecting approximately 3% of children with localized solid tumors and 7% of those with known metastatic disease.[5] The most common primary tumor giving rise to brain metastases is non-small cell lung cancer, followed by small cell lung cancer and breast cancer (Figure 92.1).[6] The median time from diagnosis of the primary tumor to development of brain metastases is approximately 8 months.[7]

The number of brain metastases identified at diagnosis is highly dependent on the imaging modality utilized. Multiple brain metastases were identified in 47% of newly diagnosed patients using computed tomography (CT) studies. This percentage increases to 75% with gadolinium contrast-enhanced magnetic resonance imaging (MRI).[6–11] Patients with prostate, unknown primary, and gastrointestinal cancers present with a higher proportion of single brain metastases than multiple metastases (Figure 92.2).[6]

Brain metastases appear to preferentially localize to certain portions of the brain in relationship to their relative blood flow. Brain metastases are usually found at gray–white matter *watershed* areas because of decreases in superficial artery sizes at these junctions that trap metastatic emboli.[9] Approximately 80% of brain metastases are supratentorial, with 15% to 17% in the cerebellum and 3% to 5% in the brainstem.[7] Patients with single brain metastases from pelvic primaries (prostate, uterine, ovarian) appear to have a predilection for the posterior fossa 50% of the time, whereas single nonpelvic primary metastases localize to the supratentorial region 80% to 90% of the time.[6,7]

Diagnosis

Two-thirds of patients present with neurologic symptoms at diagnosis, with the majority of the remainder diagnosed incidentally at time of staging evaluation. The most common neurologic symptoms are headaches or changes in mental status (Figure 92.3).[6] Five percent to 10% of patients present symptoms of secondary hemorrhage or infarction at time of diagnosis.[12] Melanoma, choriocarcinoma, renal cell carcinoma, and thyroid carcinoma brain metastases have a higher than average risk of associated hemorrhage.[6,12,13]

Twenty percent of brain metastases are diagnosed synchronously with a new extracranial malignancy; 80% are diagnosed metachronously after the primary diagnosis.[2] In the absence of a known primary, a metastatic workup should be performed, including history and physical examination, CT of the chest, abdomen, and pelvis, and bone scan. Sixty percent to 70% of synchronously diagnosed brain metastases originate from a primary lung cancer.[14–16] In a study of patients without an initially detectable primary at the time of brain metastasis diagnosis, prospective surveillance screening shows the primary to be of lung origin 82% of the time.[17]

Contrast-enhanced MRI has supplanted CT as the imaging modality of choice for the diagnosis of brain metastases because of its higher sensitivity, as previously mentioned. Figure 92.4 shows typical gadolinium-contrast enhanced T_1 and T_2 sequences from the MRI of patients with single and multiple brain metastases. Brain metastases are typically identified as spherical, multiple ring-enhancing lesions on T_1 images with surrounding edema often larger than the lesion on T_2 images.[10,11] Increased doses of gadolinium (double or triple dose) appear to be more beneficial than single doses in identifying smaller lesions.[18,19] Diffusion-weighted MRI imaging and MR spectroscopy may also aid in identifying hemorrhage within a brain metastasis and differentiate it from an abscess.[20]

Despite characteristic imaging features, a differential diagnosis should be considered for a suspected brain metastasis in the absence of a known malignancy. This is especially critical for patients with a solitary brain metastasis (a single brain lesion representing the only evidence of metastatic disease throughout the body) versus a single brain metastasis (a single brain lesion in addition to other known extracranial metastases). This differential includes primary brain tumors, abscesses, infarctions, nonmalignant hemorrhage, demyelinating diseases, or leukoencephalopathy.[13] As shown by selected randomized trials in Table 92.1, the surgically proven false-positive rate of suspected single brain metastases detected by CT or MRI in patients with known malignancies, ranges from 2% to 11%, supporting the role of biopsy for any questionable lesion before treatment.[21–23] Treatment of presumed brain metastases without a brain biopsy has routinely been delivered at most centers and on national protocols for patients with multiple suggestive lesions on MRI and known

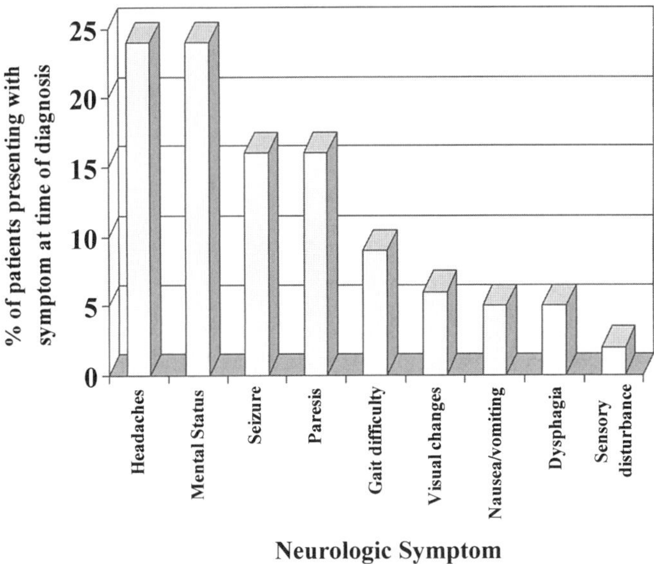

FIGURE 92.1. Frequency of brain metastases by primary tumor site.

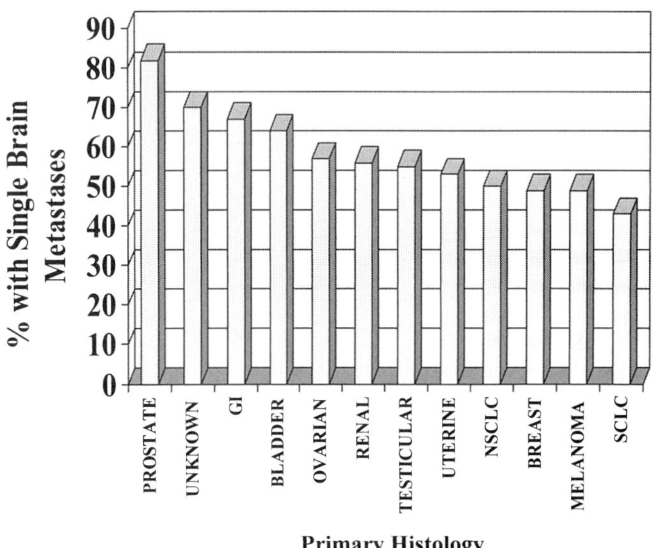

FIGURE 92.2. Frequency of single brain metastases for a given primary tumor site.

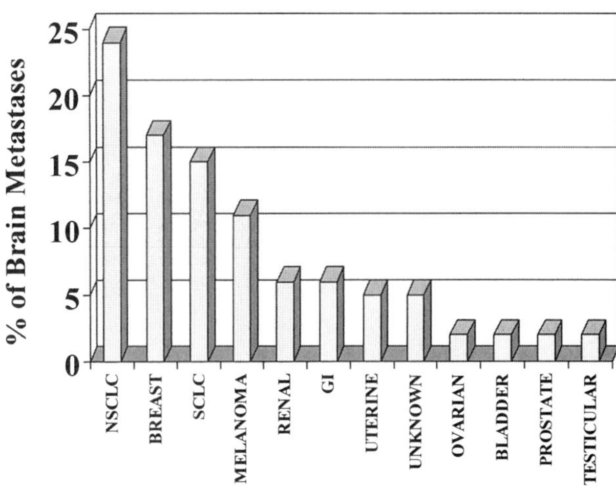

FIGURE 92.3. Frequency of neurologic symptoms at time of brain metastasis diagnosis.

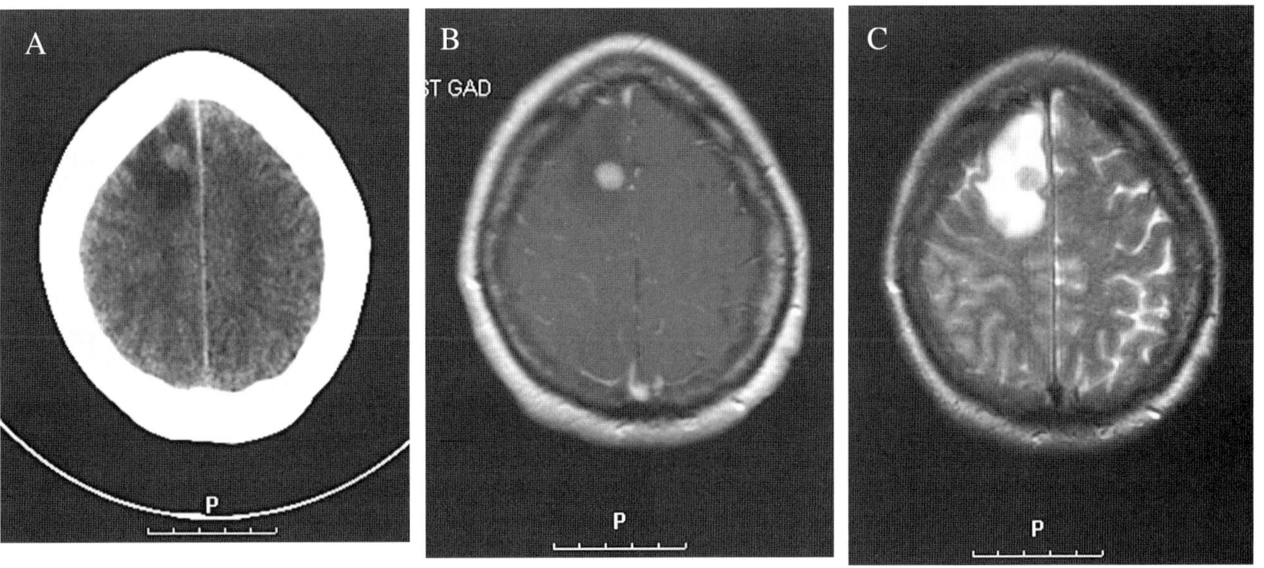

FIGURE 92.4. Contrast-enhanced axial computed tomography (CT) slices (A), gadolinium-contrast enhanced T_1 axial (B), and T_2 axial (C) sequences of a patient with brain metastases.

TABLE 92.1. False-positive rate of patients with suspected single brain metastases.

Study	*N*	*Imaging modality*	*No. of patients with nonbrain metastasis diagnosis at surgery*	*False-positive rate*
Mintz[21]	41	CT	1	2%
Noordijk[22]	32	CT	1 (at time of recurrence)	3%
Patchell[23]	54	MRI	6	11%

CT, computed tomograpy; MRI, magnetic resonance imaging.

extracranial biopsy-proven metastatic disease diagnosed within 5 years.[21–25] However, any patient with MRI imaging-equivocal single or multiple lesions should have a stereotactic biopsy or resection of the brain lesion before treatment.

Prognostic Factors

The largest study to date investigating the pretreatment prognostic factors affecting the survival of patients with brain metastases was performed by the Radiation Therapy Oncology Group (RTOG),[26] a study of 1,200 patients from three large RTOG trials. Several prognostic factors were found to be significant by univariate analysis (Table 92.2). Recursive partitioning analysis (RPA), a statistical methodology that creates a regression tree according to factors identified as significant in univariate analysis, was used to further analyze these data. Three RPA classes of patients were identified stratified by Karnofsky Performance Score (KPS), age, and extent of extracranial disease, with significantly different expected survival times (Table 92.3). These RPA classes have been borne out on analyses of other large (more than 500 patients) patient data sets (Table 92.4). It has also been proposed in a study of 916 patients[27] that RPA class 3 patients be segregated into 3A (age less than 65, controlled primary, single brain metastasis), 3B (not B or C), and 3C (age greater than 65, uncontrolled primary, multiple brain metastasis) as these three subsets have low but different median survivals of 3.2, 1.9, and 1.2 months, respectively (P less than 0.0001). The RPA classification scheme has been utilized to aid in determining which patients may benefit from more aggressive treatment of their brain metastases.

The number of lesions identified by CT imaging was also shown to have prognostic significance in an analysis of a large RTOG database of 779 patients.[28] For patients with characteristics similar to RPA class I patients (age less than 60, KPS 70 or greater, controlled extracranial disease), those patients with fewer than four lesions had a statistically significantly prolonged survival over those with four or more lesions (4.0 months versus 3.2 months; $P = 0.001$). Mass effect as evidenced by midline shift was also found to be a prognostic factor in this study. These patients, however, were imaged by CT rather than MRI, raising the possibility that the number of larger, CT-identifiable metastases may be a more important prognostic factor than the absolute number of lesions.

The Mini-Mental State Examination (MMSE), a rapid 10-question examination tool with a maximum score of 30, has also been shown to have prognostic significance for patients with brain metastases. In a study of 445 patients in a RTOG trial,[29] a decline in pretreatment MMSE score (especially less than 23) was associated with a decrease in time to death from brain metastases ($P = 0.003$). The only other factor in this study associated with an improved survival by multivariate analysis was a breast primary, which may explain some reports of gender as a prognostic factor.

TABLE 92.2. Prognostic factors identified in Radiation Therapy Oncology Group (RTOG) trials by univariate analysis.

Factor	*P value*
Solitary brain metastasis	<0.0001
KPS >70	<0.0001
Age <65 years	<0.0001
Controlled primary lesion	<0.0001
Squamous or small cell histology	<0.0001
No neurologic dysfunction	<0.0001
Total radiation dose >52 Gy	<0.0001
Breast primary	0.001
No headache	0.003
More than 2 years after primary diagnosis	0.004
Surgical resection	0.005
Complete tumor response	0.019
Noncerebellum or brainstem location	0.033
Nonmidline brain lesion	0.038

KPS, Karnofsky Performance Status.

Management and Outcomes

Symptomatic Therapy

Initial management of the patient with brain metastases consists of symptomatic therapy that is often first focused at treating peritumoral edema, resulting in increased intracranial pressure and associated neurologic symptoms. Cortico-

TABLE 92.3. Recursive partitioning analysis (RPA) classes identified in RTOG trials.

RPA class	*RPA class*	*Median survival*
I	KPS 70 or more, age less than 65 years, controlled primary, no active extracranial metastases	7.1 months
II	Not class I or III	4.2 months
III	KPS less than 70	2.3 months

TABLE 92.4. Median survival (months) of patients with brain metastases separated by RPA class.

Study	*N*	*RPA Class 1*	*RPA Class 2*	*RPA Class 3*
Gaspar[26]	1,200	7.1	4.2	2.3
Lutterbach[27]	916	8.2	4.9	1.8
Nieder[96]	528	10.5	3.5	2.0
Sanghavi[97]	502	16.1	10.3	8.7

steroids have historically been utilized because of their ability to reduce the permeability of tumor capillaries.[13] Dexamethasone is used preferentially to other steroids because of its minimal mineralcorticoid effect, lowering the potential for fluid retention; its long half-life (plasma, 2–5 hours; biologic, 24–36 hours), allowing for twice-daily dosing; and equivalent dosing by po or IV route.[13,15,30] Typically, for the symptomatic patient, loading doses of 10 to 20 mg IV are given followed by 16 to 24 mg/day in bid or qid divided doses. For the neurologically unstable patient, higher dexamethasone doses up to 100 mg/day have been utilized.[7,15,30] Sixty-five percent to 70% of patients have symptomatic relief within 6 to 24 hours after their first dose of dexamethasone.[30,31] Steroids used as a single treatment modality increases the medial survival of patients with brain metastases from 1 month, if left untreated, to 2 months.[15,31,32]

After a patient is clinically stabilized, dexamethasone should be tapered to the lowest dose necessary to maintain neurologic status because long-term steroid use can be associated with well-known side effects, such as oral candidiasis, gastritis, myopathy, hyperglycemia, fluid retention, weight gain, sleep and personality disorders, acne, osteoporosis, and immunosuppression.[7,13] In a double-blinded randomized study of patients with stable but symptomatic brain metastases treated with 16, 8, or 4 mg dexamethasone per day, 4 mg per day was found to be equally effective as 16 mg per day in maintaining neurologic status as measured by KPS.[33] Steroid taper is often started after initiation of definitive therapy, such as surgery or radiotherapy, and typically is reduced over a 3- to 4-week period by 2 mg per 5 to 7 days to avoid steroid withdrawal symptoms and adrenal insufficiency if utilized.[7,30] To minimize acute effects of gastritis, patients should be routinely placed on prophylactic H_2 blockers. *Pneumocystis carinii* pneumonia prophylaxis can also be considered for otherwise immunocompromised patients. Patients with small (less than 1 cm), asymptomatic lesions with minimal peritumoral edema often identified during staging evaluation may require no steroids or a brief course of steroids that can be discontinued within 14 days without need for tapering.[7,30]

Anticonvulsants are recommended by the American Academy of Neurology for patients presenting with seizures at time of brain metastases diagnosis.[34] Phenytoin, carbamazepine, valproic acid, and phenobarbital are the most commonly used anticonvulsants.[7,34] Anticonvulsant side effects include cognitive impairment, myelosuppression, liver dysfunction, and dermatologic reactions (ranging from minor rashes to life-threatening Stevens–Johnson syndrome), which appear to be increased in brain tumor patients.[13,34] Phenytoin, carbamazepine, and phenobarbital can also stimulate the cytochrome P-450 system, increasing the metabolism and decreasing the efficacy of many medications, including dexamethasone.[34] Newer anticonvulsants, such as levetiracetam may be a better choice for patients with brain metastases as they have a decreased risk of dermatologic reactions and do not interfere with the P-450 system.[35,36]

For patients with newly diagnosed brain metastases who have not had a seizure, the role for prophylactic anticonvulsants is controversial. A meta-analysis of four randomized trials involving the use of prophylactic anticonvulsants was performed by the American Academy of Neurology.[34] As summarized in Table 92.5, there was no statistically significant benefit to the use of prophylactic anticonvulsants. The Academy concluded, "In patients with newly diagnosed brain tumors, anticonvulsant medications are not effective in preventing first seizures. Because of their lack of efficacy and their potential side effects, prophylactic anticonvulsants should not be used routinely in patients with newly diagnosed brain tumors." With regard to postoperative anticonvulsant duration, they concluded that "In patients with brain tumors who have not had a seizure, tapering and discontinuing anticonvulsants after the first post-operative week is appropriate, particularly in those patients who are medically stable and who are experiencing anticonvulsant-related side effects."

Whole-Brain Radiotherapy

Whole-brain radiotherapy (WBRT) has been the historical standard treatment for brain metastases. WBRT is a technique by which megavoltage irradiation is delivered to the entire brain and meninges via two opposing lateral 4- to 6-MV photon beams with custom blocking to include the retina but exclude the lenses, oral/nasal cavities, and pharynx (Figure 92.5). This technique allows for the treatment of both gross and microscopic tumor within the brain. WBRT is given in fractionated form (small doses per day for a period of several weeks) to increase the therapeutic ratio by allowing normal cells to repair radiation-induced DNA damage between fractions with much greater efficacy than tumor cells, thus minimizing normal tissue toxicity.[37]

TABLE 92.5. Randomized trials of prophylactic anticonvulsant use in patients with brain tumors.

Study	*N*	*No. (%) of drug*	*Patients with seizures/placebo*	*Odds ratio (95% CI)*
Forsyth[98]	100	11/46 (24)	15/54 (28)	0.82 (0.33–2.01)
Glantz[99]	74	13/37 (35)	9/37 (24)	1.69 (0.61–4.63)
Franceschetti[100]	63	3/41 (7)	4/22 (18)	0.36 (0.07–1.76)
North[101]	81	9/42 (21)	5/39 (13)	1.85 (0.56–6.12)
Total	318	36/166 (22)	33/152 (22)	1.09 (0.63–1.89)

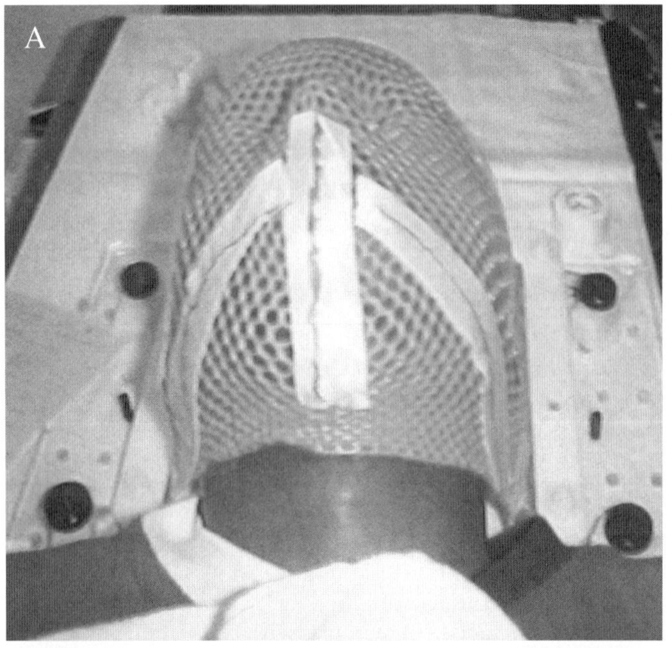

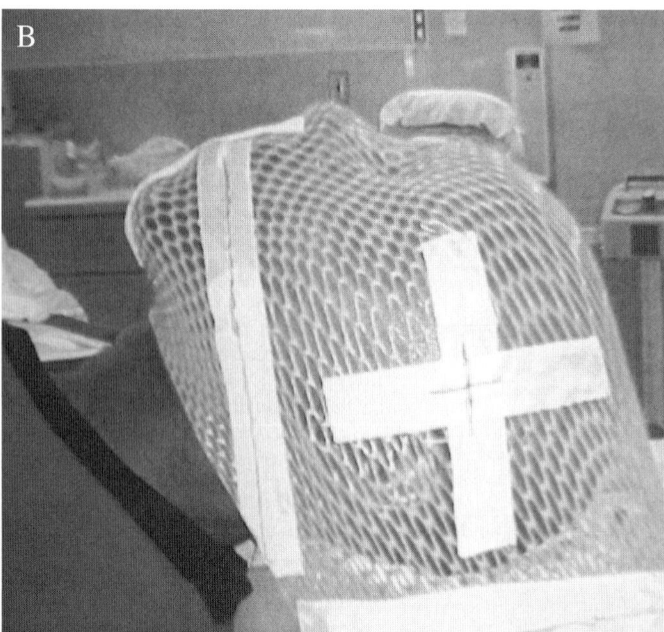

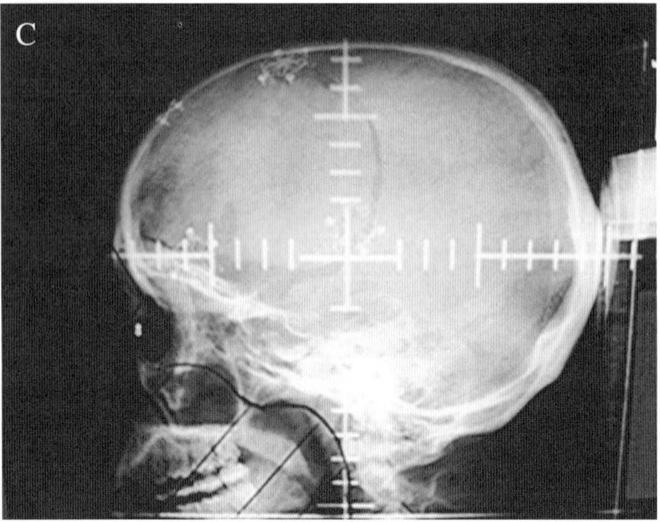

FIGURE 92.5. Typical whole-brain radiotherapy patient setup (A, B) and lateral X-ray portal (C).

Acute side effects of WBRT commonly include fatigue, a scalp skin reaction (reddening, tanning, or irritation), and hair loss. Uncommonly observed are radiation parotitis with dry mouth and change in taste sensation; otitis externa and serous otitis media with possible ear plugging, tinnitus, and drainage; possible transient increased intracranial pressure symptoms of headaches, nausea, vomiting, or seizures that may be related to increased capillary permeability; and a rare somnolence syndrome 4 to 10 weeks after WBRT with spontaneously recovering increased fatigue. Late side effects of WBRT include effects of radiation necrosis with increased peritumoral inflammation; neurocognitive impairment with decreased memory or concentration; cerebellar dysfunction with ataxia; and cataracts with a rare risk of blindness.[7,12,24]

WBRT improves the median survival of patients with brain metastases over steroid use alone to 3 to 6 months.[2,7,13,15,38] The RTOG performed the largest series of randomized trials to date investigating the optimum dose/fractionation schedule for WBRT (Table 92.6).[39–42] There was no statistically significant difference in median survival of patients treated with fractionation schemes ranging from 10 Gy in 1 fraction to 70.4 Gy in 1.6 bid fractions, with the exception of patients with solitary brain metastases treated on RTOG 85-28. Patients with solitary brain metastases treated with boost doses higher than 48 Gy had an improved median survival compared to patients treated to 48 Gy or less, although there was no dose–response differential between the three higher doses.[43] This finding led to a Phase III trial of standard WBRT versus accelerated fractionated (twice-daily) WBRT with a dose-escalated local radiation boost (RTOG 91-04).[49] This trial did not find any difference in median survival of patients treated with the dose-escalated local boost compared to lower-dose conventional daily fractionation delivered to the entire brain, supporting the use of conventional fractionation WBRT.

Although no significant differences in median survival have been produced by varying WBRT dose-fractionation schedules, there do appear to be dose-fractionation-dependent differences in quality of life and toxicity parameters. Neurologic quality of life as measured by symptom relief was ulti-

TABLE 92.6. Randomized trials of whole-brain radiotherapy alone performed by the Radiation Therapy Oncology Group (RTOG).

Trial	*N*	*Total dose (Gy)/dose per daily fraction*	*Median survival (months)*	*P value*
69-01[39]	910	30/3	5.2	
		30/2	4.5	NS
		40/2.67	4.5	
		40/2	4.0	
73-61[39]	902	20/4	4.0	
		30/3	3.7	NS
		40/2.67	4.5	
69-01/ 73-61[40]	59	10/10	3.7	NS
		12/6	3.2	
76-06[41]	255	30/3	4.5	NS
		50/2.5	4.2	
85-28[42 a]	345	48/1.6 (twice daily)	4.2	NS
		54.4/1.6 (twice daily)	5.2	Except for solitary metastases,
		64.0/1.6 (twice daily)	4.8	48 Gy vs. >48 Gy
		70.4/1.6 (twice daily)	6.4	$P = 0.05$ (48)
91-04[44]	445	30/3 (once daily)	4.5	
		54.4/1.6 (twice daily)[a]	4.5	NS

[a] Whole brain treated to 32 Gy with a reduced-field size boost beyond 32 Gy.

mately observed in 60% to 90% of patients treated in the aforementioned RTOG randomized trials. A high palliative index was also produced by WBRT alone, with patients spending 75% to 80% of their remaining life in an improved or stable neurologic state.[39–42] There was a dose-fractionation-dependent difference in the promptness of neurologic improvement. Patients receiving larger daily fraction doses reported a quicker response to neurologic improvement by the second week than those patients receiving lower daily doses (Table 92.7).[39] For patients presenting with the highest pretreatment neurologic function, total doses greater than 30 Gy were associated with a longer duration of neurologic improvement compared to lower total dose schedules (19 weeks versus 13 weeks; $P = 0.05$).[39]

Neurocognitive function also may be dependent on the daily fraction dose of WBRT. In 1 year, of long-term survivors from a widely quoted retrospective analysis of 79 patients receiving postoperative WBRT (20–40 Gy total dose in 2- to 6-Gy daily fractions) after resection of a single brain metastasis,[45] 17% of patients who received more than 3 Gy per fraction (4/23) experienced dementia versus 0% of patients who received 3 Gy per fraction or less (0/15), supporting the use of lower daily fraction size to decrease late toxicity in patients with the highest potential for long-term survival. WBRT fraction sizes of 2.5 Gy or less have also been associated with a decreased risk of late neurocognitive side effects.[46] Hyperfractionation (twice-daily radiotherapy), which has been utilized in other sites to decrease radiation side effects, did not affect neurocognitive outcome as measured by the MMSE for patients in RTOG 91-04 receiving twice-daily versus once-daily WBRT doses. The neurocognitive outcome proved to be highly dependent on tumor control with an average drop in MMSE score of 0.5 for patients with controlled brain metastases versus a drop of 6.3 in patients with uncontrolled brain metastases ($P = 0.02$).[47] Tumor growth, rather than WBRT treatment effect, was also found to be the primary factor resulting in neurocognitive decline assessed by a battery of neurocognitive tests administered before and after WBRT in another prospective trial.[48]

TABLE 92.7. Impact of daily fraction size on promptness of neurologic response after whole-brain radiation therapy (WBRT).

WBRT Dose per daily fraction	*Percent with neurologic improvement by week 2*	*P value*
<3 Gy/day	43%	
>3 Gy/day	55%	$P = 0.06$
<4 Gy/day	54%	
>4 Gy/day	64%	$P = 0.01$

TABLE 92.8. Proposed dose-fractionation schedule for whole-brain radiotherapy (WBRT) alone stratified by RPA class.

RPA class	*RPA class*	*Dose per fraction*	*Total dose*
I	KPS 70 or more, age less than 65 years, controlled primary, no active extracranial metastases	2.5 Gy	37.5 Gy
II	Not class I or III	2.5-3 Gy	30–37.5 Gy
III	KPS less than 70	3-4 Gy	20–30 Gy

The more rapid neurologic symptom improvement with higher daily fractionation schemes, combined with the longer duration of neurologic response with higher total dose and decreased late neurotoxicity in suspected longer-term survivors with lower daily doses, supports the use of stratified WBRT dose-fractionation schemes based on prognostic factors. One proposed dose-fractionation stratification based on recursive partitioning analysis (RPA) classes used at our institution is described in Table 92.8.

Surgery

Surgical intervention is indicated for patients requiring a histologic diagnosis with no known extracranial cancer, for patients requiring rapid relief from metastases causing symptomatic mass effect or obstructive hydrocephalus, and for improvement of local control.[15,49] Surgical morbidity and mortality have been improved through the use of newer advanced techniques, such as intraoperative MRI and ultrasound, functional cortical mapping, and frameless stereotaxis.[15,50] In the largest reported retrospective cohort study to date of 13,685 patients undergoing craniotomy for the resection of brain metastases from 1988 to 2000, in-hospital mortality rates decreased from 4.6% between 1988 and 1990 to 2.3% between 1997 and 2000. Mortality was dependent on hospital and surgeon volume, with lower-volume sites/surgeons associated with higher mortality rates.[51] Although surgical morbidity/mortality has been significantly reduced using advanced neurosurgical techniques, surgical therapy is often not offered for patients with extensive progressive extracranial disease, as this factor removes patients from RPA class I status and is associated with a poorer than average prognosis.[12,13]

For patients with a single brain metastasis with stable extracranial disease, surgical resection has been shown to improve survival over WBRT alone. Three randomized trials of patients with single brain metastases compared preradiotherapy surgical resection of the metastases to WBRT alone

TABLE 92.9. Randomized trials of surgical resection in addition to whole-brain radiotherapy (WBRT) for patients with a single brain metastasis.

Trial	*Randomization*	*N*	*WBRT dose (Gy)/dose per fraction*	*Median survival with progressive extracranial disease (ED)*	*P value*	*Median survival with stable ED*	*P value*	*Recurrence rate at original site*	*P value*
Patchell[52]	Surgery + WBRT	25	36/3	Not stated		40 weeks		20%	
	WBRT	23	36/3	Not stated	P = NS	15 weeks	$P < 0.01$	52%	$P < 0.02$
Noordjik[53]	Surgery + WBRT	32	40/2 bid	20 weeks		43 weeks		Not stated	
	WBRT	31	40/2 bid	20 weeks	P = NS	26 weeks	$P = 0.02$	Not stated	
Mintz[54]	Surgery + WBRT	41	30/3	12 weeks		24 weeks		Not stated	
	WBRT	43	30/3	12 weeks	P = NS	27 weeks	$P = 0.24$	Not stated	

(Table 92.9). None of the trials showed a survival advantage for patients undergoing surgery in the presence of progressive extracranial disease, again demonstrating the importance of this prognostic factor. The first two trials[52,53] found a significant increase in overall survival for patients with stable extracranial disease whose single brain metastasis was resected before WBRT. The third trial[54] failed to show a benefit for surgical resection. This may be secondary to the inclusion of patients with a KPS above 50 rather than 70 in the other trials, and a higher proportion of patients with progressive extracranial disease (45% versus 38% and 32%).[52–54]

The necessity of immediate adjuvant WBRT after surgical resection for patients with a single brain metastasis, has been investigated in several retrospective analyses with varied results,[45,55–59] but in only one prospective, randomized trial.[60] This trial randomized 95 patients with a single brain metastasis to either immediate WBRT or WBRT upon recurrence.[60] There was no difference in overall survival between the immediate WBRT group (48 weeks) and the delayed WBRT group (43 weeks). There were, however, several benefits of immediate WBRT. Immediate WBRT decreased the risk of recurrence anywhere in the brain from 70% to 18% (P less than 0.001); decreased the risk of recurrence at the site of the initial metastasis from 46% to 10% (P less than 0.001); increased the time to brain recurrence from 27 weeks to 52 weeks; and decreased death from neurologic causes from 44% to 14% ($P = 0.003$). Although delayed WBRT resulted in the same overall survival as immediate WBRT, the authors recommended the routine use of immediate WBRT to decrease brain recurrences and associated neurologic symptoms that can affect quality of life and neurologic death.

For select patients with a solitary brain metastasis from non-small cell lung cancer and resectable thoracic disease, aggressive surgical resection of gross disease at both sites has been attempted with encouraging results. In retrospective trials of patients with complete resection of both solitary brain metastases and limited (stage I or II) non-small cell lung cancer, combined resection has yielded median survivals ranging from 13 to 24 months and 5 year survival rates of 10% to 30%.[61–64] Thoracic lymph node tumor involvement was found to be the most significant negative prognostic factor for patients undergoing combined resection of their cranial and thoracic disease.[62,64]

For patients with multiple brain metastases, surgical resection has been generally limited to resection of a dominant single lesion, causing symptomatic mass effect. However, with advanced surgical techniques, the ability to resect multiple lesions has improved. Although there have been no randomized trials investigating the benefit of surgical resection of multiple brain metastases, retrospective studies of patients with multiple resected brain metastases have been reported.[65,66] The largest of these studies[65] subdivided patients undergoing resection of multiple brain metastases into three groups: group A (30 patients) had remaining metastases after resection, group B (26 patients) had all brain metastases resected, and group C patients (26 patients) were case-controlled matched patients to those in group B who underwent resection of a single brain metastasis for comparison. All patients received WBRT (30 Gy in 3-Gy daily fractions) either pre- or postoperatively. The median survival of group B patients (with all metastases resected) was 14 months, which was equivalent to those patients in group C (with a single resected metastasis), but significantly higher than the 6-month median survival of group A (with remaining unresected lesions). These authors concluded that removal of all lesions in selected patients with multiple brain metastases improves survival time, and gives a prognosis similar to that of patients with a single resected brain metastasis combined with WBRT. Although supporting surgical resection of multiple brain metastases that can be resected within a single operation, these data await validation by a prospective, randomized trial.

Stereotactic Radiosurgery

Stereotactic radiosurgery (SRS) has produced significant advances in the treatment of brain metastases over the past decade. SRS is a technique using single-fraction, high-dose megavoltage radiation directed at a discrete target identified in three-dimensional stereotactic space. Brain SRS is delivered via collimator-modified linear accelerators using multiple arcing beams intersecting at the defined target (LINAC-SRS), or via a gamma knife machine using 201 fixed cobalt sources, with the target moved into the intersection (focal point) of the beams (GK-SRS). Head position must also be fixed using stereotactic frames attached to the skull. SRS head frames, devices, and typical SRS isodose curves for brain metastases are shown in Figure 92.6.

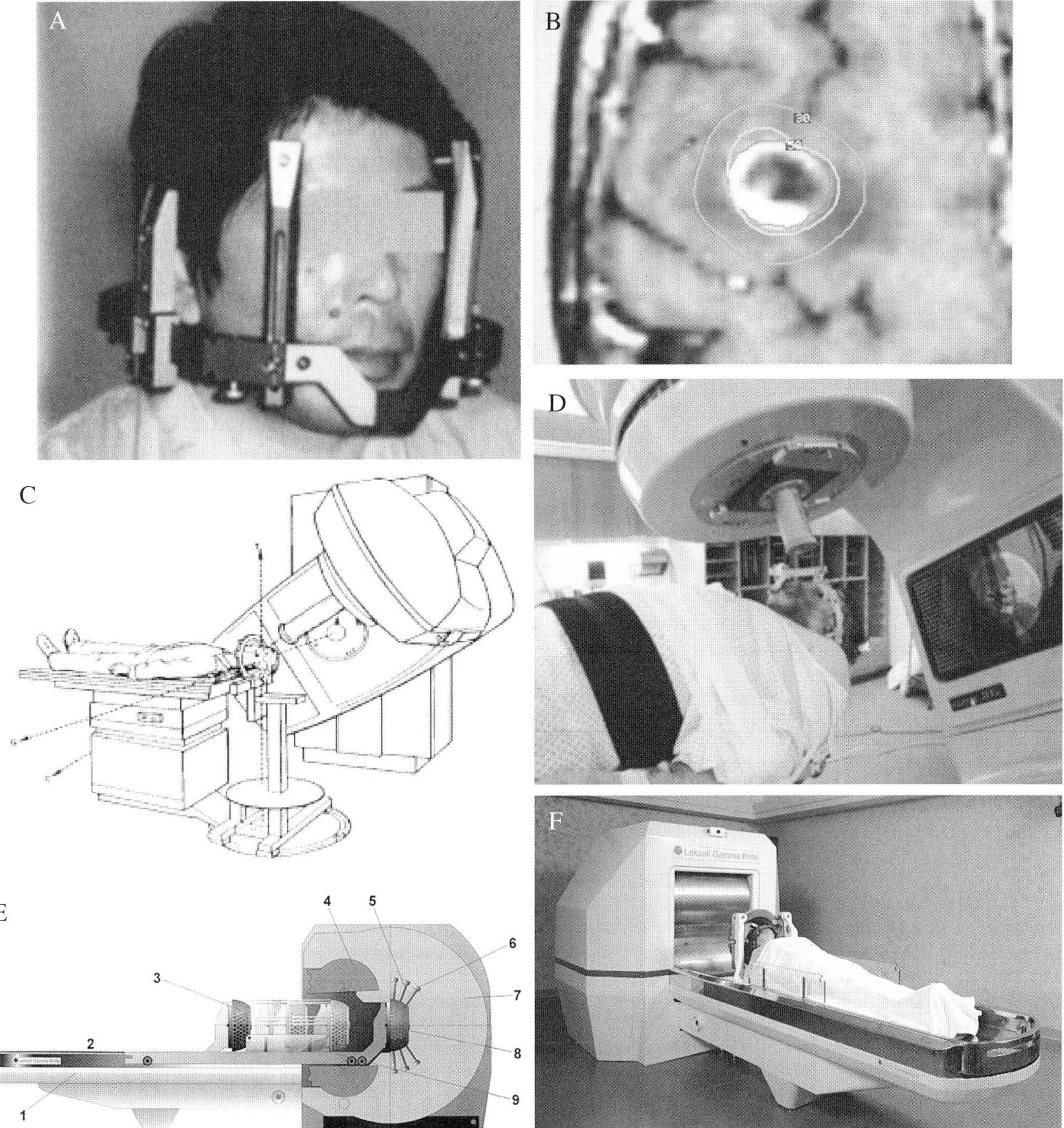

FIGURE 92.6. (A) Stereotactic radiosurgery (SRS) head immobilization frame. (B) SRS isodose curves (inner 50%, outer 30%). (C, D) LINAC stereotactic radiosurgery treatment. (E, F) Gamma knife stereotactic radiosurgery treatment.

The radiobiology of single-fraction high-dose radiation treatments allows for maximal DNA damage with minimal sublethal damage repair that normally occurs during the interfraction interval of fractionated radiotherapy treatments. Because normal tissue repair is minimized, SRS targets must be exquisitely defined to minimize the amount of normal tissue within the SRS field. Therefore, SRS is utilized, in a manner similar to surgical resection, to treat gross brain metastases that can be identified on imaging studies and is not used to treat nonvisualized microscopic metastases.

Side effects of SRS include stereotactic frame pin site issues, including transient facial swelling and rare risks of

TABLE 92.10. Radiation Therapy Oncology Group (RTOG) central nervous system (CNS) toxicity criteria.

Grade	*Definition*
1	Mild neurologic symptoms; no medication necessary
2	Moderate neurologic symptoms; outpatient medication required (e.g., steroids)
3	Severe neurologic symptoms; outpatient or inpatient medication required
4	Life-threatening neurologic symptoms (e.g., uncontrolled seizures, paralysis, or coma); includes clinically or radiographically suspected radionecrosis and histologically proven radionecrosis at the time of an operation
5	Death

TABLE 92.11. Radiosurgery maximum tolerable doses (MTDs) from RTOG 90-05.[62]

Maximum tumor diameter	*Maximum tolerable radiosurgical dose*	*Comments*
0–2.0 cm	24 Gy	MTD not reached at 24 Gy
2.1–3.0 cm	18 Gy	18 Gy based on chronic toxicity, 21 Gy based on acute toxicity
3.1–4.0 cm	15 Gy	15 Gy based on acute toxicity

bleeding or infection; radiation-induced peritumoral inflammation with risk of increased intracranial pressure symptoms, such as headaches, nausea, vomiting, or seizures within 24 to 48 hours of the radiosurgical procedure; and risk of symptomatic radiation necrosis, which can cause peritumoral edema 3 to 24 months after radiosurgery.[24] Dexamethasone and anticonvulsants delivered on the day of the procedure can decrease the risk of increased intracranial pressure (ICP) symptoms. The risk of symptomatic radiation necrosis is highly dose-volume dependent. The largest Phase I multiinstitutional trial investigating the risk of symptomatic necrosis from radiosurgery is RTOG 90-05,[67] in which 168 patients with recurrent primary brain tumors or brain metastases after large-field radiotherapy (WBRT or conformal brain radiotherapy), were entered on the protocol. Tumor diameter-dependent doses were escalated to the maximum tolerable dose (MTD) based on the incidence of acute (less than 3 months) and chronic (more than 3 months) central nervous system (CNS) toxicity as measured by RTOG CNS toxicity criteria (Table 92.10). The MTDs identified are summarized in Table 92.11. These MTDs have been used as guidelines in all subsequent RTOG radiosurgery protocols. Radiosurgical toxicity for unirradiated brain has also been investigated by the University of Pittsburgh group in their large study of 332 patients treated with SRS for arteriovenous malformations (AVMs).[68] They found a dose–volume relationship between the volume covered by the 12-Gy isodose curve and risk of symptomatic necrosis.[68]

Advantages of SRS over surgical resection include outpatient treatment with rapid recovery time, no need for general anesthesia, lower side-effect profile, easier accessibility of more eloquent regions of the brain, and less cost with the median reported cost of WBRT plus SRS of $15,102 compared to $22,018 with WBRT plus surgery.[49,69] Surgical resection remains the treatment of choice for patients who require rapid decompression of symptomatic brain metastases causing substantial mass effect, for patients requiring tissue diagnosis before treatment, and for patients with radiosurgery-ineligible tumors, that is, those larger than 4 cm, inseparable from the optic nerves or chiasm, or involving the brainstem (relative contraindication).[49]

Two randomized trials of the addition of SRS to WBRT (Table 92.12) have been conducted in a similar manner to those for the addition of surgical resection to WBRT (see Table 92.9).[70,71] The first trial by the University of Pittsburgh group[70] included 27 patients with two to four brain metastases less than 2.5 cm in diameter with a median KPS of 100 and a median age of 59 years. Most patients had active systemic disease (62% in WBRT + SRS versus 71% in WBRT alone). The trial was stopped after a planned analysis at 60% accrual that showed an improvement in 1-year local control from 8% in WBRT to 100% in WBRT + SRS ($P = 0.002$). At that level of accrual, the group found a trend in improved median overall survival from 7.5 months in the WBRT group to 11 months in the WBRT + SRS that did not reach statistical significance ($P = 0.22$). However, in the group of patients with stable extracranial disease, there was a significant improvement in overall survival from 5.5 months (with pulmonary metastases) to 7.5 months (without pulmonary metastases) to 14 months ($P = 0.02$). The difference was still significant without the pulmonary disease stratification ($P = 0.05$), emphasizing the importance of stable extracranial disease on the prognosis of patients with brain metastases.

The second trial, RTOG 95-08, is the largest multiinstitutional trial of WBRT versus WBRT + SRS to date, randomizing 333 patients with one to three brain metastases with diameters less than 4.0 cm and a KPS of 70 or more.[71,72] SRS improved survival over WBRT alone for patients with a single brain metastasis (4.9 to 6.5 months; $P = 0.04$); RPA class I patients (9.6 to 11.6 months; $P = 0.05$); and patients with non-small cell lung cancer or any squamous cell carcinoma (3.9 to 5.9 months; $P = 0.05$). All patients receiving SRS were more likely to maintain a stable or improved performance status

TABLE 92.12. Randomized trials of stereotactic radiosurgery (SRS) in addition to whole-brain radiotherapy (WBRT).

Trial	*Randomization*	*N*	*WBRT dose (Gy)/dose per fraction*	*Median survival (months) with stable extracranial disease (ED)*	*P value*	*One-year SRS in-field recurrence rate*	*P value*
Kondziolka[70]	SRS + WBRT	14	30/2.5	14 months		8%	
	WBRT	13	30/2.5	7.5 months	$P = 0.05$	100%	$P < 0.02$
RTOG 95-08[71,72]	SRS + WBRT	16 4	37.5/2.5	11.6 months		18%	
	WBRT	16 7	37.5/2.5	9.6 months	$P = 0.045$	29%	$P = 0.01$

TABLE 92.13. Retrospective studies of SRS alone versus SRS + WBRT.

Trial	*Initial treatment*	*N*	*Local control*	*P value*	*% requiring salvage therapy*	*P value*	*Median survival (months) with stable ED*	*P value*
Sneed[89]	SRS alone	268	NA		37%		8.2 months	
	SRS + WBRT	301	NA	NA	7%	*P* > 0.01	8.6 months	*P* = NS
Flickinger[102]	SRS alone	51	53%		NA		NA	
	SRS + WBRT	65	81%	*P* = 0.004	NA	NA	NA	NA
Pirzkall[103]	SRS alone	158	72%		NA		5 months	
	SRS + WBRT	78	86%	*P* = 0.13	NA	NA	6 months	*P* = NS
Sneed[105]	SRS alone	62	42%		40%		11.3 months	
	SRS + WBRT	43	63%	*P* = 0.008	19%	*P* = 0.02	11.1 months	*P* = NS
Chidel[104]	SRS alone	78	52%		NA		10.5 months	
	SRS + WBRT	57	80%	*P* = 0.034	NA	NA	6.4 months	*P* = 0.079
Shehata[106]	SRS alone	228	87%		NA		NA	
	SRS + WBRT	240	97%	*P* = 0.0001	NA	NA	NA	NA
Robinson[107]	SRS alone	68	74%		NA		5.8 months	
	SRS + WBRT	51	84%	*P* = 0.01	NA	NA	6.1 months	*P* = NS

(KPS) at 3 months (50% versus 33%; *P* = 0.02) and at 6 months (43% versus 27%; *P* = 0.03).

Thus, SRS has a proven survival benefit in addition to WBRT for all RPA class I patients and for select RPA class II patients with stable extracranial disease, young age, or single brain metastases. The benefit of SRS for RPA class III patients (KPS less than 70) has not been proven, as these patients have a historically poor prognosis and have been excluded from the aforementioned randomized trials.

Attempts have been made to delay or exclude WBRT for patients receiving initial SRS for the treatment of brain metastases to minimize treatment-related side effects of WBRT. To date, there have been no randomized trials comparing SRS alone versus SRS + WBRT, although one by the American College of Surgeons Oncology Group (ACOSOG) has recently begun accrual.[73] Based on the only randomized trial comparing surgery alone with surgery + WBRT for patients with single brain metastases,[60] one would expect similar conclusions substituting SRS for surgical resection; namely, no difference in overall survival with immediate WBRT versus WBRT upon recurrence, a decrease in future CNS failure rate with immediate WBRT, and a resultant improvement in neurologic quality of life by decreasing the risk of further symptomatic brain metastases.[60] Several retrospective studies have shown an improvement in local control with the addition of WBRT over SRS alone (Table 92.13). None of these studies, however, demonstrated a significant difference in overall survival between the SRS alone versus SRS + WBRT, presumably due to the ability to salvage recurrences with delayed WBRT or repeat SRS.

Radiosensitizing Agents

Several trials of radiosensitizing agents in conjunction with WBRT have been performed. Radiosensitizing agents, by definition, are compounds that increase the lethal effects of radiotherapy but have little activity in the absence of radiation.[37] Agents tested in trials include misonidazole (an oxygen mimetic; a hypoxic cell sensitizer), BrdU (bromodeoxyuridine; a halogenated pyrimidine), lonidamine (inhibits cellular respiration), RSR13 (increases oxygen release by hemoglobin; a hypoxic cell sensitizer), and, most recently, motexafin gadolinium (depletes reducing metabolites that may inhibit radiation-induced DNA damage). A summary of Phase II/III radiosensitizer trials is found in Table 92.14. Unfortunately,

TABLE 92.14. Phase II/III trials of WBRT with or without radiosensitizing agents.

Trial	*Phase*	*N*	*Treatment*	*Median survival*	*P value*
RTOG 79-16[108]	Phase III	190	WBRT + misonidazole	3.9 months	
		193	WBRT alone (3.0 Gy × 10 fractions)	4.5 months	*P* = NS
RTOG 79-16[108]	Phase III	196	WBRT + misonidazole	3.1 months	
		200	WBRT alone (5.0 Gy × 6 fractions)	4.1 months	*P* = NS
RTOG 89-05[109]	Phase III	30	WBRT + bromodeoxyuridine (BrdU)	4.3 months	
		34	WBRT alone (2.5 Gy × 15 fractions)	6.1 months	*P* = NS
DeAngelis[110]	Phase III	31	WBRT + lonidamine	5.4 months	
		27	WBRT alone (3.0 Gy × 10 fractions)	3.9 months	*P* = NS
Mehta[111]	Phase III	193	WBRT + motexafin gadolinium	5.2 months	
		208	WBRT alone (3 Gy × 10 fractions)	4.9 months	*P* = NS
Shaw[112]	Phase II	57	WBRT + RSR13	6.4 months	
		1,070	WBRT alone (historical from RTOG database)	4.1 months	*P* = 0.174

TABLE 92.15. Histology-specific brain metastasis response rates to chemotherapeutic agents.

Primary histology	*Response rate*	*References*
Small cell lung cancer	21%–76%	82, 83, 89
Breast cancer	38%–59%	84, 85
Non-small cell lung cancer	23%–33%	85, 86, 88
Melanoma	0%–38%	85, 87, 91

none of the randomized trials showed a benefit of the radiosensitizing agent in addition to WBRT. There was a suggestion of a benefit of RSR13, although this was only a Phase II trial, and Phase III trial results (RT-009) are pending.

Chemotherapy

Many different chemotherapeutic agents have shown activity in the treatment of brain metastases, including etoposide, cisplatin, temozolomide, thalidomide, teniposide, topotecan, vinorelbine, gemcitibine, carboplatin, IL-2, BCNU, and methyl-CCNU (chloroethylnitrosurea).[74–86] Chemotherapy has historically had limited success in the treatment of brain metastases, presumably because of blood–brain and blood–tumor barriers maintained by tight endothelial junctions and p-glycoprotein-mediated active efflux transport of chemotherapeutic agents away from the CNS.[15,74,76] Reports that some CNS-penetrating drugs, such as methyl-CCNU have failed to improve survival over WBRT alone in a randomized trial,[75] suggest that there are other factors involved in brain metastasis response to chemotherapy besides the ability to penetrate the CNS. Inherent tumor histology-specific chemosensitivity also appears to play a role in the differential response rates seen with the use of different agents in the treatment of brain metastases. Chemosensitive small cell lung cancer shows the highest response rates (Table 92.15).

One promising newer chemotherapeutic agent utilized in the treatment of brain metastases is temozolomide, an alkylating agent similar to dacarbazine (DTIC) with CNS-penetrating properties used in the treatment of malignant gliomas. A summary of Phase II/III trials of temozolomide with WBRT for newly diagnosed brain metastases is shown in Table 92.16. Although most trials have shown an increased response rate with the addition of temozolomide to WBRT in the treatment of brain metastases, none has shown a statistically significant increase in overall survival. Larger multiinstitutional trials are ongoing.

Salvage for Recurrent Brain Metastases

Options for patients with recurrent brain metastases after surgical resection/SRS, and an initial course of WBRT, include further surgical resection, repeat SRS, repeat WBRT, and chemotherapy. Surgical resection tends to be reserved for those patients with significant mass effect symptoms from their recurrent brain metastases. Several retrospective studies of patients undergoing surgical resection for recurrent brain metastases have shown encouraging median survival times after resection, ranging from 6 to 11 months.[86–88] Of the remaining options, repeat SRS to the new, previously untreated, metastasis offers the highest control rate of 60% to 90%, similar to control of initial lesions.[89–92] Lesions previously treated with SRS have been retreated with no apparent added toxicity at cumulative doses up to 39Gy with a minimum interdose interval of 4 months.[92] The largest reported study of reirradiation of recurrent brain metastases, using a repeat course of WBRT, comes from the Mayo Clinic.[93] In this retrospective study of 2,658 patients who received initial WBRT for brain metastases (median dose, 30Gy), 86 received a repeat course of WBRT (median dose, 20Gy in 10 fractions). Seventy percent of reirradiated patients had partial or complete resolution of neurologic symptoms, with a median survival of 4 months after reirradiation. Retreatment appeared to be the well tolerated, with 6% of patients developing radiographic changes consistent with reirradiation and 1 patient developing dementia believed to be secondary to reirradiation. Systemic chemotherapy for recurrent brain metastases appears to be the least successful treatment, with partial responses in 20% to 50% of patients with recurrent brain metastases. The blood–brain barrier-penetrating systemic agent temozolomide appears to have the highest activity.[73,76,94] A potentially promising chemotherapeutictreatment of recurrent brain metastases involves intraarterial delivery of chemotherapy, with regional blood–brain barrier disruption. In preliminary studies using intraarterial carboplatin and intravenous etoposide, response rates of 79% were obtained with predominantly hematologic toxicities and rare angiographic complications.[95]

TABLE 92.16. Phase II/III trials of WBRT with or without temozolomide for patients with newly diagnosed brain metastases.

Trial	*Phase*	N	*Treatment*	*Overall response*	P *value*	*Median survival*	P *value*
Antonadou[113]	Phase II	25	WBRT + temozolo mide	96%		8.6 months	
		23	WBRT alone (2.0 Gy × 20 fractions)	67%	$P = 0.017$	7.0 months	$P = 0.45$
Antonadou[114]	Phase III	67	WBRT + temozolo mide	53%		8.3 months	
		67	WBRT alone (3.0 Gy × 10 fractions)	33%	$P = 0.039$	6.3 months	$P = 0.18$
Verger[115]	Phase II/III	24	WBRT + temozolo mide	45%		18.4 weeks	
		20	WBRT alone	44%	P = NS	12.5 weeks	P = NS

References

1. Davey P. Brain metastases. Curr Probl Cancer 1999;23:59–98.
2. Patchell R. Brain metastases. Handb Neurol 1997;25:135.
3. Pikren JW, Lopez G, Tsukada Y, et al. Brain metastases: an autopsy study. Cancer Treat Symp 1983;2:295–313.
4. Sawaya R, Bindal RK. Metastatic brain tumors. In: Kaye AH, Laws, ER Jr (eds) Brain Tumors: An Encyclopedic Approach. Philadelphia: Churchill Livingstone 1995;923–946.
5. Bouffet E, Doumi N, Thiesse P, et al. Brain metastases in children with solid tumors. Cancer (Phila) 1997;79:403–410.
6. Nussbaum ES, Djalilian HR, Cho KH, Hall WA. Brain metastases. Histology, multiplicity, surgery, and survival. Cancer (Phila) 1996;78:1781–1788.
7. Mehta M, Tremont-Lukats IW. Evaluation and management of brain metastases. J Clin Oncol (ASCO Educ Book) 2002;375–382.
8. Sze G, Milano E, Johnson C, et al. Detection of brain metastasis: comparison of contrast-enhanced MR with unenhanced MR and enhanced CT. Am J Neuroradiol 1990;11:785–791.
9. Delattre JY, Krol G, Thaler HT, Posner JB. Distribution of brain metastases. Arch Neurol 1988;45:741–744.
10. Davis PC, Hudgins PA, Peterman SB, et al. Diagnosis of cerebral metastases: double-dose delayed CT vs. contrast-enhanced MR imaging. Am J Neuroradiol 1991;12:293–300.
11. Sze G, Milano E, Johnson C, Heier L. Detection of brain metastases: comparison of contrast-enhanced MR with unenhanced MR and enhanced CT. Am J Neuroradiol 1990;11:785–791.
12. Patchell RA. Treatment of brain metastases. J Clin Oncol (ASCO Educ Book) 2002;383–391.
13. Wen PY, Black PM, Loeffler JS. Treatment of metastastic brain cancer. In: Devita VT, Hellman S, Rosenberg SA (eds) Cancer: Principles and Practice of Oncology, 6th ed. Philadelphia: Lippincott, Williams, and Wilkins 2001:2655–2669.
14. Merchut MP. Brain metastases from undiagnosed systemic neoplasms. Arch Intern Med 1989;149:1076–1080.
15. Sofietti R, Ruda R, Mutani R. Management of brain metastases. J Neurol 2002;249:1357–1369.
16. Van dePol M, Van Aalst VC, Wilmink JT, Twijnstra A. Brain metastases from an unknown primary tumor: which diagnostic procedures are indicated? J Neurol Neurosurg Psychiatry 1996;61:321–323.
17. Ruda R, Borgognone M, Benech F, Vasario E, Soffietti R. Brain metastases from unknown primary tumour: a prospective study. J Neurol 2001;248:394–398.
18. VanDijk P, Sijens PD, Schmitz PI, Oudekerk M. Gd-enhanced MR imaging of brain metastases: contrast as a function of dose and lesion size. Magn Reson Imaging 1997;15:535–541.
19. Donahue BR, Goldberg JD, Golfinos JG, et al. Importance of MR technique for stereotactic radiosurgery. Neuro-oncology 2003;5:268–275.
20. Rees J. Advances in magnetic resonance imaging of brain tumors. Curr Opin Neurol. 2003;16:643–650.
21. Mintz, AH, Kestle J, Rathbone MP, et al. A randomized trial to assess the efficacy of surgery in addition to radiotherapy in patients with a single cerebral metastasis. Cancer (Phila) 1996;78:1470–1476.
22. Noordijk EM, Vecht CJ, Haaxma-Reiche H, et al. The choice of treatment of single brain metastasis should be based on extracranial tumor activity and age. Int J Radiat Biol Phys 1994;29:711–717.
23. Patchell RA, Tibbs PA, Walsh JW, et al. A randomized trial to assess the efficacy of surgery in the treatment of single metastases to the brain. N Engl J Med 1990;322:494–500.
24. Radiation Therapy Oncology Group Protocol 95-08. www.rtog.org
25. Radiation Therapy Oncology Group Protocol BR-0118. www.rtog.org
26. Gaspar L, Scott C, Rotman M, Asbell S, Phillips T, et al. Recursive partitioning analysis (RPA) of prognostic factors in three radiation therapy oncology group (RTOG) brain metastases trials. Int J Radiat Oncol Biol Phys 1997;37:745–751.
27. Lutterbach J, Bartelt S, Stancu E, Guttenberger R. Patients with brain metastases: hope for recursive partitioning analysis (RPA) class 3. Radiother Oncol 2002;63:339–345.
28. Swift PS, Phillips T, Martz K, et al. CT characteristics of patients with brain metastases treated in RTOG study 79-16. Int J Radiat Oncol Biol Phys 1993;25:209–214.
29. Murray KJ, Scott C, Zachariah B, Michalski JM, et al. Importance of the mini-mental status examination in the treatment of patients with brain metastases: a report from the radiation therapy oncology group protocol 91-04. Int J Radiat Oncol Biol Phys 2000;48:59–64.
30. Vecht CJ. Clinical management of brain metastases. J Neurol 1998;245:127–131.
31. Patchell RA. Treatment of brain metastases. Cancer Invest 1996;14:169–177.
32. Markesbery WR, Brooks WH, Gupda GD, et al. Treatment for patients with cerebral metastases. Arch Neurol 1978;35:754–756.
33. Vecht CJ, Hovestadt A, Verbiest HB, van Vliet JJ, van Putten WL. Dose-effect relationship of dexamethasone on Karnofsky performance in metastatic brain tumors: a randomized study of doses of 4, 8, and 16 mg per day. Neurology 1994;44:675–680.
34. Glantz MJ, Cole BF, Forsyth PA, et al. Practice parameter: anticonvulsant prophylaxis in patients with newly diagnosed brain tumors. Report of the Quality Standards Subcommittee of the American Academy of Neurology. Neurology 2000;54:1886–1893.
35. Patsalos PN. Pharmacokinetic profile of levetiracetam: toward ideal characteristics. Pharmacol Ther 2000;85:77–85.
36. Asconape JJ. Some common issues in the use of antiepileptic drugs. Semin Neurol 2002;22:27–39.
37. Hall E. Radiobiology for the Radiobiologist, 4th ed. Philadelphia, J.B. Lippincott Company 1994.
38. Zimm S, Wampler GL, Stablein D, Hazra T, Young HF. Intracerebral metastases in solid-tumor patients: natural history and results of treatment. Cancer (Phila) 48:384–394.
39. Borgelt B, Gelber R, Kramer S, et al. The palliation of brain metastases: final results of the first two studies of the Radiation Therapy Oncology Group. Int J Radiat Oncol Biol Phys 1980;6:1–9.
40. Borgelt B, Gelber R, Kramer S, et al. Ultra-rapid high dose irradiation scheduled for the palliation of brain metastases. Final results of the first two studies of the Radiation Therapy Oncology Group. Int J Radiat Oncol Biol Phys 1981;7:1633.
41. Kurtz J, Gelber R, Brady L, et al. The palliation of brain metastases in a favorable patient population. A randomized clinical trial by the Radiation Therapy Oncology Group. Int J Radiat Oncol Biol Phys 1981;7:891–895.
42. Sause WT, Scott C, Krisch R, et al. Phase I/II trial of accelerated fractionation in brain metastases: RTOG 85-28. Int J Radiat Oncol Biol Phys 1993;26:653–657.
43. Epstein BE, Scott CB, Sause WT, et al. Improved survival duration in patients with unresected solitary brain metastases using accelerated hyperfractionated radiation therapy at total doses of 54.4a Gy and greater. Cancer (Phila) 1993;71:1362–1367.
44. Murray KJ, Scott C, Greenberg HM, Emami B, et al. A randomized phase III study of accelerated hyperfractionation versus standard in patients with unresected brain metastases: a report of the Radiation Therapy Oncology Group (RTOG) 9104. Int J Radiat Oncol Biol Phys 1997;39:571–574.

45. Deangelis LM, Mandell LR, Thaler HT, et al. The role of postoperative radiotherapy after resection of single brain metastases. Neurosurgery 1989;24:798–805.
46. Sheline GE, Wara WM, Smith V. Therapeutic irradiation and brain injury. Int J Radiat Oncol Biol Phys 1980;6:1215–1228.
47. Regine WF, Scott C, Murray K, Curran W. Neurocognitive outcome in brain metastases treated with accelerated-fractionation vs. accelerated-hyperfractionated radiotherapy: an analysis from RTOG Study 91-04. Int J Radiat Oncol Biol Phys 2001;51: 711–717.
48. Mehta MP, Rodrigus P, Terhaard CH, et al. Survival and neurologic outcomes in a randomized trial of motexafin gadolinium and whole-brain radiation therapy in brain metastases. J Clin Oncol 2003;21:2529–2536.
49. Sawaya R. Considerations in the diagnosis and management of brain metastases. Oncology (Huntingt) 2001;15:1144–1154, 1157–1158; discussion 1158, 1163–1165.
50. Weinberg JS, Lang FF, Sawaya R. Surgical management of brain metastases. Curr Oncol Rep 2001;3(6):476–483.
51. Barker FG II. Craniotomy for the resection of metastatic brain tumors in the U.S., 1988–2000: decreasing mortality and the effect of provider caseload. Cancer (Phila) 2004;100(5):999–1007.
52. Patchell RA, Tibbs PA, Walsh JW, et al. A randomized trial of surgery in the treatment of single brain metastases to the brain. N Engl J Med 1990;322:494–500.
53. Noordijk EM, Vecht CJ, Haaxma-Reiche H, et al. The choice of treatment of single brain metastasis should be based on extracranial tumor activity and age. Int J Radiat Oncol Biol Phys 1994;29:711–717.
54. Mintz AH, Kestle J, Rathbone MP, et al. A randomized trial to assess the efficacy of surgery in addition to radiotherapy in patients with a single cerebral metastasis. Cancer (Phila) 1996; 78:470–476.
55. Dosoretz DE, Blitzer PH, Russell AH, Wang CC. Management of solitary metastases to the brain: the role of elective brain irradiation following complete surgical resection. Int J Radiat Oncol Biol Phys 1980;6:1727–1730.
56. Smalley SR, Scray MF, Laws ER, O'Fallon JR. Adjuvant radiation therapy after surgical resection of solitary brain metastasis: association with patterns of failure and survival. Int J Radiat Oncol Biol Phys 1987;13:1611–1616.
57. Hagen NA, Cirrincione C, Thaler HT, DeAngelis LM. The role of radiation therapy after resection of single brain metastasis from melanoma. Neurology 1990;40:158–160.
58. Armstrong JG, Wronski M, Galicich JH, et al. Postoperative radiation for lung cancer metastatic to the brain. J Clin Oncol 1994;12:2340–2344.
59. Skibber JM, Soong S, Austin L, et al. Cranial irradiation after surgical excision of brain metastases in melanoma patients. Ann Surg Oncol 1996;3:118–123.
60. Patchell RA, Tibbs PA, Regine WF, et al. Postoperative radiotherapy in the treatment of single metastases to the brain. JAMA 1998;280:1485–1489.
61. Kelly K, Bunn PA. Is it time to reevaluate our approach to the treatment of brain metastases in patients with non-small cell lung cancer? Lung Cancer 198;20:85–91.
62. Torre M, Quanini E, Chiesa G, et al. Synchronous brain metastases from lung cancer: result of surgical treatment in combined resection. J Thorac Cardiovasc Surg 1988;95:994–997.
63. Read RC, Boop WC, Yoder G, Schaefer R. Management of nonsmall cell lung carcinoma with solitary brain metastasis. J Thorac Cardiovasc Surg 1989;98:884–891.
64. Billing PS, Miller DL, Allen MS, et al. Surgical treatment of primary lung cancer with synchronous brain metastases. J Thorac Cardiovasc Surg 2001;112:548–553.
65. Bindal RK, Sawaya R, Leavens ME, Lee JJ. Surgical treatment of multiple brain metastases. J Neurosurg 1993;79:210–216.
66. Hazuka MB, Burleson W, Stroud DN, et al. Multiple brain metastases are associated with poor survival in patients treated with surgery and radiotherapy. J Clin Oncol 1993;11:369–373.
67. Shaw E, Scott C, Souhami L, et al. Single dose radiosurgical treatment of recurrent previously irradiated primary brain tumors and brain metastases: final report of RTOG protocol 90-05. Int J Radiat Oncol Biol Phys 2000;47:291–298.
68. Flickinger JC, Kondziolka D, Maitz AH, Lunsford LD. Analysis of neurological sequelae from radiosurgery of arteriovenous malformations: how location affects outcome. Int J Radiat Oncol Biol Phys 1998;40:273–278.
69. Boyd TS, Mehta MP. Stereotactic radiosurgery for brain metastases. Oncology (Huntingt) 1999;13:1397–1409; discussion 1409–1410, 1413.
70. Kondziolka D, Patel A, Lunsford LD, et al. Stereotactic radiosurgery plus whole brain radiotherapy versus radiotherapy alone for patients with multiple brain metastases. Int J Radiat Oncol Biol Phys 1999;45:427–434.
71. Sperduto PW, Scott C, Andrews D, et al. Preliminary report of RTOG 9508: a phase III trial comparing whole brain irradiation alone versus whole brain irradiation plus stereotactic radiosurgery for patients with two or three unresected brain metastases. Int J Radiat Oncol Biol Phys 2000;48:113.
72. Sperduto P, Scott C, Andrews D, et al. Stereotactic radiosurgery with whole brain radiation therapy improves survival in brain metastasis patients: report of the RTOG phase III study 95-08. Int J Radiat Oncol Biol Phys 2002;54:3.
73. American College of Surgeons Oncology Group Protocol Z0300. www.acosog.org.
74. Abrey LE, Mehta MP. Treatment of brain metastases: a short review of current therapies and the emerging role of temozolomide. Clin Adv Hematol Oncol 2003;1:231–235.
75. Ushio Y, Arita N, Hayakawa T, et al. Chemotherapy of brain metastases from lung carcinoma: a controlled randomized trial. Neurosurgery 1991;28:201–205.
76. Van de Bent MJ. The role of chemotherapy in brain metastases. Eur J Cancer 2003;39:2114–2120.
77. Kristensen CA, Kristjansen PE, Hansen HH. Systemic chemotherapy of brain metastases from small cell lung cancer: a review. J Clin Oncol 1992;10:1498–1502.
78. Postmus PE, Haaxma-Reiche H, Smit EF, et al. Treatment of brain metastases of small-cell lung cancer: comparing teniposide and teniposide with whole-brain radiotherapy. A phase III study of the EORTC lung cancer cooperative group. J Clin Oncol 2000;18:3400–3408.
79. Rosner D, Nemoto T, Lane WW. Chemotherapy induces regression of brain metastases in breast carcinoma. Cancer (Phila) 58:832–839.
80. Franciosi V, Cocconi G, Michiara M, et al. Front-line chemotherapy with cisplatin and etoposide for patients with brain metastases from breast carcinoma, nonsmall cell lung carcinoma, or malignant melanoma: a prospective study. Cancer 1999;85: 1599–1605.
81. Robinet G, Thomas P, Breton JL, et al. Results of a phase III study of early versus delayed whole brain radiotherapy with concurrent cisplatin and vinorelbine combination in inoperable brain metastasis of non-small-cell lung cancer: Groupe Francais de Pneumo-Cancerologie (GFPC) Protocol 95-1. Ann Oncol 2001; 12:59–67.
82. Mornex F, Thomas L, Mohr P, et al. Randomised phase III trial of fotemustine versus fotemustine plus whole brain irradiation in cerebral metastases of melanoma. Cancer Radiother 2003; 7:1–8.
83. Boogerd W, van der Sande JJ, van Zandwijk N. Teniposide sometimes effective in brain metastases from non-small cell lung cancer. J Neuro-oncol 1999;41:285–289.
84. Korfel A, Oehm C, von Pawel J, et al. Response to topotecan of symptomatic brain metastases of small-cell lung cancer also

after whole-brain irradiation. a multicentre phase II study. Eur J Cancer 2002;38:1724–1729.

85. Guirguis LM, Yang JC, White DE, et al. Safety and efficacy of high-dose interleukin-2 therapy in patients with brain metastases. J Immunother 2002;25:82–87.
86. Bafaloukos D, Gogas H, Georgoulias V, et al. Temozolomide in combination with docetaxel in patients with advanced melanoma: a phase II study of the Hellenic Cooperative Oncology Group. J Clin Oncol 2002;20:420–425.
87. Sundareasan N, Sachdev V, Digiacinto G. Reoperation for brain metastases. J Clin Oncol 1988;6:1625–1629.
88. Arbit E, Wronski M, Burt M, et al. The treatment of patients with recurrent brain metastases. Cancer (Phila) 1995;76: 765–773.
89. Sneed PK, Suh JH, Goetsch SJ, et al. A multi-institutional review of radiosurgery alone vs. radiosurgery with whole brain radiotherapy as the initial management of brain metastases. Int J Radiat Oncol Biol Phys 2002;53:519–526.
90. Sneed PK, Lamborn KR, Forstner JM, et al. Radiosurgery for brain metastases: is whole brain radiotherapy necessary? Int J Radiat Oncol Biol Phys 1999;43:549–559.
91. Chen JC, Petrovich Z, Giannotta SL, et al. Radiosurgical salvage therapy for patients presenting with recurrence of metastatic disease to the brain. Neurosurgery 2000;46:860–866.
92. Hillard VH, Shih LL, Chin S, et al. Safety of multiple stereotactic radiosurgery treatments for multiple brain lesions. J Neurooncol 2003;63:271–278.
93. Wong WW, Schild SE, Sawyer TE, Shaw EG. Analysis of outcome in patients reirradiated for brain metastases. Int J Radiat Oncol Biol Phys 1996;34:585–590.
94. Abrey LE, Olson JD, Raizer JJ, et al. A phase II trial of temozolomide for patients with recurrent or progressive brain metastases. J Neuro-oncol 2001;53:259–265.
95. Newton HB, Slivka MA, Volpi C, et al. Intra-arterial carboplatin and intravenous etoposide for the treatment of metastatic brain tumors. J Neuro-oncol 2003;61(1):35–44.
96. Neider C, Nestle U, Motaref B, et al. Prognostic factors in brain metastases: should patients be selected for aggressive treatment according to recursive partitioning analysis (RPA) class? Int J Radiat Oncol Biol Phys 2000;46:297–302.
97. Sanghavi SN, Saranarendra SM, Chappell R, et al. Radiosurgery for patients with brain metastases: a multi-institutional analysis stratified by the RTOG recursive partitioning analysis method. Int J Radiat Oncol Biol Phys 2001;51:426–434.
98. Forsyth PA, Weaver S, Fulton D, et al. Prophylactic anticonvulsants in patients with brain tumour. Can J Neurol Sci 2003;30(2):106–112.
99. Glantz MJ, Cole BF, Friedberg MH, et al. A randomized, blinded, placebo-controlled trial of divalproex sodium prophylaxis in adults with newly diagnosed brain tumors. Neurology 1996;46: 985–991.
100. Franceschetti S, Binelli S, Casazza M, et al. Influence of surgery and antiepileptic drugs on seizures symptomatic of cerebral tumors. Acta Neurochirur 1990;103:47–51.
101. North JB, Penhall RK, Hanieh A, et al. Phenytoin and postoperative epilepsy. A double-blind study. J Neurosurg 1983;58: 672–677.
102. Flickinger JC, Kondziolka D, Lunsford LD, et al. A multiinstitutional experience with stereotactic radiosurgery for solitary brain metastasis. Int J Radiat Oncol Biol Phys 1994;28:797–802.
103. Pirzkall A, Debus J, Lohr F, et al. Radiosurgery alone or in combination with whole-brain radiotherapy for brain metastases. J Clin Oncol 1998;16:3563–3569.
104. Chidel MA, Suh JH, Reddy CA, et al. Application of recursive partitioning analysis and evaluation of the use of whole brain radiation among patients treated with stereotactic radiosurgery for newly diagnosed brain metastases. Int J Radiat Oncol Biol Phys 2000;47:993–999.
105. Sneed PK, Lamborn KR, Forstner JM, et al. Radiosurgery for brain metastases: is whole brain radiotherapy necessary? Int J Radiat Oncol Biol Phys 1999;43:549–558.
106. Shehata MK, Young B, Reid BK, et al. Stereotactic radiosurgery of 468 brain metastases < or = 2 cm: implications for SRS dose and whole brain radiation therapy. Int J Radiat Oncol Biol Phys 2004;54:87–93.
107. Robinson C, Stephans K, Fu P, Pillai K, Maciunas R, Einstein DB. Impact of initial whole brain radiotherapy (WBRT) in addition to gamma knife radiosurgery (GKSRS) on the neurologic status of patients with newly diagnosed brain metastases. Int J Radiat Oncol Biol Phys 2003;57(suppl 2):S326.
108. Komarnicky LT, Phillips TL, Martz K, et al. A randomized phase III protocol for the evaluation of misonidazole combined with radiation in the treatment of patients with brain metastases (RTOG 97-16). Int J Radiat Oncol Biol Phys 1991;20:53–58.
109. Phillips TL, Scott CB, Leibel SA, Rotman M, Weigensberg IJ. Results of a randomized comparison of radiotherapy and bromodeoxyuridine with radiotherapy alone for brain metastases: report of RTOG trial 89-05. Int J Radiat Oncol Biol Phys 1995;33:339–348.
110. DeAngelis LM, Currie VE, Kim JH. The combined use of radiation therapy and lonidamine in the treatment of brain metastases. J Neuro-oncol 1989;7:241–247.
111. Mehta MP, Rodrigus P, Terhaard CH, et al. Survival and neurologic outcomes in a randomized trial of motexafin gadolinium and whole-brain radiation therapy in brain metastases. J Clin Oncol 2003;21:2529–2536.
112. Shaw E, Scott C, Suh J, et al. RSR13 plus cranial radiation therapy in patients with brain metastases: comparison with the radiation therapy oncology group recursive partitioning analysis brain metastases database. J Clin Oncol 2003;21:2364–2371.
113. Antonadou D, Paraskevaidis M, Sarris G, et al. Phase II randomized trial of temozolomide and concurrent radiotherapy in patients with brain metastases. J Clin Oncol 2002;20:3644–3650.
114. Antonadou D, Coliarakis N, Paraskevaidis M, et al. Whole brain radiotherapy alone or in combination with temozolomide for brain metastases. A phase III study. Int J Radiat Oncol Biol Phys 2002;54:93–94.
115. Verger M, Gil M, Yaya R, Vinolas N, Villa S, Pujol T, Solano M, Graus F. Concomitant temozolomide (TMZ) and radiotherapy (RT) in patients with brain metastases: randomized multicentric phase II study, a preliminary report. Proc Am Soc Clin Oncol 2002;21:78a.

93 Metastatic Cancer to Lung

Jessica S. Donington

Metastasis is the major cause of death in cancer patients. The lungs are the second most frequent site of metastatic disease for all histologies and the sole site of metastasis in 20% of autopsy cases.[1] The presence of pulmonary metastasis implies systemic dissemination of disease and was once considered beyond the realm of surgical cure. It was widely accepted that surgery could provide nothing beyond palliation. We now recognize that metastases that are isolated to the lungs are not consistently associated with the same dismal survival as metastases to multiple sites.[2] During the past 40 years, surgical resection has become a standard approach for the treatment of pulmonary metastasis in selected histologies. A multitude of series have documented the survival benefits of pulmonary metastasectomy in selected patients.

Despite the vast number of series that propose the benefit of pulmonary metastasectomy, they all share a similar weakness; data in this area are all retrospective. There are no controlled randomized trials comparing surgical metastasectomy to medical therapy or best supportive care. The definitive benefit of surgery has never been proven because no group of unresected patients has clearly been shown to be comparative. Critics of metastasectomy state that only clinically detectable disease is resected and therefore, the majority of patients will recur. This is true: more than 50% of patients will have their disease recur following resection. Critics also argue that only highly selective patients with good performance status and favorable tumor biology undergo resection and these patients would have a prolonged survival with or without surgery. Proponents of metastasectomy counter these arguments by pointing out the universally poor outcome in patients with pulmonary metastases who undergo other curative or palliative therapy.

Following metastasectomy, most patients die of recurrent pulmonary disease, but 20% to 40% of patients survive 5 years. The generally accepted selection criteria for pulmonary metastasectomy include (1) control of the primary tumor, (2) absence of extrathoracic metastasis, (3) the ability to completely resect all metastatic disease, (4) sufficient cardiopulmonary function to tolerate resection, and (5) lack of effective systemic therapy. Advancements in systemic therapy, molecular profiling of tumors, and our understanding of tumor biology continue to mold our treatment strategy.

History

Weinlecher is credited with the first pulmonary metastasectomy in 1882, when he removed a metastatic lung deposit during a chest wall resection for a rib sarcoma.[3] Divis performed the first pulmonary metastasectomy as an independent operation in 1927 in Czechoslovakia.[4] The first such resection in the United States was performed by Barney and Churchill, who performed a right lower lobectomy for metastatic kidney cancer.[5] The patient survived disease free for 23 years before dying of coronary artery disease. The success of this case and other isolated reports gave credibility to the concept of curative pulmonary metastasectomy. In 1947, Alexander and Haight published a series of 24 pulmonary metastasectomies and formally addressed appropriate selection criteria for the procedure.[6] In 1965, the Mayo Clinic published a series of more than 200 pulmonary metastasectomies and pointed out the limitations of preoperative radiologic studies in predicting the extent of metastatic disease.[7] In 1979, Memorial Sloan-Kettering Cancer Center (MSKCC) stressed the prognostic significance between metastases from sarcomas, and those from other histologies, in their series of 622 pulmonary metastasectomies.[8] Efforts to better refine selection criteria and better define prognostic variables led to the development of the International Registry of Lung Metastasis (IRLM) in 1997. The registry consists of more than 5,000 patients from major thoracic surgery groups around the world and provides the most definitive analysis of clinical prognostic factors for pulmonary metastasectomy to date.[9] Their findings guide our current treatment protocols.

Surgical Techniques

When discussing techniques for pulmonary metastasectomy, we must address the approach used to access the chest cavity and the mode of removal of the lesion from the lung parenchyma. There are a wide variety of options in surgical approach, including posterolateral thoracotomy, median sternotomy, clamshell thoracotomy (bilateral anterior thoracotomy), or, most recently, by the video-assisted thoracoscopic surgery (VATS) approach (Table 93.1).

TABLE 93.1. Approach for metastasectomy.

Approach	*Advantage*	*Disadvantage*	*Reference*
Posterior lateral thoracotomy	Excellent exposure	Unilateral access Staged operations Postoperative pain	Hazelrigg[59] Ponn[60] Rusch[10]
Median sternotomy	Bilateral access Single procedure Decreased pain	Poor exposure to left lower lobe and posterior lung fields	Hazelrigg[61] Johnston[62] Roth[11]
Clamshell (bilateral anterior thoracotomies)	Excellent exposure Bilateral access Single procedure	Increased postoperative pain Increased chest tube drainage Increased OR time	Cooper[12] Bains[14] Shimizu[13]
Video-assisted thoracoscopic surgery (VATS)	Decreased pain Decreased hospital stay	Unilateral access Staged operations No manual palpation Decreased detection of nodules	Dowling[63] Hazelrigg[64] Landrenau[15] McCormack[16]

Posterior lateral thoracotomy is the standard approach for the majority of pulmonary resections and the original approach used for pulmonary metastasectomy. The main advantage of this approach is excellent exposure to the lung and hilum. Almost any pulmonary procedure can be performed through this incision. The downside of this approach for metastasectomy is that it provides access to only one lung. Unfortunately with access to only one thoracic cavity, patients with bilateral disease are committed to two procedures. Most surgeons stage the thoracotomies from 3 days to 3 months apart. Postoperative pain issues also hamper posterior lateral thoracotomies. Pain issues are handled in the same manner as pain from posterior lateral thoracotomies for other reasons with the use of epidural analgesia and with muscle-sparing procedures. The surgeons at MSKCC advocate performing bilateral thoracotomies at a single setting and believe it can be done safely with these techniques.[10]

The median sternotomy was popularized in the 1980s as an approach for pulmonary metastasectomy. It has the advantages of access to both lung fields through a single, well-tolerated incision. The downside of this approach is that it does not provide good access to the posterior lung fields or the left lower lobe. Although most metastasectomies are performed as wedge resections, which are easily performed through a sternotomy, lobectomies can also be performed through this incision. Median sternotomy has the advantage of manual palpation of both lungs. In patients with unilateral disease on preoperative studies, up to one-third of patients can have disease on the opposite side at operation.[11]

In the 1990s, Cooper and colleagues popularized the clamshell thoracotomy (simultaneous, bilateral anterior thoracotomies) for bilateral lung transplants.[12] It provides excellent exposure to both pleural cavities while being surprisingly safe and well tolerated in even the most debilitated patients. It provides better exposure to lesions in the posterior lung fields and left lower lobe than median sternotomy. Clamshell thoracotomy has been shown to lengthen operative time and increase chest tube drainage and postoperative pain compared to median sternotomy,[13] but it has not been associated with a significant increase in morbidity or mortality compared to median sternotomy.[14]

Most recently, VATS has been advocated for pulmonary metastasectomy. VATS has the advantage of decreased pain and hospital stay compared to standard posterior lateral thoracotomy.[15] The largest disadvantage of the VATS approach is the lack of manual palpation of the lung. VATS for metastasectomy was prospectively evaluated by the MSKCC in the early 1990s.[16] Patients with one or two ipsilateral metastases on preoperative computed tomography (CT) scan were eligible for evaluation. They underwent complete resection by VATS, which was immediately followed by a thoracotomy for manual palpation of the lung. Over half of the patients had additional malignant lesions found at the thoracotomy. This study questioned the utility of VATS for metastasectomy because of the inaccuracy of preoperative staging to accurately identify all nodules. Manual palpation was thought to be vital to detecting and resecting all lesions. As radiographic technology advances with fine-cut helical CT scans, we are able to more accurately detect smaller and smaller lesions preoperatively. A more recent study found that helical CT scans are more sensitive than older scans and can accurately detect 82% of lesions and with 61.5% sensitivity for lesions less than 6mm.[17] Although a VATS trial similar to the one from MSKCC has not been repeated, many surgeons believe that as our radiographic technologies improve, VATS resection may be a viable alternative in certain histologies. Renal cell carcinomas and colorectal cancers tend to produce a smaller number of large nodules. Other histologies, especially sarcomas, may never be good candidates for VATS resection as they have a tendency to present with multiple small nodules, and may always require manual palpation to assure complete resection. It is important for the surgeon to remember that complete resection is the most important prognostic factor in patients undergoing pulmonary metastasectomy and therefore, a complete oncologic resection should never be sacrificed for the short-term benefits of a VATS approach.

Pulmonary metastasectomy should be done with the assistance of single-lung ventilation whenever possible. The lung should be thoroughly palpated, both inflated and completely deflated, to avoid missing any small nodules. The lungs should be completely examined and palpated before and after the resections by both members of the operating team. Although there is no formal margin required, 1cm circumferentially of grossly normal lung is recommended. Most metastasectomies are performed as a simple wedge resection with standard stapling device. Lesions on the flat surface of the lung, which do not lend themselves to stapled wedge resection, can be removed with precision electrocautery. With this technique, the lesion is cored out with a healthy margin, clipping and ligating large vessels during the dissection. Patients with deep lesions may require segmentectomy, lobectomy, or even pneumonectomy for complete resection.

TABLE 93.2. Long-term survival following complete resection according to disease-free interval (DFI).

DFI	N	Five-year survival (%)	Ten-year survival (%)	Median survival (months)
Overall	4,572	36	26	35
0–11 months	1,384	33	27	29
12–35 months	1,662	31	22	30
36+ months	1,416	45	29	45

Source: International Registry of Lung Metastasis (IRLM).

The value of concurrent lymph node dissection with pulmonary metastasectomy has not been well investigated. Mediastinal lymphadenectomy is a standard procedure for lung cancer resections but is not routinely performed during pulmonary metastasectomy. Mediastinal lymph node metastases, along with pulmonary metastases, carry a poor prognostic value,[18] but it is impossible to determine the true impact of lymphatic metastases on patients with resected pulmonary lesions, because lymphadenectomy has been performed in a small number of patients. If preoperative studies identify mediastinal lymph node involvement, most surgeons would agree that metastasectomy is not indicated. It is likely that PET scanning will help identify some radiographic occult lymph node metastases preoperatively to help provide improved patient selection.

International Registry of Lung Metastases (IRLM)

Over the past 40 years, pulmonary metastasectomy has become recognized as a potentially curative treatment for selected patients. To date, no controlled trial exists comparing metastasectomy to chemotherapy, radiation therapy, or best supportive care for patients with isolated pulmonary metastases, but historical data suggest that unresected lung metastases are uniformly fatal within 2 years.[19,20] IRLM pooled large numbers of unselected patients and obtained extensive follow-up from the major thoracic oncology centers worldwide. The meta-analysis of these data has helped to clarify the therapeutic benefit of pulmonary metastasectomy.

The ILMR project was launched in 1990 to combine and analyze the experience of major European and American thoracic surgery centers during the past 50 years. It created a database using a single form for each patient. The record included (1) patient identification, (2) features of the primary neoplasm, (3) description of each metastasectomy performed (sequential or staged thoracotomies were treated as a single metastasectomy), and (4) follow-up. Between 1991 and 1995, 5,290 patients were enrolled. Only 84 cases were excluded for incomplete data, leaving 5,206 evaluable patients. The largest series is from MSKCC, which submitted their consecutive series of all pulmonary metastasectomies performed in their institution from 1945 to 1995. Variables that were tested for significance included gender, age, number of resected and pathologically proven metastases, disease-free interval (DFI), histology, and site of the primary tumor. Survival was calculated from the time of the initial metastasectomy to the date of last follow-up.

Data from the registry confirmed that the morbidity from metastasectomy is very low and overall perioperative mortality was only 1%. The accuracy of preoperative radiologic testing was only 61%, with 25% of patients having more metastases at the time of resection and 14% having fewer lesions than suspected preoperatively. The accuracy of preoperative evaluation varied among histologies, with osteosarcoma frequently having a higher number of occult lesions, whereas colon cancer had the highest frequency of false-positive lesions.

Completeness of resection was the single most important prognostic factor following pulmonary metastasectomy. The actuarial survival after complete metastasectomy was 36% at 5 years, 26% at 10 years, and 22% at 15 years, with a median survival of 35 months. The median survival for patients with incomplete resections was 15 months; survival at 5 years was 13% and 7% at 10 years.

Disease-free interval (DFI) is the time between the treatment of the primary tumor and the appearance of metastases. Table 93.2 demonstrates 5- and 10-year survival according to DFI. The surprisingly good survival in patients with DFI less than 1 year is mainly due to the patients who presented with synchronous pulmonary metastases. Table 93.3 reports survival by the number of pathologically proven metastases. There was significant survival benefit for solitary lesions compared to multiple lesions. The probability of survival tends to decrease with the number of resected nodules, but very little survival difference was seen between patients who had 4 or more lesions and those with 10 or more lesions.

Table 93.4 reviews survival by primary diagnosis. Germ cell tumors had by far the best survival, 68% at 5 years and 63% at 10 years. It was apparent from the registry data that these represented a separate clinical entity because of the high frequency of complete pathologic response to chemotherapy. These patients were therefore excluded from the multivariate analysis of prognostic factors. Melanomas had the worst survival, 21% at 5 years and 14% at 10 years,

TABLE 93.3. Long-term survival following complete resection according to number of pathologically proven metastases (IRLM).

No. of metastases	N	Five-year survival (%)	Ten-year survival (%)	Median survival (months)
Overall	4,572	36	26	35
1	2,169	43	31	43
2–3	1,226	34	24	31
4+	1,123	27	19	27
10+	342	26	17	26

TABLE 93.4. Long-term survival following complete resection according to histology (International Registry of Lung Metastasis, IRLM).

Primary tumor	N	Five-year survival (%)	Ten-year survival (%)	Median survival (months)
Overall	4,572	36	26	35
Osteosarcoma	734	33	27	40
Soft tissue sarcoma	938	30	22	27
Colorectal	653	37	22	41
Breast	411	37	21	37
Renal cell	402	41	24	41
Melanoma	282	21	14	19
Germ cell	318	68	63	Not reached

with a median survival of 19 months. There was no significant difference in survival between epithelial tumors (37% at 5 years, 21% at 10 years) and sarcomas (31% at 5 years, 26% at 10 years). There were survival differences among the specific histologies of sarcoma and the various sites of epithelial cancers.

Of completely resected patients, 53% had a documented recurrence. Sarcomas (64%) and melanomas (64%) recurred more frequently than epithelial (46%) or germ cell tumors (26%). The majority of sarcomas relapsed in the lungs (66%), whereas 73% of melanoma relapses were extrathoracic. An intermediate pattern of relapse was seen in epithelial and germ cell tumors. The median time to recurrence was 10 months and was shorter in sarcomas (8 months) than epithelial tumors (12 months).

Twenty percent of patients underwent multiple metastasectomies. Repeat pulmonary metastasectomy was more common in sarcomas (53%) than in other histologies, as one might predict from their pattern of relapse. The median interval between first and second metastasectomy in sarcomas was 10 months. Long-term survival for patients who underwent repeat pulmonary metastasectomy was 44% at 5 years and 29% at 10 years. These survivals are better than those seen in patients who underwent a single operation (34% at 5 years and 25% at 10 years). Better survivals can be attributed to both the improved selection criteria of patients offered redo surgery (good performance status and limited disease) and the real salvage benefit of repeat resection.

One of the goals of the IRLM was to establish a new staging system that would be simple, discriminant, and valid across histologies. Complete resection was the single most important prognostic factor. The new classification system combined the DFI, number of nodules, and completeness of resection into a simplified reliable system that could be used to predict long-term survival across histologies. Among resectable lesions, a DFI greater than 36 months and solitary metastases were seen as independent risk factors for improved outcome. Table 93.5 demonstrates the four distinct prognostic groups based on these factors. The median survival for group I was 61 months, 34 months for group II, 24 months for group III, and 14 months for group IV (P less than 0.00001) The prognostic grouping was highly significant for the entire group and in each specific tumor histology. The log rank χ^2 was 131.8 for epithelial tumors, 118.8 for bone sarcomas, 77.4 for soft tissue sarcomas, and 29.6 for melanomas.

By combining data from the leading thoracic surgical centers, the IRLM was able to collect a large number of metastasectomies from a broad spectrum of primary diseases and with extensive follow-up. The analysis verified the low morbidity and mortality associated with metastasectomy and the inaccuracy of radiology studies to accurately stage patients. Thorough intraoperative staging by an experienced thoracic surgeon is required to optimize resection of all nodules. The proposed prognostic groups are based on easily available clinical data and represent a simple and discriminate system to classify these patients. Further confirmation of the validity of the system is planned.

TABLE 93.5. International Registry of Lung Metastasis (IRLM) system of prognostic grouping.

Group	*Description*
I	Resectable, no risk factors: DFI > 36 months and single metastasis
II	Resectable, one risk factor: DFI < 36 months *or* multiple metastases
III	Resectable, two risk factors: DFI < 36 months and multiple meastases
IV	Unresectable

Osteosarcoma

The disease model for surgical removal of pulmonary metastases is osteogenic sarcoma. High-grade osteosarcoma is a malignant bony tumor with a peak incidence in the second decade of life. Historical data demonstrate that although 80% of patients present with localized disease, 80% of those treated with amputation alone will develop pulmonary metastases within 2 years and none of those untreated will survive to 5 years.[21,22] In the absence of effective chemotherapy or radiotherapy, MSKCC led the way in developing a strategy for pulmonary metastasectomy in these young patients. In a series from 1971, 29 patients were treated with surgical metastasectomy; they demonstrated a 32% 5-year survival in the 22 patients who had a complete resection.[23]

Over the past two decades, the prognosis for patients with localized osteosarcoma has improved considerably with the development of effective chemotherapeutic regimens. The event-free survival for patients who present with localized disease, treated with neoadjuvant chemotherapy and resection, is estimated to be 44% to 78% at 5 years.[24,25] The lungs remain the most frequent site of recurrence, but an increased frequency of bony metastases is seen following chemotherapy.[26–28] Complete resection remains the most important prognostic factor following metastasectomy (Table 93.6).[25]

TABLE 93.6. Pulmonary metastasectomy for osteosarcoma.

Author	*Year*	*Institution*	*No. of patients*	*Complete resection: 5-year survival*	*Incomplete resection: 5-year survival*
Martini[23]	1971	MSKCC	140	45% (3-year)	5% (3-year)
Putnam[65]	1983	NCI	38	50%	0%
Huth[28]	1989	UCLA	77	23%	8%
Goorin[27]	1991	MIOS	52	60%	32%
Saeter[66]	1995	Norway	60	50%	0%
Thompson[67]	2002	University of Minnesota	21	38% (4-year)	10%
Ferrari[29]	2003	Italy	125	44%	0%

MSKCC, Memorial Sloan-Kettering Cancer Center; NCI, National Cancer Institute; UCLA, University of California at Los Angeles; MIOS, multiinstitutional osteosarcoma study.

TABLE 93.7. Pulmonary metastasectomy for soft tissue sarcoma.

Author	Year	Institution	No. of patients	Complete resection: 5-year survival	Incomplete resection: 5-year survival
Putman[68]	1984	NCI	67	18%	0%
Jabalons[69]	1989	NCI	57	35%	0%
Casson[70]	1992	MDACC	68	25%	NR
Verazin[71]	1992	Roswell Park	78	21%	0%
van Geel[72]	1996	EORT	255	35%	NR
Billingsley[32]	1999	MSKCC	213	37%	17%

MDACC, M.D. Anderson Cancer Center; EORT, European Organization for Research and Treatment of Cancer.

DFI and number of metastases found at resection have proven to be significant in numerous series. Neoadjuvant chemotherapy has led to an increased time to the development of lung metastases and a reduction in the number of lung lesions, helping to facilitate complete surgical resection.[26,27] The combination of effective systemic therapy and the refinement of surgical indication and techniques have greatly enhanced the outlook for these young patients. The role of second-line, salvage chemotherapy for recurrence is an area still being investigated.[29]

Soft Tissue Sarcoma

Soft tissue sarcomas are relatively uncommon, with 8,000 new cases and 4,600 deaths annually in the United States.[30] The lung is the most common site of metastases in patients with extremity soft tissue sarcomas; 20% of patients will develop isolated pulmonary metastases, and the majority of metastases occur in the first 2 years following diagnosis with a median time to development of 14 months.[31] Features of soft tissue sarcomas that are associated with a propensity to metastasize include extremity location, large size, and high grade.[32] The most common soft tissue tumors to develop pulmonary metastases are malignant fibrous histiocytoma (MFH) (23%), synovial-cell sarcoma (19%), and leiomyosarcoma (15%).[24]

Approximately one-third of patients are symptomatic at diagnosis.[33] The most common symptoms are cough and hemoptysis. The majority of patients are asymptomatic at diagnosis and have lesions detected on an abnormal chest radiograph or CT scan. Patients with soft tissue sarcomas are 10 times more likely to develop pulmonary metastases than a primary lung cancer,[34] and therefore, any new pulmonary lesions should be considered metastatic until proven otherwise.

Many series have documented survival benefit following metastasectomy in soft tissue sarcoma (Table 93.7). Complete resection is the most significant predictor of long-term survival. Attempts have been made to further identify prognostic markers in resectable patients. Factors that appear to be associated with improved survival include prolonged DFI, low histologic grade, young age, tumor depth, doubling time, number of nodules, MFH, and unilateral disease. Features associated with poor prognosis include liposarcoma, malignant peripheral nerve sheath tumor, and large tumor size.

Renal Cell Carcinoma

Renal cell carcinomas affect approximately 25,000 patients yearly in the United States, representing about 3% of all malignancies.[2] Up to one-third of patients have metastatic disease at the time of diagnosis,[35] and half of the remaining patients will develop metastases following nephrectomy.[36] The lungs are the second most common site of metastatic spread. The lack of effective chemotherapy, radiation therapy, or immunotherapy for metastatic renal cell carcinoma justifies an aggressive approach to surgical resection. Five-year survival for patients with unresected metastatic renal cell cancer is 2.7%.[37] Numerous series have been published on pulmonary metastasectomy for renal cell carcinoma, and 5-year survival rates range from 30% to 60% (Table 93.8). The studies are unanimous in the recognition that the completeness of resection is the most important factor affecting survival. The DFI, number of lesions, and lymph node involvement have less of a prognostic impact. Survival after

TABLE 93.8. Pulmonary metastasectomy for renal cell carcinoma.

Author	Year	Institution	No. of patients	Complete resection: 5-year survival	Incomplete resection: 5-year survival
Jett[2]	1983	Mayo	44	30%	25%
Pogrebniak[36]	1991	NIH/NCI	23	60%	30%
Cerfolio[73]	1994	Mayo	147	36%	NR
Fourquier[74]	1997	Marie-Lannelongue	50	44%	20%
Kavolius[75]	1998	MSKCC	211	44%	14%
Friedel[76]	1999	Gerlingen	93	39%	NR
Piltz[77]	2002	Munich	122	40%	0%
Pfannschmidt[78]	2002	Heidelberg	191	42%	22%

repeat thoracotomy for recurrent pulmonary metastases does not differ from survival following first complete resection. Pulmonary metastasectomy is a safe and effective treatment for metastatic renal cell carcinoma.

Colorectal Cancer

Colorectal cancer is one of the most common malignancies in the United States. It is the third most common cancer in both American men and women.[38] The lungs are the second most common site of metastases from colorectal cancers, but only 10% of patient with pulmonary disease have isolated pulmonary metastases and are possible candidates for resection.[39] The first pulmonary resection for metastatic colorectal cancer was performed by Blalock in 1944.[40]

There are numerous series of patients undergoing resection of pulmonary metastases from colorectal cancers with 5-year survivals ranging between 16% and 56% (Table 93.9). The most important prognostic factor in all series is the completeness of resection. Other significant predictors of survival in selected series include the number of metastases,[41–43] DFI,[44] and serum levels of carcinoembryonic antigen (CEA).[41,45] The location, stage, and grade of the primary tumor do not appear to have any influence on survival following metastasectomy.

Spread of colorectal cancers to the liver is very common, occurring in approximately 50,000 patients per year in the United States.[46] Similar to lung metastases, only a small proportion of patients with liver metastases are candidates for resection, but also similar to pulmonary metastases survival after hepatic metastasectomy is 25% to 40% at 5 years.[47] Colorectal cancer provides a unique therapeutic dilemma where patients can have surgically curable metastases in two different organs. Untreated, survival is dismal for either isolated pulmonary or hepatic metastases. Limiting surgical resection to patients with single-organ metastases may be denying some patients a chance for long-term survival. Several studies have been published addressing combined liver and lung resection for metastatic colorectal cancers (Table 93.10). The most common sequence of presentation is to have hepatic metastases that are resected and then develop lung metastases,[48] but these series also contain patients who presented with lung lesions first or simultaneous metastases. Survival following resection from both sites is comparable to survival from either site alone.

TABLE 93.9. Pulmonary metastasectomy for colorectal carcinoma.

Author	*Year*	*Institution*	*No. of patients*	*Complete resection: 5-year survival*
McCormack[79]	1992	MSKCC	144	44%
McAfee[41]	1992	Mayo	119	31%
Saclarides[43]	1993	Rush	23	16%
van Halteren[44]	1995	Netherlands	38	43%
Girard[45]	1996	France	86	24%
Okumura[42]	1996	Tokyo	111	45%
Saeter[66]	2002	Kansai	165	40%

Melanoma

Melanoma is widely recognized as the most lethal skin cancer. The lungs are the most common site of initial presentation of metastatic disease,[2] and 30% to 50% of patients with stage IV disease have pulmonary metastases.[49] Long-term survival for melanoma patients with pulmonary metastases is dismal with less than 5% surviving for 5 years.[50] Unfortunately, no effective chemotherapy, radiation, or immunotherapy exists. Surgery offers a small chance for control of disease. Numerous small series have documented occasional long-term survivors among patients who have undergone pulmonary resection for isolated metastases from melanoma (Table 93.11). The overall outcome for patients who undergo complete metastasectomy remains poor, and therefore, surgeons have continued to seek factors that will better identify patients who are likely to benefit from resection. Data from both Harpole et al.[50] and IRLM suggest that patients with complete resections, longer DFI, and solitary metastases do better overall. Progrebniak's series from the National Cancer Institute (NCI), demonstrated an important aspect of care in these patients in that 30% of patients in their series with new pulmonary nodule on serial studies were found to have nonmetastatic lesions at exploration.[36] The majority of these were benign. They thought that melanoma patients with a new pulmonary nodule who are surgical candidates should be explored for diagnosis and to attempt complete resection.

New and Evolving Treatments

Only a small proportion of patients with pulmonary metastases are candidates for metastasectomy. Many patients have disease isolated to the lungs but are either not fit candidates for thoracic surgery or have unresectable lesions. Many new and evolving treatments are being investigated for patients who are not candidates for standard resection.

TABLE 93.10. Hepatic and pulmonary metastasectomy for colorectal carcinoma.

Author	*Year*	*Institution*	*No. of patients*	*Complete resection*	*Median survival (months)*
Conlon and Minnard[88]	1996	MSKCC	33		24.5
Okumura[42]	1996	Tokyo	39	33%	30
Robinson[80]	1999	Cleveland Clinic	25	9%	16
Lehnert[81]	1999	Heidelberg	17	45% (3-year)	34
Enk[48]	2001	Mayo	58	30%	N/R

[a] Survival from time of last metastatic resection.

TABLE 93.11. Pulmonary metastasectomy for melanoma.

Author	*Year*	*Institution*	*No. of patients*	*Complete resection: 5-year survival*	*Median survival in months: complete resection*	*Incomplete resection: 5-year survival*
Mathisen[82]	1979	NIH/NCI	33	0%	12	0%
Pogrebniak[36]	1988	NIH/NCI	31	7%	13	10%
Wong[83]	1988	UCLA	47	31%	24	0%
Harpole[50]	1992	Duke	109	20%	20	10%
Leo[84]	2000	IRLM	328	22%	19	0%

Isolated Lung Perfusion

In general, systemic toxicity limits the amount of chemotherapy that can be given to an individual. New drug delivery systems, such as isolated pulmonary perfusion, may enhance chemotherapeutic treatment effects by increasing drug concentrations in the lung tissue and decreasing systemic toxicity. Isolated limb perfusion with hyperthermia and chemotherapy has become an accepted treatment strategy for locally advanced malignant melanoma. Animal studies have demonstrated that, with pulmonary artery and vein cannulation, the pulmonic vascular system can be isolated from the systemic system and chemotherapeutic agents can be infused at higher levels than systemically tolerable. This technique results in higher tissue concentrations within the lung.[51,52] Isolated pulmonary perfusion has been performed in clinical trials by using continuous infusion techniques. These procedures are cumbersome, but safe, producing elevated tissue concentration of drugs without associated systemic toxicity. Unfortunately, clinical responses have been variable (Table 93.12). Acute and late lung injury was noted in most series with a decrease in FEV_1 and diffusion capacity (DLCO). The pathophysiology of the lung injury may be secondary to elevated drug levels or to ischemia associated with the procedure. Modifications in perfusate solution could help to limit this injury.

Isolated lung perfusion may prove to be a useful system for gene delivery to the lung. Animal models have been used to study human tumor necrosis factor (TNF)-alpha gene delivery for the treatment of pulmonary sarcoma metastases.[53] The technique of isolated lung perfusion is still experimental. The ability to modulate the drug dose, concentration, and perfusate composition will help to provide safer and more effective outcomes. There remains a paucity of effective treatment for pulmonary metastases and, despite the lack of overwhelming clinical benefit to date, isolated lung perfusion warrants further clinical investigation.

Inhalation Therapy

Inhalation therapy has been used most commonly in the treatment of patients with pulmonary metastases from renal cell carcinoma. Inhaled interleukin 2 (IL-2) is given in doses of 18 to 36 million IUs, alone or in combination with other systemic therapy. It is associated with a decrease in the progression of pulmonary metastases in renal cell, ovary and breast carcinomas, and melanomas.[55] Therapy is well tolerated, the main toxicity being a dose-dependent cough. High-dose IL-2 (36 million IUs/day) with single-agent dacarbazine was studied in 27 patients with malignant melanoma.[48] Five patients had complete response and partial response was seen in 8 patients. Extrapulmonary metastases do not respond to treatment. Inhalational IL-2 appears to be a promising strategy that will allow prolonged therapeutic response and a potential long-term survival advantage to patients with isolated pulmonary metastasis with low toxicity.

Radiofrequency Ablation

Radiofrequency ablation (RFA) applies thermal energy via a catheter delivery system, resulting in coagulation necrosis. Its use is widely accepted for the treatment of unresectable liver tumors, and is now being explored for destruction of solid tumors in other locations, including the lung. Animal models investigating the histologic effects of RFA on pulmonary parenchyma revealed that tumors can be effectively ablated with minimal damage to surrounding lung.[56] A pilot study from the University of Pittsburgh, evaluated RFA in patients with unresectable lung tumors [5 with non-small cell lung cancer (NSCLC) and 13 with pulmonary metastases]. There was 1 death following treatment. A better radiographic response was seen in lesions smaller than 5 cm. After a mean follow-up of 6 months, lesions that had radiographic treatment effect did not demonstrate regrowth, but 9 of the 13 developed new sites of metastatic disease, and 6 (46%) died.[57]

TABLE 93.12. Isolated lung perfusion for pulmonary metastases.

Author	*Year*	*No. of patients*	*Agents*	*Complications*	*Response*
Johnston[54]	1995	8	Doxorubicin/CDDP	25%	0%
Ratto[85]	1996	6	Resection + CDDP	33%	N/A
Pass[86]	1996	15	TNF + interferon	20%	33%
Burt[52]	1998	8	Doxorubicin	0%	0%
Putnam[87]	2000	16	Doxorubicin	19%	6%

CDDP, cisplatin; TNF, tumor necrosis factor.

Pulmonic RFA is still new but it appears to be a promising treatment option for patients with isolated pulmonary metastases who are not resection candidates.

Stereotactic Radiosurgery

Stereotactic radiation is a method of delivering highly focused external-beam radiation using a compact fractionation schedule. The techniques are well established for intracranial neoplasms and have replaced surgical resection for many intracranial neoplasms but are a novel approach to treating tumors in the lung. Treatment uses a 6-Me LIAC (6 megavolt linear accelerator) on a robotic arm. A gold fiducial is percutaneously placed within pulmonary lesions to guide treatment and decrease treatment to surrounding tissue secondary to respiratory motion. Results from a Phase I trial at Stanford University, in patients with solitary lung tumors who were not candidates for resection (14 NSCLC, 9 metastases) show 25% stable disease, 40% partial response, and 35% complete response at median follow-up of 8 months.[58] Long-term follow-up is necessary to determine the overall toxicity and efficacy of treatment.

Conclusion

There is a wealth of retrospective data demonstrating the benefit of pulmonary metastasectomy compared to other treatment modalities for isolated pulmonary metastases, but there remains a lack of randomized clinical trials demonstrating the benefit. The IRLM has provided us with a large database with extensive follow-up to evaluate this issue. Data from the IRLM and countless smaller series demonstrate that metastasectomy can be performed with minimal morbidity and low mortality. In selected histologies, metastasectomy provides a survival advantage over other therapies. The completeness of resection is the single most significant prognostic variable across all histologies. The DFI and number of metastases appear to be the next most significant variables. Using these three variables, prognostic groups have been constructed, with patients with respectable single lesion and DFI greater than 36 months having the greatest chance for cure. The majority of patients treated with pulmonary metastasectomy will eventually die of their metastatic disease, and therefore work continues to refine selection criteria and on new treatment modalities.

References

1. Willis R. The spread of tumors in the human body. In: Pathology of Metastases. Boston: GK Hall, 1978:167–183.
2. Jett J, Hollinger CG, Zinsmeister AR, Pairolero PC. Pulmonary resection of metastatic renal cell carcinoma. Chest 1983;84(4): 442–445.
3. van Dongen JA, van Slooten EA. The surgical treatment of pulmonary metastases. Cancer Treat Rev 1978;5(1):29–48.
4. Divis G. Einbertrag zur operativen, behandlung der Lungengeschulste. Acta Chir Scand 1927;62:329–334.
5. Barney J, Churchill ED. Adenocarcinoma of the kidney with metastases to the lung cured by nephrectomy and lobectomy. J Urol 1939;42:269–276.
6. Alexander J, Haight C. Pulmonary resection for solitary metastatic sarcomas and carcinomas. Surg Gynecol Obstet 1947;85: 129–146.
7. Thromford NR, Woolner LB, Clagett OT. The surgical treatment of metastatic disease to the lungs. J Thorac Cardiovasc Surg 1965;49:357–363.
8. McCormack PM, Martini N. The changing role of surgery for pulmonary metastases. Ann Thorac Surg 1979;28(2):139–145.
9. Pastorino U, Buyse M, Friedel G, et al. Long-term results of lung metastasectomy: prognostic analyses based on 5206 cases. J Thorac Cardiovasc Surg 1997;113:37–49.
10. Rusch VW. Surgical techniques for pulmonary metastasectomy. Semin Thorac Cardiovasc Surg 2002;14(1):4–9.
11. Roth JA, Pass HI, Wesley MN, White D, Putnam JB, Seipp C. Comparison of median sternotomy and thoracotomy for resection of pulmonary metastases in patients with adult soft-tissue sarcomas. Ann Thorac Surg 1986;42(2):134–138.
12. Cooper JD. The evolution of techniques and indications for lung transplantation. Ann Surg 1990;212(3):249–255.
13. Shimizu N, Ando A, Matsutani T, Maruyama S, Date H, Teramoto S. Transsternal thoracotomy for bilateral pulmonary metastasis. J Surg Oncol 1992;50(2):105–109.
14. Bains MS, Ginsberg RJ, Jones WG, et al. The clamshell incision: an improved approach to bilateral pulmonary and mediastinal tumor. Ann Thorac Surg 1994;58(1):30–32.
15. Landreneau RJ, Hazelrigg SR, Mack MJ, et al. Postoperative pain-related morbidity: video-assisted thoracic surgery versus thoracotomy. Ann Thorac Surg 1993;56(6):1285–1289.
16. McCormack PM, Bains MS, Begg CB, et al. Role of video-assisted thoracic surgery in the treatment of pulmonary metastases: results of a prospective trial. Ann Thorac Surg 1996;62(1): 213–216.
17. Margaritora S, Porziella V, D'Andrilli A, et al. Pulmonary metastases: can accurate radiological evaluation avoid thoracotomic approach? Eur J Cardiothorac Surg 2002;21(6):1111–1114.
18. Ercan S, Nichols FC III, Trastek VF, et al. Prognostic significance of lymph node metastasis found during pulmonary metastasectomy for extrapulmonary carcinoma. Ann Thorac Surg 2004; 77(5):1786–1791.
19. Potter DA, Kinsella T, Glatstein E, et al. High-grade soft tissue sarcomas of the extremities. Cancer (Phila) 1986;58(1):190–205.
20. McCormack PM, Bains MS, Martini N. Surgical management of pulmonary metastases. In: Shui M, Brennan MF (eds) Surgical Management of Soft Tissue Sarcomas. Philadelphia: Lea & Febinger, 1989.
21. Friedman MA, Carter SK. The therapy of osteogenic sarcoma: current status and thoughts for the future. J Surg Oncol 1972; 4(5):482–510.
22. Marcove RC, Mike V, Hajek JV, Levin AG, Hutter RV. Osteogenic sarcoma under the age of twenty-one. A review of one hundred and forty-five operative cases. J Bone Joint Surg Am 1970;52(3):411–423.
23. Martini N, Huvos AG, Mike V, Marcove RC, Beattie EJ Jr. Multiple pulmonary resections in the treatment of osteogenic sarcoma. Ann Thorac Surg 1971;12(3):271–280.
24. Meyers PA, Gorlick R, Heller G, et al. Intensification of preoperative chemotherapy for osteogenic sarcoma: results of the Memorial Sloan-Kettering (T12) protocol. J Clin Oncol 1998; 16(7):2452–2458.
25. Souhami RL, Craft AW, van der Eijken JW, et al. Randomised trial of two regimens of chemotherapy in operable osteosarcoma: a study of the European Osteosarcoma Intergroup. Lancet 1997;350(9082):911–917.
26. Bacci G, Ruggieri P, Picci P, et al. Changing pattern of relapse in osteosarcoma of the extremities treated with adjuvant and neoadjuvant chemotherapy. J Chemother 1995;7(3):230–239.
27. Goorin AM, Shuster JJ, Baker A, Horowitz ME, Meyer WH, Link MP. Changing pattern of pulmonary metastases with adjuvant chemotherapy in patients with osteosarcoma: results from the

multiinstitutional osteosarcoma study. J Clin Oncol 1991;9(4): 600–605.
28. Huth JF, Eilber FR. Patterns of recurrence after resection of osteosarcoma of the extremity. Strategies for treatment of metastases. Arch Surg 1989;124(1):122–126.
29. Ferrari S, Briccoli A, Mercuri M, et al. Postrelapse survival in osteosarcoma of the extremities: prognostic factors for long-term survival. J Clin Oncol 2003;21(4):710–715.
30. Greenlee RT, Murray T, Bolden S, Wingo PA. Cancer statistics, 2000. CA Cancer J Clin 2000;50(1):7–33.
31. Gadd MA, Casper ES, Woodruff JM, McCormack PM, Brennan MF. Development and treatment of pulmonary metastases in adult patients with extremity soft tissue sarcoma. Ann Surg 1993;218(6):705–712.
32. Billingsley KG, Burt ME, Jara E, et al. Pulmonary metastases from soft tissue sarcoma: analysis of patterns of diseases and postmetastasis survival. Ann Surg 1999;229(5):602–610.
33. Whooley BP, Gibbs JF, Mooney MM, McGrath BE, Kraybill WG. Primary extremity sarcoma: what is the appropriate follow-up? Ann Surg Oncol 2000;7(1):9–14.
34. Rusch VW. Pulmonary metastasectomy. Current indications. Chest 1995;107(suppl 6):322S–331S.
35. Ritchie AW, deKernion JB. The natural history and clinical features of renal carcinoma. Semin Nephrol 1987;7(2):131–139.
36. Progrebniak HW, Hass G, Linehan M, Rosenberg SA, Pass HI. Renal cell carcinoma: Resection of solitary and multiple metastases. Ann Thorac Surg 1992;54:33–38.
37. The natural history of renal tumors. In: Riches EW (ed) Tumors of the Kidney and Ureter. Edinburgh: Churchill Livingston, 1984:124–134.
38. Skibber JM, Minsky BD, Hoff PM. Cancer of the colon. In: DeVita VT, Hellman S, Rosenberg SA (eds) Principles and Practice of Oncology. Philadelphia: Lippincott, Williams & Wilkins, 2001:1216–1271.
39. McCormack PM, Attiyeh FF. Resected pulmonary metastases from colorectal cancer. Dis Colon Rectum 1979;22(8):553–556.
40. Blalock A. Recent advances in surgery. N Engl J Med 1944;231: 261–267.
41. McAfee MK, Allen MS, Trastek VF, Ilstrup DM, Deschamps C, Pairolero PC. Colorectal lung metastases: results of surgical excision. Ann Thorac Surg 1992;53(5):780–785.
42. Okumura S, Kondo H, Tsuboi M, et al. Pulmonary resection for metastatic colorectal cancer: experiences with 159 patients. J Thorac Cardiovasc Surg 1996;112(4):867–874.
43. Saclarides TJ, Krueger BL, Szeluga DJ, Warren WH, Faber LP, Economou SG. Thoracotomy for colon and rectal cancer metastases. Dis Colon Rectum 1993;36(5):425–429.
44. van Halteren HK, van Geel AN, Hart AA, Zoetmulder FA. Pulmonary resection for metastases of colorectal origin. Chest 1995;107(6):1526–1531.
45. Girard P, Ducreux M, Baldeyrou P, et al. Surgery for lung metastases from colorectal cancer: analysis of prognostic factors. J Clin Oncol 1996;14(7):2047–2053.
46. Fong Y, Cohen AM, Fortner JG, et al. Liver resection for colorectal metastases. J Clin Oncol 1997;15(3):938–946.
47. Imamura H, Kawasaki S, Miyagawa S, Ikegami T, Kitamura H, Shimada R. Aggressive surgical approach to recurrent tumors after hepatectomy for metastatic spread of colorectal cancer to the liver. Surgery (St. Louis) 2000;127(5):528–535.
48. Enk AH, Nashan D, Rubben A, Knop J. High dose inhalation interleukin-2 therapy for lung metastases in patients with malignant melanoma. Cancer (Phila) 2000;88(9):2042–2046.
49. Coit DG. Role of surgery for metastatic malignant melanoma: a review. Semin Surg Oncol 1993;9(3):239–245.
50. Harpole DH Jr, Johnson CM, Wolfe WG, George SL, Seigler HF. Analysis of 945 cases of pulmonary metastatic melanoma. J Thorac Cardiovasc Surg 1992;103(4):743–748.
51. Li TS, Sugi K, Ueda K, Nawata K, Nawata S, Esato K. Isolated lung perfusion with cisplatin in a rat lung solitary tumor nodule model. Anticancer Res 1998;18(6A):4171–4176.
52. Weksler B, Burt M. Isolated lung perfusion with antineoplastic agents for pulmonary metastases. Chest Surg Clin N Am 1998; 8(1):157–182.
53. Brooks AD, Ng B, Liu D, et al. Specific organ gene transfer in vivo by regional organ perfusion with herpes viral amplicon vectors: implications for local gene therapy. Surgery (St. Louis) 2001;129(3):324–334.
54. Johnston MR, Minchen RF, Dawson CA. Lung perfusion with chemotherapy in patients with unresectable metastatic sarcoma. J Thorac Cardiovasc Surg 1995;110(2):368–373.
55. Huland E, Heinzer H, Huland H, Yung R. Overview of interleukin-2 inhalation therapy. Cancer J Sci Am 2000;6(suppl 1): S104–S112.
56. Putnam JB, Thomsen SL, Siegenthal M. Theraputic implications of heat-induced lung injury. Crit Rev Optical Sci Technol 2000; 75:139–160.
57. Herrera LJ, Fernando HC, Perry Y, NA et al. Radiofrequency ablation of pulmonary malignant tumors in nonsurgical candidates. J Thorac Cardiovasc Surg 2003;125(4):929–937.
58. Le Q, Ho A, Cotrutz C, et al. Single fraction stereotactic radiosurgery (SFSR) for lung tumors: a phase I dose escalation trial. Presented at American Society of Clincal Oncology 40th Annual Meeting, New Orleans, LA, June 2004.
59. Hazelrigg SR, Landreneau RJ, Boley TM, et al. The effect of muscle-sparing versus standard posterolateral thoracotomy on pulmonary function, muscle strength, and postoperative pain. J Thorac Cardiovasc Surg 1991;101(3):394–400.
60. Ponn RB, Ferneini A, D'Agostino RS, Toole AL, Stern H. Comparison of late pulmonary function after posterolateral and muscle-sparing thoracotomy. Ann Thorac Surg 1992;53(4):675–679.
61. Hazelrigg SR, Naunheim K, Auer JE, Seifert PE. Combined median sternotomy and video-assisted thoracoscopic resection of pulmonary metastases. Chest 1993;104(3):956–958.
62. Johnston MR. Median sternotomy for resection of pulmonary metastases. J Thorac Cardiovasc Surg 1983;85(4):516–522.
63. Dowling RD, Keenan RJ, Ferson PF, Landreneau RJ. Video-assisted thoracoscopic resection of pulmonary metastases. Ann Thorac Surg 1993;56(3):772–775.
64. Hazelrigg SR, Nunchuck SK, LoCicero J III. Video Assisted Thoracic Surgery Study Group data. Ann Thorac Surg 1993;56(5): 1039–1043.
65. Putnam JB Jr, Roth JA, Wesley MN, Johnston MR, Rosenberg SA. Survival following aggressive resection of pulmonary metastases from osteogenic sarcoma: analysis of prognostic factors. Ann Thorac Surg 1983;36(5):516–523.
66. Saeter G, Hoie J, Stenwig AE, Johansson AK, Hannisdal E, Solheim OP. Systemic relapse of patients with osteogenic sarcoma. Prognostic factors for long-term survival. Cancer (Phila) 1995;75(5):1084–1093.
67. Thompson RC Jr, Cheng EY, Clohisy DR, Perentesis J, Manivel C, Le CT. Results of treatment for metastatic osteosarcoma with neoadjuvant chemotherapy and surgery. Clin Orthop 2002;397: 240–247.
68. Putnam JB Jr, Roth JA, Wesley MN, Johnston MR, Rosenberg SA. Analysis of prognostic factors in patients undergoing resection of pulmonary metastases from soft tissue sarcomas. J Thorac Cardiovasc Surg 1984;87(2):260–268.
69. Jablons D, Steinberg SM, Roth J, Pittaluga S, Rosenberg SA, Pass HI. Metastasectomy for soft tissue sarcoma. Further evidence for efficacy and prognostic indicators. J Thorac Cardiovasc Surg 1989;97(5):695–705.

70. Casson AG, Putnam JB, Natarajan G, et al. Five-year survival after pulmonary metastasectomy for adult soft tissue sarcoma. Cancer (Phila) 1992;69(3):662–668.
71. Verazin GT, Warneke JA, Driscoll DL, Karakousis C, Petrelli NJ, Takita H. Resection of lung metastases from soft-tissue sarcomas. A multivariate analysis. Arch Surg 1992;127(12):1407–1411.
72. van Geel AN, Pastorino U, Jauch KW, et al. Surgical treatment of lung metastases: The European Organization for Research and Treatment of Cancer—Soft Tissue and Bone Sarcoma Group study of 255 patients. Cancer (Phila) 1996;77(4):675–682.
73. Cerfolio RJ, Allen MS, Deschamps C, et al. Pulmonary resection of metastatic renal cell carcinoma. Ann Thorac Surg 1994;57(2):339–344.
74. Fourquier P, Regnard JF, Rea S, Levi JF, Levasseur P. Lung metastases of renal cell carcinoma: results of surgical resection. Eur J Cardiothorac Surg 1997;11(1):17–21.
75. Kavolius JP, Mastorakos DP, Pavlovich C, Russo P, Burt ME, Brady MS. Resection of metastatic renal cell carcinoma. J Clin Oncol 1998;16(6):2261–2266.
76. Friedel G, Hurtgen M, Penzenstadler M, Kyriss T, Toomes H. Resection of pulmonary metastases from renal cell carcinoma. Anticancer Res 1999;19(2C):1593–1596.
77. Piltz S, Meimarakis G, Wichmann MW, Hatz R, Schildberg FW, Fuerst H. Long-term results after pulmonary resection of renal cell carcinoma metastases. Ann Thorac Surg 2002;73(4):1082–1087.
78. Pfannschmidt J, Hoffmann H, Muley T, Krysa S, Trainer C, Dienemann H. Prognostic factors for survival after pulmonary resection of metastatic renal cell carcinoma. Ann Thorac Surg 2002;74(5):1653–1657.
79. McCormack PM, Burt ME, Bains MS, Martini N, Rusch VW, Ginsberg RJ. Lung resection for colorectal metastases. 10-year results. Arch Surg 1992;127(12):1403–1406.
80. Robinson BJ, Rice TW, Strong SA, Rybicki LA, Blackstone EH. Is resection of pulmonary and hepatic metastases warranted in patients with colorectal cancer? J Thorac Cardiovasc Surg 1999;117(1):66–75.
81. Lehnert T, Knaebel HP, Duck M, Bulzebruck H, Herfarth C. Sequential hepatic and pulmonary resections for metastatic colorectal cancer. Br J Surg 1999;86(2):241–243.
82. Mathisen DJ, Flye MW, Peabody J. The role of thoracotomy in the management of pulmonary metastases from malignant melanoma. Ann Thorac Surg 1979;27:295–299.
83. Wong JH, Euhus DM, Morton DL. Surgical resection for metastatic melanoma to the lung. Arch Surg 1988;123(9):1091–1095.
84. Leo F, Cagini L, Rocmans P, et al. Lung metastases from melanoma: when is surgical treatment warranted? Br J Cancer 2000;83(5):569–572.
85. Ratto GB, Toma S, Civalleri D, et al. Isolated lung perfusion with platinum in the treatment of pulmonary metastases from soft tissue sarcomas. J Thorac Cardiovasc Surg 1996;112(3):614–622.
86. Pass HI, Mew DJ, Kranda KC, Temeck BK, Donington JS, Rosenberg SA. Isolated lung perfusion with tumor necrosis factor for pulmonary metastases. Ann Thorac Surg 1996;61(6):1609–1617.
87. Putnam JB, Benjamin RS, Rha SJ. Early results of isolated single lung perfusion for unresectable sarcomatous metastases. Presented at the American Association of Thoracic Surgery Annual Meeting, Toronto, Canada, April 2000.
88. Conlon KC, Minnard EA. The value of laparoscopic staging in upper gastrointestinal malignancy. Oncologist 1997;2:10–17.

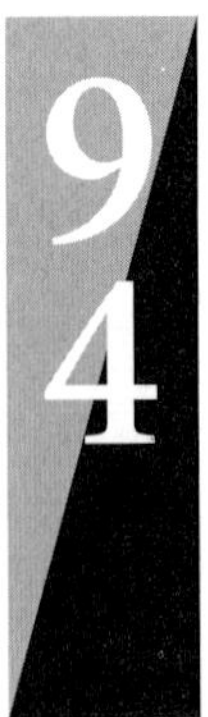

Surgical and Regional Therapy for Liver Metastases

Kenneth K. Tanabe and Sam S. Yoon

The liver is a frequent site of metastases from solid tumors and the most common site of distant metastases from colon and rectal cancer. Death from colon and rectal cancer is usually a result of metastatic disease. In one study, more than one-half of patients who died of colon and rectal cancer had liver metastases at autopsy, and the majority of these patients died as a result of their metastatic liver disease.[1] Unlike many types of cancer, however, the presence of distant metastases from colon and rectal cancer does not necessarily preclude curative treatment. Nearly 40% of patients with colon and rectal cancer and hematogenous metastases have disease that is predominantly in the liver.[2] Moreover, in a subpopulation of patients, the number of lesions is limited. Accordingly, there exists a strong rationale for regional therapies directed specifically against colon and rectal cancer liver metastases. This pattern of metastases is rarely observed in other cancers.

Resection is the most effective regional therapy for patients with colon and rectal cancer liver metastases, and this treatment leads to long-term survival in a defined subset of patients. Other regional therapies, such as cryosurgery, radiofrequency ablation (RFA), and hepatic artery infusion (HAI) chemotherapy, have been used, mainly for patients whose liver metastases are unresectable. Although ablative therapies and HAI chemotherapy hold promise, their ability to either improve quality of life or overall survival has not been convincingly demonstrated in prospective trials. Regional hepatic therapies are of much less value for patients with liver metastases from other types of cancer. Accordingly, this chapter focuses mainly on regional therapies for patients with colon and rectal cancer.

Natural History of Colon and Rectal Cancer

Understanding the natural history of colon and rectal cancer liver metastases sets a framework from which to assess the value of various treatments. Natural history data are increasingly more difficult to come by, as the vast majority of patients with this condition are treated with some form of therapy. Thus, many of the data on natural history come from studies conducted primarily in the 1960s and 1970s. Median survival for patients with colon and rectal cancer liver metastases was found to be between 5 and 9 months.[3–8] However, in these older studies, the majority of patients had advanced disease diagnosed without the advantage of modern-day imaging techniques. A few retrospective studies have assessed the survival of patients with potentially resectable colon and rectal cancer liver metastases that were left untreated. Wilson and Adson reported no 5-year survivors among patients with untreated but potentially resectable liver metastases compared to a 28% 5-year survival for patients with resected liver metastases.[9] A subsequent study found 5-year survival rates in similar groups of patients to be 2% and 25%, respectively.[10] In another study, patients with untreated but potentially resectable liver metastases had a mean survival of 21.3 months with only 1 of 13 patients surviving 5 years.[11] Wanebo et al. found that patients with an untreated single liver metastasis had a median survival of 19 months and no patients survived 5 years, whereas patients with a resected single liver metastasis had a median survival of 36 months and 25% of patients survived 5 years.[12]

Conclusions that can be reached from these studies are limited because of their retrospective patient identification and relatively insensitive methods for assessment of extent of disease. However, one can conclude that patients with a limited number of liver metastases survive longer than patients with more extensive liver metastases. Another conclusion is that 5-year survival is highly uncommon for patients with untreated liver metastases from colon and rectal cancer. Improvements in the quality of imaging in more recent years combined with more widespread use of imaging has led to earlier detection of liver metastases in the years since these original studies on natural history. Accordingly, recent "improvements" in the natural history of colon and rectal carcinoma liver metastases are expected solely as a result of earlier diagnosis.

Patient Evaluation

One of the greatest challenges to the decision-making skills of a surgeon comes with intraoperative detection of colon or rectal cancer liver metastases. The decision whether to include regional therapy during surgery for the primary tumor is a function of many variables: the surgeon's experience, the anatomic location of the liver lesions, the thoroughness and quality of intraoperative assessment of the distribution of liver metastases, the location of the primary tumor and the difficulty of the operation to remove the primary tumor, the anticipated morbidity of adding a regional therapy to the operation, and an understanding of the values and goals of the patient and family based on preoperative discussions. A decision whether or not to intraoperatively biopsy a liver lesion should be made with careful consideration of the consequences. In patients with clinically obvious liver metastases that are clearly not candidates for curative hepatectomy, core biopsy or incisional biopsy of one lesion to histologically confirm its nature is indicated. In contrast, in a patient with potentially resectable liver metastases, biopsy is not justified if the lesions appear to be obvious metastases based on clinical inspection. The risk of implanting tumor cells into the abdominal cavity or abdominal wound after an incisional biopsy, represents an unnecessary risk in a patient that has the opportunity to undergo potentially curative hepatectomy.

For patients who will undergo systemic chemotherapy rather than regional therapy as their treatment, mere confirmation of the presence and volume of metastases on computed tomography (CT) scan is sufficient. But when considering regional treatment strategies, patient evaluation necessarily focuses on evaluation of the extent and anatomic distribution of anatomic disease, the presence or absence of extrahepatic disease, underlying liver function, and medical comorbidity.

Candidates for regional therapies, including liver resection, should undergo a detailed history and physical examination, hematology and chemistry panels, liver function tests, chest X-ray, and abdominal and pelvic CT scans. Physical findings and clinical symptoms are the least reliable and least sensitive method of diagnosing liver metastases. An elevated carcinoembryonic antigen (CEA) value may be the first sign of colon or rectal cancer liver metastases and may hold prognostic value.[13,14]

In recognition that 5% of patients with colon and rectal cancer develop metachronous primary colon and rectal cancers,[15] strong consideration should be given to colonoscopy if not done within the past 12 to 24 months to exclude recurrence of the original primary colon and rectal cancer or development of a second primary colon and rectal cancer.

Chest CT scans in patients considered for regional therapy of liver metastases are of small but defined benefit in the setting of a normal chest X-ray. A retrospective study of patients with colon and rectal cancer liver metastases, without evidence of pulmonary metastases on chest X-ray, demonstrated that chest CT had a positive yield of only 4% and a positive predictive value of 36% for lung metastases.[16] However, if one modifies the manner in which these data are integrated into patient management decisions, the value to improving patient care is greater than that suggested by the authors of this study. If one sets a higher threshold for chest CT findings that alter management, the specificity will consequently improve. Along those lines, the writers of this chapter routinely obtain chest CT scans in patients considered for hepatic regional therapy. Treatment decisions are altered for findings that have a high probability of representing pulmonary metastatic disease. In patients with indeterminate findings, such as small, nonspecific lesions, management is not altered and the study serves as a baseline for future comparison.

For liver resection and ablation therapies, precise anatomic localization of liver tumors is important. Magnetic resonance imaging (MRI), CT, and intraoperative ultrasound are used frequently for this purpose and have been compared in numerous studies.[17–31] Positron emission tomography (PET) studies provide a physiologic survey for hypermetabolic tumors to complement these anatomic imaging studies. Imaging technology continues to rapidly improve. For example, faster image acquisition times, greater numbers of detectors on CT scanners (e.g., multidetector CT), postprocessing algorithms, and MRI contrast agents have dramatically improved image quality.

Abdominal CT scans remain the most commonly used modality for the assessment of the number, size, and anatomic distribution of liver metastases. Although normal liver is perfused primarily by the portal vein, liver metastases are perfused principally by the hepatic artery.[32] Therefore, on CT images obtained during the portal venous phase following intravenous contrast administration, hypoattenuated liver metastases are more easily recognized.[33]

MRI is being increasingly utilized for the diagnosis and characterization of liver lesions, particularly now that liver-specific contrast agents and dynamic scanning have been incorporated. Additional improvements in MRI, include availability of high field strength magnets, use of phased array coils, multiplanar capability, breath-hold acquisition, fat saturation, and three-dimensional imaging. Liver-specific contrast agents increase the imaging window for evaluation of liver and thus permit acquisition of high-resolution thin sections through liver. One liver-specific contrast agent, manganese pyridoxyl diphosphate (Mn-DPDP), is a paramagnetic agent taken up preferentially by hepatocytes and excreted in the bile. Normal liver parenchyma is markedly enhanced on T_1-weighted images, whereas metastases do not enhance.[34]

PET imaging has improved markedly over the past decade, and many centers routinely incorporate PET imaging results into their decisions on whether to pursue regional therapy. Many studies have focused on the diagnostic yield of fluorodeoxyglucose (FDG)-PET in staging patients with liver metastases from colon and rectal cancer, but have generally suffered from retrospective analysis concerning clinical management decisions.[24–31] In a prospective study of 51 patients analyzed for resection of colon and rectal cancer liver metastases by conventional diagnostic imaging and FDG-PET, clinical management decisions based on conventional diagnostic imaging were changed in 10 (20%) of 51 patients after FDG-PET findings were known. Eight patients were spared unwarranted liver resection or laparotomy, and 2 other patients were identified as candidates for liver resection. One patient was falsely upstaged.[35]

Transabdominal ultrasound is a relatively inexpensive modality but misses up to 50% of liver metastases.[36] It has essentially no role in the preoperative evaluation of potential liver resection candidates. However, many studies have shown the superiority of intraoperative ultrasound (IOUS) in the detection of liver lesions as compared to helical CT or MRI.[37–43] In addition, IOUS findings have been observed to change surgical management in 11% to 33% of patients.[37–43] The proportion of patients in which IOUS changes management may be dropping as a result of improvements in MRI imaging.[44,45] In a study of 79 patients treated at the Massachusetts General Hospital (MGH) who underwent

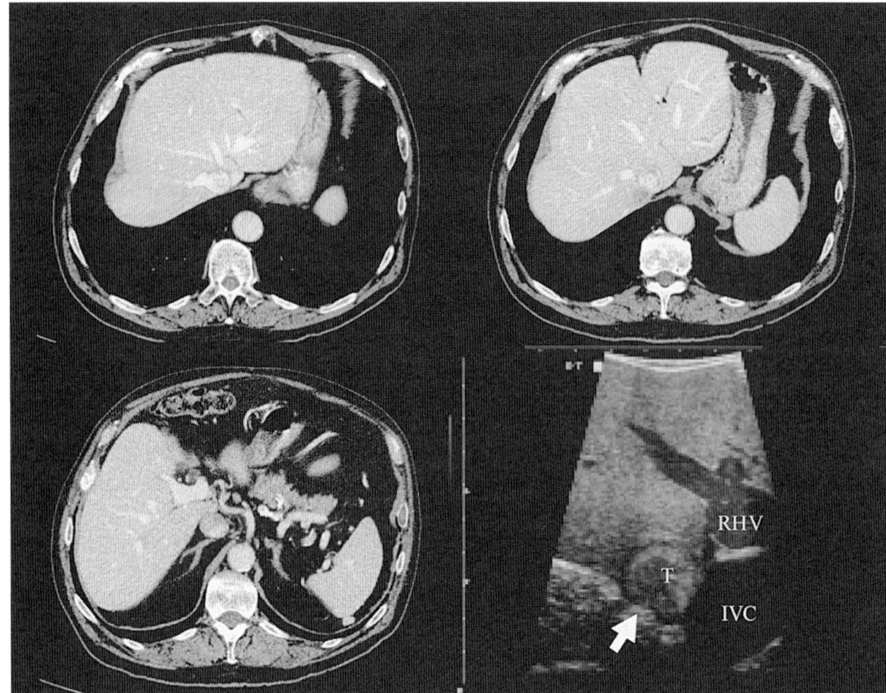

FIGURE 94.1. Intraoperative ultrasound image demonstrating the relationship between the tumor (*T*) located in segment VII and the inferior vena cava (*IVC*) and right hepatic vein (*RHV*). (By permission of Yoon SS, Tanabe KK. In: Cancer of the Lower Gastrointestinal Tract. London: Decker, 2001.)

contrast-enhanced MRI examination within 6 weeks of surgery, 10 had unsuspected liver metastases detected by IOUS examination. Surgical management was altered in only 3 of these patients by these findings.[44] Although the likelihood of new findings with IOUS examination is low, this imaging modality has other advantages. IOUS defines the location of hepatic vessels to allow segmental localization and accurately assesses the anatomic relationship between hepatic lesions and blood vessels (Figure 94.1). Additionally, small subcentimeter hepatic lesions, which could not be characterized on preoperative MRI, can be characterized on IOUS. IOUS guidance is required for RFA (see following) and aids with biopsy of small liver lesions. Most liver surgeons perform IOUS in all patients who undergo resection of colon or rectal carcinoma liver metastases.

Angiograms were once required preoperatively for patients who may undergo placement of a hepatic artery infusion pump. However, recent studies have demonstrated the accuracy of CT angiograms in which the hepatic arterial anatomy is reconstructed from either MRI or CT scans.[46,47]

Laparoscopy, sometimes combined with laparoscopic ultrasound, is increasingly used for preoperative evaluation of metastatic disease. Because the quality of liver imaging with CT or MRI scan has improved so dramatically over the past decade, the principal value of laparoscopy is now for detection of radiographically occult peritoneal metastases. Laparoscopy with laparoscopic ultrasound may change the intraoperative treatment plan.[48] In one study of 24 patients with liver tumors judged preoperatively to be resectable by conventional imaging studies, laparoscopy, combined with laparoscopic ultrasound, identified 6 patients who were in fact unresectable and avoided laparotomy in these patients.[49] The frequency with which laparoscopic findings alter intraoperative management is clearly a function of the quality of other imaging used before laparoscopy. The writers of this chapter have found a much lower incidence of unresectable metastases during laparotomy, when MRI with Mn-DPDP is used as the primary preoperative imaging study.[44]

Liver Resection

Techniques

Liver resections are performed based on the liver's functional anatomy as described by Couinaud,[50] who described anatomic division of the liver into eight segments defined by hepatic veins and portal vessels (Figure 94.2). In addition to the main hepatic veins, small hepatic veins drain directly from the posterior surface of the liver (including the caudate) directly into the inferior vena cava. The left and right triangular ligaments, coronary ligament, and the falciform ligament secure the liver to the diaphragm. Precise knowledge of the surgical anatomy of the liver, its blood vessels, and its biliary drainage system are mandatory for liver surgery.

The commonly performed major hepatic resections (Figure 94.3) include right hepatectomy, left hepatectomy, right trisegmentectomy (sparing segments II and III), left trisegmentectomy (sparing segments VI and VII), and left lateral segmentectomy (resection of segments II and III).[51,52] There is no advantage to performing a major resection when removal of one or more segments can eradicate all metastases with an adequate margin. In fact, often one or more segmental resections can spare more normal liver than a major resection or allow resection of metastases not encompassed by a traditional major resection. Anatomic segments of the liver can be delineated intraoperatively to allow removal of individual segments. In the absence of underlying liver dysfunc-

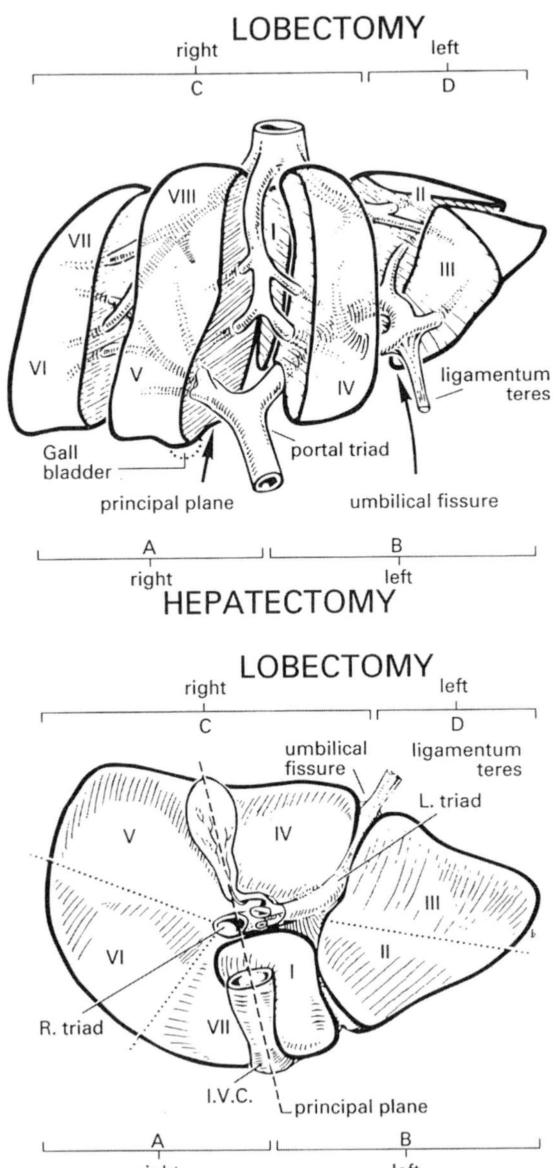

FIGURE 94.2. Functional anatomy of the liver. A schematic view of the liver demonstrates segments I–VIII, as described by Couinaud. (Adapted from Blumgart,[51] by permission of Churchill Livingstone.)

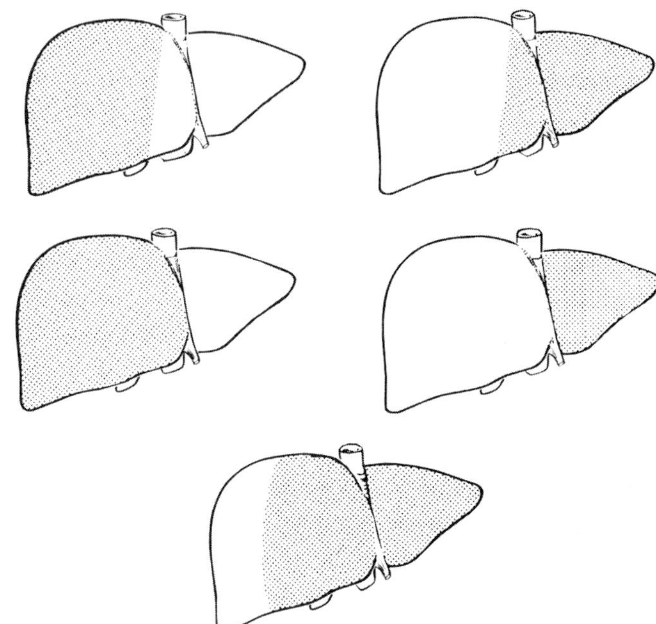

FIGURE 94.3. Commonly performed liver resections.

tion, up to 75% of the liver can be removed without subsequent hepatic failure.[53]

The operation to resect liver metastases starts with an exploratory laparotomy. Attention is paid to possible extrahepatic sites of disease, such as portal lymph nodes and peritoneum, and any suspicious areas are biopsied for frozen section analysis. The liver is then fully mobilized by dissection of its supporting ligaments and palpated to identify lesions. Intraoperative ultrasonography is performed to identify unsuspected metastases and to determine the anatomic relationship between metastases and major vascular structures.[44,45]

In situations where the tumors are located well away from the porta hepatis, the entire right or left portal pedicle may be ligated en masse away from the hepatic duct confluence, thus avoiding problems with anatomic variations in this area.[54] Following liver mobilization, the hilar plate is lowered with sharp dissection. To isolate the main right portal pedicle, incisions into the liver are made in the gallbladder fossa and in the caudate lobe immediately parallel to and 5 mm to the right of the inferior vena cava (Figure 94.4). An umbilical tape is passed around to completely encircle the portal pedicle, which may be either clamped or stapled with a TI-30 or Endo GIA stapler with a vascular cartridge (Figure 94.5). It is important to keep the umbilical tape between the stapler and the confluence of the hepatic ducts to avoid injury to the left hepatic duct. It is also important to have the right liver fully

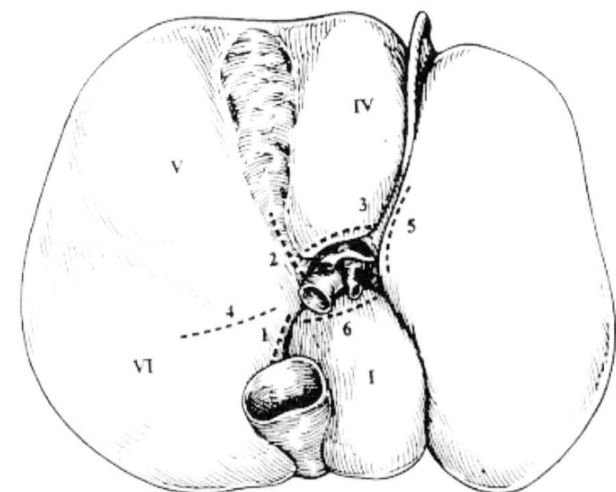

FIGURE 94.4. Sites for hepatotomy in portal pedicle isolation. The undersurface of the liver is illustrated. The *dotted lines* indicate sites for hepatotomy if control of the intrahepatic portal pedicles is desired. Incision at *3* allows lowering of the hilar plate. Incisions at *1* and *2* allow control of the main right pedicle. Incisions at *1* and *4* allow control of the right posterior pedicle. Incisions at *2* and *4* allow control of the right anterior pedicle. Incisions at *3* and *5* allow control of the left pedicle. (From Fong and Blumgart,[54] by permission of *Journal of the American College of Surgeons*.)

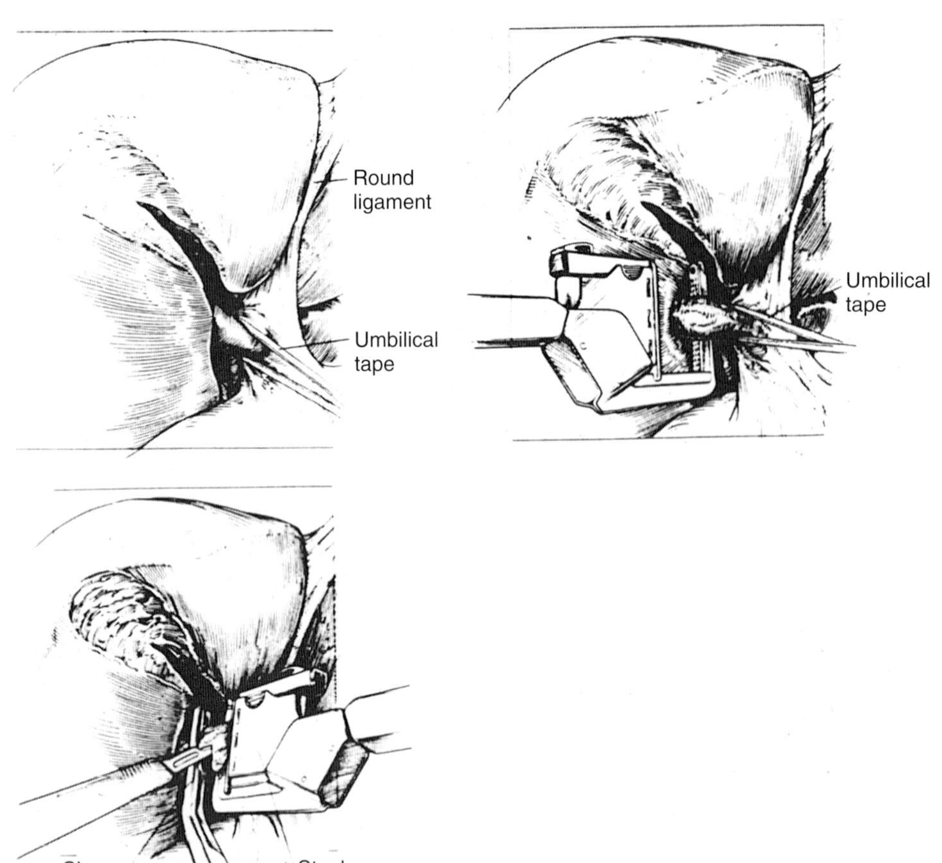

FIGURE 94.5. Control of the right portal pedicle. After an umbilical tape is passed around the main pedicle, it is retracted medially and the stapler is placed away from the bifurcation to avoid injury to the hilus. A clamp is subsequently placed to control bleeding from the specimen side. (From Fong and Blumgart,[54] by permission of *Journal of the American College of Surgeons*.)

mobilized before performing this maneuver, as it is possible to inadvertently injure a hepatic vein. The left main portal pedicle may be similarly ligated en masse by incising the liver at the base of segment IV anterior to the left portal pedicle and incising the liver in the caudate lobe posterior to the left portal pedicle.[54]

Following control of liver inflow, the liver outflow can be controlled by division of the hepatic veins. For right hepatectomy, before division of the right hepatic vein, short hepatic veins that drain directly from the caudate lobe into the vena cava are first divided. It is important to identify and avoid injury to the right adrenal vein. A ligament from the right lobe of the liver arching across the lateral aspect of the vena cava just inferior to the right hepatic vein is identified and sharply divided to gain full access to the right hepatic vein. It is safe and usually simple to divide the right hepatic vein itself using a laparoscopic Endo GIA 30 stapler with a vascular cartridge (Figure 94.6). For left hepatectomy, the left lateral segment is rotated to the right and the gastrohepatic ligament and ligamentum venosum are divided close to its entry to the left vein. A tunnel is then formed to incorporate the left hepatic vein. The laparoscopic Endo GIA 30 stapler may also be used to transect the left hepatic vein (Figure 94.7). Vascular control of the suprahepatic and infrahepatic vena cava should be obtained before isolation of the hepatic veins if the size and location of metastases reduces visualization and exposure of the hepatic veins.

Whether performing a traditional major resection or one or more segmental resections, the goal of the operation is

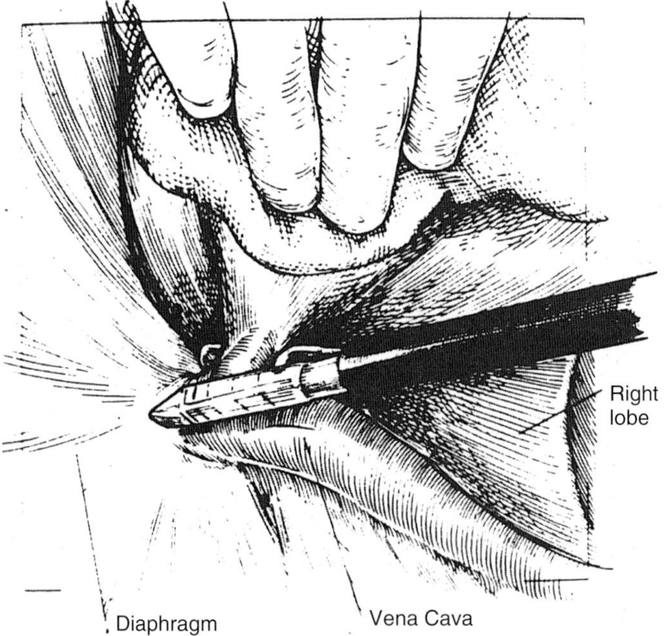

FIGURE 94.6. Stapling the right hepatic vein. The liver is rotated clockwise to provide exposure to place an Endo GIA 30 vascular stapler to the junction of the right hepatic vein and vena cava. (From Fong and Blumgart,[54] by permission of *Journal of the American College of Surgeons*.)

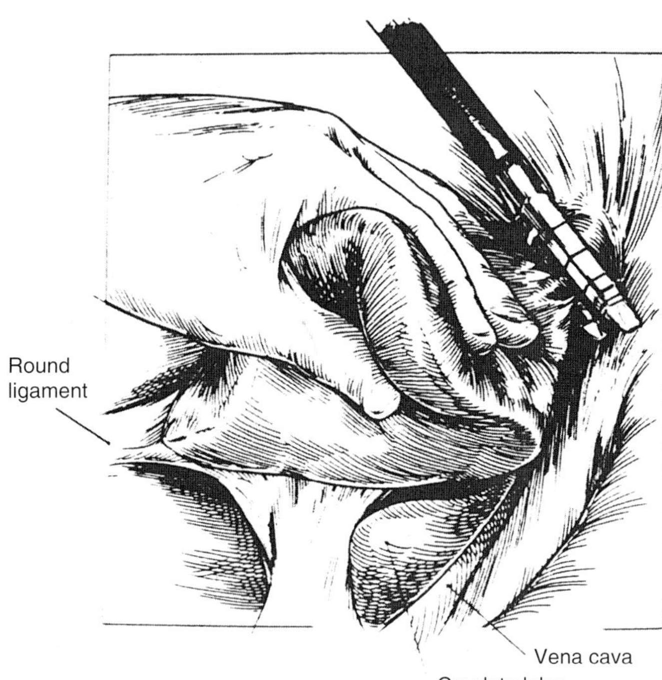

FIGURE 94.7. Stapling the left hepatic vein. The liver is rotated to the right and an Endo GIA 30 vascular stapler is applied at the junction of the left hepatic vein and the vena cava. (From Fong and Blumgart,[54] by permission of *Journal of the American College of Surgeons*.)

complete removal of all metastases with at least a 1 cm tumor-free margin. Recognition of hepatic veins is critical in determining which segments may be surgically excised. A large inferior right hepatic vein is present in approximately 20% of individuals and is usually identified on preoperative MRI or CT images (Figure 94.8). The presence of this vein permits resection of segments VII and VIII without sacrifice of segments V and VI. With the use of IOUS, the anatomic segments are quickly and accurately delineated.

There are various techniques to divide hepatic parenchyma (Table 94.1). The manner with which liver tissue is divided should achieve several objectives. The method ideally should allow visualization of blood vessels and bile ducts before their transection to allow their ligation. The method should be hemostatic and avoid bile leaks. The method should avoid devascularization of large zones of remnant liver and should allow creation of a crisply defined transection plane. Clamp fracture, ultrasonic surgical aspiration, water-jet dissection, and focused RFA dissection are methods that achieve all these goals. Finger fracture is effective but cannot create the precise transection plane that is sometimes necessary. A prospective randomized trial of clamp fracture versus ultrasonic dissection demonstrated no significant difference between the two methods in blood loss or transection time.[55]

The skill with which the liver parenchyma is transected is an important factor that influences blood loss. In addition, several surgical maneuvers can be used to minimize blood loss. Transient portal inflow occlusion during parenchymal transection is well tolerated and reduces blood loss.[56] Surgery

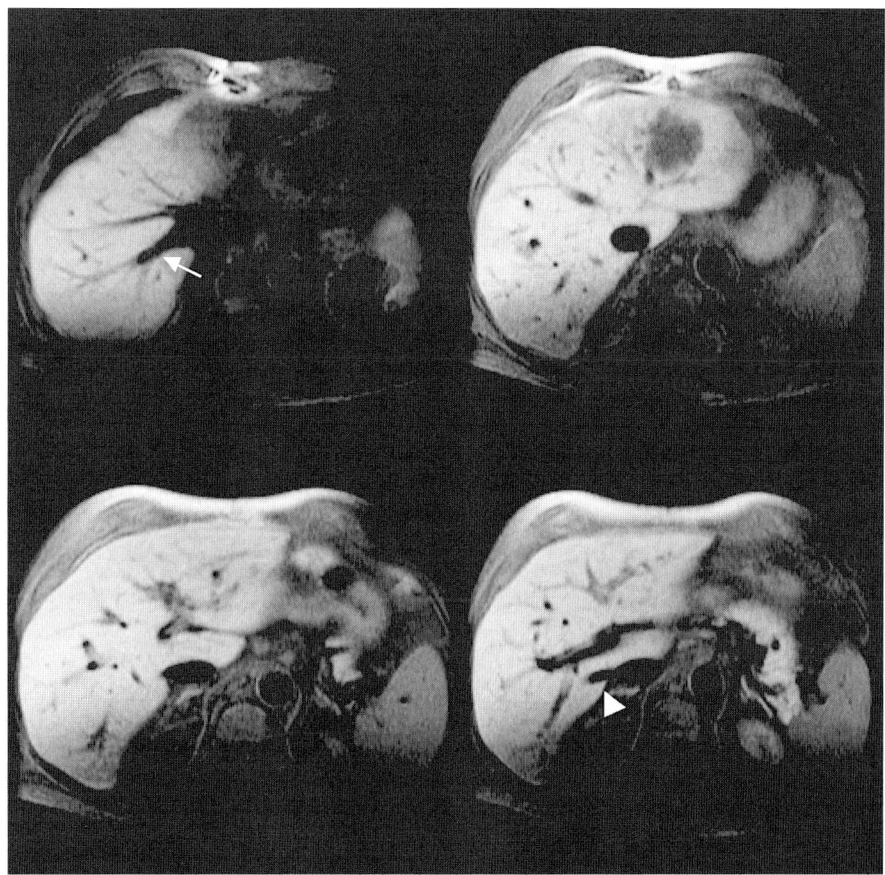

FIGURE 94.8. (A) Magnetic resonance imaging (MRI) examination demonstrates the location of the right hepatic vein (*arrow*) as well as the presence of an inferior right hepatic vein (*arrowhead*), which is present in approximately 20% of patients. (B) The presence of an inferior right hepatic vein permits resection of segments VII and VIII without resection of segments V and VI. (From Blumgart,[51] by permission of Churchill Livingstone.)

TABLE 94.1. Techniques for liver parenchymal transection.

Goals	*Methods*
Minimize blood loss	Ultrasonic dissection and aspiration
Avoid bile leaks	Water-jet dissection
Create precise line of transection	Clamp fracture
Minimize hepatic ischemia	Focused RFA Finger fracture Harmonic scalpel Compression sutures Electrocautery

RFA, radiofrequency ablation.

under low central venous pressure to reduce hepatic venous bleeding has also been demonstrated to be safe and reduces blood loss.[57] Although some anesthesiologists may feel more secure keeping the central venous pressure high during an operation that could be associated with high blood loss, this maneuver will only increase blood loss. Additionally, placement of the patient in 15° Trendelenburg position during hepatic transection will lower the hepatic vein pressure. Hemodilution is another strategy that reduces blood loss. This strategy involves removing 1 to 2 L blood in the operating room just before liver resection, with simultaneous replacement with crystalloid or colloid. The blood lost during liver transection is then more dilute. The removed blood is then reinfused following completion of the portion of the operation that is associated with blood loss. Compression of the liver edge with either a Penrose drain or a Lin liver clamp during transection reduces blood loss. Total vascular isolation is another technique that has been used to reduce intraoperative blood.[58] With this technique, vascular clamps are used to stop vascular inflow, as well as to isolate the hepatic veins from the inferior vena cava (Figure 94.9). Liver transection may then be performed with minimal blood loss.

Improvements in preoperative evaluation and imaging, surgical technique, and postoperative care have allowed liver surgeons to expand the boundaries of liver resection for colon and rectal cancer liver metastases. Liver metastases that were previously considered unresectable, such as multiple, bilobar metastases, are often now resected with multiple segmentectomies or trisegmentectomy. Strategies also have been developed to increase the volume of liver tissue that can be safely resected; these include use of sequential hepatic resections, which allows hypertrophy before removing more liver, as has been championed by Adam and Bismuth.[59] Preoperative portal vein embolization to induce hypertrophy before liver resection has been demonstrated to be safe and permits resection of larger volumes with less risk of postoperative hepatic insufficiency.[60,61]

Outcomes

The operative mortality for major hepatic resections has declined with improved operative techniques and postoperative care, but morbidity remains significant. Table 94.2 summarizes the operative mortality, morbidity, median survival, and 5-year survival in 10 published series.[14,62–70] It is important to point out that these studies all reported 5-year *actuarial* overall survival rates. Rare reports of *actual* 5-year survival rates suggest that 5-year actual survival rates are generally lower than actuarial 5-year survival rates. Operative mortality in these studies ranges from 2.8% to 7%, and causes of death include hemorrhage, sepsis, and hepatic failure. Morbidity is observed to range between 11% and 34%, and common causes of morbidity include hemorrhage, biliary leak or fistula, hepatic failure, perihepatic abscess, wound infection, pneumonia, and myocardial infarction. Median survival ranges from 28 to 46 months, and 5-year survival was between 24% and 38%.

Criteria for patient selection for liver resection have been influenced significantly by numerous retrospective studies conducted to identify prognostic factors. Hughes et al.[70a] published a multicenter retrospective review of 859 patients who had undergone resection of colon and rectal cancer liver

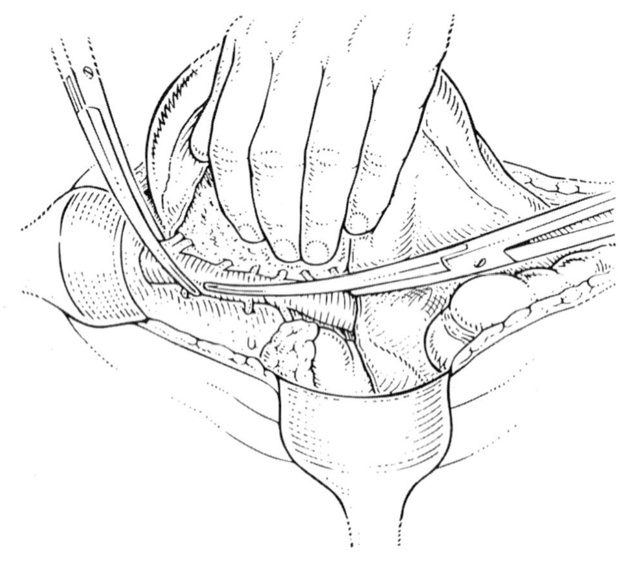

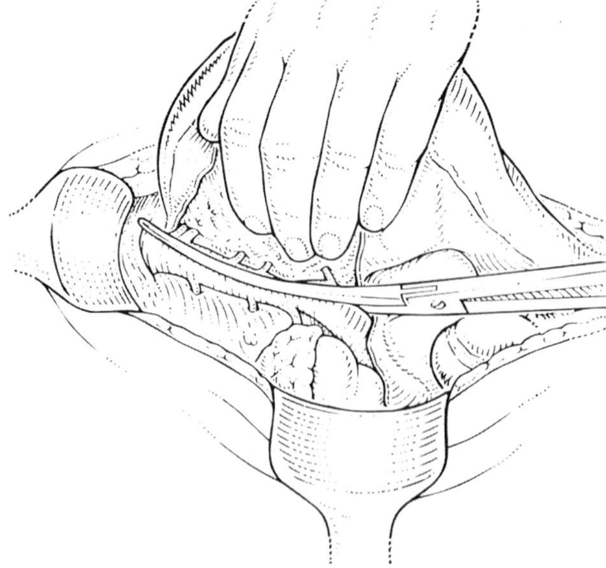

FIGURE 94.9. Hepatic vascular isolation requires positioning of either one or two vascular clamps for control of the retrohepatic vena cava. (Adapted from Blumgart,[51] by permission of Churchill Livingstone; and by permission of Hansen PD, Isla AM, Habib NA. *Journal of Gastrointestinal Surgery* 1999;3:537–542.)

TABLE 94.2. Results of resection of colon and rectal carcinoma liver metastases.

Study	*No. of patients*	*Operative mortality (%)*	*Operative morbidity (%)*	*Median survival (months)*	*Five-year survival (%)*
Schlag[62] (1990)	122	4	34	28	30
Doci[63] (1991)	100	5	11		30
Rosen[64] (1992)	116	4		33.6	25
Gajowski[65] (1994)	204				32
Scheele[66] (1995)	434	4.4	16	39.6	31
Wanebo[67] (1996)	74	7		35	24
Fong[68] (1997)	456	2.8	24	46	38
Bakalakos[69] (1998)	238	1.1		23	29
Ambiru[70] (1999)	168	3.5			26
Fong[14] (1999)	1,001	2.8		42	37

Source: Adapted from Fong et al.,[68] by permission of *Journal of Clinical Oncology.*

metastases. The overall actuarial 5-year survival was 33%. No patients with portal or lymph node metastases or with extrahepatic disease survived 5 years, and few patients with four or more metastases survived 5 years. Other less significant prognostic factors associated with a worse outcome were a surgical resection margin of less than 1 cm, advanced stage of the primary colon and rectal cancer, and short disease-free interval. Many other studies have examined prognostic factors, which are summarized in Table 94.3.[14,63–70,71]

In a large single-institution retrospective study of 456 consecutive patients with colon and rectal cancer liver metastases who underwent resection, perioperative mortality was 2.8%, perioperative morbidity was 24%, median hospital stay was 10 days, median survival was 46 months, and 5-year survival was 38%.[68] The authors concluded that the only factors that are absolute contraindications to resection are the presence of extrahepatic metastases and tumors larger than 10 cm in diameter. These factors were associated with only 13% and 14% 5-year survival rates, respectively. A reasonable percentage of patients with other negative prognostic factors, such as bilobar tumor distribution and four or more tumors, survived 5 years, and thus, the authors concluded that these factors should not be considered absolute contraindications to surgical resection. In an attempt to account for numerous prognostic factors in a formula to estimate outcome following liver resection, some investigators have developed mathematical formulas. One such example is shown in Table 94.4.

Despite careful selection, a majority of patients who undergo resection of colon and rectal cancer liver metastases will have recurrence of their cancer. The most common sites of recurrence following resection of colon and rectal cancer liver metastases are the liver and lung (Table 94.5).[14] Repeat liver resections for colon and rectal cancer liver metastases are feasible and have been reported by several groups.[72–80] In a large series, median survival reported following repeat hepatic resection in 170 patients was 34 months and 5-year survival was 32%. The only significant negative prognostic factor was an incomplete resection. Median follow-up, however, was only 25 months.[80] The number of patients who have undergone repeat hepatectomies for metastases is far fewer than the number who have had only one hepatectomy, and so the available literature is limited. In general, prognostic factors that predict outcome following repeat resection are similar to those which predict outcome following the initial liver resection. Thus, indications for repeat hepatectomy are similar to the indications for initial hepatectomy.

A few groups have reported on the resection of initially nonresectable colon and rectal cancer liver metastases following tumor regression from chemotherapy given by either systemic administration or hepatic intraarterial administration.[81–83] In a series of 53 patients with a mean follow-up of greater than 2 years, 5-year survival was 40% with 15 cases of repeat liver resection for liver recurrence.[83] In a subsequent publication, these authors reported 87 patients followed 5 years after liver resection following neoadjuvant chemotherapy, and the overall survival is 35% from the time of resection.[84] The value of this strategy for improving resectability rates or survival is currently under prospective examination in a randomized trial sponsored by the European Organiza-

TABLE 94.3. Negative prognostic factors after surgical resection of colon and rectal cancer liver metastases.

Primary colon and rectal cancer characteristics	*Metastases characteristics*	*Surgical resection characteristics*
Advanced stage	Lymph node involvement	Less than 1 cm tumor-free margin
High grade	Extrahepatic metastases	Extensive resection
	Larger size	
	Increased number	
	Satellitosis	
	Bilobar distribution	
	Short disease-free interval	
	Synchronous metastases	
	Elevated CEA level	

Source: Data from references 14, 62–70.

TABLE 94.4. Prognosis following resection of colon or rectal carcinoma.

Factor				Points[a]
Node metastases in primary tumor				1
Disease free interval <12 months				1
More than one liver metastasis				1
Preoperative CEA >200 ng/mL				1
Largest tumor >5 cm				1
Score	*One year*	*Three years*	*Five years*	*Median (months)*
0	93%	72%	60%	74
1	91%	66%	44%	51
2	89%	60%	40%	47
3	86%	42%	20%	33
4	70%	38%	25%	20
5	71%	27%	14%	22

CEA, carcinoembryonic antigen.

[a] One point is assigned for each adverse prognostic factor, and survival based on score is shown in the bottom half of the table.

Source: From Fong et al.,[14] by permission of *Annals of Surgery*.

TABLE 94.5. Patterns of first recurrence after liver resection.

Site	% of recurrences	% of all patients
Liver	48%	24%
Liver alone	41%	21%
Liver/peritoneum	2%	1%
Liver/lung	5%	3%
Other abdominal/pelvic	26%	13%
Lung (total)	26%	13%
Bone	4%	2%
Brain	2%	1%

Source: Adapted from Fong et al.,[68] by permission of *Journal of Clinical Oncology*.

tion for Research and Treatment of Cancer (EORTC), in which patients with resectable colon or rectal carcinoma liver metastases are randomized to undergo resection or neoadjuvant chemotherapy followed by resection.

Adjuvant Therapy Following Resection of Colon or Rectal Carcinoma Liver Metastases

As evidenced by 5-year survival rates averaging 35% following resection of liver metastases, two-thirds of patients develop some type of recurrence following hepatic resection. Although several retrospective studies have examined the utility of systemic chemotherapy in patients following resection of colon and rectal cancer liver metastases, most prospective studies have focused on regional, liver-directed chemotherapy.[85–91] Four small, single-arm studies have examined hepatic artery infusion (HAI) chemotherapy after liver resection.[85–87] In addition, one small[88] and three large randomized studies[89–91] of HAI chemotherapy after liver resection have been completed (Table 94.6). The largest study of adjuvant therapy following liver resection was a multicenter European study comparing HAI of 5-fluorouracil (5-FU) and folinic acid (leucovorin) to observation.[91] No differences in survival were observed between patients in these two arms, but there were several problems with this study. The use of 5-FU rather than floxuridine (FUDR) did not capitalize on the significant regional exposure advantages of FUDR (see following). In addition, the use of subcutaneous ports rather than pumps and technical problems led to termination of adjuvant therapy before completion of the planned treatment courses in many patients. Only 84 of 107 patients randomized to adjuvant chemotherapy received any chemotherapy, and only 34 finished the planned treatment.

The Eastern Cooperative Oncology Group (ECOG) and the Southwest Oncology Group (SWOG) sponsored a study in which 77 patients with fewer than four liver metastases resected were randomized to treatment with HAI FUDR and systemic 5-FU versus observation.[89] Although disease-free survival was improved by adjuvant therapy ($P = 0.03$), mainly as a result of reduced relapses in the liver, the difference in overall survival was not statistically significant.

A recently completed, single-center study randomized 156 patients to systemic 5-FU and leucovorin or to HAI FUDR and dexamethasone combined with systemic 5-FU after resection of liver metastases from colon or rectal cancer.[90] The study was designed to examine 2-year survival and patterns of recurrence at 2 years. Local recurrences in the liver were significantly reduced by regional plus systemic chemotherapy. Survival at 2 years was improved in patients randomized to combined HAI and intravenous chemotherapy; however, differences at 5 years were not statistically significant.

Newer combinations of HAI and systemic chemotherapy may be more active, such as the combination of HAI FUDR plus systemic irinotecan (CPT-11).[92] However, such newer combinations will have to be assessed in relation to newer systemic regimens for metastatic colon and rectal cancer, such as the FOLFOX (5-FU, leucovorin, oxaliplatin) and FOLFIRI (5-FU, leucovorin, and irinotecan) regimens, which have demonstrated better efficacy than systemic 5-FU and leucovorin alone.

TABLE 94.6. Selected published prospective randomized clinical trials of adjuvant hepatic arterial infusion (HAI) chemotherapy following liver resection for colon and rectal cancer liver metastases.

Trial author	Year	No. of Patients	Randomized	Stage	Intervention/design	P value	Median or overall survival
Lorenz[91]	1998	226	Yes	IV	HAI 5-FU + FA or surgery alone	0.53	MS 34.5 vs. 40.8 months
Kemeny[90]	1999	156	Yes	IV	HAI FUDR/dex + IV 5-FU or IV 5-FU	0.03	2-year OS 86% vs. 72%
Kemeny[92]	2002	75	Yes	IV	HAI FUDR + IV 5-FU or surgery alone	0.15	4-year OS 61.5% vs. 52.7%

5-FU, 5-fluorouracil; FA, folinic acid; FUDR, floxuridine; dex, dexamethasone; MS, median survival; OS, overall survival.

Hepatic Tumor Ablation

Several techniques of in situ liver tumor ablation by local destruction have been developed, including cryosurgical ablation, RFA, microwave ablation, laser ablation, and alcohol injection. These techniques are used mainly in patients whose tumors are considered unresectable, although some have used cryosurgical ablation for resectable colon and rectal cancer metastases.[93] Real-time imaging of the zone of ablated tissue is typically accomplished with MRI or ultrasound; however, the inability of these techniques to accurately assess areas of incompletely ablated tumors remains problematic.

Cryosurgical Ablation

Hepatic cryosurgery involves the freezing and thawing of liver tumors by means of a cryoprobe inserted into the tumor. Liquid nitrogen is circulated through the cryoprobe, and the subsequent iceball formation is observed by ultrasound. Freezing is continued until the iceball is at least 1 cm beyond the tumor. During freeze–thaw cycles, intracellular and extracellular ice formation occurs, leading to tumor destruction.[94] Some centers perform two or three freeze/thaw cycles or combine freezing with hepatic inflow occlusion to increase tumor destruction and iceball size.[94,95]

Hepatic cryosurgery is generally reserved for patients with colon and rectal cancer liver metastases in whom one or more lesions are not surgically resectable, although certain centers have offered hepatic cryosurgery as an alternative to surgical resection.[93] Cryosurgery can treat multiple lesions and salvages more uninvolved liver parenchyma than surgical resection. Cryosurgery may also be used to treat tumors intimately associated with major blood vessels, but large blood vessels may serve as "heat sinks" and prevent adequate freezing of immediately adjacent tumor.[96] Hepatic inflow occlusion or hepatic vein occlusion may reduce the incidence of inadequate freezing of tumor adjacent to blood vessels,[97] but recurrence of tumor adjacent to large blood vessels remains a problem.[98] In addition, many surgeons avoid hepatic inflow occlusion for fear of blood vessel wall destruction and subsequent hemorrhage. Cryosurgery may also help in treating patients who are left with a positive surgical margin after hepatic resection, as well as patients in whom underlying illness or hepatic insufficiency precludes surgical resection.

Complications associated with cryosurgery include arrhythmia, cracking of frozen liver with subsequent hemorrhage, right-sided pleural effusion, subphrenic or hepatic abscess, bile collection, biliary fistula, thrombocytopenia, myoglobinuria, acute renal failure, and cryoshock phenomenon (multisystem organ failure and disseminated intravascular coagulation).[93,97,99,100] Measures to reduce complications include packing the cryoprobe site with Gelfoam to prevent hemorrhage and postoperative administration of lasix, mannitol, and sodium bicarbonate to promote diuresis and alkalinize the urine. Overall morbidity rates range widely, from 6%[93] to 49%[100] with aggressive treatment. Mortality rates range from 0% to 8% with an overall mortality rate in reported series of 1.6%.[98] Median survival in reported series has ranged from 8 to 33 months.[98]

Hepatic cryosurgery is clearly an option for patients with isolated colon and rectal cancer liver metastases that are not surgically resectable, but limited enough to allow cryoablation of all lesions. In general, these patients' tumors usually have unfavorable tumor biology, and it is unclear whether cryoablation improves survival. It is also unclear whether hepatic cryosurgery will lead to equivalent survival in patients with more limited disease who currently undergo surgical resection. Well-controlled studies are required to address these questions. Although this technique gained popularity in the 1980s and 1990s, its usage has become much more restricted with the development of RFA.

Radiofrequency Ablation

Among the more promising experimental therapies for colon and rectal cancer liver metastases is RFA. This technique involves percutaneous or intraoperative insertion of a RFA electrode into the center of a hepatic tumor under ultrasound or CT guidance. RFA energy is then emitted from the electrode and absorbed by the surrounding tissue. This process generates extreme heat leading to coagulative necrosis of treated tissue.[101]

The initial limitation of this therapy was the small (1.5-cm) diameter of necrosis achievable with a single RF electrode. Strategies to increase this treatment area include multiprobe arrays,[102] saline infusion with RFA application,[103] and internal cooling of the tip of the RFA electrode.[103] One type of multiprobe array deploys multiple curved stiff wires in the shape of an umbrella from a single 14- or 16-gauge cannula. Studies using a 12-hook "umbrella" array in porcine liver in vivo produced spherical regions of coagulation necrosis measuring up to 3.5 cm in diameter.[104] Another type of RFA probe allows infusion of low volumes of saline during RFA that increases the volume of coagulation necrosis.[103,105,106,107] Injection of ethanol has also been demonstrated to increase the volume of coagulation necrosis achieved by RFA in animal models.[108] Another tactic to increase coagulation volume has been the development of internally cooled RF electrodes. With internal electrode tip cooling, which avoids desiccation of tissue adjacent to the electrode and rises in impedance, radiofrequency-induced coagulation necrosis is greater than that achieved with noncooled electrodes.[109]

Blood flow serves as a "heat sink," such that tumors located in vascular environments are less susceptible to thermal destruction as perfusion-mediated tissue cooling reduces the extent of coagulation necrosis. Greater coagulation is observed in vivo when radiofrequency energy is delivered during occlusion of the portal vein than when energy is delivered during normal blood flow.[110,111] Finally, pulsed current may increase the extent of coagulation necrosis as compared to continuous current.[112,113]

Techniques

Radiofrequency ablation can be performed percutaneously by means of interventional radiology or surgically, either by laparoscopic or open techniques. When performing RFA during open laparotomy, careful planning of ablation zones is necessary to achieve complete necrosis of the target lesion. Current technology allows for effective ablation of tumors up to 3 cm with an adequate margin. Tumor sizes larger than 4 to 5 cm are associated with increased incidence of local recurrence.[114,115] The location of a tumor near the main portal pedicles is considered a relative contraindication to RFA. In addition to the inability to achieve an effective ablation because of the high blood flow, ablation near the porta hepatis can result in stricture and liver failure from injury to a central bile duct.[116]

Once the target lesion is identified, the RFA electrode needle is inserted under ultrasound guidance. Optimally, the electrode is advanced in a track parallel and within the plane of the transducer, so the entire path of the needle can be visualized. When using a multielectrode needle, the array is deployed within the tumor and position is confirmed ultrasonographically. Monitoring during thermal ablation can be performed using a variety of methods. Some RFA devices have the capacity to measure tissue temperatures using thermisters located at the tips of the electrodes. Alternatively, tissue impedance and current can be monitored during treatment. With some devices, the power output is adjusted automatically to control impedance and maintain tissue temperature between 70° and 105°C. The ablation zone is visualized by ultrasound during treatment (Figure 94.10). Typically, local minuscule gas bubble formation results in hyperechogenicity within the treated tissue.

Laparoscopic RFA offers the advantage of a minimally invasive procedure with the ability to visualize the abdominal cavity and perform the therapy using IOUS. With this approach, patients are treated under general endotracheal anesthesia, typically in the supine position. In most cases, the procedure can be done with two or three ports.[117] The liver is typically partially mobilized, and viscera within 2 cm of the intended ablation zone are mobilized out of the way. The RFA electrode is placed into the abdominal cavity through a percutaneous approach and does not require the placement of an additional port. The needle is placed within the tumor under US guidance, and ablation is performed and monitored as with the open technique.

Serial follow-up imaging of the liver is recommended after RFA treatment. However, as with other ablative approaches, interpretation of these images can at times be difficult, as a hypoattenuating lesion may persist for months to years despite complete tumor destruction. In most cases, a local recurrence is characterized by an increase in the lesion size on serial scans, or evidence of new areas of contrast enhancement.[118] CT or MRI is the most useful method for follow-up imaging, emphasizing the importance of comparing images to previous ones.[119,120] The role of FDG-PET in assessing local residual or recurrent disease following RFA is yet to be defined.

Operative Versus Percutaneous Radiofrequency Ablation

Many of the published reports evaluating RFA of liver metastases have relied upon percutaneous electrode insertion under image guidance.[103,121] The principal advantage of the percutaneous approach compared to operative approaches is the lower associated morbidity and cost. A second advantage of a percutaneous approach is the ability to use either ultrasound, MRI, or CT guidance, whereas imaging of RFA performed during laparotomy or laparoscopy is for the most part limited to ultrasound guidance (Figure 94.11).

However, there are several advantages to performance of ablation during laparotomy or laparoscopy. The first benefit is that of enhanced staging, as laparotomy and laparoscopy afford the opportunity to identify both hepatic and extrahepatic metastases not visualized on preoperative imaging. Ten percent to 20% of patients who undergo exploration for intent to resect colorectal cancer liver metastases are found at laparotomy to have additional metastases that either preclude or significantly alter the planned resection. Many of these operative findings can be detected via laparoscopy as well. In addition, IOUS can frequently detect lesions that are not seen with transabdominal ultrasound, CT, or MRI.

Second, laparotomy affords the opportunity to combine ablation with surgical resection. It is important to point out that following ablation of tumors larger than 5 cm, the local recurrence rate is unacceptably high.[122] Accordingly, a significant fraction of patients with "unresectable" liver tumors can be fully treated only by the combination of resection of larger lesions and ablation of smaller lesions. For example, a patient with a 7 cm tumor occupying the left hepatic lobe and a 2 cm tumor straddling segments 6 and 7 is an ideal candi-

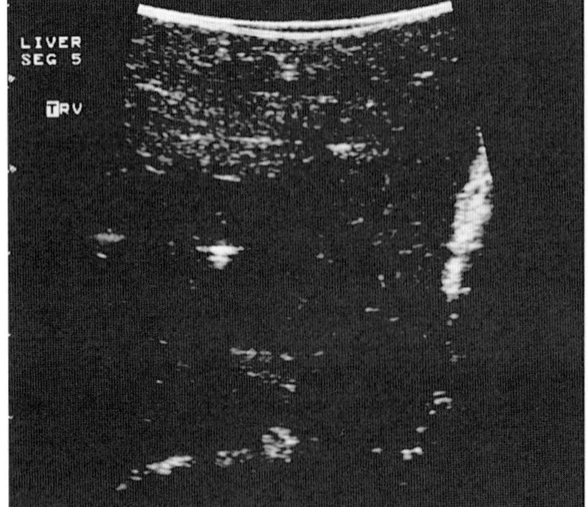

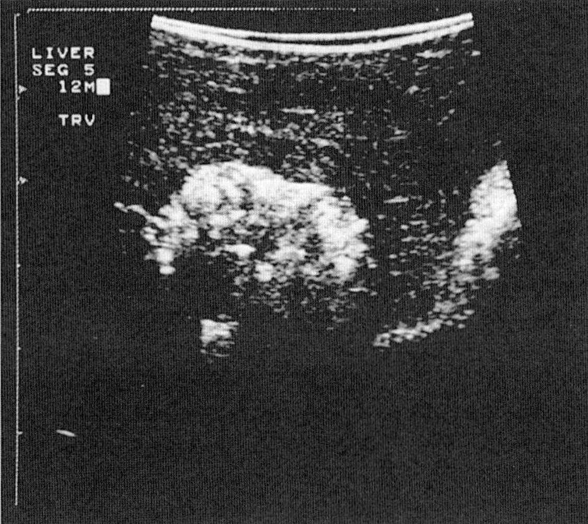

FIGURE 94.10. Placement of an electrode into the center of a liver tumor intraoperatively under ultrasound guidance (*left*). Delivery of radiofrequency (RF) energy to the tumor is associated with significantly increased echogenicity in the treated area (*right*). This typically resolves within 15 minutes. (By permission of Yoon SS, Tanabe KK. In: Cancer of the Lower Gastrointestinal Tract. London: Decker, 2001.)

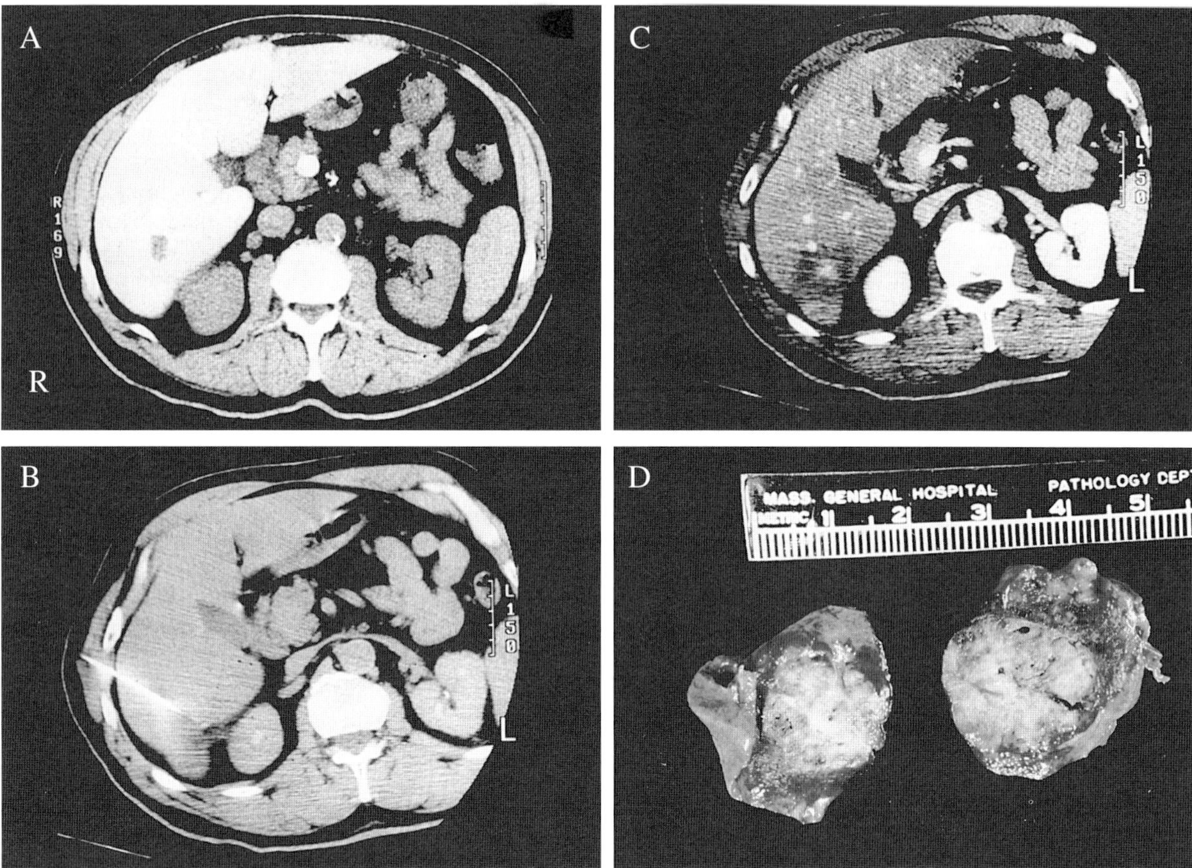

FIGURE 94.11. CT scan of a colon carcinoma liver metastasis in the right lobe before (A), during (B), and following (C) RF ablation. The tumor was resected several days later (D), and coagulation necrosis was observed throughout the tumor.

date for treatment with a combination of left hepatic lobectomy for the larger left lobe tumor and RFA of the smaller right lobe tumor.

Third, hepatic blood flow creates a "heat sink" that reduces the efficacy of thermal ablation. Ablation during laparotomy or laparoscopy can be performed with a vascular clamp occluding hepatic arterial and portal venous blood flow. This technique has been demonstrated to safely and reproducibly increase the size of the zone of ablation.[110,111,123,124] Although this can also be accomplished using percutaneous techniques, it adds negligible morbidity when performed during laparotomy or laparoscopy.

Fourth, laparotomy or laparoscopy affords excellent access to tumors in the dome of the liver or in other locations that are difficult to accurately target percutaneously. This location is difficult to access with precision using a path for the electrode that does not violate the pleura. In addition, motion of the liver caused by respiration creates further problems that can be better managed during an open laparotomy.

Fifth, operative approaches permit mobilization of structures away from a surface tumor that may be thermally injured during RFA. For example, the transverse colon may be adherent to a tumor in the inferior portion of the liver. Effective thermal ablation of the entire tumor would risk injury to the colon unless it was first dissected free from the tumor.

Finally, laparotomy affords the opportunity to implant a hepatic arterial infusion pump for postoperative administration of regional chemotherapy. The most common pattern of relapse following treatment of both primary and secondary hepatic malignancies is within the liver. A prospective, randomized trial comparing intravenous chemotherapy to HAI chemotherapy combined with intravenous chemotherapy following curative liver resection, demonstrated enhanced survival at 2 years in patients treated with the combination of hepatic arterial infusion and intravenous chemotherapy.[90] The majority of the benefit was obtained by marked reduction in hepatic recurrences observed in patients who received hepatic arterial infusion chemotherapy. This study remains the only prospective randomized trial to demonstrate a survival benefit to adjuvant therapy following curative resection of colon or rectal carcinoma liver metastases. The American College of Surgeons Oncology Group is currently conducting a clinical trial of operative RFA combined with hepatic arterial infusion of floxuridine and intravenous administration of CPT-11.

Outcomes

The analysis of clinical results achieved by RFA for the treatment of hepatic colorectal metastases has been hampered by lack of appropriate controls and relatively short follow-up times. As technical improvements have occurred, investigators have used different devices and techniques. In addition, inclusion of heterogeneous patient populations, the difficulty in defining true local recurrences, and the significant impact of distant recurrence on survival have made assessment of the efficacy of RFA challenging.

Curley et al. reported the largest series to date of operative RFA of unresectable primary and metastatic hepatic malignancies in 123 patients.[115] In these patients, RFA was used to treat 169 tumors with a median diameter of 3.4 cm. Primary liver cancer was treated in 48 patients and metastatic liver tumors were treated in 75 patients. Percutaneous and intraoperative RFA was performed in 31 patients and 92 patients, respectively. No treatment-related deaths occurred, and the complication rate was only 2.4%. All treated tumors were completely necrotic on imaging studies after completion of the RFA treatments. With a median follow-up of 15 months, tumor had recurred in 3 of 169 treated lesions (1.8%), but metastatic disease had developed at other sites in 34 patients. Based on these results, these investigators concluded that RFA is a safe, well-tolerated, and effective treatment in patients with unresectable hepatic malignancies. RFA may not cure most patients with primary or malignant metastatic disease, as witnessed by the 34 patients with disease found at extrahepatic sites, but initial disease-free rates of 20% to 50%, justify continued investigation into aggressive treatment of isolated hepatic disease with a multimodality approach including RFA. Another large series was reported by Wood et al., in which 231 tumors in 84 patients were treated in 91 procedures.[125] Thirty-nine procedures were performed via laparotomy and 27 were performed via laparoscopy. Of note, intraoperative ultrasound detected intrahepatic tumors that were not evident on preoperative scans in 38% of patients who underwent either laparotomy or laparoscopy. In 45% of patients, RFA was combined with resection or cryosurgical ablation. Median hospital stay overall was 3.6 days. Eight percent of patients had complications, and 1 patient died as a result of the procedure. With a median follow-up of 9 months, 18% of patients experienced a local recurrence at a RFA site.

In a large series from Italy of 117 patients with colorectal cancer, 179 liver metastases were treated with RFA.[122] The tumors ranged in size from 0.9 to 9.6 cm and all were percutaneously treated using internally cooled 17-gauge electrodes under image guidance. The estimated median survival was 36 months, with 1-, 2-, and 3-year survival rates of 93%, 69%, and 46%, respectively. Two-thirds of patients developed recurrences at a median time of 12 months following treatment. Seventy (39%) of 179 treated lesions developed local recurrence, and of these, 54 were observed by 6 months and 67 by 1 year. No local recurrence was observed after 18 months, although the median follow-up time for the entire study population is not reported. As expected, the incidence of local recurrence differed by size of lesion. The local recurrence rates were 22%, 53%, and 68% for lesions measuring less than 2.5 cm, 2.6 to 4.0 cm, and more than 4.1 cm, respectively.

Hepatic Arterial Infusion Chemotherapy

In patients with liver metastases from colon and rectal cancer that are not amenable to surgical resection, HAI chemotherapy can be used. HAI chemotherapy has received considerable attention over the years, and is based upon two primary concepts: (1) liver metastases larger than a few millimeters derive most of their blood supply from the hepatic arterial circulation, whereas the normal liver derives most of its blood supply from the portal circulation,[126] and (2) clearance of chemotherapeutic agents by first pass through the liver can increase drug level in the liver and limit systemic toxicity.[127] FUDR is the most commonly used agent for HAI chemotherapy. Hepatic venous levels of FUDR have been documented to be four times higher following hepatic intraarterial administration than following systemic administration, whereas systemic FUDR levels following hepatic intraarterial administration are one-fourth FUDR levels following intravenous infusion.[128] It is estimated that hepatic intraarterial administration of FUDR allows a level of liver exposure 100 to 400 times greater than with intravenous administration.[129]

HAI chemotherapy is generally reserved to patients without evidence of extrahepatic metastases. Rare exceptions are made for patients with a good performance status who have minimal extrahepatic metastases, but have substantial liver tumor burden. In the past, patients considered for HAI chemotherapy would first undergo a preoperative angiogram to define arterial anatomy because about 37% of patients have variant arterial anatomy.[130] In recent years, CT angiography has largely replaced conventional hepatic arteriography in many centers. Subsequently, an operation is performed in which a cannula is placed into the hepatic arterial circulation and attached to an infusion pump. The pump is implanted into a subcutaneous pocket in the abdominal wall.

Once appropriate hepatic perfusion is verified and the patient has recovered from the operative procedure, HAI chemotherapy is initiated. A typical infusion regimen involves a 28-day cycle of continuous infusion of FUDR for 14 days at a dose of 0.15 mg/kg/day, leucovorin 8 mg/m^2/day, and decadron 20 mg/14 days, followed by a 14-day continuous infusion of heparinized saline.[131] Hepatic toxicity is not uncommon with HAI FUDR, and liver function tests should be obtained every 2 weeks to allow dose adjustments that will reduce the chances of biliary sclerosis. FUDR infusion is generally withheld for any liver function test that exceeds twice the baseline value and resumed at one-half or one-third the original dose when the liver function tests return to baseline.[131,132] After three cycles of HAI chemotherapy, an abdominal CT scan is obtained to assess response. In patients with stable disease or disease regression, cycles can be continued and reevaluated periodically for response. Patients with disease progression during therapy should have treatment discontinued.

There have been several randomized trials comparing HAI chemotherapy with FUDR to systemic chemotherapy with FUDR or 5-fluorouracil (5-FU) (Table 94.7).[133,134–139] Median survival ranged from 12.6 to 17 months. Response rates for HAI chemotherapy ranged from 43% to 62% compared to 10% to 21% for systemic chemotherapy. The increased response rate for HAI chemotherapy did not translate into significantly increased survival in any of the studies. There are several reasons that may explain why no difference between treatment arms was observed in survival in these studies. First, colon and rectal cancer may be a systemic disease in many patients such that regional therapy will not affect survival. Second, some of the trials allowed cross-over.[134,136] Third, the high incidence of biliary sclerosis precluded full and prolonged HAI therapy in the earlier trials. Fourth, complications related to pump placement were common in the

TABLE 94.7. Selected published prospective randomized clinical trials of HAI chemotherapy compared to systemic chemotherapy.

Trial author	*Year*	*No. of patients*	*Randomized*	*Stage*	*Intervention/design*	*P value*	*Median survival (months)*	*Comments*
Kemeny[134]	1987	99	Yes	IV	HAI FUDR or systemic FUDR	0.424	17 vs. 12	Crossover allowed
Chang[135]	1987	64	Yes	IV	HAI FUDR or systemic FUDR	0.27	17 vs. 12	No crossover
Hohn[136]	1989	143	Yes	IV	HAI FUDR or systemic FUDR	NS	15.45 vs. 15.81	Crossover allowed
Martin[133]	1990	69	Yes	IV	HAI FUDR or systemic 5-FU	0.53	12.6 vs. 10.5	No crossover

FUDR, floxuridine; 5-FU, 5-fluorouracil; NS, not significant.
Source: Adapted from Harmantas et al.,[140] by permission of *Cancer*.

early trials, and this problem prevented many patients from receiving HAI therapy.[133] Subsequent improvements in surgical technique, combined with improvements in HAI chemotherapy regimens, have resulted in renewed interest in this approach in recent years.

A meta-analysis of six prospective randomized trials published by Harmantas et al.,[140] demonstrated a statistically significant survival advantage of HAI chemotherapy over systemic chemotherapy, but this analysis included one study in which some patients in the control group received no treatment.[139] Two randomized trials evaluating HAI therapy have been conducted and recently reported. A multicenter trial was recently reported in which the one group received IV leucovorin followed by HIA 5-FU every 2 weeks and the control group received systemic 5-FU and leucovorin.[141] Thirty-seven percent of patients randomized to HAI chemotherapy did not receive therapy because of technical complications. HAI chemotherapy was not associated with better median progression-free survival (7.7 versus 6.7 months) or overall survival (14.7 versus 14.8 months).

The Cancer and Leukemia Group B recently reported results of a randomized trial comparing patients treated with HAI chemotherapy with FUDR, leucovorin, and dexamethasone to patients treated with systemic 5-FU and leucovorin (Mayo regimen).[142] The trial was closed before achieving its accrual goals due to poor enrollment. An early analysis demonstrated that HAI chemotherapy was associated with a significantly higher response rate (48% versus 25%) and median survival (22.7 versus 129.8 months).

Despite better disease control in the liver, about 56% of patients receiving HAI chemotherapy, subsequently develop extrahepatic disease compared to 37% of patients receiving systemic FUDR.[134] One approach has been to combine HAI chemotherapy with systemic chemotherapy. Several centers are presently exploring the combination of FUDR-based HAI chemotherapy and intravenous CPT-11.[113] Similar to the use of HAI chemotherapy in the adjuvant setting, HAI chemotherapy for unresectable colon and rectal liver metastases needs to be compared to newer systemic regimens for metastatic colon and rectal cancer, such as the FOLFOX and FOLFIRI regimens, which have demonstrated better response rates for liver metastases than older systemic regimens.

Resection of Liver Metastases from Tumors Other Than Colon and Rectal Carcinoma

The paradigm of resection for liver metastases was established with colon and rectal cancer metastases, principally to take advantage of the known biology of this cancer, where it is not uncommon to harbor a limited number of liver metastases in the absence of extrahepatic metastases. Surgeons have exploited this knowledge to cure patients with colon and rectal cancer liver metastases. For patients with liver metastases from other cancers, the statistical likelihood that a patient actually has isolated liver metastases in the absence of extrahepatic metastases is much lower.

In one selected report concerning resection of breast cancer metastases from Duke University, 17 patients underwent resection of breast cancer liver metastases following neoadjuvant high-dose chemotherapy over a 10-year period.[143] The 5-year actuarial survival rate was calculated at 22%, and 7 of 17 patients are alive with follow-up of up to 12 years. Four of these survivors had no measurable disease and were 6 months, 17 months, 6 years, and 12 years out from their resections. This report is not an outlier, as is shown in Table 94.8, demonstrating that several centers have reported 5-year actuarial survivals of 18% to 51% following resection of breast cancer liver metastases. Probably the most important information from these studies is gained by noting the interval over which these patients were accumulated; each center reports on average 1 or 2 patients per *year*. This finding underscores two points. First, a favorable tumor biology for liver resection (i.e., isolated liver metastases) is rare with breast cancer. And second, such tumor biology does indeed exist in some patients with breast cancer.

Retrospective reports in the literature also address the issue of resection of neuroendocrine cancer liver metastases. Chen et al. reported on 15 patients over an 11-year period who underwent complete resection of their liver metastases from neuroendocrine tumors. Following complete surgical resection, patients were noted to have an actuarial 5-year survival of 73%.[144] Yao et al. identified 16 patients over a 9-year period with neuroendocrine carcinoma liver metastases who underwent resection for whom a 70% actuarial 5-year survival is reported.[152] These reports originate from a high-volume tertiary care institution, and yet they report on average 1 or 2 patients per year whom they have selected for resection. Similar patterns are observed in an analysis of published

TABLE 94.8. Selected published series of resection for breast cancer liver metastases.

Author	*Year*	*N*	*Time interval of study*	*Five-year actuarial survival*
Raab[149]	1998	34	11 years	18%
Selzner[143]	2000	17	10 years	22%
Carlini[150]	2002	17	10 years	46%
Maksan[151]	2000	9	14 years	51%

TABLE 94.9. Selected published series of resection for sarcoma liver metastases.

Author	*Year*	*N*	*Time interval of study*	*Five-year survival*
Jacques[153]	1995	14	6 years	0%
DeMatteo[154]	2001	56	19 years	30%
Hafner[155]	1995	4	19 years	33%

reports of surgery for patients with sarcoma liver metastases (Table 94.9).[153–155]

The tumor biology involving isolated liver metastases that justify regionally intensive therapy is even more rare (possibly nonexistent) for gastric cancer, esophageal cancer, pancreatic cancer, and melanoma. Although metastases from ocular melanoma commonly manifest in the liver, patients with this disease commonly also harbor metastases in other sites, such as the bone, lung, or lymph nodes.[144]

Hyperthermic Isolated Liver Perfusion

Isolated hepatic perfusion has been under clinical evaluation for four decades.[145] In this procedure, the circulation of the liver is isolated completely from the systemic circulation using an extracorporeal circuit driven by a heart–lung bypass machine. This approach has not gained widespread or consistent clinical application, because it is a complex treatment to administer, has been associated with significant morbidity, and has not demonstrated adequate efficacy to justify such aggressive treatment.

The Surgery Branch at the National Cancer Institute initiated clinical trials of isolated hepatic perfusion with several refinements and modifications to improve the potential safety and efficacy of this treatment technique. Over 200 patients have been treated on protocols designed to systematically evaluate refinements in this treatment strategy using tumor necrosis factor, melphalan, and hyperthermia as the therapeutic components of treatment. Initially, a Phase I study of escalating dose of tumor necrosis factor (TNF) alone was conducted, and the maximum safe tolerated dose defined as 1.5 mg/kg TNF administered into the perfusate during a 60-minute hyperthermic perfusion.[146] Subsequently, patients were treated on a Phase I trial of alternating escalating dose melphalan and TNF for unresectable malignancies confined to the liver.[146] In that trial, the maximum safe-tolerated dose of the agents used in combination was 1 mg TNF and 1.5 mg/kg melphalan. The dose-limiting toxicity of TNF was coagulopathy and the dose-limiting toxicity of melphalan was hepatic veno-occlusive disease. Subsequently, a Phase II trial of isolated hepatic perfusion was performed using the maximum safe-tolerated doses of these agents in patients with malignancies confined to the liver.[147] The overall response rate in that trial was approximately 75% and was consistently observed in patients with colorectal cancer, ocular melanoma, and other histologies. In addition, the response rates were observed in patients who had failed previous systemic or regional therapy, patients who had large (greater than 10 cm) lesions, patients who had multiple (more than nine) lesions, and patients who had greater than 30% hepatic replacement by tumor. Although the median duration of response was only 8 months, some patients had sustained responses that are ongoing at 3 years of follow-up. Subsequent to these studies, pharmacologic grade TNF became unavailable in the United States. Another study designed to incorporate postperfusion hepatic intraarterial FUDR and leucovorin following hyperthermic isolated liver perfusion with melphalan alone, demonstrated that hepatic arterial infusion of FUDR lengthened the duration of response.[148] Objective response rates of 75% and a median duration of response of 8 to 14 months were observed following treatment of liver metastases from a variety of cancers, including colon and rectal cancer, ocular melanoma, islet cell cancers, and cholangiocarcinomas.[146–148]

References

1. Edmondson HA, Craig JR. Neoplasms of the liver. In: Schiff L, Schiff ER (eds). Diseases of the Liver (8th ed). Philadelphia: JB Lippincott, 1987:1109–1158.
2. Weiss L, Grundmann E, Torhorst J, et al. Haematogenous metastatic patterns in colonic carcinoma: an analysis of 1541 necropsies. J Pathol 1986;150:195–203.
3. Pestana C, Reitemeier RJ, Moertel CG, Judd ES, Dockerty MB. The natural history of carcinoma of the colon and rectum. Am J Surg 1964;108:826–829.
4. Jaffe BM, Donegan WL, Watson F, Spratt JS. Factors influencing survival in patients with untreated hepatic metastases. Surg Gynecol Obstet 1968;127(1):1–11.
5. Oxley EM, Ellis H. Prognosis of carcinoma of the large bowel in the presence of liver metastases. Br J Surg 1969;56(2):149–152.
6. Bengmark S, Hafstrom L. The natural history of primary and secondary malignant tumors of the liver. Cancer (Phila) 1969; 23(1):198–202.
7. Abrams MS, Lerner HJ. Survival of patients at Pennsylvania Hospital with hepatic metastases from carcinoma of the colon and rectum. Dis Colon Rectum 1971;14(6):431–434.
8. Bengtsson G, Carlsson G, Hafstrom L, Jonsson P-E. Natural history of patients with untreated liver metastases from colorectal cancer. Am J Surg 1981;141:586–589.
9. Wilson SM, Adson MA. Surgical treatment of hepatic metastases from colorectal cancer. Arch Surg 1976;111:330–333.
10. Wagner JS, Adson MA, Van Heerden JA, Adson MH, Ilstrup DM. The natural history of hepatic metastases from colorectal cancer. Ann Surg 1984;199(5):502–508.
11. Wood CB, Gillis CR, Blumgart LH. A retrospective study of the natural history of patients with liver metastases from colorectal cancer. Clin Oncol 1976;2:285–288.
12. Wanebo HJ, Semoglou C, Attiyeh F, Stearns MJ. Surgical management of patients with primary operable colorectal cancer and synchronous liver metastases. Am J Surg 1978;135:81–85.
13. Wanebo HJ, Rao B, Pinsky CM, et al. Preoperative carcinoembryonic antigen level as a prognostic indicator in colorectal cancer. N Engl J Med 1978;299(9):448–451.
14. Fong Y, Fortner J, Sun RL, Brennan MF, Blumgart LH. Clinical score for predicting recurrence after hepatic resection for metastatic colorectal cancer: analysis of 1001 consecutive cases. Ann Surg 1999;230(3):309–318; discussion 318–321.
15. Evans JT, Dayton MT. Colon, rectum, and anus. In: Lawrence PF (ed) Essentials of General Surgery, 2nd ed. Baltimore: Williams & Wilkins, 1992:219–243.
16. Povoski SP, Fong Y, Sgouros SC, Kemeny NE, Downey RJ, Blumgart LH. Role of chest CT in patients with negative x-rays referred for hepatic colorectal metastases. Ann Surg Oncol 1998;5(1):9–15.
17. Zerhouni EA, Rutter C, Hamilton SR, et al. CT and MR imaging in the staging of colorectal carcinoma: report of the

Radiology Diagnostic Oncology Group II. Radiology 1996;200(2): 443–451.
18. Rummeny EJ, Wernecke K, Saini S, et al. Comparison between high-field-strength MR imaging and CT for screening of hepatic metastases: a receiver operating characteristic analysis. Radiology 1992;182(3):879–886.
19. Semelka RC, Worawattanakul S, Kelekis NL, et al. Liver lesion detection, characterization, and effect on patient management: comparison of single-phase spiral CT and current MR techniques. J Magn Reson Imaging 1997;7(6):1040–1047.
20. Fretz CJ, Stark DD, Metz CE, et al. Detection of hepatic metastases: comparison of contrast-enhanced CT, unenhanced MR imaging, and iron oxide-enhanced MR imaging. AJR Am J Roentgenol 1990;155(4):763–770.
21. Hagspiel KD, Neidl KF, Eichenberger AC, Weder W, Marincek B. Detection of liver metastases: comparison of superparamagnetic iron oxide-enhanced and unenhanced MR imaging at 1.5 T with dynamic CT, intraoperative US, and percutaneous US. Radiology 1995;196(2):471–478.
22. Muller RD, Vogel K, Neumann K, et al. SPIO-MR imaging versus double-phase spiral CT in detecting malignant lesions of the liver. Acta Radiol 1999;40(6):628–635.
23. Ward J, Naik KS, Guthrie JA, Wilson D, Robinson PJ. Hepatic lesion detection: comparison of MR imaging after the administration of superparamagnetic iron oxide with dual-phase CT by using alternative-free response receiver operating characteristic analysis. Radiology 1999;210(2):459–466.
24. Beets G, Penninckx F, Schiepers C, et al. Clinical value of whole-body positron emission tomography with [^{18}F]fluorodeoxyglucose in recurrent colorectal cancer. Br J Surg 1994;81(11):1666–1670.
25. Lai DT, Fulham M, Stephen MS, et al. The role of whole-body positron emission tomography with [^{18}F]fluorodeoxyglucose in identifying operable colorectal cancer metastases to the liver. Arch Surg 1996;131(7):703–707.
26. Ogunbiyi OA, Flanagan FL, Dehdashti F, et al. Detection of recurrent and metastatic colorectal cancer: comparison of positron emission tomography and computed tomography [see comments]. Ann Surg Oncol 1997;4(8):613–620.
27. Abdel-Nabi H, Doerr RJ, Lamonica DM, et al. Staging of primary colorectal carcinomas with fluorine-18 fluorodeoxyglucose whole-body PET: correlation with histopathologic and CT findings. Radiology 1998;206(3):755–760.
28. Delbeke D, Martin WH, Sandler MP, Chapman WC, Wright JK Jr, Pinson CW. Evaluation of benign vs malignant hepatic lesions with positron emission tomography. Arch Surg 1998;133(5):510–515.
29. Flanagan FL, Dehdashti F, Ogunbiyi OA, Kodner IJ, Siegel BA. Utility of FDG-PET for investigating unexplained plasma CEA elevation in patients with colorectal cancer [see comment]. Ann Surg 1998;227(3):319–323.
30. Fong Y, Saldinger PF, Akhurst T, et al. Utility of ^{18}F-FDG positron emission tomography scanning on selection of patients for resection of hepatic colorectal metastases. Am J Surg 1999; 178(4):282–287.
31. Whiteford MH, Whiteford HM, Yee LF, et al. Usefulness of FDG-PET scan in the assessment of suspected metastatic or recurrent adenocarcinoma of the colon and rectum. Dis Colon Rectum 2000;43(6):759–767.
32. Haugeberg G, Strohmeyer T, Lierse W, Bocker W. The vascularization of liver metastases. J Cancer Res Clin Oncol 1988;114: 415–419.
33. Paley MR, Ros PR. Hepatic metastases. Radiol Clin N Am 1998;36(2):349–363.
34. Hamm B, Vogl TJ, Branding G, et al. Focal liver lesions: MR imaging with Mn-DPDP. Initial clinical results in 40 patients. Radiology 1992;182:167–174.
35. Ruers TJ, Langenhoff BS, Neeleman N, et al. Value of positron emission tomography with [F-18]fluorodeoxyglucose in patients with colorectal liver metastases: a prospective study. J Clin Oncol 2002;20(2):388–395.
36. Wernecke K, Rummeny E, Bongartz G, et al. Detection of hepatic masses in patients with carcinoma: comparative sensitivities of sonography, CT, and MR imaging. AJR Am J Roentgenol 1991;157:731–739.
37. Kane RA, Hughes LA, Cua EJ, Steele GD, Jenkins RL, Cady B. The impact of intraoperative ultrasonography on surgery for liver neoplasms. J Ultrasound Med 1994;13(1):1–6.
38. Conlon R, Jacobs M, Dasgupta D, Lodge JP. The value of intraoperative ultrasound during hepatic resection compared with improved preoperative magnetic resonance imaging. Eur J Ultrasound 2003;16(3):211–216.
39. Ozsunar Y, Skjoldbye B, Court-Payen M, Karstrup S, Burcharth F. Impact of intraoperative ultrasonography on surgical treatment of liver tumours. Acta Radiol 2000;41(1):97–101.
40. Awad SS, Fagan S, Abudayyeh S, Karim N, Berger DH, Ayub K. Preoperative evaluation of hepatic lesions for the staging of hepatocellular and metastatic liver carcinoma using endoscopic ultrasonography. Am J Surg 2002;184(6):601–614.
41. Zacherl J, Pokieser P, Wrba F, et al. Accuracy of multiphasic helical computed tomography and intraoperative sonography in patients undergoing orthotopic liver transplantation for hepatoma: what is the truth? Ann Surg 2002;235(4):528–532.
42. Gaitini D, Kopelman D, Soudak M, et al. Impact of intraoperative sonography on resection and cryoablation of liver tumors. J Clin Ultrasound 2001;29(5):265–272.
43. Kopelman D, Beny A, Assalia A, Gaitini D, Klein Y, Hashmonai M. [Combined treatment of hepatic tumors by cryosurgery and resection: first results]. Harefuah 1998;134(11):835–837.
44. Sahani D, Saini S, Pena C, et al. Using multidetector CT for preoperative vascular evaluation of liver neoplasms: technique and results. AJR Am J Roentgenol 2002;179:53–59.
45. Jarnagin WR, Bach AM, Winston CB, et al. What is the yield of intraoperative ultrasonography during partial hepatectomy for malignant disease? J Am Coll Surg 2001;192(5):577–583.
46. Spielmann AL. Liver imaging with MDCT and high concentration contrast media. Eur J Radiol 2003;45(suppl 1):S50–S52.
47. Hong KC, Freeny PC. Pancreaticoduodenal arcades and dorsal pancreatic artery: comparison of CT angiography with three-dimensional volume rendering, maximum intensity projection, and shaded-surface display. AJR Am J Roentgenol 1999;172(4): 925–931.
48. Kolecki R, Schirmer B. Intraoperative and laparoscopic ultrasound. Surg Clin N Am 1998;78(2):251–271.
49. Barbot DJ, Marks JH, Feld RI, Liu JB, Rosato FE. Improved staging of liver tumors using laparoscopic intraoperative ultrasound. J Surg Oncol 1997;64(1):63–67.
50. Couinaud C. Le Foie. Etudes Anatomiques et Chirurgicales. Paris: Masson, 1957.
51. Blumgart LH. Liver resection: liver and biliary tumours. In: Blumgart LH (ed). Surgery of the Liver and Biliary Tract, 2nd ed. Edinburgh: Churchill Livingstone, 1994:1495–1535.
52. Iwatsuki S, Sheahan DG, Starzl TE. The changing face of hepatic resection. Curr Probl Surg 1989;26:291–379.
53. Melendez J, Ferri E, Zwillman M, et al. Extended hepatic resection: a 6-year retrospective study of risk factors for perioperative mortality. J Am Coll Surg 2001;192(1):47–53.
54. Fong Y, Blumgart LH. Useful stapling techniques in liver surgery. J Am Coll Surg 1997;185(1):93–100.
55. Takayama T, Makuuchi M, Kubota K, et al. Randomized comparison of ultrasonic vs. clamp transection of the liver. Arch Surg 2001;136(8):922–928.
56. Man K, Fan ST, Ng IO, Lo CM, Liu CL, Wong J. Prospective evaluation of Pringle maneuver in hepatectomy for liver tumors by a randomized study. Ann Surg 1997;226(6):704–711.

57. Melendez JA, Arslan V, Fischer ME, et al. Perioperative outcomes of major hepatic resections under low central venous pressure anesthesia: blood loss, blood transfusion, and the risk of postoperative renal dysfunction. J Am Coll Surg 1998;187(6):620–625.
58. Bismuth H, Castaing D, Garden OJ. Major hepatic resection under total vascular exclusion. Ann Surg 1989;210(1):13–19.
59. Adam R, Laurent A, Azoulay D, Castaing D, Bismuth H. Two-stage hepatectomy: a planned strategy to treat irresectable liver tumors. Ann Surg 2000;232:777–785.
60. Azoulay D, Castaing D, Smail A, et al. Resection of nonresectable liver metastases from colorectal cancer after percutaneous portal vein embolization. Ann Surg 2000;231:480–486.
61. Hemming AW, Reed AI, Howard RJ, et al. Preoperative portal vein embolization for extended hepatectomy. Ann Surg 2003;237(5):686–691.
62. Schlag P, Hohenberger P, Herfarth C. Resection of liver metastases in colorectal cancer: competitive analysis of treatment results in synchronous versus metachronous metastases. Eur J Surg Oncol 1990;16:360–365.
63. Doci R, Gennari L, Bignami P, Montalto F, Morabito A, Bozzetti F. One hundred patients with hepatic metastases from colorectal cancer treated by resection: analysis of prognostic determinants. Br J Surg 1991;78:797–801.
64. Rosen CB, Nagorney DM, Taswell HF, et al. Perioperative blood transfusion and determinants of survival after liver resection for metastatic colorectal carcinoma. Ann Surg 1992;216(4):493–505.
65. Gajowski TJ, Iwatsuki S, Madariaga JR, et al. Experience in hepatic resection for metastatic colorectal cancer: analysis of clinical and pathologic risk factors. Surgery (St. Louis) 1994;116(4):703–711.
66. Scheele J, Stang R, Altendorf-Hofmann A, Paul M. Resection of colorectal liver metastases. World J Surg 1995;19:59–71.
67. Wanebo HJ, Chu QD, Vezeridis MP, Soderberg C. Patient selection for hepatic resection of colorectal metastases. Arch Surg 1996;131:322–329.
68. Fong Y, Cohen AM, Fortner JG, et al. Liver resection for colorectal metastases. J Clin Oncol 1997;15(3):938–946.
69. Bakalakos EA, Kim JA, Young DC, Martin EW Jr. Determinants of survival following hepatic resection for metastatic colorectal cancer. World J Surg 1998;22(4):399–404.
70. Ambiru S, Miyazaki M, Isono T, et al. Hepatic resection for colorectal metastases: analysis of prognostic factors. Dis Colon Rectum 1999;42(5):632–639.
70a. Hughes KS, Simon R, Songhorabodi S, et al. Resection of the liver for colorectal carcinoma metastases: a multi-institutional study of patterns of recurrence. Surgery 1986;100:278–284.
71. Younes RN, Rogatko A, Brennan MF. The influence of intraoperative hypotension and perioperative blood transfusion on disease-free survival in patients with complete resection of colorectal liver metastases. Ann Surg 1991;214(2):107–113.
72. O'Dwyer PJ, O'Riordain DS, Martin EW. Second hepatic resection for metastatic colorectal cancer. Eur J Surg Oncol 1991;17:403–404.
73. Lange JF, Leese T, Castaing D, Bismuth H. Repeat hepatectomy for recurrent malignant tumors of the liver. Surg Gynecol Obstet 1989;169:119–126.
74. Andersson R, Tranberg KG, Bengmark S. Resection of colorectal liver secondaries: a preliminary report. HPB Surg 1990;2:69–72.
75. Dagradi AD, Mangiante GL, Marchiori LAM, Nicoli NM. Repeat hepatic resection. Int Surg 1987;72:87–92.
76. Stone MD, Cady B, Jenkins RL, McDermott WV, Steele GD Jr. Surgical therapy for recurrent liver metastases from colorectal cancer. Arch Surg 1990;125(6):718–721.
77. Fortner JG. Recurrence of colorectal cancer after hepatic resection. Am J Surg 1988;155:378–382.
78. Fong Y, Blumgart LH, Cohen A, Fortner J, Brennan MF. Repeat hepatic resections for metastatic colorectal cancer. Ann Surg 1994;220:657–662.
79. Nordlinger B, Jaeck D, Guiguet M, Vaillant J, Balladur P, Schaal J. Surgical resection of hepatic metastases: multicentric retrospective study by the French Association of Surgery. In: Nordlinger B, Jaeck D (eds) Treatment of Hepatic Metastases of Colorectal Cancer. New York: Springer-Verlag, 1992:129–146.
80. Fernandez-Trigo V, Shamsa F, Sugarbaker PH. Repeat liver resection from colorectal metastasis. Surgery (St. Louis) 1995;117(3):296–304.
81. Elias D, Lasser P, Rougier P, Ducreux M, Bognel C, Roche A. Frequency, technical aspects, results, and indications of major hepatectomy after prolonged intra-arterial hepatic chemotherapy for initially unresectable hepatic tumors. J Am Coll Surg 1995;180:213–219.
82. Fowler WC, Eisenberg BL, Hoffman JP. Hepatic resection following systemic chemotherapy for metastatic colorectal carcinoma. J Surg Oncol 1995;51:122–125.
83. Bismuth H, Adam R, Levi F, et al. Resection of nonresectable liver metastases from colorectal cancer after neoadjuvant chemotherapy. Ann Surg 1996;224:509–522.
84. Adam R, Avisar E, Ariche A, et al. Five-year survival following hepatic resection after neoadjuvant therapy for nonresectable colorectal. Ann Surg Oncol 2001;8(4):347–353.
85. Moriya Y, Sugihara K, Hojo K, Makuuchi M. Adjuvant hepatic intra-arterial chemotherapy after potentially curative hepatectomy for liver metastases from colorectal cancer: a pilot study. Eur J Surg Oncol 1991;17(5):519–525.
86. Curley SA, Roh MS, Chase JL, Hohn DC. Adjuvant hepatic arterial infusion chemotherapy after curative resection of colorectal liver metastases. Am J Surg 1993;166(6):743–746.
87. Nonami T, Takeuchi Y, Yasui M, et al. Regional adjuvant chemotherapy after partial hepatectomy for metastatic colorectal carcinoma. Semin Oncol 1997;24(2 suppl 6):S6-130–S6-134.
88. Kemeny MM, Goldberg D, Beatty JD, et al. Results of a prospective randomized trial of continuous regional chemotherapy and hepatic resection as treatment of hepatic metastases from colorectal primaries. Cancer (Phila) 1986;57(3):492–498.
89. Kemeny MM, Adak S, Gray B, et al. Combined-modality treatment for resectable metastatic colorectal carcinoma to the liver: surgical resection of hepatic metastases in combination with continuous infusion of chemotherapy. An intergroup study [see comment]. J Clin Oncol 2002;20(6):1499–1505.
90. Kemeny N, Huang Y, Cohen AM, et al. Hepatic arterial infusion of chemotherapy after resection of hepatic metastases from colorectal cancer [see comment]. N Engl J Med 1999;341(27):2039–2048.
91. Lorenz M, Muller HH, Schramm H, et al. Randomized trial of surgery versus surgery followed by adjuvant hepatic arterial infusion with 5-fluorouracil and folinic acid for liver metastases of colorectal cancer. German Cooperative on Liver Metastases (Arbeitsgruppe Lebermetastasen). Ann Surg 1998;228(6):756–762.
92. Kemeny N, Gonen M, Sullivan D, et al. Phase I study of hepatic arterial infusion of floxuridine and dexamethasone with systemic irinotecan for unresectable hepatic metastases from colorectal cancer. J Clin Oncol 2001;19(10):2687–2695.
93. Ravikumar TS, Kane R, Cady B, Jenkins R, Clouse M, Steele G. A 5-year study of cryosurgery in the treatment of liver tumors. Arch Surg 1991;126(12):1520–1523.
94. Whittaker DK. Mechanisms of tissue destruction following cryosurgery. Ann R Coll Surg Engl 1984;66:313–318.
95. Dilley AV, Warlters A, Dy D, et al. Hepatic cryotherapy: is portal clamping worth it? Aust N Z J Surg 1991;61:A522.

96. Ravikumar TS, Steele G, Kane R, King V. Experimental and clinical observations on hepatic cryosurgery for colorectal metastases. Cancer Res 1991;51:6323–6327.
97. Kane RA. Ultrasound-guided hepatic cryosurgery for tumour ablation. Semin Intervent Radiol 1993;10:132–142.
98. Seifert JK, Junginger T, Morris DL. A collective review of the world literature on hepatic cryotherapy. J R Coll Surg Edinb 1998;43:141–154.
99. Weaver ML, Atkinson D, Zemel R. Hepatic cryosurgery in treating colorectal metastases. Cancer (Phila) 1995;76(2):210–214.
100. Morris DL, Ross WB, Iqbal J, McCall JL, King J, Clingan PR. Cryoablation of hepatic malignancy: an evaluation of tumour marker data and survival in 110 patients. GI Cancer 1996;1: 247–251.
101. Cosman ER, Nashold BS, Ovelman-Levitt J. Theoretical aspects of radiofrequency lesions in the dorsal root entry zone. Neurosurgery 1984;15(6):945–950.
102. Goldberg SN, Gazelle GS, Dawson SL, Rittman WJ, Mueller PR, Rosenthal DI. Tissue ablation with radiofrequency using multiprobe arrays. Acad Radiol 1995;2:670–674.
103. Livraghi T, Goldberg SN, Monti F, et al. Saline-enhanced radiofrequency tissue ablation in the treatment of liver metastases. Radiology 1997;202:205–210.
104. Goldberg SN, Gazelle GS, Solbiati L, Rittman WJ, Mueller PR. Radiofrequency tissue ablation: increased lesion diameter with a perfusion electrode. Acad Radiol 1996;3(8):636–644.
105. Siperstein AE, Rogers SJ, Hansen PD, Gitomirsky A. Laparoscopic thermal ablation of hepatic neuroendocrine tumor metastases. Surgery (St. Louis) 1997;122:1147–1155.
106. Mittleman RS, Huang SK, de Guzman WT, Cuenoud H, Wagshal AB, Pires LA. Use of the saline infusion electrode catheter for improved energy delivery and increased lesion size in radiofrequency catheter ablation. Pacing Clin Electrophysiol 1995;18: 1022–1027.
107. Miao Y, Ni Y, Yu J, Zhang H, Baert A, Marchal G. An ex vivo study on radiofrequency tissue ablation: increased lesion size by using an "expandable-wet" electrode. Eur Radiol 2001;11(9): 1841–1847.
108. Goldberg SN, Kruskal JB, Oliver BS, Clouse ME, Gazelle GS. Percutaneous tumor ablation: increased coagulation by combining radio-frequency ablation and ethanol instillation in a rat breast tumor model. Radiology 2000;217(3):827–831.
109. Lorentzen T. A cooled needle electrode for radiofrequency tissue ablation: thermodynamic aspects of improved performance compared with conventional needle design. Acad Radiol 1996; 3(7):556–563.
110. Goldberg SN, Gazelle GS, Compton CC, Mueller PR, Tanabe KK. Treatment of intrahepatic malignancy with radiofrequency ablation: radiologic-pathologic correlation. Cancer (Phila) 2000; 88:2452–2463.
111. Goldberg SN, Hahn PF, Tanabe KK, et al. Percutaneous radiofrequency tissue ablation: does perfusion-mediated tissue cooling limit coagulation necrosis? J Vasc Intervent Radiol 1998;9(1 pt 1):101–111.
112. Goldberg SN, Gazelle GS, Solbiati L, Mullin K. Large volume radiofrequency tissue ablation: increase coagulation with pulsed technique. Radiology 1997;205:P258 (abstract).
113. Goldberg SN, Stein MC, Gazelle GS, Sheiman RG, Kruskal JB, Clouse ME. Percutaneous radiofrequency tissue ablation: optimization of pulsed-radiofrequency technique to increase coagulation necrosis. J Vasc Intervent Radiol 1999;10(7):907–916.
114. Bowles BJ, Machi J, Limm WM, et al. Safety and efficacy of radiofrequency thermal ablation in advanced liver tumors. Arch Surg 2001;136(8):864–869.
115. Curley SA, Izzo F, Delrio P, et al. Radiofrequency ablation of unresectable primary and metastatic hepatic malignancies: results in 123 patients. Ann Surg 1999;230(1):1–8.
116. Rossi S, Buscarini E, Garbagnati F, et al. Percutaneous treatment of small hepatic tumors by an expandable RF needle electrode. AJR Am J Roentgenol 1998;170(4):1015–1022.
117. Lencioni R, Cioni D, Bartolozzi C. Percutaneous radiofrequency thermal ablation of liver malignancies: techniques, indications, imaging findings, and clinical results. Abdom Imaging 2001; 26(4):345–360.
118. Kuszyk BS, Choti MA, Urban BA, et al. Hepatic tumors treated by cryosurgery: normal CT appearance. AJR Am J Roentgenol 1996;166(2):363–368.
119. Chopra S, Dodd GD III, Chintapalli KN, Leyendecker JR, Karahan OI, Rhim H. Tumor recurrence after radiofrequency thermal ablation of hepatic tumors: spectrum of findings on dual-phase contrast-enhanced CT. AJR Am J Roentgenol 2001; 177(2):381–387.
120. Berber E, Foroutani A, Garland AM, et al. Use of CT Hounsfield unit density to identify ablated tumor after laparoscopic radiofrequency ablation of hepatic tumors. Surg Endosc 2000; 14(9):799–804.
121. Solbiati LG, Tiziana I, Livraghi T, et al. Hepatic metastases: percutaneous radio-frequency ablation with cooled-tip electrodes. Radiology 1997;205:367–373.
122. Solbiati L, Livraghi T, Goldberg SN, et al. Percutaneous radiofrequency ablation of hepatic metastases from colorectal cancer: long-term results in 117 patients. Radiology 2001;221(1): 159–166.
123. Patterson EJ, Scudamore CH, Owen DA, Nagy AG, Buczkowski AK. Radiofrequency ablation of porcine liver in vivo: effects of blood flow and treatment time on lesion size. Ann Surg 1998; 227(4):559–565.
124. Chinn SB, Lee FT Jr, Kennedy GD, et al. Effect of vascular occlusion on radiofrequency ablation of the liver: results in a porcine model. AJR Am J Roentgenol 2001;176(3):789–795.
125. Wood TF, Rose DM, Chung M, Allegra DP, Foshag LJ, Bilchik AJ. Radiofrequency ablation of 231 unresectable hepatic tumors: indications, limitations, and complications. Ann Surg Oncol 2000;7(8):593–600.
126. Breedis C, Young G. The blood supply of neoplasms in the liver. Am J Pathol 1954;30:969–985.
127. Collins JM. Pharmacologic rationale for regional drug delivery. J Clin Oncol 1984;2(5):498–504.
128. Ensminger WD, Rosowsky A, Raso V, et al. A clinical-pharmacological evaluation of hepatic arterial infusions of 5-fluoro-2′-deoxyuridine and 5-fluorouracil. Cancer Res 1978;38: 3784–3792.
129. Ensminger WD, Gyves JW. Clinical pharmacology of hepatic arterial chemotherapy. Semin Oncol 1983;10:176–182.
130. Curley SA, Chase JL, Roh MS, Hohn DC. Technical considerations and complications associated with the placement of 180 implantable hepatic arterial infusion devices. Surgery (St. Louis) 1993;114(5):928–935.
131. Kemeny N, Conti JA, Cohen A, et al. Phase II study of hepatic arterial floxuridine, leucovorin, and dexamethasone for unresectable liver metastases from colorectal carcinoma. J Clin Oncol 1994;12:2288–2295.
132. Stagg RJ, Venook AP, Chase JL, et al. Alternating hepatic intra-arterial floxuridine and fluorouracil: a less toxic regimen for treatment of liver metastases from colorectal cancer. J Natl Cancer Inst 1991;83:423–428.
133. Martin KJ, O'Connell MJ, Wieand HS, et al. Intra-arterial floxuridine vs. systemic fluorouracil for hepatic metastases from colorectal cancer. Arch Surg 1990;125:1022–1027.
134. Kemeny N, Daly J, Reichman B, Geller N, Botet J, Oderman P. Intrahepatic or systemic infusion of fluorodeoxyuridine with in liver metastases from colorectal carcinoma. Ann Intern Med 1987;107:459–465.

135. Chang AE, Schneider PD, Sugarbaker PH, Simpson C, Culnane M, Steinberg SM. A prospective randomized trial of regional versus systemic continuous 5-fluorodeoxyuridine chemotherapy in the treatment of colorectal liver metastases. Ann Surg 1987; 206(6):685–693.
136. Hohn DD, Stagg RJ, Friedman MS, et al. A randomized trial of continuous intravenous versus hepatic intraarterial floxuridine in patients with colorectal cancer metastatic to the liver: the Northern California Oncology Group Trial. J Clin Oncol 1989;7(11):1646–1654.
137. Wagman LD, Kemeny MM, Leong G, et al. A prospective randomized evaluation of the treatment of colorectal cancer metastatic to the liver. J Clin Oncol 1990;8(11):1885–1893.
138. Allen-Mersh TG, Earlam S, Fordy C, Abrams K, Houghton J. Quality of life and survival with continuous hepatic-artery floxuridine infusion for colorectal liver metastases [see comment]. Lancet 1994;344(8932):1255–1260.
139. Rougier P, Laplanche A, Huguier M, et al. Hepatic arterial infusion of floxuridine in patients with liver metastases from colorectal carcinoma: long-term results of a prospective randomized trial. J Clin Oncol 1992;10(7):1112–1118.
140. Harmantas A, Rotstein LE, Langer B. Regional versus systemic chemotherapy in the treatment of colorectal carcinoma liver metastatic to the liver. Cancer (Phila) 1996;78(8):1639–1645.
141. Kerr DJ, McArdle CS, Ledermann J, et al. Intrahepatic arterial versus intravenous fluorouracil and folinic acid for colorectal cancer liver metastases: a multicentre randomised trial [see comment]. Lancet 2003;361(9355):368–373.
142. Kemeny N, Niedzwiecki D, Hollis DR, et al. Hepatic arterial infusion (HAI) versus systemic therapy for hepatic metastases from colorectal cancer; a CALGB randomized trial of efficacy, quality of life (QOL), cost effectiveness, and molecular markers. Proc Am Soc Clin Oncol 2003;22:1010A.
143. Selzner M, Morse MA, Vredenburgh JJ, Meyers WC, Clavien PA. Liver metastases from breast cancer: long-term survival after curative resection. Surgery (St. Louis) 2000;127(4):383–389.
144. Chen H, Hardacre JM, Uzar A, Cameron JL, Choti MA. Isolated liver metastases from neuroendocrine tumors: does resection prolong survival? J Am Coll Surg 1998;187(1):88–92.
145. Ausman R. Development of a technique for isolated perfusion of the liver. N Y State Med J 1961;61:3393–3397.
146. Alexander HR Jr, Bartlett DL, Libutti SK. Current status of isolated hepatic perfusion with or without tumor necrosis factor for the treatment of unresectable cancers confined to liver. Oncologist 2000;5(5):416–424.
147. Alexander HR, Bartlett DL, Libutti SK, Fraker DL, Moser T, Rosenberg SA. Isolated hepatic perfusion with tumor necrosis factor and melphalan for unresectable cancers confined to the liver. J Clin Oncol 1998;16(4):1479–1489.
148. Bartlett DL, Libutti SK, Figg WD, Fraker DL, Alexander HR. Isolated hepatic perfusion for unresectable hepatic metastases from colorectal cancer. Surgery (St. Louis) 2001;129(2):176–187.
149. Raab R, Nussbaum KT, Behrend M, Weimann A. Liver metastases of breast cancer: results of liver resection. Anticancer Res 1998;18(3C):2231–3233.
150. Carlini M, Lonardo MT, Carboni F, et al. Liver metastases from breast cancer. Results of surgical resection. Hepato-Gastroenterology 2002;49(48):1597–1601.
151. Maksan SM, Lehnert T, Bastert G, Herfarth C. Curative liver resection for metastatic breast cancer. Eur J Surg Oncol 2000; 26(3):209–222.
152. Yao KA, Talamonti MS, Nemcek A, et al. Indications and results of liver resection and hepatic chemoembolization for metastatic gastrointestinal neuroendocrine tumors. Surgery, 2001;130:677–682.
153. Jaques DP, Coit DG, Casper ES, Brennan MF. Hepatic metastases from soft-tissue sarcoma. Ann Surg 1995;221:392–397.
154. DeMatteo RP, Shah A, Fong Y, Jarnagin WR, Blumgart LH, Brennan MF. Results of hepatic resection for sarcoma metastatic to liver. Ann Surg 2001;234:540–547; discussion 7–8.
155. Hafner GH, Rao U, Karakousis CP. Liver metastases from soft tissue sarcomas. J Surg Oncol 1995;58:12–16.

95

Metastatic Cancer to Bone

Patrick J. Getty, Jeffrey L. Nielsen, Thomas Huff, Mark R. Robbin, and Beth A. Overmoyer

Metastatic disease to bone is the most common malignancy of bone. The American Cancer Society estimated that in 2004 there will have been 1,368,030 new cases of cancer in the United States.[1] Of these, they estimated that approximately 2,400 will be new cases of primary bone malignancy; that is, compared with over 230,000 new cases of prostate carcinoma, 217,000 cases of breast carcinoma, and 173,000 cases of lung carcinoma. Those three diagnoses, along with kidney cancer and thyroid carcinoma, represent 80% of metastases to the skeleton.[2] Autopsy studies have shown that 50% to 70% of patients with prostate cancer develop metastases and 85% of patients with breast cancer develop skeletal metastases. The skeleton is surpassed only by the lungs and liver for incidence of metastatic disease. Any bone of the skeleton can be involved; however, the axial skeleton is most commonly involved. Involvement of the appendicular skeleton most commonly involves the proximal portion of the lower extremities. Within the spine, it is primarily the anterior and middle columns that are involved.[3]

Presentation of patients with skeletal metastases takes many forms. Metastases may be found on routine staging studies, including bone scan. They typically become clinically evident as a result of pain and dysfunction. Spinal metastases can present because of pain with or without pathologic fracture as well as spinal instability or compression of the spinal cord. Metastases to the long bones of the extremities typically present secondary to pain or pathologic fracture.

Diagnosis of metastatic disease to bone requires an organized approach and, if necessary, a well-planned biopsy. Appropriate treatment options, including medical management, radiation therapy, and surgical treatment, can then be considered.

Mechanisms of Osseous Metastases

The development of metastatic disease to bone is a complex interaction between the neoplastic cells and the host organism. In 1889, Paget described the seed and soil hypothesis of tumor metastasis.[4] Although the exact mechanisms remain elusive, increased understanding of the mechanism of metastasis has occurred via both anatomic and molecular studies. The mechanism of metastasis to bone involves both the generalized steps required at the primary site for all metastases as well as specialized interactions at the bone end organ.[5] At the primary site of disease, the tumor cells must induce neovascularization, following which there must be alterations in the expression of cell adhesion molecules, followed by the expression of collagenases and metalloproteinases to allow the tumor cell to leave the primary site and invade the bloodstream for hematogenous spread. The tumor cells must then evade the host immune mechanisms to arrive intact at the bone end organ.

The most common sites of skeletal metastasis are the spine, pelvis, and proximal femur.[6] It is believed that these represent receptive anatomic sites due to the presence of hematopoietic marrow, which contains vascular sinuses that allow circulating tumor cells to pass from the bloodstream into the bone marrow space. Another site of valveless blood flow was described by Batson with reference to the venous plexus surrounding the spine and high incidence of spinal metastasis.[7] Once within bone, the tumor cells must adopt a mechanism for bone lysis to create the space needed for tumor growth. It is believed that tumor cells do not cause direct bone lysis, but rather induce the host osteoclasts to perform lysis of bone.[5] It is thought that tumor cells do this primarily by producing parathyroid hormone-related protein, possibly under the stimulation of transforming growth factor-beta (TGF-β.) The parathyroid hormone-related protein then stimulates the osteoclasts to perform lysis of bone. This exogenous stimulus places the normal homeostatic mechanism of bone metabolism out of balance to produce overall bone lysis and allow for increased tumor growth.

Pathophysiology of Osseous Metastasis

Both osteolytic and osteoblastic bone metastasis can be viewed as part of the spectrum of dysregulation of bone remodeling that occurs with the development of osseous metastasis. Occasionally, both types of metastasis occur in association with the same malignancy, such as with breast cancer; however, in general, breast cancer is associated with primarily osteolytic disease, contrasting with prostate cancer that has primarily osteoblastic features.[8] The skeleton is a common site of metastasis because of significant access to blood flow, and the ability of marrow stromal cells to bind to circulating tumor cells via the presence of adhesion molecules, for example, integrin $\alpha\alpha_v\beta_3$, which also function to bind osteoclasts to bone surfaces.[9–12] The microenvironment of the bone matrix facilitates tumor expansion via the paracrine production of growth factors, such as TGF-β, platelet-derived growth factor (PDGF), insulin-like growth factor I and II, and calcium. The favorable combination of these factors enhances the capacity of solid tumors to use bone as a frequent target for metastasis.[13]

Understanding the metabolic functions involved in the balance of osteoclast and osteoblast activity within the marrow stroma will help support the rationale behind newer therapies in the treatment of bone metastasis discussed later in this chapter. Osteoclasts arise from the monocyte-macrophage lineage, and are induced by macrophage colony-stimulating factor (M-CSF), and by binding to the receptor activator of nuclear factor-κB (RANK) ligand (RANKL) present on the surface of osteoblasts and stromal cells.[10,14] Osteoblastic secretion of cytokines, such as interleukin 6 (IL-6), IL-1, and prostaglandin E_2, also aids in the induction of osteoclast formation. Osteoclasts adhere to the surface of the bone via integrins, where they control osseous resorption by protease secretion. Osteoblasts arise from mesenchymal cells, and their differentiation is controlled by several of the growth factors produced by the stromal cells, such as TGF-β and PDGF.[9]

Within the bone matrix, most metastatic solid tumors secrete parathyroid hormone-related peptide, which binds to the parathyroid hormone receptor (PTHR1) and stimulates osteoclast development.[15,16] The activation of PTHR1 also stimulates expression of RANKL on stromal cells, which has been shown to induce formation of osteoclasts. Osteoclast-induced resorption of bone results in the local increase in calcium concentration, which in turn stimulates tumor growth and parathyroid hormone-related protein production. Therefore, a significant relationship appears to exist between bone destruction and metastatic tumor growth mediated through cell signaling involving the microenvironment. This phenomenon has been viewed as a "vicious cycle."[9,10]

This "vicious cycle" may also exist in the development of osteoblastic metastasis, such as that seen with prostate cancer; however, the mechanisms related to osteoblastic metastasis are less recognized. Paracrine factors, such as endothelin 1 and PDGF, also appear to stimulate osteoblastic metastasis and tumor growth.[8,9,10,17] In addition, prostate cancer cells secrete both prostate-specific antigen (PSA) and urokinase-type plasminogen activator (u-PA), which activate growth factors within the marrow stroma, such as TGF-β and insulin-like growth factors I and II that, in turn stimulate osteoblastic activity.[9]

Clinical Presentation

The principal presenting symptom of metastatic cancer to the bone is pain. The pain can have both biologic and mechanical components.[18] The biologic component refers to pain associated with growth of the tumor itself. Tumor growth must be accompanied by angiogenesis and hyperemia. Along with the increased blood flow come cytokines, which are thought to be important mediators of the pain response.[19] This biologic component to the pain is often described as a deep, dull, ache in the bone that is unrelated to activity. This type of pain is often responsive to nonsurgical management, such as radiation and chemotherapy.[20]

The mechanical aspects of the pain, on the other hand, are strain related. This pain is aggravated by weight-bearing activities and is relieved by rest. This pattern of pain results from the loss of structural integrity of the bone.[20] As already stated, for the metastatic tumor to grow within the bone there must be a mechanism for bone lysis, which is thought to occur secondary to effects on the host osteoclasts and osteoblasts, rather than by a direct effect of the tumor cells themselves. Typically, osteoclast stimulation outweighs osteoblast stimulation, and a lytic lesion of bone results.[21] This net bone loss reduces bone strength and stiffness, thereby leading to pain with weightbearing. Pain of this character is less likely to be immediately responsive to medical management. Increasing mechanical symptoms may signal impending pathologic fracture and warrant protected weight-bearing as well as a consideration of prophylactic operative stabilization.

Many metastatic tumors to bone have no presenting symptoms. These lesions may come to medical attention as an incidental finding on plain radiographs or, more commonly, by bone scintigraphy in the setting of staging of a known primary tumor.

Radiologic Evaluation of Skeletal Metastases

Radiography

The sensitivity of plain radiographs to detect metastatic lesions is low. Studies have shown that more than 50% to 70% of cancellous bone must be destroyed to be reliably detected by plain radiographs.[22] Although involvement of the cortex may be detectable much earlier (i.e., with a lesser degree of destruction), it is an uncommon site of early metastatic involvement. Cortical bone, which is much denser than cancellous bone, masks subtle foci of abnormal trabecular bone, leaving them much less conspicuous (Figure 95.1).

Appearance of the metastatic lesion also affects its detectability by radiography. Permeative lesions can be particularly difficult to detect until a large area of medullary bone is involved. Similarly, purely lytic metastases may be radiographically occult until large unless they involve the cortex (Figure 95.2). Cortical involvement of a trabecular lesion can be perceived as endosteal scalloping along the inner margin. In lesions of mixed lytic/blastic appearance, adjacent areas of sclerosis depict reaction of the adjacent normal bone in an attempt to "wall off" the metastasis. Purely blastic lesions are often more readily detectable, with areas of sclerosis often demonstrating ill-defined margins. These lesions are likely caused by reaction to osteoblast-like factors made by the tumor, attempts by the surrounding normal bone to isolate the abnormal focus, or a combination of the two processes. In the event of a direct cortical metastasis, a well-defined focal cortical defect can be seen, which can give the false impression of a benign lesion.

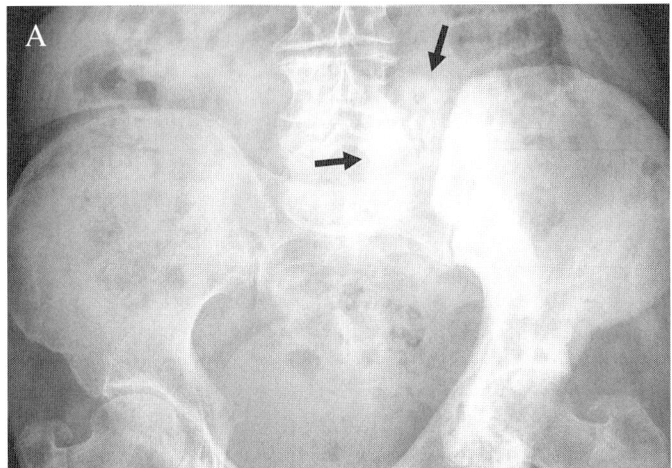

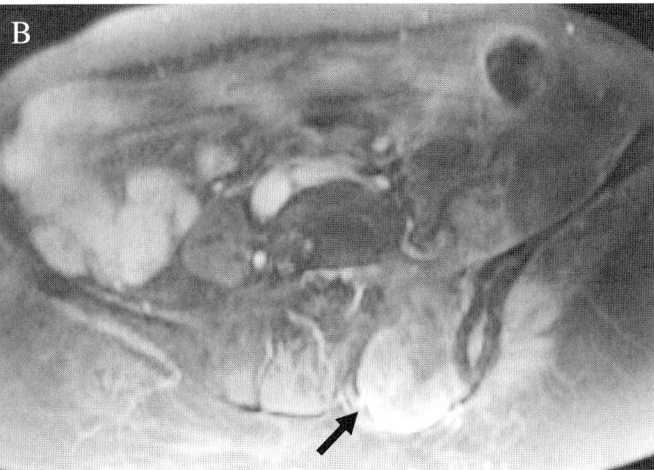

FIGURE 95.1. Anteroposterior (AP) view of the pelvis (A) in a 76-year-old patient with a history of Paget's disease shows bony expansion and trabecular thickening involving the right hemipelvis, consistent with this history. Additionally, the superior margin of the left sacrum is not seen, and there is suggestion of a soft tissue mass in this location. Dense osteoid matrix is identified within the soft tissue mass. In this setting, findings are suggestive of sarcomatous transformation in the setting of Paget's disease. (B) Axial post-gadolinium T_1-weighted magnetic resonance imaging (MRI) of the pelvis better demonstrates the extensive involvement of the left sacrum by the heterogeneously enhancing soft tissue mass.

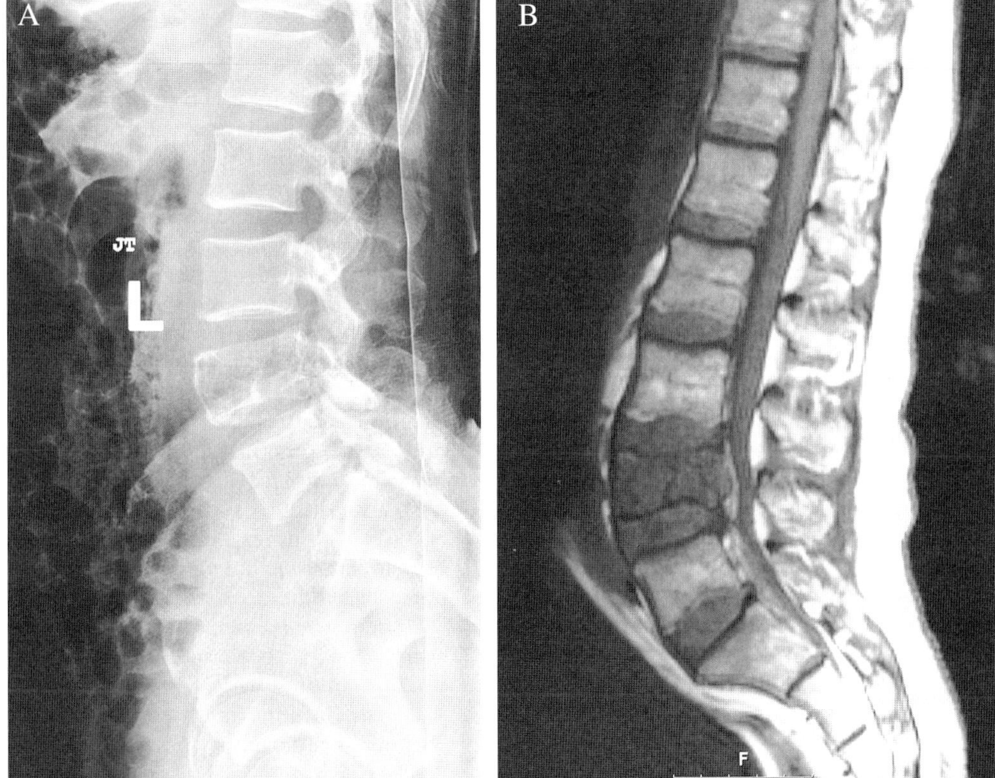

FIGURE 95.2. Lateral view of the lumbar spine (A) demonstrates lytic replacement of the L4 vertebral body in this 53-year-old patient. Sagittal T_1-weighted MRI of the spine (B) shows diffuse marrow replacement. Subsequent computed tomography (CT)-guided biopsy (not shown) confirmed the presence of a plasmacytoma.

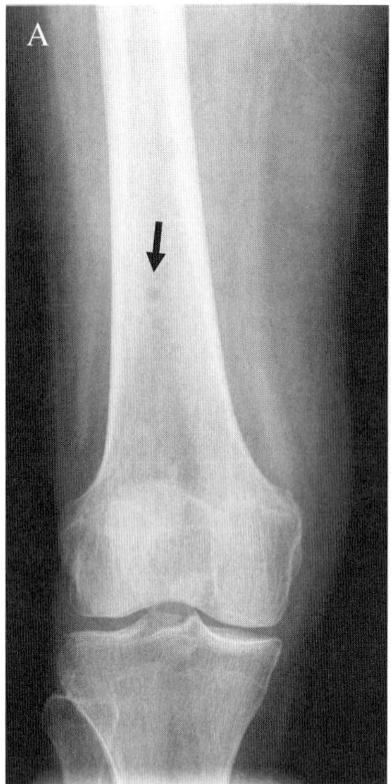

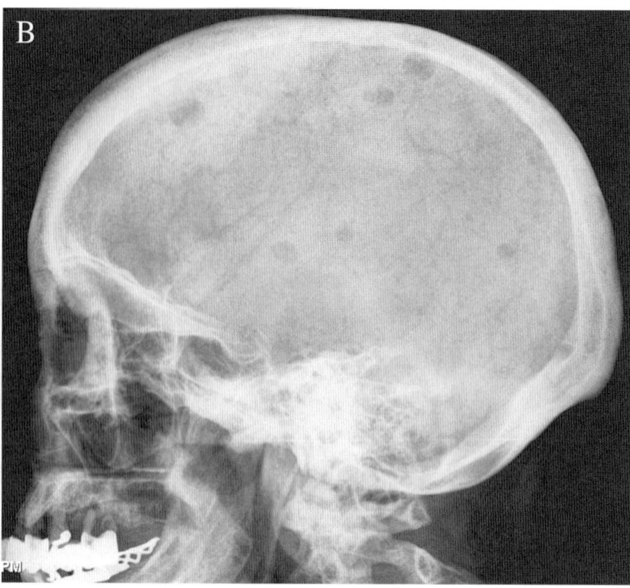

FIGURE 95.3. AP view of the right femur (A) and lateral view of the skull (B) in a patient with a history of multiple myeloma demonstrate the classic "punched-out" lytic lesions associated with this malignancy.

Because of its low sensitivity for most metastatic lesions, radiography is best used as an adjunct to other imaging modalities. Plain films can also be helpful in the evaluation of symptomatic sites. Additionally, radiography has been used in an attempt to assess the risk of pathologic fracture in long bone metastases. Fidler et al. proposed that pathologic fracture was unlikely if less than 50% of the cortex was destroyed, likely if 50% to 75% was destroyed, and expected if greater than 75% was destroyed.[23] Given the limitations of plain film radiography, this is likely only an approximation.

A related clinical presentation in which radiography is still the imaging modality of choice is multiple myeloma. Lesions associated with myeloma are notorious for their low conspicuity on conventional bone scintigraphy, such that the bone survey is still used for staging and evaluation in this disease. Plain film usually demonstrates a "punched-out" lytic lesion (Figure 95.3). Nevertheless, evaluation of these surveys is difficult, with the inherent limitations of radiography meaning that significant disease can be missed.

Nuclear Medicine

In most cases, nuclear medicine scans using Tc-99m phosphate compounds represent the preferred method of evaluating skeletal metastases in both symptomatic and asymptomatic patients. Although they represent a powerful tool in the staging of metastatic disease due to their high sensitivity, a basic understanding of their mechanism of action is important when interpreting results. The radioactive complexes are incorporated into areas of bone formation or increased osteoblast activity. This process can lead to areas of increased radiopharmaceutical activity in the presence of tumor, with a sensitivity reported at 50% to 80% greater than radiography. However, virtually any pathologic process can yield a similar appearance.[24] Foci of abnormally increased activity can be seen in the presence of fracture, infection, inflammation, surgery, and degenerative changes. Plain film correlation is indicated in situations or at sites where these processes may give the false impression of tumor spread.

In bone scintigraphy, the pattern of abnormal foci of activity may suggest the diagnosis of skeletal metastases. Multiple areas of increased activity of varying size, with a propensity for the axial skeleton, most likely represent metastatic disease (Figure 95.4). However, clinical correlation with the patient's symptoms is necessary because the aforementioned mimics can coexist with metastatic disease. It has been estimated that only 50% of solitary "hot" lesions on bone scan indicate metastasis, even in the setting of a known malignancy[25]; this underscores the importance of plain film correlation in characterizing bone scan abnormalities. Because plain film findings of metastasis can lag behind scintigraphic abnormalities, a negative plain film in the presence of an abnormality on nuclear scanning does not exclude the possibility of a metastasis.

Among metastases shown by bone scintigraphy, 39% were seen in the vertebrae, 38% in the ribs and sternum, 12% in the pelvis, with only 10% in the skull and long bones.[26] This propensity for the axial skeleton makes bone scanning particularly attractive as an initial evaluation, as it simplifies the evaluation of those parts of the skeleton that are more difficult to visualize by plain film: the scapula, sternum, ribs, and spine. Evaluation of the pelvis is sometimes complicated by pooling of the excreted radiopharmaceutical in the bladder.

The ribs are also sometimes difficult to evaluate. Areas of increased activity that parallel the long axis of the rib likely indicate metastasis, whereas more focal lesions, especially when arranged in a linear orientation in adjacent ribs, often indicate fracture. Although 80% of solitary foci of activity in a series of proven metastatic disease to bone were found to correspond to true metastatic lesions, only 17% of solitary "hot spots" in the ribs were the result of metastasis.[27]

As tracer activity is dependent on the presence of bone turnover, photopenic or "cold" lesions can be seen in the presence of particularly aggressive tumors, where the growth is too rapid for sufficient reactive bone growth. This presentation can be seen in metastases from carcinoma of the breast or lung. Additionally, diffuse metastatic involvement throughout the skeleton can lead to a relatively homogeneous appearance, yielding a false impression of a normal scan. This entity, termed the "super scan," should be suspected in the setting of intense skeletal activity in the absence of renal, bladder, or soft tissue uptake. The appearance is due to the increased extraction of the radiopharmaceutical by the reactive bone compared to the soft tissues and kidneys.

Bone marrow scanning has been advocated as an alternative to phosphate compound methods in the evaluation of some malignancies. In one study, bone marrow scanning with a monoclonal antibody complex detected almost twice the

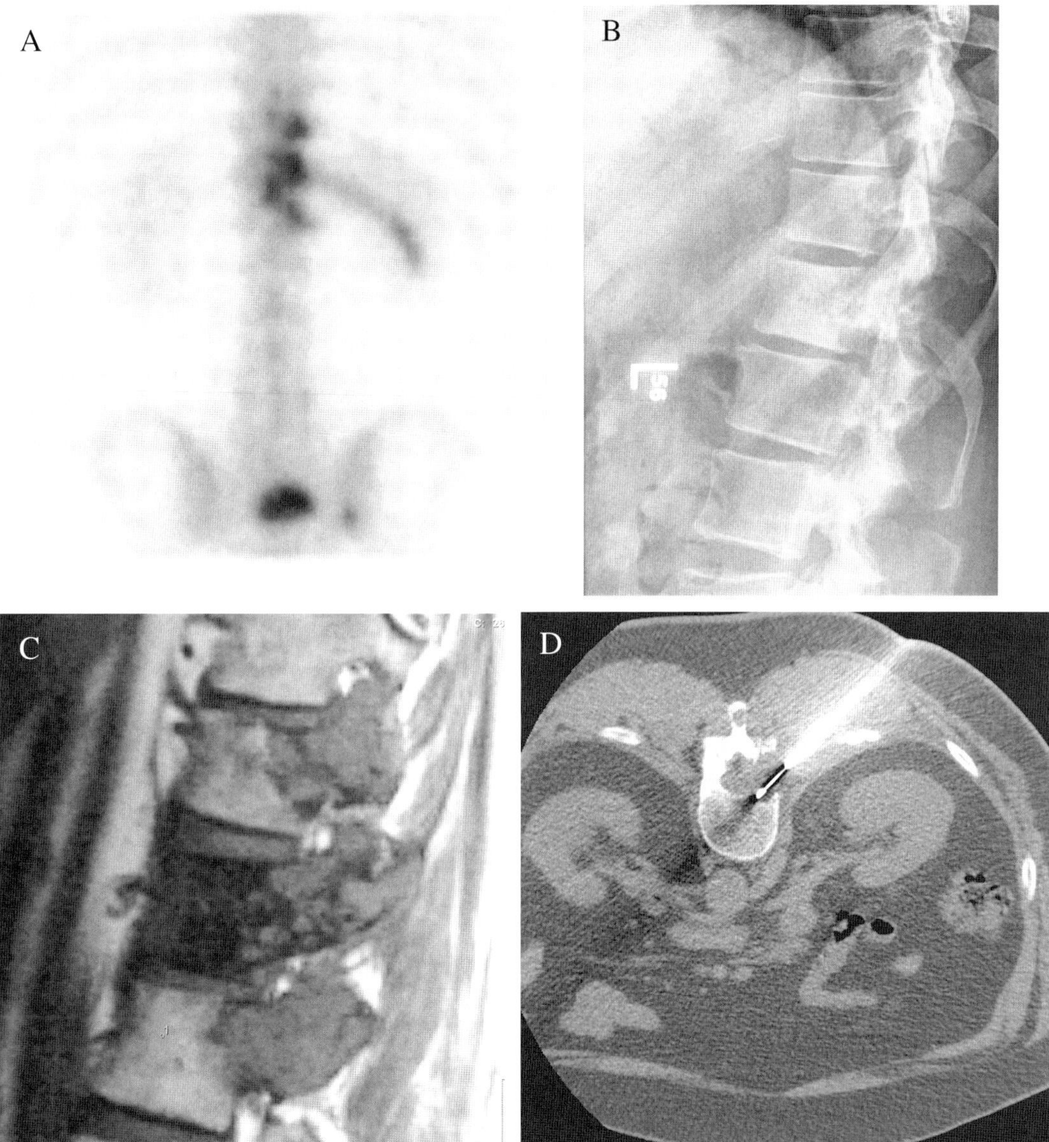

FIGURE 95.4. (A) Posterior tomographic image from a technetium-99m-MDP bone scan in a 55-year-old patient with a history of breast carcinoma, shows abnormally increased radiopharmaceutical activity on the right at the T11, T12, and L1 vertebral body levels. (B) Lateral film of the thoracolumbar spine in the same patient demonstrates lytic lesions at the same levels, which appear centered at the junction of the pedicles with the vertebral bodies. (C) Sagittal T_1-weighted noncontrast MRI through the same region demonstrates abnormal marrow replacement centered at the vertebral body–pedicle junction. This case illustrates the improved marrow resolution of MRI relative to plain film. (D) Axial CT image in the same patient showing CT-guided core biopsy of the T12 lesion via a transpedicular approach.

number of metastases as conventional bone scanning. However, the number of patients identified as having skeletal metastatic involvement was the same with both methods, suggesting that management would not have been changed.[28]

For screening in patients with papillary and follicular variants of thyroid carcinoma, ^{131}I whole-body scans are preferred over Tc-99 studies. One study found that 78% of thyroid metastases visualized by radiography or ^{131}I scans were undetectable or "minimally abnormal" on technetium bone scans.[29]

Positron emission tomography (PET) scanning has gained widespread acceptance in the evaluation and staging of metastatic disease in recent years, having lately been approved for the evaluation of breast and lung carcinomas. PET has been shown to be moderately sensitive in the detection of prostatic carcinoma metastatic to the spine (sensitivity, 65%), but with high specificity (98%).[30] PET appears to be useful in separating Paget's disease and other benign entities (which demonstrate low uptake) from bone metastases or sarcomatous degeneration of Paget's.[31,32]

Evaluation of Response to Therapy

Skeletal metastases may respond to chemotherapy, radiation therapy, and bone agents, such as the bisphosphonate class of drugs. This response may be detected through imaging studies. On plain radiographs, an increase in sclerosis may be seen, with progression of the sclerosis from the periphery toward the center of the lesion. Increasing sclerosis may make previously undetectable lesions visible radiographically. This misleading appearance may give the false impression of worsening disease. An increase in size of either a sclerotic or lytic lesion, as well as increased lysis in a previously blastic site, suggest failure of therapy and progression of metastatic disease.[33]

Similarly, radioisotope bone scans may show an increase in tracer activity shortly after administration of chemotherapeutic drugs.[34] This so-called flare phenomenon is believed to represent increased radionuclide deposition secondary to bone healing and a resultant increase in bone formation. Additionally, an increase in the number of "hot spots" in the setting of therapy may represent previously undetectable lesions being made visible by the increase in bone formation. Such appearances must be correlated with the clinical history of therapy in order to avoid a false impression of worsening disease. If followed, healing lesions will eventually demonstrate decreased radiopharmaceutical uptake and should eventually take on a normal or near-normal appearance. In equivocal cases, radiographs can offer evidence of subtle changes that may not be manifest on bone scanning.[33]

Computed Tomography

Computed tomography (CT) is useful as an adjunct to other imaging modalities in the evaluation of metastases. While CT is capable of demonstrating abnormalities before they are seen on radiography, it is a cumbersome tool for screening the skeleton. CT can delineate abnormalities seen on bone scan when they cannot be corroborated by plain film evaluation. CT can also depict subtle areas of cortical involvement in long bones better than radiography. It can demonstrate spinal metastases better than plain film, and can be used in conjunction with nuclear medicine scans to more clearly elucidate specific sites of involvement, such as the pedicles.[35,36] Similarly, the complex bony anatomy of the pelvis is better evaluated by CT. Quantitative CT has been used to detect marrow replacement in long bones before bone destruction is noted. Increased attenuation compared with the normal fatty marrow suggests the abnormality. A difference between the right and left sides of 20 Hounsfield units is considered abnormal.[37]

Perhaps the most potentially useful aspect of CT in the evaluation of metastatic disease is as a means of directing biopsy. CT-guided biopsy of suspected areas of tumor involvement has been shown to be a safe and effective means of reaching a diagnosis and, in the setting of metastatic disease, provides staging information as well.[38,39] Although image-guided biopsies of bone lesions have been performed for over 60 years, CT allows improved precision of needle placement over previous fluoroscopic techniques (Figure 95.4D). Modern techniques allow most procedures to be performed on an outpatient basis and under local anesthesia, thereby decreasing the cost and potential morbidity compared with surgical biopsy.[39–42]

Most skeletal lesions can be reached under CT guidance. This ability to make a tissue diagnosis has wide-ranging implications in guiding subsequent management. CT-guided biopsy can also identify alternative diagnoses, such as infection and primary tumors of bone. Percutaneous biopsy of metastatic lesions has been shown to have a higher accuracy than biopsies of infections and primary tumors.[43] Nonetheless, this information can drastically alter management.

Image-guided biopsy of spinal lesions under CT guidance has been shown to have an overall accuracy of 71% to 100%.[39] In an early study, 78% of clinically or histologically confirmed bone malignancies were correctly identified by CT-guided fine-needle aspiration.[40] More recent studies have reported successful diagnoses by CT-guided bone biopsy in 71% to 89% of cases.[38,39,40,44] CT-guided biopsy has also proven useful in the diagnosis of benign lesions, which can give the false impression of malignancy.[44]

In addition to CT-guided biopsy as a means of diagnosis and staging, recent work has studied the potential for percutaneous treatment of lesions. Techniques have involved alcohol injections and ablation, for the purpose of palliation. In one study, 25 patients with painful skeletal metastases that were previously unsuccessfully treated, received image-guided injection of 95% alcohol; 74% of these patients reported decreased analgesic requirements within 2 days of the procedure.[45] Painful vertebral body fractures have also been treated by vertebroplasty under fluoroscopic or CT guidance.

Magnetic Resonance Imaging

Skeletal metastases lead to infiltration or replacement of normal marrow. This propensity for marrow involvement underlies the usefulness of magnetic resonance imaging (MRI) in the identification of metastatic lesions. The fact that the majority of red marrow in adults is located within the axial skeleton, where metastases most commonly occur, makes this an ideal technique.

MRI is used most often to evaluate metastatic disease of the spine, where it has proven superior to CT and myelography.[46,47] The superior soft tissue detail of MRI allows it to demonstrate paravertebral extension of tumor as well as canal involvement, whether the spinal cord is compressed or not. In the setting of extradural masses, MRI is more sensitive than CT myelography.[48] The excellent marrow detail achievable by MRI also makes it a useful adjunct to conventional bone scans. MRI has been shown to be more sensitive to spinal metastases than bone scintigraphy, although bone scanning is probably more practical as an initial screening method at this time, with MRI used to further evaluate equivocal nuclear medicine findings.[49,50]

Faster MRI sequences under development may make screening with MRI feasible, obviating the need for scintigraphy in many circumstances. These methods employ sequences designed to highlight sites of marrow infiltration. Early studies comparing MRI marrow screening of the axial skeleton to whole-body bone scintigraphy, showed no significant difference in accuracy when evaluating breast and prostate cancer patients for skeletal metastases. In this study, 2% had isolated metastatic involvement of the appendicular skeleton. Nevertheless, 75% of patients with isolated peripheral involvement experienced pain, with subsequent plain films showing the metastatic lesions.[51] A more recent study used turbo-STIR (short tau inversion recovery) imaging of the whole body to evaluate metastatic involvement in a small group of patients with breast cancer. Comparison showed an 88% concordance rate between the two modalities, with MRI showing an additional lesion not evident on scintigraphy and subsequently shown by biopsy to be malignant.[52] MRI techniques, such as these, provide the additional potential benefit of evaluating the liver and brain. While initial results appear promising, larger studies will be required before scintigraphy is likely to be replaced.

Normal bone marrow (including hematopoietic marrow) contains a high percentage of fat, making it high in signal on T_1-weighted spin echo images. Metastatic foci in adults characteristically demonstrate areas of decreased signal on T_1-weighted images relative to the high signal of normal fatty marrow (see Figure 95.2B). These lesions often demonstrate increased signal on STIR or T_2-weighted spin echo images, owing to their high water content, and often have a surrounding area of bright T_2 signal (known as the "halo" sign).[53] Variable enhancement is seen following gadolinium administration, and different metastatic foci within the same patient can demonstrate vastly different enhancement patterns. Lesion conspicuity on gadolinium-enhanced scans can be improved by employing fat suppression techniques (see Figure 95.1B). Use of fat suppression on precontrast images can actually lower sensitivity, however, because of the loss of the otherwise noticeable fat–soft tissue interface.

MRI can be useful in distinguishing osteoporotic vertebral body compression fractures from those arising secondary to metastases. In the setting of an osteoporotic compression fracture, marrow signal intensity should follow that of normal marrow in adjacent vertebral bodies. Metastatic foci will demonstrate findings of marrow replacement, as already noted, and may show enhancement following gadolinium administration. Additional findings suggestive of metastatic compression fracture on MRI include a convex posterior border of the vertebral body, abnormal signal intensity involving the pedicle or posterior elements (Figure 95.4B,C), and the presence of an epidural or paraspinal mass.[54] The presence of multiple lesions also suggests metastatic involvement.

Acute benign compression fractures can have a similar appearance to metastatic lesions, making this differential diagnosis particularly difficult.[55] Findings suggestive of acute osteoporotic compression fracture are low signal intensity on both T_1- and T_2-weighted images, spared bone marrow signal within the vertebral body, retropulsion of bone fragments, and the presence of multiple compression fractures.[54] The use of gadolinium also may be helpful, with metastatic lesions expected to show enhancement relative to the adjacent marrow.[55]

Many of the techniques employed in MR imaging lack specificity with respect to the evaluation of metastases. Infection, as well as several benign tumors, can mimic the appearance of metastases on imaging studies. MRI is also subject to decreased sensitivity in the setting of diffuse metastatic involvement, similar to the so-called "super scan" encountered in nuclear medicine.

Diagnostic Evaluation

In general, patients presenting for evaluation of a metastatic lesion to bone fall into three categories.[56] The first category is a patient with a known primary tumor who presents with bone pain and a lesion on plain radiographs or with pathologic fracture. The second category is the asymptomatic patient with a known primary lesion who is found to have areas of increased uptake on scintigraphic evaluation. The third category is a patient who does not have a known diagnosis of cancer and presents with pain or pathologic fracture and a suspicious lesion on plain radiographs. Each patient deserves an organized approach to their management. A systematic approach can shorten the time to and improve the accuracy of the diagnosis and eliminate pitfalls in treatment.

The evaluation of the patient should begin with a thorough history and physical examination. Focused questioning in the history of present illness will often reveal symptoms of mechanical pain before pathologic fracture, which can be particularly helpful in the patient with an unknown primary. Patients should be asked directly whether they have had a diagnosis of cancer. Often patients with a history of cancer followed by a prolonged disease-free interval do not consider the previous diagnosis as pertinent. However, bone metastases may present after a decade or more of remission from, for example, breast cancer. Social and occupational history should be focused to reveal any exposure to possible carcinogens. The sexual history may also be contributory, as human immunodeficiency virus/acquired immunodeficiency syndrome (HIV/AIDS) carries an increased risk of certain neoplasms. A thorough review of systems should include specific questions regarding respiratory, endocrine, genitourinary, and integumentary systems. Patients should be asked directly about persistent cough or hemoptysis that may be associated with a lung carcinoma. The patients should be questioned directly about flank pain or hematuria, which may be related to a renal cell carcinoma. Symptoms typically associated with prostate enlargement, such as voiding hesitancy, frequency, and nocturia may be secondary to prostate carcinoma. Patients should be asked about suspicious lesions found on their skin or any history of biopsy. Patients should be asked whether they have ever had a breast mass or biopsy. All these areas should be covered directly, because the association is often not apparent to the patient.

Physical examination, as always, should be complete. If the patient is presenting without an underlying diagnosis of a primary tumor, the physical examination should not be limited to the musculoskeletal system. Breast, intraabdominal, or prostate masses may indicate the primary site of disease.

Laboratory evaluation can be diagnostic in some cases of metastatic bone disease. Serum and urine protein electrophoresis studies can be diagnostic of multiple myeloma. A markedly elevated prostate-specific antigen (PSA) can lead to the diagnosis of prostate cancer. In most cases, however, laboratory workup is relatively nonspecific and therefore nondiagnostic. Nonetheless, a general laboratory workup, including complete blood count with differential, serum chemistries, and erythrocyte sedimentation rate, can help guide the management of the patient with suspected metastatic bone disease. Elevated white count may be indicative of infection or lymphoma. Leukocytosis may also be present in other marrow cell tumors, such as Ewing's sarcoma, multiple myeloma, histiocytosis, or leukemia. Erythrocyte sedimentation rate may also be elevated in these settings.[57] The utility of serum tumor markers has been established in the setting of known primary disease; however, they are of little value in the diagnostic workup of suspected metastatic disease to bone in the setting of an unknown primary tumor.[58]

After a thorough history and physical examination and the appropriate laboratory studies, an algorithmic approach to the evaluation of suspected metastatic bone disease splits into two categories based on whether the patient has a known primary or not. Asymptomatic patients with a known primary malignancy typically present following a bone scan that demonstrates an area of increased metabolic activity. If this is the case, the next study obtained should be a plain radiograph of the area in question. If plain radiographs reveal a lesion that is nonaggressive in appearance and demonstrates diagnostic characteristics, it may represent an enchondroma or other benign bone tumor. The lesion can be followed with serial radiographs over time. Experience in recognizing such lesions may save the patient an unnecessary biopsy.[56]

If the plain radiograph reveals a suspicious lesion, then bone scans should be reviewed to determine whether the patient has monostotic or polyostotic involvement. Metastatic disease to bone is commonly polyostotic; therefore, a monostotic lesion warrants advanced imaging before further workup. Advanced imaging would consist of CT and/or MRI. These studies can be diagnostic for certain primary tumors of bone and also are helpful in planning a biopsy.[59–61] Options for biopsy include CT-guided core needle biopsy, incisional biopsy, and excisional biopsy.

The issue of biopsy technique is important. The biopsy tract must be placed in such a way that it can be resected with the tumor in cases in which the final diagnosis is primary sarcoma of bone. Also, excessive dissection and tissue contamination should be avoided while meticulous hemostasis must be maintained. Mankin et al. have shown that poorly placed and poorly performed biopsies can result in a higher incidence in the need for amputation.[60,61] Pathologic analysis is necessary to determine definitively whether a lesion represents a primary bone tumor, such as sarcoma, or metastatic disease. It must be remembered that patients with a history of cancer elsewhere can have a second primary malignancy. The clinician must be particularly concerned about the patient with monostotic disease and no previous history of metastasis. However, in the setting of metastatic disease, pathologic analysis of the biopsy specimen is often unable to provide the primary diagnosis.[62] Once the diagnosis has been established, treatment can proceed as indicated.

The patient with a known primary malignancy who presents with a bone scan that demonstrates polyostotic disease, should obtain plain radiographs of each involved area. If there is no area of impending pathologic fracture identified on plain radiograph, the patient can be followed with observation or treated medically and/or with radiation. If the diagnosis is in doubt, biopsy can be performed at the most accessible site. If radiographs do reveal an impending fracture, surgical treatment should be considered.

Diagnosing the patient with an unknown primary can present a more daunting clinical dilemma. However, an organized approach can produce a diagnosis of the primary site of disease in the majority of cases.[62] A thorough history and physical, along with laboratory evaluation, in some cases will reveal the primary diagnosis. Serum or urine protein electrophoresis may lead to a diagnosis of myeloma. In these cases, a skeletal survey should be obtained and the patient should be referred to a medical oncologist. If history, physical, and laboratory findings fail to identify a primary diagnosis, the workup should proceed with a bone scan to look for polyostotic disease. CT images of the chest, abdomen, and pelvis also should be obtained as a screening for primary tumors.[56,62] If the CT scan identifies a primary tumor, the patient should then be staged and treated as indicated. If the CT scan fails to identify a primary tumor and the bone scan reveals polyostotic disease, biopsy should then be performed on the most appropriate and accessible site. Treatment can then proceed as indicated. If the CT scan is negative and the bone scan reveals monostotic disease, the lesion should be assumed to be sarcoma until proven otherwise, and the patient should be referred to an orthopedic oncologist.

Rougraff et al. conducted a study of 40 consecutive patients with metastasis of unknown origin.[62] The patients were evaluated with history and physical, routine serum laboratory studies, plain radiographs of the involved bones and chest, whole-body bone scintigraphy, and CT of the chest, abdomen, and pelvis. The most accessible bone lesion was then biopsied. Serum laboratory studies were nondiagnostic. History and physical revealed the primary site in 3 patients (1 each with carcinoma of the breast, kidney, and bladder). Plain chest radiographs established the diagnosis of lung carcinoma in 17 patients whereas chest CT made that diagnosis in an additional 6 cases. CT of the abdomen and pelvis established the diagnosis in 5 patients (3 with kidney carcinoma and 1 each with carcinoma of the liver and colon). Examination of the bone biopsy specimen established the diagnosis in 3 additional patients (1 with melanoma and 1 each with carcinoma of the lung and thyroid) and confirmed the primary diagnosis in 11 others. Therefore, with this strategy, the authors were able to identify the primary site of disease in 34 of 40 patients who presented with metastasis of unknown origin. Of interest, the most common primary site of disease was the lung (24 cases) followed by the kidney (3 cases). Breast carcinoma only accounted for 1 case, whereas prostate carcinoma accounted for no cases. Also of interest, histologic review of the biopsy specimen alone was able to identify the primary site in only 14 cases, whereas the prebiopsy workup identified the primary site in 31 cases.

Once the diagnosis has been established, there are three primary modes of treatment: medical management, radiation, and surgical treatment. These modes of treatment are addressed in the following sections.

Treatment Options

Radiation Treatment

External-Beam Radiation Therapy

Although the specific cause of cancer-related bone pain may differ, that is, mechanical, inflammatory, muscle spasm, or nerve compromise, more than 75% of patients with osseous metastasis will develop pain as their most important cause of reduced quality of life.[63] Radiation therapy has been the mainstay of relieving pain associated with bone metastasis. Unfortunately, this modality is used for localized palliation and is often used in conjunction with other systemic means of pain control. Data supporting wide-field radiation therapy, or "half-body" irradiation, do exist; however, this modality is not generally used in the United States. Regardless, there are several randomized trials providing Level 1 evidence concerning the optimal schedule of local radiation treatment (Table 95.1).

The primary endpoint in all these studies is pain relief. Keep in mind that differences exist in the mechanism of ascertaining pain relief, for example, physician assessment versus patient assessment, and that often, patients are given concurrent analgesia, which complicates the conclusions. The major question that is addressed in these trials is whether a shorter radiation therapy schedule results in comparable pain relief compared to the conventional schedule. Five prospective randomized trials performed during the 1980s to 1990s, examined variations in duration of treatment. Various treatment programs were compared, ranging from 30 Gy in 2 to 3 weeks (daily dose of 2–3 Gy) as the standard approach, with shorter durations of treatment utilizing three to five fractions of 15 to 20 Gy total. Overall, each study concluded that significant differences in pain relief did not occur with shorter duration of treatment. Clearly, these studies varied in sample size (57 to 759), performance status, and whether concurrent systemic antineoplastic therapy was permitted; however, these studies supported the trend in reducing duration of radiation treatment for palliation of osseous metastasis.[64–68] Only one study performed by the Radiation Therapy Oncology Group (RTOG) was large enough to support Level 1 evidence; however, the remaining studies can be classified as having Level 2 scientific evidence.[68,69]

Five additional prospective randomized trials compared the outcome of "conventional" duration of radiation treatment for bone metastasis with a single treatment fraction of 8 Gy. Again, these studies provide Level 1 evidence supporting equivalency in symptom relief with a single treatment dose. Two studies randomized a total of 1,200 patients to either a single dose of 8 Gy or a total of 24 Gy given in 6 fractions, and found no difference in pain scores.[70,71] These results were supported by three prospective randomized trials involving a total of 1,294 patients receiving treatment, either with a single fraction of 8 Gy or 20 to 30 Gy given over 5 to 10 frac-

TABLE 95.1. Radiation schedule and the treatment of osseous metastasis.

Trial	*Year*	*No. of patients*	*Randomized*	*Disease*	*Design*	*Median follow-up*	*Results*	*Conclusions*
Bone[73] Pain Trial Working Party	1999	765	Prospective	All	8 Gy single fraction vs. 20 Gy/5 fractions or 30 Gy/10 fractions	12 months	No difference in pain relief or overall survival	Single-fraction treatment is comparable to multifraction treatment
Gaze[75]	1997	245	Prospective	All	10 Gy single vs. 22.5 Gy/5 fractions	2 years	Median duration of pain relief: 13.5 weeks (single) vs. 14 weeks (multi)	Single-fraction treatment is comparable to multifraction treatment
Nielsen[72]	1998	241	Prospective, Phase III	All	8 Gy single vs. 20 Gy/4 fractions	2 years	At 20 weeks follow-up: 72% pain relief (single) vs. 82% (multi); duration of relief is same	Single-fraction treatment is comparable to multifraction treatment
Steenland[71]	1999	1171	Prospective	All	8 Gy single vs. 24 Gy/6 fractions	4 months	Time to pain relief is same, 3 weeks; no difference in pain scores ($P = 0.24$)	Single-fraction treatment is comparable to multifraction treatment
Price[74]	1986	288	Prospective	All	8 Gy single vs. 30 Gy/10 fractions	3 months	Incidence of complete relief at 4 weeks = 27% (same); same duration of relief	Single-fraction treatment is comparable to multifraction treatment

TABLE 95.2. Efficacy of radioisotopes in the treatment of osseous metastasis.

Trial	*Year*	*No. of patients*	*Randomized*	*Disease*	*Design*	*Median follow-up*	*Results*	*Conclusions*
Serafini[92]	1998	118	Double-blind	All	^{153}Sm-EDTMP 0.5 vs. 1.0 mCi/kg or placebo	16 wks	31% pain relief by week 4	Benefit in higher-dose ^{153}Sm
Lewington[91]	1991	32	Double-blind, crossover	Prostate	^{89}Sr 150 MBq vs. placebo	5 wks	Only patients receiving ^{89}Sr were pain free	Benefit with ^{89}Sr
Porter[90]	1993	126	Double-blind	Prostate	^{89}Sr 10.8 mCi vs. placebo	6 mo	At 3 months follow-up: 40% pain free with ^{89}Sr vs. 23% placebo	Reduced pain-score in 70% ^{89}Sr vs. 55% placebo; benefit with ^{89}Sr
Buchali[89]	1988	49	Double-blind	Prostate	75 MBq ^{89}Sr vs. placebo	5 wks	No difference in pain; increased survival with ^{89}Sr: 46% vs. 4% 2-year OS	Survival benefit with ^{89}Sr

OS, overall survival.

tions. Pain relief was comparable between the two regimens.[72–74] A single trial using 10 Gy as its single treatment fraction supported the previous results when compared with a 22.5 Gy treatment given over 5 fractions.[75] Two additional randomized trials investigated the optimal single fraction dose of radiation therapy; 4 Gy versus 6 Gy versus 8 Gy. In general, 8 Gy was considered the "lowest" dose that would result in adequate pain control of bone metastasis.[76,77]

Three systematic reviews of the literature describing randomized trials comparing short versus long duration of radiation therapy for palliation have concluded that shorter therapy (single fraction of 6–10 Gy) is comparable to longer treatment.[78–80] Overall, there is sufficient Level 1 evidence to support single-fraction therapy for the palliation of bone metastasis.[81] An additional benefit of single-dose therapy that was discussed within these randomized trials was the ability of retreating the disease site if symptoms reoccurred. This action was deemed acceptable in the majority of studies, yet clearly the need for retreatment suggests an inadequate disease response to the original radiation received. These difficulties in comparing pain relief due to radiation therapy among the various studies is being addressed by a task force (International Bone Metastasis Consensus Working Party) that will enable further prospective randomized trials utilizing radiation therapy to be performed in a more consistent fashion and support stronger evidence for treatment strategies.[82]

Systemic Radionuclide Therapy

Several radiopharmaceuticals are approved for palliative treatment of bone metastasis in the United States; however, the Level 1 and Level 2 data are scarcer than those available for conventional radiation therapy. The characteristics of all radionuclides used in this setting are the need for the nuclide to be preferentially deposited in the bone, and that the product emits particulate radiation that is locally absorbed.[83] Phosphorus-32 has been widely used for the control of myeloproliferative diseases because it is also preferentially incorporated into bone marrow; however, it can also be used to effectively control pain caused by osseous metastasis from solid tumors.[84]

Physician practice is not as supportive of radionuclide therapy for palliation, and specifically, ^{32}P is used less than newer approved treatments because of concerns with myelosuppression.[85] This concern was supported in a randomized trial of 31 patients receiving either ^{32}P or ^{89}Sr, a radioactive calcium analogue that is a beta emitter which has less hematologic toxicity and is effective in the treatment primarily of blastic metastasis.[86,87] More than 90% of the patients in each group achieved pain relief; however, bone marrow suppression was slightly more common in the ^{32}P-treated patients.[88] Three randomized control trials with ^{89}Sr and one trial with samarium-153 (both approved for use in the United States) provide Level 1 evidence supporting the use of radionuclides in reducing pain due to osseous metastasis.[89,90,91,92] Two systematic reviews lend Level 1 support and confirm the optimal dose of ^{89}Sr (150–200 MBq) and ^{153}Sm (1.0 mCi/kg) that result in pain relief after approximately 1 to 2 weeks, lasting for approximately 2 to 4 months in 60% to 80% of patients treated with a single administration of nuclide.[78,93] Caution must be used in the application of these therapies because of the potential for bone marrow suppression; repeated administration of nuclide has not been thoroughly investigated. Patients with multiple osteoblastic metastasis or mixed lesions that have not been extensively pretreated with radiation therapy and chemotherapy offer the optimal patient population for response with minimal toxicity with radiopharmaceuticals.[94] These results are presented in Table 95.2.

Medical Treatment

Bisphosphonate Therapy

Bisphosphonates are analogues of pyrophosphate wherein a carbon atom replaces the central oxygen atom. This structure permits binding to hydroxyapatite within bone and results in an increased resistance to hydrolysis and consequent reduction in bone mineral dissolution because of their phosphorus–carbon–phosphorus bond. For this reason, bisphosphonates are extremely effective in the treatment of hypercalcemia that occurs in approximately 10% to 20% of patients with cancer. In addition, bisphosphonates have been shown to inhibit osteoclast activity, lessen chemotaxis of osteoclasts to sites of bone resorption, and induce osteoclast apoptosis by inhibiting the enzyme farnesyl diphosphate synthetase and inhibiting cytokine synthesis by stromal cells, for example, IL-6 production.[95–97] Consequently, the use of bisphosphonates is effective in reducing the morbidity of skeletal events associated with metastatic disease, such as fracture and pain, and may contribute to the delay in the progression of osseous metastasis by interfering with tumor cell adhesion to bone or directly inducing tumor apoptosis.[98,99] Although the majority of data supporting the use of bisphosphonates primarily involve patients with metastatic breast and prostate cancer or multiple myeloma, several recent trials also support the use of this class of drugs for adjunctive treatment of osseous metastasis due to other solid tumors.

Hypercalcemia

Level 1 evidence does exist that supports the use of bisphosphonates in the treatment of hypercalcemia of malignancy.[100] However, these studies are very heterogeneous and they could not be analyzed in a meta-analysis. Overall, the randomized trials demonstrate that the administration of bisphosphonates (pamidronate, clodronate, etidronate, ibandronate) resulted in greater than 70% incidence of normalization of calcium levels within 2 to 6 days, which is significantly superior to either saline infusion or mithramycin.[101–105] There is a single randomized trial involving 71 patients that demonstrated superiority of gallium nitrate compared with etidronate in controlling hypercalcemia.[106]

A summary of the randomized trials presented in Table 95.3 demonstrates nonstatistically significant superiority by

TABLE 95.3. Comparisons of bisphosphonates in the treatment of cancer-related hypercalcemia.

Trial	*Year*	*No. of patients*	*Randomized*	*Disease*	*Design*	*Median follow-up*	*Results*	*Conclusions*
Gucalp[107]	1992	65	Randomized after 24h IV hydration	All	60mg IV pamidronate vs. 7.5mg/kg IV etidronate × 3	7 days	Pamidronate normalized calcium in 70% vs. 41% ($P = 0.26$)	Pamidronate normalizes calcium more frequently than etidronate
Purohit[108]	1995	41	Randomized after 48h IV hydration	All	90mg IV pamidronate vs. 1,500mg IV clodronate	28 days	Pamidronate normalized calcium in 100% vs. 80% (NS) Median duration of normalization 28 days pamidronate vs. 14 days ($P < 0.01$)	Pamidronate results in a longer duration of normal calcium levels than clodronate
Ralston[109]	1989	48	Randomized after 48h IV hydration	All	30mg IV pamidronate vs. 600mg IV clodronate vs. 7.5mg/kg IV etidronate × 3	9 days	At day 6, calcium levels were lower with pamidronate vs. clodronate ($P = 0.01$) vs. etidronate ($P = 0.001$) Longer median time to relapse with pamidronate, 29 days vs. 12 days vs. 10.5 days	Pamidronate results in a longer duration of normal calcium levels than clodronate or etidronate
Major[112]	2001	287	Two identical parallel concurrent double-blind, double-dummy	All	90mg IV pamidronate vs. 4mg or 8mg IV zoledronic acid	56 days	Zoledronic acid normalized calcium within 10d in 88.4% (4mg, $p = 0.002$), 86.7% (8mg $p = 0.015$) vs. 69.7% pamidronate. Median duration of normalization 30d (4mg, $p = 0.001$), 40d (8mg, $p = 0.007$) vs. 17d pamidronate	Zoledronic acid results in a longer duration of normal calcium levels than pamidronate

pamidronate in the time to normalization of calcium levels and prolongation of the time to relapse of hypercalcemia compared with etidronate and clodronate.[107–111] Two parallel multicenter double-blind, double-dummy randomized trials, involving a total of 275 patients, compared two dose levels of zoledronic acid (4 mg and 8 mg) to pamidronate (90 mg) in the treatment of malignancy-induced hypercalcemia. Interestingly, both dose levels of zoledronic acid were superior to pamidronate in both response rates, resulting in normalization of calcium levels and duration of normocalcemia.[112]

Several other studies investigated the optimal dose of each bisphosphonate, including pamidronate and zoledronic acid. A well-designed randomized trial demonstrated a dose–response relationship using pamidronate, with the optimal dose equaling 90 mg IV. There did not appear to be any advantage among the various dosing durations or schedules.[113] The toxicity associated with bisphosphonate use in this setting is minimal. Self-limiting fever appears to be the most common effect, followed by hypocalcaemia and hypophosphatemia, which did not require metabolic correction.

Skeletal Morbidity

Several bisphosphonates have demonstrated the ability to reduce the incidence of bone pain and fracture due to metastatic disease. Most of the current evidence supports the use of intravenous administration, because approximately 5% of bisphosphonates are absorbed with oral administration, and this absorption is quite variable depending upon concurrent intake with other medicines and food. Level 1 evidence supports the inclusion of bisphosphonates as adjunctive therapy in the treatment of osseous metastasis to reduce skeletal morbidity. This Level 1 evidence is presented in the form of a meta-analysis involving 18 randomized clinical trials that compare bisphosphonate use with placebo and result in a statistically significant reduction in the odds ratio (OR) for vertebral fractures of 0.692 [95% confidence interval (CI), 0.570–0.840], nonvertebral fractures of 0.653 (95% CI, 0.540–0.791), combined fractures of 0.653 (95% CI, 0.547–0.780), and need for radiation therapy of 0.674 (95% CI, 0.573–0.791).[100] Several bisphosphonates were included in this analysis, including zoledronic acid, pamidronate, and clodronate, administered either orally or intravenously.

Among those randomized placebo-controlled studies included in the meta-analysis, the majority of trials involved patients with metastatic breast cancer, evaluating the efficacy of either adjunctive pamidronate or clodronate versus placebo.[114–119] Again, a dose response was demonstrated with regard to skeletal-related events, and the administration of bisphosphonates orally was problematic due to gastrointestinal (GI) toxicity.[120–124] The efficacy of zoledronic acid compared with placebo was examined among patients with metastatic prostate cancer, lung cancer, and other malignancies.[125,126] In two very large randomized trials comparing zoledronic acid with pamidronate, they appear to have equal efficacy in the reduction of skeletal events among a total of 2,128 patients with breast cancer or multiple myeloma.[127,128] This Level 1 evidence establishes the role of bisphosphonates in the reduction of the incidence of skeletal-related events compared with placebo, regardless of the type of underlying cancer.

Although the majority of skeletal-related events discussed in the foregoing section referred to bone fractures, skeletal pain has been significantly reduced with the administration of bisphosphonates, and is often included in the description of "skeletal-related events" identified in clinical trials. Level 1 evidence exists supporting the addition of bisphosphonates as adjunct therapy to reduce the level of pain and to prolong the time to progression of pain associated with bone metastasis, regardless of the concurrent use of antineoplastic therapy.[129] Two randomized trials involving a total of 465 patients with metastatic breast cancer determined that pamidronate administration statistically significantly increased the time to progression of tumor pain and resulted in a significant reduction of bone pain.[130,131] Identical results were demonstrated in a randomized trial of 55 patients with metastatic breast cancer treated with oral clodronate.[132] The administration of zoledronic acid among 635 patients with metastatic prostate cancer resulted in lower pain and analgesic scores compared with placebo.[133]

Tumor Progression

One large, placebo-controlled trial has specifically investigated the benefit of adding bisphosphonates to systemic therapy for the treatment of metastatic osseous neoplasm and its impact upon disease progression (Level 2 evidence). This European Phase III trial involved 295 patients with metastatic breast cancer, and it showed that the addition of a bisphosphonate to traditional systemic therapy, whether it is chemotherapy or hormonal therapy, will result in a statistically significant delay in the progression of disease. These 295 patients were concurrently receiving chemotherapy and were randomized to either placebo or pamidronate, 45 mg intravenously, every 3 weeks. The group receiving the pamidronate had a 48% increase in the median time to bone progression: 249 days versus 168 days in the control arm ($P = 0.02$).[134,135] Other randomized trials did not specifically address the issue of disease progression and its association with bisphosphonate use; however, they clearly demonstrate that the addition of bisphosphonate therapy did not affect overall survival.

Emerging Medical Therapy

Although there are good evidence-based data supporting several adjunctive therapies available for supportive treatment of osseous metastasis, many questions remain unanswered. We have yet to determine the optimal bisphosphonate, or whether it should be used in prevention strategies to reduce the risk of developing bone metastasis. It also is unclear as to what the optimal duration of bisphosphonate therapy is, or whether bisphosphonates in fact affect tumor growth and impact on survival. These are questions that future clinical trials need to address, and fortunately, the American Society of Clinical Oncology has presented some guidelines to aid the clinician in the application of bisphosphonate therapy in the treatment of breast cancer.[136] Increasing knowledge of the underlying pathogenesis of osseous metastasis has prompted several new therapies that target the biologic mechanisms responsible for the development of osteolytic bone metastasis and subsequent hypercalcemia. Biologic tumor necrosis factor-alpha antagonists, such as etanercept, are currently being investigated as therapies that relieve painful metastasis that are otherwise refractory to treatment.[137] Col-3 is a modified form of tetracycline and its inhibitory effects on matrix metalloproteinases are currently being explored as a potential treatment for osseous metastasis. A similar mechanism of action has been noted with doxycycline, which also suppresses osteoclast differentiation and consequent survival.[138] Recent studies using calcitonin to reduce bone pain and the incidence of pathologic fractures have not been very encouraging, and the use of gene therapy, specifically targeting osteocalcin, continues to require ongoing investigation.[139,140] Promising investigation is continuing using a humanized monoclonal antibody to parathyroid hormone-related protein that does not cross-react with parathyroid hormone.[141] These are just some of the current clinical investigations in the pursuit of controlling the adverse consequences of metastatic disease involving bone.

Image-Guided Treatment

Approximately 50% of patients who develop metastatic disease have poorly controlled pain, and management of pain in patients with metastatic disease can be difficult.[142] Traditional treatment modalities, such as radiation therapy, chemotherapy, surgery, and analgesic medication, may not satisfactorily address the needs of patients with skeletal metastases. Both radiation and chemotherapy have thresholds above which their toxic side effects become too severe to continue therapy. Additionally, side effects of conventional opioid analgesics can have a detrimental effect on the patient's quality of life.

Early research into image-guided, site-specific therapies has shown promise in the management of pain and immobility related to skeletal metastatic involvement. Initial studies involving injection of 95% ethanol into bone metastases under CT guidance led to decreased analgesic requirements in 60% of patients within 2 weeks.[45]

More recent work has focused on the use of radiofrequency ablation of tumors as an additional option for pain management in metastatic disease. This research has borrowed from the collective experience using ablation to treat solid tumors of the abdomen and pelvis, especially the liver.[143,144] This experience led to use of the technique to treat benign primary neoplasms of bone, such as osteoid osteoma and chondroblastoma, a practice that has since gained widespread acceptance.[145–147]

Applying radiofrequency (RF) ablation to painful skeletal metastatic lesions represents an exciting new option for patients for whom conventional therapies have been exhausted. Callstrom et al. demonstrated significant decreases in the pain scores and pain interference with daily activity in a series of patients treated with ablation. Eighty percent of patients using analgesic medication reported a decrease in use after the treatment.[148] In another study, 10 patients with unresectable spine metastases were treated with RF ablation. The patients reported an average of 74% decrease in pain scores, with 9 of 10 patients reporting an improvement in symptoms. Postprocedure MRI showed no further tumor growth at a mean follow-up time of 5.8 months.[149]

Several studies have reported the use of cementoplasty under image guidance as a potential treatment for pathologic fractures. Conventionally used to prevent further collapse in the setting of osteoporotic compression fractures, this technique is being applied to existing and potential sites of pathologic fracture as well. Most reports concern treatment of sites of vertebral body involvement, with marked improvement in pain management, stability, and patient mobility.[150–153] Significant pain relief and improved mobility were seen in 70% to 80% of patients treated with vertebroplasty in various studies.[150] In these patients, pain relief was apparent within 1 to 2 days of the procedure and persisted for several months to several years. Complications reported have been rare, with occasional symptoms related to extrusion of cement and subsequent compression of neural structures. When compared to the relatively higher cost and risk associated with spinal surgery, vertebroplasty may by an increasingly viable option in these settings.[150] Although most studies have dealt with treatment of spinal lesions, cementoplasty in combination with RF ablation has even been used to treat long bone metastases.[154]

Although these findings represent the potential of new, more effective treatment of skeletal tumors, the number of patients studied remains low. Also, the small number of patients with various histopathologic diagnoses makes it impossible to determine whether certain types of malignancies are more susceptible than others to RF ablation.

Surgical Treatment

Indications for Operative Treatment

Patients with cancer metastatic to bone often present with pathologic fracture. Pathologic fracture of vertebral bodies and flat bones can often be treated nonsurgically. Pathologic fractures of long bones, however, are associated with significant morbidity and are often best managed with surgical intervention (Figure 95.5). If the patient's general medical status does not prohibit the risk of anesthesia, open reduction

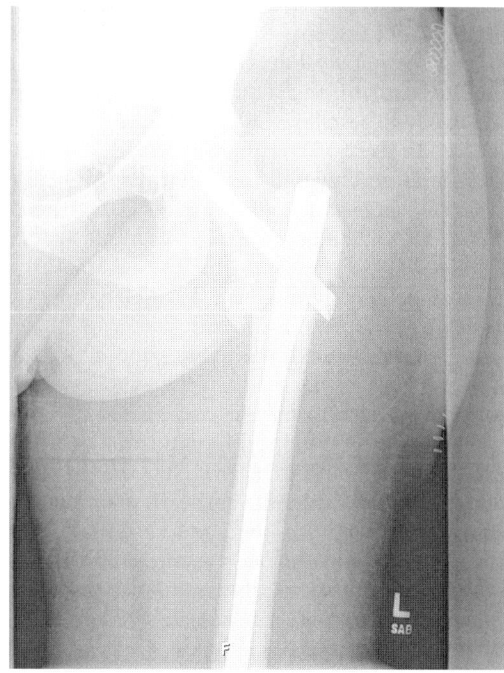

FIGURE 95.5. AP radiograph of a peritrochanteric left femur pathologic fracture secondary to metastatic breast carcinoma in a 79-year-old woman stabilized with a cephalomedullary nail.

and rigid internal fixation or resection and reconstruction should be considered. There are also many cases in which prophylactic stabilization should be considered. Prophylactic stabilization of impending fracture can spare the patient significant morbidity. The difficulty lies in deciding which lesions represent impending fracture.[23] The decision of whether to perform prophylactic surgery should depend on several factors, including (1) the biologic activity of the lesion, as demonstrated by serial radiographs over time; (2) how the lesion responds to nonsurgical management, such as chemotherapeutics and radiation therapy; (3) the location of the lesion, for example, a periarticular lesion in the weight-bearing long bone demands stronger consideration than a lesion in a non-weight-bearing bone; and (4) the overall health and expectations of the individual patient.[155]

Any cortical defect in a bone compromises its biomechanical properties, making it more prone to fracture. Cortical defects lead to an uneven distribution of stresses and are therefore, termed stress risers. Stress risers created by cortical screw holes were studied by Burstein et al. in a rabbit model. In their study, they demonstrated a 70% decrease in energy storage capacitance created by a single drill hole. The loss of bone strength is most significant in torsion.[156]

Lesions creating cortical defects are generally divided into two categories, based on the relationship between the diameter of the involved bone and the maximum dimension of the lesion. Smaller lesions are simply referred to as stress risers, whereas larger lesions are termed open-section defects. Frankel and Burstein demonstrated through biomechanical testing of cadaveric bone that, by creating stress risers, the bone strength in torsion decreased by 60%, whereas open-section defects can decrease the load to failure of a bone by 90%.[157]

These in vitro studies correlate with clinical findings and have led to some recommendations regarding prophylactic treatment. It has been recommended that for lesions greater than 2.5 cm in maximum dimension or lesions that are greater than 50% of the cross-sectional area of the bone, prophylactic treatment may be warranted.[158] Plain radiographs can be used to measure the maximum linear dimension and can also be used with orthogonal views to estimate the cross-sectional area involved. CT will give more accurate measures of cross-sectional involvement. Even with advanced imaging, however, interobserver variability exists. Using the criterion of a 2.5-cm or larger defect, Hipp et al. found up to a 42% probability of clinical errors on predicting fracture risk in metastatic lesions in 60 femurs (i.e., 19 of 60 femurs that were predicted not to fracture, did fracture), and up to 10% error in predicting fracture based on the criterion of 50% of cross-sectional area.[23,159]

The clinical symptom of pain and specifically, the character of the pain, can be helpful in determining the need for prophylactic fixation. Pain that is worsened with activity and particularly, weightbearing, is suggestive of compromised mechanical integrity of the bone and potential for fracture. On the other hand, pain that is present at all times and not affected by activity is more likely associated with the biologic activity of the tumor and not necessarily a lack of mechanical integrity of the bone. Nonetheless, pain is a subjective factor, and as reported by Keene et al., there has been no study that has shown any value in the use of pain scores alone in estimating risk for pathologic fracture.[160]

TABLE 95.4. Mirels objective scoring system.

Score	*1*	*2*	*3*
Site of lesion	Upper extremity	Lower extremity	Peritrochanteric
Pain	Mild	Moderate	Functional
Lesion	Blastic	Mixed	Lytic
Size	Less than 1/3	1/3 to 2/3	More than 2/3

Data from Mirels.[163]

The biologic activity of the metastatic lesion, as best demonstrated by serial radiographs, can be very useful in predicting impending fracture. Serial radiographs should be used whenever possible to monitor the response of a lesion to conservative treatment. It is important to remember that bone is a living tissue, the form and function of which is a result of dynamic interplay among many factors. In the case of lytic metastatic lesions to bone, it is thought that the tumor cells tip the balance in favor of osteoclasis; not all metastatic lesions are purely lytic, however. They may be lytic or blastic or mixed lytic and blastic. Zickel and Mouradian reported that purely lytic lesions were the most likely to fracture, whereas purely blastic lesions were the least likely to fracture.[161,162]

With the foregoing in mind, it is important to treat each patient on an individual basis. The patient must have sufficient life expectancy to consider undergoing surgical treatment. The outcome of the surgical intervention must be expected to expedite mobilization or facilitate the general care of the patient, barring any complication. Mirels created a scoring system to help predict the need for prophylactic fixation and retrospectively applied the system to 78 metastatic lesions to bone that were treated with radiation and without surgery.[163] Through his review, he was able to estimate pathologic fracture risk based on his objective scoring system. The scoring system rates four criteria from 1 to 3: anatomic site, pain level, lesion type, and fraction of cortex destroyed (Table 95.4). Mirels recommended prophylactic fixation of patients with a score of 8 or greater (Table 95.5). By his scoring system, a patient with functional pain (described as severe pain at rest, or pain with use of the extremity) in a weightbearing bone, automatically scores at least 8. This scoring system can be used as a guideline; however, it was created before bisphosphonates and some other nonsurgical treatment options were available.

TABLE 95.5. Risk of pathologic fracture by Mirels objective scoring system.

Score	*Fracture (%)*
Less than 6	0
7	4
8	15
9	33
10	72
11	96
12	100

Data from Mirels.[163]

Perioperative Considerations

The typical cancer patient with disease metastatic to bone is elderly, malnourished if not cachectic, and has a limited physiologic reserve. The majority of these patients have significant medical comorbidities, including cardiovascular, respiratory, and metabolic disturbances. Careful preoperative medical evaluation and optimization are necessary to minimize the risk of operative and postoperative complications.[164] Preoperative assessment will identify patients that simply do not have the medical reserve to tolerate the anesthetic event or the surgical insult. Careful screening will identify these patients and direct them toward other treatment modalities. Special attention should be paid to patients who have been treated with chemotherapeutic agents with cardiotoxic side effects, or patients who have received radiation therapy that has exposed the heart or great vessels. Cancer patients are also prone to electrolyte disturbances and deep venous thrombosis.[165] These problems should be identified and managed appropriately preoperatively.

Metastatic tumors of certain origin, particularly kidney cancer, or in specific locations, are notorious for hypervascularity. These tumors should be considered for preoperative arteriogram followed by embolization before undergoing a planned resection. Sun and Lang reported a 40% decrease in operative blood loss achieved by preoperative embolization.[166] This successful use of preoperative embolization has been reported in metastatic lesions from renal cell, breast, thyroid, and bronchogenic carcinomas.[167–169] Periacetabular lesions of any origin should be considered for preoperative embolization. Preoperative embolization should be performed within 24 to 36 hours of surgery. Embolization procedures are not without complication, however. Reported complications include transient lower extremity paresis, local muscle and soft tissue flap necrosis, cardiac arrest, and sciatic nerve impairment.[170] Tumor embolization has also been used as a palliative treatment for unresectable bone metastases and has demonstrated significant decreases in pain and improvement in patient mobility.[171–173]

Operative Treatment

It is important to address the goals of surgery before outlining the different options in operative management. It is critical that both the surgeon and the patient understand the goals and expectations of operative treatment. The goals fall into the following general categories: palliation, fracture stabilization and healing, ease in patient care, maintenance of limb function, and restoration of the ability to ambulate. Underlying all these goals is the basic principle to do no harm. The patient must be expected to have the physiologic reserve to tolerate the planned procedure. This concern creates a difficult balance between sparing the patient with a poor prognosis from extensive surgery and rehabilitation that they may not tolerate, and undertreating patients who might have the quality of their remaining life improved by operative intervention. Schneiderbauer et al. recently published a retrospective study of 306 patients who underwent hip arthroplasty for treatment of pathologic or impending pathologic hip fracture. In their series, the median duration of survival after arthroplasty was 8.6 months, with a range from 0 days to 19 years. The survival rate reported was 78% at 3 months, 60% at 6 months, 40% at 1 year, 21% at 2 years, and 6% at 5 years postarthroplasty. Only 17 patients were alive after 5 years.[174]

There are a number of surgical options available, which include fracture fixation with plates and screws or intramedullary rods. This fixation can be accompanied by resection of the lesion and allograft bone grafting or by augmentation of stabilization with methylmethacrylate cement. Resection of the lesion may require an intercalary prosthesis or bone graft for reconstruction. Periarticular lesions may be treated by resection arthroplasty, or resection and reconstruction with standard endoprostheses or mega-metallic endoprostheses.

In general, the operative treatment of metastatic bone disease can be categorized according to the site of the lesion. Lesions of flat bones that are symptomatic and refractory to conservative treatment can be treated with resection alone. Lesions involving the diaphysis of long bones are often optimally treated with intramedullary or plate fixation with or without cementation of the defect left by curettage of the lesion. Periarticular lesions often require reconstruction with endoprostheses. Depending on the extent of bone loss, complex reconstruction may be required; this may include a long-stemmed endoprosthesis in combination with a periarticular allograft in an attempt to preserve muscle attachments. Another alternative is to use an endoprosthesis designed to include segmental metallic replacement of the involved bone.

Many operative considerations are specific to the anatomic site of metastatic disease. Some site-specific considerations follow.

The axial skeleton is more commonly affected by metastatic disease than the appendicular skeleton. The axial skeleton consists of the spine and pelvis. The spine is particularly vulnerable to metastatic disease because of the anatomic relationship of the venous plexus of Batson,[7] as previously described. Autopsy studies have reported that from 36% to 70% of patients who die with cancer have spinal metastasis.[175] Many spinal metastases are not detectable on plain radiographs. Spinal metastases most often occur in the anterior and middle columns.[176] Harrington devised a classification scheme for metastatic disease of the spine that is useful in formulating treatment plans[177,178] This classification scheme places patients into one of five classes. In class I, there is no significant neurologic involvement. In class II, there is bony involvement without any collapse. In class III, there is neurologic impairment and the absence of vertebral body involvement. In class IV, there is vertebral collapse or instability without significant neurologic involvement. In class V, there is vertebral collapse with major neurologic impairment. Typically, only patients with Harrington class IV or V spine disease are indicated for surgical intervention. In general terms, surgical treatment consists of neurologic decompression and stabilization of any mechanical instability. The decompression is typically achieved through an anterior approach. Stabilization of mechanical instability often requires structural grafting anteriorly combined with posterior instrumentation.[179–181] The majority of metastatic disease to the spine, however, can be managed nonoperatively.

The bony pelvis is the second most common site of metastatic disease to bone.[6] Metastatic disease to the bony pelvis is often amenable to nonoperative treatment.[182] However, many patients with periacetabular lesions will develop progressive functional pain or pathologic fracture

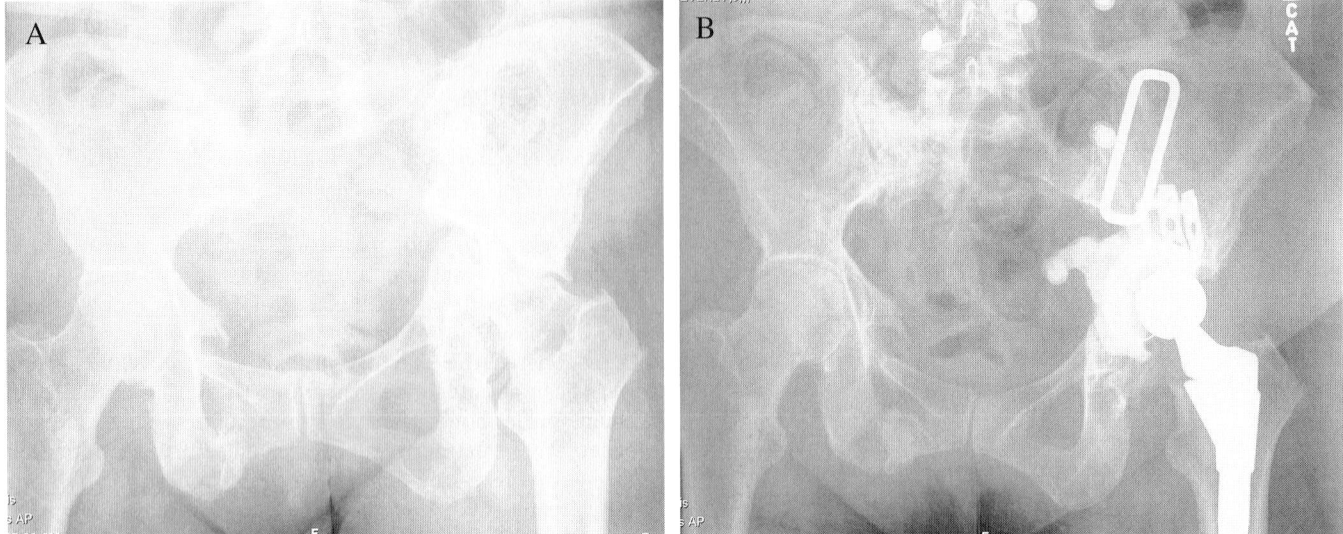

FIGURE 95.6. Preoperative (A) and postoperative (B) AP pelvis radiographs of a 46-year-old woman with metastatic breast carcinoma to her left acetabulum. Because of the destruction of the medial wall of the acetabulum, the hip was reconstructed with a cemented acetabular cup and protrusio plate reinforcement.

accompanied by the inability to ambulate; these patients' conditions can often be improved by operative reconstruction (Figure 95.6). Harrington devised a classification of acetabular insufficiency secondary to metastatic disease that helps direct the type of reconstruction the patient will need.[183] Class I acetabular insufficiency is one in which the lateral cortices, the superior and medial walls, are structurally intact; these lesions are amenable to conventional total hip arthroplasty. Class II insufficiencies include a deficient medial wall with a resulting hip protrusio. Class II deficiencies require a protrusio cup and cemented total hip arthroplasty. Class III insufficiencies include a deficient lateral and superior acetabulum. Harrington recommended a Steinmann pin-reinforced protrusio cup along with cemented total hip arthroplasty for these deficiencies. Class IV acetabular insufficiency is reserved for lesions for which complete resection is desirable, for example, renal cell carcinoma or thyroid carcinoma. These lesions require resection with reconstruction with saddle prostheses or custom implants, or resection without reconstruction could be considered (resection arthroplasty). Any reconstruction for an acetabular lesion should allow for immediate weightbearing.

The most common site of metastasis in the appendicular skeleton is the proximal femur.[6] According to Ward et al., the femur is the most common site affected by metastatic disease of the bone that requires surgical treatment.[184] As alluded to previously, treatment options are based on the site of disease within the femur. Diaphyseal lesions may be treated by curettage and cementing with plate and screw fixation or with an intramedullary device (Figure 95.7). Advantages to the use of plate and screws include direct exposure of the tumor site, which allows for open biopsy and confirmation of diagnosis. The major disadvantage of plate and screw fixation is that it only stabilizes the bone across the plate fixation. Intramedullary nailing has the advantage of providing a load-sharing device that can stabilize the entire length of the bone, including the lesion in question as well as any future lesions that might develop. A disadvantage to intramedullary nailing is the potential to spread the tumor locally along the extent of the bone during the reaming process. Ward recommends curettage of large lytic lesions before nail placement to minimize the risk of this complication.[184] Ward also recommends the use of a cephalomedullary nail as opposed to a standard intramedullary femoral nail to stabilize the femoral head and neck in the event of future spread to these areas.[184]

Lesions at the proximal end of the femur, including the femoral head, neck, and intertrochanteric area, are often treated with arthroplasty. Depending on the extent of involvement, the reconstruction may involve a standard hemiarthroplasty or total hip arthroplasty, whereas extensive involvement of the proximal end of the femur may require proximal femoral resection and reconstruction with a customized megaprosthesis (Figure 95.8).[185–187] Distal femoral

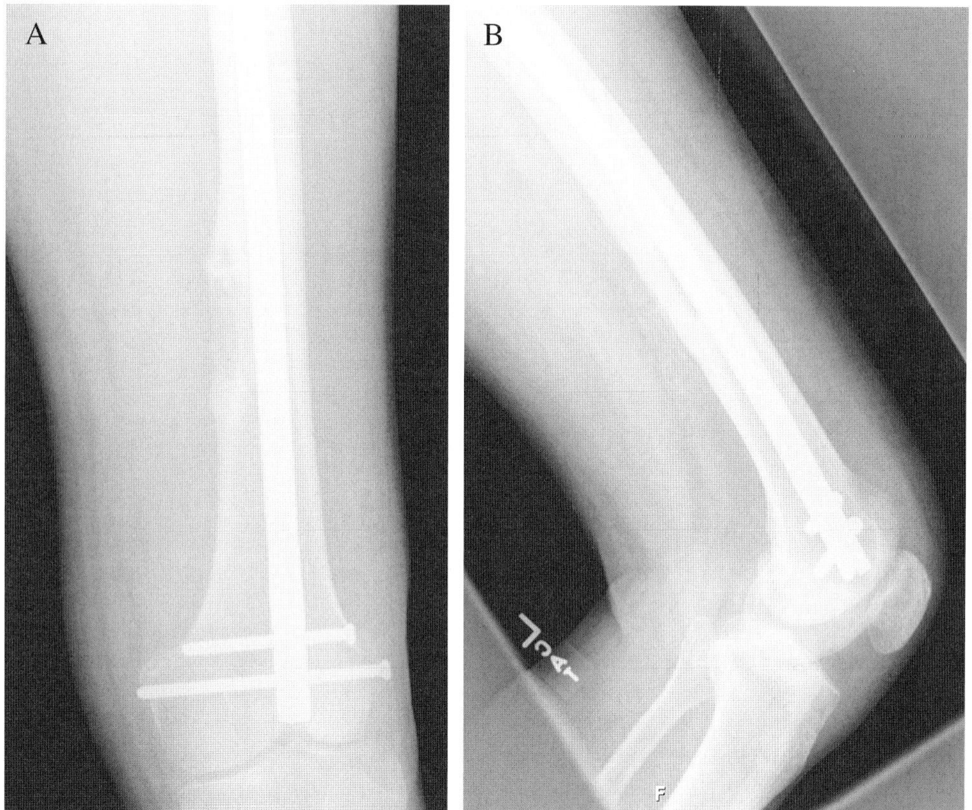

FIGURE 95.7. AP (A) and lateral (B) distal left femoral radiographs of a 65-year-old man with an intracortical metastasis from lung carcinoma. He underwent prophylactic fixation with a retrograde intramedullary femoral nail.

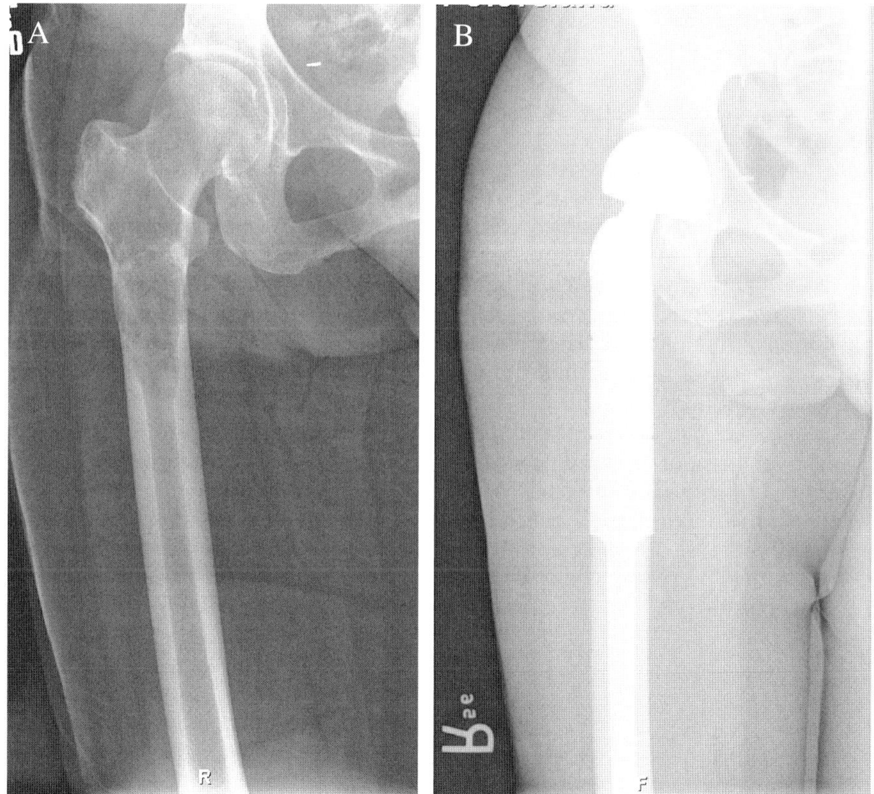

FIGURE 95.8. Preoperative (A) and postoperative (B) AP right hip radiographs of a 56-year-old woman with metastatic kidney carcinoma. Because this was her only known site of disease, she was treated with a proximal femoral resection and prosthetic reconstruction.

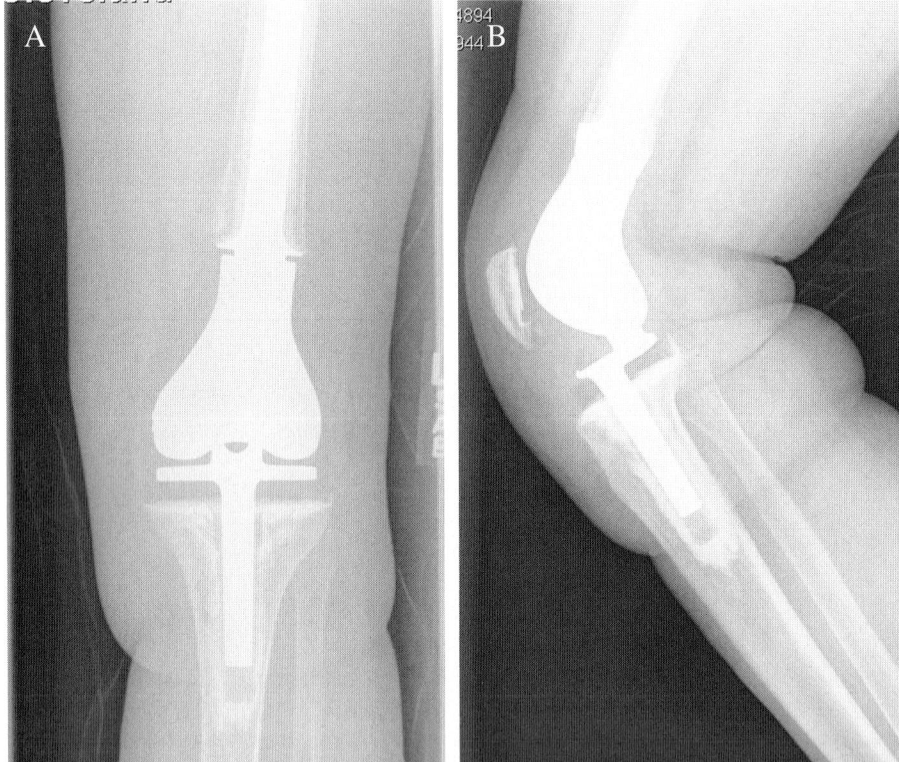

FIGURE 95.9. Postoperative AP (A) and lateral (B) radiographs of a 64-year-old woman with metastatic lung carcinoma to the distal femur. Because of extensive bone destruction, she was treated with distal femoral resection and prosthetic reconstruction.

metaphyseal lesions can occasionally be treated with a periarticular plate and screw construct along with curettage and cementing. If the lesion involves the articular surface, this can be treated with distal femoral resection and reconstruction, along with total joint replacement (Figure 95.9). Reconstructions of this type use a rotating-hinge total knee due to the loss of ligamentous attachments. Customized or modular megaprostheses can be utilized to reconstruct large intercalary segments of lost bone in the diaphysis, the proximal femur, the distal femur, or, in cases of massive involvement of the entire femur, the entire femur can be replaced with a megametallic prosthesis along with a proximal tibia replacement. Resection arthroplasty and amputation are very rarely required for treatment of metastatic disease to bone.

The treatment of metastatic disease to the humerus can be approached in a fashion similar to the treatment of the femur. Diaphyseal lesions may be treated with intramedullary nailing or with plate and screw fixation (Figure 95.10). Intercalary prosthetic reconstruction is an option for cases requiring diaphyseal resection or revision of failed fixation with segmental bone loss (Figure 95.11). Lesions in the proximal humerus may be amenable to periarticular plate and screw fixation with local curettage and cementing or may require proximal humeral resection and reconstruction with a megametallic prosthesis (Figure 95.12).

Lesions that have not been radiated before surgery should receive postoperative external-beam radiation. In a retrospective study, Townsend et al. demonstrated a 15% failure rate requiring reoperation in patients treated with surgery alone. Only 3% of patients treated with surgery and postoperative radiation required reoperation.[188]

Regardless of the location of the operative treatment, there is a constant goal of rapid return to weightbearing and functional rehabilitation.

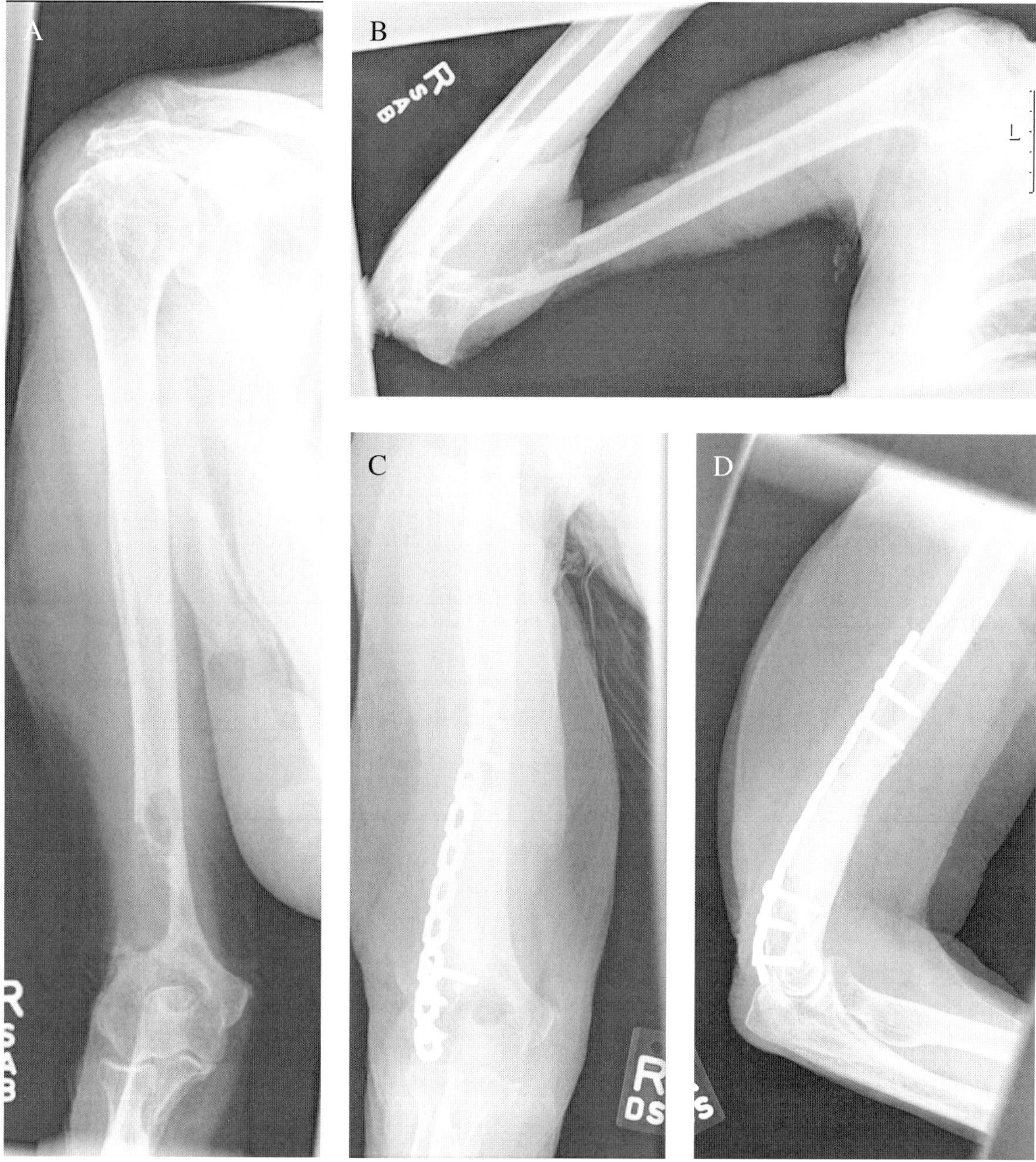

FIGURE 95.10. AP (A) and lateral (B) right humerus radiographs of a 72-year-old woman with metastatic breast carcinoma showing a lytic lesion at risk for pathologic fracture. Postoperative AP (C) and lateral (D) radiographs demonstrate curettage and cementation of the lesion with prophylactic plate fixation.

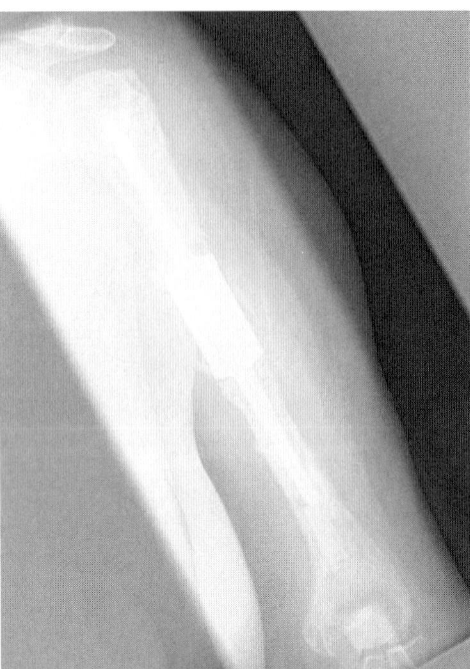

FIGURE 95.11. AP radiograph demonstrating intercalary prosthetic reconstruction of the left humerus in a 52-year-old woman with metastatic breast carcinoma following failed fixation and segmental bone loss.

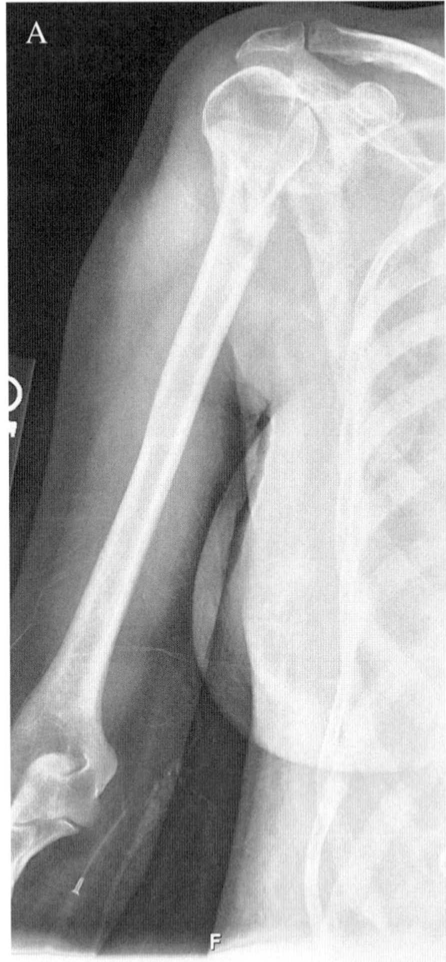

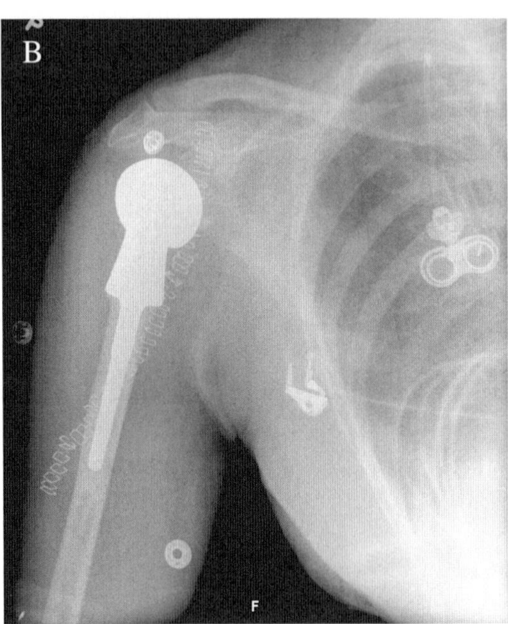

FIGURE 95.12. Preoperative (A) and postoperative (B) AP right shoulder radiographs of a 68-year-old woman with metastatic breast carcinoma refractory to radiation treatment. She was treated with proximal humeral resection and prosthetic reconstruction.

References

1. Cancer Facts and Figures. Atlanta, GA: American Cancer Society, 2004:1–16.
2. Buckwalter JA, Brandser EA. Metastatic disease of the skeleton. Am Fam Physician 1997;55:1761–1768.
3. Hage WD, Aboulafia AJ, Aboulafia DM. Incidence, location and diagnostic evaluation of metastatic bone disease. Orthop Clin N Am 2000;31:515–528.
4. Paget S. The distribution of secondary growths in cancer of the breast. Lancet 1889;1:571.
5. Mollabarsky A, Scarborough M. The mechanisms of metastasis. Orthop Clin N Am 2000;31:529–535.
6. Clain A. Secondary malignant disease of bone. Br J Cancer 1965;19:15–29.
7. Batson OV. The function of the vertebral veins and their role in the spread of metastases. Ann Surg 1940;112:138–149.
8. Mohammad K, Guise T. Mechanisms of osteoblastic metastases: role of endothelin. 1. Clin Orthop Relat Res 2003;415S:S67–S74.
9. Roodman G. Mechanisms of bone metastasis. N Engl J Med 2004;350:1655–1664.
10. Mohla S, Weilbacher K, Cher M, et al. Third North American symposium on skeletal complications of malignancy. Cancer (Phila) 2003;97(suppl 3):719–725.
11. Aebi M. Spinal metastasis in the elderly. Eur Spine J 2003; 12(suppl 2):S202–S213.
12. Kahn D, Weiner G, Ben-Haim S, et al. Positron emission tomographic measurement of bone marrow blood flow to the pelvis and lumbar vertebrae in young normal adults. Blood 1994;83: 958–963.
13. Orr F, Lee J, Duivenvoorden W, et al. Pathophysiologic interactions in skeletal metastasis. Cancer (Phila) 2000;88:2912–2918.
14. Yasuda H, Shima N, Nakagawa N, et al. Osteoclast differentiation factor is a ligand for osteoprotegerin/osteoclastogenesis-inhibitory factor and is identical to TRANCE/RANKL. Proc Natl Acad Sci USA 1998;95:3597–3602.
15. Powell G, Southby J, Danks J, et al. Localization of parathyroid hormone-related protein in breast cancer metastases: increased incidence in bone compared with other sites. Cancer Res 1991;51:3059–3061.
16. Henderson M, Danks J, Moseley J, et al. Parathyroid hormone-related protein production by breast cancers, improved survival and reduced bone metastases. J Natl Cancer Inst 2001;93: 234–237.
17. Brown J, Coleman R. Assessment of the effects of breast cancer on bone and the response to therapy. Breast 2002;11:375–385.
18. Coleman E. Skeletal complications of malignancy. Cancer (Phila) 1997;80:1588–1594.
19. Bjurholm A, Kreicbergs A, Brodin E, Schultzberg M. Substance P- and CGRP-immunoreactive nerves in bone. Peptides 1988;9:165–171.
20. Healey JH. The mechanism and treatment of bone pain. In: Arbit E (ed) Management of Cancer-Related Pain. Mount Kisco, NY: Futura, 1993:515.
21. Mundy GR. Mechanisms of bone metastasis. Cancer (Phila) 1997;80(suppl 8):1546–1556.
22. Edelstyn GA, Gillespie PJ, Grebbell FS. The radiological demonstration of osseous metastases: experimental observations. Clin Radiol 1967;18:158–162.
23. Fidler M. Incidence of fracture through metastases in long bones. Acta Orthop Scand 1981;52:623–627.
24. de Santos LA, Libshitz HI. Adult bone. In: Libshitz HI (ed) Diagnostic Roentgenology of Radiotherapy Change. Baltimore: Williams & Wilkins, 1979:137–150.
25. Rosenthal DI. Radiologic diagnosis of bone metastases. Cancer (Phila) 1997;80:1595–1607.
26. Vande Streek PR. Nuclear medicine approaches to musculoskeletal disease. Radiol Clin N Am 1994;32:243–253.
27. Corcoran RJ, Thrall JH, Kyle RW, et al. Solitary abnormality in bone scans of patients with extraosseous malignancies. Radiology 1976;121:663–667.
28. Zoeller G, Sandrock D, Munz DL, et al. Bone marrow immunoscintigraphy versus conventional bone scintigraphy in the diagnosis of skeletal metastases in urogenital malignancies. Eur Urol 1994;26:141–144.
29. Castillo LA, Yeh SDJ, Leeper RD, et al. Bone scans in bone metastases from functioning thyroid carcinoma. Clin Nucl Med 1980;5:200–209.
30. Shreve PD, Grossman HB, Gross MD, et al. Metastatic prostate cancer: initial findings of PET with 2-deoxy2-[F-18]fluoro-D-glucose. Radiology 1996;199:751–756.
31. Ryan PJ, Fogelman I. The bone scan: where are we now? Semin Nucl Med 1995;25:76–91.
32. Dedashti F, Siegel BA, Griffeth LK, et al. Benign versus malignant intraosseous lesions: discrimination by means of PET with 2[F-18]fluoro-2-deoxy-D-glucose. Radiology 1996;200:243–247.
33. Pagani JJ, Libshitz HI. Imaging bone metastases. In: Radiologic Clinics of North America. Philadelphia: Saunders, 1982: 545–560.
34. Ciray I, Astrom G, Andreasson I, et al. Evaluation of new sclerotic bone metastases in breast cancer patients during treatment. Acta Radiol 2000;41:178–182.
35. Braunstein EM, Kuhns LR. Computed tomographic demonstration of spinal metastases. Spine 1983;8:912–915.
36. Redmond J III, Spring DB, Munderloh SH, et al. Spinal computed tomography scanning in the evaluation of metastatic disease. Cancer (Phila) 1984;54:253–258.
37. Helms CA, Cann CE, Brunelle FO, et al. Detection of bone marrow metastases using quantitative computed tomography. Radiology 1981;140:745–750.
38. Kang M, Gupta S, Khandelwal S, et al. CT-guided fine needle aspiration biopsy of spinal lesions. Acta Radiol 1999;40:474–478.
39. Kornblum MB, Wesolowski DP, Fischgrund JS, et al. Computed tomography-guided biopsy of the spine: a review of 103 patients. Spine 1998;23:81–85.
40. Philips J, Waugh R, Ng AB. Radiologically-guided percutaneous fine needle aspiration biopsies of abdominal and osseous lesions. Aust N Z J Med 1984;14:260–263.
41. Murphy WA, Destouet JM, Gilula LA. Percutaneous skeletal biopsy 1981: a procedure for radiologists. Results, review and recommendations. Radiology 1981;139:545–549.
42. Stoker DJ, Kissin CM. Percutaneous vertebral biopsy: a review of 135 cases. Clin Radiol 1985;36:569–577.
43. Kattapuram SV, Rosenthal DI. Percuatneous biopsy of skeletal lesions. AJR 1991;157:935–942.
44. Ciray I, Astrom G, Sundstrom C. Assessment of suspected bone metastases: CT with and without clinical information compared to CT-guided bone biopsy. Acta Radiol 1997;38:890–895.
45. Gangi A, Kastler B, Klinkert A, et al. Injection of alcohol into bone metastases under CT guidance. J Comput Assist Tomogr 1994;18:932–935.
46. Zimmer WD, Berquist TH, McLeod RA, et al. Bone tumors: magnetic resonance imaging versus computed tomography. Radiology 1985;155:709–718.
47. Smoker WRK, Godersky JC, Knutzon RK, et al. The role of MR imaging in evaluating metastatic spinal disease. AJR 1987;149:1241–1248.
48. Lien HH, Blomlie V, Heimdal K. Magnetic resonance imaging of malignant extradural tumors with acute spinal cord compression. Acta Radiol 1990;31:187–190.
49. Frank JA, Ling A, Patronas NJ, et al. Detection of malignant bone tumors: MR imaging versus scintigraphy. AJR 1990;155: 1043–1048.
50. Algra PR, Bloem JL, Tissing H, et al. Detection of vertebral metastases: comparison between MR imaging and bone scintigraphy. Radiographics 1991;11:219–232.

51. Traill ZC, Talbot D, Golding S, et al. Magnetic resonance imaging versus radionuclide scintigraphy in screening for bone metastases. Clin Radiol 1999;54:448–451.
52. Walker R, Kessar P, Blanchard R, et al. Turbo STIR magnetic resonance imaging as a whole-body screening tool for metastases in patients with breast carcinoma: preliminary clinical experience. J Magn Reson Imaging 2000;11:343–350.
53. Schweitzer ME, Levine C, Mitchell DG, et al. Bull's eyes and halos: useful discriminators of osseous metastases. Radiology 1993;188:249–252.
54. Jung HS, Jee WH, McCauley TR, et al. Discrimination of metastatic from acute osteoporotic compression fractures with MR imaging. Radiographics 2003;23:179–187.
55. Baker LL, Goodman SB, Perkash I, et al. Benign versus pathologic compression fractures of vertebral bodies: assessment with conventional spin-echo, chemical-shift, and STIR MR imaging. Radiology 1990;174:495–502.
56. Hage W, Aboulafin A, Aboulafin D. Incidence, location and evaluation of metastatic bone disease. Orthop Clin N Am 2000;31:515–528.
57. Simon MA, Finn HA. Diagnostic strategy for bone and soft-tissue tumors. J Bone Joint Surg Am 1993;75:622–631.
58. Bates SE. Clinical applications of serum tumor markers. Ann Intern Med 1991;115:623–638.
59. Aboulafia AJ. Biopsy. Instr Course Lect 1999;48:587–590.
60. Mankin HJ, Lange TA, Spanier SS. The hazards of biopsy in patients with malignant primary bone and soft-tissue tumors. J Bone Joint Surg Am 1982;64:1121–1127.
61. Mankin HJ, Mankin CJ, Simon MA. The hazards of biopsy, revisited. Members of the Musculoskeletal Tumor Society. J Bone Joint Surg Am 1996;78:656–663.
62. Rougraff BT, Kneisl JS, Simon MA. Skeletal metastases of unknown origin: a prospective study of a diagnostic strategy. J Bone Joint Surg Am 1993;75:1276–1281.
63. ASCO Ad Hoc Committee on Cancer Pain. Cancer pain assessment and treatment curriculum guidelines. J Clin Oncol 1992; 10:1976–1982.
64. Niewald M, Tkocz H, Abel U, et al. Rapid course radiation therapy vs. more standard treatment: a randomized trial for bone metastases. Int J Radiat Oncol Biol Phys 1996;36:1085–1089.
65. Rasmusson B, Vejborg I, Jensen A, et al. Irradiation of bone metastases in breast cancer patients: a randomized study with 1 year follow-up. Radiother Oncol 1995;34:179–184.
66. Okawa T, Kita M, Goto M, et al. Randomized prospective clinical study of small, large and twice-a-day fraction radiotherapy for painful bone metastases. Radiother Oncol 1988;13:99–104.
67. Madsen E. Painful bone metastasis: efficacy of radiotherapy assessed by the patients: a randomized trial comparing 4 Gy × 6 versus 10 Gy × 2. Int J Radiat Oncol Biol Phys 1983;9:1775–1779.
68. Blitzer P. Reanalysis of the RTOG study of the palliation of symptomatic osseous metastasis. Cancer (Phila) 1985;55: 1468–1472.
69. Tong D, Gillick L, Hendrickson F. The palliation of symptomatic osseous metastases: final results of the Study by the Radiation Therapy Oncology Group. Cancer (Phila) 1982;50:893–899.
70. Cole D. A randomized trial of a single treatment versus conventional fractionation in the palliative radiotherapy of painful bone metastases. Clin Oncol (R Coll Radiol) 1989;1:59–62.
71. Steenland E, Leer J, van Houwelingen H, et al. The effect of a single fraction compared to multiple fractions on painful bone metastases: a global analysis of the Dutch Bone Metastasis Study. Radiother Oncol 1999;52:101–109.
72. Nielsen O, Bentzen S, Sandberg E, et al. Randomized trial of single dose versus fractionated palliative radiotherapy of bone metastases. Radiother Oncol 1998;47:233–240.
73. Bone Pain Trial Working Party. 8 Gy single fraction radiotherapy for the treatment of metastatic skeletal pain: randomized comparison with a multifraction schedule over 12 months of patient follow-up. Radiother Oncol 1999;52:111–121.
74. Price P, Hoskin P, Easton D, et al. Prospective randomized trial of single and multifraction radiotherapy schedules in the treatment of painful boney metastases. Radiother Oncol 1986;6: 247–255.
75. Gaze M, Kelly C, Kerr G, et al. Pain relief and quality of life following radiotherapy for bone metastases: a randomised trial of two fractionation schedules. Radiother Oncol 1997;45:109–116.
76. Jeremic B, Shibamoto Y Acimovic L, et al. A randomized trial of three single-dose radiation therapy regimens in the treatment of metastatic bone pain. Int J Radiat Oncol Biol Phys 1998; 42:161–167.
77. Hoskin P, Price P, Easton D, et al. a prospective randomized trial of 4 Gy or 8 Gy single doses in the treatment of metastatic bone pain. Radiother Oncol 1992;23:74–78.
78. Falkmer U, Järhult J, Wersäll P, et al. A systematic overview of radiation therapy effects in skeletal metastases. Acta Oncol 2003;42:620–633.
79. Sze W, Shelley M, Held I, et al. Palliation of metastatic bone pain: single fraction versus multifraction radiotherapy. A systematic review of randomized trials. Clin Oncol 2003;15: 345–352.
80. The Breast Specialty Group of the British Association of Surgical Oncology. The management of metastatic bone disease in the United Kingdom. Eur J Surg Oncol 1999;25:3–23.
81. McQuay HJ, Collins SL, Moore RA. Radiotherapy for the palliation of painful bone metastasis (Cochrane Review). In: The Cochrane Library, vol 2. Chichester, UK: Wiley, 2004.
82. International Bone Metastases Consensus on endpoint measurements for future clinical trials. Proceedings of the first survey and meeting (work in progress) International Bone Metastases Consensus Working Party. Clin Oncol 2001;13:82–84.
83. Ackery D, Yardley J. Radionuclide-targeted therapy for the management of metastatic bone pain. Semin Oncol 1993;20 (suppl 2):27–31.
84. Silberstein EB. The treatment of painful osseous metastases with phosphorus-32-labeled phosphates. Sem Oncol 1993; 20(suppl 2):10–21.
85. Papatheofanis F. Variation in oncologic opinion regarding management of metastatic bone pain with systemic radionuclide therapy. J Nucl Med 1999;40:1420–1423.
86. Dickinson C, Hendrix N. Strontium-89 therapy in painful bony metastases. J Nucl Med Technol 1993;21:133–137.
87. Robinson R. Strontium-89: precursor targeted therapy for pain relief of blastic metastatic disease. Cancer (Phila) 1993; 72:3433–3435.
88. Nair N. Relative efficacy of ^{32}P and ^{89}Sr in palliation in skeletal metastases. J Nucl Med 1999;40:256–262.
89. Buchali K, Correns HJ, Schuerer M, et al. Results of a double blind study of 89-strontium therapy of skeletal metastases of prostatic carcinoma. Eur J Nucl Med 1988;44:349–351.
90. Porter AT, McEwan AJB. Strontium-89 as an adjuvant to external beam radiation improves pain relief and delays disease progression in advanced protate cancer: results of a randomized controlled trial. Semin Oncol 1993;20(suppl 2):38–43.
91. Lewington VJ, McEwan AJ, Ackery DM, et al. A prospective randomised double-blind crossover study to examine the efficacy of strontium-89 in pain palliation in patients with advanced prostate cancer metastatic to bone. Eur J Cancer 1991;27: 954–958.
92. Serafini AN, Houston SJ, Resche I, et al. Palliation of pain associated with metastatic bone cancer using samarium-153 lexidronam: a double-blind placebo-controlled clinical trial. J Clin Oncol 1998;16:1574–1581.
93. Roqué M, Martinez M, Alonso-Coello P, et al. Radioisotopes for metastatic bone pain (Cochrane Review). In: The Cochrane Library, issue 1. Chichester, UK: Wiley, 2004.
94. Serafini A. Systemic metabolic radiotherapy with samarium-153 EDTMP for the treatment of painful bone metastasis. Q J Nucl Med 2001;45:91–99.

95. Fitton A, McTavish D. Pamidronate: a review of its pharmacological properties and therapeutic efficacy in resorptive bone disease. Drugs 1991;41:289–318.
96. Benford HL, Frith JC, Auriola S, et al. Farnesol and geranylgeraniol prevent activation of caspases by aminiobisphosphonates: evidence for two distinct pharmacological classes of bisphosphonate drugs. Mol Pharmacol 1999;56:131–140.
97. Derenne S, Amiot M, Barill S, et al. Zoledronate is a potent inhibitor of myeloma cell growth and secretion of IL-6 and MMP-1 by the tumoral environment. J Bone Miner Res 1999;14: 2048–2056.
98. Boissier S, Magnetto S, Frappart L, et al. Bisphosphonates inhibit prostate and breast carcinoma cell adhesion to unmineralized and mineralized bone extracellular matrix. Cancer Res 1997:57: 3890–3894.
99. Senaratne SG, Pirianov G, Mansi JL, et al. Bisphosphonates induce apoptosis in human breast cancer cell lines. Br J Cancer 2000;82:1459–1468.
100. Ross JR, Saunders Y, Edmonds PM, et al. A systemic review of the role of bisphosphonates in metastatic disease. Health Technol Assess 2004;8:1–176.
101. Østenstad B, Andersen OK. Disodium pamidronate versus mithramycin in the management of tumour-associated hypercalcemia. Acta Oncol 1992;31:861–864.
102. Hasling C, Charles P, Mosekilde L. Etidronate disodium for treating hypercalcaemia of malignancy: a double blind, placebo-controlled study. Eur J Clin Invest 1986;16:433–437.
103. Rotstein, S, Glas U, Eriksson M, et al. Intravenous clodronate for the treatment of hypercalcaemia in breast cancer patients with bone metastases: a prospective randomized placebo-controlled multicenter study. Eur J Cancer 1992;28A:890–893.
104. Gucalp R, Theriault R, Gill I, et al. Treatment of cancer-associated hypercalcemia: double-blind comparison of rapid and slow intravenous infusion regimens of pamidronate disodium and saline alone. Arch Intern Med 1994;154:1935–1944.
105. Syrigos KN, Michalaki V, Mitromaras A, et al. Safety and efficacy of the new bisphosphonate ibandronate in the management of bone metastasis following rapid infusion. In Vivo 2002;16: 361–364.
106. Warrell RP, Murphy WK, Schulman P, et al. A randomized double-blind study of gallium nitrate compared with etidronate for acute control of cancer-related hypercalcemia. J Clin Oncol 1991;9:1467–1475.
107. Gucalp R, Ritch P, Wiernik P, et al. Comparative study of pamidronate disodium and etidronate disodium in the treatment of cancer-related hypercalcemia. J Clin Oncol 1992;10:134–142.
108. Purohit OP, Radstone CR, Anthony C, et al. A randomized double-blind comparison of intravenous pamidronate and clodronate in the hypercalcaemia of malignancy. Br J Cancer 1995; 72:1289–1293.
109. Ralston SH, Gallacher SJ, Patel U, et al. Comparison of three intravenous bisphosphonates in cancer-associated hypercalcaemia. Lancet 1989;ii:1180–1182.
110. Vinholes J, Guo CY, Purohit OP, et al. Evaluation of new bone resorption markers in a randomized comparison of pamidronate or clodronate for hypercalcemia of malignancy. J Clin Oncol 1997;15:131–138.
111. Rizzoli R, Buchs B, Bonjour JP. Effect of a single infusion of alendronate in malignant hypercalcaemia: dose dependency and comparison with clodronate. Int J Cancer 1992;50:706–712.
112. Major P, Lortholary A, Hon J, et al. Zoledronic acid is superior to pamidronate in the treatment of hypercalcemia of malignancy: a pooled analysis of two randomized, controlled clinical trials. J Clin Oncol 2001;19:558–567.
113. Nussbaum SR, Younger J, Vandepol CJ, et al. Single-dose intravenous therapy with pamidronate for the treatment of hypercalcemia of malignancy: comparison of 30-, 60-, and 90-mg dosages. Am J Med 1993;95:297–304.
114. Hultborn R, Gundersen S, Ryden S, et al. Efficacy of pamidronate in breast cancer with bone metastases: a randomized double-blind placebo controlled multicenter study. Acta Oncol 1996; 35(S5):73–74.
115. van Holten-Verzantvoort A, Zwinderman A, Aaronson N, et al. The effect of supportive pamidronate treatment on aspects of quality of life of patients with advanced breast cancer. Eur J Cancer 1991;27:544–549.
116. Cleton FJ, van Holten-Verzantvoort A, Bijvoet O. Effect of long-term bisphosphonate treatment on morbidity due to bone metastases in breast cancer patients. Recent Results Cancer Res 1989;116:73–78.
117. Hortobagyi GN, Theriault RL, Lipton A, et al. Long-term prevention of skeletal complications of metastatic breast cancer with pamidronate. J Clin Oncol 1998;16:2038–2044.
118. Hortobagyi GN, Theriault RL, Porter L, et al. Efficacy of pamidronate in reducing skeletal complications in patients with breast cancer and lytic bone metastasis. N Engl J Med 1996; 335:1785–1791.
119. Theriault RL, Lipton A, Hortobagyi GN, et al. Pamidronate reduces skeletal morbidity in women with advanced breast cancer and lytic bone lesions: a randomized, placebo-controlled trial. J Clin Oncol 1999;17:846–854.
120. Kristensen B, Ejlertsen B, Groenvold M, et al. Oral clodronate in breast cancer patients with bone metastasis: a randomized study. Ann Intern Med 1999;246:67–74.
121. Paterson AHG, Powles TJ, Kanis JA, et al. Double-blind controlled trial of oral clodronate in patients with bone metastases from breast cancer. J Clin Oncol 1993;11:59–65.
122. Tubiana-Hulin M, Beuzeboc P, Mauriac L, et al. [Double-blinded controlled study comparing clodronate versus placebo in patients with breast cancer bone metastases.] Bull Cancer 2001;88:701–707.
123. van Holten-Verzantvoort ATM, Kroon HM, Bijvoet OLM, et al. Palliative pamidronate treatment in patients with bone metastases from breast cancer. J Clin Oncol 1993;11:491–498.
124. van Holten-Verzantvoort AT, Bijvoet OLM, Cleton FJ, et al. Reduced morbidity from skeletal metastases in breast cancer patients during long-term bisphosphonate (ADP) treatment. Lancet 1987;2(8566):983–985.
125. Saad F, Gleason DM, Murray R, et al. Long-term efficacy of zoledronic acid for the prevention of skeletal complications in patients with metastatic hormone-refractory prostate cancer. J Natl Cancer Inst 2004;96:879–882.
126. Rosen LS, Gordon D, Tchekmedyian S, et al. Zoledronic acid versus placebo in the treatment of skeletal metastases in patients with lung cancer and other solid tumors: a phase III, double-blind, randomized trial. The zoledronic acid lung cancer and other solid tumors study group. J Clin Oncol 2003;21: 3150–3157.
127. Rosen LS, Gordon D, Kaminski M, et al. Zoledronic acid versus pamidronate in the treatment of skeletal metastases in patients with breast cancer or osteolytic lesions of multiple myeloma: a phase III, double-blind, comparative trial. Cancer J 2001;7: 377–387.
128. Berenson JR, Rosen LS, Howell A, et al. Zoledronic acid reduces skeletal-related events in patients with osteolytic metastasis: a double-blind, randomized dose-response study. Cancer (Phila) 2001;91:1191–1200.
129. Theriault R. Pamidronate in the treatment of osteolytic bone metastases in breast cancer patients. Br J Clin Pract 1996; 87(suppl):8–12.
130. Hultborn R, Gundersen S, Ryden S, et al. Efficacy of pamidronate in breast cancer with bone metastasis: a randomized, double-blind placebo-controlled multicenter study. Anticancer Res 1999;19:3383–3392.
131. Glover D, Lipton A, Keller A, et al. Intravenous pamidronate disodium treatment of bone metastases in patients with breast cancer. Cancer (Phila) 1994;74:2949–2955.

132. Robertson AG, Reed NS, Ralston SH. Effect of oral clodronate on metastatic bone pain: a double-blind, placebo-controlled study. J Clin Oncol 1995;13:2427–2430.
133. Saad F, Gleason DM, Murray R, et al. A randomized, placebo-controlled trial of zoledronic acid in patients with hormone-refractory metastatic prostate carcinoma. J Natl Cancer Inst 2002;94:1458–1468.
134. Conte PF, Giannessi PG, Latreille J, et al. Delayed progression of bone metastases with pamidronate therapy in breast cancer patients: a randomized, multicenter phase III trial. Ann Oncol 1994;5(S7):S41–S44.
135. Conte PF, Latreille J, Mauriac L, et al. Delay in progression of bone metastases in breast cancer patients treated with intravenous pamidronate: results from a multinational randomized controlled trial. J Clin Oncol 1996;14:2552–2559.
136. Hillner BE, Ingle JN, Chlebowski RT, et al. American Society of Clinical Oncology 2003 update on the role of bisphosphonates and bone health issues in women with breast cancer. J Clin Oncol 2003;21:4042–4057.
137. Tobinick EL. Targeted etanercept for treatment-refractory pain due to bone metastasis: two case reports. Clin Ther 2003;25: 2279–2288.
138. Saikali Z, Singh G. Doxycycline and other tetracyclines in the treatment of bone metastasis. Anti-Cancer Drugs 2003;14: 773–778.
139. Martinez MJ, Roqué M, Alonso-Coello P, et al. Calcitonin for metastatic bone pain (Cochrane Review). In: The Cochrane Library, issue 1. Chichester, UK: Wiley, 2004.
140. Koeneman KS, Kao C, Ko SC, et al. Osteocalcin-directed gene therapy for prostate-cancer bone metastasis. World J Urol 2000; 18:102–110.
141. CAL-03. Humanized monoclonal antibody to parathyroid hormone related protein. Chugai Pharma USA, LLC, 2002.
142. Cleeland CS, Gonin R, Hatfield AK, et al. Pain and its treatment in outpatients with metastatic cancer. N Engl J Med 1994;330:592–596.
143. McGahan JP, Dodd GD. Radiofrequency ablation of the liver: current status. AJR 2001;176:3–16.
144. Solbiati L, Goldberg SN, Ierace T, et al. Hepatic metastases: percutaneous radio-frequency ablation with cooled-tip electrodes. Radiology 1997;205:367–373.
145. Rosenthal DI, Alexander A, Rosenberg AE, et al. Ablation of osteoid osteomas with a percutaneously placed electrode: a new procedure. Radiology 1992;183:29–33.
146. Rosenthal DI, Springfield DS, Gebhardt MC, et al. Osteoid osteoma: percutaneous radiofrequency ablation. Radiology 1995;197:451–454.
147. Rosenthal DI, Hornicek FJ, Wolfe MW, et al. Percutaneous radiofrequency coagulation of osteoid osteoma compared with operative treatment. J Bone Joint Surg Am 1998;80:815–821.
148. Callstrom MR, Charboneau WJ, Goetz MP, et al. Painful metastases involving bone: feasibility of percutaneous CT- and US-guided radio-frequency ablation. Radiology 2002;224:87–97.
149. Gronemeyer DHW, Schirp S, Gevargez A. Image-guided radiofrequency ablation of spinal tumors: preliminary experience with an expandable array electrode. Cancer J 2002;8:33–39.
150. Levine SA, Perin LA, Hayes D, et al. An evidence-based evaluation of percutaneous vertebroplasty. Manag Care 2000;9:56–60, 63.
151. Weill A, Chiras J, Simon J, et al. Spinal metastases: indications for and results of percutaneous injection of acrylic surgical cement. Radiology 1996;199:241–247.
152. Fourney DR, Schomer DF, Nader R, et al. Percutaneous vertebroplasty and kyphyoplasty for painful vertebral body fractures in cancer patients. J Neurosurg 2003;98:21–30.
153. Kaufmann TJ, Jensen ME, Schweickert PA, et al. Age of fracture and clinical outcomes of percutaneous vertebroplasty. Am J Neuroradiol 2001;22:1860–1863.
154. Schaefer O, Lohrmann C, Herling M, et al. Combined radiofrequency thermal ablation and percutaneous cementoplasty treatment of a pathologic fracture. J Vasc Intervent Radiol 2002;13: 1047–1050.
155. Rougraff B. Indications for operative treatment. Orthop Clin N Am 2000;31:567–575.
156. Burstein AH, Currey J, Frankel VH, et al: Bone strength: the effect of screw holes. J Bone Joint Surg 1972;54:1143–1156.
157. Frankel BH, Burstein AH. Orthopaedic Biomechanics. Malvern, PA: Lea & Febiger, 1970.
158. Parrish FF, Murray JA. Surgical treatment for secondary neoplastic fractures: a retrospective study of ninety-six patients. J Bone Joint Surg 1970;52:665–686.
159. Hipp JA, Springfield DS, Hayes WC. Predicting pathologic fracture risk in the management of metastatic bone defects. Clin Orthop 1995;312:120–135.
160. Keene JS, Sellinger DS, McBeath AA, et al: Metastatic breast cancer in the femur: a search for the lesion at risk of fracture. Clin Orthop 1986;203:282–288.
161. Zickel RG, Mouradian WH. Intramedullary fixation of pathologic fractures and lesions of the subtrochanteric region of the femur. J Bone Joint Surg 1976;58:1061–1066.
162. Harrington KD. Orthopaedic management of extremity and pelvic lesions. Clin Orthop 1995;312:136–147.
163. Mirels H. Metastatic disease in long bones: a proposed scoring system for diagnosing impending pathologic fractures. Clin Orthop 1989;249:256–264.
164. Nierman E, Zakrzewski K. Recognition and management of preoperative risk. Rheum Dis Clin N Am 1999;25:585–622.
165. Kopec IC, Groeger JS. Life-threatening fluid and electrolyte abnormalities associated with cancer. Crit Care Clin 1988;4: 81–105.
166. Sun S, Lang EV. Bone metastases from renal cell carcinoma: preoperative embolization. J Vasc Intervent Radiol 1998;9:263–269.
167. Gellad FE, Sadato N, Numaguchi Y, et al. Vascular metastatic lesions of the spine: preoperative embolization. Radiology 1990;176:683–686.
168. Keller FS, Rosch J, Bird CB. Percutaneous embolization of bony pelvic neoplasms with tissue adhesive. Radiology 1983; 147:21–27.
169. Layalle I, Flandroy P, Trotteur G, et al. Arterial embolization of bone metastases: is it worthwhile? J Belg Radiol 1998;81: 223–225.
170. Barton PP, Waneck RE, Karnel FJ, et al. Embolization of bone metastases. J Vasc Intervent Radiol 1996;7:81–88.
171. Breslau J, Eskridge JM. Preoperative embolization of spinal tumors. J Vasc Intervent Radiol 1995;6:871–875.
172. Chuang VP, Wallace S, Swanson D, et al. Arterial occlusion in the management of pain from metastatic renal carcinoma. Radiology 1979;133:611–614.
173. Varma J, Huben RP, Wajsman Z, et al. Therapeutic embolization of pelvic metastases of renal cell carcinoma. J Urol 1984;131: 647–649.
174. Schneiderbauer MM, Von Knoch M, Schleck CD, et al. Patient survival after hip arthroplasty for metastatic disease of the hip. J Bone Joint Surg Am 2004;86:1684–1689.
175. Wong DA, Fornasier VL, MacNab I. Spinal metastases: the obvious, the occult, and the impostors. Spine 1990;15: 1–4.
176. Weinstein JN. Differential diagnosis and surgical treatment of pathologic spine fractures. Instr Course Lect 1992;41:301–315.
177. Harrington KD. Anterior cord decompression and spinal stabilization for patients with metastatic lesions of the spine. J Neurosurg 1984;61:107–117.
178. Harrington KD. Metastatic disease of the spine. J Bone Joint Surg Am 1986;68:1110–1115.

179. Siegal T, Tiqva P, Siegal T. Vertebral body resection for epidural compression by malignant tumors. J Bone Joint Surg Am 1985;67:375–382.
180. Weinstein JN. Spine neoplasms. In: Weinstein SL (ed) The Pediatric Spine: Principles and Practice. New York: Raven Press, 1994:887.
181. Weinstein JN, McLain RF. Tumors of the spine. In: Rothman RA, Simeone FA (eds) The Spine, 3rd ed. Philadelphia: Saunders, 1992:1279.
182. Patterson FR, Peabody TD. Operative management of metastases to the pelvis and acetabulum. Orthop Clin N Am 2000;31:623–631.
183. Harrington KD. The management of acetabular deficiency secondary to metastatic malignant disease. J Bone Joint Surg Am 1981;63:653–664.
184. Ward WG, Spang J, Howe D. Metastatic disease of the femur: surgical management. Orthop Clin N Am 2000;31:633–645.
185. Lane JM, Sculco TP, Zolan SG. Treatment of pathological fractures of the hip by endoprosthetic replacement. J Bone Joint Surg Am 1980;62:954–959.
186. Ward WG, Dorey F, Eckardt JJ. Total femoral endoprosthetic reconstruction. Clin Orthop 1995;316:195–206.
187. Ward WG, Eckardt JJ. Endoprosthetic reconstruction of the femur following massive bone resections. J Bone Orthop Assoc 1994;3:108.
188. Townsend PW, Rosenthal HG, Smalley SR, et al. Impact of postoperative radiation therapy and other perioperative factors on outcome after orthopedic stabilization of impending or pathologic fractures due to metastatic disease. J Clin Oncol 1994;12:2345–2350.

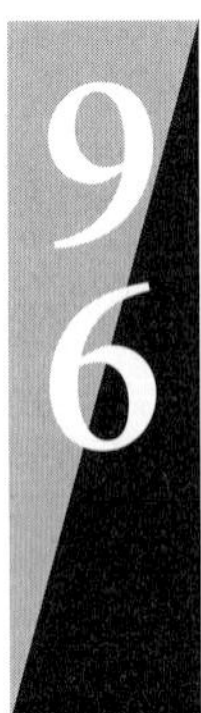

Cancer in the Immunosuppressed Patient

Patrick Whelan and David T. Scadden

During the 1960s, as oncology research was rapidly expanding, MacFarlane Burnett's idea that cancer resulted from a failure of tumor surveillance by the aging immune system was broadly acknowledged. The development of cancer genetics focused the field on mutational causes of tumorigenesis. However, a new appreciation for the role that a well-functioning immune system plays in protecting against virally induced tumors was brought to light in the 1980s with the acquired immunodeficiency syndrome (AIDS) epidemic. The phenomenon of the human immunodeficiency virus (HIV)-associated cancer epidemic within defined populations, particularly due to the recent dramatic responses to treatment of the underlying immunodeficiency, has given insight into other etiologic factors for a variety of tumors.

A greater appreciation of the elevated lymphoma risk for children with congenital immunodeficiencies developed in association with the early literature in this area. The advent of solid organ and bone marrow transplantation in the 1960s and 1970s added pressure to more quickly reach an understanding of the relationship between immunosuppression and cancer. Careful epidemiologic studies to delineate increased cancer risks for patients with more complex immune dysfunction, such as thyroiditis, celiac sprue, and Sjögren's disease, have begun only in this past decade.

The inability to control viruses with a direct transforming capability, such as Epstein–Barr virus (EBV), is just a part of the explanation. Persistent immune stimulation by chronic viral or microbial infection, or as a result of the loss of normal lymphocyte homeostatic mechanisms, may play a crucial role, particularly with regard to hematologic malignancies. The newly recognized role of the hepatitis C virus and gastric *Helicobacter pylori* infection in the eruption of characteristic lymphomas, are the only prototypes to date. Treatment of these two infections can often lead to regression of the related lymphomas.[1,2] This chapter examines some of the unique considerations that influence the diagnosis and treatment of cancer in the immunocompromised patient. Generally, these immunodeficiencies are divided into inherited and acquired forms. Among the acquired deficiencies are the special cases of malignancy in the posttransplant period, in adults with common variable immunodeficiency, and finally, in people suffering from infection with HIV/AIDS.

Congenital Immunodeficiency

Congenital immunodeficiency-associated lymphoproliferative disorders share several characteristics that differentiate them from spontaneous non-Hodgkin's lymphoma (NHL) and other lymphoproliferative disease[3] (Table 96.1). First, lymphoma is disproportionately represented among all cancers in this population. Between 50% and 65% of cancers among children with immunodeficiency diseases are lymphomas, compared to about 12% of cancers in the general pediatric population. Children who are posttransplant fall in between, with lymphoma constituting about a third of malignancies in this group.

Second, one might expect impairment of specific immune defenses to predispose to certain kinds of infections. In general, impaired immune defenses against EBV appear to result in a high rate of B-cell transformation. With the exception of ataxia telangiectasia (AT), congenital immunodeficiency patients frequently develop EBV-infected lymphoproliferative lesions, either secondary to natural infection or potentially from graft-derived virus in those who undergo stem cell transplantation.

Third, these children develop lymphoma in a distinct anatomic distribution compared to other children with lymphoma. Most of these tumors occur outside of lymph nodes, particularly in the central nervous system and in the gastrointestinal tract. For example, a pediatric cancer registry in Britain, studying 51 children who developed lymphoproliferative disorders secondary to congenital or acquired immunodeficiency, found 32 nonlocalized tumors compared to 10 that were localized.[4] AT-related NHL may be mostly extranodal, similar to other immunodeficiency-related NHL.[5]

Finally, the histology of these lymphomas is typically of the diffuse large cell type and is associated with rapid clinical progression in untreated patients. Lymphoproliferative disease is the second leading cause of death, after opportunistic infection, for children with congenital immunodeficiency. The risk of lymphoproliferative disease may approach 10,000-fold compared with the general pediatric population,[6] and risk of death exceeds three times that of children who develop these lymphomas posttransplantation.[4] The one silver lining may be that, as in posttransplant lymphoma pediatric patients, those with congenital immunodeficiency

TABLE 96.1. Lymphoma in congenital versus sporadic immunosuppression.

	Congenital immunodeficiency	*Sporadic childhood cancer*
Lymphoma as percent of all cancers	50%–65%	12% (ALL and brain tumors are more prevalent)
Role of EBV in lymphomagenesis	Prevalent[a]	Rare
Anatomic localization of lymphoma	Predominantly extranodal	More lymph node centered[b]
Predominant lymphoma type	Diffuse large cell	Burkitt's and lymphoblastic types are more common

EBV, Epstein–Barr virus.

[a] Except for ataxia telangiectasia.

[b] Adult lymphoma generally more nodal than childhood disease.

have a risk of death that largely evaporates about 18 months after diagnosis, probably because of compensatory increases in the remaining elements of the immune system.

Ataxia Telangiectasia

Defects in the ataxia telangiectasia mutated (ATM) gene, when inherited from both parents, result in dysfunctional angiogenesis in the ocular and cutaneous circulation, immune impairment with sinus and pulmonary infection susceptibility, and an ataxic gate secondary to a spinocerebellar neurodegenerative process. Children with AT also represent the largest subpopulation of congenital immunodeficiency patients with lymphoma in a national cancer registry for these patients.[7] AT patients are thought to have a risk for leukemia about 70-fold over the general pediatric population, and the risk for lymphoma may approach 300-fold.[8] African-Americans with AT appear disproportionately affected by cancer in general and lymphoma in particular. One retrospective study of 263 ATM homozygotes found a 184-fold-increased incidence of cancer and a 750-fold increased risk for lymphoma among black patients, compared with 61-fold and 252-fold, respectively, for homozygotes of European descent compared to the general population.[8]

More than 10% of ATM homozygotes develop some form of malignancy, most in the lymphoid lineages.[9,10] After age 20, the incidence of lymphoid malignancies drops to less than half and the incidence of solid tumors rises. The solid tumors most commonly described, include gastric adenocarcinomas, astrocytomas, medulloblastomas, and cancers of the oral cavity, pancreas, breast, ovary, and bladder. The relationship between *Helicobacter pylori* and development of gastric carcinoma in AT patients is unclear, but there appears to be an important link in patients with common variable immunodeficiency and gastric cancer.[11]

The increased incidence of breast cancer in female relatives of AT patients led to studies suggesting that ATM missense mutations may be involved in up to 5% of all breast cancer in the general population.[12,13] Some controversy persists on this point, because the truncation mutants that appear to predominate in AT patients may not predispose to breast cancer in heterozygotes[14] in the same way that dominant negative missense mutations apparently do.[15] ATM mutations are found in as many as 2% of the U.S. population.[16] Furthermore, ATM carriers are thought to have an increased risk of cancer, with a relative risk of cancer death before age 80 estimated at 2.6-fold compared to noncarriers[10] and as high as 5-fold before age 45.[17]

The ATM gene is composed of 66 exons on chromosome 11q22-23 and has sequence homology to an enzyme involved in intermediary metabolism, phosphatidylinositol-3-kinase (Table 96.2). The PI-3-kinase family is perhaps best known for its role in transmembrane signal transduction in response to a number of extracellular growth factors, but plays an important related role in cell-cycle regulation. ATM mutations inherited from both parents lead to inefficient DNA repair and dysfunctional cellular immunity,[18] resulting in a combination of genetic instability and potential impairment of putative immune surveillance. ATM is believed to function normally as part of the sensing mechanism for double-stranded breaks in DNA, which rapidly activate its kinase activity and lead to repair by homologous recombination or nonhomologous end-joining. Mutations may serve to disrupt the kinase activity and subsequent signaling to other proteins involved in DNA repair, resulting in dysfunctional cell-cycle checkpoint regulation and DNA repair.

The immune dysfunction is a combination of abnormal B-cell and T-cell receptor rearrangement and disrupted thymic organogenesis. γ/δ T-cell numbers are within the normal range, but α/β T-cells are significantly reduced.[19] Because ATM knockout mice frequently develop thymomas with rearrangements in the TCR α/δ locus, it had been assumed that lymphomagenesis in these patients represented an ATM-dependent disruption of VDJ recombination.[20,21] However, both the Rag-1 and Rag-2 genes, essential components of the VDJ recombination machinery, are dispensable for thymoma development in ATM knockout mice.[22] This finding suggests that the inability to deal with double-stranded DNA breaks is likely to represent the more central defect predisposing to the development of lymphoma.

ATM-deficient mice are markedly sensitive to gamma irradiation.[23] As noted previously, studies of the recurrence of breast cancer in women treated with radiation, have failed to show a predisposition to second cancers among women with ATM mutations.[14] Inhibition of homologous recombination in ATM-deficient mice partially rescues them from lymphoma development, suggesting that excessive homologous recombination is at least partially responsible for the propensity toward lymphomagenesis.[24]

Among the ATM homozygotes who develop cancer, lymphoma and leukemia in the lymphocytic lineages predominate. Those with NHL have presented with diverse histologic

TABLE 96.2. Pathways involved in congenital immunodeficiency.

Disease	*Molecular defect*	*Clinical manifestations*	*Cancer risk*	*Tumor type*
Ataxia telangiectasia	*atm* gene, 11q22-23	Sinopulmonary infection Ocular telangiectasiae Spinocerebellar ataxia	10%	Early NHL Solid tumors later
X-linked lymphoproliferative	Sh2D1A, Xq25	Severe mononucleosis	>30%	Burkitt-type lymphoma
X-linked agammaglobulinemia	*btk* gene, Xq22	Sinopulmonary infection		Lymphoma Gastric/colon cancer
Wiskott–Aldrich	*wasp* gene, Xp11.22	Thrombocytopenia Eczema Autoimmune sequelae Recurrent infection	16%	Large cell immunoblastic lymphoma
Severe combined immunodeficiency	*ADA* gene, others	Recurrent infection		Non-Hodgkin's lymphoma
Autoimmune lymphoproliferative syndrome	*Fas* gene, others	Hepatosplenomegaly Cytopenias Glomerulonephritis	8%	Hodgkin's > NHL
Chediak–Higashi	*lyst* gene, 1q42-43	Bacterial infection Hypopigmentation Thrombocytopenia Peripheral neuropathy	Majority	T-cell infiltrative disease
Common variable immunodeficiency	Acquired	Recurrent infection Intestinal lymphoid hyperplasia Splenomegaly Autoimmune cytopenias	Variable	NHL, gastric adenocarcinoma

NHL, non-Hodgkin's lymphoma.

phenotypes, in contrast to the overrepresented subtypes typical of other childhood immunodeficiencies.[25] The ATM gene product appears to act early in the response to DNA damage, initiating a pause in cell-cycle progression and then facilitating the repair of double-stranded DNA breaks. Apart from patients with congenital AT, inactivation of the ATM gene has been found in cases of mantle cell lymphoma and in both B-cell and T-cell leukemias.

At least five different functional domains have been identified in addition to the critical kinase domain in the ATM gene.[26] This multifunctionality, and the identification of more than 100 distinct ATM mutations scattered throughout the gene, may explain the considerable phenotypic heterogeneity among affected homozygotes. Curiously, most mutations appear to be frame-shift and nonsense mutations, predicted to cause truncation of the ATM protein, and relatively few are base-pair substitutions.[27]

As suggested previously, the biology of ATM-associated lymphoma differs from that of other immunodeficiencies. Most are not EBV-infected and do not have characteristic c-*myc* translocations. More than 80% of these lymphomas are T-cell derived, in stark contrast to the B-cell predominance seen in other immunodeficiencies and among sporadic cases in the general population. Ataxia telangiectasia patients appear to have a preferential disruption of the VDJ recombination process in the T-cell lineage, although functional ATM is required for receptor gene rearrangement in both T cells and B cells.[28] Myeloid malignancies are not overrepresented in this population.

Does the development of malignancies in children with AT result from a relative decline in immune function over time? Patients with AT demonstrate a variety of immune defects. B and T lymphocytes are severely depleted, and functional tests reveal poor proliferative responses to antigens and mitogens,[29,30] leading to prominent deficiencies in serum IgA, IgG2, IgG4, and IgE. Although AT patients have a rising susceptibility to lower respiratory infections with age, nonrespiratory infections are not increased. Upper respiratory infections may actually decline with age, as in the general population, and AT patients are not susceptible to chronic upper respiratory infections.[31] The function of natural killer and lymphokine-activated killer cells appears to be maintained.[32] Furthermore, AT patients do not demonstrate progression of their lymphopenia or hypogammaglobulinemia with age.[31] If an age-related decline in immune function contributes to the cancer risk, it would have to be a somewhat specific element of antitumor immunity that has not been identified to date.

X-Linked Lymphoproliferative Syndrome

X-linked lymphoproliferative (XLP) syndrome, also referred to as Duncan disease after one of the first described patients, is an immunodeficiency associated with mutation in the SLAM-associated protein (SAP, also known as SH2D1A) gene on chromosome Xq25.[33] These boys have a marked susceptibility to EBV infection, and a resulting hepatonecrosis is a significant cause of death.[34] About half develop severe mononucleosis during the first decade of life, with pronounced pharyngitis, hepatosplenomegaly, diffuse lymphadenopathy, hepatitis, and occasionally, aplastic anemia. Lymph nodes showing an immunoblastic appearance, and circulating atypical lymphocytes, can be mistaken for signs of acute leukemia in these very ill mononucleosis patients. Among the important immune defects are severe hypogammaglobulinemia and a loss of cytotoxic T-lymphocyte-derived interferon-gamma production and cytotoxic activity toward EBV-infected cells.[35] Interestingly, the SAP protein is not physiologically expressed in activated B cells, which are presumably the precursors for development of the B-cell-predominant lymphomas that afflict XLP patients.[36]

SAP functions as an adaptor protein, binding via an Src-homology domain (SH2) to a common motif in the cytoplasmic domain of the CD2 and SLAM family of cell-surface signaling molecules (CD84, CD150, CD229, CD244, and NTB-A).[37] Because SAP is expressed only physiologically in activated T cells and NK cells, the inability of these cells to regulate B cells is suspected to be at the heart of lymphomagenesis in XLP. As many as a third of patients are thought to develop lymphoma eventually, including some who are not infected with EBV.[34,38] The most common presenting symptoms are nausea, emesis, and abdominal pain, and most have prominent constitutional symptoms, including fever.

The small, noncleaved type (Burkitt) predominates with a risk estimated at 200-fold that of the general population, although multiple other lymphoma types have been described.[39] Anatomically, these lymphomas are extranodal, arising in the small bowel most of the time (commonly in the iliocecal area). Lymph node pathology shows effacement of the normal architecture by uniform-appearing lymphoblasts that are predominantly of follicular center cell origin, in contrast to the infectious mononucleosis process that typically preserves lymph node architecture amid polymorphous lymphoid elements.[40] In an early series of 17 patients,[41] the median age at diagnosis was 4 years (range, 2 to 19 years) with a median survival of 12 months. The 40% of patients with the Burkitt's phenotype had the worst prognosis, despite treatment, representing 7 of 9 deaths among these 17 boys; most deaths were attributable to bacterial infection. The series included single cases of lymphoma in the lung, liver, and central nervous system (CNS),[41] and renal involvement has also been described.[42]

Hematopoietic stem cell transplantation (HSCT) is thought to be the best chance for remission in XLP patients with Burkitt-type tumors.[43] The largest study to date was also the earliest, reporting a series of seven XLP patients who received allogeneic HSCT.[44] All seven had HLA-identical donors, six from siblings (five bone marrow and one cord blood), and one bone marrow transplant from an unrelated donor. All the patients successfully engrafted, with six demonstrating low-grade graft-versus-host reactions without any attributable deaths. Two patients died of infectious complications posttransplant and one of multiorgan failure. The other four were healthy at the time of publication, more than 3 years after HSCT. Risk factors for poor HSCT outcome were age greater than 15 years, preconditioning with total-body irradiation, and significant infection problems pretransplant. More recently, success has been reported using unrelated umbilical cord stem cell transplantation.[45]

X-Linked Agammaglobulinemia

Bruton's agammaglobulinemia is an immunodeficiency manifested only after maternal immunoglobulin begins to wane, typically presenting with recurrent otitis in the absence of obvious tonsils or cervical lymph nodes. Patients often develop sinus and pulmonary infections because they lack circulating B cells, fail to form B-cell follicles in the lymph node and spleen, and thus fail to generate a good antibody response to bacterial infection.[46] Affected children may suffer onset of lymphoma in late infancy,[47] and an increased incidence of gastric and colorectal cancer has been reported in older children.[48,49] A contributing factor to colorectal cancer susceptibility may be a decreased expression of distal colonic glutathione-S-transferase in these patients, resulting in decreased detoxification of bacterial products of metabolism.[50]

Most affected individuals have a mutation in the btk gene on chromosome Xq22, which is critical for intracellular signaling by surface immunoglobulin and for early B-cell development. Btk is a member of the TEC family of tyrosine kinases. Immunoglobulin ligation results in mobilization of btk into a signaling complex at the cell membrane, where it is activated by src family kinases. Btk then acts in part by phosphorylating key residues within phospholipase C-gamma-2, an enzyme critical to the release of inositol trisphosphate and the early intracellular calcium flux.[51] Activation of cellular calcium channels is essential to the phosphorylation of IkB, resulting in disinhibition of the critical transcriptional factor NF-kB that translocates to the nucleus and activates several families of immune-related genes in response to antigen.[52,53] Other activation pathways are also affected, namely, interleukin (IL)-5, IL-10, and CD38 signaling.[54–56] The CD40–CD40 ligand interaction that partly mediates T-cell help for B-cell differentiation may also be impaired by btk mutation.[57] Consequently, boys lacking functional btk are unable to form germinal centers, have markedly decreased levels of serum immunoglobulin, and are significantly impaired in mounting T-cell-dependent humoral immune responses. Their state of immune compromise results in susceptibility to infection with the common encapsulated bacterial pathogens of infancy (e.g., *Hemophilus influenzae* and *Streptococcus pneumoniae*), mycoplasma pneumonia, and common enteroviruses.

The pathogenesis of lymphoma development in these patients remains a mystery, in part, because healthy older X-linked agammaglobulinemia patients lack evidence for infection with the Epstein–Barr virus.[58] EBV may lack sufficient target cells for infection in these patients, who have minimally detectable B cells in their peripheral circulation and an absence of pharyngeal tonsils. Compromised antibody production in these patients may possibly impair homeostatic mechanisms that normally control EBV or other viral factors that contribute to lymphomagenesis. Another possibility is a role for btk as a tumor suppressor gene. Mutated btk has not to date been shown to act as an oncogene, but the btk protein has been shown to be capable of nuclear translocation and to function in both up- and downregulation of apoptosis.[59] Thus, Btk loss may result indirectly in an increased susceptibility to lymphoma by playing a role in either regulation of apoptosis or transcriptional activation.

Wiskott–Aldrich Syndrome

Children with a mutation in the Wiskott–Aldrich-associated protein (WASP) gene present in late infancy with eczema, low platelets, and functional deficiencies in their T cells, B cells, and neutrophils. About one in six also develop lymphoma, most commonly, large cell immunoblastic non-Hodgkin's lymphoma,[60] at a median age of 6.5 years.[61] The WASP gene is located on Xp11.22. WASP is a cytoskeletal protein that is phosphorylated in B cells by btk (Bruton's defect) in the immunoglobulin signaling pathway,[62] and in T cells by fyn in response to TCR cross-linking.[63] When T cells interact with their cognate antigens on antigen-presenting cells, the TCR signal results in a WASP-dependent reorganization of the actin cytoskeleton and formation of an "immunologic synapse" between the two cells.[64] Deficiency of WASP appears to compromise the ability to fully polarize T-cell cytoskeletal elements at low doses of antigen, although production of IL-2 is substantially impaired even at saturating antigen levels.[65] The defect appears to be in directional secretion of cytokines, though not in chemokines that have been studied.[66]

Historically, more than 10% of WAS patients eventually contracted some form of cancer, with median onset at age 6[67] and an incidence estimated to climb by 2% per year.[61] Competing pressures on these rates include the increased cancer risk created as patients live longer, and the increasing number of children who are transplanted early in life for nonneoplastic complications. About 40% of patients develop some autoimmune manifestations (i.e., immune cytopenias, nephritis, inflammatory bowel disease, uveitis, and occasionally, arthritis), and these individuals appear to be at increased risk for subsequent development of cancer[68]; this may be because those with autoimmune symptoms typically have more severe disease in general. CNS involvement appears to predominate among the diffuse, high-grade lymphomas that constitute at least half of all malignancies in WAS patients. The tumors are almost exclusively extranodal with a large cell immunoblastic phenotype, and are distinctly lacking in Burkitt or lymphoblastic histology.[69] One survey found these lymphomas to be universally infected with EBV.[67] Nonsense and frame-shift mutations in the WASP gene, which usually result in nonexpression of the protein, are associated with more severe disease and with at least a threefold-greater risk for lymphoma compared with patients who have missense mutations.[70] Some of the clinical heterogeneity in the disease may result from differing levels of WASP expression in different cell types, with lower expression correlating with greater dysfunction.[71]

Bone marrow transplantation is an effective treatment for the thrombocytopenia and immunosuppressive elements of WAS, which is probably the second most common immunodeficiency indication for transplantation.[72] In a study of 170 transplants accumulated in the International Bone Marrow Transplant Registry and/or National Marrow Donor Program, WAS patients achieved a 5-year probability of survival that was 87% for HLA-identical sibling donors, 52% for other related donors, and 71% for unrelated donors.[73] Boys younger than age 5 who received an unrelated donor transplant had survival similar to those receiving HLA-identical sibling transplants, so good survival outcomes are possible with unrelated donors in younger children. Cord blood stem cells may be particularly useful in younger children who are cytomegalovirus (CMV) negative, and five reported cases have offered good outcomes to date.[74–76] EBV-induced B-cell proliferative disorders, and other viral infections, are a significant cause of mortality in this transplanted population, developing most prominently in those children with slower development of full T- and B-cell functions and subsequent severe infectious complications.[77]

Severe Combined Immunodeficiency

The severe combined immunodeficiency (SCID) term covers an array of different genetic defects that impair some combination of cellular and humoral immunity, resulting in severe infections after maternal transplacental antibody wanes.[78] Many of these children died before the era of immune reconstitution. Following bone marrow or stem cell transplantation, a susceptibility emerges to lymphoproliferative disease, often related to naturally acquired or transplant-transmitted EBV infection.[79] As in Wiskott–Aldrich syndrome, lymphoma represents 75% of all malignancies in SCID patients and almost universally demonstrates EBV infection.[47]

Children with an unusually aggressive variant of SCID, termed Omenn syndrome, die early in life if not recognized and treated for their severe hypogammaglobulinemia. These patients present with rash, elevated IgE levels, swollen lymph nodes, and hepatosplenomegaly. Stem cell transplantation is required to avoid fatal complications.

Autoimmune Lymphoproliferative Syndrome (ALPS)

Also known as Canale–Smith syndrome, autoimmune lymphoproliferative syndrome (ALPS) usually results from inherited mutations in the CD95 (Fas) gene.[80] Less common mutations in the Fas ligand, caspase 8, and caspase 10 genes have been described with a similar phenotype. Fas is a member of the tumor necrosis factor receptor family and is critical to normal apoptosis during development and postinfection immune senescence. The Fas defect results in reduced apoptosis and increased proliferation of T cells. Consequently, lymph node pathology shows marked paracortical hyperplasia, expanded interfollicular areas, follicular hyperplasia, and a polyclonal plasmacytosis. The paracortical lymphoid cells have a high proliferative index and frequent mitoses.[81]

These patients develop massive splenomegaly and liver infiltration with a unique subpopulation of T cells akin to those in the lymph nodes and peripheral blood. These α/β-TCR-bearing T cells, lacking both the CD4 and CD8 markers, are normally found as minor populations in the thymus, skin, and spleen.[82] Although in vitro studies have suggested that these cells are poorly responsive to mitogens or antigen,[83] their expansion in patients with lupus has fueled speculation that they may help drive some of the autoimmune phenomena observed in ALPS patients.[84] Also seen in the peripheral circulation, is a polyclonal expansion of CD5+ B cells, which produce most of the circulating IgM antibody. ALPS patients are frequently misdiagnosed as having systemic lupus, particularly given their propensity to hemolytic anemia, thrombocytopenia, neutropenia, and glomerulonephritis.[81] The prognosis in this condition is not necessarily that of progressive disease.[85]

Fas germ-line mutations, mostly in the cytoplasmic "death domain," impose a risk estimated at 14-fold for non-Hodgkin's lymphomas and as high as 51-fold for Hodgkin's disease. These numbers were based on a series of 10 patients with lymphoma among 130 with heterozygous germ-line Fas mutations.[86] Among those with Hodgkin's lymphoma, the atypical nodular lymphocyte predominant form was particularly prominent, having been reported in three separate families with ALPS cases.[87] Aside from patients with ALPS, somatic mutations in Fas have been identified in sporadic cases of non-Hodgkin's lymphomas. These constituted about 11% in one series of 150 cases and may represent a higher percentage of MALT-type lymphomas. Similarly, somatic mutations in the caspase 10 gene have been found in a significant number of NHLs.[88] B cells often develop missense mutations in the Fas gene, as they do in the Bcl-6 gene, once they become germinal center centroblasts.[89] Consequently, the relationship of these mutations to lymphomagenesis is unclear.

Chediak–Higashi Syndrome

This autosomal recessively inherited immunodeficiency is characterized by oculocutaneous hypopigmentation, abnormal platelets, and susceptibility to bacterial infections. At a molecular level, many of these patients' cells display exaggerated lysosomes and melanosomes. The neutrophils in particular, show impaired degranulation, resulting from mutations in the lysosomal trafficking regulator (LYST) gene that appear to be present in all affected patients.[90] This cytoplasmic protein has been shown to interact with other proteins important in vesicular transport and signal transduction (among others, the casein kinase II protein, the SNARE complex protein HRS, and the 14-3-3 adaptor protein).[91] Among the immune defects, is difficulty controlling EBV replication in infected individuals, with abnormal serologic responses to EBV resulting in a chronic active EBV infection that may predispose to lymphoproliferative disease.[92] These patients experience what is frequently referred to as an accelerated phase, with a lymphocyte and macrophage infiltration of bone marrow, spleen, lymph nodes, liver, and central nervous system that resembles lymphoma and can lead to significant functional compromise.

Chemotherapy with combinations of etoposide, glucocorticoids, methotrexate, cyclophosphamide, and vincristine can restrain the accelerated phase, but relapses are common.[93] Allogeneic bone marrow transplant, particularly from HLA-identical related donors, has shown good success in reconstituting immune function and controlling recurrence of the accelerated phase.[94]

Acquired Immunodeficiency

Three forms of acquired immunodeficiency have offered accelerating clarity as to the causes and predisposing factors to cancer. In the 1950s and 1960s, it was appreciated that loss of the ability to make immunoglobulin during adulthood was a relatively common immunodeficiency, and that it predisposed to cancer.[95,96] The advent of the 1970s brought a wide expansion of organ transplantation, and a new appreciation for cancer risk in individuals whose immunity was iatrogenically suppressed. Of course, the HIV epidemic in the 1980s ultimately revealed how important immune function is to controlling the development of cancer. Studies on these three categories of illness have served to highlight the interplay of genetic, infectious, and immunologic phenomena in the genesis of cancer. A fourth category of acquired immune dysfunction, namely the rheumatic or autoimmune diseases, has reinforced an appreciation of the complexity that surrounds susceptibility to cancer in general and lymphoma in particular.

Common Variable Immunodeficiency

Common variable immunodeficiency (CVID) is the most common cause of non-HIV-related immunodeficiency, associated with low levels of immunoglobulin and poor humoral responses to vaccination. The pathophysiology may be secondary to a variety of other observed deficiencies, including low NK cell levels,[97] reduced T-cell expression of CD40L, relative CD4 T-cell lymphopenia, and poor T-cell responses to mitogen.[98–100] A defect in B-cell generation of somatic hypermutation may also contribute.[101] Disease onset is usually after age 20 but has been described in toddlers.[102] Most patients have no identifiable genetic defect, but mutations have been found in the CD40 ligand, btk (Bruton's), and SAP (X-linked lymphoproliferative syndrome) genes.[103] Affected individuals have an increased susceptibility to otitis and sinusitis problems caused by encapsulated organisms, such as *Streptococcus pneumoniae* and *Haemophilus influenzae*, akin to the susceptibility seen in early childhood and in splenectomized adults.[104] Beyond respiratory infections, some patients present with diarrhea and crampy abdominal pain. Some cases of irritable bowel syndrome have turned out to be CVID on immunologic testing. Patients experience an increased incidence of immune cytopenias, inflammatory arthritis, and granulomatous vasculitis.

A high incidence of atrophic gastritis, possibly related to *H. pylori* infection, appears to contribute to these patients' increased risk for gastric carcinoma.[105] CVID patients in general, are at increased risk for lymphomas of the CNS and gastrointestinal tract. The risk of lymphoma has been estimated at 8.5% in those diagnosed with CVID as adults.[106] One registry of 120 CVID patients with malignancies demonstrated a breakdown showing 46% of cancers were NHL, 16% gastric carcinoma, and 7.5% Hodgkin's disease.[107] Clinical presentation crosses a spectrum from atypical or reactive lymphoid hyperplasia to malignancy, with a predominance of benign disease.[108] The elevated lymphoma risk has diverged widely in different studies, from 12.0-fold among the 176 patients in the Scandanavian cohort[109] to 30-fold in a British study of 220 CVID subjects,[49] to 259-fold among 98 patients followed at Sloan-Kettering in New York.[110] Women with CVID may have a particularly pronounced susceptibility to lymphoma.[110]

The pathology of these tumors is largely that of postgerminal center B cells, or centrocytes,[111] with a diffuse large cell phenotype and frequent mutations and rearrangements within the Bcl-6 locus.[112] Similar pathology is seen in HIV-related and posttransplant lymphoma, although in contrast, the CVID-related tumors are EBV negative.[112] Reexamination of these lymphomas has led to speculation that a significant percentage of CVID-related NHL may be lymphomas of the mucosa-associated lymphoid tissue (MALT),[113] also referred to in the REAL classification as marginal zone B-cell lymphomas. From a mechanistic standpoint, it is appealing to think that chronic antigenic stimulation in the absence of effective humoral immunity could lead to a type of lymphoma that has been associated specifically with certain chronic infections (e.g., *H. pylori*-associated gastric lymphoma, HCV-associated MALT lymphoma). Perhaps more aggressive treatment of underlying chronic infections could serve to prevent the development of these tumors or retard their growth once diagnosed.

The increased risk for gastric carcinoma has been confirmed in several studies, with a standardized incidence ratio of 10.3 in the largest study.[109] Two women in their thirties have been described with CVID and breast cancer,[114] but no cases were seen in a retrospective study of 176 CVID patients.[109] Similarly, 2 cases of thymoma were described from one center's experience with 36 Dutch CVID patients, but other larger series did not identify such patients.[109]

Acquired Immunodeficiency Syndrome

According to the Joint United Nations Program on HIV/AIDS, an estimated 40 million people are living with HIV infection, with close to 20 million deaths attributable to the virus since its discovery in 1984. Most cases are in Africa, but Asia may represent the part of the world with the most explosive HIV problem.[115,116] Malignancy is probably the most difficult complication of HIV in the developed world from a treatment standpoint. The relative risk of death from opportunistic infection has declined for many infectious complications and for Kaposi's sarcoma, but has remained stubbornly persistent for AIDS-related lymphoma. The characteristic features of both these opportunistic neoplasms have changed in the context of antiretroviral therapy.

Kaposi's Sarcoma

Among the first clues to the emerging AIDS epidemic was the diagnosis of clusters of Kaposi's sarcoma (KS) among young men in California. At the time, the three primary populations to present with this intermittently aggressive tumor of skin and visceral organs included elderly men of Mediterranean origin, an endemic form prevalent in Central Africa that affects both men and women, and posttransplant patients under immunosuppression. Ten years after the discovery of HIV, the Kaposi's sarcoma-associated herpesvirus (KSHV), also referred to as human herpesvirus 8 (HHV-8), was identified as an etiologic agent strongly connected with all forms of Kaposi's sarcoma, including the HIV-associated cases.[117] In addition, primary effusion lymphoma (PEL) and multicentric Castleman's disease were two other HIV-associated illnesses to be quickly linked to KSHV infection.[118] KSHV appears to represent a sexually transmitted cancer threat that is exposed by subsequent HIV infection or immunosuppressive therapy, although the exact route of KSHV transmission has not been definitively demonstrated.

Serology and Epidemiology

KSHV is a sizeable double-stranded DNA virus (165 kb).[119] Closely related viruses have been found in three monkey species, the horse, cow, rabbit, and mouse, and together comprise the rhabdinoviridae genus of the gamma herpesviruses. The most closely related human pathogen is the Epstein–Barr virus (EBV), a lymphocryptogenous gamma herpesvirus that shares a similar genomic structure with three large regions of conserved, mostly lytic cycle genes (Figure 96.1). Chang and colleagues first described KSHV in 1994.[118] This group was motivated to search for the virus by circumstantial epidemiologic evidence of a transmissible agent for KS.[120] Among HIV-infected people in the West, for example, KS is uncom-

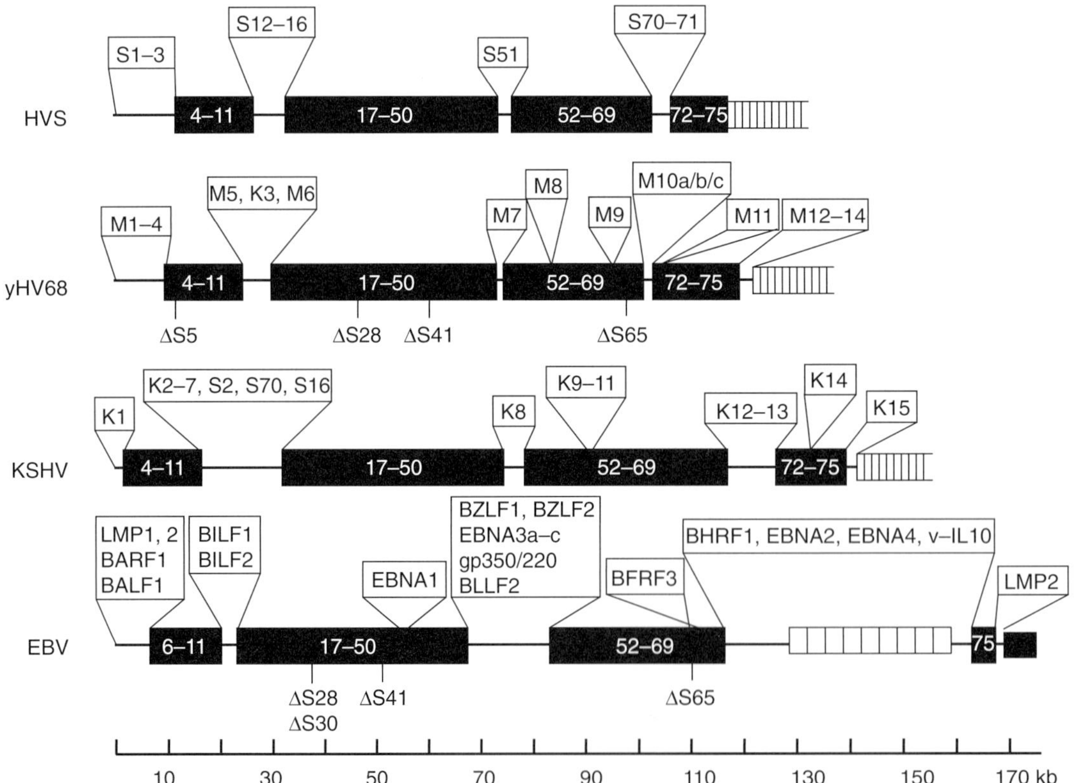

FIGURE 96.1. Comparative maps of KSHV, EBV, HSV, and GHV68 genomes. (By permission of Virgin et al. J Virol 1997;71:5894–5904.)

mon in women, and spares almost completely, patients with transfusion-acquired HIV infection.[121] KS is principally found in HIV-infected persons whose HIV risk group is men having sexual relations with men. Accordingly, a second transmissible agent was long hypothesized, and growing evidence strongly indicates that this agent is KSHV[120,122]: infection precedes tumor formation, the prevalence of KSHV infection tightly correlates with the epidemiology of the disease,[121] and the virus infects the cell types implicated in tumor formation.[123]

Found in about 80% of HIV-infected KS patients,[121] are antibodies directed against a latency-associated nuclear antigen (LANA) that have been the basis for the first generation of serologic tests available to detect previous exposure or active infection with KSHV. The incidence of infection appears to be at least 1% to 2% in the healthy HIV-negative U.S. blood donor population, compared with 2% of people with hemophilia, 3% to 4% of HIV-positive women,[124] and 25% to 30% of HIV-positive gay men by that assay.[125] A new enzyme-linked immunosorbent assay (ELISA), based on a whole virus lysate from the KS-1 cell line, may be even more sensitive[126]: 92% of 134 KS patients, independent of HIV status, were shown to have positive titers for anti-KSHV antibodies, compared with 11% of 91 healthy blood donors. Another study analyzing antibodies to lytic antigens in 1,400 serum samples, may suggest an even higher exposure rate in the U.S. general population: 25% of nonselected individuals were positive, as were 90% of HIV-infected homosexual men assessed by this method.[127] The sensitivity and specificity of these various assays, however, need additional definition and a standardized test developed to better evaluate this issue.

Detailed epidemiologic studies of the prevalence and mode of viral spread among various susceptible populations around the world have been made possible through the availability of specific oligonucleotide primers and of these serologic tests. Research in Italy, involving a cohort of healthy individuals and non-KS dermatology patients, showed 24% to have KSHV sequences in their peripheral blood.[128] In Sardinia, a region where classic KS is particularly prevalent, KS patients were shown to be seropositive for antibodies against a minor capsid antigen in 95% of individuals. Additionally, 39% of their family members were also positive, compared with 11% of age- and sex-matched controls.[129] Therefore, in Mediterranean countries, where cases of classic KS are focused, the prevalence of KSHV infection appears to be higher. Vertical transmission is suggested by the evidence that communicability of the virus may occur preferentially among family members, although recent evidence suggests that breast milk is not a vector.[130]

Among the endemic KSHV-infected populations of sub-Saharan Africa, where children contract a less aggressive form of Kaposi's sarcoma both with and without coincident HIV infection, vertical or paravertical transmission is also evident. In some studies, KSHV appears to be independently associated with hepatitis B infection,[131] and seropositivity to LANA and the open reading frame (ORF) 65 proteins reached adult levels of about 50% before puberty. Vertical and multiple modes of horizontal transmission may be prevalent in endemic populations of southern Europe and in Africa, although detailed mechanisms of transmission remain to be defined.

The role of sexual transmission is clear and has been best demonstrated in a cohort of men from whom serum samples were gathered over a 10-year period. The frequency of seroconversion was linearly related to male sexual intercourse contacts, with no seropositivity among 195 exclusively heterosexual men.[125] The seropositivity rate reached 65% among men with more than 250 sexual partners in the preceding 2 years. Where the virus resides within the male genitourinary tract, if indeed this is a route of transmission, is not clear. Studies have supported[132] or contradicted[133] the presence of KSHV in semen, and one report found KSHV in glandular epithelial cells of the prostate.[123]

Clinical Manifestations

Kaposi's sarcoma represented the AIDS-defining illness in more than 10% of HIV-infected individuals, and ultimately occurred in approximately 20% of the HIV-infected population before the availability of potent anti-HIV therapy. Among those HIV-positive patients who are seropositive for KSHV, the risk of developing KS was noted to be 50% at 10 years in one large study.[125] Interestingly, that risk is expected to be much lower in the era of highly active antiretroviral therapy (HAART), as discussed next.

Erythematous or violaceous macules or nodules on any mucocutaneous surface in the body may occur in isolation or in clusters. Cutaneous KS lesions are found more often on the lower extremities, where they can become confluent and circumferential, and on the face with a particular predilection for the ears and nose. The heterogeneity of their appearance covers a spectrum from faint salmon-colored macules to plaques, prominent nodular densities in some patients, and occasionally ulceration with superinfection. In dark-complexioned individuals, KS lesions may be somewhat more subtle. The highly vascular nature of the macules lends a characteristic reddish-blue tint that blanches minimally, if at all, on palpation. The natural history may vary widely, ranging from spontaneous remission in some individuals to explosive, fatal progression in others.

Edema is also frequently seen and may be distant from any cutaneous KS lesions. One-third of KS patients present with edema localized to affected extremities,[134] frequently in the legs. A peau d'orange appearance may result from obstruction of dermal lymphatics locally, or lymph node enlargement may be seen with attendant distal edema. In addition to mechanical causes of edema induced by obstructing lymphatic flow, KS lesions are composed of abnormal vessels with poor integrity. Surrounding the vessels in lesions are extravasated red blood cells that account for the pigmentation of the lesions. A KSHV viral protein has been shown to induce local vascular endothelial growth factor (VEGF),[135] a known permeability factor. Therefore, normal vessels surrounding KS lesions may also be altered in their integrity, contributing to interstitial fluid in KS lesions or affected limbs.[135] Lower extremity involvement can lead to disabling loss of joint mobility. Considerable morbidity can occur when peculiar syndromes of periorbital edema or peripubic edema are seen.

In addition to skin and lymphatics, KS can involve any epithelial surface in the body, including the oral cavity, pulmonary tree, and gastrointestinal tract. In one report, patients with cutaneous KS had a 50% incidence of coexistent oral involvement, 30% had pulmonary lesions, and 10% had KS in the gastrointestinal (GI) tract.[134] Many patients have GI lesions noted on endoscopic procedures, but clinical consequences are infrequent. Chronic or acute blood loss or protein-losing enteropathy is occasionally caused by GI involvement.

One particular type of KS that is life threatening and mandates aggressive therapy, is pulmonary parenchymal involvement. Chest X-rays are routinely performed on patients initially diagnosed with cutaneous KS to assess the possibility of lung lesions. Other screening studies for organ involvement are targeted to symptoms and are not recommended simply for observation.

The differential diagnosis for nonblanching lesions resembling KS includes[136] hematoma, purpura, sarcoid plaques, lichen planus, pyogenic granuloma,[137] mycosis fungoides, bacillary angiomatosis (usually due to *Bartonella* infection, with increased frequency in advanced HIV patients), secondary syphilis, pityriasis rosea (possibly associated with HHV-7 reactivation),[138] drug-related erythema multiforme, prurigo nodularis, nevi, vascular lesions of the phakomatoses (e.g., neurofibromatosis), epithelioid hemangioendothelioma, angiosarcoma, melanoma, and basal cell carcinoma. The potential for processes requiring entirely different therapeutic approaches strongly supports the need for histologic confirmation upon initial presentation, even though the CDC definition of KS does not require biopsy.

With the pervasiveness of KSHV infection in the general population, the virus is presumed to spread insidiously with disease manifestations occurring only in the context of some form of immunosuppression. However, a possible acute viral syndrome caused by KSHV in an HIV-positive patient has been described.[139] Kikuchi's disease, a cervical lymph node hyperplasia syndrome seen predominantly in women in the Far East, is another systemic syndrome that has been associated with KSHV. These patients typically present with fever, flu-like symptoms, neutropenia, an atypical lymphocytosis, and an elevated erythrocyte sedimentation rate (ESR). One retrospective analysis of 26 lymph node biopsies found polymerase chain reaction (PCR) evidence of KSHV sequences in 23%, with none in 40 controls.[140]

Pathology and Pathogenesis

The KS lesion can best be described as a complex array of endothelial cells, surrounded by spindle cells and extravasated blood elements. The spindle cell mass typically forms a cluster around slitlike endothelium-lined vascular spaces in the dermis, and becomes more densely packed in nodular lesions; both the spaces and the spindle cells characteristically lie parallel to the epidermis.[141] The spindle cell mass is thought to produce paracrine cytokines, which recruit neoangiogenic elements and inflammatory cells.[120] Spindle cells are not themselves infected with HIV, but KSHV sequences can often be amplified from them.[123,142] The origin of the spindle cells is controversial, alternately being viewed as having mesenchymal or endothelial cell features. One report demonstrated a phenotype more typical of the sinus-lining cells of spleen and lymph nodes than of other vascular or lymphatic endothelium.[143] These investigators and others have suggested that the cells of origin may be circulating in the blood. Expression of the mannose receptor and CD68 by these cells suggests that the spindle cells may derive from a macrophage-like population in the sinuses of secondary lymphoid organs that enter the bloodstream, and spread hematologically to the epithelial surfaces where KS lesions are found. This origin may explain the peculiar histology of KS lesions, with vascular spaces reminiscent of splenic sinuses. A newer marker, the VEGR-C receptor that appears specific for lymphatic endothelium, has been reported to be expressed in KS biopsy tissue.[144] In contrast, endothelial nitric oxide synthase, expressed in vascular endothelium, is not detectable in KS cells.[145]

An autocrine or paracrine secretion of cytokines, such as VEGF and basic fibroblast growth factor (bFGF), appear to maintain the spindle cells. The absence of a signal sequence in bFGF motivated one group to postulate that its export from KS cells may be mediated by one of the ATP-binding cassette transport proteins.[146] They showed that the multidrug resistance gene (MDR) is expressed in KS cells, and that the secretion of bFGF can be blocked by the MDR inhibitor probenecid. Furthermore, probenecid induced apoptosis in these cells in vitro. These data are compatible with an MDR or other probenecid-sensitive channel mediating an essential secretion of bFGF that then protects virally infected cells from apoptosis.

Even in the presence of exogenous growth factors, such as the IL-6–IL-6R complex, IL-1b, TNF-α, and oncostatin M, antibodies[147] to bFGF block the proliferation of KS cells and prevent them from entering the S phase of the cell cycle. However, exogenous growth factors do not completely explain the phenotype and growth potential of KS cells, which have been shown to overexpress the antiapoptotic bcl-2 gene independently of any factors contained in conditioned medium from these cells.[148]

Regardless of the HIV-1 status of the patients,[149] the phenotype of the tumor-infiltrating lymphocytes in KS lesions is CD8+ T-cell predominant. Other significant populations include CD4+ T cells and CD4/CD8 double-negative T cells. Compared to biopsy-derived lymphocytes in other dermatologic conditions, stimulation of KS-derived leukocytes in culture results in high levels of IFN-γ but no IL-2. CD68/CD14+ cells of the monocyte lineage are a minority population, but also contribute to this strong IFN-γ production.[150] These monocytic cells produce a variety of other proinflammatory cytokines, including IL-1 and TNF-α, which in turn induce the KS spindle cells to produce bFGF and VEGF. These latter factors have been shown to induce angiogenic lesions resembling KS in nude mice, and cause increased vascular permeability and edema in guinea pigs.[151]

Regardless of whether the underlying context is HIV disease, organ transplantation, or endemic KS, KSHV appears necessary for the induction of KS and is found in KS lesions. The exact mechanisms, however, by which the virus participates in the oncogenic process are uncertain.

The methods of cell transformation seem to be unique among human viruses. None of the EBV genes expressed in its latent phase of infection has a homologue in KSHV, even though KSHV is closely related to the known transforming virus EBV.[122] Four open reading frames in KSHV have been identified as having the ability to transform mammalian cells when expressed (K1, K9, K12, and CRF74), but whether they participate in vivo is not entirely clear.[152–155]

Several other genes have also been isolated for their possible role in host cell transformation. These genes can be divided into three classes of KSHV homologues to known mammalian genes: (1) apoptosis: ORF 16 (related to human Bcl-2); (2) cell-cycle interference: ORF 72 (cyclin D) binds and activates human cdk-6, making it resistant to the normal inhibition of the CDK inhibitors p16(Ink4a), p27Kip1, and p21Cip1[44,156]; and (3) immunomodulating cytokines: K2 (IL-6), K4 (MIP-II), and K6 (MIP-I). Subsequently, viral proteins could possibly act in a paracrine manner and affect neighboring cells. In addition, viral gene products in the infected cell may affect its growth, apoptotic potential, or vulnerability to immune defense targeting.

The pervasiveness of KS in populations that are HIV infected, post-solid organ transplant, of elderly Mediterranean extraction, or in economically disadvantaged tropical Africa, suggests that expression of a KS disease phenotype requires a degree of immunosuppression. The introduction of HAART for HIV treatment offers remarkable support to a central role for immunosuppression: complete remissions of cutaneous[157] and pulmonary KS are well recognized in the context of increases in CD4 count and declines in HIV viral load induced by HAART.[158]

Treatment

Over the past several years, the treatment of KS has changed dramatically. Antiretroviral therapy has had a major impact on the natural history of HIV disease, reducing its incidence and inducing regression in some patients with established disease. Specific therapies for KS have also improved dramatically, and most patients can anticipate a satisfactory outcome with limited treatment toxicity. One issue of which patients and providers need to be mindful is that even with regression of lesions, a disfiguring pigmentation can remain. The prominent extravasation of red blood cells in active KS lesions leads to hemosiderin deposition that can leave gray-brown macules when KS can no longer be histologically identified. Therefore, even successful treatment for KS masses may leave a residual stain that fades only after prolonged intervals. Laser therapy has been used to hasten the process for some with particularly disfiguring macules.

Quantitative methods have been developed for monitoring KSHV viral loads in patients under treatment. KSHV DNA level has been shown in transplant patients to increase with time after transplantation, and to correlate with progression of KS, stage of disease, and loss of the graft. In one multivariate analysis, the clinical activity of the tumor independently correlated with levels of KSHV DNA in the blood ($P = 0.01$).[159] KSHV viral loads may have more limited utility in HIV-infected individuals under treatment but do correlate with HIV viral load, CD4 cell counts, and the serologic response to KSHV lytic antigens.[160]

Anti-HIV Therapy

Extraordinary declines in HIV-related mortality in the Western world have occurred since the advent of HIV-1 protease inhibitors and combination therapy for HIV. The rate of death fell by 70% among those with AIDS following the introduction of HAART in one U.S. study.[161] Declines in opportunistic diseases associated with advanced immunosuppression have correspondingly been observed. Clinical entities, such as CMV retinitis, disseminated atypical mycobacterial disease, and *Pneumocystis* pneumonia are increasingly unusual events among patients on HAART. KS is the opportunistic neoplasm with the most dramatic decrease in incidence.[162] Table 96.3 presents a summary of the

TABLE 96.3. Effect of highly active antiretroviral therapy (HAART) on incidence of cancer in AIDS patients.

Study authors	*Year*	*Data source*	*N*	*Disease*	*Pre-HAART*	*HAART era*	*P value*
Besson et al.[202]	2001	French Hospital Database	80,000+	Total lymphoma CNS lymphoma	8.6 2.78	4.29 0.97	<0.001 <10e–11
International Collaboration[200]	2000	Meta-analysis	47,936	Total cancer	6.2	3.6	<0.001
Jones et al.[315]	1998	U.S. Centers for Disease Control Surveillance	37,303	Kaposi's sarcoma[a]	41	7	<0.001
Jones et al.[163]	1999	U.S. Centers for Disease Control Surveillance	19,684	Kaposi's sarcoma[b] CNS lymphoma	49.9 8	25.7 2.1	0.001 0.01
Grulich et al.[199]	2001	Australian HIV Database	9,209	Total lymphoma Kaposi's sarcoma	7.5 6.1	4.3 2.1	0.012 0.045
Kirk et al.[201]	2001	EuroSIDA	8,556	Systemic NHL	19.9	3	<0.001
Matthews et al.[251]	2000	Chelsea and Westminster Hospital (London)	7,840	Systemic NHL	5.3	4.7	0.933
Rabkin et al.[192]	1999	AIDS Clinical Trials Group (ACTG)	6,587	Total NHL Kaposi's sarcoma	31 96	4 3	nc nc
Dean et al.[193]	1999	Multicenter AIDS Cohort Study	5,622	Total NHL Kaposi's sarcoma	5.2 25.6	7.5 7.5	<0.001 0.003
Buchbinder et al.	1999	SF City Clinic Cohort	622	Total lymphoma Kaposi's sarcoma	14 35	19 0	0.19 0.07

NHL, non-Hodgkin's lymphoma; CNS, central nervous system; KS, Kaposi's sarcoma; nc, not calculated.

Incidence values are per 1000 person-years.

[a] Comparing KS incidence in 1990 to 1998.

[b] Comparing 1994 to 1997; decline occurred in both treated and untreated groups ($P = 0.8$).

Source: Adapted from Cheung TW. Cancer Invest 2004;22:774–786, with permission.

largest studies to date. The first large survey study of KS among HIV patients found that incidence dropped by half when comparing the period before 1994 to the first half of 1997.[163] Although fewer cases were seen for both treated and untreated patients among the nearly 20,000 patients studied, HAART-treated patients experienced a more dramatic decline.

There is a well-recognized clinical phenomenon of established KS responding to HAART, in addition to the decrease in new cases of KS. This anti-KS effect has been demonstrated in four small series reported to date. A Swiss study of 9 individuals with cutaneous KS who were treated for a median 7 months with a protease inhibitor showed partial response in 6, stabilization in 2, and progression in 1 noncompliant patient.[164] In another trial examining 8 HIV-infected men with cutaneous disease, 4 experienced a complete remission following a mean of 12 months of HAART.[165] Another study of 10 KS patients showed a decrease to undetectable in the anti-KSHV peripheral blood titer following HAART in 7 of the 8 patients who showed partial or complete regression of KS.[166]

Although most likely due to the recovery of immune function rather than a direct inhibitory effect on KSHV replication, KSHV sequences have been noted to disappear from peripheral blood following commencement of HAART.[167] There is no known impact of HIV therapy on KSHV directly. The effects of anti-HIV treatment are likely similar to the KS remission seen in posttransplant patients following withdrawal of their immunosuppression. KS is an immunologically responsive tumor, and the partial restoration of immune function with HAART is sufficient for tumor regression in many, but not all, patients.

Antiherpesviral Therapy

KSHV replication can be inhibited in vitro by the antiherpes drugs foscarnet, ganciclovir, and cidofovir.[168] Quantitation of KSHV copy number in peripheral blood of individuals on ganciclovir or foscarnet for other reasons has shown a decrease in KSHV viral load.[169] Although some studies have indicated a response,[170–173] most results have been disappointing.[172–174] Currently available antiherpesvirus drugs are too toxic to be considered a reasonable part of the therapeutic armamentarium.

Local Antitumor Chemotherapy

KS therapy is either local or systemic. Small, singular lesions on the trunk or an extremity may be more appropriate for local therapy. Local therapy is either liquid nitrogen, intralesional injection of vinblastine, topical 9-*cis*-retinoic acid, or radiation therapy.

Intralesional vinblastine is particularly useful for palatal or buccal mucosa lesions with a response rate estimated at 90%.[134] Vinblastine can be administered at 0.1 to 0.4 mg/mL, injecting approximately 0.1 to 0.2 mL into a 1-cm^2 lesion. As with liquid nitrogen, local discomfort is common and skin breakdown may occur. Regrowth of lesions is common.

Radiotherapy has taken on a new role in the treatment of KS in the HIV population, being used principally in the treatment of anal and cervical cancer with the advent of the HAART era.[175] However, orthovoltage irradiation and electron beam radiotherapy have been shown to be effective for treatment of larger dermal KS plaques.[134] In France, 643 HIV-infected patients with KS showed a complete response rate of 92% from 20 Gy over 2 weeks, followed 2 weeks later by 10 GY over 1 week.[176] Other studies have shown a response rate of 77% with a single dose of 8 Gy.[177] Radiation therapy generally can be useful for large or clustered lesions but can cause severe mucositis. HIV-infected individuals appear to have a heightened sensitivity to radiation injury of mucosa.

Topical use of 9-*cis*-retinoic acid cream was approved after a placebo-controlled, randomized trial of 82 patients.[178] Responses were sixfold higher in retinoic acid-treated patients, but the local side effects were often substantial. Patients often have discomfort and erythema at the site of application.[178] Open label trials of the same compound given systemically showed partial or complete responses in 37%.[179,180] Tolerability was limited by complications that included dry skin, rash, alopecia, exfoliation, and headache (70%).[179]

Systemic Antitumor Chemotherapy

Among the first agents available for treatment of KS were type I interferons, and their use has been comprehensively reviewed.[181] Interferon-α_2 has been shown to induce remission of KS in a dose-dependent fashion when given in combination with AZT, with 31% of 54 patients responding to 8 million units given daily subcutaneously.[74,182] Interferon therapy is most effective in those with relative preservation of immune function, generally reserved for those with 100 CD4 cells/mm^3 or more. The use of interferon is limited by its slow commencement of action (median time to response of 10 weeks in some studies) and the numerous and troubling side effects. Initially, and most prominent, are flu-like symptoms, followed by depression and fatigue after prolonged use.

For patients with advanced symptomatic KS, particularly those patients with edema, extensive mucocutaneous disease, and pulmonary or GI involvement, chemotherapy is recommended. Symptomatic pulmonary disease can be rapidly fatal and is particularly important to treat aggressively. Combination cytotoxic therapy with vincristine, bleomycin, and doxorubicin has served as a standard for comparison for newer treatment regimens, having demonstrated a 40% KS regression rate. The treatment involves a variety of difficult side effects, including nausea, alopecia, fatigue, peripheral neuropathy, acral cyanosis, and Raynaud's phenomenon.[183] Two Phase III studies, with about 250 HIV-related KS patients each, found a 25% response rate to this triple therapy or to bleomycin + vincristine; this compared to 46% and 58% for liposomal doxorubicin in the two studies, respectively.[184,185] In contrast, a large, randomized study comparing the BVD triple combination to liposomal daunorubicin found them to be of comparable efficacy.[186] Whether liposomal doxorubicin is truly superior to liposomal daunorubicin is unclear. These agents have different kinetic profiles, and the longer half-life of liposomal doxorubicin may account for its differential activity and association with the hand-foot syndrome. Many practitioners use these agents interchangeably for first-line therapy of patients with advanced, symptomatic KS, although current U.S. Food and Drug Administration (FDA) approval for liposomal doxorubicin is for use only in refractory or relapsed KS.

One newer class of agents being examined is the taxane tubulin stabilizers. Paclitaxel, for instance, was shown in a Phase I trial involving 28 patients to induce a major response in 71%,[187] including those previously and unsuccessfully treated with anthracyclines. This treatment appears to have both profound activity and highly durable responses. Tumor breakthrough is relatively rare and patients can tolerate low-dose paclitaxel (100 mg/m^2 every 2 weeks) extremely well. Some patients have received this therapy for over 2 years at our center, with cessation of therapy resulting in prompt regrowth of tumors.

KS lesions are highly vascular, which has led to the investigation of antiangiogenic therapies. Thalidomide was studied in a Phase II trial of 20 patients, with 8 of them achieving partial responses and 2 with stable disease; other than drowsiness and depression, the drug was well tolerated over a median 6-month treatment period.[188] Fumagillin (TNP-470) was well tolerated in a study of 38 patients but had poor activity.[189] In an effort to bridge the gap between antiretroviral regimens and systemic chemotherapy, halofuginon and other agents are all currently under in-depth investigation.

Summary

The identification of the human pathogen KSHV has been a major boon to understanding the basis of KS. This newest of human tumor-associated viruses appears to act via unique means of cell transformation, the understanding of which is likely to contribute novel paradigms for viral oncogenesis. In addition, virus-related antibodies may ultimately provide a means of screening for KS risk among immunosuppressed patients, and the virus itself may represent a target for future therapies. At present, the treatment of choice for AIDS-related KS is potent anti-HIV therapy. Those patients with advanced KS who require prompt improvement in symptoms, or who fail anti-HIV therapy, have a number of active chemotherapy options. Those who are not appropriate for cytotoxic agents still await a satisfactory systemic treatment, but local therapies can provide temporary improvement and the antiangiogenesis compounds offer promise that this gulf may soon be bridged.

AIDS-Associated Lymphoma

Epidemiology

The risk of developing lymphoma for HIV patients is estimated to be 60- to 110-fold higher than that of the general population. Genetic background, use of HAART, and subtype of lymphoma greatly influence the development and course of AIDS-related lymphoma (ARL). ARL is about twice as common among people of European ancestry compared with African-Americans and among men as compared with women.[190] It is the most common malignant complication of AIDS in children, representing 42 of 64 cancer cases in a British registry.[4] These are generally high-grade tumors, though a minority are low-grade lymphomas of the mucosa-associated lymphoid tissue termed maltomas. The estimated incidence of ARL in patients with symptomatic HIV infection is 1.6% per year.[191]

Specific genotypes appear to alter the risk of ARL. Specifically, polymorphisms in the 3′-region of the gene encoding the chemokine SDF-1 were associated with a higher risk of AIDS-related lymphoma.[192] Those heterozygous for the polymorphism had a twofold increase in risk whereas homozygous individuals had a fourfold-increased risk of lymphoma. The polymorphism was detected in 37% of whites, but only 11% of African-Americans, possibly accounting for the noted infrequency of this complication in black Americans with HIV. Other chemokine alterations also may affect lymphoma incidence, including a reduced incidence of ARL among those with a deletion within the CCR5 chemokine receptor gene (CCR5-delta32) that has been shown to be protective against HIV-1 infection. A threefold reduction in risk of ARL was noted in individuals with the CCR5 deletion. CCR5-delta32 is thought to affect the sensitivity of cells to the chemokine ligand of CCR5, RANTES, possibly causing altered B-cell function, either directly or through T-cell-mediated events.[193] The polymorphism in SDF-1 may change expression of RANTES, which is a known B-cell growth factor. Therefore, regulatory genes of the immune system may enhance or decrease an individual's likelihood of developing a lymphoproliferative disease.

Primary CNS lymphoma has been most dramatically altered in incidence since the advent of HAART therapy. It is a complication of far-advanced HIV disease that is now rarely seen, and generally only among those who have either failed antiretroviral therapy or for whom it is not available.

Among the ARL, primary CNS lymphoma in AIDS closely resembles posttransplant lymphoproliferative disease (PTLPD). Both tumors manifest a type II pattern of EBV latent gene expression (EBNA1-6 and LMP1-2).[194,195] EBNA-2 and -3 gene products are those generally well targeted by cytotoxic T lymphocytes (CTL), and the reduced incidence of primary CNS lymphoma with HAART may reflect an improved anti-EBV immune response. Of note, even among HIV-infected individuals with relatively normal numbers of EBV-specific CTL, there are abnormalities in cell function that have been linked to the development of EBV-associated lymphoproliferation.[196]

Systemic lymphomas have been less markedly reduced in the era of HAART than has ARL, the primary CNS lymphoma subset of AIDS-related lymphomas, in which the risk of systemic lymphomas is less dramatically reduced by HAART.[197,198] Systemic ARLs have a more complex pathophysiology, discussed next, that likely accounts for this less dramatic decrease in incidence since the advent of HAART. The estimated decline in systemic lymphoma incidence is approximately two- to sevenfold since the introduction of potent antiretroviral therapy (see Table 96.3).[199–202] An observational cohort analysis of 8,500 HIV-positive individuals across Europe (EuroSIDA),[201] demonstrated a significant decrease in the incidence of all subtypes of lymphoma after 1999, when the use of combination antiretroviral therapy was widespread compared with the period before HAART.[200] Similarly, an international multicohort study found a reduced incidence of ARL of approximately twofold following the introduction of HAART. Subtypes of lymphomas were also investigated in this study, and the greatest difference in incidence was observed in immunoblastic and primary CNS lym-

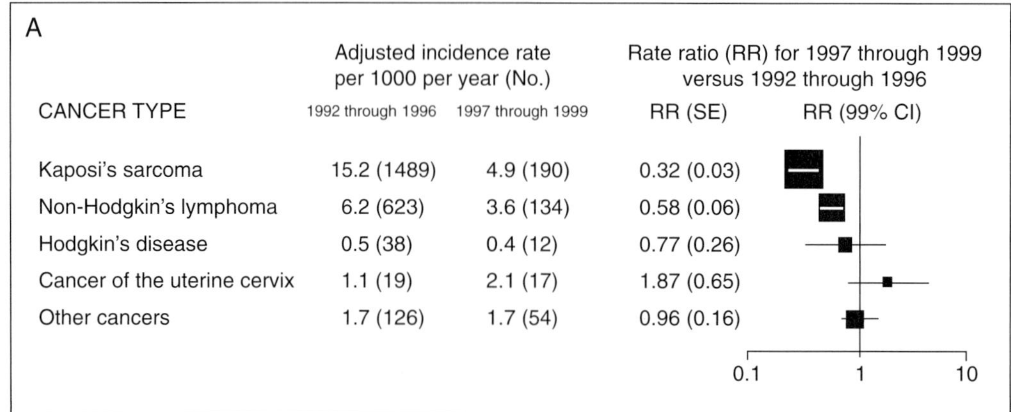

A

CANCER TYPE	Adjusted incidence rate per 1000 per year (No.) 1992 through 1996	1997 through 1999	Rate ratio (RR) for 1997 through 1999 versus 1992 through 1996 RR (SE)
Kaposi's sarcoma	15.2 (1489)	4.9 (190)	0.32 (0.03)
Non-Hodgkin's lymphoma	6.2 (623)	3.6 (134)	0.58 (0.06)
Hodgkin's disease	0.5 (38)	0.4 (12)	0.77 (0.26)
Cancer of the uterine cervix	1.1 (19)	2.1 (17)	1.87 (0.65)
Other cancers	1.7 (126)	1.7 (54)	0.96 (0.16)

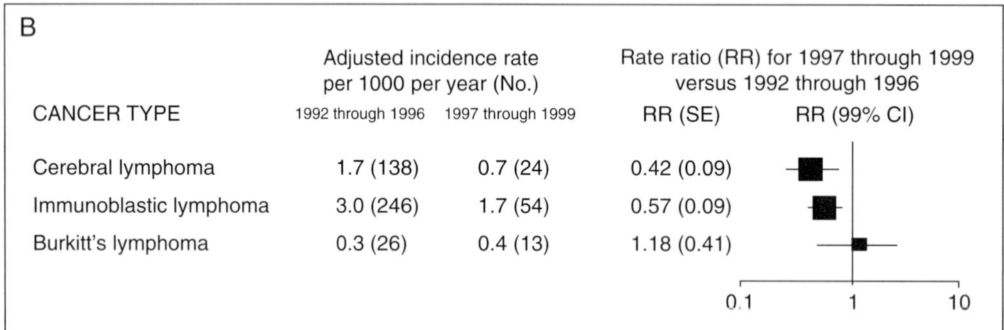

B

CANCER TYPE	Adjusted incidence rate per 1000 per year (No.) 1992 through 1996	1997 through 1999	Rate ratio (RR) for 1997 through 1999 versus 1992 through 1996 RR (SE)
Cerebral lymphoma	1.7 (138)	0.7 (24)	0.42 (0.09)
Immunoblastic lymphoma	3.0 (246)	1.7 (54)	0.57 (0.09)
Burkitt's lymphoma	0.3 (26)	0.4 (13)	1.18 (0.41)

FIGURE 96.2. Meta-analysis of highly active antiretroviral therapy (HAART) effect on (A) cancer incidence and (B) certain non-Hodgkin's lymphoma subtypes in HIV-infected adults, comparing pre-HAART to the treatment era. Rate ratios are adjusted for factors including study type, age, gender and transmission group. (From the International Collaboration on HIV and Cancer,[200] by permission of *Journal of the National Cancer Institute*.)

phoma. Both those lymphomas are closely associated with EBV, although EBV DNA in the tumor specimens was not specifically assessed in this study. In contrast, as noted in Figure 96.2, a large meta-analysis found there was no change in incidence of either Burkitt's lymphoma or Hodgkin's disease.[200] Therefore, the effect of antiretroviral therapy and the resultant improvement in immune function were not globally effective. Thus, although poor control of EBV plays a critical role in the genesis of ARL, susceptibility represents a complex interplay of immunity and other factors, such as lymphocyte growth control.

Non-Hodgkin's Lymphoma

Pathophysiology

The simplest scenario by which altered immunity could affect lymphoma occurrence is that in which an infectious agent directly alters the molecular basis of cell growth regulation. One rare example of this is HIV itself. HIV is tropic for CD4+ T cells and within that subset HIV has been implicated in rarely inducing T-cell non-Hodgkin's lymphomas.[203,204] Some of these tumors have been molecularly analyzed and noted to have an insertion site for HIV-1 in the host genome that juxtaposes HIV with the *c-fes/fps* protooncogene.[205] Dysregulated expression of c-fes/fps by the presence of HIV may result in altered cell proliferation or survival.

In contrast to HIV, gammaherpesviruses are commonly implicated in ARL. Within the gammaherpesvirus family, two have been implicated in AIDS-related lymphomas and in immunodeficiency-related lymphomas generally: EBV and the Kaposi's sarcoma-associated herpesvirus (KSHV). Two distinct subsets of AIDS-related lymphomas are directly linked to one or both of these viruses. Primary CNS lymphomas are infected with EBV, whereas primary effusion lymphomas uniformly have the KSHV genome present in tumor tissue. The EBV latent membrane protein 1 (LMP-1) is the gene most directly associated with transforming capability and is widely expressed in primary CNS lymphomas.[206,207] LMP-1 activates the tumor necrosis receptor-associated factor (TRAF) family signaling pathway,[208] resulting in enhanced expression of the transcription factor NF-κB and in transformation of B lymphocytes.

The mechanism of KSHV-mediated transformation remains controversial, although a number of viral gene products, such as IL-6, have been implicated. In addition, KSHV encodes an interferon regulatory factor homologue (vIRF1 or K9) that is capable of repressing interferon-induced host genes and inhibiting pathways of apoptosis normally enhanced by interferon, thereby further impairing a critical host antiviral defense mechanism.[152,209]

KSHV may be capable of altering immune recognition of virus-infected cells through inhibition of the MHC class I-dependent pathway of antigen presentation by preventing attachment to NK cells. Although EBV and KSHV may directly alter target cell growth in the genesis of CNS NHL and PEL, respectively, other mechanisms are clearly at work in the majority of AIDS-related lymphomas. Aside from these two minor subsets, other lymphomas in AIDS patients are often negative for EBV, which, for example, infects only about 30% of AIDS-related Burkitt lymphomas.[210] Of those tumors that are EBV infected, the type III latent gene pattern seen in infectious mononucleosis and low-grade B lymphoproliferative disorders is not consistently observed.[211–213] These lymphomas often express a type II profile of EBV genes more consistent with that seen in Hodgkin's disease. Among those ARL without EBV DNA, there are often genetic abnormalities. Large cell histology ARL demonstrate EBV infection in approximately 80% of tumors but show other genetic abnormalities that include nonoverlapping subsets with rearrangements of the Bcl-6 (21%) and c-*myc* (21%) transcription factor genes. p53 tumor suppressor gene rearrangements are generally not present.[214] The pattern is somewhat different in AIDS-related lymphoma of Burkitt histology, with c-*myc* rearrangements being almost universal (as in non-HIV-associated forms of Burkitt lymphoma), p53 mutations seen in 61%, and Bcl-6 rearrangements very uncommon. There is no clear link between EBV and any specific genetic mutation.[215–218]

Large cell lymphomas, whether in endemic or HIV-associated settings, are thought to be germinal center in origin. The Bcl-6 gene expressed in these tumors is characteristic of germinal center cells.[219] Burkitt cells are also a mature B-cell lymphoma thought to represent a transformed germinal center blast cell. They have c-*myc* translocations into either the heavy- or light-chain immunoglobulin gene loci. The translocation of the HIV-associated Burkitt tumor is distinct from endemic Burkitt's. In the HIV patients, c-*myc* has translocated into the immunoglobulin heavy-chain gene switch region rather than the joining region of the immunoglobulin locus that is characteristic of the endemic tumors.[220] This finding suggests that the rearrangement in the HIV-associated tumors occurred at a later time in B-cell maturation when heavy-chain class switching was occurring rather than during early B-cell differentiation when VDJ recombination takes place.

Although direct effects of herpesviruses may be relevant for transformation, and the interaction with other somatic mutations in host cells may enhance tumorigenicity, these events alone would be unlikely to account for the high incidence of lymphoma in AIDS patients. HIV-induced impairment of the immune system is likely to provide the critical context in which lymphoma can emerge. HIV-induced impairment of the immune system first enables transforming herpesviruses to propagate but may facilitate secondary transforming events by other means. B-cell proliferation is common in HIV infection independent of secondary herpesvirus, as is clinically manifest as the frequent lymphadenopathy and hypergammaglobulinemia seen in HIV-infected individuals. HIV may directly contribute to the process through antigenic drive, and the HIV envelope glycoprotein has also been reported to directly enhance B-cell activation.[221,222] Further, the HIV gp120 engages with the CXCR-4 chemokine receptor and may directly alter B-cell proliferation, as this receptor is known to provide a growth-promoting signal to B-cell subsets akin to the SDF-1 discussed earlier.[223–227] B-cell proliferation may be further augmented by viral perturbation of the T-cell compartment, with expansion of the Th2 subpopulation that releases B-cell stimulatory factors, such as IL-10 and IL-4.[228,229] HAART may reduce the incidence of ARL partly through reverting these direct and indirect mechanisms driving B-cell proliferation.

Clinical Biology

Virtually all ARL are high grade and of mature B-cell origin. The histology is usually either large cell anaplastic or small cell (Burkitt), and these are thought to be either germinal center or postgerminal center B cell in origin. Subsets of tumors have been more finely divided into other stages of B-cell differentiation as well. For example, by staining with antibodies against Bcl-6 (associated with germinal center cells), MUM1/IRF4 (associated with late or postgerminal center cells). and CD138/syndican-1 (associated with postgerminal center cells), Carbone et al. noted that the majority of large cell or Burkitt lymphomas were germinal center. In contrast, immunoblastic histology was described as late germinal center and primary CNS, primary effusion, plasmablastic, Hodgkin's, and some large immunoblastic lymphomas were characterized as postgerminal center.[230]

The localization of systemic AIDS-related lymphomas frequently extends beyond involved lymph nodes and affects extranodal tissues. Extranodal sites that are particularly common are the gastrointestinal tract, bone marrow and central nervous system, although virtually any tissue may be involved.[201,231–248] The tumor histology significantly influences its localization. In particular, large cell tumors preferentially involve the gastrointestinal tract, whereas Burkitt tumors often involve the bone marrow and meninges. The presenting symptoms of ARL can be very variable and do not appear to be appreciably affected by HAART.[250,251]

The different histologic subtypes of systemic ARL may occur in different settings and have unique features. AIDS-related Burkitt's lymphoma usually arises in patients with a less severe degree of immunosuppression than other histologic subtypes.[252] In those cases of Burkitt's that are EBV infected, only two EBV-encoded RNAs and only a single protein-encoding gene (EBNA-1) are expressed; this is the type I program of latent gene expression.[253] Immune reconstitution of EBV-infected cells typically does not include EBNA-1 because infected cells cannot process this protein and therefore, cannot present the antigens on class I MHC.[254] The basis for the approximately 1000-fold increase in risk for Burkitt's lymphoma among HIV-infected individuals compared with other immunosupressed populations remains an unresolved mystery.

CNS involvement with ARLs was noted early in the HIV epidemic with up to 20% incidence reported.[236] That has resulted in an emphasis on aggressively evaluating the CNS in patients with systemic AIDS-related lymphoma, including imaging and cerebrospinal fluid sampling studies. Some centers prophylactically treat all patients with intrathecal therapy, but data suggest EBV in the primary tumor is of strong predictive value for an increased risk of CNS relapse (P = 0.003).[255] Extranodal involvement has also been noted as a strong predictive factor for CNS involvement (P = 0.006).[255,256]

The prognosis for patients with AIDS-related lymphoma has been markedly affected by HAART. Prognostic factors defined before the advent of HAART need to be revised, but one large multivariate analysis indicated that CD4 count less than 100 cells/mm^3, age greater than 35 years, intravenous drug use, and stage III/IV disease, were negative prognostic factors. When only one or none of these factors was present, the overall survival was 46 weeks; when two factors were present, 44 weeks; and when three or four factors were present, 18 weeks.

The International Prognostic Index (IPI)[258] has been validated in the context of AIDS,[259] and other studies have indicated that factors used in the IPI, such as elevated lactate dehydrogenase (LDH)[258] or age more than 40 years do provide independent prognostic information in ARL. Curiously, given its impact outside the setting of HIV, Burkitt histology has not been consistently found to be of prognostic significance. Similarly, treatment protocols have not specifically evaluated this subset, and it remains unclear whether they do better with a more aggressive regimen in the setting of HIV.

Primary effusion lymphoma is a very unusual subset of systemic ARL. It is a liquid-phase tumor that rarely involves the blood, lymph nodes, or solid organs. Body cavity effusions[261–263] laden with large anaplastic or immunoblastic-appearing cells are characteristic. The cells can be identified as hematologic by staining for surface CD45 (common leukocyte antigen), but antibodies specific for B cells (CD20 or CD19) or T cells (CD3) generally do not stain the tumor cells. Molecular analysis of tumor cells is required to demonstrate VDJ rearrangement of the immunoglobulin locus, thereby defining the cells as being of B-cell origin. These cells also uniformly are infected with KSHV and are frequently coinfected with EBV. These tumors are not restricted to HIV-related immunodeficiency and may be found in other immunodeficient states. They provide a unique and intriguing paradigm for virus-induced human malignancy.

Another rare form of systemic AIDS-related lymphoma is that of plasmablastic lymphoma of the oral cavity.[264] This is an aggressive B-cell lymphoma that is distinct from other HIV-related large cell lymphomas in their presentation, histology, and immunohistochemistry (CD20 is not expressed). EBV is often, but not uniformly, present in these tumors.

Treatment

The ability to effectively treat ARL has long been complicated by the coincident presence of other complications of immunosuppression, which led to an approach of compromised dose chemotherapy early in the HIV epidemic. Although such therapies were found to result in comparable response rates to full-dose chemotherapy,[265] they are generally now reserved for those patients who have failed HAART or for whom it is not available. The introduction of HAART has resulted in far superior tolerance of chemotherapy, and full-dose regimens are now the standard of care. The specific regimen remains controversial. Full-dose CHOP or infusional regimens, such as modified-dose EPOCH have both been shown to be effective.[266,267] The response rate of the infusional EPOCH regimen was particularly impressive, with 74% of patients achieving a complete remission. Overall and disease-free survival were 92% and 60%, respectively, at a median of 53 months of follow-up. However, this was a single-center trial and validation in a larger, multicenter setting is currently being tested through the U.S. AIDS Malignancy Consortium (AMC).

The issue of whether rituximab adds benefit when added to standard chemotherapy is also still unclear in the setting of ARL. Preliminary data from a randomized trial comparing CHOP versus CHOP plus rituximab by the AMC, suggest that there may be an increased risk of infectious death in those patients receiving the rituximab without any clear improvement in tumor outcomes (Kaplan, in press). If rituximab is used, these data would indicate that it is prudent to include antibiotic prophylaxis; an intervention currently being tested in an EPOCH plus rituximab trial.

Whether specific subsets of tumors require distinct therapies has not been well defined. The numbers of patients have generally been too small to run histology-specific trials, and subgroup analysis of larger trials has not provided clear indication of histology-specific outcomes. Given the uniquely aggressive nature of Burkitt histology outside the setting of HIV, however, many centers employ a treatment regimen designed for Burkitt histology rather than using a more conventional CHOP-like regimen. One study of hyper-CVAD in AIDS-related Burkitt lymphoma demonstrated a 92% complete remission rate with tolerable toxicity and some long-term disease-free survivors.[268] Primary effusion lymphomas generally do poorly regardless of regimen, but again the data are mostly anecdotal, and no systematic evaluation has been performed.

For patients who have relapsed beyond initial therapy, the potential for high-dose chemotherapy with stem cell rescue was thought prohibitively toxic until recently. There have now been several trials that have indicated the tolerability of this approach and the potential for durable tumor control for those with ARL.[269–272] Somewhat unexpectedly, hematopoietic engraftment or infectious complication have not been problematic. Long-term outcomes remain poorly defined, but this therapy appears to be a useful intervention in the setting of lymphoma relapse and HIV disease.

Managing antiretroviral therapy during cancer chemotherapy is an issue that has been addressed by clinical trials. In one study by the AMC, a set regimen of HAART (indinivir, d4T, and 3TC) was prescribed for those receiving CHOP or modified CHOP, and it was maintained throughout the chemotherapy program.[266] No unusual or unusually severe toxic reactions were noted, and there was no change in the pharmacokinetics of either daunorubicin or indinivir. There was, however, a prolonging of the area under the curve for cyclophosphamide levels, although this did not have apparent clinical consequences. This approach was generally well accepted by patients, but only a small number of the now wide range of antiretroviral agents available have been studied. It remains possible that untoward drug–drug interactions will emerge if cancer and antiretroviral therapies are given concurrently. Taking the opposite tack to entirely avoid this issue, Little and colleagues suspended all antiretrovirals during dose-adjusted EPOCH therapy and noted that CD4 and viral loads returned to baseline when HAART was reinitiated after the completion of cancer treatments.[267] Stopping anti-HIV medications can be particularly difficult for patients to accept, however. The decision of whether to continue or interrupt HAART is a complicated one with limited available data; many centers proceed only after extensive open discussion with the patient weighing the relative likelihood of adverse effects from pharmacologic principles of the drugs in question. If anti-HIV medications are to be continued, compromised dosing or schedule should be avoided to reduce the likelihood of resistant viral strains emerging.

Hodgkin's Disease

The incidence of Hodgkin's disease has been estimated to be increased 2.5- to 8.5-fold above that of the uninfected population,[273–278] with certain geographic groups reporting an increase of up to 18.3-fold.[275] The risk of Hodgkin's disease appears to be uniformly increased across the risk groups for HIV infection, and independent of age or gender.[278] The clinical features of the disease in HIV-positive persons are substantially different from uninfected counterparts with a higher incidence of advanced-stage disease, B symptoms, and extranodal disease.[279–282] Stage III or IV disease was reported in 91% of HIV-infected patients compared with 46% in individuals without HIV.[283] Bone marrow may be involved in up to 50% of patients,[284–286] in addition to less common extranodal sites, such as the tongue, rectum, skin, and lung. Staging procedures should follow guidelines in the HIV-uninfected population, but with particular care to assess for coincident infectious causes of B symptoms.

Pathologic features of Hodgkin's disease are also different in the HIV-infected individual, with mixed cellularity histology more commonly noted.[279–281,287] EBV is also much more frequently detected in the tumor specimens. EBV has been estimated to be present in 80% to 100% of Hodgkin's tumors from individuals with HIV,[287–290] typically expressing LMP-1 but not EBNA2.[290] The transcription factor Bcl-6, expressed as noted earlier in germinal center B cells, is present in Reed–Sternberg cells from both HIV-1-infected and uninfected individuals. However, syndecan 1 (a proteoglycan associated with the postgerminal center) is restricted to the HIV-1-positive population,[291,292] suggesting that the postgerminal center B cell may be the cell of origin in HIV-1-related Hodgkin's disease. In contrast, the germinal center cell is considered to be the source of Reed–Sternberg cells in HIV-negative patients with Hodgkin's disease.

Treatment guidelines for patients with Hodgkin's disease in the setting of HIV should be the same as those without HIV. The one caveat is that HIV patients with CD4 depression should receive prophylaxis for PCP during therapy.

Posttransplant Lymphoproliferative Disease

Epidemiology

Posttransplant lymphoproliferative disease (PTLPD) is a severe complication of organ transplantation resulting from iatrogenic immunosuppression. PTLPD is the most common malignancy in the posttransplantation population; the other major complicating neoplasms are Kaposi's sarcoma, basal cell carcinoma, and cutaneous squamous cell carcinomas, which are generally less frequent or severe. PTLPD is seen both early and late after transplantation, with distinct pathophysiologic factors distinguishing these two settings. In the immediate posttransplant setting, PTLPD is uniformly EBV related. The median time to onset of PTLPD has been variably reported, but was 10 months after surgery in a series of 4,000 consecutive liver transplants in one retrospective series.[293] PTLPD is rarely seen after 5 years posttransplantation, and its frequency and perhaps time to occurrence are related to the magnitude of immunosuppression.[294] For this reason, lung and multiorgan transplants are generally associated with a higher incidence and more rapid onset of disease than kidney transplants. European centers using regimens that are less immunosuppressive, generally see less PTLPD than centers in the United States. In one multicenter study of more than 50,000 patients, the incidence of PTLPD during the first posttransplant year was 1.2%, with subsequent years estimated at 0.3% per year in cardiac transplant recipients, but these rates vary considerably depending upon the center.[295]

A number of features factor into the risk of developing PTLPD. Perhaps most important is whether the organ recipient is EBV seropositive before transplant and whether the recipient is a child or an adult. The incidence of PTLPD is significantly greater (~3-fold) in children, probably because of the lower incidence of preceding EBV infection, and is approximately 24-fold higher in EBV-seronegative versus EBV-seropositive recipients.[293,296,297] In those not previously exposed to EBV, primary EBV infection via the graft or from transfusions during surgery can result in florid lymphoproliferative disease that is generally polymorphic and polyclonal and responds to reduction in immunosuppression.[298] Although often mentioned in conjunction with PTLPD in previously EBV-infected adults or children, the pathophysiology of disease in patients with perioperatively acquired EBV is distinct, as discussed next.

The extent of immunosuppression is one of several reported risk factors, and studies have indicated that the therapeutic use of antibodies directed against T cells (for graft rejection) provide a particular enhancement of risk.[299] Alcoholic cirrhosis, and notably, the presence of hepatitis C, as a cause of liver failure in liver transplants, also appear to increase the risk of PTLPD, for reasons that are not clear.[300]

When assessing patients in the posttransplant setting, it has been reported that elevated titers of EBV viral load in the blood (more than 25,000 copies/μg DNA) are associated with the development of PTLPD and have been correlated with a suppression of EBV-reactive T cells.[297,301] Inversion of these parameters has been associated with improvement in PTLPD, usually seen in conjunction with a decrease in therapeutic immunosuppression.

The late-occurring lymphoproliferative disorders seen in the posttransplant patient are not EBV associated, may be either B or T cell in origin, and are generally similar to lymphoma in the immunocompetent population.

Pathophysiology

Posttransplantation lymphoproliferative disorders often have a polymorphic histologic appearance that may complicate diagnosis and likely reflect some of the underlying pathophysiologic differences within this group. Knowles has advocated dividing PTLPD into plasmacytic hyperplasias, polymorphic lymphoproliferative disorders, and malignant lymphomas/multiple myeloma.[302] The plasmacytic hyperplasias are polyclonal and generally regress spontaneously following withdrawal of immunosuppression. The malignant lymphomas are monoclonal, possess a variety of genetic alterations, and generally progress despite aggressive therapy. The polymorphic lymphoproliferative disorders are also monoclonal but display variable clinical behavior, their progression and response to chemotherapy apparently correlating with Bcl-6 gene mutation.[302–304] These correlations between clonality and mutation, with responsiveness to alteration of immunosuppression, support the following model. In the posttransplant setting, EBV reactivation induces a reactive lymphoid hyperplasia. The lifting of pharmacologic suppression results in restoration of the ability to control the consequences of EBV lytic replication through rejuvenated CTL responsiveness. The recalcitrance of some more blastoid PTLPD tumor types to the lifting of immunosuppression supports the notion that these tumors represent a fundamentally different disease process. EBV may serve as an initiation factor in this subset, but progression may be secondary to genomic mutation and resultant dysregulation of the cell cycle; thus, restoration of an anti-EBV CTL response may no longer be sufficient to control a rapidly progressive tumor.

Overall, PTLPD may be regarded as a relatively straightforward failure of immune control of EBV. Pharmacologically induced immunosuppression is clearly the central factor in the susceptibility, and may serve as a model for the genesis of similar lymphomas in the broader context of autoimmune disease and congenital immunodeficiency. Other genetic traits (e.g., a polymorphism in the hMSH2 DNA mismatch repair gene)[305] and environmental factors (e.g., alcohol use)[306] likely also contribute to lymphomagenesis in these patients, but any discussion of causation must begin with a focus on the host interaction with chronic EBV infection.

Despite its ubiquity as a chronic infecting agent in more than 90% of adults worldwide, EBV was first identified in 1964 by a British team[307] that found viral particles in tumor biopsies from patients with the endemic non-Hodgkin's lymphoma subtype first identified in African children by Burkitt in 1958.[308] B lymphocytes appear to be the most important targets of primary infection through exposure to oral secretions. Patients with the infectious mononucleosis symptom complex demonstrate activated B-cell blasts in the paracortical region of the tonsils.[309] EBV-infected T cells and oropharyngeal epithelial cells are only rarely identified during acute mononucleosis.[310] Viral particles release their double-stranded linear DNA in the B-cell cytoplasm, subsequently circularizing and surreptitiously assuming control of cellular replication. This viral episome is transcriptionally active in as few as 3 of the 90+ viral genes.[311] As many as 10 latency genes are active in in vitro transformed B cells, which are sufficient to cause a relative immortalization of the host cell. This parsimony of viral gene expression is believed to contribute significantly to the ability of the virus to hide from immune recognition in the normal host.

Independent of the immunosuppression factor, the specific steps leading to transformation of infected B lymphocytes are still poorly understood. Three different latency gene expression patterns have been described in most EBV-related lymphomas as previously noted, constituted by different combinations of the 10 genes expressed in B-cell lines transformed in vitro. All three patterns are represented among PTLPD patients, with the full complement expressed in polymorphic lymphoproliferative disease and a more restricted expression profile in monoclonal lymphomas.[310]

Successful suppression of viral replication is maintained in large part by the generation of cytotoxic T cells directed against several splice products of the Epstein–Barr nuclear antigen (EBNA) genes. The ability of renal transplant patients who develop PTLPD to respond to therapy (acyclovir treatment and a decrease in immunosuppression) has been shown to correlate with the recovery of the CD8+ CTL population.[312] This finding suggests that the mechanism behind regression of PTLPD in the setting of the withdrawal of immunosuppression is the release of pharmacologic impairment of CTL function. Because of the ubiquity of EBV infection in PTLPD, it is tempting to speculate that the invigoration of CTL function restores a previously suppressed ability to control EBV in these patients. Indeed, administration of autologous EBV-specific CTL has also been shown to induce regression of PTLPD in both renal transplant patients[313] and following allogeneic bone marrow transplantation.[314] One of these studies[313] found that in three patients with EBV reactivation in association with lymphoproliferation, serum EBV DNA concentrations dropped as much as three logs, back to the control range, within a month after CTL infusion.

Although PTLPD is generally due to EBV if seen in the first 2 years posttransplant, there can be rare cases of EBV-negative tumors, including KSHV-related primary effusion lymphomas. Primary effusion lymphoma associated with KSHV in the tumor has been reported in the heart allograft of a patient who had a prior history of Kaposi's sarcoma.[315]

Clinical Biology

PTLPD after solid organ transplantation often presents as lymphadenopathy or a mass. As with AIDS-related lymphomas, extranodal involvement is common. Sites of particular proclivity are the CNS and the gastrointestinal tract. A site not uncommonly involved is that of the allograft itself, where presumably the antigenic stimulation is greatest in magnitude and perturbations in immune regulation may be most dramatic. The transplanted organ has been estimated to be involved in about 20% of cases involving heart, lung, or liver transplants. Depending on the nature of the lymphomatous infiltration, distinguishing between PTLPD and graft rejection may be difficult and may require biopsy and supportive clinical information, such as EBV viral load.

The clinical approach to patients with PTLPD is generally multistep and involves reduction in immunosuppression, as tolerated. Antiherpesvirus agents are often given, though their use outside the context of primary EBV infection is highly controversial. These antiviral medications generally target the viral thymidine kinase, a gene expressed only during the lytic replication phase of the viral life cycle. Consequently, use of these drugs is appropriate in PTLPD resulting from primary EBV infection in recipients who were EBV seronegative at the time of transplant. In contrast, these antivirals are unlikely to affect the predominantly latent viral gene expression seen in PTLPD of the polymorphic or monoclonal type. In patients who do not respond to reduction in immunosuppressive drugs or are critically ill at presentation, treatment with the anti-CD20 monoclonal antibody rituximab may be highly successful.[316–318] The use of rituximab has been reported only in limited studies to date, but the results are highly encouraging. The apparent toxicities are relatively few, although hypogammaglobulinemia is an expected and potentially important clinical outcome. Interestingly, rituximab induces a reduction in EBV viral load, but this reduction does not exactly correlate with antitumor effect. Quite probably different populations of B cells are producing EBV versus those that are malignant.[319] For those patients who are refractory to anti-CD20, other antibody therapies may be useful, but no published results are available. Cytotoxic chemotherapy is another alternative, although the sensitivity of patients to the toxic side effects of these agents is increased.[320]

Drug-Associated Risk for Lymphoma in Autoimmune Disease Patients

The relationship between treatment for rheumatoid arthritis and the development of lymphoproliferative disorders is controversial, with numerous suggestive case reports[321] but no validation in large series.[322] Early studies had shown an increased risk in patients receiving cyclophosphamide[323] or chlorambucil,[324] but neither of these drugs has been widely used in rheumatoid arthritis since the advent of methotrexate therapy in the 1980s and the very effective biologic agents in the late 1990s. As indicated in Figure 96.3, these agents are associated with some risk for development of lymphoma.

The possibility of treatment-associated lymphoma has been a cause of great recent concern, particularly that associated with the most frequently used drug in rheumatoid arthritis, methotrexate.[325] The dilemma at the heart of this analysis has been whether methotrexate use is a surrogate marker for those patients with the most severe disease and thus possibly the highest risk of disease-associated lymphoma. However, many of these NHL cases have demonstrated a tumor regression following cessation of methotrexate therapy. If not a causative relationship, this observation suggests that there is something unique about the immunosuppression induced by the drug that leads to lymphoma in this disease context. One analysis of 9 new cases and review of 28 published cases[326] found that 10 of 16 patients who were diagnosed with lymphoma at the time of methotrexate discontinuation, subsequently experienced a complete or partial spontaneous remission with no other therapy. Of these responders, 8 of the 9 who were studied showed evidence of EBV infection in the tumor. Only 1 of 6 without evidence of EBV responded to methotrexate withdrawal. A more recent prospective study was performed seeking to identify all rheumatoid arthritis patients in France over a 3-year period who developed lymphoma while on methotrexate.[327,328] The estimated annual incidence of NHL was 33.3 per 100,000 population for male rheumatoid arthritis patients treated with methotrexate and 16.7 per 100,000 for women. The standardized mortality ratio was 1.07, based on the observed NHL incidence in the general French population when adjusted for age and gender, suggesting no increased risk of NHL for these rheumatoid arthritis patients. In contrast, the standardized mortality ratio for Hodgkin's disease was 7.4, with 27.8 cases per 100,000 treated male patients and 2.8 per 100,000 women. The number of cases identified in this study was much higher than those expected, based on U.S. population incidence of Hodgkin's disease, and this association has not been previously reported.

One is tempted to speculate that the success of methotrexate in treating the systemic inflammation in rheumatoid arthritis patients could decrease the established risk of NHL generally, while causing a small increase in the

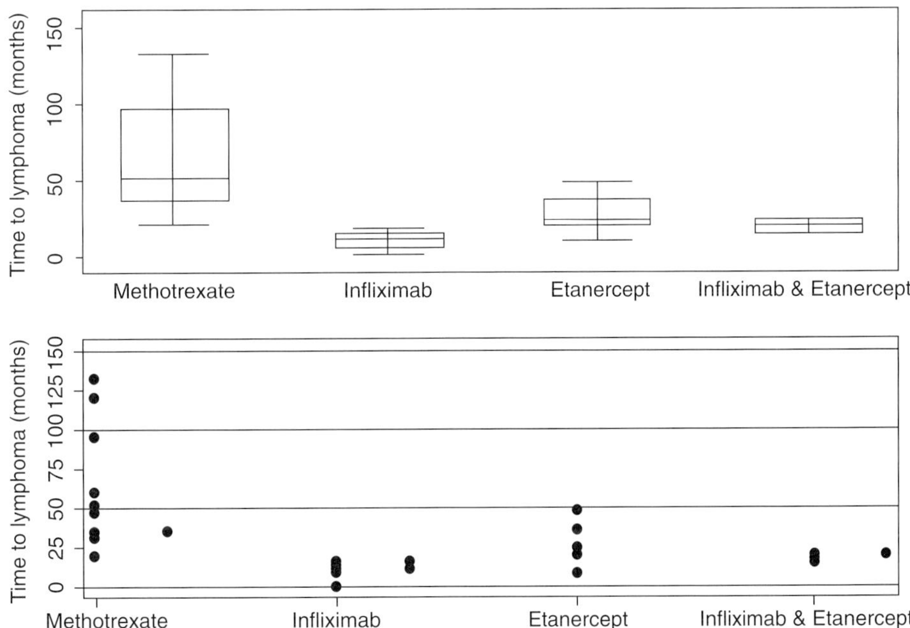

FIGURE 96.3. Lymphoma development in rheumatoid arthritis (RA) patients treated with immune-modulating therapy. Figure depicts the number of months from the start of therapy to the development of lymphoma, with bars showing the 5th and 95th percentiles. Lymphoma incidence in this study of 18,572 RA patients in the National Data Bank for Rheumatic Diseases, at the University of Kansas School of Medicine, showed overall standard incidence ratio (SIR) for lymphoma of 1.9 (95% CI, 1.3–2.7). SIR for lymphoma was 2.9 (95% CI, 1.7–4.9) in patients receiving biologics, 2.6 (95% CI, 1.4–5.0) in those receiving infliximab, with or without etanercept, and 3.8 (95% CI, 1.9–7.5) in patients treated with etanercept, with or without infliximab. Results do not show an increased SIR in patients receiving MTX compared with those who were never exposed to MTX. (From Wolfe,[330] by permission of *Arthritis Rheumatism*.)

risk for both Hodgkin's disease and NHL associated with dysregulation of anti-EBV immunity. The overall result might be neutral with regard to the lymphoma incidence in methotrexate-treated patients, at least as concerns NHL. An important new study has suggested that all-cause mortality is strongly decreased in rheumatoid arthritis patients who are treated with methotrexate, particularly cardiac-related death.[329] All in all, cytotoxic treatments for rheumatoid arthritis are unlikely to play a significant role in the genesis of the increased susceptibility to non-Hodgkin' lymphoma, and the balance of benefit for disease activity and overall mortality strongly favor the use of drugs, such as methotrexate.

Since the 1990s, rheumatologists have achieved dramatic success in treating many types of inflammatory arthritis with a new class of biologic agents that block the effects of TNF-α. Roughly 80% of patients experience significant responses in the first week of therapy with these agents, compared with the 6 to 8 weeks that typically elapse before the first benefits of methotrexate therapy. However, MedWatch postmarketing surveillance for adverse events among patients with either rheumatoid arthritis or Crohn's disease, identified 26 cases of lymphoproliferative disorders following treatment with etanercept (18 cases) or infliximab (8 cases). A third drug, adalimumab, was more recently FDA approved (December 2002), and has been reported preliminarily to be similarly associated with increased risk[330]; 81% of these cases were non-Hodgkin's lymphomas, primarily diffuse large cell phenotype. Lymphoma-related symptoms typically developed in only a median of 8 weeks after initiation of etanercept or 6 weeks after starting infliximab therapy. In 2 cases, 1 apiece for each drug, lymphoma regression occurred (similar to the experience with methotrexate) following discontinuation of anti-TNF therapy without specific cytotoxic lymphoma therapy. Besides the 16 etanercept-treated patients with NHL, 1 case each of thymoma and Hodgkin's disease was reported. Also of note, 13 of 18 patients were simultaneously or previously treated with methotrexate. Among the infliximab patients, most of whom were being treated for Crohn's disease, 5 developed NHL, and the other 3 had Hodgkin's. In the year following publication of this report, the authors noted an additional 68 case reports, with 54 classified as probable medication-associated lymphomas (29 infliximab, 25 etanercept), and 14 as possible medication-associated lymphomas (10 infliximab, 4 etanercept).[331]

More recently, another group studied 18,572 patients with rheumatoid arthritis (RA) enrolled in a national databank for rheumatic disease. About a third of the lymphoma cases were logged prospectively. The overall standard incidence ratio (SIR) for lymphoma was 1.9 [95% confidence interval (CI), 1.3–2.7]. The SIR for biologic agent use was 2.9 (95% CI, 1.7–4.9), for etanercept was 3.8 (95% CI, 1.9–7.5), and for infliximab was 2.6 (95% CI, 1.4–4.5). They found a SIR for methotrexate of 1.7 (95% CI, 0.9–3.2). Duration of RA did not influence lymphoma risk. Factors predisposing to lymphoma in this patient group were increasing age [odds ratio (OR), 1.7 for each 10 years], male gender (OR, 2.6), and to a minor degree, the level of education (a variable that correlated with likelihood of receiving TNF blockers).

There is a biologically plausible explanation for an association between TNF inhibition and tumor development. TNF knockout mice that are transgenic for a B-cell differentiation factor (BAFF), have a significantly increased incidence of lymphoma compared with the transgenic mice alone.[332] This finding may reflect the several decades of work in tumor immunology that had suggested that TNF is part of the body's armamentarium in fighting tumor development. Treatment with these agents is clearly a surrogate marker for the sicker patients, but also appears to represent an independent risk factor for lymphoma.[330]

Looking prospectively at the use of another class of biologic agents, the IL-1 receptor antagonists, preliminary data with relatively short follow-up for 233 patients, found no cases of lymphoma. Similarly, there were no cases among patients treated with leflunamide, a newer cytotoxic agent used in place of methotrexate but sullied by problems with comparatively greater hepatotoxicity.[330]

References

1. Wotherspoon AC, Ortiz-Hidalgo C, Falzon MR, Isaacson PG. *Helicobacter pylori*-associated gastritis and primary B-cell gastric lymphoma. Lancet 1991;338:1175–1176.
2. Willis TG, Jadayel DM, Du MQ, et al. Bcl10 is involved in t(1;14)(p22;q32) of MALT B cell lymphoma and mutated in multiple tumor types. Cell 1999;96:35–45.
3. Oertel SH, Riess H. Immunosurveillance, immunodeficiency and lymphoproliferations. Recent Results Cancer Res 2002; 159:1–8.
4. Pinkerton CR, Hann I, Weston CL, et al. Immunodeficiency-related lymphoproliferative disorders: prospective data from the United Kingdom Children's Cancer Study Group Registry. Br J Haematol 2002;118:456–461.
5. Murphy RC, Berdon WE, Ruzal-Shapiro C, et al. Malignancies in pediatric patients with ataxia telangiectasia. Pediatr Radiol 1999;29(4):225–230.
6. Mueller BU, Pizzo PA. Cancer in children with primary or secondary immunodeficiencies. J Pediatr 1995;126:1–10.
7. Elenitoba-Johnson KS, Jaffe ES. Lymphoproliferative disorders associated with congenital immunodeficiencies. Semin Diagn Pathol 1997;14:35–47.
8. Morrell D, Cromartie E, Swift M. Mortality and cancer incidence in 263 patients with ataxia-telangiectasia. J Natl Cancer Inst 1986;77:89–92.
9. Morrell D, Chase CL, Swift M. Cancers in 44 families with ataxia-telangiectasia. Cancer Genet Cytogenet 1990;50:119–123.
10. Su Y, Swift M. Mortality rates among carriers of ataxia-telangiectasia mutant alleles. Ann Intern Med 2000;133: 770–778.
11. Zullo A, Romiti A, Rinaldi V, et al. Gastric pathology in patients with common variable immunodeficiency. Gut 1999;45:77–81.
12. Inskip HM, Kinlen LJ, Taylor AM, Woods CG, Arlett CF. Risk of breast cancer and other cancers in heterozygotes for ataxia-telangiectasia. Br J Cancer 1999;79:1304–1307.
13. Geoffroy-Perez B, Janin N, Ossian K, et al. Cancer risk in heterozygotes for ataxia-telangiectasia. Int J Cancer 2001;93: 288–293.
14. Shafman TD, Levitz S, Nixon AJ, et al. Prevalence of germline truncating mutations in ATM in women with a second breast cancer after radiation therapy for a contralateral tumor. Genes Chromosomes Cancer 2000;27:124–129.
15. Khanna KK. Cancer risk and the ATM gene: a continuing debate. J Natl Cancer Inst. 2000;92:795–802.
16. Swift M, Morrell D, Cromartie E, Chamberlin AR, Skolnick MH, Bishop DT. The incidence and gene frequency of ataxia-telangiectasia in the United States. Am J Hum Genet 1986; 39:573–583.
17. Swift M, Sholman L, Perry M, Chase C. Malignant neoplasms in the families of patients with ataxia-telangiectasia. Cancer Res 1976;36:209–215.

18. Boultwood J. Ataxia telangiectasia gene mutations in leukaemia and lymphoma. J Clin Pathol 2001;54:512–516.
19. Carbonari M, Cherchi M, Paganelli R, et al. Relative increase of T cells expressing the gamma/delta rather than the alpha/beta receptor in ataxia-telangiectasia. N Engl J Med 1990;322:73–76.
20. Hollis RJ, Kennaugh AA, Butterworth SV, Taylor AM. Growth of large chromosomally abnormal T cell clones in ataxia telangiectasia patients is associated with translocation at 14q11. A model for other T cell neoplasia. Hum Genet 1987;76:389–395.
21. Heppell A, Butterworth SV, Hollis RJ, Kennaugh AA, Beatty DW, Taylor AM. Breakage of the T cell receptor alpha chain locus in nonmalignant clones from patients with ataxia telangiectasia. Hum Genet 1988;79:360–364.
22. Petiniot LK, Weaver Z, Vacchio M, et al. RAG-mediated V(D)J recombination is not essential for tumorigenesis in Atm-deficient mice. Mol Cell Biol 2002;22:3174–3177.
23. Barlow C, Hirotsune S, Paylor R, et al. Atm-deficient mice: a paradigm of ataxia telangiectasia. Cell 1996;86:159–171.
24. Treuner K, Helton R, Barlow C. Loss of Rad52 partially rescues tumorigenesis and T-cell maturation in Atm-deficient mice. Oncogene. 2004;23:4655–4661.
25. Kersey JH, Shapiro RS, Filipovich AH. Relationship of immunodeficiency to lymphoid malignancy. Pediatr Infect Dis J 1988; 7(suppl 5):S10–12.
26. Gronbaek K, Worm J, Ralfkiaer E, Ahrenkiel V, Hodland P, Guldberg P. ATM mutations are associated with inactivation of the ARF-TP53 tumor suppressor pathway in diffuse large B-cell lymphoma. Blood 2002;100:1430–1437.
27. Li A, Swift M. Mutations at the ataxia-telangiectasia locus and clinical phenotypes of A-T patients. Am J Med Genet 2000;92: 170–177.
28. Taylor AM, Metcalfe JA, Thick J, Mak YF. Leukemia and lymphoma in ataxia telangiectasia. Blood 1996;87:423–438.
29. Fiorilli M, Businco L, Pandolfi F, Paganelli R, Russo G, Aiuti F. Heterogeneity of immunological abnormalities in ataxia-telangiectasia. J Clin Immunol 1983;3:135–141.
30. Sanal O, Ersoy F, Tezcan I, et al. Antibody response to a seven-valent pneumococcal conjugated vaccine in patients with ataxia-telangiectasia. J Clin Immunol 2004;24:411–417.
31. Nowak-Wegrzyn A, Crawford TO, Winkelstein JA, Carson KA, Lederman HM. Immunodeficiency and infections in ataxia-telangiectasia. J Pediatr 2004;144:505–511.
32. Tsuge I, Matsuoka H, Torii S, et al. Preservation of natural killer and interleukin-2 activated killer cell activity in ataxia-telangiectasia with T cell deficiency. J Clin Lab Immunol 1987;23:7–13.
33. Coffey AJ, Brooksbank RA, Brandau O, et al. Host response to EBV infection in X-linked lymphoproliferative disease results from mutations in an SH2-domain encoding gene. Nat Genet 1998;20:129–135.
34. Schuster V, Kreth HW. X-linked lymphoproliferative disease is caused by deficiency of a novel SH2 domain-containing signal transduction adaptor protein. Immunol Rev 2000;178:21–28.
35. Sharifi R, Sinclair JC, Gilmour KC, et al. SAP mediates specific cytotoxic T-cell functions in X-linked lymphoproliferative disease. Blood 2004;103:3821–3827. (Epub 2004 Jan 3815.)
36. Nagy N, Mattsson K, Maeda A, Liu A, Szekely L, Klein E. The X-linked lymphoproliferative disease gene product SAP is expressed in activated T and NK cells. Immunol Lett 2002; 82:141–147.
37. Parolini O, Kagerbauer B, Simonitsch-Klupp I, et al. Analysis of SH2D1A mutations in patients with severe Epstein–Barr virus infections, Burkitt's lymphoma, and Hodgkin's lymphoma. Ann Hematol 2002;81:441–447. (Epub 2002 Jul 2020.)
38. Brandau O, Schuster V, Weiss M, et al. Epstein–Barr virus-negative boys with non-Hodgkin lymphoma are mutated in the SH2D1A gene, as are patients with X-linked lymphoproliferative disease (XLP). Hum Mol Genet 1999;8:2407–2413.
39. Purtilo DT, Sakamoto K. Immunodeficiency as a factor in lymphomagenesis. Perspect Pediatr Pathol 1984;8:181–191.
40. Weisenburger DD, Purtilo DT. Failures in immunological control of Epstein–Barr virus infection: fatal infectious mononucleosis. In: Epstein MA, Achong BG (eds) The Epstein–Barr Virus: Recent Advances. London: Heinemann, 1986:127–161.
41. Harrington DS, Weisenburger DD, Purtilo DT. Malignant lymphoma in the X-linked lymphoproliferative syndrome. Cancer (Phila) 1987;59:1419–1429.
42. MacGinnitie AJ, Geha R. X-linked lymphoproliferative disease: genetic lesions and clinical consequences. Curr Allergy Asthma Rep 2002;2:361–367.
43. Kawa K, Okamura T, Yasui M, Sato E, Inoue M. Allogeneic hematopoietic stem cell transplantation for Epstein–Barr virus-associated T/NK-cell lymphoproliferative disease. Crit Rev Oncol Hematol 2002;44:251–257.
44. Gross TG, Filipovich AH, Conley ME, et al. Cure of X-linked lymphoproliferative disease (XLP) with allogeneic hematopoietic stem cell transplantation (HSCT): report from the XLP registry. Bone Marrow Transplant 1996;17:741–744.
45. Ziegner UH, Ochs HD, Schanen C, et al. Unrelated umbilical cord stem cell transplantation for X-linked immunodeficiencies. J Pediatr 2001;138:570–573.
46. Maas A, Hendriks RW. Role of Bruton's tyrosine kinase in B cell development. Dev Immunol 2001;8:171–181.
47. Filipovich A, Gross T, Jyonouchi H, Shapiro RS. Immune-mediated hematologic oncologic disorders, including Epstein–Barr virus infection. In: Stiehm E (ed) Immunologic Disorders in Infants and Children, 3rd ed. Philadelphia: Saunders, 1996:855–889.
48. van der Meer JW, Weening RS, Schellekens PT, van Munster IP, Nagengast FM. Colorectal cancer in patients with X-linked agammaglobulinaemia. Lancet 1993;341:1439–1440.
49. Kinlen LJ, Webster AD, Bird AG, et al. Prospective study of cancer in patients with hypogammaglobulinaemia. Lancet 1985; 1:263–266.
50. Grubben MJ, van den Braak CC, Peters WH, van der Meer JW, Nagengast FM. Low levels of colonic glutathione S-transferase in patients with X-linked agammaglobulinaemia. Eur J Clin Invest 2000;30:642–645.
51. Humphries LA, Dangelmaier C, Sommer K, et al. Tec kinases mediate sustained calcium influx via site-specific tyrosine phosphorylation of the phospholipase Cgamma Src homology 2-Src homology 3 linker. J Biol Chem 2004;279(36):37651–37661.
52. Petro JB, Rahman SMJ, Ballard DW, Khan WN. Bruton's tyrosine kinase is required for activation of I{kappa}B kinase and nuclear factor {kappa}B in response to B cell receptor engagement. J Exp Med 2000;191:1745–1754.
53. Bajpai UD, Zhang K, Teutsch M, Sen R, Wortis HH. Bruton's tyrosine kinase links the B cell receptor to nuclear factor {kappa}B activation. J Exp Med 2000;191:1735–1744.
54. Hitoshi Y, Sonoda E, Kikuchi Y, Yonehara S, Nakauchi H, Takatsu K. IL-5 receptor positive B cells, but not eosinophils, are functionally and numerically influenced in mice carrying the X-linked immune defect. Int Immunol 1993;5:1183–1190.
55. Santos-Argumedo L, Lund FE, Heath AW, et al. CD38 unresponsiveness of xid B cells implicates Bruton's tyrosine kinase (btk) as a regular of CD38 induced signal transduction. Int Immunol 1995;7:163–170.
56. Go NF, Castle BE, Barrett R, et al. Interleukin 10, a novel B cell stimulatory factor: unresponsiveness of X chromosome-linked immunodeficiency B cells. J Exp Med 1990;172:1625–1631.
57. Brunner C, Avots A, Kreth HW, Serfling E, Schuster V. Bruton's tyrosine kinase is activated upon CD40 stimulation in human B lymphocytes. Immunobiology 2002;206:432–440.
58. Faulkner GC, Burrows SR, Khanna R, Moss DJ, Bird AG, Crawford DH. X-Linked agammaglobulinemia patients are not

infected with Epstein–Barr virus: implications for the biology of the virus. J Virol 1999;73:1555–1564.
59. Uckun FM, Waddick KG, Mahajan S, et al. BTK as a mediator of radiation-induced apoptosis in DT-40 lymphoma B cells. Science 1996;273:1096–1100.
60. Cotelingam JD, Witebsky FG, Hsu SM, Blaese RM, Jaffe ES. Malignant lymphoma in patients with the Wiskott–Aldrich syndrome. Cancer Invest 1985;3:515–522.
61. Perry GS III, Spector BD, Schuman LM, et al. The Wiskott–Aldrich syndrome in the United States and Canada (1892–1979). J Pediatr 1980;97:72–78.
62. Baba Y, Nonoyama S, Matsushita M, et al. Involvement of Wiskott–Aldrich syndrome protein in B-cell cytoplasmic tyrosine kinase pathway. Blood 1999;93:2003–2012.
63. Badour K, Zhang J, Shi F, Leng Y, Collins M, Siminovitch KA. Fyn and PTP-PEST-mediated regulation of Wiskott–Aldrich syndrome protein (WASp) tyrosine phosphorylation is required for coupling T cell antigen receptor engagement to WASp effector function and T cell activation. J Exp Med 2004;199: 99–112.
64. Badour K, Zhang J, Siminovitch KA. The Wiskott–Aldrich syndrome protein: forging the link between actin and cell activation. Immunol Rev 2003;192:98–112.
65. Cannon JL. Differential roles for Wiskott–Aldrich syndrome protein in immune synapse formation and IL-2 production. J Immunol 2004;173:1658–1662.
66. Morales-Tirado V, Johannson S, Hanson E, et al. Cutting edge: selective requirement for the Wiskott–Aldrich syndrome protein in cytokine, but not chemokine, secretion by CD4(+) T cells. J Immunol 2004;173:726–730.
67. Filipovich AH, Mathur A, Kamat D, Shapiro RS. Primary immunodeficiencies: genetic risk factors for lymphoma. Cancer Res 1992;52:5465s–5467s.
68. Sullivan KE, Mullen CA, Blaese RM, Winkelstein JA. A multi-institutional survey of the Wiskott–Aldrich syndrome. J Pediatr 1994;125:876–885.
69. Cotelingam JD, Witebsky FG, Hsu SM, Blaese RM, Jaffe ES. Malignant lymphoma in patients with the Wiskott–Aldrich syndrome. Cancer Invest 1985;3:515–522.
70. Shcherbina A, Candotti F, Rosen FS, Remold-O'Donnell E. High incidence of lymphomas in a subgroup of Wiskott–Aldrich syndrome patients. Br J Haematol 2003;121:529–530.
71. Shcherbina A, Rosen FS, Remold-O'Donnell E. WASP levels in platelets and lymphocytes of Wiskott-Aldrich syndrome patients correlate with cell dysfunction. J Immunol 1999;163: 6314–6320.
72. Buckley RH. A historical review of bone marrow transplantation for immunodeficiencies. J Allergy Clin Immunol 2004; 113:793–800.
73. Filipovich AH, Stone JV, Tomany SC, et al. Impact of donor type on outcome of bone marrow transplantation for Wiskott–Aldrich syndrome: collaborative study of the International Bone Marrow Transplant Registry and the National Marrow Donor Program. Blood 2001;97:1598–1603.
74. Knutsen AP, Steffen M, Wassmer K, Wall DA. Umbilical cord blood transplantation in Wiskott–Aldrich syndrome. J Pediatr 2003;142:519–523.
75. Kernan NA, Schroeder ML, Ciavarella D, Preti RA, Rubinstein P, O'Reilly RJ. Umbilical cord blood infusion in a patient for correction of Wiskott–Aldrich syndrome. Blood Cells 1994;20: 245–248.
76. Kaneko M, Watanabe T, Watanabe H, et al. Successful unrelated cord blood transplantation in an infant with Wiskott–Aldrich syndrome following recurrent cytomegalovirus disease. Int J Hematol 2003;78:457–460.
77. Filipovich AH. Unrelated cord blood transplantation for correction of genetic immunodeficiencies. J Pediatr 2001;138: 459–461.
78. Buckley RH. Advances in the understanding and treatment of human severe combined immunodeficiency. Immunol Res 2000; 22:237–251.
79. Shearer WT, Ritz J, Finegold MJ, et al. Epstein-Barr virus-associated B-cell proliferations of diverse clonal origins after bone marrow transplantation in a 12-year-old patient with severe combined immunodeficiency. N Engl J Med 1985;312: 1151–1159.
80. Bleesing JJ. Autoimmune lymphoproliferative syndrome (ALPS). Curr Pharm Des 2003;9:265–278.
81. Lim MS, Straus SE, Dale JK, et al. Pathological findings in human autoimmune lymphoproliferative syndrome. Am J Pathol 1998;153:1541–1550.
82. Bleesing JJ, Brown MR, Novicio C, et al. A composite picture of TcR alpha/beta(+) CD4(–)CD8(–) T cells (alpha/beta-DNTCs) in humans with autoimmune lymphoproliferative syndrome. Clin Immunol 2002;104:21–30.
83. Fuss I, Strober W, Dale J, et al. Characteristic T helper 2 T cell cytokine abnormalities in autoimmune lymphoproliferative syndrome, a syndrome marked by defective apoptosis and humoral autoimmunity. J Immunol 1997;158:1912–1918.
84. Shivakumar S, Tsokos G, Datta S. T cell receptor alpha/beta expressing double-negative (CD4-/CD8-) and CD4+ T helper cells in humans augment the production of pathogenic anti-DNA autoantibodies associated with lupus nephritis. J Immunol 1989;143:103–112.
85. Infante AJ, Britton HA, DeNapoli T, et al. The clinical spectrum in a large kindred with autoimmune lymphoproliferative syndrome caused by a Fas mutation that impairs lymphocyte apoptosis. J Pediatr 1998;133:629–633.
86. Straus SE, Jaffe ES, Puck JM, et al. The development of lymphomas in families with autoimmune lymphoproliferative syndrome with germline Fas mutations and defective lymphocyte apoptosis. Blood 2001;98:194–200.
87. van den Berg A, Maggio E, Diepstra A, de Jong D, van Krieken J, Poppema S. Germline FAS gene mutation in a case of ALPS and NLP Hodgkin lymphoma. Blood 2002;99:1492–1494.
88. Shin MS, Kim HS, Kang CS, et al. Inactivating mutations of CASP10 gene in non-Hodgkin lymphomas. Blood 2002;99: 4094–4099.
89. Muschen M, Re D, Jungnickel B, Diehl V, Rajewsky K, Kuppers R. Somatic mutation of the CD95 gene in human B cells as a side effect of the germinal center reaction. J Exp Med 2000; 192:1833–1840.
90. Certain S, Barrat F, Pastural E, et al. Protein truncation test of LYST reveals heterogeneous mutations in patients with Chediak–Higashi syndrome. Blood 2000;95:979–983.
91. Tchernev VT, Mansfield TA, Giot L, et al. The Chediak–Higashi protein interacts with SNARE complex and signal transduction proteins. Mol Med 2002;8:56–64.
92. Merino F, Henle W, Ramirez-Duque P. Chronic active Epstein–Barr virus infection in patients with Chediak–Higashi syndrome. J Clin Immunol 1986;6:299–305.
93. Mottonen M, Lanning M, Baumann P, Saarinen-Pihkala UM. Chediak–Higashi syndrome: four cases from Northern Finland. Acta Paediatr 2003;92:1047–1051.
94. Haddad E, Le Deist F, Blanche S, et al. Treatment of Chediak–Higashi syndrome by allogenic bone marrow transplantation: report of 10 cases. Blood 1995;85:3328–3333.
95. Gatti RA, Good RA. Occurrence of malignancy in immunodeficiency diseases. A literature review. Cancer (Phila) 1971;28: 89–98.
96. Schroeder HW Jr, Schroeder HW III, Sheikh SM. The complex genetics of common variable immunodeficiency. J Invest Med 2004;52:90–103.
97. Aspalter RM, Sewell WA, Dolman K, Farrant J, Webster AD. Deficiency in circulating natural killer (NK) cell subsets in

common variable immunodeficiency and X-linked agammaglobulinaemia. Clin Exp Immunol 2000;121:506–514.
98. Oliva A, Scala E, Quinti I, et al. IL-10 production and CD40L expression in patients with common variable immunodeficiency. Scand J Immunol 1997;46:86–90.
99. Brugnoni D, Airo P, Lebovitz M, et al. CD4+ cells from patients with common variable immunodeficiency have a reduced ability of CD40 ligand membrane expression after in vitro stimulation. Pediatr Allergy Immunol 1996;7:176–179.
100. Farrington M, Grosmaire LS, Nonoyama S, et al. CD40 ligand expression is defective in a subset of patients with common variable immunodeficiency. Proc Natl Acad Sci USA 1994;91: 1099–1103.
101. Levy Y, Gupta N, Le Deist F, et al. Defect in IgV gene somatic hypermutation in common variable immunodeficiency syndrome. Proc Natl Acad Sci USA 1998;95:13135–13140.
102. Cunningham-Rundles C, Bodian C. Common variable immunodeficiency: clinical and immunological features of 248 patients. Clin Immunol 1999;92:34–48.
103. Morra M, Silander O, Calpe S, et al. Alterations of the X-linked lymphoproliferative disease gene SH2D1A in common variable immunodeficiency syndrome. Blood 2001;98:1321–1325.
104. Van der Hilst JC, Smits BW, van der Meer JW. Hypogammaglobulinaemia: cumulative experience in 49 patients in a tertiary care institution. Neth J Med 2002;60:140–147.
105. Zullo A, Romiti A, Rinaldi V, et al. Gastric pathology in patients with common variable immunodeficiency. Gut 1999;45:77–81.
106. Groopman JE, Broder S. Cancers in AIDS and other immunodeficiency states. In: DeVita VT, Hellman S, Rosenbert SA (eds) Cancer: Principles and Practice of Oncology, 3rd ed. Philadelphia: Lipincott, 1989:1958–1959.
107. Filipovich AH, Mathur A, Kamat D, Kersey JH, Shapiro RS. Lymphoproliferative disorders and other tumors complicating immunodeficiencies. Immunodeficiency 1994;5:91–112.
108. Sander CA, Medeiros LJ, Weiss LM, Yano T, Sneller MC, Jaffe ES. Lymphoproliferative lesions in patients with common variable immunodeficiency syndrome. Am J Surg Pathol 1992;16:1170–1182.
109. Mellemkjaer L, Hammarstrom L, Andersen V, et al. Cancer risk among patients with IgA deficiency or common variable immunodeficiency and their relatives: a combined Danish and Swedish study. Clin Exp Immunol 2002;130:495–500.
110. Cunningham-Rundles C, Siegal FP, Cunningham-Rundles S, Lieberman P. Incidence of cancer in 98 patients with common varied immunodeficiency. J Clin Immunol 1987;7:294–299.
111. Ariatti C, Rossi D, Vivenza D, et al. Molecular characterization of common variable immunodeficiency-related lymphomas. Ann Ital Med Int 2001;16:163–169.
112. Ariatti C, Vivenza D, Capello D, et al. Common-variable immunodeficiency-related lymphomas associate with mutations and rearrangements of BCL-6: pathogenetic and histogenetic implications. Hum Pathol 2000;31:871–873.
113. Cunningham-Rundles C, Cooper DL, Duffy TP, Strauchen J. Lymphomas of mucosal-associated lymphoid tissue in common variable immunodeficiency. Am J Hematol 2002;69:171–178.
114. Mehta AC, Faber-Langendoen K, Duggan DB. Common variable immunodeficiency and breast cancer. Cancer Invest 2004;22: 93–96.
115. Steinbrook R. The AIDS epidemic in 2004. N Engl J Med 2004; 351:115–117.
116. Chaisson RE. HIV becomes world's leading infectious cause of death. Hopkins HIV Rep 1999;11:1.
117. Chang Y, Cesarman E, Pessin MS, et al. Identification of herpesvirus-like DNA sequences in AIDS-associated Kaposi's sarcoma [see comments]. Science 1994;266:1865–1869.
118. Knowles DM, Cesarman E. The Kaposi's sarcoma-associated herpesvirus (human herpesvirus-8) in Kaposi's sarcoma, malignant lymphoma, and other diseases. Ann Oncol 1997;8(suppl 2:123–129.
119. Russo JJ, Bohenzky RA, Chien MC, et al. Nucleotide sequence of the Kaposi sarcoma-associated herpesvirus (HHV8). Proc Natl Acad Sci USA 1996;93:14862–14867.
120. Moore PS, Chang Y. Kaposi's sarcoma (KS), KS-associated herpesvirus, and the criteria for causality in the age of molecular biology. Am J Epidemiol 1998;147:217–221.
121. Kedes DH, Operskalski E, Busch M, Kohn R, Flood J, Ganem D. The seroepidemiology of human herpesvirus 8 (Kaposi's sarcoma-associated herpesvirus): distribution of infection in KS risk groups and evidence for sexual transmission [see comments] [published erratum appears in Nat Med 1996;2(9):1041]. Nat Med 1996;2:918–924.
122. Ganem D. KSHV and Kaposi's sarcoma: the end of the beginning? Cell 1997;91:157–160.
123. Staskus KA, Zhong W, Gebhard K, et al. Kaposi's sarcoma-associated herpesvirus gene expression in endothelial (spindle) tumor cells. J Virol 1997;71:715–719.
124. Min J, Katzenstein D. Detection of human herpesvirus 8 DNA in peripheral blood mononuclear cells of HIV+ subjects, with and without KS. 5th Conf Retrovir Oppor Infect 1998;160(abstract 432).
125. Martin JN, Ganem DE, Osmond DH, Page-Shafer KA, Macrae D, Kedes DH. Sexual transmission and the natural history of human herpesvirus 8 infection. N Engl J Med 1998;338:948–954.
126. Chatlynne LG, Lapps W, Handy M, et al. Detection and titration of human herpesvirus-8-specific antibodies in sera from blood donors, acquired immunodeficiency syndrome patients, and Kaposi's sarcoma patients using a whole virus enzyme-linked immunosorbent assay. Blood 1998;92:53–58.
127. Lennette ET, Blackbourn DJ, Levy JA. Antibodies to human herpesvirus type 8 in the general population and in Kaposi's sarcoma patients [see comments]. Lancet 1996;348:858–861.
128. Cattani P, Capuano M, Lesnoni La Parola I, et al. Human herpesvirus 8 in Italian HIV-seronegative patients with Kaposi sarcoma [see comments]. Arch Dermatol 1998;134:695–699.
129. Angeloni A, Heston L, Uccini S, et al. High prevalence of antibodies to human herpesvirus 8 in relatives of patients with classic Kaposi's sarcoma from Sardinia [see comments]. J Infect Dis 1998;177:1715–1718.
130. Brayfield BP, Kankasa C, West JT, et al. Distribution of Kaposi sarcoma-associated herpesvirus/human herpesvirus 8 in maternal saliva and breast milk in Zambia: implications for transmission. J Infect Dis 2004;189:2260–2270.)
131. Mayama S, Cuevas LE, Sheldon J, et al. Prevalence and transmission of Kaposi's sarcoma-associated herpesvirus (human herpesvirus 8) in Ugandan children and adolescents. Int J Cancer 1998;77:817–820.
132. Monini P, de Lellis L, Fabris M, Rigolin F, Cassai E. Kaposi's sarcoma-associated herpesvirus DNA sequences in prostate tissue and human semen [see comments]. N Engl J Med 1996; 334:1168–1172.
133. Diamond C, Huang ML, Kedes DH, et al. Absence of detectable human herpesvirus 8 in the semen of human immunodeficiency virus-infected men without Kaposi's sarcoma. J Infect Dis 1997; 176:775–777.
134. Kroll M, Shandera W. AIDS-associated Kaposi's sarcoma. Hosp Pract 1998;33:85–102.
135. Bais C, Santomasso B, Coso O, et al. G-protein-coupled receptor of Kaposi's sarcoma-associated herpesvirus is a viral oncogene and angiogenesis activator [see comments] [published erratum appears in Nature 1998;392(6672):210]. Nature (Lond) 1998; 391:86–89.

136. Hennessey N, Friedman-Kien A. Clinical simulators of the lesions of Kaposi's sarcoma. In: Friedman-Kien AE (ed) Color Atlas of AIDS. Philadelphia: Saunders, 1989:49–70.
137. Wyatt ME, Finlayson CJ, Moore-Gillon V. Kaposi's sarcoma masquerading as pyogenic granuloma of the nasal mucosa. J Laryngol Otol 1998;112:280–282.
138. Drago F, Ranieri E, Malaguti F, Losi E, Rebora A. Human herpesvirus 7 in pityriasis rosea [letter]. Lancet 1997;349: 1367–1368.
139. Oksenhendler E, Cazals-Hatem D, Schulz TF, et al. Transient angiolymphoid hyperplasia and Kaposi's sarcoma after primary infection with human herpesvirus 8 in a patient with human immunodeficiency virus infection. N Engl J Med 1998;338: 1585–1590.
140. Huh J, Kang GH, Gong G, Kim SS, Ro JY, Kim CW. Kaposi's sarcoma-associated herpesvirus in Kikuchi's disease. Hum Pathol 1998;29:1091–1096.
141. Silvers D. The microscopic diagnosis of classical and epidemic Kaposi's sarcoma. In: Friedman-Kien AE (ed) Color Atlas of AIDS. Philadelphia: Saunders, 1989:71–82.
142. Boshoff C, Schulz TF, Kennedy MM, et al. Kaposi's sarcoma-associated herpesvirus infects endothelial and spindle cells. Nat Med 1995;1:1274–1278.
143. Uccini S, Sirianni MC, Vincenzi L, et al. Kaposi's sarcoma cells express the macrophage-associated antigen mannose receptor and develop in peripheral blood cultures of Kaposi's sarcoma patients. Am J Pathol 1997;150:929–938.
144. Jussila L, Valtola R, Partanen TA, et al. Lymphatic endothelium and Kaposi's sarcoma spindle cells detected by antibodies against the vascular endothelial growth factor receptor-3. Cancer Res 1998;58:1599–1604.
145. Weninger W, Rendl M, Pammer J, et al. Nitric oxide synthases in Kaposi's sarcoma are expressed predominantly by vessels and tissue macrophages. Lab Invest 1998;78:949–955.
146. Gupta S, Aggarwal S, Nakamura S. A possible role of multidrug resistance-associated protein (MRP) in basic fibroblast growth factor secretion by AIDS-associated Kaposi's sarcoma cells: a survival molecule? J Clin Immunol 1998;18:256–263.
147. Murakami-Mori K, Mori S, Nakamura S. Endogenous basic fibroblast growth factor is essential for cyclin E-CDK2 activity in multiple external cytokine-induced proliferation of AIDS-associated Kaposi's sarcoma cells: dual control of AIDS-associated Kaposi's sarcoma cell growth and cyclin E-CDK2 activity by endogenous and external signals. J Immunol 1998;161:1694–1704.
148. Simonart T, Degraef C, Noel JC, et al. Overexpression of Bcl-2 in Kaposi's sarcoma-derived cells. J Invest Dermatol 1998; 111:349–353.
149. Sirianni MC, Vincenzi L, Fiorelli V, et al. Ggamma-interferon production in peripheral blood mononuclear cells and tumor infiltrating lymphocytes from Kaposi's sarcoma patients: correlation with the presence of human herpesvirus-8 in peripheral blood mononuclear cells and lesional macrophages. Blood 1998;91:968–976.
150. Fiorelli V, Gendelman R, Sirianni MC, et al. Gamma-interferon produced by CD8+ T cells infiltrating Kaposi's sarcoma induces spindle cells with angiogenic phenotype and synergy with human immunodeficiency virus-1 Tat protein: an immune response to human herpesvirus-8 infection? Blood 1998;91: 956–967.
151. Samaniego F, Markham PD, Gendelman R, et al. Vascular endothelial growth factor and basic fibroblast growth factor present in Kaposi's sarcoma (KS) are induced by inflammatory cytokines and synergize to promote vascular permeability and KS lesion development. Am J Pathol 1998;152:1433–1443.
152. Li M, Lee H, Guo J, et al. Kaposi's sarcoma-associated herpesvirus viral interferon regulatory factor. J Virol 1998;72: 5433–5440.
153. Zimring JC, Goodbourn S, Offermann MK. Human herpesvirus 8 encodes an interferon regulatory factor (IRF) homolog that represses IRF-1-mediated transcription. J Virol 1998;72: 701–707.
154. Gao SJ, Boshoff C, Jayachandra S, Weiss RA, Chang Y, Moore PS. KSHV ORF K9 (vIRF) is an oncogene which inhibits the interferon signaling pathway. Oncogene 1997;15:1979–1985.
155. Muralidhar S, Pumfery AM, Hassani M, et al. Identification of kaposin (open reading frame K12) as a human herpesvirus 8 (Kaposi's sarcoma-associated herpesvirus) transforming gene [published erratum appears in J Virol 1999;73(3):2568]. J Virol 1998;72:4980–4988.
156. Swanton C, Mann DJ, Fleckenstein B, Neipel F, Peters G, Jones N. Herpes viral cyclin/Cdk6 complexes evade inhibition by CDK inhibitor proteins. Nature (Lond) 1997;390:184–187.
157. Murphy M, Armstrong D, Sepkowitz KA, Ahkami RN, Myskowski PL. Regression of AIDS-related Kaposi's sarcoma following treatment with an HIV-1 protease inhibitor [letter]. AIDS 1997;11:261–262.
158. Aboulafia D. Regression of AIDS-related pulmonary Kaposi's sarcoma after highly active antiretroviral therapy. Mayo Clin Proc 1998;73:439–443.
159. Pellet C, Chevret S, Frances C, et al. Prognostic value of quantitative Kaposi sarcoma-associated herpesvirus load in post-transplantation Kaposi sarcoma. J Infect Dis 2002;186:110–113. (Epub 2002 Jun 2003.)
160. Tedeschi R, Enbom M, Bidoli E, Linde A, De Paoli P, Dillner J. Viral load of human herpesvirus 8 in peripheral blood of human immunodeficiency virus-infected patients with Kaposi's sarcoma. J Clin Microbiol 2001;39:4269–4273.
161. Palella FJ Jr, Delaney KM, Moorman AC, et al. Declining morbidity and mortality among patients with advanced human immunodeficiency virus infection. HIV Outpatient Study Investigators [see comments]. N Engl J Med 1998;338:853–860.
162. Rabkin CS, Testa MA, Fischl MA, Roenn JV. Declining incidence of Kaposi's sarcoma in ACTG trials. J Acquir Immune Defic Syndr Hum Retrovirol 1998;17.
163. Jones JL, Hanson DL, Dworkin MS, Ward JW, Jaffe HW. Effect of antiretroviral therapy on recent trends in selected cancers among HIV-infected persons. Adult/Adolescent Spectrum of HIV Disease Project Group. J Acquir Immune Defic Syndr 1999;21(suppl 1):S11–S17.
164. Krischer J, Rutschmann O, Hirschel B, Vollenweider-Roten S, Saurat JH, Pechere M. Regression of Kaposi's sarcoma during therapy with HIV-1 protease inhibitors: a prospective pilot study. J Am Acad Dermatol 1998;38:594–598.
165. Dupin N, Rubin De Cervens V, Gorin I, et al. The influence of highly active antiretroviral therapy on AIDS-associated Kaposi's sarcoma. Br J Dermatol 1999;140:875–881.
166. Lebbe C, Blum L, Pellet C, et al. Clinical and biological impact of antiretroviral therapy with protease inhibitors on HIV-related Kaposi's sarcoma. AIDS 1998;12:F45–F49.
167. Rizzieri DA, Liu J, Traweek ST, Miralles GD. Clearance of HHV-8 from peripheral blood mononuclear cells with a protease inhibitor [letter]. Lancet 1997;349:775–776.
168. Kedes DH, Ganem D. Sensitivity of Kaposi's sarcoma-associated herpesvirus replication to antiviral drugs. Implications for potential therapy. J Clin Invest 1997;99:2082–2086.
169. Low P, Neipel F, Rascu A, et al. Suppression of HHV-8 viremia by foscarnet in an HIV-infected patient with Kaposi's sarcoma and HHV-8 associated hemophagocytic syndrome. Eur J Med Res 1998;3:461–464.
170. Hammoud Z, Parenti DM, Simon GL. Abatement of cutaneous Kaposi's sarcoma associated with cidofovir treatment [see comments]. Clin Infect Dis 1998;26:1233.
171. Simonart T, Noel JC, De Dobbeleer G, et al. Treatment of classical Kaposi's sarcoma with intralesional injections of cidofovir: report of a case. J Med Virol 1998;55:215–218.

172. Mocroft A, Youle M, Gazzard B, Morcinek J, Halai R, Phillips AN. Anti-herpesvirus treatment and risk of Kaposi's sarcoma in HIV infection. Royal Free/Chelsea and Westminster Hospitals Collaborative Group. AIDS 1996;10:1101–1105.
173. Glesby MJ, Hoover DR, Weng S, et al. Use of antiherpes drugs and the risk of Kaposi's sarcoma: data from the Multicenter AIDS Cohort Study. J Infect Dis 1996;173:1477–1480.
174. Little RF, Merced-Galindez F, Staskus K, et al. A pilot study of cidofovir in patients with Kaposi sarcoma. J Infect Dis 2003;187:149–153. (Epub 2002 Dec 2013.)
175. Lukawska J, Cottrill C, Bower M. The changing role of radiotherapy in AIDS-related malignancies. Clin Oncol (R Coll Radiol) 2003;15:2–6.
176. Belembaogo E, Kirova Y, Frikha H, Yu SJ, Piedbois P, Le Bourgeois JP. Radiotherapy of epidemic Kaposi's sarcoma: the experience of the Henri-Mondor Hospital (643 patients). Cancer Radiother 1998;2:49–52.
177. Harrison M, Harrington KJ, Tomlinson DR, Stewart JS. Response and cosmetic outcome of two fractionation regimens for AIDS-related Kaposi's sarcoma. Radiother Oncol 1998;46: 23–28.
178. Bodsworth NJ, Bloch M, Bower M, Donnell D, Yocum R. Phase III vehicle-controlled, multi-centered study of topical alitretinoin gel 0.1% in cutaneous AIDS-related Kaposi's sarcoma. Am J Clin Dermatol 2001;2:77–87.
179. Walmsley S, Northfelt DW, Melosky B, Conant M, Friedman-Kien AE, Wagner B. Treatment of AIDS-related cutaneous Kaposi's sarcoma with topical alitretinoin (9-cis-retinoic acid) gel. Panretin Gel North American Study Group. J Acquir Immune Defic Syndr 1999;22:235–246.
180. Miles SA, Dezube BJ, Lee JY, et al. Antitumor activity of oral 9-cis-retinoic acid in HIV-associated Kaposi's sarcoma. AIDS 2002;16:421–429.
181. Krown SE. Interferon-alpha: evolving therapy for AIDS-associated Kaposi's sarcoma. J Interferon Cytokine Res 1998; 18:209–214.
182. Shepherd FA, Beaulieu R, Gelmon K, et al. Prospective randomized trial of two dose levels of interferon alfa with zidovudine for the treatment of Kaposi's sarcoma associated with human immunodeficiency virus infection: a Canadian HIV Clinical Trials Network study. J Clin Oncol 1998;16:1736–1742.
183. Reiser M, Bruns C, Hartmann P, Salzberger B, Diehl V, Fatkenheuer G. Raynaud's phenomenon and acral necrosis after chemotherapy for AIDS-related Kaposi's sarcoma. Eur J Clin Microbiol Infect Dis 1998;17:58–60.
184. Northfelt DW, Dezube BJ, Thommes JA, et al. Pegylated-liposomal doxorubicin versus doxorubicin, bleomycin, and vincristine in the treatment of AIDS-related Kaposi's sarcoma: results of a randomized phase III clinical trial. J Clin Oncol 1998;16:2445–2451.
185. Stewart S, Jablonowski H, Goebel FD, et al. Randomized comparative trial of pegylated liposomal doxorubicin versus bleomycin and vincristine in the treatment of AIDS-related Kaposi's sarcoma. International Pegylated Liposomal Doxorubicin Study Group. J Clin Oncol 1998;16:683–691.
186. Gill PS, Wernz J, Scadden DT, et al. Randomized phase III trial of liposomal daunorubicin versus doxorubicin, bleomycin, and vincristine in AIDS-related Kaposi's sarcoma. J Clin Oncol 1996;14:2353–2364.
187. Welles L, Saville MW, Lietzau J, et al. Phase II trial with dose titration of paclitaxel for the therapy of human immunodeficiency virus-associated Kaposi's sarcoma. J Clin Oncol 1998; 16:1112–1121.
188. Little RF, Wyvill KM, Pluda JM, et al. Activity of thalidomide in AIDS-related Kaposi's sarcoma. J Clin Oncol 2000;18: 2593–2602.
189. Dezube BJ, Von Roenn JH, Holden-Wiltse J, et al. Fumagillin analog in the treatment of Kaposi's sarcoma: a phase I AIDS Clinical Trial Group study. AIDS Clinical Trial Group No. 215 Team. J Clin Oncol 1998;16:1444–1449.
190. Beral V, Peterman T, Berkelman R, Jaffe H. AIDS-associated non-Hodgkin lymphoma [see comments]. Lancet 1991;337:805–809.
191. Moore RD, Chaisson RE. Natural history of HIV infection in the era of combination antiretroviral therapy. AIDS 1999;13: 1933–1942.
192. Rabkin CS, Yang Q, Goedert JJ, Nguyen G, Mitsuya H, Sei S. Chemokine and chemokine receptor gene variants and risk of non-Hodgkin's lymphoma in human immunodeficiency virus-1-infected individuals. Blood 1999;93:1838–1842.
193. Dean M, Jacobson LP, McFarlane G, et al. Reduced risk of AIDS lymphoma in individuals heterozygous for the CCR5-delta32 mutation. Cancer Res 1999;59:3561–3564.
194. Young L, Alfieri C, Hennessy K, et al. Expression of Epstein–Barr virus transformation-associated genes in tissues of patients with EBV lymphoproliferative disease. N Engl J Med 1989;321: 1080–1085.
195. Sample J, Kieff E. Transcription of the Epstein–Barr virus genome during latency in growth-transformed lymphocytes. J Virol 1990;64:1667–1674.
196. van Baarle D, Hovenkamp E, Callan MF, et al. Dysfunctional Epstein–Barr virus (EBV)-specific CD8(+) T lymphocytes and increased EBV load in HIV-1 infected individuals progressing to AIDS-related non-Hodgkin lymphoma. Blood 2001;98: 146–155.
197. Biggar RJ. AIDS-related cancers in the era of highly active antiretroviral therapy. Oncology (Huntingt) 2001;15:439–448; discussion 448–449.
198. Grulich AE. AIDS-associated non-Hodgkin's lymphoma in the era of highly active antiretroviral therapy. J Acquir Immune Defic Syndr 1999;21(suppl 1):S27–S30.
199. Grulich AE, Li Y, McDonald AM, Correll PK, Law MG, Kaldor JM. Decreasing rates of Kaposi's sarcoma and non-Hodgkin's lymphoma in the era of potent combination anti-retroviral therapy. AIDS 2001;15:629–633.
200. International Collaboration on HIV and Cancer. Highly active antiretroviral therapy and incidence of cancer in human immunodeficiency virus-infected adults. J Natl Cancer Inst 2000;92:1823–1830.
201. Kirk O, Pedersen C, Cozzi-Lepri A, et al. Non-Hodgkin lymphoma in HIV-infected patients in the era of highly active antiretroviral therapy. Blood 2001;98:3406–3412.
202. Besson C, Goubar A, Gabarre J, et al. Changes in AIDS-related lymphoma since the era of highly active antiretroviral therapy. Blood 2001;98:2339–2344.
203. Herndier BG, Shiramizu BT, Jewett NE, Aldape KD, Reyes GR, McGrath MS. Acquired immunodeficiency syndrome-associated T-cell lymphoma: evidence for human immunodeficiency virus type 1-associated T-cell transformation. Blood 1992;79: 1768–1774.
204. Lust JA, Banks PM, Hooper WC, et al. T-cell non-Hodgkin lymphoma in human immunodeficiency virus-1-infected individuals. Am J Hematol 1989;31:181–187.
205. Shiramizu B, Herndier BG, McGrath MS. Identification of a common clonal human immunodeficiency virus integration site in human immunodeficiency virus-associated lymphomas. Cancer Res 1994;54:2069–2072.
206. Liebowitz D. Epstein–Barr virus and a cellular signaling pathway in lymphomas from immunosuppressed patients [see comments]. N Engl J Med 1998;338:1413–1421.
207. Camilleri-Broet S, Camparo P, Mokhtari K, et al. Overexpression of BCL-2, BCL-X, and BAX in primary central nervous system lymphomas that occur in immunosuppressed patients. Mod Pathol 2000;13:158–165.
208. Izumi KM, Kieff ED. The Epstein–Barr virus oncogene product latent membrane protein 1 engages the tumor necrosis factor receptor-associated death domain protein to mediate B lympho-

cyte growth transformation and activate NF-kappaB. Proc Natl Acad Sci USA 1997;94:12592–12597.
209. Seo T, Lee D, Shim YS, et al. Viral interferon regulatory factor 1 of Kaposi's sarcoma-associated herpesvirus interacts with a cell death regulator, GRIM19, and inhibits interferon/retinoic acid-induced cell death. J Virol 2002;76:8797–8807.
210. Neri A, Barriga F, Inghirami G, et al. Epstein–Barr virus infection precedes clonal expansion in Burkitt's and acquired immunodeficiency syndrome-associated lymphoma. Blood 1991;77:1092–1095.
211. Levine AM. Acquired immunodeficiency syndrome-related lymphoma. Blood 1992;80:8.
212. Hamilton-Dutoit SJ, Pallesen G, Franzmann MB, et al. AIDS-related lymphoma. Histopathology, immunophenotype, and association with Epstein–Barr virus as demonstrated by in situ nucleic acid hybridization. Am J Pathol 1991;138:149–163.
213. Hamilton-Dutoit SJ, Pallesen G, Karkov J, Skinhoj P, Franzmann MB, Pedersen C. Identification of EBV-DNA in tumour cells of AIDS-related lymphomas by in-situ hybridisation [letter]. Lancet 1989;1:554–552.
214. Gaidano G, Lo Coco F, Ye BH, et al. Rearrangements of the BCL-6 gene in acquired immunodeficiency syndrome-associated non-Hodgkin's lymphoma: association with diffuse large-cell subtype. Blood 1994;84:397–402.
215. Shiramizu B, Herndier B, Meeker T, Kaplan L, McGrath M. Molecular and immunophenotypic characterization of AIDS-associated, Epstein-Barr virus-negative, polyclonal lymphoma. J Clin Oncol 1992;10:383–389.
216. Pelicci PG, Knowles DM, Arlin ZA, et al. Multiple monoclonal B cell expansions and c-myc oncogene rearrangements in acquired immune deficiency syndrome-related lymphoproliferative disorders. Implications for lymphomagenesis. J Exp Med 1986;164:2049–2060.
217. Ballerini P, Gaidano G, Gong JZ, et al. Multiple genetic lesions in acquired immunodeficiency syndrome-related non-Hodgkin's lymphoma. Blood 1993;81:166–176.
218. Levine A, Shibata D, Weiss L. Molecular characteristics of intermediate/high (I/H) grade lymphomas (NHL) arising in HIV-positive vs. HIV-negative PTS: preliminary data from a population (POP) based study in the county of Los Angeles. Blood 1992;80:1028.
219. Gaidano G, Carbone A, Dalla-Favera R. Genetic basis of acquired immunodeficiency syndrome-related lymphomagenesis. J Natl Cancer Inst Monogr 1998;23:95–100.
220. Neri A, Barriga F, Knowles DM, Magrath IT, Dalla-Favera R. Different regions of the immunoglobulin heavy-chain locus are involved in chromosomal translocations in distinct pathogenetic forms of Burkitt lymphoma. Proc Natl Acad Sci USA 1988;85:2748–2752.
221. Kehrl JH, Rieckmann P, Kozlow E, Fauci AS. Lymphokine production by B cells from normal and HIV-infected individuals. Ann N Y Acad Sci 1992;651:220–227.
222. Yarchoan R, Redfield RR, Broder S. Mechanisms of B cell activation in patients with acquired immunodeficiency syndrome and related disorders. Contribution of antibody-producing B cells, of Epstein–Barr virus-infected B cells, and of immunoglobulin production induced by human T cell lymphotropic virus, type III/lymphadenopathy-associated virus. J Clin Invest 1986; 78:439–447.
223. Davis CB, Dikic I, Unutmaz D, et al. Signal transduction due to HIV-1 envelope interactions with chemokine receptors CXCR4 or CCR5. J Exp Med 1997;186:1793–1798.
224. Madani N, Kozak SL, Kavanaugh MP, Kabat D. gp120 envelope glycoproteins of human immunodeficiency viruses competitively antagonize signaling by coreceptors CXCR4 and CCR5. Proc Natl Acad Sci USA 1998;95:8005–8010.
225. Popik W, Pitha PM. Early activation of mitogen-activated protein kinase kinase, extracellular signal-regulated kinase, p38 mitogen-activated protein kinase, and c-Jun N-terminal kinase in response to binding of simian immunodeficiency virus to Jurkat T cells expressing CCR5 receptor. Virology 1998;252: 210–217.
226. Popik W, Hesselgesser JE, Pitha PM. Binding of human immunodeficiency virus type 1 to CD4 and CXCR4 receptors differentially regulates expression of inflammatory genes and activates the MEK/ERK signaling pathway. J Virol 1998;72:6406–6413.
227. Su SB, Gong W, Grimm M, et al. Inhibition of tyrosine kinase activation blocks the down-regulation of CXC chemokine receptor 4 by HIV-1 gp 120 in CD4+ T cells. J Immunol. 1999;162: 7128–7132.
228. Clerici M, Wynn TA, Berzofsky JA, et al. Role of interleukin-10 in T helper cell dysfunction in asymptomatic individuals infected with the human immunodeficiency virus. J Clin Invest 1994;93:768–775.
229. Muller F, Aukrust P, Nordoy I, Froland SS. Possible role of interleukin-10 (IL-10) and CD40 ligand expression in the pathogenesis of hypergammaglobulinemia in human immunodeficiency virus infection: modulation of IL-10 and Ig production after intravenous Ig infusion. Blood 1998;92:3721–3729.
230. Carbone A, Gloghini A, Larocca LM, et al. Expression profile of MUM1/IRF4, BCL-6, and CD138/syndecan-1 defines novel histogenetic subsets of human immunodeficiency virus-related lymphomas. Blood 2001;97:744–751.
231. Katler SP, Riggs SA, Cabanillas F. Aggressive non-Hodgkin's lymphoma in immunocompromised homosexual males. Blood 1985;66.
232. Ioachim HL, Dorsett B, Cronin W, Maya M, Wahl S. Acquired immunodeficiency syndrome-associated lymphomas: clinical, pathologic, immunologic, and viral characteristics of 111 cases. Hum Pathol 1991;22:659–673.
233. Ziegler JL, Beckstead JA, Volberding PA, et al. Acquired immunodeficiency syndrome-associated lymphomas: clinical, pathologic, immunologic, and viral characteristics of 111 cases. N Engl J Med 1984;311:565–570.
234. Lowenthal DA, Straus DJ, Campbell SW, Gold JW, Clarkson BD, Koziner B. AIDS-related lymphoid neoplasia. The Memorial Hospital experience. Cancer (Phila) 1988;61:2325–2337.
235. National Cancer Institute sponsored study of classifications of non-Hodgkin's lymphomas: summary and description of a working formulation for clinical usage. The Non-Hodgkin's Lymphoma Pathologic Classification Project. Cancer (Phila) 1982;49:2112–2135.
236. Levine AM, Wernz JC, Kaplan L. Low-dose chemotherapy with central nervous system prophylaxis and zidovudine maintenance in AIDS-related lymphoma. JAMA 1991;266:84–88.
237. Gill PS, Levine AM, Meyer PR, et al. Primary central nervous system lymphoma in homosexual men. Clinical, immunologic, and pathologic features. Am J Med 1985;78:742–748.
238. Gill PS, Levine AM, Krailo M. AIDS-related malignant lymphoma: results of prospective treatment trials. J Clin Oncol 1987;5:1322–1328.
239. Knowles DM, Chamulak GA, Subar M. Lymphoid neoplasia associated with the acquired immunodeficiency syndrome (AIDS): The New York University Medical Center experience with 105 patients. Ann Intern Med 1988;108:744–753.
240. Bermudez MA, Grant KM, Rodvien R, Mendes F. Non-Hodgkin's lymphoma in a population with or at risk for acquired immunodeficiency syndrome: indications for intensive chemotherapy. Am J Med 1989;86:71.
241. Kaplan LD, Abrams DI, Feigal E. AIDS-associated non-Hodgkin's lymphoma in San Francisco. JAMA 1989;261:719–724.
242. Kaplan MH, Susin M, Pahwa SG, et al. Neoplastic complications of HTLV-III infection. Lymphomas and solid tumors. Am J Med 1987;82:389–396.
243. Kaplan LD, Kahn JO, Crowe S, et al. Clinical and virologic effects of recombinant human granulocyte-macrophage colony-

stimulating factor in patients receiving chemotherapy for human immunodeficiency virus-associated non-Hodgkin's lymphoma: results of a randomized trial. J Clin Oncol 1991;9: 929–940.

244. Remick SC, McSharry JJ, Wolf BC. Novel oral combination chemotherapy in the treatment of intermediate-grade and high-grade AIDS-related non-Hodgkin's lymphoma. J Clin Oncol 1993;11:1691–1702.
245. Freter CE. Acquired immunodeficiency syndrome-associated lymphomas. J Natl Cancer Inst Monogr 1990;10:45–54.
246. von Gunten CF, Von Roenn JH. Clinical aspects of human immunodeficiency virus-related lymphoma. Curr Opin Oncol 1992;4:894–899.
247. Raphael M, Gentilhomme O, Tulliez M, Byron PA, Diebold J. Histopathologic features of high-grade non-Hodgkin's lymphomas in acquired immunodeficiency syndrome. The French Study Group of Pathology for Human Immunodeficiency Virus-Associated Tumors. Arch Pathol Lab Med 1991;115:15–20.
248. Burkes RL, Meyer PR, Gill PS, Parker JW, Rasheed S, Levine AM. Rectal lymphoma in homosexual men. Arch Intern Med 1986;146:913–915.
249. Ziegler JL, Beckstead JA, Volberding PA, et al. Non-Hodgkin's lymphoma in 90 homosexual men. Relation to generalized lymphadenopathy and the acquired immunodeficiency syndrome. N Engl J Med 1984;311:565–570.
250. Levine AM, Seneviratne L, Espina BM, et al. Evolving characteristics of AIDS-related lymphoma. Blood 2000;96:4084–4090.
251. Matthews GV, Bower M, Mandalia S, Powles T, Nelson MR, Gazzard BG. Changes in acquired immunodeficiency syndrome-related lymphoma since the introduction of highly active antiretroviral therapy. Blood 2000;96:2730–2734.
252. Gabarre J, Raphael M, Lepage E, et al. Human immunodeficiency virus-related lymphoma: relation between clinical features and histologic subtypes. Am J Med 2001;111:704–711.
253. Rowe M, Rowe DT, Gregory CD, et al. Differences in B cell growth phenotype reflect novel patterns of Epstein–Barr virus latent gene expression in Burkitt's lymphoma cells. EMBO J 1987;6:2743–2751.
254. Levitskaya J, Sharipo A, Leonchiks A, Ciechanover A, Masucci MG. Inhibition of ubiquitin/proteasome-dependent protein degradation by the Gly-Ala repeat domain of the Epstein–Barr virus nuclear antigen 1. Proc Natl Acad Sci USA 1997;94: 12616–12621.
255. Cingolani A, Gastaldi R, Fassone L, et al. Epstein–Barr virus infection is predictive of CNS involvement in systemic AIDS-related non-Hodgkin's lymphomas. J Clin Oncol 2000;18: 3325–3330.
256. Scadden DT. Epstein–Barr virus, the CNS, and AIDS-related lymphomas: as close as flame to smoke. J Clin Oncol 2000; 18:3323–3324.
257. Straus DJ, Huang J, Testa MA, Levine AM, Kaplan LD. Prognostic factors in the treatment of human immunodeficiency virus-associated non-Hodgkin's lymphoma: analysis of AIDS Clinical Trials Group protocol 142: low-dose versus standard-dose m-BACOD plus granulocyte-macrophage colony-stimulating factor. National Institute of Allergy and Infectious Diseases. J Clin Oncol 1998;16:3601–3606.
258. Shipp MA, Harrington DP, Klatt MM, et al. Identification of major prognostic subgroups of patients with large-cell lymphoma treated with m-BACOD or M-BACOD. Ann Intern Med 1986;104:757–765.
259. Navarro JT, Ribera JM, Oriol A, et al. International prognostic index is the best prognostic factor for survival in patients with AIDS-related non-Hodgkin's lymphoma treated with CHOP. A multivariate study of 46 patients. Haematologica 1998;83: 508–513.
260. Vaccher E, Tirelli U, Spina M, et al. Age and serum lactate dehydrogenase level are independent prognostic factors in human immunodeficiency virus-related non-Hodgkin's lymphomas: a single-institute study of 96 patients. J Clin Oncol 1996;14: 2217–2223.
261. Cesarman E, Chang Y, Moore PS, Said JW, Knowles DM. Kaposi's sarcoma-associated herpesvirus-like DNA sequences in AIDS-related body-cavity-based lymphomas [see comments]. N Engl J Med 1995;332:1186–1191.
262. Nador RG, Cesarman E, Chadburn A, et al. Primary effusion lymphoma: a distinct clinicopathologic entity associated with the Kaposi's sarcoma-associated herpes virus. Blood 1996; 88:645–656.
263. Karcher DS, Alkan S. Human herpesvirus-8-associated body cavity-based lymphoma in human immunodeficiency virus-infected patients: a unique B-cell neoplasm. Hum Pathol 1997; 28:801–808.
264. Delecluse HJ, Anagnostopoulos I, Dallenbach F, et al. Plasmablastic lymphomas of the oral cavity: A new entity associated with the human immunodeficiency virus infection. Blood 1997;89:1413–1420.
265. Kaplan LD, Straus DJ, Testa MA, et al. Low-dose compared with standard-dose m-BACOD chemotherapy for non-Hodgkin's lymphoma associated with human immunodeficiency virus infection. N Eng J Med 1997;336:1641–1648.
266. Ratner L, Lee J, Tang S, et al. Chemotherapy for human immunodeficiency virus-associated non-Hodgkin's lymphoma in combination with highly active antiretroviral therapy. J Clin Oncol 2001;19:2171–2178.
267. Little RF, Pittaluga S, Grant N, et al. Highly effective treatment of acquired immunodeficiency syndrome-related lymphoma with dose-adjusted EPOCH: impact of antiretroviral therapy suspension and tumor biology. Blood 2003;101:4653–4659.
268. Cortes J, Thomas D, Rios A, et al. Hyperfractionated cyclophosphamide, vincristine, doxorubicin, and dexamethasone and highly active antiretroviral therapy for patients with acquired immunodeficiency syndrome-related Burkitt lymphoma/ leukemia. Cancer (Phila) 2002;94:1492–1499.
269. Molina A, Krishnan AY, Nademanee A, et al. High dose therapy and autologous stem cell transplantation for human immunodeficiency virus-associated non-Hodgkin lymphoma in the era of highly active antiretroviral therapy. Cancer (Phila) 2000;89: 680–689.
270. Gabarre J, Marcelin AG, Azar N, et al. High-dose therapy plus autologous hematopoietic stem cell transplantation for human immunodeficiency virus (HIV)-related lymphoma: results and impact on HIV disease. Haematologica 2004;89:1100–1108.
271. Re A, Cattaneo C, Michieli M, et al. High-dose therapy and autologous peripheral-blood stem-cell transplantation as salvage treatment for HIV-associated lymphoma in patients receiving highly active antiretroviral therapy. J Clin Oncol 2003;21: 4423–4427.
272. Krishnan A, Molina A, Zaia J, et al. Autologous stem cell transplantation for HIV-associated lymphoma. Blood 2001;98: 3857–3859.
273. Reynolds P, Saunders LD, Layefsky ME, Lemp GF. The spectrum of acquired immunodeficiency syndrome (AIDS)-associated malignancies in San Francisco, 1980–1987. Am J Epidemiol 1993;137:19–30.
274. Lyter DW, Bryant J, Thackeray R, Rinaldo CR, Kingsley LA. Incidence of human immunodeficiency virus-related and nonrelated malignancies in a large cohort of homosexual men. J Clin Oncol 1995;13:2540–2546.
275. Grulich A, Wan X, Law M, Coates M, Kaldor J. Rates of non-AIDS defining cancers in people with AIDS. J AIDS Human Retrovirol 1997;14:A18.
276. Serraino D, Pezzotti P, Dorrucci M, Alliegro MB, Sinicco A, Rezza G. Cancer incidence in a cohort of human immunodeficiency virus seroconverters. HIV Italian Seroconversion Study Group [see comments]. Cancer (Phila) 1997;79:1004–1008.

277. Goedert JJ, Cote TR, Virgo P, et al. Spectrum of AIDS-associated malignant disorders [see comments]. Lancet 1998;351:1833–1839.
278. Franceschi S, Dal Maso L, Arniani S, et al. Risk of cancer other than Kaposi's sarcoma and non-Hodgkin's lymphoma in persons with AIDS in Italy. Cancer and AIDS Registry Linkage Study. Br J Cancer 1998;78:966–970.
279. Scheib RG, Siegel RS. Atypical Hodgkin's disease and the acquired immunodeficiency syndrome. Ann Intern Med 1985; 102:554.
280. Schoeppel SL, Hoppe RT, Dorfman RF, et al. Hodgkin's disease in homosexual men with generalized lymphadenopathy. Ann Intern Med 1985;102:68–70.
281. Robert NJ, Schneiderman H. Hodgkin's disease and the acquired immunodeficiency syndrome. Ann Intern Med 1984;101: 142–143.
282. Levine AM. Hodgkin's disease in the setting of human immunodeficiency virus infection. J Natl Cancer Inst Monogr 1998; 23:37–42.
283. Kieff E. Current perspectives on the molecular pathogenesis of virus-induced cancers in human immunodeficiency virus infection and acquired immunodeficiency syndrome. J Natl Cancer Inst Monogr 1998;23:7–14.
284. Andrieu JM, Roithmann S, Tourani JM, et al. Hodgkin's disease during HIV1 infection: the French registry experience. French Registry of HIV-associated Tumors. Ann Oncol 1993;4:635–641.
285. Monfardini S, Tirelli U, Vaccher E, Foa R, Gavosto F. Hodgkin's disease in 63 intravenous drug users infected with human immunodeficiency virus. Gruppo Italiano Cooperativo AIDS & Tumori (GICAT). Ann Oncol 1991;2(suppl 2):201–205.
286. Serrano M, Bellas C, Campo E, et al. Hodgkin's disease in patients with antibodies to human immunodeficiency virus. A study of 22 patients. Cancer (Phila) 1990;65:2248–2254.
287. Tirelli U, Errante D, Dolcetti R, et al. Hodgkin's disease and human immunodeficiency virus infection: clinicopathologic and virologic features of 114 patients from the Italian Cooperative Group on AIDS and Tumors. J Clin Oncol 1995;13: 1758–1767.
288. Carbone A, Weiss LM, Gloghini A, Ferlito A. Hodgkin's disease: old and recent clinical concepts. Ann Otol Rhinol Laryngol 1996;105:751–758.
289. Carbone A, Dolcetti R, Gloghini A, et al. Immunophenotypic and molecular analyses of acquired immune deficiency syndrome-related and Epstein–Barr virus-associated lymphomas: a comparative study. Hum Pathol 1996;27:133–146.
290. Spina M, Sandri S, Tirelli U. Hodgkin's disease in HIV-infected individuals. Curr Opin Oncol 1999;11:522–526.
291. Carbone A, Gloghini A, Larocca LM, et al. Human immunodeficiency virus-associated Hodgkin's disease derives from post-germinal center B cells. Blood 1999;93:2319–2326.
292. Carbone A, Gloghini A, Gaidano G, et al. Expression status of BCL-6 and syndecan-1 identifies distinct histogenetic subtypes of Hodgkin's disease. Blood 1998;92:2220–2228.
293. Jain A, Nalesnik M, Reyes J, et al. Posttransplant lymphoproliferative disorders in liver transplantation: a 20-year experience. Ann Surg 2002;236:429–436; discussion 436–437.
294. Ramalingam P, Rybicki L, Smith MD, et al. Posttransplant lymphoproliferative disorders in lung transplant patients: the Cleveland Clinic experience. Mod Pathol 2002;15:647–656.
295. Opelz G, Henderson R. Incidence of non-Hodgkin lymphoma in kidney and heart transplant recipients. Lancet 1993;342: 1514–1516.
296. Allen U, Hebert D, Moore D, Dror Y, Wasfy S. Epstein–Barr virus-related post-transplant lymphoproliferative disease in solid organ transplant recipients, 1988–97: a Canadian multi-centre experience. Pediatr Transplant 2001;5:198–203.
297. Smets F, Sokal EM. Epstein–Barr virus-related lymphoproliferation in children after liver transplant: role of immunity, diagnosis, and management. Pediatr Transplant 2002;6:280–287.
298. Hayashi RJ, Kraus MD, Patel AL, et al. Posttransplant lymphoproliferative disease in children: correlation of histology to clinical behavior. J Pediatr Hematol Oncol 2001;23:14–18.
299. Duvoux C, Pageaux GP, Vanlemmens C, et al. Risk factors for lymphoproliferative disorders after liver transplantation in adults: an analysis of 480 patients. Transplantation 2002;74: 1103–1109.
300. McLaughlin K, Wajstaub S, Marotta P, et al. Increased risk for posttransplant lymphoproliferative disease in recipients of liver transplants with hepatitis C. Liver Transplant 2000;6:570–574.
301. Stevens SJ, Verschuuren EA, Verkuujlen SA, Van Den Brule AJ, Meijer CJ, Middeldorp JM. Role of Epstein–Barr virus DNA load monitoring in prevention and early detection of post-transplant lymphoproliferative disease. Leuk Lymphoma 2002;43:831–840.
302. Knowles DM. Immunodeficiency-associated lymphoproliferative disorders. Mod Pathol 1999;12:200–217.
303. Chadburn A, Chen JM, Hsu DT, et al. The morphologic and molecular genetic categories of posttransplantation lymphoproliferative disorders are clinically relevant. Cancer (Phila) 1998;82: 1978–1987.
304. Cesarman E, Chadburn A, Liu YF, Migliazza A, Dalla-Favera R, Knowles DM. BCL-6 gene mutations in posttransplantation lymphoproliferative disorders predict response to therapy and clinical outcome. Blood 1998;92:2294–2302.
305. Paz-y-Mino C, Perez JC, Fiallo BF, Leone PE. A polymorphism in the hMSH2 gene (gIVS12-6T>C) associated with non-Hodgkin lymphomas. Cancer Genet Cytogenet 2002;133:29–33.
306. Chiu BC, Weisenburger DD, Cantor KP, et al. Alcohol consumption, family history of hematolymphoproliferative cancer, and the risk of non-Hodgkin's lymphoma in men. Ann Epidemiol 2002;12:309–315.
307. Epstein MA, Achong BG, Barr YM. Virus particles in cultured lymphoblasts from Burkitt's lymphoma. Lancet 1964;1:702–703.
308. Burkitt DA. Sarcoma involving the jaws in African children. Br J Surg 1958;45:218–223.
309. Niedobitek G, Hamilton-Dutoit S, Herbst H, et al. Identification of Epstein–Barr virus-infected cells in tonsils of acute infectious mononucleosis by in situ hybridization. Hum Pathol 1989; 20:796–799.
310. Niedobitek G, Meru N, Delecluse H. Epstein–Barr virus infection and human malignancies. Int J Exp Pathol 2001;82:149–170.
311. Tierney RJ, Steven N, Young LS, Rickinson AB. Epstein–Barr virus latency in blood mononuclear cells: analysis of viral gene transcription during primary infection and in the carrier state. J Virol 1994;68:7374–7385.
312. Porcu P, Eisenbeis CF, Pelletier RP, et al. Successful treatment of posttransplantation lymphoproliferative disorder (PTLD) following renal allografting is associated with sustained CD8+ T-cell restoration. Blood 2002;100:2341–2348.
313. Rooney CM, Smith CA, Ng CYC, et al. Use of gene-modified virus-specific T lymphocytes to control Epstein–Barr-virus-related lymphoproliferation. Lancet 1995;345:9–13.
314. Rooney CM, Smith CA, Ng CY, et al. Infusion of cytotoxic T cells for the prevention and treatment of Epstein–Barr virus-induced lymphoma in allogeneic transplant recipients. Blood 1998;92:1549–1555.
315. Jones D, Ballestas ME, Kaye KM, et al. Primary-effusion lymphoma and Kaposi's sarcoma in a cardiac-transplant recipient [see comments]. N Engl J Med 1998;339:444–449.
316. Faye A, Quartier P, Reguerre Y, et al. Chimaeric anti-CD20 monoclonal antibody (rituximab) in post-transplant B-lymphoproliferative disorder following stem cell transplantation in children. Br J Haematol 2001;115:112–118.
317. Milpied N, Vasseur B, Parquet N, et al. Humanized anti-CD20 monoclonal antibody (Rituximab) in post-transplant B-lymphoproliferative disorder: a retrospective analysis on 32 patients. Ann Oncol 2000;11:113–116.

318. Berney T, Delis S, Kato T, et al. Successful treatment of posttransplant lymphoproliferative disease with prolonged rituximab treatment in intestinal transplant recipients. Transplantation 2002;74:1000–1006.
319. Yang J, Tao Q, Flinn IW, et al. Characterization of Epstein–Barr virus-infected B cells in patients with posttransplantation lymphoproliferative disease: disappearance after rituximab therapy does not predict clinical response. Blood 2000;96:4055–4063.
320. Swinnen LJ, Mullen GM, Carr TJ, Costanzo MR, Fisher RI. Aggressive treatment for postcardiac transplant lymphoproliferation. Blood 1995;86:3333–3340.
321. Abu-Shakra M, Buskila D, Shoenfeld Y. Rheumatoid arthritis and cancer. In: Shoenfeld Y, Gershwin ME (eds) Cancer and Autoimmunity. Amsterdam: Elsevier, 2000:19–30.
322. Kinlen LJ. Malignancy in autoimmune diseases. J Autoimmun 1992;5:363–371.
323. Baker GL, Kahl LE, Zee BC, Stolzer BL, Agarwal AK, Medsger TA. Malignancy following treatment of rheumatoid arthritis with cyclophosphamide. Am J Med 1987;83:1–9.
324. Patapanian H, Graham S, Sambrook PN, et al. The oncogenicity of chlorambucil in rheumatoid arthritis. Br J Rheumatol 1988;27:44–47.
325. Kremer JM. Is methotrexate oncogenic in patients with rheumatoid arthritis? Semin Arthritis Rheum 1997:785–787.
326. Salloum E, Cooper DL, Howe G, et al. Spontaneous regression of lymphoproliferative disorders in patients treated with methotrexate for rheumatoid arthritis and other rheumatic diseases. J Clin Oncol 1996;14:1943–1949.
327. Sibilia J, Mariette X. Methotrexate treatment and mortality in rheumatoid arthritis. Lancet 2002;360:1096–1097.
328. Mariette X, Cazals-Hatem D, Warszawki J, Liote F, Balandraud N, Sibilia J. Lymphomas in rheumatoid arthritis patients treated with methotrexate: a 3-year prospective study in France. Blood 2002;99:3909–3915.
329. Choi HK, Hernan MA, Seeger JD, Robins JM, Wolfe F. Methotrexate and mortality in patients with rheumatoid arthritis: a prospective study. Lancet 2002;359:1173–1177.
330. Wolfe F, Michaud K. Lymphoma in rheumatoid arthritis: the effect of methotrexate and anti-tumor necrosis factor therapy in 18,572 patients. Arthritis Rheum 2004;50:1740–1751.
331. Brown SL, Greene MH, Gershon SK, Edwards ET, Braun MM. Tumor necrosis factor antagonist therapy and lymphoma development: twenty-six cases reported to the Food and Drug Administration. Arthritis Rheum 2002;46:3151–3158.
332. Batten M, Fletcher C, Ng LG, et al. TNF deficiency fails to protect BAFF transgenic mice against autoimmunity and reveals a predisposition to B cell lymphoma. J Immunol 2004;172: 812–822.

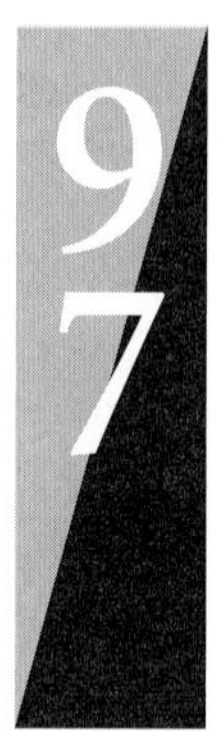

Cancer in the Older Population

Karim S. Malek and Rebecca A. Silliman

Epidemiology

Cancer Burden in the Older Population

Advancing age comes bundled with increased cancer incidence and mortality.[1,2] Indeed, the median age at diagnosis of all cancers combined is 69 years for men and 67 for women.[3] Age-adjusted cancer incidence is 10 times higher in the 65+ population compared to their younger counterparts (2,151.2 versus 208.8/100,000 persons).[2] Similarly, age-adjusted cancer mortality is 15-fold higher in the 65+ population (1,068.2 versus 67.3/100,000 persons).[2] Figure 97.1 illustrates the proportions of the commonest cancers incidence and mortality in the 65+ population.[4] As a result, although the total U.S. population is expected to grow by 9% between 1990 and 2010, the incidence of cancer is expected to increase by a disproportionate 32% in the same time frame.[5,6] These trends are mirrored in countries across the globe.[7,8]

These figures have pressed many private and public institutions to sponsor the development of geriatric oncology as a separate subspecialty. Recent literature has seen a surge in the number of seminal publications specifically devoted to the management of older patients with cancer.[9–12] Geriatric oncology is a rapidly growing field and, although not exhaustive, this chapter outlines the challenges that are unique to this new discipline and briefly explores future research directions.

How Old Is Old?

Physiologically, however, there are no data to favor one particular age cutoff over the other. Although chronologic aging and organ function decline with advancing age are undeniable realities, individual organ functions decline at different rates in different persons.

Practical Approach to Geriatric Oncology

Geriatric oncologists are faced with a two-sided challenge: on the one hand, they have to carefully select evidence-based data that are applicable to older cancer patients from an ever-expanding oncology literature addressed to a wider audience. This is a difficult task given the limited representation of older individuals in cancer clinical trials.[13] Indeed, even after removing age as an exclusion criterion from collaborative group trials, only 13% of all participants in Southwest Oncology Group (SWOG) and 8% of all participants in European Organization for Research and Treatment of Cancer (EORTC) clinical trials are older than 70 years[14,15] compared to 47% of the total U.S. population with cancer in the same age group.[14] A retrospective review of National Cancer Institute (NCI)-sponsored clinical trials active between 1997 and 2000 yielded similar conclusions.[16] On the other hand, treating cancer in older patients requires that four unique points be addressed: (1) estimating the patient's life expectancy; (2) evaluating the patient's comorbidities and functional status; (3) increased susceptibility to treatment toxicity in older patients; and (4) putting treatment benefits in perspective: absolute versus relative gains.

Estimating the Patient's Life Expectancy

Although the *average* life expectancy of the general population has doubled in the last century, it is important to note that those who live close to or beyond the *average* expectancy are not condemned to imminent death but, on the contrary, have the highest odds of surviving even longer.[17] The average life expectancy at ages 65, 75, and 85 years is respectively, 17.5, 11.2, and 6 years.[18] This concept is key in avoiding the temptation of undertreating older patients based solely on their advanced age.[12,19]

Evaluating the Patient's Comorbidities and Functional Status

Eighty percent of individuals who are 65 years of age and older have at least one comorbidity.[20] The interaction of comorbidity and cancer is a very complex one and is the subject of the following detailed discussion. Comorbidities are independent predictors of survival in cancer patients.[21,22] Accounting for them is an essential step in the management of older patients with cancer.

There are many tools to assess comorbidity with variable content and different goals,[23–26] but there is no consensus on which one to use in routine geriatric oncology. Additionally, these tools often require lengthy administration, rendering them less practical for regular use in a busy oncology practice. For example, the Multidimensional Assessment of Cancer in the Elderly (MACE), although specifically developed to evaluate comorbidity in older cancer patients, requires 27 ± 7 minutes for scoring.[27] We and others have implemented shorter screening questionnaires as a practical substitute to exhaustive geriatric assessment scales (Table 97.1).[28,29] This screening questionnaire can often be self-

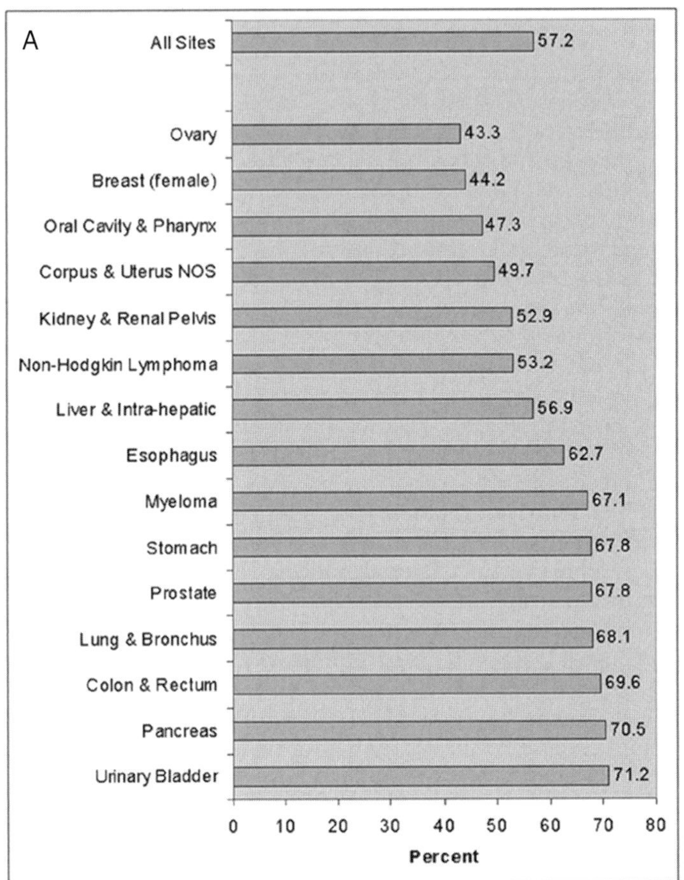

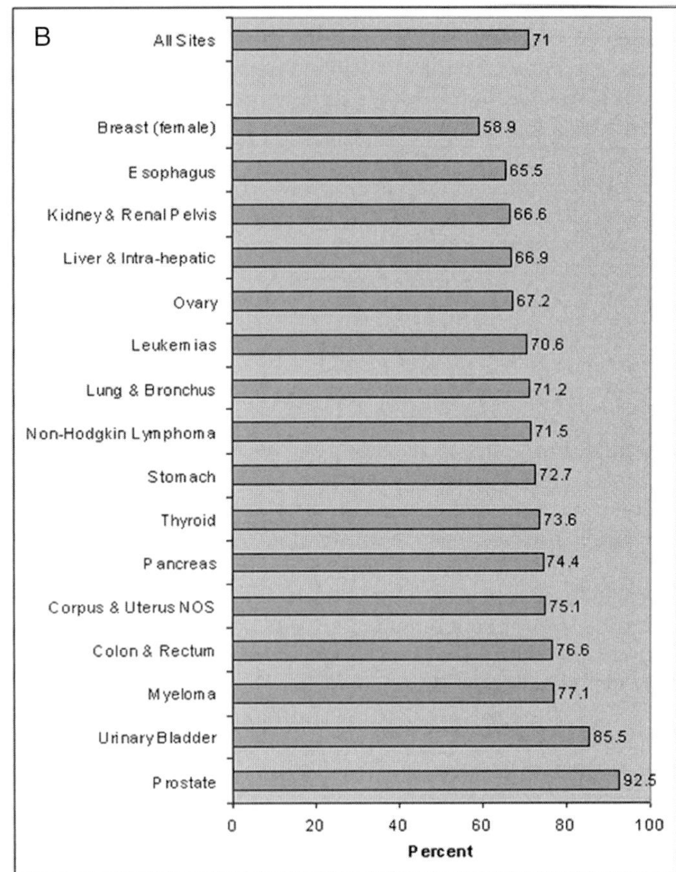

FIGURE 97.1. (A) Age-adjusted cancer incidence in the 65+ population. (B) Age-adjusted cancer mortality in the 65+ population. [Data from Ries et al. (eds) SEER Cancer Statistics Review, 1975–2000. Bethesda, MD: National Cancer Institute, 2003. http://seer.cancer.gov/csr/1975_2000.]

TABLE 97.1. Geriatric screening questionnaire.

To be filled by the patient (Yes/No)
1. Have you lost 10 pounds or more in the last 6 months without trying to do so?
2. How are you able to walk? Independent _________ Assist _________ Cane _________ Walker _________ Dependent _________
3. (A) In the past year, have you ever lost your urine and gotten wet? (B) If you have answered "Yes" to the above question, have you lost urine on at least 6 separate days?
4. Are you able to: • Do strenuous activities, like fast walking or biking? • Do heavy work around the house like washing windows, walls or floors? • Go shopping for groceries or clothes? • Get to places out of walking distances? • Bathe (either a sponge bath or tub bath) or shave? • Dress, like putting on a shirt, buttoning or zipping, or putting on shoes?
5. Do you feel that your needs at home are not being met?
To be filled by healthcare professional
6. Do you feel unsafe or threatened by someone around you?
7. Do you often feel sad or depressed?
8. I am going to give you the names of three objects. Please repeat them after me: "Apple, penny, table". Recall at 1 minute: _________ (of 3)

Source: Adapted from Reuben and Moore et al.[28,30]

administered by the patient with minimal help from family members. The sensitivity, specificity, positive, and negative predictive values of the questionnaire items are well established.[30] Results of the screening test are reported as part of the initial geriatric oncology evaluation, and the test can be subsequently repeated at the physician's discretion. Patients who perform poorly in the initial screening test are candidates for referral to a geriatrician who would then perform a comprehensive geriatric assessment.

Increased Susceptibility to Treatment Toxicity in Older Patients

This susceptibility is the subject of ongoing research and is one of the main barriers to extrapolating clinical trial data obtained from younger trial participants to older cancer patients. Older patients are more susceptible to the side effects of chemotherapeutic agents.[31] Additionally, cancer treatment modalities may affect older patients in a unique fashion. For example, a chemotherapeutic agent that causes peripheral neuropathy may worsen imbalance in an older individual and increase his or her risks of falling and the subsequent morbidity that ensues. Increased treatment toxicity may also negatively affect an often-compromised quality of life. The common problem of polypharmacy in older age increases the likelihood of drug–drug and/or drug–food interactions.[32–34] The impact of treatment modalities on older cancer patients is detailed below.

Putting Treatment Benefits in Perspective: Absolute Versus Relative Gains

Barring untoward side effects, a treatment that offers a 25% relative reduction of mortality at 10 years may be an attractive modality for a 65-year-old patient, whose average life expectancy is otherwise 17.5 years. The same relative risk reduction may not, however, represent a significant survival gain in an 85-year-old with the same disease stage and whose life expectancy is limited to 6 years. Treatment gains and side effects should be carefully weighed against the individual's life expectancy *and* quality of life. How comorbidities affect life expectancy is also an integral part of the equation.[21,22]

Comorbidity and Cancer

Importance of Integrating Comorbidity and Cancer

Comorbidity is defined as the presence of more than one concomitant chronic health condition in an individual. Conditions, such as diabetes, hypertension, and/or other age-related conditions, such as limited self-reliance, dementia, malnutrition, or incontinence, represent a problem of significant magnitude while managing older patients. Eighty percent of individuals who are 65 and older have at least one comorbidity; 30% have three or four and 15% have seven or more such conditions.[20,21] Comorbidity and cancer interact intimately. On one hand, comorbidities affect cancer in multiple ways: They influence survival, independent of patients' age and/or tumor stage.[22,35] They compete with cancer as a cause of death and increase the risks of disability among cancer patients.[21,36] Their presence is often associated with the receipt of less definitive cancer therapy,[37] which in turn leads to poorer treatment outcomes.[12] On the other hand, cancer and its treatment modalities, even the adjunct ones, may affect preexisting morbidities. For example, steroids are potent antiemetics but they can wreak havoc on diabetic control. Similarly, erythropoietin is an effective treatment for cancer-related anemia, but it can worsen hypertension. This is especially true given that older patients are generally more susceptible to developing treatment-related side effects.[31] The concomitant management of comorbidities and cancer presents its own challenges, because primary and specialty care may not always be well coordinated. Patients themselves may not think that the continued management of other conditions is as important after a cancer diagnosis is established.

An important aspect of integrating comorbidities and cancer is the understanding of their impact on clinical trials in older cancer patients. Patients with severe organ dysfunction are often excluded from clinical trials, limiting the applicability of the trial results to such groups of patients. Comorbidities may also introduce a confounding bias in the results of cancer clinical trials.[38] The presence of multiple comorbidities may increase morbidity and mortality in any given trial, outweighing its projected benefits. Care should therefore be exercised in the extrapolation of trial outcomes to older cancer patients. The interaction of cancer and comorbidity can be better accounted for through patient stratification by severity and/or number of existing morbidities and/or balanced randomization.[38]

Sources of Comorbidity Data

Multiple sources could be exploited to collect comorbidity data and they should ideally be used in a complementary fashion: (1) medical records, (2) medical interviews, and (3) administrative datasets. The computerization of billing information has resulted in large databases, often coded using ICD-9-CM nomenclatures.

Note should be made that some comorbidities are often overlooked and therefore underrecorded in routine clinical practice. Depression and anxiety are classic examples of under-recognized morbidities.[39,40] Others include fatigue, malnutrition, pain, and/or anemia.

Comorbidity Indices

There are multiple tools to evaluate and score morbidities, each with different goals and outcomes.[22,25,27,41–45] Their description is outlined in Table 97.2. As stated earlier, there is no consensus on which tool is best adapted to routine clinical practice.[24,26]

Quantification of the Impact of Comorbidities on Cancer

This area has largely benefited from the work of Yancik et al.[21] Using an established model of high-, moderate-, and low-impact comorbidities,[46,47] the relationship between select comorbidities and increased mortality risk was examined in a cohort of colon cancer patients who were 55 years and older (Table 97.3).[21] Patients with five or more comorbidities were also found to have lower survival rates than those with four or fewer (Table 97.4). Other studies had also reached similar

TABLE 97.2. Commonly used comorbidity indices.

	Description	*Advantages*	*Disadvantages*
Charlson Index[25]	Provides an overall score based on a composite of values assigned to 19 comorbidity conditions; estimates risk of death from comorbid conditions	Shorter administration time than ICED Validated in breast cancer patients Derived from medical records	No measure of severity of comorbidity No functional evaluation Dichotomous
Satariano and Ragland[22,23]	Modified Charlson index providing survival estimates in breast cancer	Validated in breast cancer patients	No measure of severity of comorbidity No functional evaluation
Index of Co-Existing Diseases (ICED)[44]	Integrates measures of 10 functional areas, each divided into three levels of severity; chart-based review	Provides functional evaluation Provides an estimate of severity of disease	Average overall reliability (kappa, 0.5–0.6) and Index of Disease Severity subindex (kappa, 0.4–0.5)
Kaplan and Feinstein[43]	Assigns scores from 1 to 3 to comorbidity in various organ systems	Provides and estimate of severity of disease Validated in several cancers, including breast, prostate, and head and neck	No functional evaluation
Multidimensional Assessment of Cancer in the Elderly (MACE)[27]	Integrates measures of comorbidity, functional status, depression, balance, physical function and disability	Validated in cancer patients Provides a structured evaluation of functional status	Lengthy administration (27 ± 7 min)
Multiple Informants Analysis[42]	Combined scoring of the Charlson, ICED, PS and American Society of Anesthesiologists Index	Superior in estimating the overall effect of comorbidity than separate models that included only one index	Lengthy administration (average, 30 minutes[a])

[a] T. Lash, personal communication.

Source: Data from Charlson et al.,[25] Greenfield et al.,[44] Feinstein et al.,[41,43] Satariano et al.,[22,23] Monfardini et al.,[27] and Lash et al.[42]

conclusions in breast cancer patients, where those with an increasing number of comorbidities had a progressively lower relative risk of dying of their breast cancer compared to all other causes combined.[22]

Cancer Screening in Older Individuals

Cancer screening in older individuals comes with its own sets of problems and characteristics.[48] (1) The characteristics of a given screening test may change with age. For example, the sensitivity and specificity of mammography gradually increases with advancing age.[49] Similarly, the specificity of prostate-specific antigen (PSA) screening for prostate cancer decreases with age because of the increased prevalence of benign prostatic hyperplasia. (2) Tumors may have a different biology in older patients (e.g., slower growth rate),[50] leading to an increased detection of slowly growing tumors, known as *length–time bias*. (3) Older individuals have a shorter life expectancy compared to younger counterparts, by virtue of their advanced age or associated comorbidities. The detection of an asymptomatic tumor may not translate into a longer survival in the older individual, therefore questioning the rationale of screening at extremes of age. In general terms, the effect of screening is evident 3 to 5 years later, and the value of screening may be therefore limited in individuals with shorter life expectancy.[51,52] (4) This *overdetection* of clinically nonsignificant tumors may lead to treatments that adversely

TABLE 97.3. Relationship of overall survival to total comorbidity in a cohort of colon cancer patients.[a]

No. of comorbidities	*Risk ratio*	*95% confidence interval*
0–2	(Reference group)	
3	1.33	(0.98, 1.80)
4	0.96	(0.68, 1.36)
5–6	1.44	(1.10, 1.90)
7–14	1.85	(1.39, 2.46)

[a]Adjusted for age group, gender and colon cancer stage.

Source: From *Cancer* Vol. 82, 1998, pp. 2123–2134.[21] Copyright 1998 American Cancer Society. Reprinted by permission of Wiley-Liss, Inc., a subsidiary of John Wiley & Sons, Inc.

TABLE 97.4. Specific comorbidities and mortality risk ratio in a cohort of colon cancer patients.

Comorbidity	*Mortality risk ratio*	*95% confidence interval*
Liver disease	3.04	(1.74, 5.30)
Other serious comorbidity	2.33	(1.53, 3.55)
Alcohol abuse	2.20	(1.23, 3.93)
Deep vein thrombosis	2.06	(1.23, 3.47)
Renal failure	1.99	(1.21, 3.29)
COPD	1.67	(1.34, 2.08)
Depression	1.63	(1.12, 2.38)
Thyroid/glandular disease	1.49	(1.09, 2.03)
Heart disease (high-impact)	1.48	(1.21, 1.82)
Diabetes mellitus	1.37	(1.05, 1.79)
Anemia	1.25	(1.04, 1.51)

Source: Data from Yancik R, Wesley M, Ries L. Comorbidity and age as predictors of risk for early mortality in male and female colon cancer patients: A population-based study. Cancer 1998;82:2123–2134. Copyright 1998 American Cancer Society.

affect the quality of life of the older individual and may represent an unjustified healthcare cost to the community.[51]

Breast Cancer Screening in Older Individuals

Breast cancer remains the leading cancer by incidence in women in the United States. Annual incidence is expected to top 217,000 new cases in 2004, and 48,000 women are expected to die of their disease in the same time period, making breast cancer-specific mortality second only to lung cancer. Breast cancer screening is an attractive intervention in an attempt to reduce breast cancer mortality, but data are restricted to mammography.

Mammography

Mammography is considered the standard approach to breast cancer screening and is thought to reduce breast cancer mortality by 20% to 40% in women who are 50 to 70 years of age at the time of their first screening.[53–56] Fewer studies have, however, looked at the impact in women in the 70 or older age group. One retrospective, one case-control and two randomized clinical trials did include patients who were 70 years or older (Table 97.5). The case-control Dutch study suggested that screening mammography was associated with reduced breast cancer mortality in women who were 65 to 74 years of age [relative risk (RR), 0.34; 95% confidence interval (CI), 0.12–0.97], but not in women who were older than 75.[57] Similarly, the large retrospective SEER study showed that screening mammography reduces the relative risk of breast cancer mortality by about one-half.[58] In women who were at least 69 years of age, mammography screening in the 2 years preceding a diagnosis of breast cancer was also found to eliminate the age-related disparities in size and stage of the breast tumor at diagnosis.[59] The results of the two randomized trials were less conclusive, with a meta-analysis showing that the relative risk of breast cancer mortality is 0.94 (95% CI, 0.6–1.6) in women aged 70 to 75 years.[56] In addition to the reduction in breast cancer mortality, a retrospective cohort of more than 690,000 women aged 66 to 79 years, showed that screening mammography was associated with a decreased risk of detecting metastatic breast cancer (RR, 0.57; 95% CI, 0.45–0.72) and increased chances of detecting localized breast cancer (RR, 3.3; 95% CI, 3.1–3.5).

The U.S. Preventive Services Task Force analyzed the cost-effectiveness of continued screening after age 65. It was estimated that extending the biennial screening to age 75 or 80 years costs between $34,000 and $80,000 per life-year gained, compared to stopping the screening at age 65. This was thought to be a reasonable cost and that targeting healthy older women may be more cost-effective than extending screening to those with multiple competing causes of death.[60,61]

Overall, evidence-based data support screening mammograms at least until the age of 75. The absence of data in older women should not be interpreted that no such benefit exists, at least on an individual basis. It is the authors' opinion that mammograms should continue to be offered based on individual life expectancy and associated morbidities.

Screening for Colorectal Cancers

Fecal Occult Blood Testing

Three randomized controlled trials have previously demonstrated that annual or biennial fecal occult blood testing (FOBT) reduces colorectal cancer mortality in patients who are 50 to 80 years of age.[62–65] One prospective study followed 46,551 individuals for an average of 18 years and demonstrated that annual and biennial FOBT significantly also reduce the *incidence* of colorectal cancer (0.80 and 0.83 for annual and biennial screening, respectively).[66] *One-time* screening with FOBT and sigmoidoscopy still failed to detect 24% of colorectal cancer in 2,885 individuals who were 50 to 75 years of age.[67] There are no data on the value of screening in individuals who are older than 80 years. Similar to breast cancer patients reaching an extreme age, individualized decision should be made regarding screening based on life expectancy and existing comorbidities.

Endoscopy Screening

The value of endoscopy screening has been elegantly outlined elsewhere.[68,69] Two case-controlled trials showed that serial flexible sigmoidoscopies or colonoscopies are associated with reduced colorectal cancer mortality.[70,71] The value of colonoscopy over sigmoidoscopy in detecting advanced colorectal cancer has been demonstrated in the study of 3,121 patients with a mean age of 62.9 years, of whom 19% were older than 69. Patients with small (less than 10mm) or large (10mm or larger) distal adenomas were more likely to have a proximal colon cancer than those who did not have any distal lesion [odds ratio (OR), 2.6; 95% CI, 1.7–4.1 and OR, 3.4; 95% CI, 1.8–6.5, respectively].[72] Colonoscopy every 10 years is also more cost-effective than sigmoidoscopy every 5 years.[73]

Prostate Cancer Screening

Digital Rectal Examination (DRE)

Annual DRE has long been part of prostate cancer screening. It remains, however, operator dependent, and two prospective

TABLE 97.5. Mammography screening for breast cancer in the older population.

Study	*Design*	*Age of population screened (years)*	*Screening interval (number of examinations)*	*Risk ratio (RR) of breast cancer mortality*
Kopparberg	Randomized controlled	40–74	24–33 months (5–6)	0.64
Ostergotland	Randomized controlled	40–74	24–3 months (5–6)	0.74
Dutch	Case-control	70–75	—	0.58
SEER	Retrospective	≥70	≥10 months (0–2)	0.4

Source: Data from Nystrom et al.,[53] van Dijck et al.,[57] and McCarthy et al.[58]

TABLE 97.6. Age-related changes and increased surgical risks.

Organ system	*Physiologic and pathologic age-related changes*	*Surgical risks*
Cardiovascular	Increased atherosclerosis Increased risk of arrhythmias Decreased ventricular distensibility Increased dependence on pre-load	Increased sensitivity to fluid shifts Increased risk of cardiac ischemia Increased risk of congestive heart failure
Kidney	Decreased renal mass Decreased renal blood flow Decreased glomerular filtration rate (GFR)	Risks of acid–base balance disturbances Risk of electrolytes imbalance Increased sensitivity to renally cleared drugs Increased risk of renal ischemia
Liver	Decreased hepatic mass Decreased hepatic blood flow	Increased sensitivity to hepatically cleared drugs
Pulmonary	Decreased pulmonary volumes Decreased compliance Decreased ciliary function	Risk of postoperative atelectasis Risk of postoperative pneumonia
Central nervous system	Decreased cerebral mass Decreased cerebral blood flow Dementia	Difficulty obtaining informed consent Risk of postoperative delirium Slow postoperative recovery and prolonged hospitalization

studies have demonstrated its inferiority to annual PSA measurements.[74,75] No study has yet demonstrated that DRE reduces prostate cancer mortality.

Prostate-Specific Antigen (PSA)

Two randomized controlled trials have demonstrated the value of PSA in reducing prostate cancer mortality.[76,77] PSA is usually performed annually; however, less frequent screening may be as effective in select cases (every 5 years in men with PSA less than 1 ng/ml and every 2 years in men with PSA in the 1- to 2-ng/ml range). Ultrasound-guided prostate biopsy is recommended once PSA is higher than 4.0 ng/ml; however, this cutoff was demonstrated to miss an impressive 65% of prostate cancers in older individuals.[78] The use of the percentage of free PSA level was proposed as a means to increase the test specificity in men with benign prostatic hyperplasia.[79]

Specific Cancer Management Issues in the Older Population: Treatment Modalities

Older cancer patients benefit from the same treatment modalities widely used in the management of cancer, including surgery, radiation therapy, and chemotherapy. The following section highlights how these modalities are applied to older cancer patients. It is important to note, however, that treatment choices in older patients go beyond the mere age-associated physiologic and/or pathologic changes. Older patients often have a different outlook on life, caring more about their quality of life rather than longevity; how they opt for one therapeutic modality over the other has not been fully studied. Additionally, social and/or financial considerations may ultimately affect their choice. For example, lumpectomy followed by radiation therapy for breast cancer has yielded similar survival results as a more extensive mastectomy; however, older patients may still opt for mastectomy because it obviates the need for postoperative radiation therapy, which would requires additional logistic arrangements over several weeks.

Cancer Surgery in the Older Patient

Surgery is an integral part of a multimodality approach to the treatment of most cancers; its use is very frequently a prerequisite for treatment plans with a curative intent. Geriatric surgery has been the subject of excellent reviews elsewhere.[80–82] The following section highlights some of its most salient aspects.

Increased Operative Risks in Older Age

Age-related physiologic changes and accumulating comorbidities continue, however, to expose older patients to specific risks.[83–86] These changes involve all major organ systems, as summarized in Table 97.6. The mortality risks of a select number of surgical interventions in older patients are outlined in Table 97.7.

Preoperative Risk Assessment

Careful preoperative evaluation of older patients is a crucial step in estimating operative risk and planning interventions to reduce it to a minimum.[87] Controversy persists on how extensive preoperative risk assessments should be.[88–91] Of interest, several preoperative risk assessment scales consider age per se as a factor that increases the risks of an adverse

TABLE 97.7. Mortality from select surgical procedures in older patients.

Surgical procedure	*Average mortality risk (%)*
Breast cancer surgery[158]	0.5–1.5
Elective colorectal cancer surgery[159–161]	6–15
Emergent colorectal cancer surgery[160,161]	15–53.5
Gastric resection[162–164]	5–15
Liver resection (primary or secondary tumors)[165]	4
Pancreatic resection[175]	6

Source: Data from Busch et al.,[158] Hesterberg et al.,[159] Arnaud et al.,[160] Mulcahy et al.,[161] and Bonenkamp et al.[162] Viste et al.,[163] Tsujitani et al.,[164] Fong et al.[165]

cardiac event in noncardiac surgical interventions. For example, age greater than 70 years contributes 5 points to the Goldman index of cardiac risk in noncardiac surgical procedures.[92,93] Similarly, being 80 years of age or older automatically puts a patient in class II (of a possible V) in the American Society of Anesthesia (ASA) scale.[94] However, these scales remain heavily weighted by the presence or absence of comorbid conditions, rather than by age alone. For example, clinical evidence of congestive heart failure and a history of recent myocardial infarction contribute 11 and 10 points, respectively, to the Goldman index,[92] overshadowing the more limited contribution of age to the final score.

Reduction of Operative Risks

Multiple interventions have been advocated to reduce operative risks in older patients: these include (1) correction of reversible metabolic parameters,[95] (2) use of beta-blockers to reduce perioperative mortality from cardiac events,[87] (3) adequate blood pressure control,[87] (4) close monitoring of volume status using invasive pulmonary artery catheters,[96] although their benefit is contested,[97] and (5) most importantly, avoiding the delay in surgery that exposes the patient to higher risks of needing an emergent intervention[81] or a more extensive surgery secondary to tumor progression.

In conclusion, surgical risks related to aging are mostly related to coexisting morbidities, rather than to age by itself. Therefore, older patients should not be denied a chance at curative treatment based on their age alone.

Radiation Therapy in Older Cancer Patients

Similar to surgery, radiation therapy plays a central role in the treatment of older cancer patients, both as part of a multimodality approach and/or with a palliative intent.[98] There are no convincing data that tissue tolerance to radiation therapy is different in older than in younger patients. Most laboratory data were obtained in rapidly growing tissue cultures and apply only to acute radiation toxicity.[99] Tolerance of radiation therapy in older patients is modulated by existing comorbidities. Specifics of radiation treatment in older patients with breast, lung, gastrointestinal, and genitourinary cancers are beyond the scope of this chapter and have been extensively reviewed elsewhere.[100,101] Radiation therapy improves the quality of life in older patients and it has proven a special efficacy in controlling tumor-induced pain.[102–104] Social issues, such as transportation continue to pose a significant logistic and financial burden on those who have lost their physical and/or financial independence.

Chemotherapy in Older Cancer Patients

Chemotherapy is a mainstay treatment of many types of cancer. Two retrospective trials showed that chemotherapy toxicity does not differ between older and younger patients.[105,106] Results of these trials, however, should be carefully interpreted, because stringent exclusion criteria may preclude their generalization to the average older patient. The pharmacology of individual antineoplastic agents in older patients is extensively reviewed elsewhere.[107]

Every aspect of drug pharmacokinetics is potentially affected in older patients, in part, explaining why they have an increased rate of chemotherapy toxicity.

Absorption

Mucosal atrophy, decreased gastrointestinal motility, and splanchnic blood flow are all documented changes in older patients and can account for decreased absorption of drugs in the older population.[108] This limitation is especially important, given that an increasing number of new chemotherapeutic agents, such as capecitabine and imatinib, are orally administered.

Distribution

Several factors affect drug distribution in older patients: (1) decreased body water by about 20% in older patients leads to decreased volume of distribution of polar drugs, such as methotrexate and mitomycin-C; (2) plasma albumin is decreased by an average of 15% to 20% in older patients, leading an increase in the unbound fraction of protein-bound drugs, such as etoposide, anthracyclines, and taxanes[109]; (3) increased body fat leads to increased half-life and lower clearance of fat-soluble agents; (4) changes in the shape of the area under the curve (AUC), with water soluble drugs showing higher plasma concentrations and shorter half-lives, while fat-soluble drugs show lower plasma concentrations and prolonged half-lives, changes affecting both drug efficacy and toxicity profile; and (5) anemia can significantly increase the toxicity of red blood cell-bound drugs, such as taxanes and anthracyclines.

Hepatic Clearance

Decreased liver size and reduced hepatic blood flow both contribute to reduced clearance of hepatically cleared chemotherapeutic agents.[110] Several of the cytochrome P-450 enzyme activities decline with age, leaving the patient at risk of increased toxicity from delayed clearance.[111,112] Moreover, older patients are commonly subject to polypharmacy. CYP3A4 is inhibited by a large number of commonly prescribed drugs, leaving patients at risk for increased toxicity from CYP3A4-dependent chemotherapy agents, such as cyclophosphamide, ifosfamide, taxanes, tamoxifen, and vinca alkaloids.

Renal Clearance

Glomerular filtration rate (GFR) steadily decreases at the rate of 1 mL/year in individuals who are 40 years or older.[113] This decrease is not proportionally translated into an increased serum creatinine value because of the parallel reduction in muscle mass. Serum creatinine and estimates of creatinine clearance such as the Cockroft–Gault formula may therefore overestimate the renal GFR.[114] This in turn may result in increased serum levels and toxicity of any of the renally excreted agents. Doses of drugs, such as carboplatinum and bleomycin, should be reduced by 25% to 30% in moderate renal insufficiency (creatinine clearance of 10–30 mL/min), whereas the use of other agents, such as cisplatinum, methotrexate, and nitrosoureas should be completely avoided.

Prevention of Chemotherapy-Induced Toxicity in Older Patients

Neutropenia

Older patients are at a higher risk of hematopoietic toxicity because of limited hematopoietic reserves and decreased response to hematopoietic growth factors.[115] Older patients are more liable to develop clinically significant neutropenia, although this finding was contested by other studies.[106,116] Several trials have demonstrated the value of adding a granulocyte colony-stimulating factor (G-CSF) to moderately myelosuppressive chemotherapy regimens.[117–119] These trials serve as a sufficient basis for the regular use of G-CSF in older patients receiving such chemotherapy. Although G-CSF use is associated with reduced neutropenia and risk of sepsis, complete remissions and overall survival remain generally unchanged.[120]

Anemia

Anemia of chronic disease is a common complication of cancer and its various treatment modalities. Several studies have shown that anemia is an independent predictor of survival in older individuals.[121–123] Anemia significantly affects quality of life, with increased fatigue,[124] difficulty in concentration, impaired memory,[125] and increased susceptibility to complications from red blood cell-bound chemotherapy agents.[126] Synthetic erythropoietin use has been associated with relief of anemia of chronic disease and improved quality of life.[127] Newer agents, such as glycosylated erythropoietin, have a very long half-life that allows their administration on a bimonthly basis. Interestingly, concomitant G-CSF administration may augment erythropoietin efficacy in treating anemia in diseases, such as myelodysplastic syndromes.[128]

Mucositis and Diarrhea

Two reports have yielded contrasting results regarding the incidence of mucositis in older cancer patients, one arguing for an increased incidence, while the other stating that there was no age-associated differences in the incidence of gastrointestinal toxicities.[129,130]

Interventions to reduce oral mucositis include oral cryotherapy and careful oral hygiene. The use of G-CSF is associated with reduced mucosal ulcerations, presumably through its effect in increasing salivary neutrophils.

Although this section discussed the physical brunt of various treatment modalities, older cancer patients are further confronted with complex psychosocial and social functioning challenges, which are detailed in the following section.

Psychosocial Issues in Older Cancer Patients

Psychologic Issues in Older Cancer Patients

Forty-seven percent of cancer patients suffer from a form of psychiatric disorder. The majority of these (32%) present with adjustment disorder, while the remainder is divided between major depressive disorder (6%), mood disorder secondary to medical conditions (4%), personality disorders (3%), and anxiety (2%).[131]

Older cancer patients suffer less from depression and psychosocial distress compared to their younger counterparts.[132] These findings remain true even after adjusting for physical impairment and symptoms severity.[133] It is unclear, however, whether these are related to better adaptation and fewer psychologic needs in older adults or whether they result from underreporting of depressive symptoms in this age group.[134,135]

Social Isolation

Psychiatric disorders, physical impairment, and social isolation are often intricately related[136–138]; all three can feed into each other, leading the patient into a downward-spiraling path. For example, 48% and 49% of older cancer patients have difficulty with at least one activity of daily living (ADL) and one instrumental activity of daily living (IADL), respectively.[139] Additionally, more than 33 million of the 65+ population live below the poverty line.[140] These factors increase patients' *need* for social support. Unfortunately, the same factors *predispose* to social isolation. This dual relationship makes older cancer patients particularly vulnerable. The recognition of such an interaction is key in managing older cancer patients because social isolation is associated with an increased mortality in this population (age-adjusted relative risk of death = 2.3 in men and 2.8 in women).[141] This was found to be independent of self-reported physical health, socioeconomic status, and associated morbidities.

Evaluation of Psychosocial Needs in Older Cancer Patients

This is an integral part of the initial Geriatric Oncology evaluation. A number of self-administered tools can be routinely implemented, even in a busy practice. Several dimensions are typically assessed:

1. *Emotional needs:* Several tools can be used to evaluate depression in older patients. The self-administered Beck Depression Inventory is a simple screening tool that can be routinely used as part of the initial Geriatric Oncology evaluation.[142] More extensive testing includes the Hamilton Depression Rating Scale (HAM-D), Geriatric Depression Scale (GDS), and Inventory for Depressive Symptomatology (IDS).[143–145]
2. *Cognitive impairment:* The incidence and prevalence of cognitive impairment increases with advancing age and significantly complicates several aspects of cancer management, not the least of which are building the direct doctor–patient relationship and issues pertaining to informed consent. The Modified Mini-Mental State Examination (MMMSE) is a simple test that translates patient-specific performance into age-matched percentile.[146,147]
3. *Comorbid conditions*: These have been discussed in detail earlier. Their functional impact can be assessed using the Activities of Daily Living (ADL) and Instrumental Activities of Daily Living (IADL) tools.[148]
4. *Other issues*, such as stressful life events, the presence of a structured social support, and economic resources, should be tactfully probed.

Management of Psychosocial Distress in Older Cancer Patients

Complexly ill older cancer patients—those with multiple comorbidities, cognitive and functional impairments, and psychosocial needs—can benefit from involvement of geriatricians and their interdisciplinary teams. Patients with major depression, a history of major psychiatric disorders earlier in life, and/or those with depression and dementia can also benefit from the involvement of a geropsychiatric team. However, even less complexly ill patients are likely to need comprehensive psychosocial support as they progress from diagnosis, to treatment, and on to posttreatment management. As no one resource can single-handedly provide this, it represents one of the strongest arguments for developing a "case management" approach that incorporates geriatric oncologists, specialized geriatric oncology nurses, and social workers.

1. *Symptoms management*: Particular attention should be devoted to this issue, whether the symptoms are cancer or treatment related. Pain control, management of nausea, vomiting, mucositis, anemia, malnutrition, and other potential side effects are all key components that have been extensively addressed elsewhere.[149] This care results not only in improved quality of life but also in improved physical function.
2. *Patient–doctor communication*: Caring for older cancer patients is inherently more time-consuming than for younger ones. Older patients cannot—and should not—be rushed. Physicians' interpersonal skills are associated with better psychologic adjustment in cancer patients.[150,151] Ideally, geriatric oncology clinics should be places where pace is dictated by patients rather than by scheduling constraints. Medicare and other insurers are pressed to recognize the management of cancer in the older population as a highly complex encounter.
3. *Counseling*: Patient-tailored services and coordination of existing support structures by a social worker or other professional case manager can be particularly helpful. For example, such interventions have been shown to reduce depression in older cancer patients and improve psychologic adaptation to cancer.[152,153]
4. *Psychologic support:* Psychotherapy, provided by a social worker, psychologist, psychiatrist, and/or other mental health professionals, should be routinely offered to older cancer patients. This is especially true in view of the older patients' tendency to stoicism and underreporting their symptoms. Nonetheless, many older adults are reluctant to use such services, recalling the stigmatization associated with such services earlier in their lives. In such instances, the care team will need to provide such care as best as possible, including psychotropic medication management. Several volunteer and professional organizations that provide cancer support groups in many areas of the United States may be particularly helpful in these instances.[154]

Future Considerations and Research Venues

Geriatric oncology is a field in full expansion. Integrated research agendas are needed to challenge the limitations of the single-specialty approach to the complex problem of aging.[155] A comprehensive research map of aging and cancer has been elegantly outlined in the National Cancer Institute/National Institute on Aging common workshop, and includes the study of the biology of aging and cancer, patterns of care, risk assessment and cancer prevention, palliative care, psychologic issues, and pain relief.[156] The study of the intricate relationship between comorbidity and cancer deserves special attention.[157] This research will benefit the growing number of older cancer patients in America and the world.

References

1. Smith D. Changing causes of death of elderly people in the United States, 1950–1990. Gerontology 1998;44:331–335.
2. Ries L, Kosary C, Hankey B. SEER Cancer Statistics Review, 1973–1996. Bethesda, MD: National Cancer Institute, 1999.
3. Miller B, Ries L, Hankey B, et al. Cancer Statistics Review 1973–1989. Bethesda, MD: National Cancer Institute, 1992.
4. Ries L, Eisner M, Kosary C, et al. Surveillance, Epidemiology and End Results (SEER) Cancer Statistics Review 1975–2000. Bethesda, MD: National Cancer Institute, 2003. Available from: URL: http://seer.cancer.gov/csr/1975_2000
5. Kennedy B, Bushhouse S, Benber A. Minnesota population cancer risks. Cancer (Phila) 1994;73:724–729.
6. Mettlin C. New evidence of progress in the National Cancer Program. Cancer (Phila) 1996;78:2043–2044.
7. Levi F, Vecchia CL, Lucchini F, et al. Worldwide trends in cancer mortality in the elderly, 1955–1992. Eur J Cancer 1996;32A: 652–672.
8. Vecchia CL, Levi F, Lucchini F, et al. International perspectives of cancer and aging. In: Ershler WB (ed) Comprehensive Geriatric Oncology. Amsterdam: Harwood, 1998:19–93.
9. Sargent D, Goldberg R, Jacobson S, et al. A pooled analysis of adjuvant chemotherapy for resected colon cancer in elderly patients. N Engl J Med 2001;345:1091–1097.
10. Schild S, Stella P, Geyer S, et al. The outcome of combined-modality therapy for stage III non-small cell lung cancer in the elderly. J Clin Oncol 2003;21:3201–3206.
11. Silliman RA. What constitutes optimal care for older women with breast cancer? J Clin Oncol 2003;21:3554–3556.
12. Bouchardy C, Rapiti E, Fioretta G, et al. Undertreatment strongly decreases prognosis of breast cancer in elderly women. J Clin Oncol 2003;21:3580–3587.
13. Yee K, Pater J, Pho L, et al. Enrollment of older patients in cancer treatment trials in Canada: why is age a barrier? J Clin Oncol 2003;21:1618–1623.
14. Hutchins L, Unger J, Crowley J, et al. Underrepresentation of patients 65 years of age or older in cancer-treatment trials. N Eng J Med 1999;341:2061–2067.
15. Monfardini S, Sorio R, Boes G, et al. Entry and evaluation of elderly patients in European Organization for Research and Treatment of Cancer (EORTC) new drug development studies. Cancer (Phila) 1995;76:333–338.
16. Lewis JH, Kilgore ML, Goldman DP, et al. Participation of patients 65 years of age or older in cancer clinical trials. J Clin Oncol 2003;21:1383–1389.
17. United States life tables, 2000. Natl Vital Stat Rep 2002;51:1–38.
18. Record high life expectancy. Stat Bull Metrop Insur Co 1993;74: 28–35.
19. Moroff S, Pauker S. What to do when the patient outlives the literature, or DEALE-ing with a full deck. Med Decision Making 1983;3:313–338.
20. Fried L, Wallace R. The complexity of chronic illness in the elderly: from clinic to community. In: Wallace R, Woolson R (eds) The Epidemiologic Study of the Elderly. New York: Oxford University Press, 1992:10–19.

21. Yancik R, Wesley M, Ries L. Comorbidity and age as predictors of risk for early mortality in male and female colon cancer patients: a population-based study. Cancer (Phila) 1998;82: 2123–2134.
22. Satariano W, Ragland D. The effect of comorbidity on 3-year survival of women with primary breast cancer. Ann Intern Med 1994;120:104–110.
23. Satariano W. Comorbidities and cancer. In: Muss HB (ed) Cancer in the Elderly. New York: Dekker, 2000:477–499.
24. Mandeblatt J, Bierman A, Gold K, et al. Constructs of burden of illness in older patients with breast cancer: a comparison of measurement methods. Health Serv Res 2001;36:1085–1107.
25. Charlson M, Pompei P, Ales K, et al. A new method of classifying prognostic comorbidity in longitudinal studies: development and validation. J Chronic Dis 1987;40:373–383.
26. Wang P, Walker A, Tsuang M, et al. Strategies for improving comorbidity measures based on Medicare and Medicaid claims data. J Clin Epidemiol 2000;53:571–578.
27. Monfardini S, Ferrucci L, Fratino L, et al. Validation of a multidimensional evaluation scale for use in elderly cancer patients. Cancer (Phila) 1996;77:395–401.
28. Reuben D. Principles of geriatric assessment. In: Tinetti M (ed) Principles of Geriatric Medicine and Gerontology. New York: McGraw-Hill, 2003:99–110.
29. Balducci L, Yates J. General guidelines for the management of older patients with cancer. Oncology (Huntingt) 2000;14: 221–227.
30. Moore AA, Siu AL. Screening for common problems in ambulatory elderly: clinical confirmation of a screening instrument [see comment]. Am J Med 1996;100:438–443.
31. Chen H, Cantor A, Meyer J, et al. Can older cancer patients tolerate chemotherapy? A prospective pilot study. Cancer (Phila) 2003;97:1107–1114.
32. Greenblatt D, Sellers E, Shader R. Drug therapy: drug disposition in old age. New Engl J Med 1982;306:1018–1028.
33. Shaw P. Common pitfalls in geriatric drug prescribing. Drugs 1982;23:324–328.
34. Beers M, Ouslander J. Risk factors in geriatric drug prescribing: a practical guide to avoid problems. Drugs 1989;37:105–112.
35. West D, Satariano W, Ragland D. Comorbidity and breast cancer survival: a comparison between black and white women. Ann Intern Med 1996:413–419.
36. Fleming S, Rastogi A, Dmitrienko A, Johnson KD. A comprehensive prognostic index to predict survival based on multiple comorbidities: a focus on breast cancer. Med Care 1999;37(6): 601–614.
37. Yancik R, Wesley M, Ries M, et al. Effect of age and comorbidity in postmenopausal breast cancer patients aged 55 years and older. JAMA 2001;285:885–892.
38. Schneeweiss S, Maclure M. Use of comorbidity scores for the control of confounding in studies using administrative databases. Int J Epidemiol 2000;29:891–898.
39. Small GW. Recognizing and treating anxiety in the elderly. J Clin Psychiatry 1997;58:41–47.
40. Osborn DP, Fletcher AE, Smeeth L, et al. Factors associated with depression in a representative sample of 14 217 people aged 75 and over in the United Kingdom: results from the MRC trial of assessment and management of older people in the community. Int J Geriatr Psychiatry 2003;18:623–630.
41. Feinstein A. The pre-therapeutic classification of comorbidity in chronic diseases. J Chronic Dis 1970;23:455–469.
42. Lash T, Thwin S, Horton N, et al. Multiple informants: a new method to assess comorbidity in breast cancer patients. Am J Epidemiol 2003;157:249–257.
43. Kaplan M, Feinstein A. The importance of classifying initial comorbidity in evaluating the outcome of diabetes mellitus. J Chronic Dis 1974;27:387–404.
44. Greenfield S, Blanco D, Elashoff R, et al. Patterns of care related to age of breast cancer patients. JAMA 1987;257:2766–2770.
45. Bennett C, Greenfield S, Aronow H, et al. Patterns of care related to age of men with prostate cancer. Cancer (Phila) 1991;67: 2633–2441.
46. Ienozzi L, Ash A, Coffman G, et al. Predicting in-hospital mortality: a comparison of severity measurement approaches. Med Care 1992;30:347–359.
47. Ienozzi L, Moskowitz M. A clinical assessment of Medis-Groups. JAMA 1988;260:3159–3163.
48. Lyman G. Decision analysis: a way of thinking about health care in the elderly. In: Ershler WB (ed) Geriatric Oncology. Philadelphia: Lippincott, 1992:5–14.
49. Carney P, Miglioretti D, Yankaskas B, et al. Individual and combined effects of age, breast density, and hormone replacement therapy use on the accuracy of screening mammography. Ann Intern Med 2003;138:168–175.
50. Diab S, Elledge R, Clark G. Tumor characteristics and clinical outcome of elderly women with breast cancer. J Natl Cancer Inst 2000;92:550–556.
51. Walter L, Covinsky K. Cancer screening in the elderly patients. A framework for individualized decision making. JAMA 2001; 285:2750–2756.
52. Law M. Screening without evidence of efficacy [see comment]. BMJ 2004;328:301–302.
53. Nystrom L, Rutqvist L, Wall S, et al. Breast cancer screening with mammography: overview of Swedish randomized trials. Lancet 1993;341:973–978.
54. Olsen O, Gotzsche P. Cochrane review on screening for breast cancer with mammography. Lancet 2001;358:1340–1342.
55. Duffy S, Tabar L, Chen H-H, et al. The impact of organized mammography service screening on breast carcinoma mortality in seven Swedish counties: a collaborative evaluation. Cancer (Phila) 2002;95:458–469.
56. Kerlikowske K, Grady D, Rubin S, et al. Efficacy of screening mammography: a meta-analysis. JAMA 1995;273:149–154.
57. van Dijck J, Holland R, Verbeek A, et al. Efficacy of mammographic screening of the elderly: a case-referent study in the Nijmegen program in The Netherlands. J Natl Cancer Inst 1994;86:934–938.
58. McCarthy E, Burns R, Freund K, et al. Mammography use, breast cancer stage at diagnosis and survival among older women. J Am Geriatr Soc 2000;48:1226–1233.
59. Randolph W, Goodwin J, Mahnken J, et al. Regular mammography use is associated with elimination of age-related disparities in size and stage of breast cancer at diagnosis. Ann Intern Med 2002;137:783–790.
60. Mandelblatt J, Saha S, Teutsch S, et al. The cost-effectiveness of screening mammography beyond age 65 years: a systematic review for the U.S. Preventive Service Task Force. Ann Intern Med 2003;139:835–842.
61. Zappa M, Visioli C, Ciatto S. Mammography screening in elderly women: efficacy and cost-effectiveness. Crit Rev Oncol Hematol 2002;46:235–239.
62. Mandel J, Bond J, Church T. Reducing mortality from colorectal cancer by screening for fecal occult blood. N Engl J Med 1993; 328:1365–1371.
63. Hardcastle J, Chamberlain J, Robinson M, et al. Randomised controlled trial of faecal-occult-blood screening for colorectal cancer. Lancet 1996;348:1472–1477.
64. Kronborg O, Fenger C, Olsen J, et al. Randomized study of screening for colorectal cancer with faecal-occult-blood test. Lancet 1996;348:1467–1471.
65. Mandel J, Church T, Ederer F, et al. Colorectal cancer mortality: effectiveness of biennial screening for fecal occult blood. J Natl Cancer Inst 1999;91:434–437.

66. Mandel JS, Church TR, Bond JH, et al. The effect of fecal occult-blood screening on the incidence of colorectal cancer. N Engl J Med 2000;343:1603–1607.
67. Lieberman DA, Harford WV, Ahnen DJ, et al. One-time screening for colorectal cancer with combined fecal occult-blood testing and examination of the distal colon. N Engl J Med 2001;345:555–560.
68. Winawer S, Fletcher R, Miller L, et al. Colorectal cancer screening: clinical guidelines and rationale. Gastroenterology 1997; 112:594–642.
69. Ransohoff DF, Sandler RS. Screening for colorectal cancer. N Engl J Med 2002;346:40–44.
70. Selby J, Friedman G, Queensburry C, et al. A case-controlled study of screening sigmoidoscopy and mortality from colorectal cancer. N Engl J Med 1992;326:653–657.
71. Muller A, Sonnenberg A. Protection by endoscopy against death from colorectal cancer: a case-control study among veterans. Arch Intern Med 1995;155:1741–1748.
72. Lieberman DA, Weiss DG, Bond JH, et al. Use of colonoscopy to screen asymptomatic adults for colorectal cancer. N Engl J Med 2000;343:162–168.
73. Sonnenberg A, Delco F, Inadomi J, et al. Cost-effectiveness of colonoscopy screening for colorectal cancer. Ann Intern Med 2000;133:573–584.
74. Crawford E, Leewansangtong S, Goktas S, et al. Efficiency of prostate specific antigen and digital rectal examination in screening using 4.0ng/ml and age-specific reference range as cut-off for abnormal values. Prostate 1999;38:296–302.
75. Schroder F, Maas P, Beemsterboer P, et al. Evaluation of the digital rectal examination as a screening test for prostate cancer: Rotterdam section of the European Randomized Study of Screening for Prostate Cancer. J Natl Cancer Inst 1998; 1998:1817–1823.
76. Labrie F, Candas B, Dupont A, et al. Screening decreases prostate cancer death: first analysis of the Quebec randomized controlled trial. Prostate 1999;38:83–91.
77. Horninger W, Reisigl A, Rogatsch H, et al. Prostate cancer screening in Tyrol, Austria: experience and results. Eur J Cancer 2000;2000:1322–1335.
78. Punglia RS, D'Amico AV, Catalona WJ, et al. Effect of verification bias on screening for prostate cancer by measurement of prostate-specific antigen. N Engl J Med 2003;349:335–342.
79. Catalona W, Partin A, Slawin K, et al. Use of percentage of free prostate-specific antigen to enhance differentiation of prostate cancer from benign prostatic disease: A prospective multicenter clinical trial. JAMA 1998;279:1542–1547.
80. In: Katlic MR (ed) Principles and Practice of Geriatric Surgery. New York: Springer-Verlag, 2001:1098.
81. Pofahl WE, Pories WJ. Current status and future directions of geriatric general surgery. J Am Geriatr Soc 2003;51:S351–S354.
82. Devereaux E, Kemeny M. Surgery in the elderly oncology patient. In: Muss HB (ed) Cancer in the Elderly. New York: Dekker, 2000:153–186.
83. Evans B, Townsend C, Thompson J. Organ physiology of aging. Surg Clin N Am 1994;74:23–29.
84. Wynne H, Cope L, Mutch E, et al. The effect of aging upon liver volume and apparent liver blood flow in healthy men. Hepatology 1989;1989:297–301.
85. Mooney H, Roberts R, Cooksley W, et al. Alterations in the liver with ageing. Clin Gastroenterol 1985;14:757–771.
86. Rocca R. Psychosocial aspects of surgical care in the elderly patient. Surg Clin N Am 1994;74:223–243.
87. Fleisher L, Eagle K. Lowering cardiac risk in non-cardiac surgery. N Engl J Med 2001;345:1677–1682.
88. Marcello P, Roberts P. "Routine" preoperative studies: which studies in which patients? Surg Clin N Am 1996;76:11–23.
89. Velanovich V. Preoperative laboratory evaluation. J Am Coll Surg 1996;183:79–87.
90. Kaplan E, Sheiner L, Boeckmann A, et al. The usefulness of preoperative laboratory screening. JAMA 1985;253:3576–3581.
91. Roizen M, Kaplan E, Schreider B, et al. The relative roles of the history and physical examination, and laboratory testing in preoperative evaluation for outpatient surgery: the "Starling" curve of preoperative laboratory testing. Anesthesiol Clin N Am 1987;5:15.
92. Goldman L, Caldera D, Nussbaum S. Multifactorial index of cardiac risk in noncardiac surgical procedures. N Engl J Med 1977;297:845–850.
93. Goldman L. Cardiac risks and complications of noncardiac surgery. Ann Intern Med 1983;98:504–513.
94. Owens W, Felts J Jr. ASA physical status classifications: a study of consistency of ratings. Anesthesiology 1978;49:239–243.
95. Evans T. Hemodynamic and metabolic therapy in critically ill patients. N Engl J Med 2001;345:1417–1418.
96. Cooper A, Doig G, Sibbald W. Pulmonary artery catheters in the critically ill: an overview using the methodology of evidence-based medicine. Crit Care Clin 1996;12:777–794.
97. Sandman J, Hull R, Brant R, et al. A randomized, controlled trial of the use of pulmonary-artery catheters in high-risk surgical patients. N Engl J Med 2003;348:5–14.
98. Tobias J. Clinical practice of radiotherapy. Lancet 1992;339: 159–163.
99. Sargent E, Burns F. Repair of radiation-induced DNA damage in rat epidermis as function of age. Radiat Res 1985;102:176–181.
100. Scalliet P, Pignon T. Radiotherapy in the elderly. In: Ershler WB (ed) Comprehensive Geriatric Oncology. Amsterdam: Harwood, 2000:421–427.
101. Mundt A. Radiation therapy and the elderly. In: Muss HB (ed) Cancer in the Elderly. New York: Dekker, 2000:187–216.
102. Isenring E, Bauer J, Capra S. The scored Patient-generated Subjective Global Assessment (PG-SGA) and its association with quality of life in ambulatory patients receiving radiotherapy. Eur J Clin Nutr 2003;57:305–309.
103. Nag S, Ellis RJ, Merrick GS, et al. American Brachytherapy Society recommendations for reporting morbidity after prostate brachytherapy. Int J Radiat Oncol Biol Phys 2002;54:462–470.
104. Janda M, Johnson D, Woelfl H, et al. Measurement of quality of life in head and neck cancer patients utilizing the quality of life radiation therapy questionnaire. Strahlenther Onkol 2002;178: 153–158.
105. Berg C, Carbone P. Clinical trials and drug toxicity in the elderly: the experience of the Eastern Cooperative Oncology Group. Cancer (Phila) 1983;52:1986–1992.
106. Christman K, Muss H, Case L, et al. Chemotherapy of metastatic breast cancer in the elderly: the Piedmont Oncology Association experience. JAMA 1992;268:57–62.
107. Lichtman S, Skirvin J, Vemulapalli S. Pharmacology of antineoplastic agents in older cancer patients. Clin Rev Oncol Hematol 2003;46:101–114.
108. Yuen G. Altered pharmacokinetics in the elderly. Clin Geriatr Med 1990;6:257–267.
109. Wallace S, Whiting B. Factors affecting drug binding in plasma of elderly patients. Br J Clin Pharmacol 1976;3:327–330.
110. Woodhouse K, Wynne H. Age-related changes in liver size and hepatic blood flow: the influence on drug metabolism in the elderly. Clin Pharmacokinet 1998;15:287–294.
111. Soteniemi E, Arranto A, Pelkonen O, et al. Age and cytochrome P450-linked drug metabolism in humans: an analysis of 226 subjects with equal histopathologic conditions. Clin Pharmacol Ther 1997;61:331–339.
112. Vestal R. Aging and pharmacology. Cancer (Phila) 1997;80: 1302–1310.
113. Lindeman R, Tobin J, Shock N, et al. Longitudinal studies on the rate of decline in renal function with age. J Am Geriatr Soc 1985;33:278–285.

114. Cockroft D, Gault M. Prediction of creatinine clearance from serum creatinine. Nephron 1976;16:31–42.
115. Lipschitz D. Age-related declines in hematopoietic reserve capacity. Semin Oncol 1995;22(suppl):3–5.
116. Ibrahim N, Frye D, Buzdar A, et al. Doxorubicin-based chemotherapy in elderly patients with metastatic breast cancer: tolerance and outcome. Arch Intern Med 1996;156:882–888.
117. Fisher R, Graynor E, Dahlberg S, et al. Comparison of a standard regimen (CHOP) with three intensive chemotherapy regimens for advanced non-Hodgkin's lymphoma. N Engl J Med 1993; 328:1002–1006.
118. Lyman G, Kuderer D, Djulbegovic B. Prophylactic granulocyte colony-stimulating factors in patients receiving dose-intensive cancer chemotherapy: a meta-analysis. Am J Med 2002;112: 406–411.
119. Balducci L, Lyman G. Patients aged ≥70 are at high risk for neutropenic infection and should receive hematopoietic growth factors when treated with moderately toxic chemotherapy. J Clin Oncol 2001;19:1583–1585.
120. Ozer H, Armitage J, Bennett C, et al. 2000 Update of recommendations for the use of hematopoietic colony-stimulating factors: evidence-based, clinical practice guidelines. J Clin Oncol 2000;18:3558–3585.
121. Chavez P, Volpato S, Fried L. Challenging the World Health Organization criteria for anemia in older women. J Am Geriatr Soc 2001;49(suppl 3):10.
122. Izaks G, Westendorp R, Knoot D. The definition of anemia in older persons. JAMA 1999;281:1714–1717.
123. Kikuchi M, Inagaki T, Shinagawa N. Five-year survival of older people with anemia: variation with hemoglobin concentration. J Am Geriatr Soc 2001;49:1226–1228.
124. Gutstein H. The biologic basis of fatigue. Cancer (Phila) 2001; 92(suppl):1678–1683.
125. Nissenson A. Epoetin and cognitive function. Am J Kidney Dis 1992;20(suppl):21–24.
126. Shrijvers D, Highley M, Bruyn ED, et al. Role of red blood cells in pharmacokinetics of chemotherapeutic agents. Anticancer Drugs 1999;10:147–153.
127. Rizzo J, Lichtin A, Woolf S, et al. Use of epoetin in patients with cancer: evidence-based clinical practice guidelines of the American Society of Clinical Oncology and the American Society of Hematology. J Clin Oncol 2002;19:4083–4107.
128. Hellstrom-Lindberg E, Ahlgren T, Begguin Y, et al. Treatment of the anemia of myelodysplastic syndromes with G-CSF plus erythoropoietin: results of a randomized phase II study and long-term follow-up of 71 patients. Blood 1998;92:68–75.
129. Popescu R, Norman A, Ross P, et al. Adjuvant or palliative chemotherapy for colorectal cancer in patients 70 years or older. J Clin Oncol 1999;17:2412–2418.
130. Sargent D, Goldberg R, MacDonald J, et al. Adjuvant chemotherapy for colon cancer (CC) is beneficial without significant incrased toxicity in elderly patients: results from 3351 Pt meta-analysis. Proc Am Soc Clin Oncol 2000;19:241a (abstract 933).
131. Derogatis L. The prevalence of psychiatric disorders among patients with cancer. JAMA 1983;249:751–757.
132. Sanson-Fisher R, Girgis A, Boyes A, et al. Supportive Care Review Group. The unmet supportive care needs of patients with cancer. Cancer (Phila) 2000;88:225–236.
133. Mor V, Allen S, Malin M. The psychological impact of cancer on older versus younger patients. Cancer (Phila) 1994;74:2118–2127.
134. Lyness J, Cox C, Curry J, et al. Older age and the underreporting of depressive symptoms. J Am Geriatr Soc 1995;43:216–221.
135. Cassileth B, Lusk E, Strouse T, et al. Psychological status in chronic illness: a comparative analysis of six diagnostic groups. N Engl J Med 1984;311:506–511.
136. Willey C, Silliman R. The impact of disease on social support experiences of patients with cancer. J Psychol Oncol 1990;8: 79–95.
137. Goodwin J, Hunt W, Samet J. A population-based study of functional status and social support networks of elderly patients newly diagnosed with cancer. Arch Intern Med 1991;151: 366–370.
138. Kurtz M, Kurtz J, Stommel M, et al. The influence of symptoms, age, comorbidity and cancer site on physical functioning and mental health in geriatric women patients. Women Health 1999;29:1–12.
139. Stafford R, Cyr P. The impact of cancer on the physical function of the elderly and their utilization of health care. Cancer (Phila) 1980;80:1973–1980.
140. Dalaker J. People 65 years and over by ratio of income to poverty and state: 1999–2001 averages. U.S. Government Printing Office, 2003. Available from: URL: http://www.census.gov/hhes/poverty/65+inctopov.html
141. Berkman L, Syme S. Social networks, host resistance and mortality: a nine-year follow-up study of Alameda County residents. Am J Epidemiol 1979;109:186–204.
142. Beck A, Ward C, Mendelson M. An inventory for measuring depression. Arch Gen Psychiatry 1961;4:561–571.
143. Hamilton M. The development of a rating scale for primary depressive illness. Br J Soc Clin Psychol 1967;6:278–296.
144. Rush A, Giles D, Schlesser M. The Inventory for Depressive Symptomatology (IDS): preliminary findings. Psychiatry Res 1986;18:65–87.
145. Sheikh J, Yesavage J. Geriatric Depression Scale [GDS]: recent evidence and development of a shorter version. In: Brink TL (ed) Clinical Gerontology: A Guide to Assessment and Intervention. New York: Haworth Press, 1986:165.
146. Folstein M, Folstein S, McHugh P. "Mini-mental state." A practical method for grading the cognitive state of patients for the clinician. J Psychiatr Res 1875;12:189–198.
147. Crum R, Anthony J, Bassett S, et al. Population-based norms for the Mini-Mental State Examination by age and educational level. JAMA 1993;269:2386–2391.
148. Crooks V, Waller S, Smith T, et al. The use of the Karnofsky Performance Scale in determining outcomes and risks in geriatric outpatients. J Gerontol 1991;46:M139–M144.
149. Optimizing cancer care: the importance of symptom management. In: von Gunten CF (ed) ASCO Curriculum, vol I. Dubuque, IA: Kendall/Hunt, 2003.
150. Roberts C, Cox C, Reintgen D, et al. Influence of physician communication on newly diagnosed breast cancer patients' psychological adjustment and decision making. Cancer (Phila) 1994; 74:157–164.
151. Eide H, Graugaard P, Holgersen K, et al. Physician communication in different phases of a consultation at an oncology outpatient clinic related to patient satisfaction. Patient Educ Counsel 2003;51:259–266.
152. Hann D, Oxman T, Ahles T, et al. Social support adequacy and depression in older patients with metastatic cancer. Psycho-Oncology 1995;4:213–221.
153. Northouse L. Social support in patients' and husbands' adjustment to breast cancer. Nurs Res 1988;37:91–95.
154. Spiegel D, Bloom J, Krawmer H, et al. Effect of psychosocial treatment on survival of patients with metastatic breast cancer. Lancet 1989;2:888–891.
155. Callahan C, McHorney C, Mulrow C, et al. Determinants of successful aging: Developing an integrated research agenda for the 21st century. Ann Intern Med 2003;139(suppl):389–462.
156. Exploring the role of cancer centers for integrating aging and cancer research. Workshop report. Bethesda, MD: National Institute on Aging and National Cancer Institute, June 13–15, 2001: 36–40.

157. Yancik R, Ganz P, Varricchio C, et al. Perspectives on comorbidity and cancer in older patients: approaches to expand the knowledge base. J Clin Oncol 2001;19:1147–1115.
158. Busch E, Kemeny M, Fremgen A, et al. Patterns of breast cancer care in the elderly. Cancer (Phila) 1996;78:101–111.
159. Hesterberg R, Schmidt W, Ohmann C, et al. Risk of elective surgery in colorectal carcinoma in the elderly. Dig Surg 1991; 8:2–27.
160. Arnaud J, Schloegel M, Ollier J. Colorectal cancer in patients over 80 years of age. Dis Colon Rectum 1991;34:896–898.
161. Mulcahy H, Patchett S, Daly L, et al. Prognosis of patients with large bowel cancer. Br J Surg 1994;81:736–738.
162. Bonenkamp J, Songun I, Hermans J, et al. Randomized comparison of morbidity after D1 and D2 dissection for gastric cancer in 996 Dutch patients. Lancet 1995;345:745–748.
163. Viste A, Haugstvedt T, Eide G, et al. Postoperative complications and mortality after surgery for gastric cancer. Ann Surg 1998; 207:7–13.
164. Tsujitani S, Katano K, Oka A, et al. Limited operation for gastric cancer in the elderly. Br J Surg 1996;83:836–839.
165. Fong Y, Blumgart L, Fortner J, et al. Pancreatic or liver resection is safe and effective in the elderly. Ann Surg 1995;222:426–434.

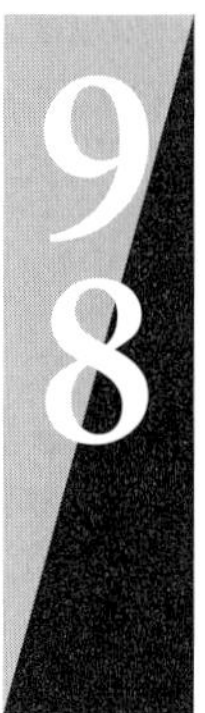

Chemotherapy in Patients with Organ Dysfunction

John L. Marshall, Jimmy Hwang, Shakun Malik, and Asim Amin

Clinical studies of chemotherapy, or other antineoplastic therapies, are usually conducted in physiologically otherwise normal patients with cancer. As a result, limited information is typically available about the optimal dosage and schedule of chemotherapy for patients with organ dysfunction and the impact of chemotherapy in such patients. This is a potentially important problem, because most chemotherapies, as with other pharmacologic agents, are metabolized by the liver or kidney. Over the past decade, a concerted effort has been made to focus on chemotherapy in this patient population. The new generation of biologic therapies may not possess this difficulty, as the monoclonal antibodies that, to date, comprise the most successful of these agents are metabolized by the reticuloendothelial system and may not require these modifications. However, these concerns regarding the appropriate administration of antineoplastic agents will persist with the new small molecule inhibitors, including tyrosine kinase inhibitors, which also may require individual evaluation in patients with organ dysfunction.

This chapter focuses on the administration of chemotherapy in patients with organ dysfunction. Given the limitations in the available data regarding the correct dosing in these settings, we briefly review the methods of evaluating organ function, the drugs metabolized or excreted predominantly by those pathways, disease-specific studies, and finally the Phase I studies that may help guide recommendations for treatment in these patients.

Chemotherapy-Specific Trials in End-Organ Dysfunction

Paclitaxel

The taxoids comprise a class of antineoplastic agents originally derived from several plants in the yew family, but some of which are now synthetically derived. Paclitaxel is metabolized hepatically by the cytochrome P-450 system. Therefore, the Cancer and Leukemia Group B (CALGB) performed a Phase I study in 87 patients with varying levels of hepatic dysfunction (trial 9264).[1] Patients with a primary hepatic tumor, or metastatic solid tumors and evidence of hepatic insufficiency, were enrolled in this study in one of three cohorts, each of which participated in a separate dose-escalation program. Cohort I included patients with aspartate serum transaminase (AST) of at least twice the upper limit of normal (ULN), and a total bilirubin of 1.5 mg/dL or less. Cohorts II and III had AST, but the former included patients with a total bilirubin of 1.6 to 3.0 mg/dL, and cohort III patients had a total bilirubin of greater than 3.0 mg/dL. At the time this study was designed, paclitaxel infusion was typically accomplished (60 patients) over 24 hours, with cycles repeated every 3 weeks. As the study proceeded, the typical administration of paclitaxel became intravenously over 3 hours, and several cohorts of patients on this study, primarily cohorts II and III, were treated accordingly.

In the CALGB studies, dose-limiting toxicities were defined as grade 4 nonhematologic toxicities, grade 3 neurotoxicity, grade 3 stomatitis, esophagitis, or dysphagia of more than 3 days duration, and grade 4 neutropenia or thrombocytopenia lasting more than 3 days. The determination of the maximum tolerated dose (MTD) was based upon toxicities encountered in the first cycle of therapy only.

Somewhat surprisingly, in all cohorts of patients, the doses administered had to be serially deescalated. In cohort I (elevated ALT [alanine aminotransferase]), evaluation started at 200 mg/m^2, but the eventual dose recommended was 50 mg/m^2. All except 1 of the 36 patients treated on this level received paclitaxel over 24 hours, and no recommendations could be made for patients who received the shorter infusion of paclitaxel. Similarly, cohort II patients were evaluated at decreasing doses of paclitaxel from 150 mg/m^2 to the recommended 75 mg/m^2. Two-thirds of the 24 patients on this level received paclitaxel over 24 hours. In cohort III (total bilirubin greater than 3.0 mg/dL), most patients (12 of 21) were given paclitaxel with the shorter infusion, but the results were similar to the other cohorts, with the doses administered being decreased from 75 mg/m^2 to 50 mg/m^2. The authors recommended a dose of 50 to 75 mg/m^2 of paclitaxel over 24 hours for patients with a bilirubin of more than 1.5 mg/dL. With a limited number of patients overall receiving a 3-hour infusion of paclitaxel, the recommendations carry less strength, but the authors considered a dose of 75 mg/m^2 of paclitaxel reasonable for patients with hyperbilirubinemia. Because granulocyte colony-stimulating factor (G-CSF) was not employed in this study, the authors acknowledge that the doses recommended could be somewhat conservative. However, the hepatic metabolism of paclitaxel clearly requires a modification of the doses of paclitaxel employed when treating patients with biochemical evidence of hepatic dysfunction.

Across the cohorts, the dose-limiting toxicity (DLT) was similar, primarily myelosuppression in 27 patients and thrombocytopenia in 3, with grade 4 fatigue occurring in 2 patients. Four patients died during the first cycle of therapy, 2 of sepsis. Although grade 3 fatigue was not considered to be a DLT, it occurred in 15 patients who received the 24-hour infusion of paclitaxel.

Pharmacokinetic studies were obtained from 56 of the participating patients. The results were similar to historical controls who were treated with similar doses of paclitaxel, with no apparent difference in the free paclitaxel detected in the plasma. In the latter part of the study, with the increasing use of 3-hour infusions, and the recognition of the potential importance of the duration of time of paclitaxel concentrations exceeding 0.05 μmol/L, the latter parameter was evaluated in a limited subset of patients. The results suggested that in patients with hepatic dysfunction the duration of paclitaxel concentrations exceeding 0.05 μmol/L was higher than that expected for patients with normal hepatic function. With only 9 patients having both detailed pharmacokinetic information and neutrophil data, no correlation of these parameters was performed. In 4 patients who had external biliary drains, the excretion of paclitaxel and its metabolites detected in the biliary fluid ranged from 2.3% to 50.1% of the administered dose, primarily as 6-α-hydroxypaclitaxel.

Despite the relatively low doses of paclitaxel, the therapy was not bereft of anti-tumor activity, with three partial responses noted, two in breast cancer (cohort I at 150 mg/m^2 over 24 hours, and cohort II at a dose of 125 mg/m^2 over 3 hours), and one in a woman with germ cell tumor (100 mg/m^2 over 24 hours in cohort II). However, all these doses exceed the recommended doses.

Because paclitaxel is not excreted renally, it has been assumed that paclitaxel can be administered in patients with renal insufficiency without significant difficulty. However, Conley et al. reported a series of four patients with renal dysfunction, as defined by a creatinine clearance of less than 60 mL/min (0–58), who were treated with paclitaxel at a dose of 135 mg/m^2 over 3 hours.[2] The mean duration of a paclitaxel concentration exceeding 0.05 μmol/L was 37.7 hours, which is slightly higher than historical reports. In addition, a single case report of a patient with recurrent ovarian cancer and chronic renal insufficiency who worsened with the use of both cisplatin and later, carboplatin, in conjunction with cyclophosphamide, confirmed this finding. At the time of treatment with paclitaxel, 157 mg/m^2 (a 10% dose reduction from the authors' usual dose of 175 mg/m^2) over 3 hours (cycles repeated every 3 weeks), the patient's creatinine clearance was 20 mL/min.[3] During the third cycle of therapy, the patient was administered G-^{3}H-paclitaxel. In this single patient, the disposition half-life was 29 hours, about 50% longer than in patients with normal renal function. In addition, the authors reported a "surprisingly high" plasma AUC (area under the curve) of about 26. The clearance of paclitaxel was primarily fecal, with only 1.58% of paclitaxel excreted unchanged in the urine at 24 hours. The pharmacokinetic parameters of Cremphor were similar to historical controls. Despite these changes in pharmacokinetic parameters of paclitaxel in this patient with renal insufficiency, no significant toxicity aside from severe fatigue occurred, and she was able to attain a partial response to therapy. Thus, the authors recommended that paclitaxel could be safely administered in patients with renal insufficiency, with a 10% dose reduction.

Gemcitabine

The CALGB has also performed a Phase I and pharmacokinetic study in 43 patients with hepatic or renal dysfunction evaluating gemcitabine (CALGB 9565).[4] Broadly, the schema was similar to the paclitaxel study, but with cohorts defined differently. The first two escalation cohorts were in patients with hepatic dysfunction. Cohort I included patients with AST that was more than 2× ULN, but with normal bilirubin and creatinine, whereas in cohort II patients had a total bilirubin between 1.6 and 7.0, and AST. In cohort III, patients could potentially have a serum creatinine between 1.6 and 5.0, but required normal liver function tests. In fact, all the patients in cohort III had a relatively mild to moderate renal dysfunction, with serum creatinine between 1.6 and 3.2.

Gemcitabine was administered intravenously over 30 minutes on days 1, 8, and 15, with cycles repeated every 28 days. The starting dose in each cohort was 800 mg/m^2. In cohort I, the initial 3 patients tolerated therapy well, with no DLT, and at 950 mg/m^2, 1 of the 4 patients enrolled had DLT, and elevation in AST. However, because of results in the concurrently enrolled cohort II, the dose escalation was halted. In cohort II, however, DLT was reported in 3 of 8 patients treated with 800 mg/m^2 of gemcitabine, and in 8 of 10 patients who received 950 mg/m^2 of gemcitabine. Seven of these DLT were elevations in the bilirubin, and another was a rise in the serum transaminases. Two DLT were grade 3 diarrhea, and 1 patient experienced angina. In the patients with renal insufficiency who were enrolled in cohort III, 3 of 9 patients who were treated at the initial dose level of gemcitabine experienced DLT, including 2 with a severe rash and 1 with hepatic transaminase elevation. Doses were then decreased to 650 mg/m^2, at which level only 1 of 6 patients had a DLT.

Pharmacokinetic studies were performed in 36 of the patients. The concentrations of gemcitabine and its inactive metabolite 2′,2′-difluorodeoxyuridine (dFdU) were not significantly different among the cohorts and doses evaluated.

Again, an important conclusion from these investigators is that there is much heterogeneity among patients with organ dysfunction, and that all patients must be considered individually. The results of this study demonstrate that, in patients with hepatic insufficiency as manifested by a total bilirubin between 1.5 and 7.0 or an AST greater than 2× ULN, gemcitabine can be safely administered at a dose of 800 mg/m^2 when it is infused over 30 minutes, weekly for 3 consecutive weeks, with cycles repeated every 4 weeks. In patients with renal insufficiency, as determined by a serum creatinine between 1.6 and 3.2, although the data, as derived from this study, suggest that gemcitabine can be delivered safely on the same schedule at a dose of 650 mg/m^2, and despite the fact that there was no clear difference in pharmacokinetics in patients with renal insufficiency, the authors concluded that no dose of gemcitabine could be safely recommended because of the variability in toxicities.

Fludarabine

There is little information available regarding the administration of other nucleoside analogues. Martell et al. performed a retrospective analysis regarding the toxicity of fludarabine in chronic lymphocytic leukemia. They reported that the renal insufficiency, as determined by an estimated creatinine clearance less than 80 mL/min, was associated with an increased incidence of toxicity, particularly anemia. However, given the nature of the study, no recommendation was made regarding dose modification of fludarabine in patients with renal insufficiency.[5]

Campothecins

Irinotecan

Irinotecan has now been well characterized to be metabolized by the liver and may serve as one of the early models of pharmacogenomics in oncology. Initially, Wasserman et al. reported life-threatening neutropenia and diarrhea in two patients with Gilbert's syndrome who were treated with irinotecan.[6] This finding was provocative because patients with Gilbert's syndrome present with asymptomatic unconjugated hyperbilirubinemia as a result of deficiency in UGT1A1. This result was further highlighted by Gupta et al.[7] In patients treated on a dose-escalation study of irinotecan, the glucuronidation of irinotecan's active metabolite, SN-38, was inversely correlated with higher biliary concentration. Thus, patients with impaired glucuronidation suffered from greater diarrhea. It has subsequently been reported that patients with Gilbert's syndrome may also suffer from a higher incidence of diarrhea than other patients.[8] The enzyme UGT1A1 was subsequently targeted as the putative gene that most affected the metabolism of irinotecan, and in particular, the presence of the 7/7 genotype has been demonstrated to result in an impaired glucuronidation, and therefore, the greater toxicity of irinotecan.

In an attempt to formalize recommendations regarding the administration of irinotecan in patients with hepatic dysfunction, Raymond et al. categorized 33 patients into four groups: I, total bilirubin within the range of normal; II, total bilirubin 1.1–1.5× ULN; III, total bilirubin 1.51–3.0 × ULN; IV, total bilirubin 3.01× ULN, or greater. Patients were then treated with irinotecan every 3 weeks.[9] In the first two cohorts, the standard dose (350 mg/m^2) of irinotecan was well tolerated. In patients with moderate hepatic dysfunction in cohort III, the initial dose of 175 mg/m^2 every 3 weeks was well tolerated. However at the next planned dose, 240 mg/m^2, three of the six patients treated experienced DLT, including grade 4 diarrhea in two patients, and one with grade 4 neutropenia. Thus, an intermediate dose of 200 mg/m^2 was explored, with DLT in only one (grade 4 neutropenia) in five patients. In addition, in cohort IV, three patients were treated with 100 mg/m^2, with no dose-limiting toxicity, but all these patients had a rapid decline in performance status, and no dose escalation was performed.

Pharmacokinetic studies were also performed in this study, and demonstrated that in all the groups with bilirubin elevation, the clearances of irinotecan diminished and the AUC of its active metabolite, SN-38, increased. Indeed, the irinotecan clearance was inversely correlated with the level of bilirubin, but plateaued at 40 μmol/L of bilirubin. The clearance of irinotecan was also correlated with the alkaline phosphatase and γ Glutamyl Transferase (GGTP), but not AST, ALT, albumin, or prothrombin time. Very little of the irinotecan (15%) and SN-38 (less than 0.3%) was excreted renally, and this finding was similar in all the cohorts.

Based upon these results, the authors recommended that no modification in the dose of irinotecan, when administered every 3 weeks, was necessary for patients with a total bilirubin less than 1.5× ULN. For patients with a total bilirubin 1.5–3.0× ULN, the recommended dose of irinotecan is 200 mg/m^2. However, too limited data were available to make a recommendation for therapy in patients with a total bilirubin of more than 3× ULN.

The CALGB has also performed a dose-escalation study in patients with hepatic or renal dysfunction.[10] Liver dysfunction, as defined by AST, of more than 2× ULN (cohort I) or direct bilirubin 1.6–7.0 mg/dL (cohort II) was evaluated. Cohort III was composed of patients with renal insufficiency as defined by a serum creatinine of 1.6 to 5.0 mg/dL. A fourth cohort (IV) included patients who had received prior pelvic radiation. As with prior CALGB studies, doses were escalated individually in separate cohorts.

Given the heterogeneous population of patients, the authors did not make any recommendations regarding the dosage of irinotecan in these diverse populations of patients with organ dysfunction, either measured by laboratory studies or potential, as indicated by prior pelvic radiation. Taken together, the data demonstrate that patients with renal insufficiency, as defined by an elevated bilirubin, should receive, at best, attenuated doses of irinotecan.

Topotecan

Investigators from the Johns Hopkins University have performed dose-escalation studies of topotecan in patients with hepatic or renal insufficiency. In the former study, 14 patients with hepatic dysfunction, as defined by a total bilirubin greater than 1.2 mg/dL, and 7 patients with normal hepatic function, were treated with topotecan intravenously for 5 days, with cycles repeated every 21 days.[11] In both groups, the standard dose of topotecan, 1.5 mg/m^2 daily, was well tolerated, with similar pharmacokinetic results, and no changes in the dose of topotecan administered was deemed necessary to compensate for hepatic dysfunction. Moreover, no concomitant increase in renal elimination was noted.

In the companion to this study, O'Reilly et al. treated 28 patients with renal insufficiency and 14 with normal renal function (creatinine clearance 60 mL/min or greater, as defined by 24-hour urine collection) with the daily × five schedule of topotecan.[12] The patients with renal insufficiency were divided into three separate cohorts (by creatinine clearances of 40–59, 20–39, and less than 20 mL/min, respectively), which were dose escalated individually. In this study, different MTDs were ultimately determined for patients who were heavily and minimally pretreated. Patients with mild renal impairment (creatinine clearance, 40–59 mL/min) were primarily heavily pretreated but were able to receive the standard dose of topotecan. However, patients with moderate renal insufficiency (creatinine clearance, 20–39 mL/min) were able to receive significantly lower doses of topotecan. In patients who were heavily pretreated were recommended to receive 0.5 mg/m^2, but those who were minimally pretreated were able to tolerate 0.75 mg/m^2. These investigators were unable to recommend any dose of topotecan for patients with severe renal dysfunction, as both patients enrolled on this study experienced dose-limiting thrombocytopenia at the initial dose of 0.5 mg/m^2.

The toxicities that were reported in this study were similar to those reported in patients with normal renal function, mainly myelosuppression. With renal impairment, the clearance of topotecan was clearly diminished, with a direct association with creatinine clearance. Interestingly, the pharmacokinetic studies also demonstrated a second peak of topotecan, suggesting the possibility of enterohepatic circulation, although the authors' companion study in hepatic dysfunction did not report a major impact of hepatic metabolism upon topotecan disposition.

Platinums: Oxaliplatin

The platinums comprise a pharmacologically interesting family of agents. It is well known that one of the primary toxicities of cisplatin is nephrotoxicity, which can be ameliorated by hyperhydration and forced diuresis. As noted earlier in this chapter, the second-generation platinum carboplatin can be safely dosed in a fashion to accommodate renal insufficiency. The third-generation platinum oxaliplatin, a DACH platinum, has been approved for use in colorectal cancer and has been demonstrated to have antitumor activity in other malignancies, including breast and prostate cancer. In Phase I and II studies, the appropriate dose of oxaliplatin has been determined to be 85 mg/m^2 every 14 days, or 130 mg/m^2 every 3 weeks. The impact of hepatic and renal dysfunction on the toxicity and pharmacokinetics of oxaliplatin have been evaluated in several Phase I studies.

In a dose-escalation study, 37 patients with various advanced solid malignancies were enrolled.[13] Twelve patients had normal renal function, defined as a creatinine clearance of 60 or more mL/min, and all were treated at 130 mg/m^2 every 3 weeks. Patients with renal insufficiency were assigned cohorts (B, 40–59 mL/min; C, 20–39 mL/min; D, less than 20 mL/min) based upon the level of their renal function, and then dose escalation was performed within each cohort. Ten patients with "mild" insufficiency in cohort B could be escalated from 105 to 130 mg/m^2 without any occurrence of severe toxicities. In cohort C, 14 patients were treated at doses that were successfully increased from 80 to 105 to 130 mg/m^2. At the usual dose of 130 mg/m^2, 3 patients experienced severe, non-dose-limiting thrombocytopenia. No other severe toxicities were reported. With repeated dosing in this cohort, 2 patients did experience a worsening of serum creatinine, but both cases were attributed to progressive disease and obstructive uropathy. Only 1 patient with severe renal impairment (cohort D) was treated. He experienced a nonneutropenic urosepsis with the first dose (60 mg/m^2) of therapy, and was withdrawn from the study. Although the systemic platinum exposure increased with worsening renal insufficiency, there was no significant difference in the toxicity profile of oxaliplatin in the different cohorts of patients treated on this protocol. Thus, the authors recommended that oxaliplatin could be administered at the full dose of 130 mg/m^2 every 3 weeks in patients with a creatinine clearance of 20 mL/min or greater.

The same group of investigators performed a similar study in patients with liver dysfunction.[14] Forty-three patients were treated in the report, 11 of whom had normal hepatic function. Liver dysfunction was defined as mildly impaired [cohort B: normal bilirubin; serum glutamic-oxaloacetic transaminase (SGOT), less than 2.5× ULN; alkaline phosphatase, less than 5× ULN], moderately impaired (cohort C: total bilirubin less than 3; SGOT, less than 2.5× ULN; alkaline phosphatase, less than 5× ULN), and severely impaired (cohort D: total bilirubin of 3, but any level of SGOT or alkaline phosphatase). One patient who had a prior orthotopic liver transplant (cohort E) was also treated. Doses were escalated from 60 mg/m^2 to the full dose of 130 mg/m^2, if possible. The dose of oxaliplatin was successfully escalated to the full dose in cohorts A, B, and C. In these groups, only one DLT occurred, with grade 3 neurotoxicity in one of seven patients in cohort C treated with 80 mg/m^2. Seven patients with severe liver dysfunction were enrolled in this study, with no DLT at 60 or 80 mg/m^2. In addition, no DLT was noted in the single patient who had a prior liver transplant and was treated with 60 mg/m^2 of oxaliplatin. Pharmacokinetic studies were performed on 15 of the patients who were enrolled in this study. They demonstrated a decrease in the clearance of ultrafilterable platinum with increasing hepatic dysfunction, as indicated by total bilirubin and alkaline phosphatase, with the patients in cohort C having a clearance of 35% less than the patients with normal hepatic function. This finding was not accompanied by any difference in toxicity, however. Thus, the authors of this study recommended that the full dose of oxaliplatin can be administered to patients with moderate hepatic dysfunction, as defined by a total bilirubin of 3.0, SGOT 2.5× ULN, and alkaline phosphatase of 5.0× ULN or less.

Antifolates

The fluoropyrimidines have long been available as an important component of therapy for gastrointestinal malignancies and breast cancers. Because of the broad spectrum of activity of these agents and the schedule-dependent nature of antitumor activity, fluoropyrimidines are an area of extensive investigation and development, in particular, the oral fluoropyrimidines. Although 5-fluorouracil (5-FU) has been available for more than 40 years, limited information is available regarding the dosing of 5-FU in patients with organ dysfunction.

5-Fluorouracil

In patients with renal or hepatic dysfunction, Fleming et al. have performed a dose-escalation study of infusional (weekly 24-hour infusion) 5-FU from 1,000 to 18,000 to 2,600 mg/m^2, admixed with 500 mg/m^2 leucovorin.[15] Patients were divided into three groups: Cohort I was composed of 16 patients with renal insufficiency as defined by a serum creatinine of 1.5 to 3.0 mg/dL. Cohorts II and III included patients with a total bilirubin of greater than 1.5 to less than 5.0 mg/dL, and 5.0 mg/dL or greater, respectively. In all the cohorts, the typical doses of 5-FU (2,600 mg/m^2 over 24 hours) and leucovorin (500 mg/m^2 over 24 hours) were safely attainable. The dose-limiting toxicities that were encountered were the expected ones of fatigue, diarrhea, anemia, and thrombocytopenia. The pharmacokinetic results for 5-FU were similar to those reported by others evaluating a 24-hour infusion of the drug, with no clear evidence of any relationship between 5-FU clearance and either bilirubin or creatinine. However, the authors pointed out that given the pharmacokinetic differences between bolus and infusional 5-FU, it cannot be assumed that bolus 5-FU can be administered safely to patients with hepatic or renal insufficiency. This recommendation has been buttressed by some of the findings from studies with the oral fluoropyrimidines, which may act more like multiple "mini-boluses" of 5-FU, rather than a continuous infusion of 5-FU.

Supporting this concern were the results of a retrospective analysis of a pair of studies in patients with metastatic colorectal cancer who were randomly assigned to receive either capecitabine or 5-FU/leucovorin by IV bolus according to the Mayo clinic schedule.[16] A total of 1,207 patients were enrolled in the study and 605 were randomly assigned to receive 5-FU/leucovorin. Patients and their toxicities were analyzed according to calculated creatinine clearance (by the Cockroft–Gault formula). Of the patients who received 5-FU/leucovorin, the incidence of any grade 3 or 4 toxicity was higher among the patients with moderate renal insufficiency (creatinine clearance, 30–50 mL/min) than in patients with mild renal insufficiency (51–80 mL/min) or normal renal function, at 51%, 35%, and 31% of patients, respectively. The primary difference was in the occurrence of severe stomatitis 26%, compared to 16% and 11%. The difference in the toxicities were reflected in the fact that 30% of patients with moderate renal insufficiency withdrew from therapy because of toxicity, compared to 14% of patients with mild renal dysfunction, and 10% of patients with normal renal function.

Capecitabine

The only oral fluoropyrimidine that has been approved by the U.S. Food and Drug Administration (FDA) for use in the United States is capecitabine. It is also the member of this class that has been most extensively evaluated in the setting of organ dysfunction.

Poole et al. performed a study in 27 patients, all of whom were given the standard dose of capecitabine, 1,250 mg/m^2 twice daily for 14 days, with cycles repeated every 3 weeks.[17] Six (group A) had normal renal function, as defined by a creatinine clearance of greater than 80 mL/min. The other patients were divided into mild impairment (group B, 8 patients; creatinine clearance, 51–80 mL/min), moderate impairment (group C, 6 patients; creatinine clearance, 30–50 mL/min), and severe impairment (group D, 4 patients; creatinine clearance, less than 30 mL/min).

In this study, there was no significant impact of creatinine clearance upon the systemic exposure to capecitabine in any of the groups. In contrast, patients with moderate and severe renal insufficiency (creatinine clearance, 50 mL/min or less) had lower day 14 AUC of the metabolite 5′-DFCR and higher levels of 5′-DFUR and FBAL. The AUC of 5-FU was elevated only in patients in group D. The half-life and C_{max} of these agents were generally similar among the groups. However, all four of the patients with severe renal insufficiency experienced toxicity, including one patient who died (sepsis) and another who discontinued therapy as a result of toxicity. Patients with mild and moderate renal insufficiency had toxicity profiles similar to those of patients with normal renal function.

As a result of these findings, the investigators recommended that capecitabine could safely be administered to patients with mild renal insufficiency (creatinine clearance of 50 mL/min or greater) at the full dose but should not be prescribed to patients with severe renal dysfunction. Although patients with moderate renal insufficiency (creatinine clearance, 30–50 mL/min) did not experience any greater toxicity than patients within other cohorts, based on the pharmacokinetic studies, the authors recommended the administration of capecitabine with an initial dose reduction of 25%, which should result in a system exposure similar to that in patients without renal dysfunction.

Bolstering these data were the results of a retrospective analysis of a pair of studies in patients with metastatic colorectal cancer who were randomly assigned to receive either capecitabine or 5-FU/leucovorin by IV bolus.[15] A total of 1,207 patients were enrolled in the study and 603 were randomly assigned to receive capecitabine. Patients and their toxicities were analyzed according to calculated creatinine clearance (by the Cockroft–Gault formula). About 10% of patients who received capecitabine had moderate renal insufficiency (creatinine clearance, 30–50 mL/min), and 5 patients had severe insufficiency. The patients who had moderate renal insufficiency experienced more severe toxicities (54%), especially hand-foot syndrome (25.4%), than those with mild renal impairment (41% and 18.3%) or normal renal function (36% and 12.3%). This difference resulted in a more frequent incidence of dose reduction of capecitabine in patients with moderate renal insufficiency (44% of patients, compared to 32% and 33%), and a greater likelihood of withdrawing from therapy because of toxicity, especially diarrhea. However, the objective response rates were similar among these subgroups of patients.

The pharmacokinetics of capecitabine have also been explored in 16 patients with hepatic dysfunction that resulted from liver metastases and compared to results in patients with normal hepatic function.[18] Hepatic dysfunction was graded by serum total bilirubin, transaminases, and alkaline phosphatase in a unique scale, and the patients in this study were determined to have had "mild-to-moderate hepatic dysfunction." Patients were treated with a single dose of capecitabine at a dose of 1,255 mg/m^2. The patients with hepatic dysfunction attained higher plasma concentrations of capecitabine, 5′-DFUR, and 5-FU but lower levels of 5′-DFCR. Similarly, the C_{max} and AUC of capecitabine, 5′-DFUR, and 5-FU were lower, but higher with 5′-DFCR in patients with hepatic dysfunction. Despite the differences that were detected, none were found to be statistically significant, and overall results were similar to the results for patients with normal hepatic function. There did not appear to be any compensatory changes in the urinary excretion of capecitabine or its metabolites. No significant differences in the toxicity profiles in the two groups were noted, although this was a single-dose study of capecitabine. As a result of these findings, Twelves et al. recommended that, in patients with mild and moderate hepatic insufficiency, capecitabine can be cautiously administered at full doses. However, no comment can be made regarding patients with severe hepatic dysfunction.

S-1

S-1 is another oral fluoropryimidine that is composed of a combination of tegafur, a prodrug of 5-fluorouracil, with a drug that inhibits dihydropyrimidine dehydrogenase (5-chloro-2,4-dihydroxypyridine, CDHP) and another that reduces gastrointestinal toxicity (potassium oxonate) in a 1:0.4:1 ratio. Based on the findings from an animal model of induced renal failure that suggested that the clearance of both 5-FU and CDHP were correlated with the degree of renal failure, Ikeda et al. treated four patients with unresectable gastric cancer and renal insufficiency with S-1.[19] Three of the patients had a relatively mild renal insufficiency, with a creatinine clearance greater than 50mL/min, and were treated with 20mg/m^2/day of S-1, half the usual dose. The fourth patient, with a creatinine clearance of 36mL/min, received one-third the usual dose of S-1. In the patients with minimal renal insufficiency (creatinine clearance, 75mL/min or greater) demonstrated no differences in single- and multiple-dose pharmacokinetics of any of the drugs in S-1. However, in the two patients with mild and moderate renal insufficiency, there was a notably longer half-life of both 5-FU and CDHP with multiple-dose administrations when compared to a single dose. Despite these findings, no serious toxicities were reported in any patient when receiving S-1 with these dose modifications. Based on these findings, the authors suggest that S-1 may be administered to patients with renal insufficiency, but only with close monitoring, and no specific dosing recommendations could be made.

5-FU/Eniluracil

An important limitation to the administration of oral 5-FU as a single agent appears to be its metabolism by dihydropyrimidine dehydrogenase (DPD). Eniluracil is an inhibitor of DPD, which may then allow the administration of oral 5-FU by increasing the latter's bioavailability. The combination has been evaluated in patients with metastatic colorectal cancer. O'Donnell et al. have also performed a study of this combination in 17 patients with refractory solid tumors.[20] Nine patients had renal insufficiency (creatinine clearance, less than 50mL/min), and the others were considered to have "normal" renal function (group A). Treatment was divided into a test period and treatment period. Based on the pharmacokinetic results from the test period, patients with renal insufficiency were then subsequently treated with the eniluracil/5-FU. The patients in group A received eniluracil 50mg on days 1 to 7 and 5-FU 20mg/m^2 on days 1 to 5. The clearance of 5-FU and eniluracil decreased with worsening renal function. However, there did not appear to be an increase in toxicity in the patients with renal impairment, suggesting that the test dose strategy was successful, but would be necessary for eniluracil/5-FU.

Pemetrexed (MTA, LY231514)

Pemetrexed disodium is a new multitargeted antifolate that inhibits thymidylate synthase, dihydrofolate reductase, and glycinamide ribonucleotide formyl transferase. It has demonstrated notable antitumor activity in combination with cisplatin in mesothelioma and promising antitumor activity in other solid tumors. Takimoto et al. performed a dose-escalation study in 29 patients with renal insufficiency.[21] Renal function was determined by technetium 99m-DPTA glomerular filtration rates. Cohort 1B included patients with creatinine clearance of 60 to 79mL/min; cohort 2, 40–59mL/min; cohort 3, 20–39mL/min; and cohort 4, 19mL/min, or less. Eighteen patients with normal renal function were also treated (cohort 1A). In cohort 1B, myelosuppressive DLT were found with pemetrexed in 3 of 5 patients who were treated with a higher than standard dose of pemetrexed (600mg/m^2). At the standard dose of 500mg/m^2, pemetrexed was well tolerated. Patients with creatinine clearance of 40 to 59mL/min were also able to receive the standard dose of pemetrexed. No patients were enrolled in cohort 3, but 1 patient with severe renal insufficiency died with febrile neutropenia, and no further accrual was performed in either arm. In this study, the clearance of pemetrexed was strongly correlated with glomerular filtration rate (GFR). Based on these results, the investigators recommended that, with vitamin B_{12} and folic acid supplementation, the standard dose of pemetrexed, 500mg/m^2 every 21 days, could be administered to patients with mild renal dysfunction, as defined by a creatinine clearance of greater than 40mL/min.

Raltitrexed

Thymidylate synthase (TS) has proven to be a fruitful target in the therapy of many different tumors, including colorectal cancers. Raltitrexed is a synthetic TS inhibitor that can be administered intravenously once every 3 weeks. An important limitation of raltitrexed is that it cannot be administered to patients with significant effusions. Because of these considerations, raltitrexed has undergone limited evaluation in patients with renal insufficiency.[22] Judson et al. treated 8 patients with renal insufficiency (creatinine clearance, 25–65mL/min) and 8 with "normal" renal function with ralitrexed at 3mg/m^2 every 21 days. The $t_{1/2}\gamma$ and AUC of raltitrexed were significantly greater in the patients with renal insufficiency. The clearance of raltitrexed was clearly related to creatinine clearance. Given these findings, and that the doses of raltitrexed were similar in the two groups, it is not surprising that the patients with renal insufficiency had substantially more toxicity, with 6 patients requiring hospitalization (compared to 2 of the patients with normal renal function). Based on these results, Judson et al. recommended that if raltitrexed is being administered to patients with a creatinine clearance of 25 to 65mL/min, the dose be decreased by 50%, and the interval between treatments be increased to 4 weeks, rather than the usual 3 weeks. Moreover, they recommended that raltitrexed not be administered to patients with severe renal insufficiency, as indicated by a creatinine clearance less than 25mL/min.

Anthracyclines

Anthracyclines were among the first agents to have demonstrated a clear propensity to have greater toxicity in patients who had organ dysfunction, in particular, hepatic insufficiency. As a result, some of the first evidence-based recommendations were with doxorubicin.

Adriamycin

Benjamin et al. performed a pharmacologic study of adriamycin 60mg/m^2 every 3 weeks in 96 patients with a variety of malignancies.[23] Eight of the patients had hepatic insufficiency, and these patients experienced significantly more toxicity than the patients with normal hepatic function. For example, all 8 had severe pancytopenia, 3 had severe mucositis, and 3 died (37.5%). In five patients with hepatic insufficiency, the plasma levels of adriamycin and its metabolites were four to five times as great as those for patients with normal hepatic function, with significantly delayed excretion. By comparison, the 79 patients with normal hepatic function experienced less toxicity with no cases of severe mucositis and 3 drug-related deaths (3.8%). As the result of these experiences, 9 further patients with abnormal liver function studies, as defined by bilirubin, were treated with a lower dose of adriamycin. Patients with a bilirubin of 1.2 to 3.0 mg/dL received a 50% reduction in the dose of adriamycin (30 mg/m^2), and those with a bilirubin of greater than 3.0 mg/dL received adriamycin with a 75% dose reduction (15 mg/m^2). After receiving adriamycin with these dose modifications, the toxicity profile of adriamycin in these patients was similar to that in patients with normal hepatic function. An additional patient with severe renal insufficiency (serum creatinine, 9.0 mg/dL) received a full dose of adriamycin, with only mild toxicity reported. This result likely reflected the fact that the urinary excretion of adriamycin was "limited." Based on these results, these dose modifications for patients with hyperbilirubinemia have been employed for adriamycin.

However, in some contrast to these results, Brenner et al. treated 64 patients with acute nonlymphocytic leukemia with adriamycin and cytosine arabinoside.[24] Hepatic function was determined by bromsulphalein (BSP) retention, a functional test. The standard dose of adriamycin in this study was 30 mg/m^2 for 3 consecutive days. This dose was administered to 28 patients with normal hepatic function (group I) and 26 patients with mild hepatic dysfunction by BSP retention (greater than 5% over 45 minutes). In the other 10 patients, who had an elevated BSP retention, adriamycin was delivered at a 50% to 67% dose reduction (10–15 mg/m^2/day). In groups I and II, which were treated with similar doses of adriamycin, there was no significant difference in acute toxicity, as defined by mucositis, patient outcomes, or in pharmacokinetic profiles. The patients in group III, receiving a lower dose of adriamycin because of hepatic insufficiency, had perhaps less toxicity, but were found to have a significantly lower drug exposure, and possibly shorter survivals, than the patients treated at the higher doses. The authors believe that, based on these results, perhaps the recommendations from Benjamin et al. require further validation before widespread application.

Epirubicin

Epirubicin is a derivative of adriamycin that may have somewhat less cardiotoxicity at equipotent doses. As a derivative of adriamycin, several studies have evaluated the administration of epirubicin in patients with hepatic insufficiency, believing that a dose reduction may be necessary for such patients. These expectations have indeed been borne out by the study results.

Camaggi et al. performed a study with epirubicin in 22 patients with previously treated advanced solid tumors.[25] Half the patients, who had normal hepatic and renal function, received 90 mg/m^2 epirubicin intravenously, and were used as controls. Five patients had an elevated serum creatinine, which suggested renal insufficiency, and 6 patients had abnormal liver function studies as a result of hepatic metastases. All except 1 (with normal bilirubin, but other elevated transaminases and alkaline phosphatase) of these patients received 35.7 mg/m^2 epirubicin. The patients with hepatic insufficiency demonstrated a decrease in the plasma clearance and increase in the area under the curve, but similar half-life of epirubicin. The patient with a liver function study abnormality who received the full dose of epirubicin had higher epirubicin and epidoxorubicinol levels than those patients who had normal liver function. Based on these findings, in conjunction with previously reported results with the parent compound doxorubicin, the authors suggested that a 50% dose reduction of epirubicin be considered for patients with liver metastases, even in the absence of overt hepatic dysfunction. However, they also recommended that further studies be conducted to refine the recommendations, given the small number of patients evaluated in this study. With regard to the patients with renal insufficiency, who received a lower dose of epirubicin, the pharmacokinetic parameters of epirubicin were similar to those in patients without renal insufficiency; this confirms the finding that renal excretion is a minor pathway of elimination for epirubicin. Thus, the authors concluded that epirubicin may be administered without dose modification in patients with renal dysfunction.

Furthering the studies of epirubicin and hepatic function, Twelves et al. evaluated the drug in 52 women with advanced breast cancer.[26] These patients were divided into three populations. The first group comprised women with normal hepatic function, and they were treated with varying doses of epirubicin (12.5–120 mg/m^2) every 3 weeks. Twenty-two patients in group 2 had elevated AST, but normal bilirubin, and 8 patients in group 3 had elevations in both AST and bilirubin. Most of the women in these groups received epirubicin 25 mg/m^2 weekly. The authors found that the patients in groups 2 and 3 had decreased epirubicin clearance and a prolonged terminal half-life of epirubicin compared to the patients in group 1 (normal hepatic biochemistry studies). The strongest correlation was between AST elevation and clearance.

Based on these findings, this group then attempted to derive a more specific dose modification plan in women with breast cancer.[27] Again, group 1 included 15 patients with normal liver biochemistry studies (AST less than 2× ULN and bilirubin less than 2.0 μmol/L) served as the controls, receiving various doses of epirubicin (25–120 mg/m^2) to define a "high" and "low" AUC (2,400 mg/mL/h and 1,600 mg/mL/h, respectively) that would correspond to epirubicin doses of 90 and 60 mg/m^2, respectively. The formula that was derived was dose = AUC × [87.5 − (34.2 × $\log_{10}$AST)]. Group 2 consisted of 16 patients with abnormal liver function who were treated with epirubicin 25 mg/m^2 to confirm the results in this population. In this population, the clearance of epirubicin was again correlated with the $\log_{10}$ of AST.

A third group then included 41 women with abnormal liver function who were prospectively treated with epirubicin that was dosed according to the AST, targeted to attain either the "high" AUC in 25 patients or "low" AUC in the other 16. Finally, the fourth group of patients was composed of 25 patients with hepatic metastases and abnormal hepatic transaminases who were treated with epirubicin 25 mg/m^2

weekly. In the last two groups of patients, epirubicin therapy was well tolerated. However, the median survival in these patients with hepatic dysfunction and breast cancer was only 14 weeks. Ten of the 38 evaluable patients had a partial response to therapy, and all had some improvement in their liver biochemistries, including two who had an initial worsening of these studies.

As a result of these findings, the authors concluded that the epirubicin could be dosed safely according to a target AUC, with the actual dose dependent on the pretreatment AST. Doing so appears to decrease the pharmacokinetic variability of the administered epirubicin in comparison to the patients treated with a fixed dose regardless of hepatic function. However, the potential benefits of these recommendations await confirmation by a randomized study.

Etoposide

Similar to the anthracyclines, etoposide is an inhibitor of topoisomerase II. Its administration has also been explored in several studies in patients with hepatic and renal insufficiency. In the mid-1980s, the initial reports were made by D'Incalci and Arbuck, respectively. In the first report, D'Incalci et al. treated 15 patients with hepatic insufficiency, as defined by a total bilirubin greater than 1.2, GGTP greater than 28, or alkaline phosphatase greater than 170, and compared pharmacokinetic results to a control population of 18 patients.[28] Both groups of patients received varying doses and schedules of etoposide, sometimes in combination with other drugs. Overall, the pharmacokinetic results in the two populations were similar, but with somewhat more interpatient variability in the patients with hepatic dysfunction.

Arbuck et al. observed eight patients with hepatic insufficiency (total bilirubin, greater than 1.0, including six values greater than 3.0) with etoposide.[29] As in the prior study, these patients often also received other chemotherapy drugs, and on varying schedules. Very little (less than 3%) of the etoposide was excreted in the bile, but much of the clearance of etoposide was unaccountable. Etoposide clearance in patients with hepatic insufficiency appeared to be similar to historic control patients with normal renal function.

More recently, Hande et al. treated 11 patients with obstructive jaundice and total bilirubin greater than 2.0 mg/dL, comparing the results to 23 control patients with normal hepatic function (including bilirubin less than 1.4 mg/dL).[30] Again, patients received varying doses of etoposide (100–800 mg/m^2), many in combination with other drugs. There was no significant difference in the pharmacokinetic profiles and urinary excretion in the two populations. Thus, the authors recommended that dose modifications are not necessary for patients with obstructive jaundice or hepatic dysfunction, if they have normal renal function.

However, Stewart et al. reported some interesting findings that, although consistent with the others, also raise interesting questions.[31] They treated 21 patients with etoposide 100 mg/m^2 intravenously over 1 hour on days 1, 3, and 5, with cisplatin 70 mg/m^2 IV on day 1. Fourteen patients had liver metastases, but only 6 patients had a total bilirubin greater than 1, including 4 with a total bilirubin greater than 2, 4 with ascites, and 6 had a creatinine clearance less than 70 mL/min. The authors specifically reported on the results in the patients with hepatic dysfunction. They found that the clearance of total etoposide was similar in patients with hepatic dysfunction, hepatic metastases, ascites, and normal hepatic function. The clearance of unbound etoposide was significantly lower, resulting in a higher AUC in the patients with hyperbilirubinemia than in the other patients. Toxicity was not reported, so it is unclear if this increase in the exposure to unbound etoposide has any clinical impact. Overall, these data suggest that perhaps the dose of etoposide should be decreased in patients with an elevated bilirubin. This finding requires confirmation, and was not explored in the other studies.

Taken together, the burden of the data suggests that in patients with hepatic dysfunction, etoposide can probably be administered safely without dose modification. However, the study reported by Stewart et al. certainly indicates that caution must continue to be used when administering etoposide in patients with hepatic insufficiency.

Less information is available regarding the administration of etoposide in patients with renal insufficiency. D'Incalci also treated eight patients with normal hepatic function, but impaired renal function, as defined by a serum creatinine greater than 1.5 or creatinine clearance less than 60 mL/min.[27] Five of these patients had renal dysfunction from cisplatin. In this small group of patients, 2% to 23% of the dose was recovered in the urine, which was less than in the control group of 18 patients (40%) with normal organ function. In addition, the plasma clearance and half-life of etoposide were significantly less in the patients with renal dysfunction than the control patients. Arbuck also treated nine patients with renal insufficiency (creatinine clearance less than 70 mL/min, but only three less than 50 mL/min).[28] Although the pharmacokinetic findings in the patients with renal insufficiency were similar to those in the patients with hepatic dysfunction, creatinine clearance was found to be the strongest predictor of etoposide clearance. Thus, the results from these limited studies suggest that etoposide clearance is correlated with creatinine clearance, and both sets of authors suggested that the dose of etoposide be decreased in patients with renal insufficiency.

Targeted Therapy

Imatinib Mesylate (Gleevec, STI 571)

Imatinib was the first oral "targeted therapy" to be approved for use in the United States. It is metabolized in the liver, which suggests that its toxicity profile may be altered in patients who have hepatic insufficiency. However, two reports, each composed of two patients, suggested that despite the hepatic metabolism of the drug, imatinib can be given safely to patients with gastrointestinal stromal tumors and hepatic dysfunction, as deteremined by bilirubin and hepatic transaminases, with no clear worsening of drug toxicity.[32,33]

The administration of imatinib in patients with organ dysfunction has been explored more formally through the National Cancer Institute Cancer Therapy Evaluation Program (NCI CTEP) in a pair of studies that have been reported in preliminary form. Ramanathan et al. reported on the administration of imatinib in patients with hepatic dysfunction, primarily the result of liver metastases, or 15 patients with normal liver function.[34] The severity of hepatic dysfunction was defined by total bilirubin and SGOT, in reference to laboratory normals. Thus, the mild hepatic dysfunction cohort included patients with total bilirubin less than 1.5× ULN, or SGOT above normal. Moderate dysfunction encompassed patients with a total bilirubin 1.5–3.0× ULN, but any SGOT, whereas severe hepatic dysfunction included patients with a total bilirubin 3–10× ULN, and any SGOT. At the time of the abstract presentation, 13, 9, and 12 patients had been enrolled in the study, with only 1 DLT (vomiting/diarrhea in 1 patient in the mild hepatic dysfunction cohort at 400mg daily). Generally, therapy was well tolerated, and the toxicity profile was similar to that reported in gastrointestinal stromal tumors, including nausea/vomiting, edema/weight gain, fatigue, and elevation in liver function studies. Preliminary evaluation of the pharmacokinetic studies that have been performed demonstrated a large interpatient variability, but also with a 50% increase in steady-state levels of imatinib in the patients with hepatic dysfunction compared to the normal patients. However, as the dose escalation was continuing, no specific recommendations have yet been made.

For the same consortium, Remick et al. reported on a similar study in patients with renal dysfunction.[35] Again, four cohorts of patients underwent parallel dose escalations. These cohorts were patients with normal renal function and patients with mild (creatinine clearance between 40 and 59mL/min), moderate (20–39mL/min), or severe (less than 20mL/min) renal dysfunction. At the time of the report, therapy had been well tolerated, with patients again having typical toxicities for imatinib. The clearance of imatinib declined with creatinine clearance, and appeared to be inversely correlated with plasma alpha-1-acid glycoprotein. However, in patients with mild and moderate renal insufficiency, the toxicity profile did not appear to be significantly different than for patients with normal renal function. Only one DLT was reported (nausea/vomiting) in a patient with moderate renal dysfunction who received imatinib at 200mg daily. Dose escalation was continuing in this study as well, and again, no specific dose recommendations were made for patients with renal insufficiency.

Gefitinib (Iressa, ZD 1839)

Another in the new generation of targeted therapy is gefitinib, which inhibits the tyrosine kinase of epidermal growth factor receptors and has demonstrated antitumor activity, with suggested symptomatic benefit in patients with non-small cell lung cancer. Twelves et al. evaluated the role of hepatic insufficiency in patients who were treated with gefitinib at the standard dose of 250mg daily.[36] Hepatic insufficiency was defined by serum aspartate aminotransferase and total bilirubin. Forty-one patients were treated in this study, including 18 with normal hepatic function, 16 with moderate hepatic insufficiency, and 7 with severe hepatic dysfunction. No significant differences in systemic exposure, as defined by AUC and C_{max}, or toxicities were noted among the groups.

Vincristine

Although the vinca alkaloids have been used as antineoplastic therapy for several decades, limited information is available regarding the administration of these microtubule inhibitors in patients with organ dysfunction. Van den Berg et al. reported on a series of 39 patients who received vincristine at various doses, usually in combinations with other drugs.[37] Fifteen patients had elevated alkaline phosphatase, 3 of whom had elevated bilirubin, and 7 also had elevated GGTP. In these patients, the half-life and AUC of vincristine were elevated. With the limitations of this study, no recommendations regarding dosing of vincristine in patients with elevated alkaline phosphatase and likely, impaired hepatic function.

Renal Dysfunction

Our knowledge of the elimination of drugs remains incomplete, which makes dose modifications for end-organ dysfunction difficult (Tables 98.1, 98.2). The narrow therapeutic index of antineoplastic drugs makes a solid understanding of drug metabolism critical when administering chemotherapy in patients with renal dysfunction. In this section, we review the available evidenced-based recommendations for chemotherapy administration in renal dysfunction to serve as a reference for treatment decision making.

Disease-Specific Trials in Renal Dysfunction

Few disease-specific studies exist in the literature addressing the role of chemotherapy in patients with renal dysfunction. The majority of the trials have been performed in genitourinary cancer, as renal insufficiency is commonly observed in this patient population. Transitional cell carcinoma of the urinary bladder is a moderately chemosensitive tumor with published response rates of 60% to 70% and complete responses in 20% to 30% using cisplatin-based chemotherapy.[38–40] Almost half the patients presenting with advanced bladder malignancies have compromised clinical status due to advanced age, comorbidities, and renal dysfunction, making the delivery of full-dose cisplatin-based chemother-

TABLE 98.1. Chemotherapeutic agents metabolized or excreted by the kidneys.

Azathioprine
Busulfan
Bleomycin
Capecitabine
Carboplatin
Cisplatin
Cytarabine
Dacarbazine
Etoposide
Fludarabine
Hydroxyurea
Ifosfamide
Melphalan
Methotrexate
Mitomycin C
Oxaliplatin
Pentostatin
Streptozocin
Temozolomide
Topotecan

TABLE 98.2. Recommendations by trial for patients with renal dysfunction.

Author	*Year*	*N*	*Renal function*	*Chemotherapy*	*Relative risk (RR)*	*Complete response (CR)*	*Partial response (PR)*	*Grade 3/4 toxicity*
Dreicer[42]	1996	9	2.25 (1.9–3.2)	Taxol 24-h CIV	56%	—	5	Leukopenia, neutropenia
Vaughn[45]	1998	17	1.1 (0.7–2.7) Cr Cl, 52 (24–110)	Carbo AUC 6 Taxol 225 mg/m^2	50%			Neutropenia, neuropathy
Dimopoulos[43]	1998	11	2.6	Docetaxel 100 mg/m^2	—		5	Neutropenia
Small[47]	2000	29	Cr Cl, 61 (36–125)	Carbo AUC 5 Taxol 200 mg/m^2	20.7%	—	6	Neutropenia, anemia, pain, thrombocytopenia, cardiac, pulmonary, neurologic, GI, metabolic, infection, renal
Llado[51]	2000	16	5 > 55 7, 30–55 4 < 30	Carbo AUC 4.5 Gem 1,000 mg/m^2	43.7%	1	6	Anemia, neutropenia, thrombocytopenia
Shannon[52]	2001	17	Cr Cl, 56 (34–90)	Carbo AUC 5 Gem 1,000 mg/m^2	58.8%	3	7	Neutropenia, anemia, thrombocytopenia
Vaughn[46]	2002	42	1.7 (1.5–3)	Taxol 225 mg/m^2 Carbo AUC 6	24.3%	3	6	Neutropenia
Ricci[56]	2002	38	1.3 (0.6–2.6) Cr Cl <60–30	Gem 1,000 mg/m^2 Epirubicin 70 mg/m^2	39.5%	2	13	Neutropenia, anemia Thrombocytopenia
Nogué-Aliguer[55]	2003	41	Cr Cl <60–22 Cr Cl >60–19	Carbo AUC 5 Gem 1,000 mg/m^2	56.1%	6	17	Neutropenia, anemia Thrombocytopenia

R, renal dysfunction; H, hepatic dysfunction; ULN, upper limit of laboratory normals; CrCl, creatinine clearance, as measured by mL/min; PCr, serum creatinine, as measured by mg/dL; Tbili, total bilirubin, as measured by mg/dL; AST, aspartate serum transaminase; AUC, area under the curve; CrCl, creatinine clearance.
Source: Standard recommendations derived from *Drugs Facts and Comparisons 2004*, 58th edition. St. Louis: Facts & Comparisons, 2004.

apy difficult if not dangerous. This issue has thus led to several initiatives exploring systemic chemotherapy in the presence of renal dysfunction and perhaps representing genitourinary (GU) malignancies, giving us the most extensive body of literature in a disease-specific setting.

Paclitaxel, primarily metabolized by the liver, has been evaluated in several studies of patients with renal insufficiency.[41] Dreicer et al. treated six chemotherapy-naïve bladder cancer patients with renal insufficiency defined by median serum creatinine of 2.25 mg/dL (range, 1.6–3.2), with paclitaxel 175–250 mg/m^2 over 24 hours every 21 days.[42] Four of the patients had a documented partial response while another had stabilization of disease. Three of the patients had experienced neutropenia with an associated fever, and 2 had severe neurotoxicity. This toxicity profile is similar to that reported with paclitaxel when used as a single agent in patients with normal renal function.

Dimopoulos et al. treated a similar group of 11 patients with docetaxel 100 mg/m^2 every 21 days, with G-CSF support.[43] Five of the patients had an objective response and 3 had stable disease. Three of the responding patients normalized their renal function after relief of ureteral obstruction. The median survival in these patients was 11 months. The regimen was considered to be safe. Five patients experienced severe neutropenia, including two episodes of neutropenic fever; no other severe toxicities were reported.

Having exhibited activity with acceptable toxicity in patients with mild renal insufficiency, taxanes were then studied in combination with carboplatin, adjusting for renal function. Bekele et al. reported a case of a patient with metastatic transitional cell carcinoma and chronic renal insufficiency (baseline serum creatinine, of 6.6 mg/dL) secondary to poststreptococcal glomerulonephritis.[44] The patient was treated with carboplatin (AUC = 5) and paclitaxel 135 mg/m^2 every 3 weeks. This chemotherapy combination induced a partial regression of disease and was well tolerated. The patient experienced grade 2 anemia, grade 1 neuropathy, did not require hemodialysis, and died 17 months later with progressive disease.

Vaughn et al. reported a Phase I/II study of carboplatin and paclitaxel in 33 patients with a median creatinine clearance of 52 mL/min (range, 24–100). Sixteen patients were accrued in Phase I and administered carboplatin AUC 6 and paclitaxel 150 to 225 mg/m^2 IV over 3 hours.[45] Subsequently, 17 patients were treated with carboplatin AUC 6 and paclitaxel 225 mg/m^2 IV over 3 hours. Although responses were observed at all dose levels, an objective response rate of 50% was documented in this Phase II setting.

Drawing from this experience, the Eastern Cooperative Oncology Group carried out a Phase II study (E2896) of carboplatin and paclitaxel in 42 patients with advanced urothelial cancer and renal dysfunction.[46] A serum creatinine between 1.6 and 4.0 mg/dL was required for study entry. Nine of the 37 evaluable patients had an objective response (24.3%); 3 complete responses were observed. The median survival was 7.1 months and the median progression-free survival 3.0 months. The toxicity profile of the combination in this study was typical for the regimen, with severe neutropenia observed in 60% and anemia in 18% of the 40 evaluable patients. Severe neurotoxicity was reported in 35% and nausea/vomiting in 10% of the patients. Of note, 4 patients died on therapy; 1 with neutropenic sepsis, 1 with gastrointestinal bleeding in the setting of grade 4 thrombocytopenia, 1 with pulmonary embolism, and 1 of an unknown cause. The authors concluded that the combination of carboplatin and paclitaxel could be administered safely to patients with renal insufficiency and should be subjected to further evaluation as an optimal therapeutic option.

The Southwest Oncology Group (SWOG) replicated this study, treating 29 patients with a median creatinine clearance of 61 mL/min with carboplatin at AUC 5 and paclitaxel 200 mg/m^2 every 21 days.[47] Six partial responses with an overall response rate of 20.7% were observed. Toxicity was primarily hematologic, with 38% experiencing grade 4 neutropenia. Neurologic toxicity was observed in 16 patients; grade 1 in 4, grade 2 in 5; grade 3 in 6; and grade 4 in 1 patient. Although the regimen was deemed to be well tolerated, the response proportion in this study was considerably lower than prior studies.

Single-agent gemcitabine has been shown to have activity and excellent tolerance in patients with transitional cell carcinoma.[48,49] Gemcitabine in combination with cisplatin has been shown to have equivalent activity compared to methotrexate, vinblastine, doxorubicin, and cisplatin (MVAC) in advanced urothelial cancer.[50] Llado et al. treated 16 patients with renal insufficiency, substituting carboplatin AUC 4.5 in combination with gemcitabine 1,000 mg/m^2 with an overall response rate of 43.7%. One patient had a complete response while 6 had partial responses.[51] Toxicity was primarily hematologic. The combined regimen with carboplatin (AUC = 5, on day 1) and gemcitabine (1,000 mg/m^2 over 30 minutes on days 1 and 8), repeated every 21 days, has been studied by several investigators. Shannon et al. administered this combination to 17 patients with poor prognostic factors; 13 of these patients had a creatinine clearance less than 60 mL/min.[52] Overall, 10 patients had an objective response (58.8%). The median survival was 10.5 months and the median time to progression 4.6 months. As expected, the primary toxicity was myelosuppression; 12 patients (70%) experienced severe neutropenia without neutropenic fever, 8 (47%) had thrombocytopenia, and 3 (18%) had anemia. Severe nonhematologic toxicity was relatively uncommon, with 2 patients experiencing nausea/vomiting and 1 mucositis. It was concluded that this combination was active, with acceptable toxicity. Carles et al. treated 17 patients with median creatinine clearance of 45 mL/min (range, 20–55 mL/min) using the same regimen.[53,54] An objective response of 56% was observed; the median survival was 10 months. Overall, this schedule of carboplatin/gemcitabine was tolerated well; severe neutropenia occurred in 4 patients (23.5%) and thrombocytopenia and anemia in 18% each. The authors concluded that this combination is active in patients with renal insufficiency and had similar antitumor efficacy as observed in patients with normal renal function.

The largest series of patients treated with this schedule of carboplatin and gemcitabine was reported by Nogue-Aliguer et al.[55] Twenty-two of the 41 patients in this series had renal insufficiency as defined by a creatinine clearance between 30 and 60 mL/min. The remainder of the patients were considered to be poor candidates for cisplatin-based chemotherapy because of age or performance status. The results mirrored those from the reports from Shannon and Carles, with a response rate of 56.1%, median survival of 10.1 months, and median progression-free survival of 7.2 months. Unfortunately, the results for the patients with renal insufficiency were not reported separately from the poor performance status patients. The toxicity profile was again similar to the previous reports. Severe myelosuppression was the primary toxicity, with neutropenia in 63% of patients (including 3 episodes of neutropenic fever), anemia in 54%, and thrombocytopenia in 32%. Twenty percent of patients had severe asthenia and 7% severe nausea/vomiting. One patient had an increase in serum creatinine.

Seeking to avoid the use of any platinums in patients who may be poor candidates for such therapy, Ricci et al. investigated a combination of epirubicin and gemcitabine.[56] Epirubicin was administered on day 1 at a dose of 70 mg/m^2 and gemcitabine 1,000 mg/m^2 on days 1 and 8, with cycles every 21 days. Thirty of the 38 patients enrolled had a creatinine clearance of less than 60 mL/min. Fifteen of the patients (39.5%) had an objective response. The median survival was 8.0 months, with a 1-year survival of 38% and median progression-free survival of 4.8 months. The combination was well tolerated, with severe neutropenia in 22% of all cycles, and 2 episodes of neutropenic fever. Severe anemia occurred in 11% of cycles, and thrombocytopenia in 7% of cycles; no severe nonhematologic toxicities were noted. The authors concluded that this regimen could have potential utility for patients with advanced urothelial carcinoma who are considered to be suboptimal candidates for platinum-based therapy, including those with renal insufficiency.

Taken together, these series of studies suggest that taxanes, platinums, gemcitabine, and epirubicin may be administered safely in patients with mild renal insufficiency without compromising antitumor activity or increased toxicity, alone or in combination.

Chemotherapy and Hemodialysis

With the improvement in hemodialysis techniques and supportive care, the prognosis of patients with chronic renal failure has improved. The improvement in survival in turn, has led to the increased number of hemodialysis patients with development of various types of cancers.[57] Many chemotherapeutic agents are dependent on renal excretion, and the role of chemotherapy in adult patients who require hemodialysis has rarely been reported.

The impact of chemotherapy in adult patients who require hemodialysis has rarely been reported, and specific recommendations cannot be made for most agents. The literature reveals only case reports and small series. The largest of these series was performed in lung cancer. Watanabe et al. treated five patients with increasing doses of cisplatin on day 1, and etoposide on days 1, 3, and 5.[58] Hemodialysis was performed within an hour after completion of chemotherapy. Two patients were treated with an intrapatient dose escalation to determine the toxicity of the regimen in these patients. Full doses of cisplatin (80 mg/m^2) and etoposide (100 mg/m^2) could be administered in the other three patients. Four of the patients had partial responses, two of two in small cell and two of three in non-small cell lung cancer. The toxicity profile was similar to other series of patients with normal renal function. All the patients had severe grade 3/4 anemia and neutropenia. Two each had severe thrombocytopenia and nausea/vomiting. The pharmacokinetic results in this study were similar to those from patients with normal renal function, although the free platinum was somewhat higher in the patients on hemodialysis. These findings suggest that full doses of cisplatin and etoposide could be administered safely to patients requiring hemodialysis.

Two case reports have also been published suggesting the safety of paclitaxel in patients requiring hemodialysis. One woman with ovarian cancer was treated with escalating doses of paclitaxel, from 175 to 300 mg/m^2 over 3 hours, on nondialysis days. Pharmacokinetic studies were performed, and demonstrated nonlinear pharmacokinetics with the high doses, similar to other studies. Paclitaxel could not be dialyzed. Similar results were reported in an iatrogenically anephric child requiring hemodialysis who received paclitaxel at 250 and 350 mg/m^2 over 24 hours. The peak concentration and systemic exposure of paclitaxel was similar to historically reported values in children. Again, paclitaxel could not be detected in the dialysate. Taken together, these results suggest that paclitaxel can be safely administered in full doses to patients requiring hemodialysis.

There also have been two cases of the use of gemcitabine in patients requiring hemodialysis. An 81-year-old man with metastatic pancreatic adenocarcinoma received gemcitabine 650 mg/m^2 on days 1, 8, and 15 every 28 days. Hemodialysis was performed 5.5 hours after completion of the infusion. No significant toxicities were reported. The C_{max}, AUC, and clearance of gemcitabine were similar to prior reports of gemcitabine in patients without renal dysfunction. However, the metabolite dFdU did not decrease until dialysis started. However, upon the initiation of dialysis, the dFdU levels decreased by 46%. Kiani et al.[59] reported a 64-year-old man with locally advanced pancreatic cancer who received gemcitabine 1,000 mg/m^2 on days 1 and 10 every 28 days. Hemodialysis was performed 24 hours after completion of the chemotherapy. Again, the pharmacokinetics of gemcitabine were similar to those for patients with normal renal function. The half-life of dFdU was prolonged, but without apparent clinical consequence. These reports also suggest that gemcitabine may also be administered at the full doses to patients who are undergoing hemodialysis.

Cisplatin and Paclitaxel

Most of the cases reports using carboplatin and paclitaxel combinations in dialysis patients have been patients with gynecologic malignancies. A high proportion of the carboplatin administered remains free in plasma. Because the major route of elimination of carboplatin is through glomerular filtration and tubular secretion, it has high dialysis efficacy. By contrast, the majority of cisplatin is rapidly protein bound, and renal excretion accounts for a minority of the elimination of free platinum.[60] Thus, due to its predictable kinetics, similar efficacy, and limited toxicity, carboplatin is usually preferable to cisplatin in patients with gynecologic malignancies on hemodialysis.

The carboplatin AUC observed in a hemodialysis patients is not only dependent on the dose and GFR but also on the interval between the drug administration and hemodialysis. Kurata et al. compared the AUC of carboplatin followed by hemodialysis 1 and 2 hours after administration.[61] Although the predicted AUC was 9.6 mg/min/mL after administration of carboplatin at the dose of 240 mg/m^2, the observed AUC was 3.1 mg/min/mL for 1 hour and 5.1 mg/min/mL for 2 hours after the dose. Niikura et al. reported three cases of long-term dialysis patients with gynecologic malignancies. They chose the dose of 200 mg/m^2 for the initial administration of carboplatin with expectation of an AUC of 4 mg/min/mL during hemodialysis 2 hours after administration based on pharmacokinetic data.[62] Severe or prolonged thrombocytopenia during chemotherapy in two of three patients was observed, and thus the authors suggest that a dose of 200 mg/m^2 may be too high in these patients. Clinically complete remission was observed in a patient receiving a carboplatin dose of 100 mg/m^2 in this series. Similarly, a case report by Chatelut et al. noted a complete response in an advanced ovarian cancer patient on hemodialysis with carboplatin at the dose of 100 to 150 mg/m^2.[63] The authors thus recommend 100 to 150 mg/m^2 of carboplatin as an appropriate dose for patients undergoing hemodialysis in spite of a low AUC achieved pharmacokinetically. Patients on long-term hemodialysis may have an abnormal bone marrow function and therefore, the dose of carboplatin may need to be reduced in spite of reported pharmacokinetic data.

Watanabe et al. reported a case of stage III ovarian cancer treated with carboplatin/paclitaxel combination chemotherapy after debulking surgery.[64] Paclitaxel was administered at 150 mg/m^2 and carboplatin at AUC 5, according to the Calvert formula. Chemotherapy was given on nondialysis days and an acceptable degree of thrombocytopenia and neutropenia was noted. The patient had a complete response after five cycles and remained disease free for 8 months after completion of the therapy. The authors suggest administering chemotherapy at least 16 hours before the scheduled hemodialysis.

Furuya et al. reported a case of a dialysis patient with metastatic urothelial carcinoma treated with a combination of carboplatin dosed at AUC of 5 mg/min/mL, calculated according to the Calvert formula, and a full dose of paclitaxel, 175 mg/m^2.[65] The patient was able to tolerate four courses of chemotherapy with minimal toxicity (grade 3 neutropenia and grade 1 thrombocytopenia) while achieving a 20% tumor regression.

Paclitaxel is extensively metabolized by the liver and secreted in bile, with less than 10% extracted by the kidneys.[66,67] Paclitaxel is not eliminated by hemodialysis; no dose adjustment has been required based on renal failure alone.[68] Tomita et al. collected dialysate samples 30 min after the start of hemodialysis for measurement of paclitaxel concentration, but none was identified.[69]

Cisplatin and Etoposide

Several small case series have been reported with use of attenuated doses of cisplatin in hemodialysis patients. Tomita et al. reported a case of a recurrent ovarian cancer patient undergoing hemodialysis treated with cisplatin and paclitaxel.[69] At a dose of cisplatin 30 mg/m^2 and paclitaxel 150 mg/m^2, a 42% tumor size reduction was noted after two cycles; however, grade IV neutropenia and grade 3 thrombocytopenia were noted. Similar case studies have been reported with use of cisplatin in hemodialysis patients in testicular cancer, bladder cancer, gastric cancer, and lung cancer.[70–73]

Kamizuru et al. reported a pharmacokinetic study in a hemodialysis patient with stage IIIA seminoma treated with cisplatin at 7 mg/m^2 on days 1, 3, and 5, 14 mg/m^2 cisplatin on days 2 and 4, with etoposide 70 mg/m^2 on days 1 to 5.[70] They noticed a high degree of myelosuppression and thus had to attenuate their chemotherapy doses of cisplatin to 14 mg/m^2 on days 1, 3, and 5 and etoposide to 35 mg/m^2 on days 1 to 5 for the next three cycles. The AUC of free cisplatin found on pharmacokinetic study was 6.82 µg/h/min in the first course, and 4.07 µg/h/min in the second course. The AUC of etoposide was 241.9 µg/h/mL in the first course and 216.9 µg/h/mL in the second course. A complete response was achieved, and the patient did not have any recurrence for 5 years. The authors concluded that the cisplatin and etoposide could be given to the patients receiving hemodialysis, and suggested the use of lower doses to prevent side effects.

Obana et al. reported three cases of small cell lung cancer patients with underlying renal failure treated with carboplatin and etoposide.[73] Hemodialysis was used in two of three cases. Two of the three patients had a partial response and there was improvement in quality of life in the third. The need for selection of suitable chemotherapy regimens, their optimal dose, and the timing of hemodialysis was raised by the authors. A recent case series by Watanabe et al., was published in the *British Journal of Cancer*.[58] They reported a dose-escalation study of cisplatin and etoposide for hemodialysis patients with lung cancer. A starting dose of cisplatin at 40 mg/m^2 on day 1, and etoposide at 50 mg/m^2 on days 1, 3, and 5, was escalated course by course and patient by patient by monitoring toxicity and pharmacokinetic data. In their series of five patients they were able to give the full dose of cisplatin at 80 mg/m^2 on day 1 and 100 mg/m^2 etoposide on days 1, 3, and 5. Pharmacokinetic data were comparable to those from the patients with normal renal function except for uncleared free platinum in renal insufficiency patients. All patients in their series developed anemia, neutropenia, and prolonged thrombocytopenia. The authors concluded that, in this small number of patients, further studies in larger patient populations are warranted, even though dose escalation showed that full-dose chemotherapy administration in hemodialysis patients was possible.

Hepatic Dysfunction

Evaluating Hepatic Function

One of the primary difficulties in the evaluation of the appropriate role and dose of chemotherapy in patients with hepatic dysfunction is determining an appropriate definition of hepatic insufficiency. The liver is an organ with multiple functions, and as one of the largest organs in the body, one with great reserve. Different medical disciplines have evaluated hepatic function differently, based on biochemical function (synthetic or metabolic), or more grossly, as with the Childs' classification. Similarly, there is no agreement on what constitutes hepatic dysfunction in regard to pharmacology. Even within a relatively uniform and consistent group of investigators, such as the Cancer and Leukemia Group B Pharmacology and Experimental Therapy group, the definition of hepatic dysfunction used in protocols has evolved.

Some studies have based the definition of hepatic insufficiency upon function studies. Most protocols have defined laboratory values, some based upon synthetic function, and others related to metabolism, or the transaminases.

Disease-Specific Trials in End-Organ Dysfunction, Primarily Hepatocellular Carcinoma

As with renal dysfunction, few disease-specific studies have been conducted for patients with hepatic dysfunction (Table 98.3). The studies that have been reported are primarily with anthracyclines, which require dose modification in the setting of hepatic insufficiency, in patients with hepato-

TABLE 98.3. Chemotherapeutic agents metabolized or excreted by the liver.

Capecitabine
Chlorambucil
Cyclophosphamide
Dacarbazine
Daunorubicin
Docetaxel
Doxorubicin
Epirubicin
Etoposide
Fluorouracil
Gefitinib
Hydroxyurea
Idarubicin
Imatinib
Irinotecan
Lomustine
Methotrexate
Mitomycin C
Mitoxantrone
Paclitaxel
Vinblastine
Vincristine
Vinorelbine

cellular cancer (HCC). This disease often occurs in the setting of cirrhosis, and the dysfunction is often not a specific reflection of the malignancy.

Chan et al.[74] treated 7 patients with hepatocellular carcinoma, three of whom had biopsy-proven cirrhosis, but normal LFTs with various doses of doxorubicin (10–45 mg/m^2) and methyl CCNU. The pharmacokinetic results in these patients were compared to the results in 10 patients with other malignancies who received the same combination. The results were similar in the two populations, suggesting that cirrhosis does not inherently change the clearance of doxorubicin.

Similarly, Johnson et al.[75] evaluated 30 consecutive patients with hepatocellular cancer who were treated with doxorubicin, 60 mg/m^2. Sixteen of the patients had hyperbilirubinemia, defined by a total bilirubin greater than 1.7.

TABLE 98.4. Recommendations for dose modifications in hepatic or renal dysfunction, based on clinical data, compared with "Standard Recommendations."

Agent	*Standard recommendations for dose modifications*	*Recommendations for modification based on clinical studies*
Capecitabine	R: CrCl 30–50: 25% reduced	R: CrCl 30–50: 25% reduced
Carboplatin	R: Area under the curve (AUC)	R: AUC
Docetaxel	H: Transaminase >1.5 × ULN, and alkaline phosphatase >2.5 × ULN: do not administer	H: No recommendations
Doxorubicin	H: Tbili 1.2–3.0: 50% reduced Tbili >3.0–5.0: 75% reduced Tbili >3.0: 75% reduced Tbili >5: Do not administer R: CrCl <10: 25% reduced	H: Tbili 1.2–3.0: 50% reduced
Epirubicin	H: Tbili 1.2–3.0: 50% reduced Tbili >3.0–5.0: 75% reduced AST 2–4 × ULN: 50% reduced AST >4 × ULN: 75% reduced	H: 50% reduced Maybe, AUC guided
Etoposide	H: Tbili 1.5–3.0: 50% reduced Tbili >3.0: 75% reduced R: CrCl 10–50: 25% reduced CrCl <10: 50% reduced	H: None needed R: No recommendations possible
Fluorouracil	R: No recommendations H: Tbili 3.0–5.0: 50% reduced Tbili >5.0: Do not administer	R: PCr 1.5–3.0: 100% if 24-h infusion H: 100%, if 24-h infusion
Gefitinib	No recommendations	H: No changes necessary
Gemcitabine	H: "with caution" R: "with caution"	H: TBili 1.5–7.0; AST >2x ULN: 800 mg/m^2 IV over 30 min days 1, 8, 15 q 28 d R: PCr 1.6–5.0: 650 mg/m^2 IV Over 30 min days 1, 8, 15 q 28 d
Imatinib	No recommendations	H: Studies ongoing, no recommendations R: Studies ongoing, no recommendations
Irinotecan	H: Tbili >2: "use lower doses"	H: Tbili 1.5–3.0 × ULN: 200 mg/m^2 IV over 90 min, q 21 d
Oxaliplatin	H: No recommendations made R: "Severe": "with caution"	H: Tbili <3, AST <2.6 × ULN, AP <5 × ULN: 100% of dose R: CrCl >20: 100% of dose
Paclitaxel	H: "with caution" R: No recommendations	H: Incomplete AST: 50 mg/m^2 IV over 24 h q 21 d Tbili >1.5: 50–75 mg/m^2 IV over 24 h q 21 d R: 10% dose reduction
Pemetrexed	No recommendations	R: CrCl >40: 500 mg/m^2 IV q 21 d
Raltitrexed	No recommendations in U.S.	R: CrCl 25–65: 50% dose reduction
Topotecan	H: No recommendations R: CrCl 20–39: 50% reduced CrCl <20: Do not administer	H: Tbili >1.2 × ULN: 100% of dose R: CrCl 20–39: 0.5–0.75 mg/m^2/d × 5, q 21 d
Vinblastine	H: Tbili >3.0: 50% reduced	No recommendations
Vincristine	H: Tbili >3.0: 50% reduced	H: No recommendations possible
Vinorelbine	H: Tbili 2.1–3.0: 50% reduced Tbili >3.0: 75% reduced	No recommendations

R, renal dysfunction; H, hepatic dysfunction; ULN, upper limit of laboratory normals; CrCl, creatinine clearance, as measured by mL/min; PCr, serum creatinine, as measured by mg/dL; Tbili, total bilirubin, as measured by mg/dL; AST, aspartate serum transaminase.

These patients had a greater AUC but similar terminal half-life as those with normal hepatic function. The antitumor efficacy was similar (2/11 evaluable patients) in each group. The patients with hyperbilirubinemia were significantly more likely to have leukopenia on day 7, however.

Subsequent explorations have involved liposomal formulations of anthracyclines. Hong et al.[76] reported a single case of a patient with inoperable hepatocellular cancer, and severe hepatic dysfunction, as indicated by an abnormally increased indocyanine green clearance (ICG) study: 30 mg/m^2 of pegylated liposomal doxorubicin was given every 3 to 4 weeks. The patient tolerated therapy well, with grade 2 stomatitis and grade 2 and 3 leukopenia, and he was able to receive therapy for eight cycles, with an initial partial response. The pharmacokinetic studies were compared to results from eight patients with normal hepatic function and found that the volume of distribution and clearance of doxorubicin were higher, and AUC lower, in this patient. Based on this result, the authors then performed a Phase II study with this drug and dose in this population. Forty patients with hepatocellular cancer were enrolled; they were required to have a total bilirubin of 3.0 mg/dL or less. The overall response rate was 10%, with a median survival of 3.0 months. The toxicity was acceptable, with severe neutropenia in 9% of cycles and stomatitis in 7% of cycles. The results from the pharmacokinetic studies were variable, with no clear correlation to toxicity. Hepatic function as determined by ICG studies also did not correlate with pharmacokinetic or toxicity results. Compared to the results from a Phase I study, the results from this study again suggested a lower initial concentration of doxorubicin, larger volume of distribution, and more rapid clearance of doxorubicin in these patients with hepatocellular carcinoma.

Daniele et al.[77] planned a dose-escalation study of liposomal daunorubicin in patients with hepatocellular carcinoma and cirrhosis. However, because of the toxicity encountered in this study, dose deescalation, from 80 to 60 to 40 mg/m^2 every 21 days, occurred. Indeed, even at the lowest level, three of the four patients encountered dose-limiting toxicity. No objective responses were noted. The primary toxicity in this study, however, was elevations in bilirubin and other hepatic biochemical studies. This study was ultimately also discontinued in part because of the finding of significant uptake of the liposomes in the "normal" liver parenchyma. Specific recommendations based on the previous discussion are presented in Table 98.4.

References

1. Venook AP, Egorin MJ, Rosner GL, et al. Phase I and pharmacokinetic trial of paclitaxel in patients with hepatic dysfunction: Cancer and Leukemia Group B 9264. J Clin Oncol 1998; 16(5):1811–1819.
2. Conley BA, Zaharski D, Kearns CM, et al. Paclitaxel (P) pharmacokinetic (PK)/pharmacodynamic (PD) relationships in patients (pts) with renal dysfunction (RD). Proc Am Soc Clin Oncol 1997;16:223A.
3. Gelderblom H, Verweij J, Brouwer E, et al. Disposition of [G-^{3}H] paclitaxel and cremophor EL in a patient with severely impaired renal function. Drug Metab Dispos 1999;27(11): 1300–1305.
4. Venook AP, Egorin MJ, Rosner GL, et al. Phase I and pharmacokinetic trial of gemcitabine in patients with hepatic or renal dysfunction: Cancer and Leukemia Group B 9565. J Clin Oncol 2000;18(14):2780–2787.
5. Martell RE, Peterson BL, Cohen HJ, et al. Analysis of age, estimated creatinine clearance and pretreatment hematologic parameters as predictors of fludarabine toxicity in patients treated for chronic lymphocytic leukemia: a CALGB (9011) coordinated intergroup study. Cancer Chemother Pharmacol 2002;50:37–45.
6. Wasserman E, Myara A, Lokiec F, et al. Severe CPT-11 toxicity in patients with Gilbert's syndrome: two case reports. Ann Oncol 1987;8:1049–1051.
7. Gupta E, Lestingi TM, Mick R, et al. Metabolic fate of irinotecan in humans: correlation of glucuronidation with diarrhoea. Cancer Res 1994;54:3723–3725.
8. Van Groeningen CJ, Van der Vijgh WJF, Baars JJ, et al. Altered pharmacokinetics and metabolism of CPT-11 in liver dysfunction: a need for guidelines. Clin Cancer Res 2000;6(4):1342–1346.
9. Raymond E, Boige V, Faivre S, et al. Dosage adjustment and pharmacokinetic profile of irinotecan in cancer patients with hepatic dysfunction. J Clin Oncol 2002;20(21):4304–4312.
10. Venook AP, Enders Klein C, Fleming G, et al. A Phase I and pharmacokinetic study of irinotecan in patients with hepatic or renal dysfunction or with prior pelvic radiation: CALGB 9863. Ann Oncol 2003;14(12):1783–1790.
11. O'Reilly S, Rowinsky EK, Slichenmyer W, et al. Phase I and pharmacologic studies of topotecan in patients with impaired hepatic function. J Natl Cancer Inst 1996;88:817–824.
12. O'Reilly S, Rowinsky EK, Slichenmyer W, et al. Phase I and pharmacologic study of topotecan in patients with impaired renal function. J Clin Oncol 1996;14(12):3062–3073.
13. Takimoto C, Remick SC, Sharma S, et al. Dose-escalating and pharmacological study of oxaliplatin in adult patients with impaired renal function: a National Cancer Institute Organ Dysfunction Working Group Study. J Clin Oncol 2003; 21(14):2664–2672.
14. Doroshow JH, Synold T, Longmate J, et al. Phase I pharmacokinetic (PK) trial of oxaliplatin (OX) in solid tumor patients (Pts) with varying degrees of liver dysfunction (LD). Proc Am Soc Clin Oncol 2001;22 (abstract 449).
15. Fleming GF, Schilsky RL, Schumm LP, et al. Phase I and pharmacokinetic study of 24-hour infusion of 5-fluorouracil in patients with organ dysfunction. Ann Oncol 2003;14(7): 1142–1147.
16. Cassidy J, Twelves C, Van Cutsem E, et al. First-line oral capecitabine in metastatic colorectal cancer: a favorable safety profile compared with intravenous 5-fluorouracil/leucovorin. Ann Oncol 2003;13: 566–575.
17. Poole C, Gardiner J, Twelves C, et al. Effect of renal impairment on the pharmacokinetics and tolerability of capecitabine (Xeloda) in cancer patients. Cancer Chemother Pharmacol 2002;49:225–234.
18. Twelves C, Glynne-Jones R, Cassidy J, et al. Effect of hepatic dysfunction due to liver metastases on the pharmacokinetics of capecitabine and its metabolites. Clin Cancer Res 1999; 5(7):1696–1702.
19. Ikeda M, Furukawa H, Imamura H, et al. Pharmacokinetic study of S-1, a novel oral fluorouracil antitumor agent in animal model and in patients with impaired renal function. Cancer Chemother Pharmacol 2002;50:25–32.
20. O'Donnell A, Punt CJA, Judson I, et al. A study to evaluate the pharmacokinetics of oral 5-fluorouracil and eniluracil after concurrent administration to patients with refractory solid tumors and varying degrees of renal impairment (FUMA1005). Cancer Chemother Pharmacol 2003;51:58–66.
21. Takimoto CH, Forero L, Baker SD, et al. Phase I & pharmacokinetic study of LY231514 (pemetrexed disodium, MTA) in renal dysfunction patients (pts). Ann Oncol 2002;13(suppl 5):12 (abstract 41PD).

22. Judson I, Maughan T, Beale P, et al. Effects of impaired renal function on the pharmacokinetics of raltitrexed (Tomudex ZD1694). Br J Cancer 1998;78(9):1188–1193.
23. Benjamin RS, Wiernik PH, Bachur NR. Adriamycin chemotherapy—efficacy, safety, and pharmacologic basis of an intermittent single high-dosage schedule. Cancer (Phila) 1974;33(1):19–27.
24. Brenner DE, Wiernik PH, Wesley M, et al. Acute doxorubicin toxicity. Relationship to pretreatment liver function, response, and pharmacokinetics in patients with acute nonlymphocytic leukemia. Cancer (Phila) 1984;53(5):1042–1048.
25. Camaggi CM, Strocchi E, Tamassia V, et al. Pharmacokinetic studies of 4′-epi-doxorubicin in cancer patients with normal and impaired renal function and with hepatic metastases. Cancer Treat Rep 1982;66:1819–1824.
26. Twelves CJ, Dobbs NA, Michael Y, et al. Clinical pharmacokinetics of epirubicin: the importance of liver biochemistry tests. Br J Cancer 1992;66:765–769.
27. Dobbs NA, Twelves CJ, Gregory W, et al. Epirubicin in patients with liver dysfunction: development and evaluation of a novel dose modification scheme. Eur J Cancer 2003;39:580–586.
28. D'Incalci M, Rossi C, Zucchetti M, et al. Pharmacokinetics of etoposide in patients with abnormal renal and hepatic function. Cancer Res 1986;46:2566–2571.
29. Arbuck SG, Douglass H, Crom WR, et al. Etoposide pharmacokinetics in patients with normal and abnormal organ functions. J Clin Oncol 1986;4(11):1690–1695.
30. Hande KR, Wolff SN, Greco FA, et al. Etoposide kinetics in patients with obstructive jaundice. J Clin Oncol 1990;8(6):1101–1108.
31. Stewart CF, Arbuck SG, Fleming RA, et al. Changes in the clearance of total and unbound etoposide in patients with liver dysfunction. J Clin Oncol 1990;8(11):1874–1879.
32. Bauer S, Hagen V, Pielken HJ, et al. Imatinib mesylate therapy in patients with gastrointestinal stromal tumors and impaired liver function. Anticancer Drugs 2002;13(8):847–849.
33. DePas T, Danesi R, Catania C, et al. Imatinib administration in two patients with liver metastases from GIST and severe jaundice. Br J Cancer 2003;89:1403–1404.
34. Ramanathan RK, Remick SC, Mulkerin D, et al. P-5331: a phase I pharmacokinetic (PK) study of STI571 in patients (pts) with advanced malignancies and varying degrees of liver dysfunction (LD). Proc Am Soc Clin Oncol 2003; (abstract 502).
35. Remick SC, Ramanathan RK, Mulkerin D, et al. P-5340: a phase I pharmacokinetic (PK) study of STI571 in patients (pts) with advanced malignancies and varying degrees of renal dysfunction. Proc Am Soc Clin Oncol 2003;22 (abstract 503).
36. Twelves C, White J, Harris A, et al. The pharmacokinetics and tolerability of ZD 1839 in hepatically impaired patients with solid tumors. Ann Oncol 2002;13(suppl 5):27 (abstract 96P).
37. Van den Berg HW, Desai ZR, Wilson R, et al. The pharmacokinetics of vincristine in man: reduced drug clearance associated with raised serum alkaline phosphatase and dose-limited elimination. Cancer Chemother Pharmacol 1982;8:215–219.
38. Sternberg CN, Yagoda A, Scher HI, et al. Preliminary results of M-VAC (methotrexate, vinblastine, doxorubicin and cisplatin) for transitional cell carcinoma of the urothelium. J Urol 1985;133(3):403–407.
39. Sternberg CN, Yagoda A, Scher HI, et al. Methotrexate, vinblastine, doxorubicin, and cisplatin for advanced transitional cell carcinoma of the urothelium. Efficacy and patterns of response and relapse. Cancer (Phila) 1989;64(12):2448–2458.
40. Sternberg CN, De Mulder PH, Schornagel JH, et al. Randomized phase III trial of high-dose-intensity methotrexate, vinblastine, doxorubicin, and cisplatin (MVAC) chemotherapy and recombinant human granulocyte colony-stimulating factor versus classic MVAC in advanced urothelial tract tumors: European Organization for Research and Treatment of Cancer Protocol No. 30924. J Clin Oncol 2001;19(10):2638–2646.
41. Roth BJ, Dreicer R, Einhorn LH, et al. Significant activity of paclitaxel in advanced transitional-cell carcinoma of the urothelium: a phase II trial of the Eastern Cooperative Oncology Group. J Clin Oncol 1994;12(11):2264–2270.
42. Dreicer R, Gustin DM, See WA, et al. Paclitaxel in advanced urothelial carcinoma: its role in patients with renal insufficiency and as salvage therapy. J Urol 1996;156(5):1606–1608.
43. Dimopoulos MA, Deliveliotis C, Moulopoulos LA, et al. Treatment of patients with metastatic urothelial carcinoma and impaired renal function with single-agent docetaxel. Urology 1998;52(1):56–60.
44. Bekele L, Vidal Vazquez M, et al. Systemic chemotherapy in patients with renal failure. Am J Clin Oncol 2001;24(4):382–384.
45. Vaughn DJ, Malkowicz SB, Zoltick B, et al. Paclitaxel plus carboplatin in advanced carcinoma of the urothelium: an active and tolerable outpatient regimen. J Clin Oncol 1998;16(1):255–260.
46. Vaughn DJ, Manola J, Dreicer R, et al. Phase II study of paclitaxel plus carboplatin in patients with advanced carcinoma of the urothelium and renal dysfunction (E2896): a Trial of the Eastern Cooperative Oncology Group. Cancer 2002;95(5):1022–1027.
47. Small EJ, Lew D, Redman BG, et al. Southwest Oncology Group Study of paclitaxel and carboplatin for advanced transitional-cell carcinoma: the importance of survival as a clinical trial end point. J Clin Oncol 2000;18(13):2537–2544.
48. Stadler WM, Kuzel T, Roth B, et al. A phase II study of single-agent gemcitabine in previously untreated patients with metastatic urothelial cancer. J Clin Oncol 1997;15(11):3394–3398.
49. Lorusso V, Pollera CF, Antimi M, et al. A phase II study of gemcitabine in patients with transitional cell carcinoma of the urinary tract previously treated with platinum. Italian Co-Operative Group on Bladder Cancer. Eur J Cancer 1998;34(8):1208–1212.
50. von der Maase H, Hansen SW, Roberts JT, et al. Gemcitabine and cisplatin versus methotrexate, vinblastine, doxorubicin, and cisplatin in advanced or metastatic bladder cancer: results of a large, randomized, multinational, multicenter, phase III Study. J Clin Oncol 2000;18(17):3068–3077.
51. Llado A, Bellmunt J, Kaiser G, et al. A dose finding study of carboplatin with fixed doses of gemcitabine in "unfit" patients with advanced bladder cancer. ASCO 2000;19:344a (abstract 1354).
52. Shannon C, Crombie C, Brooks A, et al. Carboplatin and gemcitabine in metastatic transitional cell carcinoma of the urothelium: effective treatment of patients with poor prognostic features. Ann Oncol 2001;12(7):947–952.
53. Carles J, Nogue M, Domenech M, et al. Carboplatin-gemcitabine treatment of patients with transitional cell carcinoma of the bladder and impaired renal function. Oncology 2000;59(1):24–27.
54. Carles J, Nogue M. Gemcitabine/carboplatin in advanced urothelial cancer. Semin Oncol 2001;28(3 suppl 10):19–24.
55. Nogue-Aliguer M, Carles J, Arrivi A, et al. Gemcitabine and carboplatin in advanced transitional cell carcinoma of the urinary tract: an alternative therapy. Cancer (Phila) 2003;97(9):2180–2186.
56. Ricci S, Galli L, Chioni A, et al. Gemcitabine plus epirubicin in patients with advanced urothelial carcinoma who are not eligible for platinum-based regimens. Cancer (Phila) 2002;95(7):1444–1450.
57. Maisonneuve P, Agodoa L, Gellert R, et al. Cancer in patients on dialysis for end-stage renal disease: an international collaborative study. Lancet 1999;354:93–99.
58. Watanabe R, Takiguchi Y, Moriya T, et al. Feasibility of combination chemotherapy with cisplatin and etoposide for hemodialysis patients with lung cancer. Br J Cancer 2003;88:25–30.
59. Kiani A, Kohne CH, Franz T, et al. Pharmacokinetics of gemcitabine in a patient with end-stage renal disease: effective clearance of its main metabolite by standard hemodialysis treatment. Cancer Chemother Pharmacol 2003;51(3):266–270.

60. Motzer RJ, Niedzwiecki D, Isaacs M, et al. Carboplatin-based chemotherapy with pharmacokinetic analysis for patients with hemodialysis-dependent renal insufficiency. Cancer Chemother Pharmacol 1990;27:234–238.
61. Kurata H, Yoshiya N, Ikarashi H, et al. Pharmacokinetics of carboplatin in a patient undergoing hemodialysis. Jpn J Cancer Chemother 1994;21:547–550.
62. Niikura H, Koizumi T, Ito K, et al. Carboplatin-based chemotherapy in patients with gynecological malignancies on long-term dialysis. Anti-Cancer Drugs 2003;14:735–738.
63. Chatelut E, Rostaing L, Gualano V, et al. Pharmacokinetics of carboplatin in a patient suffering from advanced ovarian carcinoma with hemodialysis-dependent renal insufficiency. Nephron 1994;66:157–161.
64. Watanabe M, Aoki Y, Tomita M, et al. Paclitaxel and carboplatin combination chemotherapy in a hemodialysis patient with advanced ovarian cancer. Gynecol Oncol 2002;84(2):335–338.
65. Furuya Y, Takihana Y, Araki I, et al. Pharmacokinetics of paclitaxel and carboplatin in a hemodialysis patient with metastatic urothelial carcinoma—a case report (Japanese). Gan To Kagaku Ryoho 2003;7:1017–1020.
66. Weirnik PH, Schwartz ELLL, Strauman JJ, et al. Phase I clinical and pharmacokinetic study of taxol. Cancer Res 1987;47: 2486–2493.
67. Longnecker SM, Donehower RC, Cates AE, et al. High performance liquid chromatographic assay for taxol in human plasma and urine pharmacokinetics in a phase I trial. Cancer Treat Rep 1987;71:53–59.
68. Woo MH, Greggornik D, Shearer PD, et al. Pharmacokinetics of paclitaxel in an anephric patient. Cancer Chemother Pharmacol 1999;43:92–96.
69. Tomita M, Kurata H, Aoki Y, et al. Pharmacokinetics of paclitaxel and cisplatin in a hemodialysis patient with recurrent ovarian cancer. Anti-Cancer Drugs 2001;12:485–487.
70. Kamizuru M, Iwata H, Terada T, et al. Chemotherapy in hemodialysis patient with metastatic testicular cancer; pharmacokinetics of etoposide and cisplatin. Nippon Hinyokika Gakkai Zasshi 2000;91:599–603.
71. Tokunaga J, Kikukawa H, Nishi K, et al. Pharmacokinetics of cisplatin and methotrexate in a patient suffering from advanced ureteral tumor accompanied by chronic renal failure, undergoing combined hemodialysis and systemic M-VAC chemotherapy. Gan To Kagaku Ryoho 2000;27:2079–2085.
72. Cho H, Imada T, Masudo K, et al. Combined 5-FU and CDDP in a gastric cancer patient undergoing hemodialysis-pharmacokinetics of 5-FU and CDDP. Gan To Kagaku Ryoho 2000;27:2135–2138
73. Obana T, Tanio Y, Takenaka M, et al. Chemotherapy for small-cell lung cancer (SCLC) patients with renal failure. Gan To Kagaku Ryoho 2002;29:435–438.
74. Chan KK, Chlebowski RT, Tong M, et al. Clinical Pharmacokinetics of Adriamycin in Hepatoma Patients with Cirrhosis. Cancer Res 1980;40:1263–1268.
75. Johnson PJ, Dobbs N, Kalayci C, et al. Clinical efficacy and toxicity of standard dose Adriamycin in hyperbilirubinemic patients with hepatocellular carcinoma—relation to liver tests and pharmacokinetic parameters. Br J Cancer 1992;65:751–755.
76. Hong R-L, Tseng Y-L, Chang F-H. Pegylated liposomal doxorubicin in treating a case of advanced hepatocellular carcinoma with severe hepatic dysfunction and pharmacokinetic study. Ann Oncol 2000;22:349–353.
77. Daniele B, De Vivo R, Perrone F, et al. Phase I Clinical Trial of Liposomal Daunorubicin in Hepatocellular Carcinoma Complicating Liver Cirrhosis. Anticancer Research. 2000;20:1249–1252.

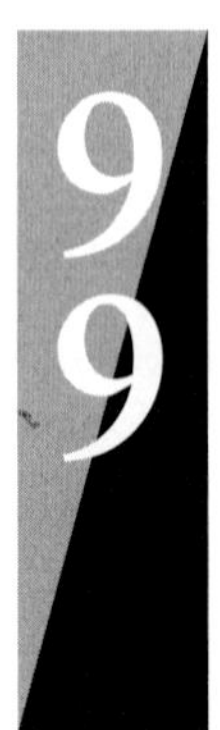

Management of the Pregnant Cancer Patient

Deepjot Singh and Paula Silverman

One in every 1,000 pregnant women will be diagnosed with cancer.[1] Despite this fact, the level of evidence-based medicine[2] available in the field of cancer during pregnancy is low. Randomized controlled trials in this area do not exist. Instead, retrospective collections of patients treated with varying treatment regimens and strategies, collected case reports, studies based on events, such as the Japanese atomic bomb experience, and, for rare malignancies, isolated case reports generally constitute the medical literature on pregnancy and cancer. Nonetheless, this chapter may guide oncologists facing patients in this relatively uncommon, but serious position. We discuss the use of the major diagnostic and treatment modalities in oncology during pregnancy: surgery, diagnostic imaging and therapeutic radiation, and antineoplastic agents. Therapeutic strategies for malignancies seen most frequently during pregnancy are addressed: these include breast cancer, cancer of the uterine cervix, Hodgkin's disease, and non-Hodgkin's lymphoma. Medical management of symptoms of malignancy and its treatment that are unique to the pregnant patient are discussed.

Cancer is the second leading cause of death in women between the ages of 20 and 39, following closely behind accidents.[3] The most frequent cancer deaths in this age group are cancers of the breast, lung, colon, and rectum, leukemia, and nervous system cancers. Because of differences between incidence and mortality, the malignancies seen most often in conjunction with pregnancy are lymphoma, leukemia, melanoma, and cancers of the breast, cervix, ovary, thyroid, and colon.[1] Evidence does not support an increased incidence of cancer during pregnancy. The coincidence of pregnancy and cancer does not influence the biology of cancer, nor does it worsen the prognosis of cancer, except when it delays diagnosis or alters therapy. No firm data exist supporting a greater likelihood of a previously treated cancer relapsing during pregnancy. Cancer itself rarely affects the fetus, with only rare reports of placental metastases or fetal malignancy.[4] The impact on mother and fetus may, however, be profound. Diagnostic and therapeutic interventions that are selected may affect the fetus and may even include terminating the pregnancy. Delays in diagnosis or alterations in treatment based on the coincidence of cancer and pregnancy may affect maternal outcome.

The optimal management of a cancer associated with pregnancy requires cooperation and collaboration with a multidisciplinary team that may include obstetricians, gynecologists, medical and radiation oncologists, surgeons, neonatologists, psychologists, nurses, and social workers. It demands intensive interaction between the patient and her care team, and increases the burden of education of the patient and her family members. *Ideally*, a desired pregnancy will continue without fetal injury or interruption, with delivery of a normal infant at term. *Ideally*, the mother will receive optimal cancer treatment without delay. Balancing these ideals and making reasonable compromises constitute the crux of medical decision making when cancer is diagnosed during pregnancy.

The management of malignancy in the pregnant woman depends on factors including the type of cancer, its stage, maternal and fetal prognosis, and the week of gestation.[5] The need for therapy may be deemed "relative" or "absolute" depending on the urgency of treatment with regard to maternal well-being. Figure 99.1 illustrates one author's overview of potential therapeutic choices.[5] With some malignancies (e.g., low-grade lymphoma), treatment may be delayed until week 24 of gestation or longer, when early cesarean section or cancer therapy can be more safely performed. In other cases (e.g., acute leukemia), delay will endanger the mother's life. Diagnosis early in pregnancy of a life-threatening malignancy requires consideration of therapeutic abortion and careful assessment of treatment-related risks to the fetus. Diagnosis in late trimesters may allow treatment during pregnancy with less fetal risk.

Use of Specific Treatment Modalities in Pregnant Patients

Surgery During Pregnancy

Surgical interventions and procedures may be indicated for cancer diagnosis, staging, or treatment. For the most part, uncomplicated surgery or anesthetic procedures do not increase the risk of an adverse pregnancy outcome.

Although primarily nononcologic, the largest report and analysis of surgical and anesthetic risk to pregnancy is from the Swedish Birth Registry.[6] The authors found increases in perinatal morbidity associated with nonobstetric surgery during pregnancy. The significant adverse outcomes were low birth weight and increased early infant mortality. The authors concluded that the morbidity was most likely attributable to the disease prompting surgery, rather than the adverse effects of surgery or anesthesia. An updated report by the same group[7] linked three Swedish healthcare registries and reviewed outcomes after surgery during pregnancy. They

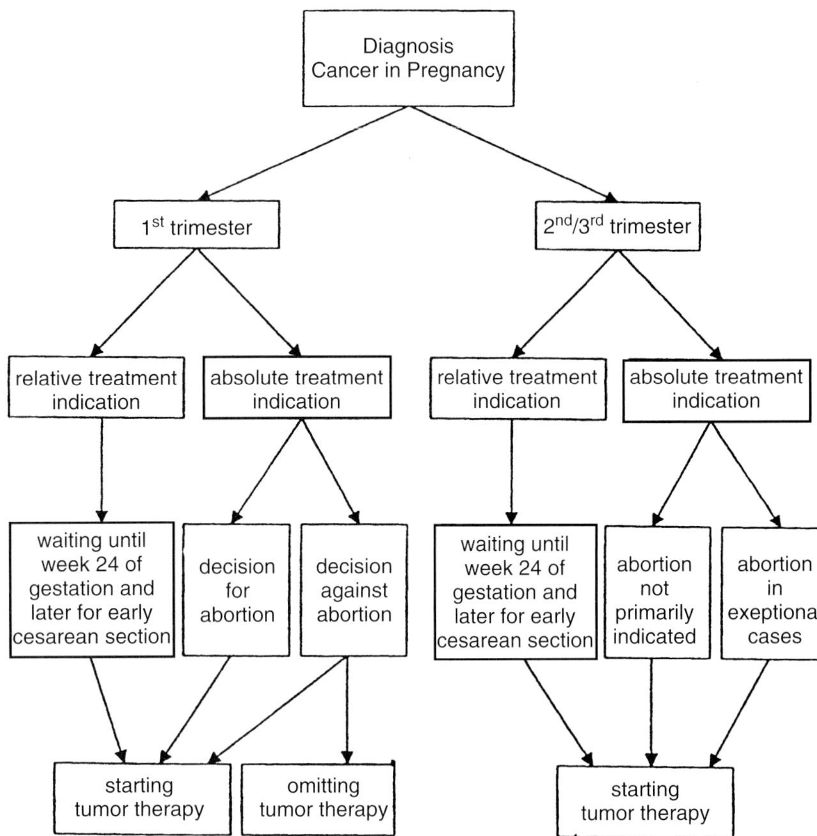

FIGURE 99.1. Potential treatment options during different stages of pregnancy. For Oduncu et al.,[5] the distinction between the terms *absolute* and *relative* treatment indication refers to the therapeutic necessity with regards to the mother's well-being. (From Oduncu et al.,[5] by permission of *Journal of Cancer Research and Clinical Oncology*.)

found that offspring of mothers who had undergone surgery in the first trimester had increased neural tube defects (6 versus expected number, 2.5). The significance of this finding is greater because five of the six mothers with affected offspring had surgery during the fourth or fifth week of gestation, the period of neural tube formation. However, the association between neural tube defects and maternal surgery during the period of neural tube formation was thought by the authors to be unclear and hypothetical.

Based on these findings, Sylvester et al.[8] used the Atlanta Birth Defects Registry to do a population-based case control study that evaluated whether general anesthesia exposure during the first trimester of pregnancy is associated with increased central nervous system defects (Table 99.1). They found a strong association between exposure and the combination of hydrocephalus and eye defects. The limitation of this study is the self-reporting of anesthesia exposure, which is subject to recall bias.

Laparotomy during pregnancy has become safer in recent years. In 1987, Kort et al.[9] reported a fetal death rate of 3.8% after major intraabdominal or extraabdominal surgery, with no postoperative fetal deaths after 60 laparotomies. This result was comparable to a fetal death rate of 2% in pregnancy controls not undergoing surgery, and superior to studies from the 1960s and 1970s, where the fetal wastage after surgery was four to six times higher.[10] However, in Kort's study, premature deliveries were 21.8% after major surgery, twice the rate seen in controls.[9] Another series, reported by Duncan and

TABLE 99.1. Association between multiple central nervous system defects and first-trimester exposure to general anesthesia: Atlanta Birth Defects Case-Control Study, 1968–1990.

	N	*Exposed number (%)*	*Odds ratio*	*95% confidence interval (CI)*
Mothers of control infants	2,846	32 (1.1)	1.0	Reference
Mothers of infants with central nervous system defects	204	7 (3.4)	2.9	1.2, 6.8
Neural tube defects	70	0 (0.0)	0.0	0.0, 4.0
Microcephaly	41	0 (0.0)	0.0	0.0, 7.0
Hydrocephalus				
All	70	7 (10.0)	9.6	3.8, 24.6
Eye defects	8	3 (37.5)	39.6	7.5, 209.2
Cataracts	2	2 (100.0)	Infinity	1,329, infinity

Source: From Sylvester et al.,[8] by permission of *American Journal of Public Health*.

colleagues in 1986,[11] compared 2,565 pregnant women who underwent surgery with pregnant controls who did not. No increase in congenital anomalies was observed. The greatest risk of spontaneous preterm birth or pregnancy occurred with intraabdominal surgery, especially in the presence of infection.

Laparoscopy is a safe surgical option during pregnancy. It has been used for the exploration and treatment of adnexal masses, cholecystectomy, and appendectomy. Reedy et al.[12] used the Swedish Birth Registry to study the impact of laparoscopy on pregnancy. They compared the outcomes of more than 2 million pregnancies, of whom 2,181 had laparoscopy and 1,522 had laparotomy. Nearly all the laparoscopic procedures were in the first trimester, whereas the laparotomies were evenly distributed throughout, with fewer in weeks 32 to 40. The authors found an increased risk of low birth weight infants, preterm delivery, and fetal growth retardation in the operative group compared to pregnancies without surgery. However, there was no increased risk when laparoscopy was compared with laparotomy.

Fine-needle aspiration, core needle, or excisional biopsy under local anesthesia pose essentially no risk to the fetus.[5,13] Modified radical mastectomies have been performed during pregnancy without fetal compromise or preterm labor.[14] Mastectomy with axillary dissection is considered the treatment of choice for operable breast cancer in the pregnant woman.[14,15] Breast reconstruction should be delayed until after delivery.

Antineoplastic Agents During Pregnancy

Drug metabolism is altered by several mechanisms during pregnancy.[4,16] Delayed gastric emptying during late pregnancy may alter the rate of oral drug absorption. Plasma volume increases by approximately 50%, allowing a greater space for drug dilution. Plasma unbound drug concentration is altered as albumin concentration decreases and plasma protein levels increase. Both the hepatic drug metabolism and glomerular filtration rate increase during pregnancy. It is unknown whether the amniotic fluid acts as a functional third space. These changes may alter the narrow therapeutic window of cancer chemotherapy and potentially have an impact on its efficacy.

Before the thalidomide disaster of the early 1960s, the placenta was believed to be an effective barrier, protecting the fetus from drugs given to the mother.[17] Placental transfer is now understood to depend on maternal metabolism, protein binding and storage, molecular size, electrical charge, and lipid solubility.[18] Many antineoplastic agents share properties that permit placental transfer. Because of immaturity of the fetal metabolic and excretory processes, drugs that do cross the placenta may cause severe toxicity in the fetus.

A brief review of fetal development[18] underscores the potential effects of chemotherapy on the fetus. The first phase of gestation is preimplantation, occurring in the first 2 weeks following conception. Administration of chemotherapy during this time period may cause spontaneous abortion. All major organs and organ systems are formed during the period of organogenesis in the second to eighth week of gestation (first trimester). Most congenital malformations caused by drugs occur because of injury during this critical period. Although the development of many organ systems is completed during this period, the nervous system, eye, respiratory, and hematopoietic systems continue to develop throughout gestation. These systems may continue to be susceptible to damage from antineoplastic agents. The final phase of fetal development is characterized by growth and maturation of tissues, beginning with the third month of pregnancy. Growth retardation and low birth weight are the major effects of insults from drugs or disease during this period.

A birth defect is defined as a major deviation from normal morphology or function that is congenital in origin. Birth defects are common, and 3% of children born in the United States have a birth defect.[18] A teratogen is any agent that acts during embryonic or fetal development to produce a permanent alteration of form or function. Only 10% of malformations identified at birth are caused by teratogens.

The U.S. Food and Drug Administration (FDA) developed a rating system to provide guidance to drug use during pregnancy. In this system, drugs are divided into five categories depending on the fetal risk demonstrated in animal or human studies. A summary of these categories is provided in Table 99.2. Most antineoplastic drugs are classified as category D, drugs that have fetal risk, but benefit is thought to outweigh these risks. Updates to the FDA ratings are somewhat slow, and information that is more current may be obtained through online services, such as reprotox (http://reprotox.org).

Much of the medical literature on chemotherapy during pregnancy consists of retrospective series of patients with varying diseases treated with different multidrug regimens at times throughout pregnancy. Only limited information exists on outcomes of children exposed to chemotherapy in utero. For example, one of the larger series is that of Aviles et al.[19] The authors reported a series from Mexico, examining the growth and development of 43 children of mothers treated with chemotherapy during pregnancy. The mothers had hematologic malignancies and were treated with a variety of antineoplastic agents. Drug exposure for the leukemia patients included combinations of vincristine, prednisone, doxorubicin, 6-mercaptopurine, methotrexate, cyclophosphamide, busulfan, and cytosine arabinoside. Lymphoma patients were given cyclophosphamide, doxorubicin, vincristine, and prednisone (CHOP), or CHOP with bleomycin, some with the addition of etoposide and methotrexate. Hodgkin's disease patients were given mechlorethamine

TABLE 99.2. U.S. Food and Drug Administration (FDA) classification of therapeutic agents based on fetal risk.

Category A	Drugs have shown no fetal risks in controlled studies in humans
Category B	Drugs do not show fetal risks in animal studies but human studies do not exist; or adverse effects have been demonstrated in animals but not in well-controlled human studies
Category C	No adequate animal or human studies, or there are adverse fetal effects in animal studies but no available human data
Category D	Fetal risk present, but benefits are thought to outweigh these risks
Category X	Drugs for which the proven fetal risks clearly outweigh any benefits

Source: From Briggs et al.,[15] by permission of Lippincott, Wilkins & Williams, 2002.

(nitrogen mustard), vincristine, prednisone, and procarbazine (MOPP), or doxorubicin, bleomycin, vinblastine, and dacarbazine (ABVD) or a combination of both. Nineteen of the 43 mothers received treatment during the first trimester. Children were examined from ages 3 to 19 for physical, neurologic, psychologic, hematologic, and immune functions and cytogenetics. All children were found to be normal, leading the authors to conclude that chemotherapy during pregnancy, including the first trimester, is safe. In another report, Reynoso and colleagues reported the effects of intrapartum combination chemotherapy for acute leukemia in seven children.[20] The drugs used included vincristine, cytarabine, prednisone, cyclophosphamide, 6-thioguanine, and daunorubicin. With a follow-up interval ranging from 1 to 17 years, growth and development were reported as normal. No evidence of malignancy was found in any of the seven children.

Other authors do not concur with Aviles or Reynoso, and chemotherapy is generally avoided during the first trimester of pregnancy to reduce the risk of fetal loss and teratogenesis. In a retrospective review of 217 pregnant women treated with a variety of systemic therapies, there were 2 spontaneous abortions, 1 stillbirth, and 3 infants born with congenital anomalies. The majority of complications occurred when the chemotherapy was administered during the first trimester.[21] During the second or third trimester, there does not appear to be an increased risk of teratogenesis. However, there is a risk of central nervous system or other major organ toxicity and intrauterine growth retardation, and the potential for premature labor.[22] The timing of chemotherapy given late in pregnancy should be coordinated to avoid delivery during the nadir in the mother's blood count. This practice reduces the fetal risk of myelosuppression with resultant infectious complications or hemorrhage from thrombocytopenia.

Specific Antineoplastic Agents in Pregnancy

Cyclophosphamide and Other Alkylating Agents

The alkylating agents, such as busulfan, chlorambucil, cyclophosphamide, and nitrogen mustard, show a rate of fetal malformation of approximately 13% with first-trimester exposure, compared with 4% with exposure in the later trimesters.[16] Cyclophosphamide may inflict a chemical insult on developing fetal tissues, resulting in cell death and heritable DNA alterations in surviving cells.[18] Anomalies of the extremities, including absent toes and fingers, palatal grooves and other facial abnormalities, microcephaly, and hernias have been attributed to cyclophosphamide exposure in early pregnancy.[23] Later in pregnancy, the drug is without significant reported fetal abnormalities and can therefore be given during the second and third trimester.[15,18] Growth retardation has been reported with cyclophosphamide late in pregnancy.[24] The use of busulfan in pregnancy has been linked to a variety of fetal abnormalities.[15] The use of chlorambucil during pregnancy has been associated with both normal and abnormal outcomes.[15]

Methotrexate and Other Antimetabolites

Methotrexate is a folic acid antagonist; exposure to this drug during pregnancy is associated with fetal loss and a distinct pattern of fetal abnormalities. The principal features of the abnormalities include growth restriction, failure of calvarial ossification, craniosynostosis, hypoplastic supraorbital ridges, micrognathia, and external ear and severe limb abnormalities.[18] Methotrexate crosses the placenta[15]and has been found in cord serum and fetal red cells. Inhibition of dihydrofolate reductase in fetal tissues is thought to be responsible for methotrexate-induced embryopathy.[25] Feldcamp and Carey stress that in cases of inadvertent methotrexate exposure during unanticipated pregnancy, it is important to define the period of drug exposure and the dose to avoid an unnecessary recommendation for abortion of a potentially healthy fetus.[26] The critical period of exposure to this drug appears to be weeks 6 through 8 from conception, with a teratogenic dose probably above 10 mg per week.[26]

Other antimetabolites, such as 5-fluoruracil and cytosine arabinoside are less frequently associated with malformations.[16] Although hydroxyurea is teratogenic in animals, no fetal abnormalities have been observed in 13 human pregnancies that resulted in live infants when the drug was used to treat maternal disease.[15]

Doxorubicin and Other Antitumor Antibiotics

Bleomycin, doxorubicin, dactinomycin, and daunorubicin infrequently cause fetal abnormalities. Doxorubicin has been used in breast cancer patients during second and third trimesters with infrequent adverse outcome.[14,27] A number of reports support the use of anthracycline-based chemotherapy in pregnancy, but patients should be informed that long-term follow-up data on large numbers of children exposed to chemotherapy in utero are not available.[28] No reports have linked bleomycin use with congenital defects in humans.[15] In six pregnancies, dactinomycin was administered in the second and third trimesters with delivery of normal infants.[15]

Other Chemotherapeutic Agents

Cisplatin use has been reported infrequently in pregnancy, but no fetal abnormalities have been identified.[15] Vinca alkaloids (vincristine, vinorelbine, and vinblastine) have been associated with fetal abnormalities, spontaneous abortions, and low birth weight.[15] Asparaginase use during pregnancy is limited, but it has been reported in combination with other agents.[15] In six cases of exposure during the second trimester, no fetal abnormalities were noted.[15] Two infants did suffer drug-induced bone marrow suppression.

The safety of the taxanes in pregnancy is unknown. The use of paclitaxel and docetaxel during pregnancy is limited to isolated case reports and case series.[29–31] In rats, the use of paclitaxel in early pregnancy has been associated with craniofacial malformations, diaphragmatic hernias, and kidney and cardiovascular defects.[29] The taxanes have been used mainly as part of combination chemotherapy regimens in the treatment of breast cancer and gynecologic cancers. Gaducci et al.[32] used sequential epirubicin with paclitaxel from the 14th to 32nd weeks of gestation with no reported side effects in the patients or the fetus and normal development and growth at 36 months of follow-up. De Santis et al.[30] reported the use of docetaxel in the treatment of metastatic breast cancer in a pregnant patient during the second trimester. No adverse effects were noted in either the patient or the infant. Sood et al.[29] used cisplatin and paclitaxel in the case of a pregnant woman with advanced ovarian epithelial cancer with resultant maternal neutropenia. Similarly, Méndez et al.[31]

reported the use of combined paclitaxel and carboplatin in a woman with Stage IIIc ovarian cancer without any adverse effects on the infant.

Immunomodulating Agents

Interferon Alpha

Interferon alpha is a family of similar subtypes of immunomodulating human proteins and glycoproteins. Interferon alpha does not appear to transfer across the placenta to the fetus. There are reports describing the use of interferon alpha in all phases of pregnancy without adverse fetal outcome.[15] This agent is not thought to pose a significant risk when used during pregnancy. Interferon alpha is a class C agent.

Thalidomide

The evidence implicating thalidomide as a teratogen is overwhelming. In pregnant women, exposure to even a single dose, from the 20th to the 35th day after conception, produced a unique syndrome characterized principally by deformities of the arms, legs and face, often with other more widespread abnormalities.[17]

Thalidomide was unavailable until recently, when applications for it were found in the immunomodulation of patients with neoplastic and immunologic diseases.[33,34] Thalidomide has shown activity in the treatment of multiple myeloma and other lymphoproliferative and myeloproliferative disorders, malignant melanoma, glioblastoma multiforme, and renal cell carcinoma. Thalidomide is contraindicated throughout pregnancy. Its use is additionally prohibited by the manufacturer in women of childbearing age who are not using two reliable methods of contraception for 1 month before starting therapy, during therapy, and 1 month after stopping therapy.[35] Special precautions are taken in labeling and distribution to be sure no women of childbearing potential are exposed to thalidomide.[36]

Monoclonal Antibodies

Limited information exists regarding the use of monoclonal antibodies, such as trastuzumab or rituximab in malignancy associated with pregnancy. However, immunoglobulins appear safe and several are indicated for conditions occurring in pregnancy.[15] Intramuscular immunoglobulin is recommended for postexposure prophylaxis for hepatitis A and measles.[37] Intravenous immunoglobulin is indicated in pregnancy for common variable immunodeficiency and in autoimmune diseases, such as immune thrombocytopenia and alloimmune diseases, such as severe Rh immunization.[38] Immunoglobulin crosses the human placenta if the gestational age is greater than 32 weeks.

Trastuzumab is a recombinant DNA-derived humanized monoclonal antibody that selectively binds to the extracellular domain of the human epidermal growth factor receptor 2 protein, HER2. Trastuzumab has proven efficacy in HER-2-overexpressing metastatic breast cancer both as a single agent and in combination with chemotherapeutic agents.[39] Trastuzumab is classified as a category B drug, having shown no adverse effects when tested in monkeys during pregnancy.[40] However, the HER2 protein expression is high in many embryonic tissues in early gestation.[41] Placental transfer of trastuzumab has been observed in monkeys.[40] There are no adequate or well-controlled studies in pregnant women.

Rituximab is a genetically engineered chimeric murine/human antibody directed against the CD20 antigen found on the surface of normal and malignant B lymphocytes.[42] Rituximab is indicated for the treatment of patients with CD20-positive, B-cell non-Hodgkin's lymphoma, and is used as a single agent and in conjunction with chemotherapy. Rituximab has efficacy in both indolent and aggressive lymphomas. Recent studies have demonstrated efficacy in a variety of other B-cell-mediated disorders.[43] Rituximab is classified as a category C drug because animal studies in pregnancy have not been performed.[42] It is not known whether rituximab can cause fetal harm when administered to a pregnant woman or whether it can affect reproductive capacity. A concern is that because human immunoglobulin is known to pass the placental barrier, rituximab could potentially cause fetal B-cell depletion.

Hormonal Agents

Tamoxifen is a selective estrogen receptor-modulating agent that acts primarily as an antiestrogen but has some estrogenic properties. There are limited data pertaining to human fetal exposure. In a reported case in which tamoxifen was inadvertently used in all three trimesters, the fetus was born with a syndrome of ambiguous genitalia.[15,21] Because of its long half-life, women should be informed that a pregnancy occurring within 8 weeks of stopping the drug could expose the fetus to tamoxifen.

Other hormonal agents primarily used to treat breast cancer include gonadotropin-releasing hormone agonists, aromatase inhibitors (e.g., letrozole, anastrazole, and exemestane), and progestins, primarily megestrol acetate. The gonadotropin-releasing hormone agonist leuprolide may theoretically cause spontaneous abortions because it suppresses endometrial proliferation. Its manufacturer maintains a registry of inadvertent human exposures during pregnancy and, with more than 100 cases reported, has found no congenital defects attributable to the drug.[15] However, the numbers of cases are too few to draw conclusions regarding safety or risk. Aromatase inhibitors are recommended only for postmenopausal women, as they act by preventing the peripheral conversion of circulating androgens to estrogen. No information is available regarding their use in pregnancy. All progestins have had an FDA-mandated deletion of pregnancy-related indications because of a possible association with congenital abnormalities.[15] Cases of ambiguous genitalia have been reported to the FDA, and a paired analysis of first-trimester fetal exposure has shown an increase in cardiovascular defects and hypospadias.[15]

Prednisone and other corticosteroids are widely used in treatment regimens for leukemia, lymphoma, and Hodgkin's disease. They appear to pose only small risks to the fetus, but may increase the incidence of orofacial clefts.[15] The risk is greatest in the first trimester.

Ionizing Radiation and Diagnostic Imaging During Pregnancy

Ionizing radiation techniques are used during pregnancy both for diagnosis and staging of cancer and as a treatment modality. Ionizing radiation refers to waves or particles of sufficient energy to break chemical bonds, such as those in DNA, or

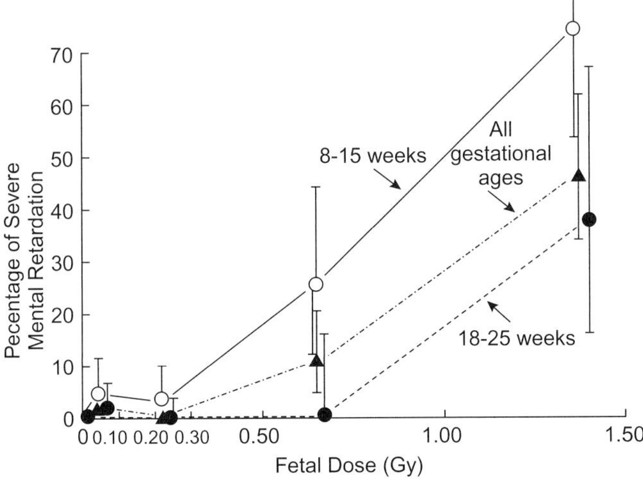

FIGURE 99.2. Effects of ionizing radiation on severe mental retardation in fetuses exposed at various gestational ages to the atomic bomb in Hiroshima and Nagasaki (1 Gy = 100 rad). The *bar lines* represent 90%. (From Sacher and King,[38] by permission of *Obstetrical & Gynecological Survey*.)

create free radicals that can cause tissue damage. The potential harmful effects on a fetus from ionizing radiation exposure are (1) cell death, affecting embryogenesis, (2) growth restriction, (3) congenital malformation, (4) carcinogenesis, (5) microcephaly and neonatal mental retardation, and (6) sterility.[44] Much of the pertinent research has been performed in animals. Human data have been obtained largely from studies of atomic bomb survivors from Hiroshima and Nagasaki.

Significant radiation exposure during preimplantation, the period in human development corresponding to the first 9 or 10 days after conception, results in prenatal death.[45] Preimplantation is the most sensitive time with respect to fetal death from radiation. Mouse and rat studies constitute the bulk of evidence for prenatal or neonatal death caused by ionizing radiation.[46,47] The consequences of radiation of the fetus during the period of major organogenesis may include teratogenic effects on various organs, as shown in many experimental animal studies.[45] In humans, effects on the central nervous system are the best documented. Japanese atomic bomb survivors irradiated in utero show an increased risk of microcephaly and severe mental retardation with high prenatal exposure. The risk is greatest at 8 to 15 weeks of gestation, with even very low doses causing a slight increase in the risk of mental retardation. As shown in Figure 99.2, this risk is probably a nonthreshold linear function of dose, with the risk of severe mental retardation being as low as 4% for 10 cGy and as high as 60% 150 cGy.[44,48] After 16 weeks, the risk is less, and there is no proven risk between 0 to 8 weeks or after 25 weeks. Fortunately, 10 cGy is many times higher than exposure seen from diagnostic radiation.

It is controversial whether there is an association between in utero diagnostic radiation exposure and an increased risk of childhood cancers. Some investigators have found an increased risk of leukemia and other cancers; others have not.[18] A major positive study used concordance data on twins exposed to diagnostic X-rays in utero; this led to a finding by the National Research Council Committee on Biological Effects of Ionizing Radiation to conclude that there is an association, with the estimated risk per unit absorbed dose to be about 200 to 250 excess cancer deaths per 10,000 person-Gy in the first 10 years of life.[49] Animal studies suggest that there are late-occurring cancers following prenatal exposure, but long-term studies of atomic bomb survivors are not available.[44] Retardation of growth has also been shown over a broad range of gestational ages in animal models and in humans.[49]

Diagnostic Imaging

How then, do the doses of radiation delivered during a single exam or series of diagnostic X-rays compare with those doses that increase the risk of the effects discussed previously? Which of our diagnostic procedures involves exposure to ionizing radiation? Imaging modalities, including ultrasound, magnetic resonance imaging (MRI), and X-rays, are all used as adjuncts to the diagnosis and staging of cancer in pregnancy. Most diagnostic imaging procedures, even those involving X-rays, are associated with little or no known fetal risks. Fetal anomalies, growth restriction, or abortions are not increased with radiation exposure of less than 5 cGy, which is above the range of exposure for diagnostic procedures.[50] The estimated fetal exposure from common radiologic procedures that involve ionizing radiation is summarized in Table 99.3. The uterus should be shielded for nonpelvic procedures during pregnancy.

Nuclear studies are performed by *tagging* a chemical agent with a radioisotope for tests, such as pulmonary ventilation-perfusion, thyroid, and bone scans. Bone scans that use technetium (^{99m}Tc) result in a fetal exposure of less than 0.5 cGy.[51] One of the more common nuclear medicine studies performed during pregnancy is the ventilation-perfusion scan for suspected pulmonary embolism. Both intravenous ^{99m}Tc and inhaled xenon gas are used. Nonetheless, in total, the fetal exposure is approximately 0.05 cGy.[51] Radioactive iodine readily crosses the placenta and can adversely affect the fetal thyroid, especially after 10 to 12 weeks of gestation. If a diagnostic scan of the thyroid is essential, ^{123}I or ^{99m}Tc should be used instead of ^{131}I.[51]

Ultrasound uses sound waves and is not a form of ionizing radiation. Ultrasound appears to present minimal or no

TABLE 99.3. Estimated fetal exposure from common radiologic procedures.

Procedure	*Fetal exposure (cGy)*
Chest X-ray (two views)	0.00002–0.00007
Abdominal film (single view)	0.1
Intravenous pyelogram	≥1[a]
Hip film (single view)	0.2
Mammography	0.007–0.02
Barium enema or small bowel series	2–4
CT scan of head or chest	<1
CT scan of abdomen and lumbar spine	3.5
CT pelvimetry	0.25

CT, computed tomography.

[a] Exposure depends on number of films.

Source: Adapted from Committee on Obstetric Practice, American College of Obstetricians and Gynecologists. *Guidelines for Diagnostic Imaging During Pregnancy*. Washington, DC: Copyright Clearance Center, 1995:158.

risks to the fetus,[50] and there are no contraindications to ultrasound procedures during pregnancy.[51] MRI employs magnets that alter the energy state of hydrogen protons to create diagnostic images. No documented adverse effects to the fetus have been reported. MRI has been proven useful for evaluation of maternal pelvic masses.[51] Noncontrasted MRI can be used for detection of liver metastases in several malignancies. However, it is thought that there are insufficient data on fetal safety during the first trimester of pregnancy.[52]

There are no known adverse effects to the fetus from use of either ionic or nonionic intravenous contrast media used in computerized tomography.[53] Iodinated contrast agents have not been studied in pregnant women. Gadolinium-based contrast medium used for MRI is not recommended for use during pregnancy. Gadolinium crosses the placenta, is filtered through the fetal kidneys, and then reingested through the amniotic fluid.[53]

Therapeutic Radiation

Experience is greatest with therapeutic radiation used to treat cervical cancer, breast cancer, and Hodgkin's disease. Alternatives to radiation therapy during pregnancy should always be sought, recalling that fetal radiation doses above 10cGy increase the risk of malformations and nervous system damage during organogenesis. Options include delaying treatment until after fetal maturity to allow safer delivery, abortion, or alternative treatment that may include surgery or chemotherapy. If no alternatives exist that do not compromise maternal prognosis, radiation therapy may be used during pregnancy. The risk falls if treatment is delayed until fetal maturity passes the period of organogenesis (through week 8 of development). Risk to the developing nervous system appears to extend through the early and midfetal stages of development.

Radiation therapy for cancer generally uses a man-made source of ionizing radiation, including the linear accelerator, radioisotope, cyclotron, or nuclear reactor. Whatever the source of ionizing radiation, the pathway to both cellular damage and treatment effectiveness is through ionization of matter. The effects of cellular damage vary from none, when damage is repaired, to mutagenesis, carcinogenesis, or cell death. The benefits of radiation therapy are always balanced against the risk of ionization of normal tissues. These concerns also exist when the developing fetus is considered. The period of fetal development during which the conceptus is radiated, the dosage of ionizing radiation received, and the type of radiation given modify the risk.

Medical physicists must perform a fetal dose estimate before initiation of radiation therapy. Dose is estimated to the fundus, pubic symphysis, and umbilicus.[54] Dose measurements are repeated following modification of the treatment plan or application of appropriate shielding. Modifications of standard treatment plans to reduce fetal dose include using the smallest field possible, and minimizing the lead blocking and eliminating wedges used for field shaping as these increase radiation scatter. Collimating the field as close to the patient as possible, selecting photon energy between 4 and 10MV, directing field angles away from the pelvis, and minimizing the use of and field size of portal films all decrease the fetal dose.[47] Additional techniques include shielding by placing heavy lead barriers above and below the abdomen and pelvis. Several designs have been published; each allows fetal dose reduction as well as patient and therapist safety.

Management and Outcome of Specific Malignancies During Pregnancy

Breast Cancer

Breast cancer is the second most common cancer in pregnant, lactating, or postpartum women, with an incidence of 1 in 3,000 pregnancies. The median age at diagnosis is between 32 and 38 years.[55] The incidence of pregnancy-associated breast cancer is projected to increase as more women choose to delay childbearing into their forties, a reflection of the increased incidence of breast cancer with advancing age.[56] One study suggested a genetic predisposition to pregnancy-associated breast cancer, as the authors found that 80% of these patients had allelic deletion and loss of heterozygosity at the hereditary BRCA2 locus compared with 20% of patients with sporadic breast cancer.[57]

During pregnancy, marked lobuloalveolar growth in the breast results in engorgement and hypertrophy. The resultant dense, multinodular consistency of breast tissue makes clinical palpation of masses or thickening difficult, resulting in diagnostic delays.[58] Although 70% to 80% of breast biopsies performed in pregnant women reveal a benign diagnosis, all palpable masses persisting for 2 to 4 weeks warrant evaluation by biopsy.[58] Diagnostic mammography with abdominal shielding can be performed with minimal risk to the fetus, although the test's sensitivity is reduced by the higher density, water content, and loss of contrasting fat in breasts of pregnant or lactating women. Breast sonography is a safe, rapid, and accurate method of differentiating cystic from solid masses during pregnancy.[59] Gupta[60] demonstrated that fine-needle aspiration is highly accurate in the diagnosis of breast lesions in pregnant women. Core-biopsies have rarely resulted in milk-fistula formation.[61] Although breast biopsies can be safely performed during pregnancy, the increased breast vascularity at this time may increase risk of hemorrhage.[62]

Retrospective series have shown that breast cancers detected during pregnancy are larger and have a greater likelihood of nodal involvement than those diagnosed in non-pregnant women. Fifty-six percent of pregnant women have positive axillary lymph nodes compared with 38% to 54% positive nodes in their nonpregnant counterparts.[27] Between 25% and 33% of pregnancy-associated breast cancer is estrogen- and progesterone-receptor positive.[63–65] Overexpression of the human epidermal growth factor receptor, HER2/neu, was seen in 58% of breast cancers in pregnancy compared to 16% in a nonpregnant control group. Higher rates of the markers associated with rapidly proliferating breast cancers, Ki-67 and p53, have been seen in breast cancers associated with pregnancy.[63]

Reported case series have shown that survival in pregnant women is not improved by abortion, and therefore, this is not routinely recommended.[65] Approximately 60% of pregnancy-associated breast cancer is diagnosed in stage I or II (early stage) and should be approached with curative intent. Modified radical mastectomy with axillary lymph node dissection can be performed with minimal risk to the developing fetus during any trimester of pregnancy.[63]

Radiation therapy to the breast is a standard part of breast-conserving therapy. Chest wall radiation is indicated post-mastectomy for patients with large tumors, positive margins, or extensive lymph node involvement. Breast-conserving treatment during pregnancy has been considered contraindicated because mastectomy is equally curative and does not pose a risk to the fetus through radiation therapy.[47,66] However, exceptions to this contraindication exist when radiation therapy can be delayed until after the fetus is delivered. Although delaying radiation raises concern for compromising local control, it is important to remember that a delay of up to 6 months during adjuvant chemotherapy has been found to be associated with maintained disease control.[67] In fact, there was a similar disease-free and overall survival when breast-conserving therapy and mastectomy were compared in early-stage breast cancer diagnosed during pregnancy.[68]

When breast radiation is needed during pregnancy, information to estimate dose received by a fetus from tangential breast irradiation is provided by Mazonakis et al.[69] Using anthropomorphic phantoms, they found that a treatment course delivering 50 Gy to the breast gave an estimated conceptus dose in the first trimester of 2.1 to 7.6 cGy. During the second and third trimesters, the estimated dose increases to 2.2 to 24.6 cGy and 2.2 to 58.6 cGy, respectively. These estimates do not include shielding of the uterus, which would further reduce conceptus dose. The authors suggest that delivered doses would, in many cases, be below the threshold doses that cause adverse effects in the middle fetal period.

Most women with pregnancy-associated breast cancer are candidates for systemic adjuvant chemotherapy, during or after the completion of the pregnancy. If chemotherapy is indicated, it may be delivered preoperatively (neoadjuvant) to more optimally treat the mother for locally advanced disease or to delay exposure to the fetus to the risk of surgery, anesthesia, and/or radiation. Methotrexate is contraindicated in all stages of pregnancy because of its abortifacient effects, teratogenic potential, and delayed elimination from sequestered spaces.[22] Chemotherapy is inadvisable during the first trimester of pregnancy until fetal organogenesis is complete, as there is a substantial risk of fetal loss and teratogenesis. In a retrospective review of 217 pregnant women (14 with breast cancer), treated with a variety of systemic therapies, there were two spontaneous abortions, one stillborn, and three infants born with congenital anomalies. The majority of complications occurred when the chemotherapy was administered during the first trimester.[21] During the second or third trimester, there does not appear to be an increased risk of teratogenesis. However, there is a risk of central nervous system or other major organ toxicity and intrauterine growth retardation, and the potential for premature labor is present.[22]

The combination of doxorubicin, cyclophosphamide, and 5-flurouracil has been evaluated in one prospective trial of 24 women with pregnancy-associated breast cancer at M.D. Anderson Medical Center.[14] Patients were treated in their second and third trimesters with 5-fluorouracil (100 mg/m^2), doxorubicin (50 mg/m^2 continuous infusion over 72 hours), and cyclophosphamide (500 mg/m^2) given every 3 weeks for a median of four cycles. No maternal or fetal deaths were observed. Three patients had preterm labor and 1 patient had severe preeclampsia requiring early delivery. The only complication attributable to chemotherapy occurred after preterm delivery of an infant 2 days after the last chemotherapy dose. The infant had transient leukopenia without infectious complications.

The doxorubicin and cyclophosphamide (AC) combination regimen for 12 weeks is comparable in efficacy to 6 months of CMF (cyclophosphamide, methotrexate, and fluorouracil). The shorter duration and absence of methotrexate in the regimen makes AC safer in the treatment of the pregnant breast cancer patient. Standard doses of AC should be adequate, because this combination is not influenced by distribution into a third space (i.e., ascites, pleural or amniotic fluid).

Women with breast cancer in pregnancy have the same survival as nonpregnant women with breast cancer.[63] In a comparison of 56 pregnant patients and 166 nonpregnant controls, there was no statistically significant difference in survival.[70] The pregnant patients had a 5-year survival rate of 82% when lymph nodes were negative and 47% when positive. However, patients with pregnancy-associated breast cancer had more advanced disease at diagnosis.[70] Other series have shown similar results. Patients with breast cancer diagnosed during pregnancy may do more poorly because they present with more advanced disease.

Cervical Cancer

Invasive carcinoma of the cervix is the most frequent cancer associated with pregnancy in the United States. It occurs in approximately 1 in 2,200 pregnancies,[1] with an average age at diagnosis of 32 years. This rate may be falling because of improved screening leading to treatment of noninvasive lesions. Maternal prognosis in cervical cancer is not altered by pregnancy, but the fetus may suffer morbidity or mortality from treatment.[71] Early diagnosis of cervical cancer in pregnant women is three times more likely than in their non-pregnant counterparts because of the frequent and detailed gynecologic examinations that are a part of routine prenatal care.[72] The majority of women with early cervical cancer are asymptomatic, although a few may report vaginal bleeding, discharge, or pain.[73]

Approximately 5% of all Papanicolaou (Pap) smears are abnormal,[74] usually representing cervical dysplasia. The cytopathologist should be notified that the Pap smear is from a pregnant patient because physiologic changes of pregnancy may alter the pathologist's interpretation.[73] Pregnant women with an abnormal Pap test should undergo colposcopy with punch biopsies to exclude invasive carcinoma.[73,74] Conization is performed to rule out invasion when the colposcopic biopsy shows microinvasive disease or if the procedure is unsatisfactory.[75,76] Conization is safest early in pregnancy. In a minority of patients (3% to 6%), this procedure may be associated with significant bleeding, infection, pregnancy loss, and preterm birth. Patients diagnosed with low- or high-grade dysplasia, carcinoma in situ, or microinvasive squamous carcinoma (up to 3 mm in depth) can be followed to term and allowed to deliver vaginally.[77] Reevaluation and treatment are done at 6 weeks postpartum.

When invasive cervical cancer is diagnosed in the pregnant patient, staging procedures are modified to minimize radiation exposure to the developing fetus. Magnetic resonance imaging is a safe and noninvasive modality to assess tumor extent, volume, and to monitor response to therapy.[78]

The prognosis of early-stage cervical cancer appears similar in pregnant women and nonpregnant controls.[71] Traditionally, if the diagnosis is made before 20 weeks of gestation, immediate radical hysterectomy with pelvic and paraaortic lymphadenectomy is advised to avoid delay in treatment. For women with stage Ia or Ib cancer diagnosed after 20 weeks of gestation, several small series have shown that a delay in therapy of up to 17 weeks to achieve fetal lung maturity is reasonable.[79] In a retrospective series of 27 pregnant women with stage Ia or Ib cervical cancer, 8 patients waited for fetal lung maturity before delivery (mean diagnosis to treatment interval, 144 days). Fetal outcome was good in this group, and all women were disease free 2 years following treatment.[80] No randomized trials have evaluated the benefits of vaginal delivery versus cesarean section in pregnant women with cervical cancer. Jones et al.[81] reported a poorer 5-year cumulative survival with vaginal delivery in comparison with cesarean section (55% versus 75%). In addition, rare recurrences of the cancer at the episiotomy site have been reported following vaginal delivery.[77] For these reasons, cesarean section is the preferred mode of delivery in pregnant women with cervical cancer.[82]

For stage IIb or higher-stage cervical cancer, treatment is limited to radiation therapy. When the fetus is viable, delivery should be performed before the initiation of therapy. If the fetus is not considered viable, external-beam radiation therapy can be started before delivery. Patients will abort 20 to 24 days after the start of the radiation therapy, after a mean dose of 34 to 40 Gy.[79]

Hodgkin's Disease and Non-Hodgkin's Lymphoma

The mean age of patients with Hodgkin's disease (HD) is 27 years, whereas that of those with non-Hodgkin's lymphoma (NHL) is 42 years. The incidence of pregnancy-associated lymphoma, both HD and NHL, is similar and ranges from 1 in 1,000 to 1 in 6,000. Most of the patients are diagnosed at stages II to IV, and on average at 22 weeks of gestation.[83,84] In a series of 48 women with HD, the median age was 26 years, which is similar to other series.[83–85] When matched with nonpregnant controls, there was no significant difference in the clinical presentation of HD.[85] Most pregnant patients present without B symptoms.[83–85]

Several studies have suggested that neither HD nor pregnancy has an independent impact on either condition.[84,86–88] Barry et al.[86] evaluated 347 women with HD and found that the survival curves were similar in pregnant and nonpregnant women. There was no difference in survival between patients who underwent a therapeutic abortion and those who did not.[86] Lishner et al. obtained similar results[85] when cause-specific survival was compared in 33 pregnant women and 67 case-matched controls. No significant effect of age or stage at diagnosis on maternal or pregnancy outcome was seen. Infants did not have a higher risk of premature birth or intrauterine growth retardation. At 25 years of follow-up, 70% of patients were alive. Anselmo et al.[88] also reported that women with HD safely carry their pregnancy to term, giving birth to healthy children.

Most pregnancy-associated NHLs have an aggressive histologic subtype and present with advanced-stage disease.[89–91] In a retrospective review of 96 women with pregnancy-associated NHL, 60% of the patients presented with stage III/IV disease.[92] An unusually high incidence of breast, uterine, cervical, and ovarian involvement is seen and has been attributed to changes in hormones and/or increased blood flow to these organs during pregnancy.[90] Some series report a stable course of the NHL in women while pregnant, followed by rapid progression postpartum.[89,91] Others report a similar response to treatment, failure of treatment, and rate of progression in pregnant and nonpregnant patients. NHL has been reported by some to affect the pregnancy adversely by causing maternal death.[90] Others conclude that NHL does not have an effect on premature birth, spontaneous abortion, or malformations.[91]

Chemotherapy should be avoided when possible during the first trimester. The standard treatment for newly diagnosed HD is ABVD (doxorubicin, bleomycin, vinblastine, and dacarbazine) and for diffuse large B-cell lymphoma is CHOP (cyclophosphamide, doxorubicin, vincristine, and prednisone).[93,94] Treatment of HD and NHL during pregnancy carries risks, but as discussed next, retrospective series substantiate the safety and efficacy of its use.

In reviews of chemotherapy during pregnancy, the incidence of fetal malformations after exposure during the first trimester was about 15%.[22,95] This risk was greatest with alkylating agents and antimetabolites (such as methotrexate) and lowest with vinblastine (1 of 14 first-trimester treated patients). The risk of fetal malformations decreased to 1.3% when chemotherapy was administered during the second or third trimester, which is similar to the 3.1% risk seen in the general population.

In one series of 14 women with HD treated with MOPP and ABVD (5 in the first trimester), all had full-term pregnancy without any congenital anomalies, and 11 remained in complete remission at 3 to 17+ years follow-up.[96] Another 18 women with NHL in the same series received CHOP (9 in the first trimester). No congenital malformations were noted on successful delivery at 35 to 40 weeks.

In a review of 24 pregnant women receiving chemotherapy for HD, Ebert et al.[21] reported multiple fetal anomalies in some but not all of the infants exposed to MOPP (mechlorethamine, vincristine, procarbazine, and prednisone), ABVD, or cyclophosphamide with radiation in utero. In another series, 43 children exposed to chemotherapy during pregnancy were compared to a group of 25 case-control children. Fourteen of the pregnant women with HD received MOPP and/or ABVD (5 during the first trimester). At the time of evaluation, all 43 children, ranging in age from 3 to 19 years, were developmentally normal.[19] Sutcliffe[97] treated three women with stage II nodular sclerosing HD with ABVD chemotherapy during the second and third trimester with normal fetal outcome in all, at 1+, 5+, and 7+ years follow-up.

In a series of 16 pregnant women with HD treated at the M.D. Anderson Cancer Center,[98] 2 patients received involved-field radiation to the neck (3,500 cGy), 3 patients received extended-field radiation to the neck or mediastinum (4,000 cGy), and the remaining 11 patients received full mantle irradiation (4,000 cGy). Four to five half-value layers of lead maximized uterine shielding. It was estimated that the fetal dose was 140 to 550 cGy with 6 MV photons and 10–13.6 cGy for cobalt 60. All offspring were reported as being physically and mentally normal with a 10-year-survival of 83%.

A number of authors have suggested treatment guidelines for pregnancy-associated lymphoma.[44,91,92,99] Patients with HD presenting in the first trimester with B symptoms, bulky disease, advanced stage, or rapid progression require therapy. Therapeutic abortion should be recommended to enable treatment. If the patient desires to continue the pregnancy and is willing to accept the risks of therapy to the fetus and to herself, single-agent vinblastine can be used until disease progression or the second trimester. ABV in the first trimester, followed by ABVD in the second and third trimester, is given if combination chemotherapy is needed. If possible, patients presenting in their second or third trimester should be observed and treatment delayed until postpartum. If treatment is necessary, ABVD is given. Patients with clinical stage IA lymphocyte predominant disease or progression on chemotherapy may be offered mantle radiotherapy with extensive abdominal blocking.

Women with low-grade/indolent lymphomas, relatively normal complete blood counts, and without impending organ compromise may be safely observed until delivery or disease progression. In the aggressive histologic subtypes of NHL, treatment with CHOP should be instituted promptly. Successful treatment of Burkitt's lymphoma requires high-dose methotrexate. Patients presenting with this disease in the first trimester should have a therapeutic abortion.[92]

Symptom Management During Cancer Treatment

A great concern to patients, families, and the care team is which drugs can be used during pregnancy for symptom control. Pain management and control of nausea are as important in the pregnant as the nonpregnant patient. Physicians may need to manage anxiety or depression in young women with a newly diagnosed cancer. Bracken and Holford[100] performed a case-control study of deliveries with ($n = 1{,}427$) and without ($n = 3{,}001$) congenital malformations in Connecticut between 1974 and 1976. They examined prescription drug use in each trimester for cases and controls. Three classes of agents were found associated with congenital malformations when used in the first trimester of pregnancy: narcotic analgesics, tranquilizers, and antidepressants. Antiemetics were not associated with congenital malformations in their study. Recent retrospective and prospective studies have shown that a newer class of antidepressants, that is, the selective serotonin reuptake inhibitors, may be safer than the antidepressants studied previously.[15] Table 99.4 lists many of the drugs commonly used for symptom control in cancer, along with their FDA risk classification.[15]

TABLE 99.4. Drugs used in symptom management by pharmacologic type and FDA fetal risk category.

Anesthetics	Lidocaine (B)
Antihistamines	Chlorpheniramine (B) Cyproheptadine (B) Diphenhydramine (B) Meclizine (B) Promethazine (C)
Analgesics and antipyretics	Acetaminophen (B) Phenacetin (B)
Antidepressants	Amitriptyline (C) Amoxapine (C) Bupropion (B) Citalopram (C) Desipramine (D) Doxepin (C) Fluoxetine (C) Imipramine (D) Mirtazapine (C) Nortriptyline (D)
Narcotic analgesics (D) NSAIDs	Aspirin (D) Celecoxib (D) Diflunisal (D) Ibuprofen (D) Ketoprofen (D) Antiemetics Dimenhydrinate (B) Dolasetron (B) Droperidol (C) Doxylamine (A) Meclizine (B) Granisetron (B) Metoclopramide (B) Ordansetron (B) Prochlroperazine (C)

Source: From Briggs et al.,[15] by permission of Lippincott, Wilkins & Williams, 2002.

Dolasetron and ondansetron, selective serotonin subtype 3 receptor antagonists used in the treatment of chemotherapy-associated nausea and vomiting, are considered class B agents by the FDA. Neither causes fetal harm in rats or rabbits, but only ondansetron has been studied in pregnant women.[15] Prochlorperazine readily crosses the placenta and has been used to treat nausea and vomiting in pregnancy. It is considered safe for this indication when used occasionally and in low doses.[15]

Acetaminophen is routinely used during all stages of pregnancy for pain relief and to control fever.[15,18] Pregnant women also frequently use salicylates. There is a theoretical risk of prostaglandin inhibitors, such as aspirin, causing premature closure of the ductus arteriosus, resulting in cardiovascular abnormalities. However, no adverse fetal outcomes have been reported after exposure to low-dose aspirin.[15] Ibuprofen and other nonsteroidal antiinflammatory drugs (NSAIDs) are without apparent teratogenicity, but may have reversible fetal effects when used in the third trimester.[15] NSAIDs cause decreased urine output and reduced amniotic fluid volume after prolonged usage.[101] Meperidine and morphine are not associated with fetal abnormalities,[17] nor are codeine, propoxyphene, oxycodone, or hydrocodone.[100] Maternal addiction to narcotics with subsequent neonatal narcotic withdrawal syndrome has been well described.[15]

Depression may be controlled with selective serotonin reuptake inhibitors, such as fluoxetine and sertraline. Fluoxetine does not have teratogenic effects and may be used in pregnancy. Sertraline is also an option, has a shorter half-life, and may be preferred over fluoxetine.[15] The effects of the anxiolytic benzodiazepines, including diazepam and lorazepam, on the human embryo and fetus are controversial. A number of studies have reported an association with congenital defects while other studies have not.[15] The risk, if present, appears to be low. Neonatal withdrawal has followed continuous use of diazepam during pregnancy, and a dose-related sedation of the infant is apparent if the drug is used close to delivery.[15]

Fatigue is a common symptom during chemotherapy and may be exacerbated by anemia. Epoetin alpha, recombinant human erythropoietin, is indicated for chemotherapy-associated anemia. The drug has been studied in pregnant patients with renal disease and other disorders and does not appear to present a major risk to the fetus.[15] It should be recalled, however, that mild anemia is physiologic during pregnancy and that iron deficiency is common. The latter should be corrected before epoetin alpha is added.

Conclusion

The coincidence of pregnancy and cancer poses challenges for caregivers, patients, and families. The survival of two patients, the mother and the fetus, is at risk. Randomized controlled trials are not available to guide practice. Even more than in other areas of oncology, the patient's personal values and religion may play a role in choosing the appropriate course of treatment. All options, including delaying treatment or abortion to allow immediate treatment, must be carefully considered. Patients must be given the best estimates of risks to mother and fetus for each possible treatment strategy.

In general, diagnostic imaging to accomplish anatomic staging does not increase fetal risk and may aid in appropriate maternal risk assessment. Therefore, staging should not be neglected in the pregnant patient. Radiation therapy can be used as a treatment modality, either when treatment planning is carefully performed to minimize fetal risk, or when sacrifice of the fetus is anticipated. Fetal doses of ionizing radiation less than 5 cGy do not appear to cause fetal injury, whereas more than 10 cGy exposure in early pregnancy is teratogenic. Chemotherapy during the first trimester of pregnancy poses the greatest risk of fetal loss and birth defects. Risks decrease thereafter, depending on the specific drugs employed and the timing during the pregnancy. During the third trimester, chemotherapy is associated with fetal growth restriction, whereas peripartum chemotherapy poses a risk for myelosuppression in the newborn. Supportive care needs should not be ignored during pregnancy, and analgesics, antidepressants, and antiemetics can and should be used.

References

1. Antonelli N, Dotters D, Katz V, et al. Cancer in pregnancy: a review of the literature. Part I. Obstet Gynecol Surg 1996;51: 125–134.
2. The Canadian Task Force on Periodic Health Examination. The periodic health examination. Can Med Assoc J 1979;121: 1187–1154.
3. Greenlee RT, Murray T, Bolden S, et al. Cancer statistics, 2000. Ca Cancer J Clin 2000;50:7–33.
4. Doll DC, Ringenberg S, Yarbro JW. Management of cancer during pregnancy. Arch Intern Med 1988;148:2058–2064.
5. Oduncu FS, Phil MA, Kimming R, et al. Cancer in pregnancy: maternal-fetal conflict. J Cancer Res Clin Oncol 2003;129: 133–146.
6. Mazze RI, Kallen B. Reproductive outcome after anesthesia and operation during pregnancy: a registry study of 5405 cases. Am J Obstet Gynecol 1989;161:1178–1185.
7. Kallen B, Mazze RI. Neural tube defects and first trimester pregnancy. Teratology 1990;41:717–720.
8. Sylvester GC, Khoury MJ, Lu X, et al. First-trimester anesthesia exposure and the risk of central nervous system defects: a population-based case-control study. Am J Public Health 1994;84: 1757–1760.
9. Kort B, Katz VL, Watson WJ. The effect of non-obstetric operation during pregnancy. Surg Gynecol Obstet 1987;177: 3717–3176.
10. Cappell MS. Colon cancer during pregnancy. Gastroenterol Clin N Am 2003;32:341–383.
11. Duncan P, Pope W, Cohen M, et al. Fetal risk of anesthesia and surgery during pregnancy. Anesthesiology 1986;64:790–794.
12. Reedy MB, Kallen B, Kuehl TJ. Laparoscopy during pregnancy: a study of five fetal outcome parameters with use of the Swedish Health Registry. Am J Obstet Gynecol 1997;177:673–679.
13. Melnick D. Management of general surgical problems in the pregnant patient. Am J Surg 2004;187:170–180.
14. Berry D, Theriault R, Holmes F, et al. Management of breast cancer during pregnancy using a standardized protocol. J Clin Oncol 1999;17:855–861.
15. Briggs GG, Freeman RK, Yaffe SJ. A Reference Guide to Fetal and Neonatal Risk: Drugs in Pregnancy and Lactation, 6th ed. Philadelphia: Lippincott, Wilkins & Williams, 2002.
16. Williams SF, Schilsky RL. Antineoplastic drugs administered during pregnancy. Semin Oncol 2000;27:618–622.
17. Heinohen OP, Slone D, Shapiro S. Birth defects and drugs in pregnancy. Cleveland, Littleton: Publishing Sciences Group, 1977.
18. Cunningham FG, Gant NF, Leveno, KJ, et al. (eds). Teratology, drugs and medications. In: Williams Obstetrics, 21st ed. New York: McGraw-Hill, 2001:1005–1038.
19. Aviles A, Diaz-Maqueo J, Talavera A, et al. Growth and development of children of mothers treated with chemotherapy during pregnancy: current status of 43 children. Am J Hematol 1991;36:243–248.
20. Reynoso EE, Shepherd FA, Messner HA, et al. Acute leukemia during pregnancy: The Toronto Leukemia Study Group experience with long-term follow-up of children exposed in utero to chemotherapeutic agents. J Clin Oncol 1987;5:1098–1106.
21. Ebert U, Loeffler H, Kirch W. Cytotoxic therapy and pregnancy. Pharmacol Ther 1997;74:207–220.
22. Doll DC, Ringenberg S, Yarbro J. Antineoplastic agents and pregnancy. Semin Oncol 1989;16:337–346.
23. Kirshon B, Wasserstrum N, Willis R, et al. Teratogenic effects of first-trimester cyclophosphamide therapy. Obstet Gynecol 1988; 72:462–464.
24. Glantz JC. Reproductive toxicology of alkylating agents. Obstet Gynecol Surv 1994;49:709–715.
25. Sutton C, McIvor RS, Vagt M, et al. Methotrexate-resistant form of dihydrofolate reductase protects transgenic murine embryos from teratogenic effects of methotrexate. Pediatr Dev Pathol 1998;1:503–512.
26. Feldkamp M, Carey JC. Clinical teratology counseling and consultation case report: low dose methotrexate exposure in the early weeks of pregnancy. Teratology 1987;47:533–539.
27. Woo J, Taechin Y, Hurd T. Breast cancer in pregnancy. Arch Surg 2003;138:91–99.
28. Turchi J, Villasis C. Anthracyclines in the treatment of malignancy in pregnancy. Cancer (Phila) 1988;61:435–440.
29. Sood A, Shahin M, Sorosky J. Paclitaxel and platinum chemotherapy for ovarian carcinoma during pregnancy. Gynecol Oncol 2001;83:599–600.
30. De Santis M, Lucchese A, De Carolis S. Metastatic breast cancer in pregnancy: first case of chemotherapy with docetaxel. Eur J Cancer Care 2000;9:235–237.
31. Méndez L, Mueller A, Salom E et al. Paclitaxel and carboplatin chemotherapy administered during pregnancy for advanced epithelial ovarian cancer. Obstet Gynecol 2003;102:1200–1202.
32. Gadducci A, Cosio S, Fanucchi A, et al. Chemotherapy with epirubicin and paclitaxel for breast cancer during pregnancy: case report and review of the literature. Anticancer Res 2003;23: 5225–5259.

33. Matthews SJ, McCoy C. Thalidomide: a review of approved and investigational uses. Clin Ther 2003;25:342–395.
34. Fanelli M, Sarmiento R, Gattuso C, et al. Thalidomide: a new anticancer drug? Expert Opin Invest Drugs 2003;12:1211–1225.
35. Product information. Thalidomide. Celgene Corporation, 2000.
36. Public Affairs Committee, Teratology Society. Teratology Society Public Affairs Committee position paper: thalidomide. Teratology 2000;62:172–173.
37. American College of Obstetricians and Gynecologists. Immunization during pregnancy. Technical Bulletin No. 160, October 1991.
38. Sacher RA, King JC. Intravenous gamma-globulin in pregnancy: a review. Obstet Gynecol Surv 1988;44:25–34.
39. Untch M, Ditsch N, Hermelink K. Immunotherapy: new options in breast cancer treatment. Expert Rev Anticancer Ther 2003;3: 403–448.
40. Product information. Herceptin. Genentech, Inc. 2002.
41. Lee KS. Requirement for neuroregulin receptor, erbB2, in neural and cardiac development. Nature (Lond) 1995;379:394–396.
42. Product information. Rituxan. IDEC Pharmaceuticals Corp., 2002.
43. Bosly A, Keating MJ, Stasil R, et al. Rituximab in B-cell disorders other than non-Hodgkin's lymphoma. Anticancer Drugs 2003;13(suppl):S25–S33.
44. Cunningham FG, Gant NF, Leveno, KJ, et al. (eds). General considerations and maternal evaluation. In: Williams Obstetrics, 21st ed. New York: McGraw-Hill, 2001:1143–1158.
45. Hall EJ. Scientific view of low-level risks. Radiographics 1991;11:509–518.
46. Roux C, Horvath C, Depuis R. Effects of pre-implantation low-dose radiation on rat embryos. Health Phys 1983;45:987–999.
47. Greskovich JF, Macklis RM. Radiation therapy in pregnancy: risk calculation and risk minimization. Semin Oncol 2000;27: 633–645.
48. Otake M, Yoshimaru H, Schull WJ. Severe mental retardation among the prenatally exposed survivors of the atomic bombing of Hiroshima and Nagasaki: a comparison of the old and new dosimetry systems. Radiation Effects Research Foundation, Technical Report no. 6–87, 1987.
49. Committee on Biological Effects of Ionizing Radiation, National Research Council. Other somatic and fetal effects. In: Beir V (ed) Effects of Exposure to Low Levels of Ionizing Rradiation. Washington, DC: National Academy Press, 1990:352–370.
50. Brent RL. The effect of embryonic and fetal exposure to x-ray, microwaves, and ultrasound: counseling the pregnant and non-pregnant patient about these risks. Semin Oncol 1989;16: 347–368.
51. Committee on Obstetric Practice, American College of Obstetricians and Gynecologists. Guidelines for Diagnostic Imaging During Pregnancy. Washington, DC: Copyright Clearance Center, 1995:158.
52. Kanal E. Pregnancy and the safety of magnetic resonance imaging. Magn Reson Imaging Clin N Am 1994;2:309–317.
53. Nicklas AH, Baker ME. Imaging strategies in the pregnant cancer patient. Semin Oncol 2000;27:623–632.
54. Stovall M, Blackwell C, Cundiff J, et al. Fetal dose from radiotherapy with photon beams: report of AAPM Radiation Therapy Committee Task Group No. 36. Med Phys 1995;22:63–82.
55. Anderson JM. Mammary cancer and pregnancy. Br Med J 1979; 1:1124–1127.
56. Kelsey JL, Berkowitz GS. Breast cancer Epidemiology. Cancer Res 1988;48:5615–5623.
57. Shen T, Vortmeyer AO, Zhuang Z, et al. High frequency of allelic loss of BRCA2 gene in pregnancy-associated breast carcinoma. J Natl Cancer Inst 1999;91:1686–1687.
58. Carol EH, Conner S, Schorr S. The diagnosis and management of breast problems during pregnancy and lactation. Am J Surg 1995;170:401–404.
59. Liberman L, Giesss CS, Dershaw DD, et al. Imaging of pregnancy-associated breast cancer. Radiology 1994;191:245–248.
60. Gupta RK. The diagnostic impact of aspiration cytodiagnosis of breast masses in association with pregnancy and lactation with the emphasis on clinical decision making. Breast J 1997;3: 131–134.
61. Schackmuth EM, Harlow CL, Norton LW. Milk fistula: a complication after core breast biopsy. Am J Roentgenol 1987;161: 961–962.
62. Collins J, Liao S, Wile A. Surgical management of breast masses in pregnant women. J Reprod Med 1995;40:785–788.
63. Keleher A, Theriault R, Gwyn K, et al. Multidisciplinary management of breast cancer concurrent with pregnancy. Am Coll Surg 2001;194(1):54–64.
64. Elledge R, Ciocca D, Langone G, et al. Estrogen receptor, progesterone receptor, and HER-2/neu protein in breast cancers from pregnant patients. Cancer (Phila) 1987;71:2499–2506.
65. Holleb A, Farrow J. The relation of carcinoma of the breast and pregnancy in 283 patients. Surg Gynecol Obstet 1962;115: 65–71.
66. Fisher B, Anderson S, Redmond C, et al. Reanalysis and results after 12 years of follow-up in a randomized trial comparing total mastectomy with lumpectomy with or without irradiation in the treatment of breast cancer. N Engl J Med 1997;337:956–962.
67. Metz J, Schultz D, Fox K, et al. Analysis of outcomes for high-risk breast cancer based on interval from surgery to post-mastectomy radiation therapy. Cancer J 2000;6:324–330.
68. Kuerer H, Cunningham J, Bleiweiss I, et al. Conservative breast surgery for breast carcinoma associated with pregnancy. Breast J 1998;4:761–767.
69. Mazonakis M, Varveris H, Damilakis J, et al. Radiation dose to conceptus resulting from tangential breast irradiation. Int J Radiat Oncol Biol Phys 2003;55:386–391.
70. Petrek JA, Dukoff R, Rogatko A. Prognosis of pregnancy associated breast cancer. Cancer (Phila) 1991;67:869–872.
71. Van der Vange N, Weverling G, Keting B, et al. The prognosis of cervical cancer associated with pregnancy: a matched cohort study. Obstet Gynecol 1996;85:1022–1026.
72. Zemlickis D, Lishner M, Degendorfer P, et al. Maternal and fetal outcome after invasive cervical cancer in pregnancy. J Clin Oncol 1991;9:1956–1961.
73. Brotzman G. Abnormal pap smears and lower genital tract neoplasia in pregnancy. Clin Fam Pract 2001;3(2):333–335.
74. Campion M, Sedlacek T. Colposcopy in pregnancy. Obstet Gynecol Clin N Am 1987;20:153–163.
75. Connor J. Noninvasive cervical cancer complicating pregnancy. Obstet Gynecol Clin N Am 1998;25:331–342.
76. Wright T, Cox, J, Massad, L, et al. 2001 Consensus Guidelines for the management of women with cervical intraepithelial neoplasia. Am J Obstet Gynecol 2003;189(1):295–304.
77. Committee on Practice Bulletins: Gynecology. Diagnosis and treatment of cervical carcinomas, number 35, May 2002. Obstet Gynecol 2002;99:855.
78. Mayr N, Magnotta V, Wheeler J, et al. Usefulness of tumor volumetry by magnetic resonance MR imaging in assessing response to radiation therapy in carcinoma of the uterine cervix. Int J Radiat Oncol Biol Phys 1996;35:915–924.
79. Sood A, Sorosky J. Invasive cancer complicating pregnancy. How to manage the dilemma. Obstet Gynecol Clin N Am 1998;25: 343–352.
80. Duggan B, Muderspach L, Roman L, et al. Cervical cancer in pregnancy: reporting on planned delay in therapy. Obstet Gynecol 1987;82:598–602.
81. Jones WB, Shingleton HM, Russell A, et al. Cervical carcinoma and pregnancy: a national pattern of care study of the American College of Surgeons. Cancer (Phila) 1996;77:1479–1488.

82. Sood A, Sorosky J, Mayr N, et al. Radiotherapeutic management of cervical carcinoma that complicates pregnancy. Cancer (Phila) 1997;80:1073–1078.
83. Stewart H, Monto R. Hodgkin's disease and pregnancy. Am J Obstet Gynecol 1992;63:570–578.
84. Gelb A, Van de Rijn M, Warnke R, et al. Pregnancy-associated lymphomas. A clinicopathologic study. Cancer (Phila) 1996;78: 304–310.
85. Lishner M, Zemlickis, D, Degendorfer, P, et al. Maternal and foetal outcome following Hodgkin's disease. Br J Cancer 1992;65: 114–117.
86. Barry R, Diamond D, Graver L. Influence of pregnancy on the course of Hodgkin's disease. Am J Obstet Gynecol 1962;84: 445–454.
87. Hennessy J, Rottino A. Hodgkin's disease and pregnancy. Hematologica 1963;97:851–853.
88. Anselmo A, Cavalieri E, Maurizi Enrici R, et al. Hodgkin's disease during pregnancy: diagnosis and therapeutic management. Fetal Diagn Ther 1999;14:102–105.
89. Ward F, Weiss R. Lymphoma and pregnancy. Semin Oncol 1989;16:397–409.
90. Dhedin N, Coiffier B. Lymphoma in the elderly and in pregnancy. In: Canellos GP, Liter TA, Sklar JL (eds) The Lymphomas. Philadelphia: Saunders, 1998:549–556.
91. Zuazu J, Julia A, Sierra J, et al. Pregnancy outcome in hematologic malignancies. Cancer (Phila) 1991;67:703–709.
92. Pohlman B, Macklis R. Lymphoma and pregnancy. Semin Oncol 2000;27:657–667.
93. Canellos G, Anders J, Propert K, et al. Chemotherapy of advanced Hodgkin's disease with MOPP, ABVD, or MOPP alternating with ABVD. N Engl J Med 1992;327:1278–1284.
94. Fisher R, Gaynor K, Dahlberg S, et al. Comparison of a standard regimen (CHOP) with three intensive chemotherapy regimens for advanced non-Hodgkin's lymphoma. N Engl J Med 1987; 328:1002–1006.
95. Barnicle M. Chemotherapy and pregnancy. Semin Oncol Nurs 1992;8:124–132.
96. Becker M, Hyman G. Management of Hodgkin's disease coexistent with pregnancy. Radiology 1965;85:725–728.
97. Sutcliffe S. ABVD chemotherapy for Hodgkin's disease in pregnancy: a report of three cases and cytogenetic and clinical follow-up at 1, 5, and 7 years. Ann Oncol 1996;7(suppl 3):113 (abstract).
98. Woo S, Fuller L, Cardiff J, et al. Radiotherapy during pregnancy for clinical stages IA–IIA Hodgkin's disease. Int J Oncol Biol Phys 1992;23:407–412.
99. Jacobs C, Donaldson SS, Rosenberg S, et al. Management of the pregnant patient with Hodgkin's disease. Ann Intern Med 1981; 95:669–675.
100. Bracken M, Holford T. Exposure to prescribed drugs in pregnancy and association with congenital malformations. Obstet Gynecol 1981;58:336–344.
101. Hickok DE, Hollenbach, KA, Reilly SF, Nyberg DA. The association between decreased amniotic fluid volume and treatment with nonsteroidal anti-inflammatory agents for preterm labor. Am J Obstet Gynecol 1989;160:1525–1530.

SECTION EIGHT

Cancer Survivorship

100

Survivorship Research: Past, Present, and Future

Julia H. Rowland

Origins of Cancer Survivorship Research

In 1884, an official ceremony was held and the cornerstone laid for an ornate and turreted building in New York City that would for many years house the first cancer treatment center in the country. The site, located on the upper west side of Central Park, then a virtual wilderness area on the larger island of Manhattan, was selected because the belief at the time was that cancer was contagious. The rounded design of the towers, where patient beds were to be located, was intended to discourage the risk of germs, which were thought to lurk in corners. Named The New York Cancer Hospital, this institution would later be moved in 1948 to its current east side location where it was, until 1960, called the Memorial Hospital for Cancer and Allied Diseases. The history of this leading center for cancer care and research, known today as the Memorial Sloan-Kettering Cancer Center, a sprawling multisite enterprise, is illustrative of where we have come in viewing cancer.[1]

At the turn of the 20th century, cancer was largely incurable, poorly understood, and associated with treatments that were often as dire as the disease itself. By midcentury, with the advent of anesthesia, antibiotics, and the introduction of multimodal cancer therapies, the number of individuals living longer (beyond 5 years) with cancer had slowly increased. However, it was not until the latter part of the 1900s that the nationally estimated 5-year cancer prevalence figures (prevalence being defined as the number of people alive at a given point in time with a history of cancer) reached 50%. From an evidence perspective, this event, which occurred between 1974 and 1976,[2] might in hindsight be considered a turning point in what would soon become the field of cancer survivorship. Arguably, without substantial numbers of survivors, issues of "survivorship" would never have become of interest; the focus of research would have remained, as it had in the past, largely on trying simply to enable an individual to become a survivor, not what the future of that person's life might be like.

The first glimpse at this new world came from pediatric oncology where, seemingly overnight, a death sentence was being converted into long-term cure. This point is well illustrated in the steady upward curve in pediatric cancer survival rates from 1950 to 1998 depicted in Figure 100.1. Introduction in the late 1960s of therapies to prevent central nervous system relapse in survivors of childhood lymphoblastic leukemia (ALL) was among several key treatment changes that would lead to a revised perspective on this disease (Figure 100.2). Because ALL is the most common form of childhood cancer, accounting today for approximately 30% of cancer cases diagnosed in children before the age of 14,[3] the impact of this breakthrough produced a dramatic shift in 5-year survival rates for pediatric cancer as a whole. It also spawned the first generation of articles calling for attention by the medical community to issues that went beyond merely curing a child to those affecting his or her quality of life after treatment.[4–6] This same process was slower to evolve in the adult cancer arena.

Development of Survivorship Researcher and Assessment Tools

Others, and most notably Jimmie Holland,[7,8] have written in detail about the confluence of both medical and societal factors that led to the recognition of the field of psychosocial oncology. Three elements essential to the growth of the field were the change within the medical community toward disclosing a cancer diagnosis, training of a cadre of researchers to address posttreatment issues related to quality of life (QOL), and development of assessment tools to measure and describe the survivorship experience. Of these, the movement toward disclosing a cancer diagnosis was the most critical.

Throughout most of the 1960s, the practice in the United States was not to tell patients their diagnosis, "never tellers" constituting an estimated 90% of physicians surveyed in a report by Oken.[9] A report published by Novack and colleagues revealed that this policy reversed in the course of a brief 10 years. By 1977, 97% of physicians stated that they told patients they had cancer at the time of diagnosis.[10] This change in practice was important because it opened the door for researchers to approach and ask patients directly about their understanding of their illness and its impact on their lives. The shift in candor about a cancer diagnosis was consequent to growing attention in the United States to patients' rights, particularly in the health arena. However, physicians' willingness to adopt this practice was also a reflection of the greater optimism about survival prospects for those diagnosed with cancer. It should be noted that sharing the diagnosis is not a universal practice. In many countries around the world, including several industrialized nations, physicians still hide this information, sometimes at the request of family members.[11–13] In Third World countries, where access to curative therapies is more limited and hence prognosis is grim,

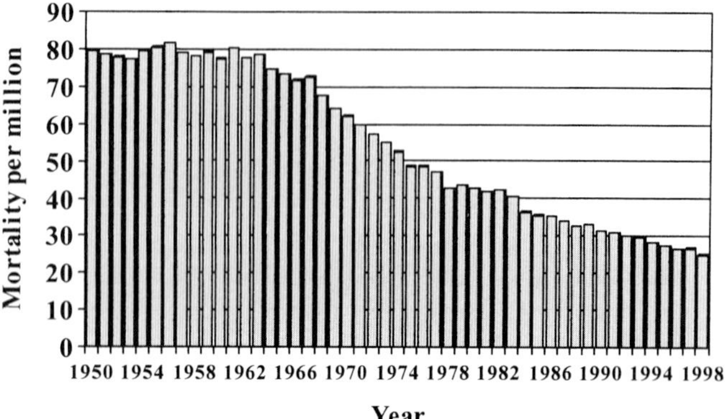

FIGURE 100.1. Remarkable past progress: childhood cancer mortality, 1950–1998.

protecting patients from learning their diagnosis is considered more humane.[14] Even in many European countries, cancer still carries a significant social stigma. As part of its year-long study of cancer survivorship in the United States, the President's Cancer Panel held a meeting in Lisbon, Portugal, in May 2003. The purpose of this meeting was "to learn about the health services and survivorship activities in diverse European nations and health systems that might benefit survivors in this country".[15] The Panel found that the term survivor was rarely used, and in some countries no linguistic equivalent existed. It was common for European survivors, the testimony from many of whom is included in transcripts and the final report from this meeting,[15] to feel they could not publicly reveal their cancer history, or discuss their illness experience, even with family. In contrast to the situation in the United States, few prominent Europeans have disclosed their status as cancer survivors.

Early pioneers in the field of psychosocial oncology often came from mental health or nursing backgrounds. Few, however, had formal training in psycho-oncology, as dedicated educational programs in this field did not appear until the late 1970s and early 1980s.[7,16] Today, a number of the National Cancer Institute (NCI)-designated clinical and comprehensive cancer centers offer 2- to 3-year training programs for MDs and PhDs who wish to specialize in this area of research or care. Many also provide access to courses in psychosocial aspects of cancer research to a diversity of healthcare professionals. It also is increasingly common to see position openings for psychosocial oncology specialists announced on association-based online listserves, such as that supported by the American Psychological Association's Division 38 Health Psychology forum.

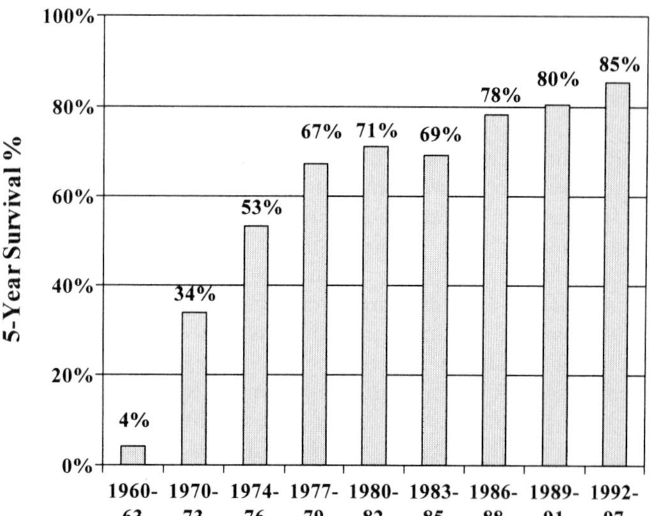

FIGURE 100.2. Remarkable past progress: childhood acute lymphoblastic anemia (ALL) survival rates, 1960–1997.

Paralleling the expertise of the early researchers, the tools used for QOL assessment of survivors' outcomes were drawn initially from the psychiatric or mental health field. Examples of frequently used instruments included the Hopkin's Symptom Checklist (better known to many as the SCL-90),[17] the Profile of Mood States,[18] and the Center for Epidemiologic Studies Depression Scale (CES-D).[19] It quickly became apparent that these measures were not well suited to the cancer survivor population, which, although experiencing distress, generally did not report symptoms at psychiatric or pathologic levels. At the same time, teasing apart symptoms that might be caused by the effects of treatment (e.g., fatigue/lack of energy, sleep disruption, problems concentrating) from signs of emotional distress created a challenge to score interpretation.[20–22] Further, many of the experiences of those treated were poorly captured by the questions asked in these tools. Frustration with the limits of these more-generic tools resulted in the birth of cancer-specific measurements, an enterprise that, although starting slowly, burgeoned in the 1980s to produce many of the QOL measures, or at least their sophisticated variants, most commonly used today.[23–26]

Role of Advocacy in the Growth of the Field

Defining the Domain

The shift in focus and language to recognition of people with a history of cancer as "survivors" and their health and social outcomes as constituting "survivorship research" has its own history. In 1985, a young pediatrician working for the Public Health Service, Fitzhugh Mullan, wrote about his experience of living with cancer in a short piece for the *New England Journal of Medicine*. He referred to his journey as the "Seasons of Survival" and in his text first gave name to issues of survivorship.[27] In October 1986, he and an intrepid group of about two dozen fellow survivors, cancer healthcare providers and advocates, met in Albuquerque, New Mexico, and established the National Coalition for Cancer Survivorship (NCCS).[28] The standard medical definition of a survivor at the time of that gathering, and the only definition commonly applied, held that only those individuals who remained disease free for a minimum of 5 years could be labeled as survivors. At the founding NCCS meeting, the group declared that a person should be viewed as, and was entitled to call himself or herself, a survivor, "from the moment of diagnosis and for the balance of his or her life, regardless of the ultimate cause of death."

The group's argument for advancing this new definition was that it was only by endorsing such thinking that survivors would be able to significantly alter the prevailing medical culture. Specifically, they sought to encourage the cancer practitioner community to move away from its more narrow focus on starting treatment as quickly as possible to one that recognized that a person's unique needs, desires, and ultimate health and life outcomes must be acknowledged in this process. Ideally this would start on day 1, after diagnosis. Although controversial at the time, and certainly not uniformly embraced even today, this broader definition of a cancer survivor has taken hold, at least in the United States. In a search of *Pub Med* from 1981 to 1985, the 5-year period before the founding of the NCCS, 28 research articles (among humans, published in English), were identified using the terms cancer survivorship. Using the same approach to examine the "hits" in 5-year increments since then yielded the following: 1986–1990, 1,700 citations; 1991–1995, 8,417; 1996–2000, 10,574; 2001 to current (with 16 months still remaining to come during this 5-year period), 7,673. Although many of the citations identified would not be classified by many as addressing issues related to living with or beyond cancer (i.e., many still focus on survival, not survivorship), the numbers speak for themselves. On the public side, since 1987 the first Sunday in June has been celebrated as National Cancer Survivors' Day. Many of the large cancer centers in major cities now hold their own "Cancer Survivors Day" celebrations, often in association with special presentations by survivors, scientists, and advocates. The most significant evidence that the field of cancer survivorship had finally come into its own was the creation of an Office of Cancer Survivorship within the world's premier cancer research center, the U.S. National Cancer Institute.

A Brief History of the Office of Cancer Survivorship

Had NCCS members decided to stop at endorsing a new definition of survivor, it is not clear how rapidly the broader field of survivorship research might have progressed. Fortunately, they were not content to merely draw attention to the needs of those living with a history of cancer. NCCS members began to advocate for specific resources to further identify and address these needs. In anticipation of what would become the first NCCS Congress, held in Washington, D.C., in November 1995, the Coalition sought the input of scores of researchers, clinicians, and survivors on what questions remained unanswered, who should be charged with addressing these, and how best were we going to achieve optimal cancer care for all. Response to this inquiry was combined in a white paper entitled Imperatives for Quality Cancer Care: Access, Advocacy, Action & Accountability. In spring 1996, Ellen Stovall, Executive Director for NCCS, gave a copy of this document to the director of the NCI, Dr. Richard Klausner. After reading this paper, Dr. Klausner called for the creation of the Office of Cancer Survivorship (OCS).

Formally inaugurated at a ceremony held in the Rose Garden of the White House in October 1996, the OCS was established in recognition of the growing population of cancer survivors and their unique and poorly understood needs.[29] The overall mission of the office is to enhance the length and quality of survival of all those diagnosed with cancer. The OCS achieves this by serving as a focus for the support and direction of research that will lead to a clearer understanding of, and the ultimate prevention of, or reduction in, the adverse psychosocial, physical, and economic outcomes of cancer and its treatment. Survivorship research is seen as encompassing the medical, functional, and health-related QOL of children and adults diagnosed with cancer, as well as that of their families. It also includes within its domain issues related to healthcare delivery, access, and follow-up care as they relate to survivors. Because considerable work had been done in elucidating the needs and care of those newly diagnosed and in active treatment, particular emphasis in creating the OCS was placed on developing and supporting research that addresses the health and well-being of individuals who are posttreatment or in remission. The OCS also has as its purview a commitment to educating healthcare providers, as well as survivors themselves, about issues and practices critical to their patients (or in the case of survivors, their own) optimal well-being. Finally, the OCS works to foster and promote the training of the next generation of survivorship researchers and clinicians.

In 2001, members of the OCS, the NCI Director's Consumer Liaison Group, and a number of community researchers and advocates independently suggested that NCI leadership consider advancing cancer survivorship as an area for special focus along with other previously identified topics such as Genes and the Environment, Cancer Imaging, Research on Tobacco and Tobacco-Related Cancers, and Cancer Communications. This recommendation met with approval and elevated Cancer Survivorship to special status in NCI's Fiscal Year 2004 and 2005 budgets[31,32] (pp 88–93 and 66–71, respectively). Successful adoption of cancer survivorship as an extraordinary opportunity for investment by the NCI was in significant measure due to the specific intercession of Dr. Andrew von Eschenbach. Dr. von Eschenbach's appointment as NCI Director by the President of the United States brought to the Institute in February 2002, for the first time, a cancer survivor as its director. Throughout his leadership, Dr. von Eschenbach has been outspoken about his own cancer experience as a three-time survivor and an unflagging champion for survivorship research.

The breadth of attention to cancer survivorship as an area of public health interest is reflected in a number of recent events at the national level. These events include the release in 2002 by the Institute of Medicine's National Cancer Policy Board of its report *Childhood Cancer Survivorship: Improving Care and Quality of Life* (the adult cancer companion for which is expected to appear in late 2005)[32]; the decision by the President's Cancer Panel to pursue cancer survivorship as a theme for its planned hearings in 2003 and 2004, the report from which activities, *Living Beyond Cancer: Finding a New Balance*, was released at the annual meetings of the American Society of Clinical Oncology held in New Orleans in June 2004[33]; and the publication in April 2004 of *A National Action Plan for Cancer Survivorship: Advancing Public Health Strategies* by the Centers for Disease Control and Prevention (CDC) and the Lance Armstrong Foundation.[34] The latter two initiatives bear the important contribution of Lance Armstrong. Lance, seven-time winner of the world's most grueling bicycle race, the Tour de France, an accomplishment achieved after his diagnosis with and treatment for metastatic testicular cancer, was nominated in 2002 by President

Bush to serve as one of three members of the President's Cancer Panel. The foundation that bears his name underwrote the CDC effort to produce the *National Action Plan* document. During this same period, 2002–2004, five separate bills were introduced in Congress that included language identifying cancer survivorship as an area warranting more attention and funds from the U.S. Department of Health and Human Services (DHHS); one of these would have formally authorized the office by an act of Congress. None of these bills ultimately became law. However, the fact that they were put forward (with others of similar intent likely to follow) is strong evidence that the nation acknowledges that it is not enough for our scientists to find a cure for cancer; we must also, as a country, ensure the quality of the lives of those treated. In the Congressional appropriations document for 2003 (Senate Report 107-216; Department of Labor, Health and Human Services, and Education, and Related Agencies Appropriation Bill), members of the Senate wrote "... More must be done to improve the understanding of the growing cancer survivorship population, including determinations of the physiological and psychological late effects, prevalence of secondary cancers, as well as further development of effective survivorship interventions. The Committee supports an aggressive expansion of the NCI Office of Cancer Survivorship activities ...".

Function of Survivorship Research in Cancer Control and Care

The world of cancer survivorship research has expanded far beyond that originally envisioned. In the early 1970s, the function of such research was largely limited to describing the "terrain" of survival. By the early 1980s, researchers sought not simply to elucidate the impact of cancer on the lives of individuals and their families but to use this information to develop interventions to help survivors cope better with their illness.[35,36] In the case of pediatrics, the findings from survivorship research were being used to refine cancer therapies so as to reduce their associated morbidity without diminishing the gains achieved in reduced mortality.[37] As we race into the new millennium, this vision, along with the approach to as well as application of survivorship research, has vastly expanded and come to encompass the entire cancer control continuum (Figure 100.3). Originally occupying just one part of the continuum, cancer survivorship research and care now have the potential to address and affect issues along the entire continuum. For example, with more young survivors expected to live full or lengthened lifetimes, they need to be counseled to reduce the risk of (primary prevention) and screened for (secondary prevention) other unrelated malignancies for which they would be at risk across the course of life/normal aging.[38]

Clinically, the primary function of survivorship research is fivefold. Information about survivors is critical if we are to help patients make decisions now about treatment options that will affect their future; understand the action of and tailor therapies to maximize cure while minimizing adverse treatment-related effects; develop and disseminate evidence-based interventions that reduce cancer morbidity as well as mortality and facilitate adaptation among cancer survivors; improve quality of care and control costs; and equip the next generation of physicians, nurses, and other healthcare professionals to provide not just the science but also the art of comprehensive cancer medicine.

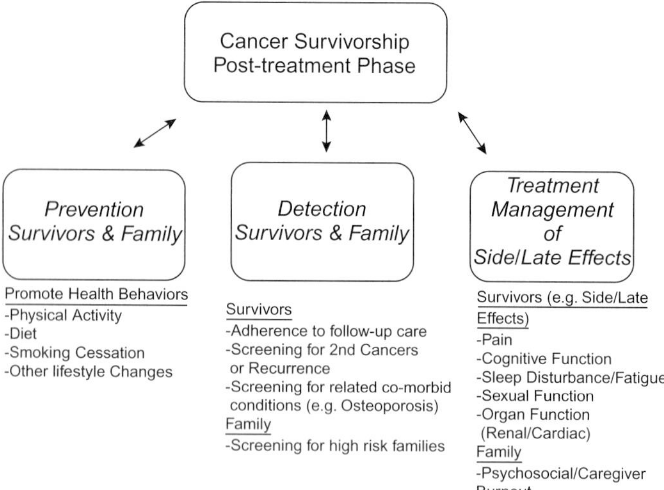

FIGURE 100.3. Aspects of cancer survivorship interventions.

The New Generation of Survivors: Who are They?

Profile of the Current Survivor Population

"The new population of survivors hanging in there can be found everywhere ... in offices and factories, on bicycles and cruise ships, on tennis courts and beaches, and in bowling alleys. You see them in all ages, shapes, sizes, colors, usually unremarkable in their appearance, sometimes remarkable for the way they learn to live with disabilities." (Natalie Davis Spingarn,[39] p. 69)

In 1982, Natalie Davis Spingarn became one of a feisty vanguard of cancer survivors, and vocal patient advocates, to publish a book about their encounter with cancer. Her volume, titled *Hanging in There, Living Well on Borrowed Time*,[39] chronicled her experience of being diagnosed as a young woman (under age 50) and living long term with metastatic breast cancer. A journalist and investigative reporter by training, Natalie provided information often hard for fellow cancer travelers to find and encouraged them to become active participants in their care, a quite provocative message for those more comfortable operating in the paternalistic model of care of the times. In 1999 she published an update of this journey in a book titled *The New Cancer Survivors: Living with Grace, Fighting with Spirit*.[40] In this second volume she describes what she recognized as a new and emerging generation of survivors who come from all walks of life, seek an equal or at a minimum a partnership role in their health-related decision making and care, and expect to be treated as whole persons, not as a particular disease (cancer) or body site (breast patient).

The main driver behind interest in issues of cancer survivorship is necessarily the growing population of survivors. Cancer survival in the United States has risen steadily over the past three decades for all cancers combined. When Nixon declared "the war" on cancer in 1971, there were only

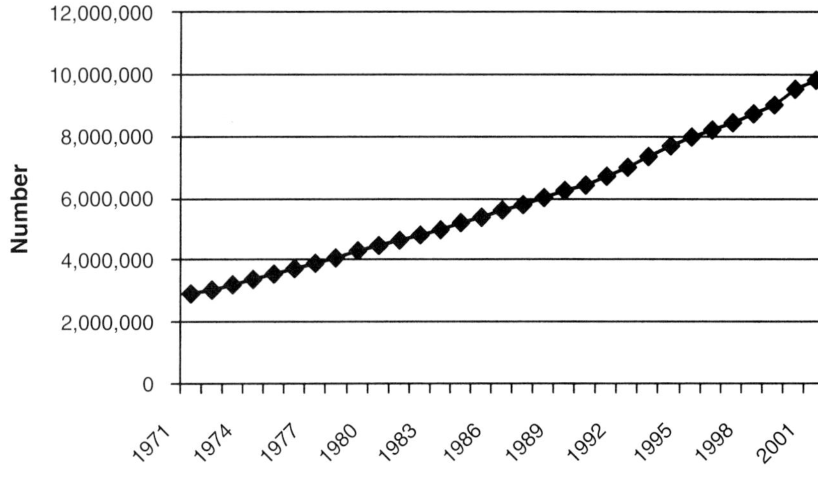

FIGURE 100.4. Estimated number of cancer survivors in the United States from 1971 to 2001. U.S. estimated prevalence counts were estimated by applying U.S. populations to Surveillance Epidemiology and End Results (SEER) 9 Limited Duration Prevalence proportions. Populations from January 2000 were based on the average of the July 1999 and July 2000 population estimates from the U.S. Bureau of Census. (*Source:* November 2002 submission.)

3 million survivors. Today, there are approximately 22.4 million cancer survivors worldwide; an estimated 9.8 million of these live in the United States alone, representing between 3% and 4% of the population (Figure 100.4).[41] In the absence of other competing causes of death, current figures indicate that for adults diagnosed during 1995 to 2000, 64% could expect to be alive in 5 years; this is up from 50% estimated for those diagnosed during 1974 to 1976. The relative 5-year survival rate for those diagnosed as children (less than 19 years of age) is even higher. Of children diagnosed with cancer between 1974 and 1976, while 80% survived beyond 1 year, little more than half (56%) were still alive 5 years later. Today, 79% of childhood cancer survivors will be alive at 5 years, and the 10 year survival is approaching 75%. If these trends in survival continue, we may reasonably expect to reach the *2010 Healthy People* goal of 70% 5-year survival for all those diagnosed with cancer.

Of the 9.8 million survivors in the United States, an impressive 14% were diagnosed 20 or more years ago (Figure 100.5). More women than men are survivors. The higher proportion of men who are within 5 years of diagnosis is consistent with the larger number of males versus females diagnosed annually with cancer. At the other end of the survivorship continuum, more women survive longer than men due to the higher proportion found to have more readily detected and treatable cancers (e.g., breast, gynecologic), the fact that fewer women (n = 80,660) than men (n = 93,110) develop lung cancer or die of it (females, 68,510 versus males, 91,930) annually,[3] and the generally lower all-cause mortality rate among women versus men in this country.

Of the prevalent cancer population, the largest constituent group comprises breast cancer survivors (22%), followed by survivors of prostate cancer (17%), colorectal cancer (11%), and gynecologic cancer (10%) (Figure 100.6). Consonant with the fact that cancer is a disease associated with aging [median age of cancer patients at diagnosis based on

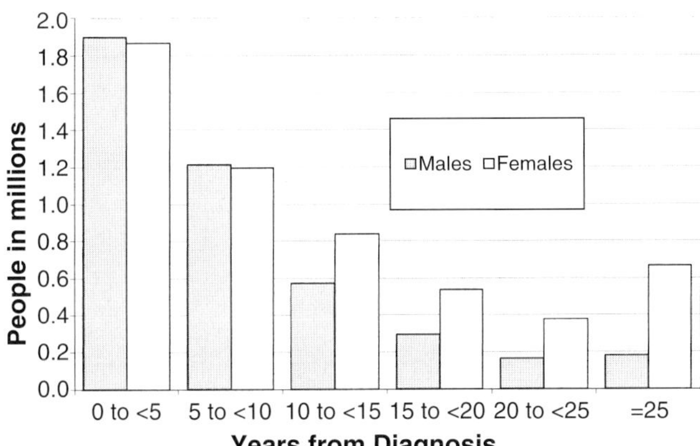

FIGURE 100.5. Estimated number of persons alive in the United States diagnosed with cancer on January 1, 2001, by time from diagnosis and gender (invasive/first primary cases only; n = 9.8 million survivors). U.S. prevalence counts were estimated by applying U.S. populations to SEER-9 Limited Duration Prevalence proportions. Populations from January 2001 were based on the average of the July 2000 and July 2001 population estimates from the U.S. Bureau of Census. (*Source:* November 2003 submission.)

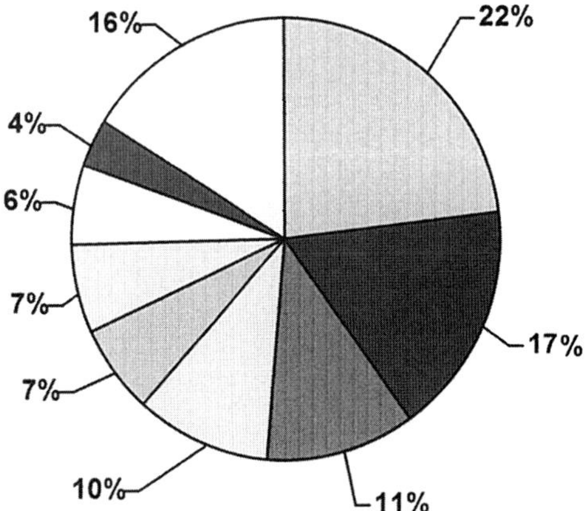

FIGURE 100.6. Estimated number of persons alive in the United States diagnosed with cancer by site. Starting *clockwise from 12:00 position:* female breast (22%), prostate (17%), colorectal (11%), gynecologic (10%), other genitourinary (GU, bladder and testis) (7%), hematologic [Hodgkin's Disease (HD), non-Hodgkin's lymphoma (NHL), leukemia] (7%), melanoma (6%), lung (4%), and other (16%). U.S. Estimated Prevalence counts were estimated by applying U.S. populations to SEER 9 for All Races, White, and Black, SEER 11 for Asian/Pacific Islander, and SEER 11 (excluding Hawaii and Detroit for Hispanic) Limited Duration Prevalence proportions. Populations from January 2001 were based on the average of the July 2000 and July 2001 population estimates from the U.S. Bureau of Census. (*Source:* November 2003 submission.)

SEER (Surveillance, Epidemiology, and End Results) 12 data from 1997 to 2001 was 67 years; an estimated 56.8% of new cancers are diagnosed in patients 65 and older],[42] the majority (61%) of our survivors are aged 65 or older, while 33% are between ages 40 and 64, 5% are aged from 20 to 39 years, and fewer than 1% are 19 or younger. It is currently estimated that one of every six persons over the age of 65 is living with a history of cancer. Although it is unknown what impact the use of chemopreventive agents such as tamoxifen will have on the larger figures for breast cancer incidence, as past and future advances in cancer detection, treatment, and care diffuse into clinical practice, the number of survivors can be expected to increase. Fewer deaths from cardiovascular disease and the aging of the population will contribute to this trend.

Projected Population of the Future

Realization that the world's population is aging is sobering.[43] In 2011, the first members of the baby boomer generation (those born between 1946 and 1964) will turn 65. It is estimated that by the year 2030 one in five individuals will be age 65 or older and 40% will be from minority groups. At the same time, it is recognized that older cancer patients tend to be in poorer health (34% versus 10% of the general population), often have two or more chronic medical conditions (16% versus 4%), report functional limitations (nearly 70% versus less than 30%), and experience more limitations in activities of daily living (ADL) or instrumental ADL (17% versus 3%).[44] Given these figures, it is clear that planning for the care and ongoing health of our aging population, many of whom will become cancer survivors, constitutes a critical public health challenge for the future.[43]

The OCS includes family or caregivers as "secondary" survivors in its definition of survivors. This concept reflects the growing appreciation of the critical role they play in a loved one's or family member's illness. The American Cancer Society (ACS) in its *Facts and Figures* publication for 1996 estimated that three of every four families would have an affected family member. Recent data on caregiving in America suggest that 21% of those over the age of 18 provide unpaid care for an adult 18 and older. The second most common reason for a recipient to need care, after old age, is cancer.[45] Data obtained from cancer survivors identified by the National Health Interview Survey in 1992 indicated that approximately 24% of adult cancer survivors (1.3 million) had a child 18 years of age or younger living in the home.[46] To date, relatively little is known about the impact of living with someone who has cancer on other family members in general; even less is known about cancer's impact on the current or future health behaviors and well-being of younger and potentially highly vulnerable family members.

With advances in our understanding of genomics and proteomics and the application of novel delivery systems, many project that future antineoplastic therapies will be more targeted to cancer cells and less toxic to normal tissue, resulting in significant reductions in treatment-associated morbidity. This is not to say cancer therapy will be entirely benign, as few pharmacological treatments are ever entirely without side effects. Monitoring for the novel, potentially subtle, and late-appearing or unexpected effects of newer approaches to cure represents a challenge to future researchers. Of equal importance will be our ability to assess the impact of delivery of these molecularly targeted treatments. Many agents will be administered orally, shifting the responsibility for delivery and monitoring away from the medical team and to the patient. Appreciating the obstacles faced by patients and families to understand and adhere to regimens will be critical if we are to understand not just drug effectiveness but also survivors' QOL and health-related outcomes.

Domains of Survivorship Research: Multidimensionality

In the early era of research on the psychosocial and physical impact of cancer, the common practice was to use global (e.g., Karnofsky) or summary scores representing overall function across a range of activities of daily living activities (e.g., FLIC, functional living index-cancer; LASA, linear analog self assessment). Perhaps unique to cancer QOL studies (as opposed to those for other chronic illnesses) is their history of emphasis on the importance of patient-based outcomes. What was quickly apparent in instrument selection and development was the need for patient (versus physician)-based measures.[47–49] The few clinician-rated scales still commonly in use represent measures to assess patient status for clinical trials (e.g., ECOG, Easterm Collaborative Oncology Group, status) or were designed for use when a patient might be too sick to complete a self-assessment, e.g., the Spitzer Quality of Life Index.[50]

As clinicians began looking more closely at patient-focused outcomes and more behavioral scientists joined the field of inquiry, four primary areas of QOL impact emerged: physical (symptoms), functional (capacity to engage in activities of daily living), emotional (mood/affective and cognitive status), and social (role functioning and/or support, financial burden). Examples of early scales with these four domains include the Quality of Life Index[51] and the Sickness Impact Profile.[52] These four domains remain at the core of contemporary scales.

An early challenge for the field was the need to develop and test cancer-specific tools. As already noted, initial studies of mental health outcomes for survivors relied heavily on the use of instruments borrowed from the psychiatric arena, for example, the Hopkins Symptom Checklist (SCL-90) and the Profile of Mood States (POMS). Even when studies became more sophisticated and expanded to include such domains as sexual functioning, the available measures (e.g., Derogatis Sexual Functioning Inventory) were often poorly designed to assess cancer patients' functioning or unique areas or types of dysfunction. It is of note that the recent interest in examining benefit finding among survivors led clinical researchers to reflexively go back to the psychiatric literature for tools (e.g., posttraumatic stress scale, civilian version; posttraumatic growth inventory) before realizing that they would need to develop measures better suited to capturing the cancer experience.

The most recent generation of cancer-specific measures is designed to assess domains of well-being that represent newer foci of attention. These measures include, for example, items or scales to assess fatigue, cognitive dysfunction, and menopausal or hot flash symptoms, as well as bowel and urologic status in colorectal, select gynecologic, and prostate cancer survivors. (See the Cancer Outcomes Measurement Working group-generated publication for an excellent review of current measurement tools.[53]) The two newest areas of attention in measurement development are long-term survivorship scales[54–56] and measures of postcancer health behaviors.[57–60] Curiously, although fear of recurrence is probably the single most common concern of those living with a history of cancer, efforts to create instruments designed specifically to measure this domain have languished.[61–63]

There has been considerable debate as to whether current measures assess QOL or simply health-related quality of life (HRQOL).[64,65] Many argue that individual QOL is intangible and almost impossible to meaningfully measure. Although the majority of survivorship researchers today use the terms QOL and HRQOL interchangeably, when pressed most agree that our common assessment tools are most accurate in providing (and often specifically designed to generate or elicit) information on survivors' perception of their health-related quality of life than QOL per se. One of the more recently appreciated challenges to the field of QOL assessment among cancer survivors is interpreting the impact cancer has over time in individuals' lives. Cancer researchers are (re)learning what others have reported for decades,[66] that humans are incredibly adaptable and, given time and support, can adapt to considerable limitations. The manifestation of this resilience is seen in what researchers now refer to as "response shift" in subjects' report of functioning and well-being when measured over time.[67] In this paradigm, respondents, as they accommodate to a loss or disability, are less likely to report being upset by it, even though the impairment may continue to cause the same level of, and sometimes greater, disability over time. Trying to make sense of this phenomenon while teasing out what health-promoting interventions may or may not be most helpful for survivors' recovery has become a respected field of inquiry in itself.

Trends in Survivorship Research

Past

The historical research on survivorship has been well reviewed by others.[35,36] General themes have evolved over time. In the early era of survivorship research, most studies focused on the psychological impact of cancer or the delineation of specific sequelae of treatment (e.g., impact of stomas, lymphedema, amputation).[68,69] As the number of survivors grew and length of survival increased, attention expanded to include examination of the social (interpersonal, family, work, school) and sexual well-being of survivors.[6,70–72] By the mid-1980s, researchers, responding to the observation by many survivors that they continued to reexperience aspects of the events associated with their diagnosis and treatment, began to conceptualize cancer as a "traumatic event." A new wave of studies sought to determine the extent to which cancer produced symptoms of posttraumatic stress disorder (PTSD).[73,74] In pursuing this path, investigators began to hear from survivors, particularly in studies that contained qualitative analyses or open-ended formats, that cancer also caused them to recognize the positive aspects of their lives. The consequence of this observation is that a current trend in research is to examine the role of benefit finding in promoting and/or mediating and moderating survivorship outcomes.[75–77]

Since the establishment of psychosocial oncology as a field of its own in the early 1970s, clinical researchers have actively sought to take what they learned in their surveys and apply it to interventions that would reduce cancer's toll on survivors and their families. Relatively little of this research, however, was designed exclusively to meet the needs of those posttreatment.[78,79] This picture is slowly changing.

Present

Since 2000, the NCI's Office of Cancer Survivorship has conducted annual analyses of the number and types of grants in the area of cancer survivorship funded across the National Institutes of Health. (These data are updated and posted yearly online.[80]) Included in this analysis are grants that examine the health or behavior of individuals after treatment for cancer or that of their family members. Excluded from this review are studies that consider patients solely during active treatment or early posttreatment (less than 2 months follow-up) or survivors with recurrent or advanced disease. When the OCS was originally established in 1996, only 24 National Institutes of Health (NIH) grants could be identified that met these narrower criteria. In the philosophy of "build it and they will come," the NCI's commitment to this area of science, with the creation of the OCS, appears to have been successful.

Judging by the numbers, the research community is slowly being enticed to advance its expertise to tackle issues further along the cancer control continuum. In fiscal year 2003 (encompassing October 2002 through September 2003), the period for which most complete data exist, a total of 179 grants were identified as addressing survivorship issues. Of these, 154 (86%) were funded through the NCI. The remainder were supported by the National Institute for Nursing Research ($n = 14$), National Institutes of Mental Health ($n = 5$), National Institute on Aging ($n = 4$), and the National Institute of Dental and Craniofacial Research ($n = 2$). That many grants end up at institutes other than the NCI reflects the fact that many of the issues faced by survivors (e.g., depression, aging, family challenges, pain syndromes) are not always unique to cancer. In keeping with past patterns, the majority of studies supported were descriptive or analytic in nature (54%). However, 42% of the funded research projects contained an intervention component designed to improve the psychosocial well-being, physical status, and/or health behaviors of survivors and/or their family members. This latter figure is important as it denotes the transition that is occurring in the research arena away from mere identification of problems (discovery) to the development and testing of interventions designed to reduce posttreatment morbidity and mortality (development). Most of the studies continue to be unique to or include samples of breast cancer survivors ($n = 79$, 44%), who, for a variety of reasons, have historically been the focus of the majority of the psychosocial research conducted in cancer.[81] Other leading cancer sites represented in this work include hematologic, prostate, and colorectal.

A clear testament to the success of the NCI's efforts to grow in survivorship research, and the readiness of the research community to pursue questions in this area, is reflected in the response to its request for applications (RFA) for studies addressing long-term cancer survivorship (defined as studies among cancer survivors diagnosed 5 or more years ago). In 1997 the OCS presented its first such RFA (CA 97-018), which attracted 79 applications. In 2003, the RFA was reissued (CA 04-003). A total of 125 applications were received in response to this second call. Of the 125 grants received, 50 (40%) were from investigators new to the field of cancer survivorship research.

One of the reasons that the NCI reissued the Long-Term Survivors RFA was that without this impetus few investigators appeared willing to take on the additional challenges of studying individuals years posttreatment. A review of the research portfolio conducted before the RFA reissuance revealed that only 27 of 126 grants analyzed were studying survivors 5 or more years postdiagnosis; 21 of these were developed in response to the initial RFA. Critical barriers to long-term survivorship research include finding this population, obtaining access to them, including negotiating the many hurdles consequent to the recently implemented Health Insurance Portability and Accountability Act (HIPAA) regulations, developing tools that measure outcomes of relevance to the long-term survivorship experience, identifying appropriate control or comparison groups, and coordinating a team invested in addressing these issues.

Future

Staff at the American Cancer Society took advantage of the opportunity to poll investigators engaged in behavioral, psychosocial, and policy research in cancer about their current interests and expectations for future research foci when compiling a directory of these individuals in 1997 and again when they updated the directory for release in 2002.[82] Addressing psychosocial issues and treatment and outcomes remained key interest areas over time, a finding not altogether surprising given the target survey participants. However, two important areas for future research emerged in this report: the need to address special populations, a future direction voiced by members of all five of the disciplines represented (behavioral scientist, epidemiologist, nurse, physician, psychologist), and growing attention to health education and communication. Interesting in this study was the low endorsement of interest in survivorship research. Less than 10% said they were engaged in this type of research in 1997 (7.3%), and only 1.5% in 2002. However, in 2002, 11.7% thought it was going to be an important area of research in the future.

Ongoing analysis of the NIH-wide survivorship portfolio highlights a number of areas where our knowledge is lacking. Two of these areas echo themes identified for future targeting by Nehl and colleagues[82]: (1) the exploration of outcomes for our diverse population of survivors, specifically those from ethnoculturally diverse backgrounds, those from low-income or low educational backgrounds, rural survivors, elderly survivors, and survivors from common cancer sites under-represented in the literature (lung, colorectal, gynecologic, hematologic)[83]; and (2) effective communication about survivorship-related issues. To these, four more areas are added, including (3) research on the impact of cancer on the family or caregiver; (4) studies addressing the economic impact of cancer on survivors and survivorship; (5) assessment of the nature, delivery, and outcomes of follow-up care to survivors; and (6) measurement tool development, including that which would enable us to compare survivors with those without a cancer history while also controlling for other comorbid illness states.

As the field of survivorship research has matured, change has occurred not only in the focus of the research being conducted but also in how and by whom this research is being carried out. The typical published cancer survivorship study has evolved from a largely descriptive outcome report based on a small single institution sample[84,85] to one involving multidisciplinary teams accruing large cohorts and applying complex outcome and intervention assessments.[86,87] A concrete measure of the growing sophistication of this body of research is the expectation by standing members of study sections (peer review groups) to see power analyses, detailed rationales for measurement choices, adequate representation by appropriate diverse scientific experts, and demonstrated sensitivity to the unique needs and experience of the target survivor group in grants submitted for review, with general impatience with studies that appear to "rediscover" what is already documented. Table 100.1 provides an overview of some of these trends over time.

Looking to the future, it is expected that a healthy balance needs to be maintained between the identification of problematic long-term and late effects of cancer and our ability to address these. The roughly 60%/40% split in current NIH-funded research between studies aimed at identifying problem areas and those designed to develop and test interventions that reduce the negative effects of cancer is probably a reasonable balance. With respect to the intervention arena, two new trends are of note. It is increasingly apparent that to be successful this research must (a) attempt to explain the biopsychosocial interaction between what is being delivered and its impact on health outcomes[88,89] and (b) control or account for the costs associated with its delivery.[90] Although psychoneuroimmunology (PNI) research in cancer is by no means new,[91–93] attention to mind–body links is expanding as researchers seek to explain what is going on inside the proverbial "black box," in particular, in the context of psychosocial interventions that might mediate or moderate the impact of these trials on cancer recurrence or survival. Further, although drug interventions are relatively low cost, most psychosocial or behavioral interventions are labor intensive and hence more expensive to deliver. Despite this, there is good evidence to suggest they can reduce medical costs.[94] In recognition of this, investigators are working hard to design interventions that can be either self-administered,[90,95] delivered readily by available healthcare staff with minimal training,[96] and/or, the newest piece in these models, made available online.[97,98] This last point is critical if we are to have any hope of taking into the broader community interventions that hold the promise of significantly reducing the burden of cancer on individuals and society.

TABLE 100.1. Trends in cancer survivorship research design.

	Past	*Present*	*Future*
Target samples	Generally small convenience samples, often single institution based and mainly white, middle class, and middle age; largely breast cancer, or mixed, some colorectal, gynecologic; also pediatric, but largely leukemia	Moderate to large samples; often multiinstitutional; some clinical trials and population- or registry-based; increasing diversity of survivor groups by age and site (especially prostate, Hodgkin's disease, other gynecologic); still limited ethnocultural, income, and geographic diversity; more focus on family/caregivers	Mix of large (e.g., cohort, population-based) and moderate size; largely multiinstitutional; greater representation of more diverse cancer sites and previously neglected populations (e.g., by ethnic/income/geographic/age groups); more use of clinical trials samples
Team	Physicians, nurses, and some mental health professionals	Multidisciplinary teams; behavioral scientists leading in many areas; nurses with strong role as well; increasing role of advocates/survivors in research design	Truly multidisciplinary teams; attention to addition of basic scientists and psychoneuroimmunology (PNI) researchers to understand mind–body implications and impact of research findings for recurrence/survival, risk, and treatments; customary role for advocates/ survivors in research
Basic design	Descriptive; limited interventions; often atheoretical and exploratory in nature; almost exclusively cross-sectional designs	Increase in hypothesis- and model-driven designs; complex multicomponent interventions growing; replication studies appearing; longitudinal studies increasing	Sophisticated model building and hypothesis testing; emphasis on building on prior studies, including research to take interventions to different audiences, settings, deliverers; intervention designs incorporating biologic markers and/or economic and health services endpoints or outcomes; longitudinal/ cohort research
Topic	Focus almost exclusively on documenting dysfunction: distress, disability, impairment; a few coping studies; limited risk modeling	HRQOL instrument development; shift to evaluate both benefits and deficits of illness; modeling of risk for poor outcomes; examining role of caregivers in survivor outcomes and vice versa; growing attention to treatment effects and focused attention to specific problems, e.g., sexual dysfunction, fatigue, cognitive impairment; beginning attention to health after treatment	HRQOL development for long-term survivors (including comparison to other chronic illness groups and controlling for comorbid conditions); identifying/describing late, as yet unknown effects of cancer and novel problems associated with newer treatments and risk for these; targeting and tailoring interventions to survivors; identifying who may need what delivered by whom and when in the course of care; establishing the unique human and economic burden of cancer (versus other chronic illnesses); health promotion, follow-up care studies

HRQOL, health-related quality of life.

Challenges for the Future

Looking to the future, investigators face a number of challenges in advancing cancer survivorship research.[99] These challenges can be seen as falling into three broad categories: (1) identifying the most salient topics for study, (2) creating or enhancing the resources necessary to conduct the research, and (3) developing ways to make use of what is discovered.

Discovery

One of the greatest challenges to engaging in survivorship research is keeping up with the rapid pace of change in cancer treatments and care, as is particularly well illustrated in the context of breast cancer. In the past 10 years we have seen the uptake into standard practice of the use of sentinel node biopsies (replacing axillary node dissections), neoadjuvant (presurgical administration of) chemotherapy for large tumors, dose-intense and dense regimens of adjuvant chemotherapy with their greater attendant exposure to growth factors, testing for Her2 and consideration of herceptin, autologous tissue implants (over saline or silicone implants) for breast reconstruction, and aromatase inhibitors in the adjuvant setting, as well as a shift away from use of stem cell transplant as a treatment option. Each of these alterations in practice has implications for QOL outcomes for women treated. For example, elimination for many women of the need for axillary node dissection may result in far fewer women developing lymphedema as a consequence of their breast cancer therapy.[100,101] Nevertheless, greater exposure to more-intense chemotherapy regimens will likely increase the number of women at risk for persistent problems with pain (related to the accompanying use of growth factors)[102] and memory problems (or chemo brain).[103] Meanwhile, continued changes in the healthcare delivery system are transforming significantly the availability of and access to resources that have been shown to buffer the adverse effects of care (e.g., access to social support, information and education, and rehabilitation services). In an effort to control rising medical costs and respond to diminished insurance reimbursements, many hospitals and medical centers have sought to decrease the number of patient hospitalizations and length of stay, eliminate or downsize the types of support services as well as the number of social workers in their systems, and shift the delivery of oncology care largely to the outpatient setting.[104,105] Third-party payers in turn have placed constraints on patients' ability to use specialized providers and/or services. Combined, these changes in the delivery of cancer care have put enormous pressure on cancer survivors and their family members or caregivers to be more self-sufficient or in some cases to do without the support or services they might wish to have in facilitating optimal recovery.[106] This burden is borne disproportionately by minority and underserved members of our society.[107] Curiously, while research consistently shows that providing education and support is important for survivors' capacity to cope with cancer, access to this help is diminishing.

The implication of these changes for researchers is that what may have been critically important for one cohort of survivors may be less relevant to the next generation of individuals treated. For example, body image was a major focus of research in early studies of breast cancer outcomes when mastectomy was the treatment of choice.[68] Today, most women have a choice (often involving several options) in how to treat the breast and deal with the cosmetic impact of breast cancer. As a consequence, body image disruption is less salient as either an outcome or research issue. Of more concern is how breast cancer treatment may alter sexual function and/or menopausal symptoms, given that more than 50% of women diagnosed now receive some form of adjuvant chemotherapy or hormonal therapy.[108] Increasingly, researchers are finding themselves caught between the need to identify emerging chronic or late effects of newer therapies and chronicling and addressing the long-term effects of older ones. This dilemma can become problematic if, at review, scientific peers around the table cannot see the relevance of long-term outcomes studies (given this picture), or when forced to make a choice about limited funding dollars, opt to support studies about current therapies only.

Some of the more recently identified "hot" areas of symptom research include a focus on memory problems, fatigue, weight gain, long-term cardiac health, osteoporosis, and persistent pain syndromes (associated with exposure to taxanes and/or use of growth factors). Interest in all these concerns has occurred in direct response to survivors' accounts of specific problems with these conditions (e.g., memory problems, fatigue, weight gain, pain), or clinicians' concerns about known potential toxicities of treatment (e.g., second malignancies, cardiac dysfunction, osteoporosis). As already observed, the recent advances in modern computer and laboratory technology and the associated explosion of discovery in the molecular sciences lend hope that future therapies can be designed to have fewer adverse effects on healthy tissue. Nevertheless, listening carefully to patients' experience of these new approaches is critical if we are to identify and evaluate in future generations of survivors the impact of cancer on health.

On a larger scale, with so many individuals living longer following a diagnosis of cancer, growing attention is being given to researching the efficacy of more generic interventions in improving the future health of survivors, not merely in diminishing their current symptoms. There is a growing movement in particular to develop interventions that include elements with the potential to be generalized to other noncancer conditions. Two good examples of this are the work being done by Antoni and colleagues in the area of stress management[109,110] and that of Courneya and colleagues on delivery of physical activity interventions.[111,112] With the baby boomers fast entering the years of greatest cancer risk, understanding the role of comorbidities on cancer outcomes and care is critical to both evaluating and reducing the burden of cancer.[43,44,113,114] At the same time, a pressing need continues for us to understand the enormous and growing divide between survival—and necessarily the survivorship experience—of our communities of color, low income, low education, and rural status, versus the Caucasian and Asian survivor populations about whom we have the most data.[83,115]

Development

To accomplish any of this work will take some very specific resources and infrastructure or capacity building. First is access to relevant study samples. A continuing challenge for many researchers is identifying and reaching long-term survivors, in particular those diagnosed more than 5 years earlier.[116] Tumor registries can help,[117] but loss to follow-up is common. Clinical trials groups, an obvious place to partner to obtain long-term follow-up data, also often lose track of their participants over time.[118] The introduction of new federal privacy laws (Health Insurance Portability and Accountability Act, or HIPAA), by requiring individual consent for the conduct of specific studies and data sharing, has made access to survivors and their medical records even more cumbersome. This problem is not unique to the United States.[119] Establishment of the NCI-supported Childhood Cancer Survivor Study cohort currently provides a rich resource for survivorship information generated from its ascertained sample of roughly 14,000 survivors of childhood cancer diagnosed between 1978 and 1986 and the companion sample of more than 3,800 siblings.[120] To date, no such repository exists for survivors of adult cancer.

A second critical need is a steady flow of researchers. Despite the fact that the field of psycho-oncology (or psychosocial oncology), and the more-specific area of posttreatment survivorship research, has grown steadily in the past two decades, the number of researchers devoted to this science is still very limited. Further, there continue to be only a handful of training centers across the country devoted to the education and support of the next generation of researchers invested in survivorship research. With the recent creation of the American Society of Psychosocial Oncology (APOS), now independent from the older International Psycho-Oncology Society, there is hope that this picture may change. Further, the advances in computer technology, use of self-training programs for credit, and online access to a world of expertise may help close this gap in investigator resources. In this regard, APOS and the American Society of Clinical Oncology are pioneering efforts to promote the pursuit of continuing education by members in this and related symptom management and assessment domains.[121,122] Further, colleagues around the world are beginning to develop programs that promise to ensure a future cadre of talented clinicians and researchers.[123,124]

A third area of necessary development is on the provider side. Some in the pediatric oncology community have been heard to lament that fewer physicians are choosing to pursue careers in this specialty, assuming (incorrectly) that with survival figures already so high, few challenges or opportunities remain to make breakthroughs in this field. Adult oncology, by contrast, continues to offer diverse challenges; one of these being to better understand the long-term and late consequences of treatment as a way to improve cancer diagnosis, treatment, and care. Inadequate support for young physicians to engage in research remains a barrier to ensuring more oncologists will seek to expand their expertise in the survivorship arena. In a 2002 review of professional education and training in cancer survivorship commissioned by the National Cancer Policy Board (NCPB), Roger Winn found that although oncology textbooks were beginning to incorporate pieces about this aspect of care (in particular, the incidence and pathophysiology of chronic or late effects), often the material was fragmented and provided few guidelines for evaluation and care. There were, however, notable exceptions to this, including the Harris et al. volume *Diseases of the Breast*, and the monograph produced for the benefit of its members by the American Association of Family Practitioners on *Cancer Survivors*.

The picture in nursing appears to be quite different. Nurses were among the leaders in pioneering psychosocial research and QOL instrument development in cancer.[51,54–56] In a review also commissioned in 2002 by the NCPB, Betty Ferrell and Rose Virani found that all the major nursing textbooks of oncology nursing had sections or information on cancer survivorship and addressing late and long-term effects of disease. The Oncology Nursing Society has had a Special Interest Group in this area for several years.

Engaging the entire medical community (including nurses, primary care physicians, mental health professionals, and rehabilitation specialists) is necessary to ensure that we ask the right questions in survivorship research and use the best approaches to conduct this science. All this activity will require fiscal resources. Already there has been a rapid growth in the number of federal dollars being expended on survivorship research. This amount of money remains small, nevertheless, when compared to that being invested in cancer biology, detection, and treatment. In 2003, the OCS supported $17 million in grant-related research; NCI-wide investment in survivorship research, broadly defined to include studies among individuals across the survivorship continuum from diagnosis to end of life, was estimated at $160 million, less than 4% of the NCI budget for that year. Further, the end of the doubling of the NIH budget with FY 2004 and expected spending limits projected for the near future threaten to make competition for this still-nascent area of research a critical source of challenge.

On the positive side, a number of additional funders committed to supporting research on survivors' outcomes have appeared on the scene; these include the Lance Armstrong Foundation, the Avon Foundation, the Susan G. Komen Foundation, and the California Breast Cancer Research Program. Recently reframed as constituting a public health issue,[34] cancer survivorship is also beginning to appear on the agenda of the Center for Disease Control and Prevention. In addition, as noted earlier, Congress has put forward a number of bills in the past 2 years indicating their intention that the NIH in general and NCI in particular continue to invest in this science. The creation of the Office of Cancer Survivorship at the NCI provided a critical infrastructure and platform from which to oversee, track, and direct cancer survivorship research at the Federal level. Its existence within the NCI serves as a reminder of the importance of this aspect of the cancer control continuum both across NCI and nationally. Staff from the CDC, National Association of American Cancer Registries, ACS, NCI, and American College of Surgeons recently put forward recommendations for elements of the framework necessary to move cancer control forward in the next 20 years.[125] Similarly, members of NCI's Division of Cancer Control and Population Sciences have outlined where we need to go in the future to advance quality of cancer care across the continuum.[126]

Delivery

The final challenge faced is how best to disseminate and use the information gleaned from the growing body of cancer survivorship research. To date, this process has been painstakingly slow, in particular in the adult oncology arena. Delivering on what we already know represents, both historically[127] and at the present time, the least developed area of cancer survivorship research and constitutes one of the most significant challenges for the future.[128–130] This problem is well illustrated in a recent publication of the Institute of Medicine (IOM) entitled *Meeting the Psychosocial Needs of Women with Breast Cancer*.[131] In this volume, the multiple authors provide a wealth of evidence indicating that we already understand the kinds of problems faced by women treated for this disease, the handful of risk factors that increase risk for poor QOL, and the types of interventions that may help improve women's outcomes. Translating this into practice remains the biggest hurdle. This need includes educating healthcare providers about the psychosocial and behavioral effects of cancer and training them to incorporate psychosocial concerns into standard treatment planning and posttreatment monitoring, as well as designing and funding healthcare delivery systems that support this activity.[128] It is of note that, even in the nation's comprehensive cancer centers, programs for survivors who have completed their cancer therapy remain limited.[132] In addition, in many of these centers, researchers engaged in survivorship research are not routinely connected with the clinics or care centers.

These same kinds of struggles play out differently in the area of childhood cancer. In pediatrics, attention to the "total child" and his or her family is simply part of standard care.[133] Further, most pediatric care, whether in the cancer or noncancer setting, is designed around promoting normal development and preventing or minimizing risk of disease. Pediatric oncologists, perhaps because of the dramatic advances made in curing childhood cancers, have been at the forefront of efforts to tailor therapies to reduce morbidity without compromising cure. For example, once trials began to show that use of central nervous system prophylaxis dramatically altered the survival for children with ALL in the late 1960s and early 1970s, clinicians quickly turned their attention to finding less-toxic ways to provide this coverage that would eliminate the need for or reduce the dose of cranial radiation to which children would be exposed.[37] Equivalent evidence for this approach in adult oncology is harder to identify. The movement away from more-radical excisions to greater tissue-sparing approaches to surgery, as seen in breast and colorectal cancer, are good examples of efforts to modify treatment to improve QOL without adversely affecting cure. These surgical oncology examples notwithstanding, the general trend in adult oncology remains heavily focused on delivering more, not less, treatment, even if the length of time over which these therapies are administered is shrinking.

More recently, both the pediatric and adult oncology communities have engaged in efforts to decide how best to follow themselves, or engage the larger adult healthcare delivery system to care for, the growing population of young and maturing adults previously treated as children.[134,135] The Children's Oncology Group (COG) has taken a leadership role in shaping this effort. In spring 2004 COG publicly released the first set of comprehensive, long-term follow-up guidelines.[136] Unique to this document is its attention to the long-term and late sequelae of curative therapies. Unlike currently available guidelines for adult survivors who are posttreatment (e.g., as developed by ASCO, American Society of Clinical Oncology, and NCCN, National Comprehensive Cancer Network) that focus exclusively on cancer surveillance, the childhood cancer follow-up guidelines are constructed around identification and management of risk-based, exposure-related problems that may be screened for and potentially addressed after treatment. Largely unknown is how nononcology professionals view and care for the survivors in their patient population.[137] What evidence we have suggests that many survivors are not receiving care that might be expected for peers without a cancer history.[38,59,138,139] In this regard, data from two NCI-led SEER-based research studies on hematologic (non-Hodgkin's lymphoma, NHL) and selected solid tumor (breast, colorectal, prostate, gynecologic) survivors' experience of posttreatment care that will be available starting in 2005 should be informative.

A final criterion for the success of what one might call the cancer survivorship research enterprise is whether it is having an impact on the outcomes of present and future survivors and/or their families and caregivers. This aspect of survivorship research is as yet the least developed of all. Benchmarks for success exist in other realms of cancer control. For example, one can track the reduction in smoking rates to assess prevention efforts, the uptake of screening modalities (e.g., mammography, colonoscopy) by the appropriate populations to monitor inroads in promoting early detection, and survival curves to determine global cancer control. However, it is not clear what the markers of success are for improved survivorship (not to be confused with survival) outcomes.[140] Should this be return to school for children? Return to work for younger adults? Self-reported QOL compared to the general population for cohorts of survivors? Decrease in medical care use among survivors receiving a supportive intervention? If we have learned anything from survivors it is that being disease free does not mean being free of your disease. It is not enough to cure or enable individuals to live long term with a chronic illness without attending to what they are being returned. Because so many cancer survivors are older and present with a history of other comorbid conditions and experience, determining and alleviating what may be the unique burden of cancer is an area that remains to be fully addressed.[44,113,114,141] At a minimum, we need to be able to provide more than an estimate of the number of individuals who are living beyond a diagnosis of cancer. Finding ways to quantify how those individuals are faring in the main, and where they are on the cancer trajectory (i.e., recently diagnosed, in active treatment, posttreatment, living with or dying of progressive disease) is critical, particularly if we are to establish benchmarks against which to measure our progress. Efforts to do this are under way in Europe[142] and here in the United States.[143,144]

In summary, the evidence is clear that cancer survivorship, once merely a nascent field, is fast entering its adolescence, its pace of maturation driven by the progress made in controlling the many diseases we call cancer. Although still modest for most cancers, the body of research identifying the long-term and late effects of illness, as detailed in Chapter 101 by Aziz in this volume, is growing rapidly. At the same time, investment in the study of interventions to eliminate or reduce adverse cancer- or treatment-related outcomes is increasing. The cancer advocacy community has matured and provides an invaluable resource for ensuring continued attention to survivorship issues.[145–147] However, it is becoming apparent daily that improvements in cancer survivors' outcomes will likely be affected most by what happens to our healthcare delivery system in the years to come. We already know a great deal about what harms or helps those diagnosed and treated for cancer; delivering on the promise of care that conforms to that knowledge should be our most significant overarching goal for the foreseeable future.

References

1. A History of Commitment: 1884–Today. New York: Memorial Sloan-Kettering Cancer Center, Public Affairs Department booklet, 1994.
2. Jemal A, Clegg LX, Ward E, et al. Annual report to the nation on the status of cancer, 1975–2001, with a special feature regarding survival. Cancer (Phila) 2004;101:3–27.
3. Cancer Facts and Figures 2004. Atlanta, GA: American Cancer Society, 2004.
4. D'Angio GJ. Pediatric cancer in perspective: cure is not enough. Cancer (Phila) 1975;35:866–870.
5. Meadows AT, D'Angio GJ, Evans AE, et al. Oncogenesis and other late effects of cancer treatment in children. Radiology 1975;114:175–180.
6. Koocher G, O'Malley J. The Damocles Syndrome. New York: McGraw-Hill, 1981.
7. Holland JC. Historical overview. In: Holland JC, Rowland JH (eds). Handbook of Psychooncology: Psychological Care of the Patient with Cancer. Oxford: Oxford University Press, 1989:3–12.
8. Dolbeault S, Szporn A, Holland JC. Psycho-oncology: where have we been? Where are we going? Eur J Cancer 1999;35: 1554–1558.
9. Oken D. What to tell cancer patients: a study of medical attitudes. JAMA 1961;175:1120–1128.
10. Novack DH, Plumer R, Smith RL, et al. Changes in physicians' attitudes toward telling the cancer patient. JAMA 1979;241: 897–900.
11. Mystakidou K, Parpa E, Tsilila E, et al. Cancer information disclosure in different cultural contexts. Support Care Cancer 2004;12(3):147–154.
12. Surbone A. Persisting differences in truth telling throughout the world. Support Care Cancer 2004;12(3):143–146.
13. Wang S-Y, Chen C-H, Chen Y-S, Huang H-L. The attitude toward truth telling of cancer in Taiwan. J Psychosom Res 2004;57:53–58.
14. Holland JC. IPOS Sutherland Memorial Lecture: An international perspective on the development of psychosocial oncology: overcoming cultural and attitudinal barriers to improve psychosocial care. Psycho-Oncology 2004;13(7):445–459.
15. Reuben SH (ed). Living Beyond Cancer: A European Dialogue. President's Cancer Panel 2003–2004 Annual Report Supplement. Bethesda, MD: U.S. Department of Health and Human Services, NIH, NCI, May 2004.
16. Die-Trill M, Holland JC. A model curriculum for training in psycho-oncology. Psycho-Oncology 1995;4:169–182.

17. Derogatis LR, Lipman RS, Covi L. SCL-90: an outpatient psychiatric rating scale: preliminary report. Psychopharmacol Bull 1973;9:13–28.
18. NcNair DM, Lorr M, Droppleman R. EITS Manual for the Profile of Mood States. San Diego, CA: Educational and Industrial Testing Service, 1971.
19. Radloff LS. The CES-D scale: a self-report depression scale for research in the general population. Appl Psychol Meas 1977;1:385–401.
20. Endicott J. Measurement of depression in patients with cancer. Cancer (Phila) 1984;53:2243–2249.
21. Kathol RG, Noyes R, Williams J, et al. Diagnosing depression in patients with medical illness. Psychosomatics 1990;31(4): 434–440.
22. Cohen-Cole SA, Brown FW, McDainel JS. Assessment of depression and grief reactions in the medically ill. In: Stoudemire A, Fogel BS (eds). Psychiatric Care of the Medical Patient. New York: Oxford University Press, 1993:53–69.
23. Schipper H, Clinch J, McMurray A, Levitt M. Measuring the quality of life of cancer patients: The Functional Living Index—Cancer: development and validation. J Clin Oncol 1984;2(5):475–483.
24. Schag CAC, Heinrich RL. Development of a comprehensive quality of life measurement tool: CARES. Oncology 1990;4(5): 135–138.
25. Aaronson NK, Ahmedzai S, Bergman B, et al. The European Organization for Research and Treatment of Cancer QLQ-C30: a quality of life instrument for use in international clinical trials in oncology. J Natl Cancer Inst 1993;85(5):365–376.
26. Cella DF, Tulsky DS, Gray G, et al. The Functional Assessment of Cancer Therapy Scale: development and validation of the general measure. J Clin Oncol 1993;11(3):570–579.
27. Mullan F. Seasons of survival: reflections of a physician with cancer. N Engl J Med 1985;313:270–273.
28. Hoffman B (ed) National Coalition for Cancer Survivorship. A cancer survivor's almanac. Charting your journey. Minneapolis: Chronimed Publishing, 1996:XII–XIII. http://www.canceradvocacy.org
29. http://www.survivorship.cancer.gov
30. The Nation's Investment in Cancer Research: A plan and budget proposal for fiscal year 2004. NIH Publication No. 03-4373. Prepared by the Director, National Cancer Institute. Bethesda, MD: National Institutes of Health, USDHHS, October 2002.
31. The Nation's Investment in Cancer Research: A plan and budget proposal for fiscal year 2005. NIH Publication No. 03-5446. Prepared by the Director, National Cancer Institute. Bethesda: National Institutes of Health, USDHHS, October 2003.
32. Hewitt M, Weiner SL, Simone JV (eds). Childhood Cancer Survivorship. Improving Care and Quality of Life. Washington, DC: National Academies Press, 2003.
33. Living Beyond Cancer: Finding a New Balance. President's Cancer Panel 2003 Annual Report. Bethesda, MD: U.S. Department of Health and Human Services, NIH, NCI, May 2004.
34. CDC, Lance Armstrong Foundation. A national action plan for cancer survivorship: advancing public health strategies. Atlanta, GA: U.S. Department of Health and Human Services, CDC, 2004.
35. Tross S, Holland JC. Psychological sequelae in cancer survivors. In: Holland JC, Rowland JH (eds). Handbook of Psychooncology: Psychological Care of the Patient with Cancer. Oxford: Oxford University Press, 1989:101–116.
36. Kornblith AB. Psychosocial adaptation of cancer survivors. In: Holland JC (ed). Psycho-Oncology. New York: Oxford University Press, 1998:223–241.
37. Meadows AT. Pediatric cancer survivors: past history and future challenges. Curr Probl Cancer 2003;27:112–126.
38. Yeazel MW, Oeffinger KC, Gurney JG, et al. The cancer screening practices of adult survivors of childhood cancer: a report from the Childhood Cancer Survivors Study. Cancer (Phila) 2004;100:631–640.
39. Spingarn ND. Hanging in There: Living Well on Borrowed Time. New York: Stein & Day, 1982.
40. Spingarn ND. The New Cancer Survivors: Living With Grace, Fighting with Spirit. Baltimore: Johns Hopkins University Press, 1999.
41. Cancer survivorship–United States, 1971–2001. MMWR 2004;53(24):526–529.
42. http://www.seer.cancer.gov/seerstat
43. Yancik R, Ries LA. Cancer in older persons: an international issue in an aging world. Semin Oncol 2004;31:128–136.
44. Hewitt M, Rowland JH, Yancik R. Cancer survivors in the United States: age, health, and disability. J Gerontol A Biol Sci Med Sci 2003;58(1):82–91.
45. Caregiving in the U.S. A report by the National Alliance for Caregiving and AARP, 2004, http://www.caregiving.org/pubs/data.htm
46. Hewitt M, Breen N, Devesa S. Cancer prevalence and survivorship issues: analyses of the 1992 National Health Interview Survey. J Natl Cancer Inst 1999;91:1480–1486.
47. Cella DF, Tulsky DS. Quality of life in cancer: definition, purpose and method of measurement. Cancer Invest 1993;11: 327–336.
48. Sprangers MAG, Aaronson NK. The role of health care providers and others in evaluating the quality of life of patients with chronic disease: a review. J Clin Epidemiol 1992;45:743–760.
49. Fromme EK, Eilers KM, Mori M, et al. How accurate is clinician reporting of chemotherapy adverse effects? A comparison with patient-reported symptoms from the Quality-of-Life Questionnaire C30. J Clin Oncol 2004;22:3485–3490.
50. Sptizer QO, Dobson AJ, Hall J, et al. Measuring the quality of life of cancer patients: a concise QL-Index for use by physicians. J Chron Dis 1981;34:585–597.
51. Padilla GV, Presant C, Grant MM, et al. Quality of Life Index for patients with cancer. Res Nurs Health 1983;6:117–126.
52. Bergner M, Bobbitt RA, Careter WB, Gilson BS. The Sickness Impact Profile: development and final revision of a health status measure. Med Care 1981;19:787–806.
53. Lipscomb J, Gotay CC, Snyder CF. Outcomes Assessment in Cancer: Measures, Methods, and Applications. Cambridge, England: Cambridge University Press, 2005.
54. Ferrell BR, Dow KH, Grant M. Measurement of quality of life in cancer survivors. Qual Life Res 1995;4:523–531.
55. Wyatt GK, Friedman LL. Development and testing of a quality of life model for long-term female cancer survivors. Qual Life Res 1996;5:387–394.
56. Ferrans CE, Power MJ. Quality of life index: development and psychometric properties. Ann Nurs Sci 1995;8:15–24.
57. Pinto B, Eakin E, Maruyama N. Health behavior changes after a cancer diagnosis: what do we know and where do we go from here? Ann Behav Med 2000;22:38–52.
58. Blanchard CM, Denniston M, Baker F, et al. Do adults change their lifestyle behaviors after a cancer diagnosis? Am J Health Behav 2003;27:246–256.
59. Oeffinger KC, Mertens AC, Hudson MM, et al. Health care of young adult survivors of childhood cancer; a report from the Childhood Cancer Survivor Study. Ann Fam Med 2004;2:61–70.
60. Holmes MD, Kroenke CH. Beyond treatment: lifestyle choices after breast cancer to enhance quality of life and survival. Womens Health Issues 2004;14:11–13.
61. Northouse LL. Mastectomy patients and the fear of cancer recurrence. Cancer Nurs 1981;4:213–220.
62. Lee-Jones C, Humphris G, Dixon R, Hatcher M. Fear of cancer recurrence: a literature review and proposed cognitive formulation to explain exacerbation of recurrence fears. Psycho-Oncology 1997;6:95–105.

63. Vickberg SM. The Concerns About Recurrence Scale (CARS): a systematic measure of women's fears about the possibility of breast cancer recurrence. Ann Behav Med 2003;25(1):16–24.
64. Doward LC, McKennssa SP. Evolution of quality of life assessment. In: Rajagopalan R, Sheretz EF, Anderson RT (eds). Care Management of Skin Disease: Life Quality and Economic Impact. New York: Dekker, 1997:9–33.
65. Guyatt GH, Feeny DH, Patrick DL. Measuring health-related quality of life. Ann Intern Med 1993;118:622–629.
66. Bonanno GA. Loss, trauma and human resilience. Have we underestimated the human capacity to thrive after extremely aversive events? Am Psychol 2004;59:20–28.
67. Sprangers MA. Quality-of-life assessment in oncology. Achievements and challenges. Acta Oncol 2002;41:229–237.
68. Bard M, Sutherland AM. The psychological impact of cancer and its treatment: IV. Adaptation to radical mastectomy. Cancer (Phila) 1955;8:656–672.
69. Holmes HA, Holmes FF. After ten years, what are the handicaps and life styles of children treated for cancer? Clin Pediatr 1975;14:819–823.
70. Rieker P, Edbril SD, Garnick MB. Curative testis cancer therapy: psychosocial sequelae. J Clin Oncol 1985;3:1117–1126.
71. Cella DF, Tross S. Psychological adjustment to survival from Hodgkin's disease. J Consult Clin Psychol 1986;54:616–622.
72. Rapoport Y, Keritler S, Chaitchik S, et al. Psychosocial problems in head-and-neck cancer patients and their change with time since diagnosis. Ann Oncol 1993;4:69–73.
73. Green BL, Krupnick JL, Rowland JH, et al. Trauma history as a predictor of psychologic symptoms in women with breast cancer. J Clin Oncol 2000;18:1084–1093.
74. Cordova MJ, Andrykowski MA. Responses to cancer diagnosis and treatment: posttraumatic stress and posttraumatic growth. Semin Clin Neuropsychiatry 2003;8:286–296.
75. Lechner SC, Zakowski SG, Antoni MH, et al. Do sociodemographic and disease-related variables influence benefit-finding in cancer patients? Psycho-Oncology 2003;12:491–499.
76. Sears SR, Stanton AL, Danoff-Burg S. The yellow brick road and the emerald city: benefit finding, positive reappraisal coping and post-traumatic growth in women with early-stage breast cancer. Health Psychol 2003;22:487–497.
77. Tomich PL, Helgeson VS. Is finding something good in the bad always good? Benefit finding among women with breast cancer. Health Psychol 2004;23:16–23.
78. Meyer TJ, Mark MM. Effects of psychosocial interventions with adult cancer patients. A meta-analysis of randomized experiments. Health Psychol 1995;14:101–108.
79. Devine EC, Westlake SK. The effects of psychoeducational care provided to adults with cancer: metaanalysis of 116 studies. Oncol Nurs Forum 1995;22:1369–1381.
80. http://dccps.nci.nih.gov/ocs/portfolio.asp
81. Rowland JH. Psycho-oncology and breast cancer: a paradigm for research and intervention. Breast Cancer Res Treat 1994;31(2–3):315–324.
82. Nehl EJ, Blanchard CM, Stafford JS, et al. Research interests in the field of behavioral, psychosocial, and policy cancer research. Psycho-Oncology 2003;12:385–392.
83. Aziz NM, Rowland JH. Cancer survivorship research among ethnic minority and medically underserved groups. Oncol Nurs Forum 2002;29(5):789–801.
84. Schottenfeld D, Robbins GF. Quality of survival among patients who have had radical mastectomy. Cancer (Phila) 1970;26: 650–654.
85. Li FP, Stone R. Survivors of cancer in childhood. Ann Intern Med 1976;84:551–553.
86. Ganz PA, Kwan L, Stanton AL, et al. Quality of life at the end of primary treatment of breast cancer: first results from the moving beyond cancer randomized trial. J Natl Cancer Inst 2004;96:376–387.
87. Kroenke CH, Rosner B, Chen WY, et al. Functional impact of breast cancer by age at diagnosis. J Clin Oncol 2004;22: 1849–1856.
88. Andersen BL, Farrar WB, Golden-Kreutz DM, et al. Psychological, behavioral, and immune changes after a psychological intervention: a clinical trial. J Clin Oncol 2004;22:3570–3580.
89. Abercrombie HC, Giese-Davis J, Sephton S, et al. Flattened cortisol rhythms in metastatic breast cancer patients. Psychoneuroendocrinology 2004;29:1082–1092.
90. Jacobsen PB, Meade CD, Stein KD, et al. Efficacy and costs of two forms of stress management training for cancer patients undergoing chemotherapy. J Clin Oncol 2002;20:2851–2862.
91. Bovbjerg D. Psychoneuroimmunology and cancer. In: Holland JC, Rowland JH (eds). Handbook of Psychooncology. Psychological Care of the Patient with Cancer. New York: Oxford University Press, 1989:727–734.
92. Bauer-Wu SM. Psychoneuroimmunology. Part II: Mind-body interventions. Clin J Oncol Nurs 2002;6:243–246.
93. Antoni MH. Psychoneuroendocrinology and psychoneuroimmunology of cancer: plausible mechanisms worth pursuing? Brain Behav Immun 2003(suppl 1):S84–S91.
94. Sobel DS. The cost-effectiveness of mind-body medicine interventions. Prog Brain Res 2000;122:393–412.
95. Angell KL, Kreshka MA, McCoy R, et al. Psychosocial intervention for rural women with breast cancer: the Sierra–Stanford Partnership. J Gen Intern Med 2003;18:499–507.
96. Fawzy NW. A psychoeducational nursing intervention to enhance coping and affective state in newly diagnosed malignant melanoma patients. Cancer Nurs 1995;18:427–438.
97. Gustafson DH, Hawkins RP, Boberg EW, et al. CHESS: 10 years of research and development in consumer health informatics for broad populations, including the underserved. Int J Med Inform 2002;65:169–177.
98. Lierberman MA, Golant M, Giese-Davis J, et al. Electronic support groups for breast carcinoma: a clinical trial of effectiveness. Cancer (Phila) 2003;97:920–925.
99. Aziz NM, Rowland JH. Trends and advances in cancer survivorship research: challenge and opportunity. Semin Radiat Oncol 2003;13:248–266.
100. Schijven MP, Vingerhoets AJ, Rutten HJ, et al. Comparison of morbidity between axillary lymph node dissection and sentinel node biopsy. Eur J Surg Oncol 2003;29(4):341–350.
101. Blanchard DK, Donohue JH, Reynolds C, Grant CS. Relapse and morbidity in patients undergoing sentinel lymph node biopsy alone or with axillary dissection for breast cancer. Arch Surg 2003;138(5):482–487.
102. Ingham J, Seidman A, Yao TJ, et al. An exploratory study of frequent pain measurement in a cancer clinical trial. Qual Life Res 1996;5:503–507.
103. Tannock IF, Ahles TA, Ganz PA, van Dam FS. Cognitive impairment associated with chemotherapy for cancer: report of a workshop. J Clin Oncol 2004;22:2233–2239.
104. Hewitt M, Simone JV (eds) Ensuring Quality Cancer Care. Washington, DC: National Academy Press, 1999.
105. Chassin MR, Galvin RW. The urgent need to improve health care quality. Institute of Medicine National Roundtable on Health Care Quality. JAMA 1998;280:1000–1005.
106. Hewitt M, Rowland JH. Mental health service use among adult cancer survivors: analyses of the National Health Interview Survey. J Clin Oncol 2002;20(23):4581–4590.
107. Freeman HP, Reuben SH (eds) Voices of a Broken System: Real People, Real Problems. President's Cancer Panel Report of the Chairman, 2000–2001. NIH Publication No. 03-5301. Bethesda, MD: National Institutes of Health, National Cancer Institute, December 2002.

108. Rowland JH, Desmond KA, Meyerowitz BE, et al. Role of breast reconstructive surgery in physical and emotional outcomes among breast cancer survivors. J Natl Cancer Inst 2000;92(17):1422–1429.
109. McGregor BA, Antoni MH, Boyers A, et al. Cognitive-behavioral stress management increases benefit finding and immune function among women with early-stage breast cancer. J Psychosom Res 2004;56:1–8.
110. Antoni MH. Stress Management Intervention for Women with Breast Cancer (accompanied by Therapist's Manual and Participant's Workbook). Washington, DC: American Psychological Association Press, 2003.
111. Courneya KS, Mackey JR, Bell GJ, et al. Randomized controlled trial of exercise training in postmenopausal breast cancer survivors: cardiopulmonary and quality of life outcomes. J Clin Oncol 2003;21(9):1660–1668.
112. Courneya KS. Exercise in cancer survivors: an overview of research. Med Sci Sports Exerc 2003;35(11):1846–1852.
113. Piccirillo JF, Tierney RM, Costas I, et al. Prognostic importance of comorbidity in a hospital-based cancer registry. JAMA 2004;291:2441–2447.
114. Yabroff KR, Lawrence WF, Clauser S, et al. Burden of illness in cancer survivors; findings from a population-based national sample. J Natl Cancer Inst 2004;96:1322–1330.
115. Meyerowitz BE, Richardson J, Hudson S, Leedham B. Ethnicity and cancer outcomes: behavioral and psychosocial considerations. Psychol Bull 1998;123:47–70.
116. Ganz PA. Why and how to study the fate of cancer survivors: observations from the clinic and the research laboratory. Eur J Cancer 2003;39(15):2136–2141.
117. Pakilit AT, Kahn BA, Petersen L, et al. Making effective use of tumor registries for cancer survivorship research. Cancer (Phila) 2001;92:1305–1314.
118. Robison L. Research involving long-term survivors of childhood and adolescent cancer: methodologic considerations. Curr Probl Cancer 2003;27:212–224.
119. Ward HJT, Cousens SN, Smith-Bathgate B, et al. Obstacles to conducting epidemiological research in the UK general population. BMJ 2004;329:277–279.
120. http://www.cancer.umn.edu/ltfu
121. http://www.apos-society.org/webcasts.asp
122. http://www.asco.org/ac/1,1003,_12-002303-00_18-0012404,00.asp
123. Loiselle CG, Bottorff JL, Butler L Degner LF. PORT: Psychosocial oncology research training: a newly funded strategic initiative in health research. Can J Nurs Res, 2004;36:159–164.
124. Fallowfield L, Jenkins V, Farewell V, Solis-Trapala I. Enduring impact of communication skills training: results of a 12-month follow-up. Br J Cancer 2003;20:1445–1449.
125. Wingo PA, Howe HL, Thun MJ, et al. A national framework for cancer surveillance in the United States. Cancer Causes Control 2005;16:151–170.
126. Lipscomb J, Donaldson MS, Arora NK, et al. Cancer outcomes Research. Natl Cancer Inst Momogr 2004;33:178–192.
127. Greer S. Psycho-oncology: its aims, achievements and future tasks. Psycho-Oncology 1994;3:87–101.
128. Holland JC. Psychological care of patients: psycho-oncology's contribution. J Clin Oncol 2003;21:253s–265s.
129. Greer S. Psychological intervention. The gap between research and practice. Acta Oncol 2002;41:238–243.
130. Nicassio PM, Meyerowitz BE, Kerns RD. The future of health psychology interventions. Health Psychol 2004;23:132–137.
131. Hewitt M, Herdman R, Holland J (eds). Meeting the Psychosocial Needs of Women with Breast Cancer. Washington, DC: National Academies Press, 2004.
132. Tesauro GM, Rowland JH, Lustig C. Survivorship resources for post-treatment cancer survivors. Cancer Pract 2002;10: 277–283.
133. Rowland JH. Looking beyond cure: pediatric cancer as a model. J Pediatr Psychol 2005;30:1–3.
134. Mertens AC, Cotter LK, Foster BM, et al. Improving health care for adult survivors of childhood cancer: recommendations from a Delphi panel of health policy experts. Health Policy 2004;69:169–178.
135. Kattlove H, Winn RJ. Ongoing care of patients after primary treatment for their cancer. CA Cancer J Clin 2003;54:172–196.
136. http://www.survivorshipguidelines.org
137. McMurchie M. Life after cancer. Aust Fam Physician 1991;20:1444–1451.
138. Earle CC, Burstein JH, Winer EP, Weeks JC. Quality of non-breast cancer health maintenance among elderly breast cancer survivors. J Clin Oncol 2003;21:1447–1451.
139. Earle CC, Neville BA. Under use of necessary care among cancer survivors. Cancer (Phila) 2004;101:1712–1719; 2004; epub.
140. Ganz PA. What outcomes matter to patients: a physician-researcher point of view. Med Care 2002;40(6 suppl):III-1–III-9.
141. Yancik R, Ganz PA, Varricchio CG, Conley B. Perspectives on comorbidity and cancer in older patients; approaches to expand the knowledge base. J Clin Oncol 2001;19:1147–1151.
142. Gatta G, Capocaccia R, Berrino F, et al., and EUROPREVAL Working Group. Colon cancer prevalence and estimation of differing care needs of colon cancer patients. Ann Oncol 2004;15:1136–1142.
143. Earle CC, Nattinger AB, Potosky AL, et al. Identifying cancer relapse using SEER-Medicare data. Med Care 2002;40:5–81.
144. Mariotto A. Surveillance Research Program, Division of Cancer Control and Population Sciences. National Cancer Institute, NIH/DHHS, Bethesda, MD. Personal communication.
145. Leigh S. The culture of survivorship. Semin Oncol Nurs 2001;17:234–235.
146. Zebrack B. An advocate's perspective on cancer survivorship. Semin Oncol Nurs 2001;17:284–287.
147. Stovall E, Gesme D. Coming together to conquer cancer. J Clin Oncol 1999;17:730.

101

Late Effects of Cancer Treatments

Noreen M. Aziz

Background and Significance

With continued advances in strategies to detect cancer early and treat it effectively, along with the aging of the population, the number of individuals living years beyond a cancer diagnosis can be expected to continue to increase. Statistical trends show that, in the absence of other competing causes of death, 64% of adults diagnosed with cancer today can expect to be alive in 5 years.[1–4] Relative 5-year survival rates for those diagnosed as children (age less than 19 years) are even higher, with almost 79% of childhood cancer survivors estimated to be alive at 5 years and 75% at 10 years.[5]

Survival from cancer has seen dramatic improvements over the past three decades, mainly as a result of advances in early detection, therapeutic strategies, and the widespread use of combined modality therapy (surgery, chemotherapy, and radiotherapy).[6–10] Medical and sociocultural factors such as psychosocial and behavioral interventions, active screening behaviors, and healthier lifestyles may also play an integral role in the length and quality of that survival.[11]

Although beneficial and often lifesaving against the diagnosed malignancy, most therapeutic modalities for cancer are associated with a spectrum of late complications ranging from minor and treatable to serious or, occasionally, potentially lethal.[2,6,12–15] While living for extended periods of time beyond their initial diagnosis, many cancer survivors often face various chronic and late physical and psychosocial sequelae of their disease or its treatment. Additionally, as the number of survivors and their length of survival expand, long-term health issues specific to cancer survival are also fast emerging as a public health concern. Questions of particular importance to cancer survivors include surveillance for the adverse sequelae, or late and long-term effects, of treatment; the development of new (second) cancers; and recurrence of their original cancer. One-fourth of *late deaths* occurring among survivors of childhood cancer during the extended survivorship period, when the chances of primary disease recurrence are negligible, can be attributed to a treatment-related effect such as a second cancer or cardiac dysfunction.[16] The most *frequently observed* medical sequelae among pediatric cancer survivors include endocrine complications, growth hormone deficiency, primary hypothyroidism, and primary ovarian failure. Also included within the rubric of late effects are second cancers arising as a result of genetic predisposition (e.g., familial cancer syndromes) or the mutagenic effects of therapy. These factors may act independently or synergistically. Synergistic effects of mutagenic agents such as cigarette smoke or toxins such as alcohol are largely unknown.[2,6,12]

Thus, there is today a greater recognition of symptoms that persist after the completion of treatment and which arise years after primary therapy. Both acute organ toxicities such as radiation pneumonitis and chronic toxicities such as congestive cardiac failure, neurocognitive deficits, infertility, and second malignancies are being described as the price of cure or prolonged survival.[2,6,12] The study of late effects, originally within the realm of pediatric cancer, is now germane to cancer survivors at all ages because concerns may continue to surface throughout the life cycle.[2,6] These concerns underscore the need to follow up and screen survivors of cancer for toxicities such as those mentioned and also to develop and provide effective interventions that carry the potential to prevent or ameliorate adverse outcomes.

The goal of survivorship research is to focus on the *health and life* of a person with a history of cancer *beyond* the acute diagnosis and treatment phase. Survivorship research seeks to examine the causes of, and to prevent and control the adverse effects associated with, cancer and its treatment and to optimize the physiologic, psychosocial, and functional outcomes for cancer survivors and their families. A hallmark of survivorship research is its emphasis on understanding the integration/interaction of multidisciplinary domains.

This chapter presents definitional issues relevant to cancer survivorship; examines late effects of cancer treatment among survivors of pediatric and adult cancer; and articulates gaps in knowledge and emerging research priorities in cancer survivorship research relevant to late effects of cancer treatment. It draws heavily from pediatric cancer survivorship research because a paucity of data continue to exist for medical late effects of treatment for survivors of cancer diagnosed as adults. Research on late effects of cancer treatment began in the realm of pediatric cancer and continues to yield important insights for the impact of cancer therapies among those diagnosed as adults.

Definitional Issues

Fitzhugh Mullan, a physician diagnosed with and treated for cancer himself, first described cancer survivorship as a concept.[17] Definitional issues for cancer survivorship encompass three related aspects:[2,6] *(1) Who is a cancer survivor?* Philosophically, anyone who has been diagnosed with cancer is a survivor, from the time of diagnosis to the end of life.[1] Caregivers and family members are also included within this definition as secondary survivors. *(2) What is cancer survivorship?* Mullan described the survivorship experience as similar to the seasons of the year. Mullan recognized three seasons or phases of survival: acute (extending from diagnosis to the completion of initial treatment, encompassing issues dominated by treatment and its side effects); extended (beginning with the completion of initial treatment for the primary disease, remission of disease, or both, dominated by watchful waiting, regular follow-up examinations, and, perhaps, intermittent therapy); and permanent survival (not a single moment; evolves from extended disease-free survival when the likelihood of recurrence is sufficiently low). An understanding of these phases of survival is important for facilitating an optimal transition into and management of survivorship. *(3) What is cancer survivorship research?* Cancer survivorship research seeks to identify, examine, prevent, and control adverse cancer diagnosis and treatment-related outcomes (such as late effects of treatment, second cancers, and quality of life); to provide a knowledge base regarding optimal follow-up care and surveillance of cancer survivors; and to optimize health after cancer treatment.[2,6]

Other important definitions include those for long-term cancer survivorship and late versus long-term effects of cancer treatment. Generally, *long-term cancer survivors* are defined as those individuals who are 5 or more years beyond the diagnosis of their primary disease and embody the concept of permanent survival described by Mullan. *Late effects* refer specifically to unrecognized toxicities that are absent or subclinical at the end of therapy and become manifest later with the unmasking of hitherto unseen injury caused by any of the following factors: developmental processes; the failure of compensatory mechanisms with the passage of time; or organ senescence. *Long-term effects* refer to any side effects or complications of treatment for which a cancer patient must compensate; also known as persistent effects, they begin during treatment and continue beyond the end of treatment. Late effects, in contrast, appear months to years after the completion of treatment. Some researchers classify cognitive problems, fatigue, lymphedema, and peripheral neuropathy as long-term effects while others classify them as late effects.[18–21]

This chapter focuses largely on the *physiologic* or *medical* long-term and late effects of cancer treatment. Physiologic sequelae of cancer treatment can also be further classified as follows:

a. System-specific (e.g., organ damage, failure, or premature aging, immunosuppression or issues related to compromised immune systems, and endocrine damage);
b. Second malignant neoplasms (such as an increased risk of recurrent malignancy, increased risk of a certain cancer associated with the primary malignancy, and/or increased risk of secondary malignancies associated with cytotoxic or radiologic cancer therapies (this topic is not covered in detail in this chapter as it is reviewed comprehensively elsewhere in this book); and
c. Functional changes such as lymphedema, incontinence, pain syndromes, neuropathies, fatigue; cosmetic changes such as amputations, ostomies, and skin/hair alterations; and comorbidities such as osteoporosis, arthritis, and hypertension.

[1]From the National Coalition for Cancer Survivorship.

Late and Long-Term Effects of Cancer and Its Treatment: Overview and Generalizations

Consequent to the phenomenal success in treating cancer effectively and detecting it early, we are faced today with an increasing population of individuals who, although cancer free for many years, have issues and concerns regarding the persistent (chronic) and the late (delayed) effects of cancer therapies on their health, longevity, and quality of life. The long-term impact of cancer and its treatment can include premature mortality and long-term morbidity. The two most frequent causes of premature mortality in disease-free cancer survivors are (1) cardiac disease and (2) second malignant neoplasms.[22,23] The subject of late effects among children treated for cancer has been the topic of numerous reviews.[21,24–28] To varying degrees, it has been shown that disease- or treatment-specific subgroups of long-term survivors are at risk of developing adverse outcomes. These adverse consequences of cancer treatment include early death, second neoplasms, organ dysfunction (e.g., cardiac, pulmonary, gonadal), reduced growth and development, decreased fertility, impaired intellectual function, difficulties obtaining employment and insurance, and a decreased quality of life. This chapter summarizes selected aspects of the spectrum of outcomes relating to the late effects of therapy among individuals (adults, children, and adolescents) treated for cancer.

Generalizations About Late Effects

Several generalizations can be made.[2,6,29] It is now possible to anticipate certain types of late effects on the basis of specific therapies to which the survivor was exposed, the age of the survivor at the time of treatment, combinations of treatment modalities used, and the dosage administered. There are differences in susceptibility between pediatric and adult patients. Generally, chemotherapy results in acute toxicities that can persist whereas radiation leads to sequelae that are not apparent immediately and surface after a latent period. Combinations of chemotherapy and radiation therapy are more often associated with late effects in the survivorship period.[2,6,29]

Toxicities related to chemotherapy, especially those of an acute but possibly persistent nature, may be related to proliferation kinetics of individual cell populations as these drugs are usually cell cycle dependent. Thus, organs or tissues most susceptible are those with high cell proliferation (turnover) rates such as the skin (epidermis), bone marrow, gastrointestinal mucosa, liver, and testes. Theoretically, the least susceptible organs and tissues are those that replicate very slowly or not at all and include muscle cells, neurons, and the connective tissue.[2,6,29]

Issues Unique to Certain Cancer Sites

Late effects have been studied in greater depth for certain cancer sites. The examination of late effects for childhood cancers such as acute lymphoblastic leukemia, Hodgkin's disease, and brain tumors have provided the foundation for this area of research. A body of knowledge on late effects of radiation and/or chemotherapy is subsequently being developed for adult sites such as breast cancer. For example, recent studies have evaluated and reported on the development of neurocognitive deficits after chemotherapy for breast cancer, a late effect that was initially observed among survivors of childhood cancer receiving cranial irradiation and/or chemotherapy. Late effects of bone marrow transplant have been studied for both adult and childhood cancer survivors, as have sequelae associated with particular chemotherapeutic regimens such as those for Hodgkin's disease or breast cancer.

Chemotherapeutic drugs for which late effects have been reported most frequently include adriamycin, bleomycin, vincristine, methotrexate, cytoxan, and many others (Table 101.1).

The side effects of radiotherapy, both alone and in conjunction with chemotherapy, have been reported fairly comprehensively for most childhood cancer sites associated with good survival rates. It is important to bear in mind that most cancer treatment regimens consist of chemotherapy in conjunction with surgery and/or radiation, and multidrug chemotherapeutic regimens are the rule rather the exception. As such, the risk of late effects must always be considered in light of all other treatment modalities to which the patient has been exposed.

Special Considerations of Primary Diagnosis and Treatment in Childhood

Cancer therapy may interfere with development in terms of physical and musculoskeletal growth, neurocognitive/intellectual growth, and pubertal development. These effects may be most *notable* during the adolescent growth spurt, even though they occur during the childhood period. These specific sequelae are covered in greater detail in the chapter by Bhatia et al. (see Chapter 102) and are not discussed here. A brief classification follows.

a. Alterations in physical growth
   i. Linear growth effects[30–32]
   ii. Impact of early puberty on growth[33,34]
   iii. Hypoplasia[35]
b. Alterations in intellectual development[36–39]
c. Altered pubertal development[40]
d. Obesity[41–43]

Special Considerations of Primary Diagnosis and Treatment During Adulthood

Some late effects of chemotherapy may assume special importance depending on the adult patient's age at the time of diagnosis and treatment. Diagnosis and treatment during the *young adult or reproductive years* may call for a special cognizance of the importance of maintaining reproductive func-

TABLE 101.1. Possible late effects of radiotherapy and chemotherapy.

Organ system	*Late effects/sequelae of radiotherapy*	*Late effects/sequelae of chemotherapy*	*Chemotherapeutic drugs responsible*
Bone and soft tissues	Short stature; atrophy, fibrosis, osteonecrosis	Avascular necrosis	Steroids
Cardiovascular	Pericardial effusion; pericarditis; CAD	Cardiomyopathy; CHF	Anthracylines Cyclophosphamide
Pulmonary	Pulmonary fibrosis; decreased lung volumes	Pulmonary fibrosis; interstitial pneumonitis	Bleomycin, BCNU Methotrexate, adriamycin
Central nervous system (CNS)	Neuropsychologic deficits, structural changes, hemorrhage	Neuropsychologic deficits, structural changes Hemiplegia; seizure	Methotrexate
Peripheral nervous system		Peripheral neuropathy; hearing loss	Cisplatin, vinca alkaloids
Hematologic	Cytopenia, myelodysplasia	Myelodyplastic syndromes	Alkylating agents
Renal	Decreased creatinine clearance Hypertension	Decreased creatinine clearance Increased creatinine Renal filtration Delayed renal filtration	Cisplatin Methotrexate Nitrosoureas
Genitourinary	Bladder fibrosis, contractures	Bladder fibrosis; hemorrhagic cystitis	Cyclophosphamide
Gastrointestinal	Malabsorption; stricture; abnormal LFT	Abnormal LFT; hepatic fibrosis; cirrhosis	Methotrexate, BCNU
Pituitary	Growth hormone deficiency; pituitary deficiency		
Thyroid	Hypothyroidism; nodules		
Gonadal	Men: risk of sterility, Leydig cell dysfunction. Women: ovarian failure, early menopause	Men: sterility Women: sterility, premature menopause	Alkylating agents Procarbazine
Dental/oral health	Poor enamel and root formation; dry mouth		
Opthalmologic	Cataracts; retinopathy	Cataracts	Steroids

CAD, coronary artery disease; CCF, congestive cardiac failure; LFT, liver function tests; BCNU, carmustine.

Source: Data from Ganz (1998, 2001)[12,13] and Aziz (2002, 2003).[2,6]

tion and the prevention of second cancers. These are also key issues for children whose cancers are diagnosed during childhood.

Cancer patients diagnosed and treated during *middle age* may need specific attention to sequelae such as premature menopause, issues relating to sexuality and intimacy, pros and cons of using estrogen replacement therapy (ERT), prevention of neurocognitive, cardiac, and other sequelae of chemotherapy, and the prevention of coronary artery disease and osteoporosis. It has been reported that sexual dysfunction persists after breast cancer treatment, despite recovery in other domains, and includes vaginal discomfort, hot flashes, and alterations in bioavailable testosterone, luteinizing hormone, and sex hormone-binding globulin.[44] Menopausal symptoms such as hot flashes, vaginal dryness, and stress urinary incontinence are very common in breast cancer survivors and cannot be managed with standard estrogen replacement therapy.[45] The normal life expectancy of survivors of early-stage cancers during these years of life underscores the need to address their long-term health and quality of life issues.

Although *older patients* (65 years and over) bear a disproportionate burden of cancer, advancing age is associated with increased vulnerability to other age-related health problems and concurrent ailments such as diabetes, chronic obstructive pulmonary disease, heart disease, arthritis, and/or hypertension. Any of these could potentially affect treatment choice, prognosis, and survival. Hence, cancer treatment decisions may need to be made in the context of the older individual's preexisting health problems (comorbidities). Measures that can help evaluate the existence, nature, and severity of comorbidities among older cancer patients in a reliable manner are needed. Currently, there is little information on how comorbid age-related conditions influence treatment decisions, the subsequent course of the disease, the way that already-compromised older cancer patients tolerate the stress of cancer and its treatment, and how concomitant comorbid conditions are managed.[46]

Review of Late and Long-Term Effects by Organ System or Tissues Affected[(2)]

System-Specific Physiologic Sequelae[(3)]

Cardiac Sequelae

The heart may be damaged by both therapeutic irradiation and chemotherapeutic agents commonly used in the treatment for cancer. Several types of damage have been reported, including pericardial, myocardial, and vascular. Cardiac damage is most pronounced after treatment with the anthracycline drugs doxorubicin and daunorubicin, used widely in the treatment of most childhood cancers and adjuvant chemotherapy for breast and many other adult cancers. An additive effect has also been reported when anthracyclines are used in conjunction with cyclophosphamide and radiation therapy. Anthracyclines cause myocardial cell death, leading to a diminished number of myocytes and compensatory hypertrophy of residual myocytes.[47] Major clinical manifestations include reduced cardiac function, arrhythmia, and heart failure. Chronic cardiotoxicity usually manifests itself as cardiomyopathy, pericarditis, and congestive heart failure.

Cardiac injury that becomes clinically manifest during or shortly after completion of chemotherapy may progress, stabilize, or improve after the first year of treatment. This improvement may either be of a transient nature or last for a considerable length of time. There is also evidence of a continuum of injury that will manifest itself throughout the lives of these patients.[48] From a risk factor perspective, patients who exhibit reduced cardiac function within 6 months of completing chemotherapy are at increased risk for the development of late cardiac failure.[49] However, a significant incidence of late cardiac decompensation manifested by cardiac failure or lethal arrhythmia occurring 10 to 20 years after the administration of these drugs has also been reported.[50]

In a recent study of Hodgkin's disease (HD) survivors, investigators reported finding cardiac abnormalities in the majority of the participants.[51] This is an important finding especially because the sample consisted of individuals who did not manifest symptomatic heart disease at screening and described their health as "good." Manifestations of cardiac abnormalities included (a) restrictive cardiomyopathy (suggested by reduced average left ventricular dimension and mass without increased left ventricular wall thickness); (b) significant valvular defects; (c) conduction defects; (d) complete heart block; (e) autonomic dysfunction (suggested by a monotonous heart rate in 57%); (f) persistent tachycardia; and (g) blunted hemodynamic responses to exercise. The peak oxygen uptake (VO_{2max}) during exercise, a predictor of mortality in heart failure, was significantly reduced (less than 20 mL/kg/m^2) in 30% of survivors and was correlated with increasing fatigue, increasing shortness of breath, and a decreasing physical component score on the SF-36. Given the presence of these clinically significant cardiovascular abnormalities, investigators recommend serial, comprehensive cardiac screening of HD survivors who fit the profile of having received mediastinial irradiation at a young age.

Congestive cardiomyopathy is directly related to the total dose of the agent administered; the higher the dose, the greater the chance of cardiotoxicity. Subclinical abnormalities have also been noted at lower doses. The anthracyclines doxorubicin and daunorubicin are well-known causes of cardiomyopathy that can occur many years after completion of therapy. The incidence of anthracycline-induced cardiomyopathy, which is dose dependent, may exceed 30% among patients receiving cumulative doses in excess of 600 mg/m^2. A cumulative dose of anthracyclines greater than 300 mg/m^2 has been associated with an 11-fold-increased risk of clinical heart failure, compared with a cumulative dose of less than 300 mg/m^2, the estimated risk of clinical heart failure increasing with time from exposure and approaching 5% after 15 years.

A reduced incidence and severity of cardiac abnormalities was reported in a study of 120 long-term survivors of acute lymphoblastic leukemia (ALL) who had been treated with lower anthracycline doses (90–270 mg/m^2), compared with previous reports in which subjects had received moderate

[(2)]Common to both children and adults depending on cancer site and treatment(s) received.

[(3)]These include organ damage, failure, or premature aging resulting from chemotherapy, hormone therapy, radiation, surgery, or any combination thereof.

anthracycline doses (300–550 mg/m²).[52,53] Twenty-three percent of the patients were found to have cardiac abnormalities, 21% had increased end-systolic stress, and only 2% had reduced contractility. The cumulative anthracycline dose within the 90 to 270 mg/m² range did not relate to cardiac abnormalities. The authors concluded that there may be no safe anthracycline dose to completely avoid late cardiotoxicity. A recent review of 30 published studies in childhood cancer survivors found that the frequency of clinically detected anthracycline cardiac heart failure ranged from 0% to 16%.[54] In an analysis of reported studies, the type of anthracycline (e.g., doxorubicin) and the maximum dose given in a 1-week period (e.g., more than 45 mg/m²) was found to explain a large portion of the variation in the reported frequency of anthracycline-induced cardiac heart failure.

Cyclophosphamide has been associated with the development of congestive cardiomyopathy, especially when administered at the high doses used in transplant regimens. Cardiac toxicity may occur at lower doses when mediastinal radiation is combined with the chemotherapeutic drugs mentioned above. Late onset of congestive heart failure has been reported during pregnancy, rapid growth, or after the initiation of vigorous exercise programs in adults previously treated for cancer during childhood or young adulthood as a result of increased afterload and the impact of the additional stress of such events on marginal cardiac reserves. Initial improvement in cardiac function after completion of therapy appears to result, at least in part, from compensatory changes. Compensation may diminish in the presence of stressors such as those mentioned earlier and myocardial depressants such as alcohol.

The incidence of subclinical anthracycline myocardial damage has been the subject of considerable interest. Steinherz et al. found 23% of 201 patients who had received a median cumulative dose of doxorubicin of 450 mg/m² had echocardiographic abnormalities at a median of 7 years after therapy.[55] In a group of survivors of childhood cancer who received a median doxorubicin dose of 334 mg/m², it was found that progressive elevation of afterload or depression of left ventricular contractility was present in approximately 75% of patients.[47] A recent review of the literature on subclinical cardiotoxicity among children treated with an anthracycline found that the reported frequency of subclinical cardiotoxicity varied considerably across the 25 studies reviewed (frequency ranging from 0% to 57%).[56] Because of marked differences in the definition of outcomes for subclinical cardiotoxicity and the heterogeneity of the patient populations investigated, it is difficult to accurately evaluate the potential long-term outcomes within anthracycline-exposed patient populations or the potential impact of the subclinical findings.

Effects of radiation on the heart may be profound, and include valvular damage, pericardial thickening, and ischemic heart disease. Patients with radiation-related cardiac damage have a markedly increased relative risk of both angina and myocardial infarction [relative risk (RR), 2.56] years after mediastinal radiation for Hodgkin's disease in adult patients, whereas the risk of cardiac death is 3.1.[57] This risk was greatest among patients receiving more than 30 Gy of mantle irradiation and those treated before 20 to 21 years of age. Blocking the heart reduced the risk of cardiac death due to causes other than myocardial infarction.[58]

In general, among anthracycline-exposed patients, the risk of cardiotoxicity can be increased by mediastinal radiation,[59] uncontrolled hypertension,[60,61] underlying cardiac abnormalities,[62] exposure to nonanthracycline chemotherapeutic agents (especially cyclophosphamide, dactinomycin, mitomycin C, dacarbazine, vincristine, bleomycin, and methotrexate),[63,64] female gender,[65] younger age,[66] and electrolyte imbalances such as hypokalaemia and hypomagnesaemia.[67] Previous reports have suggested that doxorubicin-induced cardiotoxicity can be prevented by continuous infusion of the drug.[68] However, Lipshultz et al. compared cardiac outcomes in children receiving either bolus or continuous infusion of doxorubicin, and reported that continuous doxorubicin infusion over 48 hours for childhood leukemia did not offer a cardioprotective advantage over bolus infusion.[69] Both regimens were associated with progressive subclinical cardiotoxicity, thus suggesting that there is no benefit from continuous infusion of anthracyclines.

Chronic cardiotoxicity associated with radiation alone most commonly involves pericardial effusions or constrictive pericarditis, sometimes in association with pancarditis. Although a dose of 40 Gy of total heart irradiation appears to be the usual threshold, pericarditis has been reported after as little as 15 Gy, even in the absence of radiomimetic chemotherapy.[70,71] Symptomatic pericarditis, which usually develops 10 to 30 years after irradiation, is found in 2% to 10% of patients.[72] Subclinical pericardial and myocardial damage, as well as valvular thickening, may be common in this population.[73,74] Coronary artery disease has been reported after radiation to the mediastinum, although mortality rates have not been significantly higher in patients who receive mediastinal radiation than in the general population.[58]

Given the known acute and long-term cardiac complications of therapy, prevention of cardiotoxicity is a focus of active investigation. Several attempts have been made to minimize the cardiotoxicity of anthracyclines, such as the use of liposomal-formulated anthracyclines, less-cardiotoxic analogues, and the additional administration of cardioprotective agents. The advantages of these approaches are still controversial, but there are ongoing clinical trials to evaluate the long-term effects. Certain analogues of doxorubicin and daunorubicin, with decreased cardiotoxicity but equivalent antitumour activity, are being explored. Agents such as dexrazoxane, which are able to remove iron from anthracyclines, have been investigated as cardioprotectants. Clinical trials of dexrazoxane have been conducted in children, with encouraging evidence of short-term cardioprotection[75]; however, the long-term avoidance of cardiotoxicity with the use of this agent has yet to be sufficiently determined. The most recent study by Lipshultz et al. reported that dexrazoxane prevents or reduces cardiac injury, as reflected by elevations in troponin T, that is associated with the use of doxorubicin for childhood ALL without compromising the antileukemic efficacy of doxorubicin. Longer follow-up will be necessary to determine the influence of dexrazoxane on echocardiographic findings at four years and on event-free survival.[76]

Another key emerging issue is the interaction of taxanes with doxorubicin. Epirubicin–taxane combinations are active in treating metastatic breast cancer, and ongoing research is focusing on combining anthracyclines with taxanes in an effort to continue to improve outcomes following adjuvant therapy.[77] Clinically significant drug interactions have been reported to occur when paclitaxel is administered with doxorubicin, cisplatin, or anticonvulsants (phenytoin, carbamazepine, and phenobarbital), and pharmacodynamic interactions have been reported to occur with these agents that are sequence- or schedule dependent.[78] Because the taxanes undergo hepatic oxidation via the cytochrome P-450 system, pharmacokinetic interactions from enzyme induction or inhibition can also occur. A higher than expected myelotoxicity has been reported. However, there is no enhanced doxorubicinol formation in human myocardium, a finding consistent with the cardiac safety of the regimen.[79] Investigators have suggested that doxorubicin and epirubicin should be administered 24 hours before paclitaxel and the cumulative anthracycline dose be limited to $360\,mg/m^2$, thereby preventing the enhanced toxicities caused by sequence- and schedule-dependent interactions between anthracyclines and paclitaxel.[78] Conversely, they also suggest that paclitaxel should be administered at least 24 hours before cisplatin to avoid a decrease in clearance and increase in myelosuppression. With concurrent anticonvulsant therapy, cytochrome P-450 enzyme induction results in decreased paclitaxel plasma steady-state concentrations, possibly requiring an increased dose of paclitaxel. A number of other drug interactions have been reported in preliminary studies for which clinical significance has yet to be established.[78]

The human epidermal growth factor receptor (HER) 2 is overexpressed in approximately 20% to 25% of human breast cancers and is an independent adverse prognostic factor. Targeted therapy directed against this receptor has been developed in the form of a humanized monoclonal antibody, trastuzumab. Unexpectedly, cardiac toxicity has developed in some patients treated with trastuzumab, and this has a higher incidence in those treated in combination with an anthracycline.[80,81] Both clinical and in vitro data suggest that cardiomyocyte HER2/erbB2 is uniquely susceptible to trastuzumab.[82] Tratuzumab has shown activity as a single agent in metastatic breast cancer both before chemotherapy and in heavily pretreated patients, and its use in combination with an anthracycline or paclitaxel results in a significant improvement in survival, time to progression, and response.[80] The HER2 status of a tumor is a critical determinant of response to trastuzumab-based treatment; those expressing HER2 at the highest level on immunohistochemistry, 3+, derive more benefit from treatment with trastuzumab than those with overexpression at the 2+ level. Interactions between the estrogen receptor and HER2 pathway has stimulated interest in using trastuzumab in combination with endocrine therapy. Current clinical trials are investigating the role of this agent in the adjuvant setting.

Neurocognitive Sequelae

Long-term survivors of cancer may be at risk of neurocognitive and neuropsychologic sequelae. Among survivors of childhood leukemia, neurocognitive late effects represent one of the more intensively studied topics. Adverse outcomes are generally associated with whole-brain radiation and/or therapy with high-dose systemic or intrathecal methotrexate or cytarabine.[83–85] High-risk characteristics, including higher dose of central nervous system (CNS) radiation, younger age at treatment, and female sex, have been well documented. Results from studies of neurocognitive outcomes are directly responsible for the marked reduction (particularly in younger children) in the use of cranial radiation, which is currently reserved for treatment of very high risk subgroups or patients with CNS involvement.[86]

A spectrum of clinical syndromes may occur, including radionecrosis, necrotizing leukoencephalopathy, mineralizing microangiopathy and dystropic calcification, cerebellar sclerosis, and spinal cord dysfunction.[87] Leukoencephalopathy has been primarily associated with methotrexate-induced injury of white matter. However, cranial radiation may play an additive role through the disruption of the blood–brain barrier, thus allowing greater exposure of the brain to systemic therapy.

Although abnormalities have been detected by diagnostic imaging studies, the abnormalities observed have not been well demonstrated to correlate with clinical findings and neurocognitive status.[88,89] Chemotherapy- or radiation-induced destruction in normal white matter partially explains intellectual and academic achievement deficits.[90] Evidence suggests that direct effects of chemotherapy and radiation on intracranial endothelial cells and brain white matter as well as immunologic mechanisms could be involved in the pathogenesis of central nervous system damage.

Neurocognitive deficits, as a general rule, usually become evident within several years following CNS radiation and tend to be progressive in nature. Leukemia survivors treated at a younger age (i.e., less than 6 years of age) may experience significant declines in intelligence quotient (IQ) scores.[91] However, reductions in IQ scores are typically not global, but rather reflect specific areas of impairment, such as attention and other nonverbal cognitive processing skills.[92] Affected children may experience information-processing deficits, resulting in academic difficulties. These children are particularly prone to problems with receptive and expressive language, attention span, and visual and perceptual motor skills, most often manifested in academic difficulties in the areas of reading, language, and mathematics. Accordingly, children treated with CNS radiation or systemic or intrathecal therapy with the potential to cause neurocognitive deficits should receive close monitoring of academic performance. Referral for neuropsychologic evaluation with appropriate intervention strategies, such as modifications in curriculum, speech and language therapy, or social skills training, implemented in a program tailored for the individual needs and deficits of the survivor should be taken into consideration.[93] Assessment of educational needs and subsequent educational attainment have found that survivors of childhood leukemia are significantly more likely to require special educational assistance, but have a high likelihood of successfully completing high school.[37,94] However, when compared with siblings, survivors of leukemia and non-Hodgkin's lymphoma (NHL) are at greater risk of not completing high school. As would be anticipated from the results of neurocognitive studies, it has been shown that survivors, particularly those under 6 years of age at treatment, who received cranial radiation and/or intrathecal chemotherapy were significantly more likely to require special education services and least likely to complete a formal education.[86,95,96]

Progressive dementia and dysfunction have been reported in some long-term cancer survivors as a result of whole-brain radiation with or without chemotherapy, and occur most often in brain tumor patients and patients with small cell lung cancer who have received prophylactic therapy. Neuropsychologic abnormalities have also been reported after CNS prophylaxis utilizing whole-brain radiation for leukemia in childhood survivors. In fact, cognitive changes in children began to be recognized as treatments for childhood cancer, especially ALL, became increasingly effective. These observations have resulted in changes in treatment protocols for childhood ALL.[97,98]

Several recent studies have reported cognitive dysfunction in women treated with adjuvant therapy for breast cancer.[99,100] In one study,[101] investigators compared the neuropsychologic performance of long-term survivors of breast cancer and lymphoma treated with standard-dose chemotherapy who carried the epsilon 4 allele of the apolipoprotein E (APOE) gene to those who carry other APOE alleles. Survivors with at least one epsilon 4 allele scored significantly lower in the visual memory (P less than 0.03) and the spatial ability (P less than 0.05) domains and tended to score lower in the psychomotor functioning (P less than 0.08) domain as compared to survivors who did not carry an epsilon 4 allele. No group differences were found on depression, anxiety, or fatigue. The results of this study provide preliminary support for the hypothesis that the epsilon 4 allele of APOE may be a potential genetic marker for increased vulnerability to chemotherapy-induced cognitive decline.

Although cranial irradiation is the most frequently identified causal factor in both adults and children, current work in adults indicates that cognitive problems may also occur with surgery, chemotherapy, and biologic response modifiers.[102–104] These findings need to be validated in prospective studies along with the interaction between treatment with chemotherapeutic agents, menopausal status, and hormonal treatments. Emotional distress also has been related to cognitive issues in studies of patients beginning cancer treatment.

Patients have attributed problems in cognition to fatigue, and others have reported problems with concentration, short-term memory, problem-solving, and concerns about "chemobrain" or "mental pause."[105] Comparisons across studies are difficult because of different batteries of neuropsychologic tests used, and differences among patient samples by diagnosis, age, gender, or type of treatment received, and, finally, inconsistency in the timing of measures in relation to treatment landmarks. Despite these methodologic issues, studies have shown impairments in verbal information processing, complex information processing, concentration, and visual memory.[106–109]

Current studies indicate that cognitive deficits are often subtle but are observed consistently in a proportion of patients, may be durable, and can be disabling.[110] Deficits have been observed in a range of cognitive functions. Although underlying mechanisms are unknown, preliminary studies suggest a genetic predisposition. Cognitive impairment may be accompanied by changes in the brain detectable by neuroimaging. Priorities for future research include (1) large-scale clinical studies that use both a longitudinal design and concurrent evaluation of patients with cancer who do not receive chemotherapy—such studies should address the probability and magnitude of cognitive deficits, factors that predict them, and underlying mechanisms; (2) exploration of discrepancies between subjective reports of cognitive dysfunction and the objective results of cognitive testing; (3) studies of cognitive function in patients receiving treatment for diseases other than breast cancer, and in both men and women, to address the hypothesis that underlying mechanisms relate to changes in serum levels of sex hormones and/or to chemotherapy-induced menopause; (4) development of interventions to alleviate these problems; and (5) development of animal models and the use of imaging techniques to address mechanisms that might cause cognitive impairment.

Endocrinologic Sequelae

Thyroid

Radiation exposure to the head and neck is a known risk factor for subsequent abnormalities of the thyroid. Among survivors of Hodgkin's disease and, to a lesser extent, leukemia survivors, abnormalities of the thyroid gland, including hypothyroidism, hyperthyroidism, and thyroid neoplasms, have been reported to occur at rates significantly higher than found in the general population.[111–114] Hypothyroidism is the most common nonmalignant late effect involving the thyroid gland. Following radiation doses above 15 Gy, laboratory evidence of primary hypothyroidism is evident in 40% to 90% of patients with Hodgkin's disease, NHL, or head and neck malignancies.[113,115,116] In a recent analysis of 1,791 5-year survivors of pediatric Hodgkin's disease (median age at follow-up, 30 years), Sklar et al. reported the occurrence of at least one thyroid abnormality in 34% of subjects.[114] The risk of hypothyroidism was increased 17 fold compared with sibling control subjects, with increasing dose of radiation, older age at diagnosis of Hodgkin's disease, and female sex as significant independent predictors of an increased risk. The actuarial risk of hypothyroidism for subjects treated with 45 Gy or more was 50% at 20 years following diagnosis of their Hodgkin's disease. Hyperthyroidism was reported to occur in only 5%.

Hormones Affecting Growth

Poor linear growth and short adult stature are common complications after successful treatment of childhood cancers.[117] The adverse effect of CNS radiation on adult final height among childhood leukemia patients has been well documented, with final heights below the fifth percentile occurring in 10% to 15% of survivors.[43,118,119] The effects of cranial radiation appear to be related to age and gender, with children younger than 5 years at the time of therapy and female patients being more susceptible. The precise mechanisms by which cranial radiation induces short stature are not clear. Disturbances in growth hormone production have not been found to correlate well with observed growth patterns in these patients.[31,120] The phenomenon of early onset of puberty in girls receiving cranial radiation may also play some role in the reduction of final height.[33,121] In childhood leukemia survivors not treated with cranial radiation, there are conflicting results regarding the impact of chemotherapy on final height.[122]

Hormonal Rationale for Obesity

An increased prevalence of obesity has been reported among survivors of childhood ALL.[123–125] Craig et al. investigated the relationship between cranial irradiation received during treatment for childhood leukemia and obesity.[126] Two hundred thirteen (86 boys and 127 girls) irradiated patients and 85 (37 boys and 48 girls) nonirradiated patients were enrolled. For cranially irradiated patients, an increase in the body mass index (BMI) Z score at the final height was associated with female sex and lower radiation dose but not with age at diagnosis. Severe obesity, defined as a BMI Z score greater than 3 at final height, was only present in girls who received 18 to 20 Gy irradiation at a prevalence of 8%. Both male and female nonirradiated patients had raised BMI Z scores at latest follow-up, and there was no association with age at diagnosis. The authors concluded that these data demonstrated a sexually dimorphic and dose-dependent effect of cranial irradiation on BMI. In a recent analysis from the Childhood Cancer Survivor Study, Oeffinger et al. compared the distribution of BMI of 1,765 adult survivors of childhood ALL with that of 2,565 adult siblings of childhood cancer survivors.[127] Survivors were significantly more likely to be overweight (BMI, 25–30) or obese (BMI, 30 or more). Risk factors for obesity were cranial radiation, female gender, and age from 0 to 4 years at diagnosis of leukemia. Girls diagnosed under the age of 4 years who received a cranial radiation dose greater than 20 Gy were found to have a 3·8-fold-increased risk of obesity.

Gonadal Dysfunction

Treatment-related gonadal dysfunction has been well documented in both men and women following childhood malignancies.[128] However, survivors of leukemia and T-cell non-Hodgkin's lymphoma treated with modern conventional therapy are at a relatively low risk of infertility and delayed or impaired puberty. Treatment-related gonadal failure or dysfunction, expressed as amenorrhea or azoospermia, can lead to infertility in both male and female cancer survivors, and may have its onset during therapy.[129] Infertility can be transient, especially in men, and may recover over time after therapy. Reversibility is dependent on the dose of gonadal radiation or alkylating agents. Ovarian function is unlikely to recover long after the immediate treatment period because long-term amenorrhea commonly results from loss of ova. Cryopreservation of sperm before treatment is an option for men,[130] but limited means are available to preserve ova or protect against treatment-related ovarian failure for women.[131–133] A successful live birth after orthotopic autotransplantation of cryopreserved ovarian tissue has been recently reported.[134–137] A reasonable body of research on topics relating to the long-term gonadal effects of radiation and chemotherapy exists[138–161] and provides a basis for counseling patients and parents of the anticipated outcomes on pubertal development and fertility. For greater detail on this topic, please see Chapter 90.

Among survivors of adult cancer, the risk of premature onset of menopause in women treated with chemotherapeutic agents such as alkylating agents and procarbazine or with abdominal radiation therapy is age related, with women older than age 30 at the time of treatment having the greatest risk of treatment-induced amenorrhea and menopause, and sharply increased rates with chemotherapy around the age of 40 years. Tamoxifen has not been associated with the development of amenorrhea so far.[162] Cyclophosphamide at doses of 5 g/m^2 is likely to cause amenorrhea in women over 40, whereas many adolescents will continue to menstruate even after more than 20 g/m^2.[163] Although young women may not become amenorrheic after cytotoxic therapy, the risk of early menopause is significant. Female disease-free survivors of cancer diagnosed at ages 13 to 19 who were menstruating at age 21 were at fourfold-higher risk of menopause compared to controls.[140]

Fertility and Pregnancy Outcomes

Fertility The fertility of survivors of childhood cancer, evaluated in the aggregate, is impaired. In one study, the adjusted relative fertility of survivors compared with that of their siblings was 0.85 [95% confidence interval (CI), 0.78, 0.92]. The adjusted relative fertility of male survivors (0.76; 95% CI, 0.68, 0.86) was slightly lower than that of female survivors (0.93; 95% CI, 0.83, 1.04). The most significant differences in the relative fertility rates were demonstrated in male survivors who had been treated with alkylating agents with or without infradiaphragmatic irradiation.[164]

Fertility can be impaired by factors other than the absence of sperm and ova. Conception requires delivery of sperm to the uterine cervix and patency of the fallopian tubes for fertilization to occur and appropriate conditions in the uterus for implantation. Retrograde ejaculation occurs with a significant frequency in men who undergo bilateral retroperitoneal lymph node dissection. Uterine structure may be affected by abdominal irradiation. Uterine length was significantly reduced in 10 women with ovarian failure who had been treated with whole-abdomen irradiation. Endometrial thickness did not increase in response to hormone replacement therapy in 3 women who underwent weekly ultrasound examination. No flow was detectable with Doppler ultrasound through either uterine artery of 5 women and through one uterine artery in 3 additional women.[165,166] Similarly, 4 of 8 women who received 1,440 cGy total-body irradiation had reduced uterine volume and undetectable uterine artery blood flow.[167] These data are pertinent when considering the feasibility of assisted reproduction for these survivors.

Pregnancy Most chemotherapeutic agents are mutagenic, with the potential to cause germ cell chromosomal injury. Possible results of such injury include an increase in the frequency of genetic diseases and congenital anomalies in the offspring of successfully treated childhood and adolescent cancer patients. Several early studies of the offspring of patients treated for diverse types of childhood cancer identified no effect of previous treatment on pregnancy outcome and no increase in the frequency of congenital anomalies in the offspring.[168–170] However, a study of offspring of patients treated for Wilm's tumor demonstrated that the birth weight of children born to women who had received abdominal irradiation was significantly lower than that of children born to women who had not received such irradiation,[171] a finding that was confirmed in several subsequent studies.[172–174] The abnormalities of uterine structure and blood flow reported after abdominal irradiation might explain this clinical finding.

Prior studies of offspring of childhood cancer survivors were limited by the size of the population of offspring and the number of former patients who had been exposed to mutagenic therapy. Several recent studies that attempted to address some of these limitations did not identify an increased frequency of major congenital malformations,[175–180] genetic disease, or childhood cancer[181,182] in the offspring of former pediatric cancer patients, including those conceived after bone marrow transplantation.[183] However, there are data suggesting a deficit of males in the offspring of the partners of male survivors in the Childhood Cancer Survivor Study cohort,[184] as well as an effect of prior treatment with doxorubicin or daunorubicin on the percentage of offspring with a birth weight less than 2,500 g born to female survivors in the Childhood Cancer Survivor Study who were treated with pelvic irradiation.[185]

Pulmonary Sequelae

The *acute* effects of chemotherapy on the lungs may be lethal, may subside over time, may progress insidiously to a level of clinical pulmonary dysfunction, or may be manifested by abnormal pulmonary function tests. Classically, high doses of bleomycin have been associated with pulmonary toxicity. However, drugs such as alkylating agents, methotrexate, and nitrosoureas may also lead to pulmonary fibrosis, especially when combined with radiation therapy. Radiation is thus an important contributor to pulmonary sequelae of chemotherapy.[186] Alkylating agents can injure the lung parenchyma, cause restrictive lung disease by inhibiting chest wall growth, and lead to thin anteroposterior chest diameters even 7 years after completion of therapy. Bleomycin may cause pulmonary insufficiency and interstitial pneumonitis.[187]

Pulmonary fibrosis can cause late death in the survivorship period. Among children treated for brain tumors with high doses of nitrosurea and radiotherapy, 35% died of pulmonary fibrosis, 12% within 3 years and 24% after a symptom-free period of 7 to 12 years.[188] The risk for overt decompensation continues for at least 1 year after cessation of therapy and can be precipitated by infection or exposure to intraoperative oxygen. In terms of long-term outcomes, a recent study noted that 22% of Hodgkin's disease patients with normal pulmonary function tests at the end of therapy (three cycles each of mechlorethamine (nitrogen mustard), vincristine, procarbazine, prednisone (MOPP) and adriamycin (doxovubicin), bleomycin, vinblastic, dacarbazine (ABVD) or two cycles of each plus 2,550 cGy of involved-field radiotherapy) developed abnormalities with follow-up of 1 to 7 years.

The long-term outcome of pulmonary toxicity is determined by factors such as the severity of the acute injury, the degree of tissue repair, and the level of compensation possible. Pulmonary dysfunction is usually subclinical and may be manifested by subconscious avoidance of exercise owing to symptoms. Premature respiratory insufficiency, especially with exertion, may also become evident with aging. Recent aggressive lung cancer treatment regimens consisting of surgery, radiation, and chemotherapy may well put patients at high risk for decreased pulmonary function and respiratory symptoms.

Genitourinary Tract

Several drugs such as cisplatin, methotrexate, and nitrosoureas have been associated with both acute and chronic toxicities such as glomerular and tubular injury.[189] Glomerular injury may recover over time whereas tubular injury generally persists. Hemodialysis to counteract the effects of chronic renal toxicity may be warranted for some patients. Ifosfamide may cause Fanconi's syndrome with glycosuria, phosphaturia, and aminoaciduria, and may affect glomerular filtration. Hypophosphatemia may result in slow growth with possible bone deformity if untreated.

Radiation therapy may cause tubular damage and hypertension as a result of renal artery stenosis, especially in doses greater than 20 Gy, especially among children.[190] Radiation and chemotherapy may act synergistically, the dysfunction occurring with only 10 to 15 Gy.

The bladder is particularly susceptible to certain cytotoxic agents. Acrolein, a metabolic by-product of cyclophosphamide and ifosfamide, may cause hemorrhagic cystitis, fibrosis, and occasionally diminished bladder volume. An increased risk of developing bladder cancer also exists. Radiation may lead to bladder fibrosis, diminished capacity, and decreased contractility, the severity proportional to dose and area irradiated. The resultant scarring may diminish urethral and ureteric function.

Gastrointestinal/Hepatic

There are few studies describing long-term effects to this system, either due to underdetection or to a longer latency period than for other organs. Hepatic effects may result from the deleterious effects of many chemotherapeutic agents and radiotherapy. Transfusions may increase the risk of viral hepatitis. Hepatitis C has also been identified in increasing numbers of survivors, 119 of 2,620 tested. Of these patients, 24 of 56 who agreed to participate in a longitudinal study underwent liver biopsy. Chronic hepatitis was noted in 83%, fibrosis in 67%, and cirrhosis in 13%. Fibrosis and adhesions are known to occur after radiotherapy to the bowel.

Compromised Immune System

Hematologic and immunologic impairments can occur after either chemotherapy or radiation and are usually acute in nature. They are temporally related to the cancer treatment. Occasionally, persistent cytopenias may persist after pelvic radiation or in patients who have received extensive therapy with alkylating agents. Alkylating agents may cause myelodysplastic syndrome or leukemia as a late sequela. Immunologic impairment is seen as a long-term problem in Hodgkin's disease, relating to both the underlying disease and the treatments used. Hodgkin's disease patients are also at risk for serious bacterial infections if they have undergone splenectomy.

Peripheral Neuropathies

These effects are particularly common after taxol, vincristine, and cisplatin. However, despite the frequent use of such chemotherapeutic agents, few studies have characterized the nature and course of neuropathies associated with these drug regimens or dose levels.[191,192] Peripheral neuropathy may or may not resolve over time, and potential residual deficits are possible. Clinical manifestations include numbness and tingling in the hands and feet years after completion of cancer treatment.

Second Malignant Neoplasms and Recurrence

Second malignant neoplasms occur as result of an increased risk of second primary cancers associated with (a) the primary malignancy or (b) the iatrogenic effect of certain cancer therapies.[193–196] Examples include the development of breast cancer after Hodgkin's disease, ovarian cancer after primary breast cancer, and cancers associated with the HNPCC gene. Survivors of childhood cancer have an 8% to 10% risk of developing a second malignant neoplasm within 20 years of the primary diagnosis[197,198]; this is attributable to the mutagenic risk of both radiotherapy and chemotherapy.[199–213] This increased risk may be further potentiated in patients with genetic predispositions to malignancy.[214–220] The risk of secondary malignancy induced by cytotoxic agents is related to the cumulative dose of drug or radiotherapy (dose dependence). The risk of malignancy with normal aging results from the risk of cumulative cellular mutations. Compounding the normal aging process by exposure to mutagenic cytotoxic therapies results in an increased risk of secondary malignancy, particularly after radiotherapy, alkylating agents, and podophyllotoxins. Commonly cited secondary malignancies include (a) leukemia after alkylating agents and podophyllotoxins[221]; (b) solid tumors such as breast, bone, and thyroid cancer in the radiation fields in patients treated with radiotherapy[222]; (c) bladder cancer after cyclophosphamide; (d) a higher risk of contralateral breast cancer after primary breast cancer; and (e) ovarian cancer after breast cancer. Please refer to Chapter 111 for a detailed discussion of this significant issue.

Ancillary Sequelae

Lymphedema

Lymphedema can occur as a persistent or late effect of surgery and/or radiation treatment, and has been reported most commonly after breast cancer treatment, incidence rates ranging between 6% and 30%.[223] Lymphedema can occur in anyone with lymph node damage or obstruction to lymphatic drainage. Women undergoing axillary lymph node dissection and high-dose radiotherapy to the axilla for breast cancer are regarded as the highest risk group. Clinically, lymphedema symptoms may range from a feeling of fullness or heaviness in the affected limb to massive swelling and major functional impairment. Recommendations from the American Cancer Society conference on lymphedema in 1998 emphasize the need for additional research on prevention, monitoring, early intervention, and long-term treatment. Treatments suggested encompass multiple treatment modalities including skin care, massage, bandaging for compression, and exercise. Intermittent compression pumps were recommended only when used as an adjunct to manual approaches within a multidisciplinary treatment program, and routine use of medications such as diuretics, prophylactic antibiotics, bioflavinoids, and benzopyrones was discouraged in the absence of additional research. The impact of sentinel node biopsy in lieu of extensive axillary node dissection procedures for breast cancer on the incidence of lymphedema is not known at this time. A recent review by Erickson et al. found that arm edema was a common complication of breast cancer therapy, particularly when axillary dissection and axillary radiation therapy were used, and could result in substantial functional impairment and psychologic morbidity.[224] The authors note that although recommendations for "preventive" measures (e.g., avoidance of trauma) are anecdotally available, these measures have not been well studied. They found that nonpharmacologic treatments, such as massage and exercise, have been shown to be effective therapies for lymphedema, but the effect of pharmacologic interventions remains uncertain.

Fatigue

Fatigue has been reported as persistent side effect of treatment in many studies.[225–228] This is especially true among patients who have undergone bone marrow transplant.[229] Treatment-related fatigue may be associated with various factors such as anemia, infection, changes in hormonal levels, lack of physical activity, cytokine release, and sleep disorders.[230] The impact of exercise interventions on fatigue is a promising area of research. Fatigue is an important influence on quality of life for both the patient and the family and needs to be managed effectively.

Sexuality and Intimacy

Sexuality encompasses a spectrum of issues ranging from how one feels about one's body to the actual ability to function as a sexual being and has been reported as a persistent effect of treatment. In a recent study on breast, colon, lung, and prostate cancer survivors, issues related to sexual functioning were among the most persistent and severe problems reported. Preexisting sexual dysfunction may also be exacerbated by cancer and its treatment.[231] Please refer to Chapter 90 for further details.

Surgical and Radiation-Induced Toxicities

Surgical effects include increased risk of infections and physiologic comprise associated with nephrectomy (lifestyle changes to prevent trauma to remaining kidney), splenectomy (increased risk for sepsis resulting from encapsulated bacteria), and limb amputation.

Radiation therapy may especially exert effects on the musculoskeletal system and soft tissues among children and young adults, causing injury to the growth plates of long bones and muscle atrophy, osteonecrosis, and fractures.[2,5] Short stature can occur as a result of direct bone injury or pituitary radiation and resultant growth hormone deficiency. Chronic pain, the result of scarring and fibrosis in soft tissues surrounding the joints and large peripheral nerves, is a particularly distressing problem among patients who have received moderately high doses of radiation. Soft tissue sarcomas, skin cancers at previously irradiated sites, and pregnancy loss due to decreased uterine capacity in young girls after abdominal radiation are also possible.

Cancer Survivors, Healthcare Utilization, and Comorbid Conditions

Cancer survivors are high healthcare utilizers affecting distinct healthcare domains.[232,233] Data clearly show that cancer survivors are at greater risk for developing secondary cancers, late effects of cancer treatment, and chronic comorbid conditions. Exposures leading to these risks include cancer treatment, genetic predisposition and/or common lifestyle factors.[234–236] Although the threat of progressive or recurrent disease is at the forefront of health concerns for a cancer survivor, increased morbidity and decreased functional status and disability that result from cancer, its treatment, or health-related sequelae also are significant concerns. The impact of chronic comorbid conditions on cancer and its treatment is heightened more so among those diagnosed as adults and those who are elderly at the time of diagnosis.

Presented next is a brief overview of some factors potentiating the risk for chronic comorbid conditions among cancer survivors. A brief discussion of the major comorbid illnesses observed among survivors is also presented.

Metabolic Syndrome-Associated Diseases: Obesity, Diabetes, and Cardiovascular Disease

Obesity is a well-established risk factor for cancers of the breast (postmenopausal), colon, kidney (renal cell), esophagus (adenocarcinoma), and endometrium; thus, a large proportion of cancer patients are overweight or obese at the time of diagnosis.[237,238] Additional weight gain also can occur during or after active cancer treatment, an occurrence that has been frequently documented among individuals with breast cancer, but recently has been reported among testicular and gastrointestinal cancer patients as well.[239,240] Given data that obesity is associated with cancer recurrence in both breast and prostate cancer, and reduced quality of life among survivors, there is compelling evidence to support weight control efforts in this population.[14,15,241] Also, gradual weight loss has proven benefits in controlling hypertension, hyperinsulinemia, pain, and dyslipidemia and in improving levels of physical functioning, conditions that reportedly are significant problems in the survivor population.[14,15,21,242] Accordingly, the ACS Recommendations for Cancer Survivors list the "achievement of a healthy weight" as a primary goal.[14]

Obesity represents one of several metabolic disorders that are frequently manifest among cancer survivors, disorders that are grouped under the umbrella of "the metabolic syndrome" and include diabetes and cardiovascular disease (CVD). Insulin resistance is the underlying event associated with the metabolic syndrome, and either insulin resistance, co-occurring hyperinsulinemia, or diabetes have been reported as health concerns among cancer survivors.[243–245] As Brown and colleagues observed,[234] diabetes may play a significant role in the increased number of noncancer-related deaths among survivors; however, its role in progressive cancer is still speculative.

Although there is one study that suggests that older breast cancer patients derive a cardioprotective benefit from their diagnosis and/or associated treatments (most likely tamoxifen),[246] most reports indicate that CVD is a major health issue among survivors, evidenced by mortality data that show that half of noncancer-related deaths are attributed to CVD.[10] Risk is especially high among men with prostate cancer who receive hormone ablation therapy, as well as patients who receive adriamycin and radiation treatment to fields surrounding the heart.[247] Although more research is needed to explore the potential benefits of lifestyle interventions specifically within survivor populations, the promotion of a healthy weight via a low saturated fat diet with ample amounts of fruits and vegetables and moderate levels of physical activity is recommended.[14,15]

Osteoporosis

Osteoporosis and osteopenia are prevalent conditions in the general population, especially among women. Despite epidemiologic findings that increased bone density and low fracture risk are associated with increased risk for breast cancer,[248–256] clinical studies suggest that osteoporosis is still a prevalent health problem among survivors.[257–260] Data of Twiss et al.[258] indicate that 80% of older breast cancer patients have T-scores less than –1 and thus have clinically confirmed osteopenia at the time of their initial appointment. Other cancer populations, such as premenopausal breast and prostate cancer patients, may possess good skeletal integrity at the onset of their disease, but are at risk of developing osteopenia that may ensue with treatment-induced ovarian failure or androgen ablation.

Decreased Functional Status

Previous studies indicate that functional status is lowest immediately after treatment and tends to improve over time; however, the presence of pain and co-occurring diseases may affect this relationship.[261] In the older cancer survivor, regardless of duration following diagnosis, the presence of comorbidity, rather than the history of cancer per se, correlates with impaired functional status.[262] Cancer survivors have almost a twofold increase in having at least one functional limitation; however, in the presence of another comorbid condition, the odds ratio increases to 5.06 (95% CI, 4.47–5.72).[263] These findings have been confirmed by other studies in diverse populations of cancer survivors.[264–266] A cost analysis by Chirikos et al.[266] indicates that "the economic consequence of functional impairment exacts an enormous toll each year on cancer survivors, their families and the American economy at large."

Grading of Late Effects

The assessment and reporting of toxicity, based on the toxicity criteria system, plays a central role in oncology. Grading of late effects can provide valuable information for systematically monitoring the development and/or progression of late effects.[267] Although multiple systems have been developed for grading the adverse effects[(4)] of cancer treatment, there is, to date, no universally accepted grading system.[3] In contrast to the progress made in standardizing acute effects, the use of multiple late effects grading systems by different groups hinders the comparability of clinical trials, impedes the development of toxicity interventions, and encumbers the proper recognition and reporting of late effects. The wide adoption of a standardized criteria system can facilitate comparisons between institutions and across clinical trials.

[(4)]Any new finding or undesirable event that may or may not be attributed to treatment.

Some adverse events are clinical changes or health problems unrelated to the cancer diagnosis or its treatment.

A definitive assignment of attribution cannot always be rendered at the time of grading.

Multiple systems have been developed and have evolved substantially since being first introduced more than 20 years ago.[268] Garre et al. developed a set of criteria to grade late effects by degree of toxicity as follows: grade 0 (no late effect), grade 1 (asymptomatic changes not requiring any corrective measures, and not influencing general physical activity), grade 2 (moderate symptomatic changes interfering with activity), grade 3 (severe symptomatic changes that require major corrective measures and strict and prolonged surveillance), and grade 4 (life-threatening sequelae).[269] The SPOG (Swiss Pediatric Oncology Group) grading system has not been validated so far. It also ranges from 0 to 4: grade 0, no late effect; grade 1, asymptomatic patient requiring no therapy; grade 2, asymptomatic patient, requires continuous therapy, continuous medical follow-up, or symptomatic late effects resulting in reduced school, job, or psychosocial adjustment while remaining fully independent; grade 3, physical or mental sequelae not likely to be improved by therapy but able to work partially; and grade 4, severely handicapped, unable to work independently).[270]

The National Cancer Institute Common Toxicity Criteria (CTC) system was first developed in 1983. The most recent version, CTCAE v3.0 (Common Terminology Criteria for Adverse Events version 3.0) represents the first comprehensive, multimodality grading system for reporting *both* acute and late effects of cancer treatment. This new version requires changes in two areas: (1) application of adverse event criteria (e.g., new guidelines regarding late effects, surgical and pediatric effects, and issues relevant to the impact of multimodal therapies); and (2) reporting of the *duration* of an effect. This instrument carries the potential to facilitate the standardized reporting of adverse events and a comparison of outcomes between trials and institutions.

It is important to be aware that tools for grading late effects of cancer treatment are available, to validate them in larger populations, and to examine their utility in survivors of adult cancers. Oncologists, primary care physicians, and ancillary providers should be educated and trained to effectively monitor, evaluate, and optimize the health and well-being of a patient who has been treated for cancer. Additional research is needed to provide adequate knowledge about symptoms that persist following cancer treatment or those that arise as late effects, especially among survivors diagnosed as adults. Prospective studies that collect data on late effects will provide much needed information regarding the temporal sequence and timing of symptoms related to cancer treatment. It may be clinically relevant to differentiate between onset of symptoms during treatment, immediately posttreatment, or months later. Continued, systematic follow-up of survivors will result in information about the full spectrum of damage caused by cytotoxic and/or radiation therapy and possible interventions that may mitigate these adverse effects. We also need to examine the role of comorbidities on the risk for, and development of, late effects of cancer treatment among, especially, adult cancer survivors. Practice guidelines for follow-up care of cancer survivors and evaluation and management of late effects need to be developed so that effects can be mitigated when possible. Clearly, survivors can benefit from guidelines established for the primary prevention of secondary cancers as well as continued surveillance.[271,272]

Follow-Up Care for Late and Long-Term Effects

Optimal follow-up of survivors includes both ongoing monitoring and assessment of persistent and late effects of cancer treatment and the successful introduction of appropriate interventions to ameliorate these sequelae. The achievement of this goal is challenging, and inherent in that challenge is the recognition of the importance of preventing premature mortality from the disease and/or its treatment and the prevention or early detection of both the physiologic and psychologic sources of morbidity. The prevention of late effects, second cancers, and recurrences of the primary disease requires watchful follow up and optimal utilization of early detection screening techniques. Physical symptom management is as important in survivorship as it is during treatment, and effective symptom management during treatment may prevent or lessen lasting effects.

Regular monitoring of health status after cancer treatment is recommended, because this should (1) permit the timely diagnosis and treatment of long-term complications of cancer treatment; (2) provide the opportunity to institute preventive strategies such as diet modification, tobacco cessation, and other lifestyle changes; (3) facilitate screening for, and early detection of, a second cancer; (4) timely diagnosis and treatment of recurrent cancer; and (5) the detection of functional or physical or psychologic disability.

There has been no consensus on overall recommendations for routine follow-up after cancer therapy for *all* cancer survivors. A recent review by Kattlove and Winn can help guide oncologists in providing quality continuing care for their patients—care that spans a broad spectrum of medical areas ranging from surveillance to genetic susceptibility.[273] Health promotion is a key concern of patients once acute management of their disease is complete. Increasingly, cancer survivors are looking to their oncology care providers for counsel and guidance with respect to lifestyle change that will improve their prospects of a healthier life and possibly a longer one as well. Although complete data regarding lifestyle change among cancer survivors have yet to be determined, and there remains an unmet need for behavioral interventions with proven efficacy in various cancer populations,[274] the oncologist can nonetheless make use of extant data to inform practice and also should be attentive to new developments in the field.

Follow-up care and monitoring for late effects is usually done more systematically and rigorously for survivors of childhood cancer while they continue to be part of the program or clinic where they were treated. The monitoring of adult cancer sites for the development of late effects, particularly outside the oncology practice, is neither thorough nor systematic. It is important that survivors of both adult and childhood cancers be monitored for the late and long-term effects or treatment, as discussed in preceding sections, at regular intervals.

It is now recognized that cancer survivors may experience various late physical and psychologic sequelae of treatment and that many healthcare providers may be unaware of actual or potential survivor problems.[275] Until recently, there were no clearly defined, easily accessible risk-based guidelines for cancer survivor follow-up care. Such clinical practice guidelines can serve as a guide for doctors, outline appropriate methods of treatment and care, and address specific clinical situations (disease-oriented) or use of approved medical products, procedures, or tests (modality-oriented). In response to this growing mandate, the Children's Oncology Group has now developed and published its guidelines for long-term follow-up for Survivors of Childhood, Adolescent, and Young Adult Cancers.[275] These risk-based, exposure-related clinical practice guidelines are intended to promote earlier detection of and intervention for complications that may potentially arise as a result of treatment for pediatric malignancies, and are both evidence based (utilizing established associations between therapeutic exposures and late effects to identify high-risk categories) and grounded in the collective clinical experience of experts (matching the magnitude of risk with the intensity of screening recommendations). Importantly, they are intended for use beginning 2 or more years following the completion of cancer therapy and are not intended to provide guidance for follow-up of the survivor's primary disease.

Of great significance to survivors of adult cancer, using the best available evidence, the American Society of Clinical Oncology (ASCO) expert panels have also identified and developed practice recommendations for posttreatment follow-up of specific cancer sites (breast and colorectal; source: www.asco.org). In addition, ASCO has also created an expert panel tasked with the development of follow-up care guidelines geared toward the prevention or early detection of late effects among survivors diagnosed and treated as adults.

To facilitate optimal follow-up during the posttreatment phase, the patient's age at diagnosis, side effects of treatment reported or observed during treatment, calculated cumulative doses of drugs or radiation, and an overview of late effects most likely for a given patient given the treatment history should be summarized and kept on file. A copy of this summary should be provided to the patient or to the parent of a child who has undergone treatment for cancer. The importance of conveying this detailed treatment history to primary care providers should be clearly communicated, especially if follow-up will occur in the primary/family care setting. Finally, screening tests that may help detect subclinical effects that could become clinically relevant in the future should be listed.

Recommendations for regular, ongoing follow-up of cancer survivors are summarized in Table 101.2. For the prevention or early detection of second malignant neoplasms occurring as a late effect of treatment, providers should remain ever vigilant for the possibility. A detailed history and physical examination is always appropriate, in conjunction with screening at age-appropriate intervals or as outlined by consensus panel recommendations.

Physicians, caregivers, and the family must be able to hear and observe what the patient is trying to communicate, reduce fear and anxiety, counter feelings of isolation, correct misconceptions, and obtain appropriate symptom relief. Practitioners inheriting care for child or adult survivors need to understand the effects of cytotoxic therapies on the growing child or the adult at varying stages/ages of life and be knowledgeable about interventions that may mitigate the effects of these treatments.

Patient education should guide lifestyle and choices for follow-up care, promote adaptation to the disease or relevant sequelae, and help the patient reach an optimal level of wellness and functioning, both physical and psychologic, within the context of the disease and treatment effects.

Research Implications of Long-Term and Late Effects of Cancer

Cancer survivorship research continues to provide us with a growing body of evidence regarding the unique and uncharted consequences of cancer and its treatment among those diagnosed with this disease. It is becoming an acknowledged fact that most cancer treatment options available and in use today will affect the future health and life of those diagnosed with this disease. Adverse cancer treatment-related sequelae thus carry the potential to contribute to the ongoing burden of illness, health care costs, and decreased length and quality of survival.

Data and results from ongoing survivorship studies, examining outcomes among both adult and pediatric cancer survivors, are continuing to demonstrate that (a) there may be long latencies for potentially life-threatening late effects (e.g., cardiac failure secondary to the cardiotoxic effects of cancer treatment); (b) both late and chronic toxicities (e.g., fatigue, sexual dysfunction, cognitive impairment, neuropathies) are persistent, worsen over time, and carry significant potential to adversely affect the health and well being of survivors; (c) early interventions may hold the promise of reducing adverse outcomes; and (d) there may be a continued need for extended follow-up of survivors to prevent, detect early, control, or manage adverse sequelae of cancer or its treatment.

Among childhood cancer survivors, residual endocrine disorders have been shown to be as high as 40%.[276] A recent study found the cumulative frequency of congestive heart failure to be 17.4% at 20 years after diagnosis[277, (5)] and that risk factors such as female gender, higher cumulative doxorubicin doses, and lung and left abdominal irradiation increased the likelihood of heart failure in this population, variables that may affect practice in terms of initial cancer treatment, recommendations for posttreatment follow-up care, and interventions (behavioral, medical, or pharmacologic) to decrease future risk. Others have reported that there may be an increased risk of fetal malposition and premature labor among girls who received flank radiation therapy as part of their treatment for Wilm's tumor, and, among their offspring, an elevated risk for low birth weight, premature birth (less than 36 weeks gestation), and congenital malformations. These risks carry distinct implications for the obstetrical management of female survivors of Wilm's tumor.[278] Finally, data continue to show that survivors of acute lymphoblastic leukemia are at significant risk of being overweight or obese when compared to sibling controls.[125] Because premature coronary artery disease has been reported in this population, these findings underscore the importance of lifestyle and health promotion interventions.

Studies have also begun to demonstrate the deleterious impact of cancer treatment among those diagnosed with this disease as adults. Even after adjustment for age, baseline functional health status, and multiple covariates, long-term breast

[(5)]Among survivors of Wilm's tumor treated with doxorubicin.

TABLE 101.2. Follow-up care and surveillance for late effects.

Follow-up visit	*Content of clinic visit*	*Suggested evaluative procedures and ancillary actions*
Chemotherapy treatment cessation visit	1. Review complete treatment history 2. Calculate cumulative dosages of drugs 3. Document regimen(s) administered 4. Radiation ports, dosage, machine 5. Document patient age at diagnosis/ treatment 6. Side effects during treatment 7. Identify likely late effects 8. Baseline "grading" of late effects (Garre or SPOG)	Develop late effect risk profile Summarize all information in previous column Provide copy to patient (or parent if minor child) Instruct that this summary should be provided to primary care or other healthcare providers Keep copy of summary in patient chart
General measures at every visit	1. Detailed history 2. Complete physical examination 3. Review systems 4. Meds, maintenance, prophylactic antibiotics 5. Education: GPA, school performance 6. Employment history 7. Menstrual status/cycle 8. Libido, sexual activity 9. Pregnancy and outcome	Evaluate symptomatology, patient reports of issues Review any intercurrent illnesses Evaluate for disease recurrence, second neoplasms Systematic evaluation of long-term (persistent) and late effects (see specific measures) Grade long-term and late effects: Garre or SPOG criteria CBC; urinalysis; other tests depending on exposure history and late effect risk profile
Specific measures to evaluate late effects Relevance differs by: 1. Age at diagnosis/treatment 2. Specific drugs, regimens 3. Combinations of treatment modalities 4. Dosages administered 5. Expected toxicities (based on mechanics of action of cytotoxic drugs (cell-cycle-dependent; proliferation kinetics) 6. Exceptions occur to the theoretical assumption that least susceptible organs/tissues are those that replicate slowly or not at all (vinca, methotrexate, adriamycin) 7. Combinations of radiation/ chemotherapy more often associated with late effects	Growth: includes issues such as short stature, scoliosis, hypoplasia	Monitor growth (growth curve); sitting height, parental heights, nutritional status/diet, evaluate scoliosis, bone age, growth hormone assays, thyroid function, endocrinologist consult; orthopedic consult
	Cardiac	EKG, echo, afterload reduction, cardiologist consult Counsel against isometric exercises if high risk, advise ob/gyn risk of cardiac failure in pregnancy
	Neurocognitive	History and exam Communicate: school, family, special education Compensatory remediation techniques Neuropsychology consult; CT or MRI; CSF; basic myelin protein Written instructions, appointment cards
	Neuropathy	History/exam: neurologic exam, sensory changes hands/feet, paresthesias, bladder, gait, vision, muscle strength Neurologist consult
	Gonadal toxicity	History for primary vs. secondary dysfunction, gonadal function (menstrual cycle, pubertal development/delay, libido); hormone therapy; interventions (bromocriptine) Premature menopause: hormone replacement unless contraindicated; DXA scans for osteoporosis; calcium Endocrinologist consult Reproductive technologies
	Pulmonary	Chest X-ray; pulmonary function tests; pulmonologist consultation
	Urinary	Urinalysis; BUN/creatinine; urologist if hematuria
	Thyroid	Annual TSH; thyroid hormone replacement; endocrinologist
	Weight history	Evaluate dietary intake (food diary)/physical activity Nutritionist and/or endocrinologist consult
	Lymphedema	History/exam: swelling, sensations of heaviness/fullness
	Fatigue	Rule out hypothyroidism; anemia, cardiac/pulmonary sequelae; evaluate sleep habits Evaluate physical fitness and activity levels Regular physical activity unless contraindicated
	Surgical toxicity	Antibiotic prophylaxis (splenectomy)
	Gastrointestinal/hepatic	Liver function, hepatitis screen, gastroenterologist consult
Screening for second malignant neoplasms	Screening guidelines differ by age	Follow guidelines for age-appropriate cancer screening (mammogram, Pap smear, FOBT/flexible sigmoidoscopy)
	Oncologist consult	Mammogram at age 30 if history of mantle radiation for Hodgkins Screen for associated cancers in HNPCC family syndrome Screen for ovarian cancer if history of breast cancer and BRCAI II.
Assess/manage comorbidities	Osteoporosis; heart disease; arthritis, etc.	History/exam; be cognizant of risk; appropriate consult

Evaluations are suggestions only. Relevance will differ by treatment history and late effect risk profile.

Source: Data from Aziz (2002, 2003).[2,6]

cancer survivors are more likely to experience persistent significant declines in *physical* health status when compared to cancer-free controls, with younger or socially isolated survivors faring worse than those middle-aged or older in both physical and psychosocial dimensions.[279] These findings have been substantiated by another recent study where breast cancer survivors were found to be at significantly higher risk of physical declines in health status compared to age-matched controls.[280]

Outcomes of cancer and its treatment may be even more complex among medically underserved or ethnoculturally diverse populations. It has been reported that African-American survivors experience poorer functional health and consistently higher levels of comorbidities, decreased physical functioning, and general health vulnerability after cancer diagnosis and treatment compared to age-matched Caucasian patients.[281] From an economic standpoint, survivors working at the time of diagnosis may experience a significant reduction in annual market earnings,[(6)] the adverse economic impact being worse among survivors with the greatest declines in health status.[282] Long reported as a late effect among pediatric survivors, the adverse neurocognitive impact of cancer treatment is now increasingly reported as a potentially devastating outcome among adult survivors. Breast and lymphoma survivors exposed to systemic chemotherapy are at increased risk for neurocognitive deficits affecting memory, concentration, and attention. Diffuse white and gray matter changes have been reported in magnetic resonance imaging studies, and early data indicate that APOEe4 may be a potential genetic marker for risk.[283,284] Sexual dysfunction continues to be a persistent finding among both men and women years after cancer treatment.[285,286] Finally, the extent to which women's daily living is affected by lymphedema is not recognized routinely by healthcare providers even today.[287]

There are promising findings from intervention studies among both adult and childhood cancer survivors. Daily consumption of aspirin may result in a significant reduction in relative risk of death from breast cancer.[(7)] Dexrazoxane (DEXRA or Zinecard) administered during active treatment may prevent or reduce acute cardiac injury associated with doxorubicin therapy.[288,289] Methylphenidate (Ritalin) may provide at least a short-term benefit in childhood cancer survivors who experience clinically significant learning problems and deficits in attention and memory.[290]

Home-based educational interventions can help to improve cancer knowledge, self-efficacy (coping), and awareness of resources among both white and African-American breast cancer survivors.[291]

Self-reported depression burden may significantly influence the severity and number of side effects experienced by breast cancer survivors, and self-help interventions may reduce fatigue, pain, and nausea burden in women with breast cancer.[292] Last but not least, cognitive-behavioral stress management interventions may successfully reduce the prevalence of moderate depression and increase generalized optimism and positive reframing, lending support to the importance of examining positive responses to traumatic events.[293]

Thus, research that examines the effects of cancer and its treatment among individuals diagnosed with the disease and their family members is critical if we are to help patients make decisions about treatment options that could affect their future. Cancer survivorship research carries the potential to enable providers of care to tailor therapies to maximize cure while minimizing adverse treatment-related effects. The development and dissemination of evidence-based interventions may help us to reduce cancer morbidity as well as mortality and facilitate adaptation among cancer survivors. Finally, knowledge gained from survivorship research could help improve quality of care, control costs, and equip the next generation of physicians, nurses, and other healthcare professionals to provide not just the science but also the art of comprehensive cancer medicine.

Conclusions

A large and growing community of cancer survivors is one of the major achievements of cancer research during the past three decades. Both length and quality of survival are important endpoints. Many cancer survivors are at risk for, and develop, physiologic late effects of cancer treatment that may lead to premature mortality and morbidity. As in the past when treatments were modified to decrease the chance of developing toxicities among survivors of childhood cancer, the goal of future research and treatment should also be to evaluate late effects systematically and further modify toxicities without diminishing cures. Interventions and treatments that can ameliorate or manage effectively both persistent and late physical effects of treatment should be developed and promoted for use in this population. Oncologists, primary care physicians, and ancillary providers should be educated and trained to effectively monitor, evaluate, and optimize the health and well-being of a patient who has been treated for cancer.

Additional research is needed to provide adequate knowledge about symptoms that persist following cancer treatment or those that arise as late effects. Prospective studies that collect data on late effects prospectively are needed as most of the literature on late effects is derived from cross-sectional studies in which it is not clear if the symptom began during treatment or immediately after treatment. Continued, systematic follow-up of survivors will provide information about the full spectrum of damage caused by cytotoxic or radiation therapy and possible interventions that may mitigate the effects. Interventions, therapeutic or lifestyle, that can treat or ameliorate these late effects need to be developed. Practice guidelines for follow-up care of cancer survivors and evaluation and management of late effects need to be developed so that effects can be mitigated when possible.

Our knowledge about the late effects of cancer treatment, in large part, comes from studies conducted among survivors of pediatric cancer. We need to explore further the impact cancer treatment on late effects in survivors diagnosed as adults. We also need to examine the role of comorbidities on the risk for, and development of, late effects of cancer treatment among these adult cancer survivors.

[(6)]Compared to age-matched cancer free controls.
[(7)]Holmes MA. Personal communication.

Although there has been considerable research on the late outcomes among survivors of cancer, future research must be directed toward identification of risks associated with more-recent treatment regimens, as well as the very late occurring outcomes resulting from treatment protocols utilized three or more decades ago. As treatment- and patient-related factors impact the subsequent risk of late-occurring adverse outcomes, clear delineation of those survivors who are at high risk of specific adverse outcomes is essential for the rational design of follow-up guidelines, prevention, and intervention strategies.

Each person with cancer has unique needs based on the extent of the disease, effects of treatment, prior health, functional level, coping skills, support systems, and many other influences. This complexity requires an interdisciplinary approach by all health professionals that is organized, systematic, and geared toward the provision of high-quality care. This ambience may facilitate the adaptation of cancer survivors to temporary or permanent sequelae of the disease and its treatment.

References

1. American Cancer Society. Cancer Facts and Figures, 2003. Atlanta, GA: American Cancer Society, 2004.
2. Aziz N, Rowland J. Trends and advances in cancer survivorship research: challenge and opportunity. Semin Radiat Oncol 2003; 13:248–266.
3. Jemal A, Clegg LX, Ward E, et al. Annual report to the nation on the status of cancer, 1875–2001, with a special feature regarding survival. Cancer (Phila) 2004;101:3–27.
4. Rowland J, Mariotto A, Aziz N, et al. Cancer survivorship—United States, 1971–2001. MMWR 2004;53:526–529.
5. Ries LAG, Smith MA, Gurney JG, et al. (eds). Cancer incidence and survival among children and adolescents: United States SEER program 1975–1995. NIH Publication 99–4649. Bethesda, MD: National Cancer Institute, 1996.
6. Aziz NM. Long-term survivorship: late effects. In: Berger AM, Portenoy RK, Weissman DE (eds). Principles and Practice of Palliative Care and Supportive Oncology, 2nd ed. Philadelphia: Lippincott Williams & Wilkins, 2002:1019–1033.
7. Chu KC, Tarone RE, Kessler LG. Recent trends in U.S. breast cancer incidence, survival, and mortality rates. J Natl Cancer Inst 1996;88:1571–1579.
8. McKean RC, Feigelson HS, Ross RK. Declining cancer rates in the 1990s. J Clin Oncol 2000;18:2258–2268.
9. Ries LAG, Wing PA, Miller DS. The annual report to the nation on the status of cancer, 1973–1997, with a special section on colorectal cancer. Cancer (Phila) 2000;88:2398–2424.
10. Shusterman S, Meadows AT. Long term survivors of childhood leukemia. Curr Opin Hematol 2000;7:217–220.
11. Demark-Wahnefried W, Peterson B, McBride C. Current health behaviors and readiness to pursue life-style changes among men and women diagnosed with early stage prostate and breast carcinomas. Cancer (Phila) 2000;88:674–684.
12. Ganz PA. Late effects of cancer and its treatment. Semin Oncol Nurs 2001;17(4):241–248.
13. Ganz PA. Cancer Survivors: Physiologic and Psychosocial Outcomes. Alexandria, VA: American Society of Clinical Oncology, 1998:118–123.
14. Schwartz CL. Long-term survivors of childhood cancer: the late effects of therapy. Oncologist 1999;4:45–54.
15. Brown ML, Fintor L. The economic burden of cancer. In: Greenwald P, Kramer BS, Weed DL (eds). Cancer Prevention and Control. New York: Dekker, 1995:69–81.
16. Sklar CA. Overview of the effects of cancer therapies: the nature, scale and breadth of the problem. Acta Paediatr (Suppl) 1999;88: 1–4.
17. Mullan F. Seasons of survival: reflections of a physician with cancer. N Engl J Med 1995;313:270–273.
18. Loescher LJ, Welch-McCaffrey D, Leigh SA. Surviving adult cancers. Part 1: Physiologic effects. Ann Intern Med 1989;111: 411–432.
19. Welch-McCaffrey D, Hoffman B, Leigh SA. Surviving adult cancers. Part 2: Psychosocial implications. Ann Intern Med 1989;111:517–524.
20. Herold AH, Roetzheim RG. Cancer survivors. Primary Care 1992;19:779–791.
21. Marina N. Long-term survivors of childhood cancer. The medical consequences of cure. Pediatr Clin N Am 1997;44: 1021–1041.
22. Green DM. Late effects of treatment for cancer during childhood and adolescence. Curr Probl Cancer 2003;27(3):127–142.
23. Mertens AC, Yasui Y, Neglia JP, et al. Late mortality experience in five-year survivors of childhood and adolescent cancer: The Childhood Cancer Survivor Study. J Clin Oncol 2001;19: 3163–3172.
24. Robison LL, Bhatia S. Review: Late-effects among survivors of leukaemia and lymphoma during childhood and adolescence. Br J Haematol 2003;122:345–356.
25. Boulad F, Sands S, Sklar C. Late complications after bone marrow transplantation in children and adolescents. Curr Probl Pediatr 1998;28:273–304.
26. Bhatia S, Landier W, Robison LL. Late effects of childhood cancer therapy. In: DeVita VT, Hellman S, Rosenberg SA (eds). Progress in Oncology. Sudbury: Jones and Bartlett, 2002:171–213.
27. Dreyer ZE, Blatt J, Bleyer A. Late effects of childhood cancer and its treatment. In: Pizzo PA, Poplack DG (eds). Principles and Practice of Pediatric Oncology, 4th ed. Philadelphia: Lippincott, Williams & Wilkins, 2002:1431–1461.
28. Hudson M. Late complications after leukemia therapy. In: Pui CG (ed). Childhood Leukemias. Cambridge: Cambridge University Press, 1991:463–481.
29. Blatt J, Copeland DR, Bleyer WA. Late effects of childhood cancer and its treatment. In: Pizzo PA, Poplack DG (eds). Principles and Practice of Pediatric Oncology, revised ed. Philadelphia: Lippincott, 1997:1091–1114.
30. Kirk JA, Raghupathy P, Stevens MM, et al. Growth failure and growth-hormone deficiency after treatment for acute lymphoblastic leukemia. Lancet 1987;1:190–193.
31. Blatt J, Bercu BB, Gillin JC, et al. Reduced pulsatile growth hormone secretion in children after therapy for acute lymphoblastic leukemia. J Pediatr 1984;104:182–186.
32. Silber JH, Littman PS, Meadows AT. Stature loss following skeletal irradiation for childhood cancer. J Clin Oncol 1990; 8:304–312.
33. Leiper AD, Stanhope R, Preese MA, et al. Precocious or early puberty and growth failure in girls treated for acute lymphoblastic leukemia. Horm Res 1988;30:72–76.
34. Ogilvy-Stuart AL, Clayton PE, Shalet SM. Cranial irradiation and early puberty. J Clin Endocrinol Metab 1994;78:1282–1286.
35. Furst CJ, Lundell M, Ahlback SO. Breast hypoplasia following irradiation of the female breast in infancy and early childhood. Acta Oncol 1989;28(4):519–523.
36. Meyers CA, Weitzner MA. Neurobehavioral functioning and quality of life in patients treated for cancer of the central nervous system. Curr Opin Oncol 1995;7:197–200.
37. Haupt R, Fears TR, Robeson LL, et al. Educational attainment in long-term survivors of childhood acute lymphoblastic leukemia. JAMA 1994;272:1427–1432.
38. Stehbens JA, Kaleih TA, Noll RB, et al. CNS prophylaxis of childhood leukemia: what are the long-term neurological,

neuropsychological and behavioral effects? Neuropsychol Rev 1991;2:147–176.
39. Ochs J, Mulhern RK, Faircough D et al. Comparison of neuropsychologic function and clinical indicators of neurotoxicity in long-term survivors of childhood leukemia given cranial irradiation or parenteral methotrexate: a prospective study. J Clin Oncol 1991;9:145–151.
40. Ash P. The influence of radiation on fertility in man. Br J Radiol 1990;53:155–158.
41. Didi M, Didcock E, Davies HA, et al. High incidence of obesity in young adults after treatment of acute lymphoblastic leukemia in childhood. J Pediatr 1995;127:63–67.
42. Oberfield SE, Soranno D, Nirenberg A, et al. Age at onset of puberty following high-dose central nervous system radiation therapy. Arch Pediat Adolesc Med 1996;150:589–592.
43. Sklar C, Mertens A, Walter A, et al. Final height after treatment for childhood acute lymphoblastic leukemia: comparison of no cranial irradiation with 1,800 and 2,400 centigrays of cranial irradiation. J Pediatr 1993;123:59–64.
44. Greendale GA, Petersen L, Zibecchi L, Ganz PA. Factors related to sexual function in postmenopausal women with a history of breast cancer. Menopause 2001;8:111–119.
45. Ganz PA, Greendale GA, Petersen L, Zibecchi L, Kahn B, Belin TR. Managing menopausal symptoms in breast cancer survivors: results of a randomized controlled trial. J Natl Cancer Inst 2000;5:1054–1064.
46. Yancik R, Ganz PA, Varricchio CG, Conley B. Perspectives on comorbidity and cancer in older patients: approaches to expand the knowledge base. J Clin Oncol 2001;19:1147–1151.
47. Lipshultz SE, Colan SD, Gelber RD, et al. Late cardiac effects of doxorubicin therapy for acute lymphoblastic leukemia in childhood. N Engl J Med 1991;324:808–814.
48. Bu'Lock FA, Mott MG, Oakhill A, et al. Left ventricular diastolic function after anthracycline chemotherapy in childhood: relation with systolic function, symptoms and pathophysiology. Br Heart J 1995;73:340–350.
49. Goorin AM, Borow KM, Goldman A, et al. Congestive heart failure due to adriamycin cardiotoxicity: its natural history in children. Cancer (Phila) 1981;47:2810–2816.
50. Steinherz LJ, Steinherz PG. Cardiac failure and dysrhythmias 6–19 years after anthracycline therapy: a series of 15 patients. Med Pediatr Oncol 1995;24:352–361.
51. Adams MJ, Lipsitz SR, Colan SD, et al. Cardiovascular status in long-term survivors of Hodgkin's disease treated with chest radiotherapy. J Clin Oncol 2004;22(15):3139–3148.
52. Kremer LCM, van Dalen EC, Offringa M, Otenkamp J, Voute PA. Anthracycline-induced clinical heart failure in a cohort of 607 children: long-term follow-up study. J Clin Oncol 2001;19: 191–196.
53. Sorensen K, Levitt G, Chessells J, Sullivan I. Anthracycline dose in childhood acute lymphoblastic leukemia: issues of early survival versus late cardiotoxicity. J Clin Oncol 1997;15:61–68.
54. Kremer LCM, van Dalen EC, Offringa M, Voute PA. Frequency and risk factors of anthracycline-induced clinical heart failure in children: a systematic review. Ann Oncol 2002;13:503–512.
55. Steinherz LJ, Steinherz PG, Tan CT, Heller G, Murphy ML. Cardiac toxicity 4–20 years after completing anthracycline therapy. JAMA 1991;266:1672–1677.
56. Kremer LCM, van der Pal HJH, Offringa M, van Dalen EC, Voute PA. Frequency and risk factors of subclinical cardiotoxicity after anthracycline therapy in children: a systematic review. Ann Oncol 2002;13:819–829.
57. Hancock SL, Tucker MA, Hoppe RT. Factors affecting late mortality from heart disease after treatment of Hodgkin's disease. JAMA 1993;270:1949–1955.
58. Hancock SL, Donaldson SS, Hoppe RT. Cardiac disease following treatment of Hodgkin's disease in children and adolescents. J Clin Oncol 1993;11:1199–1203.
59. Fajardo L, Stewart J, Cohn K. Morphology of radiation-induced heart disease. Arch Pathol 1968;86:512–519.
60. Minow RA, Benjamin RS, Gottlieb JA. Adriamycin (NSC-123127) cardiomyopathy: an overview with determination of risk factors. Cancer Chemother Rep 1975;6:195–201.
61. Prout MN, Richards MJ, Chung KJ, Joo P, Davis HL Jr. Adriamycin cardiotoxicity in children: case reports, literature review, and risk factors. Cancer (Phila) 1977;39:62–65.
62. Von Hoff DD, Layard MW, Basa P, et al. Risk factors for doxorubicin-induced congestive heart failure. Ann Intern Med 1979;91:710–717.
63. Kushner JP, Hansen VL, Hammar SP. Cardiomyopathy after widely separated courses of adriamycin exacerbated by actinomycin-D and mithramycin. Cancer (Phila) 1975;36:1577–1584.
64. Von Hoff DD, Rozencweig M, Piccart M. The cardiotoxicity of anticancer agents. Semin Oncol 1982;9:23–33.
65. Lipshultz SE, Lipsitz SR, Mone SM, et al. Female sex and drug dose as risk factors for late cardiotoxic effects of doxorubicin therapy for childhood cancer. N Engl J Med 1995;332:1738–1743.
66. Pratt CB, Ransom JL, Evans WE. Age-related adriamycin cardiotoxicity in children. Cancer Treat Rep 1978;62:1381–1385.
67. Pai VB, Nahata MC. Cardiotoxicity of chemotherapeutic agents: incidence, treatment and prevention. Drug Saf 2000;22:263–302.
68. Legha SS, Benjamin RS, Mackay B, et al. Reduction of doxorubicin cardiotoxicity by prolonged continuous intravenous infusion. Ann Intern Med 1982;96:133–139.
69. Lipshultz SE, Giantris AL, Lipsitz SR, et al. Doxorubicin administration by continuous infusion is not cardioprotective: the Dana-Farber 91-01 Acute Lymphoblastic Leukemia Protocol. J Clin Oncol 2002;20:1677–1682.
70. Marks RD Jr, Agarwal SK, Constable WC. Radiation induced pericarditis in Hodgkin's disease. Acta Radiol Ther Phys Biol 1973;12:305–312.
71. Martin RG, Ruckdeschel JC, Chang P, Byhardt R, Bouchard RJ, Wiernik PH. Radiation-related pericarditis. Am J Cardiol 1975; 35:216–220.
72. Ruckdeschel JC, Chang P, Martin RG, et al. Radiation-related pericardial effusions in patients with Hodgkin's disease. Medicine (Baltim) 1975;54:245–259.
73. Perrault DJ, Levy M, Herman JD, et al. Echocardiographic abnormalities following cardiac radiation. J Clin Oncol 1985;3: 546–551.
74. Kadota RP, Burgert EO Jr, Driscoll DJ, Evans RG, Gilchrist GS. Cardiopulmonary function in long-term survivors of childhood Hodgkin's lymphoma: a pilot study. Mayo Clin Proc 1988;63: 362–367.
75. Wexler LH. Ameliorating anthracycline cardiotoxicity in children with cancer: clinical trials with dexrazoxane. Semin Oncol 1998;25:86–92.
76. Lipshultz SE, Rifai N, Dalton VM, et al. The effect of dexrazoxane on myocardial injury in doxorubicin-treated children with acute lymphoblastic leukemia. N Engl J Med 2004;351(2): 145–153.
77. Gluck S. The expanding role of epirubicin in the treatment of breast cancer. Cancer Control 2002;9(suppl 2):16–27.
78. Baker AF, Dorr RT. Drug interactions with the taxanes: clinical implications. Cancer Treat Rev 2001;27(4):221–233.
79. Sessa C, Perotti A, Salvatorelli E, et al. Phase IB and pharmacological study of the novel taxane BMS-184476 in combination with doxorubicin. Eur J Cancer 2004;40(4):563–570.
80. Jones RL, Smith IE. Efficacy and safety of trastuzumab. Expert Opin Drug Saf 2004;3(4):317–327.
81. Schneider JW, Chang AY, Garratt A. Trastuzumab cardiotoxicity: speculations regarding pathophysiology and targets for further study. Semin Oncol 2002;29(3 suppl 11):22–28.
82. Schneider JW, Chang AY, Rocco TP. Cardiotoxicity in signal transduction therapeutics: erbB2 antibodies and the heart. Semin Oncol 2001;28:18–26.

83. Meadows AT, Gordon J, Massari DJ, Littman P, Fergusson J, Moss K. Declines in IQ scores and cognitive dysfunctions in children with acute lymphocytic leukaemia treated with cranial irradiation. Lancet 1981;2:1015–1018.
84. Jankovic M, Brouwers P, Valsecchi MG, et al. Association of 1800 cGy cranial irradiation with intellectual function in children with acute lymphoblastic leukaemia. ISPACC. International Study Group on Psychosocial Aspects of Childhood Cancer. Lancet 1994;344:224–227.
85. Hertzberg H, Huk WJ, Ueberall MA, et al. CNS late effects after ALL therapy in childhood. Part I. Neuroradiological findings in long-term survivors of childhood ALL: an evaluation of the interferences between morphology and neuropsychological performance. The German Late Effects Working Group. Medical and Pediatric Oncology, 1997;28:387–400.
86. Green DM, Zevon MA, Rock KM, Chavez F. Fatigue after treatment for Hodgkin's disease during childhood or adolescence. Proc Am Soc Clin Oncol 2002;21:396a.
87. Price R. Therapy-related central nervous system diseases in children with acute lymphocytic leukemia. In: Mastrangelo R, Poplack DG, Riccardi R (eds). Central Nervous System Leukemia: Prevention and Treatment. Boston: Martinus-Nijhoff, 1983:71–83.
88. Peylan-Ramu N, Poplack DG, Pizzo PA, Adornato BT, Di Chiro G. Abnormal CT scans of the brain in asymptomatic children with acute lymphocytic leukemia after prophylactic treatment of the central nervous system with radiation and intrathecal chemotherapy. N Engl J Med 1978;298:815–818.
89. Riccardi R, Brouwers P, Di Chiro G, Poplack DG. Abnormal computed tomography brain scans in children with acute lymphoblastic leukemia: serial long-term follow-up. J Clin Oncol 1985;3:12–18.
90. Mulhern RK, Reddick WE, Palmer SL, et al. Neurocognitive deficits in medulloblastoma survivors and white matter loss. Ann Neurol 1999;46:834–841.
91. Packer RJ, Sutton LN, Atkins TE, et al. A prospective study of cognitive function in children receiving whole-brain radiotherapy and chemotherapy: 2-year results. J Neurosurg 1989;70: 707–713.
92. Peckham VC, Meadows AT, Bartel N, Marrero O. Educational late effects in long-term survivors of childhood acute lymphocytic leukemia. Pediatrics 1988;81:127–133.
93. Moore IM, Packer RJ, Karl D, Bleyer WA. Adverse effects of cancer treatment on the central nervous system. In: Schwarta CL, Hobbie WL, Constine WL, Ruccione KS (eds). Survivors of Childhood Cancer: Assessment and Management. St. Louis: Mosby, 1994:81–95.
94. Mitby PA, Robison LL, Whitton JA, et al. Utilization of special education services among long-term survivors of childhood cancer: a report from the Childhood Cancer Survivor Study. Cancer (Phila) 2003;97:1115–1126.
95. Loge JH, Abrahamsen AF, Ekeberg O, Kaasa S. Hodgkin's disease survivors more fatigued than the general population. J Clin Oncol 1999;17:253–261.
96. Knobel H, Loge JH, Lund MB, Forfang K, Nome O, Kaasa S. Late medical complications and fatigue in Hodgkin's disease survivors. J Clin Oncol 2001;19:3226–3233.
97. Chessells JM. Recent advances in the management of acute leukaemia. Arch Dis Child 2000;82:438–442.
98. Pui CH. Acute lymphoblastic leukemia in children. Curr Opinion Oncol 2000;12:2–12.
99. van Dam FS, Schagen SB, Muller MJ, et al. Impairment of cognitive function in women receiving adjuvant treatment for high-risk breast cancer: high-dose versus standard-dose chemotherapy. JNCI 1998;90:210–218.
100. Brezden CB, Phillips KA, Abdolell M, et al. Cognitive function in breast cancer patients receiving adjuvant chemotherapy. J Clin Oncol 2000;18:2695–2701.
101. Ahles TA, Saykin AJ, Noll WW, et al. The relationship of APOE genotype to neuropsychological performance in long-term cancer survivors treated with standard dose chemotherapy. Psychooncology 2003;12(6):612–619.
102. Ganz PA. Cognitive dysfunction following adjuvant treatment of breast cancer: a new dose-limiting toxic effect? JNCI 1998;90:182–183.
103. Hjermstad M, Holte H, Evensen S, Fayers P, Kaasa S. Do patients who are treated with stem cell transplantation have a health-related quality of life comparable to the general population after 1 year? Bone Marrow Transplant 1999;24:911–918.
104. Walker LG, Wesnes KP, Heys SD, Walker MB, Lolley J, Eremin O. The cognitive effects of recombinant interleukin-2 therapy: a controlled clinical trial using computerised assessments. Eur J Cancer 1996;32A:2275–2283.
105. Curt GA, Breitbart W, Cella D, et al. Impact of cancer related fatigue on the lives of patients: new findings from the Fatigue Coalition. Oncologist 2000;5:353–360.
106. Ahles TA, Tope DM, Furstenberg C, Hann D, Mill L. Psychologic and neuropsychologic impact of autologous bone marrow transplantation. J Clin Oncol 1996;14:1457–1462.
107. Ahles TA, Silberfarb PM, Maurer LH, et al. Psychologic and neuropsychologic functioning of patients with limited small-cell lung cancer treated with chemotherapy and radiation therapy with or without warfarin: a study by the Cancer and Leukemia Group B. J Clin Oncol 1998;16:1954–1960.
108. Mulhern RK, Kepner JL, Thomas PR, Armstrong FD, Friedman HS, Kun LE. Neuropsychologic functioning of survivors of childhood medulloblastoma randomized to receive conventional or reduced-dose craniospinal irradiation: a Pediatric Oncology Group study. Clin Oncol 1998;16:1723–1728.
109. Raymond-Speden E, Tripp G, Lawrence B, Holdaway D. Intellectual, neuropsychological, and academic functioning in long-term survivors of leukemia. J Pediatr Psychol 2000;25:59–68.
110. Tannock IF, Ahles TA, Ganz PA, Van Dam FS. Cognitive impairment associated with chemotherapy for cancer: report of a workshop. J Clin Oncol 2004;22(11):2233–2239.
111. Shalet SM, Beardwell CG, Twomey JA, Jones PH, Pearson D. Endocrine function following the treatment of acute leukemia in childhood. J Pediatr 1977;90:920–923.
112. Robison LL, Nesbit ME Jr, Sather HN, Meadows AT, Ortega JA, Hammond GD. Height of children successfully treated for acute lymphoblastic leukemia: a report from the Late Effects Study Committee of Childrens Cancer Study Group. Med Pediatr Oncol 1985;13:14–21.
113. Hancock SL, Cox RS, McDougall IR. Thyroid diseases after treatment of Hodgkin's disease. N Engl J Med 1991;325:599–605.
114. Sklar C, Whitton J, Mertens A, et al. Abnormalities of the thyroid in survivors of Hodgkin's disease: data from the Childhood Cancer Survivor Study. J Clin Endocrinol Metab 2000;85: 3227–3232.
115. Glatstein E, McHardy-Young S, Brast N, Eltringham JR, Kriss JP. Alterations in serum thyrotropin (TSH) and thyroid function following radiotherapy in patients with malignant lymphoma. J Clin Endocrinol Metab 1971;32:833–841.
116. Rosenthal MB, Goldfine ID. Primary and secondary hypothyroidism in nasopharyngeal carcinoma. JAMA 1976;236: 1591–1593.
117. Sklar CA. Growth and neuroendocrine dysfunction following therapy for childhood cancer. Pediatr Clin N Am 1997;44: 489–503.
118. Berry DH, Elders MJ, Crist W, et al. Growth in children with acute lymphocytic leukemia: a Pediatric Oncology Group study. Med Pediatr Oncol 1983;11:39–45.
119. Papadakis V, Tan C, Heller G, Sklar C. Growth and final height after treatment for childhood Hodgkin disease. J Pediatr Hematol/Oncol 1996;18:272–276.

120. Shalet SM, Price DA, Beardwell CG, Jones PH, Pearson D. Normal growth despite abnormalities of growth hormone secretion in children treated for acute leukemia. J Pediatr 1979;94:719–722.
121. Didcock E, Davies HA, Didi M, Ogilvy Stuart AL, Wales JK, Shalet SM. Pubertal growth in young adult survivors of childhood leukemia. J Clin Oncol 1995;13:2503–2507.
122. Katz JA, Pollock BH, Jacaruso D, Morad A. Final attained height in patients successfully treated for childhood acute lymphoblastic leukemia. J Pediatr 1993;123:546–552.
123. Odame I, Reilly JJ, Gibson BE, Donaldson MD. Patterns of obesity in boys and girls after treatment for acute lymphoblastic leukaemia. Arch Dis Child 1994;71:147–149.
124. Van Dongen-Melman JE, Hokken-Koelega AC, Hahlen K, De Groot A, Tromp CG, Egeler RM. Obesity after successful treatment of acute lymphoblastic leukemia in childhood. Pediatr Res 1995;38:86–90.
125. Sklar CA, Mertens AC, Walter A, et al. Changes in body mass index and prevalence of overweight in survivors of childhood acute lymphoblastic leukemia: role of cranial irradiation. Med Pediatr Oncol 2000;35:91–95.
126. Craig F, Leiper AD, Stanhope R, Brain C, Meller ST, Nussey SS. Sexually dimorphic and radiation dose dependent effect of cranial irradiation on body mass index. Arch Dis Child 1999;81:500–510.
127. Oeffinger KC, Mertens AC, Sklar CA, et al. Obesity in adult survivors of childhood acute lymphoblastic leukemia: a report from the Childhood Cancer Survivor Study. J Clin Oncol 2003; 21:1359–1365.
128. Thomson AB, Critchley HOD, Wallace WHB. Fertility and progeny. Eur J Cancer 2002;38:1634–1644.
129. Lamb MA. Effects of cancer on the sexuality and fertility of women. Semin Oncol Nurs 1995;11:120–127.
130. Brougham MF, Kelnar CJ, Sharpe RM, Wallace WH. Male fertility following childhood cancer: current concepts and future therapies. Asian J Androl 2003;5(4):325–337.
131. Wallace WH, Anderson R, Baird D. Preservation of fertility in young women treated for cancer. Lancet Oncol 2004;5(5): 269–270.
132. Opsahl MS, Fugger EF, Sherins RJ. Preservation of reproductive function before therapy for cancer: new options involving sperm and ovary cryopreservation. Cancer J 1997;3:189–191.
133. Oktay K, Newton H, Aubard Y, Salha O, Gosden RG. Cryopreservation of immature human oocytes and ovarian tissue: an emerging technology? Fertil Steril 1998;69:1–7.
134. Donnez J, Dolmans MM, Demylle D, et al. Livebirth after orthotic transplantation of cryopreserved ovarian tissue. Lancet 2004;364(9443):1405–1410.
135. Wallace WH, Pritchard J. Livebirth after cryopreserved ovarian tissue autotransplantation. Lancet 2004;364(9451):2093–2094.
136. Bath LE, Tydeman G, Critchley HO, Anderson RA, Baird DT, Wallace WH. Spontaneous conception in a young woman who had ovarian cortical tissue cryopreserved before chemotherapy and radiotherapy for a Ewing's sarcoma of the pelvis: case report. Hum Reprod 2004;19(11):2569–2572.
137. Wallace WH, Kelsey TW. Ovarian reserve and reproductive age may be determined from measurement of ovarian volume by transvaginal sonography. Hum Reprod 2004;19(7):1612–1617.
138. Chapman RM, Sutcliffe SB, Malpas JS. Cytotoxic-induced ovarian failure in Hodgkin's disease. II. Effects on sexual function. JAMA 1979;242:1882–1884.
139. Waxman JHX, Terry YA, Wrigley PFM, et al. Gonadal function in Hodgkin's disease: long-term follow-up of chemotherapy. Br Med J 1982;285:1612–1613.
140. Byrne J, Fears TR, Gail MH, et al. Early menopause in long-term survivors of cancer during adolescence. Am J Obstet Gynecol 1992;166:788–793.
141. Madsen BL, Giudice L, Donaldson SS. Radiation-induced premature menopause: a misconception. Int J Radiat Oncol Biol Phys 1995;32:1461–1464.
142. Li FP, Gimbreke K, Gelber RD, et al. Outcome of pregnancy in survivors of Wilms' tumor. JAMA 1987;257:216–219.
143. Constine LS, Rubin P, Woolf PD, et al. Hyperprolactinemia and hypothyroidism following cytotoxic therapy for central nervous system malignancies. J Clin Oncol 1987;5:1841–1851.
144. Lushbaugh CC, Casarett GW. The effects of gonadal irradiation in clinical radiation therapy: a review. Cancer (Phila) 1976;37: 1111–1125.
145. Stillman RJ, Schinfeld JS, Schiff I, et al. Ovarian failure in long-term survivors of childhood malignancy. Am J Obstet Gynecol 1981;139:62–66.
146. Wallace WHB, Thomson AB, Kelsey TW. The radiosensitivity of the human oocyte. Hum Reprod 2003;18:117–121.
147. DaCunha MF, Meistrich ML, Fuller LM, et al. Recovery of spermatogenesis after treatment for Hodgkin's disease: limiting dose of MOPP chemotherapy. J Clin Oncol 1984;2:571–577.
148. Narayan P, Lange PH, Fraley EE. Ejaculation and fertility after extended retroperitoneal lymph node dissection for testicular cancer. J Urol 1982;127:685–688.
149. Schlegel PN, Walsh PC. Neuroanatomical approach to radical cystoprostatectomy with preservation of sexual function. J Urol 1987;138:1402–1406.
150. Rowley MJ, Leach DR, Warner GA, Heller CG. Effect of graded doses of ionizing radiation on the human testis. Radiat Res 1974;59:665–678.
151. Speiser B, Rubin P, Casarett G. Aspermia following lower truncal irradiation in Hodgkin's disease. Cancer (Phila) 1973;32: 692–698.
152. Shamberger RC, Sherins RJ, Rosenberg SA. The effects of postoperative adjuvant chemotherapy and radiotherapy on testicular function in men undergoing treatment for soft tissue sarcoma. Cancer (Phila) 1981:47:2368–2374.
153. Green DM, Brecher ML, Lindsay AN, et al. Gonadal function in pediatric patients following treatment for Hodgkin disease. Med Pediatr Oncol 1981;9:235–244.
154. Sklar C. Reproductive physiology and treatment-related loss of sex hormone production. Med Pediatr Oncol 1999;33:2–8.
155. Shalet SM, Horner A, Ahmed SR, Morris-Jones PH. Leydig cell damage after testicular irradiation for lymphoblastic leukaemia. Med Pediatr Oncol 1985;13:65–68.
156. Leiper AD, Grant DB, Chessells JM. Gonadal function after testicular radiation for acute lymphoblastic leukaemia. Arch Dis Child 1986;61:53–56.
157. Sklar CA, Robison LL, Nesbit ME, et al. Effects of radiation on testicular function in long-term survivors of childhood acute lymphoblastic leukemia: a report from the Children Cancer Study Group. J Clin Oncol 1990;8:1981–1987.
158. Chapman RM, Sutcliffe SB, Malpas JS. Cytotoxic-induced ovarian failure in women with Hodgkin's disease. I. Hormone function. JAMA 1979;242:1877–1881.
159. Whitehead E, Shalet SM, Jones PH, Beardwell CG, Deakin DP. Gonadal function after combination chemotherapy for Hodgkin's disease in childhood. Arch Dis Child 1982;57: 287–291.
160. Ortin TT, Shostak CA, Donaldson SS. Gonadal status and reproductive function following treatment for Hodgkin's disease in childhood: the Stanford experience. Int J Radiat Oncol Biol Phys 1990;19:873–880.
161. Mackie EJ, Radford M, Shalet SM. Gonadal function following chemotherapy for childhood Hodgkin's disease. Med Pediatr Oncol 1996;27:74–78.
162. Goodwin PJ, Ennis M, Pritchard KI, et al. Risk of menopause during the first year after breast cancer diagnosis. J Clin Oncol 1999;17:2365–2370.

163. Koyama H, Wada T, Nishzawa Y, et al. Cyclophosphamide induced ovarian failure and its therapeutic significance in patients with breast cancer. Cancer (Phila) 1977;39:1403–1409.
164. Byrne J, Mulvihill JJ, Myers MH, et al. Effects of treatment on fertility in long-term survivors of childhood or adolescent cancer. N Engl J Med 1987;317:1315–1321.
165. Critchley HOD, Wallace WHB, Shalet SM, et al. Abdominal irradiation in childhood: the potential for pregnancy. Br J Obstet Gynecol 1992;99:392–394.
166. Critchley HOD. Factors of importance for implantation and problems after treatment for childhood cancer. Med Pediatr Oncol 1999;33:9–14.
167. Bath LE, Critchley HO, Chambers SE, et al. Ovarian and uterine characteristics after total body irradiation in childhood and adolescence: response to sex steroid replacement. Br J Obstet Gynaecol 1999;106:1265–1272.
168. Li FP, Fine W, Jaffe N, et al. Offspring of patients treated for cancer in childhood. J Natl Cancer Inst 1979;62:1193–1197.
169. Hawkins MM, Smith RA, Curtice LJ. Childhood cancer survivors and their offspring studied through a postal survey of general practitioners: preliminary results. J R Coll Gen Pract 1988;38:102–105.
170. Byrne J, Rasmussen SA, Steinhorn SC, et al. Genetic disease in offspring of long-term survivors of childhood and adolescent cancer. Am J Hum Genet 1998;62:45–52.
171. Green DM, Fine WE, Li FP. Offspring of patients treated for unilateral Wilms' tumor in childhood. Cancer (Phila) 1982;49: 2285–2288.
172. Byrne L, Mulvihill JJ, Connelly RR, et al. Reproductive problems and birth defects in survivors of Wilms' tumor and their relatives. Med Pediatr Oncol 1988;16:233–240.
173. Li FP, Gimbrere K, Gelber RD, et al. Outcome of pregnancy in survivors of Wilms' tumor. JAMA 1987;257:216–219.
174. Hawkins MM, Smith RA. Pregnancy outcomes in childhood cancer survivors: probable effects of abdominal irradiation. Int J Cancer 1989;43:399–402.
175. Hawkins MM. Is there evidence of a therapy-related increase in germ cell mutation among childhood cancer survivors? J Natl Cancer Inst 1991;83:1643–1650.
176. Green DM, Zevon MA, Lowrie G, et al. Pregnancy outcome following treatment with chemotherapy for cancer in childhood and adolescence. N Engl J Med 1991;325:141–146.
177. Nygaard R, Clausen N, Siimes MA, et al. Reproduction following treatment for childhood leukemia: a population-based prospective cohort study of fertility and offspring. Med Pediatr Oncol 1991;19:459–466.
178. Dodds I, Marrett LD, Tomkins DJ, et al. Case-control study of congenital anomalies in children of cancer patients. Br Med J 1993;307:164–168.
179. Kenny LB, Nicholson HS, Brasseux C, et al. Birth defects in offspring of adult survivors of childhood acute lymphoblastic leukemia. Cancer (Phila) 1996;78:169–176.
180. Green DM, Fiorello A, Zevon MA, et al. Birth defects and childhood cancer in offspring of survivors of childhood cancer. Arch Pediatr Adolesc Med 1997;151:379–383.
181. Mulvihill JJ, Myers MH, Connelly RR, et al. Cancer in offspring of long-term survivors of childhood and adolescent cancer. Lancet 1987;2:813–817.
182. Hawkins JJ, Draper GJ, Smith RA. Cancer among 1,348 offspring of survivors of childhood cancer. Int J Cancer 1989;43:975–978.
183. Sanders JE, Hawley J, Levy W, et al. Pregnancies following high-dose cyclophosphamide with or without high-dose busulfan or total-body irradiation and bone marrow transplantation. Blood 1996;87:3045–3052.
184. Green DM, Whitton JA, Stovall M, et al. Pregnancy outcome of partners of male survivors of childhood cancer. A report from the Childhood Cancer Survivor Study. J Clin Oncol 2003;21: 716–721.
185. Green DM, Whitton JA, Stovall M, et al. Pregnancy outcome of female survivors of childhood cancer. A report from the Childhood Cancer Survivor Study. Am J Obstet Gynecol 2002; 187:1070–1080.
186. Horning SJ, Adhikari A, Rizk N. Effect of treatment for Hodgkin's disease on pulmonary function: results of a prospective study. J Clin Oncol 1994;12:297–305.
187. Samuels ML, Douglas EJ, Holoye PV, et al. Large dose bleomycin therapy and pulmonary toxicity. JAMA 1976;235:1117–1120.
188. O'Driscoll BR, Hasleton PS, Taylor PM, et al. Active lung fibrosis up to 17 years after chemotherapy with carmustine (BCNU) in childhood. N Engl J Med 1990;323:378–382.
189. Vogelzang NJ. Nephrotoxicity from chemotherapy: prevention and management. Oncology 1991;5:97–112.
190. Dewit L, Anninga JK, Hoefnagel CA, et al. Radiation injury in the human kidney: a prospective analysis using specific scintigraphic and biochemical endpoints. Int J Radiat Oncol Biol Phys 1990;19:977–983.
191. Hilkens PHE, Verweij J, Vecht CJ, Stoter G, Bent MHvd. Clinical characteristics of severe peripheral neuropathy incuded by docetaxel, taxotere. Ann Oncol 1997;8:187–190.
192. Tuxen MK, Hansen SW. Complications of treatment: neurotoxicity secondary to antineoplastic drugs. Cancer Treat Rev 1994; 20:191–214.
193. Bhatia S, Robison LL, Meadows AT, LESG Investigators. High risk of second malignant neoplasms (SMN) continues with extended follow-up of childhood Hodgkin's disease (HD) cohort: report from the Late Effects Study Group. Blood 2001;98: 768a.
194. van Leeuwen FE, Klokman WJ, Stovall M, et al. Roles of radiotherapy and smoking in lung cancer following Hodgkin's disease. J Natl Cancer Inst 1995;87:1530–1537.
195. Kreiker J, Kattan J. Second colon cancer following Hodgkin's disease. A case report. J Med Libanais 1996;44:107–108.
196. Deutsch M, Wollman MR, Ramanathan R, Rubin J. Rectal cancer twenty-one years after treatment of childhood Hodgkin disease. Med Pediatr Oncol 2002;38:280–281.
197. Hawkins MM, Draper GJ, Kingston JE. Incidence of second primary tumors among childhood cancer survivors. Br J Cancer 1984;56:339–347.
198. Meadows AT, Baum E, Fossati-Bellani F, et al. Second malignant neoplasms in children: an update from the Late Effects Study Group. J Clin Oncol 1985;3:532–538.
199. Bhatia S, Robison LL, Oberlin O, et al. Breast cancer and other second neoplasms after childhood Hodgkin's disease. N Engl J Med 1996;334:745–751.
200. Malkin D, Li FP, Strong LC, et al. Germline p53 mutations in a familial syndrome of breast cancer, sarcomas, and other neoplasms. Science 1990;250:1333–1338.
201. Neglia JP, Friedman DL, Yasui Y, et al. Second malignant neoplasms in five-year survivors of childhood cancer: childhood cancer survivor study. J Natl Cancer Inst 2001;93:618–629.
202. Bhatia S, Sather HN, Pabustan OB, Trigg ME, Gaynon PS, Robison LL. Low incidence of second neoplasms among children diagnosed with acute lymphoblastic leukemia after 1983. Blood 2002;99:4257–4264.
203. Neglia JP, Meadows AT, Robison LL, et al. Second neoplasms after acute lymphoblastic leukemia in childhood. N Engl J Med 1991;325:1330–1336.
204. Relling MV, Rubnitz JE, Rivera GK, et al. High incidence of secondary brain tumours after radiotherapy and antimetabolites. Lancet 1999:354:34–39.
205. Hawkins MM, Wilson LM, Stovall MA, et al. Epipodophyllotoxins, alkylating agents, and radiation and risk of secondary leukaemia after childhood cancer. Br Med J 1992;304:951–958.
206. Tucker MA. Solid second cancers following Hodgkin's disease. Hematol-Oncol Clin N Am 1993;7:389–400.

207. Beatty O III, Hudson MM, Greenwald C, et al. Subsequent malignancies in children and adolescents after treatment for Hodgkin's disease. J Clin Oncol 1995;13:603–609.
208. Bhatia S, Robison LL, Oberlin O, et al. Breast cancer and other second neoplasms after childhood Hodgkin's disease. N Engl J Med 1996;334:745–751.
209. Jenkin D, Greenberg M, Fitzgerald A. Second malignant tumours in childhood Hodgkin's disease. Med Pediatr Oncol 1996;26: 373–379.
210. Sankila R, Garwicz S, Olsen JH, et al. Risk of subsequent malignant neoplasms among 1,641 Hodgkin's disease patients diagnosed in childhood and adolescence: a population-based cohort study in the five Nordic countries. Association of the Nordic Cancer Registries and the Nordic Society of Pediatric Hematology and Oncology. J Clin Oncol 1996;14:1442–1446.
211. Wolden SL, Lamborn KR, Cleary SF, Tate DJ, Donaldson SS. Second cancers following pediatric Hodgkin's disease. J Clin Oncol 1998;16:536–544.
212. Green DM, Hyland A, Barcos MP, et al. Second malignant neoplasms after treatment for Hodgkin's disease in childhood or adolescence. J Clin Oncol 2000;18:1492–1499.
213. Metayer C, Lynch CF, Clarke EA, et al. Second cancers among long-term survivors of Hodgkin's disease diagnosed in childhood and adolescence. J Clin Oncol 2000;18:2435–2443.
214. Wrighton SA, Stevens JC. The human hepatic cytochromes P450 involved in drug metabolism. Crit Rev Toxicol 1992;22: 1–21.
215. Hayes JD, Pulford DJ. The glutathione S-transferase supergene family: regulation of GST and the contribution of the isoenzymes to cancer chemoprotection and drug resistance. Crit Rev Biochem Mol Biol 1995;30:445–600.
216. Raunio H, Husgafvel-Pursiainen K, Anttila S, Hietanen E, Hirvonen A, Pelkonen O. Diagnosis of polymorphisms in carcinogen-activating and inactivating enzymes and cancer susceptibility: a review. Gene (Amst) 1995;159:113–121.
217. Smith G, Stanley LA, Sim E, Strange RC, Wolf CR. Metabolic polymorphisms and cancer susceptibility. Cancer Surv 1995; 25:27–65.
218. Felix CA, Walker AH, Lange BJ, et al. Association of CYP3A4 genotype with treatment-related leukemia. Proc Natl Acad Sci U S A 1998;95:13176–13181.
219. Naoe T, Takeyama K, Yokozawa T, et al. Analysis of genetic polymorphism in NQO1, GST-M1, GST-T1, and CYP3A4 in 469 Japanese patients with therapy-related leukemia/myelodysplastic syndrome and de novo acute myeloid leukemia. Clin Cancer Res 2000;6:4091–4095.
220. Blanco JG, Edick MJ, Hancock ML, et al. Genetic polymorphisms in CYP3A5, CYP3A4 and NQO1 in children who developed therapy-related myeloid malignancies. Pharmacogenetics 2002;12:605–611.
221. Zim S, Collins JM, O'Neill D, et al. Inhibition of first-pass metabolism in cancer chemotherapy: interaction of 6-mercaptopurine and allopurinol. Clin Pharmacol Ther 1983; 34:810–817.
222. Hildreth NG, Shore RE, Dvortesky PM. The risk of breast cancer after irradiation of the thymus in infancy. N Engl J Med 1989;321:1281–1284.
223. Petrek JA, Heelan MC. Incidence of breast carcinoma-related lymphedema. Cancer (Phila) 1998;83(suppl 12):2776–2781.
224. Erickson VS, Pearson ML, Ganz PA, Adams J, Kahn KL. Arm edema in breast cancer patients. JNCI 2004;93:96–111.
225. Andrykowski MA, Curran SL, Lightner R. Off-treatment fatigue in breast cancer survivors: a controlled comparison. J Behav Med 1998;21:1–18.
226. Broeckel JA, Jacobsen PB, Horton J, Balducci L, Lyman GH. Characteristics and correlates of fatigue after adjuvant chemotherapy for breast cancer. J Clin Oncol 1998;16: 1689–1696.
227. Greenberg DB, Kornblith AB, Herndon JE, et al. Quality of life for adult leukemia survivors treated on clinical trials of Cancer and Leukemia Group B during the period 1971–1988. Cancer (Phila) 1997;80:1936–1944.
228. Loge JH, Abrahamsen AF, Ekeberg O, Kaasa S. Hodgkin's disease survivors more fatigued than the general population. J Clin Oncol 1999;17:253–261.
229. Bush NE, Haberman M, Donaldson G, Sullivan KM. Quality of life of 125 adults surviving 6–18 years after bone marrow transplant. Social Sci Med 1995;40:479–490.
230. Mock V, Piper B, Escalante C, Sabbatini P. National Comprehensive Cancer Network practice guidelines for the management of cancer-related fatigue. Oncologist 2000;14(11A):151–161.
231. Ganz PA, Schag CAC, Lee JJ, et al. The CARES: a generic measure of health-related quality of life for cancer patients. Qual Life Res 1992;1:19–29.
232. Demark-Wahnefried W, Aziz NM, Rowland JH, Pinto BM. Riding the Crest of the Teachable Moment: Promoting Long-Term Health after the Diagnosis of Cancer. J Clin Oncol, 2005.
233. Day RW. Future need for more cancer research. J Am Diet Assoc 1998;98:523.
234. Brown BW, Brauner C, Minnotte MC. Noncancer deaths in white adult cancer patients. JNCI 1993;85:979–997.
235. Meadows AT, Varricchio C, Crosson K, et al. Research issues in cancer survivorship. Cancer Epidemiol Biomarkers Prev 1998;7: 1145–1151.
236. Travis LB. Therapy-associated solid tumors. Acta Oncol 2002; 41:323 333.
237. Bergstrom A, Pisani P, Tenet V, et al. Overweight as an avoidable cause of cancer in Europe. Int J Cancer 2001;91:421–430.
238. World Health Organization. IARC Handbook of Cancer Prevention, vol 6. Geneva: World Health Organization, 2002.
239. Chlebowski RT, Aiello E, McTiernan A. Weight loss in breast cancer patient management. J Clin Oncol 2002;20:1128–1143.
240. Nuver J, Smit AJ, Postma A, et al. The metabolic syndrome in long-term cancer survivors, an important target for secondary measures. Cancer Treat Rev 2002;28:195–214.
241. Freedland SJ, Aronson WJ, Kane CJ, et al. Impact of obesity on biochemical control after radical prostatectomy for clinically localized prostate cancer: a report by the Shared Equal Access Regional Cancer Hospital database study group. J Clin Oncol 2004;22:446–453.
242. Argiles JM Lopez-Soriano FJ. Insulin and cancer. Int J Oncol 2001;18:683–687.
243. Bines J, Gradishar WJ. Primary care issues for the breast cancer survivor. Compr Ther 1997;23:605–611.
244. Yoshikawa T, Noguchi Y, Doi C, et al. Insulin resistance in patients with cancer: relationships with tumor site, tumor stage, body-weight loss, acute-phase response, and energy expenditure. Nutrition 2001;17:590–593.
245. Balkau B, Kahn HS, Courbon D, et al. Paris Prospective Study. Hyperinsulinemia predicts fatal liver cancer but is inversely associated with fatal cancer at some other sites: the Paris Prospective Study. Diabetes Care 2001;24:843–849.
246. Lamont EB, Christakis NA, Lauderdale DS. Favorable cardiac risk among elderly breast carcinoma survivors. Cancer (Phila) 2003;98:2–10.
247. Hull MC, Morris CG, Pepine CJ, et al. Valvular dysfunction and carotid, subclavian, and coronary artery disease in survivors of Hodgkin lymphoma treated with radiation therapy. JAMA 2003; 290:2831–2837.
248. Buist DS, LaCroix AZ, Barlow WE, et al. Bone mineral density and endogenous hormones and risk of breast cancer in postmenopausal women (United States). Cancer Causes Control 2001;12:213–222.
249. Buist DS, LaCroix AZ, Barlow WE, et al. Bone mineral density and breast cancer risk in postmenopausal women. J Clin Epidemiol 2001;54:417–422.

250. Cauley JA, Lucas FL, Kuller LH, et al. Bone mineral density and risk of breast cancer in older women: the study of osteoporotic fractures. Study of Osteoporotic Fractures Research Group. JAMA 1996;276:1404–1408.
251. Lamont EB, Lauderdale DS. Low risk of hip fracture among elderly breast cancer survivors. Ann Epidemiol 2003;13: 698–703.
252. Lucas FL, Cauley JA, Stone RA, et al. Bone mineral density and risk of breast cancer: differences by family history of breast cancer. Study of Osteoporotic Fractures Research Group. Am J Epidemiol 1998;148:22–29.
253. Newcomb PA, Trentham-Dietz A, Egan KM, et al. Fracture history and risk of breast and endometrial cancer. Am J Epidemiol 2001;153:1071–1078.
254. van der Klift M, de Laet CE, Coebergh JW, et al. Bone mineral density and the risk of breast cancer: the Rotterdam Study. Bone (NY) 2003;32:211–216.
255. Zhang Y, Kiel DP, Kreger BE, et al. Bone mass and the risk of breast cancer among postmenopausal women. N Engl J Med 1997;336:611–617.
256. Zmuda JM, Cauley JA, Ljung BM, et al. Study of Osteoporotic Fractures Research Group. Bone mass and breast cancer risk in older women: differences by stage at diagnosis. JNCI 2001;93: 930–936.
257. Schultz PN, Beck ML, Stava C, et al. Health profiles in 5836 long-term cancer survivors. Int J Cancer 2003;104:488–495.
258. Twiss JJ, Waltman N, Ott CD, et al. Bone mineral density in postmenopausal breast cancer survivors. J Am Acad Nurse Pract 2001;13:276–284.
259. Ramaswamy B, Shapiro CL. Osteopenia and osteoporosis in women with breast cancer. Semin Oncol 2003;30:763–775.
260. Diamond TH, Higano CS, Smith MR, et al. Osteoporosis in men with prostate carcinoma receiving androgen-deprivation therapy: recommendations for diagnosis and therapies. Cancer (Phila) 2004;100:892–899.
261. Ko CY, Maggard M, Livingston EH: Evaluating health utility in patients with melanoma, breast cancer, colon cancer, and lung cancer: a nationwide, population-based assessment. J Surg Res 2003;114:1–5.
262. Garman KS, Pieper CF, Seo P, et al. Function in elderly cancer survivors depends on comorbidities. J Gerontol A Biol Sci Med Sci 2003;58:M1119–M1124.
263. Hewitt M, Rowland JH, Yancik R. Cancer survivors in the U.S.: age, health and disability. J Gerontol Biol Sci Med Sci 2003; 58:82–91.
264. Ashing-Giwa K, Ganz PA, Petersen L. Quality of life of African-American and white long term breast carcinoma survivors. Cancer (Phila) 1999;85:418–426.
265. Baker F, Haffer S, Denniston M. Health-related quality of life of cancer and noncancer patients in Medicare managed care. Cancer (Phila) 2003;97:674–681.
266. Chirikos TN, Russell-Jacobs A, Jacobsen PB. Functional impairment and the economic consequences of female breast cancer. Womens Health 2002;36:1–20.
267. Trotti A. The evolution and application of toxicity criteria. Semin Radiat Oncol 2002;12(1 suppl 1):1–3.
268. Hoeller U, Tribius S, Kuhlmey A, Grader K, Fehlauer F, Alberti W. Increasing the rate of late toxicity by changing the score? A comparison of RTOG/EORTC and LENT/SOMA scores. Int J Radiat Oncol Biol Phys 2003;55(4):1013–1018.
269. Garre ML, Gandus S, Cesana B, et al. Health status of long term survivors after cancer in childhood. Am J Pediatr Hematol Oncol 1994;16:143–152.
270. Von der Weid N, Beck D, Caflisch U, Feldges A, Wyss M, Wagner HP. Standardized assessment of late effects in long term survivors of childhood cancer in Switzerland: results of a Swiss Pediatrics Oncology Group (SPOG) study. Int J Pedatr Hematol Oncol 1996;3:483–490.
271. Brown JK, Byers T, Doyle C, et al. Nutrition and physical activity during and after cancer treatment: an American Cancer Society guide for informed choices. CA Cancer J Clin 2003;53: 268–291.
272. Rock CL, Demark-Wahnefried W. Nutrition and survival after the diagnosis of breast cancer: a review of the evidence. J Clin Oncol 2002;20:3302–3316.
273. Kattlove H, Winn RJ. Ongoing care of patients after primary treatment for their cancer. CA Cancer J Clin 2003;53:172–196.
274. Robison LL. Cancer survivorship: Unique opportunities for research. Cancer Epidemiol Biomarkers Prev 2004;13:1093.
275. Eshelman D, Landier W, Sweeney T, Hester AL, Forte K, Darling J, Hudson MM. Facilitating care for childhood cancer survivors: integrating children's oncology group long-term follow-up guidelines and health links in clinical practice. J Pediatr Oncol Nurs 2004;21:271–280.
276. Oberfield SE, Sklar CA. Endocrine sequelae in survivors of childhood cancer. Adolesc Med 2002;13:161–169.
277. Green DM, Grigoriev YA, Nan B, et al. Congestive heart failure after treatment for Wilms' tumor: a report from the National Wilms' Tumor Study group. J Clin Oncol 2001;19:1926–1934.
278. Green DM, Peabody EM, Nan B, Peterson S, Kalapurakal JA, Breslow NE. Pregnancy outcome after treatment for Wilms tumor: a report from the National Wilms Tumor Study Group. J Clin Oncol 2002;20:2506–2513.
279. Michael YL, Kawachi I, Berkman LF, et al. The persistent impact of breast carcinoma on functional health status. Cancer (Phila) 2000;89:2176–2186.
280. Chirikos TN, Russell-Jacobs A, Jacobsen PB. Functional impairment and the economic consequences of female breast cancer. Women Health 2002;36:1–20.
281. Deimling GT, Schaefer ML, Kahana B, Bowman KF, Reardon J. Racial differences in the health of older adult long-term cancer survivors. Psychosoc Oncol (in press).
282. Chirikos TN, Russell-Jacobs A, Cantor AB. Indirect economic effects of long-term breast cancer survival. Cancer Pract 2002;10:248–255.
283. Ahles TA, Saykin AJ, Furstenberg CT, et al. Neuropsychologic impact of standard-dose systemic chemotherapy in long-term survivors of breast cancer and lymphoma. J Clin Oncol 2002; 20:485–493.
284. Ahles TA, Saykin AJ, Noll WW, et al. The relationship of APOE genotype to neuropsychological performance in long-term cancer survivors treated with standard dose chemotherapy. J Clin Oncol 2002;20(2):485–493.
285. Syrjala KL, Schroeder TC, Abrams JR, Atkins TZ, Sanders JE, Brown W, Heiman JR. Sexual function measurement and outcomes in cancer survivors and matched controls. J Sex Research 2000;37(3):213–225.
286. Syrjala KL, Roth SL, Abrams JR, Chapko MK, Visser S, Sanders JE. Prevalence and predictors of sexual dysfunction in long-term survivors of bone marrow transplantation. J Clin Oncol 1998; 16:3148–3157.
287. Paskett ED, Stark N. Lymphedema: knowledge, treatment, and impact among breast cancer survivors. Breast J 2000;6(6):373–378.
288. Simbre VC II, Admas MJ, Deshpande SS, Duffy SA, Miller TL, Lipshultz SE. Cardiomyopathy caused by antineoplastic therapies. Curr Treat Options Cardiovasc Med 2001;3:493–505.
289. Lipshultz SE, Lipsitz SR, Sallan SE, et al. Long-term enalapril therapy for left ventricular dysfunction in doxorubicin-treated survivors of childhood cancer. J Clin Oncol 2002;20:4517–4522.
290. Thompson SJ, Leigh L, Christensen R, et al. Immediate neurocognitive effects of methylphenidate on learning-impaired survivors of childhood cancer. J Clin Oncol 2001;19:1802–1808.
291. Longman AJ, Braden CJ, Mishel MH. Side-effects burden, psychological adjustment, and life quality in women with breast

cancer: pattern of association over time. Oncol Nurs Forum 1999;26:909–915.

292. Badger TA, Braden CJ, Mishel MH. Depression burden, self-help interventions, and side effect experience in women receiving treatment for breast cancer. Oncol Nurs Forum 2001;28(3):567–574.

293. Antoni MH, Lehman JM, Kilbourn KM, et al. Cognitive-behavioral stress management intervention decreases the prevalence of depression and enhances benefit finding among women under treatment for early-stage breast cancer. Health Psychol 2001;20:20–32.

102

Medical and Psychosocial Issues in Childhood Cancer Survivors

Smita Bhatia, Wendy Landier, Jacqueline Casillas, and Lonnie Zeltzer

More than 12,000 children and adolescents younger than 20 years are diagnosed with cancer each year in the United States.[1] With the use of risk-based therapies, the overall 5-year survival rate is approaching 80%, resulting in a growing population of childhood cancer survivors.[1] In 1997, there were an estimated 270,000 survivors of childhood cancer; over two-thirds of these were older than 20 years of age.[2] This figure translates into 1 in 810 individuals under the age of 20 and 1 in 640 individuals between the ages of 20 and 39 years having successfully survived childhood cancer (see Chapter 62).

Unlike an adult, the growing child tolerates the acute side effects of therapy relatively well. However, the use of cancer therapy at an early age can produce complications that may not become apparent until years later as the child matures. The resulting complications are related to the specific therapy employed and the age of the child at the time the therapy was administered. A *late effect* is defined as a late-occurring or chronic outcome—either physical or psychologic—that persists or develops beyond 5 years from the diagnosis of cancer. These late effects include complications such as cognitive impairment, cardiopulmonary compromise, endocrine dysfunction, renal impairment, chronic hepatitis, and subsequent malignancies. As many as two-thirds of survivors experience at least one late effect as a result of treatment for cancer during childhood.[3–7] Therefore, ongoing evaluation of childhood cancer survivors is an essential component of follow-up. This chapter discusses the long-term complications that can occur among pediatric patients treated for cancer, along with recommendations for follow-up. Table 102.1 summarizes the data on the magnitude of risk and associated risk factors for select long-term outcomes.

Neurocognitive Sequelae

Neurocognitive sequelae of treatment for childhood cancer occur as a consequence of radiation to the whole brain and/or therapy with high-dose methotrexate, cytarabine, and/or intrathecal methotrexate. Children with a history of brain tumors, acute lymphoblastic leukemia (ALL), or non-Hodgkin's lymphoma (NHL) are most likely to be affected. Risk factors include increasing radiation dose, young age at the time of treatment, therapy with both cranial radiation and systemic or intrathecal chemotherapy, and female sex.[8] Severe deficits are most frequently noted in children with brain tumors, especially those who were treated with radiation therapy, and in children who were less than 5 years of age at the time of treatment.[9]

Neurocognitive deficits usually become evident within 1 to 2 years following radiation and are progressive in nature.[10] Affected children may experience information-processing deficits, resulting in academic difficulties. These children are particularly prone to problems with receptive and expressive language, attention span, and visual and perceptual motor skills. They most often experience academic difficulties in the areas of reading, language, and mathematics. Children in the younger age groups and those treated for brain tumors may experience significant drops in intelligence quotient (IQ) scores, with irradiation- or chemotherapy-induced destruction in normal white matter partially explaining intellectual and academic achievement deficits.[9,11–13]

Cardiovascular Function

Chronic cardiotoxicity usually manifests itself as cardiomyopathy, pericarditis, and congestive heart failure. The anthracyclines are well-known causes of cardiomyopathy.[14–17] The incidence of cardiomyopathy is dose dependent and may exceed 30% among patients who received cumulative doses of anthracyclines in excess of 600 mg/m^2 (daunorubicin/doxorubicin equivalent).[18] With a total dose of 500 to 600 mg/m^2, the incidence is 11%, falling to less than 1% for cumulative doses less than 500 mg/m^2.[19] These data have formed the basis for the use of a threshold of 500 mg/m^2 as the cumulative dose for cardiotoxicity. However, Kremer et al.[20] reported that a cumulative dose of anthracyclines greater than 300 mg/m^2

TABLE 102.1. Clinical characteristics and risk factors for select long-term sequelae after treatment for childhood cancer.

Long-term sequelae	*Cumulative probability*	*Risk factors*
Congestive heart failure	4%–17% at 20 years (risk increasing with increasing therapeutic exposures)	• Higher cumulative dose of anthracyclines • Female sex • Younger age at exposure to anthracyclines • Black race • Presence of trisomy 21 • Radiation therapy involving the heart • Exposure to cyclophosphamide, ifosfamide, or amsacrine
Myocardial infarction	21% at 20–25 years	• Radiation therapy to the mediastinum • Dose >30 Gy • Increasing time since irradiation • Younger age at irradiation (<20 years) • Hypertension/hypercholesterolemia/DM/smoking/obesity
Ischemic stroke	12% at 15 years (among patients exposed to neck radiation)	• Radiation therapy to the head and neck • Younger age at irradiation (<20 years) • Hypertension/hypercholesterolemia/DM/smoking
Subsequent malignant neoplasms	3% at 20 years	• HD, soft tissue sarcoma, hereditary retinoblastoma • Younger age at exposure to therapeutic agents • Female sex • Radiation therapy • Exposure to alkylating agents or topoisomerase • II inhibitors

DM, diabetes mellitus; HD, Hodgkin's disease.

was associated with an increased risk of clinical heart failure (relative risk, 11.8) compared with a cumulative dose lower than 300 mg/m^2. Thus, a lower cumulative dose of anthracyclines may place children at increased risk for cardiac compromise.[20]

Cardiomyopathy can occur many years after completion of therapy, and the onset may be spontaneous or coincide with exertion or pregnancy. Risk factors known to be associated with anthracycline-related cardiac toxicity include mediastinal radiation;[21] uncontrolled hypertension;[17,18] exposure to other chemotherapeutic agents, especially cyclophosphamide,[18] dactinomycin,[22] mitomycin,[18] decarbazine,[23] vincristine, bleomycin, and methotrexate;[24] female sex;[25] younger age;[17,26,27] and electrolyte imbalance such as hypokalemia and hypomagnesemia.[16]

Chronic cardiac toxicity associated with radiation alone most commonly manifests as pericardial effusions or constrictive pericarditis, sometimes in association with pancarditis. Although 4,000 cGy of total heart radiation dose appears to be the usual threshold, pericarditis has been reported after as little as 1,500 cGy, even in the absence of radiomimetic chemotherapy.[28,29] Symptomatic pericarditis, which usually develops 10 to 30 months after radiation, is found in 2% to 10% of patients.[28–30] Subclinical pericardial and myocardial damage as well as valvular thickening may be common in this population,[31,32] and symptomatic pericarditis may first appear as late as 45 years after therapy.[33,34] Coronary artery disease has been reported following radiation to the mediastinum.[35]

Prevention of cardiotoxicity is a primary focus of investigation. Liposomal anthracyclines are being explored to reduce cardiotoxicity. The anthracyclines chelate iron, and the anthracycline–iron complex catalyzes the formation of extremely hydroxyl radicals. Agents such as dexrazoxane that are able to remove iron from the anthracyclines have been investigated as cardioprotectants. Clinical trials of dexrazoxane have been conducted in children, with encouraging evidence of short-term cardioprotection.[36,37] The long-term avoidance of cardiotoxicity with the use of this agent needs to be determined.[38] Smaller doses and reduced port sizes of radiation therapy may also help in decreasing the incidence of carditis.

Pulmonary Function

Radiation-induced restrictive lung disease is seen in patients who received whole-lung radiation at a dose of 1,100 to 1,400 cGy and results primarily from a proportionate interference with the growth of both the lung and the chest wall.[39–41] Children under 3 years of age at time of therapy appear to be more susceptible to chronic toxicity. Obstructive changes are also reported after conventional radiation therapy and have been reported after 1,000 cGy total-body irradiation for hematopoietic cell transplant (HCT).[42] A cohort of 12,390 childhood cancer survivors participating in the Childhood Cancer Survivor Study (CCSS)[43] had a statistically significantly increased risk of lung fibrosis, recurrent pneumonia, chronic cough, pleurisy, use of supplemental oxygen, abnormal chest wall, exercise-induced shortness of breath, bronchitis, recurrent sinus infection, and tonsillitis when compared with sibling controls.[44] Statistically significant associations were identified for lung fibrosis and chest radiation, and for supplemental oxygen use and chest radiation, BCNU (carmustine), bleomycin, busulfan, CCNU (lomustine), and cyclophosphamide. Chest radiation was associated with a 3.5% cumulative incidence of lung fibrosis at 20 years after diagnosis.

Several chemotherapeutic agents have been associated with pulmonary disease in long-term survivors. Bleomycin toxicity is the prototype for chemotherapy-related lung injury. The chronic lung toxicity is dose dependent above a threshold cumulative dose of 400 units/m^2 and is exacerbated by previous or concurrent radiation therapy,[45] cyclophosphamide,[46] or subsequent oxygen therapy.[47] At doses exceeding 400 units/m^2, 10% of the patients experience fibrosis, and 35% to 55% suffer severe symptoms in the face of combinations of other injuries.[48] Other chemotherapeutic agents associated with chronic lung injury include BCNU,[49] busulfan, and CCNU.

Symptoms of pulmonary dysfunction include chronic cough or dyspnea, and close evaluation should be performed during yearly follow-up. All patients must be educated about the risks of smoking. The best possible approach to chronic pulmonary toxicity of anticancer therapy is preventive and includes the following: careful monitoring of pulmonary function and chest radiographs before and during bleomycin and radiation; respecting cumulative dose restrictions on bleomycin administration; and limiting radiation dosage and port sizes.

Endocrine Function

Thyroid

Hypothyroidism is the most common nonmalignant late effect involving this gland and is almost always caused by radiation of the head and neck for a nonthyroid malignancy. Laboratory evidence of primary hypothyroidism is evident in 40% to 90% of patients receiving radiation doses in excess of 1,500 cGy.[50–52] The actuarial risk of clinical hypothyroidism for subjects treated with 4,500 Gy or more is 50% at 20 years from diagnosis. Childhood brain tumor survivors were compared with siblings as part of the CCSS study, and were found to be at a 14.3-fold-increased risk of developing hypothyroidisms.[53] Risk factors associated with the development of hypothyroidism include increasing dose of radiation (higher risk associated with conventionally fractionated radiotherapy as compared with hyperfractionated radiotherapy), thyroidectomy, use of iodide-containing contrast material as in lymphangiography, older age at irradiation, and female gender.[54,55]

Hyperthyroidism has been reported in up to 5% of the survivors of Hodgkin's disease (HD) and is associated with radiation doses exceeding 3,500 cGy.[54] Thyroid nodules are observed among patients exposed to radiation. Female gender and radiation doses exceeding 2,500 cGy have been identified as risk factors.[54] The actuarial risk of female survivors of HD developing a thyroid nodule is 20% at 20 years from diagnosis. Patients with HD receiving radiation to the thyroid gland have been reported to be at an 18-fold-increased risk of developing thyroid cancer when compared with the general population.

Growth

Poor linear growth and short adult stature are common complications following successful treatment for childhood cancer.[56] Although in some children catch-up growth may occur, short stature may be permanent or even progressive. Severe growth retardation, defined as a standing height below the fifth percentile, has been observed in as many as 30% to 35% of survivors of childhood brain tumors[57–59] and 10% to 15% of patients treated for leukemia.[60,61] Whole-brain irradiation has been identified as the principal cause of short stature.[60] Compared with siblings, childhood brain tumor survivors participating in the CCSS study were at a 277.8-fold-increased risk of developing growth hormone deficiency.[53] The effects of cranial irradiation appear to be related to age and sex, with children younger than 5 years at time of therapy and girls being more susceptible to the radiation effect.[62–64] The effects of radiation are also dose dependent, with doses exceeding 3,000 cGy associated with growth retardation in 50% of the patients.[58,59] The mechanism by which cranial irradiation induces short stature is not clear. Growth hormone deficiency and early onset of puberty in girls may contribute to loss of final height.[65] Direct inhibition of vertebral growth by spinal irradiation often contributes to short stature.

Body Mass Index

An increased prevalence of obesity has been reported among survivors of childhood ALL, with the prevalence increasing with increasing dose of cranial radiation. In a study conducted by Sklar et al.,[66] the percentage of subjects who were overweight at attainment of final height was 10.5%, 40%, and 38% for subjects treated with no cranial radiation, 18 Gy of cranial radiation, and 24 Gy of cranial radiation, respectively. This study documented that children with ALL given cranial radiation develop increases in their body mass index early on during their treatment and remain at significant risk for becoming overweight as young adults. A recent report has shown that the age-and race-adjusted odds ratio (OR) for being obese in ALL survivors treated with cranial radiation doses of 20 Gy or more in comparison with siblings was 2.6 for females and 1.9 for males.[67] Furthermore, the OR for obesity was greatest among girls diagnosed at 0 to 4 years of age and treated with radiation doses of 20 Gy or more. Thus, this study clearly demonstrated in a large cohort of ALL survivors that 20 Gy or more is associated with an increased prevalence of obesity, especially in females treated at a young age. It is therefore important for healthcare professionals to recognize this risk and to address it in the long-term follow-up of the survivors.

Gonadal Function

Males

Male survivors of childhood cancer may experience germ cell depletion and abnormalities of gonadal endocrine function. These abnormalities may be secondary to radiation, chemotherapy, or surgery, with the effects of therapy varying depending on age at treatment. In patients who receive testicular radiation doses of 400 to 600 cGy, azoospermia may persist for 3 to 5 years, and at doses above 600 cGy, germinal loss with resulting increases in follicle-stimulating hormone (FSH) and decreases in testicular volume usually appears to be irreversible.[68,69] Prepubertal testicular germ cells also appear to be radiosensitive, although tubular damage may be difficult to assess until the patient has progressed through puberty. Radiation therapy at doses of 2,000 cGy or higher is also toxic to Leydig cells, with resulting inadequate production of testosterone.[70]

Chemotherapy can also interfere with testicular function. Alkylating agents decrease spermatogenesis in long-term survivors of cancer. The effects of cyclophosphamide and chlorambucil are dose dependent but are reversible in up to 70%

of patients after several years.[71] Among pubertal boys treated for HD with six cycles of mechlorethamine, vincristine, prednisone, and procarbazine (MOPP), azoospermia is found in 80% to 100%, and is reversible in only 20% of cases.[72] After adriamycin, bleomycin, vinblastine, and dacarbazine (ABVD), the incidence of azoospermia was 36%, with 100% recovery.[73] The effect of MOPP on Leydig cell function appears to be age related, with normal pubertal progression after therapy for patients treated before the onset of puberty, gynecomastia with low testosterone and increased luteinizing hormone (LH) in patients treated during adolescence, and compensated Leydig cell failure without gynecomastia in adults.[71]

Females

Radiation therapy effects on the ovary are both age- and dose dependent. Amenorrhea develops in only 68% of prepubescent girls treated with higher doses of radiation (1,200–1,500 cGy).[74] Spinal irradiation for the treatment of ALL and brain tumors appears to result in clinically significant ovarian damage in some young women, although the majority of these women go on to experience normal puberty and menarche, generally at a slightly older age. Girls treated with whole abdominal and/or pelvic irradiation for HD or Wilm's tumor or other solid tumors are at a high risk of ovarian failure. Patients who receive HCT with total-body irradiation, both single-dose and fractionated, are at a high risk of developing permanent ovarian failure. Almost all patients who undergo HCT after the age of 10 years will develop premature ovarian failure, whereas only 50% of girls transplanted before the age of 10 years will.[75]

Ovarian failure has also been observed after chemotherapy, in particular, with alkylating agents. Toxicity is, again, dose- and age dependent. Only 30% of women and girls younger than 35 years of age at exposure to MOPP chemotherapy develop temporary amenorrhea, with irreversible ovarian failure seen in a small minority.[76] Females who receive high-dose, myeloablative therapy with alkylating agents in the context of allogeneic or autologous HCT are at high risk of developing ovarian failure.[76]

Pregnancy Outcomes of Childhood Cancer Survivors

Radiation therapy and many of the chemotherapeutic agents used in the treatment of childhood cancer could potentially be mutagenic and have an adverse effect on the health of the offspring of the survivors. Green et al.[77] evaluated the health of the offspring of partners of male childhood cancer survivors participating in the CCSS and demonstrated that the proportion of pregnancies of the partners of male survivors that ended with a liveborn infant was significantly lower than for the partners of male siblings of the survivors who served as controls. This study of male survivors did not identify adverse pregnancy outcomes for the partners of male survivors treated with most chemotherapeutic agents. A similar study focusing on offspring of the female survivors failed to identify adverse pregnancy outcomes for female survivors treated with most chemotherapeutic agents. The offspring of women who received pelvic irradiation were at risk for low birth weight.[78]

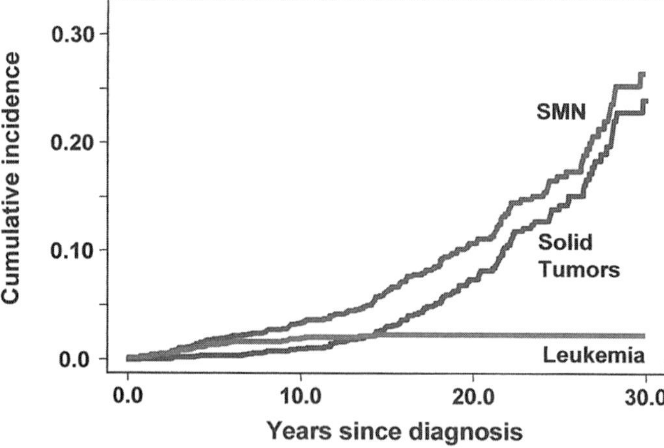

FIGURE 102.1. Cumulative incidence of subsequent malignant neoplasms after extended follow-up of Hodgkin's disease in childhood. (Adapted from Bhatia et al.,[81] by permissions of *Journal of Clinical Oncology*.)

Second Malignant Neoplasms

Several studies following large cohorts of childhood cancer survivors have reported a threefold- to sixfold-increased risk of a second cancer, when compared with the general population, and this risk continues to increase as the cohort ages[79–83] (Figure 102.1; see Chapter 111).

Late Mortality Among Childhood Cancer Survivors

Several investigators have shown a 10-fold excess in overall mortality among 5-year childhood cancer survivors when compared with the general population.[84,85] The excess mortality was due to death from primary cancer, second cancer, cardiotoxicity, and noncancer death.

Psychosocial Issues of Childhood Cancer Survivors

There is a large body of scientific literature addressing the subject of psychosocial outcomes for childhood cancer survivors. Findings are varied in part as a result of differing definitions for psychosocial outcomes among the studies. For example, in some studies the outcomes are defined in terms of psychologic health (e.g., depression, anxiety, posttraumatic stress, posttraumatic growth, and somatization). In other studies, the outcomes are defined in terms of social health (e.g., employment, education, and marriage). In addition, many pediatric cancer survivorship studies focusing on psychosocial outcomes are limited because of small sample size and/or lack of a comparison group. Many of the studies are from the health-related quality of life (HRQOL) literature because assessment of psychosocial outcomes is often included as part of a global HRQOL assessment. Notwithstanding these differences in definitions of study outcomes and study designs, the scientific literature concerning psychosocial outcomes in childhood cancer survivors is summarized in the following sections.

Psychologic Health

An emerging body of literature indicates that childhood cancer survivors are experiencing good psychologic health years after completion of their cancer treatment. One of the earliest studies, done by Teta et al.,[86] assessed the prevalence of major depression in 450 long-term childhood cancer survivors and found no difference in depression between survivors, their siblings, and general population norms. Elkin et al.,[87] using a standardized self-report measure (the Symptom Checklist-90-Revised or SCL-90-R), assessed psychologic functioning in adolescent and young adult survivors who attended a long-term follow-up clinic for pediatric cancer survivors at a single institution. Results of this study indicated that the study population was significantly psychologically healthier than age- and gender-matched norms for the general population based on SCL-90 scores. For the small percentage of survivors who displayed some psychologic symptoms, three factors were associated with an increased risk of maladjustment: older patient age at follow-up, greater number of relapses, and presence of severe functional impairment (defined as requiring frequent assistance with activities of daily living). The findings from these earlier studies were confirmed in a recently reported study by Zebrack et al.[88] on psychological outcomes in survivors of childhood leukemia and lymphoma, using data from the Childhood Cancer Survivor Study (CCSS).

Systematic literature reviews of the smaller studies published on this topic have also reported psychological wellbeing following treatment for childhood cancer; however, there are subgroups of survivors who may be at risk for poorer psychosocial health outcomes.[89–94] The largest and most recent of these studies to date was reported by Hudson et al.,[95] who analyzed data from the 9,535 adult survivors in the CCSS cohort compared with a randomly selected cohort of the survivors' siblings ($n = 2{,}916$). When compared with siblings, survivors in this study were significantly more likely to report adverse general health and moderate to severe impairment in mental health across all diagnostic groups. However, although general health was reported to be very good, with only 10.9 percent reporting fair or poor health, specific adverse effects were relatively common, as reflected by 43.6% of the cohort reporting impairment in one or more of the health domains evaluated in the study. Specifically, three diagnostic groups (survivors of Hodgkin's disease, sarcomas, or bone tumors) were found to be at increased risk for continued cancer-related anxiety.[95] Furthermore, the authors emphasize that these three diagnoses are more common in the adolescent age group. Because adolescence is the developmental period during which abstract thinking develops, adolescents diagnosed with cancer may have a better understanding of the meaning of their diagnosis and the risks of treatment. The findings of this study confirmed the results of earlier studies[96–98] (Table 102.2). Thus, these studies suggest that there are certain at-risk groups of survivors who may be experiencing negative psychosocial sequelae and therefore may benefit from targeted psychosocial support interventions during long-term follow-up care.

The childhood cancer survivorship literature also suggests that use of a posttraumatic stress model is helpful in elucidating the long-term psychosocial sequelae for certain subsets of childhood cancer survivors[99–102] (Table 102.3). Family members, friends, and caregivers are also affected by the survivorship experience and are therefore included in the definition of survivorship.[2] It is, therefore, not surprising that there are reports of family members being affected by posttraumatic stress disorder (PTSD). Kazak et al.[94] did not find an increased prevalence of PTSD in a cohort of 133 childhood leukemia survivors when compared with a control group, but did find more PTSD symptoms in their mothers and fathers. Barakat et al.[93] found that past perceived life threat and family social support resources contributed to PTSD symptoms in both parents and survivors. All these studies suggest that the childhood cancer experience is complex and extends beyond the survivor, even years after the completion of therapy.

Social Health

Review of the childhood cancer survivorship literature indicates that overall this population is doing well in terms of social and emotional adjustment. Differences in educational needs, behavioral adjustment, employment status, and marriage rate for certain populations of childhood cancer survivors do occur. A recent longitudinal study of the social functioning of childhood cancer survivors 2 years following completion of therapy was conducted by Reiter-Purtill et al.[103] Children who completed cancer treatment were compared

TABLE 102.2. Summary of additional studies demonstrating adverse psychologic outcomes in childhood cancer survivors.

Study	*Sample size*	*Primary disease*	*Comparison group*	*Adverse outcomes*	*Risk factors*
Zeltzer et al.[96]	500	ALL, treated on CCG protocols	Siblings	Depression, tension, anger, and confusion	Females, minorities, unemployed
Mulhern et al.[97]	183	Any pediatric malignancy	Normative data from the general population	Deficits in social competence and behavioral abnormalities	Presence of functional impairments, older age at evaluation, treatment with cranial irradiation, residence in a single-parent household
Glover et al.[98]	555	Leukemia	Siblings	Mood disturbance	Females, nonwhite males, females with a special education history, high school dropouts with a special education history, age younger than 12.5 years of age at diagnosis, survivors with negative perceptions of current health

ALL, acute lymphoblastic leukemia; CCG, Children's Cancer Group.

TABLE 102.3. Studies supporting the posttraumatic stress model in childhood cancer survivors.

Study	*Sample size*	*Age range*	*Percent with posttraumatic stress symptoms or disorder*	*Risk factors*
Stuber et al.[99]	64	7–19 years	13%	Symptoms of increased anxiety and reexperiencing traumatic incidents, which persisted many years after the end of treatment without evidence of decrement over time
Hobbie et al.[101]	78	18–40 years	20.5%	Anxiety and other psychologic distress
Meeske et al.[102]	51	18–37 years	20%	Poorer QOL (as measured by the SF-36), increased psychologic distress

QOL, quality of life; SF-36, Short Form-36.

with children who were not chronically ill. The children's self-reports, as well as peer and teacher assessments of social functioning, were obtained while children were on therapy and then 2 years following completion of therapy. Findings of this study indicated minimal impact on the social functioning of the majority of childhood cancer survivors, but certain subpopulations were found to be vulnerable. Specifically, children who underwent high-intensity treatment were perceived by their peers as more "prosocial and less aggressive," although they had fewer nominations as "best friends." The authors hypothesized that this group of survivors may be less assertive about making and/or maintaining friendships or that their less-aggressive behavior may be due to fatigue. A study by Spirito et al.[104] reported similar findings when they compared 56 children (aged 5–12 years) to healthy controls using questionnaires assessing social adjustment, including the Self-Perception Profile. In this study, the only reported difference was of greater feelings of isolation in the childhood cancer survivors compared with the controls.

Conversely, reports of lower social competence were demonstrated by Mulhern et al.[105] In a cohort of survivors ($n = 183$) 2 or more years off-therapy, social competence and behavioral adjustment were assessed using a standardized questionnaire (The Child Behavior Checklist). Functional (but not cosmetic) impairments were found to increase the risk for academic and adjustment problems. Other risk factors for social and emotional problems included: older age at assessment (correlated with time since diagnosis and time since completion of therapy), treatment with cranial irradiation, and living in a single-parent household. Similarly, a study by Pendley et al.[106] found that adolescent survivors who had been off treatment for longer periods of time reported more social anxiety as well as more-negative body image and lower self-worth.

Educational attainment as an outcome of social health has also been assessed in the leukemia survivor study[107] and in the CCSS[108,109] (Table 102.4). The findings from these studies indicate that survivors are more likely to use special educational services, but overall are just as likely to graduate from high school when compared with their siblings.

Multiple studies have assessed the vocational status of childhood cancer survivors. One of the earliest studies assessing occupational status was completed by Meadows et al.[110] The cohort of survivors demonstrated no differences in educational achievement or occupational status by diagnostic group, age at diagnosis, or treatment received. Nicholson et al.[111] compared osteosarcoma and Ewing sarcoma survivors with sibling controls and found that employment status and annual income were similar in the two groups despite the physical impairments following limb amputation for many of the sarcoma survivors. Hays et al.[112] reported similar employment findings in more than 200 childhood cancer survivors. Specifically, the employment status of the survivors was similar to individually matched controls. There were, however, findings of employment discrimination for entry into the military for survivors during the initial years following completion of therapy. The authors concluded that childhood cancer survivors who were treated in the era between 1945 and 1975 had few economic sequelae that extended beyond the first decades after treatment.

TABLE 102.4. Childhood Cancer Survivor Study (CCSS) studies assessing educational attainment as an outcome measure for social health.

Study	*Sample size*	*Primary disease*	*Comparison group*	*Educational outcome assessed*	*Findings*	*Risk factors*
Mitby et al.[108]	12,000	Any pediatric malignancy	3,000 siblings	Use of special education services	23% of survivors compared with 8% of siblings used special education services	Diagnosis <6 years of age; brain tumor, leukemia, and HD survivors; treatment variables of use of IT MTX and CXRT (with a positive dose–response relationship found)
Nagarajan et al.[109]	694	Osteosarcoma or Ewing's sarcoma	Age at diagnosis (≤12 years compared with >12 years), type of surgery (amputation vs. limb-sparing), and 2,667 siblings	Graduation from high school or college	No differences found between the different age or surgery groups.	More than 12 years/amputation group was less likely to graduate from high school and college compared with siblings, but there were still high rates of reports of graduation from high school in the survivors group (93%) and for those survivors older than 25 years of age, and 50% reported being a college graduate

HD, Hodgkin disease; IT MTX, intrathecal methotrexate; CXRT, cranial irradiation.

The literature regarding employment outcome for childhood cancer survivors yields mixed conclusions. For example, a study by Novakovic et al.[113] found that although nearly 90 survivors of Ewing's sarcoma did not differ in educational achievement, they were less likely to be employed full time when compared with sibling controls. Conversely, Evans and Radford[114] assessed educational achievement and employment in a small group of survivors and found that survivors were significantly less likely to complete higher education than their siblings, but had similar rates of employment and were earning similar salaries. The differences in the findings may represent the small sample sizes in the various studies.

Marital status has also been assessed as a measure of social well-being for survivors of childhood cancer. In one of the earlier studies, Makipernaa[115] interviewed 94 survivors of solid tumors diagnosed between 1960 and 1976. When the survivor population was compared with the general Finnish population, fewer female survivors were married. Green et al.[116] found that the percentages of married male and female survivors were both significantly lower than the U.S. population norms. Byrne et al.[117] studied a much larger population of childhood cancer survivors and found that both male and female survivors were less likely to be married when compared with a sibling control group. The study also demonstrated that survivors of central nervous system (CNS) malignancies accounted for the majority of unmarried survivors, with the males in this diagnostic group having the greatest relative risk. The findings of these two earlier studies were also confirmed more recently in a large CCSS cohort. Rauck et al.[118] described the marital status of more than 10,000 childhood cancer survivors within the CCSS cohort and compared them to the U.S. population according to age-specific groups. Compared with the U.S. population, childhood cancer survivors, particularly females and Caucasians, were less likely to have ever been married. CNS tumor survivors as a subgroup, and particularly males within this group, were less likely to have ever been married and were more likely to divorce or separate when compared with childhood cancer survivors who had other diagnoses, as well as with the general U.S. population. Felder-Puig et al.[119] also found a lower incidence of marriage in survivors of bone cancer. Interestingly, survivors in this study reported staying home longer after reaching adulthood than did the control group of a similar age. The investigators postulated that the survivors would, therefore, postpone marriage for a longer time than their peers. A study by Gray et al.[120] yields further insight regarding interpersonal relationships in survivors of childhood cancer. In this study, survivors reported higher intimacy motivation, but were more likely to express dissatisfaction with important relationships, when compared with a peer group. Nonetheless, despite differences in marriage rates, studies support the fact that, overall, survivors of pediatric malignancies are doing well in terms of psychosocial functioning and that only certain subgroups are at greatest risk for adverse psychosocial sequelae.

Special Populations

Two special populations of survivors (childhood acute lymphoblastic leukemia and brain tumors) warrant special attention due to their increased risk for adverse psychosocial outcomes as a result of previous CNS treatment: Acute lymphoblastic leukemia (ALL) is the most commonly diagnosed pediatric malignancy, with an annual incidence of 3,250 children and adolescents diagnosed each year in the United States and a survival rate of approximately 85%.[1] Brain tumors are the second most commonly diagnosed pediatric malignancy, and the most common solid neoplasm. Approximately 2,200 children and adolescents under 20 years of age are diagnosed within the United States each year. The overall survival rate is approximately 68%.[1] Thus, there are rapidly growing numbers of survivors treated for both of the most commonly diagnosed pediatric malignancies.

Acute Lymphoblastic Leukemia Survivors

Improvement in the survival rates for ALL in the 1980s and 1990s has resulted in the emergence of studies focused on the neuropsychologic consequences in this population. Brown et al.[121] followed a small cohort of ALL survivors who received prophylactic chemotherapy to the CNS. Survivors, when compared with their siblings, showed impairment in right hemispheric simultaneous processing when evaluated at the off-therapy time point. These differences were not found while the patient was actively undergoing treatment for ALL, a finding that illustrates the importance of continued long-term neuropsychologic evaluation for this group of survivors, as deficits may not be evident on initial assessments. Cetingul et al.[122] studied a small sample of 5-year Turkish survivors of childhood ALL and compared them to their siblings. In this study, total IQ scores of survivors were significantly lower than the sibling control group, although small numbers limit the conclusions drawn from this study. Kingma et al.[123] also studied academic performance in a small sample of Dutch ALL survivors who were treated with cranial irradiation (18 or 25 Gy) and intrathecal methotrexate as CNS prophylaxis, and compared them to siblings. Survivors were more likely to be placed in special education programs than were siblings, although there was no effect of sex or irradiation dose. The investigators concluded that cranial irradiation and chemotherapy administered at a young age were associated with poorer academic career outcomes for survivors. Haupt et al.[107] completed a large multicenter retrospective trial of adult survivors of childhood ALL with sibling controls, assessing practical, easily understandable educational outcomes that included "enrollment in special programs, grades during high school, graduation from high school, college admission, and college graduation."[107] Similar to the findings of smaller studies, ALL survivors in this study were more likely to enter special education or learning-disabled programs when compared with siblings. Higher doses of cranial irradiation (24 Gy versus 18 Gy versus none) and young age (less than 6 years of age) at diagnosis were found to be the most important predictors for poor educational outcomes, defined as a lesser likelihood of entering college.

It should also be noted that craniospinal irradiation, used in early treatment regimens for ALL to prevent CNS leukemia, resulted in neurodevelopmental delays in children. In the early 1980s, Robison et al.[124] and Moss et al.[125] demonstrated that prophylactic treatment of the CNS with craniospinal irradiation was associated with decreased IQ scores. These early studies documenting the risk of neurocognitive late effects, coupled with the high cure rates, have led to the elimination of prophylactic craniospinal irradiation from most current ALL treatment regimens. Therefore, the importance of assessing long-term psychosocial outcomes of childhood cancer treatment cannot be overemphasized, because there may be direct and practical applications for intervention and long-term follow-up care.

Brain Tumor Survivors

The second special population of childhood cancer survivors who warrant further discussion regarding psychosocial outcomes are those treated for pediatric brain tumors. Roman and Sperduto[126] reviewed the literature on the neuropsychologic effects of cranial radiation. Research on low-dose whole-brain radiation (such as that used for childhood ALL patients) was compared with studies on high-dose focal or whole-brain radiation used in the treatment of brain lesions. In this review, the investigators found that the low-dose whole-brain radiation (18–24 Gy) resulted in the mild decline of IQ and that subsequent learning disabilities may be the result of poor attention and memory instead of low intellectual level. Conversely, pediatric survivors who received higher-dose radiation for the treatment of brain tumors, particularly those who received whole-brain radiation, were found to be at risk for poorer cognitive outcomes. In a subsequent study by Anderson et al.,[127] higher-dose radiation used for treatment of brain tumors (when compared with that used for other malignancies) was more often found to be associated with late cognitive effects. Further research has shown that neurocognitive deficits occurring among brain tumor survivors most commonly involve the areas of memory, attention, and academic achievement.[126,128] Whether cognitive deficits in these brain tumor survivors are primarily caused by disruption of "executive function" (ability to organize and prioritize activities to be functionally effective) is suspected but not yet proven. Data forthcoming from the CCSS will help to answer this question.

A study by Glaser et al.[129] evaluated school behavior in a small sample of brain tumor survivors compared with a control group of school-age siblings. The brain tumor survivors had good social reintegration but also had evidence of impaired cognition, emotion, and lower self-esteem. Even though they worried more than the control group, the brain tumor survivors attended school willingly and interacted with their peers normally. Zebrack et al.[88] assessed psychologic outcomes in more than 1,000 adult long-term survivors of childhood brain tumors within the CCSS cohort and compared them with almost 3,000 sibling controls and normative data from the general population. The majority of survivors and siblings reported few symptoms of psychologic distress 5 or more years after the original cancer diagnosis. The prevalence of psychologic distress was similar to that found in the general population. Yet, when accounting for significant sociodemographic, socioeconomic, and health status variables, survivors of childhood brain cancer, in aggregate, appear to report significantly higher global distress and depression scores than do siblings. Factors associated with higher levels of psychologic distress for both survivors and siblings included female sex, low household income, lower educational attainment, being unmarried, having no employment in the past 12 months, and poor physical health status. There were no diagnostic- or treatment-related variables that were associated with an increase in distress symptoms for this group of childhood brain tumor survivors.

Providing Follow-Up Care for Childhood Cancer Survivors

Essential Elements of Follow-Up Care

General agreement exists that survivors of childhood cancer require ongoing lifelong follow-up to provide early intervention for, or prevention of, potential late effects of treatment.[130–134] The Children's Oncology Group (COG) has developed systematic evidence-based, exposure-related guidelines for ongoing follow-up of pediatric cancer survivors. These guidelines allow the clinician to determine a specific follow-up plan for each survivor, tailored to risk of late effects based on therapeutic exposures. A comprehensive treatment summary (Table 102.5) is also an essential tool for providing

TABLE 102.5. Components of a comprehensive treatment summary.

Essential elements	*Details*
Demographics	Treating institution, treatment team
Diagnosis	Date, site(s), stage
Relapse(s)	Date(s)
Subsequent malignant neoplasms	Date(s), types
Protocol(s)	Title(s)/number(s), dates initiated and completed
Completion of therapy	Date
Chemotherapy	Names and administration routes for all agents Cumulative doses (per m^2) for alkylators, anthracyclines, and bleomycin Determination of intermediate/high (≥1,000 mg/m^2) dose vs. standard dose for cytarabine and methotrexate
Radiation	Dates, type, fields, total dose, number of fractions/dose per fraction
Surgical procedures	Type(s), date(s)
Hematopoietic cell transplant	Type(s), date(s), GVHD prophylaxis/treatment
Major medical events	Events with potential for residual/late effects
Adverse drug reactions/allergies	Name of drug, type of reaction

GVHD, graft-versus-host disease.

comprehensive survivorship care. The Children's Oncology Group Long-Term Follow-Up Guidelines, accompanying health education materials (known as "Health Links"), and a model comprehensive treatment summary form are available to clinicians free of charge on the Children's Oncology Group website at www.survivorshipguidelines.org.

Models of Clinical Care Delivery

In 1997, the American Academy of Pediatrics mandated that children with cancer should be treated in specialized centers for pediatric oncology care[135]; between 1989 and 1991, 94% of children diagnosed with cancer under the age of 15 in the United States were seen at an institution that was affiliated with the cooperative pediatric oncology clinical trials groups.[136] Specialized pediatric oncology centers that are members of the Children's Oncology Group are required to provide long-term follow-up services for survivors of pediatric cancer[137]; this can be accomplished in a variety of ways.[11,134,138–142]

Specialized Long-Term Follow-Up Clinics

In some pediatric oncology centers, the original treatment team, or a designated multidisciplinary long-term follow-up team at the treatment center, continue to provide life long follow-up to the childhood cancer survivor. Generally, the ongoing follow-up is limited to an annual comprehensive multidisciplinary health evaluation, and the survivor is encouraged to establish an ongoing relationship with a primary healthcare provider in their local community for routine healthcare needs. The long term follow-up care is often directed by a nurse practitioner specializing in healthcare for childhood cancer survivors. Benefits of this approach are that the patient remains in contact with a team that is knowledgeable and committed to long-term follow-up care, contact with the original treatment center is maintained, opportunities for research are optimized, and multidisciplinary referrals are usually available within the healthcare system (although referrals for patients who are beyond the pediatric age range may be limited in pediatric centers). Disadvantages of this approach include the unfamiliarity of the pediatric treatment team with the healthcare issues that arise as the survivor ages, reluctance of the older patient to return to a pediatric facility (especially if pediatric patients are present in the clinic/waiting room at the time of the long-term follow-up clinic), problems with reimbursement for specialized services not covered by insurance companies, and, often, problems of access due to long distances between the medical center and the survivor's residence. An example of successful implementation of this model is the Survivorship Clinic at the City of Hope National Medical Center in Duarte, California. As an NIH-designated Comprehensive Cancer Center, City of Hope provides specialized cancer-related care to patients throughout the lifespan, allowing ongoing long-term follow-up of patients with pediatric malignancies as they enter and progress through adulthood.

Transition Models

Pediatric oncology centers, often as a result of institutional policies with an upper age limit for care, may require transition of young adult survivors to adult care providers. In some instances, institutions have established formalized transition programs with specialized long-term follow-up programs for adult survivors of childhood cancer [e.g., Children's Medical Center of Dallas transitions its survivors to the ACE (After the Cancer Experience) Program for Young Adult Survivors at the University of Texas Southwestern, and Children's Memorial Hospital in Chicago transitions its survivors to the STAR (Survivors Taking Action and Responsibility) Program for Young Adult Survivors at Northwestern University]. Transition programs often use collaborative practice models, drawing on expertise from both oncology and primary care providers, and maintain many of the benefits of the specialized long-term follow-up clinics, with the added benefit of care providers with expertise in adult medicine. Affiliation of these programs with academic institutions usually provides access to multidisciplinary referrals; however, because the setting is academic and the focus is on survivorship care, ongoing primary care is often not accessible through these specialized programs, and distance to the center may remain problematic for some survivors.

Adult Oncology Directed Care

In this model, when the survivor reaches adulthood, the pediatric provider makes a referral to an adult oncologist for ongoing follow-up. Advantages of this system include ongoing monitoring for disease recurrence in a system designed for adult medical care, and accessibility to care in the local community. Disadvantages include the unfamiliarity of most adult oncologists with the long-term follow-up evaluations indicated for childhood cancer survivors, and the likelihood of early discharge from specialty care once there is minimal risk of disease recurrence. However, with appropriate education and collaboration, this model has been used successfully to provide ongoing long-term follow-up care for childhood cancer survivors. An example of this model is the cooperative agreement between the Children's Hospital of Philadelphia and the oncology service of the University of Pennsylvania Medical Center.

Community-Based Care

In this model, follow-up care is provided by an adult primary care provider (e.g., internist, family practitioner), who ideally is in ongoing communication with the original pediatric oncology treatment team or long-term follow-up center. Advantages of this system include seamless care for the patient, who can see their local primary care provider for most healthcare services and develop an ongoing relationship with a provider who is familiar with their specialized healthcare needs. Disadvantages include the primary care provider's lack of familiarity with the potential late effects for which the survivor is at risk, the considerable effort required for the primary care provider to determine appropriate follow-up care for the survivor, the survivor's potential lack of access to multidisciplinary specialty care providers, and the potential loss of contact with the survivor. The community-based system of care has been used successfully by St. Jude Children's Research Hospital (Memphis, TN) to provide care for survivors who are more than 10 years posttreatment. In this setting, potential disadvantages of this system have been addressed by providing a dedicated staff at St. Jude to track the status of these survivors and to provide ongoing consultation with community healthcare providers as required.

Acknowledgment. Supported in part by 5 U10 CA13539-26S2.

References

1. Reis LAG, Eisner MP, Kosary CL, et al. SEER Cancer Statistics Review, 1973–1998. Bethesda, MD: National Cancer Institute, MD, 2001.
2. Hewitt M, Weiner SL, Simone JV. Childhood Cancer Survivorship: Improving Care and Quality of Life. Washington, DC: National Academies Press, 2003.
3. Sklar CA. An overview of the effects of cancer therapies: the nature, scale, and breadth of the problem. Acta Paediatr Scand Suppl 1999;433:1–4.
4. Garré ML, Gandus S, Cesana B, et al. Health status of long-term survivors after cancer in childhood. Am J Pediatr Hematol Oncol 1994;16:143–152.
5. Oeffinger KC, Eshelman DA, Tomlinson GE, et al. Grading of late effects in young adult survivors of childhood cancer followed in an ambulatory adult setting. Cancer (Phila) 2000;88:1687–1695.
6. Stevens MCG, Mahler H, Parkes S. The health status of adult survivors of cancer in childhood. Eur J Cancer 1998;34:694–698.
7. Vonderweid N, Beck D, Caflisch U, et al. Standardized assessment of late effects in long-term survivors of childhood cancer in Switzerland: results of a Swiss Pediatric Oncology Group (SPOG) pilot study. Int J Pediatr Hematol/Oncol 1996;3:483–490.
8. Brown RT, Sawyer MB, Antoniou G, et al. A 3-year follow-up of the intellectual and academic functioning of children receiving central nervous system prophylactic chemotherapy for leukemia. J Dev Behav Pediatr 196;17(6):392–398.
9. Kramer J, Moore IM. Late effects of cancer therapy on the central nervous system. Semin Oncol Nurs 1989;5:22–28.
10. Moore IM, Packer RJ, Karl D, et al. Adverse effects of cancer treatment on the central nervous system. In: Schwartz CL HW, Constine LS, Ruccione KS (eds). Survivors of Childhood Cancer: Assessment and Management. St. Louis: Mosby, 1994:81–95.
11. Fochtman D. Follow-up care for survivors of childhood cancer. Nurse Pract Forum 1996;6:194–200.
12. Packer RJ, Sutton LN, Atkins TE, et al. A prospective study of cognitive function in children receiving whole-brain radiotherapy and chemotherapy: 2-year results. J Neurosurg 1989;70:707–713.
13. Mulhern RK, Reddick WE, Palmer SL, et al. Neurocognitive deficits in medulloblastoma survivors and white matter loss. Ann Neurol 1999;46:834–841.
14. Shan K, Lincoff AM, Young JB. Anthracycline-induced cardiotoxicity. Ann Intern Med 1966;125:47–58.
15. Grenier MA, Lipshultz SE. Epidemiology of anthracycline cardiotoxicity in children and adults. Semin Oncol 1998;25:72–85.
16. Pai VB, Nahata MC. Cardiotoxicity of chemotherapeutic agents: incidence, treatment and prevention. Drug Saf 2000;22:263–302.
17. Prout MN, Richards MJS, Chung KJ, et al. Adriamycin cardiotoxicity in children. Cancer (Phila) 1977;39:62.
18. Minow RA, Benjamin RS, Gottlieb JA. Adriamycin (NSC-123127) cardiotoxicity: a clinicopathologic correlation. Cancer Chemother Rep 1975;6:195.
19. Bossi G, Lanzarini L, Laudisa ML, et al. Echocardiographic evaluation of patients cured of childhood cancer: a single center study of 117 subjects who received anthracyclines. Med Pediatr Oncol 2001;36:593–600.
20. Kremer LCM, van Dalen EC, Offringa M, et al. Anthracycline-induced clinical heart failure in a cohort of 607 children: long-term follow-up study. J Clin Oncol 2001;19:191–196.
21. Fajardo L, Stewart J, Cohn K. Morphology of radiation-induced heart disease. Arch Pathol 1968;86:512–519.
22. Kushner JR, Hansen VL, Hammar SP. Cardiomyopathy after widely separated courses of Adriamycin exacerbated by actinomycin D and mithramycin. Cancer (Phila) 1975;36:1577.
23. Smith PJ, Eckert H, Waters KD, et al. High incidence of cardiomyopathy in children treated with Adriamycin and DTIC in combination chemotherapy. Cancer Treat Rep 1977;61:1736.
24. Von Hoff D, Rozencweig M, Piccart M. The cardiotoxicity of anticancer agents. Semin Oncol 1982;9:23.
25. Lipshultz SE, Lipshultz SR, Mone SM, et al. Female sex and higher drug dose as risk factors for late cardiotoxic effects of doxorubicin therapy for childhood cancer. N Engl J Med 1995;332:1738–1743.
26. Pratt CB, Ransom JL, Evans WE. Age-related Adriamycin cardiotoxicity in children. Cancer Treat Rep 1978;62:1381.
27. Von Hoff DD, Rozencweig M, Layard M, et al. Daunomycin induced cardiotoxicity in children and adults. Am J Med 1977;62:200.
28. Martin RG, Rukdeschel JC, Chang P, et al. Radiation-related pericarditis. Am J Cardiol 1975;35:216.
29. Marks RDJ, Agarwal SK, Constable WC. Radiation induced pericarditis in Hodgkin's disease. Acta Radiol Ther Phys Biol 1973;12:305.
30. Mill WB, Baglan RJ, Kurichetz P, et al. Symptomatic radiation induced pericarditis in Hodgkin's disease. Int J Radiat Oncol Biol Phys 1984;10:2061.
31. Kadota RP, Burgert EO, Driscoll DJ, et al. Cardiopulmonary function in long-term survivors of childhood Hodgkin's lymphoma: a pilot study. Mayo Clin Proc 1988;63:362.
32. Perraut DJ, Levy M, Herman JD, et al. Echocardiac abnormalities following cardiac radiation. J Clin Oncol 1985;3:546.
33. Scott DL, Thomas RD. Late onset constrictive pericarditis after thoracic radiotherapy. Br Med J 1978;1:341.
34. Haas JM. Symptomatic constrictive pericarditis developing 45 years after radiation therapy to the mediastinum: a review of radiation pericarditis. Am Heart J 1969;77:89.
35. Boivin JF, Hutchinson GB, Lubin JH, et al. Coronary artery disease in patients treated for Hodgkin's disease. Cancer (Phila) 1992;69:1241–1247.
36. Bu'Lock FA, Gabriel HM, Oakhill A, et al. Cardioprotection by ICRF187 against high dose anthracycline toxicity in children with malignant disease. Br Heart J 1993;70:185–188.
37. Wexler L. Ameliorating anthracycline cardiotoxicity in children with cancer: clinical trials with dexrazoxane. Semin Oncol 1998;25:86–92.
38. Iarussi D, Indolfi P, Coppolino P, et al. Recent advances in the prevention of anthracycline cardiotoxocity in childhood. Curr Med Chem 2001;8:1667–1678.
39. Littman P, Meadows AT, Polgar G, et al. Pulmonary function in survivors of Wilm's tumor: patterns of impairment. Cancer (Phila) 1976;37:2773.
40. Benoit MR, Lemerle J, Jean R, et al. Effects on pulmonary function of whole lung irradiation for Wilms' tumor in children. Thorax 1982;37:175.
41. Miller RW, Fusner JE, Fink RJ, et al. Pulmonary function abnormalities in long-term survivors of childhood cancer. Med Pediatr Oncol 1986;14:202.
42. Springmeyer SC, Flourney N, Sullivan KM, et al. Pulmonary function changes in long-term survivors of allogeneic marrow transplantation. In: Gale RP (ed). Recent Advances in Bone Marrow Transplantation. New York: Liss, 1983:343.
43. Robison LL, Mertens AC, Boice JD Jr, et al. Study design and cohort characteristics of the Childhood Cancer Survivor Study:

a multi-institutional collaborative project. Med Pediatr Oncol 2002;38(4):229–339.
44. Mertens AC, Yasui Y, Liu Y, et al. Pulmonary complications in survivors of childhood and adolescent cancer. A report from the Childhood Cancer Survivor Study. Cancer (Phila) 2002;95: 2431–2441.
45. Gisberg SJ, Comis RL. The pulmonary toxicity of antineoplastic agents. Semin Oncol 1982;9:34.
46. Bauer KA, Sskarin AT, Balikian JP, et al. Pulmonary complications associated with combination chemotherapy programs containing bleomycin. Am J Med 1983;74:557.
47. Goldiner PL, Schweizer O. Hazards of anesthesia and surgery in bleomycin-treated patients. Semin Oncol 1979;6:121.
48. Samuels ML, Johnson DE, Holoye PY, et al. Large doses of bleomycin therapy and pulmonary toxicity: a possible role of prior radiotherapy. JAMA 1976;235:1117.
49. Aronin PA, Mahaley MSJ, Rudnick SA, et al. Prediction of BCNU pulmonary toxicity in patients with malignant gliomas: an assessment of risk factors. N Engl J Med 1980;303:183.
50. Hancock S, Cox R, McDougall I. Thyroid diseases after treatment of Hodgkin's disease. N Engl J Med 1991;325:599.
51. Glatstein E, McHardy-Young S, Brast N, et al. Alterations in serum thyrotropin (TSH) and thyroid function following radiotherapy in patients with malignant lymphoma. J Clin Endocrinol Metab 1971;32:833.
52. Rosenthal MB, Goldfine ID. Primary and secondary hypothyroidism in nasophanryngeal carcinoma. JAMA 1976;236:1591.
53. Gurney JG, Kadan-Lottick NS, Packer RJ, et al. Endocrine and cardiovascular late effects among adult survivors of childhood brain tumors: Childhood Cancer Survivor Study. Cancer (Phila) 2003;97:663–673.
54. Sklar C, Whitton J, Mertens A, et al. Abnormalities of the thyroid in survivors of Hodgkin's disease: data from the Childhood Cancer Survivor Study. J Clin Endocrinol Metab 2000;85: 3227–3232.
55. Chin D, Sklar C, Donahue B, et al. Thyroid dysfunction as a late effect in survivors of pediatric medulloblastoma/primitive neuroectodermal tumors: a comparison of hyperfractionated versus conventional radiotherapy. Cancer (Phila) 1997;80:798–804.
56. Sklar CA. Growth and neuroendocrine dysfunction following therapy for childhood cancer. Pediatr Clin N Am 1997;44: 489–503.
57. Danoff BF, Cowchock FS, Marquette C, et al. Assessment of the long-term effects of primary radiation therapy for brain tumors in children. Cancer (Phila) 1982;49:1580.
58. Onoyama Y, Mitsuyuki A, Takahashi M, et al. Radiation therapy of brain tumors in children. Radiology 1977;115:687.
59. Oberfield SE, Allen JC, Pollack J, et al. Long-term endocrine sequelae after treatment of medulloblastoma: prospective study of growth and thyroid function. J Pediatr 1986;108:219.
60. Oliff A, Bode U, Bercu BB, et al. Hypothalamic-pituitary dysfunction following CNS prophylaxis in acute lymphocytic leukemia: correlation with CT scan abnormalities. Med Pediatr Oncol 1979;7:141.
61. Robison LL, Nesbit ME, Sather HN, et al. Height of children successfully treated for acute lymphoblastic leukemia: a report from the late effects study committee of Children's Cancer Study Group. Med Pediatr Oncol 1985;13:14.
62. Berry DH, Elders MJ, Crist W, et al. Growth in children with acute lymphocytic leukemia: a Pediatric Oncology Group study. Med Pediatr Oncol 1983;11:39.
63. Papadakis V, Tan C, Heller G, et al. Growth and final height after treatment for childhood Hodgkin's disease. J Pediatr Hematol Oncol 1996;18:272–276.
64. Sklar C, Mertens A, Walter A, et al. Final height after treatment for childhood acute lymphoblastic leukemia: comparison of no cranial irradiation with 1800 and 2400 centigrays of cranial irradiation. J Pediatr 1993;123:59–64.
65. Blatt J, Bercu BB, Gillin JC, et al. Reduced pulsatile growth hormone secretion in children after therapy for acute lymphocytic leukemia. J Pediatr 1984;104:182.
66. Sklar CA, Mertens AC, Walter A, et al. Changes in body mass index and prevalence of overweight in survivors of childhood acute lymphoblastic leukemia: role of cranial irradiation. Med Pediatr Oncol 2000;35:91–95.
67. Oeffinger KC, Mertens AC, Sklar CA, et al. Obesity in adult survivors of childhood acute lymphoblastic leukemia: a report from the Childhood Cancer Survivor Study. J Clin Oncol 2003;21:1359–1365.
68. Cifton DK, Bremmer WJ. The effect of testicular x-irradiation on spermatogenesis in man. J Androl 1983;4:387.
69. Rowley MM, Leach DR, Warner GA, et al. Effect of graded doses of ionizing radiation on the human testes. Radiat Res 1974; 59:665.
70. Blatt J, Sherins RJ, Niebrugge D, et al. Leydig cell function in boys following treatment for testicular relapse of acute lymphoblastic leukemia. J Clin Oncol 1985;3:1227.
71. Sherins RJ, DeVita VT. Effects of drug treatment for lymphoma on male reproductive capacity. Ann Intern Med 1973;79:216.
72. da Cunha MF, Meisrich ML, Fuller LM, et al. Recovery of spermatogenesis after treatment for Hodgkin's disease with limiting dose of MOPP chemotherapy. J Clin Oncol 1984;2:571.
73. Santaro A, Bonadonna G, Valagussa P, et al. Long-term results of combined chemotherapy-radiotherapy approach in Hodgkin's disease: superiority of ABVD plus radiotherapy versus MOPP plus radiotherapy. J Clin Oncol 1987;5:27.
74. Stillman RJ, Schilfeld JS, Schiff I, et al. Ovarian failure in long-term survivors of childhood malignancy. Am J Obstet Gynecol 1981;139:62.
75. Sarafoglou K, Boulad F, Gillio A, et al. Gonadal function after bone marrow transplantation for acute leukemia during childhood. J Pediatr 1997;130:210–216.
76. Sklar C. Reproductive physiology and treatment-related loss of sex hormone production. Med Pediatr Oncol 1999;33:2–8.
77. Green D, Whitton J, S M, et al. Pregnancy outcomes of partners of male survivors of childhood cancer: a report from the Childhood Cancer Survivor Study. J Clin Oncol 2003;21:716–721.
78. Green D, Whitton JA, Stovall M, et al. Pregnancy outcome of female survivors of childhood cancer: A report from the childhood cancer survivor study. Am J Obstet Gynecol 2002;187:1070–1080.
79. Neglia JP, Friedman DL, Yutaka Y, et al. Second malignant neoplasms in five-year survivors of childhood cancer: childhood cancer survivor study. J Natl Cancer Inst 2001;93:618–629.
80. Olsen JH, Garwicz S, Hertz H, et al. Second malignant neoplasms after cancer in childhood or adolescence. Nordic Society of Paediatric Haematology and Oncology Association of the Nordic Cancer Registries. BMJ 1993;307:1030–1036.
81. Bhatia S, Yasui Y, Robison LL, et al. High risk of subsequent neoplasms continues with extended follow-up of childhood Hodgkin's disease: report from the Late Effects Study Group. J Clin Oncol 2003;21:4386–4394.
82. Bhatia S, Ramsay NKC, Steinbuch M, et al. Malignant neoplasms following bone marrow transplantation. Blood 1996;87: 3633–3639.
83. Darrington DL, Vose JM, Anderson JR, et al. Incidence and characterization of secondary myelodysplastic syndrome and acute myelogenous leukemia following high-dose chemoradiotherapy and autologous stem cell transplantation for lymphoid malignancies. J Clin Oncol 1994;12:2527–2534.
84. Mertens AC, Yasui Y, Neglia JP, et al. Late mortality experience in five-year survivors of childhood and adolescent cancer: the childhood cancer survivors study. J Clin Oncol 2001;19: 3163–3172.
85. Moller TR, Garwicz S, Barlow L, et al. Decreasing late mortality among five-year survivors of cancer in childhood and ado-

lescence: a population-based study in the Nordic countries. J Clin Oncol 2001;19:3173–3181.
86. Teta MJ, Del Po MC, Kasl SV, et al. Psychosocial consequences of childhood and adolescent cancer survival. J Chronic Dis 1986; 39:751–759.
87. Elkin T, Phipps S, Mulhern R. Psychological functioning of adolescent and young adult survivors of pediatric malignancy. Med Pediatr Oncol 1997;29:582–588.
88. Zebrack BL, Zeltzer LK, Whitton J, et al. Psychological outcomes in long-term survivors of childhood leukemia, Hodgkin's disease, and non-Hodgkin's lymphoma: a report from the Childhood Survivor Study. Pediatrics 2002;110:42–52.
89. Eiser C, Hill J, Vance YH. Examining the psychological consequences of surviving childhood cancer: systematic review as a research method in pediatric psychology. J Pediatr Psychol 2000; 25:449–460.
90. Zeltzer LK. Cancer in adolescents and young adults psychosocial aspects. Long term survivors. Cancer (Phila) 1993;15: 3463–3468.
91. Chang PN. Psychosocial needs of long-term childhood cancer survivors: a review of the literature. Pediatrician 1991;18:20–24.
92. Fritz GK, Williams JR, Amylon MD. After treatment ends: psychosocial sequelae in pediatric cancer survivors. Am J Orthopsychiatry 1988;58:552–561.
93. Barakat LP, Kazak AE, Meadows AT, et al. Families surviving childhood cancer: a comparison of posttraumatic stress symptoms with familes of healthy children. J Pediatr Psychol 1997;22:843–859.
94. Kazak AE, Barakat LP, Meeske K, et al. Post traumatic stress, family functioning and social support in survivors of childhood leukemia and their mothers and fathers. J Consult Clin Psychol 1997;65:120–129.
95. Hudson MM, Mertens AC, Yasui Y, et al. Health status of adult long-term survivors of childhood cancer. A report from the childhood cancer survivor study. JAMA 2003;290:1583–1592.
96. Zeltzer LK, Chen E, Weiss R, et al. Comparison of psychologic outcome in adult survivors of childhood acute lymphoblastic leukemia versus sibling controls: a cooperative Children's Cancer Group and National Institutes of Health study. J Clin Oncol 1997;15:547–556.
97. Mulhern RK, Wasserman AL, Friedman AG, et al. Social competence and behavioral adjustment of children who are long-term survivors of cancer. Pediatrics 1989;83:18–25.
98. Glover DA, Byrne J, Mills JL, et al. Impact of CNS treatment on mood in adult survivors of childhood leukemia: a report from the Children's Cancer Group. J Clin Oncol 2003;21:4395–4401.
99. Stuber ML, Christakis DA, Houskamp B, et al. Posttrauma symptoms in childhood leukemia survivors and their parents. Psychosomatics 1996;37:254–261.
100. Stuber ML, Kazak AE, Meeske K, et al. Predictors of posttraumatic stress symptoms in childhood cancer survivors. Pediatrics 1997;100:958–964.
101. Hobbie WL, Stuber M, Meeske K, et al. Symptoms of posttraumatic stress in young adult survivors of childhood cancer. J Clin Oncol 2000;18:4060–4066.
102. Meeske KA, Ruccione K, Globe DR, et al. Posttraumatic stress, quality of life, and psychological distress in young adult survivors of childhood cancer. Oncol Nurs Forum 2001;28:481–489.
103. Reiter-Purtill J, Vannatta K, Gerhardt CA, et al. A controlled longitudinal study of the social functioning of children who completed treatment of cancer. J Pediatr Hematol/Oncol 2003; 25:467–473.
104. Spirito A, Stark LJ, Cobiella C, et al. Social adjustment of children successfully treated for cancer. J Pediatr Psychol 1990; 15:359–371.
105. Mulhern R, Wasserman A, Friedman A, et al. Social competence and behavioral adjustment of children who are long-term survivors of cancer. Pediatrics 1989;83:18–25.
106. Pendley JS, Dahlquist LM, Dreyer ZA. Body image and psychosocial adjustment in adolescent cancer survivors. J Pediatr Psychol 1997;22:29–43.
107. Haupt R, Fears TR, Robison LL, et al. Educational attainment in long-term survivors of childhood acute lymphoblastic leukemia. JAMA 1994;272:1134–1135.
108. Mitby PA, Robison LL, Whitton JA, et al. Utilization of special education services and educational attainment among long-term survivors of childhood cancer: a report from the Childhood Cancer Survivor Study. Cancer (Phila) 2003;97: 1115–1126.
109. Nagarajan R, Neglia JP, Clohisy DR, et al. Education, employment, insurance, and marital status among 694 survivors of pediatric lower extremity bone tumors: a report from the childhood cancer survivor study. Cancer (Phila) 2003;97: 2554–2564.
110. Meadows AT, McKee L, Kazak AE. Psychosocial status of young adult survivors of childhood cancer: a survey. Med Pediatr Oncol 1989;17:466–470.
111. Nicholson HS, Mulvihill JJ, Byrne J. Late effects of therapy in adult survivors of osteosarcoma and Ewing's sarcoma. Med Pediatr Oncol 1992;20:6–12.
112. Hays DM, Landsverk J, Sallan SE, et al. Educational, occupational, and insurance status of childhood cancer survivors in their fourth and fifth decades of life. J Clin Oncol 1992;10: 1397–1406.
113. Novakovic B, Fears TR, Horowitz ME, et al. Late effects of therapy in survivors of Ewing's sarcoma family of tumors. J Pediatr Hematol Oncol 1997;19:220–225.
114. Evans SE, Radford M. Current lifestyle of young adults treated for cancer in childhood. Arch Dis Child 1995;72:423–426.
115. Makipernaa A. Long-term quality of life and psychosocial coping after treatment of solid tumours in childhood. A population-based study of 94 patients 11–28 years after their diagnosis. Acta Paediatr Scand Suppl 1989;78:728–735.
116. Green DM, Zevon MA, Hall B. Achievement of life goals by adult survivors of modern treatment for childhood cancer. Cancer (Phila) 1991;67:206–213.
117. Byrne J, Fears TR, Steinhorn SC, et al. Marriage and divorce after childhood and adolescent cancer. JAMA 1989;262:2693–2699.
118. Rauck AM, Green DM, Yasui Y, et al. Marriage in the survivors of childhood cancer: a preliminary description from the Childhood Cancer Survivor Study. Med Pediatr Oncol 1999;33:60–63.
119. Felder-Puig R, Formann AK, Mildner A, et al. Quality of life and psychosocial adjustment of young patients after treatment of bone cancer. Cancer (Phila) 1998;83:69–75.
120. Gray RE, Doan BD, Shermer P, et al. Psychologic adaptation of survivors of childhood cancer. Cancer (Phila) 1992;70: 2713–2721.
121. Brown RT, Madan-Swain A, Pais R, et al. Cognitive status of children treated with central nervous system prophylactic chemotherapy for acute lymphocytic leukemia. Arch Clin Neuropsychol 1992;7:481–497.
122. Cetingul N, Aydinok Y, Kantar M, et al. Neuropsychologic sequelae in the long-term survivors of childhood acute lymphoblastic leukemia. Pediatr Hematol Oncol 1999;16: 213–220.
123. Kingma A, Rammeloo LAJ, van der Does-van den Berg A, et al. Academic career after treatment for acute lymphoblastic leukemia. Arch Dis Child 2000;82:353–357.
124. Robison LL, Nesbit MEJ, Sather HN, et al. Factors associated with IQ scores in long-term survivors of childhood acute lymphoblastic leukemia. Am J Pediatr Hematol Oncol 1984;6: 115–121.
125. Moss HA, Nannis ED, Poplack DG. The effects of prophylactic treatment of the central nervous system on the intellectual functioning of children with acute lymphocytic leukemia. Am J Med 1981;71:47–52.

126. Roman DD, Sperduto PW. Neuropsychological effects of cranial radiation: current knowledge and future directions. Int J Radiat Oncol Biol Phys 1995;31:983–998.
127. Anderson DM, Rennie KM, Ziegler RS, et al. Medical and neurocognitive late effects among survivors of childhood central nervous system tumors. Cancer (Phila) 2001;92:2709–2719.
128. Johnson DL, McCabe MA, Nicholson HS, et al. Quality of long-term survival in young children with Medulloblastoma. J Neurosurg 1994;80:1004–1010.
129. Glaser AW, Abdul Rashid NF, Walker DA. School behavior and health status after central nervous system tumours in childhood. Br J Cancer 1997;76:643–650.
130. Arceci RJ, Reaman GH, Cohen AR, et al. Position statement for the need to define pediatric hematology/oncology programs: a model of subspecialty care for chronic childhood diseases. Health Care Policy and Public Issues Committee of the American Society of Pediatric Hematology/Oncology. J Pediatr Hematol Oncol 1998;20:98–103.
131. Bleyer WA, Smith RA, Green DM, et al. American Cancer Society Workshop on Adolescents and Young Adults with Cancer. Workgroup #1: Long-term care and lifetime follow-up. Cancer (Phila) 1993;71:2413.
132. Masera G, Chesler M, Jankovic M, et al. SIOP Working Committee on psychosocial issues in pediatric oncology: guidelines for care of long-term survivors. Med Pediatr Oncol 1996;27:1–2.
133. Wallace WH, Blacklay A, Eiser C, et al. Developing strategies for long term follow up of survivors of childhood cancer. BMJ 2001;323:271–274.
134. Hollen PJ, Hobbie WL. Establishing comprehensive specialty follow-up clinics for long-term survivors of cancer. Providing systematic physiological and psychosocial support. Support Care Cancer 1995;3:40–44.
135. American Academy of Pediatrics Section on Hematology/Oncology. Guidelines for the pediatric cancer center and role of such centers in diagnosis and treatment. Pediatrics 1997;99:139–141.
136. Ross JA, Severson RK, Robison LL, et al. Pediatric cancer in the United States. A preliminary report of a collaborative study of the Childrens Cancer Group and the Pediatric Oncology Group. Cancer (Phila) 1993;71:3415–3421.
137. Children's Oncology Group. Requirements for Institutional Membership. Arcadia: COG, 2001.
138. Hobbie WL, Ogle S. Transitional care for young adult survivors of childhood cancer. Semin Oncol Nurs 2001;17:268–273.
139. Konsler GK, Jones GR. Transition issues for survivors of childhood cancer and their healthcare providers. Cancer Pract 1993;1:319–324.
140. Oeffinger KC, Eshelman DA, Tomlinson GE, et al. Programs for adult survivors of childhood cancer. J Clin Oncol 1998;16:2864–2867.
141. Richardson RC, Nelson MB, Meeske K. Young adult survivors of childhood cancer: attending to emerging medical and psychosocial needs. J Pediatr Oncol Nurs 1999;16:136–144.
142. Rigon H, Lopes LF, do Rosario Latorre M, et al. The GEPETTO program for surveillance of long-term survivors of childhood cancer: preliminary report from a single institution in Brazil. Med Pediatr Oncol 2003;40:405–406.

103

Medical and Psychosocial Issues in Hodgkin's Disease Survivors

Jon Håvard Loge and Stein Kaasa

The first attempts to treat Hodgkin's disease by radiotherapy were conducted at the beginning of the last century. The prognosis for survival was poor but slowly improved by the use of radiotherapy and some chemotherapy until 1960. For example, in 1939 a 20-year survival rate of 17% was reported.[1]

During the 1960s the prognosis for survival vastly improved, which was mainly related to the introduction of improved staging systems, better understanding of the spread and course of the disease, improved diagnostic methods, and refined therapy. The latter included improved radiotherapy and the introduction of chemotherapeutic regimens such as the MOPP (mechlorethamine, vincristine, procarbazine, prednisone) in 1967.[2] The therapeutic pessimism turned into optimism, and the clinicians dared to speak of a cure. Cure was defined as follows: "We can speak of a cure when in time, probably a decade or so after treatment, there remains a group of disease-free survivors whose progressive *death rate* from all causes is similar to that of a normal population of the same sex and age constitution"[3,4] (see Chapter 67).

This chapter is about the price of cure in terms of medical late effects and psychosocial issues related to survivorship. To speak of a price of cure first became relevant when death no longer was the predominant outcome. The improved prognosis for survival achieved during the 1960s created an increasing number of survivors, and studies of possible late effects thereby became possible. For the clinician, a patient consulting for late effects, medical or psychosocial, probably has now become a more commonly encountered clinical problem than a patient presenting with Hodgkin's disease itself.

Late effects can mainly be divided into three categories. First, there are the late medical effects, which include secondary cancers or ill effects on of one or more organ systems. Second, there are the late effects in subjective health, which include symptoms such as fatigue or pain as well as psychologic phenomena such as anxiety and depression. Third, there are the late effects encountered as difficulties in returning to normal life such as resuming work or difficulties in partnership or in participation in leisure activities. The definition of a late effect is not commonly agreed upon, but it is reasonable to separate late effects from acute effects by both duration and time of debut. Some late effects such as fatigue might be traced back to the period of active disease. Other late effects such as secondary cancers might present after a shorter or longer period without symptoms or signs of disease.

Challenges in Clinics and Research

The late effects represent several challenges for the researcher as well as for the clinician. In the investigation of late effects the researcher is challenged by the complexity of the late effects, but also by the effects of aging, environment, lifestyle, behavior, etc. upon health. Consequently, it may be difficult to find causal factors related to the outcomes observed. For the clinicians (as well as for the researcher) the challenge is to understand what the needs of the survivors are. An increased understanding of long-term effects of somatic, psychologic, and social nature will, it is hoped, help healthcare providers to better deliver follow-up programs and patients and family members to better understand their needs.

The low incidence of Hodgkin's disease generates relatively few survivors and consequently a relative scarcity of data. The social mobility in many Western countries is high, and many survivors are lost to follow-up or are even impossible to locate several years after treatment. Furthermore, the treatment regimens are under constant revision, and late effects caused by one regimen may not necessarily be caused by another type of treatment. Some late effects are relevant only for subgroups of survivors such as breast cancer affecting females irradiated by fields including their breast during their reproductive years. Such factors further add to the scarcity of data. Additionally, some late affects such as secondary cancers first become manifest several years after termination of treatment. A long latency period between active disease and debut of late effects might also generate findings, which are not necessarily related to Hodgkin's disease or its treatment. For example, is symptomatic coronary heart disease 30 years after termination of treatment to be looked upon as a late effect, as related to nutrition, smoking habits, and physical exercise, after termination of treatment, or as a combination of all these factors? To answer such a question the researcher needs large samples (i.e., statistical power), advanced medical technology, and skilled experienced clinicians to evaluate the patients, and from a design point of view controlled groups are needed. The distinction between late effects and morbidity related to increasing age becomes increasingly blurred as the observation time increases. At present there is a scarcity of prospectively collected data, which limits the possibility of drawing valid conclusions about causality. Ideally, one should therefore have comparative data to identify the late effects of Hodgkin's disease. Lack of a comparison group is of particular concern regarding subjective outcomes such as fatigue, which is frequently found in a general population, and may be caused by a series of factors during a lifetime observation.[5] The optimal study design is a prospective follow-up of the survivors from the time of diagnoses through the treatment and into the follow-up phase for many years. In such nonrandomized designs, valid control groups are needed, which should be age- and gender matched and generated by random draws from the general population. In cross-sectional designs, subjective health outcomes from the general population may serve as valid comparisons and will definitely strengthen the conclusions, while the validity of "ad hoc-generated comparisons groups" should be questioned. Volunteer bias is an example that may represent a serious threat to the internal validity of studies with ad hocgenerated comparison groups such as relatives or hospital visitors.

The constitution of a survivor population might also be biased. For example, the patients treated at the Norwegian Radium Hospital (NRH) were assumed to be representative of the Norwegian population of Hodgkin's disease survivors. After survival of the NRH cohorts was investigated, it was concluded that patients with a better prognosis for survival were found in this sample, as compared with the national sample.[6]

The choice of outcome measures may also represent a challenge. For example, the current most commonly used measures for late effects such as psychologic distress and fatigue have limitations with regard to content, reliability, and validity. Another major limitation is the lack of standardization of outcome measures. Different outcome measures have been used to measure the same phenomenon such as fatigue and pain. On the other hand, prospective studies might *lock* the data collection to measurement techniques that become obsolete during the observation period.

Given an accumulating prevalence of late effects, content and organization of the follow-ups should be discussed and ideally investigated in research and in quality assurance programs, and an increasing emphasis on economic effects on the healthcare system should be questioned. Furthermore, it should be questioned: What part of the healthcare system is best suited for conducting surveillance, what is a reasonable price for a surveillance program, and should the optimal program be individualized? Finally, how are medical students and future oncologists/radiotherapists best trained to detect and treat late effects? In sum, these challenges also raise ethical dilemmas related to what to tell the patients about late effects and the possibility of creating lifelong patients under continuous observation for possible late effects that might never even occur.

Epidemiology

Incidence of Hodgkin's Disease

The incidence of Hodgkin's disease (HD) varies across countries but is at a comparable level (approximately 2 to 3 per 100,000) in the Western countries.[7] Generally, more males than females are affected (M/F ratio, approximately 60:40). Incidence in the Western world was stable until 1980, slowly decreased during the period 1980–1990, and thereafter it has slightly increased.[8] The decreased incidence was mostly due to a decreasing number of patients above 60 years of age with non-Hodgkin's lymphomas earlier being misclassified as Hodgkin's disease.[6,8,9] More than 50% of the patients are 39 years of age or younger at time of diagnosis.[7]

Prevalence of Survivorship

A disease mainly affecting young adults combined with a good prognosis for survival (best among the younger patients) generates a population of survivors with a long life expectancy. In general, the 5-year survival for all patients with Hodgkin's disease exceeds 80%, and for patients 39 years of age or younger, more than 90% are expected to live for 5 years or more.[10,11] Consequently, the prevalence of survivorship has steadily increased over the past three to four decades. The long life expectancy of the survivors permits long-term follow-up studies but also makes control for expected diseases necessary. As indicated earlier, it is therefore urgent to design prospective and large enough follow-up studies of Hodgkin's disease survivors. Without conducting such studies our follow-up programs may not only be burdensome to the healthcare system, but many patients may be offered invalid follow-up.

The latest Norwegian data illustrate this point clearly. Although the yearly incidence of Hodgkin's disease has been around 80 new cases per year (2/100,000) during the past two decades, the number of Norwegians alive and having had Hodgkin's disease has been steadily increasing and now exceeds 1,500.[12] In 1990 the prevalence of survivorship was 1,100 in a population of about 4.5 million.[13]

Advanced disease and B symptoms in addition to age predict incomplete remission, relapse, and shortened survival after first-line treatment.[14,15] Age is at present the single most important predictor for survival. Advanced disease and relapse both increase the treatment burden. Some survivors have therefore received intensive treatment (chemotherapy and radiotherapy) in several cycles eventually supplemented with high-dose chemotherapy and bone marrow transplantation. In general, the most recent improvement in survival is therefore a consequence of more-intensive treatment. Potentially the more-intensive treatment may affect the prevalence of long-term medical and/or psychosocial effects. Subgroups of survivors might therefore be of special interest for future assessments of late effects. However, such groups must be considered relatively small, which affects whether proper follow-up studies can be performed, unless such studies are conducted as multicenter studies with a sufficient number of patients.

Medical Issues

About the Treatment

Treatment with radiotherapy has during the past decades been partly replaced and/or combined with chemotherapy. Radiotherapy as a single modality is today given only to a subgroup of patients with limited disease.

In the 1960s, fractionated large fields were irradiated with the consequence of a substantially increased survival rate. Continuous research on radiotherapy techniques has resulted in more individualized treatment, and today more often smaller fields are delivered as compared to the standard mantle fields used at the start of the radiotherapy era. To reduce radiotherapy-related acute and late toxicity, the total dose in many programs has been reduced from a standard total dose of 40 Gy treated in 3 Gy per fraction to a dose of 30 to 35 Gy with reduced single fraction to a proximately 1.75 Gy. Critical organs are sometimes included in the fields, such as lung, heart, thyroid, major blood vessel, and bone marrow, which may give long-term side effects.

Combination chemotherapy was introduced into the treatment plans of Hodgkin's disease in the mid-1960s with the so-called MOPP regimens (mechlorethamine, vincristine, procarbazine, prednisone) as the gold standard in most countries.[2] Other combinations of chemotherapy have been in use as well as various ways of escalating doses to improve survival and reduce acute toxicity and long-term morbidity.

Both treatment modalities, that is, radiotherapy and chemotherapy or combinations, can potentially give the patients medical (somatic) long-term side effects. Furthermore, the cancer itself may also have and will alter the biology of the host (i.e., the patient). So, consequently, either of these factors, separately or in combination, may result in late morbidity for HD survivors.

Long-Term Morbidity: General Considerations

The most frequent causes of death other than Hodgkin's disease itself are cardiac disease and secondary malignancy, while infertility, thyroid abnormalities, and pulmonary disease may cause serious late effects of various prevalences in Hodgkin's disease survivors.[16] The most commonly encountered late medical effects are presented in Table 103.1. In a recent review it was concluded that secondary malignancies and ischemic heart disease are the two most frequent causes of death.[17] However, it must be kept in mind that, in patients with good prognoses, the actual overall survival at 20 years is about 93%,[11] and that treatment-related mortality exceeds the mortality from Hodgkin's disease 12 to 15 years after the primary treatment.[18]

TABLE 103.1. Main medical late effects of Hodgkin's lymphoma and its treatment.

- Secondary cancers
- Cardiac disease
- Endocrine dysfunction
  —Hypothyroidism
  —Hypogonadism
- Lung damage
- Dental caries

Cardiac Late Effects

An increased incidence of coronary heart disease, specifically in patients less than 40 years of age, has been attributed to radiotherapy. The expected number of cardiovascular deaths in age- and sex-matched population was similar to the cardiovascular deaths in Hodgkin's disease populations.[19] The history of myocardial infarction was no more frequent after mantle field irradiation than in HD patients who received chemotherapy,[20] whereas others have reported an increased risk of myocardial infarction after mediastinal irradiation.[21,22] Up to a threefold increase in the relative risk of cardiac deaths has been reported.[23] In another retrospective review, coronary artery disease occurred in patients who were treated at the ages of 16, 21, 35, and 48 years with latency periods of 19, 12, 7, and 3 years, respectively.[24]

The technology used to evaluate morbidity, such as valvular dysfunction, may have major impact on the findings. Before Doppler technology was used, valvular dysfunction was considered a rare finding in survivors of Hodgkin's disease. By using Doppler echo cardiography, aortic and/or mitral valvular regurgitation and valve thickness have been observed at rates of 24% to 40% of patients treated successfully for Hodgkin's disease.[25–27] The clinical implications of these findings are at present unknown.

Endocrine Dysfunction

The prevalence of hypothyroidism varies substantially between studies. As for most of the other medical side effects as well as for the subjective ones, sample selection, definition of cases, etc. have a major influence on the results. The rate of hypothyroidism seems to be influenced by observation time, irradiation (field and amount), and the definition of hypothyroidism.[28–30] In a sample from Norway where 221 patients were observed, 55% developed biochemical hypothyroidism 3 to 23 years after treatment.[20]

In the Stanford study the actual risk of thyroid disease was 52% after 20 years and rose to 67% after a follow-up of 26 years.[16] In this study, younger patients, women, combined-modality treatment, and time since radiation were associated with a high incidence of thyroid disease, whereas other studies from Europe have not confirmed these findings.[20,31]

Although thyroid abnormality is prevalent in HD survivors, the early use of thyroid supplementation in patients with elevated thyroid-stimulating hormone (TSH) level has greatly reduced the risk of overt clinical hypothyroidism when compared with earlier studies.[32] However, no consensus seems to have been reached with regard to when and on which indications to start hormonal substitution in patients with biochemical hypothyroidism.

Lung Damage

Dyspnea is a subjective phenomenon experienced by the patients as shortness of breath. Consequently it is recommended that dyspnea as well as other subjective symptoms should be assessed by the patients themselves by means of questionnaires or other subjective measures. Dyspnea is frequently reported in HD survivors in approximately 30% of the cases.[20] In the Norwegian study, dyspnea was not associated with sex, age, or chemotherapy.[20] Pulmonary complications after radiotherapy are first observed clinically as an acute radiation pneumonitis, followed by radiation fibrosis, which evolves over time and seems to reach a stable appearance after 9 to 12 months.[33] Pulmonary toxicity secondary to chemotherapy is rare; however, bleomycin may enhance pulmonary dysfunction when given in conjunction with radiotherapy.[34]

In one study consisting of a selected cohort of 116 patients treated with mediastinal radiotherapy alone or in combination with chemotherapy, 30% of the patients had pulmonary dysfunction and associated reductions in total lung capacity, forced vital capacity, forced expiratory volume in 1 second, and gas transfer impairment.[35] The size of the radiation fields has been found to be related to the extent of fibrosis, and the most dramatic changes were observed in patients treated simultaneously with bleomycin and anthracyclines.[35] In single cases major interindividual variations have been found with respect to the sensitivity of the lung parenchyma to develop radiation fibrosis.

In conclusion, a consistent finding is that the severity of the fibrosis is related to the volume of irradiation, the presence of parenchymal involvement in the disease itself, and the use of bleomycin and anthracyclines.

Comments

Most studies assessing medical morbidity in HD survivors have either a retrospective design and/or a cross-sectional design. The studies are performed ad hoc, with few upfront hypotheses stated, and how to define the level of morbidity and which indicators to use to define morbidity varies considerably. Scientific discussions of possible confounding factors are rarely presented, and few studies have comparison groups. Based on the findings in one of the studies including a comparison group, it has been, for example, suggested that the incidence of cardiac death is not any higher than in the matched population.[19] However, details on how these comparisons were performed were not given. A similar criticism can be raised for treatment of symptoms and biochemical findings of hypothyroidism. Most studies have an ad hoc retrospective design, and consequently it is difficult to draw valid conclusions with regard to treatment proposals.

Psychosocial Issues

Historical Perspective and General Points

The first descriptions of the psychosocial aspects of cancer survivorship were conflicting. Case observations led to the postulation of a Damocles syndrome in which the survivors lived their lives under the constant threat of a relapse.[36] The syndrome was characterized as a specific psychologic state with tension, emptiness, and lack of pleasure and direction of life. The other position, in general held by epidemiologists, stated that the cancer survivors lived well-adjusted lives and were as satisfied with their lives as the general population.[37] It is now obvious that the two concepts were equally wrong and that both positions were based on methodologic shortcomings. The epidemiologists based their statements on too-general outcome measures and the psychologists based their postulation of a specific syndrome upon case observations without sufficient perspective on the generalizability of their observations.

From a psychiatric point of view, one can hypothesize that the psychologic burden of survivorship per se would be more of a posttraumatic stress disorder than depression. Being cured is difficult to characterize as a loss with subsequent potential for development of depression. However, reduced health status after cure, either objectively or subjectively, might represent a loss and thereby a potential for development of depression. Premorbid characteristics as well as social and psychologic support during and after the disease will always interact with the stressor (i.e., the disease and the treatment). No published studies have investigated these variables systematically.

Most published studies of psychosocial aspects of cancer survivorship have been descriptive and lacking a specific hypothesis. The study by Cella and Tross from 1986 is one exception, and three possible psychologic sequelae were proposed (anticipatory, residual, and current) and explored with generally negative findings.[38] Facing death and receiving burdensome treatment during a period of life when friends fulfill education and establish themselves in jobs and families may be regarded as a longlasting trauma, and the model of a posttraumatic stress disorder may apply for this population. Such a specific model for development of late psychosocial effects has not been tested, except for the study by Cella and Tross.[38] Generally, the studies of psychologic late effects have used self-report measures of psychologic distress as outcomes, and none has looked for specific psychiatric diagnoses. There have been several methodologic limitations, among which selection bias is probably the most serious and difficult to handle. It is reasonable to assume that late effects might increase the response rates, and this is of particular concern in cross-sectional studies relying on one single data collection. Still, it is reasonable to conclude that psychosocial late effects in survivors of Hodgkin's disease are the exception rather than the rule.

Quality of Life

Quality of life (QOL) reflects the definition of health as proposed by the World Health Organization in 1947 with emphasis on the subjective aspect of health and not only the absence of disease.[39] During the 1980s and 1990s, the concept of QOL became more directed toward health by the introduction of the term Health-Related Quality of Life. The latter operationalizes health as encompassing a social, a physical, and a mental dimension. It should be regarded as a narrowing of the concept QOL, and some therefore prefer the term subjective health. The distinction is not only of academic interest. Figure 103.1 demonstrates the responses from survivors of Hodgkin's disease and normal controls to a single question about satisfaction with life, which is close to the more global concept of QOL. More of the survivors reported being very satisfied with their lives than the normal controls, in spite of more health problems among the survivors. This is in line with findings reported by Cella and Tross.[38] In spite of the possible existential dimension of this finding, overall QOL does not seem to capture the health-related aspects of the survivors' quality of life (i.e., their subjective health status).

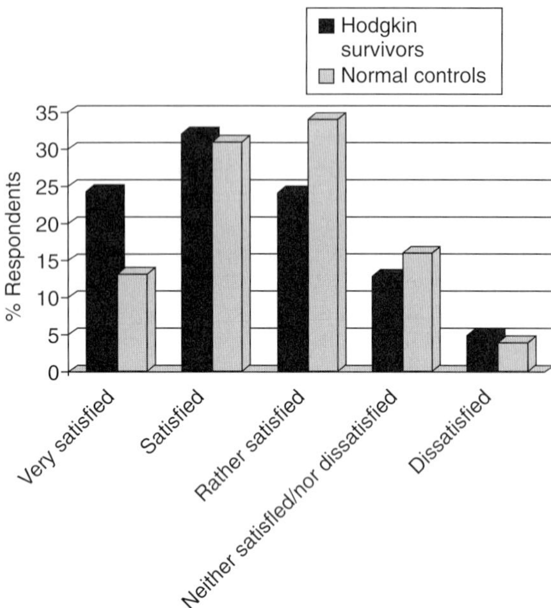

FIGURE 103.1. Satisfaction with life in Norwegian survivors of Hodgkin's disease ($n = 453$) and in normal control subjects ($n = 2323$). (Unpublished data from the authors.)

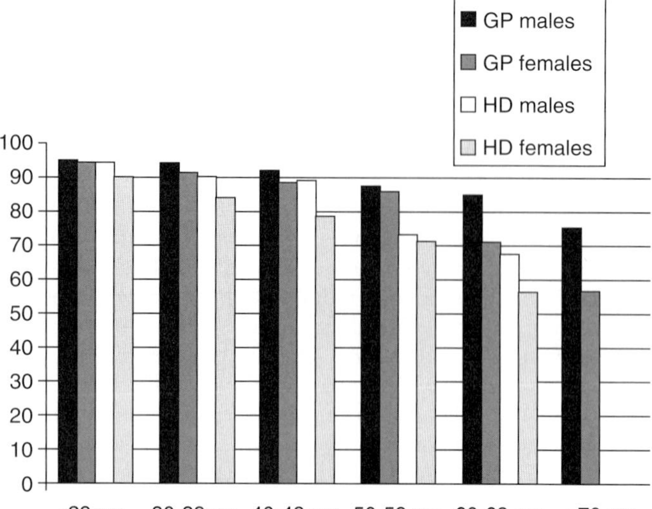

FIGURE 103.2. Physical functioning as measured by the Physical Functioning Scale of the SF-36 in the general Norwegian population (*GP*) (Norwegian norm data; $n = 2263$) and survivors of Hodgkin's disease (*HD*; $n = 459$). (Data from references 48, 49.)

Subjective Health Status: Early Findings

The first studies of subjective health status in survivors of Hodgkin's disease were published in 1986.[38,40] As demonstrated in Table 103.2, the first studies included quite different sample sizes, and the findings were inconsistent, partly reflecting different measures of subjective health. Only two studies included comparison groups. In these studies, selected cohorts of U.S. patients from controlled clinical trials were included. A minority of all U.S. cancer patients are included in clinical trials, and the generalizability of the findings can therefore be questioned.

Subjective Health Status: Physical Health

Physical health is about physical symptoms such as pain, dyspnea, and nausea in addition to physical functioning, which generally includes different physical activities commonly performed during a day. Present subjective health status measures such as the SF-36, the European Organization for Research and Treatment of Cancer Core Quality of Life Questionnaire (EORTC QLQ C-30), and the Functional Assessment of Cancer Therapy-General (FACT-G) all put a great emphasis on physical functioning, which generally is affected by somatic health events and has low correlation with mental health.[45–47] In the SF-36, 10 of 36 items are about physical functioning.[47] However, the content of physical functioning scales varies among the instruments, and this hinders comparisons across the instruments. Physical functioning in the general population is related to age and gender (Figure 103.2).[48,49] The decline by age reflects increasing morbidity with increasing age and needs to be controlled for in studies of cancer survivors.[48]

The first studies of Hodgkin's disease survivors indicated problems with the survivors' physical health, but standardized measures were not applied.[41,50,51] Three studies from the 1990s included both standardized measures of physical functioning (the EORTC QLQ C-30 and the SF-36) and comparison groups.[42,44,49] The findings were surprisingly similar in that physical functioning was reduced by approximately 0.5 SD compared to the control groups.[42,44,49] None of the studies demonstrated any robust associations between disease characteristics, treatment, and reduced physical functioning. Some later studies have failed to replicate this finding, but the design of these studies limits the possibility of drawing firm conclusions.[52,53]

Clinicians report stiffness and pain from the musculoskeletal system as common among the survivors.[20] However, compared with healthy controls, no differences in pain level between survivors and controls have been detected.[42,44,49] Another somatic symptom, dyspnea, is included the cancer-specific instrument EORTC QLQ C30 but not in the generic instrument SF-36. Joly et al. compared

TABLE 103.2. Early studies of health-related quality of life among survivors of Hodgkin's disease.

Study	*Year*	*Country*	*N*	*Origin of sample*	*Mean observation period (years)*	*Effect stage/ treatment*	*Comparison group*
Cella[38]	1986	USA	60	Hospital	Unknown	Yes	Yes
Fobair[40]	1986	USA	403	Clinical trials	9	Yes	No
Kornblith[41]	1992	USA	273	Advanced disease/clinical trials	6	No	No
van Tulder[42]	1994	Netherlands	81	Hospital	14	No	Yes
Norum[43]	1996	Norway	42	Hospital	4	Yes	No
Joly[44]	1996	France	93	Region	10	No	Yes

French survivors with randomly selected and matched controls and found nearly three times higher levels of dyspnea in the survivors than in the controls.[44] A Spanish study from 2003 also found higher levels of dyspnea in the survivors than in healthy controls.[54] Given the difficulties patient have in distinguishing dyspnea from fatigue and the association between fatigue and gas transfer impairment, a further elaboration on this point seems warranted.[55]

The French study by Joly et al. found very low levels of nausea and vomiting as measured by the EORTC QLQ C30 and no difference between the survivors and the age- and gender-matched healthy controls.[44] Cameron et al. also reported low levels of nausea and vomiting but pointed to the possibility of classical conditioning as the mechanism underlying persisting symptoms such as distress in the survivors.[56] By exploring and confirming a specific mechanism, this study yielded knowledge that is directly applicable in the prevention and/or treatment of persisting symptoms by use of psychologic techniques.

There are some main limitations to our present knowledge on the physical health of the survivors. On a group level their physical health is lowered, and the reduction is of clinical significance.[57] Still, the majority enjoys a physical health similar to the general population of same age. The survivors with reduced physical health have not been clearly identified, and how the survivors' physical health is affected by time since termination of primary treatment is not documented. The mechanisms underlying the survivors' reduced physical health are unknown, and this lack hinders efforts to prevent and treat. The reduced physical health might reflect the total sum of negative health events such as gas transfer impairment, muscular waste, and hypothyrosis. Another explanation might be an association between reduced physical health and other subjective late effects such as fatigue.[58] However, none of the published studies on physical health has controlled for the level of fatigue.

Subjective Health Status: Fatigue

The first report on fatigue among Hodgkin's disease survivors was published by Fobair et al. in 1986, and fatigue was a major problem as 37% had not regained their energy.[40] Patients with self-reported energy loss were more likely to be depressed.[40] Another early study demonstrated that Hodgkin's disease survivors were more fatigued than survivors of testicular cancer.[51] A British study of lymphoma patients off treatment described mental and physical fatigue as major concerns.[59,60] However, in all the earliest studies published before 1997 fatigue was measured by single questions (i.e., not validated and reliability tested questionnaires), and such single questions have disputable validity and reliability.[61] Further, none of the early studies took into account the high prevalence of fatigue in the general population (11%–45%).[61,62] The main studies on fatigue in the survivors are presented in Table 103.3.

Newer studies employing standardized measures and comparison groups have confirmed that fatigue is a major problem among the survivors compared to healthy subjects and more of a problem among survivors of Hodgkin's disease than among survivors of other cancer types.[63–68] The prevalence of fatigue is clearly related to the measurement technique, and the exact magnitude of this problem is therefore not known.[61]

Attempts to relate persisting fatigue to disease and treatment characteristics have yielded conflicting results. The close connection between disease burden and type of treatment also hinders analyses of separate effects of the two. However, a recent prospective study demonstrated that combined treatment yielded higher levels of fatigue only during the first year as compared to radiation therapy.[63] Thereafter, the two groups reported similar levels of fatigue, which was significantly higher than in the general population (Figure 103.3).[63]

A cross-sectional study reported an association between late pulmonary sequelae (in particular, gas transfer impairment) and fatigue.[55] A significant association between psychologic distress and fatigue has been demonstrated.[40,69] However, a review strongly supported a differentiated view on fatigue and depression in cancer patients.[70] Some authors have proposed a common mechanism underlying the symptoms of cancer and cancer treatment, namely, cytokines, which induce sickness behavior in animal models including

TABLE 103.3. Fatigue in survivors of Hodgkin's disease: main studies.

Author	*Year*	*Sample (N)*	*Main finding*	*Comparison group (N)*	*Type of measurement*
Fobair[40]	1986	403	37% tired	—	Single item
Devlen[59,60]	1987	90/120[a]	30%/42% tired	—	Single item
Bloom[51]	1993	85	22% energy not returned	Testicular survivors	Single item
van Tulder[42]	1994	81	No significant difference	Healthy controls	SF-36
Loge[65b]	1999	458	24%–27% chronic fatigued	General population norms	Fatigue Questionnaire
Kornblith[64]	1998	273	More fatigued than controls	Acute leukemia survivors	POMS
Wettergren[67]	2003	121	Worries about fatigue	Healthy controls	SEIQoL-DW
Fosså[68]	2003	458	24% chronic fatigued	Testicular survivors	Fatigue Questionnaire
Ganz[63]	2003	247	Persistent fatigue > population norms	—	SF-36
Ruffer[66]	2003	836	21% higher level	Healthy controls	MFI

SF-36, Short Form 36; POMS, Profile of Mood States; SEIQoL-DW, Schedule for the Evaluation of the Individual Quality of Life-Direct Weighting.

[a] Two studies; retrospective and prospective including Hodgkin's disease and non-Hodgkin lymphomas.

[b] Identical sample of Hodgkin's disease survivors.

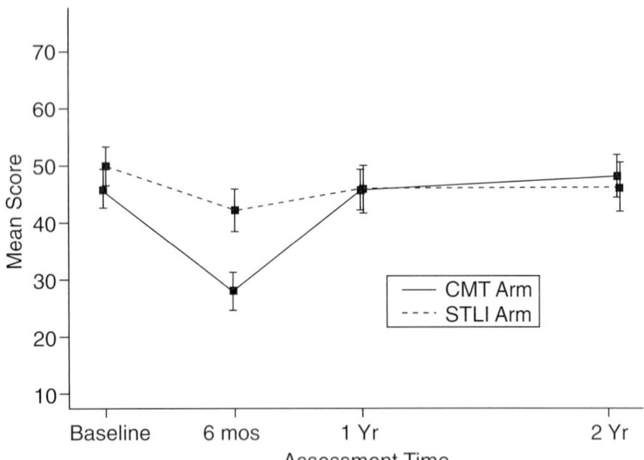

FIGURE 103.3. Average SF-36 Vitality Scale scores (mean with 95% CI) by assessment time and treatment arm. Lower scores reflect greater fatigue. *STLI*, subtotal lymphoid irradiation; *CMT*, combined-modality therapy. For healthy men aged 35 to 44 years, the mean Vitality Scale score is 65.5. For women aged 35 to 44 years, it is 59.4. (From Ganz et al.,[63] by permission of *Journal of Clinical Oncology*.)

fatigued behavior.[71] However, attempts to correlate some of the relevant cytokines to fatigue have failed.[72]

Except for the study by Ganz, all studies on fatigue in Hodgkin's disease survivors were cross-sectional, which limits the possibility of inferences about causality. No prospective longitudinal studies to investigate the course of fatigue among Hodgkin's disease survivors have been published. This lack of knowledge limits the clinician's ability to give valid and reliable information to individual patients on the expected course of their fatigue.

At present we can therefore only hypothesize about the mechanisms underlying fatigue in the survivors. In some, as in the general population, fatigue is probably part of being psychologically distressed.[73] However, as compared to sufferers of the chronic fatigue syndrome, the survivors have significantly lower levels of psychologic distress as measured by the Hospital Anxiety and Depression Scale.[69,73] Second, fatigue might reflect the combined burden of the late complications after having had Hodgkin's disease. Fatigue is by many considered a final common endpoint that is associated with most diseases; this indicates that fatigue is an "unclean" endpoint affected by most altered health states. Third, fatigue might be a specific late effect after Hodgkin's disease and related to some specific mechanisms characteristic of this disease; this might include the cytokines, which is supported by the altered immunity found in many of the survivors. At present, none of these seems more strongly supported than the others, and given the complexity of fatigue all might be correct in subgroups of fatigued survivors.

Subjective Health Status: Mental Health

Some of the earliest studies indicated rather great psychologic problems among the survivors. For example, Kornblith et al. reported in 1992 psychologic distress one SD above that of healthy subjects, and 22% met the criterion suggested for a psychiatric diagnosis.[41] Later studies from the 1990s did not confirm this finding. Three studies used health-related quality of life (HRQOL) measures and different comparison groups, and none reported any deviances in mental health (SF-36) or emotional functioning (EORTC QLQ C-30) between the survivors and the controls.[42,44,49] The first comparative study between Hodgkin's disease survivors and testicular cancer survivors did not find any significant difference in psychologic outcomes between the two groups of survivors.[51]

One study from the last part of the 1990s identified as many as 27% of the survivors as probable anxiety and depression cases, but no comparison group was included.[74] Previous psychiatric problems, psychiatric problems during the treatment phase, and low education were identified as risk factors. The most intensive treatment regimen was associated with increased risk for probable anxiety.[74] This study employed the Hospital Anxiety and Depression Scale (the HADS), which generally tends to produce high levels of anxiety and higher prevalences of anxiety cases than depression cases.[75] This finding was confirmed by the most recent study, which found no differences in the level of depression between Hodgkin's disease survivors, testicular cancer survivors, and the general Norwegian population.[68] The levels of anxiety in both groups of survivors (4.7 in testicular cancer survivors and 4.6 in Hodgkin's disease survivors) were slightly elevated as compared to the general population (3.9).[68] In sum, these studies indicate that the level of depressive symptoms is not elevated in the survivors, that anxiety symptoms are just slightly elevated, and that we do not know whether these symptoms are part of a specific psychiatric condition.

Some other psychologic symptoms have been assessed and reported as more prevalent than expected. Cella et al. in 1986 reported no elevated level of psychologic distress, but indication of psychosocial dysfunction in areas such as intimacy motivation, increased avoidant thinking about disease, and illness-related concerns.[38] These findings may be of clinical relevance, for example, as effectors on partnership and illness behavior but have to our knowledge not been addressed in later studies.

Social Functioning

Three aspects of social functioning have received special attention in the literature: divorce rate, difficulties in returning to ordinary work, and difficulties in getting health insurance/borrowing from banks. Additional aspects of social life such as participation in leisure activities, sexual activity, sexual interest, and reproduction have also been included in some studies.

In general it is reasonable to state that the social consequences of survivorship from cancer are influenced by social mechanisms that may vary considerably across culturally relatively comparable nations, as is in accordance with the handicap model as proposed by the WHO.[76] For example, in the Scandinavian countries health insurance is public and granted to every citizen. Life insurance is partly private and partly public, and in sum insurance is probably of lesser relevance in these countries than in the United States. An early U.S. study demonstrated difficulties in getting health insurance.[41] The lack of a comparison group hinders estimation of the clinical significance of this possible late effect.

In general, the relationship between cancer, cancer treatment, late medical or late subjective health effects, and social consequences is complex and relatively poorly understood.

Type of treatment seems to be of lesser relevance, while subjective late effects was associated with poorer social functioning.[63,77]

Difficulties returning to an ordinary job are also affected by country-specific variables in addition to the labor market in general. The earliest U.S. studies indicated various work-related problems such as getting a job or working at a former pace.[38,40,41] The Norwegian data demonstrated that the majority of the survivors with a mean follow-up time of 12 years were in full-time work at follow-up.[77] However, about 20% were permanently disabled, compared with 10% of the general Norwegian population of similar age at the time of the follow-up study.[77] Predictors of disablement were increasing age, low education, combined-treatment modality, and high levels of anxiety, depression, and fatigue.[77] The French study by Joly et al. did not demonstrate lower proportions of survivors at work, but they had less ambitious professional plans.[44] The latter finding was replicated by the Norwegian study.[77]

Divorce is generally a common event in most Western countries. The earliest studies found divorce rates up to 32% among the survivors.[40] Among the French survivors studied by Joly et al., the divorce rate was lower among the survivors than among the controls but length of the marriage was not controlled for.[44] Generally, several methodologic aspects hinder interpretation of whether the divorce rate deviates from the general population. The age of the survivors and controls at time of data collection, the different divorce rates across different age groups, and the effect of marriage duration upon divorce rate all add to the uncertainty of the published data on divorce rates. Additionally, one could also hypothesize different mechanisms for divorce between spouses being married during the treatment phase and between spouses who marry after termination of treatment. A couple living through the treatment of Hodgkin's disease faces serious and long-lasting stressors. Generally such strain may strengthen bonds in some couples but also represent tensions that subsequently end up in divorce in others. The modern tendency to involve the family including the children during the treatment phase may have positive effects for the family as a whole, but this has not been addressed in published studies until now. On the other hand, one may also speculate that such a practice increases the total burden on the family and particularly on the healthy spouse. No studies until now have addressed the burden of disease and treatment on the family, but one might speculate that the stress on the family is affected by the quality of care which the family receives during and after the treatment phase. For example, a recent study has demonstrated much less psychologic distress among the relatives of patients included in a palliative program as compared to the relatives of patients receiving standard care.[78]

The prevalence of sexual problems among Hodgkin's disease survivors has been reported to be between 12% and 20%, whereas infertility among women and men has been reported to be less than 10% and less than 20%, respectively.[40,41,44,64,77] In the Norwegian sample, the great majority of the men reporting infertility had received treatment known to reduce fertility (chemotherapy containing an alkylating agent and procarbazine). One single study reported difficulties in participation in leisure activities, and this was related to fatigue.[37]

Treatment

Medical Late Effects

Treatment of late medical effects after curative treatment of Hodgkin's disease has, to our knowledge, not been systematically investigated. For patients with symptoms from heart, lung, and/or thyroid gland, general guidelines on how to treat or relieve symptoms have been followed. For patients with hypothyroidism, general international accepted treatment guidelines seem advisable to follow. Similar approaches have also been used by cardiologists and lung physicians. However, it is reasonable to assume that the pathophysiology for these conditions in many cases is different in Hodgkin's disease survivors than in other groups of patients. If these assumptions are correct, one may argue that at least patients need to be followed systematically and prospectively after treatment is initiated to evaluate both immediate and long-term effects of the intervention. Furthermore, one may also expect that the condition itself, for example, cardiac sequelae after radiotherapy, may have a different "natural cause" than what is expected in patients with the same condition, but with other causes. Additionally, one may also expect that in many patients with Hodgkin's disease a combination of factors may cause the condition itself.

For patients with no symptoms, but with pathologic blood markers, X-rays, or physiologic tests, no clear treatment guidelines are established to our knowledge. For these patients one may possibly overtreat some patients who are nonsymptomatic if the treatment itself does not prevent the development of the disease or undertreat patients if the treatment itself is effective to prevent the development of symptoms.

Taking all these uncertainties under consideration, we therefore argue that multicenter treatment studies are needed to establish sufficient knowledge so it may become possible to establish international guidelines, not only on the diagnostic level in this cohort of patients, but also on the treatment level.

Subjective Late Effects

Generally, specific treatment studies of subjective late effects have not been published and the clinician must therefore rely on general knowledge from other fields of medicine. An open pilot study on the effects of physical exercise upon fatigue in survivors supported the findings of a meta-analysis on the treatment of the chronic fatigue syndrome (CFS).[79,80] The fatigue level was reduced by 50% after an intervention of 12 weeks duration.[79] CFS differs from chronic fatigue in the survivors on several variables, including level of psychologic distress,[69] but physical exercise has multiple effects including lowered anxiety, depression, and fatigue levels. The exact mechanism for this effect in the survivors and in other patient groups is not known. The other type of therapy with effect on CFS, cognitive behavioral therapy, has not been tested on survivors specifically. However, it is reasonable to assume that physical exercise also has cognitive effects, that is, the subjects gain other cognitions about their physical capacity during such a training period. Oldervoll et al. also demonstrated that aerobic exercise improved subjective physical functioning and aerobic capacity.[79]

The high prevalence of hypothyroidism among the survivors and the tendency to substitute with thyroxin yield many survivors on thyroxin substitution therapy for long periods. It is reasonable to assume that fatigue is a central symptom when substitution is started. However, the clinical effect of such substitution is questionable, at least in terms of reduced fatigue-level. Knobel et al. demonstrated a significant higher level of fatigue among patients receiving thyroxin substitution than among unsubstituted patients with biochemical hypothyroidism.[55]

Anecdotally, fatigued survivors are offered antidepressants. In sufferers of the CFS, antidepressants have no effect unless fatigue is part of a depressive disorder.[80] A recent study of the effects of an antidepressant upon fatigue and depression in cancer patients demonstrated that fatigue was not improved (i.e., serotonin was not the mediator of fatigue in cancer patients) while depressive symptoms improved.[81] In sum, these findings indicate that fatigue in the survivors should not be treated with antidepressants unless fatigue is part of a depressive condition characterized by lowered mood and other depressive symptoms.

Treatment of psychologic symptoms should be based on a psychiatric diagnosis. Conditioned responses are best treated by unconditioning if the symptoms need to be treated. Whether to treat such symptoms depends on the subjects' wishes and the symptom burden. Conditioned responses only experienced at the sight of the hospital are probably less burdensome than responses triggered by food or beverages.[56] Anxiety may reflect quite different disorders: posttraumatic stress disorder (PTSD), panic disorder, or generalized anxiety disorder. Both pharmacologic and psychotherapeutic interventions differ among the three, and treatment must follow the general outlines for treatment of these conditions. For example, PTSD can be treated with exposure therapy, cognitive therapy, selective seratonin reuptake inhibitors (SSRIs), or combinations of the three.[82] Treatment of depression in somatically ill patients principally equals treatment of depression in "pure" psychiatric patients, although the presence of other somatic symptoms such as nausea can be of importance for the patients' compliance with the treatment.[83]

Conclusions

Present Level of Knowledge

Our present level of knowledge on late medical effects is characterized by uncertainties regarding prevalence and clinical significance of reported findings. The distinction between late effects and age- and lifestyle-related morbidity is unclear and generally is not properly controlled for. However, there is an increased risk for secondary cancers and particularly breast cancer in women irradiated by fields involving their breast during their reproductive years. Fatigue seem to be the most consistently reported subjective late effect, and survivors of Hodgkin's disease seem to be at particular risk for this late effect compared to other cancer survivors.

Treatment of late effects generally follows the general guidelines for treatment of the specific condition at stake, and the need for specific treatment studies may seem disputable. Some special considerations regarding volume of irradiation might indicate a need for specialized studies of optimal adjuvant treatment of breast cancer, for example. Given the prevalence of persisting fatigue and the uncertainty related to the treatment of fatigue, there seems to be a need for controlled trials on the treatment of this symptom.

Future

Future research on late effects should ideally be based upon larger data sets collected prospectively as part of multicenter studies, and the data collection should ideally start when treatment starts. Smaller or medium-sized cross-sectionally designed studies with retrospective data collection without specified hypotheses have been dominating until now, and such studies will probably be of lesser relevance in the future. There is also a need for representative comparison groups that make it possible to specifically estimate if there is an increase in specific disorders and symptoms. At present the cancer registers have this function regarding the secondary cancers, and this advantage has made the prevalence estimates of secondary cancers the most reliable among the reported late medical effects. An optimal strategy can be establishment of surveillance programs for the most prevalent and/or disabling late effects. There is also a definite need for improvement of measurement techniques for subjective late effects, but this is not a challenge for studies of cancer survivors in particular but rather a general challenge for the assessment of subjective health status. A better understanding of biologic mechanisms related to late subjective effects and particularly fatigue is warranted. Such knowledge can improve prevention as well as therapy.

In sum, the ideal goal should be to have sufficient knowledge to identify which patients are at risk for developing which late effects so that preventive measures can be taken at the earliest possible time or that optimal treatment can be offered before the late effects become a health problem of significant magnitude.

References

1. Gilbert R. Radiotherapy in Hodgkin's disease (malignant granulomatosis): anatomic and clinical foundations, governing principles, results. Am J Roentgenol 1939;41:198–241.
2. De Vita VT, Serpick AA, Carbone PP. Combination chemotherapy in the treatment of advanced Hodgkin's disease. Ann Intern Med 1970;73:881–895.
3. Easson EC, Russel MH. The cure of Hodgkin's disease. Br Med J 1963;1:1704–1707.
4. Easson EC. Possibilities for the cure of Hodgkin's disease. Cancer (Phila) 1966;19:345–350.
5. Wessely S, Hotopf M, Sharpe M. Chronic fatigue and its syndromes. Oxford: Oxford University Press, 1999.
6. Foss AA, Egeland T, Hansen S, Langholm R, Holte H, Kvaloy S. Hodgkin's disease in a national and hospital population: trends over 20 years. Eur J Cancer 1997;33(14):2380–2383.
7. Thomas RK, Re D, Zander T, Wolf J, Diehl V. Epidemiology and etiology of Hodgkin's lymphoma. Ann Oncol 2002;13(suppl 4): 147–152.
8. Glaser SL, Swartz WG. Time trends in Hodgkin's disease incidence. The role of diagnostic accuracy. Cancer (Phila) 1990; 66(10):2196–2204.
9. Glaser SL. Recent incidence and secular trends in Hodgkin's disease and its histologic subtypes. J Chronic Dis 1986;39(10): 789–798.

10. Aleman BM, van den Belt-Dusebout AW, Klokman WJ, Van't Veer MB, Bartelink H, van Leeuwen FE. Long-term cause-specific mortality of patients treated for Hodgkin's disease. J Clin Oncol 2003;21(18):3431–3439.
11. Vaughan HB, Vaughan HG, Linch DC, Anderson L. Late mortality in young BNLI patients cured of Hodgkin's disease. Ann Oncol 1994;5(suppl 2)0:65–66.
12. The Cancer Registry of Norway. Cancer in Norway 2001. Oslo: The Cancer Registry of Norway, 2004.
13. The Cancer Registry of Norway. Cancer in Norway 1992. Oslo: The Cancer Registry of Norway, 1992.
14. Canellos GP. Primary treatment of Hodgkin's disease. Ann Oncol 2002;13(suppl 4):153–158.
15. Josting A, Engert A, Diehl V, Canellos GP. Prognostic factors and treatment outcome in patients with primary progressive and relapsed Hodgkin's disease. Ann Oncol 2002;13(suppl 1): 112–116.
16. Donaldson SS, Hancock SL, Hoppe RT. The Janeway lecture. Hodgkin's disease: finding the balance between cure and late effects. Cancer J Sci Am 1999;5(6):325–333.
17. Yung L, Linch D. Hodgkin's lymphoma. Lancet 2003;361(9361): 943–951.
18. Ng AK, Bernardo MP, Weller E, et al. Long-term survival and competing causes of death in patients with early-stage Hodgkin's disease treated at age 50 or younger. J Clin Oncol 2002;20(8): 2101–2108.
19. van Rijswijk RE, Verbeek J, Haanen C, Dekker AW, van Daal WA, van Peperzeel HA. Major complications and causes of death in patients treated for Hodgkin's disease. J Clin Oncol 1987;5(10):1624–1633.
20. Abrahamsen AF, Loge JH, Hannisdal E, et al. Late medical sequelae after therapy for supradiaphragmatic Hodgkin's disease. Acta Oncol 1999;38(4):511–515.
21. Boivin JF, Hutchison GB, Lubin JH, Mauch P. Coronary artery disease mortality in patients treated for Hodgkin's disease. Cancer (Phila) 1992;69(5):1241–1247.
22. Cosset JM, Henry-Amar M, Pellae-Cosset B, et al. Pericarditis and myocardial infarctions after Hodgkin's disease therapy. Int J Radiat Oncol Biol Phys 1991;21(2):447–449.
23. Hancock SL, Tucker MA, Hoppe RT. Factors affecting late mortality from heart disease after treatment of Hodgkin's disease. JAMA 1993;270(16):1949–1955.
24. Sears JD, Greven KM, Ferree CR, D'Agostino RB Jr. Definitive irradiation in the treatment of Hodgkin's disease. Analysis of outcome, prognostic factors, and long-term complications. Cancer (Phila) 1997;79(1):145–151.
25. Lund MB, Ihlen H, Voss BM, et al. Increased risk of heart valve regurgitation after mediastinal radiation for Hodgkin's disease: an echocardiographic study. Heart 1996;75(6):591–595.
26. Gustavsson A, Eskilsson J, Landberg T, et al. Late cardiac effects after mantle radiotherapy in patients with Hodgkin's disease. Ann Oncol 1990;1(5):355–363.
27. Glanzmann C, Huguenin P, Lutolf UM, Maire R, Jenni R, Gumppenberg V. Cardiac lesions after mediastinal irradiation for Hodgkin's disease. Radiother Oncol 1994;30(1):43–54.
28. Hancock SL, Cox RS, McDougall IR. Thyroid diseases after treatment of Hodgkin's disease. N Engl J Med 1991;325(9): 599–605.
29. Peerboom PF, Hassink EA, Melkert R, DeWit L, Nooijen WJ, Bruning PF. Thyroid function 10–18 years after mantle field irradiation for Hodgkin's disease. Eur J Cancer 1992;28A(10): 1716–1718.
30. Brierley JD, Rathmell AJ, Gospodarowicz MK, et al. Late effects of treatment for early-stage Hodgkin's disease. Br J Cancer 1998; 77(8):1300–1310.
31. Bethge W, Guggenberger D, Bamberg M, Kanz L, Bokemeyer C. Thyroid toxicity of treatment for Hodgkin's disease. Ann Hematol 2000;79(3):114–118.
32. Mauch P, Tarbell N, Weinstein H, et al. Stage IA and IIA supradiaphragmatic Hodgkin's disease: prognostic factors in surgically staged patients treated with mantle and paraaortic irradiation. J Clin Oncol 1988;6(10):1576–1583.
33. Hassink EA, Souren TS, Boersma LJ, et al. Pulmonary morbidity 10–18 years after irradiation for Hodgkin's disease. Eur J Cancer 1993;29A(3):343–347.
34. Loyer E, Fuller L, Libshitz HI, Palmer JL. Radiographic appearance of the chest following therapy for Hodgkin disease. Eur J Radiol 2000;35(2):136–148.
35. Lund MB, Kongerud J, Nome O, et al. Lung function impairment in long-term survivors of Hodgkin's disease. Ann Oncol 1995;6(5):495–501.
36. Koocher G, O'Malley J. The Damocles Syndrome: Psychosocial Consequences of Surviving Childhood Cancer. New York: McGraw-Hill, 1981.
37. Tross S, Holland JC. Psychological sequelae in cancer survivors. In: Holland JC, Rowland JH (eds). Handbook of Psychooncology. London: Oxford University Press, 1990:101–116.
38. Cella DF, Tross S. Psychological adjustment to survival from Hodgkin's disease. J Consult Clin Psychol 1986;54(5):616–622.
39. The Constitution of the World Health Organisation. WHO Chronicle 1947;29.
40. Fobair P, Hoppe RT, Bloom J, Cox R, Varghese A, Spiegel D. Psychosocial problems among survivors of Hodgkin's disease. J Clin Oncol 1986;4(5):805–814.
41. Kornblith AB, Anderson J, Cella DF, et al. Hodgkin disease survivors at increased risk for problems in psychosocial adaptation. The Cancer and Leukemia Group B. Cancer (Phila) 1992;70(8): 2214–2224.
42. van Tulder MW, Aaronson NK, Bruning PF. The quality of life of long-term survivors of Hodgkin's disease. Ann Oncol 1994; 5(2):153–158.
43. Norum J, Wist EA. Quality of life in survivors of Hodgkin's disease. Qual Life Res 1996;5(3):367–374.
44. Joly F, Henry-Amar M, Arveux P, et al. Late psychosocial sequelae in Hodgkin's disease survivors: a French population-based case-control study. J Clin Oncol 1996;14(9):2444–2453.
45. Aaronson NK, Cull A, Kaasa S. The EORTC modular approach to quality of life assessment in oncology. Int J Ment Health 1994;23:75–96.
46. Cella DF, Tulsky DS, Gray G, et al. The Functional Assessment of Cancer Therapy scale: development and validation of the general measure. J Clin Oncol 1993;11(3):570–579.
47. Ware JE. The SF-36 health survey. In: Spilker B (ed). Quality of Life and Pharmaeconomics in Clinical Trials. Philadelphia: Lippincott-Raven, 1996:337–346.
48. Loge JH, Kaasa S. Short form 36 (SF-36) health survey: normative data from the general Norwegian population. Scand J Soc Med 1998;26(4):250–258.
49. Loge JH, Abrahamsen AF, Ekeberg O, Kaasa S. Reduced health-related quality of life among Hodgkin's disease survivors: a comparative study with general population norms. Ann Oncol 1999;10(1):71–77.
50. Bloom JR, Gorsky RD, Fobair P, et al. Physical performance at work and at leisure: validation of a measure of biological energy in survivors of Hodgkin's disease. J Psychosocial Oncol 1990; 8(1):49–63.
51. Bloom JR, Fobair P, Gritz E, et al. Psychosocial outcomes of cancer: a comparative analysis of Hodgkin's disease and testicular cancer. J Clin Oncol 1993;11(5):979–988.
52. Greil R, Holzner B, Kemmler G, et al. Retrospective assessment of quality of life and treatment outcome in patients with Hodgkin's disease from 1969 to 1994. Eur J Cancer 1999;35(5): 698–706.
53. Olweny CL, Juttner CA, Rofe P, et al. Long-term effects of cancer treatment and consequences of cure: cancer survivors enjoy

quality of life similar to their neighbours. Eur J Cancer 1993; 29A(6):826–830.
54. Gil-Fernandez J, Ramos C, Tamayo T, et al. Quality of life and psychological well-being in Spanish long-term survivors of Hodgkin's disease: results of a controlled pilot study. Ann Hematol 2003;82(1):14–18.
55. Knobel H, Havard LJ, Brit LM, Forfang K, Nome O, Kaasa S. Late medical complications and fatigue in Hodgkin's disease survivors. J Clin Oncol 2001;19(13):3226–3233.
56. Cameron CL, Cella D, Herndon JE, et al. Persistent symptoms among survivors of Hodgkin's disease: an explanatory model based on classical conditioning. Health Psychol 2001;20(1): 71–75.
57. Osoba D, Rodrigues G, Myles J, Zee B, Pater J. Interpreting the significance of changes in health-related quality-of-life scores. J Clin Oncol 1998;16(1):139–144.
58. Lee JQ, Simmonds MJ, Wang XS, Novy DM. Differences in physical performance between men and women with and without lymphoma. Arch Phys Med Rehabil 2003;84(12): 1747–1752.
59. Devlen J, Maguire P, Phillips P, Crowther D. Psychological problems associated with diagnosis and treatment of lymphomas. II: Prospective study. Br Med J (Clin Res Ed) 1987;295(6604): 955–957.
60. Devlen J, Maguire P, Phillips P, Crowther D, Chambers H. Psychological problems associated with diagnosis and treatment of lymphomas. I: Retrospective study. Br Med J (Clin Res Ed) 1987; 295(6604):953–954.
61. Lewis G, Wessely S. The epidemiology of fatigue: more questions than answers. J Epidemiol Community Health 1992;46(2): 92–97.
62. Pawlikowska T, Chalder T, Hirsch SR, Wallace P, Wright DJ, Wessely SC. Population based study of fatigue and psychological distress [see comments]. BMJ 1994;308(6931):763–766.
63. Ganz PA, Moinpour CM, Pauler DK, et al. Health status and quality of life in patients with early-stage Hodgkin's disease treated on Southwest Oncology Group Study 9133. J Clin Oncol 2003;21(18):3512–3519.
64. Kornblith AB, Herndon JE, Zuckerman E, et al. Comparison of psychosocial adaptation of advanced stage Hodgkin's disease and acute leukemia survivors. Cancer and Leukemia Group B. Ann Oncol 1998;9(3):297–306.
65. Loge JH, Abrahamsen AF, Ekeberg O, Kaasa S. Hodgkin's disease survivors more fatigued than the general population. J Clin Oncol 1999;17(1):253–261.
66. Ruffer JU, Flechtner H, Tralls P, et al. Fatigue in long-term survivors of Hodgkin's lymphoma: a report from the German Hodgkin Lymphoma Study Group (GHSG). Eur J Cancer 2003; 39(15):2179–2186.
67. Wettergren L, Bjorkholm M, Axdorph U, Bowling A, Langius-Eklof A. Individual quality of life in long-term survivors of Hodgkin's lymphoma: a comparative study. Qual Life Res 2003; 12(5):545–554.
68. Fossa SD, Dahl AA, Loge JH. Fatigue, anxiety and depression and mental health in long-term survivors of testicular cancer. J Clin Oncol 2003;21:1249–1254.
69. Loge JH, Abrahamsen AF, Ekeberg, Kaasa S. Fatigue and psychiatric morbidity among Hodgkin's disease survivors. J Pain Symptom Manag 2000;19(2):91–99.
70. Visser MR, Smets EM. Fatigue, depression and quality of life in cancer patients: how are they related? Support Care Cancer 1998;6(2):101–108.
71. Cleeland CS, Bennett GJ, Dantzer R, et al. Are the symptoms of cancer and cancer treatment due to a shared biologic mechanism? A cytokine-immunologic model of cancer symptoms. Cancer (Phila) 2003;97(11):2919–2925.
72. Knobel H, Loge JH, Nordoy T, et al. High level of fatigue in lymphoma patients treated with high dose therapy. J Pain Symptom Manag 2000;19(6):446–456.
73. Wessely S, Chalder T, Hirsch S, Wallace P, Wright D. Psychological symptoms, somatic symptoms, and psychiatric disorder in chronic fatigue and chronic fatigue syndrome: a prospective study in the primary care setting. Am J Psychiatry 1996;153(8): 1050–1059.
74. Loge JH, Abrahamsen AF, Ekeberg O, Hannisdal E, Kaasa S. Psychological distress after cancer cure: a survey of 459 Hodgkin's disease survivors. Br J Cancer 1997;76(6):791–796.
75. Herrmann C. International experiences with the Hospital Anxiety and Depression Scale: a review of validation data and clinical results. J Psychosom Res 1997;42(1):17–41.
76. Minaire P. Disease, illness and health: theoretical models of the disablement process. Bull WHO 1992;70(3):373–379.
77. Abrahamsen AF, Loge JH, Hannisdal E, Holte H, Kvaloy S. Socio-medical situation for long-term survivors of Hodgkin's disease: a survey of 459 patients treated at one institution. Eur J Cancer 1998;34(12):1865–1870.
78. Ringdal GI, Ringdal K, Jordhoy MS, Ahlner-Elmqvist M, Jannert M, Kaasa S. Health-related quality of life (HRQOL) in family members of cancer victims: results from a longitudinal intervention study in Norway and Sweden. Palliat Med 2004;18(2): 108–120.
79. Oldervoll LM, Kaasa S, Knobel H, Loge JH. Exercise reduces fatigue in chronic fatigued Hodgkin's disease survivors: results from a pilot study. Eur J Cancer 2003;39(1):57–63.
80. Whiting P, Bagnall AM, Sowden AJ, Cornell JE, Mulrow CD, Ramirez G. Interventions for the treatment and management of chronic fatigue syndrome: a systematic review. JAMA 2001; 286(11):1360–1368.
81. Morrow GR, Hickok JT, Roscoe JA, et al. Differential effects of paroxetine on fatigue and depression: a randomized, double-blind trial from the University of Rochester Cancer Center community clinical oncology program. J Clin Oncol 2003;21(24): 4635–4641.
82. Yehuda R. Post-traumatic stress disorder. N Engl J Med 2002; 346(2):108–114.
83. Gill D, Hatcher S. Antidepressants for depression in people with physical illness. Cochrane Database Syst Rev 2000;2:CD001312.

104

Medical and Psychosocial Issues in Testicular Cancer Survivors

Sophie D. Fosså, Lois B. Travis, and Alvin A. Dahl

Testicular cancer (TC) is the most frequent malignancy in men between 20 and 40 years of age, and the annual incidence rates are continuously increasing in the Western world.[1] Since the introduction of cisplatin-based chemotherapy, at least 90% of the patients are cured,[2] and testicular cancer survivors (TCSs) currently have a life expectancy similar to that of age-matched normal men, with posttreatment life spans of 30 to 50 years. Thus, an increasing number of TCSs experience survivorship problems related to the malignancy, its treatment, or both.

Treatment

Unilateral orchiectomy is the primary treatment of TC and yields the histologic diagnosis of seminoma and nonseminoma with equal frequency (see Chapter 49). Modern postorchiectomy therapy of TC is based on the histologic type and the extent of disease. Risk-adapted treatment is based on a balance between malignancy-related risk factors, expected side effects, the likelihood of regular follow-up, and, not least, the patient's preference. As effective chemotherapy is available to salvage most of the patients who relapse, today's clinicians tend to administer the least toxic treatment schedule to both low-risk patients without metastases and to the good prognosis metastatic group.[3]

In patients with nonmetastatic seminoma, the standard adjuvant radiotherapy field currently comprises the intradiaphragmatic paraaortic lymph nodes,[4] which are irradiated to 20Gy.[5] Surveillance[6] is a valid alternative, or the use of one cycle of chemotherapy.[7] *Surveillance* is also the standard policy in patients with nonmetastatic, nonseminomatous germ cell tumors,[8] with nerve-sparing retroperitoneal lymph node dissection (RPLND), or two cycles of chemotherapy as alternatives in selected patients.[9,10] In patients with metastatic disease, the standard *chemotherapy* regimen is cisplatin based, most often containing etoposide and bleomycin,[11,12] eventually modified by ifosfamide[13] or taxol in high-risk patients or used as salvage chemotherapy.[14] In patients with metastatic disease, induction chemotherapy is frequently followed by surgical resection of residual masses.[15]

Each of the foregoing principal therapeutic modalities (surgery, radiotherapy, chemotherapy) leads to transient short-term (less than 1 year) and long-term (1 year or more) side effects, and their severity often increases with combined treatment. Previous cross-sectional studies on long-term side effects in TCSs have predominantly examined the side effects within the first 5 years posttreatment. Relatively few studies have follow-up times beyond 5 years.

Not all long-term sequelae in TCSs are caused by treatment. Impaired posttreatment endocrine and exocrine gonadal function, for example, is related both to the germ cell malignancy itself and to its treatment. The development of a contralateral testicular tumor is treatment independent and represents primary germ cell carcinogenesis at another site. The diagnosis of a second, possibly treatment-related, malignancy must be clearly separated from a late relapse with non-germ cell differentiation. Leukemia in patients with mediastinal germ cell tumor may thus be treatment related or may arise on the background of the extragonadal germ cell malignancy,[16] recognizable by modern molecular biologic techniques.[17]

Second Malignancies

Solid Tumors

The most serious late toxicity of therapy for TC is the development of a non-germ cell malignancy, for simplicity referred to as second cancer. Although several investigations[18,19] have evaluated the risk of second cancers among patients with TC, few studies have estimated long-term risks among large numbers of TCSs, taking into consideration both histology and initial treatment. The largest study to date comprised more than 28,000 1-year TCSs (1935–1993) reported to population-based cancer registries in North America and Europe.[18] Second cancers were diagnosed in 1,406 patients [observed to expected ratio (O/E), 1.43; 95% confidence interval (CI), 1.36–1.51; absolute excess risk, 16 excess cancers per 10,000 men per year]. Second cancer risk was similar following seminomas (O/E, 1.4) and nonseminomatous tumors (O/E, 1.5).

TABLE 104.1. Relative risk of second malignancies following treatment of testicular cancer.

	No. of second cancers	*Relative risk*		
		All	*Seminoma*	*Nonseminoma*
All second cancers	1,406	1.43	1.42	1.50
All solid tumours	1,251	1.35	1.35	1.36
Stomach	93	1.95	1.73	2.95
Small intestine	12	3.18	4.35	—
Colon	105	1.27	1.30	1.32*
Rectum	77	1.41	1.58	0.92*
Pancreas	66	2.21	2.35	1.85*
Kidney	55	1.50	1.50	1.41*
Bladder	154	2.02	2.12	1.85
Melanoma	58	1.69	1.57	1.74
Thyroid	19	2.92	2.61	3.82
Connective tissue	22	3.16	3.46	2.40*
Non-Hodgkin's lymphoma	68	1.88	1.83	2.09
All leukemias**	64	2.13	1.92	2.78

*Nonsignificant.

**Statistical significance restricted to acute leukemia.

Source: Modified from Travis et al.,[18] by permission of *Journal of the Naional Cancer Institute*, with emphasis on statistically significant ($P < 0.05$) observations.

Among all TCSs, significantly increased risks were observed for all malignancies taken together: malignant melanoma, acute lymphoblastic leukemia, acute nonlymphocytic leukemia, non-Hodgkin's lymphoma, and cancers of the stomach, colon, rectum, pancreas, kidney, bladder, thyroid, and connective tissue (Table 104.1). The risk of solid tumors increased with follow-up time since the diagnosis of TC and reached 1.5 after two decades (*P* trend, 0.00002). Twenty-year survivors of TC remained at significantly increased risk for cancers of stomach (O/E, 2.3), colon (O/E, 1.7), pancreas (O/E, 3.2), kidney (O/E, 2.3), bladder (O/E, 2.8), and connective tissue (O/E, 4.7). The cumulative risk of any second cancer 25 years after TC diagnosis was 15.7% (Figure 104.1, Table 104.2). The larger risk for seminoma patients (18.2%; 95% CI, 16.8–19.6) than for those with nonseminomatous tumors (11.1%; 95% CI, 9.3–12.9) most likely reflects the older mean age of the former group (39.2 years versus 29.8 years), given the similarity in the excess cumulative risks. The temporal distribution of increased risks and apportionment between treatment groups were consistent with the late sequelae of radiation for cancers of stomach, bladder, and possibly pancreas. These findings were thus consistent with the location of these organs in the infradiaphragmatic radiotherapy fields administered for TC. Although information on radiotherapy fields and dose are not registered in cancer registry records, Travis et al.[18] provided estimates of the average radiation doses received by stomach (mean, 13–26 Gy), bladder (mean, 22.4–45 Gy), and pancreas (mean, 16.7–33.8 Gy) at treatment doses of 25 and 50 Gy for seminomas and nonseminomatous germ cell cancer, respectively, using standard anteroposterior (AP)/posteroanterior paraaortic or inguinal iliac fields.[4]

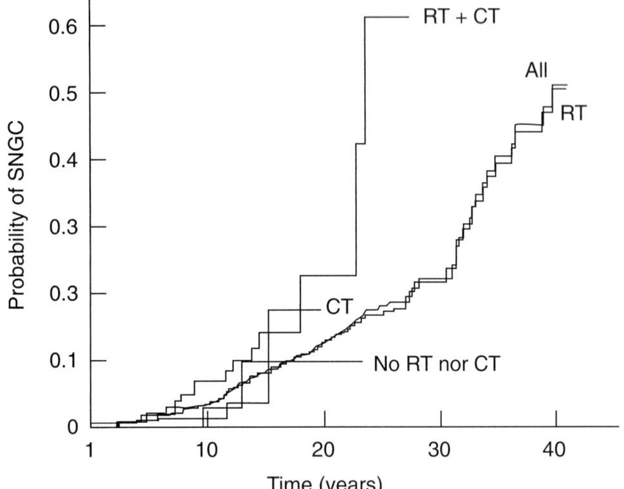

FIGURE 104.1. Cumulative risk of any second non-germ cell cancer by time from primary diagnosis for different treatment groups. (See Table 104.2.) *RT*, radiotherapy; *CT*, chemotherapy. (From Hoff Wanderas et al.,[23] by permission of *European Journal of Cancer*.)

Previous clinical series have found significantly eightfold-increased risks of stomach cancer ($n = 2$) following infra- and supradiaphragmatic irradiation for testicular tumors[20] and a four- to fivefold risk with abdominal radiotherapy ($n = 10$).[21] There are few data, however, that quantify the relationship between radiation dose and the risk of gastric cancer.[22] In particular, the precise impact of radiation field size and/or dose is not clearly defined for current infradiaphragmatic adjuvant

TABLE 104.2. Patients at risk at start of interval.[a]

Time from diagnosis (years)	*Treatment category (n)* *RT*	*CT*	*RT + CT*	*No RT or CT*	*All*
1–9	1,194	346	277	189	2,006
10–19	827	112	83	59	1,081
20–29	365	2	7	5	379
30–39	92	—	—	—	92

[a] See Figure 104.1 for further information and definitions.

radiotherapy. Therefore, the NCRI (National Cancer Research Institute, UK) Testis Cancer Clinical Studies Group has initiated a long-term follow-up study of 2,500 patients with stage I TC treated between 1962 and 1994 with infradiaphragmatic radiotherapy, recording the individual target fields and doses, and any salvage treatment as predictors of development of second cancer.

Before the use of cisplatin in TC therapy, few patients treated with chemotherapy only lived long enough to develop a secondary malignancy. To date, modern chemotherapy alone (e.g., bleomycin, etoposide, and cisplatin, or BEP) has not, to our knowledge, been associated with an increased risk of secondary solid tumors. The number of patients observed for more than 10 years after cisplatin-based chemotherapy is limited, however, and further follow-up will be required.

There is also little information on whether TC patients treated with both radiotherapy and chemotherapy are at greater risk of solid tumors than those who received radiation alone. Van Leeuwen et al.[21] found that the risk of all gastrointestinal cancers following radiotherapy alone (O/E, 2.9; 95% CI, 1.8–4.4; observed, 22) did not differ significantly from the risk (O/E, 5.5; 95% CI 1.1–15.9; observed, 3) in patients given both radiotherapy and chemotherapy, but low numbers in the latter group limit the statistical power to detect any difference.

Hoff Wanderas et al.[23] showed that the risk of all second non-germ cell cancers following radiotherapy alone (O/E, 1.58; 95% CI, 1.3–1.9; observed, 130) was significantly larger than the risk (O/E, 3.54; 95% CI, 2.0–5.8; observed, 15) after radiotherapy plus chemotherapy, but also pointed out that patients in the latter group frequently received multiple irradiation fields and larger doses. Further, many patients who received combined-modality therapy also received chemotherapy regimens that included doxorubicin.[23] Breslow and colleagues[24] reported that children (n = 234) given doxorubicin and more than 35 Gy of abdominal radiation for Wilm's tumor were at 36-fold risk (95% CI, 16–72; observed, 8) of second solid tumors, compared with no second tumors observed among children (n = 291) given doxorubicin alone.[24] These investigators[24] hypothesized that doxorubicin might inhibit the repair of radiation-induced damage, perhaps through its effects on topo-isomerase II. Evidence with regard to the human carcinogenicity of doxorubicin itself remains conflicting.[20]

Leukemias

TCS patients are at increased risk of leukemia[18,21,25–29]; however, there are few analytical studies that characterize in detail the contribution of both radiotherapy and chemotherapy to these cancers. Travis and colleagues[16] conducted an international case-control investigation of secondary myelodysplastic syndrome or leukemia within a cohort of 18,567 1-year TCSs survivors of TC diagnosed between 1970 and 1993 and reported to eight population-based cancer registries in North America and Europe. For all patients (36 cases, 106 controls), detailed information on all treatment was gathered for chemotherapy drugs including cumulative dose and duration of chemotherapy. External-beam radiotherapy, usually to paraaortic and pelvic regions, was administered to 101 patients. Radiotherapy for 17 patients (restricted to 1970–1980) included mediastinal irradiation (mean dose, 35.0 Gy), in addition to abdominal and pelvic fields; 3 additional patients were given extended-field (abdomen/pelvis/chest) radiotherapy and alkylating agent chemotherapy. For patients who received radiation limited to abdomen and pelvis without alkylating agents, larger mean treatment doses were used for nonseminomatous tumors (35.4 Gy) than for seminomas (30.7 Gy). Daily radiotherapy logs for each patient were used to calculate an average dose to the active bone marrow.

For all TC patients, leukemia risk increased with increasing radiation dose to active bone marrow (P = 0.02), with patients given chest radiotherapy in addition to abdominal/pelvic fields accounting for much of the risk at higher doses.[16] A nonsignificant 3-fold-increased relative risk of leukemia was demonstrated after pelvic-abdominal radiotherapy (mean dose to bone marrow, 10.9 Gy) without alkylating agent chemotherapy; for patients who received additional supradiaphragmatic irradiation (mean dose to bone marrow 19.5 Gy), a significantly increased 11-fold risk was apparent. For patients given radiotherapy limited to abdomen and pelvis, the estimated relative risk (RR) of leukemia associated with a treatment dose of 25, 30, and 35 Gy was 2.2, 2.5, and 2.9, respectively; none of these estimates was statistically significant.

Radiation dose to active bone marrow and cumulative dose of cisplatin to treat TC were both predictive of elevated risks of leukemia (P = 0.001) in a statistical model that took into account all treatment parameters.[16] The highly significant dose–response relationship observed for total amount of cisplatin and leukemia risk was in accord with results in a study of women treated with platinum-based chemotherapy for ovarian cancer.[30]

Although the cumulative dose of etoposide used to treat TC did not contribute to leukemia risk when doses of cisplatin and radiation were taken into account, patients given etoposide also received larger amounts of cisplatin, making it difficult to tease apart any individual contributions to leukemia risk.[16] The predicted risk of leukemia associated with a cumulative cisplatin dose of 650 mg was 3.2 (95% CI, 1.5–8.4); larger cumulative doses (1,000 mg cisplatin) were associated with significantly increased sixfold risks. In terms of absolute risk, Travis et al.[16] estimated that of 10,000 testicular cancer patients treated with cisplatin-based chemotherapy with a cumulative cisplatin dose of about 650 mg and followed for 15 years, 16 excess leukemias might result.

Based on small numbers, prior studies have linked etoposide and cisplatin for TC with excess leukemias,[26–29] usually at high cumulative doses of etoposide (3,000 mg/m^2)[26] in contrast to the lower total doses administered in the study by Travis et al.,[30] which are similar to the dose of less than 2,000 mg/m^2 (33) used today. Smith et al.[31] reported that the 6-year cumulative risk of secondary leukemia among patients who received 1,500 to 2,999 mg/m^2 etoposide was small (0.7%), based on a survey of clinical trials. In a recent review of the literature, Kollmannsberger et al.[32] concluded that the cumulative incidence of leukemia for TC patients given etoposide at cumulative doses of less than 2,000 mg/m^2 and more than 2,000 mg/m^2 was 0.5% and 2% at a median of 5 years follow-up.

Whether combined radiochemotherapy for TC results in a larger risk of leukemia than chemotherapy alone has not been well-studied. Van Leeuwen et al.[21] found no significant difference between the risk of leukemia following chemotherapy alone (one case) and combined modality therapy (two cases), but the small numbers precluded any opportunity to detect a difference. Similarly, in the case-control study by Travis et al.,[16] only a small number of patients were given combined-modality therapy (two cases and four controls), and the risk of leukemia (fivefold) was nearly identical for all investigated patients.

Contralateral TC

Three percent to 5% of the patients with unilateral TC develop a germ cell malignancy of the contralateral testicle.[33] The increased risk of contralateral TC in men with TC has generally been thought to reflect shared etiologic influences.[34] Few large studies,[33,35] however, have provided estimates of the risk for contralateral TC. The largest investigation[35] to date, based on 60 cases occurring in 2,201 men diagnosed with a first primary germ cell cancer (1953–1990), reported that the cumulative risk of a contralateral testicular cancer at 15 years of follow-up was 3.9% (95% CI, 2.8%–5.0%). The investigators also concluded that the risk was not significantly altered by treatment of the first cancer. Patients with a contralateral testicular cancer usually undergo a second orchiectomy with the subsequent need of lifelong androgen substitution.

Patients with extragonadal germ cell tumors (EGCT) are at a significantly elevated risk for subsequently developing TC, most probably based on the existence of carcinoma in situ in one or both testicles.[36,37] In a large, international study of 635 patients with EGCT conducted by Hartmann and colleagues,[36] the cumulative risk of developing a metachronous TC was 10.3% at 10 years. The treatment follows the risk-adapted strategies as for TC with principally the same long-term sequelae.

Based on the increased risk of developing a new gonadal germ cell tumor, TCSs and patients with a cured extragonadal tumor are recommended to perform regular testicular self-examination.

Gonadal Toxicity

Spermatogenesis and Leydig Cell Function

According to today's most relevant hypothesis, germ cell carcinogenesis starts in the primordial cells during the 8th week of embryonic life.[38] Deleterious environmental influences may result in aberrant gonadal development that subsequently manifests as testicular maldescent, testicular atrophy, reduced Lydig cell function, impaired spermatogenesis, or even germ cell malignancy. These etiologic factors together with tumor-related influences are the reasons why about 60% of unilaterally orchiectomized patients with newly diagnosed TC have impaired spermatogenesis before any additional treatment.[39–43] Impaired Leydig cell function and reduced sperm cell production may be found even in patients with TC before orchiectomy of the affected testicle.[41–43] Further, this etiologic hypothesis also explains why 10% to 15% of TCSs have permanently reduced exocrine and endocrine gonadal function even without having received chemotherapy or radiotherapy.[44,45]

The exocrine long-term gonadal function in TCSs has been extensively studied, although the available investigations do not clearly differentiate between cisplatin-based chemotherapy containing vinblastine from those containing etoposide or ifosfamide. Carboplatin seems to be less gonadotoxic than cisplatin.[46] Standard cisplatin-based chemotherapy (four cycles) and infradiaphragmatic radiotherapy (36 Gy or less) transiently reduces or abolishes spermatogenesis (low sperm counts; high serum follicle-stimulating hormone, FSH) with recovery starting 6 to 8 months after treatment discontinuation. These effects are dependent on the type of the radiation target field as well as types of cytotoxic drugs, number of cycles, and cumulative doses[4,39,40,42,47–59] (Figure 104.2, Table 104.3). Age above 35 years and reduced pretreatment gonadal function reduce the ability for such recovery.[52]

The Leydig cell function is affected by radiotherapy or chemotherapy at a lesser degree than spermatogenesis, but Nord et al.[45] demonstrated an increasing number of hypogonadal long-term TCSs in relation to treatment type and treatment intensity. According to this study 16% of the long-term TCSs are hypogonadal, most often subclinically, but 25% of these TCSs need androgen substitution.

There is no effective treatment available for TCSs who have become oligo- or azospermic as a result of cytotoxic treatment. Moreover, treatment with luteinizing hormone-releasing hormone (LH-RH) analogues together with chemotherapy has not shown sufficient gonadal protection either.[60] Pretreatment cryopreservation of sperm cells[61] and exogenous androgen substitution[62] thus remain the only means to ameliorate gonadotoxic long-term sequelae.

Somatic Aspects of Fertility

Posttreatment fertility is threatened by ejaculatory dysfunction, permanent azospermia, or high-grade oligospermia, and psychosocial distress.

After bilateral radical template RPLND[63,64] almost all TCSs have to face infertility problems as a result of postoperative "dry ejaculation." The introduction of unilateral and/or nerve-sparing procedures[10] has reduced this proportion to 10% to 15% even when the operation is performed following chemotherapy.[65] However, even though statistical analyses have proven that fertility-saving strategies have been successful in groups of patients prediction of posttreatment fertility is difficult in the *individual patient*. It is, therefore,

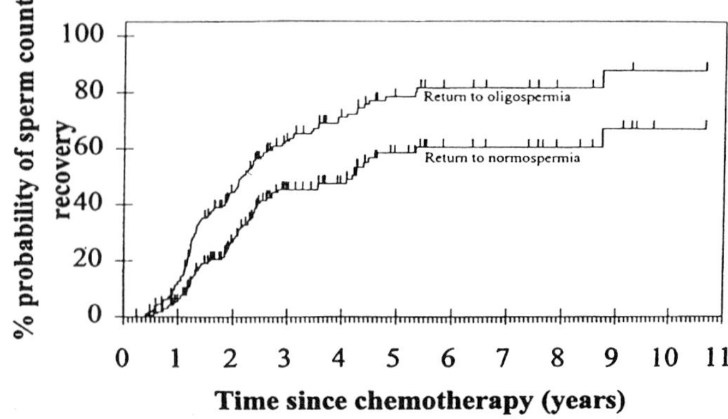

FIGURE 104.2. Recovery to oligospermia and normospermia in 178 patients after chemotherapy for testicular cancer. (From Lampe et al.,[47] by permission of *Journal of Clinical Oncology*.)

TABLE 104.3. Long-term gonadal function in testicular cancer survivors.[a]

Author		*No. of patients*	*Observation time (months)*	*Sperm count (10^6/mL)*	*Azospermia*	*Elevated* LH	*Elevated* FSH	*Sub-normal testosterone*
Surgery only								
Aass (1991)		33	24–48b	20[c]	11/24	1	8	5
Jacobsen (2000)		60	63	(0–222)[b]			10	
				37				
				(0–243)				
Radiotherapy								
Aass (1991)		36	24–48	11 (0–76)	9/22	2	13	4
Jacobsen (1997)								
Dog-leg		44	12	20 ± 14, 0[d]				
Paraaortic		24	12	49 ± 35, 6[d]				
Fosså (1999)								
Dog-leg		48	18		17/48			
Paraaortic		54	18		6/54			
Chemotherapy								
Cisplatin-based								
Standard								
Aass (1991)		42	24–48	65	5/17	5	17	6
Petersen (1994)		33	79	(0–166)	5/27	8	8	1
Stephenson (1995)		30	>24	6 (0–83)	6/30			
Palmieri (1996)		28	37		6/28	4	11	3
				35 (0–90)				
High dose or combined with radiotherapy	Aass (1991)	19	24–48			3	12	4
	Peterson (1994)	21	58	0 (0–70)	8/17	8	22	2
	Palmieri (1996)	10	36	8 (0–18)	3/10	6	8	2
Carboplatin	Reiter (1998)	22	48	(35–128)				
	Lampe (1999)	59	30		12/59			
Not specified	Bokemeyer (1996)	63	58			21	40	6
	Lampe (1999)	119	30		50/119			
	Strumberg (2002)	30	15			13	22	2

Blank spaces indicate that information is not provided.

[a] Limited to reports published after 1990.

[b] Range.

[c] Median.

[d] Mean ± standard deviation (only patients with pretreatment sperm count ≥10).

recommended that sperm banking[61] with the possibility of assisted fertilization[66] is offered to all patients with newly diagnosed TC who do not explicitly exclude future fatherhood. (See also Chapter 90).

Gonadal Long-Term Effects of Treatment for Bilateral TC

Testicular radiotherapy (18–20 Gy) usually prevents the development of an invasive cancer in TCSs with cancer in situ in the contralateral testicle,[67] although with an increased risk of hypogonadism. Surgical testicle-saving strategies are recommended in case of small tumors.[68]

Neurologic Morbidity

Peripheral Neurotoxicity

Cisplatin-based chemotherapy leads to dose-dependent peripheral sensory neuropathy (paraesthesiae, pain) with a peak occurrence about 6 months after treatment initiation and a slight decrease thereafter.[53,69–73] Vinblastine displays an at least additive effect, whereas VP-16 is less neurotoxic.[11] About 20% of TCSs report peripheral sensory neuropathy ("quite a bit," "very much") 2 years after three or four cycles of BEP chemotherapy,[73] although objective measurements reveal persistent peripheral neuropathy in 70% to 80% of the patients.[74] The long-term peripheral sensory neuropathy is, however, only rarely handicapping, and most TCSs have "become used" to this problem at long-term follow-up.

Ototoxicity

Ototoxicity represents a specific long-term sequela in TCSs after cisplatin-containing chemotherapy,[53,57,69,73,75,76] with tinnitus and hearing loss in about 25% and 20% of the patients, respectively.[53,69,73] Audiograms indicate that cisplatin mostly decreases the auditory acuity above 4,000 Hz.[57] To decrease long-term ototoxicity, each cycle of standard chemotherapy (BEP) should be given during 5 days, in particular if more than three cycles are planned.[73]

Autonomic Neuropathy

The resection of sympathetic nerve fibers may lead to considerable persistent disturbance of blood flow and temperature sense in the legs.[77] The possibility exists that chemotherapy-induced long-term autonomic neurotoxicity contributes to vascular dysfunction.[78,79]

Because no effective treatment exists for cisplatin-induced peripheral neuropathy or ototoxicity, prevention of these late effects is essential by adequate hydration during drug administration and possibly by the supportive use of amifosfine.[80]

Nephrotoxicity

Cisplatin is highly nephrotoxic if sufficient hydration and diuresis are not provided during the drug's administration. Even then, four cycles of standard BEP may lead to chronic dose-dependent, though often subclinical, decrease of the glomerular function.[81]

Several authors have described persistent low serum magnesium and/or low phosphate levels after standard chemotherapy,[53,69] although not all investigators have been able to confirm these findings.[81,82] Carboplatin is less nephrotoxic than cisplatin, but doses of 1,500 mg/m^2 or more given over 3 days have a comparable effect as cisplatin 50 mg/m^2 applied on 1 day.[83]

Radiation target fields always include parts of the renal arteries, with the risk of postradiation subintimal fibrosis and reduction of the arterial flow. Fosså et al.[81] showed that infradiaphragmatic radiotherapy (30–40 Gy) leads to subclinical nephrotoxicity after a mean observation time of 11 years, in particular if combined with chemotherapy.

Cardiovascular Toxicity

Raynaud's Phenomenon

About 20% to 30% of TCSs report the development of Raynaud-like phenomenon after standard BEP chemotherapy that peak at 6 months after chemotherapy and subsequently slightly decrease to a persistent pathologic level.[53,56,73,76,84] These side effects are related to disturbance of autonomous innervation as well as thickening of the intima in small arteries with reduction of the blood vessel volume. Most studies point to bleomycin as an important etiological agent.[69] Interestingly, TCSs complaining of postchemotherapy Raynaud's phenomenon display an increased risk for erectile dysfunction.[78]

Cardiovascular Risk Factors and Major Events

Increased risk of postchemotherapy cardiovascular morbidity in TCSs as compared with TCSs on surveillance or men from the general population is evidenced in several studies[53,85–87] (Tables 104.4, 104.5). Today's chemotherapy for TC may even represent a high-risk factor for the development of a "metabolic syndrome" (diabetes mellitus, hypertension, hypercholesterolemia, obesity) and myocardial infarction.[86,88]

Huddart et al.[82] point out the possibility that partial heart irradiation during adjuvant radiotherapy may increase the risk of life-threatening cardiac events, as portions of the heart receive radiation doses of 30 to 90 cGy during current routine radiotherapy. TCSs having received former times mediastinal radiotherapy (30–40 Gy) for stage II or III TC represent a high-risk group for cardiac events and should be monitored accordingly.[89] These observations are in line with the findings of Fosså et al.[90] of an increased relative risk of cardiovascular mortality in TCSs treated from 1962 to 1993, most of them having received radiotherapy.

TABLE 104.4. Cardiovascular risk factors in TCSs.

Author	*No. of patients*	*Observation time (years)*[a]	*High cholesterol*[b]	*Reduced renal function*[c]	*Low Mg*[c]	*Hypertension*[b]	*Abnormal body mass index (BMI) increase*
Surgery only							
Meinardi (2002)	40	8	58%			8%	28%
Fosså (2003)	14	11		14%	7%		
Huddart (2003)	24	10	1%	8%	0%	9%	
Radiotherapy							
Fosså (2003)	18	11		28%	0%		
Huddard (2003)	230	10	3%	13%	0%	12%	
Chemotherapy							
Boyer (1992)	497			8–43%			
Osanto (1992)	43	4		15%			
Bokemeyer (2000)	63	5	32%	19%	18%	15%	32%
Meinardi (2000)	62	8	79%	31%	8%	39%	21%
Strumberg (2002)	32	15	81%			25%	48%
Fosså (2003)	44	11		30%	5%		
Huddard (2003)	390	10	2%	14%	0%	21%	
Chemotherapy + Radiotherapy							
Fosså (2003)	9	11		56%	0%		
Huddard (2003)	130	10	0%	27%	2%	13%	

[a] Median.

[b] Above.

[c] Below the institution's normal range.

TABLE 104.5. Cardiovascular events in TCSs: angina pectoris, myocardial infarction, cerebrovascular hemorrhage, cardiovascular death.

Author	*No. of patients*	*Median observation time (years)*	*No. of events*	*Age-adjusted RR*
Chemotherapy				
Boyer (1992)[a]	480	≥1	23	
Bokemeyer (1996)	63	5	2	
Meinardi (2000)[86]	62	8	5	7.1 (1.9–18.3)[c]
Strumberg (2002)	32	15	1	
Cardiovascular mortality				
Huddart (2003)[b82]	992	10	68	
All treatment	242		9	Reference
Surgery only	230		22	2.40 (1.04–5.49)
Radiotherapy	390		26	2.59 (1.15–5.84)
Chemotherapy	130		11	2.78 (1.09–7.07)
Chemotherapy + radiotherapy				
Lagars (2004)	211	>15	23	1.95 (1.24–2.94)
Fosså (2004)[d90]				
Not specified	3,378	1962–1997	107	1.2 (1.0–1.5)

[a] Review.

[b] Mono-institutional.

[c] Numbers in parentheses, 95% confidence interval.

[d] Cancer Registry based.

Gastrointestinal Toxicity

With the target doses and target fields administered today,[4,91] the prevalence of slight gastrointestinal (GI) symptoms among TCSs[70,91,92] is only marginally above the proportion reported by the general population.[93] Major long-term GI problems such as peptic ulcer are observed in only 3% to 5% of the TCSs.[94,95] Target doses of 36 Gy or more or the combination of radiotherapy with radiosensitizing cytostatic drugs (adriamycin, cisplatin) increase the risk of persistent diarrhea and malabsorption.[70,96] Increased retroperitoneal fibrosis has occasionally been observed causing ureteric or biliary stenosis[97] or mimicking pancreatic cancer.[98]

Other Long-Term Toxicities

The typical acute toxicities of bleomycin of the skin and the lungs do not, in general, remain as long-term morbidities, whereas corticosteroid-related aseptic osteonecrosis represents a rare long-term complication in TCSs.[99]

Psychosocial and Quality of Life Issues

Introduction

Psychologic distress, health-related quality of life, as well as sexual dysfunctions and paternity distress, have all been the focus for several quantitative and a few qualitative investigations in TCSs. Hardly any of these studies have randomized controlled designs.

TC involves an organ intrinsically associated with reproduction, sexuality, and masculine self-image, issues of importance to ill and healthy men alike. Global health-related quality of life (HRQoL) as assessed by available instruments does not cover these functions. The only available TC module[100] has not been completely validated. Paternity issues are regularly rated with unvalidated questions, whereas mental health and issues of sexuality have been studied by psychometrically validated and nonvalidated forms.

TCSs, similar to men in the general population, may have significant pretreatment problems such as unemployment, economical worries, mental disorders, relational problems, and other physical illnesses. The influence of such pretreatment issues on posttreatment adaptation is not well known because of the lack of prospective studies with sufficient sample sizes. Sociocultural differences in relationship to masculinity, sexuality, fertility, and employment should also be kept in mind when findings are compared across studies. Long-term TCSs also have problems in common with cancer patients in general, such as fear of recurrence and death. Coping ability has not been studied in either short- or long-term TCSs.

The overall conclusion so far is that long-term TCSs in general show good psychosocial adaptation; the mean HRQoL is at the level of the general male population. However, TCSs show a higher prevalence of anxiety disorders and some sexual dysfunctions.

Partnered Relationship in TCSs

In most studies, the majority of TCSs (70% to 90%) were in partnered relationships when TC was diagnosed. The rate of divorce and broken relationships for TCSs is 5% to 10% in most follow-up studies. Those couples that did separate saw the cancer as a significant factor in their breakup.[101,102]

Few wives found their husbands less attractive or masculine as TCSs, and in the few studies of wives, the majority found their sexual satisfaction unchanged.[103] The main concern of the wives was to have children, particularly if the couple had not achieved parenthood before the TC was diagnosed. Moynihan[104] found that 22% of partners had psychiatric morbidity, mainly anxiety and fertility worries.

Changes in Body Image

The studies published so far do not confirm any devastating effects on body image or feelings of masculinity as suggested by van Basten et al.[105] However, Gritz et al.[103] reported that 23% of patients perceived a permanent decrease in overall attractiveness. Rudberg et al.[84] reported that 15% of Swedish TCSs felt less attractive, whereas 33% was found in a sample from Japan.[106] No negative impact of orchidectomy was reported in a Scottish[107] and in an Italian sample.[108] These differences could reflect different cultural attitudes toward orchiectomy.

Health-Related Quality of Life

Posttreatment HRQoL is not identical to therapy-related psychologic or somatic morbidity, but relates to the patient's overall perception of physical and psychosocial well-being, including family life, leisure activity, and occupational situation. Older studies found that TCSs generally were strong, fit, and satisfied compared with controls.[103,109–111] Newer studies with validated instruments have confirmed that HRQoL generally is as good in TCSs as in the general male population.[112,113] Data from Norwegian TCSs (n = 1,409) with a mean follow-up age of 11 years show minimal differences on the eight dimensions of Short Form 36 (SF-36) compared with the general male population (n = 2673)[114] (Figure 104.3).

The influence of treatment modalities on HRQoL is still unsettled, mostly due to small samples with lack of statistical power. Joly et al.[113] found no differences (n = 71), while Rudberg et al.[112] (n = 277) found that those treated with intensive chemotherapy scored less favorably concerning HRQoL. In initially metastatic patients postchemotherapy RPLND did not worsen HRQoL as compared with chemotherapy alone.[115] Recently, Fosså et al.[73] reported that 2 years after chemotherapy, 36% of TCSs displayed improved and 13% deteriorated HRQoL, compared with baseline.

Mental Health

Most studies report a higher level of anxiety symptoms and higher prevalence of anxiety disorders among TCSs (20%) compared with controls and in the general population.[104,116,117] There is indication that a considerable proportion of TCSs live with a low feeling of safety.[117] It is unclear if there is more mental morbidity associated with the more-intensive treatment regimens. If the prevalence of depression is increased, it is also unsettled due to considerable overlap between depression and fatigue. The level of fatigue, but not of depression, was reported to be higher than in the general population, but lower than among male patients with Hodgkin's disease.[117] Fatigue was considered a major problem by many TCSs.[118]

During recent years, increasing attention has been paid to postchemotherapy cognitive mental disturbances in cancer patients.[119,120] In the European experience about 20% of the TCSs report decreased cognitive functions 2 years after four cycles of BEP.[73] In the future, prospective studies are highly needed to assess changes of cognitive functions in TCSs.

Social Functioning

The continuation of planned education and professional life after treatment obviously is of great importance for TCSs, but only few reports have dealt with this issue. Studies indicate that most TCSs continue in work.[105,108] Kaasa et al.[116] reported even greater work satisfaction in TCSs in general than in an age-matched population sample. There appears to be little change in relation to friends and social contacts.[112]

Obtaining bank loans and life insurance is a common problem for TCSs,[113] although national policies vary considerably.

Sexual Dysfunctions

Two systematic reviews of sexual functioning in TCSs[121,122] emphasize the considerable methodologic problems in the field. TC treatment can result in both physiologic changes in sexual functioning and trigger emotional reactions (e.g., sexual performance anxiety, fear of loss of control, uncertainty about the future). Fatigue and general malaise can have profound effect on libido, as can hair loss and weight loss. Emotional factors such as uncertainty about the future, anxiety, and loss of control may also inhibit libido. Generally,

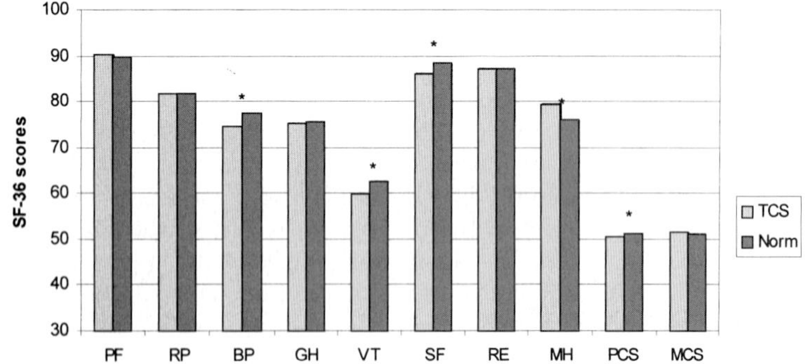

FIGURE 104.3. Health-related quality of life (SF-36) in testicular cancer survivors (TCSs) versus age-matched men from the general population. PF, physical functioning; RP, role physical; BP, bodily pain; GH, general health; VT, vitality; SF, social functioning; RE, role emotional; MH, mental health; PCS, physical composite score; MCS, mental composite score. Norm data are age adjusted to mach the TCS. *P less than 0.05.

TABLE 104.6. Future directions.

Healthcare professionals	*Patients*
Clinical routine 1. Thorough pretreatment counseling and information on expected unavoidable side effects 2. Use of risk-adapted therapy 3. Organization of long-term follow-up 4. Evidence-based treatment of side effects, including psychosocial support, and structured intervention trials	1. Psychologic acceptance of being a TCS, sometimes with unavoidable side effects 2. Adoption of a healthy lifestyle (nonsmoking, weight control, physical activity) 3. Testicular self-examination
Research 1. Prospective studies 2. Biochemical pharmacokinetic and pharmacogenetic analyses 3. Epidemiologic investigations comparing TCSs with other cancer survivors and the general population	

there seems to be a high correlation between sexual functioning before and after treatment for TC, whereas the relation to treatment modality is less clear.[123–125] Findings must be considered in relation to age[123] and to the prevalence in the general population.[126] Erectile dysfunction is, for example, reported at the same level as in the general population (approximately 10%).[127]

Thirty per cent to 50% of TCSs report a decrease in sexual functioning compared with before treatment for TC.[112,123–125,127] Two-thirds reported decreased sexual activity, and one-third was dissatisfied with their sexual functioning.[127]

Psychologic and behavioral features such as desire, orgasmic pleasure, sexual activity, and satisfaction are affected by all treatment modalities, even surveillance. Reduction or loss of orgasm, loss of desire, and sexual dissatisfaction all show a prevalence of approximately 20%, which is significantly higher than in the general population.[127] Even in the surveillance group, 25% of TCSs report negative changes, which is the same proportion as in the radiation group, whereas those with chemotherapy reported more dysfunctions.[122] Psychologic functions play a strong role for these sexual dysfunctions.[128,129]

Fertility Issues

Biologic inability to father a child presents a serious challenge to a man's perception of his masculinity, to his self-esteem, and to his intimate relations, although the inability to achieve paternity evokes different responses at various points in a man's life.

Rieker et al.[130] found that fertility distress was common, but was a major problem only among those childless and those with ejaculatory dysfunction. No significant relationship was, however, found between TC-related infertility and marital separation.[101,104]

Psychologic Interventions

A randomized controlled trial of psychologic support in relation to primary treatment of TC showed an effectiveness that hardly differed from that of nonintervention.[131] Treatment for sexual dysfunctions in TCSs has been scarcely described, but seems to follow general principles for such dysfunctions.

Summary and Future Directions

The introduction of cisplatin-based chemotherapy into the treatment of testicular cancer has been one of the largest successes during the past three decades in oncology. Both oncologists and TCSs, however, must accept that long-term toxicity cannot completely be avoided: 10% to 20% of TCSs develop long-term health problems, most of them only slightly interfering with the patients' quality of life.

To minimize treatment-induced side effects, oncologists should follow evidence-based risk-adapted therapeutic guidelines, thus avoiding over- and undertreatment (Table 104.6). Furthermore, TCSs must be educated about the importance of adopting a healthy lifestyle (smoking cessation, weight control, physical activity) to minimize life-threatening side effects such as cardiovascular toxicity. They should be offered long-term follow-up in specialized multidisciplinary cancer survivor clinics that follow structured clinical and research programs with the aim at an early phase to recognize side effects and, if possible, to intervene (for example, testosterone substitution in hypogonal TCSs). Such long-term follow-up of TCSs and other cancer survivors will enable large-scale comparative epidemiologic investigations. Avoiding unnecessary anxiety, a former TC patient should also be made aware of his increased risk of tumor development in the contralateral testicle, warranting regular self-examination. Only rarely the oncologist will have to discuss the excess risk of subsequent non-germ cell cancer, although this risk should always be considered by healthcare professionals seeing TCSs with "unusual" symptoms.

Many of the reports on TCSs' long-term toxicity rely on the patients' responses to questionnaires. However, during recent years clinical investigators increasingly have validated these responses by objective measures, such as clinical examinations and organ-specific functional tests.[45,79,82,86] Interestingly, such studies have demonstrated that, for example, cisplatin or cisplatin adducts are retained in the human body (plasma, liver, muscle) for at least 20 years.[132,133] Whether an association exists between such cisplatin retention and long-term toxicity should be studied in future analyses, which should also take into account pharmacogenetic and molecular biologic parameters. The results of such investigations will increase our understanding of the considerable variability of physical and psychosocial long-term toxicity and will assist the identification of risk groups.

So far, the medical literature on long-term survivorship in TC patients almost exclusively contains cross-sectional studies. Prospective investigations are needed to identify premorbid risk factors of physical and psychosocial long-term toxicity.

References

1. Engeland A, Haldorsen T, Tretli S, et al. Prediction of cancer incidence in the Nordic countries up to the years 2000 and 2010. A Collaborative Study of the Five Nordic Cancer Registries. APMIS 1993;101(suppl 38):1–124.
2. Einhorn LH, Williams SD, Loehrer PJ, et al. Evaluation of optimal duration of chemotherapy in favorable-prognosis disseminated germ cell tumours: a Southeastern Cancer Study Group protocol. J Clin Oncol 1989;7:387–391.
3. International Germ Cell Cancer Collaborative Group (IGCCCG). The International Germ Cell Consensus Classification: a prognostic factor-based staging system for metastatic germ cell cancers. J Clin Oncol 1997;15:594–603.
4. Fosså SD, Horwich A, Russell JM, et al. Optimal planning target volume for stage I testicular seminoma: A Medical Research Council Testicular Tumour Working Group. J Clin Oncol 1999; 17:1146–1154.
5. Fosså SD, Jones WG, Stenning SP, for the TE18 Collaborators; MRC Clinical Trials Unit, London. Quality of life (QL) after radiotherapy (RT) for stage I seminoma: results from a randomised trial of two RT schedules (MRC TE18). Proc Am Soc Clin Oncol 2002;21:188.
6. Warde P, Specht L, Horwich A, et al. Prognostic factors for relapse in stage I Seminoma managed by surveillance: a pooled analysis. J Clin Oncol 2002;20:4448–4452.
7. Oliver RTD, Edmonds PM, Ong JYH, et al. Pilot studies of 2 and 1 course carboplatin as adjuvant for stage I seminoma: should it be tested in a randomized trial against radiotherapy? Int J Radiat Oncol Biol Phys 1994;29:3–8.
8. Read G, Stenning SP, Cullen MH, et al. Medical Research Council Prospective study of surveillance for stage I testicular teratoma. J Clin Oncol 1992;10:1762–1768.
9. Cullen MH, Stenning SP, Parkinson MC, et al. for the Medical Research Council Testicular Tumour Working Party. Short-course adjuvant chemotherapy in high-risk stage I nonseminomatous germ cell tumors of the testis: a Medical Research Council report. J Clin Oncol 1996;14:1106–1113.
10. Donohue JP, Foster RS, Rowland RG, et al. Nerve-sparing retroperitoneal lymphadenectomy with preservation of ejaculation. J Urol 1990;144:287–292.
11. Williams SD, Birch R, Einhorn LH, et al. Treatment of disseminated germ-cell tumours with cisplatin, bleomycin, and either vinblastin or eroposide. N Engl J Med 1987;316:1435–1440.
12. de Wit R, Roberts JT, Wilkinson PM, et al. Equivalence of three or four cycles of bleomycin, etoposide, and cisplatin chemotherapy and of a 3- or 5-day schedule in good-prognosis germ cell cancer: a randomized study of the European Organization for Research and Treatment of Cancer Genitourinary Tract Cancer Cooperative Group and the Medical Research Council. J Clin Oncol 2001;19:1629–1640.
13. Nichols CR, Catalano PJ, Crawford ED, et al. Randomized comparison of cisplatin and etoposide and either bleomycin or ifosfamide in treatment of advanced disseminated germ cell tumours: an Eastern Cooperative Oncology Group, Southwest Oncology Group, and Cancer and Leukemia Group B Study. J Clin Oncol 1998;16:1287–1293.
14. Motzer RJ, Sheinfeld J, Mazumdar M, et al. Paclitaxel, ifosfamide and cisplatin second-line therapy for patients with relapsed testicular germ cell cancer. J Clin Oncol 2000;18:2413–2418.
15. Toner G, Panicek D, Heelan R, et al. Adjuvant surgery after chemotherapy for nonseminomatous germ cell tumors: recommendations for patient selection. J Clin Oncol 1990;8: 1683–1694.
16. Travis LB, Andersson M, Gospodarowicz M, et al. Treatment-associated leukemia following testicular cancer. J Natl Cancer Inst 2000;92:1165–1171.
17. Bosl GJ, Ilson DH, Rodriguez E, et al. Clinical relevance of the i(12P) marker chromosome in germ cell tumours. J Natl Cancer Inst 1994;86:349–355.
18. Travis LB, Curtis RE, Storm H, et al. Risk of second malignant neoplasms among long-term survivors of testicular cancer. J Natl Cancer Inst 1997;89:1429–1439.
19. Van Leeuwen FE, Travis LB. Second cancers. In: Devitz VT, et al. (eds). Cancer: Principles and Practice of Oncology, 6th ed. Philadelphia: Lippincott Williams & Wilkins, 2001:2939–2964.
20. Fosså SD, Langmark F, Aass N, et al. Second non-germ cell malignancies after radiotherapy of testicular cancer with or without chemotherapy. Br J Cancer 1990;61:639–643.
21. Van Leeuwen FE, Stiggelbout AM, van den Belt-Dusebout AW, et al. Second cancer risk following testicular cancer: a follow-up study of 1,909 patients. J Clin Oncol 1993;11:415–424.
22. United Nations Scientific Committee on the Effects of Atomic Radiation (UNSCEAR). Report to the General Assembly, with Scientific Annexes. Sources and Effects of Ionizing Radiation, UNSCEAR. New York: United Nations, 2000.
23. Hoff Wanderas E, Fosså SD, Tretli S. Risk of subsequent non-germ cell cancer after treatment of germ cell cancer in 2006 Norwegian male patients. Eur J Cancer 1997;33:253–262.
24. Breslow NE, Takashima JR, Whitton JA, et al. Second malignant neoplasms following treatment for Wilm's tumor: a report from the National Wilms' Tumor Study Group. J Clin Oncol 1995; 13:1851–1859.
25. Redman JR, Vugrin D, Arlin ZA, et al. Leukemia following treatment of germ cell tumors in men. J Clin Oncol 1984;2: 1080–1087.
26. Pedersen-Bjergaard J, Daugaard G, et al. Increased risk of myelodysplasia and leukaemia after etoposide, cisplatin, and bleomycin for germ-cell tumours. Lancet 1991;338:359–363.
27. Nichols CR, Breeden ES, Loehrer PJ, et al. Secondary leukemia associated with a conventional dose of etoposide: review of serial germ cell tumor protocols. J Natl Cancer Inst 1993;85: 36–40.
28. Bokemeyer C, Schmoll HJ, Kuczyk MA, et al. Risk of secondary leukemia following high cumulative doses of etoposide during chemotherapy for testicular cancer (letter). J Natl Cancer Inst 1995;87:58–60.
29. Boshoff C, Begent RH, Oliver RT, et al. Secondary tumours following etoposide containing therapy for germ cell cancer. Ann Oncol 1995;6:35–40.
30. Travis LB, Holowaty E, Hall P, et al. Risk of leukemia following platinum-based chemotherapy for ovarian cancer. N Engl J Med 1999;340:351–357.
31. Smith MA, Rubinstein L, Anderson JR, et al. Secondary leukemia or myeloodysplastic syndrome after treatment with epipodophyllotoxins. J Clin Oncol 1999;17:569–577.
32. Kollmannsberger C, Hartmann JT, Kanz L, et al. Therapy-related malignancies following treatment of germ cell cancer. Int J Cancer 1999;83:860–863.
33. von der Maase H, Rørth M, Walbom-Jørgensen S, et al. Carcinoma in situ of contralateral testis in patients with testicular germ cell cancer: study of 27 cases in 500 patients. Br Med J 1986;293:1398–1401.
34. Sokal M, Peckham MJ, Hendry WF. Bilateral germ cell tumours of the testis. Br J Urol 1980;52:158–162.
35. Hoff Wanderas E, Fosså SD, Tretli S. Risk of a second germ cell cancer after treatment of a primary germ cell cancer in 2201 Norwegian male patients. Eur J Cancer 1997;33:244–252.

36. Hartmann JG, Fosså SD, Nichols CR, et al. Incidence of metachronous testicular cancer in patients with extragonadal germ cell tumors. J Natl Cancer Inst 2001;93:1733–1738.
37. Fosså SD, Aass N, Heilo A, et al. Testicular carcinoma in situ in patients with extragonadal germ cell tumours: the clinical role of pre-treatment biopsy. Ann Oncol 2003;14:1412–1418.
38. Oosterhuis JW, Looijenga LHJ. The biology of human germ cell tumours: retrospective speculations and new prospectives. Eur Urol 1993;23:245–250.
39. Fosså SD, Åbyholm T, Aakvaag A. Spermatogenesis and hormonal status after orchiectomy for cancer and before supplementary treatment. Eur Urol 1984;10:173–177.
40. Hansen PV, Trykker H, Andersen J, et al. Germ cell function and hormonal status in patients with testicular cancer. Cancer (Phila) 1989;64:956–961.
41. Petersen PM, Skakkebaek NE, Vistisen K, et al. Semen quality and reproductive hormones before orchiectomy in men with testicular cancer. J Clin Oncol 1999;17:941–947.
42. Petersen PM, Skakkebæk NE, Rørth M, et al. Semen quality and reproductive hormones before and after orchiectomy in men with testicular cancer. J Urol 1999;161:822–826.
43. Carroll PR, Whitmore Jr WF, Herr HW, et al. Endocrine and exocrine profiles of men with testicular tumours before orchiectomy, J Urol 1987;137:420–423.
44. Jacobsen KD, Theodorsen L, Fosså SD. Spermatogenesis after unilateral orchiectomy for testicular cancer in patients following surveillance policy. J Urol 2001;165:93–96.
45. Nord C, Bjøro T, Ellingsen D, et al. Gonadal hormones in long-term survivors 10 years after treatment for unilateral testicular cancer. Eur Urol 2003;44:322–328.
46. Reiter WJ, Kratzik C, Brodowicz T, et al. Sperm analysis and serum follicle-stimulating hormone levels before and after adjuvant single-agent carboplatin therapy for clinical stage I seminoma. Urol 1998;52:117–119.
47. Lampe H, Horwich A, Norman A, et al. Fertility after chemotherapy for testicular germ cell cancers. J Clin Oncol 1997;15:239–245.
48. Drasga RE, Einhorn LH, Williams SD, et al. Fertility after chemotherapy for testicular cancer. J Clin Oncol 1983;1:179–183.
49. Taksey J, Bissada NK, Chaudhary UB. Fertility after chemotherapy for testicular cancer. Arch Androl 2003;49:389–395.
50. Petersen PM, Skakkebæk NE, Giwercman A. Gonadal function in men with testicular cancer: biological and clinical aspects. APMIS 1998;106:24–36.
51. Palmieri G, Lotrecchiano G, Ricci G, et al. Gonadal function after multimodality treatment in men with testicular germ cell cancer. Eur J Endocrinol 1996;134:431–436.
52. Aass N, Fosså SD, Theodorsen L, et al. Prediction of long-term gonadal toxicity after standard treatment for testicular cancer. Eur J Cancer 1991;27:1087–1091.
53. Bokemeyer C, Berger CC, Kuczyk MA, et al. Evaluation of long-term toxicity after chemotherapy for testicular cancer. J Clin Oncol 1996;14:2923–2932.
54. Fosså SD, Ous S, Abyholm T, et al. Post-treatment fertility in patients with testicular cancer. II. Influence of cisplatin-based combination chemotherapy and of retroperitoneal surgery on hormone and sperm cell production. Br J Urol 1985;57:210–214.
55. Petersen PM, Hansen SW, Giwercman A, et al. Dose-dependent impairment of testicular function in patients treated with cisplatin-based chemotherapy for germ cell cancer. Ann Oncol 1994;5:355–358.
56. Stephenson WT, Poirier SM, Rubin L, et al. Evaluation of reproductive capacity in germ cell tumor patients following treatment with cisplatin, etoposide, and bleomycin. J Clin Oncol 1995;13:2278–2280.
57. Strumberg D, Brügge S, Korn MW, et al. Evaluation of long-term toxicity in patients after cisplatin-based chemotherapy for non-seminomatous testicular cancer. Ann Oncol 2002;13:229–236.
58. Jacobsen KD, Olsen DR, Fosså K, et al. External beam abdominal radiotherapy in patients with seminoma stage I: field type, testicular dose, and spermatogenesis. Int J Radiat Oncol Biol Phys 1997;38:95–102.
59. Hansen PV, Trykker H, Svennekjær IL, et al. Long-term recovery of spermatogenesis after radiotherapy in patients with testicular cancer. Radiat Oncol 1990;18:117–125.
60. Kreuser ED, Klingmüller D, Thiel E. The role of LHRH-Analogues in protecting gonadal function during chemotherapy and irradiation. Eur Urol 1993;23:157–164.
61. Hallak J, Hendin BN, Thomas AJ, et al. Investigation of fertilizing capacity of cryopreserved spermatozoa from patients with cancer. J Urol 1998;159:1217–1220.
62. Fosså SD, Opjordsmoen S, Haug E. Androgen replacement and quality of life in patients treated for bilateral testicular cancer. Eur J Cancer 1999;35:1220–1225.
63. Whitmore WE Jr. Surgical treatment of adult germinal testis tumours. Semin Oncol 1979;6:55–68.
64. Nijman JM, Jager S, Boer PW, et al. The treatment of ejaculation disorders after retroperitoneal lymph node dissection. Cancer (Phila) 1982;50:2967–2971.
65. Jacobsen KD, Ous S, Wæhre H, et al. Ejaculation in testicular cancer patients after post-chemotherapy retroperitoneal lymph node dissection. Br J Cancer 1999;80:249–255.
66. Jacobsen KD, Fosså SD. Fatherhood in testicular cancer patients with carcinoma in situ in the contralateral testicle. Eur Urol 2000;38:725–727.
67. Giwercman A, von der Maase H, Berthelsen JG, et al. Localized irradiation of testis with carcinoma in situ: effects on Leydig cell function and eradication of malignant germ cell in 20 patients. J Clin Endocrinol Metab 1991;73:596–603.
68. Heidenreich A, Weizbach L, Höltl W, et al. Organ sparing surgery for malignant germ cell tumor of the testis. J Urol 2001;166: 2161–2165.
69. Boyer M, Raghavan D. Toxicity of treatment of germ cell tumours. Semin Oncol 1992;19:128–142.
70. Aass N, Kaasa S, Lund E, et al. Long-term somatic side-effects and morbidity in testicular cancer patients. Br J Cancer 1990; 61:151–155.
71. Petersen PM, Hansen SW. The course of long-term toxicity in patients treated with cisplatin-based chemotherapy for non-seminomatous germ-cell cancer. Ann Oncol 1999;10:1475–1483.
72. von Schlippe M, Fowler CJ, Harland SJ. Cisplatin neurotoxicity in the treatment of metastatic germ-cell tumour: time course and prognosis. Br J Cancer 2001;85:823–826.
73. Fosså SD, de Wit R, Roberts T, et al. Quality of life in good prognosis patients with metastatic germ cell cancer: a prospective study of the European Organization for Research and Treatment of Cancer Genitourinary Group/Medical Research Council Testicular Cancer Study Group (30941/TE20). J Clin Oncol 2003;21:1107–1118.
74. Hansen SW, Helweg-Larsen S, Trojaborg W. Long-term neurotoxicity in patients treated with cisplatin, vinblastine, and bleomycin for metastatic germ cell cancer. J Clin Oncol 1989; 7:1457–1461.
75. Osanto S, Bukman A, van Hoek F, et al. Long-term effects of chemotherapy in patients with testicular cancer. J Clin Oncol 1992;10:574–579.
76. Stoter G, Koopman A, Vendrik CPJ, et al. Ten-year survival and late sequelae in testicular cancer patients treated with cisplatin, vinblastine and bleomycin. J Clin Oncol 1989;7:1099–1104.
77. Skard Heier M, Aass N, Ous S, et al. Asymmetrical autonomic dysfunction of the feet after retroperitoneal surgery in patients with testicular cancer: 2 case reports. J Urol 1992;147:470–471.
78. van Basten JP, Hoekstra HJ, van Driel MF, et al. Sexual dysfunction in nonseminoma testicular cancer patients is related to chemotherapy-induced angiopathy. J Clin Oncol 1997;15: 2442–2448.

79. Hansen SW. Autonomic neuropathy after treatment with cisplatin, vinblastin, and bleomycin for germ cell cancer. Br Med J 1990;3000:511–512.
80. Koukourakis MI. Amifostine in clinical oncology: current use and future applications. Anti-Cancer Drugs 2002;13:181–209.
81. Fosså SD, Aass N, Winderen M, et al. Long-term renal function after treatment for malignant germ cell tumours. Ann Oncol 2002;13:222–228.
82. Huddart RA, Norman A, Shahidi M, et al. Cardiovascular disease as a long-term complication of treatment for testicular cancer. J Clin Oncol 2003;21:1513–1523.
83. Kollmannsberger C, Kuzcyk M, Mayer F, et al. Late toxicity following curative treatment of testicular cancer. Semin Surg Oncol 1999;17:275–281.
84. Rudberg L, Carlsson M, Nilsson S, et al. Self-perceived physical, psychologic, and general symptoms in survivors of testicular cancer 3 to 13 years after treatment. Cancer Nurs 2002;25: 187–195.
85. Fosså SD, Lehne G, Heimdal K, et al. Clinical and biochemical long-term toxicity after postoperative cisplatin-based chemotherapy in patients with low-stage testicular cancer. Oncology 1995;52:300–305.
86. Meinardi MT, Gietema JA, van der Graaf WTA, et al. Cardiovascular morbidity in long-term survivors of metastatic testicular cancer. J Clin Oncol 2000;18:1725–1732.
87. Raghavan D, Cox K, Childs A, et al. Hypercholesterolemia after chemotherapy for testis cancer. J Clin Oncol 1992;10:1386–1389.
88. Nord C, Fosså SD, Egeland T. Excessive annual BMI increase after chemotherapy among young survivors of testicular cancer. Br J Cancer 2003;88:36–41.
89. Zagars GK, Ballo MT, Lee AK, Strom SS. Mortality after cure of testicular seminoma. J Clin Oncol 2004;22:640–647.
90. Fosså SD, Aass N, Harvei S, et al. Increased mortality rates in young and middle-aged patients with malignant germ cell tumours. Br J Cancer 2004;90:607–612.
91. Bamberg M, Schmidberger H, Meisner C, et al. Radiotherapy for stages I and IIA/B testicular seminoma. Int J Cancer 1999;83: 823–827.
92. Yeoh E, Horowitz M, Russo A, et al. The effects of abdominal irradiation for seminoma of the testis on gastrointestinal function. J Gastroenterol Hepatol 1995;10:125–130.
93. Haug TT, Mykletun A, Dahl AA. Are anxiety and depression related to gastrointestinal symptoms in the general population? Scand J Gastroenterol 2002;37:294–298.
94. Fosså SD, Aass N, Kaalhus O. Radiotherapy for testicular seminoma stage I: treatment results and long-term post-irradiation morbidity in 365 patients. Int J Radiat Oncol Biol Phys 1989; 16:383–388.
95. Hamilton CR, Horwich A, Bliss JM, et al. Gastrointestinal morbidity of adjuvant radiotherapy in stage I malignant teratoma of the testis. Radiother Oncol 1987;10:85–90.
96. Hoff Wanderås E, Fosså SD, Tretl, S, Klepp O. Toxicity in long-term survivors after adriamycin containing chemotherapy of malignant germ cell tumours. Int J Oncol 1994;4:681–688.
97. Moul JW. Retroperitoneal fibrosis following radiotherapy for stage I testicular seminoma. J Urol 1992;147:124–126.
98. Stensvold E, Aass N, Gladhaug I, et al. Erroneous diagnosis of pancreatic cancer: a possible pitfall after radiotherapy of testicular cancer. Eur J Surg Oncol 2004;30:352–355.
99. Winquist EW, Bauman GS, Balogh J. Nontraumatic osteonecrosis after chemotherapy for testicular cancer systematic review. Am J Clin Oncol 2001;24:603–606.
100. Fosså SD, Moynihan C, Serbouti S. Patients' and doctors' perception of long-term morbidity in patients with testicular cancer clinical stage I. A descriptive pilot study. Support Care Cancer 1996;4:118–128.
101. Schover LR, von Eschenbach AC. Sexual and marital relationships after treatment for nonseminomatous testicular cancer. Urology 1985;25:251–255.
102. Rieker PP, Edbril SD, Garnick MB. Curative testis cancer therapy: psychosocial sequelae. J Clin Oncol 1985;3:1117–1126.
103. Gritz ER, Wellisch DK, Wang H-J, et al. Long-term effects of testicular cancer on sexual functioning in married couples. Cancer (Phila) 1989;64:1560–1567.
104. Moynihan C. Testicular cancer: the psychosocial problems of patients and their relatives. Cancer Surv 1987;6:477–510.
105. van Basten JP, Jonker-Pool G, van Driel MF, et al. Fantasies and facts of the testes. Br J Urol 1996;78:756–762.
106. Arai Y, Kawakita M, Hida S, et al. Psychosocial aspects in long-term survivors of testicular cancer. J Urol 1996;155:574–578.
107. Blackmore C. The impact of orchiectomy upon the sexuality of the man with testicular cancer. Cancer Nurs 1988;11:33–40.
108. Caffo O, Amichetti M. Evaluation of sexual life after orchidectomy followed by radiotherapy for early stage seminoma of the testis. BJU Int 1999;83:462–468.
109. Fosså SD, Aass N, Kaalhus O. Testicular cancer in young Norwegians. J Surg Oncol 1988;39:43–63.
110. Fosså SD, Aass N, Ous S, et al. Long-term morbidity and quality of life in testicular cancer patients. Scand J Urol Nephrol 1991;138(suppl):241–246.
111. Douchez J, Droz JP, Desclaux B, et al. Quality of life in long-term survivors of nonseminomatous germ cell testicular tumors. J Urol 1993;149:498–501.
112. Rudberg L, Nilsson S, Wikblad K. Health-related quality of life in survivors of testicular cancer 3 to 13 years after treatment. J Psychosoc Oncol 2000;18:19–31.
113. Joly F, Héron JF, Kalusinski L, et al. Quality of life in long-term survivors of testicular cancer: a population-based case-control study. J Clin Oncol 2002;20:73–80.
114. Mykletun A, Dahl AA, Haaland CF, et al. Side-effects and cancer-related stress determine quality of life on long-term survivors of testicular cancer. J Clin Oncol 2005;23(13):3061–3068.
115. Weissbach L, Bussar-Maatz R, Flechtner H, et al. RPLND or primary chemotherapy in clinical stage IIA/B non-seminomatous germ cell tumours. Eur Urol 2000;37:582–594.
116. Kaasa S, Aass N, Mastekaasa A, et al. Psychosocial well-being in testicular cancer patients. Eur J Cancer 1991;27:1091–1095.
117. Fosså SD, Dahl AA, Loge JH. Fatigue, anxiety, and depression in long-term survivors of testicular cancer. J Clin Oncol 2003;21: 1249–1254.
118. Jones GY, Payne S. Searching for safety signals: the experience of medical surveillance among men with testicular teratomas. Psycho-Oncology 2000;9:385–394.
119. Ozen H, Sahin A, Toklu C, et al. Psychosocial adjustment after testicular cancer treatment. J Urol 1998;159:1947–1950.
120. Schagen SB, Muller MJ, Boogerd W, et al. Late effects of adjuvant chemotherapy on cognitive function: a follow-up study in breast cancer patients. Ann Oncol 2002;13:1387–1397.
121. Nazareth I, Lewin J, King M. Sexual dysfunction after treatment for testicular cancer: a systematic review. J Psychosom Res 2001;51:735–743.
122. Jonker-Pool G, Van de Wiel HBM, Hoekstra HJ, et al. Sexual functioning after treatment for testicular cancer: review and meta-analysis of 36 empirical studies between 1975 and 2000. Arch Sex Behav 2001;30:55–74.
123. Aass N, Grünfeld B, Kaalhus O, et al. Pre- and posttreatment sexual life in testicular cancer patients: a descriptive investigation. Br J Cancer 1993;67:1113–1117.
124. Tinkler SD, Howard GCW, Kerr GR. Sexual morbidity following radiotherapy for germ cell tumours of the testis. Radiat Oncol 1992;25:207–212.
125. Incrocci L, Hop WCJ, Wijnmaalen A, et al. Treatment outcome, body image, and sexual functioning after orchiectomy and radio-

therapy for stage I-II testicular seminoma. Int J Radiat Oncol Biol Phys 2002;53:1165–1173.

126. Laumann EO, Paik A, Rosen RC. Sexual dysfunction in the United States. Prevalence and predictors. JAMA 1999;281:537–544.
127. Jonker-Pool G, van Basten JP, Hoekstra HJ, et al. Sexual functioning after treatment for testicular cancer. Cancer (Phila) 1997;80:454–464.
128. van Basten JPA, van Driel HJ, Hoekstra D, et al. Objective and subjective effects of treatment for testicular cancer on sexual function. BJU Int 1999;84:671–678.
129. Schover LR, von Eschenbach AC. Sexual and marital counselling in men treated for testicular cancer. J Sex Marit Ther 1984;10: 29–40.
130. Rieker PP, Fitzgerald EM, Kalish LA. Adaptive behavioral responses to potential infertility among survivors of testis cancer. J Clin Oncol 1990;8:347–355.
131. Moynihan C, Bliss JM, Davidson J, et al. Evaluation of adjuvant psychosocial therapy in patients with testicular cancer: randomised controlled trial. BMJ 1998;316:429–435.
132. Gerl A, Schierl R. Urinary excretion of platinum in chemotherapy-treated long-term survivors of testicular cancer. Acta Oncol 2000;39:519–522.
133. Gelevert T, Messerschmidt J, Meinardi MT, et al. Adsorptive Voltametry to determine platinum levels in plasma from testicular cancer patients treated with cisplatin. Ther Drug Monit 2001;23:169–173.

105

Medical and Psychosocial Issues in Gynecologic Cancer Survivors

Karen Basen-Engquist and Diane C. Bodurka

An emerging body of research has documented the quality of life of women with gynecologic cancer around the time of diagnosis and during treatment. However, we know much less about the quality of life and psychosocial and medical needs of gynecologic cancer survivors after treatment.[1,2] In particular, there are very few studies documenting the risk of possible late medical effects of gynecologic cancer treatment such as osteoporosis and second primary cancers. More is known about self-reported symptoms and psychosocial sequelae, such as sexual functioning and psychologic distress, but even these studies rarely focus on survivors more than 5 years after diagnosis. Additionally, much of the extant research has limitations such as small sample sizes, nonstandardized measures, and cross-sectional designs, often without appropriate comparison groups. Finally, there is a dearth of research testing interventions to ameliorate problems experienced by gynecologic cancer survivors. While in some areas additional research is needed to better describe the sequelae and determine who is at risk for adverse late effects, in others areas (e.g., sexual functioning), adequate data describing the problem are available, and a stronger focus on treatment interventions is needed. (See also Chapter 90, Reproductive Complications and Sexual Dysfunction in the Cancer Patient.)

The shortage of research contributes to several clinical challenges in the health care of gynecologic cancer survivors. Without adequate research on the long-term late effects of gynecologic cancer, appropriate follow-up care is difficult to establish. For example, should screening tests for other cancers or for conditions such as osteoporosis be started at an earlier age or done on a different schedule? The lack of an evidence base from which to make such decisions hampers effective health care for long-term survivors. We also have limited data on potential interventions for ameliorating certain late effects. For example, the data to support clinician and patient decision making about hormone replacement therapy for gynecologic cancer survivors do not exist, particularly for those who are premenopausal at diagnosis. This situation forces providers and survivors to extrapolate data on the risks and benefits of hormone replacement in healthy postmenopausal women to women who experience premature menopause as a result of cancer treatment.

A further challenge in the care of long-term survivors of gynecologic cancer is to identify not only what the healthcare system can provide to help survivors maintain their health but what they themselves can do. Research on improving health behaviors in cancer survivors, for example, increasing physical activity, is in its infancy. Early studies show that exercise benefits quality of life and functional capacity in breast cancer survivors[3,4] and decreases fatigue in prostate cancer survivors.[5] There have been no trials in the gynecologic cancer survivor population to test the effects of changes in health behaviors such as diet, exercise, and smoking cessation on potential late effects such as chronic fatigue, osteoporosis, second primary cancers, or recurrence. Such interventions could also benefit women with comorbid conditions that are either coincidental to their cancer or risk factors for the development of gynecologic cancer, such as the obesity, hypertension, and diabetes that are prevalent among endometrial cancer survivors.[6–8]

Characteristics of Gynecologic Cancer Survivors

The three major gynecologic cancers (endometrial, cervical, ovarian) differ in terms of their risk factors, median age at diagnosis, ethnic distribution, type of treatment, and survival probability. The characteristics of survivors, therefore, vary as a function of these factors as well. Table 105.1 provides information about the three diseases that impact the characteristics of the survivor population.

Endometrial cancer is the most common gynecologic cancer in the United States, followed by ovarian and cervical.[9,10] By contrast, however, cervical cancer is more common in developing countries; worldwide it is the second most common cancer among women.[11] Despite the fact that ovarian cancer is a more common diagnosis in the United States than cervical cancer, there are more cervical cancer survivors because ovarian cancer has a relatively low overall

TABLE 105.1. Variables related to gynecologic cancers that influence the characteristics of the survivor population.

	Endometrial	*Ovarian*	*Cervical*
Projected number of cases in U.S. in 2004[9]	40,320	25,580	10,520
Percentage diagnosed with localized disease[10]	73%	29%	54%
Average 5-year survival[10]	84%	53%	71%
Median age at diagnosis[10]	65	59	47
Number of survivors in U.S.[10]	556,640	202,949	231,064
Percentage of survivors within 10 years of diagnosis[10]	44%	55%	37%
Ethnic distribution of survivors within 10 years of diagnosis[a10]			
• White	92%	89%	77%
• African-American	5%	7%	14%
• Asian/Pacific Islander	2%	3%	4%
• Hispanic[b]	4%	6%	16%
Risk factors[6–8,13–17,63–65]	Obesity Diabetes (among obese women) Hypertension Nulliparity	Family history Nulliparity Use of talc Oral Contraceptives (protective) Tubal ligation and hysterectomy (protective)	Early initiation of sexual intercourse More than four sexual partners Smoking

[a] Information on ethnicity of survivors is available only for those diagnosed in past 10 years.

[b] Percentages total to more than 100 because the ethnic group Hispanic is not mutually exclusive of the other racial/ethnic categories.

survival. On average, cervical cancer is diagnosed at a younger age than ovarian and endometrial cancer, so survivors of cervical cancer are more likely to be dealing with family and work responsibilities in addition to cancer survivorship issues.

The ethnic distribution of each survivorship group also varies, with endometrial and ovarian cancer survivors being predominantly white. Among cervical cancer survivors, the proportion of minority ethnicity women is higher.[10] Because many cases of invasive cervical cancer are prevented by screening and treatment of preinvasive lesions, a number of invasive cervical cancers arise in women who have not had adequate screening,[12] either by choice or because of lack of access. Thus, women of lower socioeconomic status, who have poorer access to health care, may be overrepresented among cervical cancer patients and survivors.

The behavioral risk factors for the gynecologic cancer differ, and many of these behaviors may be continued after diagnosis and treatment, putting survivors at additional risk of second primaries or other comorbid conditions. Smoking, for example, is a risk factor for cervical cancer,[13–15] and one study has found that few cervical cancer survivors quit smoking after diagnosis.[16] Obesity is a risk factor for endometrial cancer,[6,7,17] indicating relatively low levels of physical activity relative to calorie consumption before diagnosis. Data are emerging that indicate endometrial cancer survivors also have low levels of physical activity.[18,19]

Medical Issues

Survivors of gynecologic cancer report lingering symptoms and treatment side effects even after treatment has concluded. Most studies of medical sequelae are limited to survivor self-report of symptoms, rather than medical evaluations. Although the self-report data are valuable, more data are needed on conditions that may not cause immediately observable symptoms, such as osteoporosis, second cancers, and cardiovascular disease.

Gastrointestinal Symptoms

Gynecologic cancer survivors, particularly those who are treated with pelvic radiation, report more gastrointestinal symptoms than women from the general population, even several years after treatment. Li et al.[18] studied 61 five-year endometrial cancer survivors (47% of whom received radiation therapy) and found that they reported more gastrointestinal symptoms (stomach ache, diarrhea, and nausea) than a comparison group of women of comparable age. A similar study of 46 cervical cancer survivors (who had not received radiation) found that they reported a similar degree of gastrointestinal distress to the same comparison group.[20] Klee and Machin also found that endometrial[21] and cervical[22] cancer survivors treated with radiation therapy reported more diarrhea than population-based controls matched for age and partner status; the group differences in diarrhea were present out to the final evaluation point, 24 months from diagnosis, although levels of diarrhea were low (average score between "not at all" and "a little"). Bye studied 79 survivors of endometrial and cervical cancer who were 3 to 4 years from their radiation treatment and found that diarrhea was their most common symptom. They reported more diarrhea than the general population, and experiencing frequent diarrhea was associated with higher fatigue and poorer social functioning.[23] Acute bowel toxicity during radiation treatment increases the probability of late bowel toxicity,[24] indicating that effective interventions to reduce bowel toxicity may have beneficial long-term effects as well.[23]

Neurotoxicity

Women with advanced cervical and endometrial cancer and most ovarian cancer patients receive neurotoxic chemotherapy regimens.[25] Although in many cases neurotoxicity remits after the conclusion of treatment, some survivors continue to experience neurotoxic effects. A study of 49 early-stage ovarian cancer survivors who were between 5 and 10 years from diagnosis found that a significant proportion still reported symptoms of neurotoxicity: numbness in the hands was reported by 10%; trouble walking, 16%, discomfort in hands, 23%; ringing in ears, 29%, discomfort in feet, 29%; trouble hearing, 35%; and muscle cramps, 39%.[26] Neurotoxicity symptoms were associated with poor physical and psychologic well-being, depression, sexual discomfort, and low confidence for managing cancer.

Pain

Approximately half of the 200 ovarian cancer survivors (no evidence of disease, 2 or more years from diagnosis) in one study reported pain or discomfort that they attributed to ovarian cancer or its treatment. Pain was located mainly in the bowel, pelvis, bladder, or groin. Of those who reported pain, 46% rated it as mild, 21.1% as severe. Approximately half of those with pain reported that it had a low impact on their lives.[27] Various somatic pains (e.g., headache, leg and back pain) were reported by 30% to 50% of cervical cancer survivors[20]; however, several studies found that pain levels of endometrial and cervical cancer survivors are similar to, or even lower than, those of controls.[18,20–23] Continued pain naturally has an impact on overall quality of life; Bye et al.[23] found that pain in endometrial cancer survivors 3 to 4 years after treatment was associated with lower quality of life and higher fatigue.

Menopausal Symptoms

Women who are premenopausal when diagnosed with gynecologic cancer often suffer a loss of ovarian function and experience premature menopause. Andersen's study of gynecologic cancer survivors in the year after diagnosis indicates that menopausal symptoms among the survivors remain higher than those of healthy controls up to 12 months from diagnosis.[28] Other studies of endometrial and cervical cancer survivors have also noted significant problems with menopausal symptoms (e.g., hot flashes, vaginal dryness/irritation[18,20,21]). However, two studies of cervical cancer survivors did not find the prevalence of hot flashes to be higher than that of a comparison group, possibly because of the use of hormone replacement therapy.[20,22] Among endometrial survivors, younger women report more hot flashes and other menopausal symptoms than older survivors.[18] In a study of ovarian cancer survivors, Carmack Taylor et al.[29] found that those who were off treatment reported less vaginal dryness and pain during intercourse than patients receiving treatment, but more than breast cancer survivors or women who had not had cancer.

Another implication of early ovarian failure, especially for younger survivors, is the increased risk of osteoporosis. This problem has not been well studied in gynecologic cancer patients, to determine either the prevalence of the problem or effective strategies to treat and/or prevent osteoporosis. One pilot study of 27 breast cancer survivors found that those who became permanently amenorrheic after chemotherapy had a 14% lower bone mineral density than breast cancer survivors who maintained or resumed menses.[30] Although this is a potentially serious problem, particularly for those survivors who have their ovaries removed or experience ovarian failure at a young age, many healthcare providers do not routinely recommend screening for osteoporosis in this population. A survey of outpatient oncology nurses indicated that bone mineral density testing is one of the least frequently performed screening tests for cancer survivors.[31]

Fatigue

Fatigue is a significant problem for many cancer patients during treatment, and it can last beyond the acute treatment phase.[32] In a longitudinal study of gynecologic patients in the year after diagnosis, Lutgendorf et al.[33] found that most aspects of survivors' mood were similar to healthy individuals, but that fatigue was elevated above norms for survivors of both early-stage and advanced disease. The study by Ersek and colleagues[32] of ovarian cancer survivors found that fatigue was the most severe physical symptom experienced by the sample. Qualitative data indicated that fatigue interfered with general activities, employment, relationships, and ability to enjoy life. Li et al.[18] found that their sample of 5-year endometrial cancer survivors reported less energy, poorer memory, and less patience than age-matched population controls, whereas Klee and Machin[21,22] found no differences in the level of tiredness between controls and survivors of endometrial and cervical cancer, and Bye et al.[23] found higher levels of fatigue in controls than survivors.

Psychosocial Issues

Despite losses inherent in gynecologic cancer and treatment, reports of overall quality of life are good.[34] The psychosocial issues that have been most frequently studied in gynecologic cancer survivors are psychologic distress and sexuality.

Psychologic Distress

Although the reported prevalence of psychologic distress among gynecologic cancer survivors varies depending on the population and the measure used, several studies have followed survivors longitudinally from diagnosis and have found that the distress experienced by gynecologic cancer survivors after diagnosis and during treatment abates over time.[21,33,35–37] A study that followed women with gynecologic cancer for 1 year after diagnosis found that their mood disturbance was not significantly different from that of women receiving surgical intervention for benign gynecologic conditions or healthy women 8 and 12 months posttreatment.[35] The majority of cross-sectional studies have found that long-term survivors report levels of psychologic distress that are comparable to women who have not had cancer,[26,33,38–41] although one study reported elevated levels of distress for survivors.[42] Wenzel's study of long-term survivors of early-stage ovarian cancer found that only 6% scored above the cutpoint for the Center for Epidemiologic Studies—Depression (CESD)

Scale.[26] Bodurka-Bevers et al.[38] found that 15% of posttreatment survivors were above the CESD cutpoint (compared to 15%–19%) for the healthy population[43,44] and that only 22% were above the 75th percentile for anxiety.[45] Congruent with findings of lower psychologic distress for long-term survivors, they also appear to be less interested in psychologic services, particularly individual counseling.[46] One study indicated that anxiety may be a bigger problems for gynecology cancer survivors than depression. Paraskevaidis et al.[47] found, in a sample of gynecologic cancer survivors (median time since diagnosis, 25 months), that 21% had clinically significant anxiety while 4% reported high levels of depression.

Psychologic concerns can persist for gynecologic cancer survivors, however, particularly those who are at high risk for recurrence or suffer lingering physical problems as a result of the cancer or its treatment. While not reporting a high prevalence of major psychiatric disorder, survivors do describe continued distress related to fears of second cancers, recurrence, and diagnostic tests.[2,26,32,39,42] This distress has been labeled the Damocles syndrome, referring to the story of Damocles, first told by Cicero, who must enjoy a grand banquet with a sword hanging by a single horsehair over his head. Cancer survivors, particularly those who have survived advanced disease, often report feeling that they have the 'sword' of recurrence hanging above them. Survivors who are at increased risk of recurrent or persistent disease, such as those with advanced gynecologic cancer, have been reported to experience higher levels of anxiety and depression.[33] Ovarian cancer, in particular, has a high risk of recurrence, and the diagnosis of persistent disease after conventional treatment appears to be more stressful than the initial diagnosis.[48]

Some studies report that younger survivors experience more severe psychologic symptoms than those who are older.[20,38] One study of long-term cervical cancer survivors of childbearing age found that while their overall quality of life was good, they were more likely to be in the lowest quartile on general health, vitality, and mental health subscales than expected based on normative data. They reported more problems with social and emotional well-being, sexual discomfort, and gynecologic symptoms compared to women who have had gestational trophoblastic disease or lymphoma.[49]

Sexual Functioning

Gynecologic cancer and its treatment often has serious, long-term effects on the sexual functioning of survivors. In 1962, Decker and Schwartzman noted that "The deprivation of sexual function may have serious sequelae . . . it appears that little attention has been given to the problem of sexual function following treatment for cervical carcinoma".[50] These authors studied 78 patients at one point in time 6 to 10 years after treatment and noted that 31% experienced partial or complete loss of sexual function. In one study that prospectively assessed sexual functioning in women with gynecologic cancer, women having surgery for benign gynecologic conditions, and healthy women, Andersen et al.[28] found numerous sexual difficulties among gynecologic cancer survivors in the year after diagnosis. Cancer survivors reported greater difficulty with sexual desire, excitement, orgasm, and resolution. Although the women who received surgery for benign conditions also reported some sexual functioning problems, they were less severe than those reported by the cancer survivors.

Carmack Taylor and colleagues[29] found lower levels of sexual activity and sexual pleasure, and higher sexual discomfort, among 248 ovarian cancer patients and survivors as compared to data from samples of healthy women and breast cancer survivors reported in other studies using the same questionnaire. Ovarian cancer survivors were also less likely to be sexually active than healthy women, regardless of whether the healthy women were pre- or postmenopausal, or on hormone replacement therapy. Patients and survivors were more likely to be sexually active if they were married, happy with their body's appearance, younger, and not on active treatment. In two additional cross-sectional studies of long-term ovarian cancer survivors, problems in sexual functioning emerged as a major concern. In a study of long-term survivors of early-stage ovarian cancer, respondents reported difficulties with decreased libido (37%) and arousal (28%), problems with orgasm (13%), and difficulty with intercourse as a result of treatment (20%). Only 12 of 49 survivors were sexually active (25%), although 51% were married.[26] Stewart and colleagues[27] reported that a significant number of the 200 ovarian cancer survivors who responded to their survey had problems with sexuality; these reports were highest among women who were treated with radiation therapy. Over half of the survivors reported that their sex lives had been negatively affected by cancer and/or its treatment. Although 64% reported that their sex lives were average to excellent before diagnosis, only 25% reported average to excellent sex lives currently. Before cancer, 36% reported their sex lives were poor to adequate, whereas now 75% rated their sex lives as poor to adequate. However, only about 20% of the sample reported a moderate to great sense of loss associated with the decline in their sexual functioning.

Survivors of cervical and endometrial cancer also experience declines in sexual functioning, and those who receive radiation therapy report more sexual difficulties.[51,52] A study of 221 indigent women treated with radiation therapy for invasive cervix cancer reported an 88% incidence of vaginal stenosis; however, sexual functioning was not evaluated in this study.[53] A decrease in sexual function in irradiated patients was reported by Seibel et al., who compared 22 patients radiated for cervical cancer versus 20 patients undergoing hysterectomy for preinvasive disease 1 year posttreatment.[54]

Schover et al.[52] conducted the first prospective evaluation of sexual function, frequency, and behavior, as well as marital happiness and psychologic distress, in 61 patients treated for early-stage cervical cancer in the United States. Although the surgical and radiation treatment groups appeared similar post-treatment and at 6-month follow-up, by 1-year women treated with radiation had more dyspareunia and problems with sexual desire and arousal than women who underwent radical hysterectomy. Pelvic examinations were performed, and a rating scale used to assess vaginal atrophy correlated with women's reports of dyspareunia, but no specific vaginal measurements were obtained. This study remains one of the few to compare the specific sexual impact of surgery versus radiation therapy.

Bruner et al. evaluated vaginal stenosis, sexual activity, and satisfaction in 90 patients treated with intracavitary radiation for endometrial or cervical cancer.[55] The authors noted a correlation between decrease in vaginal length and decrease in sexual satisfaction, but a cause-and-effect relationship was not demonstrated. Most recently, Bergmark and colleagues studied vaginal changes and sexuality in Swedish women 4 or more years after completion of treatment for cervical cancer. When compared to controls, patients with a history of cervical cancer noted similar frequency of sexual intercourse, but reported decreased vaginal lubrication and a reduction in perceived vaginal length and elasticity during intercourse. A large proportion of these women also reported that they were distressed by these changes and their effects on sexual function.[56] Although this study was described as one focusing on the impact of radical hysterectomy, the majority of women had also had radiation therapy, a likely confounding variable.

Women treated for vulvar cancer may have the most severe sexual functioning problems because of the radical surgery they often receive. A cross-sectional study of 105 survivors of vulvar and cervical cancer (average of 28 months from diagnosis)[39] found that most women who were sexually active before cancer diagnosis had resumed sexual intercourse, with the exception of older women who had received radical vulvectomies and the 3 women who received pelvic exenterations. Frequency of sexual intercourse was reduced, however. Approximately three-fourths of the women experienced sexual problems during the year following diagnosis, and 66% reported continued problems. In a study of 42 women treated for in situ vulvar cancer, Andersen and colleagues found that these women experienced more disruption in sexual functioning compared to healthy women, and that these disruptions increased over time. In addition, increasing numbers of survivors discontinued sexual activity over time. Degree of sexual dysfunction was related to the extensiveness of the treatment.[57]

Interventions

The literature includes no published trials of interventions to address late psychosocial or medical effects of gynecology cancer and its treatment. There is a small number of studies testing interventions delivered during cancer treatment that may influence long-term sequelae in survivors. These studies are reviewed here to provide information regarding what interventions might benefit gynecologic cancer survivors. Several of the studies assess outcomes 12 months or more from diagnosis. We focus on these longer-term outcomes where available (Table 105.2).

Psychosocial Issues

Four studies were identified that evaluated interventions to improve psychosocial functioning of gynecologic cancer survivors. Three of these focused primarily on sexuality[58–60] and one was concerned with a broader range of psychosocial issues.[61] All four programs used fairly standard psychoeducational approaches, providing information and opportunities for emotional expression and problem solving. Two of the studies used group interventions.[60,61] The treatments focusing on sexuality appear to have some positive effects on sexual functioning, including resuming sexual activity,[58] returning to usual frequency of sexual activity,[59] decreasing sexual fears,[60] and increasing dilator use (among younger women).[60] The intervention with the broader psychosocial focus decreased psychologic distress and improved adjustment to cancer.[61] These results indicate that psychoeducational interventions can be helpful to gynecologic cancer survivors up to a year from diagnosis and may provide benefits beyond that point. Studies by Wenzel and colleagues[26,49] indicated that a high percentage of long-term (greater than 5 years) ovarian (43%) and cervical (60%) cancer survivors would be interested in participating in programs offering psychosocial support. Given that sexual dysfunction seems to be a very prevalent problem for long-term gynecologic cancer survivors, interventions that focus on sexuality are particularly appropriate. More research is needed to refine interventions such as those tested in these studies to produce programs that can be disseminated and implemented by physician extenders and/or survivor organizations.

Medical Issues

Only one study was identified that tested an intervention for its ability to reduce late medical effects of gynecologic cancer. Bye et al.[23,62] tested a dietary intervention to reduce diarrhea in cervical and endometrial cancer patients receiving radiation therapy. The intervention (recommendation of a low-fat, low-lactose diet during radiation therapy and for 6 weeks after treatment) was effective during treatment[62]; 3 to 4 years after treatment some positive effects were still present.[23] While these results are intriguing, more research is needed to replicate this finding.

Emerging Areas

It is critical that the study of cancer survivorship in gynecology advance beyond small descriptive studies of the sequelae of gynecologic cancer. The field needs more carefully controlled longitudinal studies of late effects, using standardized measures, triangulation of self-report measures with clinical evaluation, and adequate sample sizes. Additionally, input from survivors themselves is needed to determine what sequelae and late effects of cancer are salient to them. For example, although the prevalence of clinically significant psychologic distress appears to be fairly low in gynecologic cancer survivors, some studies indicate that long-term survivors feel they would benefit from additional psychosocial services.[26,49]

Additional research data would guide clinical care of long-term cancer survivors and would identify areas in which interventions are needed. The existing research base indicates that treatment to address menopausal symptoms, sexual functioning, anxiety about recurrence and follow-up visits, fatigue, pain, gastrointestinal symptoms, and health behaviors such as physical activity and smoking cessation would be helpful to gynecologic cancer survivors. More careful longitudinal research would identify which survivors need intervention and elucidate optimal timing for providing assistance in these areas.

TABLE 105.2. Studies evaluating interventions for gynecologic cancer survivors.

Author	*Year*	*Intervention focus*	*Type of trial*	*No. of participants*	*Type of participants*	*Type of treatment*	*Length of follow-up*	*Results*
Lamont et al.[58]	1978	Psychosexual rehabilitation after pelvic exenteration	Case series	12	Gynecologic cancer patients receiving pelvic exenteration	Team approach to treatment including sex therapist meetings with patient and partner before surgery, in hospital, and after discharge as needed Provides information and counseling	6 months	Of the 12 women receiving treatment with the team approach, 8 were thought to have good adjustment before surgery. Seven of these women resumed sexual activity. Six were having orgasms within 6 months; the 7th was still recovering from surgery at the time of article publication. Decreased sexual desire and difficulty using dilators was a common concern.
Capone et al.[59]	1980	Psychosocial rehabilitation and sexuality (for sexually active patients)	Quasi-experimental	97	Gynecologic cancer patients	Counseling by psychologist during initial hospitalization, minimum of four sessions	12 months	Women in experimental group more likely to have returned to usual frequency of sexual activity at 12 months than women in control group. Experimental group twice as likely to have returned to work at 12 months, but differences not significant. No significant differences between groups in emotional functioning at 12 months.
Cain et al.[61]	1986	Individual and group counseling	Randomized	80 (60 with 1-year follow-up)	Gynecologic cancer patients	Patients randomized to group or individual counseling, or standard care Counseling consisted of eight weekly sessions focusing on predetermined themes Techniques included providing information, emotional expression, problem-solving, and relaxation	12 months	Survivors in both the individual and group counseling conditions had less anxiety and depression and better adjustment to their illness than the standard care group at the final (12-month) assessment.
Robinson et al.[60]	1999	Sexuality and use of vaginal dilators	Randomized	32	Cervix and endometrial cancer patients receiving radiotherapy	Two 1.5-hour group sessions presented information about sexuality and cancer, promoted the idea that sex is pleasurable, and taught behavioral skills in communication about sexuality, using dilators and lubricants, and performing Kegel exercises	12 months	No impact on Sexual History Form scores (overall sexual functioning); intervention group had significantly lower scores on scale measuring sexual fears, intervention improved knowledge in older group but not younger group. Intervention increased dilator use in younger group but not older group.
Bye et al.[23]	2000	Diet to reduce diarrhea during radiation treatment	Randomized	143 in initial trial, 79 (43 intervention, 36 control) in 3- to 4-year follow-up	Cervix and endometrial cancer patients receiving radiation therapy	Low-fat, low-lactose diet during radiation therapy and for 6 weeks after the end of treatment	3–4 years	7% of the intervention group and 22% of the control group reported diarrhea at follow-up ($P = 0.05$), although difference in diarrhea score was not statistically significant (Intervention group, M = 19.4; Control group, M = 29.6; $P = 0.09$). In original study, 23% of intervention group and 48% of control group reported diarrhea during radiation therapy. Diarrhea during radiation was associated with diarrhea at follow-up for the control group only. There were no differences at follow-up in quality of life.

References

1. Anderson B, Lutgendorf S. Quality of life in gynecologic cancer survivors. CA Cancer J Clin 1997;47:218–225.
2. Auchincloss SS. After treatment: psychosocial issues in gynecologic cancer survivorship. Cancer (Phila) 1995;76(suppl 10): 2117–2124.
3. Segal R, Evans W, Johnson D, et al. Structured exercise improves physical functioning in women with stage I and II breast cancer: results of a randomized controlled trial. J Clin Oncol 2001;19: 657–665.
4. Courneya KS, Mackey JR, Bell GJ, Jones LW, Field CJ, Fairey AS. Randomized controlled trial of exercise training in postmenopausal breast cancer survivors: Cardiopulmonary and quality of life outcomes. J Clin Oncol 2003;21:1660–1668.
5. Segal RJ, Reid RD, Courneya KS, et al. Resistance exercise in men receiving androgen deprivation therapy for prostate cancer. J Clin Oncol 2003;21:1653–1659.
6. Kaaks R, Lukanova A, Kurzer MS. Obesity, endogenous hormones, and endometrial cancer risk: a synthetic review. Cancer Epidemiol Biomarkers Prev 2002;11:1531–1543.
7. Goodman MT, Hankin JH, Wilkens LR, et al. Diet, body size, physical activity, and the risk of endometrial cancer. Cancer Res 1997;57:5077–5085.
8. Bristow RE. Endometrial cancer. Curr Opin Oncol 1999;11: 388–393.
9. Jemal A, Tiwari RC, Murray T, et al. Cancer statistics, 2004. CA Cancer J Clin 2004;54:8–29.
10. Ries LAG, Eisner MP, Kosary CL, et al. SEER Cancer Statistics Review, 1975–2000. Bethesda, MD: National Cancer Institute, 2003.
11. Waggoner SE. Cervical cancer. Lancet 2003;361:2217–2225.
12. Sung HY, Kearney KA, Miller M, Kinney W, Sawaya GF, Hiatt RA. Papanicolaou smear history and diagnosis of invasive cervical carcinoma among members of a large prepaid health plan. Cancer (Phila) 2000;88:2283–2289.
13. Kjaer SK, Engholm G, Dahl C, Bock JE. Case-control study of risk factors for cervical squamous cell neoplasia in Denmark. IV: Role of smoking habits. Eur J Cancer Prev 1996;5:359–365.
14. Wilkenstein W. Smoking and cervical cancer—current status: a review. J Epidemiol 1990;131:945–957.
15. Daling JR, Madeleine MM, McKnight B, et al. The relationship of human papillomavirus-related cervical tumors to cigarette smoking, oral contraceptive use, and prior herpes simplex virus type 2 infection. Cancer Epidemiol Biomarkers Prev 1996;5: 541–548.
16. Waggoner S, Fuhrman B, Monk B, et al. Influence of smoking on progression-free and overall survival in stage II-B, III-B and IV-A cervical carcinoma: a gynecologic or (GOG) study. Society of Gynecologic Oncologists, New Orleans, LA, January 31 to February 4 2003.
17. Furberg AS, Thune I. Metabolic abnormalities (hypertension, hyperglycemia and overweight), lifestyle (high energy intake and physical inactivity) and endometrial cancer risk in a Norwegian cohort. Int J Cancer 2003;104:669–676.
18. Li C, Samsioe G, Iosif C. Quality of life in endometrial cancer survivors. Maturitas 1999;31:227–236.
19. Scruggs S, Carmack Taylor C, Jhingran A, et al. Obesity and physical functioning in endometrial cancer survivors. Presented at the Annual Meeting of the Society of Behavioral Medicine, Baltimore, MD, 2004.
20. Li C, Samsioe G, Iosif C. Quality of life in long-term survivors of cervical cancer. Maturitas 1999;32:95–102.
21. Klee M, Machin D. Health-related quality of life of patients with endometrial cancer who are disease-free following external irradiation. Acta Oncol 2001;40:816–824.
22. Klee M, Thranov I, Machin D. The patients' perspective on physical symptoms after radiotherapy for cervical cancer. Gynecol Oncol 2000;76:14–23.
23. Bye A, Trope C, Loge JH, Hjermstad M, Kaasa S. Health-related quality of life occurrence of intestinal side effects after pelvic radiotherapy. Evaluation of long-term effects of diagnosis and treatment. Acta Oncol 2000;39:173–180.
24. Jereczek-Fossa BA. Postoperative irradiation in endometrial cancer: still a matter of controversy. Cancer Treat Rev 2001; 27:19–33.
25. DiSaia PJ, Creasman WT. Clinical Gynecologic Oncology. St. Louis: Mosby, 2002:675.
26. Wenzel LB, Donnelly JP, Fowler JM, et al. Resilience, reflection, and residual stress in ovarian cancer survivorship: a gynecologic oncology group study. Psycho-Oncology 2002;11:142–153.
27. Stewart DE, Wong F, Duff S, Melancon CH, Cheung AM. "What doesn't kill you makes you stronger": an ovarian cancer survivor survey. Gynecol Oncol 2001;83:537–542.
28. Andersen BL, Anderson B, deProsse C. Controlled prospective longitudinal study of women with cancer: I. Sexual functioning outcomes. J Consult Clin Psychol 1989;57:683–691.
29. Carmack Taylor C, Basen-Engquist K, Shinn EH, Bodurka DC. Predictors of sexual functioning in ovarian cancer patients. J Clin Oncol 2004;22:881–889.
30. Headley JA, Theriault RL, LeBlanc AD, Vassilopoulou-Sellin R, Hortobagyi GN. Pilot study of bone mineral density in breast cancer patients treated with adjuvant chemotherapy. Cancer Invest 1998;16:6–11.
31. Mahon SM, Williams MT, Spies MA. Screening for second cancers and osteoporosis in long-term survivors. Cancer Pract 2000;8:282–290.
32. Ersek M, Ferrell BR, Dow KH, Melancon CH. Quality of life in women with ovarian cancer. West J Nurs Res 1997;19:334–350.
33. Lutgendorf SK, Anderson B, Ullrich P, et al. Quality of life and mood in women with gynecologic cancer: a one year prospective study. Cancer (Phila) 2002;94:131–140.
34. McCartney CF, Larson DB. Quality of life in patients with gynecologic cancer. Cancer (Phila) 1987;60:2129–2136.
35. Andersen BL, Anderson B, deProsse C. Controlled prospective longitudinal study of women with cancer: II. Psychological outcomes. J Consult Clin Psychol 1989;57:692–697.
36. Klee M, Thranov I, Machin D. Life after radiotherapy: the psychological and social effects experienced by women treated for advanced stages of cervical cancer. Gynecol Oncol 2000;76: 5–13.
37. Greimel E, Thiel I, Peintinger F, Cegnar I, Pongratz E. Prospective assessment of quality of life of female cancer patients. Gynecol Oncol 2002;85:140–147.
38. Bodurka-Bevers D, Basen-Engquist K, Carmack CL, et al. Depression, anxiety and quality of life in patients with epithelial ovarian cancer. Gynecol Oncol 2000;78:302–308.
39. Corney RH, Everett H, Howells A, Crowther ME. Psychosocial adjustment following major gynaecological surgery for carcinoma of the cervix and vulva. J Psychosom Res 1992;36:561–568.
40. Andersen BL, Hacker NF. Psychosexual adjustment after vulvar surgery. Obstet Gynecol 1983;62:457.
41. Miller BE, Pittman B, Case D, McQuellon RP. Quality of life after treatment for gynecologic malignacies: A pilot study in an outpatient clinic. Gynecol Oncol 2002;87:178–184.
42. Cull A, Cowie VJ, Farquharson DI, Livingstone JR, Smart GE, Elton RA. Early stage cervical cancer: psychosocial and sexual outcomes of treatment. Br J Cancer 1993;68:1216–1220.
43. Radloff LS. The CES-D scale: a self-report depression scale for research in the general population. Appl Psychol Measure 1977; 1:385–401.
44. Roberts RE, Vernon SW. The center for epidemiologic studies depression scale: its use in a community sample. Am J Psychiatry 1983;140:41–46.
45. Spielberger CD, Gorsuch RL, Lushene R, Vagg PR, Jacobs GA. State-Trait Anxiety Inventory for Adults: Sampler Set Manual, Test, Scoring Key, vol 1. Palo Alto, CA: Consulting Psychologists Press, 1983:70.

46. Pistrang N, Winchurst C. Gynaecological cancer patients' attitudes towards psychological services. Psychol Health Med 1997; 2:135–147.
47. Paraskevaidis E, Kitchener HC, Walker LG. Doctor-patient communcation and subsequent mental health in women with gynaecological cancer. Psycho-Oncology 1993;2:195–200.
48. Guidozzi F. Living with ovarian cancer. Gynecol Oncol 1993; 50:202–207.
49. Basen-Engquist K, Paskett ED, Buzaglo J, et al. Cervical cancer: behavioral factors related to screening, diagnosis, and survivors' quality of life. Cancer (Suppl) 2003;98:2009–2014.
50. Decker WH, Schwartzman E. Sexual function following treatment for carcinoma of the cervix. Am J Obstet Gynecol 1962; 83:401–405.
51. Juraskova I, Butow P, Robertson R, Sharpe L, McLeod C, Hacker N. Post-treatment sexual adjustment following cervical and endometrial cancer: a qualitative insight. Psycho-Oncology 2003;12:267–279.
52. Schover LR, Fife M, Gershenson DM. Sexual dysfunction and treatment for early stage cervical cancer. Cancer (Phila) 1989; 63:204–212.
53. Hartman P, Diddle AW. Vaginal stenosis following irradiation therapy for carcinoma of the cervix uteri. Cancer (Phila) 1972; 30:426–429.
54. Seibel MM, Freeman MG, Graves WL. Carcinoma of the cervix and sexual function. Obstet Gynecol 1980;55:484–487.
55. Bruner DW, Lanciano R, Keegan M, Corn B, Martin E, Hanks GE. Vaginal stenosis and sexual function following intracavitary radiation for the treatment of cervical and endometrial carcinoma. Int J Radiat Oncol Biol Phys 1993;27:825–830.
56. Bergmark K, Avall-Lundqvist E, Dickman PW, Henningsohn L, Steineck G. Vaginal changes and sexuality in women with a history of cervical cancer. N Engl J Med 1999;340:1383–1389.
57. Andersen BL, Turnquist, Dawn, et al. Sexual functioning after treatment of in situ vulvar cancer: preliminary report. Obstet Gynecol 1988;71:15–19.
58. Lamont JA, De Petrillo AD, Sargeant EJ. Psychosexual rehabilitation and exenterative surgery. Gynecol Oncol 1978;6:236–242.
59. Capone MA, Good RS, Westie KS, Jacobson AF. Psychosocial rehabilitation of gynecologic oncology patients. Arch Phys Med Rehabil 1980;61:128–132.
60. Robinson JW, Faris PD, Scott CB. Psychoeducational group increases vaginal dilation for younger women and reduces sexual fears for women of all ages with gynecological carcinoma treated with radiotherapy. Int J Radiat Oncol Biol Phys 1999;44:497–506.
61. Cain EN, Kohorn EI, Quinlan DM, Latimer K, Schwartz PE. Psychosocial benefits of a cancer support group. Cancer (Phila) 1986;57:183–189.
62. Bye A, Kaasa S, Ose T, Sundfor K, Trope C. The influence of low-fat, low lactose diet on radiation induced diarrhoea. Clin Nutr 1992;11:147–153.
63. Brekelmans CT. Risk factors and risk reduction of breast and ovarian cancer. Curr Opin Obstet Gynecol 2003;15:63–68.
64. Gershenson DA, Tortolero-Luna G, Malpica A, et al. Ovarian intraepithelial neoplasia and ovarian cancer. Gynecol Cancer Prev 1996;23:475–543.
65. Edmondson RJ, Monaghan JM. The epidemiology of ovarian cancer. Int J Gynecol Cancer 2001;11:423–429.

106

Medical, Psychosocial, and Health-Related Quality of Life Issues in Breast Cancer Survivors

Julie Lemieux, Louise J. Bordeleau, and Pamela J. Goodwin

Women with breast cancer account for the largest group of female cancer survivors. It is estimated that there are currently 8.9 million cancer survivors in the United States; 41% of the female subjects are breast cancer survivors.[1] The growing number of breast cancer survivors reflects increasing incidence of the disease, diagnosis at earlier stages when outcome is better, and widespread adoption of effective adjuvant treatment (see Chapter 28 and Chapter 54).

Methodologic Issues in Survivorship Research

The Office of Cancer Survivorship of the National Cancer Institute (U.S.) defines a survivor as follows: "An individual is considered a cancer survivor from the time of cancer diagnosis, through the balance of his or her life. Family members, friends and caregivers are also impacted by the survivorship experience and are therefore included in this definition."[1] This is a very broad definition; most survivorship research in breast cancer focuses on the experience of individuals with cancer after they have completed their primary therapy, usually while they are free of recurrent disease. Some studies have focused on women who are 1, 3, 5, or more years postdiagnosis. In breast cancer, where long-term survival is becoming increasingly common, this variable definition may account for some of the inconsistencies in the literature. In this chapter, we have not adopted a single definition of survivorship but have tried to relate results to the definition used in each study.

Definition, recruitment, and identification of study populations are among the most challenging aspects of breast cancer survivorship research. Ideally, if the objective is to examine long-term outcomes, an inception cohort identified at a uniform time early in the course of the disease should be assembled (e.g., women with locoregional breast cancer in the immediate postoperative period, before adjuvant therapy). Prospective recruitment of a sample such as this is costly and time consuming. An alternative approach involves the use of administrative databases (including tumor registries) that retrospectively identify women diagnosed years earlier; however, careful attention must be paid to refusers and nonresponders, who may differ in important ways from responders. Investigators often conducted cross-sectional surveys of breast cancer patients attending follow-up clinics, or in a community. The populations thus assembled may not be representative of all breast cancer survivors, particularly when response rates are low, or well women have been discharged from follow-up clinics. Convenience samples, drawn from breast cancer advocacy groups or other sources, were recruited in some studies. This approach may lead to systematic overestimation or underestimation of the long-term impact of breast cancer and its treatment, because participation of women in these groups may be related to their survivorship experience.

Inclusion of a control population without cancer should be considered in breast cancer survivorship research. This condition allows the effects of aging and comorbid conditions to be differentiated from those of prior breast cancer and its treatment, important for many of the medical concerns of breast cancer survivors (e.g., menopause, osteoporosis, heart disease). Although inclusion of a noncancer control group is often desirable, it increases costs and complexity of research. Instead, investigators may opt to use measurement instruments for which population-based norms are available, comparing the results obtained in the breast cancer survivors with published results in age-matched controls.

Breast cancer survivorship studies often examine a broad variety of attributes: medical status, psychosocial issues, health-related quality of life (HRQOL), and sexuality, for example. Some of these attributes are readily measurable (e.g., bone density after chemotherapy-induced early menopause) while others are not (e.g., the social impact of breast cancer diagnosis). It is important that measurement instruments be valid and reliable and that they measure key areas of interest. A wide variety of standardized, validated instruments are available to measure many of the important psychosocial issues and health-related quality of life (HRQOL) in breast cancer survivors. When valid instruments are not available for key attributes, such as body image postmastectomy, investigators may need to develop new instruments and validate these instruments during the course of the research. In selecting questionnaires, investigators should avoid overburdening respondents.

It is likely that not all salient issues in breast cancer survivors have been identified. Recent evidence that cognitive dysfunction may occur in women receiving adjuvant chemotherapy is a prime example. Investigators should be aware of new and ongoing research and be prepared to examine newly emerging concepts.

Statistical analysis should include the use of appropriate statistical tests, with adjustment for the effects of age because it could be an important confounder. The use of baseline information, which allows evaluation of change over time, can provide valuable insights into the breast cancer survivorship process. As noted previously, comparison of study data with population-based norms also provides insight into the impact of aging versus the impact of prior breast cancer diagnosis.

In the remainder of this chapter, we review the survivorship literature in breast cancer, first as it relates to medical status and then as it relates to psychosocial status and HRQOL. This separation is somewhat artificial; there is overlap between the sections. Because most studies are observational, grading of evidence regarding efficacy of interventions is usually not possible.

Medical Status

Arm Symptoms/Upper Body Function

Treatment for breast cancer can be associated with a number of localized physical sequelae including arm edema (AE), impaired shoulder mobility, pain, neurologic deficits, and reduced upper body function. The literature assessing arm symptoms and limitations is summarized in Table 106.1.

There are three approaches to arm measurement: (1) circumference at various points (with bony landmarks as references), (2) volumetric measurements using limb submersion in water, and (3) skin and soft tissue tonometry.[2] Tape-measured circumference (10cm above and below the olecranon or the lateral epicondyle) has been the traditional method but can be imprecise. Volumetric measurements are more accurate but have limited availability. Tonometry is not used clinically.

The occurrence of, and risk factors for, AE have been reviewed by Erickson et al.[3] The reported incidence of AE has ranged from 0% after partial or total mastectomy with sentinel node biopsy to 56% after modified radical mastectomy (MRM) or breast-conserving surgery (BCS) with both axillary lymph node dissection (ALND) and axillary radiation therapy (XRT).[4,5] Werner et al.[6] reported that the median time to development of AE in patients treated with BCS, ALND (almost one-third had level 3 ALND), and breast XRT (with or without axillary XRT) was 14 months (range, 2–92 months); 97% of those who developed AE did so by 4 years.

The association between the extent of breast surgery and AE is less clear. Tasmuth et al. reported AE to be significantly more frequent in a prospective cohort study of 93 women treated with MRM versus BCS; however, women undergoing MRM had axillary XRT (also associated with AE) more commonly than those undergoing BCS.[7] Paci et al.[8] reported the odds ratio of chronic AE to be slightly, but not significantly, higher after MRM [odds ratio (OR), 1.62; 95% confidence interval (CI), 0.91–2.88] than after BCS (XRT was not examined). In a randomized trial comparing MRM to BCS with XRT to the breast and internal mammary and supraclavicular nodes, Gerber et al. reported the rate of AE did not differ between the two groups; however, axillary XRT (given if the dissection was inadequate or there was extracapsular extension) was not considered in the analysis.[5]

The risk of AE increases with the extent of axillary dissection. Yeoh et al.[9] reported frequency of AE to be 25% with no axillary surgery, 50% after axillary sampling, and 84% after ALND. The risk of AE was higher with an increasing number of axillary lymph nodes resected (more than 15 nodes[10]; more than 40 nodes[11]) in two studies. Schrenk et al. reported AE did not occur in a small cohort of patients undergoing sentinel lymph node dissection.[4] In a prospective randomized trial of sector resection and ALND with or without breast XRT, young age [relative risk (RR), 0.93 per year of increasing age; 95% CI, 0.91–0.97) and number of lymph nodes resected (RR, 1.11 per lymph node resected; 95% CI, 1.05–1.18) were significantly associated with any arm symptoms (not necessarily AE).[12]

Axillary XRT has been associated with AE. Senofsky et al., in a cohort of 264 patients treated with total ALND, found AE to occur in 6% of those not treated with XRT, 14.7% of those receiving XRT to the breast only, and 29.6% of those receiving XRT to the breast and regional nodes.[13] Furthermore, Keramopoulos et al. reported AE to be significantly more frequent when XRT was delayed (6 months postoperatively) than when it was given immediately postoperatively (4% versus 27%).[11]

The combination of XRT and ALND further increases the risk of AE. Kissin et al.[14] reported AE in 8.3% of women treated with breast surgery and axillary XRT, 9.1% undergoing axillary sampling and XRT, and 7.4% undergoing ALND only (7.4%). However, AE occurred in 38.3% of women undergoing both ALND and axillary XRT. In a randomized trial comparing ALND to axillary sampling, a significant increase in arm volume was experienced in 14 (12 of whom received axillary XRT) of 47 (29.8%) patients treated with ALND.[15] None of the 48 patients undergoing axillary sampling experienced AE (regardless of XRT).

The occurrence of other reduced upper body function, pain, neurologic deficits, and restricted shoulder mobility has also been evaluated. In a prospective cohort study, decline in upper body function was substantially higher during the first year after MRM or BCS with or without XRT than in the subsequent 4 years.[16] Cardiopulmonary comorbidity significantly increased the risk of decline in upper body function at 5 months (OR, 2.8; 95% CI, 1.3–5.7). Cardiopulmonary

TABLE 106.1. Arm symptoms in treatment for breast cancer.

Reference	*Primary objective(s)*	*Study population and follow-up (years)*	*No. of patients*	*Type of local treatment*	*Instruments*	*Response rate*	*Results and conclusions*
Kissin et al. 1986[14]	Compare the incidence of AE by subjective and objective methods; identify independent risk for late AE; compare the incidence of AE after different treatments	Cohort (clinic) diagnosed at least 1 year prior	200 patients	BCS or MRM with no axillary surgery, sampling or ALND	• Subjective: graded as no difference, moderate AE, or severe AE (patient + observer) • Objective: (1) arm circumference measured 15 cm above and 10 cm below the lateral epicondyle, (2) volume measured by water immersion		Objective AE more frequent (25.5%) than subjective AE (14%). Subjective AE was significantly more common after ALND with XRT (38.3%), axillary XRT alone (8.3%), axillary sampling with XRT (9.1%), and ALND alone (7.4%).
Yeoh et al. 1986[9]	Assess the complications following surgery and postoperative XRT	Cohort assessed median F/U of 1.7–3.24 years	187 patients	Surgical management of the axilla: none, sampling, or ALND with three different XRT dose fractionation	• Physical exam: (1) arm circumference measured 7.5 cm above the olecranon process, (2) shoulder movement and degree of restriction		Complication rates similar with three different XRT schedules. AE ± restriction of shoulder movements were different at 30 months with no surgery (25%), sampling (50%), and ALND (84%).
Borup Christensen et al. 1989[15]	Compare the sequelae of ALND vs. axillary sampling ± XRT	Prospective randomized trial with assessment at 14 days, 3, 6, and 12 months postoperative	100 patients	BCS or MRM ± XRT, randomization to ALND vs. axillary sampling	• Physical exam: (1) arm volume (measured by water displacement and corrected for changes in body weight), (2) shoulder mobility using 360 scale • Questionnaire re: arm swelling, shoulder mobility, and loss of sensibility.		AE (≥10% volume increase) in 14 pts (all with ALND), 12 received XRT. Impairment of shoulder mobility was more frequent after axillary XRT ($P = 0.07$).

Satariano et al. 1990[138]	Assess physical functioning	Case control (3 and 12 months post diagnosis) (Metropolitan Detroit Cancer Surveillance System)	571 cases (breast cancer) 647 controls (no breast cancer)	Not mentioned	• Structured interview with items from (1) Massachusetts Health Care Panel Study, (2) Framingham Disability Study, and (3) the National Institute on Aging EPESE	Cases: 81.1% 3 months, 95.1% 12 months Controls: 83.3% 3 months, 90.9% 12 months	At 3 months, cases age 55–74 had greater difficulty completing tasks requiring upper body strength. At 12 months, upper body strength remained diminished in cases aged 65–74, more so than cases aged 55–64.
Senofsky G.M. et al. 1991[13]	Assess the effects of TAL	Prospective cohort, median follow-up of 41 months	264 patients	BSC or MRM + TAL ± XRT	• Medical records review • Clinical examination: AE graded I–IV (method of measurement not stated).		AE in 9.4% of patients. Breast and nodal XRT significantly associated with AE. Breast edema associated with XRT.
Segerstrom et al. 1991[18]	Study the natural history of pain and functional impairment after surgery and XRT	Prospective cohort assessed at 1–23 months and 1 week–24 months after exam 1	100 patients	MRM + ALND + high-dose XRT (±XRT to axilla)	• Questionnaire • Physical exam: (1) arm edema (water displacement method), (2) ROM (inspection)	93 patients (93%)	AE observed in 43% of patients; AE disappeared in 8 patients at follow-up (all had slight to moderate edema). Stiffness and edema good predictors of subjective functional impairment.
Werner et al. 1991[6]	Assess predictors of AE	Cohort of patients receiving XRT, median F/U of 37 months	282 patients	BCS + ALND (30.5% had level I, II, and III dissected) + XRT	• Arm circumference measured 13 cm above and 10 cm below the olecranon on both arms		Transient AE in 7.4%, chronic arm edema in 12.1%. Persistent AE at 5 years in 16%. Body mass index strongly associated with AE.
Sneeuw et al. 1992[139]	Assess the cosmetic and functional outcomes of BCS and relationship to psychosocial functioning	Cohort, mean 4 years (2–11 years)	160 patients eligible	BCS + XRT; most patients had ALND	• In-home interview: GHQ, QOL • Physical exam	76 (47.5%) patients	High levels of psychologic distress, disturbance of body image, and decreased sexual functioning ~25%. Patient ratings of overall cosmesis and AE significantly associated with body image.
Gerber et al. 1992[5]	To compare pain, motion, and edema after MRM vs. BCS with ALND and XRT	Prospective randomized trial, annual evaluation	247 patients	MRM vs. BCS + XRT with ALND	• Physical exam: (1) functional ROM (goniometry), (2) chest wall tenderness, (3) arm circumference at ulnar styloid, olecranon, and 35 cm proximal to the ulnar styloid, (4) cosmetic outcome	165 patients (66.8%) had pre-op and post-op ROM, 131 (53%) patients had pre-op and 1 yr post-op arm circumference	Greater chest wall tenderness post-XRT. Slower recovery of pre-operative ROM post MRM. No difference in arm circumference.

(continued)

TABLE 106.1. Arm symptoms in treatment for breast cancer. (continued)

Reference	*Primary objective(s)*	*Study population and follow-up (years)*	*No. of patients*	*Type of local treatment*	*Instruments*	*Response rate*	*Results and conclusions*
Lin et al. 1993[19]	Assess impact of ALND	Retrospective review	283 patients	BCS or MRM + ALND	• Chart review • Physical examination 1 year: arm circumference, ROM, numbness, and pain.		Arm swelling (≥2 cm) in 16% of women, ≥15 degrees of restriction in 17%, numbness in the distribution of the intercostals brachial nerve in 78%, and numbness and pain in 22%.
Keramopoulos et al. 1993[11]	Assess arm morbidity following treatment	Clinic population over a 6-month window	104 patients	BCS or MRM with ALND	• Interview • Physical examination: arm circumference measured at 15 cm above and 10 cm below the lateral epicondyles in both hands.		Late AE (>3 months postsurgery) occurred in 17%; more frequent when XRT <6 months postoperative or >40 LN resected. Limb pain was more frequent >60 years old or after MRM.
Kiel et al. 1996[10]	Incidence of AE after BCS and XRT	Cohort q 6 mo for up to 3 years	402 women	BCS + XRT (±AND)	• Physical examination: arm circumference measured 15 cm above and 10 cm below the olecranon process.	183 included in the study	Axillary dissection (>15 LN) and age (>55 years) are predictors of AE.
Paci et al. 1996[8]	Assess long-term sequelae of breast cancer surgery	Cohort of 5-year survivors	346 survivors	BCS or MRM	• Interview • Physical exam: arm circumference measured at six points	238 women (68.8%)	30.2% had a chronic lymphedema and 18.9% a shoulder deficit. Chronic lymphedema greater after MRM vs. BCS. Early lymphedema more frequent after BCS.
Tasmuth et al. 1996[7]	Assess physical symptoms and anxiety/depression	Prospective cohort day—1, 1 month, 6 months, and 1 year after surgery	105 women	MRM vs. BCS with ALND ± XRT	• Interview • Neurologic examination • Grip strength • Arm circumference • STAI + 2 additional questions re depression	93 women (89%)	Incidence of chronic posttreatment pain higher after BCS vs. MRM. Phantom sensations in 25%. Psychologic morbidity highest before surgery and decreased with time.

Liljegren et al. 1997[12]	Assess arm morbidity after sector resection and ALND ± XRT	Prospective randomized trial 3, 12, 24, and 36 months after surgery	381 women	Sector resection and ALND ± XRT	• Arm circumference 10 cm above and below the elbow on both arms • Subjective arm symptoms (graded as none, moderate, or severe)	Arm circumference: 273 pts at 3–12 mo., 270 pts at 13–36 mo., <50 pts at >36 mo. Arm symptoms: 368 pts at 3–12 mo., 335 pts at 13–36 mo., 115 pts >36 mo.	Extent of surgical procedure and young age are determinants of arm morbidity. Arm symptoms are most common during the first year.
Silliman et al. 1999[17]	To identify risk factors for decline in upper body function	Cross-sectional observational study 3–5 months postoperative	300 women	BCS or MRM ± XRT	• Review of medical records • Telephone interview	213 women (71%)	Extent and type of primary therapy and cardiopulmonary comorbidity associated with a decline in upper body function.
Schrenk et al. 2000[4]	Assess postoperative morbidity of the operated arm	Prospective cohort 15–17 months F/U	35 women	BCS or MRM ± XRT with ALND or SN dissection	• Physical exam: arm circumference (15 cm above and 10 cm below the lateral epicondyle), numbness, mobility, strength, stiffness • Interview	35 patients (100%)	SN associated with negligible morbidity compared with ALND.
Lash et al. 2000[16]	Assess the effect of patient characteristics and therapy on self-reported upper-body function and discomfort	Prospective cohort 5 and 21 months postoperative	388 invited, 303 interviewed	MRM or BCS ± XRT	• Review of medical records • Computer-assisted telephone interviews		Cardiopulmonary comorbidity associated with decline at 5-month interview (OR 2.8, 95% CI 1.3–5.7). ALND associated with axillary numbness, pain.
Lash et al. 2002[140]	Characterize the incidence and predictors of upper body function decline and recovery	Cohort for 5 years	303 women	BCS ± XRT or MRM	• Review of medical records • Telephone interviews • SF-36	82 met case definition for upper-body function decline. 32 met the definition for recovery.	The incidence of decline in the first year was substantially higher than in the subsequent 4 years. Women with less than a high school education had an increased risk of decline (HR 2.3). Recovery was higher for women followed by breast cancer specialist.

BCS, breast-conserving surgery; XRT, radiation therapy; HR, hazard ratio; OR, odds ratio; ALND, axillary lymph node dissection; SN, sentinel node dissection; AE, arm edema; F/U, follow-up; TAL, total axillary lymphadenectomy; EPESE, Established Populations for the Epidemiological Study of the Elderly; GHQ, General Health Questionnaire; STAI, State Trait Anxiety Inventory; SF-36, Medical Outcomes Study Short Form—36 Items.

morbidity was an independent predictor of upper body function decline ($P = 0.006$) in a second study[17]; mastectomy and XRT were also associated with significant declines in upper body function. Women treated with an ALND were more likely to report numbness or pain in the axilla (OR, 6.4; 95% CI, 0.2–33).[16]

In a prospective cohort study, Segerstrom et al.[18] reported 35 of 93 (37.6%) patients had restricted shoulder range of motion during the first 2 years after surgery; this increased to 49.5% up to 2 years later. Paci et al.[8] reported that 18.9% of patients experienced shoulder deficit as assessed by physical examination performed 5 or more years after diagnosis. Lin et al.[19] reported 15° or greater loss of ROM in 17% of the patients and 30° or more loss in 4% at 1 or more years after ALND. In contrast, Gerber et al.[5] found no significant loss in functional ROM (assessed using goniometry) 1 year postoperatively; however, patients undergoing MRM reached their preoperative ROM more slowly than those undergoing BCS.[5] Pain and chest wall tenderness have been reported following breast surgery.[5,7,11] Pain was more frequent after BCS in one study[7] and after mastectomy in another.[11]

Arm symptoms have been associated with psychologic, social, sexual, and functional morbidity.[20] In two case-control studies, women experiencing AE after treatment for breast cancer showed greater psychologic morbidity and greater impact of illness measured using the Psychosocial Adjustment to Illness Scale (PAIS), effects that remained stable over a 6-month period, even if AE was being treated.[21,22] Maunsell et al. also reported the proportion of women experiencing psychological distress as measured by the Psychiatric Symptom Index (PSI) increased significantly with an increased number of problems in the affected arm.[23]

In summary, significant physical and functional sequelae in the arm and upper body may occur as a result of local therapy, especially ALND and axillary XRT. Prospective, population-based studies that include an assessment of patient demographics, risk factors, stage, and treatment coupled with outcome evaluation that involves standardized, blinded assessment of arm symptoms and function preoperatively and during long-term follow-up would expand available information; intervention research to identify effective management approaches is urgently needed.

Menopause

Women with breast cancer may experience early menopause as a result of their treatment. They report a higher frequency of menopausal symptoms than women in the general population.[24] The high frequency of menopausal symptoms in breast cancer survivors is caused by several factors[25]: (1) age at diagnosis (frequently over 50 years), (2) abrupt discontinuation of hormone replacement therapy (HRT) at the time of breast cancer diagnosis, (3) induction of premature menopause by therapy (i.e., chemotherapy and ovarian ablation), and (4) induction of estrogen deficiency symptoms by therapy (e.g., tamoxifen and aromatase inhibitors) (Table 106.2). Chemotherapy is frequently associated with either temporary or permanent amenorrhea. The incidence of amenorrhea is related to the type of chemotherapy regimen, the cumulative dose (particularly cyclophosphamide), and the age of the patient.[26,27] Surgically induced menopause and premature menopause have been associated with more severe symptoms than natural menopause.[28,29] The health consequences of menopause can be divided into four categories: vasomotor symptoms, genitourinary signs and symptoms, skeletal effects, and cardiovascular effects.[30] In a survey of 190 breast cancer survivors, the most common symptoms experienced were hot flashes (65%), night sweats (44%), vaginal dryness (44%), difficulty sleeping (44%), depression (44%), and dyspareunia (26%).[31] Hot flashes (HF) are more frequent, severe, distressing, and of greater duration in breast cancer survivors compared with controls without breast cancer.[32]

Before 2002, HRT was frequently prescribed to healthy women for the control of menopausal symptoms and primary prevention of disease (i.e., cardiovascular disease and osteoporosis). In 2002, the Women's Health Initiative (WHI), a large randomized trial of HRT versus placebo in healthy women, was stopped early because overall health risks of combined estrogen plus progesterone exceeded benefits at an average 5.2-year follow-up.[33] Risks of coronary heart disease, stroke, pulmonary embolism, and invasive breast cancer were increased, whereas risks of colon cancer and hip fracture were minimally decreased. Results for estrogen alone versus placebo are pending.

The use of HRT in breast cancer survivors has been controversial.[34,35] Four case series,[36–39] three case-control studies,[40–43] and one cohort study[44] failed to identify an increased risk in women who chose to take HRT; two additional studies reported a lower risk of recurrence and death when HRT was used.[42,43] The studies are susceptible to selection bias, particularly in view of the reluctance of many breast cancer survivors to accept HRT.[45,46] One randomized clinical trial of HRT in 434 breast cancer survivors was recently stopped for safety reasons because of an unacceptably high risk of breast cancer events [hazard ratio (HR), 3.5; 95% CI, 1.5–8.1] in women receiving HRT.[47] Women on HRT were advised to discontinue the treatment. Current guidelines[34,48] that recommend postmenopausal breast cancer survivors be encouraged to consider alternatives to HRT but state that minimal HRT use may be considered in a well-informed patient with severe symptoms will likely be modified in view of these results, with a greater focus on recommending nonhormonal approaches to symptom management.

Vasomotor symptoms are the most common complaint of perimenopausal and postmenopausal women. More than 60% of postmenopausal women experience hot flashes, and one-third of those find them nearly intolerable.[49] HRT relieves HF in 80% to 90% of women who initiate treatment.[50–52]

Progestational agents (e.g., megestrol acetate, medroxyprogesterone acetate, and depo-Provera) decrease HF by 85%.[53–57] Herbal remedies, including soy products and black cohosh, have been reported to minimally decrease HF or have no effect. Vitamin E (800 IU/day) minimally decreases HF (i.e., one fewer HF/day). Clonidine is modestly active in reducing hot flashes. Selective serotonin reuptake inhibitors (SSRIs) such as venlafaxine and paroxetine have also been shown to significantly reduce HF. Possible interactions between SSRIs and selective estrogen receptor modulators (SERMS) are being evaluated. Gabapentin (widely used in neurologic disorders) has been recently reported to reduce HF scores.[58] Most of these trials have evaluated the short-term effect (e.g., 4–12 weeks); long-term effects have not been addressed.

Severe symptoms of urogenital atrophy occur in nearly half of postmenopausal women surviving breast cancer.

Lubricants and moisturizers have been shown to be helpful but do not completely relieve symptoms. Very low dose vaginal estrogen creams can reverse atrophy but systemic absorption of estrogen may occur. Newer methods of estrogen delivery include a ring device (Estring; Pfizer, New York, NY). This device provides almost complete relief of symptoms and minimal systemic absorption[48]; however, recent evidence that lipid levels may be altered[59] raises concerns about its use.

One randomized trial[60] evaluated the use of a comprehensive menopause assessment program in breast cancer survivors; the intervention (which did not involve use of estrogen but permitted megestrol acetate and nonhormonal agents such as clonidine) reduced menopausal symptoms and improved sexual functioning when compared with a control arm.

Bone loss occurs at a rate of 1% to 5% per year and is greatest during the first 5 years after natural menopause.[61] Chemotherapy-induced ovarian failure causes more rapid and significant bone loss.[62] Tamoxifen in premenopausal, but not postmenopausal, women and aromatase inhibitors have also been associated with increased bone loss. Bone density should be monitored in survivors.[63] Preventive measures such as proper intake of vitamin D and calcium, regular exercise, and counseling about the relationship between cigarette smoking, alcohol, and bone loss should be initiated in all patients. Pharmacologic approaches currently recommended for survivors include (1) bisphosphonates (alendronate, risedronate), (2) SERMs (raloxifene), and (3) calcitonin.

The risk of coronary heart disease increases with increasing age.[64,65] HRT in the primary and secondary prevention of coronary heart disease has not been shown to reduce cardiac events in four large randomized clinical trials.[33,66,67] Management of known risk factors and encouragement of lifestyle modification are warranted.[68]

Pregnancy

Limited data exist on the effect of pregnancy on breast cancer outcome. Based on the experience at major institutions[68–71] and population-based registries,[68,72,73] women who become pregnant after a diagnosis of breast cancer appear to have similar breast cancer outcomes to those who do not. Selection biases may be responsible for these results. Prior chemotherapy does not appear to have teratogenic effects in future pregnancies[74,75]; however, local breast cancer treatment (i.e., surgery and XRT) may affect the ability to lactate after BCS.[68,76,77] Breast cancer and pregnancy have been recently reviewed (see Chapter 99).[78,79]

Fatigue

Fatigue is often experienced during, and shortly after, cancer treatment. The level of fatigue in a large survey of breast cancer survivors (1–5 years after initial diagnosis) was comparable with that of age-matched controls using the RAND-36 questionnaire.[80,81] However, severe and persistent fatigue was experienced in a subgroup of survivors and was related to depression and pain. In a second smaller cohort study, fatigue (measured using a number of fatigue questionnaires including the RAND-36) was more common in breast cancer survivors than in age-matched controls.[81,82]

Second Malignancies

Second malignancies (e.g., angiosarcoma, sarcoma, and skin cancer) at the site of previous local treatment for breast cancer occur in less than 1% of survivors (see Chapter 111).[68]

Cardiac Toxicity

The most common form of anthracycline-induced cardiotoxicity is chronic cardiomyopathy.[83] The risk of cardiomyopathy is principally dependent on the cumulative anthracycline dose and may occur years after therapy.[84] Prospective monitoring of signs and symptoms of congestive heart failure (CHF) revealed a 9% risk of CHF after 450 mg/m^2 doxorubicin and 25% after 500 mg/m^2 [85]; this risk may be higher when doxorubicin is used in combination with paclitaxel.[86] Prospective cardiac monitoring using MUGA scans has been included in more recent clinical trials of breast cancer treatment including anthracyclines, taxanes, and herceptin. Based on a recent randomized trial,[87] cardiotoxicity is particularly pronounced when herceptin is combined with either adriamycin or epirubicin plus cyclophosphamide (any cardiotoxicity = 27%, grade 3–4 cardiotoxicity = 10%). Bradycardia has been reported with the use of paclitaxel alone.

Surveillance

Evidence-based surveillance strategies for breast cancer survivors have been established.[63] There are sufficient data to recommend monthly breast self-examination, annual mammography of the preserved and contralateral breast, as well as a careful history and physical examination every 3 to 6 months for 3 years, then every 6 to 12 months for 2 years, then annually. Data are not sufficient to recommend routine radiologic investigations or blood work (including tumor markers). Primary care of breast cancer survivors has also been reviewed.[68] Grunfeld et al.[88] conducted a large randomized trial of specialist versus general practitioner care in Great Britain; patients were more satisfied with care provided by the latter, with no differences in medical outcomes being observed, although only a small number of medical events were reported.

Psychosocial Status and HRQOL

Breast cancer is a stressful event that can perturb psychologic equilibrium and reduce HRQOL in the short-term[89–92]; recent survivorship research has evaluated long-term sequelae. Early studies involved mainly small convenience samples (maximum, 61 survivors), descriptive designs, and interview-based measurements.[93–97] Key results of these studies include observations that the majority of survivors are fairly to very satisfied with their lives 8 years after diagnosis despite thoughts of recurrence reported by 50%[93]; that survivors have a positive perception of life and attach less importance to trivial stressors even though fear of recurrence is a major concern[94]; and that the majority of survivors thrive despite experiencing problems related to breast cancer and its treatment.[95] Several ongoing issues were identified in a focus group of 10-year survivors: integration of disease into current life, change in relationship with others, restructuring life perspective, and unresolved issues.[96]

TABLE 106.2. Menopause in breast cancer survivors.

Reference	*Primary objective(s)*	*Study population and follow-up (years)*	*No. of patients*	*Instruments*	*Response rate*	*Results and conclusions*
Guidozzi et al. 1999[141]	Determine whether ERT adversely affects outcome of survivors	Prospective descriptive study of women 8–91 months postdiagnosis treated with oral continuous opposed ERT observed for 24–44 months	24	• History and physical exam 3×/year • Mammogram yearly. • BSE taught to the patient. • Appointment with surgeon annually.		No recurrences.
Brewster et al. 1999[142]	Evaluate the outcome of patients who elected ERT	Convenience sample treated with oral continuous ERT for at least 3 months starting 41 months (range 0–401 months) postdiagnosis; median F/U 30 months	145	• Routine surveillance by an oncologist	145/168	13 recurrences (9%).
Vassilopoulou-Sellin et al. 1999[44]	Determine whether ERT alters the development of new or recurrent breast cancer	Prospective randomized study of ERT, cohort of nonparticipants	319	• Monitor clinical outcome for new or recurrent cancer	319/331	ERT does not seem to increase events. Events during follow-up: 20/280 in controls vs. 1/39 in ERT group.
Ganz et al. 1999[45]	Assess willingness to undergo HRT in survivors	Sample of survivors from a previous survey an average of 3.1 years postdiagnosis	39	• Interview • Standardized health-related instruments including the RAND Health Survey • Decision analysis interview.		Older survivors are reluctant to take estrogen. Increased willingness to consider therapy if multiple symptoms coexisted and the risk of recurrence was small.
Ganz et al. 2000[60]	Assess the efficacy of a comprehensive menopausal assessment (CMA) intervention program in achieving relief of symptoms, improvement in QOL, and sexual functioning in survivors	Randomized controlled design of postmenopausal breast cancer survivors (8 months to 5 years after diagnosis)	72	• Menopausal symptom scale score adapted from the Breast Cancer Prevention Trial Symptom Checklist • Vitality Scale from the RAND Health Survey 1.0 • Sexual Summary Scale from the Cancer Rehabilitation Evaluation System.	72/197	A clinical assessment and intervention program for menopausal symptom management is feasible and acceptable to patients, leading to reduction in symptoms and improvement in sexual functioning.
Peters et al. 2001[143]	Define the prevalence of ERT usage, identify risks	Cohort of survivors (ER+ in 74%), median disease-free 46.7 months (range, 0–448 months), followed for ≥60 months, treated with ERT	56	• Review of medical records Routine surveillance by an oncologist including history and physical examinations every 3–6 months, annual mammograms and CXR, and evaluation of liver chemistries at each visit.	56/607 interviewed	Use of ERT was not associated with increased events.

O'Meara et al. 2001[43]	Evaluate the impact of HRT on recurrence and mortality	Record-based study of women 35–74 years identified in the SEER records (1977–1994) (1 user matched to 4 nonusers) (48% of users/59% of nonusers ER+)	2,755	Data obtained from: • The Cancer Surveillance System • Group Health Cooperative pharmacy • Medical records		Lower risks of recurrence and mortality observed with HRT.
Harris et al. 2002[24]	Assess the burden of menopausal symptoms, HRT use, and alternative treatments in recent survivors	Population-based, case-control study of survivors (8–11 months postdiagnosis) and age-matched controls	183	• Standardized telephone questionnaire • F/U 10-minute telephone questionnaire on HRT and menopause	93% cases, 95% controls	Cases more likely to experience menopausal symptoms, less likely to use HRT, more likely to use alternative therapies (soy, vitamin E, and herbal remedies).
Durna et al. 2002[144]	Compare the QOL of survivors who received HRT and those who did not	Nonrandomized qualitative study of women from a cancer registry. QOL was compared for 3 groups based on the time since diagnosis: <4 years, 4–8 years and >8 years	123	Questionnaires including: • Demographic data • QOL Breast Cancer version Questionnaire • QOL Self Evaluation Questionnaire	123/190 (64.8%)	No significant difference between users and nonusers. Near-normal QOL after a 4-year adjustment period.
Carpenter et al. 2002[32]	Compare the HF symptom experience and related outcomes between survivors and healthy women	Descriptive, cross-sectional, comparative study of survivors (mean of 39 months postdiagnosis) and age-matched healthy female volunteers	69 survivors/ 63 age-matched	Questionnaires: • Demographic and disease/ treatment information • Gynecologic and reproductive history form • Hot flash questionnaire and diary • POMS-SF • PANAS • HFRDIS	69/207 survivors	Hot flashes are a significant problem for survivors. Survivors with severe hot flashes reported significantly greater mood disturbance, higher negative affect, more interference with daily activities (sleep, concentration, and sexuality), and decreased QOL.
Biglia et al. 2003[46]	Determine the prevalence of menopausal symptoms, explore attitudes toward HRT or other treatments and the willingness to take estrogen	Convenience sample (early breast cancer) Mean F/U not stated	250	• 35-item questionnaire formulated for this study	Not stated	Survivors are interested in treatments that may improve their QOL, but fear of HRT persists among survivors and their doctors.
Holmberg 2004[47]	To examine impact of HRT on events in survivors	RCT of HRT vs. no therapy in survivors	434	• Clinical examination, mammography	345 had ≥1 follow-up	RCT stopped early because of excess events in survivors treated with HRT (relative hazard 3.5, 95% CI 1.5–8.1).

HRT, hormone replacement therapy; ERT, estrogen replacement therapy; RCT, randomized clinical trial; F/U, follow-up; POMS-SF, Profile of Mood States-Short Form; PANAS, Positive and Negative Affect Scale; HFRDIS, Hot Flash-Related Daily Interference Scale; BSE, breast self-examination; QOL, quality of life.

Second-generation studies used stronger designs, more standardized measurement approaches, and larger sample sizes. They were more often population based and/or used control groups of women without breast cancer. They frequently used generic instruments (applicable to healthy and medically ill individuals) for which normative data are available. One generic instrument that has been widely used in survivorship research is the Medical Outcomes Study Short Form—36 (MOS SF-36), a reliable and valid measure of HRQOL. It has 36 items rated on a 5-point Likert scale. There are eight subscales grouped in two composite scales: Physical Component Summary (PCS) and Mental Component Summary (MCS). Cancer-specific instruments, which measure attributes that are specific or unique to cancer patients, were also used in a large number of studies. Due to their nature, normative data for the general population are not available for these instruments. Nonetheless, they provide data that can be used to describe groups of survivors, evaluate change in their status over time, or compare different groups of survivors. Specific examples of these instruments are discussed.

Psychologic Status and Overall HRQOL

Many studies have examined psychosocial status and HRQOL in breast cancer survivors as a single group. Results of these studies are reviewed first, followed by a discussion of the status of defined subgroups of survivors.

Several cross-sectional, case-control, and cohort studies using the MOS SF-36 have reported scores on the Mental Component Summary scale or one of its subscales in breast cancer survivors 2 to 8 years postdiagnosis to be comparable with, or better than, scores obtained from either the general population or individuals with other chronic illnesses[80,98–102] (Table 106.3). Dorval et al.[103] used the Psychiatric Symptom Index (PSI), another generic instrument that measures the presence and intensity of four psychologic dimensions (depression, anxiety, cognitive impairment, and irritability) in a case-control study; no difference was found between 8-year survivors and controls randomly matched for age and residence. Studies using the generic measure of mood, the Profile of Mood States (POMS), reported women with breast cancer who were 2 years postdiagnosis to have scores comparable to published norms[80] or to a control group.[104] Taken together, these observations using generic instruments provide little evidence of impaired long-term HRQOL or psychologic status in breast cancer survivors compared to the general population.

A cancer-specific instrument, the QOL Cancer Survivors Tool (QOL-CS), yielded psychologic subscale scores that were worse than those for the social, spiritual well-being, and physical subscales 5.7 years postdiagnosis.[105] The inclusion of specific questions related to fear of recurrence of the cancer, which are not explicitly evaluated in generic questionnaires, and the specific population studied (members of the National Coalition for Cancer Survivorship) may have contributed to this result. Mosconi et al.[102] used the European Organization for Research and Treatment of Cancer Quality of Life Questionnaire Core-30 (EORTC QLQ-C30), a multidimensional cancer-specific questionnaire, to study Italian breast and colon cancer survivors. Overall HRQOL was reported to be good, and scores for emotional functioning did not differ between the two groups of survivors.

Physical Functioning

Earlier, we discussed specific physical symptoms in breast cancer survivors. The MOS SF-36 has been employed to measure general physical functioning. Physical functioning scores in survivors have been reported to be similar to,[102] or better than, published norms for individuals with other chronic illnesses[80,106] or the general population.[106] However, some studies[98,99,101] reported physical functioning scores in survivors that were lower than norms for the general population. A modest decline in physical functioning over time (mean, 6.3 years) has been reported by Ganz et al.[99]; the magnitude of the decline was small and was thought to be related to aging. Dow et al.[105] studied members of the National Coalition for Cancer Survivorship, a group that may not be representative of all cancer survivors. Overall physical well-being scores were good compared with other domains (e.g. psychologic); however, problems with components of physical well-being (i.e., pain, energy) were identified.

Thus, evaluation of general physical functioning in breast cancer survivors has yielded inconsistent results in comparison with published norms for the general population. However, differences from general population norms are small and may be due to effects of age.

Sexual Functioning

Breast cancer diagnosis and treatment can adversely affect sexuality. Surgical treatment of the primary tumor can affect body image, while systemic therapy can cause premature menopause or vaginal dryness. Measurement of the impact of breast cancer and its treatment on sexual functioning is challenging because few instruments specifically address this aspect of HRQOL. These measurement challenges may be compounded by a reporting bias if survivors are reluctant to respond to questions about sexual functioning. The use of specific questionnaires (e.g., the Sexual Activity Questionnaire, SAQ) in recent studies permits a more detailed assessment than is possible using more general multidimensional questionnaires.

Matthews et al.[98] administered the Satisfaction with Life Domains Scale for Cancer (SLDS-C) to breast cancer survivors (American Cancer Society Reach to Recovery volunteers) a mean of 8.6 years postdiagnosis. Scores for sexual functioning were worse than for other aspects of functioning. Dow et al.[105] also reported that satisfaction with sex life was the worst of all domains on the Functional Assessment of Cancer Therapy—General (FACT-G) in 294 survivors taking part in a peer-support group 5.7 years postdiagnosis. In contrast, Kurtz et al.[107] reported 5- to 10-year breast cancer survivors had high levels of sexual satisfaction on the Long Term Quality of Life Instrument.

Ganz et al.[99,106] used questionnaires that specifically address sexual functioning in two recent studies. In a cross-sectional study of 864 women,[106] use of the Watts Sexual Functioning Questionnaire identified modest increases in sexual dysfunction with aging but use of the Cancer

TABLE 106.3. Psychosocial status and health-related quality of life (HRQOL) overall associations in breast cancer survivors.

Reference	*Primary objective(s)*	*Study population and follow-up (years)*	*No. of subjects*	*Instrument(s)*	*Response rate*	*Results and conclusions*
Vinokur et al. 1989[120]	To assess the effect of age, time since diagnosis and disease severity	Case-control (population-based screening program) 53% > 5 years	178 survivors 176 controls	• HSC • PM • SE • ICO • PQOL • PREF • SC • Others	91%	Comparable QOL (physical, mental, health, and emotional well-being) in survivors and controls. Severity and recency of diagnosis were independent predictors of adverse effects on mental and physical well-being in survivors. Younger survivors with recent diagnosis have psychosocial concerns. Older with recent diagnosis have physical concerns.
Ellman et al. 1995[145]	To measure anxiety and depression	Case-control (screening clinic registry) 13 years	331 survivors 584 controls	• HADS	76% (survivors) 75% (controls)	Significantly more cases of depression and anxiety in controls. Time since diagnosis did not affect depression or anxiety except for the first anniversary.
Kurtz et al. 1995[107]	To explore six aspects of QOL	Hospital based tumor registry >5 years	191	• LTQL • CARES	55%	Best scores on psychologic domain and sexual satisfaction. Good psychologic state highly correlated with low somatic concerns and sexual satisfaction. Middle-aged: more positive philosophical/spiritual outlook.
Ganz et al. 1996[80]	To describe psychosocial concerns and QOL among survivors	Participants in rehabilitation RCT 2–3 years	139 (12 had recurrence)	• FLIC • CARES • SF-36 • POMS	77%	FLIC-POMS: no difference at 2–3 years versus 1 year. CARES: decline in global QOL, sexual and marital functioning at 3 vs. 1 year. Sexual functioning difficulties persisted from diagnosis to 3 years. Arms symptoms persist. Maximum recovery in QOL 1 year after treatment.
Dow et al. 1996[105]	To describe QOL in survivors including positive and negative outcomes	Convenience sample (mailed questionnaire to national coalition for cancer survivorship-peer support) 5.7 years	294 BCS (56 had recurrence)	• QOL-CS • FACT-G	56%	Fatigue, aches, sleep problems, fear of recurrence, family distress, sex life problems persisted over time. Physical QOL better than emotional/social QOL.
Saleeba et al. 1996[146]	To compare emotional status of survivors to screening population	Case-control (MDACC, screening clinic) >5 years	Survivors = 52 Control = 88	• BDI • STAI	Not stated	Mean depression score higher in survivors (within normal range). Survivors seek more frequent counseling (29% vs. 16%).
Weitzner et al. 1997[147]	To compare mood and QOL of survivors to screening population	Case-control, clinic samples >5 years	Survivors = 60 Controls = 93	• BDI • STAI • FPQLI	Not stated	No difference between cases and controls. Worse mood score correlated with lower QOL in survivors.
Lee 1997[148]	To examine social support, type of surgery, geographic location, and QOL	Convenience sample (Reach for Recovery volunteers) 14.1 years	100	• FPQLI	88%	QOL not associated with number of support persons, mental status, time from surgery, or type of surgery.
Ganz et al. 1998[106]	To describe survivorship in relation to age, menopausal status, treatment	Cross-sectional (random selection from two large metropolitan areas; tumor registry, clinics, hospitals) 3.1 years	864	• SF-36 • CES-D • DAS • CARES • WSFQ • Others	39%	Survivors had more frequent physical symptoms. Worse sexual functioning in survivors with chemo, menopause. and age <50, but no difference in sexual satisfaction and marital/partner adjustment. Unpartnered women have concerns about dating. Body image worse with MT.

(continued)

TABLE 106.3. Psychosocial status and health-related quality of life (HRQOL) overall associations in breast cancer survivors. (continued)

Reference	*Primary objective(s)*	*Study population and follow-up (years)*	*No. of subjects*	*Instrument(s)*	*Response rate*	*Results and conclusions*
Ganz et al. 1998[100]	To describe QOL related to adjuvant treatment	Cross-sectional (mailed survey, tumor registry, clinics, hospitals) 2.7–3.1 years	1,098	• SF36 • CES-D • CARES • LLS • Others	35%	No difference in mental-psychologic (SF-36, CES-D) and global QOL according to treatment. Physical and sexual: worse functioning in adjuvant therapy. Small adverse impact of adjuvant treatment on physical functioning but no impact on overall QOL.
Dorval et al. 1998[103]	To compare QOL in 8-year survivors	Survivors cohort assembled from seven hospitals, random digit dialing age-matched control, random digit dialing age-matched control 8.8 years	124 survivors (26 had new events) 427 controls	• PSI • LWMAT • MOS SSS • Others	96% (survivors) 61% (controls)	No difference in QOL. Arm problems and sexual satisfaction worse in survivors.
Dorval et al. 1999[108]	To examine marital breakdown	Survivors cohort assembled from seven hospitals 3 months–8 years	366	• SLES • LWMA • Others	89%–95%	Marital breakdown similar in survivors and controls. Marital satisfaction: predictor of marital breakdown in both groups.
Joly et al. 2000[135]	To evaluate long-term QOL in relation to chemo	Inception cohort (from a RCT on chemo) 9.6 years	119	• EORTC QLQ-C30 • Others	68%	No difference in functioning scales, body image, sex life, breast symptoms, social or professional life; trend for poorer cognitive functioning in CMF.
Montazeri et al. 2001[149]	To assess QOL at two time points	Members of the three support groups 1–5 years (54%)	56	• HADS	100%	29% and 14% scored above "case" cutpoint for anxiety and depression at baseline; significant improvement at 1 year.
Holzner et al. 2001[136]	To evaluate the effect of time on QOL	Convenience sample (outpatient)	87	• EORTC QLQ-C30 • FACT-B	Not stated	Worse emotional, cognitive, sexual functioning, global QOL >5 years vs. 2–5 years posttreatment. Better global QOL, social, emotional functioning >5 years vs. 1–2 years post Rx. Highest QOL in the period between 2–5 year post Rx.
Matthews et al. 2002[98]	To compare health status, life satisfaction, and QOL	Convenience sample (peer support-volunteers) 8.6 years	586	• SF-36 • SLDS-C	63%	Survivors reported higher emotional well-being, social functioning, and vitality but lower physical functioning compared to population-based norms. Worse sexual satisfaction, body image, physical strength for survivors. Younger women had better physical functioning but lower emotional well-being and vitality.
Tomich et al. 2002[101]	To compare QOL and psychologic well-being in BCS and controls	Survivors from RCT of peer and education groups; neighborhood controls >5.5 years	BCS = 164 Control = 164	• WAS • SWBS • FACI • SF-36 • PANAS	61%	Overall HRQOL similar in survivors and controls; no-intervention survivors had worse physical functioning. Poor QOL associated with beliefs of lasting harmful effect of treatment, low level of personal control, lack of sense of purpose in life.

Kessler et al. 2002[137]	To assess HRQOL	Convenience sample (ACS Reach for Recovery program) Mean 3.5 years (<0.1 to >10 years)	148 (23 had metastasis)	• PANAS • QOLM (Selby and Boyd) • Others	71%	QOL improved with increasing time from diagnosis and less extensive disease. More positive and less negative affect associated with better QOL.
Mosconi et al. 2002[102]	To assess long-term HRQOL of survivors	Survivors in a RCT of F/U testing (colon cancer survivors also studied) 8.3 years	433	• SF-36 • EORTC QLQ-C30	52%	Long-term survivors have HRQOL comparable to age/sex-matched norms. HRQOL lower with comorbidities or chemo. Physical functioning lower in breast vs. colon survivors.
Cimprich et al. 2002[121]	To assess age, duration of survival, and QOL	Tumor registry of Midwestern comprehensive cancer center 11.5 years	105	• QOL-CS	54%	Lower QOL on physical domain in older survivors. Lower QOL on social domain in younger survivors. Best QOL (overall and physical) in middle-aged survivors.
Ganz et al. 2002[99]	To evaluate long-term survivorship	5- to 10-year F/U of earlier cohort (population-based tumor registries, clinics, and hospitals) 6.3 years.	817 (*54 had recurrence and were excluded)	• SF-36 • LLS • CES-D$ • PANAS • RDAS • SAQ • CARES • MOS-SSS • Others	61%	Excellent physical and emotional well-being (minimal declines reflected expected age-related changes). No change in sexual interest but sexual activities declined. Stable energy level and social functioning. Some symptoms improved; others worsened. Survivors not receiving chemo had better overall QOL, physical functioning, less sexual discomfort.
Ganz et al. 2003[122]	To evaluate QOL and reproductive health in younger survivors	Cohort (two hospitals tumor registries) 5.9 years	577	• SF-36 • LLS • CES-D • PANAS • SAQ • Others	56%	High level of physical functioning. Youngest: Decrement in vitality, lowest score in social and emotional functioning, more depressive symptomatology, lower positive affect, and more negative affect. Amenorrhea frequent in women age ≥40 and associated with poorer health perception.
Ganz et al. 2003[123]	To examine HRQOL in older survivors	Cohort (identified through pathology reports, tumor registries) 3–5, 6–8, and 15–17 months	691	• PF10 • MHI-5 • CARES-SF-36 • MOS-SSS • Others	43%	Physical and mental health score decreased significantly at 15 months (SF-36). Improvement at 15 months in CARES.

Response rate: as stated in the paper or if not, the percentage of eligible patients who completed the study.

*, Valid and reliable instruments.

QOL, quality of life; BC, breast cancer; F/U, follow-up; Rx, treatment; ACS, American Cancer Society; HSC, Hopkins Symptom Checklist*; PM, positive morale, based from Bradburn's positive affect scale; SE, self-esteem: based on Rosenberg's scale of self esteem; ICO, internal control orientation, based on Rotter's scale; PQOL, perceived QOL, based on scale developed by Andrews and Withey; PREF, perceived role and emotional functioning; SC, social contacts, from Berkman's Social Network Index; HADS, Hospital Anxiety and Depression Scale*; LTQL, long-term quality of life*; CARES, Cancer Rehabilitation Evaluation System*; FLIC, Functional Living Index–Cancer*; SF-36, RAND or MOS Short-Form-36*; POMS, Profile of Mood States*; QOL-CS, Quality of Life–Cancer Survivors*; FACT, Functional Assessment of Cancer Therapy*; BDI, Beck Depression Inventory*; STAI, State-Trait Anxiety Inventory*; FPQLI, Ferrans and Powers Quality of Life Index*; CES-D, Center of Epidemiologic Studies–Depression Scale*; DAS, Dyadic Adjustment Scale*; WSFQ, Watts Sexual Function Questionnaire*; PSI, Psychiatric Symptom Index*; LWMAT, Locke–Wallace Marital Adjustment Test*; MOS SSS, MOS Social Support Survey*; SLES, Stressful Life Event Scale*; EORTC-QLQ C-30, European Organization for Research and Treatment of Cancer–Quality of Life Questionnaire C-30*; SLDS-C, Satisfaction with Life Domains Scales for Cancer; WAS, Words Assumption Scale; SWBS, Spiritual Well-Being Scale of FACI (Functional Assessment of Chronic Illness therapy); PANAS, Positive and Negative Affect Schedule*; QOLM, WOL Measurement, Selby and Boyd*; RDAS, Revised Dyadic Adjustment Scale*; SAQ, Sexual Activity Questionnaire*; LLS, Ladder of Life scale*; PF-10, 10-item functioning scale from SF-36; MHI-5, Mental Health Inventory, from the SF-36.

Rehabilitation Evaluation System (CARES) identified no impairment in sexual satisfaction. Sexual functioning was significantly worse in those who received chemotherapy (but not tamoxifen), particularly in women who were menopausal (either naturally or secondary to treatment) and in women under 50 years of age. Using the SAQ in their cohort study of 763 long-term breast cancer survivors, this group also reported sexual discomfort to be greatest in women who received chemotherapy but identified no differences in sexual pleasure or sexual habits.[99] In summary, sexual functioning appears to be adversely impacted in breast cancer survivors, particularly in younger women who receive adjuvant chemotherapy.

Social Functioning and Marital Status

Studies evaluating social functioning in breast cancer survivors have usually shown little evidence of impairment. The social functioning subscale of the MOS SF-36 has yielded similar scores in breast cancer survivors and in the general population in the majority of studies.[80,98–102] Use of the EORTC QLQ-C30 has also demonstrated high level of social functioning in breast cancer survivors.[102] Use of the MOS Social Support Measure also showed no difference between breast cancer patients with a control population[99,103] and no change according to time elapsed since diagnosis.[99]

In a cohort of 763 survivors, there was no significant change in marital status over 5 years of follow-up.[99] In another cohort followed for 8 years, no difference in divorce or separation rates at 12 months, 18 months, and 8 years after diagnosis was identified in survivors compared to age-/residence-matched women.[108] In survivors, low marital satisfaction at 3 months predicted future marital difficulties (16.7% divorced at 1 year versus 2.1% in those with high marital satisfaction; $P = 0.02$). Women not in a partnered relationship expressed concerns about dating, telling about cancer, and fear of initiating sexual relationship.[80,106]

Finally, in their follow-up of 817 long-term breast cancer survivors, Ganz et al. reported more than two-thirds had stable household income and 20% had increased income (versus 12% who had decreased income) since diagnosis.[99] Eighty percent reported no change in employment status; a minority moved from full- to part-time work or retired. Marital status did not change. In a separate study, this group reported that 90% of survivors had health insurance 2 or 3 years postdiagnosis, although some had their premiums increased or had switched to a spouse's plan.[80] Most (65%) were working or doing volunteer work.

Thus, there is little evidence that social or marital functioning or employment is adversely affected in survivors. Specific concerns about dating have been reported, especially in young, unpartnered women.

Cognitive Functioning

In 1995, Wieneke and Dienst[109] published the first report of cognitive dysfunction in women with breast cancer (Table 106.4). To date, four reports have evaluated cognitive functioning during and within the first 2 years postchemotherapy using a battery of neuropsychologic tests[109–111] or the High Sensitivity Cognitive Screen,[104] a valid reliable instrument that predicts overall qualitative results of formal neuropsychologic testing. All four studies identified significantly lower cognitive functioning in women receiving adjuvant chemotherapy (with or without anthracyclines) compared with those not receiving chemotherapy or to a control group without breast cancer. Cognitive dysfunction was more prevalent in women who received high-dose chemotherapy in one study.[111] Interestingly, there appears to be little correlation between cognitive functioning as assessed by the test battery and self-reported by the patient.[110,111]

Studies evaluating cognitive dysfunction beyond 2 years have yielded conflicting results. Schagen et al.[112] reported improvement in performance in all chemotherapy groups between 2 and 4 years posttreatment. Ahles et al.[113] reported patients who had been diagnosed at least 5 years earlier had greater cognitive impairment on a battery of neuropsychologic tests and were more likely to report memory problems on the Squire Memory Self-Rating Questionnaire if they had received adjuvant chemotherapy.

Cognitive dysfunction in women receiving adjuvant chemotherapy is an emerging area of interest in survivorship research. Future research should identify risk factors for this complication and evaluate potential interventions to minimize its impact.

Spirituality

Spirituality is often poorly addressed in multidimensional questionnaires. Based on the holistic Ferrell[114] model of QOL in breast cancer survivors (physical, psychologic, social, spiritual), Wyatt et al. developed the Long-Term Quality of Life (LTQL) instrument, which includes a philosophical/spiritual view dimension.[115] Kurtz et al.,[107] using this instrument in long-term (more than 5 years) survivors, reported a positive spiritual outlook to be associated with good health habits and an increased likelihood of being supportive of others. In their cohort of long-term survivors (6.3 years), Ganz et al.[99] reported a positive impact of breast cancer on religious beliefs and activities, an effect that tended to be more pronounced in young survivors. Dow et al.[105] used the QOL-CS to evaluate spiritual well-being in members of the National Coalition for Cancer Survivorship. Although fears about future cancer and uncertainty about the future were identified as important concerns, beneficial spiritual outcomes including hopefulness and having a purpose in life as well as positive and spiritual change were also reported. Further research is needed to confirm these early observations, using population-based controls as a comparison group.

Diet and Complementary and Alternative Medicine

Maunsell et al.[116] evaluated diet during the first year after breast cancer diagnosis in a group of 250 women who were surveyed with a standardized interview about diet changes. Forty-one percent of women reported a change in their diet; these changes were positive (i.e., healthy) in over 90%. Women under 50 years and those who were more distressed

TABLE 106.4. QOL and cognitive dysfunction in breast cancer survivors.

Reference	*Primary objective(s)*	*Study population and follow-up (years)*	*No. of subjects*	*Instruments*	*Response rate*	*Results and conclusions*
Wieneke et al. 1995[109]	To evaluate cognitive functioning after adjuvant chemo	Convenience sample (clinic) 6.6 months post chemo	28	• Neuropsychologic tests	84%	Cognitive deficit related to tests norms (adjusted for age, education, gender) in 5 of 7 domains assessed. 75% had moderate impairment on at least 1 test. Level of impairment unrelated to depression, type of chemo, time since treatment; positively related to the length of chemo.
van Dam et al. 1998[111]	To assess the prevalence of cognitive deficit after adjuvant chemo	RCT of high-dose vs. standard dose chemo Control group were BCS who did not received chemo 2 years	34 high dose 36 standard dose 34 no chemo	• Neuropsychologic tests • Semistructured interview for self-reported cognitive functioning • EORTC QLQ-C30 • HSCL-25	84%–85% (chemo treated) 68% (controls)	Lower global QOL and higher score on depression subscale with high dose. Cognitive impairment: 32% high dose, 17% standard dose, 9% no chemo ($P = 0.043$).
Schagen et al. 1999[110]	To assess neuropsychologic functioning following CMF vs. no chemo	Consecutive series 2 years	39 chemo 34 control	• Neuropsychologic test • Semistructured interview • EORTC QLQ-C30 • HSCL-25	78% (chemo) 68% (control)	Higher IQ at baseline in CMF group. Neuropsychologic tests: 28% of patients in chemo cognitively impaired vs. 12% in control. Self-reported problems: in chemo group, more problems with concentration and memory. No relation between reported complaints and neuropsychologic testing. Chemo: lower QOL (physical, cognitive), greater depression.
Brezden et al. 2000[104]	To assess cognitive function in chemo vs. control patients	Convenience sample (two academic hospitals) 2.1 years for the group post chemo	Chemo: 31 Postchemo: 40 Controls: 36	• HSCS • POMS	Not stated	More patients with cognitive impairment during or after chemo vs. controls. No difference in mood status in the three groups.
Schagen et al. 2002[112]	To assess long-term neuropsychologic sequelae following chemo	Follow-up of earlier cohort[120,121] 4 years	103	• Neuropsychologic tests • EORTC QLQ-C30 • HSCL	84%–96%	Improvement in performance in all chemo group (FEC, high-dose, CMF) and a slight deterioration in controls. Cognitive dysfunction following adjuvant chemo may be transient.
Ahles et al. 2002[113]	To compare neuropsychologic functioning of long-term survivors	Tumor registry 9.7 years for BC	BC = 70 Lymphoma = 58	• Neuropsychologic tests • SMSRQ • CES-D • STAI • FSI	75%	Neuropsychologic test and SMSRQ: chemo group score lower than local therapy group (adjusted for age and education). No other differences.

Response rate: as stated in the paper or if not, the percentage of eligible patients who completed the study.

*, Valid and reliable instruments.

CMF, cyclophosphamide, methotrexate, 5-flouuracil; Chemo, chemotherapy; RCT, randomized controlled trial; FEC, 5-flouuracil, epirubicin, cyclophosphamide; BC, breast cancer; neuropsychologic tests, a battery of tests were used; Cf., see reference for more details; EORTC-QLQC-30, European Organization for Research and Treatment of Cancer–Quality of Life Questionnaire C-30*; HSCL, Hopkins Symptom Checklist-25; HSCS, High Sensitivity Cognitive Screen*; POMS, Profile of Mood States*; SMSRQ, Squire Memory Self-Rating Questionnaire; CES-D, Center for Epidemiological Study-Depression*; STAI, State-Trait Anxiety Inventory*; FSI, Fatigue Symptom Inventory*.

at diagnosis were most likely to change their diets (P = 0.0001).

Burstein et al.[117] evaluated complementary and alternative medicine (CAM) use during the first 12 months after breast cancer diagnosis (see Chapter 15). Twenty-eight percent of 480 women began an alternative therapy after diagnosis; these women tended to be younger and more educated. Ganz et al.[99] reported vitamins and herbal preparations were used by 86.6% and 49.3% of breast cancer survivors, respectively. More than half (60.7%) altered diet or used dietary supplements. Few women were using psychosocial or counseling therapies (13%) or attending a cancer support group (5.5%). More than one-third reported enhanced physical activity postdiagnosis. Lee et al.[118] conducted telephone interviews in 379 women (black, Chinese, Latino, white) 3 to 6 years after breast cancer diagnosis. At least one alternative therapy was used by 48.3%. Most common approaches therapies were dietary change (26.6%), herbal/homeopathic medication (13.5%), psychologic or spiritual healing (30.1%), and physical approaches such as yoga or acupuncture (14.2%). Therapies were used for brief periods, usually for 3 to 6 months. Women who used alternative therapies were younger and more educated.

Thus, more than one-third of breast cancer survivors use at least one kind of alternative therapy. Nonpharmacologic supplements appear to be most commonly used. Further research is needed to evaluate duration of use and changes over time in use of CAMS, comparing survivors to healthy controls.

Psychosocial Status and HRQOL in Defined Subgroups

Consideration of breast cancer survivors as a group may mask important differences in subgroups and over time. In this section we summarize research examining subgroups defined by age, ethnicity, and treatment (surgery, adjuvant therapy) and according to time elapsed since diagnosis.

Age at Diagnosis

Age at diagnosis appears to be an important determinant of survivorship. This may be due, in part, to treatment: women who receive chemotherapy, many of whom are younger, experience greater long-term physical and sexual sequelae (see following discussion); psychosocial effects of mastectomy may also differ with age, especially in the short term.[119] However, Ganz et al.[106] reported poorer sexual functioning in younger survivors who became menopausal, regardless of whether they received chemotherapy. Vinokur et al.[120] compared survivors (50% of whom were followed more than 5 years) to controls participating in a breast cancer screening program; younger survivors had more problems in psychosocial adjustment while older survivors had more physical difficulties. Cimprich et al.[121] reported similar findings in 105 survivors using the QOL-CS. Women over 65 at diagnosis had worse scores in the physical domain while those diagnosed before 44 years of age had poorer scores in the social domain. Women diagnosed between 45 and 65 years of age had the best overall HRQOL. Two pivotal studies examining survivorship issues in younger[122] and older women[123] have been reported recently. In the first of these, a cohort of 577 patients diagnosed at age 50 or younger was assembled for the Cancer and Menopause Study a mean of 5.9 years postdiagnosis.[122] Most had received adjuvant chemotherapy. Physical functioning was good. The youngest women reported poor mental health, less vitality, and poorer social and emotional functioning (MOS SF36). In the second study, 691 women aged 65 years of age or more at diagnosis were evaluated 3, 6, and 15 months after surgery.[123] Physical and mental functioning (MOS SF-36) showed significant declines during the year of follow-up. Declines in the former were associated with greater comorbidity and receipt of adjuvant chemotherapy. In contrast, the CARES Psychosocial Summary and Medical Interaction Scales showed significant improvement over time. Social support was lowest in women over 75 years. The discrepant results obtained with the MOS SF-36 Mental Health Inventory and the CARES Psychosocial Summary Scale were explored: the former appeared to be influenced to a greater extent by declines in physical functioning and the latter appeared to reflect adaptation and adjustment to cancer-specific concerns. In summary, younger age is associated with lower mental and emotional wellbeing. Older women experience more physical problems, partly the result of aging.

Ethnicity

The impact of ethnicity on survivorship has been poorly studied. Ashing-Giwa et al.[124] investigated HRQOL in white and African-American survivors. Response rate among African-Americans was significantly lower than among whites (44% versus 65%). The former were more often single, had a lower income, and lower HRQOL. Multivariate analyses revealed that 45% of the variance in HRQOL was accounted for by general health perception, life stress, partnership status, and income; ethnicity was not a significant contributor. The authors concluded that African-American and white report favorable overall QOL; differences are secondary to life burden and socioeconomic factors but not to ethnicity per se.

Primary Surgical Procedure

The primary surgical procedure performed also appears to impact survivorship (Table 106.5). Maunsell et al.[119] reported that psychologic distress (measured using the PSI) at 3 months was worse in women undergoing BCS; this difference was not present at 18 months. Age modified this effect; the greater psychologic distress at 3 months was not present in women under 40 years. Follow-up 8 years after diagnosis found that psychologic distress declined over time and was similar to that in the general population.[125] Ganz et al.,[126] using a battery of general questionnaires, reported few differences in HRQOL with respect to type of surgery; however, women undergoing mastectomy had more problems with clothing and body image than those undergoing BCS. Mosconi et al.[102] found none of the EORTC QLQ C-30 domains to be affected by the type of surgery. Janni et al.[127] studied 76 pairs of patients who had undergone either a mastectomy or BCS a mean of 3.8 years earlier; women undergoing mastectomy were significantly less satisfied with their cosmetic result and change in appearance and were twice as likely to be stressed by their physical appearance secondary to the surgery. No

TABLE 106.5. Survivorship and surgery in breast cancer survivors.

Reference	*Primary objective(s)*	*Study population and follow-up (in years)*	*No. of subjects*	*Instruments*	*Response rate*	*Results and conclusions*
Schain et al. 1983[130]	To compare QOL after MRM vs. BCS	RCT of MRM vs. BCS 11.3 months	38	• Others	97%	No difference in psychosocial outcomes, except greater concerns about seeing oneself naked in MRM. 69% of BCS vs. 28% of MT had limited arm motion.
Meyer et al. 1989[131]	To compare long-term psychosocial and sexual adaptation after MRM vs. BCS	Convenience sample (one center) 5 years	58	• Interview	68%	No differences in psychiatric state, marital adjustment, fear of recurrence. BCS preserves female identity and acceptance of body image.
Maunsell et al. 1989[119]	To describe psychologic distress after MRM vs. BCS	Cohort (consecutive cases from seven hospitals) 3 and 18 months	227 at 3 months and 205 at 18 months	• PSI • LES (modified) • DSI • Others	97%	At 3 months, greater psychologic distress (PSI) in BCS vs. MRM but no difference at 18 months. Age modified the relation: BCS was protective for women <40 years of age.
Ganz et al. 1992[126]	To evaluate QOL and psychologic adjustment after MRM vs. BCS	RCT testing (two rehabilitation programs) 1 year	109	• FLIC • CARES • Karnofsky (PS) • POMS • GAIS	44%	No difference in mood disturbance, QOL, performance status, global adjustment. MRM associated with more difficulties with clothing and body image.
Mock 1993[150]	To compare body image with MRM, MRM + delayed R, MRM + immediate R, BCS	Clinical sample from four hospitals 14 months	257	• BIS • TSCS • BIVAS	57%	Body image was more positive after BCS (when measured by BIVAS but not by BIS). No difference in self-concept.
Omne-Pontén et al. 1994[128]	To assess psychosocial adjustment after MRM vs. BCS	Consecutive clinic patients 6 years	66	• Interview • Others	80% (of the first study)	No impact of the surgery on psychosocial adjustment.
Dorval et al. 1998[125]	To assess psychosocial adjustment after MRM vs. BCS	Cohort (seven hospitals) 3 months, 18 months, 8 years	235 at 3 months 211 at 18 months 124 at 8 years	• PSI • MOS-SSS • LES • LWMAT	97% 3 months 97% 18 months 96% 8 years	At 8 years no difference in QOL. BCS protected women against distress if they were <50 years of age at diagnosis (short and long term).
Curran et al. 1998[129]	To describe QOL after MRM vs. BCS	Sample from EORTC trial 10801 2 years	278	• Newly constructed questionnaire	14%–64% (between different countries)	BCS gives a better body image with no increase in fear of recurrence. Cosmetic results: patient rating superior to the surgeon.
Rowland et al. 2000[133]	To evaluate women's adaptation to different types of surgery	Two cohorts (from two large metropolitan areas) 2.7 and 3.2 years	1,957	• SF-36 • MOS SSS • CES-D • RDAS • WSFQ • CARES	54%	Fewer problems with body image and sexual attractiveness after BCS vs. MRM ± R. MT + R: report more negative impacts on sex life. MRM ± R vs. BCS: more physical symptom and discomfort at the surgical site. No difference in emotional, social, role function (CES-D, SF-36).
Janni et al. 2001[127]	To compare impact of BCS vs. MRM	Convenience sample (one hospital) 3.8 years	152 pairmatched patients	• EORTC QLQ C-30 • Other	Not stated	No difference for QOL between the two groups. MRM women had less satisfaction with cosmetic results, appearance, and were more emotionally distressed by these issues.
Nissen et al. 2001[134]	To compare QOL after BCS, MRM, MRM ± R	RCT of effect of advanced practice nursing 2 years	198	• MUIS • POMS • FACT-B	94%	BCS vs. MRM: no difference in well-being. More mood disturbance and poorer well-being in MRM + R vs. MRM alone.

Response rate: reported by the author or calculated as the percentage of eligible patients who completed the study.

*, Valid and reliable instruments.

MRM, modified radical mastectomy; BCS, breast-conserving surgery; R, reconstruction; PSI, Psychiatric Symptom Index*; LES, Life Events Schedule*; DSI, Diagnostic Interview Schedule*; FLIC, Functional Living Index–Cancer*; CARES, Cancer Rehabilitation Evaluation System*; POMS, Profile of Mood States*; GAIS, Global Adjustment to Illness Scale*; SBAS, Social Behaviour Assessment Schedule*; BIS, Body Image Scale*; TSCS, Tennessee Self-Concept Scale*; BIVAS, Body Image Visual Analogue Scale; MOS-SSS, MOS Social Support Survey*; LES, Life Experience Survey*; LWMAT, Locke–Wallace Marital Adjustment Test* ; SF-36, RAND or MOS Short-Form-36*; CES-D, Center of Epidemiologic Studies–Depression Scale*; RDAS, Revised Dyadic Adjustment Scale*; WSFQ, Watts Sexual Function Questionnaire*; EORTC-QLQ C-30, European Organization for Research and Treatment of Cancer–Quality of Life Questionnaire C-30*; MUIS, Mishel Uncertainty in Illness Scale*; FACT, Functional Assessment of Cancer Therapy*.

differences were seen in EORTC QLQ-C30 scores. Psychosocial adjustment measured using the Social Adjustment Scale was similar in the mastectomy and BCS treatment groups; however, women undergoing mastectomy felt mutilated and less attractive.[128] A companion study to EORTC trial 10801 comparing mastectomy to BCS and radiotherapy surveyed 278 patients 2 years after treatment.[129] Body image and satisfaction with treatment were better in the BCS. There was no difference in fear of recurrence. Patients considered their cosmetic results to be more acceptable than the surgeon did at several time points. Other studies have reported beneficial effects of BCS on body image.[130,131] In summary, BCS leads to enhanced body image and, in younger women (less than 40), it may protect against psychologic distress. No differences in depression were identified in one study of spouses of women undergoing mastectomy or BCS.[132]

Breast Reconstruction

Breast reconstruction is offered to reduce the adverse impact of mastectomy. Rowland et al.[133] studied a cohort of 1,957 long-term (1 to 5 years) survivors in Los Angeles and Washington. Women undergoing mastectomy had more physical symptoms related to the surgery regardless of whether they had reconstruction. No differences in overall HRQOL or worry about cancer returning were identified in women undergoing BCS, mastectomy alone, or mastectomy with reconstruction. Body image and feelings of sexual attractiveness were significantly better after BCS compared with mastectomy with or without reconstruction. Women who had reconstruction were younger and better educated than those in the other two groups. They also expressed greater concern that their cancer had a negative impact on their sex life. Nissen et al.[134] reported that women who had a mastectomy with reconstruction had greater mood disturbance and poorer well-being 18 months after surgery compared with those who did not undergo reconstruction.

Adjuvant Therapy

There is growing evidence that adjuvant therapy adversely affects survivors' HRQOL. In a cross-sectional survey, Ganz et al.[100] reported global HRQOL (measured using the Ladder of Life and the MOS SF-36) to be similar 1 to 5 years postdiagnosis in women who received chemotherapy and/or tamoxifen compared with those who received no adjuvant therapy. However, physical and sexual functioning were worse in women receiving adjuvant therapy. A mean of 6.3 years postdiagnosis, the no-adjuvant treatment group reported more favorable scores for global HRQOL (Ladder of Life) and most domains of the MOS SF-36 than those who received adjuvant therapy.[99] There were no differences in emotional functioning (MOS SF-36, Center for Epidemiology Study—Depression). The sexual discomfort scale (SAQ) and sexual functioning (CARES) were significantly worse in women who received adjuvant chemotherapy compared to those who received either tamoxifen or no therapy. Mosconi et al.[102] reported slightly better HRQOL (EORTC QLQ-C30) in women treated with tamoxifen versus those who received either chemotherapy or no adjuvant therapy. In contrast, participants of an adjuvant trial of chemotherapy versus no treatment who were 9.6 years postdiagnosis reported no differences in sexual functioning/enjoyment according to treatment arm.[135] Small sample size (119 patients) and the long interval after diagnosis may account for these results. In summary, the majority of studies have identified long-term adverse effects of adjuvant therapy, notably chemotherapy.

Time Elapsed Since Diagnosis

The status of survivors also varies according to time elapsed since diagnosis. Ganz et al.[99] re-evaluated a cross-sectional sample of survivors who had been recruited 1 to 5 years postdiagnosis when they were a mean of 6.3 (minimum, 5) years postdiagnosis. Small decreases in physical functioning, role functioning-physical, bodily pain, and general health (MOS SF-36) over time were thought to be related to aging. Sexual activity with a partner declined significantly and specific symptoms persisted, especially in women receiving chemotherapy. In an earlier cohort study, Ganz et al.[80] compared HRQOL measured using the POMS and Functional Living Index for Cancer at 2 and 3 years after surgery to that between 1 month and 1 year after surgery. Most scores improved between 1 month and 1 year,[126] but there was no subsequent improvement. This might reflect ongoing rehabilitation problems, as most CARES scores worsened between 1 and 3 years postdiagnosis. Holzner et al.[136] evaluated 87 breast cancer survivors using two cancer-specific questionnaires. Women who were more than 5 years postdiagnosis had significantly worse global QOL, role functioning, sexual functioning, and enjoyment than those 1 to 2 or 2 to 5 years postdiagnosis. However, women more than 5 years postdiagnosis were slightly older than those 1 to 2 and 2 to 5 years postdiagnosis (55.1 years old versus 52.9 and 52.5 years old, respectively). Women 2 to 5 years postdiagnosis had less impairment in emotional and social functioning than those diagnosed earlier or later. In contrast, Kessler et al.,[137] studying a convenience sample of 148 breast cancer survivors 0.3 to 19 years postdiagnosis, reported that overall QOL and life satisfaction were high and that greater time since diagnosis and lesser extent of disease were associated with improved global QOL. Thus, HRQOL and most aspects of physical and psychosocial functioning improve during the first few years after breast cancer diagnosis. However, specific treatment-related problems and symptoms persist long term, and there is some evidence of HRQOL decline 2 to 5 years after diagnosis, possibly related to aging.

Conclusions

Long-term survivors have a high level of functioning and good HRQOL, often comparable to that of the general population. However, many survivors experience physical symptoms (notably arm symptoms and early menopause) and reduced sexual functioning related to their diagnosis and treatment. Young women, those receiving chemotherapy, and those with comorbidity may be at greatest risk. Younger women experience greater psychologic distress. Cognitive dysfunction has recently been identified in women receiving adjuvant chemotherapy. BCS leads to enhanced body image; however, reconstruction does not add a major benefit in terms of QOL. Quality of survivorship in different ethnic groups has been inadequately investigated.

A considerable body of observational research has been conducted in breast cancer survivors. Although there are knowledge gaps that should be addressed in further observational research, there is also a need for research to develop and evaluate interventions that will reduce the adverse impact of breast cancer diagnosis and treatment which has been identified in research to date. Primary areas for intervention research include psychologic distress and sexual dysfunction in younger women; cognitive dysfunction, sexual dysfunction, and fatigue in women receiving chemotherapy; and body image in women undergoing mastectomy with or without reconstruction.

References

1. http://survivorship.cancer.gov.
2. Gerber LH. A review of measures of lymphedema. Cancer (Phila) 1998;83:2803–2804.
3. Erickson VS, Pearson ML, Ganz PA, Adams J, Kahn KL. Arm edema in breast cancer patients. J Natl Cancer Inst 2001;93: 96–111.
4. Schrenk P, Rieger R, Shamiyeh A, Wayand W. Morbidity following sentinel lymph node biopsy versus axillary lymph node dissection for patients with breast carcinoma. Cancer (Phila) 2000;88:608–614.
5. Gerber L, Lampert M, Wood C, et al. Comparison of pain, motion, and edema after modified radical mastectomy vs. local excision with axillary dissection and radiation. Breast Cancer Res Treat 1992;21:139–145.
6. Werner RS, McCormick B, Petrek J, et al. Arm edema in conservatively managed breast cancer: obesity is a major predictive factor. Radiology 1991;180:177–184.
7. Tasmuth T, von Smitten K, Kalso E. Pain and other symptoms during the first year after radical and conservative surgery for breast cancer. Br J Cancer 1996;74:2024–2031.
8. Paci E, Cariddi A, Barchielli A, et al. Long-term sequelae of breast cancer surgery. Tumori 1996;82:321–324.
9. Yeoh EK, Denham JW, Davies SA, Spittle MF. Primary breast cancer. Complications of axillary management. Acta Radiol Oncol 1986;25:105–108.
10. Kiel KD, Rademacker AW. Early-stage breast cancer: arm edema after wide excision and breast irradiation. Radiology 1996;198: 279–283.
11. Keramopoulos A, Tsionou C, Minaretzis D, Michalas S, Aravantinos D. Arm morbidity following treatment of breast cancer with total axillary dissection: a multivariated approach. Oncology 1993;50:445–449.
12. Liljegren G, Holmberg L. Arm morbidity after sector resection and axillary dissection with or without postoperative radiotherapy in breast cancer stage I. Results from a randomised trial. Uppsala-Orebro Breast Cancer Study Group. Eur J Cancer 1997; 33:193–199.
13. Senofsky GM, Moffat FL Jr, Davis K, et al. Total axillary lymphadenectomy in the management of breast cancer. Arch Surg 1991;126:1336–1341; discussion 1341–1342.
14. Kissin MW, Querci della Rovere G, Easton D, Westbury G. Risk of lymphoedema following the treatment of breast cancer. Br J Surg 1986;73:580–584.
15. Borup Christensen S, Lundgren E. Sequelae of axillary dissection vs. axillary sampling with or without irradiation for breast cancer. A randomized trial. Acta Chir Scand 1989;155:515–519.
16. Lash TL, Silliman RA. Patient characteristics and treatments associated with a decline in upper-body function following breast cancer therapy. J Clin Epidemiol 2000;53:615–622.
17. Silliman RA, Prout MN, Field T, Kalish SC, Colton T. Risk factors for a decline in upper body function following treatment for early stage breast cancer. Breast Cancer Res Treat 1999; 54:25–30.
18. Segerstrom K, Bjerle P, Nystrom A. Importance of time in assessing arm and hand function after treatment of breast cancer. Scand J Plast Reconstr Surg Hand Surg 1991;25:241–244.
19. Lin PP, Allison DC, Wainstock J, et al. Impact of axillary lymph node dissection on the therapy of breast cancer patients. J Clin Oncol 1993;11:1536–1544.
20. Passik SD, McDonald MV. Psychosocial aspects of upper extremity lymphedema in women treated for breast carcinoma. Cancer (Phila) 1998;83:2817–2820.
21. Woods M, Tobin M, Mortimer P. The psychosocial morbidity of breast cancer patients with lymphoedema. Cancer Nurs 1995;18:467–471.
22. Tobin MB, Lacey HJ, Meyer L, Mortimer PS. The psychological morbidity of breast cancer-related arm swelling. Psychological morbidity of lymphoedema. Cancer (Phila) 1993;72:3248–3252.
23. Maunsell E, Brisson J, Deschenes L. Arm problems and psychological distress after surgery for breast cancer. Can J Surg 1993; 36:315–320.
24. Harris PF, Remington PL, Trentham-Dietz A, Allen CI, Newcomb PA. Prevalence and treatment of menopausal symptoms among breast cancer survivors. J Pain Symptom Manag 2002;23:501–509.
25. Ganz PA. Menopause and breast cancer: symptoms, late effects, and their management. Semin Oncol 2001;28:274–283.
26. Goodwin PJ, Ennis M, Pritchard KI, Trudeau M, Hood N. Risk of menopause during the first year after breast cancer diagnosis. J Clin Oncol 1999;17:2365–2370.
27. Bines J, Oleske DM, Cobleigh MA. Ovarian function in premenopausal women treated with adjuvant chemotherapy for breast cancer. J Clin Oncol 1996;14:1718–1729.
28. Bachmann GA. Vasomotor flushes in menopausal women. Am J Obstet Gynecol 1999;180:S312–S316.
29. Schwingl PJ, Hulka BS, Harlow SD. Risk factors for menopausal hot flashes. Obstet Gynecol 1994;84:29–34.
30. Theriault RL, Sellin RV. Estrogen-replacement therapy in younger women with breast cancer. J Natl Cancer Inst Monogr 1994;16:149–152.
31. Mortimer JE. Hormone replacement therapy and beyond. The clinical challenge of menopausal symptoms in breast cancer survivors. Geriatrics 2002;57:25–31.
32. Carpenter JS, Johnson D, Wagner L, Andrykowski M. Hot flashes and related outcomes in breast cancer survivors and matched comparison women. Oncol Nurs Forum 2002;29: E16–E25.
33. Rossouw JE, Anderson GL, Prentice RL, et al. Risks and benefits of estrogen plus progestin in healthy postmenopausal women: principal results. From the Women's Health Initiative randomized controlled trial. JAMA 2002;288:321–333.
34. Pritchard KI, Khan H, Levine M. Clinical practice guidelines for the care and treatment of breast cancer: 14. The role of hormone replacement therapy in women with a previous diagnosis of breast cancer. Can Med Assoc J 2002;166:1017–1022.
35. Marsden J. Hormone-replacement therapy and breast cancer. Lancet Oncol 2002;3:303–311.
36. DiSaia PJ, Grosen EA, Kurosaki T, Gildea M, Cowan B, Anton-Culver H. Hormone replacement therapy in breast cancer survivors: a cohort study. Am J Obstet Gynecol 1996;174: 1494–1498.
37. Decker D, Cox T, Burdakin J. Hormone replacement therapy (HRT) in breast cancer survivors. Proc Am Soc Clin Oncol 1996;15:209.
38. Bluming AZ, Waisman JR, Dosik GM. Hormone replacement therapy (HRT) in women with previously treated breast cancer, update IV. Proc Am Soc Clin Oncol 1998;17:496.
39. Powles TJ, Hickish T, Casey S, O'Brien M. Hormone replacement after breast cancer. Lancet 1993;342:60–61.

40. Wile AG, Opfell RW, Margileth DA. Hormone replacement therapy does not affect breast cancer outcome. Proc Am Soc Clin Oncol 1991;10:58.
41. Wile AG, Opfell RW, Margileth DA. Hormone replacement therapy in previously treated breast cancer patients. Am J Surg 1993;165:372–375.
42. Eden JA, Wren BG, Dew J. Hormone replacement therapy after breast cancer. Educational book. Alexandria (VA): American Society of Clinical Oncology, 1996:187–189.
43. O'Meara ES, Rossing MA, Daling JR, Elmore JG, Barlow WE, Weiss NS. Hormone replacement therapy after a diagnosis of breast cancer in relation to recurrence and mortality. J Natl Cancer Inst 2001;93:754–762.
44. Vassilopoulou-Sellin R, Asmar L, Hortobagyi GN, et al. Estrogen replacement therapy after localized breast cancer: clinical outcome of 319 women followed prospectively. J Clin Oncol 1999;17:1482–1487.
45. Ganz PA, Greendale GA, Kahn B, O'Leary JF, Desmond KA. Are older breast carcinoma survivors willing to take hormone replacement therapy? Cancer (Phila) 1999;86:814–820.
46. Biglia N, Cozzarella M, Cacciari F, et al. Menopause after breast cancer: a survey on breast cancer survivors. Maturitas 2003;45:29–38.
47. Holmberg L, Anderson H. HABITS (hormonal replacement therapy after breast cancer—is it safe?): a randomised comparison: trial stopped. Lancet 2004;363:453–455.
48. Treatment of estrogen deficiency symptoms in women surviving breast cancer. Part 6: Executive summary and consensus statement. Proceedings of a conference held at Boar's Head Inn, Charlottesville, Virginia, September 21–23, 1997. Oncology (Huntingt) 1999;13:859–861, 865–866, 871–872 passim.
49. Kronenberg F. Hot flashes: epidemiology and physiology. Ann N Y Acad Sci 1990;592:52–86; discussion 123–133.
50. Notelovitz M, Lenihan JP, McDermott M, Kerber IJ, Nanavati N, Arce J. Initial 17beta-estradiol dose for treating vasomotor symptoms. Obstet Gynecol 2000;95:726–731.
51. Rabin DS, Cipparrone N, Linn ES, Moen M. Why menopausal women do not want to take hormone replacement therapy. Menopause 1999;6:61–67.
52. Stearns V, Hayes DF. Approach to menopausal symptoms in women with breast cancer. Curr Treat Options Oncol 2002;3: 179–190.
53. Loprinzi CL, Michalak JC, Quella SK, et al. Megestrol acetate for the prevention of hot flashes. N Engl J Med 1994;331: 347–352.
54. Bullock JL, Massey FM, Gambrell RD Jr. Use of medroxyprogesterone acetate to prevent menopausal symptoms. Obstet Gynecol 1975;46:165–168.
55. Morrison JC, Martin DC, Blair RA, et al. The use of medroxyprogesterone acetate for relief of climacteric symptoms. Am J Obstet Gynecol 1980;138:99–104.
56. Schiff I, Tulchinsky D, Cramer D, Ryan KJ. Oral medroxyprogesterone in the treatment of postmenopausal symptoms. JAMA 1980;244:1443–1445.
57. Bertelli G, Venturini M, Del Mastro L, et al. Intramuscular depot medroxyprogesterone versus oral megestrol for the control of postmenopausal hot flashes in breast cancer patients: a randomized study. Ann Oncol 2002;13:883–888.
58. Guttuso T Jr, Kurlan R, McDermott MP, Kieburtz K. Gabapentin's effects on hot flashes in postmenopausal women: a randomized controlled trial. Obstet Gynecol 2003;101: 337–345.
59. Naessen T, Rodriguez-Macias K, Lithell H. Serum lipid profile improved by ultra-low doses of 17 beta-estradiol in elderly women. J Clin Endocrinol Metab 2001;86:2757–2762.
60. Ganz PA, Greendale GA, Petersen L, Zibecchi L, Kahn B, Belin TR. Managing menopausal symptoms in breast cancer survivors: results of a randomized controlled trial. J Natl Cancer Inst 2000; 92:1054–1064.
61. Basil JB, Mutch DG. Role of hormone replacement therapy in cancer survivors. Clin Obstet Gynecol 2001;44:464–477.
62. Shapiro CL, Manola J, Leboff M. Ovarian failure after adjuvant chemotherapy is associated with rapid bone loss in women with early-stage breast cancer. J Clin Oncol 2001;19:3306–3311.
63. Recommended breast cancer surveillance guidelines. American Society of Clinical Oncology. J Clin Oncol 1997;15:2149–2156.
64. Barrett-Connor E, Bush TL. Estrogen and coronary heart disease in women. JAMA 1991;265:1861–1867.
65. Colditz GA, Willett WC, Stampfer MJ, Rosner B, Speizer FE, Hennekens CH. Menopause and the risk of coronary heart disease in women. N Engl J Med 1987;316:1105–1110.
66. Effects of estrogen or estrogen/progestin regimens on heart disease risk factors in postmenopausal women. The Postmenopausal Estrogen/Progestin Interventions (PEPI) Trial. The Writing Group for the PEPI Trial. JAMA 1995;273:199–208.
67. Hulley S, Grady D, Bush T, et al. Randomized trial of estrogen plus progestin for secondary prevention of coronary heart disease in postmenopausal women. Heart and Estrogen/progestin Replacement Study (HERS) Research Group. JAMA 1998;280: 605–613.
68. Burstein HJ, Winer EP. Primary care for survivors of breast cancer. N Engl J Med 2000;343:1086–1094.
69. Surbone A, Petrek JA. Childbearing issues in breast carcinoma survivors. Cancer (Phila) 1997;79:1271–1278.
70. Collichio FA, Agnello R, Staltzer J. Pregnancy after breast cancer: from psychosocial issues through conception. Oncology (Huntingt) 1998;12:759–765, 769; discussion 770, 773–775.
71. Blakely LJ, Buzdar AU, Lozada JA, et al. Effects of pregnancy after treatment for breast carcinoma on survival and risk of recurrence. Cancer (Phila) 2004;100:465–469.
72. Kroman N, Jensen MB, Melbye M, Wohlfahrt J, Mouridsen HT. Should women be advised against pregnancy after breast-cancer treatment? Lancet 1997;350:319–322.
73. Velentgas P, Daling JR, Malone KE, et al. Pregnancy after breast carcinoma: outcomes and influence on mortality. Cancer (Phila) 1999;85:2424–2432.
74. Sutton R, Buzdar AU, Hortobagyi GN. Pregnancy and offspring after adjuvant chemotherapy in breast cancer patients. Cancer (Phila) 1990;65:847–850.
75. Mulvihill JJ, McKeen EA, Rosner F, Zarrabi MH. Pregnancy outcome in cancer patients. Experience in a large cooperative group. Cancer (Phila) 1987;60:1143–1150.
76. Higgins S, Haffty BG. Pregnancy and lactation after breast-conserving therapy for early stage breast cancer. Cancer (Phila) 1994;73:2175–2180.
77. Tralins AH. Lactation after conservative breast surgery combined with radiation therapy. Am J Clin Oncol 1995;18:40–43.
78. Moore HC, Foster RS Jr. Breast cancer and pregnancy. Semin Oncol 2000;27:646–653.
79. Rosner D, Yeh J. Breast cancer and related pregnancy: suggested management according to stages of the disease and gestational stages. J Med 2002;33:23–62.
80. Ganz PA, Coscarelli A, Fred C, Kahn B, Polinsky ML, Petersen L. Breast cancer survivors: psychosocial concerns and quality of life. Breast Cancer Res Treat 1996;38:183–199.
81. Bower JE, Ganz PA, Desmond KA, Rowland JH, Meyerowitz BE, Belin TR. Fatigue in breast cancer survivors: occurrence, correlates, and impact on quality of life. J Clin Oncol 2000;18: 743–753.
82. Andrykowski MA, Curran SL, Lightner R. Off-treatment fatigue in breast cancer survivors: a controlled comparison. J Behav Med 1998;21:1–18.
83. Hochster H, Wasserheit C, Speyer J. Cardiotoxicity and cardioprotection during chemotherapy. Curr Opin Oncol 1995;7: 304–309.
84. Steinherz LJ, Steinherz PG, Tan CT, Heller G, Murphy ML. Cardiac toxicity 4 to 20 years after completing anthracycline therapy. JAMA 1991;266:1672–1677.

85. Swain SM. Adult multicenter trials using dexrazoxane to protect against cardiac toxicity. Semin Oncol 1998;25:43–47.
86. Sparano JA. Doxorubicin/taxane combinations: cardiac toxicity and pharmacokinetics. Semin Oncol 1999;3(suppl 9):14–19.
87. Slamon DJ, Leyland-Jones B, Shak S, et al. Use of chemotherapy plus a monoclonal antibody against HER2 for metastatic breast cancer that overexpresses HER2. N Engl J Med 2001;344: 783–792.
88. Grunfeld E, Fitzpatrick R, Mant D, et al. Comparison of breast cancer patient satisfaction with follow-up in primary care versus specialist care: results from a randomized controlled trial. Br J Gen Pract 1999;49:705–710.
89. Zabora J, BrintzenhofeSzoc K, Curbow B, Hooker C, Piantadosi S. The prevalence of psychological distress by cancer site. Psycho-Oncology 2001;10:19–28.
90. Gallagher J, Parle M, Cairns D. Appraisal and psychological distress six months after diagnosis of breast cancer. Br J Health Psychol 2002;7:365–376.
91. Kissane DW, Clarke DM, Ikin J, et al. Psychological morbidity and quality of life in Australian women with early-stage breast cancer: a cross-sectional survey. Med J Aust 1998;169:192–196.
92. Aragona M, Muscatello MR, Mesiti M. Depressive mood disorders in patients with operable breast cancer. J Exp Clin Cancer Res 1997;16:111–118.
93. Halttunen A, Hietanen P, Jallinoja P, Lonnqvist J. Getting free of breast cancer. An eight-year perspective of the relapse-free patients. Acta Oncol 1992;31:307–310.
94. Fredette SL. Breast cancer survivors: concerns and coping. Cancer Nurs 1995;18:35–46.
95. Ferrans CE. Quality of life through the eyes of survivors of breast cancer. Oncol Nurs Forum 1994;21:1645–1651.
96. Wyatt G, Kurtz ME, Liken M. Breast cancer survivors: an exploration of quality of life issues. Cancer Nurs 1993;16:440–448.
97. Carter BJ. Long-term survivors of breast cancer. A qualitative descriptive study. Cancer Nurs 1993;16:354–361.
98. Matthews BA, Baker F, Hann DM, Denniston M, Smith TG. Health status and life satisfaction among breast cancer survivor peer support volunteers. Psycho-Oncology 2002;11:199–211.
99. Ganz PA, Desmond KA, Leedham B, Rowland JH, Meyerowitz BE, Belin TR. Quality of life in long-term, disease-free survivors of breast cancer: a follow-up study. J Natl Cancer Inst 2002; 94:39–49.
100. Ganz PA, Rowland JH, Meyerowitz BE, Desmond KA. Impact of different adjuvant therapy strategies on quality of life in breast cancer survivors. Recent Results Cancer Res 1998;152:396–411.
101. Tomich PL, Helgeson VS. Five years later: a cross-sectional comparison of breast cancer survivors with healthy women. Psycho-Oncology 2002;11:154–169.
102. Mosconi P, Apolone G, Barni S, Secondino S, Sbanotto A, Filiberti A. Quality of life in breast and colon cancer long-term survivors: an assessment with the EORTC QLQ-C30 and SF-36 questionnaires. Tumori 2002;88:110–116.
103. Dorval M, Maunsell E, Deschenes L, Brisson J, Masse B. Long-term quality of life after breast cancer: comparison of 8-year survivors with population controls. J Clin Oncol 1998;16:487–494.
104. Brezden CB, Phillips KA, Abdolell M, Bunston T, Tannock IF. Cognitive function in breast cancer patients receiving adjuvant chemotherapy. J Clin Oncol 2000;18:2695–2701.
105. Dow KH, Ferrell BR, Leigh S, Ly J, Gulasekaram P. An evaluation of the quality of life among long-term survivors of breast cancer. Breast Cancer Res Treat 1996;39:261–273.
106. Ganz PA, Rowland JH, Desmond K, Meyerowitz BE, Wyatt GE. Life after breast cancer: understanding women's health-related quality of life and sexual functioning. J Clin Oncol 1998;16: 501–514.
107. Kurtz ME, Wyatt G, Kurtz JC. Psychological and sexual well-being, philosophical/spiritual views, and health habits of long-term cancer survivors. Health Care Women Int 1995;16: 253–262.
108. Dorval M, Maunsell E, Taylor-Brown J, Kilpatrick M. Marital stability after breast cancer. J Natl Cancer Inst 1999;91:54–59.
109. Wieneke MH, Dienst ER. Neuropsychological assessment of cognitive functioning following chemotherapy for breast cancer. Psycho-Oncology 1995;4:61–66.
110. Schagen SB, van Dam FS, Muller MJ, Boogerd W, Lindeboom J, Bruning PF. Cognitive deficits after postoperative adjuvant chemotherapy for breast carcinoma. Cancer (Phila) 1999;85: 640–650.
111. van Dam FS, Schagen SB, Muller MJ, et al. Impairment of cognitive function in women receiving adjuvant treatment for high-risk breast cancer: high-dose versus standard-dose chemotherapy. J Natl Cancer Inst 1998;90:210–218.
112. Schagen SB, Muller MJ, Boogerd W, et al. Late effects of adjuvant chemotherapy on cognitive function: a follow-up study in breast cancer patients. Ann Oncol 2002;13:1387–1397.
113. Ahles TA, Saykin AJ, Furstenberg CT, et al. Neuropsychologic impact of standard-dose systemic chemotherapy in long-term survivors of breast cancer and lymphoma. J Clin Oncol 2002;20: 485–493.
114. Ferrell BR. Overview of breast cancer: quality of life. Oncology Patient Care 1993;3:7–8.
115. Wyatt G, Kurtz ME, Friedman LL, Given B, Given CW. Preliminary testing of the Long-Term Quality of Life (LTQL) instrument for female cancer survivors. J Nurs Meas 1996;4:153–170.
116. Maunsell E, Drolet M, Brisson J, Robert J, Deschenes L. Dietary change after breast cancer: extent, predictors, and relation with psychological distress. J Clin Oncol 2002;20:1017–1025.
117. Burstein HJ, Gelber S, Guadagnoli E, Weeks JC. Use of alternative medicine by women with early-stage breast cancer. N Engl J Med 1999;340:1733–1739.
118. Lee MM, Lin SS, Wrensch MR, Adler SR, Eisenberg D. Alternative therapies used by women with breast cancer in four ethnic populations. J Natl Cancer Inst 2000;92:42–47.
119. Maunsell E, Brisson J, Deschenes L. Psychological distress after initial treatment for breast cancer: a comparison of partial and total mastectomy. J Clin Epidemiol 1989;42:765–771.
120. Vinokur AD, Threatt BA, Caplan RD, Zimmerman BL. Physical and psychosocial functioning and adjustment to breast cancer. Long-term follow-up of a screening population. Cancer (Phila) 1989;63:394–405.
121. Cimprich B, Ronis DL, Martinez-Ramos G. Age at diagnosis and quality of life in breast cancer survivors. Cancer Pract 2002;10: 85–93.
122. Ganz PA, Greendale GA, Petersen L, Kahn B, Bower JE. Breast cancer in younger women: reproductive and late health effects of treatment. J Clin Oncol 2003;21:4184–4193.
123. Ganz PA, Guadagnoli E, Landrum MB, Lash TL, Rakowski W, Silliman RA. Breast cancer in older women: quality of life and psychosocial adjustment in the 15 months after diagnosis. J Clin Oncol 2003;21:4027–4033.
124. Ashing-Giwa K, Ganz PA, Petersen L. Quality of life of African-American and white long term breast carcinoma survivors. Cancer (Phila) 1999;85:418–426.
125. Dorval M, Maunsell E, Deschenes L, Brisson J. Type of mastectomy and quality of life for long term breast carcinoma survivors. Cancer (Phila) 1998;83:2130–2138.
126. Ganz PA, Schag AC, Lee JJ, Polinsky ML, Tan SJ. Breast conservation versus mastectomy. Is there a difference in psychological adjustment or quality of life in the year after surgery? Cancer (Phila) 1992;69:1729–1738.
127. Janni W, Rjosk D, Dimpfl TH, et al. Quality of life influenced by primary surgical treatment for stage I-III breast cancer-long-term follow-up of a matched-pair analysis. Ann Surg Oncol 2001;8:542–548.
128. Omne-Ponten M, Holmberg L, Sjoden PO. Psychosocial adjustment among women with breast cancer stages I and II: six-year follow-up of consecutive patients. J Clin Oncol 1994;12: 1778–1782.

129. Curran D, van Dongen JP, Aaronson NK, et al. Quality of life of early-stage breast cancer patients treated with radical mastectomy or breast-conserving procedures: results of EORTC Trial 10801. The European Organization for Research and Treatment of Cancer (EORTC), Breast Cancer Co-operative Group (BCCG). Eur J Cancer 1998;34:307–314.
130. Schain W, Edwards BK, Gorrell CR, et al. Psychosocial and physical outcomes of primary breast cancer therapy: mastectomy vs excisional biopsy and irradiation. Breast Cancer Res Treat 1983;3:377–382.
131. Meyer L, Aspegren K. Long-term psychological sequelae of mastectomy and breast conserving treatment for breast cancer. Acta Oncol 1989;28:13–18.
132. Omne-Ponten M, Holmberg L, Bergstrom R, Sjoden PO, Burns T. Psychosocial adjustment among husbands of women treated for breast cancer; mastectomy vs. breast-conserving surgery. Eur J Cancer 1993;29A:1393–1397.
133. Rowland JH, Desmond KA, Meyerowitz BE, Belin TR, Wyatt GE, Ganz PA. Role of breast reconstructive surgery in physical and emotional outcomes among breast cancer survivors. J Natl Cancer Inst 2000;92:1422–1429.
134. Nissen MJ, Swenson KK, Ritz LJ, Farrell JB, Sladek ML, Lally RM. Quality of life after breast carcinoma surgery: a comparison of three surgical procedures. Cancer (Phila) 2001;91: 1238–1246.
135. Joly F, Espie M, Marty M, Heron JF, Henry-Amar M. Long-term quality of life in premenopausal women with node-negative localized breast cancer treated with or without adjuvant chemotherapy. Br J Cancer 2000;83:577–582.
136. Holzner B, Kemmler G, Kopp M, et al. Quality of life in breast cancer patients—not enough attention for long-term survivors? Psychosomatics 2001;42:117–123.
137. Kessler TA. Contextual variables, emotional state, and current and expected quality of life in breast cancer survivors. Oncol Nurs Forum 2002;29:1109–1116.
138. Satariano WA, Ragheb NE, Branch LG, Swanson GM. Difficulties in physical functioning reported by middle-aged and elderly women with breast cancer: a case-control comparison. J Gerontol 1990;45:M3–M11.
139. Sneeuw KC, Aaronson NK, Yarnold JR, et al. Cosmetic and functional outcomes of breast conserving treatment for early stage breast cancer. 2. Relationship with psychosocial functioning. Radiother Oncol 1992;25:160–166.
140. Lash TL, Silliman RA. Long-term follow-up of upper-body function among breast cancer survivors. Breast J 2002;8:28–33.
141. Guidozzi F. Estrogen replacement therapy in breast cancer survivors. Int J Gynaecol Obstet 1999;64:59–63.
142. Brewster WR, DiSaia PJ, Grosen EA, McGonigle KF, Kuykendall JL, Creasman WT. An experience with estrogen replacement therapy in breast cancer survivors. Int J Fertil Womens Med 1999;44:186–192.
143. Peters GN, Fodera T, Sabol J, Jones S, Euhus D. Estrogen replacement therapy after breast cancer: a 12-year follow-up. Ann Surg Oncol 2001;8:828–832.
144. Durna EM, Crowe SM, Leader LR, Eden JA. Quality of life of breast cancer survivors: the impact of hormonal replacement therapy. Climacteric 2002;5:266–276.
145. Ellman R, Thomas BA. Is psychological wellbeing impaired in long-term survivors of breast cancer? J Med Screen 1995;2: 5–9.
146. Saleeba AK, Weitzner MA, Meyers CA. Subclinical psychological distress in long-term survivors of breat cancer: a preliminary communication. J Psychosocial Oncol 1996;14:83–93.
147. Weitzner MA, Meyers CA, Stuebing KK, Saleeba AK. Relationship between quality of life and mood in long-term survivors of breast cancer treated with mastectomy. Support Care Cancer 1997;5:241–248.
148. Lee CO. Quality of life and breast cancer survivors. Psychosocial and treatment issues. Cancer Pract 1997;5:309–316.
149. Montazeri A, Jarvandi S, Haghighat S, et al. Anxiety and depression in breast cancer patients before and after participation in a cancer support group. Patient Educ Couns 2001;45:195–198.
150. Mock V. Body image in women treated for breast cancer. Nurs Res 1993;42:153–157.

107

Medical and Psychosocial Issues in Prostate Cancer Survivors

Tracey L. Krupski and Mark S. Litwin

Of the more than 200,000 men diagnosed each year with prostate cancer in the United States,[1] most live with their disease or the effects of treatment for many years.[2] Although many men remain asymptomatic throughout their lives, others face a multitude of physical and psychosocial challenges. Because the duration of survival is typically long, patients and their families are particularly interested in optimizing their quality of life. At the generic level, health-related quality of life (HRQOL) encompasses an individual's perceptions of his or her own health and ability to function in the physical, emotional, and social domains.[3,4] In prostate cancer survivors, the medical outcomes of urinary, bowel, and sexual impairments that result from treatment will influence the rest of the patient's life. The psychosocial aspects of HRQOL are impacted by the intimate nature of these medical side effects. Urinary leakage and erectile dysfunction may cause both private and public social embarrassment. In addition, such treatment-related complications may be compounded by the additional stressors associated with aging, such as retirement or death of peers.[5] Nearly one-third of men diagnosed with prostate cancer in a genitourinary clinic had levels of psychologic distress that met criteria for anxiety disorder.[6]

This chapter examines the medical and psychosocial issues impacting men with early- and late-stage prostate cancer. Late-stage patients are included because the course of prostate cancer recurrence is often indolent. Therefore, men with prostate cancer typically "survive" to require secondary treatments that compound existing medical problems. For men with early-stage tumors, the focus is on the repercussions of treatment decision on medical outcomes, the partner, decisional regret, and fear of recurrence. For men with advanced disease, the focus is on these issues with the addition of end-of-life decisions. The chapter concludes with emerging research challenges.

Early-Stage Medical Issues

Survivor Demographics

The strongest risk factors for prostate cancer are age and positive family history.[7,8] When survival rates are compared without controlling for stage, Caucasian men have improved survival rate compared to African-American, Hispanic, and American Indian men.[9–11] Survival rates are favorably influenced by higher socioeconomic status and the presence of a spouse or partner.[12,13] African American and Hispanic men bear a disproportionately high prostate cancer burden when compared to Caucasians.[14] Numerous studies have confirmed that both African-American and Hispanic men present with more-advanced [higher initial prostate-specific antigen (PSA) and T stage] prostate cancer than do non-Hispanic white men.[1,10,15–17] Debate exists as to whether this is a function of underlying differences in biology or disparities in access to health care. Ross et al.[18] found African-American men to have testosterone levels that were 15% higher than white men, suggesting a possible endocrine explanation for their increased risk. Because access to the healthcare system is influenced by socioeconomic parameters such as income and insurance status, African-American and Hispanic men often lack consistent high-quality medical care.[19,20]

Treatment Decision Making and the Effect on Survivorship

The impact of treatment effects on HRQOL is the major issue affecting posttreatment psychosocial quality of survivorship. Since the advent of prostate-specific antigen (PSA) screening in the early 1990s, most men present with early-stage disease, leading them to consider a variety of issues related to treatment. Those diagnosed with early-stage prostate cancer are challenged to choose among several treatment options (radical prostatectomy, radiation therapy, or watchful waiting) because studies have not yet proven an overall survival benefit of one treatment option over another.[21,22] The cure rates, defined as no evidence of biochemical (PSA) recurrence, for early-stage disease following radiation therapy or surgery range from 70% to 94%.[23–26] However, the medical outcomes do differ among these treatment options.

Medical Outcomes

Prostate cancer survivors face three long-term medical problems following primary treatment: incontinence, erectile dysfunction, and recurrence. The likelihood of these side effects will vary depending on the primary treatment chosen, stage of disease, and need for additional treatments. However, to date, no randomized controlled trials evaluating brachytherapy versus prostatectomy have been performed. The American College of Surgeons Oncology Group initiated such a trial but it was closed in 2004 for lack of enrollment. Cancer control outcomes and complication rates are inferred from predominantly retrospective, single-institution studies using different endpoints.

Postsurgical Incontinence

Even with improved surgical technique, urinary leakage after operative intervention persists (Table 107.1). Centers of excellence often report high rates of continence and potency whereas community-based outcomes may be different.[27–30] Causative factors for disparate outcomes include differences in patient selection, surgical volume, surgical skill, and definitions used for particular outcomes.[30–34] Further, the reporting of symptoms has been shown to be most accurate when elicited with written, confidential surveys that are self-administered and submitted to third parties, rather than by physician assessment.[35,36]

Time to recovery varies for each condition and may continue for at least 2 years after therapy.[37–39] Talcott et al.[40–42] reported that 12 months after prostatectomy 35% of patients were wearing pads, whereas Walsh et al.[40–42] reported this rate to be only 7%, despite using what appears to be the same definition and time point. These differences could be due to surgical technique, but the disparity is striking. Using yet another definition, Catalona and colleagues[43] also reported at 12 months that 45% of men under 70 years old claimed total urinary continence. Indeed, several authors have found that the definition itself influences continence rates. Wei[41] reported continence rates that varied from 43% to 84% depending on whether the definition was total urinary control or zero to one pad per day. Similarly, Krupski et al. found that among men claiming total urinary control, 98% also claimed no pads; however, among those reporting no pads, only 47% reported total control. Hence, total control is the stricter definition.[44] By 2 years postsurgery, further improvement in urinary control is unlikely. Therefore, men must learn to adapt with any residual incontinence for the rest of their lives. Table 107.1 depicts surgical rates of incontinence.

Management

Posttreatment incontinence may be secondary to bladder dysfunction or sphincteric insufficiency.[45] The former of these is treated with anticholinergic therapy, timed voiding, and fluid restriction in the evening.[46] If the etiology of the incontinence is from an incompetent sphincter, bulking agents may be attempted, although long-term results have been mixed at best. Collagen and Durasphere are agents that, if injected in the periurethral space, will increase sphincter competence.[47] Smith et al.[48] treated 62 postprostatectomy patients with multiple collagen injections, and one-third achieved social continence. Patients experiencing minimal incontinence (fewer than three pads/day) have the greatest chance of benefiting from a bulking agent.[49] The definitive therapy for patients with severe incontinence is an artificial urinary sphincter (AUS). After placement of an AUS, 76% were dry.[50] Appropriate patient selection is important, as mechanical failure, infection, and erosion are known complications.[51]

Postsurgical Potency

All surgical series have demonstrated that men undergoing radical prostatectomy have more sexual impairment than do age-matched controls.[43,52,53] The spectrum of reported potency using a similar definition, erections sufficient for intercourse, ranges from 87% to 21% to 14%[40,54,55] (Table 107.2).

Because the cavernosal nerves provide the innervation required for erections, the logical assumption would be that preservation of both sets of nerves would lead to higher potency rates. As familiarity and acceptance of nerve-sparing techniques developed, potency rates increased. A community-based urologist employed chart review techniques and reported 71% potency rates after bilateral nerve-sparing

TABLE 107.1. Postsurgical continence.

	N	*Definition of incontinence*	*% incontinent*	*Time from procedure*
Assessment of treating physician				
Zincke et al. 1994[128]	1,728	Uses three or more pads/day	5	5 years
Eastham et al. 1996[28]	581	Leaks with moderate activity	9	2 years
Murphy et al. 1994[176]	1,796	Requires a pad	19	
		Complete incontinence	4	
Survey data				
Talcott et al. 1998[177]	279	Wears an absorptive pad	35	1 year
Stanford et al. 2000[178]	1,291	Requires a pad	21	1.5 years
		Severe leaking	8.4	1.5 years
Smith et al. 2000[43]	941	Less than total urinary control	65	1 year
		Occasional dribbling	14	1 year
Walsh et al. 2000[40]	64	Using pads	7	1.5 years
Potosky et al. 2000[115]	1,156	Wearing a pad	9	2 years

TABLE 107.2. Postsurgical potency.

	N	*Definition of potency*	*% potent*	*Time from procedure*
Cohn et al. 2002[a 55]	199	Erections rigid enough for vaginal penetration	71	1.5 years
Murphy et al. 1994[a 176]	1059	Capable of full erection	35	1 year
Smith et al. 2000[43]	941	Sufficient for intercourse, <70 years old	25	1 year
Walsh et al. 2000[40]	64	Unassisted intercourse ± phosphodiesterase (PDE) inhibitor	86	1.5 years
Moul et al. 1998[54]	374	Full erections when stimulated	13	10 months
Potosky et al. 2000[115]	1156	Erection sufficient for intercourse	20	2 years

[a]Assessment by treating physician.

prostatectomy, which is similar to the 86% reported by centers of excellence.[40,55]

Management

The treatment of erectile dysfunction consists of a stepwise approach beginning with the least invasive therapies progressing to surgical options. The type 5 phosphodiesterase inhibitors (PDEs) constitute the first line of therapy because they are an oral medication. The largest body of evidence surrounds sildenafil, as it has been marketed the longest, and suggests that PDEs increase penile nitric oxide, leading to cavernosal smooth muscle dilation and engorgement.[56] Younger men who have undergone unilateral or bilateral nerve sparing appear to benefit the most.[57] Zagaja et al.[58] found that postprostatectomy patients enjoyed an increasing response rate with highest satisfaction 18 to 24 months after surgery. Local medical therapies require an intraurethral suppository or needle injection into the cavernosal bodies (ICI). The success rate of the intraurethral suppository as measured by successful intercourse at home is reported at 40%.[59] ICI in postsurgical patients results in 60% to 90% of men developing an erection, but many patients conceptually have difficulty undertaking this therapy.[60,61] Third-line therapy is a vacuum device; an external vacuum device generates negative pressure, leading to penile engorgement. Soderdahl et al.[62] randomized groups of men to ICI or an external vacuum device and found a statistical difference in preference for ICI (50%) compared to the vacuum device (27%). Last, a penile prosthesis can result in an active sex life. Although no data specifically relate to postsurgical patients, general function and satisfaction have been reported as around 85%.[63] An industry-sponsored multicenter trial demonstrated 5- and 10-year reliability rates of 85% and 71%, respectively.[64]

Urethral Stricture

Anastomotic stricture has been reported in 0.5% to 10% of patients following surgical treatment of prostate cancer.[65] Patients will typically present with a decreased force of urinary stream. If left untreated, urinary obstruction and urinary retention may result. Gentle dilation in the clinic is often sufficient, but for more-severe strictures an endoscopic operative procedure is necessary.[66]

External-Beam Radiation

For prostate cancer, the traditional target radiation dose with a four-field box is 70 Gy. The advent of three-dimensional (3-D) conformal therapy allowed radiation oncologists to increase the dose to 78 Gy. However, several studies documented that morbidity is both dose- and volume dependent.[67] Although the higher dose results in improved biochemical recurrence for men with high-risk disease, increased complications are also seen.[67,68] The late complications (2–5 years postprocedure) associated with such dosing follow: persistent incontinence, 29%; grade 2 to 3 bladder toxicity, 9% to 20%; grade 2 or higher rectal toxicity, 14% to 26%; and only 51% retained erections adequate for intercourse.[67,69,70] Ensuring that less than 25% of the rectum receives the higher dose minimizes these complications. Fowler et al.[30] assessed complication rates in Medicare beneficiaries treated with external-beam radiation and compared these rates to a previously published sample of Medicare surgery patients. They noted that radiation patients experienced less incontinence (7% versus 32%), more erections (77% versus 44%), and greater bowel dysfunction (10% versus 4%). Tables 107.3 through 107.5 summarize the complication rates by radiation type. An additional side effect of external radiation not seen with

TABLE 107.3. Postradiation bladder complications.

	N	*Definition of bladder symptom*	*% affected*	*Time from procedure*
Brachytherapy				
Wallner et al. 2002[73]	380	Grade 1–2 toxicity	19	1 year
Talcott et al. 2001[93]	105	Daily leakage	11	5 years
		Wearing a pad	16	
External beam				
Fowler et al. 1996[30]	621	Pads for wetness	7	5 years
Potosky et al. 2000[115]	435	Wearing a pad	3	2 years
Storey et al. 2000[70] (70 Gy vs. 78 Gy)	189	Grade 2 or higher	20 and 9	5 years
External-beam + brachytherapy				
Ghaly et al. 2003[94]	51	Grade 1–2	7	6 months
Zeitlin et al. 1998[86]	212	Any leakage of urine	4	2 years

TABLE 107.4. Postradiation potency.

	N	Definition of potency	% potent	Time from procedure
Brachytherapy				
Stutz et al. 2003[83]	148	Score of 22 on Sexual Health Inventory	69	2 years
Raina et al. 2003[85]	79	Erections sufficient for vaginal penetration − PDE	29	4 years
		Erections sufficient for vaginal penetration + PDE	70	
Potters et al. 2001[82]	482	Erection suitable for intercourse + PDE	76	3 years
External beam				
Fowler et al. 1996[30]	621	Ability to achieve erection	77	5 years
Potosky et al. 2000[115]	435	Erection sufficient for intercourse	39	2 years
External beam + brachytherapy				
Potters et al. 2001[82]	482	Erection suitable for intercourse + PDE	56	3 years
Zeitlin et al. 1998[86]	212	Ability to have satisfactory vaginal intercourse	62	2 years

surgery is fatigue. Immediately after initiation of radiotherapy, patients experience increasing symptoms of fatigue. Longer follow-up reveals the fatigue is temporary, with most men returning to baseline by 6 months.[71,72]

Brachytherapy

Brachytherapy (BT) is touted as having a very low rate of acute or long term complications. In thc initial 6 months all patients suffer from obstructive or irritative symptoms as a consequence of the radiation prostatitis. A randomized prospective comparison of iodine-125 (^{125}I) and palladium-103 (^{103}Pd) found that American Urologic Association symptom scores (now called the International Prostate Symptom Score, IPSS) peaked at 1 month and were generally higher in the ^{125}I patients. ^{125}I patients also experienced slightly higher grade 1 and grade 2 urinary and rectal morbidity.[73] The literature, in general, suggests that 2% to 18% of patients experience grade 2 or 3 urinary or rectal morbidity. Examples of such complications include stricture, urethritis, cystitis, proctitis, and rectal ulceration.[74–79] Urinary retention has been reported at 10% and incontinence was as high as 6% in the Medicare population.[80,81] Potency with implants alone is 69% to 76% at 1 to 3 years after implantation.[82,83] Because even the longest modern BT series span only 12 to 15 years, very little literature exists on long-term complications from BT. Merrick et al. commented that long-term urinary morbidity is restricted to patients having a prior transurethral resection of the prostate. Long-term erectile dysfunction ranges from as low as 29% without use of a phosphodiesterase inhibitor to as high as 70% at 5 years. The most serious and difficult to treat of the reported complications is a prostatourethral–rectal fistula.[84–88]

External-Beam Therapy Combined with Brachytherapy

Controversy still exists over the role for combined radiotherapy in prostate cancer.[76] Patients at low risk for extracapsular disease (Gleason less than 7, PSA less than 10 ng/dL, clinical stage less than T2b) are excellent candidates for brachytherapy monotherapy.[89,90] However, patients at intermediate or high risk for extracapsular disease may be better served by combined radiotherapy or either form of radiotherapy with the addition of androgen ablation.[24,91,92] The Radiation Therapy Oncology Group has initiated trial P-0232 [external-beam radiation therapy (EBRT) + BT versus BT] to assess these issues.[93,94]

Management

Following EBRT or BT, patients are started prophylactically on alpha-blockers to decrease the expected side effects of dysuria and frequency that result from radiation prostatitis. Select patients may stay on the alpha-blocker for 6 to 12 months. Nonsteroidals and antiinflammatory suppositories are used to treat proctitis. For a patient with a large prostate gland (more than 50 mm^3), androgen deprivation therapy is

TABLE 107.5. Postradiation bowel complications.

	N	Definition of bowel toxicity	% affected	Time from procedure
Brachytherapy				
Wallner et al. 2002[73]	380	Grade 1	20	1 year
Talcott et al. 2001[93]	105	Diarrhea or watery stool several times/week	6	
External beam				
Potosky et al. 2000[115]	435	Bowel urgency	36	2 years
Storey et al. 2000[70] (70 Gy vs. 78 Gy)	189	Grade 2 or 3	14 and 21	5 years
Kuban et al. 2003[67] (70 Gy vs. 78 Gy)	1,087	Grade 2 or 3	12 and 26	5 years
External beam + brachytherapy				
Zeitlin et al. 1998[86]	212	Blood per rectum (proctitis)	21	2 years

employed to "downsize" the prostate, facilitating BT.[95] The added benefit of androgen deprivation therapy is to decrease the risk of postoperative urinary retention. Sacco et al. have also demonstrated that dexamethasone (4 mg twice daily for 1 week then 2 mg twice daily) instead of androgen ablation also decreases the risk of retention in these patients.[96] Erectile dysfunction is treated in the same manner as for postsurgical patients as already described.

Prostate-Specific Health-Related Quality of Life

Several cross-sectional surveys have compared health-related quality of life outcomes after brachytherapy, external-beam radiation, and radical prostatectomy. Two studies reported that overall HRQOL was similar between brachytherapy and radical prostatectomy patients, with those undergoing brachytherapy having better urinary control but similar bother.[97,98] However, in a study of 1,400 patients, Wei et al.[99] found that men receiving brachytherapy experienced worse outcomes in the areas of urinary, bowel, and sexual HRQOL than did those undergoing either of the other two treatments. This finding contrasts with that of Eton et al.,[100] who reported that brachytherapy patients had the least sexual dysfunction and the best physical functioning of all treatment groups, and with that of Davis et al.[101] who reported that bowel bother was worst after external-beam therapy. Direct comparison of such studies is difficult because demographic characteristics, clinical factors, and measurement instruments vary from one investigator to another. Van Andel et al.[102] reported that radiation patients, on average, are 7.9 years older, have lower socioeconomic status, and more often have a higher tumor stage. They also found that radiation patients reported more pain and fatigue, lower overall HRQOL, and worse sexual function than men undergoing surgery.

Early-Stage Psychosocial Issues

Partners

Cancer affects family members as well as patients. Prostate cancer, more so than other malignancies, has been labeled a "relationship disease" because it so profoundly impacts both partners.[103,104] In fact, studies have found that psychologic distress is equivalent in the prostate cancer patient and his partner.[105] Clearly, once the cancer is discovered, both partners experience increased levels of anxiety compared with healthy couples.[106]

Although there is evidence that marital status impacts prostate cancer outcomes, the direction of the effect is mixed. The diagnosis of prostate cancer may evoke anxiety or depression in both partners. The response to this stress can nurture or undermine the relationship. A good relationship can foster healthy coping skills, alleviate distress, and encourage optimism. Increased optimism has been shown to correlate with improved cancer outcomes and survival.[107]

Depression/Distress

Being diagnosed with cancer naturally evokes a sense of sadness.[108] The difficulty is to distinguish the normal response from a clinical disorder. Symptoms indicative of a clinical disorder include a sense of failure, social withdrawal, suicidal ideation, and indecision.[109–111] Few studies have examined depression in patients with early-stage disease. Kornblith et al. studied 163 men with localized prostate cancer and found that 29% reported "worry" and 21% complained of depression. Patients and spouses both had frequent intrusive thoughts and images.[112]

Psychologic distress is complicated in prostate cancer because of the dual implications of treatment and distress. Prostate cancer treatment may itself induce sexual dysfunction, which adds further to such distress. Studying traumatic distress in men newly diagnosed with early-stage disease, Bisson et al.[113] found very few depressive symptoms. Instead, patients demonstrated higher anxiety and traumatic stress symptoms. The authors postulated that older men may be more likely to use denial as a defense mechanism. A more-holistic approach by the physician, incorporating attention to both psychologic and physical needs, benefits the patient and his spouse. Emotional support allows both members of the couple to target their energies on preparing for the treatment process.

Regret

Decisional regret relates to the notion that another treatment might have been preferable. Davison et al.[114] undertook a study to assess how factors such as HRQOL and level of patient involvement in medical decision making impact decisional regret. Higher regret scores did correlate with poorer emotional and urinary function. Although not a direct measure of decisional regret, the Prostate Cancer Outcomes Study that found 92% of patients who chose surgery or radiation would do so again.[115] In contrast, Hu et al.[116] used the two-item Clark regret scale[117,118] and discerned that 16% of men with localized prostate cancer experienced decisional regret. College education and worse HRQOL appeared to foster regret, but treatment type did not have an effect.

Fear of Recurrence

Using the CaPSURE database, Mehta et al.[119] identified more than 500 men with pre- and posttreatment questionnaires to measure fear of recurrence. All patients, regardless of treatment type, reported the most severe fear of recurrence before treatment. Their levels of fear improved after treatment and remained constant over the next 2 years. Another study utilized the Profile of Mood States (POMS)[120] in men with and without biochemical recurrence. Urinary tract symptoms were associated with increased cancer fear, but biochemical recurrence alone was not associated. However, men with both urinary tract symptoms and biochemical recurrence reported the highest level of cancer fear.[121] In an attempt to elucidate better the problems faced by men with prostate cancer, Roth et al. developed a new scale to measure anxiety in prostate cancer patients. The Memorial Anxiety Scale for Prostate Cancer (MAX-PC)[122] comprises three subsections including a prostate cancer anxiety scale, PSA anxiety scale, and fear of recurrence scale. The authors identify the prostate cancer anxiety subscale as being most specific to cancer anxiety while the fear of recurrence captures general distress. Loneliness and general uncertainty about the future heighten anxiety in prostate cancer survivors. Men who have elected to undergo no treatment (watchful waiting) also experience PSA anxiety. Wallace[123] identified 19 men on watchful waiting and found they experienced heightened uncertainty, leading to a higher perception of danger, which impaired their quality of life. Discussions with other men facing similar clinical scenarios promote positive coping skill and diminish anxiety. National and local support groups can help meet the emotional and educational needs of patients concerned with facing a recurrence.[124,125]

Late-Stage Medical Issues

Demographics

African-American men have a significantly higher mortality rate from prostate cancer than do non-Hispanic white men.[126] However, the traditional 5-year survival rates are almost irrelevant to men with prostate cancer, given that this rate approaches 100%, regardless of treatment.[2] This figure includes the 15% to 35% of men who will experience biochemical progression within 10 years of treatment.[25,127,128] The natural history of disease recurrence following radical prostatectomy was characterized by Pound et al.,[23] who showed that the median time to development of metastatic disease was 8 years and death followed at a median of 5 additional years. The risk factors for progression were time to biochemical progression, Gleason score, and PSA doubling time. The earlier the PSA recurrence, the higher the Gleason score, and the faster the doubling time, the worse the prognosis. No patients placed on early hormone ablation were included in the study.

Definition of Recurrence

After a radical retropubic prostatectomy, PSA levels should be undetectable. Original assays utilized a threshold level of 0.2ng/dL, and values less than this constituted freedom from disease. Although more-recent assays have lowered this threshold, the PSA should still be undetectable. A detectable PSA preceded clinical recurrence by 6 to 8 years.[129,130] The definition of recurrence after radiation therapy is three successive rises in PSA based on American Society for Therapeutic Radiology and Oncology (ASTRO) criteria.[131] However, because recurrent patients after either treatment will survive for many years, secondary treatment in the form of hormonal therapy results in additional medical problems.

Androgen Ablation

Medical induction of castration can be obtained through drugs affecting the production of luteinizing hormone-releasing hormone (LHRH), blocking the peripheral effects of androgens (steroidal and nonsteroidal antiandrogens), eliminating all steroid hormone production, and estrogens. The luteinizing hormone-releasing hormone agonists (which paradoxically lower LHRH levels) are typically administered by injection every 3 to 4 months whereas peripheral blocking agents are taken orally every day. However, once androgens are ablated, the prostate cancer begins an inexorable change to hormone independence.[132] Once a hormone refractory state has developed, few effective treatment options exist. Therefore, questions arise regarding the timing of androgen ablation and which agents to use.

Hormonal Complications

The predominant treatments are LHRH agonists and nonsteroidal antiandrogens, but these are not without side effects. LHRH agonists cause hot flashes, loss of libido and potency, anemia, fatigue, weight gain, depression, and decreased bone mineral density.[133,134] Antiandrogens maintain potency in a subset of patients but lead to gynecomastia and nipple tenderness.[135] Controversy remains over whether these agents are as effective when used alone as when used in combination with LHRH agonists. Two large trials demonstrated prolonged time to progression (by 2 months) in patients with modest disease; however, meta-analysis and other small studies have failed to demonstrate a significant advantage to combined androgen blockade.[136–138] Once metastatic bone deposits develop, LHRH agonists appear to be the most cost-effective, efficacious treatment.[139] However, men with high-risk disease or rising PSA are often started on hormone ablation.[140,141] To decrease the side effects, intermittent hormone ablation is increasingly being utilized.

Bone Complications

Hypogonadal men are at risk for potentially debilitating bone complications such as osteoporosis and hip fractures.[142,143] In patients with prostate cancer on androgen ablation, Hatano et al. reported a 6% nonpathologic fracture rate while Townsend et al. found a 9% overall fracture rate.[144,145] A smaller retrospective studies found even higher fracture rates of 40% after 15 years in 161 men after bilateral orchiectomy.[146] Daniell analyzed 59 men who had undergone bilateral orchiectomy for prostate cancer and found 8 (13.6%) with osteoporotic fractures of the femur or vertebra. However, when he analyzed the 17 patients still alive 5 to 12 years later, he noted that 38% had had one or more osteoporotic fractures.[147]

According to the World Health Organization, osteopenia denotes a bone mineral density between 1.0 and 2.5 standard deviations below the mean for young adults and osteoporosis is greater than 2.5 standard deviations below the mean.[148] Using this definition, Finkelstein et al. documented cortical bone density loss at least 2 standard deviations below normal in men with isolated gonadotropin-releasing hormone deficiency.[149] These changes in bone mineral density have been confirmed in men with therapeutic hypogonadism from prostate cancer treatment.[150,151] Smith et al. reported that trabecular bone mineral density of the spine decreased by 8.6% during the first year of androgen-deprivation therapy (ADT) for nonmetastatic prostate cancer.[151] With aging itself leading to decreased bone mineral density, the addition of ADT further places these men at risk.[152,153]

Management

The agents used in the treatment of osteoporosis and osteopenia depend on whether the etiology of the bone loss is from a benign or malignant process. Disease of benign etiology has been successfully treated with calcitonin, oral bisphosphonates, and a combination of vitamin D and calcium.[154,155]

However, the bone loss associated with prostate cancer and androgen deprivation therapy is accelerated, requiring additional therapeutic options.[153,156,157] A prospective randomized controlled trial revealed that intravenous bisphosphonate was effective in increasing bone mineral density in men on androgen deprivation therapy for prostate cancer.[158] Therefore, men with D0 disease as well as metastatic prostate cancer on ADT are candidates for intravenous bisphosphonates.

Fatigue

Throughout the disease trajectory, cancer patients experience fatigue, which is recognized to have a significant impact on quality of life.[159] Indeed, clinical experience with fatigue in hypogonadal men indicates that androgen deprivation therapy should lead to some degree of fatigue.[160] Stone et al.[161] used the Fatigue Severity Scale[162] to follow patients before and after treatment with goserelin and cyproterone. Fatigue worsened in 66% of patients after 3 months of androgen deprivation therapy. All patients responded to the therapy with decreasing PSA levels, eliminating disease progression as a possible source of fatigue. On multivariate analysis, only depression remained a significant predictor of fatigue.[163] The depression literature supports this association.[164] This study did not find any association with anemia, but others suggest that fatigue in prostate cancer patients on androgen deprivation therapy may be because of anemia, a well-known side effect of therapeutic hypogonadism.[165] Patients on androgen deprivation therapy experience not only the expected physical side effects such as hot flashes, loss of libido and potency, weight gain, and anemia but also the psychosocial changes of depression and fatigue. Close monitoring of all these parameters is critical.

Health-Related Quality of Life

The clinical rationale for selecting the method and agent for androgen ablation is controversial. Therefore, the physician must engage the patient in a discussion to decide what balance of side effects, cost, and risk of progression is optimal. Because the patient will likely survive for many years before developing bone metastasis or other evidence of clinical progression, the potential cost in quality of life may be great. Additionally, when the physical side effects of fatigue, sexual dysfunction, and weight are considered, deferment of this potentially emotionally debilitating therapy may promote HRQOL in men living daily with prostate cancer.

Late-Stage Psychosocial Issues

Partners

Researchers have used focus groups to describe the impact of prostate cancer on the couple as a unit. Both patients and partners feel unprepared to manage treatment- and prostate-related changes as they arise. The spousal role is increasingly difficult as the cancer progresses. Often the role shifts to that of a caregiver focusing on three major areas of concern. Caregivers contend with fear of cancer and its spread, helping patients respond to the emotional ramifications of the disease, and managing the disruptions caused by cancer.[166] For survivors of prostate cancer with late-stage disease, uncertainty prevails. Men with partners may benefit from physical assistance from their partner but bear additional emotional weight from their sense of being a burden. Men without partners experience more of a physical decline and loneliness.[166–168]

Depression

The concept that depression is linked to testosterone has been explored in the psychiatric literature. Studies have examined the treatment of elderly males with major depressive disorders with testosterone replacement. The therapy appears to be effective in men with late-onset depression.[169] Therefore, older men receiving androgen deprivation therapy for prostate cancer are an at-risk population. Among 45 men receiving androgen deprivation therapy (ADT) as prostate cancer treatment, the prevalence of major depressive disorder was eight times the national rate.[170] Although cancer progression was not the primary cause of the depression, history of depression was a strong risk factor. Involving experts in depression and palliative care can provide social support and help patients confront end-of-life issues.

Regret

Regret has been evaluated in men who developed metastasis and had initiated androgen deprivation therapy. Almost one-fourth of these men expressed regret. The demographics and time since diagnosis with metastatic disease were similar between men who were and were not regretful; however, men who had undergone orchiectomy were more likely to express regret.[119] Clark et al.[118] did find that men expressing regret were more likely to have poorer quality of life, particularly in the role and emotional limitations subscales. These men did not have more treatment-induced side effects, yet they perceived themselves as having worse functional status.

End of Life

Quality of life steadily descends in the final months of life.[171] Marriage appears to protect men from rapid decline in the physical domains but surprisingly does not offer protection in the emotional domains. Single men may feel the persistent effects of loneliness, while married men may sense being a burden. Higher socioeconomic status has been associated with a slower decline in physical domains but a more acute decline in the emotional domains.[172] Other studies in terminally ill cancer patients have found accelerated HRQOL declines at 1 to 3 weeks before death.[173] Because prostate cancer death can be so delayed, patients, family, and physicians often neglect to address end-of-life planning issues. Steinhauser et al.[174] evaluated factors considered important for a "good death," emphasizing that this is highly idiosyncratic. Control of symptoms, preparation for death, opportunity for closure, and good relationship with healthcare professionals were factors considered crucial to easing the end-of-life transition for patients and families. One responsibility of the physician is to consider what the patient and caregiver need emotionally and psychologically. This need includes assessing what interventions might be used for long-

or short-term gain or discussing transfer to a hospice or palliative care program. When these issues are adequately addressed, terminally ill patients feel more prepared for death and are better able to live to the fullest degree possible.[175]

Conclusion

The high prevalence of prostate cancer and the impact on the partner make the psychosocial aspects of prostate cancer particularly relevant to long-term survivorship. A man's masculinity is intricately intertwined with his personal identity. Therefore, the intimate nature of the treatment-related side effects of early- or late-stage prostate cancer may have far-reaching emotional consequences for these men. They are at risk for anxiety, depression, distress, fatigue, and bone complications at many stages of the disease trajectory. The most effective tool against these sequelae is awareness on the part of physicians and other health professionals in identifying psychosocial needs and directing patients to the appropriate resources.

References

1. Jemal A, Murray T, Samuels A, Ghafoor A, Ward E, Thun MJ. Cancer statistics, 2003. CA Cancer J Clin 2003;53(1):5–26.
2. Greenlee RT, Murray T, Bolden S, Wingo PA. Cancer statistics, 2000. CA Cancer J Clin 2000;50(1):7–33.
3. Osoba D. Measuring the effect of cancer on quality of life. In: Osoba D (ed). Effect of Cancer on Quality of Life. Boca Raton: CRC Press, 1991:25–40.
4. Penson DF, Litwin MS. The Impact of Urologic Complications on Quality of Life. In: Taneja SS, Smith RB, Ehrlich RM, (eds). Complications of Urologic Surgery, 3rd edition. Philadelphia PA: WB Saunders and Co., 2000:56–66.
5. Roth AJ, Kornblith AB, Batel-Copel L, Peabody E, Scher HI, Holland JC. Rapid screening for psychologic distress in men with prostate carcinoma: a pilot study. Cancer (Phila) 1998; 82(10):1904–1908.
6. Roth A, Scher H. Genitourinary malignancies. In: Holland JC (ed). Psycho-oncology. New York: Oxford University Press, 1998: 39–358.
7. Spitz MR, Currier RD, Fueger JJ, Babaian RJ, Newell GR. Familial patterns of prostate cancer: a case-control analysis. J Urol 1991;146(5):1305–1307.
8. Parker SL, Tong T, Bolden S, Wingo PA. Cancer statistics, 1996. CA Cancer J Clin 1996;46(1):5–27.
9. Gilliland FD, Key CR. Prostate cancer in American Indians, New Mexico, 1969 to 1994. J Urol 1998;159(3):893–897; discussion 897–898.
10. Hoffman RM, Gilliland FD, Eley JW, et al. Racial and ethnic differences in advanced-stage prostate cancer: the Prostate Cancer Outcomes Study. J Natl Cancer Inst 2001;93(5):388–395.
11. Underwood W, De Monner S, Ubel P, Fagerlin A, Sanda MG, Wei JT. Racial/ethnic disparities in the treatment of localized/ regional prostate cancer. J Urol 2004;171(4):1504–1507.
12. Nayeri K, Pitaro G, Feldman JG. Marital status and stage at diagnosis in cancer. N Y State J Med 1992;92(1):8–11.
13. Harvei S, Kravdal O. The importance of marital and socioeconomic status in incidence and survival of prostate cancer. An analysis of complete Norwegian birth cohorts. Prev Med 1997;26(5 pt 1):623–632.
14. ACS. Cancer Facts and Figures. Washington, DC: American Cancer Society, 2003.
15. Zietman A, Moughan J, Owen J, Hanks G. The Patterns of Care Survey of radiation therapy in localized prostate cancer: similarities between the practice nationally and in minority-rich areas. Int J Radiat Oncol Biol Phys 2001;50(1):75–80.
16. Ries LA, Wingo PA, Miller DS, et al. The annual report to the nation on the status of cancer, 1973–1997, with a special section on colorectal cancer. Cancer (Phila) 2000;88(10):2398–2424.
17. Hankey BF, Ries LA, Edwards BK. The surveillance, epidemiology, and end results program: a national resource. Cancer Epidemiol Biomarkers Prev 1999;8(12):1117–1121.
18. Ross R, Bernstein L, Judd H, Hanisch R, Pike M, Henderson B. Serum testosterone levels in healthy young black and white men. J Natl Cancer Inst 1986;76(1):45–48.
19. Hargraves JL, Hadley J. The contribution of insurance coverage and community resources to reducing racial/ethnic disparities in access to care. Health Serv Res 2003;38(3):809–829.
20. Cunningham PJ, Kemper P. The uninsured getting care: where you live matters. Issue Brief Cent Stud Health Syst Change 1998(15):1–6.
21. D'Amico AV, Whittington R, Malkowicz SB, et al. Biochemical outcome after radical prostatectomy, external beam radiation therapy, or interstitial radiation therapy for clinically localized prostate cancer. JAMA 1998;280(11):969–974.
22. Holmberg L, Bill-Axelson A, Helgesen F, et al. A randomized trial comparing radical prostatectomy with watchful waiting in early prostate cancer. N Engl J Med 2002;347(11):781–789.
23. Pound CR, Partin AW, Eisenberger MA, Chan DW, Pearson JD, Walsh PC. Natural history of progression after PSA elevation following radical prostatectomy. JAMA 1999;281(17):1591–1597.
24. D'Amico AV, Moul J, Carroll PR, Sun L, Lubeck D, Chen MH. Cancer-specific mortality after surgery or radiation for patients with clinically localized prostate cancer managed during the prostate-specific antigen era. J Clin Oncol 2003;21(11):2163–2172.
25. Catalona WJ, Smith DS. 5-year tumor recurrence rates after anatomical radical retropubic prostatectomy for prostate cancer. J Urol 1994;152(5 pt 2):1837–1842.
26. Sylvester JE, Blasko JC, Grimm PD, Meier R, Malmgren JA. Ten-year biochemical relapse-free survival after external beam radiation and brachytherapy for localized prostate cancer: the Seattle experience. Int J Radiat Oncol Biol Phys 2003;57(4):944–952.
27. Catalona WJ, Ramos CG, Carvalhal GF. Contemporary results of anatomic radical prostatectomy. CA Cancer J Clin 1999;49(5): 282–296.
28. Eastham JA, Kattan MW, Rogers E, et al. Risk factors for urinary incontinence after radical prostatectomy. J Urol 1996;156(5): 1707–1713.
29. Walsh PC, Partin AW, Epstein JI. Cancer control and quality of life following anatomical radical retropubic prostatectomy: results at 10 years. J Urol 1994;152(5 pt 2):1831–1836.
30. Fowler FJ Jr, Barry MJ, Lu-Yao G, Wasson JH, Bin L. Outcomes of external-beam radiation therapy for prostate cancer: a study of Medicare beneficiaries in three surveillance, epidemiology, and end results areas. J Clin Oncol 1996;14(8):2258–2265.
31. Begg CB, Riedel ER, Bach PB, et al. Variations in morbidity after radical prostatectomy. N Engl J Med 2002;346(15):1138–1144.
32. Hu JC, Gold KF, Pashos CL, Mehta SS, Litwin MS. Role of surgeon volume in radical prostatectomy outcomes. J Clin Oncol 2003;21(3):401–405.
33. Walsh PC, Partin AW. Treatment of early stage prostate cancer: radical prostatectomy. Important Adv Oncol 1994:211–223.
34. Wei JT, Montie JE. Comparison of patients' and physicians' rating of urinary incontinence following radical prostatectomy. Semin Urol Oncol 2000;18(1):76–80.
35. Litwin MS, McGuigan KA. Accuracy of recall in health-related quality-of-life assessment among men treated for prostate cancer. J Clin Oncol 1999;17(9):2882–2888.
36. Litwin MS, Lubeck DP, Henning JM, Carroll PR. Differences in urologist and patient assessments of health related quality of life in men with prostate cancer: results of the CaPSURE database. J Urol 1998;159(6):1988–1992.

37. Litwin MS, Flanders SC, Pasta DJ, Stoddard ML, Lubeck DP, Henning JM. Sexual function and bother after radical prostatectomy or radiation for prostate cancer: multivariate quality-of-life analysis from CaPSURE. Cancer of the Prostate Strategic Urologic Research Endeavor. Urology 1999;54(3):503–508.
38. Litwin MS, Pasta DJ, Yu J, Stoddard ML, Flanders SC. Urinary function and bother after radical prostatectomy or radiation for prostate cancer: a longitudinal, multivariate quality of life analysis from the Cancer of the Prostate Strategic Urologic Research Endeavor. J Urol 2000;164(6):1973–1977.
39. Fulmer BR, Bissonette EA, Petroni GR, Theodorescu D. Prospective assessment of voiding and sexual function after treatment for localized prostate carcinoma: comparison of radical prostatectomy to hormonobrachytherapy with and without external beam radiotherapy. Cancer (Phila) 2001;91(11):2046–2055.
40. Walsh PC, Marschke P, Ricker D, Burnett AL. Patient-reported urinary continence and sexual function after anatomic radical prostatectomy. Urology 2000;55(1):58–61.
41. Wei JT, Dunn RL, Marcovish R, et al. Prospective assessment of patient reported urinary continence after radical prostatectomy. J Urol 2000;164(3):744–748.
42. Talcott JA, Rieker P, Propert KJ, et al. Patient-reported impotence and incontinence after nerve-sparing radical prostatectomy. J Natl Cancer Inst 1997;89(15):1117–1123.
43. Smith DS, Carvalhal GF, Schneider K, Krygiel J, Yan Y, Catalona WJ. Quality-of-life outcomes for men with prostate carcinoma detected by screening. Cancer (Phila) 2000;88(6):1454–1463.
44. Krupski TL, Saigal CS, Litwin MS. Variation in continence and potency by definition. J Urol 2003;170(4 pt 1):1291–1294.
45. Leach GE, Trockman B, Wong A, Hamilton J, Haab F, Zimmern PE. Post-prostatectomy incontinence: urodynamic findings and treatment outcomes. J Urol 1996;155(4):1256–1259.
46. Haab F, Yamaguchi R, Leach GE. Postprostatectomy incontinence. Urol Clin N Am 1996;23(3):447–457.
47. Lightner DJ. Review of the available urethral bulking agents. Curr Opin Urol 2002;12(4):333–338.
48. Smith DN, Appell RA, Rackley RR, Winters JC. Collagen injection therapy for post-prostatectomy incontinence. J Urol 1998;160(2):364–367.
49. Cross CA, English SF, Cespedes RD, McGuire EJ. A follow-up on transurethral collagen injection therapy for urinary incontinence. J Urol 1998;159(1):106–108.
50. Montague DK, Angermeier KW. Postprostatectomy urinary incontinence: the case for artificial urinary sphincter implantation. Urology 2000;55(1):2–4.
51. Montague DK, Angermeier KW. Artificial urinary sphincter troubleshooting. Urology 2001;58(5):779–782.
52. Litwin MS, Hays RD, Fink A, et al. Quality-of-life outcomes in men treated for localized prostate cancer. JAMA 1995;273(2):129–135.
53. Fowler FJ Jr, Barry MJ, Lu-Yao G, Roman A, Wasson J, Wennberg JE. Patient-reported complications and follow-up treatment after radical prostatectomy. The National Medicare Experience: 1988–1990 (updated June 1993). Urology 1993;42(6):622–629.
54. Moul JW, Mooneyhan RM, Kao TC, McLeod DG, Cruess DF. Preoperative and operative factors to predict incontinence, impotence and stricture after radical prostatectomy. Prostate Cancer Prostatic Dis 1998;1(5):242–249.
55. Cohn JH, El-Galley R. Radical prostatectomy in a community practice. J Urol 2002;167(1):224–228.
56. Uckert S, Hedlund P, Waldkirch E, et al. Interactions between cGMP- and cAMP-pathways are involved in the regulation of penile smooth muscle tone. World J Urol 2004;22(4):261–266.
57. Zippe CD, Jhaveri FM, Klein EA, et al. Role of Viagra after radical prostatectomy. Urology 2000;55(2):241–245.
58. Zagaja GP, Mhoon DA, Aikens JE, Brendler CB. Sildenafil in the treatment of erectile dysfunction after radical prostatectomy. Urology 2000;56(4):631–634.
59. Costabile RA, Spevak M, Fishman IJ, et al. Efficacy and safety of transurethral alprostadil in patients with erectile dysfunction following radical prostatectomy. J Urol 1998;160(4):1325–1328.
60. Rodriguez VGI, Bona, AA, Benejam GJ, Cuesta P, Jioja Sanz LA. Erectile dysfunction after radical prostatectomy etiopathology and treatment. Acta Urol Esp 1997;21:909–921.
61. Fallon B. Intracavernous injection therapy for male erectile dysfunction. Urol Clin N Am 1995;22(4):833–845.
62. Soderdahl DW, Thrasher JB, Hansberry KL. Intracavernosal drug-induced erection therapy versus external vacuum devices in the treatment of erectile dysfunction. Br J Urol 1997;79(6):952–957.
63. Meuleman EJ, Mulders PF. Erectile function after radical prostatectomy: a review. Eur Urol 2003;43(2):95–101; discussion 101–102.
64. Carson CC, Mulcahy JJ, Govier FE. Efficacy, safety and patient satisfaction outcomes of the AMS 700CX inflatable penile prosthesis: results of a long-term multicenter study. AMS 700CX Study Group. J Urol 2000;164(2):376–380.
65. Geary ES, Dendinger TE, Freiha FS, Stamey TA. Incontinence and vesical neck strictures following radical retropubic prostatectomy. Urology 1995;45(6):1000–1006.
66. Kochakarn W, Ratana-Olarn K, Viseshsindh V. Vesicourethral strictures after radical prostatectomy: review of treatment and outcome. J Med Assoc Thai 2002;85(1):63–66.
67. Kuban D, Pollack A, Huang E, et al. Hazards of dose escalation in prostate cancer radiotherapy. Int J Radiat Oncol Biol Phys 2003;57(5):1260–1268.
68. Dale E, Olsen DR, Fossa SD. Normal tissue complication probabilities correlated with late effects in the rectum after prostate conformal radiotherapy. Int J Radiat Oncol Biol Phys 1999;43(2):385–391.
69. Nguyen LN, Pollack A, Zagars GK. Late effects after radiotherapy for prostate cancer in a randomized dose-response study: results of a self-assessment questionnaire. Urology 1998;51(6):991–997.
70. Storey MR, Pollack A, Zagars G, Smith L, Antolak J, Rosen I. Complications from radiotherapy dose escalation in prostate cancer: preliminary results of a randomized trial. Int J Radiat Oncol Biol Phys 2000;48(3):635–642.
71. Jereczek-Fossa BA, Marsiglia HR, Orecchia R. Radiotherapy-related fatigue: how to assess and how to treat the symptom. A commentary. Tumori 2001;87(3):147–151.
72. Janda M, Gerstner N, Obermair A, et al. Quality of life changes during conformal radiation therapy for prostate carcinoma. Cancer 2000;89(6):1322–1328.
73. Wallner K, Merrick G, True L, Cavanagh W, Simpson C, Butler W. I-125 versus Pd-103 for low-risk prostate cancer: morbidity outcomes from a prospective randomized multicenter trial. Cancer J 2002;8(1):67–73.
74. Stone NN, Stock RG. Complications following permanent prostate brachytherapy. Eur Urol 2002;41(4):427–433.
75. Peschel RE, Chen Z, Roberts K, Nath R. Long-term complications with prostate implants: iodine-125 vs. palladium-103. Radiat Oncol Invest 1999;7(5):278–288.
76. Peschel RE, Colberg JW. Surgery, brachytherapy, and external-beam radiotherapy for early prostate cancer. Lancet Oncol 2003;4(4):233–241.
77. Gelblum DY, Potters L, Ashley R, Waldbaum R, Wang XH, Leibel S. Urinary morbidity following ultrasound-guided transperineal prostate seed implantation. Int J Radiat Oncol Biol Phys 1999;45(1):59–67.
78. Gelblum DY, Potters L. Rectal complications associated with transperineal interstitial brachytherapy for prostate cancer. Int J Radiat Oncol Biol Phys 2000;48(1):119–124.
79. Snyder KM, Stock RG, Hong SM, Lo YC, Stone NN. Defining the risk of developing grade 2 proctitis following ^{125}I prostate brachytherapy using a rectal dose-volume histogram analysis. Int J Radiat Oncol Biol Phys 2001;50(2):335–341.

80. Merrick GS, Butler WM, Tollenaar BG, Galbreath RW, Lief JH. The dosimetry of prostate brachytherapy-induced urethral strictures. Int J Radiat Oncol Biol Phys 2002;52(2):461–468.
81. Benoit RM, Naslund MJ, Cohen JK. Complications after prostate brachytherapy in the Medicare population. Urology 2000;55(1): 91–96.
82. Potters L, Torre T, Fearn PA, Leibel SA, Kattan MW. Potency after permanent prostate brachytherapy for localized prostate cancer. Int J Radiat Oncol Biol Phys 2001;50(5):1235–1242.
83. Stutz MA, Gurel MH, Moran BJ. Potency preservation after prostate brachytherapy. Int J Radiat Oncol Biol Phys 2003; 57(suppl 2):S393–S394.
84. Merrick GS, Butler WM, Lief JH, Dorsey AT. Is brachytherapy comparable with radical prostatectomy and external-beam radiation for clinically localized prostate cancer? Tech Urol 2001;7(1):12–19.
85. Raina R, Agarwal A, Goyal KK, et al. Long-term potency after iodine-125 radiotherapy for prostate cancer and role of sildenafil citrate. Urology 2003;62(6):1103–1108.
86. Zeitlin SI, Sherman J, Raboy A, Lederman G, Albert P. High dose combination radiotherapy for the treatment of localized prostate cancer. J Urol 1998;160(1):91–95; discussion 95–96.
87. Jordan GH, Lynch DF, Warden SS, McCraw JD, Hoffman GC, Schellhammer PF. Major rectal complications following interstitial implantation of ^{125}iodine for carcinoma of the prostate. J Urol 1985;134(6):1212–1214.
88. Theodorescu D, Gillenwater JY, Koutrouvelis PG. Prostatourethral-rectal fistula after prostate brachytherapy. Cancer 2000;89(10):2085–2091.
89. Blasko JC, Grimm PD, Sylsvester JE, Cavanagh W. The role of external beam radiotherapy with I-125/Pd-103 brachytherapy for prostate carcinoma. Radiother Oncol 2000;57(3):273–278.
90. D'Amico AV, Whittington R, Malkowicz SB, et al. Biochemical outcome after radical prostatectomy or external beam radiation therapy for patients with clinically localized prostate carcinoma in the prostate specific antigen era. Cancer (Phila) 2002;95(2): 281–286.
91. D'Amico AV, Schultz D, Loffredo M, et al. Biochemical outcome following external beam radiation therapy with or without androgen suppression therapy for clinically localized prostate cancer. JAMA 2000;284(10):1280–1283.
92. D'Amico AV, Schultz D, Schneider L, Hurwitz M, Kantoff PW, Richie JP. Comparing prostate specific antigen outcomes after different types of radiotherapy management of clinically localized prostate cancer highlights the importance of controlling for established prognostic factors. J Urol 2000;163(6): 1797–1801.
93. Talcott JA, Clark JA, Stark PC, Mitchell SP. Long-term treatment related complications of brachytherapy for early prostate cancer: a survey of patients previously treated. J Urol 2001; 166(2):494–499.
94. Ghaly M, Wallner K, Merrick G, et al. The effect of supplemental beam radiation on prostate brachytherapy-related morbidity: morbidity outcomes from two prospective randomized multicenter trials. Int J Radiat Oncol Biol Phys 2003;55(5): 1288–1293.
95. Wang H, Wallner K, Sutlief S, Blasko J, Russell K, Ellis W. Transperineal brachytherapy in patients with large prostate glands. Int J Cancer 2000;90(4):199–205.
96. Sacco DE, Daller M, Grocela JA, Babayan RK, Zietman AL. Corticosteroid use after prostate brachytherapy reduces the risk of acute urinary retention. BJU Int 2003;91(4):345–349.
97. Krupski T, Petroni GR, Bissonette EA, Theodorescu D. Quality of life comparison of radical prostatectomy and interstitial brachytherapy in the treatment of clinically localized prostate cancer. Prostate Cancer Prostatic Dis 1999;2(S3):S32.
98. Downs TM, Sadetsky N, Pasta DJ, et al. Health related quality of life patterns in patients treated with interstitial prostate brachytherapy for localized prostate cancer: data from CaPSURE. J Urol 2003;170(5):1822–1827.
99. Wei JT, Dunn RL, Sandler HM, et al. Comprehensive comparison of health-related quality of life after contemporary therapies for localized prostate cancer. J Clin Oncol 2002;20(2):557–566.
100. Eton DT, Lepore SJ, Helgeson VS. Early quality of life in patients with localized prostate carcinoma: an examination of treatment-related, demographic, and psychosocial factors. Cancer (Phila) 2001;92(6):1451–1459.
101. Davis JW, Kuban DA, Lynch DF, Schellhammer PF. Quality of life after treatment for localized prostate cancer: differences based on treatment modality. J Urol 2001;166(3):947–952.
102. Van Andel G, Visser AP, Hulshof MC, Horenblas S, Kurth KH. Health-related quality of life and psychosocial factors in patients with prostate cancer scheduled for radical prostatectomy or external radiation therapy. BJU Int 2003;92(3):217–222.
103. Saigal CS, Gornbein J, Reid K, Litwin MS. Stability of time trade-off utilities for health states associated with the treatment of prostate cancer. Qual Life Res 2002;11(5):405–414.
104. Gray RE, Fitch MI, Phillips C, Labrecque M, Klotz L. Presurgery experiences of prostate cancer patients and their spouses. Cancer Pract 1999;7(3):130–135.
105. Baider L, Walach N, Perry S, Kaplan De-Nour A. Cancer in married couples: higher or lower distress? J Psychosom Res 1998;45(3):239–248.
106. Hagedoorn M, Buunk BP, Kuijer RG, Wobbes T, Sanderman R. Couples dealing with cancer: role and gender differences regarding psychological distress and quality of life. Psycho-Oncology 2000;9(3):232–242.
107. Funch DP, Marshall J. The role of stress, social support and age in survival from breast cancer. J Psychosom Res 1983;27(1): 77–83.
108. Greer S, Watson M. Towards a psychobiological model of cancer: psychological considerations. Soc Sci Med 1985;20(8):773–777.
109. Massie MJ, Shakin EJ. Management of depression and anxiety in the cancer patient. In: Breitbart W, Holland JC (eds). Psychiatric Aspects of Symptoms Management in Cancer Patients. Washington, DC: American Psychiatric Press, 1993:1–21.
110. McDaniel JS, Musselman DL, Porter MR, Reed DA, Nemeroff CB. Depression in patients with cancer. Diagnosis, biology, and treatment. Arch Gen Psychiatry 1995;52(2):89–99.
111. Bukberg J, Penman D, Holland JC. Depression in hospitalized cancer patients. Psychosom Med 1984;46(3):199–212.
112. Kornblith AB, Herr HW, Ofman US, Scher HI, Holland JC. Quality of life of patients with prostate cancer and their spouses. The value of a data base in clinical care. Cancer (Phila) 1994; 73(11):2791–2802.
113. Bisson JI, Chubb HL, Bennett S, Mason M, Jones D, Kynaston H. The prevalence and predictors of psychological distress in patients with early localized prostate cancer. BJU Int 2002; 90(1):56–61.
114. Davison BJ, Goldenberg SL. Decisional regret and quality of life after participating in medical decision-making for early-stage prostate cancer. BJU Int 2003;91(1):14–17.
115. Potosky AL, Legler J, Albertsen PC, et al. Health outcomes after prostatectomy or radiotherapy for prostate cancer: results from the Prostate Cancer Outcomes Study. J Natl Cancer Inst 2000; 92(19):1582–1592.
116. Hu JC, Kwan L, Saigal CS, Litwin MS. Regret in men treated for localized prostate cancer. J Urol 2003;169(6):2279–2283.
117. Clark JA, Wray NP, Ashton CM. Living with treatment decisions: regrets and quality of life among men treated for metastatic prostate cancer. J Clin Oncol 2001;19(1):72–80.
118. Clark JA, Wray N, Brody B, Ashton C, Giesler B, Watkins H. Dimensions of quality of life expressed by men treated for metastatic prostate cancer. Soc Sci Med 1997;45(8):1299–1309.

119. Mehta SS, Lubeck DP, Pasta DJ, Litwin MS. Fear of cancer recurrence in patients undergoing definitive treatment for prostate cancer: results from CaPSURE. J Urol 2003;170(5):1931–1933.
120. McNair DM, Lorr M, Droppleman CF. Manual: Profile of Mood States, 2nd ed. San Diego: Educational and Industrial Testing Service, 1981.
121. Ullrich PM, Carson MR, Lutgendorf SK, Williams RD. Cancer fear and mood disturbance after radical prostatectomy: consequences of biochemical evidence of recurrence. J Urol 2003; 169(4):1449–1452.
122. Roth AJ, Rosenfeld B, Kornblith AB, et al. The memorial anxiety scale for prostate cancer: validation of a new scale to measure anxiety in men with prostate cancer. Cancer (Phila) 2003; 97(11):2910–2918.
123. Wallace M. Uncertainty and quality of life of older men who undergo watchful waiting for prostate cancer. Oncol Nurs Forum 2003;30(2):303–309.
124. Kaps EC. The role of the support group, "Us Too". Cancer (Phila) 1994;74(suppl 7):2188–2189.
125. Kunkel EJ, Bakker JR, Myers RE, Oyesanmi O, Gomella LG. Biopsychosocial aspects of prostate cancer. Psychosomatics 2000;41(2):85–94.
126. Austin JP, Aziz H, Potters L, et al. Diminished survival of young blacks with adenocarcinoma of the prostate. Am J Clin Oncol 1990;13(6):465–469.
127. Trapasso JG, deKernion JB, Smith RB, Dorey F. The incidence and significance of detectable levels of serum prostate specific antigen after radical prostatectomy. J Urol 1994;152(5 pt 2): 1821–1825.
128. Zincke H, Oesterling JE, Blute ML, Bergstralh EJ, Myers RP, Barrett DM. Long-term (15 years) results after radical prostatectomy for clinically localized (stage T2c or lower) prostate cancer. J Urol 1994;152(5 pt 2):1850–1857.
129. Abi-Aad AS, Macfarlane MT, Stein A, deKernion JB. Detection of local recurrence after radical prostatectomy by prostate specific antigen and transrectal ultrasound. J Urol 1992;147(3 pt 2): 952–955.
130. Paulson DF. Impact of radical prostatectomy in the management of clinically localized disease. J Urol 1994;152(5 pt 2):1826–1830.
131. ASTRO. Consensus Statement: Guidelines for PSA following radiation therapy. Int J Radiat Oncol Biol Phys 1997;37: 1035–1041.
132. Noble RL. Hormonal control of growth and progression in tumors of Nb rats and a theory of action. Cancer Res 1977; 37(1):82–94.
133. Schroder FH. Endocrine treatment of prostate cancer: recent developments and the future. Part 1: maximal androgen blockade, early vs. delayed endocrine treatment and side-effects. BJU Int 1999;83(2):161–170.
134. Kaisary AV, Tyrrell CJ, Peeling WB, Griffiths K. Comparison of LHRH analogue (Zoladex) with orchiectomy in patients with metastatic prostatic carcinoma. Br J Urol 1991;67(5):502–508.
135. Iversen P. Quality of life issues relating to endocrine treatment options. Eur Urol 1999;36(suppl 2):20–26.
136. Denis LJ, Carnelro de Moura JL, Bono A, et al. Goserelin acetate and flutamide versus bilateral orchiectomy: a phase III EORTC trial (30853). EORTC GU Group and EORTC Data Center. Urology 1993;42(2):119–129; discussion 129–130.
137. Crawford ED, Eisenberger MA, McLeod DG, et al. A controlled trial of leuprolide with and without flutamide in prostatic carcinoma. N Engl J Med 1989;321(7):419–424.
138. Denis L, Murphy GP. Overview of phase III trials on combined androgen treatment in patients with metastatic prostate cancer. Cancer (Phila) 1993;72(suppl 12):3888–3895.
139. Seidenfeld J, Samson DJ, Aronson N, et al. Relative effectiveness and cost-effectiveness of methods of androgen suppression in the treatment of advanced prostate cancer. Evid Rep Technol Assess (Summ) 1999(4):i–x, 1–246, I241–236, passim.
140. Bolla M, de Reijke TM, Zurlo A, Collette L. Adjuvant hormone therapy in locally advanced and localized prostate cancer: three EORTC trials. Front Radiat Ther Oncol 2002;36:81–86.
141. Messing EM, Manola J, Sarosdy M, Wilding G, Crawford ED, Trump D. Immediate hormonal therapy compared with observation after radical prostatectomy and pelvic lymphadenectomy in men with node-positive prostate cancer. N Engl J Med 1999; 341(24):1781–1788.
142. Orwoll ES, Klein RF. Osteoporosis in men. Endocr Rev 1995; 16(1):87–116.
143. Niewoehner CB. Osteoporosis in men. Is it more common than we think? Postgrad Med 1993;93(8):59–60, 63–70.
144. Townsend MF, Sanders WH, Northway RO, Graham SD Jr. Bone fractures associated with luteinizing hormone-releasing hormone agonists used in the treatment of prostate carcinoma. Cancer (Phila) 1997;79(3):545–550.
145. Hatano T, Oishi Y, Furuta A, Iwamuro S, Tashiro K. Incidence of bone fracture in patients receiving luteinizing hormone-releasing hormone agonists for prostate cancer. BJU Int 2000;86(4):449–452.
146. Melton LJ III, Alothman KI, Khosla S, Achenbach SJ, Oberg AL, Zincke H. Fracture risk following bilateral orchiectomy. J Urol 2003;169(5):1747–1750.
147. Daniell HW. Osteoporosis after orchiectomy for prostate cancer. J Urol 1997;157(2):439–444.
148. Kanis JA, Melton LJ III, Christiansen C, Johnston CC, Khaltaev N. The diagnosis of osteoporosis. J Bone Miner Res 1994;9(8): 1137–1141.
149. Finkelstein JS, Klibanski A, Neer RM, Greenspan SL, Rosenthal DI, Crowley WF Jr. Osteoporosis in men with idiopathic hypogonadotropic hypogonadism. Ann Intern Med 1987;106(3): 354–361.
150. Berruti A, Dogliotti L, Terrone C, et al. Changes in bone mineral density, lean body mass and fat content as measured by dual energy x-ray absorptiometry in patients with prostate cancer without apparent bone metastases given androgen deprivation therapy. J Urol 2002;167(6):2361–2367; discussion 2367.
151. Smith MR, McGovern FJ, Zietman AL, et al. Pamidronate to prevent bone loss during androgen-deprivation therapy for prostate cancer. N Engl J Med 2001;345(13):948–955.
152. Orwoll ES. Osteoporosis in men. Endocrinol Metab Clin N Am 1998;27(2):349–367.
153. Daniell HW. Osteoporosis due to androgen deprivation therapy in men with prostate cancer. Urology 2001;58(2 suppl 1): 101–107.
154. Higano CS. Management of bone loss in men with prostate cancer. J Urol 2003;170(6 pt 2):S59–S63; discussion S64.
155. Orwoll E, Ettinger M, Weiss S, et al. Alendronate for the treatment of osteoporosis in men. N Engl J Med 2000;343(9):604–610.
156. Diamond T, Campbell J, Bryant C, Lynch W. The effect of combined androgen blockade on bone turnover and bone mineral densities in men treated for prostate carcinoma: longitudinal evaluation and response to intermittent cyclic etidronate therapy. Cancer (Phila) 1998;83(8):1561–1566.
157. Higano CS. Bone loss and the evolving role of bisphosphonate therapy in prostate cancer. Urol Oncol 2003;21(5):392–398.
158. Smith MR, Eastham J, Gleason DM, Shasha D, Tchekmedyian S, Zinner N. Randomized controlled trial of zoledronic acid to prevent bone loss in men receiving androgen deprivation therapy for nonmetastatic prostate cancer. J Urol 2003;169(6): 2008–2012.
159. Vogelzang NJ, Breitbart W, Cella D, et al. Patient, caregiver, and oncologist perceptions of cancer-related fatigue: results of a tripart assessment survey. The Fatigue Coalition. Semin Hematol 1997;34(3 suppl 2):4–12.
160. Engelson ES, Rabkin JG, Rabkin R, Kotler DP. Effects of testosterone upon body composition. J Acquir Immune Defic Syndr Hum Retrovirol 1996;11(5):510–511.

161. Stone P, Hardy J, Huddart R, A'Hern R, Richards M. Fatigue in patients with prostate cancer receiving hormone therapy. Eur J Cancer 2000;36(9):1134–1141.
162. Krupp LB, LaRocca NG, Muir-Nash J, Steinberg AD. The fatigue severity scale. Application to patients with multiple sclerosis and systemic lupus erythematosus. Arch Neurol 1989;46(10):1121–1123.
163. Stone P, Richards M, A'Hern R, Hardy J. Fatigue in patients with cancers of the breast or prostate undergoing radical radiotherapy. J Pain Symptom Manag 2001;22(6):1007–1015.
164. Pawlikowska T, Chalder T, Hirsch SR, Wallace P, Wright DJ, Wessely SC. Population based study of fatigue and psychological distress. BMJ 1994;308(6931):763–766.
165. Strum SB, McDermed JE, Scholz MC, Johnson H, Tisman G. Anaemia associated with androgen deprivation in patients with prostate cancer receiving combined hormone blockade. Br J Urol 1997;79(6):933–941.
166. Herr HW, Kornblith AB, Ofman U. A comparison of the quality of life of patients with metastatic prostate cancer who received or did not receive hormonal therapy. Cancer (Phila) 1993;71(suppl 3):1143–1150.
167. Blanchard CG, Albrecht TL, Ruckdeschel JC. The crisis of cancer: psychological impact on family caregivers. Oncology (Williston Park) 1997;11(2):189–194; discussion 196, 201–202.
168. Valdimarsdottir U, Helgason AR, Furst CJ, Adolfsson J, Steineck G. The unrecognised cost of cancer patients' unrelieved symptoms: a nationwide follow-up of their surviving partners. Br J Cancer 2002;86(10):1540–1545.
169. Perry PJ, Yates WR, Williams RD, et al. Testosterone therapy in late-life major depression in males. J Clin Psychiatry 2002;63(12):1096–1101.
170. Pirl WF, Siegel GI, Goode MJ, Smith MR. Depression in men receiving androgen deprivation therapy for prostate cancer: a pilot study. Psycho-Oncology 2002;11(6):518–523.
171. Litwin MS, Lubeck DP, Stoddard ML, Pasta DJ, Flanders SC, Henning JM. Quality of life before death for men with prostate cancer: results from the CaPSURE database. J Urol 2001;165(3):871–875.
172. Melmed GY, Kwan L, Reid K, Litwin MS. Quality of life at the end of life: trends in patients with metastatic prostate cancer. Urology 2002;59(1):103–109.
173. Morris JN, Suissa S, Sherwood S, Wright SM, Greer D. Last days: a study of the quality of life of terminally ill cancer patients. J Chronic Dis 1986;39(1):47–62.
174. Steinhauser KE, Christakis NA, Clipp EC, McNeilly M, McIntyre L, Tulsky JA. Factors considered important at the end of life by patients, family, physicians, and other care providers. JAMA 2000;284(19):2476–2482.
175. Saunders Y, Ross JR, Riley J. Planning for a good death: responding to unexpected events. BMJ 2003;327(7408):204–206; discussion 206–207.
176. Murphy GP, Mettlin C, Menck H, Winchester DP, Davidson AM. National patterns of prostate cancer treatment by radical prostatectomy: results of a survey by the American College of Surgeons Commission on Cancer. J Urol 1994;152(5 pt 2):1817–1819.
177. Talcott JA, Rieker P, Clark JA, et al. Patient-reported symptoms after primary therapy for early prostate cancer: results of a prospective cohort study. J Clin Oncol 1998;16(1):275–283.
178. Stanford JL, Feng Z, Hamilton AS, et al. Urinary and sexual function after radical prostatectomy for clinically localized prostate cancer: the Prostate Cancer Outcomes Study. JAMA 2000;283(3):354–360.

108

Physical and Psychosocial Issues in Lung Cancer Survivors

Linda Sarna, Frederic W. Grannis, Jr., and Anne Coscarelli

Lung cancer emerged during the 20th century as an epidemic of enormous proportions.[1] A rare disease at the beginning of the past century, lung cancer continues to be one of the most common cancers in the world, affecting 173,700 Americans (93,110 men and 80,660 women) in 2004.[2] Mirroring changes in smoking patterns, the incidence of lung cancer among men continues to decline. Large-scale smoking among women occurred almost 20 years after men in the United States, with a subsequent delay in increased cases, peaking in the 1990s. Encouragingly, the most recent evidence demonstrates that lung cancer incidence among women is declining, as are death rates.[3] In 2000, approximately 13% of men and 17% of women (age-adjusted, 15% overall) diagnosed with lung cancer were expected to survive at least 5 years (an estimated 26,065 Americans each year).[2]

There has been minimal (albeit statistically significant) increase in the overall percentage of survivors over the past 30 years (13%, 1974–1976; 14%, 1983–1985; 15%, 1992–1999).[2] The focus of this chapter is on the emerging data describing the long-term medical and psychosocial consequences of survival from lung cancer and its treatment. In addition to length of survival, the physical, psychologic, social, and existential components of heath-related quality of life (QOL) data have been recognized as important outcome measures of lung cancer treatment for more than 30 years.[4,5] These measures are now a common part of clinical trials of patients with lung cancer,[6] but there is limited information about QOL of long-term survivors. In an extensive review of literature on QOL in patients with lung cancer, 151 studies were identified covering 1970–1995.[7] Almost all these studies focused on patients in treatment. Only one focused on patients with early-stage disease treated by surgery,[8] and only one study was identified with long-term survivors.[9] Since that review, there have been several additional reports[10–14] on survivors of lung cancer who were disease free and off treatment at the time of the data collection. Details of these studies and others focused on recovery after curative treatment are displayed in Table 108.1.

Lung cancer survivorship, in contrast to breast cancer survivorship, which has shaped the quantity and quality of survivorship research, is in its infancy. For the purposes of this chapter, studies published (in English) since 1980 that provide data about the physical functional status, QOL, symptoms, and other issues experienced by survivors after curative treatment are reviewed. Studies that only addressed cardiopulmonary function in the brief postoperative period are not included.

Survivorship and Lung Cancer

There are many survivors of lung cancer as a result of the high incidence of this disease when using the National Coalition of Cancer Survivors' definition, which is "from the point of diagnosis forward." However, with a definition that sets a defined time frame of "5-year survival" or "disease-free survival," the field of survivors is narrowed to a smaller number of patients and, thus, a more-limited opportunity for research. Survival following a diagnosis of non-small cell lung cancer depends primarily upon stage and effective treatment. Only 16% of patients are diagnosed with localized disease, 36% with regional disease, and 38% with distant metastasis.[3] Although more than 80% of patients with surgically resected stage IA disease may have 5-year disease-free survival, expectation of survival diminishes progressively through stages II and III and is rare in stage IV. If untreated, few patients, even with small peripheral stage IA tumors, survive 5 years.[15,16] The statistics for long-term survivors of limited-stage small cell lung cancer are even less optimistic. Only 6% of 144 patients with limited-stage disease treated in Canada survived longer than 5 years.[17]

Long-Term Impact of Curative Surgical Interventions

The majority of QOL studies including patients with lung cancer have focused on symptoms of and issues facing patients with advanced disease.[7] The quality of lung cancer survivorship and resulting physical impairment has been minimally addressed. The majority of medical issues surrounding lung cancer survivorship are related to curative surgical therapy and tend to be short term. A major consequence of the successful treatment of lung cancer arises from the

TABLE 108.1. Studies documenting symptoms, functional status, and quality of life of lung cancer survivors since 1980 (in chronologic order).

Author	*Sample[a] characteristics: mean age[b], sex, ethnicity[c], education, marital status, health status*	*Disease characteristics/treatment/ follow-up period*	*Purpose/method Comparison group*	*Findings related to survivorship*
Nou and Aberg[71]	N = 69 (34% of whom received surgery for cure, n = 21, 30%, survivors) Age: 62 years Ethnicity: Swedish Health status: ND	Histology: bronchial carcinoma (1967 WHO classification) Stage: mixed Surgery: 27% pneumonectomy, 62% lobectomy, 13% nonresectional thoracotomies Follow up: 3–8 years Disease-free status not clear	Purpose: describe QOL and symptoms postthoracotomy, 1-month and at 3-month intervals Method: prospective evaluation of performance status by physicians Instruments: Carlens vitagram index (performance level, including working capacity, ambulation, symptoms, hospital treatment) Comparison groups: 28% nonresectional thoracotomy, 72% deceased patients	Good QOL among 5-year survivors: most capable of full-time work Initial preop QOL highest for long-term survivors Noncurative resection associated with lower QOL Specific information about symptoms not provided
Pelletier et al.[33]	N = 47 Age: 58 Sex: majority male Ethnicity: Canadian Health status: ND	Histology: ND Stage: ND Surgery: 43% pneumonectomy, 57% lobectomy Follow-up: approximately 3 months (mean 73 days postlobectomy, 62 days postpneumonectomy, range 29–200 days)	Purpose: evaluate impact of lung resection on pulmonary and exercise capacity Method: prospective pre- and 3 months postop Instruments: Borg scale Spirometry, exercise testing Comparison: No	Lobectomy: 20% reduction in exercise capacity Pneumonectomy: 28% reduction in exercise capacity due to dyspnea Leg discomfort contributed to decreased exercise capacity postop; none were limited by thoracic pain Decrease in PF is a poor predictor of exercise capacity
Dajczman et al.[40]	N = 56 (91% with malignant disease) Age: 62 Sex: 50% male Health status: ND	Histology: ND Stage: ND Surgery: lateral thoracotomy by 1 surgeon; 13% received postoperative radiation Rx Follow-up: median 19.5 months (range 2 months–5 years), disease free at time of interview	Purpose: describe prevalence and impact of postop pain Method: cross-sectional Instrument: interview about presence, intensity, functional impact of postthoracotomy pain, and influencing factors; VAS for pain Comparison: none	Persistent pain: 55% 1 year, 45% >2 years postsurgery, 38% >3 years, 30% >4 years Pain group: 33% had constant pain, 43% numbness, 23% shoulder pain Pain interfered with daily lives (44%) Five used medication, 3 had undergone nerve block NS differences in demographic or disease/ treatment variables in groups with or without pain Patients with no pain reported functional limitations, numbness
Dales et al.[8]	N = 91 with lung cancer (of 117) Age: 65 Sex: 71% male Ethnicity: Canadian Health status: 14% had moderate/severe dyspnea preoperatively Tobacco use: 25% current smokers, 72% former smokers	Histology: ND Stage: ND Surgery: 73% Lobectomy, 20% Pneumonectomy Follow-up: up to 9 months	Purpose: compare pre and post (1, 3, 6, and 9 months) operative QOL Method: Prospective self-report Instruments: QL-Index, Sickness Impact Profile Clinical Dyspnea Index, Pneumonconiosis Research Unit Index Comparison: n = 26 who underwent thoracotomy without lung cancer	Dyspnea peaked at 3-months (34%), but continued for 10% at 6 and 9 months Patients with cancer had 2× decrease in QOL at 1, 3 months postop ADL returned to baseline at 6, 9 months QOL scores similar for all groups preop, patients with cancer had significantly greater deterioration postop Extent of resection and cancer dx associated with deterioration in QOL in SIP Older age associated with poorer scores on QL-Index

Schag et al.[9]	$N = 57$ Mean age: 62 Sex: 56% male Ethnicity: 93% white Education: 68% ≥ HS Marital status: 61% married Health status: 41% hypertension, 32% heart disease, 11% diabetes, 7% skin cancer, 11% alcohol use	Histology: ND Stage: disease-free Surgery: 84% had surgery (details not described) Follow up: Mean 3.4 years since diagnosis, $n = 33$ short-term (>2–5 years), $n = 24$ long-term (>5 years) survivors	Purpose: describe and compare QOL among lung, colon, and prostate cancer survivors Method: cross-sectional, self-report Instruments: Cancer Rehabilitation Evaluation System (CARES), QOL–LASA Comparison: survivors of colon ($n = 117$) and prostate cancer ($n = 104$)	Lung cancer survivors had more problems than other cancer survivors Disruptions in physical function and pain were frequent and severe problems (46% chronic pain from scars) Short-term survivors noted depression (51%) and anxiety (63%), and distress with body changes (35%), 28% report feeling overwhelmed by cancer 17%–45% report difficulties with partners (e.g., communication, expressions of affection), 79% decreased sexual contact and problems, 7%–27% difficulty in dating, 63% difficulty with memory, 25%–32% with difficulty with thinking clearly Of the 1/4 working at the time of diagnosis, 96% of short-term survivors quit work due to disease and treatment
Cull et al.[48]	$N = 64$, >2 years in remission Age: 61 (median) Sex: 51% male Ethnicity: Scottish Education: 19% > HS Health status: ND	Histology: SCLC Stage: 95% limited-stage disease Treatment: 80% PCI (50% with concurrent chemo) Follow-up: 2 to >8 years	Purpose: describe QOL and prevalence of neuropsychologic disturbances in long-term survivors Method: Instruments: clinical and neurologic examination, CT scan, neuropsychologic testing, QOL (RSC, HADS)	Abnormal neuro exams (24% of $n = 37$), 16% with ataxia, 11% cognitive deficits; no association with abnormalities found on neuropsych testing: 81% (of 59) impaired on ≥1 exam, 54% ≥ 2 Most common QOL disruptions: fatigue (64%), lack of energy (59%), difficulty sleeping (54%), problems with concentration (54%); >1/3 had dryness of mouth, tingling hands/feet, pain/burning in eyes; psychologic distress similar to normative data for cancer survivors HADS (borderline/case level): 19% anxiety, 15% depression
Landreneau et al.[39]	$N = 142$ VATS, $N = 97$ thoracotomy (<1 year) $n = 36$ VAT, $n = 68$ thoracotomy (>1 year postoperative) Age: 60 (VATS), 59 (thoracotomy) Sex: 56% men (VATS), 42% men (thoracotomy) Health status: ND	Histology: malignant group: 66% of thoracotomy patients, 42% VATS Stage: ND Surgery: VATS, thoracotomy Follow-up: <1 year postop, >1 year postop	Purpose: compare prevalence and severity of chronic pain post-VATS vs. lateral thoracotomy Method: cross-sectional Instruments: Visual analogue scale to assess presence and intensity of discomfort, and shoulder limitations on the side of the operation Use of medication: Comparison: None	<1 year postop, VATS group had significantly less pain and shoulder dysfunction, but similar use of pain meds No significant differences >1 year postop
Hendriks et al.[23]	$N = 100$, $N = 31$ with QOL data (48%) response ND for QOL subset	ND for subset	Purpose: describe QOL 2.5 months postthoracotomy Methods: mailed questionnaire Instruments: EORTC QLQ = 30 Comparison: none	Good/excellent global QOL (56%) Poor/very poor QOL (26%) Higher percent of patients with pneumonectomy had lower scores Dyspnea (29%), pain (29%) no clear relationship of sx to extent of resection

(continued)

TABLE 108.1. Studies documenting symptoms, functional status, and quality of life of lung cancer survivors since 1980 (in chronologic order). (continued)

Author	*Sample[a] characteristics: mean age[b], sex, ethnicity[c], education, marital status, health status*	*Disease characteristics/treatment/ follow-up period*	*Purpose/method Comparison group*	*Findings related to survivorship*
Zieren et al.[34]	N = 52 (12 months postoperative), n = 20 (pre- and postoperative data) Age: 61 years Sex: 73% male Ethnicity: German Marital status: 12% partnered Health status: ND	Histology: NSCLC Stage: ND Treatment Surgery: 81% Lobectomy, 10% pneumonectomy Adjuvant treatment: 25% radiation therapy Follow-up period: 1 year, 19% with recurrence	Purpose: describe QOL post surgery Method: mix of cross-sectional and prospective Instruments: EORTC QOL, Psychologist-rated Spitzer QOL Index Comparison: none	Dyspnea at exertion and pain continued at 12 months Physical dysfunction returned to preoperative level at 12 months postsurgery Emotional, social, and financial dysfunction was less severe, but continued postop Pneumonectomy was associated with more symptom distress and limitations in physical function, but not with greater emotional, social, or financial dysfunction NS differences based upon adjuvant treatment. QOL rated as higher by the external rater as compared to the patient. 12% employed full time Recurrence negatively impacted postop QOL
Bolliger et al.[30]	N = 68 Age: 61 Sex: 84% males Ethnicity: Swiss Health status: Preoperative FEV_1 = 2.38 (lobectomy), 2.50 (pneumonectomy)	Histology: ND Stage: ND Surgery: 74% lobectomy, 26% pneumonectomy Follow-up: 3 and 6 months postop	Purpose: compare effect of lobectomy and pneumonectomy on PFT, exercise capacity, and perception of symptoms Method: prospective, pre, 3, 6 months postsurgery Instruments: PFT Comparison group: none	Lobectomy: no change in exercise capacity; PFT significant decreased at 3 months and significant increased at 6 months (10% permanent loss) Exercise capacity limited by leg muscle fatigue and deconditioning Pneumonectomy: 20% reduction in exercise capacity; PFT significant lower at 3 months and did not recover at 6 months (30% permanent loss); significantly lower than lobectomy, exercise capacity limited by Dyspnea
Larsen et al.[28]	N = 57 with pre and post assessments Age: 59 (pneumonectomy); 67 (lobectomy) Sex: 72% male Ethnicity: Danish Health status: ND	Histology: NSCLC Stage: ND Surgery: 28% pneumonectomy, 72% lobectomy	Purpose: describe postop changes in cardiopulmonary function Methods Instruments: exercise testing, pulmonary function, arterial blood gas	Lobectomy: minimal change in lung function or exercise capacity Pneumonectomy: decrease in PF, but compensation due to better oxygen uptake; decrease in exercise values less than expected Change in FEV_1 was a poor predictor of change in exercise capacity Variable changes in PF and exercise capacity with some patient improving postop, some worsening, and some with little change
Mangione et al.[42]	N = 123 with lung cancer Age: 64 Sex: 54% male Ethnicity: 97% white Health status: 94% with at least 1 comorbid condition, 49% with >3	Histology: NSCLC Stage: ND Surgery: thoracotomy Follow-up: 6 and 12 months postsurgery	Purpose: examine QOL changes over time and compare QOL of patients undergoing elective surgery Method: prospective, pre- and postsurgery Instruments: SF-36, Specific Activity Scale, health transition questions and rating of general health Comparison: n = 236, with total hip arthroplasty, n = 95, repair of abdominal aortic aneurysm	Significant declines in health perceptions, physical function, role-physical, bodily pain, vitality, social function at 6 and 12 months after surgery Improvement in mental health and role-mental function over time By 12 months, physical function, bodily pain, health perceptions were lower than preop levels, but similar to population-based norms Compared to other groups, lung cancer patients continued to have the lowest health perceptions, lower role-physical and social function ratings

Nezu et al.[26]	N = 82 (including n = 10 undergoing lobectomy with hemodynamic data) Lobectomy: Age: 64 Sex: 84% male Ethnicity: Japanese Pneumonectomy: Age: 62 Sex: 90% male Ethnicity: Japanese Health status: FEV_1% predicted: 86 (lobectomy) n = 6 hypertension, n = 2 chronic bronchitis	Histology: ND Stage: "operable" Surgery: n = 20 pneumonectomy, n = 62 lobectomy Follow-up: 3, >6 months postop	Purpose: assess effects of resection on exercise limitation Method: prospective, pre- and postop Instruments: exercise testing, spirometry, Borg scale (dyspnea) Comparison: none	Improvement in exercise capacity 3–6 months postop for lobectomy but not pneumonectomy patients Mean loss of exercise capacity (VO_2 max) after 6 months: 28% pneumonectomy, 13% lobectomy Changes in PF did not correlate with exercise capacity Dyspnea was a limiting factor in exercise testing for pneumonectomy (65% at 3 months, 60% after 6 months), leg discomfort continued as the limiting factor for the lobectomy group (58% at 3 months, 64% after 6 months)
Nugent et al.[36]	N = 106, n = 53 with follow-up data Age: 61–64 (by surgical procedure) Ethnicity: Irish sample Health status: Preoperative FEV_1 % predicted ranged from 71% to 82%	Histology: not reported Stage: ND Surgery: n = 13, pneumonectomy, n = 26, lobectomy/wedge resection, n = 13 thoracotomy (inoperable tumor) Follow-up: 3 and 6 months	Purpose: describe and compare the effects of different types of lung resections and thoracotomy alone (inoperable tumor) on exercise capacity Method: prospective, pre-, postsurgery Instruments: PF, exercise testing, Borg dyspnea scale Comparison:	Thoracotomy alone did not significantly affect exercise capacity Pneumonectomy: exercise capacity reduced by 28% Lobectomy: exercise capacity unchanged No significant difference in Borg dyspnea rating pre and post any procedures
Miyazawa et al.[27]	N = 8 Age: 67 Health status: FEV_1% predicted = 67.2, VC = 3.47 Tobacco use: all had quit smoking after surgery (never smokers were excluded); smoking "piece-years" range 600–1,600	Histology: ND Stage: potentially resectable Surgery: lobectomy Follow-up: 4–6 months, 42–48 months	Purpose: to examine postop changes in cardiopulmonary function Method: prospective Instruments: PF, exercise testing, hemodynamic monitoring, Fletcher, Hugh–Jones' dyspnea index Comparison: none	None had any symptoms before surgery 63% had increased dyspnea scores at 4–6 months; at 42–48 months, all had decreased to preop levels except for 1 patient Symptoms not directly related to physiologic outcomes FEV_1% predicted increased postop (77% at 4–6 months; at 72% 42–48 months); airway resistance at preop levels over time Long-term decrease in cardiopulmonary function
Sugiura et al.[41]	N = 22 VATS, N = 22 thoracotomy Age: 62 (VATS), 61 (thoracotomy) Sex: 83% men (VATS), 38% thoracotomy Health status: ND	Histology: NSCLC Stage: stage I Surgery: VATS, thoracotomy Follow-up: mean 21 months (VATS), 30 months (thoracotomy)	Purpose: describe and compare QOL post-VAT with thoracotomy Method: prospective; Instruments: self-report questionnaire regarding chest pain, arm/shoulder limitations, time to return to preop activity, satisfaction Comparison: none	NS differences in patient characteristics Significantly decreased in chronic pain, return to ADL, and improved satisfaction with VATS At 12 months, no patient who received the VATS reported postthoracotomy pain; 4 patients in thoracotomy group required narcotics at 12 months
Uchitomi et al.[14]	N = 223 with successful surgical resection Age: 63 years Ethnicity: Japanese Marital status: 82% married Education: 21% ≥ HS Health status: 23% < 70% predicted FEV_1 6% history of depression Tobacco use: 41% current smokers, 24% former smokers	Histology: 68% adenocarcinoma, 21% squamous carcinoma; Stage: 92% stage I or II Treatment: 96% lobectomy, 5% pneumonectomy Follow-up: 1 and 3 months postresection	Purpose: to describe depression at 1, 3 months post curative resection Method: prospective; Instruments: Psychiatric interview at baseline using criteria from the DSMMD, Profile of Mood States	Major or minor depressions: at 1 month (9.0%), at 2 months (9.4%), at 3 months (5.8%) Education level related to depression in the perioperative phase Depression preop was related to subsequent depression Lack of confidence in confidants (social support), pain and diminished performance status significantly associated with depression at 3 months

(continued)

TABLE 108.1. Studies documenting symptoms, functional status, and quality of life of lung cancer survivors since 1980 (in chronologic order). (continued)

Author	*Sample[a] characteristics: mean age[b], sex, ethnicity[c], education, marital status, health status*	*Disease characteristics/treatment/ follow-up period*	*Purpose/method Comparison group*	*Findings related to survivorship*
Uchitomi et al.[60]	N = 226 patients with curative disease Age: 62 years Sex: 61% male Ethnicity: Japanese Education: 66% > JHS Marital status: 82% married Health status: 22% < 70 & FEV_1% predicted 31% with prior history of depression, 43% with moderate/severe dyspnea	Histology: NSCLC, Stage: 76% stage I, 16% stage II Surgery: curative resection Follow-up: 3 months	Purpose: describe impact of physician support on psychologic responses post curative surgery Method: prospective; Instruments: Structured interviews 1 and 3 months after surgery using DSM-III-R, Profile of Mood States, Mental Adjustment to Cancer	Depression: 9% at 1 month, 6% at 3 months postop; 26% had hx of depression History of depression was related to psychologic distress postsurgery Dyspnea, FEV_1, and PS related to psychologic distress at 3 months 24% used the physician and 4% used nurses for social support Physician support related to decreased psychologic distress, helplessness/ hopelessness, and increased fighting spirit, not related to depression Physician support was the sole factor in a multivariate regression related to increased fighting spirit for females and patients with no hx of depression
Handy et al.[29]	N = 139, n = 103 with 6-month data Age: 62 years Sex: 59% male Health status: Respiratory function: mean predicted FEV_1 76% Comorbid conditions: 30%, cardiac, 16% diabetes, 15% peripheral vascular disease Tobacco use: 40% smoking within 8 weeks of surgery	Histology: ND Stage: 67% had stage I or II Surgery: pneumonectomy (8%), lobectomy (78%) 58% had open thoracotomy, 1% video-assisted thoracotomy, 5% muscle-sparing thoracotomy Follow-up: 6 months (12% died within 6 months), includes 7 with metastatic disease	Purpose: compare functional status and QOL preop and 6-month post lung resection. Design: prospective Methods: prospective; Instruments: Short-Form 36, Ferrans and Powers Quality of Life Index Control: Age-matched healthy controls	Functional health status impaired Preop pain, impaired physical status, role function, social functioning, and mental health were present 6 months postsurgery Dyspnea significantly worse postop General health status, energy level unchanged Postthoracotomy/neuropathic pain was an issue for 8 subjects No age or gender differences Pre-operative DLCO (<45% predicted), not FEV_1, predicted postop QOL Adjuvant treatment, 6-minute walk, extent of resection, complications did not predict QOL 6 months after surgery
Li et al.[44]	N = 51 Age: 63 years (VATS), 67 years (thoracotomy) Sex: 74% male Ethnicity: Chinese Marital status: 71% married	Histology: 55% adenocarcinoma, 20% squamous Surgery: VATS (n = 27), thoracotomy (n = 24) Follow-up: minimum of 6-months postsurgery (range 6–75 months: for VAT (mean 34 months), for thoracotomy (mean 39 months)	Purpose: compare QOL and symptoms between VATS and thoracotomy Design: cross-sectional Instruments: EORTC-C30 core questionnaire, EORTC QLQ-LC13 (Chinese versions) Investigator developed additional surgery-related questions	NS differences in QOL or symptoms between VATS group and open thoracotomy group According to EORTC ratings: good to high level of functioning Symptoms continued, including fatigue, coughing, dyspnea, thoracotomy pain (74% VATS, thoracotomy, 75%) Most severe symptoms included coughing, fatigue, and arm/shoulder pain; 44% reported financial difficulties
Sarna et al.[10]	N = 142 (5-year minimum disease-free survivors of NSCLC) Age: 71 years Sex: 46% male Ethnicity: 83% Caucasian Marital status: 47% married Education: 28% ≥ HS Health status: 50% FEV_1 < 70% 60% had at least 1 comorbid condition, 50% reported 2 conditions (heart disease, 29% and cataracts, 35%, most	Histology: 59% adenocarcinoma; 35% squamous Stage: 80% stage I and II Surgery: 12% pneumonectomy, 74% lobectomy, 11% segmental/wedge Follow-up period: 10 years, range 5–21 years	Purpose: describe QOL Method: cross-sectional Instruments: QOL-Survivor, SF-36, CES-D, spirometry Comparison group: population-based norms	Majority reported positive attitudes: 71% described as hopeful; 50% described cancer as contributing to positive life experiences; 22% depressed (CES-D ≥ 16) Most serious issues: fatigue (27%), pain (24%), anxiety (30%), changes in self-concept (21%), changes in appearance (20%), 34% reported families experienced significant distress Lower QOL associated with depressed mood and being Caucasian Lower physical QOL linked to older age, poorer PF, living alone, longer time since diagnosis, depressed mood, more comorbid conditions

	common); 9% with second primary lung cancer, 17% with history of other cancers Tobacco use: 76% former smokers, 13% current smokers			
Evangelista et al.[13]	As described above	As described above	Purpose: describe health perceptions and risk behaviors of survivors Method: cross-sectional Instruments: Perceived health status item (from Short-Form 36), self-report and biochemical verification of tobacco use, self-reported alcohol use, spirometry, BMI Comparison group: none	Most survivors had healthy lifestyles. Good/excellent health (37%), fair/poor health (30%) NS difference based upon clinical or demographic characteristics. 67% of smokers quit after diagnosis; 16% never smokers Current smokers (13%) more likely to be male (32%) and single (60%), 28% exposed to secondhand smoke, 58% used alcohol (16% quit after diagnosis), 51% overweight (BMI ≥ 25); 16% obese (BMI ≥ 30) Current smoking, exposure to second-hand smoke, current drinking, and BMI ≥ 25 were significant predictors of poor health perceptions
Maliski et al.[12]	I = 29 survivors within another study[10] Age 72, 55% men Marital status: 55% married Ethnicity: 69% white Education: 52% >HS Health status: FEV_1 % predicted, 59.8% Average of 1.75 comorbid conditions Tobacco use: 10% current smoking, 79% former smokers	Histology: 48% adenocarcinoma, 48% squamous cell, Stage: 72% stage I, 10% stage II Surgery: 79%, lobectomy/wedge resection Follow-up period: mean 11 years	Purpose: describe the survivorship experience in long-term survivors Method: cross-sectional, qualitative interviews, self-report questionnaires, pulmonary function Instruments: Interview questions about survivorship experience CES-D Spirometry Comparison group: none	Themes related to physical and emotional well-being: (1) appreciation for life and a changed outlook, (2) taking control and appreciation of health, (3) overcoming and rationalizing changes in physical ability, (4) changed lifestyle, (5) giving and receiving support. 31% met CES-D criteria for potential depression and those in that group had more negative views of survivorship
Myrdal et al.[35]	$N = 112$, NSCLC Age 67 Sex: 57% male Ethnicity: Swedish Health status: Preoperative pulmonary function: 33% < 60% FEV_1 Tobacco use: 70% former, 11% current smokers	Histology: ND Stage: 67% stage I, 17% stage II. Surgery: 22% pneumonectomy, 76% lobectomy Follow-up: mean 48 months, range, 4–48 months	Purpose: describe symptoms and QOL postsurgery Method: cross-sectional, mailed survey. Instruments SF-36, HADS, assessment of pulmonary symptoms Comparison group: $N = 121$ post-CABG	Bodily pain was the only SF-36 subscale similar to a normative cohort QOL scores comparable to patients who underwent CABG except for physical function, which was significantly lower Social and mental health scores similar to normative standards Dyspnea on exertion higher among those with lung cancer. 20% of patients had possible depression Compared to never and former smokers, smokers had lower mental health (SF-36) and higher ratings of depression and anxiety
De Leyn et al.[20]	$N = 77$ Age: ND Sex: ND Ethnicity: Belgian Health status: ND	Histology: bronchogenic ca Stage: Surgery: sleeve-lobectomy Follow-up: early postop recovery, 45.6% at 5 years	Purpose: to describe postop complications Instruments: medical record Comparison: none	Exercise tolerance and QOL acceptable and better than that reported for pneumonectomy Five developed an anastomotic suture and required subsequent pneumonectomy

(continued)

TABLE 108.1. **Studies documenting symptoms, functional status, and quality of life of lung cancer survivors since 1980 (in chronologic order).** (continued)

Author	Sample[a] characteristics: mean age[b], sex, ethnicity[c], education, marital status, health status	Disease characteristics/treatment/ follow-up period	Purpose/method Comparison group	Findings related to survivorship
Welcker et al.[135]	$N = 65$ ($n = 22$ with 1-year follow-up data) Age: 65 Sex: 71% male Ethnicity: German Health status: ND	Histology: NSCLC Stage: surgery for surgical intent Surgery: variety of surgical procedures ($n = 2$ pneumonectomy, $n = 36$ lobectomy) Follow-up: 1+ year postsurgery	Purpose: to examine cost and quality of life after thoracic surgery Methods: retrospective, cross-sectional, mailed survey Instruments: SF-36, cost indicators, Qualys Comparison: none	SF-36 ratings for 2-year survivors generally lower than normative scores for those with COPD and with cancer Gain of 4.62 Qualys, with higher costs associated with resection with more-advanced stages and complexity of surgery
Nomori et al.[32]	$N = 220$ VATS: 28 ALT: 28 AAT: 28 PLT: 28 Age: 61–62/group Sex: 71% male	Histology Stage: 65% stage I, 10% stage II Surgery: VATS, ALT, AAT, PLT Follow-up: pre-, 1, 2, 4, 12, 24 weeks postsurgery for PF; 1	Purpose: compare differences in functional impairment by type of surgery Methods: retrospective Instruments: PFT, 6MW Comparison:	VC in all groups increased over time PLT had the greatest impairment in VC 24 weeks after surgery and in 6MW 1 week postsurgery; better functional recovery was associated with VATS and ALT procedures
Pompeo et al.[21]	$N = 16$ Age: 65 Ethnicity: Italian Health status: All had severe and diffuse emphysema before surgery	Histology: 9 adenocarcinoma, 5 squamous, 2 large cell Stage: 11 (T1N)M0, 5, T2N0M0 Surgery: VATS ($n = 5$ LVR, $n = 3$ wedge resections, $n = 2$ segmentectomy), open thoracotomy ($n = 6$ lobectomy) Follow-up: 46 months	Purpose: describe QOL in lung cancer patients with emphysema who underwent resection plus lung volume reduction Method: prospective assessments: preop, 6 ($n = 16$), 12 ($n = 15$), 24 ($n = 13$), 36 months ($n = 9$) Instruments: SF-36, Medical Research Council Dyspnea Index, 6-minute walk test, self-report postthoracotomy pain Spirometry Control: $n = 16$ healthy adults	Patients with end-stage emphysema and stage 1 lung cancer benefited from surgical resection Significant improvement QOL domains and dyspnea at 6 months, continuing through 36 months Some differences based upon type of resection No differences between lobectomy and VATS patients Pain peaked at 6 months and continued for a small subset throughout the assessment period 68% 5-year survival Analysis includes patients with recurrence and metastasis
Sarna et al.[11]	As described above[10]	As described above[10]	Purpose: describe respiratory symptoms and PF of long-term survivors Method: cross-sectional Instruments: self-report of respiratory symptoms, spirometry, SF-36 Control: none	2/3 of survivors reported respiratory symptoms: 39% dyspnea, 31% wheezing, 28% phlegm, 25% cough; 21% reported that they stayed most of the day in bed because of symptoms % predicted FEV_1 68%; 21% % predicted <50% FEV_1 36% moderate/severe obstructive and/or restrictive ventilatory impairment Survivors exposed to secondhand smoke 3× more likely to have respiratory symptoms Respiratory symptoms related to reduced physical function, role-limits physical, vitality, social functioning, general health, and increased bodily pain

ND, no data; NS, not significant, ADL, activities of daily living; SF-36, Short form-36; PF, pulmonary function, VAS, visual analogue scale; Qualys; quality-adjusted life years; VATS; video-assisted thoracoscopic surgery; MST, muscle-sparing thoracotomy; AAT, anteroaxillary thoracotomy; ALT, anterior limited thoracotomy; PLT, posterolateral thoracotomy; 6MW, 6-minute walk; SCLC, small cell lung cancer; PCI, prophylactic cranial irradiation; CT, computed tomography; neuropsych, neuropsychometric testing; QOL, quality of life; RSC, Rotterdam Symptom Checklist; HADS, Hospital Anxiety Depression Scale.

[a] All available data reported.

[b] Mean age.

[c] In most cases denotes country of study.

requirement for partial ablation of a vital organ. The pneumonectomy has been used successfully for lung cancer treatment since the 1930s.[18] Evidence-based strategies to enhance QOL, improve symptom control, and support recovery after curative surgery for lung cancer are almost nonexistent. Although the normal healthy individual can sustain the loss of one entire lung (pneumonectomy), most patients with lung cancer have comorbid illness. Many patients have sustained cardiopulmonary damage from long-term smoking and have increased risk of mortality following pneumonectomy (or in some cases even after lobectomy or limited resection). When comparing sleeve lobectomy with pneumonectomy, a meta-analysis of published studies from 1990 to 2003, using quality-adjusted life years (QUALYS) as one of the outcomes, found that sleeve lobectomy resulted in better survival, and for patients who did not have recurrence, better QOL.[19] Other studies also support the superiority of lobectomy over pneumonectomy in terms of physical recovery.[20]

One recent advance in the treatment of early-stage lung cancer is limited resection performed by video-assisted thoracoscopic techniques (VAT) in patients with poor lung function. Patients with limited respiratory reserve are at increased risk for perioperative respiratory complications. Recent experience with the use of thoracoscopic procedures in benign lung disorders, especially emphysema, confirms that limited thoracoscopic lung resections can be performed safely in this setting, under select circumstances. Thoracoscopic pulmonary resection requires less time in hospital and reduces the duration of postoperative pain and disability. Better understanding of pulmonary function tests (PFTs) and limits of resection now allow resection of small peripheral tumors in patients with poor pulmonary function via open segmental resection, thoracoscopic wedge resection, or a combination of reduction pneumoplasty with wedge resection in carefully selected patients. The lung cancer surgery can even serve as a lung volume reduction intervention for these compromised patients. In a small study of 16 stage I non-small cell lung cancer survivors with severe emphysema who underwent a variety of surgical resections, including lung volume reduction, 68% had 5-year survival. These carefully selected patients had improved QOL (as measured by the SF-36), especially in physical functioning and reduction in dyspnea 2 years after surgery.[21]

As displayed in Table 108.1, a number of studies have identified lingering symptoms and issues faced by lung cancer survivors in the months and years after potentially curative treatment. Some prospective studies suggest a pattern of symptom resolution with full recovery 6 months after surgery, but others point to ongoing problems years later. Some studies have included comparison groups of patients with other forms of cancer or patients without cancer who underwent similar surgical procedures (e.g., thoracotomy). Although some studies have included mixed stage and histology of patients with lung cancer, the majority of studies address the issues of survivors of non-small cell lung cancer who underwent surgical resection with minimal attention to those with small cell lung cancer or those who have undergone adjuvant treatment. These posttreatment data, including both physical as well as emotional well-being, identify a range of issues faced by survivors of lung cancer and underscore the need to develop supportive care interventions. The perceptions of QOL by survivors are important, as they are linked to severity of symptom distress and have been associated with long-term survival.[22] Pneumonectomy has been more clearly associated with ongoing symptoms and reduced QOL.[23] Because of the lack of prospective data, few studies have reported patterns of symptom occurrence and resolution after curative treatment. A cross-sectional study of patterns of symptom distress studied 117 patients with lung cancer, enrolled within 100 days of diagnosis and receiving a variety of treatments. It found that those patients receiving surgery (n = 45) were noted to have decreased symptoms over a 6-month period.[24]

Available data describing the prevalence and patterns of lingering symptoms (dyspnea, pain, altered functional status/fatigue, emotional distress, cognitive difficulties, relationships, sexual dysfunction, and alterations in communication abilities) reported in long-term lung cancer survivors are described next.

Dyspnea and Pulmonary Impairment

The loss of functional lung tissue as a result of lung cancer surgery may result in transitory and permanent reductions in pulmonary function and, for some, physical disability. Pulmonary function can be affected by lung cancer and its treatment, by the consequences of the patient's past tobacco use, and by comorbid disease.[25] Changes in pulmonary function are variable and not a clear predictor of exercise capacity,[26] severity of dyspnea,[27] patients' perceptions of physical disruptions in day-to-day activities,[28] or even QOL outcomes.[10,29,30] Larsen et al.[28] note the variability of performance of lung cancer patients after resection. Based upon physiologic differences, resection of the right lung (contributing to 55% of overall lung function) might lead to more severe pulmonary consequences.[18] There are clear differences based upon the extent of resection. Bolliger et al.[31] reported reduction in PFT in the immediate postoperative period with recovery at the 6-month period for patients who underwent lobectomy. This recovery was not seen for patients who underwent pneumonectomy, similar to findings by Nezu et al.[26] Several studies support the benefit of the VATS procedure in improved functional recovery as compared to other approaches.[32]

Although dyspnea is not always a consequence of surgical treatment, the majority of studies reported ongoing problems of breathlessness in some survivors, often linked with reduction in exercise capacity.[8,21,23,26,27,29,30,33–35] Dales et al.[8] reported an increase in the prevalence of severe dyspnea in the first 3 months postthoracotomy, with reductions at 6 and 9 months, but with the continuance of severe dyspnea for 10% of the patients. Nugent et al.[36] reported long-term deficits in exercise performance in patients undergoing a pneumonectomy, with limited changes after lobectomy. The symptom dyspnea was the limiting factor in performance in exercise tests for the pneumonectomy group. Pelletier et al.[33] cited dyspnea as a factor attributing to dropout in exercise programs postthoracotomy. Zieren et al.[34] also reported continued dyspnea at exertion 1 year after surgery. However, Nugent et al.[36] reported no changes in dyspnea after surgery.

In a study comparing VATS to thoractomy, dyspnea (85% versus 75%) and cough (82% versus 75%) were continuing problems more than a year after surgery for both groups. Aging, tobacco use and comorbid conditions, in particular, may influence respiratory symptoms and level of pulmonary function. Uchitomi et al.[37] report the significant relationship of dyspnea to emotional distress in the postoperative period. This relationship was also reported by Sarna et al.[10] However, there is little research specifically looking at these issues in a systematic way. In addition to dyspnea, respiratory symptoms such as cough, phlegm, and wheezing continue to plague some long-term survivors and diminish QOL.[11]

Pain

In a recent review,[38] Rogers et al. reported on the incidence of chronic mild to moderate postthoracotomy pain, which was described as "under-rated" and affecting approximately 50% of patients. Chronic postthoracotomy pain along the incision line often has neuropathic features. It is less often associated with initial lung cancer surgery, but has been linked with tumor recurrence.[38] The etiology of long-term pain is not well established but may be caused by intercostal nerve damage. Several of the studies reviewed (see Table 108.1) describe persistent pain for some long-term survivors.[9,10,21,23,29,34,35,39–42] Not all studies are limited to patients with lung cancer; some included others who received a thoracotomy. Reports of lingering pain vary. Schag et al.[9] reported that 46% of survivors experience pain from scars postsurgery and 24% report aches and pains. In a study of 85 patients, 26 had moderate to severe pain 1 month after surgery. Gotoda and colleagues[43] reported that female gender and pain immediately postthoracotomy were predictive of pain 1 month and 1 year after surgery. Handy et al.[29] reported continued pain 6 months after surgery. Similarly, Pompeo et al.[21] and Zieren et al.[34] reported continued pain for some patients even 1 year after surgery. Pompeo et al.[21] also identified a subset of patients who continued to have lingering pain. However, Mangione et al.[42] and Myrdal et al.[35] reported that pain scores after surgery were similar to population norms 1 to 2 years after surgery.

Although the prevalence of chronic pain may be expected to differ by surgical procedure, especially with the emergence of the muscle- and nerve-sparing VATS procedure, reports do not consistently support significant differences. Landreneau et al.[39] reported less pain and shoulder dysfunction, but not a difference in use of pain medication.[44] Pain was reported by 71% of the thoracotomy group and 67% of the VATS group. Comparing the VATS with thoracotomy, specific type of pain included thoracotomy pain (74% versus 75%), chest pain (48% versus 29%), and arm or shoulder pain (59% versus 46%). One-third of both groups (33%) reported shoulder dysfunction. Neither Pompeo et al.[21] or Li et al.[44] report significant differences in pain when comparing lobectomy and VATS procedures. However, another study did support a beneficial difference.[41] Treatment strategies of postthoracotomy pain vary,[45] and reports for definitive treatment from clinical trials are not available.

Another painful and disabling condition is frozen shoulder, a potential postsurgical risk[46] affecting lung cancer survivors. However, there are no known studies describing the prevalence of this condition among survivors of lung cancer.

Altered Functional Status/Fatigue

Level of postoperative physical disability is an important consideration in examining the QOL of survivors. Although it is often related to dyspnea, decreased functional status may have other contributing factors as well, and the measurement is different. In fact, in surveying the views of a patient population at risk for lung cancer surgery ($n = 64$), many stated they would not undergo life-saving surgery if it resulted in permanent physical disability.[47] Early studies considering recovery from lung cancer surgery focused almost exclusively on pulmonary and cardiovascular function, exercise capacity, and predictors of those at risk for severe disability. Mangione et al.[42] note recovery of physical function after thoracotomy at 12 months, but never to preoperative levels. Compared to other surgical groups (hip replacement, repair of aortic aneurysm), survivors of lung cancer had lower physical function. In a small prospective study of recovery after lobectomy, Miyazawa et al.[27] reported that recovery to preoperative levels occurred approximately 1 year after surgery for most, but not all, patients. Improvement in exercise capacity also was noted by Nezu et al.,[26] but not for those who underwent pneumonectomy.

Many of these studies are limited in that a preoperative assessment was lacking and time since surgery in the postoperative assessment varied. Additionally, multiple factors, including comorbid conditions (e.g., emphysema) and impairments (e.g., arthritis), were not considered as contributors to physical function after surgery. When exercise performance is limited, deconditioning (often described as leg cramps) as well as dyspnea are factors.[33] In an older population of lung cancer survivors, comparison of physical function with other patient populations or normative standards is useful. In the 5-year survival group,[10] QOL scores for physical components showed a somewhat poorer status compared to norms of patients with cancer, older adults, and those with other chronic lung disease.

In addition to functional decline, fatigue has been identified as a troublesome symptom. It is unclear if these are associated with aging or comorbidity because few studies have comparison groups. In the study by Li and colleagues,[44] fatigue was the most commonly reported symptom more than 1 year postsurgery for patients who underwent a VATS (74%) or thoracotomy (92%), as was the case with long-term survivors of small cell lung cancer.[48] Fatigue also may accompany other symptoms. In a cross-sectional study assessing symptom distress in women with primary or recurrent lung cancer within the past 5 years, Sarna[49] found that when fatigue was present, 41% experienced frequent pain, 31% insomnia, 23% breathing difficulties, and 21% cough. No studies have reported fatigue after lung cancer surgery with adjuvant chemotherapy.

There appears to be a subset of survivors that reports reduction in energy and increased fatigue. In a cross-sectional study of 130 older patients with lung cancer 3 months after diagnosis (including 34 treated with surgery), risk for impaired physical functioning was strongly linked to preexisting physical impairment and symptom distress.[50] In Schag et al.'s study of lung cancer survivors,[9] almost all the shorter-term survivors reported significant decreases in their energy (84%). Fatigue also was the most common symptom reported by Sarna et al.[10] With the lack of age-matched comparison groups, it is difficult to tell how dissimilar these reports are from the population of older adults without cancer and with/or without other chronic illnesses. Schag reported on this issue comparing cancer patients to health controls using the same instrument. She notes that 84% of survivors had problems with functional health status compared to 22% of healthy controls in a previous study.[51]

Emotional Distress

Presenting evidence on the psychosocial issues and concerns of survivors of lung cancer is both a simple and complicated task. It is simple because there is a paucity of information and it is complicated by the absence of data and the clear definitions of survivor. It is important to note that positive as well as negative consequences may result from the experience of lung cancer.[52] In the qualitative study,[12] survivors described existential changes prompting them to "seeing life as a gift," "appreciating the little things in life," and "trying to live life to its fullest." However, some reflect that life after lung cancer is not a normal life, and there were multiple statements related to uncertainty. A review of available data provides support for the hypothesis that a subset of survivors experience ongoing psychologic distress such as anxiety and depression. Handy et al.[29] reported impaired mental health 6 months posttreatment, but Mangione et al.[42] noted improvement in mental health over time. Different measures were used to measure depression in the studies reviewed, and it is difficult to know whether the responses reflect a diagnosable depression (major or minor) or reflect a state of depressed feelings. Interestingly, in contrast to differences in physical function, pneumonectomy was not necessarily associated with greater emotional or social dysfunction.[34]

Depression

It may seem surprising to find reports of depression among the "fortunate few" who do survive lung cancer. The findings of disease-free survivors are surprisingly consistent with other studies that have looked at the global population of lung cancer patients which includes all stages of disease. Depression and emotional distress have been reported as higher among people with lung cancer than people with other cancers.[53] It is estimated that the incidence of depression in patients with lung cancer of all stages ranges from 15% to 44%.[7,14,54–57] Depressed mood in patients with cancer has been linked to increased reporting of symptoms.[8,57] In a study of 95 patients with newly diagnosed lung cancer of all stages, depression was linked to poorer prognosis.[58]

Interestingly, in a prospective study of survival and positive attitude (optimism) before a randomized clinical trial of chemotherapy and radiation therapy for unresectable non-small cell lung cancer,[59] mood did not influence or correlate with overall survival. According to Uchitomi's findings, depression did decrease over the year after surgery.[14,37,60] However Sarna et al.[10] reported that one of five long-term survivors required further workup for depression because of high CES-D scores and this score was also a major predictor of ratings of QOL. These reports underscore the importance of screening for depression as part of follow-up care. Depression is treatable, but it is unknown how many lung cancer survivors have this clinical diagnosis and are treated.

Anxiety and Fears of Recurrence

Many patients who survive a first lung cancer develop a second cancer, either a second primary lung cancer or a local recurrence. Additionally, patients with prior lung cancer are at high risk of development of second tobacco-caused cancers other than lung cancer. A few prospective studies[34] have noted significantly lower QOL scores for survivors who experienced recurrence compared to scores of those who remained disease free. The threat of recurrence is not unique to lung cancer survivors, and this fear has been noted in studies of disease-free survivors. In Schag et al.'s study,[9] 63% of lung cancer survivors reported anxiety, and 58% had worries about a cancer recurrence. Sarna et al.[10] reported 30% with anxiety, with 12% of survivors fearful of a second cancer, 11% fearful of a recurrence, and 11% fearful of metastatic disease.

Ongoing and quality communication with the healthcare team is essential throughout to course of treatment and during recovery. Because lung cancer has been so frequently fatal for patients, communications around survivorship issues and QOL may seem less important than for other patients with a better prognosis. However, it is important to recognize that there are phases of treatment, and it may be important to identify fears and issues facing survivors that lead to education, information, and interventions. For example, discussions about the potential consequences of curative treatment do not have to be limited to informing patients of potential risks.[61,62] It also can be an opportunity to prepare patients for survivorship. Resources available for rehabilitative support, including psychologic support, can be included in the plan for care.

Cognitive Difficulties

A meta-analysis of seven clinical trials demonstrated that prophylactic cranial irradiation (PCI) increased disease-free survival and decreased risk of brain metastasis for patients with small cell lung cancer.[63] Since the 1980s neurologic toxicity has emerged as a concern for some long-term survivors.[64] These problems include a range of abnormalities including problems with memory, concentration, parasthesias, and gait.[48,65–67] However, the etiology of cognitive impairment is not clear, with suggestions of abnormalities present before treatment.[17,67] Comprehensive information about the impact of cognitive impairment on QOL is needed in this population.

Cognitive problems also have been reported in survivors of non-small cell lung cancer. In Schag's study[9] (including patients with both small cell and non-small cell lung cancer), the majority (63%) of the short-term survivors noted that they had difficulty remembering things. Diminished ability to think clearly was associated with a diminished interest or pleasure in a recent study evaluating somatic symptoms of patients with lung cancer with major depression.[68] Sorting out cognitive difficulties from the effects of depression is an ongoing issue in cancer research but may be particularly relevant for this population.

Relationships

There are limited data describing the impact of lung cancer on marital and other relationships. In many studies information about marital status or living situations is unknown. Difficulties with relationships with families and friends were uncovered both by Schag et al.[9] and Sarna et al.,[10] but it is hard to determine if social support changed and whether there is an ongoing impact. This is clearly an area that could use additional investigation. Additionally, information about the impact of lung cancer on employment is limited.

Sexual Dysfunction

Disruptions in sexual function may be an issue for survivors of lung cancer as a result of diminished physical functional status, but data are practically nonexistent. Schag's study[9] reported on a range of activities related to intimacy among married and single individuals. In a study of 69 women with lung cancer,[69] including 38% treated with curative intent, sexual disruptions were reported by more than 20% of the sample.

Communication Ability

Complications of surgical treatment of lung cancer also could include vocal cord paralysis, although data about the prevalence of this condition among long-term survivors are lacking. Recurrent laryngeal nerve damage resulting from pneumonectomy, mediastinoscopy, or tumor invasion can result in laryngeal paralysis or paresis, causing hoarseness and soft whispery voice. This problem can have a profound impact on communication and ultimately QOL. In a rare study of 28 patients with vocal cord paralysis from cancer or its treatment (including 25% with lung cancer), QOL improved after thryoplasty.[70] Cancer patients had QOL and voice improvement similar to that of patients who received treatment for benign conditions. Improvements in QOL included physical function aspects that could be negatively affected by glottic incompetency.

Economic Impact

A few studies reviewed noted employment status and the impact of the disease on work situation, although many patients were retired at the time of diagnosis.[9,10] In some studies, return to work was viewed as a proxy for QOL among long-term survivors.[71,72] The impact of altered physical functional capacity after curative treatment and the long-term economic consequences on these survivors are unknown.

Support and Psychosocial Intervention

There is limited evidence as to the impact of community resources on the recovery and adaptation of lung cancer survivors. Community-based and philanthropic organizations have historically provided cancer patients and their families with essential services that have been unavailable from traditional medical sources, and reliance on these organizations is growing. A recent study[73] evaluated the resources that are available nationwide to provide support for patients with cancer and their family members, how these resources are used, and whom they serve. The primary mission of the organizations that participated in the study (32 of the 41 identified) was information/referral centered. Of the 31 organizations reviewed, not 1 was devoted to patients with lung cancer, although two-thirds were specifically dedicated to patients with cancers other than lung. Problems identified for the one database of patients indicated that there is a strong need for assistance with personal adjustment to illness, financial concerns, home care, and transportation. The study also noted that the patients that are at the highest risk for developing cancer and dying of it are the least likely to utilize formal support networks. In addition, there were gaps noted in service provision. As medical environments provide less assistance for psychosocial needs, it will become incumbent upon these communities to provide assistance for patients, especially for those with lung cancer.

The Ted Mann Family Resource Center at UCLA's Jonsson Comprehensive Cancer Center has developed an approach to helping patients cope with the diagnosis of lung cancer at all phases of the disease. Funded by the surviving spouse of a patient who died of lung cancer, the Ann and John Nickoll Lung Cancer Support Program has established a variety of services for patients and family members. Patients and family members receive individual contact and psychosocial evaluation by a psychologist or social worker. Patients are offered a variety of services, including informational booklets with a library of resources, a support group for patients with lung cancer and their family members, lectures by healthcare professionals on the topic of lung cancer, individual and group programs to teach relaxation exercises and cognitive coping skills, and assistance with access to reliable web sites. Patients who are depressed receive individual counseling and are referred to psychiatry for medication evaluation if they are amenable to this type of intervention. Patients have welcomed this program of support. Some of the patients have commented, "Now we have what the breast cancer patients have," the standard by which all cancers are currently measured. The greatest difficulty that patients with lung cancer face, however, is the fact that so many cancers are found at a late stage, and patients must not only deal with the diagnosis of cancer but may have to grapple with declining function and the loss of their life in a relatively short period of time after the diagnosis. Although as yet untested, this resource may provide a model for comprehensive support for people living with lung cancer.

There is a small, but growing, network of patients and families who are participating in advocacy efforts that are primarily Internet based, as displayed in Table 108.2. Each of these organizations provides information about disease and treatment, organizes political advocacy efforts, and has a mission oriented toward better care and research for patients with lung cancer and links to other resources. These resources offer tips and suggest areas of need and intervention for survivors of lung cancer.

Although research on psychosocial interventions for a variety of types of cancer patients is not reviewed here, there is an extensive literature documenting the efficacy of a variety of interventions in diverse patient populations. These interventions are oriented toward improving the quality of life of patients with cancer through education, individual support, and groups. A recent meta-analysis of 37 published controlled studies that investigated the effectiveness of psychosocial interventions on QOL in adult cancer patients found that psychosocial interventions with durations of more

TABLE 108.2. Resources for lung cancer survivors.

Organization	*Web site*	*Purpose/mission*
Alliance for Lung Cancer Advocacy, Support, and Education	www.alcase.org	National not-for-profit organization dedicated solely to helping people with lung cancer, and those who are at risk for the disease, to improve quality of life through advocacy, support, and education
American Cancer Society	www.cancer.org	Nonprofit provides general cancer educational and support services, including a Lung Cancer Resource Center that describes lung cancer, its risk factors, prevention, causes, detection, symptoms, diagnosis, staging, and treatment
American Society of Clinical Oncology	www.asco.org; www.plwc.org	Site run by the American Society of Clinical Oncology; provides up-to-date scientific information about lung cancer treatment, including links to many patient-focused resources
Cancer Care	www.lungcancer.org	Informational website sponsored CancerCare
Lung Cancer Online Foundation	www.lungcanceronline.org	Focus on improving the quality of care and quality of life for people with lung cancer by funding lung cancer research and providing information to patients and families; provides a comprehensive, annotated directory to Internet information and resources for patients and families
Lung Cancer Survivors for Change	www.lchelp.com/mambo	An organization composed of ordinary people who have survived lung cancer as well as family members of people living with lung cancer
National Coalition of Lung Cancer Survivors (NCCS)	www.canceradvocacy.org	Survivor-led advocacy organization working exclusively on behalf of this country's more than 9 million cancer survivors and the millions more touched by this disease; founded in 1986, NCCS continues to lead the cancer survivorship movement
Roy Castle Foundation	www.roycastle.org	Provides patient support and information network throughout Great Britain; every lung cancer patient and their family will have access to a comprehensive support, information, and advocacy service for all issues concerning lung cancer
Ted Mann Family Resource Center, UCLA Jonsson Comprehensive Cancer Center	www.CancerResources.mednet.ucla.edu	Provides education through streaming video as well as articles on all phases of the disease, including survivorship, and caregiver-oriented materials
Women Against Lung Cancer	www.4walc.org	Special focus on women with lung cancer, educates the public and health care professionals about women and lung cancer; provides a web listing of many lung cancer resources

than 12 weeks were more effective than interventions of shorter duration.[74]

Health Behaviors

Little is known about the health behaviors (tobacco use, alcohol use, nutrition/weight) and changes that may occur in response to the diagnosis or the perceived health status of lung cancer survivors. In an analysis of these factors, Evangelista et al.[13] reported that 70% of 5-year survivors reported their health to be good to excellent. Continued smoking, exposure to second-hand smoke, current alcohol use, and being overweight (body mass index of 25 or more) were significant predictors of poor health perceptions.

Tobacco Use and Cessation

Assessment of current and former smoking of lung cancer survivors is relevant because of the potential impact on recurrence, second primaries,[75–80] and comorbid conditions. Smoking cessation can slow the decline in pulmonary function, and if smokers quit before extensive pulmonary damage, they may never develop clinically significant chronic obstructive pulmonary disease (COPD).[81] Approximately 90% of lung cancer cases are attributed to lifetime smoking.[82,83] Smoking continues to be the leading cause of preventable death in the United States,[84] and tobacco control is a priority for the American Society of Clinical Oncology.[85]

Rarely included in analysis of clinical trial data on survivorship are data about tobacco use. Amount of smoking (30 or more pack-years) has been shown to be an independent prognostic factor in a study of 375 patients who underwent complete surgical resection for stage I non-small cell lung cancer from 1981 to 1993.[86] Smoking is receiving special attention during clinical trials investigating efficacy of lung cancer screening.[87] At the time of surgery for lung cancer, many smokers may quit. However, some are unable to do so,[78,88–94] and others restart smoking during recovery. In Dresler et al.'s report,[93] 23% of patients who quit within the 2 weeks before surgery relapsed, and 61% who did not quit before surgery continued to smoke. She reports that 89% of smokers acknowledged receiving physician advice to stop smoking. Patients at highest risk for return to smoking were those with the briefest quit time before surgery. In a study of long-term survivors,[13] 13% continued to smoke after curative surgery. There have been several attempts to provide targeted smoking cessation interventions for survivors of cancer, including lung cancer.[79,95,96] However, it is important to note that former smokers continue to be at lifelong increased risk for lung cancer.[78,97] Minimal attention has been given to the risks of exposure to second-hand smoke, also a risk factor for lung cancer. This exposure was reported among 28% of disease-free survivors.[13]

Patients with lung cancer, including long-term survivors, may receive more attributions of blame and responsibility for their disease because of their smoking behavior. Clinically, patients have noted that they feel a judgment that comes from others (healthcare providers, family members, and friends) that they are responsible for their disease if they smoked. Additionally, patients who never smoked or who quit long before their diagnosis may feel unfairly judged. In a qualitative study of 45 patients with lung cancer, patients reported feeling stigmatized because of their smoking. Regardless of current smoking status, patients believed that that past or current smoking affected their quality of care, and for this reason, some concealed their diagnosis.[98] The individual smoker is blamed for his or her illness; even though he or she may have become addicted as a youth, little blame is aimed at the tobacco industry that misled the public about health risks. Only a few studies have explored causal attributions that might affect a patient's response to the diagnosis of lung cancer, especially in the case of a smoking history. There are data to suggest that medical staff's attitudes toward patients may be influenced by these factors as well.[99] In a study that looked at lung cancer patients' own attributions for the cause of their illness, it was found that while smoking cigarettes was the most frequently suggested causal factor, patients also tried to minimize the impact.[100] Eighty-one percent of patients put forward at least one statement that served to qualify or argue the relevance of smoking as the cause. For example, 41% of the patients indicated that "they didn't really know where the disease came from," others argued "they had always led a normal/healthy life, that non-smokers also got lung cancer, that there must be other causes for lung cancer, and that they had always been healthy." Patients are able to reduce their sense of guilt by diluting the cause of the disease; this allows the person to feel some responsibility without shouldering the full sense of blame. Despite the potential causes and responsibilities, there is a need to understand more about these processes and their impact on coping; however, understanding what patients must cope with is a significant concern.

Alcohol Use and Substance Abuse

Although tobacco use is associated with increased risk of alcohol use, few studies have reported on alcohol use or substance abuse among people with cancer, including lung cancer survivors. Among 5-year survivors,[13] 58% were reported to have had a drink in the previous month, with 3% reporting more than 8 drinks in one sitting. As described previously, alcohol use among survivors was associated with poorer perceptions of health.

Nutrition and Weight

There are limited data about weight, nutritional intake, and physical activity that can be used to recommend lifestyle changes for lung cancer survivors. Evangelista et al.[13] reported that 51% of survivors were overweight, including 23% with a body mass index of 30 or more. Recently, a panel of experts convened by the American Cancer Society reviewed the available scientific evidence regarding the benefit of nutritional and activity interventions to decrease recurrence, improve overall survival, and increase QOL. They concluded (with an indication of the strength of the evidence as "probable" or "possible" benefit) that lung cancer survivors should strive for a healthy weight during treatment and recovery, and increase fruit, vegetable, and omega 3 fatty acids uptake (especially in the face of weight loss).[101] Additionally, increased activity after treatment was recommended to increase overall survival and QOL. There was insufficient evidence for recommendations regarding total fat intake or intake of fiber or soy. The negative impact of tobacco use on decreasing nutrition was noted. Limited information is available about nutritional supplements and the lung cancer survivor, although two previous trials of beta-carotene pills demonstrated an increased risk of lung cancer in smokers.[102,103] A current clinical trial is investigating the potential benefit of selenium supplements in reducing risk of lung cancer recurrence.[104]

Factors Associated with Increased Problems

Although prognostic variables associated with survival have been well studied, factors associated with increased morbidity and diminished QOL among disease-free survivors have received limited attention. Age, sex, race/ethnicity, socioeconomic status, and comorbidity have been suggested to contribute to differences.

Age

Older age at diagnosis may influence recovery needs as well as occurrence of long-term sequelae. With the growing number of older Americans, many of whom have had a lifetime of tobacco use and exposure, lung cancer incidence among the elderly can be expected to climb along with the burden of other tobacco-related comorbidities.[84] In a study of patients with limited small cell lung cancer, older patients were more likely to have poorer performance status, more likely to experience poorer survival, and less likely to receive the full extent of optimal treatment.[105] However, older age and comorbidity were not directly related to survival. In Sarna's study,[10] older age was associated with poorer physical function. In a study of physical functioning among older cancer patients, patients who were 3 to 6 weeks post lung cancer surgery ($n = 32$) had significantly lower physical function and more limitations than older patients who had undergone surgery for breast, colon, or prostate surgery.[106] In a cross-sectional study of 133 older patients with lung cancer (over 65 years of age) with various stages of disease and treatment ($n = 26$, including 11 with adjuvant treatment), prior physical function, symptom severity, and older age were predictors of diminished physical functioning.[107]

Sex Differences

As reviewed by Patel et al.,[108] there are important sex differences in lung cancer that may affect survivorship, including the generally female advantage for long-term survival, and differential response to treatment. However, women may be at increased susceptibility to the carcinogens of tobacco[109] and are more likely to be diagnosed with adenocarcinoma.[108,110] Additionally, younger female nonsmokers appear to be at increased risk for lung cancer.[111] However, sex differences in physical and psychologic dimensions of QOL are less clear among long-term survivors. None of the studies reviewed supported sex differences in pulmonary function of exercise capacity, although many had only a small subset of women. Sarna et al.[10] reported that women survivors were more likely to live alone and had significantly higher ratings in the existential/spiritual domain of QOL as compared to men. In the study by Uchitomi et al.,[60] findings indicate that female patients, but not male patients, did benefit from physicians' social support.

Race/Ethnicity and Socioeconomic Status

Lung cancer incidence varies by race/ethnicity and social status, and these differences have been attributed to differences in lung cancer survivorship.[112] Over 45 million Americans continue to smoke. The gap between smoking among the higher and lower socioeconomic classes is widening, with 32.9% of those below the poverty line smoking as compared to 22.2% at or above the poverty level.[113] Lung cancer is fast becoming a cancer of the impoverished, poorly educated, and ethnic minorities,[114,115] but it is not clear how these factors influence survivorship. Tobacco use has been suggested as a cause of the large differential in male black cancer deaths over the past several decades.[116] African-Americans are less likely to be diagnosed with localized disease as compared to whites (14% versus 16%), and there has been minimal change in survivorship over time (1974–1976, 11%; 1983–1985, 11%; 1992–1999, 12%).[2] A variety of factors have been suggested to account for this disturbing difference, including differences in access to care. Using Surveillance, Epidemiology, and End Results (SEER) data between 1985 and 1993 for black (n = 860) and white (n = 10,124) patients with resectable non-small cell lung cancer, 12.7% fewer black patients in comparison with white patients received potentially curative resection.[117] This unequal treatment resulted in racial differences in survival, as has been reported by others.[118]

Long-term survivors of lung cancer are more likely to come from higher socioeconomic groups.[112] Socioeconomic status has been related to stage at diagnosis and, thus, survivorship.[118,119] Using SEER data for all races from 1995–1999, for those below the poverty rate, 25.3% and 59% of lung cancer patients were diagnosed with regional and distant disease, respectively. Additionally, in a prospective cross-sectional study of 129 newly diagnosed patients with non-small cell lung cancer (including 6 who received surgery), those with lower socioeconomic status, regardless of clinical status, had more health problems and poorer quality of life than those who were affluent.[120]

Comorbidity

In evaluating the QOL and health status of survivors, the presence of comorbid conditions, especially those associated with tobacco-related illnesses, may more directly affect QOL ratings than the cancer or its treatment. However, there has been limited investigation in this area. Few studies reviewed have adequately documented comorbid conditions among patients who have undergone surgery for lung cancer.[121] In a survey (including preoperative patient history) of 2,189 patients who underwent surgery for lung cancer in Spain, 73% reported at least one comorbid condition, including 50% COPD, 16.5% hypertension, 13.5% heart disease, 10% peripheral vascular disease, and 9% diabetes. Comorbidity was higher in older age groups, but smoking status was not reported. These findings of comorbidity were similar to findings of Sarna et al.[10] among 142 disease-free survivors, in which 70% reported one or more conditions: 28.9% heart disease, 17.6% COPD, 16.9% peptic ulcer disease, 13.4% diabetes, and 16% with reports of other cancers. Fewer comorbid conditions were significantly related to higher physical QOL scores, especially for survivors with known heart disease, and contributed to the statistical model for overall QOL. Schag et al.[9] found similar results: 32% cardiovascular disease, 41% hypertension, 11% diabetes, and 28% other illnesses; however, a comorbidity index was not predictive of QOL for the lung cancer survivors. The Karnofsky performance status was significant, which may be in part a surrogate for the combined effect of comorbid illnesses.

Long-term tobacco use can complicate recovery from lung cancer and its treatment[122] and increase the potential for other and tobacco-related comorbid conditions. Because smoking is a major risk for cardiovascular disease and increases the risk of disease in the presence of other risk factors (e.g., untreated hypertension),[123] the assessment of the impact of tobacco-related comorbidity is essential to survivorship concerns. Additionally, chronic obstructive pulmonary disease (COPD), now the fourth leading cause of death in the United States, continues to increase, especially among women.[123] Similar to lung cancer, more than 90% of cases of COPD are due to smoking; 15% of smokers develop significant COPD.[81] Additionally, COPD has been postulated as a risk factor for lung cancer.[124] Lung function declines more rapidly in smokers as compared to nonsmokers and is associated with progressive disability.[125] Twenty-five percent of patients with small cell lung cancer were noted to have COPD at diagnosis, and 15% had heart disease; however, the prevalence among the 60 long-term survivors is not reported.[72] In a cross-sectional study of 129 older patients with lung cancer at various stages of disease, an average of 3.1 comorbid conditions was reported.[107]

Limits to Current Studies of Lung Cancer Survivors

There are numerous limitations to the current studies describing issues facing lung cancer survivors. A variety of instruments have been used, limiting comparisons across studies. Several have used standardized instruments such as the Center for Epidemiology Status-Depression (CES-D) to assess depression that allow score comparison with normal populations. Other studies have allowed comparison of scores across cancer survivors. Comparing survivors of lung cancer to other populations of survivors of cancer and to populations without major illness is essential in evaluating generalizability of research among survivors. However, further qualitative studies also are needed that provide details about the survivors' lives, identifying positive and negative outcomes.

To determine if these findings are different from or similar to those in others with chronic illness or others with cancer, comparison groups are important. This differences are beyond the extent of surgery alone, as long-term survivors were noted to have higher preoperative QOL, when compared to those who suffered recurrence.[71] A health utility score, a global indicator of health reflecting QOL, allows for comparisons across studies. This strategy was used in a study using population-based cross-sectional data from the National Health Interview Survey (1998 cohort) of 692 long-term survivors recovering from surgical cancer treatment: breast (n = 377), colon (n = 169), melanoma (n = 92), and lung cancer (n = 54, 50% females). In the acute less than 1-year time period, the scores for the lung cancer survivors (0.42, with 1.0 indicating perfect health), were significantly lower than for the other survivor groups.[126] However, the scores in the longer term cohort (more than 5 years) increased by 47% to 0.62. The presence of pain and angina contributed to poorer scores in long-term survivors. In Schag's study,[9] there was a greater frequency of psychologic distress in patients with lung cancer than the survivors of colon and prostate cancer.

Recommendations to Support Recovery of Lung Cancer Survivors

Based on the available evidence, several interventions are essential to decrease morbidity and promote QOL among lung cancer survivors. As a diagnosis of any life-threatening illness such as lung cancer offers clinicians a "teachable moment", recovery can be the impetus for important life changes and behavioral interventions. (1) All lung cancer survivors who smoke must be offered/referred to support and resources to promote tobacco cessation. (2) Because a significant number of survivors experience serious emotional distress in the face of curative treatment, vigilant attention is needed in the ongoing assessment to detect psychosocial problems and to ensure referral for subsequent treatment of those with clinical symptomatology. (3) There should be ongoing assessment and treatment of postthoracotomy pain. (4) Physical rehabilitation must be promoted, especially among those with evidence of disability before curative treatment. (5) Interventions to provide interventions to support relief of dyspnea should be offered to those with this symptom. (6) Changes in lifestyle including healthy diet and activity to promote QOL and reduce disability should be supported. (7) There should be identification of and intervention with high-risk patients with known risk factors for morbidity after curative treatment.

A comprehensive wellness approach to survivorship requires that clinicians challenge existing nihilistic views of the curability of lung cancer in general, including negative attitudes toward investing in efforts to support QOL regardless of the length of survival. Many of these interventions may be synergistic, such as the decrease in depression associated with exercise. Additionally, those with stable disease may live for many years with lung cancer. Although they may not be "disease free," they should not be neglected in the efforts to improve coping and living with uncertainty while reducing physical and emotional distress.

Future Research

The excellent survival of individuals treated with adequate surgical resection in stage 1 non-small cell lung cancer suggests that increasing survivorship is linked with early detection. Henschke and her colleagues at Cornell University conducted a prospective single-arm trial of low-dose noncontrast spiral computerized tomography (CT) in high-risk patients and demonstrated that CT is three times as sensitive in the detection of small pulmonary nodules as chest roentgenogram and that 80% of lung cancer is detected by this methodology in stage IA.[127]

The National Lung Screening Trial is underway to evaluate current and former smokers aged 55 to 74 at risk for cancer.[128] Findings from standard chest X-rays will be compared with spiral computed tomography (CT) scans to see if early detection of small potentially curable lesions will result in reduced deaths from lung cancer. Thus, an increased number of disease-free survivors might be anticipated, making information about the issues associated with survivorship all the more important. Regardless of efforts to prevent tobacco use and to support cessation, former smokers will continue at higher risk. Hundreds of thousands of Americans will be at risk for lung cancer in the next decades. It is also important to acknowledge the lack of information about long-term survivors with advanced-stage disease. For example, in a few selected cases of patients with isolated brain metastasis, long term survival (more than 10 years) occurred after surgical removal of tumor.[129]

Much more evidence is needed to provide a clear understanding and support for interventions to prevent or reduce physical and psychosocial sequelae of lung cancer and its treatment.[130] Further research is needed to monitor the course of symptoms post treatment and to evaluate strategies for reducing overall symptom burden and improving QOL. The studies reviewed are limited primarily because of small sample size and the cross-sectional nature of the design. There are almost no prospective studies documenting the course of survivors who have received adjuvant treatment. Although Schumacher et al. reported that preoperative chemoradiation did not significantly reduce QOL in 54 patients in the immediate posttreatment time frame, data for long-term survivors were not available.[131] There is almost no information available about the issues of survivors of small cell lung cancer. Although smoking cessation is included in recommendations for follow-up and surveillance,[132] it is clear from this review of the literature that there is strong evidence to support monitoring physical and emotional well-being after treatment as well.

There are minimal reports of efforts to promote wellness after curative treatment or to examine the efficacy of rehabilitation programs for lung cancer survivors. Future research needs to address the wide range of problems with an eye toward developing a body of literature in which one study can be compared with another. Further research is needed to evaluate available instruments and determine how to get the most information, to provide opportunities for comparison and generalizations across studies, and to not overburden respondents. The work to date represents a start in the understanding of the needs of lung cancer survivors, but it raises more questions than it answers. Some have expressed concerns that if the perception of the physician is that surgery would result in substantial reduction in QOL, curative treatment would not be offered, regardless of the patient's view.[133] There are subsets of patients who have significant difficulties in a range of areas. More research is needed in nonwhite samples, from a variety of socioeconomic strata, and the inclusion of family members will provide a more complete view of the impact and needs of survivors.

Intervention studies such as targeting depressed patients might involve both psychologic interventions oriented toward cognitive coping as well as medication trials. The role of multidisciplinary care teams involved in the coaching, support, and physical reconditioning posttreatment need to be explored. The interaction between beliefs and behaviors on the part of the medical team with the patients' belief systems may lead to ways to create greater support and interaction. Additionally, the involvement of survivor participants in the development and monitoring of this research would be useful.

Limiting research for survivors of lung cancer to the disease-free period after 5 years is far too narrow. There is limited knowledge about the period after treatment is completed and before recurrence or second primaries. Newer therapies for advanced non-small cell lung cancer have resulted in improved QOL and symptom relief.[134] These needs and issues faced by these survivors with stable disease also need attention.

The evidence base for frequency and type of screening test is important. This information is important in exploring the need for rehabilitation and support. According to findings from available research, lung cancer survivors are diverse, with different profiles of comorbidity, and different vulnerabilities and needs for rehabilitation. Future studies are needed to explore the need to test tailored assessments and interventions so that those at highest risk are appropriately treated to prevent unnecessary short- and long-term morbidity. Because of the relatively small number of lung cancer survivors, the development of a database through a clinical trial mechanism would be useful. Additionally, the quality and the impact of the explosion of web-based sources for cancer survivors, including lung cancer survivors, on QOL has not been evaluated.

References

1. Centers for Disease Control. Ten great public health achievements—United States, 1900–1999. MMWR (Morb Mortal Wkly Rep) 1999;48:241–243.
2. Jemal A, Murray T, Samuels A, et al. Cancer statistics, 2003. CA Cancer J Clin 2004;54:8–29.
3. Jemal A, Clegg LX, Ward E, et al. Annual report to the nation on the status of cancer, 1975–2001, with a special feature regarding survival. Cancer (Phila) 2004;101:3–27.
4. Carlens EDG, Nou E. Comparative measurements of quality of survival of lung cancer patients after diagnosis. Scand J Respir Dis 1970;51:268–275.
5. Carlens EDG, Nou E. An attempt to include "quality of life" in evaluation of survival in bronchial cancer therapy. Bronches 1971;21:215–219.
6. Sarna L, Reidinger MS. Assessment of quality of life and symptom improvement in lung cancer clinical trials. Semin Oncol 2004;31(suppl 9):1–10.
7. Montazeri A, Gillis CR, McEwen J. Quality of life in patients with lung cancer: a review of literature from 1970 to 1995. Chest 1998;113:467–481.
8. Dales RE, Belanger R, Shamiji FM, et al. Quality of life following thoracotomy for lung cancer. J Clin Epidemiol 1994;47: 1443–1449.
9. Schag CAC, Ganz PA, Wing DS, et al. Quality of life in adult survivors of lung, colon and prostate cancer. Qual Life Res 1994;3:127–141.
10. Sarna L, Padilla G, Holmes C, et al. Quality of life of long-term survivors of non-small cell lung cancer. J Clin Oncol 2002;20: 2920–2929.
11. Sarna L, Evangelista L, Tashkin D, et al. Impact of respiratory symptoms and pulmonary function on quality of life of long-term survivors of non-small cell lung cancer. Chest 2004;125: 439–445.
12. Maliski SL, Sarna L, Evangelista L, et al. The aftermath of lung cancer: balancing the good and bad. Cancer Nurs 2003;26: 237–244.
13. Evangelista LS, Sarna L, Brecht ML, et al. Health perceptions and risk behaviors of lung cancer survivors. Heart Lung 2003;32: 131–139.
14. Uchitomi Y, Mikami I, Kugaya A, et al. Depression after successful treatment for nonsmall cell lung carcinoma. A 3-month follow-up study. Cancer (Phila) 2000;89:1172–1179.
15. Motohiro A, Ueda H, Komatsu H, et al. Prognosis of non-surgically treated, clinical stage I lung cancer patients in Japan. Lung Cancer 2002;36:65–69.
16. McGarry RC, Song G, des Rosiers P, et al. Observation-only management of early stage, medically inoperable lung cancer: poor outcome. Chest 2002;2002:1155–1158.
17. Tai THP, Yu E, Dickof P, et al. Prophylactic cranial irradiation revisited: cost-effectiveness and quality of life in small-cell lung cancer. Int J Radiat Oncol Biol Phys 2002;52:68–74.
18. Fuentes PA. Pneumonectomy: historical perspective and prospective insight. Eur J Cardiothorac Surg 2003;23:439–445.
19. Ferguson MK, Lehman AG. Sleeve lobectomy or pneumonectomy: optimal management strategy using decision analysis techniques. Ann Thorac Surg 2003;76:1782–1788.
20. De Leyn P, Rots W, Deneffe G, et al. Sleeve lobectomy for non-small cell lung cancer. Acta Chir Belg 2003;103:570–576.
21. Pompeo E, De Dominicis E, Ambrogi V, et al. Quality of life after tailored combined surgery for stage 1 non-small-cell lung cancer and severe emphysema. Ann Thorac Surg 2003;76:1821–1827.
22. Montazeri A, Milroy R, Hole D, et al. Anxiety and depression in patients with lung cancer before and after diagnosis: findings from a population in Glasgow, Scotland. J Epidemiol Community Health 1998;52(3):203–204.
23. Hendriks J, Van Schil P, Van Meerbeeck J, et al. Short-term survival after major pulmonary resections for bronchogenic carcinoma. Acta Chir Belg 1996;96:273–279.
24. Cooley M. Patterns of symptom distress in adults receiving treatment for lung cancer. J Palliat Care 2002;18:150–159.
25. Pelkonen M, Notkola I-L, Tukianinen H, et al. Smoking cessation, decline in pulmonary function and total mortality: a 30 year follow up study among the Finnish cohorts of the Seven Counties Study. Thorax 2001;56:703–707.
26. Nezu K, Kushibe K, Tojo T, et al. Recovery and limitation of exercise capacity after lung resection for lung cancer. Chest 1998;113:1511–1516.

27. Miyazawa M, Haniuda M, Nishimura H, et al. Long-term effects of pulmonary resection on cardiopulmonary function. J Am Coll Surg 1999;189:26–33.
28. Larsen KR, Svendsen UG, Milman N, et al. Cardiopulmonary function at rest and during exercise for bronchial resection for bronchial carcinoma. Ann Thorac Surg 1997;64:960–964.
29. Handy JR, Asaph JW, Skokan L, et al. What happens to patients undergoing lung cancer surgery? Outcomes and quality of life before and after surgery. Chest 2002;122:21–30.
30. Bolliger CT, Jordan P, Soler M, et al. Pulmonary function and exercise capacity after lung resection. Eur Respir J 1996;9:415–421.
31. Bolliger CT, Zellweger JJP, Danielsson T, et al. Influence of long-term smoking reduction on health risk markers and quality of life. Nicotine Tobacco Res 2002;4:433–439.
32. Nomori H, Ohtsuka T, Horio H, et al. Difference in the impairment of vital capacity and 6-minute walking after a lobectomy performed by thoracoscopic surgery, an anterior limited thoracotomy, an anteroaxillary thoracotomy, and a posterolateral thoracotomy. Surg Today 2003;33:7–12.
33. Pelletier C, Lapointe L, LeBlanc P. Effects of lung resection on pulmonary function and exercise capacity. Thorax 1990; 1990:497–502.
34. Zieren HU, Muller JM, Hamberger U, et al. Quality of life after surgical therapy of bronchogenic carcinoma. Eur J Cardiothorac Surg 1996;10:233–237.
35. Myrdal G, Valtysdottir S, Lambe M, et al. Quality of life following lung cancer surgery. Thorax 2003;58:194–197.
36. Nugent AM, Steele IC, Carragher AM, et al. Effect of thoracotomy and lung resection on exercise capacity in patients with lung cancer. Thorax 1999;54:334–338.
37. Uchitomi Y, Mikami I, Nagai K, et al. Depression and psychological distress in patients during the year after curative resection of non-small cell lung cancer. J Clin Oncol 2003;21:69–77.
38. Rogers ML, Duffy JP. Surgical aspects of chronic post-thoracotomy pain. Eur J Cardiothorac Surg 2000;19:711–716.
39. Landreneau RJ, Mack MJ, Hazelrigg SR, et al. Prevalence of chronic pain after pulmonary resection by thoracotomy or video-assisted thoracic surgery. J Cardiovasc Surg 1995;109:1085–1086.
40. Dajczman E, Gordon A, Kreisman H, et al. Long-term postthoracotomy pain. Chest 1991;99:270–274.
41. Sugiura H, Morikawa T, Kaji M, et al. Long-term benefits for the quality of life after video-assisted thoracoscopic lobectomy in patients with lung cancer. Surg Laparosc Endosc Percutan Tech 1999;9:403–408.
42. Mangione CM, Goldman L, Orav J, et al. Health-related quality of life after elective surgery. J Gen Intern Med 1997;12:686–697.
43. Gotoda Y, Kambara N, Sakai T, et al. The morbidity, time course and predictive factors for persistent post-thoracotomy pain. Eur J Pain 2001;5:89–96.
44. Li WW, Lee TW, Lam SS, et al. Quality of life following lung cancer resection: video-assisted thoracic surgery versus thoracotomy. Chest 2002;122:584–589.
45. d'Amours RH, Riegler FX, Little AG. Pathogenesis and management of persistent postthoracotomy pain. Chest Surg Clin N Am 1998;8:703–722.
46. Goldberg BA, Scarlat MM, Harryman DT. Management of the stiff shoulder. J Orthop Sci 1999;4:462–471.
47. Cykert S, Kissling G, Hansen CJ. Patient preferences regarding possible outcomes of lung resection. Chest 2000;117:1551–1559.
48. Cull A, Gregor A, Hopwood P, et al. Neurological and cognitive impairment in long-term survivors of small cell lung cancer. Eur J Cancer 1994;30A:1067–1074.
49. Sarna L. Correlates of symptom distress in women with lung cancer. Cancer Pract 1993;1:21–28.
50. Kurz ME, Kurtz JC, Stommel M, et al. Predictors of physical functioning among geriatric patients small cell or non-small cell lung cancer 3 months after diagnosis. Support Care Cancer 1999; 7:328–331.
51. Schag CC, Heinrich RL. The impact of cancer on daily living. A comparison with cardiac patients and health controls. Rehabil Psychol 1986;31:157–167.
52. Zebrack BJ. Cancer survivor identity and quality of life. Cancer Pract 2000;8:238–242.
53. Zabora J, Brintzenhofeszoc K, Curbow B, et al. The prevalence of psychological distress by cancer site. Psycho-Oncology 2001; 10:19–28.
54. Ginsberg ML, Quirt C, Ginsberg AD, et al. Psychiatric illnesses and psychosocial concerns of patients with newly diagnosed lung cancer. Can Med Assoc J 1995;152:1961–1963.
55. Hopwood PS. Depression in patients with lung cancer: prevalence and risk factors. J Clin Oncol 2000;18:893–903.
56. Hughes JE. Depressive illness and lung cancer. II. Follow-up of inoperable patients. Eur J Surg Oncol 1985;11:21–24.
57. Kurtz ME, Kurtz JC, Stommel M, et al. Predictors of depressive symptomatology of geriatric patients with lung cancer: a longitudinal analysis. Psycho-Oncology 2002;11:12–22.
58. Buccheri G. Depressive reactions to lung cancer are common and often followed by poor outcome. Eur Respir J 1998;11: 173–178.
59. Schofield P, Ball D, Smith JG, et al. Optimism and survival in lung carcinoma patients. Cancer (Phila) 2004;100:1276–1282.
60. Uchitomi Y, Mikami I, Kugaya A, et al. Physician support and patient psychologic responses after surgery for non-small cell lung carcinoma: a prospective observational study. Cancer (Phila) 2001;92:1926–1935.
61. Dowie J, Wildman M. Choosing the surgical mortality threshold for high risk patients with stage Ia non-small cell lung cancer: insights from decision analysis. Thorax 2002;57:7–10.
62. Treasure T. Whose lung is it anyway? Thorax 2002;57:3–4.
63. Auperin A, Arriagada R, Pignon JP, et al. Prophylactic cranial irradiation for patients with small-cell lung cancer in complete remission. Prophylactic cranial irradiation overview collaborative group. N Engl J Med 1999;12:476–484.
64. Turrisi AT, Sherman CA. The treatment of limited small cell lung cancer: a report of the progress made and future prospects. Eur J Cancer 2002;38:279–291.
65. Johnson BE, Becker B, Goff WB, et al. Neurologic, neuropsychologic, computed cranial tomography scan abnormalities in 2- to 10-year survivors of small-cell lung cancer. J Clin Oncol 1985;3:1659–1667.
66. Albain KS, Crowley JJ, Livingston RB. Long-term survival and toxicity in small cell lung cancer. Chest 1991;99:1425–1432.
67. van Oosterhout AGM, Ganzevles PGJ, Wilmink JT, et al. Sequelae in long-term survivors of small cell lung cancer. Int J Radiat Oncol Biol Phys 1996;34:1037–1044.
68. Akechi T, Akizuke N, Sakuma K, et al. Somatic symptoms for diagnosing major depression in cancer patients. Psychosomatics 2003;44:244–248.
69. Sarna L. Women with lung cancer: impact on quality of life. Qual Life Res 1993;2:13–22.
70. Billante CR, Specto B, Hudson M, et al. Voice outcome following thyroplasty in patients with cancer-related vocal fold paralysis. Auris Nasus Larnyx 2001;28:315–321.
71. Nou E, Aberg T. Quality of survival in patients with surgically treated bronchial carcinoma. Thorax 1980;35:255–263.
72. Lassen U, Osterlind K, Hansen M, et al. Long-term survival in small-cell lung cancer: posttreatment characteristics in patients surviving 5 to 18+ years. An analysis of 1,714 consecutive patients. J Clin Oncol 1995;13:1215–1220.
73. Shelby RA, Taylor KL, Kerner JF, et al. The role of community-based and philanthropic organizations in meeting cancer patient and caregiver needs. CA Cancer J Clin 2002;52:229–246.
74. Pukrop R, Rehse B. Effects of psychosocial interventions on quality of life in adult cancer patients: meta analysis of 37 published controlled outcome studies. Patient Educ Counsel 2003; 50:179–186.

75. Johnson BE. Second lung cancers in patients after treatment for an initial lung cancer. JNCI 1998;90:1335–1345.
76. Johnson-Early A, Cohen MH, Minna JD, et al. Smoking abstinence and small cell lung cancer survival: an association. JAMA 1980;244:2175–2179.
77. Kawahara M, Ushijima S, Kamimori T, et al. Second primary tumours in more than 2-year disease-free survivors of small-cell lung cancer in Japan: the role of smoking cessation. Br J Cancer 1998;78:409–412.
78. Richardson GE, Tucker MA, Venzon DJ. Smoking cessation after successful treatment of small-cell lung cancer is associated with fewer smoking-related second primary cancers. Ann Intern Med 1993;119:383–390.
79. Gritz E, Vidrine DJ, Lazev AB. Smoking cessation in cancer patients: never too late to quit. In: Given B, Given CW, Champion V, et al. (eds). Evidence-Based Interventions in Oncology. New York: Springer, 2004.
80. Videtic GMM, Stitt LW, Dar R, et al. Continued cigarette smoking by patients receiving concurrent chemoradiotherapy for limited-stage small-cell lung cancer is associated with decreased survival. J Clin Oncol 2003;21:1544–1549.
81. Anthonisen N, Connett JE, Kiley JP, et al. Effects of smoking intervention and the use of an inhaled anticholinergic bronchodilator on the rate of decline of FEV1. The Lung Health Study. JAMA 1994;272:1497–1505.
82. Peto R, Darby S, Deo H, et al. Smoking, smoking cessation, and lung cancer in the UK since 1950: combination of national statistics with two case control studies. BMJ 2000;321:323–329.
83. Doll R, Peto R, Boreham J, et al. Mortality in relation to smoking: 50 years' observation on male British doctors. BMJ 2004. doi: 10.1136/bmj.38142.554479.AE, retrieved July 15, 2004.
84. Mokdad AH, Marks JS, Stroup DF, et al. Actual causes of death in the United States, 2000. JAMA 2004;291:1238–1245.
85. American Society of Clinical Oncology. American Society of Clinical Oncology Policy Statement Update: Tobacco control—reducing cancer incidence and saving lives. J Clin Oncol 2003; 21:2777–2786.
86. Fujisawa T, Iizasa T, Saitoh Y, et al. Smoking before surgery predicts poor long-term survival in patients with stage I non-small cell lung carcinomas. J Clin Oncol 1999;17:2086–2091.
87. Clarke MM, Cox LS, Jett JR, et al. Effectiveness of smoking cessation self-help materials in a lung cancer screening population. Lung Cancer 2004;44:13–21.
88. Cox L, Africano N, Tercyak K, et al. Nicotine dependence treatment for patients with cancer: review and recommendations. Cancer (Phila) 2003;98:632–644.
89. Cox LS, Sloan JA, Patten CA, et al. Smoking behavior of 226 patients with diagnosis of stage IIIA/IIIB non-small cell lung cancer. Psycho-Oncology 2002;11:472–478.
90. Davison G, Duffy M. Smoking habits of long-term survivors of surgery for lung cancer. Thorax 1982;37:331–333.
91. Gritz ER, Nisenbaum R, Elashoff RE, et al. Smoking behavior following diagnosis in patients with stage I non-small cell lung cancer. Cancer Causes Control 1991;2:105–112.
92. Sridhar KS, Raub WA Jr. Present and past smoking history and other predisposing factors in 100 lung cancer patients. Chest 1992;101:19–25.
93. Dresler CM, Bailey M, Roper CR, et al. Smoking cessation and lung cancer resection. Chest 1996;110:1199–1202.
94. Grannis FW. The lung cancer and cigarette smoking web page: a pilot study in telehealth promotion on the World Wide Web. Can Respir J 2001;8:333–337.
95. Browning KK, Ahijevych KA, Ross P, et al. Implementing the Agency for Health Care Policy and Research's Smoking Cessation Guideline in a Lung Cancer Surgery Clinic. Oncol Nurs Forum 2000;27:1248–1254.
96. Wewers ME, Jenkins L, Mignery T. A nurse-managed smoking cessation during diagnostic testing for lung cancer. Oncol Nurs Forum 1997;24:1419–1422.
97. Ebbert JO, Yang P, Vachon CM, et al. Lung cancer risk reduction after smoking cessation: observations from a prospective cohort of women. J Clin Oncol 2003;21:921–926.
98. Chapple A, Ziebland S, McPherson A. Stigma, shame, and blame experienced by patients with lung cancer: a qualitative study. BMJ 2004. doi: 10.1136/bmj.38111.639734.7c (published June 11), retreived July 15, 2004.
99. Marteu T, Riordan DC. Staff attitudes towards patients: the influence of causal attributions for illness. Br J Clin Psychol 1992;31:107–110.
100. Faller H, Schilling S, Lang H. Causal attribution and adaptation among lung cancer patients. J Psychosom Res 1995;39:619–627.
101. Brown JK, Byers T, Doyle C, et al. Nutrition and physical activity during and after cancer treatment: an American Cancer Society guide for informed choices. CA A Cancer J Clin 2003;53:268–291.
102. The Alpha Tocopherol Betacarotene Prevention Study Group. The effect of vitamin E and betacarotene on the incidence of lung cancer and other cancers in male smokers. N Engl J Med 1994;330:1029–1035.
103. Omenn G, Goodman G, Thornquist M, et al. Effects of a combination of betacarotene and vitamin A on lung cancer and cardiovascular disease. N Engl J Med 1996;334:1150–1155.
104. Phase III randomized chemoprevention study of selenium in participants with previously resected stage I non-small cell lung cancer (Protocol ID E-5597). http://www.cancer.gov/ClinicalTrials/, retreived July 15, 2004.
105. Ludbrook JJ, Truong PT, MacNeil MV, et al. Do age and comorbidity impact treatment allocation and outcomes in limited stage small-cell lung cancer? A community-based population analysis. Int J Radiat Oncol Biol Phys 2003;55:1321–1330.
106. Kurz ME, Kurtz JC, Stommel M, et al. Loss of physical functioning among geriatric cancer patients: relationships to cancer site, treatment, comorbidity and age. Eur J Cancer 1997;33: 2352–2358.
107. Kurtz ME, Kurtz JC, Stommel M, et al. Symptomatology and loss of physical functioning among geriatric patients with lung cancer. J Pain Symptom Manag 2000;19:249–256.
108. Patel JD, Bach PB, Kris MG. Lung cancer in US women: a contemporary epidemic. JAMA 2004;291:1763–1768.
109. Henschke CI, Miettinen OS. Women's susceptibility to tobacco carcinogens. Lung Cancer 2004;43:1–5.
110. Thun M, Lally C, Flannery J, et al. Cigarette smoking and changes in histopathology of lung cancer. JNCI 1997;89: 1580–1586.
111. Lienert T, Serke N, Schofeld N, et al. Lung cancer in young females. Eur Respir J 2000;16:986–990.
112. Singh GK, Miller BA, Hankey BF. Changing area socioeconomic patterns in U.S. cancer mortality, 1950–1998. Part II: Lung and colorectal cancers. JNCI 2002;94:916–925.
113. Centers for Disease Control and Prevention. Cigarette smoking among adults: United States, 2002. MMWR 2004;53:427–431.
114. Barbeau EM, Krieger N, Soobader MJ. Working class matters: socioeconomic disadvantage, race/ethnicity, gender, and smoking in NHIS 2000. Am J Public Health 2003;94:269–278.
115. Centers for Disease Control and Prevention. Prevalence of cigarette use among 14 racial/ethnic populations—United States, 1999–2001. MMWR (Morbid Mort Wkly Rep) 2004;53: 49–52.
116. Leisktikow B. Lung cancer rates as an index of tobacco smoke exposures: validation against black male–non-lung cancer death rates, 1969–2000. Prev Med 2004;38:511–515.
117. Bach PB, Cramer LD, Warren JL, et al. Racial differences in the treatment of early-stage lung cancer. N Engl J Med 1999;341: 1198–1205.

118. Greenwald HP, Polissar NH, Borgatta EF, et al. Social factors, treatment, and survival in early-stage non-small cell lung cancer. Am J Public Health 1998;88:1681–1684.
119. Ward E, Jemal A, Cokkinides V, et al. Cancer disparities by race/ethnicity and socioeconomic status. CA A Cancer J Clin 2004; 54:78–93.
120. Montazeri A, Hole DJ, Milroy R, et al. Quality of life in lung cancer patients: does socioeconomic status matter? Health Qual Life Outcomes 2003;1:19–24.
121. Lopez-Encuentra A. Bronchogenic Carcinoma Co-Operative Group: comorbidity inoperable lung cancer. A multicenter descriptive study on 2992 patients. Lung Cancer 2002;35:263–269.
122. Gritz E. Facilitating smoking cessation in cancer patients. Tobacco Control 2000;i50(suppl 1):50.
123. U.S. Department of Health and Human Services. The health consequences of tobacco use: a report of the Surgeon General. Atlanta, GA: U.S. Department of Health and Human Services, Public Health Service, Centers for Disease Control and Prevention, National Center for Chronic Disease Prevention and Health Promotion, Office on Smoking and Health, 2003.
124. Nakayma M, Satoh H, Sekizawa K. Risk of cancers in COPD patients. Chest 2003;123:1775.
125. Beck GJ, Doyle CA, Schachter EN. Smoking and lung function. Am Rev Respir Dis 1981;123:149–155.
126. Ko CY, Maggard M, Livingston EH. Evaluating health utility in patients with melanoma, breast cancer, colon cancer, and lung cancer. A nationwide, population-based assessment. J Surg Res 2003;114:1–5.
127. Henschke CI, McCauley DI, Yankelevitz DF, et al. Early lung cancer action project: overall design and findings from baseline screening. Lancet 1999;354:99–105.
128. Patz EF, Swensen SJ, Herndon RE. Estimate of lung cancer mortality from low-dose spiral computed tomography screening trials: implications for current mass screening recommendations. J Clin Oncol 2004;22:2202–2206.
129. Shahidi H, Kvale PA. Long-term survival following surgical treatment of solitary brain metastasis in non-small cell lung cancer. Chest 1996;109:271–276.
130. Dow KH. Challenges and opportunities in cancer survivorship research. Oncol Nurs Forum 2003;30:455–469.
131. Schumacher A, Riesenbeck D, Braunheim M, et al. Combined modality treatment for locally advanced non-small cell lung cancer: preoperative chemoradiation does not result in poorer quality of life. Lung Cancer 2004;44:89–97.
132. Colice GL, Rubins J, Unger M. Follow-up and surveillance of the lung cancer patient following curative-intent therapy. Chest 2003;123:272S–283S.
133. McManus K. Concerns of poor quality of life should not deprive patients of the opportunity for curative surgery. Thorax 2003; 58:189.
134. Natale RB. Effects of ZD 1839 (Iressa, Gefitinib) treatment on symptoms and quality of life in patients with advanced non-small cell lung cancer. Semin Oncol 2004;31:23–30.
135. Welcker K, Marian P, Thetter O, et al. Cost and quality of life in thoracic surgery. Thorac Cardiovasc Surg 2003;51:260–266.

109

Cancer Survivorship Issues in Colorectal Cancer

Clifford Y. Ko and Patricia A. Ganz

Epidemiologic Trends That Will Influence the Number of Colon and Rectal Cancer Survivors

Colon and rectal cancers (CRC) are among the most common adult malignancies worldwide, and for a variety of reasons, the numbers of survivors of colorectal cancer are likely to increase in coming years. The incidence of these cancers doubles with each successive decade of life beyond 50 years, and with the expansion of the older population in the coming years, the absolute numbers of CRC patients in the United States will grow substantially.[1] It is estimated that by the year 2030 the number of persons over the age of 65 years will have doubled and the number of persons over the age of 85 years will have quadrupled.[2] Given this expanding and aging population, projections suggest that the numbers of CRC patients may increase by as much as 30%.[3] Thus, with these profound demographic changes, it will be imperative to have a better understanding of the late effects and health care needs of long-term CRC survivors.

In addition to the increased incidence of colorectal cancer, advances in the detection and treatment are contributing to improved survival outcomes for patients with this disease. Earlier detection of CRC leads to better survival through downstaging of the disease. Several large population-based studies have demonstrated that increasingly more colon and rectal cancers are being detected at an earlier stage through screening.[4–9] Data from the Surveillance, Epidemiology, and End Results (SEER) program[10] demonstrate an increasing proportion of localized colon cancers for the population 65 years and older: in the 1970s, 36% of tumors were localized; in the 1980s, 39% were localized; and in the 1990s, this increased to 42%. Similarly, the proportion of localized rectal cancers has increased from 46% to 49% from the 1970s to the 1990s.

In addition, there is an anticipated growth for the number of CRC survivors secondary to secular trends in screening for this disease. As CRC screening becomes more widespread through current health promotion campaigns, there will be an accelerated shift to earlier-stage disease, contributing further to a stage-related increase in the numbers of long-term survivors. The benefits of earlier stage on survival are demonstrated by looking at data on survival by stage (1992–1998): the 5-year survival for regional tumors (i.e., AJCC stage III) is 65.2%, while for localized colon and rectal cancers (i.e., AJCC stage I and II) the survival rate is 90.1%.[10] Overall, we can be optimistic about better outcomes and long-term survival for CRC patients in the decades ahead.

Finally, there are increasing numbers of CRC survivors because of advances in medical treatments. For example, the surgical technique of total mesorectal excision for rectal cancers has significantly decreased the likelihood of local recurrence,[11] and the use of radiation therapy in the disease both decreases local recurrence and improves overall survival.[12,13] Studies have also demonstrated the efficacy of various adjuvant chemotherapy regimens for improving survival in colon cancer patients.[14–16] The benefits of these improvements in detection and treatment are also reflected in population-based survival rates for CRC. In reviewing the latest data from the SEER program database, the overall 5-year survival rate for colon and rectal cancer for all races and both sexes is 61.9%.[10] This rate is significantly better than 1974–1976, which was 49.8% (P less than 0.05). Furthermore, the survival for patients under 65 years of age versus over 65 years is not dramatically different (63% versus 61.3%), which shows that the elderly with colorectal cancer achieve long-term survival as well. Data for survival beyond 5 years are also available through SEER and have shown similar improvements. For example, the 10-year survival for colon and rectal cancer patients improved from 44.7% in 1975 to 55.3% in 1989. For all these cited reasons, there will be a growing number of CRC survivors in the decades ahead.

Given that the number of CRC survivors is increasing, there are a number of important issues pertinent solely to this cancer site—some that are related to the CRC treatments, and others that are related to specific characteristics of the population that survives colorectal cancer (e.g., the level of comorbidity in this elderly population). The following sections address these survivorship issues. First, the treatment-related issues are discussed, including prevalence, symptomology, and quality of life. The subsequent sections examine issues related to the comorbidity and use of medical services for the CRC survivors population as a whole. The last part of this chapter discusses strategies that may help to improve survivorship outcomes now and in the future.

Treatment-Specific Survivorship Issues

Treatment of colorectal cancer is often multidisciplinary, depending on the stage of disease and whether or not the cancer arises in the colon or the rectum. More specifically, the treatment modalities can include surgical resection and chemotherapy for colon cancer and surgical resection, chemotherapy, and radiation therapy for rectal cancer. Although the current first-line chemotherapeutics do not have appreciable long-term effects on survivors, surgery and radiation therapy can have associated lasting morbidities that affect the function and quality of life of survivors long after the cancer is treated. A description of the pertinent effects related to surgical resection and radiation therapy is presented next.

Survivorship Issues Related to Surgery

Surgical resection is the mainstay of curative treatment for colon and rectal cancers.[17] The surgical procedure requires removal of a segment of colon and/or rectum where the tumor is located, as well as the associated blood vessels and draining lymph nodes.[11,18] In addition, if there is evidence of metastatic disease, this tissue (e.g., liver, omentum) is also removed or biopsied at the time of initial surgery.[19] Currently, most operations are performed through an open vertical incision up to 30 to 40cm in length through the abdominal wall. This open approach has associated risks of complications that may be important for colorectal cancer survivors in relation to function status and quality of life. Of note, trials have been reported regarding laparoscopic colon cancer resections. This latter issue is discussed at the end of the chapter.

Long-Term Complications of Abdominal Surgery

Several possible surgery-associated problems can occur in the short and long term that will affect colorectal cancer survivors. In the acute period, clinical complications may include wound infections (3%–26%), intraabdominal infections (2%–5%), and anastomotic leaks (2%–10%), all of which may require rehospitalization and possible additional invasive (e.g., surgical) procedures.[20–22]

However, more important for longer-term survivors of CRC are the issues that occur beyond the acute period: three important issues are bowel obstructions, abdominal wall hernias, and functional problems. Complications from bowel obstruction can occur any time after surgery (e.g., weeks to years), and the presentation can range from imminent bowel necrosis that requires immediate surgery to chronic cyclic episodes of debilitating pain that may require hospitalization, intravenous hydration, and gastrointestinal decompression with use of nasogastric drainage. In one study of 472 consecutive patients operated on for colorectal cancer who were followed for a median period greater than 5 years, small bowel obstruction necessitating an operation occurred in 10% after resection with curative intent and in 4% after a palliative operation.[23] Obstruction is particularly relevant to survivors of CRC because it always has the potential of being a sign of tumor recurrence. In this same study, although benign adhesions accounted for 51% of the obstructions, local tumor recurrence and carcinomatosis accounted for 49%.

Another potential surgical complication for colorectal cancer survivors is an *abdominal wall hernia*. Abdominal wall hernias can potentially lead to pain, limitation of activities, and the need for emergent surgery for possible bowel strangulation. It has been estimated that hernias at the incision site (i.e., incisional hernias) occur in approximately 4% to 10% of patients after open surgical procedures.[24,25] However, the rate increases to as high as 20% for patients whose wounds are infected. As only 50% of incisional hernias become evident within 6 months after an operation, many will continue to have this problem much beyond the acute recovery of their surgery. Overall, more than 100,000 incisional hernia repairs are performed each year in the United States, and the rate of reoperation for such repairs is high (the 5-year reoperative rate was 24% after an initial operation).[26,27]

Although intestinal obstruction and incision hernias are two of the most common (and generic) potentially chronic problems associated with open colon or open rectal cancer surgery, there are some unique factors that are specifically pertinent to survivors of rectal cancer who have undergone complete or partial proctectomy, especially if radiation therapy is also used. These issues include functional problems in three areas: fecal dysfunction and incontinence, sexual dysfunction, and urinary bladder dysfunction. These areas, which may substantially affect survivors, are discussed next.

Bowel Changes/Dysfunction

One role of the rectum is storage of fecal material. When the rectum is resected for cancer, the storage capacity of the rectum's replacement, the colon (e.g., usually the descending or sigmoid colon), is substantially less, and therefore frequent, clustered, and/or incomplete bowel movements can ensue.[28] Also, because of possible nerve damage from surgery or radiation therapy, anal sphincter function may be further affected, and the degree of incontinence may be worsened.[29]

Many providers and patients alike strongly prefer a sphincter-sparing procedure; however, it is necessary for the patient/survivor to understand that bowel dysfunction may occur even in the presence of sphincter preservation. In part, the level of the anastomosis is extremely relevant to subsequent function. A low colorectal or a coloanal anastomosis (i.e., an anastomosis performed immediately adjacent to the sphincter muscles) is associated with a higher frequency of defecation and more fecal leakage and incontinence than a high colorectal anastomosis. In addition, defecatory problems can occur as a result of surgical trauma or the effects of radiation therapy to the anal sphincter and its innervation, even when sphincter preservation is performed.

Overall, the most common bowel-related symptoms following rectal resection are increased frequency of bowel motion, urgency, fecal leakage, and incontinence. However, also reported by patients to some degree are diarrhea, constipation, and excessive flatus. These are clearly important issues for rectal cancer survivors because even though their cancer may be cured, their function and quality of life may be severely diminished as a result of bowel-related symptoms, even if the anal sphincter is spared.

A short-term single-institution series recently reported that 56% of patients who underwent sphincter preservation for rectal cancer reported unfavorable function and were all

TABLE 109.1. Bowel dysfunction in rectal cancer survivors.

Bowel dysfunction (overall)	*56%–60%*
Fecal leakage	44%–64%
Pad usage	18%–39%
Four or more bowel movements/day	16%–22%
Urgency	22%–24%
Unable to defer defecation 15 min	73%
Unable to defer defecation 5 min	27%
Bowel dysfunction requiring ostomy	5%

Source: References 28–30.

dissatisfied with their quality of life.[30] Although few long-term data are available, small case series have shown that bowel dysfunction and incontinence is often a chronic issue for many rectal cancer survivors who undergo sphincter preservation. Table 109.1 highlights some of the functional outcomes in rectal cancer survivors.

Ostomy Issues

In patients who undergo abdominoperineal resection, not only do pelvic dissection and rectal resection influence survivorship issues, but the presence of a permanent colostomy also has strong influence on survivors. First, stoma-related problems are common. In a series of 203 patients with end sigmoid colostomies, the 13-year actuarial risk of paracolostomy complications was 58%. Paracolostomy hernia was the most common complication (36% at 10 years).[31] Other stoma-related complications may occur in survivors, including stomal prolapse (12%), skin-related problems (e.g., excoriation) (12%), and stenosis of the stomal opening (7%).[31,32] In a survey study of almost 400 ostomates, 51% had skin problems (e.g., rashes) and 36% had leakage; 80% reported some change in lifestyle[33] (Table 109.2).

In addition to complications, several studies have compared postoperative psychosocial adjustment and quality of life in ostomy and nonostomy patients, including concerns regarding sexuality, limitations of activity, and bowel function. These quality of life issues related to ostomy are discussed later in this chapter. It is important that clinicians make use of referral of patients to enterostomal therapists who are able to address both the physical and psychosocial sequelae of having a stoma. Their consultation is valuable throughout the course of survivorship from preoperative to short- and long-term periods. Stoma support groups exist in many communities and are another resource.[34,35]

Sexual Dysfunction

Sexual problems are associated with surgical and radiation therapies that affect the tissues/organs of the pelvis and the nerves that innervate them (Table 109.3). The potential sexual dysfunctions for males include erectile dysfunction and ejaculatory difficulties (inability to ejaculate or retrograde ejaculation).[36] Disruption of the parasympathetic nerve network interferes with penile erection, and sympathetic nerve disruption impairs normal ejaculation. The incidence of sexual dysfunction increases with advancing patient age and is higher after abdominoperineal resection (i.e., removal of the rectum and placement of a permanent colostomy) than after anterior resection. A conventional rectal cancer resection in men is associated with postoperative impotence and retrograde ejaculation or both in 25% to 100% of cases.[37–39]

In females, the most common postoperative sexual complaint is dyspareunia, which may include loss of vaginal lubrication and inability to achieve orgasm. Although somewhat difficult to objectively assess, sexual activity has been used as a surrogate measure. Of those women who are sexually active before surgery, 47% to 86% remain sexually active after surgery. Other studies have demonstrated that while 55% to 58% of women remain sexually active after sphincter preservation surgery, only 10% to 39% remain sexually active after an abdominoperineal resection.[37,38,40] In some women who have undergone a posterior vaginectomy in addition to an abdominoperineal dissection, sexual intercourse may be impossible because of a stenotic vaginal introitus.

Havenga et al.[38] surveyed 54 women after total mesorectal excision (i.e., a surgical technique that removes the rectal mesentery and is associated with lower cancer recurrence rates) with autonomic nerve preservation for carcinoma of the rectum (44 low anterior resection, 10 abdominoperineal resection) and found that 95% of women remained interested in sex, 86% remained sexually active, 85% continued to experience vaginal lubrication during arousal, and 91% maintained their ability to achieve orgasm postoperatively. Although the most common postoperative sexual complaint was dyspareunia, the incidence was not significantly changed from the preoperative to postoperative periods.[38] Just as with men, the best possible outcome is achieved by careful sharp dissection with preservation of the pelvic autonomic nerves. Additional data regarding nerve-preserving surgery are presented at the end of the chapter.

TABLE 109.2. Colostomy problems in rectal cancer survivors.

Colostomy problems (overall)	*21%–76%*
Parastomal hernia	37%
Leakage	36%
Prolapse	12%
Skin problems	12%
Stomal stenosis	7%

Source: References 31, 33.

TABLE 109.3. Sexual dysfunction in rectal cancer survivors.

Sexual dysfunction (overall)	*14%–95%*
Male	33%–95%
Female	14%–67%
Low anterior resection	42%–45%
Abdominal perineal resection	25%–90%
Sexual dysfunction following autonomic nerve preservation surgery	4%–14%

Source: References 36–40.

Urologic Dysfunction

Bladder dysfunction has been reported to occur in 7% to 68% of patients after low rectal cancer resection; however, the incidence is generally quoted to be around 30% in most series.[41] Urologic dysfunction includes problems such as incomplete emptying, urgency, overflow or stress incontinence, loss of bladder sensation, dysuria, and chronic urinary tract infections. Similar to sexual dysfunction, the majority of voiding difficulties have been shown to be neurogenic in origin. Parasympathetic denervation is specific to urologic dysfunction in this setting. Although a neurogenic bladder may occur in as many as 50% of men after abdominoperineal resection, voiding difficulties resolve in the majority within 3 to 6 months after surgery.[41,42] In addition to neurogenic problems, mechanical and physiologic issues plays a role as bladder neck angulation following surgery, and the presence of benign prostatic hypertrophy (particularly in this age group) also contributes to urologic dysfunction.

As with sexuality, urinary difficulties are more often associated with abdominoperineal resection than with anterior resection. Balslev and Harling[43] identified urologic symptoms such as dysuria and incontinence in 29 of 31 patients who underwent abdominoperineal resection. As with sexual dysfunction, favorable outcomes may be achieved by careful sharp dissection with preservation of pelvic anastomotic nerves.

Survivorship Issues Regarding Radiation Therapy

According to National Cancer Institute (NCI)-developed guidelines, stage II and III rectal cancer patients should receive radiation therapy.[44] Studies have subsequently shown that radiation therapy decreases local recurrence as well as increases survival.[12] However, radiation therapy can have potentially serious late effects for the rectal cancer survivor. While short-term (acute) complications of radiotherapy may include lethargy, nausea, diarrhea, and skin changes (i.e., erythema and/or desquamation), and also develop to some degree in the majority of patients during treatment, they are generally self-limiting.[45]

For the long-term rectal cancer survivor who underwent radiation therapy, it is important to evaluate the morbidity, pelvic floor function, and quality of life. In this regard, delayed radiation toxicities have been reported and include radiation enteritis (4%), small bowel obstruction (5%), and rectal stricture (5%); this is in addition to the bowel, sexual, and urinary dysfunction discussed earlier that may be compounded by radiation-induced pelvic nerve injuries.[46] Regarding the latter two issues, although sexual and urologic function is poorly studied, data suggest that radiation has a negative impact in both men and women.[47]

Bowel function after radiation therapy is an important functional issue. There are several studies that are generally consistent and show that bowel function, as measured by frequency, urgency, evacuation, sensation, and/or continence, is impaired after radiation therapy when compared with patients not treated with radiation.[47]

The Swedish Rectal Cancer randomized controlled trial[12] has shown that preoperative high-dose radiotherapy improves survival and decreases local recurrence; they have also studied the long-term bowel function following radiation therapy (XRT) and anterior resection. The authors found that the median frequency of bowel movements was higher in the XRT plus surgery group versus the surgery-only group (20 versus 10 bowel movements per week; P less than 0.0001).[12,48] Additionally, urgency, emptying difficulties, and incontinence for loose stools were more common in the XRT plus surgery group (all P less than 0.0001). In terms of quality of life, 30% of the XRT plus surgery group stated that their social life was impaired because of bowel dysfunction compared to 10% of the surgery-only group (P less than 0.01).[48]

TABLE 109.4. Bowel issues in rectal cancer patients following radiation.

Diarrhea	39%
Nocturnal defecation	36%
Use of pad/diaper	32%
Number of bowel movements per day	0.5–3.5

Source: References 45–50, 84.

Another study of rectal cancer patients undergoing surgical resection with or without radiation therapy found similar results that the irradiated group had more diarrhea (39% versus 13%; $P = 0.005$) and more nocturnal defecation (36% versus 15%; $P = 0.03$) compared with the nonirradiated group.[49]

Looking at slightly longer outcomes, a recent study examined rectal cancer patients between 2 and 8 years following surgical resection with no radiation, preoperative radiation, or postoperative radiation.[50] They found that the postoperative radiation group had more episodes of clustered bowel movements (P less than 0.02) than either the preoperative radiation group or the no-radiation group. The authors attributed the adverse effects of postoperative radiation therapy to irradiation of the neorectum, which is spared when radiation is given preoperatively (Table 109.4).

Along these same lines, manometric studies of low anterior resection patients with and without chemoradiation shows that resting pressure, resting volume, and maximal tolerable volume of the neorectum was significantly worsened in the irradiated group after radiation compared with before radiation. These same parameters did not change in the nonirradiated group.[51]

Quality of Life in Colorectal Cancer Survivors

Some of the earliest studies of quality of life (QOL) in cancer patients were done by Ganz and colleagues using a newly developed instrument called the Cancer Inventory of Problem Situations (CIPS), which was later renamed the Cancer Rehabilitation Evaluation System (CARES).[52–56] These studies were conducted with heterogeneous samples of cancer patients and survivors, with several common cancers being represented, including 277 CRC patients and survivors.[55] In one of the first published studies to examine quality of life in adult cancer survivors, Schag et al.[53] reported on a sample of lung, colon, and prostate cancer disease-free survivors that compared QOL outcomes across disease sites as well as by length of survivorship (short-term, less than 2 years after diagnosis; intermediate-term, 2–5 years after diagnosis; long-term, more than 5 years after diagnosis). This particular study included a total of 117 CRC survivors, with 27 of them being long-term survivors. In comparing the CRC survivors across the three time periods of survivorship, the long-term survivors reported significantly better QOL on a global single-item rating of QOL, as well as better psychosocial functioning on the CARES, compared with the short- and intermediate-term survivors. Specific problems that were frequent and severe in CRC survivors were difficulty in doing physical activities, reduction

TABLE 109.5. Proportion of colon cancer survivors with issues rated as frequent/severe.

Difficulty with bending or lifting	42%
Difficulty with walking/moving around	26%
Difficulty doing physical activities	50%
Difficulty driving	5%
Not engaged in recreational activities	33%
Has frequent pain	30%
Difficulty thinking clearly	45%

Source: Reference 53.

in energy, difficulty doing recreational activities, having trouble gaining weight, worry about whether treatments worked, body image problems, problems with sexual interest and functioning, and at-work concerns such as difficulty talking to others about the cancer, difficulty asking for time off from work for treatment, and worrying about being fired (Table 109.5). Across all the CRC survivors, significant predictors of QOL were the Karnofsky Performance Status score, type of hospital setting in which treatment was received (higher QOL in a private hospital in comparison to a VA, teaching hospital, public hospital, or HMO), gender (males better QOL than females), and work status (nonworking survivors reported better QOL). In this model, comorbid conditions nearly reached significance, with better QOL associated with fewer comorbid conditions.[53] These findings suggest that a variety of factors influence QOL in CRC survivors and that they are important to address in treatment planning (Table 109.6).

A more-recent study of 227 colorectal cancer survivors by Ramsey et al. examined the quality of life after more than 5 years of survivorship. They found that survivors report a relatively uniform and high QOL. In addition, the presence and severity of comorbid conditions and low income status were more predictive of overall QOL than the stage of cancer. Interestingly, compared to age-matched controls, long term survivors reported higher overall QOL, although problems remained such as frequent bowel movements (16%), diarrhea (49%), and depression.[57]

With the advent of new surgical techniques that allow for the performance of lower-level anastomoses for rectal cancer resection, there has been a strong push for sphincter-sparing procedures. In a review of quality of life articles regarding the presence of an ostomy, Sprangers[58] identified studies that addressed at least one of four aspects (i.e., physical, psychologic, social, and sexual) for stoma versus nonstoma patients. The authors found that both patient cohorts were troubled by frequent or irregular bowel movements and diarrhea. Also, although both patient groups reported restrictions in their social functioning, colostomy patients reported a higher prevalence of these problems. Finally, stoma patients reported higher levels of psychologic distress as well as more impaired sexual dysfunction. Overall, this review shows that although both stoma and nonstoma survivors have impaired function and quality of life, nonstoma patients might fare better than do stoma patients.

TABLE 109.6. Treatment strategies for improving survivorship quality of life, function, and outcomes.

1. Informed discussion of expectations following treatment
2. Address coexistent disease throughout care and survivorship
3. Consider laparoscopic approach if appropriate
4. If colostomy will be performed, consider marking the site preoperatively.
5. Consider ostomy support group.
6. Consider transanal excision if appropriate
7. Consider neoadjuvant radiation (vs. adjuvant)
8. Autonomic nerve preservation techniques
9. Create neorectum with coloplasty or colonic J pouch

Increasingly more sphincter-preserving procedures are being performed, but other recent studies show that it remains unclear whether quality of life has definitively improved.[59] It should be noted that these studies comparing sphincter-sparing resection with abdominoperineal resection/permanent colostomy are nonrandomized and therefore may be biased with regard to patient selection. The results are nonetheless interesting, particularly because a randomized controlled trial will likely never be performed.

A study by Grumann et al.[60] examined 73 rectal cancer patients and compared quality of life in patients undergoing anterior resection (AR; e.g., sphincter preservation) or abdominoperineal resection (APR). All patients were treated for cure and were disease free throughout the study. QOL was evaluated before surgery and at two time points following surgery (6–9 months, and 14–15 months). The findings revealed that on most scales the rectal cancer survivors who had an APR had superior, although not significantly better, scores than the AR patients. Of note, APR patients had significantly less constipation and diarrhea than AR patients, and also had significantly less sleeplessness; for example, the AR patients reported significantly more sleep disturbances than APR patients. On further comparison of low anterior resection versus high anterior resection, low anterior resection patients had significantly lower total QOL, role function, social function, body image, and future perspective, and more gastrointestinal- and defecation-related symptoms, than patients undergoing high anterior resection.

In another quality of life study of ostomates versus nonostomate rectal cancer survivors, a 4-year prospective study by Engel et al. examined 329 rectal cancer patients in Germany and demonstrated somewhat different findings.[61] Overall, survivors who underwent anterior resection had better QOL scores than APR patients (i.e., stoma patients had significantly worse QOL scores than nonstoma patients). High anterior resection patients had significantly better scores than both low anterior resection patients and APR patients. Interestingly, APR patients' QOL scores did not improve over time.

The somewhat inconsistent findings of these studies highlight the likely selection bias that is inherent in nonrandomized observational studies. These studies do illustrate, however, the importance of having informed discussions between the patient and provider regarding options, benefits, risks, and overall expectations.

Role of Comorbid Conditions in CRC Survivors

With the earlier detection of colorectal cancer due to improved screening, there will be increasing numbers of older survivors who have a greater likelihood of comorbid conditions. Healthcare providers for these survivors will have to address the disease of colorectal cancer (including the follow-up surveillance) as well as issues related to comorbid diseases. Coordinating the efforts of disease prevention, disease surveillance, and addressing the active issues of comorbidities is a complex task that requires good coordination among healthcare providers.

Few studies are available that have specifically characterized the burden of comorbid conditions in colorectal cancer survivors, partly because of the difficulty of obtaining this type of data. One study of colorectal cancer survivors (5+ years following diagnosis) using a mailed survey found the most common comorbid conditions were arthritis/rheumatism (20%), congestive heart failure (6%), hypertension (5%), angina (5%), and myocardial infarction (4%).[57]

In another study using a large population-based, nationwide, patient interview, comorbidities and use of services were characterized in colon cancer patients who were 1 to 3 years past diagnosis.[62] The study showed that 75% of survivors had reported having a major comorbid disease. The most common comorbid condition was cardiovascular related (55%), followed by hypertension (46%), arthritis (44%), coronary heart disease (13%), and pulmonary-related comorbidity (11%). Of note, almost 1 of 10 survivors reported having a history of a myocardial infarction. Also prevalent was diabetes, which was present in 14% of survivors, of which 57% were insulin dependent.

The potential significance of having diabetes is seen in a study by Meyerhardt et al.,[63] which showed that at 5 years, colon cancer patients with diabetes mellitus, compared with colon cancer patients without diabetes, had a significantly worse disease-free survival, overall survival, and recurrence-free survival. Median survival was 6 years and 11.3 years for diabetics and nondiabetics, respectively. Although cause of death was not explicitly studied in detail, compared with patients without a history of diabetes, those with diabetes had a 42% increased risk of death from any cause (P less than 0.0001). Further studies are needed to determine if better management of a comorbid condition such as diabetes will influence survival after a diagnosis of colon cancer.

While the available evidence in this regard is sparse, these studies highlight the potential issues related to the prevalence, detection, and need for treatment of comorbid conditions in a colorectal cancer survivor cohort. This is especially relevant as survival times increase from colorectal cancer; it is likely that the comorbidity prevalence and severity will increase as well.

Healthcare Utilization in CRC Survivors

There have been relatively few studies that have characterized the colorectal cancer patient's use of healthcare services following treatment of the cancer. One important study has examined the use of surveillance related to colorectal cancer survivors. A study by Lafata et al. examined the use of CRC surveillance tests in more than 250 colorectal cancer survivors enrolled in a large managed care organization.[64] The specific surveillance tests included colonic examinations, carcinoembryonic antigen (CEA) testing, and metastatic disease testing. The study demonstrated that within 18 months of treatment, 55% of the cohort received a colon examination, 71% received CEA testing, and 59% received metastatic disease screening tests. While it may be difficult to evaluate these findings without the breakdown of cancer stage, it is noteworthy that race/ethnicity disparities were demonstrated. Whites were more likely than minorities to receive CEA testing ($P = 0.04$) and also tended to be more likely to receive a colon examination ($P = 0.09$). Moreover, socioeconomic disparities were apparent. As the median household income increased, so too did the likelihood of colon examination and metastatic disease testing ($P = 0.03$, $P = 0.01$, respectively). The presence of disparate care is an important issue for colorectal cancer survivors.

One other study provides limited characterization of the use of services of colon cancer patients 1 to 3 years after diagnosis.[62] In this survey-based study, the report showed that 95% of the cohort had a usual source of care and that 66% saw a primary care provider in the past 12 months. Of note, 84% saw a specialist in the past 12 months, and 68% were in the emergency room at least once during that same time period. Eighteen percent reported having had home care in the prior year. It is evident that these survivors need and obtain medical care, both for cancer surveillance as well as the comorbid conditions. It appears, however, that there may be room for improvements. Using the receipt of preventive care measures as a rough proxy for appropriate receipt of health care, the study found that only 53% of the survivors received a flu shot in the past year. Moreover, further pulmonary and/or new cancer concerns arise because the study shows that 33% still smoked tobacco, with 27% overall reported to smoke daily.

Ongoing Issues: Changes in Treatments to Minimize Treatment Morbidity

From the discussions presented here, one can see that there are considerable short- and long-term problems associated with CRC treatment. As such, there is great interest in using efficacious treatments with less morbidity. Treatment modifications that are continually being clinically defined and used include laparoscopic-assisted surgery, the use of local excision of rectal cancers, the use of nerve-sparing surgical techniques, possibly using radiation therapy less frequently, and the use of chemoprevention. The following section briefly summarizes the current issues that surround these treatments.

Laparoscopic Surgery

Although an open approach has been the traditional method of performing colorectal cancer surgery, recently there have been studies that have demonstrated the advantages of laparoscopic resection. In brief, the advantages are smaller incisions, less pain, decreased length of stay, a decrease in the incisional hernia rate, and possible less adhesion formation. A recent randomized controlled trial (RCT) compared the efficacy of laparoscopic-assisted colectomy with open colectomy and found that patients having the former approach recovered faster, had lower blood loss, and had lower morbidity (P less than 0.001). Finally, the authors report that the probability of cancer-related survival was higher in the laparoscopic-assisted group ($P = 0.02$), as the Cox model showed that laparoscopic-assisted approach was independently associated with reduced risk of tumor relapse, death from any cause, and death from a cancer-related cause compared to open colectomy.[65]

A trial of the laparoscopic versus open approach for colon cancer treatment has also been performed in North America. Regarding quality of life issues, Weeks et al. demonstrated that the global quality of life was significantly higher at 2 weeks following the laparoscopic approach.[66] Additionally, the laparoscopic patients required significantly fewer days of parenteral and oral narcotics. Of note, however, is that no differences in QOL were demonstrated at 2 months following surgery. Importantly, the survival and recurrence results of this trial were not statistically different, which thus suggests that in appropriately performed operations, laparoscopic colon cancer resections can be performed safely.[67]

In the future, it is likely that increasingly more laparoscopically assisted surgical resections of colon and rectal cancers will be performed; however, it remains a priority that, with the laparoscopic approach, appropriately indicated and safe cancer resections are performed.

Local Excision for Rectal Cancer

Several researchers have reported that local excision with or without chemoradiation therapy is an alternative approach for sphincter preservation in patients with locally invasive rectal carcinoma.[68–71] While local excision has been performed in the past for early-stage rectal cancers, complete indications, appropriateness, and long-term results have not been finalized at this point. Local excision is performed transanally and is fundamentally a wide excisional biopsy. The rationale for this procedure is that for those patients with favorable prognosis rectal tumors confined to the bowel wall where removal of the draining lymphatic tissue would not add any oncologic benefit, local excision would be adequate and appropriate.

The technique can be relatively simple or very difficult, depending on such things as body habitus and the location and size of the tumor. In brief, using retractors or an operating proctoscope, the lesion is excised transanally with an adequate margin of normal tissue. Currently, local excision of T1 lesions with good prognostic factors (e.g., well differentiated) yields good results, and the use of adjuvant therapy in T2 lesions and lesions with high-risk factors has also been associated with favorable results. This literature is discussed in further detail in other chapters. Regarding survivors, however, meticulous follow-up is essential for early detection of local recurrences, which possibly allows for good results from salvage surgery.

In terms of function and quality of life, what is clearly advantageous regarding a transanal excision of a rectal cancer is that the potential morbidity associated with either a low anterior resection, coloanal, or an abdominoperineal resection (e.g., fecal incontinence, sexual and urologic dysfunction) is virtually eliminated (unless adjuvant radiation therapy is also performed).

Surgical Creation of a Neorectum to Improve Bowel-Related Function

One of the functions of the rectum is storage, and in this regard the rectum is a capacitance organ. When the rectum is resected for rectal cancer and the colon is put in its place, it is understandable that bowel function is worsened. In this regard, to overcome the functional deficiencies attributed to the loss of rectal capacity and decrease in compliance, studies have demonstrated how the creation of a neorectum improves bowel function. The two most common techniques to create a neorectum are the colonic J pouch and the coloplasty.

Creation of a J pouch involves folding over the lower 6 to 8 cm of the colon to make a "J" configuration. This J pouch basically doubles the lumen diameter over the straight colon. The J pouch has been compared to straight colon anastomoses in several RCTs and has been shown to result in better function. Bowel movement frequency, continence to liquids and gas, and cancer-specific quality of life are better with the J pouch.[28,72,73]

Another option is the coloplasty, which has been described and primarily developed in the past 5 years. Creation of a coloplasty involves making a 6- to 8-cm longitudinal incision in the lower colon and then suturing the incision closed in a transverse direction. This technique creates a larger pouch toward the lower end of the colon, just above the site of the anastomosis. RCTs of coloplasty versus J pouch have basically demonstrated an equivalent outcome in terms of bowel function (stool frequency, clustering of bowel movements, and urgency), continence, and quality of life.[73,74] What may be advantageous for the coloplasty is the maintenance of bowel length for performance of an anastomosis and a less bulky neorectum for patients with an especially narrow pelvis. In an unpublished review, the use of neorectal pouches in rectal cancer patients is below 25%.

Necessity of Radiation Therapy: When Not to Use It

The excellent results reported by Heald[11,75] and others utilizing "optimal surgery" (i.e., total mesorectal excision) without routine adjuvant therapy, the results of the NSABP R-02 trial, and other work bring to the forefront the controversy of omitting radiation therapy in the face of optimal surgery. Because the main purpose of radiation therapy is to improve local control, can optimally performed surgery in appropriately selected patients obviate the need for radiation therapy?

Heald examined this issue performing total mesorectal excisions for his patients with rectal cancer.[11,75] Total mesorectal excision involves complete removal of all the rectal mesentery, which includes the lymph nodes adjacent to the rectum. In a series of 419 consecutive rectal cancer patients, cancer-specific survival of all surgically treated patients was 68% at 5 years and 66% at 10 years. The local recurrence rate was 6% at 5 years and 8% at 10 years. In 405 "curative" resections, the local recurrence rate was 3% at 5 years and 4% at 10 years. Disease-free survival in this group was 80% at 5 years and 78% at 10 years. In his series overall, Heald found that rectal cancer can be cured by surgical therapy alone in 2 of 3 patients undergoing surgical excision in all stages and in 4 of 5 patients having curative resections [it should be noted that a small percentage of the series did receive chemotherapy (6%) and preoperative radiation (9%)].

A similar case series study of a specific tumor stage (i.e., T3N0M0) has demonstrated that adequate surgery will result in superb oncological outcomes, without use of adjuvant radiation therapy. In a single institutional series, Merchant et al.

showed that sharp mesorectal excision for T3N0M0 rectal cancers results in a local recurrence rate of less than 10% without the use of adjuvant therapy.[76]

Although not specifically tested, the National Surgical Adjuvant Bowel Program's R-02 trial is consistent with the nonuse of adjuvant radiation therapy. In this RCT, eligible patients ($n = 694$) with Dukes' B or C carcinoma of the rectum were randomly assigned to receive either postoperative adjuvant chemotherapy alone ($n = 348$) or chemotherapy with postoperative radiotherapy ($n = 346$).[77] The results showed that postoperative radiotherapy resulted in no beneficial effect on disease-free survival ($P = 0.90$) or overall survival ($P = 0.89$), regardless of chemotherapy. It should be noted, however, that radiation therapy did reduce the cumulative incidence of locoregional relapse from 13% to 8% at 5-year follow-up ($P = 0.02$).

In a review of the literature, Meagher et al.[78] reported that radiotherapy has only been demonstrated to significantly improve survival in one individual study and one recent meta-analysis. Although the local recurrence rates in the no-radiotherapy arm of these studies were 27% and 21% to 36.5%, respectively, in more-recent studies, with lower local recurrence rates reflecting modern surgical standards, no survival advantage has been found. While it is currently unknown whether radiotherapy improves patients' quality of life, studies have demonstrated that radiotherapy does bring about both acute and long-term detrimental effects on quality of life. Finally, these authors report that 17 to 20 patients need to undergo adjuvant radiotherapy to prevent 1 local recurrence,[78] questioning the appropriateness of radiation therapy as a general rule.

Data are available that supports the opposite sentiment. In contrast to the foregoing views, an important and recently published interim report from the Dutch Colorectal Cancer Group compared preoperative radiotherapy (20 Gy over 5 days) followed by total mesorectal resection (924 patients) with total mesorectal excision alone (937 patients), that is, no radiation therapy.[13] At 2 years, no difference in overall survival was demonstrated; however, the rate of local recurrence at 2 years was significantly lower in the radiation group (2.4% versus 8.2%; P less than 0.0001). This study demonstrates that local recurrence is lessened with adjuvant radiation therapy, even with the use of "optimal surgery."

Overall, several issues remain regarding the use of radiation therapy in rectal cancer. First, will differences in local recurrence rates affect survival rates when examined in the long term? Second, is the toxicity of radiation therapy warranted with a decrease in local recurrence? Finally, can we select patients based on preoperative stage or tumor grade who should (and should not) receive radiation therapy?

Surgical Nerve-Sparing Techniques

Nerve preservation is important when performing rectal cancer surgery. Havenga et al.[37] evaluated sexual and urinary function after total mesorectal excision with autonomic nerve preservation was performed in patients with tumors situated within 12 cm of the anal verge. The ability to engage in intercourse was maintained by 86% of the male patients under 60 years of age and 67% of those age over 60 or undergoing APR, with a mean of 80% of preoperative penile rigidity. The ability to achieve orgasm was retained in 87% of men and 91% of women, with arousal and lubrication present in 85% of the women. There were no severe urinary dysfunctions.

Masui et al.[79] evaluated sexual function in 134 men who had histologically curative resections with varying degrees of autonomic nerve preservation. All were under 65 years of age and all were sexually active preoperatively; 49% had tumors above the peritoneal reflection and 52% below. These patients were interviewed at least 1 year after surgery. Erection was maintained in 93% of those with complete nerve preservation, 82% when there was a hemilateral nerve preservation, and 61% with only pelvic plexus preservation. The respective proportions with erectile rigidity and duration sufficient for vaginal insertion were 90%, 53%, and 26%. Ejaculation potencies were 82%, 47%, and 0%. Although 96% of patients reported orgasm preoperatively, 94% of men with complete preservation, 65% with hemilateral preservation, and 22% with plexus preservation reported orgasm postoperatively. The combining of total mesorectal incision with autonomic nerve preservation is essential to reducing the long-term genitourinary morbidity of rectal cancer resection. These results suggest that preservation of sexual function is dependent on careful operative technique with preservation of the pelvic autonomic nerves. The low incidence of injury after curative total mesorectal incision also stands in contradiction to earlier admonitions that if erection and ejaculation were maintained then the operation was not curative.

Chemoprevention for Survivors

An important area of cancer research that may potentially impact the mecial treatment for colorectal cancer survivors is chemoprevention. Chemoprevention is the use of specific agents to prevent, inhibit, or reverse tumorigenic progression to invasive cancer. It is not intended to treat invasive carcinomas and therefore should be clearly distinguished from chemotherapy. The main goals of chemoprevention are to block the original initiation of the carcinogenic process, to arrest or reverse further progression of premalignant cells into becoming invasive or metastatic. Agents that have been investigated for chemopreventative activity in CRC include NSAIDs, calcium, antioxidant vitamins, and selenium.

Most of the work in chemoprevention of CRC has been performed in NSAIDs because of biologic evidence of the role of the cyclooxygenase pathway in CRC pathogenesis. More specifically, animal studies have demonstrated that NSAIDs function to stop colorectal carcinogenesis by blocking prostaglandin synthesis. Of the various available NSAIDs, sulindac is the most extensively studied. One study by Waddell et al. demonstrated that at doses ranging from 150 to 400 mg per day, colorectal polyps in FAP were eliminated. Importantly, the polyps regrew after sulindac was stopped, but then the polyps disappeared again after sulindac was reinstituted.[80]

Other studies have shown contrary results. A more recent RCT of 41 young (age 8 to 25 years) familial adenomatous polyposis (FAP) patients who were phenotypically unaffected received either 75 or 150 mg sulindac orally twice a day or identical-appearing placebo tablets for 48 months. This study found that after 4 years of treatment, adenomas developed in 9 of 21 subjects (43%) in the sulindac group and 11 of 20 subjects in the placebo group (55%) ($P = 0.54$). There were no significant differences in the mean number ($P = 0.69$) or size ($P = 0.17$) of polyps between the groups. While this study was performed in FAP patients and not in survivors, it did demonstrate that standard doses of sulindac did not prevent the development of adenomas.[81]

The role and effect of NSAIDs are still to be determined. Important to their use of NSAIDs for chemoprevention is the level of associated toxicity. A recent Japanese study of sulindac 300 mg per day showed that five of six patients had drug related complications, which ranged from severe nausea and vomiting to multiple ulcers of the small bowel and stomach.[82]

Recently, aspirin, which irreversibly affects the cyclooxygenase pathway, has been reported to decrease adenoma formation. In a randomized controlled study, 1,121 patients with a history of biopsy-proven adenomas were randomized to receive placebo (372 patients), 81 mg aspirin (377 patients), or 325 mg aspirin (372 patients) daily. Follow-up colonoscopy demonstrated that the incidence of one or more adenomas was 47% in the placebo group, 38% in the group given 81 mg aspirin per day, and 45% in the group given 325 mg aspirin per day (global $P = 0.04$). Unadjusted relative risks of any adenoma (as compared with the placebo group) were 0.81 in the 81-mg group (95% confidence interval, 0.69–0.96) and 0.96 in the 325-mg group (95% confidence interval, 0.81–1.13). For advanced neoplasms (adenomas measuring at least 1 cm in diameter or with tubulovillous or villous features, severe dysplasia, or invasive cancer), the respective relative risks were 0.59 (95%, 0.38–0.92) and 0.83 (95% confidence interval, 0.55–1.23).[83]

A separate randomized controlled trial of 635 colorectal cancer survivors who were randomized to receive either 325 mg aspirin per day or placebo corroborates these findings. The mean (±SD) number of adenomas was lower in the aspirin group than the placebo group (0.30 ± 0.87 versus 0.49 ± 0.99; $P = 0.003$ by the Wilcoxon test). The adjusted relative risk of any recurrent adenoma in the aspirin group, as compared with the placebo group, was 0.65 (95% confidence interval, 0.46–0.91). The time to the detection of a first adenoma was longer in the aspirin group than in the placebo group (hazard ratio for the detection of a new polyp, 0.64; 95% confidence interval, 0.43–0.94; $P = 0.022$).[84]

For colorectal cancer survivors in the future, chemoprevention appears to be a promising modality. There are ongoing large randomized controlled trials to address these issues and define the optimal prevention strategy.

Future Work

It is clear that there is a paucity of good evidence regarding colorectal cancer survivorship issues. Because the number of survivors will be increasing, this will be an important topic of study in the future. Specific issues include addressing the morbidities associated with the different treatment modalities, identifying and focusing on the presence of comorbidities in this elderly patient population, and improving the performance of CRC surveillance (without disparities).

References

1. Jemal A, Murray T, Samuels A, Ghafoor A, Ward E, Thun MJ. Cancer statistics, 2003. CA Cancer J Clin 2003;53:5–26.
2. Hutchins LF, Unger JM, Crowley JJ, Coltman CA Jr, Albain KS. Underrepresentation of patients 65 years of age or older in cancer-treatment trials. N Engl J Med 1999;341:2061–2067.
3. Etzioni DA, Liu JH, Maggard MA, Ko CY. The aging population and its impact on the surgery workforce. Ann Surg 2003;238: 170–177.
4. Mandel JS, Bond JH, Church TR, et al. Reducing mortality from colorectal cancer by screening for fecal occult blood. Minnesota Colon Cancer Control Study. N Engl J Med 1993;328:1365–1371.
5. Mandel JS, Church TR, Bond JH, et al. The effect of fecal occult-blood screening on the incidence of colorectal cancer. N Engl J Med 2000;343:1603–1607.
6. Kronborg O, Fenger C, Olsen J, Jorgensen OD, Sondergaard O. Randomised study of screening for colorectal cancer with faecal-occult-blood test. Lancet 1996;348:1467–1471.
7. Hardcastle JD, Chamberlain JO, Robinson MH, et al. Randomised controlled trial of faecal-occult-blood screening for colorectal cancer. Lancet 1996;348:1472–1477.
8. Ransohoff DF, Sandler RS. Clinical practice. Screening for colorectal cancer. N Engl J Med 2002;346:40–44.
9. Troisi RJ, Freedman AN, Devesa SS. Incidence of colorectal carcinoma in the U.S.: an update of trends by gender, race, age, subsite, and stage, 1975–1994. Cancer (Phila) 1999;85:1670–1676.
10. SEER. www.seer.cancer.gov 2004.
11. Heald RJ, Moran BJ, Ryall RD, Sexton R, MacFarlane JK. Rectal cancer: the Basingstoke experience of total mesorectal excision, 1978–1997. Arch Surg 1998;133:894–899.
12. Improved survival with preoperative radiotherapy in resectable rectal cancer. Swedish Rectal Cancer Trial. N Engl J Med 1997; 336:980–987.
13. Kapiteijn E, Marijnen CA, Nagtegaal ID, et al. Preoperative radiotherapy combined with total mesorectal excision for resectable rectal cancer. N Engl J Med 2001;345:638–646.
14. Rao S, Cunningham D. Adjuvant therapy for colon cancer in the new millennium. Scand J Surg 2003;92:57–64.
15. O'Connell MJ, Laurie JA, Kahn M, et al. Prospectively randomized trial of postoperative adjuvant chemotherapy in patients with high-risk colon cancer. J Clin Oncol 1998;16:295–300.
16. Arkenau HT, Bermann A, Rettig K, Strohmeyer G, Porschen R. 5-Fluorouracil plus leucovorin is an effective adjuvant chemotherapy in curatively resected stage III colon cancer: long-term follow-up results of the adjCCA-01 trial. Ann Oncol 2003;14: 395–399.
17. Schwartz SI, Shires GT, Spencer FC, Daly JM, Fischer JE, Galloway AC (eds). Principles of Surgery, 7th ed. New York: McGraw Hill, 1999.
18. Joseph NE, Sigurdson ER, Hanlon AL, et al. Accuracy of determining nodal negativity in colorectal cancer on the basis of the number of nodes retrieved on resection. Ann Surg Oncol 2003; 10:213–218.
19. Kemeny N, Huang Y, Cohen AM, et al. Hepatic arterial infusion of chemotherapy after resection of hepatic metastases from colorectal cancer. N Engl J Med 1999;341:2039–2048.
20. Gordon PH, Nivatvongs S. Surgery of the Colon, Rectum, and Anus. London: Saunders, 2001.
21. Corman MC. Surgery of the Colon and Rectum. Philadelphia: Lippincott Williams & Wilkins. 2001.
22. Smith R, Bohl J, McElearney S, et al. Wound infection after elective colorectal resection. Ann Surg 2004;239:599–605.
23. Edna TH, Bjerkeset T, Loe B. Small bowel obstruction in patients previously operated on for colorectal cancer. Eur J Surg 1998; 164:587–592.
24. Cameron J ed). Current Surgical Therapy, 7th ed. St. Louis: Mosby, 2001.
25. Cahalane MJ, Shapiro ME, Silen W, et al. Abdominal incision: decision or indecision? Lancet 1989;1:146–148.
26. Millikan KW. Incisional hernia repair. Surg Clin N Am 2003; 83:1223–1234.

27. Flum DR, Horvath K, Koepsell T. Have outcomes of incisional hernia repair improved with time? A population-based analysis. Ann Surg 2003;237:129–135.
28. Sailer M, Fuchs KH, Fein M, Thiede A. Randomized clinical trial comparing quality of life after straight and pouch coloanal reconstruction. Br J Surg 2002;89:1108–1117.
29. Mancini R, Cosimelli M, Filippini A, et al. Nerve-sparing surgery in rectal cancer: feasibility and functional results. J Exp Clin Cancer Res 2000;19:35–40.
30. Chatwin NA, Ribordy M, Givel JC. Clinical outcomes and quality of life after low anterior resection for rectal cancer. Eur J Surg 2002;168:297–301.
31. Londono-Schimmer EE, Leong AP, Phillips RK. Life table analysis of stomal complications following colostomy. Dis Colon Rectum 1994;37:916–920.
32. Makela J, Turku P, Laitinen S. Analysis of late stomal complications following ostomy surgery. Ann Chir Gynaecol 1997; 86:305–310.
33. Nugent KP, Daniels P, Stewart B, Patankar R, Johnson CD. Quality of life in stoma patients. Dis Colon Rectum 1999;42: 1569–1574.
34. Bass EM, Del Pino A, Tan A, Pearl RK, Orsay CP, Abcarian H. Does preoperative stoma marking and education by the enterostomal therapist affect outcome? Dis Colon Rectum 1997;40: 440–442.
35. Sprangers MA, Taal BG, Aaronson NK, te Velde A. Quality of life in colorectal cancer. Stoma vs. nonstoma patients. Dis Colon Rectum 1995;38:361–369.
36. Beck D, Wexner SD eds) Fundamentals of Anorectal Surgery. London: Saunders, 1998.
37. Havenga K, DeRuiter MC, Enker WE, Welvaart K. Anatomical basis of autonomic nerve-preserving total mesorectal excision for rectal cancer. Br J Surg 1996;83:384–388.
38. Havenga K, Enker WE, McDermott K, Cohen AM, Minsky BD, Guillem J. Male and female sexual and urinary function after total mesorectal excision with autonomic nerve preservation for carcinoma of the rectum. J Am Coll Surg 1996;182:495–502.
39. Enker WE, Havenga K, Polyak T, Thaler H, Cranor M. Abdominoperineal resection via total mesorectal excision and autonomic nerve preservation for low rectal cancer. World J Surg 1997;21:715–720.
40. van Driel MF, Weymar Schultz WC, van de Wiel HB, Hahn DE, Mensink HJ. Female sexual functioning after radical surgical treatment of rectal and bladder cancer. Eur J Surg Oncol 1993; 19:183–187.
41. Rothenberger DA, Wong WD. Abdominoperineal resection for adenocarcinoma of the low rectum. World J Surg 1992;16: 478–485.
42. Havenga K, Enker WE, Norstein J, et al. Improved survival and local control after total mesorectal excision or D3 lymphadenectomy in the treatment of primary rectal cancer: an international analysis of 1411 patients. Eur J Surg Oncol 1999; 25:368–374.
43. Balslev I, Harling H. Sexual dysfunction following operation for carcinoma of the rectum. Dis Colon Rectum 1983;26:785–788.
44. NIH CC. Adjuvant therapy for patients with colon and rectal cancer. JAMA 1990;264:1444–1450.
45. Guren MG, Dueland S, Skovlund E, Fossa SD, Poulsen JP, Tveit KM. Quality of life during radiotherapy for rectal cancer. Eur J Cancer 2003;39:587–594.
46. Ooi BS, Tjandra JJ, Green MD. Morbidities of adjuvant chemotherapy and radiotherapy for resectable rectal cancer: an overview. Dis Colon Rectum 1999;42:403–418.
47. Temple LK, Wong WD, Minsky B. The impact of radiation on functional outcomes in patients with rectal cancer and sphincter preservation. Semin Radiat Oncol 2003;13:469–477.
48. Dahlberg M, Glimelius B, Graf W, Pahlman L. Preoperative irradiation affects functional results after surgery for rectal cancer: results from a randomized study. Dis Colon Rectum 1998;41: 543–549; discussion 549–551.
49. Dehni N, McNamara DA, Schlegel RD, Guiguet M, Tiret E, Parc R. Clinical effects of preoperative radiation therapy on anorectal function after proctectomy and colonic J-pouch-anal anastomosis. Dis Colon Rectum 2002;45:1635–1640.
50. Nathanson DR, Espat NJ, Nash GM, et al. Evaluation of preoperative and postoperative radiotherapy on long-term functional results of straight coloanal anastomosis. Dis Colon Rectum 2003;46:888–894.
51. Ammann K, Kirchmayr W, Klaus A, et al. Impact of neoadjuvant chemoradiation on anal sphincter function in patients with carcinoma of the midrectum and low rectum. Arch Surg 2003; 138:257–261.
52. Schag CA, Ganz PA, Heinrich RL. Cancer Rehabilitation Evaluation System–short form (CARES-SF). A cancer specific rehabilitation and quality of life instrument. Cancer (Phila) 1991;68:1406–1413.
53. Schag CA, Ganz PA, Wing DS, Sim MS, Lee JJ. Quality of life in adult survivors of lung, colon and prostate cancer. Qual Life Res 1994;3:127–141.
54. Schag CA, Heinrich RL, Aadland RL, Ganz PA. Assessing problems of cancer patients: psychometric properties of the cancer inventory of problem situations. Health Psychol 1990; 9:83–102.
55. Ganz PA, Schag CA, Lee JJ, Sim MS. The CARES: a generic measure of health-related quality of life for patients with cancer. Qual Life Res 1992;1:19–29.
56. Heinrich RL, Schag CC, Ganz PA. Living with cancer: the Cancer Inventory of Problem Situations. J Clin Psychol 1984; 40:972–980.
57. Ramsey SD, Berry K, Moinpour C, Giedzinska A, Andersen MR. Quality of life in long term survivors of colorectal cancer. Am J Gastroenterol 2002;97:1228–1234.
58. Sprangers MA. Quality-of-life assessment in colorectal cancer patients: evaluation of cancer therapies. Semin Oncol 1999;26: 691–696.
59. Allal A, Bieri S, Pelloni A, et al. Sphincter-sparing surgery after preoperative radiotherapy for low rectal cancers: feasibility, oncologic results and quality of life outcomes. Br J Cancer 2000; 82:1131–1137.
60. Grumann MM, Noack EM, Hoffmann IA, Schlag PM. Comparison of quality of life in patients undergoing abdominoperineal extirpation or anterior resection for rectal cancer. Ann Surg 2001;233:149–156.
61. Engel J, Kerr J, Schlesinger-Raab A, Eckel R, Sauer H, Holzel D. Quality of life in rectal cancer patients: a four-year prospective study. Ann Surg 2003;238:203–213.
62. Ko C, Chaudhry S. The need for a multidisciplinary approach to cancer care. J Surg Res 2002;105:53–57.
63. Meyerhardt JA, Catalano PJ, Haller DG, et al. Impact of diabetes mellitus on outcomes in patients with colon cancer. J Clin Oncol 2003;21:433–440.
64. Lafata JE, Johnson CC, Ben-Menachem T, Morlock RJ. Sociodemographic differences in the receipt of colorectal cancer surveillance care following treatment with curative intent. Med Care 2001;39:361–372.
65. Lacy AM, Garcia-Valdecasas JC, Delgado S, et al. Laparoscopy-assisted colectomy versus open colectomy for treatment of non-metastatic colon cancer: a randomised trial. Lancet 2002;359: 2224–2229.
66. Weeks JC, Nelson H, Gelber S, Sargent D, Schroeder G. Short-term quality-of-life outcomes following laparoscopic-assisted colectomy vs. open colectomy for colon cancer: a randomized trial. JAMA 2002;287:321–328.

67. Group COoSTS. A comparison of laparoscopically assisted and open colectomy for colon cancer. N Engl J Med 2004;350: 2050–2059.
68. Paty PB, Nash GM, Baron P, et al. Long-term results of local excision for rectal cancer. Ann Surg 2002;236:522–529; discussion 529–530.
69. Saclarides TJ. Transanal endoscopic microsurgery: a single surgeon's experience. Arch Surg 1998;133:598–599.
70. Rothenberger DA, Garcia-Aguilar J. Role of local excision in the treatment of rectal cancer. Semin Surg Oncol 2000;19: 367–375.
71. Blair S, Ellenhorn JD. Transanal excision for low rectal cancers is curative in early-stage disease with favorable histology. Am Surg 2000;66:817–820.
72. Furst A, Burghofer K, Hutzel L, Jauch KW. Neorectal reservoir is not the functional principle of the colonic J-pouch: the volume of a short colonic J-pouch does not differ from a straight coloanal anastomosis. Dis Colon Rectum 2002;45:660–667.
73. Furst A, Suttner S, Agha A, Beham A, Jauch KW. Colonic J-pouch vs. coloplasty following resection of distal rectal cancer: early results of a prospective, randomized, pilot study. Dis Colon Rectum 2003;46:1161–1166.
74. Ho YH, Brown S, Heah SM, et al. Comparison of J-pouch and coloplasty pouch for low rectal cancers: a randomized, controlled trial investigating functional results and comparative anastomotic leak rates. Ann Surg 2002;236:49–55.
75. Heald RJ. Total mesorectal exsicion (TME). Acta Chir Iugosl 2000;47:17–18.
76. Merchant NB, Guillem JG, Paty PB, et al. T3N0 rectal cancer: results following sharp mesorectal excision and no adjuvant therapy. J Gastrointest Surg 1999;3:642–647.
77. Wolmark N, Wieand HS, Hyams DM, et al. Randomized trial of postoperative adjuvant chemotherapy with or without radiotherapy for carcinoma of the rectum: National Surgical Adjuvant Breast and Bowel Project Protocol R-02. J Natl Cancer Inst 2000; 92:388–396.
78. Meagher AP, Ward RL. Current evidence does not support routine adjuvant radiotherapy for rectal cancer. ANZ J Surg 2002;72:835–840.
79. Masui H, Ike H, Yamaguchi S, Oki S, Shimada H. Male sexual function after autonomic nerve-preserving operation for rectal cancer. Dis Colon Rectum 1996;39:1140–1145.
80. Waddell WR, Ganser GF, Cerise EJ, Loughry RW. Sulindac for polyposis of the colon. Am J Surg 1989;157:175–179.
81. Giardiello FM, Yang VW, Hylind LM, et al. Primary chemoprevention of familial adenomatous polyposis with sulindac. N Engl J Med 2002;346:1054–1059.
82. Ishikawa H, Akedo I, Suzuki T, Narahara H, Otani T. Adverse effects of sulindac used for prevention of colorectal cancer. J Natl Cancer Inst 1997;89:1381.
83. Baron JA, Cole BF, Sandler RS, et al. A randomized trial of aspirin to prevent colorectal adenomas. N Engl J Med 2003;348(10): 891–899.
84. Sandler RS, Halabi S, Baron JA, et al. A randomized trial of aspirin to prevent colorectal adenomas in patients with previous colorectal cancer. N Engl J Med 2003;348:883–890.

110

Medical and Psychosocial Issues in Transplant Survivors

Karen L. Syrjala, Paul Martin, Joachim Deeg, and Michael Boeckh

Survival rates for hematopoietic cell transplantation (HCT) have improved with advances in supportive care that have reduced acute, transplant-related mortality. More than 40,000 transplants were performed worldwide in 2002, mostly for the treatment of leukemia, lymphoma, or multiple myeloma[1] (see Chapters 63 through 69 for discussions of specific diseases). The probability of successful transplantation is generally greater for patients transplanted early in their disease course, for younger patients, and for patients who receive stem cells from donors whose human leukocyte antigens (HLA) match the patient's. For survivors who receive HCT for acute leukemia or chronic myeloid leukemia and who remain free of disease after 2 years, the probability of living 5 or more years is 89%.[2]

HCT survivors experience short and long-term problems similar to those of many other cancer survivors who receive systemic high-dose therapy. In addition, patients receiving stem cells from a related or unrelated donor (allogeneic) rather than receiving their own stem cells (autologous) experience complications related to the immunologic reaction of donor cells against the patient's cells and tissues. Chronic graft-versus-host disease (GVHD) occurs in about 60% of patients who survive the acute transplant-related toxicities and can persist for years. It is generally treated with immunosuppressive medications, often including high-dose glucocorticoids. Extended immunosuppression leads to several other vulnerabilities in allogeneic HCT recipients beyond that which is seen in other cancer survivors. Some of these effects result from GVHD itself; others are a consequence of the treatments used for GVHD.

Although evidence-based conclusions from HCT clinical trials are plentiful, research on survivor medical and quality of life issues is limited and largely descriptive. Randomized controlled trials are few, in part because they are difficult to accomplish with widely dispersed patients who, until recently, represented a small percentage of the cancer survivor population. Effective treatment of chronic GVHD without dependence on high-dose glucocorticoids is a primary need for improving both survival and quality of life for allogeneic transplant survivors. Evidence is needed regarding the risks and effective treatments for fungal and pulmonary complications as well as bone- and joint-related problems such as osteoporosis and avascular necrosis.

Chronic Graft-Versus-Host Disease

Chronic GVHD is a pleiotropic syndrome with onset generally occurring between 3 and 24 months after HCT from an allogeneic donor.[3–5] Clinical manifestations of chronic GVHD are highly variable and resemble an overlap of several collagen vascular diseases, with frequent involvement of the skin, liver, eyes, mouth, sinuses, and esophagus, and less-frequent involvement of serosal surfaces, lungs, lower gastrointestinal tract, female genitalia, and fascia. Major causes of morbidity include scleroderma, contractures, ulceration, keratoconjunctivitis, esophageal and vaginal strictures, obstructive pulmonary disease, and weight loss with or without malabsorption. Uncontrolled chronic GVHD interferes with immune reconstitution and is strongly associated with increased risks of opportunistic infections and death.

Studies have provided a good understanding of risk factors for development of chronic GVHD and risk factors for mortality among patients with newly diagnosed GVHD. Five-year survival rates for patients with newly diagnosed *standard-risk* chronic GVHD have remained at approximately 70%, and 5-year survival rates for those with "high-risk" chronic GVHD have remained at 40% to 50%. In aggregate, only 50% of patients with chronic GVHD are able to discontinue immunosuppressive treatment within 5 years after the diagnosis, and 10% require continued treatment beyond 5 years. The remaining 40% die or develop recurrent malignancy before chronic GVHD resolves. Prolonged treatment with high-dose glucocorticoids causes considerable morbidity, leading to a desperate need for agents that can decrease the dependence on steroids for controlling the disease.

Prevention of Chronic GVHD

Results of retrospective analyses and Phase 3 clinical trials have identified a variety of risk factors for the development of chronic GVHD after allogeneic HCT (Table 110.1). Risk factors that cannot be controlled as part of medical management include older age of the patient, the use of a female donor, and the use of an unrelated donor or HLA-mismatched related donor as opposed to an HLA-identical sibling.[3,5] Risk factors that can be controlled as part of medical management are related to the use of marrow versus growth factor-mobilized blood as the source of hematopoietic cells, the numbers of T cells and CD34-positive cells in the graft, the use of prednisone for prevention of GVHD after the transplant, and the duration of cyclosporine administration.

The use of growth factor-mobilized peripheral blood as opposed to marrow as a source of stem cells clearly increases the risk of chronic GVHD[6] and may prolong the duration of immunosuppression needed to control chronic GVHD.[7] These results are consistent with findings that the risk of chronic GVHD increases after administration of nonmobilized buffy coat cells to prevent rejection after marrow transplantation for treatment of aplastic anemia.[8] Despite these observations, the choice between mobilized blood cells and marrow depends primarily on the evaluation of other endpoints, such as survival or relapse-free survival, which are more important than the risk of chronic GVHD per se.

The increased risk of chronic GVHD after transplantation with mobilized blood could reflect the 10-fold-higher number of T cells in the graft as compared to marrow. However, results of retrospective studies that correlated the cellular composition of mobilized apheresis products with a variety of outcomes after transplant did not support this interpretation. Instead, chronic GVHD was associated with high numbers of CD34-positive cells in the graft.[9,10] Mechanisms to explain this unexpected association remain to be defined.

Results of an early randomized trial[11] and many Phase 2 studies have suggested that depletion of T cells from the graft decreases the risk of chronic GVHD, and this suggestion was initially confirmed by results from a large retrospective review of data from the International Bone Marrow Transplant Registry (IBMTR).[12] A subsequent review of data in the IBMTR, however, unexpectedly showed a higher risk of chronic GVHD among patients who received HLA-mismatched marrow treated with "narrow specificity" antibodies compared to those who received marrow that was treated by other methods or that was not treated.[13] Preliminary results of a recent randomized controlled trial showed that T-cell depletion did not decrease the risk of chronic GVHD.[14] Recent evidence has suggested that depletion of donor T cells by in vivo administration of rabbit antithymocyte globulin (ATG) may reduce the risk of chronic GVHD.[15]

Taken together, the T-cell depletion trials and ATG trials have produced inconsistent results regarding the relationship between the T-cell content of the graft and risk of chronic GVHD, making it difficult to reach a general conclusion. The possible association between the number of CD34 cells in the graft and risk of chronic GVHD needs confirmation from additional studies.

Four randomized clinical trials have evaluated the effects of prophylactic glucocorticoid administration after allogeneic marrow transplantation.[16–19] In each of these studies, the primary endpoint was the development of acute GVHD, and chronic GVHD was a secondary endpoint. Results with respect to chronic GVHD were inconsistent, despite enrollment of 108 to 186 patients in each study. The weight of the evidence suggests that prophylactic administration of glucocorticoids after marrow transplantation is likely to increase rather than decrease the risk of chronic GVHD.

Two randomized trials[20,21] and one sequential cohort study[22] have evaluated the risk of chronic GVHD as related to the duration of cyclosporine administration. Taken together, the consistent results of these trials suggest that prolonged administration of cyclosporine might yield a modest reduction in the risk of chronic GVHD, but the effect was too small to reach statistical significance in the two randomized trials.

Results from Phase 2 studies suggested that thalidomide might be effective for treatment of chronic GVHD, but results from a Phase 3 study showed that mortality was increased when thalidomide was administered before the onset of chronic GVHD.[23]

Treatment of Chronic GVHD

Anecdotal experience and retrospective reviews during the 1970s and early 1980s demonstrated that untreated clinical extensive chronic GVHD generally causes severe disability related to scleroderma, contractures, strictures, pulmonary disease, and keratoconjunctivitis (Table 110.2).[3–5] Administration of prednisone late in the natural history of the disease provided little benefit. Early administration of prednisone appeared to prevent disability but did not greatly affect survival. Retrospective reviews have identified a variety of factors associated with an increased risk of mortality from causes other than recurrent malignancy among patients with chronic GVHD.[3,5] The most consistently reported findings indicate an increased risk of transplant-related mortality among patients who have direct progression from acute to chronic GVHD or a platelet count less than 100,000/μL at the diagnosis of GVHD. The term high-risk chronic GVHD has been used to describe cases with either of these characteristics, whereas standard-risk chronic GVHD excludes cases with either of these characteristics.

An early double-blind randomized trial was carried out to determine whether administration of azathioprine together with prednisone might be more effective than prednisone alone for treatment of newly diagnosed chronic GVHD.[24] The results unexpectedly showed inferior outcomes for patients in the azathioprine arm. The difference in survival was attributed to an increased incidence of infections in the azathioprine arm.

Results of sequential Phase 2 studies suggested that survival among patients with high-risk chronic GVHD might be improved by combined treatment with cyclosporine and prednisone.[24,25] In a subsequent randomized prospective trial, however, cyclosporine did not provide a survival benefit, although the incidence of avascular necrosis was decreased in the cyclosporine arm, suggesting a steroid-sparing effect.[26]

Results of several Phase 2 studies suggested that thalidomide might be effective for treatment of steroid-refractory chronic GVHD, but subsequent randomized trials showed no benefit with the use of thalidomide.[27,28]

TABLE 110.1. Clinical trials of prevention of chronic graft-versus-host disease.

Author	*Reference*	*Year*	*No. of patients*	*Randomized (Y/N)*	*Diagnosis/ stage of disease*	*Intervention/design*	*Follow-up*	*Relative risk/outcomes*	*Survival statistics*	*Conclusions/ comments*
Mitsuyasu et al.	11	1986	40	Y	Leukemia	T-cell-depleted marrow compared with unmodified marrow; methotrexate or cyclosporine also given to prevent GVHD; RCT	1–2 years	Decreased incidence of chronic GVHD with T-cell-depleted marrow (5% versus 25%)	No significant difference between arms	T-cell depletion increased the risk of recurrent malignancy after the transplant
Marmont et al.	12	1991	3,211	N	Leukemia	T-cell-depleted marrow compared with unmodified marrow; retrospective multicenter cohort study	3–8 years	Relative risk of chronic GVHD = 0.56 with T-cell depletion compared to unmodified marrow ($P < 0.0001$)	Decreased leukemia-free survival with T-cell depletion	T-cell depletion increased the risk of recurrent malignancy after the transplant
Champlin et al.	13	2000	1,868	N	Leukemia	T-cell-depleted marrow compared with unmodified marrow; depletion with "narrow specificity" antibodies compared to other methods; retrospective multicenter cohort study	4 months to 11 years	Relative risk of chronic GVHD = 1.5 for marrow treated with "narrow specificity" antibodies compared to untreated marrow ($P < 0.0003$)	Leukemia-free survival better after T-cell depletion with "narrow specificity" antibodies compared to other methods; no significant difference in leukemia-free survival with "narrow specificity" antibodies compared to unmodified marrow	The use of "broad specificity" methods that deplete natural killer cells and T cells from HLA-mismatched donor marrow appeared to have detrimental effects on outcome
Wagner et al.	14	2002	410	Y	Mostly leukemia	T-cell-depleted marrow and immunosuppression with cyclosporine compared with unmodified marrow and immunosuppression with methotrexate and cyclosporine; multicenter RCT	2–6 years	Incidence of chronic GVHD = 24% with T-cell depletion and 29% with unmodified marrow	T-cell depletion was associated with an increased risk of recurrent malignancy among patients with chronic myeloid leukemia; leukemia-free survival was similar in the two arms for patients with other diseases	T-cell depletion decreased the risk of severe acute GVHD but did not improve survival
Bacigalupo et al.	15	2001	109	Y	Hematologic malignancies	Conventional pretransplant conditioning with or without rabbit antithymocyte globulin administered at two different doses; two consecutive RCT		Incidence of chronic GVHD = 39% with ATG and 62% without ($P = 0.04$)	No difference in survival between arms	Use of ATG at the higher dose was associated with an increased risk of infections
Storb et al.	16	1990	147	Y	Mostly leukemia	Posttransplant immunosuppression using methotrexate plus cyclosporine, with or without prednisone administered throughout the first 35 days after transplant; two studies, one RCT and the other a prospective cohort study	1.5–3 years	Incidence of chronic GVHD = 62% with prednisone and 40% without ($P = 0.01$)	No difference in survival between arms	Use of prednisone increased the risk of chronic GVHD

Deeg et al.	180	1997	122	Y	Hematologic malignancy	Posttransplant immunosuppression with cyclosporine with or without methylprednisolone administered between days 7 and 72 after transplant; RCT	0.5–3.5 years	Incidence of chronic GVHD = 44% with methylprednisolone and 21% without ($P = 0.02$)	No difference in survival between arms	Incidence of acute GVHD was 60% with methylprednisolone and 73% without ($P = 0.01$)
Chao et al.	18	2000	193	Y	Leukemia	Posttransplant immunosuppression using methotrexate plus cyclosporine with or without prednisone administered between days 7 and 180 after transplant; RCT	1–6 years	Incidence of chronic GVHD = 46% with prednisone and 52% without ($P = 0.38$)	No difference in survival between arms	Incidence of acute GVHD was 18% with prednisone and 20% without ($P = 0.6$)
Ruutu et al.	181	2000	108	Y	Hematologic malignancy	Posttransplant immunosuppression using methotrexate plus cyclosporine with or without methylprednisolone administered between days 14 and 110 after transplant; RCT	4–9 years	Incidence of chronic GVHD = 35% with methylprednisolone and 48% without ($P = 0.17$)	No difference in survival between arms	Incidence of acute GVHD was 19% with methylprednisolone and 56% without ($P = 0.0001$)
Storb et al.	20	1997	103	Y	Mostly leukemia	Posttransplant immunosuppression using methotrexate plus cyclosporine administered to day 60 or day 180 among patients who did not have GVHD on day 60; RCT	1–10 years	Incidence of chronic GVHD = 54% in the day 60 arm and 43% in the day 180 arm ($P = 0.26$)	Possible increase in transplant-related mortality in day 60 arm among patients with GVHD before day 60	No benefit from prolonged administration of cyclosporine among patients who did not have acute GVHD
Kansu et al.	21	2001	162	Y	Mostly leukemia	Patients eligible if they had a prior history of acute GVHD or if skin biopsy showed histologic evidence of GVHD on day 80; RCT comparing administration of cyclosporine for 6 or 24 months	2–9 years	Incidence of chronic GVHD = 39% in the 24-month arm and 51% in the 6-month arm ($P = 0.24$); hazard ratio = 0.76 ($P = 0.25$)	No difference in survival	Prolonged administration of cyclosporine did not greatly decrease the incidence of chronic GVHD
Mengarelli et al.	22	2003	57	N	Hematologic malignancy	Patients received peripheral blood cells from an HLA-identical sibling, and cyclosporine was administered for either 6 or 12 months in two consecutive retrospective cohorts	1–4 years	Incidence of chronic GVHD = 25% in the 12-month group and 69% in the 6-month group; hazard ratio = 0.2 (adjusted $P = 0.008$)	No difference in survival	Prolonged administration of cyclosporine appeared to decrease the incidence of chronic GVHD
Chao et al.	23	1996	59	Y	Hematologic malignancy	Administration of thalidomide or placebo beginning at day 80 after transplant; double-blind RCT	6 months to 3 years	Incidence of chronic GVHD = 64% with thalidomide and 38% with placebo ($P = 0.06$)	Increased mortality in the thalidomide arm ($P = 0.006$)	Administration of thalidomide was unexpectedly found to be harmful

GVHD, graft-versus-host disease; RCT, randomized controlled trial; ATG, antithymocyte globulin.

TABLE 110.2. Clinical trials of chronic graft-versus-host disease.

Author	Reference	Year	No. of patients	Randomized (Y/N)	Diagnosis/stage of disease	Intervention/design	Follow-up	Relative risk/ outcomes	Survival statistics	Conclusions/comments
Sullivan et al.	25	1988	126	Y	Newly diagnosed chronic GVHD and platelet count >100,000/µL	Prednisone with or without azathioprine; double-blind RCT	Minimum of 3.8 years	Not stated	47% survival at 5 years with prednisone plus azathioprine, 61% with prednisone plus placebo ($P = 0.03$)	Results demonstrate inferior outcomes when azathioprine was used to treat chronic GVHD
Koc et al.	26	2002	287	Y	Newly diagnosed chronic GVHD and platelet count >100,000/µL	Prednisone with or without continued administration of cyclosporine; RCT	4–14 years	Incidence of nonrelapse mortality at 5 years = 17% with prednisone plus cyclosporine, 13% with prednisone; hazard ratio = 1.55 ($P = 0.11$)	67% survival at 5 years with prednisone plus cyclosporine, 72% with prednisone; hazard ratio = 1.35 ($P = 0.13$) 61% survival without recurrent malignancy at 5 years with prednisone plus cyclosporine, 71% with prednisone; hazard ratio = 1.51 ($P = 0.03$)	Subset analysis suggested increased mortality among patients with chronic GVHD that evolved directly from acute GVHD Incidence of avascular necrosis was lower with prednisone plus cyclosporine than with prednisone alone
Arora et al.	27	2001	54	Y	Newly diagnosed chronic GVHD	Prednisone and cyclosporine with or without thalidomide (200–800 mg/day); double-blind RCT	0.5–4.8 years	Incidence of partial or complete response at 2, 6, and 12 months = 83%, 88% and 85% with thalidomide, 89%, 84%, and 73% without thalidomide	66% at 2 years with thalidomide, 54% without thalidomide ($P = 0.85$)	High response rate was observed in both groups; study was terminated early due to low accrual rate
Koc et al.	28	2000	52	Y	Newly diagnosed chronic GVHD with platelet count <100,000/µL or progressive onset from acute GVHD as high-risk features	Prednisone and cyclosporine or tacrolimus with or without thalidomide (200–800 mg /day); double-blind RCT	Not reported	No statistically significant difference in transplant-related mortality	49% survival at 4 years with thalidomide, 47% without thalidomide ($P = 0.87$)	Thalidomide caused intolerable side effects, leading to premature discontinuation of administration in 92% of patients; the duration of thalidomide administration was not sufficient to allow assessment of efficacy

Phase 2 studies have been carried out to evaluate the use of many immunosuppressive agents for treatment of steroid-refractory chronic GVHD. The small number of enrolled patients, the widely divergent enrollment criteria and poorly defined efficacy criteria, and the lack of controls hamper the interpretation of these studies. Efficacy is generally reported as improvement in symptoms or signs of chronic GVHD at any time after introduction of the additional immunosuppressive treatment. The duration of clinical improvement is typically not taken into account, and survival data are difficult to interpret because of variable follow-up and possible selection biases in enrollment. In the absence of pharmacokinetic evaluation, studies of this type typically do not add useful information to the available safety profile of approved immunosuppressive agents. Trial designs with prior specification of criteria for judging efficacy according to robust and meaningful endpoints would help to make the results of Phase 2 studies more informative.

Emerging Challenges in Chronic GVHD

Advances in supportive care have reduced morbidity, but survival for patients with newly diagnosed chronic GVHD has not changed since the mid-1980s.[3,5] In the past, investigators have taken the highly empirical approach of testing virtually any available immunosuppressive agent for treatment of chronic GVHD, because the pathophysiology of chronic GVHD is complex and poorly understood. Development of a more-direct approach will require an improved understanding of the pathophysiologic mechanisms leading to chronic GVHD.

Infections

A susceptibility to late infectious complications persists because of residual immunodeficiency that is observed in all HCT recipients, not only those with allogeneic donors,[29] although infection risk is increased with the additional immunosuppression associated with chronic GVHD and its treatment (Table 110.3).

Bacterial

There is a significant risk for severe infection with encapsulating bacteria (*Streptococcus pneumoniae, Haemophilus influenzae*) after HCT in the setting of chronic GVHD.[30] Patients may develop rapidly progressive disease, which is often fatal. The presumed explanation for bacteremic pneumococcal infections is that HCT patients lose and do not subsequently make opsonizing antibody to encapsulated gram-positive organisms, even after recovery from infection.[30] Patients also respond poorly to immunization with prototype pneumococcal vaccines for the first 1 to 2 years after transplant, although response again improves with time.[31,32] Immunization with the available pneumococcal vaccines provides incomplete protection for those most in need, that is, patients with chronic GVHD.[33]

Antibacterial prophylaxis is recommended in patients with chronic GVHD to prevent both bacteremic pneumococcal and other infection, although no randomized placebo-controlled trials have been performed.[34] The 23-valent pneumococcal polysaccharide vaccine (12 and 24 months after transplantation) and the *Haemophilus influenzae* B conjugate vaccine (12, 14, and 24 months after transplantation) are recommended in standard guidelines.[34] However, these vaccinations are not 100% protective; the 7-valent conjugated pneumococcal vaccine has not been evaluated in transplant recipients.

Althouogh penicillin appears to work for this indication, the recent emergence of penicillin-resistant pneumococci make it a less preferable choice.[35] Rather, trimethoprim-sulfamethoxazole (TMP-SMX) given once daily (80mg TMP component) provides protection both against *Pneumocystis jiroveci* pneumonia (PCP), encapsulated bacteria, and possibly also against toxoplasmosis. Controlled trial data are not available to evaluate the efficacy of such prophylaxis, but retrospective study of nonrandomized treatment groups indicates that patients with chronic GVHD who receive TMP-SMX prophylaxis have a significantly lower incidence of infection.[29] Oral penicillins should be reserved for patients who are unable to tolerate daily TMP-SMX. No reports exist about new quinolones or macrolides for this indication.

Because infection with other organisms including both *Staphylococcus* species and gram-negative aerobic bacteria also occurs, empirical antibiotic treatment of HCT patients admitted with clinical sepsis should include broad-spectrum coverage until the identity of the infecting organisms is known.

Viral

Varicella-zoster virus (VZV) disease is the most common viral infection late after HCT.[36–40] Median time of onset is 5 months after transplant, and most cases occur within the first year. However, VZV disease can occur up to several years after transplantation, especially in the setting of chronic GVHD. A subgroup at particularly high risk for VZV infection is VZV-seropositive allogeneic transplant recipients of age greater than 10 years who received total-body irradiation (TBI). In one study, the risk of VZV disease was 44% during the first 3 years after transplant among these patients.[41] Abdominal infections without skin manifestations are observed occasionally. These manifestations carry a high mortality, and the clinical hallmark is rapidly rising transaminases. In an unpublished randomized double-blind trial, oral acyclovir at a dose of 800mg twice daily for 1 year prevented VZV infection after HCT without rebound disease after discontinuation of prophylaxis. This treatment may be particularly useful in patients with continued chronic GVHD.[37] Strategies that used lower doses for a shorter duration resulted in a high number of infections after discontinuation of prophylaxis.[42]

Cytomegalovirus (CMV) seropositive transplant recipients and recipients of stem cell products from a seropositive donor continue to be at risk for late CMV disease if they have chronic GVHD and/or have reactivated CMV during the first 100 days after transplantation.[43–46] The majority of late disease occurs during the first year after transplantation, but there may be cases until 3 years after transplant if immunosuppression continues. Clinical manifestation of late CMV disease may differ from the typical pneumonia and gastrointestinal disease seen earlier. Cases of retinitis, late marrow failure, and encephalitis have been described.[47] Outcome of late CMV disease is poor, with pneumonia having the highest

TABLE 110.3. Infections after hematopoietic cell transplantation (HCT).

Author	*Reference*	*Year*	*No. of patients*	*Randomized (Y/N)*	*Diagnosis/ stage of disease*	*Intervention/design RCT*	*Median follow-up 12 months*	*Relative risk/hazard ratio*	*Conclusions/results*
Ljungman et al.	42	1986	42	Y	Various			Not reported	Acyclovir prophylaxis given for 6 months leads to prevention of HSV and VZV infection during prophylaxis but frequent recurrence of VZV after discontinuation
Locksley et al.	36	1985	1,394	N	Various	Cohort study	NR	3.6 (allogeneic transplantation) 1.6 (chronic GVHD) 1.5 (ATG)	Risk factors for dissemination of VZV or death: GVHD (all deaths within 9 months after transplantation)
Han et al.	37	1994	1,186	N	Various	Cohort study	NR	Not reported	VZV seropositive + age > 10 years + radiation pretransplant: 44% VZV infection
Boeckh et al.	46	2003	146	N	Allogeneic, CMV seropositive	Cohort study	NR	3.3 (CMV reactivation <day 100 for late CMV disease)	Late CMV disease common Late viremia associated with poor survival
Peggs et al.	48	2000	81	N	Allogeneic, CMV seropositive	Prospective cohort study	13.5 months	Not reported	No late CMV disease with PCR-based surveillance and preemptive therapy for 6 months
Marr et al.	49	2002	1,682	N	All types of transplants	Retrospective cohort study	NR	6.7 (GVHD) 6.6 (CMV disease)	Late aspergillosis common GVHD, CMV disease increase risk of aspergillosis >6 months
Fukuda et al.	50	2003	163	N	Nonmyeloma blative conditioning	Cohort study	23 months	2.8 (acute GVHD) 3.7 (chronic GVHD) 13.3 (CMV disease)	15% invasive mold infection 5% invasive candidiasis Steroids associated with poor outcome of disease

HSV, herpes simplex virus; VZV, varicella-zoster virus; CMV, cytomegalovirus; PCR, polymerase chain reaction; NR, not reported.

mortality.[46] About one-third of patients who survive the first episode of late disease will suffer a relapse after a median of 3 months.[46] Continued monitoring [pp65 antigenemia, polymerase chain reaction (PCR) for CMV DNA] and use of preemptive therapy in high-risk patients is useful in the management of patients at risk for late CMV disease.[46,48]

HCT recipients with chronic GVHD continue to be at risk for acquisition of respiratory virus infections such as respiratory syncytial virus, influenza viruses, and parainfluenza viruses. Seasonal vaccination of close contacts with the inactivated vaccine is recommended.[34] Recipient vaccination starting at 6 months after transplantation is also recommended.[34] Less commonly, late impaired graft function has been described in association with human herpes virus (HHV)-6 and human parvovirus B 19.

Fungal

Late invasive aspergillosis is an increasingly frequent event in allogeneic graft recipients with chronic GVHD and preceding viral infections (i.e., CMV, respiratory viruses), possibly due to an immunosuppressive effect of these viruses.[49] Recipients of lower-dose conditioning regimens who have GVHD are also at risk for late mold infections.[50] In contrast, invasive candidiasis occurs infrequently after day 100.[50,51] The outcomes of both mold and candidal infections in this setting remain poor. Mold-active drugs are now available (itraconazole, voriconazole). However, the efficacy and toxicity of long-term prophylaxis have not been tested in randomized fashion in this setting. Sensitive diagnostic tests (aspergillus galactomannan assay, PCR) can be used for early diagnosis of disease.

Pneumocystis jiroveci Pneumonia (PCP)

With the availability of effective prophylaxis, early cases of *Pneumocystis jiroveci* pneumonia (PCP) are only rarely seen late after transplant.[52] Most cases occur in a setting of poor adherence or in patients who are unable to tolerate TMP-SMX because of side effects or allergy, or who received ineffective alternative prophylaxis regimens.[53] Standard guidelines following allogeneic transplantation recommend prophylaxis for the duration of drug-induced immunosuppression.[34] However, the optimal duration of prophylaxis after autologous transplant is currently poorly defined, as recent data suggest that there is late PCP in autologous graft recipients as well.[54] Approximately 15% to 30% of HCT recipients require alternative prophylaxis regimens at some time after transplantation.[55] Reasons for requiring alternative prophylaxis include allergy to TMP-SMX, gastrointestinal intolerance, increased transaminases, and neutropenia. Very few data exist on the efficacy and toxicity of alternative prophylaxis regimens. Daily dapsone appears to be superior to inhaled pentamidine.[55] As it has overall superior results, TMP-SMX should be given whenever possible. Desensitization should be attempted in all patients with allergy to TMP-SMX.[52] Only limited data exist on atovaquone.[56]

The clinical syndrome of PCP is indistinguishable both clinically and radiologically from other nonbacterial pneumonias. The diagnosis is established either by bronchoalveolar lavage (BAL), induced sputum, or thoracoscopic or open lung biopsy. The treatment of choice is high-dose intravenous TMP-SMX in combination with a short course of corticosteroids based on results in human immunodeficiency virus (HIV)-infected patients.[57] Of the alternative agents used in the HIV setting (intravenous pentamidine, atovaquone, clindamycin/primaquine, dapsone/trimethoprim, and trimetrexate), clindamycin/primaquine appears to be most effective for treatment of disease.[58]

Distinctions in Adult and Pediatric Presentation, Course, and Treatment

Virtually no data exist on differences in infection risk and outcome among survivors of HCT. Whether immune reconstitution is faster in younger individuals has not been studied. However, if chronic GVHD is present, all available data suggest that children have the same infectious risk as adults. The exposure to respiratory viruses may even be higher if children are exposed to group settings. Certain contraindications for use of antimicrobials (e.g., quinolones) should be considered in the management of children.

Emerging Challenges in Infection

The major challenge is to design infection prevention strategies for survivors of HCT with persistent severe immunosuppression. These patients are not only at risk for VZV, PCP, and encapsulated bacteria but also for CMV and invasive mold infections. Strategies need to be easy to administer, effective, and well tolerated. With increasing long-term use of antimicrobials, resistance may become a challenge in the future.

Other Medical Complications

Pulmonary

Chronic pulmonary complications affect at least 15% to 20% of patients after HCT, and pulmonary dysfunction is an important risk factor for delayed mortality. However, current knowledge is based exclusively on retrospective analyses (Table 110.4).

Late-Onset Pneumonitis

Late-onset interstitial pneumonitis usually occurs in patients with chronic GVHD.[59] Most require therapy with immunosuppressive agents; treatment with bronchodilators is usually ineffective. However, late pneumonias occur also in the absence of GVHD, and even after autologous transplantation in patients who have not previously had pulmonary disease, with an incidence of 31% at 4 years. The prognosis is generally good with bacterial etiology, but mortality reaches 80% with fungal or polymicrobial pneumonia.[54]

Restrictive Pulmonary Disease

Pretransplant and posttransplant abnormal pulmonary function tests (PFTs), in particular decreased diffusing capacity (DLCO) and increased oxygen gradient [P(A-a) O_2], are associated with higher posttransplant mortality than seen in

TABLE 110.4. Pulmonary complications after HCT.

Author	Reference	Year	No. of patients	Randomized (Y/N)	Diagnosis/stage of disease	Intervention/ design	Follow-up	Relative risk/outcomes/predictors	Disease-free survival (or survival statistics)	Conclusions/results
Chien et al.	63	2003	1,131	N	Various	Retrospective cohort study	1–11 years	AFO associated with decrease in FEV_1 >5%/year, decreased pretransplant FEV_1/FVC, acute and chronic GVHD, respiratory virus infection Among patients with chronic GVHD, those with AFO have a higher risk of mortality (HR 2.3, 95% CI 1.63.3) than patients without AFO Risk increases with increasing age (RR 1.7–2.5) for patients more than 20 to more than 60 years of age and patients with quiescent (RR 1.6) or progressive onset (RR 1.9) of chronic GVHD	AFO attribution to mortality, all patients (those with chronic GVHD): 9% (22), 12% (27), 18% (40) at 3, 5, and 10 years, respectively	75% of AFO occurred in patients with chronic GVHD AFO is more frequent than previously reported and has a major negative impact on long-term survival, particularly in patients with chronic GVHD
Chen et al.	54	2003	1,359	N	Various	Retrospective cohort study	0.01–5 years	Risk factors include: patient age, HLA non-identity, and chronic GVHD among allogeneic recipients (none identified for autologous)	Cumulative incidence of first pneumonia at 4 years was 31% (18% for autologous, 34% for HLA-identical allogeneic, 39% for other allogeneic/ unrelated) Survival rates were best with bacterial (71%), and worst with multimicrobial pneumonias (8%)	Pneumonia is frequent, even late after transplantation and poses a significant risk, particularly among patients more than 40 years of age, and in patients with chronic GVHD

Crawford et al.	60	1995	906	N	Various	Retrospective cohort study	1–9 years	Restrictive lung defect at 3 months after transplant or ≥15% decline in total lung capacity from baseline was associated with a twofold increase in risk of nonrelapse mortality (respiratory failure)	Death from respiratory failure occurred in 1.9% of patients with normal or unchanging total lung capacity, compared to 5.3% in patients with restrictive ventilatory defects; chronic GVHD did not appear to influence the rate of death with respiratory failure	Impaired total lung capacity, impaired airflow, and decreased diffusing capacity all had a negative impact on survival
Sullivan et al.	68	1996	250	Y	Various	IV immunoglobulin (500 mg/kg/month) between days 90 and days xvs. none; RCT		No difference in systemic infections; localized infections marginally more frequent in controls ($P = 0.07$); after 2 years total infections less common in controls ($P = 0.03$)	No difference	Prophylactic administration of IV immunoglobulin, in the absence of in the absence of hypogammaglobulin emia, has no demonstrable benefit, and in fact may delay endogenous immune recovery
Freudenberger et al.	69	2003	49 patients 161 controls	N	Various	Case-control study	Sequentially	Risk factors for bronchiolitis obliterans organizing pneumonia (BOOP): acute ($P = 0.002$) and chronic ($P = 0.02$) GVHD; progressive onset chronic GVHD ($P = 0.001$); skin involvement with acute (HR 4.6), and oral (HR 5.9) and gut involvement (HR 6.6)	5-year survival 31% in patients with BOOP vs. 45% in controls ($P = 0.05$)	BOOP is more frequent in patients with acute or chronic GVHD Steroid treatment has no recognizable therapeutic effect

AFO, air flow obstruction.

patients with normal tests.[60] Restrictive defects, defined as a decrease in total lung capacity to less than 80% of predicted values, are present in one-third of all patients studied. Changes are not correlated with the type of conditioning regimen or with chronic GVHD and generally do not produce severe symptoms. However, becuase they are associated with an increase in late mortality, routine evaluation of lung function after HCT is warranted.[61] Aggressive therapy of any infection of the respiratory tract is indicated.

Obstructive Pulmonary Disease

Air flow obstruction (AFO), defined as decreased expiratory airflow, in particular, a decrease in the proportion of air that can be exhaled over the first second of expiration, may represent sequelae to extensive restrictive changes in the small airways or may be related to small airway destruction.[62] Both acute and chronic GVHD are important risk factors for AFO, and thereby affect long-term survival, with 75% of AFO cases occurring among patients with chronic GVHD, particularly those with quiescent or progressive onset (see Table 110.4).[63] There is generally no response to bronchodilator treatment; 30% to 40% of patients improve on glucocorticoids. Few patients with end-stage disease have been treated successfully with cadaveric lung transplants.[64,65]

Bronchiolitis Obliterans

Progressive bronchiolitis obliterans has been reported in 10% of patients with chronic GVHD.[66,67] Chest radiographs may show hyperinflation of the lungs and flattening of the diaphragm, but abnormalities are best identified by high-resolution computed tomography (CT) scans (inspiratory and expiratory cuts). PFTs show a reduction in forced midexpiratory flow to 10% or 20% of predicted values and moderate to severe reduction in forced vital capacity. The diffusion capacity is usually normal. Pulmonary ventilation scans show decreased activity patterns corresponding to areas of obliteration of bronchiolar walls along with atelectatic areas. Histologic changes are thought to be due to a graft-versus-host reaction, possibly aggravated by infections.

The clinical course of bronchiolitis varies from mild, with slow deterioration, to diffuse necrotizing fatal bronchiolitis. Severe disease may not respond to glucocorticoids, but corticosteroids in combination with calcineurin inhibitors or possibly azathioprine can stabilize PFTs and improve outcome. It is of note that a randomized trial examining the effect of intravenous immunoglobulin on chronic GVHD and bronchiolitis showed a marked decrease in the incidence of obliterative bronchiolitis in all patients such that an effect of intravenous Ig was not apparent.[68]

Bronchiolitis obliterans organizing pneumonia (BOOP) histologically shows polypoid masses of granulation tissue in the bronchioles and alveolar sacs as well as infiltration of alveolar septa by mononuclear cells. A recent analysis of results in 6,523 patients transplanted at the Fred Hutchinson Cancer Research Center revealed 51 cases of BOOP, all but 2 after allogeneic transplants.[69,70] BOOP was diagnosed at 5 to 2,819 (median, 108) days after HCT. The chest radiograph was abnormal in 47 patients. Most patients presented with fever, dyspnea, or cough, but 23% were asymptomatic. Most patients respond to glucocorticosteroids (1–2 mg/kg), which often must be continued for 6 months or longer.

Osteoporosis

Dual-energy X-ray absorptiometry (DEXA), a semiquantitative method to assess bone mineral density (BMD), is a validated method commonly used to detect osteoporosis [as defined by a Z-score of less than or equal to 2.5 standard deviations (SD) below sex- and age-related mean bone mineral density (BMD)] and osteopenia (defined by a Z-score of 1.0 to 2.4 SD below sex- and age-related mean BMD). Reduction of bone mass using DEXA has been reported in approximately 40% of men and women at 1 year after allogeneic HCT, with nontraumatic fractures in 11% by 3 years.[71] Risk factors include number of days and dose of glucocorticoids and number of days of cyclosporine or tacrolimus used for treating chronic GVHD.

In women, supplementation with estrogens and medroxyprogesterone can increase bone mass after HCT.[72] However, there may be increased risks of cardiovascular diseases (venous thrombosis, strokes, pulmonary emboli) and breast cancer in postmenopausal women given conjugated equine estrogen (0.625 mg) with medroxyprogesterone (2.5 mg).[73] This possibility is of concern because HCT recipients are at risk for secondary malignancies even without hormone therapy. Thus, the overall risks and benefits of hormone replacement in this situation remain to be determined. Lower doses of estrogen alone (after hysterectomy) or combined with progestin (in women with uterus intact) have been used for the management of bone loss in other patient populations.[74] Alternative regimens of bisphosphonates or hormone therapy have not been tested in clinical trials for efficacy or safety in women after HCT either for osteoporosis prevention or for postmenopausal symptoms.

Aseptic Necrosis

Avascular necrosis, especially in weight-bearing joints, is a classic side effect of glucocorticoid therapy and has been reported in 4% to 10% of allogeneic HCT survivors as early as 2 months and as late as 10 years posttransplant.[75–77] The hip is the joint most frequently affected (two-thirds of all cases). In most patients more than one joint is affected. One-third of patients with this disease required joint replacement at 2 to 42 months.[76] A case-control study of 87 patients with avascular necrosis found that posttransplant glucocorticoid use and TBI given in preparation for HCT were significant risk factors.[78] In addition to glucocorticoid therapy, male gender (relative risk, 4.2) and age greater than 15 years (relative risk, 3.8) were risk factors.

Endocrinology

Thyroid

Overt or compensated hypothyroidism and the "euthyroid sick syndrome" [ETS; low free triiodothyronine, free thyroxine, or both, along with normal or low thyroid-stimulating hormone (TSH)] are the most frequent thyroid abnormalities following transplantation (Table 110.5).[79] In one study ETS was associated with a significantly lower survival than observed in patients not affected by ETS (34.5% versus 96.2%; P less than 0.0001).[80,81] The risk of hypothyroidism is increased in patients who received pretransplant cranial

TABLE 110.5. Endocrine function, and growth and development.

Author	*Reference*	*Year*	*No. of patients*	*Randomized (Y/N)*	*Diagnosis/stage of disease*	*Intervention/design*	*Follow-up*	*Relative risk/outcomes/predictors*	*Conclusions/results*
Leung et al.	182	2000	43	N	Various with chemotherapy alone vs. chemo + cranial irradiation vs. chemo +TBI HCT	Retrospective cohort study	Median 13 years	Decreased height by 0.21 SD with chemo vs. 1.2 with chemo + cranial vs.1.33 with HCT	Importance of irradiation; growth hormone deficiency only with HCT
Thomas et al.	183	1993	49	N	Various	Retrospective cohort study	1–3 years	TBI 1,000 cGy single vs. 1,200–1,440 cGy fractionated dose; decrease in height of 0.2–0.9 SD vs. 0.09–0.2 SD; accentuated by cranial irradiation	Irradiation impairs growth; more so as single dose, and even further with cranial irradiation; growth hormone is helpful; should be instituted early (before the growth lag is >1.5 SD); dose should be adjusted for puberty
Sanders	184	1991	63 (55) (154)	N	Various	Retrospective cohort study	>12 years	Cyclophosphamide alone leads to little delay; TBI, single dose (71%; 83%) more than fractionated (49%; 58%) delays development	Cyclophosphamide by itself is well tolerated; little if any delay and normal rates of pregnancy Busulfan has intermediate effect TBI results in marked impairment
Sanders	83	2004	145/93 128/98	N	Various	Retrospective cohort study	1–12 years	Cyclophosphamide alone, 54% of women recover normal function; among men, 95% normal Sertoli cellfunction, 61% normal FSH; with busulfan/cyclophosphamide, only 2 of 93 women recovered ovarian function. Among men 65% showed azoospermia	Significant impairment of gonadal function with busulfan-containing regimens; less so with cyclophosphamide
Sanders	83	2004	562 498	N	Various	Retrospective cohort study	1–14 years	1,000 cGy single or 1,200–1,575 fractionated TBI; 83 women recovered ovarian function at 3–7 years; in men Leydig cell function was generally preserved, but Sertoli cell function was impaired in the majority	TBI has major impact; high frequency of sexual dysfunction, decrease in libido (associated with decreased testosterone in men) Chronic GVHD further impairs function. In women, systemic and topical vaginal hormone application is indicated

TBI, total-body irradiation; FSH, follicle-stimulating hormone.

irradiation or irradiation to the neck (e.g., for Hodgkin's disease).[82] All patients who have received irradiation to the thyroid should be followed for life with annual physical evaluation and thyroid function studies as indicated.[82]

Adrenal Glands

Many HCT patients receive glucocorticoid therapy. Endogenous cortisol production is suppressed, and any superimposed stress may cause a relative adrenal insufficiency. However, lasting adrenal dysfunction appears to be uncommon. One study in 78 patients showed 24% to have subnormal 11-deoxycortisol levels following discontinuation of glucocorticoid therapy at 1 to 8 years posttransplant. No patient was symptomatic, and the proportion of patients affected did not increase with time posttransplant.[83,84]

Hypothalamic–Pituitary Axis

Cranial irradiation, with or without TBI, affects the pituitary gland.[85–87] Thyrotropin-releasing hormone (TRH) may be low early posttransplant, and TRH-induced TSH responses may be subnormal and delayed.[85] Release of gonadotropin in response to luteinizing hormone-releasing hormone (LHRH) may be elevated.[85] Prolactin secretion and the pituitary–adrenal axis are usually intact. Growth hormone levels are decreased after cranial irradiation, and deficiency becomes apparent earlier with younger age at transplant.[83,86]

Gonadal Function, Puberty, and Fertility

Chemotherapy and TBI regimens used before hematopoietic transplantation for malignancies usually cause gonadal failure. Puberty and menarche are markedly delayed or may not occur, and fertility is infrequently regained in either men or women.

In men, testosterone levels usually decline as a result of transplant conditioning, but recover by 1 year posttransplant. Decreased libido, reduced bone mineral density, and low testosterone levels after transplant are indications for testosterone replacement unless contraindicated for other reasons. Risk for short stature is increased in males and those who are younger if they also receive TBI.[88]

Permanent ovarian failure invariably occurs in women who receive busulfan and cyclophosphamide pretransplant, whereas recovery of ovarian function has been observed after transplant in 54% of younger patients less than 26 years conditioned with cyclophosphamide only, and in 10% of younger patients who received more than 1,000 cGy TBI with cyclophosphamide. Pregnancy, although not common, has occurred following high-dose HCT, with increased risk for spontaneous abortion after TBI and preterm delivery of low birth weight babies. However, no increased risk of congenital abnormalities has been observed.[89,90] Lack of hormone therapy by 1 year after HCT for women with ovarian failure is a risk factor for sexual dissatisfaction at 3 years after HCT.[91] Vasomotor and sexual complaints 6 months after HCT improve after the start of hormone therapy, based on results from a nonrandomized pre–post cohort study.[92]

Safety of hormone therapy after transplantation has not been reported; thus, hormone replacement for survivors must be individualized. Males treated with testosterone may be at increased risk for prostate hypertrophy and prostate carcinoma. A nonrandomized cohort study has reported that hormone therapy in women does not influence chronic GVHD activity between 3 and 24 months after starting the hormone therapy (most of whom were also receiving cyclosporine) after allogeneic HCT.[93] Unfortunately, combined estrogen and progestin was recently found to increase the risk of cardiovascular disease and to increase the risk of invasive breast cancer after 3 years of therapy in naturally postmenopausal older women who had not had transplants, but no effect on survival was observed.[73] Human pituitary growth hormone replacement has been associated with increased risk of mortality from colorectal and Hodgkin's disease in a cohort study, a study not conducted in survivors of HCT.[94] These relative risks versus the consequences of delayed pubertal development, extremely short stature, attainment of peak bone mass, osteoporosis, and other quality of life factors need to be weighed along with hormone alternatives. If hormone therapy is elected, duration of treatment and a monitoring plan for complications should be part of the treatment plan.

Emerging Challenges in Medical Complications

Most treatment strategies for pulmonary, bone, and endocrine complications in transplant survivors are empirical rather than evidence based. Safety and toxicity of hormone therapies and efficacy of treatments for all medical complications need to be examined further, but in general are those that apply to the population at large.

Late Medical Complications

As large numbers of survivors live longer, late complications are being recognized. With fractionated TBI, 30% to 47% of HCT recipients have cataracts by 5 to 7 years; without TBI, 10% to 16% have cataracts, most often those who received corticosteroids for longer than 3 months.[95,96] Keratoconjunctivitis sicca syndrome is seen in up to 40% of patients with chronic GVHD. Other risk factors include female gender, older age, and methotrexate for GVHD prophylaxis.[97] Other than hepatitis, iron overload is the primary identified hepatic late effect; 22% of survivors showed fibrosis at a median follow-up of 5 years.[98] After mean follow-up of 7 years for four randomized trials comparing busulfan plus cyclophosphamide regimens with cyclophosphamide plus TBI in 488 survivors, late complications have not been noted to differ, with the exceptions of cataracts (more common after busulfan) and alopecia (more common after TBI).[96] Of greatest concern because of their potential lethality are second cancers and cardiovascular effects of transplantation.

Second Cancers

Lymphoproliferative disorders after HCT [posttransplant lymphoproliferative disorder (PTLD)], generally of B-cell lineage, occur mostly in allogeneic transplant recipients.[99,100] T-cell PTLD, non-Hodgkin's lymphoma and Hodgkin's disease have also been reported (Table 110.6). More than 80% of cases of PTLD are diagnosed within 1 year of transplantation, with peak occurrence (120 cases/10,000 patients/year) at 2 to 5 months.[101] The incidence is highest in patients

TABLE 110.6. Malignancies after HCT.

Author	*Reference*	*Year*	*No. of patients*	*Randomized (Y/N)*	*Diagnosis/ stage of disease*	*Intervention/ design*	*Duration of follow-up*	*Relative risk/outcomes/ predictors*	*Conclusions/results*
Metayer et al.	109	2003	56 patients, 168 controls	N	Hodgkin's disease; non-Hodgkin's lymphoma	Multicenter retrospective case-control study	Not reported	Pretransplant use of mechlorethamine (P = 0.04) or chlorambucil (P = 0.009) significantly increased the risk of MDS/AML after autologous transplantation; conditioning with TBI ≥1,320 cGy increased risk (P = 0.03)	The risk of MDS/AML after autologous transplants for Hodgkin's disease or non-Hodgkin's lymphoma is significantly increased with pretransplant use of alkylating agents and high-dose TBI in preparation for transplantation
Curtis et al.	110	1997	19,229	N	Various	Retrospective multicenter cohort study	Median 3.5 years	Ratio of observed/ expected cases was 2.7. The risk was 8.3 fold increased in patients surviving >10 years. Younger age, higher doses of TBI, chronic GVHD, and male sex were risk factors	Solid tumors, in particular malignant melanoma, cancers of the buccal cavity, liver, brain, thyroid, bone, and connective tissue were increased. Cancers of the buccal cavity were prominent among male patients and patients with chronic GVHD. Lifelong surveillance is indicated
Curtis et al.	101	1999	18,014	N	Various	Retrospective multicenter cohort study	<1 month to >10 years	Cumulative incidence 1% at 10 years. Unrelated or HLA non-identical transplants, T-cell depletion of donor marrow, use of ATG or anti-CD3 monoclonal antibody, acute GVHD, and conditioning with TBI were risk factors	Most lymphopro-liferative disorders occurred within 5 months of transplantation; late cases rare. Risk factors are cumulative. The use of broadly reactive monoclonal antibodies was associated with a lower risk than narrowly reactive anti-T-cell antibodies

DS, myelodysplasias; AML, acute myeloid leukemia.

transplanted for immunodeficiency disorders. Risk factors include the use of ATG or anti-CD3 monoclonal antibody (MAB) for acute GVHD prophylaxis or in the preparative regimen, use of TBI in the conditioning regimen, T-cell depletion of donor marrow, unrelated donor or HLA nonidentical-related donor, and primary immunodeficiency disease. The impact of risk factors is additive (or synergistic). Increasing intensity of posttransplant immunosuppression in patients who are otherwise at low risk significantly increases the incidence of PTLD.[100] The best approach to prevent Epstein–Barr virus (EBV)-related PTLD currently is close monitoring and preemptive therapy with anti-CD20 monoclonal antibody (325 mg) in patients with rising EBV titers. Additional doses of anti-CD20 antibody can be given if high EBV titers persist.

Rare T-cell proliferative disorders with or without EBV association have been reported.[102] None was associated with HTLV1, HIV, or HHV-6 infection. Several cases of late-occurring lymphomas have been reported,[103–105] some linked to EBV infection (just as early-onset PTLD), and others associated with T-cell depletion of the graft.

"Secondary" myelodysplasias (MDS) and acute myeloid leukemia (AML) occur after conventional chemotherapy with or without radiotherapy for Hodgkin's disease, non-Hodgkin's lymphoma, and solid tumors,[106] as well as after autologous HCT.[103,107,108] After autologous HCT, incidence rates of 4% to 18% have been reported.

A case-control study analyzed data on 56 patients who developed MDS/leukemia and 168 controls within a cohort of 2,739 patients with Hodgkin's disease or non-Hodgkin's lymphoma transplanted at 12 institutions.[109] MDS/AML was significantly correlated with the intensity of pretransplant chemotherapy, specifically mechlorethamine [relative risk (RR), 2.0 and 4.3 for doses of less than 50 or 50 mg/m^2 or more, respectively], and chlorambucil (RR, 3.8 and 8.4 for duration of less than 10 or 10 months or more; $P = 0.0009$) compared to cyclophosphamide. Also, higher doses of TBI (more than 1,200 cGy) used for transplant conditioning tended to carry a higher risk (RR, 4.7).

A spectrum of tumors including glioblastoma, melanoma, squamous cell carcinoma, adenocarcinoma, hepatoma, and basal cell carcinoma has been reported. A recent study analyzed results in 19,220 patients (97.2% allogeneic, 2.8% syngeneic recipients) transplanted between 1964 and 1992.[110] There were 80 solid tumors for an observed/expected (O:E) ratio of 2.7 (P less than 0.001). In 10-year survivors, the risk increased eightfold. The tumor incidence was 2.2% at 10 years and 6.7% at 15 years. The risk increased significantly for melanoma (O:E, 5.0), cancers of the oral cavity (11.1), liver (7.5), central nervous system (CNS) (7.6), thyroid (6.6), bone (13.4), and connective tissue (8.0). The risk was highest for the youngest patients and declined with age. Preliminary data from an ongoing nested case-control study in a cohort of 29,737 patients suggest that duration of chronic GVHD for more than 2 years and prolonged therapy are risk factors, in particular for the development of squamous cell carcinoma.

Cardiovascular Effects

Cardiac insufficiency and coronary artery disease are known complications of intensive cytotoxic therapy, in particular, high-dose anthracycline and mediastinal irradiation. Cardiac insufficiency may also be seen in patients conditioned with cyclophosphamide 200 mg/kg, usually early, sometimes before conditioning is completed, although the overall incidence is low and approximately 0.7% are life threatening or fatal.[111] Late cardiomyopathy has occasionally been observed and treated successfully by orthotopic cardiac transplantation.[112]

Coronary artery disease and thrombotic events have been reported at various time intervals after HCT.[113,114] Hyperlipidemia and hyperglycemia are common in patients treated with calcineurin inhibitors, rapamycin, and glucocorticosteroids. Although data are lacking, potential risk factors for the development of coronary disease in long-term survivors of HCT include treatment with estrogen/progesterone and inactivity due to fatigue or other causes.

Functional and Quality of Life Outcomes

Many cross-sectional cohort studies, and a smaller number of prospective longitudinal cohort or case-control studies, have defined functional and psychosocial outcomes after HCT. These investigations consistently find that 85% to 90% of survivors of HCT do well in their return to "normal" life in the domains of physical, psychologic, social, existential, and overall subjective quality of life, although specific residual problems remain for many.[2,115,116] Physical recovery returns to pretransplant levels by 1 year for most survivors. However, return to work and emotional recovery may take longer.[117–119] Although physical recovery is more rapid for autologous transplant recipients, results are inconsistent as to whether function continues better for autologous survivors after 1 year.[118,120] Risk factors for poorer quality of life include older age, being female, and chronic GVHD.[118,121–124] Specifically, females have a more difficult time in the areas of sexuality, fatigue, emotional adaptation, and return to work.[116,123–126] After resolution of chronic GVHD, survivor function seems to be equal to those patients who did not have chronic GVHD.[118,127] Cross-sectional studies of survivors 5 to 18 years after HCT do not suggest deterioration over time in quality of life.[124,128,129] Residual symptoms that are most common and remain after 5 years in at least a third of survivors, based on a survey of 125 adults, include sexual dysfunction, emotional reactivity and fears, fatigue, joint and muscle pains, eye problems, sleep disruption, financial and insurance worries, cognitive concerns, and social roles and relationships.[128] Only 7% of this cohort was disabled and 74% was employed; the number who considered home-making their job was not reported, but only 3 survivors were seeking employment.

Rates of return to work continue to rise until 5 years after HCT. By 3 or more years after HCT, between 72% and 89% of patients have returned to full-time work or school.[96,119,124,127] Survivors who are older, female, have had chronic myeloid leukemia, or have had extensive chronic GVHD are at risk for incomplete resumption of work or school activity after 5 years.[124,127] A nonrandomized cohort-controlled trial found that HCT survivors who received a 3- to 4-week inpatient rehabilitation program demonstrated no difference in employment when compared with a group of patients who did not receive this rehabilitation.[130]

Pediatric survivor quality of life is similar to adults. A cohort study compared 120 survivors who had HCT as children 5 or more years previously, with 114 survivors of childhood leukemia who had received chemotherapy without transplant, and 149 age- and gender-matched nontransplanted comparison subjects.[131] The HCT survivors reported more major illness, physician visits, diabetes, second malignancies, and poorer physical health than participants in either of the other two cohorts. Both survivor groups reported more health or life insurance refusals (25% and 33% versus 3% for comparison subjects). Marital status and mental health did not differ between cohorts, and other psychosocial factors also did not differ.[131] Other researchers have found comparable results. Investigators who compared adolescents and young adults 2 to 13 years after HCT or bone cancer found that[132] the groups did not differ in adjustment or perceived quality of life, with the exception that HCT survivors reported higher anxiety and feelings of sensitivity and vulnerability. Other researchers have reported that pediatric survivors do better than their peers in psychosocial domains.[133] The rate of successful return to school (85% to 95%) is similar to rates of return to work in adult survivors.[134]

Fatigue

Fatigue is the one of the most persistent symptoms beyond the first year after HCT. A multicenter longitudinal cohort study of fatigue and sleep disturbance in 172 adult survivors more than 12 months after HCT, followed again 18 months after the first assessment, found that a majority reported at least mild problems at both time points, with 15% to 20% reporting moderate to severe problems.[135] Risk factors for sleep but not fatigue included older age, receipt of TBI, and female sex. Problems did not resolve over time, and no specific risk factors for fatigue were identified. Other studies have reported age to be a risk factor for fatigue.[128] A cohort study of breast cancer 20-month survivors after autologous HCT found significantly higher levels of fatigue than in a matched noncancer cohort of women,[136] and another longitudinal cohort study reported that more than 80% of survivors at both 100 days and 1 year reported "I tire easily".[137] Many biologic mechanisms have been postulated to explain fatigue following HCT or other cancer treatments. Considered among potential causes are effects of interleukins and interferons, anemia, metabolic abnormalities, infection, immunosuppression, gonadal insufficiency, TBI, sleep disruption, lack of physical activity, depression, systemic medications such as corticosteroids, and other medications. However, evidence does not clearly support any of these causes over others in HCT survivors.[138] Treatments for fatigue and physical strength have been tested in randomized or nonrandomized trials using exercise, erythropoietin, or coping skills that included relaxation training. Results show improved fatigue and reduced medical complications.[139–141] However, these studies have focused on the acute phase of treatment, not fatigue in survivors.

Neurologic and Cognitive Deficits

Neurologic complications are numerous during acute treatment and as a consequence of chronic GVHD treatment. Neuroradiologic studies have determined that changes such as cortical atrophy and ventricular enlargement occur in some patients after HCT conditioning chemotherapy or total body irradiation.[142] Chronic GVHD-related CNS neurotoxicities seem to resolve with discontinuation of the drug causing the problems unless stroke or other permanent brain events occur.[143–146] An adult cohort study[146] tested 66 patients with neurologic examination, magnetic resonance imaging, and neuropsychologic exams from 8 months to 5 years after transplant. Neuropsychologic deficits did not correlate with pathology seen in neurologic or imaging tests. Pathology on neuroradiologic examination was greater for patients with progressive-onset chronic GVHD or corticosteroid or cyclosporine use. Meanwhile, long-term cyclosporine use and age increased the risk for neuropsychologic impairment.

Twenty percent to 56% of patients enter transplant with cognitive deficits that could interfere with function.[147–149] Thus, without knowing the pretransplant function of a patient, it is not possible to determine whether long-term problems are a consequence of transplantation, or of treatment predating HCT, or instead are outcomes of depression, anxiety, or fatigue. Patient complaints about cognitive difficulties following transplantation are prevalent. However, complaints do not always match objective neuropsychologic test results[150,151] and more likely correlate with subjective anxiety, depression, and fatigue.

Mechanisms underlying cognitive impairment related to chemotherapy remain uncertain but include (1) direct neurotoxic injury, (2) secondary inflammatory response, (3) microvascular injury leading to obstruction, and (4) altered neurotransmitter levels.[152] Data indicate that TBI has significant diffuse effects on neuropsychologic function in the short term, but toxicities resolve with time if doses are 12 Gy or less.[153–156] A study of patients tested pretransplant and at 80 days and 1 year after transplantation found major decrements at 80 days, but recovery of function to pretransplant levels by 1 year, in most neuropsychologic areas tested.[149] A cross-sectional study reported impairment in 25% of allogeneic transplant recipients 2 or more years posttransplant.[151]

Among survivors of pediatric transplantation, a prospective longitudinal cohort study of 102 pediatric survivors found no declines at 1- or 3-year follow-up testing of patients over the age of 5 at the time of transplant.[157] However, younger patients, particularly those under 3 years of age, do have some risk of IQ decline over time posttransplant.[157–159] Testing of children before and at 1 year and 3 years after transplant indicates no difference in performance based on whether the child received TBI.[159,160]

To date there is no indication that adult cognitive abilities decline more rapidly after HCT when compared with nontransplanted adults.[155] By 1 or 2 years posttransplant, approximately 55% to 60% of adult allogeneic HCT survivors and 32% of autologous breast cancer survivors have some evidence of neuropsychologic impairment on objective tests versus 17% of standard-dose chemotherapy recipients.[149–151] Surprisingly, few risk factors specific to HCT have been identified as predictors of long-term deficits. Rather, accumulated difficulties in overall health, fatigue, mood, and physical function predict deficits (Table 110.7).

Sexual Function

Both men and women report lower rates of sexual activity and satisfaction after HCT than before transplantation and in comparison with either the general population or patients who receive chemotherapy without transplantation (Table 110.8). This result is consistent across time points after

TABLE 110.7. Neuropsychologic function after HCT.

Author	Reference	Year	No. of patients	Disease/stage	Intervention/ design	Follow-up	Relative risk/outcomes	Conclusions/results
Arvidson et al.	158	1999	26	Pediatric hematologic malignancies with autologous HCT	Cohort study	8–10 years post-HCT	Risk for impairment increased with younger age, longer follow-up time	Children treated with auto HCT had average IQ; however, deficits in memory and attention were seen
Harder et al.	151	2002	40	Progression-free adult survivors of allogeneic HCT including TBI	Cohort study	22–82 months after HCT	Predictors of poor performance included fatigue, global health, educational level, subjective cognitive complaints, physical functioning, social functioning, mood, employment status	Mild to moderate cognitive impairment found in 60% Compared with healthy population norms, areas most likely to be affected were selective attention and executive function, information processing speed, verbal learning, and verbal and visual memory HCT may lead to cognitive complaints and late cognitive deficits in long-term adult survivors
Kramer et al.	159	1997	67: 1 year after HCT 26: 3 years after HCT	Pediatric HCT	Prospective cohort study	1 year or 3 years	Not reported	Significant decline in IQ was seen between baseline and 1 year Although IQ was lower at 1 year, no further changes were evident at 3-year follow-up
Padovan et al.	146	1998	66	Various adults	Cohort study	Mean 34 months post-HCT	Risk factors for neuropsychologic impairment were age, long time post-HCT, intrathecal methotrexate, long-term cyclosporine, progressive chronic GVHD	Mild cognitive deficit, especially impaired memory, seen in more than 1/3 of allogeneic-HCT patients; lower risk of pathologic neurologic exam after auto-HCT
Peper et al.	154	2000	14: before TBI and HCT, 20: after TBI and autologous HCT 11: controls with renal insufficiency	Adult acute leukemias, lymphoma	Cohort and case-control study	32 months and 8.8 years	Brain atrophy increase was associated primarily with pretransplant irradiation or methotrexate No medical factors were associated with cognitive deficits	Neurologic deficits seen in one new case after HCT All brain atrophy measures were within normal range, but were slightly increased after TBI Cognitive deficit levels were not significant Power may have been inadequate to detect clinically meaningful differences Some tests were associated with ventricle index results No decline in cognitive function seen long term

Phipps et al.	157	2000	102 survivors to 1 year with 54 followed to 3 years	Pediatric HCT	Prospective cohort study	3 years	Younger age showed more decline over time; <3 years particularly vulnerable	No significant changes on global measures of VC intelligence or academic achievement at either 1 or 3 years after an HCT HCT with or without TBI entails minimal risk of late neurocognitive sequelae in patients who are 6 years of age or older
Simms et al.	160	1998	122	Pediatric HCT recipients with no previous cranial irradiation	Prospective cohort study	1 year	None identified	No statistically significant differences between the two groups Regression analysis failed to identify treatment, age, or gender effects Suggests that neuropsychologic functioning 1 year after HCT was not detrimentally affected by chemotherapy or TBI
Syrjala et al.	149	2004	142	Adults with malignancy receiving first allogeneic HCT	Prospective cohort study	80 days and 1 year	2.76 RR (CI = 1.01–7.55) for impaired motor dexterity in patients actively receiving cyclosporine, tacrolimus or my cophenolate mofetil vs. not 2.99 RR (CI = 1.08–8.30) for impairment on any test pretransplant in patients with no previous chemotherapy, or only hydroxyurea before HCT	Performance on all tests declined from pretransplant to 80 days and improved by 1 year to pretransplant levels on all tests except strength and dexterity Verbal fluency and memory recovered by 1 year but remained below norms suggesting that these long term cognitive decrements were not a result of HCT treatment in most patients
van Dam et al.	150	1998	34: autologous HCT 36: standard dose 34: controls, stage I, no chemotherapy	Adult breast cancer	Case-control and cohort study	Mean 2 years, minimum 6 months	8.2 RR (CI = 1.8–37.7) for HCT vs. control 3.5 RR (CI = 1.1–12.8) for HCT vs. standard chemotherapy	Patients with high-dose chemo have a greater risk of cognitive impairment than patients with standard dose
Wenz et al.	155	2000	58	Adult hyperfractionated TBI with autologous HCT	Prospective cohort study	Median 27 months	None found	No measurable radiation damage found

TABLE 110.8. Sexual function after HCT.

Author	Reference	Year	No. of patients	Randomized (Y/N)	Diagnosis/stage of disease	Intervention/ design	Follow-up	Relative risk/outcomes	Conclusions/results
Balleari et al.	93	2002	39 received hormone therapy; 32 controls	N	Premenopausal women treated with autologous transplant for hematologic malignancies	Case-control study	24 months	No increased risk of chronic GVHD activity with hormone therapy	No differences observed in chronic GVHD activity score between HRT and controls after 3, 6, 12, and 24 months
Chatterjee et al.	169	2002	8	N	Males after HCT for lymphoma, with hypogonadism, erectile dysfunction, diminished libido and ejaculatory disorders; all had Leydig cell insufficiency with or without frank serum testosterone insufficiency; all but one had cavernosal arterial insufficiency	Case series Patients received intramuscular testosterone cypionate (250 mg 4× weekly) and 50–100 mg of sildenafil orally one to two times per week for 6 months	6 months	Not reported	All patients responded favorably; results suggest therapy is a safe and effective approach in recipients of high-dose therapy with erectile dysfunction after HCT
Chatterjee et al.	185	2000	24 HCT survivors 10 healthy controls	N	Males after HCT with hypogonadism and erectile dysfunction	Case-control study	Mean 34 months	TBI increases risk for Leydig cell insufficiency; cavernosal vascular insufficiency increased risk of erectile dysfunction	Testosterone levels were lower than controls but within normal range Cavernosal arterial insufficiency found in 11/14 of TBI-treated and 3/10 chemotherapy treated patients Testosterone therapy improved libido but not erectile dysfunction
Molassiotis et al.	164	1995	29 HCT survivors 30 non-HCT cancer survivors 119 controls	N	Males after autologous and allogeneic HCT	Case-control study	Mean 35.6 months	Risk increased with TBI	FSH and LH increased throughout years after HCT Hyperprolactinemia observed only in the second year after HCT; testosterone levels were normal Long-term HCT survivors had similar psychosexual adjustment to non-HCT cancer survivors Major problems were erectile difficulties (37.9%), low sexual desire (37.9%), altered body image (20.7%)

Mumma et al.	186	1992	26 HCT survivors 33 non-HCT survivors	N	Acute leukemia	Cohort study	Mean 47 months for HCT; 64 months for non-HCT	Longer time since cancer treatment predicted greater frequency of sexual activity in women but poorer body image for both men and women	No differences between HCT and conventional chemotherapy Compared with controls, women had decreased sexual frequency and satisfaction; both men and women had poorer body image
Syrjala et al.	91	1998	407	N	Various	Prospective cohort study	1 and 3 years	Male sexual dissatisfaction at 3 years was predicted by older age, not being married, pretransplant sexual dissatisfaction, and poorer psychologic function Females were more dissatisfied at 3 years if they did not receive hormone therapy by 1 year and if they were less satisfied at 1 year	Pretransplant men and women did not differ in sexual satisfaction. After 1 and 3 years women were more dissatisfied and had more problems. No pretransplant factors predicted 3-year outcomes for women. At 3 years, 80% of women and 29% of men had at least one sexual problem
Syrjala et al.	166	2000	185 HCT survivors 94 non-HCT survivors 121 controls	N	Various	Cohort study	1–10 years	Risk of poorer sexual function for: HCT survivors vs. controls, females, shorter time since HCT for females, postmenopausal status for females, extensive chronic GVHD for males	Hormone therapy was not associated with sexual function. HCT survivors and females have high levels of sexual dysfunction
Watson et al.	165	1999	168 HCT, 311 non-HCT	N	AML	Cohort study	Median 14 months	Sexual function worse in HCT, females, older	Sexual function correlated with fatigue and emotional function
Wingard et al.	163	1992	126	N	Various HCT survivors	Cohort study	Mean 47 months	Sexual satisfaction correlated with serum estrogen or testosterone levels though levels were within normal range Satisfaction increased with younger age and satisfaction with appearance, life, and partner relationship	22% were dissatisfied with sexual function. 24% of men had erectile difficulty; 13% had ejaculation difficulty For women, hormone therapy was not associated with satisfaction

HCT, and across ages at time of transplantation, in both prospective longitudinal and cohort comparison studies.[91,115,120,123,161–165] Before HCT, 42% of females and 14% of males report one or more sexual problems, compared with 17% to 35% of the general population of females and up to 19% of males.[91] By 3 years after HCT, the prevalence of problems increases to 80% of females and 29% of males. Risk factors include, for women, initiation of hormone therapy after 1 year posttransplantation and chronic GVHD, and, for men, older age, chronic GVHD, and psychologic function before HCT.[91,165,166]

Long-term problems for females are presumably caused by ovarian failure and consequent endocrine changes or by chronic GVHD-related vaginal introital stenosis and mucosal changes.[167] Prospective cohort studies indicate that hormone therapy with oral estrogen improves or prevents more serious decline in sexual function in women after HCT but does not eliminate problems.[91,93] Because hormone replacement has been widely prescribed after HCT, vasomotor symptoms and other menopausal syndromes have been less commonly reported than sexual dysfunction. However, with new concerns about the long-term risks of hormone therapy, menopausal symptoms and hormone alternatives need to be reconsidered. We have found no clinical trials comparing treatments for female sexual dysfunction after HCT despite the well-recognized prevalence of problems. Descriptions of clinical interventions for women recommend vaginal lubricants to improve comfort as well as counseling with sexual partners. Some couples do well after brief counseling that provides education, facilitates communication, and encourages gradually increasing intimacy behaviors and relearning pleasurable sexual strategies rather than avoiding sexual activity.[168]

Male sexual problems have been attributed to gonadal and cavernosal arterial insufficiency, with resulting libido and erectile dysfunction.[169] Results from a small case-series of eight patients 6 months after HCT suggested that testosterone injections and sildenafil one to two times per week improved sexual performance for men with erectile dysfunction, low libido, and ejaculatory disorders.[169] However, other data indicate that most males recover testosterone levels and sexual function between 6 months and 1 year after transplantation.[170] Thus, without controlled clinical trials, it is unclear whether sexual function in the treated men would have recovered without treatment.

Psychologic Adaptation

Rates of depression and anxiety among HCT recipients are higher than population norms. Prospective studies have reported depressive symptoms in 43% to 53% of survivors at some time during or after HCT.[127,137] Rates of both general anxiety and depression decline from pretransplant to 1 year and then stabilize.[117,127] Depression is of particular concern because studies have found it to be a risk factor for mortality and poorer long-term physical and psychologic functioning after HCT.[117,127,171,172] More prevalent than clinical syndromes of depression or anxiety are subclinical elevations in emotions that continue long term.[128] Worries and concerns related to health and survival decline gradually between discharge and 3 years.[127,173] However, other concerns increase after the first year, including work, relationships, finances, and social and family issues.[137] Children, similar to adults, appear to be distressed during treatment but then to recover psychologically.[174]

Emerging Challenges in Functional and Quality of Life Outcomes

Evidence related to functional and quality of life outcomes indicate that physical capability improves within 1 year whereas treatment-related distress and return to work resolve by 2 to 3 years. Other problems do not resolve without treatment; for instance, sexual dysfunction, fatigue, and reduced social activities persist past 5 years. Long-term impact of HCT on cognitive function remains undefined for adults. The clearest challenge is to increase testing of treatments to improve outcomes for those problems that persist.

Emerging Issues

Nonmyeloablative Transplants

Both the pretransplant conditioning regimen and posttransplant donor immune-mediated mechanisms account for elimination of malignant cells in the recipient. Conventional high-dose, myeloablative pretransplant conditioning regimens have been designed to prevent graft rejection and to eliminate as many malignant cells as possible, but these regimens are not well tolerated in older patients or in those who are not in good medical condition at the time of the transplant. During the past 5 years, improvements have been made in posttransplant immunosuppressive regimens so that low-dose, nonmyeloablative pretransplant conditioning regimens are sufficient to prevent graft rejection. This treatment strategy relies heavily on immune-mediated mechanisms to eliminate malignant cells when immunosuppressive medications are gradually withdrawn after the transplant.

Results from many Phase 2 studies have suggested that low-dose, nonmyeloablative pretransplant conditioning regimens cause much less posttransplant morbidity than conventional, high-dose myeloablative conditioning regimens during the first month after the transplant. This impression has been confirmed by comparing skin, liver, and gastrointestinal morbidity between two cohorts of patients who had either a myeloablative or nonmyeloablative conditioning regimen.[175] Morbidity after the first month, however, was similar in the two groups. The proportion of patients who needed treatment for either acute or chronic GVHD was lower among patients who received a nonmyeloablative conditioning regimen, and the time to onset of GVHD was delayed. Randomized trials have not yet been carried out to compare results with the two types of conditioning regimens.

Caregiver and Family Needs

Caregiving by a spouse, parent, or other family member or friend is vital to recovery after HCT. Longitudinal studies find that emotional distress in caregivers peaks during the first 2 weeks of treatment[176] while fatigue peaks at 3 months.[177] Mothers of pediatric HCT patients seem to suffer the greatest emotional strain in the course of their child's treatment.[178] In a case-matched, longitudinal, prospective cohort study that also included nontransplant controls, spouse caregivers reported greater depression and anxiety than patients throughout the first year after HCT.[179] Female caregivers also were at higher risk of marital dissatisfaction than male caregivers. Little else has been published about the financial or family costs of HCT. Particularly lacking is information on family responses after an HCT recipient dies.

Conclusions

Medical and quality of life issues facing survivors of HCT have been well described, as have risk factors for major medical complications. In contrast, few randomized controlled trials have tested efficacy of treatments for chronic GVHD or infectious, pulmonary, endocrine, or functional problems. For most medical complications, treatment choices are based on Phase 2 data or historical case-control studies. Evidence for treatment of functional or quality of life problems such as fatigue, sexual dysfunction, or cognitive deficits must be extrapolated either from studies during the acute phase of treatment, as for fatigue, or from research with other populations of patients, as with sexual dysfunction, cognitive deficits, or psychosocial adaptation.

The foremost risk factors for mortality and morbidity in survivors are chronic GVHD and its treatment, infection, or malignancy recurrence. However, if transplant recipients survive without malignancy recurrence, their physical and psychosocial quality of life is excellent for more than 80%, whether they have autologous or allogeneic transplant, whether or not they have clinical extensive chronic GVHD, and regardless of age. Although males have higher rates of mortality, female survivors are at greater risk for functional and psychosocial complications. Recent descriptive studies indicate that most survivors perceive long-term benefits as well as losses as a consequence of their disease and HCT. Although second cancers are more prevalent in survivors and problems with insurance and cataracts have been documented, few other late effects of HCT have been detected thus far.

Acknowledgments. This work was supported by grants from the National Cancer Institute CA63030, CA79880, CA102542, and CA18029. We thank Ashley Walter, Bonnie Larson, and Helen Crawford for assistance with the research review and manuscript preparation.

References

1. Loberiza F. Report on state of the art in blood and marrow transplantation: part I of the IBMTR/ABMTR summary slides with guide. IBMTR/ABMTR Newsl 2003;10:7–10.
2. Socie G, Stone JV, Wingard JR, et al. Long-term survival and late deaths after allogeneic bone marrow transplantation: late effects working committee of the International Bone Marrow Transplant Registry. N Engl J Med 1999;341:14–21.
3. Sullivan KM. Graft-versus-host disease. In: Thomas ED, Blume KG, Forman SJ (eds). Hematopoietic Cell Transplantation, 2nd ed. Boston: Blackwell Science, 1999:515–536.
4. Vogelsang GB. How I treat chronic graft-versus-host disease. Blood 2001;97:1196–1201.
5. Lee SJ, Vogelsang G, Flowers MED. Chronic graft-versus-host disease. Biol Blood Marrow Transplant 2003;9:215–233.
6. Cutler C, Giri S, Jeyapalan S, et al. Acute and chronic graft-versus-host disease after allogeneic peripheral-blood stem-cell and bone marrow transplantation: a meta-analysis. J Clin Oncol 2001;19:3685–3691.
7. Flowers MED, Parker PM, Johnston LJ, et al. Comparison of chronic graft-versus-host disease after transplantation of peripheral blood stem cells versus bone marrow in allogeneic recipients: long-term follow-up of a randomized trial. Blood 2002;100:415–419.
8. Storb R, Doney KC, Thomas ED, et al. Marrow transplantation with or without donor buffy coat cells for 65 transfused aplastic anemia patients. Blood 1982;59:236–246.
9. Zaucha JM, Gooley T, Bensinger WI, et al. CD34 cell dose in granulocyte colony-stimulating factor-mobilized peripheral blood mononuclear cell grafts affects engraftment kinetics and development of extensive chronic graft-versus-host disease after human leukocyte antigen-identical sibling transplantation. Blood 2001;98:3221–3227.
10. Przepiorka D, Anderlini P, Saliba R, et al. Chronic graft-versus-host disease after allogeneic blood stem cell transplantation. Blood 2001;98:1695–1700.
11. Mitsuyasu RT, Champlin RE, Gale RP, et al. Treatment of donor bone marrow with monoclonal anti-T-cell antibody and complement for the prevention of graft-versus-host disease. Ann Intern Med 1986;105:20–26.
12. Marmont AM, Horowitz MM, Gale RP, et al. T-cell depletion of HLA-identical transplants in leukemia. Blood 1991;78:2120–2130.
13. Champlin RE, Passweg JR, Zhang MJ, et al. T-cell depletion of bone marrow transplants for leukemia from donors other than HLA-identical siblings: advantage of T-cell antibodies with narrow specificities. Blood 2000;95:3996–4003.
14. Wagner JE, Thompson JS, Carter S, et al. Impact of graft-versus-host disease (GVHD) prophylaxis on 3-year disease-free survival (DFS): results of a multi-center, randomized phase II–III trial comparing T cell depletion/cyclosporine (TCD) and methotrexate/cyclosporine (M/C) in 410 recipients of unrelated donor bone marrow (BM). Blood 2002;100:75a–76a.
15. Bacigalupo A, Lamparelli T, Bruzzi P, et al. Antithymocyte globulin for graft-versus-host disease prophylaxis in transplants from unrelated donors: 2 randomized studies from Gruppo Italiano Trapianti Midollo Osseo (GITMO). Blood 2001;98:2942–2947.
16. Storb R, Pepe M, Anasetti C, et al. What role for prednisone in prevention of acute graft-versus-host disease in patients undergoing marrow transplants? Blood 1990;76:1037–1045.
17. Deeg HJ, Lin D, Leisenring W, et al. Cyclosporine or cyclosporine plus methylprednisolone for prophylaxis of graft-versus-host disease: a prospective, randomized trial. Blood 1997;89:3880–3887.
18. Chao NJ, Snyder DS, Jain M, et al. Equivalence of 2 effective graft-versus-host disease prophylaxis regimens: results of a prospective double-blind randomized trial. Biol Blood Marrow Transplant 2000;6:254–261.
19. Ruutu T, Volin L, Parkkali T, et al. Cyclosporine, methotrexate, and methylprednisolone compared with cyclosporine and methotrexate for the prevention of graft-versus-host disease in bone marrow transplantation from HLA-identical sibling donor: a prospective randomized study. Blood 2000;96:2391–2398.
20. Storb R, Leisenring W, Anasetti C, et al. Methotrexate and cyclosporine for graft-vs.-host disease prevention: what length of therapy with cyclosporine? Biol Blood Marrow Transplant 1997;3:194–201.
21. Kansu E, Gooley T, Flowers MED, et al. Administration of cyclosporine for 24 months compared with 6 months for prevention of chronic graft-versus-host disease: a prospective randomized clinical trial [brief report]. Blood 2001;98:3868–3870.

22. Mengarelli A, Iori AP, Romano A, et al. One-year cyclosporine prophylaxis reduces the risk of developing extensive chronic graft-versus-host disease after allogeneic peripheral blood stem cell transplantation. Haematologica 2003;88:315–323.
23. Chao NJ, Parker PM, Niland JC, et al. Paradoxical effect of thalidomide prophylaxis on chronic graft-vs.-host disease. Biol Blood Marrow Transplant 1996;2:86–92.
24. Sullivan KM, Witherspoon RP, Storb R, et al. Prednisone and azathioprine compared with prednisone and placebo for treatment of chronic graft-versus-host disease: prognostic influence of prolonged thrombocytopenia after allogeneic marrow transplantation. Blood 1988;72:546–554.
25. Sullivan KM, Witherspoon RP, Storb R, et al. Alternating-day cyclosporine and prednisone for treatment of high-risk chronic graft-versus-host disease. Blood 1988;72:555–561.
26. Koc S, Leisenring W, Flowers MED, et al. Therapy for chronic graft-versus-host disease: a randomized trial comparing cyclosporine plus prednisone versus prednisone alone. Blood 2002; 100:48–51.
27. Arora M, Wagner JE, Davies SM, et al. Randomized clinical trial of thalidomide, cyclosporine, and prednisone versus cyclosporine and prednisone as initial therapy for chronic graft-versus-host disease. Biol Blood Marrow Transplant 2001;7: 265–273.
28. Koc S, Leisenring W, Flowers MED, et al. Thalidomide for treatment of patients with chronic graft-versus-host disease. Blood 2000;96:3995–3996.
29. Storek J, Dawson MA, Storer B, et al. Immune reconstitution after allogeneic marrow transplantation compared with blood stem cell transplantation. Blood 2001;97:3380–3389.
30. Winston DJ, Schiffman G, Wang DC, et al. Pneumococcal infections after human bone marrow transplantation. Ann Intern Med 1979;91:835–841.
31. Witherspoon RP, Storb R, Ochs HD, et al. Recovery of antibody production in human allogeneic marrow graft recipients: influence of time posttransplantation, the presence or absence of chronic graft-versus-host disease, and antithymocyte globulin treatment. Blood 1981;58:360–368.
32. Storek J, Viganego F, Dawson MA, et al. Factors affecting antibody levels after allogeneic hematopoietic cell transplantation. Blood 2003;101:3319–3324.
33. Singhal S, Mehta J. Reimmunization after blood or marrow stem cell transplantation. Bone Marrow Transplant 1999;23:637–646.
34. Centers for Disease Control and Prevention, Infectious Disease Society of America, American Society of Blood and Marrow Transplantation. Guidelines for preventing opportunistic infections among hematopoietic stem cell transplant recipients. MMWR (Morbid Mort Wkly Rep) 2000;49:1–125.
35. D'Antonio D, Di Bartolomeo P, Iacone A, et al. Meningitis due to penicillin-resistant *Streptococcus pneumoniae* in patients with chronic graft-versus-host disease. Bone Marrow Transplant 1992;9:299–300.
36. Locksley RM, Flournoy N, Sullivan KM, et al. Infection with varicella-zoster virus infection after marrow transplantation. J Infect Dis 1985;152:1172–1181.
37. Han CS, Miller W, Haake R, et al. Varicella zoster infection after bone marrow transplantation: incidence, risk factors and complications. Bone Marrow Transplant 1994;13:277–283.
38. Koc Y, Miller KB, Schenkein DP, et al. Varicella zoster virus infections following allogeneic bone marrow transplantation: frequency, risk factors, and clinical outcome. Biol Blood Marrow Transplant 2000;6:44–49.
39. Bilgrami S, Chakraborty NG, Rodriguez-Pinero F, et al. Varicella zoster virus infection associated with high-dose chemotherapy and autologous stem-cell rescue. Bone Marrow Transplant 1999; 23:469–474.
40. Schuchter LM, Wingard JR, Piantadosi S, et al. Herpes zoster infection after autologous bone marrow transplantation. Blood 1989;74:1424–1427.
41. Bowden RA, Roger KS, Meyers JD. Oral acyclovir for the long-term suppression of varicella zoster virus infection after marrow transplantation. In: 29th Interscience Conference on Antimicrobial Agents and Chemotherapy 1989, p 62.
42. Ljungman P, Wilczek H, Gahrton G, et al. Long-term acyclovir prophylaxis in bone marrow transplant recipients and lymphocyte proliferation responses to herpes virus antigens *in vitro*. Bone Marrow Transplant 1986;1:185–192.
43. Boeckh M, Gooley TA, Myerson D, et al. Cytomegalovirus pp65 antigenemia-guided early treatment with ganciclovir versus ganciclovir at engraftment after allogeneic marrow transplantation: a randomized double-blind study. Blood 1996;88:4063–4071.
44. Krause H, Hebart H, Jahn G, et al. Screening for CMV-specific T cell proliferation to identify patients at risk of developing late onset CMV disease. Bone Marrow Transplant 1997;19: 1111–1116.
45. Zaia JA, Gallez-Hawkins GM, Tegtmeier BR, et al. Late cytomegalovirus disease in marrow transplantation is predicted by virus load in plasma. J Infect Dis 1997;176:782–785.
46. Boeckh M, Leisenring W, Riddell SR, et al. Late cytomegalovirus disease and mortality in recipients of allogeneic hematopoietic stem cell transplants: importance of viral load and T-cell immunity. Blood 2003;101:407–414.
47. Crippa F, Corey L, Chuang EL, et al. Virological, clinical, and ophthalmologic features of cytomegalovirus retinitis after hematopoietic stem cell transplantation. Clin Infect Dis 2001; 32:214–219.
48. Peggs KS, Preiser W, Kottaridis PD, et al. Extended routine polymerase chain reaction surveillance and pre-emptive antiviral therapy for cytomegalovirus after allogeneic transplantation. Br J Haematol 2000;111:782–790.
49. Marr KA, Carter RA, Boeckh M, et al. Invasive aspergillosis in allogeneic stem cell transplant recipients: changes in epidemiology and risk factors. Blood 2002;100:4358–4366.
50. Fukuda T, Boeckh M, Carter RA, et al. Risks and outcomes of invasive fungal infections in recipients of allogeneic hematopoietic stem cell transplants after nonmyeloablative conditioning. Blood 2003;102:827–833.
51. Marr KA, Seidel K, Slavin M, et al. Prolonged fluconazole prophylaxis is associated with persistent protection against candidiasis-related death in allogeneic marrow transplant recipients: long-term follow-up of a randomized, placebo-controlled trial. Blood 2000;96:2055–2061.
52. Souza JP, Boeckh M, Gooley TA, et al. High rates of *Pneumocystis carinii* pneumonia in allogeneic blood and marrow transplant recipients receiving dapsone prophylaxis. Clin Infect Dis 1999;29:1467–1471.
53. Tuan I-Z, Dennison D, Weisdorf DJ. *Pneumocystis carinii* pneumonitis following bone marrow transplantation. Bone Marrow Transplant 1992;10:267–272.
54. Chen C-S, Boeckh M, Seidel K, et al. Incidence, risk factors and mortality from pneumonia developing late after hematopoietic stem cell transplantation. Bone Marrow Transplant 2003;32: 515–522.
55. Vasconcelles MJ, Bernardo MV, King C, et al. Aerosolized pentamidine as pneumocystis prophylaxis after bone marrow transplantation is inferior to other regimens and is associated with decreased survival and an increased risk of other infections. Biol Blood Marrow Transplant 2000;6:35–43.
56. Colby C, McAfee S, Sackstein R, et al. A prospective randomized trial comparing the toxicity and safety of atovaquone with trimethoprim/sulfamethoxazole as *Pneumocystis carinii* pneumonia prophylaxis following autologous peripheral blood stem cell transplantation. Bone Marrow Transplant 1999;24: 897–902.
57. Gagnon S, Boota AM, Fischl MA, et al. Corticosteroids as adjunctive therapy for severe Pneumocystis carinii pneumonia in the acquired immunodeficiency syndrome. A double-blind, placebo-controlled trial. N Engl J Med 1990;323:1444–1450.

58. Smego RA Jr, Nagar S, Maloba B, et al. A meta-analysis of salvage therapy for *Pneumocystis carinii* pneumonia. Arch Intern Med 2001;161:1529–1533.
59. Kantrow SP, Hackman RC, Boeckh M, et al. Idiopathic pneumonia syndrome: changing spectrum of lung injury after marrow transplantation. Transplantation 1997;63:1079–1086.
60. Crawford SW, Pepe M, Lin D, et al. Abnormalities of pulmonary function tests after marrow transplantation predict nonrelapse mortality. Am J Respir Crit Care Med 1995;152:690–695.
61. Crawford SW. Respiratory infections following organ transplantation. Curr Opin Pulmonary Med 1995;1:209–215.
62. Clark JG, Schwartz DA, Flournoy N, et al. Risk factors for airflow obstruction in recipients of bone marrow transplants. Ann Intern Med 1987;107:648–656.
63. Chien JW, Martin PJ, Gooley TA, et al. Airflow obstruction after myeloablative allogeneic hematopoietic stem cell transplantation. Am J Respir Crit Care Med 2003;168:208–214.
64. Boas SR, Noyes BE, Kurland G, et al. Pediatric lung transplantation for graft-versus-host disease following bone marrow transplantation. Chest 1994;105:1584–1586.
65. Spray TL, Mallory GB, Canter CB, Huddleston CB. Pediatric lung transplantation. Indications, techniques, and early results. J Thorac Cardiovasc Surg 1994;107:990–999; discussion 999–1000.
66. Sullivan KM, Mori M, Witherspoon R, et al. Alternating-day cyclosporine and prednisone (CSP/PRED) treatment of chronic graft-vs.-host disease (GVHD): Predictors of survival. Blood 1990;76(suppl 1):568a.
67. Philit F, Wiesendanger T, Archimbaud E, et al. Post-transplant obstructive lung disease ("bronchiolitis obliterans"): a clinical comparative study of bone marrow and lung transplant patients. Eur Resp J 1995;8:551–558.
68. Sullivan KM, Storek J, Kopecky KJ, et al. A controlled trial of long-term administration of intravenous immunoglobulin to prevent late infection and chronic graft-vs.-host disease after marrow transplantation: clinical outcome and effect on subsequent immune recovery. Biol Blood and Marrow Transplant 1996;2:44–53.
69. Freudenberger TD, Madtes DK, Curtis JR, et al. Association between acute and chronic graft-versus-host disease and bronchiolitis obliterans organizing pneumonia in recipients of hematopoietic stem cell transplants. Blood 2003;102:3822–3828.
70. Palmas A, Tefferi A, Myers JL, et al. Late-onset noninfectious pulmonary complications after allogeneic bone marrow transplantation. Br J Haematol 1998;100:680–687.
71. Stern JM, Sullivan KM, Ott SM, et al. Bone density loss after allogeneic hematopoietic stem cell transplantation: a prospective study. Biol Blood Marrow Transplant 2001;7:257–264.
72. Castelo-Branco C, Rovira M, Pons F, et al. The effect of hormone replacement therapy on bone mass in patients with ovarian failure due to bone marrow transplantation. Maturitas 1996;23:307–312.
73. Rossouw JE, Anderson GL, Prentice RL, et al. Risks and benefits of estrogen plus progestin in healthy postmenopausal women. JAMA 2002;288:321–333.
74. Lindsay R, Gallagher JC, Kleerekoper M, et al. Effect of lower doses of conjugated equine estrogens with and without medroxyprogesterone acetate on bone in early postmenopausal women. JAMA 2002;287:2668–2676.
75. Fink JC, Leisenring WM, Sullivan KM, et al. Avascular necrosis following bone marrow transplantation: a case-control study. Bone (NY) 1998;22:67–71.
76. Socié G, Cahn JY, Carmelo J, et al. Avascular necrosis of bone after allogeneic bone marrow transplantation: analysis of risk factors for 4,388 patients by the Societe Francaise de Greffe de Moelle (SFGM). Br J Haematol 1997;97:865–870.
77. Fletcher BD, Crom DB, Krance RA, et al. Radiation-induced bone abnormalities after bone marrow transplantation for childhood leukemia. Radiology 1994;191:231–235.
78. Fink JC, Leisenring WM, Sullivan KM, et al. Avascular necrosis following bone marrow transplantation: a case-control study. Bone (NY) 1998;22:67–71.
79. Toubert ME, Socié G, Gluckman E, et al. Short- and long-term follow-up of thyroid dysfunction after allogeneic bone marrow transplantation without the use of preparative total body irradiation. Br J Haematol 1997;98:453–457.
80. Thomas BC, Stanhope R, Plowman PN, et al. Endocrine function following single fraction and fractionated total body irradiation for bone marrow transplantation in childhood. Acta Endocrinol 1993;128:508–512.
81. Boulad F, Bromley M, Black P, et al. Thyroid dysfunction following bone marrow transplantation using hyperfractionated radiation. Bone Marrow Transplant 1995;15:71–76.
82. Neglia JP, Nesbit ME, Jr. Care and treatment of long-term survivors of childhood cancer [review]. Cancer (Phila) 1993;71: 3386–3391.
83. Sanders JE. Growth and development after hematopoietic cell transplantation. In: Blume KG, Forman SJ, Appelbaum FR (eds). Thomas' Hematopoietic Cell Transplantation, 3rd ed. Oxford: Blackwell, 2004:929–943.
84. Sierra J, Bjerke J, Hansen J, et al. Marrow transplants from unrelated donors as treatment for acute leukemia. Leuk Lymphoma 2000;39:495–507.
85. Kubota C, Shinohara O, Hinohara T, et al. Changes in hypothalamic-pituitary function following bone marrow transplantation in children. Acta Paediatr Jpn 1994;36:37–43.
86. Brauner R, Adan L, Souberbielle JC, et al. Contribution of growth hormone deficiency to the growth failure that follows bone marrow transplantation. J Pediatr 1997;130:785–792.
87. Clement-De Boers A, Oostdijk W, Van Weel-Sipman MH, et al. Final height and hormonal function after bone marrow transplantation in children. J Pediatr 1996;129:544–550.
88. Cohen A, Rovelli A, Bakker B, et al. Final height of patients who underwent bone marrow transplantation for hematological disorders during childhood: a study by the Working Party for Late Effects–EBMT. Blood 1999;93:4109–4115.
89. Sanders JE, Hawley J, Levy W, et al. Pregnancies following high-dose cyclophosphamide with or without high-dose busulfan or total-body irradiation and bone marrow transplantation. Blood 1996;87:3045–3052.
90. Salooja N, Szydlo RM, Socie G, et al. Pregnancy outcomes after peripheral blood or bone marrow transplantation: a retrospective survey. Lancet 2001;358:271–276.
91. Syrjala KL, Roth-Roemer SL, Abrams JR, et al. Prevalence and predictors of sexual dysfunction in long-term survivors of marrow transplantation. J Clin Oncol 1998;16:3148–3157.
92. Spinelli S, Chiodi S, Bacigalupo A, et al. Ovarian recovery after total body irradiation and allogeneic bone marrow transplantation: long-term follow up of 79 females. Bone Marrow Transplant 1994;14:373–380.
93. Balleari E, Garre S, van Lint MT, et al. Hormone replacement therapy and chronic graft-versus-host disease activity in women treated with bone marrow transplantation for hematologic malignancies. Ann NY Acad Sciences 2002;966:187–192.
94. Swerdlow AJ, Higgins CD, Adlard P, et al. Risk of cancer in patients treated with human pituitary growth hormone in the UK, 1959–85: a cohort study. Lancet 2002;360:273–277.
95. Benyunes MC, Sullivan KM, Deeg HJ, et al. Cataracts after bone marrow transplantation: long-term follow-up of adults treated with fractionated total body irradiation. Int J Radiat Oncol Biol Phys 1995;32:661–670.
96. Socie G, Clift RA, Blaise D, et al. Busulfan plus cyclophosphamide compared with total-body irradiation plus cyclophosphamide before marrow transplantation for myeloid leukemia: long-term follow-up of 4 randomized studies. Blood 2001;98: 3569–3574.

97. Tichelli A, Duell T, Weiss M, et al. Late-onset keratoconjunctivitis sicca syndrome after bone marrow transplantation: incidence and risk factors. European Group on Blood and Marrow Transplantation (EBMT) Working Party on Late Effects. Bone Marrow Transplant 1996;17:1105–1111.
98. Strasser SI, Sullivan KM, Myerson D, et al. Cirrhosis of the liver in long-term marrow transplant survivors. Blood 1999;93: 3259–3266.
99. Shepherd JD, Gascoyne RD, Barnett MJ, et al. Polyclonal Epstein–Barr virus-associated lymphoproliferative disorder following autografting for chronic myeloid leukemia. Bone Marrow Transplant 1995;15:639–641.
100. O'Reilly RJ, Lacerda JF, Lucas KG, et al. Adoptive cell therapy with donor lymphocytes for EBV-associated lymphomas developing after allogeneic marrow transplants. In: DeVita VT, Jr., Hellman S, Rosenberg SA (eds). Important Advances in Oncology. Philadelphia: Lippincott, 1996:149–166.
101. Curtis RE, Travis LB, Rowlings PA, et al. Risk of lymphoproliferative disorders after bone marrow transplantation: a multi-institutional study. Blood 1999;94:2208–2216.
102. Hanson MN, Morrison VA, Peterson BA, et al. Posttransplant T-cell lymphoproliferative disorders–an aggressive, late complication of solid-organ transplantation. Blood 1996;88:3626–3633.
103. Deeg HJ, Socié G. Malignancies after hematopoietic stem cell transplantation: many questions, some answers. Blood 1998; 91:1833–1844.
104. Meignin V, Devergie A, Brice P, et al. Hodgkin's disease of donor origin after allogeneic bone marrow transplantation for myelogenous chronic luekiemia [review]. Transplantation 1998; 65:595–597.
105. Schouten HC, Hopman AH, Haesevoets AM, et al. Large-cell anaplastic non-Hodgkin's lymphoma originating in donor cells after allogeneic bone marrow transplantation. Br J Haematol 1995;91:162–166.
106. Travis LB, Curtis RE, Stovall M, et al. Risk of leukemia following treatment for non-Hodgkin's lymphoma. J Natl Cancer Inst 1994;86:1450–1457.
107. Chao NJ, Nademanee AP, Long GD, et al. Importance of bone marrow cytogenetic evaluation before autologous bone marrow transplantation for Hodgkin's disease. J Clin Oncol 1991; 9:1575–1579.
108. Stone RM. Myelodysplastic syndrome after autologous transplantation for lymphoma: the price of progress? Blood 1994;83:3437–3440.
109. Metayer C, Curtis RE, Vose J, et al. Myelodysplastic syndrome and acute myeloid leukemia after autotransplantation for lymphoma: a multicenter case-control study. Blood 2003;101: 2015–2023.
110. Curtis RE, Rowlings PA, Deeg HJ, et al. Solid cancers after bone marrow transplantation. N Engl J Med 1997;336:897–904.
111. Murdych T, Weisdorf DJ. Serious cardiac complications during bone marrow transplantation at the University of Minnesota, 1977–1997. Bone Marrow Transplant 2001;28:283–287.
112. Ramrakha PS, Marks DI, O'Brien SG, et al. Orthotopic cardiac transplantation for dilated cardiomyopathy after allogeneic bone marrow transplantation. Clin Transplant 1994;8:23–26.
113. Kakavas PW, Ghalie R, Parrillo JE, et al. Angiotensin converting enzyme inhibitors in bone marrow transplant recipients with depressed left ventricular function. Bone Marrow Transplant 1995;15:859–861.
114. Hochster H, Wasserheit C, Speyer J. Cardiotoxicity and cardioprotection during chemotherapy [review]. Curr Opin Oncol 1995;7:304–309.
115. Bush NE, Donaldson GW, Haberman MH, et al. Conditional and unconditional estimation of multidimensional quality of life after hematopoietic stem cell transplantation: a longitudinal follow-up of 415 patients. Biol Blood Marrow Transplant 2000; 6:576–591.
116. Wingard JR, Curbow B, Baker F, et al. Health, functional status, and employment of adult survivors of bone marrow transplantation. Ann Intern Med 1991;114:113–118.
117. Broers S, Kaptein AA, Cessie SL, et al. Psychological functioning and quality of life following bone marrow transplantation: a 3-year follow-up study. J Psychosom Res 2000;48:11–21.
118. Lee SJ, Fairclough D, Parsons SK, et al. Recovery after stem-cell transplantation for hematologic diseases. J Clin Oncol 2001;19: 242–252.
119. Syrjala KL, Chapko MK, Vitaliano PP, et al. Recovery after allogeneic marrow transplantation: prospective study of predictors of long-term physical and psychosocial functioning. Bone Marrow Transplant 1993:11:319–327.
120. Zittoun R, Suciu S, Watson M, et al. Quality of life in patients with acute myelogenous leukemia in prolonged first complete remission after bone marrow transplantation [allogeneic or autologous] or chemotherapy: a cross-sectional study of the EORTC-GIMEMA AML 8 A trial. Bone Marrow Transplant 1997;20:307–315.
121. Andrykowski MA, Bruehl S, Brady MJ, et al. Physical and psychosocial status of adults one year after bone marrow transplantation: a prospective study. Bone Marrow Transplant 1995;15:837–844.
122. Brezden CB, Phillips KA, Abdolell M, et al. Cognitive function in breast cancer patients receiving adjuvant chemotherapy. J Clin Oncol 2000;18:2695–2701.
123. Chiodi S, Spinelli S, Ravera G, et al. Quality of life in 244 recipients of allogeneic bone marrow transplantation. Br J Haematol 2000;110:614–619.
124. Duell T, van Lint MT, Ljungman P, et al. Health and functional status of long-term survivors of bone marrow transplantation. Ann Intern Med 1997;126:184–192.
125. Heinonen H, Volin L, Uutela A, et al. Quality of life and factors related to perceived satisfaction with quality of life after allogeneic bone marrow transplantation. Ann Hematol 2001;80: 137–143.
126. Prieto JM, Saez R, Carreras E, et al. Physical and psychosocial functioning of 117 survivors of bone marrow transplantation. Bone Marrow Transplant 1996;17:1133–1142.
127. Syrjala KL, Langer SL, Abrams JR, et al. Recovery and long-term function after hematopoietic cell transplantation for leukemia or lymphoma. JAMA 2004;291(19):2335–2343.
128. Bush NE, Haberman M, Donaldson G, et al. Quality of life of 125 adults surviving 6–18 years after bone marrow transplantation. Soc Sci Med 1995;40:479–490.
129. Kiss TL, Abdolell M, Jamal N, et al. Long-term medical outcomes and quality of life assessment of patients with chronic myeloid leukemia followed at least 10 years after allogeneic bone marrow transplantation. J Clin Oncol 2002;20:2334–2343.
130. Hensel M, Egerer G, Schneeweiss A, et al. Quality of life and rehabilitation in social and professional life after autologous stem cell transplantation. Ann Oncol 2002;13:209–217.
131. Sanders JE, Syrjala KL, Hoffmeister PA, et al. Quality of life (QOL) of adult survivors of childhood leukemia treated with chemotherapy (CT) or bone marrow transplant (BMT). Blood 2001;98:741a.
132. Felder-Puig R, Peters C, Matthes-Martin S, et al. Psychosocial adjustment of pediatric patients after allogeneic stem cell transplantation. Bone Marrow Transplant 1999;24:75–80.
133. Badell I, Igual L, Gomez P, et al. Quality of life in young adults having received a BMT during childhood: a GETMON study. Bone Marrow Transplant 1998;21(suppl 2):S68–S71
134. Schmidt GM, Niland JC, Forman SJ, et al. Extended follow-up in 212 long-term allogeneic bone marrow transplant survivors. Transplantation 1993;55:551–557.
135. Andrykowski MA, Carpenter JS, Greiner CB, et al. Energy level and sleep quality following bone marrow transplantation. Bone Marrow Transplant 1997;20:669–679.

136. Hann DM, Jacobsen PB, Martin SC, et al. Fatigue in women treated with bone marrow transplantation for breast cancer: a comparison with women with no history of cancer. Support Care Cancer 1997;5:44–52.
137. McQuellon RP, Russell GB, Rambo TD, et al. Quality of life and psychological distress of bone marrow transplant recipients: the "time trajectory" to recovery over the first year. Bone Marrow Transplant 1998;21:477–486.
138. Knobel H, Loge JH, Nordøy T, et al. High level of fatigue in lymphoma patients treated with high dose therapy. J Pain Symptom Manag 2000;19:446–456.
139. Baron F, Sautois B, Baudoux E, et al. Optimization of recombinant human erythropoietin therapy after allogeneic hematopoietic stem cell transplantation. Exp Hematol 2002;30:546–554.
140. Dimeo FC, Stieglitz RD, Novelli-Fischer U, et al. Effects of physical activity on the fatigue and psychologic status of cancer patients during chemotherapy. Cancer (Phila) 1999;85: 2273–2277.
141. Gaston-Johansson F, Fall-Dickson JM, Nanda J, et al. The effectiveness of the comprehensive coping strategy program on clinical outcomes in breast cancer autologous bone marrow transplantation. Cancer Nurs 2000;23:277–285.
142. Jager HR, Williams EJ, Savage DG, et al. Assessment of brain changes with registered MR before and after bone marrow transplantation for chronic myeloid leukemia. Am J Neurorad 1996;17:1275–1282.
143. Provenzale JM, Graham ML. Reversible leukoencephalopathy associated with graft-versus-host disease: MR findings. Am J Neurorad 1996;17:1290–1294.
144. Openshaw H, Slatkin NE, Smith E. Eye movement disorders in bone marrow transplant patients on cyclosporin and ganciclovir. Bone Marrow Transplant 1997;19:503–505.
145. Shah AK. Cyclosporine A neurotoxicity among bone marrow transplant recipients [review]. Clin Neuropharmacol 1999;22: 67–73.
146. Padovan CS, Yousry TA, Schleuning M, et al. Neurological and neuroradiological findings in long-term survivors of allogeneic bone marrow transplantation. Ann Neurol 1998;43:627–633.
147. Andrykowski MA, Schmitt FA, Gregg ME, et al. Neuropsychologic impairment in adult bone marrow transplant candidates. Cancer (Phila) 1992;70:2288–2297.
148. Meyers CA, Weitzner M, Byrne K, et al. Evaluation of the neurobehavioral functioning of patients before, during, and after bone marrow transplantation. J Clin Oncol 1994;12:820–826.
149. Syrjala KL, Dikmen S, Roth-Roemer S. Neuropsychological changes from pretransplant to one year in patients receiving myeloablative allogeneic hematopoietic cell transplant. Blood 2004;104:3386–3392.
150. van Dam FS, Schagen SB, Muller MJ, et al. Impairment of cognitive function in women receiving adjuvant treatment for high-risk breast cancer: high-dose versus standard-dose chemotherapy. J Natl Cancer Inst 1998;90:210–218.
151. Harder H, Cornelissen JJ, Van Gool AR, et al. Cognitive functioning and quality of life in long-term adult survivors of bone marrow transplantation. Cancer (Phila) 2002;95:183–192.
152. Saykin A, Ahles T, McDonald BC. Mechanisms of chemotherapy-induced cognitive disorders: neuropsychological, pathophysiological, and neuroimaging perspectives. Semin Clin Neuropsychol 2003;8:201–216.
153. Andrykowski MA, Altmaier EM, Barnett RL, et al. Cognitive dysfunction in adult survivors of allogeneic marrow transplantation: relationship to dose of total body irradiation. Bone Marrow Transplant 1990;6:269–276.
154. Peper M, Steinvorth S, Schraube P, et al. Neurobehavioral toxicity of total body irradiation: a follow-up in long-term survivors. Int J Radiat Oncol Biol Phys 2000;46:303–311.
155. Wenz F, Steinvorth S, Lohr F, et al. Prospective evaluation of delayed central nervous system [CNS] toxicity of hyperfractionated total body irradiation [TBI]. Int J Radiat Oncol Biol Phys 2000;48:1497–1501.
156. Fann JR, Roth-Roemer S, Burington BE, et al. Delirium in patients undergoing hematopoietic stem cell transplantation. Cancer (Phila) 2002;95:1971–1981.
157. Phipps S, Dunavant M, Srivastava DK, et al. Cognitive and academic functioning in survivors of pediatric bone marrow transplantation. J Clin Oncol 2000;18:1004–1011.
158. Arvidson J, Kihlgren M, Hall C, et al. Neuropsychological functioning after treatment for hematological malignancies in childhood, including autologous bone marrow transplantation. Pediatr Hematol Oncol 1999;16:9–21.
159. Kramer JH, Crittenden MR, DeSantes K, et al. Cognitive and adaptive behavior 1 and 3 years following bone marrow transplantation. Bone Marrow Transplant 1997;19:607–613.
160. Simms S, Kazak AE, Gannon T, et al. Neuropsychological outcome of children undergoing bone marrow transplantation. Bone Marrow Transplant 1998;22:181–184.
161. Howell SJ, Radford JA, Smets EM, et al. Fatigue, sexual function and mood following treatment for haematological malignancy: the impact of mild Leydig cell dysfunction. Br J Can 2000; 82:789–793.
162. Schimmer AD, Ali V, Stewart AK, et al. Male sexual function after autologous blood or marrow transplantation. Biol Blood Marrow Transplant 2001;7:279–283.
163. Wingard JR, Curbow B, Baker F, et al. Sexual satisfaction in survivors of bone marrow transplantation. Bone Marrow Transplant 1992;9:185–190.
164. Molassiotis A, van den Akker OB, Milligan DW, et al. Gonadal function and psychosexual adjustment in male long-term survivors of bone marrow transplantation. Bone Marrow Transplant 1995;16:253–259.
165. Watson M, Wheatley K, Harrison GA, et al. Severe adverse impact on sexual functioning and fertility of bone marrow transplantation, either allogeneic or autologous, compared with consolidation chemotherapy alone: analysis of the MRC AML 10 trial. Cancer (Phila) 1999;86:1231–1239.
166. Syrjala KL, Schroeder TC, Abrams JR, et al. Sexual function measurement and outcomes in cancer survivors and matched controls. J Sex Res 2000;37:213–225.
167. Schubert MA, Sullivan KM, Schubert MM, et al. Gynecological abnormalities following allogeneic bone marrow transplantation. Bone Marrow Transplant 1990;5:425–430.
168. Syrjala KL, Powell-Emsbo S, Garrett K, et al. Focus Forward: Recovery Tips and Tools for Transplant Recipients and Caregivers. Seattle: Fred Hutchinson Cancer Research Center, 2002.
169. Chatterjee R, Kottaridis PD, McGarrigle HH, et al. Management of erectile dysfunction by combination therapy with testosterone and sildenafil in recipients of high-dose therapy for haematological malignancies. Bone Marrow Transplant 2002; 29:607–610.
170. Kauppila M, Viikari J, Irjala K, et al. The hypothalamus-pituitary-gonad axis and testicular function in male patients after treatment for haematological malignancies. J Intern Med 1998;244:411–416.
171. Loberiza FR Jr, Rizzo JD, Bredeson CN, et al. Association of depressive syndrome and early deaths among patients after stem-cell transplantation for malignant disease. J Clin Oncol 2002;20:2118–2126.
172. Molassiotis A, van den Akker OB, Milligan DW, et al. Symptom distress, coping style and biological variables as predictors of survival after bone marrow transplantation. J Psychosom Res 1997;42:275–285.
173. Fife BL, Huster GA, Cornetta KG, et al. Longitudinal study of adaptation to the stress of bone marrow transplantation. J Clin Oncol 2000;18:1539–1549.
174. Phipps S, Dunavant M, Garvie PA, et al. Acute health-related quality of life in children undergoing stem cell transplant: I.

Descriptive outcomes. Bone Marrow Transplant 2002;29: 425–434.
175. Mielcarek M, Martin PJ, Leisenring W, et al. Graft-versus-host disease after nonmyeloablative versus conventional hematopoietic stem cell transplantation. Blood 2002;100:175a.
176. Foxall M, Gaston-Johansson F. Burden and health outcomes of family caregivers of hospitalized bone marrow transplant patients. J Adv Nurs 1996;24:915–923.
177. Zabora JR, Smith ED, Baker F, et al. The family: the other side of bone marrow transplantation. J Psychosoc Oncol 1992;10: 35–46.
178. Manne S, DuHamel K, Nereo N, et al. Predictors of PTSD in mothers of children undergoing bone marrow transplantation: the role of cognitive and social processes. J Pediatr Psychol 2002;27:607–617.
179. Langer SL, Abrams JR, Syrjala KL. Caregiver and patient marital satisfaction and affect following hematopoietic stem cell transplantation: a prospective, longitudinal investigation. Psycho-Oncology 2003;12:239–253.
180. Deeg HJ, Lin D, Leisenring W, et al. Cyclosporine or cyclosporine plus methylprednisolone for prophylaxis of graft-versus-host disease: a prospective, randomized trial. Blood 1997;89: 3880–3887.
181. Ruutu T, Volin L, Parkkali T, et al. Cyclosporine, methotrexate, and methylprednisolone compared with cyclosporine and methotrexate for the prevention of graft-versus-host disease in bone marrow transplantation from HLA-identical sibling donor: a prospective randomized study. Blood 2000;96:2391–2398.
182. Leung W, Hudson M, Zhu Y, et al. Late effects in survivors of infant leukemia. Leukemia 2000;14:1185–1190.
183. Thomas BC, Stanhope R, Plowman PN, et al. Growth following single fraction and fractionated total body irradiation for bone marrow transplantation. Eur J Pediatr 1993;152:888–892.
184. Sanders JE, and the Seattle Marrow Transplant Team. The impact of marrow transplant preparative regimens on subsequent growth and development. Semin Hematol 1991;28: 244–249.
185. Chatterjee R, Andrews HO, McGarrigle HH, et al. Cavernosal arterial insufficiency is a major component of erectile dysfunction in some recipients of high-dose chemotherapy/chemoradiotherapy for haematological malignancies. Bone Marrow Transplant 2000;25:1185–1189.
186. Mumma GH, Mashberg D, Lesko LM. Long-term psychosexual adjustment of acute leukemia survivors: impact of marrow transplantation versus conventional chemotherapy. Gen Hosp Psychiatry 1992;14(1):43–55.

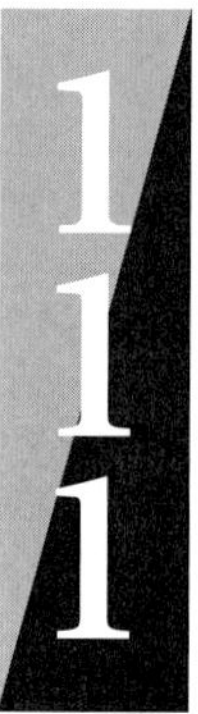

Second Malignancies After Radiation Treatment and Chemotherapy for Primary Cancers

Lydia B. Zablotska, Matthew J. Matasar, and Alfred I. Neugut

Cancer survivors have been shown to have an increased risk for second malignant neoplasms (SMN). These increased risks result from genetic predisposition, harmful environmental exposures, or cancer treatment therapies. Regardless of their cause, SMNs now comprise the sixth most common group of malignancies after skin, prostate, breast, lung, and colorectal cancers.[1] It is important to emphasize that the fear of SMN related to the treatment of the first cancer diagnosis should not outweigh the positive effects of curative therapy for the first cancer. Both physicians and patients should, however, be aware of the consequences of the cancer treatment regimens, specifically radiation therapy (RT) and chemotherapy, and consider them while devising follow-up plans.

Radiation Therapy

The following are general criteria for attributing a malignancy to the effects of radiation, defined by Goolden in 1951: (a) a history of prior irradiation; (b) malignancy occurring within the prior irradiation field; (c) gross or microscopic pathologic evidence of radiation damage to the surrounding tissues; and (d) a long, latent interval between the prior irradiation and the development of the malignancy.[2–5] Only the first two criteria are considered essential.

External-beam radiation therapy has the potential for the induction of mutations in normal cells because of the harmful effects of the radiation used to kill cancer cells. Years or decades later, such mutated cells may give rise to new primary cancers.

Although ionizing radiation has been shown to cause most types of cancer, some organs and tissues appear to be more susceptible than others. Based on radiation epidemiologic studies, the most radiation-sensitive solid tissues and organs are the bone marrow, thyroid, and female breast. Bone and soft tissue sarcomas also can occur following radiation therapy.[6] In addition, cancers of the lung, stomach, colon, bladder, and esophagus have been conclusively associated with ionizing radiation exposure. Possible links have been described for cancers of the kidney, ovary, brain, and central nervous system (CNS). Cancers of other sites have not been correlated with radiation exposure.[7]

In addition to individual susceptibility, the risk of second cancers after radiation therapy depends on the total dose of radiation delivered during the course of treatment, as well as on the type and energy of the radiation. Megavoltage treatments currently in use deliver concentrated high energy to tumors, with low scatter of the radiation to areas outside of the treatment field (low peripheral doses). Orthovoltage treatments, which were used in previous decades, on the other hand, frequently injured the skin and delivered higher doses of radiation to the bone than to the surrounding tissues, and in the process produced substantial peripheral doses.

The type of dose delivery (protracted or instantaneous) also plays a role in the carcinogenesis of second malignancies. It is generally recognized that, as the exposure time for a given total dose is extended, the biologic effect is reduced. Protracted delivery of a dose over hours or days, in general, will result in less severe consequences because of reduced tumorigenic effectiveness as compared to the instantaneous delivery of the total dose.

Finally, the risks of second cancers depend on the volume of irradiated tissues and organs. Current treatment guidelines recommend that smaller fractions should be used when larger volumes need to be irradiated to decrease the acute side effects of radiation treatment. The late effects of radiotherapy could be lessened by "hyperfractionation" of radiation therapy (smaller doses twice per day over the same treatment period).[6]

Recent technologic advances (shielding, collimation of the radiation beam, use of multivoltage beams, more precise localization of tumors) have significantly reduced the irradiation of normal tissues and the risk of posttherapy new cancers. However, because radiation-associated cancers tend to appear at the same age as spontaneous cancers, patients who were exposed many years ago at young ages may, potentially, be at risk of developing SMN cancers due to radiation exposure.

Individual risks for patients are modified by such factors as their age at the time of exposure, time since exposure/survival time, gender, exposure to other carcinogens (including chemotherapy), as well as by immune and hormonal status. Although the risks associated with radiation exposure are substantially less than the risks posed by the initial tumor, it is important to know them before the start of the radiation therapy to make informed decisions about treatment regimens that might minimize the side effects of radiation therapy. This information is also important for counseling patients who are at increased risk of developing second malignancies due to other risk factors, as well as for continuing surveillance of those treated. Our knowledge of the possible adverse effects associated with radiation therapy should be used for the development of surveillance programs aimed at the early detection of cancers and campaigns to decrease negative behaviors and exposures that have been shown to promote the development of second cancers after radiation therapy.

Individual Cancers

In our review, we look at the subjects who received irradiation for treatment of nine specific primary malignant diseases and summarize the evidence from the descriptive (case reports and case series) and analytical (case-control, cohort, and randomized controlled trials) epidemiologic studies to show the current state of knowledge on the consequences of the treatment for each of the nine diseases.

After reviewing epidemiologic studies for the nine primary cancers, we compare and contrast their findings. We show that they add to our knowledge of the effects of high-dose exposures and can be used for risk estimation purposes as well as to provide both physicians and patients with the necessary information to make informed decisions regarding radiation therapy for primary cancer.

Pediatric Cancers

Various epidemiologic studies have shown that the incidence of the majority of cancers increases with age. Based on data from the Japanese survivors of the atomic bombings of Hiroshima and Nagasaki, the effect of radiation exposure is to multiply age-specific solid cancer rates by a constant radiation dose-dependent factor through lifetime. Thus, those with absorbed dose of 0.20 Sv experience a 10% increase in the risk of solid cancer above background rates. Estimates of risk also depend on age at exposure (increase by 10 years decreases relative risk for solid cancers by 130%).[8] Based on the same data, most organizations have adopted a multiplicative risk model for most solid cancers, which states that after a specified latency period, "the excess cancer risk is given by a constant factor applied to the age-dependent incidence of natural cancers in the population"[9] (p. 108) (in other words, the relative risk remains constant as subjects are followed over time).

The majority of cancers that are associated with radiation exposure, thus, will appear at the same time when spontaneous cancers of the same organ appear. The difference between exposed and unexposed populations, then, will be in the number of new incident cases. Researchers, therefore, have combined subjects with specific types of first childhood cancers and studied them as a group named "pediatric cancers."

The significance of the problem of second malignancies after pediatric cancers is underscored by the fact that survival following childhood cancer has improved markedly and now approaches 70%.[1] Thus, it is important to compare the carcinogenic potential of different treatments for primary pediatric cancers. Some pediatric cancers are more likely to be treated with radiation than others and, as a consequence, they are associated with second malignancies within the radiation field. First reports about second cancers following primary pediatric cancers started appearing in the late 1970s with the advent of new radiation treatment regimens. A large study of pediatric patients who were followed for at least 2 years after initial treatment of the primary tumor showed no association between RT and the subsequent development of leukemia.[10] Although large, this study had a very small proportion of subjects who received only RT; the majority of subjects also received chemotherapy. Thus, the effects of RT could have been obscured by the effects of treatment by various alkylating agents. In a more-recent study of childhood cancer survivors, the risk of second leukemia after RT was significantly increased eightfold.[11] The difference between the two studies could be explained by the size of the irradiation field. Patients with HD usually receive more targeted radiation treatment, whereas the cumulative doses for radiotherapy for NHL are usually smaller than the doses delivered for treatment of HD. Nevertheless, in the process of treatment, larger areas of radiosensitive tissues, such as bone marrow, are exposed to radiation.

Other second cancers that have been associated with RT for primary childhood cancers include cancers of the bone,[12] skin,[13] nervous system,[14] and thyroid gland.[15] As one would expect with solid cancer, in these studies the incidence increased with time since treatment. For example, in The Late Effects Study Group, which followed 9,000 survivors of childhood cancer, a lifetime risk of thyroid gland cancer after RT for primary childhood cancer was almost 4% after 26 years of follow-up.[15] To avoid problems associated with low power of individual studies, Ron et al. pooled data from seven individual studies to evaluate the risk of thyroid cancer following exposure to external radiation. Individual estimates of increased risk of thyroid cancer varied from 1.4 to 33.5 per Gy[16]; that is, those who were exposed to 1 Gy of radiation during RT for primary cancer had a much higher risk of developing second primary thyroid cancer compared to those who did not receive RT. This study provided strong evidence that, along with the breast and bone marrow, the thyroid gland is one of the most radiosensitive organs.

Population-based study of the occurrence of second cancers following primary childhood cancer in the five Nordic countries showed that childhood cancer survivors have a fourfold-higher risk of second cancers compared to the general population.[17] The largest increase was observed during the first 10 years following RT; however, risks remained increased throughout their lifetimes and the absolute excess of second cancers increased with time. This result probably reflects the promotional effect of radiation on the carcinogenic effects of environmental exposures.

Several publications from the large Childhood Cancer Survivor Study cohort show an increased risk of second malignant neoplasms more than 20 years after RT for primary childhood cancer. In comparison with the general population, their risk of bone second cancers, in particular bone sarcomas and breast cancer, was increased sixfold.[18]

In summary, the effects of radiation treatment for childhood cancers start to increase in early adolescence and early adulthood and continue to be increased later in life. Bone marrow, bone and soft tissues, and breast and thyroid gland appear to be the most radiosensitive. Risk of second tumors depends on the age at exposure (the risk is greatest among those exposed at the youngest ages) and on the time since exposure. Current knowledge of the effects of ionizing radiation had an important influence on RT practices. Specifically, lead aprons and shields are currently being used to protect the most radiation-sensitive organs and tissues. In addition, advances in technology, such as utilization of wedge compensators or half-beam blocks, minimize scattering of radiation to adjacent tissues. Finally, because of the greater awareness of the effects of radiation, survivors of childhood cancers are being constantly monitored and screened for second cancers during follow-up.

Bone Marrow Transplantation

High-dose total-body irradiation (TBI) is part of the conditioning regimen for bone marrow transplantation used for treatment of leukemia and other diseases. One of the mechanisms of development of second cancers following TBI is thought to be due to radiation-induced immunosuppression.[19] In addition to radiation-associated effects, it is also necessary to consider the effects of immunosuppressive drugs that are used concomitantly with radiation. Curtis et al. showed that patients who received TBI had an increased risk of subsequent new solid cancers compared to those who did not receive radiation treatment.[20] High doses of TBI were associated with increased risks of melanoma and cancers of the brain and thyroid. The risk was higher for recipients who were younger at the time of transplantation than for those who were older (P for trend less than 0.001).

Another registry-based study found that high-dose TBI increased the risk of subsequent solid tumors threefold [95% confidence interval (CI), 1.1, 10.3].[21] Younger age at the time of treatment increased the risk of brain and thyroid tumors. In addition, cancers of the salivary gland, bone, and connective tissues were also increased.

In summary, various studies show the trend toward an increased risk over time after transplantation and the greater risk among younger patients. Second cancers could be related to both transplant therapy and to chemotherapy treatments given before it. All these factors indicate the need for lifelong surveillance of the patients who received irradiation as part of the bone marrow transplantation.

Hodgkin's Disease

Introduction of intensive radiotherapy and chemotherapy to treat Hodgkin's disease (HD) three decades ago dramatically changed survival times and prognosis for patients with this disorder. Long-term sequelae of treatment have become increasingly important as patients now survive for several decades. HD is a systemic cancer and radiation treatment frequently consists of irradiation of mantle fields, including all lymph node regions ('total lymphoid irradiation' with cumulative doses 20–40 Gy) or only some regions ('subtotal lymphoid irradiation' with doses less than 20 Gy), by external-radiation beams.[22] Dose–response analysis of the effects of radiation is frequently confounded by the concurrent chemotherapy in the majority of patients.

Several studies looked at breast cancer incidence and mortality, the most frequently seen second malignancy following treatment for HD. Table 111.1 summarizes the results of the most influential studies. In general, risk of breast cancer was increased and ranged from 2 to 75 times compared to the risk in the general population. Most cancers appeared within or at the margin of the radiation field, and the risk increased with dose. Investigators from the Late Effects Study Group estimated that the cumulative probability of breast cancer at age 40 following radiation exposure for HD in childhood is close to 35% (following a median dose of radiotherapy of 40 Gy).[23]

Clemons et al.[22] reviewed 18 epidemiologic studies on the risk of breast cancer in patients treated with radiation for Hodgkin's disease. They concluded that women between the ages of puberty and 30 years are at the highest risk. Data on the use of exogenous estrogen hormones, age at first pregnancy, and prevalence of early menopause were not available

TABLE 111.1. Studies of breast cancer risk among patients treated for primary Hodgkin's disease.

Reference	*Year*	*RT and follow-up*	*Age at the time of first treatment*	*SIR and 95% CI*
Hancock et al.[114]	1993	1961–1989	Mean age 25 years	SIR = 4.1 (2.5, 5.7)
Bhatia et al.[23]	1996	1955–1986, follow-up till 1996	Younger than 16 years old	SIR = 75.3 (44.9, 118.4)
Tinger et al.[115]	1997	1966–1974 treatment era	Mean age 30 years	4.7
Tinger et al.[115]	1997	1974–1985 treatment era	Mean age 28 years	2.2
Hudson et al.[116]	1998	1968–1990	—	SIR = 1.33 (1.12, 1.72)
Wolden et al.[117]	1998	1960–1995	Younger than 21 years	SIR = 1.26 (1.15, 1.42)
Swerdlow et al.[27]	2000	1963–1993	60% younger than 35 years old	SIR = 2.5 (1.4, 4.0)
Van Leeuwen et al.[70]	2000	1966–1986	Younger than 40 years old	SIR = 7.7 (4.3, 12.7)

RT, radiotherapy; SIR, standardized incidence ratio; CI, confidence interval.

to control for possible confounding effects of these variables. Breast cancers due to irradiation tend to appear after a 15-year latency period at the age from 30 to 40. Breast cancer risk is highly dependent on age at irradiation, time since irradiation, dose, and concurrent chemotherapy. These findings, along with the finding that no cases of breast cancer after radiation therapy for HD have been reported in men, suggest that the actively growing and differentiating cells of female breast tissue are particularly vulnerable to radiation exposure.

A nested case-control study of lung cancer among patients previously treated for HD found that radiation doses greater than 5 Gy increased the risk sixfold (95% CI, 2.7, 13.5).[24] Smoking acted in a multiplicative way with radiation exposure [relative risk (RR) comparing moderate-heavy smokers to nonsmokers and light smokers among those without radiation treatment was 6.0; RR comparing those with radiation treatment to those without among nonsmokers and light smokers was 7.2; RR comparing those with radiation treatment to those without among all subjects adjusting for smoking was 20.2]. Treatment with alkylating agents, on the other hand, acted additively with radiation therapy (individual risks added up to perfect additivity). Similar to other studies, increased age at diagnosis of HD was associated with an increased risk of lung cancer.

Birdwell et al.[25] noticed that high doses to the abdomen from radiation for HD cause multiple gastrointestinal (GI) cancers, including stomach, pancreas, and small intestine (RR for all GI cancers, 2.0, 95% CI, 1.0, 3.4). Risks started to increase after a latency period of 10 years and were highest among younger patients. GI cancers were similarly increased in the large study based on the International Database on HD (more than 12,000 cases)[25] and in the study of atomic bomb survivors (53% of all incident cancers in the atomic bomb study were due to cancers of the digestive system).[26]

Findings of increased risk of second cancers are further supported by the largest current study of 5,519 British patients with HD who were followed for more than 30 years.[27] Irradiated patients had a 1.7 fold (95% CI, 1.0, 2.5) higher incidence of GI cancers, 2.5 fold (95% CI, 1.4, 4.0) higher incidence of breast cancer, and 2.9 fold (95% CI, 1.9, 4.1) higher incidence of lung cancer than the general population. Risk of leukemia was increased in patients who received combined modality treatment (chemotherapy with radiotherapy) or chemotherapy alone compared to those who received RT alone. Similar to previous studies, relative risks tended to increase 5 to 10 years after treatment and decreased with increasing age at first treatment. Women older than 25 years were not at risk of increased breast cancer [$RR_{<25\ years}$, 14.4 (95% CI, 5.7, 29.3) and $RR_{25\text{–}44\ years}$, 1.6 (95% CI, 0.5, 3.7)]. A combined study of 16 population-based cancer registries in Europe and North America, which included HD patients diagnosed before the age of 21 years, also found that the risk of second malignancy decreased with increasing age at HD diagnosis and treatment on a relative scale.[28] High estimates of relative risks of second cancers in this cohort were due to low background rates in the relatively young cohort.

In summary, it appears that radiation treatment for HD increases the risk of second malignancies. Long-term risks depend on age at exposure and time since exposure. Latency periods differ from study to study, but a major increase in risks appears at 10 to 14 years of follow-up. Second cancers sometimes appear at a much younger age than similar cancers. Radiation treatment for HD is linked to cancers of the GI tract, breast, lung, bone, and soft tissue, melanoma, and thyroid gland (Table 111.2).

Breast Cancer

Standard treatment for invasive breast cancer includes high, concentrated doses of radiation to the chest and to the lymph nodes (about 40–60 Gy total).[29] Initially, localized radiotherapy was combined with radical mastectomy, but since the mid-1980s treatment consists of breast-conserving surgery and radiotherapy. Women irradiated before the mid-1980s received higher doses of radiation to the lungs, contralateral breast, thoracic bone, and bone marrow. A small increase in risk of leukemia was shown in a cohort of women from the Connecticut Tumor Registry irradiated between 1935 and 1972.[29] Following an average dose of 5.3 Gy to the bone marrow, the risk was 16% higher in irradiated women than in nonirradiated women (90% CI, 0.6, 2.1). A larger study based on five population-based cancer registries in the United States (1973–1985)[30] found a 2.4 times increased risk (95% CI, 1.0, 5.8) of acute nonlymphocytic leukemia after radiation treatment with an average dose of 7.5 Gy over the total active bone marrow. They observed a positive dose–response relation in the data (those exposed to doses higher than 9 Gy had a 7-fold-higher risk). Increase in risk was first seen 2 years after initial treatment, and it persisted, albeit at a much lower level, 7 years after treatment. The authors described a statistical multiplicative interaction effect of radiotherapy and treatment with alkylating agents on the development of ANLL (RR for radiotherapy alone, 2.4; RR for alkylating agents therapy, 10.0; RR for combined therapy, 17.4).

Boice et al.[31] described an increase in the risk of cancer in the contralateral breast in patients from the Connecticut Tumor Registry diagnosed between 1935 and 1982. An average dose of 2.8 Gy was associated with a twofold increase in risk in 10-year survivors. Risk was significantly higher among women who were younger than 45 years at the time of radiation treatment. The investigators estimated that the absolute excess risk of contralateral breast cancer was 4.4 cases per 10,000 person-years per Gy (compared to 6.7 cases per 10,000 person-years per Gy for atomic bomb survivors).[26]

Several studies have shown a significantly increased risk of lung cancer following radiation therapy (RT) after total mastectomy. Ten-year survivors from the Connecticut Tumor Registry who were diagnosed with histologically confirmed primary invasive breast cancer between 1935 and 1971 had an 80% higher risk (95% CI, 0.8, 3.8) of developing lung cancer if they received radiotherapy as part of their initial treatment regimen compared to those not receiving initial RT (mean dose to both lungs, 9.8 Gy).[32] Risk continued to increase with time and after 15 years reached 2.8 (95% CI, 1.0, 8.2). The excess relative rate was 0.20 per Gy (95% CI, −0.62, 1.03) compared to an estimate of 0.95 per Gy (95% CI, 0.60, 1.4) for trachea, bronchus, and lung in the atomic bomb study.[26] In a case-control study from this cohort, Neugut et al.[33] assessed risk of lung cancer in relation to radiation treatment and smoking in 10-year survivors. They observed a multiplicative interaction effect if both exposures were present (OR for RT alone, 3.2; OR for smoking and no RT, 17.7; OR for both RT and smoking, 32.7).

TABLE 111.2. Studies of risks of second malignant neoplasms (SMNs) among patients treated for primary Hodgkin's disease.

Reference	*Year*	*Design*	*Median follow-up, years*	*Site(s) of SMN*	*Primary treatment modalities*	*Estimates of risk and 95% CI*
Swerdlow et al.[27]	2000	Cohort	8.5	Gastrointestinal	ChT	SIR = 1.5 (0.8, 2.5; $P > 0.05$)*
					ChT + RT	SIR = 3.3 (2.1, 4.8; $P < 0.001$)
				Lung	ChT	SIR = 3.3 (2.2, 4.7; $P < 0.001$)
					ChT + RT	SIR = 4.3 (2.9, 6.2; $P < 0.001$)
				NHL	ChT	SIR = 14.8 (8.7, 23.3; $P < 0.001$)
Swerdlow et al.[71]	2001	Nested case-control	8.5	Lung	MOPP + RT (vs. RT)	OR = 2.41 (1.33, 4.51; $P = 0.004$)
Dores et al.[18]	2002	Cohort	25	Cumulative solid tumor	ChT	RR = 2.1 (n/a; $P < 0.05$)
					ChT + RT	RR = 2.0 (1.9, 2.0; $P < 0.05$)
				Acute nonlymphcytic leukemia	ChT	RR = 36.1 (25.6, 49.3; $P < 0.05$)
van Leeuwen et al.[70]	2000	Cohort	14.1	Breast	RT	RR = 7.7 (4.3, 12.7)
					ChT + RT	RR = 7.5 (2.7, 16.3)
					ChT + RT + salvage	RR = 1.4 (0.2, 5.1)
				Nonbreast solid tumor	RT	RR = 4.9 (3.0, 7.4)
					ChT + RT	RR = 4.4 (2.0, 8.3)
					ChT + RT + salvage	RR = 10.0 (6.8, 14.3)
				Gastrointestinal	RT	RR = 3.7 (1.0, 9.5)
					ChT + RT	RR = 7.8 (2.1, 20.0)
					ChT + RT + salvage	RR = 13 (6.2, 23.9)
Neglia et al.[18]	2001	Cohort	5	Cumulative SMN	Not specified	RR = 2.34 (1.44, 3.81)
				Breast		RR = 4.89 (0.95, 25.24)
				Leukemia		RR = 3.99 (0.84, 18.88)
				Soft tissue sarcoma		RR = 10.32 (1.18, 90.18)
				Thyroid		RR = 1.74 (0.50, 6.01)
Bhatia et al.[23]	1996	Cohort	11.4	Cumulative SMN	Not specified	SIR 18.1 (14.3, 22.3)
				Breast		SIR 75.3 (44.9, 118.4)
				Leukemia		SIR 78.8 (56.6, 123.2)
				Leukemia	ChT	RR = 1,091 (344, 2256)
					ChT + RT	RR = 439 (270, 645)
				Non-Hodgkin's lymphoma	ChT	RR = 60 (0.02, 235)
					ChT + RT	RR = 23 (6, 50)
Metayer et al.[28]	2000	Cohort	10.5	Cumulative SMN	Not specified	RR = 7.7 (6.6, 8.8)
				Breast		RR = 14.1 ($P < 0.05$)
				Thyroid		RR = 13.7 (8.6, 20.7)
				Leukemia		RR = 20.9 (13.9, 30.3)
				Non-Hodgkin's lymphoma		RR = 27.4 (17.9, 40.2)
Green et al.[69]	2000	Cohort	17.1	*Cumulative SMN (male)	Not specified	RR = 9.39 (4.05, 18.49, $P < 0.00001$)
					RT	RR = 12.32 (2.54, 36.01, $P < 0.005$)
					ChT + RT	RR = 8.64 (2.81, 20.16, $P < 0.001$)
				Cumulative SMN (female)	Not specified	RR = 10.16 (5.56, 17.05, $P < 0.00001$)
					RT	RR = 4.46 (0.92, 13.02, $P = 0.062$)
					ChT + RT	RR = 15.93 (7.95, 28.51, $P < 0.00001$)

OR, odds ratio; NHL, non-Hodgkin's lymphoma; RR, relative risk; ChT, chemotherapy; RT, radiation therapy; SMN, second malignant neoplasm.
*P value of significance.

As was noted earlier, radiation treatment regimens have changed over the past two decades, lowering radiation doses to the lungs.[34] In a large population-based study from the SEER (Surveillance, Epidemiology, and End Results) database of subjects diagnosed and followed up from 1973 till the end of 1998, the risk of cancer in the ipsilateral lung 10 to 14 years after RT and radical mastectomy was increased by 2.06 (95% CI, 1.53, 2.78), whereas the risk of ipsilateral lung cancer 10 to 14 years after conservative surgery (lumpectomy) and adjuvant RT was not increased (RR, 0.80; 95% CI, 0.23, 2.84).[35]

Studies of other cohorts also showed increased risk of second cancers following breast cancer.[36] Another SEER-based study showed that the standardized incidence ratio (SIR) of esophageal cancer after RT for primary breast cancer was 54% higher than in the general population (95% CI, 1.27, 1.84).[37] Risk increased with time, reaching 5.42 (95% CI, 2.33, 10.68) for esophageal squamous cell carcinoma 10 years after radiotherapy. No information on smoking or alcohol consumption was available.

Gynecologic Cancers

Hormones, in general, in these cancers could play an important role in the timing of late effects of radiation treatment, their dependence on the age at exposure, and time since exposure. Some studies do not have data on the use of exogenous estrogen hormones, age at first pregnancy, time of menopause, and other factors related to hormonal status. Therefore, possible confounding effects of these variables could not be evaluated.

Cancer of the Uterus

Curtis et al. examined the relationship of leukemia risk to radiation dose following radiotherapy of the uterine corpus in a nested case-control study based on a cohort of women drawn from nine population-based registries in the United States and Europe.[38] After external-beam therapy (mean dose, 9.88 Gy), cases were two times more likely to develop leukemia (excluding chronic lymphocytic leukemia) than matched controls (ERR, 0.13 per Gy; 95% CI, 0.04, 0.27).

Based primarily on data from the cohort of atomic bomb survivors, the association between radiation exposure and development of leukemia appears to depend on total dose to the bone marrow, total percent of the person's bone marrow exposed to radiation, and the dose rate at which radiation was delivered. As was mentioned earlier, the dose response for atomic bomb survivors is linear-quadratic for doses below 4 Gy (ERR, 4.8 per Sv).[39] The difference between the estimates from the Curtis et al. study and the estimate from the LSS cohort can be partly explained by the killing of stem cells of the bone marrow at high doses. Treatment regimens with low-dose-rate radiation (e.g., brachytherapy) were more leukemogenic per unit dose than external-beam therapy, perhaps due to the repair of radiation damage in protracted exposure regimens.

As a result of a wide field of radiation encompassed by the partial-body radiation treatment (only parts of the body are irradiated as opposed to the total-body irradiation as in bone marrow transplantation) of cancer of the corpus uteri, patients are also at risk of developing second solid cancers. Subjects with primary cancer of the uterine cervix from a Swedish cancer registry had a 20% higher risk of developing a second malignancy compared to the population rates.[40] Organs situated in the immediate proximity to the radiation field had the highest risk of second cancer (colon, vulva, and bladder) 9 years after initial treatment. A fourfold increase in leukemia was observed 3 to 9 years after exposure, but it was based on a small number of cases (95% CI, 1.68, 8.59).

Ovarian Cancer

A SEER-based study of long-term survivors of ovarian cancer found a twofold-increased risk of leukemia 5 to 9 years after radiotherapy,[41] although several case-control studies did not.[42,43] A twofold increase in risk was also observed for all solid cancers 10 to 14 years after exposure (P less than 0.05).[41] Significant associations were seen for cancers of connective tissue, bladder, and pancreas. A case-control study of ovarian cancer survivors who later developed bladder tumor showed that those treated with radiotherapy alone had a twofold-higher risk (95% CI, 0.77, 4.9).[44]

In summary, RT for gynecologic cancers has been linked to the development of various second primary malignancies. They mainly experience increased risks of second malignancies of the organs situated in immediate proximity to the radiation field as well as leukemia.

Testicular Cancer

Testicular cancer is the most common cancer in men in the age group 20 to 44 years.[1] Early reports showed that these patients are at increased risk of second cancers following 10 to 15 years after radiotherapy.[45] Significant increases were observed for all solid cancers (RR, 1.6; 95% CI, 1.3, 2.1), gastrointestinal cancers (RR, 2.6; 95% CI, 1.7, 3.9), and leukemia (RR, 5.1; 95% CI, 1.4, 13.0).

A large population-based study of testicular cancer survivors in 1997 confirmed an increased risk of stomach, bladder, and pancreatic cancers by twofold. Overall risk was similar after seminomas (SIR, 1.42) or nonseminomatous tumors (SIR, 1.50). The largest investigation to date of leukemia following testicular cancer was done in the follow-up of the same cohort.[46] Those treated with radiotherapy had a three times higher risk of developing leukemia (95% CI, 0.7, 22.0). This risk is similar to the risks estimated after radiation therapy for cancers of the cervix,[47] breast,[30] or Hodgkin's disease.[48] Although atomic bomb survivors received lower doses of radiation, they experienced higher risks than medically irradiated subjects mainly because the dose was delivered to the entire body without dose fractionation.[49]

In summary, because testicular cancer is a disease of men under the age of 40 years, they are at increased risk of developing second malignancies later in life. In particular, both physicians and patients should be aware of increased risks of second cancers located in the bladder, lungs, connective tissue, and stomach. These patients should be under continuous surveillance for possible second cancer. In addition, because of the high risks of lung cancer, patients should be advised to quit smoking.

Prostate Cancer

In a large population-based retrospective cohort study of survivors of first primary prostate cancer in the Detroit metropolitan area who were diagnosed between 1973 and 1982, the overall risk of second malignancies was similar to the rates of cancer in the general population.[50] Subanalyses, however, showed that prostate cancer survivors were at increased risk of bladder cancer (SIR, 1.49; 95% CI, 1.07–2.02) when compared to the Detroit-area male population. Researchers concluded that the magnitude of relative and absolute risks did not suggest the presence of large risks associated with radiation treatment. In another large population-based study from the database of the Connecticut Tumor Registry, comparison of the risk of developing a SMN cancer following prostate irradiation compared to the underlying risk in patients with prostate cancer showed that the risks were not significantly different, at any time period and in all age groups, between the two groups of patients.[51] Short follow-up (mean follow-up under 4 years) could have contributed to these negative findings. However, more careful investigation of the cases who survived more than 10 years again showed no significantly increased risk of second malignancy following radiation therapy for primary prostate cancer.[52]

In the largest to date epidemiologic study of second cancers after prostate cancer based on the SEER database, a cohort of patients who received radiation treatment sometime between 1973 and 1990 showed a significant 50% increase in risk of second primary bladder cancer.[53] Risk remained increased for at least 8 years after initial radiation treatment. There was no increased risk of rectal carcinoma or leukemia after this type of radiation exposure.

In summary, prostate cancer is the most common male cancer in the United States, with nearly 200,000 men diagnosed annually.[1] Findings regarding the effect of RT for prostate cancer have been conflicting. If present, risks are probably significantly lower than risks described for other first cancers. This fact could be explained by smaller doses and less-aggressive treatments.

Lung Cancer

In a large retrospective cohort study of 2-year survivors of primary small cell lung cancer, patients who received RT experienced a 13-fold increase in the risk of second primaries among those who received chest irradiation, whereas nonirradiated patients experienced only a 7-fold increase compared to that of the general population.[54] The highest risk was observed among those who continued smoking, with evidence of an interaction between chest irradiation and continued smoking (RR, 21). Risks continued to increase with time after radiation treatment.

In a large population-based study based on the Finnish Tumor Registry lung cancer patients treated with RT between 1953 and 1989, there was a significant increase in the risk of esophageal cancer and leukemia among lung cancer patients subject to radiotherapy.[55] The risk of a second cancer among lung cancer patients increased with the length of follow-up.

Colorectal Cancer

In the past, radiotherapy was not widely used to treat colorectal cancer. There are, consequently, only a few epidemiologic studies of the effects of radiation in colorectal cancers. These studies have shown that patients with primary cancers of the colon and rectum have small increases in risks of SMN cancers as a result of radiation therapies. In particular, irradiation increases the risk of second primaries of the breast, uterus, ovaries, and other pelvic organs in the radiation field.[1,56]

Chemotherapy

That only a small percentage of individuals receiving a given chemotherapeutic regimen will go on to develop a SMN suggests that individual variations play a role in this process. Indeed, it has become apparent that a number of individual factors contribute in part to this risk. Germ-line mutations have long been recognized to predispose to primary malignancies; indeed, more than 40 genes have been cloned that, when mutated from the wild-type, are known to increase the susceptibility to malignancy.[57] Although the mechanisms of this increased susceptibility are variable, it has become apparent that many individuals with these germ-line mutations are at heightened risk of SMN and, specifically, treatment-associated malignancies.

Next we explore the various factors that contribute to the risk of SMN among patients treated with systemic chemotherapy, including the organ affected by the primary cancer, the chemotherapeutic agents employed, and host factors such as environmental exposures and immune status.

Individual Cancers

Although the use of chemotherapeutic alkylating agents imparts a risk of secondary malignancy, particularly secondary leukemia, the concern regarding SMNs is not restricted to their use alone. Indeed, for many of the hematologic and solid malignancies, there are concerns about the potential for patients to experience treatment-related neoplasms. Evidence for such an association is stronger for some malignancies, weaker for others; in some malignancies, there are as yet no convincing data regarding an elevated risk of SMN as a result of treatment. Whether this lack of effect is due to an inability of cancer chemotherapy to significantly prolong life, or whether it reflects a truly low oncogenic potential of the agents employed, is difficult to determine; what is clear, however, is that as chemotherapeutic regimens continue to become both more complex and more effective, the challenge of treatment-related SMN will require ongoing vigilance.

Pediatric Cancers

Acute Lymphocytic Leukemia

A number of reports have been published regarding the risk of treatment-associated malignancies following treatment of childhood acute lymphocytic leukemia (ALL). Children treated with all the most common protocols in ALL therapy, including the Berlin–Frankfurt–Munster (BFM) protocol, Children's Cancer Group protocol, and the Dana–Farber protocol, experience an estimated risk of SMN within 15 years of treatment ranging from 2.5% to 3.3%, although children receiving weekly or twice-weekly epipodophyllotoxin have been found to have a 12% cumulative incidence of secondary myelogenous leukemia.[14,58–60] Despite these concerning statistics, the BFM study failed to find an association between a specific chemotherapeutic agent and subsequent acute myeloid leukemia (AML); 12 of the 16 cases of secondary AML they report had not received epipodophyllotoxin.[60] Patients in these groups who also received craniospinal radiation were found to be at an increased risk of a number of radiation-induced SMNs, including primary CNS malignancy, thyroid cancer, and skin cancers; more-recent ALL protocols have rejected craniospinal radiotherapy in favor of intrathecal chemotherapy for younger patients without evidence of CNS involvement at initiation of therapy.

An additional risk of SMN among patients treated during childhood for ALL is that of malignant melanoma. It had been reported that patients receiving monthly maintenance therapy of vincristine and prednisone, weekly methotrexate, and daily 6-mercaptopurine (6-MP) were found to have an increased number of melanocytic nevi and dysplastic nevi; on this basis, concern was raised that these patients may be at higher risk of subsequent malignant melanoma than the general population.[61] Whether such an effect will be seen with more modern maintenance regimens has not yet been determined.

Sarcoma

In contrast to the specific case of RB-associated sarcoma, the treatment and sequelae from therapy of primary pediatric sarcoma have been well studied. Among these patients, a consistent and long-lasting rate of SMN following intensive chemotherapy of sarcoma has been identified. The reported cumulative incidence of solid SMN among patients treated for Ewing's sarcoma ranges from 5% at 15 years of follow-up to more than 20% at 20 years, whereas the risk of leukemia has been estimated in the range of 2%.[62–64] These patients went on to develop a variety of hematologic complications, including myelodysplasia (MDS) as well as AML and ALL, between 1 and 8 years after therapy for Ewing's sarcoma. Secondary sarcomas within the field of radiotherapy have been described as well; no clear association with systemic chemotherapy has yet been established for these SMNs.

Treatment of pediatric rhabdomyosarcoma has also been associated with the development of SMNs. The latency period for these patients appears to be slightly longer, with a median time to diagnosis of between 5 and 11 years following initial treatment.[65,66] The cumulative incidence of SMN following rhabdomyosarcoma appears to be similar to that found in Ewing's sarcoma, but unlike the case of Ewing's sarcoma, this risk seems to be at least in part attributable to a potentiating effect of systemic chemotherapy.[62,67] Although solid tumor SMNs appear to be salvageable with multimodal therapy, hematologic SMNs following treatment for pediatric sarcoma appear to share the generally poor prognosis of secondary leukemias more commonly seen with epipodophyllotoxins and alkylating agents.[64,66]

Wilm's Tumor

Long-term follow-up data gathered by the National Wilms Tumor Study Group (NWTSG) demonstrated that, between 1969 and 1991, patients treated in childhood for Wilm's tumor went on to develop an eightfold-greater risk of SMN.[68] These malignancies consisted of both solid tumors, largely within the field of irradiation, and hematologic malignancies, including both lymphomas and leukemias. The NWTSG reported that their cohort had developed carcinomas of the breast, thyroid, colon, and parotid gland, hepatocellular carcinoma, and primary CNS malignancies. The study group concluded that it appeared that treatment of these patients with doxorubicin increased the risk of SMN, potentiating the oncogenic effect of the administered ionizing radiation.

Hodgkin's Disease

Patients treated for Hodgkin's disease with chemotherapy, ionizing radiation, or both have a risk of developing a variety of SMNs that, cumulatively, is 2 to 4 times greater than unaffected individuals.[23,27,28,48,69–71] The relative risk of developing specific solid tumors as SMNs shows a great variability, ranging from 2 to more than 50 times greater, depending upon the tissue of origin as well as the chemotherapeutic agents used and whether ionizing radiation was administered concomitantly. The cumulative incidence of SMN following the treatment of Hodgkin's disease thus shows a great variability as well, from as low as 2% to as high as 27% within 30 years of treatment.

Specific tissues of origin for these secondary SMNs include thyroid, breast, and skin (melanoma and nonmelanoma). Thyroid cancer remains the most common SMN following the treatment of Hodgkin's and is affected by both chemotherapeutic agents as well as the dose of ionizing radiation.[18] And, although the risks associated with ionizing radiation have already been discussed, the risks associated with alkylating agents apply to patients treated for Hodgkin's disease as well. Indeed, up to 25% of SMNs among these patients are either lymphomas or leukemias.[27,28,48,69,70] The risk of hematologic malignancy as an SMN is, in large part, attributable to the chemotherapeutic agents included in the management of the disease, that is, alkylators versus others. Risks of leukemia, demonstrating the dose–response relationship as discussed, continue to rise with additional chemotherapy, and thus patients requiring retreatment for recurrence of Hodgkin's disease are at higher risk yet of SMN. Given the significant concerns regarding long-term risk of SMNs from therapy, pediatric oncologists have begun modifying treatment regimens, with boys receiving fewer alkylating agents and girls receiving less chest wall irradiation.

Breast Cancer

Women with breast cancer are known to be at higher risk for SMN malignancies within the contralateral breast, as well as at least a slightly elevated risk of primary malignancies of many other organs, including the ovaries, endometrium, and lower gastrointestinal tract; this risk elevation, however, appears to be independent of the treatment modalities used in the primary malignancy.[72–74] These associations suggest that these organs share one or more common risk factors for malignancy with the breast, including hormonal status, diet, and adiposity. A subset of patients with breast cancer carries a heritable risk due to mutations in *BRCA1* and *BRCA2*; these patients are also at greatly increased risk for ovarian neoplasms and second primary breast cancer. Among patients with a history of breast cancer, rigorous screening for SMN within the breast is universally advocated, and many experts argue for screening for both ovarian and endometrial neoplasms as well.[31,74]

The modalities employed in the treatment of breast cancer have the ability to impact the frequency of SMNs within and beyond the breast. However, unlike each of the organs discussed so far, treatments of breast cancer can either raise or lower this risk. There appears to be an increased risk among patients receiving radiotherapy administered for breast cancer of ipsilateral lung cancer, particularly among smokers.[33,75] When alkylating agents or anthracyclines are used in the adjuvant setting, an increased risk of treatment-associated leukemia has been seen, an effect that appears to be augmented by concomitant radiotherapy.[30,76]

Antiestrogenic therapy has been well documented in its ability to both decrease the mortality from primary breast cancer as well as diminish the frequency of second breast cancers.[77–79] This chemoprotective effect has been observed in the high-risk subgroup of patients with *BRCA1* and *BRCA2* mutation-associated primary malignancies, with odds ratios of between 0.4 and 0.6, odds that approach those seen with prophylactic oophorectomy.[80] Data from the largest randomized clinical trial, however, have to date been unable to confirm this observation. Although limited by an extremely small number of incident cancers among *BRCA* mutation carriers in the trial, the investigators were unable to show a protective effect among *BRCA1*-positive patients (RR, 1.67; 95% CI, 0.32, 10.7) and only found a trend toward efficacy among *BRCA2*-positive patients (RR, 0.38; 95% CI, 0.06, 1.56).[81] Newly emerging data suggest that the protective benefit of tamoxifen's antiestrogenic effect on breast tissue can be further prolonged by the use of aromatase inhibitors after the discontinuation of tamoxifen. Tamoxifen, however, acts in certain tissues, such as breast tissue, as an estrogen receptor antagonist, whereas in others as an estrogen receptor agonist, tissues that include the ovaries and endometrium.[82] Research has consistently found that women who undergo long-term tamoxifen therapy are at approximately twice the risk of endometrial cancer, or about 80 excess cases per 10,000 tamoxifen-treated individuals.[83–85] Early suggestions that tamoxifen may confer an additional risk of ovarian, colorectal, and stomach cancers as SMNs have not been borne out by additional investigation.[82,85] Although there is some debate concerning the potential value of screening for endometrial cancer via transvaginal ultrasonography or endometrial biopsy among breast cancer patients taking tamoxifen, experts agree on the value of annual visits to an experienced gynecologist for these patients and on the importance of an expeditious evaluation of abnormal vaginal bleeding.[1,86]

Testicular Cancer

Etoposide is a mainstay of chemotherapy in testicular malignancies, often at high doses, and it comes as little surprise that long-term survivors demonstrate an elevated risk of hematologic malignancy. Estimates have placed the cumulative incidence of AML or non-Hodgkin's lymphoma as SMNs following treatment of testicular cancer at between 1.3% and 2%.[46,87–89] Although the development of metachronous contralateral testicular cancer remains a concern for patients cured of a primary unilateral cancer, the incidence of contralateral testicular cancer as an SMN does not appear to be influenced by the treatments chosen for the first primary malignancy.[90]

Survivors of primary testicular cancer have also been described as having an increased incidence of solid tumors involving the stomach, colon, rectum, pancreas, prostate, kidney, bladder, and thyroid, as well as soft tissue sarcomas and cutaneous malignancies. All of these, with the possible exception of cutaneous malignancies, have been found to be solely associated with the dose of ionizing radiation administered.[91] The association of both melanoma and nonmelanoma skin cancers with chemotherapy of testicular cancer has been reported but remains incompletely elucidated.[92]

Lung Cancer

Both non-small cell lung cancer (NSCLC) and small cell lung cancer (SCLC) have been clearly associated with an increased risk of developing SMNs. However, the elevated risk of second upper aerodigestive tract tumors, including head and neck tumors, esophageal cancers, and second primary lung cancers, has been clearly and closely linked to smoking status[93,94] and the field cancerization that can ensue following continuous exposure to the carcinogens present in cigarette smoke.[95,96] No association has been identified to link the treatment of a primary NSCLC with an increased risk of SMN. This stands in contrast to the case of SCLC, for which such an association does appear to exist.

Although long-term survival in SCLC patients with extensive disease (ED) rarely exceeds 5 years, more-favorable results have been reported in patients with limited disease (LD); disease-free survival at 2 years in some reports has approached or exceeded 50%.[97–99] Among SCLC survivors, there has been noted a markedly greater risk of subsequent development of an SMN, as has been noted. However, this risk is not limited to those patients undergoing therapeutic irradiation. An early retrospective analysis of long-term SCLC survivors had found a markedly elevated risk of SMN, with an overall risk of 10.3% per person-year and an 8-year actuarial risk of 50.3%.[100] Although all SCLC patients have an increased rate of second lung cancers (typically NSCLC in histology), this risk rises from approximately 7 times that of unaffected patients to approximately 13 times among patients treated with any of a number of combination chemotherapy protocols.[54]

Prostate Cancer

Although some reports concerning the risk of therapy-associated SMN with radiotherapy of prostate cancer have emerged, far less attention has been either merited or received from the risk of SMN from chemotherapy for prostate cancer. While systemic chemotherapy has a limited role in the treatment of prostate cancer, there is some use of nitrogen mustard, which has been associated with increased risk of myelodysplastic syndrome in patients receiving it for the treatment of prostate cancer.[92] The use of antiandrogenic therapy in controlling this malignancy is far more common than traditional chemotherapeutic agents, and the theoretical possibility exists that such agents could predispose to tumors that are suppressed by the androgenic state. Suggestion of such a possible phenomenon can be found in a recent report of an increased risk of male breast cancer among patients treated for prostate cancer.[101]

Gastrointestinal Cancers

It is interesting to note that among the most prevalent gastrointestinal cancers—colorectal cancer, gastric cancer, and pancreatic cancer—there are no convincing data suggesting linkage between chemotherapy and SMN. The reasons underlying this lack of convincing connections undoubtedly vary by malignancy (see Chapters 41 and 43).

Gynecologic Cancers

Analyses of the common gynecologic malignancies—cervical, uterine, and ovarian—have established some patterns of increased risk of SMNs. However, there lacks a robust literature addressing the attributable risk of systemic chemotherapy in patients with cancer of either the uterine cervix or the corpus uteri; that chemotherapy has at this time a limited role in the treatment of these malignancies both makes the identification of such an association difficult and renders any findings clinically unimportant.

Ovarian cancer presents a different scenario altogether, as it is often treated with a multimodal regimen that includes systemic chemotherapy. Historically, associations had been seen between melphalan-based chemotherapeutic regimens that would now be considered outdated and risk of secondary leukemia in patients treated for ovarian cancer.[43,102] A Swedish record-linkage study from 1995 found a relative risk of 7 for leukemia among patients with ovarian cancer, likely reflecting the common use of melphalan during the time period under investigation, 1958–1992.[40] Although an elevated risk of acute nonlymphocytic leukemia has been suggested to exist for patients treated for ovarian cancer with cyclophosphamide, chlorambucil, or regimens containing doxorubicin and cisplatin,[102–105] a retrospective analysis stratified by decade demonstrated that the risk of leukemia following treatment of ovarian cancer has decreased from 40 during the 1970s to 17 from 1980 to 1992.[41] While this suggests that more modern regimens, largely cisplatin based, may be less leukemogenic, clearly more data are needed to more thoroughly clarify this risk relationship more thoroughly.

Transplantation and Oncogenesis

An additional predisposing factor toward treatment-induced SMN that has recently emerged is immunosuppression. Over the past two decades we have seen a dramatic improvement in the ability to suppress immunologic transplant rejection thanks to new, potent immunosuppressive agents, including cyclophosphamide, cyclosporine A, tacrolimus, and mycophenolate mofetil, but it has become apparent that the long-term administration of such medications can dramatically increase the risk of developing late neoplasia, both hematologic and solid malignancies.[106,107]

Risk of hematologic malignancy has been noted to be dramatically elevated among transplant recipients, both allogeneic bone marrow transplant (BMT) recipients as well as patients receiving solid organ donation. Indeed, the name posttransplantation lymphoproliferative disorder (PTLD) has emerged in the literature to report and describe such patients. PTLD as a diagnostic category includes a spectrum of pathology ranging from atypical marrow hyperplasia to frank non-Hodgkin's lymphoma; what the constituent diagnoses share is a common association with Epstein–Barr virus infection, either acute seroconversion or reactivation of latent infection.[107] Rates of lymphoma are dramatically increased by bone marrow ablation and hematopoietic stem cell transplant in the treatment of malignancy; these rates are higher yet when the stem cell transplant was given for an indication of an underlying immunocompromised condition, such as Hodgkin's disease or chronic myelogenous leukemia (CML).[108] These PTLDs can occur quite rapidly following BMT, with a median time to onset of 2.5 months, whereas secondary leukemias have an almost equally rapid arrival, with a median time to onset of 6.7 months.[109,110] PTLD complicates solid organ transplant as well; while most studies place the cumulative "de novo" tumor incidence among recipients of solid organs at between 5% and 15%, PTLD accounts for 15% to 25% of these malignancies, a marked elevation of risk as compared to the general population.[111,112]

Although the rise in risk of lymphoproliferative disorders among transplant recipients is striking, there have been noted elevated risks of a number of solid tumors as well in this population. Kaposi's sarcoma, another malignancy with a viral pathogenesis (human herpesvirus 8), is seen among transplant recipients, as are hepatomas among patients with chronic infection by hepatitis B or C virus. And while some solid tumors (renal carcinoma in renal transplant patients, for example) are largely attributable to the underlying conditions necessitating transplantation (e.g., analgesic nephropathy), it is clear that others are strongly associated with the induction of an immunocompromised state. This connection is most clear in the case of squamous cell skin cancer: the cumulative incidence of this malignancy 10 years after transplant is 10% and 20 years after transplant rises to 40%. In Australia, where the baseline incidence is higher than that in the United States because of more-intense solar UV exposure, these numbers rise to 45% and 70%, respectively.[113]

References

1. Neugut AI, Meadows AT, Robinson E (eds). Multiple primary cancers. Philadelphia: Lippincott Williams & Wilkins, 1999.
2. Goolden WG. Radiation cancer of the pharynx. Br Med J 1951;2:1110–1117.
3. Sherrill DJ, Grishkin BA, Galal FS, Zajtchuk R, Graeber GM. Radiation associated malignancies of the esophagus. Cancer (Phila) 1984;54(4):726–728.
4. Shimizu T, Matsui T, Kimura O, Maeta M, Koga S. Radiation-induced esophageal cancer: a case report and a review of the literature. Jpn J Surg 1990;20(1):97–100.
5. Ribeiro U Jr, Posner MC, Safatle-Ribeiro AV, Reynolds JC. Risk factors for squamous cell carcinoma of the oesophagus. Br J Surg 1996;83(9):1174–1185.
6. Neugut AI, Weinberg MD, Ahsan H, Rescigno J. Carcinogenic effects of radiotherapy for breast cancer. Oncology (Huntingt) 1999;13(9):1245–1256; discussion 57, 61–65.
7. Boice JD Jr. Studies of atomic bomb survivors. Understanding radiation effects. JAMA 1990;264(5):622–623.
8. Pierce DA, Preston DL. Radiation-related cancer risks at low doses among atomic bomb survivors. Radiat Res 2000;154(2): 178–186.
9. UNSCEAR (United Nations Scientific Committee on the Effects of Atomic Radiation). 2000 Report to the General Assembly, with Scientific Annexes. Volume II: Effects. New York: United Nations, 2000.
10. Tucker MA, Meadows AT, Boice JD Jr, et al. Leukemia after therapy with alkylating agents for childhood cancer. J Natl Cancer Inst 1987;78(3):459–464.
11. Hawkins MM, Wilson LM, Stovall MA, et al. Epipodophyllotoxins, alkylating agents, and radiation and risk of secondary leukaemia after childhood cancer. BMJ 1992;304(6832):951–958.
12. Tucker MA, D'Angio GJ, Boice JD Jr, et al. Bone sarcomas linked to radiotherapy and chemotherapy in children. N Engl J Med 1987;317(10):588–593.
13. de Vathaire F, Francois P, Hill C, et al. Role of radiotherapy and chemotherapy in the risk of second malignant neoplasms after cancer in childhood. Br J Cancer 1989;59(5):792–796.
14. Neglia JP, Meadows AT, Robison LL, et al. Second neoplasms after acute lymphoblastic leukemia in childhood. N Engl J Med 1991;325(19):1330–1336.

15. Tucker MA, Jones PH, Boice JD Jr, et al. Therapeutic radiation at a young age is linked to secondary thyroid cancer. The Late Effects Study Group. Cancer Res 1991;51(11):2885–2888.
16. Ron E, Lubin JH, Shore RE, et al. Thyroid cancer after exposure to external radiation: a pooled analysis of seven studies. Radiat Res 1995;141(3):259–277.
17. Olsen JH, Garwicz S, Hertz H, et al. Second malignant neoplasms after cancer in childhood or adolescence. Nordic Society of Paediatric Haematology and Oncology Association of the Nordic Cancer Registries. BMJ 1993;307(6911):1030–1036.
18. Neglia JP, Friedman DL, Yasui Y, et al. Second malignant neoplasms in five-year survivors of childhood cancer: childhood cancer survivor study. J Natl Cancer Inst 2001;93(8):618–629.
19. Boice JD Jr. Radiation and non-Hodgkin's lymphoma. Cancer Res 1992;52(19 suppl):5489s–5491s.
20. Curtis RE, Rowlings PA, Deeg HJ, et al. Solid cancers after bone marrow transplantation. N Engl J Med 1997;336(13):897–904.
21. Socie G, Curtis RE, Deeg HJ, et al. New malignant diseases after allogeneic marrow transplantation for childhood acute leukemia. J Clin Oncol 2000;18(2):348–357.
22. Clemons M, Loijens L, Goss P. Breast cancer risk following irradiation for Hodgkin's disease. Cancer Treat Rev 2000;26(4): 291–302.
23. Bhatia S, Robison LL, Oberlin O, et al. Breast cancer and other second neoplasms after childhood Hodgkin's disease. N Engl J Med 1996;334(12):745–751.
24. Travis LB, Gospodarowicz M, Curtis RE, et al. Lung cancer following chemotherapy and radiotherapy for Hodgkin's disease. J Natl Cancer Inst 2002;94(3):182–192.
25. Birdwell SH, Hancock SL, Varghese A, Cox RS, Hoppe RT. Gastrointestinal cancer after treatment of Hodgkin's disease. Int J Radiat Oncol Biol Phys 1997;37(1):67–73.
26. Ron E, Preston DL, Mabuchi K, Thompson DE, Soda M. Cancer incidence in atomic bomb survivors. Part IV: Comparison of cancer incidence and mortality. Radiat Res 1994;137(2 suppl): S98–S112.
27. Swerdlow AJ, Barber JA, Hudson GV, et al. Risk of second malignancy after Hodgkin's disease in a collaborative British cohort: the relation to age at treatment. J Clin Oncol 2000;18(3): 498–509.
28. Metayer C, Lynch CF, Clarke EA, et al. Second cancers among long-term survivors of Hodgkin's disease diagnosed in childhood and adolescence. J Clin Oncol 2000;18(12):2435–2443.
29. Curtis RE, Boice JD Jr, Stovall M, Flannery JT, Moloney WC. Leukemia risk following radiotherapy for breast cancer. J Clin Oncol 1989;7(1):21–29.
30. Curtis RE, Boice JD Jr, Stovall M, et al. Risk of leukemia after chemotherapy and radiation treatment for breast cancer. N Engl J Med 1992;326(26):1745–1751.
31. Boice JD Jr, Harvey EB, Blettner M, Stovall M, Flannery JT. Cancer in the contralateral breast after radiotherapy for breast cancer. N Engl J Med 1992;326(12):781–785.
32. Inskip PD, Stovall M, Flannery JT. Lung cancer risk and radiation dose among women treated for breast cancer. J Natl Cancer Inst 1994;86(13):983–988.
33. Neugut AI, Murray T, Santos J, et al. Increased risk of lung cancer after breast cancer radiation therapy in cigarette smokers. Cancer (Phila) 1994;73(6):1615–1620.
34. Travis LB, Curtis RE, Inskip PD, Hankey BF. Re: Lung cancer risk and radiation dose among women treated for breast cancer. J Natl Cancer Inst 1995;87(1):60–61.
35. Zablotska LB, Neugut AI. Lung carcinoma after radiation therapy in women treated with lumpectomy or mastectomy for primary breast carcinoma. Cancer (Phila) 2003;97(6):1404–1411.
36. Rubino C, de Vathaire F, Diallo I, Shamsaldin A, Le MG. Increased risk of second cancers following breast cancer: role of the initial treatment. Breast Cancer Res Treat 2000;61(3): 183–195.
37. Ahsan H, Neugut AI. Radiation therapy for breast cancer and increased risk for esophageal carcinoma. Ann Intern Med 1998;128(2):114–117.
38. Curtis RE, Boice JD Jr, Stovall M, et al. Relationship of leukemia risk to radiation dose following cancer of the uterine corpus. J Natl Cancer Inst 1994;86(17):1315–1324.
39. BEIR V (Committee on the Biological Effects of Ionizing Radiations). Health effects of exposure to low levels of ionizing radiation. Washington, DC: National Academy Press, 1990.
40. Bergfeldt K, Einhorn S, Rosendahl I, Hall P. Increased risk of second primary malignancies in patients with gynecological cancer. A Swedish record-linkage study. Acta Oncol 1995;34(6): 771–777.
41. Travis LB, Curtis RE, Boice JD Jr, Platz CE, Hankey BF, Fraumeni JF Jr. Second malignant neoplasms among long-term survivors of ovarian cancer. Cancer Res 1996;56(7):1564–1570.
42. Travis LB, Holowaty EJ, Bergfeldt K, et al. Risk of leukemia after platinum-based chemotherapy for ovarian cancer. N Engl J Med 1999;340(5):351–357.
43. Kaldor JM, Day NE, Pettersson F, et al. Leukemia following chemotherapy for ovarian cancer. N Engl J Med 1990;322(1):1–6.
44. Kaldor JM, Day NE, Kittelmann B, et al. Bladder tumours following chemotherapy and radiotherapy for ovarian cancer: a case-control study. Int J Cancer 1995;63(1):1–6.
45. van Leeuwen FE, Stiggelbout AM, van den Belt-Dusebout AW, et al. Second cancer risk following testicular cancer: a follow-up study of 1,909 patients. J Clin Oncol 1993;11(3):415–424.
46. Travis LB, Andersson M, Gospodarowicz M, et al. Treatment-associated leukemia following testicular cancer. J Natl Cancer Inst 2000;92(14):1165–1171.
47. Boice JD Jr, Blettner M, Kleinerman RA, et al. Radiation dose and leukemia risk in patients treated for cancer of the cervix. J Natl Cancer Inst 1987;79(6):1295–1311.
48. Kaldor JM, Day NE, Clarke EA, et al. Leukemia following Hodgkin's disease. N Engl J Med 1990;322(1):7–13.
49. Preston DL, Kusumi S, Tomonaga M, et al. Cancer incidence in atomic bomb survivors. Part III. Leukemia, lymphoma and multiple myeloma, 1950–1987. Radiat Res 1994;137(2 suppl): S68–S97.
50. Pawlish KS, Schottenfeld D, Severson R, Montie JE. Risk of multiple primary cancers in prostate cancer patients in the Detroit metropolitan area: a retrospective cohort study. Prostate 1997; 33(2):75–86.
51. Movsas B, Hanlon AL, Pinover W, Hanks GE. Is there an increased risk of second primaries following prostate irradiation? Int J Radiat Oncol Biol Phys 1998;41(2):251–255.
52. Johnstone PA, Powell CR, Riffenburgh R, Rohde DC, Kane CJ. Second primary malignancies in T1-3N0 prostate cancer patients treated with radiation therapy with 10-year followup. J Urol 1998;159(3):946–949.
53. Neugut AI, Ahsan H, Robinson E, Ennis RD. Bladder carcinoma and other second malignancies after radiotherapy for prostate carcinoma. Cancer (Phila) 1997;79(8):1600–1604.
54. Tucker MA, Murray N, Shaw EG, et al. Second primary cancers related to smoking and treatment of small-cell lung cancer. Lung Cancer Working Cadre. J Natl Cancer Inst 1997;89(23): 1782–1878.
55. Salminen E, Pukkala E, Teppo L, Pyrhonen S. Risk of second cancers among lung cancer patients. Acta Oncol 1995; 34(2):165–169.
56. Hoar SK, Wilson J, Blot WJ, McLaughlin JK, Winn DM, Kantor AF. Second cancer following cancer of the digestive system in Connecticut, 1935–82. Natl Cancer Inst Monogr 1985;68:49–82.
57. Knudson AG. Karnofsky Memorial Lecture. Hereditary cancer: theme and variations. J Clin Oncol 1997;15(10):3280–3287.
58. Pui CH, Ribeiro RC, Hancock ML, et al. Acute myeloid leukemia in children treated with epipodophyllotoxins for acute lymphoblastic leukemia. N Engl J Med 1991;325(24):1682–1687.

59. Kimball Dalton VM, Gelber RD, Li F, Donnelly MJ, Tarbell NJ, Sallan SE. Second malignancies in patients treated for childhood acute lymphoblastic leukemia. J Clin Oncol 1998;16(8): 2848–2853.
60. Loning L, Zimmermann M, Reiter A, et al. Secondary neoplasms subsequent to Berlin-Frankfurt-Munster therapy of acute lymphoblastic leukemia in childhood: significantly lower risk without cranial radiotherapy. Blood 2000;95(9):2770–2775.
61. Relling MV, Yanishevski Y, Nemec J, et al. Etoposide and antimetabolite pharmacology in patients who develop secondary acute myeloid leukemia. Leukemia 1998;12(3):346–352.
62. Meadows AT, Baum E, Fossati-Bellani F, et al. Second malignant neoplasms in children: an update from the Late Effects Study Group. J Clin Oncol 1985;3(4):532–538.
63. Kuttesch JF Jr, Wexler LH, Marcus RB, et al. Second malignancies after Ewing's sarcoma: radiation dose-dependency of secondary sarcomas. J Clin Oncol 1996;14(10):2818–2825.
64. Dunst J, Ahrens S, Paulussen M, et al. Second malignancies after treatment for Ewing's sarcoma: a report of the CESS-studies. Int J Radiat Oncol Biol Phys 1998;42(2):379–384.
65. Rich DC, Corpron CA, Smith MB, Black CT, Lally KP, Andrassy RJ. Second malignant neoplasms in children after treatment of soft tissue sarcoma. J Pediatr Surg 1997;32(2):369–372.
66. Raney RB, Asmar L, Vassilopoulou-Sellin R, et al. Late complications of therapy in 213 children with localized, nonorbital soft-tissue sarcoma of the head and neck: A descriptive report from the Intergroup Rhabdomyosarcoma Studies (IRS)-II and -III. IRS Group of the Children's Cancer Group and the Pediatric Oncology Group. Med Pediatr Oncol 1999;33(4):362–371.
67. Heyn R, Haeberlen V, Newton WA, et al. Second malignant neoplasms in children treated for rhabdomyosarcoma. Intergroup Rhabdomyosarcoma Study Committee. J Clin Oncol 1993; 11(2):262–270.
68. Breslow NE, Takashima JR, Whitton JA, Moksness J, D'Angio GJ, Green DM. Second malignant neoplasms following treatment for Wilm's tumor: a report from the National Wilms' Tumor Study Group. J Clin Oncol 1995;13(8):1851–1859.
69. Green DM, Hyland A, Barcos MP, et al. Second malignant neoplasms after treatment for Hodgkin's disease in childhood or adolescence. J Clin Oncol 2000;18(7):1492–1499.
70. van Leeuwen FE, Klokman WJ, Veer MB, et al. Long-term risk of second malignancy in survivors of Hodgkin's disease treated during adolescence or young adulthood. J Clin Oncol 2000; 18(3):487–497.
71. Swerdlow AJ, Schoemaker MJ, Allerton R, et al. Lung cancer after Hodgkin's disease: a nested case-control study of the relation to treatment. J Clin Oncol 2001;19(6):1610–1618.
72. Boice JD Jr, Storm H, Curtis RE. Multiple primary cancers in Connecticut and Denmark. Monogr Natl Cancer Inst 1985; 68(1):1–437.
73. Schatzkin A, Baranovsky A, Kessler LG. Diet and cancer. Evidence from associations of multiple primary cancers in the SEER program. Cancer (Phila) 1988;62(7):1451–1457.
74. Bergfeldt K, Nilsson B, Einhorn S, Hall P. Breast cancer risk in women with a primary ovarian cancer: a case-control study. Eur J Cancer 2001;37(17):2229–2234.
75. Inskip PD, Boice JD Jr. Radiotherapy-induced lung cancer among women who smoke. Cancer (Phila) 1994;73(6):1541–1543.
76. Saso R, Kulkarni S, Mitchell P, et al. Secondary myelodysplastic syndrome/acute myeloid leukaemia following mitoxantrone-based therapy for breast carcinoma. Br J Cancer 2000;83(1): 91–94.
77. Cook LS, Weiss NS, Schwartz SM, et al. Population-based study of tamoxifen therapy and subsequent ovarian, endometrial, and breast cancers. J Natl Cancer Inst 1995;87(18):1359–1364.
78. Curtis RE, Boice JD Jr, Shriner DA, Hankey BF, Fraumeni JF Jr. Second cancers after adjuvant tamoxifen therapy for breast cancer. J Natl Cancer Inst 1996;88(12):832–834.
79. Li CI, Malone KE, Weiss NS, Daling JR. Tamoxifen therapy for primary breast cancer and risk of contralateral breast cancer. J Natl Cancer Inst 2001;93(13):1008–1013.
80. Narod SA, Brunet JS, Ghadirian P, et al. Tamoxifen and risk of contralateral breast cancer in BRCA1 and BRCA2 mutation carriers: a case-control study. Hereditary Breast Cancer Clinical Study Group. Lancet 2000;356(9245):1876–1881.
81. King MC, Wieand S, Hale K, et al. Tamoxifen and breast cancer incidence among women with inherited mutations in BRCA1 and BRCA2: National Surgical Adjuvant Breast and Bowel Project (NSABP-P1) Breast Cancer Prevention Trial. JAMA 2001;286(18):2251–2256.
82. Rutqvist LE, Johansson H, Signomklao T, Johansson U, Fornander T, Wilking N. Adjuvant tamoxifen therapy for early stage breast cancer and second primary malignancies. Stockholm Breast Cancer Study Group. J Natl Cancer Inst 1995;87(9):645–651.
83. Fisher B, Costantino JP, Redmond CK, Fisher ER, Wickerham DL, Cronin WM. Endometrial cancer in tamoxifen-treated breast cancer patients: findings from the National Surgical Adjuvant Breast and Bowel Project (NSABP) B-14. J Natl Cancer Inst 1994;86(7):527–537.
84. Fisher B, Costantino JP, Wickerham DL, et al. Tamoxifen for prevention of breast cancer: report of the National Surgical Adjuvant Breast and Bowel Project P-1 Study. J Natl Cancer Inst 1998;90(18):1371–1388.
85. Fisher B, Dignam J, Wolmark N, et al. Tamoxifen in treatment of intraductal breast cancer: National Surgical Adjuvant Breast and Bowel Project B-24 randomised controlled trial. Lancet 1999;353(9169):1993–2000.
86. Shapiro CL, Recht A. Side effects of adjuvant treatment of breast cancer. N Engl J Med 2001;344(26):1997–2008.
87. Kollmannsberger C, Beyer J, Droz JP, et al. Secondary leukemia following high cumulative doses of etoposide in patients treated for advanced germ cell tumors. J Clin Oncol 1998;16(10): 3386–3391.
88. Kollmannsberger C, Hartmann JT, Kanz L, Bokemeyer C. Therapy-related malignancies following treatment of germ cell cancer. Int J Cancer 1999;83(6):860–863.
89. Ruther U, Dieckmann K, Bussar-Maatz R, Eisenberger F. Second malignancies following pure seminoma. Oncology 2000;58(1): 75–82.
90. Hale GA, Marina NM, Jones-Wallace D, et al. Late effects of treatment for germ cell tumors during childhood and adolescence. J Pediatr Hematol Oncol 1999;21(2):115–122.
91. Travis LB, Curtis RE, Storm H, et al. Risk of second malignant neoplasms among long-term survivors of testicular cancer. J Natl Cancer Inst 1997;89(19):1429–1439.
92. Hartmann JT, Nichols CR, Droz JP, et al. The relative risk of second nongerminal malignancies in patients with extragonadal germ cell tumors. Cancer (Phila) 2000;88(11):2629–2635.
93. Warren S, Gates DC. Multiple primary malignant tumors: a survey of the literature and statistical study. Am J Cancer 1932; 16:1358–1414.
94. Lippman SM, Lee JJ, Karp DD. Phase III intergroup trial of 13-cis-retinoic acid to prevent second primary tumors in stage I non-small cell lung cancer (SNCLC): interim report of NCI No. I19-0001. Proc Am Soc Clin Oncol 1998;17:1753.
95. Vokes EE, Weichselbaum RR, Lippman SM, Hong WK. Head and neck cancer. N Engl J Med 1993;328(3):184–194.
96. Tepperman BS, Fitzpatrick PJ. Second respiratory and upper digestive tract cancers after oral cancer. Lancet 1981; 2(8246):547–549.
97. Johnson BE, Bridges JD, Sobczeck M, et al. Patients with limited-stage small-cell lung cancer treated with concurrent twice-daily chest radiotherapy and etoposide/cisplatin followed by cyclophosphamide, doxorubicin, and vincristine. J Clin Oncol 1996; 14(3):806–813.

98. Jeremic B, Shibamoto Y, Acimovic L, Milisavljevic S. Carboplatin, etoposide, and accelerated hyperfractionated radiotherapy for elderly patients with limited small cell lung carcinoma: a phase II study. Cancer (Phila) 1998;82(5):836–841.
99. Turrisi AT III, Kim K, Blum R, et al. Twice-daily compared with once-daily thoracic radiotherapy in limited small-cell lung cancer treated concurrently with cisplatin and etoposide. N Engl J Med 1999;340(4):265–271.
100. Heyne KH, Lippman SM, Lee JJ, Lee JS, Hong WK. The incidence of second primary tumors in long-term survivors of small-cell lung cancer. J Clin Oncol 1992;10(10):1519–1524.
101. Thellenberg C, Malmer B, Tavelin B, Gronberg H. Second primary cancers in men with prostate cancer: an increased risk of male breast cancer. J Urol 2003;169(4):1345–1348.
102. Greene MH, Harris EL, Gershenson DM, et al. Melphalan may be a more potent leukemogen than cyclophosphamide. Ann Intern Med 1986;105(3):360–367.
103. Kaldor JM, Day NE, Pettersson F, et al. Leukemia following chemotherapy for ovarian cancer. N Engl J Med 1990;322(1):1–6.
104. Haas JF, Kittelmann B, Mehnert WH, et al. Risk of leukaemia in ovarian tumour and breast cancer patients following treatment by cyclophosphamide. Br J Cancer 1987;55(2):213–218.
105. Greene MH, Boice JD Jr, Greer BE, Blessing JA, Dembo AJ. Acute nonlymphocytic leukemia after therapy with alkylating agents for ovarian cancer: a study of five randomized clinical trials. N Engl J Med 1982;307(23):1416–1421.
106. Ciancio G, Siquijor AP, Burke GW, et al. Post-transplant lymphoproliferative disease in kidney transplant patients in the new immunosuppressive era. Clin Transplant 1997;11(3):243–249.
107. Andreone P, Gramenzi A, Lorenzini S, et al. Posttransplantation lymphoproliferative disorders. Arch Intern Med 2003;163(17):1997–2004.
108. Gross TG, Steinbuch M, DeFor T, et al. B cell lymphoproliferative disorders following hematopoietic stem cell transplantation: risk factors, treatment and outcome. Bone Marrow Transplant 1999;23(3):251–258.
109. Deeg HJ, Socie G. Malignancies after hematopoietic stem cell transplantation: many questions, some answers. Blood 1998;91(6):1833–1844.
110. Socie G, Kolb HJ. Malignant diseases after bone marrow transplantation: the case for tumor banking and continued reporting to registries. EBMT Late-Effects Working Party. Bone Marrow Transplant 1995;16(4):493–495.
111. Catena F, Nardo B, Liviano d'Arcangelo G, et al. De novo malignancies after organ transplantation. Transplant Proc 2001;33(1–2):1858–1859.
112. Valero JM, Rubio E, Moreno JM, Pons F, Sanchez-Turrion V, Cuervas-Mons V. De novo malignancies in liver transplantation. Transplant Proc 2003;35(2):709–711.
113. Dreno B. Skin cancers after transplantation. Nephrol Dial Transplant 2003;18(6):1052–1058.
114. Hancock SL, Tucker MA, Hoppe RT. Breast cancer after treatment of Hodgkin's disease. J Natl Cancer Inst 1993;85(1):25–31.
115. Tinger A, Wasserman TH, Klein EE, et al. The incidence of breast cancer following mantle field radiation therapy as a function of dose and technique. Int J Radiat Oncol Biol Phys 1997;37(4):865–870.
116. Hudson MM, Poquette CA, Lee J, et al. Increased mortality after successful treatment for Hodgkin's disease. J Clin Oncol 1998;16(11):3592–3600.
117. Wolden SL, Lamborn KR, Cleary SF, Tate DJ, Donaldson SS. Second cancers following pediatric Hodgkin's disease. J Clin Oncol 1998;16(2):536–544.
118. Dores GM, Metayer C, Curtis RE, et al. Second malignant neoplasms among long-term survivors of Hodgkin's disease: a population-based evaluation over 25 years. J Clin Oncol 2002;20(16):3484–3494.

112

Psychosocial Rehabilitation in Cancer Care

Richard P. McQuellon and Suzanne C. Danhauer

Prevalence data on psychosocial morbidity indicate that from 30% to 50% of cancer patients may experience distress significant enough to warrant professional intervention at some time during survivorship.[1,2] These patients may require professional attention to manage the debilitating effects of diagnosis, treatment, and morbidity that can wax and wane over time depending upon a host of other variables. It is in this group that some form of psychosocial rehabilitation may be useful.[3,4]

Psychosocial Rehabilitation in Cancer Care

The formal definition of rehabilitation is "the process by which physical, sensory and mental capacities are restored or developed in (for) people with disabling conditions."[5] This definition implies some type of disabling condition that requires rehabilitation. Not all cancer patients experience a disability and not all cancer patients require rehabilitation of any sort. The founders of cancer rehabilitation were physicians trained in rehabilitative medicine largely focused on physical needs of cancer patients with interdisciplinary teams.[6,7] The Oncology Nursing Society in 1989 defined cancer rehabilitation as "a process by which individuals within their environments are assisted to achieve optimal functioning within limits imposed by cancer."[8] Psychosocial rehabilitation in cancer care has a more specific focus than rehabilitation in general[9] and is often described by the broader term psychosocial intervention.

The diagnosis, treatment and survivorship of cancer often involves much more varied rehabilitation needs than those experienced following most other medical problems.[10] There are more than 100 cancer diagnoses that can elicit a multitude of psychosocial responses. Hence, there may be wide variability in the needs for rehabilitative intervention in the psychosocial area. For example, the patient with radical head and neck surgery left with significant disfiguration is very different than the early-stage breast cancer patient expected to have complete cure with no significant appearance alteration who may require minimal or no psychosocial intervention. The irony of this situation is that although we would expect one patient to experience intensive psychosocial distress and the other not, depending upon a host of mediating variables (social support, natural resilience, effective communication with healthcare team, etc.), the outcome may be not what one would predict. This variability of psychosocial needs and experiences illustrates but one challenge for the psychosocial care of patients: How can patients who need and want services be identified?

The National Comprehensive Cancer Center Network has developed definitions and guidelines to help treat distressed cancer patients.[11] Distress has been defined as "a multifactorial, unpleasant experience of an emotional, psychological, social, or spiritual nature that interferes with the ability to cope with cancer, its physical symptoms, and its treatment. Distress extends along a continuum ranging from normal feelings of vulnerability, sadness and fear to disabling conditions such as clinical depression, anxiety, panic, isolation and existential or spiritual crisis" (p. 369). In the context of cancer care, the term psychosocial refers to the psychologic and social adaptation and reaction of the patient to the diagnosis of cancer, treatment, and survivorship.[12]

Scope of the Field

Psychosocial rehabilitation could include all psychosocial interventions that are designed to positively influence patient psychosocial adaptation and adjustment to diagnosis, treatment, and survivorship. For example, physical and occupational therapists play a significant role with patients undergoing debilitating treatment. To illustrate, bone marrow transplantation and cytoreductive surgery plus intraperitoneal hyperthermic chemotherapy often leave patients deconditioned physically and distressed psychologically.[13,14] Such patients might benefit significantly from a physical rehabilitation program without explicit emphasis on psychosocial care or intervention. An example of a physical rehabilitation program (walking) following bone marrow transplantation has been reported as effective.[15] Such interventions do not explicitly focus on psychologic outcomes with the use of targeted psychosocial interventions but may measure them as secondary endpoints. This chapter focuses primarily on randomized clinical trials specifically designed

patients.[33] The stated hypothesis was that cancer patients treated with adjuvant psychosocial intervention experienced a higher level of subjective quality of life (QOL) compared to those without additional psychosocial intervention. The authors identified 37 studies that included a total of 3,120 cancer patients. The overall effect size on QOL in this study was 0.31 [95% confidence interval (CI), 0.13 ≤ 0.31 ≤ 0.75). The authors concluded that psychosocial interventions have a positive impact on quality of life in adult cancer patients, and the effect was moderated by duration of treatment, suggesting that psychosocial interventions should be planned for at least 12 weeks.

A study of psychological interventions for patients with symptoms of anxiety and depression has particular relevance for this chapter.[28] In this study, two meta-analyses were conducted with anxiety and depression examined as separate outcome measures. Even though the majority of trials included in the analysis were preventive (i.e., not targeted to patients with identified abnormal symptoms of anxiety or depression), these studies can shed some light on the rehabilitation process. Nineteen trials on anxiety had a combined effect size of 0.42 favoring treatment against "no treatment controls" (95% CI, 0.08–0.74; n = 1,023). Twenty trials on depression had a combined effect size of 0.36 as well, favoring the treatment (95% CI, 0.06–0.66; n = 1,101). Four trials focusing on patients who were identified as "at risk" had particularly significant effects, suggesting that targeted interventions were more likely to demonstrate beneficial effects. However, the mean effect size for depression was weak to negligible (0.19), prompting the authors to state that preventive psychological interventions with cancer patients may have a moderate effect on anxiety but little effect on depression. The authors concluded that resources should be directed toward those patients demonstrating psychological or psychosocial deficits, and that group therapy trials appear to be equally effective relative to individual interventions and are likely more economical. Finally, relatively short, intensive interventions delivered by more-experienced counselors appear to be more effective than interventions delivered by less-experienced counselors over a long period of time.

Measurement Tools in Psychosocial Rehabilitation

A number of assessment tools are widely used by researchers and clinicians for examining the psychosocial impact of cancer and its treatment as well as the impact of psychosocial interventions on patient functioning. These tools include measures of general mood (e.g., Profile of Mood States, Positive and Negative Affect Scale), depression (e.g., Center for Epidemiologic Studies Depression, Beck Depression Inventory, Hamilton Depression Inventory), anxiety (e.g., State-Trait Anxiety Inventory), and general mental health symptoms (e.g., Brief Symptom Inventory).[22] These instruments have been used largely because of their psychometric properties and ease of administration.

The interest in overall patient QOL has spawned the Functional Assessment of Cancer Therapy (FACT) and the European Organization for Research and Treatment of Cancer (EORTC) questionnaires. These methods include modules that measure symptoms of specific cancers or characteristics of treatment situations (e.g., bone marrow transplantation). For example, the FACT includes many disease site-related subscales (breast, colon, brain, etc.)[34,35] and treatment- or symptom-related modules (bone marrow transplantation, etc.).[36–38] The SF-36 has also been used in the assessment of cancer patients because it provides normative values for the nonmedical patient population;[39] this allows for comparison of patients undergoing treatment with normative samples in the U.S. adult population. Such comparisons can be helpful when patients ask what they might expect in terms of healthy functioning following specific treatments.[40–42] These instruments have been particularly useful as they allow for comparisons over time because of their sensitivity to change. Thus, one would be able to look at baseline levels of emotional well-being with the FACT or mental health functioning on the EORTC and compare these with posttreatment functioning in longitudinal studies. These instruments, however, were not developed with the intent of measuring outcomes of psychosocial rehabilitation following cancer treatment.

In contrast, the Cancer Rehabilitation Evaluation System (CARES) allows patients to identify problems and to indicate with which problems they want help.[43] For example, one item on the CARES reads something like the following, "I have difficulty doing physical activity such as running." Patients are asked to answer on a 5-point scale from "not at all" to "very much" and then to indicate "yes" or "no" to the question, "Do you want help?" The 139 items on the CARES cover nearly every conceivable problem situation. It has been used in a number of studies attempting to assess rehabilitation needs and success in patients.[44–46] Because of the depth of coverage of items in the CARES, it is not typically used in clinical trials where the emphasis must necessarily be on rapid assessment and fewer items, but one of the most significant strengths of the CARES is that it directs patients to identify problems (including psychosocial problems) that they want to address. This coverage can be very useful to providers trying to focus scarce resources, because as few as one-third of patients actually are interested in a counseling intervention[47] even though a significant number of cancer patients may experience psychosocial distress.[1]

Randomized Controlled Trials

We systematically searched Pub Med and PsychInfo with the following descriptors: psychosocial rehabilitation and cancer, psychosocial intervention and cancer, psychological intervention and cancer, and behavioral intervention and cancer. After compiling this list we also looked for relevant studies in the reference sections of studies identified in the searches. We selected studies based on two criteria: (1) for the most part, the intervention was targeted toward a current or anticipated need or deficit exhibited by the patient (e.g., high distress, anxiety, or depression); and (2) assignment to treatment was made randomly. We have selected representative studies that provide evidence for the effectiveness of psychosocial interventions in modifying and potentially improving outcomes for patients in the psychological and social domains. The studies reviewed, including caregiver studies, are summarized in Table 112.2.

TABLE 112.2. Randomized control trials.

Reference	*Year*	*n/dx*	*Intervention/source/duration*	*Measures/timing*	*Outcomes*
Gordon et al.[48]	1980	217/Breast = 71 Lung = 37 Melanoma = 109	Three interventions: (1) patient education re: how to live with disease; (2) general counseling; (3) environmental manipulation, e.g., consultation with other professionals vs. usual care/a single oncology counselor Average of 11 20-minute sessions	Problems (number, intensity severity); MAACL; LPIS; SREs; HLC; ADL (modified version); API. Hospital admit., hosp. d/c, 3 and 6 months post d/c.	Intervention group showed improvement of some problems, more rapid decline of neg. affect, more realistic outlook, return to previous vocational status and more active pattern of time usage.
Cheung et al.[49]	2003	59/Colorectal	Progressive muscle relaxation training (PMRT) vs. standard care/therapist and audiotape/two face-to-face teaching sessions before intervention of listening to tape Two to three times/1-week interval period	STAI; QOL-Colostomy; WHO QOL measure abbreviated version (all instruments Chinese version for Chinese population). Within 1 week of surgery, week 5, and week 10 postsurgery.	Reduced state anxiety; no significant difference between groups over time on disease-specific QOL; both groups improved with time. Improved general QOL for experimental group.
Mishel et al.[51]	2002	239/Prostate	Three intervention groups: uncertainty management direct, uncertainty management supplemented (family support person received phone call also), and control/trained nurse Eight consecutive weekly phone calls	Mishel Uncertainty in Illness scale, Self-Control scale (problem solving and cognitive reframing subscales), the Symptom distress scale, and two study specific measures, i.e., the Cancer Knowledge Scale and a measure of patient–provider communication. Baseline, 4 and 7 months.	Improvement in cognitive reframing and problem solving at 4 mos. for intervention groups; decrease in symptom intensity for all groups, no difference by intervention. Impact of impotence was modified for some in intervention group. Some differences between African-Americans and Caucasians described.
Lepore et al.[52]	2003	250/prostate	Three groups: group education (GE); group education + discussion (GED); usual care control/ content experts, i.e., oncologist, urologist, etc. Six weekly 1-hour sessions	Prostate cancer knowledge; ratings of lectures; health behavior index; SF-36; CES-D; UCLA Prostate Cancer Index. Baseline, 2 weeks, 6 months, and 12 months.	Both interventions increased prostate ca. knowledge. GED group had fewer sexual problems than controls. Among noncollege graduates, GED and GE results in better physical functioning than controls and GED resulted in more positive health behaviors. No differences in these variables for college graduates.
Goodwin et al.[53]	2001	235/breast	Two groups: supportive expressive group therapy or usual care control/two professional counselors Weekly group sessions of 90 minutes for 1 year	POMS; LASA pain; EORTC-QLQ-30; Survival. Baseline, 4, 8, and 12 months.	No increased survival; improved mood and reduced pain for intervention group.
Molassiotis et al.[55]	2002	71/breast	Two groups: progressive muscle relaxation training, including individual audiocassettes and 30-minute video training program or control/ therapist trained in PMRT Thirty-minute sessions daily beginning 1 hour before chemotherapy and for 6 days following	POMS; STAI; MANE; Karnofsky Performance Index/ baseline (POMS, STAI, Karnofsky). At 7 and 14 days postchemotherapy (MANE).	Significant decrease in duration and trend toward lower frequency of N/V in intervention group; significant decrease in total mood disturbance.

TABLE 112.2. (continued)

Reference	*Year*	*n/dx*	*Intervention/source/duration*	*Measures/timing*	*Outcomes*
McArdle et al.[56]	1996	272/breast	Three groups: support from breast care nurse; support from voluntary organization; support from both nurse and organization; routine care control/breast care nurse and Tak Tent (Take Care) volunteer organization Variable	GHQ; HADS. First postoperative visit, 3, 6, and 12 months.	Psychological morbidity fell for all groups over 12 months. Compared to other groups, support from breast care nurse resulted in significant declines in depression, anxiety, and insomnia.
Winzelberg et al.[57]	2003	72/breast	Two groups: internet-based social support group with moderator; wait-list control health care professional Twelve weeks	CES-D, PCL-C, STAI, PSS, Cancer Behavior Inventory, Mini-MAC. Baseline (before randomization), post termination of group session.	Significantly greater decreases in depression, cancer-related trauma, and perceived stress in intervention compared to control group.
Helgeson et al.[58]	2001	312/ breast	Four groups: education; peer discussion; education + peer discussion; control/ facilitators and content experts Eight weekly 45-minute sessions	SF-36/six assessments. Baseline (after diagnosis, before randomization). Time 6 was mean 3.6 years postdiagnosis.	Long-term follow-up (mean, 3.6 years): higher vitality and physical functioning and lower bodily pain in education group. No long-term benefits on health-related QOL in peer discussion or education + peer discussion groups.
Antoni et al.[59]	2001	100/ breast	Two groups: cognitive-behavioral stress management group (intervention) and seminar (control)/postdoctoral fellows and graduate students Ten weekly 2-hour sessions (intervention) and 1 day (control)	POMS-SF; CES-D; IES; LOT-R; novel measures of perceived benefits and emotional processing. Baseline; postintervention; 3 and 9 months postintervention.	No overall effects of intervention on distress for intervention group; however, reduced depressive symptoms for those with higher depressive symptoms at baseline. Intervention group increased in benefit finding and optimism, particularly those with lower scores at baseline.
Edelman et al.[60]	1999	121/ breast	Two groups: cognitive-behavioral group intervention; control group/professional therapists Twelve 2-hour sessions	POMS; Coopersmith Self-Esteem Inventory; Survival. Baseline, immediately postintervention, and 3, 6, and 12 months postintervention.	Reduced depression and total mood and disturbance and increased self-esteem in intervention compared to control group. No group differences at 3- or 6-month follow-up. No survival effects.
Fukui et al.[61]	2000	50/ breast	Two groups: cognitive-behavioral therapy group; wait-list control group/ one psychologist and one psychiatrist Six weekly 90-minute sessions	POMS; MAC; HADS Baseline, 6 weeks (postintervention), and 6 months.	Significant decreases in anxiety and depression for tx group but no group differences for these outcomes. Tx group had lower mood disturbance, greater vigor, and greater fighting spirit at both follow-ups compared to control group.
Edmonds et al.[62]	1999	66/ breast	Two groups: psychological intervention, (supportive therapy + cognitive-behavioral techniques); control group (received information on coping and relaxation audio tapes)/ trained therapists Weekly 2-hour sessions for 35 weeks + one weekend	POMS; POMS-SF; FLIC; MAC; RED; DUFSS; RED; M-C. Baseline, 4, 8, and 14 months.	No group differences for mood, QOL, social support, or repression. In intervention group, greater anxious preoccupation and less helplessness; no survival effects.

TABLE 112.2. Randomized control trials. (continued)

Reference	*Year*	*n/dx*	*Intervention/source/duration*	*Measures/timing*	*Outcomes*
Classen et al.[63]	2001	125/ breast	Two groups: supportive-expressive group + educational materials; educational materials only (control)/a psychiatrist, psychologists, and social workers Weekly 90-minute sessions for 1 year	POMS; IES. Baseline, every 4 months for 1 year, every 6 months thereafter.	Greater decline in traumatic stress symptoms for intervention group but no group difference for mood at 1 year. When data excluded in year preceding death, mood disturbance and traumatic stress symptoms declined more for treatment group.
Bultz et al.[64]	2000	36 breast cancer partners	Two groups: psychoeducational and control/cofacilitated by two psychologists Six weekly 1.5- to 2-hour sessions	POMS; Index of Marital Satisfaction; DUFSS; MAC. Pre- and postintervention, 3 months postintervention.	Partners in intervention group had less mood disturbance than controls 3 months post-intervention. Women whose partners received the intervention reported less mood disturbance, and greater confidant support and marital satisfaction.
Toseland et al.[65]	1995	40 cancer patients and spouses	Two groups: intervention (support, problem-solving, coping skills) and usual treatment (control)/ experienced oncology social worker Six 1-hour sessions with patient's spouse	For caregivers: CES-D; STAI; Dyadic Adjustment Scale; Social Functioning Subscale from Health & Daily Living Form; SF-20; Zarit Burden Inventory; Help-Seeking Coping Index; Index of Coping Responses; Pressing problems (cancer caregiving); drug/EtOh use; Personal Change Scale. For patients: FLIC; ECOG Global Performance Scale. Baseline, postintervention.	No significant between-group differences found for any measures. Intervention appeared to be effective only for distressed subsample of caregivers.

n/dx, number of patients/diagnosis; MAACL, Multiple Affect Adjective Checklist—state form; LPIS, Langer Psychiatric Impairment Scale; SRE, Schedule of recent events; HLC, Health Locus of Control; ADL, activities of daily living; ADPI, Activity Pattern Indicators; STAI, State-Trait Anxiety inventory; QOL, quality of life; WHO, World Health Organization; SF-36, Short Form 36 (Rand Medical Outcomes Study); CES-D, Center for Epidemiologic Studies–Depression scale; POMS, Profile of Mood States; LASA, Linear Analog Scale Assessment; EORTC-QLQ-30, European Organization for Research and Treatment of Cancer—Quality of Life Questionnaire–30; PMRT, progressive muscle relaxation training; MANE, Morrow Assessment of Nausea and Emesis; GHQ, General Health Questionnaire; HADS, Hospital Anxiety and Depression Scale; PCL-C, posttraumatic stress disorder (PTSD) Checklist—Civilian Version; PSS, Perceived Stress Scale; Mini-MAC, mini-mental adjustment to cancer scale; SF-36, Medical Outcomes Study Short-Form 36; SF-20, Medical Outcomes Study—20; IES, Impact of Events Scale; LOT-R, Life Orientation Test–Revised; MAC, Mental Adjustment to Cancer Scale; FLIC, Functional Living Index for Cancer; ECOG, Eastern Cooperative Oncology Group performance status scale; DUFSS, Duke-UNC Functional Social Support Questionnaire; RED, Rationality/Emotional Defensiveness Scale; M-C, Marlowe Crowne Social Desirability Scale; N/V, nausea/vomiting.

In one of the earliest randomized clinical trials measuring the efficacy of a psychosocial intervention, cancer patients with diagnoses of breast or lung cancer or melanoma were studied.[48] The intervention group ($n = 157$) was given one of three types of psychosocial intervention: (1) patient education about how to live with the disease effectively; (2) a more generic counseling intervention focusing on patients' reactions to and feelings about their disease; and (3) environmental manipulation, including consultations with other healthcare personnel and referral for additional services as necessary. The control group ($n = 151$) received usual care and evaluations only. The most notable effects of the intervention included amelioration of psychosocial problems reported by the patient, a more-rapid decline of negative affect (anxiety, hostility, and depression), a more realistic outlook on life, a greater proportion of return to previous vocational status, and a more-active pattern of time usage.

Another study examined the effect of progressive muscle relaxation training (PMRT) on anxiety and quality of life following stoma surgery in Chinese colorectal cancer patients.[49] Subjects were randomly assigned to a control group ($n = 30$) and the experimental group utilizing PMRT ($n = 29$). This procedure significantly decreased state anxiety and improved overall quality of life in the experimental group. These findings are notable particularly because patient baseline state anxiety scores were higher than reported norms.[50] Thus, this sample would constitute one that needed psychosocial rehabilitation, assuming that premorbid state anxiety was lower than that reported at baseline here.

In a unique study with prostate cancer patients, Mishel et al. examined effects of a nurse-delivered psychoeducational intervention over the telephone in helping patients to manage uncertainty and treatment side effects.[51] A total of 239 men were randomly assigned to one of the three treatment conditions: (1) uncertainty management with the patient, (2) uncertainty management with the patient and a family member (supplemented group), and (3) the control group. The intervention consisted of eight weekly telephone calls by a nurse who was trained in this specific intervention. Patients in each of the two treatment groups (individual or supplemented) received the same intervention. However, in the supplemented group, a spouse or designated significant other from the family also received a weekly telephone call and a similar intervention was applied. The majority of intervention effects were seen at 4 months after baseline, a time when treatment side effects were also most intense. Both uncertainty management approaches were useful in producing cognitive reframing and problem solving. When both individual and supplemented intervention groups were combined for analysis, there was measured improvement in control of incontinence at the 4-month assessment. Furthermore, the negative impact of impotence could be modified for some of the men who had received the intervention. This study represents an economical and convenient intervention in a population with significant morbidity, particularly in terms of sexual functioning and incontinence following treatment for localized prostate cancer. The telephone intervention method is also portable and has great potential for psychosocial interventions with cancer patients.

Lepore et al. attempted to improve the QOL of men recently treated for prostate cancer.[52] Two hundred and fifty patients were randomly assigned to a control group, a group education intervention (GE), or a group education-plus-discussion intervention (GED). Both GE and GED increased prostate cancer knowledge. In the year following the intervention, men in the GED condition were less bothered by sexual problems than men in the control condition, and they were more likely to remain steadily employed than men in the GE or control conditions. Both the Mishel and Lepore studies support the idea that relatively straightforward interventions can be useful for improving psychosocial functioning in prostate cancer patients.

Breast Cancer Studies

Breast cancer patients are the most extensively studied group in randomized clinical trials conducted in the area of psychosocial rehabilitation. The literature is extensive, and we only cite representative studies here. There is an excellent review of health-related QOL results that does include 20 studies with psychosocial outcomes in breast cancer.[53]

In a study of women with newly diagnosed breast cancer ($n = 96$) about to begin chemotherapy, patients were randomized to an intervention (standard care plus relaxation training and imagery) or to a control condition (standard care only).[54] The goal of this study was to develop and evaluate a simple and easily administered intervention to help women cope with the diagnosis and treatment of breast cancer. Those in the intervention group practiced relaxation and imagery daily for the 18 weeks of their chemotherapy. No significant between-group differences were noted for anxiety and depression. Using intention-to-treat analyses, between-group effects were found with women in the intervention group reporting fewer psychologic symptoms and higher quality of life during chemotherapy.

Molassiotis and colleagues assessed the effectiveness of progressive muscle relaxation training (PMRT) in the management of chemotherapy-related nausea and vomiting, mood disturbance and anxiety.[55] Women diagnosed with nonmetastatic breast cancer ($n = 71$) were randomized to the PMRT intervention or to a control condition. The PMRT intervention was administered by a trained therapist six times for 30 minutes before receiving chemotherapy. The total mood disturbance score of the POMS decreased in the intervention group and increased in the control group when assessed at 7 and 14 days postintervention. No between-group differences were observed for POMS subscales or for anxiety.

McArdle et al. examined the effects of support from a nurse specialist and from a volunteer support organization in breast cancer.[56] Women under 70 years of age diagnosed with breast cancer ($n = 272$) were randomized to one of four groups before undergoing surgery for breast cancer: (1) standard support from ward staff and information booklet; (2) standard support from ward staff plus support from a specialist breast care nurse; (3) standard support from ward staff plus support from a voluntary organization (included any combination of information, counseling, and group meetings); and (4) standard support from ward staff plus support from a specialist breast care nurse and from a voluntary organization. Individuals in the treatment group receiving support mainly from the nurse specialist reported improved depressive symptoms, anxiety symptoms, somatic symptoms, and social dysfunction compared to all other groups, including the group that had support from *both* the nurse specialist and the voluntary organization.

Another RCT employed a newer technologic approach to providing psychosocial support to women with breast cancer.[57] Women with breast cancer ($n = 72$) were randomly assigned to a 12-week internet-based social support group moderated by a healthcare professional or to a wait-list control group. Participants in the intervention group reported significantly decreased depressive symptoms, cancer-related traumatic stress, and perceived overall stress when compared to the control group. No changes were found for anxiety or coping measures.

Helgeson and colleagues examined the long-term effects of participation in a psychosocial group intervention on health-related quality of life (measured with the SF-36)[58] in which 312 women with early-stage breast cancer were randomly assigned to one of four conditions: education, peer discussion, education plus peer discussion, and control. The length of the intervention was 8 weeks with participants meeting once each week. The education group focused on the provision of information to enhance sense of control while the peer discussion group focused on the expression of feelings and self-disclosure. Intent-to-treat analysis was used in this study. Follow-up with those who had no recurrent disease at 3 years revealed that the women in the education-only group retained higher levels of vitality (energy and lack of fatigue) and physical functioning and lower bodily pain than women in the control group. No benefits of the peer discussion group or the education plus peer discussion group were observed at 3-year follow-up.

Antoni et al. examined distress as well as positive outcomes in women who had recently been treated for early-stage breast cancer.[59] Patients were randomly assigned to take part in a 10-week cognitive-behavioral stress management intervention (met weekly for 2 hours over 10 weeks) or to a more-limited control condition (1-day informational seminar). Findings showed that while there were no overall effects of the intervention on measures of distress, participation in the 10-week intervention reduced the prevalence of moderate depressive symptoms for those whose levels were higher at baseline. Also, benefit-finding and optimism increased for those taking part in the intervention, with the effects most pronounced in women with low baseline scores. Findings from this study underscore the notion that psychosocial rehabilitation is most likely to be useful for those patients who report the most psychosocial distress and/or the least psychosocial resources.

In a study with metastatic breast cancer patients, 124 patients were randomized to take part in a group cognitive behavioral therapy (CBT) intervention or to a no-therapy control group condition.[60] Participants in the CBT group attended eight weekly group sessions, followed by a family night and three additional monthly sessions. Immediately following participation in the CBT group, data indicated significant improvements in depression, total mood disturbance, and self-esteem. However, no significant differences between the CBT and control groups were evident at 3- or 6-month follow-up.

A similar study of a short-term psychosocial intervention was conducted with lymph node-positive breast cancer patients in Japan.[61] Patients ($n = 50$) were randomized to a 6-week structured psychosocial group intervention (included health education, coping skills training, stress management, and support) or to a wait-list control group. Analyses were conducted on the 46 women who completed the intervention. Anxiety and depression decreased significantly over the course of the study for the treatment group; however, no significant between-group differences emerged for these outcomes. Significant between-group differences were found for POMS total mood disturbance score at both the 6-week (immediately following the intervention) and 6-month assessments. The experimental group had significantly lower scores than the controls for total mood disturbance and significantly higher scores for vigor on the POMS, and significantly higher scores for fighting spirit on the MAC at the end of the 6-week intervention. These improvements were sustained over 6 months of follow-up.

Several of the previously described studies demonstrated that short-term psychosocial interventions resulted in improvement in quality of life and psychosocial distress. There has been little evidence, however, for the efficacy of longer-term psychosocial interventions. In a study of longer duration, patients with metastatic breast cancer were randomized to an 8-month weekly psychologic intervention ($n = 36$; group discussion, emotional support, coping skills training, and relaxation) or to a control group ($n = 30$; received information on coping and relaxation audio tapes).[62] Study outcomes included mood, quality of life, and adjustment to cancer measured at baseline, 4 months, 8 months, and 14 months. Participation in the long-term psychologic intervention did not result in significantly improved mood or quality of life in comparison to those in the control group, although there were short-term clinical gains reported by therapists that were not quantified.

A group of 125 metastatic breast cancer patients was randomized to a 1-year weekly supportive-expressive group psychotherapy intervention with additional educational materials or to a control group offered only educational materials.[63] Data from all participants who completed at least one follow-up assessment ($n = 102$) regardless of level of group attendance were included in study analyses. Women in the group intervention reported a significantly greater decline in traumatic stress symptoms at 1 year, but no difference in overall mood when compared with women randomized to the control condition. However, when data from final assessments that took place during the year before participants' deaths were excluded, both mood disturbance and traumatic stress symptoms declined significantly more for those in the treatment compared to the control condition.

Caregiver Studies

The patient has long been the primary focus for psychosocial rehabilitation or psychosocial interventions. However, the diagnosis and treatment of cancer can have far-reaching effects, evoking distress and feelings of helplessness in spouses/partners and other close family members. Role transitions in spousal and family relationships are often required. Relatively few interventions and even fewer RCTs to date have focused on psychosocial rehabilitation issues in close family members of cancer patients. The following several studies are representative examples of high-quality research that has sought to empirically validate methods for helping family members increase their understanding of cancer and treatment, normalize their responses to a loved one's cancer, and provide a safe place for relatives to express emotional distress.

One RCT examined the effects of a brief psychoeducational support group intervention for male partners of women with early-stage breast cancer ($n = 36$ pairs).[64] The intervention was offered to partners of breast cancer patients weekly for six sessions by two experienced psychologists and focused on two primary components: education and support. Results indicated that total mood disturbance score had improved by 3-month follow-up for both patients and partners who in the intervention group; however, these findings did not reach statistical significance.

Another RCT offered a six-session intervention to spouses ($n = 40$ male, $n = 40$ female) of patients with various types of cancer.[65] Spouses were randomly assigned to the intervention that included support, problem-solving, and coping skills or to a usual care condition. At baseline and within 2 weeks of completing the intervention, spousal caregivers completed measures of depression, anxiety, marital satisfaction, social support, health status, burden, help-seeking behavior, coping (perceived stressfulness of 17 cancer-related caregiving problems), and drug/alcohol use. At the same time points, patients completed measures of functional and physical status. Taking part in the group did not significantly improve any of the psychosocial outcomes for those in the intervention versus the control group. However, post hoc subgroup analyses revealed that for those caregivers who were more distressed at baseline (lower marital satisfaction, higher burden), greater improvements were found in the intervention group compared to the control group. This type of result, once again, highlights the usefulness of targeting psychosocial rehabilitation interventions to those individuals most in need of them.

Rehabilitation Programs

A number of programs have been developed and tested over the past 15 years directed at psychosocial care of patients.[66–68] Examples of such programs include Gilda's House, The Wellness Community, and the Commonweal Help Program. Even though there are programs for posttreatment cancer survivors that have a psychosocial component (e.g., the posttreatment resource center at Memorial Sloan Kettering Cancer Center), there is a need for dissemination of research outcomes so that programs can integrate evidence-based rehabilitation strategies. Additionally, specific programs have been developed to attend to particular difficulties of patients.

In a review article, Ronson and Body described the psychosocial rehabilitation of cancer patients after curative therapy.[69] They reported that even though the majority of cancer survivors do quite well, there is a substantial minority of patients who have significant psychosocial distress and/or psychiatric disturbance. A number of factors seem to predict psychosocial difficulty or adjustment, including a past history of psychiatric disturbance (especially depression), comorbid physical problems, poor social support, low social or economic status, and individual psychologic factors (including certain coping styles and personality traits). An important observation they make is that "no effective psychosocial rehabilitation can be achieved without simultaneous efforts to promote improvement of the physical condition." Physical and psychosocial functioning may be so closely related that it is impossible to talk about one without reference to the other. It is safe to say that patients returning to predisease physical functioning are less likely to experience severe psychosocial distress, although this cannot be stated with 100% certainty. Under the best of conditions, when patients return to health, fear and anxiety can act to rob the patient of the present when a feared future looms ahead in the form of recurrent disease.

Specific psychologic disorders and symptom entities that were summarized from the literature by Ronson and Body with estimated prevalence rates were posttraumatic stress disorder (as high as 14% to 21%), fear of recurrence (ranging from 10% to 89%), conditioned nausea/vomiting (no estimates given; highly dependent on emetogenic potential of chemotherapy and antiemetic agents used), treatment-related body image disturbances (no estimates given; related to area of surgery, timing of assessment, and premorbid functioning), and general psychosocial functioning (ranging from 18% to 40% depending on tumor type and treatment). They also identified aspects of physical functioning that have a psychosocial impact. Although attention to the literature on physical functioning is beyond the scope of this paper, it is important that the reciprocal relationship between physical and psychosocial functioning in general be understood, as well as the psychosocial issues related to specific tumor types and their treatment.

There are few randomized prospective studies of rehabilitation programs described in the literature. One such study is the "Starting Again Group Rehabilitation Program"[67] that enrolled a total of 199 patients ($n = 98$ intervention; $n = 101$ control) in the program. The intervention (called the "Starting Again Program") consisted of eleven 2-hour sessions that emphasized physical training, information, and coping skills. Outcomes that improved following the intervention included appraisal of having received sufficient information, physical strength, and fighting spirit. The psychosocial area of this study consisted of coping skills training and role playing (employed to help study participants understand the issues of returning to work, as well as problem situations that may arise with return medical appointments). One session devoted to anxiety management included coping strategies such as relaxation, distraction, and cognitive techniques. Depressive symptoms for program participants diminished significantly over time. The authors pointed out that the study included patients at low risk for psychosocial disturbance, thereby making it more difficult to measure appreciable change. Furthermore, spontaneous recovery is common for those experiencing psychosocial morbidity in low-risk patients, and it would be difficult for an intervention to achieve superior results under these circumstances. In other words, many people simply improve with time with regard to sadness and depressive symptoms related to the diagnosis and treatment of cancer.

The Tapestry Program is an example of a novel method for providing psychosocial support for persons living with cancer.[68] It consists of a 5-day residential retreat program focusing on the following areas: creating a safe environment for patients, providing a daily narrative group, the use of arts and medicine therapy, providing yoga and meditation sessions, discussions about complementary therapies and pain control, death and dying, and use of rituals to foster a supportive collegial atmosphere. A primary method within this group involves general support provided by patients undergoing similar difficulties together. The Tapestry group has attempted to measure patient improvement following participation in the program with pre- and posttest measures that generally favor the impact of this program. There have been other promising reports of the effectiveness of these types of programs.[70]

Returning to Normal

Returning to "normal" is a prominent theme in the clinical care of patients. Although there has been some work in this area,[71] there is little research on returning to normal from a psychosocial standpoint only. Indeed, some patients comment that "things will never be normal again," because the issue of recurrence is always present even after a declaration of survival at the 5-year posttreatment time point. However, although some patients may carry a constant sense of foreboding and worry about cancer recurring, others may claim not only a return to normality but a deeper appreciation for life.[72–74] Such patients not only return to normal but actually find some benefits and, perhaps, improved psychosocial functioning in the form of deeper appreciation and meaning in everyday living. This finding has been incidental, although researchers are now focusing more on benefits that patients experience following a cancer diagnosis and treatment.[74] Typically, such benefit finding is in the area attitudinal shifts and/or improved social relations. For example, one attitudinal shift might be reflected in a change of career or a change of work habits in the direction of increasing time with family or friends as a consequence of recognition of mortality. Even though benefit finding is not a particularly common approach in psychosocial rehabilitation, it is an important area to consider because it could be that one psychosocial deficit such as fear of recurrence is balanced by a benefit in the form of deeper meaning noted by the patient or other family members.

Concluding Comments

There is a growing body of literature supporting the effectiveness of psychosocial interventions in the rehabilitation of cancer patients. Interest in this area is driven by the increasing number of cancer survivors living 5 years or longer, less stigma attached to utilizing psychosocial services such as support groups or individual coaching/counseling, research initiatives of the National Cancer Institute (NCI) emphasizing psychosocial care, efforts of the National Coalition for Cancer Survivorship and Office of Cancer Survivorship of the NCI, growing consumer interest, effective intervention techniques, and validated measurement tools for assessing the usefulness of such interventions. Another force operating within the community of cancer medicine is the emphasis on quality of life as an important outcome in addition to survival.

There are specific types of treatments that have been shown to be effective for a variety of patients for reasons of their ease of administration as well as face validity. These interventions include cognitive behavioral therapy, progressive muscle relaxation, structured psychoeducational interventions including problem solving, and supportive-expressive therapy. For the most part, such interventions have been demonstrated with breast cancer patients, possibly because of funding opportunities provided by the Department of Defense and the Komen Foundation. There are few RCTs with psychosocial interventions in most other cancer sites. Patients with head and neck and pancreatic cancer, as well as those with brain tumors, remain little researched for a variety of reasons. Most of the excellent randomized clinical trials that have been conducted are associated with major medical centers. However, the vast majority of cancer care is delivered in communities. Patients treated in community settings are most likely to find psychosocial care with mental health counselors and the clergy, American Cancer Society programs, and in Wellness Communities. These settings are hard pressed to devote the resources necessary to conduct a clinical trial on psychosocial care.

If psychosocial rehabilitation is to move forward, more clinical trials with a broader range of patients need to be developed and conducted. There has been progress made. Cognitive behavior therapy and structured supportive educational approaches have promise, as do telephone interventions. Yet, the central question remains: What interventions for what patients along what point of their trajectory of survivorship and care, delivered by what type of professional, can offer the promise of reduced suffering and return to full-quality living following the diagnosis and treatment for cancer?

References

1. Zabora J, BrintzenhofeSzoc K, Curbow B, Hooker C, Piantadosi S. The prevalence of psychological distress by cancer site. Psycho-Oncology 2001;10(1):19–28.
2. Derogatis LR, Morrow GR, Fetting J, et al. The prevalence of psychiatric disorders among cancer patients. JAMA 1983; 249(6):751–757.
3. American Cancer Society: Facts and Figures. Atlanta, GA: American Cancer Society, 2003.
4. Psychosocial care improves quality of life but half of US cancer patients do not receive essential interventions. In: The Clinical Cancer Letter: A Research Guide for Clinicians. The Cancer Letter, Inc. 1995:1–9.
5. Enabling America: Assessing the Role of Rehabilitation, Science and Engineering. Washington, DC: National Academy Press, 1997.
6. Dietz JH. Rehabilitation Oncology. New York: Wiley, 1981.
7. Gunn AE. Cancer Rehabilitation. New York: Raven, 1984.
8. Mayer D, O'Connor L. Rehabilitation of persons with cancer: an ONS position statement. Oncol Nurs Forum 1989;16(3):433.
9. Ganz PA. Current issues in cancer rehabilitation. Cancer (Phila) 1990;65(3 suppl):742–751.
10. McQuellon RP, Hurt GJ. The psychosocial impact of the diagnosis and treatment of laryngeal cancer. Otolaryngol Clin N Am 1997;30(2):231–241.
11. Distress management: clinical practice guidelines. J Natl Comprehens Cancer Network 2003;1(3):344–374.
12. Holland JC. Update: NCCN Practice Guidelines for the Management of Psychosocial Distress. Oncology 1999;13(5A): 113–147.
13. McQuellon RP, Russell GB, Rambo TD, et al. Quality of life and psychological distress of bone marrow transplant recipients: the "time trajectory" to recovery over the first year. Bone Marrow Transplant 1998;21(5):477–486.
14. McQuellon RP, Loggie BW, Fleming RA, Russell GB, Lehman AB, Rambo TD. Quality of life after intraperitoneal hyperthermic chemotherapy (IPHC) for peritoneal carcinomatosis. Eur J Surg Oncol 2001;27(1):65–73.
15. Dimeo F, Bertz H, Finke J, Fetscher S, Mertelsmann R, Keul J. An aerobic exercise program for patients with haematological malignancies after bone marrow transplantation. Bone Marrow Transplant 1996;18(6):1157–1160.
16. Engel GL. The need for a new medical model: a challenge for biomedicine. Science 1977;196(4286):129–136.
17. Kornblith AB. Psychosocial adaptation of cancer survivors. In: Holland JC, Breitbart W, Jacobsen PB, et al. (eds). Psycho-Oncology. New York: Oxford University Press, 1998:223–254.
18. Fallowfield L, Jenkins V. Effective communication skills are the key to good cancer care. Eur J Cancer 1999;35(11):1592–1597.
19. Lehmann JF, DeLisa JA, Warren CG, deLateur BJ, Bryant PL, Nicholson CG. Cancer rehabilitation: assessment of need, development, and evaluation of a model of care. Arch Phys Med Rehabil 1978;59(9):410–419.
20. Barofsky I. The status of psychosocial research in the rehabilitation of the cancer patient [review]. Semin Oncol Nurs 1992; 8(3):190–201.
21. Andersen BL, Kiecolt-Glaser JK, Glaser R. A biobehavioral model of cancer stress and disease course [review]. Am Psychologist 1994;49(5):389–404.
22. Zabora JR, Smith-Wilson R, Fetting JH, Enterline JP. An efficient method for psychosocial screening of cancer patients. Psychosomatics 1990;31(2):192–196.
23. Zabora JR. "Development of a self-administered psychosocial cancer screening tool" [letter]. Cancer Pract 1995;3(2):117–118.
24. Newell SA, Sanson-Fisher RW, Savolainen NJ. Systematic review of psychological therapies for cancer patients: overview and recommendations for future research. J Natl Cancer Inst 2002;94(8):558–584.
25. Andersen BL. Psychological interventions for cancer patients to enhance the quality of life. J Consult Clin Psychol 1992;60(4): 552–568.
26. Fawzy FI, Fawzy NW, Arndt LA, Pasnau RO. Critical review of psychosocial interventions in cancer care [review]. Arch Gen Psychiatry 1995;52(2):100–113.
27. Meyer TJ, Mark MM. Effects of psychosocial interventions with adult cancer patients: a meta-analysis of randomized experiments [see comments]. Health Psychol 1995;14(2):101–108.

28. Sheard T, Maguire P. The effect of psychological interventions on anxiety and depression in cancer patients: results of two meta-analyses. Br J Cancer 1999;80(11):1770–1780.
29. Rehse B, Pukrop R. Effects of psychosocial interventions on quality of life in adult cancer patients: meta analysis of 37 published controlled outcome studies. Patient Educ Counsel 2003;50(2):179–186.
30. Mulrow CD OA. Cochrane Collaboration Handbook. Oxford (UK): Cochrane Collaboration, 1997.
31. Wells ME, McQuellon RP, Hinkle JS, Cruz JM. Reducing anxiety in newly diagnosed cancer patients: a pilot program. Cancer Pract 1995;3(2):100–104.
32. McQuellon RP, Wells M, Hoffman S, et al. Reducing distress in cancer patients with an orientation program. Psycho-Oncology 1998;7(3):207–217.
33. Rehse B, Pukrop R. Effects of psychosocial interventions on quality of life in adult cancer patients: meta analysis of 37 published controlled outcome studies. Patient Educ Counsel 2003;50(2):179–186.
34. Brady MJ, Cella DF, Mo F, et al. Reliability and validity of the Functional Assessment of Cancer Therapy-Breast quality-of-life instrument. J Clin Oncol 1997;15(3):974–986.
35. Cella DF, Bonomi AE, Lloyd SR, Tulsky DS, Kaplan E, Bonomi P. Reliability and validity of the Functional Assessment of Cancer Therapy–Lung (FACT-L) quality of life instrument. Lung Cancer 1995;12:199–220.
36. Cella DF. Manual for the Functional Assessment of Cancer Therapy (FACT) Measurement System (version 3): 1994. Chicago: Rush Cancer Center, 1994.
37. Yellen SB, Cella DF, Webster K, Blendowski C, Kaplan E. Measuring fatigue and other anemia-related symptoms with the Functional Assessment of Cancer Therapy (FACT) measurement system. J Pain Symptom Manag 1997;13(2):63–74.
38. Cella DF, Tulsky DS, Gray G, et al. The Functional Assessment of Cancer Therapy scale: development and validation of the general measure. J Clin Oncol 1993;11(3):570–579.
39. Ware JE Jr, Snow KK, Kosinski M, Gandek B. SF-36 health survey. Manual and interpretation guide. Boston: Nimrod Press, 1993.
40. Hann DM, Jacobsen PB, Martin SC, Kronish LE, Azzarello LM, Fields KK. Quality of life following bone marrow transplantation for breast cancer: a comparative study. Bone Marrow Transplant 1997;19(3):257–264.
41. Hann DM, Jacobsen PB, Martin SC, Kronish LE, Azzarello LM, Fields KK. Fatigue in women treated with bone marrow transplantation for breast cancer: a comparison with women with no history of cancer. Support Care Cancer 1997;5(1):44–52.
42. McQuellon RP, Loggie BW, Lehman AB, et al. Long-term survivorship and quality of life after cytoreductive surgery plus intraperitoneal hyperthermic chemotherapy for peritoneal carcinomatosis. Ann Surg Oncol 2003;10(2):155–162.
43. Ganz PA, Schag CA, Lee JJ, Sim MS. The CARES: a generic measure of health-related quality of life for patients with cancer. Qual Life Res 1992;1(1):19–29.
44. Schag CA, Ganz PA, Polinsky ML, Fred C, Hirji K, Petersen L. Characteristics of women at risk for psychosocial distress in the year after breast cancer. J Clin Oncol 1993;11(4):783–793.
45. Ganz PA, Greendale GA, Petersen L, Zibecchi L, Kahn B, Belin TR. Managing menopausal symptoms in breast cancer survivors: results of a randomized controlled trial. J Natl Cancer Inst 2000;92(13):1054–1064.
46. Schag CA, Ganz PA, Wing DS, Sim MS, Lee JJ. Quality of life in adult survivors of lung, colon and prostate cancer. Qual Life Res 1994;3(2):127–141.
47. Worden JW, Weisman AD. Do cancer patients really want counseling? Gen Hosp Psychiatry 1980;2(2):100–103.
48. Gordon WA, Freidenbergs I, Diller L, et al. Efficacy of psychosocial intervention with cancer patients. J Consult Clin Psychol 1980;48(6):743–759.
49. Cheung YL, Molassiotis A, Chang AM. The effect of progressive muscle relaxation training on anxiety and quality of life after stoma surgery in colorectal cancer patients. Psycho-Oncology 2003;12(3):254–266.
50. Spielberger CD, Gorsuch RL, Lushene RD. STAI: Manual for the State-Trait Anxiety Inventory. Palo Alto: Consulting Psychologists Press, 1970.
51. Mishel MH, Belyea M, Germino BB, et al. Helping patients with localized prostate carcinoma manage uncertainty and treatment side effects: nurse-delivered psychoeducational intervention over the telephone. Cancer (Phila) 2002;94(6):1854–1866.
52. Lepore SJ, Helgeson VS, Eton DT, Schulz R. Improving quality of life in men with prostate cancer: a randomized controlled trial of group education interventions. Health Psychol 2003;22(5):443–452.
53. Goodwin PJ, Black JT, Bordeleau LJ, Ganz PA. Health-related quality-of-life measurement in randomized clinical trials in breast cancer: taking stock. J Natl Cancer Inst 2003;95(4):263–281.
54. Walker LG, Walker MB, Ogston K, et al. Psychological, clinical and pathological effects of relaxation training and guided imagery during primary chemotherapy. Br J Cancer 1999;80(1–2):262–268.
55. Molassiotis A, Yung HP, Yam BM, Chan FY, Mok TS. The effectiveness of progressive muscle relaxation training in managing chemotherapy-induced nausea and vomiting in Chinese breast cancer patients: a randomised controlled trial. Support Care Cancer 2002;10(3):237–246.
56. McArdle JM, George WD, McArdle CS, et al. Psychological support for patients undergoing breast cancer surgery: a randomised study. BMJ 1996;312(7034):813–816.
57. Winzelberg AJ, Classen C, Alpers GW, et al. Evaluation of an internet support group for women with primary breast cancer. Cancer (Phila) 2003;97(5):1164–1173.
58. Helgeson VS, Cohen S, Schulz R, Yasko J. Long-term effects of educational and peer discussion group interventions on adjustment to breast cancer. Health Psychol 2001;20(5):387–392.
59. Antoni MH, Lehman JM, Kilbourn KM, et al. Cognitive-behavioral stress management intervention decreases the prevalence of depression and enhances benefit finding among women under treatment for early-stage breast cancer. Health Psychol 2001;20(1):20–32.
60. Edelman S, Bell DR, Kidman AD. A group cognitive behaviour therapy programme with metastatic breast cancer patients. Psycho-Oncology 1999;8(4):295–305.
61. Fukui S, Kugaya A, Okamura H, et al. A psychosocial group intervention for Japanese women with primary breast carcinoma. Cancer (Phila) 2000;89(5):1026–1036.
62. Edmonds CV, Lockwood GA, Cunningham AJ. Psychological response to long-term group therapy: a randomized trial with metastatic breast cancer patients. Psycho-Oncology 1999;8(1):74–91.
63. Classen C, Butler LD, Koopman C, et al. Supportive-expressive group therapy and distress in patients with metastatic breast cancer: a randomized clinical intervention trial. Arch Gen Psychiatry 2001;58(5):494–501.
64. Bultz BD, Speca M, Brasher PM, Geggie PH, Page SA. A randomized controlled trial of a brief psychoeducational support group for partners of early stage breast cancer patients. Psycho-Oncology 2000;9(4):303–313.
65. Toseland RW, Blanchard CG, McCallion P. A problem solving intervention for caregivers of cancer patients. Soc Sci Med 1995;40(4):517–528.
66. McQuellon RP, Hurt GJ, DeChatelet P. Psychosocial care of the patient with cancer: a model for organizing services. Cancer Pract 1996;4(6):304–311.
67. Berglund G, Bolund C, Gustafsson UL, Sjoden PO. One-year follow-up of the "Starting Again" group rehabilitation programme for cancer patients. Eur J Cancer 1994;30A(12):1744–1751.

68. Angen MJ, MacRae JH, Simpson JS, Hundleby M. Tapestry: a retreat program of support for persons living with cancer. Cancer Pract 2002;10(6):297–304.
69. Ronson A, Body JJ. Psychosocial rehabilitation of cancer patients after curative therapy. Support Care Cancer 2002;10(4):281–291.
70. Walsh-Burke K. Family communication and coping with cancer: impact of the We Can Weekend. J Psychosocial Oncol 1992; 10(1):63–81.
71. Andrykowski MA, Brady MJ, Greiner CB, et al. 'Returning to normal' following bone marrow transplantation: outcomes, expectations and informed consent. Bone Marrow Transplant 1995;15(4):573–581.
72. Andrykowski MA, McQuellon RP. Readaptation to normal life following bone marrow transplantation. In: Barrett J, Treleaven J (eds). The Clinical Practice of Stem Cell Transplantation. Oxford: Isis Medical Media, 1997:828–835.
73. Fromm K, Andrykowski MA, Hunt J. Positive and negative psychosocial sequelae of bone marrow transplantation: implications for quality of life assessment. J Behav Med 1996;19(3): 221–240.
74. Sears SR, Stanton AL, Danoff-Burg S. The yellow brick road and the emerald city: benefit finding, positive reappraisal coping and posttraumatic growth in women with early-stage breast cancer. Health Psychol 2003;22(5):487–497.

113

Cancer Advocacy

Ellen L. Stovall

Thousands of individual citations using the expression *cancer advocacy* can be found in contemporary medical and scientific literature as well as in the popular press and on Internet websites. For purposes of this chapter, the term *cancer advocacy* is used to describe a skill set that has been documented in previously published work by Clark and Stovall.[1] This chapter also includes specific examples of how self-described advocacy organizations are involved with research organizations and how they influence cancer research and related health policy.

In 1996, Clark and Stovall described a cancer-related advocacy skill set that could be acquired through a learning process and would ideally be incorporated into care plans for cancer patients. Their article proposed a definition of cancer advocacy that most easily correlated with the terms "cancer survivor" and "cancer survivorship" first used by the founders of the National Coalition for Cancer Survivorship (NCCS) in 1986.[2] NCCS defines a cancer survivor as anyone with a diagnosis of cancer—from the time of its discovery and for the balance of life. NCCS further defines cancer survivorship as a process that begins when an individual is diagnosed with cancer and continues until their death. NCCS believes that, at the time of diagnosis, an individual with cancer [and/or a significant person in his or her life—known as the "other survivor"(s)] can play a very active role in assuring that they receive quality care. This is the first step in the cancer advocacy continuum and is further defined by Clark and Stovall as "personal advocacy or self-advocacy." The next step in the continuum is "advocacy for others." This is where some of the most effective advocacy occurs for individuals with cancer, and it is where many people with cancer find a role for themselves as advocates in their own community. The third part of the advocacy paradigm described by Clark and Stovall is national advocacy, or public interest advocacy.

Over the past decade, relative survival data for all cancer types have ranged from 6 to 10 million survivors in any given year, and estimates are that of that number, more than half are living 5 years or more postdiagnosis.[3] With this epidemiology alone, it is likely that this cohort (and their primary caregivers and healthcare providers) could be the most likely beneficiaries of a greater understanding of the role that advocacy can play as part of a successful adjustment to a cancer diagnosis. To accept the notion that advocacy can play a role in enhancing the quality of one's survivorship, a shared understanding of cancer advocacy and its relationship to cancer survivorship among healthcare professionals and significant others involved with a cancer patient's adjustment postdiagnosis is desirable.

The term *cancer survivorship* was a term of art rather than science when the founders of NCCS used it to describe the condition of living with the consequences of a diagnosis of cancer. Now commonly referred to as the cancer survivorship movement, several of its early founders and adopters crafted the language and gave definition to terminology frequently used today for what has become a burgeoning field of study called *cancer survivorship research*. Mullan wrote about cancer survivorship as the "act of living on."[4] Carter and Leigh have written about survivorship in terms of "going through" and "the experience of living with, through or beyond cancer."[5,6] These dynamic concepts of survivorship suggested that more research was needed to focus on cancers whose prognosis could be defined as protracted and/or episodic, rather than as an acute diagnosis followed by death. It was also noted that the degree to which a history of cancer affects the life of an individual is largely dependent on many qualitative variables with respect to how they experience their illness. These variables include, but are not limited to, their familial and cultural relationships, their religious beliefs, how their cancer is treated, and how their disease progresses or is resolved.

Previous chapters in of this section elaborate on the survivorship issues and deal specifically with the myriad of medical and psychosocial sequelae of many cancers. The challenges posed by these changes in one's biologic and psychologic condition suggest that although each person's cancer is an individual experience, there are overarching issues with which many survivors contend.[7] We also know from the literature and from the cancer survivorship movement that the skills necessary for positive adaptation to cancer have been identified and that survivors must become self-advocates and viewed by health professionals as partners in making the very important decisions that will impact on their medical, social, psychologic, and vocational well-being. What follows is a suggestion by Clark and Stovall that successful adaptation to cancer involves acquiring advocacy skills that will enhance each survivor's sense of self-determination throughout his or her survivorship. The skill set is neither gender- nor age-specific and does not suggest an impact on longevity, but rather on quality of life across several domains.

Using advocacy as an approach to adjusting to cancer calls for establishing a competency model that has skill-building and coping strategies at its core. This approach is suggested as a way of preventing or overcoming psychosocial limitations and promoting expectations for effective living.[8,9] The notion of learning an advocacy skill set is especially useful if one agrees that the psychosocial dimensions of a cancer diagnosis may cause a time-limited state of diminished functioning. Maher[10] defines a diagnosis of cancer as an anomic situation for many, suggesting it is "a temporary state of mind occasioned by a sudden alteration in one's life situation, and characterized by confusion and anxiety, uncertainty, loss of purpose, and a sense of separateness from one's usual social support system." Clark[11] suggests that the concept of crisis is useful for adaptation to cancer in terms of both situational requirements and the various phases over time of the mobilization of resources. The tasks facing the individual, as well as the strategies selected for attempted management of these tasks, become important parts of the process for resolving crises. These tasks and the strategies for managing them, such as seeking information or support, can be integrated into a method of skills training.

Skills training is used across many diverse professional settings, including education, psychology, sociology, and social work, and is distinguished from competence by McFall,[12,13] who associates skills with the specific underlying component processes that enable a person to perform in a manner which has been identified as competent. Skills are task specific and are acquired through a learning process.

Skills training is especially useful because of the complexities of the cancer experience. Drawing from a body of evidence found largely in the psychosocial research literature and derived from educational programs developed by cancer advocacy organizations, four interrelated skills have been identified as integral to the advocacy skills model: (1) information-seeking skills,[14–16] (2) communication skills,[17–21] (3) problem-solving skills,[22–28] and (4) negotiation skills.[29–31]

The founders of many patient advocacy organizations widely agree that providing reliable and timely information as well as providing decision support to people with cancer are among the most pressing needs of the public who are in touch with them when dealing with a diagnosis of cancer. Information needs are variable among cancer patients and change over the course of their illness. Also variable are the methods used by people when they seek health- and medical-related information. Books and articles about cancer can be found in public, university, hospital, and medical school libraries, and public access to the Internet is widely available. If anything, the amount of cancer information is daunting, and there are few compendia that annotate the information available, often making it difficult to identify what are the most suitable and reliable cancer-related resources. The Internet Health Care Coalition[32] offers an excellent guide for evaluating the reliability of online health information and advice, including cancer information. Being a wise medical consumer involves asking questions, seeking answers, gathering and organizing data, and the ability to access resources. Training for the development of information-seeking skills involves well-developed communication and negotiation skills.

Communication skills-building is an aspect of medical consumerism that is frequently complicated by the patient's need to learn a new lexicon of terms to increase his or her comprehension and understanding of cancer. At the critical time of learning about and understanding the diagnosis, the goals of treatment, and decision making about which treatment is most suitable, shared responsibility for communicating clearly between the healthcare provider and patient is important. The quality of communication should be characterized by equity, reciprocity, and a mutual understanding of hope and goals, wherein both patient and professional have input into care decisions.[33]

The literature on effective communication skills is widely available and adaptable to a clinical setting. The American Society of Clinical Oncology (ASCO) and the Oncology Nursing Society (ONS) are excellent resources of information on patient/provider communications skills building, and both associations provide workshops to their members on effective communication strategies.

Problem-solving skills are especially helpful when utilized to more carefully consider a situation with no clear and evident resolution. A diagnosis of cancer is one of those situations that can benefit from employing a number of problem-solving methods including modeling and role-playing.[34] Modeling is a form of observational learning in which the behavior of an individual or group acts as a stimulus for similar thoughts, attitudes, and behavior on the part of another individual. Role-playing relies on the re-creation of real or hypothetical situations. Cancer survivors use role-playing effectively in group settings where peer support and critique for their interactions with role-playing professionals can be supported.

It is common to hear cancer survivors use words such as "powerless" or "out of control" when describing how they felt when diagnosed with cancer. Because these feelings of temporary impotence frequently accompany a diagnosis of cancer, how one advocates for one's own needs during this time may be compromised. Especially relevant to a diagnosis of cancer is negotiation skills training if one must contend with employment, insurance, and financial institutions. Advocating in the occupational setting or with insurers often includes negotiations that go beyond anyone's ordinary mastery of skills and requires the involvement of legal counsel.[35,36] Because conflict is inherent in many well-intended interactions, conflict resolution through negotiation bears attention as part of a good self-advocacy model. Effective communication, resourcefulness, open-mindedness, and understanding alternative positions are central to all negotiation efforts.[37]

The advocacy continuum as described by Clark and Stovall may begin at a personal level wherein the previously outlined skill sets are most relevant. As the survivorship continuum changes, so do the advocacy needs of the individual and his/her support system. Self-advocacy may evolve into wanting to participate or interact with small groups or organizations at the community level, and, for some, public policy activities at the national level. Succinctly stated, Clark and Stovall describe an advocacy paradigm as follows: (1) Personal Advocacy; (2) Advocacy for Others; and (3) Public Interest Advocacy.

Personal advocacy or self-advocacy is a way of taking charge in an otherwise portentous environment of tests, surgery, radiation, chemotherapy, and office visits. From arming oneself with good information about one's diagnosis, to seeking second opinions, to locating resources for identifying and obtaining support, to knowing how to ask the right questions and negotiate the terms of one's employment while undergoing treatment, a cancer patient can become self-efficacious. This type of self-determination can mean the difference between maintaining a positive future outlook and enhancing one's quality of life or feeling helpless and less certain of the desirability of survival.[38,39]

For many cancer survivors, the 5 years following diagnosis and treatment mark a time of reentry and reevaluation of one's life. Many significant relationships in the lives of survivors change during this time as family and friends cannot understand why survivors are not simply jubilant with their survival. Support systems that were intact during the initial workup and treatment period may diminish or disappear. It is at this time in survivorship that many seek out others with whom they can identify. This transitional period, whether at age 20 or 70, calls for another kind of self-advocacy. With the notion that they may want to "give something back" in gratitude for their survival, many survivors seek to share their experiences with others.[40] The idea that shared information can be both powerful and validating—the veteran helping the rookie—is what the survivorship movement is largely about. When occurring in the context of a support group, this transmission of wisdom from a more-seasoned survivor to the newcomer provides a strong foundation for people who have had cancer to play a more-proactive role in making the myriad decisions that will follow them the rest of their lives.

The second part of the advocacy paradigm is characterized by cancer survivors going on to relay their experiences beyond one-on-one counseling interventions or small group interactions. Involvement in one's community can range from speaking to civic or religious groups and to the local media, participating in runs/walks for cancer awareness and cancer research, enrolling in advocacy training courses such as the National Breast Cancer Coalition's Project LEAD, to inquiring about participation on local Institutional Review Boards, etc. By speaking about one's experience to groups of medical students, for example, cancer survivors have an opportunity to educate them about the complex interpersonal and psychosocial issues that dominate their lives after treatment. This public speaking becomes a testimony that affirms one's survival, defies the myths and stigmas about cancer, and perhaps reaches others who are silently struggling with similar issues.

The last part of the cancer advocacy paradigm is Public Interest Advocacy. Largely a consequence of improved diagnostic tools and treatments for cancer that resulted in months and years of survival beyond initial diagnosis, issues related to adult cancer survivorship emerged as an agenda for advocacy and activism in the mid-1980s. These issues principally fall into three areas: economic/vocational, psychosocial/spiritual, and physiologic.

Compared with the number of cancer survivors, relatively very few engage in this type of advocacy, although breast cancer survivors have been visible and notable in the way they have brought about policy change through political advocacy and activism. A distinction is being made between the visibility or awareness of breast and other cancers through mass cause-related marketing campaigns and the work of cancer advocates and activists who participate in focused activities to change or initiate public policies.

Although *cancer advocacy* is not a contemporary phenomenon and includes much public education and outreach to diverse constituencies, *cancer activism* is in its relative infancy. Cancer survivors as advocates became very visible during the mid-1980s and 1990s when national breast cancer activists petitioned the federal government to target research in breast cancer and petitioned Congress to earmark funds through an unprecedented appropriation from the Department of Defense. Their petitioning not only increased federal funding for research, but led to a change in the peer-review process for granting monies to research under this program. The distinguishing characteristic of this example was the involvement of cancer survivors at every step of designing the Department of Defense Breast Cancer Program. Their activism laid the groundwork and set an example for participation of advocates at all levels of government-funded cancer research programs.

The 1990s and the new millennium ushered in an era that witnessed the creation of many organizations that self-identify themselves as cancer advocacy groups. Often founded by survivors and/or their supporters, these groups represent the voices of people with commonly diagnosed cancers, for example, breast, colon, lung, lymphatic, and prostate, as well as less-common cancers, such as ovarian, head and neck, brain, pancreatic, and kidney, and provide a valuable resource for people with cancer and their families. Increasingly, their representation can be found sitting on review groups, on the boards of cancer centers, on federal advisory commissions, and walking the halls of Congress to educate their elected officials about the needs of those they represent.

References

1. Clark EJ, Stovall E. Advocacy: the cornerstone of cancer survivorship. Cancer Pract 1996;5:239–244.
2. National Coalition for Cancer Survivorship. Charter. Silver Spring, MD: National Coalition for Cancer Survivorship, 1986.
3. American Cancer Society. Cancer Facts and Figures: 1994–2003. Atlanta, GA: The American Cancer Society, 2003.
4. Mullan F, Hoffman B (eds). Charting the Journey: An Almanac of Practical Resources for Cancer Survivors. Mount Vernon, NY: Consumers Union, 1990.
5. Carter B. Going through: a critical theme in surviving breast cancer. Innov Oncol Nurs 1989;5:2–4.
6. Leigh S. Myths, monsters, and magic: personal perspectives and professional challenges of survival. Oncol Nurs Forum 1992;19: 1475–1480.
7. Loescher L, Clark L, Atwood J, Leigh S, Lawl G. The impact of the cancer experience on long-term survivors. Oncol Nurs Forum 1990;17:223–229.
8. Rowland JH. Intrapersonal resources: coping. In: Holland JC, Rowland JH (eds). Handbook of Psychooncology. New York: Oxford University Press, 1990:44–57
9. Seeman J. Toward a model of positive health. Am Psychologist 1989;44:1099–1109.
10. Maher EL. Anomic aspects of recovery from cancer. Soc Sci Med 1982;16:907–912.
11. Clark EJ. Social assessment of cancer patients. Proceedings of the National Conference on Practice, Education, and Research in Oncology Social Work—1984. Philadelphia: American Cancer Society, 1984.
12. McFall R, Dodge K. Self-management and interpersonal skills learning. In: Karoly P, Kanfer F (eds). Self-Management and Behavior Change. New York: Pergamon Press, 1982:353–392.
13. McFall R. A review and reformulation of the concept of social skills. Behav Assess 1082;4:1–33.
14. Tabak ER. Encouraging patient question-asking: a clinical trial. Patient Educ Counsel 1988;12:37–49.
15. Blanchard CG, Labrecque MS, Ruckdeschel JC, Blanchard EB. Information and decision-making preferences of hospitalized adult cancer patients. Soc Sci Med 1988;27:1139–1145.

16. Messerli M, Garamendi C, Romano J. Breast cancer information as a technique of crisis intervention. Am J Orthopsychiatry 1980;50:728–731
17. Mullan F, Hoffman B (eds). Charting the Journey: An Almanac of Practical Resources for Cancer Survivors. Mount Vernon, NY: Consumers Union, 1990.
18. Sharf B. Teaching patients to speak up: past and future trends. Patient Educ Counsel 1988;11:95–108.
19. Knapp ML, Miller GR. Handbook of Interpersonal Communication. Newbury Park, CA: Sage Publications, 1994.
20. Moore LG. Teamwork: The Cancer Patient's Guide To Talking With Your Doctor (booklet). Silver Spring, MD: National Coalition for Cancer Survivorship, 1991.
21. Telch C, Telch M. Group coping skills instruction and supportive group therapy for cancer patients: a comparison of strategies. J Consult Clin Psychol 1986;54:802–808.
22. Mullan F, Hoffman B (eds). Charting the Journey: An Almanac of Practical Resources for Cancer Survivors. Mount Vernon, NY: Consumers Union, 1990.
23. Gray RE, Doan B, Church K. Empowerment issues in cancer. Health Values 1991;15:22–28.
24. Tabak ER. Encouraging patient question-asking: a clinical trial. Patient Educ Counsel 1988;12:37–49.
25. Hoffman B. Employment discrimination: another hurdle for cancer survivors. Cancer Invest 1991;9:589–595.
26. Fawzy F, Cousins N, Fawzy N, Kemeny M, Elashoff R, Morton D. A structured psychiatric intervention for cancer patients: changes over time in methods of coping and affective disturbance. Arch Gen Psychiatry 1990;47:720–725.
27. Roter D. An exploration of health education responsibility for a partnership model of client-provider relations. Patient Educ Counsel 1987;9:25–31.
28. Welch-McCaffrey D, Hoffman B, Leigh S, Loescher L, Meyskans F. Surviving adult cancers. Part 2: psychosocial implications. Ann Intern Med 1989;111:517–524.
29. Kauffman DB. Surviving Cancer. Washington, DC: Acropolis, 1989.
30. Rowland JH. Intrapersonal resources: coping. In: Holland JC, Rowland JH (eds). Handbook of Psychooncology. New York: Oxford University Press, 1990:44–57.
31. Callan DB. Hope as a clinical issue in oncology social work. J Psychosoc Oncol 1989;7:31–46.
32. http://www.ihealthcoalition.org/.
33. Thoits P. Stressors and problem-solving: the individual as social activist. J Health Soc Behav 1994;35:293–304.
34. Anderson L, DeVellis B, DeVellis F. Effects of modeling on patient communication, satisfaction, and knowledge. Med Care 1987;25:1044–1056.
35. Hoffman B. Working It Out: Your Employment Rights As A Cancer Survivor (booklet). Silver Spring, MD: National Coalition for Cancer Survivorship, 2002.
36. Calder K, Pollitz K. What Cancer Survivors Need To Know About Health Insurance (booklet). Silver Spring, MD: National Coalition for Cancer Survivorship, 2002.
37. Volpe M, Maida P. Sociologists and the processing of conflicts. Sociol Pract 1992;10:13–25.
38. Clark EJ. You Have The Right To Be Hopeful (booklet). Silver Spring, MD: National Coalition for Cancer Survivorship, 1995.
39. Farran CJ, Herth KA, Popovich JM. Hope and Hopelessness: Critical Clinical Constructs. Thousand Oaks, CA: Sage, 1995.
40. Ferrell BR, Dow KH. Portraits of cancer survivorship: a glimpse through the lens of survivors' eyes. Cancer Pract 1996;4:76–80.

Index